# Foreword

## THE NATIONAL CONSENSUS

A generation before American physicians joined together to form a national organization to promote and protect medicine as a profession, they joined together to create a national pharmacopeia to promote and protect the public health.

A generation before pharmacists joined together to form a national organization to promote and protect pharmacy as a profession, they joined the physicians in the work of the Pharmacopeia.

This magnificent record of public service of the health professions results now in the establishment of legally recognized national standards of quality for drugs and this national consensus on the clinically relevant drug use information needed by the patient and needed by those practitioners caring for the patient who is taking the medicine.

*The national consensus.* A proud claim. It is based on the comprehensiveness of the involvement of all interested parties, the unbiased structure of the system, and the constant public access to the system.

• An extensive expert advisory panel system reaching across the entire health field; a cross-fertilized matrix of:

—medical specialty panels, which consider drug use information from the standpoint of its scientific accuracy and clinical relevance in each of the therapeutic or medical specialty areas;

—practice oriented panels, which review drug use information from the standpoint of its utility in each of the professions that care for patients who use the drug;

—a panel of consumers who watch over language, format, and general approach;

—and an international health advisory panel to reflect drug information needs and use in other countries and to enrich the database with the experience of those countries.

• The system is designed to secure an evidence-based, unbiased consensus or, more properly, to secure a balance of biases, because no human or human endeavor is ever totally unbiased:

—USP Committee of Revision members are elected for their individual expertise, regardless of their current place of employment or organizational memberships;

—electors in this nationwide election procedure include members of the U.S. Pharmacopeial Convention (USP) from each college and state association in medicine and pharmacy; national scientific, professional, and trade associations and agencies of the federal government that are concerned with drugs; consumer organizations; international organizations and foreign government; and members at large;

—panelists, all of whom are volunteers, are selected by the USP Committee of Revision member who has been elected to represent that particular area or specialty, and consented to by the USP Nominating Committee;

—freedom from influence resulting from financial interests in organizations that manufacture and market drugs is guaranteed by a conflict-of-interest program that protects the integrity of the consensus process.

• Opportunity for input from all interested parties and public review of the text that is proposed by the Panels for adoption by the Committee of Revision:

—several hundred reviewers are designated by colleges, associations, and government agencies, including the U.S. Food and Drug Administration and Canada's Drugs Directorate;

—researchers and manufacturers involved with the individual drug provide review;

—review and comment by any interested member of the public of draft text for USP DI monographs as listed in *USP DI Review*, a special section of the monthly *USP DI Update,* is encouraged;

—meetings of all advisory panels are open to the public;

—review and revision are continuous, with the electronic database updated daily and representing the most current information and print publications representing the official text at the time of publication.

*The national consensus.* Why is such an extensive and costly system needed? Because practitioners and patients need *up-to-date* information about *all* drugs; because patients need consistency and reinforcement in the information given to them; because the health professions and the public need confidence in the authoritativeness of the information they give and get; and because the provision of patient information about prescription drugs breaks and bends a number of outdated legal and professional boundaries.

• Confidence in the *authoritativeness* of the information requires that USP DI information is accurate and can be relied upon by health care practitioners and patients.

• Confidence in the *credibility* of the process by which USP DI is assembled requires confidence in the *integrity* of the people who operate it.

• Consistency and reinforcement are accepted principles of education. It is important, therefore, that the patient receive essentially the same information from both the prescriber and the dispenser.

• Confidence by the professions is exemplified by USP's strategic alliance with the American Medical Association (AMA) whereby USP has taken over repsonsibility for the AMA Drug Evaluations (AMA DE) database, in the acceptance of *USP DI* as a practice parameter by the AMA/Specialty Society Practice Parameter Forum, and in the use of *USP DI* information by numerous pharmacy associations and practice sites.

• Confidence by the Federal government is shown in the recognition of *USP DI* in the 1990 and 1993 federal Omnibus Budget Reconciliation Acts (OBRA '90 and '93) as an "official" compendium for use by state Medicaid agencies for drug utilization review (DUR) and patient counseling, and information on medically accepted unlabeled uses of medications, and recognized under the Medicare provisions of OBRA '93 as a source of medically accepted indications or "off label" uses of anticancer drugs.

• Legal barriers and legal threats based on decades of non-information and misinformation are shifting before the increasing demand for patient drug use information:

—pharmacists, who in some states previously were prohibited from discussing a prescription drug with the patient, are now legally required to offer counseling and to give patient information for certain drugs and are proclaimed by leaders in pharmacy as the source of patient information on any drug;

—physicians, who have been the gate-keepers of prescription drugs, are being urged by leaders in medicine to open the gates wider and provide more information to patients about the medicines they are prescribing;

—and pharmaceutical manufacturers, who have fulfilled their legal obligation by providing information only to the prescriber (the government generally did not allow them to do more), are now being encouraged by the government voluntarily to provide information to patients. The issue at hand is how to do it in a way that balances patients' needs for accurate, understandable information within the legal requirements.

The shifting of these legal barriers and regulatory requirements should be less litigious with the presence of this USP-developed, strong national consensus on what generally is the appropriate content of information for today's patient. Of course, the shift can work both ways. The practitioner who ignores it, or who continues the tradition of providing no information, is at increasing risk. The practitioner who bases his or her information on the national consensus and then individualizes it for the patient will have a better defense.

Jerome A. Halperin
Executive Vice President

Rockville, Maryland
January 2, 1997

# Preface

Since 1820, the United States Pharmacopeia has set standards for the medications used by the American public. In establishing the Pharmacopeia, the founders were reacting to an unmet need of the professions and their patients—that is, the need for generally accepted procedures for the preparation of medications which would allow for confidence in their use.

The need for quality standards remains, and the work of USP in establishing those standards continues. However, additional needs regarding the use of medications have arisen, within both the health care provider and health care recipient populations. Some of these newly recognized needs relate to information sources. *USP DI* is one reaction to these previously unmet needs.

At the 1970 meeting of the Pharmacopeial Convention, a resolution to increase in the Pharmacopeia or in a companion volume the amount of information that would be useful to pharmacists and others was adopted. In response to this, the 1970-1975 Subcommittee on Posology and Related Information, under the chairmanship of John A. Owen, Jr., M.D., expanded the category and dose information and introduced in the *USP XIX* monographs of many dosage forms a section entitled Dispensing Information. This information served as a basic reminder or general guide to the pharmacist, who could vary or omit it in accordance with the best interests of the patient or the particular circumstances involved.

Continuing this development, the 1975-1980 Subcommittee, under the chairmanship of Harry C. Shirkey, R.Ph., M.D., greatly expanded the amount and kinds of information in the USP DI database, focusing on that believed to enhance the safe and effective use of a medication once it was prescribed. This included drug use information relating to dispensing, administration, monitoring, and/or patient consultation. The work of the Subcommittee resulted in the first edition (1980) of *USP DI*. From one book in 1980, it grew to two volumes in 1983, and three volumes in 1989.

*USP DI* is, and it always will be, a work in progress. The information is under constant revision. This seventeenth edition incorporates the experiences and comments generated by previous editions. New drug monographs and information have been added, and the existing text has been reviewed for changes and revised accordingly.

*USP DI* is an ongoing publication. The main volumes are supplemented by publication of an update every month. *USP DI Update* presents monographs on selected, newly marketed drugs as well as selected changes in the information base of drugs already in the data base. Not all new drugs and not all new information on drugs already in *USP DI* will appear in *USP DI Update*. *Updates*, therefore, are only an interim partial supplement to the most recent *USP DI* annual volumes.

## Development of *USP DI*

The *USP DI* is a comprehensive collection of clinically relevant, established information about each drug. However, it is far more than that. It is a continuous collection of the current judgments of experts in the use of drugs. The information included is the result of a planned, organized, nationwide consensus-generating system (with worldwide input). This system has been designed to involve not only the experts but all interested parties through open public review and comment.

Using the parameters established by the USP Division of Information Development Executive Committee, staff develops draft monographs for each drug selected for inclusion in *USP DI*. These initial drafts are reviewed by the appropriate Advisory Panel(s) and other designated reviewers and are revised accordingly. Re-drafted text may again be reviewed by Advisory Panel(s) as many times as necessary to achieve an initial consensus. Proposed monographs are then made available for general public review and comment. Announcement of availability is made in the *USP DI Review* listing as published in the monthly *USP DI Update*.

The comments generated by the public review process are fed back into the USP Advisory Panel system. If substantive changes result, the monograph is again listed in *USP DI Review* announcing additional proposed changes. The process is repeated as required to develop final consensus.

Of course, the consensus can change from one edition to the next, and users of *USP DI* are encouraged to submit comments at any time to:

USP
Division of Information Development
12601 Twinbrook Parkway
Rockville, Maryland 20852
Telephone: (301) 816-8351
Telefax: (301) 816-8374
E-mail: jar@usp.org

## Organization of *USP DI*

*USP DI* comprises three distinct sections. The first volume, *Drug Information for the Health Care Professional*, includes the DI monographs arranged in alphabetic order. The Volume I general index includes established names, cross-references by brand names (both U.S. and Canadian), and older nonproprietary names. In addition, an indications index and appendixes presenting categories of use and other useful information are included. The second volume, *Advice for the Patient,* includes the lay language versions of the patient consultation guidelines found in Volume I. These lay language versions are intended to be used at the discretion of the health care provider as an aid to patient consultation if written information would be of benefit or if it is requested by the prescriber. Brand and generic names are cross-referenced in the index of *Advice for the Patient*. The third volume, *Approved Drug Products and Legal Requirements*, reproduces information from the Food and Drug Administration on therapeutic equivalence and other requirements relating to drug product selection. It includes USP and NF legal requirements for labeling, storage, packaging, and quality for drugs. It also contains those portions of the federal Controlled Substances Act Regulations, the Poison Prevention

Packaging Act and Regulations, and the FD&C Act provisions relating to drugs for human use, and the Current Good Manufacturing Practice Regulations that are most relevant to the physician, pharmacist, nurse, and other health care professionals.

The individual Volume I monograph covers the basic information which is applicable to that substance when used for a specific area of effect (e.g., Systemic). Information that is unique for a specific dosage form of the base substance is then included under that specific dosage form heading. To illustrate this approach, assume that DRUG X is used for its systemic effects and its topical effects. Also assume that the drug is available in the following dosage forms: cream, injection, ointment, syrup, and tablet. The *USP DI* Volume I monographs for DRUG X would be organized as follows:

DRUG X (Systemic)
[General information applicable to Drug X's systemic use.]
  Drug X Syrup
  Drug X Tablets
  Drug X Injection
  [Specific information applicable to each of the systemic dosage forms.]

DRUG X (Topical)
[General information applicable to Drug X's topical use.]
  Drug X Cream
  Drug X Ointment
  [Specific information applicable to each of the topical dosage forms.]

Where appropriate, other major headings based on specific area of effect are used for Dental, Inhalation-Local, Intracavernosal, Mucosal-Local, Nasal-Local, Ophthalmic, Oral-Local, Otic, Parenteral-Local, Rectal-Local, Transdermal-Systemic, or Vaginal use.

Whenever feasible, monographs are grouped under family headings. This permits a sizable saving of space and also allows the practitioner to readily identify differences among agents of the same family. Significant differences are addressed in charts and in Summary of Differences sections.

The following headings and subheadings are employed, where appropriate, in organizing the information for each Volume I monograph:

Category
Indications
  General considerations
  Accepted
  Acceptance not established
  Unaccepted
Pharmacology/Pharmacokinetics
  Physicochemical characteristics
    Source
    Molecular weight
    pKa
    Solubility
    Partition coefficient
    Other characteristics
  Mechanism of action/Effect
  Other actions/effects
  Absorption
  Distribution
  Protein binding
  Biotransformation
  Half-life
  Onset of action

Time to peak concentration
Peak serum concentration
Time to peak effect
Duration of action
Elimination
  In dialysis
Precautions to Consider
  Cross-sensitivity and/or related problems
  Carcinogenicity
  Tumorigenicity
  Mutagenicity
  Pregnancy/Reproduction
    Fertility
    Pregnancy
    Labor
    Delivery
    Postpartum
  Breast-feeding
  Pediatrics
  Adolescents
  Geriatrics
  Pharmacogenetics
  Dental
  Surgical
  Critical/Emergency care
  Drug interactions and/or related problems
  Laboratory value alterations
    With diagnostic test results
    With physiology/laboratory test values
  Medical considerations/Contraindications
  Patient monitoring
Side/Adverse Effects
  Those indicating need for medical attention
  Those indicating need for medical attention only if they continue or are bothersome
  Those not indicating need for medical attention
  Those indicating need for medical attention if they occur after medication is discontinued
Overdose
  Clinical effects of overdose
  Treatment of overdose

Patient Consultation
  Before using this medication
  Proper use of this medication
  Precautions while using this medication
  Side/adverse effects
General Dosing Information
  Diet/Nutrition
  Bioequivalence information
  Safety considerations for handling this medication
  For treatment of adverse effects
Dosage forms (each separate)
  Usual adult dose
  Usual adult prescribing limits
  Usual pediatric dose
  Usual pediatric prescribing limits
  Usual geriatric dose
  Strengths usually available
  Packaging and storage
  Preparation of dosage form
  Stability
  Incompatibilities
  Auxiliary labeling

viii

Caution

Additional information

Selected Bibliography

## Description and Limitations of Information Included

*USP DI* contains selected information and takes into account practice concerns. Selection is based on what is considered by the Committee of Revision and its Advisory Panels to be practical, clinically significant information needed to help assure that a drug is being safely and effectively used. It is meant to aid the health care professional and the patient in minimizing the risks and enhancing the benefits of the drugs used. Collectively, it is valuable in assessing the quality of care through drug utilization review programs. Ultimately, the information required is defined by the practice standards of medicine, pharmacy, nursing, dentistry, and the other health professions as well as by the information needs of the patient.

*USP DI* is not intended to be "full disclosure" information.

Readers are advised that the information in *USP DI* may contain statements that differ from those in the "full disclosure" information labeling approved or required by the United States or Canadian governments. On the other hand, readers should remember that FDA-approved full disclosure information can differ from brand to brand of the same generic drug product. It should not be inferred that the inclusion of information that is not in the approved labeling has been sought or agreed to by the manufacturer.

Selected brand names are included in the monographs as well as in the indexes of both volumes I and II for ease of reference purposes only. The inclusion of a brand name is not intended as an endorsement of a particular product. The omission of a particular brand name does not indicate that the article was judged to be inferior or inadequate. The inclusion of various brands in volumes I and II bears no relationship to and is not intended to affect any applicable brand interchange requirements.

The Veterans Administration medication classification codes (primary and secondary assignments) are included at the beginning of each monograph. See the VA Medication Classification System appendix in *USP DI* Volume I for a detailed description as well as a complete listing of primary and secondary classifications.

Where appropriate, controlled substance classifications are included at the beginning of the monograph. United States schedules include:

Schedule I—No legal medical use is recognized by the U.S. Controlled Substances Act. Use of Schedule I substances for research purposes is permitted with proper registration. Schedule I substances are not included in *USP DI*. Examples: Heroin, LSD, peyote.

Schedule II—The most stringent classification for drugs recognized by the U.S. Controlled Substances Act as having a legitimate medical use; these drugs are characterized by a very high abuse potential and/or potential for severe physical and psychic dependency. Distribution and inventory are highly controlled; prescriptions are non-refillable. Emergency telephone orders for limited quantities of these drugs are authorized but the prescriber must provide a written, signed prescription order to the pharmacy within 72 hours. Examples: Amphetamines, anabolic steroids, meperidine, morphine, short-acting barbiturates.

Schedule III—Includes drugs having significant abuse potential, but to a lesser degree than Schedule II substances. Prescriptions can be refilled up to five times within six months after the date of issue if authorized by the prescriber. Telephone orders are permitted. Examples: Certain barbiturates not included in Schedule II, opiates in combination with other substances such as acetaminophen or aspirin.

Schedule IV—Includes drugs having a low abuse potential. Prescriptions can be refilled up to five times within six months after the date of issue if authorized by the prescriber. Telephone orders are permitted. Examples: Benzodiazepines, certain long-acting barbiturates, chloral hydrate, pentazocine, propoxyphene.

Schedule V—Includes products having the lowest abuse potential of the controlled substances. No limitations on refills other than those imposed by the prescriber. Some Schedule V products may be available without a prescription (for example, certain cough preparations and antidiarrheal preparations containing limited amounts of an opiate).

In addition to the federal Controlled Substances Act, most states have controlled substances acts similar to the federal requirements. In some instances, the state regulations may be more restrictive. These differences are not addressed in *USP DI* monographs.

Canadian controlled substance classifications (and the designations used in this publication) include:

Narcotics (N)—Includes products containing a narcotic. Within this broad classification, there are several levels of regulatory control. These levels range from strict controls for the most abusable of the substances (for example, single-entity narcotics; products containing a narcotic with one active non-narcotic ingredient; any preparation containing heroin, hydrocodone, or oxycodone) to lesser controls for preparations containing one narcotic and two active non-narcotic ingredients and exempt codeine preparations (those containing a limited amount of codeine plus two active non-narcotic ingredients).

Controlled Drugs (C)—Includes non-narcotic preparations with abuse potential. As with narcotics, different regulations apply depending on specific content. Examples: Amphetamines, barbiturates.

**Category/Indications**—Statements of categories of use and indications are provided for each article.

The category of use indicates the area of therapeutic utility for which the drug was included and generally represents an application of the best known pharmacologic action of the article or its active ingredient. The statement is not intended to be all inclusive nor to indicate that the article may have no other activity or utility.

Indications of use stated in manufacturers' labeling and approved by the U.S. Food and Drug Administration (FDA) or Canada's Health Protection Branch (HPB) are generally included, as well as additional unlabeled indications selected as appropriate by USP Advisory Panels. These two types of indications are included under an *Accepted* subheading. An *Unaccepted* indications section identifies uses of a drug that are considered by USP Advisory Panels to be inappropriate, obsolete, or unproven. For certain drugs whose place in therapy has not been determined and the use does not clearly fall into the "Accepted" or "Unaccepted" categorization, information is included under an *Acceptance not established* subheading.

A *General considerations* subsection is included in the Indications section for some drugs, such as antibiotics, to give the reader more complete information about the drug (e.g., the activity spectrum of antibiotics).

New uses for approved products that are not reflected in a product's labeling are often discovered after marketing. Before a pharmaceutical manufacturer may include any new indications in the labeling for a particular drug (and to promote the product for those uses), it must obtain the government's approval for the uses. Such approval requires the completion of adequate and well-controlled clinical trials to document the drug's safety and efficacy for the new uses. Since the clinical trials required for approval may take considerable time and effort, manufacturers, in some cases, may not seek or obtain approval for new uses since there may not be sufficient economic incentive for the product sponsor to perform the necessary research or to make application to the agency. In other cases, of course, the research may have been carried out by the manufacturer but the new proposed use found to be unsupported.

In an attempt to be of assistance to practitioners, USP Advisory Panels have been requested to include those unlabeled or off-label indications (i.e., not included in the labeling of *any* brand) which they believe represent reasonable, current prescribing practices based on their knowledge of the drug, the literature, and of current prescribing and utilization practices which practitioners should be prepared to address. In certain instances, particularly life-threatening diseases for which a definitive cure is not available (e.g., some cancers), unlabeled uses may be included as acceptable although experimental because other therapy is either unavailable or has been tried and has failed.

Medically accepted unlabeled indications are identified in the *Indications* section by brackets for the U.S. and/or a superscript 1 for Canada. The unlabeled indication may be followed by a brief explanatory statement.

The legality of the prescribing of approved drugs for uses not included in their official labeling is sometimes a cause for concern and confusion among practitioners. The appropriateness of prescribing or dispensing an approved drug for an unlabeled indication would ultimately be judged in accordance with normal legal principles governing professional activities such as negligence or strict liability in the event of a question of liability to an injured patient. In the U.S., the Federal Food, Drug, and Cosmetic Act does not prohibit practitioners from prescribing nor pharmacists from dispensing a drug product for a particular patient for an indication not contained in its approved labeling.

Another point of concern to practitioners relates to differences in approved labeled indications for different brands of the same generic drug product. Because of the legalities involved, it is possible for different manufactured products of the same generic product to have in their labeling different indications (as well as different precautions, side effects, dosage schedules, etc.). *USP DI* indications are not directed to a specific brand product unless a particular characteristic of a brand must be taken into account.

**Pharmacology/Pharmacokinetics**—A brief statement of physicochemical characteristics and pharmacologic actions includes, whenever appropriate and available, source, molecular weight, pKa, solubility, partition coefficient, mechanism of action, actions other than the therapeutic actions, absorption, distribution in the body, protein-binding characteristics, biotransformation, half-life, onset of action, time to peak concentration, peak serum concentration, time to peak effect, duration of action, and elimination. The information is not intended to be inclusive. In some cases, protein binding is expressed in general terms with ranges as follows, rather than in terms of specific percentages:

Very high: >90%
High: 65–90%
Moderate: 35–64%
Low: 10–34%
Very low: <10%

**Precautions to Consider**—The precautions to consider in using a specific drug, as listed under this heading, are not intended to provide "full disclosure" information. Instead, precautions have been selected on the basis of their common or usual clinical significance to the population as a whole. It cannot be assumed that the omission of a precaution in *USP DI* means that such a precaution may not be of clinical significance for a specific patient. In many cases, there is a lack of scientifically valid information to support inclusion in *USP DI*. As in all aspects of medical care, risk-benefit considerations must be made on an individual basis, which may, in fact, supersede general precautions to the use of any medication.

*Cross-sensitivity and/or related problems*—Where known, potential for cross-sensitivity with other drugs is included.

*Carcinogenicity*—Where known, reference is made to the cancer-causing potential of a drug. Not all such precautions may necessarily be listed.

*Tumorigenicity*—Where known, reference is made to the tumor-causing potential of a drug. Not all such precautions may necessarily be listed.

*Mutagenicity*—Where known, reference is made to the mutagenic potential of a drug. Not all such precautions may necessarily be listed.

*Pregnancy/Reproduction*—Documented problems in humans with the use of a drug during pregnancy are included. Where appropriate, information is included on fertility, pregnancy, labor, delivery, and postpartum effects. In addition, reference is made to problems documented in animal studies even though the significance of such findings to humans may not be known. FDA-assigned pregnancy categories are included whenever available. These categories are:

A: Adequate and well-controlled studies have failed to demonstrate a risk to the fetus in the first trimester of pregnancy (and there is no evidence of risk in later trimesters).

B: Animal reproduction studies have failed to demonstrate a risk to the fetus and there are no adequate and well-controlled studies in pregnant women.

C: Animal reproduction studies have shown an adverse effect on the fetus and there are no adequate and well-controlled studies in humans, but potential benefits may warrant use of the drug in pregnant women despite potential risks.

D: There is positive evidence of human fetal risk based on adverse reaction data from investigational or marketing experience or studies in humans, but potential benefits may warrant use of the drug in pregnant women despite potential risks.

X: Studies in animals or humans have demonstrated fetal abnormalities and/or there is positive evidence of human fetal risk based on adverse reaction data from investigational or marketing experience, and the risks involved in use of the drug in pregnant women clearly outweigh potential benefits.

*Breast-feeding*—Documented problems in humans associated with the use of a drug while breast-feeding are included. Where appropriate, reference is also made to problems documented in animal studies even though the significance of such findings to humans may not be known.

*Pediatrics*—Selected precautions relating to use of an agent in the pediatric patient are included. Not all precautions relevant to such use may necessarily be listed. If no information about the use of a drug in the pediatric patient is known, this is so stated.

*Adolescents*—Selected precautions relating to use of an agent in the adolescent patient are included. Not all precautions relevant to such use may necessarily be listed.

*Geriatrics*—Selected precautions relating to use of an agent in the geriatric patient are included. Not all precautions relevant to such use may necessarily be listed. If no information about the use of a drug in the geriatric patient is known, this is so stated.

*Pharmacogenetics*—Selected precautions relating to genetic factors and potential responses to drugs are included. Not all such potential effects may necessarily be listed.

*Dental*—Selected precautions relating to potential dental effects of an agent are included. Not all such potential effects may necessarily be listed.

*Surgical*—Selected precautions relating to potential effects of an agent on surgery are included. Not all precautions relevant to surgery may necessarily be listed.

*Critical/Emergency care*—Selected precautions relating to potential effects of an agent in a critical/emergency care situation are included. Not all such precautions may necessarily be listed.

*Drug interactions and/or related problems*—Drug and/or food interactions have been selected on the basis of their potential clinical significance. Those considered to have greater significance are identified with a chevron (») to the left of the drug entry. In some cases, an interaction appearing in one monograph may not be cross-referenced in the corresponding monograph. Since each monograph is finalized individually, such inconsistencies are constantly in the process of resolution in preparation for the next update or edition of *USP DI*.

*Laboratory value alterations*—This section includes effects of the drug on laboratory test values. No attempt has been made to provide a complete listing of effects on the normal or diseased body or interferences with other tests that may be required if proper diagnosis is to be expected. The information included in this section is broken down into two subsections:

With diagnostic test results—Includes changes in laboratory test values caused by effects of the drug in the body or on the test materials or procedure that may produce inaccurate results (e.g., diagnostic tests for which the results may be false-positive or false-negative in patients receiving the drug).

With physiology/laboratory test values—Includes changes in laboratory test values that may occur because of the physiologic effects of the drug (for example, increases or decreases in serum electrolytes).

Effects listed have been selected on the basis of potential clinical significance. The list is not necessarily inclusive.

*Medical considerations/Contraindications*—Some medical conditions, the presence of which may alter the decision to prescribe a drug for a given patient or may affect the dosage, are listed. As a general rule, the list is compiled from the approved labeling and covers precautions, warnings, and contraindications. Those conditions considered to be of greater importance are identified by a chevron (») to the left of the specific medical problem. Contraindications that are considered to be absolute, except under special circumstances, are listed first. Relative contraindications are included for those problems requiring risk-benefit consideration.

*Patient monitoring*—To exercise judgment in refilling prescriptions and to monitor continuing use of a medication, patient examinations that may be particularly important are listed. The list is not meant to be a complete listing of the check-ups a patient may require nor is it meant to imply that all check-ups listed are necessarily required for every patient taking the medication.

**Side/Adverse Effects**—Selected side effects are listed. Selection is based on seriousness (e.g., agranulocytosis), frequency of occurrence, effect on life style (e.g., drowsiness), and/or likelihood that a nonthreatening side effect might cause concern to the patient if he or she were not aware that the effect might occur (e.g., rapid pulse). Wherever possible, side effects are grouped according to reported incidence—i.e., incidence more frequent, incidence less frequent, or incidence rare; or by percentages, if available. Not all such side/adverse effects may necessarily be listed.

The side effects are listed by effect with presenting symptom(s) in parentheses.

**Overdose**—This section includes selected information on therapeutic and toxic concentrations of the drug, time to onset of overdose symptoms, clinical effects of overdose, and treatment of overdose.

The *Overdose* section of the monographs is currently in the process of being phased in. For some monographs, the relevant information may still be included under *Side/Adverse Effects* and *General Dosing Information*.

**Patient Consultation**—Current medical practice embraces the belief that patient compliance and the effectiveness of therapy can be advanced in certain clinical situations if the prescriber provides, or asks the dispenser to provide, written drug use information of the type contained in *USP DI*. To help ensure patient understanding, the prescriber and dispenser should, in turn, translate the essence of this information in words suitable to the ability of the individual patient to understand.

Prior to providing oral consultation, health care professionals should apprise themselves of the entire monograph for the indicated medication. The patient consultation section is provided as a reminder, highlighting a limited, selected number of items peculiar to the medication for oral discussion and, in general, assumes more complete written information can be made available.

Suggested guidelines for patient consultation are listed. The statements marked with a chevron (») are considered to be of greatest importance. If written information is desired, the health care provider may refer to the corresponding lay language monograph in *Advice for the Patient*.

The information provided is intended to aid efforts to advance patient compliance and the effectiveness of the therapy selected by the prescriber. The information provided is not complete, but is intended to serve as a basic reminder or general guide to the health care provider who may vary or omit it in accordance with professional judgment taking into account the best interests of the patient, the request of the prescriber, or the particular circumstances involved. It is not intended as a substitute for professional judgment or to modify any legal requirements imposed on the dispenser. It serves also as a general reminder to the prescriber of the concerns of the dispenser in the dispenser-patient relationship.

Some drugs are not amenable to general rules since they may be prescribed for various purposes not necessarily known to the dispenser, to the person administering the drug, or to other physicians caring for the patient; also, the differences in their utilization might affect the advice to be given. However, where it is clear how a drug is being utilized, it may be helpful to reinforce the prescriber's instructions or to provide such additional advice as would assist the patient.

Occasionally, a dispenser or person administering a drug may have particular knowledge of problems peculiar to the patient that justifies giving exceptional instructions. The fact that *USP DI* makes no mention of such unusual or exceptional circumstances is not intended to limit or influence professional judgment in conveying to the patient information that is deemed to be correct and proper under the circumstances.

**General Dosing Information**—Dosing information of a general nature which may be applicable to the usual dispensing or administration situation and guidelines relating to diet/nutrition and bioequivalence are included, where appropriate. The information is meant to supplement the dosing information included under each specific dosage form and the two sets of information must be used together.

Information relating to safety considerations for handling a medication and the treatment of adverse effects is also included in this section.

**Dosage Forms**—The following information is listed separately for each dosage form, whenever appropriate:

*Summary of differences*—In family monographs, a summary of differences for each individual family member is included. Not all differences are necessarily included. The fact that this section does not include certain information does not necessarily indicate that the point in question does not occur with that particular family member. It may, instead, reflect a lack of information. Users of *USP DI* must exercise caution and not use the information included in family monographs as the sole basis of comparison between agents.

*Usual adult dose*—The usual adult dose given for each article is that which may ordinarily be expected to produce in adults with normal renal/hepatic function, following administration in the manner indicated, at such time intervals as may be specified, the diagnostic, therapeutic, prophylactic, or other effect for which the article is recognized. The usual adult dose is intended to serve only as a guide and it may be varied in the best interests of the patient and in accordance with the variables that affect the action of the drug.

The statements of dosage in the case of capsules and tablets are in terms of the content of active ingredient and rarely represent the total weight of the capsule contents or of the tablets.

In some instances, the dosage may be stated in terms of the pharmacologically active portion (moiety) of the molecule in order to permit the prescriber or dispenser to correlate the weight equivalent for salts, esters, or other chemical forms of the drug moiety. However, it is not to be inferred that all chemical forms in which the active moiety may be presented are therapeutically equivalent. Neither are different dosage forms administered by the same route always therapeutically equivalent, e.g., tablets vs. syrups or creams vs. ointments.

*Usual adult prescribing limits*—The usual adult prescribing limits subsection is intended primarily to guide the dispenser with respect to seeking confirmation of prescription orders calling for unusually small or large doses. In some cases, it may take into account some uses in addition to those implied in the statement of category. The time schedule and route of administration where given for the usual adult dose apply also to the usual adult prescribing limits unless otherwise specified.

The limits statement does not address the issue of toxicity levels but instead focuses on the generally accepted lower and/or upper ranges of dosage believed to be used in medical practice.

*Usual pediatric dose*—The usual pediatric dose generally given in the monograph is that which may ordinarily be expected to produce in infants and children with normal renal/hepatic function, following administration in the manner indicated, at such time intervals as may be designated, the diagnostic, therapeutic, or prophylactic effect for which the article is recognized.

The provision of the usual pediatric dose is not a recommendation or indication that the drug should be utilized in the pediatric patient, but is intended to serve only as a guide. It should be emphasized that metabolism and elimination of many drugs, including the "inactive" ingredients in the dosage forms, are markedly different in full-term newborn infants, and even more so in premature infants, from those in older children and adults.

*Usual pediatric prescribing limits*—The usual pediatric prescribing limits subsection is intended primarily to guide the dispenser with respect to seeking confirmation of prescription orders calling for unusually small or large doses. In some cases, it may take into account some uses in addition to those implied in the statement of category. The time schedule and route of administration where given for the usual pediatric dose apply also to the usual pediatric prescribing limits unless otherwise specified.

*Usual geriatric dose*—A usual geriatric dose statement is included if current knowledge allows. It is to be emphasized that metabolism and elimination of many drugs, including the "inactive" ingredients in the dosage forms, may be markedly different in the geriatric patient.

The provision of the usual geriatric dose is not a recommendation or indication that the drug should be utilized in the geriatric patient. It is intended to serve only as a guide and it may be varied in the best interests of the patient and in accordance with the variables that affect the action of the drug.

*Strength(s) usually available*—The statement on strengths usually available for a dosage form, given in the individual monograph, is not necessarily complete and is intended solely as information to physicians, pharmacists, nurses, and others concerned with the manner in which dosage forms are commercially supplied.

If a specific drug product is known to contain sulfites, large amounts of lactose, or other inactive ingredients known to cause allergic reactions in large numbers of patients, this information has been included for selected medications.

*Packaging and storage*—Information concerning packaging and storage of medications as applicable to the dispenser is provided in this section. The labeling of the brand product selected may contain additional or other packaging and storage information specific to that product.

The information included in this section is not intended to replace more definitive requirements that may be contained in the official *USP* monographs. For those dosage forms included in *USP*, compendial requirements for packaging and storage apply to the dispenser.

For those products not covered by *USP*, the packaging and storage recommendations found in *USP DI* are usually those recommended by the manufacturer(s).

*Preparation of dosage form*—Instructions on constitution and/or dilution of a dosage form for administration are included. Information on the extemporaneous preparation of certain drugs, for example, for pediatric use, is also included, where deemed appropriate.

*Stability*—Included is information concerning beyond-use dates for constituted solutions or suspensions, along with special stability problems associated with certain drug products (for example, nitroglycerin tablets). The labeling of the brand product selected may contain specific stability information which differs from that stated in *USP DI*.

*Incompatibilities*—Chemical and physical incompatibilities of certain admixtures (e.g., intravenous preparations) are included, where deemed appropriate.

*Auxiliary labeling*—Auxiliary information (in addition to the prescription labeling) that is suggested for consideration of placement on the actual prescription container in accordance with applicable practice requirements is specified in this section.

Recommended labeling that relates to physical properties of the product (e.g., "shake well" for suspensions) can be considered to be universally applicable.

Suggested labeling that relates to therapy (e.g., take on an empty stomach) and would be appropriate for most, but not necessarily all patients, must be considered on an individual basis by the dispenser.

*Caution*—Information on potential medication errors, where known, and steps to help minimize occurrence of such errors are included as appropriate.

*Additional information*—Additional information relating to the specific drug product is included if necessary, especially as this information relates to the act of dispensing the medication.

**Advice for the Patient**—*Advice for the Patient* (Volume II) presents in lay language the concepts listed in the Patient Consultation guidelines of Volume I. It is meant to reinforce the oral consultation and to be provided in written form at the discretion of the health care provider. In general, statements that warrant a chevron (») in Patient Consultation are printed in *italic* type for immediate notice in *Advice for the Patient*.

Physicians, dentists, pharmacists, nurses, and other health care practitioners are given permission to reproduce a limited number of pages of Volume II but only when for direct distribution, without charge, to their patients or clients receiving the prescribed drug, provided that such reproduction shall include the copyright notice on each page.

The information presented under the section entitled *Additional Information* includes information related to medically accepted unlabeled uses of the drug. This section is intended for use where the health care provider has knowledge that the medication has been prescribed for a particular purpose referred to therein. It is intended as an aid to providing individualized patient education and is not for use when providing the general population with information about the drug. Since the section may contain information which may be or seem to be contradictory or confusing to the patient receiving the drug for its labeled purposes, the health care provider should consider not including this section if photocopies of the information are given to patients routinely.

**Approved Drug Products and Legal Requirements**—The United States Pharmacopeial Convention is the publisher of the *United States Pharmacopeia* and the *National Formulary*. These texts are recognized as official compendia by the pharmacy and medical professions. They contain standards, specifications, and other requirements relating to drugs and other articles used in medical and pharmacy practice that may be enforceable under various statutes. These requirements are applicable not only when drugs are in the possession of the manufacturer, but at the practice level as well.

Although the standards continue to be applicable when drugs are dispensed or sold, it must also be recognized that most prescriptions today are filled with manufactured products and for the most part physicians and pharmacists no longer compound or analyze drug products. On the other hand, dispensers need to be aware of the quality attributes of products, their packaging and storage requirements, and the other applicable standards to which legal consequences may attach.

In recognition of this need, Volume III provides abstracts of *USP-NF* standards. Similarly, selected portions of the *USP-NF* General Notices and Chapters that are deemed to be especially relevant are reprinted in Volume III.

The incorporation of these official *USP-NF* materials into *USP DI* is for informational purposes only. Because of varying publication schedules, there may occasionally be a time difference between publication of revisions in the *USP-NF* and the appearance of these changes in *USP DI*. Readers are advised that only the standards as written in the *USP-NF* are regarded as official.

The *USP-NF* material included in *USP DI* is not intended to represent nor shall it be interpreted to be the equivalent of or a substitute for the official *United States Pharmacopeia* and/ or *National Formulary*. In the event of any difference or discrepancy between the current official *USP* or *NF* standards and the information contained herein, the context and effect of the official compendia shall prevail.

Volume III also contains federal and state requirements relevant to the dispensing situation, including:

• the entire text of FDA's "Orange Book," *Approved Drug Products with Therapeutic Equivalence Evaluations;*
• separate listings of B-rated drugs from the FDA "Orange Book" and pre-1938 drugs ("grandfathered" drugs not included in the "Orange Book");
• selected portions of the federal Controlled Substance Act Regulations;
• the federal Food, Drug and Cosmetic Act requirements as they relate to human drugs, including the recent drug diversion and sampling amendments;
• FDA's Current Good Manufacturing Practice Regulations for Finished Pharmaceuticals.

Selected portions of each state's pharmacy practice act and regulations for dispensing, including product selection regulations, are included individually in a special *State Supplement* to the subscribers in that state.

*USP DI* Volume III is updated monthly, as is Volume I, *Drug Information for the Health Care Professional*, and Volume II, *Advice for the Patient*, as part of the regular *USP DI Update* service.

### Appendixes

To help the user of *USP DI*, numerous appendixes have been included in both Volume I and Volume II.

**Volume I**—Volume I includes the following additional material as appendixes:

*Additional Products and Indications* (Appendix I)—Newly marketed and other products not included in the main text of *USP DI* are referenced in this appendix in order to provide as much useful information as possible. The information included has not gone through the USP DI review process and is based simply on the product's package insert.

*Selected List of Drug-induced Effects* (Appendix II)—A list of selected drug-induced side effects has been compiled for use primarily in conjunction with the drug interactions section of *USP DI* monographs. The listing of drugs is not meant to be inclusive.

*Therapeutic Guidelines* (Appendix III)—This appendix provides selected general therapeutic guidelines for the health care professional.

*VA Medication Classification System* (Appendix IV)—The Veterans Administration Medication Classification system was developed to provide a systematic and management approach to the classification of medications, investigational drugs, prosthetic items, and expendable supplies for hospital patients. Primary and secondary VA codes are included in each *USP DI* monograph and in this appendix. In addition, codes for new products are included in the Additional Products and Indications chart (Appendix I).

*Orphan Drug and Biological Listing* (Appendix V)—As a service to users of the USP DI data base, this appendix reproduces the list of orphan drug and biological designations as issued by the U.S. Food and Drug Administration. This list includes the names of the substances, designated uses, and the names and addresses of sponsors. The information is inclusive for all orphan drug/biological designations made since the inception of the program. Some of these products have since been fully approved by the Food and Drug Administration and are currently being marketed. Others remain under investigation or are no longer being actively studied. The current status of each orphan drug/biological, where known, is included in the listing.

It should be noted that the names used in this listing for products that have not been approved for marketing may not be the established names approved by FDA for these products if they are eventually approved for marketing. Since these products are investigational, some may not have been reviewed for purposes of assigning the most appropriate name.

*Poison Control Center Listing* (Appendix VI)—Includes a listing of certified regional U.S. poison control centers.

*The Medicine Chart* (Appendix VII)—The Medicine Chart presents photographs of many of the most frequently prescribed medicines in the United States. In general, commonly used brand names and a representative sampling of generic products have been included. Only solid oral dosage forms (tablets and capsules) have been included. Since color and size variations may exist and since product changes may have subsequently been adopted by a manufacturer, the chart should be used only as an initial guide, with verification of product identity being made before any further actions are taken.

*The USP-Practitioners' Reporting Network* (Appendix VIII)—To assist health care professionals in their responsibility to report reactions to or problems with medications, the appropriate reporting forms are reproduced in this appendix.

**January *USP DI* Update**—The following supplemental information is included in the *USP DI Update* for January 1997, with page references to this book (i.e., Volume I):

*Category of Use Listing*—The category designations for each drug in the *USP DI* database are listed.

*Pregnancy Precaution Listing*—To assist the user of the *USP DI* database, this list includes those *USP DI* monographs that have a specific precaution as to use during pregnancy. Since the clinical significance of the precaution varies from drug to drug, the individual monograph should be consulted for additional information. The absence of a drug from the list is not meant to imply that that drug is necessarily known to be safe for use in pregnant patients.

*Breast-feeding Precaution Listing*—This list includes those *USP DI* monographs that have a specific precaution as to use of a drug while breast-feeding. Since the clinical significance of the precaution varies from drug to drug, the individual monograph should be consulted for additional information. The absence of a drug from the list is not meant to imply that that drug is necessarily known to be safe for use in women who are breast-feeding.

*Pediatrics Precaution Listing*—This list includes those *USP DI* monographs that have a specific precaution as to use of a drug in pediatric patients. Since the clinical significance of the precaution varies from drug to drug, the individual monograph should be consulted for additional information. The absence of a drug from the list is not meant to imply that that drug is necessarily known to be safe for use in pediatric patients.

*Geriatrics Precaution Listing*—This list includes those *USP DI* monographs that have a specific precaution as to use of a drug in geriatric patients. Since the clinical significance of the precaution varies from drug to drug, the individual monograph should be consulted for additional information. The absence of a drug from the list is not meant to imply that that drug is necessarily known to be safe for use in geriatric patients.

*Dental Precaution Listing*—This list includes those *USP DI* monographs that have a specific precaution as to dental effects. Since the type of effect and the clinical significance varies from drug to drug, the individual monograph should be consulted.

*Athletes Precautions*—Examples of drug substances that are banned and tested for in athletic competitions by the United States Olympic Committee (USOC), the National Collegiate Athletic Association (NCAA), and/or the International Olympic Committee (IOC) are listed. Not all such precautions may necessarily be listed. Official listings are maintained by the various athletic competition authorities.

*Drug Utilization Review*—The Drug Utilization Review (DUR) chapter includes a DUR process description, definitions, bibliography, framework for criteria development, and selected case studies.

*Total Parenteral Nutrition*—The Total Parenteral Nutrition/Total Nutrient Admixture (TPN/TNA) chapter includes information on stability, calcium/phosphate precipitates, medication compatibility, container recommendations, compounding guidelines, filtration recommendations, and environmental exposure risks.

*Introductory Version Monographs*—This section includes monographs on newly approved drugs based primarily on the manufacturer's package insert and reviewed by selected members of the appropriate USP DI Advisory Panels. Introductory Version Monographs fill the immediate need for information until a full monograph for a given drug has been developed and assessed by the advisory panels.

**Volume II**—As in Volume I, *The Medicine Chart* is included in Volume II in the front of the book. In addition, Volume II includes:

*General Information* (Appendix I)—This appendix includes sections on General Information about Use of Medicines, Avoiding Medicine Mishaps, Getting the Most Out of Your Medicines, and About the Medicines You Are Taking.

*Additional Products and Uses* (Appendix II)—Newly marketed and other products not included in the main text of *USP DI* are referenced in this appendix in order to provide as much useful information as possible. The information included has not gone through the *USP DI* review process and is based simply on the product's package insert.

*Poison Control Center Listing* (Appendix III)—Includes a listing of certified regional U.S. poison control centers.

*USP People* (Appendix IV)—This appendix lists USP Officers, Board of Trustees, Committees, Panels, and Members.

*Athletes Precautions* (Appendix V)—This appendix provides a selected list of those substances in *USP DI* that are banned and tested for in athletes by the United States Olympic Committee (USOC), the National Collegiate Athletic Association (NCAA), and/or the International Olympic Committee

(IOC). Not all such substances may necessarily be listed. Official listings are maintained by the various athletic competition authorities. Substances or drugs whose effects may be detrimental to an athlete or whose therapeutic effects may be affected by exercise are not addressed.

*Pictograms* (Appendix VI)—Visual images, or pictograms, which represent selected commonly used patients' directions are included in this appendix. The pictograms are intended to be used in a fashion that will reinforce other printed or oral instructions and as a reminder to patients as to the proper way to take or store their medication. They should not be used as the sole means of transferring information to the patient because of the potential for misinterpretation.

Although pictograms are copyrighted by the USPC, the USP has no objection to their use in accordance with the conditions described herein, provided the pictogram is accompanied by the indication of USP copyright ownership. USP assumes no responsibility for any misinterpretation or adverse results or effects resulting from the uses to which they may be put.

*Categories of Use* (Appendix VII)—A listing of drugs by their category of use is included in this appendix only as a useful reference. It should not be used to make decisions concerning the appropriateness of therapy. In addition, the drugs included under each entry should not be considered interchangeable for any given patient since in many instances the drugs will differ significantly with regard to effectiveness, seriousness of side effects, and other critical considerations.

*Pregnancy Precaution Listing* (Appendix VIII)—To assist the user of the *USP DI* database, this appendix provides a list of those *USP DI* monographs that have a specific precaution included as to use during pregnancy. Since the clinical significance of the precaution varies from drug to drug, the individual monograph should be consulted for additional information. The absence of a drug from the list is not meant to imply that the drug is necessarily known to be safe for use in pregnant patients.

*Breast-feeding Precaution Listing* (Appendix IX)—This appendix provides a list of those *USP DI* monographs that have a specific preaution included as to use of a drug while breast-feeding. Since the clinical significance of the precaution varies from drug to drug, the individual monograph should be consulted for additional information. The absence of a drug from the list is not meant to imply that the drug is necessarily known to be safe for use in women who are breast-feeding.

Volume II also includes a glossary of drug and medical terminology to help the consumer better understand the information presented in the *Advice for the Patient* monographs.

# USP PEOPLE 1995–2000

Stanley van den Noort, M.D., Irvine, CA
Joseph C. Veltri, Pharm.D., Salt Lake City, UT
Robert E. Vestal, M.D., Boise, ID
Irving W. Wainer, Ph.D., Montreal, PO
Philip D. Walson, M.D., Columbus, OH
Elliott T. Weisman, Philadelphia, PA
Paul F. White, Ph.D., M.D., Dallas, TX
Richard J. Whitley, M.D., Birmingham, AL
Robert J. Wolfangel, Ph.D., St. Louis, MO
Manfred E. Wolff, Ph.D., Laguna Beach , CA
Marie Linda A. Workman, Ph.D., R.N., Bay Village, OH
Wesley E. Workman, Ph.D., Chesterfield, MO
Timothy J. Wozniak, Ph.D., Indianapolis, IN
Dale Eric Wurster, Ph.D., Iowa City, IA
John W. Yarbro, M.D., Columbia, MO
Lynn C. Yeoman, Ph.D., Houston, TX
Thom J. Zimmerman, M.D., Ph.D., Louisville, KY

## EXECUTIVE COMMITTEE OF REVISION
Jerome A. Halperin, *Chair*
Lester Chafetz, Ph.D.
Joseph F. Gallelli, Ph.D.
Gordon L. Klein, M.D., M.P.H.
Robert D. Lindeman, M.D.
Carol S. Marcus, Ph.D., M.D.
Joseph R. Robinson, Ph.D.

## DIVISION OF INFORMATION DEVELOPMENT EXECUTIVE COMMITTEE
Robert E. Vestal, M.D., *Chair*
Ann B. Amerson, Pharm.D.
James C. Boylan, Ph.D.
Culley C. Carson, M.D.
Sebastian G. Ciancio, D.D.S.
Evelyn V. Hess, M.D., F.A.C.P., M.A.C.R.
V. Cory Langston, D.V.M., Ph.D. Diplomate ACVCP
Catherine M. MacLeod, M.D.
Carol S. Marcus, Ph.D., M.D.
Rosemary C. Polomano, Ph.D., M.S.N., R.N.
Thomas P. Reinders, Pharm.D.
Dan M. Roden, M.D.

Gordon D. Schiff, M.D.
Robert S. Stern, M.D.
Joseph C. Veltri, Pharm.D.

## DIVISION OF STANDARDS DEVELOPMENT EXECUTIVE COMMITTEE
Thomas P. Layloff, Ph.D., *Chair*
Gregory E. Amidon, Ph.D.
Judy P. Boehlert, Ph.D.
James C. Boylan, Ph.D.
William H. Briner
Herbert S. Carlin, D.Sc.
Zak T. Chowhan, Ph.D.
Everett Flanigan, Ph.D.
Thomas S. Foster, Pharm.D.
Robert L. Garnick, Ph.D.
Dennis K.J. Gorecki, Ph.D.
Stanley L. Hem, Ph.D.
Joseph E. Knapp, Ph.D.
Thomas Medwick, Ph.D.
Sharon J. Northup, Ph.D., M.B.A.
Ralph F. Shangraw, Ph.D.
E. John Staba, Ph.D.
James T. Stewart, Ph.D.
Henry S.I. Tan, Ph.D.
Elliott T. Weisman

## DRUG NOMENCLATURE COMMITTEE
Herbert S. Carlin, D.Sc., *Chair*
Ann B. Amerson, Pharm.D.
Lester Chafetz, Ph.D.
Stephanie Y. Crawford, Ph.D.
Everett Flanigan, Ph.D.
Douglas D. Glover, M.D., R.Ph.
Richard D. Johnson, Ph.D., Pharm D.
Edward G. Lovering, Ph.D.
Rosemary C. Polomano, Ph.D., M.S.N., R.N.
Thomas P. Reinders, Pharm.D.
Eric B. Sheinin, Ph.D.
Thomas D. Thomson, Ph.D., V.M.D.
Philip D. Walson, M.D.

# DIVISION OF INFORMATION DEVELOPMENT ADVISORY PANELS

Members who serve as Chairs are listed first.

The information presented in this text represents an ongoing review of the drugs contained herein and represents a consensus of various viewpoints expressed. The individuals listed below have served on the USP Advisory Panels for the 1995–1996 revision period and have contributed to the development of the 1997 USP DI database. Such listing does not imply that these individuals have reviewed all of the material in this text or that they individually agree with all statements contained herein.

## Anesthesiology
Paul F. White, Ph.D., M.D., *Chair*, Dallas, TX; Charles J. Coté, M.D., Chicago, IL; Peter S.A. Glass, M.D., Durham, NC; Michele E. Gold, Ph.D., C.R.N.A., Beverly Hills, CA; Frederick J. Goldstein, Ph.D., Philadelphia, PA; Thomas K. Henthorn, M.D., Chicago, IL; Michael B. Howie, M.D., Columbus, OH; Robert J. Hudson, M.D., Winnipeg, Manitoba; Scott D. Kelley, M.D., San Francisco, CA; Susan K. Palmer, M.D., Aurora, CO; Carl E. Rosow, M.D., Ph.D., Boston, MA; Mark A. Schumacher, Ph.D., M.D., San Francisco, CA; Peter S. Sebel, Ph.D., Atlanta, GA; Mehernoor F. Watcha, M.D., Dallas, TX; Matthew B. Weinger, M.D., San Diego, CA; Richard B. Weiskopf, M.D., San Francisco, CA; David H. Wong, Pharm.D., M.D., Long Beach, CA

## Blood and Blood Products
Harvey G. Klein, M.D., *Chair*, Bethesda, MD; James P. AuBuchon, M.D., Lebanon, NH; Morris A. Blajchman, M.D., Hamilton, Ontario; Marcela Contreras, M.D., FRCP, London, England; Alfred J. Grindon, M.D., Atlanta, GA; Douglas A. Kennedy, Ph.D., Ottawa, Ontario; Craig M. Kessler, M.D., Washington, DC; Jukka Koistinen, M.D., Ph.D., Helsinki, Finland; Volker Kretschmer, M.D., Ph.D.,

Marburg, Germany; Margot S. Kruskall, M.D., Boston, MA; Naomi L.C. Luban, M.D., Washington, DC; Jay E. Menitove, M.D., Cincinnati, OH; Paul M. Ness, M.D., Baltimore, MD; Henk W. Reesink, M.D., Ph.D., Amsterdam, The Netherlands; Karen A. Skalla, R.N., M.S.N., OCN, Windsor, VT; Ronald G. Strauss, M.D., Iowa City, IA

## Cardiovascular and Renal Drugs
Dan M. Roden, M.D., *Chair*, Nashville, TN; Jonathan Abrams, M.D., Albuquerque, NM; Joseph S. Alpert, M.D., Tucson, AZ; Jerry L. Bauman, Pharm.D., Chicago, IL; Ellen D. Burgess, M.D., Calgary, Alberta; James H. Chesebro, M.D., New York, NY; Moses Chow, Pharm.D., Hartford, CT; Joseph Cinanni, M.D., Ottawa, Ontario; Peter B. Corr, Ph.D., St. Louis, MO; David J. Driscoll, M.D., Rochester, MN; Dwain L. Eckberg, M.D., Richmond, VA; Andrew E. Epstein, M.D., Birmingham, AL; Arthur M. Feldman, M.D., Ph.D., Pittsburgh, PA; Michael P. Frenneaux, M.D., Herston Queensland, Australia; William H. Frishman, M.D., Bronx, NY; Edward D. Frohlich, M.D., New Orleans, LA; Donald B. Hunninghake, M.D., Minneapolis, MN; Joseph L. Izzo, Jr., M.D., Buffalo, NY; Norman M. Kaplan, M.D., Dallas, TX; Peter R. Kowey, M.D., Wynnewood, PA; Joseph Loscalzo, M.D., Ph.D., Boston, MA; Patrick A. McKee, M.D.,

xvii

Oklahoma City, OK; Juan Carlos Prieto, M.D., Santiago, Chile; Jane F. Schultz, R.N., B.S.N., Rochester, MN; Alexander M.M. Shepherd, M.D., San Antonio, TX; Burton E. Sobel, M.D., Burlington, VT; Raymond L. Woosley, M.D., Ph.D., Washington, DC

## Children and Medicines (Ad Hoc)
Janice M. Ozias, Ph.D., *Chair*, Austin, TX; Anna Birna Almarsdottir, Ph.D., Copenhagen, Denmark; Pilar Aramburuzabala, Ph.D., New York, NY; Roger Bibace, Ph.D., Worcester, MA; Renee R. Jenkins, M.D., Washington, DC; Margo Kroshus, B.S.N., Rochester, MN; Colleen Lum Lung, R.N., Englewood, CO; Carolyn H. Lund, R.N., San Francisco, CA; Robert O'Brien, Ph.D., Chevy Chase, MD; Robert H. Pantell, M.D., San Francisco, CA; Susan Schneider, M.P.H., Bethesda, MD; Bernard A. Sorofman, Ph.D., Iowa City, IA; Wayne A. Yankus, M.D., Midland Park, NJ

## Clinical Toxicology/Substance Abuse
Joseph C. Veltri, Pharm.D., *Chair*, Salt Lake City, UT; Neal L. Benowitz, M.D., San Francisco, CA; Usoa E. Busto, Pharm.D., Toronto, Ontario; Timothy R. Dring, Woodbridge, NJ; David J. George, Ph.D., R.Ph., Madison, NJ; Edward P. Krenzelok, Pharm.D., Pittsburgh, PA; David C. Lewis, M.D., Providence, RI; Michael Montagne, Ph.D., Boston, MA; Claudio A. Naranjo, M.D., North York, Ontario; Edward J. Otten, M.D., Cincinnati, OH; Paul Pentel, M.D., Minneapolis, MN; Lorie G. Rice, San Francisco, CA; Elizabeth J. Scharman, Pharm.D., Charleston, WV; Michael W. Shannon, M.D., Boston, MA; Rose Ann G. Soloway, RN, MSEd, ABAT, Washington, DC; Anthony C. Tommasello, M.S., Baltimore, MD; Theodore G. Tong, Pharm.D., Tucson, AZ; Alison M. Trinkoff, ScD, RN, Baltimore, MD; William A. Watson, Pharm.D., Kansas City, MO; Julian White, M.D., Australia

## Consumer Interest/Health Education
Gordon D. Schiff, M.D., *Chair*, Chicago, IL; Michael J. Ackerman, Ph.D., Bethesda, MD; Frank J. Ascione, Pharm.D., Ph.D., Ann Arbor, MI; Roger Bibace, Ph.D., Worcester, MA; Allan H. Bruckheim, M.D., Harrison, NY; Mary E. Carman, B.Sc., Ottawa, Ontario; Margaret A. Charters, Ph.D., Syracuse, NY; Laura J. Cranston, Fairfax Station, VA; Jennifer Cross, San Francisco, CA; David A. Danielson, Roxbury, MA; Sandra M. Fabregas, R.Ph., San Juan, PR; Sophia Jones-Redmond, Chicago, IL; Louis H. Kompare, Nashville, TN; Margo Kroshus, B.S.N., Rochester, MN; Bruce L. Lambert, Ph.D., Chicago, IL; Arthur Levin, New York, NY; Roberto Lopez Linares, Chimbote, Peru; Janet M. Manuel, Halifax, Nova Scotia; Frederick S. Mayer, Sausalito, CA; Jacqueline D. McLeod, New York, NY; Charles Medawar, London, England; Nancy Milio, Ph.D., Chapel Hill, NC; Michael A. Mone', Tallahassee, FL; Janet Ohene-Frempong, Philadelphia, PA; James C. Wohlleb, Little Rock, AR

## Critical Care Medicine
Catherine M. MacLeod, M.D., *Chair*, Chicago, IL; Robert A. Balk, M.D., Chicago, IL; Philip S. Barie, M.D., New York, NY; Thomas P. Bleck, M.D., Charlottesville, VA; Eugene Y. Cheng, M.D., Milwaukee, WI; Susan S. Fish, Pharm.D., Boston, MA; Edgar R. Gonzalez, Pharm.D., Richmond, VA; Angela M. Hadbavny, Pharm.D., Pittsburgh, PA; John W. Hoyt, M.D., Pittsburgh, PA; Louis J. Ling, M.D., Minneapolis, MN; Sheldon A. Magder, M.D., Canada; Daniel A. Notterman M.D., Princeton, NJ; Sharon D. Peters, M.D., CANADA; Domenic A. Sica, M.D., Richmond, VA; George A. Skowronski, New South Wales, Australia; Andrea L. Strayer, CNRN, Madison, WI; Martin G. Tweeddale, Ph.D., Vancouver, British Columbia

## Dentistry
Sebastian G. Ciancio, D.D.S., *Chair*, Buffalo, NY; B. Ellen Byrne, D.D.S., Ph.D., Richmond, VA; Barbara R. Clark, Pharm.D., Kansas City, MO; Frederick Curro, D.M.D., Ph.D., Jersey City, NJ; Tommy W. Gage, D.D.S., Ph.D., Dallas, TX; Daniel A. Haas, D.D.S., Ph.D., Toronto, Ontario; Richard E. Hall, D.D.S., Ph.D., Buffalo, NY; John T. Hamilton, Ph.D., London, Ontario; Angelo J. Mariotti, D.D.S., Ph.D., Columbus, OH; Linda C. Niessen, D.M.D., Dallas, TX; Clarence L. Trummel, D.D.S., Farmington, CT; Joel. M. Weaver, II, D.D.S., Ph.D., Columbus, OH; Clifford W. Whall, Jr., Ph.D., Chicago, IL; Raymond P. White, Jr., D.D.S., Ph.D., Chapel Hill, NC; Richard L. Wynn, Ph.D., Baltimore, MD; John A. Yagiela, D.D.S., Ph.D., Los Angeles, CA

## Dermatology
Robert S. Stern, M.D., *Chair*, Boston, MA; Beatrice B. Abrams, Ph.D., East Hanover, NJ; Richard D. Baughman, M.D., Lebanon, NH; Mary-Margaret Chren, M.D., Shaker Heights, OH; Diane M. Cooper, Ph.D., R.N., Bay Pines, FL; Ponciano D. Cruz, M.D., Dallas, TX; Vincent Falanga, M.D., Miami, FL; James J. Ferry, Ph.D., Kalamazoo, MI; Vincent C. Ho, M.D., Vancouver, British Columbia; Donald P. Lookingbill, M.D., Hershey, PA; Stuart Maddin, M.D., Vancouver, British Columbia; Milton Orkin, M.D., Minneapolis, MN; Amy S. Paller, M.D., Chicago, IL; Jean-Claude Roujeau, M.D., Paris, France; Neil H. Shear, M.D., Toronto, Ontario; Celia A. Viets, M.D., Ottawa, Ontario; Dennis P. West, Ph.D., Chicago, IL

## Diagnostic Agents--Nonradioactive
Robert L. Siegle, M.D., *Chair*, San Antonio, TX; Leonard M. Baum, R.Ph., Princeton, NJ; Martin J. K. Blomley, M.B., London, England; Robert C. Brasch, M.D., San Francisco, CA; Olivier Clement, M.D., Ph.D., Paris, France; Sachiko T. Cochran, M.D., Los Angeles, CA; Kathryn L. Grant, Pharm.D., Tucson, AZ; Kenneth D. Hopper, M.D., Hershey, PA; Fred T. Lee, Jr., M.D., Madison, WI; Robert F. Mattrey, M.D., San Diego, CA; James A. Nelson, M.D., Seattle, WA; Jovitas Skucas, M.D., Rochester, NY; Gerald L. Wolf, Ph.D., M.D., Charlestown, MA

## Drug Utilization Review
Terrence F. Blaschke, M.D., *Chair*, Stanford, CA; David M. Angaran, R.Ph., Columbus, OH; Edward P. Armstrong, Pharm.D., Tucson, AZ; Jim L. Blackburn, Pharm.D., Saskatoon, Saskatchewan; Catherine E. Burley, M.D., Fayetteville, GA; Patricia J. Byrns, M.D., Denver, CO; Elizabeth A. Chrischilles, Ph.D., Iowa City, IA; Theodore M. Collins, R.Ph., Madison, WI; Robert P. Craig, Pharm.D., Scottsdale, AZ; W. Gary Erwin, Pharm.D., Philadelphia, PA; Stan N. Finklestein, M.D., Cambridge, MA; Catherine A. Harrington, Pharm.D., Ph.D., Fairfax, VA; Joel W. Hay, Ph.D., Los Angeles, CA; Mark L. Horn, M.D., New York, NY; Judith K. Jones, M.D., Ph.D., Arlington, VA; Michael L. Kelly, R.Ph., Jackson, MS; Duane M. Kirking, Pharm.D., Ph.D., Ann Arbor, MI; Ann M. Koeniguer, R.Ph., Summerfield, NC; David Lee, M.D., Arlington, VA; Gary M. Levine, R.Ph., St. Louis, MO; Gladys Peachey, RN, MEd, MHSc, Dundas, Ontario; Eleanor M. Perfetto, Ph.D., Radnor, PA; T. Donald Rucker, Ph.D., River Forest, IL; Daniel W. Saylak, D.O., Bryan, TX; Fredrica E. Smith, M.D., Los Alamos, NM; Brian L. Strom, M.D., Philadelphia, PA; Ilene H. Zuckerman, Pharm.D., Batimore, MD

## Endocrinology
David S. Cooper, M.D., *Chair*, Baltimore, MD; Robert L. Barbieri, M.D., Wellesley, MA; Stuart J. Brink, M.D., Waltham, MA; R. Keith Campbell, Pharm.D., Pullman, WA; Ernesto Canalis, M.D., Hartford, CT; Betty J. Dong, Pharm.D., San Francisco, CA; Shereen Ezzat, M.D., Toronto, Ontario; Lawrence A. Frohman, M.D., Chicago, IL; Steven R. Goldring, M.D., Boston, MA; Jerome M. Hershman, M.D., Los Angeles, CA; Robert G. Josse, M.B., Toronto, Ontario; Michael M. Kaplan, M.D., West Bloomfield, MI; Selna Kaplan, M.D., Ph.D., San Francisco, CA; Marvin E. Levin, M.D., Chesterfield, MO; Marvin M. Lipman, M.D., Scarsdale, NY; Daniel J. Marante, M.D., Caracas, Venezuela; Robert Marcus, M.D., Palo Alto, CA; Barbara J. Maschak-Carey, RNCS, Philadelphia, PA; Shlomo Melmed, M.D., Los Angeles, CA; Ronald P. Monsaert, M.D., Danville, PA; John E. Morley, M.B., B.Ch., St. Louis, MO; Paul Saenger, M.D., Bronx, NY; Mary Lee Vance, M.D., Charlottesville, VA; Leonard Wartofsky, M.D., Washington, DC

## Family Practice
Robert M. Guthrie, M.D., *Chair*, Columbus, OH; John A. Brose, D.O., Athens, OH; Mark E. Clasen, M.D., Ph.D., Dayton, OH; Yves Gariepy, B.Sc., Ste-Foy, Quebec; Sloan Karver, M.D., Wyomissing, PA; Joseph A. Lieberman, III, M.D., Wilmington, DE; Charles D. Ponte, Pharm.D., Morgantown, WV; John W. Robinson, M.D., Salt Lake City, UT; Jack M. Rosenberg, Pharm.D., Ph.D., Hillsdale, NJ; Jorge E. Sanchez, M.D., San Salvador, El Salvador; May S.M. Smith, Ottawa, Ontario; John E. Thornburg, D.O., Ph.D., East Lansing, MI; Richard A. Wherry, M.D., Dahlonega, GA; Theodore L. Yarboro, Sr., M.D., M.P.H., Sharon, PA

## Gastroenterology
Gordon L. Klein, M.D., *Chair*, Galveston, TX; Karl E. Anderson, M.D., Galveston, TX; Paul Bass, Ph.D., Madison, WI; Adrian M. Di Bisceglie, M.D., St. Louis, MO; Jack A. DiPalma, M.D., Mobile, AL;

Thomas Q. Garvey III, M.D., Potomac, MD; Flavio Habal, M.D., Ph.D., Toronto, Ontario; Eric G. Hassall, M.D., Vancouver, British Columbia; Alan F. Hofmann, M.D., La Jolla, CA; Paul E. Hyman, M.D., Orange, CA; Agnes V. Klein, M.D., Ottawa, Ontario; James H. Lewis, M.D., Washington, DC; Bernard Mehl, D.P.S., New York, NY; Joel E. Richter, M.D., Cleveland, OH; William J. Snape, Jr., M.D., Long Beach, CA; C. Noel Williams, M.D., Halifax, Nova Scotia; Hyman J. Zimmerman, M.D., Bethesda, MD

### Geriatrics
Robert E. Vestal, M.D., *Chair*, Boise, ID; Darrell R. Abernethy, M.D., Washington, DC; Mark H. Beers, M.D., West Point, PA; Robert A. Blouin, Pharm.D., Lexington, KY; S. George Carruthers, M.D., London, Ontario; Martin J. Connolly, M.D., Cheshire, England; Madeline Feinberg, Pharm.D., Silver Spring, MD; Jerry H. Gurwitz, M.D., Worcester, MA; Geri R. Hall, Ph.D.(c), ARNP, CS, Coralville, IA; Martin D. Higbee, Pharm.D., Tucson, AZ; Brian B. Hoffman, M.D., Palo Alto, CA; Barbara A. Liu, M.D., North York, Ontario; Ann Miller, Morro Bay, CA; Paul A. Mitenko, M.D., Nanaimo, British Columbia; Janice B. Schwartz, M.D., Chicago, IL; Joanne G. Schwartzerg, M.D., Chicago, IL; William Simonson, Pharm.D., Portland, OR; Daniel S. Sitar, Ph.D., Winnipeg, Manitoba; Alastair J.J. Wood, M.D., Nashville, TN

### Hematologic and Oncologic Disease
John W. Yarbro, M.D., Ph.D., *Chair*, Columbia, MO; Joseph S. Bailes, M.D., Dallas, TX; Laurence H. Baker, D.O., Ann Arbor, MI; Edward Braud, M.D., Springfield, IL; Donald C. Doll, M.D., Columbia, MO; Ross C. Donehower, M.D., Baltimore, MD; Janet M. Ellerhorst-Ryan, R.N., Cincinnati, OH; Martha Harczy, M.D., Ottawa, Ontario; David T. Harris, M.D., Wynewood, PA; Connie Henke Yarbro, R.N., Columbia, MO; Charles Hoppel, M.D., Cleveland, OH; B. J. Kennedy, M.D., Minneapolis, MN; Barnett S. Kramer, M.D., Bethesda, MD; Celeste Lindley, Pharm.D., Chapel Hill, NC; Michael J. Mastrangelo, M.D., Philadelphia, PA; Paulette Mehta, M.D., Gainesville, FL; Perry D. Nisen, M.D., Ph.D., Dallas, TX; David S. Rosenthal, M.D., Cambridge, MA; Roy L. Silverstein, M.D., New York, NY; Ellen L. Stovall, Silver Spring, MD; Samuel G. Taylor, M.D., Chicago, IL; Raymond B. Weiss, M.D., Rockville, MD

### Infectious Disease Therapy
William A. Craig, M.D., *Chair*, Madison, WI; P. Joan Chesney, M.D., Memphis, TN; C. Glenn Cobbs, M.D., Birmingham, AL; Courtney V. Fletcher, Pharm.D., Minneapolis, MN; H. Hunter Handsfield, M.D., Seattle, WA; Frederick G. Hayden, M.D., Charlottesville, VA; Carol A. Kauffman, M.D., Ann Arbor, MI; Marc LeBel, Pharm.D., Ste-Foy, Quebec; S. Ragnar Norrby, M.D., Ph.D., Lund, Sweden; Laszlo Palkonyay, M.D, Ottawa, Ontario; Douglas D. Richman, M.D., La Jolla, CA; Xavier Saez-Llorens, M.D., Panama City, Panama; Roy T. Steigbigel, M.D., Stony Brook, NY; Richard J. Whitley, M.D., Birmingham, AL

### Information Science [or Informatics]
Ann B. Amerson, Pharm.D., *Chair*, Lexington, KY; Marie A. Abate, Pharm.D., Morgantown, WV; Wesley G. Byerly, Pharm.D., Winston-Salem, NC; Teresa Dowling, Pharm.D., Wilmington, DE; Thomas M. Gesell, Pharm.D., Abbott Park, IL; Stephen R. Kaplan, M.D., Buffalo, NY; Ossy M J Kasilo, Ph.D., Harare, Zimbabwe; Aishah A. Latiff, Ph.D., Penang, Malaysia; Leslie A. Lenert, M.D., Stanford, CA; Dr. Hubert G.M. Leufkens, Utrecht, The Netherlands; M. Laurie Mashford, M.D., Victoria, Australia; Louise Matte, B.Sc., B.Pharm., Montreal, Quebec; Kurt A. Proctor, Ph.D., Alexandria, VA; Carol A. Romano, Ph.D., R.N., Bethesda, MD; Cedric M. Smith, M.D., Buffalo, NY; Gary H. Smith, Pharm.D., Tucson, AZ; Dennis F. Thompson, Pharm.D., Oklahoma City, OK; William G. Troutman, Pharm.D., Albuquerque, NM; Gordon J. Vanscoy, Pharm.D., Irwin, PA; Valentin A. Vinogradov, M.D., Ph.D., Moscow, Russia; Lee A. Wanke, Seattle, WA; Antonio Carlos Zanini, M.D., Ph.D., Sao Paulo, Brazil

### International Health
Eugenie Brown, Pharm.D., Kingston, Jamaica; Laura Ceron, Pharm.D., Lima, Peru; Albin Chaves Matamoros, M.D., San Jose, Costa Rica; Gabriel Daniel, Washington, DC; Enrique Fefer, Ph.D., Rockville, MD; Peter H.M. Fontilus, Curacao, Netherlands Antilles; Reginald F. Gipson, M.D., MPH, Atlanta, GA; Mariatou Tala Jallow, Pharm.D., Banjul, The Gambia; Mohan P. Joshi, M.D., Kathmandu,

Nepal; Rosalyn C. King, Pharm.D., Silver Spring, MD; David E. Kuhl, Pharm.D., Albuquerque, NM; Richard O. Laing, M.D., Boston, MA; Thomas Lapnet-Moustapha, Pharm.D., Yaounde, Cameroon; Denise Leclerc, Ph.D., Montreal, Quebec; Aissatou Lo, Dakar, Dakar, Senegal; David Ofori-Adjei, M.D., Accra, Ghana; Dr. S. Ofosu-Amaah, Legon, Accra, Ghana; James Rankin, Arlington, VA; Dennis Ross-Degnan, Boston, MA; Budiono Santoso, M.D., Ph.D., Yogyakarta, Indonesia; Fela Viso Gurovich, Ph.D., Mexico City, Mexico; Krisantha Weerasuriya, M.D., Colombo, Sri Lanka; Albert I. Wertheimer, Ph.D., Glen Allen, VA

### Medication Counseling Behavior Guidelines (Ad Hoc)
Frank J. Ascione, Pharm.D., Ph.D., *Chair*, Ann Arbor, MI; John E. Arradondo, M.D., Nashville, TN; Candace Barnett, Atlanta, GA; Allan H. Bruckheim, M.D., Harrison, NY; Mark E. Clasen, M.D., Ph.D., Dayton, OH; Frederick Curro, D.M.D., Ph.D., Jersey City, NJ; Robin DiMatteo, Ph.D., Riverside, CA; Diane B. Ginsburg, Austin, TX; Denise Grimes, Jackson, MI; Richard Herrier, Tucson, AZ; Barry Kass, R.Ph., Boston, MA; Thomas Kellenberger, Pharm.D., Montvale, NJ; Alice Kimball, Darnestown, MD; Patricia A. Kramer, B.S., Bismarck, ND; Patricia Kummeth, Rochester, MN; Ken Leibowitz, Philadelphia, PA; Colleen Lum Lung, R.N., Englewood, CO; Louise Matte, B.Sc., B.Pharm., Montreal, Quebec; Amy Outlaw,Pharm.D., Stone Mountain, GA; Constance Pavlides, R.N., Rockville, MD; Scotti Russell, Richmond, VA; Lisa Tedesco, Ph.D., Ann Arbor, MI

### Neurology
Stanley van den Noort, M.D., *Chair*, Irvine, CA; A. Leland Albright, M.D., Pittsburgh, PA; Elizabeth U. Blalock, M.D., Anaheim, CA; Mitchell F. Brin, M.D., New York, NY; Louis R. Caplan, M.D., Boston, MA; James C. Cloyd, Pharm.D., Minneapolis, MN; David M. Dawson, M.D., West Roxbury, MA; Mark J. Fisher, M.D., Los Angeles, CA; Kathleen M. Foley, M.D., New York, NY; Robert A. Gross, M.D., Ph.D., Rochester, NY; Stanley Hashimoto, M.D., Vancouver, British Columbia; William C. Koller, M.D., Ph.D., Kansas City, KS; Ilo E. Leppik, M.D., Minneapolis, MN; Ira T. Lott, M.D., Orange, CA; Susan McMillan, R.N., Ph.D., Temple Terrace, FL; T.J. Murray, M.D., Halifax, Nova Scotia; Judith A. Paice, Ph.D., R.N., Chicago, IL; Richard D. Penn, M.D., Chicago, IL; Roger J. Porter, M.D., Philadelphia, PA; Neil H. Raskin, M.D., San Francisco, CA; James F. Toole, M.D., Winston-Salem, NC; Howard L. Weiner, M.D., Boston, MA

### Nursing Practice
Rosemary C. Polomano, Ph.D., R.N., *Chair*, Pottstown, PA; Bonnie J. Adamson, R.N., London, Ontario; Ramona A. Benkert, M.S.N., R.N., Plymouth, MI; Mecca S. Cranley, Ph.D., R.N., Buffalo, NY; Linda Felver, Ph.D., R.N., Portland, OR; Hector Hugo Gonzalez, Ph.D., R.N., San Antonio, TX; Theodore L. Goodfriend, M.D., Madison, WI; Ada K. Jacox, R.N., Ph.D., Detroit, MI; Daisy M. Jones, R.N., Chicago, IL; Patricia Kummeth, Rochester, MN; Ida S. Martinson, Ph.D., R.N., San Francisco, CA; Ginette A. Pepper, Ph.D., R.N., Denver, CO; Geraldine A. Peterson, M.A., R.N., Potomac, MD; Linda C. Pugh, Ph.D., Hershey, PA; Sharon S. Rising, R.N., Chesire, CT; April H. Vallerand, Ph.D., R.N., Manalapan, NJ

### Nutrition and Electrolytes
Robert D. Lindeman, M.D., *Chair*, Albuquerque, NM; Jeffrey P. Baker, M.D., Toronto, Ontario; Connie W. Bales, Ph.D., R.D., Durham, NC; Dennis M. Bier, M.D., Houston, TX; Gladys Block, Ph.D., Berkeley, CA; Karim Anton Calis, Pharm.D., M.P.H., Rockville, MD; David F. Driscoll, Ph.D., Boston, MA; P.W.F. Fischer, Ph.D., Ottawa, Ontario; Dr. Nigel Gericke, Cape Town, South Africa; Walter H. Glinsmann, M.D., Washington, DC; Helen A. Guthrie, Ph.D., State College, PA; John N. Hathcock, Ph.D., Washington, DC; Ronald M. Isaac, M.D., Round Lake, IL; Leslie M. Klevay, M.D., Grand Forks, ND; Linda S. Knox, Ph.D., R.N., Philadelphia, PA; Bonnie Liebman, M.S., Washington, DC; Sohrab Mobarhan, M.D., Maywood, IL; Robert M. Russell, M.D., Boston, MA; Harold H. Sandstead, M.D., Galveston, TX; Benjamin Torun, M.D., Ph.D., Guatemala City, Guatemala; Carlos A. Vaamonde, M.D., Miami, FL; Stanley Wallach, M.D., New York, NY

### Obstetrics and Gynecology
Douglas D. Glover, M.D., *Chair*, Morgantown, WV; Rudi Ansbacher, M.D., Ann Arbor, MI; James E. Axelson, Ph.D., Aldergrove, British

## Rheumatology-Clinical Immunology

Evelyn V. Hess, M.D., *Chair*, Cincinnati, OH; Donato Alarcon-Segovia, M.D., Mexico City, Mexico; John Baum, M.D., Rochester, NY; David H. Campen, M.D., Santa Clara, CA; Paul Emery, M.D., Leeds, England; Daniel E. Furst, M.D., Seattle, WA; Jean G. Gispen, M.D., Oxford, MS; Esther Gonzales-Pares, M.D., San Juan, PR; Donna J. Hawley, R.N., Ed.D., Wichita, KS; Israeli A. Jaffe, M.D., New York, NY; Daniel J. Lovell, M.D., M.P.H., Cincinnati, OH; Walter P. Maksymowych, M.D., Edmonton, Alberta; Donald R. Miller, Pharm.D., Fargo, ND; Ivan G. Otterness, Ph.D., Groton, CT; Robert L. Rubin, Ph.D., La Jolla, CA; Lee S. Simon, M.D., Boston, MA; Daniel J. Stechschulte, M.D., Kansas City, KS; Michael E. Weinblatt, M.D., Boston, MA; Michael H. Weisman, M.D., San Diego, CA; William S. Wilke, M.D., Cleveland, OH; David E. Yocum, M.D., Tucson, AZ

## Surgical Drugs and Devices

Lary A. Robinson, M.D., *Chair*, Tampa, FL; Kay A. Ball, M.S.A., R.N., Lewis Center, OH; Alan R. Dimick, M.D., Birmingham, AL; G. Douglas Letson, M.D., Tampa, FL; H. Kim Lyerly, M.D., Durham, NC; Henry J. Mann, Pharm.D., Minneapolis, MN; Joseph A. Moylan, M.D., Miami, FL; Ronald Lee Nichols, M.D., New Orleans, LA; Hiram C. Polk, Jr., M.D., Louisville, KY; Robert P. Rapp, Pharm.D., Lexington, KY; Ronald Rubin, M.D., West Newton, MA

## Transplant Immunology

Thomas E. Starzl, M.D., Ph.D., *Chair*, Pittsburgh, PA; Clyde F. Barker, M.D., Philadelphia, PA; Gilbert J. Burckart, Pharm.D., Pittsburgh, PA; Paul M. Colombani, M.D., Baltimore, MD; Allan P. Donner, Ph.D., London, Ontario; Robert A. Good, Ph.D., M.D., St. Petersburg, FL; Carl C. Groth, M.D., Ph.D., Huddinge, Sweden; John A. Hansen, M.D., Seattle, WA; Roger L. Jenkins, M.D., Boston, MA; John R. Lake, M.D., San Francisco, CA; Leonard Makowka, M.D., Ph.D., Los Angeles, CA; Suzanne V. McDiarmid, M.D., Los Angeles, CA; Charles Miller, M.D., New York, NY; Ali Naji, M.D., Ph.D., Philadelphia, PA; David H. Sachs, M.D., Boston, MA; Joseph A. Tami, Pharm.D., Carlsbad, CA; Angus W. Thomson, Ph.D., Pittsburgh, PA; Raman Venkataramanan, Ph.D., Pittsburgh, PA; Prof. Roger Williams, CBE, London, England

## Urology

Culley C. Carson, M.D., *Chair*, Chapel Hill, NC; John A. Belis, M.D., Hershey, PA; B. J. Reid Czarapata, Rockville, MD; Sam D. Graham, Jr., M.D., Atlanta, GA; Mireille Gregoire, M.D., Quebec, Quebec; Wayne Hellstrom, M.D., New Orleans, LA; Joseph M. Khoury, M.D., Chapel Hill, NC; Marguerite C. Lippert, M.D., Charlottesville, VA; Michael G. Mawhinney, Ph.D., Morgantown, WV; Nelson Rodrigues Netto Jr., M.D., Sao Paulo, Brazil; Mariano Rosello-Barbera, M.D., Palma de Mallorca, Spain; Randall G. Rowland, M.D., Ph.D., Indianapolis, IN; J. Patrick Spirnak, M.D., Cleveland, OH; William F. Tarry, M.D., Morgantown, WV; Chris M. Teigland, M.D., Charlotte, NC; Robert M. Weiss, M.D., New Haven, CT

## Veterinary Medicine

V. Cory Langston, D.V.M., Ph.D., *Chair*, Mississippi State, MS; Michael D. Apley, D.V.M., Ph.D., Ames, IA; Gordon W. Brumbaugh, D.V.M., Ph.D., College Station, TX; Thomas J. Burkgren, D.V.M., M.B.A., Perry, IA; Cynthia T. Culmo, R.Ph., Austin, TX; Lloyd E. Davis, Ph.D., D.V.M., Champaign, IL; Joseph A. DiPietro, D.V.M., M.S., Urbana, IL; Patricia M. Dowling, D.V.M., M.S., Saskatoon, Saskatchewan; Stuart D. Forney, M.S., Fort Collins, CO; Antoinette D. Jernigan, D.V.M., Ph.D., Groton, CT; Mark G. Papich, D.V.M., Raleigh, NC; Thomas E. Powers, D.V.M., Ph.D., Columbus, OH; Jim E. Riviere, D.V.M., Ph.D., Raleigh, NC; Charles R. Short, D.V.M., Ph.D., Baton Rouge, LA; Hector Sumano Lopez, D.V.M., Ph.D., M.D., Mexico City, Mexico; Jeffrey R. Wilcke, D.V.M., Blacksburg, VA;

---

# DIVISION OF INFORMATION DEVELOPMENT
# ADDITIONAL CONTRIBUTORS

The information presented in this text represents an ongoing review of the drugs contained herein and represents a consensus of various viewpoints expressed. In addition to the individuals listed below, many schools, associations, pharmaceutical companies, and governmental agencies have provided comment or otherwise contributed to the development of the 1997 USP DI data base. Such listing does not imply that these individuals have reviewed all of the material in this text or that they individually agree with all statements contained herein.

Donald I. Abrams, M.D., San Francisco, CA
Werner Apt, M.D., Santiago, Chile
Philip L. Ballard, M.D., Philadelphia, PA
Rick A. Barbarash, Pharm.D., St. Louis, MO
Patsy Barnett, Pharm.D., Birmingham, AL
Norman W. Barton, M.D., Phoenix, MD
LuAnne Barron, Birmingham, AL
Guy Beaulieu, Ph.D., Ottawa, Ontario
Robert W. Beightol, Pharm.D., Roanoke, VA
William Bell, M.D., Baltimore, MD
Dr. Bruno Bembi, Trieste, Italy
Ernest Beutler, M.D., La Jolla, CA
Martin Black, M.D., Philadelphia, PA
Robert Blizzard, M.D., Charlottesville, VA
Mark Blumenthal, Austin, TX
Richard Bockman, M.D., Ph.D., New York, NY
Bertha A. Bouroncle, M.D., Columbus, OH
Wayne Bradley, Duluth, GA
Michael Brady, M.D., Columbus, OH
Lewis E. Braverman, M.D., Worcester, MA
Aodan S. Breathnach, M.D., London, England
Prof. Martin J. Brodie, Glasgow, Scotland
Dr. Anthony F.T. Brown, Herston, Queensland, Australia
Beverly S. Brozanski, M.D., Pittsburgh, PA
William Budris, BSPharm, Chicago, IL
Bruce Burgess, M.S., N. Billerica, MA
William Busse, M.D., Madison, WI
Wesley G. Byerly, Pharm.D., Winston-Salem, NC
Michael Camilleri, M.D., Rochester, MN
Marcel Casavant, M.D., Columbus, OH
Bartolome R. Celli, M.D., Boston, MA
Chih Wen Chang, Pharm.D., Maywood, IL
Kenneth R. Chapman, M.D., Toronto, Ontario

Dr. Souchai Chazasousobhon, Anaheim, CA
Neil S. Cherniak, M.D., Cleveland, OH
Bruce D. Cheson, M.D., Bethesda, MD
Dr. Guy Chovinard, Montreal, Quebec
Debbie Cipoletti, Pharm.D., Phoenix, AZ
Robert Clemons, M.D., Phoenix, AZ
Donald Cockcroft, M.D., Hamilton, Ontario
Dr. R.E. Coleman, Sheffield, England
R. Edward Coleman, M.D., Durham, NC
Jackson Como, Pharm.D., Birmingham, AL
James W. Cooper, Ph.D., Athens, GA
Clinton N. Corder, Ph.D., M.D., Oklahoma City, OK
Lawrence Corey, M.D., Seattle, WA
Dr. Jim Correia, N. Billerica, MA
Deborah Cotton, M.D., Boston, MA
Timothy Cox, M.D., Cambridge, England
Arthur L. Craigmill, Ph.D., Davis, CA
Dr. Bart Currie, Darwin, Australia
Dr. Anthony J. Cutie, Brooklyn, NY
Dr. H.G. Cutler, Athens, GA
Pamela B. Davis, M.D. , Ph.D., Cleveland, OH
Tom Day, D.V.M., M.S., Mississippi State, MS
Thomas D. DeCillis, North Port, FL
Louis Diamond, Ph.D., Denver, CO
Michael S. Dunn, M.D., Toronto, Ontario
Sue Duran, R.Ph., M.S., Auburn University, AL
Deborah Elstein, M.D., Jerusalem, Israel
Elihu H. Estey, M.D., Houston, TX
Edward R. Faught, M.D., Birmingham, AL
William Feldman, M.D., Toronto, Ontario, Canada
Duncan Ferguson, Athens, GA
Durland Fish, Ph.D., New Haven, CT
Maria Font, Vicenza, Italy

Jonathan Foster, M.D., Waterbury, CT
Kenneth Fotherby, M.D., London, England
Dr. Ruth Francis-Floyd, Gainesville, FL
Mitchell Friedman, M.D., New Orleans, LA
William A. Gahl, M.D., Bethesda, MD
Jose P.B. Gallardo, R.Ph., Iowa City, IA
Gary F. Gates, M.D., Portland, OR
Edward Genton, M.D., New Orleans, LA
Dr. Joe Glajch, N. Billerica, MA
W. Paul Glezen, M.D., Houston, TX
Harvey M. Golomb, M.D., Chicago, IL
Michelle Goodman, RN, MS, Chicago, IL
Maj. John D. Grabenstein, M.S., Chapel Hill, NC
Gregory A. Grabowski, M.D., Cincinnati, OH
David A. Grimes, M.D., San Francisco, CA
Jack M. Gwaltney, Jr., M.D., Charlottesville, VA
Carla Hallak, M.D., Amsterdam, The Netherlands
John J. Halperin, M.D., Manhasset, NY
Ada Hamosh, M.D., M.P.H., Baltimore, MD
Edward A. Hartshorn, Ph.D., League City, TX
Duncan H. Haynes, Ph.D., Miami, FL
Cleopatra L. Hazel, Pharm.D., Netherland Antilles
Melvin B. Heyman, M.D., San Francisco, CA
Laura A. Hillman, M.D., Columbia, MO
E. M. Hilton, M.D., Cleveland, OH
M.E. Hoar, Springfield, MA
Hans Hogerzeil, M.D., Geneva, Switzerland
Dr. Richard Holmes, N. Billerica, MA
William Hopkins, Pharm.D., Atlanta, GA
Peter Houghton, London, England
Gary Hunninghake, M.D., Iowa City, IA
Moe Hussain, M.D., Ottawa, Ontario
B. Thomas Hutchinson, M.D., Boston, MA
Rodney D. Ice, Ph.D., Atlanta, GA
Richard S. Irwin, M.D., Worcester, MA
Mark Jacobson, M.D., San Francisco, CA
Ann L. Janer, Auburn, AL
Alan H. Jobe, M.D., Torrance, CA
Hugh F. Kabat, Ph.D., Albuquerque, NM
Allen Kaplan, M.D., Phoenix, AZ
Barbara Kaplan, Pharm.D., Charleston, WV
Michael Kelley, M.D., Columbus, OH
Alan Knight, M.D., North York, Ontario
John Koepke, Pharm.D., Columbus, OH
Stephen Krane, M.D., Boston, MA
Eric H. Kraut, M.D., Columbus, OH
Daryl E. Krepps, B.S.P., Ottawa, Ontario
Paul A. Krusinski, M.D., Burlington, VT
Paul B. Kuehn, Ph.D., Woodinville, WA
Thomas L. Kurt, M.D., Dallas, TX
Belle Lee, Pharm.D., San Francisco, CA
Robert L. Lesser, M.D., New Haven, CT
Joseph Levy, M.D., New York, NY
Paul Lin, M.D., Phoenix, AZ
Timothy O. Lipman, M.D., Washington, DC
Michael L. Macknin, M.D., Cleveland, OH
Louis A. Magnarelli, Ph.D., New Haven, CT
Howard I. Maibach, M.D., San Francisco, CA
Jean-Luc Malo, M.D., Montreal, Quebec
Victor J. Marder, M.D., Rochester, NY
Joseph E. Margarone, D.D.S., Buffalo, NY
Saul Markman, M.D., Ottawa, Ontario
Iris P. Masucci, Pharm.D., Bethesda, MD
Katherine E. McArthur, M.D., Dallas, TX
Patricia McCartney, R.N., Ph.D., Buffalo, NY
Debra McCauley, Rochester, MN
Norman L. McElroy, San Jose, CA
Ross E. McKinney, M.D., Durham, NC
Michael I. McLean, M.D., Nashville, TN
Rima McLeod, M.D., Chicago, IL
Anne McNulty, M.D., Waterbury, CT
John A. Messenheimer, M.D., Chapel Hill, NC
Craig S. Miller, D.D.S., Lexington, KY
John Mills, M.D., Fairfield, Victoria, Australia
Lynne M. Mofenson, M.D., Bethesda, MD
Garreth A. Moore, D.V.M., Blacksburg, VA
Laura Morales, Pharm.D., Little Rock, AR
Doris Hupfeld Moreno, M.D., Sao Paulo, Brazil
Dr. Raymond G. Morris, Woodville South, South Australia, Australia
Richard B. Moss, M.D., Palo Alto, CA
Arno Motulsky, M.D., Seattle, WA

Robert Naclerio, M.D., Chicago, IL
Peadar Noone, M.D., Chapel Hill, NC
Sven A. Normann, Pharm.D., Tampa, FL
Cheryl Nunn-Thompson, Pharm.D., West Zundee, IL
Patience Obih, M.D., New Orleans, LA
Edward J. O'Connell, M.D., Rochester, MN
R.I. Ogilvie, M.D., Toronto, Ontario
Susan Orenstein, M.D., Pittsburgh, PA
Judith M. Ozbun, R.Ph., M.S., Fargo, ND
Jenni Pandak, B.S., Pharm.D., Glen Allen, VA
Michael F. Para, M.D., Columbus, OH
Dra. Carmen Alerany Pardo, Barcelona, Spain
Robert C. Park, M.D., Washington, DC
Gregory M. Pastores, M.D., New York, NY
Albert Patterson, Hines, IL
Herbert Patrick, M.D., Philadelphia, PA
Page Pigg, B.S., Pharm.D., Glen Allen, VA
Philip A. Pizzo, M.D., Bethesda, MD
Therese Poirier, Pharm.D., Pittsburgh, PA
Daniel H. Polk, M.D., Torrance, CA
Michael Postelnick, BSPharm, Chicago, IL
Colin Powell, M.D., Halifax, Nova Scotia
R. Eugene Ramsay, M.D., Miami, FL
Terry D. Rees, D.D.S., M.S.D., Dallas, TX
Alfred J. Remillard, Pharm.D., Saskatoon, Saskatchewan
Stephen I. Rennard, M.D., Omaha, NE
Joseph G. Reves, M.D., Durham, NC
Ann Richards, Pharm.D., San Antonio, TX
Andrew L. Ries, M.D., San Diego, CA
Daniel C. Robinson, Pharm.D., Los Angeles, CA
Ken Rockwood, M.D., Halifax, Nova Scotia
Alice L. Rogers-McAfee, Pharm.D., San Pedro, CA
Sheldon H. Roth, Ph.D., Calgary, Alberta
Evelyn Salerno, Pharm.D., Hialeah, FL
Jay P. Sanford, M.D., Dallas, TX
Anthony J. Schaeffer, M.D., Chicago, IL
Irwin A. Schaffer, M.D., Cleveland, OH
Linda Schlaeffer, M.D., New Haven, CT
Steven M. Schnittman, M.D., Rockville, MD
Charles F. Seifert, Pharm.D., Rapid City, SD
Allen Shaughnessy, Pharm.D., Harrisburg, PA
Yvonne M. Shevchuk, Pharm.D., Saskatoon, Saskatchewan
Leonard Sigal, M.D., New Brunswick, NJ
Alan E. Smith, Ph.D., Framingham, MA
Carl V. Smith, M.D., Omaha, NE
Samuel Smith, M.D., Baltimore, MD
Michael B.H. Smith, M.D., Halifax, Nova Scotia
Elliott M. Sogol, Ph.D., Research Triangle Park, NC
Sunil K. Sood, M.D., New Hyde Park, NY
William N. Speliacy, M.D., Tampa, FL
Leon Speroff, M.D., Portland, OR
Joan Stachnik, Chicago, IL
Allen C. Steere, M.D., Boston, MA
David C. Stuhr, Denver, CO
Linda Gore Sutherland, Pharm.D., Laramie, WY
Dr. Straun Sutherland, Melbourne, Victoria, Australia
Carl Swanson, Kalamazoo, MI
Lynn M. Taussig, M.D., Denver, CO
Daniel Thiebeaud, M.D., Lausanne, Switzerland
Eric J. Topol, M.D., Ann Arbor, MI
Julia Vertrees, Pharm.D., San Antonio, TX
Donald G. Vidt, M.D., Cleveland, OH
Paul A. Volberding, M.D., San Francisco, CA
William Warner, Ph.D., New York, NY
Raymond Warrell, M.D., New York, NY
Miles M. Weinberger, M.D., Iowa City, IA
Robert S. Weinstein, M.D., Little Rock, AR
G. John Weir, M.D, Marshfield, WI
Timothy E. Welty, Pharm.D., Cincinnati, OH
Catherine Wilfert, M.D., Durham, NC
Craig C. Williams, R.Pharm., Flagstaff, AZ
James M. Wilson, M.D., Ph.D., Philadelphia, PA
Donna Wohlhuter, D.D.S., Rochester, MN
Robert G. Wolfangel, Ph.D., St. Louis, MO
M. Michael Wolfe, M.D., Boston, MA
Seth W. Wright, M.D., Nashville, TN
J. Richard Wuest, Pharm.D., Cincinnati, OH
Corinne Zara Yahni, Barcelona, Spain
Marc Yudkoff, M.D., Philadelphia, PA
Ari Zimran, M.D., Jerusalem, Israel
Frederic J. Zucchero, M.A., R.Ph., Chesterfield, MO

# HEADQUARTERS STAFF

## DIVISION OF INFORMATION DEVELOPMENT

**Director:** Keith W. Johnson
**Assistant Director:** Georgie M. Cathey
**Administrative Staff:** Jaime A. Ramirez (*Administrative Assistant*), Albert Crucillo, Maureen Rawson, Mayra L. Rios
**Senior Drug Information Specialists:** Ann Corken (*Nutrition Information Coordinator*), Nancy Lee Dashiell, Debra E. Boxwell (*Supervisor*), Angela Méndez Mayo (*Supervisor* and *Spanish Publications Coordinator*)
**Drug Information Specialists:** Rizwan Ahmad, Katherine M. Bennett, Susan Braun, Robyn C. Tyler, Jymeann King, Esther Klein, Denise S. Penn, Bridget Petry, Kathleen M. Phelan, Robin S. Isham-Schermerhorn, Daniel W. Seyoum, Susanne Streety, Ronald T. Wassel, Joyce P. Weaver
**Drug Utilization Review Program Director:** Thomas R. Fulda
**Medical Information Program Director:** David C. Pang
**Medical Information Specialists:** Joyce Carpenter, Rosaly Correa de Araujo, Fay Menacker, Monique Parr
**Veterinary Drug Information Specialists:** Kathyrn Meyer, Amy Neal
**Coordinator, Patient Counseling and Education Programs:** Stacy M. Hartranft
**Computer/Database Applications:** Anna Poker, Darcy Schwartz, Bernard G. Silverstein (*Manager, Database Development*), Jenny Tao
**Consumer Information Development:** Diana M. Blais (*Manager*), Bandana Das (*Assistant*), Marilyn L. Foster (*Associate*), Lauren E. O'Connor (*Assistant*), Dorothy Raymond (*Assistant*), Janet E. Schmidt (*Associate*)
**Technical Editors:** Anne M. Lawrence, Carol N. Hankin, Alessandra M. Potter, Jody Vilschick
**Library Services:** Florence A. Hogan (*Manager*), Terri Rikhy (*Associate*), Madeleine Welsch (*Assistant*)
**International Programs:** Kirill A. Burimski (*Russia Project Coordinator*), David D. Housley (*Coordinator*)
**Research Assistants:** Maria C. Robie, Annamarie J. Sibik
**Consultants:** Sandra Lee Boyer, Patricia J. Bush, David W. Hughes, Marcelo Vernengo
**Medical Consultants:** William P. Baker, M.D., Ph.D.; Donald R. Bennett, M.D., Ph.D.; Carol Proudfit, Ph.D.
**Scholar in Residence:** Albin Chaves Matamoras, San José, Costa Rica
**Student Interns/Externs:** Laurence Lamaitre, Catholic University of Leuven, Belgium; Nadia Minian, Clark University, School of Public Health; Madalena Rodrigues, University of Oporto, Portugal; Robert Smith, George Washington University, School of Public Health; Ellen Striebel, Johns Hopkins University, School of Nursing
**Visiting Scholars:** Marja Airaksinen, Finland; Eiichi Akaho, Japan; Sally-Ann Cryan, Ireland; Filiz Hincal, Turkey; Eustace Orleans-Linday, Ghana

## USP ADMINISTRATIVE STAFF

**Executive Vice President:** Jerome A. Halperin
**Senior Vice President and General Counsel:** Joseph G. Valentino
**Vice President, External Affairs:** Jacqueline L. Eng
**Vice President, Information Systems:** Joseph Knudson
**Senior Vice President, Business Operations and Development:** J. Robert Strang
**Director, Personnel:** Arlene Bloom
**Director, Finance:** Abe Brauner
**Director, Fulfillment/Facilities:** Drew J. Lutz
**Legal:** Kim Keller Reid (*Staff Attorney*), Ken Alexander (*Associate Legal Counsel for Business Affairs*), Colleen Ottoson (*Staff Attorney*)

## DIVISION OF STANDARDS DEVELOPMENT

**Vice President and Director:** Lee T. Grady
**Assistant Directors:** Charles H. Barnstein (*Revision*), Barbara B. Hubert, (*DSD*)
**Senior Scientists:** Roger Dabbah, V. Srinivasan, William W. Wright
**Scientists:** Frank P. Barletta, Vivian A. Gray, W. Larry Paul
**Senior Scientific Associates:** Todd L. Cecil, Terry H. Mainprize, Claudia C. Okeke
**Scientific Associate:** Horacio Pappa
**Senior Technical Editor:** Ann K. Ferguson
**Senior Translator:** Maria T. Gil-Montero
**Technical Editors:** Keith A. Seabaugh, Melissa M. Smith
**Supervisor of Administration:** Anju K. Malhotra
**Support Staff:** Gerald L. Anderson, Angela M. Healey, Cecilia Luna, Sonya M. Smoot
**Drug Research and Testing Laboratory:** Richard F. Lindauer (*Director*)
**Reference Standards Operations:** Robert H. King (*Director*)
**Hazard Communications:** Linda Shear
**Consultants:** J. Joseph Belson, Gabriel Giancaspro, Martin Golden, Aubrey S. Outschoorn

## MARKETING

**Director:** Joan R. Blitman
**Assistant Director:** Mark A. Sohasky (*Electronic Products*)
**Product Manager:** Joan April
**Associate Product Manager:** Jennifer C. Glenn
**Marketing Associates:** Pam Nelson, Matthew Yalleskey
**Senior Account Manager:** Susan M. Williams (*Electronic Applications*)
**Account Managers:** Charlotte McKany, Richard Charlton
*Technical Support Specialist:* Dennis Vich

## PRODUCTION SERVICES

**Director:** Carolyn A. Fleeger
**Production Managers/Managing Editors:** A. V. Precup (*USP DI*), Sandra Boynton (*USP-NF*)
**Applications Specialist, SGML:** Linda M. Guard
**Senior Editorial Associates:** Jesusa D. Cordova (*USP-NF*), Harriet S. Nathanson (*USP DI*)
**Editorial Associates:** *USP DI*—Susan J. Detwiler, Ellen D. Smith, Barbara A. Visco; *USP-NF*—Ellen Elovitz, Keith D. Gentile, Margaret Kay Walshaw
**Typesetting Staff:** Susan L. Entwistle (*Supervisor/Applications Analyst*), Deborah R. Connelly, Lauren Taylor Davis, Deborah James, M. T. Samahon, Donna Singh, Micheline Tranquille
**Consultants:** Don Barker of Spectrum Computer Services, Inc., Data Programming and Conversion; Mary Coe and Suzanne Peake, Indexing; Melvin Vaughn, Data Programming
**Also Contributing:** Doris Mullen and Gretchen Peeler of Editech Services, Inc., Proofreading; Doug Bushnell, Clerical Assistance

## CREATIVE SERVICES

**Director:** Gail M. Oring
**Graphics:** Derik Rice (*Senior Project Manager*), Cristy Gonzalez (*Project Manager*), Tia C. Morfessis and Randy White (*Senior Designers*), Rodney Warren (*Designer*)
**Word Processing:** Barbara A. Bowman (*Supervisor*), Olivia Hebron

## PRACTITIONER REPORTING PROGRAMS

**Vice President, Practitioner Reporting Programs:** Diane D. Cousins
**Manager, Program Development:** Shawn C. Becker
**Manager, Program Operations:** Rita Calnan, Dorothy Kolsky, Ilze Mohseni, Lata Rao, Elinor Skinner, Mary Susan Zmuda

# MEMBERS OF THE UNITED STATES
# PHARMACOPEIAL CONVENTION
## as of September 15, 1996

**U.S. Colleges and Schools of Medicine**

*Albany Medical College, Albany, NY:* Daniel S. Stein, M.D.

*Boston University School of Medicine, Boston, MA:* J. Worth Estes, M.D.

*Brown University School of Medicine, Providence, RI:* Edward Hawrot, Ph.D.

*Case Western Reserve University School of Medicine, Cleveland, OH:* Charles L. Hoppel, M.D.

*Columbia University College of Physicians and Surgeons, New York, NY:* Brian F. Hoffman, M.D.

*Creighton University School of Medicine, Omaha, NE:* Peter W. Abel, Ph.D.

*Duke University Medical Center School of Medicine, Durham, NC:* James C. McAllister, III, M.S.

*East Carolina University School of Medicine, Greenville, NC:* Donald W. Barnes, Ph.D.

*East Tennessee State University James H. Quillen College of Medicine, Johnson City, TN:* Ernest A. Daigneault, Ph.D.

*Emory University School of Medicine, Atlanta, GA:* Yung-Fong Sung, M.D.

*Georgetown University School of Medicine, Washington, DC:* Arthur Raines, Ph.D.

*Harvard Medical School, Boston, MA:* David E. Golan, M.D., Ph.D.

*Howard University College of Medicine, Washington, DC:* Robert E. Taylor, M.D., Ph.D.

*Indiana University School of Medicine, Indianapolis, IN:* D. Craig Brater, M.D.

*Johns Hopkins University School of Medicine, Baltimore, MD:* E. Robert Feroli, Pharm.D.

*Louisiana State University School of Medicine, New Orleans, LA:* Paul L. Kirkendol, Ph.D.

*Loyola University of Chicago Stritch School of Medicine, Maywood, IL:* Stanley A. Lorens, Ph.D.

*Marshall University School of Medicine, Huntington, WV:* John L. Szarek, Ph.D.

*Mayo Medical School, Rochester, MN:* James J. Lipsky, M.D.

*Medical College of Ohio School of Medicine, Toledo, OH:* Robert D. Wilkerson, Ph.D.

*Medical College of Pennsylvania and Hahnemann University School of Medicine, Philadelphia, PA:* Edward J. Barbieri, Ph.D.

*Medical College of Wisconsin, Milwaukee, WI:* Garrett J. Gross, Ph.D.

*Meharry Medical College School of Medicine, Nashville, TN:* Dolores Shockley, Ph.D.

*Mount Sinai School of Medicine, New York, NY:* Christopher Cardozo, M.D.

*New York Medical College, Valhalla, NY:* Mario A Inchiosa, Jr., Ph.D.

*Northwestern University Medical School, Chicago, IL:* Marilynn C. Frederiksen, M.D.

*Oregon Health Sciences University School of Medicine, Portland, OR:* Hall Downes, M.D., Ph.D.

*Ponce School of Medicine, Ponce, PR:* Arthur L. Hupka, Ph.D.

*Rush Medical College, Chicago, IL:* Paul G. Pierpaoli, M.S.

*St. Louis University Health Sciences Center School of Medicine, St. Louis, MO:* Alvin H. Gold, Ph.D.

*Stanford University School of Medicine, Stanford, CA:* Leslie A. Lenert, M.D.

*SUNY at Buffalo School of Medicine and Biomedical Sciences, Buffalo, NY:* Cedric M. Smith, M.D.

*SUNY Health Science Center at Syracuse, Syracuse, NY:* Oliver M. Brown, Ph.D.

*Temple University School of Medicine, Philadelphia, PA:* Ronald J. Tallarida, Ph.D.

*The Bowman Gray School of Medicine of Wake Forest University, Winston-Salem, NC:* Jack W. Strandhoy, Ph.D.

*The Medical College of Georgia School of Medicine, Augusta, GA:* David W. Hawkins, Pharm.D.

*The Ohio State University College of Medicine, Columbus, OH:* Robert M. Guthrie, M.D.

*The Pennsylvania State University College of Medicine, Hershey, PA:* Cheston M. Berlin, Jr., M.D.

*The University of Iowa College of Medicine, Iowa City, IA:* John E. Kasik, M.D., Ph.D.

*The University of Michigan Medical School, Ann Arbor, MI:* Edward F. Domino, Ph.D.

*The University of Mississippi Medical Center, Jackson, MS:* George W. Moll, Jr., M.D., Ph.D.

*Tufts University School of Medicine, Boston, MA:* John M. Mazzullo, M.D.

*Tulane University School of Medicine, New Orleans, LA:* Floyd R. Domer, Ph.D.

*Uniformed Services University of the Health Sciences, Bethesda, MD:* Louis R. Cantilena, M.D., Ph.D.

*University of Alabama School of Medicine, Birmingham, AL:* Robert B. Diasio, M.D.

*University of California, Davis School of Medicine, Davis, CA:* Larry G. Stark, Ph.D.

*University of California, San Diego School of Medicine, La Jolla, CA:* Harold J. Simon, M.D., Ph.D.

*University of California, San Francisco School of Medicine, San Francisco, CA:* Mark A. Schumacher, Ph.D., M.D.

*University of Chicago Pritzker School of Medicine, Chicago, IL:* Patrick Horn, M.D.

*University of Cincinnati College of Medicine, Cincinnati, OH:* Leonard T. Sigell, Ph.D.

*University of Colorado School of Medicine, Denver, CO:* Alan S. Hollister, M.D., Ph.D.

*University of Connecticut Health Center School of Medicine, Farmington, CT:* Paul F. Davern, M.B.A.

*University of Florida College of Medicine, Gainesville, FL:* Lal C. Garg, Ph.D.

*University of Hawaii John A. Burns School of Medicine, Honolulu, HI:* Bert K.B. Lum, Ph.D., M.D.

*University of Illinois at Chicago School of Medicine, Chicago, IL:* Lawrence Isaac, Ph.D.

*University of Kansas Medical Center School of Medicine, Kansas City, KS:* Harold N. Godwin, M.S.

*University of Louisville School of Medicine, Louisville, KY:* Peter P. Rowell, Ph.D.

*University of Massachusetts Medical School, Worcester, MA:* Glenn R. Kershaw, M.D.

*University of Medicine and Dentistry of New Jersey New Jersey Medical School, Newark, NJ:* Mohamed S. Abdel-Rahman, Ph.D.

*University of Medicine and Dentistry of New Jersey Robert Wood Johnson Medical School, New Brunswick, NJ:* Richard D. Huhn, M.D.

*University of Missouri-Columbia School of Medicine, Columbia, MO:* John W. Yarbro, M.D.

*University of Missouri-Kansas City School of Medicine, Kansas City, MO:* Paul G. Cuddy, Pharm.D.

*University of Nebraska College of Medicine, Omaha, NE:* Manuchair Ebadi, Ph.D.

*University of Nevada School of Medicine, Reno, NV:* John Q. Adams, Pharm.D.

*University of New Mexico School of Medicine, Albuquerque, NM:* Jane E. Henney, M.D.

*University of North Dakota School of Medicine, Grand Forks, ND:* David W. Hein, Ph.D.

*University of Oklahoma College of Medicine, Oklahoma City, OK:* Patrick A. McKee, M.D.

*University of Pennsylvania School of Medicine, Philadelphia, PA:* Marilyn E. Hess, Ph.D.

*University of Rochester School of Medicine and Dentistry, Rochester, NY:* Ira Shoulson, M.D.

*University of South Florida College of Medicine, Tampa, FL:* Joseph J. Krzanowski, Ph.D.

*University of Tennessee, Memphis College of Medicine, Memphis, TN:* Murray Heimberg, M.D., Ph.D.

*University of Texas Health Science Center at San Antonio Medical School, San Antonio, TX:* Alexander M.M. Shepherd, M.D., Ph.D.

*University of Texas Houston Medical School, Houston, TX:* Timothy P. Bohan, M.D.

*University of Texas Southwestern Medical Center at Dallas, Dallas, TX:* Paul F. White, Ph.D., M.D.

*University of Washington School of Medicine, Seattle, WA:* Georgiana K. Ellis, M.D.

*Vanderbilt University School of Medicine, Nashville, TN:* Dan M. Roden, M.D.

*Wayne State University School of Medicine, Detroit, MI:* Deborah G. May, M.D.

*West Virginia University Robert C. Byrd Health Sciences Center, Morgantown, WV:* Douglas D. Glover, M.D., R.Ph.

*Wright State University School of Medicine, Dayton, OH:* Robert L. Koerker, Ph.D.

*Yale University School of Medicine, New Haven, CT:* Florence Comite, M.D.

**State Medical Societies**

*Alaska State Medical Association, Anchorage, AK:* Keith M Brownsberger, M.D.

*Connecticut State Medical Society, New Haven, CT:* James E. O'Brien, M.D., Ph.D.

*Florida Medical Association, Jacksonville, FL:* Robert E. Windom, M.D.

*Idaho Medical Association, Boise, ID:* Lawrence L. Knight, M.D.

*Indiana State Medical Association, Indianapolis, IN:* Daria Schooler, M.D., R.Ph.

*Kentucky Medical Association, Louisville, KY:* Ellsworth C. Seeley, M.D.

*Louisiana State Medical Society, Metairie, LA:* Merlin H. Allen, M.D.

Massachusetts Medical Society, Waltham, MA: Errol Green, M.D.
Medical Association of Georgia, Atlanta, GA: Edwin D. Bransome, M.D.
Medical Association of the State of Alabama, Montgomery, AL: James R. Reed, M.D., Ph.D.
Medical Society of Delaware, Wilmington, DE: Michael J. Pasquale, M.D.
Medical Society of New Jersey, Lawrenceville, NJ: Joseph N. Micale, M.D.
Medical Society of the District of Columbia, Washington, DC: Wayne D. Blackmon, M.D.
Medical Society of the State of New York, Lake Success, NY: Richard Blum, M.D.
Missouri State Medical Association, Jefferson City, MO: C.C. Swarens,
North Dakota Medical Association, Bismarck, ND: William W. Barnes, M.D.
Ohio State Medical Association, Columbus, OH: Janet K. Bixel, M.D.
Oklahoma State Medical Association, Oklahoma City, OK: Clinton N. Cordon, M.D.
Pennsylvania Medical Society, Harrisburg, PA: Benjamin Calesnick, M.D.
South Dakota State Medical Association, Sioux Falls, SD: Thomas C. Johnson, M.D.
Utah Medical Association, Salt Lake City, UT: Douglas E. Rollins, M.D., Ph.D.
Washington State Medical Association, Seattle, WA: William O. Robertson, M.D.
Wyoming Medical Society, Inc., Cheyenne, WY: Richard W. Johnson, Jr.

### U.S. Colleges and Schools of Pharmacy
Albany College of Pharmacy, Albany, NY: Andrew B.C. Yu, Ph.D.
Auburn University School of Pharmacy, Auburn, AL: Kenneth N. Barker, Ph.D.
Butler University College of Pharmacy and Health Sciences, Indianapolis, IN: Jayesh Vora, Ph.D.
Campbell University School of Pharmacy, Buies Creek, NC: Antoine Al-Achi, Ph.D.
Creighton University School of Pharmacy and Allied Health Professions, Omaha, NE: Kenneth R. Keefner, Ph.D.
Drake University College of Pharmacy and Health Sciences, Des Moines, IA: Sidney Finn, Ph.D.
Duquesne University School of Pharmacy, Pittsburgh, PA: Lawrence H. Block, Ph.D.
Ferris State University College of Pharmacy, Big Rapids, MI: Kenneth J. McMullen,
Howard University College of Pharmacy and Pharmaceutical Sciences, Washington, DC: Eucharia E. Nnadi-Okolo, Ph.D.
Idaho State University College of Pharmacy, Pocatello, ID: Eugene I. Isaacson, Ph.D.
Long Island University Arnold & Marie Schwartz College of Pharmacy and Health Sciences, Brooklyn, NY: Jack Rosenberg, Pharm.D., Ph.D.
Massachusetts College of Pharmacy and Allied Health Sciences, Boston, MA: Sumner M. Robinson, Ph.D.
Mercer University Southern School of Pharmacy, Atlanta, GA: J. Grady Strom, Jr., Ph.D.
Midwestern University Chicago College of Pharmacy, Downers Grove, IL: Mary W.L. Lee, Pharm.D.
Northeast Louisiana University School of Pharmacy, Monroe, LA: William M. Bourn, Ph.D.
Northeastern University School of Pharmacy, Boston, MA: Mehdi Boroujerdi, Ph.D.
NOVA Southeastern University College of Pharmacy, North Miami Beach, FL: William D. Hardigan, Ph.D.
Ohio Northern University College of Pharmacy, Ada, OH: Metta Lou Henderson, Ph.D.
Philadelphia College of Pharmacy and Science, Philadelphia, PA: Alfonso R. Gennaro, Ph.D.
Purdue University School of Pharmacy, West Lafayette, IN: Stephen R. Byrn, Ph.D.
Rutgers-The State University of New Jersey College of Pharmacy, Piscataway, NJ: Leonard C. Bailey, Ph.D.
Samford University School of Pharmacy, Birmingham, AL: Hilmer (Tony) A. McBride, Ph.D.
South Dakota State University College of Pharmacy, Brookings, SD: Chandradhar Dwivedi, Ph.D.
Southwestern Oklahoma State University School of Pharmacy, Weatherford, OK: Keith W. Reichmann, Ph.D.
St. Louis College of Pharmacy, St. Louis, MO: John W. Zuzack, Ph.D.
Temple University School of Pharmacy, Philadelphia, PA: Reza Fassihi, Ph.D.
Texas Southern University College of Pharmacy and Health Sciences, Houston, TX: William B. Harrell, Ph.D.
The Ohio State University College of Pharmacy, Columbus, OH: Sylvan G. Frank, Ph.D.
The University of Arizona College of Pharmacy, Tucson, AZ: Michael Mayersohn, Ph.D.
The University of Georgia College of Pharmacy, Athens, GA: Stuart Feldman, Ph.D.
University at Buffalo School of Pharmacy, Buffalo, NY: Howard Forman, Pharm.D.

University of Arkansas for Medical Sciences College of Pharmacy, Little Rock, AR: Jonathan J. Wolfe, Ph.D.
University of California San Francisco, School of Pharmacy, San Francisco, CA: Emil T. Lin, Ph.D.
University of Cincinnati College of Pharmacy, Cincinnati, OH: Henry S.I. Tan, Ph.D.
University of Colorado School of Pharmacy, Denver, CO: Louis Diamond, Ph.D.
University of Connecticut School of Pharmacy, Storrs, CT: Michael C. Gerald, Ph.D.
University of Florida College of Pharmacy, Gainesville, FL: Michael A. Schwartz, Ph.D.
University of Houston College of Pharmacy, Houston, TX: Mustafa F. Lokhandwala, Ph.D.
University of Iowa College of Pharmacy, Iowa City, IA: Gilbert S. Banker, Ph.D.
University of Kansas School of Pharmacy, Lawrence, KS: John Stobaugh, Ph.D.
University of Kentucky College of Pharmacy, Lexington, KY: Paul M. Bummer, Ph.D.
University of Maryland at Baltimore School of Pharmacy, Baltimore, MD: Larry Augsburger, Ph.D.
University of Michigan School of Pharmacy, Ann Arbor, MI: Duane M. Kirking, Ph.D.
University of Minnesota College of Pharmacy, Minneapolis, MN: James C. Cloyd, Pharm.D.
University of Mississippi School of Pharmacy, University, MS: Alan B Jones, Ph.D.
University of Missouri-Kansas City School of Pharmacy, Kansas City, MO: William A. Watson, Pharm.D.
University of Montana School of Pharmacy and Allied Health Professions, Missoula, MT: Todd G. Cochran, Ph.D.
University of Nebraska College of Pharmacy, Omaha, NE: Clarence T. Ueda, Pharm D., Ph.D.
University of New Mexico College of Pharmacy, Albuquerque, NM: William M. Hadley, Ph.D.
University of North Carolina School of Pharmacy, Chapel Hill, NC: Richard J. Kowalsky, Pharm.D.
University of Oklahoma College of Pharmacy, Oklahoma City, OK: Loyd V. Allen, Jr., Ph.D.
University of Pittsburgh School of Pharmacy, Pittsburgh, PA: Dennis P. Swanson, M.S.
University of Rhode Island College of Pharmacy, Kingston, RI: Hossein Zia, Ph.D.
University of South Carolina College of Pharmacy, Columbia, SC: Bozena B. Michniak, Ph.D.
University of Southern California School of Pharmacy, Los Angeles, CA: Robert T. Koda, Pharm.D., Ph.D.
University of Tennessee College of Pharmacy, Memphis, TN: Dick R. Gourley, Pharm.D.
University of Texas College of Pharmacy, Austin, TX: James T. Doluisio, Ph.D.
University of the Pacific School of Pharmacy, Stockton, CA: Ravindra Vasavada, Ph.D.
University of Toledo College of Pharmacy, Toledo, OH: Paul W. Erhardt, Ph.D.
University of Utah College of Pharmacy, Salt Lake City, UT: David B. Roll, Ph.D.
University of Washington School of Pharmacy, Seattle, WA: Danny D. Shen, Ph.D.
University of Wisconsin School of Pharmacy, Madison, WI: Melvin H. Weinswig, Ph.D.
University of Wyoming School of Pharmacy, Laramie, WY: Kenneth F. Nelson, Ph.D.
Virginia Commonwealth University/Medical College of Virginia School of Pharmacy, Richmond, VA: Susanna Wu-Pong, Ph.D.
Washington State University College of Pharmacy, Pullman, WA: Mahmoud M. Abdel-Monem, Ph.D.
Wayne State University College of Pharmacy and Allied Health Professions, Detroit, MI: Craig K. Svennson, Pharm.D., Ph.D.
West Virginia University School of Pharmacy, Morgantown, WV: Arthur I. Jacknowitz, Pharm.D.
Xavier University of Louisiana College of Pharmacy, New Orleans, LA: Merrill A. Patin, Pharm.D.

### State Pharmacy Associations
Alabama Pharmacy Association, Montgomery, AL: David L. Laven,
Arizona Pharmacy Association, Tempe, AZ: Edward P. Armstrong, Ph.D.
California Pharmacists Association, Sacramento, CA: R. David Lauper, Pharm.D.
Colegio de Farmaceuticos de Puerto Rico, Hato Rey, PR: Luz C. Rivera, R.Ph.
Colorado Pharmacists Association, Inc., Englewood, CO: Thomas G. Arthur, R.Ph., M.S.A.
Connecticut Pharmacists Association, Rocky Hill, CT: Henry A. Palmer, Ph.D.
Delaware Pharmaceutical Society, Wilmington, DE: Kenneth Musto, Jr.,
Florida Pharmacy Association, Tallahassee, FL: Michael A. Mone, B.S., J.D.
Georgia Pharmacy Association, Inc., Atlanta, GA: Larry L. Braden, R.Ph.

# ABCIXIMAB    Systemic†

VA CLASSIFICATION (Primary/Secondary): BL700/CV900

Another commonly used name is c7E3 Fab.

Note: For a listing of dosage forms and brand names by country availability, see *Dosage Forms* section(s). For a listing of brand names for the articles in this monograph, refer to the General Index.

---

†Not commercially available in Canada.

---

## Category

Antithrombotic; monoclonal antibody (antithrombotic); platelet aggregation inhibitor.

## Indications

### Accepted

Thrombosis, percutaneous transluminal coronary angioplasty or atherectomy (PTCA)–related (prophylaxis)—Abciximab is indicated as an adjunct to aspirin and heparin for the prevention of acute cardiac ischemic complications in patients undergoing PTCA who are at high risk for abrupt closure of the treated coronary vessel. Patients considered to be at high risk for abrupt vessel closure include those undergoing PTCA with at least one of the following conditions:
• Unstable angina or non-Q-wave myocardial infarction
• Acute Q-wave myocardial infarction within 12 hours of onset of symptoms or
• Clinical and/or angiographic characteristics indicating high risk as adapted from the criteria of the American Heart Association and the American College of Cardiology, including two type B lesion characteristics in the artery to be dilated, one type B lesion characteristic in the artery to be dilated in a female 65 years of age or older, one type B lesion characteristic in the artery to be dilated in a patient with diabetes mellitus, one type C lesion characteristic in the artery to be dilated, or angioplasty of an infarct-related lesion within seven days of myocardial infarction.

## Pharmacology/Pharmacokinetics

### Physicochemical characteristics

Source—Derived from the murine immunoglobulin $G_1$ monoclonal antibody, m7E3.

Molecular weight—Approximately 47,600 daltons.

### Mechanism of action/Effect

Abciximab is a chimeric human-murine monoclonal antibody Fab (fragment antigen binding) fragment. It inhibits platelet aggregation by specifically binding to the glycoprotein GPIIb/IIIa receptor, the major surface receptor involved in the final common pathway for platelet aggregation. Inhibition of platelet aggregation occurs in a dose-dependent manner. Abciximab binding to the GPIIb/IIIa receptor prevents fibrinogen, von Willebrand factor, vitronectin, and other adhesive molecules from binding to the receptor, thereby inhibiting platelet aggregation. Abciximab is thought to block access of large molecules to the receptor by steric hindrance and/or conformational effects rather than interacting directly with the arginine-glycine-aspartic acid binding site of GPIIb/IIIa.

### Other actions/effects

Abciximab may also bind to the vitronectin receptor and to the Mac-1 integrin receptor on activated monocytes. However, resulting clinical effects have not been identified.

### Half-life

Cleared rapidly from plasma, with an initial phase half-life of less than 10 minutes and a second phase half-life of 30 minutes.

### Duration of action

Platelet function generally recovers within 48 hours; however, low levels of GPIIb/IIIa receptor blockade are present for up to 10 days after discontinuation of the infusion.

### Elimination

In general, Fab fragments are cleared more rapidly by the kidneys than are whole antibodies. Abciximab is probably catabolized in a manner similar to that of other natural proteins.

## Precautions to Consider

### Cross-sensitivity and/or related problems

Patients with known sensitivity to murine monoclonal antibodies may also be sensitive to abciximab. Patients who develop human anti-chimeric antibody (HACA) titers after abciximab therapy may have allergic or hypersensitivity reactions when treated with other diagnostic or therapeutic monoclonal antibodies.

### Carcinogenicity

Long-term studies evaluating the carcinogenic potential of abciximab have not been performed.

### Mutagenicity

*In vitro* and *in vivo* mutagenicity studies have not demonstrated any mutagenic effect.

### Pregnancy/Reproduction

Fertility—Studies evaluating abciximab's effect on fertility in male or female animals have not been done.

Pregnancy—Studies have not been done in humans.
Studies have not been done in animals.

FDA Pregnancy Category C.

### Breast-feeding

It is not known whether abciximab is distributed into breast milk.

### Pediatrics

No information is available on the relationship of age to the effects of abciximab in pediatric patients. Safety and efficacy have not been established.

### Geriatrics

There may be an increased risk of major bleeding in patients over 65 years of age. Caution is recommended.

### Drug interactions and/or related problems

The following drug interactions and/or related problems have been selected on the basis of their potential clinical significance (possible mechanism in parentheses where appropriate)—not necessarily inclusive (» = major clinical significance):

Note: Combinations containing any of the following medications, depending on the amount present, may also interact with this medication.

» Anticoagulants, oral
   (administration within 7 days of abciximab is not recommended unless the prothrombin time is ≤ 1.2 times control because of the increased risk of bleeding)

   Anti-inflammatory drugs, nonsteroidal or
   Cefamandole or
   Cefoperazone or
   Cefotetan or
» Dipyridamole or
» Platelet aggregation inhibitors (See *Appendix II*) or
» Ticlopidine
   (concurrent use with abciximab may increase the risk of bleeding; caution is recommended during concurrent use)

» Dextran
   (concurrent or sequential use with abciximab may increase the risk of bleeding; concurrent use is not recommended)

» Thrombolytic agents
   (there are limited data evaluating the concurrent administration of abciximab with thrombolytic agents; because of the potential for bleeding, caution is recommended during concurrent or sequential use)

### Medical considerations/Contraindications

The medical considerations/contraindications included here have been selected on the basis of their potential clinical significance (reasons given in parentheses where appropriate)—not necessarily inclusive (» = major clinical significance).

*Except under special circumstances, this medication should not be used when the following medical problems exist:*

» Aneurysm, intracranial or
» Arteriovenous malformation, intracranial or
» Bleeding, active or
» Bleeding, gastrointestinal or genitourinary, recent (within 6 weeks) or
» Bleeding diathesis or
» Cerebrovascular accident (CVA), history of (within 2 years) or
» CVA with significant residual neurological deficit or
» Hypertension, severe, uncontrolled or
» Neoplasm, intracranial or
» Surgery, major, recent (within 6 weeks) or
» Thrombocytopenia (< 100,000 cells per microliter) or
» Trauma, major, recent (within 6 weeks) or
» Vasculitis, presumed or documented history of
   (increased risk of bleeding with abciximab)

*Risk-benefit should be considered when the following medical problems exist:*

» Age over 65 years or
» Gastrointestinal disease, history of or
» Weight < 75 kg
(increased risk of major bleeding with abciximab)
» PTCA, failed or
» PTCA, prolonged (lasting more than 70 minutes) or
» PTCA within 12 hours of the onset of symptoms for acute myocardial infarction
(increased risk of bleeding that may be additive to that of abciximab)
Sensitivity to abciximab or to murine proteins

### Patient monitoring

The following may be especially important in patient monitoring (other tests may be warranted in some patients, depending on condition; » = major clinical significance):

» Activated clotting time (ACT)
(recommended during and following therapy)
» Activated partial thromboplastin time (APTT) and
» Prothrombin time (PT)
(recommended at baseline prior to initiation of abciximab therapy, during, and following therapy)
» Monitoring of potential bleeding sites
(careful attention to all potential bleeding sites, including catheter insertion sites, arterial and venous puncture sites, cutdown sites, needle puncture sites, and gastrointestinal, genitourinary, and retroperitoneal sites is recommended)
» Platelet counts
(recommended at baseline prior to initiation of abciximab therapy, at 2 to 4 hours following the initial intravenous injection dose, and at 24 hours or prior to discharge, whichever is first. Additional platelet counts should be determined if a patient experiences an acute platelet decrease; if thrombocytopenia is verified, abciximab therapy should be discontinued immediately)

## Side/Adverse Effects

Note: Human anti-chimeric antibody (HACA) development may occur secondary to abciximab therapy. In the Evaluation of platelet IIb/IIIa antibody for Preventing Ischemic Complications of high-risk angioplasty (EPIC) trial, HACA's were detected in 6.5% of patients receiving an initial intravenous injection plus infusion of abciximab, 5.2% of patients receiving an initial intravenous injection of abciximab plus a placebo infusion, and 0% of patients receiving placebo. There was no excess hypersensitivity or allergic reactions related to abciximab treatment compared to placebo treatment. Patients who develop HACA titers may have allergic or hypersensitivity reactions when treated with other diagnostic or therapeutic monoclonal antibodies.

The following side/adverse effects have been selected on the basis of their potential clinical significance (possible signs and symptoms in parentheses where appropriate)—not necessarily inclusive:

### Those indicating need for medical attention
Incidence more frequent
*Bleeding; hypotension*
Note: *Bleeding* is the most common complication of abciximab therapy. In the EPIC trial, *major bleeding* was defined as an intracranial hemorrhage or a decrease in hemoglobin greater than 5 grams per dL. Major bleeding occurred in 14% of patients receiving abciximab intravenous injection plus infusion versus 7% of patients receiving placebo. In the lightest (by weight) third of patients, major bleeding occurred in 21% of those receiving both the initial intravenous injection plus the infusion. Approximately 70% of abciximab-treated patients with major bleeding had bleeding at the arterial access site in the groin. An increased incidence of major bleeding from retroperitoneal, gastrointestinal, genitourinary, and other sites also occurred in abciximab-treated patients.

If serious uncontrolled *bleeding* or the need for surgery occurs, an Ivy bleeding time determination is recommended. Preliminary evidence suggests that platelet function may be partly restored with platelet transfusions.

Percutaneous transluminal coronary angioplasty (PTCA) within 12 hours of the onset of symptoms for acute myocardial infarction, prolonged PTCA, or failed PTCA may be associated with an increased risk of *bleeding* in the angioplasty setting that may be additive to that of abciximab.

*Hypotension* is often related to bleeding complications associated with abciximab.
Incidence less frequent
*Thrombocytopenia*
Note: In the EPIC trial, *thrombocytopenia* (<100,000 platelets per microliter) and *severe thrombocytopenia* (<50,000 platelets per microliter) occurred in 5.2% and 1.6%, respectively, of patients receiving an initial intravenous injection plus infusion of abciximab, 3.6% and 0.3%, respectively, of patients receiving an initial intravenous injection of abciximab plus placebo infusion, and 3.4% and 0.7%, respectively, of placebo recipients.

Incidence rare
*Anemia; bradycardia; edema, peripheral; leukocytosis; pleural effusion or pleurisy; pneumonia*

### Those indicating need for medical attention only if they continue or are bothersome
Incidence less frequent or rare
*Abnormal vision; confusion; hypesthesia; nausea; vomiting*

## General Dosing Information

Administration of abciximab through a continuous infusion pump equipped with an in-line sterile, non-pyrogenic, low-protein binding 0.2 or 0.22 micrometer filter is recommended.

There are no data evaluating readministration of abciximab. Abciximab administration may result in human anti-chimeric antibody (HACA) formation. Therefore, readministration of abciximab may cause hypersensitivity reactions (including anaphylaxis), thrombocytopenia, or diminished benefit of abciximab.

Hypersensitivity or anaphylaxis may occur at any time during abciximab administration.

Because of the risk of bleeding, arterial and venous punctures, intramuscular injections, and use of urinary catheters, nasotracheal tubes, nasogastric tubes, and automatic blood pressure cuffs should be minimized. Noncompressible sites, such as subclavian or jugular veins, should be avoided when obtaining intravenous access.

If serious uncontrolled bleeding or the need for surgery occurs, an Ivy bleeding time determination is recommended. Preliminary evidence suggests that platelet function may be partly restored with platelet transfusions.

Since abciximab is associated with an increased bleeding rate, particularly at the site of arterial access for femoral sheath placement, care should be taken when attempting vascular access that only the anterior wall of the femoral artery is punctured, avoiding a Seldinger technique for obtaining sheath access. Femoral vein sheath placement is not recommended, unless needed. While the vascular sheath is in place, patients should be maintained on complete bed rest with the head of the bed placed at an angle of 30° or less and the affected limb kept in a straight position. Heparin should be discontinued at least 4 hours prior to arterial sheath removal. After the sheath is removed, pressure should be applied to the femoral artery for at least 30 minutes using either manual compression or a mechanical device for hemostasis. A pressure dressing should be applied following hemostasis and the patient maintained on bed rest for 6 to 8 hours following sheath removal or discontinuation of abciximab therapy, whichever is later.

The sheath insertion site and distal pulses of affected leg (s) should be checked frequently while the femoral artery sheath is in place and for 6 hours after the sheath is removed. Any hematoma should be measured and monitored for enlargement.

Careful attention to all potential bleeding sites, including catheter insertion sites, arterial and venous puncture sites, cutdown sites, needle puncture sites, and gastrointestinal, genitourinary, and retroperitoneal sites is recommended.

### For treatment of adverse effects
Recommended treatment consists of the following—
For anaphylaxis:
• Stopping the infusion immediately.
• Symptomatic and supportive treatment. Epinephrine, dopamine, theophylline, antihistamines, and corticosteroids should be readily available.
For bleeding:
• Stopping the infusion immediately.
• Symptomatic and supportive treatment.

## Parenteral Dosage Forms

### ABCIXIMAB INJECTION

**Usual adult dose**
Prophylaxis of percutaneous transluminal coronary angioplasty or atherectomy (PTCA)–related thrombosis—
Initial: Intravenous, 250 mcg (0.25 mg) per kg of body weight administered ten to sixty minutes prior to the start of PTCA.
Maintenance: Intravenous infusion, 10 mcg (0.01 mg) per minute for twelve hours.

Note: Abciximab has been studied only with concomitant administration with heparin and aspirin.

The continuous infusion of abciximab should be stopped in cases of failed PTCA, since there is no evidence for the efficacy of abciximab in that setting.

If serious bleeding that cannot be controlled by compression occurs, abciximab and heparin should be discontinued immediately.

**Usual pediatric dose**
Safety and efficacy have not been established.

**Strength(s) usually available**
U.S.—
2 mg per mL (single-use vial) (Rx) [*ReoPro* (buffered solution of 0.01 molar sodium phosphate; 0.15 molar sodium chloride; 0.001% polysorbate 80 in Water for Injection)].
Canada—
Not commercially available.

**Packaging and storage**
Store at 2 to 8°C (36 to 46°F). Protect from freezing.

**Preparation of dosage form**
For the intravenous infusion solution, 4.5 mL of abciximab should be added to 250 mL of 0.9% sodium chloride injection or 5% dextrose injection. Administration at a rate of 17 mL per hour provides 10 mcg per minute of abciximab.

**Stability**
Discard any unused portion of the infusion solution.

**Incompatibilities**
Abciximab should be administered through a separate intravenous line. No other medications should be added to the infusion solution.

**Auxiliary labeling**
• Do not shake.

### Selected Bibliography

The EPIC Investigators. Use of a monoclonal antibody directed against the platelet glycoprotein IIb/IIIa receptor in high-risk coronary angioplasty. N Engl J Med 1994; 330: 956-61.

Faulds D, Sorkin EM. Abciximab (c7E3 Fab). A review of its pharmacology and therapeutic potential in ischemic heart disease. Drugs 1994; 48 (4): 583-98.

Developed: 07/05/95
Interim revision: 08/15/95

---

**ACEBUTOLOL**—See *Beta-adrenergic Blocking Agents (Systemic)*

---

# ACETAMINOPHEN Systemic

INN: Paracetamol

VA CLASSIFICATION (Primary/Secondary): CN103/CN850

Note: For information on acetaminophen combinations that are used for antacid as well as analgesic effects, see *Acetaminophen, Sodium Bicarbonate, and Citric Acid (Systemic)*.

Other commonly used names are APAP and paracetamol.

Note: For a listing of dosage forms and brand names by country availability, see *Dosage Forms* section(s). For a listing of brand names for the articles in this monograph, refer to the General Index.

## Category

Analgesic; antipyretic.

## Indications

**Accepted**
Pain (treatment);
Pain, arthritic, mild (treatment); or
Fever (treatment)—Acetaminophen is indicated to relieve mild to moderate pain and reduce fever. It provides symptomatic relief only; additional therapy to treat the cause of the pain or fever should be instituted when necessary.

Acetaminophen has minimal anti-inflammatory activity and does not relieve redness, swelling, or stiffness due to arthritis; it cannot be used in place of aspirin or other salicylates or other nonsteroidal anti-inflammatory drugs (NSAIDs) in the treatment of rheumatoid arthritis. However, it may be used to relieve pain due to mild osteoarthritis.

Acetaminophen may be used when aspirin therapy is contraindicated or inadvisable, e.g., in patients receiving anticoagulants or uricosuric agents, patients with hemophilia or other bleeding problems, and those with upper gastrointestinal disease or intolerance or hypersensitivity to aspirin. However, chronic, high-dose acetaminophen therapy may require adjustment of anticoagulant dosage based on increased monitoring of prothrombin time in patients receiving a coumarin- or indandione-derivative anticoagulant.

Note: The FDA has proposed that caffeine (present as an analgesic adjuvant in some products) be classified as a Category III ingredient (i.e., lacking documentation of efficacy) in OTC products containing acetaminophen as the sole analgesic/antipyretic agent.

## Pharmacology/Pharmacokinetics

**Physicochemical characteristics**
Molecular weight—151.16.

**Mechanism of action/Effect**
*For acetaminophen—*
Analgesic:
The mechanism of analgesic action has not been fully determined. Acetaminophen may act predominantly by inhibiting prostaglandin synthesis in the central nervous system (CNS) and, to a lesser extent, through a peripheral action by blocking pain-impulse generation. The peripheral action may also be due to inhibition of prostaglandin synthesis or to inhibition of the synthesis or actions of other substances that sensitize pain receptors to mechanical or chemical stimulation.
Antipyretic:
Acetaminophen probably produces antipyresis by acting centrally on the hypothalamic heat-regulating center to produce peripheral vasodilation resulting in increased blood flow through the skin, sweating, and heat loss. The central action probably involves inhibition of prostaglandin synthesis in the hypothalamus.
*For caffeine—*
Caffeine is a mild CNS stimulant. Caffeine-induced constriction of cerebral blood vessels, which leads to a decrease in cerebral blood flow and in the oxygen tension of the brain, may contribute to relief of some types of headache.
It has been suggested that the addition of caffeine to acetaminophen may provide a more rapid onset of action and/or enhanced pain relief with lower doses of the analgesic. However, the FDA has determined that studies performed to date have not demonstrated that caffeine is an effective analgesic adjuvant or that it does not interfere with acetaminophen's efficacy as an antipyretic.

**Absorption**
Oral—Rapid and almost complete; may be decreased if acetaminophen is taken following a high-carbohydrate meal.
Rectal—The rate and extent of absorption from the suppository dosage form may vary, depending on the composition of the base.

**Distribution**
In breast milk—Peak concentrations of 10 to 15 mcg per mL (66.2 to 99.3 micromoles/L) have been measured 1 to 2 hours following maternal ingestion of a single 650-mg dose. The half-life in breast milk is 1.35 to 3.5 hours.

**Protein binding**
Not significant with doses producing plasma concentrations below 60 mcg per mL (397.2 micromoles/L); may reach moderate levels with high or toxic doses.

**Biotransformation**
Approximately 90 to 95% of a dose is metabolized in the liver, primarily by conjugation with glucuronic acid, sulfuric acid, and cysteine. An intermediate metabolite, which may accumulate in overdosage after the primary metabolic pathways become saturated, is hepatotoxic and possibly nephrotoxic.

**Half-life**
1 to 4 hours; does not change with renal failure but may be prolonged in acute overdosage, in some forms of hepatic disease, in the elderly, and in the neonate; may be somewhat shortened in children.

**Time to peak concentration**
0.5 to 2 hours

**Peak plasma concentration**
5 to 20 mcg per mL (33.1 to 132.4 micromoles/L), with doses up to 650 mg.

**Time to peak effect**
1 to 3 hours

**Duration of action**
3 to 4 hours

**Elimination**
Renal, as metabolites, primarily conjugates; 3% of a dose may be excreted unchanged.
> In dialysis—
>> Hemodialysis: 120 mL per minute (for unmetabolized drug); metabolites are also cleared rapidly.
>> Hemoperfusion: 200 mL per minute.
>> Peritoneal dialysis: <10 mL per minute.

## Precautions to Consider

### Cross-sensitivity and/or related problems
Patients sensitive to aspirin may not be sensitive to acetaminophen; however, mild bronchospastic reactions with acetaminophen have been reported in some aspirin-sensitive asthmatics (less than 5% of those tested).

### Pregnancy/Reproduction
Fertility—Chronic toxicity studies in animals have shown that high doses of acetaminophen cause testicular atrophy and inhibition of spermatogenesis; the relevance of this finding to use in humans is not known.

Pregnancy—Problems in humans have not been documented. Although controlled studies have not been done, it has been shown that acetaminophen crosses the placenta.

### Breast-feeding
Problems in humans have not been documented. Although peak concentrations of 10 to 15 mcg per mL (66.2 to 99.3 micromoles/L) have been measured in breast milk 1 to 2 hours following maternal ingestion of a single 650-mg dose, neither acetaminophen nor its metabolites were detected in the urine of the nursing infants. The half-life in breast milk is 1.35 to 3.5 hours.

### Pediatrics
Studies performed to date have not demonstrated pediatrics-specific problems that would limit the usefulness of acetaminophen in children. However, some products intended for pediatric use contain aspartame, which is metabolized to phenylalanine, and must be used with caution, if at all, in children with phenylketonuria.

### Geriatrics
Appropriate studies performed to date have not demonstrated geriatrics-specific problems that would limit the usefulness of acetaminophen in the elderly.

### Drug interactions and/or related problems
The following drug interactions and/or related problems have been selected on the basis of their potential clinical significance (possible mechanism in parentheses where appropriate)—not necessarily inclusive (» = major clinical significance):

Note: Combinations containing any of the following medications, depending on the amount present, may also interact with this medication.

*For acetaminophen*
» Alcohol, especially chronic abuse of or
  Hepatic enzyme inducers (See *Appendix II*) or
  Hepatotoxic medications, other (See *Appendix II*)
      (risk of hepatotoxicity with single toxic doses or prolonged use of high doses of acetaminophen may be increased in alcoholics or in patients regularly taking other hepatotoxic medications or hepatic enzyme inducers)
      (chronic use of barbiturates [except butalbital] or primidone has been reported to decrease the therapeutic effects of acetaminophen, probably because of increased metabolism resulting from induction of hepatic microsomal enzyme activity; the possibility should be considered that similar effects may occur with other hepatic enzyme inducers)
  Anticoagulants, coumarin- or indandione-derivative
      (concurrent chronic, high-dose administration of acetaminophen may increase the anticoagulant effect, possibly by decreasing hepatic synthesis of procoagulant factors; anticoagulant dosage adjustment based on increased monitoring of prothrombin time may be necessary when chronic, high-dose acetaminophen therapy is initiated or discontinued; however, this does not apply to occasional use, or to chronic use of doses below 2 grams per day, of acetaminophen)
  Anti-inflammatory drugs, nonsteroidal (NSAIDs) or
  Aspirin or other salicylates
      (prolonged concurrent use of acetaminophen and a salicylate is not recommended because recent evidence suggests that chronic, high-dose administration of the combined analgesics [1.35 grams daily, or cumulative ingestion of 1 kg annually, for 3 years or longer] significantly increases the risk of analgesic nephropathy, renal papillary necrosis, end-stage renal disease, and cancer of the kidney or urinary bladder; also, it is recommended that for short-term use, the combined dose of acetaminophen plus salicylate not exceed that recommended for acetaminophen or a salicylate given alone)
      (prolonged concurrent use of acetaminophen and NSAIDs other than aspirin may also increase the risk of adverse renal effects; it is recommended that patients be under close medical supervision while receiving such combined therapy)
      (diflunisal may increase the plasma concentration of acetaminophen by 50%, leading to increased risk of acetaminophen-induced hepatotoxicity)

*For formulations containing caffeine (in addition to those interactions listed above)*
  CNS stimulation–producing medications, other (See *Appendix II*)
      (concurrent use with caffeine may result in excessive CNS stimulation, leading to unwanted effects such as nervousness, irritability, insomnia, or possibly convulsions or cardiac arrhythmias; close observation is recommended)

  Lithium
      (caffeine increases urinary excretion of lithium, and may thereby reduce its therapeutic effect)

  Monoamine oxidase (MAO) inhibitors, including furazolidone, procarbazine, and selegiline
      (the sympathomimetic side effects of caffeine may produce dangerous cardiac arrhythmias or severe hypertension when large doses of caffeine are used concurrently with MAO inhibitors)

### Laboratory value alterations
The following have been selected on the basis of their potential clinical significance (possible effect in parentheses where appropriate)—not necessarily inclusive (» = major clinical significance):

With diagnostic test results
  Glucose, blood, determinations
      (acetaminophen may cause falsely decreased values when the glucose oxidase/peroxidase method is used, but probably not when the hexokinase/glucose-6-phosphate dehydrogenase [G6PD] method is used)
      (values may be falsely increased when certain instruments are used in glucose analysis if high acetaminophen concentrations are present; instrument manufacturer's instruction manual should be consulted)

  5-Hydroxyindoleacetic acid (5-HIAA), serum, determinations
      (acetaminophen may cause false-positive results in qualitative screening tests using nitrosonaphthol reagent; the quantitative test is unaffected)

  Myocardial perfusion imaging, radionuclide, when adenosine or dipyridamole is used as an adjunct to the radiopharmaceutical
      (the caffeine in specific formulations may reverse the effects of adenosine or dipyridamole on myocardial blood flow, thereby in-

terfering with test results; patients should be advised to avoid caffeine for 8 to 12 hours prior to the test)

Pancreatic function test using bentiromide
(administration of acetaminophen prior to the bentiromide test will invalidate test results because acetaminophen is also metabolized to an arylamine and will thus increase the apparent quantity of para-aminobenzoic acid [PABA] recovered; it is recommended that acetaminophen be discontinued at least 3 days prior to administration of bentiromide)

Uric acid, serum, determinations
(acetaminophen may cause falsely increased values when the phosphotungstate uric acid test method is used)

With physiology/laboratory test values
Bilirubin concentrations, serum and
Lactate dehydrogenase activity, serum and
Prothrombin time and
Transaminase activity, serum
(may be increased, indicating hepatotoxicity, especially in alcoholics, patients taking other hepatic enzyme inducers, or patients with pre-existing hepatic disease, when single toxic doses [> 8 to 10 grams] of acetaminophen are taken or with prolonged use of lower doses [> 3 to 5 grams a day])

## Medical considerations/Contraindications

The medical considerations/contraindications included here have been selected on the basis of their potential clinical significance (reasons given in parentheses where appropriate)—not necessarily inclusive (» = major clinical significance).

**Risk-benefit should be considered when the following medical problems exist:**

» Alcoholism, active or
» Hepatic disease or
» Viral hepatitis
(increased risk of hepatotoxicity)

Phenylketonuria
(products that contain aspartame, which is metabolized to phenylalanine, may be hazardous to patients with phenylketonuria, especially young children; caution is recommended)

Renal function impairment, severe
(risk of adverse renal effects may be increased with prolonged use of high doses; occasional use is acceptable)

Sensitivity to acetaminophen or aspirin
(increased risk of allergic reaction)

### Patient monitoring

The following may be especially important in patient monitoring (other tests may be warranted in some patients, depending on condition; » = major clinical significance):

Hepatic function determinations
(may be required at periodic intervals during high-dose or long-term therapy, especially in patients with pre-existing hepatic disease)

## Side/Adverse Effects

The following side/adverse effects have been selected on the basis of their potential clinical significance (possible signs and symptoms in parentheses where appropriate)—not necessarily inclusive:

### Those indicating need for medical attention
Incidence rare
*Agranulocytosis* (fever with or without chills; sores, ulcers or white spots on lips or in mouth; sore throat); *anemia* (unusual tiredness or weakness); *dermatitis, allergic* (skin rash, hives or, itching); *hepatitis* (yellow eyes or skin); *renal colic* (pain, severe and/or sharp, in lower back and/or side)—with prolonged use of high doses in patients with severe renal function impairment; *renal failure* (sudden decrease in amount of urine); *sterile pyuria* (cloudy urine); *thrombocytopenia* (rarely, unusual bleeding or bruising; black, tarry stools; blood in urine or stools; pinpoint red spots on skin)—usually asymptomatic
Note: Acetaminophen-induced *renal function impairment* may be sufficiently severe to result in *uremia*, especially with prolonged use of high doses in patients with pre-existing renal impairment. Also, although a causal association has not been established, a retrospective study has suggested that long-term daily use of acetaminophen may be associated with an increased risk of *chronic renal failure* (analgesic nephropathy) in individuals without pre-existing renal function impairment.

## Overdose

For specific information on the agents used in the management of acetaminophen overdose, see:
• *Acetylcysteine (Systemic)* monograph; and/or
• *Charcoal, Activated (Oral-Local)* monograph.

For more information on the management of overdose or unintentional ingestion, **contact a Poison Control Center** (see *Poison Control Center Listing*).

### Clinical effects of overdose
The following effects have been selected on the basis of their potential clinical significance (possible signs and symptoms in parentheses where appropriate)—not necessarily inclusive:

Acute
***Gastrointestinal upset*** (diarrhea, loss of appetite, nausea or vomiting, stomach cramps or pain); ***increased sweating***
Note: Although *gastrointestinal upset* and *increased sweating* often do not occur, they sometimes occur within 6 to 14 hours after ingestion of an overdose and persist for about 24 hours.

Chronic
***Hepatotoxicity*** (pain, tenderness, and/or swelling in upper abdominal area)—may occur 2 to 4 days after the overdose is ingested
Note: The first indications of overdosage may be signs and symptoms of possible *liver damage* and abnormalities in liver function tests, which may not occur until 2 to 4 days after ingestion of the overdose. Maximal changes in liver function tests usually occur 3 to 5 days after ingestion of the overdose.

Overt *hepatic disease or failure* may occur 4 to 6 days after ingestion of the overdose. *Hepatic encephalopathy* (with mental changes, confusion, agitation, or stupor), *convulsions, respiratory depression, coma, cerebral edema, coagulation defects, gastrointestinal bleeding, disseminated intravascular coagulation, hypoglycemia, metabolic acidosis, cardiac arrhythmias,* and *cardiovascular collapse* may occur.

*Renal tubular necrosis* leading to *renal failure* (signs may include bloody or cloudy urine and sudden decrease in amount of urine) has also been reported in acetaminophen overdose, usually, but not exclusively, in conjunction with acetaminophen-induced *hepatotoxicity*.

### Treatment of overdose
To decrease absorption—May include emptying the stomach via induction of emesis or gastric lavage.

Removing activated charcoal (if used) by gastric lavage may be advisable. Although activated charcoal is recommended in cases of mixed drug overdose, it may interfere with absorption of orally administered acetylcysteine (antidote used to protect against acetaminophen-induced hepatotoxicity) and decrease its efficacy.

To enhance elimination—Instituting hemodialysis or hemoperfusion to remove acetaminophen from the circulation may be beneficial if acetylcysteine administration cannot be instituted within 24 hours following ingestion of a massive acetaminophen overdose. However, the efficacy of such treatment in preventing acetaminophen-induced hepatotoxicity is not known.

Specific treatment—Use of acetylcysteine. *It is recommended that acetylcysteine administration be instituted as soon as possible after ingestion of an overdose has been reported,* without waiting for the results of plasma acetaminophen determinations or other laboratory tests. Acetylcysteine is most effective if treatment is started within 10 to 12 hours after ingestion of the overdose; however it may be of some benefit if treatment is started within 24 hours. See the package insert or *Acetylcysteine (Systemic)* monograph for specific dosing guidelines for use of this product.

Monitoring—May include determining plasma acetaminophen concentration at least 4 hours following ingestion of the overdose. Determinations performed prior to this time are not reliable for assessing potential hepatotoxicity. Initial plasma concentrations above 150 mcg per mL (993 micromoles/L) at 4 hours, 100 mcg per mL (662 micromoles/L) at 6 hours, 70 mcg per mL (463.4 micromoles/L) at 8 hours, 50 mcg per mL (331 micromoles/L) at 10 hours, 20 mcg per mL (132.4 micromoles/L) at 15 hours, 8 mcg per mL (53 micromoles/L) at 20 hours, or 3.5 mcg per mL (23.2 micromoles/L) at 24 hours postingestion indicate possible hepatotoxicity and the need for completing the full course of acetylcysteine treatment. If the initial determination indicates a plasma concentration below those listed at the times indicated, cessation of acetylcysteine therapy can be considered. However, some clinicians advise that more than one determination should be performed to ascertain peak absorption and half-life of acetaminophen prior to considering discontinuation of acetylcysteine.

Performing liver function tests (serum aspartate aminotransferase [AST; SGOT], serum alanine aminotransferase [ALT; SGPT], prothrombin time, and bilirubin) at 24-hour intervals for at least 96 hours post-ingestion if the plasma acetaminophen concentration indicates potential hepatotoxicity. If no abnormalities are detected within 96 hours, further determinations are not needed.

Monitoring renal and cardiac function and administering appropriate therapy as required.

Supportive care—May include maintaining fluid and electrolyte balance, correcting hypoglycemia, and administering vitamin K₁ (if prothrombin time ratio exceeds 1.5) and fresh frozen plasma or clotting factor concentrate (if prothrombin time ratio exceeds 3.0). Patients in whom intentional overdose is known or suspected should be referred for psychiatric consultation.

## Patient Consultation

As an aid to patient consultation, refer to *Advice for the Patient, Acetaminophen (Systemic)*.

In providing consultation, consider emphasizing the following selected information (» = major clinical significance):

### Before using this medication
» Conditions affecting use, especially:
    Sensitivity to acetaminophen or aspirin
    Use in children—Aspartame-containing chewable tablets must be used with caution, if at all, in children with phenylketonuria
    Other medical problems, especially alcoholism (active), hepatic disease, or viral hepatitis

### Proper use of this medication
» Importance of not taking more medication than the amount recommended because acetaminophen may cause kidney or liver damage with long-term use or greater-than-recommended doses
» Unless otherwise directed by physician, children should not receive more than 5 doses per day
» Proper administration of:
    Acetaminophen oral granules
    Acetaminophen oral powders
    Acetaminophen suppositories
» Proper dosing
» Proper storage

### Precautions while using this medication
Regular visits to physician to check progress if long-term therapy is prescribed
Checking with physician because additional treatment may be needed:
    —if taking for pain, including arthritic pain, and pain persists for longer than 10 days for adults or 5 days for children, condition becomes worse, new symptoms occur, or the painful area is red or swollen
    —if taking for fever, and fever persists for longer than 3 days, condition becomes worse, or new symptoms occur
    —if taking for sore throat, and sore throat is severe, persists for longer than 2 days, or occurs together with or is followed by fever, headache, rash, nausea, or vomiting
» Risk of overdose if other medications containing acetaminophen are used
» Avoiding use of alcohol if taking more than an occasional 1 or 2 doses of this medication; increased risk of liver toxicity, especially in alcoholics, with high doses or prolonged use
Not using a salicylate or a nonsteroidal anti-inflammatory drug together with acetaminophen for more than a few days, unless directed by physician
Possible interference with some laboratory tests; preferably discussing use of the medication with physician in charge 3 to 4 days ahead of time; if this is not possible, informing physician in charge if acetaminophen taken within the past 3 or 4 days
Diabetics: Possible false results with blood glucose tests; checking with physician, nurse, or pharmacist if changes in test results noted
Not taking caffeine-containing formulations for 8 to 12 hours prior to adenosine- or dipyridamole-assisted myocardial perfusion imaging test
» Suspected overdose: Getting emergency help at once even if no symptoms apparent; symptoms of severe overdosage may be delayed, but treatment must be begun as soon as possible; treatment started 24 hours or more after the overdose may be ineffective in preventing liver damage or fatality

### Side/adverse effects
Signs and symptoms of potential side effects, especially adverse renal effects, allergic dermatitis, hepatotoxicity, agranulocytosis, and thrombocytopenia

## General Dosing Information

The doses are based on the FDA's proposed labeling requirements for over-the-counter (OTC) internal analgesic, antipyretic, and antirheumatic products. The dosage unit of 80 mg (1.23 grains) is used for pediatric doses; the dosage unit of 325 mg (5 grains) is used for adult doses. The conversion factor of 1 grain equal to 65 mg is used. The doses recommended by manufacturers of individual products, and the strengths of individual products, may not conform to the recommended doses.

One retrospective study has suggested that long-term daily use of acetaminophen may be associated with an increased risk of chronic renal disease (analgesic nephropathy). The results of this study are not considered conclusive, and further investigation is required to establish a causal association. However, until more definitive information is available, prolonged daily administration of acetaminophen should probably be limited to patients who are receiving appropriate medical supervision.

## Oral Dosage Forms
### ACETAMINOPHEN CAPSULES USP

**Usual adult and adolescent dose**
Analgesic and
Antipyretic—
    Oral, 325 to 500 mg every three hours, 325 to 650 mg every four hours, or 650 mg to 1 gram every six hours as needed, while symptoms persist.

Note: For patient self-medication, it is recommended that a physician be consulted if pain is not relieved within ten days, fever within three days, or sore throat within two days.

**Usual adult prescribing limits**
For short-term therapy (up to ten days)—Up to 4 grams daily.
For long-term therapy—Up to 2.6 grams daily, unless chronic treatment with higher doses is prescribed and monitored by a physician.

**Usual pediatric dose**
Analgesic and
Antipyretic—
    Oral, 1.5 grams per square meter of body surface a day in divided doses; or for
    Infants up to 3 months of age—Oral, 40 mg every four hours as needed.
    Infants 4 to 12 months of age—Oral, 80 mg every four hours as needed.
    Children 1 to 2 years of age—Oral, 120 mg every four hours as needed.
    Children 2 to 4 years of age—Oral, 160 mg every four hours as needed, while symptoms persist.
    Children 4 to 6 years of age—Oral, 240 mg every four hours as needed, while symptoms persist.
    Children 6 to 9 years of age—Oral, 320 mg every four hours as needed, while symptoms persist.
    Children 9 to 11 years of age—Oral, 320 to 400 mg every four hours as needed, while symptoms persist.
    Children 11 to 12 years of age—Oral, 320 to 480 mg every four hours as needed, while symptoms persist.

Note: It is recommended that children up to 12 years of age receive no more than five doses in each twenty-four-hour period, unless otherwise directed by a physician, and that a physician be consulted if pain is not relieved within five days, fever within three days, or sore throat within two days.

    Dosage recommendations for children younger than 2 years of age do not appear on OTC packaging.

    Administration of an individual product to a pediatric patient depends upon ability to achieve suitable dosage for the age of the child. Liquid dosage forms (oral solution or suspension), granules, powders, or chewable tablets are usually used.

**Strength(s) usually available**
U.S.—
    325 mg (OTC) [GENERIC].
    500 mg (OTC) [*Apacet Capsules; Dapa X-S;* GENERIC].
Canada—
    Not commercially available.

**Packaging and storage**
Store below 40 °C (104 °F), preferably between 15 and 30 °C (59 and 86 °F), unless otherwise specified by manufacturer. Store in a tight container.

**Auxiliary labeling**
• Avoid alcoholic beverages.

# ACETAMINOPHEN ORAL GRANULES

**Usual adult and adolescent dose**
See *Acetaminophen Capsules USP.*

**Usual pediatric dose**
See *Acetaminophen Capsules USP.*

**Strength(s) usually available**
U.S.—
　80 mg (in individual packets) (OTC) [*Snaplets-FR*].
Canada—
　Not commercially available.

**Packaging and storage**
Store below 40 °C (104 °F), preferably between 15 and 30 °C (59 and 86 °F), unless otherwise specified by manufacturer.

**Preparation of dosage form**
Single dose—The contents of the packets are to be mixed with a small quantity of soft food, such as applesauce, ice cream, or jam immediately prior to ingestion.

# ACETAMINOPHEN ORAL POWDERS

**Usual adult and adolescent dose**
See *Acetaminophen Capsules USP.*

**Usual pediatric dose**
See *Acetaminophen Capsules USP.*

**Strength(s) usually available**
U.S.—
　80 mg (in capsules) (OTC) [*Feverall Sprinkle Caps, Children's*].
　160 mg (in capsules) (OTC) [*Feverall Sprinkle Caps Junior Strength*].
Canada—
　Not commercially available.

**Packaging and storage**
Store below 40 °C (104 °F), preferably between 15 and 30 °C (59 and 86 °F), unless otherwise specified by manufacturer.

**Preparation of dosage form**
Single dose—The capsules are not intended to be swallowed whole. They are to be opened and the contents sprinkled over a small quantity (< 5 mL) of water or other liquid immediately prior to ingestion. Alternatively, the contents of the capsules may be mixed with a small quantity of soft food, such as applesauce, ice cream, or jam, immediately prior to ingestion.

# ACETAMINOPHEN ORAL SOLUTION USP

**Usual adult and adolescent dose**
See *Acetaminophen Capsules USP.*

**Usual adult prescribing limits**
See *Acetaminophen Capsules USP.*

**Usual pediatric dose**
See *Acetaminophen Capsules USP.*

**Strength(s) usually available**
U.S.—
　100 mg per mL (80 mg per 0.8-mL dropperful) (OTC) [*Apacet, Infants'; Genapap, Infants'; Panadol, Infants'; St. Joseph Aspirin-Free Fever Reducer for Children; Tempra, Infants'; Tylenol Infants' Drops;* GENERIC].
　80 mg per 5 mL (OTC) [GENERIC].
　120 mg per 5 mL (OTC) [*Aceta Elixir* (alcohol 7%); *Oraphen-PD* (alcohol 5%); GENERIC].
　130 mg per 5 mL (OTC) [GENERIC].
　160 mg per 5 mL (OTC) [*Apacet Elixir; Genapap Children's Elixir; Liquiprin Children's Elixir; Panadol, Children's; St. Joseph Aspirin-Free Fever Reducer for Children; Tempra Syrup; Tylenol Children's Elixir* (sugar); GENERIC].
　　Note: Also available generically in unit-dose cups containing 325 mg per 10.15 mL and 650 mg per 20.3 mL.
　500 mg per 15 mL (OTC) [*Tylenol Extra Strength Adult Liquid Pain Reliever* (alcohol 7%)].
Canada—
　80 mg per mL (OTC) [*Atasol Drops; Panadol; Tempra Drops* (alcohol 10%); *Tylenol Drops;* GENERIC].
　80 mg per 5 mL (OTC) [*Atasol Oral Solution; Panadol* (sodium); *Robigesic* (alcohol 8.5%); *Tempra Syrup*].
　160 mg per 5 mL (OTC) [*Tempra Syrup; Tylenol Elixir;* GENERIC].
Note: The strengths of specific products may not conform to some of the recommended pediatric dosages.

**Packaging and storage**
Store below 40 °C (104 °F), preferably between 15 and 30 °C (59 and 86 °F), unless otherwise specified by manufacturer. Store in a tight container. Protect from freezing.

**Auxiliary labeling**
• Avoid alcoholic beverages.

# ACETAMINOPHEN ORAL SUSPENSION USP

**Usual adult and adolescent dose**
See *Acetaminophen Capsules USP.*

**Usual pediatric dose**
See *Acetaminophen Capsules USP.*

**Strength(s) usually available**
U.S.—
　48 mg per mL (120 mg per 2.5-mL dropperful) (OTC) [*Liquiprin Infants' Drops*].
　100 mg per mL (80 mL per 0.8-mL dropperful) (OTC) [*Tylenol Infants' Suspension Drops*].
　160 mg per 5 mL (OTC) [*Tylenol Children's Suspension Liquid*].
Canada—
　80 mg per mL (OTC) [*Actimol Infants' Suspension*].
　80 mg per 5 mL (OTC) [*Actimol Children's Suspension*].

**Packaging and storage**
Store below 40 °C (104 °F), preferably between 15 and 30 °C (59 and 86 °F), unless otherwise specified by manufacturer. Store in a tight container. Protect from freezing.

**Auxiliary labeling**
• Shake well.

# ACETAMINOPHEN TABLETS USP

**Usual adult and adolescent dose**
See *Acetaminophen Capsules USP.*

**Usual adult prescribing limits**
See *Acetaminophen Capsules USP.*

**Usual pediatric dose:**
See *Acetaminophen Capsules USP.*

**Strength(s) usually available**
U.S.—
　120 mg (OTC) [GENERIC].
　160 mg (OTC) [*Panadol Junior Strength Caplets; Tylenol Junior Strength Caplets* (scored)].
　325 mg (OTC) [*Aceta Tablets; Actamin; Aminofen; Apacet Regular Strength Tablets; Dapa; Genapap Regular Strength Tablets; Genebs Regular Strength Tablets; Phenaphen Caplets; Tylenol Regular Strength Caplets; Tylenol Regular Strength Tablets* (scored); *Valorin;* GENERIC].
　　Note: In Canada, *Phenaphen* is available as capsules containing aspirin (ASA) and phenobarbital.
　500 mg (OTC) [*Aceta Tablets; Actamin Extra; Aminofen Max; Apacet Extra Strength Caplets; Apacet Extra Strength Tablets; Aspirin Free Anacin Maximum Strength Caplets; Aspirin Free Anacin Maximum Strength Gel Caplets; Aspirin Free Anacin Maximum Strength Tablets; Banesin; Datril Extra-Strength; Genapap Extra Strength Caplets; Genapap Extra Strength Tablets; Genebs Extra Strength Caplets; Genebs X-Tra; Panadol Maximum Strength Caplets; Panadol Maximum Strength Tablets; Redutemp; Tapanol Extra Strength Caplets; Tapanol Extra Strength Tablets; Tylenol Extra Strength Caplets; Tylenol Extra Strength Gelcaps; Tylenol Extra Strength Tablets; Valorin Extra;* GENERIC].
　650 mg (OTC) [GENERIC].
Canada—
　160 mg (OTC) [*Actimol Junior Strength Caplets* (scored); *Tempra Caplets; Tylenol Junior Strength Caplets*].
　325 mg (OTC) [*Anacin-3; Apo-Acetaminophen* (scored); *Atasol Caplets* (scored); *Atasol Tablets* (scored); *Exdol* (scored); *Panadol; Robigesic* (scored); *Rounox; Tylenol Caplets; Tylenol Tablets;* GENERIC].
　500 mg (OTC) [*Anacin-3 Extra Strength; Apo-Acetaminophen* (scored); *Atasol Forte Caplets; Atasol Forte Tablets* (scored); *Exdol Strong* (scored); *Panadol Extra Strength; Tylenol Caplets; Tylenol Gelcaps; Tylenol Tablets;* GENERIC].

**Packaging and storage**
Store below 40 °C (104 °F), preferably between 15 and 30 °C (59 and 86 °F), unless otherwise specified by manufacturer. Store in a tight container.

**Auxiliary labeling**
• Avoid alcoholic beverages.

## ACETAMINOPHEN TABLETS (CHEWABLE) USP

**Usual adult and adolescent dose**
See *Acetaminophen Capsules USP.*

**Usual pediatric dose**
See *Acetaminophen Capsules USP.*

**Strength(s) usually available**
U.S.—
　80 mg (OTC) [*Genapap Children's Tablets; Panadol, Children's* (scored); *St. Joseph Aspirin-Free Fever Reducer for Children; Tempra; Tylenol Children's Chewable Tablets* (scored); GENERIC].
　120 mg (OTC) [GENERIC].
　160 mg (OTC) [*Tempra D.S* (scored); *Tylenol Junior Strength Chewable Tablets* (scored)].
Canada—
　80 mg (OTC) [*Actimol Chewable Tablets; Panadol* (scored); *Tempra Chewable Tablets; Tylenol Children's Chewable Tablets* (scored); GENERIC].
　160 mg (OTC) [*Tempra Chewable Tablets*].

**Packaging and storage**
Store below 40 °C (104 °F), preferably between 15 and 30 °C (59 and 86 °F), unless otherwise specified by manufacturer. Store in a tight container.

**Auxiliary labeling**
• Avoid alcoholic beverages.
• May be chewed.

## ACETAMINOPHEN AND CAFFEINE TABLETS USP

**Usual adult and adolescent dose**
See *Acetaminophen Capsules USP.* Dosage is based on acetaminophen only.

**Usual adult prescribing limits**
See *Acetaminophen Capsules USP.* Dosage is based on acetaminophen only.

**Usual pediatric dose**
See *Acetaminophen Capsules USP.* Dosage is based on acetaminophen only.

**Strength(s) usually available**
U.S.—
　500 mg of acetaminophen and 65 mg of caffeine (OTC) [*Aspirin-Free Excedrin Caplets; Bayer Select Maximum Strength Headache Pain Relief Formula*].
　500 mg of acetaminophen and 65.4 mg of caffeine (OTC) [*Actamin Super*].
Canada—
　325 mg of acetaminophen and 65 mg of caffeine (OTC) [*Excedrin Caplets*].
　500 mg of acetaminophen and 65 mg of caffeine (OTC) [*Excedrin Extra Strength Caplets*].
　Note: In the U.S., *Excedrin* contains aspirin, in addition to acetaminophen and caffeine. See *Acetaminophen and Salicylates (Systemic)*. The U.S. product corresponding to the Canadian *Excedrin* formulation is *Aspirin-Free Excedrin*.

**Packaging and storage**
Store below 40 °C (104 °F), preferably between 15 and 30 °C (59 and 86 °F), unless otherwise specified by manufacturer.

**Auxiliary labeling**
• Avoid alcoholic beverages.

# Rectal Dosage Forms

## ACETAMINOPHEN SUPPOSITORIES USP

**Usual adult and adolescent dose**
Analgesic and
Antipyretic—
　Rectal, 325 to 500 mg every three hours, 325 to 650 mg every four hours, or 650 mg to 1 gram every six hours as needed, while symptoms persist.
　Note: For patient self-medication, it is recommended that a physician be consulted if pain is not relieved within ten days, fever within three days, or sore throat within two days.

**Usual adult prescribing limits**
For short-term therapy (up to ten days)—Up to 4 grams daily.
For long-term therapy—Up to 2.6 grams daily, unless chronic treatment with higher doses is prescribed and monitored by a physician.

**Usual pediatric dose**
Analgesic and
Antipyretic—
　Rectal, 1.5 grams per square meter of body surface a day in divided doses; or for
　Children up to 2 years of age—Dosage must be individualized by physician.
　Children 2 to 4 years of age—Rectal, 160 mg every four hours as needed, while symptoms persist.
　Children 4 to 6 years of age—Rectal, 240 mg every four hours as needed, while symptoms persist.
　Children 6 to 9 years of age—Rectal, 320 mg every four hours as needed, while symptoms persist.
　Children 9 to 11 years of age—Rectal, 320 to 400 mg every four hours as needed, while symptoms persist.
　Children 11 to 12 years of age—Rectal, 320 to 480 mg every four hours as needed, while symptoms persist.
Note: It is recommended that children up to 12 years of age receive no more than five doses in each twenty-four-hour period, unless otherwise directed by a physician, and that a physician be consulted if pain is not relieved within five days, fever within three days, or sore throat within two days.

**Strength(s) usually available**
U.S.—
　80 mg (OTC) [*Feverall, Infants'*].
　120 mg (OTC) [*Acetaminophen Uniserts; Feverall, Children's; Neopap* (scored); *Suppap-120;* GENERIC].
　300 mg (OTC) [GENERIC].
　325 mg (OTC) [*Acetaminophen Uniserts; Feverall Junior Strength; Suppap-325*].
　650 mg (OTC) [*Acetaminophen Uniserts; Suppap-650;* GENERIC].
Canada—
　120 mg (OTC) [*Abenol*].
　325 mg (OTC) [*Abenol*].
　650 mg (OTC) [*Abenol*].
Note: The strengths of the specific products may not conform to the recommended pediatric doses.

**Packaging and storage**
Store below 40 °C (104 °F), preferably between 15 and 30 °C (59 and 86 °F), in a well-closed container, unless otherwise specified by manufacturer. Protect from freezing.

**Auxiliary labeling**
• Avoid alcoholic beverages.

Revised: 07/12/94

# ACETAMINOPHEN-CONTAINING COMBINATIONS—

Acetaminophen and Aspirin (Systemic)—See *Acetaminophen and Salicylates (Systemic)*
Acetaminophen, Aspirin, and Caffeine (Systemic)—See *Acetaminophen and Salicylates (Systemic)*
Acetaminophen, Aspirin, and Caffeine, Buffered (Systemic)—See *Acetaminophen and Salicylates (Systemic)*
Acetaminophen, Aspirin, and Salicylamide, Buffered (Systemic)—See *Acetaminophen and Salicylates (Systemic)*
Acetaminophen, Aspirin, Salicylamide, and Caffeine (Systemic)—See *Acetaminophen and Salicylates (Systemic)*
Acetaminophen and Caffeine (Systemic)—See *Acetaminophen (Systemic)*
Acetaminophen and Codeine (Systemic)—See *Opioid (Narcotic) Analgesics and Acetaminophen (Systemic)*
Acetaminophen, Codeine, and Caffeine (Systemic)—See *Opioid (Narcotic) Analgesics and Acetaminophen (Systemic)*
Acetaminophen and Salicylamide (Systemic)—See *Acetaminophen and Salicylates (Systemic)*
Acetaminophen, Salicylamide, and Caffeine (Systemic)—See *Acetaminophen and Salicylates (Systemic)*
Acetaminophen, Sodium Bicarbonate, and Citric Acid (Systemic)
Brompheniramine, Phenylpropanolamine, and Acetaminophen (Systemic)—See *Antihistamines, Decongestants, and Analgesics (Systemic)*
Brompheniramine, Pseudoephedrine, and Acetaminophen (Systemic)—See *Antihistamines, Decongestants, and Analgesics (Systemic)*
Butalbital and Acetaminophen (Systemic)—See *Barbiturates and Analgesics (Systemic)*
Butalbital, Acetaminophen, and Caffeine (Systemic)—See *Barbiturates and Analgesics (Systemic)*
Chlorpheniramine, Dextromethorphan, and Acetaminophen (Systemic)—See *Cough/Cold Combinations (Systemic)*

Chlorpheniramine, Phenindamine, Phenylephrine, Dextromethorphan, Acetaminophen, Salicylamide, Caffeine, and Ascorbic Acid (Systemic)—See *Cough/Cold Combinations (Systemic)*

Chlorpheniramine, Phenylephrine, and Acetaminophen (Systemic)—See *Antihistamines, Decongestants, and Analgesics (Systemic)*

Chlorpheniramine, Phenylephrine, Acetaminophen, and Salicylamide (Systemic)—See *Antihistamines, Decongestants, and Analgesics (Systemic)*

Chlorpheniramine, Phenylephrine, Acetaminophen, Salicylamide, and Caffeine (Systemic)—See *Antihistamines, Decongestants, and Analgesics (Systemic)*

Chlorpheniramine, Phenylephrine, Dextromethorphan, Acetaminophen, and Salicylamide (Systemic)—See *Cough/Cold Combinations (Systemic)*

Chlorpheniramine, Phenylephrine, Hydrocodone, Acetaminophen, and Caffeine (Systemic)—See *Cough/Cold Combinations (Systemic)*

Chlorpheniramine, Phenylephrine, Phenylpropanolamine, Dextromethorphan, Guaifenesin, and Acetaminophen (Systemic)—See *Cough/Cold Combinations (Systemic)*

Chlorpheniramine, Phenylpropanolamine, and Acetaminophen (Systemic)—See *Antihistamines, Decongestants, and Analgesics (Systemic)*

Chlorpheniramine, Phenylpropanolamine, Acetaminophen, and Caffeine (Systemic)—See *Antihistamines, Decongestants, and Analgesics (Systemic)*

Chlorpheniramine, Phenylpropanolamine, Codeine, Guaifenesin, and Acetaminophen (Systemic)—See *Cough/Cold Combinations (Systemic)*

Chlorpheniramine, Phenylpropanolamine, Dextromethorphan, and Acetaminophen (Systemic)—See *Cough/Cold Combinations (Systemic)*

Chlorpheniramine, Phenylpropanolamine, Dextromethorphan, Acetaminophen, and Caffeine (Systemic)—See *Cough/Cold Combinations (Systemic)*

Chlorpheniramine, Phenyltoloxamine, Phenylpropanolamine, and Acetaminophen (Systemic)—See *Antihistamines, Decongestants, and Analgesics (Systemic)*

Chlorpheniramine, Pseudoephedrine, and Acetaminophen (Systemic)—See *Antihistamines, Decongestants, and Analgesics (Systemic)*

Chlorpheniramine, Pseudoephedrine, Dextromethorphan, and Acetaminophen (Systemic)—See *Cough/Cold Combinations (Systemic)*

Chlorpheniramine, Pseudoephedrine, Dextromethorphan, Acetaminophen, and Caffeine (Systemic)—See *Cough/Cold Combinations (Systemic)*

Chlorpheniramine, Pyrilamine, Phenylephrine, and Acetaminophen (Systemic)—See *Antihistamines, Decongestants, and Analgesics (Systemic)*

Chlorpheniramine, Pyrilamine, Phenylephrine, Phenylpropanolamine, and Acetaminophen (Systemic)—See *Antihistamines, Decongestants, and Analgesics (Systemic)*

Chlorzoxazone and Acetaminophen (Systemic)

Dexbrompheniramine, Pseudoephedrine, and Acetaminophen (Systemic)—See *Antihistamines, Decongestants, and Analgesics (Systemic)*

Dextromethorphan and Acetaminophen (Systemic)—See *Cough/Cold Combinations (Systemic)*

Dihydrocodeine, Acetaminophen, and Caffeine (Systemic)—See *Opioid (Narcotic) Analgesics and Acetaminophen (Systemic)*

Diphenhydramine, Pseudoephedrine, and Acetaminophen (Systemic)—See *Antihistamines, Decongestants, and Analgesics (Systemic)*

Diphenhydramine, Pseudoephedrine, Dextromethorphan, and Acetaminophen (Systemic)—See *Cough/Cold Combinations (Systemic)*

Diphenylpyraline, Phenylpropanolamine, Acetaminophen, and Caffeine (Systemic)—See *Antihistamines, Decongestants, and Analgesics (Systemic)*

Doxylamine, Pseudoephedrine, Dextromethorphan, and Acetaminophen (Systemic)—See *Cough/Cold Combinations (Systemic)*

Hydrocodone and Acetaminophen (Systemic)—See *Opioid (Narcotic) Analgesics and Acetaminophen (Systemic)*

Isometheptene, Dichloralphenazone, and Acetaminophen (Systemic)

Oxycodone and Acetaminophen (Systemic)—See *Opioid (Narcotic) Analgesics and Acetaminophen (Systemic)*

Pentazocine and Acetaminophen (Systemic)—See *Opioid (Narcotic) Analgesics and Acetaminophen (Systemic)*

Pheniramine, Phenylephrine, and Acetaminophen (Systemic)—See *Antihistamines, Decongestants, and Analgesics (Systemic)*

Pheniramine, Pyrilamine, Phenylpropanolamine, Codeine, Acetaminophen, and Caffeine (Systemic)—See *Cough/Cold Combinations (Systemic)*

Phenylephrine and Acetaminophen (Systemic)—See *Decongestants and Analgesics (Systemic)*

Phenylephrine, Guaifenesin, Acetaminophen, Salicylamide, and Caffeine (Systemic)—See *Cough/Cold Combinations (Systemic)*

Phenylpropanolamine and Acetaminophen (Systemic)—See *Decongestants and Analgesics (Systemic)*

Phenylpropanolamine, Acetaminophen, and Aspirin (Systemic)—See *Decongestants and Analgesics (Systemic)*

Phenylpropanolamine, Acetaminophen, and Caffeine (Systemic)—See *Decongestants and Analgesics (Systemic)*

Phenylpropanolamine, Acetaminophen, Salicylamide, and Caffeine (Systemic)—See *Decongestants and Analgesics (Systemic)*

Phenylpropanolamine, Dextromethorphan, and Acetaminophen (Systemic)—See *Cough/Cold Combinations (Systemic)*

Phenyltoloxamine, Phenylpropanolamine, and Acetaminophen (Systemic)—See *Antihistamines, Decongestants, and Analgesics (Systemic)*

Propoxyphene and Acetaminophen (Systemic)—See *Opioid (Narcotic) Analgesics and Acetaminophen (Systemic)*

Pseudoephedrine and Acetaminophen (Systemic)—See *Decongestants and Analgesics (Systemic)*

Pseudoephedrine, Dextromethorphan, and Acetaminophen (Systemic)—See *Cough/Cold Combinations (Systemic)*

Pseudoephedrine, Dextromethorphan, Guaifenesin, and Acetaminophen (Systemic)—See *Cough/Cold Combinations (Systemic)*

Pyrilamine, Phenylephrine, Dextromethorphan, and Acetaminophen (Systemic)—See *Cough/Cold Combinations (Systemic)*

Pyrilamine, Phenylpropanolamine, Acetaminophen, and Caffeine (Systemic)—See *Antihistamines, Decongestants, and Analgesics (Systemic)*

Pyrilamine, Pseudoephedrine, Dextromethorphan, and Acetaminophen (Systemic)—See *Cough/Cold Combinations (Systemic)*

Triprolidine, Pseudoephedrine, and Acetaminophen (Systemic)—See *Antihistamines, Decongestants, and Analgesics (Systemic)*

Triprolidine, Pseudoephedrine, Dextromethorphan, and Acetaminophen (Systemic)—See *Cough/Cold Combinations (Systemic)*

# ACETAMINOPHEN AND SALICYLATES   Systemic

This monograph includes information on the following: Acetaminophen and Aspirin; Acetaminophen, Aspirin, and Salicylamide; Acetaminophen and Salicylamide

INN: Acetaminophen—Paracetamol.

VA CLASSIFICATION (Primary/Secondary): CN103/CN850

**NOTE:**  The *Acetaminophen and Salicylates (Systemic)* monograph is maintained on the USP DI electronic data base. For a printed copy of the most recent revision of the complete monograph, contact the USP Division of Information Development, 12601 Twinbrook Parkway, Rockville, MD 20852.

For information on the specific components of this combination, see the *USP DI* monographs for *Acetaminophen (Systemic), Caffeine (Systemic),* and *Salicylates (Systemic).*

The information that follows is selectively abstracted from the complete monograph and is provided to facilitate drug use review and patient counseling.

Note: For a listing of dosage forms and brand names by country availability, see *Dosage Forms* section(s). For a listing of brand names for the articles in this monograph, refer to the General Index.

## Category

Analgesic; antipyretic.

## Indications

### Accepted

Pain (treatment)

Pain, arthritic, mild (treatment) or

Fever (treatment)—Acetaminophen and salicylate combinations are indicated to relieve mild to moderate pain and reduce fever. Salicylamide is less effective than acetaminophen or aspirin. These medications provide only symptomatic relief; additional therapy to treat the cause of the pain or fever should be instituted when necessary.

Acetaminophen and salicylate combinations are indicated to provide temporary relief of pain caused by mild inflammation or arthritis. Although acetaminophen may be effective in relieving pain caused by mild osteoarthritis, it has minimal anti-inflammatory activity. Salicylamide also has minimal anti-inflammatory activity. Therefore, efficacy in relieving pain caused by inflammation or arthritis may depend upon the quantity of aspirin present in the individual product.

Note: The FDA has proposed that salicylamide be classified as a Category III ingredient (i.e., lacking documentation of efficacy) in OTC analgesic/antipyretic products.

### Unaccepted

Acetaminophen and salicylate combinations are not recommended for the treatment of severe inflammation or severe arthritic pain, or for long-term treatment of chronic arthritis. Achieving and maintaining therapeutically effective salicylate plasma concentrations may require ingestion of undesirably large daily doses of other ingredients present in these formulations. Also, prolonged high-dose administration of these combinations is not recommended because of the risk of analgesic nephropathy.

## Patient Consultation

As an aid to patient consultation, refer to *Advice for the Patient, Acetaminophen and Salicylates (Systemic).*

In providing consultation, consider emphasizing the following selected information (» = major clinical significance):

### Before using this medication

» Conditions affecting use, especially:

   Sensitivity to acetaminophen, aspirin, or nonsteroidal anti-inflammatory drugs (NSAIDs)

   Pregnancy—Not taking aspirin in third trimester unless prescribed by physician; high-dose chronic use or abuse of aspirin in third trimester may be hazardous to the mother as well as the fetus and/or neonate, causing heart problems in fetus or neonate and/or bleeding in mother, fetus, or neonate; high-dose chronic use or abuse may also prolong and complicate labor and delivery; large quantities of caffeine may cause arrhythmias and growth retardation in the fetus

   Use in children—Checking with physician before giving a salicylate to children with symptoms of acute febrile illness, especially influenza or varicella, because of the risk of Reye's syndrome; also, increased susceptibility to aspirin toxicity in children, especially with fever and dehydration

   Use in teenagers—Checking with physician before giving a salicylate to teenagers with symptoms of acute febrile illness, especially influenza or varicella, because of the risk of Reye's syndrome

   Use in the elderly—Increased risk of aspirin toxicity and of combination analgesic–induced adverse renal effects

   Other medications, especially anticoagulants, antidiabetic agents (oral), those cephalosporins that may cause hypoprothrombinemia, methotrexate, NSAIDs, platelet aggregation inhibitors, plicamycin, probenecid, sulfinpyrazone, and urinary alkalizers and, for buffered formulations, fluoroquinolone antibiotics, itraconazole, ketoconazole, and oral tetracyclines

   Other medical problems, especially alcoholism (active), coagulation or platelet function disorders, gastrointestinal problems such as ulceration or erosive gastritis (especially a bleeding ulcer), and hepatic disease or viral hepatitis

### Proper use of this medication

» Taking with food or a full glass (240 mL) of water to minimize gastrointestinal irritation

» Importance of not taking more medication than recommended on package label, unless otherwise directed by physician, because of risk of acetaminophen-induced liver damage with long-term use or greater-than-recommended doses, gastrointestinal toxicity with salicylates, and acetaminophen or salicylate overdose

» Importance of children not receiving more than 5 doses per day unless otherwise directed by physician

» Not taking for chronic or severe inflammatory or rheumatic conditions without first checking with physician because prolonged treatment may be necessary and medication may not be effective unless extremely high doses are taken

» Not taking combinations containing aspirin if a strong vinegar-like odor is present

» Proper dosing

» Proper storage

### Precautions while using this medication

» Regular visits to physician to check progress if long-term or high-dose therapy is prescribed

   Checking with physician because additional treatment may be needed:
   —if taking for pain or fever, and pain persists for longer than 10 days (5 days for children) or fever persists for longer than 3 days,

if condition becomes worse, if new symptoms occur, or if the painful area is red or swollen
   —if taking for sore throat, and sore throat is severe, persists for longer than 2 days, or occurs together with or is followed by fever, headache, rash, nausea, or vomiting

   Not taking products containing aspirin for 5 days prior to any kind of surgery, unless otherwise directed by physician

» Caution if other medications containing acetaminophen, aspirin, or other salicylates (including diflunisal) are used

» Avoiding alcoholic beverages if taking more than an occasional 1 or 2 doses of these medications; alcohol consumption may increase risk of salicylate-induced gastrointestinal toxicity and acetaminophen-induced liver toxicity

   Not using an NSAID together with this medication for more than a few days, unless directed by physician or dentist

   Not taking buffered formulations within 6 hours before or 2 hours after ciprofloxacin or lomefloxacin, 8 hours before or 2 hours after enoxacin, 2 hours after itraconazole, 3 hours before or after ketoconazole, 2 hours before or after norfloxacin or ofloxacin, 3 to 4 hours before or after an oral tetracycline, or 1 to 2 hours before or after other oral medications

   Not taking a cellulose-containing laxative within 2 hours of aspirin-containing medications

   Possible interference with some laboratory tests; preferably discussing use of the medication with physician in charge 3 to 4 days ahead of time; if this is not possible, informing physician in charge if medication taken within the past 3 or 4 days

   Diabetics: Possible false results with blood and urine glucose tests; checking with physician, nurse, or pharmacist if changes in test results noted

   Not taking caffeine-containing formulations for 8 to 12 hours prior to adenosine- or dipyridamole-assisted myocardial perfusion imaging test

» Suspected overdose: Getting emergency help at once

### Side/adverse effects

   Signs of potential side effects, especially allergic reactions, anemia, gastrointestinal toxicity, agranulocytosis, hepatotoxicity, renal failure, sterile pyuria, and thrombocytopenia.

---

## *ACETAMINOPHEN AND ASPIRIN*

## Oral Dosage Forms

### ACETAMINOPHEN AND ASPIRIN TABLETS USP

**Usual adult and adolescent dose**

Analgesic or
Antipyretic—
   Oral, up to a total of approximately 650 mg of acetaminophen and aspirin (combined) every four to six hours as needed, while symptoms persist.

Note: For patient self-medication, it is recommended that a physician be consulted if pain is not relieved within ten days, fever within three days, or sore throat within two days.

   For geriatric patients, it may be advisable that acetaminophen and salicylate combinations not be used for longer than five days at a time, because such patients may be more susceptible to adverse renal effects.

**Usual adult prescribing limits**

For short-term therapy (up to ten days)—Up to a total of approximately 4 grams of acetaminophen and aspirin (combined) daily.

For long-term therapy—Up to a total of approximately 2.6 grams of acetaminophen and aspirin (combined) daily, unless chronic treatment with higher doses is prescribed and monitored by a physician.

**Usual pediatric dose**

Product of suitable strength not available.

**Usual geriatric dose**

See *Usual adult and adolescent dose.*

Note: Because geriatric patients may be more susceptible to adverse renal effects, it may be advisable that they not use acetaminophen and salicylate combinations for longer than five days at a time.

**Strength(s) usually available**

U.S.—
   325 mg of acetaminophen and 325 mg of aspirin (OTC) [*Gemnisyn*].
Canada—
   Not commercially available.

**Auxiliary labeling**
- Avoid alcoholic beverages.
- Take with food or a full glass of water.

## ACETAMINOPHEN, ASPIRIN, AND CAFFEINE ORAL POWDERS

**Usual adult and adolescent dose**
See *Acetaminophen and Aspirin Tablets USP.* Dosing is based only on the analgesic ingredients.

**Usual adult prescribing limits**
See *Acetaminophen and Aspirin Tablets USP.* Dosing is based only on the analgesic ingredients.

**Usual pediatric dose**
Product of suitable strength not available.

**Usual geriatric dose**
See *Acetaminophen and Aspirin Tablets USP.* Dosing is based only on the analgesic ingredients.

**Strength(s) usually available**
U.S.—
    260 mg of acetaminophen, 500 mg of aspirin, and 32.5 mg of caffeine (OTC) [*Goody's Headache Powders* (lactose)].
Canada—
    Not commercially available.

**Auxiliary labeling**
- Avoid alcoholic beverages.
- Take with a full glass of water or other liquid.

## ACETAMINOPHEN, ASPIRIN, AND CAFFEINE TABLETS USP

**Usual adult and adolescent dose**
See *Acetaminophen and Aspirin Tablets USP.* Dosing is based only on the analgesic ingredients.

**Usual adult prescribing limits**
See *Acetaminophen and Aspirin Tablets USP.* Dosing is based only on the analgesic ingredients.

**Usual pediatric dose**
Analgesic or
Antipyretic—
    Children up to 9 years of age: Product of suitable strength not available.
    Children 9 to 11 years of age: Oral, up to a total of approximately 400 mg of acetaminophen and aspirin (combined) every four hours as needed, while symptoms persist.
    Children 11 to 12 years of age: Oral, up to a total of approximately 480 mg of acetaminophen and aspirin (combined) every four hours as needed, while symptoms persist.
Note: Administration of a specific product to a pediatric patient depends upon ability to achieve suitable dosage for the age of the child.

    It is recommended that children up to 12 years of age receive no more than five doses in each twenty-four-hour period, unless otherwise directed by a physician, and that a physician be consulted if pain is not relieved within five days, fever within three days, or sore throat within two days.

**Usual geriatric dose**
See *Acetaminophen and Aspirin Tablets USP.* Dosing is based only on the analgesic ingredients.

**Strength(s) usually available**
U.S.—
    130 mg of acetaminophen, 260 mg of aspirin, and 16.25 mg of caffeine (OTC) [*Goody's Extra Strength Tablets*].
    180 mg of acetaminophen, 230 mg of aspirin, and 15 mg of caffeine (OTC) [*Duradyne*].
    250 mg of acetaminophen, 250 mg of aspirin, and 65 mg of caffeine (OTC) [*Excedrin Extra-Strength Caplets; Excedrin Extra-Strength Tablets*].
Canada—
    Not commercially available.
    Note: In Canada, *Excedrin* contains only acetaminophen and caffeine. See *Acetaminophen (Systemic).*

**Auxiliary labeling**
- Avoid alcoholic beverages.
- Take with food or a full glass of water.

## BUFFERED ACETAMINOPHEN, ASPIRIN, AND CAFFEINE TABLETS

**Usual adult and adolescent dose**
See *Acetaminophen and Aspirin Tablets USP.* Dosing is based only on the analgesic ingredients.

**Usual adult prescribing limits**
See *Acetaminophen and Aspirin Tablets USP.* Dosing is based only on the analgesic ingredients.

**Usual pediatric dose**
See *Acetaminophen, Aspirin, and Caffeine Tablets USP.* Dosing is based only on the analgesic ingredients.

**Usual geriatric dose**
See *Acetaminophen and Aspirin Tablets USP.* Dosing is based only on the analgesic ingredients.

**Strength(s) usually available**
U.S.—
    125 mg of acetaminophen, 240 mg of aspirin, 32 mg of caffeine, and buffering agents (OTC) [*Gelpirin*].
    160 mg of acetaminophen, 230 mg of aspirin, 33 mg of caffeine, and 60 mg of calcium gluconate (OTC) [*Supac* (scored)].
    162 mg of acetaminophen, 226.8 mg of aspirin, 32.4 mg of caffeine, and 50 mg of aluminum hydroxide (OTC) [*Buffets II*].
    194 mg of acetaminophen, 227 mg of aspirin, 33 mg of caffeine, 50 mg of magnesium hydroxide, and 25 mg of aluminum hydroxide (OTC) [*Vanquish Caplets*].
Canada—
    Not commercially available.

**Auxiliary labeling**
- Avoid alcoholic beverages.
- Take with food or a full glass of water.

---

### *ACETAMINOPHEN, ASPIRIN, AND SALICYLAMIDE*

## Oral Dosage Forms

### ACETAMINOPHEN, ASPIRIN, SALICYLAMIDE, AND CAFFEINE TABLETS

**Usual adult and adolescent dose**
Analgesic or
Antipyretic—
    Oral, up to a total of approximately 325 to 500 mg of acetaminophen, aspirin, and salicylamide (combined) every three hours, 325 to 650 mg of acetaminophen, aspirin, and salicylamide (combined) every four hours, or 650 mg to 1 gram of acetaminophen, aspirin, and salicylamide (combined) every six hours as needed, while symptoms persist.
Note: For patient self-medication, it is recommended that a physician be consulted if pain is not relieved within ten days, fever within three days, or sore throat within two days.

    For geriatric patients, it may be advisable that these medications not be used for longer than five days at a time, because such patients may be more susceptible to adverse renal effects.

**Usual adult prescribing limits**
For short-term therapy (up to ten days)—Up to a total of approximately 4 grams of acetaminophen, aspirin, and salicylamide (combined) daily.
For long-term therapy—Up to a total of approximately 2.6 grams of acetaminophen, aspirin, and salicylamide (combined) daily, unless chronic treatment with higher doses is prescribed and monitored by a physician.

**Usual pediatric dose**
Analgesic or
Antipyretic—
    Children up to 9 years of age: Product of suitable strength not available.
    Children 9 to 11 years of age: Oral, up to a total of approximately 320 to 400 mg of acetaminophen, aspirin, and salicylamide (combined) every four hours as needed, while symptoms persist.
    Children 11 to 12 years of age: Oral, up to a total of approximately 320 to 480 mg of acetaminophen, aspirin, and salicylamide (combined) every four hours as needed, while symptoms persist.
Note: Administration of a specific product to a pediatric patient depends upon ability to achieve suitable dosage for the age of the child.

It is recommended that children up to 12 years of age receive no more than five doses in each twenty-four-hour period, unless otherwise directed by a physician, and that a physician be consulted if pain is not relieved within five days, fever within three days, or sore throat within two days.

**Usual geriatric dose**
See *Usual adult and adolescent dose.*

Note: Because geriatric patients may be more susceptible to adverse renal effects, it may be advisable that they not use acetaminophen and salicylate combinations for longer than five days at a time.

**Strength(s) usually available**
U.S.—
   115 mg of acetaminophen, 210 mg of aspirin, 65 mg of salicylamide, and 16 mg of caffeine (OTC) [*Saleto*].
   162 mg of acetaminophen, 162 mg of aspirin, 162 mg of salicylamide, and 16.2 mg of caffeine (OTC) [*Tri-Pain Caplets*].
Canada—
   Not commercially available.

**Auxiliary labeling**
• Avoid alcoholic beverages.
• Take with food or a full glass of water.
• May cause drowsiness.

## BUFFERED ACETAMINOPHEN, ASPIRIN, AND SALICYLAMIDE TABLETS

**Usual adult and adolescent dose**
See *Acetaminophen, Aspirin, Salicylamide, and Caffeine Tablets.* Dosing is based only on the analgesic ingredients.

**Usual adult prescribing limits**
See *Acetaminophen, Aspirin, Salicylamide, and Caffeine Tablets.* Dosing is based only on the analgesic ingredients.

**Usual pediatric dose**
Product of suitable strength not available.

**Usual geriatric dose**
See *Acetaminophen, Aspirin, Salicylamide, and Caffeine Tablets.* Dosing is based only on the analgesic ingredients.

**Strength(s) usually available**
U.S.—
   120 mg of acetaminophen, 260 mg of aspirin, 120 mg of salicylamide, and 100 mg of aluminum hydroxide (OTC) [*Presalin*].
Canada—
   Not commercially available.

**Auxiliary labeling**
• Avoid alcoholic beverages.
• Take with food or a full glass of water.
• May cause drowsiness.

---

### *ACETAMINOPHEN AND SALICYLAMIDE*

# Oral Dosage Forms
## ACETAMINOPHEN AND SALICYLAMIDE CAPSULES

**Usual adult and adolescent dose**
Analgesic
or Antipyretic—
   Oral, 500 mg of acetaminophen and salicylamide (combined) every four hours, or 1 gram of acetaminophen and salicylamide (combined) every six hours as needed, while symptoms persist.

Note: For patient self-medication, it is recommended that a physician be consulted if pain is not relieved within ten days, fever within three days, or sore throat within two days.

   For geriatric patients, it may be advisable that these medications not be used for longer than five days at a time, because such patients may be more susceptible to adverse renal effects.

**Usual adult prescribing limits**
For short-term therapy (up to ten days)—Up to a total of approximately 4 grams of acetaminophen and salicylamide (combined) daily.
For long-term therapy—Up to a total of approximately 2.6 grams of acetaminophen and salicylamide (combined) daily, unless chronic treatment with higher doses is prescribed and monitored by a physician.

**Usual pediatric dose**
Product of suitable strength not available.

**Usual geriatric dose**
See *Usual adult and adolescent dose.*

Note: Because geriatric patients may be more susceptible to adverse renal effects, it may be advisable that they not use acetaminophen and salicylate combinations for longer than five days at a time.

**Strength(s) usually available**
U.S.—
   250 mg of acetaminophen and 250 mg of salicylamide (OTC) [*Duoprin*].
Canada—
   Not commercially available.

**Auxiliary labeling**
• Avoid alcoholic beverages.
• Take with food or a full glass of water.
• May cause drowsiness.

## ACETAMINOPHEN, SALICYLAMIDE, AND CAFFEINE CAPSULES

**Usual adult and adolescent dose**
See *Acetaminophen and Salicylamide Capsules.* Dosing is based only on the analgesic ingredients.

**Usual adult prescribing limits**
See *Acetaminophen and Salicylamide Capsules.* Dosing is based only on the analgesic ingredients.

**Usual pediatric dose**
Analgesic or
Antipyretic—
   Children up to 6 years of age: Product of suitable strength not available.
   Children 6 to 9 years of age: Oral, up to a total of approximately 320 mg of acetaminophen and salicylamide (combined) every four hours as needed, while symptoms persist.
   Children 9 to 11 years of age: Oral, up to a total of approximately 320 to 400 mg of acetaminophen and salicylamide (combined) every four hours as needed, while symptoms persist.
   Children 11 to 12 years of age: Oral, up to a total of approximately 320 to 480 mg of acetaminophen and salicylamide (combined) every four hours as needed, while symptoms persist.

Note: Administration of a specific product to a pediatric patient depends upon ability to achieve suitable dosage for the age of the child.

   It is recommended that children up to 12 years of age receive no more than five doses in each twenty-four-hour period, unless otherwise directed by a physician, and that a physician be consulted if pain is not relieved within five days, fever within three days, or sore throat within two days.

**Usual geriatric dose**
See *Acetaminophen and Salicylamide Capsules.* Dosing is based only on the analgesic ingredients.

**Strength(s) usually available**
U.S.—
   226.8 mg of acetaminophen, 97.2 mg of salicylamide, and 32.4 mg of caffeine (OTC) [*Rid-A-Pain Compound*].
Canada—
   Not commercially available.

**Auxiliary labeling**
• Avoid alcoholic beverages.
• Take with food or a full glass of water.
• May cause drowsiness.

## ACETAMINOPHEN, SALICYLAMIDE, AND CAFFEINE TABLETS

**Usual adult and adolescent dose**
See *Acetaminophen and Salicylamide Capsules.* Dosing is based only on the analgesic ingredients.

**Usual adult prescribing limits**
See *Acetaminophen and Salicylamide Capsules.* Dosing is based only on the analgesic ingredients.

**Usual pediatric dose**
Analgesic or
Antipyretic—
   Children up to 9 years of age: Product of suitable strength not available.
   Children 9 to 12 years of age: See *Acetaminophen and Salicylamide Capsules.* Dosing is based only on the analgesic ingredients.

**Usual geriatric dose**
See *Acetaminophen and Salicylamide Capsules.* Dosing is based only on the analgesic ingredients.

**Strength(s) usually available**
U.S.—
  150 mg of acetaminophen, 230 mg of salicylamide, and 30 mg of caffeine (OTC) [S-A-C].
Canada—
  Not commercially available.

**Auxiliary labeling**
- Avoid alcoholic beverages.
- Take with food or a full glass of water.
- May cause drowsiness.

Revised: 07/12/94

---

# ACETAMINOPHEN, SODIUM BICARBONATE, AND CITRIC ACID    Systemic

INN: Acetaminophen—Paracetamol
VA CLASSIFICATION (Primary): CN103
**NOTE:** The *Acetaminophen, Sodium Bicarbonate, and Citric Acid (Systemic)* monograph is maintained on the USP DI electronic data base. For a printed copy of the most recent revision of the complete monograph, contact the USP Division of Information Development, 12601 Twinbrook Parkway, Rockville, MD 20852.

For information on the specific components of this combination, see the *USP DI* monographs for *Acetaminophen (Systemic), Sodium Bicarbonate (Systemic),* and *Citrates (Systemic).*

The information that follows is selectively abstracted from the complete monograph and is provided to facilitate drug use review and patient counseling.

Note: For a listing of dosage forms and brand names by country availability, see *Dosage Forms* section(s). For a listing of brand names for the articles in this monograph, refer to the General Index.

## Category
Analgesic-antacid.

## Indications
### Accepted
Pain and upset stomach (treatment)—Acetaminophen, sodium bicarbonate, and citric acid combination is indicated for relief of mild to moderate pain, primarily when an upset stomach is also present. However, it is recommended that this medication be used only on an occasional or short-term basis; long-term use is not recommended because of the high sodium bicarbonate content.

## Patient Consultation
As an aid to patient consultation, refer to *Advice for the Patient, Acetaminophen, Sodium Bicarbonate, and Citric Acid (Systemic).*

In providing consultation, consider emphasizing the following selected information (» = major clinical significance):

### Before using this medication
» Conditions affecting use, especially:
  Allergic reaction to acetaminophen, aspirin, or sodium bicarbonate, history of
  Pregnancy—Acetaminophen crosses the placenta; sodium may cause edema and weight gain
  Use in the elderly—Because of the very high sodium content, use of this acetaminophen and antacid combination should preferably be limited to 5 days at a time, unless more prolonged therapy is prescribed and monitored by a physician
  Other medications, especially alcohol (especially chronic abuse of), mecamylamine, methenamine, oral ciprofloxacin, enoxacin, itraconazole, ketoconazole, lomefloxacin, norfloxacin, ofloxacin, and tetracyclines
  Other medical problems, especially alcoholism (active), symptoms of appendicitis or, hepatic disease or viral hepatitis, conditions in which sodium may be detrimental, and intestinal obstruction.

### Proper use of this medication
» Following physician's or manufacturer's directions; not taking more medication than the amount recommended because acetaminophen may cause liver damage with long-term use or greater-than-recommended doses and because of the very high sodium content of this medication
  Proper administration:
    Dissolving granules in water prior to ingestion: Pouring measured dose into glass, then adding ½ glass (120 mL) cool water
    Drinking while solution is still effervescing, or after it has settled
    Drinking entire amount, then rinsing glass with a little more water and drinking that, to ensure receiving full dosage
» Proper dosing

Missed dose (if on scheduled dosing): Taking as soon as possible; not taking if almost time for next dose; not doubling doses
» Proper storage

### Precautions while using this medication
Regular visits to physician to check progress if long-term therapy is prescribed
Checking with physician, because additional treatment may be needed, if symptoms persist for longer than 10 days, condition becomes worse, new symptoms occur, or the painful area is red or swollen
» Not taking this medication within:
    —6 hours before or 2 hours after ciprofloxacin or lomefloxacin
    —8 hours before or 2 hours after enoxacin
    —2 hours after itraconazole
    —3 hours before or after ketoconazole
    —2 hours before or after norfloxacin or ofloxacin
    —3 to 4 hours before or after an oral tetracycline
    —1 or 2 hours before or after any other oral medication
» Caution if other medications containing acetaminophen or significant quantities of sodium are used
  Not using a salicylate or a nonsteroidal anti-inflammatory drug together with acetaminophen for longer than a few days, unless otherwise directed by physician
  If taking more than an occasional 1 or 2 doses of this medication:
» Avoiding alcoholic beverages; increased risk of liver toxicity, especially in alcoholics, with high doses or prolonged use of acetaminophen
» Avoiding large amounts of milk or milk products
  Possible need for sodium restriction
  Possible interference with some laboratory tests; preferably checking with laboratory 3 to 4 days ahead of time; if this is not possible, informing physician in charge if acetaminophen taken within the past 3 or 4 days
  Diabetics: Possible false results with blood glucose tests; checking with physician, nurse, or pharmacist if changes in test results noted
» Suspected overdose: Getting emergency help at once even if no symptoms apparent; symptoms of severe acetaminophen overdosage may be delayed, but treatment must be begun as soon as possible; treatment started 24 hours or more after the overdose may be ineffective in preventing liver damage or fatality

### Side/adverse effects
Signs of potential side effects, especially edema, hypercalcemia associated with milk-alkali syndrome, increased blood pressure, metabolic alkalosis, agranulocytosis, anemia, allergic dermatitis, hepatitis, renal colic, renal failure, sterile pyuria, and thrombocytopenia

## Oral Dosage Forms
### ACETAMINOPHEN FOR EFFERVESCENT ORAL SOLUTION USP

#### Usual adult and adolescent dose
Analgesics-antacid—
Oral, 325 to 650 mg of acetaminophen every four hours as needed.

Note: It is recommended that a physician be consulted if symptoms are not relieved within ten days. However, geriatric patients should preferably not self-medicate with this product for longer than five days at a time, because of the very high sodium content.

#### Usual pediatric dose
Dosage has not been established.

#### Strength(s) usually available
U.S.—
  325 mg of acetaminophen with 2.781 grams of sodium bicarbonate and 2.224 grams of citric acid per ¾-capful measured dose (OTC) [*Bromo-Seltzer* (sodium 761 mg [33.08 mmol] per 325-mg dose)].

#### Preparation of dosage form
The measured dose is to be dissolved in 120 mL of cool water just prior to administration.

**Auxiliary labeling**
• Avoid alcoholic beverages.
• Keep container tightly closed.

Revised: 07/12/94

---

**ACETAZOLAMIDE**—See *Carbonic Anhydrase Inhibitors (Systemic)*

---

**ACETIC ACID–CONTAINING COMBINATIONS—**

Desonide and Acetic Acid (Otic)—See *Corticosteroids and Acetic Acid (Otic)*

Hydrocortisone and Acetic Acid (Otic)—See *Corticosteroids and Acetic Acid (Otic)*

---

**ACETOHEXAMIDE**—See *Antidiabetic Agents, Sulfonylurea (Systemic)*

---

# ACETOHYDROXAMIC ACID  Systemic†

**VA CLASSIFICATION (Primary):** GU900

Note: For a listing of dosage forms and brand names by country availability, see *Dosage Forms* section(s). For a listing of brand names for the articles in this monograph, refer to the General Index.

†Not commercially available in Canada.

## Category

Antiurolithic (struvite calculi); urinary tract infection treatment adjunct.

## Indications

### Accepted

Renal calculi, struvite (prophylaxis)—Acetohydroxamic acid is indicated in the prophylaxis of struvite calculi formation that is promoted by urease-producing bacteria such as *Proteus*. Its use may enhance effectiveness of urinary antibacterials, especially following surgical removal of existing stones. Use of acetohydroxamic acid also improves the possibility of reducing the frequency and rate of new stone formation.

Urinary tract infections, bacterial (treatment adjunct)—Acetohydroxamic acid is indicated as an adjunct in the treatment of chronic, urea-splitting urinary tract infections caused by urease-producing bacteria. Its inhibition of urease activity decreases the urinary ammonia and alkalinity produced from the enzyme hydrolysis of urea.

### Unaccepted

Acetohydroxamic acid is *not* indicated for dissolution of existing calculi, replacement of indicated surgical treatment, urinary tract infections controllable by culture-specific oral antibacterials, or urinary tract infections caused by nonurease producing organisms.

## Pharmacology/Pharmacokinetics

### Physicochemical characteristics

Molecular weight—75.07.
pKa—9.32.

### Mechanism of action/Effect

Inhibits the hydrolysis of urea and production of ammonia in urine infected with urea-splitting bacteria, by reversible inhibition of the bacterial enzyme urease, and by the chelation of nickel, an essential component of urease enzymes. Such enzyme inhibition results in reduction of both urine alkalinity and ammonia concentration. The effectiveness of antibacterial medication is then enhanced and the formation of urinary calculi reduced.

### Absorption

Well absorbed from gastrointestinal tract.

### Distribution

Well distributed throughout body fluids.

### Biotransformation

Hepatic, partial. Acetamide is active metabolite.

### Half-life

Plasma—
Acetohydroxamic acid: 5 to 10 hours (normal renal function), dose-related.
Acetamide: 23.4 ± 5.6 hours.

### Time to peak serum concentration

15 minutes to 1 hour after ingestion.

### Therapeutic urine concentration

Not completely determined, but 8 mcg/mL has been effective. Higher concentrations, such as 30 mcg/mL, are expected to provide increased

results; concentration of unchanged medication is dose-related; only the unchanged form of acetohydroxamic acid is therapeutically active.

### Elimination

Renal—Unchanged, 36 to 65%; as acetamide, 9 to 14%.
Respiratory—As carbon dioxide, 20 to 40%.

## Precautions to Consider

### Carcinogenicity

Well-controlled, long-term animal studies have not been conducted. Acetamide, a metabolite of acetohydroxamic acid, has been shown to cause hepatocellular carcinoma in rats when used in very high doses.

### Mutagenicity

Acetohydroxamic acid was positive for mutagenicity in the Ames test.

### Pregnancy/Reproduction

Pregnancy—Studies have not been done in humans.

However, use of acetohydroxamic acid is contraindicated during pregnancy since studies in animals have shown it to cause leg deformities at doses of 750 mg per kg of body weight (mg/kg) and above. At doses of 1500 mg/kg, exencephaly and encephalocele occurred. Also, cardiac, coccygeal, and abdominal-wall anomalies developed in pups of beagle dogs given 25 mg/kg a day during pregnancy.

Adequate contraceptive methods must be utilized by women of child-bearing potential during therapy.

FDA Pregnancy Category X.

### Breast-feeding

It is not known if acetohydroxamic acid is distributed into breast milk. Although problems in humans have not been documented, its use is not recommended in breast-feeding mothers because of the potential for serious adverse effects in the nursing infant.

### Pediatrics

Appropriate studies on the relationship of age to the effects of acetohydroxamic acid have not been performed in the pediatric population. However, no pediatrics-specific problems have been documented to date.

### Geriatrics

No information is available on the relationship of age to the effects of acetohydroxamic acid in geriatric patients.

### Drug interactions and/or related problems

The following drug interactions and/or related problems have been selected on the basis of their potential clinical significance (possible mechanism in parentheses where appropriate)—not necessarily inclusive (» = major clinical significance):

Note: Combinations containing any of the following medications, depending on the amount present, may also interact with this medication.

Alcohol
(concurrent use of alcoholic beverages with acetohydroxamic acid has resulted in a nonpruritic, reddish, macular skin rash about 30 to 45 minutes after ingestion. The rash may be associated with a general feeling of warmth and tingling, and usually disappears spontaneously in 30 to 60 minutes)

» Iron and other heavy metals
(acetohydroxamic acid chelates iron and possibly other heavy metals with concurrent oral administration; this may result in reduced intestinal absorption of both; if iron therapy is indicated, parenteral administration of iron is recommended)

### Medical considerations/Contraindications

The medical considerations/contraindications included here have been selected on the basis of their potential clinical significance (reasons given

in parentheses where appropriate)—not necessarily inclusive (» = major clinical significance).

*Except under special circumstances, this medication should not be used when the following medical problem exists:*

» Renal function impairment with creatinine clearance less than 20 mL per minute or serum creatinine concentration greater than 2.5 mg per deciliter
(excessive accumulation of acetohydroxamic acid may result)

*Risk-benefit should be considered when the following medical problems exist:*

Anemia, hypochromic
(acetohydroxamic acid may make this condition worse)

» Phlebitis, or history of, or
» Phlebothrombosis, or history of, or
» Thrombophlebitis, or history of
(increased risk of recurrence)

Renal function impairment with creatinine clearance not less than 20 mL per minute
(risk of excessive accumulation of acetohydroxamic acid)

Sensitivity to acetohydroxamic acid

### Patient monitoring

The following may be especially important in patient monitoring (other tests may be warranted in some patients, depending on condition; » = major clinical significance):

Coagulation tests, especially platelet counts and plasma fibrinopeptide A concentrations
(periodic monitoring and observation is recommended for clinical signs of thrombotic activity due to low-grade diffuse intravascular coagulation syndrome induced by acetohydroxamic acid)

Complete blood cell count, including reticulocytes
(recommended after 2 weeks of therapy and at 3-month intervals during treatment; close monitoring of children's clinical and hematologic status is recommended)

Hepatic function determinations
(close monitoring is recommended since the possibility of significant liver function impairment exists because of the chlorobenzene derivative)

Renal function determinations, especially serum creatinine
(close monitoring of patients with significantly impaired renal function is recommended; the daily dose of acetohydroxamic acid should not exceed 1 gram for patients with serum creatinine concentrations greater than 1.8 mg per deciliter [159 micromoles per liter], and dosage should be at 12-hour intervals; dosage reduction may be necessary)

Urinary pH
(periodic monitoring by physician or patient, using pH indicator strips, recommended to assess degree of urinary acidification achieved with therapy)

## Side/Adverse Effects

The following side/adverse effects have been selected on the basis of their potential clinical significance (possible signs and symptoms in parentheses where appropriate)—not necessarily inclusive:

### Those indicating need for medical attention
Incidence more frequent
*Anemia, hemolytic* (loss of appetite; nausea or vomiting; unusual tiredness or weakness); *anxiety, confusion, or mental depression; nervousness, shakiness, or tremors; phlebitis or thrombosis* (severe headaches of sudden onset; sudden loss of coordination; pains in chest, groin, or legs, especially calves of legs; sudden onset of shortness of breath for no apparent reason; sudden onset of slurred speech; sudden vision changes)

### Those indicating need for medical attention only if they continue or are bothersome
Incidence more frequent
*Gastrointestinal effects, specifically anorexia* (loss of appetite); *malaise* (general feeling of discomfort or illness); *nausea and vomiting; mild headache*

Incidence less frequent or rare
*Hair loss; non-itching skin rash on arms and face*

## Overdose

For more information on the management of overdose or unintentional ingestion, **contact a Poison Control Center** (see *Poison Control Center Listing*).

### Clinical effects of overdose
The following effects have been selected on the basis of their potential clinical significance—not necessarily inclusive:
Acetohydroxamic acid overdose has not been reported. However, if it should occur, concomitant reduction in platelets and/or white blood cells should be anticipated; reticulocyte count is likely to be elevated; and severe hemolysis may occur.

### Treatment of overdose
Administration should be stopped. There is no known specific antidote for acetohydroxamic acid overdose.
Recommended treatment consists of the following:
  • Monitoring—Close monitoring of hematologic status.
  • Specific treatment—Symptomatic treatment as necessary. Blood transfusions if required. Dialysis (considered possible but not yet proven).

## Patient Consultation

As an aid to patient consultation, refer to *Advice for the Patient, Acetohydroxamic Acid (Systemic)*.

In providing consultation, consider emphasizing the following selected information (» = major clinical significance):

### Before using this medication
» Conditions affecting use, especially:
Sensitivity to acetohydroxamic acid
Pregnancy—Contraindicated in pregnant patients because animal studies have shown leg deformities, and cardiac, coccygeal, and abdominal-wall anomalies; adequate contraception necessary for women of child-bearing potential
Breast-feeding—Not recommended because of potential adverse effects in infant
Other medications, especially oral iron supplements
Other medical problems, especially severe renal function impairment or history of phlebitis, phlebothrombosis, or thrombophlebitis

### Proper use of this medication
» Taking medication on an empty stomach, 1 hour before or 2 hours after meals
» Compliance with therapy; importance of taking medication exactly as directed by physician
» Importance of using an effective method of contraception during therapy in women of child-bearing potential
» Not missing doses; stone formation and growth may recur
» Proper dosing
Missed dose: Taking as soon as remembered; going back to regular dosing schedule; not doubling doses
» Proper storage

### Precautions while using this medication
Regular visits to physician to check progress of therapy
» Not taking oral iron preparations concurrently with acetohydroxamic acid
» Avoiding the use of alcoholic beverages during treatment with acetohydroxamic acid; flushing and skin rash may result
» Stopping medication immediately and checking with doctor if pregnancy occurs

### Side/adverse effects
» Stopping medication and notifying physician immediately if symptoms of blood clots occur, such as severe headaches of sudden onset, sudden loss of coordination, pains in chest, groin, or legs, especially calves of legs, sudden onset of shortness of breath for no apparent reason, sudden onset of slurred speech, sudden vision changes

## General Dosing Information

Acetohydroxamic acid should not be used in place of surgical treatment when surgery is indicated.

Existing calculi are unlikely to be reduced or dissolved by acetohydroxamic acid therapy.

### Diet/Nutrition
Acetohydroxamic acid is administered on an empty stomach.

Dietary iron is chelated and its absorption inhibited by acetohydroxamic acid, possibly leading to hypochromic anemia.

## Oral Dosage Forms

### ACETOHYDROXAMIC ACID TABLETS USP

**Usual adult and adolescent dose**
Antiurolithic—
Oral, 250 mg three or four times a day at six- to eight-hour intervals.

Note: Dosage must be proportionately reduced and individually adjusted for patients with renal function impairment.

**Usual adult prescribing limits**
Up to 1.5 grams.

**Usual pediatric dose**
Antiurolithic—
　Oral, initially 10 mg per kg of body weight a day, the dosage being adjusted as needed and tolerated.

**Strength(s) usually available**
U.S.—
　250 mg (Rx) [*Lithostat* (scored)].
Canada—
　Not commercially available.

**Packaging and storage**
Store below 40 °C (104 °F), preferably between 15 and 30 °C (59 and 86 °F), unless otherwise specified by manufacturer. Store in a tight container.

**Auxiliary labeling**
• Avoid alcoholic beverages.
• Take 1 hour before or 2 hours after meals.

**Note**
Unit-of-use package. Include patient instructions when dispensing.

Revised: 12/11/92
Interim revision: 06/13/94

# ACETONE-CONTAINING COMBINATIONS—
Alcohol and Acetone (Topical)

# ACETOPHENAZINE—See *Phenothiazines (Systemic)*

# ACETYLCYSTEINE　Inhalation-Local

VA CLASSIFICATION (Primary/Secondary): RE400/DX900
Note: For a listing of dosage forms and brand names by country availability, see *Dosage Forms* section(s). For a listing of brand names for the articles in this monograph, refer to the General Index.

## Category
Mucolytic; diagnostic aid (bronchial studies).

## Indications
Note: Bracketed information in the *Indications* section refers to uses that are not included in U.S. product labeling.

**Accepted**
Amyloidosis, primary, of lung (treatment adjunct)
Bronchiectasis (treatment adjunct)
Bronchitis (treatment adjunct)
Bronchitis, asthmatic (treatment adjunct)
Cystic fibrosis, pulmonary complications of (treatment adjunct)
Emphysema, pulmonary (treatment adjunct)
[Lung abscess (treatment adjunct)]
Pneumonia (treatment adjunct)
Tracheobronchitis (treatment adjunct)
Tracheostomy care, adjunct or
Tuberculosis (treatment adjunct)—Acetylcysteine is indicated as adjuvant therapy for abnormal, viscid, or inspissated mucous secretions in acute bronchopulmonary disease (pneumonia, bronchitis, and tracheobronchitis); chronic bronchopulmonary disease (chronic pulmonary emphysema, emphysema with bronchitis, chronic asthmatic bronchitis, [lung abscess], tuberculosis, bronchiectasis, and primary amyloidosis of the lung); and pulmonary complications of cystic fibrosis. It is also used as an adjunct in tracheostomy care.
Atelectasis due to mucous obstruction (treatment adjunct)—Acetylcysteine is indicated as adjuvant therapy for abnormal, viscid, or inspissated mucous secretions in atelectasis due to mucous obstruction. However, acetylcysteine is of no proven value in atelectasis due to simple hypoventilation, such as postoperative hypoventilation.
Bronchial studies—Acetylcysteine is indicated as a diagnostic aid in bronchial studies, such as bronchograms, bronchospirometry, and bronchial wedge catheterization.

## Pharmacology/Pharmacokinetics

**Physicochemical characteristics**
Molecular weight—163.19.

**Mechanism of action/Effect**
The viscosity of pulmonary mucous secretions depends on the concentrations of mucoproteins and, to a lesser extent, of deoxyribonucleic acid (DNA). Acetylcysteine decreases the viscosity of pulmonary secretions and facilitates their removal by coughing, postural drainage, or mechanical means. It exerts its mucolytic action through its free sulfhydryl group, which acts directly on the mucoproteins to open the disulfide bonds and lower the viscosity of the mucus. This action increases with increasing pH and is most significant at pH 7 to 9. The mucolytic action of acetylcysteine is not affected by the presence of DNA.

**Other actions/effects**
Acetylcysteine has no effect on fibrin, blood clots, or living tissue.

**Absorption**
Most of an acetylcysteine dose participates in the sulfhydryl-disulfide reaction; the remainder is absorbed from the pulmonary epithelium.

**Biotransformation**
Hepatic. Acetylcysteine undergoes rapid deacetylation *in vivo* to yield cysteine or oxidation to yield diacetylcystine.

**Onset of action**
Inhalation—Within 1 minute.
Direct instillation—Immediate.

**Time to peak effect**
Inhalation—5 to 10 minutes.

## Precautions to Consider

**Carcinogenicity**
Studies have not been done to determine the carcinogenic potential of acetylcysteine.

**Mutagenicity**
In the Ames test, both with and without metabolic activation, acetylcysteine was not shown to be mutagenic.

**Pregnancy/Reproduction**
Fertility—A reproduction toxicity study in rats given acetylcysteine with isoproterenol by inhalation showed no adverse effects on fertility. In reproduction toxicity studies in rats given acetylcysteine orally at doses up to 5.2 times the human dose, one study showed only a slight non–dose-related reduction in fertility.
Pregnancy—Adequate and well-controlled studies in humans have not been done.
Reproduction studies in rats given acetylcysteine with isoproterenol and in rabbits given acetylcysteine alone at doses up to 2.6 times the human dose have shown no evidence of teratogenicity or harm to the fetus.
FDA Pregnancy Category B.

**Breast-feeding**
It is not known whether acetylcysteine is distributed into breast milk. However, problems in humans have not been documented.

**Pediatrics**
Appropriate studies on the relationship of age to the effects of acetylcysteine inhalation have not been performed in the pediatric population. However, no pediatrics-specific problems have been documented to date.

**Geriatrics**
Appropriate studies on the relationship of age to the effects of acetylcysteine inhalation have not been performed in the geriatric population. However, no geriatrics-specific problems have been documented to date.

**Medical considerations/Contraindications**

The medical considerations/contraindications included here have been selected on the basis of their potential clinical significance (reasons given in parentheses where appropriate)—not necessarily inclusive (» = major clinical significance).

*Risk-benefit should be considered when the following medical problems exist:*

» Asthma, bronchial, or

» Respiratory insufficiency, severe

(obstruction of bronchial airways may be increased, especially in debilitated patients; if acetylcysteine is used in these patients, pretreatment with a bronchodilator may be indicated)

Sensitivity to acetylcysteine

## Side/Adverse Effects

The following side/adverse effects have been selected on the basis of their potential clinical significance (possible signs and symptoms in parentheses where appropriate)—not necessarily inclusive:

**Those indicating need for medical attention**

Incidence less frequent

*Hemoptysis* (spitting up blood); *increased airways obstruction,* (wheezing, tightness in chest, or difficulty in breathing)—especially in asthma patients; more frequent with the 20% solution

Incidence rare

*Sensitization* (skin rash or other irritation)—with frequent and prolonged exposure

**Those indicating need for medical attention only if they continue or are bothersome**

Incidence less frequent

*Clammy skin; fever; increase in bronchial secretions; irritation of throat or lungs; nausea or vomiting; rhinorrhea* (runny nose); *stomatitis* (irritation or soreness of mouth)

**Those not indicating need for medical attention**

Incidence more frequent

*Stickiness on face, after nebulization using a face mask; unpleasant odor during administration, transient*

## Patient Consultation

As an aid to patient consultation, refer to *Advice for the Patient, Acetylcysteine (Inhalation).*

In providing consultation, consider emphasizing the following selected information (» = major clinical significance):

**Before using this medication**

» Conditions affecting use, especially:

Sensitivity to acetylcysteine

Other medical problems, especially bronchial asthma or other severe respiratory insufficiency

**Proper use of this medication**

» Importance of not using more medication than the amount prescribed

Proper administration: Knowing correct administration technique; checking with physician if necessary

After using medication, coughing up loosened mucus to prevent excessive accumulation in lungs; mechanical suction may be necessary if cough inadequate to remove mucus

» Proper dosing

Missed dose: Using as soon as possible; using any remaining doses for that day at regularly spaced intervals

» Proper storage

**Precautions while using this medication**

» Checking with physician if condition does not improve or if it becomes worse

**Side/adverse effects**

Signs of potential side effects, especially hemoptysis, increased airways obstruction, and sensitization

Possibility of stickiness on face after nebulization using a face mask; removing by washing with water

Possibility of acetylcysteine having a transient unpleasant odor during administration

## General Dosing Information

The method of acetylcysteine administration depends on the condition being treated. Acetylcysteine, usually as a 10 to 20% solution, may be administered by nebulization, direct instillation, or intratracheal instillation.

Acetylcysteine is usually administered by nebulization, using conventional nebulizers made of plastic or glass. Certain materials used in nebuli-

zation equipment react with acetylcysteine, especially iron, copper, and rubber.

When acetylcysteine is administered by nebulization, compressed tank gas (air) or an air compressor should be used to provide pressure for nebulizing the solution. Oxygen may also be used; however, it should be used with the usual precautions in patients with severe respiratory disease and carbon dioxide retention. Acetylcysteine may also be administered by ultrasonic nebulization.

The nebulizer used should be capable of providing optimal quantities of a suitable range of particle sizes. Commercially available nebulizers will produce nebulae of acetylcysteine satisfactory for retention in the respiratory tract, usually providing a high proportion of the acetylcysteine solution as particles of less than 10 microns in diameter.

The nebulized solution may be inhaled directly from the nebulizer or the nebulizer may be attached to a plastic face mask or tent, plastic mouthpiece, conventional plastic oxygen tent, or head tent. Suitable nebulizers may also be fitted for use with the various intermittent positive pressure breathing (IPPB) machines.

Acetylcysteine should not be placed directly into the chamber of a heated (hot pot) nebulizer. A heated nebulizer may be part of the nebulization assembly to provide a warm saturated atmosphere if the acetylcysteine aerosol is introduced by means of a separate unheated nebulizer. The usual precautions for administration of warm saturated nebulae should be followed.

The nebulizing equipment should be cleaned immediately after use because the residues may clog the smaller orifices or corrode metal parts.

Hand bulb nebulizers are not recommended for nebulizing acetylcysteine because their output is generally too small and some of them deliver particles that are larger than optimum for inhalation therapy.

When acetylcysteine is nebulized for a prolonged period of time with a dry gas, the solution may become overconcentrated (due to evaporation) and nebulization may be impaired. After three-fourths of the initial volume of solution has been nebulized, the remaining solution in the nebulizer should be diluted with an approximately equal volume of sterile water for injection.

After administration of acetylcysteine, an increase in volume of liquefied bronchial secretions may occur. This may produce breathing difficulty in patients who have poor ventilatory mechanics and/or poor cough, such as postoperative or trauma patients. When the cough is inadequate to maintain an open airway, mechanical suction or endotracheal aspiration should be used if necessary.

Nebulization with a face mask may leave a sticky residue on the face. This can be removed by washing with water.

When acetylcysteine inhalation is administered to patients with asthma or hyperactive airways disease, a bronchodilator should be administered prior to acetylcysteine to protect against bronchospasm.

**For treatment of adverse effects**

Bronchospasm may be relieved by the administration of a bronchodilator by nebulization. If bronchospasm continues, acetylcysteine should be discontinued.

## Inhalation Dosage Forms

### ACETYLCYSTEINE SOLUTION USP

**Usual adult and adolescent dose**

Mucolytic—

Nebulization via face mask, mouth piece, or tracheostomy:

Inhalation, 3 to 5 (range, 1 to 10) mL of a 20% solution or 6 to 10 (range, 2 to 20) mL of a 10% solution three or four times a day (range, every two to six hours).

Nebulization via tent or croupette:

Inhalation, a sufficient volume of a 10 or 20% solution to maintain a very heavy mist in the tent or croupette for the period of time necessary.

Note: The method of nebulization, via tent or croupette, must be individualized according to the available equipment and the patient's condition. Very large volumes of the solution are required, occasionally as much as 300 mL during a single treatment period.

Instillation, direct:

1 to 2 mL of a 10 to 20% solution every hour, if necessary.

For routine care of patients with tracheostomy—Intratracheal, 1 to 2 mL of a 10 to 20% solution every one to four hours.

For instillation into a particular segment of bronchopulmonary tree via small plastic catheter into trachea—Intratracheal, 2 to 5 mL of a 20% solution instilled by means of a syringe connected to the catheter.

For instillation via percutaneous intratracheal catheter—Intratracheal, 2 to 4 mL of a 10% solution or 1 to 2 mL of a 20%

solution every one to four hours administered by a syringe attached to the catheter.

Diagnostic aid (bronchial studies)—
Inhalation or intratracheal instillation, 1 to 2 mL of a 20% solution or 2 to 4 mL of a 10% solution for two or three doses prior to the procedure.

**Usual pediatric dose**
See *Usual adult and adolescent dose.*

**Usual geriatric dose**
See *Usual adult and adolescent dose.*

**Strength(s) usually available**
U.S.—
   10% (Rx) [*Mucomyst-10; Mucosil-10;* GENERIC].
   20% (Rx) [*Mucomyst; Mucosil-20;* GENERIC].
Canada—
   20% (Rx) [*Mucomyst*].

**Packaging and storage**
Store below 40 °C (104 °F), preferably between 15 and 30 °C (59 and 86 °F), unless otherwise specified by manufacturer. Store in a tight container with a glass or polyethylene or polytef-coated elastomeric closure.

**Preparation of dosage form**
The 10% solution may be used undiluted.
The 20% solution may be used undiluted or diluted to a lesser concentration with 0.9% sodium chloride injection, sodium chloride inhalation solution, sterile water for injection, or sterile water for inhalation.

**Stability**
Acetylcysteine solution does not contain an antimicrobial agent; therefore, care must be taken to minimize contamination of the sterile solution.

After opening, the vial should be stored in the refrigerator; the opened vial should be discarded after 96 hours.

A color change may occur in acetylcysteine after the bottle has been opened. The light purple color results from a chemical reaction that does not significantly affect the safety or mucolytic efficacy of acetylcysteine.

If an admixture with acetylcysteine is necessary, it should be administered as soon as possible after preparation; unused admixtures should not be stored.

**Incompatibilities**
Acetylcysteine reacts with certain materials, such as iron, copper, and rubber, used in nebulization equipment. Where materials may come into contact with acetylcysteine solution, parts made of the following materials should be used: glass, plastic, aluminum, anodized aluminum, chromed metal, tantalum, sterling silver, or stainless steel. Silver may become tarnished after exposure but this does not affect the efficacy of acetylcysteine or harm the patient.

Acetylcysteine has been shown to be incompatible, when mixed in the same solution, with amphotericin B, chlortetracycline hydrochloride, erythromycin lactobionate, oxytetracycline hydrochloride, ampicillin sodium, or tetracycline hydrochloride. These agents should be administered as separate solutions if administration is necessary.

Acetylcysteine is also incompatible with iodized oil (contrast media), hydrogen peroxide, chymotrypsin, and trypsin.

**Auxiliary labeling**
• Store in refrigerator after opening.
• Discard opened vial after 96 hours.

Revised: 08/03/93
Interim revision: 04/29/94

# ACETYLCYSTEINE   Systemic

JAN: *N*-Acetyl-L-Cysteine.

VA CLASSIFICATION (Primary/Secondary):
   Oral—RE400/AD900
   Parenteral—AD900

Note: For a listing of dosage forms and brand names by country availability, see *Dosage Forms* section(s). For a listing of brand names for the articles in this monograph, refer to the General Index.

## Category

Antidote (to acetaminophen overdose).

## Indications

**Accepted**
Toxicity, acetaminophen (treatment)—Acetylcysteine is indicated in the treatment of acetaminophen overdose to protect against hepatotoxicity.

## Pharmacology/Pharmacokinetics

**Physicochemical characteristics**
Molecular weight—163.19.

**Mechanism of action/Effect**
Acetylcysteine may protect against acetaminophen overdose–induced hepatotoxicity by maintaining or restoring hepatic concentrations of glutathione. Glutathione is required to inactivate an intermediate metabolite of acetaminophen that is thought to be hepatotoxic. In acetaminophen overdose, excessive quantities of this metabolite are formed because the primary metabolic (glucuronide and sulfate conjugation) pathways become saturated. Acetylcysteine may act by reducing the metabolite to the parent compound and/or by providing sulfhydryl for conjugation of the metabolite. Experimental evidence also suggests that a sulfhydryl-containing compound such as acetylcysteine may also directly inactivate the metabolite.

**Biotransformation**
Deacetylated by the liver to cysteine and subsequently metabolized.

## Precautions to Consider

**Carcinogenicity**
Studies have not been done to determine the carcinogenic potential of acetylcysteine.

**Mutagenicity**
In the Ames test, both with and without metabolic activation, acetylcysteine was not shown to be mutagenic.

**Pregnancy/Reproduction**
Fertility—Reproductive studies performed in rats given oral doses of up to 1000 mg per kg of body weight (mg/kg) of acetylcysteine per day showed a slight reduction in fertility with doses of 500 or 1000 mg/kg per day (2.6 and 5.2 times the human dose, respectively). Studies in rabbits given up to 500 mg/kg per day (2.6 times the human dose) revealed no evidence of impaired fertility.

Pregnancy—Adequate and well-controlled studies in humans have not been done. However, several reports have indicated that use of acetylcysteine to treat acetaminophen overdose in pregnant women is safe and effective, and may prevent hepatotoxicity in the fetus as well as in the mother.

Studies in rabbits given oral doses of 500 mg/kg per day on Day 6 through Day 16 of gestation and in rabbits given 10% acetylcysteine plus 0.5% isoproterenol by inhalation for 30 or 35 minutes twice a day on Day 16 through Day 18 of gestation showed no evidence of teratogenicity or harm to the fetus. Also, studies in rats administered acetylcysteine and isoproterenol by inhalation showed no evidence of teratogenicity or harm to the fetus.

FDA Pregnancy Category B.

**Breast-feeding**
It is not known whether acetylcysteine is distributed into breast milk. However, problems in humans have not been documented.

**Pediatrics**
Appropriate studies on the relationship of age to the effects of acetylcysteine have not been performed in the pediatric population. However, no pediatrics-specific problems have been documented to date.

**Geriatrics**
No information is available on the relationship of age to the effects of acetylcysteine in geriatric patients being treated for acetaminophen overdose.

**Medical considerations/Contraindications**
The medical considerations/contraindications included here have been selected on the basis of their potential clinical significance (reasons given in parentheses where appropriate)—not necessarily inclusive (» = major clinical significance).

*Risk-benefit should be considered when the following medical problems exist:*

Asthma, history of
    (risk of bronchospastic reactions—with intravenous administration)

Conditions predisposing to gastrointestinal hemorrhage, such as:
    Esophageal varices
    Peptic ulceration
    (acetylcysteine-induced vomiting may increase the risk of hemorrhage)

Sensitivity to acetylcysteine

## Side/Adverse Effects

The following side/adverse effects have been selected on the basis of their potential clinical significance (possible signs and symptoms in parentheses where appropriate)—not necessarily inclusive:

### Those indicating need for medical attention
Incidence rare
> *Bronchospastic allergic reaction* (shortness of breath, troubled breathing, tightness in chest, or wheezing); *dermatitis, allergic* (skin rash or hives); *facial edema*
>
> Note: *Bronchospasm* may also occur in conjunction with a generalized *anaphylactoid reaction*. These allergic reactions and *facial edema* have been reported only with intravenous administration.

### Those indicating need for medical attention only if they continue or are bothersome
> *Drowsiness; fever; nausea or vomiting*

## General Dosing Information

Because an injectable dosage form of acetylcysteine is not commercially available in the U.S., some emergency care practitioners have advocated that the oral solution be diluted and given by intravenous infusion when necessary. Oral administration is preferred because of the risk of bronchospastic or anaphylactoid reactions associated with intravenous administration of acetylcysteine. Also, the fact must be kept in mind that the oral solution available in the U.S., although sterile, is not required to be pyrogen-free.

Administration of acetylcysteine is only part of an overall regimen for the treatment of acetaminophen overdose. Other measures include emptying the stomach via induction of emesis or gastric lavage; monitoring plasma acetaminophen concentration, liver function, renal function, and fluid and electrolyte balance; and supportive treatment as described below. Administration of activated charcoal as part of the treatment regimen may be needed. Although its use has been recommended primarily in cases of mixed overdose, one study has shown that administration of activated charcoal plus acetylcysteine may be more effective than acetylcysteine alone in preventing hepatotoxicity after an acetaminophen overdose.

Acetylcysteine therapy should be initiated within 24 hours after ingestion of an acetaminophen overdose. If initiation of treatment will not be delayed beyond 10 to 12 hours after ingestion of the overdose, acetylcysteine therapy may be withheld until the results of plasma acetaminophen determinations are available. Otherwise, *an initial dose of acetylcysteine should be administered immediately*, without waiting for the results of acetaminophen determinations or other laboratory tests.

The plasma acetaminophen concentration should be determined not less than 4 hours following ingestion of the overdose. Concentrations determined prior to this time are not reliable for assessing potential hepatotoxicity. The following table shows plasma concentrations of acetaminophen that are potentially hepatotoxic if they are measured at the listed times after ingestion of a possible overdose. If the initial determination shows a higher concentration, a full course of acetylcysteine should be administered. If a lower plasma concentration is reported, initiation or continuation of acetylcysteine treatment is not necessary.

| Time after Ingestion of Overdose (hr) | Acetaminophen Concentration | |
|---|---|---|
| | mcg/mL | micromoles/L |
| 4 | 150 | 993 |
| 6 | 100 | 662 |
| 8 | 70 | 463.4 |
| 10 | 50 | 331 |
| 15 | 20 | 132.4 |
| 20 | 8 | 53 |
| 24 | 3.5 | 23.2 |

Liver function tests (serum aspartate aminotransferase [AST; SGOT], serum alanine aminotransferase [ALT; SGPT], prothrombin time, and

bilirubin) should be performed at 24-hour intervals for at least 96 hours postingestion if the plasma acetaminophen concentration indicates potential hepatotoxicity. If no abnormalities are detected within 96 hours, further determinations are not needed.

Renal and cardiac function should be monitored and appropriate therapy instituted if necessary.

Supportive treatment includes maintaining fluid and electrolyte balance, correcting hypoglycemia, and administering vitamin $K_1$ (if prothrombin time ratio exceeds 1.5) and fresh frozen plasma or clotting factor concentrate (if prothrombin time ratio exceeds 3).

Administration of diuretics and forced diuresis are not recommended.

Additional therapy to treat mixed overdose with other agents (i.e., naloxone for an opioid analgesic) may be needed, especially if symptoms of central nervous system (CNS) depression occur within a few hours after ingestion of the overdose.

Discontinuation of acetylcysteine therapy should be considered if generalized urticaria or other symptoms of an allergic reaction occur and cannot be controlled by other means.

### For oral dosage form only
Acetylcysteine solution must be diluted prior to administration because of its unpleasant odor and its irritating or sclerosing properties. Dilution may also reduce the risk of vomiting. Also, the medication may be tolerated better if the diluted solution is administered well chilled (over ice, if necessary) and sipped from a covered container through a drinking straw. If necessary, an antiemetic may be used concurrently or acetylcysteine can be given via nasogastric tube.

## Oral Dosage Forms

Note: The dosage form administered orally is the same solution that is administered via inhalation as a mucolytic (see *Acetylcysteine [Inhalation-Local]*).

### ACETYLCYSTEINE SOLUTION USP

#### Usual adult and adolescent dose
Antidote (to acetaminophen overdose)—
> Oral, 140 mg per kg of body weight initially, followed by 70 mg per kg of body weight every four hours for seventeen additional doses.

Note: Any dose vomited within one hour of administration must be repeated. If necessary, an antiemetic may be given concurrently and/or acetylcysteine, diluted with water, may be given via nasogastric tube.

#### Usual pediatric dose
See *Usual adult and adolescent dose.*

#### Strength(s) usually available
U.S.—
> 10% (100 mg per mL) (Rx) [*Mucomyst; Mucosil;* GENERIC].
> 20% (200 mg per mL) (Rx) [*Mucomyst; Mucosil;* GENERIC].

Canada—
> 20% (200 mg per mL) (Rx) [*Mucomyst*].

#### Packaging and storage
Store below 40 °C (104 °F), preferably between 15 and 30 °C (59 and 86 °F), unless otherwise specified by manufacturer. Keep container tightly closed. Protect from freezing.

#### Preparation of dosage form
For patients weighing up to 20 kg (usually children younger than 6 years of age)—Dilute each mL of acetylcysteine solution with 3 mL of cola or other soft drinks.

For patients weighing 20 kg or more—Dilute the required quantity of acetylcysteine solution with enough cola or other soft drinks to make a 5% solution. The following quantities of acetylcysteine (20% solution) and diluent are needed to prepare a 5% solution containing the required initial dose and subsequent doses for patients weighing up to 110 kg:

| Body weight (kg) | Acetylcysteine | | mL of diluent | mL of 5% solution |
|---|---|---|---|---|
| | Grams | mL of 20% solution | | |
| **Loading dose** | | | | |
| 100–110 | 15 | 75 | 225 | 300 |
| 90–100 | 14 | 70 | 210 | 280 |
| 80–90 | 13 | 65 | 195 | 260 |
| 70–80 | 11 | 55 | 165 | 220 |
| 60–70 | 10 | 50 | 150 | 200 |
| 50–60 | 8 | 40 | 120 | 160 |
| 40–50 | 7 | 35 | 105 | 140 |
| 30–40 | 6 | 30 | 90 | 120 |
| 20–30 | 4 | 20 | 60 | 80 |

| Body weight (kg) | Acetylcysteine | | | |
| | Grams | mL of 20% solution | mL of diluent | mL of 5% solution |
|---|---|---|---|---|
| **Maintenance dose** | | | | |
| 100–110 | 7.5 | 37 | 113 | 150 |
| 90–100 | 7.0 | 35 | 105 | 140 |
| 80–90 | 6.5 | 33 | 97 | 130 |
| 70–80 | 5.5 | 28 | 82 | 110 |
| 60–70 | 5.0 | 25 | 75 | 100 |
| 50–60 | 4.0 | 20 | 60 | 80 |
| 40–50 | 3.5 | 18 | 52 | 70 |
| 30–40 | 3.0 | 15 | 45 | 60 |
| 20–30 | 2.0 | 10 | 30 | 40 |

## Stability

Because the solution contains no preservative, partially used vials should be refrigerated; opened vials should be discarded after 96 hours.
Diluted solutions should be freshly prepared and used within one hour.

## Incompatibilities

Acetylcysteine reacts with certain metals, especially iron, nickel, and copper, and with rubber. Contact with these substances should be avoided.

## Auxiliary labeling

• Store in refrigerator after opening.
• Discard opened vial after 96 hours.

# Parenteral Dosage Forms

## ACETYLCYSTEINE INJECTION

### Usual adult and adolescent dose

Antidote (to acetaminophen overdose)—
Intravenous, 300 mg per kg of body weight administered over twenty and one-fourth hours, divided as follows:
Initial loading dose—150 mg per kg of body weight in up to 200 mL of 5% dextrose injection, administered over fifteen minutes.
Second infusion—50 mg per kg of body weight in 500 mL of 5% dextrose injection, administered over four hours.
Third infusion—100 mg per kg of body weight in 1000 mL of 5% dextrose injection, administered over the next sixteen hours.

### Usual pediatric dose

See *Usual adult and adolescent dose.*

Note:  The volumes and rates of infusion administered to children must be adjusted according to the medical circumstances and any restrictions in the volumes of parenteral fluids administered, as applicable to the individual patient.

### Strength(s) usually available

U.S.—
Not commercially available.
Canada—
20% (200 mg per mL) (Rx) [*Mucomyst; Parvolex*].

## Preparation of dosage form

Initial loading dose (to be administered over fifteen minutes):
Add the required quantity of acetylcysteine injection to the following quantities of 5% dextrose injection:
For patients weighing 10 to 15 kg—40 mL.
For patients weighing 15 to 20 kg—50 mL.
For patients weighing 20 to 30 kg—75 mL.
For patients weighing 30 to 40 kg—100 mL.
For patients weighing 40 kg and over—200 mL.
Second infusion (to be administered over four hours)—
Add the required quantity of acetylcysteine injection to 500 mL of 5% dextrose injection.
Third infusion (to be administered over sixteen hours)—
Add the required quantity of acetylcysteine injection to 1 liter of 5% dextrose injection.
Note:  The following quantities of acetylcysteine injection and 5% dextrose injection are needed for preparing initial and subsequent infusion solutions for administration to patients of various weights:

| Body weight (kg) | 20% Acetylcysteine (mL) | | |
| | First infusion/ 5% dextrose injection (mL) | Second infusion* | Third infusion† |
|---|---|---|---|
| 100–110 | 82.5/200 | 27.5 | 55 |
| 90–100 | 75/200 | 25 | 50 |
| 80–90 | 67.5/200 | 22.5 | 45 |
| 70–80 | 60/200 | 20 | 40 |
| 60–70 | 52.5/200 | 17.5 | 35 |
| 50–60 | 45/200 | 15 | 30 |
| 40–50 | 37.5/200 | 12.5 | 25 |
| 30–40 | 30/100 | 10 | 20 |
| 25–30 | 22.5/75 | 7.5 | 15 |
| 20–25 | 18.75/75 | 6.25 | 12.5 |
| 15–20 | 15/50 | 5 | 10 |
| 10–15 | 11.25/40 | 3.75 | 7.5 |

*Add to 500 mL of 5% dextrose injection.
†Add to 1000 mL of 5% dextrose injection.

## Incompatibilities

Acetylcysteine reacts with certain metals, especially iron, nickel, and copper, and with rubber. Contact with these substances should be avoided.

Revised: 07/29/94

# ACRIVASTINE—See *Antihistamines (Systemic)*

# ACRIVASTINE-CONTAINING COMBINATIONS—

Acrivastine and Pseudoephedrine (Systemic)—See *Antihistamines and Decongestants (Systemic)*

# ACYCLOVIR   Systemic

INN: Aciclovir
VA CLASSIFICATION (Primary): AM800
Note: For a listing of dosage forms and brand names by country availability, see *Dosage Forms* section(s). For a listing of brand names for the articles in this monograph, refer to the General Index.

## Category

Antiviral (systemic).

## Indications

Note:  Bracketed information in the *Indications* section refers to uses that are not included in U.S. product labeling.

### Accepted

Herpes genitalis (treatment)—Oral acyclovir is indicated in the treatment of initial episodes and management of recurrent, severe herpes genitalis infections in immunocompromised and nonimmunocompromised patients. Parenteral acyclovir is indicated in the treatment of severe initial herpes genitalis infections in immunocompromised and non-

immunocompromised patients, and in patients who are unable to take (or absorb) oral acyclovir.

Herpes genitalis (prophylaxis)—Oral acyclovir is indicated in the prophylaxis of frequently recurrent (≥ 6 episodes per year) herpes genitalis infections in immunocompromised and nonimmunocompromised patients.

Herpes simplex (treatment)—Parenteral [and oral] acyclovir are indicated in the treatment of initial and recurrent mucocutaneous herpes simplex (HSV-1 and HSV-2) infections in immunocompromised patients.

[Herpes simplex (prophylaxis)][1]—Parenteral and oral acyclovir are used in the prophylaxis of herpes simplex virus (HSV) infections in patients who are immunocompromised, including transplant patients receiving immunosuppressant therapy, human immunodeficiency virus (HIV)-infected patients, and patients receiving chemotherapy.

Herpes simplex encephalitis (treatment)[1]—Parenteral acyclovir is indicated in the treatment of herpes simplex encephalitis.

Herpes zoster (treatment)—Oral acyclovir is indicated in the treatment of herpes zoster infections (shingles) caused by varicella-zoster virus (VZV) in any adult patient with herpes zoster. Therapy is most effective when started within 48 hours of the onset of rash. Parenteral acyclovir is indicated in the treatment of herpes zoster infections (shingles) caused by VZV in immunocompromised patients and disseminated herpes zoster in nonimmunocompromised patients.

[Herpes zoster (prophylaxis)][1]—Oral acyclovir is used in the prophylaxis of herpes zoster infections (shingles) caused by VZV, after an initial period of parenteral acyclovir, in any immunocompromised patient, including transplant patients receiving immunosuppressant therapy, HIV-infected patients, and patients receiving chemotherapy.

Herpes zoster ophthalmicus (treatment)—Oral and parenteral acyclovir are indicated in the treatment of herpes zoster ophthalmicus.

[Herpes simplex virus, disseminated neonatal infection (treatment)][1]—Parenteral acyclovir is used in the treatment of disseminated HSV in neonates.

Varicella (treatment)—Oral acyclovir is indicated in the treatment of varicella infections (chickenpox) in nonimmunocompromised patients when started within 24 hours of the onset of a typical chickenpox rash. [Parenteral acyclovir is used in the treatment of varicella infections (chickenpox) caused by VZV in immunocompromised patients.]

Although acyclovir is indicated for the treatment of varicella infections in nonimmunocompromised patients, the American Academy of Pediatrics does not recommend its use for the treatment of uncomplicated chickenpox in healthy children. It is recommended for certain groups at increased risk of severe varicella or its complications, such as otherwise healthy, nonpregnant persons 13 years of age or older; children older than 12 months of age with a chronic cutaneous or pulmonary disorder; and children receiving short, intermittent or aerosolized courses of corticosteroids. If possible, steroids should be discontinued after known exposure to varicella.

Resistance of HSV and VZV to acyclovir has been reported to develop with prolonged treatment or repeated therapy in severely immunocompromised patients. Resistance may occasionally develop as quickly as within a few weeks. If lesions due to herpes simplex virus fail to respond to acyclovir therapy, especially with continued viral shedding, viral isolates should be tested for susceptibility to acyclovir.

### Unaccepted
Oral acyclovir is not indicated in the suppression of recurrent herpes genitalis in patients with infrequent recurrences.

---

[1]Not included in Canadian product labeling.

## Pharmacology/Pharmacokinetics

### Physicochemical characteristics
Molecular weight—Acyclovir: 225.21.
Acyclovir sodium: 247.19.
pH—Reconstituted acyclovir (50 mg per mL): Approximately 11.

### Mechanism of action/Effect
Acyclovir is converted to acyclovir monophosphate, a nucleotide, by the viral thymidine kinases of herpes simplex virus (HSV) and varicellazoster virus (VZV). Acyclovir monophosphate is converted to the diphosphate by cellular guanylate kinase and to the triphosphate by a number of cellular enzymes. Acyclovir triphosphate interferes with HSV and VZV DNA polymerase and inhibits viral DNA replication. The triphosphate can be incorporated into growing chains of DNA by viral DNA polymerase, resulting in termination of the DNA chain.

### Absorption
Oral—Bioavailability 20% (range, 15 to 30%). Poorly absorbed from the gastrointestinal tract. Not significantly affected by food.

### Distribution
Widely distributed to tissues and body fluids, including brain, kidneys, lungs, liver, aqueous humor, tears, intestines, muscle, spleen, breast milk, uterus, vaginal mucosa, vaginal secretions, semen, amniotic fluid, cerebrospinal fluid (CSF), and herpetic vesicular fluid. Highest concentrations are found in kidneys, liver, and intestines. CSF concentrations are approximately 50% of plasma concentrations. Crosses the placenta, also.

Vol$_D$ (steady state)—
    Adults: Approximately 48 liters (L) per square meter of body surface (m²) (range, 37 to 57 L per m²).
    Children and adolescents (1 to 18 years old): Approximately 45 L per m².
    Neonates (0 to 3 months old): Approximately 28 L per m² (range, 24 to 30 L per m²).
    End-stage renal disease: Approximately 41 L per m².

### Protein binding
Low (9 to 33%).

### Biotransformation
Hepatic; only major metabolite found in urine is 9-carboxymethoxymethylguanine, which accounts for approximately 9 to 14% of the dose. This metabolite has no known antiviral activity.

### Half-life
Intravenous—
    Adults: Approximately 2.5 hours.
    Children (1 to 18 years old): Approximately 2.6 hours.
    Neonates (0 to 3 months old): Approximately 4 hours.
Renal impairment (adults)—

| Creatinine Clearance (mL/min)/ (mL/sec) | Half-life (hr) |
|---|---|
| >80/1.33 | 2.5 |
| 50–80/0.83–1.33 | 3.0 |
| 15–50/0.25–0.83 | 3.5 |
| Anuric | 19.5 |
| During hemodialysis | 5.7 |
| Continuous ambulatory peritoneal dialysis | 14–18 |

Oral—
    3.3 hours.

### Time to peak serum concentration
Intravenous—End of infusion (approximately 1 hour).
Oral—1.7 hours.

### Mean peak serum concentration (steady-state)
Oral—Adults—
    200 mg every 4 hours:
        0.6 mcg/mL (2.5 micromoles/L).
    400 mg every 4 hours:
        1.2 mcg/mL (5.3 micromoles/L).
    800 mg every 4 hours:
        1.6 mcg/mL (6.9 micromoles/L).
Intravenous—
    Adults:
        5 mg per kg (over 1 hour) every 8 hours—9.8 mcg/mL (43.5 micromoles/L).
        10 mg per kg (over 1 hour) every 8 hours—22.9 mcg/mL (101.7 micromoles/L).
    Children (1 to 18 years old):
        250 mg per m² (over 1 hour) every 8 hours—10.3 mcg/mL (45.8 micromoles/L).
        500 mg per m² (over 1 hour) every 8 hours—20.7 mcg/mL (91.9 micromoles/L).
    Neonates (0 to 3 months old):
        5 mg per kg (over 1 hour) every 8 hours—6.8 mcg/mL (30 micromoles/L).
        10 mg per kg (over 1 hour) every 8 hours—13.8 mcg/mL (61.2 micromoles/L).

### Elimination
Renal—
    Excreted by both glomerular filtration and tubular secretion.
    Oral: Approximately 14% of total dose excreted unchanged in urine.
    Intravenous: Approximately 45 to 79% excreted unchanged in urine.
Fecal—
    Insignificant amounts (<2%).
Lungs—
    Trace amounts in exhaled $CO_2$.
Dialysis—
    Hemodialysis: A single 6-hour period of hemodialysis reduces plasma acyclovir concentrations by approximately 60%.
    Peritoneal dialysis: Peritoneal dialysis does not substantially alter acyclovir clearance.

## Precautions to Consider

### Cross-sensitivity and/or related problems
Patients allergic to ganciclovir may also be allergic to acyclovir because of the chemical similarity of the two medications.

### Carcinogenicity
Life-time bioassays in rats and mice given daily doses of 50, 150, and 450 mg per kg of body weight (mg/kg) by gavage have not shown any evidence of carcinogenicity. However, *in vitro* cell transformation assays have given conflicting results, being positive at the highest dose used in one system. The resulting morphologically transformed cells induced tumors when inoculated into immunosuppressed, syngeneic, weanling mice, although results were negative in another transformation assay.

**Mutagenicity**

Oral acyclovir has been shown to be mutagenic at high concentrations in some acute animal studies. However, no chromosomal damage was noted at maximum tolerated parenteral doses (100 mg/kg) in rats or Chinese hamsters. Higher doses (500 and 1000 mg/kg) were clastogenic in Chinese hamsters. No problems were reported in dominant lethal studies in mice. Also, there was no evidence of mutagenicity in 9 out of 11 microbial and mammalian cell assays. In 2 of the mammalian cell assays, a positive response for mutagenicity and chromosomal damage was noted, but only at concentrations at least 25 times the usual plasma concentrations achieved in humans.

**Pregnancy/Reproduction**

Fertility—Impairment of spermatogenesis, sperm motility, or morphology has not been documented in humans. However, high doses of parenteral acyclovir have caused testicular atrophy in rats and dogs. Some evidence of sperm production recovery was evident 30 days post-dose. Studies in mice given oral doses of up to 450 mg/kg per day have shown that acyclovir does not impair fertility or reproduction. Studies in female rabbits given acyclovir subcutaneously subsequent to mating have shown a significant decrease in implantation efficiency, but no decrease in litter size at doses of 50 mg/kg per day.

Pregnancy—Acyclovir crosses the placenta. Acyclovir has been used in all stages of pregnancy, most commonly in the third trimester. No adverse fetal effects have been reported. One small, controlled study found that pre-partum treatment of women with recurrent genital herpes helped prevent symptomatic recurrences and viral shedding at the time of delivery, reducing the risk of the infant being exposed to the virus. Adequate and well-controlled studies in humans have not been done.

Studies in mice given oral doses of 450 mg/kg per day and studies in rats and rabbits given subcutaneous doses of 50 mg/kg per day have shown that acyclovir does not cause adverse effects in the fetus.

FDA Pregnancy Category C.

**Breast-feeding**

Acyclovir passes into breast milk at concentrations from 0.6 to 4.1 times the corresponding plasma concentration. A very small amount of acyclovir has been measured in one nursing infant's urine; no toxicity was observed.

**Pediatrics**

Limited data are available about the use of oral acyclovir in children younger than 2 years of age. However, no unusual toxicity or pediatrics-specific problems have been observed in studies done in children using doses of up to 3000 mg per square meter of body surface area ($mg/m^2$) per day and 80 mg/kg per day. Intravenous acyclovir should be used with greater caution in neonates due to their age-related decrease in clearance. The half-life and clearance of intravenous acyclovir in children older than 1 year of age is similar to that seen in adults with normal renal function.

**Geriatrics**

Studies performed to date have not demonstrated geriatric-specific problems that would limit the usefulness of acyclovir in the elderly. However, elderly patients are more likely to have an age-related decrease in renal function, which may require an adjustment of acyclovir dosage or dosing interval.

**Drug interactions and/or related problems**

The following drug interactions and/or related problems have been selected on the basis of their potential clinical significance (possible mechanism in parentheses where appropriate)—not necessarily inclusive (» = major clinical significance):

Note: Combinations containing any of the following medications, depending on the amount present, may also interact with this medication.

» Nephrotoxic medications, other (See *Appendix II*)
(concurrent use with intravenous acyclovir may increase the potential for nephrotoxicity, especially in the presence of renal function impairment)

Probenecid
(may decrease renal tubular secretion of intravenous acyclovir when used concurrently, resulting in increased acyclovir serum and cerebrospinal fluid [CSF] concentrations, prolonged elimination half-life in the serum and CSF, and, potentially, increased toxicity)

**Laboratory value alterations**

The following have been selected on the basis of their potential clinical significance (possible effect in parentheses where appropriate)—not necessarily inclusive (» = major clinical significance):

With physiology/laboratory test values
» Blood urea nitrogen (BUN) and
» Creatinine, serum
(concentrations may be increased because of renal tubular obstruction caused by intravenous acyclovir; no increase generally occurs with proper dosage and adequate hydration)

**Medical considerations/Contraindications**

The medical considerations/contraindications included here have been selected on the basis of their potential clinical significance (reasons given in parentheses where appropriate)—not necessarily inclusive (» = major clinical significance).

*Risk-benefit should be considered when the following medical problems exist:*

» Dehydration or
» Renal function impairment, pre-existing
(intravenous acyclovir may increase the potential for nephrotoxicity; it is recommended that acyclovir be administered in a reduced dosage to patients with impaired renal function)

Hypersensitivity to acyclovir or ganciclovir

Neurological abnormalities or
Prior neurologic reactions to cytotoxic medications
(intravenous acyclovir may increase the potential for neurologic side effects)

**Patient monitoring**

The following may be especially important in patient monitoring (other tests may be warranted in some patients, depending on condition; » = major clinical significance):

Papanicolaou (Pap) test
(although a clear association has not been shown to date, patients with genital herpes may be at increased risk of developing cervical cancer; Pap test should be done at least once a year to detect early cervical changes)

» Blood urea nitrogen (BUN) and
» Creatinine, serum
(concentrations required prior to and during therapy since intravenous acyclovir may be nephrotoxic; if acyclovir is given by rapid intravenous injection or its urine solubility is exceeded, precipitation of acyclovir crystals may occur in renal tubules; renal tubular damage may occur and may progress to acute renal failure)

# Side/Adverse Effects

Note: Acute renal insufficiency may occur due to precipitation of acyclovir in the renal tubules. It is most likely to occur if acyclovir is given by rapid intravenous injection, concurrently with known nephrotoxic medications, to patients who are inadequately hydrated, or to patients with renal function impairment without appropriate dosage reduction. However, acute renal failure has also been reported in patients receiving oral acyclovir.

Neuropsychiatric toxicity has been associated with high plasma acyclovir concentrations—which may occur when high doses are used, or when patients with renal function impairment are not given an appropriately lowered dose. Neuropsychiatric toxicity may also be more likely to occur in immunocompromised patients and geriatric patients.

The following side/adverse effects have been selected on the basis of their potential clinical significance (possible signs and symptoms in parentheses where appropriate)—not necessarily inclusive:

**Those indicating need for medical attention**

Incidence more frequent
*For parenteral acyclovir*
**Phlebitis or inflammation at the injection site** (pain, swelling, or redness)

Incidence less frequent
*For parenteral acyclovir—more common with rapid intravenous injection*
**Acute renal failure** (abdominal pain; decreased frequency of urination or amount of urine; increased thirst; loss of appetite; nausea; vomiting; unusual tiredness or weakness)

Incidence rare
> For parenteral acyclovir only
>> *Encephalopathic changes* (coma; confusion; hallucinations; seizures; tremors)

**Those indicating need for medical attention only if they continue or are bothersome**
Incidence more frequent—especially with high doses
> For parenteral acyclovir
>> *Gastrointestinal disturbances* (loss of appetite; nausea or vomiting); *lightheadedness*
Incidence less frequent—with long-term use or high doses
> For oral acyclovir
>> *Gastrointestinal disturbances* (nausea or vomiting; diarrhea; abdominal pain); *headache; lightheadedness*

## Patient Consultation
As an aid to patient consultation, refer to *Advice for the Patient, Acyclovir (Systemic)*.

In providing consultation, consider emphasizing the following selected information (» = major clinical significance):

**Before using this medication**
» Conditions affecting use, especially:
   Hypersensitivity to acyclovir or ganciclovir
   Pregnancy—Acyclovir crosses the placenta
   Breast-feeding—Acyclovir is distributed into breast milk at concentrations from 0.6 to 4.1 times the corresponding plasma concentration
   Use in children—Neonates have an age-related decrease in acyclovir clearance
   Other medications, especially nephrotoxic medications
   Other medical problems, especially dehydration or pre-existing renal function impairment

**Proper use of this medication**
   Supplying patient information about herpes simplex or varicella-zoster infections
   For treatment of recurrent herpes simplex infections, initiating use of the medication as soon as possible after symptoms of recurrence begin to appear
   For treatment of chickenpox (varicella), initiating use of oral acyclovir at the earliest sign or symptom; it is most effective when started within 24 hours of the onset of a typical chickenpox rash
   Capsules, tablets, and oral suspension may be taken with meals
   Taking with full glass of water
   Proper administration technique for oral liquids
» Compliance with full course of therapy; not using more often or for longer than prescribed
» Proper dosing
   Missed dose: Taking as soon as possible; not taking if almost time for next dose; not doubling doses
» Proper storage

**Precautions while using this medication**
» Women with herpes genitalis may have an increased risk of developing cervical cancer; annual Pap tests may be required
   Checking with physician if no improvement within a few days
   Keeping affected areas as clean and dry as possible; wearing loose-fitting clothing to avoid irritation of lesions
» Use of acyclovir has not been shown to prevent the transmission of herpes simplex virus to sexual partners
» Herpes genitalis may be sexually transmitted even if partner is asymptomatic; sexual activity should be avoided if either partner has signs and symptoms of herpes genitalis; use of a condom may help prevent transmission of herpes; however, spermicidal jellies or diaphragms probably will not be adequately protective

**Side/adverse effects**
   Signs of potential side effects, especially phlebitis or inflammation at site of injection, acute renal failure, and encephalopathic changes

## General Dosing Information
Therapy should be initiated as soon as possible following the onset of signs and symptoms of herpes simplex or varicella zoster infections.

Because it may take longer for lesions to heal in immunocompromised patients (an average of 2 weeks of therapy for herpes simplex infections), the duration of therapy may need to be prolonged beyond the recommended number of days until the lesions are crusted over or epithelialized.

**For oral dosage forms only**
Acyclovir capsules, tablets, and oral suspension may be taken with meals since absorption has not been shown to be significantly affected by food.

Intermittent short-term treatment of recurrent herpes genitalis infections may be effective for some patients, especially when treatment is patient-initiated during the prodrome or first sign of lesion formation.

**For parenteral dosage forms only**
Sterile acyclovir sodium should be administered by intravenous infusion only. It should not be administered topically, intramuscularly, orally, subcutaneously, or ophthalmically.

Intravenous infusions of acyclovir should be administered at a constant rate over at least a 1-hour period to avoid renal tubular obstruction. Rapid injection must be avoided since precipitation of acyclovir crystals in the tubules may occur and may result in renal function impairment in up to 10% of patients receiving intravenous acyclovir.

Obese patients should be dosed based on ideal body weight.

Since maximum urinary concentrations of acyclovir are achieved within 2 hours, patients receiving intravenous infusions and high oral doses must be adequately hydrated during this period to prevent precipitation of acyclovir in renal tubules.

The dose of acyclovir should be adjusted so that a dose is repeated after hemodialysis since each 6-hour hemodialysis period results in approximately a 60% reduction in acyclovir plasma concentrations.

**For treatment of adverse effects**
Since there is no specific antidote, treatment of adverse effects should be symptomatic and supportive with possible utilization of the following:
• Adequate hydration to prevent precipitation of acyclovir in the renal tubules.
• Hemodialysis to aid in the removal of acyclovir from the blood, especially in patients with acute renal failure and anuria.

## Oral Dosage Forms
Note: Bracketed uses in the *Dosage Forms* section refer to categories of use and/or indications that are not included in U.S. product labeling.

### ACYCLOVIR CAPSULES

**Usual adult and adolescent dose**
Genital herpes infections—
   Initial therapy: Oral, 200 mg every four hours while awake, five times a day, for ten days.
   Recurrent infections, intermittent therapy: Oral, 200 mg every four hours while awake, five times a day, for five days.
   Recurrent infections, chronic suppressive therapy: Oral, 400 mg twice a day; or 200 mg three to five times a day.
Herpes zoster—
   Oral, 800 mg every four hours while awake, five times a day, for seven to ten days.
Varicella—
   Oral, 20 mg per kg of body weight, up to 800 mg per dose, four times a day for five days. Treatment should be initiated at the earliest sign or symptom of chickenpox.
[Herpes simplex, mucocutaneous (treatment)]—
   Oral, 200 to 400 mg five times a day for ten days in immunocompromised patients.
[Herpes simplex, mucocutaneous (prophylaxis)][1]—
   Oral, 400 mg every twelve hours.
Note: Adults with acute or chronic renal impairment require a reduction in dose.

The recommended dose for initial therapy and intermittent therapy of herpes infections in patients with renal function impairment is:

| Creatinine Clearance (mL/min)/ (mL/sec) | Dose (mg) | Dosing Interval (hr) |
|---|---|---|
| Genital herpes: | | |
| Initial/intermittent therapy | | |
| >10/0.17 | 200 | 4 |
| | | (5 times daily) |
| 0–10/0–0.17 | 200 | 12 |
| Chronic suppressive | | |
| >10/0.17 | 400 | 12 |
| 0–10/0–0.17 | 200 | 12 |
| Herpes zoster (shingles): | | |
| >25/0.42 | 800 | 4 |
| | | (5 times daily) |
| 10–25/0.17–0.42 | 800 | 8 |
| 0–10/0–0.17 | 800 | 12 |

### Usual pediatric dose
Children up to 2 years of age—Dosage has not been established. However, no unusual toxicity or pediatrics-specific problems have been observed in studies done in children using doses of up to 3000 mg per square meter of body surface area per day and 80 mg per kg of body weight per day.

Children 2 to 12 years old—Varicella: Oral, 20 mg per kg of body weight, up to 800 mg per dose, four times a day for five days. Treatment should be initiated at the earliest sign or symptom of chickenpox.

### Strength(s) usually available
U.S.—

200 mg (Rx) [*Zovirax* (lactose)].

Canada—

200 mg (Rx) [*Avirax; Zovirax* (lactose; parabens)].

### Packaging and storage
Store between 15 and 25 °C (59 and 77 °F), in a tight container, unless otherwise specified by manufacturer. Protect from light and moisture.

### Auxiliary labeling
• Continue medicine for full time of treatment.

## ACYCLOVIR ORAL SUSPENSION
### Usual adult and adolescent dose
See *Acyclovir Capsules.*

### Usual pediatric dose
See *Acyclovir Capsules.*

### Strength(s) usually available
U.S.—

200 mg per 5 mL (Rx) [*Zovirax*].

Canada—

200 mg per 5 mL (Rx) [*Avirax; Zovirax*].

### Packaging and storage
Store between 15 and 25 °C (59 and 77 °F), in a tight container, unless otherwise specified by manufacturer. Protect from light.

### Stability
Suspension retains its potency for 24 months from date of manufacture. Does not require reconstitution or refrigeration.

### Auxiliary labeling
• Continue medicine for full time of treatment.
• Shake well.
• Take with water.
• Beyond-use date.

### Note
When dispensing, include a calibrated liquid-measuring device.

## ACYCLOVIR TABLETS
### Usual adult and adolescent dose
See *Acyclovir Capsules.*

### Usual pediatric dose
See *Acyclovir Capsules.*

### Strength(s) usually available
U.S.—

400 mg (Rx) [*Zovirax*].
800 mg (Rx) [*Zovirax*].

Canada—

200 mg (Rx) [*Avirax; Zovirax* (lactose)].
400 mg (Rx) [*Avirax; Zovirax* (lactose)].
800 mg (Rx) [*Avirax; Zovirax* (lactose)].

### Packaging and storage
Store between 15 and 25 °C (59 and 77 °F), in a tight container, unless otherwise specified by manufacturer. Protect from light.

### Auxiliary labeling
• Continue medicine for full time of treatment.

## Parenteral Dosage Forms
Note: Bracketed uses in the *Dosage Forms* section refer to categories of use and/or indications that are not included in U.S. product labeling.

The dosing and strength of the dosage forms available are expressed in terms of acyclovir base.

### STERILE ACYCLOVIR SODIUM
#### Usual adult and adolescent dose
Genital herpes infections, severe, initial—

Intravenous infusion, 5 mg (base) per kg of body weight every eight hours for five days. Administer at a constant rate over at least a one-hour period.

Herpes simplex (HSV-1 and HSV-2) infections, mucocutaneous, in immunocompromised patients—

Intravenous infusion, 5 to 10 mg (base) per kg of body weight every eight hours for seven to ten days. Administer at a constant rate over at least a one-hour period.

Herpes simplex encephalitis[1]—

Intravenous infusion, 10 mg (base) per kg of body weight every eight hours for ten days. Administer at a constant rate over at least a one-hour period.

Varicella zoster in immunocompromised patients—

Intravenous infusion, 10 mg (base) per kg of body weight every eight hours for seven days. Administer at a constant rate over at least a one-hour period.

Note: Adults with acute or chronic renal impairment require a reduction in dose and/or dosing interval as follows:

| Creatinine Clearance (mL/min)/ (mL/sec) | Dose (base) | Dosing Interval (hr) |
|---|---|---|
| >50/0.83 | 100% | 8 |
| 25–50/0.42–0.83 | 100% | 12 |
| 10–25/0.17–0.42 | 100% | 24 |
| 0–10/0–0.17 | 50% | 24 |

#### Usual adult prescribing limits
Up to 30 mg (base) per kg of body weight or 1.5 grams per square meter of body surface daily.

#### Usual pediatric dose
Herpes genitalis infections, severe, initial—

Intravenous infusion, Infants and children up to 12 years of age—250 mg (base) per square meter of body surface every eight hours for five days. Administer at a constant rate over at least a one-hour period.

Children 12 years of age and over—See *Usual adult and adolescent dose.*

Herpes simplex (HSV-1 and HSV-2) infections, mucocutaneous, in immunocompromised patients—

Infants and children up to 12 years of age—Intravenous infusion, 250 mg (base) per square meter of body surface every eight hours for seven days. Administer at a constant rate over at least a one-hour period.

Children 12 years of age and over—See *Usual adult and adolescent dose.*

Herpes simplex encephalitis[1]—

Intravenous infusion, 10 mg (base) per kg of body weight, or 500 mg per square meter, every eight hours for ten days. Administer at a constant rate over at least a one-hour period.

Varicella zoster in immunocompromised children—

Intravenous infusion, 500 mg (base) per square meter every eight hours for seven days. Administer at a constant rate over at least a one-hour period.

[Disseminated HSV in neonates][1]—

Intravenous infusion, 10 mg (base) per kg of body weight every eight hours for ten to fourteen days. Administer at a constant rate over at least a one-hour period.

#### Strength(s) usually available
U.S.—

500 mg (base) (Rx) [*Zovirax*].
1 gram (base) (Rx) [*Zovirax*].

Canada—

500 mg (base) (Rx) [*Zovirax*].
1 gram (base) (Rx) [*Avirax*].

**Packaging and storage**
Prior to reconstitution, store between 15 and 30 °C (59 and 86 °F), unless otherwise specified by manufacturer.

**Preparation of dosage form**
To prepare initial dilution for intravenous infusion, add 10 or 20 mL of sterile water for injection or bacteriostatic water for injection to each 500-mg or 1-gram vial, respectively, to provide a concentration of 50 mg per mL. Do not use bacteriostatic water for injection containing benzyl alcohol. To ensure complete dissolution, shake vial well until solution is clear. The resulting solution should be further diluted with a suitable diluent (standard electrolyte- and dextrose-containing solutions) to at least 100 mL. Final concentrations of 7 mg per mL or less are recommended. Higher concentrations (e.g., 10 mg per mL) may cause phlebitis or inflammation at the injection site upon inadvertent extravasation.

**Stability**
After reconstitution with sterile water for injection, solutions at concentrations of 50 mg per mL retain their potency for 12 hours at controlled room temperature (15 to 25 °C [59 to 77 °F]).

After further dilution with standard electrolyte- and dextrose-containing solutions for intravenous infusion, solutions retain their potency for 24 hours at controlled room temperature (15 to 25 °C [59 to 77 °F]). Refrigeration of reconstituted solutions may result in the formation of a precipitate, which will redissolve when warmed to room temperature.

**Incompatibilities**
Sterile acyclovir sodium is incompatible with biological or colloidal solutions (e.g., blood products, protein-containing solutions).
Parabens are incompatible with sterile acyclovir sodium and may cause precipitation.

---

[1]Not included in Canadian product labeling.

## Selected Bibliography

Wagstaff AJ, Faulds D, Goa KL. Aciclovir. A reappraisal of its antiviral activity, pharmacokinetic properties, and therapeutic efficacy. Drugs 1994; 47 (1): 153-205.
Whitley RJ, Gnann JW. Acyclovir: a decade later. N Engl J Med 1992; 327 (11): 782-9.

---

Revised: 06/22/94

---

# ACYCLOVIR   Topical

INN: Aciclovir
VA CLASSIFICATION (Primary): DE103
A commonly used name is acycloguanosine.
Note: For a listing of dosage forms and brand names by country availability, see *Dosage Forms* section(s). For a listing of brand names for the articles in this monograph, refer to the General Index.

## Category

Antiviral (topical).

## Indications

Note: Bracketed information in the *Indications* section refers to uses that are not included in U.S. product labeling.

**Accepted**
Herpes simplex (treatment)—Topical acyclovir is indicated in the treatment of limited non–life-threatening initial and recurrent mucocutaneous herpes simplex (HSV-1 and HSV-2) infections in immunocompromised patients; however, systemic acyclovir is more effective and may be preferred.

[Herpes zoster (treatment adjunct)]—Topical acyclovir is used as adjunctive therapy to improve cutaneous healing of localized herpes zoster in immunosuppressed persons being treated systemically with other treatment regimens for herpes zoster.

Resistance to acyclovir, although currently of minor clinical significance, has been reported to develop with prolonged treatment in immunocompromised patients. Resistance does not appear to be significant in patients with normal immune function.

**Unaccepted**
Herpes genitalis (treatment)—Although topical acyclovir is FDA approved for the treatment of *initial* herpes genitalis infections caused by herpes simplex virus (HSV), the Centers for Disease Control (CDC) and USP medical experts do not recommend it for use, because oral acyclovir is considerably more effective.

Topical acyclovir is not effective in the treatment of *recurrent* herpes genitalis or herpes febrilis (labialis) infections in nonimmunocompromised patients, although topical acyclovir may cause some reduction in the duration of viral shedding. Also, there is no evidence that topical acyclovir will prevent the transmission of herpes infection to others or that it will prevent recurrent infections in the absence of signs and symptoms of infection.

## Pharmacology/Pharmacokinetics

**Physicochemical characteristics**
Molecular weight—225.21.

**Mechanism of action/Effect**
Acyclovir is converted to acyclovir monophosphate, a nucleotide, by herpes simplex virus (HSV)–coded thymidine kinase. Acyclovir monophosphate is converted to the diphosphate by cellular guanylate kinase and to the triphosphate by a number of cellular enzymes. Acyclovir triphosphate interferes with HSV DNA polymerase and inhibits viral DNA replication. The triphosphate can be incorporated into growing chains of DNA by viral DNA polymerase, resulting in termination of the DNA chain. Since acyclovir is preferentially taken up and selectively converted to the active triphosphate form by HSV-infected cells, it is much less toxic to normal uninfected cells.

**Absorption**
Intact skin—Minimal; acyclovir not detected in blood or urine.
Diseased skin (herpes zoster)—Moderate; serum concentrations up to 0.28 mcg per mL have been reported in patients with normal renal function and up to 0.78 mcg per mL in patients with impaired renal function.

**Elimination**
Renal—Up to approximately 9% of the total daily dose may be excreted in the urine.

## Precautions to Consider

**Carcinogenicity**
Lifetime bioassays in rats and mice given daily doses of 50, 150, and 450 mg per kg of body weight (mg/kg) by gavage have not shown any evidence of carcinogenicity. However, *in vitro* cell transformation assays have given conflicting results, being positive at the highest dose used in one system. The resulting morphologically transformed cells induced tumors when inoculated into immunosuppressed, syngeneic, weanling mice, although results were negative in another animal system.

**Tumorigenicity**
Studies in rats and mice have not shown any statistically significant difference between the incidence of benign tumors produced in drug-treated animals and that produced in control animals.

**Mutagenicity**
No chromosomal damage was noted at maximum tolerated parenteral doses (100 mg/kg) in rats or Chinese hamsters. Higher doses (500 and 1000 mg/kg) were clastogenic in Chinese hamsters. No problems were reported in dominant lethal studies in mice. Also, there was no evidence of mutagenicity in 9 out of 11 microbial and mammalian cell assays. In 2 of the mammalian cell assays, a positive response for mutagenicity and chromosomal damage was noted, but only at concentrations at least 1000 times the usual plasma concentrations in humans following topical application.

**Pregnancy/Reproduction**
Fertility—Studies in mice given oral doses of up to 450 mg/kg per day have not shown that acyclovir impairs fertility or reproduction. Studies in female rabbits given acyclovir subcutaneously subsequent to mating have shown a significant decrease in implantation efficiency, but no decrease in litter size at doses of 50 mg/kg per day.

Pregnancy—Adequate and well-controlled studies in humans have not been done.
Studies done in rats and rabbits given subcutaneous doses of up to 50 mg/kg daily and in mice given oral doses of up to 450 mg/kg daily have not shown that acyclovir causes adverse effects on the fetus.

FDA Pregnancy Category C.

**Breast-feeding**

It is not known whether topical acyclovir is distributed into breast milk. However, acyclovir is unlikely to be distributed into breast milk in significant amounts following topical administration, since the total daily dose is small, even though absorption through diseased skin is moderate.

**Pediatrics**

Appropriate studies on the relationship of age to the effects of topical acyclovir have not been performed in the pediatric population. However, limited data are available about the use of oral acyclovir in the pediatric population, and no unusual toxicity or pediatrics-specific problems have been observed in studies done in children using doses of up to 3000 mg per square meter of body surface per day and 80 mg/kg per day.

**Geriatrics**

Appropriate studies on the relationship of age to the effects of topical acyclovir have not been performed in the geriatric population. However, no geriatrics-specific problems have been documented to date.

**Medical considerations/Contraindications**

The medical considerations/contraindications included here have been selected on the basis of their potential clinical significance (reasons given in parentheses where appropriate)—not necessarily inclusive (» = major clinical significance).

*Risk-benefit should be considered when the following medical problem exists:*

Sensitivity to topical acyclovir

**Patient monitoring**

The following may be especially important in patient monitoring (other tests may be warranted in some patients, depending on condition; » = major clinical significance):

Papanicolaou (Pap) test

(although a clear association has not been shown to date, patients with genital herpes may be at increased risk of developing cervical cancer; Pap tests should be done at least once a year to detect early cervical changes)

## Side/Adverse Effects

The following side/adverse effects have been selected on the basis of their potential clinical significance (possible signs and symptoms in parentheses where appropriate)—not necessarily inclusive:

**Those indicating need for medical attention only if they continue or are bothersome**

Incidence more frequent—Approximately 28%
   *Mild pain, burning, or stinging*

Incidence less frequent—Approximately 4%
   *Pruritus* (itching)

Incidence rare—Approximately 0.3%
   *Skin rash*

## Patient Consultation

As an aid to patient consultation, refer to *Advice for the Patient, Acyclovir (Topical).*

In providing consultation, consider emphasizing the following selected information (» = major clinical significance):

**Proper use of this medication**

Reading patient information about herpes simplex infections
» Avoiding contact with eyes
» Using medication as soon as possible after symptoms of herpes begin to appear
» Proper administration technique

*To use*

Using a finger cot or rubber glove to prevent autoinoculation

Applying sufficient medication to cover affected areas; a 1.25-cm strip of ointment per 25 cm² of affected skin is usually sufficient
» Compliance with full course of therapy; not using more often or longer than prescribed

» Proper dosing

Missed dose: Applying as soon as possible; not applying if almost time for next dose
» Proper storage

**Precautions while using this medication**

» Women with herpes genitalis may be more likely to develop cervical cancer; annual or more frequent Pap tests may be required

Checking with physician if no improvement within 1 week

Keeping affected areas as clean and dry as possible; wearing loose-fitting clothing to avoid irritation of lesions
» Herpes genitalis may be sexually transmitted, even if sexual partner is asymptomatic; avoiding sexual activity if either partner has symptoms of herpes genitalis; use of condom may help prevent transmission of herpes; however, topical acyclovir or the use of spermicidal jellies or diaphragms will not prevent transmission of herpes to others

## General Dosing Information

Use of topical antivirals may lead to skin sensitization, resulting in hypersensitivity reactions with subsequent topical or systemic use of the medication.

Topical acyclovir is for cutaneous use only; it should not be used in the eyes.

Therapy should be initiated as soon as possible following the onset of signs and symptoms of herpes infection.

A 1.25-cm (½-inch) strip of ointment should be applied per 25 cm² (4 inches²) of affected skin. A finger cot or rubber glove should be used to prevent autoinoculation of other body sites.

The recommended dose, frequency of application, and length of treatment should not be exceeded.

## Topical Dosage Forms

### ACYCLOVIR OINTMENT

**Usual adult and adolescent dose**

Antiviral—

Topical, to the skin and mucous membranes, every three hours, six times a day, for seven days. Apply a sufficient quantity to cover all lesions adequately.

**Usual pediatric dose**

See *Usual adult and adolescent dose.*

**Strength(s) usually available**

U.S.—

5% (Rx) [*Zovirax*].

Canada—

5% (Rx) [*Zovirax*].

**Packaging and storage**

Store between 15 and 25 °C (59 and 78 °F) in a dry place, unless otherwise specified by manufacturer.

**Auxiliary labeling**
• For external use only.
• Do not use in the eye.
• Continue medicine for full time of treatment.

**Note**

Acyclovir ointment has a polyethylene glycol base.

Although herpes virus may theoretically persist for up to 24 hours on any fomite, it is unlikely that herpes infections can be transmitted via contaminated ointment tubes.

## Selected Bibliography

Pariser DM. Cutaneous viral infections: herpes simplex and varicella-zoster. Prim Care 1989 Sep;16 (3): 577-89.

Revised: 01/15/92
Interim revision: 05/10/94

# ADENOSINE Systemic†

VA CLASSIFICATION (Primary/Secondary): CV300/DX900

Note: For a listing of dosage forms and brand names by country availability, see *Dosage Forms* section(s). For a listing of brand names for the articles in this monograph, refer to the General Index.

†Not commercially available in Canada.

## Category

Antiarrhythmic; diagnostic aid adjunct (ischemic heart disease).

## Indications

Note: Bracketed information in the *Indications* section refers to uses that are not included in U.S. product labeling.

### Accepted

Tachycardia, supraventricular, paroxysmal (treatment)—Adenosine is indicated for conversion to sinus rhythm of paroxysmal supraventricular tachycardia, including those due to atrioventricular (AV) node reentry and associated with accessory bypass tracts (Wolff-Parkinson-White syndrome), after appropriate vagal maneuvers (e.g., Valsalva maneuver) have been attempted.

[Myocardial perfusion imaging, radionuclide (adjunct)][1]; or

[Stress echocardiography (adjunct)][1]—Adenosine is used to induce coronary artery vasodilation in conjunction with myocardial perfusion imaging or two-dimensional echocardiography for the detection of perfusion defects or regional contraction abnormalities associated with coronary artery disease.

[1]Not included in Canadian product labeling.

## Pharmacology/Pharmacokinetics

### Mechanism of action/Effect

Antiarrhythmic—Slows impulse formation in the sinoatrial (SA) node, slows conduction time through the atrioventricular (AV) node, and can interrupt reentry pathways through the AV node. Adenosine depresses left ventricular function, but because of its short half-life, the effect is transient, allowing use in patients with existing poor left ventricular function.

Diagnostic aid—The precise mechanism of coronary vasodilation is not completely understood. However, it is speculated that adenosine may have a direct effect on smooth muscle receptors and may influence cellular calcium dynamics. Coronary vasodilation by adenosine contributes to the creation of heterogeneity of myocardial blood flow. The difference in coronary reserve in the vascular bed distal to a critical coronary stenosis versus that supplied by normal coronary arteries accounts for a significantly greater, 3- to 5-fold, increase in regional myocardial blood flow to normal epicardial vessels.

### Other actions/effects

Administration of doses larger than 12 mg by intravenous infusion decreases blood pressure by reducing peripheral vascular resistance. Physiologically, naturally occurring adenosine functions as an intermediate metabolite in a number of processes including regulation of coronary and systemic vascular tone, platelet function, lipolysis in fat cells, and intracardiac conduction.

### Biotransformation

Very rapid, by circulating enzymes in erythrocytes and vascular endothelial cells, by deamination, primarily to inactive inosine (further degraded to hypoxanthine and then to uric acid) and by phosphorylation to adenosine monophosphate (AMP).

### Half-life

Less than 10 seconds.

### Onset of action

Immediate.

### Elimination

Principal elimination routes are cellular uptake and metabolism. Metabolites excreted renally. The predominant final excretory metabolite is uric acid.

## Precautions to Consider

### Carcinogenicity

Studies have not been done.

### Mutagenicity

Mutagenicity tests in the Salmonella/mammalian microsome assay (Ames test) were negative. However, adenosine causes chromosomal alterations.

### Pregnancy/Reproduction

Fertility—In rats and mice, intraperitoneal administration of 50, 100, and 150 mg per kg of body weight (mg/kg) per day for 5 days caused decreased spermatogenesis and increased numbers of abnormal sperm.

Pregnancy—Studies have not been done in humans. Because adenosine occurs naturally in the body, problems are not expected. Scant reports of adenosine use in pregnant women have not revealed fetal or maternal sequelae.

Studies have not been done in animals.

FDA Pregnancy Category C.

### Breast-feeding

Because of rapid removal from circulation, adenosine is not expected to be distributed into breast milk.

### Pediatrics

Studies performed to date on adenosine's use as an antiarrhythmic have not demonstrated pediatrics-specific problems that would limit the usefulness of this medication in the pediatric population.

### Geriatrics

Appropriate studies on the relationship of age to the effects of adenosine have not been performed in the geriatric population. However, geriatrics-specific problems that would limit the usefulness of this medication in the elderly are not expected.

### Drug interactions and/or related problems

The following drug interactions and/or related problems have been selected on the basis of their potential clinical significance (possible mechanism in parentheses where appropriate)—not necessarily inclusive (» = major clinical significance):

Note: Combinations containing any of the following medications, depending on the amount present, may also interact with this medication.

Carbamazepine
(may increase heart block caused by adenosine)

Dipyridamole
(potentiates the effects of adenosine by inhibiting cellular uptake; dosage reduction is recommended)

Xanthines, especially caffeine and theophylline
(antagonize the effects of adenosine; larger doses of adenosine may be required or alternative therapy should be used)

(concurrent use with xanthines may invalidate test when adenosine is used as a diagnostic aid)

### Medical considerations/Contraindications

The medical considerations/contraindications included here have been selected on the basis of their potential clinical significance (reasons given in parentheses where appropriate)—not necessarily inclusive (» = major clinical significance).

*Except under special circumstances, this medication should not be used when the following medical problem exists:*

» Atrioventricular (AV) block, pre-existing second or third degree without pacemaker
(risk of complete heart block)

*Risk-benefit should be considered when the following medical problems exist:*

Asthma
(although problems have not been reported with adenosine injection, inhaled adenosine has been reported to cause bronchoconstriction in asthmatic patients but not in normal individuals)

Sensitivity to adenosine

» Sick sinus syndrome
(sinus node recovery time prolonged; sinus bradycardia, sinus pause, or sinus arrest may occur)

### Patient monitoring

The following may be especially important in patient monitoring (other tests may be warranted in some patients, depending on condition; » = major clinical significance):

» Blood pressure and

» Heart rate
(determinations recommended every 15 to 30 seconds for several minutes)

» Electrocardiogram (ECG)
(recommended to confirm efficacy of adenosine)

## Side/Adverse Effects

Note: Side/adverse effects are usually transient, generally lasting less than one minute. However, loss of consciousness and prolonged hypotension have been reported rarely.

The following side/adverse effects have been selected on the basis of their potential clinical significance (possible signs and symptoms in parentheses where appropriate)—not necessarily inclusive:

**Those indicating need for medical attention**
Incidence more frequent
*Arrhythmias, new, including premature ventricular contractions, atrial premature contractions, sinus bradycardia, sinus tachycardia, and skipped beats; chest, jaw, throat, or arm pain; dyspnea* (shortness of breath)

Note: *New arrhythmias* usually last only a few seconds.

Incidence rare
*Heart block, first-, second-, or third-degree*

Note: *Heart block* is usually of short duration and may occur more frequently in patients who receive a rapid intravenous dose of adenosine. Episodes of transient asystole have been reported.

**Those indicating need for medical attention only if they continue or are bothersome**
Incidence more frequent
*Flushing of face; headache*
Incidence less frequent
*Cough; dizziness or lightheadedness; nausea; numbness or tingling in arms*

## General Dosing Information

If high-level heart block occurs after one dose of adenosine, it is recommended that additional doses not be given. The effect usually resolves quickly because of adenosine's short duration of action.

Rapid intravenous administration of adenosine is recommended to achieve the desired negative chronotropic and dromotropic activity. Slow administration may result in an increase in heart rate in response to vasodilation.

### For treatment of adverse effects and/or overdose

Because of adenosine's extremely short duration of action, adverse effects are usually self-limiting. Treatment of prolonged adverse effects should be individualized. Xanthines (e.g., caffeine, theophylline) are competitive antagonists of adenosine.

## Parenteral Dosage Forms

Note: Bracketed uses in the *Dosage Forms* section refer to categories of use and/or indications that are not included in U.S. product labeling.

### ADENOSINE INJECTION

**Usual adult dose**
Antiarrhythmic—
Intravenous, rapid (over one to two seconds), 6 mg. If the first dose is not effective within one to two minutes, a rapid intravenous dose of 12 mg may be given, and repeated if necessary.

[Diagnostic aid adjunct][1]—
Intravenous, 140 mcg (0.14 mg) per kg of body weight per minute given for six minutes.

Note: In patients at increased risk for side/adverse effects, the dose may be titrated from 50 mcg (0.05 mg) per kg of body weight per minute up to 140 mcg (0.14 mg) per kg of body weight per minute at one-minute intervals. If side/adverse effects are severe, the infusion rate may be reduced to a more tolerable level. Doses of 75 and 100 mcg (0.075 and 0.1 mg) per kg of body weight per minute can adequately increase coronary blood flow.

Thallium injection should be given into a separate vein and is usually injected at the three- or four-minute mark of the adenosine infusion.

Note: To ensure that adenosine injection reaches the systemic circulation, it should be given directly into a vein or, if given into an intravenous line, be given as proximally as possible and followed by a rapid saline flush.

**Usual adult prescribing limits**
Up to 12 mg per dose.

**Usual pediatric dose**
Antiarrhythmic—
Intravenous, 50 mcg (0.05 mg) per kg of body weight. Dose may be increased in increments of 50 mcg (0.05 mg) per kg of body weight given every two minutes up to a maximum dose of 250 mcg (0.25 mg) per kg of body weight.

**Strength(s) usually available**
U.S.—
3 mg per mL (Rx) [*Adenocard*].
Canada—
Not commercially available.

**Packaging and storage**
Store between 15 and 30 °C (59 and 86 °F), unless otherwise specified by manufacturer. Do not refrigerate. Protect from freezing.

**Stability**
Because adenosine injection contains no preservatives, any unused portion should be discarded.
Crystallization may occur if adenosine injection is refrigerated. If that occurs, the crystals may be dissolved by warming the injection to room temperature. The solution must be clear before use.

---

[1]Not included in Canadian product labeling.

## Selected Bibliography

Parker RB, McCollam PL. Adenosine in the episodic treatment of paroxysmal supraventricular tachycardia. Clin Pharm 1990 Apr; 9: 261-71.

Gupta NC, Esterbrooks DJ, Hilleman DE, Mohiuddin SM. Comparison of adenosine and exercise thallium-201 single-photon emission computed tomography (SPECT) myocardial perfusion imaging. J Am Coll Cardiol 1992; 19: 248-57.

Rankin AC, Brooks R, Ruskin JN. Adenosine and the treatment of supraventricular tachycardia. Am J Med 1992; 92: 655-64.

Revised: 07/12/94

---

# ALBENDAZOLE Systemic*†

VA CLASSIFICATION (Primary): AP200
Note: For a listing of dosage forms and brand names by country availability, see *Dosage Forms* section(s). For a listing of brand names for the articles in this monograph, refer to the General Index.

---

*Not commercially available in the U.S.
†Not commercially available in Canada.

---

## Category
Anthelmintic (systemic).

## Indications

Note: Because albendazole is not commercially available in the U.S. or Canada, the bracketed information and the use of the superscript 1

in this monograph reflect the lack of labeled (approved) indications for this medication in these countries.

### General considerations

Albendazole is a broad-spectrum anthelmintic. It is structurally related to mebendazole and has similar anthelmintic activity against many helminths.

### Accepted

[Ascariasis (treatment)][1]—Albendazole is used in the treatment of ascariasis caused by *Ascaris lumbricoides* (roundworm).

[Capillariasis (treatment)][1]—Albendazole is used as a secondary agent in the treatment of capillariasis caused by *Capillaria philippinensis*. Mebendazole is preferred for the treatment of capillariasis.

[Enterobiasis (treatment)][1]—Albendazole is used in the treatment of enterobiasis (oxyuriasis) caused by *Enterobius vermicularis* (pinworm).

[Hookworm infections (treatment)][1]—Albendazole is used in the treatment of hookworm infections, such as ancylostomiasis caused by *Ancylostoma duodenale* (common hookworm; Old World hookworm) and necatoriasis caused by *Necatur americanus* (American hookworm; New World hookworm).

[Hydatid disease (treatment)][1]—Albendazole is used in the treatment of hydatid disease (echinococcosis) caused by *Echinococcus granulosus* or *E. multilocularis*. It is also used as an adjunct to surgery of hydatid cysts, either preoperatively or postoperatively, to reduce the risk of recurrence due to operative spillage.

[Neurocysticercosis (treatment)][1]—Albendazole is used in the treatment of neurocysticercosis caused by the larval form of *Taenia solium* (pork tapeworm). It is the only drug used in the treatment of ocular neurocysticercosis.

[Strongyloidiasis (treatment)][1]—Albendazole is used in the treatment of strongyloidiasis caused by *Strongyloides stercoralis*.

[Taeniasis (treatment)][1]—Albendazole is used as an alternative treatment for taeniasis caused by *Taenia solium* (pork tapeworm) or *T. saginata* (beef tapeworm). Niclosamide or praziquantel is preferred for the treatment of taeniasis. Although albendazole is known to offer little therapeutic advantage in the treatment of taeniasis, it is generally preferred in developing countries because it is cheaper and has a broader spectrum of anthelmintic activity than niclosamide or praziquantel.

[Trichostrongyliasis (treatment)][1]—Albendazole is used as a secondary agent in the treatment of trichostrongyliasis caused by *Trichostrongylus* species. Pyrantel pamoate is preferred for the treatment of trichostrongyliasis.

[Trichuriasis (treatment)][1]—Albendazole is used in the treatment of trichuriasis caused by *Trichuris trichiura* (whipworm).

### Acceptance not established

Preliminary studies suggest albendazole may be used as an alternative agent to treat *giardiasis* caused by *Giardia* species. However, data are limited and results of recent clinical evaluations have shown variable efficacy of albendazole for this indication. Metronidazole or quinacrine is generally preferred in the treatment of giardiasis.

Albendazole is used as an experimental therapeutic agent in *trichinosis* caused by *Trichinella spiralis*. Currently, there are insufficient data to establish efficacy of albendazole for this indication. Mebendazole is preferred for the treatment of trichinosis.

---

[1]Not included in Canadian product labeling.

## Pharmacology/Pharmacokinetics

### Physicochemical characteristics
Molecular weight—265.34.

### Mechanism of action/Effect
Vermicidal; albendazole causes degenerative alterations in the tegument and intestinal cells of the worm by binding to the colchicine-sensitive site of tubulin, thus inhibiting its polymerization or assembly into microtubules. The loss of the cytoplasmic microtubules leads to impaired uptake of glucose by the larval and adult stages of the susceptible parasites, and depletes their glycogen stores. Degenerative changes in the endoplasmic reticulum, the mitochondria of the germinal layer, and the subsequent release of lysosomes result in decreased production of adenosine triphosphate (ATP), which is the energy required for the survival of the helminth. Due to diminished energy production, the parasite is immobilized and eventually dies.

Albendazole also has been shown to inhibit the enzyme fumarate reductase, which is helmint-specific. This action may be considered secondary to the effect on the microtubules due to the decreased absorption of glucose. This action occurs in the presence of reduced amounts of nicotinamide-adenine dinucleotide in reduced form (NADH), which is a coenzyme involved in many cellular oxidation-reduction reactions.

Albendazole has larvicidal effects in necatoriasis and ovicidal effects in ascariasis, ancylostomiasis, and trichuriasis.

### Absorption
Poorly and erratically absorbed from the gastrointestinal tract. Absorption of albendazole is greatly increased if the medication is taken with food containing relatively high concentrations of fat.

### Distribution
Distributed into bile, cerebrospinal fluid (CSF), fluid in hydatid cysts, and serum.

### Protein binding
High (70%).

### Biotransformation
Hepatic; rapidly and extensively metabolized mainly to the active metabolite, albendazole sulfoxide, which appears in the systemic circulation at detectable concentrations. Albendazole is also metabolized to the 6-hydroxy sulfoxide and sulfone metabolites, but not in sufficient quantities to be detected consistently in the plasma.

### Half-life
Single dose—
    400 mg: Approximately 8 to 9 hours.
    15 mg/kg: Approximately 10 to 15 hours.

### Time to peak concentration
Single dose—
    400 mg: Approximately 2 to 3 hours.
    15 mg/kg: Approximately 4 hours.

### Peak serum concentration
Single dose—
    400 mg: Approximately 0.20 to 0.94 mcg/mL.
    15 mg/kg: Approximately 0.45 to 2.96 mcg/mL.

### Elimination
Renal—Approximately 0.1 to 0.9% is excreted in the urine as albendazole sulfoxide during the first 24 hours. Other metabolites also are renally excreted.
Fecal—A small amount is found in the feces.

## Precautions to Consider

### Carcinogenicity/Mutagenicity
Albendazole has been tested in different species of animals and has not been found to be carcinogenic or mutagenic.

### Pregnancy/Reproduction
Fertility—Albendazole has not been shown to cause adverse effects on fertility.

Pregnancy—Adequate and well-controlled studies in humans have not been done. However, albendazole is not recommended for use in pregnant women because of its teratogenic effects in animals. For women of childbearing age (15 to 40 years), it is recommended that albendazole be administered within 7 days after the start of normal menstruation. Following a negative pregnancy test, contraceptive measures must be used for the duration of treatment and for one month after cessation of treatment.

Albendazole was embryotoxic and teratogenic in rats and rabbits given an oral dose of 30 mg per kg of body weight per day for 10 and 13 days, respectively.

### Breast-feeding
It is not known whether albendazole is distributed into breast milk. However, problems in humans have not been documented.

### Pediatrics
Appropriate studies on the relationship of age to the effects of albendazole have not been performed in the pediatric population. However, no pediatrics-specific problems have been documented to date.

### Geriatrics
Appropriate studies on the relationship of age to the effects of albendazole have not been performed in the geriatric population. However, no geriatrics-specific problems have been documented to date.

### Laboratory value alterations
The following have been selected on the basis of their potential clinical significance (possible effect in parentheses where appropriate)—not necessarily inclusive (» = major clinical significance):

With physiology/laboratory test values
»  Alanine aminotransferase (ALT [SGPT]), serum and
»  Aspartate aminotransferase (AST [SGOT]), serum
    (values may be transiently elevated)

»  Leukocytes (neutrophils [WBC])
    (concentration may be transiently decreased)

### Medical considerations/Contraindications
The medical considerations/contraindications included here have been selected on the basis of their potential clinical significance (reasons given in parentheses where appropriate)—not necessarily inclusive (» = major clinical significance).

*Risk-benefit should be considered when the following medical problems exist:*

»  Hepatic function impairment, such as in hepatic cirrhosis (albendazole is extensively metabolized in the liver; intrahepatic hemodynamics caused by a disordered liver architecture as in hepatic cirrhosis may impair the rate of hepatic clearance, thereby resulting in albendazole accumulation and an increased incidence of side effects)

    Hypersensitivity to albendazole

**Patient monitoring**

The following may be especially important in patient monitoring (other tests may be warranted in some patients, depending on condition; » = major clinical significance):

*For ascariasis, hookworm infections, and trichuriasis*
» Stool examinations

(may be required prior to treatment to detect the presence of eggs, and approximately 1 to 3 weeks following treatment with albendazole to determine efficacy of medication or establish proof of cure)

*For enterobiasis*
» Perianal examinations

(cellophane tape swabbing of the perianal area to detect the presence of eggs may be required prior to treatment to confirm the diagnosis of pinworms, and starting 1 week following treatment with albendazole, especially in patients with persisting symptoms; swabbing should be done every morning after getting out of bed and prior to defecation and bathing for at least 3 days to determine efficacy of medication or establish proof of cure; perianal examinations also may be required to detect the presence of adult worms in the perianal area; perianal swabbings should be negative for 7 consecutive days for the patient to be considered cured)

*For strongyloidiasis*
» Stool examinations

(routine stool examinations and special concentration examinations, preferably the Baermann technique [which is especially useful when there is a high index of suspicion for strongyloidiasis and when routine stool examinations are negative for the organism], may be required prior to treatment to detect the presence of larvae, and repeated at intervals of 3 months along with clinical assessment of the patient, beginning at 6 weeks after completion of treatment with albendazole, to determine efficacy of the medication or establish proof of cure; however, determination of cure may be difficult since the parasite is not easily eradicated and therefore, retreatment may be necessary)

*For taeniasis*
» Cellophane tape swabbing or
» Stool examinations

(may be required prior to treatment to detect the presence of eggs or proglottids, and approximately 3 and 6 months following treatment to determine efficacy of medication or establish proof of cure)

*For patients on long-term therapy*
» Complete blood counts (CBCs) and
» Liver function tests

(since albendazole may cause a reduction in total white cell counts and an elevation in hepatic enzymes with prolonged use, it is recommended that blood counts and liver function tests be carried out prior to treatment and every 2 weeks during treatment with albendazole; retreatment should not be initiated if significant depression in total white cell counts or elevation in liver enzymes persists)

## Side/Adverse Effects

The following side/adverse effects have been selected on the basis of their potential clinical significance (possible signs and symptoms in parentheses where appropriate)—not necessarily inclusive:

**Those indicating need for medical attention**
Incidence rare
*Hypersensitivity* (fever; skin rash or itching); *neutropenia* (sore throat and fever; unusual tiredness and weakness)—with high doses, reversible

**Those indicating need for medical attention only if they continue or are bothersome**
Incidence less frequent
*CNS effects* (dizziness; headache); *gastrointestinal disturbances* (abdominal pain; diarrhea; nausea; vomiting)
Incidence rare
*Alopecia* (thinning of hair or moderate hair loss)—reversible

## Overdose

For more information on the management of overdose or unintentional ingestion, **contact a Poison Control Center** (see *Poison Control Center Listing*).

**Treatment of overdose**
Since no specific antidote is known, recommended treatment of albendazole overdose consists of the following:
To decrease absorption—Gastric lavage may be undertaken within the first 2 to 3 hours after ingestion.

Symptomatic treatment may be given.
Supportive measures such as maintaining an open airway, respiration, and circulation may be instituted. Patients in whom intentional overdose is confirmed or suspected should be referred for psychiatric consultation.

## Patient Consultation

As an aid to patient consultation, refer to *Advice for the Patient, Albendazole (Systemic)*.

In providing consultation, consider emphasizing the following selected information (» = major clinical significance):

**Before using this medication**
» Conditions affecting use, especially:
Hypersensitivity to albendazole
Pregnancy—Not recommended for use in pregnancy because albendazole has been found to be teratogenic in animals; for women of childbearing age (15 to 40 years), taking the medication within 7 days after the start of normal menstruation; after a negative pregnancy test, using contraceptive measures during treatment and for one month after cessation of treatment
Other medical problems, especially hepatic function impairment

**Proper use of this medication**
No specific procedures such as fasting or purging or other measures are required before, during, or immediately after treatment with albendazole
» Taking with food containing fat to increase absorption
Proper administration for tablet dosage form—Chewing tablets, swallowing whole, or crushing tablets and mixing with food
» Compliance with full course of therapy; treatment program may be repeated in 2 to 3 weeks for heavy infection
» Proper dosing
Missed dose: Taking as soon as possible; not taking if almost time for next dose; not doubling doses
» Proper storage
*For pinworms*
Treating all household members simultaneously

**Precautions while using this medication**
Regular visits to physician to check progress
Checking with physician if no improvement after the full course of treatment or if symptoms persist
For women of childbearing age, using contraception since albendazole has been found to be embryotoxic and teratogenic in animals
*For hookworms*
For anemic patients, importance of taking supplementary iron salts daily during and after treatment, for at least 3 to 6 months, even after the hemoglobin concentration has regained the threshold of 12 grams per mL
*For pinworms*
Wearing pajamas and underwear to sleep; taking daily baths; washing (not shaking) all bedding and nightclothes after treatment to prevent reinfection; treating all household members simultaneously; repeating treatment in 3 weeks

**Side/adverse effects**
Signs of potential side effects, especially hypersensitivity and neutropenia

## General Dosing Information

Patients who are heavily infected with helminths may require a second treatment.

If using albendazole to treat *giardiasis*, asymptomatic patients may be treated to prevent spread of infection to others. Parasitologic and clinical relapse of *giardiasis* may occur after the completion of therapy; long-term follow-up with the physician may be necessary.

If using albendazole to treat *trichinosis*, concurrent use of corticosteroids may be required to alleviate the allergic and inflammatory symptoms.

**For enterobiasis**
Because of the high probability of transfer of pinworms, it is usually recommended that all members of the household be treated simultaneously.

**For neurocysticercosis**
Corticosteroids have been shown to increase the plasma levels of albendazole. Concurrent use may be required to relieve the exacerbated symptoms due to the inflammatory response around the dying parasites. However, use of corticosteroids with albendazole in neurocysticercosis has not been adequately studied and remains controversial.

# Oral Dosage Forms

Note: Because albendazole is not commercially available in the U.S. or Canada, the bracketed uses and the use of the superscript 1 in this monograph reflect the lack of labeled (approved) indications for this medication in these countries.

## ALBENDAZOLE ORAL SUSPENSION

### Usual adult and adolescent dose

[Ascariasis][1] or
[Enterobiasis][1] or
[Hookworm infections][1] or
[Trichuriasis][1]—
    Oral, 400 mg as a single dose for one day. Treatment may be repeated in three weeks.
[Capillariasis][1]—
    Oral, 200 mg two times a day for ten days.
[Hydatid disease][1]—
    Oral, 800 mg per day for twenty-eight days. Treatment may be repeated as necessary. Up to two or three cycles of albendazole treatment may be given. For inoperable hydatid cysts, up to five cycles may be given.
    Note: In hydatid disease, the dose of albendazole for patients under 60 kg of body weight is 12 mg per kg of body weight per day.
[Neurocysticercosis][1]—
    Oral, 15 mg per kg of body weight per day for thirty days. Treatment may be repeated as necessary.
[Strongyloidiasis][1] or
[Taeniasis][1]—
    Oral, 400 mg as a single dose per day for three days. Treatment may be repeated in three weeks.
[Trichostrongyliasis][1]—
    Oral, 400 mg as a single dose.
    Note: In the treatment of *giardiasis,* an oral dose of 400 mg per day for five days has been used.

### Usual pediatric dose

[Ascariasis][1] or
[Enterobiasis][1] or
[Hookworm infections][1] or
[Trichuriasis][1]—
    Children up to 2 years of age: Oral, 200 mg as a single dose for one day. Treatment may be repeated in three weeks.
    Children 2 years of age and over: See *Usual adult and adolescent dose.*
[Capillariasis][1] or
[Neurocysticercosis][1] or
[Trichostrongyliasis][1]—
    See *Usual adult and adolescent dose.*
[Hydatid disease][1]—
    Children up to 6 years of age: Dosage has not been established.
    Children 6 years of age and over: Oral, 10 to 15 mg per kg of body weight per day for twenty-eight days. Treatment may be repeated as necessary.
[Strongyloidiasis][1] or
[Taeniasis][1]—
    Children up to 2 years of age: Oral, 200 mg as a single dose per day for three consecutive days. Treatment may be repeated in three weeks.
    Children 2 years of age and over: See *Usual adult and adolescent dose.*
    Note: In the treatment of *giardiasis,* see *Usual adult and adolescent dose.*

### Strength(s) usually available

U.S.—
    Not commercially available.
    Note: Although albendazole is not commercially available in the U.S., the manufacturer makes it available for compassionate use only (tel. no.: 215-751-4000).
Canada—
    Not commercially available.
United Kingdom—
    100 mg per 5 mL (Rx) [*Zentel*].

### Packaging and storage

Store below 40 °C (104 °F), preferably between 15 and 30 °C (59 and 86 °F), unless otherwise specified by manufacturer. Protect from freezing and direct sunlight.

### Auxiliary labeling

- Shake well.
- Take with meals.
- Continue medication for full time of treatment.

## ALBENDAZOLE TABLETS

### Usual adult and adolescent dose

[Ascariasis][1] or
[Capillariasis][1] or
[Enterobiasis][1] or
[Hookworm infections][1] or
[Hydatid disease][1] or
[Neurocysticercosis][1] or
[Strongyloidiasis][1] or
[Taeniasis][1] or
[Trichostrongyliasis][1] or
[Trichuriasis][1]—
    See *Albendazole Oral Suspension.*
Note: In the treatment of *giardiasis,* see *Albendazole Oral Suspension.*

### Usual pediatric dose

[Ascariasis][1] or
[Capillariasis][1] or
[Enterobiasis][1] or
[Hookworm infections][1] or
[Hydatid disease][1] or
[Neurocysticercosis][1] or
[Strongyloidiasis][1] or
[Taeniasis][1] or
[Trichostrongyliasis][1] or
[Trichuriasis][1]—
    See *Albendazole Oral Suspension.*
Note: In the treatment of *giardiasis,* see *Albendazole Oral Suspension.*

### Strength(s) usually available

U.S.—
    Not commercially available.
    Note: Although albendazole is not commercially available in the U.S., the manufacturer makes it available for compassionate use only (tel. no.: 215-751-4000).
Canada—
    Not commercially available.
United Kingdom—
    200 mg (Rx) [*Zentel*].
    400 mg (Rx) [*Eskazole* (scored)].

### Packaging and storage

Store below 40 °C (104 °F), preferably between 15 and 30 °C (59 and 86 °F), in a well-closed container, unless otherwise specified by manufacturer. Protect from direct sunlight.

### Auxiliary labeling

- May be chewed, crushed, or swallowed whole.
- Take with meals.
- Continue medication for full time of treatment.

---

[1]Not included in Canadian product labeling.

## Selected Bibliography

Teggi A, Lastilla MG, De Rosa F. Therapy of human hydatid disease with mebendazole and albendazole. Antimicrob Agents Chemother 1993; 1679-84.

Todorov T, Vutova K, Mechkov G, et al. Chemotherapy of human cystic echinococcosis: comparative efficacy of mebendazole and albendazole. Ann Trop Med Parasitol 1992 Feb; 86 (1): 59-66.

---

Revised: 04/19/96

# ALBUMIN HUMAN   Systemic

VA CLASSIFICATION (Primary): BL800

Note: For a listing of dosage forms and brand names by country availability, see *Dosage Forms* section(s). For a listing of brand names for the articles in this monograph, refer to the General Index.

## Category

Blood volume expander; antihyperbilirubinemic.

## Indications

### Accepted

**Hypovolemia (treatment)**—The 5 and 25% concentrations of albumin are indicated in the emergency treatment of hypovolemia with or without shock. Albumin restores intravascular volume and maintains cardiac output and colloid oncotic pressure. If blood loss is severe, a transfusion of whole blood or red blood cells may be indicated to restore the hemoglobin concentration and improve oxygen transport.

**Hypoproteinemia (treatment)**—The 5 and 25% concentrations of albumin are indicated in the treatment of hypoproteinemia caused by loss of plasma proteins. Loss of plasma proteins may occur through decreased absorption in gastrointestinal disorders, inadequate synthesis in chronic liver disease, or excessive urinary loss and increased catabolism in chronic kidney disease. This loss of protein leads to edema secondary to a fluid shift from the intravascular space to the interstitium and a compensatory increase in salt and water retention. Albumin serves to restore colloid oncotic pressure and, in conjunction with a diuretic, promote diuresis.

**Burns, severe (treatment adjunct)**—The 5 and 25% concentrations of albumin are indicated, in conjunction with large volumes of crystalloid injection, to maintain plasma volume and protein concentration and to prevent the intravascular hemoconcentration accompanying severe burns.

**Hyperbilirubinemia, neonatal (treatment)**—The 25% albumin injection is indicated in the treatment of hyperbilirubinemia whether or not it is associated with hemolytic disease. It may be used prior to or during an exchange transfusion to bind free bilirubin and to enhance its removal.

**Respiratory distress syndrome, adult (ARDS) (treatment adjunct)**—The 25% albumin injection may be indicated, in conjunction with diuretics, to correct the fluid volume overload associated with ARDS.

**Cardiopulmonary bypass (treatment adjunct)**—The 5 and 25% concentrations of albumin may be indicated as adjuncts to provide hemodilution in cardiopulmonary bypass procedures.

**Ascites (treatment adjunct)[1]**—The 5 and 25% concentrations of albumin may be used to maintain cardiovascular function following the removal of large volumes of ascitic fluid.

**Nephrosis, acute (treatment adjunct) or**
**Nephrotic syndrome, acute (treatment adjunct)**—The 25% albumin injection may be indicated as an adjunct in the control of edema in patients refractory to cyclophosphamide and corticosteroid therapy.

**Hemodialysis**—The 25% albumin injection may be used as an adjunct in patients who are undergoing long-term hemodialysis and are susceptible to shock and hypotension, or in dialysis patients who are hypervolemic and may not tolerate large volumes of crystalloid injection as treatment for shock or hypotension.

**Pancreatitis (treatment adjunct) or**
**Intra-abdominal infections (treatment adjunct)**—The 5 and 25% concentrations of albumin may be indicated, along with crystalloids, as fluid replacement in the treatment of shock associated with acute hemorrhagic pancreatitis or peritonitis when there is loss of fluid into the third space.

**Liver failure, acute (treatment adjunct)**—The 5 and 25% concentrations of albumin may be indicated as adjuncts in the treatment of acute liver failure to stabilize the circulation, maintain plasma colloid oncotic pressure, and bind excess bilirubin.

**Red blood cell resuspension**—Albumin may be indicated to provide sufficient volume and to prevent excessive hypoproteinemia during certain types of exchange transfusions or during the administration of large volumes of previously frozen or washed red blood cells.

### Unaccepted

Albumin has not been shown to be effective in the treatment of chronic cirrhosis or nephrosis.

Albumin does not contain all the essential amino acids and is, therefore, not an appropriate source of protein in the treatment of malnutrition.

Given in excessive amounts, albumin may increase the catabolism of endogenous albumin.

[1]Not included in Canadian product labeling.

## Pharmacology/Pharmacokinetics

### Physicochemical characteristics

**Source**—Obtained from source blood, plasma, serum, or placentas of healthy human donors by fractionation according to the Cohn cold ethanol process.

Albumin is heat pasteurized for 10 hours at 60 °C to inactivate human immunodeficiency virus (HIV) and hepatitis viruses; sodium caprylate and sodium acetyltryptophanate are added to prevent denaturation during this process.

**Molecular weight**—66,300 to 69,000.

**pH**—6.4 to 7.4

### Mechanism of action/Effect

**Blood volume expander**—Albumin is an important regulator of the volume of circulating blood. It accounts for 70 to 80% of the colloid oncotic pressure of plasma. An infusion of albumin 5% is oncotically equivalent to an equal volume of human plasma and increases blood volume by an amount approximately equal to the volume of albumin infused; albumin 25% is oncotically equivalent to approximately 5 times the volume of human plasma and draws into the circulation an amount of fluid approximately 3.5 times the volume of albumin infused. Albumin provides a temporary increase in blood volume, which reduces hemoconcentration and blood viscosity.

**Antihyperbilirubinemic**—Albumin is a transport protein that reversibly binds both endogenous and exogenous substances including bilirubin, fatty acids, hormones, enzymes, drugs, dyes, and trace metals.

### Distribution

Albumin is distributed throughout the extracellular water; more than 60% is located in the extravascular fluid compartment.

### Half-life

**Elimination**—15 to 20 days.

**Other**—Intravascular: 24 hours.

### Onset of action

**Blood volume expansion**—With albumin 25% injection: 15 minutes, provided the patient is well hydrated.

### Duration of action

Dependent upon the initial blood volume of the patient. If blood volume is reduced, volume expansion persists for many hours; however, if blood volume is normal, the effect lasts a shorter time.

## Precautions to Consider

### Pregnancy/Reproduction

**Pregnancy**—Studies have not been done in humans.
Studies have not been done in animals.
FDA Pregnancy Category C.

### Breast-feeding

It is not known whether albumin is distributed into breast milk. However, problems in humans have not been documented.

### Pediatrics

Appropriate studies performed to date have not demonstrated pediatrics-specific problems that would limit the usefulness of albumin in children.

### Geriatrics

No information is available on the relationship of age to the effects of albumin in geriatric patients.

### Medical considerations/Contraindications

The medical considerations/contraindications included here have been selected on the basis of their potential clinical significance (reasons given in parentheses where appropriate)—not necessarily inclusive (» = major clinical significance).

*Except under special circumstances, this medication should not be used when the following medical problems exist:*
» Anemia, severe or
» Cardiac failure or
» Hypervolemia or
» Pulmonary edema
    (these medical problems may increase the risk of and/or be exacerbated by circulatory overload)

*Risk-benefit should be considered when the following medical problems exist:*

Hypertension or
Normal serum albumin concentrations
    (increased plasma volume may lead to circulatory overload; hypertension may be exacerbated)

Renal function impairment
    (aluminum, sometimes present as a contaminant in albumin injections, may accumulate, leading to anemia, dialysis encephalopathy, hypercalcemia, or vitamin D–refractory osteomalacia)

Sensitivity to albumin

## Patient monitoring

The following may be especially important in patient monitoring (other tests may be warranted in some patients, depending on condition; » = major clinical significance):

Aluminum concentrations, serum
    (recommended in patients with renal function impairment, who are infused repeatedly with large volumes of albumin)

» Blood pressure measurements
    (a rapid rise in blood pressure may reveal bleeding that was not apparent at the lower blood pressure)

Pulmonary wedge pressure determinations
    (recommended to guard against circulatory overload)

## Side/Adverse Effects

The following side/adverse effects have been selected on the basis of their potential clinical significance (possible signs and symptoms in parentheses where appropriate)—not necessarily inclusive:

### Those indicating need for medical attention

Incidence less frequent
  *Congestive heart failure*—especially in patients with compromised cardiovascular function; *decreased myocardial contractility; pulmonary edema; salt and water retention*

  Note: These side effects are more likely to occur in patients given large volumes of crystalloids prior to the administration of albumin.

Incidence rare
  *Changes in blood pressure, pulse, and respiration; chills; fever; increased salivation; nausea or vomiting; skin rash or hives; tachycardia*

## General Dosing Information

Albumin contains no blood group isoagglutinins and, therefore, may be given without regard to the blood group of the patient.

Albumin must be administered by intravenous infusion. It may be administered without dilution or diluted with 0.9% sodium chloride injection, 5% dextrose injection, or sodium lactate injection. It also may be administered with plasma, packed red blood cells, or whole blood; however, except when used as a red blood cell resuspension medium, albumin should not be added directly to any of these three components.

Albumin may be administered at a rate of 1 to 2 mL per minute; however, the rate of infusion and the total volume of albumin administered ultimately must be guided by the hemodynamic response of the patient.

Patients with marked dehydration given 25% albumin injection require administration of additional fluids.

Transfusions of whole blood or packed red blood cells may be necessary following administration of large volumes of albumin to restore hemoglobin concentration and to prevent anemia.

## Parenteral Dosage Forms

### ALBUMIN HUMAN USP

#### Usual adult dose

Hypovolemia—
  Intravenous infusion, 25 grams as a 5 or 25% injection, administered as rapidly as tolerated by the patient. If an adequate response is not achieved within fifteen to thirty minutes, an additional dose may be given.

Hypoproteinemia—
  Intravenous infusion, 50 to 75 grams as a 25% injection, administered at a rate of 100 mL over thirty to forty minutes. For slow infusion, 50 grams in 300 mL of 10% dextrose injection, administered at a rate of 100 mL per hour.

Burns—
  Therapy is usually begun with the administration of large volumes of crystalloid injection to maintain plasma volume. After 24 hours, albumin may be added at an initial dose of 25 grams, with the dose adjusted thereafter to maintain a plasma albumin concentration of 2.5 grams per 100 mL (25 grams/L), or a total serum protein concentration of 5.2 grams per 100 mL (52 grams/L).

Cardiopulmonary bypass—
  Intravenous infusion, as a 5 or 25% injection, with crystalloid as a pump prime to achieve plasma albumin and hematocrit concentrations of 2.5 grams per 100 mL (25 grams/L) and 20%, respectively.

Nephrosis, acute or
Nephrotic syndrome, acute—
  Intravenous infusion, 25 grams as a 25% injection, administered with an appropriate diuretic once a day for seven to ten days.

Hemodialysis—
  Intravenous infusion, 25 grams as a 25% injection.

Red blood cell resuspension—
  20 to 25 grams as a 25% injection, per liter of red blood cells.

#### Usual adult prescribing limits

Up to 2 grams per kg of body weight within twenty-four hours.

#### Usual pediatric dose

Hypovolemia—
  Intravenous infusion, 2.5 to 12.5 grams, or 0.5 to 1 gram per kg of body weight, administered as rapidly as tolerated by the patient. If an adequate response is not achieved within fifteen to thirty minutes, an additional dose may be given.

Burns—
  Therapy is usually begun with the administration of large volumes of crystalloid injection to maintain plasma volume. After 24 hours, albumin may be added at an initial dose of 25 grams, with the dose adjusted thereafter to maintain a plasma albumin concentration of 2 to 2.5 grams per 100 mL (20 to 25 grams/L), or a total serum protein concentration of 5.2 grams per 100 mL (52 grams/L).

Hyperbilirubinemia, neonatal—
  Intravenous infusion, 1 gram per kg of body weight as a 25% injection, administered during, or one to two hours prior to exchange transfusion.

#### Strength(s) usually available

U.S.—

5% in 50 mL (Rx) [*Albuminar-5* (sodium ion 130–160 mEq per L; potassium ion ≤ 1 mEq per L); *Plasbumin-5;* GENERIC (sodium ion 130–160 mEq per L)].

5% in 250 mL (Rx) [*Albuminar-5* (sodium ion 130–160 mEq per L; potassium ion ≤ 1 mEq per L); *Albutein 5%* (sodium ion 130–160 mEq per L); *Buminate 5%* (sodium ion 130–160 mEq per L); *Plasbumin-5;* GENERIC (sodium ion 130–160 mEq per L)].

5% in 500 mL (Rx) [*Albuminar-5* (sodium ion 130–160 mEq per L; potassium ion ≤ 1 mEq per L); *Albutein 5%* (sodium ion 130–160 mEq per L); *Buminate 5%* (sodium ion 130–160 mEq per L); *Plasbumin-5;* GENERIC (sodium ion 130–160 mEq per L)].

5% in 1000 mL (Rx) [*Albuminar-5* (sodium ion 130–160 mEq per L; potassium ion ≤ 1 mEq per L)].

25% in 20 mL (Rx) [*Albuminar-25* (sodium ion 130–160 mEq per L; potassium ion ≤ 1 mEq per L); *Albutein 25%* (sodium ion 130–160 mEq per L); *Buminate 25%* (sodium ion 130–160 mEq per L); *Plasbumin-25;* GENERIC (sodium ion 130–160 mEq per L)].

25% in 50 mL (Rx) [*Albuminar-25* (sodium ion 130–160 mEq per L; potassium ion ≤ 1 mEq per L); *Albutein 25%* (sodium ion 130–160 mEq per L); *Buminate 25%* (sodium ion 130–160 mEq per L); *Plasbumin-25;* GENERIC (sodium ion 130–160 mEq per L)].

25% in 100 mL (Rx) [*Albuminar-25* (sodium ion 130–160 mEq per L; potassium ion ≤ 1 mEq per L); *Albutein 25%* (sodium ion 130–160 mEq per L); *Buminate 25%* (sodium ion 130–160 mEq per L); *Plasbumin-25;* GENERIC (sodium ion 130–160 mEq per L)].

Canada—

5% in 50 mL (Rx) [*Plasbumin-5*].
5% in 250 mL (Rx) [*Plasbumin-5*].
5% in 500 mL (Rx) [*Plasbumin-5*].
25% in 20 mL (Rx) [*Plasbumin-25*].
25% in 50 mL (Rx) [*Plasbumin-25*].
25% in 100 mL (Rx) [*Plasbumin-25*].

#### Packaging and storage

Store at 15 to 30 °C (59 to 86 °F), unless otherwise specified by manufacturer. Protect from freezing.

#### Stability

Should not be used if solution is turbid or contains a precipitate. Albumin contains no preservative and should be used within 4 hours after the vial is opened. Partially used vials should be discarded.

#### Incompatibilities

Albumin is incompatible with verapamil hydrochloride, alcohol-containing solutions, amino acid solutions, fat emulsions, and protein hydrolysates.

## Selected Bibliography

Tullis JL. Albumin 1. Background and use. JAMA 1977; 237: 355-60.

Tullis JL. Albumin 2. Guidelines for clinical use. JAMA 1977; 237: 460-3.

Van Der Weyden MB, Trinker FR, Hemming M, Rush B, McGrath KM, Hargreaves AP. Human albumin solutions: Consensus statements for use in selected clinical situations. Med J Aust 1992; 157: 340-3.

Revised: 08/17/93

---

**ALBUTEROL**—See *Bronchodilators, Adrenergic (Systemic)*

---

**ALCLOMETASONE**—See *Corticosteroids (Topical)*

---

# ALCOHOL AND ACETONE    Topical†

VA CLASSIFICATION (Primary): DE752

Note: For a listing of dosage forms and brand names by country availability, see *Dosage Forms* section(s). For a listing of brand names for the articles in this monograph, refer to the General Index.

---

†Not commercially available in Canada.

---

## Category

Antiacne agent (topical); cleansing agent (astringent; defatting).

## Indications

### Accepted

Acne vulgaris (treatment) or

Oily skin (treatment)—Alcohol and acetone combination is indicated as an aid in the treatment of mild acne vulgaris and oily skin.

## Pharmacology/Pharmacokinetics

### Physicochemical characteristics

Molecular weight—
    Alcohol: 46.07.
    Acetone: 58.08.

### Mechanism of action/Effect

Alcohol and acetone aid in the removal of sebum (oil) from the surface of the skin.

## Precautions to Consider

### Pregnancy/Reproduction

Problems in humans have not been documented.

### Breast-feeding

Problems in humans have not been documented.

### Pediatrics

Appropriate studies on the relationship of age to the effects of alcohol and acetone have not been performed in the pediatric population. However, it is recommended that alcohol and acetone combination not be used on children up to 8 years of age. Pediatrics-specific problems that would limit the usefulness of this medication in older children are not expected.

### Geriatrics

Appropriate studies on the relationship of age to the effects of alcohol and acetone have not been performed in the geriatric population. However, geriatrics-specific problems that would limit the usefulness of this medication in the elderly are not expected.

### Drug interactions and/or related problems

The following drug interactions and/or related problems have been selected on the basis of their potential clinical significance (possible mechanism in parentheses where appropriate)—not necessarily inclusive (» = major clinical significance):

Note: Combinations containing any of the following medications, depending on the amount present, may also interact with this medication.

    Abrasive or medicated soaps or cleansers or
    Acne preparations or preparations containing a peeling agent, such as:
        Benzoyl peroxide
        Resorcinol
        Salicylic acid
        Sulfur
        Tretinoin or

Acne preparations, topical, other or
Alcohol-containing preparations, topical, such as
    After-shave lotions
    Astringents
    Perfumed toiletries
    Shaving creams or lotions or
Cosmetics or soaps with a strong drying effect or
Isotretinoin or
Medicated cosmetics or ''cover-ups''
    (concurrent use with alcohol and acetone combination may cause a cumulative irritant or drying effect, especially with the application of peeling, desquamating, or abrasive agents, resulting in excessive irritation of the skin)

### Medical considerations/Contraindications

The medical considerations/contraindications included here have been selected on the basis of their potential clinical significance (reasons given in parentheses where appropriate)—not necessarily inclusive (» = major clinical significance).

*This medication should not be used when the following medical problems exist:*

» Burns or wounds
    (use may cause severe irritation)

*Risk-benefit should be considered when the following medical problem exists:*

Sensitivity to this medication
    (may cause allergic contact dermatitis, contact urticaria syndrome, sensitive skin [i.e., easily irritated], or subjective irritation [i.e., burning, stinging, and itching without objective signs])

## Side/Adverse Effects

The following side/adverse effects have been selected on the basis of their potential clinical significance (possible signs and symptoms in parentheses where appropriate)—not necessarily inclusive:

### Those indicating need for medical attention

*Hypersensitivity* (irritation, pain, redness, or swelling of skin); *skin infection*

### Those indicating need for medical attention only if they continue or are bothersome

*Burning or stinging of skin*

## Patient Consultation

As an aid to patient consultation, refer to *Advice for the Patient, Alcohol and Acetone (Topical).*

In providing consultation, consider emphasizing the following selected information (» = major clinical significance):

### Before using this medication

» Conditions affecting use, especially:
        Sensitivity to alcohol or acetone
        Use in children—Not using on children up to 8 years of age
        Other medical problems, especially burns or wounds

### Proper use of this medication

» Avoiding contact with the eyes, nostrils, and lips
    Medication is flammable; not using near heat or open flame or while smoking
    Proper administration
        Applying the lotion by putting a small amount on a gauze pad or cotton ball and wiping or rubbing over face and other affected areas
        Using the pledget by wiping or rubbing over face and other affected areas
        Not rinsing after application

» Proper dosing
  Missed dose: If on scheduled dosing regimen—Applying as soon as possible
» Proper storage

### Precautions while using this medication
» Avoiding simultaneous use with other topical acne preparations or preparations containing peeling agents, other alcohol-containing preparations, abrasive soaps or cleansers, cosmetics or soaps with drying effect, medicated cosmetics, or other topical skin medications, unless otherwise directed by physician

### Side/adverse effects
Signs of potential side effects, especially hypersensitivity or skin infection

## Topical Dosage Forms

### ALCOHOL AND ACETONE DETERGENT LOTION

#### Usual adult and adolescent dose
Acne vulgaris (treatment) or
Oily skin (treatment)—
  Topical, to the skin, two to four times a day as needed.

#### Usual pediatric dose
Acne vulgaris (treatment) or
Oily skin (treatment)—
  Children up to 8 years of age: Use is not recommended.
  Children 8 years of age and older: See *Usual adult and adolescent dose.*

#### Strength(s) usually available
U.S.—
  Alcohol 49.7% and acetone 18% (OTC) [*Seba-Nil Liquid Cleanser*].
  Alcohol 50% and acetone 10% (OTC) [*Tyrosum Liquid*].
Canada—
  Not commercially available.

### Packaging and storage
Store below 40 °C (104 °F), preferably between 15 and 30 °C (59 and 86 °F), in a tight container, unless otherwise specified by manufacturer.

### Auxiliary labeling
• For external use only.
• Keep container tightly closed.
• Flammable.

### Additional information
The lotion should be applied using a gauze pad or cotton ball.

### ALCOHOL AND ACETONE PLEDGETS

#### Usual adult and adolescent dose
See *Alcohol and Acetone Detergent Lotion.*

#### Usual pediatric dose
See *Alcohol and Acetone Detergent Lotion.*

#### Strength(s) usually available
U.S.—
  Alcohol 50% and acetone 10% (OTC) [*Tyrosum Packets*].
Canada—
  Not commercially available.

### Packaging and storage
Store below 40 °C (104 °F), preferably between 15 and 30 °C (59 and 86 °F), in a well-closed container, unless otherwise specified by manufacturer.

### Auxiliary labeling
• For external use only.
• Flammable.

Revised: 01/15/92
Interim revision: 06/08/94

# ALCOHOL AND SULFUR   Topical

VA CLASSIFICATION (Primary/Secondary): DE752/DE500
Note: For a listing of dosage forms and brand names by country availability, see *Dosage Forms* section(s). For a listing of brand names for the articles in this monograph, refer to the General Index.

## Category
Antiacne agent (topical); cleansing agent (astringent; defatting)-keratolytic.

## Indications
### Accepted
Acne vulgaris (treatment) or
Oily skin (treatment)—Topical alcohol and sulfur combination is indicated as an aid in the treatment of acne vulgaris and oily skin.

## Pharmacology/Pharmacokinetics
### Physicochemical characteristics
Molecular weight—Alcohol: 46.07.
Sulfur: 32.06.

### Mechanism of action/Effect
Alcohol—Aids in the removal of sebum (oil) from the surface of the skin.
Sulfur—Acts as a keratolytic and promotes drying and peeling of the skin. Sulfur also has germicidal action, which results from its conversion to pentathionic acid presumably by epidermal cells or certain microorganisms.

## Precautions to Consider
### Pregnancy/Reproduction
Problems in humans have not been documented.

### Breast-feeding
Problems in humans have not been documented.

### Pediatrics
Appropriate studies on the relationship of age to the effect of alcohol and sulfur have not been performed in the pediatric population. However, it is recommended that alcohol and sulfur combination not be used on children up to 8 years of age. In older children, pediatrics-specific

problems that would limit the usefulness of this medication are not expected.

### Geriatrics
Appropriate studies on the relationship of age to the effect of alcohol and sulfur have not been performed in the geriatric population. However, geriatrics-specific problems that would limit the usefulness of this medication in the elderly are not expected.

### Drug interactions and/or related problems
The following drug interactions and/or related problems have been selected on the basis of their potential clinical significance (possible mechanism in parentheses where appropriate)—not necessarily inclusive (» = major clinical significance):

Note: Combinations containing any of the following medications, depending on the amount present, may also interact with this medication.

Abrasive or medicated soaps or cleansers or
Acne preparations or preparations containing a peeling agent such as
  Benzoyl peroxide
  Resorcinol
  Salicylic acid
  Tretinoin or
Acne preparations, topical, other or
Alcohol-containing preparations, topical such as
  After-shave lotions
  Astringents
  Perfumed toiletries
  Shaving creams or lotions or
Cosmetics or soaps with a strong drying effect or
Isotretinoin or
Medicated cosmetics or ''cover-ups''
  (concurrent use with alcohol and sulfur combination may cause a cumulative irritant or drying effect, especially with the application of peeling, desquamating, or abrasive agents, resulting in excessive irritation of the skin)

Mercury compounds, topical
  (concurrent use with sulfur may result in a chemical reaction releasing hydrogen sulfide, which has a foul odor, may be irritating, and may stain the skin black)

**Medical considerations/Contraindications**

The medical considerations/contraindications included here have been selected on the basis of their potential clinical significance (reasons given in parentheses where appropriate)—not necessarily inclusive (» = major clinical significance).

*Risk-benefit should be considered when the following medical problem exists:*

Sensitivity to this medication
(may cause allergic contact dermatitis, contact urticaria syndrome, sensitive skin [i.e., easily irritated], or subjective irritation [i.e., burning, stinging, or itching without objective signs])

## Side/Adverse Effects

The following side/adverse effects have been selected on the basis of their potential clinical significance (possible signs and symptoms in parentheses where appropriate)—not necessarily inclusive:

**Those indicating need for medical attention**
*Hypersensitivity* (skin irritation not present before therapy)

**Those indicating need for medical attention only if they continue or are bothersome**
*Burning or stinging of skin; dryness or peeling of skin*—may occur after a few days

## Patient Consultation

As an aid to patient consultation, refer to *Advice for the Patient, Alcohol and Sulfur (Topical).*

In providing consultation, consider emphasizing the following selected information (» = major clinical significance):

**Before using this medication**
» Conditions affecting use, especially:
Sensitivity to alcohol or sulfur
Use in children—Not using on children up to 8 years of age

**Proper use of this medication**
Proper administration: Before using, washing or cleansing affected areas thoroughly and patting dry; applying small amount of medication to affected area (s) of skin and rubbing in gently
» Avoiding contact with the eyes, nostrils, and lips; flushing thoroughly with water if medication accidentally gets into eyes or nostrils or on lips
Medication is flammable; not using near heat or open flame or while smoking
» Using only as directed; importance of not using more medication than the amount recommended
» Proper dosing
Missed dose: Applying as soon as possible
» Proper storage

**Precautions while using this medication**
» Avoiding simultaneous use with other topical acne preparations or preparations containing peeling agents, other alcohol-containing preparations, abrasive soaps or cleansers, cosmetics or soaps with

drying effect, medicated cosmetics, or other topical skin medications, unless prescribed by physician
» Avoiding concurrent use with topical mercury-containing preparations

**Side/adverse effects**
Signs of potential side effects, especially hypersensitivity

## General Dosing Information

Some alcohol and sulfur combination products are tinted a flesh color and can be used as a makeup or cover-up.

Since this medication is an effective drying agent, it should be used sparingly when therapy is initiated, especially for those patients with sensitive skin.

The frequency of applications may be increased gradually up to three times a day as tolerated.

In dry or cold climates, the skin may be more sensitive to this medication, and the frequency of use should be reduced. During warm, humid weather, frequency of use may be increased.

**For treatment of adverse effects**
If the medication comes in contact with the eyes, flush the eyes with water.

## Topical Dosage Forms
### ALCOHOL AND SULFUR LOTION

**Usual adult and adolescent dose**
Acne vulgaris (treatment) or
Oily skin (treatment)—
Topical, to the skin, one or two times a day.

**Usual pediatric dose**
Acne vulgaris (treatment) or
Oily skin (treatment)—
Children up to 8 years of age: Use is not recommended.
Children 8 years of age and older: See *Usual adult and adolescent dose.*

**Strength(s) usually available**
U.S.—
22% alcohol and 5% sulfur (OTC) [*Liquimat Light; Liquimat Medium*].
22.5% alcohol and 10% sulfur (OTC) [*Acne Lotion 10*].
Canada—
20% alcohol and 2% colloidal sulfur (OTC) [*Postacne* (butylparaben; methylparaben; sodium metabisulfite)].

**Packaging and storage**
Store below 40 °C (104 °F), preferably between 15 and 30 °C (59 and 86 °F), in a well-closed container, unless otherwise specified by manufacturer. Protect from freezing.

**Auxiliary labeling**
• Shake well.
• For external use only.

Revised: 08/02/95

---

# ALDESLEUKIN   Systemic†

VA CLASSIFICATION (Primary): AN900

Other commonly used names are interleukin-2, recombinant, and rIL-2.

Note: For a listing of dosage forms and brand names by country availability, see *Dosage Forms* section(s). For a listing of brand names for the articles in this monograph, refer to the General Index.

†Not commercially available in Canada.

## Category
Biological response modifier; antineoplastic.

## Indications

**Accepted**
Carcinoma, renal cell (treatment)—Aldesleukin is accepted for treatment of metastatic renal carcinoma, based on reports of objective remissions (most of which were partial) observed in some patients.
*Because of its potential life-threatening toxicities, USP DI Advisory Panels recommend that this medication be used only after careful consideration of risk-benefit.* It is recommended that aldesleukin be used

only by qualified specialists who are fully aware of and equipped to monitor and treat the potential toxicities of this medication.

## Pharmacology/Pharmacokinetics

Note: Pharmacokinetics can be described by a 2-compartment model.

**Physicochemical characteristics**
Source—Synthetic. Produced by a recombinant DNA process involving genetically engineered *Escherichia coli* containing an analog of the human interleukin-2 gene. Genetic engineering techniques used to modify the human interleukin-2 gene result in an expression clone that encodes a modified human interleukin-2. Aldesleukin differs from naturally occurring interleukin-2 in that it is not glycosylated because it is derived from *Escherichia coli*, the molecule has no *N*-terminal alanine (the codon for this amino acid was deleted during the genetic engineering process), the molecule has serine substituted for cysteine at amino acid position 125 (this was accomplished by site specific manipulation during the genetic engineering process), and the aggregation state of aldesleukin is likely to be different from that of native interleukin-2. The manufacturing process involves fermentation in a

defined medium containing tetracycline hydrochloride; the presence of the antibiotic is not detectable in the final product.

Chemical group—Related to naturally occurring interleukins, which are lymphokines, a subgroup of the hormone-like glycoprotein growth factors also known as cytokines.

Molecular weight—Approximately 15,300 daltons.

### Mechanism of action/Effect

The exact mechanism of the antineoplastic action of aldesleukin is unknown, although it is postulated that stimulation of an immunological host reaction to the tumor is involved.

Interleukins facilitate communication among leukocytes. In general, endogenous interleukin-2 (first known as T-cell growth factor), which is secreted by activated T cells, has immunoregulatory properties, including enhancement of lymphocyte mitogenesis and stimulation of long-term growth of human interleukin-2 dependent cell lines, enhancement of lymphocyte toxicity, induction of killer cell (lymphokine-activated [LAK] and natural [NK]) activity, and induction of interferon-gamma production. Recombinant interleukin-2 has the same biological activity as the endogenous cytokine.

The effects of aldesleukin include activation of cellular immunity with profound lymphocytosis, eosinophilia, and thrombocytopenia, and the production of cytokines including tumor necrosis factor, interleukin-1, gamma interferon, and granulocyte-macrophage colony stimulating factor (GM-CSF).

### Other actions/effects

Aldesleukin causes a capillary leak syndrome (CLS) as a result of increased capillary permeability, leading to extravasation of plasma proteins and fluid into the extravascular space and contributing to loss of vascular resistance. Interleukin-2 has been reported to reversibly decrease serum cholesterol concentrations. Interleukin-2 has been reported to transiently decrease serum testosterone and dihydroepiandrosterone concentrations and to transiently increase plasma estradiol concentrations. It has also been reported to transiently increase adrenal secretion of ACTH and cortisol.

### Distribution

Interleukin-2 activity has been measured in cerebrospinal fluid of patients after intravenous administration.

### Biotransformation

Renal. Greater than 80% of the amount of aldesleukin distributed to plasma, cleared from the circulation, and presented to the kidney is metabolized to amino acids in the cells lining the proximal convoluted tubules.

### Half-life

Distribution—13 minutes.

Elimination—85 minutes.

### Duration of action

Tumor regression may continue for up to 12 months following initiation of therapy.

### Elimination

Renal. Cleared from the circulation by both glomerular filtration and peritubular extraction in the kidney. The mean clearance rate in cancer patients is 268 mL per minute.

## Precautions to Consider

Note: In general, risks associated with aldesleukin therapy are dose- and schedule-related; toxicity of the high-dose regimen currently recommended is high.

### Cross-sensitivity and/or related problems

Patients sensitive to *Escherichia coli*–derived proteins may also be sensitive to aldesleukin.

### Carcinogenicity/Mutagenicity

Studies have not been done.

### Pregnancy/Reproduction

Fertility—Studies have not been done.

Pregnancy—Studies in humans have not been done.

Hazards to the fetus include adverse reactions seen in adults.

In general, use of a contraceptive is recommended during antineoplastic therapy.

Studies in animals have not been done.

FDA Pregnancy Category C.

### Breast-feeding

It is not known whether aldesleukin is distributed into breast milk.

### Pediatrics

No information is available on the relationship of age to the effects of aldesleukin in pediatric patients. However, preliminary studies seem to indicate no difference in responsiveness to or toxicity from inter-

leukin-2 between children and adults. Safety and efficacy have not been established.

### Geriatrics

Although appropriate studies on the relationship of age to the effects of aldesleukin have not been performed in the geriatric population, clinical trials have included elderly patients. There is some evidence that elderly patients do not tolerate aldesleukin's toxicity as well. Cardiac status is of particular concern. In addition, elderly patients are more likely to have age-related renal function impairment, which may require caution in patients receiving aldesleukin.

### Dental

The impairment of neutrophil function caused by aldesleukin may result in an increased incidence of microbial infection, delayed healing, and gingival bleeding. Dental work, whenever possible, should be completed prior to initiation of therapy or deferred until blood counts have returned to normal. Patients should be instructed in proper oral hygiene during treatment, including caution in use of regular toothbrushes, dental floss, and toothpicks.

Aldesleukin also commonly causes stomatitis, and less commonly causes glossitis, which may be associated with considerable discomfort.

### Drug interactions and/or related problems

The following drug interactions and/or related problems have been selected on the basis of their potential clinical significance (possible mechanism in parentheses where appropriate)—not necessarily inclusive (» = major clinical significance):

Note: Combinations containing any of the following medications, depending on the amount present, may also interact with this medication.

Blood dyscrasia–causing medications (See *Appendix II*)
(leukopenic and/or thrombocytopenic effects of aldesleukin may be increased with concurrent or recent therapy if these medications cause the same effects)

» Bone marrow depressants, other (See *Appendix II*) or
Radiation therapy
(additive bone marrow depression may occur)

» Cardiotoxic medications, other, including daunorubicin or doxorubicin
(concurrent use may result in increased cardiotoxicity)

Central nervous system (CNS) depressants
(concurrent use may result in increased CNS depression)

Contrast media, iodinated
(incidence of delayed [more than 1 hour after administration] reactions to intravenous iodinated contrast media [e.g., hypersensitivity, fever, skin rash, flu-like symptoms, joint pain, flushing, pruritus, emesis, hypotension, dizziness] may be increased in patients who have received interleukin-2; some symptoms may resemble a "recall" reaction to interleukin-2; supportive medical treatment may be necessary if symptoms are significant; there is some evidence that incidence of this reaction is reduced if contrast media administration is delayed until 6 weeks after interleukin-2 administration)

» Corticosteroids, glucocorticoid, systemic
(although glucocorticoids, especially dexamethasone, have been shown to reduce some adverse effects of aldesleukin, including fever, renal insufficiency, hyperbilirubinemia, confusion, and dyspnea, there is some evidence that concurrent use may reduce the antitumor efficacy of aldesleukin; therefore, it is generally recommended that dexamethasone be avoided, except in cases of life-threatening aldesleukin toxicity)

» Hepatotoxic medications, other (See *Appendix II*) or
» Nephrotoxic medications, other (See *Appendix II*)
(concurrent and/or sequential administration should be avoided since the potential for hepatotoxicity or nephrotoxicity may be increased, especially in the presence of hepatic or renal function impairment that may be caused by aldesleukin)

» Hypotension-producing medications, other (See *Appendix II*)
(concurrent use may result in increased hypotension)

### Laboratory value alterations

The following have been selected on the basis of their potential clinical significance (possible effect in parentheses where appropriate)—not necessarily inclusive (» = major clinical significance):

With physiology/laboratory test values
Alanine aminotransferase (ALT [SGPT]) and
Alkaline phosphatase and
Aspartate aminotransferase (AST [SGOT]) and
Bilirubin and
Lactate dehydrogenase (LDH)
(serum values are increased in most patients)

Albumin and
Protein
    (plasma concentrations may be decreased and urinary concentrations increased as a sign of renal toxicity)
Bicarbonate and
Calcium and
Magnesium and
Phosphate and
Potassium and
Sodium
    (serum concentrations may be decreased but return to normal shortly after withdrawal of interleukin-2)
Blood urea nitrogen (BUN) and
Creatinine concentrations, serum
    (dose-related increases commonly occur, indicating renal toxicity)
Creatine kinase (CK)
    (serum concentrations may be increased with or without symptoms of cardiotoxicity and may be associated with nonischemic myocardial injury or myocarditis rather than myocardial ischemia or infarction)
Electrocardiogram (ECG) changes, including:
    QRS voltage reductions
    ST segment changes
    T-wave changes
    (may occur as signs of cardiotoxicity)
Left ventricular ejection fraction and
Left ventricular stroke work index
    (frequently decreased in cardiotoxicity; these effects resemble septic shock)
Prothrombin time
    (may be prolonged)
Uric acid
    (concentrations in blood and urine may be increased, possibly as a result of catabolism of lymphokine-activated killer [LAK] cells and natural killer [NK] cells)

## Medical considerations/Contraindications
The medical considerations/contraindications included here have been selected on the basis of their potential clinical significance (reasons given in parentheses where appropriate)—not necessarily inclusive (» = major clinical significance).

*Except under special circumstances, high-dose regimens of this medication should not be used when the following medical problems exist:*
» Cardiac function impairment, as determined by thallium stress test
» Organ allograft
    (enhancement of cellular immune function by aldesleukin may increase the risk of allograft rejection)
» Pulmonary function impairment
» Because aldesleukin may exacerbate symptoms of clinically unrecognized or untreated central nervous system (CNS) metastases, generally treatment with aldesleukin should not begin until a patient has had thorough evaluation and treatment of CNS metastases, resulting in neurologic stability and a negative computed tomography (CT) scan.

*Risk-benefit should be considered when the following medical problems exist:*
Autoimmune disease, including autoimmune thyroiditis
    (aldesleukin-associated hypothyroidism may be an autoimmune effect; autoimmune thyroiditis may be exacerbated)
» Bone marrow depression
» Cardiac function impairment, history of, even if function tests are normal
    (may be exacerbated)
» Hepatic function impairment
    (may be exacerbated)
Hypothyroidism, uncontrolled
    (aldesleukin can cause hypothyroidism; no problems are anticipated in patients who are euthyroid as a result of thyroid hormone replacement therapy)
» Infection
    (should be treated before initiation of aldesleukin therapy)
» Mental status impairment
    (may be exacerbated)
Psoriasis
    (may be exacerbated)

» Pulmonary function impairment, history of, even if function tests are normal
    (may be exacerbated)
» Renal function impairment
    (reduced elimination of aldesleukin, which may result in increased toxicity; impairment may be exacerbated by aldesleukin; patients with nephrectomy are eligible for high-dose aldesleukin therapy if their serum creatinine concentrations are less than or equal to 1.5 mg per deciliter)
» Seizure disorder, history of
    (aldesleukin may cause seizures)
» Sensitivity to aldesleukin
» Caution should be used also in patients who have had previous cytotoxic drug therapy or radiation therapy.

## Patient monitoring
The following are especially important in patient monitoring (other tests may be warranted in some patients, depending on condition; » = major clinical significance):
» Body weight and
» Electrolytes, serum and
» Vital signs, including temperature, pulse, blood pressure, and respiratory rate
    (recommended daily; if blood pressure decreases to less than 90 mm Hg, constant cardiac rhythm monitoring, hourly vital signs, and central venous pressure [CVP] checks are recommended; if an abnormal complex or rhythm is seen, performance of an ECG and determination of cardiac enzymes are recommended)
» Cardiac function, including thallium stress test
    (determination recommended prior to initiation of therapy; ejection fraction should be normal and wall function unimpaired; in patients with minor wall motion abnormalities of questionable significance suggested by the thallium stress test, a stress echocardiogram to document normal wall motion and exclude significant coronary disease may be useful; during treatment, cardiac function should be assessed daily by clinical examination and assessment of vital signs, adding ECG examination and creatine kinase [CK] evaluation for patients exhibiting signs or symptoms of chest pain, murmurs, gallops, irregular rhythm, or palpitations; a repeat thallium stress test is recommended if there is evidence of cardiac ischemia or congestive heart failure; use of a cardiac monitor is recommended if patients require pressor support)
» Hematocrit or hemoglobin and
» Leukocyte count, total and, if appropriate, differential and
» Platelet count
    (determinations recommended prior to initiation of therapy and at periodic intervals during therapy; frequency varies according to clinical state, agent, dose, and other agents being used concurrently)
» Hepatic function and
» Renal function
    (determinations recommended prior to initiation of therapy and daily during therapy)
» Pulmonary function, including arterial blood gases
    (determination recommended prior to initiation of therapy; adequate pulmonary function, as defined by FEV₁ of greater than 2 liters or 75% or more of that predicted for height and age, should be present; during treatment, pulmonary function should be routinely monitored by clinical examination, assessment of vital signs, and pulse oximetry, adding arterial blood gas determination for patients exhibiting dyspnea or clinical signs of respiratory impairment [tachypnea or rales])
Thyroid function
    (determinations recommended at periodic intervals during therapy)

# Side/Adverse Effects

Note: High-dose aldesleukin causes frequent, often serious, and sometimes fatal toxicity. Fatalities have occurred as a result of hepatic or renal failure, cardiac arrest, intestinal perforation, malignant hyperthermia, pulmonary edema, respiratory failure or arrest, pulmonary embolism, stroke, or severe depression leading to suicide.

Toxicity of aldesleukin is dose-related and schedule-dependent. Incidence of toxicity is probably increased in patients with a poor initial performance status.

Patient tolerance to interleukin-2 toxicity has been reported to decline with successive courses.

Most side/adverse effects are reversible within 2 or 3 days after aldesleukin is discontinued. However, permanent damage may result from myocardial infarction, bowel perforation or infarction, and gangrene.

Aldesleukin causes a dose-related capillary leak syndrome (CLS) as a result of increased capillary permeability, leading to extravasation of plasma proteins and fluid into the extravascular space and contributing to loss of vascular resistance. It is believed that hypotension and reduced organ perfusion that occur as a result of CLS are at least partially responsible for many of the toxicities of aldesleukin, including cardiac arrhythmias (supraventricular and ventricular), angina, myocardial infarction, respiratory insufficiency requiring intubation, gastrointestinal bleeding or infarction, renal insufficiency, and some mental status changes. The effects of CLS may be severe or fatal. CLS begins immediately after initiation of treatment, resulting initially, in most patients, in a decline in mean arterial blood pressure within 2 to 12 hours. Clinically significant hypotension (systolic blood pressure below 90 millimeters of mercury [mm Hg] or a 20 mm Hg decline from baseline systolic pressure) and hypoperfusion will occur with continued therapy. Protein and fluid extravasation will also cause edema and effusions; some patients may develop ascites or pleural effusions. Recovery from CLS begins soon after the end of aldesleukin therapy. Usually within a few hours, blood pressure rises, organ perfusion is restored, and resorption of extravasated fluid and protein begins.

In addition to CLS, other possible causes of interleukin-2 toxicity include growth of lymphocytes in visceral organs, which has been described in animal toxicology studies, and stimulation of secretion of other cytokines (e.g., tumor necrosis factor [TNF]) by cells of the immune system. For example, TNF and interleukin-1 secretion may be responsible for hemodynamic effects, which resemble septic shock.

Intravenous or subcutaneous aldesleukin administration frequently results in formation of low titers of non-neutralizing anti-interleukin-2 antibodies. Neutralizing antibodies have been detected in less than 1% of patients treated with aldesleukin. Evidence to date does not appear to indicate that antibody formation impairs response to aldesleukin.

It has been postulated that some toxicities (e.g., hypothyroidism, dermatologic effects) indicate a possible autoimmune effect of interleukin-2.

Hemodynamic and cardiac changes (e.g., peripheral vascular resistance, blood pressure, stroke index, left ventricular stroke volume, heart rate, ECG, creatine kinase) usually return to normal within a few days after interleukin-2 is discontinued.

The following side/adverse effects have been selected on the basis of their potential clinical significance (possible signs and symptoms in parentheses where appropriate)—not necessarily inclusive:

## Those indicating need for medical attention
Incidence more frequent

*Anemia* (asymptomatic); *arrhythmias, especially sinus tachycardia* (usually asymptomatic; less frequently, fast or irregular heartbeat); *diarrhea; dizziness; edema, including peripheral edema with symptomatic nerve or vessel compression* (tingling of hands or feet); *eosinophilia; fever and/or chills; hepatotoxicity* (usually asymptomatic; seen as changes on hepatic function tests that are attributable to severe cholestasis; less frequently, yellow eyes and skin); *hypotension* (usually asymptomatic; less frequently, faintness); *hypothyroidism* (usually asymptomatic; rarely, changes in menstrual periods; clumsiness; coldness; dry, puffy skin; headache; listlessness; muscle aches; sleepiness; tiredness; weakness; goiter [swelling in the front of the neck]); *infection* (fever or chills); *leukopenia* (usually asymptomatic; less frequently, fever or chills; cough or hoarseness; lower back or side pain; painful or difficult urination); *lymphocytosis; nausea and vomiting; neuropsychiatric effects, including mental status changes* (agitation; confusion; mental depression; drowsiness; unusual tiredness); *pulmonary toxicity, including pulmonary congestion, pulmonary edema, pleural effusion* (shortness of breath); *renal toxicity, including oliguria and anuria* (unusual decrease in urination); *stomatitis* (sores in mouth and on lips); *thrombocytopenia* (usually asymptomatic; less frequently, unusual bleeding or bruising; black, tarry stools; blood in urine or stools; pinpoint red spots on skin); *weight gain of 5 to 10 pounds or more*

Note: *Anemia* usually requires blood transfusions.

Supraventricular *arrhythmias* usually resolve after treatment has ended. Potentially fatal ventricular arrhythmias have been reported.

*Diarrhea* occurs in most patients. Severe diarrhea can lead to hypokalemia or acidosis.

*Dizziness* is a neurologic effect.

*Eosinophilia*, which can be pronounced, tends to occur near the end of therapy, during the first 5 days after treatment. Eosinophilic myocarditis has been reported.

*Fever, chills, rigors,* or *malaise* usually occurs within hours after administration.

*Hepatic* function tests usually return to normal within several days after treatment has ended.

Mean arterial pressure begins to decline within 2 to 12 hours after initiation of therapy, necessitating intravenous administration of fluids (to correct hypovolemia) and pressors (to maintain blood pressure and perfusion). *Hypotension* is accompanied by an increase in heart rate.

*Hypothyroidism* may require thyroid replacement therapy. A hyperthyroid phase may precede hypothyroidism. Thyroid function tests usually return to normal within a few days or weeks after therapy, although effects have been reported to persist for several months. In some patients, presence of antibodies to thyroglobulin suggests exacerbation or initiation of autoimmune thyroiditis.

Impaired neutrophil function (reduced chemotaxis) may also increase the risk of disseminated *infection*. Infection may include urinary tract, injection site, or central venous catheter tip infections, as well as bacterial endocarditis, phlebitis, or sepsis. Positive cultures may be found without symptomatic infection. Infections are usually gram-positive, although gram-negative infection has also been reported. Early signs and symptoms of sepsis (e.g., hypotension) may be masked by prophylactic medication for systemic effects.

*Mental status changes*, which appear after several days of treatment, may be signs of bacteremia or early bacterial sepsis, as well as cerebral edema or immune effects. Changes due solely to aldesleukin are usually reversible on withdrawal, although they may continue to progress for several days before recovery begins.

*Nausea and vomiting* occur in most patients.

*Oliguria* is accompanied by reversible prerenal azotemia (increased serum creatinine and BUN), hypoalbuminemia, and proteinuria. Fractional sodium excretion is also decreased. In a small percentage of patients, *renal toxicity* may require dialysis. Renal function tests usually return to normal within 7 to 30 days, although recovery may sometimes be prolonged or incomplete. Interstitial nephritis and glomerulonephritis have been reported.

*Stomatitis* may be severe enough to necessitate a liquid diet.

*Weight gain* may be 10% or more of pretreatment body weight. Reversal of weight gain may take up to 1 to 2 weeks after therapy, as patients diurese fluid.

Incidence less frequent

*Ascites* (bloating and stomach pain); *aphasia* (trouble in speaking); *exfoliative dermatitis* (blisters on skin); *gastrointestinal bleeding* (blood in stools; bloody vomit); *glossitis* (redness, swelling, and soreness of tongue); *intestinal ischemic necrosis or perforation* (bloody vomit; severe stomach pain); *myocardial ischemia or myocardial infarction* (chest pain); *pulmonary toxicity, including respiratory failure, tachypnea, and wheezing* (rapid breathing; severe shortness of breath); *sensory neurologic effects* (blurred or double vision; loss of taste)

Note: *Exfoliative dermatitis* can be fatal. Life-threatening bullous drug eruptions, resembling toxic epidermal necrolysis, have also been reported.

In a small percentage of patients, *gastrointestinal bleeding* may require surgery.

Frequency of *myocardial ischemia or infarction* can be reduced by careful patient screening before interleukin-2 treatment and monitoring during treatment.

Evidence of *pulmonary* infiltration may become apparent by the fourth day of therapy and usually resolves within a few weeks after therapy. Intubation may be required for *respiratory failure*.

*Vision* problems usually begin shortly after interleukin-2 administration and are reversible, although they may persist for several weeks.

Incidence rare

*Cardiovascular effects, other, including congestive heart failure, endocarditis, myocarditis, cardiomyopathy, gangrene, stroke, and thrombosis* (swelling of feet or lower legs; sudden weakness or inability to move); *coma; injection site reaction* (pain or redness at site of injection); *pericardial effusion; seizures*

**Those indicating need for medical attention only if they continue or are bothersome**
Incidence more frequent
   *Dry skin; loss of appetite; macular erythema* (skin rash or redness with burning or itching, followed by peeling); *malaise* (unusual feeling of discomfort or illness); *weakness*

   Note: *Macular erythema*, which seems to be an immunological effect, begins 2 to 3 days after initiation of treatment and usually begins to resolve, with desquamation, within 2 to 3 days after interleukin-2 is discontinued. Peeling of skin is most pronounced on palms and soles; skin appears normal within 2 to 3 weeks. It recurs with each cycle. Other dermatological effects, including angioedema, urticaria, and erythema nodosum, have also been reported.

Incidence less frequent
   *Arthralgia or myalgia* (joint pain; muscle pain); *constipation; headache*

## Overdose

For more information on the management of overdose or unintentional ingestion, **contact a Poison Control Center** (see *Poison Control Center Listing*).

### Treatment of overdose
Treatment consists of withdrawal of aldesleukin and supportive therapy. Life-threatening toxicities have been ameliorated by the intravenous administration of dexamethasone; however, this may result in loss of aldesleukin's therapeutic effect.

## Patient Consultation

As an aid to patient consultation, refer to *Advice for the Patient, Aldesleukin (Systemic)*.

In providing consultation, consider emphasizing the following selected information (» = major clinical significance):

**Before using this medication**
» Conditions affecting use, especially:
   Sensitivity to aldesleukin
   Pregnancy—Use not recommended; advisability of using contraception; telling physician immediately if pregnancy is suspected
   Breast-feeding—Not recommended because of risk of serious side effects
   Other medications, especially other bone marrow depressants, other cardiotoxic medications, systemic glucocorticoids, other hepatotoxic medications, other hypotension-producing medications, other nephrotoxic medications, or other cytotoxic drug or radiation therapy
   Other medical problems, especially cardiac function impairment, organ allograft, pulmonary function impairment, hepatic function impairment, infection, mental status impairment, renal function impairment, or history of seizure disorder

**Proper use of this medication**
» Proper dosing

**Precautions while using this medication**
*Caution if impaired neutrophil function or thrombocytopenia occurs*
» Avoiding exposure to persons with bacterial infections, especially during periods of low blood counts; checking with physician immediately if fever or chills, cough or hoarseness, lower back or side pain, or painful or difficult urination occur
» Checking with physician immediately if unusual bleeding or bruising; black, tarry stools; blood in urine or stools; or pinpoint red spots on skin occur
   Caution in use of regular toothbrush, dental floss, or toothpick; physician, dentist, or nurse may suggest alternatives; checking with physician before having dental work done
   Not touching eyes or inside of nose unless hands washed immediately before
   Using caution to avoid accidental cuts with use of sharp objects such as safety razor or fingernail or toenail cutters
   Avoiding contact sports or other situations where bruising or injury could occur

**Side/adverse effects**
   Importance of discussing possible life-threatening toxicity with physician
   Signs of potential side effects, especially arrhythmias, diarrhea, dizziness, edema, fever and/or chills, jaundice, faintness, hypothyroidism, infection, leukopenia, nausea and vomiting, mental status

changes, pulmonary toxicity, renal toxicity, stomatitis, thrombocytopenia, weight gain, ascites, aphasia, exfoliative dermatitis, gastrointestinal bleeding, glossitis, intestinal ischemic necrosis or perforation, myocardial ischemia or myocardial infarction, blurred or double vision, loss of taste, other cardiovascular effects, injection site reaction, and seizures
   Asymptomatic side effects, including anemia, cardiotoxicity, hepatotoxicity, hypotension, hypothyroidism, eosinophilia, leukopenia, renal toxicity, and thrombocytopenia
   Physician or nurse can help in dealing with side effects

## General Dosing Information

Patients receiving aldesleukin should be under supervision of a physician experienced in cancer chemotherapy.

It is recommended that high-dose aldesleukin be administered in a tertiary care hospital setting, with an intensive care facility and specialists skilled in cardiopulmonary and intensive care medicine readily available.

Dosage of interleukin-2 is usually expressed in units of activity in promoting proliferation in a responsive cell line; conversion to Units from mg of protein varies somewhat, depending on the source of interleukin-2. In the literature, dosage of aldesleukin is expressed in terms of Cetus units; dosage of teceleukin, another form of recombinant interleukin-2, is expressed in Roche units or Nutley units. However, strength and dosage of commercially available aldesleukin are expressed in International Units (IU). Conversion to IU is as follows:
   1 Cetus Unit = 6 International Units.
   1 Roche Unit or Nutley Unit = 3 International Units.
In addition:
   18 million IU = 1.1 mg protein.

It is recommended that acetaminophen and a nonsteroidal anti-inflammatory drug (NSAID) such as indomethacin be administered prior to initiation of aldesleukin therapy, to reduce fever. The increased risk of nephrotoxicity with concurrent use of indomethacin must be kept in mind. Meperidine may be added to control the rigors associated with fever.

Ranitidine or cimetidine may be given for prophylaxis of gastrointestinal irritation and bleeding.

Dosage adjustment of high-dose aldesleukin in response to toxicity is accomplished by withholding the medication rather than by decreasing the dosage. Toxicity usually reverses promptly (within several hours) on withdrawal of aldesleukin. It is recommended that aldesleukin be held and restarted according to the following guidelines:
• Atrial fibrillation, supraventricular tachycardia, or bradycardia that requires treatment or is recurrent or persistent—Hold dose. Obtain EKG and cardiac enzymes. Subsequent doses may be given if patient is asymptomatic with full recovery to normal sinus rhythm.
• Systolic blood pressure less than 90 mm Hg with increasing requirement for pressors—Hold dose. Subsequent doses may be given if systolic blood pressure becomes greater than or equal to 90 mm Hg and stable, or requirements for pressors are improving.
• Any ECG change consistent with myocardial infarction or ischemia with or without chest pain; suspicion of cardiac ischemia—Hold dose. Subsequent doses may be given if patient is asymptomatic, myocardial infarction has been ruled out, or clinical suspicion of angina and/or myocarditis is low.
• Oxygen saturation of less than 90% with 2 liters $O_2$ by nasal prongs—Hold dose. Subsequent doses may be given if $O_2$ saturation becomes greater than or equal to 90% with 2 liters $O_2$ by nasal prongs.
• Mental status changes, including moderate confusion or agitation—Hold dose. Subsequent doses may be given if mental status changes are completely resolved.
• Sepsis syndrome, where patient is clinically unstable—Hold dose. Subsequent doses may be given if sepsis syndrome has resolved, patient is clinically stable, and infection is under treatment.
• Serum creatinine greater than or equal to 5.0 mg per deciliter or serum creatinine of any level in the presence of severe volume overload, acidosis, or hyperkalemia—Hold dose. Subsequent doses may be given if serum creatinine is less than 4 mg per deciliter and fluid and electrolyte status is stable.
• Signs of hepatic failure including encephalopathy, increasing ascites, liver pain, hypoglycemia—Discontinue all treatment for that course. Consider starting a new course of treatment at least 7 weeks after cessation of adverse event and hospital discharge if all signs of hepatic failure have resolved.
• Stool guaiac repeatedly greater than 3-4+—Hold dose. Subsequent doses may be given if stool guaiac is negative.
• Bullous dermatitis or marked worsening of pre-existing skin condition—Hold dose. Subsequent doses may be given upon resolution of all signs of bullous dermatitis. Avoid topical steroid therapy.

High-dose aldesleukin therapy should also be withheld for oliguria unresponsive to fluid replacement or diuretics and for respiratory distress.

It is recommended that aldesleukin be permanently discontinued in patients who experienced the following toxicities in an earlier course of therapy:
- Sustained ventricular tachycardia (5 beats or more)
- Cardiac rhythm disturbances not controlled or unresponsive to management
- Recurrent chest pain with ECG changes consistent with angina or myocardial infarction
- Pericardial tamponade
- Intubation required for more than 72 hours
- Renal function impairment requiring dialysis for more than 72 hours
- Coma or toxic psychosis lasting more than 48 hours
- Repetitive or difficult to control seizures
- Bowel ischemia/perforation
- Gastrointestinal bleeding requiring surgery.

Special precautions are recommended in patients who develop thrombocytopenia as a result of administration of aldesleukin. These may include extreme care in performing invasive procedures; regular inspection of intravenous sites, skin (including perirectal area), and mucous membrane surfaces for signs of bleeding or bruising; limiting frequency of venipuncture and avoiding intramuscular injections; testing urine, emesis, stool, and secretions for occult blood; care in use of regular toothbrushes, dental floss, toothpicks, safety razors, and fingernail and toenail cutters; avoiding constipation; and using caution to prevent falls and other injuries. Such patients should avoid alcohol and aspirin intake because of the risk of gastrointestinal bleeding. Platelet transfusions may be required.

Patients should be observed carefully for signs of infection. Antibiotic support may be required. Because of the risk of infection, it is recommended that all patients with indwelling central lines receive antibiotic prophylaxis against *Staphylococcus aureus*, along with meticulous catheter care.

### For treatment of adverse effects

Antiemetics and antidiarrheals may be given as needed to treat gastrointestinal effects. They usually are discontinued 12 hours after the last dose of aldesleukin.

Hydroxyzine or diphenhydramine and emollients may be used to prevent or control symptoms from pruritic rashes and are continued until resolution of pruritus. Some clinicians recommend that use of topical or systemic corticosteroids be avoided because of the risk of diminishing aldesleukin's therapeutic effect.

Supraventricular arrhythmias usually respond to conventional treatment (digoxin or verapamil).

Debilitating mental status changes may respond to low doses of haloperidol.

For capillary leak syndrome—

Capillary leak syndrome (CLS) is initially managed with careful monitoring of the patient's fluid and organ perfusion status by means of frequent determination of blood pressure and pulse and monitoring of organ function, including assessment of mental status and urine output. Hypovolemia is assessed by catheterization and central pressure monitoring. Because flexibility in fluid and pressor management is essential for maintaining organ perfusion and blood pressure, extreme caution is recommended in treating patients with fixed requirements for large volumes of fluid (e.g., patients with hypercalcemia).

Hypovolemia is managed by administration of intravenous fluids, either colloids or crystalloids, which are usually given when the central venous pressure (CVP) is below 3 to 4 mm $H_2O$. Although correction of hypovolemia may require large volumes of fluids, caution is necessary because of the risk that unrestrained fluid administration may exacerbate problems associated with concomitant edema or effusions. A diuretic such as furosemide may be administered to reduce edema or pulmonary infiltration.

Management of edema, ascites, or pleural effusions depends on a careful balancing of the effects of fluid shifts so that neither the consequences of hypovolemia (e.g., impaired organ perfusion) nor the consequences of fluid accumulation (e.g., pulmonary edema) exceed the patient's tolerance.

Early administration of dopamine (1 to 5 mcg per kg of body weight [mcg/kg] per minute), before the onset of hypotension, may help maintain organ perfusion, particularly to the kidney, and preserve urine output. Weight and urine output should be carefully monitored. If this dose of dopamine fails to sustain organ perfusion and blood pressure, some clinicians increase the dose of dopamine to 6 to 10 mcg/kg per minute or add

phenylephrine (1 to 5 mcg/kg per minute) to the lower dose of dopamine. However, prolonged use of pressors, either individually or in combination, at relatively high doses may be associated with cardiac rhythm disturbances.

If organ perfusion cannot be maintained (demonstrated by altered mental status, reduced urine output, reduction in blood pressure below 90 mm Hg, or onset of cardiac arrhythmias), it is recommended that subsequent doses of aldesleukin be withheld until recovery of organ perfusion and return of systolic pressure to above 90 mm Hg.

Once recovery from CLS begins and blood pressure has normalized, use of diuretics may hasten recovery in patients in whom there has been excessive weight gain or edema formation, particularly if associated with shortness of breath from pulmonary congestion.

Oxygen is administered if pulmonary function monitoring confirms that $P_a O_2$ is decreased.

For relief of anemia and to ensure maximal oxygen carrying capacity, administration of packed red cells may be used.

To resolve absolute thrombocytopenia and reduce the risk of gastrointestinal bleeding, platelet transfusions may be given.

## Parenteral Dosage Forms
### ALDESLEUKIN FOR INJECTION

**Usual adult dose**

Renal carcinoma, metastatic—

High dose therapy: Intravenous infusion (over fifteen minutes), 600,000 International Units (IU) per kg of body weight (0.037 mg per kg of body weight) every eight hours for a total of fourteen doses. Following nine days of rest, the schedule is repeated for another fourteen doses, for a maximum of twenty-eight doses per course.

Note: Although aldesleukin has been given in lower doses and by other routes (e.g., continuous intravenous infusion, subcutaneous) by some investigators to reduce toxicity, relative efficacy of these regimens compared to the high-dose regimen has not been established.

Although glass bottles and plastic (polyvinyl chloride) bags have been used in clinical trials with comparable results, the manufacturer recommends that plastic bags be used as the dilution container since experimental studies suggest that use of plastic containers results in more consistent drug delivery.

Use of in-line filters is not recommended during aldesleukin administration because of the risk of adsorption of aldesleukin to the filter.

If the aldesleukin solution has been refrigerated, it should be brought to room temperature before administration.

Each treatment period should be separated by a rest period of at least seven weeks from the date of hospital discharge.

Dose modification in response to toxicity is accomplished by holding or interrupting a dose rather than reducing the dose. Some toxicities necessitate permanent withdrawal of aldesleukin. For recommendations concerning toxicities requiring either permanent withdrawal or holding of a dose, see *General Dosing Information*.

**Usual pediatric dose**

Safety and efficacy have not been established.

**Size(s) usually available**

U.S.—

22 million IU (1.3 mg) (Rx) [*Proleukin* (mannitol; sodium dododecyl sulfate; monobasic sodium phosphate; dibasic sodium phosphate)].

Canada—

Not commercially available.

**Packaging and storage**

Store between 2 and 8 °C (36 and 46 °F), unless otherwise specified by manufacturer. Protect from freezing.

**Preparation of dosage form**

Aldesleukin for injection is reconstituted for intravenous or subcutaneous administration by adding 1.2 mL of sterile water for injection to the vial (directing the diluent at the side of the vial and swirling the contents gently to avoid excess foaming), to produce a clear and colorless to slightly yellow solution containing 18 million Units (1.1) mg per mL. The vial should not be shaken.

For administration by rapid intravenous infusion, the reconstituted solution is further diluted in 50 mL of 5% dextrose injection.

**Stability**

Reconstituted and diluted solutions should be stored in the refrigerator, since the product contains no preservative. Reconstituted solutions should be used within forty-eight hours. Any unused portion should be discarded.

### Incompatibilities
Bacteriostatic water for injection or 0.9% sodium chloride injection should not be used for reconstitution because of increased aggregation.

### Auxiliary labeling
- Do not shake.
- Do not freeze.

## Selected Bibliography
Kintzel PE, Calis KA. Recombinant interleukin-2: a biological response modifier. Clin Pharm 1991 Feb; 10: 110-28.

Williams TM, Fox KR, Kant JA. Interleukin-2: basic biology and therapeutic use. Hematol Pathol 1991; 5 (2): 45-55.
Rosenberg SA. The immunotherapy and gene therapy of cancer. J Clin Oncol 1992 Feb; 10: 180-99.

Developed: 09/15/93
Interim revision: 08/08/94

---

**ALFACALCIDOL**—See *Vitamin D and Analogs (Systemic)*

---

**ALFENTANIL**—See *Fentanyl and Derivatives (Systemic)*

---

# ALGLUCERASE   Systemic

VA CLASSIFICATION (Primary): BL900
Note: For a listing of dosage forms and brand names by country availability, see *Dosage Forms* section(s). For a listing of brand names for the articles in this monograph, refer to the General Index.

## Category
Enzyme (glucocerebrosidase) replenisher.

## Indications
### Accepted
Gaucher's disease, due to deficiency of glucocerebrosidase (treatment)—
Alglucerase is indicated as enzyme replacement therapy in Type I Gaucher's disease, where glucocerebrosidase is absent or deficient, resulting in an accumulation of glycolipids in the spleen, liver, and bone marrow. Symptoms requiring treatment include moderate to severe anemia, thrombocytopenia with bleeding tendency, bone disease, and/or significant hepatomegaly or splenomegaly.

## Pharmacology/Pharmacokinetics
### Physicochemical characteristics
Source—Alglucerase is prepared from pooled human placental tissue
Molecular weight—59,300.

### Mechanism of action/Effect
Alglucerase catalyzes the hydrolysis of the glycolipid glucocerebroside to glucose and ceramide as part of the normal degradation pathway for membrane lipids.

### Distribution
$Vol_D$—49.4 to 282.1 mL per kilogram.

### Half-life
Elimination—3.6 to 10.4 minutes.

### Time to peak concentration
60 minutes following an intravenous infusion of 0.6 to 234 Units per kilogram of body weight over 4 hours.

## Precautions to Consider
### Pregnancy/Reproduction
Pregnancy—Studies have not been done in humans.
Studies have not been done in animals.
FDA Pregnancy Category C.

### Breast-feeding
It is not known whether alglucerase is distributed into breast milk.

### Pediatrics
Appropriate studies performed to date have not demonstrated pediatrics-specific problems that would limit the usefulness of alglucerase in children.

### Geriatrics
No information is available on the relationship of age to the effects of alglucerase in geriatric patients.

### Medical considerations/Contraindications
The medical considerations/contraindications included here have been selected on the basis of their potential clinical significance (reasons given in parentheses where appropriate)—not necessarily inclusive (» = major clinical significance).

*Except under special circumstances, this medication should not be used when the following medical problem exists:*
» Sensitivity to alglucerase

### Patient monitoring
The following may be especially important in patient monitoring (other tests may be warranted in some patients, depending on condition; » = major clinical significance):
Acid phosphatase, serum
  (determinations recommended every 2 months by some clinicians; values should decrease with alglucerase treatment)
Chemistry panel
  (some clinicians may recommend monitoring every six months)
Hemoglobin and
Platelet count
  (recommended monthly to assess effectiveness of alglucerase therapy; if hemoglobin falls below 7 grams% and platelet count is under 50,000 then monitoring at 2-week intervals may be recommended; both values should increase with alglucerase treatment)
Liver size and
Spleen size
  (recommended every 6 months to assess effectiveness of therapy; liver and spleen should decrease in size with alglucerase treatment)

## Side/Adverse Effects
Note: Alglucerase is prepared from pooled human placental tissue collected from selected donors. Each lot is tested for hepatitis B surface antigen and antigens of the human immunodeficiency virus (HIV). The risk of contamination from slow-acting or latent viruses is believed to be remote but has not been tested.

The following side/adverse effects have been selected on the basis of their potential clinical significance (possible signs and symptoms in parentheses where appropriate)—not necessarily inclusive:

**Those indicating need for medical attention only if they continue or are bothersome**
Incidence less frequent
  *Abdominal discomfort; chills; fever; nausea and vomiting; swelling at injection site*

## Patient Consultation
As an aid to patient consultation, refer to *Advice for the Patient, Alglucerase (Systemic)*.

In providing consultation, consider emphasizing the following selected information (» = major clinical significance):

**Before using this medication**
» Conditions affecting use, especially:
    Sensitivity to alglucerase

**Proper use of this medication**
  Does not cure, but helps control Gaucher's disease; possible need for lifelong therapy; serious consequences of untreated Gaucher's disease
» Proper dosing

**Precautions while receiving this medication**
  Importance of monitoring by the physician

## Parenteral Dosage Forms

### ALGLUCERASE FOR INJECTION—CONCENTRATE

#### Usual adult and adolescent dose

Enzyme replenisher—Intravenous infusion, the individualized dose given over one to two hours. The initial dose may be as little as 1.15 Units per kilogram of body weight three times a week up to as much as 60 Units per kilogram of body weight as frequently as once a week or as infrequently as every four weeks. Dosage may be raised or lowered at 3- to 6-month intervals while monitoring response parameters.

Note: The manufacturer's product labeling recommends an initial dose of up to 60 Units per kilogram of body weight. More recent and ongoing trials are looking at low-dose treatment regimens. For example, one small clinical trial found that most patients responded to an initial dose as small as 1.15 Units per kilogram of body weight. Several additional trials found that most patients responded to an initial dose of 2.3 Units per kilogram of body weight. Patients vary considerably in their response to alglucerase therapy; therefore, the dose must be individualized. Varying degrees of clinical responses have been observed with all dosage regimens tested. Patients receiving low-dose alglucerase therapy may respond more slowly, but response may be slow regardless of dose. The National Institutes of Health Technology Assessment Conference on Gaucher Disease recommends that the goal of initial and maintenance alglucerase therapy is sustained benefit using the lowest possible dose.

#### Usual pediatric dose

See *Usual adult and adolescent dose.*

### Strength(s) usually available

U.S.—
    10 Units per mL (Rx) [*Ceredase*].
    80 Units per mL (Rx) [*Ceredase*].
Canada—
    80 Units per mL (Rx) [*Ceredase*].

Note: Alglucerase is a monomeric glycoprotein of 497 amino acids with carbohydrates making up approximately 6% of the molecule. The product contains 1% human albumin.

### Packaging and storage

Store at 4 °C (39 °F).

### Preparation of dosage form

On the day of use, the appropriate patient dose is diluted with preservative-free normal saline to a final volume not to exceed 100 mL.

### Stability

Alglucerase does not contain a preservative. The product information for alglucerase states that the diluted product is stable for up to 18 hours at a temperature of 2 to 8° C; however, some clinicians store the diluted product at 4° C for up to 2 weeks. Do not use any bottles that are discolored or contain particulate matter.

### Auxiliary labeling

• Do not shake.

### Additional information

Shaking alglucerase may denature the glycoprotein, rendering it inactive. Use of a saline diluent that contains a preservative may inactivate the enzyme.

Revised: 01/18/93
Interim revision: 09/15/95; 09/05/96

---

# ALLOPURINOL   Systemic

VA CLASSIFICATION (Primary/Secondary): MS400/GU900
Note: For a listing of dosage forms and brand names by country availability, see *Dosage Forms* section(s). For a listing of brand names for the articles in this monograph, refer to the General Index.

---

## Category

Antihyperuricemic; antigout agent; antiurolithic (uric acid calculi; calcium oxalate calculi)..

Note: Antihyperuricemic is the basic category; the other categories are specific categories of use.

## Indications

Note: Bracketed information in the *Indications* section refers to uses that are not included in U.S. product labeling.

### Accepted

Gouty arthritis, chronic (treatment)—Allopurinol is indicated for the long-term management of hyperuricemia associated with primary or secondary gout. The aim of allopurinol therapy is to reduce the number of acute gout attacks and decrease the risk of uric acid calculi and urate nephropathy in patients with chronic gout.

Allopurinol is recommended for patients in whom treatment with uricosuric antigout agents such as probenecid or sulfinpyrazone would be ineffective or inadvisable (e.g., patients who are hyperuricemic as a result of overproduction of urate, patients with extensive tophi or who are otherwise at risk for urate nephropathy, and patients with moderate to severe renal function impairment). Both allopurinol and the uricosuric antigout agents are effective in patients whose 24-hour renal excretion of uric acid is 800 mg (4.8 mmol) or less, i.e., individuals who are hyperuricemic as a result of underexcretion of uric acid. However, the uricosuric agents are less toxic than allopurinol and should be considered for use when appropriate.

Allopurinol has no anti-inflammatory activity and should not be used for the treatment of acute attacks of gouty arthritis. An anti-inflammatory agent, preferably a nonsteroidal anti-inflammatory drug (NSAID) or a corticosteroid (preferably via intrasynovial injection, when feasible), should be used to treat acute attacks. Also, initiation of antihyperuricemic therapy may lead to fluctuations in urate concentration that may result in prolongation of an acute attack or initiation of new attacks. The patient should be receiving appropriate anti-inflammatory therapy when allopurinol treatment is initiated.

Hyperuricemia (prophylaxis and treatment)—Allopurinol is indicated to control hyperuricemia secondary to blood dyscrasias, such as polycythemia vera or myeloid metaplasia, or their treatment. It is also indicated to prevent or treat hyperuricemia secondary to tumor lysis induced by cancer chemotherapy with cytotoxic antineoplastic agents or radiation therapy in patients with leukemias, lymphomas, or other neoplastic disease. [Allopurinol is also used to treat hyperuricemia secondary to the neoplastic disease itself.] Allopurinol prevents complications of hyperuricemia (e.g., acute uric acid nephropathy or renal calculi, tissue urate deposition, or gouty arthritis) in these patients. However, allopurinol may increase the toxicity of several antineoplastic agents, and some clinicians have questioned its routine administration during cancer chemotherapy.

[Allopurinol is also used to control hyperuricemia in patients with Lesch-Nyhan syndrome. However, it does not improve neurologic or behavioral abnormalities or affect the course of the disease in these patients.]

Nephropathy, uric acid (prophylaxis and treatment)—Allopurinol is indicated in the treatment of primary or secondary uric acid nephropathy (with or without accompanying symptoms of gouty arthritis) to prevent progression of the condition. However, this medicine will not reverse severe renal damage that has already occurred. Allopurinol is also indicated to prevent uric acid nephropathy in certain patients as described under *Hyperuricemia,* above.

Renal calculi, uric acid (prophylaxis)—Allopurinol is indicated to prevent recurrence of uric acid stone formation in patients with a history of recurrent uric acid calculi. It is also indicated to prevent uric acid calculi in certain other patients as described under *Hyperuricemia,* above.

Renal calculi, calcium oxalate, recurrence (prophylaxis)—Allopurinol is indicated to prevent recurrence of calcium stone formation in patients with a history of recurrent calcium oxalate calculi associated with hyperuricosuria (i.e., uric acid excretion 800 mg [4.8 mmol] per day in males or 750 mg [4.5 mmol] per day in females).

### Unaccepted

*Allopurinol is not recommended for treatment of asymptomatic hyperuricemia* associated with conditions or induced by medications other than those described above.

# Pharmacology/Pharmacokinetics

## Physicochemical characteristics
Chemical group—A structural analog of hypoxanthine.
Molecular weight—136.11.
pKa—10.2.

## Mechanism of action/Effect
Allopurinol and its metabolite, oxipurinol (alloxanthine), decrease the production of uric acid by inhibiting the action of xanthine oxidase, the enzyme that converts hypoxanthine to xanthine and xanthine to uric acid. Also, allopurinol increases reutilization of hypoxanthine and xanthine for nucleotide and nucleic acid synthesis via an action involving the enzyme hypoxanthine-guanine phosphoribosyltransferase (HGPRTase). The resultant increase in nucleotide concentration leads to feedback inhibition of de novo purine synthesis. Allopurinol thereby decreases uric acid concentrations in both serum and urine.

By lowering both serum and urine concentrations of uric acid below its solubility limits, allopurinol prevents or decreases urate deposition, thereby preventing the occurrence or progression of both gouty arthritis and urate nephropathy. In patients with chronic gout, allopurinol may prevent or decrease tophi formation and chronic joint changes, promote resolution of existing urate crystals and deposits, and, after several months of therapy, reduce the frequency of acute gout attacks. Also, reductions in urine urate concentration prevent or decrease the formation of uric acid or calcium oxalate calculi.

## Other actions/effects
Allopurinol inhibits hepatic microsomal enzyme activity.

Allopurinol increases plasma and urine concentrations of xanthine and hypoxanthine. Although the concentrations of these oxypurines usually remain within their solubility limits, xanthine renal stones have been reported very rarely in patients with HGPRTase deficiency or very high pretreatment uric acid concentrations.

## Absorption
About 80 to 90% of a single 300-mg dose is absorbed from the gastro-intestinal tract.

## Protein binding
Neither allopurinol nor its metabolite, oxipurinol, is bound to plasma proteins.

## Biotransformation
Primarily hepatic. About 70% of a dose is metabolized to the active metabolite, oxipurinol. One study indicates that allopurinol may also be taken up by, and metabolized in, red blood cells.

## Half-life
Allopurinol—1 to 3 hours

Oxipurinol—12 to 30 hours (average about 15 hours); may be greatly prolonged in patients with renal function impairment.

## Onset of action
A significant reduction of serum uric acid concentration usually occurs within 2 or 3 days.

Note: In some patients, especially those with severe tophaceous deposits or those who are underexcretors of uric acid, significant reduction of serum and urine uric acid concentrations may be substantially delayed, possibly because of mobilization of urate from existing tissue deposits.

## Time to peak serum concentration
Allopurinol—0.5 to 2 hours following a single 300-mg dose.
Oxipurinol—4.5 to 5 hours

## Peak serum concentration
Following a single 300-mg dose—
Allopurinol: About 2 to 3 mcg per mL (14.7 to 22.05 micromoles/L).
Oxipurinol: About 5 to 6.5 mcg per mL (32.85 to 42.7 micromoles/L); may be increased to 30 to 50 mcg per mL (197.1 to 328.5 micromoles/L) in patients with renal function impairment.

## Time to peak effect
Reduction of serum uric acid concentration to normal range—1 to 3 weeks.

Reduction of frequency of acute gout attacks—Several months of therapy may be required, even though the serum uric acid concentration returns to normal values, possibly because of mobilization and recrystallization of urate as serum concentrations fluctuate.

## Duration of action
The serum uric acid concentration usually returns to the pretreatment value 1 to 2 weeks after discontinuation of therapy.

## Elimination
Renal—Up to 10% of a dose is excreted as unchanged allopurinol and about 70% as oxipurinol.

Fecal—About 20% of a dose.
In dialysis—Both allopurinol and oxipurinol are dialyzable.

# Precautions to Consider

## Pregnancy/Reproduction
Fertility—No impairment of fertility was observed in rats or rabbits given up to 20 times the usual human dose.

Pregnancy—Although adequate and well-controlled studies in humans have not been done, 3 reports indicate no evidence of birth defects in offspring of women receiving allopurinol during pregnancy.

In a study in mice, administration of 100 mg of allopurinol per kg of body weight (mg/kg) intraperitoneally on Day 10 or Day 13 of gestation caused an increased number of fetal deaths; no such effect was seen with a dose of 50 mg/kg. In the same study, 50 or 100 mg/kg caused external fetal malformations when administered intraperitoneally on Day 10 of gestation and skeletal malformations when administered intraperitoneally on Day 13 of gestation. Whether these effects were due to maternal toxicity or a direct effect on the fetus has not been determined. However, other studies in rats and rabbits given up to 20 times the usual human dose have not shown that allopurinol affects the fetus adversely.

FDA Pregnancy Category C.

## Breast-feeding
Allopurinol and oxipurinol are distributed into breast milk. Whether this toxic medication may cause adverse effects in the nursing infant has not been determined. However, problems in humans have not been documented.

## Pediatrics
Appropriate studies performed to date have not demonstrated pediatrics-specific problems that would limit the usefulness of allopurinol in children. However, use of allopurinol in pediatric patients has been limited to children with certain rare inborn errors of purine metabolism or hyperuricemia secondary to a malignancy or cancer therapy.

## Geriatrics
No information is available on the relationship of age to the effects of allopurinol in geriatric patients. However, elderly patients are more likely to have age-related renal function impairment, which may require adjustment of the dose and/or dosing interval in patients receiving allopurinol.

## Drug interactions and/or related problems
The following drug interactions and/or related problems have been selected on the basis of their potential clinical significance (possible mechanism in parentheses where appropriate)—not necessarily inclusive (» = major clinical significance):

Note: Combinations containing any of the following medications, depending on the amount present, may also interact with this medication.

Acidifiers, urinary, such as:
  Ammonium chloride
  Ascorbic acid
  Potassium or sodium phosphate
    (urinary acidification by these medications may increase the possibility of allopurinol-induced xanthine kidney stone formation)

Alcohol or
Diazoxide or
Mecamylamine or
Pyrazinamide
    (these medications may increase serum uric acid concentrations; dosage adjustment of allopurinol may be necessary to control hyperuricemia and gout)

Amoxicillin or
Ampicillin or
Bacampicillin or
Hetacillin
    (concurrent use with allopurinol may significantly increase the possibility of skin rash; however, it has not been established that allopurinol, rather than the presence of hyperuricemia, is responsible for this effect)

» Anticoagulants, coumarin- or indandione-derivative
    (allopurinol may inhibit enzymatic metabolism of the anticoagulant, leading to potentiation of the anticoagulant effect; dosage adjustments based on increased monitoring of prothrombin time may be necessary during and after concurrent use)

Antineoplastics
    (rapidly cytolytic antineoplastic agents may increase serum uric acid concentrations; prophylactic administration of allopurinol may be indicated to prevent complications associated with antineoplastic agent–induced hyperuricemia; also, patients receiving allopu-

rinol to treat pre-existing hyperuricemia or gout may require allopurinol dosage adjustment during and following concurrent therapy with one of these agents)

(concurrent use of allopurinol with cyclophosphamide and possibly other antineoplastic agents may increase the potential for bone marrow depression; although studies of this possibility have reported conflicting results, it is recommended that patients receiving allopurinol concurrently with antineoplastic agents, especially cyclophosphamide, be carefully monitored)

» Azathioprine or
» Mercaptopurine

(allopurinol-induced inhibition of xanthine oxidase decreases metabolism of these medications and may potentiate therapeutic and toxic effects, especially bone marrow depression; the effect on azathioprine metabolism is especially critical in renal transplant patients because of the high risk of oxipurinol accumulation and consequent azathioprine toxicity if the transplanted kidney is rejected; if concurrent use is essential, it is recommended that azathioprine or mercaptopurine dosage be reduced to one-third to one-fourth of the usual dosage, that the patient be carefully monitored, and that subsequent dosage adjustments be based on patient response and evidence of toxicity)

(mercaptopurine may increase serum uric acid concentration in some patients; patients receiving allopurinol to treat pre-existing hyperuricemia or gout may require allopurinol dosage adjustment when mercaptopurine therapy is initiated or discontinued)

Chlorpropamide
(allopurinol may inhibit renal tubular secretion of chlorpropamide; patients receiving the medications concurrently should be monitored for possible increased hypoglycemic effect)

Dacarbazine
(dacarbazine inhibits xanthine oxidase and may cause additive hypouricemic effects when used concurrently with allopurinol)

Diuretics, thiazide
(caution and careful monitoring of the patient are advised when allopurinol and thiazide diuretics are used concurrently, especially in patients with known or possible renal function impairment, because severe hypersensitivity reactions to allopurinol may occur; although it has been suggested that compromised renal function, rather than the combination of medications, may be responsible for the adverse reactions, it has also been proposed that thiazide diuretics may increase serum oxipurinol concentrations by decreasing its renal excretion)

Probenecid
(probenecid increases urinary excretion of oxipurinol; however, the antihyperuricemic effects of the medications are additive, and increased therapeutic benefit has been reported with concurrent use)

Sulfinpyrazone
(the antihyperuricemic effects of allopurinol and sulfinpyrazone are additive; increased therapeutic benefit has been reported with concurrent use)

Vidarabine, systemic
(concurrent use with allopurinol may increase the risk of neurotoxicity and other side effects such as anemia, nausea, pain, and pruritus; caution is recommended if concurrent use is necessary)

Xanthines, such as:
  Aminophylline
  Oxtriphylline
  Theophylline
(concurrent use of large doses [600 mg per day] of allopurinol with the xanthines [except dyphylline] may decrease theophylline clearance, resulting in increased serum theophylline concentrations; when steady-state theophylline concentration is 13 mcg per mL [72.15 micromoles/L] or higher and 600 mg of allopurinol per day is required, serum theophylline concentrations should be monitored and theophylline dosage adjusted if necessary)

**Laboratory value alterations**
The following have been selected on the basis of their potential clinical significance (possible effect in parentheses where appropriate)—not necessarily inclusive (» = major clinical significance):

With physiology/laboratory test values
Alkaline phosphatase activity, serum and
Bilirubin concentrations, serum and
Transaminase activity, serum
(may be increased, indicating hepatotoxicity, especially in patients with pre-existing hepatic or renal disease)

Blood urea nitrogen (BUN) and
Creatinine, serum
(concentrations may be increased, indicating nephrotoxicity, especially in patients with pre-existing renal disease)

**Medical considerations/Contraindications**
The medical considerations/contraindications included here have been selected on the basis of their potential clinical significance (reasons given in parentheses where appropriate)—not necessarily inclusive (» = major clinical significance).

*Risk-benefit should be considered when the following medical problems exist:*
Renal function impairment or any illness that may predispose to a change in renal function, such as:
  Congestive heart disease
  Diabetes mellitus
  Hypertension
    (oxipurinol may accumulate; risk of severe allergic reactions and other adverse effects is increased; a reduction in dosage may be required)
    (risk of renal failure may be increased, especially when allopurinol is being used for hyperuricemia secondary to neoplastic disease or urate nephropathy; monitoring of renal function may be especially important when these conditions exist)
Sensitivity to allopurinol, history of

**Patient monitoring**
The following may be especially important in patient monitoring (other tests may be warranted in some patients, depending on condition; » = major clinical significance):
Complete blood counts and
Hepatic function determinations and
Renal function determinations
  (recommended at periodic intervals during therapy, especially during the first few months)
» Uric acid, serum
  (monitoring may be required for proper dosing; the upper limit of normal is about 7 mg per 100 mL [416.36 micromoles/L] for males and postmenopausal females and about 6mg per 100 mL [356.88 micromoles/L] for premenopausal females but may vary, depending on the patient and laboratory methodology)

# Side/Adverse Effects

Note: Following initiation of allopurinol therapy for gouty arthritis, the most commonly encountered adverse effect is a temporary increase in the frequency of acute gout attacks. The occurrence of such reactions may be reduced by initiating therapy with a low dose that is gradually increased until the desired effect is obtained and by administration of prophylactic doses of colchicine or a nonsteroidal anti-inflammatory drug.

The following side/adverse effects have been selected on the basis of their potential clinical significance (possible signs and symptoms in parentheses where appropriate)—not necessarily inclusive:

**Those indicating need for medical attention**
Incidence more frequent
  *Dermatitis, allergic* (skin rash, hives, or itching)
  Note: *Maculopapular skin rash* occurs most often; however, *eczematoid, exfoliative, urticarial, vesicular bullous,* or *purpuric lesions* and *lichen planus* have also been reported rarely.

    Very rarely, *skin rash* may be followed by more severe allergic reactions, usually in patients with renal function impairment and/or those receiving thiazide diuretics. *Generalized vasculitis, hepatotoxicity, and/or acute renal failure* may occur. Laboratory studies may indicate *eosinophilia* and *leukopenia* or *leukocytosis.* Several deaths have been attributed to these reactions.

Incidence rare
  *Agranulocytosis* (fever with or without chills; sores, ulcers, or white spots on lips or in mouth; sore throat); *anemia* (unusual tiredness and/or weakness); *angiitis [vasculitis], hypersensitivity* (chills, fever, and sore throat; muscle aches, pains, or weakness; shortness of breath, troubled breathing, tightness in chest, or wheezing); *aplastic anemia* (shortness of breath, troubled breathing, tightness in chest, and/or wheezing; sores, ulcers, or white spots on lips or in mouth; swollen and/or painful glands; unusual bleeding or bruising; unusual tiredness or weakness); *dermatitis, exfoliative* (possible prodrome of chills, fever, sore throat, muscle aches or pains, and/or nausea with or without vomiting; red, thickened, scaly skin); *erythema multiforme* (possible prodrome of chills, fever, sore throat, muscle aches or pains, and/or nausea with or without vomiting; sores, ulcers, or white spots in mouth

or on lips; skin rash or sores, hives, and/or itching); *hepatotoxicity* (swelling in upper abdominal area; yellow eyes or skin); *hypersensitivity reaction, allopurinol-induced* (initially skin rash immediately preceding or concurrent with chills, fever, and sore throat; muscle aches or pains; and/or nausea with or without vomiting; followed by signs and symptoms of angiitis [vasculitis], hepatotoxicity, and/or acute renal failure); *loosening of fingernails; necrolysis, toxic epidermal* (possible prodrome of chills, fever, sore throat, muscle aches or pains, and/or nausea with or without vomiting; redness, tenderness, itching, burning, or peeling of skin; red or irritated eyes); *neuritis, peripheral* (numbness, tingling, pain, or weakness in hands or feet); *renal calculus, xanthine* (blood in urine, difficult or painful urination, pain in lower back and/or side); *renal failure, acute* (sudden decrease in amount of urine; swelling of face, fingers, feet, and/or lower legs; weight gain, rapid); *Stevens-Johnson syndrome* (possible prodrome of chills, fever, sore throat, muscle aches and pains, and/or nausea with or without vomiting; sores, ulcers, or white spots in mouth or on lips; bleeding sores on lips); *thrombocytopenia* (usually asymptomatic; rarely, unusual bleeding or bruising; black, tarry stools; blood in urine or stools; pinpoint red spots on skin); *unexplained nosebleeds*

Note: *Bone marrow depression* has been reported to occur 6 weeks to 6 years after initiation of allopurinol therapy. Most of the affected patients were also receiving other medications with the potential for causing this reaction. However, *bone marrow depression* affecting one or more cell lines has rarely occurred in patients receiving allopurinol alone.

*Hepatotoxicity* may be hypersensitivity-mediated; hepatic necrosis, granulomatous hepatitis, and cholestatic jaundice have been reported.

*Renal failure* associated with allopurinol therapy has been reported in patients being treated for hyperuricemia secondary to neoplastic diseases or gouty nephropathy as well as in patients experiencing *hypersensitivity reactions* to the medication.

**Those indicating need for medical attention only if they continue or are bothersome**
Incidence less frequent or rare
*Diarrhea; drowsiness; headache; indigestion; nausea or vomiting without symptoms of skin rash, chills or fever, or muscle aches and pains; stomach pain; unusual hair loss*

## Overdose

For more information on the management of overdose or unintentional ingestion, **contact a Poison Control Center** (see *Poison Control Center Listing*).

**Treatment of overdose**
Immediate discontinuation of allopurinol.

To decrease absorption—Gastric lavage, if very large quantities have been ingested.

To enhance elimination—Although allopurinol and oxipurinol are dialyzable, the value of hemodialysis or peritoneal dialysis in the management of allopurinol overdose has not been established.

Monitoring—May include observing the patient and treating the observed symptoms.

Supportive care—Maintaining hydration. Patients in whom intentional overdose is known or suspected should be referred for psychiatric consultation.

## Patient Consultation

As an aid to patient consultation, refer to *Advice for the Patient, Allopurinol (Systemic)*.

In providing consultation, consider emphasizing the following selected information (» = major clinical significance):

**Before using this medication**
» Conditions affecting use, especially:
   Other medications, especially coumarin- or indandione-derivative anticoagulants, azathioprine, and mercaptopurine

**Proper use of this medication**
   Taking after meals, if necessary, to minimize gastrointestinal irritation
» Compliance with therapy
   Importance of high fluid intake during therapy and compliance with therapy for alkalinization of urine, if prescribed, to help prevent kidney stones
   Several months of continuous therapy may be required for maximum effectiveness in patients with chronic gout
» Medication helps prevent, but does not relieve, acute gout attacks; need to continue taking allopurinol with medication prescribed for gout attacks

» Proper dosing
   Missed dose: Taking as soon as possible; not taking if almost time for next dose; not doubling doses
» Proper storage

**Precautions while using this medication**
   Regular visits to physician to check progress during therapy; possible need for periodic blood tests to determine efficacy of therapy and/or occurrence of side effects
   Avoiding large amounts of alcohol, which may increase uric acid concentrations and reduce effectiveness of medication
   Possibility that vitamin C taken in large amounts may increase the potential for kidney stone formation
» Notifying physician immediately if skin rash occurs or if influenza-like symptoms (chills, fever, muscle aches and pains, or nausea or vomiting) occur concurrently with or shortly after skin rash; these symptoms may rarely indicate onset of severe hypersensitivity reaction
» Caution if drowsiness occurs

**Side/adverse effects**
   Signs of potential adverse effects, especially allergic dermatitis, agranulocytosis, anemia, angiitis, aplastic anemia, exfoliative dermatitis, erythema multiforme, hepatotoxicity, hypersensitivity reaction, loosening of fingernails, toxic epidermal necrolysis, peripheral neuritis, renal caluli, renal failure, Stevens-Johnson syndrome, thrombocytopenia, and unexplained nosebleeds

## General Dosing Information

Allopurinol may be administered after meals to lessen gastrointestinal irritation.

An increase in the frequency of acute attacks of gouty arthritis may occur during the early months of allopurinol therapy. The risk of precipitating acute gout attacks may be reduced by initiating allopurinol therapy with a low dose, then gradually increasing dosage until the desired effect is obtained. Also, it is recommended that prophylactic doses of colchicine (or, if the patient cannot take colchicine, a nonsteroidal anti-inflammatory drug [NSAID]) be administered concurrently during the first 3 to 6 months of allopurinol therapy.

Acute attacks of gout may occur during allopurinol therapy, even with colchicine or NSAID prophylactic therapy. During an attack, allopurinol therapy should be continued at the same dose while an appropriate anti-inflammatory agent (preferably an NSAID or a corticosteroid [preferably via intrasynovial injection, when feasible]) is administered to relieve the attack. Because of the toxicity associated with therapeutic doses of colchicine, its use for treatment of an acute attack of gout should be reserved for patients in whom the preferred medications are contraindicated or ineffective.

The total daily dose may be administered in divided doses or as a single dose. Each single dose should not exceed 300 mg. Daily dosage requirements exceeding 300 mg should be administered in divided doses.

Monitoring of serum uric acid concentrations may be necessary for proper dosing.

To reduce the risk of xanthine calculi formation, and to help prevent renal precipitation of urates in patients receiving concomitant uricosuric agents, a high fluid intake (no less than 2.5 to 3 liters daily) and maintenance of a neutral, or preferably slightly alkaline, urine are recommended.

When uricosuric therapy is being changed to allopurinol therapy, the dose of the uricosuric agent should be reduced gradually over a period of several weeks and the dose of allopurinol increased gradually to the dose required for maintenance of normal serum uric acid concentrations.

It is recommended that allopurinol therapy be discontinued at once if a skin rash or any other sign of adverse reaction occurs. Skin rash may be followed by more severe hypersensitivity reactions. After a severe reaction, therapy should be discontinued permanently. However, after a mild reaction, it may be possible to reinstate therapy at a lower dosage (50 mg per day initially and increased very gradually) after the reaction has subsided. If skin rash recurs, therapy should be discontinued permanently.

**For treatment of adverse effects**

Hypersensitivity reactions—Administer glucocorticoids. Prolonged administration may be required after a severe reaction.

## Oral Dosage Forms
### ALLOPURINOL TABLETS USP
**Usual adult and adolescent dose**
Antigout agent—
  Initial—Oral, 100 mg once a day, to be increased by 100 mg per day at one-week intervals until the desired serum uric acid concentration is attained, not to exceed the maximum recommended dosage of 800 mg per day.
  Maintenance—Oral, 100 to 200 mg two or three times a day; or 300 mg as a single dose once a day. The usual maintenance dose is 200 to 300 mg per day in mild gout or 400 to 600 mg per day in moderately severe tophaceous gout.
Neoplastic disease therapy—
  Initial—Oral, 600 to 800 mg per day starting twelve hours to three days (preferably two to three days) prior to initiation of chemotherapy or radiation therapy.
  Maintenance—Dosage should be based on serum uric acid determinations performed approximately forty-eight hours after initiation of allopurinol therapy and periodically thereafter. Allopurinol should be discontinued following the period of tumor regression.
Antiurolithic (uric acid calculi)—
  Oral, 100 to 200 mg one to four times a day; or 300 mg as a single dose once a day.
Antiurolithic (calcium oxalate calculi)—
  Oral, 200 to 300 mg a day as a single dose or in divided doses.
Note: Because oxipurinol is excreted primarily by the kidneys, accumulation may occur in patients with renal failure. Patients receiving dialysis may require usual therapeutic doses of allopurinol; however, in patients not receiving dialysis, it is recommended that the dosage be reduced as follows:

| Creatinine Clearance (mL/min) | Dose |
|---|---|
| 10 to 20 | 200 mg daily |
| 3 to 10 | no more than 100 mg daily |
| < 3 | 100 mg at intervals of more than 24 hours may be necessary |

  Some patients with renal function impairment may require even lower doses or longer intervals between doses. In some cases, 300 mg twice a week, or even less, may suffice.

**Usual adult prescribing limits**
300 mg per dose; 800 mg per day.

**Usual pediatric dose**
Antihyperuricemic, in neoplastic disease therapy—
  Children up to 6 years of age: Oral, 50 mg three times a day.
  Children 6 to 10 years of age: Oral, 100 mg three times a day; or 300 mg as a single dose once a day.
Note: Dosage adjustment may be necessary after approximately forty-eight hours of therapy, depending on the patient's response.

**Strength(s) usually available**
U.S.—
  100 mg (Rx) [*Lopurin* (scored); *Zyloprim* (scored); GENERIC].
  300 mg (Rx) [*Lopurin* (scored); *Zyloprim* (scored); GENERIC].
Canada—
  100 mg (Rx) [*Apo-Allopurinol* (scored); *Purinol* (scored); *Zyloprim* (scored)].
  200 mg (Rx) [*Apo-Allopurinol* (scored); *Purinol* (scored); *Zyloprim* (scored)].
  300 mg (Rx) [*Apo-Allopurinol* (scored); *Purinol* (scored); *Zyloprim* (scored)].

**Packaging and storage**
Store below 40 °C (104 °F), preferably between 15 and 25 °C (59 and 77 °F). Store in a well-closed container.

**Auxiliary labeling**
• Drink large amounts of fluids.

## Selected Bibliography
Ettinger B, Tang A, Citron JT, Livermore B, Williams T. Randomized trial of allopurinol in the prevention of calcium oxalate calculi. N Engl J Med 1986; 315: 1386-9.
Lupton GP, Odom RB. The allopurinol hypersensitivity syndrome. J Am Acad Dermatol 1979; 1: 365-74.

Revised: 08/25/94

# ALPHA₁-PROTEINASE INHIBITOR, HUMAN    Systemic

VA CLASSIFICATION (Primary): RE900
Another commonly used name is alpha₁-antitrypsin.
Note: For a listing of dosage forms and brand names by country availability, see *Dosage Forms* section(s). For a listing of brand names for the articles in this monograph, refer to the General Index.

## Category
Alpha₁-antitrypsin replenisher.

## Indications
### Accepted
Emphysema, panacinar, due to alpha₁-antitrypsin deficiency (treatment)—Human alpha₁-proteinase inhibitor (alpha₁-PI) is indicated for chronic replacement therapy in individuals with clinically apparent panacinar emphysema due to a congenital deficiency of alpha₁-antitrypsin.

Because panacinar emphysema does not develop in some individuals who have alpha₁-antitrypsin deficiency, chronic replacement therapy with alpha₁-PI should be used only in those individuals with evidence of the disease.

Alpha₁-PI is indicated for use only in patients with PiZZ, PiZ (null), Pi (null) (null), or other phenotypes associated with serum alpha₁-antitrypsin concentrations of less than 50 mg per deciliter (dL). It should not be used in individuals with the PiMZ or PiMS phenotypes of alpha₁-antitrypsin deficiency because these individuals appear to be at small risk of developing panacinar emphysema.

In some adults, alpha₁-antitrypsin deficiency is complicated by cirrhosis.

The long-term effects of chronic replacement therapy with alpha₁-PI in individuals having emphysema due to alpha₁-antitrypsin deficiency are not known because of inadequate clinical data (the number of patients is small and the course of the disease is variable and slowly progressive).

## Pharmacology/Pharmacokinetics
**Physicochemical characteristics**
Source—Prepared from pooled human plasma of normal donors by modification and refinements of the cold ethanol method of Cohn.
Other characteristics—When alpha₁-PI is reconstituted, it has a pH of 6.6 to 7.4.

**Mechanism of action/Effect**
Alpha₁-proteinase inhibitor (alpha₁-PI), a plasma protein and the principal inhibitor of neutrophil elastase, increases the plasma concentration of alpha₁-PI and the concentration of functionally active alpha₁-PI in the epithelial lining of the lower respiratory tract to provide adequate antineutrophil elastase activity, and thus protection, in the lungs of individuals with alpha₁-antitrypsin deficiency.
In patients with alpha₁-antitrypsin deficiency, the cause of the development of emphysema is not well understood; however, it is believed to be due to a chronic biochemical imbalance between elastase (an enzyme capable of degrading elastin tissues, released by inflammatory cells, primarily neutrophils, in the lower respiratory tract) and alpha₁-PI (the principal inhibitor of neutrophil elastase) that is deficient in alpha₁-antitrypsin disease. This imbalance appears to result in alveolar structures being unprotected from chronic exposure to elastase released from a chronic, low-level burden of neutrophils in the lower respiratory tract and, subsequently, progressive degradation of elastin tissues. Replacement therapy with alpha₁-PI reverses the biochemical abnormalities and brings the antineutrophil elastase capacity of the serum into the normal range in direct proportion to the serum concentrations of alpha₁-PI.

**Half-life**
*In vivo*—Approximately 4.5 days.

**Onset of action**
Within a few weeks.

**Therapeutic blood concentration**
In clinical studies, blood concentrations of alpha₁-PI above 80 mg per deciliter (dL) significantly increased concentrations of alpha₁-PI and functional antineutrophil elastase capacity in the epithelial lining fluid of the lower respiratory tract of the lungs, as compared to concentrations prior to replacement therapy with human alpha₁-PI.

Note: Although there are many phenotypic variants of alpha₁-antitrypsin deficiency, the individuals most severely affected are those with the PiZZ variant that is characterized by alpha₁-PI concentrations <35% normal. Epidemiologic studies have shown that individuals with endogenous serum concentrations of alpha₁-PI ≤50 mg per dL have a risk >80% of developing emphysema over a lifetime. In individuals with endogenous alpha₁-PI concentrations >80 mg per dL, there is generally no increased risk for development of emphysema above the general population risk. Therefore, it appears that the concentration of alpha₁-PI in the serum required to provide adequate anti-elastase action in the lungs of individuals with alpha₁-antitrypsin deficiency is approximately 80 mg per dL (based on commercial standards for immunologic assay of alpha₁-PI).

## Precautions to Consider

### Carcinogenicity/Mutagenicity
Long-term studies in animals to determine the carcinogenic and mutagenic potential of alpha₁-proteinase inhibitor (alpha₁-PI) have not been done.

### Pregnancy/Reproduction
Fertility—Long-term studies in animals to determine fertility impairment potential of alpha₁-PI have not been done.

Pregnancy—Studies have not been done in humans.
Studies have not been done in animals.

FDA Pregnancy Category C.

### Breast-feeding
It is not known whether alpha₁-proteinase inhibitor is distributed into breast milk. However, problems in humans have not been documented.

### Pediatrics
Appropriate studies on the relationship of age to the effects of alpha₁-proteinase inhibitor have not been performed in the pediatric population. Safety and efficacy have not been established.

### Geriatrics
No information is available on the relationship of age to the effects of alpha₁-proteinase inhibitor in geriatric patients.

### Medical considerations/Contraindications
The medical considerations/contraindications included here have been selected on the basis of their potential clinical significance (reasons given in parentheses where appropriate)—not necessarily inclusive (» = major clinical significance).

*Except under special circumstances, this medication should not be used when the following medical problem exists:*
» Immunoglobulin antibody (IgA) deficiency, selective, in patients with known antibody against IgA (anti-IgA antibody)
(patients may experience severe reactions, including anaphylaxis, to IgA, which may be present in human alpha₁-proteinase inhibitor)

*Risk-benefit should be considered when the following medical problem exists:*
Sensitivity to alpha₁-proteinase inhibitor

### Patient monitoring
The following may be especially important in patient monitoring (other tests may be warranted in some patients, depending on condition; » = major clinical significance):

Alpha₁-PI concentrations, serum
(determinations may be useful in monitoring serum concentrations of alpha₁-PI in patients receiving the medication, using currently available commercial assays of antigenic activity; however, results of these assays should not be used to determine the required therapeutic dosage)

## Side/Adverse Effects

Note: Because alpha₁-proteinase inhibitor (alpha₁-PI) is prepared from large pools of fresh human plasma obtained from donors, each unit of plasma has been tested, using FDA-approved tests, and found negative for human immunodeficiency virus (HIV) antibody and nonreactive for hepatitis B surface antigen (HBsAg). However, hepatitis viruses may be present in such human plasma pools.

Also, human alpha₁-PI has been heat-treated in solution at 60 ± 0.5 °C for not less than 10 hours to reduce the potential risk of transmission of infectious agents; however, no procedure has been found to be totally effective in removing viral infectivity from plasma products.

Although no cases of hepatitis, either hepatitis B or non-A, non-B hepatitis have been reported in individuals who have received alpha₁-PI, all individuals should receive prophylaxis against hepatitis B prior to administration of alpha₁-PI because the potential for transmission of hepatitis B virus is not known.

The following side/adverse effects have been selected on the basis of their potential clinical significance (possible signs and symptoms in parentheses where appropriate)—not necessarily inclusive:

**Those indicating need for medical attention only if they continue or are bothersome**
Incidence less frequent or rare
*Leukocytosis* (chills and fever); *dizziness or lightheadedness; fever up to 38.9 °C (102 °F), delayed*

Note: Mild transient *leukocytosis* may occur several hours after infusion.
*Fever* may occur up to 12 hours after infusion; disappears over 24 hours.

## Patient Consultation
As an aid to patient consultation, refer to *Advice for the Patient, Alpha₁-proteinase Inhibitor, Human (Systemic)*.

In providing consultation, consider emphasizing the following selected information (» = major clinical significance):

**Before receiving this medication**
» Conditions affecting use, especially:
Sensitivity to alpha₁-proteinase inhibitor
Other medical problems, especially immunoglobulin antibody (IgA) deficiency, selective, in patients with known antibody against IgA (anti-IgA antibody)

**Proper use of this medication**
» Compliance with therapy
» Proper dosing

**Side/adverse effects**
Fever may occur up to 12 hours after infusion
Mild transient leukocytosis (chills and fever) may occur several hours after infusion

## General Dosing Information

Prior to administration of human alpha₁-proteinase inhibitor (alpha₁-PI), it is recommended that patients be immunized against hepatitis B by administration of a licensed hepatitis B vaccine according to the manufacturer's recommendations. However, if it is necessary to treat an individual with alpha₁-PI and there is insufficient time for an adequate antibody response to the vaccination, a single dose of hepatitis B immune globulin (human), 0.06 mL per kg of body weight, should be administered intramuscularly at the time of administration of the initial dose of hepatitis B vaccine.

Prior to administration, parenteral alpha₁-PI should be inspected visually for particulate matter and discoloration if possible.

Alpha₁-PI is for intravenous use only.

Following administration of alpha₁-PI, the administration equipment and any unused reconstituted human alpha₁-PI should be appropriately discarded.

Following intravenous administration of alpha₁-proteinase inhibitor, plasma volume will usually be increased (as with any colloid solution); therefore, caution should be used in patients who are at risk of circulatory overload.

## Parenteral Dosage Forms

### ALPHA₁-PROTEINASE INHIBITOR, HUMAN, FOR INJECTION

**Usual adult dose**
Alpha₁-antitrypsin replenisher—
Intravenous infusion, 60 mg per kg of body weight, administered at a rate of 0.08 mL (approximately 1.6 mg) per kg of body weight per minute or greater, once a week.

**Usual pediatric dose**
Alpha₁-antitrypsin replenisher—
Safety and efficacy have not been established.

**Usual geriatric dose**
See *Usual adult dose.*

**Size(s) usually available**
U.S.—
    500 mg with 20 mL of diluent (Rx) [*Prolastin*].
    1 gram with 40 mL of diluent (Rx) [*Prolastin*].
Canada—
    500 mg with 20 mL of diluent (Rx) [*Prolastin*].
    1 gram with 40 mL of diluent (Rx) [*Prolastin*].

Note: Each vial contains the labeled amount of total functional alpha$_1$-proteinase inhibitor (alpha$_1$-PI) activity, in mg, as determined by capacity to neutralize porcine pancreatic elastase.

Prior to reconstitution, the specific activity of alpha$_1$-PI is $\geq 0.35$ mg functional alpha$_1$-PI per mg of protein.

When reconstituted, the concentration of alpha$_1$-PI is $\geq 20$ mg per mL (sodium 100 to 210 mEq per L; chloride 60 to 180 mEq per L; sodium phosphate 0.015 to 0.025 M; polyethylene glycol not more than 5 ppm; sucrose not more than 0.1%).

Human alpha$_1$-PI contains small amounts of other plasma proteins including alpha$_2$-plasmin inhibitor, alpha$_1$-antichymotrypsin, C$_1$-esterase inhibitor, haptoglobin, antithrombin III, alpha$_1$-lipoprotein, albumin, and IgA.

**Packaging and storage**
Prior to reconstitution, store between 2 and 8 °C (35 and 46 °F), unless otherwise specified by manufacturer. Protect diluent from freezing.
After reconstitution, medication should not be refrigerated.

**Preparation of dosage form**
To prepare an intravenous infusion solution of human alpha$_1$-PI, use the diluent, Sterile Water for Injection USP, supplied by the manufacturer.

**Stability**
Alpha$_1$-PI, human, for injection contains no preservative.
After reconstitution, medication should be administered within 3 hours.
Any unused reconstituted human alpha$_1$-PI should be appropriately discarded.

**Incompatibilities**
Alpha$_1$-PI should be administered alone, without mixing with other agents or diluting solutions. However, if required, alpha$_1$-PI may be diluted with normal saline.

## Selected Bibliography

Pierce JA. Antitrypsin and emphysema: perspective and prospects. JAMA 1988 May 20; 259 (19): 2890-5.
Hubbard RC, Crystal RG. Alpha-1-antitrypsin augmentation therapy for alpha-1-antitrypsin deficiency. In: Proceedings of a symposium on alpha-1-antitrypsin deficiency; usage of alpha-1-proteinase inhibitor concentrate in replacement therapy. Am J Med 1988 June 24; 84 (suppl 6A): 52-62.

Revised: 08/09/94

**ALPRAZOLAM**—See *Benzodiazepines (Systemic)*

---

# ALPROSTADIL   Intracavernosal

VA CLASSIFICATION (Primary/Secondary): HS875/CV500; GU900
Note: For information pertaining to the use of alprostadil for other indications, see *Alprostadil (Systemic).*

Other commonly used names are PGE$_1$ and prostaglandin E$_1$.

Note: For a listing of dosage forms and brand names by country availability, see *Dosage Forms* section(s). For a listing of brand names for the articles in this monograph, refer to the General Index.

## Category
Impotence therapy.

## Indications
Note: Bracketed information in the *Indications* section refers to uses that are not included in U.S. product labeling.

**Accepted**
[Impotence (treatment)][1]—Alprostadil is used by intracavernosal injection to facilitate erections in men with impotence. In general, it is most useful in patients with organic impotence (neurogenic and, to a lesser extent, vascular). It is less useful in patients with impotence due to endocrine problems (hypogonadism, hyper- or hypothyroidism) or medications.

[Impotence (diagnosis)][1]—Alprostadil is used by intracavernosal injection as an aid in the evaluation of penile vasculature, alone or prior to angiography, cavernosography, or cavernosometry.

**Unaccepted**
Use of alprostadil to enhance erections in men who are not impotent is not recommended because of the risk of priapism and permanent damage to penile tissues.

[1]Not included in Canadian product labeling.

## Pharmacology/Pharmacokinetics

**Physicochemical characteristics**
Molecular weight—354.49.
pKa—6.3.

**Mechanism of action/Effect**
Alprostadil is one of a family of naturally occurring prostaglandins, which causes vasodilation by means of a direct effect on vascular smooth muscle. It is present naturally in the seminal vesicle and seminal plasma.
When administered by intracavernous injection, it is thought to cause relaxation of the trabecular cavernous smooth muscles and vasodilation of the penile arteries. This results in increased arterial blood flow into the corpus cavernosa, and swelling and elongation of the penis; the glans and corpus spongiosum also swell.
Venous outflow is also reduced, possibly as a result of increased venous resistance.

**Biotransformation**
Local, rapid.

**Onset of action**
5 to 10 minutes.

**Time to peak effect**
Within 20 minutes.

**Duration of action**
1 to 3 hours; dose-related.

## Precautions to Consider

**Carcinogenicity**
Studies have not been done.

**Mutagenicity**
According to results of Ames and Alkaline Elution assays, alprostadil has no potential for mutagenicity.

**Pregnancy/Reproduction**
Problems in humans have not been documented.

**Geriatrics**
No information is available on the relationship of age to the effects of alprostadil used intracavernosally in geriatric patients. However, elderly patients are more likely to have peripheral vascular disease, which may result in a decreased response to intracavernosal alprostadil; dosage adjustment may be necessary.

**Drug interactions and/or related problems**
The following drug interactions and/or related problems have been selected on the basis of their potential clinical significance (possible mechanism in parentheses where appropriate)—not necessarily inclusive ($\gg$ = major clinical significance):

Note: Combinations containing any of the following medications, depending on the amount present, may also interact with this medication.

Sympathomimetics, alpha-adrenergic, especially metaraminol, epinephrine, and phenylephrine
    (reverse the vasodilating effect of alprostadil; may be used to treat priapism or overdose)

**Medical considerations/Contraindications**
The medical considerations/contraindications included here have been selected on the basis of their potential clinical significance (reasons given

in parentheses where appropriate)—not necessarily inclusive (» = major clinical significance).

***Risk-benefit should be considered when the following medical problems exist:***

»  Coagulation defects, severe or
»  Liver disease, severe
      (risk of bleeding at injection site; alprostadil inhibits platelet aggregation)
»  Priapism, history of or
»  Sickle cell disease
      (increased risk of priapism)
      Sensitivity to alprostadil

### Patient monitoring

The following may be especially important in patient monitoring (other tests may be warranted in some patients, depending on condition; » = major clinical significance):

Palpation of penis
      (recommended at regular intervals by both the patient and the physician to check for developing fibrosis or curvature)

## Side/Adverse Effects

The following side/adverse effects have been selected on the basis of their potential clinical significance (possible signs and symptoms in parentheses where appropriate)—not necessarily inclusive:

**Those indicating need for medical attention**
Incidence rare
    *Priapism* (erection, continuing for more than 4 hours)
    Note: Usually due to excessive dosage. Prolonged erection may resolve spontaneously, but in some cases will require treatment.

**Those indicating need for medical attention only if they continue or are bothersome**
Incidence more frequent
    *Pain at site of injection; pain during erection* (burning or aching)—may be severe
Incidence rare
    *Superficial hematoma* (bruising or bleeding at site of injection)

## Patient Consultation

As an aid to patient consultation, refer to *Advice for the Patient, Alprostadil (Intracavernosal)*.

In providing consultation, consider emphasizing the following selected information (» = major clinical significance):

**Before using this medication**
»  Conditions affecting use, especially:
    Sensitivity to alprostadil
    Other medical problems, especially severe coagulation defects, history of priapism, or sickle cell disease

**Proper use of this medication**
*Proper administration*
»  Cleansing injection site with alcohol; injecting slowly and directly into corpus cavernosum at base or midshaft of penis; avoiding subcutaneous administration; if inadvertently injected subcutaneously (as evidenced by pain at injection site), stopping, withdrawing, and repositioning needle
    Putting pressure on injection site for 5 minutes to prevent bruising; massaging penis, as directed by physician, to distribute medication
    Effect begins in about 5 to 10 minutes; attempting intercourse within 10 to 30 minutes after administration
    Alternating puncture (injection) sites
»  Proper dosing
»  Proper storage

**Precautions while using this medication**
»  Compliance with therapy; importance of not exceeding prescribed dosage and frequency of use; risk of priapism, tissue ischemia, and permanent damage with overdose
»  Telling physician immediately if erection persists longer than 4 hours or becomes painful
    If bleeding occurs at injection site, applying pressure; checking with physician if bleeding persists

**Side/adverse effects**
    Signs of potential side effects, especially excessive dosage or priapism

## General Dosing Information

Patients receiving intracavernosal alprostadil should be under supervision of a physician experienced in its use and familiar with proper management of sustained erection and priapism.

Dosage adjustment should be made carefully, based on the degree and duration of tumescence achieved with the previous dose. In general, patients with neurogenic impotence may be more sensitive to the effects of intracavernosal vasodilators and may require lower doses.

Intracavernosal alprostadil may be self-administered by the patient, but only after careful training in the technique to reduce the incidence of inadvertent subcutaneous administration, ecchymosis, and urethral injury.

For treatment of impotence, alprostadil is injected slowly (over 1 to 2 minutes), directly into the the corpus cavernosum at the base or midshaft of the penis. A characteristic give should be noticed as the needle penetrates the tunica albuginea and enters the corpus cavernosum. Proper injection technique is necessary to avoid injury or injection of the urethra or vessels on the dorsal aspect of the penis.

After completion of the injection, pressure is applied to the injection site to prevent bleeding. Then the entire length of the corpus cavernosum should be squeezed firmly to distribute medication to the other side, followed by the same procedure on the other side. The penis should then be pinched transversely in several places to distribute medication to both ends of the corpus cavernosa.

If a sustained erection or pain at the site of injection occurs, the next dose of alprostadil should be reduced.

Intercourse should be attempted within 10 to 30 minutes after administration.

Alternate puncture (injection) sites.

**For treatment of prolonged erection or priapism**
A sustained erection should be treated if it persists for longer than 4 hours; priapism should be treated promptly. If tumescence is not reversed, interruption of blood flow may result in penile tissue ischemia and permanent damage.

Depending on the severity, treatment may include:
    • Aspiration of intracavernous blood.
    • Irrigation of the corpus cavernosa with saline to remove clotted blood.
    • Intracavernous administration of an alpha-adrenergic agonist, such as metaraminol, epinephrine, or phenylephrine.
    • Surgery.

## Parenteral Dosage Forms

Note: Bracketed information in the *Dosage Forms* section refers to uses that are not included in U.S. product labeling.

### ALPROSTADIL INJECTION USP

**Usual adult dose**
[Impotence therapy][1]—
    Intracavernosal, 2.5 to 20 mcg (0.0025 to 0.02 mg), the dosage being adjusted according to response.

Note: Patients with neurogenic impotence may require lower doses.

**Usual adult prescribing limits**
Impotence therapy—
    Up to 40 mcg (0.04 mg) of alprostadil per dose. The injection should not be given more than three times weekly or two days in succession.

**Strength(s) usually available**
U.S.—
    500 mcg (0.5 mg) per mL (Rx) [*Prostin VR Pediatric* (in dehydrated alcohol)].
Canada—
    500 mcg (0.5 mg) per mL (Rx) [*Prostin VR* (in dehydrated alcohol)].

**Packaging and storage**
Store between 2 and 8 °C (36 and 46 °F), unless otherwise specified by manufacturer. Protect from freezing.

**Preparation of dosage form**
Alprostadil injection is prepared for intracavernosal use by diluting the desired dose in 0.5 to 3.0 mL of 0.9% sodium chloride injection.

**Stability**
Stability after dilution is unknown.

---

[1]Not included in Canadian product labeling.

## Selected Bibliography

Bernard F, Lue TF. Self-administration in the pharmacological treatment of impotence. Drugs 1990; 39 (3): 394-8.

Lue TF, Tanagho EA. Physiology of erection and pharmacological management of impotence. J Urol 1987; 137: 829-36.

Morley JE. Impotence. Am J Med 1986 May; 80: 897-905.

Sidi AA, Lange PH. Recent advances in the diagnosis and management of impotence. Urol Clin N Am 1986 Aug; 13 (3): 489-500.

Revised: 04/08/92
Interim revision: 06/29/94

---

# ALPROSTADIL    Systemic

---

VA CLASSIFICATION (Primary): HS875

Note: For information pertaining to use of alprostadil for diagnosis and treatment of impotence, see *Alprostadil (Intracavernosal)*.

Other commonly used names are PGE$_1$ and prostaglandin E$_1$.

Note: For a listing of dosage forms and brand names by country availability, see *Dosage Forms* section(s). For a listing of brand names for the articles in this monograph, refer to the General Index.

---

## Category
Ductus arteriosus patency adjunct.

## Indications
Note: Bracketed information in the *Indications* section refers to uses that are not included in U.S. product labeling.

### Accepted
Ductus arteriosus, patent (maintenance)—Alprostadil is indicated for palliative, not definitive, therapy in neonates born with various congenital heart defects, including pulmonary atresia, pulmonary stenosis, tricuspid atresia, tetralogy of Fallot, interruption of the aortic arch, coarctation of the aorta, transposition of the great vessels with or without other defects, [hypoplastic left heart syndrome][1], and [critical aortic valve stenosis][1]. The medication is used to maintain the patency of the ductus arteriosus (DA), thereby improving circulation and oxygenation until corrective or palliative surgery can be performed. Although alprostadil treatment is intended primarily as a short-term measure, longterm (up to several months) therapy may be needed, for example, when surgery must be delayed until a very small infant has grown sufficiently to undergo the procedure.

In infants with cyanotic congenital heart disease (for example, pulmonary atresia or stenosis, tricuspid atresia, tetralogy of Fallot, or transposition of the great vessels) in which there is a severe or complete obstruction to right ventricular outflow, patency of the DA is necessary to provide adequate pulmonary blood flow (and, therefore, an adequate oxygen supply) and to prevent or reverse acidemia. In infants with restricted pulmonary blood flow, the best results have generally been attained in patients with low pretreatment blood Po$_2$ who were 4 days old or less; little response was attained in patients with initial Po$_2$ values of 40 torr or more. In infants with acyanotic congenital heart disease (for example, with aortic arch anomalies such as aortic arch interruption or severe coarctation of the aorta) in which there is obstructed systemic outflow, partial or complete patency of the DA is necessary to provide adequate systemic blood flow and to prevent or reverse acidemia.

---

[1]Not included in Canadian product labeling.

## Pharmacology/Pharmacokinetics

### Physicochemical characteristics
Chemical group—Prostaglandins.
Molecular weight—354.49.
pKa—6.3.

### Mechanism of action/Effect
Alprostadil is one of a family of naturally occurring prostaglandins. It causes vasodilation by means of a direct effect on vascular and ductus arteriosus (DA) smooth muscle.
Ductus arteriosus (DA) patency maintenance—
By its effect on DA smooth muscle, alprostadil prevents or reverses the functional closure of the DA that occurs shortly after birth, which results in increased pulmonary or systemic blood flow in infants with impairment of this blood flow. A reduction in pulmonary vascular resistance has also been postulated, which may improve pulmonary perfusion in neonates in whom congenital heart disease is associated with increased pulmonary vascular resistance.

In cyanotic congenital heart disease, alprostadil's actions result in an increased oxygen supply to the tissues.

In infants with interrupted aortic arch or very severe aortic coarctation, alprostadil maintains distal aortic perfusion by permitting blood flow through the DA from the pulmonary artery to the aorta. In infants with aortic coarctation, alprostadil reduces aortic obstruction either by relaxing ductus tissue in the aortic wall or by increasing effective aortic diameter by dilating the DA. In infants with these aortic arch anomalies, systemic blood flow to the lower body is increased, improving tissue oxygen supply and renal perfusion.

### Other actions/effects
Alprostadil has been reported to inhibit macrophage activation, neutrophil chemotaxis, and release of oxygen radicals and lysosomal enzymes. Inhibition of neutrophil chemotaxis has the potential to impair defense mechanisms and increase the risk of bacterial infection.

Alprostadil inhibits coagulation by inhibiting platelet aggregation and possibly by inhibiting activation of factor X (by increasing the concentration of cyclic adenosine monophosphate [cAMP]). Alprostadil may also promote fibrinolysis by stimulating production of tissue plasminogen activator, which converts plasminogen to the fibrinolytic enzyme plasmin. Stimulation of cellular adenylate cyclase may initiate this effect.

Other effects of prostaglandins include stimulation of intestinal and uterine smooth muscle.

### Protein binding
High to very high (81 to 99%), depending on the method of measurement, to albumin.

### Biotransformation
Pulmonary. In patients with normal respiratory function, up to 80% of a dose may be metabolized in one pass through the lungs.

### Half-life
5 to 10 minutes (after a single dose), in healthy adults. Although the half-life in premature neonates has not been determined, a short half-life would be expected in these patients also.

### Time to peak effect
Acyanotic congenital heart disease—
    Coarctation of the aorta: Usually about 3 hours (range, 15 minutes to 11 hours).
    Interruption of aortic arch: Usually about 1.5 hours (range, 15 minutes to 4 hours).
Cyanotic congenital heart disease—
    Approximately 30 minutes.

### Duration of action
Ductus arteriosus (DA) patency maintenance—As long as the infusion is continued; closure of the DA usually begins within 1 to 2 hours after the infusion is discontinued.

### Elimination
Renal (as metabolites); elimination is virtually complete within 24 hours after administration.

## Precautions to Consider

### Carcinogenicity
Studies have not been done.

### Mutagenicity
According to results of Ames and Alkaline Elution assays, alprostadil has no potential for mutagenicity.

### Drug interactions and/or related problems
The following drug interactions and/or related problems have been selected on the basis of their potential clinical significance (possible mechanism in parentheses where appropriate)—not necessarily inclusive (» = major clinical significance):

Note: In addition to the interactions listed below, the possibility should be considered that multiple effects leading to further impairment of blood clotting and/or increased risk of bleeding may occur if alprostadil is administered to a patient receiving any medication having a significant potential for causing hypoprothrombinemia, thrombocytopenia, or gastrointestinal ulceration or hemorrhage.

Anticoagulants, coumarin-derivative, or
Cefamandole or
Cefoperazone or
Cefotetan or
Heparin or
Moxalactam or
Platelet aggregation inhibitors, other (See *Appendix II*), or
Thrombolytic agents
(these medications may cause one or more interferences with blood clotting; concurrent use with alprostadil may increase the risk of bleeding)

Sympathomimetics, alpha-adrenergic, especially metaraminol, epinephrine, and phenylephrine
(these medications reverse the vasodilating effect of alprostadil)

Vasodilators, other
(concurrent use with alprostadil may increase the risk of vasodilation-associated side effects such as hypotension)

### Laboratory value alterations
The following have been selected on the basis of their potential clinical significance (possible effect in parentheses where appropriate)—not necessarily inclusive (» = major clinical significance):

With physiology/laboratory test values
Bilirubin concentrations
(may be increased—incidence less than 1%)

Calcium concentrations, serum
(may be decreased—incidence about 15%)

Glucose concentrations, blood
(may be decreased—incidence less than 1%)

Potassium concentrations, serum
(may be decreased or increased—incidence 1% or less)

### Medical considerations/Contraindications
The medical considerations/contraindications included here have been selected on the basis of their potential clinical significance (reasons given in parentheses where appropriate)—not necessarily inclusive (» = major clinical significance).

*Except under special circumstances, this medication should not be used when the following medical problem exists:*

» Respiratory distress syndrome, neonatal
(closure of the ductus arteriosus [DA] is necessary to prevent overload of pulmonary circulation; a differential diagnosis between cyanotic heart disease [restricted pulmonary blood flow] and neonatal respiratory distress syndrome [hyaline membrane disease] is essential prior to administration)

*Risk-benefit should be considered when the following medical problems exist:*

Bleeding disorders
(increased risk of bleeding because alprostadil inhibits platelet aggregation and may promote fibrinolysis)

Conditions in which increased pulmonary blood flow may result in pulmonary edema

Sensitivity to alprostadil, history of

### Patient monitoring
The following may be especially important in patient monitoring (other tests may be warranted in some patients, depending on condition; » = major clinical significance):

*For all infants with congenital heart defects*
Blood gases (Po$_2$, Pco$_2$), arterial, measurement of
(recommended at intermittent intervals throughout the infusion)

Blood pH, arterial, measurement of
(recommended at frequent intervals during infusion)

Blood pressure, arterial, measurement of by umbilical artery catheter, auscultation, or Doppler transducer, and
Electrocardiogram (ECG) and
Heart rate, measurement of, and
Respiratory rate, measurement of, and
Temperature, rectal, measurement of, and
Respiratory status
(monitoring is recommended throughout therapy for maintaining neonatal ductus arteriosus patency; continuous monitoring is recommended initially, and may be continued throughout short-term therapy, but intermittent monitoring is usually sufficient when treatment is to be continued for an extended period after the patient's condition has stabilized)

Note: In infants with restricted pulmonary blood flow, efficacy of alprostadil may be determined by monitoring improvement in blood oxygenation. In infants with restricted systemic blood flow, improvement of systemic blood pressure and blood pH confirms efficacy.

*For infants with aortic arch anomalies (in addition to those listed above)*
Blood pressure, measured in descending aorta or lower extremity, and
Femoral pulse, palpation for, and
Renal output, measurement of
(recommended at periodic intervals during infusion to confirm efficacy)

## Side/Adverse Effects

Note: Cardiovascular side effects (especially cutaneous vasodilation) have been reported more frequently in infants with cyanotic lesions than in those with aortic lesions (possibly because the intra-aortic route [no longer recommended] was used more often in these patients).
Cardiovascular side effects are more frequent in infants weighing less than 2 kg or with infusions of greater than 48 hours' duration. Respiratory depression occurs more commonly in patients weighing less than 2 kg at birth and in cyanotic infants. Central nervous system (CNS) side effects are more frequent in neonates with preinfusion pH of 7.1 or less and with infusions of greater than 48 hours' duration.
Damage to the ductus, pulmonary artery, and aorta (weakening of the wall, leading to edema, laceration, and possible aneurysm) has been reported with long-term use.

The following side/adverse effects have been selected on the basis of their potential clinical significance (possible signs and symptoms in parentheses where appropriate)—not necessarily inclusive:

### Those indicating need for medical attention
Incidence more frequent
*Apnea*—incidence 10 to 12%; generally occurs within the first hour of infusion; the incidence is greatest in neonates weighing less than 2 kg at birth and is also increased if a rapid or large infusion is given initially (e.g., to purge the intravenous line); *fever*—incidence 14%, primarily a CNS effect, infection occurs in about 2% of patients; *flushing of face or arm*—incidence about 10%, especially with intra-arterial or intra-aortic administration, which is no longer recommended, may indicate misplacement of the catheter and introduction of alprostadil into the subclavian or carotid artery; *hypocalcemia*

Incidence less frequent
*Bradycardia*—incidence 7%; *diarrhea*—incidence 2%; *hypotension*—incidence 4%; *seizures*—incidence 4%; *tachycardia*—incidence 3%

Incidence rare—1% or less
*Anemia; anuria; bleeding; bradypnea, tachypnea, or bronchial wheezing; cardiac arrest; cerebral bleeding; congestive heart failure; cortical hyperostosis*—with long-term therapy, regresses after discontinuation of therapy; *disseminated intravascular coagulation; edema; gastric regurgitation; second degree heart block; hematuria; hypercapnia; hyperemia; hyperextension of the neck; ketotic hyperglycemia*—when given to an infant born to an insulin-dependent diabetic patient; *hyperirritability; hyperkalemia or hypokalemia; hypoglycemia; hypothermia; jitteriness; lethargy; peritonitis; respiratory distress, including respiratory depression; shock; spasm of right ventricle infundibulum; stiffness; supraventricular tachycardia; thrombocytopenia; ventricular fibrillation*

## Overdose

For more information on the management of overdose or unintentional ingestion, **contact a Poison Control Center** (see *Poison Control Center Listing*).

The following effects have been selected on the basis of their potential clinical significance (possible signs and symptoms in parentheses where appropriate)—not necessarily inclusive:

*Apnea; bradycardia; fever; flushing of skin; hypotension*

## General Dosing Information

Because of the risk of apnea, it is recommended that alprostadil be administered in an area with trained personnel and facilities necessary to provide pediatric intensive care. Respiratory support should be immediately available.

In patients with cyanotic heart defects, alprostadil is effective only if it is administered before permanent closure of the ductus arteriosus (DA) occurs. In normal-term infants, functional closure of the DA is usually complete within 10 to 15 hours after birth, and the DA is usually completely sealed off within 2 to 3 weeks. In clinical studies, the greatest response to alprostadil in patients with cyanotic heart defects was achieved in infants 4 days old or less. In infants with acyanotic heart defects, DA closure may be delayed, or the age of the patient and/or the extent of DA closure may be less critical. Beneficial responses to alprostadil may be achieved in infants up to 2 weeks of age, and occasionally in even older patients.

Because of its rapid metabolism, alprostadil must be diluted and administered by infusion. Use of a constant-rate infusion pump is recommended to avoid inadvertent rapid administration, because of the risk of apnea.

Alprostadil may be administered by intravenous infusion (peripheral or central) or intra-arterial infusion (through the pulmonary artery or an umbilical arterial catheter positioned at the level of the DA). The medication has also been administered via intra-aortic infusion, into the descending aorta adjacent to the DA. Theoretically, intra-aortic or intra-arterial administration should provide the greatest concentration to the DA and allow for rapid deactivation in the lungs, thereby reducing the risk of side effects. However, intra-arterial or intra-aortic administration has not proved more efficacious than intravenous administration, nor has it decreased the occurrence of side effects. Intravenous administration is now preferred for maintaining DA patency.

If fever or hypotension occurs, the rate of alprostadil infusion should be reduced

If a significant reduction of arterial blood pressure occurs, alprostadil should be discontinued immediately and appropriate treatment measures (e.g., volume replacement, administration of vasopressors) instituted. After the patient's blood pressure has stabilized, therapy may be reinstituted cautiously.

If apnea occurs, alprostadil should be discontinued or respiratory support instituted if continued use of alprostadil may be life saving.

If bradycardia occurs, alprostadil should be discontinued and appropriate medical treatment provided.

Flushing (peripheral arterial vasodilation) is usually the result of incorrect intra-arterial catheter placement and usually responds to repositioning of the catheter.

Alprostadil infusion may be continued during cardiac catheterization and may even facilitate the procedure.

Alprostadil infusion is usually continued until surgical repair is completed, usually within 24 to 48 hours after initiation of therapy, although it is sometimes continued postoperatively. Alprostadil should be administered for the shortest time and in the lowest dose that will produce the desired effect. However, long-term treatment may be required for some patients, especially very small infants who cannot undergo surgery until sufficient growth has taken place. The risks of long-term use (e.g., vascular damage, cortical proliferation of the long bones) must be weighed against the possible benefits. However, infants with severe cyanotic congenital heart disease have been treated for up to 3 months without adverse effects occurring.

## Parenteral Dosage Forms

### ALPROSTADIL INJECTION USP

**Usual pediatric dose**
Ductus arteriosus patency adjunct—
  Initial: Intravenous, into a large vein (preferred) or intra-arterial (via umbilical arterial catheter placed at the ductal opening), 0.05 to 0.1 mcg per kg of body weight per minute. However, if the ductus arteriosus is nonrestrictive at the time of diagnosis, an initial dose as low as 0.01 mcg per kg of body weight per minute may be effective. The rate of infusion may gradually be increased to up to 0.4 mcg per kg of body weight per minute, if necessary, although

doses higher than 0.1 mcg per kg of body weight per minute have not been shown to produce greater effects. After a satisfactory response is obtained, the rate of infusion may be reduced to the minimum level that will maintain the response. Dosage reduction is usually accomplished by progressively halving the previous dose, e.g., from 0.1 to 0.05 to 0.025 to 0.01 mcg per kg of body weight per minute.

  Maintenance: Intravenous, into a large vein (preferred) or intra-arterial (via umbilical arterial catheter placed at the ductal opening), infused at the minimum rate that will maintain the desired response. Doses as low as 0.002 mcg per kg of body weight per minute have been effective in some infants. However, maintenance dosage requirements may vary, and the infusion rate should be adjusted (increased or decreased) as necessary.

**Strength(s) usually available**
U.S.—
  500 mcg (0.5 mg) per mL (Rx) [*Prostin VR Pediatric* (in dehydrated alcohol)].
Canada—
  500 mcg (0.5 mg) per mL (Rx) [*Prostin VR* (in dehydrated alcohol)].

**Packaging and storage**
Store between 2 and 8 °C (36 and 46 °F), unless otherwise specified by manufacturer. Protect from freezing.

**Preparation of dosage form**
Alprostadil infusions are prepared by diluting 1 mL of the injection with a volume of 0.9% sodium chloride injection or 5% dextrose injection suitable for the pump delivery system available. For example, to provide 0.1 mcg per kg of body weight per minute, the following dilutions and infusion rates could be used:

| Amount of Diluent (mL) for each mL (500 mcg) of Alprostadil | Approximate Concentration of Resulting Solution (mcg/mL) | Infusion Rate (mL/min per kg of body weight) |
|---|---|---|
| 250 | 2 | 0.05 |
| 100 | 5 | 0.02 |
| 50 | 10 | 0.01 |
| 25 | 20 | 0.005 |

Caution: Use of diluents containing benzyl alcohol is not recommended for preparation of medications for use in neonates. A fatal toxic syndrome consisting of metabolic acidosis, CNS depression, respiratory problems, renal failure, hypotension, and possibly seizures and intracranial hemorrhages has been associated with this use.

**Stability**
Alprostadil infusions should be discarded 24 hours after they are prepared.

## Selected Bibliography

Roehl Sl, Townsend RJ. Alprostadil (Prostin VR Pediatric sterile solution, the Upjohn Company). Drug Intel Clin Pharm 1982 Nov; 16: 821-32.

Heymann MA, Clyman RI. Evaluation of alprostadil (prostaglandin E1) in the management of congenital heart disease in infancy. Pharmacotherapy 1982; 2: 148-55.

Bhatt V, Nahata MC. Pharmacologic management of patent ductus arteriosus. Clin Pharm 1989; 8: 17-33.

Revised: 04/09/92

---

## ALTEPLASE, RECOMBINANT—See *Thrombolytic Agents (Systemic)*

---

# ALTRETAMINE   Systemic

VA CLASSIFICATION (Primary): AN900
Another commonly used name is hexamethylmelamine.

Note: For a listing of dosage forms and brand names by country availability, see *Dosage Forms* section(s). For a listing of brand names for the articles in this monograph, refer to the General Index.

## Category
Antineoplastic.

## Indications

**Accepted**
Carcinoma, ovarian (treatment)—Altretamine is indicated for use as a single agent in the palliative treatment of patients with persistent or recurrent ovarian cancer following first-line therapy with a cisplatin- and/or alkylating agent–based combination.

## Pharmacology/Pharmacokinetics

Note: Pharmacokinetic studies have been done in only a limited number of patients; figures below are based on a study in 11 patients.

## Physicochemical characteristics
Source—Synthetic.
Chemical group—S-triazine derivative.

## Mechanism of action/Effect
The exact mechanism of action is unknown. Although altretamine structurally resembles an alkylating agent, it has not been found to have alkylating activity *in vitro*. There is some evidence that it may inhibit DNA and RNA synthesis.

## Absorption
Rapidly and well-absorbed following oral administration; however, because of rapid hepatic metabolism, peak plasma concentrations are variable.

## Distribution
Because it is highly lipid-soluble, altretamine is distributed to tissues with a high lipid component (e.g., omentum and subcutaneous tissues).

## Protein binding
Free fractions—
    Altretamine: 6%.
    Pentamethylmelamine: 25%.
    Tetramethylmelamine: 50%.

## Biotransformation
Hepatic. Metabolism is required for activity. Altretamine undergoes rapid and extensive demethylation, catalyzed by cytochrome P450 enzymes.

## Half-life
Elimination—Beta-phase: Range, 4.7 to 10.2 hours.

## Time to peak concentration
Plasma—0.5 to 3 hours.

## Elimination
Renal, less than 1% unchanged.

# Precautions to Consider

## Carcinogenicity
Secondary malignancies are potential delayed effects of many antineoplastic agents, although it is not clear whether the effect is related to their mutagenic or immunosuppressive action. The effect of dose and duration of therapy is also unknown, although risk seems to increase with long-term use. Although information is limited, available data seem to indicate that the carcinogenic risk is greatest with the alkylating agents.
One case of acute myelocytic leukemia has been reported in a patient treated with altretamine.
Studies with altretamine in animals have not been done.

## Mutagenicity
Altretamine was weakly mutagenic in strain TA100 of *Salmonella typhimurium*.

## Pregnancy/Reproduction
Fertility—Gonadal suppression, resulting in amenorrhea or azoospermia, may occur in patients taking antineoplastic therapy, especially with the alkylating agents. In general, these effects appear to be related to dose and length of therapy and may be irreversible. Prediction of the degree of testicular or ovarian function impairment is complicated by the common use of combinations of several antineoplastics, which makes it difficult to assess the effects of individual agents.
No adverse effect on fertility was found in female rats when altretamine was administered from 14 days prior to breeding through the gestation period. Administration to male rats in doses of 120 mg per square meter of body surface per day for 60 days prior to mating resulted in testicular atrophy, reduced fertility, and a possible dominant lethal mutagenic effect; doses of 450 mg per square meter of body surface per day for 10 days caused decreased spermatogenesis, atrophy of testes, seminal vesicles, and ventral prostate.
Pregnancy—Studies have not been done in humans.
First trimester: It is usually recommended that use of antineoplastics, especially combination chemotherapy, be avoided whenever possible, especially during the first trimester. Although information is limited because of the relatively few instances of antineoplastic administration during pregnancy, the mutagenic, teratogenic, and carcinogenic potential of these medications must be considered.
Other hazards to the fetus include adverse reactions seen in adults.
In general, use of a contraceptive is recommended during cytotoxic drug therapy.
Altretamine is embryotoxic and teratogenic in rats and rabbits given 2 to 10 times the human dose.
FDA Pregnancy Category D.

## Breast-feeding
Although very little information is available regarding distribution of antineoplastic agents into breast milk, breast-feeding is not recommended during chemotherapy because of the potential risks to the infant (adverse effects, mutagenicity, carcinogenicity). It is not known whether altretamine or its metabolites are distributed into breast milk.

## Pediatrics
No information is available on the relationship of age to the effects of altretamine in pediatric patients. Safety and efficacy have not been established.

## Geriatrics
Although appropriate studies on the relationship of age to the effects of altretamine have not been performed in the geriatric population, clinical trials have included elderly patients and geriatrics-specific problems that would limit the usefulness of this medication in the elderly are not expected. However, elderly patients are more likely to have age-related renal function impairment, which may require caution in patients receiving altretamine.

## Dental
The bone marrow depressant effects of altretamine may result in an increased incidence of microbial infection, delayed healing, and gingival bleeding. Dental work, whenever possible, should be completed prior to initiation of therapy or deferred until blood counts have returned to normal. Patients should be instructed in proper oral hygiene during treatment, including caution in use of regular toothbrushes, dental floss, and toothpicks.

## Drug interactions and/or related problems
The following drug interactions and/or related problems have been selected on the basis of their potential clinical significance (possible mechanism in parentheses where appropriate)—not necessarily inclusive (» = major clinical significance):

Note: Combinations containing any of the following medications, depending on the amount present, may also interact with this medication.

Blood dyscrasia–causing medications (See *Appendix II*)
    (leukopenic and/or thrombocytopenic effects of altretamine may be increased with concurrent or recent therapy if these medications cause the same effects; dosage adjustment of altretamine, if necessary, should be based on blood counts)

» Bone marrow depressants, other (See *Appendix II*) or
   Radiation therapy
    (additive bone marrow depression may occur; dosage reduction may be required when two or more bone marrow depressants, including radiation, are used concurrently or consecutively)

Cimetidine
    (inhibition of the cytochrome-P450 enzyme system by cimetidine would be expected to cause a decrease in the hepatic metabolism of altretamine, which could result in delayed elimination and increased blood concentrations)

» Monoamine oxidase (MAO) inhibitors, including furazolidone, procarbazine, and selegiline
    (concurrent use may result in severe orthostatic hypotension)

Vaccines, killed virus
    (because normal defense mechanisms may be suppressed by altretamine therapy, the patient's antibody response to the vaccine may be decreased. The interval between discontinuation of medications that cause immunosuppression and restoration of the patient's ability to respond to the vaccine depends on the intensity and type of immunosuppression-causing medication used, the underlying disease, and other factors; estimates vary from 3 months to 1 year)

» Vaccines, live virus
    (because normal defense mechanisms may be suppressed by altretamine therapy, concurrent use with a live virus vaccine may potentiate the replication of the vaccine virus, may increase the side/adverse effects of the vaccine virus, and/or may decrease the patient's antibody response to the vaccine; immunization of these patients should be undertaken only with extreme caution after careful review of the patient's hematologic status and only with the knowledge and consent of the physician managing the altretamine therapy. The interval between discontinuation of medications that cause immunosuppression and restoration of the patient's ability to respond to the vaccine depends on the intensity and type of immunosuppression-causing medication used, the underlying disease, and other factors; estimates vary from 3 months to 1 year. Patients with leukemia in remission should not receive live virus vaccine until at least 3 months after their last chemotherapy. In addition, immunization with oral poliovirus vaccine should be

postponed in persons in close contact with the patient, especially family members)

**Laboratory value alterations**

The following have been selected on the basis of their potential clinical significance (possible effect in parentheses where appropriate)—not necessarily inclusive (» = major clinical significance):

With physiology/laboratory test values

Alkaline phosphatase
(increases in serum values have been reported)

Blood urea nitrogen (BUN) and
Creatinine concentrations, serum
(moderate increases have been reported)

**Medical considerations/Contraindications**

The medical considerations/contraindications included here have been selected on the basis of their potential clinical significance (reasons given in parentheses where appropriate)—not necessarily inclusive (» = major clinical significance).

*Risk-benefit should be considered when the following medical problems exist:*

» Bone marrow depression
(lower dosage may be necessary)

» Chickenpox, existing or recent (including recent exposure) or
» Herpes zoster
(risk of severe generalized disease)

» Infection
Hepatic function impairment, severe
(reduced activation or metabolism)

» Neurologic toxicity, severe
Renal function impairment
(reduced elimination)

» Sensitivity to altretamine
» Tumor cell infiltration of the bone marrow
» Caution should be used also in patients who have had previous cytotoxic drug therapy or radiation therapy.

**Patient monitoring**

The following may be especially important in patient monitoring (other tests may be warranted in some patients, depending on condition; » = major clinical significance):

» Hematocrit or hemoglobin and
» Platelet count and
» Leukocyte count, total and, if appropriate, differential
(determinations recommended prior to initiation of therapy and at periodic intervals during therapy; frequency varies according to clinical state, agent, dose, and other agents being used concurrently)

» Neurologic examinations
(recommended at regular intervals during therapy)

# Side/Adverse Effects

Note: Many "side effects" of antineoplastic therapy are unavoidable and represent the medication's pharmacologic action. Some of these (for example, leukopenia and thrombocytopenia) are actually used as parameters to aid in individual dosage titration.

Toxicity is dose-related and cumulative.

Altretamine causes mild to moderate myelosuppression and neurotoxicity.

The following side/adverse effects have been selected on the basis of their potential clinical significance (possible signs and symptoms in parentheses where appropriate)—not necessarily inclusive:

**Those indicating need for medical attention**

Incidence more frequent
*Anemia* (often asymptomatic; less commonly or rarely, unusual tiredness); *leukopenia* (often asymptomatic; less commonly or rarely, fever or chills; cough or hoarseness; lower back or side pain; painful or difficult urination); *neurotoxicity, including central nervous system (CNS) effects* (anxiety; clumsiness; confusion; dizziness; mental depression; weakness; rarely, seizures); *neurotoxicity, including peripheral neuropathy* (numbness in arms or legs); *thrombocytopenia* (often asymptomatic; less commonly or rarely, unusual bleeding or bruising; black, tarry stools; blood in urine or stools; pinpoint red spots on skin)

Note: In *leukopenia*, with intermittent dosing (e.g., 8 to 12 mg per kg of body weight [mg/kg] per day for 21 days), the nadir of leukocyte counts occurs at about 3 to 4 weeks, with recovery by 6 weeks; with continuous dosing, the nadir occurs at 6 to 8 weeks (median).

Incidence of *neurotoxicity* is greater with daily high-dose therapy than with intermittent moderate-dose therapy. Neurotoxicity is reversible on withdrawal of altretamine.

In *thrombocytopenia*, with intermittent dosing (e.g., 8 to 12 mg/kg per day for 21 days), the nadir of platelet counts occurs at about 3 to 4 weeks, with recovery by 6 weeks; with continuous dosing, the nadir occurs at 6 to 8 weeks (median).

Incidence rare
*Hepatotoxicity* (asymptomatic); *skin rash or itching*

**Those indicating need for medical attention only if they continue or are bothersome**

Incidence more frequent
*Nausea and vomiting*

Note: *Nausea* and *vomiting* are usually mild to moderate, although they may be dose-limiting. The mechanism of the effect may be central because they usually do not occur until several days after initiation of treatment.

Incidence less frequent
*Diarrhea; loss of appetite; stomach cramps*

# Patient Consultation

As an aid to patient consultation, refer to *Advice for the Patient, Altretamine (Systemic)*.

In providing consultation, consider emphasizing the following selected information (» = major clinical significance):

**Before using this medication**

» Conditions affecting use, especially:
Sensitivity to altretamine
Pregnancy—Use not recommended because of mutagenic, teratogenic, and carcinogenic potential; advisability of using contraception; telling physician immediately if pregnancy is suspected
Breast-feeding—Not recommended because of risk of serious side effects
Other medications, especially other bone marrow depressants, monoamine oxidase (MAO) inhibitors, or other cytotoxic drug or radiation therapy
Other medical problems, especially chickenpox, herpes zoster, renal function impairment, infection, or severe neurotoxicity

**Proper use of this medication**

Frequency of nausea and vomiting; importance of continuing medication despite stomach upset; taking after meals to reduce stomach upset

» Proper dosing
Missed dose: Taking as soon as possible; however, if almost time for next dose, not taking missed dose; not doubling doses

» Proper storage

**Precautions while using this medication**

» Importance of close monitoring by the physician
» Avoiding immunizations unless approved by physician; other persons in patient's household should avoid immunizations with oral poliovirus vaccine; avoiding other persons who have taken oral poliovirus vaccine or wearing a protective mask that covers nose and mouth

*Caution if bone marrow depression occurs:*

» Avoiding exposure to persons with bacterial infections, especially during periods of low blood counts; checking with physician immediately if fever or chills, cough or hoarseness, lower back or side pain, or painful or difficult urination occur
» Checking with physician immediately if unusual bleeding or bruising; black, tarry stools; blood in urine or stools; or pinpoint red spots on skin occur

Caution in use of regular toothbrush, dental floss, or toothpick; physician, dentist, or nurse may suggest alternatives; checking with physician before having dental work done

Not touching eyes or inside of nose unless hands washed immediately before

Using caution to avoid accidental cuts with use of sharp objects such as safety razor or fingernail or toenail cutters

Avoiding contact sports or other situations where bruising or injury could occur

**Side/adverse effects**

May cause adverse effects such as blood problems; importance of discussing possible effects with physician

Signs of potential side effects, especially leukopenia, neurotoxicity, and thrombocytopenia

Physician or nurse can help in dealing with side effects

## General Dosing Information

Patients receiving altretamine should be under supervision of a physician experienced in cancer chemotherapy.

Dosage must be adjusted to meet the individual requirements of each patient, on the basis of clinical response and degree of bone marrow depression and neurotoxicity.

A variety of dosage schedules and regimens of altretamine, alone or in combination with other antitumor agents, are used. The prescriber may consult the medical literature as well as the manufacturer's literature in choosing a specific dosage.

Altretamine therapy should be temporarily withheld if any of the following occur:

Gastrointestinal intolerance unresponsive to symptomatic measures

Leukocyte count less than 2000 per cubic millimeter or granulocyte count less than 1000 per cubic millimeter

Platelet count less than 75,000 per cubic millimeter

Progressive neurotoxicity

After a period of at least 14 days, therapy may be reinitiated at a reduced dose of 200 mg per square meter of body surface per day.

If neurotoxicity continues even after dosage reduction, it is recommended that altretamine be discontinued.

Special precautions are recommended in patients who develop thrombocytopenia as a result of administration of altretamine. These may include extreme care in performing invasive procedures; regular inspection of intravenous sites, skin (including perirectal area), and mucous membrane surfaces for signs of bleeding or bruising; limiting frequency of venipuncture and avoiding intramuscular injections; testing urine, emesis, stool, and secretions for occult blood; care in use of regular toothbrushes, dental floss, toothpicks, safety razors, and fingernail and toenail cutters; avoiding constipation; and using caution to prevent falls and other injuries. Such patients should avoid alcohol and aspirin intake because of the risk of gastrointestinal bleeding. Platelet transfusions may be required.

Patients who develop leukopenia should be observed carefully for signs of infection. Antibiotic support may be required. In neutropenic patients who develop fever, broad-spectrum antibiotic coverage should be initiated empirically, pending bacterial cultures and appropriate diagnostic tests.

### Diet/Nutrition

It is recommended that altretamine be taken after meals to reduce nausea and vomiting.

## Oral Dosage Forms

### ALTRETAMINE CAPSULES

**Usual adult dose**
Carcinoma, ovarian—

Oral, 260 mg per square meter of body surface per day, in four divided daily doses after meals and at bedtime, for either fourteen or twenty-one consecutive days in a twenty-eight–day cycle.

Note: If excessive nausea and vomiting, leukopenia, thrombocytopenia, or neurotoxicity occur, it is recommended that altretamine be withheld for at least 14 days and then reinstituted at a dose of 200 mg per square meter of body surface per day.

**Usual pediatric dose**
Safety and efficacy have not been established.

**Strength(s) usually available**
U.S.—

50 mg (Rx) [*Hexalen* (lactose)].

Canada—

50 mg (Rx) [*Hexastat*].

100 mg (Rx) [*Hexastat*].

**Packaging and storage**
Store below 40 °C (104 °F), preferably between 15 and 30 °C (59 and 86 °F), unless otherwise specified by manufacturer.

**Auxiliary labeling**
• Take after meals.

## Selected Bibliography

Hansen LA, Hughes TE. Altretamine. DICP Ann Pharmacother 1991 Feb; 24: 146-52.

Hellmann K (ed). Hexamethylmelamine. Cancer Treat Rev 1991 Mar; 18 (Suppl A): entire issue. (Supported by a grant from U.S. Bioscience.)

Revised: 07/23/92
Interim revision: 04/29/94

## ALUMINA-CONTAINING COMBINATIONS—

Acetaminophen, Aspirin, and Salicylamide, Buffered (Systemic)—See *Acetaminophen and Salicylates (Systemic)*

Alumina and Magnesia (Oral-Local)—See *Antacids (Oral-Local)*

Alumina, Magnesia, and Calcium Carbonate (Oral-Local)—See *Antacids (Oral-Local)*

Alumina, Magnesia, Calcium Carbonate, and Simethicone (Oral-Local)—See *Antacids (Oral-Local)*

Alumina, Magnesia, and Simethicone (Oral-Local)—See *Antacids (Oral-Local)*

Alumina and Magnesium Carbonate (Oral-Local)—See *Antacids (Oral-Local)*

Alumina and Magnesium Trisilicate (Oral-Local)—See *Antacids (Oral-Local)*

Alumina, Magnesium Trisilicate, and Sodium Bicarbonate (Oral-Local)—See *Antacids (Oral-Local)*

Aspirin, Buffered (Systemic)—See *Salicylates (Systemic)*

Aspirin and Codeine, Buffered (Systemic)—See *Opioid (Narcotic) Analgesics and Aspirin (Systemic)*

Simethicone, Alumina, Magnesium Carbonate, and Magnesia (Oral-Local)—See *Antacids (Oral-Local)*

## ALUMINUM CARBONATE, BASIC—See *Antacids (Oral-Local)*

## ALUMINUM HYDROXIDE—See *Antacids (Oral-Local)*

# AMANTADINE   Systemic

VA CLASSIFICATION (Primary/Secondary): AM800/AU350; CN900

Note: For a listing of dosage forms and brand names by country availability, see *Dosage Forms* section(s). For a listing of brand names for the articles in this monograph, refer to the General Index.

## Category

Antiviral (systemic); antidyskinetic; antifatigue, specifically in multiple sclerosis.

## Indications

Note: Bracketed information in the *Indications* section refers to uses that are not included in U.S. product labeling.

**Accepted**

Influenza A (prophylaxis and treatment)—Amantadine is indicated as a primary agent in the prophylaxis and treatment of respiratory tract infections caused by influenza A virus strains in high-risk patients (including those with pulmonary or cardiovascular disease, the elderly, and residents of nursing homes and other chronic care facilities who have chronic medical conditions), hospital ward contacts of high-risk patients, immunocompromised patients, those in critical public service positions (e.g., police, firefighters, medical personnel), in high-risk patients for whom the influenza vaccine is contraindicated, and patients with severe influenza A viral infections. It is effective against all strains of influenza A virus that have been tested to date, including Russian, Brazilian, Texan, London, and others. It may be given as chemoprophylaxis concurrently with inactivated influenza A virus vaccine until protective antibodies develop. However, it should be emphasized that vaccination of high-risk persons each year is the single most important measure for reducing the impact of influenza. No well-controlled studies have examined whether amantadine prevents complications of influenza A in high-risk persons.

Resistant strains of influenza A have been reported in patients receiving rimantadine; these resistant strains were also apparently transmitted to household contacts. Rimantadine has a similar chemical structure, spectrum of activity, and mechanism of action to amantadine, and drug-resistant strains of virus have cross-resistance to amantadine and rimantadine.

**Extrapyramidal reactions, drug-induced (treatment) or**
**Parkinsonism (treatment)**—Amantadine is indicated in the treatment of idiopathic parkinsonism (paralysis agitans; shaking palsy), postencephalitic parkinsonism, drug-induced extrapyramidal reactions, symptomatic parkinsonism following injury to the nervous system caused by carbon monoxide intoxication, and parkinsonism associated with cerebral arteriosclerosis in the elderly.

**[Fatigue, multiple sclerosis–associated (treatment)][1]**—Amantadine is used in the management of certain aspects of fatigue associated with multiple sclerosis, including lowered energy level, decreased sense of well-being, decreased perceived attention and memory, and diminished problem solving ability.

### Unaccepted

Amantadine is not effective against other respiratory viral infections, including influenza B and parainfluenza.

---

[1]Not included in Canadian product labeling.

## Pharmacology/Pharmacokinetics

### Physicochemical characteristics
Molecular weight—187.71.

### Mechanism of action/Effect
Antiviral (systemic)—Not completely understood; amantadine appears to block the uncoating of influenza A virus and the release of viral nucleic acid into respiratory epithelial cells. May also affect early replicative phase of viruses that have already penetrated cells.
Antidyskinetic—Unknown; amantadine causes an increase in dopamine release in the animal brain. Probably increases release of dopamine and norepinephrine from central nerve terminals; also inhibits the reuptake of dopamine and norepinephrine.

### Absorption
Rapidly and almost completely absorbed from gastrointestinal tract.

### Distribution
Distributed to saliva, tear film, and nasal secretions; in animals, tissue (especially lung) concentrations higher than serum concentrations. Crosses the placenta and blood-brain barrier; excreted in breast milk. Cerebral spinal fluid concentrations were 52% of corresponding plasma concentrations in one patient.
$Vol_D =$
    $4.4 \pm 0.2$ liters per kg (normal renal function).
    $5.1 \pm 0.2$ liters per kg (renal failure).

### Protein binding
Normal renal function—Approximately 67%.
Hemodialysis patients—Approximately 59%.

### Biotransformation
No appreciable metabolism. Small amounts of an acetyl metabolite identified.

### Half-life
Normal renal function—11 to 15 hours.
Elderly patients—24 to 29 hours.
Renal function impairment, severe—7 to 10 days.
Hemodialysis—24 hours.

### Onset of action
Antidyskinetic—Usually within 48 hours.

### Time to peak serum concentration
2 to 4 hours (range, 1 to 8 hours); steady-state concentrations achieved within 2 to 3 days of daily administration.

### Peak serum concentration
Approximately 0.3 mcg per mL; steady-state trough concentrations after 50, 200, and 300 mg per day are approximately 0.1, 0.3, and 0.6 mcg per mL, respectively. Plasma concentrations exceeding 1.0 mcg per mL are considered to be in the toxic range.

### Elimination
Renal; 90% excreted unchanged in urine by glomerular filtration and renal tubular secretion. Rate of excretion rapidly increased in acid urine.
In dialysis—Only small amounts (approximately 4%) removed from the blood by hemodialysis.

## Precautions to Consider

### Carcinogenicity
Long-term studies have not been done in animals.

### Mutagenicity
Studies have not been done.

### Pregnancy/Reproduction
Pregnancy—Amantadine crosses the placenta. However, adequate and well-controlled studies in humans have not been done.
Studies in animals have shown that amantadine is embryotoxic and teratogenic in rats at doses of 50 mg per kg of body weight (mg/kg) per day. No adverse effects were seen in rats at doses of 37 mg/kg per day.
FDA Pregnancy Category C.

### Breast-feeding
Amantadine is excreted in breast milk. However, the effects of amantadine in neonates and infants are not known.

### Pediatrics
Appropriate studies on the relationship of age to the effects of amantadine have not been performed in neonates and infants up to one year of age. However, use of amantadine in children older than 1 year of age has not been shown to cause any pediatrics-specific problems that would limit its usefulness in children.

### Geriatrics
Geriatric patients may exhibit increased sensitivity to the anticholinergic-like side effects of amantadine, including confusion. A dosage reduction of 50% ($\leq$ 100 mg per day) appears to reduce the frequency of side effects without compromising antiviral prophylactic effectiveness. In addition, elderly patients are more likely to have an age-related decline in renal function, which may require a dosage reduction of greater than 50% in patients receiving amantadine, depending on the extent of renal dysfunction.

### Dental
Prolonged use of amantadine may decrease or inhibit salivary flow, thus contributing to the development of caries, periodontal disease, oral candidiasis, and discomfort.

### Drug interactions and/or related problems
The following drug interactions and/or related problems have been selected on the basis of their potential clinical significance (possible mechanism in parentheses where appropriate)—not necessarily inclusive (» = major clinical significance):

Note: Combinations containing any of the following medications, depending on the amount present, may also interact with this medication.

» Alcohol
    (concurrent use with amantadine is not recommended since this may increase the potential for CNS effects such as dizziness, lightheadedness, orthostatic hypotension, or confusion)

» Anticholinergics (See *Appendix II*), or other medications with anticholinergic activity, or
Antidepressants, tricyclic, or
Antidyskinetics, other, or
Antihistamines or
Phenothiazines
    (concurrent use with amantadine may potentiate the anticholinergic-like side effects, especially those of confusion, hallucinations, and nightmares; dosage adjustments of these medications or of amantadine may be necessary; also, patients should be advised to report occurrence of gastrointestinal problems promptly since paralytic ileus may occur with concurrent therapy)

Antidiarrheals, opioid- and anticholinergic-containing
    (concurrent use with amantadine may potentiate the anticholinergic-like side effects; although significant interaction is unlikely with usual doses of opioid- and anticholinergic-containing antidiarrheals, significant interaction may occur if these medications are abused)

Carbidopa and levodopa combination or
Levodopa
    (concurrent use with amantadine may result in increased efficacy of carbidopa and levodopa combination, and levodopa; however, concurrent use is not recommended if there is a history of psychosis)

» CNS stimulation–producing medications, other (See *Appendix II*)
    (concurrent use with amantadine may result in additive CNS stimulation to excessive levels, which may cause unwanted effects such as nervousness, irritability, or insomnia, and possibly seizures or cardiac arrhythmias; close observation is recommended)

Hydrochlorothiazide and
Triamterene
(one or both of these drugs may reduce the renal clearance of
amantadine, resulting in increased plasma concentrations and possible amantadine toxicity)

### Medical considerations/Contraindications
The medical considerations/contraindications included here have been selected on the basis of their potential clinical significance (reasons given
in parentheses where appropriate)—not necessarily inclusive (» =
major clinical significance).

*Risk-benefit should be considered when the following medical problems
exist:*

Eczematoid rash, recurrent, history of
» Edema, peripheral, or
» Heart failure, congestive
(amantadine may cause congestive heart failure and peripheral
edema; presumed to be due to redistribution of fluid, not a gain of
body water)
» Epilepsy, history of, or other seizure disorders
(amantadine may cause increased seizure activity; it may be necessary to reduce the dosage by 50% [≤ 100 mg per day]; this
appears to reduce the frequency of side effects without compromising antiviral prophylactic effectiveness)

Hypersensitivity to amantadine

Psychosis or severe psychoneurosis
(anticholinergic-like side effects of amantadine may result in confusion, hallucinations, and nightmares; it may be necessary to reduce the dosage by 50% [≤ 100 mg per day]; this appears to
reduce the frequency of side effects without compromising antiviral prophylactic effectiveness)
» Renal function impairment
(since amantadine is not metabolized and is excreted primarily in
the urine, toxic concentrations may accumulate in patients with
impaired renal function; it may be necessary to reduce the dosage
by 50% [≤ 100 mg per day in such patients]; this appears to reduce
the frequency of side effects without compromising antiviral prophylactic effectiveness)

## Side/Adverse Effects

Note: In controlled studies, side effects, including nausea, dizziness, insomnia, nervousness, and impaired concentration, were reported in
5 to 10% of young healthy adults taking the standard adult dosage
of 200 mg per day. Side effects may diminish or cease after the
first week of use. Serious, less frequent central nervous system
(CNS) side effects, such as confusion or seizures, have usually only
affected elderly patients, and patients with renal disease, seizure
disorders, or altered mental/behavioral conditions. Reducing the
dosage by 50% (≤ 100 mg per day) appears to reduce the frequency of side effects without compromising antiviral prophylactic
effectiveness.

The following side/adverse effects have been selected on the basis of their
potential clinical significance (possible signs and symptoms in parentheses where appropriate)—not necessarily inclusive:

### Those indicating need for medical attention
Incidence less frequent
*Anticholinergic-like effects* (blurred vision; confusion; difficult urination; hallucinations); *orthostatic hypotension* (fainting)
Incidence rare
*CNS toxicity* (impaired coordination; mental depression; seizures);
*congestive heart failure* (swelling of feet or lower legs; unexplained
shortness of breath)—usually only with chronic therapy; *corneal deposits* (irritation and swelling of the eye; decreased vision or any
change in vision); *skin rash*

### Those indicating need for medical attention only if they continue
### or are bothersome
Incidence more frequent
*CNS toxicity* (difficulty concentrating; dizziness or lightheadedness;
headache; insomnia; irritability; nervousness; nightmares); *gastrointestinal disturbances* (loss of appetite; nausea); *livedo reticularis* (purplish red, net-like, blotchy spots on skin)—usually only with chronic
therapy
Incidence less frequent or rare
*Anticholinergic-like effects* (constipation; dry mouth, nose, and
throat)—especially in elderly patients, patients receiving higher doses,
and patients with renal dysfunction; *vomiting*

## Overdose
For more information on the management of overdose or unintentional
ingestion, **contact a Poison Control Center** (See *Poison Control Center Listing*).

### Clinical effects of overdose
The following effects have been selected on the basis of their potential
clinical significance (possible signs and symptoms in parentheses
where appropriate)—not necessarily inclusive:
Symptoms of overdose
*Arrhythmias; pulmonary edema; status epilepticus; toxic psychosis*
(hallucinations; aggressive and violent behavior)

### Treatment of overdose
There is no specific antidote for the treatment of amantadine overdose.
Recommended treatment consists of the following:
To decrease absorption—
Gastric decontamination with activated charcoal; gastric lavage may be
performed if the ingestion was very recent.
Vomiting should not be induced due to the risk of seizures after the
overdose.
Supportive care—Supportive therapy. Patients in whom intentional over-
dose is known or suspected should be referred for psychiatric
consultation.

## Patient Consultation
As an aid to patient consultation, refer to *Advice for the Patient,
Amantadine (Systemic).*
In providing consultation, consider emphasizing the following selected
information (» = major clinical significance):

### Before using this medication
» Conditions affecting use, especially:
Hypersensitivity to amantadine
Pregnancy—Amantadine crosses the placenta
Breast-feeding—Amantadine is excreted in breast milk
Use in the elderly—Geriatric patients may exhibit increased sen-
sitivity to the anticholinergic-like side effects of amantadine
Other medications, especially alcohol, anticholinergics or other
medications with anticholinergic activity, or other CNS stim-
ulation–producing medications
Other medical problems, especially congestive heart failure, pe-
ripheral edema, renal function impairment, seizure disorders,
or a history of epilepsy

### Proper use of this medication
» Proper storage
» Proper dosing
Missed dose: Taking as soon as possible; not taking if almost time for
next dose; not doubling doses
*For use as an antiviral*
Receiving a flu shot if have not already done so
» Taking before exposure or as soon as possible after exposure
» Compliance with full course of therapy
» Importance of not missing doses and taking at evenly spaced times
Proper administration technique for oral liquid
*For use as an antidyskinetic*
» Not taking more medication than the amount prescribed; not missing
doses
May require up to 2 weeks for full benefit

### Precautions while using this medication
» Avoiding alcoholic beverages
» Caution if mental acuity or eyesight is impaired
Caution when getting up suddenly from a lying or sitting position
Possible dryness of mouth, nose, and throat; using sugarless candy or
gum, ice, or saliva substitute for relief of dry mouth; checking with
physician or dentist if dry mouth continues for more than 2 weeks
Possible appearance of livedo reticularis; gradual disappearance within
2 to 12 weeks after stopping medication
*For use as an antiviral*
Checking with physician if no improvement within a few days
*For use as an antidyskinetic*
» Resuming physical activities gradually as condition improves
Checking with physician if medication gradually loses its effectiveness
» Checking with physician before discontinuing medication; gradual
dosage reduction may be necessary

### Side/adverse effects
Signs of potential side effects, especially anticholinergic-like effects,
orthostatic hypotension, CNS toxicity, congestive heart failure,
corneal deposits, and skin rash

# General Dosing Information

In controlled studies, side effects, including nausea, dizziness, insomnia, nervousness, and impaired concentration, were reported in 5 to 10% of young healthy adults taking the standard adult dosage of 200 mg per day. Data suggest that comparable protection may be provided by a daily prophylactic dosage of 100 mg, but with fewer side effects. No studies have been done comparing 100-mg and 200-mg doses for the treatment of influenza A infection.

Patients receiving doses exceeding 200 mg per day should be closely observed for signs of increased incidence of side effects or toxicity. Monitoring of such patients for blood pressure, pulse, respiration, and temperature should be considered, especially for a few days following the increase in dose. Patients with active seizure disorders may be at increased risk for seizures while receiving amantadine.

Changing from once-a-day to twice-a-day administration may eliminate or reduce the severity of side effects such as lightheadedness, insomnia, and nausea.

If possible, plasma concentrations should be monitored in patients with end-stage renal disease since a single dose may provide adequate concentrations for as long as 7 to 10 days.

## For use in the prophylaxis and treatment of influenza type A virus infection

Chemoprophylactic administration should be started in anticipation of contact with, or as soon as possible after exposure to, persons having influenza A virus infections. Administration should be continued for at least 10 days following exposure. In influenza epidemics, amantadine should be given daily during the epidemic (usually 6 to 8 weeks in most communities) or until active immunity can be expected from administration of inactivated influenza A virus vaccine. However, rimantadine, chemically similar to amantadine, has been reported to be ineffective when used prophylactically in household members while concurrently treating index cases for influenza A. This was apparently due to transmission of drug-resistant strains of the virus.

If administered concurrently with inactivated influenza A virus vaccine until protective antibodies develop, amantadine should be continued chemoprophylactically for 2 to 3 weeks after the vaccine has been administered. Amantadine may then be discontinued. However, since the vaccine is only 70 to 80% effective, more prolonged administration of amantadine may be beneficial in elderly or high-risk patients. If the vaccine is unavailable or contraindicated, amantadine should be administered for up to 90 days in cases of possible repeated or unknown exposure.

Treatment of the symptoms of influenza A virus infections should be started within 24 to 48 hours after their onset and should be continued for 48 hours after their disappearance. Cough may persist for several weeks.

## For use in the treatment of parkinsonism

Patients initially benefiting from the continuous administration of amantadine may experience a decline in effectiveness after a few months. Effectiveness may be restored by increasing the dose to 300 mg daily or temporarily discontinuing amantadine therapy for several weeks, and then resuming it.

Patients who have concurrent serious illnesses or are receiving high doses of other antiparkinsonian medications may be started on 100 mg of amantadine once a day. After one to several weeks, the dose may be increased to 100 mg two times a day, if necessary. If response is still not optimal, patients may benefit from a further increase to 400 mg daily in divided doses.

Concurrent administration of anticholinergic antiparkinsonian medications or levodopa with amantadine may provide additional benefit, including reduction in fluctuations in improvement occurring with levodopa alone. If dosage reductions of levodopa are required because of side effects, the benefit lost by the reduction may be restored by the concurrent administration of amantadine.

If carbidopa and levodopa combination or levodopa is initially being administered concurrently with amantadine, the dose of amantadine should be maintained at 100 mg one or two times a day while the dose of carbidopa and levodopa combination, or levodopa is gradually increased to provide optimal benefit.

Patients who have drug-induced extrapyramidal reactions may be started on 100 mg of amantadine two times a day. If response is not optimal, dose may be increased to 300 mg daily in divided doses.

When amantadine is to be discontinued, dosage should be reduced gradually in order to prevent a sudden increase in parkinsonian symptoms.

# Oral Dosage Forms

Note: Bracketed uses in the *Dosage Forms* section refer to categories of use and/or indications that are not included in U.S. product labeling.

## AMANTADINE HYDROCHLORIDE CAPSULES USP

### Usual adult and adolescent dose
Antiviral (systemic)—
    Oral, 200 mg once a day; or 100 mg every twelve hours.
    Oral, 100 mg one or two times a day.
[Antifatigue, multiple sclerosis–associated][1]—
    Oral, 200 mg once a day; or 100 mg two times a day.

Note: Adults with impaired renal function may require a reduction in dose as noted below. Elderly patients, and patients with seizure disorders, or altered mental/behavioral conditions may require even further dose reductions.

| Creatinine Clearance (mL/min)/ (mL/sec) | Dose |
|---|---|
| >50/0.83 | See *Usual adult and adolescent dose* |
| 30–50/0.50–0.83 | 200 mg the first day, then 100 mg once a day |
| 15–29/0.25–0.48 | 200 mg the first day, then 100 mg every other day |
| <15/0.25 | 200 mg once every 7 days |
| Hemodialysis patients | 200 mg once every 7 days |

### Usual adult prescribing limits
Antiviral (systemic)—
    Up to 200 mg daily.
Antidyskinetic—
    Up to 400 mg daily.

### Usual pediatric dose
Antiviral (systemic)—
    Neonates and infants up to 1 year of age: Dosage has not been established.
    Children 1 to 9 years of age: Oral, 1.5 to 3 mg per kg of body weight every eight hours; or 2.2 to 4.4 mg per kg of body weight every twelve hours. Maximum daily dose should not exceed 150 mg.
    Children 9 to 12 years of age: Oral, 100 mg every twelve hours.
    Children 12 years of age and over: See *Usual adult and adolescent dose.*

Note: For children 10 years of age or older weighing less than 45 kg of body weight, it may be advisable to use a dosage of 2.2 mg per kg of body weight every twelve hours.

    Some references recommend doses as low as 1.5 mg per kg of body weight every twelve hours in children 1 to 9 years of age.

### Usual geriatric dose
Antiviral (systemic)—
    Oral, 100 mg once a day.
Antidyskinetic—
    Oral, 100 mg once a day to start, titrating the dose to 100 mg two or three times a day.

Note: A daily dose of amantadine exceeding 100 mg should be used with caution in persons 65 years of age or older for influenza prophylaxis or treatment. If the patient has any renal function impairment, the dose should be reduced further.

### Strength(s) usually available
U.S.—
    100 mg (Rx) [*Symadine; Symmetrel;* GENERIC].
Canada—
    100 mg (Rx) [*Symmetrel*].

### Packaging and storage
Store below 40 °C (104 °F), preferably between 15 and 30 °C (59 and 86 °F), unless otherwise specified by manufacturer. Store in a tight container.

### Auxiliary labeling
• May cause dizziness or blurred vision.
• Avoid alcoholic beverages.
• Continue medicine for full time of treatment (antiviral).

## AMANTADINE HYDROCHLORIDE SYRUP USP

### Usual adult and adolescent dose
See *Amantadine Hydrochloride Capsules USP.*

### Usual adult prescribing limits
See *Amantadine Hydrochloride Capsules USP.*

### Usual pediatric dose
See *Amantadine Hydrochloride Capsules USP.*

**Usual geriatric dose**
See *Amantadine Hydrochloride Capsules USP*.

**Strength(s) usually available**
U.S.—
50 mg per 5 mL (Rx) [*Symmetrel;* GENERIC].
Canada—
50 mg per 5 mL (Rx) [*Symmetrel*].

**Packaging and storage**
Store below 40 °C (104 °F), preferably between 15 and 30 °C (59 and 86 °F), unless otherwise specified by manufacturer. Store in a tight container. Protect from freezing.

**Auxiliary labeling**
• May cause dizziness or blurred vision.
• Avoid alcoholic beverages.
• Continue medicine for full time of treatment (antiviral).

**Note**
When dispensing, include a calibrated liquid-measuring device for antiviral use.

Revised: 02/23/93

---

**AMBENONIUM**—See *Antimyasthenics (Systemic)*

---

**AMCINONIDE**—See *Corticosteroids (Topical)*

---

**AMIKACIN**—See *Aminoglycosides (Systemic)*

---

**AMILORIDE**—See *Diuretics, Potassium-sparing (Systemic)*

---

**AMILORIDE-CONTAINING COMBINATIONS**—

Amiloride and Hydrochlorothiazide (Systemic)—See *Diuretics, Potassium-sparing, and Hydrochlorothiazide (Systemic)*

---

# AMINOBENZOATE POTASSIUM   Systemic

VA CLASSIFICATION (Primary): DE890

Other commonly used names are KPAB, potassium aminobenzoate, and potassium para-aminobenzoate.

Note: For a listing of dosage forms and brand names by country availability, see *Dosage Forms* section(s). For a listing of brand names for the articles in this monograph, refer to the General Index.

## Category
Antifibrotic.

## Indications

**Accepted**
Dermatomyositis, fibrosis and/or nonsuppurative inflammation in (treatment)
Morphea, fibrosis and/or nonsuppurative inflammation in (treatment)
Pemphigus, fibrosis and/or nonsuppurative inflammation in (treatment)[1]
Peyronie's disease, fibrosis and/or nonsuppurative inflammation in (treatment)
Scleroderma, fibrosis and/or nonsuppurative inflammation in (treatment) or
Scleroderma, linear, fibrosis and/or nonsuppurative inflammation in (treatment)—The U.S. Food and Drug Administration (FDA) has classified aminobenzoate potassium as being possibly effective in the treatment of dermatomyositis, morphea, pemphigus, Peyronie's disease, scleroderma, and linear scleroderma, involving fibrosis and/or nonsuppurative inflammation. This classification requires the submission of adequate and well-controlled studies to provide substantial evidence of effectiveness.

[1]Not included in Canadian product labeling.

## Pharmacology/Pharmacokinetics

**Physicochemical characteristics**
Molecular weight—175.23.

**Mechanism of action/Effect**
The mechanism by which aminobenzoate potassium exerts its antifibrotic effect is not known. It has been postulated that fibrosis results from an imbalance of serotonin and monoamine oxidase (MAO) mechanisms at the tissue level. Fibrosis is believed to occur when an excessive serotonin effect is sustained over a period of time. This could be the result of too much serotonin or too little MAO activity. Aminobenzoate potassium increases oxygen utilization at the tissue level. It has been suggested that this increased oxygen utilization could enhance the degradation of serotonin by enhancing MAO activity or other activities that decrease the tissue concentration of serotonin.

**Onset of action**
Improvement in fibrosis usually occurs within the first 3 months of therapy.

## Precautions to Consider

**Cross-sensitivity and/or related problems**
Patients sensitive to aminobenzoic acid (PABA) may be sensitive to potassium aminobenzoate also, since this medication is the potassium salt of PABA.

**Pregnancy/Reproduction**
Pregnancy—Studies have not been done in humans.
Studies have not been done in animals.

**Breast-feeding**
Problems in humans have not been documented.

**Pediatrics**
Appropriate studies on the relationship of age to the effects of aminobenzoate potassium have not been performed in the pediatric population. However, pediatrics-specific problems that would limit the usefulness of this medication in children are not expected.

**Geriatrics**
In the elderly, the hypoglycemia that may occur if this medication is continued through several days of inadequate food intake may be more difficult to recognize and may cause more neurological symptoms than physical ones. In addition, elderly patients are more likely to have age-related renal function impairment, which may require adjustment in dosage in patients receiving aminobenzoate potassium.

**Drug interactions and/or related problems**
The following drug interactions and/or related problems have been selected on the basis of their potential clinical significance (possible mechanism in parentheses where appropriate)—not necessarily inclusive (» = major clinical significance):

Note: Combinations containing any of the following medications, depending on the amount present, may also interact with this medication.

» Aminosalicylates or
» Sulfonamides, systemic
(concurrent use with aminobenzoate potassium may inhibit the action of these medications because aminobenzoate potassium is absorbed by bacterial pathogens preferentially over sulfonamides and aminosalicylates; concurrent use is not recommended)

**Laboratory value alterations**
The following have been selected on the basis of their potential clinical significance (possible effect in parentheses where appropriate)—not necessarily inclusive (» = major clinical significance):

With physiology/laboratory test values
Glucose concentration, blood
(may be decreased; hypoglycemia may occur when aminobenzoate potassium therapy is continued through several days of inadequate food intake)

White blood cell counts
(may be temporarily decreased; there is usually a return to normal values despite continued administration of medication)

**Medical considerations/Contraindications**
The medical considerations/contraindications included here have been selected on the basis of their potential clinical significance (reasons given in parentheses where appropriate)—not necessarily inclusive (» = major clinical significance).

*Risk-benefit should be considered when the following medical problems exist:*
Diabetes mellitus or
Hypoglycemia
   (may predispose the patient to, or cause potentiation of, drug-induced hypoglycemia, especially if medication is continued through several days of inadequate food intake)
Renal function impairment
   (since aminobenzoate potassium is excreted by the kidneys, impaired renal function may cause accumulation of this medication in the blood, thereby increasing the chance of side effects)
Sensitivity to aminobenzoate potassium

**Patient monitoring**
The following may be especially important in patient monitoring (other tests may be warranted in some patients, depending on condition; » = major clinical significance):

White blood cell counts
   (may be performed prior to initiation of therapy, and at periodic intervals during therapy if signs of leukopenia occur)

## Side/Adverse Effects

The following side/adverse effects have been selected on the basis of their potential clinical significance (possible signs and symptoms in parentheses where appropriate)—not necessarily inclusive:

**Those indicating need for medical attention**
Incidence less frequent or rare
   *Allergic reaction* (fever; skin rash); *hypoglycemia* (anxiety; chills; cold sweats; confusion; cool pale skin; difficulty in concentration; drowsiness; excessive hunger; fast heartbeat; headache; nervousness; shakiness; unsteady walk; unusual tiredness or weakness)—may occur if aminobenzoate potassium therapy is continued through several days of inadequate food intake; *leukopenia* (fever and chills; sore throat)

**Those indicating need for medical attention only if they continue or are bothersome**
Incidence more frequent
   *Anorexia* (loss of appetite); *nausea*
   Note: If *anorexia, nausea,* or any other problem prevents the patient from eating normally, therapy with aminobenzoate potassium should be interrupted until the patient is eating normally again, to prevent the possible development of hypoglycemia.

## Patient Consultation

As an aid to patient consultation, refer to *Advice for the Patient, Aminobenzoate Potassium (Systemic)*.

In providing consultation, consider emphasizing the following selected information (» = major clinical significance):

**Before using this medication**
» Conditions affecting use, especially:
   Sensitivity to aminobenzoate potassium or aminobenzoic acid (PABA)
   Use in the elderly—Elderly people may be more sensitive to certain symptoms of the hypoglycemia side effect. These symptoms include confusion, difficulty in concentration, and headache. In addition, these symptoms may be harder to detect in elderly persons than in younger adults. Also, elderly people are more likely to have age-related renal function impairment. This may increase the chance of problems during treatment with this medication
   Other medications, especially aminosalicylates and sulfonamides

**Proper use of this medication**
Taking with meals or snacks to minimize stomach upset; checking with physician if stomach upset continues
*Proper administration of capsule or tablet dosage form*
   Taking each dose with a full glass (240 mL) of water or milk to minimize stomach upset
   If taking the tablets, dissolving them in water first to minimize stomach upset
*Proper administration of powder dosage form*
   Not taking in dry form; mixing with water or citrus juice

Masking taste of medication by dissolving medication in citrus juice instead of in water, or by drinking citrus juice or carbonated beverage after taking medication in water
   Chilling solution before taking to improve flavor
*Preparation of solutions*
*Using individual 2-gram packets of powder to make solution*
   Dissolving one packet (2 grams) of powder in a full glass (8 ounces) of water or citrus juice; stirring well to dissolve powder
*Using bulk powder to make a 10% solution*
   Using a light-resistant container, such as an amber glass, opaque plastic, or stainless steel container, that is large enough to measure 1 liter (L) (approximately 1 quart)
   Using a specially marked measuring device for measuring out the bulk powder
   Measuring out 100 grams (approximately 3 ounces) of powder and placing in container
   Adding enough water or citrus juice to make 1 L (approximately 1 quart) of solution; stirring well to dissolve powder; discarding unused portion after 1 week
   Storing in a light-resistant container, such as an amber glass, opaque plastic, or stainless steel container
   Stirring well before pouring each dose
» Compliance with therapy; 3 or more months may be required before improvement in condition is noticed
» Proper dosing
   Missed dose: Taking as soon as possible; not taking if within 2 hours of next dose; not doubling doses
» Proper storage

**Precautions while using this medication**
Regular visits to your physician to check progress of therapy
» Notifying physician immediately if unable to eat normally for any reason, such as nausea or loss of appetite; hypoglycemia may occur if medication is continued through a period of several days of inadequate food intake
» If symptoms of hypoglycemia occur
   Stopping medication
   Taking sugar and notifying physician immediately
   Instructing someone ahead of time to take you to your physician or hospital immediately if you begin to feel that you may pass out, or to get emergency help immediately in case you do pass out
   Calling physician immediately even if you start to feel better; blood sugar–lowering effects of medication may last for a few days and may recur frequently during this period of time

**Side/adverse effects**
Signs of potential side effects, especially allergic reaction, hypoglycemia, and leukopenia
   Hypoglycemia may occur if aminobenzoate potassium therapy is continued through a period of several days of inadequate food intake
   If hypoglycemia occurs in the elderly, the neurological signs, such as confusion, difficulty in concentration, or headache, are more likely to occur

## General Dosing Information

The exact dosing schedule depends on what is convenient for the patient.

The doses of this medication should be spread over each day as much as possible, with the first dose being taken at breakfast or upon arising and the last dose at bedtime.

Patients tolerate the powder for oral solution best and the capsules second best. The tablets are the least tolerated dosage form; they should be dissolved in an adequate amount of liquid to prevent gastrointestinal upset.

If the patient is not eating normally for any reason, such as nausea or loss of appetite, therapy should be interrupted until the patient is eating normally again, to prevent the possible development of hypoglycemia.

Desensitization should be considered if side/adverse effects prevent the patient from continuing therapy.

**Diet/Nutrition**
The medication should be taken with food or snacks to minimize stomach upset.

**For treatment of adverse effects**
If symptoms of hypoglycemia appear, patient should discontinue medication, eat or drink a source of sugar, and obtain medical assistance immediately.

Good sources of sugar are table sugar mixed in water, sugar cubes, orange juice, corn syrup, or honey. A popular source of sugar is a glassful of orange juice containing 2 or 3 teaspoonfuls of table sugar.

Severe hypoglycemic reactions with coma, seizures, or other neurological impairment can occur. If hypoglycemic coma is diagnosed or suspected, the patient should be given a rapid intravenous injection of 50% glucose solution. This should be followed by a continuous infusion of a 10% glucose solution at a rate that will maintain the blood glucose at a level above 100 mg/dL. Patients should be closely monitored for at least 24 to 48 hours in the hospital.

## Oral Dosage Forms

### AMINOBENZOATE POTASSIUM CAPSULES USP

**Usual adult and adolescent dose**
Dermatomyositis or
Morphea or
Pemphigus[1] or
Peyronie's disease or
Scleroderma or
Scleroderma, linear—
   Oral, 12 grams a day, usually in four to six divided doses, with meals or snacks.

**Usual pediatric dose**
Dermatomyositis or
Morphea or
Pemphigus[1] or
Peyronie's disease or
Scleroderma or
Scleroderma, linear—
   Oral, 220 mg per kg of body weight a day, usually in four to six divided doses, with meals or snacks.

Note: Aminobenzoate Potassium for Oral Solution USP may be a more easily administered dosage form for children.

**Strength(s) usually available**
U.S.—
   500 mg (Rx) [*Potaba*].
Canada—
   500 mg (Rx) [*Potaba*].

**Packaging and storage**
Store between 8 and 15 °C (46 and 59 °F), in a well-closed container, unless otherwise specified by manufacturer.

**Auxiliary labeling**
• Take with full glass (8 ounces) of water or milk after meals or snacks.

### AMINOBENZOATE POTASSIUM FOR ORAL SOLUTION USP

**Usual adult and adolescent dose**
See *Aminobenzoate Potassium Capsules USP*.

**Usual pediatric dose**
See *Aminobenzoate Potassium Capsules USP*.

**Size(s) usually available**
U.S.—
   2 grams (individual powder packets) (Rx) [*Potaba Envules*].
   100 grams (bulk powder) (Rx) [*Potaba Powder*].
   454 grams (bulk powder) (Rx) [*Potaba Powder*].
Canada—
   2 grams (individual powder packets) (Rx) [*Potaba Envules*].
   100 grams (bulk powder) (Rx) [*Potaba Powder*].

**Packaging and storage**
Prior to constitution, store between 8 and 15 °C (46 and 59 °F), unless otherwise specified by manufacturer. After constitution, store between 2 and 8 °C (36 and 46 °F), unless otherwise specified by manufacturer. Store in a tight container. Protect from light.

**Preparation of dosage form**
The oral solution is usually administered as a 10% aqueous solution.
To prepare a 10% solution, dissolve 100 grams of aminobenzoate potassium powder in sufficient water to make 1 L of solution.
The taste of the powder can be improved if it is dissolved in citrus drinks, such as lemon, orange, or grapefruit juice.

**Stability**
Constituted solutions should be stored in the refrigerator and discarded after one week.
Solutions are light sensitive and should be mixed and stored in amber glass or other light-resistant containers.

**Auxiliary labeling**
• Refrigerate solution.
• Stir well before pouring each dose.
• Take after meals or snacks.
• Discard unused portion after one week.

### AMINOBENZOATE POTASSIUM TABLETS USP

**Usual adult and adolescent dose**
See *Aminobenzoate Potassium Capsules USP*.

Note: The tablets should be dissolved in an adequate amount of liquid to prevent gastrointestinal upset.

**Usual pediatric dose**
See *Aminobenzoate Potassium Capsules USP*.

Note: Aminobenzoate Potassium for Oral Solution USP may be a more easily administered dosage form for children.

   If the tablets are used, they should be dissolved in an adequate amount of liquid to prevent gastrointestinal upset.

**Strength(s) usually available**
U.S.—
   500 mg (Rx) [*Potaba*].
Canada—
   500 mg (Rx) [*Potaba*].

**Packaging and storage**
Store between 8 and 15 °C (46 and 59 °F), in a well-closed container, unless otherwise specified by manufacturer.

**Auxiliary labeling**
• Take with full glass (8 ounces) of water or milk with meals or snacks.

Revised: 07/06/94

---

## AMINOBENZOIC ACID-CONTAINING COMBINATIONS—

Aminobenzoic Acid, Padimate O, and Oxybenzone (Topical)—See *Sunscreen Agents (Topical)*
Aminobenzoic Acid and Titanium Dioxide (Topical)—See *Sunscreen Agents (Topical)*

---

# AMINOCAPROIC ACID   Systemic

JAN: Epsilon-aminocaproic acid
VA CLASSIFICATION (Primary): BL300
Note: For a listing of dosage forms and brand names by country availability, see *Dosage Forms* section(s). For a listing of brand names for the articles in this monograph, refer to the General Index.

## Category
Antifibrinolytic; antihemorrhagic.

## Indications
Note: Bracketed information in the *Indications* section refers to uses that are not included in U.S. product labeling.

**Accepted**
Hemorrhage, hyperfibrinolysis-induced (treatment)

Hemorrhage, postsurgical (prophylaxis and treatment) or
[Hemorrhage, following dental surgery, in hemophiliacs (prophylaxis and treatment)]—Aminocaproic acid is indicated for treatment of severe bleeding that may occur following heart surgery (with or without cardiac bypass procedures) and portacaval shunt, prostatectomy, or nephrectomy, and in association with hematologic disorders (such as aplastic anemia), abruptio placentae (with laboratory confirmation of hyperfibrinolysis), hepatic cirrhosis, neoplastic disease, and polycystic or neoplastic diseases of the genitourinary system.

[Aminocaproic acid is used in the management of hemophilic patients (i.e., patients with Factor VIII or Factor IX deficiency) undergoing surgery, including tooth extractions or other dental surgical procedures. The medication prevents or decreases hemorrhaging during and following surgery in these patients and reduces the need for administration of clotting factors.]

[Aminocaproic acid is also used to prevent intra- and postoperative hemorrhaging in patients with clotting defects other than hemophilia (including von Willebrand disease or deficiencies of factors other than Factor VIII or Factor IX).][1]

[Aminocaproic acid is used to treat severe hemorrhaging caused by thrombolytic agents (alteplase [tissue-type plasminogen activator, recombinant], anistreplase [anisoylated plasminogen-streptokinase activator complex], streptokinase, or urokinase). However, controlled studies to demonstrate its efficacy for this use have not been done in humans.][1]

[Hemorrhage, subarachnoid, recurrence (prophylaxis)]—Aminocaproic acid is used to prevent recurrence of subarachnoid hemorrhage, especially when surgery is delayed.

Note: In some patients receiving treatment for hemorrhaging, other emergency measures including transfusion of whole blood, fresh frozen plasma, specific clotting factors, or fibrinogen may be needed.

Aminocaproic acid is ineffective in bleeding caused by loss of vascular integrity; a definite clinical diagnosis or laboratory findings indicative of hyperfibrinolysis (hyperplasminemia) is essential prior to initiation of aminocaproic acid therapy. However, some conditions and laboratory findings suggestive of hyperfibrinolysis are also present in disseminated intravascular coagulation; differentiation between the 2 conditions is essential because aminocaproic acid may promote thrombus formation in patients with disseminated intravascular coagulation and must *not* be used unless heparin is administered concurrently. The following criteria may be useful in differential diagnosis:

| Test | Primary Hyperfibrinolysis Results | Disseminated Intravascular Coagulation Results |
| --- | --- | --- |
| Platelet count* | Normal | Decreased |
| Protamine paracoagulation test | Negative | Positive |
| Euglobulin clot lysis time | Decreased | Normal |

*Following extracorporeal circulation (during cardiovascular surgery), decreased platelet count may not be useful for differentiating between primary hyperfibrinolysis and disseminated intravascular coagulation; the other criteria may be more useful in differential diagnosis in these patients.

[1]Not included in Canadian product labeling.

## Pharmacology/Pharmacokinetics

### Physicochemical characteristics
Molecular weight—131.17.

### Mechanism of action/Effect
Aminocaproic acid competitively inhibits activation of plasminogen, thereby reducing conversion of plasminogen to plasmin (fibrinolysin), an enzyme that degrades fibrin clots as well as fibrinogen and other plasma proteins including the procoagulant factors V and VIII. Aminocaproic acid also directly inhibits plasmin activity, but higher doses are required than are needed to reduce plasmin formation. *In vitro*, the antifibrinolytic potency of aminocaproic acid is approximately one-fifth to one-tenth that of tranexamic acid.

### Absorption
Absorbed rapidly following oral administration.

### Protein binding
Does not appear to bind to plasma protein.

### Time to peak concentration
Within 2 hours following a single oral dose.

### Therapeutic plasma concentration
For inhibition of systemic hyperfibrinolysis—130 mcg per mL (991 micromoles/L).
For prevention of recurrent subarachnoid hemorrhage—150 to 300 mcg per mL (1143 to 2287 micromoles/L).

### Elimination
Renal. Excreted rapidly, mostly as unchanged drug.

## Precautions to Consider

### Pregnancy/Reproduction
Fertility—Studies in rodents have suggested an adverse effect on fertility, consistent with aminocaproic acid's antifibrinolytic activity.

Pregnancy—Studies have not been done in humans.

Studies have not been done in animals.
FDA Pregnancy Category C.

### Breast-feeding
It is not known whether aminocaproic acid is distributed into breast milk. However, problems in humans have not been documented.

### Pediatrics
Although studies on the relationship of age to the effects of aminocaproic acid have not been performed in the pediatric population, no pediatrics-specific problems attributed to aminocaproic acid have been documented to date. However, aminocaproic acid injections that contain benzyl alcohol should not be administered to premature neonates because the preservative has been associated with a fatal toxic syndrome consisting of metabolic acidosis, central nervous system (CNS) depression, respiratory problems, renal failure, hypotension, and possibly seizures and intracranial hemorrhages in these patients.

### Geriatrics
Although studies on the relationship of age to the effects of aminocaproic acid have not been performed in the geriatric population, no geriatrics-specific problems have been documented to date. However, elderly patients are more likely to have age-related renal function impairment, which may require dosage reduction in patients receiving aminocaproic acid.

### Drug interactions and/or related problems
The following drug interactions and/or related problems have been selected on the basis of their potential clinical significance (possible mechanism in parentheses where appropriate)—not necessarily inclusive (» = major clinical significance):

Note: Combinations containing any of the following medications, depending on the amount present, may also interact with this medication.

Anti-inhibitor coagulant complex or
Factor IX complex
  (although aminocaproic acid is often used in conjunction with clotting factor replacement for the perisurgical management of hemophilic patients, concurrent use may increase the risk of thrombotic complications; some hematologists recommend that administration of aminocaproic acid be delayed for 8 hours following injection of either of the clotting factor complexes)

Contraceptives, estrogen-containing, oral or
Estrogens
  (concurrent use with aminocaproic acid may increase the potential for thrombus formation)

Thrombolytic agents
  (the actions of aminocaproic acid and of thrombolytic agents [e.g., alteplase (tissue-type plasminogen activator, recombinant; tPA), anistreplase (anisoylated plasminogen-streptokinase activator complex; APSAC), streptokinase, or urokinase] are mutually antagonistic; although controlled studies to demonstrate its efficacy for this use have not been done in humans, aminocaproic acid may be useful in treating severe hemorrhage caused by a thrombolytic agent)

### Medical considerations/Contraindications
The medical considerations/contraindications included here have been selected on the basis of their potential clinical significance (reasons given in parentheses where appropriate)—not necessarily inclusive (» = major clinical significance).

*Except under special circumstances, this medication should not be used when the following medical problem exists:*
» Intravascular clotting, active
    (risk of serious, even fatal, thrombus formation)

*Risk-benefit should be considered when the following medical problems exist:*
  Cardiac disease
    (aminocaproic acid may cause hypotension and bradycardia, especially with rapid intravenous administration or if the patient is hypovolemic; also, endocardial hemorrhages and myocardial fat degeneration have been demonstrated in animals)
  Hematuria of upper urinary tract origin
    (risk of intrarenal obstruction secondary to clot retention in the renal pelvis and ureters)
  Hepatic disease
    (cause of bleeding may be more difficult to diagnose)
  Renal disease
    (medication may accumulate; reduction in dosage may be required; also, aminocaproic acid has caused acute renal failure in a few patients and kidney concretions in animals)

Sensitivity to aminocaproic acid

Thrombosis, predisposition to, or history of
(medication inhibits clot dissolution and may interfere with mechanisms for maintaining blood vessel patency)

## Side/Adverse Effects

Note: Patients receiving this medication must be monitored for signs of thromboembolic complications.

The following side/adverse effects have been selected on the basis of their potential clinical significance (possible signs and symptoms in parentheses where appropriate)—not necessarily inclusive:

**Those indicating need for medical attention**
Incidence less frequent
*Bladder obstruction caused by blood clot formation* (decreased urination); *decrease in blood pressure*—may reach hypotensive levels; *dizziness; headache; myopathy* (muscular pain or weakness, severe and continuing)—may be associated with necrosis of muscle fibers; *red or bloodshot eyes; renal failure* (sudden decrease in amount of urine; swelling of face, fingers, feet, or lower legs; rapid weight gain); *ringing or buzzing in ears; skin rash; slow or irregular heartbeat*—after too-rapid intravenous administration; *stomach cramps; stuffy nose; thrombosis or thromboembolism* (pains in chest, groin, or legs [especially calves]; severe, sudden headache; sudden and unexplained shortness of breath, slurred speech, vision changes, and/or weakness or numbness in arm or leg; sudden loss of coordination)—signs and symptoms depend on site of thrombus formation or embolization; *unusual tiredness or weakness*—after too-rapid intravenous administration

Incidence rare
*Rhabdomyolysis with myoglobinuria and renal failure*

**Those indicating need for medical attention only if they continue or are bothersome**
Incidence less frequent
*Diarrhea; dry ejaculation*—reported in hemophilia patients receiving the medication in conjunction with dental surgery; symptom has resolved within 24 to 48 hours after cessation of treatment in all cases reported to date; *nausea; unusual menstrual discomfort*—caused by clotting of menstrual fluid; *unusual tiredness*—with long-term use

## Patient Consultation

As an aid to patient consultation, refer to *Advice for the Patient, Antifibrinolytic Agents (Systemic)*.

In providing consultation, consider emphasizing the following selected information (» = major clinical significance):

**Before using this medication**
» Conditions affecting use, especially:
Sensitivity to aminocaproic acid
Other medical problems, especially active intravascular clotting

**Proper use of this medication**
» Importance of not using more or less medication than the amount prescribed
» Proper dosing
Missed dose: Taking as soon as possible, then returning to regular dosing schedule or doubling next dose
» Proper storage

**Side/adverse effects**
Signs and symptoms of potential side effects, especially bladder obstruction caused by blood clot formation, decrease in blood pressure, dizziness, headache, myopathy, red or bloodshot eyes, renal failure, ringing or buzzing in ears, skin rash, slow or irregular heartbeat, stomach cramps, stuffy nose, thrombosis or thromboembolism, unusual tiredness or weakness, and rhabdomyolysis with myoglobinuria and renal failure

## General Dosing Information

When aminocaproic acid is used during surgery, the bladder must first be freed of clots. Aminocaproic acid may accumulate in the clots and inhibit their dissolution.

A reduction in dosage may be required in patients with renal function impairment.

Aminocaproic acid therapy may be discontinued when there is evidence of cessation of bleeding or when laboratory determinations of fibrinolysis indicate that the medication is no longer required.

**For parenteral dosage forms only**
Intravenous injection of the undiluted aminocaproic acid solution is not recommended.

Rapid intravenous administration may induce hypotension or bradycardia and should be avoided.

To help minimize the possibility of thrombophlebitis, careful attention to the proper insertion of the needle and the fixing of its position is necessary before administration of this medication.

## Oral Dosage Forms

Note: Bracketed uses in the *Dosage Forms* section refer to categories of use and/or indications that are not included in U.S. product labeling.

### AMINOCAPROIC ACID SYRUP USP

**Usual adult dose**
Acute bleeding syndromes—
Oral, 5 grams the first hour, followed by 1 or 1.25 grams per hour for approximately eight hours or until the desired response is obtained.
Note: Following prostatic surgery, a lower dose of 6 grams in the first twenty-four hours may be sufficient, since aminocaproic acid is concentrated in the urine. Also, the lower dosage may reduce the risk of clot formation and subsequent obstruction in the bladder.
[Prevention of hemorrhage following dental surgery, in hemophiliacs]—
Oral, 6 grams immediately following surgery, then 6 grams every six hours for nine or ten days.
Note: Prior to surgery, clotting factors (Factor VIII or Factor IX) should be administered. However, because of an increased risk of thrombotic complications when aminocaproic acid and Factor IX or antiinhibitor coagulant complex are administered concurrently, some hematologists recommended that aminocaproic acid not be administered within eight hours of these clotting factor concentrates.
Another dosing regimen that has been recommended consists of an initial 2-gram dose of aminocaproic acid thirty to sixty minutes prior to surgery, with clotting factors also administered if needed. Following surgery, 2 grams of aminocaproic acid may be administered three or four times a day for three to seven days.
[Hemorrhage, subarachnoid, recurrence]—
To be administered following initial intravenous therapy: Oral, 36 grams per day (3 grams every two hours) until surgery is performed. If surgery is not performed, continue therapy with 3 grams every two hours for twenty-one days after the last bleeding episode. Dosage should then be reduced to 24 grams per day (2 grams every two hours) for three days, then to 12 grams per day (1 gram every two hours) for three days, prior to discontinuation of the medication.

**Usual adult prescribing limits**
[Hemorrhage, subarachnoid, recurrence]—36 grams per twenty-four hours.
Other indications—Up to 30 grams per twenty-four hours.

**Usual pediatric dose**
Acute bleeding syndromes—
Oral, 100 mg per kg of body weight or 3 grams per square meter of body surface the first hour, followed by 33.3 mg per kg of body weight or 1 gram per square meter of body surface per hour, not to exceed 18 grams per square meter of body surface in twenty-four hours.

**Strength(s) usually available**
U.S.—
250 mg per mL (1.25 grams per 5 mL) (Rx) [*Amicar* (potassium sorbate 0.2%; sodium benzoate 0.1%; citric acid; flavorings; sodium saccharin; sorbitol)].
Canada—
250 mg per mL (1.25 grams per 5 mL) (Rx) [*Amicar* (potassium sorbate 0.2%; sodium benzoate 0.1%)].

**Packaging and storage**
Store below 40 °C (104 °F), preferably between 15 and 30 °C (59 and 86 °F), unless otherwise specified by manufacturer. Store in a tight container. Protect from freezing.

### AMINOCAPROIC ACID TABLETS USP

**Usual adult dose**
See *Aminocaproic Acid Syrup USP*.

**Usual adult prescribing limits**
See *Aminocaproic Acid Syrup USP*.

**Usual pediatric dose**
See *AminocaproicAcid Syrup USP*.

**Strength(s) usually available**
U.S.—
500 mg (Rx) [*Amicar* (magnesium stearate; stearic acid; povidone)].
Canada—
500 mg (Rx) [*Amicar*].

## Packaging and storage

Store below 40 °C (104 °F), preferably between 15 and 30 °C (59 and 86 °F), unless otherwise specified by manufacturer. Store in a tight container.

## Parenteral Dosage Forms

Note: Bracketed uses in the *Dosage Forms* section refer to categories of use and/or indications that are not included in U.S. product labeling.

### AMINOCAPROIC ACID INJECTION USP

#### Usual adult dose

Acute bleeding syndromes—

Intravenous infusion, initially 4 to 5 grams administered over a period of one hour, followed by continuous infusion at the rate of 1 gram per hour for approximately eight hours or until the desired response is obtained.

Note: Following prostatic surgery, a lower dose of 6 grams in the first twenty-four hours may be sufficient, since aminocaproic acid is concentrated in the urine. Also, the lower dosage may reduce the risk of clot formation and subsequent obstruction in the bladder.

[Hemorrhage, subarachnoid, recurrence]—

Intravenous infusion, 36 grams per day (18 grams in 400 mL of 5% dextrose injection infused over each twelve-hour period) for ten days. Therapy is continued using orally administered aminocaproic acid.

#### Usual adult prescribing limits

[Hemorrhage, subarachnoid, recurrence]—36 grams per twenty-four hours.

Other indications—Up to 30 grams per twenty-four hours.

#### Usual pediatric dose

Acute bleeding syndromes—

Intravenous infusion, initially 100 mg per kg of body weight or 3 grams per square meter of body surface over a period of one hour, followed by continuous infusion at the rate of 33.3 mg per kg of body weight or 1 gram per square meter of body surface per hour, not to exceed 18 grams per square meter of body surface in twenty-four hours.

#### Strength(s) usually available

U.S.—

250 mg per mL (Rx) [*Amicar* (benzyl alcohol); GENERIC (may contain benzyl alcohol—see labeling for individual product)].

Canada—

250 mg per mL (Rx) [*Amicar* (benzyl alcohol)].

#### Packaging and storage

Store below 40 °C (104 °F), preferably between 15 and 30 °C (59 and 86 °F), unless otherwise specified by manufacturer. Protect from freezing.

#### Preparation of dosage form

For administration by slow intravenous infusion, the 250-mg-per-mL concentration must be diluted with a compatible intravenous vehicle such as sterile water for injection, 0.9% sodium chloride injection, 5% dextrose injection, or lactated Ringer's injection. However, dilution with sterile water for injection is not recommended when the medication is used in patients with subarachnoid hemorrhage.

Revised: 06/17/94

---

# AMINOGLUTETHIMIDE   Systemic

VA CLASSIFICATION (Primary/Secondary): HS900/AN500

Note: For a listing of dosage forms and brand names by country availability, see *Dosage Forms* section(s). For a listing of brand names for the articles in this monograph, refer to the General Index.

## Category

Antiadrenal; antineoplastic.

## Indications

Note: Bracketed information in the *Indications* section refers to uses that are not included in U.S. product labeling.

### Accepted

Cushing's syndrome (treatment)—Aminoglutethimide is indicated for temporary suppression of adrenal function in selected patients with Cushing's syndrome, including that associated with adrenal carcinoma and ectopic adrenocorticotropic hormone (ACTH)–producing tumors or adrenal hyperplasia.

[Carcinoma, breast (treatment)]—Aminoglutethimide is used to produce a "medical adrenalectomy" in the treatment of postmenopausal metastatic breast cancer, especially inoperable or recurrent breast cancer proven to be hormone-dependent.

[Carcinoma, prostatic (treatment)][1]—Aminoglutethimide is used for treatment of prostatic carcinoma unresponsive to hormonal or surgical therapy.

### Unaccepted

Aminoglutethimide is no longer used as an anticonvulsant because of its adrenal suppressant effect.

[1]Not included in Canadian product labeling.

## Pharmacology/Pharmacokinetics

### Physicochemical characteristics

Molecular weight—232.28.

### Mechanism of action/Effect

Aminoglutethimide produces suppression of the adrenal cortex by inhibiting enzymatic conversion of cholesterol to pregnenolone, thus blocking synthesis of adrenal steroids; it may also affect other steps in the synthesis and metabolism of these steroids. A compensatory increase in secretion of adrenocorticotropic hormone (ACTH) by the pituitary occurs (except in patients with ACTH-independent adenomas or carcinomas), necessitating glucocorticoid administration to maintain aminoglutethimide's effect. Aminoglutethimide also inhibits estrogen production from androgens in peripheral tissues by blocking the aromatase enzyme. An additional mechanism in breast cancer, involving enhanced metabolism of estrone sulfate, has also been proposed.

### Other actions/effects

Hepatic P-450 microsomal enzyme inducer.

### Absorption

Rapidly and completely absorbed from gastrointestinal tract.

### Protein binding

Low (20 to 25%).

### Biotransformation

Hepatic; the major metabolite is *N*-acetylaminoglutethimide and there may be genetic variation among individuals in the rate of acetylation.

### Half-life

12.5 hours; reduced to 7 hours after prolonged (2 to 32 weeks) treatment because aminoglutethimide is a hepatic enzyme inducer and accelerates its own metabolism.

### Onset of action

Suppression of adrenal function—3 to 5 days.

### Time to peak concentration

1.5 hours.

### Duration of action

Recovery of normal adrenal basal secretion and responsiveness to stress usually occurs within 36 to 72 hours after withdrawal of combined aminoglutethimide and hydrocortisone therapy; recovery may take longer after prolonged therapy (e.g., 1 year or longer).

### Elimination

Renal, 34 to 54% unchanged.
In dialysis—Removable by hemodialysis.

## Precautions to Consider

### Cross-sensitivity and/or related problems

Patients sensitive to glutethimide may be sensitive to aminoglutethimide also.

### Carcinogenicity/Mutagenicity

Studies have not been done.

### Pregnancy/Reproduction

Fertility—Studies in female rats at doses 1/2 and 1-1/4 times the maximum daily human dose found a decrease in fetal implantation.

Pregnancy—Risk-benefit must be carefully considered when this medication is required in life-threatening situations or in serious diseases for which other medications cannot be used or are ineffective.

Aminoglutethimide crosses the placenta and has been shown to cause pseudohermaphroditism in female infants whose mothers took concomitant anticonvulsants.

Aminoglutethimide has been shown to cause increased fetal deaths and teratogenic effects including pseudohermaphroditism in rats given up to three times the highest recommended human dose.

FDA Pregnancy Category D.

**Breast-feeding**

It is not known whether aminoglutethimide is distributed into breast milk. However, problems in humans have not been documented.

**Pediatrics**

Appropriate studies on the relationship of age to the effects of aminoglutethimide have not been performed in the pediatric population. However, there is a rare possibility that aminoglutethimide will induce precocious sexual development in males and masculinization and hirsutism in females.

**Geriatrics**

Appropriate studies on the relationship of age to the effects of aminoglutethimide have not been performed in the geriatric population. However, the elderly may be more sensitive to the central nervous system (CNS) effects and more likely to become lethargic with this medication. In addition, elderly patients are more likely to have age-related renal function impairment, which may require caution in patients receiving aminoglutethimide.

**Drug interactions and/or related problems**

The following drug interactions and/or related problems have been selected on the basis of their potential clinical significance (possible mechanism in parentheses where appropriate)—not necessarily inclusive (» = major clinical significance):

Note: Combinations containing any of the following medications, depending on the amount present, may also interact with this medication.

Anticoagulants, coumarin-type
(aminoglutethimide accelerates metabolism of coumarin anticoagulants; dosage adjustments should be based on monitoring of coagulation times)

Corticosteroids, mineralocorticoid
(aminoglutethimide may alter metabolism of mineralocorticoids; dosage adjustments may be required)

Corticotropin (ACTH)
(aminoglutethimide may inhibit the adrenal response to ACTH; this may interfere with the therapeutic response to ACTH)

» Dexamethasone
(aminoglutethimide accelerates metabolism of dexamethasone, possibly resulting in a two-fold reduction in dexamethasone's half-life; if glucocorticoid therapy is necessary in a patient receiving aminoglutethimide, hydrocortisone is recommended instead)

Digoxin or
Theophylline
(effects may be reduced because of induction of hepatic microsomal enzymes by aminoglutethimide; caution is recommended)

**Laboratory value alterations**

The following have been selected on the basis of their potential clinical significance (possible effect in parentheses where appropriate)—not necessarily inclusive (» = major clinical significance):

With physiology/laboratory test values
Aldosterone
(urinary concentrations may be decreased, resulting in orthostatic hypotension and hyponatremia)

Alkaline phosphatase and
Aspartate aminotransferase (AST [SGOT]) and
Bilirubin
(serum values may be increased)

Cortisol
(plasma concentrations are decreased slowly in patients with adrenal hyperfunction and rapidly in patients with breast cancer and in otherwise healthy individuals)

Thyroid-stimulating hormone (TSH)
(serum concentrations may be increased as a reflex response to reduced serum thyroxine concentrations)

Thyroxine
(serum concentrations may be decreased; hypothyroidism is infrequent because of reflex increase in TSH secretion)

**Medical considerations/Contraindications**

The medical considerations/contraindications included here have been selected on the basis of their potential clinical significance (reasons given in parentheses where appropriate)—not necessarily inclusive (» = major clinical significance).

*Risk-benefit should be considered when the following medical problems exist:*

» Chickenpox, existing or recent (including recent exposure) or
» Herpes zoster
(risk of severe generalized disease)

Hepatic function impairment
(reduced biotransformation)

Hypothyroidism
(aminoglutethimide may decrease serum thyroxine concentrations)

» Infection
(reduced adrenal responsiveness may result in acute adrenocortical insufficiency; additional steroid supplementation may be necessary)

Renal function impairment
(reduced elimination)

» Sensitivity to aminoglutethimide or glutethimide

**Patient monitoring**

The following may be especially important in patient monitoring (other tests may be warranted in some patients, depending on condition; » = major clinical significance):

Alkaline phosphatase values, serum and
» Aspartate aminotransferase (AST [SGOT]) values, serum and
Blood counts, complete and
» Thyroid function tests
(recommended at periodic intervals in patients receiving aminoglutethimide for prolonged periods)

» Blood pressure determinations, recumbent and upright
(recommended at periodic intervals to detect hypotension due to reduced aldosterone production)

» Electrolyte (sodium, potassium, chloride) and carbon dioxide concentrations, serum
(recommended at regular intervals to detect hyponatremia, ensure absence of acidosis, and make sure mineralocorticoid supply is sufficient)

*In adrenal disorders*
» Cortisol concentrations, 8 a.m. plasma or
» 17-Hydroxycorticosteroid concentrations, 24-hour urinary
(recommended at periodic intervals to aid in assessing clinical response and determine if steroid supplement therapy is necessary)

*In prostatic carcinoma*
Acid phosphatase concentrations, serum
(recommended at periodic intervals to aid in assessing clinical response; concentrations should decrease)

# Side/Adverse Effects

Note: Most side effects decrease in incidence and severity after the first 2 to 6 weeks because of accelerated metabolism of the drug with continued use.

The following side/adverse effects have been selected on the basis of their potential clinical significance (possible signs and symptoms in parentheses where appropriate)—not necessarily inclusive:

**Those indicating need for medical attention**

Incidence less frequent
*Adrenocortical insufficiency* (fever; darkening of skin; mental depression); *leukopenia or agranulocytosis* (usually asymptomatic; rarely, fever or chills; cough or hoarseness; lower back or side pain; painful or difficult urination); *thrombocytopenia* (usually asymptomatic; rarely, unusual bleeding or bruising; black, tarry stools; blood in urine or stools; pinpoint red spots on skin)

Incidence rare
*Hypersensitivity, possible* (fever; yellow eyes or skin); *hypothyroidism and goiter* (neck tenderness or swelling)

Note: A rare *hypersensitivity* or drug reaction has been reported, consisting of cholestatic jaundice, fever, skin eruptions, increased aspartate aminotransferase (AST [SGOT]), and possibly eosinophilia.

*Hypothyroidism and goiter* may occur with long-term use because aminoglutethimide blocks iodination of tyrosine.

**Those indicating need for medical attention only if they continue or are bothersome**
Incidence more frequent
   *CNS effects* (clumsiness; dizziness; drowsiness; lack of energy; uncontrolled eye movements)—*dose-related; loss of appetite or nausea*—incidence about 12%; *measles-like skin rash or itching on face and/or palms of hands*
   Note: *CNS effects* usually are reduced within 2 to 6 weeks with continued treatment, although some may be severe enough to necessitate discontinuing treatment in some patients.
       The *measles-like skin rash* is often accompanied by fever. It usually appears within 10 to 15 days after therapy is started and persists for 5 to 7 days; it is recommended that aminoglutethimide be withdrawn if mild to moderate skin rash persists for longer than 5 to 8 days or if skin rash is severe.
Incidence less frequent or rare
   *Headache; hypotension, orthostatic or persistent, due to suppression of aldosterone production* (dizziness or lightheadedness, especially when getting up from a lying or sitting position); *masculinization and hirsutism in females* (deepening of voice; increased hair growth; irregular menstrual periods); *muscle pain; vomiting*

## Overdose

For specific information on the agents used in the management of aminoglutethimide overdose, see:
   • *Corticosteroids—Glucocorticoid Effects (Systemic)* monograph; and/or
   • *Sympathomimetic Agents—Cardiovascular Use (Parenteral-Systemic)* monograph.
For more information on the management of overdose or unintentional ingestion, *contact a Poison Control Center* (see *Poison Control Center Listing*).

**Treatment of overdose**
Treatment of overdose may include:
Gastric lavage.
Symptomatic, supportive treatment.
Intravenous hydrocortisone if glucocorticoid insufficiency develops.
Intravenous norepinephrine plus rehydration if hypovolemia or hypotension occurs.
Dialysis, if toxicity is severe.

## Patient Consultation

As an aid to patient consultation, refer to *Advice for the Patient, Aminoglutethimide (Systemic).*

In providing consultation, consider emphasizing the following selected information (» = major clinical significance):

**Before using this medication**
» Conditions affecting use, especially:
       Sensitivity to aminoglutethimide or glutethimide
       Pregnancy—Teratogenic in humans and animals
       Use in children—Rare possibility of precocious sexual development in males and masculinization and hirsutism in females
       Use in the elderly—Lethargy may be more frequent
       Other medications, especially dexamethasone
       Other medical problems, especially chickenpox, herpes zoster, or infection

**Proper use of this medication**
» Importance of not taking more or less medication than the amount prescribed
» Possible nausea and vomiting; usually lessens with continued therapy; checking with physician before discontinuing medication
   Checking with physician if vomiting occurs shortly after dose is taken
» Proper dosing
       Missed dose: Taking as soon as possible if remembered within 2 to 4 hours; not taking if almost time for next dose; not doubling doses
» Proper storage

**Precautions while using this medication**
» Importance of close monitoring by physician
       Carrying medical identification card or wearing bracelet stating that medication is being used
       Caution if any kind of surgery (including dental surgery) or emergency treatment is required
» Checking with physician immediately if injury, infection, or other illness occurs, because of the risk of adrenal insufficiency; physician may prescribe steroid supplement
» Caution if drowsiness, dizziness, or hypotension occurs, especially if driving, using machines, or doing other things that require alertness

**Side/adverse effects**
   Signs of potential side effects, especially adrenocortical insufficiency, leukopenia or agranulocytosis, thrombocytopenia, hypersensitivity, and hypothyroidism and goiter
   Asymptomatic side effects, including leukopenia or agranulocytosis, and thrombocytopenia

## General Dosing Information

Patients receiving aminoglutethimide should be under the supervision of a physician experienced in cancer chemotherapy or a clinical endocrinologist.

Dosage must be adjusted to provide the desired level of adrenal suppression.

Mineralocorticoid replacement (such as fludrocortisone) may be necessary in 20 to 50% of patients because of reduction of aldosterone production caused by aminoglutethimide, which could lead to hyponatremia and orthostatic hypotension.

Patients should be monitored carefully during periods of stress such as surgery, trauma, or acute illness. Additional steroids may be required because adrenal suppression may prevent the normal response to stress. It is recommended that aminoglutethimide be temporarily withdrawn immediately following shock or severe trauma.

It is recommended that dosage be reduced if CNS side effects occur.

It is recommended that aminoglutethimide be withdrawn if mild to moderate skin rash persists for longer than 5 to 8 days or if skin rash is severe. Skin rash may respond to treatment with diphenhydramine. After a mild to moderate rash disappears, aminoglutethimide therapy may be restarted at a dose of 250 mg per day and gradually increased to the therapeutic dose.

**For use as an antineoplastic**
Inhibition of the adrenal cortex by aminoglutethimide results in a reflex increase in secretion of adrenocorticotropic hormone (ACTH) by the pituitary (except in patients with ACTH-independent adenomas or carcinomas); therefore, replacement with a glucocorticoid (usually hydrocortisone) may be necessary to maintain the desired effect of aminoglutethimide by preventing adrenal cortical hypertrophy and renewed synthesis of steroids.

Replacement glucocorticoid therapy is usually required in patients with metastatic breast cancer.

Because of the rapid return of the adrenal cortex to normal responsiveness following withdrawal of aminoglutethimide and hydrocortisone, dosage tapering is usually not necessary.

## Oral Dosage Forms

Note: Bracketed uses in the *Dosage Forms* section refer to categories of use and/or indications that are not included in U.S. product labeling.

### AMINOGLUTETHIMIDE TABLETS USP

**Usual adult dose**
Antiadrenal—
   Initial: Oral, 250 mg two or three times a day for approximately two weeks (to induce metabolism and minimize CNS side effects).
   Maintenance: Oral, 250 mg four times a day, preferably every six hours.
[Breast cancer] or
[Prostatic cancer][1]—
   Initial: Oral, 250 mg two or three times a day for approximately two weeks (to induce metabolism and minimize CNS side effects), in combination with 40 mg of hydrocortisone per day (10 mg in the morning and at 5 p.m. and 20 mg at bedtime).
   Maintenance: Oral, 250 mg four times a day, preferably every six hours, in combination with 40 mg of hydrocortisone per day (10 mg in the morning and at 5 p.m. and 20 mg at bedtime).

**Usual adult prescribing limits**
Cushing's syndrome—
   Up to 2 grams per day.
[Breast cancer] or
[Prostatic cancer][1]—
   Up to 1 gram per day.

**Usual pediatric dose**
Safety and efficacy have not been established.

**Strength(s) usually available**
U.S.—
   250 mg (Rx) [*Cytadren* (double-scored)].
Canada—
   250 mg (Rx) [*Cytadren* (scored)].

**Packaging and storage**
Store below 40 °C (104 °F), preferably between 15 and 30 °C (59 and 86 °F), unless otherwise specified by manufacturer. Store in a tight container. Protect from light.

[1]Not included in Canadian product labeling.

## Selected Bibliography

Melamed AJ. Current concepts in the treatment of prostate cancer. Drug Intell Clin Pharm 1987; 21: 247-54.

Lonning PE, Kvinnsland S. Mechanisms of action of aminoglutethimide as endocrine therapy of breast cancer. Drugs 1988; 35: 685-710.

May CA, Garnett WR. Treatment of adrenocortical carcinoma: a case report and review of the literature. Drug Intell Clin Pharm 1986 Jan; 20: 24-32.

Revised: 04/09/93
Interim revision: 04/29/94

# AMINOGLYCOSIDES   Systemic

This monograph includes information on the following: Amikacin; Gentamicin; Kanamycin†; Neomycin†; Netilmicin; Streptomycin; Tobramycin.

VA CLASSIFICATION (Primary/Secondary):
Amikacin—AM300
Gentamicin—AM300
Kanamycin—AM300
Neomycin—AM300
Netilmicin—AM300
Streptomycin—AM300/AM500
Tobramycin—AM300

Note: For a listing of dosage forms and brand names by country availability, see *Dosage Forms* section(s). For a listing of brand names for the articles in this monograph, refer to the General Index.

†Not commercially available in Canada.

## Category

Antibacterial (systemic)—Amikacin; Gentamicin; Kanamycin; Netilmicin; Streptomycin; Tobramycin.
Antibacterial (antimycobacterial)—Streptomycin.

## Indications

### General considerations

Aminoglycosides are indicated in the treatment of serious systemic infections for which less toxic antibacterials are ineffective or contraindicated. The spectrum of aminoglycosides covers aerobic gram-negative bacilli, and some gram-positive organisms. They are not active against anaerobic organisms.

The antibacterial activity of aminoglycosides against different strains of organisms varies among institutions and regions. However, aminoglycosides are generally active against most Enterobacteriaceae, including *Escherichia coli*, *Proteus mirabilis*, indole-positive *Proteus*, *Citrobacter*, *Enterobacter*, *Klebsiella*, *Providencia*, and *Serratia* species. *Acinetobacter* and *Pseudomonas* species are also usually susceptible. Although tobramycin is more potent *in vitro* against *Pseudomonas aeruginosa*, and gentamicin is more potent *in vitro* against *Serratia* species, neither has been shown to be more clinically effective than other aminoglycosides if the organism is susceptible. Aminoglycosides are used concurrently with antipseudomonal penicillins or certain cephalosporins in the treatment of serious *Pseudomonas aeruginosa* infections.

Bacterial resistance to gentamicin and tobramycin is very similar, although a few organisms resistant to gentamicin remain susceptible to tobramycin. The antibacterial activity and resistance pattern of netilmicin is very similar to those of both gentamicin and tobramycin, although there are a few gentamicin- and tobramycin-resistant strains that remain susceptible to netilmicin.

Amikacin is similar to gentamicin, tobramycin, and netilmicin in its spectrum of activity; however, amikacin has the advantage of not being inactivated by the same enzymes that render other aminoglycosides inactive against resistant organisms. Therefore, amikacin may remain active against strains of *Pseudomonas aeruginosa* that are resistant to tobramycin and netilmicin. Kanamycin use has declined over the years due to the emergence of a large number of resistant organisms. However, because of its disuse, resistance has decreased in some areas.

Streptomycin is used primarily as an antitubercular and is active against *Mycobacterium tuberculosis* and *M. bovis*. It is also considered the drug of choice for the treatment of infections caused by *Francisella tularensis* and *Yersinia pestis*, and is often used to treat *Brucella* infections. Because many other gram-negative bacilli are resistant, streptomycin is rarely used to treat those organisms.

Aminoglycosides are also active against *Staphylococcus aureus*, but are rarely used as sole therapy since other, less toxic, antibiotics are available. Amikacin, gentamicin, netilmicin, or tobramycin, administered concurrently with a penicillin, is synergistic against certain susceptible strains of *Enterococcus faecalis*. Streptomycin has been used, in combination with penicillin or vancomycin, in the treatment of endocarditis caused by *Enterococcus faecalis* or *S. viridans*.

Aminoglycosides are indicated for the treatment of serious infections caused by, or strongly suspected to be caused by, susceptible gram-negative bacilli. Some aminoglycosides, such as amikacin, gentamicin, and tobramycin, may also be given as an aerosol nebulization. This is usually as an adjunct to parenteral therapy in patients with cystic fibrosis with acute exacerbations of pulmonary infections. Aminoglycosides are used to treat central nervous system (CNS) infections mainly in neonates due to better penetration across the blood-brain barrier in this age group; gentamicin may also be given intrathecally to treat CNS infections in adults. Aminoglycosides are also used in combination with other antibacterials for a possible synergistic effect.

### Accepted

Biliary tract infections (treatment)—Amikacin, gentamicin, kanamycin, netilmicin, and tobramycin are indicated in the treatment of biliary tract infections caused by susceptible organisms.

Bone and joint infections (treatment)—Amikacin, gentamicin, kanamycin, netilmicin, and tobramycin are indicated in the treatment of bone and joint infections caused by susceptible organisms.

Brucellosis (treatment)—Streptomycin is indicated in the treatment of brucellosis caused by *Brucella* species.

Central nervous system infections (including meningitis and ventriculitis) (treatment)—Amikacin, gentamicin, kanamycin, netilmicin, and tobramycin are indicated in the treatment of central nervous system infections caused by susceptible organisms.

Granuloma inguinale (treatment)—Streptomycin is indicated in the treatment of granuloma inguinale.

Intra-abdominal infections (including peritonitis) (treatment)—Amikacin, gentamicin, kanamycin, netilmicin, and tobramycin are indicated in the treatment of intra-abdominal infections caused by susceptible organisms.

Plague (treatment)—Streptomycin is indicated in the treatment of plague.

Pneumonia, gram-negative, bacterial (treatment)—Amikacin, gentamicin, kanamycin, netilmicin, and tobramycin are indicated in the treatment of bacterial, gram-negative pneumonia caused by susceptible organisms.

Septicemia, bacterial (treatment)—Amikacin, gentamicin, kanamycin, netilmicin, and tobramycin are indicated in the treatment of bacterial septicemia caused by susceptible organisms.

Skin and soft tissue infections (including burn wound infections) (treatment)—Amikacin, gentamicin, kanamycin, netilmicin, and tobramycin are indicated in the treatment of skin and soft tissue infections caused by susceptible organisms.

Tuberculosis (treatment)—Streptomycin is indicated in the treatment of tuberculosis.

Tularemia (treatment)—Streptomycin is indicated in the treatment of tularemia.

Urinary tract infections (recurrent complicated) (treatment)—Amikacin, gentamicin, kanamycin, netilmicin, and tobramycin are indicated in the treatment of recurrent complicated urinary tract infections caused by susceptible organisms.

Not all species or strains of a particular organism may be susceptible to a specific aminoglycoside.

### Unaccepted

Aminoglycosides are not indicated routinely in the treatment of staphylococcal infections since less toxic antibacterials are available.

Aminoglycosides are not routinely indicated in the initial treatment of uncomplicated urinary tract infections unless the organism is resistant to other less toxic antibacterials.

Parenteral neomycin has been replaced by safer and more effective agents. **Because of its potential toxicity, parenteral use of neomycin is not recommended for any indication.**

# Pharmacology/Pharmacokinetics

## Physicochemical characteristics
Molecular weight—
    Amikacin sulfate: 781.75.
    Kanamycin sulfate: 582.58.
    Netilmicin sulfate: 1441.54.
    Tobramycin sulfate: 1425.39.

## Mechanism of action/Effect
Actively transported across the bacterial cell membrane, irreversibly binds to one or more specific receptor proteins on the 30 S subunit of bacterial ribosomes, and interferes with an initiation complex between messenger RNA (mRNA) and the 30 S subunit. DNA may be misread, thus producing nonfunctional proteins; polyribosomes are split apart and are unable to synthesize protein. This results in accelerated aminoglycoside transport, increasing the disruption of bacterial cytoplasmic membranes, and eventual cell death.

Note: Aminoglycosides are bactericidal, while most other antibiotics that interfere with protein synthesis are bacteriostatic.

## Absorption
All aminoglycosides—
    Intramuscular: Rapidly and completely absorbed after intramuscular administration.
    Local; topical: May also be absorbed in significant amounts from body surfaces (except urinary bladder) following local irrigation or topical application. Intraperitoneal and intrapleural administration results in rapid absorption.
    Oral: Poorly absorbed from intact gastrointestinal tract after oral administration, but may accumulate in patients with renal failure.

## Distribution
All aminoglycosides—
    Distributed to extracellular fluid, including serum, abscesses, ascitic, pericardial, pleural, synovial, lymphatic, and peritoneal fluids. High concentrations found in urine.
    Low concentrations found in bile, breast milk, aqueous humor, bronchial secretions, sputum, and cerebral spinal fluid (CSF). In adults, does not cross the blood-brain barrier (BBB) in therapeutically adequate concentrations. Small improvement in penetration with inflamed meninges. Higher levels are achieved in the CSF of newborns than in adults.
    Crosses the placenta.
    Also distributed to all body tissues, where aminoglycosides accumulate intracellularly.
    High concentrations found in highly perfused organs, such as the liver, lungs, and especially, the kidneys, where aminoglycosides accumulate in the renal cortex.
    Lower concentrations are seen in muscle, fat, and bone.
$Vol_D$—
    Adults—0.26 L per kg (range, 0.20 to 0.40 L per kg).
    Children—0.2 to 0.4 L per kg.
    Neonates—
    < 1 week old, < 1500 grams: up to 0.68 L per kg.
    < 1 week old, > 1500 grams: up to 0.58 L per kg.
    Cystic fibrosis patients—0.30 to 0.39 L per kg.

## Protein binding
All aminoglycosides—Low (0 to 10%).

## Biotransformation
Not metabolized.

## Half-life
All aminoglycosides—
    Distribution half-life:
        5 to 15 minutes.
    Elimination half-life:
        Adults—
            Normal renal function: 2 to 4 hours.
            Impaired renal function: Varies with degree of dysfunction; up to 100 hours.
            Cystic fibrosis patients: 1 to 2 hours.
            Burn patients and febrile patients: May have a shorter half-life than average due to increased clearance of the drug.

Pediatrics—
    Neonates: 5 to 8 hours.
    Children: 2.5 to 4 hours.
Terminal half-life:
    > 100 hours (release of intracellularly bound aminoglycoside).

## Time to peak concentration
All aminoglycosides—
    Intramuscular: 0.5 to 1.5 hours.
    Intravenous (time to post-distributional peak level): 30 minutes after end of 30 minute infusion, or 15 minutes after end of 1 hour infusion.

## Time to peak bile concentration
Kanamycin—Approximately 6 hours (intramuscular).

## Peak serum concentrations
In adults with normal renal function—
    Amikacin:
        Intramuscular—7.5 mg per kg of body weight (mg/kg): 21 mcg per mL.
        Intravenous over 30 minutes—7.5 mg/kg: 38 mcg per mL.
    Gentamicin:
        Intramuscular or intravenous—1.5 mg/kg: 6 mcg per mL.
    Kanamycin:
        Intramuscular or intravenous—7.5 mg/kg: 22 mcg per mL.
    Netilmicin:
        Intramuscular—2 mg/kg: 5.5 mcg per mL.
        Intravenous over 30 minutes—2 mg/kg: 11.8 mcg per mL.
    Streptomycin:
        Intramuscular—1 gram: 25 to 50 mcg per mL.
    Tobramycin:
        Intramuscular or intravenous—1 mg/kg: 4 mcg per mL.

## Bile concentration
Netilmicin—10% of serum concentrations; may vary up to 25% of serum concentrations with abnormal hepatic function.

## Elimination
Renal; excreted unchanged by glomerular filtration. 70 to 95% of aminoglycoside dose recovered in urine over 24 hours. Small amount excreted in bile.
Hemodialysis—Each 4 to 6 hour hemodialysis period decreases plasma aminoglycoside concentrations by up to 50%.
Peritoneal dialysis—Less effective than hemodialysis. Removes approximately 25% of a dose in 48 to 72 hours.

# Precautions to Consider

## Cross-sensitivity and/or related problems
Patients hypersensitive to one aminoglycoside may be hypersensitive to other aminoglycosides also.

## Carcinogenicity/Mutagenicity/Tumorigenicity
*Amikacin and kanamycin*—Studies on the carcinogenic or mutagenic effects in humans have not been done.
*Netilmicin*—Lifetime carcinogenicity studies in mice and rats have not shown any netilmicin-related tumors. Mutagenicity studies in mice and rats have shown negative results.

## Pregnancy/Reproduction
Fertility—
*Amikacin:* Reproduction studies in rats and mice have not shown that amikacin causes impaired fertility.
*Gentamicin:* Reproduction studies in rats and rabbits have not shown that gentamicin causes impaired fertility.
*Kanamycin:* Studies in rats and rabbits have not shown that kanamycin causes impaired fertility.
*Netilmicin:* Reproduction studies in rats and rabbits given intramuscular and subcutaneous doses of netilmicin approximately 13 to 15 times the highest adult human dose have not shown that netilmicin impairs fertility or causes adverse effects on the fetus.

Pregnancy—All aminoglycosides cross the placenta, sometimes resulting in significant concentrations in the cord blood and/or amniotic fluid. Aminoglycosides may be nephrotoxic in the human fetus. In addition, some aminoglycosides (e.g., streptomycin, tobramycin) have been reported to cause total irreversible, bilateral congenital deafness in children whose mothers received aminoglycosides during pregnancy.
*Amikacin:* Adequate and well-controlled studies in humans have not been done. Amikacin has not been shown to cause adverse effects on the fetus, even though peak fetal serum concentrations of amikacin average approximately 16% of peak maternal serum concentrations and amikacin may be concentrated in the fetal kidneys. However, since other aminoglycosides have been reported to cause deafness in the fetus, risk-benefit must be carefully considered

when this medication is required in life-threatening situations or in serious diseases for which other medications cannot be used or are ineffective.

FDA Pregnancy Category D.

*Gentamicin:* Adequate and well-controlled studies in humans have not been done. Since other aminoglycosides have been reported to cause deafness in the fetus, risk-benefit must be carefully considered when this medication is required in life-threatening situations or in serious diseases for which other medications cannot be used or are ineffective.

Studies in rats and rabbits have not shown that gentamicin causes adverse effects on the fetus.

FDA Pregnancy Category C.

*Kanamycin:* Fetal serum concentrations average approximately 16 to 50% of maternal serum concentrations. Adequate and well-controlled studies in humans have not been done.

Studies in rats and rabbits have not shown that kanamycin is teratogenic. However, studies in rats and guinea pigs given doses of 200 mg/kg daily have shown that kanamycin causes hearing impairment in the fetus.

FDA Pregnancy Category D.

*Netilmicin:* Netilmicin has been detected in cord blood and in the human fetus. Therefore, risk-benefit must be carefully considered when this medication is required in life-threatening situations or in serious diseases for which other medications cannot be used or are ineffective.

Studies in rats given netilmicin subcutaneously during pregnancy have not shown that netilmicin causes ototoxicity in the fetus.

FDA Pregnancy Category D.

*Streptomycin:* Adequate and well-controlled studies in humans have not been done. Fetal serum concentrations are usually less than 50% of maternal serum concentrations. Streptomycin has been shown to cause deafness in infants whose mothers received streptomycin during pregnancy. Therefore, risk-benefit must be carefully considered when this medication is required in life-threatening situations or in serious diseases for which other medications cannot be used or are ineffective.

FDA Pregnancy Category D.

*Tobramycin:* Tobramycin concentrates in the fetal kidneys and has been shown to cause total irreversible bilateral congenital deafness in the human fetus. Therefore, risk-benefit must be carefully considered when this medication is required in life-threatening situations or in serious diseases for which other medications cannot be used or are ineffective.

FDA Pregnancy Category D.

**Breast-feeding**

Aminoglycosides are excreted in breast milk in small but variable amounts (e.g., up to 18 mcg per mL for kanamycin). However, aminoglycosides are poorly absorbed from the gastrointestinal tract and problems in nursing infants have not been documented.

**Pediatrics**

*All aminoglycosides—* CNS depression, characterized by stupor, flaccidity, coma, or deep respiratory depression, has been reported in very young infants receiving streptomycin at doses that exceeded the maximum recommended amount. However, all aminoglycosides have this potential to cause neuromuscular blockade.

*Amikacin, gentamicin, kanamycin, netilmicin, and tobramycin—* These aminoglycosides should be used with caution in premature infants and neonates because of these patients' immature renal capability, which may result in prolonged elimination half-life and aminoglycoside-induced toxicity. Dosage adjustments may be required in pediatric patients. See also *Patient monitoring* and *General Dosing Information*.

**Geriatrics**

Because of their toxicity, aminoglycosides should be used with caution in elderly patients, only after less toxic alternatives have been considered and/or found ineffective. Elderly patients are more likely to have an age-related decrease in renal function. Recommended doses should not be exceeded, and the patient's renal function should be carefully monitored during therapy. Geriatric patients may require smaller daily doses of aminoglycosides in accordance with their increased age, decreased renal function, and, possibly, decreased weight. In addition, loss of hearing may result even in patients with normal renal function.

**Drug interactions and/or related problems**

The following drug interactions and/or related problems have been selected on the basis of their potential clinical significance (possible mechanism in parentheses where appropriate)—not necessarily inclusive (» = major clinical significance):

Note: Combinations containing any of the following medications, depending on the amount present, may also interact with this medication.

»  Aminoglycosides, 2 or more concurrently or
»  Capreomycin

(concurrent and/or sequential use of 2 or more aminoglycosides by any route or concurrent use of capreomycin with aminoglycosides should be avoided since the potential for ototoxicity, nephrotoxicity, and neuromuscular blockade may be increased; hearing loss may occur and may progress to deafness even after discontinuation of the drug; loss of hearing may be reversible, but usually is permanent; neuromuscular blockade may result in skeletal muscle weakness and respiratory depression or paralysis [apnea]. Also, concurrent use of 2 or more aminoglycosides may result in reduced bacterial uptake of each one since the medications compete for the same uptake mechanism)

Antimyasthenics

(concurrent use of medications with neuromuscular blocking action may antagonize the effect of antimyasthenics on skeletal muscle; temporary dosage adjustments of antimyasthenics may be necessary to control symptoms of myasthenia gravis during and following use of medications with neuromuscular blocking action)

Beta-lactam antibiotics

(aminoglycosides can be inactivated by many beta-lactam antibiotics [cephalosporins, penicillins] *in vitro* and *in vivo* in patients with significant renal failure. Degradation depends on the concentration of the beta-lactam, storage time, and temperature)

Indomethacin, intravenous

(when aminoglycosides are administered concurrently with intravenous indomethacin in the premature neonate, renal clearance of aminoglycosides may be decreased, leading to increased plasma concentrations, elimination half-lives, and risk of aminoglycoside toxicity; dosage adjustment of aminoglycosides based on measurement of plasma concentrations and/or evidence of toxicity may also be required)

»  Methoxyflurane or
»  Polymyxins, parenteral

(concurrent and/or sequential use of these medications with aminoglycosides should be avoided since the potential for nephrotoxicity and/or neuromuscular blockade may be increased; neuromuscular blockade may result in skeletal muscle weakness and respiratory depression or paralysis [apnea]; caution is also recommended when methoxyflurane or polymyxins are used concurrently with aminoglycosides during surgery or in the postoperative period)

»  Nephrotoxic medications, other (See *Appendix II*) or
»  Ototoxic medications, other (See *Appendix II*)

(concurrent or sequential use of these medications with aminoglycosides may increase the potential for ototoxicity or nephrotoxicity; hearing loss may occur and may progress to deafness even after discontinuation of the drug and may be reversible, but usually is permanent; serial audiometric function determinations may be required with concurrent or sequential use of other ototoxic antibacterials; renal function determinations may be required)

(vancomycin and aminoglycosides must often be administered concurrently in the prophylaxis of bacterial endocarditis, in the treatment of endocarditis caused by streptococci and *Corynebacteria* species, in the treatment of resistant staphylococcal infections, or in penicillin-allergic patients; appropriate monitoring will help to reduce the risk of nephrotoxicity or ototoxicity; renal function determinations, serum aminoglycoside and vancomycin concentrations, dosage reductions, and/or dosage interval adjustments, or alternate antibacterials, may be required)

»  Neuromuscular blocking agents or medications with neuromuscular blocking activity, other

(concurrent use of medications with neuromuscular blocking activity, including halogenated hydrocarbon inhalation anesthetics, opioid analgesics, and massive transfusions with citrate anticoagulated blood, with aminoglycosides should be carefully monitored since neuromuscular blockade may be enhanced, resulting in skeletal muscle weakness and respiratory depression or paralysis [apnea]; caution is recommended when these medications and aminoglycosides are used concurrently during surgery or in the postoperative period, especially if there is a possibility of incomplete reversal of neuromuscular blockade postoperatively; treatment with anticholinesterase agents or calcium salts may help reverse the blockade)

### Laboratory value alterations

The following have been selected on the basis of their potential clinical significance (possible effect in parentheses where appropriate)—not necessarily inclusive (» = major clinical significance):

With physiology/laboratory test values

Alanine aminotransferase (ALT [SGPT]), serum and
Alkaline phosphatase, serum and
Aspartate aminotransferase (AST [SGOT]), serum and
Bilirubin, serum and
Lactate dehydrogenase (LDH), serum
(values may be increased)

Blood urea nitrogen (BUN) and
Creatinine, serum
(concentrations may be increased)

Calcium, serum and
Magnesium, serum and
Potassium, serum and
Sodium, serum
(concentrations may be decreased)

### Medical considerations/Contraindications

The medical considerations/contraindications included here have been selected on the basis of their potential clinical significance (reasons given in parentheses where appropriate)—not necessarily inclusive (» = major clinical significance).

*Risk-benefit should be considered when the following medical problems exist:*

» Botulism, infant or
» Myasthenia gravis or
» Parkinsonism
(aminoglycosides may cause neuromuscular blockade, resulting in further skeletal muscle weakness)

Dehydration or
» Renal function impairment
(possible increased risk of toxicity because of elevated serum concentrations; it is recommended that aminoglycosides be administered in a reduced dosage at a fixed interval, or in normal doses at prolonged intervals, to patients with impaired renal function)

» Eighth-cranial-nerve impairment
(aminoglycosides may cause auditory and vestibular toxicity)

» Previous allergic reaction to aminoglycosides
(hypersensitivity reaction to one aminoglycoside may contraindicate the use of other aminoglycosides due to known cross-sensitivity)

### Patient monitoring

The following may be especially important in patient monitoring (other tests may be warranted in some patients, depending on condition; » = major clinical significance):

*For all aminoglycosides*

» Aminoglycoside concentrations, serum
(aminoglycoside levels should be monitored in all patients, especially neonates and the elderly, even without renal function impairment, to avoid potentially toxic concentrations from accumulation of the drug; peak levels should be drawn 30 minutes after a 30-minute aminoglycoside infusion, to allow for drug distribution, and trough levels, immediately prior to the next dose; see *General Dosing Information*)

» Audiograms and
» Renal function determinations and
» Vestibular function determinations
(may be required prior to, periodically during, and following treatment in patients with pre-existing renal or eighth-cranial-nerve impairment; twice-weekly or weekly audiometric testing to detect high-frequency hearing loss in patients old enough to be tested and daily renal function determinations may be required in patients on high-dose therapy or therapy continued for longer than 10 days, especially if renal function is changing; renal function determinations may be required to detect nephrotoxicity and to help prevent severe neurotoxic reactions; audiometric testing may also be required with concurrent or sequential administration of other ototoxic antibacterials; if renal, vestibular, or auditory function impairment occurs, reduction in dose or discontinuation of the aminoglycoside may be required)

» Urinalyses
(may be required prior to treatment and daily during treatment to detect albumin, casts, and cells in the urine, as well as decreased specific gravity)

*For streptomycin*

» Caloric stimulation tests
(may also be required prior to, periodically during, and following prolonged therapy to detect vestibular toxicity)

## Side/Adverse Effects

Note: Leg cramps, skin rash, fever, and seizures have been reported when gentamicin was administered concurrently by the systemic and intrathecal routes.

Neuromuscular blockade, respiratory paralysis, ototoxicity, and nephrotoxicity may occur following local irrigation and following topical application of aminoglycosides during surgery.

Because of its potential toxicity, use of parenteral neomycin is not recommended.

The following side/adverse effects have been selected on the basis of their potential clinical significance (possible signs and symptoms in parentheses where appropriate)—not necessarily inclusive:

### Those indicating need for medical attention

Incidence more frequent

*Nephrotoxicity* (greatly increased or decreased frequency of urination or amount of urine; increased thirst; loss of appetite; nausea; vomiting); *neurotoxicity* (muscle twitching; numbness; seizures; tingling); *ototoxicity, auditory* (any loss of hearing; ringing or buzzing, or a feeling of fullness in the ears); *ototoxicity, vestibular* (clumsiness; dizziness; nausea; vomiting; unsteadiness); *peripheral neuritis* (burning of face or mouth; numbness; tingling)—streptomycin only

Incidence less frequent

*Hypersensitivity* (skin itching, redness, rash, or swelling); *optic neuritis* (any loss of vision)—streptomycin only

Incidence rare

*Neuromuscular blockade* (difficulty in breathing; drowsiness; weakness)

### Those indicating possible ototoxicity, vestibular toxicity, or nephrotoxicity and the need for medical attention if they occur and/or progress after medication is discontinued

*Any loss of hearing; clumsiness or unsteadiness; dizziness; greatly increased or decreased frequency of urination or amount of urine; increased thirst; loss of appetite; nausea or vomiting; ringing or buzzing or a feeling of fullness in the ears*

## Overdose

For more informatin on the management of overdose or unintentional ingestion, **contact a Poison Control Center** (See *Poison Control Center Listing*).

### Treatment of overdose

Specific treatment—

Hemodialysis or peritoneal dialysis to remove aminoglycosides from the blood of patients with impaired renal function.

Anticholinesterase agents, calcium salts, or mechanical respiratory assistance to treat neuromuscular blockade, resulting in prolonged skeletal muscle weakness and respiratory depression or paralysis (apnea), that may occur when two or more aminoglycosides are given concurrently.

Supportive care—Since there is no specific antidote, treatment of aminoglycoside overdose or toxic reactions should be symptomatic and supportive. Patients in whom intentional overdose is known or suspected should be referred for psychiatric consultation.

## Patient Consultation

As an aid to patient consultation, refer to *Advice for the Patient, Aminoglycosides (Systemic)*.

In providing consultation, consider emphasizing the following selected information (» = major clinical significance):

### Before using this medication

» Conditions affecting use, especially:

Hypersensitivity to aminoglycosides

Pregnancy—May be nephrotoxic in the fetus or cause irreversible deafness in children whose mothers received aminoglycosides during pregnancy

Use in children—Premature infants and neonates may be more susceptible to renal toxicity because of their immature renal capability

Use in the elderly—Geriatric patients may be at risk of renal toxicity because of an age-related decrease in renal function

Other medications, especially 2 or more aminoglycosides used together, capreomycin, other nephrotoxic or ototoxic medications, or other neuromuscular blocking agents

Other medical problems, especially eighth-cranial-nerve impairment, infant botulism, myasthenia gravis, parkinsonism, or renal function impairment

**Proper use of this medication**

» Importance of receiving medication for full course of therapy and on regular schedule

» Proper dosing

**Side/adverse effects**

Signs of potential side effects, especially hypersensitivity, optic neuritis, neuromuscular blockade, nephrotoxicity, neurotoxicity, auditory and vestibular ototoxicity, and peripheral neuritis, which are more likely to occur in children and the elderly

## General Dosing Information

Because of the low therapeutic index of aminoglycosides, it is best to base dosage calculations on ideal body weight (IBW) as follows:

IBW (males) = 50 kg + (2.3 kg × inches over 5 feet)
IBW (females) = 45 kg + (2.3 kg × inches over 5 feet)

Serum concentrations should be monitored, especially in neonates and the elderly, even without renal function impairment, and in patients with impaired renal function to ensure adequate concentrations and to avoid potentially toxic concentrations. Therapeutic concentrations are shown in the table below. Prolonged peak (post-distributional) concentrations (measured 15 to 30 minutes after injection) and trough concentrations (measured immediately prior to the next dose) greater than those shown below should be avoided.

| Drug | Therapeutic Concentration (mcg/mL) | Maximum Peak Concentration (mcg/mL) | Maximum Trough Concentration (mcg/mL) |
|---|---|---|---|
| Amikacin | 15–25 | 35 | 5 |
| Gentamicin | 4–10 | 10 | 2 |
| Kanamycin | 15–30 | 30–35 | 5 |
| Netilmicin | 6–12 | 16 | 2 |
| Streptomycin | — | 20–25 * | — |
| Tobramycin | 4–10 | 10 | 2 |

*In patients with renal damage. Peak concentrations greater than 50 mcg per mL are associated with increased risk of toxicity.

Because of their larger volume of distribution and reduced renal development, infants may require larger doses, given at less frequent intervals, for achievement of therapeutic serum concentrations. Cystic fibrosis patients and burn patients may also require larger doses, but because they eliminate the aminoglycoside faster than average, the dosing interval may need to be decreased too.

Serum concentrations should be used whenever possible to monitor aminoglycoside therapy. Creatinine clearance may be used to help monitor therapy, in conjunction with serum levels. Creatinine clearance (in mL per minute) may be calculated as follows:

Adult males: Creatinine clearance =
$$[(140 - age) \times (ideal\ body\ weight\ in\ kg)]/$$
$$[72 \times serum\ creatinine\ (mg\ per\ dL)]$$

Adult females: Creatinine clearance =
$$[(140 - age) \times (ideal\ body\ weight\ in\ kg)]/$$
$$[72 \times serum\ creatinine\ (mg\ per\ dL)] \times 0.85$$

Creatinine clearance may also be calculated in SI units (as mL per second) as follows:

Adult males: Creatinine clearance =
$$[(140 - age) \times (ideal\ body\ weight\ in\ kg)]/$$
$$[50 \times serum\ creatinine\ (micromoles\ per\ L)]$$

Adult females: Creatinine clearance =
$$[(140 - age) \times (ideal\ body\ weight\ in\ kg)]/$$
$$[50 \times serum\ creatinine\ (micromoles\ per\ L)] \times 0.85$$

The following dosing chart by Sarubbi and Hull (Ann Intern Med 1978; 89: 612-8) may be used to provide the clinician with an *initial* loading dose and maintenance dosage regimen in adult patients. *Further dosage adjustments should be individualized and based on peak and trough serum concentrations,* which should be drawn after the third maintenance dose.

1. Select loading dose based on the patient's ideal body weight (in mg per kg of body weight [mg/kg]) to provide peak serum concentration in the range listed below for the desired aminoglycoside.

| Aminoglycoside | Usual Loading Dose (mg/kg) | Expected Peak Serum Concentrations (mcg/mL) |
|---|---|---|
| Gentamicin Tobramycin | 1.5 to 2 | 4 to 10 |
| Amikacin Kanamycin | 5 to 7.5 | 15 to 30 |
| Netilmicin | 1.3 to 3.25 | 4 to 12 |

2. Select maintenance dose (as percentage of chosen loading dose) to maintain peak serum concentrations indicated above according to desired dosing interval and the patient's corrected creatinine clearance. This chart is not applicable to neonates and children.

| CrCl (mL/min)/ (mL/sec) | Half-life (hours) | Percentage of Loading Dose Required for Dosage Interval Selected | | |
|---|---|---|---|---|
| | | 8 hours | 12 hours | 24 hours |
| 90/1.50 | 3.1 | 84% | — | — |
| 80/1.33 | 3.4 | 80 | 91% | — |
| 70/1.17 | 3.9 | 76 | 88 | — |
| 60/1.00 | 4.5 | 71 | 84 | — |
| 50/0.83 | 5.3 | 65 | 79 | — |
| 40/0.67 | 6.5 | 57 | 72 | 92% |
| 30/0.50 | 8.4 | 48 | 63 | 86 |
| 25/0.42 | 9.9 | 43 | 57 | 81 |
| 20/0.33 | 11.9 | 37 | 50 | 75 |
| 17/0.28 | 13.6 | 33 | 46 | 70 |
| 15/0.25 | 15.1 | 31 | 42 | 67 |
| 12/0.20 | 17.9 | 27 | 37 | 61 |
| 10*/0.17* | 20.4 | 24 | 34 | 56 |
| 7/0.12 | 25.9 | 19 | 28 | 47 |
| 5/0.08 | 31.5 | 16 | 23 | 41 |
| 2/0.03 | 46.8 | 11 | 16 | 30 |
| 0/0 | 69.3 | 8 | 11 | 21 |

*Dosing for patients with CrCl <10 mL/min (<0.17 mL/sec) should be assisted by measured serum levels.

After an initial full therapeutic loading dose, neonates or patients with impaired renal, vestibular, or auditory function may require (1) a reduction in the maintenance dose administered either (a) by administration of the usual dose at prolonged intervals or (b) by administration of reduced dose at fixed intervals or (2) discontinuation of the aminoglycoside. Since aminoglycosides are not metabolized and are excreted primarily in the urine, toxic concentrations may accumulate in patients with impaired renal function.

Because of the high concentrations of aminoglycosides in the urine and excretory system, patients should be well hydrated to prevent or minimize chemical irritation of the renal tubules. Therapeutic serum aminoglycoside levels are usually not needed to effectively treat urinary tract infections.

If a dose of this medication is missed, give it as soon as possible. However, if it is almost time for the next dose, skip the missed dose and go back to the regular dosing schedule. Do not double doses.

## AMIKACIN

## Additional Dosing Information

For initial dosing guidelines for patients with renal function impairment, see the Sarubbi and Hull nomogram in *General Dosing Information.*

Burn and certain other patients may require a dose of 5 to 7.5 mg per kg of body weight (mg/kg) every four to six hours because of the shorter half-life (1 to 1.5 hours) in these patients.

Amikacin sulfate injection may also be administered as an aerosol nebulization.

## Parenteral Dosage Forms

### AMIKACIN SULFATE INJECTION USP

**Usual adult and adolescent dose**

Antibacterial (systemic)—

Intramuscular or intravenous infusion, 5 mg per kg of body weight every eight hours; or 7.5 mg per kg of body weight every twelve hours for seven to ten days.

Note: Urinary tract infections, bacterial (uncomplicated)—Intramuscular or intravenous infusion, 250 mg every twelve hours.

Following hemodialysis, a supplemental dose of 3 to 5 mg per kg of body weight may be administered.

## Usual adult prescribing limits
Up to 15 mg per kg of body weight daily, but not to exceed 1.5 grams daily for more than ten days.

## Usual pediatric dose
Antibacterial (systemic):—

Intramuscular or intravenous infusion:

Premature neonates—
Initially, 10 mg per kg of body weight, then 7.5 mg per kg of body weight every eighteen to twenty-four hours for seven to ten days.

Neonates—
Initially, 10 mg per kg of body weight, then 7.5 mg per kg of body weight every twelve hours for seven to ten days.

Older infants and children—
See *Usual adult and adolescent dose.*

## Strength(s) usually available
U.S.—

50 mg per mL (Rx) [*Amikin* (sodium bisulfite 0.13%); GENERIC].

250 mg per mL (Rx) [*Amikin* (sodium bisulfite 0.66%); GENERIC].

Canada—

250 mg per mL (Rx) [*Amikin* (sodium bisulfite 0.66%)].

## Packaging and storage
Store below 40 °C (104 °F), preferably between 15 and 30 °C (59 and 86 °F), unless otherwise specified by manufacturer. Protect from freezing.

## Preparation of dosage form
To prepare initial dilution for intravenous use, add the contents of each 500-mg vial to 100 to 200 mL of 0.9% sodium chloride injection, 5% dextrose injection, or other suitable diluent. The resulting solution should be administered slowly over a 30- to 60-minute period to help avoid neuromuscular blockade. Pediatric patients may require a proportionately smaller volume of diluent.

## Stability
Intravenous infusions of amikacin retain their potency for 24 hours at room temperature at concentrations of 0.25 and 5 mg per mL in dextrose injection, dextrose and sodium chloride injection, 0.9% sodium chloride injection, lactated Ringer's injection, and other electrolyte-containing solutions (see manufacturer's package insert).

Intravenous infusions of amikacin retain their potency for 60 days at 4 °C (39 °F) at concentrations of 0.25 and 5 mg per mL in the above-listed diluents. When these solutions are then stored at 25 °C (77 °F), they retain their potency for 24 hours.

Intravenous infusions of amikacin retain their potency for 30 days when frozen at −15 °C (5 °F) at concentrations of 0.25 and 5 mg per mL in the above-listed diluents. When these solutions are thawed and stored at 25 °C (77 °F), they retain their potency for 24 hours.

Solutions may vary in color from colorless to light straw or very pale yellow; this variation does not affect their potency. Discard dark-colored solutions.

## Incompatibilities
Extemporaneous admixtures of beta-lactam antibacterials (penicillins and cephalosporins) and aminoglycosides may result in substantial mutual inactivation. If these groups of antibacterials are administered concurrently, they should be administered in separate sites. Do not mix them in the same intravenous bag or bottle.

Amikacin is incompatible with amphotericin B, cephalothin sodium, nitrofurantoin sodium, sulfadiazine sodium, and tetracyclines (in some solutions).

Since complexes form with a number of other drugs also, extemporaneous admixtures with Amikacin Sulfate Injection USP are not recommended.

## Additional information
Commercially available amikacin sulfate injection contains sodium bisulfite, an antioxidant, but no preservatives.

---

# GENTAMICIN

## Additional Dosing Information
Surgical, obstetrical, gynecological, or burn patients receiving gentamicin doses adjusted on the basis of serum concentrations may require less than the minimum recommended dose or greater than the maximum recommended dose of gentamicin because of wide interpatient varia-

bility. In patients receiving gentamicin intrathecally, CSF concentrations should also be monitored.

For initial dosing guidelines for patients with renal function impairment, see the Sarrubi and Hull nomogram in *General Dosing Information.*

Subcutaneous administration is not recommended and may be painful.

Commercially available gentamicin piggyback injections should be administered by intravenous infusion only.

Preservative-free gentamicin may also be administered directly into the subdural space, directly into the ventricles, or by means of an implanted reservoir.

Gentamicin sulfate injection may also be administered as an aerosol nebulization.

## Parenteral Dosage Forms
Note: The dosing and dosage forms available are expressed in terms of gentamicin base.

### GENTAMICIN SULFATE INJECTION USP
## Usual adult and adolescent dose
Antibacterial (systemic)—

Intramuscular or intravenous infusion, 1 to 1.7 mg (base) per kg of body weight every eight hours for seven to ten days or more.

Note: Urinary tract infections, bacterial (uncomplicated)—Intramuscular or intravenous infusion:

Adults less than 60 kg of body weight—3 mg (base) per kg of body weight once a day; or 1.5 mg per kg of body weight every twelve hours.

Adults 60 kg of body weight and over—160 mg (base) once a day; or 80 mg every twelve hours.

Following hemodialysis, a supplemental dose of 1 to 1.7 mg (base) per kg of body weight may be administered, depending on the severity of the infection.

Intralumbar or intraventricular, 4 to 8 mg (base) once a day.

## Usual adult prescribing limits
Up to 8 mg (base) per kg of body weight daily in severe, life-threatening infections.

Note: Doses up to 15 mg (base) per kg of body weight daily have been used in the treatment of intraocular infections.

## Usual pediatric dose
Antibacterial (systemic)—

Intramuscular or intravenous infusion:

Premature or full-term neonates up to 1 week of age—
2.5 mg (base) per kg of body weight every twelve to twenty-four hours for seven to ten days or more.

Older neonates and infants—
2.5 mg (base) per kg of body weight every eight to sixteen hours for seven to ten days or more.

Children—
2 to 2.5 mg (base) per kg of body weight every eight hours for seven to ten days or more.

Note: The dosing interval of gentamicin in pediatric patients may vary from every four hours to every twenty-four hours, depending on the medical condition of the patient (cystic fibrosis, burns, renal dysfunction); serum levels must be monitored.

Following hemodialysis, a supplemental dose of 2 to 2.5 mg (base) per kg of body weight may be administered, depending on the severity of the infection.

Intralumbar or intraventricular:

Infants up to 3 months of age—
Dosage has not been established.

Infants and children 3 months of age and over—
1 to 2 mg (base) once a day.

Note: Doses up to 8 mg (base) daily have been used in infants with functioning ventricular shunts.

## Strength(s) usually available
U.S.—

Intramuscular and intravenous:

10 mg per mL (base) (Rx) [*Garamycin;* GENERIC (sodium bisulfite 3.2 mg)].

40 mg per mL (base) (Rx) [*Garamycin; G-Mycin; Jenamicin;* GENERIC (sodium bisulfite 3.2 mg)].

Intrathecal:

2 mg per mL (base) (Rx) [*Garamycin*].

Canada—
Intramuscular and intravenous:
10 mg per mL (base) (Rx) [*Cidomycin* (sodium bisulfite 3.2 mg); *Garamycin* (sodium bisulfite)].
40 mg per mL (base) (Rx) [*Cidomycin* (sodium bisulfite 3.2 mg); *Garamycin* (sodium bisulfite)].

**Packaging and storage**
Store below 40 °C (104 °F), preferably between 15 and 30 °C (59 and 86 °F), unless otherwise specified by manufacturer. Protect from freezing.

**Preparation of dosage form**
Intravenous—To prepare initial dilution for intravenous use, add each dose to 50 to 200 mL of 0.9% sodium chloride injection or 5% dextrose injection to provide a concentration not exceeding 1 mg (base) per mL (0.1%). The resulting solution should be administered slowly over a 30- to 60-minute period to help decrease the chance of neuromuscular blockade. Pediatric patients may require a proportionately smaller volume of diluent.

Intralumbar and/or intraventricular (2 mg per mL)—To prepare initial dilution for intralumbar use, each dose should be drawn up into a 5- or 10-mL sterile syringe. Following lumbar puncture and the removal of a specimen of cerebrospinal fluid (CSF) for laboratory analysis, the syringe containing gentamicin is inserted into the hub of the spinal needle. A quantity of CSF equal to approximately 10% of the total estimated CSF volume is allowed to flow into the syringe and mix with the gentamicin. The resulting solution should be administered over a 3- to 5-minute period with the bevel of the spinal needle directed upward. Gentamicin may also be diluted with sodium chloride injection (without preservatives) if the CSF is grossly purulent or unobtainable. Since the 2-mg-per-mL concentration contains no preservatives, it should be used promptly after being opened; unused portions should be discarded.

**Stability**
Do not use if injection is discolored or contains a precipitate.

**Incompatibilities**
Extemporaneous admixtures of beta-lactam antibacterials (penicillins and cephalosporins) and aminoglycosides may result in substantial mutual inactivation. If these groups of antibacterials are administered concurrently, they should be administered in separate sites. Do not mix them in the same intravenous bag or bottle.

Since complexes form with a number of other drugs also, extemporaneous admixtures with Gentamicin Sulfate Injection USP are not recommended.

**Additional information**
Intrathecal gentamicin is commercially available as a preservative-free injection.

## GENTAMICIN SULFATE IN SODIUM CHLORIDE INJECTION

**Usual adult and adolescent dose**
Antibacterial (systemic)—
Intravenous infusion, 1 to 1.7 mg (base) per kg of body weight every eight hours for seven to ten days or more.

Note:  Urinary tract infections, bacterial (uncomplicated)—Intravenous infusion:
Adults less than 60 kg of body weight—3 mg (base) per kg of body weight once a day; or 1.5 mg per kg of body weight every twelve hours.
Adults 60 kg of body weight and over—160 mg (base) once a day; or 80 mg every twelve hours.
Following hemodialysis, a supplemental dose of 1 to 1.7 mg (base) per kg of body weight may be administered, depending on the severity of the infection.

**Usual adult prescribing limits**
Up to 8 mg (base) per kg of body weight daily in severe, life-threatening infections.

Note:  Doses up to 15 mg (base) per kg of body weight daily have been used in the treatment of intraocular infections.

**Usual pediatric dose**
Antibacterial (systemic)—
Intravenous infusion:
Premature or full-term neonates up to 1 week of age—
2.5 mg (base) per kg of body weight every twelve to twenty-four hours for seven to ten days or more.
Older neonates and infants—
2.5 mg (base) per kg of body weight every eight to sixteen hours for seven to ten days or more.

Children—
2 to 2.5 mg (base) per kg of body weight every eight hours for seven to ten days or more.

Note:  The dosing interval of gentamicin in pediatric patients may vary from every four hours to every twenty-four hours, depending on the medical conditions of the patient (cystic fibrosis, burns, renal dysfunction); serum levels must be monitored.
Following hemodialysis, a supplemental dose of 2 to 2.5 mg (base) per kg of body weight may be administered, depending on the severity of the infection.

**Strength(s) usually available**
U.S.—
40 mg in 50 mL (base) (Rx) [GENERIC].
40 mg in 100 mL (base) (Rx) [GENERIC].
60 mg in 50 mL (base) (Rx) [GENERIC].
60 mg in 100 mL (base) (Rx) [GENERIC].
70 mg in 50 mL (base) (Rx) [GENERIC].
80 mg in 50 mL (base) (Rx) [GENERIC].
80 mg in 100 mL (base) (Rx) [GENERIC].
90 mg in 100 mL (base) (Rx) [GENERIC].
100 mg in 50 mL (base) (Rx) [GENERIC].
100 mg in 100 mL (base) (Rx) [GENERIC].
120 mg in 100 mL (base) (Rx) [GENERIC].
160 mg in 100 mL (base) (Rx) [GENERIC].
180 mg in 100 mL (base) (Rx) [GENERIC].
Canada—
60 mg in 50 mL (base) (Rx) [GENERIC].
70 mg in 50 mL (base) (Rx) [GENERIC].
80 mg in 100 mL (base) (Rx) [GENERIC].

**Packaging and storage**
Store between 2 and 30 °C (36 and 86 °F), unless otherwise specified by manufacturer. Protect from freezing.

**Preparation of dosage form**
Commercially available gentamicin piggyback injections require no further dilution prior to administration (see manufacturer's labeling for instructions). Since these injections contain no preservatives, they should be used promptly after being opened; unused portions should be discarded.

**Stability**
Do not use if injection is discolored or contains a precipitate.

**Incompatibilities**
Extemporaneous admixtures of beta-lactam antibacterials (penicillins and cephalosporins) and aminoglycosides may result in substantial mutual inactivation. If these groups of antibacterials are administered concurrently, they should be administered in separate sites. Do not mix them in the same intravenous bag or bottle.

Since complexes form with a number of other drugs also, extemporaneous admixtures with gentamicin in sodium chloride injection are not recommended.

**Additional information**
The sodium content is approximately 19.6 mEq (450 mg) per 50 mL. This must be considered in patients on a restricted sodium intake when calculating total daily sodium intake.

---

## *KANAMYCIN*

## Additional Dosing Information

For initial dosing guidelines for patients with renal function impairment, see the Sarubbi and Hull nomogram in *General Dosing Information*.
For intravenous use only:
• Direct intravenous administration of undiluted kanamycin sulfate injection is not recommended because of the possibility of neuromuscular blockade.
For intramuscular use only:
• Inject kanamycin sulfate injection deeply into the upper outer quadrant of the gluteal muscle.
For other routes:
• Kanamycin sulfate injection may also be administered as an irrigation in a concentration of 0.25%.
• Kanamycin sulfate injection may also be administered as an aerosol nebulization.
• Kanamycin sulfate injection may also be administered intraperitoneally in a concentration of 2.5%.

# Parenteral Dosage Forms

## KANAMYCIN SULFATE INJECTION USP

### Usual adult and adolescent dose
Antibacterial (systemic)—
Inhalation treatment, 250 mg two to four times a day.
Intramuscular, 3.75 mg per kg of body weight every six hours; 5 mg per kg of body weight every eight hours; or 7.5 mg per kg of body weight every twelve hours for seven to ten days.
Intraperitoneal, 500 mg.
Intravenous infusion, 5 mg per kg of body weight every eight hours; or 7.5 mg per kg of body weight every twelve hours for seven to ten days.

### Usual adult prescribing limits
Up to 15 mg per kg of body weight daily, but not to exceed 1.5 grams daily.
Note: The total daily dose should take into account the amounts given by all routes, including intraperitoneal, inhalation, and irrigation. In intraocular infections, initial intramuscular doses of 2 grams, followed by 1 gram every twelve hours, have been used.

### Usual pediatric dose
Antibacterial (systemic)—Intramuscular or intravenous infusion: See *Usual adult and adolescent dose.*
Note: Doses up to 30 mg per kg of body weight daily have been used in children.

### Strength(s) usually available
U.S.—
37.5 mg per mL (Rx) [*Kantrex;* GENERIC (sodium bisulfite 0.099%)].
250 mg per mL (Rx) [*Kantrex;* GENERIC (sodium bisulfite 0.66%)].
333.3 mg per mL (Rx) [*Kantrex;* GENERIC (sodium bisulfite 0.45%)].
Canada—
Not commercially available.

### Packaging and storage
Store below 40 °C (104 °F), preferably between 15 and 30 °C (59 and 86 °F), unless otherwise specified by manufacturer. Protect from freezing.

### Preparation of dosage form
Intraperitoneal—To prepare dilution for intraperitoneal use, add the contents of each 500-mg vial to 20 mL of sterile water for injection. The resulting solution may be instilled postoperatively through a polyethylene catheter sutured into the wound at closure. To help prevent or minimize neuromuscular blockade, instillation of kanamycin should be postponed until the patient has fully recovered from the effects of anesthesia or neuromuscular blocking agents.
Intravenous—To prepare initial dilution for intravenous use, add the contents of each 500-mg vial to 100 to 200 mL or the contents of each 1-gram vial to 200 to 400 mL of 0.9% sodium chloride injection, 5% dextrose injection, or other suitable diluent. The resulting solution should be administered over a 30- to 60-minute period. Pediatric patients may require a proportionately smaller volume of diluent.

### Stability
Solutions may darken during storage; this darkening does not affect their potency.

### Incompatibilities
Extemporaneous admixtures of beta-lactam antibacterials (penicillins and cephalosporins) and aminoglycosides may result in substantial mutual inactivation. If these groups of antibacterials are administered concurrently, they should be administered in separate sites. Do not mix them in the same intravenous bag or bottle.
Since complexes form with a number of other drugs also, extemporaneous admixtures with kanamycin sulfate injection are not recommended.

---

## *NEOMYCIN*

### STERILE NEOMYCIN SULFATE USP
Note: Parenteral neomycin has been replaced by safer and more effective agents. **Because of its potential toxicity, the parenteral use of neomycin is not recommended for any indication.**

### Size(s) usually available
U.S.—
500 mg (Rx) [GENERIC].
Canada—
Not commercially available.

---

## *NETILMICIN*

# Additional Dosing Information

Serum concentrations of netilmicin in febrile patients may be lower than in afebrile patients receiving the same dose because of shorter half-life. The half-life may also be shorter in anemic patients. However, when the body temperature returns to normal in febrile patients, serum concentrations may increase. Dosage adjustments are not usually necessary.

For initial dosing guidelines for patients with renal function impairment, see the Sarubbi and Hull nomogram in *General Dosing Information.*

In severely burned patients, serum concentrations of netilmicin may be lower than expected from a particular dose. Serum determinations are especially important in these patients for dosage adjustment.

# Parenteral Dosage Forms

Note: The dosing and dosage forms available are expressed in terms of netilmicin base.

## NETILMICIN SULFATE INJECTION USP

### Usual adult and adolescent dose
Antibacterial (systemic)—
Intramuscular or intravenous:
Systemic infections (serious)—
1.3 to 2.2 mg (base) per kg of body weight every eight hours; or 2 to 3.25 mg (base) per kg of body weight every twelve hours for seven to fourteen days.
Urinary tract infections, bacterial (complicated)—
1.5 to 2 mg (base) per kg of body weight every twelve hours for seven to fourteen days.
Note: Following hemodialysis, a supplemental dose of 1 mg (base) per kg of body weight may be administered.

### Usual adult prescribing limits
Up to 7.5 mg (base) per kg of body weight daily.
Note: Doses up to 12 mg (base) per kg of body weight daily have been used in cystic fibrosis patients.

### Usual pediatric dose
Antibacterial (systemic)—
Intramuscular or intravenous:
Neonates up to 6 weeks of age—
2 to 3.25 mg (base) per kg of body weight every twelve hours for seven to fourteen days.
Infants and children 6 weeks to 12 years of age—
1.83 to 2.67 mg (base) per kg of body weight every eight hours; or 2.75 to 4 mg (base) per kg of body weight every twelve hours for seven to fourteen days.

### Strength(s) usually available
U.S.—
100 mg per mL (base) (Rx) [*Netromycin* (benzyl alcohol 10 mg, sodium metabisulfite 2.4 mg, sodium sulfite 0.8 mg)].
Canada—
25 mg per mL (base) (Rx) [*Netromycin* (sodium metabisulfite 2.1 mg, sodium sulfite 1.2 mg)].
50 mg per mL (base) (Rx) [*Netromycin* (sodium metabisulfite 2.1 mg, sodium sulfite 1.2 mg)].
100 mg per mL (base) (Rx) [*Netromycin* (benzyl alcohol 10 mg, sodium metabisulfite 2.4 mg, sodium sulfite 0.8 mg)].

### Packaging and storage
Store below 40 °C (104 °F), preferably between 15 and 30 °C (59 and 86 °F), unless otherwise specified by manufacturer. Protect from freezing.

### Preparation of dosage form
To prepare initial dilution for intravenous use, each dose should be diluted in 50 to 200 mL of a suitable diluent (see manufacturer's package insert). The resulting solution should be administered slowly over a 30- to 60-minute period to help avoid neuromuscular blockade. Pediatric patients may require a proportionately smaller volume of diluent.

### Stability
Intravenous infusions of netilmicin retain their potency for up to 72 hours at room temperature or when refrigerated and stored in glass containers at concentrations of 2.1 to 3 mg per mL in suitable diluents (see manufacturer's package insert).

### Incompatibilities
Extemporaneous admixtures of beta-lactam antibacterials (penicillins and cephalosporins) and aminoglycosides may result in substantial mutual

inactivation. If these groups of antibacterials are administered concurrently, they should be administered in separate sites. Do not mix them in the same intravenous bag or bottle.

## STREPTOMYCIN

## Summary of Differences

Indications: Used for the treatment of brucellosis, granuloma inguinale, plague, tuberculosis, and tularemia.
Pregnancy/Reproduction: Has been shown to cause deafness in humans.
Patient monitoring: Caloric stimulation tests may also be required.

## Additional Dosing Information

Tuberculosis therapy may have to be continued for 1 to 2 years, and may even be required for up to several years or indefinitely, although in some patients shorter treatment regimens may also be effective. However, streptomycin should be discontinued when toxicity or toxic symptoms appear or are impending, when organisms have become resistant, or when the full therapeutic effect has been achieved.

Injection sites should be alternated and concentrations greater than 500 mg per mL are not recommended.

## Parenteral Dosage Forms

Note: The dosing and dosage forms available are expressed in terms of streptomycin base.

### STREPTOMYCIN SULFATE INJECTION USP

**Usual adult and adolescent dose**
Antibacterial (antimycobacterial)—
    Tuberculosis:
        Intramuscular—
            In combination with other antimycobacterials, 1 gram (base) once a day. Dosage should be reduced to 1 gram two or three times a week as soon as clinically feasible.
Antibacterial (systemic)—
    Other infections:
        Intramuscular—
            In combination with other antibacterials, 250 mg to 1 gram (base) every six hours; or 500 mg to 2 grams every twelve hours.
Note: Plague—Intramuscular: 500 mg to 1 gram (base) every six hours; or 1 to 2 grams every twelve hours.
        Tularemia—Intramuscular: 250 to 500 mg (base) every six hours; or 500 mg to 1 gram every twelve hours for seven to ten days.

**Usual adult prescribing limits**
Tuberculosis—
    1 gram twice weekly to 2 grams (base) daily.
Other infections—
    Up to 4 grams (base) daily.

**Usual pediatric dose**
Antibacterial (antimycobacterial)—
    Tuberculosis:
        Intramuscular—
            In combination with other antimycobacterials, 20 mg (base) per kg of body weight once a day. Maximum dose per day should not exceed 1 gram.
Antibacterial (systemic)—
    Other infections:
        Intramuscular—
            In combination with other antibacterials, 5 to 10 mg (base) per kg of body weight every six hours; or 10 to 20 mg per kg of body weight every twelve hours.

**Usual geriatric dose**
Antibacterial (antimycobacterial)—
    Tuberculosis:
        Intramuscular—
            In combination with other antimycobacterials, 500 to 750 mg (base) once a day.

**Strength(s) usually available**
U.S.—
    Not commercially available.
Canada—
    500 mg per mL (base) (Rx) [GENERIC].

**Packaging and storage**
Store below 40 °C (104 °F), preferably between 15 and 30 °C (59 and 86 °F), unless otherwise specified by manufacturer. Protect from freezing.

## Stability

Solutions may vary in color from colorless to yellow and may darken on exposure to light. This variation does not affect their potency.
Solutions should not be autoclaved since loss of potency may result.

### STERILE STREPTOMYCIN SULFATE USP

**Usual adult and adolescent dose**
Antibacterial (antimycobacterial)—
    Tuberculosis:
        Intramuscular—
            In combination with other antimycobacterials, 1 gram (base) once a day. Dosage should be reduced to 1 gram two or three times a week as soon as clinically feasible.
Antibacterial (systemic)—
    Other infections:
        Intramuscular—
            In combination with other antibacterials, 250 mg to 1 gram (base) every six hours; or 500 mg to 2 grams every twelve hours.
Note: Plague—Intramuscular: 500 mg to 1 gram (base) every six hours; or 1 to 2 grams every twelve hours.
        Tularemia—Intramuscular: 250 to 500 mg (base) every six hours; or 500 mg to 1 gram every twelve hours for seven to ten days.

**Usual adult prescribing limits**
Tuberculosis—
    1 gram twice weekly to 2 grams (base) daily.
Other infections—
    Up to 4 grams (base) daily.

**Usual pediatric dose**
Antibacterial (antimycobacterial)—
    Tuberculosis:
        Intramuscular—
            In combination with other antimycobacterials, 20 mg (base) per kg of body weight once a day. Maximum dose per day should not exceed 1 gram.
Antibacterial (systemic)—
    Other infections:
        Intramuscular—
            In combination with other antibacterials, 5 to 10 mg (base) per kg of body weight every six hours; or 10 to 20 mg per kg of body weight every twelve hours.

**Size(s) usually available**
U.S.—
    1 gram (base) (Rx) [GENERIC].
Canada—
    Not commercially available.

**Packaging and storage**
Prior to reconstitution, store below 40 °C (104 °F), preferably between 15 and 30 °C (59 and 86 °F), unless otherwise specified by manufacturer.

**Preparation of dosage form**
To prepare initial dilution for intramuscular use, add 4.2 to 4.5 mL of 0.9% sodium chloride injection or sterile water for injection to each 1-gram vial, according to the manufacturer, to provide a concentration of 200 mg (base) per mL or 3.2 to 3.5 mL of diluent to provide a concentration of 250 mg per mL; and add 17 mL of diluent to each 5-gram vial to provide a concentration of 250 mg per mL or 6.5 mL of diluent to provide a concentration of 500 mg per mL.

**Stability**
After reconstitution, solutions retain their potency for 2 to 28 days at room temperature or for 14 days if refrigerated, depending on manufacturer.

## TOBRAMYCIN

## Summary of Differences

Pregnancy/Reproduction: Has been shown to cause deafness in humans.

## Additional Dosing Information

Commercially available tobramycin piggyback injections should be administered by intravenous infusion only.

Tobramycin sulfate injection may also be administered as an aerosol nebulization.

## Parenteral Dosage Forms

Note: The dosing and dosage forms available are expressed in terms of tobramycin base.

# TOBRAMYCIN SULFATE INJECTION USP

**Usual adult and adolescent dose**
Antibacterial (systemic)—
Intramuscular or intravenous infusion, 0.75 mg to 1.25 mg (base) per kg of body weight every six hours; or 1 to 1.7 mg per kg of body weight every eight hours for seven to ten days or more.

**Usual adult prescribing limits**
Up to 8 mg (base) per kg of body weight daily in severe, life-threatening infections.

**Usual pediatric dose**
Antibacterial (systemic)—
Intramuscular or intravenous infusion:
Premature or full-term neonates up to 1 week of age—
Up to 2 mg (base) per kg of body weight every twelve to twenty-four hours.
Older infants and children—
1.5 to 1.9 mg (base) per kg of body weight every six hours; or 2 to 2.5 mg per kg of body weight every eight to sixteen hours.
Note: The dosing interval of tobramycin in pediatric patients may vary from every four hours to every twenty-four hours, depending on the medical condition of the patient (cystic fibrosis, burns, renal dysfunction); serum levels must be monitored.

**Strength(s) usually available**
U.S.—
10 mg per mL (base) (Rx) [*Nebcin* (sodium bisulfite 3.2 mg); GENERIC].
20 mg per mL (base) (Rx) [GENERIC].
40 mg per mL (base) (Rx) [*Nebcin* (sodium bisulfite 3.2 mg); GENERIC].
60 mg per mL (base) (Rx) [GENERIC].
80 mg per mL (base) (Rx) [GENERIC].
Canada—
10 mg per mL (base) (Rx) [*Nebcin* (sodium bisulfite)].
40 mg per mL (base) (Rx) [*Nebcin* (sodium bisulfite)].

**Packaging and storage**
Store below 40 °C (104 °F), preferably between 15 and 30 °C (59 and 86 °F), unless otherwise specified by manufacturer. Protect from freezing.

**Preparation of dosage form**
To prepare initial dilution for intravenous use, add each dose to 50 to 200 mL of 0.9% sodium chloride injection or 5% dextrose injection to provide a concentration not exceeding 1 mg (base) per mL (0.1%). The resulting solution should be administered slowly over a 30- to 60-minute period to avoid neuromuscular blockade. In addition, infusion periods of less than 20 minutes are not recommended since peak serum concentrations may exceed 12 mcg per mL. Pediatric patients may require a proportionately smaller volume of diluent.

**Incompatibilities**
Extemporaneous admixtures of beta-lactam antibacterials (penicillins and cephalosporins) and aminoglycosides may result in substantial mutual inactivation. If these groups of antibacterials are administered concurrently, they should be administered in separate sites. Do not mix them in the same intravenous bag or bottle.
Since complexes form with a number of other drugs also, extemporaneous admixtures with tobramycin sulfate injection are not recommended.

**Additional information**
Subcutaneous administration is not recommended and may be painful.

# STERILE TOBRAMYCIN SULFATE USP

**Usual adult and adolescent dose**
Antibacterial (systemic)—
Intravenous infusion, 0.75 mg to 1.25 mg (base) per kg of body weight every six hours; or 1 to 1.7 mg per kg of body weight every eight hours for seven to ten days or more.

**Usual adult prescribing limits**
Up to 8 mg (base) per kg of body weight daily in severe, life-threatening infections.

**Usual pediatric dose**
Antibacterial (systemic)—
Intravenous infusion:
Premature or full-term neonates up to 1 week of age—
Up to 2 mg (base) per kg of body weight every twelve to twenty-four hours.
Older infants and children—
1.5 to 1.9 mg (base) per kg of body weight every six hours; or 2 to 2.5 mg per kg of body weight every eight to sixteen hours.

Note: The dosing interval of tobramycin in pediatric patients may vary from every four hours to every twenty-four hours, depending on the medical condition of the patient (cystic fibrosis, burns, renal dysfunction); serum levels must be monitored.

**Size(s) usually available**
U.S.—
1.2 grams (base) (Rx) [*Nebcin;* GENERIC].
Canada—
1.2 grams (base) (Rx) [*Nebcin*].

**Packaging and storage**
Prior to reconstitution, store below 40 °C (104 °F), preferably between 15 and 30 °C (59 and 86 °F), unless otherwise specified by manufacturer.

**Preparation of dosage form**
To prepare initial dilution for intravenous use, add 30 mL of sterile water for injection to each 1.2-gram vial to provide 40 mg (base) per mL. Withdraw each dose from the pharmacy bulk vial and add it to 50 to 200 mL of 0.9% sodium chloride injection or 5% dextrose injection to provide a final concentration not exceeding 1 mg per mL (0.1%). The resulting solution should be administered slowly over a 30- to 60-minute period to avoid neuromuscular blockade. In addition, infusion periods of less than 20 minutes are not recommended since peak serum concentrations may exceed 12 mcg per mL. Pediatric patients may require a proportionately smaller volume of diluent.

**Stability**
After reconstitution, solutions retain their potency for 24 hours at room temperature or for 96 hours if refrigerated.

**Incompatibilities**
Extemporaneous admixtures of beta-lactam antibacterials (penicillins and cephalosporins) and aminoglycosides may result in substantial mutual inactivation. If these groups of antibacterials are administered concurrently, they should be administered in separate sites. Do not mix them in the same intravenous bag or bottle.
Since complexes form with a number of other drugs also, extemporaneous admixtures with Sterile Tobramycin Sulfate USP are not recommended.

**Additional information**
Sterile Tobramycin Sulfate USP is available only in a pharmacy bulk vial (multiple-dose) and is intended for use in the extemporaneous preparation of intravenous admixtures.

# TOBRAMYCIN SULFATE IN SODIUM CHLORIDE INJECTION

**Usual adult and adolescent dose**
See *Tobramycin Sulfate Injection USP.*

**Usual adult prescribing limits**
See *Tobramycin Sulfate Injection USP.*

**Usual pediatric dose**
See *Tobramycin Sulfate Injection USP.*

**Strength(s) usually available**
U.S.—
60 mg in 50 mL (base) (Rx) [GENERIC].
80 mg in 100 mL (base) (Rx) [GENERIC].
Canada—
Not commercially available.

**Packaging and storage**
Store between 2 and 30 °C (36 and 86 °F), unless otherwise specified by manufacturer. Protect from freezing.

**Preparation of dosage form**
Commercially available tobramycin piggyback injections require no further dilution prior to administration (see manufacturer's labeling for instructions).

**Stability**
Do not use if injection is discolored or contains a precipitate.

**Incompatibilities**
Extemporaneous admixtures of beta-lactam antibacterials (penicillins and cephalosporins) and aminoglycosides may result in substantial mutual inactivation. If these groups of antibacterials are administered concurrently, they should be administered in separate sites. Do not mix them in the same intravenous bag or bottle.
Since complexes form with a number of other drugs also, extemporaneous admixtures with tobramycin in sodium chloride injection are not recommended.

**Additional information**
The sodium content is approximately 19.6 mEq (450 mg) per 50 mL. This must be considered in patients on a restricted sodium intake when calculating total daily sodium intake.

Revised: 02/23/93
Interim revision: 04/24/95; 06/20/95

**AMINOPHYLLINE**—See    *Bronchodilators,    Theophylline (Systemic)*

# AMINOSALICYLATE SODIUM   Systemic

VA CLASSIFICATION (Primary): AM500
Note: Aminosalicylate sodium, a 4-amino antimycobacterial compound, differs from 5-aminosalicylic acid (mesalamine), which is used in the treatment of nonbacterial inflammatory conditions such as ulcerative colitis, proctosigmoiditis, or proctitis.

Another commonly used name is PAS.

Note: For a listing of dosage forms and brand names by country availability, see *Dosage Forms* section(s). For a listing of brand names for the articles in this monograph, refer to the General Index.

## Category
Antibacterial (antimycobacterial)

## Indications
**Accepted**
Tuberculosis (treatment)—Aminosalicylate sodium is indicated in the treatment of pulmonary and extrapulmonary tuberculosis caused by *Mycobacterium tuberculosis*. However, aminosalicylate sodium is much less effective than other antituberculars and must be given in combination with other medications.

Since bacterial resistance may develop rapidly when aminosalicylate sodium is administered alone, it should only be administered concurrently with other antimycobacterials. Development of resistance to streptomycin and isoniazid may be delayed when these medicines are administered concurrently with aminosalicylate sodium.

**Unaccepted**
Aminosalicylate sodium has been used in the treatment of atypical mycobacterial infections; however, most atypical mycobacteria are not inhibited by this medication.

## Pharmacology/Pharmacokinetics
**Physicochemical characteristics**
Molecular weight—211.15.

**Mechanism of action/Effect**
Bacteriostatic; analog of aminobenzoic acid (PABA); believed to suppress growth and reproduction of *Mycobacterium tuberculosis* by competitively inhibiting folic acid formation.

**Absorption**
Rapidly and well absorbed from gastrointestinal tract.

**Distribution**
Diffuses readily into various body fluids, achieving high concentrations in pleural fluid, but low concentrations in the cerebrospinal fluid (CSF); diffuses readily into kidneys, lungs, and liver, achieving high concentrations in caseous tissue.

**Protein binding**
Low (15%).

**Biotransformation**
Hepatic; greater than 50% acetylation to inactive metabolites.

**Half-life**
Normal renal function—
    45 to 60 minutes.
Impaired renal function—
    Up to 23 hours.

**Time to peak serum concentration**
1 to 2 hours.

**Peak serum concentration**
Approximately 75 mcg per mL after a 4 gram oral dose.

**Elimination**
Renal; 85% of a dose is rapidly excreted within 7 to 10 hours by glomerular filtration and tubular secretion: 14 to 33% excreted unchanged in the urine, 50% as metabolites.

In dialysis—
    It is not known if aminosalicylate sodium is removed by dialysis.

## Precautions to Consider
**Cross-sensitivity and/or related problems**
Patients sensitive to other salicylates, including methyl salicylate (oil of wintergreen), or to other compounds containing a *p*-amino phenyl group (certain sulfonamides and dyes) may be sensitive to this medication also.

**Pregnancy/Reproduction**
Pregnancy—Adequate and well-controlled studies in humans have not been done. In one study, an increased malformation rate for ears and limbs, and hypospadias were reported in infants of patients taking aminosalicylates with other antitubercular medications. However, other studies have not found aminosalicylates to be teratogenic.

**Breast-feeding**
Aminosalicylate sodium is distributed into breast milk. However, problems in humans have not been documented.

**Pediatrics**
No information is available on the relationship of age to the effects of aminosalicylate sodium in pediatric patients.

**Geriatrics**
No information is available on the relationship of age to the effects of aminosalicylate sodium in geriatric patients.

**Drug interactions and/or related problems**
The following drug interactions and/or related problems have been selected on the basis of their potential clinical significance (possible mechanism in parentheses where appropriate)—not necessarily inclusive (» = major clinical significance):

Note: Combinations containing any of the following medications, depending on the amount present, may also interact with this medication.

» Aminobenzoates
    (aminobenzoates may be absorbed by bacteria preferentially over aminosalicylate sodium, thereby antagonizing the bacteriostatic effect of aminosalicylate sodium; concurrent use is not recommended)

Anticoagulants, coumarin- or indandione-derivative
    (when coumarin- or indandione-derivative anticoagulants are used concurrently with aminosalicylate sodium, their effects may be increased because of decreased hepatic synthesis of procoagulant factors; dosage adjustments may be necessary during and after aminosalicylate sodium therapy)

Probenecid or
Sulfinpyrazone
    (may decrease renal tubular secretion of aminosalicylate sodium when used concurrently, resulting in increased and prolonged serum concentrations and/or toxicity; aminosalicylate sodium dosage adjustments may be necessary during and after concurrent therapy, and patients should be monitored; however, probenecid is not currently recommended as an adjunct to therapy with aminosalicylate sodium)

Rifampin
    (aminosalicylate sodium may impair absorption of rifampin, resulting in decreased rifampin serum concentrations; patients should be advised to take aminosalicylate sodium and rifampin at least 6 hours apart)

Vitamin $B_{12}$
    (aminosalicylate sodium may impair absorption of vitamin $B_{12}$ from the gastrointestinal tract; requirements for vitamin $B_{12}$ may be increased in patients receiving aminosalicylate sodium)

## Laboratory value alterations

The following have been selected on the basis of their potential clinical significance (possible effect in parentheses where appropriate)—not necessarily inclusive (» = major clinical significance):

### With diagnostic test result

Glucose, urine

(aminosalicylate sodium may produce a false-positive test result with copper sulfate tests)

Schilling test

(aminosalicylate sodium may impair absorption of vitamin $B_{12}$ from the gastrointestinal tract; study results may be misinterpreted as pernicious anemia or other causes of malabsorption)

Urobilinogen, urine

(aminosalicylate sodium reacts with Ehrlich's reagent, producing an orange turbidity and/or yellow color; some commercially available reagent strips that use a similar reagent system are also affected)

### With physiology/laboratory test values

Alanine aminotransferase (ALT [SGPT]) and
Aspartate aminotransferase (AST [SGOT])

(values may be increased)

## Medical considerations/Contraindications

The medical considerations/contraindications included here have been selected on the basis of their potential clinical significance (reasons given in parentheses where appropriate)—not necessarily inclusive (» = major clinical significance).

*Except under special circumstances, this medication should not be used when the following medical problem exists:*

» Previous allergic reaction to aminosalicylates, other salicylates or sulfonamides

*Risk-benefit should be considered when the following medical problems exist:*

» Congestive heart failure

(high sodium concentrations may exacerbate condition because of fluid accumulation and overload)

» Gastric ulcer

(aminosalicylate sodium commonly causes gastric irritation)

Glucose-6-phosphate dehydrogenase (G6PD) deficiency

(aminosalicylate sodium may cause hemolytic anemia in G6PD-deficient patients)

Hepatic function impairment, severe

(aminosalicylate sodium may cause hepatitis)

Renal function impairment, severe

(patients with impaired renal function may require a reduction in dose or withdrawal of the medication)

## Side/Adverse Effects

The following side/adverse effects have been selected on the basis of their potential clinical significance (possible signs and symptoms in parentheses where appropriate)—not necessarily inclusive:

### Those indicating need for medical attention

Incidence more frequent

*Hypersensitivity reaction* (eosinophilia; fever; joint pains; leukopenia; skin rash or itching; unusual tiredness or weakness)

Incidence less frequent

*Crystalluria* (lower back pain; pain or burning while urinating); *goiter or myxedema*—with prolonged high-dose therapy (changes in menstrual periods; decreased sexual ability in males; dry, puffy skin; swelling of front part of neck; unusual weight gain); *hemolytic anemia* (abdominal pain; backache; paleness of skin)—with G6PD deficiency; *hepatitis or jaundice* (yellow eyes or skin); *infectious mononucleosis–like syndrome* (fever; headache; skin rash; sore throat; unusual tiredness or weakness)

### Those indicating need for medical attention only if they continue or are bothersome

Incidence more frequent

*Gastrointestinal disturbances* (abdominal pain; anorexia; diarrhea; nausea; vomiting)

## Patient Consultation

As an aid to patient consultation, refer to *Advice for the Patient, Aminosalicylate Sodium (Systemic).*

In providing consultation, consider emphasizing the following selected information (» = major clinical significance):

### Before using this medication

» Conditions affecting use, especially:

Allergies to aminosalicylates, other salicylates, or sulfonamides

Pregnancy—An increased malformation rate for ears and limbs and hypospadias were reported in patients taking aminosalicylates with other antitubercular medications; however, other studies did not find aminosalicylates to be teratogenic

Breast-feeding—Aminosalicylate sodium is distributed into breast milk

Other medications, especially aminobenzoates

Other medical problems, especially the presence of congestive heart failure or a gastric ulcer

### Proper use of this medication

Taking with or after meals or with antacid to minimize possible gastric irritation

» Compliance with full course of therapy, which may take months or years

» Importance of not missing doses and taking at evenly spaced times

» Proper dosing

Missed dose: Taking as soon as possible; not taking if almost time for next dose; not doubling doses

» Proper storage

### Precautions while using this medication

Checking with physician if no improvement within 2 or 3 weeks

Not taking aminosalicylate sodium within 6 hours of rifampin

» Diabetics: False-positive reactions with copper sulfate urine glucose tests may occur

### Side/adverse effects

Signs of potential side effects, especially hypersensitivity reactions, crystalluria, goiter, myxedema, hemolytic anemia, hepatitis or jaundice, and infectious mononucleosis–like syndrome

## General Dosing Information

Aminosalicylate sodium may be taken with or after meals or with an antacid if gastric irritation occurs. If gastric irritation persists, a temporary reduction in dose or a brief rest period of up to 2 weeks may be helpful. Aminosalicylate sodium may then be restarted in small daily doses and gradually increased to full therapeutic doses. If tolerated, the total daily dose may be given as a single dose.

If crystalluria occurs, the urine should be maintained at neutral or alkaline pH.

Therapy may have to be continued for 1 to 2 years, and may even be required for up to several years or indefinitely, although in some patients shorter treatment regimens may be effective.

Patient compliance may be poor because of gastric irritation or hypersensitivity reactions. Children may tolerate aminosalicylate sodium better than do adults.

## Oral Dosage Forms

### AMINOSALICYLATE SODIUM TABLETS USP

#### Usual adult and adolescent dose

Tuberculosis—

In combination with other antimycobacterials: Oral, 3.3 to 4 grams (aminosalicylic acid) every eight hours; or 5 to 6 grams every twelve hours.

#### Usual adult prescribing limits

Up to 20 grams (aminosalicylic acid) daily.

#### Usual pediatric dose

Tuberculosis—

In combination with other antimycobacterials: Oral, 50 to 75 mg (aminosalicylic acid) per kg of body weight every six hours; or 66.7 to 100 mg per kg of body weight every eight hours.

Note: The maximum daily dose in children should not exceed 12 grams (aminosalicylic acid).

#### Strength(s) usually available

U.S.—

500 mg (equivalent to 365 mg of aminosalicylic acid) (Rx) [*Tubasal* (sodium 2.4 mEq)].

Canada—

500 mg (equivalent to 365 mg of aminosalicylic acid) (Rx) [*Nemasol Sodium* (sodium 2.4 mEq)].

**Packaging and storage**
Store below 40 °C (104 °F), unless otherwise specified by manufacturer. Store in a tight, light-resistant container.

**Stability**
Aminosalicylates deteriorate rapidly in contact with water, heat, or sunlight.

**Auxiliary labeling**
• Continue medicine for full time of treatment.
• Keep from heat and light.

Revised: 05/02/94

---

# AMIODARONE   Systemic

VA CLASSIFICATION (Primary): CV300

Note: For a listing of dosage forms and brand names by country availability, see *Dosage Forms* section(s). For a listing of brand names for the articles in this monograph, refer to the General Index.

## Category
Antiarrhythmic.

## Indications
Note: Bracketed information in the *Indications* section refers to uses that are not included in U.S. product labeling.

**Accepted**
Arrhythmias, ventricular (prophylaxis and treatment)—Amiodarone is indicated to suppress and prevent recurrence of life-threatening ventricular arrhythmias, including hemodynamically unstable ventricular tachycardia or ventricular fibrillation.

[Arrhythmias, supraventricular (prophylaxis and treatment)][1]—Amiodarone is used to suppress and prevent recurrence of supraventricular arrhythmias refractory to conventional treatment, especially when associated with Wolff-Parkinson-White (W-P-W) syndrome, including paroxysmal atrial fibrillation, atrial flutter, ectopic atrial tachycardia, and paroxysmal supraventricular tachycardia from both atrioventricular (AV) nodal re-entrant and AV re-entrant tachycardia in patients with W-P-W syndrome.

Note: Because of its delayed onset of action, complex dosing schedule, and potentially serious side effects, amiodarone is used only when other agents are ineffective or cannot be tolerated.

[1] Not included in Canadian product labeling.

## Pharmacology/Pharmacokinetics

**Physicochemical characteristics**
Molecular weight—681.8.
pKa—5.6.
Other—Contains 37.3% iodine by weight; highly lipophilic.

**Mechanism of action/Effect**
Prolongs action potential duration and refractory period in all cardiac tissues (including the sinus node, atrium, atrioventricular [AV] node, and ventricle) by a direct action on the tissues, without significantly affecting membrane potential. Decreases sinus node automaticity and junctional automaticity, prolongs AV conduction, and slows automaticity of spontaneously firing fibers in the Purkinje system. Prolongs refractoriness and slows conduction in accessory pathway tissue in patients with Wolff-Parkinson-White (W-P-W) syndrome. Also causes noncompetitive alpha- and beta-adrenergic receptor antagonism and calcium channel inhibition and affects thyroid hormone metabolism, but relationship of these effects to its antiarrhythmic action is unknown. In the Vaughan Williams classification of antiarrhythmics, amiodarone is considered to be a predominantly class III agent, with some class I properties.

**Other actions/effects**
Has a mild negative inotropic effect, more prominent with intravenous than with oral administration, but usually does not depress left ventricular function. Causes coronary and peripheral vasodilation and therefore decreases peripheral vascular resistance (afterload), but only causes hypotension with large oral doses.

**Absorption**
Slow and variable; about 20 to 55% of an oral dose is absorbed.

**Distribution**
Large and variable volume of distribution as a result of extensive accumulation in adipose tissue and highly perfused organs (liver, lung, spleen) leads to slow achievement of steady-state and therapeutic plasma concentration and prolonged elimination.

**Protein binding**
Very high (96%).

**Biotransformation**
Hepatic, extensive; one active metabolite (desethylamiodarone); possibly also by deiodination (a dose of 300 mg releases approximately 9 mg of elemental iodine).

**Half-life**
Elimination (Biphasic)—
  Initial:
    Amiodarone: 2.5 to 10 days.
  Terminal:
    Amiodarone: 26 to 107 days (mean 53 days; 40 to 55 days in most patients).
    Desethylamiodarone: Mean 61 days.

**Onset of action**
2 to 3 days to 2 to 3 months, even with loading doses.

**Time to peak plasma concentration**
3 to 7 hours.

**Therapeutic plasma concentration**
1 to 2.5 mcg (0.001 to 0.0025 mg) per mL at steady-state (after 2 months of therapy). However, antiarrhythmic effect is difficult to predict by means of plasma concentrations, and toxicity may occur even at therapeutic concentrations.

**Duration of action**
Variable—Weeks to months; plasma concentrations are measurable for up to 9 months after amiodarone is discontinued.

**Elimination**
Biliary.
In breast milk—About 25% of maternal dose is excreted in breast milk.
In dialysis—Not removable by hemodialysis.

## Precautions to Consider

**Carcinogenicity/Tumorigenicity**
Studies in rats at doses one-half the maximum recommended human maintenance dose and greater found a dose-related increase in the incidence of thyroid follicular adenomas and/or carcinomas.

**Mutagenicity**
Mutagenicity studies (Ames, micronucleus, and lysogenic tests) with amiodarone were negative.

**Pregnancy/Reproduction**
Fertility—Studies in male and female rats at doses 8 times the maximum recommended human maintenance dose found that amiodarone reduced fertility.

Pregnancy—Amiodarone crosses the placenta; neonatal plasma concentrations of amiodarone and desethylamiodarone are 10% and 25% of maternal plasma concentrations, respectively. Although studies in humans have not been done, some reports have indicated an absence of adverse effects when amiodarone was administered late in pregnancy. However, amiodarone can cause fetal harm when administered to pregnant women. Potential adverse effects include bradycardia and effects on thyroid status (iodine is known to cause fetal goiter, hypothyroidism, and mental retardation) in the neonate. There have been a small number of reports of congenital goiter/hypothyroidism and hyperthyroidism.

Studies in rats and one strain of mice at doses 18 times and one-half the maximum recommended human maintenance dose, respectively, have shown that amiodarone is embryotoxic. Amiodarone was not embryotoxic in a second strain of mice or in rabbits at doses up to 9 times the maximum recommended human maintenance dose.

FDA Pregnancy Category D.

Labor and delivery—Although studies in humans have not been done, studies in rodents found no adverse effects of amiodarone on duration of gestation or on parturition.

**Breast-feeding**

Amiodarone is excreted in human breast milk. The infant receives approximately 25% of the maternal dose. Amiodarone has been shown to cause reduced viability and growth of offspring when used in lactating rats. Mothers should be advised to contact physician before nursing, since use by nursing mothers is not recommended.

**Pediatrics**

Appropriate studies on the relationship of age to the effects of amiodarone have not been performed in the pediatric population. However, when amiodarone is used concurrently with digoxin, the interaction has been reported to be more acute in children than in adults. In addition, onset and duration of action of amiodarone may be shorter in pediatric patients.

**Geriatrics**

Appropriate studies on the relationship of age to the effects of amiodarone have not been performed in the geriatric population. However, the elderly tend to be more sensitive to the effects of thyroid hormones and may also, therefore, be more sensitive to the effects of amiodarone on thyroid function. Thyroid function monitoring is particularly important in these patients. In addition, the elderly may experience an increased incidence of ataxia and other neurotoxic effects.

**Drug interactions and/or related problems**

The following drug interactions and/or related problems have been selected on the basis of their potential clinical significance (possible mechanism in parentheses where appropriate)—not necessarily inclusive (» = major clinical significance):

Note: Because of its slow elimination, amiodarone may interact with other medications for weeks to months after it is discontinued.

Combinations containing any of the following medications, depending on the amount present, may also interact with this medication.

Anesthetics, inhalation
(amiodarone may potentiate hypotension and atropine-resistant bradycardia)

» Antiarrhythmics, other
(amiodarone may produce additive cardiac effects with other antiarrhythmics and increase the risk of tachyarrhythmias; amiodarone increases plasma concentrations of quinidine, procainamide, flecainide, and phenytoin; concurrent use of amiodarone with quinidine, disopyramide, procainamide, or mexiletine has been reported to result in a more prolonged QT interval and, rarely, torsade de pointes, and therefore, concurrent use with all class I antiarrhythmics requires great caution; the dose of previously given antiarrhythmics should be reduced by 30 to 50% several days after initiation of amiodarone therapy and gradually withdrawn; if antiarrhythmic therapy is needed in addition to amiodarone, it should be initiated at one-half the usual recommended dose)

» Anticoagulants, coumarin-derivative
(amiodarone inhibits metabolism and potentiates the anticoagulant effect, beginning as early as 4 to 6 days after initiation of amiodarone therapy and persisting as long as weeks or months after it is withdrawn; prothrombin times may double or triple, but effect is very erratic; it is recommended that the dose of anticoagulant be reduced by one-third to one-half and prothrombin times monitored closely)

Beta-adrenergic blocking agents or
Calcium channel blocking agents
(amiodarone may cause potentiation of bradycardia, sinus arrest, and atrioventricular [AV] block, especially in patients with underlying sinus function impairment. If this occurs, dosage reduction of amiodarone or the beta-blocker or calcium channel blocker is recommended; in some cases, amiodarone therapy may be continued after insertion of a pacemaker)

» Digitalis glycosides
(amiodarone increases serum concentrations of digoxin and probably other digitalis glycosides, possibly to toxic levels; when amiodarone therapy is initiated, the digitalis glycoside should be withdrawn or the dose reduced by 50%; if digitalis glycoside therapy is continued, serum concentrations should be carefully monitored; amiodarone and digitalis glycosides may also produce additive effects on sinoatrial [SA] and AV nodes)

Diuretics, loop or
Diuretics, thiazide or
Indapamide
(concurrent use of amiodarone with potassium-depleting diuretics may lead to an increased risk of arrhythmias associated with hypokalemia)

» Phenytoin
(amiodarone may increase plasma concentrations of phenytoin, resulting in increased effects and/or toxicity)

Photosensitizing medications, other
(concurrent use with amiodarone may cause additive photosensitizing effects)

Sodium iodide I 123 or
Sodium iodide I 131 or
Sodium pertechnetate Tc 99m
(thyroidal uptake may be inhibited by amiodarone)

**Laboratory value alterations**

The following have been selected on the basis of their potential clinical significance (possible effect in parentheses where appropriate)—not necessarily inclusive (» = major clinical significance):

With physiology/laboratory test values
Alanine aminotransferase (ALT [SGPT]) and
Alkaline phosphatase and
Aspartate aminotransferase (AST [SGOT])
(serum values commonly increased; hepatotoxicity is rare)

Antinuclear antibody (ANA) titer concentrations
(may be increased but usually not symptomatic; elevated concentrations may be associated with pulmonary toxicity)

Electrocardiogram (ECG) changes, such as:
PR prolongation and
QRS widening, slight and
QT prolongation and
T-wave amplitude reduction with T-wave widening and bifurcation and
U-wave development
(occur in most patients; QT prolongation may in some cases be associated with worsening of arrhythmias)

Thyroid function changes, such as

Free and total serum thyroxine ($T_4$) concentrations
(increased in most patients, although clinical hyperthyroidism is not common; may be decreased or low normal in hypothyroidism; may be increased in hyperthyroidism)

Free and serum triiodothyronine ($T_3$) concentrations
(may be decreased; decrease in $T_3$ may occur in hypothyroidism; increase in $T_3$ is the determining sign of hyperthyroidism)

Serum reverse $T_3$ concentrations
(increased in most patients)

Serum thyroid-stimulating hormone (TSH) concentrations
(may be increased initially; increase in TSH with continued amiodarone treatment, along with a decrease in $T_3$, is the determining sign of hypothyroidism)

Note: Amiodarone inhibits peripheral conversion of $T_4$ to $T_3$, leading to increased serum $T_4$ and reverse $T_3$ and a slight decrease in serum $T_3$.

Thyroid function abnormalities are common, but clinical thyroid function impairment is not.

Thyroid function abnormalities may persist for several weeks or months after withdrawal of amiodarone.

**Medical considerations/Contraindications**

The medical considerations/contraindications included here have been selected on the basis of their potential clinical significance (reasons given in parentheses where appropriate)—not necessarily inclusive (» = major clinical significance).

*Except under special circumstances, this medication should not be used when the following medical problems exist:*

» Atrioventricular (AV) block, pre-existing 2nd or 3rd degree without pacemaker
(risk of complete heart block)

» Bradycardic episodes resulting in syncope, unless controlled by pacemaker, or

» Sinus node function impairment, severe, causing marked sinus bradycardia, unless controlled by pacemaker
(amiodarone reduces sinus node automaticity and may cause atropine-resistant sinus bradycardia)

*Risk-benefit should be considered when the following medical problems exist:*

Congestive heart failure
(mild negative inotropic effect of amiodarone usually does not cause problems; hemodynamic deterioration may occur secondary to sympatholytic blockage of augmented sympathetic drive)

Hepatic function impairment
(reduced metabolism; lower doses may be required)

Hypokalemia
(amiodarone may be ineffective or arrhythmogenic; should be corrected prior to initiation of amiodarone therapy)

Sensitivity to amiodarone

Thyroid function impairment, including goiter or nodules
(increased risk of hypothyroidism or hyperthyroidism)

Caution is recommended also during open-heart surgery in patients receiving amiodarone because of the risk of hypotension upon discontinuation of cardiopulmonary bypass.

**Patient monitoring**

The following may be especially important in patient monitoring (other tests may be warranted in some patients, depending on condition; » = major clinical significance):

» Alanine aminotransferase (ALT [SGPT]) and

» Alkaline phosphatase and

» Aspartate aminotransferase (AST [SGOT])
(serum value determinations recommended at regular intervals, especially in patients receiving high maintenance doses; dosage reduction of amiodarone is recommended if concentrations increase to 3 times normal or double in patients with elevated baseline concentrations, or if hepatomegaly occurs)

Auscultation of the chest
(recommended at periodic intervals; presence of rales, decreased breath sounds, or pleuritic friction rub may indicate pulmonary toxicity)

Bronchoscopy with lung biopsy
(may be useful if symptoms of pulmonary toxicity occur that cannot be diagnosed from a chest x-ray)

Chest x-ray
(recommended prior to initiation of therapy and at 3- to 6-month intervals during therapy to detect diffuse interstitial changes or alveolar infiltrates associated with pulmonary toxicity)

» ECG
(continuous Holter monitoring may assist in assessing efficacy and adjusting dosage; usefulness of programmed electrical stimulation in clinical management is controversial, although it may be useful for predicting efficacy of amiodarone)

Gallium radionuclide scan
(may be useful if symptoms of pulmonary toxicity occur that cannot be diagnosed from a chest x-ray; may show marked uptake in the lung)

Ophthalmologic examinations
(slit-lamp examinations recommended prior to initiation of therapy and if symptoms of ocular toxicity occur)

Plasma amiodarone determinations
(may be useful in dosage adjustment or to assess lack of response or unexpectedly severe toxicity, although correlation does not always occur, especially within first 2 months of therapy)

Pulmonary function determinations, including diffusion capacity and total lung capacity
(recommended prior to initiation of amiodarone therapy and if symptoms of pulmonary toxicity occur that cannot be diagnosed from a chest x-ray)

» Thyroid function determinations
(recommended prior to initiation and at periodic intervals during amiodarone therapy; interpretation of thyroid function tests in patients receiving amiodarone can be difficult because its effects are complex; a flat TSH response to protirelin will help confirm the presence of hyperthyroidism. If hypothyroidism occurs, dosage reduction or withdrawal of amiodarone is recommended, along with addition of thyroid hormone supplementation. If hyperthyroidism occurs, withdrawal of amiodarone and/or treatment with antithyroid medication, beta-adrenergic blocking agents, and/or temporary adrenocorticoid therapy should be considered, although the action of antithyroid medications may be delayed because of large stores of pre-formed thyroid hormones in the thyroid gland; radioiodine therapy is not useful because of low thyroidal uptake in amiodarone-induced hyperthyroidism; there is a risk of inducing thyroid storm with surgical ablation)

## Side/Adverse Effects

Note: Incidence of side/adverse effects is generally related to dose and duration of therapy. Side/adverse effects may occur even at therapeutic plasma amiodarone concentrations but are more common at concentrations over 2.5 mcg per mL and with continuous treatment for longer than 6 months.

Side/adverse effects may not appear until several days, weeks, or years after initiation of amiodarone therapy and may persist for several months after withdrawal.

Asymptomatic sinus bradycardia is common, but is symptomatic in only 2 to 4% of patients taking amiodarone. Sinus arrest and heart block occur rarely. Atrioventricular (AV) block occurs infrequently. New or exacerbated arrhythmias occur in 2 to 5% of patients and may include paroxysmal ventricular tachycardia, ventricular fibrillation, increased resistance to cardioversion, and torsade de pointes; they may be associated with marked QT prolongation. New or exacerbated arrhythmias may also be a sign of hyperthyroidism.

The following side/adverse effects have been selected on the basis of their potential clinical significance (possible signs and symptoms in parentheses where appropriate)—not necessarily inclusive:

**Those indicating need for medical attention**

Incidence more frequent

*Neurotoxicity* (trouble in walking; numbness or tingling in fingers or toes; trembling or shaking of hands; unusual and uncontrolled movements of body; weakness of arms or legs); *photosensitivity, particularly to long-wave ultraviolet-A [UVA] light* (sensitivity of skin to sunlight); *pulmonary fibrosis or interstitial pneumonitis/alveolitis* (cough; painful breathing; shortness of breath; slight fever)

Note: *Ataxia* is the most common symptom; occurs in 20 to 40% of patients, especially during administration of loading doses; may occur within 1 week to several months after initiation of therapy and may persist for more than a year after withdrawal.

*Photosensitivity* may occur even through window glass and thin cotton clothing; not dose-related. Since most sunscreens are not useful for protection because they block only ultraviolet-B [UVB] light, a barrier sun-block such as zinc or titanium oxide and protective clothing are recommended.

*Pulmonary fibrosis or interstitial pneumonitis alveolitis* is clinically significant in up to 10 to 15% of patients, but abnormal diffusion capacity occurs in much higher percentage; more frequent with doses of 400 mg per day and after several months of treatment but may also occur with small doses; usually reversible after withdrawal of amiodarone, with or without steroid treatment, but is fatal in about 10% of cases, especially when not diagnosed promptly; recurrence has been reported after withdrawal of several months of steroid therapy; often mistaken for but rarely related to congestive heart failure or pneumonic infection.

Incidence less frequent

*Arrhythmias, new or exacerbated* (fast or irregular heartbeat); *blue-gray coloring of skin on face, neck, and arms; congestive heart failure* (swelling of feet or lower legs); *hyperthyroidism* (nervousness; sensitivity to heat; sweating; trouble in sleeping; weight loss); *hypothyroidism* (coldness; dry, puffy skin; unusual tiredness; weight gain); *noninfectious epididymitis* (pain and swelling in scrotum); *ocular toxicity* (blurred vision or blue-green halos seen around objects; dry eyes; sensitivity of eyes to light); *sinus bradycardia* (slow heartbeat)

Note: *Blue-gray skin coloring* occurs with prolonged use, usually longer than 1 year, especially in patients with fair skin or with excessive sun exposure; slowly and occasionally incompletely reversible after withdrawal.

*Hyperthyroidism* occurs in about 2% of patients, although thyroid hormone concentration changes are common and may persist for several months after withdrawal of amiodarone.

*Hypothyroidism* occurs in less than 10% of patients, although thyroid hormone concentration changes are common and may persist for several months after withdrawal of amiodarone.

Bilateral and symmetric *asymptomatic corneal deposits* appearing as yellow-brown pigmentation on slit-lamp examination occur in all patients after 6 months of treatment, but may appear sooner; symptomatic corneal deposits occur in up to 10% of patients; macular degeneration and decreased visual acuity are rare; corneal deposits are reversible after withdrawal of amiodarone, although it may take up to 7 months.

*Sinus bradycardia* usually responds to dosage reduction but may require a pacemaker; atropine-resistant.

Incidence rare

*Allergic reaction* (skin rash); *hepatitis* (yellow eyes or skin)

Note: *Allergic reaction* usually occurs within the first 2 weeks of therapy.

In *hepatitis* hepatic enzymes are commonly elevated to several times normal within 2 months after initiation of therapy; deaths as a result of hepatic failure resembling alcoholic cirrhosis have occurred rarely.

**Those indicating need for medical attention only if they continue or are bothersome**
Incidence more frequent—approximately 25%, especially during administration of high doses, as during loading
   *Constipation; headache; loss of appetite*—may lead to severe weight loss; *nausea and vomiting*
Incidence less frequent
   *Bitter or metallic taste; decreased sexual ability in males; decrease in sexual interest; dizziness* (central nervous system [CNS] effect; hypotension is rare); *flushing of face*
**Those indicating possible pulmonary toxicity and the need for medical attention if they occur after medication is discontinued**
   *Cough; fever, slight; painful breathing; shortness of breath*

## Overdose

For more information on the management of overdose or unintentional ingestion, **contact a Poison Control Center** (see *Poison Control Center Listing*).

**Treatment of overdose**
Decrease absorption—Recent oral ingestion may benefit from emesis and/or lavage.
   Specific treatment—
      Primarily supportive and symptomatic.
      Monitoring of cardiac rhythm and blood pressure is important.
      For bradycardia, a beta-adrenergic agonist or pacemaker may be indicated.
      Hypotension may respond to positive inotropic and/or vasopressor agents.

## Patient Consultation

As an aid to patient consultation, refer to *Advice for the Patient, Amiodarone (Systemic)*.

In providing consultation, consider emphasizing the following selected information (» = major clinical significance):

**Before using this medication**
» Conditions affecting use, especially:
      Sensitivity to amiodarone
      Pregnancy—Potential risk of bradycardia and iodine toxicity in fetus
      Breast-feeding—Excreted in breast milk
      Use in children—Shorter onset and duration of action
      Use in the elderly—Increased sensitivity to effects on thyroid function and increased incidence of ataxia and other neurotoxic effects
      Other medications, especially other antiarrhythmics, coumarin-derivative anticoagulants, digitalis glycosides, or phenytoin
      Other medical problems, especially pre-existing AV block without pacemaker, bradycardic episodes resulting in syncope (unless controlled by pacemaker), or severe sinus node function impairment causing marked bradycardia (unless controlled by pacemaker)

**Proper use of this medication**
» Compliance with therapy; taking as directed even if feeling well
» Proper dosing
      Missed dose: Not taking at all; notifying physician if two or more doses in a row are missed; not doubling doses
» Proper storage

**Precautions while using this medication**
   Regular visits to physician to check progress
   Carrying medical identification card or bracelet
» Caution if any kind of surgery (including dental surgery) or emergency treatment is required
» Protecting skin from sunlight during and for several months following withdrawal of treatment; burns may occur even through window glass and thin cotton clothing; use of protective clothing and barrier sunscreen; checking with physician if severe burn occurs
   Checking with physician if blue-gray discoloration of skin occurs

**Side/adverse effects**
   Signs of potential side effects, especially pulmonary fibrosis; interstitial pneumonitis/alveolitis; neurotoxicity; photosensitivity; blue-gray coloring of skin on face, neck, and arms; ocular toxicity; hypothyroidism; hyperthyroidism; new or exacerbated arrhythmias; noninfectious epididymitis; sinus bradycardia; congestive heart failure; allergic reaction; and hepatitis

## General Dosing Information

Because of its delayed onset of action, difficulty in dosage adjustment, and potentially serious adverse effects, it is recommended that amiodarone administration be initiated in the hospital and that the patient remain in the hospital at least for the loading dose phase. Dosage must be adjusted to meet the individual requirements of each patient, based on clinical response, appearance or severity of toxicity, and in some cases, plasma amiodarone concentrations.

If signs or symptoms of pulmonary toxicity occur, it is recommended that amiodarone therapy be withdrawn until the cause has been determined. If pulmonary toxicity is related to amiodarone, withdrawal of amiodarone is recommended. Usefulness of steroid therapy is controversial, but such therapy may be useful for severe toxicity.

If symptoms of neurotoxicity occur, dosage reduction is recommended; rarely, withdrawal of amiodarone may be necessary.

If photosensitivity occurs, dosage reduction and use of a sunscreen are recommended.

Nausea and vomiting may be relieved by reduction of dose or administration of amiodarone in divided doses.

If epididymitis occurs, dosage reduction or withdrawal of amiodarone is recommended.

## Oral Dosage Forms

Note:   Bracketed uses in *Dosage Forms* refer to categories of use and/or indications that are not included in the U.S. product labeling.

### AMIODARONE HYDROCHLORIDE TABLETS

**Usual adult dose**
Ventricular arrhythmias—
   Loading: Oral, 800 mg to 1.6 grams per day for one to three weeks (or longer, if necessary) until an initial therapeutic response or side effects occur; may be given in divided doses with meals for doses greater than 1 gram per day or if gastrointestinal side effects occur. When adequate control or excessive side effects occur, the dose is reduced to 600 to 800 mg per day for one month and then decreased again to the lowest effective maintenance dose.
   Maintenance: Oral, approximately 400 mg per day, the dosage being increased or decreased as necessary.
[Supraventricular tachycardia][1]—
   Loading: Oral, 600 to 800 mg per day for one week or until an initial therapeutic response or side effects occur. When adequate control or excessive side effects occur, the dose is reduced to 400 mg per day for three weeks.
   Maintenance: Oral, 200 to 400 mg per day.

**Usual pediatric dose**
Ventricular arrhythmias
[Supraventricular arrhythmias][1]—
   Loading: Oral, 10 mg per kg of body weight per day or 800 mg per 1.72 square meters of body surface per day for ten days or until an initial therapeutic response or side effects occur. When adequate control or excessive side effects occur, the dose is reduced to 5 mg per kg of body weight or 400 mg per 1.72 square meters of body surface per day for several weeks and then decreased gradually to the lowest effective maintenance dose.
   Maintenance: Oral, 2.5 mg per kg of body weight per day or 200 mg per 1.72 square meters of body surface per day.

**Strength(s) usually available**
U.S.—
   200 mg [*Cordarone* (scored; lactose)].
Canada—
   200 mg [*Cordarone* (scored; lactose)].

**Packaging and storage**
Store below 40 °C (104 °F), preferably between 15 and 30 °C (59 and 86 °F), unless otherwise specified by manufacturer. Protect from light.

---

[1]Not included in Canadian product labeling.

## Selected Bibliography

Naccarelli GV, Romlemberger RL, Dougherty AH, Giebel RA. Amiodarone: pharmacology and antiarrhythmic and adverse effects. Pharmacother 1985 Nov/Dec; 5: 298-313.

Heger JJ, Prystowsky EN, Miles WM, Zipes DP. Clinical use and pharmacology of amiodarone. Med Clin N Am 1984 Sep; 68: 1339-66.

Focus on amiodarone. Drugs 1985; 29 (Suppl 3).

---

Revised: 04/13/93

**AMITRIPTYLINE**—See *Antidepressants, Tricyclic (Systemic)*

**AMITRIPTYLINE-CONTAINING COMBINATIONS**—

Chlordiazepoxide and Amitriptyline (Systemic)
Perphenazine and Amitriptyline (Systemic)

# AMLODIPINE    Systemic†

VA CLASSIFICATION (Primary/Secondary): CV200; CV250; CV490

Note: For a listing of dosage forms and brand names by country availability, see *Dosage Forms* section(s). For a listing of brand names for the articles in this monograph, refer to the General Index.

†Not commercially available in Canada.

## Category
Antianginal; antihypertensive.

## Indications

### Accepted
Angina, chronic stable (treatment)—Amlodipine is indicated for the treatment of chronic stable angina; it may be used alone or in combination with other antianginal agents.

Angina, vasospastic (treatment)—Amlodipine is indicated for the treatment of confirmed or suspected vasospastic angina. It may be used alone or in combination with other antianginal agents.

Hypertension (treatment)—Amlodipine is indicated for the treatment of hypertension; it may be used alone or in combination with other antihypertensive agents.

For additional information on initial therapeutic guidelines related to the treatment of hypertension, see *Appendix III*.

## Pharmacology/Pharmacokinetics

### Physicochemical characteristics
Molecular weight—567.05.

### Mechanism of action/Effect
Amlodipine is a dihydropyridine calcium channel blocking agent. Like the other dihydropyridine agents, amlodipine selectively inhibits calcium influx across cell membranes in cardiac and vascular smooth muscle, with a greater effect on vascular smooth muscle. Amlodipine is a peripheral arteriolar vasodilator; thus it reduces afterload.

### Other actions/effects
Amlodipine exhibits negative inotropic effects *in vivo*, but appears to have no significant effect on the sinoatrial (SA) or atrioventricular (AV) node in humans.

### Absorption
Slowly and almost completely absorbed from the gastrointestinal tract; absorption not affected by food. Bioavailability is approximately 60 to 65%.

### Distribution
$Vol_D$—21 L per kg.

### Protein binding
Very high (95 to 98%).

### Biotransformation
Undergoes minimal presystemic metabolism. Amlodipine undergoes slow but extensive hepatic metabolism, producing metabolites lacking significant pharmacological activity.

### Half-life
Elimination—Mean, 35 hours in healthy volunteers; may be prolonged to a mean of 48 hours in hypertensive patients, 65 hours in the elderly, and 60 hours in patients with hepatic function impairment. Not affected by renal function impairment.

### Time to peak concentration
Single-dose—6 to 9 hours.

### Duration of action
24 hours.

### Elimination
Renal—59 to 62% (about 5% as unchanged amlodipine).
Biliary/fecal—20 to 25%.
In dialysis—Amlodipine is not removed by hemodialysis.

## Precautions to Consider

### Carcinogenicity
No evidence of carcinogenicity was revealed in studies with rats and mice given amlodipine at dosages of 0.5, 1.25, and 2.5 mg per kg of body weight (mg/kg) per day for 2 years.

### Mutagenicity
No evidence of mutagenicity was observed at the gene or chromosome level.

### Pregnancy/Reproduction
Fertility—No impairment of fertility was observed in rats given amlodipine at doses 8 times the maximum recommended human dose prior to mating.

Pregnancy—Studies have not been done in humans.

No evidence of teratogenicity or other embryo/fetal toxicity was observed in rats or rabbits given up to 10 mg/kg during periods of major organogenesis. However, the number of intrauterine deaths increased about five-fold, and rat litter size was significantly decreased (by 50%).

FDA Pregnancy Category C.

Labor—Amlodipine has been shown to prolong the duration of labor in rats.

### Breast-feeding
It is not known whether amlodipine is distributed into breast milk.

### Pediatrics
No information is available on the relationship of age to the effects of amlodipine in pediatric patients. Safety and efficacy have not been established.

### Geriatrics
The half-life of amlodipine may be increased in the elderly. These patients may be more sensitive to the hypotensive effects of amlodipine and may require a lower initial dose.

### Dental
Gingival hyperplasia is a rare side effect that has been reported with amlodipine. It also has been reported with other calcium channel blocking agents, such as diltiazem, felodipine, verapamil, and, most commonly, nifedipine. It usually starts as gingivitis or gum inflammation in the first 1 to 9 months of treatment. Resolution of the hyperplasia and improvement of the clinical symptoms usually occur one to four weeks after discontinuation of therapy. A strictly enforced program of professional teeth cleaning combined with plaque control by the patient will minimize growth rate and severity of gingival enlargement. Periodontal surgery may be indicated in some cases, and should be followed by careful plaque control to inhibit recurrence of gum enlargement.

### Surgical
Recent evidence suggests that withdrawal of antihypertensive therapy prior to surgery may be undesirable. However, the anesthesiologist must be aware of such therapy.

### Drug interactions and/or related problems
The following drug interactions and/or related problems have been selected on the basis of their potential clinical significance (possible mechanism in parentheses where appropriate)—not necessarily inclusive (» = major clinical significance):

Note: Combinations containing any of the following medications, depending on the amount present, may also interact with this medication.

Anesthetics, hydrocarbon inhalation
(concurrent use with amlodipine may produce additive hypotension; although calcium channel blocking agents may be useful to prevent supraventricular tachycardias, hypertension, or coronary spasm during surgery, caution is recommended during use)

Anti-inflammatory drugs, nonsteroidal (NSAIDs), especially indomethacin
(NSAIDs may reduce the antihypertensive effects of amlodipine by inhibiting renal prostaglandin synthesis and/or causing sodium and fluid retention)

Beta-adrenergic blocking agents
(although reports of adverse effects resulting from concurrent use of amlodipine with the beta-adrenergic blocking agents are lacking, caution is recommended given the similarity of amlodipine to nifedipine; concurrent use of nifedipine with the beta-adrenergic blocking agents, although usually well-tolerated, may produce excessive hypotension and, in rare cases, may increase the possibility of congestive heart failure)

Estrogens
(estrogen-induced fluid retention may tend to increase blood pressure; the patient should be carefully monitored to confirm that the desired effect is being obtained)

Highly protein-bound medications, such as:
Anticoagulants, coumarin- and indandione-derivative
Anticonvulsants, hydantoin
Anti-inflammatory drugs, nonsteroidal
Quinine
Salicylates
Sulfinpyrazone
(caution is advised when these medications are used concurrently with amlodipine since amlodipine is highly protein bound; changes in serum concentrations of the free, unbound medications may occur)

Hypotension-producing medications, other (See *Appendix II*)
(antihypertensive effects may be potentiated when amlodipine is used concurrently with hypotension-producing medications; although some antihypertensive and/or diuretic combinations are frequently used for therapeutic advantage, when any of these medications are used concurrently, dosage adjustments may be necessary)

Lithium
(concurrent use with amlodipine potentially may result in neurotoxicity in the form of nausea, vomiting, diarrhea, ataxia, tremors, and/or tinnitus; caution is recommended)

Sympathomimetics
(concurrent use may reduce antihypertensive effects of amlodipine; the patient should be carefully monitored to confirm that the desired effect is being obtained)

**Medical considerations/Contraindications**
The medical considerations/contraindications included here have been selected on the basis of their potential clinical significance (reasons given in parentheses where appropriate)—not necessarily inclusive (» = major clinical significance).

*Except under special circumstances, this medication should not be used when the following medical problem exists:*
» Hypotension, severe
(amlodipine may aggravate this condition)

*Risk-benefit should be considered when the following medical problems exist:*
Aortic stenosis
(increased risk of heart failure because of fixed impedance to flow across aortic valve)

Congestive heart failure
(amlodipine should be used with caution in patients with congestive heart failure because of the slight risk for negative inotropic effect)

Hepatic function impairment
(clearance of amlodipine may be reduced since it undergoes extensive hepatic metabolism; elimination half-life may be prolonged to 60 hours)

Sensitivity to amlodipine

**Patient monitoring**
The following may be especially important in patient monitoring (other tests may be warranted in some patients, depending on condition; » = major clinical significance):
» Blood pressure determinations and
» ECG readings and
» Heart rate determinations
(recommended primarily during dosage titration or when dosage is increased from established maintenance dosage level; also recommended when other medications are added that affect cardiac conduction or blood pressure)

(blood pressure determinations are recommended at periodic intervals to monitor efficacy and safety of amlodipine therapy; selected patients may be trained to perform blood pressure measurements at home and report the results at regular physician visits)

## Side/Adverse Effects
The following side/adverse effects have been selected on the basis of their potential clinical significance (possible signs and symptoms in parentheses where appropriate)—not necessarily inclusive:

**Those indicating need for medical attention**
Incidence more frequent
*Edema, peripheral* (swelling of ankles and feet)
Incidence less frequent
*Dizziness; palpitations* (pounding heartbeat)
Incidence rare
*Angina* (chest pain); *bradycardia* (slow heartbeat); *hypotension* (dizziness); *orthostatic hypotension* (dizziness or lightheadedness when getting up from a lying or sitting position)

**Those indicating need for medical attention only if they continue or are bothersome**
Incidence more frequent
*Flushing; headache*
Incidence less frequent
*Fatigue* (unusual tiredness or weakness); *nausea*

## Patient Consultation
As an aid to patient consultation, refer to *Advice for the Patient, Amlodipine (Systemic)*.

In providing consultation, consider emphasizing the following selected information (» = major clinical significance):

**Before using this medication**
» Conditions affecting use, especially:
Use in the elderly—Half-life increased; increased sensitivity to hypotensive effects
Dental—Risk of gingival hyperplasia
Other medications
Other medical problems, especially severe hypotension

**Proper use of this medication**
» Compliance with therapy; importance of not taking more medication than amount prescribed
» Proper dosing
Missed dose: Taking as soon as possible; not taking if almost time for next scheduled dose; not doubling doses
» Proper storage
*For use as an antihypertensive*
Possible need for control of weight and diet, especially sodium intake
» Patient may not experience symptoms of hypertension; importance of taking medication even if feeling well
» Does not cure, but helps control hypertension; possible need for lifelong therapy; serious consequences of untreated hypertension

**Precautions while using this medication**
Regular visits to physician to check progress during therapy
Checking with physician before discontinuing medication; gradual dosage reduction may be necessary
» Discussing exercise or physical exertion limits with physician; reduced occurrence of chest pain may tempt patient to be overactive
Possible headache; checking with physician if continuing or severe
» Maintaining good dental hygiene and seeing dentist frequently for teeth cleaning to prevent tenderness, bleeding, and gum enlargement
*For use as an antihypertensive*
» Not taking other medications, especially nonprescription sympathomimetics, unless discussed with physician

**Side/adverse effects**
Signs of potential side effects, especially peripheral edema, dizziness, palpitations, angina, bradycardia, hypotension, or orthostatic hypotension

## General Dosing Information
Concurrent administration of sublingual nitroglycerin or long-acting nitrates with amlodipine may produce an additive antianginal effect. Sublingual nitroglycerin may be used as needed to abort acute angina attacks during amlodipine therapy. Nitrate medication may be used during amlodipine therapy for angina prophylaxis.

Although no "rebound effect" has been reported upon discontinuation of amlodipine, a gradual decrease of dosage with physician supervision is recommended.

**For treatment of overdose or acute adverse effects**
Recommended treatment consists of the following:
- Hypotension, symptomatic—Intravenous fluids, intravenous dopamine or dobutamine, calcium chloride, isoproterenol, metaraminol, or norepinephrine should be used as appropriate.
- Tachycardia, rapid ventricular rate in patients with antegrade conduction in atrial flutter fibrillation, and accessory pathway with Wolff-Parkinson-White or Lown-Ganong-Levine syndrome—Direct-current cardioversion, intravenous lidocaine, or intravenous procainamide. Intravenous fluids given by slow-drip.
- Bradycardia, rarely second or third degree atrioventricular (AV) block, with a few patients progressing to asystole—Intravenous atropine, isoproterenol, norepinephrine, or calcium chloride, or use of electronic cardiac pacemaker, as appropriate.

## Oral Dosage Forms

### AMLODIPINE BESYLATE TABLETS

**Usual adult dose**
Antianginal or antihypertensive—
    Oral, 5 to 10 mg once a day.

Note: An initial antihypertensive dose of 2.5 mg is recommended for small, fragile, or elderly patients, patients with hepatic function impairment, or when adding amlodipine to other antihypertensive therapy.

   An initial antianginal dose of 5 mg is recommended for the elderly and for patients with hepatic function impairment.

**Usual pediatric dose**
Safety and efficacy have not been established.

**Strength(s) usually available**
U.S.—
    2.5 mg (Rx) [*Norvasc*].
    5 mg (Rx) [*Norvasc*].
    10 mg (Rx) [*Norvasc*].
Canada—
    Not commercially available.

**Packaging and storage**
Store below 40 °C (104 °F), preferably between 15 and 30 °C (59 and 86 °F), in a tight, light-resistant container unless otherwise specified by manufacturer.

**Auxiliary labeling**
- Do not take other medicines without physician's advice.

## Selected Bibliography

Murdoch D, Heel RC. Amlodipine: a review of its pharmacodynamic and pharmacokinetic properties, and therapeutic use in cardiovascular disease. Drugs 1991; 41 (3): 478-505.

The fifth report of the Joint National Committee on Detection, Evaluation, and Treatment of High Blood Pressure (JNC V). Arch Intern Med 1993; 153 (2): 154-83.

Revised: 08/12/93

---

# AMMONIA N 13   Systemic*†

VA CLASSIFICATION (Primary): DX201

Note: For a listing of dosage forms and brand names by country availability, see *Dosage Forms* section(s). For a listing of brand names for the articles in this monograph, refer to the General Index.

   *Not commercially available in the U.S.
   †Not commercially available in Canada.

## Category

Diagnostic aid, radioactive (cardiac disease; hepatic disease; cerebrovascular disease).

## Indications

**Accepted**

Note: Accepted indications for positron emitters, such as ammonia N 13 ($^{13}NH_3$), are still evolving. Ongoing studies are revealing new indications for these agents.

Cardiac imaging, positron emission tomographic—Positron emission tomography (PET) using $^{13}NH_3$ is used in studies of myocardial blood flow in various physiological and pathological states. PET-$^{13}NH_3$ is currently used for the following diagnostic studies:

Cardiac wall-motion abnormalities assessment—PET using $^{13}NH_3$ to assess the distribution of myocardial blood flow in conjunction with fludeoxyglucose F 18 to estimate myocardial metabolic viability in dysfunctional myocardial segments serves to predict, preoperatively, the presence of reversible regional wall-motion abnormalities, which is helpful in the selection of patients in whom revascularization may lead to improved ventricular function.

Coronary artery disease (diagnosis)—$^{13}NH_3$ myocardial PET performed at rest and during stress (either exercise or dipyridamole or adenosine infusion) is used to detect coronary artery disease (CAD) and to identify individual stenosed vessels.

Myocardial infarction (diagnosis) and
Myocardial perfusion imaging, positron emission tomographic—PET-$^{13}NH_3$ is used in myocardial perfusion imaging for the diagnosis and localization of myocardial infarction.

Ischemia, myocardial (diagnosis)—PET-$^{13}NH_3$ is used in patients with known or suspected CAD, to define the areas of the left ventricular myocardium that have become critically ischemic during acute coronary artery occlusion.

Cardiac bypass surgery assessment—PET-$^{13}NH_3$ is used before and after aortocoronary bypass surgery to help evaluate the effect of surgery on myocardial perfusion. Also, graft patency can be established with postoperative images.

Cardiac blood pool imaging, positron emission tomographic—Dynamic cardiac PET-$^{13}NH_3$ is used to obtain cardiac blood pool images, which permit the evaluation of size and configuration of ventricles and atria.

Liver imaging, positron emission tomographic—Carcinoma, hepatocellular (diagnosis): Dynamic PET-$^{13}NH_3$ is used for the detection of primary hepatocellular carcinoma (hepatoma).

   Arterial blood flow, hepatic, regional, assessment: Dynamic PET-$^{13}NH_3$ is used to quantitate regional hepatic arterial blood flow to enhance understanding of various liver diseases.

Brain imaging, positron emission tomographic—Dynamic PET-$^{13}NH_3$ is used to locate and assess the extent of altered brain perfusion with cerebrovascular diseases.

## Physical Properties

**Nuclear data**

| Radionuclide (half-life) | Decay constant | Mode of decay | Principal emissions (keV) | Mean number of emissions/ disintegration |
|---|---|---|---|---|
| N 13 (10 min) | 0.07 min$^{-1}$ | Positron decay | Gamma (annihilation) (511) | 2.0 |

## Pharmacology/Pharmacokinetics

**Mechanism of action/Effect**
Cardiac imaging—
   Based on myocardial tissue uptake of $^{13}NH^3$, which is related to regional myocardial blood flow. In the blood, more than 90% is in the form of ammonium ($^{13}NH_4^+$); however, at 3 to 5 minutes a significant percentage of the activity is present as [$^{13}N$]glutamine and urea. Although myocardial uptake was once thought to be the result of ammonium competition with potassium transport, it is now accepted that myocardial localization is due to diffusion across capillaries and cellular membranes as ammonia ($^{13}NH_3$). Retention in myocardial cells is the result of metabolism to glutamine. In myocardial infarct patients, the slow blood pool clearance and prolonged lung retention is apparently the result of a large pulmonary distribution volume.

Liver imaging—
   Hepatocellular carcinoma: Accumulation in the hepatoma is not yet well understood. It is assumed that $^{13}NH_3$ accumulation in the tumors is governed by the capillary blood flow of the tumor and the extraction efficacy of the neoplastic tissues for $_{13}NH_3$. Localization

of $_{13}NH_3$ in hepatoma is seen in early scans. As time progresses, the radioactivity accumulation in the rest of the liver continues to increase, making the recognition of the tumor difficult. The early accumulation of $^{13}NH_3$ in the hepatoma may be due to the greater relative perfusion to the hepatoma via the hepatic artery, while the main vascular supply to the liver is from the portal vein, which results in delayed and decreased delivery of the radiotracer.

Regional hepatic arterial blood flow assessment: High first-pass extraction of $^{13}NH_3$ by the liver allows assessment of hepatic arterial blood flow.

Brain imaging—

Based on the different patterns of accumulation of radioactivity in brain tissue, which reflect differences in regional cerebral perfusion. Ischemic lesions show as areas of low perfusion. Brain localization is probably due in part to diffusion across capillaries and cellular membranes as ammonia ($^{13}NH_3$).

### Distribution

$^{13}NH_3$, in equilibrium with $^{13}NH_4^+$, is transported in arterial blood and within a few minutes after injection is rapidly converted into metabolites (e.g., $^{13}N$-glutamine [amide]) by different organs of the body. The metabolites are mainly taken up by the liver, and to a lesser extent, by the myocardium.

### Biotransformation

$^{13}NH_3$ is metabolized principally to $^{13}N$-glutamine by glutamine synthetase in skeletal muscle, brain, liver, and other organs, and to $^{13}N$-urea by a five-enzyme step in the liver.

### Radiation dosimetry

| Estimated absorbed radiation dose* | | |
|---|---|---|
| Target organ | mGy/MBq | rad/mCi |
| Bladder wall | 0.0081 | 0.030 |
| Kidneys | 0.0046 | 0.017 |
| Brain | 0.0042 | 0.016 |
| Liver | 0.0040 | 0.015 |
| Spleen | 0.0025 | 0.0092 |
| Lungs | 0.0025 | 0.0092 |
| Adrenals | 0.0023 | 0.0085 |
| Heart | 0.0021 | 0.0077 |
| Pancreas | 0.0019 | 0.0070 |
| Uterus | 0.0019 | 0.0070 |
| Breast | 0.0018 | 0.0066 |
| Small intestine | 0.0018 | 0.0066 |
| Thyroid | 0.0017 | 0.0063 |
| Stomach wall | 0.0017 | 0.0063 |
| Bone surface | 0.0016 | 0.0059 |
| Other tissue | 0.0027 | 0.0099 |

Effective dose equivalent: 0.0027mSv/MBq (0.01 rem/mCi)

*For adults; intravenous injection.

### Elimination
Renal (10–20%).

## Precautions to Consider

### Pregnancy/Reproduction

Pregnancy—The possibility of pregnancy should be assessed in women of child-bearing potential. Clinical situations exist where the benefit to the patient and fetus from information derived from radiopharmaceutical use outweighs the risks from radiation exposure to the fetus. In this situation, the physician should use discretion and reduce the radiopharmaceutical dose to the lowest possible amount. However, the effects of radiation exposure to the embryo or fetus with the use of $^{13}NH_3$ are expected to be negligible due to $^{13}NH_3$'s rapid clearance from the blood and short physical half-life.

### Breast-feeding

It is not known whether $^{13}NH_3$ is excreted in breast milk; however, it is expected that some will be present. Temporary discontinuation of nursing for a period of 1 to 2 hours is considered adequate.

### Pediatrics

Although $^{13}NH_3$ is used in children, there have been no specific studies evaluating safety and efficacy. When used in children, the diagnostic benefit should be judged to outweigh the potential risk of radiation.

### Geriatrics

Diagnostic studies performed to date using $^{13}NH_3$ have not demonstrated geriatrics-specific problems that would limit the usefulness of $^{13}NH_3$ in the elderly.

### Drug interactions and/or related problems

There are no known drug interactions and/or related problems associated with the use of $^{13}NH_3$.

### Laboratory value alterations

There is no evidence of any alteration of laboratory test results associated with the use of $^{13}NH_3$.

### Medical considerations/Contraindications

There is no information regarding medical problems that would present an increased risk or interfere with the use of $^{13}NH_3$.

## Side/Adverse Effects

There are no known side/adverse effects associated with the use of $^{13}NH_3$.

## Patient Consultation

As an aid to patient consultation, refer to *Advice for the Patient, Radiopharmaceuticals (Diagnostic)*.

In providing consultation, consider emphasizing the following selected information (» = major clinical significance):

**Description of use**

Action in the body: Concentration of radioactivity in heart, brain, and liver allows images to be obtained

Small amounts of radioactivity used in diagnosis; radiation received is low and considered safe

**Before having this test**

Conditions affecting use, especially:

Pregnancy—Risk to fetus from radiation exposure as opposed to benefit derived from use should be considered

Breast-feeding—Risk to infant from radiation exposure; temporary discontinuation of breast-feeding for 1 to 2 hours recommended

**Preparation for this test**

Special preparatory instructions may be given; patient should inquire in advance

**Precautions after having test**

No special precautions

## General Dosing Information

Radiopharmaceuticals are to be administered only by or under the supervision of physicians who have had extensive training in the safe use and handling of radionuclides and who are approved by the appropriate regulatory agency or, outside the U.S., the appropriate authority.

Imaging is usually performed 3 minutes after injection of $^{13}NH_3$, or during administration if dynamic studies are performed.

### Safety considerations for handling this radiopharmaceutical

Improper handling of this radiopharmaceutical may cause radioactive contamination. Guidelines for handling radioactive material have been prepared by scientific, professional, state, federal, and international bodies and are available to the specially qualified and authorized users who have access to radiopharmaceuticals.

## Parenteral Dosage Forms

### AMMONIA N 13 INJECTION

**Usual adult and adolescent dose**

Cardiac imaging—

Intravenous, 555 to 740 megabecquerels (15 to 20 millicuries).

Liver imaging—

Intravenous 370 to 740 megabecquerels (10 to 20 millicuries).

Brain imaging—

Intravenous, 740 to 1480 megabecquerels (20 to 40 millicuries).

**Usual pediatric dose**

Dosage has not been established.

Note: Doses of 8 megabecquerels (0.22 millicuries) per kg of body weight have been used in pediatric patients.

**Usual geriatric dose**

See *Usual adult and adolescent dose*.

**Strength(s) usually available**

U.S.—

Prepared on-site at various clinical facilities.

Canada—
Prepared on-site at various clinical facilities.

**Packaging and storage**
Store below 40 °C (104 °F), preferably between 15 and 30 °C (59 and 86 °F). Protect from freezing.

**Note**
Caution—Radioactive material.

## Selected Bibliography

Hayashi N, Tamaki N, Yonekura Y, et al. Imaging of the hepatocellular carcinoma using dynamic positron emission tomography with nitrogen-13 ammonia. J Nucl Med 1985; 26: 254-7.

Tominaga T, Inoue O, Suzuki K, et al. Evaluation of [13]N-amines as tracers. Nucl Med Biol 1987; 14 (5): 485-90.
Phelps ME, Mazziotta JC, Schelbert HR. Positron emission tomography and autoradiography. Raven Press, 1986: 593-5.
Schelbert HM, Wisenberg G, Phelps M, et al. Noninvasive assessment of coronary stenosis by myocardial imaging during pharmacologic coronary vasodilation. VI. Detection of coronary artery disease in man with intravenous [[13]NH₃] ammonia and positron computed tomography. Am J Cardiol 1982; 49: 1197.

Revised: 07/08/92
Interim revision: 08/02/94

---

# AMMONIA SPIRIT, AROMATIC   Inhalation-Systemic

VA CLASSIFICATION (Primary): RE900
Another commonly used name is smelling salts.
Note: For a listing of dosage forms and brand names by country availability, see *Dosage Forms* section(s). For a listing of brand names for the articles in this monograph, refer to the General Index.

## Category
Respiratory stimulant.

## Indications

**Accepted**
Syncope (prophylaxis and treatment)—Aromatic ammonia spirit is indicated to treat or prevent syncope (fainting).

## Pharmacology/Pharmacokinetics

**Mechanism of action/Effect**
Respiratory stimulant—Aromatic ammonia spirit is a reflex respiratory stimulant that acts by causing peripheral irritation of the sensory receptors in the nasal mucous membranes, esophageal mucosa, and fundus of the stomach.

**Other actions/effects**
Aromatic ammonia spirit has antacid and carminative properties.

## Precautions to Consider

**Pregnancy/Reproduction**
Pregnancy—Problems in humans have not been documented.

**Breast-feeding**
It is not known whether aromatic ammonia spirit is distributed into breast milk. However, problems in humans have not been documented.

**Pediatrics**
Appropriate studies performed to date have not demonstrated pediatrics-specific problems that would limit the usefulness of aromatic ammonia spirit in children. However, this medication should be used in children only when directed by a physician.

**Geriatrics**
Appropriate studies on the relationship of age to the effects of aromatic ammonia spirit have not been performed in the geriatric population. However, no geriatrics-specific problems have been documented to date.

**Medical considerations/Contraindications**
The medical considerations/contraindications included here have been selected on the basis of their potential clinical significance (reasons given in parentheses where appropriate)—not necessarily inclusive (» = major clinical significance).

*Risk-benefit should be considered when the following medical problems exist:*
Eye problems or
Respiratory disease or impairment
   (these conditions may be aggravated by the use of aromatic ammonia spirit)
» Flushed face
   (when associated with syncope, flushed face may indicate the presence of cardiovascular disease or cerebrovascular disturbance)

## Side/Adverse Effects

Note: Inhaling high concentrations of ammonia can cause severe lung damage, but the small amount of ammonia inhaled from aromatic ammonia spirit inhalants has not been reported to cause toxicity.

   If aromatic ammonia spirit comes into contact with the eyes or skin, burns and irritation may occur. Burns in the eyes may lead to blindness.

The following side/adverse effects have been selected on the basis of their potential clinical significance (possible signs and symptoms in parentheses where appropriate)—not necessarily inclusive:

**Those indicating need for medical attention**
Incidence less frequent
   *Cough; diarrhea; difficulty in breathing; headache; vomiting*

## Patient Consultation

As an aid to patient consultation, refer to *Advice for the Patient, Ammonia Spirit, Aromatic (Inhalation).*

In providing consultation, consider emphasizing the following selected information (» = major clinical significance):

**Before using this medication**
Conditions affecting use, especially:
   Sensitivity to aromatic ammonia spirit
   Use in children—Use not recommended unless directed by physician

**Proper use of this medication**
Proper dosing
Proper storage

**Precautions while using this medication**
Checking with physician if you are an older adult or have history of heart problems; fainting may signal a serious medical problem
» Keeping medication away from eyes and skin
Following eye contact, flushing eyes with a gentle stream of water for 20 minutes and calling poison control center, physician, or emergency room immediately
Following external exposure, removing contaminated clothing, flushing skin with water, not rubbing or applying ointment to skin; calling physician if skin irritation persists
Following ingestion of a large amount of solution, drinking a glass (8 ounces) of water and calling poison control center, physician, or emergency room immediately

**Side/adverse effects**
Signs of potential side effects, especially cough, diarrhea, difficulty in breathing, headache, and vomiting

## General Dosing Information

Aromatic ammonia spirit should be kept away from the eyes and should not be allowed to come into contact with the skin.

Esophagoscopy is not routinely indicated following acute ingestion of an aromatic ammonia spirit inhalant because the contact time with esophageal tissue is limited and the volume contained in the capsule is extremely small (0.33 mL).

**For treatment of adverse effects**

Recommended treatment consists of the following:

    x Following eye contact—Flushing the eye with a gentle stream of water for 20 minutes; holding the eyelid away from the eyeball to facilitate thorough rinsing.

    x Following external exposure—Removing contaminated clothing and flushing the affected area with large amounts of water. Not rubbing or applying ointment to the affected area.

    x Following ingestion of a large amount of solution—Having patient drink a glass (8 ounces) of water; evaluating for burns in the mouth and throat if a significant amount of solution has been ingested.

For more information on the management of overdose or unintentional exposure, **contact a Poison Control Center** (see *Poison Control Center Listing*).

## Inhalation Dosage Forms

### AROMATIC AMMONIA SPIRIT INHALANT

**Usual adult and adolescent dose**

Respiratory stimulant—

    Inhalation, inhalant should be held away from the face and crushed between the fingers. The inhalant should then be held approximately four inches from the nostrils, and the vapor slowly inhaled until the patient awakens or no longer feels faint.

**Usual pediatric dose**

Use is not recommended unless directed by a physician.

**Usual geriatric dose**

See *Usual adult and adolescent dose*.

**Strength(s) usually available**

U.S.—

    0.33 mL (OTC) [GENERIC (ammonia 15%; alcohol 35%)].

Canada—

    Not commercially available.

**Packaging and storage**

Store at a temperature not exceeding 30 ℃ (86 ℉) in a light-resistant container.

### AROMATIC AMMONIA SPIRIT

**Usual adult and adolescent dose**

Respiratory stimulant—

    Inhalation of vapor until the patient awakens or no longer feels faint.

**Usual pediatric dose**

Use is not recommended unless directed by a physician.

**Usual geriatric dose**

See *Usual adult and adolescent dose*.

**Strength(s) usually available**

U.S.—

    100 mL (OTC) [GENERIC (total ammonia 1.9 grams; ammonium carbonate 4 grams; lemon oil; lavender oil; nutmeg oil; alcohol 65%)].

Canada—

    Not commercially available.

**Packaging and storage**

Store at a temperature not exceeding 30 ℃ (86 ℉) in a tight, light-resistant container.

**Incompatibilities**

Aromatic ammonia spirit is incompatible with acids, aqueous preparations containing alkaloids or of low alcoholic content, halogens, hypochlorites, and sodium hydroxide.

**Auxiliary labeling**

Keep container tightly closed.

Developed: 06/23/95

---

**AMMONIATED MERCURY**—Since Ammoniated Mercury is not commercially available in the U.S. or Canada, the *Ammoniated Mercury (Topical)* monograph is not included in this published version of the USP DI database. Copies of the monograph are available on request from the USP Division of Information Development, 12601 Twinbrook Parkway, Rockville, MD 20852; telephone (301) 816-8351; telefax (301) 816-8374.

---

## AMMONIUM CHLORIDE–CONTAINING COMBINATIONS—

Bromodiphenhydramine, Diphenhydramine, Codeine, Ammonium Chloride, and Potassium Guaiacolsulfonate (Systemic)—See *Cough/Cold Combinations (Systemic)*

Chlorpheniramine, Ephedrine, Phenylephrine, Dextromethorphan, Ammonium Chloride, and Ipecac (Systemic)—See *Cough/Cold Combinations (Systemic)*

Chlorpheniramine, Phenylephrine, Codeine, and Ammonium Chloride (Systemic)—See *Cough/Cold Combinations (Systemic)*

Chlorpheniramine, Phenylephrine, Dextromethorphan, Guaifenesin, and Ammonium Chloride (Systemic)—See *Cough/Cold Combinations (Systemic)*

Chlorpheniramine, Phenylpropanolamine, Dextromethorphan, and Ammonium Chloride (Systemic)—See *Cough/Cold Combinations (Systemic)*

Codeine, Ammonium Chloride, and Guaifenesin (Systemic)—See *Cough/Cold Combinations (Systemic)*

Diphenhydramine, Codeine, and Ammonium Chloride (Systemic)—See *Cough/Cold Combinations (Systemic)*

Diphenhydramine, Dextromethorphan, and Ammonium Chloride (Systemic)—See *Cough/Cold Combinations (Systemic)*

Pheniramine, Pyrilamine, Phenylpropanolamine, Dextromethorphan, and Ammonium Chloride (Systemic)—See *Cough/Cold Combinations (Systemic)*

Pyrilamine, Phenylephrine, Hydrocodone, and Ammonium Chloride (Systemic)—See *Cough/Cold Combinations (Systemic)*

---

**AMMONIUM MOLYBDATE**—See *Molybdenum Supplements (Systemic)*

---

**AMOBARBITAL**—See *Barbiturates (Systemic)*

---

## AMOBARBITAL-CONTAINING COMBINATIONS—

Secobarbital and Amobarbital (Systemic)—See *Barbiturates (Systemic)*

---

**AMOXAPINE**—See *Antidepressants, Tricyclic (Systemic)*

---

**AMOXICILLIN**—See *Penicillins (Systemic)*

---

## AMOXICILLIN-CONTAINING COMBINATIONS—

Amoxicillin and Clavulanate (Systemic)—See *Penicillins and Beta-lactamase Inhibitors (Systemic)*

---

**AMPHETAMINE**—See *Amphetamines (Systemic)*

# AMPHETAMINES   Systemic

This monograph includes information on the following: Amphetamine†;
   Dextroamphetamine†; Methamphetamine†.

INN:
   Amphetamine—Amfetamine
   Dextroamphetamine—Dexamfetamine
   Methamphetamine—Metamfetamine

VA CLASSIFICATION (Primary): CN801

Note: Controlled substances in the U.S. and Canada as follows:

| Drug | U.S. | Canada |
|---|---|---|
| Amphetamine | II | † |
| Dextroamphetamine | II | C |
| Methamphetamine | II | † |

   †Not commercially available in Canada.

Note: For a listing of dosage forms and brand names by country availability, see *Dosage Forms* section(s). For a listing of brand names
   for the articles in this monograph, refer to the General Index.

   †Not commercially available in Canada.

## Category

Central nervous system (CNS) stimulant.

## Indications

Note: Bracketed information in the *Indications* section refers to uses that
   are not included in U.S. product labeling.

**Accepted**

Attention-deficit hyperactivity disorder (treatment)—Amphetamines are
   indicated as an integral part of a total treatment program that includes
   other remedial measures (psychological, educational, social) for a stabilizing effect in children [and adults][1] with attention-deficit hyperactivity disorder, characterized by moderate to severe distractibility,
   short attention span, hyperactivity, emotional lability, and impulsivity.
   Nonlocalizing neurological signs, learning disability, and abnormal
   electroencephalogram (EEG) may also be present. Amphetamines are
   usually not indicated when the above symptoms are associated with
   acute stress reactions.

Narcolepsy (treatment)—Amphetamine and dextroamphetamine are indicated in the treatment of well-established and proven narcolepsy.

**Unaccepted**

Due to their high potential for abuse, amphetamines are not recommended
   for use as appetite suppressants.

Amphetamines should not be used to combat fatigue or to replace rest in
   normal subjects.

   [1]Not included in Canadian product labeling.

## Pharmacology/Pharmacokinetics

**Physicochemical characteristics**

Molecular weight—
   Amphetamine sulfate: 368.49.
   Dextroamphetamine sulfate: 368.49.
   Methamphetamine hydrochloride: 185.70.

**Mechanism of action/Effect**

Amphetamines are sympathomimetic amines that increase motor activity
   and mental alertness, and diminish drowsiness and a sense of fatigue.

In attention-deficit hyperactivity disorder, amphetamines decrease motor
   restlessness and enhance the ability to pay attention.

The exact mechanism of action has not been established. However, in
   animals, amphetamines facilitate the action of dopamine and norepinephrine by blocking reuptake from the synapse, inhibit the action of
   monoamine oxidase (MAO), and facilitate the release of catecholamines. Increase in locomotor activity at relatively low doses and increase in stereotypic behavior with a concomitant decrease in activity
   at higher doses appear to be due to stimulation of mesocorticolimbic
   and nigrostriatal dopaminergic pathways. Dextroamphetamine may
   also stimulate inhibitory autoreceptors in the substantia nigra and ventral tegmentum.

Some studies support the theory that amphetamine exerts a dual effect on
   the striatal dopaminergic nerve terminal, thus explaining the paradoxical effects of amphetamines. Amphetamines may selectively facilitate
   the dopaminergic transmission by promoting the release of recently

synthesized dopamine from a reserpine-resistant pool and, in addition,
   may inhibit the classical dopaminergic neurotransmission involving
   the calcium-dependent depolarization-evoked release of dopamine
   from reserpine-sensitive storage sites.

**Other actions/effects**

Peripheral actions include elevation of both diastolic and systolic blood
   pressure, and weak bronchodilator and respiratory stimulant action.

**Biotransformation**

Hepatic.

**Half-life**

Amphetamine—
   10 to 30 hours; dependent on urinary pH.
Dextroamphetamine—
   10 to 12 hours in adults; 6 to 8 hours in children.
Methamphetamine—
   4 to 5 hours; dependent on urinary pH.

**Elimination**

Renal; dependent on urinary pH. Excretion is accelerated in acidic urine
   and slowed in alkaline urine.

## Precautions to Consider

**Cross-sensitivity and/or related problems**

Patients sensitive to other sympathomimetics (for example, ephedrine, epinephrine, isoproterenol, metaproterenol, norepinephrine, phenylephrine, phenylpropanolamine, pseudoephedrine, terbutaline) may be
   sensitive to amphetamines also.

**Carcinogenicity/Mutagenicity**

Mutagenicity and long-term carcinogenicity studies in animals have not
   been done.

**Pregnancy/Reproduction**

Pregnancy—Although adequate and well-controlled studies in humans
   have not been done, use of amphetamines during early pregnancy may
   be associated with an increased risk of congenital malformations, especially in the cardiovascular system and biliary tract.

Reproduction studies in animals have suggested both an embryotoxic and
   a teratogenic potential when amphetamines were administered at high
   multiples of the human dose.

FDA Pregnancy Category C.

Delivery—Infants born to mothers dependent on amphetamines have an
   increased risk of premature delivery and low birth weight. These infants may experience symptoms of withdrawal, including agitation and
   significant drowsiness.

**Breast-feeding**

Amphetamines are distributed into breast milk. However, problems in
   nursing infants have not been documented.

**Pediatrics**

Data suggest that prolonged administration of amphetamines to children
   may inhibit growth. Careful monitoring during treatment is
   recommended.

Psychotic children may experience exacerbation of symptoms of behavior
   disturbance and thought disorder.

Amphetamines may provoke or exacerbate motor and vocal tics and Tourette's syndrome, necessitating clinical evaluation before administration
   of amphetamines.

**Geriatrics**

No information is available on the relationship of age to the effects of the
   amphetamines in geriatric patients.

**Drug interactions and/or related problems**

The following drug interactions and/or related problems have been selected on the basis of their potential clinical significance (possible
   mechanism in parentheses where appropriate)—not necessarily inclusive (» 5 major clinical significance):

Note: Combinations containing any of the following medications, depending on the amount present, may also interact with this
   medication.

   Acidifiers, gastrointestinal, such as:
   Ascorbic acid
   Fruit juices
   Glutamic acid hydrochloride or

Acidifiers, urinary, such as:
Ammonium chloride
Sodium acid phosphate
(concurrent use may decrease the effects of amphetamines as a
result of decreased absorption and increased elimination)

Alkalizers, urinary, such as:
Antacids, calcium- and/or magnesium-containing
Carbonic anhydrase inhibitors
Citrates
Sodium bicarbonate
(concurrent use may increase the effects of amphetamines as a
result of decreased elimination caused by alkalinization of urine)

Anesthetics, inhalation
(halothane and, to a much lesser extent, enflurane, isoflurane, and
methoxyflurane, may sensitize the myocardium to the effects of
sympathomimetics, including chronic use of amphetamines prior
to anesthesia, so that the risk of severe ventricular arrhythmias is
increased; sympathomimetics should be used with caution and in
substantially reduced dosage in patients receiving these agents)

» Antidepressants, tricyclic
(although tricyclic antidepressants may be used concurrently with
amphetamines for therapeutic effect, concurrent use may potentiate
cardiovascular effects due to the release of norepinephrine, possibly resulting in arrhythmias, tachycardia, or severe hypertension
or hyperpyrexia; close monitoring is recommended and dosage adjustments may be necessary)

Antihypertensives or
Diuretics used as antihypertensives
(hypotensive effects may be reduced when these medications are
used concurrently with amphetamines; the patient should be carefully monitored to confirm that the desired effect is obtained)

» Beta-adrenergic blocking agents, including ophthalmics
(concurrent use with amphetamines may result in unopposed alpha-
adrenergic activity with a risk of hypertension and excessive bradycardia and possible heart block; risk may be less with labetalol
because of its alpha-blocking activity)

» CNS stimulation–producing medications, other (See *Appendix II*)
(additive CNS stimulation to excessive levels may result in nervousness, irritability, insomnia, or possibly seizures; close observation is recommended)

(also, concurrent use of amphetamines with other sympathomimetics may increase cardiovascular effects of either medication)

(in addition to possibly increasing CNS stimulation, concurrent use
of norepinephrine with large doses of amphetamines may enhance
the pressor response to norepinephrine; caution may also be warranted in patients receiving usual doses of amphetamines)

» Digitalis glycosides
(concurrent use with amphetamines may cause additive effects,
resulting in cardiac arrhythmias)

Ethosuximide or
Phenobarbital or
Phenytoin
(concurrent use with amphetamines may cause a delay in the intestinal absorption of ethosuximide, phenobarbital, or phenytoin)

Haloperidol or
Loxapine or
Molindone or
Phenothiazines or
Pimozide or
Thioxanthenes
(central stimulant effects of amphetamines may be inhibited be-
cause of alpha-adrenergic blockade by these agents; also, concur-
rent use with amphetamines may reduce the antipsychotic effects
of these agents)

Levodopa
(the risk of cardiac arrhythmias may be increased; dosage reduction of amphetamine is recommended)

Lithium
(central stimulant effects of amphetamines may be antagonized by
lithium)

» Meperidine
(the analgesic effects of meperidine may be potentiated by amphetamines; however, concurrent use of meperidine is not recommended, as it may potentially result in hypotension, severe respiratory depression, coma, convulsions, hyperpyrexia, vascular
collapse, and death in some patients due to the monoamine oxidase
inhibition properties of amphetamines)

Metrizamide
(intrathecal administration of metrizamide may increase the risk of
seizures because of lowered seizure threshold; it is recommended
that amphetamines be discontinued for at least 48 hours before and
24 hours after myelography)

» Monoamine oxidase (MAO) inhibitors, including furazolidone, procarbazine, and selegiline
(concurrent use may prolong and intensify cardiac stimulant and
vasopressor effects [including headache, cardiac arrhythmias, vomiting, sudden and severe hypertensive and hyperpyretic crises] of
amphetamines because of the release of catecholamines that accumulate in intraneuronal storage sites during MAO inhibitor therapy; amphetamines should not be administered during or within
14 days following the administration of an MAO inhibitor)

Propoxyphene
(overdosage of propoxyphene may potentiate central stimulant effects of amphetamines; fatal convulsions can occur)

» Thyroid hormones
(the effects of either these medications or amphetamines may be
increased; thyroid hormones enhance the risk of coronary insufficiency when amphetamines are administered to patients with coronary artery disease)

**Laboratory value alterations**
The following have been selected on the basis of their potential clinical
significance (possible effect in parentheses where appropriate)—not
necessarily inclusive (» = major clinical significance):

With diagnostic test results
Urinary steroid determinations
(may be altered, interfering with results of such tests as the metyrapone test)

With physiology/laboratory test values
Plasma corticosteroid concentrations
(may be increased, with greatest increase in evening)

**Medical considerations/Contraindications**
The medical considerations/contraindications included here have been selected on the basis of their potential clinical significance (reasons given
in parentheses where appropriate)—not necessarily inclusive (» =
major clinical significance).

*Risk-benefit should be considered when the following medical problems
exist:*
» Agitated states or
» Arteriosclerosis, advanced or
» Cardiovascular disease, symptomatic or
» Drug abuse or dependence, history of or
» Glaucoma or
» Hypertension or
» Hyperthyroidism or
Psychoses, especially in children or
» Tourette's syndrome or other motor or vocal tics
(increased risk of exacerbation)
Sensitivity to amphetamines and other sympathomimetics

**Patient monitoring**
The following may be especially important in patient monitoring (other
tests may be warranted in some patients, depending on condition;
» = major clinical significance):

Assessment of potential tolerance, dependence, or drug-seeking behavior and
Blood pressure determinations and
Cardiac rhythm determinations
(recommended at periodic intervals during therapy)

Monitoring of growth in children
(recommended during therapy since data suggest that chronic administration of amphetamines may be associated with growth
inhibition)

Monitoring for motor and vocal tics
(recommended during therapy)

Reassessment of need for therapy for attention-deficit hyperactivity
disorder in children
(interruption of therapy at periodic intervals is recommended to
determine if a recurrence of behavioral symptoms is sufficient to
continue therapy)

## Side/Adverse Effects

Note: Psychological dependence and tolerance may occur with amphetamines following prolonged use or high doses.

The following side/adverse effects have been selected on the basis of their potential clinical significance (possible signs and symptoms in parentheses where appropriate)—not necessarily inclusive:

**Those indicating need for medical attention**
Incidence more frequent
*Irregular heartbeat*
Incidence rare
*Allergic reaction* (skin rash or hives); *chest pain; CNS stimulation, severe,* or *Tourette's syndrome* (uncontrolled movements of the head, neck, arms, and legs); *hyperthermia* (extremely high body temperature)
With prolonged use or high doses
*Cardiomyopathy* (chest discomfort or pain; difficulty in breathing; dizziness or feeling faint; irregular or pounding heartbeat; unusual tiredness or weakness); *increase in blood pressure; psychotic reactions or toxic psychoses* (mood or mental changes)

**Those indicating need for medical attention only if they continue or are bothersome**
Incidence more frequent
*CNS stimulation* (false sense of well-being; irritability; nervousness; restlessness; trouble in sleeping)—drowsiness, fatigue, trembling, or mental depression may follow the stimulant effects
Incidence less frequent
*Blurred vision; changes in sexual desire or decreased sexual ability; constipation; diarrhea; loss of appetite; nausea; stomach cramps or pain; weight loss; vomiting; dizziness; lightheadedness; headache; dryness of mouth or unpleasant taste; fast or pounding heartbeat; increased sweating*

**Those indicating possible withdrawal and the need for medical attention if they occur after medication is discontinued**
*Mental depression; nausea; stomach cramps or pain; vomiting; trembling; unusual tiredness or weakness*

## Overdose

For specific information on the agents used in the management of amphetamine overdose, see:
- *Barbiturates (Systemic)* monograph;
- *Chlorpromazine* in *Phenothiazines (Systemic)* monograph; and/or
- *Phentolamine (Systemic)* monograph.

For more information on the management of overdose or unintentional ingestion, **contact a Poison Control Center** (see *Poison Control Center Listing*).

**Treatment of overdose**
Since there is no specific antidote for overdosage with amphetamines, treatment is symptomatic and supportive with possible utilization of the following:
To decrease absorption—
Induction of emesis and/or use of gastric lavage is primary.
Use of saline cathartics to hasten evacuation of sustained-release dosage forms.
To enhance elimination—
Acidification of urine to increase amphetamine excretion. Acidification is contraindicated in presence of rhabdomyolysis, myoglobinuria, or hemoglobinemia, as renal failure may result.
Forced diuresis if condition permits.
Specific treatment—
Barbiturate sedatives or chlorpromazine sometimes used to control excessive CNS stimulation.
Intravenous phentolamine to control hypertension.
Monitoring—
Cardiovascular and respiratory monitoring.
Supportive care—
Protection of patient from self-injury by use of restraints if necessary.
Intravenous fluids to control hypotension.
Patients in whom intentional overdose is confirmed or suspected should be referred for psychiatric consultation.

## Patient Consultation

As an aid to patient consultation, refer to *Advice for the Patient, Amphetamines (Systemic)*.

In providing consultation, consider emphasizing the following selected information (» = major clinical significance):

**Before using this medication**
» Conditions affecting use, especially:
Sensitivity to amphetamines and other sympathomimetics
Pregnancy—Increased risk of congenital malformations, especially in cardiovascular system and biliary tract; potential embryotoxic and teratogenic effects in animals given large doses; risk

of premature delivery and low birth weight may be increased; newborn may experience withdrawal symptoms
Breast-feeding—Not recommended since amphetamines are distributed into breast milk
Use in children—May inhibit growth; may provoke motor and vocal tics and Tourette's syndrome; may exacerbate behavior problems and thought disorder in psychotic children
Other medications, especially tricyclic antidepressants, beta-adrenergic blocking agents, digitalis glycosides, meperidine, monoamine oxidase inhibitors, other CNS stimulation–producing medications, or thyroid hormones
Other medical problems, especially agitated states, advanced arteriosclerosis or symptomatic cardiovascular disease, history of drug dependence, glaucoma, hypertension, hyperthyroidism, or Tourette's syndrome or other tics

**Proper use of this medication**
Taking the last dose of the day of the regular dosage form at least 6 hours before bedtime and the daily dose of the extended-release dosage form about 10 to 14 hours before bedtime to minimize the possibility of insomnia
Proper administration of extended-release dosage forms:
Swallowing whole
Not breaking, crushing, or chewing
» Importance of not taking more medication than the amount prescribed because of habit-forming potential
» Not increasing dose if medication becomes less effective after a few weeks; checking with physician
» Proper dosing
Missed dose: If dosing schedule is—
Once a day: Taking as soon as possible but not later than stated above; if remembered later, not taking until next day; not doubling doses
Two or three times a day: Taking as soon as possible if remembered within an hour or so; not taking if remembered later; not doubling doses
» Proper storage

**Precautions while using this medication**
Regular visits to physician to check progress during therapy
» Checking with physician before discontinuing medication after prolonged high-dose therapy; gradual dosage reduction may be necessary to avoid possibility of withdrawal symptoms
» Caution if dizziness or euphoria occurs; not driving, using machinery, or doing other activities that are potentially hazardous
Caution if any laboratory tests required; possible interference with results of metyrapone test
» Suspected psychological or physical dependence; checking with physician

**Side/adverse effects**
Signs of potential side effects, especially irregular heartbeat; allergic reaction; chest pain; tics or other signs of severe CNS stimulation; hyperthermia; cardiomyopathy; increased blood pressure; psychotic reactions
Potential unwanted effects during long-term use in children
Possibility of withdrawal effects, especially mental depression, nausea, stomach cramps or pain, vomiting, trembling, or unusual tiredness or weakness

## General Dosing Information

When the regular tablet dosage form of amphetamines is administered, the first dose should be taken on awakening, followed by 1 or 2 additional doses at intervals of 4 to 6 hours.

To reduce the possibility of insomnia, the last dose of the day of the regular dosage form should be administered at least 6 hours before bedtime, and the daily dose of the extended-release dosage form should be administered approximately 10 to 14 hours before bedtime.

The extended-release dosage form may be used for once-a-day dosing whenever it is feasible.

When symptoms of attention-deficit hyperactivity disorder are controlled in children, dosage reduction or interruption in therapy may be possible during the summer months and at other times when the child is under less stress; medication may be given on each of the 5 school days during the week, with medication-free weekends and school holidays.

Prolonged use of amphetamines may result in tolerance, extreme psychological dependence, or severe social disability.

When the medication is to be discontinued following prolonged high-dose administration, the dosage should be reduced gradually since abrupt withdrawal may result in extreme fatigue and mental depression.

## *AMPHETAMINE*

# Oral Dosage Forms

Note: Bracketed uses in the *Dosage Forms* section refer to categories of
use and/or indications that are not included in U.S. product labeling.

## AMPHETAMINE SULFATE TABLETS USP

### Usual adult dose
[Attention-deficit hyperactivity disorder] or
Narcolepsy—
  Oral, 5 to 20 mg one to three times a day.

### Usual pediatric dose
Attention-deficit hyperactivity disorder—
  Children up to 3 years of age: Use is not recommended.
  Children 3 to 6 years of age: Oral, 2.5 mg once a day, the dosage
    being increased by 2.5 mg per day at one-week intervals until the
    desired response is obtained.
  Children 6 years of age and over: Oral, 5 mg one or two times a day,
    the dosage being increased by 5 mg per day at one-week intervals
    until the desired response is obtained.
Narcolepsy—
  Children up to 6 years of age: Dosage has not been established.
  Children 6 to 12 years of age: Oral, 2.5 mg two times a day, the dosage
    being increased by 5 mg per day at one-week intervals until the
    desired response is obtained or until the adult dose is reached.
  Children 12 years of age and over: Oral, 5 mg two times a day, the
    dosage being increased by 10 mg per day at one-week intervals
    until the desired response is obtained or until the adult dose is
    reached.

### Strength(s) usually available
U.S.—
  5 mg (Rx) [GENERIC].
  10 mg (Rx) [GENERIC].
Canada—
  Not commercially available.

### Packaging and storage
Store below 40 °C (104 °F), preferably between 15 and 30 °C (59 and 86
  °F), unless otherwise specified by manufacturer. Store in a well-closed
  container.

### Note
Controlled substance in the U.S.

## *DEXTROAMPHETAMINE*

# Oral Dosage Forms

Note: Bracketed uses in the *Dosage Forms* section refer to categories of
use and/or indications that are not included in U.S. product labeling.

## DEXTROAMPHETAMINE SULFATE EXTENDED-RELEASE CAPSULES

Note: The extended-release dosage form should not be used for initiation
of dosage, nor should it be used until the conventional titrated daily
dosage is equal to or greater than the dosage provided in the extended-release dosage form.

### Usual adult dose
[Attention-deficit hyperactivity disorder][1] or
Narcolepsy—
  Oral, 5 to 60 mg once a day, or in divided doses.

### Usual pediatric dose
Attention-deficit hyperactivity disorder—
  Children up to 3 years of age: Use is not recommended.
  Children 3 to 6 years of age: Oral, initially 2.5 mg once a day, the
    dosage being increased by 2.5 mg per day at one-week intervals
    until the desired response is obtained.
  Children 6 years of age and over: Oral, 5 mg once or twice a day, the
    dosage being increased by 5 mg a day at one-week intervals until
    the desired response is obtained.
Narcolepsy—
  Children up to 3 years of age: Use is not recommended.
  Children 3 to 6 years of age: Dosage has not been established.
  Children 6 to 12 years of age: Oral, initially 5 mg once a day, the
    dosage being increased by 5 mg a day at one-week intervals until
    the desired response is obtained.
  Children 12 years of age and over: Oral, initially 10 mg once a day,
    the dosage being increased by 10 mg a day at one-week intervals
    until the desired response is obtained.

Note: The usual pediatric dose rarely exceeds 40 mg a day.

### Strength(s) usually available
U.S.—
  5 mg (Rx) [*Dexedrine Spansule* (tartrazine)].
  10 mg (Rx) [*Dexedrine Spansule* (tartrazine)].
  15 mg (Rx) [*Dexedrine Spansule* (tartrazine)].
Canada—
  10 mg (Rx) [*Dexedrine Spansule* (tartrazine)].
  15 mg (Rx) [*Dexedrine Spansule* (tartrazine)].

### Packaging and storage
Store between 15 and 30 °C (59 and 86 °F), in a tight, light-resistant
  container, unless otherwise specified by manufacturer.

### Auxiliary labeling
• Swallow capsules whole.

### Note
Controlled substance in both the U.S. and Canada.

## DEXTROAMPHETAMINE SULFATE TABLETS USP

### Usual adult dose
[Attention-deficit hyperactivity disorder][1] or
Narcolepsy—
  Oral, 5 to 60 mg a day in divided doses as needed and tolerated.

### Usual pediatric dose
Attention-deficit hyperactivity disorder—
  Children up to 3 years of age: Use is not recommended.
  Children 3 to 5 years of age: Oral, 2.5 mg once a day, the dosage
    being increased by 2.5 mg a day at one-week intervals until the
    desired response is obtained.
  Children 6 years of age and over: Oral, 5 mg one or two times a day,
    the dosage being increased by 5 mg a day at one-week intervals
    until the desired response is obtained.
Narcolepsy—
  Children up to 6 years of age: Dosage has not been established.
  Children 6 to 12 years of age: Oral, 5 mg a day, the dosage being
    increased by 5 mg a day at one-week intervals until the desired
    response is obtained or until the adult dose is reached.
  Children 12 years of age and over: Oral, 10 mg a day, the dosage
    being increased by 10 mg a day at one-week intervals until the
    desired response is obtained or until the adult dose is reached.

Note: The usual pediatric dose rarely exceeds 40 mg a day.

### Strength(s) usually available
U.S.—
  5 mg (Rx) [*Dexedrine* (tartrazine); *Dextrostat;* GENERIC].
  10 mg (Rx) [GENERIC].
Canada—
  5 mg (Rx) [*Dexedrine* (tartrazine)].

### Packaging and storage
Store below 40 °C (104 °F), preferably between 15 and 30 °C (59 and 86
  °F), unless otherwise specified by manufacturer. Store in a tight
  container.

### Note
Controlled substance in both the U.S. and Canada.

[1]Not included in Canadian product labeling.

## *METHAMPHETAMINE*

# Oral Dosage Forms

## METHAMPHETAMINE HYDROCHLORIDE TABLETS USP

### Usual pediatric dose
Attention-deficit hyperactivity disorder—
  Children up to 6 years of age: Use is not recommended.
  Children 6 years of age and over: Oral, 5 mg one or two times a day,
    the dosage being increased by 5 mg per day at one-week intervals
    until the desired response is obtained (usually 20 to 25 mg per
    day).

### Strength(s) usually available
U.S.—
  5 mg (Rx) [*Desoxyn* (lactose)].
Canada—
  Not commercially available.

### Packaging and storage
Store below 40 °C (104 °F), preferably between 15 and 30 °C (59 and 86
  °F), in a well-closed container, unless otherwise specified by
  manufacturer.

**Note**
Controlled substance in the U.S.

## METHAMPHETAMINE HYDROCHLORIDE EXTENDED-RELEASE TABLETS

Note: The extended-release dosage form should not be used for initiation of dosage or until the conventional titrated daily dosage is equal to or greater than the dosage provided in the extended-release dosage form.

**Usual pediatric dose**
Attention-deficit hyperactivity disorder—
Children up to 6 years of age: Use is not recommended.
Children 6 years of age and over: Oral, 20 to 25 mg once a day.

**Strength(s) usually available**
U.S.—
5 mg (Rx) [*Desoxyn Gradumet*].
10 mg (Rx) [*Desoxyn Gradumet*].
15 mg (Rx) [*Desoxyn Gradumet* (tartrazine)].

Canada—
Not commercially available.

**Packaging and storage**
Store below 40 °C (104 °F), preferably between 15 and 30 °C (59 and 86 °F), in a well-closed container, unless otherwise specified by manufacturer.

**Auxiliary labeling**
• Swallow tablets whole.
• Keep container tightly closed.

**Note**
Controlled substance in the U.S.

Revised: 08/18/94

---

# AMPHOTERICIN B    Systemic

VA CLASSIFICATION (Primary/Secondary): AM700/AP109

Note: For a listing of dosage forms and brand names by country availability, see *Dosage Forms* section(s). For a listing of brand names for the articles in this monograph, refer to the General Index.

## Category

Antifungal (systemic); antiprotozoal.

## Indications

Note: Bracketed information in the *Indications* section refers to uses that are not included in U.S. product labeling.

**Accepted**
Aspergillosis (treatment)—Parenteral amphotericin B is indicated in the treatment of aspergillosis caused by *Aspergillus fumigatus*. [Intracavitary amphotericin B has also been used in the treatment of pulmonary aspergilloma with hemoptysis.]

Blastomycosis (treatment)—Parenteral amphotericin B is indicated in the treatment of North American blastomycosis caused by *Blastomyces dermatitidis*.

Candidiasis, disseminated (treatment)—Parenteral amphotericin B is indicated in the treatment of disseminated candidiasis caused by *Candida* species.

Coccidioidomycosis (treatment)—Parenteral amphotericin B is indicated in the treatment of coccidioidomycosis caused by *Coccidioides immitis*.

Cryptococcosis (treatment)—Parenteral amphotericin B is indicated in the treatment of cryptococcosis caused by *Cryptococcus neoformans*.

Endocarditis, fungal (treatment)—Parenteral amphotericin B is indicated in the treatment of fungal endocarditis.

Endophthalmitis, candidal (treatment)—Parenteral and intraocular administration of amphotericin B are used in the treatment of candidal endophthalmitis.

Histoplasmosis (treatment)—Parenteral amphotericin B is indicated in the treatment of histoplasmosis caused by *Histoplasma capsulatum*.

Intra-abdominal infections (treatment)—Parenteral and intraperitoneal administration of amphotericin B, with or without concurrent administration of other antifungal medications, are used for the treatment of intra-abdominal infections, including dialysis-related and non–dialysis-related peritonitis.

Leishmaniasis, American mucocutaneous (treatment)—Parenteral amphotericin B is indicated as an alternative agent in the treatment of American mucocutaneous leishmaniasis caused by *Leishmania braziliensis* and *L. mexicana*.

Meningitis, cryptococcal (treatment) or
Meningitis, cryptococcal (suppression) or
Meningitis, fungal, other (treatment)—Parenteral amphotericin B is indicated, with or without concurrent administration of flucytosine, in the treatment and suppression of cryptococcal meningitis caused by *Cryptococcus neoformans*.

Parenteral amphotericin B is also indicated in the treatment of fungal meningitis caused by organisms such as *Coccidioides immitis*, *Candida* species, *Sporothrix schenckii*, and *Aspergillus* species.

Mucormycosis (treatment)—Parenteral amphotericin B is indicated in the treatment of mucormycosis (phycomycosis) caused by *Mucor*, *Rhizopus*, *Absidia*, *Entomophthora* and *Basidiobolus* organisms.

Septicemia, fungal (treatment)—Parenteral amphotericin B is indicated in the treatment of fungal septicemia.

Sporotrichosis, disseminated (treatment)—Parenteral amphotericin B is indicated in the treatment of disseminated sporotrichosis caused by *Sporothrix schenckii*.

Urinary tract infections, fungal (treatment)—Parenteral administration [and continuous bladder irrigation] of amphotericin B are indicated in the treatment of fungal (particularly *Candida* species) urinary tract infections.

[Meningoencephalitis, primary amebic (treatment)][1]—Parenteral amphotericin B is used in the treatment of primary amebic meningoencephalitis caused by *Naegleria* species.

[Paracoccidioidomycosis (treatment)][1]—Parenteral amphotericin B is used as a secondary agent in the treatment of paracoccidioidomycosis caused by *Paracoccidioides brasiliensis*.

Not all species or strains of a particular organism may be susceptible to amphotericin B. Because of its toxicity, amphotericin B is indicated primarily in patients with progressive, potentially fatal infections in whom the diagnosis is firmly established, preferably by positive culture or histologic study.

**Unaccepted**
Amphotericin B is not indicated in the treatment of common, clinically inapparent fungal infections that show only positive skin or serologic tests.

Amphotericin B is not effective against bacteria, rickettsiae, or viruses.

[1]Not included in Canadian product labeling.

## Pharmacology/Pharmacokinetics

**Physicochemical characteristics**
Molecular weight—924.09.

**Mechanism of action/Effect**
Antifungal (systemic)—
Fungistatic in concentrations usually obtained clinically; however, in concentrations near the upper limits of tolerance, may be fungicidal. Probably acts by binding to sterols in the fungus cell membrane, producing a change in membrane permeability that allows loss of potassium and small molecules from the cell.

**Distribution**
Distributed to lungs, liver, spleen, kidneys, adrenal glands, muscle, and other tissues (potentially therapeutic concentrations); reaches approximately two-thirds the concurrent plasma concentration in the fluids of inflamed pleura, peritoneum, synovium and aqueous humor; concentrations in cerebrospinal fluid (CSF) usually undetectable.

Vol$_D$—
    Neonates: Variable (range, 1.5 to 9.4 L per kg).
    Children: Variable (range, 0.4 to 8.3 L per kg).
    Adults: Approximately 4 L per kg.

**Protein binding**
Very high (90% or more).

**Biotransformation**
Metabolic pathways unknown.

**Half-life**
Elimination half-life—
    Neonates: Variable (range, 18.8 to 62.5 hours).
    Children: Variable (range, 5.5 to 40.3 hours).
    Adults: Approximately 24 hours.
Terminal half-life—
    Approximately 15 days.

**Peak plasma concentration**
Approximately 0.5 to 2 mcg per mL, following repeated doses of approximately 0.5 mg per kg per day.

**Elimination**
Renal—Very slow; 2 to 5% of a dose eliminated in biologically active form in urine; approximately 40% excreted over a 7-day period. May be detected in urine for at least 7 weeks after medication is discontinued.
Biliary—Minimal excretion of active form.
In dialysis—Poorly dialyzable.

## Precautions to Consider

### Carcinogenicity/Mutagenicity
Long-term studies in animals have not been done to evaluate the carcinogenic or mutagenic potential of amphotericin B.

### Pregnancy/Reproduction
Pregnancy—Amphotericin B crosses the placenta. Adequate and well-controlled studies in humans have not been done. However, no adverse fetal effects have been documented in numerous case reports where amphotericin B was used in all stages of pregnancy.
Studies in animals have not shown that amphotericin B causes adverse effects on the fetus.
FDA Pregnancy Category B.

### Breast-feeding
It is not known whether amphotericin B is excreted in breast milk. However, problems in humans have not been documented.

### Pediatrics
Appropriate studies on the relationship of age to the effects of amphotericin B have not been performed in the pediatric population. However, systemic fungal infections have been successfully treated in children and no pediatrics-specific problems have been documented to date.

### Geriatrics
No information is available on the relationship of age to the effects of amphotericin B in geriatric patients.

### Drug interactions and/or related problems
The following drug interactions and/or related problems have been selected on the basis of their potential clinical significance (possible mechanism in parentheses where appropriate)—not necessarily inclusive (» = major clinical significance):

Note: Combinations containing any of the following medications, depending on the amount present, may also interact with this medication.

Blood dyscrasia–causing medications (See *Appendix II*) or
» Bone marrow depressants (See *Appendix II*) or
» Radiation therapy
    (concurrent use of these medications or radiation therapy with amphotericin B may increase the chance of anemia or other hematologic effects; dosage reduction may be required)

Carbonic anhydrase inhibitors or
» Corticotropin (ACTH), especially with chronic use or
» Corticosteroids, glucocorticoid, especially with significant mineralocorticoid activity or
» Corticosteroids, mineralocorticoid or
    (concurrent use of these medications with parenteral amphotericin B may result in severe hypokalemia and should be undertaken with caution; patients should have serum potassium determinations at frequent intervals during concurrent therapy; cardiac function should also be monitored)

    (concurrent use of corticotropin with parenteral amphotericin B may decrease adrenocortical responsiveness to corticotropin)

» Digitalis glycosides or
Neuromuscular blocking agents, nondepolarizing
    (parenteral amphotericin B may induce hypokalemia, which may increase the potential for digitalis toxicity or enhance the blockade of nondepolarizing neuromuscular blocking agents)

    (serum potassium determinations and correction of hypokalemia may be necessary prior to administration of nondepolarizing neuromuscular blocking agents or at frequent intervals during concurrent therapy with digitalis glycosides)

» Diuretics, potassium-depleting or
» Nephrotoxic medications, other (See *Appendix II*)
    (concurrent use of diuretics and other nephrotoxic medications with amphotericin B may increase the potential for nephrotoxicity; dosage reduction or withdrawal of cyclosporine or amphotericin B may be necessary if renal impairment occurs. Concurrent use of diuretics with parenteral amphotericin B may also intensify electrolyte imbalance, particularly hypokalemia; frequent electrolyte determinations are necessary, and potassium supplementation may also be required)

Flucytosine
    (concurrent use of amphotericin B and flucytosine may have additive or slightly synergistic effects; amphotericin B–induced renal dysfunction may decrease the clearance of flucytosine, which may result in increased flucytosine adverse effects, such as bone marrow toxicity. However, 2-drug therapy may allow the total daily dose of amphotericin B to be lowered, decreasing the risk of nephrotoxicity)

### Medical considerations/Contraindications
The medical considerations/contraindications included here have been selected on the basis of their potential clinical significance (reasons given in parentheses where appropriate)—not necessarily inclusive (» = major clinical significance).

*Risk-benefit should be considered when the following medical problems exist:*
Hypersensitivity to amphotericin B
» Renal function impairment
    (although amphotericin B is not renally excreted, it can be nephrotoxic and worsen any pre-existing renal function impairment)

### Patient monitoring
The following may be especially important in patient monitoring (other tests may be warranted in some patients, depending on condition; » = major clinical significance):

» Blood urea nitrogen (BUN) and
» Creatinine, serum
    (concentrations recommended every other day while dosage is being increased and then at least twice weekly thereafter during therapy; if the BUN and/or the serum creatinine increase to clinically significant concentrations, discontinuation of the medication may be necessary until renal function is improved)

Complete blood count (CBC) and
Platelet count
    (recommended at weekly intervals during therapy)

Magnesium, serum and
» Potassium, serum
    (concentrations recommended twice weekly during therapy)

## Side/Adverse Effects

Note: Since amphotericin B is frequently the only effective treatment for certain potentially fatal fungal infections, its life-saving benefits must be balanced against its potential for dangerous side/adverse effects.

    Administration of an antipyretic, antihistamine, meperidine, and/or corticosteroid just prior to the amphotericin B infusion may decrease the fever and shaking chills that can be associated with amphotericin B administration.

The following side/adverse effects have been selected on the basis of their potential clinical significance (possible signs and symptoms in parentheses where appropriate)—not necessarily inclusive:

**Those indicating need for medical attention**
Incidence more frequent
    *With intravenous infusion*
    *Anemia* (unusual tiredness or weakness)—normocytic, normochromic; *hypokalemia* (irregular heartbeat; muscle cramps or pain; unusual tiredness or weakness); *infusion-related reaction* (fever and chills; nausea and vomiting; headache; hypotension); *renal function impairment* (increased or decreased urination); *thrombophlebitis* (pain at infusion site)

Incidence less frequent or rare

*With intravenous infusion*
**Blurred or double vision; cardiac arrhythmias** (irregular heartbeat)—usually with rapid infusion; **hypersensitivity** (skin rash; itching; shortness of breath; troubled breathing; wheezing; tightness in chest); **leukopenia** (sore throat and fever); **polyneuropathy** (numbness, tingling, pain, or weakness in hands or feet); **seizures; thrombocytopenia** (unusual bleeding or bruising)

*With intrathecal injection*
**Blurred vision or any change in vision; difficult urination; polyneuropathy** (numbness, tingling, pain, or weakness)

**Those indicating need for medical attention only if they continue or are bothersome**
Incidence more frequent

*With intravenous infusion*
**Gastrointestinal disturbance** (indigestion; loss of appetite; nausea; vomiting; diarrhea; stomach pain); **headache**

Incidence less frequent

*With intrathecal injection*
**Back, leg, or neck pain; dizziness or lightheadedness; headache; nausea or vomiting**

## Patient Consultation

As an aid to patient consultation, refer to *Advice for the Patient, Amphotericin B (Systemic).*

In providing consultation, consider emphasizing the following selected information (» = major clinical significance):

**Before using this medication**
» Conditions affecting use, especially:
Hypersensitivity to amphotericin B
Other medications, especially adrenocorticoids, corticotropin, other bone marrow depressants, digitalis glycosides, other nephrotoxic medications, potassium-depleting diuretics, or radiation therapy
Other medical problems, especially renal function impairment

**Side/adverse effects**
Signs of potential side effects, especially anemia, blurred or double vision, cardiac arrhythmias, difficult urination, hypersensitivity reactions, hypokalemia, infusion-related reaction, leukopenia, polyneuropathy, renal function impairment, seizures, thrombocytopenia, or thrombophlebitis

## General Dosing Information

Therapy interrupted for more than 7 days should be resumed by starting with the lowest dosage and gradually increasing to the desired dosage.

Therapy should be continued for a sufficient period of time to minimize the possibility of a relapse.

The intravenous administration of small doses of corticosteroids (i.e., ≤ 25 mg of hydrocortisone) just prior to or during intravenous infusion of amphotericin B may reduce the incidence of febrile reactions. Dosage and duration of concurrent corticosteroid therapy should be kept to a minimum. Also, acetaminophen, antihistamines, meperidine, and/or phenothiazines have been given empirically, just prior to the infusion, to decrease the nausea, fever, and chills associated with amphotericin B administration.

Amphotericin B should be infused over a period of 2 to 6 hours. In patients with normal renal function, rapid infusions of 1 to 2 hours have been used with infusion-related reactions similar to those associated with 4 to 6 hour infusions. However, rapid infusions have been associated with earlier infusion-related toxicity and more complaints of nausea and vomiting.

A cumulative dosage exceeding 4 grams may result in irreversible renal dysfunction.

Full dosage of amphotericin B is required even in patients with impaired renal function since the primary route of excretion is not renal. Patients should be observed closely if there is further loss of renal function. Nephrotoxicity may be decreased in sodium-depleted patients by salt loading prior to administration; however, routine prophylactic sodium loading is not recommended, especially in patients with underlying renal or cardiac disease.

Extravasation of the drug may cause severe local irritation.

To minimize local thrombophlebitis, which may occur with intravenous administration, heparin may be added to the amphotericin B infusion or the medication may be administered on alternate days. Administration on alternate days may also reduce the incidence of anorexia.

Alternate-day dosage should not exceed 1.5 mg per kg of body weight (mg/kg).

## Parenteral Dosage Forms

Note: The dosing and dosage forms available are expressed in terms of amphotericin B base.

### AMPHOTERICIN B FOR INJECTION USP

**Usual adult and adolescent dose**
Antifungal (systemic)—
Intracavitary instillation, initially 5 mg (base) in 10 to 20 mL of 5% dextrose injection administered over three to five minutes; then, 50 mg (base) of amphotericin B in 10 to 20 mL of 5% dextrose injection administered over three to five minutes each day. This is usually followed eight to twelve hours later by 20 mL of 5% N-acetylcysteine and overnight low-continuous wall suction.
Intrathecal, initially 0.01 to 0.1 mg (base) every forty-eight to seventy-two hours, the dosage being increased gradually to 0.5 mg as tolerated.
Intravenous infusion, initially 1 mg (base) as a test dose, administered in 20 to 50 mL of 5% dextrose injection over a period of ten to thirty minutes; the dosage may then be increased in 5- to 10-mg increments or more according to patient tolerance and severity of infection, up to a maximum of 50 mg per day, and administered over a period of two to six hours.
Note: In severely ill patients, some clinicians prefer to initiate therapy utilizing full dosage of amphotericin B.
Continuous bladder irrigation, 5 mg (base) of amphotericin B in 1000 mL of sterile water per day, administered at a rate of 40 mL per hour via a three-way catheter for five to ten days.

**Usual pediatric dose**
Antifungal (systemic)—
Intravenous infusion, initially 0.25 mg (base) per kg of body weight per day, administered in 5% dextrose injection over a period of six hours, the dosage being increased gradually (usually by 0.125 to 0.25 mg per kg of body weight increments every day or every other day) as tolerated, up to a maximum of 1 mg per kg of body weight or 30 mg per square meter of body surface per day.

**Size(s) usually available**
U.S.—
50 mg (base) (Rx) [*Amphocin; Fungizone Intravenous;* GENERIC].
Canada—
50 mg (base) (Rx) [*Fungizone Intravenous*].

**Packaging and storage**
Prior to reconstitution, store between 2 and 8 °C (36 and 46 °F). Protect from light.

**Preparation of dosage form**
To prepare initial dilution for intrathecal use or intravenous infusion, add 10 mL of sterile water for injection, without a bacteriostatic agent, to the vial containing 50 mg (base) of amphotericin B. For intrathecal use, the resulting solution containing 5 mg of amphotericin B per mL may be further diluted to a final concentration of 0.25 mg per mL by adding 1 mL (5 mg) of the solution to 19 mL of 5% dextrose injection with a pH above 4.2. Before injection, the dose is diluted with 5 to 30 mL of cerebrospinal fluid in the syringe. For intravenous infusion, the resulting solution containing 5 mg of amphotericin B per mL may be diluted to a final concentration of 0.1 mg per mL by adding 1 mL (5 mg) of the solution to 49 mL of 5% dextrose injection with a pH above 4.2.
The pH of the dextrose injection should be determined aseptically before the injection is used to dilute the 5-mg-per-mL concentration of the amphotericin B solution. If the pH is below 4.2, it should be adjusted. See the manufacturer's package insert for buffering procedure.
Amphotericin B should be reconstituted only with the diluents recommended, since solutions containing sodium chloride or a bacteriostatic agent (for example, benzyl alcohol) may cause precipitation of the medication.

**Stability**
After reconstitution, concentrated solutions (5 mg per mL) in sterile water for injection retain their potency for 24 hours at room temperature, protected from light, or for 1 week if refrigerated. Diluted solutions for intravenous infusion (0.1 mg per mL or less) in 5% dextrose injection should be used promptly after dilution.
The manufacturer recommends that the intravenous infusion be protected from light during administration. However, this is probably not necessary, since it has been reported that the loss of drug potency is negligible when amphotericin B infusions are exposed to normal lighting conditions in a hospital.

Do not use if the initial concentrate or the infusion is cloudy or contains a precipitate or foreign matter.

**Incompatibilities**
May be incompatible with sodium chloride or bacteriostatic agents such as benzyl alcohol.

**Additional information**
Since the reconstituted preparation is a colloidal suspension, membrane filters in intravenous infusion lines may remove clinically significant amounts of the medication. If an in-line membrane filter is used, the mean pore diameter should be no less than 1 micron.

Revised: 02/23/93
Interim revision: 04/19/95

# AMPHOTERICIN B    Topical†

VA CLASSIFICATION (Primary): DE102
Note: For a listing of dosage forms and brand names by country availability, see *Dosage Forms* section(s). For a listing of brand names for the articles in this monograph, refer to the General Index.

†Not commercially available in Canada.

## Category
Antifungal (topical).

## Indications
**Unaccepted**
Topical amphotericin B has been used for the topical treatment of cutaneous and mucocutaneous candidiasis caused by *Candida (Monilia)* species. However, in the opinion of most USP medical experts, it has been superseded by newer and more effective topical antifungal agents such as ciclopirox and the imidazoles (e.g., clotrimazole, econazole, miconazole).

Although topical amphotericin B exhibits some *in vitro* activity against ringworm, it has not demonstrated an effectiveness *in vivo*.

Topical amphotericin B has no significant effect either *in vitro* or clinically against viruses or gram-positive or gram-negative bacteria.

## Pharmacology/Pharmacokinetics
**Physicochemical characteristics**
Molecular weight—924.09.

**Mechanism of action/Effect**
Amphotericin B probably exerts its antifungal effects by binding to sterols in the fungus cell membrane, producing a change in membrane permeability that allows loss of potassium and small molecules from the cell.

## Precautions to Consider
**Pregnancy/Reproduction**
Pregnancy—Problems in humans have not been documented.

**Breast-feeding**
Problems in humans have not been documented.

**Pediatrics**
Appropriate studies on the relationship of age to the effects of amphotericin B topical preparations have not been performed in the pediatric population. However, pediatrics-specific problems that would limit the usefulness of this medication in children are not expected.

**Geriatrics**
Appropriate studies on the relationship of age to the effects of amphotericin B topical preparations have not been performed in the geriatric population. However, geriatrics-specific problems that would limit the usefulness of this medication in older persons are not expected.

**Medical considerations/Contraindications**
The medical considerations/contraindications included here have been selected on the basis of their potential clinical significance (reasons given in parentheses where appropriate)—not necessarily inclusive (» = major clinical significance).

*Risk-benefit should be considered when the following medical problem exists:*
Sensitivity to topical amphotericin B preparations

## Side/Adverse Effects
The following side/adverse effects have been selected on the basis of their potential clinical significance (possible signs and symptoms in parentheses where appropriate)—not necessarily inclusive:

**Those indicating need for medical attention**
Incidence less frequent
*Hypersensitivity or local irritation, especially in intertriginous areas* (burning, itching, redness or other signs of irritation not present before therapy)
Incidence rare
*Allergic contact dermatitis* (skin rash)

**Those indicating need for medical attention only if they continue or are bothersome**
Incidence less frequent
*Dryness of skin*—for cream dosage form

## Patient Consultation
As an aid to patient consultation, refer to *Advice for the Patient, Amphotericin B (Topical)*.

In providing consultation, consider emphasizing the following selected information (» = major clinical significance):

**Before using this medication**
» Conditions affecting use, especially:
   Sensitivity to amphotericin B

**Proper use of this medication**
   Applying sufficient medication to cover affected areas, and rubbing in gently
» Not applying an occlusive dressing or airtight covering over medication
» Compliance with full course of therapy, which may take several months or longer
» Proper dosing
   Missed dose: Applying as soon as possible
» Proper storage

**Precautions while using this medication**
   Checking with physician if no improvement within 1 to 2 weeks
   May stain skin or nails
   Cream or lotion form may stain clothing; removal of stain by handwashing clothing with soap and warm water
   Ointment form may stain clothing; removal of stain with standard cleaning fluid

**Side/adverse effects**
   Signs of potential side effects, especially hypersensitivity; local irritation, especially in intertriginous areas; and allergic contact dermatitis

## General Dosing Information
Use of topical antifungals may lead to skin sensitization, resulting in hypersensitivity reactions with subsequent topical or systemic use of the medication.

Therapy is usually necessary for a period of 1 to 3 weeks for intertriginous lesions; 1 to 2 weeks for candidiasis of the diaper area, perlèche, or glabrous skin lesions; 2 to 4 weeks for interdigital lesions or paronychia; and several months for onychomycoses that respond to treatment.

A single course of therapy may be sufficient, but additional courses may be necessary, especially in the treatment of interdigital lesions, paronychia, and onychomycoses.

Occlusive dressings should be avoided in the treatment of candidiasis since they provide conditions that favor the growth of yeast and the release of its irritating endotoxin.

# Topical Dosage Forms

## AMPHOTERICIN B CREAM USP

### Usual adult and adolescent dose
Candidiasis—
   Topical, to the skin, two to four times a day.

### Usual pediatric dose
See *Usual adult and adolescent dose.*

### Usual geriatric dose
See *Usual adult and adolescent dose.*

### Strength(s) usually available
U.S.—
   3% (Rx) [*Fungizone* (thimerosal; methylparaben; propylparaben; cetearyl alcohol)].
Canada—
   Not commercially available.

### Packaging and storage
Store below 40 °C (104 °F), preferably between 15 and 30 °C (59 and 86 °F), unless otherwise specified by manufacturer. Store in a collapsible tube or other well-closed container. Protect from freezing.

### Auxiliary labeling
• For external use only.
• Continue medication for full time of treatment.

### Note
Fabric stains caused by the cream may be removed with soap and warm water.

## AMPHOTERICIN B LOTION USP

### Usual adult and adolescent dose
See *Amphotericin B Cream USP.*

### Usual pediatric dose
See *Amphotericin B Cream USP.*

### Usual geriatric dose
See *Amphotericin B Cream USP.*

### Strength(s) usually available
U.S.—
   3% (Rx) [*Fungizone* (thimerosal; methylparaben; propylparaben; cetyl alcohol; stearyl alcohol)].
Canada—
   Not commercially available.

### Packaging and storage
Store below 40 °C (104 °F), preferably between 15 and 30 °C (59 and 86 °F), unless otherwise specified by manufacturer. Store in a well-closed container. Protect from freezing.

### Auxiliary labeling
• Shake gently.
• For external use only.
• Continue medication for full time of treatment.

### Note
Fabric stains caused by the lotion may be removed with soap and warm water.

## AMPHOTERICIN B OINTMENT USP

### Usual adult and adolescent dose
See *Amphotericin B Cream USP.*

### Usual pediatric dose
See *Amphotericin B Cream USP.*

### Usual geriatric dose
See *Amphotericin B Cream USP.*

### Strength(s) usually available
U.S.—
   3% (Rx) [*Fungizone*].
Canada—
   Not commercially available.

### Packaging and storage
Store below 40 °C (104 °F), preferably between 15 and 30 °C (59 and 86 °F), unless otherwise specified by manufacturer. Store in a collapsible tube or other well-closed container. Protect from freezing.

### Auxiliary labeling
• For external use only.
• Continue medication for full time of treatment.

### Note
Standard cleaning fluid may be used to remove fabric stains caused by the ointment.

Revised: 07/25/94

---

# AMPICILLIN—See *Penicillins (Systemic)*

---

# AMPICILLIN-CONTAINING COMBINATIONS—

Ampicillin and Sulbactam (Systemic)—See *Penicillins and Beta-lactamase Inhibitors (Systemic)*

---

# AMRINONE    Systemic

VA CLASSIFICATION (Primary): CV900

Note: For a listing of dosage forms and brand names by country availability, see *Dosage Forms* section(s). For a listing of brand names for the articles in this monograph, refer to the General Index.

---

## Category
Cardiotonic.

## Indications

### Accepted
Congestive heart failure (treatment)—Amrinone is indicated for the short-term management of congestive heart failure in patients who have not responded adequately to digitalis, diuretics, and/or vasodilators.

## Pharmacology/Pharmacokinetics

### Physicochemical characteristics
Molecular weight—187.20.

### Mechanism of action/Effect
Not precisely known; but seems to be peripheral vasodilation, reducing both preload and afterload, and possibly also direct stimulation of cardiac contractility (positive inotropic effect) as a result of phosphodiesterase inhibition.

### Other actions/effects
Slightly increases atrioventricular (AV) conduction velocity.

### Protein binding
Low to moderate (10 to 49%).

### Biotransformation
Hepatic.

### Half-life
Adults—
   Healthy volunteers: Approximately 3.6 hours.
   Congestive heart failure: Approximately 5.0 to 8.3 hours.
Neonates and infants—
   Less than 4 weeks: 12.7 to 22.2 hours.
   More than 4 weeks: 3.8 to 6.8 hours.

### Time to peak effect
Within 10 minutes.

### Duration of action
Dose-related—
   750 mcg (0.75 mg) per kg of body weight (mcg/kg): 30 minutes.
   3 mg per kg of body weight (mg/kg): 2 hours.

### Elimination
Renal—About 63%, as unchanged drug (10 to 40%) and metabolites.
Fecal—About 18%.

# Precautions to Consider

## Cross-sensitivity and/or related problems
Patients sensitive to bisulfites may also be sensitive to amrinone lactate injection, which contains sodium metabisulfite.

## Carcinogenicity
A 2-year study in rats found no evidence of carcinogenicity.

## Mutagenicity
Positive results were obtained in the mouse micronucleus test (at 7.5 to 10 times the maximum human dose) and in the Chinese hamster ovary chromosome aberration assay, indicating clastogenic potential and suppression of the number of polychromatic erythrocytes. However, negative results were obtained in the Ames Salmonella assay, mouse lymphoma study, and cultured human lymphocyte metaphase analysis.

## Pregnancy/Reproduction
Pregnancy—Adequate and well-controlled studies in humans have not been done.

Studies in New Zealand white rabbits at oral doses of 16 and 50 mg per kg of body weight (mg/kg) have shown that amrinone causes fetal skeletal and gross external malformations. These effects did not occur in French Hy/Cr rabbits at oral doses of 32 mg/kg per day or in rats receiving intravenous doses approximately equivalent to the recommended daily human dose.

In mutagenicity studies, gestation levels in rats were slightly prolonged at doses of 50 and 100 mg/kg per day. At the higher dose, dystocia occurred in dams and the incidence of stillbirths, decreased litter size, and poor pup survival was increased.

FDA Pregnancy Category C.

## Breast-feeding
It is not known whether amrinone is excreted in breast milk. However, problems in humans have not been documented.

## Pediatrics
Studies and case reports of amrinone use for pulmonary hypertension, congestive heart failure, and postoperative low cardiac output in approximately 30 neonates and infants and 6 children up to 24 months of age have not demonstrated pediatrics-specific problems that would limit the usefulness of amrinone in pediatric patients.

## Geriatrics
Although appropriate studies on the relationship of age to the effects of amrinone have not been performed in the geriatric population, no geriatrics-specific problems have been documented to date. However, elderly patients are more likely to have age-related renal function impairment, which may require adjustment of dosage in patients receiving amrinone.

## Laboratory value alterations
The following have been selected on the basis of their potential clinical significance (possible effect in parentheses where appropriate)—not necessarily inclusive (» = major clinical significance):

With physiology/laboratory test values
    Blood pressure and
    Potassium concentrations, serum
        (may be decreased)

    Hepatic enzymes
        (serum concentrations may be increased)

## Medical considerations/Contraindications
The medical considerations/contraindications included here have been selected on the basis of their potential clinical significance (reasons given in parentheses where appropriate)—not necessarily inclusive (» = major clinical significance).

*Except under special circumstances, this medication should not be used when the following medical problems exist:*
» Aortic or pulmonic valvular disease, severe
        (surgical relief of obstruction required)

*Risk-benefit should be considered when the following medical problems exist:*
    Hepatic function impairment
        (elimination reduced; dosage adjustment may be necessary)
» Hypertrophic cardiomyopathy
        (amrinone may aggravate outflow tract obstruction)
    Renal function impairment
        (elimination reduced; dosage adjustment may be necessary)
    Sensitivity to amrinone

## Patient monitoring
The following may be especially important in patient monitoring (other tests may be warranted in some patients, depending on condition; » = major clinical significance):
» Blood pressure and
» Heart rate
        (determinations at periodic intervals in patients receiving amrinone; amrinone infusion should be slowed or stopped in patients who develop an excessive fall in blood pressure)
» Body weight
        (determinations recommended at periodic intervals to confirm efficacy of amrinone)
    Cardiac index and
    Central venous pressure and
    Pulmonary capillary wedge pressure
        (determinations recommended at periodic intervals to confirm efficacy of amrinone)
    Hepatic function determinations and
    Renal function determinations and
    Serum electrolyte, especially potassium, concentrations
        (recommended at periodic intervals in patients receiving amrinone; hypokalemia secondary to improved cardiac output and resultant diuresis may contribute to risk of arrhythmias)
        (dosage adjustment may be necessary in patients with existing or developing renal or hepatic function impairment)
» Platelet counts
        (recommended prior to initiation and at periodic intervals during amrinone therapy. Dosage of amrinone may need to be reduced if thrombocytopenia occurs; in some cases, platelet levels stabilize with continuation at the same dose; any decision regarding a change in dosage should be based on monitoring of platelet counts; in some patients, withdrawal of amrinone may be necessary)

# Side/Adverse Effects
The following side/adverse effects have been selected on the basis of their potential clinical significance (possible signs and symptoms in parentheses where appropriate)—not necessarily inclusive:

## Those indicating need for medical attention
Incidence less frequent
    *Arrhythmias* (irregular heartbeat); *hypotension* (dizziness)
Incidence rare
    *Burning at site of injection; chest pain; hepatotoxicity* (yellow eyes or skin); *thrombocytopenia* (unusual bleeding or bruising; black, tarry stools; blood in urine or stools; pinpoint red spots on skin)
    Note: *Thrombocytopenia* occurs in about 2.4% of patients but is rarely symptomatic; more common with high doses or prolonged treatment.

## Those indicating need for medical attention only if they continue or are bothersome
Incidence less frequent or rare
    *Abdominal pain* (stomach pain); *fever; nausea or vomiting*

# Overdose
For more information on the management of overdose or unintentional ingestion, **contact a Poison Control Center** (see *Poison Contol Center Listing*).

## Treatment of overdose
Treatment of overdose consists of general measures for circulatory support.

# General Dosing Information
Pretreatment with digitalis is recommended in patients with atrial flutter/fibrillation since amrinone may increase ventricular response rates because of its slight enhancement of atrioventricular (AV) conduction.

Patients who have received vigorous diuretic therapy may need cautiously liberalized fluid and electrolyte intake to ensure an adequate cardiac filling pressure for response to amrinone.

Caution is recommended to avoid extravasation of amrinone infusion.

Tachyphylaxis to the hemodynamic effects of amrinone occurs commonly, usually within 72 hours of initiation of therapy.

# Parenteral Dosage Forms
Note: The dosing and strengths of the dosage forms available are expressed in terms of amrinone base (not the lactate salt).

## AMRINONE LACTATE INJECTION

### Usual adult dose

Initial—Intravenous, 750 mcg (0.75 mg) (base) per kg of body weight, undiluted, given slowly over 2 to 3 minutes; may be repeated after thirty minutes if necessary.

Maintenance—Intravenous infusion, 5 to 10 mcg (0.005 to 0.01 mg) (base) per kg of body weight per minute, the dosage being adjusted according to clinical response.

### Usual adult prescribing limits

Up to 10 mg (base) per kg of body weight per day, although some patients have been given doses up to 18 mg per kg per day for short durations.

### Usual pediatric dose

Neonates:

Initial: Intravenous, 3.0 to 4.5 mg per kg of body weight in divided doses.

Maintenance: Intravenous infusion, 3 mcg (0.003 mg) to 5 mcg (0.005 mg) per kg of body weight per minute.

Infants:

Initial: Intravenous, 3.0 to 4.5 mg per kg of body weight in divided doses.

Maintenance: Intravenous infusion, 10 mcg (0.01 mg) per kg of body weight per minute.

### Strength(s) usually available

U.S.—

5 mg (base) per mL (Rx) [*Inocor* (sodium metabisulphite)].

Canada—

5 mg (base) per mL (Rx) [*Inocor* (sodium metabisulphite)].

### Packaging and storage

Store below 40 °C (104 °F), preferably between 15 and 30 °C (59 and 86 °F), unless otherwise specified by manufacturer. Protect from light. Protect from freezing.

### Preparation of dosage form

For administration by intravenous infusion, amrinone lactate injection may be diluted in 0.45% or 0.9% sodium chloride injection, to produce a solution containing 1 to 3 mg of amrinone (base) per mL.

### Stability

Diluted solutions should be used within 24 hours.

### Incompatibilities

Amrinone lactate injection should not be diluted with solutions containing dextrose since a chemical interaction occurs, developing slowly over 24 hours. However, amrinone lactate injection may be injected into running dextrose infusions through a Y-connector or directly into the tubing where preferable.

Furosemide should not be administered in intravenous lines containing amrinone, since an immediate precipitate is formed.

## Selected Bibliography

Bottorff MB, Rutledge DR, Pieper JA. Evaluation of intravenous amrinone: the first of a new class of positive inotropic agents with vasodilator properties. Pharmacotherapy 1985; 5 (5): 227-37.

A symposium: amrinone. November 11, 1984, Miami, Florida. Am J Cardiol 1985 Jul 22; 56: 1B-42B.

Revised: 06/17/92

---

# AMYL NITRITE   Systemic

VA CLASSIFICATION (Primary): CV250

Note: For a listing of dosage forms and brand names by country availability, see *Dosage Forms* section(s). For a listing of brand names for the articles in this monograph, refer to the General Index.

## Category

Antianginal; antidote (to cyanide poisoning); diagnostic aid (cardiac function).

## Indications

Note: Bracketed information in the *Indications* section refers to uses that are not included in U.S. product labeling.

### Accepted

Angina pectoris, acute (treatment)—Amyl nitrite is indicated for treatment of attacks of acute angina pectoris. However, amyl nitrite is seldom used for this indication, and its use has generally been replaced by safer, less toxic, and more convenient antianginals such as the nitrates.

[Toxicity, cyanide (treatment)]—Amyl nitrite is used as an antidote in the treatment of cyanide poisoning.

[Cardiac function studies][1]—Amyl nitrite is used as a diagnostic aid for assessment of reserve cardiac function.

### Unaccepted

Amyl nitrite is abused to produce euphoria and as a sexual stimulant; these uses are associated with significant risk of toxicity and are not recommended.

---

[1]Not included in Canadian product labeling.

## Pharmacology/Pharmacokinetics

### Physicochemical characteristics

Molecular weight—117.15.

### Mechanism of action/Effect

Antianginal—Thought to be the result of a reduction in systemic and pulmonary arterial pressure (afterload) and decreased cardiac output because of peripheral vasodilation, rather than coronary artery dilation.

Antidote (to cyanide poisoning)—Amyl nitrite promotes formation of methemoglobin, which combines with cyanide to form nontoxic cyanmethemoglobin.

### Biotransformation

Hepatic.

### Onset of action

30 seconds.

### Duration of action

3 to 5 minutes.

### Elimination

Renal, approximately 33%.

## Precautions to Consider

### Cross-sensitivity and/or related problems

Patients sensitive to nitrates may be sensitive to this medication also, although the reaction is rare.

### Carcinogenicity

Studies in mice have found that amyl nitrite reacts with amines to form nitrosamines, which are carcinogenic.

### Pregnancy/Reproduction

Pregnancy—Studies have not been done in humans. However, reduction of maternal systemic blood pressure and blood flow to the placenta could result in harm to the fetus.

Studies have not been done in animals.

FDA Pregnancy Category X.

### Breast-feeding

It is not known whether amyl nitrite is excreted in breast milk. However, because of the potential for serious adverse effects in nursing infants, risk/benefit should be considered in the decision to nurse.

### Pediatrics

Appropriate studies on the relationship of age to the effects of amyl nitrite have not been performed in the pediatric population. Safety and efficacy have not been established.

### Geriatrics

Appropriate studies on the relationship of age to the effects of amyl nitrite have not been performed in the geriatric population. However, orthostatic hypotensive effects may be more likely to occur in the elderly, who are usually more sensitive to the effects of amyl nitrite.

### Drug interactions and/or related problems

The following drug interactions and/or related problems have been selected on the basis of their potential clinical significance (possible mechanism in parentheses where appropriate)—not necessarily inclusive (» = major clinical significance):

Note: Combinations containing any of the following medications, depending on the amount present, may also interact with this medication.

» Hypotension-producing medications, other (See *Appendix II*) (concurrent use may intensify the orthostatic hypotensive effects of amyl nitrite)

Norepinephrine (levarterenol)
(effects may be decreased when these medicines are used concurrently with amyl nitrite)

Sympathomimetics, such as phenylephrine, ephedrine, or epinephrine (concurrent use may reduce the antianginal effects of amyl nitrite; amyl nitrite may block the alpha-adrenergic effects of epinephrine, possibly resulting in severe hypotension and tachycardia)

**Laboratory value alterations**

The following have been selected on the basis of their potential clinical significance (possible effect in parentheses where appropriate)—not necessarily inclusive (» = major clinical significance):

With physiology/laboratory test values
Methemoglobin concentrations in blood
(may be increased by excessive doses of amyl nitrite)

**Medical considerations/Contraindications**

The medical considerations/contraindications included here have been selected on the basis of their potential clinical significance (reasons given in parentheses where appropriate)—not necessarily inclusive (» = major clinical significance).

*Risk-benefit should be considered when the following medical problems exist:*

» Anemia, severe
» Cerebral hemorrhage or
» Head trauma, recent
(amyl nitrite may increase cerebrospinal fluid pressure)

Glaucoma
(amyl nitrite may increase intraocular pressure)

» Hyperthyroidism
» Myocardial infarction, recent
(risk of hypotension and tachycardia with amyl nitrite treatment, which may aggravate ischemia)

Sensitivity to amyl nitrite or nitrates

**Patient monitoring**

The following may be especially important in patient monitoring (other tests may be warranted in some patients, depending on condition; » = major clinical significance):

Blood pressure determinations and
Cardiac function monitoring
(recommended at periodic intervals in patients using amyl nitrite regularly)

## Side/Adverse Effects

The following side/adverse effects have been selected on the basis of their potential clinical significance (possible signs and symptoms in parentheses where appropriate)—not necessarily inclusive:

**Those indicating need for medical attention**
Incidence rare
*Hemolytic anemia* (unusual tiredness or weakness); *skin rash*

**Those indicating need for medical attention only if they continue or are bothersome**
Incidence more frequent
*Flushing of face and neck; headache, mild; nausea or vomiting; orthostatic hypotension* (dizziness or lightheadedness, especially when getting up from a lying or sitting position); *restlessness; tachycardia* (fast pulse)

## Overdose

For more information on the management of overdose or unintentional ingestion, **contact a Poison Control Center** (see *Poison Control Center Listing*).

**Clinical effects of overdose**

The following effects have been selected on the basis of their potential clinical significance (possible signs and symptoms in parentheses where appropriate)—not necessarily inclusive:

*Cyanosis* (bluish-colored lips, fingernails, or palms of hands); *dizziness, extreme, or fainting; feeling of extreme pressure in head; shortness of breath; unusual tiredness or weakness; weak and fast heartbeat*

Note: *Cyanosis* may occur at blood methemoglobin concentrations of 1.5 grams per 100 mL. More pronounced signs occur at concentrations of 20 to 50 grams per 100 mL.

**Treatment of overdose**
Specific treatment—
For methemoglobinemia: Methemoglobin concentrations in blood should be monitored and methemoglobinemia treated with high-flow oxygen and intravenous methylene blue.
For hypotension: Hypotension may be treated by placing the patient in the head-down position; if pressor therapy is needed, epinephrine should be avoided since it aggravates the shock-like reaction.

## Patient Consultation

As an aid to patient consultation, refer to *Advice for the Patient, Amyl Nitrite (Systemic)*.

In providing consultation, consider emphasizing the following selected information (» = major clinical significance):

**Before using this medication**
» Conditions affecting use, especially:
Sensitivity to amyl nitrite or nitrates
Pregnancy—May reduce maternal systemic blood pressure and blood flow to placenta
Breast-feeding—Risk/benefit should be considered because of potential for serious adverse effects
Use in the elderly—Increased incidence of orthostatic hypotension
Other medications, especially other hypotension-producing medications
Other medical problems, especially severe anemia, cerebral hemorrhage, recent head trauma, hyperthyroidism, or recent myocardial infarction

**Proper use of this medication**
» Proper administration:
Crushing capsule between finger and thumb and holding up to nostrils
Inhaling 1 to 6 times
Remaining seated or lying down during administration because of possible dizziness
» Importance of not using more medication than the amount prescribed because of danger of overdose; notifying physician if reduced effect is observed
» Proper dosing
Relief usually occurs within 1 to 5 minutes—Dose may be repeated if pain not relieved in 5 minutes; calling physician or going to hospital emergency room if angina pain not relieved by 2 doses in 10 minutes
» Proper storage

**Precautions while using this medication**
» Flammable: Avoiding exposure to flame or heat
» Caution when getting up suddenly from a lying or sitting position
» Avoiding alcoholic beverages
Headache as a common effect

**Side/adverse effects**
Signs of potential side effects, especially hemolytic anemia, skin rash, and methemoglobinemia

## General Dosing Information

Tolerance of the antianginal effects of amyl nitrite is possible with prolonged use. To reduce development of tolerance, the smallest effective dose should be utilized and amyl nitrite may be alternated with other antianginal agents.

## Inhalation Dosage Forms

Note: Bracketed uses in the *Dosage Forms* section refer to categories of use and/or indications that are not included in U.S. product labeling.

**AMYL NITRITE INHALANT USP**

**Usual adult and adolescent dose**
Antianginal—
Inhalation, 0.18 or 0.3 mL (1 ampul); may be repeated in three to five minutes if necessary.
[Antidote (to cyanide poisoning)]—
Inhalation, as necessary, administered for thirty to sixty seconds every five minutes until the patient is conscious, then repeated at longer intervals for twenty-four hours.

**Size(s) usually available**
U.S.—
0.18 mL [GENERIC].
0.3 mL [GENERIC].
Canada—
0.3 mL [GENERIC].

**Packaging and storage**
Store below 40 °C (104 °F), preferably between 8 and 15 °C (46 and 59 °F), unless otherwise specified by manufacturer. Store in a tight container. Protect from light.

Note: Very flammable. Do not use amyl nitrite where it may be ignited.

**Auxiliary labeling**
• For inhalation only.

Revised: 04/12/93

# ANABOLIC STEROIDS    Systemic

This monograph includes information on the following: Nandrolone; Oxandrolone†; Oxymetholone; Stanozolol†.

VA CLASSIFICATION (Primary/Secondary):
    Nandrolone—HS100/AN900; BL400
    Oxandrolone—HS100
    Oxymetholone—HS100/BL400; IM900
    Stanozolol—HS100/BL400; IM900

Note: Controlled substances in the U.S.— Schedule III.

Note: For a listing of dosage forms and brand names by country availability, see *Dosage Forms* section(s). For a listing of brand names for the articles in this monograph, refer to the General Index.

†Not commercially available in Canada.

## Category

Note: All anabolic steroids are approximately equal in efficacy. Selection of a particular generic substance or dosage form is dependent upon the incidence of side effects, preferred route of administration, or the duration of action desired. Indications listed for individual generic products included are based on currently marketed product labeling.

Anabolic steroid—Nandrolone; Oxandrolone; Oxymetholone; Stanozolol.
Antianemic—Nandrolone; Oxymetholone; Stanozolol.
Antineoplastic—Nandrolone.
Antiangioedema (hereditary) agent—Oxymetholone; Stanozolol.

## Indications

Note: Bracketed information in the *Indications* section refers to uses that are not included in U.S. product labeling.

**Accepted**
Catabolic or tissue-depleting processes (treatment)—[Nandrolone decanoate, stanozolol], and oxandrolone are indicated in conditions such as chronic infections, extensive surgery, [corticosteroid-induced myopathy, decubitus ulcers, burns] , or severe trauma, which require reversal of catabolic processes or protein-sparing effects. These agents are adjuncts to, and not replacements for, conventional treatment of these disorders.

Anemia (treatment)—Nandrolone decanoate[1] is indicated for the treatment of anemia associated with renal insufficiency [and as adjuvant therapy for aplastic and sickle cell anemias] . Adequate iron intake is necessary for maximum therapeutic response.

[Nandrolone phenpropionate is indicated in the treatment of refractory deficient red cell production anemias. These may include aplastic anemia, myelofibrosis, myelosclerosis, agnogenic myeloid metaplasia, and hypoplastic anemias caused by malignancy or myelotoxic drugs. Anabolic steroid therapy should not replace other supportive measures.]

Oxymetholone is indicated in the treatment of bone marrow failure anemias and deficient red cell production anemias. Acquired and congenital aplastic anemias, myelofibrosis, and hypoplastic anemias due to myelotoxic medication often respond to oxymetholone. Oxymetholone should not replace other supportive measures such as transfusions; correction of iron, folic acid, vitamin $B_{12}$, or pyridoxine deficiency; antibacterial therapy; or the use of adrenocorticoids.

[Stanozolol is effective in raising hemoglobin levels in some cases of aplastic anemia (congenital or idiopathic).]

Carcinoma, breast (treatment)—Anabolic steroids such as [nandrolone decanoate] and nandrolone phenpropionate[1] are indicated as treatment for palliation of inoperable metastatic breast cancer in postmenopausal women. However, anabolic steroids should be considered for use only after inadequate response to newer, less toxic medications such as tamoxifen in hormonally responsive breast cancer. Anabolic steroids have also been used to treat breast cancer in premenopausal women who have undergone oophorectomy and are considered to have a hormone-responsive tumor.

Angioedema, hereditary (prophylaxis)—Stanozolol[1][and oxymetholone][1] are indicated in the prophylaxis of hereditary angioedema to decrease the frequency and severity of attacks.

[Angioedema, hereditary (treatment)][1]—Stanozolol and oxymetholone are used in the treatment of hereditary angioedema.

[Antithrombin III deficiency (treatment)] or
[Fibrinogen excess (treatment)]—Stanozolol is indicated in the treatment of conditions associated with decreased fibrinolytic activity due to antithrombin III deficiency or excess fibrinogen. These conditions may include cutaneous vasculitis, scleroderma of Raynaud's disease, vasculitis of Behcet's disease, and complications of deep vein thrombosis such as venous lipodermatosclerosis. Stanozolol is indicated in the prevention of recurrent venous thrombosis associated with antithrombin III deficiency. Stanozolol may be of benefit in patients susceptible to or with a history of thromboembolism for the treatment of vascular disorders associated with these forms of reduced fibrinolytic activity.

[Growth failure (treatment adjunct)]—Anabolic steroids may be used as an adjunct in the treatment of growth failure in children caused by pituitary growth hormone (GH) deficiency (pituitary dwarfism) or if the response to human growth hormone administration is inadequate.

[Turner's syndrome (treatment)]—Oxandrolone is used in the treatment of the short stature that accompanies Turner's syndrome (gonadal dysgenesis in females). Although the therapy is controversial, recent experimental reports seem to indicate that oxandrolone may be as effective as growth hormone and that oxandrolone may increase the efficacy of growth hormone therapy.

**Unaccepted**
Anabolic steroids have been used for the treatment of symptoms associated with osteoporosis. However, this use has largely been discontinued because the questionable efficacy of these agents for this indication does not justify the risk of serious adverse effects.

Oxandrolone and oxymetholone have been used for the treatment of alcoholic hepatitis with encephalopathy. However, there is currently insufficient evidence to establish the efficacy of these agents for this indication.

Use of anabolic steroids by athletes is not recommended. Objective evidence is conflicting and inconclusive as to whether these medications significantly increase athletic performance by increasing muscle strength. Weight gains reported by athletes are due in part to fluid retention, which is a potentially hazardous side effect of anabolic steroid therapy. The risk of other unwanted effects, such as testicular atrophy and suppression of spermatogenesis in males; menstrual disturbances and virilization, such as deepening of voice, development of acne, and unnatural growth of body hair in females; peliosis hepatis or other hepatotoxicity; and hepatic cancer outweigh any possible benefit received from anabolic steroids and make their use in athletes inappropriate.

[1]Not included in Canadian product labeling.

## Pharmacology/Pharmacokinetics

**Physicochemical characteristics**
Chemical group—
    Anabolic steroids are synthetic derivatives of testosterone, and as such have androgenic properties. The deletion of the $CH_3$ group from the C-19 position results in reduction of its androgenic properties and retention of its anabolic, tissue-building properties. Since complete dissociation of anabolic and androgenic effects is not possible, many of the actions of anabolic steroids are similar to those of androgens.
    The 17-alpha alkylated (oral methylated) anabolic steroids are oxandrolone, oxymetholone, and stanozolol.
Molecular weight—
    Nandrolone decanoate: 428.65.
    Nandrolone phenpropionate: 406.56.
    Oxandrolone: 306.44.
    Oxymetholone: 332.48.
    Stanozolol: 328.50.

## Mechanism of action/Effect

Anabolic steroid—

Reverses catabolic processes and negative nitrogen balance by promoting protein anabolism and stimulating appetite if there is concurrently a proper intake of calories and proteins.

Antianemic—

Anemias due to bone marrow failure: Increases production of erythropoietin.

Anemias due to deficient red cell production: Stimulates erythropoietin production and may have a direct action on bone marrow.

Anemias associated with renal disease: Increases hemoglobin and red blood cell volume.

Angioedema (hereditary) prophylactic—

Increases serum concentration of C1 esterase inhibitor and, as a result, C2 and C4 concentrations.

## Half-life

Oxandrolone:

Biphasic:

1st phase—0.55 hours.

2nd phase—9 hours.

## Time to peak serum concentration

Nandrolone decanoate intramuscular—100-mg dose: 3 to 6 days.

Nandrolone phenpropionate intramuscular—100-mg dose: 1 to 2 days.

## Elimination

Oxandrolone—Renal; small amount fecal.

# Precautions to Consider

## Carcinogenicity

Hepatocellular carcinoma has been associated rarely with long-term, high-dose anabolic steroid therapy.

## Tumorigenicity

Hepatic neoplasms have been associated rarely with long-term, high-dose anabolic steroid therapy.

## Mutagenicity

For oxandrolone—Animal or *in vitro* mutagenicity studies have not been done.

For stanozolol—Animal studies have not been done.

## Pregnancy/Reproduction

Pregnancy—Anabolic steroids are not recommended for use during pregnancy, since studies in animals have shown that anabolic steroids cause masculinization of the fetus. Risk-benefit must be carefully considered.

For oxandrolone: Animal studies have also shown oxandrolone to cause embryotoxicity, fetotoxicity, and infertility, in addition to masculinization, in offspring of animals receiving 9 times the human dose.

FDA Pregnancy Category X.

## Breast-feeding

It is not known whether anabolic steroids are distributed into breast milk. Problems in humans have not been documented. However, anabolic steroids are rarely used by lactating women.

## Pediatrics

Anabolic steroids should be used with caution in children and adolescents because of possible premature epiphyseal closure, precocious sexual development in males, and virilization in females. The epiphyseal maturation may be accelerated more rapidly than linear growth in children, and the effect may continue for 6 months after the medication has been discontinued.

For stanozolol—The safety and efficacy of stanozolol in children with hereditary angioedema have not been established. Attacks of hereditary angioedema may include symptoms such as life-threatening upper respiratory obstruction with or without severe gastrointestinal colic, but are generally infrequent in childhood. The risks from stanozolol therapy are substantially increased with long-term use. Therefore, long-term administration of stanozolol is generally not recommended in children, and should not be undertaken without consideration of risk-benefit involved and close follow-up for endocrine effects.

## Geriatrics

Treatment of geriatric male patients with anabolic steroids may cause increased risk of prostatic hyperplasia or prostatic carcinoma.

## Drug interactions and/or related problems

The following drug interactions and/or related problems have been selected on the basis of their potential clinical significance (possible mechanism in parentheses where appropriate)—not necessarily inclusive (» = major clinical significance):

Note: Combinations containing any of the following medications, depending on the amount present, may also interact with this medication.

Adrenocorticoids, glucocorticoid, especially with significant mineralocorticoid activity or

Adrenocorticoids, mineralocorticoid or

Corticotropin, especially prolonged therapeutic use or

Sodium-containing medications or foods

(concurrent use with anabolic steroids may increase the possibility of edema; in addition, concurrent use of glucocorticoids or corticotropin with anabolic steroids may promote development of severe acne)

» Anticoagulants, coumarin- or indandione-derivative or

Anti-inflammatory analgesics, nonsteroidal or

Salicylates, in therapeutic doses

(anticoagulant effect may be increased during concurrent use with anabolic steroids, especially 17-alpha-alkylated compounds, because of decreased procoagulant factor concentration caused by alteration of procoagulant factor synthesis or catabolism and increased receptor affinity for the anticoagulant; anticoagulant dosage adjustment based on prothrombin time determinations may be required during and following concurrent use)

Antidiabetic agents, sulfonylurea or

Insulin

(anabolic steroids may decrease blood glucose concentration; diabetic patients should be closely monitored for signs of hypoglycemia and dosage of hypoglycemic agent adjusted if necessary)

» Hepatotoxic medications, other (See *Appendix II* )

(concurrent use with anabolic steroids may result in an increased incidence of hepatotoxicity; patients, especially those on prolonged administration or those with a history of liver disease, should be carefully monitored)

Somatrem or

Somatropin

(concurrent use of anabolic steroids with somatrem or somatropin may accelerate epiphyseal maturation)

## Laboratory value alterations

The following have been selected on the basis of their potential clinical significance (possible effect in parentheses where appropriate)—not necessarily inclusive (» = major clinical significance):

With diagnostic test results

Fasting blood sugar and

Glucose tolerance test and

Metyrapone test

(may be altered)

Thyroid function tests

(radioactive iodine uptake and thyroxine-binding capacity [TBC] may be decreased; the decreased levels of thyroxine-binding globulin result in decreased total $T_3$ and $T_4$ serum levels and increased resin uptake of $T_3$ and $T_4$; altered tests usually persist for 2 to 3 weeks after stopping therapy)

With physiology/laboratory test values

Alanine aminotransferase (ALT [SGPT]) and

Alkaline phosphatase and

Aspartate aminotransferase (AST [SGOT]) and

Bilirubin and

Calcium, chloride, inorganic phosphates, potassium, and sodium

(serum concentrations may be increased)

Clotting factors II, V, VII, and X concentrations

(may be decreased)

Creatine and creatinine excretion

(may be increased; effect usually lasts up to 2 weeks after therapy is discontinued)

Lipoproteins, high-density and

Lipoproteins, low-density

(high-density lipoprotein concentration may be lowered; low-density lipoprotein concentration may be elevated)

Prothrombin time

(may be increased)

Serum lipid, especially triglyceride, concentrations and

Urinary 17-ketosteroid (17-KS) excretion

(may be decreased)

## Medical considerations/Contraindications

The medical considerations/contraindications included here have been selected on the basis of their potential clinical significance (reasons given in parentheses where appropriate)—not necessarily inclusive (» = major clinical significance).

*Except under special circumstances, these medications should not be used when the following medical problems exist:*

» Breast cancer, disseminated, in females with active hypercalcemia
» Breast cancer in males
» Hepatic function impairment, severe
» Hypercalcemia, active or history of
    (may be exacerbated or recurrence may result)
» Nephrosis or nephrotic phase of nephritis
» Prostate cancer
    (tumor growth may be promoted)

*Risk-benefit should be considered when the following medical problems exist:*

Cardiac function impairment or
Hepatic function impairment or
Renal function impairment
    (use of these medications may cause retention of sodium and water, resulting in edema, with or without congestive heart failure)
» Coronary artery disease, history of or
» Myocardial infarction, history of
    (because of hypercholesterolemic effects of anabolic steroids)
Diabetes mellitus
    (anabolic steroids may decrease blood sugar concentrations; insulin or oral hypoglycemic dosage may need to be adjusted)
Intolerance to anabolic steroids or androgens
Prostatic hyperplasia, benign
    (further enlargement may occur)

## Patient monitoring

The following may be especially important in patient monitoring (other tests may be warranted in some patients, depending on condition; » = major clinical significance):

Calcium
    (measurement of serum concentrations recommended at regular intervals during anabolic steroid therapy in females with breast cancer)
» Cholesterol
    (measurement of serum concentrations recommended at regular intervals during therapy because of possible decreased high-density lipoprotein and increased low-density lipoprotein, which may increase the risk of atherosclerosis)
» Hepatic function determinations
    (recommended at regular intervals during therapy because of possibility of hepatic dysfunction, peliosis hepatis, and liver cell tumors, especially with 17-alpha-alkylated compounds, which are more likely to cause hepatic dysfunction)
Iron and total iron-binding capacity (TIBC) determinations, serum
    (recommended at regular intervals during therapy because of possible iron deficiency anemia manifested by low serum iron and decrease in percentage of transferrin saturation)
X-ray studies
    (recommended at 6-month intervals in children and adolescents to monitor bone age in order to prevent the risk of compromising adult height)

## Side/Adverse Effects

Note: Peliosis hepatis and hepatic neoplasms, including hepatocellular carcinoma, have been associated with long-term, high-dose anabolic steroid therapy. These adverse reactions can be life-threatening or fatal.

The following side/adverse effects have been selected on the basis of their potential clinical significance (possible signs and symptoms in parentheses where appropriate)—not necessarily inclusive:

### Those indicating need for medical attention
Incidence more frequent

*In females only*
**Virilism** (acne or oily skin; enlarging clitoris; hoarseness or deepening of voice; menstrual irregularities; unnatural hair growth or loss)
    Note: *Enlarging clitoris, hoarseness or deepening of voice,* and *unnatural hair growth or loss* usually are not reversible even after prompt discontinuance of therapy. The concurrent use of estrogens will not prevent virilization in females.

*In prepubertal males only*
**Virilism** (acne; enlarging penis; increased frequency of erections; unnatural hair growth)

*In postpubertal males only*
**Bladder irritability** (frequent urge to urinate); **breast soreness; gynecomastia** (enlargement of breasts); **priapism** (frequent or continuing erections)

Incidence less frequent

*In both females and males*
**Anemia, iron deficiency** (loss of appetite; sore tongue); **edema** (swelling of feet or lower legs; rapid weight gain); **gastric irritation** (nausea; vomiting); **hepatic dysfunction** (yellow eyes or skin); **leukemia** (bone pain); **suppression of clotting factors** (unusual bleeding)

*In females only*
**Hypercalcemia** (mental depression; nausea; vomiting; unusual tiredness)

*In prepubertal males only*
**Unexplained darkening of skin**

*In geriatric males only*
**Prostatic carcinoma or prostatic hyperplasia** (difficult or frequent urination)

Incidence rare—with prolonged therapy

*In both females and males*
**Hepatic necrosis** (black, tarry stools; continuing feeling of discomfort; continuing headache; continuing unpleasant breath odor; vomiting of blood); **hepatocellular carcinoma** (abdominal or stomach pain; unexplained weight loss); **peliosis hepatis** (continuing loss of appetite; dark-colored urine; fever; hives; light-colored stools; nausea and vomiting; purple- or red-colored spots on body or inside the mouth or nose; sore throat)

### Those indicating need for medical attention only if they continue or are bothersome
Incidence more frequent

*In males only*
**Acne**

Incidence less frequent

*In both females and males*
**Chills; decrease or increase in libido; diarrhea; feeling of abdominal or stomach fullness; muscle cramps; trouble in sleeping**

*In males only*
**Decreased sexual ability**

## Overdose

For more information on the management of overdose or unintentional ingestion, **contact a Poison Control Center** (see *Poison Control Center Listing*).

The following effects have been selected on the basis of their potential clinical significance (possible signs and symptoms in parentheses where appropriate)—not necessarily inclusive:
    **Hepatotoxicity**

### Treatment of overdose
Treatment of overdose is symptomatic and supportive.

To decrease absorption—In acute oral overdose, decontamination includes induced emesis and/or gastric lavage.

Monitoring—Hepatic function.

## Patient Consultation

As an aid to patient consultation, refer to *Advice for the Patient, Anabolic Steroids (Systemic).*

In providing consultation, consider emphasizing the following selected information (» = major clinical significance):

### Before using this medication
» Conditions affecting use, especially:
    Carcinogenicity—Hepatocellular carcinoma associated with long-term, high-dose therapy
    Tumorigenicity—Hepatic neoplasms associated with long-term, high-dose therapy
    Pregnancy—Not recommended during pregnancy because of possible masculinization of fetus
    Use in children—Cautious use because of effects on growth and sexual development (precocious sexual development in males, virilization in females)
    Use in the elderly—Increased risk of prostatic hyperplasia or prostatic carcinoma
    Other medications, especially anticoagulants (coumarin- or indandione-derivatives) or hepatotoxic medications
    Other medical problems, especially breast cancer, coronary artery disease, hepatic function impairment, hypercalcemia, myocar-

dial infarction, nephrosis, nephrotic phase of nephritis, or prostatic cancer

**Proper use of this medication**

» Importance of not taking more medication than the amount prescribed; to do so may increase chance of side effects

» Importance of diet high in proteins and calories while taking this medication to achieve maximum therapeutic effect

» Proper dosing
Missed dose: If dosing schedule is
Once daily: Taking as soon as possible; if not remembered until next day, not taking at all; not doubling doses
More than once daily: Taking as soon as possible; not taking if almost time for next dose; not doubling doses

» Proper storage

**Precautions while using this medication**

Regular visits to physician to check progress during therapy
Diabetics: May decrease blood sugar concentrations

**Side/adverse effects**

*Signs of potential side effects, especially:*

In females only—Virilism or hypercalcemia

In prepubertal males only—Virilism or unexplained darkening of skin

In postpubertal males only—Bladder irritability, breast soreness, gynecomastia, or priapism

In geriatric males only—Prostatic carcinoma or prostatic hyperplasia

In all patients, in addition to those side effects listed above—Anemia, iron deficiency; edema; gastric irritation; hepatic dysfunction, necrosis, or carcinoma; leukemia; suppression of clotting factors; or peliosis hepatis

# General Dosing Information

Many of the side/adverse effects of anabolic steroids are dose related; therefore, patients should be placed on the lowest possible effective dose.

A well-balanced diet that provides adequate proteins and calories should accompany all anabolic steroid therapy to achieve a maximum therapeutic effect.

---

## *NANDROLONE*

## Summary of Differences

Category:
Nandrolone decanoate—Antianemic.
Nandrolone phenpropionate—Antineoplastic.
Indications:
Nandrolone decanoate is indicated in the treatment of anemia associated with renal insufficiency.
Nandrolone phenpropionate is indicated in the treatment of metastatic breast cancer in women.

## Additional Dosing Information

See also *General Dosing Information.*

Nandrolone injections should be administered intramuscularly, preferably deep into the gluteal muscle.

When using nandrolone decanoate injection, an adequate iron intake is required for maximum response.

## Parenteral Dosage Forms

### NANDROLONE DECANOATE INJECTION USP

**Usual adult and adolescent dose**
Females—Intramuscular, 50 to 100 mg given at one- to four-week intervals.
Males—Intramuscular, 50 to 200 mg given at one- to four-week intervals.
Note: When given at three- to four-week intervals, therapy may be continued for up to 12 weeks. If necessary, cycle may be repeated if second course is preceded by a four-week rest period.

In the treatment of severe disease states, such as metastatic breast cancer and refractory anemias, a higher dose, based on therapeutic response and the benefit-to-risk ratio, may be required.

**Usual pediatric dose**
Children up to 2 years of age—Dosage has not been established.
Children 2 to 13 years of age—Intramuscular, 25 to 50 mg every three to four weeks.
Children 14 years of age and over—See *Usual adult and adolescent dose.*

**Strength(s) usually available**
U.S.—
50 mg per mL (Rx) [*Deca-Durabolin; Hybolin Decanoate; Kabolin; Neo-Durabolic;* GENERIC].
100 mg per mL (Rx) [*Deca-Durabolin; Hybolin Decanoate; Neo-Durabolic;* GENERIC].
200 mg per mL (Rx) [*Deca-Durabolin; Neo-Durabolic;* GENERIC].
Canada—
50 mg per mL (Rx) [*Deca-Durabolin* (benzyl alcohol 10%; sesame oil)].
100 mg per mL (Rx) [*Deca-Durabolin* (benzyl alcohol 10%; sesame oil)].

**Packaging and storage**
Store below 40 °C (104 °F), preferably between 15 and 30 °C (59 and 86 °F), unless otherwise specified by manufacturer. Protect from light. Protect from freezing.

### NANDROLONE PHENPROPIONATE INJECTION USP

**Usual adult dose**
Intramuscular, 25 to 100 mg per week.
Note: Therapy may be continued for up to 12 weeks. If necessary, cycle may be repeated if second course is preceded by a four-week rest period.

**Usual pediatric dose**
Dosage has not been established.

**Strength(s) usually available**
U.S.—
25 mg per mL (Rx) [*Durabolin;* GENERIC].
50 mg per mL (Rx) [*Durabolin; Hybolin-Improved;* GENERIC].
Canada—
25 mg per mL (Rx) [*Durabolin* (benzyl alcohol 5%; sesame oil)].
50 mg per mL (Rx) [*Durabolin* (benzyl alcohol 10%; sesame oil)].

**Packaging and storage**
Store below 40 °C (104 °F), preferably between 15 and 30 °C (59 and 86 °F), unless otherwise specified by manufacturer. Protect from light. Protect from freezing.

---

## *OXANDROLONE*

## Summary of Differences

Indications: Indicated in the treatment of catabolic or tissue-depleting processes.

## Additional Dosing Information

See also *General Dosing Information.*

In adults, 2 to 4 weeks of therapy are usually adequate. In both adults and children, therapy may be repeated intermittently as needed.

## Oral Dosage Forms

Note: Bracketed uses in the *Dosage Forms* section refer to categories of use and/or indications that are not included in U.S. product labeling.

### OXANDROLONE TABLETS USP

**Usual adult and adolescent dose**
Oral, 2.5 mg two to four times a day.
Note: The dosage may range from 2.5 to 20 mg per day.

**Usual pediatric dose**
Children—Oral, 250 mcg (0.25 mg) per kg of body weight per day.
[Turner's syndrome]—
Oral, 50 mcg to 125 mcg (0.05 to 0.125 mg) per kg of body weight per day. Generally, the patient should be started and maintained on the lowest effective dose to minimize the potential for adverse effects.

**Strength(s) usually available**
U.S.—
2.5 mg (Rx) [*Oxandrin* (scored; lactose)].
Canada—
Not commercially available.

**Packaging and storage**
Store below 40 °C (104 °F), preferably between 15 and 30 °C (59 and 86 °F), unless otherwise specified by manufacturer. Store in a tight, light-resistant container.

---

## OXYMETHOLONE

### Summary of Differences

Category: Antianemic; angioedema (hereditary) agent.

Indications: Indicated in treatment of bone marrow failure anemias and in deficient red cell production anemias; also used in prophylaxis and treatment of hereditary angioedema.

### Additional Dosing Information

See also *General Dosing Information.*

Oxymetholone should be used for a minimum of 3 to 6 months, since a response is not always immediately observed.

Following remission of the anemia, some patients may be maintained without oxymetholone while others may be maintained on a low daily dose. Patients with congenital aplastic anemia usually require continued therapy with an appropriate maintenance dose.

### Oral Dosage Forms

#### OXYMETHOLONE TABLETS USP

**Usual adult and adolescent dose**

Oral, 1 to 5 mg per kg of body weight per day.

Note:  The usual effective dose is 1 to 2 mg per kg of body weight a day, but higher doses may be required in some patients. Treatment of refractory anemias may require 3 to 6 months.

**Usual pediatric dose**

Premature infants and neonates—Oral, 175 mcg (0.175 mg) per kg of body weight or 5 mg per square meter of body surface area per day as a single dose.

Infants and children—See *Usual adult and adolescent dose.*

**Strength(s) usually available**

U.S.—

50 mg (Rx) [*Anadrol-50* (scored; lactose)].

Canada—

50 mg (Rx) [*Anapolon 50* (scored; lactose)].

**Packaging and storage**

Store below 40 °C (104 °F), preferably between 15 and 30 °C (59 and 86 °F), unless otherwise specified by manufacturer. Store in a well-closed container.

---

## STANOZOLOL

### Summary of Differences

Category: Angioedema (hereditary) prophylactic.

Indications: Stanozolol is indicated in the prophylaxis of hereditary angioedema to decrease the frequency and severity of attacks and used in treatment of hereditary angioedema.

### Oral Dosage Forms

#### STANOZOLOL TABLETS USP

**Usual adult and adolescent dose**

Oral, 2 mg three times a day to 4 mg four times a day for 5 days, initially.

Note:  A dose of 2 mg two times a day may be used in young women, who are particularly susceptible to the androgenic effects of stanozolol.

The dosage for continuous treatment of hereditary angioedema should be individualized according to patient response. After a favorable response is obtained, the dose should be decreased at intervals of 1 to 3 months to a maintenance dose of 2 mg a day; some patients may respond to a maintenance dose of 2 mg every other day. During the dose-reduction phase, close monitoring of patient response is indicated, especially if the patient has a history of upper respiratory tract involvement.

**Usual pediatric dose**

Children up to 6 years of age—Oral, 1 mg a day, to be administered only during an attack.

Children 6 to 12 years of age—Oral, up to 2 mg a day, to be administered only during an attack.

**Strength(s) usually available**

U.S.—

2 mg (Rx) [*Winstrol* (scored; lactose)].

Canada—

Not commercially available.

**Packaging and storage**

Store below 40 °C (104 °F), preferably between 15 and 30 °C (59 and 86 °F), unless otherwise specified by manufacturer. Store in a tight, light-resistant container.

---

Revised: 06/20/92
Interim revision: 06/08/94

---

# ANDROGENS   Systemic

This monograph includes information on the following: Fluoxymesterone; Methyltestosterone; Testosterone.

VA CLASSIFICATION (Primary/Secondary):
Fluoxymesterone—HS100/AN900; BL400
Methyltestosterone—HS100/AN900
Testosterone—HS100/AN900
Testosterone cypionate—HS100/AN900; BL400
Testosterone enanthate—HS100/AN900; BL400
Testosterone propionate—HS100/AN900

Note:  Androgens are controlled substances in the U.S.—Schedule III

Note:  For a listing of dosage forms and brand names by country availability, see *Dosage Forms* section(s). For a listing of brand names for the articles in this monograph, refer to the General Index.

## Category

Androgen—Fluoxymesterone; Methyltestosterone; Testosterone.

Antineoplastic—Fluoxymesterone; Methyltestosterone; Testosterone.

Antianemic—Fluoxymesterone; Testosterone Cypionate; Testosterone Enanthate.

## Indications

Note:  Bracketed information in the *Indications* section refers to uses that are not included in U.S. product labeling.

**Accepted**

Androgen deficiency (treatment)—Androgens are primarily indicated in males as replacement therapy when endogenous androgen absence or

deficiency is associated with primary hypogonadal conditions such as testicular failure due to cryptorchidism, bilateral torsion, orchitis, or vanishing testis syndrome; inborn errors in testosterone biosynthesis; bilateral orchidectomy; hypogonadotropic hypogonadism (gonadotropin releasing hormone (GnRH) deficiency; or pituitary-hypothalamic injury from surgery, tumors, trauma, or radiation. Methyltestosterone, [testosterone cypionate] , [testosterone enanthate] , and [fluoxymesterone] are also used as replacement therapy in impotence or for male climacteric symptoms when these conditions are due to a measured or documented androgen deficiency. For long-term therapy, testosterone or a testosterone ester is preferred over the oral methylated androgens (fluoxymesterone and methyltestosterone), which increase the risk of hepatotoxicity.

Puberty, delayed male (treatment)—Short-term (≤ 6 months) therapy with androgens may be used to stimulate puberty when delayed puberty is not secondary to a pathological disorder and is expected to occur spontaneously at a relatively late date, and when the patient does not respond to interval psychological support.

Carcinoma, breast (treatment)—Androgens are indicated as secondary or tertiary hormonal treatment for palliation of metastatic breast cancer in women who have hormone receptor-positive tumors or who have previously demonstrated a response to hormone therapy. Androgens have also been used in the treatment of metastatic breast cancer as a supplement to chemotherapy.

[Anemia (treatment)]—Fluoxymesterone and testosterone cypionate or enanthate have been used to treat certain types of anemia. Fluoxymesterone is indicated in the treatment of refractory deficient red cell production anemias. These may include aplastic anemia, myelofibrosis, myelosclerosis, agnogenic myeloid metaplasia, and hypoplastic anemias caused by malignancy or myelotoxic drugs.

[Constitutional delay in growth (treatment)][1]—Androgens are used in the treatment of constitutional delay in growth. However, they are no longer considered the treatment of first choice for most patients.

[Gender change, female-to-male][1]—Testosterone is used for the development and maintenance of secondary sexual characteristics in female-to-male transsexuals.

[Lichen sclerosus (treatment adjunct)][1]—Extemporaneously compounded topical testosterone is used for the treatment of itching resulting from lichen sclerosus.

[Microphallus (treatment)][1]—Intramuscular preparations of testosterone and testosterone esters, and extemporaneously compounded topical testosterone are used in the treatment of microphallus.

### Unaccepted

Use of androgens to enhance athletic performance is illegal. Increases in muscle mass and muscle strength can be sufficient to enhance athletic performance. However, the risk of other unwanted effects, such as suppression of spermatogenesis, testicular atrophy, menstrual disturbances, virilization in females, peliosis hepatis, hepatotoxicity, potential adverse effects on cardiovascular health and hepatic cancer counter athletic benefits received from androgens and make their use in athletes inappropriate. Additionally, behavioral disturbances, including aggressive or violent behavior, have been reported with supraphysiological self-administered doses in athletes.

The use of androgens for the prevention of postpartum breast engorgement is not recommended. In many patients, postpartum breast engorgement is a benign, self-limited condition that may respond to breast support and mild analgesics, such as acetaminophen and ibuprofen. Evidence supporting the efficacy of androgens for this indication is lacking.

Androgens are not recommended for adjunctive treatment of osteoporosis or in the treatment of vasomotor symptoms of menopause, menorrhagia, or female hypoactive sexual desire disorder.

[1]Not included in Canadian product labeling.

## Pharmacology/Pharmacokinetics

### Physicochemical characteristics
Chemical group—
   Naturally occurring androgens include testosterone.
   Semi-synthetic androgens are testosterone cypionate, testosterone enanthate, and testosterone propionate.
   Synthetic androgens include fluoxymesterone and methyltestosterone.
   Oral methylated androgens (17-alpha-alkylated androgens) include fluoxymesterone and methyltestosterone.
Molecular weight—
   Fluoxymesterone: 336.45.
   Methyltestosterone: 302.46.
   Testosterone: 288.43.
   Testosterone cypionate: 412.61.
   Testosterone enanthate: 400.60.
   Testosterone propionate: 344.49.

### Mechanism of action/Effect
Androgen—
   Androgen secretion is regulated by gonadotropins. Androgens are responsible for stimulation of spermatogenesis, development of male secondary sex characteristics, and stimulation of sexual maturation at puberty. Androgens are highly lipid soluble and enter cells of target tissues by passive diffusion. Within the cells of the target tissues, testosterone is converted by the enzyme 5-alpha reductase to 5 alpha-dihydrotestosterone (DHT). Testosterone and DHT bind to cytosolic receptors, which are loosely bound to sites in the cell nucleus. The steroid receptor complex initiates transcription, resulting in an increase in protein production. Increased serum concentrations of androgens suppress gonadotropin-releasing hormone (GnRH), luteinizing hormone (LH), and follicle-stimulating hormone (FSH) through a negative feedback mechanism involving the hypothalamus and anterior pituitary.
   Microphallus: Intramuscular administration of testosterone or testosterone esters or local application of testosterone propionate ointment may result in an increase in circulating serum concentrations of DHT, which is principally responsible for phallic growth.
   Lichen sclerosus: The signs and symptoms of lichen sclerosus (vulvar itching, abnormal vulvar skin histology) may be the result of a deficiency of 5-alpha reductase activity and subsequently reduced local DHT concentrations. Local application of testosterone propionate ointment may correct this deficiency in 5-alpha reductase

activity. Testosterone may cause a slight increase in local DHT concentrations, which may induce 5-alpha reductase activity, and increase local DHT concentrations.
Antianemic—
   Stimulates production of red blood cells by enhancing production of erythropoietic stimulating factors.

### Absorption
Methyltestosterone—
   Absorbed from oral mucosa and gastrointestinal tract.
Testosterone—
   Oral:
      Rapidly absorbed from gastrointestinal tract. Also absorbed from oral mucosa. Clinically significant serum testosterone concentrations in target organs are not possible with oral administration because of extensive first-pass metabolism.
   Transdermal:
      Testosterone mean steady state area-under-the-curve (AUC) at 24 hours was 9132 nanograms/dL (0.312 micromoles/L) and dihydrotestosterone (DHT) mean serum concentrations ranged from 134 to 162 nanograms/dL (5.2 to 6.3 nanomoles/L) in hypogonadal men with 6 mg-dose. Normal DHT serum concentrations range from 30 to 85 nanograms/dL (1.2 to 3.3 nanomoles/L). Similar high intra- and intervariability of testosterone serum concentrations were reported in normal and hypogonadal men. Normal serum testosterone levels were maintained in patients while using the transdermal testosterone up to six years; elevated DHT serum concentrations remained stable.
      The patch must be applied to scrotal skin (5 to 30 times more permeable to testosterone than other skin sites) to produce an adequate testosterone serum concentration.

### Protein binding
Testosterone—Very high (approximately 99%; 80% to sex hormone-binding globulin, 19% to albumin, and 1% free).

### Biotransformation
Hepatic.
Fluoxymesterone; methyltestosterone—Presence of 17-alpha alkyl group reduces susceptibility to hepatic enzyme degradation, which slows metabolism and allows for oral administration.
Testosterone—Orally administered testosterone undergoes nearly complete first-pass metabolism; both intramuscular and transdermal administration avoid first-pass metabolism. Metabolized (90% of dose) primarily to etiocholanolone, androsterone, and androstanediol, which are then conjugated with glucuronic or sulfuric acid. Testosterone esters (cypionate, enanthate, propionate) first undergo hydrolysis of the ester to the active form, free testosterone, which may be converted further into two of the major active metabolites, DHT and estradiol. Elevated DHT serum concentrations have been reported with transdermal testosterone due to high conversion to DHT by 5-alpha-reductase in the scrotal tissue. Changes in the testosterone to DHT ratio (T/DHT) range in hypogonadal men from 0.7 to 12.5 as compared to normal untreated men at 3.6 to 15.2. Estradiol serum concentrations were increased in hypogonadal men to the normal range of 0.8 to 3.5 ng/dL (29.4 to 128.5 picomoles/L).

### Half-life
Fluoxymesterone—Approximately 9.2 hours.
Methyltestosterone—2.5 to 3.5 hours.
Testosterone (intramuscular)—10 to 20 minutes (plasma).
Testosterone transdermal patch (local)—10 to 100 minutes; the activity of testosterone in many tissues appears to be dependent on its reduction to DHT and sex hormone-binding globulin binding capacity (high in prepubertal children, declining through puberty and adulthood and increasing again later in life).
Testosterone cypionate (intramuscular)—Approximately 8 days.

### Time to peak concentration
Methyltestosterone—
   Buccal tablet: 1 hour.
   Oral tablet: 2 hours.
Testosterone—
   Transdermal patch: At steady state, approximately 2 to 4 hours after application.

### Peak serum concentration
Testosterone—Transdermal patch: At steady state (up to 3 weeks), approximately 60% of 30 hypogonadal males in a study reached maximal testosterone serum concentrations greater than 500 nanograms/dL (17.3 nanomoles/L), range, 11.5 to 44.9 nanomoles/L.

### Duration of action

Testosterone—Dependent upon the ester, dosage form, and route of administration; in order of decreasing duration—enanthate, cypionate, propionate, base.

### Elimination

Generally renal excretion of metabolites. Approximately 90% of administered dose is excreted in the urine, primarily as glucuronide or sulfated conjugates of the metabolites. Some fecal because of enterohepatic circulation.

Fluoxymesterone—Less than 5% is excreted in urine as free steroid and glucuronide conjugate over a 24-hour period after doses of 20 to 200 mg.

Testosterone—Approximately 6% of dose is excreted in the feces.

## Precautions to Consider

### Carcinogenicity/Tumorigenicity

Hepatic neoplasms have been associated with long-term, high-dose androgen therapy in humans; some cases were nonreversible after androgen withdrawal. This effect is more likely with oral methylated androgens.

It has been suggested that some strains of female mice injected with testosterone are at greater risk of hepatoma. Testosterone may increase the number of tumors and decrease tumor cell differentiation.

For testosterone—Studies in female mice given subcutaneous implantations of testosterone showed an increase in cervical-uterine tumors. Some of these tumors metastasized. This effect was not seen in mice and rats given subcutaneous injections of testosterone or in rats given subcutaneous implantations.

### Pregnancy/Reproduction

Fertility—In males, oligospermia, azoospermia, or reduced sperm function resulting in possible infertility may occur during high-dose therapy with androgens because of possible suppression of spermatogenesis through feedback inhibition of pituitary follicle-stimulating hormone (FSH). Fertility usually returns following cessation of high-dose therapy.

Pregnancy—Androgens are contraindicated during pregnancy. Studies in humans have shown that androgens cause masculinization of the external genitalia of the female fetus, including clitoromegaly, abnormal vaginal development, and fusion of genital folds to form a scrotal-like structure. The degree of masculinization is dose-related.

FDA Pregnancy Category X.

### Breast-feeding

It is not known whether androgens are distributed into breast milk. Problems in humans have not been documented. However, androgens are rarely used by lactating women. A potential exists for adverse effects in the infant such as precocious sexual development in males and virilization in females.

### Pediatrics

Androgens should be used with caution in children and adolescents who are still growing because of possible premature epiphyseal closure in males and females, precocious sexual development in prepubertal males, or virilization in females. Skeletal maturation should be monitored at 6-month intervals by an x-ray of the hand and wrist.

### Geriatrics

Treatment of male patients over the age of approximately 50 years with androgens should be preceded by a thorough examination of the prostate and baseline measurement of prostate-specific antigen serum concentration, since androgens may cause increased risk of prostatic hypertrophy or may stimulate the growth of occult prostatic carcinoma. Periodic evaluation of prostate function should also be performed during the course of therapy.

### Drug interactions and/or related problems

The following drug interactions and/or related problems have been selected on the basis of their potential clinical significance (possible mechanism in parentheses where appropriate)—not necessarily inclusive (» = major clinical significance):

Note: Combinations containing any of the following medications, depending on the amount present, may also interact with this medication.

» Anticoagulants, coumarin- or indandione-derivative
   (anticoagulant effect may be increased because of decreased procoagulant factor concentration caused by alteration of procoagulant factor synthesis or catabolism and increased receptor affinity for the anticoagulant; anticoagulant dosage adjustment may be required during and following concurrent use)

Antidiabetic agents, oral or
Insulin
   (androgens may decrease blood glucose concentration; diabetic patients should be closely monitored for signs of hypoglycemia and dosage of the hypoglycemic agent adjusted if necessary)

Cyclosporine
   (methyltestosterone has been reported to increase plasma concentrations of cyclosporine and may increase the risk of nephrotoxicity; other androgens may have the same effect)

» Hepatotoxic medications, other (See *Appendix II*)
   (may result in an increased incidence of hepatotoxicity; patients should be carefully monitored, especially those on prolonged administration or those with a history of liver disease)

Human growth hormone (somatrem or somatropin)
   (use of excessive doses of androgens in prepubertal males may accelerate epiphyseal maturation, although supplemental use of androgens may be necessary in patients with androgen deficiency to continue the growth response to human growth hormone)

### Laboratory value alterations

The following have been selected on the basis of their potential clinical significance (possible effect in parentheses where appropriate)—not necessarily inclusive (» = major clinical significance):

With diagnostic test results
   Fasting blood sugar (FBS) and
   Glucose tolerance test
      (may be altered)

With physiology/laboratory test values
   Alkaline phosphatase
      (value may be increased)

   Aspartate aminotransferase (AST [SGOT]), serum and
   Calcium, chloride, inorganic phosphates, potassium, and sodium, serum and
   17-Ketosteroid (17-KS), urine
      (concentrations may be increased)

   Bilirubin
      (serum concentrations may be increased)

   Clotting factors II, V, VII, and X
      (may be suppressed)

   Corticosteroid-binding globulin
      (concentration may be decreased; free hormone concentration remains unchanged)

   Creatine and
   Creatinine
      (serum concentrations may be increased; effect usually lasts up to 2 weeks after discontinuation of therapy)

   Follicle-stimulating hormone (FSH) and
   Luteinizing hormone (LH)
      (serum concentrations may be reduced)

   Glucose
      (blood concentrations may be increased, due to glucose intolerance)

   Hematocrit and
   Hemoglobin
      (values may be increased with high-dose or long-term therapy)

   High-density lipoproteins (HDL)
      (serum concentrations may be decreased)

   Low-density lipoproteins (LDL)
      (serum concentrations may be increased; one study showed a slight reduction with testosterone)

   Sex steroid-binding globulin
      (concentration may be decreased; free hormone concentration remains unchanged)

   Spermatozoa count and
   Hamster ova penetration test (HOPT)
      (may be severely reduced at high doses)

   Thyroxine-binding globulin
      (may be decreased resulting in decreased total $T_4$ serum concentrations and increased resin uptake of $T_3$ and $T_4$; free thyroid hormone levels remain unchanged)

### Medical considerations/Contraindications

The medical considerations/contraindications included here have been selected on the basis of their potential clinical significance (reasons given in parentheses where appropriate)—not necessarily inclusive (» = major clinical significance).

*Except under special circumstances, these medications should not be used when the following medical problems exist:*

» Breast cancer in males or
» Prostate cancer, known or suspected
    (tumor growth may be promoted)

*Risk-benefit should be considered when the following medical problems exist:*

» Cardiac failure or
    Cardiac function impairment or
» Cardio-renal disease, severe or
    Edema or
    Hepatic function impairment or
» Nephritis or
» Nephrosis or
    Renal function impairment
        (may cause fluid retention, resulting in edema with or without congestive heart failure; diuretics may be required before and during therapy)
    Coronary artery disease or
» Myocardial infarction, history of
        (may be worsened, due to hypercholesterolemic effects of androgens)
    Diabetes mellitus
        (use may result in loss of control of diabetes, due to an androgen-induced glucose intolerance; routine monitoring of blood glucose concentrations is recommended, especially upon initiation of therapy)
» Hepatic function impairment
        (biotransformation of androgens may be impaired, resulting in increased elimination half-life and increase in the incidence of gynecomastia)
» Hypercalcemia
        (may be exacerbated in patients with metastatic breast carcinoma)
» Prostatic hypertrophy, benign with urethral obstructive symptoms
        (further enlargement may occur)
    Sensitivity to anabolic steroids or androgens

**Patient monitoring**
The following may be especially important in patient monitoring (other tests may be warranted in some patients, depending on condition; » = major clinical significance):

Bone age determinations
    (x-rays recommended every 6 months for children and growing adolescents to determine rate of bone maturation and effects on epiphyseal centers)

Cholesterol and/or
High density lipoproteins and
Low density lipoproteins
    (serum profile determinations recommended prior to initiation of therapy and, in some patients, at regular intervals during therapy)

Hemoglobin and
Hematocrit determinations
    (recommended at regular intervals in patients receiving prolonged therapy or high doses of androgens to check for possible erythrocytosis)

Hepatic function determinations
    (recommended at regular intervals during therapy with oral methylated androgens)

Prostatic acid phosphatase and
Prostatic specific antigen
    (recommended at regular intervals during therapy with transdermal patch)

Testosterone, total, serum
    (determinations recommended after 3 to 4 weeks of transdermal patch use at 2 to 4 hours after patch application.)

*For treatment of breast carcinoma*
Alkaline phosphatase, serum values and
Physical examination and
X-rays of known or suspected metastases
    (recommended at regular intervals during therapy to monitor objective evidence of tumor response)

Calcium
    (measurement of serum concentrations recommended at regular intervals in women with disseminated breast carcinoma)

*For gender change androgen therapy*
» Luteinizing hormone
    (measurement of serum concentrations is recommended every 6 months, to monitor success of therapy)

» Alanine aminotransferase (ALT [SGPT])
    (measurement of serum concentrations is recommended every 6 months to monitor for adverse effects)

## Side/Adverse Effects

Note: The side effects of testosterone enanthate and testosterone cypionate cannot be quickly reversed by discontinuing medication because of the long durations of action of these medications.

The following side/adverse effects have been selected on the basis of their potential clinical significance (possible signs and symptoms in parentheses where appropriate)—not necessarily inclusive:

**Those indicating need for medical attention**
Incidence more frequent
    *In females only*
        **Amenorrhea or oligomenorrhea** (menstrual irregularities); *virilism* (acne; decreased breast size; oily skin; enlarged clitoris; male pattern baldness; hoarseness or deepening of voice; unnatural and excessive hair growth)
        Note: *Virilism* may occur with usual systemic doses, as well as with excessive doses of topical testosterone. Virilization has also been reported in the sexual partner of a male patient being treated with topical testosterone. Hoarseness or deepening of voice and enlarged clitoris may not be reversible even after the medication has been discontinued.

    *In males only*
        **Bladder irritability or urinary tract infection** (frequent urge to urinate); *breast soreness; gynecomastia* (enlargement of breasts); *priapism* (frequent or continuing erections)—sign of excessive dosage; temporary discontinuance of medication and immediate medical attention are required

    *In prepubertal males only*
        **Virilism** (acne; enlargement of penis; increased frequency of erections; early growth of pubic hair)

Incidence less frequent
    *In both females and males*
        **Edema** (swelling of feet or lower legs; rapid weight gain); *erythrocytosis or polycythemia* (dizziness; headache, frequent or continuing; unusual tiredness; flushing or redness of skin; unusual bleeding)—in severe cases; *gastrointestinal irritation* (nausea; vomiting); *hepatic dysfunction* (yellow eyes or skin; itching of skin)—more likely with the oral methylated androgens; *hypercalcemia* (confusion; mental depression; unusual tiredness; nausea; increased thirst; increased frequency of urination and quantity of urine; constipation; vomiting)—in females with breast cancer or immobilized patients

    *In males only*
        **Nonspecific acute epididymitis** (chills; pain in scrotum or groin); *prostatic carcinoma* (stimulation of tumor growth); *prostatic hypertrophy* (difficult urination)

Incidence rare—with long-term therapy and/or high doses
    *In both females and males*
        **Hepatic necrosis** (continuing abdominal or stomach pain; black, tarry stools; continuing malaise; continuing headache; continuing unpleasant breath odor; vomiting of blood); *hepatocellular tumor* (pain or tenderness in upper abdomen or liver area; swelling of abdomen)—more likely with the oral methylated androgens; may be life-threatening or fatal; *leukopenia* (sore throat; fever); *peliosis hepatis* (dark-colored urine; hives; light-colored stools; continuing loss of appetite; purple- or red-colored spots on body or inside the mouth or nose; sore throat; fever; nausea; vomiting)—more likely with the oral methylated androgens; may be life-threatening or fatal

**Those indicating need for medical attention only if they continue or are bothersome**
Incidence less frequent
    *In both females and males*
        **Mild acne; diarrhea; increase in pubic hair growth; infection, redness, pain, or other irritation at site of injection**—for intramuscular injection only; *decrease or increase in libido; stomach pain; stomatitis* (irritation or soreness of mouth; watering of mouth)—secondary to buccal administration; *trouble in sleeping*

    *In males only*
        **Impotence; infection, itching, redness, or other skin irritation of scrotum**—for transdermal use only; *testicular atrophy* (decrease in testicle size)

# Patient Consultation

As an aid to patient consultation, refer to *Advice for the Patient, Androgens (Systemic).*

In providing consultation, consider emphasizing the following selected information (» = major clinical significance):

**Before using this medication**
» Conditions affecting use, especially:

Sensitivity to androgens or anabolic steroids

Carcinogenicity—Hepatocellular carcinoma associated with long-term, high-dose therapy

Tumorigenicity—Hepatic neoplasms associated with long-term, high-dose therapy

Pregnancy—Contraindicated for use during pregnancy because of possible masculinization of female fetus

Use in children—Cautious use due to effects on growth and sexual development (precocious sexual development in males, virilization in females)

Use in the elderly—Increased risk of prostatic hypertrophy or prostatic carcinoma

Other medications, especially anticoagulants (coumarin- or indandione-derivatives) or hepatotoxic medications

Other medical problems, especially male breast cancer, possible prostate cancer, cardiac failure, cardio-renal disease, history of myocardial infarction, hepatic function impairment, hypercalcemia, nephritis, nephrosis, or prostatic hypertrophy

Fertility—May be severely impaired in males

## Proper use of this medication
*For fluoxymesterone, and capsule and oral tablet dosage forms of methyltestosterone*

Taking with food to minimize possible stomach upset

*For methyltestosterone buccal tablets*
» Importance of not swallowing buccal tablets

*For testosterone skin patch*

Applying to dry, clean, and hairless skin of scrotum; may be reapplied after bathing, swimming, or showering

*For all androgens*
» Importance of not taking more medication than the amount prescribed
» Proper administration
» Proper dosing

Missed dose: Taking as soon as possible; not taking if almost time for next dose; not doubling doses
» Proper storage

## Precautions while using this medication
Regular visits to physician to check progress during therapy

Diabetics: May alter blood sugar concentrations

Checking with doctor if female sexual partner develops mild virilization

## Side/adverse effects
*Signs of potential side effects, especially*

In females only—Menstrual irregularities, virilism

In males only—Bladder irritability or urinary tract infection, breast soreness, gynecomastia, priapism, epididymitis, prostatic carcinoma, prostatic hypertrophy

In prepubertal males only—Virilism

In all patients—Edema, erythrocytosis or polycythemia, gastrointestinal irritation, hepatic necrosis, hepatocellular tumor, hepatic dysfunction, hypercalcemia, leukopenia, or peliosis hepatis

# General Dosing Information

The dosage and duration of therapy depends on the patient's age, sex, diagnosis, and response to therapy, and the appearance of adverse effects.

It is usually preferable to begin treatment for anemia and carcinoma with full therapeutic doses and to adjust later to individual requirements.

## For treatment of delayed puberty
The dosage used in delayed puberty generally is in the lower range of the usual adult dose for androgen replacement therapy and is given for a limited duration, usually 3 to 6 months. The chronological and skeletal ages should be considered, both in determining the initial dose and in adjusting the dose. After three to six months of therapy, the medication should be discontinued for one to three months and x-rays taken to determine effect on bone growth or maturation.

Various dosage regimens have been used to induce pubertal changes in hypogonadal males. Some physicians prescribe a lower dose initially, gradually increase the dose as puberty progresses, and follow with a maintenance dose, which may be decreased.

## For treatment of breast cancer
To determine whether there will be an objective response to antineoplastic therapy, treatment should be continued for at least 3 months. A response to therapy is usually apparent within 3 months. Therapy should be discontinued after the disease becomes progressive again. If clinical circumstances allow for an observation period, the patient should be observed for a period of improvement known as "rebound regression."

Women should be checked for signs of virilization during androgen therapy. Some effects, such as voice changes or clitoromegaly, may not be reversible. A decision should be made by patient and physician as to how much virilization will be tolerated as a result of therapy with androgens. Alternatively, the drug should be discontinued or the dosage reduced. If irreversible virilization is to be prevented, drug must be discontinued when mild virilization becomes evident.

Women with metastatic breast cancer should be followed closely because androgen therapy occasionally accelerates the disease. A shorter acting androgen is preferred over one with prolonged activity, especially during the early stages of androgen therapy.

## For intramuscular dosage forms
The suspension dosage form is absorbed relatively slowly; therefore, frequent injections may cause overdosage.

Testosterone cypionate or testosterone enanthate should not be used interchangeably with testosterone propionate or testosterone base because of different durations of action.

The intramuscular injections should be administered deeply into the gluteal muscle or the deltoid muscle in larger men. Injections should not be administered intravenously.

## For transdermal patch dosage form
Potential for transfer of testosterone from the scrotal patch to the female sexual partner resulting in mild virilization, such as changes in body hair distribution and increase in acne.

Patch should be applied to clean, dry and dry-shaved scrotal skin for optimal skin contact. Chemical depilatories should not be used.

---

## *FLUOXYMESTERONE*

# Summary of Differences

Indications: Also used as an antianemic.

Side/adverse effects: Methylated androgens are more likely to predispose patients to jaundice.

# Oral Dosage Forms

Note: Bracketed uses in the *Dosage Forms* section refer to categories of use and/or indications that are not included in U.S. product labeling.

## FLUOXYMESTERONE TABLETS USP

**Usual adult dose**
Androgen replacement therapy, males—

Oral, 5 mg one to four times a day. Replacement therapy is usually started at 10 mg per day, with subsequent adjustments as necessary.

Breast cancer in females—

Oral, 20 to 50 mg per day.

[Antianemic]—

Oral, 20 to 50 mg per day, for minimum trial of two to six months.

**Usual pediatric dose**
Delayed puberty in males—

Oral, 2.5 to 10 mg per day for a limited duration, usually four to six months.

**Strength(s) usually available**
U.S.—

2 mg (Rx) [*Halotestin* (scored; lactose; sucrose; tartrazine); GENERIC (Bolar—scored; Bolar—lactose)].

5 mg (Rx) [*Halotestin* (scored; lactose; sucrose; tartrazine); GENERIC (Bolar—scored; Bolar—lactose; tartrazine)].

10 mg (Rx) [*Android-F* (scored); *Halotestin* (scored; lactose; sucrose; tartrazine); GENERIC (Bolar—scored)].

Canada—

5 mg (Rx) [*Halotestin* (scored; tartrazine)].

**Packaging and storage**
Store below 40 °C (104 °F), preferably between 15 and 30 °C (59 and 86 °F), unless otherwise specified by manufacturer. Store in a well-closed container. Protect from light.

**Auxiliary labeling**
• Take with food.

---

## METHYLTESTOSTERONE

## Summary of Differences

Indications:
  Also indicated for androgen replacement in impotence or for male climacteric symptoms.
Pharmacology/pharmacokinetics:
  Methyltestosterone buccal tablets are nearly twice as potent as the oral preparations.
Side/adverse effects:
  Methylated androgens more likely to predispose patients to jaundice.
  Irritation or soreness of mouth or unusual watering of mouth (stomatitis from buccal tablet administration).

## Oral Dosage Forms
### METHYLTESTOSTERONE CAPSULES USP

**Usual adult dose**
Androgen replacement therapy, males or
Climacteric or
Impotence or
Hypogonadism—
  Oral, 10 to 50 mg per day.
Cryptorchidism—
  Oral, 10 mg three times a day.
Breast cancer in females—
  Oral, 50 mg one to four times a day. After two to four weeks, dose may be decreased to 50 mg two times a day if response occurs.

**Usual pediatric dose**
Delayed puberty in males—
  Oral, 5 to 25 mg per day for a limited duration, usually four to six months.

**Strength(s) usually available**
U.S.—
  10 mg (Rx) [*Testred; Virilon*].

**Packaging and storage**
Store below 40 °C (104 °F), preferably between 15 and 30 °C (59 and 86 °F), unless otherwise specified by manufacturer. Store in a well-closed container.

**Auxiliary labeling**
• Take with food.

### METHYLTESTOSTERONE TABLETS (Buccal) USP

**Usual adult dose**
Androgen replacement therapy, males or
Climacteric or
Impotence or
Hypogonadism—
  Buccal, 5 to 25 mg per day.
Cryptorchidism—
  Buccal, 5 mg three times a day.
Breast cancer in females—
  Buccal, 25 mg one to four times a day. After two to four weeks, dose may be decreased to 25 mg two times a day if response occurs.

**Usual pediatric dose**
Delayed puberty in males—
  Buccal, 2.5 to 12.5 mg per day for a limited duration, usually four to six months.

**Strength(s) usually available**
U.S.—
  10 mg (Rx) [*Oreton;* GENERIC (Lilly—lactose, saccharin, sucrose)].
Canada—
  10 mg (Rx) [*Metandren* (scored)].
  25 mg (Rx) [*Metandren* (scored)].

**Packaging and storage**
Store below 40 °C (104 °F), preferably between 15 and 30 °C (59 and 86 °F), unless otherwise specified by manufacturer. Store in a well-closed container.

### METHYLTESTOSTERONE TABLETS (Oral) USP

**Usual adult dose**
See *Methyltestosterone Capsules USP.*

**Usual pediatric dose**
See *Methyltestosterone Capsules USP.*

**Strength(s) usually available**
U.S.—
  10 mg (Rx) [*Android-10; Oreton* (lactose); GENERIC].
  25 mg (Rx) [*Android-25;* GENERIC (Lilly—lactose, saccharin, sucrose)].
Canada—
  10 mg (Rx) [*Metandren* (scored; lactose)].
  25 mg (Rx) [*Metandren* (scored; lactose)].

**Packaging and storage**
Store below 40 °C (104 °F), preferably between 15 and 30 °C (59 and 86 °F), unless otherwise specified by manufacturer. Store in a well-closed container.

**Auxiliary labeling**
• Take with food.

---

## TESTOSTERONE

## Summary of Differences

Indications:
  Testosterone enanthate and testosterone cypionate are used as antianemics and in androgen replacement in impotence or for male climacteric symptoms. Testosterone cypionate and testosterone enanthate are also used for female-to-male gender change. Intramuscular testosterone and testosterone esters, and extemporaneously compounded testosterone propionate ointments are used in the treatment of microphallus. Extemporaneously compounded testosterone propionate ointments are used in the treatment of lichen sclerosus.
Side/adverse effects:
  Side effects of the enanthate and cypionate forms cannot be quickly reversed because of the long duration of effect of medication form.
  Hives, infection, redness, pain, or other irritation at site of injection.

## Parenteral Dosage Forms

Note: Bracketed uses in the *Dosage Forms* section refers to categories of use and/or indications that are not included in U.S. product labeling.

### STERILE TESTOSTERONE SUSPENSION USP

**Usual adult dose**
Androgen replacement therapy, males—
  Intramuscular, 25 to 50 mg two or three times a week.
Breast cancer in females—
  Intramuscular, 50 to 100 mg three times a week.

**Usual pediatric dose**
Delayed puberty in males—
  Intramuscular, 100 mg (maximum) per month for a limited duration, usually four to six months.

**Strength(s) usually available**
U.S.—
  25 mg per mL (Rx) [GENERIC (Steris—thimerosal 80 mcg [0.08 mg] per mL)].
  50 mg per mL (Rx) [*Histerone-50* (thimerosal); *Testaqua* (thimerosal); *Testoject-50* (thimerosal); GENERIC (Steris—thimerosal 80 mcg [0.08 mg] per mL)].
  100 mg per mL (Rx) [*Andro 100* (thimerosal 80 mcg [0.08 mg] per mL); *Histerone-100* (thimerosal); *Testamone 100* (thimerosal); *Testaqua* (thimerosal); GENERIC (Steris—thimerosal 80 mcg [0.08 mg] per mL)].
Canada—
  100 mg per mL (Rx) [*Malogen*].

**Packaging and storage**
Store below 40 °C (104 °F), preferably between 15 and 30 °C (59 and 86 °F), unless otherwise specified by manufacturer. Protect from freezing.

**Auxiliary labeling**
• Shake well.

### TESTOSTERONE CYPIONATE INJECTION USP

**Usual adult dose**
Androgen replacement therapy, males or
Climacteric or
Impotence or
Hypogonadism—
  Intramuscular, 50 to 400 mg every two to four weeks.
[Gender change][1]—
  Intramuscular, 200 mg every two weeks. Occasional patients may require a higher dose to cause cessation of menses.
Breast cancer in females—
  Intramuscular, 200 to 400 mg every two to four weeks.

**Usual pediatric dose**

Delayed puberty in males—

Intramuscular, 100 mg (maximum) per month for a limited duration, usually four to six months.

**Strength(s) usually available**

U.S.—

100 mg per mL (Rx) [*Andro-Cyp 100* (benzyl alcohol); *Andronate 100* (benzyl alcohol); *depAndro 100* (benzyl alcohol); *Depotest* (benzyl alcohol); *Depo-Testosterone* (benzyl alcohol 9.45 mg per mL; benzyl benzoate 0.1 mL per mL); *Duratest-100* (benzyl alcohol); *Testoject-LA* (benzyl alcohol); GENERIC (Steris—benzyl alcohol 0.9%, benzyl benzoate 20%)].

200 mg per mL (Rx) [*Andro-Cyp 200* (benzyl alcohol; benzyl benzoate); *Andronate 200* (benzyl alcohol; benzyl benzoate); *depAndro 200* (benzyl alcohol; benzyl benzoate); *Depotest* (benzyl alcohol; benzyl benzoate); *Depo-Testosterone* (benzyl alcohol 9.45 mg per mL; benzyl benzoate 0.2 mL per mL); *Duratest-200* (benzyl alcohol; benzyl benzoate); *T-Cypionate; Testa-C* (benzyl alcohol; benzyl benzoate); *Testoject-LA* (benzyl alcohol; benzyl benzoate); *Testred Cypionate 200* (benzyl alcohol 0.9%; benzyl benzoate 20%; *Virilon IM;* GENERIC (Steris—benzyl alcohol 0.9%, benzyl benzoate 20%)].

Canada—

100 mg per mL (Rx) [*Depo-Testosterone Cypionate* (benzyl alcohol; benzyl benzoate)].

**Packaging and storage**

Store below 40 °C (104 °F), preferably between 15 and 30 °C (59 and 86 °F), unless otherwise specified by manufacturer. Protect from light. Protect from freezing.

**Stability**

Crystals may form at low temperatures; warming and shaking the vial will redissolve any crystals.

Use of a wet needle or wet syringe may cause solution to cloud; however, potency of the medication will not be affected.

## TESTOSTERONE ENANTHATE INJECTION USP

**Usual adult dose**

Androgen replacement therapy, males—

Intramuscular, 50 to 400 mg every two to four weeks.

Breast cancer in females—

Intramuscular, 200 to 400 mg every two to four weeks.

[Antianemic]—

Intramuscular, 400 mg a day for one week, then 400 mg one or two times a week. The maintenance dose is 200 to 400 mg every 4 weeks.

[Gender change][1]—

Intramuscular, 200 mg every two weeks. Occasional patients may require a higher dose to cause cessation of menses.

**Usual pediatric dose**

Delayed puberty in males—

Intramuscular, 100 mg (maximum) per month for a limited duration, usually four to six months.

Microphallus (treatment)—

Intramuscular, 25 to 50 mg every month for 3 to 6 months.

**Strength(s) usually available**

U.S.—

100 mg per mL (Rx) [*Andropository 100* (chlorobutanol); *Delatest* (chlorobutanol); *Everone* (chlorobutanol); *Testone L.A. 100* (chlorobutanol); GENERIC (Quad—benzyl alcohol 2%)].

200 mg per mL (Rx) [*Andro L.A. 200* (chlorobutanol 0.5%); *Andryl 200* (chlorobutanol); *Delatestryl* (chlorobutanol 5 mg per mL); *Durathate-200* (chlorobutanol); *Everone* (chlorobutanol); *Testone L.A. 200* (chlorobutanol); *Testrin-P.A.* (chlorobutanol); GENERIC (Quad—benzyl alcohol 2%)].

Canada—

200 mg per mL (Rx) [*Delatestryl* (chlorobutanol 0.5%); *Malogex* (benzyl alcohol 2%)].

**Packaging and storage**

Store below 40 °C (104 °F), preferably between 15 and 30 °C (59 and 86 °F), unless otherwise specified by manufacturer. Protect from freezing.

**Stability**

Crystals may form at low temperatures; warming and shaking the vial will redissolve any crystals.

Use of a wet needle or wet syringe may cause solution to cloud; however, potency of the medication will not be affected.

## TESTOSTERONE PROPIONATE INJECTION USP

**Usual adult dose**

Androgen replacement therapy, males—

Intramuscular, 25 to 50 mg two or three times a week.

Breast cancer in females—

Intramuscular, 50 to 100 mg three times a week.

**Usual pediatric dose**

Delayed puberty in males—

Intramuscular, 100 mg (maximum) per month for a limited duration, usually four to six months.

**Strength(s) usually available**

U.S.—

100 mg per mL (Rx) [*Testex* (benzyl alcohol); GENERIC].

Canada—

100 mg per mL (Rx) [*Malogen*].

**Packaging and storage**

Store below 40 °C (104 °F), preferably between 15 and 30 °C (59 and 86 °F), unless otherwise specified by manufacturer. Protect from freezing.

**Stability**

Crystals may form at low temperatures; warming and shaking the vial will redissolve any crystals.

Use of a wet needle or wet syringe may cause solution to cloud; however, potency of the medication will not be affected.

# Topical Dosage Forms

## TESTOSTERONE PROPIONATE OINTMENT

**Usual adult dose**

Lichen sclerosus—

Initial, topical, to the vulva, as a 1 or 2% ointment, two times a day for six weeks or until relief of itching occurs. Dosage should be decreased to minimal effective dose.

**Usual pediatric dose**

Microphallus (treatment)—

Topical, to the penis, two times a day for three months, as a 5% ointment.

**Strength(s) usually available**

U.S.—

Not commercially available. Compounding required for prescription.

Canada—

Not commercially available. Compounding required for prescription.

**Preparation of dosage form**

Formulations that have been used for the extemporaneous compounding of testosterone propionate ointments are as follows—

For 15 grams of 2% testosterone propionate ointment—

3 mL of 100-mg-per-mL testosterone propionate injection

12 grams of white petrolatum.

For 15 grams of 5% testosterone propionate ointment—

7.5 mL of 100-mg-per-mL testosterone propionate injection

7.5 grams of white petrolatum.

## TESTOSTERONE TRANSDERMAL SYSTEM

**Usual adult dose**

Androgen replacement therapy, males—

Topical, one 6 mg transdermal dosage system (15 mg per sixty centimeters-squared patch) applied to clean, dry and hairless skin of scrotum every twenty-two to twenty-four hours. If scrotal area is inadequate, the smaller-sized 4 mg transdermal dosage system (10 mg per forty centimeters-squared patch) should be used every 22 to 24 hours.

Note: Discontinue if desired response is not reached at six to eight weeks.

**Usual pediatric dose**

Dosage has not been established.

**Strength(s) usually available**

U.S.—

4 mg delivered per day (Rx) [*Testoderm*].

6 mg delivered per day (Rx) [*Testoderm*].

Canada—
Not commercially available.

**Packaging and storage**
Store between 15 to 30 °C (86 °F).

**Auxiliary labeling**
• For external use only.
• Follow the manufacturer's directions carefully.

[1]Not included in Canadian product labeling.

Revised: 08/23/94

# ANDROGENS AND ESTROGENS   Systemic

This monograph includes information on the following: Diethylstilbestrol and Methyltestosterone; Estrogens, Conjugated, and Methyltestosterone; Estrogens, Esterified, and Methyltestosterone; Fluoxymesterone and Ethinyl Estradiol; Testosterone and Estradiol.

VA CLASSIFICATION (Primary/Secondary): HS900/GU900

**NOTE:** The *Androgens and Estrogens (Systemic)* monograph is maintained on the USP DI electronic data base. For a printed copy of the most recent revision of the complete monograph, contact the USP Division of Information Development, 12601 Twinbrook Parkway, Rockville, MD 20852.

For information on the specific components of this combination, see the *USP DI* monographs for *Androgens (Systemic)* and *Estrogens (Systemic)*.

The information that follows is selectively abstracted from the complete monograph and is provided to facilitate drug use review and patient counseling.

Note: For a listing of dosage forms and brand names by country availability, see *Dosage Forms* section(s). For a listing of brand names for the articles in this monograph, refer to the General Index.

## Category
Androgen-estrogen.

## Indications
### Unaccepted
There is conflicting evidence and opinion as to whether the possible benefits of postmenopausal androgen pharmacologic or replacement therapy outweigh the risks of the frequently occurring virilizing side effects, adverse effects on serum cholesterol profile, or hepatotoxicity. Virilization may be somewhat reduced with the concomitant use of estrogens. However, because further data are needed regarding the efficacy of androgens in combination with estrogen and because side effects are frequent, the routine use of these products for any indication is not recommended.

## Patient Consultation
As an aid to patient consultation, refer to *Advice for the Patient, Androgens and Estrogens (Systemic)*.

In providing consultation, consider emphasizing the following selected information (» = major clinical significance):

### Before using this medication
» Conditions affecting use, especially:
Sensitivity to anabolic steroids, androgens, or estrogens
Carcinogenicity/tumorigenicity—Hepatocellular carcinoma and neoplasms associated with long-term, high-dose androgen therapy; increased risk of endometrial cancer for patients with intact uteri when progestin is not used with estrogen; risk is decreased when a progestin is used with estrogen; continuous, long-term estrogen use in animal studies increased frequency of cancers of the breast, cervix, and liver
Pregnancy—Androgens are not recommended for use during pregnancy, because of possible masculinization of female fetus; suggestion that use of some estrogens may be associated with congenital abnormalities
Breast-feeding—Use is not recommended, because estrogens are distributed into breast milk and may have unpredictable effects; not known if androgens are distributed into breast milk; androgens could have adverse effects on the infant such as slowing or cessation of growth, precocious sexual development in males, or virilization in females
Other medications, especially anticoagulants (coumarin- or indandione-derivatives), cyclosporine, or hepatotoxic medications

Other medical problems, especially abnormal and undiagnosed vaginal bleeding; breast cancer; cardio-renal disease; cardiac failure; hepatic dysfunction or failure; history of myocardial infarction; nephrosis; nephritis; active thrombophlebitis or thromboembolic disorders
Reading patient package insert carefully

### Proper use of this medication
» Compliance with therapy
» Importance of not taking more medication than the amount prescribed
Taking with or immediately after food to reduce nausea
» Proper dosing
Missed dose: Taking as soon as possible; not taking if almost time for next dose; not doubling doses
» Proper storage

### Precautions while using this medication
» Regular visits to physician at least every 6 to 12 months, or more often if so directed, to check progress
Importance of mammography and regular self-breast examinations
Possibility of dental problems, such as tenderness, swelling, or bleeding of gums; brushing and flossing teeth, massaging gums, and having dentist clean teeth regularly; checking with dentist if there are questions about care of teeth or gums or if tenderness, swelling, or bleeding of gums is noticed
Diabetics: May alter blood glucose concentrations
» Stopping medication immediately and checking with physician if pregnancy is suspected
Smoking while taking oral contraceptives containing estrogens can increase risk of cardiovascular side effects; not known whether elevated risk occurs with estrogen therapy
Importance of not giving medication to anyone else

### Side/adverse effects
Withdrawal bleeding will occur in many postmenopausal patients placed on cyclic androgen and estrogen therapy with a progestin
Signs of potential side effects, especially anaphylaxis, breast tumors, chorea, peripheral edema, erythrocytosis, gallbladder obstruction, hepatic necrosis, hepatitis, hepatocellular tumor, hepatic dysfunction, leukopenia, menstrual irregularities, peliosis hepatis, polycythemia, virilism

---

### *DIETHYLSTILBESTROL AND METHYLTESTOSTERONE*

## Oral Dosage Forms
### DIETHYLSTILBESTROL AND METHYLTESTOSTERONE TABLETS
**Usual adult dose**
Menopause, vasomotor symptoms of (treatment)—
Initial dose: Oral, 250 mcg (0.25 mg) of diethylstilbestrol and 5 mg of methyltestosterone a day for twenty-one days, the dosage being repeated cyclically following seven days of no medication.
Selected patients—Oral, 500 mcg (0.5 mg) of diethylstilbestrol and 10 mg of methyltestosterone a day for two weeks or less.
Maintenance dosage: Oral, up to 125 mcg (0.125 mg) of diethylstilbestrol and 2.5 mg of methyltestosterone a day for twenty-one days, the dosage being repeated cyclically following seven days of no medication.
Note: To produce withdrawal bleeding, progesterone 5 mg per day may be given for the five days preceding the period of no medication of a cyclical schedule.

**Strength(s) usually available**
U.S.—
250 mcg (0.25 mg) of diethylstilbestrol and 5 mg of methyltestosterone (Rx) [*Tylosterone* (scored; sucrose)].

---

### ESTROGENS, CONJUGATED, AND METHYLTESTOSTERONE

---

## Oral Dosage Forms

### CONJUGATED ESTROGENS AND METHYLTESTOSTERONE TABLETS

#### Usual adult dose

Menopause, vasomotor symptoms of (treatment)—
Oral, 1.25 mg of conjugated estrogens and 10 mg of methyltestosterone a day for twenty-one days, the dosage being repeated cyclically following seven days of no medication.

#### Strength(s) usually available

U.S.—
625 mcg (0.625 mg) of conjugated estrogens and 5 mg of methyltestosterone (Rx) [*Premarin with Methyltestosterone* (lactose; sucrose)].

1.25 mg of conjugated estrogens and 10 mg of methyltestosterone (Rx) [*Premarin with Methyltestosterone* (lactose; sucrose)].

Canada—
625 mcg (0.625 mg) of conjugated estrogens and 5 mg of methyltestosterone (Rx) [*Premarin with Methyltestosterone* (lactose; propylparaben; sucrose)].

1.25 mg of conjugated estrogens and 10 mg of methyltestosterone (Rx) [*Premarin with Methyltestosterone* (lactose; sucrose; propylparaben)].

---

### ESTROGENS, ESTERIFIED, AND METHYLTESTOSTERONE

---

## Oral Dosage Forms

### ESTERIFIED ESTROGENS AND METHYLTESTOSTERONE TABLETS

#### Usual adult dose

Menopause, vasomotor symptoms of (treatment)—
Oral, 625 mcg (0.625 mg) to 2.5 mg of esterified estrogens and 1.25 to 5 mg of methyltestosterone a day for twenty-one days, the dosage being repeated cyclically following seven days of no medication.

#### Strength(s) usually available

U.S.—
625 mcg (0.625 mg) of esterified estrogens and 1.25 mg of methyltestosterone (Rx) [*Estratest H.S* (lactose; methylparaben; propylparaben; sodium benzoate; sucrose)].

1.25 mg of esterified estrogens and 2.5 mg of methyltestosterone (Rx) [*Estratest* (lactose; methylparaben; propylparaben; sodium benzoate; sucrose)].

---

### FLUOXYMESTERONE AND ETHINYL ESTRADIOL

---

## Oral Dosage Forms

### FLUOXYMESTERONE AND ETHINYL ESTRADIOL TABLETS

#### Usual adult dose

Menopause, vasomotor symptoms of (treatment)—
Oral, 1 to 2 mg of fluoxymesterone and 20 to 40 mcg (0.02 to 0.04 mg) ethinyl estradiol two times a day for twenty-one days, the dosage being repeated cyclically following seven days of no medication.

#### Strength(s) usually available

U.S.—
1 mg of fluoxymesterone and 20 mcg (0.02 mg) ethinyl estradiol (Rx) [*Halodrin* (scored; lactose; sucrose)].

---

### TESTOSTERONE AND ESTRADIOL

---

## Parenteral Dosage Forms

### TESTOSTERONE CYPIONATE AND ESTRADIOL CYPIONATE INJECTION

#### Usual adult dose

Menopause, vasomotor symptoms of (treatment)—
Intramuscular, 50 mg of testosterone cypionate and 2 mg of estradiol cypionate every four weeks.

#### Strength(s) usually available

U.S.—
50 mg of testosterone cypionate and 2 mg of estradiol cypionate per mL (Rx) [*De-Comberol; depAndrogyn* (chlorobutanol; cottonseed oil); *Depo-Testadiol* (chlorobutanol anhydrous 5.4 mg per mL; cottonseed oil 874 mg per mL); *Depotestogen* (chlorobutanol; cottonseed oil); *Duo-Cyp* (chlorobutanol; cottonseed oil); *Duratestin* (chlorobutanol 0.5%; cottonseed oil); *Menoject-L.A* (chlorobutanol; cottonseed oil); *Tes Est Cyp* (chlorobutanol 0.5%; cottonseed oil); *Test-Estro Cypionate* (chlorobutanol; cottonseed oil); GENERIC].

### TESTOSTERONE ENANTHATE AND ESTRADIOL VALERATE INJECTION

#### Usual adult dose

Menopause, vasomotor symptoms of (treatment)—
Intramuscular, 90 mg of testosterone enanthate and 4 mg of estradiol valerate every four weeks.

#### Strength(s) usually available

U.S.—
90 mg of testosterone enanthate and 4 mg of estradiol valerate per mL (Rx) [*Andrest 90-4* (chlorobutanol 0.5%; sesame oil); *Andro-Estro 90-4* (chlorobutanol; sesame oil); *Androgyn L.A* (chlorobutanol 0.5%; sesame oil); *Deladumone* (chlorobutanol 5 mg per mL; sesame oil); *Delatestadiol* (chlorobutanol; sesame oil); *Duo-Gen L.A* (chlorobutanol; sesame oil); *Dura-Dumone 90/4* (chlorobutanol 0.5%; sesame oil); *OB* (chlorobutanol 0.5%; sesame oil); *Teev* (chlorobutanol; sesame oil); *Valertest No. 1* (chlorobutanol; sesame oil); GENERIC].

180 mg of testosterone enanthate and 8 mg of estradiol valerate per mL (Rx) [*Valertest No. 2* (benzyl alcohol; sesame oil); GENERIC].

Canada—
90 mg of testosterone enanthate and 4 mg of estradiol valerate per mL (Rx) [*Duogex L.A* (benzyl alcohol 2%)].

100 mg of testosterone enanthate and 6.5 mg of estradiol valerate per mL (Rx) [*Neo-Pause* (benzyl alcohol 2%; chlorobutanol 0.5%; sesame oil)].

### TESTOSTERONE ENANTHATE BENZILIC ACID HYDRAZONE, ESTRADIOL DIENANTHATE, AND ESTRADIOL BENZOATE INJECTION

#### Usual adult dose

Menopause, vasomotor symptoms of (treatment) or
Osteoporosis, estrogen deficiency–induced (treatment)—
Intramuscular, 150 mg of testosterone enanthate benzilic acid hydrazone, 7.5 mg of estradiol dienanthate, and 1 mg of estradiol benzoate every four to eight weeks or less frequently.

#### Usual adult prescribing limits

Intramuscular, 150 mg testosterone enanthate benzilic acid hydrazone, 7.5 mg of estradiol dienanthate, and 1 mg of estradiol benzoate every four weeks.

#### Strength(s) usually available

U.S.—
Not commercially available.

Canada—
150 mg of testosterone enanthate benzilic acid hydrazone (69 mg base), 7.5 mg of estradiol dienanthate, and 1 mg of estradiol benzoate per mL (Rx) [*Climacteron* (benzoate alcohol 7.5%; benzyl benzoate)].

---

Revised: 06/30/92
Interim revision: 06/21/94

# ANESTHETICS   Mucosal-Local

This monograph includes information on the following: Benzocaine; Benzocaine, Butamben, and Tetracaine; Dibucaine; Dyclonine; Lidocaine; Pramoxine; Tetracaine.

Note: See also individual *Cocaine (Mucosal-Local)* monograph.

INN:
    Dibucaine—Cinchocaine
    Pramoxine—Pramocaine

BAN:
    Dibucaine—Cinchocaine
    Dyclonine—Dyclocaine
    Lidocaine—Lignocaine
    Tetracaine—Amethocaine

JAN:
    Benzocaine—Ethyl aminobenzoate

VA CLASSIFICATION (Primary/Secondary):

Note: Several of the dosage forms listed below are commercially available in more than one formulation. Because the vehicle into which a local anesthetic is incorporated may determine the appropriate usage and/or site(s) of application for a product, some of the VA classifications listed for a dosage form may apply only to specific formulations.

Benzocaine
    Dental paste—OR900
    Gel—NT300/GU900; OR900; RS900
    Lozenges—OR900
    Ointment—RS200/DE700; OR900; RS900
    Topical aerosol—DE700/NT300; OR900
    Topical solution—NT300/OR900
Benzocaine and Menthol
    Lozenges—OR900
Benzocaine and Phenol
    Gel—OR900
    Topical solution—OR900
Benzocaine, Butamben, and Tetracaine
    Gel—NT300/GU900; OR900; RS900
    Ointment—NT300/OR900
    Topical aerosol—NT300/OR900
    Topical solution—NT300/OR900
Dibucaine
    Ointment—RS200/DE700; RS900
Dyclonine
    Lozenges—OR900
    Topical solution—NT300/GU900; OR900; RS900
Lidocaine
    Ointment—NT300/DE700; OR900
    Oral topical solution—OR900
    Topical aerosol—NT300/OR900
Lidocaine Hydrochloride
    Jelly—NT300/GU900
    Oral topical solution—NT300/OR900
    Topical solution—NT300/OR900
    Topical spray solution—NT300
Pramoxine
    Aerosol foam—RS200/RS900
    Cream—RS200/DE700; RS900
    Ointment—RS200
Tetracaine
    Cream—RS200/DE700; RS900
    Topical aerosol—OR900
Tetracaine Hydrochloride
    Topical solution—NT300
Tetracaine and Menthol
    Ointment—RS200/DE700; RS900

Note: For information on local anesthetics applied topically to the skin to relieve minor dermatological conditions, see *Anesthetics (Topical)*.

For information on use of lidocaine hydrochloride by transtracheal injection to anesthetize the larynx and trachea, see *Anesthetics (Parenteral-Local)*.

Some other commonly used names are:

| | |
|---|---|
| Amethocaine [Tetracaine] | Ethyl aminobenzoate |
| Butylaminobenzoate | [Benzocaine] |
| [Butamben] | Lignocaine [Lidocaine] |
| Cinchocaine [Dibucaine] | Pramocaine [Pramoxine] |
| Dyclocaine [Dyclonine] | |

Note: For a listing of dosage forms and brand names by country availability, see *Dosage Forms* section(s). For a listing of brand names for the articles in this monograph, refer to the General Index.

## Category

Anesthetic (mucosal-local).

## Indications

Note: Bracketed information in the *Indications* section refers to uses that are not included in U.S. product labeling.

Gel, ointment, and topical solution dosage forms of benzocaine, ointment and topical solution dosage forms of lidocaine, and topical solution dosage forms of lidocaine hydrochloride are available in more than one formulation. The vehicles present in different formulations may determine the indication(s) for which the formulations are used. Therefore, some gel, ointment, or topical solution formulations that contain the same local anesthetic cannot be used interchangeably. For additional information regarding formulations and brand name products that may be used for specific indications, see the *Dosage Forms* section.

### Accepted

Anesthesia, local—Indicated to provide topical anesthesia of accessible mucous membranes prior to examination, endoscopy or instrumentation, or other procedures involving the:

Esophagus—Benzocaine (gel and topical solution); benzocaine, butamben, and tetracaine; dyclonine (topical solution); lidocaine hydrochloride (4% topical solution, topical spray solution, and [oral topical solution]); and tetracaine hydrochloride (topical solution).

Larynx—Benzocaine (gel and topical solution); benzocaine, butamben, and tetracaine; dyclonine (topical solution); lidocaine hydrochloride (4% topical solution and topical spray solution); and tetracaine hydrochloride (topical solution).

Mouth (in dental procedures and oral surgery)—Benzocaine (gel, topical aerosol, and topical solution); benzocaine, butamben, and tetracaine; dyclonine (topical solution); lidocaine (ointment, topical aerosol, and oral topical solution); lidocaine hydrochloride (oral topical solution and 4% topical solution); and tetracaine (topical aerosol).

Nasal cavity—Benzocaine (gel); benzocaine, butamben, and tetracaine; lidocaine hydrochloride (jelly and 4% topical solution); and tetracaine (topical solution).

Pharynx or throat—Benzocaine (gel, topical aerosol, and topical solution); benzocaine, butamben, and tetracaine; dyclonine (topical solution); lidocaine (ointment and topical aerosol); lidocaine hydrochloride (jelly, oral topical solution, and topical spray solution); and tetracaine (topical solution).

Rectum—Benzocaine (gel); benzocaine, butamben, and tetracaine (gel); and lidocaine hydrochloride (jelly).

Respiratory tract or trachea—Benzocaine (gel, topical aerosol, and topical solution); benzocaine, butamben, and tetracaine; dyclonine (topical solution); lidocaine (ointment); lidocaine hydrochloride (jelly, [oral topical solution], and 4% and 10% topical solution); and tetracaine (topical solution).

Urinary tract—Benzocaine (gel); dyclonine (topical solution); and lidocaine hydrochloride (jelly).

Vagina—Benzocaine (gel); benzocaine, butamben, and tetracaine (gel); and dyclonine (topical solution).

Gag reflex suppression—Indicated to suppress the gag reflex and/or other laryngeal and esophageal reflexes to facilitate dental examination or procedures (including oral surgery), endoscopy, or intubation: Benzocaine (gel, topical aerosol, and topical solution); benzocaine, butamben, and tetracaine (topical aerosol); dyclonine (0.5% topical solution); lidocaine (topical aerosol); lidocaine hydrochloride (oral topical solution and 10% topical solution); tetracaine (topical aerosol); and tetracaine hydrochloride (topical solution).

Anorectal disorders (treatment)—Indicated for the symptomatic relief of:
    Hemorrhoids
    Inflammation, anorectal and
    Pain, anorectal—Benzocaine (ointment); dibucaine; pramoxine; tetracaine hydrochloride (cream); and tetracaine and menthol. These medications are effective when applied to the anal, perianal, or anorectal areas. However, they are not likely to relieve symptoms associated with conditions confined to the rectum, which lacks sensory nerve fibers.

Pain, anogenital lesion–associated—Dyclonine (0.5% solution).

Pain, anogenital, external and

Pruritus, anogenital—Benzocaine (ointment); dibucaine; pramoxine (aerosol foam and cream); tetracaine hydrochloride (cream); tetracaine and menthol.

Oral cavity disorders (treatment); and

Perioral lesions (treatment)—Indicated for relief of

Canker sores or

Cold sores or

Fever blisters—Benzocaine (gel and topical solution); benzocaine and phenol (gel and topical solution); and lidocaine (2.5% topical solution).

Pain, gingival or oral mucosal (i.e., pain caused by mouth or gum irritation, inflammation, lesions, or minor dental procedures)—Benzocaine (gel, dental paste, lozenges, and topical solution); dyclonine (lozenges and 0.5% topical solution); benzocaine and phenol (gel and topical solution); lidocaine (oral topical solution); and lidocaine hydrochloride (oral topical solution).

Pain, dental prosthetic (i.e., pain or irritation caused by dentures or other dental or orthodontic appliances)—Benzocaine (dental paste, gel, ointment, and topical solution); benzocaine and phenol (gel and topical solution); and lidocaine (ointment).

Pain, teething—Benzocaine (7.5% and 10% gel).

Toothache—Benzocaine (10% and 20% gel and topical solution); and benzocaine and phenol (gel and topical solution).

Pain, esophageal (treatment)—Dyclonine (topical solution); and [lidocaine hydrochloride (oral topical solution)].

Pain, pharyngeal (treatment)—Benzocaine (lozenges); benzocaine and menthol (lozenges); dyclonine (lozenges); and lidocaine hydrochloride (oral topical solution).

Pain, vaginal (treatment)—Indicated to relieve pain following procedures such as episiotomy or perineorraphy: Benzocaine (topical aerosol and topical solution); and dyclonine (topical solution).

Urethritis (treatment)—Indicated to relieve or control pain: Lidocaine hydrochloride (jelly).

## Pharmacology/Pharmacokinetics

### Physicochemical characteristics

Chemical group—

Amides: Dibucaine, lidocaine.

Esters, aminobenzoic acid (para-aminobenzoic acid, PABA)–derivative: Benzocaine, butamben, tetracaine.

Unclassified: Dyclonine, pramoxine.

Molecular weight—

Benzocaine: 165.19.

Butamben: 193.25.

Dibucaine: 343.47.

Dyclonine hydrochloride: 325.88.

Lidocaine: 234.34.

Lidocaine hydrochloride: 288.82.

Pramoxine hydrochloride: 329.87.

Tetracaine: 264.37.

Tetracaine hydrochloride: 300.83.

pKa—

Dibucaine: 8.8.

Lidocaine: 7.9.

Tetracaine: 8.2.

### Mechanism of action/Effect

Local anesthetics block both the initiation and conduction of nerve impulses by decreasing the neuronal membrane's permeability to sodium ions. This reversibly stabilizes the membrane and inhibits depolarization, resulting in the failure of a propagated action potential and subsequent conduction blockade.

### Other actions/effects

If substantial quantities of local anesthetics are absorbed through the mucosa, actions on the central nervous system (CNS) may cause CNS stimulation and/or CNS depression. Actions on the cardiovascular system may cause depression of cardiac conduction and excitability and, with some of these agents, peripheral vasodilation.

### Absorption

Except for benzocaine, which is minimally absorbed, these agents are readily absorbed through mucous membranes into the systemic circulation. The rate of absorption is influenced by the vascularity or rate of blood flow at the site of application, the total dosage (concentration and volume) administered, and the duration of exposure. Absorption from mucous membranes of the throat or respiratory tract may be especially rapid. Addition of a vasoconstrictor to the anesthetic may not reduce or slow absorption sufficiently to protect against systemic effects.

### Protein binding

Lidocaine—Concentration-dependent, to alpha 1-acid glycoprotein; usually about 60 to 80% at concentrations of 1 to 4 mcg per mL (4.3 to 17.2 micromoles per L).

### Biotransformation

Amides—

Hepatic and some renal.

Lidocaine: Xylidide metabolites are active and toxic, but less so than the parent compound.

Esters (PABA-derivative)—

Hydrolyzed by plasma cholinesterases and, to a much lesser extent, by hepatic cholinesterases to PABA-containing metabolites.

### Onset of action

Benzocaine—About 1 minute.

Benzocaine, butamben, and tetracaine—About 30 seconds.

Dibucaine—Up to 15 minutes.

Dyclonine—Up to 10 minutes.

Lidocaine—Within 1 to 5 minutes, depending on formulation.

Pramoxine—3 to 5 minutes.

Tetracaine—3 to 10 minutes.

### Duration of action

Benzocaine—

15 to 20 minutes.

Dibucaine—

2 to 4 hours.

Dyclonine—

Approximately 30 to 60 minutes.

Lidocaine—

Approximately 30 to 60 minutes.

Lidocaine oral topical solution: 15 to 20 minutes.

Lidocaine topical aerosol: 10 to 15 minutes.

Tetracaine—

Approximately 30 to 60 minutes.

### Elimination

Amides—

Renal, primarily as metabolites.

Lidocaine: Up to 10% of a dose may be excreted unchanged.

Esters—

Renal, primarily as metabolites.

## Precautions to Consider

### Cross-sensitivity and/or related problems

Patients sensitive to one ester derivative (especially an aminobenzoic acid [para-aminobenzoic acid; PABA] derivative) may be sensitive to other ester derivatives also.

Patients sensitive to PABA, parabens, or paraphenylenediamine (a hair dye) may be sensitive to PABA-derivative local anesthetics also.

Patients sensitive to one amide derivative may rarely be sensitive to other amide derivatives also.

Cross-sensitivity between amide derivatives and ester derivatives, or between amides or esters and chemically unrelated local anesthetics (i.e., dyclonine or pramoxine), has not been reported. However, some lidocaine formulations and pramoxine cream contain parabens, to which cross-sensitivity with PABA-derivative local anesthetics may exist.

### Pregnancy/Reproduction

Fertility—

*Dyclonine*—

Studies have not been done.

*Lidocaine*—

Studies have not been done.

Pregnancy—

*Benzocaine*—

Studies in humans have not been done.

Studies in animals have not been done.

Benzocaine gel: FDA Pregnancy Category C.

*Dyclonine*—

Studies in humans have not been done.

Studies in animals have not been done.

Dyclonine topical solution: FDA Pregnancy Category C.

*Lidocaine*—

Adequate and well-controlled studies in humans have not been done.

Studies in rats given up to 6.6 times the human dose have not shown evidence of teratogenicity or harm to the fetus.

FDA Pregnancy Category B.

*Other mucosal-local anesthetics*—

Problems in humans have not been documented.

**Breast-feeding**

*Lidocaine—*
Distributed into breast milk in very small quantities that pose no risk to the infant.

*Other mucosal-local anesthetics—*
Problems in humans have not been documented.

**Pediatrics**

*Benzocaine—*
Benzocaine should be used with caution in infants and young children because increased absorption may result in methemoglobinemia. Nonprescription teething products (i.e., 7.5% or 10% benzocaine gel) should not be used in infants younger than 4 months of age unless prescribed by a physician or dentist. Other nonprescription products that contain benzocaine for relief of dental pain, perioral lesions, or sore throat (e.g., gel, lozenges, ointment, or topical solution and combinations containing benzocaine with menthol or phenol) should not be used in children younger than 2 years of age unless prescribed by a physician or dentist.

*Other mucosal-local anesthetics—*
Pediatric patients may be more susceptible to systemic toxicity with these medications. Nonprescription products that contain dyclonine or lidocaine for relief of sore throat or perioral lesions should not be used in children younger than 2 years of age unless prescribed by a physician or dentist. Dosage of other mucosal-local anesthetic formulations should be individualized, based on the child's age, weight, and physical condition.

**Geriatrics**

Systemic toxicity may be more likely to occur in geriatric patients, who may require lower concentrations and/or lower total dosages of mucosal-local anesthetics, especially for endoscopic procedures.

**Drug interactions and/or related problems**

See also *Laboratory value alterations.*

The following drug interactions and/or related problems have been selected on the basis of their potential clinical significance (possible mechanism in parentheses where appropriate)—not necessarily inclusive (» = major clinical significance):

Note: Combinations containing any of the following medications, depending on the amount present, may also interact with this medication.

*For ester derivatives only*
Cholinesterase inhibitors
(metabolism of an ester-derivative local anesthetic may be inhibited, leading to increased risk of systemic toxicity, when it is administered to a patient receiving a cholinesterase inhibitor)

Sulfonamides
(metabolites of PABA-derivative local anesthetics may antagonize antibacterial activity of sulfonamides)

*For lidocaine only*
Antiarrhythmic agents, amide local anesthetic–derivative, other, such as:
 Mexiletine
 Tocainide or
Lidocaine, systemic or parenteral-local
(risk of cardiotoxicity associated with additive cardiac effects, and, with systemic or parenteral-local lidocaine, the risk of overdose, may be increased in patients receiving these medications when lidocaine is applied to the mucosa, especially if it is applied in large quantities, used repeatedly, used in the oral or pharyngeal area, or swallowed)

Beta-adrenergic blocking agents
(concurrent use may slow metabolism of lidocaine because of decreased hepatic blood flow, leading to increased risk of lidocaine toxicity, especially if lidocaine is applied to the mucosa in large quantities, used repeatedly, used in the oral or pharyngeal area, or swallowed)

Cimetidine
(cimetidine may inhibit hepatic metabolism of lidocaine, leading to increased risk of lidocaine toxicity, especially if lidocaine is applied to the mucosa in large quantities, used repeatedly, used in the oral or pharyngeal area, or swallowed)

**Laboratory value alterations**

The following have been selected on the basis of their potential clinical significance (possible effect in parentheses where appropriate)—not necessarily inclusive (» = major clinical significance):

With diagnostic test results
Cystoscopic procedures following pyelography
(dyclonine interferes with visualization by reacting with iodine-containing contrast agents, resulting in precipitation of iodine)

Pancreatic function determination using bentiromide
(administration of PABA-derivative anesthetics or lidocaine prior to the bentiromide test will invalidate test results [if the anesthetics are absorbed in sufficient quantity] since they are also metabolized to arylamines and will thus increase the apparent quantity of PABA recovered; discontinuation of these medications at least 3 days prior to the test is recommended)

**Medical considerations/Contraindications**

The medical considerations/contraindications included here have been selected on the basis of their potential clinical significance (reasons given in parentheses where appropriate)—not necessarily inclusive (» = major clinical significance).

*Risk-benefit should be considered when the following medical problems exist:*

Hemorrhoids, bleeding—for rectal use

Local infection at area of treatment
(may alter pH at site of application, leading to decrease or loss of local anesthetic effect)

Sensitivity to the local anesthetic being considered for use and/or chemically related anesthetics or other compounds, history of

Traumatized mucosa, severe
(increased absorption of anesthetic, leading to increased risk of systemic toxicity)

Caution is also advised in pediatric, geriatric, acutely ill, or debilitated patients, who may be more susceptible to systemic toxicity with these medications.

## Side/Adverse Effects

Note: Adverse reactions are due to excessive dosage or rapid absorption, which produces high plasma concentrations, as well as to idiosyncrasy, hypersensitivity, or decreased patient tolerance.

Benzocaine and tetracaine are more likely to cause contact sensitization than are the other mucosal-local anesthetics. Also, tetracaine is more toxic than other mucosal-local anesthetics.

The following side/adverse effects have been selected on the basis of their potential clinical significance (possible signs and symptoms in parentheses where appropriate)—not necessarily inclusive:

**Those indicating need for medical attention**

Incidence less frequent
*Allergic contact dermatitis* (skin rash, redness, itching, or hives); *angioedema* (large, hive-like swellings on skin or in mouth or throat); *burning, stinging, swelling, or tenderness not present before therapy*

Incidence rare
*Urethritis* (blood in urine, increased frequency of urination, pain or burning during urination)—with urethral application

## Overdose

For specific information on the agents used in the management of an overdose, see:
• *Ascorbic Acid (Systemic)* monograph;
• *Benzodiazepines (Systemic)* monograph;
• *Methylene Blue (Systemic)* monograph; and/or
• *Sympathomimetic Agents—Cardiovascular Use (Parenteral-Systemic)* monograph.

For more information on the management of overdose or unintentional ingestion, **contact a Poison Control Center** (see *Poison Control Center Listing*).

The following effects have been selected on the basis of their potential clinical significance (possible signs and symptoms in parentheses where appropriate)—not necessarily inclusive:

Acute and chronic effects
*Cardiovascular system depression* (increased sweating, low blood pressure, pale skin, slow or irregular heartbeat)—may lead to cardiac arrest; *CNS toxicity* (blurred or double vision; confusion; convulsions; dizziness or lightheadedness; drowsiness; feeling hot, cold, or numb; ringing or buzzing in ears; shivering or trembling; unusual anxiety, excitement, nervousness, or restlessness); *methemoglobinemia* (difficulty in breathing on exertion, dizziness, headache, tiredness, weakness)

Note: Stimulant and/or depressant manifestations of *CNS toxicity* may occur. CNS stimulation usually occurs first, followed by CNS depression. However, CNS stimulation may be transient or absent so that drowsiness may be the first symptom of toxicity in some patients. CNS depression may lead to unconsciousness and respiratory arrest.

**Treatment of overdose**
Specific treatment—
    For circulatory depression—Administering a vasopressor and intravenous fluids.
    For convulsions—Administering a benzodiazepine anticonvulsant, keeping in mind that intravenously administered benzodiazepines may cause respiratory and circulatory depression, especially when administered rapidly. Medications and equipment needed for support of respiration and for resuscitation must be immediately available.
    For methemoglobinemia—Administering methylene blue (1 to 2 mg per kg of body weight, intravenously) and/or ascorbic acid (100 to 200 mg orally).
Supportive care—
    Securing and maintaining a patent airway, administering 100% oxygen, and instituting assisted or controlled respiration as required. In some patients, endotracheal intubation may be required.

## Patient Consultation

As an aid to patient consultation, refer to *Advice for the Patient, Anesthetics (Dental)* and *Anesthetics (Rectal)*.

In providing consultation, consider emphasizing the following selected information (» = major clinical significance):

**Before using this medication**
» Conditions affecting use, especially:
    Allergies to local anesthetics of the same chemical class, and, for ester derivatives only, aminobenzoic acid, parabens, or hair dye
    Use in children—Caution recommended, especially with use of benzocaine or lidocaine in infants and young children
    Use in the elderly—Increased risk of side effects

**Proper use of this medication**
    Following physician's or dentist's instructions if prescribed
    Following manufacturer's instructions if self-medicating
» Not using more, more often, or for a longer period of time than prescribed by physician or dentist or recommended on package label
» Checking with physician or dentist before using for problems other than those for which medication was prescribed or those stated on package label
Proper administration technique
*For lidocaine hydrochloride oral topical solution*
» Measuring dose accurately
    Applying with cotton swab or swishing around in mouth (for mouth or gum conditions) or gargling (for throat conditions)
» Not swallowing unless specifically directed by physician or dentist
*For benzocaine film-forming gel*
    Drying affected area with one of the swabs provided before applying
    Applying gel to a second swab, then rolling the swab over the affected area
    Keeping mouth open and dry for 30 to 60 seconds after applying, while film forms
    Not removing film, which will slowly disintegrate over 6 hours
*For other nonprescription gel and solution dosage forms*
    Applying to affected area(s) with a clean finger, a cotton-tipped applicator, or gauze
    If using for pain caused by dental appliances, applying to sore area and, after relief is obtained, rinsing mouth before reinserting appliance; not applying directly to or using under appliance unless directed to do so by dentist
*For benzocaine dental paste*
    Dabbing small amounts onto affected areas with cotton-tipped applicator; not rubbing or spreading, to prevent crumbling or grittiness
*For topical aerosol or spray dosage forms*
    Using care not to inhale medication
    Avoiding spraying back of throat or mouth unless specifically directed by physician or dentist
*For lozenges*
    Dissolving slowly in mouth; not biting or chewing lozenges or swallowing them whole
*For rectal cream or ointment*
    Reading patient directions
    If applying externally: Cleansing area with mild soap and water or a cleansing wipe, rinsing thoroughly, and drying gently before applying
    If inserting into anal canal: Using special applicator provided; lubricating applicator with a small amount of cream or ointment before inserting; washing reusable applicator after each use; discarding pre-filled disposable applicator

*For rectal aerosol foam*
    Reading patient directions before use
    Not inserting container into rectum; shaking container, attaching and filling the applicator provided, then detaching applicator from container prior to use
    Applying a small amount of foam to lubricate the applicator before inserting
    Taking applicator apart and washing thoroughly after each use
» Proper dosing
    Missed dose (if prescribed for scheduled dosing)—Using as soon as possible; not using if almost time for next dose; not doubling doses of dental-local anesthetics
» Proper storage

**Precautions while using this medication**
» Contacting physician:
    —if using for sore throat and sore throat is severe, persists for more than 2 days, or is accompanied or followed by other symptoms such as fever, headache, rash, swelling, nausea, or vomiting
    —if using for hemorrhoids or other perianal conditions and condition does not improve within 7 days, bleeding occurs, or symptoms such as redness, irritation, swelling, or pain develop or worsen during treatment
» Contacting physician or dentist if using for perioral lesions and symptoms do not improve within 7 days, irritation or pain persists or worsens, or swelling, rash, or fever develops
» Contacting dentist:
    —as soon as possible to arrange an appointment if using to relieve toothache; medication is a temporary measure only
    —at regular intervals when medication used to relieve pain during adjustment of new dentures or other dental appliances
    Not using benzocaine, lidocaine, or tetracaine for 72 hours prior to having pancreatic function test using bentiromide because of potential interference with test results
*For use in mouth or throat area*
» Not eating for one hour following use of medication because may impair swallowing, leading to risk of aspiration
» Not chewing gum or food while numbness persists because of risk of biting tongue or buccal mucosa

**Side/adverse effects**
    Signs and symptoms of potential side effects, especially allergic contact dermatitis; angioedema; and burning, stinging, swelling, or tenderness not present before therapy

## General Dosing Information

The safety and effectiveness of local anesthetics, when they are used for examination or instrumentation procedures (especially those involving the esophagus, larynx, pharynx, respiratory tract, or urinary tract) depend upon proper dosage, correct administration technique, adequate precautions, and readiness for emergencies. *Resuscitative equipment, oxygen, and other required medications should be immediately available.*

The dosage of mucosal-local anesthetics, when they are used for examination or instrumentation procedures, depends on the technique of anesthesia, the area to be anesthetized, the vascularity of the tissues at the application site, and the patient's tolerance.

For use in examination or instrumentation procedures, the recommended adult doses are given as a guideline for use in the average adult. *The actual dosage and maximum dosage must be individualized,* based on the age, size, and physical status of the patient and the expected rate of systemic absorption from the administration site.

Depending on the area to be anesthetized, lower concentrations and/or lower total dosage may be required for pediatric, geriatric, acutely ill, or debilitated patients.

A standard textbook should be consulted for specific techniques and procedures applicable to the use of mucosal-local anesthetics for individual diagnostic and treatment procedures.

---

### BENZOCAINE

## Summary of Differences

Pharmacology/pharmacokinetics:
    Physicochemical characteristics—
        Benzocaine is a PABA derivative ester-type local anesthetic.
    Absorption—
        Minimally absorbed.

Precautions:
  Cross-sensitivity and/or related problems—
    May occur with other ester-type local anesthetics, especially other PABA derivatives, parabens, and paraphenylenediamine.
  Pediatrics—
    May cause methemoglobinemia in infants.
  Drug interactions and/or related problems—
    Cholinesterase inhibitors inhibit metabolism of benzocaine.
    May antagonize antibacterial activity of sulfonamides.

Side/adverse effects:
  More likely to cause contact sensitization than most other local anesthetics.
  See also *Side/Adverse Effects*.

## Dental Dosage Forms

Note: The gel, ointment, and topical solution dosage forms included in this section are specifically formulated for application only to the gingival or buccal mucosa or to perioral tissues. Gel and topical solution formulations that may be applied to other mucosal tissues (in addition to the gingival or buccal mucosa) are included in the *Topical Dosage Forms* section.

### BENZOCAINE GEL (DENTAL)

**Usual adult and adolescent dose**
Anesthetic, mucosal-local—Topical, as a 10 or 20% gel, applied to affected area(s) up to four times a day or as directed by a physician or dentist.

Note: The medication may be applied with cotton, a cotton swab, or a fingertip.

The gel should not be applied directly to, or used beneath, a dental appliance unless the patient is under the supervision of a dentist. Patients using this medication without the supervision of a dentist for relief of dental appliance pain should apply the medication directly to the affected gum area, wait until relief is obtained, and rinse the mouth before reinserting the appliance.

**Usual pediatric dose**
Anesthetic, mucosal-local—
  For teething pain:
    Infants up to 4 months of age—Dosage must be individualized by a physician or dentist.
    Infants and children 4 months to 2 years of age—Topical, as a 7.5 or 10% gel, applied to affected area(s) up to four times a day as needed or as directed by a physician or dentist.
    Children 2 years of age and older—Topical, as a 7.5% or stronger gel, applied to affected area(s) up to four times a day or as directed by a physician or dentist.
  For toothache:
    Children 2 years of age and older—See *Usual adult and adolescent dose*.

Note: Product may be applied with cotton, a cotton swab, or a fingertip.

**Strength(s) usually available**
U.S.—
  7.5% (OTC) [*Anbesol, Baby; Num-Zit Gel; Orabase, Baby; Orajel, Baby*].
  10% (OTC) [*Numzident; Orajel; Orajel Nighttime Formula, Baby; Rid-A-Pain*].
  20% (OTC) [*Anbesol Maximum Strength Gel* (alcohol 60%); *Orajel Maximum Strength; SensoGARD Canker Sore Relief*].
Canada—
  7.5% (OTC) [*Anbesol Baby Jel*].
  20% (OTC) [*Orajel Extra Strength; Topicaine*].

**Packaging and storage**
Store below 40 °C (104 °F), preferably between 15 and 30 °C (59 and 86 °F), unless otherwise specified by manufacturer. Protect from freezing.

### BENZOCAINE FILM-FORMING GEL

**Usual adult and adolescent dose**
Anesthetic, mucosal-local—Topical, as a 15% gel, applied with a cotton swab to affected area(s) up to four times a day or as directed by a physician or dentist. The area should be dried with a cotton swab prior to application.

**Usual pediatric dose**
Anesthetic, mucosal-local—
  Infants and children up to 2 years of age: Dosage must be individualized by a physician or dentist.
  Children 2 years of age and older: See *Usual adult and adolescent dose*.

Note: To ensure that this medication is applied correctly, children up to 12 years of age should apply it under the supervision of an adult.

**Strength(s) usually available**
U.S.—
  15% (OTC) [*Oratect Gel*].

**Packaging and storage**
Store below 40 °C (104 °F), preferably between 15 and 30 °C (59 and 86 °F), unless otherwise specified by manufacturer. Protect from freezing.

### BENZOCAINE LOZENGES

**Usual adult and adolescent dose**
Anesthetic, mucosal-local—Oral, one 10-mg lozenge to be dissolved slowly in the mouth. May be repeated at two-hour intervals as needed.

**Usual pediatric dose**
Anesthetic, mucosal-local—
  Children up to 2 years of age: Dosage must be individualized by a physician.
  Children 2 years of age and older: Oral, one 5-mg lozenge to be dissolved slowly in the mouth. May be repeated at two-hour intervals, if needed.

**Usual pediatric prescribing limits**
Not to exceed twelve 5-mg lozenges per day.

**Strength(s) usually available**
U.S.—
  5 mg (OTC) [*Chloraseptic Lozenges, Children's*].
  10 mg (OTC) [*Spec-T Sore Throat Anesthetic*].

**Packaging and storage**
Store below 40 °C (104 °F), preferably between 15 and 30 °C (59 and 86 °F), unless otherwise specified by manufacturer.

### BENZOCAINE OINTMENT (DENTAL) USP

**Usual adult and adolescent dose**
Anesthetic, mucosal-local—Topical, applied to cleaned and dried dentures up to four times a day.

**Usual pediatric dose**
Dosage has not been established.

**Strength(s) usually available**
U.S.—
  20% (OTC) [*Benzodent; Dentapaine*].

**Packaging and storage**
Store below 30 °C (86 °F). Store in a tight container. Protect from light. Protect from freezing.

### BENZOCAINE DENTAL PASTE

**Usual adult and adolescent dose**
Anesthetic, mucosal-local—Topical, applied to the affected area as needed.

**Usual pediatric dose**
Anesthetic, mucosal-local—
  Children up to 6 years of age: Dosage must be individualized by physician or dentist.
  Children 6 years of age and older: See *Usual adult and adolescent dose*.

**Strength(s) usually available**
U.S.—
  20% (OTC) [*Orabase-B with Benzocaine*].

**Packaging and storage**
Store below 40 °C (104 °F), preferably between 15 and 30 °C (59 and 86 °F), unless otherwise specified by manufacturer. Protect from freezing.

### BENZOCAINE TOPICAL SOLUTION (DENTAL) USP

**Usual adult and adolescent dose**
Anesthetic, mucosal-local—Topical, as a 20% solution, applied to affected area(s) up to four times a day or as directed by a physician or dentist.

Note: The medication may be applied with cotton, a cotton swab, or a fingertip.

**Usual pediatric dose**
Anesthetic, mucosal-local—
  Infants and children up to 2 years of age: Dosage must be individualized by a physician or dentist.
  Children 2 years of age and older: See *Usual adult and adolescent dose*.

**Strength(s) usually available**
U.S.—
  0.2% (OTC) [*Num-Zit Lotion* (alcohol 12.6%)].
  5% (OTC) [*Dent-Zel-Ite* (alcohol 81%)].
  20% (OTC) [*Anbesol Maximum Strength Liquid* (alcohol 60%)].

Note: In Canada, *Anbesol Maximum Strength Liquid* also contains 0.45% of phenol. See *Benzocaine and Phenol Topical Solution*.

Canada—

6.5% (OTC) [*Dentocaine*].
7.5% (OTC) [*Orajel, Baby*].
20% (OTC) [*Orajel Liquid*].

**Packaging and storage**

Store below 30 °C (86 °F). Store in a tight container. Protect from light. Protect from freezing.

## BENZOCAINE AND MENTHOL LOZENGES

### Usual adult and adolescent dose

Anesthetic, mucosal-local—Oral, one lozenge dissolved slowly in the mouth every two hours as needed or as directed by a physician or dentist.

### Usual pediatric dose

Anesthetic, mucosal-local—

Children up to 2 years of age: Dosage must be individualized by a physician or dentist.

Children 2 years of age and older: See *Usual adult and adolescent dose*.

### Strength(s) usually available

U.S.—

6 mg of benzocaine and 10 mg of menthol (OTC) [*Chloraseptic Lozenges*].

Canada—

6 mg of benzocaine and 10 mg of menthol (OTC) [*Chloraseptic Lozenges Cherry Flavor*].

### Packaging and storage

Store below 40 °C (104 °F), preferably between 15 and 30 °C (59 and 86 °F), unless otherwise specified by manufacturer.

## BENZOCAINE AND PHENOL GEL

### Usual adult and adolescent dose

Anesthetic, mucosal-local—Topical, applied to affected area(s) up to four times a day or as directed by a physician or dentist.

Note: The medication may be applied with cotton, a cotton swab, or a fingertip.

The gel should not be applied directly to, or used beneath, a dental appliance unless the patient is under the supervision of a dentist. Patients using this medication without the supervision of a dentist for relief of dental appliance pain should apply the medication directly to the affected gum area, wait until relief is obtained, and rinse the mouth before reinserting the appliance.

### Usual pediatric dose

Anesthetic, mucosal-local—

Infants and children up to 2 years of age: Dosage must be individualized by a physician or dentist.

Children 2 years of age and older: See *Usual adult and adolescent dose*.

### Strength(s) usually available

U.S.—

6.3% of benzocaine and 0.5% of phenol (OTC) [*Anbesol Regular Strength Gel* (alcohol 70%)].

Canada—

6.4% of benzocaine and 0.5% of phenol (OTC) [*Anbesol Gel* (alcohol)].

### Packaging and storage

Store below 40 °C (104 °F), preferably between 15 and 30 °C (59 and 86 °F), unless otherwise specified by manufacturer. Protect from freezing.

## BENZOCAINE AND PHENOL TOPICAL SOLUTION

### Usual adult and adolescent dose

Anesthetic, mucosal-local—Topical, applied to affected area(s) up to four times a day or as directed by a physician or dentist.

Note: The medication may be applied with cotton, a cotton swab, or a fingertip.

### Usual pediatric dose

Anesthetic, mucosal-local—

Infants and children up to 2 years of age: Dosage must be individualized by a physician or dentist.

Children 2 years of age and older: See *Usual adult and adolescent dose*.

### Strength(s) usually available

U.S.—

6.3% of benzocaine and 0.5% of phenol (OTC) [*Anbesol Regular Strength Liquid* (alcohol 70%)].

Canada—

6.5% of benzocaine and 0.45% of phenol (OTC) [*Anbesol Liquid* (alcohol)].

20% of benzocaine and 0.45% of phenol (OTC) [*Anbesol Maximum Strength Liquid* (alcohol)].

Note: In the U.S., *Anbesol Maximum Strength Liquid* does not contain phenol. See *Benzocaine Topical Solution USP (Dental)*.

### Packaging and storage

Store below 40 °C (104 °F), preferably between 15 and 30 °C (59 and 86 °F), unless otherwise specified by manufacturer. Protect from freezing.

# Rectal Dosage Forms

## BENZOCAINE OINTMENT (RECTAL) USP

### Usual adult and adolescent dose

Anesthetic, mucosal-local—Topical, applied to the perianal area up to six times a day after the area has been cleansed and dried. Medication should not be inserted into the rectum.

### Usual pediatric dose

Dosage has not been established.

### Strength(s) usually available

U.S.—

20% (OTC) [*Americaine Hemorrhoidal*].

### Packaging and storage

Store below 30 °C (86 °F). Store in a tight container. Protect from light. Protect from freezing.

# Topical Dosage Forms

## BENZOCAINE GEL

### Usual adult and adolescent dose

Anesthetic, mucosal-local—

Dental procedures: Topical, as a 20% gel, applied to area with a cotton applicator as needed.

Other examination or instrumentation procedures: Topical, as a 20% gel, applied to area with a cotton applicator, or to instrument prior to insertion.

### Usual pediatric dose

Dosage has not been established.

### Strength(s) usually available

U.S.—

20% [*Americaine Anesthetic Lubricant* (Rx); *Hurricaine* (OTC)].

### Packaging and storage

Store below 40 °C (104 °F), preferably between 15 and 30 °C (59 and 86 °F), unless otherwise specified by manufacturer. Protect from freezing.

## BENZOCAINE TOPICAL AEROSOL USP

### Usual adult and adolescent dose

Anesthetic, mucosal-local—Topical, as a 20% solution, sprayed on area for one second. May be repeated if necessary.

### Usual pediatric dose

Dosage has not been established.

### Strength(s) usually available

U.S.—

20% (OTC) [*Americaine; Hurricaine*].

### Packaging and storage

Store below 40 °C (104 °F), unless otherwise specified by manufacturer.

## BENZOCAINE TOPICAL SOLUTION USP

### Usual adult and adolescent dose

Anesthetic, mucosal-local—Topical, as a 20% solution, applied to area with a cotton applicator as needed.

### Usual pediatric dose

Dosage has not been established.

### Strength(s) usually available

U.S.—

20% (OTC) [*Hurricaine*].

### Packaging and storage

Store below 30 °C (86 °F). Store in a tight container. Protect from light. Protect from freezing.

## BENZOCAINE, BUTAMBEN, AND TETRACAINE

## Summary of Differences

Pharmacology/pharmacokinetics:
  Physicochemical characteristics—
    Benzocaine, butamben, and tetracaine are all PABA-derivative ester-type local anesthetics.
Precautions:
  Cross-sensitivity and/or related problems—
    May occur with other ester-type local anesthetics, especially other PABA derivatives, parabens, and paraphenylenediamine.
  Drug interactions and/or related problems—
    Cholinesterase inhibitors inhibit metabolism of these local anesthetics.
    May antagonize antibacterial activity of sulfonamides.
Side/adverse effects:
  Benzocaine and tetracaine are more likely to cause contact sensitization than other local anesthetics.
  Tetracaine is more toxic than other mucosal-local anesthetics.
  See also *Side/Adverse Effects.*

## Additional Dosing Information

See also *General Dosing Information.*

In dentistry, this medication should not be used under dentures or cotton rolls, because retention under these materials may result in sloughing of tissue.

## Topical Dosage Forms

### BENZOCAINE, BUTAMBEN, AND TETRACAINE HYDROCHLORIDE GEL USP

**Usual adult and adolescent dose**
Anesthetic, mucosal-local—Topical, applied directly to desired area, or to instrument prior to insertion.

**Usual adult prescribing limits**
For the tetracaine component—20 mg.

**Usual pediatric dose**
Dosage has not been established.

**Strength(s) usually available**
U.S.—
  14% of benzocaine, 2% of butamben, and 2% of tetracaine hydrochloride (Rx) [*Cetacaine Topical Anesthetic*].

**Packaging and storage**
Store below 40 °C (104 °F), preferably between 15 and 30 °C (59 and 86 °F), unless otherwise specified by manufacturer. Protect from freezing.

### BENZOCAINE, BUTAMBEN, AND TETRACAINE HYDROCHLORIDE OINTMENT USP

**Usual adult and adolescent dose**
Anesthetic, mucosal-local—Topical, applied with a cotton pledget or directly to tissue.

Note: Cotton pledget should not be held in position for extended periods of time, because of increased risk of local reactions to the anesthetics.

**Usual adult prescribing limits**
For the tetracaine component—20 mg.

**Usual pediatric dose**
Dosage has not been established.

**Strength(s) usually available**
U.S.—
  14% of benzocaine, 2% of butamben, and 2% of tetracaine hydrochloride (Rx) [*Cetacaine Topical Anesthetic*].

**Packaging and storage**
Store below 40 °C (104 °F), preferably between 15 and 30 °C (59 and 86 °F), unless otherwise specified by manufacturer. Protect from freezing.

### BENZOCAINE, BUTAMBEN, AND TETRACAINE HYDROCHLORIDE TOPICAL AEROSOL USP

**Usual adult and adolescent dose**
Anesthetic, mucosal-local—Topical, sprayed on desired area for approximately one second or less.

**Usual adult prescribing limits**
Duration of spray should not exceed two seconds.

**Usual pediatric dose**
Dosage has not been established.

**Strength(s) usually available**
U.S.—
  14% of benzocaine, 2% of butamben, and 2% of tetracaine hydrochloride (Rx) [*Cetacaine Topical Anesthetic*].

**Packaging and storage**
Store below 40 °C (104 °F), preferably between 15 and 30 °C (59 and 86 °F), unless otherwise specified by manufacturer.

**Auxiliary labeling**
• Shake well.

## BENZOCAINE, BUTAMBEN, AND TETRACAINE HYDROCHLORIDE TOPICAL SOLUTION USP

**Usual adult and adolescent dose**
Anesthetic, mucosal-local—Topical, applied with a cotton pledget or directly to tissue.

Note: Cotton pledget should not be held in position for extended periods of time, because of increased risk of local reactions to the anesthetics.

**Usual adult prescribing limits**
For the tetracaine component—20 mg.

**Usual pediatric dose**
Dosage has not been established.

**Strength(s) usually available**
U.S.—
  14% of benzocaine, 2% of butamben, and 2% of tetracaine hydrochloride (Rx) [*Cetacaine Topical Anesthetic*].

**Packaging and storage**
Store below 40 °C (104 °F), preferably between 15 and 30 °C (59 and 86 °F), unless otherwise specified by manufacturer. Protect from freezing.

## DIBUCAINE

## Summary of Differences

Indications:
  Indicated for treatment of hemorrhoids and other anorectal disorders.
Pharmacology/pharmacokinetics:
  Physicochemical characteristics—
    Dibucaine is an amide-type local anesthetic.
Precautions:
  Cross-sensitivity and/or related problems—Rarely, may occur with other amide-type local anesthetics.
  Laboratory value alterations—No interference with pancreatic function test using bentiromide.

## Rectal Dosage Forms

### DIBUCAINE OINTMENT USP

**Usual adult and adolescent dose**
Anesthetic, mucosal-local—
  Rectal, a comfortable quantity, inserted three or four times a day, in the morning, in the evening, and after bowel movements; and/or
  Topical, to the perianal area three or four times a day, in the morning, in the evening, and after bowel movements.

**Usual pediatric dose**
Dosage has not been established.

**Strength(s) usually available**
U.S.—
  1% (OTC) [*Nupercainal* (acetone sodium bisulfite); GENERIC].
Canada—
  1% (OTC) [*Nupercainal* (bisulfite)].

**Packaging and storage**
Store below 40 °C (104 °F), preferably between 15 and 30 °C (59 and 86 °F), unless otherwise specified by manufacturer. Store in a collapsible tube or in a tight, light-resistant container. Protect from freezing.

## DYCLONINE

## Summary of Differences

Pharmacology/pharmacokinetics:
  Physicochemical characteristics—
    Dyclonine is neither an ester-type nor an amide-type local anesthetic.

Precautions:

Cross-sensitivity and/or related problems—

Does not occur with either ester-type or amide-type local anesthetics.

Laboratory value alterations—

May cause precipitation of iodine from contrast agents used in cystoscopic procedures following pyelography.

No interference with pancreatic function test using bentiromide.

## Dental Dosage Forms
### DYCLONINE HYDROCHLORIDE LOZENGES

**Usual adult and adolescent dose**

Anesthetic, mucosal-local—Oral, one 2-mg or 3-mg lozenge to be dissolved slowly in the mouth. May be repeated at two-hour intervals, if needed.

**Usual pediatric dose**

Anesthetic, mucosal-local—

Children up to 2 years of age: Dosage has not been established.

Children 2 years of age and older: Oral, one 1.2-mg lozenge to be dissolved slowly in the mouth. May be repeated at two-hour intervals, if needed.

**Strength(s) usually available**

U.S.—

1.2 mg (OTC) [*Sucrets, Children's*].

2 mg (OTC) [*Sucrets Regular Strength*].

3 mg (OTC) [*Sucrets Maximum Strength*].

**Packaging and storage**

Store below 40 °C (104 °F), preferably between 15 and 30 °C (59 and 86 °F), unless otherwise specified by manufacturer.

## Topical Dosage Forms
### DYCLONINE HYDROCHLORIDE TOPICAL SOLUTION USP

**Usual adult and adolescent dose**

Anesthetic, mucosal-local—

Topical, 40 to 200 mg as a 0.5 or 1% solution; specifically:

For anogenital pain—

Topical, as a 0.5% solution, applied with sponges or cotton pledgets.

For dental procedures—

Topical, as a 0.5% solution, used as a mouthwash or gargle and the excess expelled.

For otorhinolaryngologic examinations—

Topical, as a 0.5% solution, used as a spray or gargle.

For perioral lesion pain—

Topical, to the affected area(s), as a 0.5% solution, used as a rinse or swab.

For vaginal pain—

Topical, a 0.5 or 1% solution, applied as a wet compress or spray.

For esophageal lesion pain—

Oral, 25 to 150 mg (5 to 15 mL of a 0.5 or 1% solution).

**Usual adult prescribing limits**

Up to 300 mg (30 mL of a 1% solution) per examination, although this dose is rarely required. Adequate anesthesia is usually achieved with smaller quantities.

**Usual pediatric dose**

Dosage has not been established.

**Strength(s) usually available**

U.S.—

0.5% (Rx) [*Dyclone*].

1% (Rx) [*Dyclone*].

**Packaging and storage**

Store below 40 °C (104 °F), preferably between 15 and 30 °C (59 and 86 °F), unless otherwise specified by manufacturer. Store in a tight, light-resistant container. Protect from freezing.

---

## LIDOCAINE

## Summary of Differences

Pharmacology/pharmacokinetics:

Physicochemical characteristics—Lidocaine is an amide-type local anesthetic.

Protein binding—Concentration-dependent; 60 to 80% at nontoxic plasma concentrations.

Precautions:

Cross-sensitivity and/or related problems—Rarely, may occur with other amide-type local anesthetics.

Breast-feeding—Distributed into breast milk in very small quantities.

Drug interactions and/or related problems—Also interacts with beta-adrenergic blocking agents, cimetidine, and amide local anesthetic–derivative antiarrhythmic agents.

## Dental Dosage Forms

Note: The topical solution formulations included in this section are specifically formulated for application only to gingival or buccal mucosa or to perioral tissues. Topical solution formulations that are applied to other mucosal tissues (in addition to the gingival or buccal mucosa) are included in the *Topical Dosage Forms* section.

### LIDOCAINE TOPICAL AEROSOL USP

**Usual adult and adolescent dose**

Anesthetic, mucosal-local—Topical, to gingival and oral mucous membranes, 20 mg (two metered sprays) per quadrant of gingiva and oral mucosa.

**Usual adult prescribing limits**

Not to exceed 30 mg of lidocaine (three metered sprays) per quadrant of gingiva and oral mucosa over a one-half-hour period or 200 mg (twenty metered sprays) in twenty-four hours.

**Usual pediatric dose**

Anesthetic, mucosal-local—Topical, to gingival and oral mucous membranes, up to a total of 3 mg per kg of body weight.

**Strength(s) usually available**

U.S.—

10% (10 mg per metered spray) (Rx) [*Xylocaine*].

Canada—

10% (10 mg per metered spray) (OTC) [*Xylocaine*].

**Packaging and storage**

Store below 40 °C (104 °F), preferably between 15 and 30 °C (59 and 86 °F), unless otherwise specified by manufacturer. Protect from freezing.

**Auxiliary labeling**

• Shake well.

### LIDOCAINE ORAL TOPICAL SOLUTION USP

**Usual adult and adolescent dose**

Anesthesia, mucosal-local—

Dental procedures: Topical, 50 to 200 mg as a 5% solution, applied to the oral mucosa with a cotton applicator.

Perioral lesions: Topical, as a 2.5% solution, applied to affected area(s) with a cotton swab every one or two hours for the first three days, then as needed.

**Usual adult prescribing limits**

Dental procedures—Not to exceed a total of 250 mg (5 mL of a 5% solution) for all quadrants in a three-hour period.

**Usual pediatric dose**

Anesthesia, mucosal-local—Dental procedures: Topical, the dosage being individualized, based on the child's age, weight, and physical condition up to a maximum of 4.5 mg per kg of body weight as 5% solution.

**Strength(s) usually available**

U.S.—

2.5% (OTC) [*Zilactin-L*].

5% (Rx) [*Xylocaine*; GENERIC].

Canada—

5% (OTC) [*Xylocaine*].

**Packaging and storage**

Store below 40 °C (104 °F), preferably between 15 and 30 °C (59 and 86 °F), unless otherwise specified by manufacturer. Store in a tight container. Protect from freezing.

## Topical Dosage Forms
### LIDOCAINE OINTMENT USP

**Usual adult and adolescent dose**

Anesthetic, mucosal-local—

Oral mucosa:

Topical, as a 5% ointment, to previously dried oral mucosa.

For use during fitting of new dentures—Apply to all denture surfaces that contact the mucosa, up to a maximum of 5 grams of ointment (250 mg of lidocaine) per single dose or 20 grams of ointment (1000 mg of lidocaine) per day.

Note: The patient should be advised to consult the prescribing dentist at intervals not exceeding 48 hours throughout the fitting period.

Oropharynx:
  Topical, as a 5% ointment, applied to desired area, or to instrument prior to insertion.

**Usual pediatric dose**
Anesthetic, mucosal-local—Topical, the dosage being individualized, based on the child's age, weight, and physical condition, up to a maximum of 4.5 mg per kg of body weight or 2.5 grams of ointment in a six-hour period.

**Strength(s) usually available**
U.S.—
  5% (Rx) [*Xylocaine;* GENERIC].
Canada—
  5% (OTC) [*Xylocaine Dental Ointment*].

**Packaging and storage**
Store below 40 °C (104 °F), preferably between 15 and 30 °C (59 and 86 °F), unless otherwise specified by manufacturer. Store in a tight container. Protect from freezing.

## LIDOCAINE HYDROCHLORIDE JELLY USP

**Usual adult and adolescent dose**
Anesthetic, mucosal-local—
  Esophagus, larynx, trachea:
    Topical, as a 2% jelly, applied to the outer surface of the instrument prior to insertion.
    Note: Care should be taken to avoid depositing any of the medication on the inner surface of an endoscope or other instrument. It may dry on the inner surface and leave a residue that may cause narrowing or, rarely, occlusion of the lumen.
  Urinary tract:
    Female—
      Urethral, 3 to 5 mL, as a 2% jelly, several minutes prior to examination.
      Note: Jelly may be deposited on a cotton swab and introduced into urethra.
    Male—
      Prior to catheterization: Urethral, 100 to 200 mg (5 to 10 mL) as a 2% jelly.
      Prior to sounding or cystoscopy: Urethral, 600 mg (30 mL) to fill and dilate urethra. The medication is usually administered in two divided doses, with a penile clamp applied for several minutes between doses.

**Usual adult prescribing limits**
Not more than 600 mg (30 mL) in a twelve-hour period.

**Usual pediatric dose**
Anesthetic, mucosal-local—Topical, as a 2% jelly, dosage to be individualized, based on the child's age, weight, and physical condition, up to a maximum of 4.5 mg per kg of body weight.

**Strength(s) usually available**
U.S.—
  2% (Rx) [*Anestacon Jelly; Xylocaine;* GENERIC].
Canada—
  2% (OTC) [*Xylocaine*].

**Packaging and storage**
Store below 40 °C (104 °F), preferably between 15 and 30 °C (59 and 86 °F), unless otherwise specified by manufacturer. Store in a tight container. Protect from freezing.

## LIDOCAINE HYDROCHLORIDE ORAL TOPICAL SOLUTION USP

Note: Previous name—Lidocaine Hydrochloride Viscous Solution.

**Usual adult and adolescent dose**
Anesthetic, mucosal-local—
  Oral cavity disorders: Topical, 300 mg (15 mL) swished around in the mouth, then expelled, or applied with a cotton-tipped applicator, every three hours as needed.
  Pharyngeal pain: Topical, 300 mg (15 mL) used as a gargle every three hours as needed. May be swallowed if necessary.

**Usual adult prescribing limits**
Single dose—Not to exceed 4.5 mg per kg of body weight or 300 mg (15 mL). This dose should not be repeated more often than every three hours.
Multiple doses—Not to exceed 8 doses (2.4 grams or 120 mL) in twenty-four hours.

**Usual pediatric dose**
Anesthetic, mucosal-local—
  Infants and children up to 3 years of age:
    Topical, up to 1.25 mL of a 2% solution, applied to affected area(s) with a cotton-tipped applicator every three hours.
    Note: It is recommended that the dosage be accurately measured and applied to the immediate area or specific lesion with a cotton-tipped applicator. The risk of systemic toxicity, especially convulsions, is increased if dosage is not carefully controlled and/or if the patient swallows significant quantities of the medication.
  Children 3 years of age and older:
    Topical, the dosage being individualized, based on the child's age, weight, and physical condition, up to a maximum of 4.5 mg per kg of body weight as 2% solution in a three-hour period.

**Strength(s) usually available**
U.S.—
  2% (Rx) [*Xylocaine Viscous;* GENERIC].
Canada—
  2% (OTC) [*Xylocaine Viscous*].

**Packaging and storage**
Store below 40 °C (104 °F), preferably between 15 and 30 °C (59 and 86 °F), unless otherwise specified by manufacturer. Store in a tight container. Protect from freezing.

## LIDOCAINE HYDROCHLORIDE TOPICAL SOLUTION USP

**Usual adult and adolescent dose**
Anesthetic, mucosal-local—Oral or nasal cavity or esophagus: Topical, as a 4% solution, 600 mcg (0.6 mg) to 3 mg per kg of body weight; or 40 to 200 mg (1 to 5 mL).
Note: May be applied as a spray, with cotton applicators or packs, or instilled directly into cavity.

**Usual adult prescribing limits**
For use in oral or nasal cavities or upper gastrointestinal tract—Not to exceed 4.5 mg per kg of body weight or 300 mg (7.5 mL of a 4% solution).

**Usual pediatric dose**
Dosage must be individualized by physician.

**Strength(s) usually available**
U.S.—
  4% (Rx) [*Xylocaine;* GENERIC].
Canada—
  4% (OTC) [*Xylocaine*].

**Packaging and storage**
Store below 40 °C (104 °F), preferably between 15 and 30 °C (59 and 86 °F), unless otherwise specified by manufacturer. Store in a tight container. Protect from freezing.

## LIDOCAINE HYDROCHLORIDE TOPICAL SPRAY SOLUTION

Note: The dosing and strength of this dosage form are expressed in terms of lidocaine base.

**Usual adult and adolescent dose**
Anesthetic, mucosal-local—Endoscopic procedures: Topical, up to 20 metered sprays (200 mg [base]) as a 10% (base) solution, sprayed onto the oropharyngeal or tracheal mucosa.

**Usual pediatric dose**
Anesthetic, mucosal-local—
  Infants and children up to 3 years of age:
    Use is not recommended; a less concentrated solution should be used instead.
  Children 3 to 12 years of age:
    Larynx or trachea—Topical, up to 1.5 mg (base) per kg of body weight.
    Other mucosa—Topical, up to 3 mg (base) per kg of body weight.

**Strength(s) usually available**
U.S.—
  Not commercially available.
Canada—
  10% (base; 12 mg of lidocaine hydrochloride equivalent to 10 mg of lidocaine base per metered spray) (OTC) [*Xylocaine Endotracheal*].

**Packaging and storage**
Store below 40 °C (104 °F), preferably between 15 and 30 °C (59 and 86 °F), unless otherwise specified by manufacturer. Store in a tight container. Protect from freezing.

| | |
|---|---|
| *PRAMOXINE* | *TETRACAINE* |

## Summary of Differences

Indications:
    Indicated for the treatment of hemorrhoids and other anorectal disorders.
Pharmacology/pharmacokinetics:
    Physicochemical characteristics—
        Pramoxine is neither an amide-type nor an ester-type local anesthetic.
Precautions:
    Cross-sensitivity and/or related problems—Does not occur with either ester-type or amide-type local anesthetics.
    Laboratory value alterations—No interference with pancreatic function test using bentiromide.

## Rectal Dosage Forms

### PRAMOXINE HYDROCHLORIDE AEROSOL FOAM

**Usual adult and adolescent dose**
Anesthetic, mucosal-local—
    Rectal, one applicatorful two to three times a day; or
    Topical, to the external anorectal area two to three times a day.

**Usual pediatric dose**
Dosage has not been established.

**Strength(s) usually available**
U.S.—
    1% (OTC) [*ProctoFoam/non-steroid* (propylparaben)].

**Packaging and storage**
Store below 40 °C (104 °F), preferably between 15 and 30 °C (59 and 86 °F), unless otherwise specified by manufacturer. Protect from freezing.

**Auxiliary labeling**
• Shake well.
• For anorectal use only.

### PRAMOXINE HYDROCHLORIDE CREAM USP

**Usual adult and adolescent dose**
Anesthetic, mucosal-local—Topical, to the anorectal area, up to five times a day, after the area has been cleansed and dried.

**Usual pediatric dose**
Children up to 12 years of age—Dosage must be individualized by physician.

**Strength(s) usually available**
U.S.—
    1% (OTC) [*Tronolane; Tronothane*].
Canada—
    1% (OTC) [*Tronothane*].

**Packaging and storage**
Store below 40 °C (104 °F), preferably between 15 and 30 °C (59 and 86 °F), unless otherwise specified by manufacturer. Store in tight container. Protect from freezing.

### PRAMOXINE HYDROCHLORIDE OINTMENT

**Usual adult and adolescent dose**
Anesthetic, mucosal-local—
    Rectal, introduced into the rectum as a 1% ointment up to five times per day, in the morning, at night, and after bowel movements; or
    Topical, to the anorectal area as a 1% ointment up to five times a day.

**Usual pediatric dose**
Children up to 12 years of age—Dosage must be individualized by physician.

**Strength(s) usually available**
U.S.—
    1% (OTC) [*Fleet Relief*].
    Note: Available in tubes and in pre-filled 4-mL disposable applicators.

**Packaging and storage**
Store below 40 °C (104 °F), preferably between 15 and 30 °C (59 and 86 °F), unless otherwise specified by manufacturer. Protect from freezing.

## Summary of Differences

Pharmacology/pharmacokinetics:
    Physicochemical characteristics—
        Tetracaine is a PABA-derivative ester-type local anesthetic.
Precautions:
    Cross-sensitivity and/or related problems—
        May occur with other ester-type local anesthetics, especially other PABA derivatives, parabens, and paraphenylenediamine.
    Drug interactions and/or related problems—
        Cholinesterase inhibitors inhibit metabolism of tetracaine.
        May antagonize antibacterial activity of sulfonamides.
Side/adverse effects:
    More likely to cause contact sensitization than most other local anesthetics.
    More toxic than other mucosal-local anesthetics.
    See also *Side/Adverse Effects*.

## Dental Dosage Forms

### TETRACAINE TOPICAL AEROSOL

**Usual adult and adolescent dose**
Anesthetic, mucosal-local—Gingival and oral mucosa: Topical, 1.4 mg (two metered sprays).

**Usual adult prescribing limits**
Not to exceed 20 mg (approximately 28 metered sprays).

**Usual pediatric dose**
Dosage has not been established.

**Strength(s) usually available**
U.S.—
    Not commercially available.
Canada—
    700 mcg (0.7 mg) per metered spray (OTC) [*Supracaine*].

**Packaging and storage**
Store below 40 °C (104 °F), preferably between 15 and 30 °C (59 and 86 °F), unless otherwise specified by manufacturer. Protect from freezing.

**Auxiliary labeling**
• Shake well.

## Rectal Dosage Forms

### TETRACAINE HYDROCHLORIDE CREAM USP

Note: The dosing and strength of this dosage form are expressed in terms of tetracaine base.

**Usual adult and adolescent dose**
Anesthetic, mucosal-local—Rectal, introduced into rectum as a 1% (base) cream up to six times a day.

**Usual adult prescribing limits**
Not more than 28.35 grams in a twenty-four-hour period.

**Usual pediatric dose**
Dosage has not been established.

**Strength(s) usually available**
U.S.—
    1% (base) (OTC) [*Pontocaine Cream*].
Canada—
    Not commercially available.

**Packaging and storage**
Store below 40 °C (104 °F), preferably between 15 and 30 °C (59 and 86 °F), unless otherwise specified by manufacturer. Protect from freezing.

### TETRACAINE AND MENTHOL OINTMENT USP

**Usual adult and adolescent dose**
Anesthetic, mucosal-local—
    Rectal, introduced into rectum as a 0.5% ointment up to six times a day.
    Topical, applied as a 0.5% ointment spread with gauze or cotton, to anorectal area up to six times a day.

**Usual adult prescribing limits**
Not more than 28.35 grams in a twenty-four-hour period.

**Usual pediatric dose**
Dosage has not been established.

**Strength(s) usually available**
U.S.—
   0.5% of tetracaine and 0.5% of menthol (OTC) [*Pontocaine Ointment*].
Canada—
   Not commercially available.

**Packaging and storage**
Store below 40 °C (104 °F), preferably between 15 and 30 °C (59 and 86 °F), unless otherwise specified by manufacturer. Protect from freezing.

## Topical Dosage Forms

### TETRACAINE HYDROCHLORIDE TOPICAL SOLUTION USP

**Usual adult and adolescent dose**
Anesthetic, mucosal-local—Larynx, trachea, or esophagus—
   Topical, as a 0.25 or 0.5% solution prior to procedure; or
   Oral inhalation, as a nebulized 0.5% solution.
Note: 0.06 mL of 0.1% (1:1000) epinephrine may be added to each mL of tetracaine solution, to reduce absorption.

**Usual adult prescribing limits**
Not to exceed 20 mg.

**Usual pediatric dose**
Dosage has not been established.

**Strength(s) usually available**
U.S.—
   2% (Rx) [*Pontocaine*].
Canada—
   Not commercially available.

**Packaging and storage**
Store between 2 and 8 °C (36 and 46 °F), unless otherwise specified by manufacturer. Store in a tight, light-resistant container. Protect from freezing.

**Stability**
Do not use if solution is cloudy or discolored or contains crystals.

Revised: 09/01/94

---

# ANESTHETICS   Ophthalmic

This monograph includes information on the following: Proparacaine; Tetracaine.

INN:
   Proparacaine—Proxymetacaine.

BAN:
   Proparacaine—Proxymetacaine.
   Tetracaine—Amethocaine.

VA CLASSIFICATION (Primary): OP700

Other commonly used names are:
   Amethocaine [Tetracaine]            Proxymetacaine [Proparacaine]

Note: For a listing of dosage forms and brand names by country availability, see *Dosage Forms* section(s). For a listing of brand names for the articles in this monograph, refer to the General Index.

---

## Category
Anesthetic, local (ophthalmic).

## Indications

**Accepted**
Anesthesia, local—Proparacaine and tetracaine are indicated to produce local anesthesia of short duration for ophthalmic procedures including measurement of intraocular pressure (tonometry), removal of foreign bodies and sutures, and conjunctival and corneal scraping in diagnosis and gonioscopy.

Proparacaine and tetracaine are also indicated to produce local anesthesia prior to surgical procedures such as cataract extraction and pterygium excision, usually as an adjunct to locally injected anesthetics.

Ophthalmic solutions used for intraocular procedures should be preservative-free. Preservatives may cause damage to the corneal epithelium if a significant quantity of solution enters the eye through the incision.

**Unaccepted**
**Proparacaine and tetracaine are not indicated for chronic or repeated use because of the potential for severe corneal damage.** Severe keratitis and opacification and scarring of the cornea resulting in loss of vision have occurred with repeated use of these medications.

## Pharmacology/Pharmacokinetics

**Physicochemical characteristics**
Chemical group—
   Ester-type local anesthetics. Proparacaine is a meta-aminobenzoic acid derivative; tetracaine is an aminobenzoic acid (para-aminobenzoic acid; PABA) derivative
Molecular weight—
   Proparacaine hydrochloride: 330.85.
   Tetracaine: 264.37.
   Tetracaine hydrochloride: 300.83.
pKa—
   Tetracaine: 8.4.

**Mechanism of action/Effect**
After topical application to the eye, local anesthetics penetrate to sensory nerve endings in the corneal tissue. These medications block both the initiation and conduction of nerve impulses by decreasing the neuronal membrane's permeability to sodium ions. This reversibly stabilizes the membrane and inhibits depolarization, resulting in the failure of a propagated action potential and subsequent conduction blockade.

**Other actions/effects**
Following topical application to the eye, local anesthetics may retard epithelial regeneration by inhibiting mitosis, cellular migration, and corneal epithelial uptake and oxidation of glucose and pyruvate. With repeated or prolonged use, these agents may retard healing of existing corneal injury or cause new corneal damage.

If significant quantities of local anesthetics are absorbed, they may act on the central nervous system (CNS) to produce CNS stimulation followed by CNS depression, and on the cardiovascular system to produce depression of cardiac conduction and excitability.

**Absorption**
Rapidly absorbed via conjunctival capillaries..

**Protein binding**
Tetracaine—High.

**Biotransformation**
Proparacaine—Hydrolyzed by plasma esterases.
Tetracaine—Hydrolyzed by cholinesterases, primarily in the plasma and to a much lesser extent in the liver, to an aminobenzoic acid (PABA)–containing metabolite and diethylaminoethanol.

**Onset of action**
Proparacaine—Within 20 seconds.
Tetracaine—Approximately 15 seconds.

**Duration of action**
Proparacaine—15 minutes or longer.
Tetracaine—10 to 20 minutes; average 15 minutes.
Note: For topical application to the eye, the duration of action is not prolonged by use of concentrations greater than 0.5% of proparacaine or 1% of tetracaine, or by concurrent use of a vasoconstrictor. However, the duration of action increases with repeated applications.

**Elimination**
Tetracaine—Renal; as metabolites.

## Precautions to Consider

**Cross-sensitivity and/or related problems**
Patients sensitive to other ester-type local anesthetics (such as benzocaine, butacaine, butamben, chloroprocaine, procaine, or propoxycaine) or to aminobenzoic acid (para-aminobenzoic acid; PABA) or parabens may be sensitive to tetracaine also.
Cross-sensitivity between proparacaine and tetracaine or other local anesthetics has not been reported.

**Carcinogenicity/Tumorigenicity/Mutagenicity**
Studies with proparacaine or tetracaine have not been done.

## Pregnancy/Reproduction

Pregnancy—Problems in humans have not been documented.

Studies of the teratogenic potential of proparacaine or tetracaine have not been done in animals.

FDA Pregnancy Category C.

## Breast-feeding

It is not known whether proparacaine or tetracaine is distributed into breast milk. However, problems in humans have not been documented.

## Pediatrics

*Proparacaine*—Appropriate studies on the relationship of age to the effects of proparacaine have not been performed in the pediatric population. However, pediatrics-specific problems that would limit the usefulness of this medication in children are not expected.

*Tetracaine* —Appropriate studies on the relationship of age to the effects of tetracaine have not been performed in the pediatric population. However, the stinging that frequently occurs after application of tetracaine may upset small children.

## Geriatrics

Appropriate studies on the relationship of age to the effects of ophthalmic anesthetics have not been performed in the geriatric population. However, geriatrics-specific problems that would limit the usefulness of this medication in the elderly are not expected.

## Drug interactions and/or related problems

The following drug interactions and/or related problems have been selected on the basis of their potential clinical significance (possible mechanism in parentheses where appropriate)—not necessarily inclusive (» = major clinical significance):

*For tetracaine*

Cholinesterase inhibitors, especially demecarium, echothiophate, and isoflurophate

(metabolism of tetracaine may be inhibited, leading to prolonged ocular anesthetic effect and increased risk of toxicity, if administered to a patient receiving therapy with a cholinesterase inhibitor)

## Laboratory value alterations

The following have been selected on the basis of their potential clinical significance (possible effect in parentheses where appropriate)—not necessarily inclusive (» = major clinical significance):

With diagnostic test results

Cultures (24-hour) for detection of infection

(topical ocular anesthetics and preservatives present in the formulations may inhibit growth of organisms, including *Staphylococcus albus*, *Pseudomonas*, and *Candida albicans*)

## Medical considerations/Contraindications

The medical considerations/contraindications included here have been selected on the basis of their potential clinical significance (reasons given in parentheses where appropriate)—not necessarily inclusive (» = major clinical significance).

*Risk-benefit should be considered when the following medical problems exist:*

*For proparacaine or tetracaine*

Ocular inflammation and/or infection

(may alter pH and/or increase blood circulation at site of application, leading to decrease or loss of anesthetic effect)

*For proparacaine*

Allergic reaction to proparacaine, history of

Allergies

(proparacaine may cause an allergic reaction)

*For tetracaine*

Allergic reaction to tetracaine, history of

Plasma cholinesterase deficiency

(increased risk of toxicity because of decreased metabolism)

## Side/Adverse Effects

Note: Allergic contact dermatitis with drying and fissuring of the fingertips has been reported with these medications.

Prolonged use of topical ophthalmic anesthetics may produce severe keratitis, permanent corneal opacification, and scarring, with loss of visual acuity. Also, prolonged use of topical ophthalmic anesthetics may cause delay in corneal epithelial healing.

Proparacaine may rarely cause a severe, immediate hypersensitivity reaction that may include acute intense and diffuse epithelial keratitis; a gray, ground-glass appearance; sloughing of large areas of necrotic epithelium; corneal filaments and, sometimes, iritis with descemetitis. Rarely, proparacaine also causes a delayed hypersensitivity reaction characterized by softening and erosion of the cor-

neal epithelium, conjunctival congestion, and hemorrhage. Tetracaine may also rarely cause local hypersensitivity reactions. In addition, sensitivity reactions to the preservatives present in ophthalmic formulations may occur.

The following side/adverse effects have been selected on the basis of their potential clinical significance (possible signs and symptoms in parentheses where appropriate)—not necessarily inclusive:

### Those indicating need for medical attention

Signs and/or symptoms of systemic toxicity—very rare

*CNS depression* (drowsiness; shortness of breath or troubled breathing)—may follow CNS stimulation; *CNS stimulation* (blurred vision; convulsions; dizziness; muscle twitching or trembling; nausea or vomiting; unusual excitement, nervousness, or restlessness); *increased sweating; irregular heartbeat; unusual paleness; unusual tiredness or weakness*

### Those indicating need for medical attention only if they are severe or if they continue or are bothersome

Incidence less frequent

*Burning, stinging, redness, or other irritation of eye, mild*

Note: These effects may occur upon application of tetracaine, or up to several hours after application of proparacaine. Ocular discomfort characterized by a *burning sensation* occurs more frequently, and is more severe, with tetracaine than with proparacaine. Closing the eyes immediately after application may decrease the discomfort.

Incidence rare

*Allergic reaction* (itching, pain, redness, or swelling of eye or eyelid, severe; watering of eyes, severe and continuing)

## Patient Consultation

As an aid to patient consultation, refer to *Advice for the Patient, Anesthetics (Ophthalmic)*.

In providing consultation, consider emphasizing the following selected information (» = major clinical significance):

### Before receiving this medication

» Conditions affecting use, especially:

Allergic reaction to the anesthetic considered for use, history of, and, for tetracaine only, to any other PABA-derivative anesthetic, PABA, or parabens

### Proper use of this medication

» Proper dosing

### Precautions after receiving this medication

» Not rubbing or wiping the eye until anesthesia has worn off, to prevent damage to the eye

Possibility of rash with dryness and cracking of skin if medication comes in contact with fingers; washing hands after touching eyes following application of medication

### Side/adverse effects

» Checking with physician as soon as possible if severe symptoms indicating possible hypersensitivity occur

Signs and symptoms of potential side effects, especially hypersensitivity reactions

## General Dosing Information

Proparacaine is approximately equal in potency to tetracaine when used in equal concentrations, but is less irritating.

It is important that the eye be protected from irritating chemicals, foreign bodies, and rubbing during the period of anesthesia since the "blink" reflex is temporarily eliminated. Rubbing or touching the eye during anesthesia may damage the anesthetized cornea and conjunctiva.

When a local anesthetic is used for tonometry, the tonometer should be thoroughly rinsed with sterile distilled water prior to use, to remove any sterilizing or detergent solutions.

### For treatment of allergic reactions

Topical application of ophthalmic corticosteroids or antihistamines may be helpful.

### For treatment of systemic toxicity

Recommended treatment includes

• Securing and maintaining a patent airway, administering oxygen, and instituting assisted or controlled respiration as required. In some patients, endotracheal intubation may be needed. Respiratory stimulants should not be given because they are considered ineffective.

• For convulsions—Administering an anticonvulsant. Benzodiazepines are most commonly used. Because intravenously administered benzodiazepines may cause respiratory and circulatory de-

pression, especially when administered rapidly, medications and equipment needed for support of respiration and for resuscitation must be immediately available.
- Administering vasopressors and intravenous fluids, if necessary, to treat hypotension.

---

## PROPARACAINE

## Summary of Differences

Pharmacology/pharmacokinetics:
See *Pharmacology/Pharmacokinetics*.
Precautions:
Cross-sensitivity and/or related problems—No cross-sensitivity with tetracaine or other PABA-derivative local anesthetics, PABA, or parabens.
Drug interactions and/or related problems—No interaction with cholinesterase inhibitors.
Medical considerations/contraindications—Caution also required in allergies.
Side/adverse effects:
See *Side/Adverse Effects*.

## Ophthalmic Dosage Forms

### PROPARACAINE HYDROCHLORIDE OPHTHALMIC SOLUTION USP

**Usual adult and adolescent dose**
Anesthetic, local—
For superficial procedures (e.g., tonometry, suture removal, foreign body removal): Topical, to the conjunctiva, 1 or 2 drops of a 0.5% solution.
For deeper procedures (e.g., cataract removal): Topical, to the conjunctiva, 1 drop of a 0.5% solution every five to ten minutes for five to seven doses. A preservative-free solution should be used.

**Usual pediatric dose**
See *Usual adult and adolescent dose*.

**Strength(s) usually available**
U.S.—
0.5% (Rx) [*Ak-Taine; Alcaine; Ocu-Caine; Ophthaine; Ophthetic; Spectro-Caine;* GENERIC].
Canada—
0.5% (Rx) [*Alcaine; Diocaine; Ophthetic*].

**Packaging and storage**
Store below 40 °C (104 °F), preferably between 15 and 30 °C (59 and 86 °F), unless otherwise specified by manufacturer. Store in a tight, light-resistant container. Protect from freezing.
Note: Opened containers should be stored between 2 and 8 °C (36 and 46 °F).

**Stability**
Opened containers of proparacaine hydrochloride solution should be refrigerated to retard discoloration of the solution.
A discolored (amber) solution should not be used.

---

## TETRACAINE

## Summary of Differences

Pharmacology/pharmacokinetics:
See *Pharmacology/Pharmacokinetics*.

---

# ANESTHETICS   Parenteral-Local

This monograph includes information on the following: Bupivacaine; Chloroprocaine; Etidocaine; Lidocaine; Mepivacaine; Prilocaine; Procaine; Propoxycaine and Procaine; Tetracaine.
INN:
Lidocaine—Lignocaine
VA CLASSIFICATION (Primary): CN204
A commonly used name for lidocaine is lignocaine

Precautions:
Cross-sensitivity and/or related problems—Potential cross-sensitivity with other PABA-derivative local anesthetics, PABA, or parabens.
Drug interactions and/or related problems—Interaction with cholinesterase inhibitors.
Medical considerations/contraindications—Caution also required in plasma cholinesterase deficiency.
Side/adverse effects:
See *Side/Adverse Effects*.

## Ophthalmic Dosage Forms

### TETRACAINE OPHTHALMIC OINTMENT USP

Note: This product is no longer being manufactured in the U.S. but may still be in circulation.

**Usual adult and adolescent dose**
Anesthetic, local—
Topical, to the lower conjunctival fornix, approximately 1.3 to 2.5 cm (approximately 1/2 to 1 inch) of a 0.5% ointment.

**Usual pediatric dose**
Dosage has not been established.

**Strength(s) usually available**
U.S.—
0.5% (Rx) [*Pontocaine*].

**Packaging and storage**
Store below 40 °C (104 °F), preferably between 15 and 30 °C (59 and 86 °F), unless otherwise specified by manufacturer. Protect from freezing.

**Note**
Do not allow the tip of the tube to contact any surface that may cause contamination.

### TETRACAINE HYDROCHLORIDE OPHTHALMIC SOLUTION USP

**Usual adult and adolescent dose**
Anesthetic, local—
Topical, to the conjunctiva, 1 or 2 drops of a 0.5% or 1% solution.

**Usual pediatric dose**
Dosage has not been established.

**Strength(s) usually available**
U.S.—
0.5% (Rx) [*Ak-T-Caine; Opticaine; Pontocaine;* GENERIC].
Canada—
0.5% (Rx) [*Minims Tetracaine; Pontocaine;* GENERIC].
1% (Rx) [*Minims Tetracaine*].

**Packaging and storage**
Store below 40 °C (104 °F), preferably between 15 and 30 °C (59 and 86 °F), unless otherwise specified by manufacturer. Store in a tight, light-resistant container. Protect from freezing.

**Stability**
Do not use the solution if it contains crystals or is cloudy or discolored.

---

Revised: 08/25/94
Interim revision: 07/11/95

---

Note: For a listing of dosage forms and brand names by country availability, see *Dosage Forms* section(s). For a listing of brand names for the articles in this monograph, refer to the General Index.

## Category

Anesthetic (local).

# Indications

Note: Bracketed information in the *Indications* section refers to uses that are not included in U.S. product labeling.

## Accepted

Anesthesia, local—
    Parenteral-local anesthetics are generally employed to provide local or regional anesthesia, analgesia, and varying degrees of motor blockade prior to surgical procedures, dental procedures, and obstetrical delivery. They may also be used for other diagnostic or therapeutic purposes via routes of administration that are included in product labeling.

Mixtures or combinations of local anesthetics are sometimes used to provide a rapid onset of action and a prolonged duration of action. However, the possibility of additive toxicity must be considered when such combinations are used.

Vasoconstrictors are added to local anesthetic injections to decrease the rate of local clearance of the local anesthetic. Local anesthetic injections containing a vasoconstrictor generally have the same indications as the corresponding local anesthetic injection without a vasoconstrictor. However, additional precautions pertinent to the use of a vasoconstrictor must be considered.

Dextrose is added to anesthetic solutions for subarachnoid administration to render the solution hyperbaric (heavier than cerebrospinal fluid [CSF]); the local anesthetic will exert its effect above or below the site of injection, depending upon the position of the patient during and immediately following the injection.

*Specific indications include*:

Central neural blocks—Caudal or lumbar epidural: Bupivacaine (with or without epinephrine), chloroprocaine, etidocaine (with or without epinephrine), lidocaine (with or without epinephrine), and mepivacaine are indicated. Only single-dose vials that do not contain an antimicrobial preservative should be used.
    Subarachnoid: Bupivacaine and dextrose, lidocaine and dextrose, procaine[1], and tetracaine (with or without dextrose) are indicated. Commercially available products intended specifically for subarachnoid administration contain no antimicrobial preservatives. Solutions and diluents containing antimicrobial preservatives are not to be injected into the subarachnoid space and should not be used when preparing injections for administration via this route.

Dental infiltration or nerve block—Bupivacaine and epinephrine; chloroprocaine (with or without added epinephrine); etidocaine and epinephrine; lidocaine (with or without epinephrine); mepivacaine (with or without levonordefrin); prilocaine (with or without epinephrine); propoxycaine, procaine, and levonordefrin; and propoxycaine, procaine, and norepinephrine are indicated. Unless specifically contraindicated, a vasoconstrictor-containing solution is preferred.

Local infiltration—Bupivacaine (with or without epinephrine), chloroprocaine, etidocaine (with or without epinephrine), lidocaine (with or without epinephrine), mepivacaine, and procaine are indicated.
    Intravenous regional anesthesia (Bier block): [Chloroprocaine][1], lidocaine[1], and [mepivacaine][1] are indicated.

Peripheral nerve block—Bupivacaine (with or without epinephrine), chloroprocaine, etidocaine (with or without epinephrine), lidocaine (with or without epinephrine), mepivacaine, and procaine are indicated.
    Retrobulbar block: Bupivacaine, etidocaine, lidocaine, and [procaine][1] are indicated.

Sympathetic block—Bupivacaine (with or without epinephrine) and lidocaine (with or without epinephrine) are indicated.

Transtracheal—Lidocaine, [mepivacaine][1], and [tetracaine][1] are indicated.

## Unaccepted

For paracervical administration—Use of bupivacaine is not recommended for nonobstetrical procedures because of insufficient data concerning safety and dosage. Use of bupivacaine is not recommended in obstetrical procedures because such use has resulted in fetal bradycardia and death.

Solutions containing a vasoconstrictor should not be used for intravenous regional anesthesia (Bier block). Also, bupivacaine is not recommended for intravenous regional anesthesia.

For central neural block (peridural [lumbar or caudal epidural] or subarachnoid [spinal] administration)—Do not use solutions containing an antimicrobial preservative such as chlorobutanol or methylparaben.

Chloroprocaine and mepivacaine are not recommended for subarachnoid (spinal) administration.

___
[1]Not included in Canadian product labeling.

# Pharmacology/Pharmacokinetics

See also *Table 1*, page 142.

## Physicochemical characteristics

Chemical group—
    Amides: Bupivacaine, etidocaine, lidocaine, mepivacaine, prilocaine
    Esters, aminobenzoic acid (PABA)–derivative: Chloroprocaine, procaine, propoxycaine, tetracaine

Molecular weight—
    Bupivacaine hydrochloride: 342.91.
    Chloroprocaine hydrochloride: 307.22.
    Etidocaine hydrochloride: 312.88.
    Lidocaine hydrochloride: 288.82.
    Mepivacaine hydrochloride: 282.81.
    Prilocaine hydrochloride: 256.77.
    Procaine hydrochloride: 272.77.
    Propoxycaine hydrochloride: 330.85.
    Tetracaine hydrochloride: 300.83.

pKa—
    See *Table 1*, page 142.

Lipid solubility—
    See *Table 1*, page 142.

## Mechanism of action/Effect

Local anesthetics—Block both the initiation and conduction of nerve impulses by decreasing the neuronal membrane's permeability to sodium ions. This reversibly stabilizes the membrane and inhibits depolarization, resulting in the failure of a propagated action potential and subsequent conduction blockade.

Vasoconstrictors—Act on alpha-adrenergic receptors in the vasculature of the skin, mucous membranes, conjunctiva, and viscera to produce vasoconstriction, thereby decreasing blood flow in the area of injection. The resultant reduction in the rate of local clearance of the local anesthetic prolongs the duration of action, lowers the peak serum concentration, decreases the risk of systemic toxicity, and increases the frequency of complete conduction blocks with low concentrations of the local anesthetic. Vasoconstrictors may also reduce bleeding when injected at the site of surgery.

## Other actions/effects

Local anesthetics—Actions on the central nervous system (CNS) may cause CNS stimulation and/or CNS depression. Actions on the cardiovascular system may cause depression of cardiac conduction and excitability and, with most of these agents, peripheral vasodilation.

Vasoconstrictors—Vasoconstrictors having beta-adrenergic activity (epinephrine, levonordefrin, and norepinephrine) may cause cardiac stimulation resulting in increased heart rate, contractility, conduction velocity, and irritability. Also, when used for obstetrical anesthesia, vasoconstrictors having beta-adrenergic activity may decrease the intensity of uterine contractions and prolong labor. Phenylephrine is also rarely used as a vasoconstrictor in conjunction with local anesthesia; it has only alpha-adrenergic activity and does not have these additional effects.

## Absorption

Complete systemic absorption. The rate of absorption is influenced by the site and route of administration (especially the vascularity or rate of blood flow at the injection site), total dosage (volume and concentration) administered, physical characteristics (such as degree of protein binding and lipid solubility) of the individual agent, and whether or not a vasoconstrictor is used concurrently.

## Biotransformation

Amides—
    Hepatic
    Lidocaine: Xylidide metabolites are active and toxic, but less so than the parent compound.
    Prilocaine: May also be metabolized renally to some extent.

Esters—
    PABA derivatives: Hydrolyzed primarily in the plasma and, to a much lesser extent, in the liver, by cholinesterases. Procaine is hydrolyzed to PABA. Chloroprocaine and tetracaine are, and propoxycaine may be, hydrolyzed to PABA-containing compounds.

## Time to peak concentration

Usually 10 to 30 minutes; dependent upon factors affecting rate of absorption. May occur 1 to 3 minutes after intravascular or transtracheal injection.

## Peak serum concentration

Depends upon factors influencing the rate of absorption from the injection site and rate of metabolism and distribution volume of the individual anesthetic.

## Elimination

Renal, primarily as metabolites. For some of these agents, including lidocaine, mepivacaine, and tetracaine, renal excretion may follow biliary excretion into, and reabsorption from, the gastrointestinal tract. Quantity of dose excreted unchanged—

Bupivacaine: 6%
Etidocaine: 1%
Lidocaine: 10%
Mepivacaine: Up to 16%
Procaine: 2%.

# Precautions to Consider

## Cross-sensitivity and/or related problems

Patients sensitive to aminobenzoic acid (PABA) or parabens may be sensitive to procaine, chloroprocaine, propoxycaine, or tetracaine also. They may also be sensitive to other local anesthetic solutions containing parabens as preservatives.

Patients sensitive to one ester-type local anesthetic may be sensitive to other ester-type local anesthetics also.

Patients sensitive to one amide-type local anesthetic may rarely be sensitive to other amide-type local anesthetics also.

Cross-sensitivity between ester-type local anesthetics and amide-type local anesthetics has not been reported.

## Pregnancy/Reproduction

Pregnancy—Local anesthetics cross the placenta by diffusion. The rate and degree of diffusion vary considerably among the various agents as determined by their rate of metabolism and physical characteristics such as plasma protein binding (reduced placental transfer with highly protein-bound agents), lipid solubility (greater placental transfer with highly lipid soluble agents), and degree of ionization (greater placental transfer with nonionized form of agent).

*First trimester—*

For all parenteral-local anesthetics—Retrospective studies of pregnant women receiving local anesthetics for emergency surgery early in pregnancy have not shown that local anesthetics cause birth defects. However, risk-benefit must be considered because the possibility of other adverse effects on the fetus could not be excluded by these studies. Controlled studies in humans have not been done with any of these anesthetics.

For bupivacaine—Studies in rats and rabbits using doses 9 and 5 times the maximum recommended human dose (MRHD) respectively, have shown decreased survival in newborn rats and embryocidal effects in rabbits.

FDA Pregnancy Category C.

For chloroprocaine, mepivacaine, and tetracaine—Studies in animals have not been done.

FDA Pregnancy Category C.

For etidocaine, lidocaine, and prilocaine—Studies in rats or rabbits with etidocaine (using up to 1.7 times the MRHD), lidocaine (using up to 6.6 times the MRHD), or prilocaine (using 3 times the MRHD) have not shown adverse effects on the fetus.

FDA Pregnancy Category B.

For procaine—Studies in animals have not been done.

These findings do not preclude the use of local anesthetics during labor and delivery.

*Labor and delivery—*

Epidural, subarachnoid, paracervical, or pudendal administration of a local anesthetic may produce changes in uterine contractility and/or maternal expulsive efforts. Paracervical block may shorten the first stage of labor and facilitate cervical dilation. However, epidural or subarachnoid administration may prolong the second stage of labor by interfering with motor function or removing the patient's reflex urge to bear down. Use of a local anesthetic during delivery may increase the need for forceps-assisted delivery. Bupivacaine is not recommended for paracervical administration. Also, etidocaine may cause profound motor block; epidural administration of this agent is not recommended for normal vaginal delivery (although it may be used for cesarean section). In addition, a vasoconstrictor having beta-adrenergic activity used concurrently may decrease the intensity of uterine contractions and prolong labor.

Maternal hypotension, caused by sympathetic nerve blockade resulting in vasodilation, may occur during regional anesthesia.

Maternal convulsions and cardiovascular collapse have been reported following paracervical administration early in pregnancy (for elective abortion), suggesting rapid systemic absorption under these circumstances. Especially careful attention to dosage and technique is necessary.

Maternal fatalities due to cardiac arrest have been reported following inadvertent intravascular injection of 0.75% bupivacaine

during intended performance of an epidural block. Although the 0.75% strength is not recommended for epidural administration in obstetrics, lower concentrations of bupivacaine may be used.

Chloroprocaine, lidocaine, and mepivacaine have been shown to constrict uterine arteries, possibly leading to fetal hypoxia. Alpha-adrenergic blocking agents do not reverse this effect. A vasoconstrictor used concurrently may also cause constriction of uterine blood vessels and decreased placental circulation.

Fetal bradycardia, possibly associated with fetal acidosis, has been reported in 20 to 30% of patients receiving amide-type local anesthetics via paracervical block. Fetal bradycardia without fetal acidosis has also been reported in 5 to 10% of patients receiving chloroprocaine via paracervical block. The risk of this complication may be increased if prematurity, postmaturity, toxemia of pregnancy, pre-existing fetal distress, or uteroplacental insufficiency is present. Risk-benefit must be considered when amide-type local anesthetics are considered for paracervical block in these conditions. Paracervical block with chloroprocaine is not recommended if prematurity, pre-existing fetal distress, or toxemia of pregnancy is present because its safety in these conditions has not been established. Monitoring of fetal heart rate is recommended during paracervical block.

Postpartum—Neonatal neurological disturbances such as diminished muscle strength and tone may occur for 1 to 2 days postpartum. Marked neonatal CNS depression has been reported following paracervical block. Also, inadvertent fetal intracranial injection during intended caudal, paracervical, or pudendal administration may cause neonatal depression and convulsions.

## Breast-feeding

Although it is not known whether local anesthetics are distributed into breast milk, problems in humans have not been documented.

## Pediatrics

Although there is some evidence that systemic toxicity may be more likely to occur in pediatric patients, appropriate studies performed to date with mepivacaine have not demonstrated pediatrics-specific problems that would limit the use of the medication in children. Also, no information is available on the relationship of age to the effects of bupivacaine (with or without epinephrine or dextrose), etidocaine, lidocaine and dextrose combination, procaine, or tetracaine (with or without dextrose) in pediatric patients.

## Geriatrics

Systemic toxicity may be more likely to occur in geriatric patients.

## Drug interactions and/or related problems

The following drug interactions and/or related problems have been selected on the basis of their potential clinical significance (possible mechanism in parentheses where appropriate)—not necessarily inclusive (» = major clinical significance):

Note: Combinations containing any of the following medications, depending on the amount present, may also interact with this medication.

*For all local anesthetics*

Antimyasthenics

(inhibition of neuronal transmission by local anesthetics may antagonize the effects of antimyasthenics on skeletal muscle, especially if large quantities of the anesthetic are rapidly absorbed; temporary dosage adjustment of antimyasthenics may be necessary to control symptoms of myasthenia gravis)

» CNS depression–producing medications, including those commonly used as preanesthetic medication or for supplementation of local anesthesia (See *Appendix II* )

(concurrent use with a local anesthetic may result in additive depressant effects; caution and careful attention to dosage of each agent are recommended)

Disinfectant solutions containing heavy metals

(local anesthetics may cause release of heavy metal ions from these solutions, which, if injected along with the anesthetic, may cause severe local irritation, swelling, and edema; such solutions are not recommended for chemical disinfection of the container, and preventive measures are recommended if they are used for skin or mucous membrane disinfection prior to anesthetic administration)

Guanadrel or
Guanethidine or
Mecamylamine or
Trimethaphan

(the risk of severe hypotension and/or bradycardia may be increased if high levels of spinal or epidural anesthesia [i.e., sufficient to produce sympathetic blockade] are induced in patients receiving these ganglionic-blocking antihypertensive agents)

Monoamine oxidase (MAO) inhibitors, including furazolidone, procarbazine, and selegiline

(concurrent use in patients receiving local anesthetics via subarachnoid block may increase the risk of hypotension; discontinuation of MAO inhibitors 10 days before elective surgery may be advisable if subarachnoid block anesthesia is planned)

Neuromuscular blocking agents

(inhibition of neuronal transmission by local anesthetics may enhance or prolong the action of neuromuscular blocking agents if large quantities of the anesthetic are rapidly absorbed)

Opioid (narcotic) analgesic anesthesia adjuncts

(alterations in respiration caused by high levels of spinal or peridural blockade may be additive to opioid analgesic–induced alterations in respiratory rate and alveolar ventilation)

(the vagal effects of alfentanil, fentanyl or sufentanil may also be more pronounced in patients with high levels of spinal or epidural anesthesia, and may lead to bradycardia and/or hypotension)

» Vasoconstrictors such as epinephrine, methoxamine, or phenylephrine

(use of methoxamine in combination with local anesthetics to prolong their action at local sites is not recommended, since methoxamine's extended effect may cause excessive restriction of circulation and lead to sloughing of tissue)

(other vasoconstrictors should be used cautiously and in carefully circumscribed quantities, if at all, with local anesthetics when anesthetizing areas with end arteries [such as the fingers, toes, or penis] or with otherwise compromised blood supply; ischemia leading to gangrene may result)

*For lidocaine only (in addition to those interactions listed above)*

Beta-adrenergic blocking agents

(concurrent use may slow metabolism of lidocaine because of decreased hepatic blood flow, leading to increased risk of lidocaine toxicity)

Cimetidine

(cimetidine may inhibit hepatic metabolism of lidocaine, leading to increased risk of lidocaine toxicity)

*For ester-type local anesthetics only (in addition to those interactions listed above as applying to all local anesthetics)*

Cholinesterase inhibitors such as:

Antimyasthenics
Cyclophosphamide
Demecarium
Echothiophate
Insecticides, neurotoxic, possibly including large quantities of topical malathion
Isoflurophate
Thiotepa

(concurrent use with an ester-type local anesthetic may inhibit the metabolism of the anesthetic leading to increased risk of toxicity)

Sulfonamides

(antibacterial activity may be antagonized by ester-type local anesthetics, which are metabolized to PABA or PABA derivatives)

*For concurrent use of sympathomimetic vasoconstrictors such as epinephrine, levonordefrin, norepinephrine, or phenylephrine (in addition to those interactions listed above and applicable to the specific local anesthetic)*

Note: The risk of a significant systemic effect resulting from an interaction between any of the following and a vasoconstrictor-containing local anesthetic solution depends on the total dose (volume and concentration) of vasoconstrictor administered and on factors affecting the rate of absorption of the vasoconstrictor (site and route of administration and potential for inadvertent intravascular administration).

Alpha-adrenergic blocking agents, such as

Labetalol
Phenoxybenzamine
Phentolamine
Prazosin
Tolazoline or

Other medications with alpha-adrenergic blocking action, such as
» Droperidol
» Haloperidol
Loxapine
» Phenothiazines
Thioxanthenes or

Vasodilators, rapidly acting, such as nitrates

(these medications may reduce the efficacy of the vasoconstrictor)

(in patients receiving epinephrine, levonordefrin, or norepinephrine, but not phenylephrine, alpha-adrenergic blockade may result in unopposed beta-adrenergic activity with a risk of severe hypotension and tachycardia)

(vasoconstrictors may also decrease the therapeutic effects of vasodilators, including the antianginal effects of nitrates)

» Anesthetics, hydrocarbon inhalation

(chloroform, cyclopropane, halothane, or trichloroethylene and, to a much lesser extent, enflurane, isoflurane, or methoxyflurane may sensitize the heart to the effects of a sympathomimetic vasoconstrictor; concurrent use with a vasoconstrictor may cause dose-related cardiac arrhythmias)

» Antidepressants, tricyclic or
» Maprotiline

(concurrent use may potentiate the cardiovascular effects of the vasoconstrictor, possibly resulting in arrhythmias, tachycardia, or severe hypertension or hyperpyrexia)

Antihypertensives or

Diuretics used as antihypertensives

(antihypertensive effects may be decreased by vasoconstrictors; monitoring of blood pressure is recommended)

(in addition to a possible reduction in the antihypertensive effects of guanadrel, guanethidine, mecamylamine, methyldopa, or trimethaphan, concurrent use of any of these agents may enhance the pressor response to vasoconstrictors)

» Beta-adrenergic blocking agents, including ophthalmic agents

(concurrent use with a vasoconstrictor may result in unopposed alpha-adrenergic activity with a dose-dependent risk of hypertension and bradycardia with possible heart block)

CNS stimulation–producing medications, other, (See *Appendix II*), especially

» Cocaine, mucosal-local

(concurrent use with a vasoconstrictor may result in excessive CNS stimulation, leading to nervousness, irritability, insomnia, and possibly convulsions or cardiac arrhythmias; close observation of the patient is recommended)

(concurrent use of other sympathomimetics with vasoconstrictors also increases the risk of adverse cardiovascular effects; although vasoconstrictor-containing local anesthetic solutions are sometimes used in conjunction with low doses of cocaine for mucous membrane anesthesia, caution is recommended)

(concurrent use of doxapram, mazindol, or methylphenidate with a vasoconstrictor may also increase the pressor effects of the vasoconstrictor; concurrent use may also increase the pressor effect of doxapram)

» Digitalis glycosides or

Levodopa

(concurrent use with a vasoconstrictor may increase the risk of cardiac arrhythmias; caution and, with the digitalis glycosides, electrocardiographic monitoring are recommended)

Ergot derivatives, including antimigraine agents and oxytocics

(the vasoconstrictive effects of ergot derivatives may be additive to those of sympathomimetic vasoconstrictors; concurrent or sequential administration may cause severe, persistent hypertension; rarely, rupture of a cerebral blood vessel has occurred postpartum after an ergot-type oxytocic was administered within 3 to 4 hours following caudal block anesthesia with a vasoconstrictor)

Monoamine oxidase (MAO) inhibitors, including furazolidone, procarbazine, and selegiline

(concurrent use may prolong and intensify cardiac stimulant and vasopressor effects of phenylephrine, possibly leading to headache, cardiac arrhythmias, and/or severe, sustained hypertension)

Rauwolfia alkaloids

(in addition to possibly decreasing the antihypertensive effect of rauwolfia alkaloids, concurrent use may theoretically prolong the duration of action of the vasoconstrictor, by preventing uptake into storage granules; a "denervation supersensitivity" response is also possible; although problems with systemic vasoconstrictors have not been reported, a significant increase in blood pressure has been documented with administration of phenylephrine ophthalmic drops to patients taking reserpine; caution and close observation are recommended)

Ritodrine

(concurrent use with epinephrine, levonordefrin, or norepinephrine may increase the effect of either medication and the risk of side effects)

Thyroid hormones

(concurrent use with a sympathomimetic agent may increase the risk of coronary insufficiency in patients with coronary artery disease; dosage adjustment of the sympathomimetic is recommended, although the risk is reduced in euthyroid patients)

**Laboratory value alterations**

The following have been selected on the basis of their potential clinical significance (possible effect in parentheses where appropriate)—not necessarily inclusive (» = major clinical significance):

With diagnostic test results

Pancreatic function determinations using bentiromide

(administration of PABA-derivative local anesthetics or of lidocaine within 3 days before the bentiromide test may invalidate the test results because these anesthetics are metabolized to PABA or other arylamines and will therefore increase the true or apparent quantity of PABA recovered)

**Medical considerations/Contraindications**

The medical considerations/contraindications included here have been selected on the basis of their potential clinical significance (reasons given in parentheses where appropriate)—not necessarily inclusive (» = major clinical significance).

Note: A standard text and/or manufacturers' product information should be consulted for more specific information concerning medical problems that may apply to individual local anesthetic procedures.

*Except under special circumstances, this medication should not be used when the following medical problems exist:*

*For prilocaine only*

» Methemoglobinemia

(may be induced or exacerbated)

*For subarachnoid block*

» Complete heart block or
» Hemorrhage, severe or
» Hypotension, severe or
» Shock

(may be exacerbated by cardiac depressant effects; also, metabolism of amides may be decreased because of reduced hepatic blood flow)

» Local infection at site of proposed lumbar puncture

(lumbar puncture may spread infection into the arachnoid space; also, infection may alter pH at site of injection, resulting in decrease or loss of local anesthetic effect)

» Septicemia

(decreased patient tolerance to CNS stimulant effects)

*Risk-benefit should be considered when the following medical problems exist:*

*For all local anesthetic usage*

Any condition in which hepatic blood flow may be decreased, such as:

Congestive heart failure or

Hepatic disease or impairment

(increased risk of toxicity because of reduced clearance, especially with amides; a decrease in dosage and/or an increase in the interval between doses may be necessary, especially with lidocaine)

» Cardiovascular function impairment, especially heart block or shock

(may be exacerbated by cardiac depressant effects)

» Drug sensitivity, history of, especially to the anesthetic being considered for use and chemically related anesthetics or other compounds

(increased risk of hypersensitivity reactions)

Hyperthermia, malignant, history of or predisposition to—for amides

(possibility must be considered that amide-type local anesthetics may contribute to the development of malignant hyperthermia if supplemental general anesthesia is required)

» Inflammation and/or infection in region of injection

(may alter pH at site of injection resulting in decrease or loss of anesthetic effect)

Plasma cholinesterase deficiency—for esters

(increased risk of toxicity because of decreased metabolism)

Renal disease

(anesthetic or metabolites may accumulate)

Caution is also recommended in very young, elderly, acutely ill, or debilitated patients, who may be more susceptible to systemic toxicity induced by local anesthetics.

*For paracervical administration in obstetrics*

Fetal distress, pre-existing or

Prematurity or

Postmaturity or

Toxemia of pregnancy or

Uteroplacental insufficiency, pre-existing

(increased risk of fetal bradycardia and acidosis)

Note: Use of chloroprocaine is not recommended if prematurity, pre-existing fetal distress, or toxemia of pregnancy is present because its safety in these conditions has not been established.

*For peridural (caudal or lumbar epidural) anesthesia*

Neurological disease, pre-existing

Septicemia

(decreased patient tolerance to CNS stimulant effects)

Spinal deformity that may interfere with administration and/or effectiveness of local anesthetic

*For subarachnoid anesthesia*

Backache, chronic

(may be exacerbated)

» CNS disease, pre-existing, attributable to infection, tumor or other causes

» Coagulation defects induced by anticoagulant therapy or hematologic disorders

(trauma to a blood vessel during administration may result in uncontrollable CNS or soft tissue hemorrhage)

Headache, pre-existing, especially history of migraine

(may be induced or exacerbated)

Hemorrhagic spinal fluid

(risk of inadvertent intravascular administration)

Hypertension

Hypotension

(may be exacerbated by cardiac depressant and vasodilating effects)

Paresthesias, persistent

Psychosis, hysteria or uncooperative patient

Spinal conditions or deformities that may interfere with administration and/or effectiveness of anesthetic

*For vasoconstrictor-containing preparations*

Asthma

(increased risk of anaphylactic or bronchospastic allergic reactions induced by the sulfites in commercially available solutions)

» Cardiac disease or arrhythmias or
» Hyperthyroidism

(cardiac stimulant effects detrimental to patients with these conditions)

» Hypertension or
» Vascular disease, peripheral

(exaggerated vasoconstrictor response may occur, leading to increased risk of severe hypertension or ischemic injury or necrosis)

**Patient monitoring**

The following may be especially important in patient monitoring (other tests may be warranted in some patients, depending on condition; » = major clinical significance):

Cardiovascular status and

Respiratory status and

State of consciousness

(should be monitored after each local anesthetic injection to detect impending CNS and/or cardiovascular toxicity)

Fetal heart rate

(should be monitored during paracervical administration in obstetrics to detect fetal bradycardia)

## Side/Adverse Effects

Note: Adverse reactions are generally dose-related and may result from high plasma concentrations of anesthetic caused by inadvertent intravascular administration, excessive dosage, or rapid absorption from the injection site as well as reduced patient tolerance, idiosyncrasy, or hypersensitivity.

Adverse effects are also related to the specific local anesthetic used and the route and site of administration. Small doses of local anesthetics injected into the head and neck area (including retrobulbar, dental, and stellate ganglion blocks) or in the tracheobronchial area may produce adverse reactions similar to those caused by inadvertent intravascular injection of larger doses. Also, unintentional subarachnoid administration during intended performance of a peridural block or a nerve block near the vertebral column (especially in the head and neck area) may result in adverse effects that depend at least partially on the quantity of anesthetic administered subdurally.

Systemic reactions may occur rapidly or may be delayed for up to 30 minutes following administration.

Many of the neurological adverse effects may be related to the local anesthetic technique; the anesthetic used may or may not be a contributing factor in the development of these effects.

The following side/adverse effects have been selected on the basis of their potential clinical significance (possible signs and symptoms in parentheses where appropriate)—not necessarily inclusive:

**Those indicating need for medical attention**
Incidence less frequent or rare
  *For all routes*
    *Allergic reaction* (skin rash, redness, hives, and/or itching; sneezing; large, hive-like swellings on face, lips, tongue or in mouth or throat)—may be accompanied by nausea with or without vomiting; allergic reactions are much more likely to occur with esters than with amides; *cardiac depression*—if not treated promptly, may result in hypoxia, acidosis, heart block, and cardiac arrest; prolonged myocardial depression and arrhythmias have been reported with bupivacaine; *CNS toxicity*—CNS stimulation, which may lead to convulsions, usually occurs first, followed by CNS depression, which may lead to unconsciousness and respiratory arrest; however, CNS stimulation may be transient or absent so that drowsiness may be the first sign of toxicity in some patients, especially in children and with lidocaine; *methemoglobinemia* (cyanosis [if relatively mild, may be only symptom]; fatigue, weakness, breathing problems, tachycardia, headache, dizziness, or collapse [if severe and/or the patient cannot tolerate the reduced oxygen-carrying capacity of the blood])—may occur rarely with any local anesthetic but may be more likely with prilocaine; *nausea or vomiting; vasodilation, peripheral*

    Note: Anaphylactoid reactions, including shock, have also been reported rarely. The effectiveness of a small test dose in predicting the risk of allergic reactions has not been determined.

  *For central neural blocks*
    *Neurologic effects, including high or total spinal block, such as; arachnoiditis; backache; bradycardia; cranial nerve palsies; fecal and/or urinary incontinence [although urinary retention has also been reported]; headache; hypotension; loss of perineal sensation and sexual function; meningismus; paralysis of legs; paresthesia; persistent anesthesia; respiratory paralysis; septic meningitis; unconsciousness*—hypotension and respiratory paralysis may lead to cardiac arrest if not successfully treated

    Note: *High or total spinal block* may occur following inadvertent subarachnoid administration during intended performance of a peridural block as well as following intended subarachnoid administration. Persistent motor, sensory, and autonomic deficits of some lower spinal segments with slow (several months) or incomplete recovery have been reported rarely. Chloroprocaine may be especially likely to cause neuropathies.

    Inadvertent intravascular administration during intended performance of a subarachnoid block may lead to dose-related convulsions and cardiovascular collapse.

  *For dental anesthesia*
    *Allergic reaction* (swelling of lips and/or mouth); *numbness or tingling of lips and mouth, prolonged; trismus of facial muscles* (difficulty in opening the mouth)

  *For vasoconstrictors*
    *Sympathomimetic effects* (chest pain; dizziness; fast, pounding, or irregular heartbeat; headache; hypertension; trembling; unusual anxiety, nervousness, or restlessness)

## Overdose

For specific information on the agents used in the management of a local anesthetic overdose, see:
  • *Benzodiazepines (Systemic)* monograph;
  • Ephedrine in *Sympathomimetic Agents—Cardiovascular Use (Parenteral-Systemic)*;
  • Mephentermine in *Sympathomimetic Agents—Cardiovascular Use (Parenteral-Systemic)*;
  • Metaraminol in *Sympathomimetic Agents—Cardiovascular Use (Parenteral-Systemic)*;
  • *Neuromuscular Blocking Agents (Systemic)* monograph; and/or
  • Thiopental in *Anesthetics, Barbiturate (Systemic)* monograph.

For more information on the management of overdose or unintentional ingestion, **contact a Poison Control Center** (see *Poison Control Center Listing*).

The following effects have been selected on the basis of their potential clinical significance (possible signs and symptoms in parentheses where appropriate)—not necessarily inclusive:
Acute
  *Circulatory depression; convulsions*

**Treatment of overdose**
Specific treatment—
  For circulatory depression—Administering a vasopressor (preferably ephedrine, metaraminol, or mephentermine) and intravenous fluids is recommended. For maternal hypotension during obstetrical anesthesia, elevating the patient's legs or positioning the patient on her left side to displace the uterus may be sufficient to correct hypotension. Intravenous fluids and a vasoconstrictor should be administered if necessary; however, a vasoconstrictor should not be administered if the patient has received an ergot-type oxytocic agent.
  For convulsions—If convulsions do not respond to respiratory support, administering a benzodiazepine such as diazepam or an ultrashort-acting barbiturate such as thiopental or thiamylal intravenously is recommended. The fact that these agents, especially the barbiturates, may cause circulatory depression when administered intravenously must be kept in mind. A neuromuscular blocking agent may also be used to decrease the muscular manifestations of persistent convulsions; artificial respiration is mandatory if such an agent is used.
Supportive care—
  Securing and maintaining a patent airway, administering oxygen, and instituting assisted or controlled respiration as required. In some patients, endotracheal intubation may be required.

## Patient Consultation

As an aid to patient consultation, refer to *Advice for the Patient, Anesthetics (Parenteral-Local).*

In providing consultation, consider emphasizing the following selected information (» = major clinical significance):

**Before receiving this medication**
» Conditions affecting use, especially:
    Allergies to the anesthetic considered for use, related anesthetics, other related compounds, and additives (methylparaben, sulfites)
    Pregnancy—Potential rare unwanted effects with obstetrical use
    Use in children—Increased risk of systemic toxicity
    Use in the elderly—Increased risk of systemic toxicity
    Other medications
    Other medical problems

**Proper use of this medication**
  Proper dosing

**Precautions after receiving this medication**
  Caution that injury may occur undetected while numbness persists in the affected area; using care to prevent injury, including not eating or chewing gum following dental anesthesia (to prevent biting trauma)

**Side/adverse effects**
  Signs and/or symptoms of potential side effects, especially delayed skin rash, hives, or itching

## General Dosing Information

The safety and effectiveness of local anesthetics depends upon proper dosage, correct technique, adequate precautions, and readiness for emergencies. *Resuscitative equipment, oxygen, and other resuscitative drugs should be immediately available when any local anesthetic is used.*

A standard text should be consulted for specific techniques and procedures for administering local anesthetics.

The dosage of local anesthetics depends on the specific anesthetic procedure; vascularity of the tissues at or near the site of injection; specific nerve, plexus, or fiber to be blocked; type of surgery being performed (number of neuronal segments to be blocked, depth of anesthesia and degree of muscle relaxation required, and duration of anesthesia desired); and patient variables such as age and weight.

The recommended adult doses are given as a guideline for use in the average adult. *The actual dosage and maximum dosage must be individualized,* based on the age, size, and physical status of the patient and the expected rate of systemic absorption from the injection site. The lowest dosage (volume and concentration) that produces the desired results should be used.

Lower doses should be used for pediatric, geriatric, acutely ill, or debilitated patients and patients with cardiac or hepatic disease. Lower doses are also required for repeated injections (as for multiple nerve blocks or continuous catheter [intermittent] administration techniques), and for nerve blocks in highly vascular areas, in order to prevent excessively high plasma concentrations.

In patients receiving a CNS depressant, careful attention to the dosage of each agent is recommended to prevent possible additive depressant effects.

Local anesthetics may be administered as single injections or continuously or intermittently through an indwelling catheter. Fractional doses are especially recommended for peridural blocks.

Local anesthetics should be injected slowly, with frequent aspirations before and during the injection, to reduce the risk of inadvertent intravascular administration. Additional aspirations should be performed before and during each supplemental injection via an indwelling catheter. However, the fact that intravascular administration is possible even when aspiration for blood is negative must be kept in mind.

For central neural blocks in obstetrical anesthesia, the anesthetic should not be injected during a strong uterine contraction or while the patient is bearing down because excessively high levels of anesthesia may result.

For peridural blocks, injection of a small test dose (usually 2 to 5 mL of solution; consult manufacturers' product information for details) is recommended so that the patient can be monitored for signs of inadvertent subarachnoid or intravascular administration. If clinical conditions permit, the use of a vasoconstrictor-containing solution is recommended because circulatory changes produced by a vasoconstrictor may indicate intravascular administration. The test dose should be repeated if a patient is moved in any manner that may cause displacement of the catheter.

For retrobulbar block, lack of corneal sensation should not be relied upon to determine readiness for surgery because lack of corneal sensation usually precedes clinically acceptable external ocular muscle akinesia.

The extent and degree of subarachnoid block depend on the position of the patient during and immediately after injection, dosage, specific gravity of the solution, volume of solution used, force of injection, and the level of puncture. Hyperbaric solutions (with dextrose added to render the solution heavier than cerebrospinal fluid [CSF]) are usually used for low spinal anesthesia. Isobaric solutions (having the same specific gravity as CSF) produce anesthesia at the level of intrathecal injection. Hypobaric solutions (diluted to have a lower specific gravity than CSF) are used to produce anesthesia of thoracic structures and for low spinal anesthesia. A standard text and/or manufacturers' product information may be consulted for details concerning dilution and positioning of patient during and following administration.

Vasoconstrictors decrease the rate of local clearance of the local anesthetic, thereby reducing the risk of systemic toxic reactions, prolonging the anesthetic effect, increasing the frequency of complete conduction blocks at low anesthetic concentrations, and permitting larger maximum single doses of anesthetic to be administered. Epinephrine 1:200,000 is the most commonly used vasoconstrictor for most purposes; levonordefrin, norepinephrine, and phenylephrine may also be used. In dentistry, epinephrine 1:100,000 and levonordefrin 1:20,000 are the most commonly used vasoconstrictors.

Solutions containing a vasoconstrictor should be used cautiously and in carefully circumscribed quantities, if at all, in tissues supplied by end arteries (such as the fingers, toes, or penis) or having otherwise compromised blood supply; ischemia leading to gangrene may result. Also, a vasoconstrictor should not be injected repeatedly at the same site for dental procedures because reduced blood flow and increased oxygen consumption in the affected tissues may cause tissue anoxia, delayed healing, edema, or necrosis at the injection site.

**For treatment of adverse effects**

Recommended treatment consists of the following:
- For convulsions—If convulsions do not respond to respiratory support, administering a benzodiazepine such as diazepam (in 2.5-mg increments) or an ultrashort-acting barbiturate such as thiopental or thiamylal (in 50- to 100-mg increments) intravenously every 2 to 3 minutes is recommended. The fact that these agents, especially the barbiturates, may cause circulatory depression when administered intravenously must be kept in mind. A neuromuscular blocking agent may also be used to decrease the muscular manifestations of persistent convulsions; artificial respiration is mandatory if such an agent is used.
- For methemoglobinemia—If methemoglobinemia does not respond to administration of oxygen, administration of methylene blue (intravenous, 1 to 2 mg per kg of body weight (mg/kg) as a 1% solution, over a 5-minute period) is recommended.

## BUPIVACAINE

## Summary of Differences

Indications:
    Except as noted below, indicated (without epinephrine) for retrobulbar block; indicated (with or without epinephrine) for caudal or lumbar epidural block, local infiltration, peripheral nerve block, and sympathetic block; indicated (with epinephrine) for dental infiltration or nerve block; and indicated (with dextrose) for subarachnoid block.
    Paracervical administration not recommended.
    Not recommended for intravenous regional anesthesia (Bier block).
Pharmacology/pharmacokinetics:
    Physicochemical characteristics—
        Chemical group: Amide-type local anesthetic.
        Molecular weight: 342.91
        pKa: 8.1
        Lipid solubility: High.
    Protein binding—
        Very high.
    Half-life—
        2.7–3.5 hours (adults); 6–10 hours (neonates).
    Onset of action—
        Intermediate to slow.
    Duration of action—
        Long (3–10 hours; via nerve block, even longer).
    Elimination—
        6% of a dose may be excreted unchanged.
Precautions:
    Cross-sensitivity and/or related problems—
        May occur rarely with other amide-type local anesthetics.
    Pregnancy—
        Embryocidal effects have been demonstrated in rats and rabbits.
Side/adverse effects:
    Prolonged cardiovascular depression and arrhythmias have been reported.

## Additional Dosing Information

See also *General Dosing Information*.

Bupivacaine 0.25% generally produces incomplete motor block and is used when muscle relaxation is not important. However, intercostal nerve block with this strength of bupivacaine may produce complete motor block for intra-abdominal surgery in some patients.

Bupivacaine 0.5% produces motor block and some muscle relaxation when used for caudal, epidural, or nerve block. With continuous catheter (intermittent) administration techniques, repeat doses increase the degree of motor block. The first repeat dose of 0.5% bupivacaine may produce complete motor block.

Bupivacaine 0.75% produces complete motor block and complete muscle relaxation. When used for epidural block, the 0.75% solution is intended for single-dose administration only; it should not be used for intermittent administration techniques.

In obstetrics only, bupivacaine 0.75% is not recommended for epidural block because inadvertent intravascular injection has caused maternal cardiac arrest. However, lower concentrations may be used.

## Parenteral Dosage Forms

### BUPIVACAINE HYDROCHLORIDE INJECTION USP

**Usual adult and adolescent dose**

Caudal anesthesia—
    Moderate motor block: 37.5 to 75 mg (15 to 30 mL) as a 0.25% solution, repeated once every three hours as needed.
    Moderate to complete motor block: 75 to 150 mg (15 to 30 mL) as a 0.5% solution, repeated once every three hours as needed.
Epidural anesthesia—
    Partial to moderate motor block: 25 to 50 mg (10 to 20 mL) as a 0.25% solution, repeated once every three hours as needed.
    Moderate to complete motor block: 50 to 100 mg (10 to 20 mL) as a 0.5% solution, repeated once every three hours as needed.
    Complete motor block: 75 to 150 mg (10 to 20 mL) as a 0.75% solution.
Local infiltration—
    Single dose: Up to 175 mg (70 mL) as a 0.25% solution.
Peripheral nerve block—
    Moderate to complete motor block: 12.5 to 175 mg (5 to 70 mL) as a 0.25% solution; or 25 to 175 mg (5 to 37.5 mL) as a 0.5% solution. Dosage may be repeated every three hours if necessary.

Retrobulbar block—
    15 to 30 mg (2 to 4 mL) as a 0.75% solution.
Sympathetic block—
    50 to 125 mg (20 to 50 mL) as a 0.25% solution, repeated once every
        three hours as needed.

**Usual adult prescribing limits**
Up to 175 mg as a single dose or 400 mg per day.

**Usual pediatric dose**
Children up to 12 years of age—Dosage has not been established.

**Strength(s) usually available**
U.S.—
    With preservative (methylparaben 1 mg per mL)
        0.25% (2.5 mg per mL) (Rx) [*Marcaine; Sensorcaine;* GENERIC].
        0.5% (5 mg per mL) (Rx) [*Marcaine; Sensorcaine;* GENERIC].
    Without preservative
        0.25% (2.5 mg per mL) (Rx) [*Marcaine; Sensorcaine-MPF;*
            GENERIC].
        0.5% (5 mg per mL) (Rx) [*Marcaine; Sensorcaine-MPF;*
            GENERIC].
        0.75% (7.5 mg per mL) (Rx) [*Marcaine; Sensorcaine-MPF;*
            GENERIC].
Canada—
    With preservative (methylparaben 1 mg per mL)
        0.25% (2.5 mg per mL) [*Marcaine*].
        0.5% (5 mg per mL) [*Marcaine*].
    Without preservative
        0.25% (2.5 mg per mL) [*Marcaine*].
        0.5% (5 mg per mL) [*Marcaine*].
        0.75% (7.5 mg per mL) [*Marcaine*].
    Note: In Canada, this medication has not been assigned Rx status.
        However, it may not be sold or dispensed directly to the
        patient.

**Packaging and storage**
Store below 40 °C (104 °F), preferably between 15 and 30 °C (59 and 86
    °F), unless otherwise specified by manufacturer. Protect from freezing.

**Stability**
May be autoclaved.
For chemical disinfection of container surface, 91% isopropyl alcohol or
    70% ethyl alcohol without denaturants is recommended; solutions con-
    taining heavy metals should not be used.
Unused portions of solutions without a preservative must be discarded.

## BUPIVACAINE AND EPINEPHRINE INJECTION USP

**Usual adult and adolescent dose**
Dental—
    For infiltration and nerve block in maxillary and mandibular area: 9
        mg (1.8 mL) of bupivacaine hydrochloride as a 0.5% solution with
        epinephrine 1:200,000 per injection site. A second dose may be
        administered if necessary to produce adequate anesthesia after al-
        lowing up to 10 minutes for onset.
Other indications—
    See *Bupivacaine Hydrochloride Injection USP.* Administration of ep-
        inephrine concurrently with the local anesthetic may permit use of
        doses somewhat larger than those listed.

**Usual adult prescribing limits**
In dentistry—
    Up to 90 mg of bupivacaine hydrochloride per dental appointment.
Other indications—
    Up to 225 mg as a single dose or 400 mg per day of bupivacaine
        hydrochloride.

**Usual pediatric dose**
Children up to 12 years of age—
    Dosage has not been established.

**Strength(s) usually available**
U.S.—
    With preservative (methylparaben 1 mg per mL)
        0.25% (2.5 mg per mL), with epinephrine 1:200,000 (Rx) [*Mar-
            caine* (sodium metabisulfite 0.5 mg per mL; edetate calcium
            disodium); *Sensorcaine* (sodium metabisulfite 0.5 mg per mL);
            GENERIC].
        0.5% (5 mg per mL), with epinephrine 1:200,000 (Rx) [*Marcaine*
            (sodium metabisulfite 0.5 mg per mL; edetate calcium diso-
            dium); *Sensorcaine* (sodium metabisulfite 0.5 mg per mL);
            GENERIC].
    Without preservative
        0.25% (2.5 mg per mL), with epinephrine 1:200,000 (Rx) [*Mar-
            caine* (sodium metabisulfite 0.5 mg per mL; edetate calcium

disodium); *Sensorcaine-MPF* (sodium metabisulfite 0.5 mg per
            mL); GENERIC].
        0.5% (5 mg per mL), with epinephrine 1:200,000 (Rx) [*Marcaine*
            (sodium metabisulfite 0.5 mg per mL; edetate calcium diso-
            dium); *Sensorcaine-MPF* (sodium metabisulfite 0.5 mg per
            mL); GENERIC].
        0.75% (7.5 mg per mL), with epinephrine 1:200,000 (Rx) [*Mar-
            caine* (sodium metabisulfite 0.5 mg per mL; edetate calcium
            disodium); *Sensorcaine-MPF* (sodium metabisulfite 0.5 mg per
            mL); GENERIC].
    For dental use
        0.5% (5 mg per mL; 9 mg per 1.8-mL dental cartridge), with ep-
            inephrine 1:200,000 (Rx) [*Marcaine* (sodium metabisulfite 0.5
            mg per mL; edetate calcium disodium)].
Canada—
    Without preservative
        0.25% (2.5 mg per mL), with epinephrine 1:200,000 [*Marcaine*
            (sodium bisulfite 0.5 mg per mL; edetate calcium disodium)].
        0.5% (5 mg per mL), with epinephrine 1:200,000 [*Marcaine* (so-
            dium bisulfite 0.5 mg per mL; edetate calcium disodium)].
    Note: In Canada, this medication has not been assigned Rx status.
        However, it may not be sold or dispensed directly to the
        patient.

**Packaging and storage**
Store below 40 °C (104 °F), preferably between 15 and 30 °C (59 and 86
    °F), unless otherwise specified by manufacturer. Protect from light.
    Protect from freezing.

**Stability**
On removal of doses from the vial, air is introduced, which slowly oxi-
    dizes the epinephrine causing discoloration of the solution and possible
    loss of potency. Do not use if solution is discolored or contains a
    precipitate.
Should not be autoclaved. For chemical disinfection of the container sur-
    face, 91% isopropyl alcohol or 70% ethyl alcohol without denaturants
    is recommended; solutions containing heavy metals are not
    recommended.
Unused portions of solutions without a preservative must be discarded.

## BUPIVACAINE IN DEXTROSE INJECTION USP

**Usual adult dose**
Hyperbaric spinal anesthesia—
    Obstetrical anesthesia:
        Normal vaginal delivery—6 mg (0.8 mL) of bupivacaine hydro-
            chloride as a 0.75% solution.
        Cesarean section—7.5 to 10.5 mg (1 to 1.4 mL) of bupivacaine
            hydrochloride as a 0.75% solution.
    Surgical anesthesia:
        Lower extremity and perineal procedures—7.5 mg (1 mL) of bu-
            pivacaine hydrochloride as a 0.75% solution.
        Lower abdominal procedures—12 mg (1.6 mL) of bupivacaine hy-
            drochloride as a 0.75% solution.

**Usual pediatric dose**
Dosage has not been established.

**Strength(s) usually available**
U.S.—
    Without preservative
        0.75% (7.5 mg per mL), with dextrose 8.25% (82.5 mg per mL)
            (Rx) [*Marcaine Spinal; Sensorcaine-MPF Spinal;* GENERIC].
Canada—
    Without preservative
        0.75% (7.5 mg per mL), with dextrose 8.25% (82.5 mg per mL)
            [*Marcaine*].
    Note: In Canada, this medication has not been assigned Rx status.
        However, it may not be sold or dispensed directly to the
        patient.

**Packaging and storage**
Store below 40 °C (104 °F), preferably between 15 and 30 °C (59 and 86
    °F), unless otherwise specified by manufacturer. Protect from freezing.

**Stability**
May be autoclaved once; with repeated autoclaving or prolonged storage,
    caramelization of the dextrose may occur, leading to discoloration.
    Discolored solutions should not be used.
Do not use if solution contains a precipitate.

## CHLOROPROCAINE

## Summary of Differences

Indications:
  Indicated for caudal or lumbar epidural block, dental infiltration or nerve block, local infiltration, peripheral nerve block, and intravenous regional anesthesia (Bier block).
  Not recommended for subarachnoid administration.

Pharmacology/pharmacokinetics:
  Physicochemical characteristics—
    Chemical group: Ester-type local anesthetic.
    Molecular weight: 307.22
    pKa: 9.0
  Biotransformation—
    Metabolized to a PABA derivative.
  Half-life—
    19–26 seconds (adults); 41–45 seconds (neonates).
  Onset of action—
    Rapid.
  Duration of action—
    Short (30–60 minutes).

Precautions:
  Cross-sensitivity and/or related problems—
    May occur with PABA, parabens, or other ester-type local anesthetics.
  Pregnancy—
    Paracervical administration not recommended if prematurity, pre-existing fetal distress, or toxemia of pregnancy present, because safety in these conditions has not been established.
    May cause uterine artery constriction.
  Drug interactions and/or related problems—
    Interaction with cholinesterase inhibitors.
    Interaction with sulfonamides.

Side/adverse effects:
  May be especially likely to cause neuropathies.
  More likely than amide-type local anesthetics to cause hypersensitivity reactions.

## Additional Dosing Information

See also *General Dosing Information*.

Epinephrine 1:200,000 may be added to chloroprocaine *without* preservatives to prolong the duration of anesthetic effect.

## Parenteral Dosage Forms

### CHLOROPROCAINE HYDROCHLORIDE INJECTION USP

**Usual adult and adolescent dose**
Caudal anesthesia—
  300 to 500 mg (15 to 25 mL) as a 2% solution; or 450 to 750 mg (15 to 25 mL) as a 3% solution, repeated at forty- to sixty-minute intervals as needed.
Epidural anesthesia (lumbar and sacral regions)—
  40 to 50 mg (2 to 2.5 mL) as a 2% solution per segment; or 60 to 75 mg (2 to 2.5 mL) as a 3% solution per segment. The usual total dose is 300 to 750 mg (15 to 25 mL as a 2 or 3% solution). May be repeated at forty- to fifty-minute intervals using 40 to 120 mg (2 to 6 mL) less than original total dose as a 2% solution or 60 to 180 mg (2 to 6 mL) less than original total dose as a 3% solution.
Local infiltration—
  Depends on site to be infiltrated and extent of surgical procedure.
Nerve block—
  Brachial plexus:
    600 to 800 mg (30 to 40 mL) as a 2% solution.
  Digital:
    30 to 40 mg (3 to 4 mL) as a 1% solution.
  Infraorbital:
    10 to 20 mg (0.5 to 1 mL) as a 2% solution.
  Mandibular:
    40 to 60 mg (2 to 3 mL) as a 2% solution.
  Obstetrics:
    Paracervical block—30 mg (3 mL) as a 1% solution per each of four sites.
    Pudendal block—200 mg (10 mL) as a 2% solution per side.

**Usual adult prescribing limits**
Without epinephrine—
  800 mg per dose.
With added epinephrine 1:200,000—
  1 gram per dose.

**Usual pediatric dose**
Local infiltration—
  Up to 20 mg per kg of body weight as a 0.5 to 1% solution.
Nerve block—
  Up to 20 mg per kg of body weight as a 1 to 1.5% solution.
Note: Dosage must be individualized, based on the age and weight of the patient.

**Strength(s) usually available**
U.S.—
  With preservative (methylparaben 1 mg per mL)
    1% (10 mg per mL) (Rx) [*Nesacaine* (edetate disodium)].
    2% (20 mg per mL) (Rx) [*Nesacaine* (edetate disodium)].
  Without preservative
    2% (20 mg per mL) (Rx) [*Nesacaine-MPF* (edetate disodium); GENERIC].
    3% (30 mg per mL) (Rx) [*Nesacaine-MPF* (edetate disodium); GENERIC].
Canada—
  Without preservative
    2% (20 mg per mL) [*Nesacaine-CE* (edetate calcium disodium; sodium bisulfite 0.7 mg per mL)].
    3% (30 mg per mL) [*Nesacaine-CE* (edetate calcium disodium; sodium bisulfite 0.7 mg per mL)].
  Note: In Canada, this medication has not been assigned Rx status. However, it may not be sold or dispensed directly to the patient.

**Packaging and storage**
Store below 40 °C (104 °F), preferably between 15 and 30 °C (59 and 86 °F), unless otherwise specified by manufacturer. Protect from freezing.

**Preparation of dosage form**
For administration to pediatric patients in concentrations lower than those commercially available—Dilute available concentrations with the quantity of 0.9% sodium chloride injection needed to obtain the required final concentration of local anesthetic solution.

**Stability**
May be autoclaved (prior to addition of epinephrine, if added).
Sterilization of vials with ethylene oxide is not recommended because absorption through the closure may occur.
Solutions may become discolored after prolonged exposure to light. Protection from direct sunlight is recommended. The solution should not be used if discoloration occurs.
Exposure to low temperatures may cause precipitation of chloroprocaine hydrochloride crystals. These crystals usually redissolve when the solution is returned to room temperature. Solutions containing undissolved material should not be used.
Unused portions of solutions without a preservative must be discarded.

## ETIDOCAINE

## Summary of Differences

Indications:
  Indicated (without epinephrine) for retrobulbar block; indicated (with or without epinephrine) for caudal or lumbar epidural block, local infiltration, and peripheral nerve block; and indicated (with epinephrine) for dental infiltration or nerve block.

Pharmacology/pharmacokinetics:
  Physicochemical characteristics—
    Chemical group: Amide-type local anesthetic.
    Molecular weight: 312.88
    pKa: 7.7
    Lipid solubility: High.
  Protein-binding—
    Very high.
  Half-life—
    2.7 hours (adults); 4–8 hours (neonates).
  Onset of action—
    Rapid
  Duration of action—
    Long (3 to 10 hours).
  Elimination—
    1% of a dose may be excreted unchanged.

Precautions:
  Cross-sensitivity and/or related problems—
    May occur rarely with other amide-type local anesthetics.
  Pregnancy—
    Studies in animals have not shown adverse effects on the fetus.
    Epidural administration not recommended for normal vaginal delivery.

# Parenteral Dosage Forms

## ETIDOCAINE HYDROCHLORIDE INJECTION

**Usual adult and adolescent dose**
See *Etidocaine Hydrochloride and Epinephrine Injection*. Doses somewhat smaller than those listed may be required when epinephrine is not used concurrently with the local anesthetic.

**Usual adult prescribing limits**
4 mg per kg of body weight or 300 mg per injection.

**Usual pediatric dose**
Dosage has not been established.

**Strength(s) usually available**
U.S.—
   Without preservative
      1% (10 mg per mL) (Rx) [*Duranest-MPF*].

**Packaging and storage**
Store below 40 °C (104 °F), preferably between 15 and 30 °C (59 and 86 °F), unless otherwise specified by manufacturer. Protect from freezing.

**Stability**
May be autoclaved.
Unused portions of solutions must be discarded because they contain no preservative.

## ETIDOCAINE HYDROCHLORIDE AND EPINEPHRINE INJECTION

**Usual adult and adolescent dose**
Caudal anesthesia—
   50 to 150 mg (10 to 30 mL) of etidocaine hydrochloride as a 0.5% solution; or 100 to 300 mg (10 to 30 mL) of etidocaine hydrochloride as a 1% solution. Additional incremental doses may be administered at two- to three-hour intervals as needed.
Lumbar peridural anesthesia—
   Cesarean section or
   Intra-abdominal or pelvic surgery or
   Lower-limb surgery: 100 to 300 mg (10 to 30 mL) of etidocaine hydrochloride as a 1% solution; or 150 to 300 mg (10 to 20 mL) of etidocaine hydrochloride as a 1.5% solution. Additional incremental doses may be administered at two- to three-hour intervals as needed.
   Gynecological procedures: 50 to 150 mg (10 to 30 mL) of etidocaine hydrochloride as a 0.5% solution; or 50 to 200 mg (5 to 20 mL) of etidocaine hydrochloride as a 1% solution. Additional incremental doses may be administered at two- to three-hour intervals as needed.
Dental infiltration or nerve block—
   15 to 75 mg (1 to 5 mL) as a 1.5% solution.
Percutaneous infiltration—
   5 to 400 mg (1 to 80 mL) of etidocaine hydrochloride as a 0.5% solution.
Peripheral nerve block—
   25 to 400 mg (5 to 80 mL) of etidocaine hydrochloride as a 0.5% solution; or 50 to 400 mg (5 to 40 mL) of etidocaine hydrochloride as a 1% solution. Additional incremental doses may be administered at two- to three-hour intervals as needed.

**Usual adult prescribing limits**
5.5 mg per kg of body weight or 400 mg per injection of etidocaine hydrochloride with epinephrine 1:200,000.

**Usual pediatric dose**
Dosage has not been established.

**Strength(s) usually available**
U.S.—
   Without preservative
      1% (10 mg per mL), with epinephrine 1:200,000 (Rx) [*Duranest-MPF* (sodium metabisulfite 0.5 mg per mL)].
      1.5% (15 mg per mL), with epinephrine 1:200,000 (Rx) [*Duranest-MPF* (sodium metabisulfite 0.5 mg per mL)].
   For dental use
      1.5% (15 mg per mL; 27 mg per 1.8-mL dental cartridge), with epinephrine 1:200,000 (Rx) [*Duranest* (sodium metabisulfite 0.5 mg per mL)].

**Packaging and storage**
Store below 40 °C (104 °F), preferably between 15 and 30 °C (59 and 86 °F), unless otherwise specified by manufacturer. Protect from freezing.

**Stability**
Do not autoclave.
Do not use if solution is discolored.

Unused portions of solutions not containing a preservative must be discarded.

---

### LIDOCAINE

# Summary of Differences

Indications:
   Indicated (without epinephrine) for retrobulbar block, transtracheal anesthesia, and intravenous regional anesthesia (Bier block); indicated (with or without epinephrine) for caudal or lumbar epidural block, dental infiltration or nerve block, local infiltration, peripheral nerve block, and sympathetic block; and indicated (with dextrose) for subarachnoid block.
Pharmacology/pharmacokinetics:
   Physicochemical characteristics—
      Chemical group: Amide-type local anesthetic.
      Molecular weight: 288.82
      pKa: 7.9
      Lipid solubility: Medium.
   Protein-binding—
      Moderate.
   Biotransformation—
      Xylidide metabolites are active and toxic, but less so than the parent compound.
   Half-life—
      1.5–1.8 hours (adults); 3 hours (neonates).
   Onset of action—
      Rapid.
   Duration of action—
      Intermediate (1–3 hours).
   Relative toxicity (compared to procaine)—
      2
   Elimination—
      10% of a dose may be excreted unchanged.
Precautions:
   Cross-sensitivity and/or related problems—
      May occur rarely with other amide-type local anesthetics.
   Pregnancy—
      Studies in animals have not shown adverse effects on the fetus.
      May cause uterine artery constriction.
Side/adverse effects:
   Usually does not cause CNS stimulation prior to CNS depression.

# Additional Dosing Information

See also *General Dosing Information*.

Solutions containing epinephrine should be used when large doses are required.

A reduction in the dose of lidocaine, or an increase in the interval between doses, may be necessary in patients with decreased hepatic blood flow or hepatic function impairment.

For intravenous regional anesthesia, proper tourniquet technique is essential. Only the single-dose containers designated for intravenous regional anesthesia should be used. A vasoconstrictor should not be used.

Solutions containing dextrose are hyperbaric and are indicated for subarachnoid (spinal) anesthesia.

# Parenteral Dosage Forms

## LIDOCAINE HYDROCHLORIDE INJECTION USP

**Usual adult and adolescent dose**
Caudal anesthesia—
   Obstetrical analgesia: 200 to 300 mg (20 to 30 mL) as a 1% solution.
   Surgical analgesia: 225 to 300 mg (15 to 20 mL) as a 1.5% solution.
   Note: For continuous catheter (intermittent administration) techniques, the maximum dose should not be administered at intervals of less than 90 minutes.
Epidural anesthesia—
   Lumbar:
      Analgesia—250 to 300 mg (25 to 30 mL) as a 1% solution.
      Anesthesia— 225 to 300 mg (15 to 20 mL) as a 1.5% solution; or 200 to 300 mg (10 to 15 mL) as a 2% solution.
      Thoracic: 200 to 300 mg (20 to 30 mL) as a 1% solution.
   Note: Dosages given for epidural anesthesia are usual total doses; actual dosage must be based on the number of dermatomes to be anesthetized (2 to 3 mL of the indicated concentration per dermatome).

For continuous catheter (intermittent administration) techniques, the maximum dose should not be administered at intervals of less than 90 minutes.

Infiltration—
Intravenous regional: 50 to 300 mg (10 to 60 mL) as a 0.5% solution.
Percutaneous: 5 to 300 mg (up to 60 mL as a 0.5% solution; up to 30 mL as a 1% solution).
Peripheral nerve block—
Brachial: 225 to 300 mg (15 to 20 mL) as a 1.5% solution.
Dental: 20 to 100 mg (1 to 5 mL) as a 2% solution.
Intercostal: 30 mg (3 mL) as a 1% solution.
Paracervical: 100 mg (10 mL) per side as a 1% solution; may be repeated if necessary at intervals of not less than 90 minutes.
Paravertebral: 30 to 50 mg (3 to 5 mL) as a 1% solution.
Pudendal: 100 mg (10 mL) per side as a 1% solution.
Retrobulbar—
120 to 200 mg (3 to 5 mL) as a 4% solution.
Sympathetic nerve block—
Cervical (stellate ganglion): 50 mg (5 mL) as a 1% solution.
Lumbar: 50 to 100 mg (5 to 10 mL) as a 1% solution.
Transtracheal—
80 to 120 mg (2 to 3 mL) as a 4% solution. In addition, topical administration of the 4% solution to the pharynx (as a spray) may be required to achieve complete analgesia. For combined use of injection and spray, it should rarely be necessary to administer more than 200 mg (5 mL) or 3 mg per kg of body weight.

**Usual adult prescribing limits**
Not to exceed 4.5 mg per kg of body weight or 300 mg per dose, except as noted below—
Intravenous regional anesthesia: Do not exceed 4 mg per kg of body weight.
Dental: Do not exceed 6.6 mg per kg of body weight or 300 mg per dental appointment.

**Usual pediatric dose**
Local infiltration—
Up to 4.5 mg per kg of body weight as a 0.25 to 0.5% solution.
Intravenous regional anesthesia: Up to 3 mg per kg of body weight as a 0.25 to 0.5% solution.
Nerve block—
Up to 4.5 mg per kg of body weight as a 0.5 to 1% solution.
Note: Dosage must be individualized by physician, based on patient's age and weight. For local infiltration, concentrations of 0.25% to 0.5% are recommended for use in infants; concentrations of 0.5% are recommended for other pediatric patients.

**Strength(s) usually available**
U.S.—
With preservative (methylparaben 1 mg per mL)
0.5% (5 mg per mL) (Rx) [*Xylocaine*].
1% (10 mg per mL) (Rx) [*Dilocaine; L-Caine; Lidoject-1; Nervocaine; Xylocaine;* GENERIC].
2% (20 mg per mL) (Rx) [*Dilocaine; L-Caine; Lidoject-2; Nervocaine; Xylocaine;* GENERIC].
Without preservative
0.5% (5 mg per mL) (Rx) [*Xylocaine-MPF*].
1% (10 mg per mL) (Rx) [*Xylocaine-MPF;* GENERIC].
1.5% (15 mg per mL) (Rx) [*Xylocaine-MPF*].
2% (20 mg per mL) (Rx) [*Dalcaine; Xylocaine-MPF;* GENERIC].
4% (40 mg per mL) (Rx) [*Xylocaine-MPF;* GENERIC].
For dental use
2% (20 mg per mL; 36 mg per 1.8-mL dental cartridge) (Rx) [*Xylocaine*].
Canada—
With preservative (methylparaben 1 mg per mL)
0.5% (5 mg per mL) [*Xylocaine;* GENERIC].
1% (10 mg per mL) [*Xylocaine;* GENERIC].
2% (20 mg per mL) [*Xylocaine;* GENERIC].
Without preservative
1% (10 mg per mL) [*Xylocaine*].
1.5% (15 mg per mL) [*Xylocaine;* GENERIC].
2% (20 mg per mL) [*Xylocaine;* GENERIC].
Note: In Canada, this medication has not been assigned Rx status. However, it may not be sold or dispensed directly to the patient.

**Packaging and storage**
Store below 40 °C (104 °F), preferably between 15 and 30 °C (59 and 86 °F), unless otherwise specified by manufacturer. Protect from freezing.

**Preparation of dosage form**
For administration to pediatric patients in concentrations lower than those commercially available—Dilute available concentrations with the

quantity of 0.9% sodium chloride injection needed to obtain the required final concentration of local anesthetic solution.

**Stability**
May be autoclaved.
For chemical disinfection of the container surface, 91% isopropyl alcohol or 70% ethyl alcohol without denaturants is recommended; solutions containing heavy metals are not recommended.
Dental cartridges sealed with aluminum caps should not be kept in solutions made from antirust tablets or solutions containing quaternary ammonium salts such as benzalkonium chloride.
Unused portions of solutions without a preservative must be discarded.

## LIDOCAINE HYDROCHLORIDE AND DEXTROSE INJECTION USP

**Usual adult dose**
Obstetrical low spinal (saddle block) anesthesia—
Normal vaginal delivery: 9 to 15 mg (0.6 to 1 mL) of lidocaine hydrochloride as a 1.5% solution; or 50 mg (1 mL) of lidocaine hydrochloride as a 5% solution.
Cesarean section and deliveries requiring intrauterine manipulation: 75 mg (1.5 mL) of lidocaine hydrochloride as a 5% solution.
Surgical anesthesia
Abdominal—
75 to 100 mg (1.5 to 2 mL) of lidocaine hydrochloride as a 5% solution.

**Usual pediatric dose**
Children and adolescents up to 16 years of age—Dosage has not been established.

**Strength(s) usually available**
U.S.—
Without preservative
1.5% (15 mg per mL), with dextrose 7.5% (75 mg per mL) (Rx) [*Xylocaine-MPF*].
5% (50 mg per mL), with dextrose 7.5% (75 mg per mL) (Rx) [*Xylocaine-MPF with Glucose;* GENERIC].
Canada—
Without preservative
5% (50 mg per mL), with dextrose 7.5 % (75 mg per mL) [*Xylocaine with Glucose*].
Note: In Canada, this medication has not been assigned Rx status. However, it may not be sold or dispensed directly to the patient.

**Packaging and storage**
Store below 40 °C (104 °F), preferably between 15 and 30 °C (59 and 86 °F), unless otherwise specified by manufacturer. Protect from freezing.

**Stability**
May be autoclaved once; with repeated autoclaving or prolonged storage, caramelization of the dextrose may occur, leading to discoloration. Discolored solutions should not be used.
Do not use if solution contains a precipitate.
For chemical disinfection of the container surface, 91% isopropyl alcohol or 70% ethyl alcohol without a denaturant is recommended; solutions containing heavy metals are not recommended.
Unused portions of solutions must be discarded because they contain no preservative.

## LIDOCAINE AND EPINEPHRINE INJECTION USP

**Usual adult and adolescent dose**
Dental anesthesia (for infiltration or nerve block)—
20 to 100 mg (1 to 5 mL) of lidocaine hydrochloride as a 2% solution with epinephrine 1:100,000 or 1:50,000.
Other indications—
See *Lidocaine Hydrochloride Injection USP*. Administration of epinephrine concurrently with the local anesthetic may permit use of doses somewhat larger than those listed.

**Usual adult prescribing limits**
Dental anesthesia—
Up to 6.6 mg per kg of body weight or 300 mg of lidocaine hydrochloride and 3 mcg (0.003 mg) of epinephrine per kg of body weight per appointment.
Other indications—
Up to 7 mg of lidocaine hydrochloride per kg of body weight but not exceeding 300 mg as a single dose.

**Usual pediatric dose**
Dental anesthesia—
20 to 30 mg (1 to 1.5 mL) of lidocaine hydrochloride as a 2% solution with epinephrine 1:100,000.

Local infiltration—
  Dosage must be individualized by physician, based on patient's age and weight. Concentrations of 0.25 to 0.5% of lidocaine hydrochloride are recommended for use in infants; concentrations of 0.5% of lidocaine hydrochloride are recommended for other pediatric patients.

Nerve block—
  Dosage must be individualized by physician, based on patient's age and weight. Concentrations of 0.5 to 1% of lidocaine hydrochloride should suffice for most nerve blocks.

**Usual pediatric prescribing limits**
Dental anesthesia—
  4 to 5 mg of lidocaine hydrochloride per kg of body weight or 100 to 150 mg as a single dose.
Local infiltration or
Nerve block—7 mg of lidocaine hydrochloride per kg of body weight as a 0.25 to 0.5% solution with epinephrine 1:200,000.

**Strength(s) usually available**
U.S.—
  With preservative (methylparaben 1 mg per mL)
    0.5% (5 mg per mL), with epinephrine 1:200,000 (Rx) [*Xylocaine* (sodium metabisulfite 0.5 mg per mL)].
    1% (10 mg per mL), with epinephrine 1:100,000 (Rx) [*Xylocaine* (sodium metabisulfite 0.5 mg per mL); GENERIC].
    2% (20 mg per mL), with epinephrine 1:100,000 (Rx) [*Xylocaine* (sodium metabisulfite 0.5 mg per mL); GENERIC].
  Without preservative
    1% (10 mg per mL), with epinephrine 1:100,000 (Rx) [GENERIC].
    1% (10 mg per mL), with epinephrine 1:200,000 (Rx) [*Xylocaine-MPF* (sodium metabisulfite 0.5 mg per mL)].
    1.5% (15 mg per mL), with epinephrine 1:200,000 (Rx) [*Xylocaine-MPF* (sodium metabisulfite 0.5 mg per mL)].
    2% (20 mg per mL), with epinephrine 1:200,000 (Rx) [*Xylocaine-MPF* (sodium metabisulfite 0.5 mg per mL)].
  For dental use
    2% (20 mg per mL; 36 mg per 1.8-mL dental cartridge), with epinephrine 1:100,000 (Rx) [*Octocaine* (sodium metabisulfite); *Xylocaine* (sodium metabisulfite 0.5 mg per mL)].
    2% (20 mg per mL; 36 mg per 1.8-mL dental cartridge), with epinephrine 1:50,000 (Rx) [*Octocaine* (sodium metabisulfite); *Xylocaine* (sodium metabisulfite 0.5 mg per mL)].
Canada—
  With preservative (methylparaben)
    0.5% (5 mg per mL), with epinephrine 1:100,000 [*Xylocaine* (sodium metabisulfite)].
    1% (10 mg per mL), with epinephrine 1:200,000 [*Xylocaine* (sodium metabisulfite)].
    1% (10 mg per mL), with epinephrine 1:100,000 [*Xylocaine* (sodium metabisulfite)].
    2% (20 mg per mL), with epinephrine 1:100,000 [*Xylocaine* (sodium metabisulfite)].
  Without preservative
    0.5% (5 mg per mL), with epinephrine 1:200,000 [*Xylocaine* (sodium metabisulfite)].
    1.5% (15 mg per mL), with epinephrine 1:200,000 [*Xylocaine* (sodium metabisulfite); *Xylocaine Test Dose* (sodium metabisulfite)].
    2% (20 mg per mL), with epinephrine 1:200,000 [*Xylocaine* (sodium metabisulfite)].
    2% (20 mg per mL), with epinephrine 1:100,000 [*Xylocaine* (sodium metabisulfite)].
  For dental use
    2% (20 mg per mL; 36 mg per 1.8-mL dental cartridge), with epinephrine 1:100,000 [*Octocaine-100* (sodium metabisulfite); *Xylocaine* (sodium metabisulfite)].
    2% (20 mg per mL; 36 mg per 1.8-mL dental cartridge), with epinephrine 1:50,000 [*Octocaine-50* (sodium metabisulfite); *Xylocaine* (sodium metabisulfite)].
  Note: In Canada, this medication has not been assigned Rx status. However, it may not be sold or dispensed directly to the patient.

**Packaging and storage**
Store below 40 °C (104 °F), preferably between 15 and 30 °C (59 and 86 °F), unless otherwise specified by manufacturer. Protect from freezing.

**Preparation of dosage form**
For administration to pediatric patients in concentrations lower than those commercially available—Dilute available concentrations with the quantity of 0.9% sodium chloride injection needed to obtain the required final concentration of local anesthetic solution.

**Stability**
Should not be autoclaved.
Do not use if solution is discolored or contains a precipitate.
For chemical disinfection of the container surface, 91% isopropyl alcohol or 70% ethyl alcohol without denaturants is recommended; solutions containing heavy metals are not recommended.
Dental cartridges sealed with aluminum caps should not be kept in solutions made from antirust tablets or solutions containing quaternary ammonium salts such as benzalkonium chloride.
Unused portions of solutions without a preservative must be discarded.

---

### *MEPIVACAINE*

## Summary of Differences

Indications:
  Indicated for caudal or lumbar epidural block, local infiltration, intravenous regional anesthesia (Bier block), peripheral nerve block, and transtracheal anesthesia; and indicated (with or without levonordefrin) for dental infiltration or nerve block.
  Not recommended for subarachnoid administration.
Pharmacology/pharmacokinetics:
  Physicochemical characteristics—
    Chemical group: Amide-type local anesthetic.
    Molecular weight: 282.81
    pKa: 7.6
    Lipid solubility: Medium.
  Protein-binding—High.
  Half-life—2–3 hours (adults); 9 hours (neonates).
  Onset of action—Rapid to intermediate.
  Duration of action—Intermediate (1–3 hours).
  Relative toxicity (compared to procaine)—2
  Elimination—16% of a dose may be excreted unchanged.
Precautions:
  Cross-sensitivity and/or related problems—
    May occur rarely with other amide-type local anesthetics.
  Pregnancy—
    May cause uterine artery constriction.
  Pediatrics—
    Appropriate studies have not shown pediatrics-specific problems.

## Additional Dosing Information

See also *General Dosing Information.*
Mepivacaine 1, 1.5, and 2% are not intended for dental use.

## Parenteral Dosage Forms

### MEPIVACAINE HYDROCHLORIDE INJECTION USP

**Usual adult and adolescent dose**
Brachial
Cervical
Intercostal
Pudendal nerve block—
  50 to 400 mg (5 to 40 mL) as a 1% solution; or 100 to 400 mg (5 to 20 mL) as a 2% solution.
Caudal and lumbar epidural block—
  150 to 300 mg (15 to 30 mL) as a 1% solution; or 150 to 375 mg (10 to 25 mL) as a 1.5% solution; or 200 to 400 mg (10 to 20 mL) as a 2% solution.
Dental—
  Single site in upper or lower jaw: 54 mg (1.8 mL) as a 3% solution. Infiltration and nerve block of entire oral cavity—270 mg (9 mL) as a 3% solution.
  Larger doses required for an extensive procedure should be calculated according to the patient's weight, and the injections spread out over time as required.
Local infiltration (other than in dentistry)—
  Up to 400 mg (up to 40 mL) as a 0.5% or 1% solution.
Paracervical block—
  Up to 100 mg (up to 10 mL) as a 1% solution per side; may be repeated if necessary in not less than 90 minutes.
Therapeutic block (management of pain)—
  10 to 50 mg (1 to 5 mL) as a 1% solution; or 20 to 100 mg (1 to 5 mL) as a 2% solution.
Transvaginal (paracervical plus pudendal) block—
  Up to 150 mg (up to 15 mL) as a 1% solution per side.

**Usual adult prescribing limits**
Dental—
  Up to 6.6 mg per kg of body weight but not to exceed 300 mg per appointment.

Other indications—
    Up to 7 mg per kg of body weight or 400 mg per procedure.
Note: Although doses of 550 mg have been administered without adverse effects, they are not recommended. If doses of 550 mg are needed, they should not be given at intervals of less than 1½ hours nor should more than 1 gram be given in 24 hours.

**Usual pediatric dose**
Up to 5 to 6 mg per kg of body weight.
Note: Dosage must be individualized based on the patient's age and weight. For local infiltration, concentrations of 0.2 to 0.5% are recommended for infants and children up to 3 years of age; concentrations of 0.5 to 1% are recommended for children over 3 years of age and weighing more than 13.65 kg. For nerve block in children, concentrations of 0.5 to 1% are recommended.

    Maximum pediatric dosage in dentistry must be carefully calculated on the basis of the patient's weight but must not exceed 270 mg (9 mL) of the 3% solution.

**Strength(s) usually available**
U.S.—
    With preservative (methylparaben 1 mg per mL)
    1% (10 mg per mL) (Rx) [*Carbocaine; Polocaine;* GENERIC].
    2% (20 mg per mL) (Rx) [*Carbocaine; Polocaine;* GENERIC].
    Without preservative
    1% (10 mg per mL) (Rx) [*Carbocaine; Polocaine-MPF*].
    1.5% (15 mg per mL) (Rx) [*Carbocaine; Polocaine-MPF*].
    2% (20 mg per mL) (Rx) [*Carbocaine; Polocaine-MPF*].
    For dental use
    3% (30 mg per mL; 54 mg per 1.8-mL dental cartridge) (Rx) [*Carbocaine; Isocaine; Polocaine;* GENERIC].
Canada—
    With preservative (methylparaben 1 mg per mL)
    1% (10 mg per mL) [*Carbocaine*].
    Without preservative
    1% (10 mg per mL) [*Carbocaine*].
    2% (20 mg per mL) [*Carbocaine*].
    For dental use
    3% (30 mg per mL; 54 mg per 1.8-mL dental cartridge) [*Isocaine 3%; Polocaine*].
Note: In Canada, this medication has not been assigned Rx status. However, it may not be sold or dispensed directly to the patient.

**Packaging and storage**
Store below 40 °C (104 °F), preferably between 15 and 30 °C (59 and 86 °F), unless otherwise specified by manufacturer. Protect from freezing.

**Preparation of dosage form**
For administration to pediatric patients in concentrations lower than those commercially available—Dilute available concentrations with the quantity of 0.9% sodium chloride injection needed to obtain the required final concentration of local anesthetic solution.

**Stability**
May be autoclaved (except for dental cartridges).
Dental cartridges sealed with aluminum caps should not be kept in solutions made from antirust tablets or solutions containing quaternary ammonium salts such as benzalkonium chloride.
Unused portions of solutions not containing a preservative must be discarded.

## MEPIVACAINE HYDROCHLORIDE AND LEVONORDEFRIN INJECTION USP

**Usual adult and adolescent dose**
Dental infiltration and nerve block—
    Single site: 36 mg (1.8 mL) of mepivacaine hydrochloride as a 2% solution with levonordefrin 1:20,000.
    Entire oral cavity: 180 mg (9 mL) of mepivacaine hydrochloride as a 2% solution with levonordefrin 1:20,000.
Note: Larger doses required for an extensive procedure should be calculated according to the patient's weight, and the injections spread out over time as required.

**Usual adult prescribing limits**
Up to 6.6 mg per kg of body weight but not to exceed 400 mg of mepivacaine hydrochloride per appointment.

**Usual pediatric dose**
Dental infiltration and nerve block—
    Must be individualized according to patient's weight.

**Usual pediatric prescribing limits**
Maximum dosage must be carefully calculated on the basis of the patient's weight, but should not exceed 6.6 mg per kg of body weight or 180

mg of mepivacaine hydrochloride as a 2% solution with levonordefrin 1:20,000.

**Strength(s) usually available**
U.S.—
    For dental use
    2% (20 mg per mL; 36 mg per 1.8-mL dental cartridge), with levonordefrin 1:20,000 (Rx) [*Carbocaine with Neo-Cobefrin* (acetone sodium bisulfite 2 mg per mL); *Isocaine* (sodium bisulfite); *Polocaine* (sodium metabisulfite 0.5 mg per mL); GENERIC].
Canada—
    For dental use
    2% (20 mg per mL; 36 mg per 1.8-mL dental cartridge), with levonordefrin 1:20,000 [*Isocaine 2%* (sodium bisulfite 1 mg per mL); *Polocaine* (sodium metabisulfite 0.5 mg per mL)].
Note: In Canada, this medication has not been assigned Rx status. However, it may not be sold or dispensed directly to the patient.

**Packaging and storage**
Store below 40 °C (104 °F), preferably between 15 and 30 °C (59 and 86 °F), unless otherwise specified by manufacturer. Protect from freezing.

**Stability**
Do not autoclave dental cartridges.
Dental cartridges sealed with aluminum caps should not be kept in solutions made from antirust tablets or solutions containing quaternary ammonium salts such as benzalkonium chloride.
Unused portion of solution must be discarded.

---

### *PRILOCAINE*

## Summary of Differences

Indications—Indicated only for dental use.
Pharmacology/pharmacokinetics:
    Physicochemical characteristics—
        Chemical group: Amide-type local anesthetic.
        Molecular weight: 256.77
        pKa: 7.9
        Lipid solubility: Medium.
    Protein-binding—Moderate.
    Biotransformation—Also metabolized renally to some extent.
    Half-life—1.25 hours.
    Onset of action—Rapid.
    Duration of action—Intermediate (1–3 hours).
    Relative toxicity (compared to procaine)—1.7
Precautions:
    Cross-sensitivity and/or related problems—
        May occur rarely with other amide-type local anesthetics.
    Pregnancy—
        Studies in animals have not shown adverse effects on the fetus with doses up to 3 times the maximum human dose.
Side/adverse effects:
    More likely than other local anesthetics to cause methemoglobinemia.

## Parenteral Dosage Forms

### PRILOCAINE HYDROCHLORIDE INJECTION USP

**Usual adult and adolescent dose**
Dental anesthesia—
    For local infiltration or nerve block: 40 to 80 mg (1 to 2 mL) as a 4% solution initially.

**Usual adult prescribing limits**
Dental—
    Up to 400 mg (10 mL) as a 4% solution within a two-hour period.

**Usual pediatric dose**
Dental—
    Children up to 10 years of age: Doses greater than 40 mg (1 mL) as a 4% solution per procedure are rarely needed.

**Strength(s) usually available**
U.S.—
    For dental use
    4% (40 mg per mL; 72 mg per 1.8-mL dental cartridge) (Rx) [*Citanest Plain*].
Canada—
    For dental use
    4% (40 mg per mL; 72 mg per 1.8-mL dental cartridge) [*Citanest Plain*].
Note: In Canada, this medication has not been assigned Rx status. However, it may not be sold or dispensed directly to the patient.

**Packaging and storage**
Store below 40 °C (104 °F), preferably between 15 and 30 °C (59 and 86 °F), unless otherwise specified by manufacturer. Protect from freezing.

**Stability**
Dental cartridges should not be autoclaved.

For chemical disinfection of the container surface, 91% isopropyl alcohol or 70% ethyl alcohol without denaturants is recommended; solutions containing heavy metals are not recommended.

Dental cartridges are sealed with aluminum caps and therefore should not be kept in solutions made from antirust tablets or solutions containing quaternary ammonium salts such as benzalkonium chloride.

## PRILOCAINE AND EPINEPHRINE INJECTION USP

**Usual adult and adolescent dose**
Dental infiltration and nerve block—
    40 to 80 mg (1 to 2 mL) of prilocaine hydrochloride as a 4% solution with epinephrine 1:200,000 initially.

**Usual adult prescribing limits**
Up to 400 mg (10 mL) of prilocaine hydrochloride within a two-hour period.

**Usual pediatric dose**
Dental infiltration and nerve block in children up to 10 years of age—
    Doses greater than 40 mg (1 mL) of prilocaine hydrochloride as a 4% solution with epinephrine 1:200,000 are rarely needed.

**Strength(s) usually available**
U.S.—
    For dental use
    4% (40 mg per mL; 72 mg per 1.8-mL dental cartridge), with epinephrine 1:200,000 (Rx) [*Citanest Forte* (sodium metabisulfite 0.5 mg per mL)].
Canada—
    For dental use
    4% (40 mg per mL; 72 mg per 1.8-mL dental cartridge), with epinephrine 1:200,000 [*Citanest Forte* (sodium metabisulfite 0.5 mg per mL); GENERIC].

    Note: In Canada, this medication has not been assigned Rx status. However, it may not be sold or dispensed directly to the patient.

**Packaging and storage**
Store below 40 °C (104 °F), preferably between 15 and 30 °C (59 and 86 °F), unless otherwise specified by manufacturer. Protect from freezing.

**Stability**
Do not autoclave.

Do not use if solution is discolored.

For chemical disinfection of the container surface, 91% isopropyl alcohol or 70% ethyl alcohol without denaturants is recommended; solutions containing heavy metals are not recommended.

Dental cartridges are sealed with aluminum caps and therefore should not be kept in solutions made from antirust tablets or solutions containing quaternary ammonium salts such as benzalkonium chloride.

Unused portion of solution must be discarded.

---

### *PROCAINE*

---

# Summary of Differences

Indications:
    Indicated for subarachnoid block, local infiltration, peripheral nerve block, and retrobulbar block.
Pharmacology/pharmacokinetics:
    Physicochemical characteristics—
        Chemical group: An ester-type local anesthetic.
        Molecular weight: 272.77
        pKa: 8.9
        Lipid solubility: Low.
    Protein-binding—Very low.
    Biotransformation—Metabolized to PABA.
    Half-life—30–50 seconds (adults); 54–114 seconds (neonates).
    Onset of action—Slow.
    Duration of action—Short (30 to 60 minutes).
    Relative toxicity—1. Procaine is the standard against which other local anesthetics are compared.
    Elimination—2% of a dose may be excreted unchanged.
Precautions:
    Cross-sensitivity and/or related problems—
        May occur with PABA, parabens, or other ester-type local anesthetics.
    Drug interactions and/or related problems—
        Interaction with cholinesterase inhibitors.

Interaction with sulfonamides.
Side/adverse effects:
    More likely than amide-type local anesthetics to cause hypersensitivity reactions.

# Additional Dosing Information

See also *General Dosing Information*.

For peripheral nerve block, the 2% solution of procaine should be reserved for cases requiring a small volume of solution (up to 25 mL).

Epinephrine 1:200,000 or epinephrine 1:100,000 (0.5 to 1 mL of epinephrine 1:1000 per 100 mL of anesthetic solution) may be added to solutions of procaine hydrochloride for vasoconstrictive effect.

Procaine 10% is indicated for subarachnoid administration. The solution is to be diluted with 0.9% sodium chloride injection, sterile water for injection, CSF, or, for hyperbaric techniques, 10% dextrose injection. Consult a standard text or manufacturer's product information for details concerning dilution and injection sites.

# Parenteral Dosage Forms

## PROCAINE HYDROCHLORIDE INJECTION USP

**Usual adult and adolescent dose**
Infiltration—
    350 to 600 mg as a 0.25 or 0.5% solution.
Peripheral nerve block—
    500 mg as a 0.5, 1, or 2% solution.
Subarachnoid—
    Perineum: 50 mg (0.5 mL) as a 10% solution diluted with an equal volume of diluent.
    Perineum and lower extremities: 100 mg (1 mL) as a 10% solution diluted with an equal volume of diluent.
    Up to costal margin: 200 mg (2 mL) as a 10% solution diluted with 1 mL of diluent.

**Usual adult prescribing limits**
Not to exceed 1 gram initially.

**Usual pediatric dose**
Dosage has not been established.

**Strength(s) usually available**
U.S.—
    With preservative (chlorobutanol 2.5 per mL)
    1% (Rx) [*Novocain* (acetone sodium bisulfite 2 mg per mL); GENERIC].
    2% (Rx) [*Novocain* (acetone sodium bisulfite 2 mg per mL); GENERIC].
    Without preservative
    1% (Rx) [*Novocain* (acetone sodium bisulfite 2 mg per mL); GENERIC].
    10% (Rx) [*Novocain* (acetone sodium bisulfite 2 mg per mL)].
Canada—
    With preservative (chlorobutanol 2.5 mg per mL)
    2% [*Novocain* (acetone sodium bisulfite 2 mg per mL)].

    Note: In Canada, this medication has not been assigned Rx status. However, it may not be sold or dispensed directly to the patient.

**Packaging and storage**
Store below 40 °C (104 °F), preferably between 15 and 30 °C (59 and 86 °F), protected from light, unless otherwise specified by manufacturer. Protect from freezing.

**Preparation of dosage form**
For 0.25 or 0.5% concentrations for infiltration or nerve block—Dilute available concentration with enough sterile water for injection to provide the desired quantity and concentration of solution.

**Stability**
May be autoclaved (prior to addition of epinephrine, if added); however, repeated autoclaving is not recommended because of the increased likelihood of crystal formation. Autoclaving of the solution following dilution with dextrose injection may result in discoloration of the solution caused by caramelization of the dextrose.

Do not use if solution is cloudy or discolored or contains a precipitate.

For chemical disinfection of the container surface, 91% isopropyl alcohol or 70% ethyl alcohol without denaturants is recommended; solutions containing heavy metals are not recommended. Immersion of the container in antiseptic solution is not recommended.

Unused portions of solutions not containing a preservative must be discarded.

## PROPOXYCAINE AND PROCAINE

## Summary of Differences

Indications:
  Indicated for dental anesthesia.
Pharmacology/pharmacokinetics:
  Physicochemical characteristics—
    Chemical group:
      Propoxycaine and procaine are both ester-type local anesthetics.
    Molecular weight:
      Procaine hydrochloride—272.77
      Propoxycaine hydrochloride—330.85
    pKa:
      Procaine hydrochloride—8.9
      Propoxycaine hydrochloride—9.0
    Lipid solubility:
      Procaine hydrochloride—Very low.
  Protein-binding—
    Procaine hydrochloride:
      Very low.
  Biotransformation—
    Procaine metabolized to PABA.
  Half-life—
    Procaine hydrochloride:
      30–50 seconds (adults); 54–114 seconds (neonates).
  Onset of action—
    Procaine:
      Slow.
    Propoxycaine:
      Rapid.
  Duration of action—
    Procaine:
      Short (30–60 minutes).
    Propoxycaine:
      Intermediate (1–3 hours).
Precautions:
  Cross-sensitivity and/or related problems—
    May occur with PABA, parabens, or other ester-type local anesthetics.
  Drug interactions and/or related problems—
    Interaction with cholinesterase inhibitors.
    Interaction with sulfonamides.
Side/adverse effects:
  More likely than amide-type local anesthetics to cause hypersensitivity reactions.

## Parenteral Dosage Forms

### PROPOXYCAINE AND PROCAINE HYDROCHLORIDES AND LEVONORDEFRIN INJECTION USP

**Usual adult and adolescent dose**
Dental infiltration and nerve block—
  Single site: 1.8 mL (43.2 mg total anesthetics).
  Entire oral cavity: 9 mL (216 mg total anesthetics).

**Usual adult prescribing limits**
Up to 6.6 mg total anesthetics per kg of body weight per procedure.

**Usual pediatric dose**
6.6 mg total anesthetics per kg of body weight, but must not exceed 216 mg total anesthetics (9 mL) per procedure.

**Strength(s) usually available**
U.S.—
  For dental use
  0.4% of propoxycaine hydrochloride and 2% of procaine hydrochloride (4 mg of propoxycaine hydrochloride and 20 mg of procaine hydrochloride per mL; 7.2 mg of propoxycaine hydrochloride and 36 mg of procaine hydrochloride per 1.8-mL dental cartridge), with levonordefrin 1:20,000 (Rx) [*Ravocaine and Novocain with Neo-Cobefrin* (acetone sodium bisulfite 2 mg per mL)].

**Packaging and storage**
Store below 40 °C (104 °F), preferably between 15 and 30 °C (59 and 86 °F), unless otherwise specified by manufacturer. Protect from freezing.

### PROPOXYCAINE AND PROCAINE HYDROCHLORIDES AND NOREPINEPHRINE BITARTRATE INJECTION USP

**Usual adult and adolescent dose**
Dental infiltration and nerve block—
  Single site: 1.8 mL (43.2 mg total anesthetics).
  Entire oral cavity: 9 mL (216 mg total anesthetics).

**Usual adult prescribing limits**
Up to 6.6 mg total anesthetics per kg of body weight per procedure.

**Usual pediatric dose**
6.6 mg total anesthetics per kg of body weight but must not exceed 216 mg total anesthetics (9 mL) per procedure.

**Strength(s) usually available**
U.S.—
  For dental use
  0.4% of propoxycaine hydrochloride and 2% of procaine hydrochloride (4 mg of propoxycaine hydrochloride and 20 mg of procaine hydrochloride per mL; 7.2 mg of propoxycaine hydrochloride and 36 mg of procaine hydrochloride per 1.8-mL dental cartridge), with norepinephrine 1:30,000 (Rx) [*Ravocaine and Novocain with Levophed* (acetone sodium bisulfite 2 mg per mL)].

**Packaging and storage**
Store below 40 °C (104 °F), preferably between 15 and 30 °C (59 and 86 °F), unless otherwise specified by manufacturer. Protect from freezing.

## TETRACAINE

## Summary of Differences

Indications:
  Indicated (with or without dextrose) for subarachnoid block; and indicated (without dextrose) for transtracheal anesthesia.
Pharmacology/pharmacokinetics:
  Physicochemical characteristics—
    Chemical group: Ester-type local anesthetic.
    Molecular weight: 300.83
    pKa: 8.2
    Lipid solubility: High.
  Protein-binding—
    High.
  Biotransformation—
    Metabolized to a PABA derivative.
  Onset of action—
    Rapid.
  Duration of action—
    Intermediate to long (1–>3 hours).
  Relative toxicity (compared to procaine)—
    10.
Precautions:
  Cross-sensitivity and/or related problems—
    May occur with PABA, parabens, or other ester-type local anesthetics.
  Drug interactions and/or related problems—
    Interaction with cholinesterase inhibitors.
    Interaction with sulfonamides.
Side/adverse effects:
  More likely than amide-type local anesthetics to cause hypersensitivity reactions.

## Additional Dosing Information

See also *General Dosing Information.*

Tetracaine hydrochloride injection 1% is isobaric. When used for isobaric spinal anesthesia, the solution is to be diluted with CSF prior to administration. Also, it may be diluted with 10% dextrose injection to provide a hyperbaric solution.

Isobaric or hyperbaric solutions prepared using sterile tetracaine hydrochloride are to be diluted with CSF prior to administration. A hypobaric solution may also be prepared using sterile tetracaine hydrochloride.

Consult a standard text and/or manufacturer's product information for preparation and administration techniques and for proper injection sites.

## Parenteral Dosage Forms

### TETRACAINE HYDROCHLORIDE INJECTION USP

**Usual adult and adolescent dose**
Spinal anesthesia—
  Low spinal (saddle block) anesthesia for vaginal delivery: 2 to 5 mg (0.2 to 0.5 mL) as a 1% solution, to be diluted with 10% dextrose injection.
  Perineum: 5 mg (0.5 mL) as a 1% solution, to be diluted with CSF or 10% dextrose injection, depending upon technique used.
  Perineum and lower extremities: 10 mg (1 mL) as a 1% solution, to be diluted with CSF or 10% dextrose injection, depending upon technique used.

Up to costal margin: 15 to 20 mg (1.5 to 2 mL) as a 1% solution diluted with CSF.

Doses greater than 15 mg are rarely required.

**Usual pediatric dose**
Dosage has not been established.

**Strength(s) usually available**
U.S.—

Without preservative
1% (10 mg per mL) (Rx) [*Pontocaine* (acetone sodium bisulfite 2 mg per mL)].

**Packaging and storage**
Store between 2 and 8 °C (36 and 46 °F). (Exception: Injections supplied as a component of spinal anesthesia trays may be stored at room temperature for 12 months.) Protect from light. Protect from freezing.

**Preparation of dosage form**
For isobaric techniques—Dilute with an equal volume of CSF.
For hyperbaric techniques—Dilute with an equal volume of 10% dextrose injection.

**Stability**
May be autoclaved once; repeated autoclaving is not recommended because of the increased likelihood of crystal formation. Unused autoclaved ampuls should be discarded.

Do not use if solution is cloudy or discolored or contains crystals prior to diluting with CSF.

Immersion of the container in an antiseptic solution is not recommended.

Unused portion of the solution must be discarded because it contains no preservative.

## STERILE TETRACAINE HYDROCHLORIDE USP

**Usual adult and adolescent dose**
Spinal anesthesia—
Low spinal (saddle block) anesthesia for vaginal delivery: 2 to 5 mg.
Perineum: 5 mg.
Perineum and lower extremities: 10 mg.
Up to costal margin: 15 to 20 mg.
Doses exceeding 15 mg are rarely required.

**Usual pediatric dose**
Dosage has not been established.

**Size(s) usually available**
U.S.—
Without preservative
20 mg (Rx) [*Pontocaine*].
Canada—
Without preservative
20 mg [*Pontocaine*].
Note: In Canada, this medication has not been assigned Rx status. However, it may not be sold or dispensed directly to the patient.

**Packaging and storage**
Prior to reconstitution, store below 40 °C (104 °F), preferably between 15 and 30 °C (59 and 86 °F), unless otherwise specified by manufacturer.

**Preparation of dosage form**
For isobaric techniques—Dissolve in CSF to give a concentration of 5 mg per mL.
For hyperbaric techniques—Dissolve 10 mg of sterile tetracaine hydrochloride in 1 mL of 10% dextrose injection. Dilute further with 1 mL of CSF to give a final concentration of 5 mg of tetracaine hydrochloride per mL and 5% of dextrose.
For hypobaric techniques—Dissolve the sterile tetracaine hydrochloride in enough sterile water for injection to provide a concentration of 1 mg per mL.

**Stability**
May be autoclaved. Autoclaving may cause the powder to undergo a change in appearance and to adhere to the sides of the ampul. This may slightly decrease the rate of dissolution of the powder but does not affect anesthetic potency.

## TETRACAINE HYDROCHLORIDE IN DEXTROSE INJECTION USP

**Usual adult and adolescent dose**
Obstetrical low spinal (saddle block) anesthesia—
2 to 4 mg (1 to 2 mL) of tetracaine hydrochloride as a 0.2% solution.
Spinal anesthesia—
Lower abdomen: 9 to 12 mg (3 to 4 mL) of tetracaine hydrochloride as a 0.3% solution.
Perineal: 3 to 6 mg (1 to 2 mL) of tetracaine hydrochloride as a 0.3% solution.
Upper abdomen: 15 mg (5 mL) of tetracaine hydrochloride as a 0.3% solution.

**Usual pediatric dose**
Dosage has not been established.

**Strength(s) usually available**
U.S.—
Without preservative
0.2% of tetracaine hydrochloride (2 mg per mL) and 6% of dextrose (60 mg per mL) (Rx) [*Pontocaine*].
0.3% of tetracaine hydrochloride (3 mg per mL) and 6% of dextrose (60 mg per mL) (Rx) [*Pontocaine*].
Canada—
Not commercially available.

**Packaging and storage**
Store below 40 °C (104 °F), preferably between 15 and 30 °C (59 and 86 °F), protected from light, unless otherwise specified by manufacturer. Protect from freezing.

**Stability**
May be autoclaved once; repeated autoclaving is not recommended because of the increased likelihood of crystal formation. Also, with repeated autoclaving, caramelization of the dextrose may occur, leading to discoloration. Unused autoclaved ampuls should be discarded.

Do not use if solution is cloudy or discolored or contains crystals.

Unused portions of solutions must be discarded because they contain no preservative.

Revised: 01/30/92
Interim revision: 08/14/94

## Table 1. Pharmacology/Pharmacokinetics—Anesthetics (Parenteral-Local)

| Drug | pKa | Lipid Solubility (pH 7.4) | Protein Binding | Half-life adult/neonate | Onset of Action* | Duration of Action† | Relative Toxicity‡ |
|---|---|---|---|---|---|---|---|
| Bupivacaine | 8.1 | High | Very high | 2.7–3.5 hr/ 6–10 hr | Intermediate to Slow | Long§ | |
| Chloroprocaine | 9.0 | | | 19–26 sec/ 41–45 sec | Rapid | Short | |
| Etidocaine | 7.7 | High | Very high | 2.7 hr/ 4–8 hr | Rapid | Long | |
| Lidocaine | 7.9 | Medium | Moderate | 1.5–1.8 hr/ 3 hr | Rapid# | Intermediate | 2 |
| Mepivacaine | 7.6 | Medium | High | 2–3 hr/9 hr | Rapid to Intermediate# | Intermediate | 2 |
| Prilocaine | 7.9 | Medium | Moderate | 1.25 hr | Rapid | Intermediate | 1.7 |

## Table 1. Pharmacology/Pharmacokinetics—Anesthetics (Parenteral-Local) *(continued)*

| Drug | pKa | Lipid Solubility (pH 7.4) | Protein Binding | Half-life adult/neonate | Onset of Action* | Duration of Action† | Relative Toxicity‡ |
|---|---|---|---|---|---|---|---|
| Procaine | 8.9 | Low | Very low | 30–50 sec/ 54–114 sec | Slow | Short | 1 |
| Propoxycaine | 9.0 | | | | Rapid | Intermediate | |
| Tetracaine | 8.2 | High | High | | Rapid | Intermediate to Long | 10 |

*Influenced by the site, route, and technique of administration; dosage (volume and concentration) administered; pH at injection site; physical characteristics, such as lipid solubility, molecular size, and pKa of the individual anesthetic; and individual patient.

†Short=30 to 60 minutes; Intermediate=1 to 3 hours; Long=3 to 10 hours. Influenced by factors affecting rate of clearance from the injection site and individual patient.

‡As compared with procaine (the least toxic of these agents).

§Via nerve block, may produce analgesia for considerably longer than 10 hours.

#Adjustment of pH with 1 mEq (1 mmol) of sodium bicarbonate per 10 mL may increase the onset of conduction blocks (lidocaine hydrochloride injection, lidocaine and epinephrine injection, or mepivacaine hydrochloride injection).

---

# ANESTHETICS   Topical

This monograph includes information on the following: Benzocaine; Benzocaine and Menthol; Butamben; Dibucaine; Lidocaine; Pramoxine; Pramoxine and Menthol; Tetracaine†; Tetracaine and Menthol†.

Note: See also individual *Lidocaine and Prilocaine (Topical)* monograph.

INN:
　　Dibucaine—Cinchocaine
　　Pramoxine—Pramocaine

BAN:
　　Dibucaine—Cinchocaine
　　Lidocaine—Lignocaine
　　Tetracaine—Amethocaine

JAN:
　　Benzocaine—Ethyl aminobenzoate

VA CLASSIFICATION (Primary/Secondary):

Note: Several of the dosage forms listed below are commercially available in more than one formulation. Because the vehicle into which a local anesthetic is incorporated may determine the appropriate usage and/or site(s) of application of a product, some of the VA classifications listed for a dosage form may apply only to specific formulations.

　　Benzocaine
　　　　Cream—DE700
　　　　Ointment—RS200/DE700; RS900
　　　　Topical Aerosol—DE700/NT300; OR900
　　　　Topical Spray Solution—DE700
　　Benzocaine and Menthol—DE700
　　Butamben—DE700
　　Dibucaine
　　　　Cream—DE700
　　　　Ointment—RS200/DE700; RS900
　　Lidocaine
　　　　Ointment 2.5%—DE700
　　　　Ointment 5%—NT300/DE700; OR900
　　　　Topical Spray Solution—DE700
　　Lidocaine Hydrochloride
　　　　Topical Aerosol—DE700
　　　　Film-forming Gel—DE700
　　　　Jelly—NT300/GU900; DE700
　　　　Ointment—DE700
　　Pramoxine
　　　　Cream—RS200/DE700; RS900
　　　　Lotion—DE700
　　Pramoxine and Menthol
　　　　Gel—DE700
　　　　Lotion—DE700
　　Tetracaine
　　　　Cream—RS200/DE700; RE900
　　Tetracaine and Menthol
　　　　Ointment—RS200/DE700; RE900

Note: For information on local anesthetics applied topically to the oral, rectal, or other mucosa, see *Anesthetics (Mucosal-Local)*.

In Canada, *Nupercainal Cream* contains domiphen bromide in addition to dibucaine.

Other commonly used names are: Amethocaine [Tetracaine] , Butyl aminobenzoate [Butamben] , Cinchocaine [Dibucaine], Ethyl aminobenzoate [Benzocaine], Lignocaine [Lidocaine], Pramocaine [Pramoxine]

Note: For a listing of dosage forms and brand names by country availability, see *Dosage Forms* section(s). For a listing of brand names for the articles in this monograph, refer to the General Index.

†Not commercially available in Canada.

---

## Category
Anesthetic, local.

## Indications

### Accepted
Skin disorders, minor (treatment)—Topical anesthetics are indicated to relieve pain, pruritus, and inflammation associated with minor skin disorders, including:
　Burns, minor, including sunburn.
　Bites (or stings), insect.
　Dermatitis, contact, including poison ivy, poison oak, or poison sumac.
　Wounds, minor, such as cuts and scratches.

## Pharmacology/Pharmacokinetics

### Physicochemical characteristics
Chemical group—
　Amides: Dibucaine, lidocaine.
　Esters, aminobenzoic acid (para-aminobenzoic acid, PABA)–derivative: Benzocaine, butamben, tetracaine.
　Unclassified: Pramoxine.
Molecular weight—
　Benzocaine: 165.19.
　Butamben picrate: 615.60.
　Dibucaine: 343.47.
　Lidocaine: 234.34.
　Lidocaine hydrochloride: 288.82.
　Pramoxine hydrochloride: 329.87.
　Tetracaine: 264.37.
　Tetracaine hydrochloride: 300.83.
pKa—
　Dibucaine: 8.8.
　Lidocaine: 7.9.
　Tetracaine: 8.2.

### Mechanism of action/Effect
Local anesthetics block both the initiation and conduction of nerve impulses by decreasing the neuronal membrane's permeability to sodium ions. This reversibly stabilizes the membrane and inhibits depolarization, resulting in the failure of a propagated action potential and subsequent conduction blockade.

**Other actions/effects**

If significant quantities of topical anesthetics are absorbed, actions on the central nervous system (CNS) may lead to CNS stimulation and/or CNS depression. Actions on the cardiovascular system may cause depression of cardiac conduction and excitability, and possibly peripheral vasodilation.

**Absorption**

Absorption is variable; dependent on specific drug and/or its specific salt. Benzocaine is minimally absorbed. In general, ionized forms (salts) of local anesthetics are not readily absorbed through intact skin. However, both nonionized (bases) and ionized forms of local anesthetics are readily absorbed through traumatized or abraded skin into the systemic circulation.

**Biotransformation**

Amides—
  Hepatic and some renal.
  Lidocaine: Xylidide metabolites are active and toxic, but less so than the parent compound.
Esters, PABA-derivative—
  Hydrolyzed by plasma cholinesterases, and to a much lesser extent by hepatic cholinesterases, to PABA-containing metabolites.

**Onset of action**

Dibucaine—Up to 15 minutes.
Pramoxine—3 to 5 minutes.
Tetracaine—Slow.

**Duration of action**

Lidocaine—Approximately 45 minutes.
Tetracaine—Approximately 30 to 45 minutes.

**Elimination**

Amides—
  Renal, primarily as metabolites.
  Lidocaine: Up to 10% of an absorbed dose may be excreted unchanged.
Esters—
  Renal, as metabolites.

# Precautions to Consider

**Cross-sensitivity and/or related problems**

Patients sensitive to one ester-derivative (especially a PABA-derivative) local anesthetic may be sensitive to other ester derivatives also.

Patients sensitive to PABA, parabens, or paraphenylenediamine (a hair dye) may be sensitive to PABA-derivative topical anesthetics also.

Patients sensitive to one amide derivative may rarely be sensitive to other amide derivatives also.

Cross-sensitivity between amide derivatives and ester derivatives, or between amides or esters and the chemically unrelated pramoxine, has not been reported.

**Pregnancy/Reproduction**

Pregnancy—Problems in humans with topical anesthetics have not been documented.
  *Benzocaine, butamben, dibucaine, and pramoxine—*
    Studies in humans have not been done.
    Studies in animals have not been done.
  *Lidocaine—*
    Adequate and well-controlled studies in humans have not been done.
    Studies in animals given up to 6.6 times the human dose have shown no adverse effects on the fetus.
    Lidocaine ointment 5%—FDA Pregnancy Category B.
  *Tetracaine—*
    Studies in humans have not been done.
    Studies in animals have not been done.
    FDA Pregnancy Category C.

**Breast-feeding**

Problems in humans have not been documented.

**Pediatrics**

*Benzocaine*—Benzocaine should be used with caution in infants and young children because increased absorption through the skin (with excessive use) may result in methemoglobinemia. Benzocaine-containing topical formulations should not be used in children younger than 2 years of age unless prescribed by a physician.

*Other topical anesthetics*—No information is available on the relationship of age to the effects of these medications in pediatric patients following application to the skin. However, it is recommended that a physician be consulted before any topical local anesthetic is used in children younger than 2 years of age.

**Geriatrics**

No information is available on the relationship of age to the effects of topical anesthetics in geriatric patients following application to the skin.

**Drug interactions and/or related problems**

The following drug interactions and/or related problems have been selected on the basis of their potential clinical significance (possible mechanism in parentheses where appropriate)—not necessarily inclusive (» = major clinical significance):

Note: Combinations containing any of the following medications, depending on the amount present, may also interact with this medication.

*For ester derivatives*
  Cholinesterase inhibitors such as
    Antimyasthenics
    Cyclophosphamide
    Demecarium
    Echothiophate
    Insecticides, neurotoxic, possibly including large quantities of topical malathion
    Isoflurophate
    Thiotepa
    (these agents may inhibit metabolism of ester derivatives; absorption of significant quantities of ester derivatives in patients receiving a cholinesterase inhibitor may lead to increased risk of toxicity)
  Sulfonamides
    (metabolites of PABA-derivative topical anesthetics may antagonize antibacterial activity of sulfonamides, especially if the anesthetics are absorbed in significant quantities over prolonged periods of time)

*For lidocaine*
  Antiarrhythmic agents, amide local anesthetic–derivative, other, such as
    Mexiletine
    Tocainide or
  Lidocaine, systemic or parenteral-local
    (risk of cardiotoxicity associated with additive cardiac effects, and, with systemic or parenteral-local lidocaine, the risk of overdose, may be increased in patients receiving these medications if large quantities of topically applied lidocaine are absorbed)
  Beta-adrenergic blocking agents
    (concurrent use may slow metabolism of lidocaine because of decreased hepatic blood flow, leading to increased risk of lidocaine toxicity if large quantities are absorbed)
  Cimetidine
    (cimetidine inhibits hepatic metabolism of lidocaine; concurrent use may lead to lidocaine toxicity if large quantities are absorbed)

**Laboratory value alterations**

The following have been selected on the basis of their potential clinical significance (possible effect in parentheses where appropriate)—not necessarily inclusive (» = major clinical significance):

With diagnostic test results
  Pancreatic function determinations using bentiromide
    (use of PABA-derivative topical anesthetics or lidocaine prior to the bentiromide test may invalidate test results since these medications are also metabolized to PABA or other arylamines and will thus increase the real or apparent quantity of PABA recovered; patients should be advised to discontinue use of these anesthetics 3 days prior to bentiromide administration)

**Medical considerations/Contraindications**

The medical considerations/contraindications included here have been selected on the basis of their potential clinical significance (reasons given in parentheses where appropriate)—not necessarily inclusive (» = major clinical significance).

*Risk-benefit should be considered when the following medical problems exist:*

Local infection at site of application
  (infection may alter the pH at the treatment site, leading to decrease or loss of local anesthetic effect)

Sensitivity to the topical anesthetic being considered for use or to chemically related anesthetics and, for the ester derivatives, to PABA, parabens, or paraphenylenediamine, or

Sensitivity to other ingredients in the formulation

Skin disorders, severe or extensive, especially if skin is abraded or broken
  (increased absorption of anesthetic)

## Side/Adverse Effects

Note: Adverse reactions are due to excessive dosage or rapid absorption, which produces high plasma concentrations, as well as to idiosyncrasy, hypersensitivity, or decreased patient tolerance.

Benzocaine and tetracaine are more likely to cause contact sensitization than are the other local anesthetics.

The following side/adverse effects have been selected on the basis of their potential clinical significance (possible signs and symptoms in parentheses where appropriate)—not necessarily inclusive:

**Those indicating need for medical attention**
Incidence less frequent
*Angioedema* (large, hive-like swellings on skin, mouth, or throat); *dermatitis, contact* (skin rash, redness, itching, or hives; burning, stinging, swelling, or tenderness not present before therapy)

## Overdose

For specific information on the agents used in the management of topical anesthetics overdose, see:
- *Ascorbic Acid (Systemic)* monograph;
- *Benzodiazepines (Systemic)* monograph;
- *Sympathomimetic Agents—Cardiovascular Use (Parenteral-Systemic)* monograph; and/or
*Methylene Blue (Systemic)* monograph.

For more information on the management of overdose or unintentional ingestion, **contact a Poison Control Center** (see *Poison Control Center Listing*).

**Clinical effects of overdose**
The following effects have been selected on the basis of their potential clinical significance if excessive systemic absorption occurs (possible signs and symptoms in parentheses where appropriate)—not necessarily inclusive:

*Cardiovascular system depression* (low blood pressure; slow or irregular heartbeat; unusual paleness; increased sweating)—may lead to cardiac arrest; *CNS toxicity* (blurred or double vision; confusion; convulsions; dizziness or lightheadedness; drowsiness; feeling hot, cold, or numb; ringing or buzzing in the ears; shivering or trembling; unusual anxiety, excitement, nervousness, or restlessness); *methemoglobinemia* (difficulty in breathing on exertion; dizziness; headache; unusual tiredness or weakness)

Note: Stimulant and/or depressant manifestations of *CNS toxicity* may occur. CNS stimulation usually occurs first, followed by CNS depression. However, CNS stimulation may be transient or absent, so that drowsiness may be the first symptom of toxicity in some patients. CNS depression may lead to unconsciousness and respiratory arrest.

**Treatment of overdose**
Recommended treatment includes:
Specific treatment—
For methemoglobinemia—Administering methylene blue (1 to 2 mg per kg of body weight, intravenously) and/or ascorbic acid (100 to 200 mg orally).
For circulatory depression—Administration of a vasopressor and intravenous fluids is recommended.
For convulsions—Administering an anticonvulsant, usually a benzodiazepine, keeping in mind that benzodiazepines may cause respiratory and circulatory depression, especially when administered rapidly. Medications and equipment needed for support of respiration and for resuscitation must be immediately available.
Supportive Care—
For systemic reactions caused by excessive absorption—Securing and maintaining a patent airway, administering oxygen, and instituting assisted or controlled respiration as required. In some patients, endotracheal intubation may be required.

## Patient Consultation

As an aid to patient consultation, refer to *Advice for the Patient, Anesthetics (Topical)*.

In providing consultation, consider emphasizing the following selected information (» = major clinical significance):

**Before using this medication**
» Conditions affecting use, especially:
Sensitivity to local anesthetics of the same chemical class, and, for ester derivatives only, aminobenzoic acid, parabens, or hair dye
Use in children—Caution that excessive quantities of benzocaine may cause methemoglobinemia in children younger than 2

years of age; consulting physician before using any topical local anesthetic in children younger than 2 years of age

**Proper use of this medication**
Following physician's instructions if prescribed
Following manufacturer's instructions if self-medicating
» Not using on large areas, especially if skin broken or abraded, or for prolonged periods of time, without physician's advice
» Checking with physician before using for problems other than prescribed or recommended on package label, or if any suspicion of infection
» Not using products containing alcohol, which is flammable, near fire or open flame or while smoking; not smoking until area completely dry
» Using care not to get in eyes, mouth, or nose; if using topical aerosol or spray dosage forms, applying to face with hand or other suitable applicator
» Proper dosing
Missed dose (if on scheduled dosing): Applying as soon as possible; not applying if almost time for next dose
» Proper storage
*For butamben*
Butamben may permanently stain clothing and hair; covering area with a loose bandage after application to protect clothing and not allowing hair to come into contact with the medication
*For lidocaine film-forming gel*
Proper application technique: Drying area before applying; applying medication, then waiting 60 seconds until transparent film forms

**Precautions while using this medication**
» Taking precautions to prevent children from transferring medication to their mouths after application
*Discontinuing use and checking with physician*
If condition does not improve within 7 days or worsens
If problem area becomes infected
If rash, irritation, or other symptoms not present before use occur
If medication is swallowed

**Side/adverse effects**
Signs and symptoms of potential side effects, especially angioedema, contact dermatitis, and overdose

## General Dosing Information

These medications should not be applied over large areas, or for prolonged periods of time, especially to broken or abraded skin, because of the increased risk of systemic absorption and toxicity.

Topical anesthetic–containing medications may be sprayed or applied directly to the affected area, or applied with a suitable applicator (for example, a sterile gauze pad or cotton swab).

---

### *BENZOCAINE*

## Summary of Differences

Physicochemical characteristics:
An ester-type (PABA-derivative) local anesthetic.
Precautions:
Cross-sensitivity and/or related problems—
May occur with other ester-type anesthetics, especially other PABA derivatives, with PABA or parabens, and with paraphenylenediamine.
Pediatrics—
Excessive use may cause methemoglobinemia in infants and young children.
Drug interactions and/or related problems—
Cholinesterase inhibitors may inhibit metabolism of benzocaine.
Benzocaine may antagonize antibacterial activity of sulfonamides.
Side/adverse effects:
More likely to cause contact sensitization than most other topical anesthetics.
See also *Side/Adverse Effects*.

## Topical Dosage Forms

### BENZOCAINE CREAM USP

**Usual adult and adolescent dose**
Anesthetic, local—
Topical, to the affected area three or four times a day as needed.

**Usual pediatric dose**

Anesthetic, local—

Children up to 2 years of age: Dosage must be individualized by a physician.

Children 2 years of age and older: See *Usual adult and adolescent dose.*

**Strength(s) usually available**

U.S.—

5% (OTC) [GENERIC].

**Packaging and storage**

Store below 30 °C (86 °F). Store in a tight container. Protect from light. Protect from freezing.

**Auxiliary labeling**

• For external use only.

## BENZOCAINE OINTMENT USP

**Usual adult and adolescent dose**

Anesthetic, local—

Topical, to the affected area three or four times a day as needed.

**Usual pediatric dose**

Anesthetic, local—

Children up to 2 years of age: Dosage must be individualized by a physician.

Children 2 years of age and older: See *Usual adult and adolescent dose.*

**Strength(s) usually available**

U.S.—

5% (OTC) [*Lagol*].

20% (OTC) [*Americaine Topical Anesthetic First Aid Ointment*].

**Packaging and storage**

Store below 30 °C (86 °F). Store in a tight container. Protect from light. Protect from freezing.

**Auxiliary labeling**

• For external use only.

## BENZOCAINE TOPICAL AEROSOL USP

**Usual adult and adolescent dose**

Anesthetic, local—

Topical, sprayed on or applied to affected area three or four times a day as needed.

**Usual pediatric dose**

Anesthetic, local—

Children up to 2 years of age: Dosage must be individualized by a physician.

Children 2 years of age and older: See *Usual adult and adolescent dose.*

**Strength(s) usually available**

U.S.—

20% (OTC) [*Americaine Topical Anesthetic Spray*].

**Packaging and storage**

Store below 40 °C (104 °F), preferably between 15 and 30 °C (59 and 86 °F), unless otherwise specified by manufacturer.

**Auxiliary labeling**

• Shake well.

• For external use only.

## BENZOCAINE TOPICAL SPRAY SOLUTION

**Usual adult and adolescent dose**

Anesthetic, local—

Topical, sprayed on or applied to affected area three or four times a day as needed.

**Usual pediatric dose**

Anesthetic, local—

Children up to 2 years of age: Dosage must be individualized by a physician.

Children 2 years of age and older: See *Usual adult and adolescent dose.*

**Strength(s) usually available**

Canada—

2% (OTC) [*Shield Burnasept Spray*].

20% (OTC) [*Endocaine*].

**Packaging and storage**

Store below 40 °C (104 °F), preferably between 15 and 30 °C (59 and 86 °F), unless otherwise specified by manufacturer.

**Auxiliary labeling**

• For external use only.

## BENZOCAINE AND MENTHOL LOTION

**Usual adult and adolescent dose**

Anesthetic, local—

Topical, to the affected area three or four times a day as needed.

**Usual pediatric dose**

Anesthetic, local—

Children up to 2 years of age: Dosage must be individualized by a physician.

Children 2 years of age and older: See *Usual adult and adolescent dose.*

**Strength(s) usually available**

U.S.—

8% of benzocaine and 0.5% of menthol (OTC) [*Dermoplast* (methylparaben)].

**Packaging and storage**

Store below 30 °C (86 °F). Protect from freezing.

**Auxiliary labeling**

• For external use only.

## BENZOCAINE AND MENTHOL TOPICAL AEROSOL

**Usual adult and adolescent dose**

Anesthetic, local—

Topical, sprayed on or applied to affected area three or four times a day as needed.

**Usual pediatric dose**

Anesthetic, local—

Children up to 2 years of age: Dosage must be individualized by a physician.

Children 2 years of age and older: See *Usual adult and adolescent dose.*

**Strength(s) usually available**

U.S.—

8% of benzocaine and 0.5% of menthol (OTC) [*Dermoplast* (methylparaben)].

Canada—

4.5% of benzocaine and 0.5% of menthol (OTC) [*Dermoplast* (methylparaben; isopropyl alcohol)].

**Packaging and storage**

Store below 40 °C (104 °F), preferably between 15 and 30 °C (59 and 86 °F), unless otherwise specified by manufacturer.

**Auxiliary labeling**

• Shake well.

• For external use only.

---

*BUTAMBEN*

## Summary of Differences

Physicochemical characteristics:

Butamben is an ester-type (PABAderivative) local anesthetic.

Precautions:

Cross-sensitivity and/or related problems—

May occur with other ester-type anesthetics, especially other PABA derivatives, with PABA or parabens, and with paraphenylenediamine.

Drug interactions and/or related problems—

Cholinesterase inhibitors may inhibit metabolism of butamben.

Butamben may antagonize antibacterial activity of sulfonamides.

## Topical Dosage Forms

### BUTAMBEN PICRATE OINTMENT

**Usual adult and adolescent dose**

Anesthetic, local—

Topical, to the skin, as a 1% ointment three or four times a day as needed.

Note: Area should be loosely bandaged to protect clothing from staining.

**Usual pediatric dose**

Dosage has not been established.

**Strength(s) usually available**

U.S.—

1% (OTC) [*Butesin Picrate*].

**Packaging and storage**

Store below 25 °C (77 °F), unless otherwise specified by manufacturer. Protect from freezing.

**Auxiliary labeling**
• For external use only.

---

## DIBUCAINE

## Summary of Differences

Physicochemical characteristics:
    Dibucaine is an amide-type local anesthetic.
Precautions:
    Cross-sensitivity and/or related problems—Rarely, may occur with
        other amide-type local anesthetics.
    Laboratory value alterations—No interference with bentiromide test
        for pancreatic function.

## Topical Dosage Forms

### DIBUCAINE CREAM USP

**Usual adult and adolescent dose**
Anesthetic, local—
    Topical, to the skin, as a 0.5% cream three or four times a day as
        needed.

**Usual pediatric dose**
Anesthetic, local—
    Children up to 2 years of age: Dosage must be individualized by a
        physician.
    Children 2 years of age and older: See *Usual adult and adolescent
        dose.*

**Strength(s) usually available**
U.S.—
    0.5% (OTC) [*Nupercainal Cream* (acetone sodium bisulfite);
        GENERIC].
    Note: In Canada, *Nupercainal Cream* also contains domiphen
        bromide.

**Packaging and storage**
Store below 40 °C (104 °F), preferably between 15 and 30 °C (59 and 86
    °F), unless otherwise specified by manufacturer. Store in a collapsible
    tube or a tight, light-resistant container. Protect from freezing.

**Auxiliary labeling**
• For external use only.

### DIBUCAINE OINTMENT USP

**Usual adult and adolescent dose**
Anesthetic, local—
    Topical, to the skin, as a 1% ointment three or four times a day as
        needed.
Note: Area may be lightly covered for protection.

**Usual adult prescribing limits**
Not more than 30 grams in a twenty-four-hour period.

**Usual pediatric dose**
Anesthetic, local—
    Children up to 2 years of age: Dosage must be individualized by a
        physician.
    Children 2 years of age and older: See *Usual adult and adolescent
        dose.*

**Usual pediatric prescribing limits**
Not more than 7.5 grams in a twenty-four-hour period.

**Strength(s) usually available**
U.S.—
    1% (OTC) [*Nupercainal Ointment;* GENERIC].
Canada—
    1% (OTC) [*Nupercainal Ointment*].

**Packaging and storage**
Store below 40 °C (104 °F), preferably between 15 and 30 °C (59 and 86
    °F), unless otherwise specified by manufacturer. Store in a collapsible
    tube or in a tight, light-resistant container. Protect from freezing.

**Auxiliary labeling**
• For external use only.

---

## LIDOCAINE

## Summary of Differences

Physicochemical characteristics:
    Lidocaine is an amide-type local anesthetic.

Precautions:
    Cross-sensitivity and/or related problems—Rarely, may occur with
        other amide-type local anesthetics.
    Drug interactions—Possibility of toxicity in patients receiving local
        anesthetic–derivative antiarrhythmic agents, lidocaine via other
        routes of administration, beta-adrenergic blocking agents, or ci-
        metidine if large quantities of topically administered lidocaine are
        absorbed.

## Topical Dosage Forms

### LIDOCAINE OINTMENT USP

**Usual adult and adolescent dose**
Anesthetic, local—
    Topical, as a 2.5% or 5% ointment, to the affected area three or four
        times a day as needed.

**Usual adult prescribing limits**
For the 5% ointment—Not more than 5 grams per single application or
    20 grams per day.

**Usual pediatric dose**
Anesthetic, local—
    Dosage must be individualized, depending on the child's age, weight,
        and physical condition, up to a maximum of 4.5 mg per kg of
        body weight.

**Strength(s) usually available**
U.S.—
    2.5% (OTC) [*Xylocaine*].
    5% (Rx) [*Xylocaine;* GENERIC].
Canada—
    5% (OTC) [*Alphacaine; Xylocaine*].

**Packaging and storage**
Store below 40 °C (104 °F), preferably between 15 and 30 °C (59 and 86
    °F), unless otherwise specified by manufacturer. Store in a tight con-
    tainer. Protect from freezing.

**Auxiliary labeling**
• For external use only.

### LIDOCAINE TOPICAL SPRAY SOLUTION

**Usual adult and adolescent dose**
Anesthetic, local—
    Topical, sprayed on or applied to affected area three or four times a
        day as needed.

**Usual pediatric dose**
Dosage has not been established.

**Strength(s) usually available**
Canada—
    2% (OTC) [*Norwood Sunburn Spray*].

**Packaging and storage**
Store below 40 °C (104 °F), preferably between 15 and 30 °C (59 and 86
    °F), unless otherwise specified by manufacturer. Protect from freezing.

**Auxiliary labeling**
• For external use only.

### LIDOCAINE HYDROCHLORIDE TOPICAL AEROSOL

**Usual adult and adolescent dose**
Anesthetic, local—
    Topical, sprayed on or applied to the affected area three or four times
        a day as needed.

**Usual pediatric dose**
Dosage has not been established.

**Strength(s) usually available**
Canada—
    0.5% (OTC) [*After Burn Spray*].
    1% (OTC) [*After Burn Double Strength Spray*].

**Packaging and storage**
Store below 40 °C (104 °F), preferably between 15 and 30 °C (59 and 86
    °F), unless otherwise specified by manufacturer. Protect from freezing.

**Auxiliary labeling**
• Shake well.
• For external use only.

### LIDOCAINE HYDROCHLORIDE FILM-FORMING GEL

**Usual adult and adolescent dose**
Anesthetic, local—
    Topical, applied to affected area three or four times a day as needed.

**Usual pediatric dose**

Dosage has not been established.

**Strength(s) usually available**

U.S.—

2.5% (OTC) [*DermaFlex*].

**Packaging and storage**

Store below 40 °C (104 °F), preferably between 15 and 30 °C (59 and 86 °F), unless otherwise specified by manufacturer. Protect from freezing.

**Auxiliary labeling**

• For external use only.

## LIDOCAINE HYDROCHLORIDE JELLY USP

**Usual adult and adolescent dose**

Anesthetic, local—

Topical, to the affected area three or four times a day as needed.

**Usual pediatric dose**

Dosage has not been established.

**Strength(s) usually available**

Canada—

0.5% (OTC) [*After Burn Gel*].

1% (OTC) [*After Burn Double Strength Gel*].

**Packaging and storage**

Store below 40 °C (104 °F), preferably between 15 and 30 °C (59 and 86 °F), unless otherwise specified by manufacturer. Protect from freezing.

**Auxiliary labeling**

• For external use only.

## LIDOCAINE HYDROCHLORIDE OINTMENT

**Usual adult and adolescent dose**

Anesthetic, local—

Topical, as a 5% ointment, to the affected area three or four times a day as needed.

**Usual pediatric dose**

Anesthetic, local—

Children up to 2 years of age: Dosage has not been established.

Children 2 years of age and older: See *Usual adult and adolescent dose.*

**Strength(s) usually available**

U.S.—

5% (Rx) [GENERIC].

**Packaging and storage**

Store below 40 °C (104 °F), preferably between 15 and 30 °C (59 and 86 °F), unless otherwise specified by manufacturer. Protect from freezing.

**Auxiliary labeling**

• For external use only.

---

### *PRAMOXINE*

## Summary of Differences

Physicochemical characteristics: Pramoxine is an unclassified (neither an amide-type nor an ester-type) local anesthetic.

Precautions: Diagnostic interference—No interference with bentiromide test for pancreatic function.

## Topical Dosage Forms

### PRAMOXINE HYDROCHLORIDE CREAM USP

**Usual adult and adolescent dose**

Anesthetic, local—

Topical, as a 1% cream, every three to four hours as needed.

**Usual pediatric dose**

Anesthetic, local—

Children up to 2 years of age: Dosage has not been established.

Children 2 years of age and older: See *Usual adult and adolescent dose.*

**Strength(s) usually available**

U.S.—

1% (OTC) [*Prax; Tronothane*].

Canada—

1% (OTC) [*Tronothane*].

**Packaging and storage**

Store below 40 °C (104 °F), preferably between 15 and 30 °C (59 and 86 °F), unless otherwise specified by manufacturer. Store in tight container. Protect from freezing.

**Auxiliary labeling**

• For external use only.

## PRAMOXINE HYDROCHLORIDE LOTION

**Usual adult and adolescent dose**

Anesthetic, local—

Topical, as a 1% lotion, every three or four hours as needed.

**Usual pediatric dose**

Anesthetic, local—

Children up to 2 years of age: Dosage has not been established.

Children 2 years of age and older: See *Usual adult and adolescent dose.*

**Strength(s) usually available**

U.S.—

1% (OTC) [*Prax*].

**Packaging and storage**

Store below 40 °C (104 °F), preferably between 15 and 30 °C (59 and 86 °F), unless otherwise specified by manufacturer. Protect from freezing.

**Auxiliary labeling**

• For external use only.

## PRAMOXINE HYDROCHLORIDE AND MENTHOL GEL

**Usual adult and adolescent dose**

Anesthetic, local—

—Topical, applied to affected areas three or four times a day as needed.

**Usual pediatric dose**

Anesthetic, local—

Children up to 2 years of age: Dosage has not been established.

Children 2 years of age and older: See *Usual adult and adolescent dose.*

**Strength(s) usually available**

U.S.—

1% of pramoxine hydrochloride and 0.5% of menthol (OTC) [*Pramegel*].

Canada—

1% of pramoxine hydrochloride and 0.5% of menthol (OTC) [*Pramegel*].

**Packaging and storage**

Store below 40 °C (104 °F), preferably between 15 and 30 °C (59 and 86 °F), unless otherwise specified by manufacturer. Protect from freezing.

**Auxiliary labeling**

• For external use only.

## PRAMOXINE HYDROCHLORIDE AND MENTHOL LOTION

**Usual adult and adolescent dose**

Anesthetic, local—

Topical, applied to affected areas three or four times a day as needed.

**Usual pediatric dose**

Anesthetic, local—

Children up to 2 years of age: Dosage has not been established.

Children 2 years of age and older: See *Usual adult and adolescent dose.*

**Strength(s) usually available**

U.S.—

1% of pramoxine hydrochloride and 0.2% of menthol (OTC) [*Almay Anti-itch Lotion*].

**Packaging and storage**

Store below 40 °C (104 °F), preferably between 15 and 30 °C (59 and 86 °F), unless otherwise specified by manufacturer. Protect from freezing.

**Auxiliary labeling**

• For external use only.

---

### *TETRACAINE*

## Summary of Differences

Physicochemical characteristics:

An ester-type (PABA-derivative) local anesthetic.

Precautions:

Cross-sensitivity and/or related problems—May occur with other ester-type anesthetics, especially other PABA derivatives, with PABA or parabens, and with paraphenylenediamine.

Drug interactions and/or related problems:

Cholinesterase inhibitors may inhibit metabolism of tetracaine.

Tetracaine may antagonize antibacterial activity of sulfonamides.

Side/adverse effects:

More likely to cause contact sensitization than most other topical anesthetics.

See also *Side/Adverse Effects*.

## Topical Dosage Forms

### TETRACAINE HYDROCHLORIDE CREAM USP

**Usual adult and adolescent dose**

Anesthetic, local—

Topical, applied as a 1% cream to affected areas three or four times a day as needed.

**Usual adult prescribing limits**

Not more than 28.35 grams in a twenty-four-hour period.

**Usual pediatric dose**

Anesthetic, local—

Children up to 2 years of age: Dosage must be individualized by a physician.

Children 2 years of age and older: See *Usual adult and adolescent dose*.

**Usual pediatric prescribing limits**

Not more than 7 grams in a twenty-four-hour period.

**Strength(s) usually available**

U.S.—

1% (OTC) [*Pontocaine Cream*].

Canada—

Not commercially available.

**Packaging and storage**

Store below 40 °C (104 °F), preferably between 15 and 30 °C (59 and 86 °F), unless otherwise specified by manufacturer. Protect from freezing.

**Auxiliary labeling**

• For external use only.

### TETRACAINE AND MENTHOL OINTMENT USP

**Usual adult and adolescent dose**

Anesthetic, local—

Topical, applied to affected area as a 0.5% ointment three or four times a day as needed.

**Usual adult prescribing limits**

Not more than 28.35 grams in a twenty-four-hour period.

**Usual pediatric dose**

Anesthetic, local—

Children up to 2 years of age: Dosage must be individualized by a physician.

Children 2 years of age and older: See *Usual adult and adolescent dose*.

**Usual pediatric prescribing limits**

Not more than 7 grams in a twenty-four-hour period.

**Strength(s) usually available**

U.S.—

0.5% of tetracaine and 0.5% of menthol (OTC) [*Pontocaine Ointment*].

Canada—

Not commercially available.

**Packaging and storage**

Store below 40 °C (104 °F), preferably between 15 and 30 °C (59 and 86 °F), unless otherwise specified by manufacturer. Protect from freezing.

**Auxiliary labeling**

• For external use only.

Revised: 08/29/94

# ANESTHETICS, BARBITURATE    Systemic

This monograph includes information on the following: Methohexital; Thiopental.

BAN:

Methohexital—Methohexitone

Thiopental sodium—Thiopentone sodium

VA CLASSIFICATION (Primary): CN202

Note: Controlled substances in the U.S. and Canada as follows:

| Drug | U.S. | Canada |
|------|------|--------|
| Methohexital | IV | G |
| Thiopental | III | G |

Other commonly used names are: Methohexitone Thiopentone

Note: For a listing of dosage forms and brand names by country availability, see *Dosage Forms* section(s). For a listing of brand names for the articles in this monograph, refer to the General Index.

## Category

Anesthetic (general).

## Indications

Note: Bracketed information in the *Indications* section refers to uses that are not included in U.S. product labeling.

**Accepted**

Anesthesia, general—Methohexital and thiopental are indicated primarily for the induction of general anesthesia. They are also indicated for use alone as intravenous anesthesia for short (15-minute) surgical procedures with minimal painful stimuli; for supplementing other anesthetic agents; and to produce hypnosis during balanced anesthesia with other agents such as analgesics or muscle relaxants.

Barbiturate anesthetics may be administered in small doses and in combination with an opioid analgesic and nitrous oxide for maintenance of anesthesia in prolonged procedures.

Convulsions (treatment)—Thiopental for injection is indicated for short-term use in the control of convulsive states during or following in-halation anesthesia, local anesthesia, or other causes.

[Although parenteral thiopental has been reported to be effective in status epilepticus when used in low doses that do not depress the level of consciousness and has been used to induce general anesthesia in patients with prolonged status epilepticus who failed to respond to antiepileptic agents, including diazepam and phenytoin, these uses are controversial and further studies are needed.][1]

Hypertension, cerebral (treatment)[1]—Thiopental for injection may be indicated in the treatment of increased intracranial pressure if adequate ventilation is provided. It may be used to attenuate the increase in intracranial pressure during the use of volatile anesthetics. It may also be useful in the management of conditions associated with acutely increased intracranial pressure, such as Reye's syndrome, cerebral edema, and acute head injury.

Narcoanalysis[1]—Thiopental for injection is indicated for narcoanalysis in psychiatric disorders.

Anesthesia, basal or

Narcosis, basal—Thiopental rectal suspension may be indicated for basal anesthesia (preanesthetic sedation) or basal narcosis when administration via the rectal route is necessary, although absorption from the rectum may be unpredictable. Thiopental for rectal solution and methohexital for rectal solution also are used for basal anesthesia. Thiopental for rectal solution may be used for basal narcosis also. However, the barbiturate anesthetics generally have been superseded by other medications, such as diazepam, for sedation during short surgical operations, diagnostic procedures, or regional anesthesia.

[Hypoxia, cerebral (treatment)][1] or

[Ischemia, cerebral (treatment)][1]—Thiopental for injection is being used in high doses to protect the brain from hypoxia and ischemia following head injuries and other related conditions.

[1]Not included in Canadian product labeling.

## Pharmacology/Pharmacokinetics

**Physicochemical characteristics**

Molecular weight—

Methohexital sodium: 284.29.

Thiopental sodium: 264.32.

pKa—

Thiopental sodium: 7.4.

Oil: water partition coefficient—Thiopental sodium: 580.

Note: Methohexital is also highly lipid-soluble, but its oil: water partition coefficient is lower than that of thiopental.

## Mechanism of action/Effect

Ultra short-acting barbiturate anesthetics depress the central nervous system (CNS) to produce hypnosis and anesthesia without analgesia.

Anesthetic (general)—

The exact mechanism by which barbiturate anesthetics produce general anesthesia is not completely understood. However, it has been proposed that they act by enhancing responses to gamma-aminobutyric acid (GABA), diminishing glutamate (GLU) responses, and directly depressing excitability by increasing membrane conductance (an effect reversed by the GABA antagonist picrotoxin), thereby producing a net decrease in neuronal excitability to provide anesthetic action.

Although the mechanism of action of barbiturates as sedative-hypnotics has not been completely established, the barbiturates appear to act at the level of the thalamus where they inhibit ascending conduction in the reticular formation, thus interfering with the transmission of impulses to the cortex. Recent studies have suggested that the sedative-hypnotic effects of barbiturates may be related to their ability to enhance or mimic the inhibitory synaptic action of GABA.

The mechanism of action of barbiturate anesthetics as anticonvulsants has not been completely established; however, in recent electrophysiological studies, barbiturate anesthetics (such as parenteral thiopental) that exert clinical anticonvulsant activity only at doses producing deep sedation or anesthesia have been shown to act by producing a GABA-like effect and enhancing postsynaptic inhibition responses to GABA.

The mechanism by which thiopental reduces intracranial pressure and protects the brain from cerebral ischemia and hypoxia is not completely understood. However, it is related to thiopental's anesthetic action and results in increased cerebral vascular resistance with a decrease in cerebral blood flow and cerebral blood volume. Various mechanisms of action have been proposed, including a reduction of cerebral metabolic rate, a decrease in the functional activity of the brain, an inhibition of the brain stem neurogenic mechanism of vasoparalysis, a sealing effect on membranes, and a scavenging of free oxygen radicals.

## Other actions/effects

Barbiturate anesthetics are potent respiratory depressants; respiratory depression is dose-related and is potentiated by opioid premedication.

Laryngeal reflexes are depressed with deep levels of anesthesia.

Barbiturate anesthetics have little, if any, analgesic activity.

There is either a fall or no change in mean arterial blood pressure, the former being more pronounced in hypertensive or hypovolemic patients; a decrease in cardiac output; an increase in total calculated peripheral resistance; an increase or no change in heart rate; a considerable decrease in renal plasma flow; a decrease in intrathoracic blood volume; an increase in blood flow and volume in the extremities; a decrease or no change in the central, right atrial, and peripheral venous pressures; and a decrease in cerebral blood flow with a marked reduction in cerebrospinal fluid (CSF) pressure. Direct depression of cardiac contractility is dose-related.

Barbiturate anesthetics have no effect on uterine muscle tone.

Renal, hepatic, and gastrointestinal functions are depressed by barbiturate anesthetics, but the effects are rarely of clinical significance.

## Absorption

Thiopental rectal suspension—May be unpredictable.

## Distribution

Because of their high lipid solubility and low degree of ionization, barbiturate anesthetics rapidly cross the blood-brain barrier and are rapidly redistributed from the brain to other body tissues, first to highly perfused visceral organs (liver, kidneys, heart) and muscle, and later to fatty tissues.

When barbiturate anesthetics are administered repeatedly or by continuous infusion, accumulation in and slow release from lipoidal storage sites may result in prolonged anesthesia, somnolence, and respiratory and circulatory depression. Concentrations of thiopental in fatty tissues may be 6 to 12 times greater than in plasma. Because of methohexital's lower lipid solubility (and, consequently, lower concentrations in fatty tissues) and shorter elimination half-life, methohexital is less likely than thiopental to accumulate with repeated or continuous administration.

Barbiturate anesthetics rapidly cross the placenta and appear in cord blood. Also, after administration of large doses, thiopental is distributed into breast milk.

Volume of distribution at steady-state ($V_{DSS}$)—

Methohexital: 1.9 to 2.2 L per kg of body weight (L/kg).

Thiopental: 1.7 to 2.5 L/kg; may increase to 4.1 L/kg during pregnancy at term and to 7.9 L/kg in obese patients.

## Protein binding

Methohexital—High (3%).

Thiopental—High (72–86%).

## Biotransformation

Primarily hepatic; also, biotransformed to a small extent in other tissues, especially the kidneys and brain.

Methohexital is metabolized more rapidly than thiopental. Although most of thiopental's metabolites are inactive, about 3 to 5% of a dose is desulfurated to pentobarbital, which is cleared from the body much more slowly than thiopental. The significance of this metabolic pathway is relevant only in patients receiving large doses of thiopental.

When large quantities of thiopental are administered by continuous intravenous infusion over a prolonged period of time, progressively increasing saturation of hepatic metabolizing enzymes may occur, resulting in a rapid increase in the plasma concentration.

## Half-life

Distribution—

Rapid.

Methohexital:

5.6 ± 2.7 minutes.

Thiopental:

4.6 to 8.5 minutes.

Elimination—

Methohexital:

Adults—1.5 to 5 hours; increases with age.

Thiopental:

Adults—10 to 12 hours; increases with age. May be increased to 26.1 hours during pregnancy at term and to 27.85 hours in obese patients.

Children—6.1 hours.

Note: When low doses of thiopental (e.g., 5 mg per kg of body weight) are administered for induction of anesthesia, the elimination half-life is independent of plasma concentration.

Administration of high doses of thiopental (e.g., 300 to 600 mg per kg of body weight) results in an increase in the elimination half-life.

## Onset of action

Rapid, due to the high lipid solubility of the barbiturate anesthetics.

Anesthesia—

Methohexital:

Intravenous—Within 60 seconds.

Rectal—Within 5 to 11 minutes.

Thiopental:

Intravenous—30 to 60 seconds.

Rectal—Within 8 to 10 minutes.

Note: After intravenous administration of induction doses of thiopental, muscle relaxation occurs about 30 seconds after unconsciousness is attained.

After intravenous administration of induction doses of a barbiturate anesthetic, the depth of anesthesia may increase for up to 40 seconds and then decrease progressively until consciousness returns. This reflects rapid changes in the concentration of anesthetic at its sites of action in the brain and is a consequence of its initial distribution to the brain followed by subsequent redistribution to other tissues.

Hypnosis—

Thiopental (intravenous):

Within 10 to 40 seconds.

## Time to peak concentration

Intravenous administration—

Brain: Methohexital or thiopental—Within 30 seconds.

Muscles: Thiopental—15 to 30 minutes.

Fat: Thiopental—Several hours.

Note: Very highly perfused tissues such as the brain, heart, liver, and kidneys achieve concentrations equal to peak plasma concentrations.

## Duration of action

Intravenous administration—

Methohexital: 5 to 7 minutes.

Thiopental: 10 to 30 minutes.

Note: The brief duration of action is due to the rapid rate of redistribution and, to some extent, metabolism accompanied by a rapid fall in plasma concentration. Administration of large or repeated doses may substantially delay recovery.

**Elimination**

Renal; however, renal elimination is minimal because of extensive renal tubular reabsorption due to the high lipid solubility of barbiturate anesthetics.

Clearance—

In adults:

Methohexital—9.3 to 12.1 mL/kg per minute.

Thiopental—1.6 to 4.3 mL/kg per minute; may be increased during pregnancy at term to 286 mL per minute.

Note: When thiopental is administered in large doses by continuous infusion over a prolonged period of time, the kinetics of elimination change from first-order to nonlinear or zero-order kinetics. In low doses (e.g., 5 mg per kg of body weight) for induction of anesthesia, thiopental shows first-order kinetics and the rate of elimination is independent of plasma concentration. In higher doses (300 to 600 mg per kg of body weight) for more prolonged periods, it shows zero-order kinetics and the rate of elimination varies with the plasma concentration.

## Precautions to Consider

**Cross-sensitivity and/or related problems**

Patients sensitive to one barbiturate may be sensitive to other barbiturates also.

**Carcinogenicity/Mutagenicity**

Studies in animals have not been performed to determine the carcinogenic and mutagenic potential of methohexital or thiopental.

**Pregnancy/Reproduction**

Fertility—Studies in animals have not been performed to determine the effect of methohexital or thiopental on fertility.

Pregnancy—Use of barbiturate anesthetics during pregnancy may cause CNS depression in the fetus. Adequate and well-controlled studies in humans have not been done to determine whether barbiturate anesthetics are teratogenic.

*Methohexital—*

Methohexital crosses the placenta.

Studies in pregnant rabbits and rats given methohexital up to 4 and 7 times the human dose, respectively, produced no evidence of teratogenicity and no fetal abnormalities.

FDA Pregnancy Category B.

*Thiopental—*

Thiopental crosses the placenta. The concentration in cord vein blood is at its maximum 2 to 3 minutes after an intravenous dose is administered to the mother.

Studies in animals have not been done.

FDA Pregnancy Category C.

**Breast-feeding**

Problems in humans have not been documented. However, barbiturate anesthetics are distributed into breast milk; small amounts may appear in breast milk following administration of large doses to the nursing mother.

**Pediatrics**

Appropriate studies on the relationship of age to the effects of barbiturate anesthetics have not been performed in the pediatric population. However, no pediatrics-specific problems have been documented to date.

**Geriatrics**

Following administration of barbiturate anesthetics for short (outpatient) procedures, recovery of cognitive and psychomotor functions is generally slower in elderly patients than in younger adults. In addition, elderly patients are more likely to have age-related hepatic function impairment, which may require reduction of dosage in patients receiving barbiturate anesthetics, and age-related renal function impairment, which may prolong the effects of these medications.

**Drug interactions and/or related problems**

The following drug interactions and/or related problems have been selected on the basis of their potential clinical significance (possible mechanism in parentheses where appropriate)—not necessarily inclusive (» = major clinical significance):

Note: Combinations containing any of the following medications, depending on the amount present, may also interact with this medication.

» Alcohol or
» CNS depression–producing medications, other, including those commonly used for preanesthetic medication or induction or supplementation of anesthesia (See *Appendix II*)
(concurrent administration may increase the CNS depressant, respiratory depressant, or hypotensive effects of barbiturate anesthet-

ics as well as decreasing anesthetic requirements and prolonging recovery from anesthesia; dosage adjustments may be required)

Antihypertensives, especially diazoxide or ganglionic blockers such as guanadrel, guanethidine, mecamylamine, or trimethaphan or
Diuretics or
Hypotension-producing medications, other (See *Appendix II* )
(concurrent use of these medications with barbiturate anesthetics may result in an additive hypotensive effect, which could be severe; dosage adjustments may be necessary; patients should be monitored for excessive fall in blood pressure during and following concurrent use)

(concurrent use of antihypertensives with CNS depressant effects, such as clonidine, guanabenz, methyldopa, metyrosine, pargyline, and rauwolfia alkaloids, may increase the CNS depressant effects of barbiturate anesthetics)

Hypothermia-producing medications, other (See *Appendix II*)
(concurrent use with barbiturate anesthetics may increase the risk of hypothermia)

Ketamine
(concurrent use of ketamine, especially in high doses or when rapidly administered, with barbiturate anesthetics may increase the risk of hypotension and/or respiratory depression)

Magnesium sulfate, parenteral
(concurrent use may increase the CNS depressant effects of barbiturate anesthetics)

Phenothiazines, especially promethazine
(in addition to possibly increasing CNS depressant effects, concurrent use may potentiate the hypotensive and CNS excitatory effects of barbiturate anesthetics)

**Laboratory value alterations**

The following have been selected on the basis of their potential clinical significance (possible effect in parentheses where appropriate)—not necessarily inclusive (» = major clinical significance):

With diagnostic test results

Sodium iodide I 123 and

Sodium iodide I 131 and

Sodium pertechnetate Tc 99m
(thiopental may decrease thyroidal uptake of sodium iodide I 123 and I 131 and sodium pertechnetate Tc 99m)

**Medical considerations/Contraindications**

The medical considerations/contraindications included here have been selected on the basis of their potential clinical significance (reasons given in parentheses where appropriate)—not necessarily inclusive (» = major clinical significance).

*Except under special circumstances, this medication should not be used when the following medical problems exist:*

*For parenteral and rectal administration*

» Porphyria, acute intermittent or variegata or history of
(barbiturate anesthetics may aggravate symptoms by inducing enzymes responsible for porphyrin synthesis)

*For rectal administration*

» Inflammatory, ulcerative, bleeding or neoplastic lesions of the lower bowel
(condition may be exacerbated)

*Risk-benefit should be considered when the following medical problems exist:*

Note: Dosage should be reduced and the medication administered slowly if barbiturate anesthetics are used in the presence of the following medical problems.

*For parenteral and rectal administration*

Addison's disease or
Anemia, severe or
Hepatic function impairment or
Myxedema or
Renal function impairment
(hypnotic effect may be prolonged or potentiated)

» Cardiovascular disease, severe or
» Congestive heart failure or
» Hypotension or shock
(barbiturate anesthetics produce cardiovascular depressant effects; condition may be exacerbated)

Myasthenia gravis or
Neuromuscular disorders, other, such as muscular dystrophies and myotonias
(respiratory depression may be prolonged; dosage should be carefully titrated)

» Respiratory disease involving dyspnea or obstruction, particularly status asthmaticus
  (barbiturate anesthetics produce respiratory depressant effects)

» Sensitivity to barbiturates

  Caution should be used also in debilitated patients because respiratory depression, apnea, or hypotension may be more likely to occur in these patients.

**Patient monitoring**

The following may be especially important in patient monitoring (other tests may be warranted in some patients, depending on condition; » = major clinical significance):

» Blood pressure and
» Body temperature and
» Cardiac/pulse rate and
» Electrocardiographic evaluation and
» Oxygenation and
» Respiratory and ventilatory status

  (it is recommended that the patient's blood and tissue oxygenation, ventilation, circulation, and body temperature be monitored continuously during anesthetic administration and as required during the recovery period)

  Note: Various organizations, including medical specialty societies, and institutions have established standards for the pre-, intra-, and post-procedure care, evaluation, and monitoring of patients receiving various forms of anesthesia and/or sedation. The above recommendations represent the minimum standards established by the American Society of Anesthesiologists for monitoring the status of patients receiving general anesthesia. Individual patients may require additional monitoring.

*For thiopental only*

  Plasma thiopental concentrations

  (monitoring of plasma thiopental concentration is recommended if thiopental is administered by intravenous infusion over an extended period of time, such as in the treatment of increased intracranial pressure)

## Side/Adverse Effects

Note: Because barbiturate anesthetics are potent respiratory depressants, apnea may occur immediately after intravenous injection, especially in the presence of hypovolemia, cranial trauma, or opioid premedication.

  During induction of anesthesia or in lightly anesthetized patients, laryngeal spasm may be induced by a variety of stimuli such as surgical stimulation, the premature insertion of the laryngoscope blade or airway, and pharyngeal secretions.

  Excitatory phenomena such as involuntary muscle movements, coughing, and hiccups occur more frequently with methohexital than with thiopental.

  True anaphylaxis has been reported to occur with barbiturate anesthetics, but is rare.

  Overdosage may occur from too rapid or repeated injections. Too rapid injection may cause a severe drop in blood pressure, possibly to shock levels. Excessive or too rapid injections may result in respiratory difficulties such as laryngospasm and apnea. Repeated administration may also lead to accumulation of the barbiturate, resulting in substantial prolongation of the medication's effects.

  Impairment of psychomotor skills may occur following barbiturate anesthesia and may persist for varying lengths of time (usually about 24 hours), depending upon the anesthetic and/or combination of medications used and the total dosages administered. Possible adverse effects on the patient's ability to drive or perform other tasks requiring alertness and coordination should be kept in mind when a barbiturate anesthetic is administered for outpatient surgery.

The following side/adverse effects have been selected on the basis of their potential clinical significance (possible signs and symptoms in parentheses where appropriate)—not necessarily inclusive:

**Those indicating need for medical attention**

*Allergic reaction, acute* (abdominal pain; anxiety or restlessness; skin rash, hives, itching, or redness; swelling of eyelids, face, or lips; unusually low blood pressure; wheezing or difficulty in breathing); *cardiac arrhythmias* (fast, slow, or irregular heartbeat); *circulatory depression* (unusually low blood pressure, severe or continuing); *excitatory phenomena* (coughing, difficulty in breathing, hiccups, muscle twitching or jerking)—occurring during induction of anesthesia or in light anesthesia; *respiratory depression* (shortness of breath, slow

or irregular breathing, troubled breathing); *thrombophlebitis* (redness, swelling, or pain at injection site).
*With rectal administration only*
  *Cramping; diarrhea; rectal irritation or bleeding*

**Those occurring postsurgically and indicating need for medical attention**
Incidence rare
  *Emergence delirium* (anxiety; confusion; excitement; hallucinations; nervousness; restlessness); *immune hemolytic anemia with renal failure* (back, leg, or stomach pain; nausea, vomiting, or loss of appetite; unusual tiredness or weakness; fever; pale skin); *radial nerve palsy* (weakness of wrist and fingers)

  Note: *Immune hemolytic anemia with renal failure* and *radial nerve palsy* have occurred rarely with the use of thiopental.

**Those occurring postsurgically and indicating need for medical attention only if they continue**
Incidence more frequent
  *Increased sensitivity to cold, during recovery* (shivering or trembling)
Incidence less frequent or rare
  *Drowsiness, prolonged; headache; nausea or vomiting*

## Overdose

For more information on the management of overdose or unintentional ingestion, **contact a Poison Control Center** (see *Poison Control Center Listing*).

The following effects have been selected on the basis of their potential clinical significance (possible signs and symptoms in parentheses where appropriate)—not necessarily inclusive:

**Acute effects**

*CNS depression, severe; hypotension, severe; loss of peripheral vascular resistance; respiratory depression, severe, including apnea*

  Note: *Circulatory and respiratory depression* may result in *pulmonary edema* and/or *cardiorespiratory arrest*.

**Treatment of overdose**

Discontinuation of the anesthetic.

Specific treatment—If overdosage occurs with a rectal barbiturate anesthetic preparation, the contents of the rectum should be promptly evacuated; further dosing should be delayed until the effects of absorption of the initial dose can be determined.

Monitoring—Vital signs, blood gases, and serum electrolytes should be monitored.

Supportive care—Supportive measures such as establishing and maintaining a patent airway (by intubation if necessary), administering 100% oxygen with assisted ventilation if necessary. For hypotension—Intravenous fluids should be administered and the patients's legs raised. If a desirable increase in blood pressure is not obtained, vasopressor and/or inotropic drugs may be used as required.

## Patient Consultation

As an aid to patient consultation, refer to *Advice for the Patient, Anesthetics, General (Systemic)*.

In providing consultation, consider emphasizing the following selected information (» = major clinical significance):

**Before receiving this medication**

» Conditions affecting use, especially:
  Sensitivity to barbiturates
  Pregnancy—Crosses the placenta and may cause CNS depression in the fetus
  Other medications, especially other CNS depressants
  Other medical problems, especially acute intermittent or variegata porphyria (or history of); cardiovascular disease, severe; hypotension or shock; respiratory disease involving dyspnea or obstruction (particularly status asthmaticus); and, for rectal administration only, inflammatory, ulcerative, bleeding, or neoplastic lesions of lower bowel

**Proper use of this medication**

  Proper dosing

**Precautions after receiving this medication**

» Possibility of psychomotor impairment following use of anesthetics; for about 24 hours following anesthesia, using caution in driving or performing other tasks requiring alertness and coordination

» Avoiding use of alcohol or other CNS depressants within 24 hours following anesthesia except as directed by physician or dentist

# General Dosing Information

**Barbiturate anesthetics should be administered only by individuals qualified in the use of general anesthetics. Appropriate resuscitative and endotracheal intubation equipment, oxygen, and medications for prevention and treatment of anesthetic emergencies must be immediately available. Airway patency must be maintained at all times.**

Dosage of the barbiturate anesthetics must be individualized according to the desired depth of anesthesia, concomitant use of other medications and/or nitrous oxide, and the patient's physical condition, age, sex, and weight.

Young patients may require relatively larger doses than middle-aged or elderly patients. Prepuberty dose requirements are the same for both sexes, but adult females require smaller doses than adult males.

Care should be taken to avoid extravasation or intra-arterial injection of barbiturate anesthetics. Extravascular injection may cause pain, swelling, ulceration, and necrosis. Intra-arterial injection may produce arteritis, followed by vasospasm, edema, thrombosis, and gangrene of an extremity.

Repeated doses or continuous infusion of barbiturate anesthetics may cause cumulative effects, resulting in prolonged somnolence and respiratory and circulatory depression.

Caution is required if the patient requires a second anesthetic on the same day; a reduction in the dose of the intravenous barbiturate anesthetic may be required.

Although barbiturate anesthetics may be given in sufficient doses to produce deep surgical anesthesia in the presence of external stimulation such as surgical incision, these doses may also produce dangerous cardiovascular and respiratory depression.

Because the rapid distribution of barbiturate anesthetics out of the brain can result in light anesthesia characterized by reflex hyperactivity of the airway to stimulation (e.g., intubation, instrumentation, secretions), an adequate depth of anesthesia should be induced in patients predisposed to bronchospasm or with upper airway obstruction, when coughing and hiccupping are undesirable, and to avoid laryngospasm that may occur from direct or indirect stimulation.

To minimize mucous secretions, anticholinergics, such as atropine or glycopyrrolate, may be administered as premedication. In addition, an opiate may be administered to enhance the otherwise poor analgesic effects of the barbiturate anesthetic. The peak effects of the premedication should be attained shortly before induction of anesthesia. Also, muscle relaxants may be required and should be administered separately.

Tolerance has been reported following multiple use, as in burn patients.

Individuals tolerant to alcohol or barbiturates may require higher doses of barbiturate anesthetics.

## Treatment of adverse effects

Recommended treatment for adverse effects of barbiturate anesthetics includes:

• For laryngospasm—Positive pressure oxygen 100% should be administered; then, if necessary, a skeletal muscle relaxant may be administered; cricothyrotomy may be required in difficult cases.

• For extravasation—Procaine 1% may be administered locally to relieve pain and enhance vasodilation. Local application of heat may also help to increase local circulation and remove the infiltrate.

• For inadvertent intra-arterial injection—Treatment varies with the severity of symptoms. The injected barbiturate anesthetic should be diluted by removing the tourniquet and any restrictive garment. The needle should be left in place, if possible. A dilute solution of 1% procaine, 10 mL, may be injected into the artery to inhibit smooth muscle spasm. Sympathetic block of the brachial plexus or stellate ganglion should be performed, if necessary, to relieve pain and assist in opening collateral circulation. To prevent thrombus formation, heparinization should be instituted immediately, unless otherwise contraindicated. Local infiltration of an alpha-adrenergic blocking agent into the vasospastic area may be considered. Intra-arterial injection of a glucocorticoid at the site of injury, followed by administration of systemic corticosteroids should be considered. Also, it has been reported that intra-arterial administration of urokinase may promote fibrinolysis even if administration is late in treatment. Postinjury arterial injection of vasodilators and/or arterial infusion of parenteral fluids are generally not useful in reducing the area of necrosis.

• For shivering—Treatment includes warming the patient with blankets, maintaining room temperature at 22 °C (72 °F), and administering chlorpromazine or methylphenidate.

• For thrombophlebitis—Treatment is symptomatic and may require rest and application of heat.

---

## *METHOHEXITAL*

---

# Summary of Differences

Pharmacology/pharmacokinetics:

Physicochemical characteristics—Oil:water partition coefficient is lower than that of thiopental.

Distribution—Does not concentrate in lipids to the same extent as thiopental; less likely than thiopental to accumulate with repeated or prolonged administration.

Biotransformation—More rapid than thiopental.

Half-life—Distribution and elimination half-lives are shorter than those of thiopental.

Duration of action—Shorter than thiopental.

Side/adverse effects:

Excitatory phenomena occur more frequently than with thiopental.

# Additional Dosing Information

See also *General Dosing Information.*

Methohexital is about 2 to 3 times more potent than thiopental.

Preanesthetic medication may be advisable with methohexital. Any preanesthetic medication may be used; however, the combination of an opioid and a belladonna derivative is preferable to the phenothiazines, which have been reported to potentiate the hypotensive and CNS excitatory effects of methohexital.

A 1% solution of methohexital is recommended for induction of anesthesia and for maintenance by intermittent injection. Higher concentrations greatly increase the incidence of muscular movements and irregularities in respiration and blood pressure.

# Parenteral Dosage Forms

## METHOHEXITAL SODIUM FOR INJECTION USP

### Usual adult dose

Anesthesia, general—

Induction

Dosage must be individualized by physician; however, as a general guideline—Intravenous, 1 to 2 mg per kg of body weight as required, administered cautiously.Maintenance—

Dosage must be individualized by physician; however, as a general guideline—Intravenous (intermittent), 250 mcg (0.25 mg) to 1 mg per kg of body weight as required.

Note: Some anesthesiologists prefer the continuous drip method of maintenance with a 0.2% solution, the rate of flow being individualized for each patient.

### Usual pediatric dose

Anesthesia, general—

Induction

Dosage must be individualized by physician; however, as a general guideline—

Intramuscular, 5 to 10 mg per kg of body weight as required.

Intravenous, 1 to 2 mg per kg of body weight as required, administered cautiously.

### Size(s) usually available

U.S.—

500 mg (Rx) [*Brevital* (anhydrous sodium carbonate 30 mg)].

2.5 grams (Rx) [*Brevital* (anhydrous sodium carbonate 150 mg)].

5 grams (Rx) [*Brevital* (anhydrous sodium carbonate 300 mg)].

Canada—

500 mg (Rx) [*Brietal* (anhydrous sodium carbonate)].

2.5 grams (Rx) [*Brietal* (anhydrous sodium carbonate)].

### Packaging and storage

Prior to reconstitution, store below 40 °C (104 °F), preferably between 15 and 30 °C (59 and 86 °F), unless otherwise specified by manufacturer.

### Preparation of dosage form

Sterile water for injection, 5% dextrose injection, or 0.9% sodium chloride injection may be used as diluents. Bacteriostatic diluents and lactated Ringer's injection should not be used as diluents because they tend to cause precipitation.

For direct intravenous injection, sterile water for injection should be used as the diluent for preparation of a 1% methohexital sodium injection.

For more information on the preparation of a 1% methohexital injection, see the manufacturer's package insert.

For administration via intravenous infusion, a 0.2% injection is prepared by adding 500 mg of methohexital sodium to 250 mL of 5% dextrose injection or 0.9% sodium chloride injection; however, dextrose injections are sometimes sufficiently acid to cause precipitation. Sterile water for injection should not be used because of the resultant extreme hypotonicity, which will cause hemolysis.

**Stability**

Methohexital is stable in sterile water for injection at room temperature (25 °C [77 °F] or lower) for at least 6 weeks; solutions prepared with 5% dextrose injection or 0.9% sodium chloride injection are not stable for more than 24 hours.

Only clear injections should be used; if an injection becomes cloudy or a precipitate forms, the medication should be discarded.

**Incompatibilities**

Methohexital injections should not be mixed with acidic substances, such as atropine sulfate, metocurine iodide, and succinylcholine chloride, because precipitation will occur.

For additional information on the chemical compatibility of methohexital sodium with medications having a low (acid) pH, see the manufacturer's package insert.

Methohexital injections are incompatible with silicone and should not be allowed to come in contact with rubber stoppers or parts of disposable syringes that have been treated with silicone.

Methohexital sodium is incompatible with bacteriostatic diluents and with lactated Ringer's injection; precipitation will occur.

**Note**

Controlled substance in the U.S. and Canada.

## Rectal Dosage Forms

### METHOHEXITAL SODIUM FOR RECTAL SOLUTION

**Usual pediatric dose**

Anesthesia, basal—

Rectal, 15 to 30 mg per kg of body weight as a 5 to 10% solution.

Note: For inactive or debilitated patients—Lower dosage is advisable.

**Size(s) usually available**

U.S.—

Dosage form not commercially available. Compounding required for prescriptions.

Canada—

Dosage form not commercially available. Compounding required for prescriptions.

**Packaging and storage**

Store below 40 °C (104 °F), preferably between 15 and 30 °C (59 and 86 °F), in a well-closed container. Protect from freezing.

**Preparation of dosage form**

To prepare a 5 to 10% methohexital rectal solution, dissolve an appropriate amount of methohexital sodium for injection in warm tap water.

**Stability**

If the solution becomes cloudy or a precipitate forms, the solution should be discarded.

**Incompatibilities**

Methohexital should not be mixed with acidic substances, such as atropine sulfate, metocurine iodide, and succinylcholine chloride, because precipitation will occur.

For additional information on the chemical compatibility of methohexital sodium with medications having a low (acid) pH, see the manufacturer's package insert for methohexital sodium for injection.

Methohexital solutions are incompatible with silicone and should not be allowed to come in contact with rubber stoppers or parts of disposable syringes that have been treated with silicone.

Methohexital sodium is incompatible with bacteriostatic diluents and with lactated Ringer's injection; precipitation will occur.

---

### *THIOPENTAL*

---

## Summary of Differences

Indications:

Parenteral thiopental also indicated in the treatment of cerebral hypertension and for narcoanalysis in the treatment of psychiatric disorders; and is used in the treatment of cerebral ischemia and hypoxia.

Pharmacology/pharmacokinetics:

Physicochemical characteristics—

Oil:water partition coefficient is greater than that of methohexital.

Distribution—

Concentrates in fatty tissues to a greater extent than methohexital; risk of accumulation with repeated or prolonged administration is higher than with methohexital.

Appears in breast milk following administration of large doses.

Biotransformation—

Less rapid than methohexital.

Half-life—

Distribution and elimination half-lives longer than those of methohexital.

Duration of action—

Greater than that of methohexital.

Patient monitoring:

Monitoring of plasma concentrations is recommended if thiopental is administered by intravenous infusion over a prolonged period of time.

## Additional Dosing Information

See also *General Dosing Information*.

For parenteral dosage form only

• A test dose of 25 to 75 mg (1 to 3 mL of a 2.5% solution) may be administered to determine tolerance or unusual sensitivity to thiopental; patient reaction should be observed for at least 60 seconds.

• A 2 or 2.5% concentration of thiopental solution is used for intermittent intravenous administration.

• A 3.4% concentration of thiopental in sterile water for injection is isotonic; concentrations less than 2% in sterile water for injection should not be used because they cause hemolysis.

For rectal suspension dosage form only

• To assure easy extrusion of thiopental rectal suspension, instructions should be followed for filling the applicator and extruding a small amount before setting the stop device at the desired dose for rectal administration. Care should be taken not to use excessive pressure on the syringe plunger since this can cause the stop device to break or slip, which may result in an overdose.

• A new applicator should be used for each repeat administration.

• Unless there are unusual circumstances, such as fecal impaction, a cleansing enema is rarely required prior to administration of thiopental rectal suspension.

## Parenteral Dosage Forms

### THIOPENTAL SODIUM FOR INJECTION USP

**Usual adult dose**

Anesthesia, general—

Induction:

Dosage must be individualized by physician; however, as a general guideline—Intravenous, 50 to 100 mg (2 to 4 mL of a 2.5% solution) as required; or 3 to 5 mg per kg of body weight as a single dose.

Maintenance:

Dosage must be individualized by physician; however, as a general guideline—Intravenous (intermittent), 50 to 100 mg (2 to 4 mL of a 2.5% solution) as required.

Note: When thiopental is used as the sole anesthetic agent, the desired level of anesthesia can be maintained by injection of small repeated doses as needed. Also, 0.2 to 0.4% solutions have been administered by continuous intravenous drip for maintenance.

Hypertension, cerebral[1]—

Intravenous (intermittent), 1.5 to 3.5 mg per kg of body weight, repeated as required to reduce elevations of intracranial pressure.

Note: Adequate ventilation must be provided.

Convulsions—

Intravenous, 50 to 125 mg (2 to 5 mL of a 2.5% solution), administered as soon as possible after the convulsion begins.

Narcoanalysis[1]—

Intravenous, as a 2.5% solution, administered at a rate of 100 mg per minute with the patient counting backwards from one hundred. Injection should be discontinued after counting becomes confused but before actual sleep is produced.

Note: As alternative dosing, thiopental may be administered by rapid intravenous drip using a 0.2% concentration in 5% dextrose injection; however, the rate of administration should not exceed 50 mL per minute.

**Usual pediatric dose**

Anesthesia, general—

Induction:

Children up to 15 years of age—Dosage must be individualized by physician; however, as a general guideline: Intravenous, 3 to 5 mg per kg of body weight.

Maintenance:
Dosage must be individualized by physician; however, as a general guideline—Intravenous (intermittent), about 1 mg per kg of body weight as required.

### Size(s) usually available

U.S.—
250 mg (Rx) [*Pentothal;* GENERIC].
400 mg (Rx) [*Pentothal;* GENERIC].
500 mg (Rx) [*Pentothal;* GENERIC].
1 gram (Rx) [*Pentothal*].
2.5 grams (Rx) [*Pentothal*].
5 grams (Rx) [*Pentothal*].
10 grams (Rx) [GENERIC].

Canada—
1 gram (Rx) [*Pentothal*].
2.5 grams (Rx) [*Pentothal*].
5 grams (Rx) [*Pentothal*].

### Packaging and storage

Prior to reconstitution, store below 40 °C (104 °F), preferably between 15 and 30 °C (59 and 86 °F), unless otherwise specified by manufacturer.

### Preparation of dosage form

Sterile water for injection, 0.9% sodium chloride injection, or 5% dextrose injection should be used as the diluent.

Sterile water for injection should not be used to prepare a 0.2 or 0.4% thiopental sodium injection for intravenous infusion because of the resultant extreme hypotonicity, which will cause hemolysis.

For more information on the preparation of thiopental injections, see the manufacturer's package insert.

Since Thiopental for Injection USP contains no added bacteriostatic agent, extreme care in preparation and handling should be used at all times to prevent the introduction of microbial contaminants.

### Stability

Injections should be freshly prepared and used within 24 hours after reconstitution; discard unused portions after 24 hours.

Injections are most stable when prepared with sterile water for injection or 0.9% sodium chloride injection. They should be kept refrigerated and tightly stoppered.

Any factor or condition that tends to lower the pH of thiopental injections, such as diluents that are too acid or the absorption of carbon dioxide, which combines with water to form carbonic acid, will increase the possibility of precipitation of thiopental acid.

Sterilization by heating causes precipitation.

Injections containing a precipitate should not be administered.

### Incompatibilities

Thiopental injections should not be mixed with succinylcholine, tubocurarine, or other medications that have an acid pH, because precipitation will occur.

### Note

Controlled substance in the U.S. and Canada.

## Rectal Dosage Forms

### THIOPENTAL SODIUM FOR RECTAL SOLUTION

#### Usual adult and adolescent dose

Anesthesia, basal (preanesthetic sedation)—
Rectal, 30 mg per kg of body weight.
Narcosis, basal—
Normally active patients: Rectal, up to 9 mg per kg of body weight.
Note: For inactive or debilitated patients—Lower dosage is advisable.

#### Usual adult prescribing limits

Adults weighing 90 kg or more—
Up to a total of 3 to 4 grams.

#### Usual pediatric dose

See *Usual adult and adolescent dose*.

### Strength(s) usually available

U.S.—
Dosage form not commercially available. Compounding required for prescriptions.

Canada—
Dosage form not commercially available. Compounding required for prescriptions.

### Packaging and storage

Store below 40 °C (104 °F), preferably between 15 and 30 °C (59 and 86 °F), in a well-closed container. Protect from freezing.

### Preparation of dosage form

To prepare a thiopental rectal solution, dissolve an appropriate amount of thiopental sodium for injection in warm tap water.

### Stability

Solutions should be freshly prepared and used within 24 hours after reconstitution; unused portions should be discarded after 24 hours.

Solutions are most stable when prepared with water or isotonic saline and kept refrigerated and tightly stoppered.

Any factor or condition that tends to lower the pH of thiopental solutions, such as diluents that are too acid or the absorption of carbon dioxide, which combines with water to form carbonic acid, will increase the possibility of precipitation of thiopental acid.

Sterilization by heating causes precipitation.

Solutions containing a precipitate should not be administered.

### Incompatibilities

Thiopental solutions should not be mixed with succinylcholine, tubocurarine, or other medications that have an acid pH, because precipitation will occur.

### THIOPENTAL SODIUM RECTAL SUSPENSION

#### Usual adult and adolescent dose

Anesthesia, basal (preanesthetic sedation)—
Rectal, 30 mg per kg of body weight.
Narcosis, basal—
Normally active patients: Rectal, up to 9 mg per kg of body weight.
Note: For inactive or debilitated patients—Lower dosage is advisable.

#### Usual adult prescribing limits

Adults weighing 90 kg or more—
Up to a total of 3 to 4 grams.

#### Usual pediatric dose

See *Usual adult and adolescent dose*.

Note: For children weighing 34 kg or more, a total dose of 1 to 1.5 grams should not be exceeded.

For inactive or debilitated patients—Lower dosage is advisable.

### Strength(s) usually available

U.S.—
400 mg per gram (Rx) [*Pentothal* (mineral oil; dimethyldioctadecylammonium bentonite; anhydrous sodium carbonate 24 mg per gram)].

### Packaging and storage

Store below 40 °C (104 °F), preferably between 15 and 30 °C (59 and 86 °F), unless otherwise specified by manufacturer. Protect from freezing.

### Stability

Contains no bacteriostatic or antimicrobial agent. Intended only for one-time use.

### Auxiliary labeling

• Shake well.

### Note

Controlled substance in the U.S.

---

[1]Not included in Canadian product labeling.

---

Revised: 08/25/94

# ANESTHETICS, INHALATION    Systemic

This monograph includes information on the following: Enflurane; Halothane; Isoflurane; Methoxyflurane; Nitrous Oxide.

VA CLASSIFICATION (Primary): CN201

Note: For a listing of dosage forms and brand names by country availability, see *Dosage Forms* section(s). For a listing of brand names for the articles in this monograph, refer to the General Index.

## Category

Anesthetic (general).

## Indications

Note: Bracketed information in the *Indications* section refers to uses that are not included in U.S. product labeling.

### Accepted

Anesthesia, general—Enflurane, halothane, isoflurane, methoxyflurane, and nitrous oxide are indicated for the induction and maintenance of general anesthesia. However, inhalation anesthetic agents are rarely used alone; other medications are frequently administered to induce or supplement anesthesia.

Because of its weak anesthetic potency and muscle relaxant properties, nitrous oxide must be supplemented with another anesthetic or anesthesia adjunct (such as a barbiturate, benzodiazepine, opioid analgesic, or another inhalation anesthetic) and/or a neuromuscular blocking agent. Also, nitrous oxide is often administered concurrently with one of the other inhalation anesthetics to decrease the requirement for the more potent anesthetic.

[Enflurane][1], [isoflurane][1], methoxyflurane, and nitrous oxide are indicated in low doses to provide analgesia for procedures not requiring loss of consciousness.

Enflurane, [isoflurane][1], methoxyflurane, and nitrous oxide are indicated in low doses to provide analgesia for vaginal delivery.

For cesarean section: Enflurane, [halothane][1], [isoflurane][1], and [methoxyflurane][1] are indicated in low concentrations to supplement other general anesthetics during delivery by cesarean section.

### Unaccepted

Because of potential nephrotoxicity, administration of methoxyflurane in concentrations sufficient to produce muscle relaxation is not recommended; a neuromuscular blocking agent should be used concurrently if necessary. Also, it is recommended that methoxyflurane not be used during vascular surgery at or near renal blood vessels.

Halothane is not recommended for vaginal delivery unless uterine relaxation is required.

[1]Not included in Canadian product labeling.

## Pharmacology/Pharmacokinetics

See also *Table 1*, page 162 and *Table 2*, page 162.

### Physicochemical characteristics

Molecular weight—
  Enflurane: 184.49.
  Halothane: 197.38.
  Isoflurane: 184.49.
  Methoxyflurane: 164.97.
  Nitrous oxide: 44.01.
Other characteristics—
  Blood-to-gas partition coefficient—
  See *Table 1*, page 162.
  Oil-to-gas partition coefficient—
  See *Table 1*, page 162.

### Mechanism of action/Effect

The precise mechanism by which inhalation anesthetics produce loss of perception of sensations and unconsciousness is not known. Proposed mechanisms are based on the Meyer-Overton theory, which demonstrates the correlation between the potency of an anesthetic and its solubility in oil. Inhalation anesthetics may interfere with the physiological functioning of nerve cell membranes in the brain via an action at the lipid matrix of the membrane.

### Absorption

Inhalation anesthetics are rapidly absorbed into the circulation via the lungs.

## Precautions to Consider

### Carcinogenicity

For isoflurane: Although one study indicated that isoflurane may be carcinogenic, it is thought that exposure of the test animals to polybrominated biphenyls may have been responsible. Subsequent studies in which such exposure was avoided have not shown evidence of isoflurane-induced carcinogenicity.

For enflurane, halothane, methoxyflurane, and nitrous oxide: These anesthetics have not been shown to be carcinogenic.

### Tumorigenicity

For enflurane: Studies in mice have not shown evidence of tumorigenicity with enflurane.

### Mutagenicity

For halothane: *In vitro* testing (Ames test) has indicated that potential halothane metabolites (but not halothane itself) may be mutagenic.

For enflurane, isoflurane, methoxyflurane, and nitrous oxide: Mutagenic effects have not been observed with these inhalation anesthetics in the Ames test or the sister chromatid exchange test. However, statistically significant increases in sperm abnormalities have been observed in mice following 20 hours of exposure to 1.2% of enflurane.

### Pregnancy/Reproduction

Pregnancy—Inhalation anesthetics cross the placenta. Risk-benefit must be considered because studies (by retrospective survey) of operating room personnel chronically exposed to low concentrations of inhalation anesthetics indicate that pregnancies in female personnel and wives of male personnel may be subject to an increased incidence of spontaneous abortions, stillbirths, and possibly birth defects. However, the methods used in obtaining and interpreting the data in these studies have been questioned. Also, several animal studies (in which operating room conditions were simulated) have failed to show fetotoxic or teratogenic effects following chronic exposure of male and/or female animals to low concentrations of inhalation anesthetics prior to and/or during gestation.

First trimester: Administration of enflurane, halothane, or isoflurane early in pregnancy (for therapeutic abortion) has been reported to increase uterine bleeding. However, blood loss following enflurane administration was considered to be within acceptable limits.

For enflurane—Although studies in patients have not been done, some studies in rats and rabbits have not shown that enflurane causes adverse effects on the fetus. However, other studies in animals have shown that enflurane may be teratogenic.

FDA Pregnancy Category B.

For halothane—Although studies in patients have not been done, some animal studies have shown that halothane may be teratogenic.

For isoflurane—Although isoflurane has not been shown to cause fetal malformations in mice or rats, studies in mice receiving 7 MAC hours (the equivalent of 1 MAC [minimum alveolar concentration that prevents movement in 50% of subjects following a painful stimulus] administered for 7 hours) over a period of 10 days during gestation have indicated possible fetotoxicity as manifested by higher implantation losses and a significantly lower live birth index. Studies have not been done in patients.

For methoxyflurane—Although adequate and well-controlled studies in patients have not been done, some studies in animals have shown that methoxyflurane may be teratogenic. Also, studies in rats have indicated that exposure to doses equivalent to 67 hours of 0.2% methoxyflurane caused fetal growth retardation.

FDA Pregnancy Category C.

For nitrous oxide—Although problems in patients have not been documented, studies in rats have shown that nitrous oxide causes fetal death, growth retardation, and skeletal anomalies.

Labor and delivery—Enflurane, halothane, isoflurane, and methoxyflurane produce dose-dependent uterine relaxation, which may delay delivery and increase postpartum bleeding. Subanesthetic (analgesic) concentrations of enflurane, isoflurane, or methoxyflurane do not significantly decrease uterine contractions. Halothane is the most potent uterine relaxant; even low concentrations (< 0.5%) may decrease uterine contractions. Also, enflurane and halothane cause a dose-dependent decrease in the uterine response to oxytocics. Use of halothane during vaginal delivery is not recommended unless uterine relaxation is required (as for version or other intrauterine manipulations).

Although its safety in obstetrics has not been established by formal studies, isoflurane is used to provide obstetrical analgesia.

Postpartum—High concentrations of inhalation anesthetics administered during prolonged delivery may increase the risk of neonatal depression.

For methoxyflurane: Inorganic fluoride produced by methoxyflurane metabolism has been detected in cord blood in concentrations that are usually lower than, but sometimes equal to, the maternal blood concentration. The effect of inorganic fluoride on the neonate is not known; however, nephrotoxicity in the infant is thought to be unlikely following recommended doses of methoxyflurane.

### Breast-feeding
Problems in humans have not been documented. However, halothane is distributed into breast milk.

### Pediatrics
Studies performed to date have not demonstrated pediatrics-specific problems that would limit the usefulness of inhalation anesthetics in children. However, the minimum alveolar concentration (MAC) of inhalation anesthetics is higher in children than in adults. The MAC is highest in very young children and decreases as the age of the child increases.

### Geriatrics
The MAC (minimum alveolar concentration) of an anesthetic is decreased in geriatric patients. Also, geriatric patients may be more susceptible to anesthetic-induced hypotension and circulatory depression and to methoxyflurane-induced nephrotoxicity; especially careful attention to dosage is recommended.

### Drug interactions and/or related problems
See *Table 3*, page 163.

### Laboratory value alterations
The following have been selected on the basis of their potential clinical significance (possible effect in parentheses where appropriate)—not necessarily inclusive (» = major clinical significance):

With physiology/laboratory test values
Cerebrospinal fluid (CSF) pressure
(anesthetics may increase CSF pressure)

Liver function
(abnormalities in liver function as shown by transient, mild increases in serum transaminase and/or lactate dehydrogenase activity may occur in the absence of hepatotoxicity; with enflurane, halothane, or methoxyflurane, significant abnormalities indicating hepatotoxicity may occur rarely)

### Medical considerations/Contraindications
See *Table 4*, page 165.

### Patient monitoring
The following may be especially important in patient monitoring (other tests may be warranted in some patients, depending on condition; » = major clinical significance):

*For all inhalation anesthetics*
Blood pressure and
Cardiac/pulse rate and
Cardiac rhythm and
» Respiratory and ventilatory status
(monitoring recommended during anesthetic administration)

Body temperature
(continuous monitoring advisable)

*For methoxyflurane*
» Renal function determinations
(may be needed to detect possible nephrotoxicity if the patient's postoperative urine output is excessive)

## Side/Adverse Effects

Note: Hepatotoxicity ranging in severity from mild jaundice to hepatic necrosis has been reported following administration of enflurane, halothane, or methoxyflurane. Although a definite causal relationship has not been established, it has been proposed that a hypersensitivity reaction to the anesthetic may be involved. Hepatic damage has been reported much less frequently with enflurane or methoxyflurane than with halothane; however, the biochemical, clinical, and histologic features of the hepatotoxicity reported with each of these agents are similar. The risk of hepatotoxicity may be increased by intra- or postoperative hypoxia, repeated or sequential use of these agents, patient predisposition to hepatotoxicity, and patient history of hepatotoxicity not attributable to other causes following previous exposure to one of these anesthetics.

The risk of methoxyflurane-induced nephrotoxicity is related to the total dose (concentration and time) administered, degree of metabolism (which may be increased by hepatic enzyme induction), and

patient predisposition to nephrotoxicity. Although polyuric renal failure has been most often reported, some patients have developed oliguric renal failure. Renal tubular necrosis may occur. Laboratory findings indicative of methoxyflurane-induced nephrotoxicity include elevations of blood sodium, blood urea nitrogen, blood creatinine, serum and urine fluoride, serum chloride, urine oxalic acid, and blood uric acid concentrations, and reductions of urine specific gravity and osmolality. Isolated cases of nephrotoxicity have also been reported with enflurane (following prolonged administration to patients with impaired renal function) and halothane; however, a definite causal relationship has not been established.

Impairment of psychomotor skills may occur following anesthesia and may persist for varying lengths of time, depending upon the anesthetic and/or combination of medications used and the total dosages administered. With halothane, it is thought that the impairment may be at least partially caused by bromide metabolites. Possible adverse effects on the patient's ability to drive or perform other tasks requiring alertness and coordination should be kept in mind when anesthesia is administered for outpatient surgery.

The following side/adverse effects have been selected on the basis of their potential clinical significance (possible signs and symptoms in parentheses)—not necessarily inclusive:*

**Legend:**
**I** = Enflurane
**II** = Halothane
**III** = Isoflurane
**IV** = Methoxyflurane
**V** = Nitrous Oxide

| | I | II | III | IV | V |
|---|---|---|---|---|---|
| **Medical attention needed** | | | | | |
| *Bronchospasm* | R | X | U | R | U |
| *Cardiac arrhythmias*—Supraventricular arrhythmias and bradycardia are relatively common during induction of anesthesia and are not considered dangerous in patients with adequate cardiovascular function. Ventricular arrhythmias are rare in the absence of hypercapnea or hypoxia but may be more likely to occur with halothane. Other arrhythmias reported with halothane include nodal rhythm and atrioventricular dissociation. | R | R | R | R | R |
| *Circulatory depression* | R | R | R | R | R |
| *CNS excitation*—may lead to convulsions | R | X | X | X | X |
| *Emergence delirium, postanesthesia* | L | M | L | L | L |
| *Hepatotoxicity* (black or bloody vomit, severe or continuing headache, loss of appetite, severe or continuing nausea, pain in abdomen, yellow eyes or skin) | R | R | U | R | X |
| *Hypoxia*—with nitrous oxide, diffusion hypoxia may occur after discontinuation unless oxygen is administered | R | R | R | R | R |
| *Leukopenia†*—with prolonged use; may be first sign of reversible bone marrow depression | X | X | X | X | R |
| *Malignant hyperthermic crisis* | R | R | U | R | R |
| *Nephrotoxicity* (increased urination and rapid weight loss or decreased urination and rapid weight gain) | R | R | U | L | U |
| *Neurologic injury†*—with prolonged or repeated exposure | X | X | X | X | R |
| *Respiratory depression* | R | R | R | R | R |
| **Medical attention needed only if continuing or bothersome** | | | | | |
| *Drowsiness, prolonged* | U | U | U | L | U |
| *Headache, mild* | U | R | L | R | U |

| The following side/adverse effects have been selected on the basis of their potential clinical significance (possible signs and symptoms in parentheses)—not necessarily inclusive:* | Legend: I=Enflurane II=Halothane III=Isoflurane IV=Methoxyflurane V=Nitrous Oxide | | | | |
|---|---|---|---|---|---|
| | **I** | **II** | **III** | **IV** | **V** |
| *Nausea or vomiting, mild* | L | L | L | L | M |
| *Shivering or trembling* | M | M | M | L | L |

*Differences in frequency of occurrence may reflect either lack of clinical-use data or actual pharmacologic distinctions among agents. M=more frequent; L=less frequent; R=rare; U=unknown; X=does not occur.

†Operating room or dental office personnel may be at risk for this effect if they are chronically exposed to nitrous oxide because precautions to prevent contamination of the atmosphere in the room in which it is being used are not utilized or are inadequate.

## Overdose

For specific information on the agents used in the management of an inhalation anesthetic overdose, see:

• Atropine in *Anticholinergics/Antispasmodics (Systemic)* monograph; and/or

• *Sympathomimetic Agents—Cardiovascular Use (Parenteral-Systemic)* monograph.

For more information on the management of overdose, **contact a Poison Control Center** (see*Poison Control Center Listing*).

The following effects have been selected on the basis of their potential clinical significance (possible signs and symptoms in parentheses where appropriate)—not necessarily inclusive:

Acute

***Bradycardia; circulatory depression or hypotension, severe; respiratory depression***

**Specific treatment**

For bradycardia—Administering atropine.

For circulatory depression or severe hypotension—Discontinuing or lightening anesthesia (if still being administered) and administering plasma and/or intravenous fluids. If surgical or postsurgical conditions permit, positioning the patient to improve venous return to the heart (i.e., in the Trendelenburg position) is recommended. If necessary, a vasopressor may be administered.

For respiratory depression—Decreasing anesthetic dosage (if still being administered), establishing a clear airway, and instituting assisted or controlled respiration with pure oxygen.

## Patient Consultation

As an aid to patient consultation, refer to *Advice for the Patient, Anesthetics, General (Systemic).*

In providing consultation, consider emphasizing the following selected information (» = major clinical significance):

**Before receiving this medication**

» Conditions affecting use, especially:

Sensitivity to the anesthetic considered for use

Pregnancy—Inhalation anesthetics cross the placenta; enflurane, halothane, and isoflurane may increase the risk of bleeding when used for first trimester abortion; hydrocarbon anesthetics used during labor and delivery may slow delivery, increase bleeding, and cause neonatal depression, depending on dosage

Breast-feeding—Halothane passes into the breast milk

Use in the elderly—Increased risk of adverse effects

Any other medication, including use of "street" drugs

Other medical problems

**Proper use of this medication**

Proper dosing

**Precautions after receiving this medication**

» Possibility of psychomotor impairment following use of anesthetics; using caution in driving or performing other tasks requiring alertness and coordination for about 24 hours postanesthesia

» Avoiding use of alcohol or central nervous system (CNS) depressants within 24 hours following anesthesia unless specifically prescribed or otherwise authorized by physician or dentist

**Side/adverse effects**

Signs and symptoms of potential delayed side effects, especially hepatotoxicity and nephrotoxicity.

## General Dosing Information

Inhalation anesthetics are to be administered only by those individuals experienced in airway management and respiratory support. Equipment and personnel for support of ventilation must be immediately available.

The stated dosages are given as a guideline for use in the average adult. *The dosage of inhaled anesthetics must be individualized* according to surgical requirements; concurrent use of adjuvant medications and/or nitrous oxide; and patient variables, especially age, body temperature, and physical condition.

Anesthetic requirements are increased in very young children and decreased in geriatric patients.

Preanesthetic medications should be selected according to the needs of the individual patient and surgical requirements.

For patients who may be adversely affected by increases in intracranial pressure, measures (such as barbiturate administration or institution of hyperventilation) to reduce or abolish the increase produced by enflurane, halothane, isoflurane, or methoxyflurane should be carried out prior to or concurrently with administration of these agents. However, the fact that hyperventilation may increase the risk of enflurane-induced convulsive activity should be kept in mind.

Administration of inhalation anesthetics other than nitrous oxide to patients with known or suspected susceptibility to malignant hyperthermia should be avoided. Although prophylactic administration of dantrolene prior to anesthesia may prevent the occurrence of a malignant hyperthermic crisis during or shortly following surgery, this use of dantrolene is controversial and should be undertaken with caution. See *Dantrolene (Systemic).*

An intravenous induction agent is often administered prior to an inhalation anesthetic to facilitate induction of anesthesia and prevent the transient initial CNS excitation that may occur with some of the inhaled anesthetics.

Enflurane, halothane, isoflurane, or methoxyflurane may be vaporized in a flow of oxygen or a nitrous oxide–oxygen mixture.

During maintenance of anesthesia, the concentration of inhaled anesthetic may be progressively decreased as necessary to prevent further increases in depth of anesthesia and/or hypotension.

Assisted or controlled respiration may be necessary, especially during deep levels of anesthesia, to control respiratory depression and/or respiratory acidosis.

**For treatment of adverse effects**

Recommended treatment includes:

• For cardiac arrhythmias—Determining whether the level of anesthesia is adequate for the given surgical stimulus and adjusting (deepening or lightening) the level of anesthesia accordingly or discontinuing anesthesia. Also, determining whether the arrhythmia is caused by hypercarbia, hypocarbia, or hypoxia and correcting as required.

• For malignant hyperthermic crisis—Discontinuing administration of possible triggering agents (such as potent inhalation anesthetics, succinylcholine, or stress), managing increased oxygen requirement, cooling the patient, and correcting fluid and electrolyte imbalances and metabolic acidosis. If necessary, administering dantrolene by continuous rapid intravenous push (at least 1 mg per kg of body weight [mg/kg] initially, continued until the symptoms subside or the maximum total dose of 10 mg/kg has been administered). Intravenous dantrolene administration may be repeated if symptoms recur. Dantrolene (4 to 8 mg/kg per day in four divided doses) may be administered orally or intravenously, with caution, for 1 to 3 days postoperatively to prevent recurrence of symptoms.

• For inadequate postoperative ventilation—Decreasing anesthetic dosage (if still being administered), establishing a clear airway, and instituting assisted or controlled respiration with oxygen.

• For emergence delirium—Administering small doses of an opioid (narcotic) analgesic.

---

*ENFLURANE*

## Summary of Differences

Indications:

Indicated in low concentrations to supplement other anesthetics for cesarean section.

Also used in low doses to provide analgesia in obstetrics and for procedures not requiring loss of consciousness.

Pharmacology/pharmacokinetics:

Minimum alveolar concentration (MAC)—

In oxygen: 1.68%.

In 70% nitrous oxide: 0.57%.
Blood-to-gas partition coefficient (37° C)—
1.91.
Oil-to-gas partition coefficient (37° C)—
98.5.
Biotransformation—
2.4% of dose metabolized.
Elimination—
Primary: 80% excreted unchanged by exhalation.
Other actions/effects—
Deeper levels of enflurane anesthesia, especially in the presence of hyperventilation, may produce convulsive activity in electroencephalogram (EEG).
Precautions:
Mutagenicity—
Studies in mice have shown that enflurane may cause sperm abnormalities.
Pregnancy—
May cause dose-dependent uterine relaxation (anesthetic doses). May cause dose-dependent decrease in uterine response to oxytocics.
Drug interactions and/or related problems—
Isoniazid and possibly other hydrazine-containing compounds may increase the formation of potentially nephrotoxic inorganic fluoride metabolite when used concurrently with enflurane.

## Additional Dosing Information

See also *General Dosing Information*.

When enflurane is used for induction of anesthesia, it is recommended that the concentration be increased slowly, i.e., by 0.5% every few breaths.

When assisted or controlled respiration is required, extreme hyperventilation should be avoided in order to minimize the risk of CNS excitation and convulsions.

Following enflurane administration, little or no postoperative analgesia is produced because of its short duration of action. Therefore, earlier administration of analgesics for pain relief may be necessary after enflurane than after other inhalation anesthetics.

## Inhalation Dosage Forms
### ENFLURANE USP

**Usual adult dose**
Anesthetic (general)—
Surgical anesthesia:
Induction—Dosage must be individualized.
Maintenance—Inhalation, 0.5 to 3%.
Supplemental obstetrical anesthesia (for cesarean section):
Inhalation, 0.5 to 1%.
For vaginal delivery in obstetrics:
Inhalation, 0.25 to 1%.

**Usual adult prescribing limits**
For surgical anesthesia—
Induction: The final concentration for induction should not exceed 4.5%.
Maintenance: Maintenance concentration should not exceed 3%.

**Usual pediatric dose**
Dosage must be individualized.

**Product(s) usually available**
U.S.—
(Rx) [*Ēthrane;* GENERIC].
Canada—
(Rx) [*Ēthrane*].

**Packaging and storage**
Store below 40 °C (104 °F), preferably between 15 and 30 °C (59 and 86 °F), unless otherwise specified by manufacturer. Store in a tight, light-resistant container.

---

### HALOTHANE

## Summary of Differences

Indications:
Also used in low concentrations to supplement other anesthetics for cesarean section.
Not recommended for vaginal delivery unless uterine relaxation is required.

Pharmacology/pharmacokinetics:
Minimum alveolar concentration (MAC)—
In oxygen: 0.75%.
In 70% nitrous oxide: 0.29%.
Blood-to-gas partition coefficient (37° C)—
2.3.
Oil-to-gas partition coefficient (37° C)—
224.
Biotransformation—
Up to 20% of dose metabolized.
Elimination—
Primary: 60 to 80% excreted unchanged by exhalation.
Other actions/effects—
Cardiovascular system: Heart/pulse rate decrease.
Respiratory system secretions and salivation decrease.
Precautions:
Mutagenicity—
Potential halothane metabolites have been shown to be mutagenic in the Ames test.
Pregnancy—
May cause uterine relaxation even in low concentrations.
May cause dose-dependent decrease in uterine response to oxytocics.
Breast-feeding—
Halothane is distributed into breast milk.
Drug interactions and/or related problems—
Halothane may prevent or reduce trimethaphan-induced tachycardia.
Halothane greatly sensitizes the myocardium to the effects of sympathomimetics, especially catecholamines, so that the risk of severe ventricular arrhythmias is increased; sympathomimetics should be used with caution and in substantially reduced dosage in patients receiving halothane.
Concurrent use of phenytoin may increase the risk of halothane hepatotoxicity; also, halothane-induced hepatic function impairment may increase the risk of phenytoin toxicity.
Medical considerations/contraindications—
Caution needed in cardiac arrhythmias since halothane may induce or exacerbate arrhythmias.
In pheochromocytoma, there may be an increased risk of cardiac arrhythmias because the patient has high endogenous catecholamine concentrations.

## Inhalation Dosage Forms
### HALOTHANE USP

**Usual adult dose**
Anesthetic (general)—
Induction:
Dosage must be individualized.
Maintenance:
Inhalation, 0.5 to 1.5%.

**Usual pediatric dose**
Dosage must be individualized.

**Product(s) usually available**
U.S.—
(Rx) [*Fluothane;* GENERIC].
Canada—
(Rx) [*Fluothane; Somnothane*].
Other (U.K.)—
(Rx) [*Fluothane*].

**Packaging and storage**
Store below 40 °C (104 °F), preferably between 15 and 30 °C (59 and 86 °F), unless otherwise specified by manufacturer. Store in a tight, light-resistant container.

**Stability**
Stability of halothane is maintained by the addition of thymol and ammonia. Because the thymol does not vaporize along with the halothane, it accumulates in the vaporizer and may lead to a yellow discoloration of the remaining liquid or wick. Discolored solutions should be discarded and the vaporizer and wick cleaned by washing with diethyl ether. Complete removal of the diethyl ether is required to make certain that ether is not introduced into the system.

**Incompatibilities**
Halothane vapor, in the presence of moisture, reacts with aluminum, brass, and lead, but not copper.
Some plastics and rubber are soluble in halothane and will deteriorate rapidly in contact with halothane vapor or liquid.

## ISOFLURANE

## Summary of Differences

Indications:
  Also used in low doses to provide analgesia in obstetrics and for procedures not requiring loss of consciousness, and to supplement other anesthetics for cesarean section.
Pharmacology/pharmacokinetics:
  Minimum alveolar concentration (MAC)—
    In oxygen: 1.15%.
    In 70% nitrous oxide: 0.5%.
  Blood-to-gas partition coefficient (37° C)—
    1.43.
  Oil-to-gas partition coefficient (37° C)—
    97.8.
  Biotransformation—
    0.17% of dose metabolized.
  Elimination—
    Primary: 95% excreted unchanged by exhalation.
  Other actions/effects—
    Cardiac function: No decrease. Reduction in blood pressure is caused primarily by peripheral vasodilation rather than depression of cardiac function; however, recent evidence indicates that isoflurane decreases cardiac function and heart/pulse rate in infants.
    Heart/pulse rate: Increase.
Precautions:
  Pregnancy—
    Animal studies have indicated possible fetotoxicity.
    May cause uterine relaxation (anesthetic concentrations).
    Safety in obstetrics has not been established.

## Additional Dosing Information

See also *General Dosing Information.*

When isoflurane is used for induction of anesthesia, it is recommended that the concentration be increased slowly, i.e., by 0.1 to 0.25% every few breaths.

## Inhalation Dosage Forms
### ISOFLURANE USP

**Usual adult dose**
Anesthetic (general)—
  Induction:
    Inhalation, 1.5 to 3%.
  Maintenance:
    Inhalation, 1 to 3.5%.

**Usual pediatric dose**
Dosage must be individualized.

**Product(s) usually available**
U.S.—
  (Rx) [*Forane*].
Canada—
  (Rx) [*Forane*].
Other (U.K.)—
  (Rx) [*Forane*].

**Packaging and storage**
Store below 40 °C (104 °F), preferably between 15 and 30 °C (59 and 86 °F), unless otherwise specified by manufacturer. Store in a tight, light-resistant container.

## METHOXYFLURANE

## Summary of Differences

Indications:
  Administration of concentrations sufficient to provide muscle relaxation is not recommended.
  Not recommended for vascular surgery at or near the renal blood vessels.
  Also indicated in low doses to provide analgesia in obstetrics and for procedures not requiring loss of consciousness.
  Also used in low concentrations to supplement other anesthetics for cesarean section.
Pharmacology/pharmacokinetics:
  Minimum alveolar concentration (MAC)—
    In oxygen: 0.16%.
    In 70% nitrous oxide: 0.07%.

Blood-to-gas partition coefficient (37° C)—
    10 to 14.
Oil-to-gas partition coefficient (37° C)—
    825 to 970.
Biotransformation—
    50% of dose metabolized.
    A substantial quantity of inorganic fluoride is formed; also metabolized to other potentially nephrotoxic substances.
Time to onset of anesthesia—
    Slow.
Time to change in depth of anesthesia when administered concentration is changed—
    Slow.
Time to recovery from anesthesia—
    May be prolonged.
Elimination—
    Primary: 35% excreted unchanged by exhalation.
Other actions/effects—
    Respiratory system secretions do not increase.
Precautions:
  Pregnancy—
    May cause dose-dependent uterine relaxation.
  Drug interactions and/or related problems—
    Chronic use of hepatic enzyme–inducing agents may increase the formation of nephrotoxic metabolites, leading to increased risk of nephrotoxicity.
    Concurrent use of other nephrotoxic agents may increase the risk of severe nephrotoxicity.
  Medical considerations/contraindications—
    Caution needed in diabetes, uncontrolled or with polyuria or obesity; in renal function impairment or disease; or in toxemia of pregnancy, as methoxyflurane may increase the risk of nephrotoxicity.
  Patient monitoring—
    Monitoring of renal function may be needed to detect possible nephrotoxicity if patient's postoperative urine output is excessive.

## Additional Dosing Information

See also *General Dosing Information.*

A parenteral induction agent is recommended prior to administration of methoxyflurane.

Concurrent administration of at least 50% nitrous oxide is recommended, unless specifically contraindicated, to reduce the methoxyflurane requirement.

During long procedures, it is recommended that methoxyflurane be administered in decreasing concentrations because of the risk of nephrotoxicity. See manufacturer's prescribing information for an example of recommended concentrations at various times following initiation of methoxyflurane administration. Also, it is recommended that administration be limited to 4 hours or less.

Low doses of methoxyflurane may be self-administered using a hand-held inhaler. It is recommended that such use be limited to the briefest practical time and that the patient be under observation by trained personnel. The patient may be transferred to a conventional anesthesia machine if necessary. In obstetrics, methoxyflurane should not be self-administered until relief is necessary.

## Inhalation Dosage Forms
### METHOXYFLURANE USP

**Usual adult dose**
Anesthetic (general)—
  Inhalation, up to 2% administered with at least 50% nitrous oxide and oxygen initially, then decreased to the lowest effective concentration.
For obstetrics or procedures not requiring loss of consciousness—
  Inhalation, 0.3 to 0.8%, intermittently.
  Note: For patient self-administration, no more than a single 15-mL charge of liquid should be available to the patient.

**Usual adult prescribing limits**
For surgical anesthesia, administration should not exceed four hours of 0.25% methoxyflurane or two hours of 0.5% methoxyflurane or the equivalent total dosage.

**Usual pediatric dose**
Dosage must be individualized.

**Product(s) usually available**
U.S.—
  (Rx) [*Penthrane*].

**Packaging and storage**

Store below 40 °C (104 °F), preferably between 15 and 30 °C (59 and 86 °F). Store in a tight, light-resistant container. Protect from freezing.

**Stability**

Solutions of methoxyflurane contain an antioxidant, butylated hydroxytoluene, which may oxidize to a yellow pigment that progressively turns to brown. This substance may accumulate on the vaporizer wick. Diethyl ether may be used to clean the wick; complete removal of the diethyl ether is required to make certain that ether is not introduced into the system.

**Incompatibilities**

Methoxyflurane is very soluble in rubber and in soda lime.

Polyvinyl chloride plastics are extracted by methoxyflurane; contact with such plastics should be avoided.

---

## NITROUS OXIDE

## Summary of Differences

Indications:

Anesthetic potency relatively weak; usually must be supplemented with other agents.

Often given concurrently with one of the more potent inhalation anesthetics to reduce the requirement for the other anesthetic.

Also indicated in low doses to provide analgesia in obstetrics and for procedures not requiring loss of consciousness.

Pharmacology/pharmacokinetics:

Minimum alveolar concentration (MAC) in oxygen—
>100%.

Blood-to-gas partition coefficient (37° C)—
0.47

Oil-to-gas partition coefficient (37° C)—
1.4

Biotransformation—
None of dose metabolized.

Elimination—
Primary: 100% excreted unchanged by exhalation.

Other actions/effects—
Blood pressure generally unchanged.
Heart/pulse rate increases.
Constriction of peripheral vasculature.
No dose-related muscle relaxation.

Precautions:

Pregnancy—
Studies in animals have shown that nitrous oxide causes fetal death, growth retardation, and skeletal anomalies.

Drug interactions and/or related problems—
In addition to the increased central nervous system (CNS) depressant, respiratory depressant, and hypotensive effects that may occur when an anesthetic is used concurrently with any CNS depressant, concurrent use of high doses of fentanyl or its derivatives with nitrous oxide may decrease the heart rate and

cardiac output. These effects may be more pronounced in patients with poor left ventricular function.

Medical considerations/contraindications—
Caution needed in the presence of air-enclosing cavities (such as pulmonary, renal, or occluded middle ear air cysts or air embolism), acute intestinal obstruction, or pneumothorax, or during or recently following the procedure of pneumoencephalography, as nitrous oxide may increase pressure within rigid-walled cavities or volume within nonrigid-walled cavities.

## Additional Dosing Information

See also *General Dosing Information.*

Nitrous oxide must be administered with at least 30% of oxygen to reduce the risk of hypoxia.

**For anesthesia**

Premedication of the patient with an opioid analgesic or a barbiturate may be necessary in order to achieve induction of anesthesia.

Nitrous oxide may diffuse into the cuff of an endotracheal tube; periodic deflation of the endotracheal tube is recommended during administration.

The concentration administered during maintenance of anesthesia must be individualized, depending upon the condition of the patient and the type and quantity of supplemental medications administered.

When prolonged administration of nitrous oxide is discontinued, 100% oxygen should be administered briefly to reduce the risk of diffusion hypoxia.

## Inhalation Dosage Forms

### NITROUS OXIDE USP

**Usual adult dose**

Anesthetic (general)—
Induction:
Inhalation, 70% with 30% of oxygen.
Maintenance:
Inhalation, 30 to 70% with oxygen.

For obstetrics or procedures not requiring loss of consciousness—
Inhalation, 25 to 50% with oxygen.

**Usual pediatric dose**

Dosage must be individualized.

**Product(s) usually available**

U.S.—
(Rx) [GENERIC].

Canada—
(Rx) [GENERIC].

**Packaging and storage**

Store below 40 °C (104 °F), preferably between 15 and 30 °C (59 and 86 °F), unless otherwise specified by manufacturer.

---

Revised: 06/29/90

Interim revision: 08/23/94

## Table 1. Pharmacology/Pharmacokinetics

|  | Enflurane | Halothane | Isoflurane | Methoxyflurane | Nitrous Oxide |
|---|---|---|---|---|---|
| Minimum alveolar concentration (MAC)* | | | | | |
| In oxygen (%) | 1.68 | 0.75 | 1.15 | 0.16 | >100 |
| In 70% Nitrous Oxide (%) | 0.57 | 0.29 | 0.5 | 0.07 | — |
| Blood-to-Gas partition coefficient (37 °C)† | 1.91 | 2.3 | 1.43 | 10–14 | 0.47 |
| Oil-to-Gas partition coefficient (37 °C)‡ | 98.5 | 224 | 97.8 | 825–970 | 1.4 |
| Biotransformation§ | Hepatic | Hepatic | Hepatic | Hepatic | 0 |
| % of dose metabolized# | 2.4 | Up to 20 | 0.17 | 50 | — |
| Quantity of inorganic fluoride formed** | Small | Almost none | Very small | Substantial | — |
| Time to onset of anesthesia†† | Rapid | Rapid | Rapid | Slow | — |
| Time to change in depth of anesthesia when administered concentration changed | Rapid | Rapid | Rapid | Slow | — |
| Time to recovery from anesthesia‡‡ | Rapid | Rapid | Rapid | May be prolonged | Rapid |
| Elimination | | | | | |
| Primary—% excreted unchanged by exhalation | 80 | 60–80 | 95 | 35 | 100 |
| Secondary§§ | Renal | Renal | | Renal | |

*MAC—The minimum alveolar concentration that prevents movement in 50% of patients subjected to a painful stimulus. Slightly higher concentrations may be required to ensure immobility in all patients. MAC decreases with increasing age (being highest in very young children), pregnancy, hypothermia, hypotension, and concurrent use of other CNS depressants. The MACs of individual inhaled anesthetics are additive.

†Indicator of solubility in blood, which affects the rate at which the partial pressure of the anesthetic in the blood (and therefore in the brain) equilibrates with that in the alveoli. Low solubility results in rapid rates of induction, changes in depth of anesthesia, and recovery.

‡Indicator of solubility in fatty tissues. High solubility increases both anesthetic potency and the rate of elimination of the agent from the body.

§Via hepatic microsomal enzymes.

#For enflurane, halothane, and methoxyflurane, the percentage metabolized may be increased by induction of hepatic enzymes.

**Indicator of nephrotoxic potential of agent. For enflurane, the quantity of inorganic fluoride produced is not increased by hepatic enzyme induction, but it may be increased by chronic isoniazid administration. Peak concentrations occur 4 to 12 hours postoperatively with enflurane and 2 to 4 days postoperatively with methoxyflurane. Methoxyflurane is also metabolized to other potentially nephrotoxic substances.

††Rapid=7 to 10 minutes; slow=20 to 30 minutes. The pungent odor of enflurane or isoflurane may cause breath-holding, coughing, or laryngospasm. This may limit the rate at which the administered concentration can be increased, resulting in a slightly longer induction time.

‡‡Dependent on duration of anesthesia, administered concentration of anesthetic, and whether or not other CNS depressants are used. With isoflurane, administration for longer than 3 hours does not further prolong recovery time.

§§Primarily as metabolites. Small quantities of nitrous oxide may also be eliminated through the skin.

## Table 2. Pharmacology/Pharmacokinetics

| Other actions/effects: Action or Body System/Function Affected | Enflurane | Halothane | Isoflurane | Methoxyflurane | Nitrous Oxide |
|---|---|---|---|---|---|
| Analgesia (low concentrations) | Moderate | Relatively poor | | Good | Excellent |
| Brain | | | | | |
| Convulsive activity in electroencephalogram (EEG) | Yes* | No | No | No | No |
| Intracranial pressure† | Increase | Increase | Increase | Increase | May increase |
| Cardiovascular System | | | | | |
| Blood pressure‡ | Decrease | Decrease | Decrease | Decrease | Generally unchanged |
| Cardiac function | Decrease | Decrease | No decrease§ | Decrease | Slight decrease# |
| Circulation (high concentrations) | Depression | Depression | Depression | Depression | |
| Heart/pulse rate | May increase** | Decrease | Increase | May decrease | Increase |
| Peripheral vasculature | Dilation | Dilation | Dilation | | Constriction |
| Intraocular pressure†† | Significant decrease | Slight decrease | | | |
| Muscle relaxation (dose-dependent)‡‡ | Excellent | Moderate | Excellent | | None |
| Pharyngeal and laryngeal reflexes | Decrease | Decrease | Decrease | | |
| Renal function§§ | Decrease | Decrease | Decrease | Decrease | |
| Respiratory System | | | | | |
| Bronchi | Dilation | Dilation | | | |
| Respiration (dose-dependent)## | Depression | Depression | Depression | Depression | Depression |
| Secretions | May increase slightly | Decrease | May increase slightly | No increase | |

## Table 2. Pharmacology/Pharmacokinetics *(continued)*

| Other actions/effects:<br>Action or Body System/Function Affected | Enflurane | Halothane | Isoflurane | Methoxyflurane | Nitrous Oxide |
|---|---|---|---|---|---|
| Salivation | May increase slightly | Decrease | May increase slightly | | |

   \*EEG changes characterized by high voltage and fast frequency progressing through spike-dome complexes alternating with periods of electrical silence to frank seizure activity may occur during deeper levels of enflurane anesthesia, especially in the presence of hyperventilation.

   †With enflurane, halothane, isoflurane (concentration >1.25 MAC), and methoxyflurane, may be caused by increased cerebral blood flow secondary to cerebral vasodilation. This effect may be eliminated by hyperventilation-induced hypocapnea or reduced by barbiturate administration.

   ‡Effect on blood pressure is dose-dependent and is a useful indication of depth of anesthesia. With enflurane or isoflurane, blood pressure may return to near preanesthetic values with surgical stimulation or stress.

   §With isoflurane only, the reduction in blood pressure is caused primarily by peripheral vasodilation rather than depression of cardiac function. However, recent evidence indicates that isoflurane decreases cardiac function and heart/pulse rate in infants.

   #Nitrous oxide may attenuate the cardiovascular effects of other inhaled anesthetics by reducing the requirement for the other anesthetic.

   \*\*With enflurane, the heart rate may be decreased if the preanesthetic heart rate is rapid; however, bradycardia usually does not occur.

   ††With 1% of enflurane or 0.5% of halothane, given with nitrous oxide and oxygen.

   ‡‡Enflurane or isoflurane may produce muscle relaxation sufficient for many types of surgery when used without a neuromuscular blocking agent.

   §§Effect is dose-dependent; reduction in glomerular filtration rate, renal blood flow, and urine volume may reflect decreased mean arterial pressure.

   ##Respiratory depression may be partially reversed with surgical stimulation or stress.

## Table 3. Drug Interactions and/or Related Problems

| The following drug interactions and/or related problems have been selected on the basis of their potential clinical significance (possible mechanism in parentheses where appropriate)—not necessarily inclusive (» = major clinical significance):<br><br>Note: Combinations containing any of the following medications, depending on the amount present, may also interact with this medication. | Legend:<br>I=Enflurane<br>II=Halothane<br>III=Isoflurane<br>IV=Methoxyflurane<br>V=Nitrous Oxide |
|---|---|

| | I | II | III | IV | V |
|---|---|---|---|---|---|
| Alcohol, chronic ingestion<br>   (may increase anesthetic requirement) | ✔ | ✔ | ✔ | ✔ | ✔ |
| Alfentanil or<br>Fentanyl or<br>Sufentanil<br>   (in addition to the increased central nervous system [CNS] depressant, respiratory depressant, and hypotensive effects that may occur when an anesthetic is used concurrently with any CNS depressant, concurrent use of high doses of fentanyl or its derivatives with nitrous oxide may decrease heart rate and cardiac output; these effects may be more pronounced in patients with poor left ventricular function) | | | | | ✔ |
| » Aminoglycosides, systemic, or<br>» Capreomycin or<br>» Citrate-anticoagulated blood (massive transfusions) or<br>» Lincomycins, systemic, or<br>» Neuromuscular blocking agents, nondepolarizing, or<br>» Polymyxins, systemic<br>   (caution should be used in concurrent administration with halogenated anesthetics, especially enflurane or isoflurane, because of the possibility of additive neuromuscular blockade; although increased or prolonged skeletal muscle weakness and respiratory depression or paralysis [apnea] may occur, clinical significance is minimal if the patient is being mechanically ventilated; however, dosage of nondepolarizing neuromuscular blocking agents should be decreased to ¹/₂ to ¹/₃ of the usual dose or as determined using a peripheral nerve stimulator; treatment with anticholinesterase agents or calcium salts may help reverse the blockade, but calcium salts are not recommended if tubocurarine has been given because they may potentiate, rather than reverse, its effects) | ✔ | ✔ | ✔ | ✔ | |
| Amiodarone<br>   (concurrent use with inhalation anesthetics may potentiate hypotension and increase the risk of atropine-resistant bradycardia) | ✔ | ✔ | ✔ | ✔ | ✔ |
| Anticoagulants, coumarin- or indandione-derivative<br>   (inhalation anesthetics have been reported to increase the effects of these anticoagulants; although clinical significance has not been determined, the possibility of increased anticoagulation during or shortly following concurrent use should be considered) | ✔ | ✔ | ✔ | ✔ | ✔ |
| Antihypertensive agents, especially diazoxide or ganglionic blockers such as guanadrel, guanethidine, mecamylamine, or trimethaphan, or<br>Chlorpromazine or<br>Diuretics or<br>Hypotension-producing medications, other (See *Appendix II*)<br>   (hypotensive effects may be potentiated when these medications are used concurrently with inhalation anesthetics; patients should be monitored for excessive fall in blood pressure during and following concurrent use)<br><br>   (halothane may prevent or reduce trimethaphan-induced tachycardia) | ✔ | ✔<br><br>✔ | ✔ | ✔ | ✔ |

## Table 3. Drug Interactions and/or Related Problems *(continued)*

| | I | II | III | IV | V |
|---|---|---|---|---|---|

Legend:
**I**=Enflurane
**II**=Halothane
**III**=Isoflurane
**IV**=Methoxyflurane
**V**=Nitrous Oxide

| | I | II | III | IV | V |
|---|---|---|---|---|---|
| **Antimyasthenics**<br>(antimyasthenics, especially neostigmine and pyridostigmine, may decrease neuromuscular blocking activity of halogenated hydrocarbon anesthetics; also, the neuromuscular blocking activity of these anesthetics, especially enflurane or isoflurane, may interfere with the efficacy of antimyasthenics so that temporary dosage adjustment may be required to control symptoms of myasthenia gravis postoperatively) | ✔ | ✔ | ✔ | ✔ | |
| **Beta-adrenergic blocking agents, including ophthalmic betaxolol, levobunolol, or timolol**<br>(concurrent use with hydrocarbon inhalation anesthetics may result in prolonged severe hypotension because the beta-blockade reduces the ability of the heart to respond to beta-adrenergically mediated sympathetic reflex stimuli; if necessary to reverse the effects of beta-adrenergic blocking agents during surgery, agonists such as dobutamine, dopamine, isoproterenol, or norepinephrine may be used but should be administered with caution, especially in patients receiving halothane. Some clinicians recommend gradual withdrawal of beta-adrenergic blocking agents 48 hours prior to elective surgery; however, this recommendation is controversial) | ✔ | ✔ | ✔ | ✔ | |
| (it is recommended that high concentrations of halothane [3% or above] or other halogenated hydrocarbon anesthetics not be used when labetalol is used to produce controlled hypotension during surgery; possible additive effects may lead to excessive hypotension, large reduction in cardiac output, and increased central venous pressure) | ✔ | ✔ | ✔ | ✔ | |
| » Catecholamines such as dopamine, epinephrine, or norepinephrine, or<br>» Cocaine or<br>» Ephedrine or<br>» Levodopa or<br>» Metaraminol or<br>» Methoxamine or<br>Other sympathomimetic agents<br>(halothane greatly sensitizes the myocardium to the effects of sympathomimetics, especially catecholamines, so that the risk of severe ventricular arrhythmias is increased; sympathomimetics should be used with caution and in substantially reduced dosage in patients receiving halothane) | | ✔ | | | |
| (enflurane, isoflurane, or methoxyflurane may also cause some sensitization of the myocardium to the effects of sympathomimetics; caution is recommended during concurrent use) | ✔ | | ✔ | ✔ | |
| (levodopa increases endogenous dopamine concentration and should be discontinued 6 to 8 hours prior to anesthesia with these agents, especially halothane) | ✔ | ✔ | ✔ | ✔ | |
| **CNS depression–producing medications, other, including those commonly used for preanesthetic medication or induction or supplementation of anesthesia (See *Appendix II*)**<br>(concurrent administration may increase the CNS depressant, respiratory depressant, and hypotensive effects of inhalation anesthetics; decrease anesthetic requirement; and prolong recovery from anesthesia; careful attention to the dosage of each agent is required) | ✔ | ✔ | ✔ | ✔ | ✔ |
| **Doxapram**<br>(doxapram may cause catecholamine release; it is recommended that initiation of doxapram therapy be delayed for at least 10 minutes following discontinuation of anesthetics known to sensitize the myocardium to catecholamines) | ✔ | ✔ | ✔ | ✔ | |
| **Hepatic enzyme–inducing agents (See *Appendix II*)**<br>(chronic use of these medications prior to anesthesia may increase anesthetic metabolism leading to increased risk of hepatotoxicity) | ✔ | ✔ | | ✔ | |
| (chronic use of these medications prior to anesthesia may increase formation of nephrotoxic metabolites leading to increased risk of nephrotoxicity) | | | | ✔ | |
| **Isoniazid and possibly other hydrazine-containing compounds**<br>(may increase formation of the potentially nephrotoxic inorganic fluoride metabolite when used concurrently with enflurane) | ✔ | | | | |
| **Ketamine**<br>(volatile anesthetics may prolong elimination half-life of ketamine; recovery from anesthesia may be prolonged) | ✔ | ✔ | ✔ | ✔ | |
| **Methyldopa**<br>(concurrent use with general anesthetics may decrease the anesthetic requirement) | ✔ | ✔ | ✔ | ✔ | ✔ |
| » **Nephrotoxic agents, other (See *Appendix II*)**<br>(may increase the risk of severe nephrotoxicity if administered prior to, during, or following administration of methoxyflurane; concurrent or sequential use is generally not recommended) | | | | ✔ | |

## Table 3. Drug Interactions and/or Related Problems *(continued)*

| | Legend:<br>**I**=Enflurane<br>**II**=Halothane<br>**III**=Isoflurane<br>**IV**=Methoxyflurane<br>**V**=Nitrous Oxide | | | | |
|---|---|---|---|---|---|
| | **I** | **II** | **III** | **IV** | **V** |
| Nitrous oxide<br>(concurrent administration with another inhalation anesthetic reduces the requirement for the other anesthetic and may therefore attenuate some of its cardiovascular effects) | ✔ | ✔ | ✔ | ✔ | |
| Oxytocics<br>(enflurane [concentrations >1.5%], halothane [concentrations >1%], or possibly isoflurane produces a dose-dependent decrease in the uterine response to oxytocics and may abolish the response if sufficient concentrations [>3% of enflurane] are administered; uterine hemorrhage may result) | ✔ | ✔ | ✔ | | |
| Phenytoin<br>(concurrent use may increase the risk of halothane hepatotoxicity; also, halothane-induced hepatic function impairment may increase the risk of phenytoin toxicity) | | ✔ | | | |
| Ritodrine, intravenous<br>(concurrent use of halogenated hydrocarbon anesthetics may lead to potentiation of ritodrine's cardiovascular effects, especially cardiac arrhythmias or hypotension) | ✔ | ✔ | ✔ | ✔ | |
| Succinylcholine<br>(concurrent use with halogenated hydrocarbon anesthetics may increase the risk of malignant hyperthermia; also, repeated concurrent use may increase the risk of bradycardia) | ✔ | ✔ | ✔ | ✔ | |
| (halogenated hydrocarbon anesthetics may potentiate succinylcholine-induced neuromuscular blockade but to a lesser extent than they potentiate the effects of nondepolarizing neuromuscular blocking agents) | ✔ | ✔ | ✔ | ✔ | |
| Xanthines<br>(concurrent use with anesthetics, especially halothane, may increase the risk of cardiac arrhythmias) | ✔ | ✔ | ✔ | ✔ | ✔ |

## Table 4. Medical considerations/Contraindications

| The medical considerations/contraindications included have been selected on the basis of their potential clinical significance (reasons given in parentheses where appropriate)—not necessarily inclusive (» = major clinical significance). | Legend:<br>**I**=Enflurane<br>**II**=Halothane<br>**III**=Isoflurane<br>**IV**=Methoxyflurane<br>**V**=Nitrous Oxide | | | | |
|---|---|---|---|---|---|
| | **I** | **II** | **III** | **IV** | **V** |
| ***Except under special circumstances, these medications should not be used when the following medical problem exists:*** | | | | | |
| »   Malignant hyperthermia, history of or suspected genetic predisposition to<br>(risk of malignant hyperthermic crisis during or following anesthesia) | ✔ | ✔ | ✔ | ✔ | |
| ***Risk-benefit should be considered when the following medical problems exist:*** | | | | | |
| Air-enclosing cavities, such as pulmonary, renal, or occluded middle ear air cysts or air embolism, or<br>Intestinal obstruction, acute, or<br>Pneumoencephalography, during or recently following the procedure (pneumoencephalography), or<br>Pneumothorax<br>(may increase pressure within rigid-walled cavities or volume within nonrigid-walled cavities) | | | | | ✔ |
| Biliary tract disease or<br>»   Hepatic function impairment or disease or<br>»   Jaundice or acute hepatic damage, not attributable to other causes, following previous exposure to enflurane, halothane, or methoxyflurane<br>(increased risk of hepatotoxicity) | ✔ | ✔ | | ✔ | |
| Cardiac arrhythmias<br>(may be induced or exacerbated) | | ✔ | | | |
| Diabetes, uncontrolled or with polyuria or obesity, or<br>»   Renal function impairment or disease or<br>»   Toxemia of pregnancy<br>(increased risk of nephrotoxicity) | | | | ✔ | |

## Table 4. Medical considerations/Contraindications *(continued)*

| | Legend:<br>**I**=Enflurane<br>**II**=Halothane<br>**III**=Isoflurane<br>**IV**=Methoxyflurane<br>**V**=Nitrous Oxide | | | | |
| --- | --- | --- | --- | --- | --- |
| | **I** | **II** | **III** | **IV** | **V** |
| Head injury or<br>Increased intracranial pressure, pre-existing, or<br>Intracranial lesions, space-occupying, or tumors<br>(may increase intracranial pressure) | ✔ | ✔ | ✔ | ✔ | ✔ |
| Myasthenia gravis<br>(muscle weakness may be increased because of neuromuscular blocking effects of anesthetics, especially enflurane and isoflurane) | ✔ | ✔ | ✔ | ✔ | |
| Pheochromocytoma<br>(increased risk of cardiac arrhythmias because patient has high endogenous catecholamine concentrations) | | ✔ | | | |
| Sensitivity to the anesthetic being considered for use, history of | ✔ | ✔ | ✔ | ✔ | ✔ |

# ANGIOTENSIN-CONVERTING ENZYME (ACE) INHIBITORS    Systemic

This monograph includes information on the following: Benazepril†; Captopril; Enalapril; Fosinopril†; Lisinopril; Quinapril†; Ramipril†.

VA CLASSIFICATION (Primary/Secondary):
  Benazepril—CV800/CV490; CV900
  Captopril—CV800/CV490; CV900
  Enalapril—CV800/CV490; CV900
  Fosinopril—CV800/CV490; CV900
  Lisinopril—CV800/CV490; CV900
  Quinapril—CV800/CV490; CV900
  Ramipril—CV800/CV490; CV900

Note: For a listing of dosage forms and brand names by country availability, see *Dosage Forms* section(s). For a listing of brand names for the articles in this monograph, refer to the General Index.

  †Not commercially available in Canada.

## Category

Antihypertensive—Benazepril; Captopril; Enalapril; Fosinopril; Lisinopril; Quinapril; Ramipril.
Vasodilator, congestive heart failure—Benazepril; Captopril; Enalapril; Lisinopril; Quinapril; Ramipril.

## Indications

Note: Bracketed information in the *Indications* section refers to uses that are not included in U.S. product labeling.

### Accepted

Hypertension (treatment)—Angiotensin-converting enzyme (ACE) inhibitors are indicated, alone or in combination with a thiazide diuretic, in the treatment of hypertension.

  For additional information on initial therapeutic guidelines related to the treatment of hypertension, see *Appendix III*.

  [Captopril is also used for treatment of neonatal hypertension.][1]

  ACE inhibitors are also used for [treatment of malignant, refractory, or accelerated hypertension][1], and for treatment of renovascular hypertension (except in patients with bilateral renal artery stenoses or renal artery stenosis in a solitary kidney—See *Medical considerations/contraindications*).

Congestive heart failure (treatment)—Captopril, enalapril, lisinopril, [benazepril], [quinapril] , and [ramipril] are also indicated, in combination with diuretics and digitalis therapy, for treatment of congestive heart failure not responding to other measures.

  [Captopril is used for the treatment of congestive heart failure secondary to ventricular left-to-right shunt not responding to standard therapy in infants and neonates.]

Left ventricular dysfunction, asymptomatic (treatment)[1]—Enalapril is indicated for the treatment of left ventricular dysfunction (ejection fraction ≤ 35%) in clinically stable patients who are asymptomatic. Enalapril has been shown to decrease the rate of development of overt heart failure and decrease the frequency of hospitalization secondary to heart failure.

Left ventricular dysfunction following myocardial infarction (treatment)[1]—Captopril is indicated following myocardial infarction in clinically stable patients with left ventricular dysfunction (ejection fraction ≤ 40%) to improve survival and decrease the incidence of overt heart failure and subsequent hospitalization for congestive heart failure.

Diabetic nephropathy (treatment)[1]—Captopril may be used in the treatment of nephropathy in patients with Type I insulin-dependent diabetes mellitus (IDDM). Captopril has been shown to slow the progression of diabetic nephropathy in normotensive and hypertensive IDDM patients with documented diabetic retinopathy, a serum creatinine concentration of ≤ 2.5 mg per deciliter, and urinary protein excretion of ≥ 500 mg in 24 hours. The greatest effect has been seen in those patients with poorer renal function at baseline (mean serum creatinine concentration ≥ 1.5 mg per deciliter).

[Scleroderma, hypertension in (treatment)][1] or
[Scleroderma, renal crisis in (treatment)][1]—ACE inhibitors are also used for treatment of hypertension or renal crisis in scleroderma.

  [1]Not included in Canadian product labeling.

## Pharmacology/Pharmacokinetics

### Physicochemical characteristics

Molecular weight—
  Benazepril hydrochloride: 460.96.
  Captopril: 217.28.
  Enalapril: 492.52.
  Enalaprilat (active metabolite): 384.43.
  Fosinopril sodium: 585.65.
  Lisinopril: 441.52.
  Quinapril hydrochloride: 474.98.
  Ramipril: 416.52.
pKa—
  Captopril: 3.7 and 9.8 (apparent).

### Mechanism of action/Effect

Benazepril—Benazeprilat (active metabolite)
Captopril—Not a prodrug
Enalapril—Enalaprilat (active metabolite)
Fosinopril—Fosinoprilat (active metabolite)
Lisinopril—Not a prodrug
Quinapril—Quinaprilat (active metabolite)
Ramipril—Ramiprilat (active metabolite)
Antihypertensive—Exact mechanism of antihypertensive action is unknown but is thought to be related to competitive inhibition of angiotensin I–converting enzyme (ACE) activity, resulting in a decreased rate of conversion of angiotensin I to angiotensin II, which is a potent vasoconstrictor. Decreased angiotensin II concentrations result in a secondary increase in plasma renin activity (PRA), through removal of the negative feedback of renin release, and a direct reduction in

aldosterone secretion. ACE inhibitors may be less effective in control of blood pressures among hypertensives with low as compared to normal or high renin activity. ACE inhibitors reduce peripheral arterial resistance. In addition, a possible effect on the kallikrein-kinin system (interference with degradation and resulting increased concentrations of bradykinin) and an increase in prostaglandin synthesis have been suggested but not proven.

Vasodilator, congestive heart failure—Decrease in peripheral vascular (afterload) resistance, pulmonary capillary wedge pressure (preload), and pulmonary vascular resistance; and improved cardiac output and exercise tolerance.

## Other actions/effects

Captopril may reduce proteinuria in hypertensive patients with diabetic nephropathy. This effect may be due to the beneficial change in intrarenal hemodynamics (renal vasodilatation and reduced filtration pressure) produced by captopril resulting in decreased urinary protein excretion.

## Absorption

Benazepril—At least 37% absorbed from the gastrointestinal tract.

Captopril—Rapidly and at least 75% absorbed from the gastrointestinal tract. Absorption is reduced by 30 to 55% in the presence of food.

Enalapril—Approximately 60%; not affected by the presence of food.

Fosinopril—Slowly; about 36% absorbed from the gastrointestinal tract. Absorption rate may be decreased in presence of food, but extent of absorption is not affected.

Lisinopril—Approximately 25%, but widely variable between individuals (6 to 60%); not affected by the presence of food.

Quinapril—Approximately 60%; presence of food does not affect extent of absorption, but may increase the time to peak drug concentration. High-fat meals may moderately decrease absorption.

Ramipril—Rapidly and at least 50 to 60% absorbed from the gastrointestinal tract. Extent of absorption is not affected by the presence of food; however, the rate of absorption is reduced.

## Protein binding

Benazepril—Very high (96.7%).

Benazeprilat (active metabolite)—Very high (95.3%).

Captopril—Low (25 to 30%), primarily to albumin.

Enalaprilat—Moderate (50 to 60%).

Fosinoprilat (active metabolite)—Very high (97 to 98%).

Lisinopril—None.

Quinaprilat (active metabolite)—Very high (97%).

Ramipril—High (73%).

Ramiprilat (active metabolite)—High (56%).

## Biotransformation

Benazepril—Hepatic, to benazeprilat, the active metabolite.

Captopril—Hepatic.

Enalapril—Hepatic, by hydrolysis, to enalaprilat, the active metabolite.

Enalaprilat—None.

Fosinopril—Hepatic, gastrointestinal mucosa; by hydrolysis to fosinoprilat, the active metabolite.

Lisinopril—None.

Quinapril—Hepatic, gastrointestinal tract, extravascular tissue; by hydrolysis to quinaprilat, the active metabolite.

Ramipril—Hepatic.

## Half-life

Benazepril—0.6 hours.

Benazeprilat (active metabolite)—Effective accumulation half-life is 10 to 11 hours.

Captopril—Less than 3 hours; increased in renal failure (3.5 to 32 hours).

Enalaprilat—11 hours; increased in renal failure.

Fosinoprilat (active metabolite)—Effective accumulation half-life is approximately 11.5 hours.

Lisinopril—12 hours; increased in renal failure.

Quinapril—Approximately 1 to 2 hours.

Quinaprilat (active metabolite)—Effective accumulation half-life is approximately 3 hours.

Ramipril—5.1 hours.

Ramiprilat (active metabolite)—Effective accumulation half-life is 13 to 17 hours; increased in renal failure.

## Onset of action

Single dose—

Benazepril: Within 1 hour.

Captopril: 15 to 60 minutes.

Enalapril: 1 hour.

Enalaprilat (intravenous): 15 minutes.

Fosinopril: Within 1 hour.

Lisinopril: 1 hour.

Quinapril: Within 1 hour.

Ramipril: Within 1 to 2 hours.

## Time to peak serum concentration

Benazepril—0.5 to 1 hour.

Benazeprilat (active metabolite)—1 to 1.5 hours.

Captopril—30 to 90 minutes.

Enalapril—1 hour (3 to 4 hours for enalaprilat).

Enalaprilat (intravenous)—15 minutes.

Fosinoprilat (active metabolite)—2 to 4 hours.

Lisinopril—7 hours.

Quinapril—Within 1 hour.

Quinaprilat (active metabolite)—Within 2 hours.

Ramipril—Within 1 hour.

Ramiprilat (active metabolite)—3 hours.

## Time to peak effect

Single dose—

Benazepril: 2 to 4 hours.

Captopril: 60 to 90 minutes.

Enalapril: 4 to 6 hours.

Enalaprilat (intravenous): 1 to 4 hours.

Fosinopril: 2 to 6 hours.

Lisinopril: 6 hours.

Quinapril: 2 to 4 hours.

Ramipril: 4 to 6.5 hours.

Multiple doses—

The full therapeutic effect may not be noticed until several weeks after initiation of oral therapy.

## Duration of action

Single-dose—

Benazepril: Approximately 24 hours.

Captopril: Approximately 6 to 12 hours; dose related.

Enalapril: Approximately 24 hours.

Enalaprilat (intravenous): Approximately 6 hours.

Fosinopril: Approximately 24 hours.

Lisinopril: Approximately 24 hours.

Quinapril: Up to 24 hours; dose related.

Ramipril: Approximately 24 hours.

## Elimination

Benazepril—

Predominantly renal.

Nonrenal (biliary): 11 to 12%.

In dialysis: Benazeprilat is slightly removable by hemodialysis.

Captopril—

Renal: More than 95%; 40 to 50% unchanged (may be less in patients with congestive heart failure); remainder as metabolites.

In dialysis: Captopril is removable by hemodialysis.

Enalapril—

Renal: 60% (20% as enalapril and 40% as enalaprilat).

Fecal: 33% (6% as enalapril and 27% as enalaprilat).

In dialysis: Enalaprilat is removable by hemodialysis, at the rate of 62 mL per minute, and by peritoneal dialysis.

Enalaprilat—

Renal: 100% unchanged.

In dialysis: Enalaprilat is removable by hemodialysis at the rate of 62 mL per minute.

Fosinopril—

Renal: 44 to 50%.

Fecal: 46 to 50%.

In dialysis: Fosinopril is not well dialyzed. Fosinoprilat clearance by hemodialysis and peritoneal dialysis is approximately 2% and 7%, respectively, of urea clearance.

Lisinopril—

Renal: 100% unchanged.

In dialysis: Lisinopril is removable by hemodialysis.

Quinapril—

Renal: 61% (56% as quinapril and quinaprilat).

Fecal: 37%.

In dialysis: Minimal effect on the elimination of quinapril and quinaprilat.

Ramipril—

Renal: Approximately 60%.

Fecal: Approximately 40%.

In dialysis: It is not known whether ramipril or ramiprilat is removable by hemodialysis.

# Precautions to Consider

## Cross-sensitivity and/or related problems

Patients sensitive to one ACE inhibitor may also be sensitive to another.

## Carcinogenicity

*Benazepril*—Studies in mice and rats given doses of 150 mg per kg of body weight (mg/kg) per day (110 times the maximum recommended human dose by weight) for up to 2 years, revealed no evidence of carcinogenicity.

*Captopril*—Two-year studies in mice and rats at doses of 50 to 1350 mg/kg per day showed no evidence of carcinogenicity.

*Enalapril*—Studies in rats for 106 weeks and in mice for 94 weeks at doses up to 150 and 300 times the maximum daily human dose (based on a patient weight of 50 kg), respectively, found no evidence of tumorigenicity or carcinogenicity.

*Enalaprilat* (intravenous)—Studies have not been done. However, since actions of enalapril maleate are caused by enalaprilat, the active metabolite, the same information would be expected to apply.

*Fosinopril*—Studies in mice and rats given doses up to 400 mg/kg per day for up to 24 months, revealed no evidence of carcinogenicity. However, a slightly higher incidence of mesentery/omentum lipomas was found in male rats given the highest dose level (about 250 times the maximum human dose by weight).

*Lisinopril*—Studies in male and female rats for 105 weeks at doses up to 56 times the maximum recommended human daily dose (based on a patient weight of 50 kg) and in male and female mice for 92 weeks at doses up to 84 times the maximum recommended human daily dose (based on a patient weight of 50 kg) found no evidence of tumorigenicity.

*Quinapril*—Studies in mice and rats given doses up to 75 or 100 mg/kg per day (50 to 60 times the maximum recommended human daily dose by weight) for 104 weeks, revealed no evidence of carcinogenicity. However, female rats given the highest dose level had an increased incidence of mesenteric lymph node hemangiomas and skin/subcutaneous lipomas.

*Ramipril*—Studies in rats and mice given doses up to 500 mg/kg per day for 24 months and up to 1000 mg/kg per day for 18 months, respectively, revealed no evidence of tumorigenicity. Renal juxtaglomerular apparatus hypertrophy was found in mice, rats, dogs, and monkeys given doses greatly in excess of recommended human doses.

## Mutagenicity

*Benazepril*—No evidence of mutagenicity was found in tests including the Ames bacterial assay (with or without metabolic activation), an *in vitro* test for forward mutations in cultured mammalian cells, and a nucleus anomaly test.

*Enalapril* and *enalaprilat*—No evidence of mutagenicity was found in tests including the Ames bacterial assay with or without metabolic activation, rec-assay, reverse mutation assay with *E. coli*, sister chromatid exchange with cultured mammalian cells, the micronucleus test with mice, and in an *in vivo* cytogenic study using mouse bone marrow.

*Fosinopril*—No evidence of mutagenicity was found in tests including the Ames bacterial assay, the mouse lymphoma forward mutation assay, and a mitotic gene conversion assay. No evidence of genotoxicity was found in a mouse micronucleus test *in vivo* and a mouse bone marrow cytogenetic assay *in vivo*. An increased frequency of chromosomal aberrations was found in the Chinese hamster ovary cell cytogenetic assay at toxic cell concentrations tested without metabolic activation. However, this increase was not found at lower drug concentrations without metabolic activation or at any other concentration with metabolic activation.

*Lisinopril*—No evidence of mutagenicity was found in tests including the Ames bacterial assay with or without metabolic activation, forward mutation assay using Chinese hamster lung cells, *in vitro* alkaline elution rat hepatocyte assay, and chromosomal aberration studies *in vitro* in Chinese hamster ovary cells and *in vivo* in mouse bone marrow.

*Quinapril*—No evidence of mutagenicity was found in the Ames bacterial assay with or without metabolic activation.

*Ramipril*—No evidence of mutagenicity was found in tests including the Ames bacterial assay, the micronucleus test in mice, unscheduled DNA synthesis in a human cell line, and a forward gene-mutation assay in a Chinese hamster ovary cell line.

## Pregnancy/Reproduction

Fertility—*Benazepril:* No adverse effect on the reproductive performance of male and female rats was found.

*Captopril:* No impairment of fertility was found in rats.

*Enalapril:* No adverse effects on reproductive performance were found in male and female rats given 10 to 90 mg/kg per day of enalapril.

*Fosinopril:* No adverse reproductive effects were found in male and female rats given doses up to 60 mg/kg per day (about 38 times the maximum recommended human dose by weight). However, a slight increase in pairing time was observed in rats given a toxic dose of 240 mg/kg per day (150 times the maximum recommended human dose by weight).

*Lisinopril:* No adverse effects on reproductive performance were found in male and female rats given doses up to 300 mg/kg per day of lisinopril.

*Quinapril:* No adverse effects on fertility or reproduction were found in rats given doses up to 100 mg/kg per day (60 times the maximum daily human dose based on weight).

*Ramipril:* No impairment of fertility was found in rats given doses up to 500 mg/kg per day.

Pregnancy—In humans, ACE inhibitors can cause fetal and neonatal morbidity and mortality when administered to pregnant women. ACE inhibitors should be discontinued as soon as possible when pregnancy is detected.

ACE inhibitors cross the placenta. Fetal exposure to ACE inhibitors during the second and third trimesters can cause hypotension, renal failure, anuria, skull hypoplasia, and even death in the newborn. Maternal oligohydramnios has also been reported, probably reflecting decreasing fetal renal function.

Enalapril and lisinopril have been removed from neonatal circulation by peritoneal dialysis. Captopril is not removable by peritoneal dialysis. There are inadequate data concerning the effectiveness of hemodialysis and there is no information concerning use of exchange transfusion for removing captopril from general circulation. There has been no experience with hemodialysis, peritoneal dialysis, or exchange transfusion for removing benazepril, fosinopril, quinapril, or ramipril from neonatal circulation.

It is recommended that infants exposed in utero to ACE inhibitors be closely observed for hypotension, oliguria, and hyperkalemia. Oliguria should be treated with support of blood pressure and renal perfusion by administration of fluids and pressors as appropriate.

*Benazepril:* Studies in pregnant rats, mice, and rabbits at doses 300, 90, and more than 3 times, respectively, the maximum recommended human dose by weight, revealed no embryotoxic, fetotoxic, or teratogenic effects.

*Captopril:* Several cases of intrauterine growth retardation, fetal distress and hypotension, and one case of cranial malformation have been reported. Neonatal deaths have occurred in rats at up to 400 times the recommended human dose. Fetal deaths have occurred when rabbits were given 2 to 70 times the maximum recommended human dose and a low incidence of cranial malformations occurred in offspring. No teratogenicity has been noted in hamsters or rats.

*Enalapril:* Fetal toxicity (decrease in average fetal weight) has occurred in rats at doses of enalapril 2000 times the maximum daily human dose, and maternal and fetal toxicity has occurred in rabbits at doses almost double the maximum daily human dose. In some cases, saline supplementation prevented maternal and fetal toxicity. No teratogenicity has been noted in rabbits and neither fetal toxicity nor teratogenicity occurred in rats at doses up to 333 times the maximum daily human dose.

*Fosinopril:* Maternal toxicity was evident in pregnant rabbits given doses up to 40 mg/kg per day (about 50 times the maximum recommended human dose). Fosinopril at doses up to 40 mg/kg per day (about 50 times the maximum recommended human dose) was embryocidal in rabbits, probably due to marked decreases in blood pressure secondary to ACE inhibition in this species. There was no evidence of teratogenicity in rabbits at any dosage level. Maternal toxicity was evident in pregnant rats at all dose levels tested up to 400 mg/kg per day (about 500 times the maximum recommended human dose). Furthermore, all dose levels produced slight reductions in placental weights and some degree of skeletal ossification. High doses resulted in reduced fetal body weight. Three similar orofacial malformations and one fetus with situs inversus occurred in animals given fosinopril. It is uncertain whether these anomalies were associated with drug treatment.

*Lisinopril:* Lisinopril was not teratogenic in mice given doses up to 625 times the maximum recommended human dose on days 6 to 15 of gestation; an increase in fetal resorptions occurred at doses of 62.5 times the maximum recommended human dose, but was prevented at doses of 625 times the maximum recommended human dose by saline supplementation. No fetotoxicity or teratogenicity occurred in rats given doses up to 188 times the maximum recommended human dose on days 6 to 17 of gestation, but an increased incidence of pup deaths and a lower average birth weight (both preventable by saline supplementation) occurred postpartum in rats given lisinopril on day 15 of gestation through day 21 postpartum. Lisinopril crosses the placenta in rats but has not been found in the fetus. Lisinopril did not cause teratogenicity in saline-supplemented rabbits given doses up to 1 mg/kg per day, but did cause fetotoxicity (increased fetal resorptions, increased incidence of incomplete ossification).

*Quinapril:* Quinapril at doses as high as 300 mg/kg per day (180 times the maximum daily human dose by weight) did not produce fetotoxic or teratogenic effects in rats, despite maternal toxicity at 150 mg/kg per day. However, reduced offspring body weight was observed at doses greater than 25 mg/kg per day, and changes in renal histology (juxtaglomerular cell hypertrophy, tubular/pelvic dilation, glomerulosclerosis) were seen in dams and offspring given 150 mg/kg per day when tested later in gestation and during lactation. Quinapril did not produce teratogenic effects in rabbits. However, in some rabbits maternal toxicity and embryotoxicity were observed at doses as low as 0.5 mg/kg per day (one time the recommended human dose) and 1.0 mg/kg per day.

*Ramipril:* Studies in rats, mice, monkeys, and rabbits at doses up to 2500 times (in rats and mice), more than 12 times, and more than 2 times, respectively, the maximum recommended human dose by weight, revealed an increased incidence of dilated renal pelvises in rat fetuses and retarded birth weights in mice. However, these studies did not show ramipril to produce terata or to affect fertility, reproductive performance, or pregnancy.

*For all ACE inhibitors:*
FDA Pregnancy Category C—First trimester.
FDA Pregnancy Category D—Second and third trimesters.

### Breast-feeding

*Benazepril*—Benazepril and benazeprilat are distributed into breast milk. A nursing infant would receive less than 0.1% of the mg/kg maternal dose of benazepril and benazeprilat.

*Captopril*—Captopril is distributed into breast milk; concentrations in breast milk are approximately 1% of maternal blood concentrations. However, problems in humans have not been documented.

*Enalapril*—It is not known whether enalapril is distributed into breast milk. However, problems in humans have not been documented.

*Fosinopril*—Fosinoprilat (active metabolite) is distributed into breast milk. Detectable levels of fosinoprilat in breast milk were found following ingestion of 20 mg per day for 3 days.

*Lisinopril*—It is not known whether lisinopril is distributed into human breast milk; it appears to distribute into the milk of lactating rats. However, problems in humans have not been documented.

*Quinapril*—It is not known whether quinapril or its metabolites are distributed into human breast milk; quinapril appears to distribute into the milk of lactating rats. However, problems in humans have not been documented.

*Ramipril*—A 10-mg dose of ramipril resulted in undetectable amounts of ramipril and its metabolites in breast milk. However, multiple doses may produce low milk concentrations.

### Pediatrics

Appropriate studies on the relationship of age to the effects of ACE inhibitors have not been done in the pediatric population. However, the use of ACE inhibitors in a limited number of neonates and infants has identified some potential pediatrics-specific problems. In neonates and infants, there is a risk of oliguria and neurologic abnormalities, possibly as a result of decreased renal and cerebral blood flow secondary to marked and prolonged reductions in blood pressure caused by ACE inhibitors; a lower initial dose and close monitoring are recommended.

### Geriatrics

ACE inhibitors are thought to be most effective in reducing blood pressure in patients with normal or high plasma renin activity. Since plasma renin activity appears to decline with increasing age, elderly individuals may be less sensitive to the hypotensive effects of ACE inhibitors. However, elevated serum ACE inhibitor concentrations resulting from age-related decline in renal function may compensate for the lower renin dependence. Pharmacokinetic studies with lisinopril, quinapril, and ramipril have revealed higher peak serum concentrations and area under the curve (AUC) in elderly patients given doses similar to those given to younger adults. The net result is that no significant differences in blood pressure response or side/adverse effects have been noted in elderly patients receiving ACE inhibitors. Nevertheless, some elderly patients may be more sensitive to the hypotensive effects of these medications and may require caution when receiving an ACE inhibitor.

### Drug interactions and/or related problems

The following drug interactions and/or related problems have been selected on the basis of their potential clinical significance (possible mechanism in parentheses where appropriate)—not necessarily inclusive (» = major clinical significance):

Note: Combinations containing any of the following medications, depending on the amount present, may also interact with this medication.

*For all ACE inhibitors*
» Alcohol or
» Diuretics or
    Hypotension-producing medications, other (See *Appendix II*)
      (concurrent use with ACE inhibitors may produce additive hypotensive effects)

(antihypertensive agents that cause renin release or affect sympathetic activity have the greatest additive effect; concurrent use of captopril with beta-adrenergic blocking agents produces an increased but less than fully additive effect; although some antihypertensive and/or diuretic combinations may be used for therapeutic advantage, dosage adjustments may be necessary during concurrent use or when one drug is discontinued)

(if significant systemic absorption of ophthalmic beta-blockers occurs, hypotensive effects of ACE inhibitors may be potentiated)

(sudden and severe hypotension may occur within the first 1 to 5 hours after the initial dose of an ACE inhibitor, particularly in patients who are sodium- and volume-depleted as a result of diuretic therapy. Withdrawal of the diuretic or increase of salt intake approximately 1 week before start of captopril therapy or 2 to 3 days before start of benazepril, enalapril, fosinopril, lisinopril, quinapril, or ramipril therapy, or initiating ACE inhibitor therapy in lower doses, will minimize the reaction; this reaction does not usually recur with subsequent doses, although caution in increasing doses is recommended; diuretics may be reinstituted as necessary)

(risk of renal failure may be increased in patients who are sodium- and volume-depleted as a result of diuretic therapy)

(ACE inhibitors may reduce the secondary aldosteronism and hypokalemia caused by diuretics)

Anti-inflammatory drugs, nonsteroidal (NSAIDs), especially indomethacin
    (concurrent use of these agents may reduce the antihypertensive effects of ACE inhibitors; indomethacin, and possibly other NSAIDs, may antagonize the antihypertensive effect by inhibiting renal prostaglandin synthesis and/or causing sodium and fluid retention; the patient should be carefully monitored to confirm that the desired effect is being obtained)

Blood from blood bank (may contain up to 30 mEq [mmol] of potassium per liter of plasma or up to 65 mEq [mmol] per liter of whole blood when stored for more than 10 days) or
Cyclosporine or
» Diuretics, potassium-sparing or
» Low-salt milk (may contain up to 60 mEq [mmol] of potassium per liter) or
» Potassium-containing medications or
» Potassium supplements or substances containing high concentrations of potassium or
» Salt substitutes (most contain substantial amounts of potassium)
    (concurrent administration with ACE inhibitors may result in hyperkalemia since reduction of aldosterone production induced by ACE inhibitors may lead to elevation of serum potassium; frequent determination of serum potassium concentrations is recommended if concurrent use of these agents is necessary; concurrent use is not recommended in patients with congestive heart failure)

Bone marrow depressants (See *Appendix II*)
    (concurrent administration with an ACE inhibitor may result in an increased risk of development of potentially fatal neutropenia and/or agranulocytosis)

Estrogens
    (estrogen-induced fluid retention may increase blood pressure; the patient should be carefully monitored to confirm that the desired effect is being obtained)

Lithium
    (reversible increases in serum lithium concentrations and toxicity have been reported during concurrent use with ACE inhibitors; frequent monitoring of serum lithium concentrations is recommended during concurrent use)

Sympathomimetics
    (concurrent use of these agents may reduce the antihypertensive effects of ACE inhibitors; the patient should be carefully monitored to confirm that the desired effect is being obtained)

*For quinapril only*
Tetracyclines or
Other drugs that interact with magnesium
    (concurrent use of these agents with quinapril may reduce their absorption; absorption of tetracycline is reduced by approximately 28 to 37%, possibly due to the high magnesium content in Accupril brand of quinapril tablets)

### Laboratory value alterations

The following have been selected on the basis of their potential clinical significance (possible effect in parentheses where appropriate)—not necessarily inclusive (» = major clinical significance):

With diagnostic test results

*For all ACE inhibitors*

Iodohippurate sodium I 123/I 131 renal imaging or

Technetium Tc 99m pentetate renal imaging

(in patients with renal artery stenosis, captopril [and probably all ACE inhibitors] may cause a reversible decrease in localization and excretion of iodohippurate I 123/I 131 or technetium Tc 99m pentetate in the affected kidney; may cause confusion as to whether decreased renal function is drug-related)

*For captopril only*

Urinary acetone test

(captopril may produce false-positive results)

*For fosinopril only*

Digoxin levels

(fosinopril may cause a false low serum digoxin level with the Digi-Tab RIA Kit)

With physiology/laboratory test values

*For all ACE inhibitors*

Alkaline phosphatase, serum and

Bilirubin, serum and

Transaminases, serum

(concentration increases have been reported)

Antinuclear antibody (ANA) titer

(positive ANA has been reported)

Blood urea nitrogen (BUN) and

Creatinine, serum

(concentrations may be transiently increased, especially in patients with renal parenchymal and renovascular disease in patients who are volume- or sodium-depleted, in patients with renal artery stenosis, or after rapid reduction of long-standing or severe high blood pressure)

Hematocrit or

Hemoglobin

(may rarely be slightly decreased)

Potassium, serum

(concentrations may be slightly increased as a result of reduced circulating aldosterone concentrations and concomitant reduction in glomerular filtration rate [GFR], especially in patients with renal function impairment)

Sodium, serum

(concentrations may be slightly decreased, especially during initial therapy)

## Medical considerations/Contraindications

The medical considerations/contraindications included here have been selected on the basis of their potential clinical significance (reasons given in parentheses where appropriate)—not necessarily inclusive (» = major clinical significance).

*Risk-benefit should be considered when the following medical problems exist:*

*For all ACE inhibitors*

» Angioedema, history of, related to previous ACE inhibitor therapy or

» Hereditary angioedema or

» Idiopathic angioedema

(increased risk for development of ACE inhibitor–related angioedema)

Autoimmune disease, severe, especially systemic lupus erythematosus (SLE) or scleroderma

(increased risk for development of neutropenia or agranulocytosis)

Bone marrow depression

Cerebrovascular insufficiency or

Coronary insufficiency

(ischemia may be aggravated as a result of reduced blood pressure; cerebrovascular accident or myocardial infarction could be precipitated)

Diabetes mellitus

(increased risk of hyperkalemia)

» Hyperkalemia

» Renal artery stenosis, bilateral or in a solitary kidney or

» Renal transplant

(increased risk of renal function impairment)

» Renal function impairment

(decreased elimination of active ACE inhibitor [except fosinopril], resulting in higher plasma concentrations; increased risk of hyperkalemia, or, for captopril, proteinuria, neutropenia, and agranulocytosis. Patients with impaired renal function may require lower or less frequent doses and smaller increments in dose. However,

dosage adjustment may not be necessary with fosinopril since total body drug clearance even in severe renal function impairment is not decreased significantly, possibly due to compensatory hepatobiliary elimination. If a diuretic is also required, a loop diuretic is recommended instead of a thiazide diuretic in patients with severe renal function impairment)

Sensitivity to the ACE inhibitor prescribed, or any other ACE inhibitor

» Caution is required also in patients on severe dietary sodium restriction or dialysis; these patients may be volume-depleted, and sudden reduction by the initial dose of ACE inhibitor in the angiotensin II levels that have been maintaining them at a near-normotensive state may result in sudden and severe hypotension. In addition, the risk of ACE inhibitor–induced renal failure may be increased in patients who are sodium- and volume-depleted, especially those with congestive heart failure.

*For benazepril, captopril, enalapril, fosinopril, quinapril, and ramipril (in addition to the above)*

Hepatic function impairment

(may reduce metabolism of captopril and may reduce conversion of prodrug to active moiety with benazepril, enalapril, fosinopril, quinapril, and ramipril)

## Patient monitoring

The following may be especially important in patient monitoring (other tests may be warranted in some patients, depending on condition; » = major clinical significance):

» Blood pressure measurements

(recommended at periodic intervals in patients being treated for hypertension; selected patients may be trained to perform blood pressure measurements at home and report the results at regular physician visits)

Leukocyte count determinations, total and differential

(recommended prior to initiation of ACE inhibitor therapy and periodically thereafter; recommended every month for the first 3 to 6 months of therapy, and at periodic intervals thereafter for a period of up to 1 year in patients at increased risk for neutropenia [i.e., those with renal function impairment or collagen vascular disease] or receiving high doses; also recommended at the first sign of infection. It is recommended that ACE inhibitor therapy be withdrawn if neutropenia [neutrophil count less than 1000 per cubic millimeter ($1 \times 10^9$ /L)] is confirmed)

Renal function determinations

(recommended at periodic intervals, especially in patients who are sodium- and volume-depleted as a result of diuretic therapy or who have severe congestive heart failure)

Urinary protein estimates by means of dip-stick on first morning urine

(recommended prior to initiation of therapy and at periodic intervals thereafter for up to 1 year in patients with renal function impairment or those receiving doses of captopril greater than 150 mg per day; if excessive or increasing proteinuria occurs, it is recommended that ACE inhibitor therapy be re-evaluated)

# Side/Adverse Effects

Note: Proteinuria has occurred in about 1% of patients receiving greater than 150 mg of captopril per day. This adverse effect is thought to be due to the sulfhydryl moiety of captopril. However, whether this is a true causal relationship is unknown. Proteinuria usually occurs in patients with existing renal function impairment within 8 months of initiation of captopril therapy and usually reverses within 6 months even with continuation of therapy. Membranous glomerulopathy has been reported in some of these patients, especially with doses of captopril greater than 150 mg per day. Proteinuria has also been reported in patients receiving enalapril and lisinopril. Reported incidences range from 0% to 1.4% for enalapril and 0.7% for lisinopril.

There have been reports of reversible renal failure during ACE inhibitor therapy, especially in patients with bilateral renal artery stenoses or renal artery stenosis in a solitary kidney. There is also evidence that renal failure may be related to sodium and volume depletion from previous diuretic therapy or severe sodium restriction, especially in patients with congestive heart failure.

Hepatotoxicity has been reported rarely in patients receiving captopril, enalapril, and lisinopril. Cholestasis has been reported most frequently, although hepatic necrosis and hepatocellular injury have also been reported. The most common presenting symptoms are jaundice, pruritus, and abdominal tenderness. ACE inhibitor–associated hepatotoxicity is usually reversible upon discontinuation of therapy. Apparent cross-reactivity has been reported between captopril and enalapril and between lisinopril and enalapril.

The following side/adverse effects have been selected on the basis of their potential clinical significance (possible signs and symptoms in parentheses where appropriate)—not necessarily inclusive:

## Those indicating need for medical attention
Incidence less frequent
*Hypotension* (dizziness, lightheadedness, or fainting)—especially following the initial dose in sodium- or volume-depleted patients or in patients receiving an ACE inhibitor for congestive heart failure; *skin rash, with or without itching, fever, or joint pain*

Note: Maculopapular or, rarely, urticarial rash usually occurs during the first 4 weeks of the therapy with captopril and usually disappears with dosage reduction or withdrawal, or administration of an antihistamine; between 7 and 10% of these patients may show eosinophilia and/or positive antinuclear antibody (ANA) titers. The reaction may also occur, less frequently, with the other ACE inhibitors.

Rarely, a persistent lichenoid or pemphigoid reaction, possibly with a photosensitive factor, has been reported with captopril.

Incidence rare
*Angioedema of the extremities, face, lips, mucous membranes, tongue, glottis, and/or larynx* (sudden trouble in swallowing or breathing; swelling of face, mouth, hands, or feet; hoarseness)—especially following the initial dose; *chest pain; hyperkalemia* (confusion; irregular heartbeat; nervousness; numbness or tingling in hands, feet, or lips; shortness of breath or difficult breathing; weakness or heaviness of legs); *neutropenia or agranulocytosis* (fever and chills); *pancreatitis* (abdominal pain; nausea; vomiting; abdominal distention; fever)

Note: *Angioedema* involving the tongue, glottis, or larynx may cause airway obstruction, which could be fatal.

*Chest pain* is usually associated with severe hypotension.

Incidence of *neutropenia or agranulocytosis* is much higher in patients with renal function impairment (0.2% for captopril) or collagen vascular disease (e.g., SLE or scleroderma) (3.7% for captopril). Neutropenia appears to be dose-related and may begin within 3 months after initiation of therapy, with the nadir of the leukocyte count occurring after 10 to 30 days and persisting about 2 weeks after withdrawal. Deaths from pancytopenia and sepsis have been reported with captopril in patients with and without autoimmune disease.

## Those indicating need for medical attention only if they continue or are bothersome
Incidence more frequent
*Cough, dry, continuing; headache*

Note: *Cough* usually occurs within the first week of therapy (onset varies from 24 hours to several weeks after initiation), persists throughout therapy, and disappears within a few days after withdrawal of the ACE inhibitor. Characteristically the cough begins as a tickling sensation in the back of the throat leading to a dry, nonproductive, persistent cough; may be worse at night or in the supine position; onset can be paroxysmal and course may be episodic or intermittent; may occasionally lead to hoarseness or vomiting.

Incidence less frequent
*Diarrhea; dysgeusia* (loss of taste); *fatigue* (unusual tiredness); *nausea*

Note: *Loss of taste* is usually reversible after 2 to 3 months, even with continued treatment; may be associated with weight loss.

## Overdose
For more information on the management of overdose or unintentional ingestion, **contact a Poison Control Center** (see *Poison Control Center Listing*).

### Treatment of overdose
Treatment of overdose consists of volume expansion for correction of hypotension. Captopril, enalaprilat, and lisinopril are removable by hemodialysis. Benazeprilat is slightly removable by hemodialysis.

## Patient Consultation
As an aid to patient consultation, refer to *Advice for the Patient, Angiotensin-converting Enzyme (ACE) Inhibitors*.

In providing consultation, consider emphasizing the following selected information (» = major clinical significance):

### Before using this medication
» Conditions affecting use, especially:
    Sensitivity to any ACE inhibitor

Pregnancy—ACE inhibitors cross the placenta; ACE inhibitor-associated fetal hypotension, oliguria, and death reported in humans; fetotoxicity found in animals
Breast-feeding—Benazepril, captopril, and fosinopril are distributed into breast milk
Other medications, especially alcohol, diuretics (particularly potassium-sparing), potassium-containing medications, or potassium supplements
Other medical problems, especially angioedema related to previous ACE inhibitor therapy, hyperkalemia, renal artery stenosis, renal transplant, renal function impairment, or sodium and volume depletion
Use of low-salt milk or salt substitutes

### Proper use of this medication
Getting into the habit of taking at same time each day to help increase compliance
» Proper dosing
Missed dose: Taking as soon as possible; not taking if almost time for next dose; not doubling doses
» Proper storage
*For captopril*
For best results, taking on an empty stomach 1 hour before meals
*For use as an antihypertensive*
Possible need for control of weight and diet, especially sodium intake; risks associated with sodium depletion; not taking salt substitutes or using low-salt milk unless approved by physician
» Patient may not experience symptoms of hypertension; importance of taking medication even if feeling well
» Does not cure, but helps control hypertension; possible need for lifelong therapy; checking with physician before discontinuing medication; serious consequences of untreated hypertension

### Precautions while using this medication
Regular visits to physician to check progress
Caution when driving or doing other things requiring alertness, because of possible dizziness, especially after initial dose of ACE inhibitor in patients taking diuretics
To prevent dehydration and hypotension, checking with physician if severe nausea, vomiting, or diarrhea occurs and continues
Caution when exercising or during hot weather because of the risk of dehydration and hypotension due to reduced fluid volume
Caution if any kind of surgery (including dental surgery) or emergency treatment is required
*For use as an antihypertensive*
» Not taking other medications, especially nonprescription sympathomimetics, unless discussed with physician
*For captopril and fosinopril*
Caution if any laboratory tests required; possible interference with test results

### Side/adverse effects
Signs of potential side effects, especially hypotension, skin rash (with or without itching, fever, or joint pain), angioedema, chest pain, neutropenia or agranulocytosis, pancreatitis, and hyperkalemia

## General Dosing Information
Dosage must be adjusted to meet the individual requirements of each patient, on the basis of clinical response.

The hypotensive effect of ACE inhibitors is about the same in both standing and supine positions.

Recent evidence suggests that withdrawal of antihypertensive therapy prior to surgery may be undesirable. However, the anesthesiologist must be aware of such therapy.

If increased blood urea nitrogen (BUN) and creatinine concentrations occur, reduction in dosage of the ACE inhibitor and/or withdrawal of the diuretic may be required. The possibility of renovascular hypertension should also be considered, especially in the presence of a solitary kidney, transplanted kidney, or bilateral renal artery stenosis.

Caution is recommended in initiating ACE inhibitor therapy for congestive heart failure in patients who have been receiving digitalis glycosides and/or diuretics. If the patient is sodium- and water-depleted, a lower initial dosage should be used.

If symptomatic hypotension occurs, dosage reduction of the ACE inhibitor or withdrawal of the ACE inhibitor or diuretic may be necessary.

### For treatment of adverse effects
For angioedema with swelling confined to the face, mucous membranes of the mouth, lips, and extremities, treatment other than withdrawal of the medication is usually not necessary, although antihistamines may relieve the symptoms.

Treatment of angioedema involving the tongue, glottis, or larynx may include the following:
- Withdrawal of the ACE inhibitor and hospitalization of the patient.
- Subcutaneous (or, rarely, intravenous) epinephrine.
- Intravenous diphenhydramine hydrochloride.
- Intravenous hydrocortisone.

---

## BENAZEPRIL

## Summary of Differences

Precautions:
   Breast-feeding—Benazepril and benazeprilat are distributed into breast milk.

## Additional Dosing Information

See also *General Dosing Information*.

It is recommended that previous diuretic therapy be withdrawn 2 to 3 days before benazepril therapy is initiated, except in patients with accelerated or malignant hypertension or hypertension that is difficult to control. In these patients, benazepril may be initiated immediately at a lower dose under careful medical supervision, and doses increased cautiously.

Benazepril is usually effective in once-daily dosing. However, if the antihypertensive effect is diminished before 24 hours, the total daily dose may be given as 2 divided doses.

## Oral Dosage Forms

Note: Bracketed uses in the *Dosage Forms* section refer to categories of use and/or indications that are not included in U.S. product labeling.

   The dosing and strengths of the dosage forms available are expressed in terms of benazepril base (not the hydrochloride salt).

### BENAZEPRIL HYDROCHLORIDE TABLETS

**Usual adult dose**

Antihypertensive—
   Initial: Oral, 10 mg (base) once a day.
   Maintenance: Oral, 20 to 40 mg (base) once a day as a single dose or in two divided doses.

Note: An initial dose of 5 mg (base) should be used in patients who are sodium- and water-depleted as a result of prior diuretic therapy, patients continuing to receive diuretic therapy, or patients with renal failure (creatinine clearance less than 30 mL per minute per 1.73m²). Such patients should be kept under medical supervision for at least two hours after this initial dose (and for an additional hour after blood pressure has stabilized), to watch for excessive hypotension.

[Vasodilator, congestive heart failure]—
   Initial: Oral, 5 mg (base) once a day.
   Maintenance: Oral, 5 to 10 mg (base) once a day.

**Usual adult prescribing limits**

Doses above 80 mg per day have not been evaluated.

**Usual pediatric dose**

Safety and efficacy have not been established.

**Strength(s) usually available**

U.S.—
   5 mg (base) (Rx) [*Lotensin*].
   10 mg (base) (Rx) [*Lotensin*].
   20 mg (base) (Rx) [*Lotensin*].
   40 mg (base) (Rx) [*Lotensin*].

Canada—
   Not commercially available.

**Packaging and storage**

Store below 30 °C (86 °F), preferably between 15 and 30 °C (59 and 86 °F), unless otherwise specified by manufacturer. Store in a tight container.

**Auxiliary labeling**
- Do not take other medicines without your doctor's advice.

**Note**

Check refill frequency to determine compliance in hypertensive patients.

---

## CAPTOPRIL

## Summary of Differences

Indications:
   Captopril is used for the treatment of neonatal hypertension and neonatal and infant congestive heart failure.
Pharmacology/pharmacokinetics:
   Mechanism of action/Effect—Captopril is not a prodrug.
   Duration of action—Single dose: 6 to 12 hours.
Precautions:
   Breast-feeding—Captopril is distributed into breast milk.
   Laboratory value alterations—May produce false-positive results in urinary acetone test.
Side/adverse effects:
   Causes maculopapular or urticarial skin rash, sometimes with fever, joint pain, or elevated antinuclear antibody (ANA) titers.

## Additional Dosing Information

See also *General Dosing Information*.

It is recommended that previous antihypertensive therapy be withdrawn 1 week before captopril therapy is initiated, except in patients with accelerated or malignant hypertension or hypertension that is difficult to control. In these patients, captopril therapy may be initiated at the lowest dose immediately after previous therapy (except diuretics) is discontinued, under careful medical supervision, and the dosage increased every 24 hours or less until the medication is effective or the maximum dose is reached.

## Oral Dosage Forms

### CAPTOPRIL TABLETS USP

**Usual adult and adolescent dose**

Antihypertensive—
   Initial: Oral, 12.5 mg two or three times a day, the dosage being increased if necessary after one or two weeks to 25 mg two or three times a day.
Left ventricular dysfunction following myocardial infarction—
   Initial: Oral, a single dose of 6.25 mg. Then 12.5 mg three times a day, gradually increased to 25 mg three times a day over several days.
   Maintenance: Oral, 50 mg three times a day.
Note: Captopril therapy may be initiated as early as three days following a myocardial infarction.
Diabetic nephropathy[1]—
   Oral, 25 mg three times a day.
Vasodilator, congestive heart failure—
   Initial: Oral, 12.5 mg two or three times a day, the dosage being increased gradually as necessary on a daily basis up to 50 mg two or three times a day. If further increases in dosage are needed, it is recommended that they be made after an interval of two weeks so that the full effects of captopril will be apparent.
   Maintenance: Oral, 25 to 100 mg two or three times a day.
Note: An initial dose of 6.25 to 12.5 mg two or three times a day should be used in patients who are sodium- and water-depleted as a result of diuretic therapy, in patients continuing to receive diuretic therapy, or in patients with renal function impairment. Such patients should be kept under medical supervision for one hour after this initial dose, to watch for excessive hypotension.

   Dosage increases in patients with significant renal function impairment should proceed slowly (one- to two-week intervals), and smaller increments should be used.

**Usual adult prescribing limits**

Up to 450 mg per day.

**Usual pediatric dose**

Newborns:
   Initial: Oral, 10 mcg (0.01 mg) per kg of body weight two or three times a day, the dosage being adjusted as needed and tolerated.
Children:
   Initial: Oral, 300 mcg (0.3 mg) per kg of body weight three times a day, the dosage being increased if necessary in increments of 300 mcg (0.3 mg) per kg of body weight at intervals of eight to twenty-four hours to the minimum effective dose.
Note: An initial dose of 150 mcg (0.15 mg) per kg of body weight three times a day should be used in patients who are sodium- and water-depleted as a result of diuretic therapy, in patients continuing to receive diuretic therapy, or in patients with renal function impairment.

## Strength(s) usually available

U.S.—

12.5 mg (Rx) [*Capoten* (scored)].
25 mg (Rx) [*Capoten* (scored)].
50 mg (Rx) [*Capoten* (scored)].
100 mg (Rx) [*Capoten* (scored)].

Canada—

12.5 mg (Rx) [*Capoten*].
25 mg (Rx) [*Capoten* (scored)].
50 mg (Rx) [*Capoten* (scored)].
100 mg (Rx) [*Capoten* (scored)].

## Packaging and storage

Store below 40 °C (104 °F), preferably between 15 and 30 °C (59 and 86 °F), in a tight container, unless otherwise specified by manufacturer.

## Preparation of dosage form

For patients who cannot take oral solids—Captopril oral solution may be prepared by crushing a 25-mg tablet, dissolving it in 25 or 100 mL of water, and shaking the solution well for at least 5 minutes. After the tablet has dissolved, the clear solution is poured off for administration and the remaining filler, which doesn't dissolve, is discarded. Because captopril is very unstable when dissolved in water, the solution should be used within one-half hour after preparation.

## Auxiliary labeling

• Take on an empty stomach, one hour before meals.
• Do not take other medicines without your doctor's advice.

## Note

Tablets may have a slight sulfurous odor.

Check refill frequency to determine compliance in hypertensive patients.

---

[1]Not included in Canadian product labeling.

---

## *ENALAPRIL*

## Summary of Differences

Pharmacology/pharmacokinetics:
Onset of action—
Enalapril maleate: Oral—Single dose: 1 hour.
Enalaprilat: Intravenous—Single dose: 15 minutes.

## Additional Dosing Information

See also *General Dosing Information*.

It is recommended that previous diuretic therapy be withdrawn 2 to 3 days before enalapril therapy is initiated, except in patients with accelerated or malignant hypertension or hypertension that is difficult to control. In these patients, enalapril therapy may be initiated immediately at a lower dose under careful medical supervision, and increased cautiously.

Enalapril is usually effective in once-daily dosing. However, if the antihypertensive effect is diminished before 24 hours, the total daily dose may be given as 2 divided doses.

Hemodialysis reduces serum enalaprilat concentrations by approximately 35%.

## Oral Dosage Forms

### ENALAPRIL MALEATE TABLETS USP

#### Usual adult and adolescent dose

Antihypertensive—
Initial: Oral, 5 mg once a day, the dosage being adjusted after one or two weeks according to clinical response.
Maintenance: Oral, 10 to 40 mg per day, as a single dose or in two divided doses.

Note: An initial dose of 2.5 mg should be used in patients who are sodium- and water-depleted as a result of prior diuretic therapy, patients continuing to receive diuretic therapy, or patients with renal failure (creatinine clearance less than 30 mL per minute). Such patients should be kept under medical supervision for at least two hours after this initial dose (and for an additional hour after blood pressure has stabilized), to watch for excessive hypotension.

Vasodilator, congestive heart failure—
Initial: Oral, 2.5 mg once or twice a day, the dosage being adjusted after one or two weeks according to clinical response.
Maintenance: Oral, 5 to 20 mg per day, as a single dose or in two divided doses.

Left ventricular dysfunction, asymptomatic—
Oral, 2.5 mg two times a day titrated as tolerated up to a target dose of 20 mg a day in divided doses.

Note: Patients should be kept under medical supervision for at least two hours and until blood pressure has stabilized for an additional hour after the initial dose.

In patients with hyponatremia (serum sodium concentration less than 130 mEq per liter) or serum creatinine greater than 1.6 mg per deciliter, an initial dose of 2.5 mg once a day is recommended.

If possible, the dose of the diuretic should be reduced to decrease the likelihood of hypotension.

#### Usual adult prescribing limits

Up to 40 mg per day.

#### Usual pediatric dose

Safety and efficacy have not been established.

#### Strength(s) usually available

U.S.—

2.5 mg (Rx) [*Vasotec* (scored)].
5 mg (Rx) [*Vasotec* (scored)].
10 mg (Rx) [*Vasotec*].
20 mg (Rx) [*Vasotec*].

Canada—

2.5 mg (Rx) [*Vasotec*].
5 mg (Rx) [*Vasotec* (scored)].
10 mg (Rx) [*Vasotec*].
20 mg (Rx) [*Vasotec*].

#### Packaging and storage

Store below 40 °C (104 °F), preferably between 15 and 30 °C (59 and 86 °F), in a well-closed container, unless otherwise specified by manufacturer.

#### Auxiliary labeling

• Do not take other medicines without your doctor's advice.

#### Note

Check refill frequency to determine compliance in hypertensive patients.

## Parenteral Dosage Forms

### ENALAPRILAT INJECTION

#### Usual adult and adolescent dose

Antihypertensive—
Intravenous (over at least five minutes), 1.25 mg every six hours.

Note: An initial dose of 625 mcg (0.625 mg) should be used in patients who are sodium- and water-depleted as a result of prior diuretic therapy, patients continuing to receive diuretic therapy, or patients with renal failure (creatinine clearance less than or equal to 30 mL per minute). Such patients should be observed for one hour after this initial dose, to watch for excessive hypotension. If the clinical response is inadequate after one hour, the 625 mcg (0.625-mg) dose may be repeated, and therapy continued at a dose of 1.25 mg every six hours.

#### Usual pediatric dose

Safety and efficacy have not been established.

Note: Use of products containing benzyl alcohol is not recommended in neonates. A fatal toxic syndrome consisting of metabolic acidosis, CNS depression, respiratory problems, renal failure, hypotension, and possibly seizures and intracranial hemorrhages has been associated with this use.

#### Strength(s) usually available

U.S.—

1.25 mg per mL (Rx) [*Vasotec* (benzyl alcohol)].

Canada—

1.25 mg per mL (Rx) [*Vasotec* (benzyl alcohol)].

#### Packaging and storage

Store below 40 °C (104 °F), preferably between 15 and 30 °C (59 and 86 °F), unless otherwise specified by manufacturer.

#### Preparation of dosage form

Enalaprilat injection may be administered undiluted, or may be diluted with up to 50 mL of a compatible diluent.

#### Stability

Stable in compatible diluents (5% dextrose injection, 0.9% sodium chloride injection, 0.9% sodium chloride in 5% dextrose injection, 5% dextrose in lactated Ringer's injection) for 24 hours.

---

## *FOSINOPRIL*

## Summary of Differences

Precautions:

Breast-feeding—Fosinoprilat (active metabolite) is distributed into breast milk.

Medical considerations/contraindications—Dosage adjustment is not necessary in renal function impairment.

Laboratory value alterations—May cause a false low serum digoxin level with the Digi-Tab RIA Kit.

## Additional Dosing Information

See also *General Dosing Information*.

It is recommended that previous diuretic therapy be withdrawn 2 to 3 days before fosinopril therapy is initiated, except in patients with accelerated or malignant hypertension or hypertension that is difficult to control. In these patients, fosinopril therapy may be initiated immediately at a lower dose under careful medical supervision (for at least 2 hours and until blood pressure has stabilized for at least an additional hour), and doses increased cautiously.

Fosinopril is usually effective in once-daily dosing. However, if the antihypertensive effect is diminished before 24 hours, the total daily dose may be given as 2 divided doses.

## Oral Dosage Forms

### FOSINOPRIL SODIUM TABLETS

#### Usual adult dose
Antihypertensive—
Initial: Oral, 10 mg once a day, the dosage being adjusted according to clinical response.
Maintenance: Oral, 20 to 40 mg once a day.

Note: In patients continuing to receive diuretic therapy, an initial fosinopril dose of 10 mg may be given with careful medical supervision for several hours and until blood pressure is stabilized.

#### Usual adult prescribing limits
Up to 80 mg per day.

#### Usual pediatric dose
Safety and efficacy have not been established.

#### Strength(s) usually available
U.S.—
10 mg (Rx) [*Monopril*].
20 mg (Rx) [*Monopril*].
Canada—
Not commercially available.

#### Packaging and storage
Store below 30 °C (86 °F), preferably between 15 and 30 °C (59 and 86 °F), unless otherwise specified by manufacturer. Store in a tight container.

#### Auxiliary labeling
• Do not take other medicines without your doctor's advice.

#### Note
Check refill frequency to determine compliance in hypertensive patients.

---

## *LISINOPRIL*

## Summary of Differences

Pharmacology/pharmacokinetics:
Mechanism of action/Effect—Lisinopril is not a prodrug.
Protein binding—None.
Biotransformation—None.

## Additional Dosing Information

See also *General Dosing Information*.

It is recommended that previous diuretic therapy be withdrawn 2 to 3 days before lisinopril therapy is initiated, except in patients with accelerated or malignant hypertension or hypertension that is difficult to control. In these patients, lisinopril therapy may be initiated immediately at a lower dose under careful medical supervision (for at least 2 hours and until blood pressure has stabilized for at least an additional hour), and increased cautiously.

Lisinopril is usually effective in once-daily dosing. However, if the antihypertensive effect is diminished before 24 hours, an increase in dosage may be necessary.

## Oral Dosage Forms

### LISINOPRIL TABLETS

#### Usual adult and adolescent dose
Antihypertensive—
Initial: Oral, 10 mg once a day, the dosage being adjusted according to clinical response.
Maintenance: Oral, 20 to 40 mg once a day.

Note: An initial dose of 5 mg should be used in patients who are sodium- and water-depleted as a result of prior diuretic therapy, patients continuing to receive diuretic therapy, or patients with renal failure (creatinine clearance less than or equal to 30 mL per minute). An initial dose of 2.5 mg should be used in patients with a creatinine clearance less than 10 mL per minute. Such patients should be kept under medical supervision for at least two hours after this initial dose (and for an additional hour after blood pressure has stabilized), to watch for excessive hypotension.

Vasodilator, congestive heart failure—
Initial: Oral, 2.5 to 5 mg per day, the dosage being adjusted according to clinical response.
Maintenance: Oral, 10 to 20 mg per day.

#### Usual adult prescribing limits
Doses up to 80 mg per day have been used but do not appear to have a greater effect.

#### Usual pediatric dose
Safety and efficacy have not been established.

#### Strength(s) usually available
U.S.—
5 mg (Rx) [*Prinivil* (scored); *Zestril* (scored)].
10 mg (Rx) [*Prinivil; Zestril*].
20 mg (Rx) [*Prinivil; Zestril*].
40 mg (Rx) [*Prinivil; Zestril*].
Canada—
5 mg (Rx) [*Prinivil* (scored); *Zestril*].
10 mg (Rx) [*Prinivil; Zestril*].
20 mg (Rx) [*Prinivil; Zestril*].

#### Packaging and storage
Store below 40 °C (104 °F), preferably between 15 and 30 °C (59 and 86 °F), in a well-closed container, unless otherwise specified by manufacturer.

#### Auxiliary labeling
• Do not take other medicines without your doctor's advice.

#### Note
Check refill frequency to determine compliance in hypertensive patients.

---

## *QUINAPRIL*

## Summary of Differences

Precautions:

Drug interactions and/or related problems—Quinapril may reduce absorption of tetracycline or other drugs that interact with magnesium, since quinapril has a high magnesium content.

## Additional Dosing Information

See also *General Dosing Information*.

It is recommended that previous diuretic therapy be withdrawn 2 to 3 days before quinapril therapy is initiated, except in patients with accelerated or malignant hypertension or hypertension that is difficult to control. In these patients, quinapril therapy may be initiated immediately at a lower dose under careful medical supervision (for at least 2 hours and until blood pressure has stabilized for at least an additional hour), and doses increased cautiously.

Quinapril is usually effective in once-daily dosing. However, if the antihypertensive effect is diminished before 24 hours, an increase in dosage may be necessary or the total daily dose may be given as 2 divided doses.

## Oral Dosage Forms

Note: Bracketed uses in the *Dosage Forms* section refer to categories of use and/or indications that are not included in U.S. product labeling.

The dosing and strengths of the dosage forms available are expressed in terms of quinapril base (not the hydrochloride salt).

## QUINAPRIL HYDROCHLORIDE TABLETS

**Usual adult dose**

Antihypertensive—

Initial: Oral, 10 mg (base) once a day, the dosage being adjusted slowly (at 2-week intervals) and according to clinical response.

Maintenance: Oral, 20 to 80 mg (base) once a day or divided into two equal doses.

Note: An initial dose of 5 mg should be used in patients who are sodium- and water-depleted as a result of prior diuretic therapy, patients continuing to receive diuretic therapy, or in patients with a creatinine clearance of 30 to 60 mL per minute. An initial dose of 2.5 mg should be used in patients with a creatinine clearance of 10 to 30 mL per minute. Such patients should be kept under medical supervision for at least two hours after this initial dose (and for an additional hour after blood pressure has stabilized), to watch for excessive hypotension.

There are insufficient data for a dosage recommendation in patients with a creatinine clearance less than 10 mL per minute.

[Vasodilator, congestive heart failure]—

Initial: Oral, 2.5 mg (base) once a day.

Maintenance: Oral, 5 to 40 mg once a day or divided into two equal doses.

**Usual pediatric dose**

Safety and efficacy have not been established.

**Strength(s) usually available**

U.S.—

5 mg (Rx) [*Accupril* (scored)].

10 mg (Rx) [*Accupril* (scored)].

20 mg (Rx) [*Accupril* (scored)].

40 mg (Rx) [*Accupril* (scored)].

Canada—

Not commercially available.

**Packaging and storage**

Store below 40 °C (104 °F), preferably between 15 and 30 °C (59 and 86 °F), in a well-closed container, unless otherwise specified by manufacturer.

**Auxiliary labeling**

• Do not take other medicines without your doctor's advice.

**Note**

Check refill frequency to determine compliance in hypertensive patients.

---

### *RAMIPRIL*

## Additional Dosing Information

See also *General Dosing Information*.

It is recommended that previous diuretic therapy be withdrawn 2 to 3 days before ramipril therapy is initiated, except in patients with accelerated or malignant hypertension or hypertension that is difficult to control. In these patients, ramipril therapy may be initiated immediately at a lower dose under careful medical supervision (for at least 2 hours and until blood pressure has stabilized for at least an additional hour), and doses increased cautiously.

Ramipril is usually effective in once-daily dosing. However, if the antihypertensive effect is diminished before 24 hours, an increase in dosage may be necessary or the total daily dose may be given as 2 divided doses.

## Oral Dosage Forms

### RAMIPRIL CAPSULES

**Usual adult dose**

Antihypertensive—

Initial: Oral, 2.5 mg once a day, the dosage being adjusted according to clinical response.

Maintenance: Oral, 2.5 to 20 mg once a day or divided into two equal doses.

Note: An initial dose of 1.25 mg should be used in patients who are sodium- and water-depleted as a result of prior diuretic therapy, patients continuing to receive diuretic therapy, or in patients with a creatinine clearance less than 40 mL per minute per 1.73 m $^2$. Such patients should be kept under medical supervision for at least two hours after this initial dose (and for an additional hour after blood pressure has stabilized), to watch for excessive hypotension.

Dosage may be slowly titrated upward until adequate blood pres-

sure control is achieved or to a maximum total daily dose of 5 mg.

**Usual pediatric dose**

Safety and efficacy have not been established.

**Strength(s) usually available**

U.S.—

1.25 mg (Rx) [*Altace*].

2.5 mg (Rx) [*Altace*].

5 mg (Rx) [*Altace*].

10 mg (Rx) [*Altace*].

Canada—

Not commercially available.

**Packaging and storage**

Store below 40 °C (104 °F), preferably between 15 and 30 °C (59 and 86 °F), in a well-closed container, unless otherwise specified by manufacturer.

**Auxiliary labeling**

• Do not take other medicines without your doctor's advice.

**Note**

Check refill frequency to determine compliance in hypertensive patients.

## Selected Bibliography

**General**

Williams GH. Converting-enzyme inhibitors in the treatment of hypertension. New Engl J Med 1988 Dec 8; 1517-25.

Weber MA. Safety issues during antihypertenisve treatment with angiotensin converting enzyme inhibitors. Am J Med 1988; 84 (suppl 4A): 16-23.

Massie BM. New trends in the use of angiotensin converting enzyme inhibitors in chronic heart failure. Am J Med 1988 Apr 15; 84 (Suppl 4A): 36-46.

**For benazepril**

Balfour JA, Goa KL. Benazepril. A review of its pharmacodynamic and pharmacokinetic properties, and therapeutic efficacy in hypertension and congestive heart failure. Drugs 1991; 42 (3): 511-39.

**For captopril**

Vidt DG, Bravo EL, Fouad FM. Captopril. New Engl J Med 1982 Jan 28; 306: 214-9.

Ram CVS. Captopril. Arch Intern Med 1982 May; 142: 914-6.

**For enalapril**

Cleary JD, Taylor JW. Enalapril: a new angiotensin converting enzyme inhibitor. Drug Intell Clin Pharm Mar; 20: 177-86.

Vlasses PH, Larijani GE, Conner DP, Ferguson RK. Enalapril, a nonsulfhydryl angiotensin-converting enzyme inhibitor. Clin Pharm 1985; 4: 27-40.

**For fosinopril**

Sica DA, Cutler RE, Parmer RJ, Ford NF. Comparison of the steady-state pharmacokinetics of fosinopril, lisinopril and enalapril in patients with chronic renal insufficiency. Clin Pharmacokinet 1991; 20 (5): 420-7.

Oren S, Messerli FH, Grossman E, Garavaglia GE, Frohlich ED. Immediate and short-term cardiovascular effects of fosinopril, a new angiotensin-converting enzyme inhibitor, in patients with essential hypertension. J Am Coll Cardiol 1991; 17: 1183-7.

**For lisinopril**

Armayor GM, Lopez LM. Lisinopril: A new angiotensin-converting enzyme inhibitor. Drug Intell Clin Pharm 1988 May; 22: 365-72.

Lisinopril for hypertension. Med Lett Drugs Ther 1988 Apr 8; 30: 41-2.

Chase SL, Sutton JD. Lisinopril: A new angiotensin converting enzyme inhibitor. Pharmacother 1989; 9 (3): 120-30.

**For quinapril**

Cropp AB. Quinapril: A new second-generation ACE inhibitor. DICP 1991; 25: 499-504.

Wadworth AN, Brogden RN. Quinapril. A review of its pharmacologic properties, and therapeutic efficacy in cardiovascular disorders. Drugs 41 (3): 378-99.

**For ramipril**

Todd PA, Benfield P. Ramipril. A review of its pharmacological properties and therapeutic efficacy in cardiovascular disorders. Drugs 1990; 39 (1): 110-35.

---

Revised: 07/12/92

Interim revision: 08/04/93; 07/12/94

# ANGIOTENSIN-CONVERTING ENZYME (ACE) INHIBITORS AND HYDROCHLOROTHIAZIDE   Systemic

This monograph includes information on the following: Captopril and Hydrochlorothiazide; Enalapril and Hydrochlorothiazide; Lisinopril and Hydrochlorothiazide.

VA CLASSIFICATION (Primary/Secondary): CV400/CV490; CV900

**NOTE:**   The *Angiotensin-converting Enzyme (ACE) Inhibitors and Hydrochlorothiazide (Systemic)* monograph is maintained on the USP DI electronic data base. For a printed copy of the most recent revision of the complete monograph, contact the USP Division of Information Development, 12601 Twinbrook Parkway, Rockville, MD 20852.

For information on the specific components of this combination, see the *USP DI* monographs for *Angiotensin-converting Enzymes (ACE) Inhibitors (Systemic)* and *Diuretics, Thiazide (Systemic)*.

The information that follows is selectively abstracted from the complete monograph and is provided to facilitate drug use review and patient counseling.

Note:   For a listing of dosage forms and brand names by country availability, see *Dosage Forms* section(s). For a listing of brand names for the articles in this monograph, refer to the General Index.

## Category

Antihypertensive; vasodilator, congestive heart failure.

## Indications

Note:   Bracketed information in the *Indications* section refers to uses that are not included in U.S. product labeling.

### Accepted

Hypertension (treatment)—The combination of captopril, enalapril, or lisinopril and hydrochlorothiazide is indicated in the treatment of hypertension.

Fixed-dosage combinations generally are not recommended for initial therapy, but are utilized in maintenance therapy after the required dose is established in order to increase convenience, economy, and patient compliance.

For additional information on initial therapeutic guidelines related to the treatment of hypertension, see *Appendix III.*

[Congestive heart failure (treatment)]—Captopril, enalapril, or lisinopril plus a diuretic, such as hydrochlorothiazide, and a digitalis glycoside are also used for treatment of severe congestive heart failure not responding to other measures.

## Patient Consultation

As an aid to patient consultation, refer to *Advice for the Patient, Angiotensin-converting Enzyme (ACE) Inhibitors and Hydrochlorothiazide (Systemic).*

In providing consultation, consider emphasizing the following selected information (» = major clinical significance):

### Before using this medication
»   Conditions affecting use, especially:

Sensitivity to any ACE inhibitor, thiazide diuretic, carbonic anhydrase inhibitor, or other sulfonamide-type medications

Pregnancy—ACE inhibitor–associated fetal hypotension, oliguria, and death reported in humans; and fetotoxicity found in animals; hydrochlorothiazide may cause jaundice, thrombocytopenia, hypokalemia in infant

Breast-feeding—Captopril and hydrochlorothiazide are distributed into breast milk

Use in children—Caution if giving to infants with jaundice

Use in the elderly—May be more sensitive to hypotensive and electrolyte effects

Other medications, especially alcohol, cholestyramine, colestipol, diuretics (particularly potassium-sparing), potassium-containing medications, potassium supplements, low salt milk, salt substitutes, digitalis glycosides, lithium, cocaine, norepinephrine, or phenylephrine

Other medical problems, especially angioedema related to previous ACE inhibitor therapy, hereditary angioedema, idiopathic angioedema, hyperkalemia, renal artery stenosis, renal transplant, renal function impairment, or sodium and volume depletion

## Proper use of this medication

Getting into the habit of taking at same time each day to help increase compliance

Diuretic effects of the medication and timing of doses to minimize inconvenience of diuresis

»   Proper dosing

Missed dose: Taking as soon as possible; not taking if almost time for next dose; not doubling doses

»   Proper storage

*For captopril and hydrochlorothiazide*

For best results, taking on an empty stomach 1 hour before meals

*For use as an antihypertensive*

Possible need for control of weight and diet, especially sodium intake; risks associated with sodium depletion; not taking salt substitutes or using low-salt milk unless approved by physician

»   Patient may not experience symptoms of hypertension; importance of taking medication even if feeling well

»   Does not cure, but helps control hypertension; possible need for lifelong therapy; checking with physician before discontinuing medication; serious consequences of untreated hypertension

## Precautions while using this medication

Regular visits to physician to check progress

Caution when driving or doing other things requiring alertness, because of possible dizziness, especially with initial dose

To prevent dehydration and hypotension, checking with physician if severe nausea, vomiting, or diarrhea occurs and continues

Caution when exercising or during hot weather because of the risk of dehydration and hypotension due to reduced fluid volume

Caution if any kind of surgery (including dental surgery) or emergency treatment is required

Caution in using alcohol

Diabetics: May increase blood sugar levels

Possible photosensitivity; avoiding unprotected exposure to sun; using protective clothing and sun block product; avoiding use of sunlamp

Caution if any laboratory tests required; possible interference with test results

*For use as an antihypertensive*

»   Not taking other medications, especially nonprescription sympathomimetics, unless discussed with physician

## Side/adverse effects

Signs of potential side effects, especially hypotension, skin rash (with or without itching, fever, or joint pain), angioedema, chest pain, neutropenia or agranulocytosis, hyperuricemia or gout, cholecystitis or pancreatitis, thrombocytopenia, hepatic function impairment, and electrolyte imbalance

---

### *CAPTOPRIL AND HYDROCHLOROTHIAZIDE*

## Oral Dosage Forms

Note:   Bracketed uses in the *Dosage Forms* section refer to categories of use and/or indications that are not included in U.S. product labeling.

### CAPTOPRIL AND HYDROCHLOROTHIAZIDE TABLETS

#### Usual adult and adolescent dose

Antihypertensive or

[Vasodilator, congestive heart failure]—

Oral, 1 tablet two or three times a day, as determined by individual titration with the component agents.

Note:   Geriatric patients may be more sensitive to the effects of the usual adult dose.

#### Usual pediatric dose

Oral, as determined by individual titration with the component agents

Captopril: Oral, 300 mcg (0.3 mg) per kg of body weight three times a day, the dosage being increased if necessary in increments of 300 mcg (0.3 mg) per kg of body weight at intervals of eight to twenty-four hours to the minimum effective dose.

Hydrochlorothiazide: Oral, 1 to 2 mg per kg of body weight or 30 to 60 mg per square meter of body surface per day, as a single dose or in two divided daily doses, the dosage being adjusted according to response.

**Strength(s) usually available**
U.S.—
     25 mg of captopril and 15 mg of hydrochlorothiazide (Rx) [*Capozide* (scored; lactose)].
     25 mg of captopril and 25 mg of hydrochlorothiazide (Rx) [*Capozide* (scored; lactose)].
     50 mg of captopril and 15 mg of hydrochlorothiazide (Rx) [*Capozide* (scored; lactose)].
     50 mg of captopril and 25 mg of hydrochlorothiazide (Rx) [*Capozide* (scored; lactose)].
Canada—
     Not commercially available.

**Auxiliary labeling**
• Take on an empty stomach, 1 hour before meals.
• Avoid too much sun or use of sunlamp.
• Do not take other medicines without your doctor's advice.

---

### ENALAPRIL AND HYDROCHLOROTHIAZIDE

## Oral Dosage Forms
Note: Bracketed uses in the *Dosage Forms* section refer to categories of use and/or indications that are not included in U.S. product labeling.

### ENALAPRIL MALEATE AND HYDROCHLOROTHIAZIDE TABLETS

**Usual adult and adolescent dose**
Antihypertensive or
[Vasodilator, congestive heart failure]—
     Oral, 1 tablet per day, as determined by individual titration with the component agents.
Note: Geriatric patients may be more sensitive to the effects of the usual adult dose.

**Usual pediatric dose**
Oral, as determined by individual titration with the component agents
Enalapril: Oral, initially 100 mcg (0.1 mg) per kg of body weight per day, the dosage being adjusted as needed and tolerated, up to a maximum of 500 mcg (0.5 mg) per kg of body weight per day.
Hydrochlorothiazide: Oral, 1 to 2 mg per kg of body weight or 30 to 60 mg per square meter of body surface per day, as a single dose or in two divided doses, the dosage being adjusted according to response.

**Strength(s) usually available**
U.S.—
     10 mg of enalapril maleate and 25 mg of hydrochlorothiazide (Rx) [*Vaseretic* (lactose)].
Canada—
     Not commercially available.

**Auxiliary labeling**
• Avoid too much sun or use of sunlamp.
• Do not take other medicines without your doctor's advice.

---

### LISINOPRIL AND HYDROCHLOROTHIAZIDE

## Oral Dosage Forms
Note: Bracketed uses in the *Dosage Forms* section refer to categories of use and/or indications that are not included in U.S. product labeling.

### LISINOPRIL AND HYDROCHLOROTHIAZIDE TABLETS

**Usual adult and adolescent dose**
Antihypertensive or
[Vasodilator, congestive heart failure]—
     Oral, 1 or 2 tablets once a day, as determined by individual titration with the component agents.
Note: Geriatric patients may be more sensitive to the effects of the usual adult dose.

**Usual pediatric dose**
Dosage has not been established.

**Strength(s) usually available**
U.S.—
     20 mg of lisinopril and 12.5 mg of hydrochlorothiazide (Rx) [*Prinzide; Zestoretic*].
     20 mg of lisinopril and 25 mg of hydrochlorothiazide (Rx) [*Prinzide; Zestoretic*].
Canada—
     Not commercially available.

**Auxiliary labeling**
• Avoid too much sun or use of sunlamp.
• Do not take other medicines without your doctor's advice.

Revised: 07/28/92
Interim revision: 06/29/94

---

**ANISINDIONE**—See *Anticoagulants (Systemic)*

---

**ANISOTROPINE**—See *Anticholinergics/Antispasmodics (Systemic)*

---

**ANISTREPLASE**—See *Thrombolytic Agents (Systemic)*

---

# ANTACIDS    Oral-Local

This monograph includes information on the following: Alumina, Calcium Carbonate, and Sodium Bicarbonate*; Alumina and Magnesia; Alumina, Magnesia, Calcium Carbonate, and Simethicone†; Alumina, Magnesia, and Magnesium Carbonate*; Alumina, Magnesia, Magnesium Carbonate, and Simethicone*; Alumina, Magnesia, and Simethicone; Alumina, Magnesium Alginate, and Magnesium Carbonate*; Alumina and Magnesium Carbonate†; Alumina, Magnesium Carbonate, and Simethicone†; Alumina, Magnesium Carbonate, and Sodium Bicarbonate†; Alumina and Magnesium Trisilicate†; Alumina, Magnesium Trisilicate, and Sodium Bicarbonate†; Alumina and Simethicone†; Alumina and Sodium Bicarbonate*; Aluminum Carbonate, Basic†; Aluminum Carbonate, Basic, and Simethicone†; Aluminum Hydroxide; Calcium Carbonate‡; Calcium Carbonate and Magnesia; Calcium Carbonate, Magnesia, and Simethicone; Calcium Carbonate and Simethicone†; Calcium and Magnesium Carbonates; Magaldrate; Magaldrate and Simethicone; Magnesium Carbonate and Sodium Bicarbonate*; Magnesium Hydroxide§; Magnesium Oxide§†.

VA CLASSIFICATION (Primary/Secondary):
Alumina, Calcium Carbonate, and Sodium Bicarbonate—GA199
Alumina and Magnesia—GA103
Alumina, Magnesia, Calcium Carbonate, and Simethicone—GA199
Alumina, Magnesia, and Magnesium Carbonate—GA103
Alumina, Magnesia, Magnesium Carbonate, and Simethicone—GA199
Alumina, Magnesia, and Simethicone—GA199
Alumina, Magnesium Alginate, and Magnesium Carbonate—GA103
Alumina and Magnesium Carbonate—GA103
Alumina, Magnesium Carbonate, and Simethicone—GA199
Alumina, Magnesium Carbonate, and Sodium Bicarbonate—GA104
Alumina and Magnesium Trisilicate—GA103
Alumina, Magnesium Trisilicate, and Sodium Bicarbonate—GA104
Alumina and Simethicone—GA199
Alumina and Sodium Bicarbonate—GA199
Aluminum Carbonate, Basic—GA101
Aluminum Carbonate, Basic, and Simethicone—GA199
Aluminum Hydroxide—GA101/TN402; GA400
Calcium Carbonate—GA105/TN402
Calcium Carbonate and Magnesia—GA106
Calcium Carbonate, Magnesia, and Simethicone—GA199
Calcium Carbonate and Simethicone—GA199
Calcium and Magnesium Carbonates—GA106
Magaldrate—GA107
Magaldrate and Simethicone—GA199
Magnesium Carbonate and Sodium Bicarbonate—GA109
Magnesium Hydroxide—GA108/GU900
Magnesium Oxide—GA108

Note: For a listing of dosage forms and brand names by country availability, see *Dosage Forms* section(s). For a listing of brand names for the articles in this monograph, refer to the General Index.

---

*Not commercially available in the U.S.

†Not commercially available in Canada.

‡See *Calcium Supplements (Systemic)* for systemic use of calcium carbonate in hypocalcemia

§See *Laxatives (Local)* for laxative use of magnesium hydroxide and magnesium oxide

---

# Category

Antacid—All drugs included in this monograph are used as antacids.

Antiurolithic (phosphate calculi)—Aluminum Carbonate; Aluminum Hydroxide.

Laxative, hyperosmotic, saline—Magnesium Hydroxide; Magnesium Oxide (see *Magnesium Hydroxide* and *Magnesium Oxide, Laxatives [Local]*).

Antihyperphosphatemic—Aluminum Carbonate; Aluminum Hydroxide; Calcium Carbonate (see *Calcium Carbonate, Calcium Supplements [Systemic]*).

Antihypocalcemic—Calcium Carbonate (see *Calcium Carbonate, Calcium Supplements [Systemic]*).

Antiurolithic (calcium calculi)—Magnesium Hydroxide.

# Indications

Note: Bracketed information in the *Indications* section refers to uses that are not included in U.S. product labeling.

**Accepted**

Hyperacidity (treatment)

Ulcer, duodenal (treatment) or

Ulcer, gastric (treatment)—Antacids are indicated for relief of symptoms associated with hyperacidity (heartburn, acid indigestion, and sour stomach). In addition, antacids are used in hyperacidity associated with gastric and duodenal ulcers. However, there have been reports of increased gastrin levels and increased gastric secretion (acid rebound) associated with the use of antacids.

Some of the antacid combinations contain other ingredients that have no antacid properties. Simethicone, an antiflatulent, has been added as an aid in those conditions in which the retention of gas may be a problem; however, in the treatment of peptic ulcer diseases, the advantage of using antacid and simethicone combinations rather than antacids alone has not been clearly established.

Hypersecretory conditions, gastric (treatment adjunct)

Zollinger-Ellison syndrome (treatment adjunct)

Mastocytosis, systemic (treatment adjunct) or

Adenoma, multiple endocrine (treatment adjunct)—Antacids are indicated in conjunction with histamine H$_2$-receptor antagonists or omeprazole for transient symptomatic relief in the treatment of pathological gastric hypersecretion associated with Zollinger-Ellison syndrome (alone or as part of multiple endocrine neoplasia Type-I), systemic mastocytosis, and multiple endocrine adenoma.

Reflux, gastroesophageal (treatment)—Antacids are indicated in the symptomatic treatment of gastroesophageal reflux disease.

Stress-related mucosal damage (prophylaxis and treatment)—Antacids are indicated to prevent and treat upper gastrointestinal, stress-induced ulceration and bleeding, especially in intensive care patients.

[Hyperphosphatemia (treatment)][1]—Aluminum carbonate and aluminum hydroxide may be used in conjunction with a low-phosphate diet to reduce elevated phosphate levels and demineralization of bones in patients with renal insufficiency. However, use of aluminum-containing antacids as phosphate binders may lead to aluminum toxicity in patients with renal insufficiency. Other agents may be preferable for treating hyperphosphatemia in patients with renal insufficiency.

Hypocalcemia (treatment)—See *Calcium Carbonate, Calcium Supplements (Systemic)*.

[Aluminum hydroxide has been used in the treatment of neonatal hypocalcemia and diarrhea; however, it generally has been replaced by other agents. Aluminum carbonate and aluminum hydroxide have been used along with a low-phosphate diet to prevent formation of phosphatic (struvite) urinary stones; however, their use has been replaced by other agents. Magnesium hydroxide has been used to prevent recurrence of calcium stones; however, it has been replaced by other agents. Use of aluminum-containing antacids in young children and premature infants may lead to aluminum toxicity, especially in those patients with renal failure.][1]

**Unaccepted**

Antacids have been used in patients undergoing anesthesia or during labor to lessen the danger from aspiration of gastric contents. However, the use of antacids to prevent acid aspiration has generally been replaced by the equally or more effective histamine H$_2$-receptor antagonists or citrate solutions.

---

[1]Not included in Canadian product labeling.

# Pharmacology/Pharmacokinetics

**Physicochemical characteristics**

Molecular weight—

Aluminum hydroxide: 78.

Calcium carbonate: 100.09.

Magnesium hydroxide: 58.32.

Magnesium oxide: 40.30.

Sodium bicarbonate: 84.01.

**Mechanism of action/Effect**

Antacid—These medications react chemically to neutralize or buffer existing quantities of stomach acid but have no direct effect on its output. This action results in increased pH value of stomach contents, thus providing relief of hyperacidity symptoms. Also, these medications reduce acid concentration within the lumen of the esophagus. This causes an increase in intra-esophageal pH and a decrease in pepsin activity.

Antiurolithic—Aluminum carbonate and aluminum hydroxide bind phosphate ions in the intestine to form insoluble aluminum phosphate, which is excreted in the feces. They thereby reduce phosphates in the urine and prevent formation of phosphatic (struvite) urinary stones. Magnesium hydroxide inhibits the precipitation of calcium oxalate and calcium phosphate, thus preventing the formation of calcium stones.

Antihyperphosphatemic—Aluminum carbonate and aluminum hydroxide reduce serum phosphate levels by binding with phosphate ions in the intestine to form insoluble aluminum phosphate, which passes through the intestinal tract unabsorbed.

Antihypocalcemic—Aluminum hydroxide may increase the release of calcium from bone as a result of the decreased serum phosphate levels.

Antidiarrheal—Aluminum hydroxide's constipating properties help decrease the fluidity of stools.

**Other actions/effects**

Antacids may increase lower esophageal sphincter (LES) pressure. Aluminum-containing antacids have a cytoprotective effect on the gastric mucosa that may be associated with the stimulation of prostaglandin secretion, thus providing protection against mucosal necrosis and hemorrhage caused by corrosive agents, such as aspirin and ethanol.

**Absorption**

Aluminum-containing—Small amounts of the aluminum in aluminum hydroxide are absorbed from the intestine.

Calcium-containing—Approximately 15% of the calcium in calcium carbonate is absorbed from the intestine in normal persons. The amount of calcium absorbed from the gastrointestinal tract is determined by hormonal factors, particularly parathyroid hormone, and vitamin D.

Magnesium-containing—Approximately 10% of the magnesium in magnesium hydroxide (magnesia) is absorbed from the intestine.

**Onset and duration of action**

Onset of action is dependent upon the ability of the antacid to solubilize in the stomach and react with the hydrochloric acid. The poorly soluble antacids (e.g., magnesium trisilicate) will thus react more slowly with hydrochloric acid than will the more soluble ones. In most cases with slow-acting antacids, the onset of action is delayed and may not take place if gastric emptying is rapid.

Duration of action is determined primarily by gastric emptying time. Depending on the kind of antacid used, the duration of action in fasting patients may range from 20 to 60 minutes. However, when the antacid is given 1 hour after meals, the acid-neutralizing effect may be prolonged up to 3 hours.

The following table provides a relative comparison of onset and duration of action of different antacids.

| Antacid | Onset of action | Duration of action |
| --- | --- | --- |
| Aluminum Carbonate | Slow | Short |
| Aluminum Hydroxide | Slow | Prolonged * |
| Aluminum Phosphate | Slow | Short |
| Calcium Carbonate | Fast | Prolonged |
| Magaldrate | Intermediate | Prolonged |
| Magnesium Carbonate | Intermediate | Short |
| Magnesium Hydroxide | Fast | Short |
| Magnesium Oxide | Fast | Short |
| Magnesium Trisilicate | Slow | Prolonged † |
| Sodium Bicarbonate | Fast | Short |

*Absorptive properties of the gel prolong its duration of action
†If gastric emptying is rapid, stomach may empty before much of the acid is neutralized

**Elimination**
Renal and fecal; 15 to 30% of the salts formed are absorbed and are then excreted by the kidneys.

## Precautions to Consider

**Pregnancy/Reproduction**
Pregnancy—Antacids are generally considered safe as long as chronic high doses are avoided.
*Aluminum-, calcium-, or magnesium-containing antacids—*
   Adequate and well-controlled studies in humans have not been done; however, there have been reports of antacids causing such adverse effects as hypercalcemia, hypomagnesemia, hypermagnesemia, and increased tendon reflexes in fetuses and/or neonates whose mothers were chronic users of aluminum-, calcium-, and/or magnesium-containing antacids, especially in high doses.
   Studies have not been done in animals.
*Sodium bicarbonate–containing antacids—*
   Problems in humans have not been documented; however, risk-benefit must be considered because sodium bicarbonate is absorbed systemically. Chronic use may lead to systemic alkalosis. The sodium load that is absorbed can also cause edema and weight gain.

**Breast-feeding**
Problems in humans have not been documented; although some aluminum, calcium, and magnesium may be distributed into breast milk, the concentration is not great enough to produce an effect in the neonate.

**Pediatrics**
Antacids should not be given to young children (up to 6 years of age) unless prescribed by a physician. Since children are not usually able to describe their symptoms precisely, proper diagnosis should precede the use of an antacid. This will avoid the complication of an existing condition (e.g., appendicitis) or the appearance of severe adverse effects.
Use of magnesium-containing antacids is contraindicated in very young children because there is a risk of hypermagnesemia, especially in dehydrated children or children with renal failure.
Use of aluminum-containing antacids is contraindicated in very young children because there is a risk of aluminum toxicity, especially in dehydrated infants and children or infants and children with renal failure.

**Geriatrics**
Metabolic bone disease commonly seen in the elderly may be aggravated by the phosphorus depletion, hypercalciuria, and inhibition of absorption of intestinal fluoride caused by the chronic use of aluminum-containing antacids. Also, elderly patients are more likely to have age-related renal function impairment, which may lead to aluminum retention.
Although it is not known whether high intake of aluminum leads to Alzheimer's disease, the use of aluminum-containing antacids in Alzheimer's patients is not generally recommended. Research suggests that aluminum may contribute to the disease's development since it has been found to concentrate in neurofibrillary tangles in brain tissue.

**Drug interactions and/or related problems**
See *Table 1,* page 180.

**Laboratory value alterations**
See *Table 2,* page 183.

**Medical considerations/contraindications**
See *Table 3,* page 183.

**Patient monitoring**
See *Table 4,* page 185.

## Side/Adverse Effects
See *Table 5,* page 185.

## Patient Consultation
See *Table 6,* page 186.

## General Dosing Information

**For antacid use**
The dose of antacid needed to neutralize gastric acid varies among patients, depending on the amount of acid secreted and the buffering capacity of the particular preparation.

It is estimated that 99% of the gastric acid will be neutralized when a gastric pH of 3.3 is achieved.

The amount (in mEq) of 1 $N$ hydrochloric acid that can be titrated to pH 3.5 in 15 minutes by a certain dose of antacid is referred to as the neutralizing capacity of the antacid. Approximately 15 to 20 mEq of an aluminum- and magnesium-containing antacid are required to neutralize 1 mEq of gastric hydrochloric acid.

Patients with hypersecretory disorders (e.g., duodenal ulcer, Zollinger-Ellison syndrome, multiple endocrine adenomas, and systemic mastocytosis) may require 80 to 160 mEq of buffer at each dose for symptomatic relief; this is approximately 30 to 60 mL of most antacids. Only half of this dose is needed for patients with normal acid secretion.

The liquid dosage form of antacids is considered to be more effective than the solid or powder dosage form. In most cases, tablets must be thoroughly chewed before being swallowed; otherwise, they may not dissolve completely in the stomach before entering the small intestine.

The maximum recommended dosage should not be taken for more than 2 weeks, except under the advice or supervision of a physician.

Combinations of antacids containing aluminum and/or calcium compounds with magnesium salts may offer the advantage of balancing the constipating qualities of aluminum and/or calcium and the laxative qualities of magnesium.

**For use in peptic ulcer**
In the treatment of peptic ulcer disease, to achieve adequate antacid effect in the stomach at the optimum time, most antacids are administered 1 and 3 hours after meals for prolonged acid-neutralizing effect and at bedtime. However, when taken at bedtime, their effect is not prolonged because of rapid gastric emptying. Additional doses of antacids may be administered to relieve the pain that may occur between the regularly scheduled doses.

Antacid therapy should be continued for at least 4 to 6 weeks after all symptoms have disappeared, since there is no correlation between disappearance of symptoms and actual healing of the ulcer.
*Aluminum hydroxide—*
   In the treatment of peptic ulcer, 960 mg to 3.6 grams are given orally every one or two hours during waking hours, the dosage being adjusted as needed. For extremely severe symptoms of peptic ulcer (hospitalized patients), 2.6 to 4.8 grams diluted with two to three parts of water may be given intragastrically every thirty minutes for periods of twelve or more hours a day.

**For antihyperphosphatemic use**
*Aluminum hydroxide—*
   In adults, 1.9 to 4.8 grams of aluminum hydroxide are given orally three or four times a day in conjunction with dietary phosphate restriction. In children, a dose of 50 to 150 mg per kg of body weight is given in four to six divided doses in conjunction with dietary phosphate restriction.

**For antiurolithic use**
*Aluminum carbonate—*
   In the prevention of phosphate stones the equivalent of 1 to 3 grams of aluminum carbonate is given four times a day, one hour after meals and at bedtime.

## Oral Dosage Forms
See *Table 7,* page 189.

Revised: 08/15/95

## Table 1. Drug Interactions and/or Related Problems

| The following drug interactions and/or related problems have been selected on the basis of their potential clinical significance (possible mechanism in parentheses where appropriate)—not necessarily inclusive: (» = major clinical significance)<br><br>Note: Combinations containing any of the following medications, depending on the amount present, may also interact with this medication.<br><br>Only specific interactions between antacids and other oral medications have been identified in this monograph. However, because of antacids' ability to change gastric or urinary pH and to adsorb or form complexes with other drugs, the rate and/or extent of absorption of other medications may be increased or reduced when the medication is used concurrently with antacids. In general, patients should be advised not to take any other oral medications within 1 to 2 hours of antacids. | Legend:<br>**I**=Aluminum-containing<br>**II**=Calcium-containing<br>**III**=Magaldrate<br>**IV**=Magnesium-containing<br>**V**=Sodium Bicarbonate–containing | | | | |
|---|---|---|---|---|---|
| | **I** | **II** | **III** | **IV** | **V** |
| Acidifiers, urinary, such as:<br>Ammonium chloride<br>Ascorbic acid<br>Potassium or sodium phosphates<br>Racemethionine<br>(antacids may alkalinize the urine and counteract the effect of urinary acidifiers; frequent use of antacids, especially in high doses, is best avoided by patients receiving therapy to acidify the urine) | ✓ | ✓ | ✓ | ✓ | ✓ |
| Amphetamines or<br>Quinidine<br>(urinary excretion may be inhibited when these medications are used concurrently with antacids in doses that cause the urine to become alkaline, possibly resulting in toxicity; dosage adjustment may be needed when therapy with these antacids is initiated or discontinued or if dosage is changed) | ✓ | ✓ | ✓ | ✓ | ✓ |
| Anticholinergics or other medications with anticholinergic activity (See *Appendix II*)<br>(concurrent use with antacids may decrease absorption, reducing the effectiveness of anticholinergics; doses of these medications should be spaced 1 hour apart from doses of antacids) | ✓ | ✓ | ✓ | ✓ | ✓ |
| (urinary excretion may be delayed by alkalinization of the urine, thus potentiating the side effects of the anticholinergic) | ✓ | ✓ | ✓ | ✓ | ✓ |
| Calcitonin or<br>Etidronate or<br>Gallium nitrate or<br>Pamidronate or<br>Plicamycin<br>(concurrent use with calcium carbonate may antagonize the effect of these medications in the treatment of hypercalcemia) | | ✓ | | | |
| Calcium-containing preparations<br>(concurrent and prolonged use with sodium bicarbonate may result in the milk-alkali syndrome) | | | | | ✓ |
| » Cellulose sodium phosphate<br>(concurrent use with calcium-containing antacids may decrease effectiveness of cellulose sodium phosphate in preventing hypercalciuria) | | ✓ | | | |
| (concurrent use with magnesium-containing antacids may result in binding of magnesium; patients should be advised not to take these medications within 1 hour of cellulose sodium phosphate) | | | ✓ | ✓ | |
| Chenodiol<br>(concurrent use with aluminum-containing antacids may result in binding of chenodiol, thus decreasing its absorption) | ✓ | | ✓ | | |
| Citrates<br>(concurrent use with antacids containing aluminum, calcium carbonates, magaldrate, or sodium bicarbonate may result in systemic alkalosis) | ✓ | ✓ | ✓ | | ✓ |
| (concurrent use of sodium citrate with sodium bicarbonate may promote the development of calcium stones in patients with uric acid stones, due to sodium ion opposition to the hypocalciuric effect of the alkaline load; may also cause hypernatremia) | | | | | ✓ |
| (concurrent use of aluminum-containing antacids and magaldrate with citrate salts can increase aluminum absorption, possibly resulting in acute aluminum toxicity, especially in patients with renal insufficiency) | ✓ | | ✓ | | |
| Digitalis glycosides<br>(concurrent use with aluminum- and magnesium-containing antacids may inhibit absorption, possibly decreasing plasma concentrations of digitalis glycosides; although actual clinical importance of this interaction has not been established, it is recommended that doses of antacids and digitalis glycosides be separated by several hours) | ✓ | | ✓ | ✓ | |
| Diuretics, potassium-depleting, such as bumetanide, ethacrynic acid, furosemide, indapamide, thiazide diuretics<br>(concurrent use of thiazide diuretics with large doses of calcium carbonate may result in hypercalcemia) | | ✓ | | | |
| Enteric-coated medications, such as bisacodyl<br>(concurrent administration of antacids with enteric-coated medications may cause the enteric coating to dissolve too rapidly, resulting in gastric or duodenal irritation) | ✓ | ✓ | ✓ | ✓ | ✓ |

## Table 1. Drug Interactions and/or Related Problems *(continued)*

Legend:
**I**=Aluminum-containing
**II**=Calcium-containing
**III**=Magaldrate
**IV**=Magnesium-containing
**V**=Sodium Bicarbonate–containing

| | I | II | III | IV | V |
|---|---|---|---|---|---|
| **Ephedrine**<br>(urine alkalinization induced by sodium bicarbonate may increase the half-life of ephedrine and prolong its duration of action, especially if the urine remains alkaline for several days or longer; dosage adjustment of ephedrine may be necessary) | | | | | ✔ |
| » **Fluoroquinolones**<br>(alkalinization of the urine may reduce the solubility of ciprofloxacin and norfloxacin in the urine, especially when the urinary pH exceeds 7.0; if antacids and one of these medications are used concurrently, patients should be observed for signs of crystalluria and nephrotoxicity) | ✔ | ✔ | ✔ | ✔ | ✔ |
| (aluminum- and magnesium-containing antacids may reduce absorption of fluoroquinolones, resulting in lower serum and urine concentrations of these medications; therefore, concurrent use is not recommended; however, if aluminum- and magnesium-containing antacids must be used concurrently with these medications, it is recommended that enoxacin be taken at least 2 hours before or 8 hours after the antacid; ciprofloxacin and lomefloxacin should be taken at least 2 hours before or 6 hours after the antacid; and norfloxacin and ofloxacin should be taken at least 2 hours before or after the antacid) | ✔ | | | ✔ | ✔ |
| **Folic acid**<br>(prolonged use of aluminum- and/or magnesium-containing antacids may decrease folic acid absorption by raising the pH of the small intestine; patients should be advised to take antacids at least 2 hours after folic acid) | ✔ | | | ✔ | ✔ |
| **Histamine H₂-receptor antagonists**<br>(concurrent use with antacids may be indicated in the treatment of peptic ulcer to relieve pain; however, simultaneous administration of medium to high doses [80 mmol to 150 mmol] of antacids is not recommended since absorption of histamine H₂-receptor antagonists may be decreased; patients should be advised not to take any antacids within ½ to 1 hour of histamine H₂-receptor antagonists) | ✔ | ✔ | ✔ | ✔ | ✔ |
| **Iron preparations, oral**<br>(absorption may be decreased when these preparations are used concurrently with magnesium trisilicate or antacids containing carbonate; spacing the doses of the iron preparation as far as possible from doses of the antacid is recommended) | ✔ | ✔ | | ✔ | ✔ |
| » **Isoniazid, oral**<br>(concurrent use with aluminum-containing antacids may delay and decrease absorption of oral isoniazid; concurrent use should be avoided or the patient should be advised to take oral isoniazid at least 1 hour before the antacid) | ✔ | | ✔ | | |
| » **Ketoconazole**<br>(antacids may cause increased gastrointestinal pH; concurrent administration with antacids may result in a marked reduction in absorption of ketoconazole; patients should be advised to take antacids at least 3 hours after ketoconazole) | ✔ | ✔ | ✔ | ✔ | ✔ |
| **Lithium**<br>(sodium bicarbonate enhances lithium excretion, possibly resulting in decreased efficacy; this may be partly due to the sodium content) | | | | | ✔ |
| **Mexiletine**<br>(marked alkalinization of the urine caused by sodium bicarbonate may slow renal excretion of mexiletine) | | | | | ✔ |
| » **Mecamylamine**<br>(alkalinization of the urine may slow excretion and prolong the effects of mecamylamine; concurrent use is not recommended) | ✔ | ✔ | ✔ | ✔ | ✔ |
| » **Methenamine**<br>(concurrent use with antacids that cause the urine to become alkaline may reduce the effectiveness of methenamine by inhibiting its conversion to formaldehyde; concurrent use is not recommended) | ✔ | ✔ | ✔ | ✔ | ✔ |
| **Milk or milk products**<br>(concurrent and prolonged use with calcium carbonate or sodium bicarbonate may result in the milk-alkali syndrome) | | ✔ | | | ✔ |
| **Misoprostol**<br>(concurrent use with magnesium-containing antacids may aggravate misoprostol-induced diarrhea) | | | | ✔ | |
| **Pancrelipase**<br>(concurrent administration of antacids may be required to prevent inactivation of pancrelipase [except enteric-coated dosage forms] by gastric pepsin and acid pH; however, calcium carbonate– and/or magnesium-containing antacids are not recommended since they may decrease the effectiveness of pancrelipase) | | ✔ | ✔ | ✔ | |

## Table 1. Drug Interactions and/or Related Problems *(continued)*

| | Legend:<br>**I**=Aluminum-containing<br>**II**=Calcium-containing<br>**III**=Magaldrate<br>**IV**=Magnesium-containing<br>**V**=Sodium Bicarbonate–<br>containing | | | | |
|---|---|---|---|---|---|
| | **I** | **II** | **III** | **IV** | **V** |
| Penicillamine<br>(absorption may be reduced when penicillamine is administered concurrently with aluminum- or magnesium-containing antacids; although more studies are needed to establish the significance of this interaction, it is recommended that doses of antacids and penicillamine be separated by 2 hours) | ✔ | | | ✔ | |
| Phenothiazines, especially chlorpromazine, oral<br>(absorption may be inhibited when these medications are used concurrently with aluminum- or magnesium-containing antacids; although more studies are needed to establish the significance of this interaction, simultaneous administration should be avoided) | ✔ | | | ✔ | |
| Phenytoin<br>(concurrent use with aluminum-, magnesium-, and/or calcium carbonate–containing antacids may decrease absorption of phenytoin, thus reducing serum phenytoin concentrations; although more studies are needed to establish the significance of this interaction, it is recommended that doses of antacids and phenytoin be separated by about 2 to 3 hours) | ✔ | ✔ | ✔ | ✔ | |
| Phosphates, oral<br>(concurrent use with aluminum- or magnesium-containing antacids may bind the phosphate and prevent its absorption)<br>(concurrent use with calcium-containing antacids may increase potential of deposition of calcium in soft tissues if serum-ionized calcium is high) | ✔ | ✔ | | ✔ | |
| Quinine<br>(concurrent use with aluminum-containing antacids may decrease or delay the absorption of quinine) | ✔ | | | | |
| Salicylates<br>(alkalinization of the urine may increase renal salicylate excretion and lower serum salicylate levels; dosage adjustments of salicylates may be necessary when chronic high-dose antacid therapy is started or stopped, especially in patients receiving large doses of the salicylate, such as patients with rheumatoid arthritis or rheumatic fever) | ✔ | ✔ | ✔ | ✔ | ✔ |
| Sodium bicarbonate or<br>Vitamin D<br>(concurrent and prolonged use with calcium carbonate may result in the milk-alkali syndrome) | | ✔ | | | |
| Sodium fluoride<br>(concurrent use with aluminum hydroxide may decrease absorption and increase fecal excretion of fluoride)<br>(calcium ions may complex with and inhibit absorption of fluoride) | ✔ | ✔ | | ✔ | |
| » Sodium polystyrene sulfonate resin (SPSR)<br>(neutralization of gastric acid may be impaired when SPSR is used concurrently with calcium- or magnesium-containing antacids, possibly resulting in systemic alkalosis; concurrent use is not recommended) | | ✔ | ✔ | ✔ | |
| Sucralfate<br>(concurrent use with antacids may be indicated in the treatment of duodenal ulcer to relieve pain; however, simultaneous administration is not recommended since antacids may interfere with binding of sucralfate to the mucosa; patients should be advised not to take any antacids within 1/2 hour before or after sucralfate; concurrent use with aluminum-containing antacids may cause aluminum toxicity in patients with chronic renal failure) | ✔ | ✔ | ✔ | ✔ | ✔ |
| » Tetracyclines, oral<br>(absorption may be decreased when oral tetracyclines are used concurrently with antacids because of possible formation of nonabsorbable complexes and/or increase in intragastric pH; patients should be advised not to take antacids within 3 to 4 hours of tetracyclines) | ✔ | ✔ | ✔ | ✔ | ✔ |
| Vitamin D, including calcifediol and calcitriol<br>(concurrent use with magnesium-containing antacids may result in hypermagnesemia, especially in patients with chronic renal failure)<br>(concurrent use with calcium-containing antacids may result in hypercalcemia)) | | ✔ | | ✔ | |

## Table 2. Laboratory value alterations

| The following have been selected on the basis of their potential clinical significance (possible effect in parentheses where appropriate)—not necessarily inclusive (» = major clinical significance): | I | II | III | IV | V |
|---|---|---|---|---|---|
| | Legend:<br>**I**=Aluminum-containing<br>**II**=Calcium-containing<br>**III**=Magaldrate<br>**IV**=Magnesium-containing<br>**V**=Sodium Bicarbonate–containing | | | | |
| **With diagnostic test results** | | | | | |
| » Gastric acid secretion test<br>(concurrent use of antacids may antagonize the effect of pentagastrin and histamine in the evaluation of gastric acid secretory function; administration of antacids is not recommended on the morning of the test) | ✔ | ✔ | ✔ | ✔ | ✔ |
| Meckel's diverticulum imaging<br>(prior administration of aluminum-containing antacids may decrease stomach and bladder uptake of sodium pertechnetate Tc 99m and thus interfere with Meckel's diverticulum evaluation) | ✔ | | ✔ | | |
| Reticuloendothelial cell imaging of liver, spleen, or bone marrow with technetium Tc 99m sulfur colloid<br>(high doses of aluminum-containing antacids may impair reticuloendothelial cell imaging due to the polyvalent cations that cause agglomeration of the individual colloidal particles, thus causing them to be trapped by the pulmonary capillary bed rather than by the reticuloendothelial cells of the liver, spleen, and bone marrow) | ✔ | | ✔ | | |
| Skeletal imaging<br>(prior administration of aluminum-containing antacids may result in liver uptake of technetium Tc 99m pyrophosphate due to the formation of submicroscopic precipitates) | ✔ | | ✔ | | |
| **With physiology/laboratory test values** | | | | | |
| Calcium, serum<br>(concentrations may be increased with large doses) | | ✔ | | | |
| Gastrin, serum<br>(concentrations may be increased) | ✔ | ✔ | ✔ | ✔ | ✔ |
| Phosphate, serum<br>(concentrations may be decreased by excessive and prolonged use) | ✔ | ✔ | ✔ | | |
| Systemic and urinary pH<br>(may be increased) | ✔ | ✔ | ✔ | ✔ | ✔ |

## Table 3. Medical considerations/Contraindications

Note: A blank space usually signifies lack of information; it is not necessarily an indication that a given medical problem is of no concern. However, the pharmacologic similarity of these agents may suggest that if caution is required in particular medical problems for one agent, then it may be required for the others as well.

| The medical considerations/contraindications included have been selected on the basis of their potential clinical significance (reasons given in parentheses where appropriate)—not necessarily inclusive (» = major clinical significance). | I | II | III | IV | V |
|---|---|---|---|---|---|
| | Legend:<br>**I**=Aluminum-containing<br>**II**=Calcium-containing<br>**III**=Magaldrate<br>**IV**=Magnesium-containing<br>**V**=Sodium Bicarbonate–containing | | | | |
| ***Except under special circumstances, these medications should not be used when the following medical problems exist:*** | | | | | |
| » Hypercalcemia<br>(increased risk of exacerbation) | | ✔ | | | |
| » Intestinal obstruction | ✔ | ✔ | ✔ | ✔ | ✔ |
| » Renal function impairment, severe<br>(increased risk of hypermagnesemia) | | | | ✔ | ✔ |

*Aluminum hydroxide has the ability to form the insoluble complex of aluminum phosphate, which is excreted in the feces. This may lead to lowered serum phosphate concentrations and phosphorus mobilization from the bone. If phosphate depletion (e.g., malabsorption syndrome) is already present, osteomalacia, osteoporosis, and fracture may result, especially in patients with other bone disease. In such patients predisposed to phosphate depletion, other aluminum-containing antacids (except aluminum phosphate) will be of concern only in relation to their ability to form an aluminum phosphate complex.

†Antacids containing more than 5 mEq (115 mg) of sodium per total daily dose should not be used without first checking with physician. The usual amount of sodium allowed in restricted diets is 3 grams or less per day.

‡In patients with renal function impairment, use of antacids containing more than 50 mEq (608 mg) of magnesium per total daily dose should be carefully considered.

## Table 3. Medical considerations/Contraindications *(continued)*

| | Legend: **I**=Aluminum-containing, **II**=Calcium-containing, **III**=Magaldrate, **IV**=Magnesium-containing, **V**=Sodium Bicarbonate–containing | | | | |
|---|:---:|:---:|:---:|:---:|:---:|
| | I | II | III | IV | V |
| ***Risk-benefit should be considered when the following medical problems exist:*** | | | | | |
| » Alzheimer's disease (may be exacerbated) | ✓ | | ✓ | | |
| » Appendicitis, or symptoms of (may complicate existing condition; laxative or constipating effects may increase danger of perforation or rupture) | ✓ | ✓ | ✓ | ✓ | ✓ |
| Bleeding, gastrointestinal or rectal, undiagnosed (condition may be exacerbated) | ✓ | ✓ | ✓ | ✓ | ✓ |
| Bone fractures | * | | * | | |
| » Cirrhosis of liver or | † | † | | | ✓ |
| » Congestive heart failure or | † | † | | | ✓ |
| » Edema or | † | † | | | ✓ |
| » Toxemia of pregnancy (fluid retention may be increased; low-sodium antacids should be used) | † | † | | | ✓ |
| Colitis, ulcerative (may be aggravated by laxative effect of magnesium-containing antacids) | | | ✓ | ✓ | |
| Colostomy or Diverticulitis or » Ileostomy (increased risk of fluid or electrolyte imbalance) | | | ✓ | ✓ | |
| » Constipation or » Fecal impaction (may be exacerbated) | ✓ | ✓ | | | |
| Diarrhea, chronic (possible increased danger of phosphate depletion with aluminum-containing antacids) | ✓ | | ✓ | | |
| (possible increased laxative effect with magnesium-containing antacids) | | | | ✓ | |
| » Gastric outlet obstruction | ✓ | | ✓ | | |
| » Hemorrhoids (may be aggravated) | ✓ | ✓ | | | |
| » Hypoparathyroidism (calcium excretion may be decreased) | | ✓ | | | |
| » Hypophosphatemia | * | | * | | |
| » Renal function impairment (possible increased risk of aluminum toxicity to brain tissue, bone, and parathyroid glands; possible onset of the neurological syndrome—dialysis dementia—in dialysis patients with long-term use of aluminum-containing antacids) | ✓ | | ✓ | | |
| (possible increased danger of milk-alkali syndrome and hypercalcemia with calcium-containing antacids) | | ✓ | | | |
| (possible increased danger of hypermagnesemia) | | | ‡ | ‡ | |
| (may cause metabolic alkalosis) | | | | | ✓ |
| » Sarcoidosis (increased risk of hypercalcemia or renal disease) | | ✓ | | | |
| Sensitivity to aluminum-, calcium-, magnesium-, simethicone-, or sodium bicarbonate–containing medications | ✓ | ✓ | ✓ | ✓ | ✓ |

*Aluminum hydroxide has the ability to form the insoluble complex of aluminum phosphate, which is excreted in the feces. This may lead to lowered serum phosphate concentrations and phosphorus mobilization from the bone. If phosphate depletion (e.g., malabsorption syndrome) is already present, osteomalacia, osteoporosis, and fracture may result, especially in patients with other bone disease. In such patients predisposed to phosphate depletion, other aluminum-containing antacids (except aluminum phosphate) will be of concern only in relation to their ability to form an aluminum phosphate complex.

†Antacids containing more than 5 mEq (115 mg) of sodium per total daily dose should not be used without first checking with physician. The usual amount of sodium allowed in restricted diets is 3 grams or less per day.

‡In patients with renal function impairment, use of antacids containing more than 50 mEq (608 mg) of magnesium per total daily dose should be carefully considered.

## Table 4. Patient Monitoring

| The following may be especially important in patient monitoring (other tests may be warranted in some patients, depending on condition; » = major clinical significance): | Legend:<br>**I**=Aluminum-containing<br>**II**=Calcium-containing<br>**III**=Magaldrate<br>**IV**=Magnesium-containing<br>**V**=Sodium Bicarbonate–containing | | | | |
|---|---|---|---|---|---|
| | **I** | **II** | **III** | **IV** | **V** |
| Aluminum concentrations, serum<br>(determinations recommended at periodic intervals for patients with impaired renal function receiving aluminum-containing antacids, to prevent aluminum toxicity) | ✔ | | | | |
| Calcium concentrations, serum<br>(determinations recommended at periodic intervals for patients, especially those with impaired renal function, who are receiving chronic therapy with aluminum-containing antacids)<br>(recommended weekly when calcium-containing antacids are used in large doses) | ✔ | ✔ | ✔ | | |
| Phosphate concentrations, serum<br>(determinations recommended at periodic intervals for patients, especially those with impaired renal function, who are receiving chronic therapy with aluminum-containing antacids) | ✔ | | | | |
| Potassium concentrations, serum<br>(determinations recommended at periodic intervals for patients, especially those with impaired renal function, who are receiving antacids containing more than 25 mEq [925 mg] of potassium per daily dose) | ✔ | ✔ | ✔ | ✔ | ✔ |
| Renal function determinations<br>(recommended weekly in patients with renal function impairment, and whenever symptoms of hypercalcemia occur in patients receiving calcium-containing antacids in large doses)<br>(recommended at periodic intervals with long-term use of frequently repeated dosage) | ✔ | ✔ | ✔ | ✔ | ✔ |

## Table 5. Side/Adverse Effects*

| The following side/adverse effects have been selected on the basis of their potential clinical significance (possible signs and symptoms in parentheses where appropriate)—not necessarily inclusive: | Legend:<br>**I**=Aluminum-containing<br>**II**=Calcium-containing<br>**III**=Magaldrate<br>**IV**=Magnesium-containing<br>**V**=Sodium Bicarbonate–containing | | | | |
|---|---|---|---|---|---|
| | **I** | **II** | **III** | **IV** | **V** |
| **Medical attention needed**<br>With long-term use in chronic renal failure in dialysis patients<br>   *Neurotoxicity* (mood or mental changes) | ✔ | | ✔ | | |
| With large doses<br>   *Fecal impaction* (continuing severe constipation)<br>   *Swelling of feet or lower legs* | ✔ | ✔ | | | ✔ |
| With large doses or in renal insufficiency<br>   *Metabolic alkalosis* (mood or mental changes; muscle pain or twitching; nervousness or restlessness; slow breathing; unpleasant taste; unusual tiredness or weakness) | | ✔ | | | ✔ |

*Differences in frequency of occurrence may reflect either lack of clinical-use data or actual pharmacologic distinctions among agents (although their pharmacologic similarity suggests that side effects occurring with one may occur with the others). M = more frequent; L = less frequent; R = rare; U = unknown.

†May also occur with large doses and/or in chronic renal failure with calcium carbonate.

‡Osteomalacia and osteoporosis have been reported after chronic ingestion of large doses of aluminum hydroxide–containing antacids. Since magaldrate is converted to aluminum and magnesium hydroxides *in vivo*, it is likely that osteomalacia and osteoporosis may occur with excessive use of magaldrate.

§Chronic administration of magnesium trisilicate may infrequently produce silica renal stones.

## Table 5. Side/Adverse Effects* *(continued)*

Legend:
**I**=Aluminum-containing
**II**=Calcium-containing
**III**=Magaldrate
**IV**=Magnesium-containing
**V**=Sodium Bicarbonate–
    containing

|  | I | II | III | IV | V |
|---|---|---|---|---|---|
| **With long-term or prolonged use**<br>*Hypercalcemia associated with milk-alkali syndrome* (frequent urge to urinate; continuing headache; continuing loss of appetite; nausea or vomiting; unusual tiredness or weakness)<br>*Osteomalacia and osteoporosis due to phosphate depletion* (bone pain; swelling of wrists or ankles) | ✔ | † | ‡ |  | ✔ |
| **With overuse or prolonged use**<br>*Renal calculi* (difficult or painful urination) |  | ✔ |  | § |  |
| **With prolonged use or large doses**<br>*Phosphorus depletion syndrome* (continuing feeling of discomfort; continuing loss of appetite; muscle weakness; unusual weight loss) | ✔ |  | ✔ |  |  |
| **With prolonged use or large doses and/or in renal disease**<br>*Hypermagnesemia or other electrolyte imbalance* (dizziness or lightheadedness; irregular heartbeat; mood or mental changes; unusual tiredness or weakness) |  |  | ✔ | ✔ |  |
| **Medical attention needed only if continuing or bothersome**<br>*Chalky taste* | M | M | M | M | U |
| *Constipation, mild* | M | L | U | U | U |
| *Diarrhea or laxative effect*—with overdose | U | U | U | M | U |
| *Increased thirst* | U | U | U | U | L |
| *Nausea or vomiting* | L | U | U | L | U |
| *Speckling or whitish discoloration of stools* (concentrations of fatty acid–salts of aluminum) | L | U | U | U | U |
| *Stomach cramps* | M | U | U | L | L |

*Differences in frequency of occurrence may reflect either lack of clinical-use data or actual pharmacologic distinctions among agents (although their pharmacologic similarity suggests that side effects occurring with one may occur with the others). M = more frequent; L = less frequent; R = rare; U = unknown.

†May also occur with large doses and/or in chronic renal failure with calcium carbonate.

‡Osteomalacia and osteoporosis have been reported after chronic ingestion of large doses of aluminum hydroxide–containing antacids. Since magaldrate is converted to aluminum and magnesium hydroxides *in vivo*, it is likely that osteomalacia and osteoporosis may occur with excessive use of magaldrate.

§Chronic administration of magnesium trisilicate may infrequently produce silica renal stones.

## Table 6. Patient Consultation

Legend:
**I**=Aluminum-containing
**II**=Calcium-containing
**III**=Magaldrate
**IV**=Magnesium-containing
**V**=Sodium Bicarbonate–
    containing

As an aid to patient consultation, refer to *Advice for the Patient, Antacids (Oral).*

In providing consultation, consider emphasizing the following selected information (≫ = major clinical significance):

|  | I | II | III | IV | V |
|---|---|---|---|---|---|
| **Before using this medication**<br>≫  Conditions affecting use, especially: |  |  |  |  |  |
|     Sensitivity to aluminum-, calcium-, magnesium-, simethicone-, or sodium bicarbonate–containing medication | ✔ | ✔ | ✔ | ✔ | ✔ |
|     Pregnancy—Concern for fetus or neonate only with chronic high doses; sodium intake may cause edema and weight gain (for sodium-containing) | ✔ | ✔ | ✔ | ✔ | ✔ |
|     Use in children—Not recommended for children up to 6 years of age; proper diagnosis required to avoid medical complications | ✔ | ✔ | ✔ | ✔ | ✔ |
|     Use in the elderly— |  |  |  |  |  |
|         Possible aggravation of metabolic bone disease | ✔ |  |  |  |  |
|         Possible exacerbation of Alzheimer's disease | ✔ |  |  |  |  |

## Table 6. Patient Consultation (continued)

Legend:
**I**=Aluminum-containing
**II**=Calcium-containing
**III**=Magaldrate
**IV**=Magnesium-containing
**V**=Sodium Bicarbonate–containing

| | I | II | III | IV | V |
|---|---|---|---|---|---|
| Other medications, especially: | | | | | |
|   Cellulose sodium phosphate | | ✔ | ✔ | ✔ | |
|   Fluoroquinolones | ✔ | ✔ | ✔ | ✔ | ✔ |
|   Isoniazid, oral | ✔ | | ✔ | | |
|   Ketoconazole | ✔ | ✔ | ✔ | ✔ | ✔ |
|   Mecamylamine | ✔ | ✔ | ✔ | ✔ | |
|   Methenamine | ✔ | ✔ | ✔ | ✔ | |
|   Sodium polystyrene sulfonate resin | ✔ | ✔ | ✔ | ✔ | |
|   Tetracyclines, oral | ✔ | ✔ | ✔ | ✔ | ✔ |
| Other medical problems, especially: | | | | | |
|   Alzheimer's disease | ✔ | | | | |
|   Appendicitis, symptoms of | ✔ | ✔ | ✔ | ✔ | ✔ |
|   Constipation or fecal impaction or intestinal obstruction | ✔ | ✔ | | | |
|   Edematous conditions | ✔ | ✔ | | | ✔ |
|   Hemorrhoids | ✔ | ✔ | | | |
|   Hypercalcemia | | ✔ | | | |
|   Hypoparathyroidism | | ✔ | | | |
|   Hypophosphatemia | ✔ | | ✔ | | |
|   Ileostomy | | | ✔ | ✔ | |
|   Renal function impairment | | | ✔ | ✔ | |
|   Sarcoidosis | | ✔ | | | |
| **Proper use of this medication** | | | | | |
|   Following physician's or manufacturer's instructions | ✔ | ✔ | ✔ | ✔ | ✔ |
| »  Proper dosing | ✔ | ✔ | ✔ | ✔ | ✔ |
|   Missed dose: If on regular dosing schedule—Taking as soon as possible; not taking if almost time for next dose; not doubling doses | ✔ | ✔ | ✔ | ✔ | ✔ |
| »  Proper storage | ✔ | ✔ | ✔ | ✔ | ✔ |
| *For chewable tablet dosage form* | | | | | |
|   Chewing tablets well before swallowing for faster results and maximum effectiveness | ✔ | ✔ | ✔ | ✔ | |
| *For use in treatment of ulcers* | | | | | |
| »  Compliance with therapy | ✔ | ✔ | ✔ | ✔ | ✔ |
|   Taking 1 and 3 hours after meals and at bedtime for maximum effectiveness | ✔ | ✔ | ✔ | ✔ | ✔ |
| *For aluminum carbonate or aluminum hydroxide as an antiurolithic* | | | | | |
|   Drinking plenty of fluids for best results | ✔ | | | | |
| *For aluminum carbonate or aluminum hydroxide as an antihyperphosphatemic* | | | | | |
|   Possible need for low-phosphate diet | ✔ | | | | |
| **Precautions while using this medication** | | | | | |
|   Regular visits to physician to check progress of therapy if: | | | | | |
|     —taking large doses | | ✔ | | | |
|     —taking regularly for long period of time | ✔ | ✔ | ✔ | ✔ | ✔ |
|   Possible interference with gastric acid secretion tests; need to inform physician of use of medication | ✔ | ✔ | ✔ | ✔ | ✔ |
| »  Not taking this medication: | | | | | |
|     —if symptoms of appendicitis are present; checking with physician for proper diagnosis | ✔ | ✔ | ✔ | ✔ | ✔ |
|     —if symptoms of inflamed bowel are present | | | | ✔ | |
|     —within 1 to 2 hours of other oral medication | ✔ | ✔ | ✔ | ✔ | ✔ |
|     —with large amounts of milk or milk products | | ✔ | | | ✔ |
|   Possible need for sodium restriction | ✔ | ✔ | | ✔ | ✔ |
|   Possible interference with test using radiopharmaceutical; need to inform physician of using aluminum-containing antacid | ✔ | | ✔ | | |
| *For antacid use* | | | | | |
| »  Not taking this medication for more than 2 weeks or if problem is recurring, unless otherwise directed by physician | ✔ | ✔ | ✔ | ✔ | ✔ |
|   Alerting patients to laxative effect when taken too often or in large doses | | | | ✔ | ✔ |

## Table 6. Patient Consultation *(continued)*

| | Legend:<br>**I**=Aluminum-containing<br>**II**=Calcium-containing<br>**III**=Magaldrate<br>**IV**=Magnesium-containing<br>**V**=Sodium Bicarbonate–<br>containing | | | | |
|---|:---:|:---:|:---:|:---:|:---:|
| | **I** | **II** | **III** | **IV** | **V** |
| **Side/adverse effects** | | | | | |
| Signs of potential side effects, especially: | | | | | |
|   Neurotoxicity | ✓ | | ✓ | | |
|   Fecal impaction | ✓ | ✓ | | | |
|   Swelling of feet or lower legs | | | | | ✓ |
|   Metabolic alkalosis | | ✓ | | | ✓ |
|   Hypercalcemia | | ✓ | | | ✓ |
|   Osteomalacia and osteoporosis | ✓ | ✓ | | | |
|   Renal calculi | | ✓ | | | |
|   Phosphorus depletion syndrome | ✓ | | ✓ | | |
|   Hypermagnesemia | | | ✓ | ✓ | |

Table 7. Oral Dosage Forms

Note: Content and acid neutralizing capacity per capsule, tablet, or 5 mL, unless otherwise stated.

All products are available over-the-counter (OTC) in the U.S. and/or in Canada.

| Brand or generic name [availability] | Aluminum component | Calcium component | Magnesium component | Other ingredients | Acid neutralizing capacity | Other content information as per product label | Usual adult and adolescent dose prn† (maximum OTC dose/day) | Usual pediatric dose | Packaging, storage, and labeling§ |
|---|---|---|---|---|---|---|---|---|---|
| *Advanced Formula Di-Gel* Tablets USP (Chewable) [U.S.] | | Calcium carbonate 280 mg | Magnesium hydroxide 128 mg | Simethicone 20 mg | 10 mEq | Sodium <5 mg | 2–4 tabs q 2 hr (24 tabs) | | b, g |
| *Alamag* Oral Suspension USP [U.S.] | Aluminum hydroxide (equiv. to dried gel) 225 mg | | Magnesium hydroxide 200 mg | | | Sodium <1.25 mg Sugar free | 10–20 mL (80 mL) | ‡ | b, c, d, e |
| *Alamag Plus* Oral Suspension USP [U.S.] | Aluminum hydroxide (equiv. to dried gel) 225 mg | | Magnesium hydroxide 200 mg | Simethicone 25 mg | | Sodium <5 mg Sugar free | 10–20 mL (80 mL) | | b, c, d, e |
| *Alenic Alka* Oral Suspension [U.S.] | Aluminum hydroxide 31.7 mg | | Magnesium carbonate 137 mg | Sodium alginate | | Sodium 13 mg | 15–30 mL (120 mL) | ‡ | b, c, d, e, h |
| Chewable Tablets [U.S.] | Aluminum hydroxide (dried gel) 80 mg | | Magnesium trisilicate 20 mg | Alginic acid, Sodium bicarbonate | | Sodium 18.4 mg | 2–4 tabs (16 tabs) | | a, g, h |
| *Alenic Alka Extra Strength* Tablets USP (Chewable) [U.S.] | Aluminum hydroxide 160 mg | | Magnesium carbonate 105 mg | Alginic acid, Sodium bicarbonate | | Sodium 29.9 mg | 2–4 tabs (16 tabs) | | b, g, h |
| *Alka-Mints* Tablets USP (Chewable) [U.S.] | | Calcium carbonate 850 mg | | | 15.9 mEq | Sodium <0.5 mg | 1–2 tabs (9 tabs) | | b, g |

*Specific formulations may vary among the different manufacturers; check product labeling.

†In peptic ulcer disease, maximum therapeutic response may be obtained if taken 1 and 3 hours after meals and at bedtime. Severe symptoms may require more frequent dosing.

‡Pediatric doses may range between 5 and 15 mL every 3 to 6 hours or 1 and 3 hours after meals and at bedtime, unless otherwise stated. However, these are general guidelines; proper diagnosis and dose individualization should precede the use of an antacid in a pediatric patient.

§For appropriate *Packaging and storage* and *Label* information refer to designated letters as follows:

a–Store below 40 °C (104 °F), preferably between 15 and 30 °C (59 and 86 °F), in a well-closed container, unless otherwise specified by manufacturer.

b–Store below 40 °C (104 °F), preferably between 15 and 30 °C (59 and 86 °F), unless otherwise specified by manufacturer. Store in a tight container.

c–Protect from freezing.

d–Auxiliary labeling: • Shake well.

e–Auxiliary labeling: • Keep container tightly closed.

f–Auxiliary labeling: • May be chewed or swallowed whole.

g–Auxiliary labeling: • Chew tablets or wafers before swallowing.

h–Auxiliary labeling: • Follow with ½ to 1 glass of water or other liquid.

i–Auxiliary labeling: • May also be allowed to dissolve in mouth.

## Table 7. Oral Dosage Forms (continued)

Note: Content and acid neutralizing capacity per capsule, tablet, or 5 mL, unless otherwise stated.
All products are available over-the-counter (OTC) in the U.S. and/or in Canada.

| Brand or generic name [availability] | Aluminum component | Calcium component | Magnesium component | Other ingredients | Acid neutralizing capacity | Other content information as per product label | Usual adult and adolescent dose prm† (maximum OTC dose/day) | Usual pediatric dose | Packaging, storage, and labeling§ |
|---|---|---|---|---|---|---|---|---|---|
| *Alkets* Tablets USP (Chewable) [U.S.] | | Calcium carbonate 500 mg | | | | Sodium ≤2 mg | 1–2 tabs (16 tabs) | | b, g |
| *Alkets Extra Strength* Tablets USP (Chewable) [U.S.] | | Calcium carbonate 750 mg | | | | Sodium ≤2 mg | 1–2 tabs (10 tabs) | | b, e, g |
| *Almacone* Oral Suspension USP [U.S.] | Aluminum hydroxide (equiv. to dried gel) 200 mg | | Magnesium hydroxide 200 mg | Simethicone 20 mg | 10 mEq | Sodium 0.75 mg | 5–10 mL (120 mL) | ‡ | b, c, d, e |
| Tablets USP (Chewable) [U.S.] | Aluminum hydroxide (dried gel) 200 mg | | Magnesium hydroxide 200 mg | Simethicone 20 mg | | | 1–2 tabs (24 tabs) | | b, g |
| *Almacone II* Oral Suspension USP [U.S.] | Aluminum hydroxide 400 mg | | Magnesium hydroxide 400 mg | Simethicone 40 mg | 20 mEq | Sodium 1.5 mg | 5–10 mL (60 mL) | ‡ | b, c, d, e |
| *Almagel 200* Oral Suspension USP [Canada] | Aluminum hydroxide (equiv. to dried gel) 200 mg | | Magnesium hydroxide 200 mg | | | | 5–20 mL | | b, c, d, e |
| *AlternaGEL* Gel USP [U.S.] | Aluminum hydroxide (equiv. to dried gel) 600 mg | | | Simethicone | 16 mEq | Sodium <2.5 mg Sugar free | 5–10 mL (90 mL) See also *General Dosing Information* for other doses. | ‡ | b, c, d, e |
| *Alu-Cap* Capsules USP [U.S.] | Aluminum hydroxide (dried gel) 400 mg | | | | 8.5 mEq | | 3 caps (9 caps) | | a |
| *Aludrox* Oral Suspension USP [U.S.] | Aluminum hydroxide gel 307 mg | | Magnesium hydroxide 103 mg | Simethicone 5 mg | 12 mEq | Sodium 2 mg | 10 mL (60 mL) | ‡ | b, c, d, e |
| *Alugel* Gel USP [Canada] | Aluminum hydroxide gel 320 mg | | | | | | 10 mL (80 mL) | | b, c, d, e |

Table 7. Oral Dosage Forms (*continued*)

Note: Content and acid neutralizing capacity per capsule, tablet, or 5 mL, unless otherwise stated.

All products are available over-the-counter (OTC) in the U.S. and/or in Canada.

| Brand or generic name [availability] | Aluminum component | Calcium component | Magnesium component | Other ingredients | Acid neutralizing capacity | Other content information as per product label | Usual adult and adolescent dose prn† (maximum OTC dose/day) | Usual pediatric dose | Packaging, storage, and labeling§ |
|---|---|---|---|---|---|---|---|---|---|
| Alumina and Magnesia* Oral Suspension USP [U.S.] | Aluminum hydroxide (equiv. to dried gel) 240 mg | | Magnesium hydroxide 210 mg | | 13.3 mEq | | 5–20 mL (80 mL) | | b, c, d, e |
| Oral Suspension USP [Canada] | Aluminum hydroxide (equiv. to dried gel) 225 mg | | Magnesium hydroxide 200 mg | | | Sugar free | 10–20 mL (80 mL) | | b, c, d, e |
| Alumina, Magnesia, and Simethicone* Oral Suspension USP [U.S.] | Aluminum hydroxide (equiv. to dried gel) 213 mg | | Magnesium hydroxide 200 mg | Simethicone 20 mg | 12.7 mEq | | 5–10 mL (120 mL) | | b, c, d, e |
| Oral Suspension USP [Canada] | Aluminum hydroxide (equiv. to dried gel) 225 mg | | Magnesium hydroxide 200 mg | Simethicone 25 mg | | Sugar free | 10–20 mL (80 mL) | | b, c, d, e |
| Aluminum Hydroxide Gel* USP [U.S./Canada] | Aluminum hydroxide gel 320 mg  Aluminum hydroxide gel 450 mg  Aluminum hydroxide gel 600 mg  Aluminum hydroxide gel 675 mg | | | | | | 600 mg–1.2 grams. See also *General Dosing Information* for other doses. | ‡ | b, c, d, e |

*Specific formulations may vary among the different manufacturers; check product labeling.

†In peptic ulcer disease, maximum therapeutic response may be obtained if taken 1 and 3 hours after meals and at bedtime. Severe symptoms may require more frequent dosing.

‡Pediatric doses may range between 5 and 15 mL every 3 to 6 hours or 1 and 3 hours after meals and at bedtime, unless otherwise stated. However, these are general guidelines; proper diagnosis and dose individualization should precede the use of an antacid in a pediatric patient.

§For appropriate *Packaging and storage* and *Label* information refer to designated letters as follows:

a–Store below 40 °C (104 °F), preferably between 15 and 30 °C (59 and 86 °F), in a well-closed container, unless otherwise specified by manufacturer.

b–Store below 40 °C (104 °F), preferably between 15 and 30 °C (59 and 86 °F), unless otherwise specified by manufacturer. Store in a tight container.

c–Protect from freezing.

d–Auxiliary labeling: • Shake well.

e–Auxiliary labeling: • Keep container tightly closed.

f–Auxiliary labeling: • May be chewed or swallowed whole.

g–Auxiliary labeling: • Chew tablets or wafers before swallowing.

h–Auxiliary labeling: • Follow with ½ to 1 glass of water or other liquid.

i–Auxiliary labeling: • May also be allowed to dissolve in mouth.

## Table 7. Oral Dosage Forms (continued)

Note: Content and acid neutralizing capacity per capsule, tablet, or 5 mL, unless otherwise stated.
All products are available over-the-counter (OTC) in the U.S. and/or in Canada.

| Brand or generic name [availability] | Aluminum component | Calcium component | Magnesium component | Other ingredients | Acid neutralizing capacity | Other content information as per product label | Usual adult and adolescent dose prn† (maximum OTC dose/day) | Usual pediatric dose | Packaging, storage, and labeling§ |
|---|---|---|---|---|---|---|---|---|---|
| Aluminum Hydroxide Gel, Dried* Tablets USP [U.S./Canada] | Aluminum hydroxide (dried gel) 500 mg; Aluminum hydroxide (dried gel) 600 mg | | | | | | 600 mg–1.2 grams. See also General Dosing Information for other doses. | | a, g |
| Alu-Tab Tablets USP [U.S.] | Aluminum hydroxide (dried gel) 500 mg | | | | 10.6 mEq | | 3 tabs (9 tabs) | | a |
| Tablets USP [Canada] | Aluminum hydroxide (dried gel) 600 mg | | | | | Film-coated Tartrazine free | 1–2 tabs | | a |
| Amitone Tablets USP (Chewable) [U.S.] | | Calcium carbonate 350 mg | | | 7 mEq | Sodium <2 mg | 2 tabs (22 tabs) | | b, g |
| Amphojel Gel USP [U.S./Canada] | Aluminum hydroxide gel 320 mg | | | | 10 mEq | Sodium <2.3 mg (peppermint) | 10 mL (60 mL) | | b, c, d, e |
| Tablets USP [U.S./Canada] | Aluminum hydroxide (dried gel) 300 mg | | | | 8 mEq | Sodium 1.4 mg | 2 tabs (12 tabs) | | a, f, h |
| | Aluminum hydroxide (dried gel) 600 mg | | | | 16 mEq | Sodium 2.8 mg | 1 tab (6 tabs) | | a, g, h |
| Amphojel 500 Oral Suspension USP [Canada] | Aluminum hydroxide 500 mg | | Magnesium hydroxide 500 mg | | 37 mEq | Sodium 3 mg Tartrazine free Sugar free | 5–10 mL (40 mL) | ‡ | b, c, d, e |

## Table 7. Oral Dosage Forms (continued)

Note: Content and acid neutralizing capacity per capsule, tablet, or 5 mL, unless otherwise stated.
All products are available over-the-counter (OTC) in the U.S. and/or in Canada.

| Brand or generic name [availability] | Aluminum component | Calcium component | Magnesium component | Other ingredients | Acid neutralizing capacity | Other content information as per product label | Usual adult and adolescent dose prn† (maximum OTC dose/day) | Usual pediatric dose | Packaging, storage, and labeling§ |
|---|---|---|---|---|---|---|---|---|---|
| *Amphojel Plus* Oral Suspension USP [Canada] | Aluminum hydroxide 300 mg | | Magnesium hydroxide 300 mg | Simethicone 25 mg | | Sodium 7 mg Sugar free Tartrazine free | 5–10 mL (40 mL) | ‡ | b, c, d, e |
| Chewable Tablets [Canada] | | | Magnesium hydroxide 300 mg | Aluminum hydroxide and magnesium carbonate co-dried gel 300 mg, Simethicone 25 mg | | Sodium 10 mg Sugar free Tartrazine free | 1–2 tabs (8 tabs) | | a, g |
| *Antacid Gelcaps* Tablets USP [U.S.] | | Calcium carbonate 311 mg | Magnesium carbonate 232 mg | | | | 2–4 tabs (24 tabs) | | b |
| *Antacid Liquid* Oral Suspension USP [U.S.] | Aluminum hydroxide (equiv. to dried gel) 200 mg | | Magnesium hydroxide 200 mg | Simethicone 20 mg | | Sodium <1.25 mg | 10–20 mL (120 mL) | | b, c, d, e |
| *Antacid Liquid Double strength* Oral Suspension USP [U.S.] | Aluminum hydroxide (equiv. to dried gel) 400 mg | | Magnesium hydroxide 400 mg | Simethicone 40 mg | | Sodium <1.25 mg | 10–20 mL (60 mL) | | b, c, d, e |
| *Basaljel* Capsules [U.S.] | Dried basic aluminum carbonate gel equiv. to 500 mg of aluminum hydroxide or 608 mg of dried aluminum hydroxide gel | | | | 12 mEq | Sodium 2.76 mg | 2 caps q 2 hr (24 caps) See also *General Dosing Information* for other doses. | | a, h |

*Specific formulations may vary among the different manufacturers; check product labeling.

†In peptic ulcer disease, maximum therapeutic response may be obtained if taken 1 and 3 hours after meals and at bedtime. Severe symptoms may require more frequent dosing.

‡Pediatric doses may range between 5 and 15 mL every 3 to 6 hours or 1 and 3 hours after meals and at bedtime, unless otherwise stated. However, these are general guidelines; proper diagnosis and dose individualization should precede the use of an antacid in a pediatric patient.

§For appropriate *Packaging and storage* and *Label* information refer to designated letters as follows:

a–Store below 40 °C (104 °F), preferably between 15 and 30 °C (59 and 86 °F), in a well-closed container, unless otherwise specified by manufacturer.
b–Store below 40 °C (104 °F), preferably between 15 and 30 °C (59 and 86 °F), unless otherwise specified by manufacturer. Store in a tight container.
c–Protect from freezing.
d–Auxiliary labeling: • Shake well.
e–Auxiliary labeling: • Keep container tightly closed.
f–Auxiliary labeling: • May be chewed or swallowed whole.
g–Auxiliary labeling: • Chew tablets or wafers before swallowing.
h–Auxiliary labeling: • Follow with ¹/₂ to 1 glass of water or other liquid.
i–Auxiliary labeling: • May also be allowed to dissolve in mouth.

Table 7. Oral Dosage Forms (continued)

Note: Content and acid neutralizing capacity per capsule, tablet, or 5 mL, unless otherwise stated.

All products are available over-the-counter (OTC) in the U.S. and/or in Canada.

| Brand or generic name [availability] | Aluminum component | Calcium component | Magnesium component | Other ingredients | Acid neutralizing capacity | Other content information as per product label | Usual adult and adolescent dose prn† (maximum OTC dose/day) | Usual pediatric dose | Packaging, storage, and labeling§ |
|---|---|---|---|---|---|---|---|---|---|
| *Basaljel (continued)* | | | | | | | | | |
| Capsules [Canada] | Aluminum hydroxide (dried gel) 500 mg | | | | | Sodium <2 mg Tartrazine free | 2–3 caps (12 caps) | | a, h |
| Oral Suspension [U.S.] | Basic aluminum carbonate gel equiv. to 400 mg of aluminum hydroxide | | | Simethicone 5 mg | 11.5 mEq | Sodium 3 mg | 10 mL q 2 hr (120 mL) | ‡ | b, c, d, h |
| Tablets [U.S.] | Dried basic aluminum carbonate gel equiv. to 500 mg of aluminum hydroxide or 608 mg of dried aluminum hydroxide gel | | | | 12.5 mEq | Sodium 2.76 mg | 2 tabs q 2 hr (24 tabs) | | a, h |
| Calcium Carbonate* Oral Suspension USP [U.S.] | | Calcium carbonate 1250 mg | | | | | 5 mL | | b, c, e |
| Tablets USP [U.S.] | | Calcium carbonate 500 mg<br>Calcium carbonate 600 mg<br>Calcium carbonate 650 mg<br>Calcium carbonate 1250 mg | | | | | 1–2 tabs See also *General Dosing Information* for other doses. | | b, h |

## Table 7. Oral Dosage Forms (continued)

Note: Content and acid neutralizing capacity per capsule, tablet, or 5 mL, unless otherwise stated.
All products are available over-the-counter (OTC) in the U.S. and/or in Canada.

| Brand or generic name [availability] | Aluminum component | Calcium component | Magnesium component | Other ingredients | Acid neutralizing capacity | Other content information as per product label | Usual adult and adolescent dose prn† (maximum OTC dose/day) | Usual pediatric dose | Packaging, storage, and labeling§ |
|---|---|---|---|---|---|---|---|---|---|
| Calcium Carbonate* (continued) Tablets USP (Chewable) [U.S.] | | Calcium carbonate 500 mg<br><br>Calcium carbonate 750 mg | | | | | 1–2 tabs | | b, g |
| Calglycine Tablets USP (Chewable) [U.S.] | | Calcium carbonate 420 mg | | Glycine 150 mg | | Sugar free | 2 tabs (19 tabs) | | b, f, i |
| Chooz Chewing Gum [U.S.] | | Calcium carbonate 500 mg | | | 10 mEq | Sodium <5 mg | 1–2 tabs q 2–4 hr (14 tabs) | 6–12 yrs: 1 tab q 2–4 hr (8 tabs) | a |
| Dicarbosil Tablets USP (Chewable) [U.S.] | | Calcium carbonate 500 mg | | | 10 mEq | Sodium <2 mg | 2 tabs (16 tabs) | | b, g, i |
| Di-Gel Oral Suspension USP [U.S.] | Aluminum hydroxide (dried gel) 200 mg | | Magnesium hydroxide 200 mg | Simethicone 20 mg | > 9 mEq | Sodium ≤5 mg Sugar free | 10–20 mL q 2 hr (100 mL) | | b, c, d, e |

*Specific formulations may vary among the different manufacturers; check product labeling.
†In peptic ulcer disease, maximum therapeutic response may be obtained if taken 1 and 3 hours after meals and at bedtime. Severe symptoms may require more frequent dosing.
‡Pediatric doses may range between 5 and 15 mL every 3 to 6 hours or 1 and 3 hours after meals and at bedtime, unless otherwise stated. However, these are general guidelines; proper diagnosis and dose individualization should precede the use of an antacid in a pediatric patient.
§For appropriate *Packaging and storage* and *Label* information refer to designated letters as follows:
a–Store below 40 °C (104 °F), preferably between 15 and 30 °C (59 and 86 °F), in a well-closed container, unless otherwise specified by manufacturer.
b–Store below 40 °C (104 °F), preferably between 15 and 30 °C (59 and 86 °F), unless otherwise specified by manufacturer. Store in a tight container.
c–Protect from freezing.
d–Auxiliary labeling: • Shake well.
e–Auxiliary labeling: • Keep container tightly closed.
f–Auxiliary labeling: • May be chewed or swallowed whole.
g–Auxiliary labeling: • Chew tablets or wafers before swallowing.
h–Auxiliary labeling: • Follow with ¹/₂ to 1 glass of water or other liquid.
i–Auxiliary labeling: • May also be allowed to dissolve in mouth.

Table 7. Oral Dosage Forms (*continued*)

Note: Content and acid neutralizing capacity per capsule, tablet, or 5 mL, unless otherwise stated.
All products are available over-the-counter (OTC) in the U.S. and/or in Canada.

| Brand or generic name [availability] | Aluminum component | Calcium component | Magnesium component | Other ingredients | Acid neutralizing capacity | Other content information as per product label | Usual adult and adolescent dose prn† (maximum OTC dose/day) | Usual pediatric dose | Packaging, storage, and labeling§ |
|---|---|---|---|---|---|---|---|---|---|
| *Diovol* Oral Suspension [Canada] | Aluminum hydroxide 165 mg | | Magnesium hydroxide 200 mg | Simethicone | 11.9 mEq | Alcohol 1% Sodium <1 mg Sugar free Tartrazine free | 10–20 mL (80 mL) | | b, c, d, e |
| Chewable Tablets [Canada] | | | Magnesium hydroxide 100 mg | Aluminum hydroxide and magnesium carbonate co-dried gel 300 mg | 10 mEq | Sodium 1 mg Sugar free Tartrazine free | 2–4 tabs (16 tabs) | | a, g |
| *Diovol Caplets* Tablets [Canada] | Aluminum hydroxide (equiv. to dried gel) 200 mg | | Magnesium hydroxide 200 mg | | | Sugar free Tartrazine free | 2–4 tabs (16 tabs) | | a |
| *Diovol Ex* Oral Suspension [Canada] | Aluminum hydroxide 494 mg | | Magnesium hydroxide 300 mg | | 25 mEq | Alcohol 1% Sodium <1 mg Sugar free Tartrazine free | 5–10 mL (40 mL) | ‡ | b, c, d, e |
| Tablets (Chewable) [Canada] | Aluminum hydroxide (equiv. to dried gel) 600 mg | | Magnesium hydroxide 300 mg | | 24.6 mEq | Sodium 1 mg Sugar free Tartrazine free | 1–2 tabs (8 tabs) | | b, g |
| *Diovol Plus* Oral Suspension [Canada] | Aluminum hydroxide 165 mg | | Magnesium hydroxide 200 mg | Simethicone 25 mg | 11.9 mEq | Alcohol <1% Sodium <1 mg Sugar free Tartrazine free | 10–20 mL (80 mL) | ‡ | b, c, d, e |
| Chewable Tablets [Canada] | | | Magnesium hydroxide 100 mg | Aluminum hydroxide and magnesium carbonate co-dried gel 300 mg, Simethicone 25 mg | 10 mEq | Sodium 1 mg Sugar free Tartrazine free | 2–4 tabs (16 tabs) | | a, g, i |

## Table 7. Oral Dosage Forms (continued)

Note: Content and acid neutralizing capacity per capsule, tablet, or 5 mL, unless otherwise stated.
All products are available over-the-counter (OTC) in the U.S. and/or in Canada.

| Brand or generic name [availability] | Aluminum component | Calcium component | Magnesium component | Other ingredients | Acid neutralizing capacity | Other content information as per product label | Usual adult and adolescent dose prn† (maximum OTC dose/day) | Usual pediatric dose | Packaging, storage, and labeling§ |
|---|---|---|---|---|---|---|---|---|---|
| *Diovol Plus AF* Oral Suspension [Canada] | | Calcium carbonate 200 mg | Magnesium hydroxide 200 mg | Simethicone 25 mg | 9.8 mEq | Alcohol 1% Sodium 1 mg Sugar free Tartrazine free | 10–20 mL (80 mL) | | b, c, d |
| Chewable Tablets [Canada] | | Calcium carbonate 200 mg | Magnesium hydroxide 200 mg | Simethicone 25 mg | 10 mEq | Sodium 1 mg Sugar free Tartrazine fee | 2–4 tabs (16 tabs) | | a, g |
| *Equilet* Tablets USP [Chewable] [U.S.] | | Calcium carbonate 500 mg | | | | Sodium 0.3 mg | 2 tabs | | b, g |
| *Foamicon* Tablets USP (Chewable) [U.S.] | Aluminum hydroxide 80 mg | | Magnesium trisilicate 20 mg | Alginic acid, Sodium bicarbonate | | Sodium 18.4 mg | 2–4 tabs (16 tabs) | | a, g, h |
| *Gasmas* Chewable Tablets [Canada] | | | Magnesium hydroxide 100 mg | Aluminum hydroxide and magnesium carbonate co-dried gel 300 mg, Simethicone 25 mg | | | 2 tabs | | a, g |
| *Gaviscon* Oral Suspension USP [U.S.] | Aluminum hydroxide 31.7 mg | | Magnesium carbonate 119.3 mg | Sodium alginate | 2.5–4.3 mEq | Sodium 13 mg | 15–30 mL (120 mL) | ‡ | b, c, d, e, h |
| Tablets USP (Chewable) [U.S.] | Aluminum hydroxide (dried gel) 80 mg | | Magnesium trisilicate 20 mg | Alginic acid, Sodium bicarbonate | 0.5 mEq | Sodium 18.4 mg | 2–4 tabs (16 tabs) | | a, g, h |

*Specific formulations may vary among the different manufacturers; check product labeling.

†In peptic ulcer disease, maximum therapeutic response may be obtained if taken 1 and 3 hours after meals and at bedtime. Severe symptoms may require more frequent dosing.

‡Pediatric doses may range between 5 and 15 mL every 3 to 6 hours or 1 and 3 hours after meals and at bedtime, unless otherwise stated. However, these are general guidelines; proper diagnosis and dose individualization should precede the use of an antacid in a pediatric patient.

§For appropriate *Packaging and storage* and *Label* information refer to designated letters as follows:

a–Store below 40 °C (104 °F), preferably between 15 and 30 °C (59 and 86 °F), in a well-closed container, unless otherwise specified by manufacturer.
b–Store below 40 °C (104 °F), preferably between 15 and 30 °C (59 and 86 °F), unless otherwise specified by manufacturer. Store in a tight container.
c–Protect from freezing.     f–Auxiliary labeling: • May be chewed or swallowed whole.     h–Auxiliary labeling: • Follow with ½ to 1 glass of water or other liquid.
d–Auxiliary labeling: • Shake well.     g–Auxiliary labeling: • Chew tablets or wafers before swallowing.     i–Auxiliary labeling: • May also be allowed to dissolve in mouth.
e–Auxiliary labeling: • Keep container tightly closed.

## Table 7. Oral Dosage Forms (continued)

Note: Content and acid neutralizing capacity per capsule, tablet, or 5 mL, unless otherwise stated.
All products are available over-the-counter (OTC) in the U.S. and/or in Canada.

| Brand or generic name [availability] | Aluminum component | Calcium component | Magnesium component | Other ingredients | Acid neutralizing capacity | Other content information as per product label | Usual adult and adolescent dose prn† (maximum OTC dose/day) | Usual pediatric dose | Packaging, storage, and labeling§ |
|---|---|---|---|---|---|---|---|---|---|
| *Gaviscon-2* Tablets USP (Chewable) [U.S.] | Aluminum hydroxide (dried gel) 160 mg | | Magnesium trisilicate 40 mg | Alginic acid, Sodium bicarbonate | 1 mEq | Sodium 36.8 mg | 1-2 tabs (8 tabs) | | a, g, h |
| *Gaviscon Acid Plus Gas Relief* Oral Suspension [Canada] | | Calcium carbonate 660 mg | Magnesium hydroxide 145 mg | Simethicone 30 mg | | | 10-20 mL (60 mL) | | b, d |
| Tablets USP (Chewable) [Canada] | | Calcium carbonate 585 mg | Magnesium hydroxide 120 mg | Simethicone 30 mg | | | 2-4 tabs (13 tabs) | | b, g |
| *Gaviscon Acid Relief* Oral Suspension [Canada] | | Calcium carbonate 660 mg | Magnesium hydroxide 145 mg | | | | 10-20 mL (60 mL) | | b, d |
| Tablets USP (Chewable) [Canada] | | Calcium carbonate 585 mg | Magnesium hydroxide 120 mg | | | | 2-4 tabs (13 tabs) | | b, g |
| *Gaviscon Extra Strength Acid Relief* Oral Suspension [Canada] | | Calcium carbonate 1 gram | Magnesium hydroxide 250 mg | | | | 10-15 mL (40 mL) | | b, d |
| *Gaviscon Extra Strength Relief Formula* Oral Suspension USP [U.S.] | Aluminum hydroxide 254 mg | | Magnesium carbonate 238 mg | Sodium alginate, simethicone emulsion | 14.3 mEq | Sodium 20.7 mg | 10-20 mL (80 mL) | | b, c, d, e, h |
| Tablets USP (Chewable) [U.S.] | Aluminum hydroxide 160 mg | | Magnesium carbonate 105 mg | Alginic acid, Sodium bicarbonate | 5-7.5 mEq | Sodium 29.9 mg | 2-4 tabs (16 tabs) | | b, g, h |

## Table 7. Oral Dosage Forms (continued)

Note: Content and acid neutralizing capacity per capsule, tablet, or 5 mL, unless otherwise stated.
All products are available over-the-counter (OTC) in the U.S. and/or in Canada.

| Brand or generic name [availability] | Aluminum component | Calcium component | Magnesium component | Other ingredients | Acid neutralizing capacity | Other content information as per product label | Usual adult and adolescent dose prn† (maximum OTC dose/day) | Usual pediatric dose | Packaging, storage, and labeling§ |
|---|---|---|---|---|---|---|---|---|---|
| Gaviscon Heartburn Relief Oral Suspension USP [Canada] | Aluminum hydroxide (dried gel) 100 mg | | | Sodium alginate 250 mg | | Sodium 30 mg Alcohol free Sugar free Tartrazine free | 10–20 mL (100 mL) | | b, d, e |
| Oral Suspension [Canada] | | | Magnesium carbonate 100 mg | Sodium alginate 250 mg, Calcium carbonate, Sodium bicarbonate | | | 10–20 mL (100 mL) | | b, d |
| Tablets USP (Chewable) [Canada] | Aluminum hydroxide (dried gel) 80 mg | | | Alginic acid 200 mg | | Sodium 22 mg Tartrazine free | 2–4 tabs (20 tabs) | | a, g |
| Chewable Tablets [Canada] | | | Magnesium carbonate 40 mg | Alginic acid 200 mg, Sodium bicarbonate | | | 2–4 tabs (20 tabs) | | a, g |
| Gaviscon Heartburn Relief Extra Strength Tablets USP (Chewable) [Canada] | Aluminum hydroxide (dried gel) 160 mg | | | Alginic acid 400 mg | | Tartrazine free | 2 tabs (10 tabs) | | a, g |
| Gelusil Oral Suspension USP [Canada] | Aluminum hydroxide (equiv. to dried gel) 200 mg | | Magnesium hydroxide 200 mg | | | Sodium 0.84 mg Sugar free Tartrazine free | 10–20 mL 4 times/day | | b, c, d, e |
| Tablets USP (Chewable) [U.S.] | Aluminum hydroxide 200 mg | | Magnesium hydroxide 200 mg | Simethicone 25 mg | 11 mEq | Sodium <5 mg | 2–4 tabs (12 tabs) | | b, g |

*Specific formulations may vary among the different manufacturers; check product labeling.
†In peptic ulcer disease, maximum therapeutic response may be obtained if taken 1 and 3 hours after meals and at bedtime. Severe symptoms may require more frequent dosing.
‡Pediatric doses may range between 5 and 15 mL every 3 to 6 hours or 1 and 3 hours after meals and at bedtime, unless otherwise stated. However, these are general guidelines; proper diagnosis and dose individualization should precede the use of an antacid in a pediatric patient.
§For appropriate Packaging and storage and Label information refer to designated letters as follows:
a–Store below 40 °C (104 °F), preferably between 15 and 30 °C (59 and 86 °F), in a well-closed container, unless otherwise specified by manufacturer.
b–Store below 40 °C (104 °F), preferably between 15 and 30 °C (59 and 86 °F), unless otherwise specified by manufacturer. Store in a tight container.
c–Protect from freezing.
d–Auxiliary labeling:  •  Shake well.
e–Auxiliary labeling:  •  Keep container tightly closed.
f–Auxiliary labeling:  •  May be chewed or swallowed whole.
g–Auxiliary labeling:  •  Chew tablets or wafers before swallowing.
h–Auxiliary labeling:  •  Follow with ¹/₂ to 1 glass of water or other liquid.
i–Auxiliary labeling:  •  May also be allowed to dissolve in mouth.

# Table 7. Oral Dosage Forms (continued)

Note: Content and acid neutralizing capacity per capsule, tablet, or 5 mL, unless otherwise stated.

All products are available over-the-counter (OTC) in the U.S. and/or in Canada.

| Brand or generic name [availability] | Aluminum component | Calcium component | Magnesium component | Other ingredients | Acid neutralizing capacity | Other content information as per product label | Usual adult and adolescent dose prn† (maximum OTC dose/day) | Usual pediatric dose | Packaging, storage, and labeling§ |
|---|---|---|---|---|---|---|---|---|---|
| *Gelusil (continued)* Tablets USP (Chewable) [Canada] | Aluminum hydroxide (equiv. to dried gel) 200 mg | | Magnesium hydroxide 200 mg | | | Sodium 1.1 mg Tartrazine free | 2–4 tabs 4 times/day | | b, g |
| *Gelusil Extra Strength* Oral Suspension USP [Canada] | Aluminum hydroxide (equiv. to dried gel) 650 mg | | Magnesium hydroxide 350 mg | | | Sodium 1.4 mg Sugar free Tartrazine free | 10 mL 4 times/day | | b, c, d, e |
| Tablets USP (Chewable) [Canada] | Aluminum hydroxide (equiv. to dried gel) 400 mg | | Magnesium hydroxide 400 mg | | | Sodium 1.6 mg Tartrazine free | 2–4 tabs 4 times/day | | b, g, h |
| *Genaton* Oral Suspension USP [U.S.] | Aluminum hydroxide 31.7 mg | | Magnesium carbonate 137.3 mg | Sodium alginate | | Sodium 13 mg | 15–30 mL (120 ml) | | b, c, d, e, h |
| Tablets USP (Chewable) [U.S.] | Aluminum hydroxide 80 mg | | Magnesium trisilicate 20 mg | Alginic acid, Sodium bicarbonate | | Sodium 18.4 mg | 2–4 tabs (16 tabs) | | a, g, h |
| *Genaton Extra Strength* Tablets USP (Chewable) [U.S.] | Aluminum hydroxide 160 mg | | Magnesium carbonate 105 mg | Alginic acid, Sodium bicarbonate | | Sodium 35 mg | 2–4 tabs (16 tabs) | | b, e, g, h |
| *Kudrox Double Strength* Oral Suspension USP [U.S.] | Aluminum hydroxide 500 mg | | Magnesium hydroxide 450 mg | Simethicone 40 mg | 25 mEq | Sodium <5 mg | 10–20 mL (60 mL) | | b, c, d, e |
| *Life Antacid* Oral Suspension USP [Canada] | Aluminum hydroxide (dried gel) 228 mg | | Magnesium hydroxide 200 mg | | | Sugar free | 10–20 mL (80 mL) | | b, c, d, e |
| *Life Antacid Plus* Oral Suspension USP [Canada] | Aluminum hydroxide (dried gel) 228 mg | | Magnesium hydroxide 200 mg | Simethicone 25 mg | | Sugar free | 10–20 mL (80 mL) | | b, c, d, e |
| Tablets USP (Chewable) [Canada] | Aluminum hydroxide (dried gel) 200 mg | | Magnesium hydroxide 200 mg | Simethicone 25 mg | | | 1–4 tabs | | b, g |

Table 7. Oral Dosage Forms (continued)

Note: Content and acid neutralizing capacity per capsule, tablet, or 5 mL, unless otherwise stated.

All products are available over-the-counter (OTC) in the U.S. and/or in Canada.

| Brand or generic name [availability] | Aluminum component | Calcium component | Magnesium component | Other ingredients | Acid neutralizing capacity | Other content information as per product label | Usual adult and adolescent dose prn† (maximum OTC dose/day) | Usual pediatric dose | Packaging, storage, and labeling§ |
|---|---|---|---|---|---|---|---|---|---|
| Losopan Oral Suspension USP [U.S.] | | | | Magaldrate 540 mg | | Sodium <5 mg | 5–10 mL (90 mL) | | b, c, d, e |
| Losopan Plus Oral Suspension USP [U.S.] | | | | Magaldrate 540 mg, Simethicone 40 mg | | Sodium <5 mg | 5–10 mL (90 mL) | | b, c, d, e |
| Lowsium Plus Oral Suspension USP [U.S.] | | | | Magaldrate 540 mg, Simethicone 40 mg | | Sodium <5 mg | 5–10 mL (90 mL) | ‡ | b, c, d, e |
| Maalox Oral Suspension USP [U.S.] | Aluminum hydroxide (equiv. to dried gel) 225 mg | | Magnesium hydroxide 200 mg | | 13.3 mEq | Sodium <1.5 mg Sugar free | 10–20 mL (80 mL) | ‡ | b, c, d |
| Oral Suspension USP [Canada] | Aluminum hydroxide (equiv. to dried gel) 225 mg | | Magnesium hydroxide 200 mg | | 13.3 mEq | Sodium 0.92 mg Sugar free Tartrazine free | 10–20 mL (80 mL) | ‡ | b, c, d |
| Original Tablets USP (Chewable) [U.S.] | Aluminum hydroxide (dried gel) 200 mg | | Magnesium hydroxide 200 mg | | 9.7 mEq | Sodium 0.7 mg Sugar free | 2–4 tabs (16 tabs) | | b, e, g |
| Tablets USP (Chewable) [Canada] | Aluminum hydroxide (equiv. to dried gel) 400 mg | | Magnesium hydroxide 400 mg | | | Sodium 0.93 mg Tartrazine free | 1–2 tabs (8 tabs) | | b, g, h |

*Specific formulations may vary among the different manufacturers; check product labeling.

†In peptic ulcer disease, maximum therapeutic response may be obtained if taken 1 and 3 hours after meals and at bedtime. Severe symptoms may require more frequent dosing.

‡Pediatric doses may range between 5 and 15 mL every 3 to 6 hours or 1 and 3 hours after meals and at bedtime, unless otherwise stated. However, these are general guidelines; proper diagnosis and dose individualization should precede the use of an antacid in a pediatric patient.

§For appropriate Packaging and storage and Label information refer to designated letters as follows:

  a–Store below 40 °C (104 °F), preferably between 15 and 30 °C (59 and 86 °F), in a well-closed container, unless otherwise specified by manufacturer.

  b–Store below 40 °C (104 °F), preferably between 15 and 30 °C (59 and 86 °F), unless otherwise specified by manufacturer. Store in a tight container.

  c–Protect from freezing.

  d–Auxiliary labeling: • Shake well.

  e–Auxiliary labeling: • Keep container tightly closed.

  f–Auxiliary labeling: • May be chewed or swallowed whole.

  g–Auxiliary labeling: • Chew tablets or wafers before swallowing.

  h–Auxiliary labeling: • Follow with ½ to 1 glass of water or other liquid.

  i–Auxiliary labeling: • May also be allowed to dissolve in mouth.

Table 7. Oral Dosage Forms (continued)

Note: Content and acid neutralizing capacity per capsule, tablet, or 5 mL, unless otherwise stated. All products are available over-the-counter (OTC) in the U.S. and/or in Canada.

| Brand or generic name [availability] | Aluminum component | Calcium component | Magnesium component | Other ingredients | Acid neutralizing capacity | Other content information as per product label | Usual adult and adolescent dose prn† (maximum OTC dose/day) | Usual pediatric dose | Packaging, storage, and labeling§ |
|---|---|---|---|---|---|---|---|---|---|
| *Maalox Antacid Caplets* Tablets USP [U.S./Canada] | | Calcium carbonate 311 mg | Magnesium carbonate 232 mg | | | | 2–4 tabs (24 tabs) | | b |
| *Maalox Heartburn Relief Formula* Oral Suspension [U.S.] | | | Magnesium carbonate 175 mg | Aluminum hydroxide-magnesium carbonate co-dried gel 140 mg | 8.5 mEq | Sodium <1.5 mg Tartrazine | 10–20 mL (80 mL) | | b, c, d, e |
| *Maalox HRF* Oral Suspension [Canada] | | | Magnesium alginate 250 mg, Magnesium carbonate 175 mg | Aluminum hydroxide-magnesium carbonate codried gel 140 mg | | Sodium <5 mg Sugar free Tartrazine free | 10–20 mL (80 mL) | | b, c, d |
| Tablets (Chewable) [Canada] | | | Magnesium alginate 250 mg, Magnesium carbonate 160 mg | Aluminum hydroxide-magnesium carbonate codried gel 180 mg | | Sodium <3 mg Tartrazine free | 2–4 tabs (16 tabs) | | a, g, h |
| *Maalox Plus* Oral Suspension USP [Canada] | Aluminum hydroxide (equiv. to dried gel) 225 mg | | Magnesium hydroxide 200 mg | Simethicone 25 mg | 13.35 mEq | Sodium 0.92 mg Sugar free Tartrazine free | 10–20 mL (80 mL) | | b, c, d, e |
| Tablets USP (Chewable) [U.S.] | Aluminum hydroxide (equiv. to dried gel) 200 mg | | Magnesium hydroxide 200 mg | Simethicone 25 mg | 10.65 mEq | Sodium ⩽1 mg | 1–4 tabs (16 tabs) | | b, g |
| Tablets USP (Chewable) [Canada] | Aluminum hydroxide (dried gel) 200 mg | | Magnesium hydroxide 200 mg | Simethicone 25 mg | | Sodium 1 mg (lemon) 0.94 mg (mint) Tartrazine free | 2–4 tabs (16 tabs) | | a, g, h |
| *Maalox Plus, Extra Strength* Oral Suspension USP [U.S.] | Aluminum hydroxide (equiv. to dried gel) 500 mg | | Magnesium hydroxide 450 mg | Simethicone 40 mg | 26.1 mEq | Sodium <1 mg Sugar free | 10–20 mL (60 mL) | | b, c, d, e |

# Table 7. Oral Dosage Forms (continued)

Note: Content and acid neutralizing capacity per capsule, tablet, or 5 mL, unless otherwise stated.
All products are available over-the-counter (OTC) in the U.S. and/or in Canada.

| Brand or generic name [availability] | Aluminum component | Calcium component | Magnesium component | Other ingredients | Acid neutralizing capacity | Other content information as per product label | Usual adult and adolescent dose prn† (maximum OTC dose/day) | Usual pediatric dose | Packaging, storage, and labeling§ |
|---|---|---|---|---|---|---|---|---|---|
| *Maalox Plus, Extra Strength (continued)* Oral Suspension USP [Canada] | Aluminum hydroxide (equiv. to dried gel) 500 mg | | Magnesium hydroxide 450 mg | Simethicone 40 mg | | Sodium 1.2 mg Sugar free Tartrazine free | 10–20 mL (60 mL) | | b, c, d, e |
| Tablets USP (Chewable) [U.S./Canada] | Aluminum hydroxide (dried gel) 350 mg | | Magnesium hydroxide 350 mg | Simethicone 30 mg | 16.7 mEq | Sodium 1.4 mg Sugar 0.72 gram | 1–3 tabs (12 tabs) | | b, g |
| *Maalox TC* Oral Suspension USP [U.S.] | Aluminum hydroxide (equiv. to dried gel) 600 mg | | Magnesium hydroxide 300 mg | | 27.2 mEq | Sodium <1 mg Sugar free | 5–10 mL (40 mL) | | b, c, d, e |
| Oral Suspension USP [Canada] | Aluminum hydroxide (equiv. to dried gel) 600 mg | | Magnesium hydroxide 300 mg | | | Sodium 0.95 mg Sugar free Tartrazine free | 5–10 mL (40 mL) | | b, c, d, e |
| Tablets USP (Chewable) [Canada] | Aluminum hydroxide (dried gel) 600 mg | | Magnesium hydroxide 300 mg | | 28 mEq | Sodium 0.98 mg Tartrazine free | 1–2 tabs (8 tabs) | | b, g |
| Magaldrate* Oral Suspension USP [U.S.] | | | | Magaldrate 540 mg | | Sodium free Sugar free Dye free | 5–10 mL (100 mL) | ‡ | b, c, d |

*Specific formulations may vary among the different manufacturers; check product labeling.
†In peptic ulcer disease, maximum therapeutic response may be obtained if taken 1 and 3 hours after meals and at bedtime. Severe symptoms may require more frequent dosing.
‡Pediatric doses may range between 5 and 15 mL every 3 to 6 hours or 1 and 3 hours after meals and at bedtime, unless otherwise stated. However, these are general guidelines; proper diagnosis and dose individualization should precede the use of an antacid in a pediatric patient.
§For appropriate *Packaging and storage* and *Label* information refer to designated letters as follows:
  a—Store below 40 °C (104 °F), preferably between 15 and 30 °C (59 and 86 °F).
  b—Store below 40 °C (104 °F), preferably between 15 and 30 °C (59 and 86 °F), unless otherwise specified by manufacturer. Store in a tight container.
  c—Protect from freezing.
  d—Auxiliary labeling: • Shake well.
  e—Auxiliary labeling: • Keep container tightly closed.
  f—Auxiliary labeling: • May be chewed or swallowed whole.
  g—Auxiliary labeling: • Chew tablets or wafers before swallowing.
  h—Auxiliary labeling: • Follow with ½ to 1 glass of water or other liquid.
  i—Auxiliary labeling: • May also be allowed to dissolve in mouth.

## Table 7. Oral Dosage Forms (continued)

Note: Content and acid neutralizing capacity per capsule, tablet, or 5 mL, unless otherwise stated.
All products are available over-the-counter (OTC) in the U.S. and/or in Canada.

| Brand or generic name [availability] | Aluminum component | Calcium component | Magnesium component | Other ingredients | Acid neutralizing capacity | Other content information as per product label | Usual adult and adolescent dose prn† (maximum OTC dose/day) | Usual pediatric dose | Packaging, storage, and labeling§ |
|---|---|---|---|---|---|---|---|---|---|
| Magaldrate and Simethicone* Oral Suspension USP [U.S.] | | | | Magaldrate 540 mg, Simethicone 20 mg | | | 5–10 mL (100 mL) | ‡ | b, c, d, e |
| Magnalox Oral Suspension USP [U.S.] | Aluminum hydroxide (equiv. to dried gel) 225 mg | | Magnesium hydroxide 200 mg | Simethicone | | Sugar free | 10–20 mL (80 mL) | | b, c, d, e |
| Magnalox Plus Oral Suspension USP [U.S.] | Aluminum hydroxide (equiv. to dried gel) 500 mg | | Magnesium hydroxide 450 mg | Simethicone 40 mg | | | 10–20 mL (60 mL) | | b, c, d, e |
| Magnesium Hydroxide* Magnesia Tablets USP (Chewable) [Canada] | | | Magnesium hydroxide 385 mg | | | Sugar free | 2–4 tabs (16 tabs) | | b, f, h |
| Milk of Magnesia USP* [U.S.] | | | Magnesium hydroxide 400 mg | | 14 mEq | | 5–15 mL (60 mL) | ‡ | b, c, d, e |
| Milk of Magnesia USP* [Canada] | | | Magnesium hydroxide 440 mg | | | Sugar free | 10–20 mL | | b, c, d, e |
| Mag-Ox 400 Tablets USP [U.S.] | | | Magnesium oxide 400 mg | | 20 mEq | | 1–2 tabs/day (2 tabs) | | a |
| Mullamint Tablets USP (Chewable) [U.S.] | | Calcium carbonate 420 mg | | | | Sodium <0.1 mg Sugar free | 2 tabs | | a, g |
| Maox 420 Tablets USP [U.S.] | | | Magnesium oxide 420 mg | | 21 mEq | Tartrazine | 1 tab/day | | a |
| Marblen Oral Suspension [U.S.] | | Calcium carbonate 520 mg | Magnesium carbonate 400 mg | | 18 mEq | Sugar free | 5–10 mL (60 mL) | | c, d, e |
| Tablets USP [U.S.] | | Calcium carbonate 520 mg | Magnesium carbonate 400 mg | | 18 mEq | Sugar free | 1–2 tabs (12 tabs) | | g, i |

Table 7. Oral Dosage Forms (*continued*)

Note: Content and acid neutralizing capacity per capsule, tablet, or 5 mL, unless otherwise stated.
All products are available over-the-counter (OTC) in the U.S. and/or in Canada.

| Brand or generic name [availability] | Aluminum component | Calcium component | Magnesium component | Other ingredients | Acid neutralizing capacity | Other content information as per product label | Usual adult and adolescent dose prn† (maximum OTC dose/day) | Usual pediatric dose | Packaging, storage, and labeling§ |
|---|---|---|---|---|---|---|---|---|---|
| *Mi-Acid* Oral Suspension USP [U.S.] | Aluminum hydroxide (equiv. to dried gel) 200 mg | | Magnesium hydroxide 200 mg | Simethicone 20 mg | | Sodium <5 mg | 10–20 mL (120 mL) | ‡ | b, c, d, e |
| Tablets USP [U.S.] | | Calcium carbonate 311 mg | Magnesium carbonate 232 mg | | | | 2–4 tabs (24 tabs) | | a |
| *Mi-Acid Double Strength* Oral Suspension USP [U.S.] | Aluminum hydroxide (equiv. to dried gel) 400 mg | | Magnesium hydroxide 400 mg | Simethicone 40 mg | | Sodium <5 mg | 10–20 mL (60 mL) | | b, c, d, e |
| *Mintox* Oral Suspension USP [U.S.] | Aluminum hydroxide (equiv. to dried gel) 225 mg | | Magnesium hydroxide 200 mg | | | Sodium 1.38 mg | 10–20 mL (80 mL) | ‡ | b, c, d, e |
| Tablets USP (Chewable) [U.S.] | Aluminum hydroxide 200 mg | | Magnesium hydroxide 200 mg | | | | 2 tabs | | a, g |
| *Mintox Extra Strength* Oral Suspension USP [U.S.] | Aluminum hydroxide (equiv. to dried gel) 500 mg | | Magnesium hydroxide 450 mg | Simethicone 40 mg | | Sodium <5 mg | 10–20 mL (60 mL) | | b, c, d, e |
| Tablets USP (Chewable) [U.S.] | Aluminum hydroxide 200 mg | | Magnesium hydroxide 200 mg | Simethicone 25 mg | | | 1–2 tabs | | b, g |

*Specific formulations may vary among the different manufacturers; check product labeling.

†In peptic ulcer disease, maximum therapeutic response may be obtained if taken 1 and 3 hours after meals and at bedtime. Severe symptoms may require more frequent dosing.

‡Pediatric doses may range between 5 and 15 mL every 3 to 6 hours or 1 and 3 hours after meals and at bedtime, unless otherwise stated. However, these are general guidelines; proper diagnosis and dose individualization should precede the use of an antacid in a pediatric patient.

§For appropriate *Packaging and storage* and *Label* information refer to designated letters as follows:

a–Store below 40 °C (104 °F), preferably between 15 and 30 °C (59 and 86 °F), in a well-closed container, unless otherwise specified by manufacturer.

b–Store below 40 °C (104 °F), preferably between 15 and 30 °C (59 and 86 °F), unless otherwise specified by manufacturer. Store in a tight container.

c–Protect from freezing.

d–Auxiliary labeling: • Shake well.

e–Auxiliary labeling: • Keep container tightly closed.

f–Auxiliary labeling: • May be chewed or swallowed whole.

g–Auxiliary labeling: • Chew tablets or wafers before swallowing.

h–Auxiliary labeling: • Follow with 1/2 to 1 glass of water or other liquid.

i–Auxiliary labeling: • May also be allowed to dissolve in mouth.

Table 7. Oral Dosage Forms (*continued*)

Note: Content and acid neutralizing capacity per capsule, tablet, or 5 mL, unless otherwise stated.
All products are available over-the-counter (OTC) in the U.S. and/or in Canada.

| Brand or generic name [availability] | Aluminum component | Calcium component | Magnesium component | Other ingredients | Acid neutralizing capacity | Other content information as per product label | Usual adult and adolescent dose prn† (maximum OTC dose/day) | Usual pediatric dose | Packaging, storage, and labeling§ |
|---|---|---|---|---|---|---|---|---|---|
| *Mygel* Oral Suspension USP [U.S.] | Aluminum hydroxide (equiv. to dried gel) 200 mg | | Magnesium hydroxide 200 mg | Simethicone 20 mg | | Sodium 1.38 mg | 10–20 mL (120 mL) | ‡ | b, c, d, e |
| *Mygel II* Oral Suspension USP [U.S.] | Aluminum hydroxide (equiv. to dried gel) 400 mg | | Magnesium hydroxide 400 mg | Simethicone 40 mg | | Sodium 1.3 mg | 10–20 mL (60 mL) | ‡ | b, c, d, e |
| *Mylanta* Lozenges [U.S.] | | Calcium carbonate 600 mg | | | 11.4 mEq | | 1–2 lozenges (12 lozenges) | | a |
| Oral Suspension USP [U.S.] | Aluminum hydroxide (equiv. to dried gel) 200 mg | | Magnesium hydroxide 200 mg | Simethicone 20 mg | 12.7 mEq | Sodium 0.68 mg Sugar free | 10–20 mL (120 mL) | ‡ | b, c, d, e |
| Oral Suspension USP [Canada] | Aluminum hydroxide (equiv. to dried gel) 200 mg | | Magnesium hydroxide 200 mg | Simethicone 20 mg | | Sodium 3.2 mg Sugar free Tartrazine free | 10–20 mL 4 times/day | | b, c, d, e |
| Tablets USP (Chewable) [U.S.] | | Calcium carbonate 350 mg | Magnesium hydroxide 150 mg | | 12 mEq | Sodium 0.3 mg | 2–4 tabs (20 tabs) | | b, g |
| Tablets USP (Chewable) [Canada] | Aluminum hydroxide (dried gel) 200 mg | | Magnesium hydroxide 200 mg | Simethicone 20 mg | | Sodium 0.9 mg Tartrazine free | 2–4 tabs 4 times/day | | a, g, i |
| *Mylanta Double Strength* Oral Suspension USP [U.S.] | Aluminum hydroxide 400 mg | | Magnesium hydroxide 400 mg | Simethicone 40 mg | 25.4 mEq | Sodium 1.14 mg Sugar free | 10–20 mL (60 mL) | ‡ | b, c, d, e |
| Tablets USP (Chewable) [U.S.] | | Calcium carbonate 700 mg | Magnesium hydroxide 300 mg | | 24 mEq | Sodium 0.6 mg | 2–4 tabs (10 tabs) | | b, g |
| Tablets USP (Chewable) [Canada] | Aluminum hydroxide (equiv. to dried gel) 400 mg | | Magnesium hydroxide 400 mg | Simethicone 30 mg | | Sodium 1.5 mg Tartrazine free | 2–4 tabs 4 times/day | | b, g |

# Table 7. Oral Dosage Forms (*continued*)

Note: Content and acid neutralizing capacity per capsule, tablet, or 5 mL, unless otherwise stated.
All products are available over-the-counter (OTC) in the U.S. and/or in Canada.

| Brand or generic name [availability] | Aluminum component | Calcium component | Magnesium component | Other ingredients | Acid neutralizing capacity | Other content information as per product label | Usual adult and adolescent dose prn† (maximum OTC dose/day) | Usual pediatric dose | Packaging, storage, and labeling§ |
|---|---|---|---|---|---|---|---|---|---|
| *Mylanta Double Strength Plain* Oral Suspension USP [Canada] | Aluminum hydroxide (equiv. to dried gel) 400 mg | | Magnesium hydroxide 400 mg | | | Sodium 10 mg Sugar free Tartrazine free | 5–10 mL 4 times/day | | b, c, d, e |
| *Mylanta Extra Strength* Oral Suspension USP [Canada] | Aluminum hydroxide (equiv. to dried gel) 650 mg | | Magnesium hydroxide 350 mg | Simethicone 30 mg | | Sodium 1.8 mg Sugar free Tartrazine free | 5–10 mL 4 times/day | | b, c, d, e |
| *Mylanta Gelcaps* Tablets [U.S.] | | Calcium carbonate 550 mg | Magnesium hydroxide 125 mg | | 11.5 mEq | Benzyl alcohol, Sodium 2.5 mg | 2–4 tabs (24 tabs) | | a |
| *Nephrox* Oral Suspension [U.S.] | Aluminum hydroxide gel 320 mg | | | Mineral oil 10% | 9 mEq | Sugar free | 10 mL (60 mL) | | c, d, e |
| *Neutralca-S* Oral Suspension USP [Canada] | Aluminum hydroxide (equiv. to dried gel) 200 mg | | Magnesium hydroxide 200 mg | | | Sodium 0.6 mg Sugar free | 5–15 mL | ‡ | b, c, d |
| Tablets USP (Chewable) [Canada] | Aluminum hydroxide (dried gel) 400 mg | | Magnesium hydroxide 400 mg | | | Sodium 1.01 mg Scored | 1–2 tabs | | b, g |
| *Phillips'* Magnesia Tablets USP (Chewable) [Canada] | | | Magnesium hydroxide 311 mg | | | Low sodium Sucrose 195 mg | 2–4 tabs (16 tabs) | 7–14 yrs: 1 tab (4 tabs) | b, e, g |

*Specific formulations may vary among the different manufacturers; check product labeling.

†In peptic ulcer disease, maximum therapeutic response may be obtained if taken 1 and 3 hours after meals and at bedtime. Severe symptoms may require more frequent dosing.

‡Pediatric doses may range between 5 and 15 mL every 3 to 6 hours or 1 and 3 hours after meals and at bedtime, unless otherwise stated. However, these are general guidelines; proper diagnosis and dose individualization should precede the use of an antacid in a pediatric patient.

§For appropriate *Packaging and storage* and *Label* information refer to designated letters as follows:

a–Store below 40 °C (104 °F), preferably between 15 and 30 °C (59 and 86 °F), in a well-closed container, unless otherwise specified by manufacturer.

b–Store below 40 °C (104 °F), preferably between 15 and 30 °C (59 and 86 °F), unless otherwise specified by manufacturer. Store in a tight container.

c–Protect from freezing.

d–Auxiliary labeling: • Shake well.

e–Auxiliary labeling: • Keep container tightly closed.

f–Auxiliary labeling: • May be chewed or swallowed whole.

g–Auxiliary labeling: • Chew tablets or wafers before swallowing.

h–Auxiliary labeling: • Follow with ¹/₂ to 1 glass of water or other liquid.

i–Auxiliary labeling: • May also be allowed to dissolve in mouth.

Table 7. Oral Dosage Forms *(continued)*

Note: Content and acid neutralizing capacity per capsule, tablet, or 5 mL, unless otherwise stated.
All products are available over-the-counter (OTC) in the U.S. and/or in Canada.

| Brand or generic name [availability] | Aluminum component | Calcium component | Magnesium component | Other ingredients | Acid neutralizing capacity | Other content information as per product label | Usual adult and adolescent dose prn† (maximum OTC dose/day) | Usual pediatric dose | Packaging, storage, and labeling§ |
|---|---|---|---|---|---|---|---|---|---|
| *Phillips' (continued)* Milk of Magnesia USP [U.S.] | | | Magnesium hydroxide 400 mg | | | | 5–15 mL (60 mL) | | b, c, d, e |
| Milk of Magnesia USP [Canada] | | | Magnesium hydroxide 400 mg | | | Alcohol free Sodium <2.2 mg Sugar free (plain and mint) | 5–15 mL (60 mL) | 1–12 yrs: 1–10 mL | b, c, d, e |
| *Phillips' Chewable* Magnesia Tablets USP (Chewable) [U.S.] | | | Magnesium hydroxide 311 mg | | | | 2–4 tabs (16 tabs) | 7–14 yrs: 1 tab (4 tabs) | b, g |
| *Phillips' Concentrated Double-strength* Milk of Magnesia USP [U.S.] | | | Magnesium hydroxide 800 mg | | | | 2.5–7.5 mL (30 mL) | | b, c, d, e |
| *PMS Alumina, Magnesia, and Simethicone* Oral Suspension USP [Canada] | Aluminum hydroxide 200 mg | | Magnesium hydroxide 200 mg | Simethicone 25 mg | | Sugar free | 10–20 mL 4 times/day (80 mL) | | b, c, d, e |
| *Rafton* Oral Suspension [Canada] | Aluminum hydroxide 100 mg | | | Calcium carbonate, Sodium bicarbonate, Sodium alginate 250 mg | | Alcohol free Sodium 30 mg Sugar free Tartrazine free | 10–20 mL 1–4 times/day (80 mL) | | b, c, d, e, h |
| Chewable Tablets [Canada] | Aluminum hydroxide (equiv. to dried gel) 80 mg | | | Alginic acid 200 mg, Sodium bicarbonate | | Sodium 22 mg, Sucrose 1.2 grams, Tartrazine free | 2–4 tabs 1–4 times/day (16 tabs) | | a, g, h |

# Table 7. Oral Dosage Forms (continued)

Note: Content and acid neutralizing capacity per capsule, tablet, or 5 mL, unless otherwise stated.
All products are available over-the-counter (OTC) in the U.S. and/or in Canada.

| Brand or generic name [availability] | Aluminum component | Calcium component | Magnesium component | Other ingredients | Acid neutralizing capacity | Other content information as per product label | Usual adult and adolescent dose prn† (maximum OTC dose/day) | Usual pediatric dose | Packaging, storage, and labeling§ |
|---|---|---|---|---|---|---|---|---|---|
| *Riopan*<br>Oral Suspension USP [U.S.] | | | | Magaldrate 540 mg | 15 mEq | Sodium <0.3 mg | 5–10 mL (80 mL) | ‡ | b, c, d, e |
| Oral Suspension USP [Canada] | | | | Magaldrate 480 mg | | Alcohol free<br>Sodium <0.7 mg<br>Sugar free<br>Tartrazine free | 10–20 mL | ‡ | b, c, d, e |
| Tablets USP (Chewable) [Canada] | | | | Magaldrate 480 mg | | Sodium 0.7 mg<br>Tartrazine free | 1–4 tabs | | a, g |
| *Riopan Extra Strength*<br>Oral Suspension USP [Canada] | | | | Magaldrate 1080 mg | | Alcohol free<br>Sodium 0.3 mg<br>Sugar free<br>Tartrazine free | 5–10 mL | | b, c, d, e |
| *Riopan Plus*<br>Oral Suspension USP [U.S.] | | | | Magaldrate 540 mg, Simethicone 40 mg | 15 mEq | Sodium <0.3 mg | 5–10 mL (60 mL) | ‡ | b, c, d, e |
| Oral Suspension USP [Canada] | | | | Magaldrate 480 mg, Simethicone 20 mg | 13.5 mEq | Alcohol free<br>Sodium 0.7 mg<br>Sugar free<br>Tartrazine free | 10–20 mL | | b, c, d, e |

*Specific formulations may vary among the different manufacturers; check product labeling.
†In peptic ulcer disease, maximum therapeutic response may be obtained if taken 1 and 3 hours after meals and at bedtime. Severe symptoms may require more frequent dosing.
‡Pediatric doses may range between 5 and 15 mL every 3 to 6 hours or 1 and 3 hours after meals and at bedtime, unless otherwise stated. However, these are general guidelines; proper diagnosis and dose individualization should precede the use of an antacid in a pediatric patient.
§For appropriate *Packaging and storage* and *Label* information refer to designated letters as follows:
  a–Store below 40 °C (104 °F), preferably between 15 and 30 °C (59 and 86 °F), in a well-closed container, unless otherwise specified by manufacturer.
  b–Store below 40 °C (104 °F), preferably between 15 and 30 °C (59 and 86 °F), unless otherwise specified by manufacturer. Store in a tight container.
  c–Protect from freezing.
  d–Auxiliary labeling: • Shake well.
  e–Auxiliary labeling: • Keep container tightly closed.
  f–Auxiliary labeling: • May be chewed or swallowed whole.
  g–Auxiliary labeling: • Chew tablets or wafers before swallowing.
  h–Auxiliary labeling: • Follow with ½ to 1 glass of water or other liquid.
  i–Auxiliary labeling: • May also be allowed to dissolve in mouth.

## Table 7. Oral Dosage Forms *(continued)*

Note: Content and acid neutralizing capacity per capsule, tablet, or 5 mL, unless otherwise stated.

All products are available over-the-counter (OTC) in the U.S. and/or in Canada.

| Brand or generic name [availability] | Aluminum component | Calcium component | Magnesium component | Other ingredients | Acid neutralizing capacity | Other content information as per product label | Usual adult and adolescent dose prn† (maximum OTC dose/day) | Usual pediatric dose | Packaging, storage, and labeling§ |
|---|---|---|---|---|---|---|---|---|---|
| *Riopan Plus (continued)* Tablets USP (Chewable) [U.S./Canada] | | | | Magaldrate 480 mg, Simethicone 20 mg | 13.5 mEq | Sodium 0.1 mg | 2–4 tabs (25 tabs) | | b, g |
| *Riopan Plus Double Strength* Oral Suspension USP [U.S.] | | | | Magaldrate 1080 mg, Simethicone 40 mg | | Sodium ≤0.3 mg | 5–10 mL (60 mL) | ‡ | b, c, d, e |
| Tablets USP (Chewable) [U.S.] | | | | Magaldrate 1080 mg, Simethicone 20 mg | 30 mEq | Sodium ≤0.5 mg | 2–4 tabs (25 tabs) | | b, g |
| *Riopan Plus Extra Strength* Oral Suspension USP [Canada] | | | | Magaldrate 1080 mg, Simethicone 30 mg | | Sodium 0.3 mg Sugar free Tartrazine free | 5–10 mL | | b, c, d, e |
| *Rolaids* Tablets USP (Chewable) [U.S.] | | Calcium carbonate 550 mg | Magnesium hydroxide 110 mg | | 14.8 mEq | Sodium <0.1 mg | 1–4 tabs (12 tabs) | | b, g |
| Tablets USP (Chewable) [Canada] | | Calcium carbonate 317 mg | Magnesium hydroxide 64 mg | | | Sodium <1 mg Tartrazine free | 1–2 tabs (12 tabs) | | b, g |
| *Rolaids Extra Strength* Tablets USP (Chewable) [Canada] | | Calcium carbonate 750 mg | Magnesium hydroxide 64 mg | | | Sodium <1 mg Tartrazine free | 1–2 tabs (10 tabs) | | b, g |
| *Rulox* Oral Suspension USP [U.S.] | Aluminum hydroxide (equiv. to dried gel) 225 mg | | Magnesium hydroxide 200 mg | | 12 mEq | Sodium <1 mg | 10–20 mL (80 mL) | ‡ | b, c, d, e |
| *Rulox No. 1* Tablets USP (Chewable) [U.S.] | Aluminum hydroxide (dried gel) 200 mg | | Magnesium hydroxide 200 mg | | | | 1–2 tabs (16 tabs) | | b, e, g, h |
| *Rulox No. 2* Tablets USP (Chewable) [U.S.] | Aluminum hydroxide (dried gel) 400 mg | | Magnesium hydroxide 400 mg | | | | 1–2 tabs (8 tabs) | | b, e, g, h |

Table 7. Oral Dosage Forms (*continued*)

Note: Content and acid neutralizing capacity per capsule, tablet, or 5 mL, unless otherwise stated.

All products are available over-the-counter (OTC) in the U.S. and/or in Canada.

| Brand or generic name [availability] | Aluminum component | Calcium component | Magnesium component | Other ingredients | Acid neutralizing capacity | Other content information as per product label | Usual adult and adolescent dose prn† (maximum OTC dose/day) | Usual pediatric dose | Packaging, storage, and labeling§ |
|---|---|---|---|---|---|---|---|---|---|
| *Rulox Plus* Oral Suspension USP [U.S.] | Aluminum hydroxide (equiv. to dried gel) 500 mg | | Magnesium hydroxide 450 mg | Simethicone 40 mg | | | 10–20 mL (80 mL) | | b, c, d, e |
| *Simaal Gel* Oral Suspension USP [U.S.] | Aluminum hydroxide (equiv. to dried gel) 200 mg | | Magnesium hydroxide 200 mg | Simethicone 20 mg | | Sodium 1.4 mg Sugar free | 10–20 mL (120 mL) | | b, c, d, e |
| *Simaal 2 Gel* Oral Suspension USP [U.S.] | Aluminum hydroxide (equiv. to dried gel) 400 mg | | Magnesium hydroxide 400 mg | Simethicone 40 mg | | Sodium 1.84 mg Sugar free | 10–20 mL (60 mL) | ‡ | b, c, d, e |
| *Tempo* Tablets USP (Chewable) [U.S.] | Aluminum hydroxide 133 mg | Calcium carbonate 414 mg | Magnesium hydroxide 81 mg | Simethicone 20 mg | 14 mEq | Sodium 3 mg | 1 tab (12 tabs) | | b, g |
| *Titralac* Tablets USP (Chewable) [U.S.] | | Calcium carbonate 420 mg | | Glycine 183 mg | 7.5 mEq | Sodium 1.1 mg Sugar free | 2 tabs (19 tabs) | | b, f, i |
| *Titralac Extra Strength* Tablets USP (Chewable) [U.S.] | | Calcium carbonate 750 mg | | Glycine 321 mg | | Sodium 1.1 mg Sugar free | 1–2 tabs (10 tabs) | | b, f, h, i |
| *Titralac Plus* Oral Suspension [U.S.] | | Calcium carbonate 500 mg | | Simethicone 20 mg | | Sodium 2.5 mg Sugar free | 10 mL (80 mL) | | b, c, d |
| Chewable Tablets [U.S.] | | Calcium carbonate 420 mg | | Glycine 173 mg Simethicone 21 mg | | Sodium 1.1 mg Sugar free | 2 tabs (19 tabs) | | b, f, i |

*Specific formulations may vary among the different manufacturers; check product labeling.

†In peptic ulcer disease, maximum therapeutic response may be obtained if taken 1 and 3 hours after meals and at bedtime. Severe symptoms may require more frequent dosing.

‡Pediatric doses may range between 5 and 15 mL every 3 to 6 hours or 1 and 3 hours after meals and at bedtime, unless otherwise stated. However, these are general guidelines; proper diagnosis and dose individualization should precede the use of an antacid in a pediatric patient.

§For appropriate *Packaging and storage* and *Label* information refer to designated letters as follows:

a–Store below 40 °C (104 °F), preferably between 15 and 30 °C (59 and 86 °F), in a well-closed container, unless otherwise specified by manufacturer.

b–Store below 40 °C (104 °F), preferably between 15 and 30 °C (59 and 86 °F), unless otherwise specified by manufacturer. Store in a tight container.

c–Protect from freezing.

d–Auxiliary labeling: • Shake well.

e–Auxiliary labeling: • Keep container tightly closed.

f–Auxiliary labeling: • May be chewed or swallowed whole.

g–Auxiliary labeling: • Chew tablets or wafers before swallowing.

h–Auxiliary labeling: • Follow with ½ to 1 glass of water or other liquid.

i–Auxiliary labeling: • May also be allowed to dissolve in mouth.

Table 7. Oral Dosage Forms *(continued)*

Note: Content and acid neutralizing capacity per capsule, tablet, or 5 mL, unless otherwise stated.

All products are available over-the-counter (OTC) in the U.S. and/or in Canada.

| Brand or generic name [availability] | Aluminum component | Calcium component | Magnesium component | Other ingredients | Acid neutralizing capacity | Other content information as per product label | Usual adult and adolescent dose prn† (maximum OTC dose/day) | Usual pediatric dose | Packaging, storage, and labeling§ |
|---|---|---|---|---|---|---|---|---|---|
| *Trial* Tablets USP (Chewable) [Canada] | | Calcium carbonate 420 mg | | | | | 1–2 tabs (18 tabs) | | a, g |
| *Tums* Tablets USP (Chewable) [U.S.] | | Calcium carbonate 500 mg | | | 10 mEq | Sodium <2 mg | 2–4 tabs (16 tabs) | | b, g, i |
| Tablets USP (Chewable) [Canada] | | Calcium carbonate 500 mg | | | 10 mEq | Sodium <2 mg | 1–2 tabs (16 tabs) | | b, g |
| *Tums Anti-gas/ Antacid* Chewable Tablets [U.S.] | | Calcium carbonate 500 mg | | Simethicone 20 mg | 10 mEq | Sodium ≤2 mg | 1–2 tabs (16 tabs) | | a, g |
| *Tums E-X* Tablets USP (Chewable) [U.S.] | | Calcium carbonate 750 mg | | | 15 mEq | Sodium <2 mg | 2–4 tabs (10 tabs) | | b, g |
| *Tums Extra Strength* Tablets USP (Chewable) [Canada] | | Calcium carbonate 750 mg | | | 15 mEq | Sodium <2 mg | 1–2 tabs (10 tabs) | | b, g |
| *Tums Ultra* Tablets USP (Chewable) [U.S.] | | Calcium carbonate 1 gram | | | 20 mEq | Sodium ≤4 mg | 2–3 tabs (8 tabs) | | b, g |
| *Tums Ultra* Tablets USP (Chewable) [Canada] | | Calcium carbonate 1 gram | | | 20 mEq | Sodium ≤4 mg | 1–2 tabs (8 tabs) | | b, g |

Table 7. Oral Dosage Forms *(continued)*

Note: Content and acid neutralizing capacity per capsule, tablet, or 5 mL, unless otherwise stated.

All products are available over-the-counter (OTC) in the U.S. and/or in Canada.

| Brand or generic name [availability] | Aluminum component | Calcium component | Magnesium component | Other ingredients | Acid neutralizing capacity | Other content information as per product label | Usual adult and adolescent dose prn† (maximum OTC dose/day) | Usual pediatric dose | Packaging, storage, and labeling§ |
|---|---|---|---|---|---|---|---|---|---|
| *Univol* Oral Suspension [Canada] | Aluminum hydroxide 165 mg | | Magnesium hydroxide 200 mg | | | Alcohol 1% Sodium 1 mg Sugar free Tartrazine free | 10–20 mL (80 mL) | | b, c, d, e |
| *Uro-Mag* Capsules USP [U.S.] | | | Magnesium oxide 140 mg | | 7 mEq | | 3–4 caps/daily | | a |

*Specific formulations may vary among the different manufacturers; check product labeling.

†In peptic ulcer disease, maximum therapeutic response may be obtained if taken 1 and 3 hours after meals and at bedtime. Severe symptoms may require more frequent dosing.

‡Pediatric doses may range between 5 and 15 mL every 3 to 6 hours or 1 and 3 hours after meals and at bedtime, unless otherwise stated. However, these are general guidelines; proper diagnosis and dose individualization should precede the use of an antacid in a pediatric patient.

§For appropriate *Packaging and storage* and *Label* information refer to designated letters as follows:

a–Store below 40 °C (104 °F), preferably between 15 and 30 °C (59 and 86 °F), in a well-closed container, unless otherwise specified by manufacturer.

b–Store below 40 °C (104 °F), preferably between 15 and 30 °C (59 and 86 °F), in a tight container.

c–Protect from freezing.

d–Auxiliary labeling: • Shake well.

e–Auxiliary labeling: • Keep container tightly closed.

f–Auxiliary labeling: • May be chewed or swallowed whole.

g–Auxiliary labeling: • Chew tablets or wafers before swallowing.

h–Auxiliary labeling: • Follow with ½ to 1 glass of water or other liquid.

i–Auxiliary labeling: • May also be allowed to dissolve in mouth.

# ANTHRALIN   Topical

INN: Dithranol

VA CLASSIFICATION (Primary/Secondary): DE802/DE900

Note: For a listing of dosage forms and brand names by country availability, see *Dosage Forms* section(s). For a listing of brand names for the articles in this monograph, refer to the General Index.

## Category

Antipsoriatic (topical); hair growth stimulant, alopecia areata (topical).

## Indications

Note: Bracketed information in the *Indications* section refers to uses that are not included in U.S. product labeling.

### Accepted

Psoriasis (treatment)—Anthralin is indicated in the topical treatment of quiescent or chronic psoriasis of the skin and scalp.

[Alopecia areata (treatment)][1]—Anthralin is used in the topical treatment of alopecia areata.

### Unaccepted

Anthralin should not be used on acute or actively inflamed psoriatic eruptions.

---

[1]Not included in Canadian product labeling.

## Pharmacology/Pharmacokinetics

### Physicochemical characteristics

Molecular weight—226.23.

### Mechanism of action/Effect

Anthralin restores the normal rate of epidermal cell proliferation and keratinization by reducing the mitotic activity of the hyperplastic epidermis. It also has been shown to inhibit enzyme metabolism.

### Absorption

Anthralin is absorbed through the skin; however, absorption appears to be quite low.

### Elimination

Two studies found evidence of anthralin metabolites (mainly danthron) in the urine. However, a later study using a detection limit of 20 mcg per mL found no evidence of excretion of anthraquinones in the urine. In addition, other studies have found no evidence of systemic toxicity, even in patients with renal disease.

## Precautions to Consider

### Carcinogenicity/Tumorigenicity

Some long-term studies in mice have shown anthralin to be cocarcinogenic and tumorigenic. However, these effects have not been reported in humans.

### Pregnancy/Reproduction

Pregnancy—Anthralin may be systemically absorbed.

Studies have not been done in humans.

Studies have not been done in animals.

FDA Pregnancy Category C.

### Breast-feeding

It is not known whether anthralin is distributed into breast milk, and problems in humans have not been documented. However, anthralin may be systemically absorbed.

### Pediatrics

Appropriate studies on the relationship of age to the effects of anthralin have not been performed in the pediatric population. Safety and efficacy have not been established.

### Geriatrics

Appropriate studies on the relationship of age to the effects of anthralin have not been performed in the geriatric population. However, no geriatrics-specific problems have been documented to date.

### Drug interactions and/or related problems

The following drug interactions and/or related problems have been selected on the basis of their potential clinical significance (possible mechanism in parentheses where appropriate)—not necessarily inclusive (» = major clinical significance):

Note: Combinations containing any of the following medications, depending on the amount present, may also interact with this medication.

Photosensitizing medications, other

   (concurrent use of these medications with anthralin may cause additive photosensitizing effects)

### Medical considerations/Contraindications

The medical considerations/contraindications included here have been selected on the basis of their potential clinical significance (reasons given in parentheses where appropriate)—not necessarily inclusive (» = major clinical significance).

*Risk-benefit should be considered when the following medical problems exist:*

» Acute eruptions or presence of inflammation of skin, including folliculitis

   Sensitivity to anthralin

   (may cause allergic contact dermatitis)

## Side/Adverse Effects

Note: Severe conjunctivitis, keratitis, or corneal opacity may occur if this medication comes in contact with the eye.

The following side/adverse effects have been selected on the basis of their potential clinical significance (possible signs and symptoms in parentheses where appropriate)—not necessarily inclusive:

### Those indicating need for medical attention

Incidence more frequent

   *Redness or other skin irritation not present before therapy*

Incidence rare

   *Allergic reaction* (skin rash)

## Patient Consultation

As an aid to patient consultation, refer to *Advice for the Patient, Anthralin (Topical).*

In providing consultation, consider emphasizing the following selected information (» = major clinical significance):

### Before using this medication

» Conditions affecting use, especially:

   Sensitivity to anthralin

   Other medical problems, especially acute eruptions or presence of inflammation of skin, including folliculitis

### Proper use of this medication

» Avoiding contact with the eyes and other mucous membranes

» Not applying medication to blistered, raw, or oozing areas of skin or scalp

» Not using medication on face or sex organs or in the folds and creases of the skin; checking with physician if necessary

» Using medication only as directed; importance of not using more medication than the amount prescribed

   Knowing correct method of administration; checking with physician if necessary

*Proper administration*

   If irritation of normal skin occurs, applying petrolatum around affected areas before applying anthralin

   Applying a thin layer to only the affected areas

   Washing hands immediately after application

*For short contact anthralin therapy*

   Allowing medication to remain on affected area for 10 to 30 minutes or as prescribed by physician; then bathing, if applied to the skin, or shampooing, if applied to the scalp, to remove medication

*For patients using the cream for overnight treatment*

   If the skin is being treated—removing cream from skin by bathing the next morning

   If the scalp is being treated—shampooing to remove scales and any previous application, drying, and parting hair before application; checking with physician to see when cream should be removed

*For patients using the ointment for overnight treatment*

   If the skin is being treated—removing ointment from skin with warm liquid petrolatum the next morning, then bathing

   If the scalp is being treated—removing from scalp by shampooing the next morning

» Proper dosing

   Missed dose: Applying as soon as possible; not applying if almost time for next dose; not doubling doses

» Proper storage

## Precautions while using this medication

» *Medication may stain skin, hair, fingernails, clothing, bed linens, or bathtub or shower:*

Avoiding contact with clothing or bed linens; protective dressings may be used, unless otherwise directed by physician

Stain on skin or hair wears off in several weeks after medication is discontinued

Wearing plastic gloves to prevent staining of hands

If applied to scalp at night, checking with physician to see if plastic cap may be worn to prevent staining of pillow

Removing any medication on surface of bathtub or shower by washing with hot water immediately after bathing or showering, then using a household cleanser to remove any remaining deposit of medication on bathtub or shower

## Side/adverse effects

Anthralin has been shown to cause tumors (some cancerous) in animals. However, there have been no reports of anthralin causing tumors in humans

Signs of potential side effects, especially redness or other skin irritation not present before therapy or allergic reaction

## General Dosing Information

A short contact time and the initial use of a low concentration are recommended, with subsequent increase in contact time and/or concentration only as necessary.

Excessive concentrations of the ointment may produce irritation.

One criterion for determining the optimal concentration for use is the occurrence of erythema on normal skin adjacent to the lesions. When erythema occurs, the dosage, frequency of application, and/or duration of treatment should be reduced.

Once the optimal concentration has been determined, a protective coating of petrolatum may be applied to the normal skin around the affected areas before anthralin is applied, to minimize irritation.

The optimal period of contact will vary according to the strength used and the patient's response to anthralin therapy.

In the treatment of psoriasis, 2 types of anthralin therapy are being used:

Conventional therapy—Anthralin cream or ointment is applied once (sometimes twice) a day, preferably at night, and allowed to remain on the affected area overnight, then removed by bathing or shampooing the next morning or before the next application.

Short contact anthralin therapy (S.C.A.T.)—Anthralin 0.1 to 1% cream or ointment is applied once a day and allowed to remain on the affected area for only 10 to 30 minutes or as prescribed by physician, then removed by bathing, if applied to skin, or by shampooing, if applied to scalp.

It is recommended that anthralin not be applied to the face, genitalia, or intertriginous skin areas, since harmful irritation may occur.

## Topical Dosage Forms

Note: Bracketed uses in the *Dosage Forms* section refer to categories of use and/or indications that are not included in U.S. product labeling.

### ANTHRALIN CREAM USP

**Usual adult and adolescent dose**

Psoriasis—
Conventional therapy: Topical, to the skin, once a day, preferably at night.
Short contact therapy: Topical, to the skin, once a day for ten to thirty minutes or as prescribed by physician.

[Alopecia areata][1]—
Topical, to the skin, once a day.

**Usual pediatric dose**

Safety and efficacy have not been established.

**Usual geriatric dose**

See *Usual adult and adolescent dose.*

**Strength(s) usually available**

U.S.—
0.1% (Rx) [*Anthra-Tex; Drithocreme; Lasan 0.1* (BHT; methylparaben; propylparaben; sodium bisulfite)].
0.2% (Rx) [*Lasan 0.2* (BHT; methylparaben; propylparaben; sodium bisulfite)].
0.25% (Rx) [*Anthra-Tex; Drithocreme; Dritho-Scalp*].
0.4% (Rx) [*Lasan 0.4* (BHT; methylparaben; propylparaben; sodium bisulfite)].
0.5% (Rx) [*Anthra-Tex; Drithocreme; Dritho-Scalp*].
1% (Rx) [*Anthra-Tex; Drithocreme HP; Lasan HP-1* (BHT; methylparaben; propylparaben; sodium bisulfite)].

Canada—
0.1% (OTC) [*Anthranol 0.1*].
0.2% (OTC) [*Anthranol 0.2*].
0.4% (OTC) [*Anthranol 0.4; Anthrascalp* (parabens; bisulfite)].

**Packaging and storage**

Store between 8 and 15 °C (46 and 59 °F), unless otherwise specified by manufacturer. Store in a tight container. Protect from light. Protect from freezing.

**Auxiliary labeling**
• For external use only.

### ANTHRALIN OINTMENT USP

**Usual adult and adolescent dose**

Psoriasis—
Conventional therapy: Topical, to the skin, one or two times a day.
Short contact therapy: See *Anthralin Cream USP.*

[Alopecia areata][1]—
See *Anthralin Cream USP.*

**Usual pediatric dose**

See *Anthralin Cream USP.*

**Usual geriatric dose**

See *Usual adult and adolescent dose.*

**Strength(s) usually available**

U.S.—
0.1% (Rx) [*Anthra-Derm*].
0.25% (Rx) [*Anthra-Derm*].
0.4% (Rx) [*Lasan* (BHT)].
0.5% (Rx) [*Anthra-Derm*].
1% (Rx) [*Anthra-Derm*].

Canada—
1% (OTC) [*Anthraforte 1*].
2% (OTC) [*Anthraforte 2*].
3% (OTC) [*Anthraforte 3*].

**Packaging and storage**

Store between 8 and 15 °C (46 and 59 °F), unless otherwise specified by manufacturer. Store in a tight container. Protect from light. Protect from freezing.

**Auxiliary labeling**
• For external use only.

[1]Not included in Canadian product labeling.

Revised: 08/15/95

---

# ANTICHOLINERGICS/ANTISPASMODICS   Systemic

This monograph includes information on the following: Anisotropine†; Atropine; Belladonna†; Clidinium†; Dicyclomine; Glycopyrrolate; Homatropine; Hyoscyamine; Mepenzolate†; Methantheline†; Methscopolamine; Pirenzepine*; Propantheline; Scopolamine.

INN:
Anisotropine—Octatropine
Dicyclomine—Dicycloverine
Glycopyrrolate—Glycopyrronium Bromide
Methantheline—Methanthelinium
Methscopolamine—Hyoscine Methobromide

VA CLASSIFICATION (Primary/Secondary):
Anisotropine—AU350/GA801
Atropine
Oral—AU350/GA801; GU201; AD900
Parenteral—AU350/GA801; CV300; GU201; AD900
Belladonna—AU350/GA801
Clidinium—AU350/GA801
Dicyclomine—AU350/GA801
Glycopyrrolate
Oral—AU350/GA801; GA400
Parenteral—AU350/GA801; CV300; GA400; AD900

Homatropine—AU350/GA801
Hyoscyamine
    Oral—AU350/GA801; GU201
    Parenteral—AU350/GA801; GU201; CV300; AD900
Mepenzolate—AU350/GA801
Methantheline—AU350/GA801; GU201
Methscopolamine—AU350/GA801
Pirenzepine—AU350/GA801
Propantheline—AU350
Scopolamine
    Oral—AU350/GA801; CN550; GA700; GU201
    Parenteral—AU350/GA801; CV300; CN205; CN550; GA700
    Rectal—AU350
    Transdermal—CN550

Other commonly used names are: Dicycloverine [Dicyclomine], Glycopyrronium bromide [Glycopyrrolate], Hyoscine hydrobromide [Scopolamine], Hyoscine methobromide [Methscopolamine], Methanthelinium [Methantheline], Octatropine [Anisotropine]

Note: For a listing of dosage forms and brand names by country availability, see *Dosage Forms* section(s). For a listing of brand names for the articles in this monograph, refer to the General Index.

---

\*Not commercially available in the U.S.
†Not commercially available in Canada.

---

## Category

Note: All of these medications have anticholinergic and, to some extent, antispasmodic actions; however, the labeled indications for specific agents may vary because of minor differences in potency and/or receptor selectivity. **In general, there is a lack of specific testing and/or clinical-use data to support the indication of anticholinergics/antispasmodics in most conditions.**

Anticholinergic—Anisotropine; Atropine; Belladonna; Clidinium; Dicyclomine; Glycopyrrolate; Homatropine; Hyoscyamine; Mepenzolate; Methantheline; Methscopolamine; Pirenzepine; Propantheline; Scopolamine.
Antispasmodic, gastrointestinal—Dicyclomine; Scopolamine Butylbromide.
Antidysmenorrheal—Belladonna; Scopolamine Butylbromide.
Antiarrhythmic—Atropine (parenteral only); Glycopyrrolate (parenteral only); Hyoscyamine (parenteral only); Scopolamine (parenteral only).
Antidote (to cholinesterase inhibitors)—Atropine; Hyoscyamine (parenteral only).
Antidote (to muscarine)—Atropine; Hyoscyamine (parenteral only).
Antidote (to organophosphate pesticides)—Atropine.
Antispasmodic, urinary—Atropine; Scopolamine.
Cholinergic adjunct (curariform block)—Atropine (parenteral only); Glycopyrrolate (parenteral only); Hyoscyamine (parenteral only).
Anesthesia adjunct—Scopolamine (parenteral only).
Antiemetic—Scopolamine.
Antivertigo agent—Belladonna; Scopolamine.
Antidiarrheal—Glycopyrrolate.

## Indications

Note: Bracketed information in the *Indications* section refers to uses that are not included in U.S. product labeling.

### Accepted

Ulcer, peptic (treatment adjunct)—All anticholinergics included in this monograph, except dicyclomine and scopolamine hydrobromide, are FDA approved in conjunction with antacids or histamine H$_2$-receptor antagonists in the treatment of peptic ulcer, to reduce further gastric acid secretion and delay gastric emptying. However, the use of most anticholinergics as treatment adjunct in peptic ulcer has been replaced by the use of more effective agents. Results with anticholinergics usually are inconsistent and transient and require high doses, which result in significant side effects. Atropine, belladonna, clidinium, hyoscyamine, pirenzepine, and propantheline taken orally may be used rarely. Intravenous use of hyoscyamine may be indicated for prompt relief of pain in the treatment of both the moderately severe and the severe peptic ulcer. Anisotropine, glycopyrrolate, homatropine, mepenzolate, methantheline, and methscopolamine are generally no longer used for this indication.

Bowel syndrome, irritable (treatment)—Atropine, belladonna, [clidinium], dicyclomine, [glycopyrrolate], hyoscyamine, [propantheline], and [scopolamine] are indicated in the treatment of irritable bowel syndrome, mainly in patients in whom other therapy, such as sedation and/or change in diet, has failed. However, results usually are inconsistent and transient and require high doses, which result in significant

side effects. Anisotropine, mepenzolate, methantheline, methscopolamine, and pirenzepine are generally no longer used for this indication.

Urologic disorders, symptoms of (treatment)—Oral hyoscyamine is indicated to control hypermotility in cystitis. However, results of anticholinergic treatment usually are inconsistent and transient and require high doses, which result in significant side effects. Atropine and scopolamine butylbromide are generally no longer used for this indication.

Urinary incontinence (treatment)—[Propantheline][1] is used in the treatment of uninhibited hypertonic neurogenic bladder to increase bladder capacity by reducing amplitude and frequency of bladder contractions. Atropine and methantheline are generally no longer used for this indication.

Hypersecretory conditions, gastric, in anesthesia (prophylaxis)—Parenteral glycopyrrolate is indicated as preanesthetic medication to reduce gastric acid secretion.

Salivation and respiratory tract secretions, excessive, in anesthesia (prophylaxis)—Oral and parenteral atropine and the parenteral forms of glycopyrrolate and scopolamine[1] are indicated as antisialagogue preanesthetic medications to prevent or reduce salivation and respiratory tract secretions. Parenteral hyoscyamine is no longer used for these indications.

Arrhythmias, succinylcholine-induced (prophylaxis) or
Arrhythmias, surgical procedure–induced (prophylaxis)—The parenteral form of atropine is indicated as adjunct to anesthesia to prevent reflex bradycardia, sinus arrest, and hypotension induced by succinylcholine during intubation of the trachea or produced by certain surgical manipulations. Parenteral scopolamine is generally no longer used for these indications.

Arrhythmias, cardiac (treatment) or
Bradycardia, sinus (treatment)—Parenteral atropine is indicated to reduce severe sinus bradycardia and syncope associated with hyperactive carotid sinus reflex; and to lessen the degree of atrioventricular heart block in Type I atrioventricular (AV) conduction deficits. It is also used to treat ventricular asystole. Parenteral atropine also is indicated as an antidote for sinus bradycardia resulting from the improper administration of a choline ester medication. Parenteral hyoscyamine is generally no longer used for these indications.

Arrhythmias, in anesthesia (treatment) or
Arrhythmias, in surgery (treatment)—The parenteral form of atropine is indicated to restore cardiac rate and arterial pressure when increased vagal activity has reduced pulse rate and cardiac action. Parenteral glycopyrrolate is indicated to block cardiac vagal inhibitory reflexes during induction of anesthesia and intubation. Parenteral glycopyrrolate is also indicated intraoperatively to counteract drug-induced or vagal traction reflexes with the associated arrhythmias. Parenteral hyoscyamine and parenteral scopolamine are generally no longer used for these indications.

Toxicity, cholinesterase inhibitor (prophylaxis)—The parenteral forms of atropine and glycopyrrolate are indicated for administration prior to or concurrently with neostigmine or pyridostigmine during reversal of nondepolarizing neuromuscular blockade to protect against the muscarinic effects of these drugs, such as bradycardia and excessive secretions. Parenteral hyoscyamine is generally no longer used for this indication.

Toxicity, cholinesterase inhibitor (treatment)
Toxicity, muscarine (treatment) or
Toxicity, organophosphate pesticide (treatment)—Oral and parenteral atropine are indicated in the treatment of poisoning from cholinesterase inhibitors such as neostigmine, pilocarpine, physostigmine, and methacholine, and in the treatment of the rapid type of mushroom (muscarine) poisoning. Atropine is also indicated in the treatment of poisoning caused by pesticides that are organophosphate cholinesterase inhibitors, chemical warfare, and "nerve" gases. Parenteral hyoscyamine is generally no longer used for these indications.

Anesthesia, general, adjunct—Parenteral administration of scopolamine[1], in combination with morphine or meperidine, is indicated in preanesthesia to reduce excitement and produce amnesia. Scopolamine may also be used for opioid-induced respiratory depression. Parenteral scopolamine[1] is also indicated in conjunction with analgesics in cardiopulmonary bypass patients who cannot be deeply anesthetized because of the risk of severe hypotension or circulatory collapse.

Motion sickness (prophylaxis and treatment)—Transdermal scopolamine is indicated for prophylaxis of nausea and vomiting associated with motion sickness.

Pneumonitis, aspiration (prophylaxis)—Parenteral glycopyrrolate may provide some protection against aspiration of gastric contents during anesthesia.

[Salivation, excessive, postsurgical (prophylaxis)][1] or

[Salivation, excessive, medical condition–related (prophylaxis)][1]—Transdermal scopolamine is used for short-term control of drooling in postsurgical patients and in patients with goiter or other medical conditions in whom excessive salivation becomes a social problem.

[Salivation, excessive, in dental procedures (prophylaxis)][1]—The oral forms of atropine, glycopyrrolate, methantheline, and propantheline are used to control excessive salivation that interferes with dental procedures. Belladonna is generally no longer used for this indication.

Anticholinergics/antispasmodics listed below are FDA (U.S.) and HPB (Canada) approved for the following indications; however, they generally have been replaced by more effective agents—
• Biliary tract disorders (treatment adjunct)—Atropine, hyoscyamine, and scopolamine butylbromide.
• Radiography, gastrointestinal, adjunct—Parenteral atropine and parenteral hyoscyamine.
• Dysmenorrhea (treatment)—Belladonna and scopolamine butylbromide.
• Enuresis, nocturnal (treatment)—Belladonna and scopolamine butylbromide.
• Rhinitis, allergic, severe (treatment)—Oral hyoscyamine.

Anticholinergics/antispasmodics listed below have been used for the following indications; however, they generally have been replaced by more effective agents—
• [Diarrhea (treatment)][1]—Glycopyrrolate.
• [Parkinsonism (treatment)][1]—Oral atropine, belladonna, parenteral hyoscyamine, oral hyoscyamine and scopolamine combination, and oral scopolamine.

### Unaccepted

Hyoscyamine elixir and oral solution have been used in the treatment of infant colic. However, there is no conclusive evidence of effectiveness for this use.

---

[1]Not included in Canadian product labeling.

## Pharmacology/Pharmacokinetics

### Physicochemical characteristics

Molecular weight—
    Anisotropine methylbromide: 362.35.
    Atropine: 289.37.
    Clidinium bromide: 432.36.
    Dicyclomine hydrochloride: 345.95.
    Glycopyrrolate: 398.34.
    Homatropine methylbromide: 370.29.
    Hyoscyamine: 289.37.
    Hyoscyamine sulfate: 712.85.
    Mepenzolate bromide: 420.35.
    Methantheline bromide: 420.35.
    Methscopolamine bromide: 398.30.
    Pirenzepine: 351.41.
    Propantheline bromide: 448.40.
    Scopolamine hydrobromide: 438.31.

pKa—
    Atropine: 9.8.
    Dicyclomine: 9.0.
    Scopolamine: 7.55–7.81.

### Mechanism of action/Effect

Anticholinergic—The naturally occurring belladonna alkaloids, semisynthetic derivatives, quaternary ammonium compounds, and, to a lesser extent, the synthetic tertiary amines inhibit the muscarinic actions of acetylcholine on structures innervated by postganglionic cholinergic nerves as well as on smooth muscles that respond to acetylcholine but lack cholinergic innervation. These postganglionic receptor sites are present in the autonomic effector cells of the smooth muscle, cardiac muscle, sinoatrial and atrioventricular nodes, and exocrine glands. Depending on the dose, anticholinergics may reduce the motility and secretory activity of the gastrointestinal system, and the tone of the ureter and urinary bladder and may have a slight relaxant action on the bile ducts and gallbladder. In general, the smaller doses of anticholinergics inhibit salivary and bronchial secretions, sweating, and accommodation; cause dilatation of the pupil; and increase the heart rate. Larger doses are required to decrease motility of the gastrointestinal and urinary tracts and to inhibit gastric acid secretion.

Antispasmodic, gastrointestinal—Unproven. A local and direct action on smooth muscle, to reduce tone and motility of the gastrointestinal tract, has been suggested to explain the apparent gastrointestinal antispasmodic effect of the synthetic tertiary amine compounds.

Antidysmenorrheal—Effectiveness in relieving dysmenorrhea is due to spasmolytic action.

Antiarrhythmic—Inhibition of muscarinic actions of acetylcholine at postganglionic receptor sites present in the autonomic effector cells of the cardiac muscle, and sinoatrial and atrioventricular nodes.

Antidote (to cholinesterase inhibitors; to muscarine; to organophosphate pesticides)—Atropine and hyoscyamine antagonize the actions of cholinesterase inhibitors at muscarinic receptor sites, including increased tracheobronchial and salivary secretion, bronchoconstriction, autonomic ganglionic stimulation, and, to a moderate extent, central actions.

Cholinergic adjunct (curariform block)—Atropine and hyoscyamine antagonize the actions, such as vagal and secretory enhancing effects, of cholinesterase inhibitors used in the treatment of nondepolarizing neuromuscular blockade.

Anesthesia adjunct—Scopolamine depresses the cerebral cortex; in large doses and in conjunction with analgesics, produces loss of memory.

Antiemetic—Belladonna and scopolamine act primarily by reducing the excitability of the labyrinthine receptors and by depressing conduction in the vestibular cerebellar pathway.

Antivertigo—The exact mechanism by which belladonna and scopolamine exert their antimotion sickness and antivertigo effects is unknown; however, they probably act either on the cortex or more peripherally on the maculae of the utricle and saccule.

Antidiarrheal—Glycopyrrolate may reduce the activity of the gastrocolic reflex and the excessive peristaltic activity of both the small and large bowels.

Other actions/effects
Natural tertiary amines—
    Atropine: Stimulates or depresses the central nervous system (CNS), depending on the dose; and has a more prolonged and potent action than the other belladonna alkaloids on the heart, intestine, and bronchial muscle.
    Belladonna alkaloids: In parkinsonism, selectively depress certain central motor mechanisms in the CNS, controlling muscle tone and movement.
    Hyoscyamine: Has actions similar to those of atropine, but is more potent in both its central and peripheral effects.
    Scopolamine: Has peripheral action similar to that of atropine but, in contrast to atropine, is depressant to the CNS at therapeutic doses; it does not stimulate the medullary centers and therefore does not increase respiration or elevate blood pressure. Scopolamine has a more potent action than atropine on the sphincter muscle of the iris and the ciliary muscle of the lens, and on the secretory glands such as salivary, bronchial, and sweat glands.

Quaternary ammonium compounds, semisynthetic and synthetic—
    In contrast to atropine and scopolamine, effects of these medications on the CNS are negligible. These medications are also less likely to affect the pupil or ciliary muscle of the eye. Ganglionic blockade is attributed to some increased effects of the high dosage range, and toxic doses produce neuromuscular blockade.

Synthetic tertiary amines—
    These medications produce less prominent CNS effects than do the natural tertiary amines.

### Absorption

Tertiary amines—Rapidly absorbed from gastrointestinal tract; also enter the circulation through the mucosal surfaces of the body.

Quaternary ammonium compounds—Gastrointestinal absorption is poor and irregular. Total absorption after an oral dose is about 10 to 25%.

### Distribution

Exact distribution of anticholinergics has not been fully determined. However, tertiary amines appear to be distributed throughout the entire body and readily cross the blood-brain barrier, while quaternary ammonium compounds exhibit minimal passage across the blood-brain barrier and into the eye.

Atropine, belladonna, and hyoscyamine are distributed into breast milk.

### Protein binding

Atropine—Moderate.
Hyoscyamine—Moderate.
Scopolamine hydrobromide—Low.

### Biotransformation

Most anticholinergics—Hepatic, by enzymatic hydrolysis.

### Half-life

Elimination—
    Atropine: 2.5 hours.
    Dicyclomine hydrochloride: 1.8 hours (initial phase) and 9 to 10 hours (secondary phase).
    Glycopyrrolate: 1.7 hours (range 0.6–4.6 hours).
    Hyoscyamine: 3.5 hours.

Pirenzepine—10 to 12 hours.
Propantheline bromide—1.6 (mean) hours.
Scopolamine—8 hours.

**Time to peak effect**
Glycopyrrolate—Intramuscular: 30 to 45 minutes.

| Drug | Onset of Action | Duration of Action | Elimination (% excreted unchanged) |
|---|---|---|---|
| Anisotropine methyl-bromide | | | * |
| Atropine | | Oral: 4–6 hr Parenteral: Brief | Renal (30–50) |
| Belladonna | 1–2 hr | 4 hr | Renal (30–50 of atropine and 1 of scopolamine) |
| Clidinium bromide | 1 hr | Up to 3 hr | * |
| Dicyclomine hydrochloride | | | * |
| Glycopyrrolate | IM or SC: 15–30 min IV: 1 min | Antisialagogue: Up to 7 hr Vagal blocking effect: 2–3 hr | Renal |
| Homatropine | | | * |
| Hyoscyamine sulfate | Oral: 20–30 min Parenteral: 2–3 min | 4–6 hr | Renal (majority) |
| Mepenzolate bromide | | | Renal (3–22) |
| Methantheline bromide | | | * |
| Methscopo-lamine bromide | 1 hr | 6–8 hr | * |
| Pirenzepine hydrochloride | | | Renal/hepatic (80–90) |
| Propantheline bromide | | 6 hr | Renal (<6) |
| Scopolamine | | Transdermal: Up to 72 hr | Renal |
| Scopolamine hydrobromide | Antisialagogue— Oral: 30–60 min Parenteral: 30 min | Oral: 4–6 hr Parenteral: 4 hr | Renal (1 of oral dose) (3.4 of SC dose) |

*Assumed to be renal/fecal.

## Precautions to Consider

### Cross-sensitivity and/or related problems
For all anticholinergics—Patients sensitive to one belladonna alkaloid or derivative may be sensitive to the other belladonna alkaloids or derivatives also.

### Pregnancy/Reproduction
Pregnancy—
*For anisotropine methylbromide—*
Problems in humans have not been documented.
*For atropine—*
Atropine crosses the placenta. Well-controlled studies in humans have not been done. Intravenous administration of atropine during pregnancy or near term may produce tachycardia in the fetus.
Studies in mice have not shown that atropine given in doses of 50 mg per kg of body weight (mg/kg) has adverse effects on the fetus.
FDA Pregnancy Category C.
*For belladonna—*
Belladonna crosses the placenta. Studies with belladonna have not been done in either animals or humans.
FDA Pregnancy Category C.
*For clidinium—*
Adequate and well-controlled studies in humans have not been done.

Reproduction studies in rats have not shown that clidinium has adverse effects on the fetus.
*For dicyclomine—*
Dicyclomine has been associated in several isolated cases with human malformations; however, in retrospective studies there has been no evidence of dicyclomine having any untoward effect on the embryo.
*For glycopyrrolate—*
Controlled studies in humans have not been done.
Studies in rats and rabbits have not shown that glycopyrrolate causes teratogenic effects. However, studies in rats have shown that rates of conception and of survival at weaning decreased in a dose-related manner with glycopyrrolate. Studies in dogs with high doses of glycopyrrolate suggest that this may be caused by a decrease in seminal secretion.
FDA Pregnancy Category B.
*For hyoscyamine—*
Hyoscyamine crosses the placenta. Studies with hyoscyamine have not been done in either animals or humans. Intravenous administration of hyoscyamine during pregnancy, especially near term, may produce tachycardia in the fetus.
FDA Pregnancy Category C.
*For mepenzolate—*
Adequate and well-controlled studies in humans have not been done.
Reproduction studies in rats and rabbits have not shown that mepenzolate has adverse effects on the fetus.
*For propantheline—*
Studies have not been done in either animals or humans.
FDA Pregnancy Category C.
*For scopolamine—*
Scopolamine crosses the placenta. Studies with scopolamine have not been done in either animals or humans.
FDA Pregnancy Category C.
Labor—For scopolamine: Parenteral administration of scopolamine before the onset of labor may cause CNS depression in the neonate and may contribute to neonatal hemorrhage due to reduction in vitamin K–dependent clotting factors in the neonate.

### Breast-feeding
For all anticholinergics—Anticholinergics may inhibit lactation.
For atropine, belladonna, and hyoscyamine—These drugs are distributed into breast milk. Although amounts have not been quantified, the chronic use of these medications should be avoided during nursing since infants are usually very sensitive to the effects of anticholinergics.
For dicyclomine—Although a causal relationship has not been established, the use of dicyclomine in nursing mothers is not recommended, since respiratory distress has been reported in infants less than 3 months of age who ingested dicyclomine directly (not through breast milk).
For quaternary ammonium compounds—It is unlikely that these drugs are excreted in breast milk since they are incompletely absorbed from the gastrointestinal tract and have poor lipid solubility.

### Pediatrics
For all anticholinergics—
Infants and young children are especially susceptible to the toxic effects of anticholinergics.
Close supervision is recommended for infants and children with spastic paralysis or brain damage since an increased response to anticholinergics has been reported in these patients and dosage adjustments are often required.
When anticholinergics are given to children where the environmental temperature is high, there is risk of a rapid increase in body temperature because of these medications' suppression of sweat gland activity.
A paradoxical reaction characterized by hyperexcitability may occur in children taking large doses of anticholinergics.
For dicyclomine—
Respiratory symptoms, such as difficulty in breathing, shortness of breath, respiratory collapse and apnea; as well as seizures, syncope, asphyxia, pulse rate fluctuations, muscular hypotonia, and coma have been reported in some infants, 3 months old and under, with the use of dicyclomine syrup. These side effects occurred within minutes of ingestion and lasted 20 to 30 minutes. They are believed to have been caused by local irritation and/or aspiration rather than by a direct pharmacologic action.
For hyoscyamine—
Hyoscyamine sulfate injection contains benzyl alcohol as a preservative and should not be used in newborn and immature infants. The use of benzyl alcohol in neonates has been associated with a fatal

toxic syndrome consisting of metabolic acidosis and CNS, respiratory, circulatory, and renal function impairment.

## Geriatrics
Geriatric patients may respond to usual doses of anticholinergics with excitement, agitation, drowsiness, or confusion.

Geriatric patients are especially susceptible to the anticholinergic side effects, such as constipation, dryness of mouth, and urinary retention (especially in males). If these side effects occur and continue or are severe, medication should probably be discontinued.

Caution is also recommended when anticholinergics are given to geriatric patients, because of the danger of precipitating undiagnosed glaucoma.

Memory may become severely impaired in geriatric patients, especially those who already have memory problems, with the continued use of anticholinergics since these drugs block the actions of acetylcholine, which is responsible for many functions of the brain, including memory functions.

## Dental
Prolonged use of anticholinergics may decrease or inhibit salivary flow, thus contributing to the development of caries, periodontal disease, oral candidiasis, and discomfort.

## Drug interactions and/or related problems
The following drug interactions and/or related problems have been selected on the basis of their potential clinical significance (possible mechanism in parentheses where appropriate)—not necessarily inclusive (» = major clinical significance):

Note: Combinations containing any of the following medications, depending on the amount present, may also interact with this medication.

Only specific interactions between anticholinergics and other oral medications have been identified in this monograph. However, because of decreased gastrointestinal motility and delayed gastric emptying, absorption of other oral medications may be decreased during concurrent use with anticholinergics.

*For all anticholinergics*
> Alkalizers, urinary, such as:
> Antacids, calcium- and/or magnesium-containing
> Carbonic anhydrase inhibitors
> Citrates
> Sodium bicarbonate
> (urinary excretion of anticholinergics may be delayed by alkalinization of the urine, thus potentiating the anticholinergics' therapeutic and/or side effects)

» Antacids or
» Antidiarrheals, adsorbent
(simultaneous use of these medications may reduce absorption of anticholinergics, resulting in decreased therapeutic effectiveness; doses of these medications should be spaced 2 or 3 hours apart from doses of anticholinergics)

» Anticholinergics or other medications with anticholinergic activity, other (See *Appendix II*)
(concurrent use with anticholinergics may intensify anticholinergic effects; patients should be advised to report occurrence of gastrointestinal problems promptly since paralytic ileus may occur with concurrent therapy)

Antimyasthenics
(concurrent use with anticholinergics may further reduce intestinal motility; therefore, caution is recommended; although atropine may be used to reduce or prevent the muscarinic effects of antimyasthenics, routine concurrent use is not recommended since the muscarinic effects may be the first signs of antimyasthenic overdose, and masking such effects with atropine may prevent early recognition of cholinergic crisis)

» Cyclopropane
(concurrent intravenous administration of anticholinergics with cyclopropane anesthesia may result in ventricular arrhythmias; however, if the anticholinergic used is glycopyrrolate, the risk is reduced if glycopyrrolate is given in increments of 100 mcg [0.1 mg] or less)

Haloperidol
(antipsychotic effectiveness of haloperidol may be decreased in schizophrenic patients)

» Ketoconazole
(anticholinergics may increase gastrointestinal pH, possibly resulting in a marked reduction in ketoconazole absorption during concurrent use with anticholinergics; patients should be advised to take these medications at least 2 hours after ketoconazole)

Metoclopramide
(concurrent use with anticholinergics may antagonize metoclopramide's effects on gastrointestinal motility)

Opioid (narcotic) analgesics
(concurrent use with anticholinergics may result in increased risk of severe constipation, which may lead to paralytic ileus, and/or urinary retention)

» Potassium chloride, especially wax-matrix preparations
(concurrent use with anticholinergics may increase severity of potassium chloride–induced gastrointestinal lesions)

*For scopolamine (in addition to interactions listed above)*
» CNS depression–producing medications, other (See *Appendix II*)
(concurrent use may potentiate the effects of either these medications or scopolamine, resulting in additive sedation)

Lorazepam, parenteral
(concurrent use of scopolamine and parenteral lorazepam is reported to have no added beneficial effect and their combined effect may increase the incidence of sedation, hallucination, and irritational behavior)

## Laboratory value alterations
The following have been selected on the basis of their potential clinical significance (possible effect in parentheses where appropriate)—not necessarily inclusive (» = major clinical significance):

With diagnostic test results
*For all anticholinergics*
» Gastric acid secretion test
(concurrent use of anticholinergics may antagonize the effect of pentagastrin and histamine in the evaluation of gastric acid secretory function; administration of anticholinergics is not recommended during the 24 hours preceding the test)

Radionuclide gastric emptying studies
(use of anticholinergics may result in delayed gastric emptying)

*For atropine (in addition to those listed for all anticholinergics)*
» Phenolsulfonphthalein (PSP) excretion test
(atropine utilizes the same tubular mechanism of excretion as PSP resulting in decreased urinary excretion of PSP; concurrent use of atropine is not recommended in patients receiving PSP excretion test)

*For scopolamine (in addition to those listed for all anticholinergics)*
Neuroradiological tests
(residual cycloplegia and mydriasis following use of transdermal disk of scopolamine may affect results of neuroradiological tests for intracranial neoplasm, subdural hematoma, or aneurysm)

With physiology/laboratory test values
*For glycopyrrolate*
Serum uric acid
(may be decreased in patients with hyperuricemia or gout)

## Medical considerations/Contraindications
The medical considerations/contraindications included here have been selected on the basis of their potential clinical significance (reasons given in parentheses where appropriate)—not necessarily inclusive (» = major clinical significance).

*Risk-benefit should be considered when the following medical problems exist:*
Brain damage, in children
(CNS effects may be exacerbated)

» Cardiac disease, especially cardiac arrhythmias, congestive heart failure, coronary artery disease, and mitral stenosis
(increase in heart rate may be undesirable)

Down's syndrome
(abnormal increase in pupillary dilation and acceleration of heart rate may occur)

» Esophagitis, reflux
(decrease in esophageal and gastric motility and relaxation of lower esophageal sphincter may promote gastric retention by delaying gastric emptying and may increase gastroesophageal reflux through an incompetent sphincter)

Fever
(may be increased through suppression of sweat gland activity)

» Gastrointestinal tract obstructive disease as in achalasia and pyloroduodenal stenosis
(decrease in motility and tone may occur, resulting in obstruction and gastric retention)

» Glaucoma, angle-closure, or predisposition to
(mydriatic effect resulting in increased intraocular pressure may precipitate an acute attack of angle-closure glaucoma)

» Glaucoma, open-angle
(mydriatic effect may cause a slight increase in intraocular pressure; glaucoma therapy may need to be adjusted)

» Hemorrhage, acute, with unstable cardiovascular status
(increase in heart rate may be undesirable)

Hepatic function impairment
(decreased metabolism of anticholinergic)

» Hernia, hiatal, associated with reflux esophagitis
(anticholinergics may aggravate condition)

Hypertension
(may be aggravated)

Hyperthyroidism
(characterized by tachycardia, which may be increased)

» Intestinal atony in the elderly or debilitated patient or
» Paralytic ileus
(anticholinergic use may result in obstruction)

Lung disease, chronic, especially in infants, small children, and debilitated patients
(reduction in bronchial secretion can lead to inspissation and formation of bronchial plugs)

» Myasthenia gravis
(condition may be aggravated because of inhibition of acetylcholine action)

Neuropathy, autonomic
(urinary retention and cycloplegia may be aggravated)

» Prostatic hypertrophy, nonobstructive or
» Urinary retention, or predisposition to or
» Uropathy, obstructive, such as bladder neck obstruction due to prostatic hypertrophy
(urinary retention may be precipitated or aggravated)

» Pyloric obstruction
(may be aggravated)

Renal function impairment
(decreased excretion may increase the risk of side effects)

Sensitivity to any belladonna alkaloids or derivatives

Spastic paralysis, in children
(response to anticholinergics may be increased)

» Tachycardia
(may be increased)

Toxemia of pregnancy
(hypertension may be aggravated)

» Ulcerative colitis
(large anticholinergic doses may suppress intestinal motility, possibly causing paralytic ileus; also, use may precipitate or aggravate the serious complication, toxic megacolon)

Xerostomia
(prolonged use may further reduce limited salivary flow)

Caution in use is also recommended in patients over 40 years of age because of the danger of precipitating undiagnosed glaucoma.

**Patient monitoring**
The following may be especially important in patient monitoring (other tests may be warranted in some patients, depending on condition; » = major clinical significance):

Intraocular pressure determinations
(recommended at periodic intervals, as these medications may increase the intraocular pressure by producing mydriasis)

## Side/Adverse Effects

Note: When anticholinergics are given to patients, especially children, where the environmental temperature is high, there is risk of a rapid increase in body temperature because of suppression of sweat gland activity.

Infants, patients with Down's syndrome, and children with spastic paralysis or brain damage may show an increased response to anticholinergics, thus increasing the potential for side effects.

Geriatric or debilitated patients may respond to usual doses of anticholinergics with excitement, agitation, drowsiness, or confusion.

Following use of the transdermal disk of scopolamine, a dilated and fixed pupil has been reported on the side where the disk was worn. This condition usually resolves spontaneously within a few days, but may persist for up to 2 weeks after the disk has been removed and thus may be mistaken for a sign of intracranial neoplasm, subdural hematoma, or aneurysm. To avoid extensive neuroradiological tests, instillation of 1% pilocarpine solution is recommended as an aid in the diagnosis of non-neurogenic dilation of the pupil.

See also *Table 1,* page 230.

## Overdose

For specific information on the agents used in the management of overdose with anticholinergics/antispasmodics, see:

- *Benzodiazepines (Systemic)* monograph;
- *Charcoal, Activated (Oral-Local)* monograph;
- *Chloral Hydrate (Systemic)* monograph;
- *Neostigmine Methylsulfate* in *Antimyasthenics (Systemic)* monograph;
- *Norepinephrine Bitartrate* or *Metaraminol Bitartrate* in *Sympathomimetic Agents—Cardiovascular Use (Parenteral-Systemic)* monograph;
- *Physostigmine Salicylate (Systemic)* monograph; and/or
- *Thiopental* in *Anesthetics, Barbiturate (Systemic)* monograph.

For more information on the management of overdose or unintentional ingestion, **contact a Poison Control Center** (see *Poison Control Center Listing*).

**Clinical effects of overdose**
The following effects have been selected on the basis of their potential clinical significance (possible signs and symptoms in parentheses where appropriate)—not necessarily inclusive:

*Blurred vision, continuing, or changes in near vision; clumsiness or unsteadiness; confusion; difficulty in breathing*—may lead to respiratory paralysis with quaternary ammonium compounds because of curare-like effects; *dizziness; drowsiness, severe; dryness of mouth, nose, or throat, severe; fast heartbeat; fever; hallucinations; muscle weakness, severe*—may lead to respiratory paralysis with quaternary ammonium compounds because of curare-like effects; *seizures; slurred speech; tiredness, severe*—may lead to respiratory paralysis with quaternary ammonium compounds because of curare-like effects; *unusual excitement, nervousness, restlessness, or irritability; unusual warmth, dryness, and flushing of skin*

**Treatment of overdose**
Recommended treatment for anticholinergic overdose includes the following:

To decrease absorption—
Emesis or gastric lavage with 4% tannic acid solution.
Administration of an aqueous slurry of activated charcoal.

Specific treatment—
To reverse severe anticholinergic symptoms, slow, intravenous administration of physostigmine in doses of 0.5 to 2 mg (0.5 to 1 mg in children, up to a total dose of 2 mg), at a rate not to exceed 1 mg per minute; may be given in repeated doses of 1 to 4 mg as needed, up to a total dose of 5 mg in adults.
Or, neostigmine methylsulfate administered intramuscularly in doses of 0.5 to 1 mg, repeated every 2 to 3 hours; or intravenously in doses of 0.5 to 2 mg, repeated as needed.
To control excitement or delirium, administration of small doses of a short-acting barbiturate (100 mg thiopental sodium) or benzodiazepines, or rectal infusion of 2% solution of chloral hydrate.
To restore blood pressure, infusion of norepinephrine bitartrate or metaraminol.

Supportive care—
Artificial respiration with oxygen if needed for respiratory depression.
Adequate hydration.
Symptomatic treatment as necessary.
Patients in whom intentional overdose is confirmed or suspected should be referred for psychiatric consultation.

## Patient Consultation

As an aid to patient consultation, refer to *Advice for the Patient, Anticholinergics/Antispasmodics (Systemic)*.

In providing consultation, consider emphasizing the following selected information (» = major clinical significance):

**Before using this medication**
» Conditions affecting use, especially:
Sensitivity to any of the belladonna alkaloids or derivatives
Breast-feeding—Excreted in breast milk (except for quaternary ammonium compounds); possible inhibition of lactation
Use in children—Increased susceptibility to toxic effects of anticholinergics; increased response in infants and children with spastic paralysis or brain damage; risk of increased body temperature in hot weather; hyperexcitability (paradoxical reaction) with large doses; increased risk of respiratory depression and collapse (with dicyclomine)
Use in the elderly—Increased susceptibility to mental and other toxic effects of anticholinergics; danger of precipitating undiagnosed glaucoma; possible impairment of memory

Dental—Possible development of dental problems because of decreased salivary flow

Other medications, especially other anticholinergics, antacids, antidiarrheals, cyclopropane, ketoconazole, CNS depressants (with scopolamine), and potassium chloride

Other medical problems, especially cardiac disease, glaucoma, hemorrhage, hiatal hernia, intestinal atony or paralytic ileus, myasthenia gravis, obstruction in gastrointestinal or urinary tract, prostatic hypertrophy, reflux esophagitis, tachycardia, and ulcerative colitis

## Proper use of this medication

» Importance of not taking more medication than the amount prescribed
  Missed dose: Taking as soon as possible; not taking if almost time for next dose; not doubling doses
» Proper dosing
» Proper storage
*For oral dosage forms*
  Taking medication 30 minutes to 1 hour before meals
*For rectal dosage forms*
  Proper administration technique
*For transdermal scopolamine*
  Reading patient directions
  Washing and drying hands thoroughly before and after application
  Applying to hairless, intact area of skin behind ear; not applying over cuts or irritations

## Precautions while using this medication

» Suspected overdose: Getting emergency help at once
» Caution during exercise or hot weather; overheating may result in heat stroke
» Possible increased sensitivity of eyes to light
  Caution about abrupt withdrawal
» Caution if blurred vision occurs
» Possible dizziness or drowsiness; caution when driving or doing things requiring alertness
  Possible dizziness or lightheadedness; caution when getting up suddenly from a lying or sitting position
  Possible dryness of mouth; using sugarless candy or gum, ice or saliva substitute for relief; checking with physician or dentist if dry mouth continues for more than 2 weeks
*For scopolamine*
» Avoiding use of alcohol or other CNS depressants
*For oral dosage forms*
  Avoiding use of antacids and antidiarrheal medications within 2 or 3 hours of taking this medication

## Side/adverse effects

Signs of potential side effects, especially allergic reaction, confusion, increased intraocular pressure, orthostatic hypotension (especially with high doses of quaternary ammonium compounds)

## General Dosing Information

Tolerance to some of the adverse reactions may develop following continued use and/or smaller doses of anticholinergics, but effectiveness may also be reduced.

Dosage adjustments are often required for infants, patients with Down's syndrome, children with brain damage or spasticity, since an increased responsiveness to anticholinergics has been reported in these patients.

Geriatric and debilitated patients may respond to usual doses with excitement, agitation, drowsiness, or confusion; lower doses may be required in these patients.

Anticholinergics should not be withdrawn abruptly since withdrawal-like symptoms may occur. Vomiting, malaise, sweating, transient dizziness, and salivation have been reported after sudden withdrawal of large doses of scopolamine.

If scopolamine is used as antisialagogue preanesthetic medication in minor surgical procedures that do not require more than a few hours' stay in the hospital, the patient should be alerted at time of discharge about scopolamine's lingering detrimental effects on memory and motor tasks.

High dosage of quaternary ammonium compounds should not be given continuously for prolonged periods, since ganglionic and skeletal neuromuscular transmission may be blocked. Stimulation of the CNS and a curare-like action may result.

## For oral dosage forms only

Administration of anticholinergics 30 minutes to 1 hour before meals is recommended to maximize absorption.

## For parenteral dosage forms only

Atropine, hyoscyamine, and scopolamine may be administered by intramuscular, subcutaneous, or intravenous injection.

Glycopyrrolate may be administered by intramuscular or intravenous injection.

After parenteral administration a temporary feeling of lightheadedness and local irritation may occur.

## For transdermal dosage forms only

Transdermal application delivers reduced doses of scopolamine, which are large enough to be effective but small enough to eliminate most of the adverse effects, except drowsiness and cycloplegia.

---

### ANISOTROPINE

---

## Oral Dosage Forms

### ANISOTROPINE METHYLBROMIDE TABLETS

**Usual adult and adolescent dose**
Anticholinergic—
  Oral, 50 mg three times a day, the dosage being adjusted as needed and tolerated.

Note: Geriatric patients may be more sensitive to the effects of the usual adult dose.

**Usual pediatric dose**
Dosage has not been established.

**Strength(s) usually available**
U.S.—
  50 mg (Rx) [GENERIC].
Canada—
  Not commercially available.

**Packaging and storage**
Store between 15 and 30 °C (59 and 86 °F), unless otherwise specified by manufacturer.

**Auxiliary labeling**
• May cause blurred vision.

---

### ATROPINE

---

## Summary of Differences

Category:
  Also an antidote (to cholinesterase inhibitors; to organophosphate pesticides; to muscarine) and a urinary antispasmodic. Parenteral atropine is used as an antiarrhythmic and cholinergic adjunct (curariform block).
Indications:
  Also indicated for biliary tract disorders and duodenography. In preanesthesia and dental anesthesia, indicated as antisialagogue.
Pharmacology/pharmacokinetics:
  Protein binding—Moderate.
  Half-life (elimination)—2.5 hours.
  Duration of action—Oral, 4 to 6 hours; parenteral, brief.
  Elimination—Renal; 30 to 50% excreted unchanged.
Precautions:
  Pregnancy—Intravenous administration may produce tachycardia in fetus.
  Laboratory value alterations—May decrease excretion of phenolsulfonphthalein (PSP) during PSP excretion test.

## Additional Dosing Information

See also *General Dosing Information.*

Doses of 0.5 to 1 mg of atropine are mildly stimulating to the CNS. Larger doses may produce mental disturbances; very large doses have depressant effect.

The fatal dose of atropine in children may be as low as 10 mg.

## Oral Dosage Forms

### ATROPINE SULFATE TABLETS USP

**Usual adult and adolescent dose**
Anticholinergic—
  Oral, 300 mcg (0.3 mg) to 1.2 mg every four to six hours.
Prophylaxis of excessive salivation and respiratory tract secretions, in anesthesia—
  Oral, 2 mg.

Note: Geriatric patients may be more sensitive to the effects of the usual adult dose.

**Usual pediatric dose**
Anticholinergic—
  Oral, 10 mcg (0.01 mg) per kg of body weight, not to exceed 400 mcg (0.4 mg), or 300 mcg (0.3 mg) per square meter of body surface, every four to six hours.

**Strength(s) usually available**
U.S.—
  400 mcg (0.4 mg) (Rx) [GENERIC].
Canada—
  Not commercially available.

**Packaging and storage**
Store below 40 °C (104 °F), preferably between 15 and 30 °C (59 and 86 °F), in a well-closed container, unless otherwise specified by manufacturer.

**Auxiliary labeling**
• May cause blurred vision.

## ATROPINE SULFATE SOLUBLE TABLETS

**Usual adult and adolescent dose**
Anticholinergic—
  Oral, 300 mcg (0.3 mg) to 1.2 mg every four to six hours.
Prophylaxis of excessive salivation and respiratory tract secretions, in anesthesia—
  Oral, 2 mg.
Note: Geriatric patients may be more sensitive to the effects of the usual adult dose.

**Usual pediatric dose**
Anticholinergic—
  Oral, 10 mcg (0.01 mg) per kg of body weight, not to exceed 400 mcg (0.4 mg), or 300 mcg (0.3 mg) per square meter of body surface, every four to six hours.

**Strength(s) usually available**
U.S.—
  400 mcg (0.4 mg) (Rx) [GENERIC].
  600 mcg (0.6 mg) (Rx) [GENERIC].
Canada—
  Not commercially available.

**Packaging and storage**
Store below 40 °C (104 °F), preferably between 15 and 30 °C (59 and 86 °F), in a well-closed container, unless otherwise specified by manufacturer.

**Auxiliary labeling**
• May cause blurred vision.

# Parenteral Dosage Forms

## ATROPINE SULFATE INJECTION USP

**Usual adult and adolescent dose**
Anticholinergic—
  Intramuscular, intravenous, or subcutaneous, 400 to 600 mcg (0.4 to 0.6 mg) every four to six hours.
  Gastrointestinal radiography—
    Intramuscular, 1 mg.
Prophylaxis of excessive salivation and respiratory tract secretions, in anesthesia—
  Intramuscular, 200 to 600 mcg (0.2 to 0.6 mg) one-half to one hour before surgery.
Antiarrhythmic—
  Intravenous, 400 mcg (0.4 mg) to 1 mg every one to two hours as needed, up to a maximum of 2 mg.
Cholinergic adjunct (curariform block)—
  Intravenous, 600 mcg (0.6 mg) to 1.2 mg administered a few minutes before or concurrently with 500 mcg (0.5 mg) to 2 mg of neostigmine methylsulfate, using separate syringes.
Antidote (to cholinesterase inhibitors)—
  Intravenous, 2 to 4 mg initially, then 2 mg repeated every five to ten minutes until muscarinic symptoms disappear or signs of atropine toxicity appear.
Antidote (to muscarine in mushroom poisoning)—
  Intramuscular or intravenous, 1 to 2 mg every hour until respiratory effects subside.
Antidote (to organophosphate pesticides)—
  Intramuscular or intravenous, 1 to 2 mg, repeated in twenty to thirty minutes as soon as cyanosis has cleared. Continue dosage until definite improvement occurs and is maintained, sometimes for two days or more.

Note: Geriatric patients may be more sensitive to the effects of the usual adult dose.

**Usual pediatric dose**
Anticholinergic—
  Subcutaneous, 10 mcg (0.01 mg) per kg of body weight, not to exceed 400 mcg (0.4 mg), or 300 mcg (0.3 mg) per square meter of body surface, every four to six hours.
  Prophylaxis of excessive salivation and respiratory tract secretions, in anesthesia or
  Prophylaxis of succinylcholine- or surgical procedure–induced arrhythmias—
    Subcutaneous:
      Children weighing up to 3 kg: 100 mcg (0.1 mg).
      Children weighing 7 to 9 kg: 200 mcg (0.2 mg).
      Children weighing 12 to 16 kg: 300 mcg (0.3 mg).
      Children weighing 20 to 27 kg: 400 mcg (0.4 mg).
      Children weighing 32 kg: 500 mcg (0.5 mg).
      Children weighing 41 kg: 600 mcg (0.6 mg).
Antiarrhythmic—
  Intravenous, 10 to 30 mcg (0.01 to 0.03 mg) per kg of body weight.
Antidote (to cholinesterase inhibitors)—
  Intravenous or intramuscular, 1 mg initially, then 0.5 to 1 mg every five to ten minutes until muscarinic symptoms disappear or signs of atropine toxicity appear.

**Strength(s) usually available**
U.S.—
  50 mcg (0.05 mg) per mL (Rx) [GENERIC].
  100 mcg (0.1 mg) per mL (Rx) [GENERIC].
  300 mcg (0.3 mg) per mL (Rx) [GENERIC].
  400 mcg (0.4 mg) per mL (Rx) [GENERIC].
  500 mcg (0.5 mg) per mL (Rx) [GENERIC].
  1 mg per mL (Rx) [GENERIC].
Canada—
  400 mcg (0.4 mg) per mL (Rx) [GENERIC].
  600 mcg (0.6 mg) per mL (Rx) [GENERIC].

**Packaging and storage**
Store below 40 °C (104 °F), preferably between 15 and 30 °C (59 and 86 °F), unless otherwise specified by manufacturer. Protect from freezing.

**Additional information**
The intravenous injection of atropine should be administered *slowly*.

---

## BELLADONNA

# Summary of Differences

Category:
  Also an antidysmenorrheal and antivertigo agent.
Indications:
  Also indicated in nocturnal enuresis. In dental procedures, may be used as antisialagogue.
Pharmacology/pharmacokinetics:
  Onset of action—1 to 2 hours.
  Duration of action—4 hours.
  Elimination—Renal; 30 to 50% of atropine and 1% of scopolamine excreted unchanged.

# Oral Dosage Forms

## BELLADONNA TINCTURE USP

**Usual adult and adolescent dose**
Anticholinergic—
  Oral, 180 to 300 mcg (0.18 to 0.3 mg) three or four times a day, thirty minutes to one hour before meals and at bedtime, the dosage being adjusted as needed and tolerated.

Note: Geriatric patients may be more sensitive to the effects of the usual adult dose.

**Usual pediatric dose**
Anticholinergic—
  Oral, 9 mcg (0.009 mg) per kg of body weight or 240 mcg (0.24 mg) per square meter of body surface a day, in three or four divided doses.

**Strength(s) usually available**
U.S.—
  300 mcg (0.3 mg) per mL (Rx) [GENERIC].
  Note: Belladonna tincture contains 300 mcg (0.3 mg) of belladonna alkaloids (principally hyoscyamine and atropine) per mL.
Canada—
  Not commercially available.

**Packaging and storage**
Store below 40 °C (104 °F), preferably between 15 and 30 °C (59 and 86 °F), unless otherwise specified by manufacturer. Store in a tight, light-resistant container. Protect from freezing.

**Auxiliary labeling**
• May cause blurred vision.
• Keep container tightly closed.

---

## CLIDINIUM

## Summary of Differences
Pharmacology/pharmacokinetics:
   Onset of action—1 hour.
   Duration of action—Up to 3 hours.

## Oral Dosage Forms
### CLIDINIUM BROMIDE CAPSULES USP

**Usual adult and adolescent dose**
Anticholinergic—
   Oral, 2.5 to 5 mg three or four times a day, before meals and at bedtime, the dosage being adjusted as needed and tolerated.
Note: Geriatric or debilitated patients—Oral, 2.5 mg three times a day before meals.

**Usual pediatric dose**
Dosage has not been established.

**Strength(s) usually available**
U.S.—
   2.5 mg (Rx) [*Quarzan*].
   5 mg (Rx) [*Quarzan*].
Canada—
   Not commercially available.

**Packaging and storage**
Store below 40 °C (104 °F), preferably between 15 and 30 °C (59 and 86 °F), unless otherwise specified by manufacturer. Store in a tight, light-resistant container.

**Auxiliary labeling**
• May cause blurred vision.

---

## DICYCLOMINE

## Summary of Differences
Category:
   Also gastrointestinal antispasmodic.
Indications:
   Not indicated for peptic ulcer.
Pharmacology/pharmacokinetics:
   Half-life (elimination)—1.8 hours (initial phase) and 9 to 10 hours (secondary phase).
Precautions:
   Pediatrics—Respiratory symptoms, seizures, syncope, asphyxia, pulse rate fluctuations, muscular hypotonia, and coma reported with the use of the syrup in some infants 3 months old and under.

## Oral Dosage Forms
### DICYCLOMINE HYDROCHLORIDE CAPSULES USP

**Usual adult and adolescent dose**
Antispasmodic, gastrointestinal: Irritable bowel syndrome—
   Oral, 10 to 20 mg three or four times a day, the dosage being adjusted as needed and tolerated.
Note: Geriatric patients may be more sensitive to the effects of the usual adult dose.

**Usual adult prescribing limits**
Up to 160 mg daily.

**Usual pediatric dose**
Antispasmodic, gastrointestinal—
   Children up to 6 years of age: Product not suitable for pediatric administration. See *Dicyclomine Hydrochloride Syrup USP.*
   Children 6 years of age and over: Oral, 10 mg three or four times a day, the dosage being adjusted as needed and tolerated.

**Strength(s) usually available**
U.S.—
   10 mg (Rx) [*Bentyl; Di-Spaz;* GENERIC].
   20 mg (Rx) [GENERIC].

Canada—
   10 mg (Rx) [*Bentylol; Formulex; Lomine*].
   20 mg (Rx) [*Lomine*].

**Packaging and storage**
Store below 40 °C (104 °F), preferably between 15 and 30 °C (59 and 86 °F), unless otherwise specified by manufacturer. Store in a well-closed container.

**Auxiliary labeling**
• May cause blurred vision.

### DICYCLOMINE HYDROCHLORIDE SYRUP USP

**Usual adult and adolescent dose**
Antispasmodic, gastrointestinal: Irritable bowel syndrome—
   Oral, 10 to 20 mg three or four times a day, the dosage being adjusted as needed and tolerated.
Note: Geriatric patients may be more sensitive to the effects of the usual adult dose.

**Usual adult prescribing limits**
Up to 160 mg daily.

**Usual pediatric dose**
Antispasmodic, gastrointestinal—
   Children up to 6 months of age: Use is not recommended.
   Children 6 months to 2 years of age: Oral, 5 to 10 mg three or four times a day, the dosage being adjusted as needed and tolerated.
   Children 2 years of age and over: Oral, 10 mg three or four times a day, the dosage being adjusted as needed and tolerated.

**Strength(s) usually available**
U.S.—
   10 mg per 5 mL (Rx) [*Bentyl;* GENERIC].
Canada—
   10 mg per 5 mL (Rx) [*Bentylol* (alcohol 19%)].

**Packaging and storage**
Store below 40 °C (104 °F), preferably between 15 and 30 °C (59 and 86 °F), unless otherwise specified by manufacturer. Store in a tight container. Protect from freezing.

**Auxiliary labeling**
• May cause blurred vision.

### DICYCLOMINE HYDROCHLORIDE TABLETS USP

**Usual adult and adolescent dose**
Antispasmodic, gastrointestinal: Irritable bowel syndrome—
   Oral, 10 to 20 mg three or four times a day, the dosage being adjusted as needed and tolerated.
Note: Geriatric patients may be more sensitive to the effects of the usual adult dose.

**Usual adult prescribing limits**
Up to 160 mg daily.

**Usual pediatric dose**
Antispasmodic, gastrointestinal—
   Children up to 6 years of age: Product not suitable for pediatric administration. See *Dicyclomine Hydrochloride Syrup USP.*
   Children 6 years of age and over: Oral, 10 mg three or four times a day, the dosage being adjusted as needed and tolerated.

**Strength(s) usually available**
U.S.—
   20 mg (Rx) [*Bentyl;* GENERIC].
Canada—
   10 mg (Rx) [*Bentylol*].
   20 mg (Rx) [*Bentylol; Spasmoban*].

**Packaging and storage**
Store below 40 °C (104 °F), preferably between 15 and 30 °C (59 and 86 °F), unless otherwise specified by manufacturer. Store in a well-closed container.

**Auxiliary labeling**
• May cause blurred vision.

### DICYCLOMINE HYDROCHLORIDE EXTENDED-RELEASE TABLETS

**Usual adult and adolescent dose**
Antispasmodic, gastrointestinal—
   Oral, 30 mg two times a day.
Note: Geriatric patients may be more sensitive to the effects of the usual adult dose.

**Usual pediatric dose**

Antispasmodic, gastrointestinal—
    Product not suitable for pediatric administration. See *Dicyclomine Hydrochloride Syrup USP.*

**Strength(s) usually available**

U.S.—
    Not commercially available.

Canada—
    30 mg (Rx) [*Bentylol*].

**Packaging and storage**

Store below 40 °C (104 °F), preferably between 15 and 30 °C (59 and 86 °F), unless otherwise specified by manufacturer. Store in a tight container.

**Auxiliary labeling**

• May cause blurred vision.

## Parenteral Dosage Forms

### DICYCLOMINE HYDROCHLORIDE INJECTION USP

**Usual adult and adolescent dose**

Antispasmodic, gastrointestinal: Irritable bowel syndrome—
    Intramuscular, 20 mg every four to six hours, the dosage being adjusted as needed and tolerated.

Note:  Not for intravenous use.
    Geriatric patients may be more sensitive to the effects of the usual adult dose.

**Usual pediatric dose**

Dosage has not been established.

**Strength(s) usually available**

U.S.—
    10 mg per mL (Rx) [*Antispas; A-Spas; Bentyl; Dibent; Di-Spaz; Neoquess; Or-Tyl; Spasmoject;* GENERIC].

Canada—
    10 mg per mL (Rx) [*Bentylol*].

**Packaging and storage**

Store below 40 °C (104 °F), preferably between 15 and 30 °C (59 and 86 °F), unless otherwise specified by manufacturer. Protect from freezing.

---

### GLYCOPYRROLATE

## Summary of Differences

Category:
    Also, an [antidiarrheal]. Parenteral glycopyrrolate is used as an antiarrhythmic and cholinergic adjunct (curariform block).
Indications:
    Indicated as antisialagogue in preanesthesia. Also, indicated as antiarrhythmic in preanesthesia, anesthesia, and surgery. In addition, indicated to prevent aspiration pneumonitis during anesthesia. May be used as antidiarrheal and for cholinesterase inhibitor toxicity.
Pharmacology/pharmacokinetics:
    Half-life (elimination)—1.7 hours (range 0.6–4.6 hours).
    Onset of action—15 to 30 minutes with intramuscular or subcutaneous administration; 1 minute with intravenous administration.
    Duration of action—Antisialagogue effect up to 7 hours; vagal blocking effect 2 to 3 hours.
Precautions:
    Pregnancy—Rates of conception and survival at weaning decreased in studies with rats.
    Laboratory value alterations—Serum uric acid may be decreased in patients with hyperuricemia or gout.

## Oral Dosage Forms

### GLYCOPYRROLATE TABLETS USP

**Usual adult and adolescent dose**

Anticholinergic: Peptic ulcer—
    Oral, initially 1 to 2 mg two or three times a day and occasionally 2 mg at bedtime, then 1 mg two times a day, the dosage being adjusted as needed and tolerated.

Note:  Geriatric patients may be more sensitive to the effects of the usual adult dose.

**Usual adult prescribing limits**

Up to 8 mg daily.

**Usual pediatric dose**

Dosage has not been established.

**Strength(s) usually available**

U.S.—
    1 mg (Rx) [*Robinul;* GENERIC].
    2 mg (Rx) [*Robinul Forte;* GENERIC].

Canada—
    1 mg (Rx) [*Robinul*].
    2 mg (Rx) [*Robinul Forte*].

**Packaging and storage**

Store below 40 °C (104 °F), preferably between 15 and 30 °C (59 and 86 °F), unless otherwise specified by manufacturer. Store in a tight container.

**Auxiliary labeling**

• May cause blurred vision.

## Parenteral Dosage Forms

### GLYCOPYRROLATE INJECTION USP

**Usual adult and adolescent dose**

Anticholinergic—
    Peptic ulcer:
        Intramuscular or intravenous, 100 to 200 mcg (0.1 to 0.2 mg), the dosage being repeated, if necessary, at four-hour intervals up to a maximum of four times a day.
    Prophylaxis of excessive salivation and respiratory tract secretions, in anesthesia and:
    Prophylaxis of gastric hypersecretory conditions, in anesthesia:
        Intramuscular, 4.4 mcg (0.0044 mg) per kg of body weight one-half to one hour before induction of anesthesia or at the time the preanesthetic narcotic and/or sedative are administered.
Antiarrhythmic, in anesthesia or
Antiarrhythmic, in surgery—
    Intravenous, 100 mcg (0.1 mg), the dosage being repeated if necessary at two- to three-minute intervals.
Cholinergic adjunct (curariform block)—
    Intravenous, 200 mcg (0.2 mg) for each 1 mg of neostigmine or 5 mg of pyridostigmine given simultaneously; may be mixed in the same syringe.

Note:  Geriatric patients may be more sensitive to the effects of the usual adult dose.

**Usual pediatric dose**

Anticholinergic—
    Peptic ulcer:
        Dosage has not been established.
    Prophylaxis of excessive salivation and respiratory tract secretions, in anesthesia; and
    Prophylaxis of gastric hypersecretory conditions, in anesthesia:
        Intramuscular, 4.4 to 8.8 mcg (0.0044 to 0.0088 mg) per kg of body weight one-half to one hour before induction of anesthesia or at the time the preanesthetic narcotic and/or sedative are administered.
Antiarrhythmics, in anesthesia or
Antiarrhythmic, in surgery—
    Intravenous, 4.4 mcg (0.0044 mg) per kg of body weight up to a maximum of 100 mcg (0.1 mg), the dosage being repeated, if necessary, at two- to three-minute intervals.
Cholinergic adjunct (curariform block)—
    Intravenous, 200 mcg (0.2 mg) for each 1 mg of neostigmine or 5 mg of pyridostigmine given simultaneously; may be mixed in the same syringe.

**Strength(s) usually available**

U.S.—
    200 mcg (0.2 mg) per mL (Rx) [*Robinul*].

Canada—
    200 mcg (0.2 mg) per mL (Rx) [*Robinul*].

**Packaging and storage**

Store below 40 °C (104 °F), preferably between 15 and 30 °C (59 and 86 °F), unless otherwise specified by manufacturer.

**Preparation of dosage form**

Glycopyrrolate may be mixed and administered with glucose 5 or 10% in water or saline, meperidine injection, morphine sulfate, fentanyl plus droperidol injection, hydroxyzine injection, neostigmine injection, or pyridostigmine injection.

**Stability**

Stability of glycopyrrolate may be affected at a pH higher than 6. A pH above 6 will result when glycopyrrolate is mixed with dexamethasone sodium phosphate or a buffered solution of lactated Ringer's solution.

**Incompatibilities**

Chloramphenicol, diazepam, dimenhydrinate, methohexital sodium, pentobarbital sodium, secobarbital sodium, thiopental sodium, and sodium bicarbonate are *not* suitable for mixing in the same syringe with glycopyrrolate since a gas or a precipitate may result.

---

## *HOMATROPINE*

## Oral Dosage Forms

### HOMATROPINE METHYLBROMIDE TABLETS USP

**Usual adult and adolescent dose**

Anticholinergic—

Oral, 5 to 10 mg three or four times a day, the dosage being adjusted as needed and tolerated.

Note: Geriatric patients may be more sensitive to the effects of the usual adult dose.

**Usual pediatric dose**

Dosage has not been established.

**Strength(s) usually available**

U.S.—

5 mg (Rx) [*Homapin*].

10 mg (Rx) [*Homapin*].

Canada—

Not commercially available.

**Packaging and storage**

Store below 40 °C (104 °F), preferably between 15 and 30 °C (59 and 86 °F), unless otherwise specified by manufacturer. Store in a tight, light-resistant container.

**Auxiliary labeling**

• May cause blurred vision.

---

## *HYOSCYAMINE*

## Summary of Differences

Category:

Parenteral hyoscyamine is also an antiarrhythmic, antidote (to cholinesterase inhibitors and to muscarine), and a cholinergic adjunct (curariform block).

Indications:

Also indicated for biliary disorders, cystitis, duodenography, and acute rhinitis. In preanesthesia, indicated as antisialagogue and also as antiarrhythmic during anesthesia and surgery.

Pharmacology/pharmacokinetics:

Protein binding—Moderate.

Half-life (elimination)—3.5 hours.

Onset of action—20 to 30 minutes with oral administration of hyoscyamine sulfate; 2 to 3 minutes with parenteral administration.

Duration of action—4 to 6 hours.

Elimination—Renal; majority of drug excreted unchanged.

Precautions:

Pregnancy—Intravenous administration may produce tachycardia in fetus.

Side/adverse effects:

Constipation has been reported less often with hyoscyamine.

## Additional Dosing Information

See also *General Dosing Information*.

Hyoscyamine is effective at half the dosage of atropine.

In dehydrated patients, such as those with diarrhea and vomiting, treatment with hyoscyamine should be initiated at a lower dosage.

## Oral Dosage Forms

### HYOSCYAMINE TABLETS USP

**Usual adult and adolescent dose**

Anticholinergic—

Oral, 125 to 500 mcg (0.125 to 0.5 mg) three or four times a day, thirty minutes to one hour before meals and at bedtime, the dosage being adjusted as needed and tolerated.

Note: Geriatric patients may be more sensitive to the effects of the usual adult dose.

**Usual pediatric dose**

Dosage must be individualized by physician.

---

**Strength(s) usually available**

U.S.—

150 mcg (0.15 mg) (Rx) [*Cystospaz*].

Canada—

Not commercially available.

**Packaging and storage**

Store below 40 °C (104 °F), preferably between 15 and 30 °C (59 and 86 °F), unless otherwise specified by manufacturer. Store in a well-closed, light-resistant container.

**Auxiliary labeling**

• May cause blurred vision.

### HYOSCYAMINE SULFATE EXTENDED-RELEASE CAPSULES

**Usual adult and adolescent dose**

Anticholinergic—

Oral, 375 mcg (0.375 mg) two times a day, in the morning and at bedtime, the dosage being increased, if necessary, to obtain the desired response.

Note: Geriatric patients may be more sensitive to the effects of the usual adult dose.

**Usual pediatric dose**

Anticholinergic—

Children up to 2 years of age: Use is not recommended.

Children 2 years of age and over: Oral, 375 mcg (0.375 mg) two times a day, in the morning and at bedtime, the dosage being increased, if necessary, to obtain the desired response.

**Strength(s) usually available**

U.S.—

375 mcg (0.375 mg) (Rx) [*Cystospaz-M; Levsinex Timecaps*].

Canada—

Not commercially available.

**Packaging and storage**

Store below 40 °C (104 °F), preferably between 15 and 30 °C (59 and 86 °F), in a tight, light-resistant container, unless otherwise specified by manufacturer.

**Auxiliary labeling**

• Swallow capsules whole.

• May cause blurred vision.

### HYOSCYAMINE SULFATE ELIXIR USP

**Usual adult and adolescent dose**

Anticholinergic—

Oral, 125 to 250 mcg (0.125 to 0.25 mg) every four to six hours, the dosage being adjusted as needed and tolerated.

Note: Geriatric patients may be more sensitive to the effects of the usual adult dose.

**Usual pediatric dose**

Anticholinergic—

Oral, the following doses every four hours as needed:

Children weighing 2.3 to 3.3 kg—12.5 mcg (0.0125 mg).

Children weighing 3.4 to 4.4 kg—15.6 mcg (0.0156 mg).

Children weighing 4.5 to 6.7 kg—18.8 mcg (0.0188 mg).

Children weighing 6.8 to 9 kg—25 mcg (0.025 mg).

Children weighing 9.1 to 13.5 kg—31.3 mcg (0.0313 mg).

Children weighing 13.6 to 22.6 kg—63 mcg (0.063 mg).

Children weighing 22.7 to 33 kg—94 to 125 mcg (0.094 to 0.125 mg).

Children weighing 34 to 36 kg—125 to 187 mcg (0.125 to 0.187 mg).

**Strength(s) usually available**

U.S.—

125 mcg (0.125 mg) per 5 mL (Rx) [*Levsin*].

Canada—

Not commercially available.

**Packaging and storage**

Store between 15 and 30 °C (59 and 86 °F), unless otherwise specified by manufacturer. Store in a tight, light-resistant container. Protect from freezing.

**Auxiliary labeling**

• May cause blurred vision.

• Keep container tightly closed.

### HYOSCYAMINE SULFATE ORAL SOLUTION USP

**Usual adult and adolescent dose**

Anticholinergic—

Oral, 125 to 250 mcg (0.125 to 0.25 mg) every four to six hours, the dosage being adjusted as needed and tolerated.

Note: Geriatric patients may be more sensitive to the effects of the usual adult dose.

**Usual pediatric dose**

Anticholinergic—

Oral, the following doses every four hours as needed:

Children weighing 2.3 to 3.3 kg—12.5 mcg (0.0125 mg).
Children weighing 3.4 to 4.4 kg—15.6 mcg (0.0156 mg).
Children weighing 4.5 to 6.7 kg—18.8 mcg (0.0188 mg).
Children weighing 6.8 to 9 kg—25 mcg (0.025 mg).
Children weighing 9.1 to 13.5 kg—31.3 mcg (0.0313 mg).
Children weighing 13.6 to 22.6 kg—63 mcg (0.063 mg).
Children weighing 22.7 to 33 kg—94 to 125 mcg (0.094 to 0.125 mg).
Children weighing 34 to 36 kg—125 to 187 mcg (0.125 to 0.187 mg).

**Strength(s) usually available**

U.S.—

125 mcg (0.125 mg) per mL (Rx) [*Gastrosed; Levsin* (alcohol 5%)].

Canada—

125 mg (0.125 mg) per mL (Rx) [*Levsin* (alcohol 5%)].

Note: 1 mL = approximately 28 drops (may vary with dropper).

**Packaging and storage**

Store below 40 °C (104 °F), preferably between 15 and 30 °C (59 and 86 °F), unless otherwise specified by manufacturer. Store in a tight, light-resistant container. Protect from freezing.

**Auxiliary labeling**

• May cause blurred vision.
• Keep container tightly closed.

**Note**

Dispense in dropper bottle.

## HYOSCYAMINE SULFATE TABLETS USP

**Usual adult and adolescent dose**

Anticholinergic—

Oral or sublingual, 125 to 500 mcg (0.125 to 0.5 mg) three or four times a day, thirty minutes to one hour before meals and at bedtime, the dosage being adjusted as needed and tolerated.

Note: Geriatric patients may be more sensitive to the effects of the usual adult dose.

**Usual pediatric dose**

Anticholinergic—

Children weighing up to 22.7 kg—Product not suitable for pediatric administration. See *Hyoscyamine Sulfate Oral Solution USP.*
Children weighing 22.7 to 33 kg—Oral, 94 to 125 mcg (0.094 to 0.125 mg).
Children weighing 34 to 36 kg—Oral, 125 to 187 mcg (0.125 to 0.187 mg).

**Strength(s) usually available**

U.S.—

125 mcg (0.125 mg) (Rx) [*Anaspaz; Gastrosed; Levsin; Levsin/SL; Neoquess;* GENERIC].

Canada—

125 mg (0.125 mg) (Rx) [*Levsin*].

**Packaging and storage**

Store below 40 °C (104 °F), preferably between 15 and 30 °C (59 and 86 °F), unless otherwise specified by manufacturer. Store in a tight, light-resistant container.

**Auxiliary labeling**

• May be chewed, swallowed whole, or allowed to dissolve under the tongue.
• May cause blurred vision.

# Parenteral Dosage Forms

## HYOSCYAMINE SULFATE INJECTION USP

**Usual adult and adolescent dose**

Anticholinergic—

Intramuscular, intravenous, or subcutaneous, 250 to 500 mcg (0.25 to 0.5 mg) every four to six hours.

Gastrointestinal radiography—

Intramuscular, intravenous, or subcutaneous, 250 to 500 mcg (0.25 to 0.5 mg) five to ten minutes prior to the diagnostic procedure.

Peptic ulcer—

Initial: Intravenous, 250 to 500 mcg (0.25 to 0.5 mg).
Maintenance: Intramuscular or subcutaneous, 250 to 500 mcg (0.25 to 0.5 mg) every six hours until all pain has ceased.

Prophylaxis of excessive salivation and respiratory tract secretions, in anesthesia—

Intramuscular, intravenous, or subcutaneous, 500 mcg (0.5 mg); or 5 mcg (0.005 mg) per kg of body weight thirty to sixty minutes before induction of anesthesia.

Antiarrhythmic—

Intravenous, 125 mcg (0.125 mg), repeated as needed.

Cholinergic adjunct (curariform block)—

Intravenous, 200 mcg (0.2 mg) for each 1 mg of neostigmine or the equivalent dose of physostigmine or pyridostigmine.

Note: Geriatric patients may be more sensitive to the effects of the usual adult dose.

**Usual pediatric dose**

Anticholinergic—

Prophylaxis of excessive salivation and respiratory tract secretions, in anesthesia:

Children up to 2 years of age—Use is not recommended.
Children 2 years of age and over—Intramuscular, intravenous, or subcutaneous, 5 mcg (0.005 mg) per kg of body weight thirty to sixty minutes before induction of anesthesia.

Note: Hyoscyamine sulfate injection that contains benzyl alcohol as a preservative should not be used in newborn and immature infants. The use of benzyl alcohol in neonates has been associated with a fatal toxic syndrome consisting of metabolic acidosis and CNS, respiratory, circulatory, and renal function impairment.

**Strength(s) usually available**

U.S.—

500 mcg (0.5 mg) per mL (Rx) [*Levsin* (benzyl alcohol 1.5%)].

Canada—

500 mcg (0.5 mg) per mL (Rx) [*Levsin*].

**Packaging and storage**

Store below 40 °C (104 °F), preferably between 15 and 30 °C (59 and 86 °F), unless otherwise specified by manufacturer. Protect from freezing.

---

### *MEPENZOLATE*

# Summary of Differences

Pharmacology/pharmacokinetics:

Elimination—Renal; 3 to 22% excreted unchanged.

Precautions::

Pregnancy—Reproduction studies in rats and rabbits have not shown adverse effects on fetus.

# Oral Dosage Forms

## MEPENZOLATE BROMIDE TABLETS USP

**Usual adult and adolescent dose**

Anticholinergic—

Oral, 25 to 50 mg four times a day with meals and at bedtime, the dosage being adjusted as needed and tolerated.

Note: Geriatric patients may be more sensitive to the effects of the usual adult dose.

**Usual pediatric dose**

Dosage has not been established.

**Strength(s) usually available**

U.S.—

25 mg (Rx) [*Cantil*].

Canada—

Not commercially available.

**Packaging and storage**

Store below 40 °C (104 °F), preferably between 15 and 30 °C (59 and 86 °F), unless otherwise specified by manufacturer. Store in a well-closed container.

**Auxiliary labeling**

• May cause blurred vision.

---

### *METHANTHELINE*

# Summary of Differences

Indications:

Also indicated for urinary incontinence.

# Oral Dosage Forms

## METHANTHELINE BROMIDE TABLETS

### Usual adult and adolescent dose
Anticholinergic—
> Oral, 50 to 100 mg every six hours, the dosage being adjusted as needed and tolerated.

Note: Geriatric patients may be more sensitive to the effects of the usual adult dose.

### Usual pediatric dose
Anticholinergic—
> Children up to 1 month of age: Oral, 12.5 mg two times a day, the dosage being increased to three times a day if needed and tolerated.
> Children 1 month to 1 year of age: Oral, 12.5 mg four times a day, the dosage being increased to 25 mg four times a day if needed and tolerated.
> Children 1 year of age and over: Oral, 12.5 to 50 mg four times a day, the dosage being adjusted as needed and tolerated.

### Strength(s) usually available
U.S.—
> 50 mg (Rx) [Banthine (scored)].

Canada—
> Not commercially available.

### Packaging and storage
Store below 40 °C (104 °F), preferably between 15 and 30 °C (59 and 86 °F), unless otherwise specified by manufacturer. Store in a well-closed container.

### Auxiliary labeling
• May cause blurred vision.

---

METHSCOPOLAMINE

## Summary of Differences

Pharmacology/pharmacokinetics:
> Onset of action—1 hour.
> Duration of action—6 to 8 hours.

# Oral Dosage Forms

## METHSCOPOLAMINE BROMIDE TABLETS

### Usual adult and adolescent dose
Anticholinergic—
> Oral, 2.5 mg four times a day, one-half hour before meals and 2.5 to 5 mg at bedtime.
> For severe symptoms: Oral, initially 5 mg four times a day, one-half hour before meals and at bedtime, the dosage being increased, if necessary, to obtain the desired response.

Note: Geriatric patients may be more sensitive to the effects of the usual adult dose.

### Usual pediatric dose
Anticholinergic—
> Oral, 200 mcg (0.2 mg) per kg of body weight or 6 mg per square meter of body surface a day (in four divided doses, before meals and at bedtime).

### Strength(s) usually available
U.S.—
> 2.5 mg (Rx) [Pamine].

Canada—
> Not commercially available.

### Packaging and storage
Store between 15 and 30 °C (59 and 86 °F), unless otherwise specified by manufacturer. Store in a tight container.

### Auxiliary labeling
• May cause blurred vision.

---

PIRENZEPINE

## Summary of Differences

Pharmacology/pharmacokinetics:
> Half-life (elimination)—10 to 12 hours.
> Elimination—Renal and hepatic; 80 to 90% of drug excreted unchanged.

# Oral Dosage Forms

## PIRENZEPINE HYDROCHLORIDE TABLETS

### Usual adult and adolescent dose
Anticholinergic—
> Oral, 50 mg two times a day, in the morning and at bedtime, the dosage being increased to three times a day, if needed and tolerated.

Note: Geriatric patients may be more sensitive to the effects of the usual adult dose.

### Usual pediatric dose
Dosage has not been established.

### Strength(s) usually available
U.S.—
> Not commercially available.

Canada—
> 50 mg (Rx) [Gastrozepin].

### Packaging and storage
Store below 40 °C (104 °F), preferably between 15 and 30 °C (59 and 86 °F), unless otherwise specified by manufacturer.

### Auxiliary labeling
• May cause blurred vision.

---

PROPANTHELINE

## Summary of Differences

Indications:
> Also used for duodenography and urinary incontinence.

Pharmacology/pharmacokinetics:
> Half-life (elimination)—1.6 (mean) hours.
> Duration of action—6 hours.
> Elimination—Renal; less than 6% of drug excreted unchanged.

# Oral Dosage Forms

## PROPANTHELINE BROMIDE TABLETS USP

### Usual adult and adolescent dose
Anticholinergic—
> Oral, 15 mg three times a day, one-half hour before meals, and 30 mg at bedtime, the dosage being adjusted as needed and tolerated.

Note: Patients of less than average body weight may require only 7.5 mg three or four times a day.

### Usual adult prescribing limits
Up to 120 mg daily.

### Usual pediatric dose
Anticholinergic—
> Oral, 375 mcg (0.375 mg) per kg of body weight or 10 mg per square meter of body surface four times a day, the dosage being adjusted as needed and tolerated.

Note: Pediatric administration is limited by the available dosage form. The tablets are not suitable for subdivision.

### Usual geriatric dose
Oral, 7.5 mg three or four times a day.

### Strength(s) usually available
U.S.—
> 7.5 mg (Rx) [Pro-Banthine].
> 15 mg (Rx) [Pro-Banthine; GENERIC].

Canada—
> 7.5 mg (Rx) [Pro-Banthine].
> 15 mg (Rx) [Pro-Banthine; Propanthel].

### Packaging and storage
Store below 40 °C (104 °F), preferably between 15 and 30 °C (59 and 86 °F), unless otherwise specified by manufacturer. Store in a well-closed container.

### Auxiliary labeling
• May cause blurred vision.

---

SCOPOLAMINE

## Summary of Differences

Category:
> Also a gastrointestinal antispasmodic, antidysmenorrheal, urinary antispasmodic, antiemetic, and antivertigo agent. Parenteral scopolamine is used as an antiarrhythmic and anesthesia adjunct.

Indications—
Indicated in preanesthesia as antisialagogue. Also indicated for biliary tract disorders, nocturnal enuresis, and excessive salivation. Not indicated for peptic ulcer.

Pharmacology/pharmacokinetics:
Protein binding—
Scopolamine hydrobromide: Low.
Half-life (elimination)—
8 hours.
Onset of action—
Oral scopolamine hydrobromide:
30 to 60 minutes (antisialagogue effect).
Parenteral scopolamine hydrobromide:
30 minutes (antisialagogue effect).
Duration of action—
Scopolamine hydrobromide:
Oral—4 to 6 hours.
Parenteral—4 hours.
Scopolamine Transdermal:
Up to 72 hours.
Elimination—
Renal; 1% of oral dose excreted unchanged, and 3.4% of subcutaneous dose excreted unchanged.

Precautions:
Pregnancy—
Parenteral administration before onset of labor may cause CNS depression and hemorrhage in neonate.
Drug interactions and/or related problems—
Additive sedation with other CNS depressants.
Laboratory value alterations—
Residual cycloplegia and mydriasis with transdermal dosage form may affect results of neuroradiological tests for intracranial neoplasm, subdural hematoma, or cerebral aneurysm.

Side/adverse effects:
Scopolamine has been reported to cause paradoxical reaction (trouble in sleeping). Anxiety, irritability, nightmares, and trouble in sleeping may indicate rebound reduction in rapid eye movement (REM) time. Drowsiness and a false sense of well being are more common also.

## Additional Dosing Information

See also *General Dosing Information*.

In the presence of pain, scopolamine may act as a stimulant, often producing delirium, if used without morphine or meperidine.

Cardiac rate is much slower with low doses of scopolamine (0.1 to 0.2 mg) than with average clinical doses of atropine. With higher doses, a short-lived cardioacceleration occurs followed within 30 minutes by a return to the normal rate.

## Oral Dosage Forms

### SCOPOLAMINE BUTYLBROMIDE TABLETS

**Usual adult and adolescent dose**
Anticholinergic or
Antispasmodic, gastrointestinal or
Antidysmenorrheal—
Oral, 10 to 20 mg three or four times a day, the dosage being adjusted as needed and tolerated.

Note: Geriatric patients may be more sensitive to the effects of the usual adult dose.

**Usual pediatric dose**
Dosage has not been established.

**Strength(s) usually available**
U.S.—
Not commercially available.
Canada—
10 mg (Rx) [*Buscopan*].

**Packaging and storage**
Store below 40 °C (104 °F), preferably between 15 and 30 °C (59 and 86 °F), in a well-closed container, unless otherwise specified by manufacturer.

**Auxiliary labeling**
• May cause drowsiness or blurred vision.
• Avoid alcoholic beverages.

## Parenteral Dosage Forms

### SCOPOLAMINE BUTYLBROMIDE INJECTION

**Usual adult and adolescent dose**
Anticholinergic or
Antispasmodic, gastrointestinal—
Intramuscular, intravenous, or subcutaneous, 10 to 20 mg three or four times a day, the dosage being adjusted as needed and tolerated.

**Usual pediatric dose**
Dosage has not been established.

**Strength(s) usually available**
U.S.—
Not commercially available.
Canada—
20 mg per mL (Rx) [*Buscopan*].

**Packaging and storage**
Store below 40 °C (104 °F), preferably between 15 and 30 °C (59 and 86 °F), unless otherwise specified by manufacturer. Protect from freezing.

### SCOPOLAMINE HYDROBROMIDE INJECTION USP

**Usual adult and adolescent dose**
Anticholinergic—
Intramuscular, intravenous, or subcutaneous, 300 to 600 mcg (0.3 to 0.6 mg) as a single dose.
Prophylaxis of excessive salivation and respiratory tract secretions, in anesthesia—
Intramuscular, 200 to 600 mcg (0.2 to 0.6 mg) one-half to one hour before induction of anesthesia.
Antiemetic—
Intramuscular, intravenous, or subcutaneous, 300 to 600 mcg (0.3 to 0.6 mg) as a single dose.
Anesthesia adjunct—
Sedation-hypnosis:
Intramuscular, intravenous, or subcutaneous, 600 mcg (0.6 mg) three or four times a day.
Amnesia:
Intramuscular, intravenous, or subcutaneous, 320 to 650 mcg (0.32 to 0.65 mg).

Note: Geriatric patients may be more sensitive to the effects of the usual adult dose.

**Usual pediatric dose**
Anticholinergic or
Antiemetic—
Intramuscular, intravenous, or subcutaneous, 6 mcg (0.006 mg) per kg of body weight or 200 mcg (0.2 mg) per square meter of body surface, as a single dose.
Prophylaxis of excessive salivation and respiratory tract secretions, in anesthesia—
Intramuscular, administered forty-five minutes to one hour before induction of anesthesia for:
Children up to 4 months of age—Use is not recommended.
Children 4 to 7 months of age—100 mcg (0.1 mg).
Children 7 months to 3 years of age—150 mcg (0.15 mg).
Children 3 to 8 years of age—200 mcg (0.2 mg).
Children 8 to 12 years of age—300 mcg (0.3 mg).

**Strength(s) usually available**
U.S.—
300 mcg (0.3 mg) per mL (Rx) [GENERIC].
400 mcg (0.4 mg) per mL (Rx) [GENERIC].
500 mcg (0.5 mg) per mL (Rx) [GENERIC].
600 mcg (0.6 mg) per mL (Rx) [GENERIC].
1 mg per mL (Rx) [GENERIC].
Canada—
Not commercially available.

**Packaging and storage**
Store below 40 °C (104 °F), preferably between 15 and 30 °C (59 and 86 °F), unless otherwise specified by manufacturer. Store in a light-resistant container. Protect from freezing.

**Preparation of dosage form**
When given intravenously, scopolamine should be diluted with sterile water for injection before administration.

# Rectal Dosage Forms
## SCOPOLAMINE BUTYLBROMIDE SUPPOSITORIES

### Usual adult and adolescent dose
Anticholinergic or

Antispasmodic, gastrointestinal or

Antidysmenorrheal—

Rectal, 10 mg three or four times a day, the dosage being adjusted as needed and tolerated.

Note: Geriatric patients may be more sensitive to the effects of the usual adult dose.

### Usual pediatric dose
Dosage has not been established.

### Strength(s) usually available
U.S.—

Not commercially available.

Canada—

10 mg (Rx) [*Buscopan*].

### Packaging and storage
Store below 40 °C (104 °F), preferably between 15 and 30 °C (59 and 86 °F), unless otherwise specified by manufacturer.

### Auxiliary labeling
• May cause drowsiness or blurred vision.

### Note
Include patient instructions when dispensing.

# Transdermal Dosage Forms
## SCOPOLAMINE TRANSDERMAL SYSTEM

### Usual adult and adolescent dose
Antiemetic or

Antivertigo agent—

Topical, to the postauricular skin, 1 transdermal system delivering 500 mcg (0.5 mg) over a period of three days, applied at least four hours before antiemetic effect is required.

Note: Canadian brand product delivers 1.0 mg over a period of three days and should be applied approximately twelve hours before the antiemetic effect is required.

Geriatric patients may be more sensitive to the effects of the usual adult dose.

### Usual pediatric dose
Use is not recommended.

### Strength(s) usually available
U.S.—

1.5 mg (Rx) [*Transderm-Scoēp*].

Canada—

1.5 mg (Rx) [*Transderm-V*].

### Packaging and storage
Store below 40 °C (104 °F), preferably between 15 and 30 °C (59 and 86 °F), unless otherwise specified by manufacturer.

### Auxiliary labeling
• May cause drowsiness or blurred vision.

### Note
Include patient instructions when dispensing.

Revised: 01/29/92

Interim revision: 09/09/94; 07/19/95

## Table 1. Side/Adverse Effects*

The following side/adverse effects have been selected on the basis of their potential clinical significance (possible signs and symptoms in parentheses where appropriate)—not necessarily inclusive:

Legend:
I = Anisotropine
II = Atropine
III = Belladonna
IV = Clidinium
V = Dicyclomine
VI = Glycopyrrolate
VII = Homatropine
VIII = Hyoscyamine
IX = Mepenzolate
X = Methantheline
XI = Methscopolamine
XII = Pirenzepine
XIII = Propantheline
XIV = Scopolamine

**Medical attention needed**

**Symptoms of overdose** (applies to all agents I–XIV: ✓)
- Blurred vision, continuing, or changes in *near vision*†
- *Clumsiness or unsteadiness*†
- *Confusion*†
- *Difficulty in breathing*‡
- *Dizziness*
- *Drowsiness*†, *severe*
- *Dryness of mouth, nose, or throat, severe*
- *Fast heartbeat*
- *Fever*
- *Hallucinations*†
- *Muscle weakness*‡, *severe*
- *Seizures*†
- *Slurred speech*
- *Tiredness*‡, *severe*
- *Unusual excitement, nervousness, restlessness, or irritability*†
- *Unusual warmth, dryness, and flushing of skin*

| Effect | I | II | III | IV | V | VI | VII | VIII | IX | X | XI | XII | XIII | XIV |
|---|---|---|---|---|---|---|---|---|---|---|---|---|---|---|
| *Allergic reaction* (skin rash or hives) | R | R | R | R | R | R | R | R | R | R | R | R | R | R |
| *Confusion*# | R | R | R | R | R | R | R | R | R | R | R | R | R | R |
| *Increased intraocular pressure* (eye pain)† | R | R | R | R | R | R | R | R | R | R | R | R | R | R |
| *Orthostatic hypotension* (dizziness, feeling faint, or continuing lightheadedness) | § | § | R | § | R | § | § | R | § | § | § | § | § | R |

**Medical attention needed only if continuing or bothersome**

| Effect | I | II | III | IV | V | VI | VII | VIII | IX | X | XI | XII | XIII | XIV |
|---|---|---|---|---|---|---|---|---|---|---|---|---|---|---|
| *Bloated feeling* | R | R | R | R | R | R | R | R | R | R | R | R | R | R |
| *Constipation* | M | M | M | M | M | M | M | M | M | M | M | M | M | M |
| *Decreased flow of breast milk* | L | L | L | L | L | L | L | L | L | L | L | L | L | L |
| *Decreased salivary secretion* (difficulty in swallowing) | L | L | L | L | L | L | L | L | L | L | L | L | L | L |
| *Decreased sweating* | M | M | M | M | M | M | M | M | M | M | M | M | M | M |
| *Difficult urination*** | R | R | R | R | R | R | R | R | R | R | R | R | R | R |
| *Difficulty in accommodation of the eye* (blurred vision)† | R | L | L | R | L | L | L | L | L | L | L | L | L | L |
| *Drowsiness*†† | R | R | R | R | R | R | R | R | R | R | R | R | R | M |
| *Dryness of mouth, nose, throat, or skin* | M | M | M | M | M | M | M | M | M | M | M | M | M | M |
| *False sense of well-being* | U | U | U | U | U | U | U | U | U | U | U | U | U | U |
| *Headache* | R | R | R | R | R | R | R | R | R | R | R | R | R | R |
| *Lightheadedness, temporary*—with parenteral administration | U | U | U | U | R | R | R | R | U | U | U | U | R | R |

Table 1. Side/Adverse Effects* *(continued)*

Legend:
I=Anisotropine
II=Atropine
III=Belladonna
IV=Clidinium
V=Dicyclomine
VI=Glycopyrrolate
VII=Homatropine
VIII=Hyoscyamine
IX=Mepenzolate
X=Methantheline
XI=Methscopolamine
XII=Pirenzepine
XIII=Propantheline
XIV=Scopolamine

| | I | II | III | IV | V | VI | VII | VIII | IX | X | XI | XII | XIII | XIV |
|---|---|---|---|---|---|---|---|---|---|---|---|---|---|---|
| **Loss of memory‡‡** | R | R | R | R | R | R | R | R | R | R | R | R | R | M |
| **Mydriatic effect** (increased sensitivity of eyes to light)† | R | L | L | R | L | R | R | L | R | R | R | L | R | L |
| **Nausea or vomiting** | R | R | R | R | R | R | R | R | R | R | R | R | R | R |
| **Paradoxical reaction** (trouble in sleeping) | U | U | U | U | U | U | U | U | U | U | U | U | U | R |
| **Redness or other signs of irriation at injection site** | U | M | U | U | M | M | U | M | U | U | U | U | U | M |
| **Unusual tiredness or weakness** | R | R | R | R | R | R | U | R | R | R | R | R | R | R |
| *Medical attention needed if they occur after scopolamine is discontinued* | | | | | | | | | | | | | | |
| **Anxiety** | U | U | U | U | U | U | U | U | U | U | U | U | U | §§ |
| **Irritability** | U | U | U | U | U | U | U | U | U | U | U | U | U | §§ |
| **Nightmares** | U | U | U | U | U | U | U | U | U | U | U | U | U | §§ |
| **Trouble in sleeping** | U | U | U | U | U | U | U | U | U | U | U | U | U | §§ |

*Differences in frequency of occurrence may reflect either lack of clinical-use data or actual pharmacologic distinctions among agents (although their pharmacologic similarity suggests that side effects occurring with one may occur with the others). M=more frequent; L=less frequent; R=rare; U=unknown.

†Quaternary ammonium compounds are fully ionized in the pH range of body fluids and possess reduced lipid solubility. Therefore, they penetrate cellular barriers less effectively and only pass across the blood-brain barrier or into the eye with difficulty. Central and ocular effects are negligible and/or less likely to occur with quaternary ammonium compounds.

‡With quaternary ammonium compounds, difficulty in breathing, severe muscle weakness, and severe tiredness may occur because of the compounds' curare-like effects; these effects may lead to respiratory paralysis.

§Orthostatic hypotension, due to ganglion-blocking activity, is more likely to occur with high doses of quaternary ammonium compounds.

#Confusion may occur more frequently in geriatric patients.

**Difficult urination is more likely to occur in older men and may require medical attention in patients with symptoms of prostatism.

††More frequent with high doses of anticholinergics, but a common side effect with therapeutic doses of oral or parenteral scopolamine.

‡‡Scopolamine, administered parenterally as preanesthetic medication and/or given in large doses, may have a temporary but detrimental effect on memory. In geriatric patients, especially those who already have memory problems, the continued use of any anticholinergic may severely impair memory.

§§May indicate rebound reduction in rapid eye movement (REM) time.

# ANTICOAGULANTS    Systemic

This monograph includes information on the following: Anisindione†; Dicumarol†; Warfarin.

Note: See also individual *Heparin (Systemic)* and *Antithrombin III (Systemic)* monographs.

INN:
Dicumarol—Dicoumarol

VA CLASSIFICATION (Primary): BL100

Note: For a listing of dosage forms and brand names by country availability, see *Dosage Forms* section(s). For a listing of brand names for the articles in this monograph, refer to the General Index.

†Not commercially available in Canada.

## Category

Anticoagulant.

## Indications

Note: Bracketed information in the *Indications* section refers to uses that are not included in U.S. product labeling.

Several of the indications for coumarin- or indandione-derivative anticoagulant therapy are identical to those for thrombolytic (alteplase [tissue-type plasminogen activator, recombinant; tPA], anistreplase [anisoylated plasminogen-streptokinase activator complex; APSAC] streptokinase, or urokinase) and/or heparin therapy. Thrombolytic agents are used primarily to lyse obstructive thrombi and restore blood flow in a recently occluded blood vessel, whereas anticoagulants are used primarily to prevent thrombus formation and extension of existing thrombi. For treatment of acute deep venous thrombosis and acute pulmonary embolism, a thrombolytic agent may be the treatment of choice; however, the selection of thrombolytic therapy or anticoagulant therapy as opposed to other forms of treatment, including vascular surgery, must be based on determination of the severity of thrombotic disease and assessment of patient condition and history.

Because the therapeutic effects of coumarin- or indandione-derivative anticoagulants may not occur until after several days of therapy, heparin is the agent of choice when an immediate anticoagulant effect is required. A coumarin or indandione derivative is usually administered when an immediate anticoagulant effect is not necessary or when long-term anticoagulation is required following initial thrombolytic and/or heparin therapy.

### Accepted

Thrombosis, deep venous (prophylaxis and treatment) or
Thromboembolism, pulmonary (prophylaxis and treatment)—Anticoagulants are indicated in the treatment of patients with recent deep vein thrombosis or thrombophlebitis to prevent extension and embolization of the thrombus and to reduce the risk of pulmonary embolism or recurrent thrombus formation. In acute pulmonary embolism or venous thrombosis, anticoagulants are indicated following initial thrombolytic and/or heparin therapy to decrease the risk of extension, recurrence, or death.

Anticoagulants are indicated for prophylaxis of venous thrombosis and pulmonary embolism postoperatively or in high-risk patients, such as those with a history of thromboembolism or those requiring prolonged immobilization. However, subcutaneous administration of low-dose heparin is more commonly used to prevent postsurgical thromboembolic complications.

Thromboembolism (prophylaxis)—Anticoagulants are indicated [or used] for prophylaxis of thromboembolism associated with:
Chronic atrial fibrillation—Anticoagulants may prevent the formation of mural thrombi in the heart, which may lead to systemic thromboembolism in patients with chronic atrial fibrillation, especially those with rheumatic mitral stenosis, prosthetic heart valves, left atrial enlargement, or cardiomyopathy. In these patients, anticoagulants may decrease the risk of arterial embolism, pulmonary embolism, or subsequent stroke.

Myocardial infarction—Anticoagulants are indicated as adjunctive therapy to reduce the risk of systemic thromboembolic complications following acute myocardial infarction (especially an anterior wall myocardial infarction or a large apical infarction), primarily in high-risk patients such as those with shock, congestive heart failure, prolonged arrhythmias (especially atrial fibrillation), previous myocardial infarction, or history of thromboembolism.

[Cardioversion of chronic atrial fibrillation, electric or pharmacologic]—Anticoagulants are used to reduce the risk of postconversion emboli.

[Prosthetic heart valves]—Anticoagulants are used to reduce the risk of thromboembolic complications in patients with certain types of prosthetic heart valves. The effectiveness of these agents may be increased by concurrent use of a platelet aggregation inhibitor such as dipyridamole. Aspirin is also sometimes used concurrently with anticoagulants for this purpose; however, the risk of hemorrhage is increased.

[Thromboembolism, cerebral, recurrence (prophylaxis)]—Anticoagulants are used to reduce the risk of recurrence of cerebral embolism in patients with recent cerebral embolism, especially when the source of the embolism is thought to be the heart. The possibility that cerebral hemorrhage may be present must be ruled out before anticoagulant therapy is initiated. Although administration of an anticoagulant too soon after a cerebral embolism may increase the risk of cerebral hemorrhage, recent studies have indicated that the risk of early recurrence may be greater than the risk of anticoagulant therapy.

[Myocardial reinfarction (prophylaxis)]—Long-term use of anticoagulants following myocardial infarction to prevent reinfarction remains controversial; many clinicians report that recurrence of acute attacks and/or risk of death may not be reduced by such therapy. A few studies have indicated that long-term anticoagulation may reduce the risk of recurrent myocardial infarction and of nonhemorrhagic cerebrovascular accidents in patients older than 60 years of age. However, aspirin is also effective, and is more commonly used, for this purpose.

[Ischemic attacks, transient, in females and males (treatment)]—Warfarin has been used as an adjunct in the treatment of patients with transient ischemic attacks. It may reduce the incidence of repeat attacks and/or subsequent stroke, especially during the first few months of therapy. However, the risk of death may not be decreased. FDA has classified warfarin as being possibly effective for this indication; this classification requires the submission of adequate and well-controlled studies in order to provide substantial evidence of effectiveness. Platelet aggregation inhibitors (especially aspirin) are more commonly being used for this indication.

[Anticoagulants have also been used to reduce the risk of thrombosis and/or occlusion of the aortocoronary bypass following coronary bypass surgery. However, their efficacy has not been proven and platelet aggregation inhibitors are now being administered for this purpose.]

## Pharmacology/Pharmacokinetics

### Physicochemical characteristics

Chemical group—
Coumarin derivatives: Dicumarol, warfarin.
Indandione derivative: Anisindione.
Molecular weight—
Anisindione: 252.27.
Dicumarol: 336.30.
Warfarin sodium: 330.31.

### Mechanism of action/Effect

Both coumarin and indandione derivatives are indirect-acting anticoagulants (act only *in vivo*); they prevent the formation of active procoagulation factors II, VII, IX, and X in the liver by inhibiting the vitamin K–mediated gamma-carboxylation of precursor proteins. Full therapeutic action is delayed until circulating coagulation factors are removed by normal catabolism, which occurs at different rates for each factor. Although prothrombin time (PT) may be prolonged when factor VII (which has the shortest half-life) is depleted, it is believed that peak antithrombotic effects are not achieved until all four factors are removed. These agents have no direct thrombolytic effect, although they may limit extension of existing thrombi.

### Absorption

Anisindione and warfarin are well absorbed from the gastrointestinal tract. The rate, but not the extent, of warfarin absorption is decreased by food.

Dicumarol is slowly and incompletely absorbed from the gastrointestinal tract.

### Protein binding

Very high (99%); to albumin.

### Biotransformation

Hepatic.

**Elimination**

Via hepatic metabolism, followed by renal excretion of metabolites; following enterohepatic circulation.

| Drug | Half-life* | Onset of Action† (days) | Duration of Action‡ (days) |
|------|-----------|------------------------|---------------------------|
| Anisindione | 3–5 days | 2–3 | 1–3 |
| Dicumarol | 1–4 days§ | 1–5 | 2–10 |
| Warfarin# | 1.5–2.5 days** | 0.5–3 | 2–5 |

*Subject to intra- and inter-patient variation.

†As determined by effect on PT; may reflect early depletion of factor VII rather than peak antithrombotic effects. Also, may reflect use of initial loading doses, which is currently not recommended.

‡Time after discontinuation of therapy for prothrombin activity to return to the pretreatment value.

§Dose-dependent.

#For oral, intramuscular, or intravenous administration.

**Mean is approximately 50 hours.

## Precautions to Consider

### Pregnancy/Reproduction

Pregnancy—Coumarin- and indandione-derivative anticoagulants cross the placenta and are not recommended during pregnancy. Congenital malformations and other adverse effects on fetal development, including severe nasal hypoplasia, stippling of bones, optic atrophy, microcephaly, and growth and mental retardation have been reported in infants born to mothers taking these agents during pregnancy. This is especially critical during the first trimester. However, many clinicians recommend that these agents not be used at all during pregnancy because facial anomalies in the infant have occurred following maternal use in the third trimester. Also, fetal or neonatal hemorrhage, fetal death in utero, and increased risk of maternal hemorrhage during the second and third trimesters have been reported. However, other clinicians state that these agents may be used for brief periods in the second and third trimesters.

Women of childbearing potential should be informed of the risks of becoming pregnant while receiving a coumarin or indandione derivative and advised to use an effective (nonhormonal) method of birth control throughout therapy. Patients who wish to become pregnant during therapy should first discuss their plans with the prescriber. Also, patients should be instructed to contact the prescribing physician immediately if they suspect that they are pregnant. Some clinicians recommend that, if a woman becomes pregnant during coumarin or indandione anticoagulant therapy, termination of the pregnancy be considered.

If an anticoagulant is required during pregnancy, heparin may be preferred because it does not cross the placenta. A patient receiving a coumarin or indandione derivative who wishes to become pregnant should preferably be changed to heparin therapy prior to conception.

Labor and delivery—If a coumarin or indandione derivative is used during the third trimester, it should be discontinued after the 37th week of gestation, and heparin substituted if maternal anticoagulation is required, to reduce the risk of fetal hemorrhage during labor and of neonatal hemorrhage following delivery. Anticoagulants also increase the risk of maternal hemorrhage during or following delivery.

Postpartum—Anticoagulants may increase the risk of maternal hemorrhage if administered in the postpartum period.

### Breast-feeding

Warfarin is distributed into breast milk in extremely small quantities, if at all, and is not considered hazardous to the nursing infant. With other anticoagulants, there is a possibility of significant quantities being distributed into breast milk; the nursing infant should be monitored for evidence of hypoprothrombinemia and vitamin K administered if necessary.

### Pediatrics

Infants, especially neonates, may be more susceptible to the effects of anticoagulants because of vitamin K deficiency.

### Geriatrics

Geriatric patients may be more susceptible to the effects of anticoagulants, resulting in increased risk of hemorrhage, possibly because of the presence of advanced vascular disease resulting in altered homeostatic mechanisms, hepatic function impairment resulting in decreased procoagulant factor synthesis or anticoagulant metabolism, or renal function impairment. Lower maintenance doses than those usually recommended for adults may be required for these patients.

### Dental

Bleeding from gingival tissue may be a sign of anticoagulant overdose. Anticoagulant therapy increases the risk of localized hemorrhage during and following oral surgical procedures. Consultation with the prescribing physician may be advisable prior to oral surgery, to determine whether a temporary dosage reduction or withdrawal of anticoagulant therapy is feasible. Also, local measures to minimize bleeding should be used at the time of surgery.

### Drug interactions and/or related problems

See also _Table 1,_ page 238.

All interactions between coumarin or indandione derivatives and other medications have not been identified. Also, several medications may interact with anticoagulant therapy by more than one mechanism; in several cases, both increased anticoagulation and decreased anticoagulation have been reported for the same interacting medication. Therefore, the net effect of some concurrently used medications on anticoagulant therapy may be unpredictable. In addition, control of anticoagulant therapy may be more difficult to achieve if an interacting medication is used intermittently rather than chronically.

Because of the possible serious consequences of interference with anticoagulant therapy, increased monitoring of the prothrombin time (PT) is recommended when _any_ medication is added to or withdrawn from the regimen of a patient stabilized on a coumarin or indandione derivative, or if the dosage of a concurrently used medication is changed. Anticoagulant dosage must be adjusted as necessary to prevent hemorrhage or loss of effect. Also, substantial alteration of initial anticoagulant dosage may be necessary when anticoagulant therapy is initiated in a patient receiving a medication known to cause significant alteration of anticoagulant effect.

### Laboratory value alterations

The following have been selected on the basis of their potential clinical significance (possible effect in parentheses where appropriate)—not necessarily inclusive (» = major clinical significance):

With diagnostic test results

Urinalysis

(tests based on color changes may be interfered with because alkaline urine may turn orange following administration of anisindione; acidification of the urine eliminates this color)

### Medical considerations/Contraindications

The medical considerations/contraindications included here have been selected on the basis of their potential clinical significance (reasons given in parentheses where appropriate)—not necessarily inclusive (» = major clinical significance).

_Except under special circumstances, these medications should not be used when the following medical problems exist:_

» Abortion, threatened or incomplete or
» Aneurysm, cerebral or dissecting aorta or
» Bleeding, active or
» Cerebrovascular hemorrhage, confirmed or suspected or
» Neurosurgery, recent or contemplated or
» Ophthalmic surgery, recent or contemplated or
» Surgery, major, other, especially if resulting in large open surfaces
(increased risk of uncontrollable hemorrhage)

Note: Although anticoagulants are generally contraindicated following major surgery, they may be required following orthopedic (hip) surgery to reduce the risk of thromboembolism.

» Blood dyscrasias, hemorrhagic, such as thrombocytopenia or
» Hemophilia or
» Hemorrhagic tendency, other
(increased risk of hemorrhage)

» Hypertension, severe uncontrolled
(increased risk of cerebral hemorrhage)

» Pericardial effusion or
» Pericarditis
(increased risk of severe hemorrhagic pericardial effusions and pericardial tamponade)

_Risk-benefit should be considered when the following medical problems exist:_

Allergic or anaphylactic disorders, severe

Any condition in which increased risk of hemorrhage is present, such as:
» Childbirth, recent
» Diabetes, severe
Gastrointestinal ulceration, history of
Intrauterine contraceptive device, use of
Radiation therapy, recent
Renal function impairment, mild to moderate

» Renal function impairment, severe
» Trauma, severe, especially to the central nervous system (CNS)
Tuberculosis, active
» Ulceration or other lesions of the gastrointestinal, respiratory, or urinary tract, active
» Vasculitis, severe
Any condition that may reduce the effectiveness of the anticoagulant, such as:
Edema
Hypercholesterolemia
Hyperlipidemia
Hypothyroidism
Any condition that may directly or indirectly increase the patient's response to the anticoagulant leading to increased risk of bleeding, such as:
Biliary obstruction
» Carcinoma, visceral
Collagen disease
Congestive heart failure
Diarrhea, prolonged
Dietary insufficiency, prolonged
Fever
Hepatic function impairment, mild to moderate
» Hepatic function impairment, severe, or cirrhosis
Hepatitis, infectious
Hyperthyroidism
Pancreatic disorders
Sprue
Steatorrhea
» Vitamin C deficiency
» Vitamin K deficiency
Any condition that may result in reduced compliance by unsupervised outpatients, such as:
Alcoholism (active)
Emotional instability
Psychosis
Senility
Uncooperative patient
Any medical or dental procedure or condition in which the risk of bleeding or hemorrhage is present, such as:
» Anesthesia, regional or lumbar block
Catheters, indwelling
Drainage tubes in any orifice or wound
» Spinal puncture
» Endocarditis, subacute bacterial
(increased risk of hemorrhage into infarcted area)
Hypertension, mild to moderate
» Polyarthritis
Protein C deficiency, known or suspected, or any other condition predisposing to tissue necrosis
(increased risk of anticoagulant-induced tissue necrosis, although patients with protein C deficiency may require long-term anticoagulant therapy to prevent recurrent thrombus formation; administration of heparin during the first 5 to 7 days of coumarin or indandione anticoagulant therapy may reduce the risk of tissue necrosis)
Sensitivity to the anticoagulant prescribed, history of
Caution in use is also recommended in geriatric or very young patients, and in severely debilitated patients, who may be more sensitive to the effects of anticoagulants.

**Patient monitoring**
The following may be especially important in patient monitoring (other tests may be warranted in some patients, depending on condition; » = major clinical significance):
*For all anticoagulants*
» Prothrombin time determinations
(recommended prior to initiation of therapy, at 24-hour intervals while maintenance dosage is being established, then once or twice weekly for the following 3 to 4 weeks, then at 1- to 4-week intervals for the duration of treatment)
Stool tests for occult blood loss and
Urine tests for hematuria
(recommended at periodic intervals during therapy)
*For anisindione*
Hematopoietic function determinations and
Hepatic function determinations and

Renal function determinations and
Urine tests for proteinuria
(may be advisable at periodic intervals during anisindione therapy because of the increased risk of nephrotoxicity, hepatotoxicity, and blood dyscrasias associated with pheninidione [an anticoagulant chemically related to anisindione that is no longer available])

## Side/Adverse Effects

Note: The occurrence of gastrointestinal hemorrhage during anticoagulant therapy, especially if the prothrombin time (PT) is within the therapeutic range, may indicate the presence of an underlying occult lesion such as a tumor or ulcer.

Hemorrhagic necrosis (bleeding into the skin and subcutaneous tissue with resultant necrosis, vasculitis, and thrombosis) has been reported to occur rarely during anticoagulant therapy. This complication occurs more frequently in females than in males; the fatty tissues of the abdomen, breasts, buttocks, and thighs are most often affected. Tissue necrosis may be more likely to occur in patients with protein C deficiency. Concurrent use of heparin during the first 5 to 7 days of anticoagulant therapy may decrease the risk of tissue necrosis.

Adrenal hemorrhage resulting in acute adrenal insufficiency has been reported to occur rarely during anticoagulant therapy. Diagnosis may be difficult because the initial symptoms (abdominal pain, apprehension, diarrhea, dizziness or fainting, headache, loss of appetite, nausea or vomiting, and weakness) are nonspecific and variable. If acute adrenal insufficiency is suspected, anticoagulant therapy must be discontinued and high-dose adrenocorticoid therapy (preferably with hydrocortisone, since other glucocorticoids may not provide sufficient sodium retention) instituted immediately. Delay of treatment while laboratory confirmation of the diagnosis is awaited may prove fatal for the patient. It has been proposed that abdominal computerized axial tomographic (CAT) scanning may be of use in diagnosing this condition more rapidly.

| The following side/adverse effects have been selected on the basis of their potential clinical significance (possible signs and symptoms in parentheses where appropriate)—not necessarily inclusive:* | Legend: I=Anisindione II=Dicumarol III=Warfarin | | |
|---|---|---|---|
| | I | II | III |
| **Medical attention needed** | | | |
| *Adrenal insufficiency, acute* (diarrhea, nausea with or without vomiting, stomach cramps or pain) | R | R | R |
| *Agranulocytosis or* | U† | R | R |
| *Leukopenia* (chills, fever, sore throat, unusual tiredness or weakness) | U† | L | L |
| *Dermatitis, allergic* (skin rash, hives, and/or itching) | L | R | R |
| *Diarrhea* | U† | M | L |
| *Hepatotoxicity* (dark urine, yellow eyes or skin) | U† | R | R |
| *Nausea or vomiting* | U† | L | L |
| *Purple toes syndrome* (blue or purple toes, pain in toes) | U | R | R |
| *Renal damage with resultant edema and proteinuria* (bloody or cloudy urine; difficult or painful urination; sudden decrease in amount of urine; swelling of face, feet and/or lower legs) | U† | R | R |
| *Sores, ulcers, or white spots in mouth or throat* | U† | R | R |
| *Stomach cramps or pain* | U† | L | L |
| **Medical attention needed only if continuing or bothersome** | | | |
| *Bloated stomach or gas* | U | M | U |
| *Loss of appetite* | U | L | U |

| The following side/adverse effects have been selected on the basis of their potential clinical significance (possible signs and symptoms in parentheses where appropriate)—not necessarily inclusive:* | Legend: I=Anisindione II=Dicumarol III=Warfarin | | |
|---|---|---|---|
| | **I** | **II** | **III** |
| *Paralysis of accommodation* (blurred vision or other vision problems) | U† | U | U |
| *Unusual hair loss* | U† | L | L |

*Differences in frequency of occurrence may reflect either lack of clinical-use data or actual pharmacologic distinctions among agents. M=more frequent; L=less frequent; R=rare; U=unknown.

†Although not documented with anisindione, these effects have been reported with phenindione, an indandione derivative that is no longer commercially available. Other adverse effects or abnormalities reported with phenindione include aplastic anemia, eosinophilia, leukocytosis, thrombocytopenia, atypical mononuclear cells, red cell aplasia, presence of leukocyte agglutinins, and exfoliative dermatitis. Because anisindione is chemically related to phenindione, these side effects should be considered potential side effects of anisindione also.

**Signs and symptoms of hemorrhage indicating need for medical attention**

  *Bleeding from gums when brushing teeth; unexplained bruising or purplish areas on skin; unexplained nosebleeds; unusually heavy bleeding or oozing from cuts or wounds; unusually heavy or unexpected menstrual bleeding*

  Note: With anisindione, the possibility exists that unusual bruising or bleeding may also indicate thrombocytopenia.

**Signs and symptoms of internal bleeding indicating need for medical attention**

  *Abdominal pain or swelling; back pain or backaches; blood in urine; bloody or black tarry stools; constipation caused by hemorrhage-induced paralytic ileus or intestinal obstruction; coughing up blood; dizziness; headache, severe or continuing; joint pain, stiffness, or swelling; vomiting blood or material that looks like coffee grounds*

## Overdose

For specific information on the agents used in the management of anticoagulant overdose, see the *Vitamin K (Systemic)* monograph.

For more information on the management of overdose or unintentional ingestion, **contact a Poison Control Center** (see *Poison Control Center Listing*).

**Clinical effects of overdose**

The following effects have been selected on the basis of their potential clinical significance (possible signs and symptoms in parentheses where appropriate)—not necessarily inclusive:

Early signs of overdose

  *Bleeding from gums when brushing teeth; unexplained bruising or purplish areas on skin; unexplained nosebleeds; unusually heavy bleeding or oozing from cuts or wounds; unusually heavy or unexpected menstrual bleeding*

  Note: With anisindione, the possibility exists that unusual bruising or bleeding may also indicate thrombocytopenia.

Signs and symptoms of internal bleeding

  *Abdominal pain or swelling; back pain or backaches; blood in urine; bloody or black tarry stools; constipation caused by hemorrhage-induced paralytic ileus or intestinal obstruction; coughing up blood; dizziness; headache, severe or continuing; joint pain, stiffness, or swelling; vomiting blood or material that looks like coffee grounds*

**Treatment of overdose**

Recommended treatment of anticoagulant overdose includes withdrawing the medication temporarily if excessive prolongation of PT or minor bleeding occurs.

Specific treatment—

  Administering vitamin K₁ orally or intravenously (1 to 5 mg for mild overdosage; 20 to 40 mg for more severe overdosage) if necessary. However, the fact that vitamin K₁ may interfere with subsequent anticoagulant therapy must be kept in mind.

  Transfusing fresh frozen plasma (1 to 1.5 liters may be required) or prothrombin complex (about 1500 Units), in addition to administering vitamin K₁, if needed in severe cases. Although whole blood may be given if blood loss has been extensive, transfusion of whole blood will not elevate procoagulant factor concentrations sufficiently to eliminate the need for administration of plasma or prothrombin complex.

## Patient Consultation

As an aid to patient consultation, refer to *Advice for the Patient, Anticoagulants (Systemic)*.

In providing consultation, consider emphasizing the following selected information (» = major clinical significance):

**Before using this medication**

» Conditions affecting use, especially:

    Sensitivity to the anticoagulant considered for therapy

    Pregnancy—Not becoming pregnant during therapy without first discussing plans with physician, or informing physician immediately if any suspicion of pregnancy; these medications should not be used during the first trimester because of their teratogenic effects or after the 37th week of pregnancy because of the risk of fetal and neonatal bleeding

    Use in children—Infants, especially neonates, are especially sensitive to effects because of vitamin K deficiency

    Use in the elderly—Increased risk of bleeding

    Other medications

    Other medical problems, especially bleeding or clotting defects, or history of; recent surgery or childbirth; diabetes mellitus; severe renal or hepatic function impairment; active gastrointestinal, respiratory, or urinary tract ulceration; malignancy; recent spinal puncture; subacute bacterial endocarditis; or polyarthritis

**Proper use of this medication**

» Taking medication only as directed

» Regular prothrombin-time tests and regular visits to physician or clinic to check progress

» Proper dosing

» Missed dose: Taking as soon as possible; not taking if not remembered until next day; not doubling doses; keeping a record of doses taken to avoid mistakes; keeping record of missed doses to give physician

» Proper storage

**Precautions while using this medication**

» Need for patient to inform all physicians, dentists, and pharmacists that this medication is being used

» Not taking or discontinuing any other medication, including salicylates or any other over-the-counter (OTC) medications, without physician's permission

» Carrying identification indicating use of an anticoagulant

  Not engaging in activities that may lead to injuries

  Using care in activities that may cause a cut or bleeding (such as shaving)

  Minimizing alcohol consumption; i.e., not consuming more than an occasional drink or two

  Eating a normal, balanced diet; not changing dietary habits, taking vitamins, or using nutritional supplements without first seeking professional advice because of possible alteration of anticoagulant effect by substantial changes in intake of Vitamin K (present in some multiple vitamins and nutritional supplements as well as foods, including green, leafy vegetables [such as broccoli, cabbage, collard greens, kale, lettuce, spinach], and, to a lesser extent, meats and dairy products)

  Checking with physician if unable to eat for several days or if continuing gastric upset, diarrhea, or fever occurs

  Caution following cessation of therapy while body is recovering blood-clotting abilities

**Side/adverse effects**

» Checking with physician immediately if any symptoms of bleeding occur

  Checking with physician if anisindione turns urine orange

  Signs and symptoms of potential side effects, especially bleeding, agranulocytosis, renal damage, hepatotoxicity, and "purple toes" syndrome

## General Dosing Information

Patient compliance is essential to the safe use of these medications. The patient must be responsible and willing to carry out the demands that accompany the use of anticoagulants.

Dosage of anticoagulants must be individualized and adjusted according to prothrombin-time (PT) determinations. Determinations of clotting time, bleeding time, or anticoagulant plasma concentration are not effective measures for monitoring anticoagulant therapy. It is recommended that PT determinations be performed prior to initiation of therapy, at 24-hour intervals while maintenance dosage is being established, then once or twice weekly for the following 3 to 4 weeks, then at 1- to 4-week intervals for the duration of treatment.

PT is often reported by listing the value in seconds along with the control value in seconds. Alternately, PT may be reported as the ratio of the prolonged (therapeutic) value to the control value. In the past, the therapeutic value was considered to be $1^{1}/_{2}$ to $2^{1}/_{2}$ times the control value. Because the tissue thromboplastins currently used in the U.S. for PT determinations are less sensitive than those previously used, the therapeutic value for most patients is now considered to be 1.3 to 1.5 times the control value. However, when an especially high risk of thromboembolism exists (e.g., in patients with a history of recurrent systemic embolism or patients with mechanical heart valves), maintaining the PT at 1.5 to 2 times the control value may be necessary. Tissue thromboplastins currently used in North America for PT determinations are not identical to, and are less sensitive than, thromboplastins used in other countries. In 1983, the World Health Organization introduced a standardized system of reporting PT values that provides a common basis for communicating PT results and interpreting therapeutic ranges. This system is based on the determination of an International Normalized Ratio (INR), which is derived from calibrations of commercial thromboplastin reagents against the International Reference Preparation, a sensitive human brain thromboplastin. With the rabbit brain thromboplastins currently commercially available in North America, PT values of 1.3 to 1.5 times the control value are equivalent to INR values of 2 to 3 times the control value and PT values of 1.5 to 2 times the control value are equivalent to INR values of 3 to 4.5 times the control value. For other thromboplastins, the INR can be calculated using the International Sensitivity Index (available from the manufacturer) as a calibration factor.

Levels of anticoagulation (in terms of the desired PT and INR) that are recommended for specific indications by a panel assembled for the Second American College of Chest Physicians Conference on Antithrombotic Therapy are:

• For prevention of venous thromboembolism and pulmonary embolism in high-risk surgical patients when low-dose heparin is ineffective (e.g., surgery for fractured hip, other [elective] hip surgery, or knee reconstruction) or when heparin is contraindicated for any reason—

    Surgery for fractured hip: PT 1.3 to 1.5 (INR 2.0 to 3.0) times the control value.

    Elective hip surgery: PT 1.3 to 1.5 (INR 2.0 to 3.0) times the control value.

• For treatment of acute deep venous thrombosis of the popliteal and more proximal vessels or pulmonary embolism (following initial thrombolytic and/or heparin therapy)—PT 1.3 to 1.5 (INR 2.0 to 3.0) times the control value. The oral anticoagulant should be administered concurrently with heparin for at least four to five days, after which heparin can be discontinued (provided that prothrombin time determinations indicate an adequate response to the oral anticoagulant). Treatment with the oral anticoagulant should be continued for at least three months (indefinitely if recurrent venous thrombosis or continuing risk factors [e.g., antithrombin III deficiency, protein C or protein S deficiency, malignancy] exist).

• For treatment of isolated symptomatic calf-vein thrombosis—PT 1.3 to 1.5 (INR 2.0 to 3.0) times the control value. Therapy should be continued for three months.

• For prevention of cardiogenic systemic or cerebral embolism (either a first episode or a recurrence) in patients with the following risk factors—

    Mitral valve disease with documented systemic embolism: PT 1.5 to 2.0 (INR 3.0 to 4.5) times the control value. If embolism recurs, dipyridamole (225 to 400 mg per day) should be considered for addition to the regimen. Therapy should be continued at that level of anticoagulation for at least one year after an embolism occurs, after which dosage may be reduced to provide a PT of 1.3 to 1.5 (INR 2.0 to 3.0) times the control value. Long-term therapy is recommended.

    Mitral valve disease and associated chronic or paroxysmal atrial fibrillation: PT 1.3 to 1.5 (INR 2.0 to 3.0) times the control value. Long-term therapy is recommended.

    Mitral valve disease, when the left atrial diameter is >5.5 cm (but normal sinus rhythm is present): PT 1.3 to 1.5 (INR 2.0 to 3.0) times the control value. Long-term therapy is recommended.

    Mitral valve prolapse associated with documented, unexplained transient ischemic attacks unresponsive to a sufficient trial of aspirin therapy: PT 1.3 to 1.5 (INR 2.0 to 3.0) times the control value. Long-term therapy is recommended.

    Mitral valve prolapse and documented systemic embolism: PT 1.5 to 2.0 (INR 3.0 to 4.5) times the control value. Therapy should be continued at that level of anticoagulation for at least one year after an embolism occurs, after which dosage may be reduced to provide a PT of 1.3 to 1.5 (INR 2.0 to 3.0) times the control value. Long-term therapy is recommended.

    Mitral valve prolapse associated with chronic or paroxysmal atrial fibrillation: PT 1.3 to 1.5 (INR 2.0 to 3.0) times the control value. Long-term therapy is recommended.

    Mitral annular calcification complicated by systemic thromboembolism: PT 1.5 to 2.0 (INR 3.0 to 4.5) times the control value. Therapy should be continued at that level of anticoagulation for at least one year after an embolism occurs, after which dosage may be reduced to provide a PT of 1.3 to 1.5 (INR 2.0 to 3.0) times the control value. Long-term therapy is recommended.

    Mitral annular calcification associated with atrial fibrillation: PT 1.3 to 1.5 (INR 2.0 to 3.0) times the control value. Long-term therapy is recommended.

    Mechanical prosthetic heart valves: PT 1.5 to 2.0 (INR 3.0 to 4.5) times the control value. Dipyridamole (400 mg per day) may be added to the regimen (optional, although it is strongly recommended if an embolism occurs despite adequate anticoagulation). If the recommended level of anticoagulation is contraindicated or not tolerated, a lower dose that provides a PT of 1.3 to 1.5 (INR 2.0 to 3.0) times control should be administered concurrently with dipyridamole (400 mg per day). Long-term therapy is recommended.

    Bioprosthetic mitral heart valves: PT 1.3 to 1.5 (INR 2.0 to 3.0) times the control value for three months following insertion. However, if there is a history of systemic embolism, evidence of a left atrial thrombus, or atrial fibrillation, dosage sufficient to prolong the PT to 1.5 to 2.0 (INR 3.0 to 4.5) times the control value should be administered for three months, followed by long-term therapy at a reduced dosage that provides a PT of 1.3 to 1.5 (INR 2.0 to 3.0) times the control value.

    Atrial fibrillation and systemic embolism: PT 1.5 to 2 (INR 3.0 to 4.5) times the control value. Therapy should be continued at that level of anticoagulation for one year after an embolism occurs, after which dosage may be reduced to provide a PT of 1.3 to 1.5 (INR 2.0 to 3.0) times the control value. Long-term therapy is recommended.

    Atrial fibrillation associated with dilated and hypertrophic cardiomyopathy: PT 1.3 to 1.5 (INR 2.0 to 3.0) times the control value. Long-term therapy is recommended.

    Atrial fibrillation associated with congestive heart failure: Long-term anticoagulation providing a PT of 1.3 to 1.5 (INR 2.0 to 3.0) times the control value should be considered.

    Atrial fibrillation associated with coronary artery disease, hypertension, congenital heart disease, or other forms of nonvalvular heart disease: Although conclusive evidence indicating that anticoagulation is required in these circumstances is lacking, anticoagulation (PT 1.3 to 1.5 [INR 2.0 to 3.0] times the control value) should be considered for young patients who are not at increased risk of hemorrhagic complications.

    Atrial fibrillation associated with thyrotoxic heart disease: PT 1.3 to 1.5 (INR 2.0 to 3.0) times the control value. Treatment should be continued for four weeks after sinus rhythm and a euthyroid state have been restored.

    Atrial fibrillation, idiopathic: Long-term anticoagulation is not needed for young patients. However, for patients 60 years of age or older, long-term anticoagulation (PT 1.3 to 1.5 [INR 2.0 to 3.0] times the control value) should be considered on an individual basis.

    Cardioversion (elective) of atrial fibrillation: PT 1.3 to 1.5 (INR 2.0 to 3.0) times the control value. Therapy should be started three weeks before elective cardioversion and continued until normal sinus rhythm has been maintained for at least four weeks. Anticoagulation is not needed for cardioversion of atrial fibrillation of only one or two days' duration, or for cardioversion of atrial flutter or supraventricular tachycardia, unless other risk factors for systemic embolism exist.

    Anterior transmural myocardial infarction (following initial thrombolytic and/or heparin therapy): PT 1.3 to 1.5 (INR 2.0 to 3.0) times the control value. Therapy is generally continued for three months.

    Acute myocardial infarction with atrial fibrillation, history of previous systemic or pulmonary embolism or venous thromboembolism, persistently decreased left ventricular function, or chronic congestive heart failure (following initial thrombolytic and/or heparin therapy): PT 1.3 to 1.5 (INR 2.0 to 3.0) times the control value for at least three months. Long-term anticoagulation may not reduce the risk of recurrent acute myocardial infarction, but is recommended if a risk factor for systemic or pulmonary embolism is still present after three months of therapy.

• For prevention of recurrent cardiogenic brain emboli (following initial heparin therapy)—Anticoagulant therapy should be initiated only if the patient is not hypertensive and a computerized tomographic (CT) scan performed 24 hours or longer following the onset of the stroke shows no evidence of hemorrhagic transformation. If severe hypertension is present, or the embolic stroke is large, there is a risk of late hemorrhagic transformation; anticoagulant therapy should be delayed for several days. If hemorrhagic transformation is documented, anticoagulant therapy should be postponed for at least 8 to 10 days. Initially, the oral anticoagulant should be administered in dosage sufficient to provide a PT of 1.5 to 2.0 (INR 3.0 to 4.5) times the control value. Therapy should be continued at that level of anticoagulation for one year after the embolism, after which dosage may be reduced to provide a PT of 1.3 to 1.5 (INR 2.0 to 3.0) times the control value. Long-term therapy is recommended.

• For prevention of recurrent arterial thrombi or emboli—PT 1.5 to 2.0 (INR 3.0 to 4.5) times the control value. If no thrombus or embolism has recurred after one year of therapy, dosage may be reduced to provide a PT of 1.3 to 1.5 (INR 2.0 to 3.0) times the control value.

Increased monitoring of the PT is recommended when any new medication, including nonprescription medication, is added to or withdrawn from the regimen of a patient stabilized on a coumarin or indandione derivative, or when the dosage of a concurrently used medication is changed. Anticoagulant dosage must be adjusted as necessary to prevent hemorrhage or loss of effect. Also, substantial alteration of initial anticoagulant dosage may be necessary when anticoagulant therapy is initiated in a patient receiving a medication known to cause significant alteration of anticoagulant effect.

Lower doses may be required for geriatric patients because enhanced anticoagulant effect may occur.

Decreased sensitivity to the effects of anticoagulants may be evident during initiation of therapy in patients with edema, hyperlipidemia, hypercholesterolemia, or hypothyroidism. Loss of anticoagulant effect may occur if any of these conditions develop during therapy. Correction of these problems will increase or restore the effectiveness of the anticoagulant.

Some patients also exhibit resistance to anticoagulant therapy because of genetic variations in the vitamin K receptor site or because of an increased rate of anticoagulant metabolism and excretion. Doses much higher than those usually recommended may be required to achieve successful anticoagulation in these patients. Some patients resistant to therapy with a coumarin derivative may respond to the indandione derivative anisindione.

Increased anticoagulant effect may occur in a previously stabilized patient if prolonged fever occurs during therapy.

When anticoagulant therapy is initiated with heparin and continued with a coumarin or indandione derivative, it is recommended that both agents be given concurrently until PT determinations indicate an adequate response to the coumarin or indandione derivative. However, the fact that heparin may prolong the PT must be kept in mind. Full therapeutic doses given by subcutaneous administration or as a single intravenous injection may prolong the PT considerably because of the high concentrations of heparin in the blood, whereas therapeutic doses of heparin given by continuous intravenous infusion or low (prophylactic) doses of heparin administered subcutaneously usually do not increase the PT by more than a few seconds. To minimize problems in interpreting PT test results, draw blood for the PT test just prior to, or at least 5 hours after, a single intravenous dose or 24 hours following subcutaneous administration of a full therapeutic dose of heparin. Also, the fact that reduction in PT may reflect early depletion of factor VII rather than peak antithrombotic effects of coumarin or indandione derivatives must be kept in mind. Some clinicians recommend continuation of heparin therapy for up to 5 to 7 days after initiation of therapy with a coumarin or indandione derivative to ensure that peak antithrombogenic activity has been reached.

Manufacturers' dosage recommendations may include administration of an initial loading dose that is to be gradually reduced to the maintenance dose indicated by PT determinations. Many clinicians recommend that large loading doses of these medications be avoided because of the increased risk of hemorrhage and because a more rapid anticoagulant effect can be achieved with heparin.

It is recommended that therapy with these medications be discontinued if there is any suspicion that anticoagulant-induced tissue necrosis is developing. Anticoagulant therapy may be continued with heparin, if necessary.

## Diet/Nutrition

Loss of anticoagulant effect may occur in a previously stabilized patient if intake of vitamin K from dietary sources (green leafy vegetables such as broccoli, cabbage, collard greens, kale, lettuce, or spinach and, to a lesser extent, dairy products or meats) or vitamin K–containing multiple vitamins or nutritional supplements is increased during therapy.

Increased anticoagulant effect may occur in a previously stabilized patient if prolonged malnutrition or vitamin C deficiency develops, or if diarrhea, other illness, or changes in diet resulting in decreased intake or absorption of vitamin K occur during therapy.

---

## *ANISINDIONE*

# Summary of Differences

Physicochemical characteristics: Indandione-derivative anticoagulant.
Pharmacology/pharmacokinetics: See *Pharmacology/Pharmacokinetics.*
   Precautions:
      Drug interactions and/or related problems—Concurrent use with heparin does not lead to severe factor IX deficiency.
      Laboratory value alterations—Alkaline urine may turn orange.
      Patient monitoring—Monitoring of hematopoietic function, hepatic function, renal function, and urine protein may also be necessary.
Side/adverse effects: See *Side/Adverse Effects.*

# Oral Dosage Forms
## ANISINDIONE TABLETS

**Usual adult and adolescent dose**
Oral, 25 to 250 mg a day, as indicated by prothrombin-time determinations.

**Usual pediatric dose**
Dosage has not been established.

**Strength(s) usually available**
U.S.—
   50 mg (Rx) [*Miradon*].
Canada—
   Not commercially available.

**Packaging and storage**
Store below 40 °C (104 °F), preferably between 15 and 30 °C (59 and 86 °F), in a well-closed container, unless otherwise specified by manufacturer.

**Auxiliary labeling**
• Do not take other medicines without advice from your doctor.

---

## *DICUMAROL*

# Summary of Differences

Physicochemical characteristics: Coumarin-derivative anticoagulant.
Pharmacology/pharmacokinetics: See *Pharmacology/Pharmacokinetics.*
Side/adverse effects: See *Side/Adverse Effects.*

# Oral Dosage Forms
## DICUMAROL TABLETS USP

**Usual adult and adolescent dose**
Oral, 25 to 200 mg a day, as indicated by prothrombin-time determinations.

**Usual pediatric dose**
Dosage has not been established.

**Strength(s) usually available**
U.S.—
   25 mg (Rx) [GENERIC].
Canada—
   Not commercially available.

**Packaging and storage**
Store below 40 °C (104 °F), preferably between 15 and 30 °C (59 and 86 °F). Store in a well-closed container.

**Auxiliary labeling**
• Do not take other medicines without advice from your doctor.

## *WARFARIN*

## Summary of Differences

Indications: Also used for treatment of transient ischemic attacks in females and males.
Physicochemical characteristics: Coumarin-derivative anticoagulant.
Pharmacology/pharmacokinetics: See *Pharmacology/Pharmacokinetics*.
Side/adverse effects: See *Side/Adverse Effects*.

## Oral Dosage Forms

### WARFARIN SODIUM TABLETS USP

**Usual adult and adolescent dose**
Oral, 10 to 15 mg a day for two to four days, then 2 to 10 mg a day, as indicated by prothrombin-time determinations.

**Usual pediatric dose**
Dosage has not been established.

**Strength(s) usually available**
U.S.—
    1 mg (Rx) [*Coumadin*].
    2 mg (Rx) [*Coumadin* (scored; lactose); *Panwarfin* (lactose); *Sofarin* (scored; lactose); GENERIC].
    2.5 mg (Rx) [*Coumadin* (scored; lactose); *Panwarfin* (lactose); *Sofarin* (scored; lactose); GENERIC].
    4 mg (Rx) [*Coumadin* (scored; lactose)].
    5 mg (Rx) [*Coumadin* (scored; lactose); *Panwarfin* (lactose); *Sofarin* (scored; lactose); GENERIC].
    7.5 mg (Rx) [*Coumadin* (scored; lactose); *Panwarfin* (scored; lactose; tartrazine); GENERIC].
    10 mg (Rx) [*Coumadin* (scored; lactose); *Panwarfin* (scored; lactose); GENERIC].
Canada—
    2 mg (Rx) [*Coumadin* (scored; lactose)].
    2.5 mg (Rx) [*Coumadin* (scored; lactose)].
    4 mg (Rx) [*Coumadin* (scored; lactose)].
    5 mg (Rx) [*Coumadin* (scored; lactose); *Warfilone* (scored; tartrazine)].
    10 mg (Rx) [*Coumadin* (scored; lactose)].

**Packaging and storage**
Store below 40 °C (104 °F), preferably between 15 and 30 °C (59 and 86 °F), unless otherwise specified by manufacturer. Store in a tight, light-resistant container.

**Auxiliary labeling**
• Do not take other medicines without advice from your doctor.

## Parenteral Dosage Forms

### WARFARIN SODIUM FOR INJECTION USP

**Usual adult and adolescent dose**
Intramuscular or intravenous, 10 to 15 mg a day for two to four days, then 2 to 10 mg a day, as indicated by prothrombin-time determinations.

**Usual pediatric dose**
Dosage has not been established.

**Size(s) usually available**
U.S.—
    50 mg (Rx) [*Coumadin* (thimerosal)].
Canada—
    Not commercially available.

**Packaging and storage**
Store below 40 °C (104 °F), preferably between 15 and 30 °C (59 and 86 °F), unless otherwise specified by manufacturer. Protect from light.

**Preparation of dosage form**
Warfarin sodium for injection is reconstituted by adding 2 mL of sterile water for injection to the vial containing 50 mg of warfarin sodium to provide a solution containing 25 mg of warfarin sodium per mL.

**Stability**
Administer immediately after reconstitution.
Discard any unused solution.

Revised: June 1990
Interim revision: 07/28/94

## Table 1. Drug Interactions and/or Related Problems

The following drug interactions and/or related problems have been selected on the basis of their potential clinical significance (possible mechanism in parentheses where appropriate)—not necessarily inclusive (» = major clinical significance):

Note: In addition to the listed interactions, the possibility should be considered that the risk of hemorrhage may be increased by concurrent use of any medication that may inhibit platelet aggregation or cause hypoprothrombinemia, thrombocytopenia, or gastrointestinal ulceration.

Combinations containing any of the following medications, depending on the amount present, may also interact with this medication.

| Drug | Effect on Anticoagulant Activity | Mechanism* | Other Effects† | Additional Information |
|---|---|---|---|---|
| Acetaminophen (chronic high-dose usage) | Increase | A | | Does not apply to occasional use or chronic use of less than 2 grams per day of acetaminophen |
| Alcohol (acute intoxication) | Increase | B | | Other acute effects of alcohol on the liver may also be involved |
| (chronic abuse) | Decrease | C | | However, increased activity possible in advanced hepatic cirrhosis |
| » Allopurinol | Increase | B | | |
| Aminosalicylates | Increase | A | | |
| » Amiodarone | Increase | B | | Potentiation reported to occur in 4 to 6 days after initiation of amiodarone therapy and to persist up to 4 months following discontinuation of amiodarone |
| » Anabolic steroids | Increase | D, E | | Especially with 17-alpha-alkylated compounds |
| » Androgens | Increase | D, E | | |
| Anesthetics, inhalation‡ | Increase | Unknown | | |
| Antacids | Decrease | F | | May be avoided if medications given several hours apart |

## Table 1. Drug Interactions and/or Related Problems *(continued)*

| Drug | Effect on Anticoagulant Activity | Mechanism* | Other Effects† | Additional Information |
|---|---|---|---|---|
| Antibiotics‡ | Increase | G | | Significant potentiation very rare if dietary intake of vitamin K adequate |
| | | | | See also separate table entries for azlocillin, carbenicillin, cefamandole, cefoperazone, chloramphenicol, erythromycins, mezlocillin, piperacillin, rifampin, and ticarcillin |
| » Antidiabetic agents, oral | Increase<br>Decrease | H<br>I | | Initial effect<br>With continued concurrent use<br>Hepatic metabolism of antidiabetic agent may be decreased, leading to increased plasma concentration and half-life, hypoglycemic effect, and risk of toxicity of antidiabetic agent, especially with dicumarol |
| Ascorbic acid | Decrease | | | With large doses of ascorbic acid |
| » Aspirin | Increase | A (with large doses), H | a, b | Decreased platelet aggregation may occur with single doses as low as 40 mg |
| » Azlocillin | | | a | |
| » Barbiturates | Decrease | C | | |
| Bromelains | Increase | Unknown | | |
| » Carbamazepine | Decrease | C | | |
| » Carbenicillin (parenteral) | | | a | |
| » Cefamandole | Increase | D | a | |
| » Cefoperazone | Increase | D | a | |
| » Chloral hydrate | Increase | H | | Initial effect, usually during first 2 weeks of concurrent use; with continued concurrent use, anticoagulant activity may return to baseline level or be decreased |
| » Chloramphenicol | Increase | B | | |
| Chlorinated insecticides‡ | Decrease | C | | |
| Chlorobutanol‡ | Decrease | Unknown | | |
| » Cholestyramine | Decrease<br>Decrease<br>Increase | F<br>J<br>K | | May be avoided if medications given 6 hours apart<br>Not avoided if medications given 6 hours apart |
| Chymotrypsin‡ | Increase | Unknown | | |
| » Cimetidine | Increase | B | | |
| Cinchophen | Increase | Unknown | | |
| » Clofibrate | Increase | D, H | | Other mechanisms may also be involved |
| Colchicine | | | b | May also cause thrombocytopenia (with chronic use) and coagulation defects including disseminated intravascular coagulation (with overdose) |

*Mechanisms leading to increase or decrease in anticoagulant activity as shown by measurement of prothrombin time: (A) Decreased hepatic synthesis of procoagulant factors. (B) Inhibition of enzymatic metabolism of anticoagulant. (C) Accelerated metabolism of anticoagulant secondary to stimulation of hepatic microsomal enzyme activity. (D) Alteration of procoagulant factor synthesis or catabolism. (E) Increased receptor affinity for anticoagulant. (F) Decreased absorption of anticoagulant from gastrointestinal tract. (G) Decreased vitamin K synthesis secondary to alterations in intestinal flora. (H) Displacement of anticoagulant from protein-binding sites. (I) Increased metabolism of anticoagulant. (J) Interference with enterohepatic circulation of anticoagulant. (K) Decreased vitamin K absorption or synthesis. (L) Increased hepatic synthesis of procoagulant factors. (M) Reduction of plasma volume leading to concentration of procoagulant factors in the blood; diuretic-induced improvement of hepatic congestion may lead to improved hepatic function resulting in increased procoagulant factor synthesis. (N) Severe factor IX deficiency (with coumarin derivatives only). (O) Increased prothrombin synthesis or activation.

†Effects resulting in increased risk of hemorrhage in patients receiving anticoagulants; cannot be shown by measurement of prothrombin time: (a) Inhibition of platelet aggregation. (b) Potential occurrence of gastrointestinal ulceration or hemorrhage during therapy. (c) Adverse effect on vascular integrity. (d) Interference with platelet formation. (e) Anticoagulant activity of heparin. (f) Thrombolytic activity may lead to hemorrhage.

‡Clinical significance has not been determined.

## Table 1. Drug Interactions and/or Related Problems *(continued)*

| Drug | Effect on Anticoagulant Activity | Mechanism* | Other Effects† | Additional Information |
|------|------|------|------|------|
| » Colestipol | Decrease<br>Increase | F<br>K | | May be avoided if medications given 6 hours apart<br>Not avoided if medications given 6 hours apart |
| » Contraceptives, oral | Decrease<br>Increase | L<br>Unknown | | |
| Corticotropin | Increase<br>Decrease | Unknown<br>Unknown | b, c | |
| Cyclophosphamide | Increase<br>Decrease | A<br>Unknown | d | |
| » Danazol | Increase | A | | |
| » Dextran | | | a | |
| » Dextrothyroxine | Increase | D, E | | Effect may depend on thyroid status of patient |
| Diazoxide | Increase | H | | |
| » Diflunisal | Increase | H | a, b | Decreased platelet aggregation occurs only with greater-than-recommended daily doses |
| » Dipyridamole | | | a | With doses greater than 400 mg per day |
| Disopyramide‡ | Decrease<br>Increase | Unknown<br>Unknown | | |
| » Disulfiram | Increase | B | | May also act in the liver to increase directly the hypoprothrombinemia-inducing activity of coumarin derivatives |
| Diuretics‡ | Decrease | M | | See also separate table entry for ethacrynic acid |
| Divalproex | | | a | |
| » Erythromycins | Increase | B | | |
| » Estramustine | Decrease | L | | |
| » Estrogens | Decrease | L | | |
| Ethacrynic acid‡ | Increase | H | b | |
| » Ethchlorvynol | Decrease | C | | |
| » Fenoprofen | Increase | H | a, b | |
| » Gemfibrozil | Increase | Unknown | | |
| Glucagon‡ | Increase | Unknown | | Potentiation reported only with doses >25 mg per day for 2 or more days; however, these doses are rarely if ever used |
| Glucocorticoids | Increase<br>Decrease | Unknown<br>Unknown | b, c | |
| » Glutethimide | Decrease | C | | |
| » Griseofulvin | Decrease | C | | |
| Haloperidol‡ | Decrease<br>Increase | C<br>Unknown | | |
| Heparin | Increase | N | e | May prolong prothrombin time used to monitor therapy, especially when given as an intravenous bolus or if full therapeutic doses given subcutaneously; to minimize problems, draw blood for test just prior to, or at least 5 hours after, the intravenous bolus dose or 24 hours after subcutaneous injection of a full therapeutic dose |
| Ibuprofen | | | a, b | |
| » Indomethacin | Increase | H | a, b | |
| Influenza vaccine | Increase | B | | |
| Isoniazid | Increase | B | | |
| Ketoconazole | Increase | Unknown | | |
| Ketoprofen | | | a, b | |

## Table 1. Drug Interactions and/or Related Problems *(continued)*

| Drug | Effect on Anticoagulant Activity | Mechanism* | Other Effects† | Additional Information |
|------|------|------|------|------|
| Laxatives, bulk-forming | Decrease | F | | May be avoided if medications given several hours apart |
| Meclofenamate | Increase | H | b | |
| » Mefenamic acid | Increase | H | b | |
| Meperidine | Increase | Unknown | | |
| Mercaptopurine | Increase<br>Decrease | A<br>O | d | |
| » Methimazole | Increase | A | | Effect may also depend upon dosage and subsequent thyroid status of patient |
| Methotrexate | Increase | A | d | |
| Methyldopa | Increase | Unknown | | |
| Methylphenidate | Increase | B | | |
| » Metronidazole | Increase | B | | |
| » Mezlocillin | | | a | |
| Miconazole | Increase | Unknown | | |
| Mineral oil | Decrease<br>Increase | F<br>K | | May be avoided if medications given 6 hours apart<br>Not avoided if medications given 6 hours apart |
| Monoamine oxidase (MAO) inhibitors‡ | Increase | Unknown | | |
| » Nalidixic acid | Increase | H | | |
| Naproxen | | | a, b | |
| Nifedipine | Increase | H | | Nifedipine may also be displaced from protein-binding sites, leading to increased plasma concentrations of free [unbound] medication and risk of toxicity |
| » Phenylbutazone | Increase | B, H | a, b | |
| » Phenytoin, and possibly other hydantoin-type anticonvulsants | Increase<br><br>Decrease | H<br><br>C | | Initial effect<br>With continued concurrent use<br>Hepatic metabolism of hydantoin anticonvulsants, especially phenytoin, may be decreased, leading to increased anticonvulsant plasma concentration, half-life, and risk of toxicity, especially with dicumarol |
| » Piperacillin | | | a | |
| Piroxicam | | | a, b | Possibility that anticoagulant activity may be increased because of displacement from protein-binding sites should be considered; however, has not been demonstrated |
| » Plicamycin | Increase | A | d | |
| » Primidone | Decrease | C | | Effect caused by barbiturate metabolite |
| Propoxyphene‡ | Increase | Unknown | | |
| » Propylthiouracil | Increase | A | | Effect may also depend upon dosage and subsequent thyroid status of patient |

*Mechanisms leading to increase or decrease in anticoagulant activity as shown by measurement of prothrombin time: (A) Decreased hepatic synthesis of procoagulant factors. (B) Inhibition of enzymatic metabolism of anticoagulant. (C) Accelerated metabolism of anticoagulant secondary to stimulation of hepatic microsomal enzyme activity. (D) Alteration of procoagulant factor synthesis or catabolism. (E) Increased receptor affinity for anticoagulant. (F) Decreased absorption of anticoagulant from gastrointestinal tract. (G) Decreased vitamin K synthesis secondary to alterations in intestinal flora. (H) Displacement of anticoagulant from protein-binding sites. (I) Increased metabolism of anticoagulant. (J) Interference with enterohepatic circulation of anticoagulant. (K) Decreased vitamin K absorption or synthesis. (L) Increased hepatic synthesis of procoagulant factors. (M) Reduction of plasma volume leading to concentration of procoagulant factors in the blood; diuretic-induced improvement of hepatic congestion may lead to improved hepatic function resulting in increased procoagulant factor synthesis. (N) Severe factor IX deficiency (with coumarin derivatives only). (O) Increased prothrombin synthesis or activation.

†Effects resulting in increased risk of hemorrhage in patients receiving anticoagulants; cannot be shown by measurement of prothrombin time: (a) Inhibition of platelet aggregation. (b) Potential occurrence of gastrointestinal ulceration or hemorrhage during therapy. (c) Adverse effect on vascular integrity. (d) Interference with platelet formation. (e) Anticoagulant activity of heparin. (f) Thrombolytic activity may lead to hemorrhage.

‡Clinical significance has not been determined.

## Table 1. Drug Interactions and/or Related Problems *(continued)*

| Drug | Effect on Anticoagulant Activity | Mechanism* | Other Effects† | Additional Information |
|------|----------------------------------|------------|----------------|------------------------|
| » Quinidine | Increase | D, E | | |
| Quinine | Increase | A | | |
| Radioactive compounds | Increase | Unknown | | |
| » Rifampin | Decrease | C | | |
| » Salicylates | Increase | A (with large doses), H | b | See also separate table entries for aspirin and diflunisal |
| » Streptokinase | | | f | Concurrent use not recommended; however, sequential use may be indicated |
| » Sulfinpyrazone | Increase | B, H | a, b | Biphasic response, with decreased anticoagulation occurring following initial potentiation, reported in one patient; reason for this unclear since other reports indicate only potentiation of anticoagulant effect |
| » Sulfonamides | Increase | B, H | | |
| » Sulindac | Increase | H | a, b | |
| Testolactone | Increase | | | |
| » Thyroid hormones | Increase | D, E | | Effect may depend upon dosage and subsequent thyroid status of patient |
| » Ticarcillin | | | a | |
| Tobacco smoking | Decrease | C | | Thrombogenic potential of tobacco smoking should also be considered |
| Tolmetin | | | a, b | |
| Tricyclic antidepressants‡ | Increase | B | | Especially with amitriptyline or nortriptyline |
| » Urokinase | | | f | Concurrent use not recommended; however, sequential use may be indicated |
| Valproic acid | Increase | A | a | |
| Verapamil | Increase | H | | Verapamil may also be displaced from protein-binding sites, leading to increased plasma concentrations of free [unbound] medication and risk of toxicity |
| Vitamin A | Increase | Unknown | | With high doses of vitamin |
| Vitamin E‡ | Increase | Unknown | | With high doses of vitamin |
| » Vitamin K | Decrease | L | | |

*Mechanisms leading to increase or decrease in anticoagulant activity as shown by measurement of prothrombin time: (A) Decreased hepatic synthesis of procoagulant factors. (B) Inhibition of enzymatic metabolism of anticoagulant. (C) Accelerated metabolism of anticoagulant secondary to stimulation of hepatic microsomal enzyme activity. (D) Alteration of procoagulant factor synthesis or catabolism. (E) Increased receptor affinity for anticoagulant. (F) Decreased absorption of anticoagulant from gastrointestinal tract. (G) Decreased vitamin K synthesis secondary to alterations in intestinal flora. (H) Displacement of anticoagulant from protein-binding sites. (I) Increased metabolism of anticoagulant. (J) Interference with enterohepatic circulation of anticoagulant. (K) Decreased vitamin K absorption or synthesis. (L) Increased hepatic synthesis of procoagulant factors. (M) Reduction of plasma volume leading to concentration of procoagulant factors in the blood; diuretic-induced improvement of hepatic congestion may lead to improved hepatic function resulting in increased procoagulant factor synthesis. (N) Severe factor IX deficiency (with coumarin derivatives only). (O) Increased prothrombin synthesis or activation.

†Effects resulting in increased risk of hemorrhage in patients receiving anticoagulants; cannot be shown by measurement of prothrombin time: (a) Inhibition of platelet aggregation. (b) Potential occurrence of gastrointestinal ulceration or hemorrhage during therapy. (c) Adverse effect on vascular integrity. (d) Interference with platelet formation. (e) Anticoagulant activity of heparin. (f) Thrombolytic activity may lead to hemorrhage.

‡Clinical significance has not been determined.

---

# ANTICONVULSANTS, DIONE   Systemic

This monograph includes information on the following: Paramethadione*; Trimethadione*†.

BAN:

Trimethadione—Troxidone

VA CLASSIFICATION (Primary/Secondary):

Paramethadione—CN400

Trimethadione—CN400

Other commonly used names for trimethadione are TMO, trimethadionum, trimethinum, and troxidone.

Note: For a listing of dosage forms and brand names by country availability, see *Dosage Forms* section(s). For a listing of brand names for the articles in this monograph, refer to the General Index.

*Not commercially available in the U.S.
†Not commercially available in Canada.

# Category

Anticonvulsant.

# Indications

## Accepted

Epilepsy, absence seizure pattern (treatment)—Paramethadione and trimethadione are indicated in the control of absence (petit mal) seizures that are refractory to treatment with other medications.

Paramethadione and trimethadione should not be used unless other less toxic anticonvulsants have been ineffective in controlling seizures.

# Pharmacology/Pharmacokinetics

## Physicochemical characteristics

Chemical group—
Oxazolidinediones
Molecular weight—
Paramethadione: 157.17.
Trimethadione: 143.14.
pKa—
Dimethadione (DMO; active metabolite of trimethadione): 6.13.

## Mechanism of action/Effect

Dione anticonvulsants reduce T-type calcium currents in thalamic neurons, including thalamic relay neurons. This raises the threshold for repetitive activity in the thalamus, and inhibits corticothalamic transmission. Thus, the abnormal thalamocortical rhythmicity, which is thought to underlie the 3-Hz spike-and-wave discharge seen on electroencephalogram (EEG) with absence seizures, is dampened. The maximal seizure pattern in patients undergoing electroconvulsive therapy is not modified.

## Absorption

Rapid.

## Protein binding

Insignificant.

## Biotransformation

Hepatic; both medications almost completely demethylated to active metabolites.

## Half-life

Paramethadione—12 to 24 hours; active metabolite—unknown.

Trimethadione—11 to 16 hours; active metabolite (dimethadione)—about 10 days.

## Time to peak serum concentration

Trimethadione—30 to 60 minutes.

## Elimination

Metabolites— Renal (slow).

# Precautions to Consider

## Cross-sensitivity and/or related problems

Patients sensitive to one dione anticonvulsant may be sensitive to the other also.

## Carcinogenicity

No data are available on long-term potential for carcinogenicity in animals or humans.

## Pregnancy/Reproduction

Pregnancy—Use of dione anticonvulsants is not recommended during pregnancy.

Controlled studies in humans have not been done. However, there have been reports of congenital malformations and fetal death occurring with dione anticonvulsant use in humans. Fetal exposure to paramethadione and trimethadione has been associated with "fetal trimethadione syndrome," characterized by an increased frequency of congenital malformations including malformed ears, urogenital malformations, and skeletal abnormalities. An increase in fetal deaths and high rates of mental retardation in surviving children have also been reported. Patients should be advised that an effective means of contraception should be used during therapy, and that the physician should be informed if pregnancy occurs.

For paramethadione: FDA Pregnancy Category D.

For trimethadione: FDA pregnancy category not assigned.

Delivery—Exposure to dione anticonvulsants prior to delivery may lead to a neonatal coagulation defect characterized by decreased concentrations of vitamin K–dependent coagulation factors, and increased prothrombin times and/or increased partial thromboplastin times, resulting in an increased risk of life-threatening hemorrhage in the neonate, usually within 24 hours of birth. Dione anticonvulsants may also produce a vitamin K deficiency in the mother, causing increased bleeding during delivery. Risk may be reduced by administering vitamin K to the mother for one month prior to, and during delivery and to the neonate, intramuscularly or subcutaneously, immediately after birth.

## Breast-feeding

It is not known whether dione anticonvulsants are distributed into breast milk. However, many medications are distributed into breast milk, and, because of the high toxicity of dione anticonvulsants, breast-feeding is not recommended.

## Pediatrics

Appropriate studies on the relationship of age to the effects of the dione anticonvulsants have not been performed in the pediatric population. However, no pediatrics-specific problems have been documented to date.

## Geriatrics

Appropriate studies on the relationship of age to the effects of dione anticonvulsants have not been performed in the geriatric population. However, one small pharmacokinetic study of trimethadione found that metabolism may be decreased, and half-life increased in elderly patients.

## Dental

The leukopenic and thrombocytopenic effects of dione anticonvulsants may result in an increased incidence of microbial infection, delayed healing, and gingival bleeding. If leukopenia or thrombocytopenia occurs, dental work should be deferred until blood counts have returned to normal. Patients should be instructed in proper oral hygiene during treatment, including caution in use of regular toothbrushes, dental floss, and toothpicks.

## Drug interactions and/or related problems

The following drug interactions and/or related problems have been selected on the basis of their potential clinical significance (possible mechanism in parentheses where appropriate)—not necessarily inclusive (» = major clinical significance):

Note: Combinations containing any of the following medications, depending on the amount present, may also interact with this medication.

Acetazolamide
(concurrent use may potentiate acidosis, enhance ophthalmic toxicity, and alter the distribution and excretion of the active metabolite of trimethadione)

» Alcohol and
» Central nervous system (CNS) depression–producing medications, other (See *Appendix II*)
(CNS depression may be enhanced)

Antidepressants, tricyclic, or
Haloperidol or
Loxapine or
Maprotiline or
Molindone or
Monoamine oxidase (MAO) inhibitors, including furazolidone, procarbazine, and more than 10 mg a day of selegiline, or
Phenothiazines or
Pimozide or
Thioxanthenes
(concurrent use may lower the convulsive threshold, enhance CNS depression, and decrease the effects of the anticonvulsant medication; dosage adjustments may be necessary)

Phenacemide
(concurrent use with dione anticonvulsants may result in additive toxicity)

## Medical considerations/Contraindications

The medical considerations/contraindications included here have been selected on the basis of their potential clinical significance (reasons given in parentheses where appropriate)—not necessarily inclusive (» = major clinical significance).

*Risk-benefit should be considered when the following medical problems exist:*

» Blood dyscrasias or
» Hepatic function impairment or
Optic nerve or retinal disease or
» Renal function impairment
(risk of exacerbation of pre-existing conditions)
(decreased metabolism with hepatic function impairment)

Porphyria, acute intermittent
  (risk of exacerbation with the use of trimethadione)
» Sensitivity to dione anticonvulsants

**Patient monitoring**
The following may be especially important in patient monitoring (other tests may be warranted in some patients, depending on condition; » = major clinical significance):

» Blood cell and platelet counts
  (a complete blood count is recommended prior to start of treatment and monthly thereafter; if no abnormality appears within 12 months, frequency of monitoring may be decreased; if neutrophil count is between 2500 and 3000, blood count should be done more frequently than once a month; if neutrophil count is 2500 or less, withdrawal of dione anticonvulsant is indicated to prevent severe bone marrow depression)

» Hepatic function determinations
  (recommended prior to initiation of dione therapy, monthly for several months, then every few months thereafter; if jaundice or other signs of liver dysfunction occur, the medication should be withdrawn)

  Ophthalmological examinations
  (recommended every 6 months; hemeralopia can usually be reversed by decreasing dione dosage; if scotomata occur, medication should be withdrawn)

» Renal function determinations
  (recommended prior to initiation of therapy and, during therapy, at monthly intervals for several months, then every few months thereafter)

» Urinalysis
  (recommended prior to initiation of dione therapy and monthly thereafter; if persistent or increasing albuminuria or other significant renal abnormality occurs, medication should be withdrawn)

## Side/Adverse Effects

The following side/adverse effects have been selected on the basis of their potential clinical significance (possible signs and symptoms in parentheses where appropriate)—not necessarily inclusive:

**Those indicating need for medical attention**
Incidence more frequent
  *Hemeralopia, scotomata, or diplopia* (changes in vision, especially night blindness, glare or snowy image caused by bright light, or double vision)
Incidence rare
  *Allergic reaction* (itching of skin associated with swollen lymph nodes; enlarged liver and spleen); *blood dyscrasias, including agranulocytosis, aplastic anemia, eosinophilia, hypoplastic anemia, leukopenia, pancytopenia, and thrombocytopenia* (sore throat and fever; unusual bleeding, such as recurring nosebleeds, bleeding gums, or vaginal bleeding; red or purple spots on skin; unusual tiredness or weakness)—fatalities have occurred; *confusion; convulsions, tonic-clonic, precipitation of; hepatitis* (loss of appetite; unusual tiredness; yellow eyes or skin; weight loss; fever; skin rash or itching; nausea or vomiting; dark urine; pain in abdomen and joints); *lymphadenopathies* (swollen lymph nodes); *myasthenia gravis–like syndrome* (severe muscle weakness, including drooping eyelids; double vision; difficulty in chewing, swallowing, talking, and breathing; severe tiredness); *nephrosis* (swelling of face, hands, legs, and feet; cloudy urine)—fatalities have occurred; *skin rash; systemic lupus erythematosus (SLE)-like syndrome* (chest pain; fever; muscle or joint pain; shortness of breath or troubled breathing; skin rash; swollen lymph nodes)

  Note: If lymph node enlargement or lupus-like manifestations, or jaundice or other symptoms of liver dysfunction occur, dione anticonvulsant should be withdrawn. Patients with more severe systemic lupus-like manifestations may require moderate doses of corticosteroids until symptoms subside.

  If symptoms of *myasthenia gravis–like syndrome* occur, dione anticonvulsant should be withdrawn. The myasthenic reaction resolves slowly, and neostigmine may be used to control weakness in the interim.

  *Skin rash* is usually acneform or morbilliform. If skin rash appears, dione anticonvulsant should be withdrawn promptly to prevent exfoliative dermatitis or severe forms of erythema multiforme. After all signs of rash, even minor rash, have cleared, the dione anticonvulsant may be reinstituted cautiously.

**Those indicating need for medical attention only if they continue or are bothersome**
Incidence more frequent
  *Dizziness; drowsiness; headache; irritability; photophobia* (increased sensitivity of eyes to light)

  Note: *Drowsiness* tends to diminish with continued therapy. However, if drowsiness continues, dosage reduction may be necessary. Paramethadione may have a slightly greater sedative action than trimethadione.

Incidence less frequent
  *Anorexia* (loss of appetite); *behavior or mood changes; blood pressure changes; gastrointestinal effects, specifically abdominal or stomach pain, nausea,or vomiting; hair loss; hiccups; insomnia* (trouble in sleeping); *paresthesias* (tingling, burning, or prickly sensations); *unusual tiredness or weakness; unusual weight loss*

## Overdose

For more information on the management of overdose or unintentional ingestion, **contact a Poison Control Center** (see *Poison Control Center Listing*).

The following effects have been selected on the basis of their potential clinical significance (possible signs and symptoms in parentheses where appropriate)—not necessarily inclusive:
Acute effects
  *Ataxia* (clumsiness or unsteadiness); *coma*—following massive overdose; *dizziness, severe; drowsiness, severe; nausea, severe; visual disturbances*

**Treatment of overdose**
To decrease absorption—Immediate evacuation of stomach by induction of emesis, lavage, or both is recommended.

To enhance elimination—Alkalinization of urine is reported to enhance elimination of active metabolites.

Monitoring—Frequent monitoring of vital signs and close patient observation are required. Following recovery, a complete blood count and a careful evaluation of hepatic and renal function should be done.

Supportive care—General supportive care is necessary in dione anticonvulsant overdose treatment. Patients in whom intentional overdose is confirmed or suspected should be referred for psychiatric consultation.

## Patient Consultation

As an aid to patient consultation, refer to *Advice for the Patient, Anticonvulsants, Dione (Systemic)*.

In providing consultation, consider emphasizing the following selected information (» = major clinical significance):

**Before using this medication**
» Conditions affecting use, especially:
    Sensitivity to dione anticonvulsants
    Pregnancy and delivery—Risk of congenital malformations in the fetus; women of child-bearing potential advised to use an effective method of birth control during therapy, and to notify physician immediately if pregnancy occurs; bleeding problems may occur in mother during delivery and in baby immediately after delivery.
    Other medications, especially CNS depressants
    Other medical problems, especially blood dyscrasias, hepatic function impairment, or renal function impairment

**Proper use of this medication**
*Proper administration:*
*For paramethadione capsules*
    Swallowing whole; not breaking, chewing, or crushing before swallowing
*For trimethadione solution*
    Using an accurate measuring device, such as a specially marked measuring spoon, a plastic syringe, or a small graduated cup
*For trimethadione tablets*
    Chewing, or crushing and dissolving in small amount of water
*For all dosage forms*
    Taking with a small amount of food or milk to reduce gastric irritation

» Compliance with therapy; not taking more or less medication than prescribed
» Proper dosing
    Missed dose: Taking as soon as possible; not taking if almost time for next scheduled dose; one missed dose may be added at bedtime
» Proper storage

## Precautions while using this medication

» Regular visits to physician to check progress of therapy

» Reporting sore throat, fever, general feeling of tiredness, or any unusual bleeding or bruising to physician as soon as possible

Possible vision changes, especially intolerance to bright light; wearing sunglasses and avoiding bright light; caution when driving at night

» Avoiding use of alcohol and other CNS depressants

» Caution if drowsiness occurs; not driving or doing jobs requiring alertness

» Caution if any kind of surgery, dental treatment, or emergency treatment is required

» Informing physician as soon as possible if pregnancy occurs during therapy

» Checking with physician before discontinuing medication; gradual dosage reduction is usually needed

### Side/adverse effects

Signs of potential side effects, especially hemeralopia, scotomata, or diplopia; allergic reaction; blood dyscrasias; confusion; convulsions; hepatitis; lymphadenopathies; myasthenia gravis–like syndrome; nephrosis; skin rash; and SLE–like syndrome

## General Dosing Information

Because of the potential for severe adverse reactions with dione anticonvulsant use, strict medical supervision, especially during the first year of therapy, is recommended.

Physician should be notified immediately if signs or symptoms of infection or unusual bleeding, such as sore throat, fever, malaise, easy bruising, red or purple spots on skin, nosebleed, or bleeding gums occur.

When used to replace other anticonvulsant therapy, the dosage of this medication should be increased gradually while that of the other medication is gradually decreased, to maintain seizure control.

Dione anticonvulsants do not modify the maximal seizure pattern in patients undergoing electroconvulsive therapy.

When dione anticonvulsant therapy is to be discontinued, dosage should be reduced gradually to prevent possible occurrence of absence status.

### Diet/Nutrition

Dione anticonvulsants should be taken with a small amount of food or milk to reduce gastric irritation.

---

### PARAMETHADIONE

## Summary of Differences

Side/adverse effects: Slightly greater sedative action than trimethadione.

## Oral Dosage Forms

### PARAMETHADIONE CAPSULES

#### Usual adult and adolescent dose

Anticonvulsant—

Oral, initially 300 mg three times a day, the dosage being increased by an additional 300 mg a day at one-week intervals until seizure control is obtained or until toxic symptoms appear. The total daily dose is given in three or four divided doses.

#### Usual adult prescribing limits

Up to 2.4 grams a day.

#### Usual pediatric dose

Anticonvulsant—

Children up to 2 years of age: Oral, 100 mg three times a day.

Children 2 to 6 years of age: Oral, 200 mg three times a day.

Children 6 years of age and over: Oral, 300 mg three times a day.

#### Strength(s) usually available

U.S.—

Not commercially available.

Canada—

Not commercially available.

#### Packaging and storage

Store below 40 °C (104 °F), preferably between 15 and 25 °C (59 and 77 °F), unless otherwise specified by manufacturer. Store in a tight container.

#### Auxiliary labeling

• May cause drowsiness.

• Do not chew or crush capsule.

#### Additional information

Capsules contain an oily liquid.

---

### TRIMETHADIONE

## Summary of Differences

Side/adverse effects: Slightly less sedative action than paramethadione.

## Oral Dosage Forms

### TRIMETHADIONE CAPSULES USP

#### Usual adult and adolescent dose

Anticonvulsant—

Oral, initially 300 mg three times a day, the dosage being increased by an additional 300 mg a day at one-week intervals until seizure control is obtained or until toxic symptoms appear. The total daily dose is given in three or four divided doses.

#### Usual adult prescribing limits

Up to 2.4 grams a day.

#### Usual pediatric dose

Anticonvulsant—

Oral, 13 mg per kg of body weight or 335 mg per square meter of body surface three times a day; or for

Children up to 2 years of age: Oral, 100 mg three times a day.

Children 2 to 6 years of age: Oral, 200 mg three times a day.

Children 6 years of age and over: Oral, 300 mg three or four times a day.

#### Strength(s) usually available

U.S.—

Not commercially available.

Canada—

Not commercially available.

#### Packaging and storage

Store below 40 °C (104 °F), preferably between 15 and 25 °C (59 and 77 °F), unless otherwise specified by manufacturer. Store in a tight container.

#### Stability

Capsule contents may soften and shrink at elevated temperatures, but this will not alter the therapeutic effect.

#### Auxiliary labeling

• May cause drowsiness.

### TRIMETHADIONE ORAL SOLUTION USP

#### Usual adult and adolescent dose

See *Trimethadione Capsules USP.*

#### Usual pediatric dose

See *Trimethadione Capsules USP.*

#### Strength(s) usually available

U.S.—

Not commercially available.

Canada—

Not commercially available.

#### Packaging and storage

Store below 40 °C (104 °F), preferably between 15 and 30 °C (59 and 86 °F), unless otherwise specified by manufacturer. Store in a tight container. Protect from freezing.

#### Auxiliary labeling

• May cause drowsiness.

#### Additional information

Use a specially marked measuring spoon, a plastic syringe, or a small marked measuring cup to measure each dose accurately.

### TRIMETHADIONE TABLETS USP

#### Usual adult and adolescent dose

See *Trimethadione Capsules USP.*

#### Usual pediatric dose

See *Trimethadione Capsules USP.*

#### Strength(s) usually available

U.S.—

Not commercially available.

Canada—

Not commercially available.

#### Packaging and storage

Store in refrigerator, preferably between 2 and 8 °C (36 and 46 °F), to minimize crystallization. Store in a tight container.

**Stability**

Some crystallization, not harmful to product, may occur.

**Auxiliary labeling**

• Chew or crush tablets before swallowing.
• May cause drowsiness.
• Keep refrigerated. Do not freeze.

**Additional information**

Tablets should be crushed and given in a small amount of water or chewed.

Revised: 12/4/95

---

# ANTICONVULSANTS, HYDANTOIN      Systemic

This monograph includes information on the following: Ethotoin†; Mephenytoin; Phenytoin.

VA CLASSIFICATION (Primary/Secondary):
  Ethotoin—CN400
  Mephenytoin—CN400
  Phenytoin—CN400/CV300; MS200

Another commonly used name for phenytoin is diphenylhydantoin.

Note: For a listing of dosage forms and brand names by country availability, see *Dosage Forms* section(s). For a listing of brand names for the articles in this monograph, refer to the General Index.

  †Not commercially available in Canada.

---

## Category

Anticonvulsant—Ethotoin; Mephenytoin; Phenytoin.
Antiarrhythmic—Phenytoin.
Antineuralgic (trigeminal neuralgia)—Phenytoin.
Skeletal muscle relaxant—Phenytoin.

## Indications

Note: Bracketed information in the *Indications* section refers to uses that are not included in U.S. product labeling.

**Accepted**

Epilepsy (treatment)—Hydantoin anticonvulsants are indicated in the suppression and control of tonic-clonic (grand mal) and simple or complex partial (psychomotor or temporal lobe) seizures.

  Ethotoin may be administered as a second-line agent when seizures have not been adequately controlled by the primary anticonvulsants and before proceeding to more toxic anticonvulsants.

  Mephenytoin is also used in the treatment of simple partial (focal and Jacksonian) seizures in patients who have not responded to less toxic anticonvulsants.

Status epilepticus (treatment)—Parenteral phenytoin is indicated for the control of tonic-clonic type status epilepticus. Although diazepam is often used initially for rapid control of status epilepticus, phenytoin is indicated for sustained control of seizure activity because of the short duration of diazepam's effect.

Seizures in neurosurgery (prophylaxis and treatment)—Phenytoin is indicated for the prevention and treatment of seizures during and following neurosurgery.

[Arrhythmias, digitalis-induced (treatment)][1]—Phenytoin is used in the correction of atrial and ventricular arrhythmias, especially those caused by digitalis glycoside toxicity.

[Choreoathetosis, paroxysmal (treatment)][1]—Phenytoin may be effective in treating paroxysmal choreoathetosis, especially the kinesigenic type. This condition, which is considered a form of reflex epilepsy, is characterized by tonic, dystonic, or choreoathetoid contortions of the extremities, trunk, or face, which are usually precipitated by the patient's initiation of sudden voluntary movement.

[Episodic dyscontrol (treatment)][1]—Phenytoin has been used in the treatment of episodic dyscontrol and in some behavior disorders characterized by hyperexcitability, which include anger, anxiety, irritability, and insomnia.

[Neuralgia, trigeminal (treatment)][1]—Phenytoin is used alone or with other anticonvulsants to control paroxysmal pain in some patients with trigeminal neuralgia (tic douloureux). Carbamazepine is considered the first-line agent, effectively relieving pain in about 66% of patients. However, since phenytoin relieves pain during long-term use in approximately 20% of patients, it may be used alone in some patients or added to carbamazepine therapy when symptoms persist.

[Neuromyotonia (treatment)][1]

[Myotonia congenita (treatment)][1] or

[Myotonic muscular dystrophy (treatment)][1]—Phenytoin is effective in some patients as a muscle relaxant in the treatment of muscle hyper-

irritability, characterized by delayed relaxation of muscle after voluntary or mechanically induced contraction and by a state of continuous muscle contraction at rest. Neuromyotonia includes continuous muscle fiber activity syndrome, Isaac's syndrome, and "stiff man" syndrome.

[Toxicity, tricyclic antidepressant (treatment adjunct)][1]—Intravenous phenytoin loading is used to treat quinidine-like conduction defects, bradyarrhythmias, or heart block, in tricyclic antidepressant overdose.

**Unaccepted**

Hydantoin anticonvulsants are *not* indicated in the treatment of absence (petit mal) seizures, or as first-line treatment of febrile, hypoglycemic, or other metabolic seizures. When tonic-clonic (grand mal) seizures coexist with absence seizures, combined therapy may be necessary.

Although phenytoin has been used in patients with recessive dystrophic epidermolysis bullosa for the treatment of blistering and erosions of the skin that may result from even minor trauma or injury, it is no longer considered preferred therapy.

  [1]Not included in Canadian product labeling.

## Pharmacology/Pharmacokinetics

**Physicochemical characteristics**

Molecular weight—
  Ethotoin: 204.23.
  Mephenytoin: 218.25.
  Phenytoin: 252.27.
  Phenytoin sodium: 274.25.

pKa—
  Phenytoin: 8.06 to 8.33.

**Mechanism of action/Effect**

Anticonvulsant—The mechanism of action is not completely known, but it is thought to involve stabilization of neuronal membranes at the cell body, axon, and synapse and limitation of the spread of neuronal or seizure activity. In neurons, phenytoin decreases sodium and calcium ion influx by prolonging channel inactivation time during generation of nerve impulses. In glia and non-neuronal cell types, the efflux of sodium and the uptake of potassium may be increased. At the synapse, phenytoin decreases post-tetanic potentiation and repetitive after-discharge. Hydantoin anticonvulsants have an excitatory effect on the cerebellum, activating inhibitory pathways that extend to the cerebral cortex. This effect may also produce a reduction in seizure activity that is associated with an increased cerebellar Purkinje cell discharge.

Antiarrhythmic—Phenytoin may act to normalize influx of sodium and calcium to cardiac Purkinje fibers. Abnormal ventricular automaticity and membrane responsiveness are decreased. Also, phenytoin shortens the refractory period, and therefore shortens the QT interval and the duration of the action potential.

Antineuralgic—Exact mechanism is unknown. Phenytoin may act in the central nervous system (CNS) to decrease synaptic transmission or to decrease summation of temporal stimulation leading to neuronal discharge (antikindling). Phenytoin raises the threshold of facial pain and shortens the duration of attacks by diminishing self-maintenance of excitation and repetitive firing.

Skeletal muscle relaxant—Phenytoin's mechanism of action as a muscle relaxant is thought to be similar to its anticonvulsant action. In movement disorders, the membrane stabilizing effect reduces abnormal sustained repetitive firing and potentiation of nerve and muscle cells.

**Other actions/effects**

Hydantoins induce production of liver microsomal enzymes, thereby accelerating the metabolism of concomitantly administered drugs.

**Absorption**

Ethotoin—
  Rapid.

Mephenytoin—
  Rapid.

Phenytoin—
Oral: Slow and variable among products; poor in neonates.
Intravenous: Immediate.
Intramuscular: Very slow, but complete (92%).

### Distribution
Phenytoin—Distributed into cerebrospinal fluid, saliva, semen, gastrointestinal fluids, bile, and breast milk; also crosses the placenta, with fetal serum concentrations equal to those of the mother.

### Protein binding
Phenytoin—Very high (90% or more); may be lower in neonates (84%) and in hyperbilirubinemic infants (80%); also altered in patients with hypoalbuminemia (< 37 mg per dL), uremia, or acute trauma, and in pregnant patients.

### Biotransformation
Hepatic; rate increased in younger children, in pregnant women, in women during menses, and in patients with acute trauma; rate decreases with advancing age. The major inactive metabolite of phenytoin is 5- (*p*-hydroxyphenyl)-5-phenylhydantoin (HPPH). Phenytoin may be metabolized slowly in a small number of individuals due to genetic predisposition, which may cause limited enzyme availability and lack of induction. Mephenytoin has an active metabolite, nirvanol (5-ethyl-5-phenylhydantoin).

### Half-life
Ethotoin—3 to 9 hours.

Mephenytoin—About 7 hours, but for active metabolite, nirvanol, about 95 to 144 hours.

Phenytoin—Because phenytoin exhibits saturable or dose-dependent pharmacokinetics, the apparent half-life of phenytoin changes with dose and serum concentration. This is due to the saturation of the enzyme system responsible for metabolizing phenytoin, which occurs at therapeutic concentrations of the drug. Thus, a constant amount of drug is metabolized (capacity-limited metabolism), and small increases in dose may cause disproportionately large increases in serum concentrations and apparent half-life, possibly causing unexpected toxicity.

### Time to peak concentration
Mephenytoin—
45 minutes to 4 hours:
(nirvanol—16 to 36 hours).
Phenytoin sodium—
Extended capsules: 4 to 12 hours.
Prompt capsules: 1½ to 3 hours.
Phenytoin (tablets or oral suspension)—
1½ to 3 hours.

### Therapeutic serum concentration
Ethotoin—
15 to 50 mcg per mL (74 to 245 micromoles per L).
Mephenytoin—
25 to 40 mcg per mL (115 to 183 micromoles per L) (in combination with nirvanol).
Phenytoin—
10 to 20 mcg per mL (40 to 80 micromoles per L). Steady-state serum concentration is usually achieved in 5 to 10 days with daily oral dosage of 300 mg. Serum concentrations of 20 to 40 mcg per mL (80 to 159 micromoles per L) usually produce symptoms of toxicity; > 40 mcg per mL (159 micromoles per L) usually produce severe toxicity. The serum concentrations of phenytoin needed for efficacy may be influenced by seizure type. Higher concentrations (23 mcg per mL [91 micromoles per L] or greater) may be needed to control simple or complex partial seizures, with or without tonic-clonic seizures, or status epilepticus than are necessary for control of tonic-clonic seizures alone (10 to 20 mcg per mL [40 to 80 micromoles per L]). Occasionally, a patient may have seizure control with serum phenytoin concentrations of 6 to 9 mcg per mL (24 to 36 micromoles per L). Effective treatment, therefore, should be guided by clinical response, not drug serum concentrations. In patients who have hypoalbuminemia and/or renal failure, or who are taking other medications that displace phenytoin from binding sites, hydantoin serum concentrations of 5 to 10 mcg per mL (20 to 40 micromoles per L) may be adequate. For cardiac arrhythmias, plasma concentrations of 10 to 18 mcg per mL (40 to 71 micromoles per L) have been reported to be effective.
Therapeutic concentrations of free phenytoin, which are frequently monitored in patients with altered protein binding (e.g., in neonates and in patients with renal failure, hypoalbuminemia, or acute trauma), usually fall in the range of 0.8 to 2 mcg per mL.

### Elimination
Primarily renal as metabolites; also in feces. Phenytoin excretion is enhanced by alkaline urine.

## Precautions to Consider

### Cross-sensitivity and/or related problems
Patients sensitive to one hydantoin anticonvulsant may also be sensitive to other hydantoin anticonvulsants.

### Tumorigenicity
There have been isolated reports of malignancies, including neuroblastoma, in children whose mothers received phenytoin during pregnancy.

### Pregnancy/Reproduction
Pregnancy—Hydantoin anticonvulsants cross the placenta; risk-benefit must be considered, although a definite cause and effect relationship has not been established between the hydantoins and teratogenic effects. Reports in recent years indicate a higher incidence of congenital abnormalities in children whose mothers used anticonvulsant medication during pregnancy, although most epileptic mothers have delivered normal babies. Reported abnormalities include cleft lip, cleft palate, heart malformations, and the "fetal hydantoin syndrome" (characterized by prenatal growth deficiency, microcephaly, craniofacial abnormalities, hypoplasia of the fingernails, and mental deficiency associated with intrauterine development during therapy). Medication has not been definitively proven to be the cause of "fetal hydantoin syndrome." The reports, to date, relate primarily to the more widely used anticonvulsants, phenytoin and phenobarbital. Pending availability of more precise information, this risk-benefit consideration of anticonvulsant use during pregnancy is extended to the entire family of anticonvulsant medications.

Ethotoin, phenytoin—FDA Pregnancy Category C.

Mephenytoin—FDA pregnancy category not included in product labeling.
Because of altered absorption and protein binding and/or increased metabolic clearance of hydantoin anticonvulsants during pregnancy, pregnant women receiving these medications may experience an increased incidence of seizures. Serum hydantoin concentrations must be monitored and doses increased accordingly. A gradual resumption of the patient's usual dosage may be necessary after delivery. However, some patients may experience a rapid reduction in maternal hepatic phenytoin metabolism at time of delivery, requiring the dosage to be reduced within 12 hours postpartum.

Delivery—Exposure to hydantoins prior to delivery may lead to an increased risk of life-threatening hemorrhage in the neonate, usually within 24 hours of birth. Hydantoins may also produce a deficiency of vitamin K in the mother, causing increased maternal bleeding during delivery. Risk of maternal and infant bleeding may be reduced by administering water-soluble vitamin K to the mother during delivery and to the neonate, intramuscularly or subcutaneously, immediately after birth.

### Breast-feeding
Ethotoin and phenytoin are distributed into breast milk; significant amounts may be ingested by the infant. Information is not available for mephenytoin.

### Pediatrics
Children and young adults are more susceptible to gingival hyperplasia than older adults. See *Dental* section.
Some reports suggest that children may experience decreased school performance during long-term treatment with hydantoin anticonvulsants, especially at high therapeutic or toxic concentrations.
Coarsening of facial features and excessive body hair growth may be more pronounced in young patients.
Other anticonvulsants less likely to cause problems should be considered first.

### Geriatrics
Geriatric patients tend to metabolize hydantoins slowly, thereby increasing the possibility of the medication reaching toxic serum concentrations. Also, serum albumin may be low in older patients, causing a decrease in protein binding of phenytoin. Lower dosage and subsequent adjustments may be required. The rate of administration of intravenous dosage should be no more than 25 mg per minute, and possibly as low as 5 to 10 mg per minute.

### Dental
Gingival hyperplasia, a common complication of phenytoin or mephenytoin therapy, usually starts during the first 6 months of treatment as gingivitis or gum inflammation. The incidence is higher in patients under 23 years of age than in older patients, and severe gingival hyperplasia is less likely to occur with dosage under 500 mg per day. Anterior tissue overgrowth may be greater than posterior overgrowth, creating esthetic and psychological problems for the young patient. A strictly enforced program of teeth cleaning by a professional, combined with plaque control by the patient, if begun within 10 days of initiation of hydantoin anticonvulsant therapy, will minimize growth rate and severity of gingival enlargement. Periodontal surgery may be

indicated, and should be followed by careful plaque control to inhibit recurrence of gum enlargement. If gingival hyperplasia cannot be controlled by standard dental procedures, ethotoin may be substituted for phenytoin, without loss of seizure control, usually at doses 4 to 6 times greater than those of phenytoin.

In addition, the leukopenic effects of hydantoin anticonvulsants may result in an increased incidence of microbial infection, delayed healing, and gingival bleeding. If leukopenia occurs, dental work should be deferred until blood counts have returned to normal. Patient instruction in proper oral hygiene should include caution in use of regular toothbrushes, dental floss, and toothpicks.

## Drug interactions and/or related problems

The following drug interactions and/or related problems have been selected on the basis of their potential clinical significance (possible mechanism in parentheses where appropriate)—not necessarily inclusive (» = major clinical significance):

Note: Combinations containing any of the following medications, depending on the amount present, may also interact with this medication.

Acetaminophen
(risk of hepatotoxicity from a single toxic dose or prolonged use of acetaminophen may be increased and therapeutic efficacy may be decreased in patients regularly taking other hepatic enzyme–inducing agents such as phenytoin)

» Alcohol or
» CNS depression–producing medications (See *Appendix II*)
(CNS depression may be enhanced)

(chronic use of alcohol may decrease the serum concentrations and effectiveness of hydantoins; concurrent use of hydantoin anticonvulsants with acute alcohol intake may increase serum hydantoin concentrations)

» Amiodarone
(concurrent use with phenytoin and possibly with other hydantoin anticonvulsants may increase plasma concentrations of the hydantoin, resulting in increased effects and/or toxicity)

» Antacids, aluminum-magnesium–containing and calcium carbonate–containing
(concurrent use may decrease the bioavailability of phenytoin; doses of antacids and phenytoin should be separated by about 2 to 3 hours)

» Anticoagulants, coumarin- or indandione-derivative or
» Chloramphenicol or
» Cimetidine or
» Disulfiram or
Influenza virus vaccine or
» Isoniazid or
Methylphenidate or
» Phenylbutazone or
Ranitidine or
Salicylates or
» Sulfonamides
(serum concentrations of hydantoin anticonvulsants may be increased because of decreased metabolism, thereby increasing the hydantoins' effects and/or toxicity; dosage adjustments of the anticonvulsant may be necessary)

(in addition, the anticoagulant effect of coumarin- or indandione-derivative anticoagulants may be increased initially, but decreased with continued concurrent use)

Anticonvulsants, succinimide or
Carbamazepine or
» Contraceptives, estrogen-containing, oral or
» Corticosteroids, glucocorticoid and mineralocorticoid or
» Corticotropin (ACTH) or
Cyclosporine or
Dacarbazine or
Digitalis glycosides or
Disopyramide or
Doxycycline or
» Estrogens or
Furosemide or
Levodopa or
Mexiletine or
Quinidine
(therapeutic effects of these medications may be decreased because of increased metabolism and decreased plasma concentrations, which may result from hydantoin anticonvulsants' induction of hepatic microsomal enzymes; dosage adjustments of these medications may be necessary)

(carbamazepine may also induce metabolism of hydantoin anticonvulsants; monitoring of blood concentrations is recommended as a guide to dosage, especially when either carbamazepine or the hydantoin is added to or withdrawn from an existing regimen)

(in addition, concurrent use of hydantoin anticonvulsants with oral, estrogen-containing contraceptives may result in breakthrough bleeding and contraceptive failure due to the increased rate of hepatic enzyme metabolism of steroids induced by hydantoins; the dose of the estrogenic substance in the oral contraceptive may be increased to diminish bleeding and decrease the risk of conception)

Antidepressants, tricyclic or
Bupropion or
Clozapine or
Haloperidol or
Loxapine or
Maprotiline or
Molindone or
Monoamine oxidase (MAO) inhibitors, including furazolidone and procarbazine or
Phenothiazines or
Pimozide or
Thioxanthenes
(these medications may lower the seizure threshold and decrease the anticonvulsant effects of hydantoin anticonvulsants; CNS depression may be enhanced; dosage adjustment of the hydantoin anticonvulsant may be necessary)

(in addition, concurrent use of phenytoin with tricyclic antidepressants may lower serum concentrations of the antidepressant; dosage increases of the tricyclic antidepressant may be required to produce improvement of the depressed state)

(also, molindone contains calcium ions, which interfere with the absorption of phenytoin)

(also, concurrent use of phenothiazines may inhibit phenytoin metabolism, leading to phenytoin intoxication)

Antidiabetic agents, oral or
Insulin
(hydantoin anticonvulsants may increase serum glucose concentrations and the possibility of hyperglycemia; dosage adjustment of either or both medications may be necessary)

Barbiturates or
Primidone
(concurrent use may produce variable and unpredictable effects on hydantoin metabolism; serum hydantoin concentrations should be closely monitored)

» Calcium
(when used as an excipient in phenytoin capsules, calcium sulfate can decrease phenytoin absorption by as much as 20%)

(concurrent use of phenytoin with calcium supplements or any tablets or capsules that contain calcium sulfate as an excipient may result in formation of nonabsorbable complexes, thereby decreasing the bioavailability of both calcium and phenytoin; patients should be advised to take these medications 1 to 3 hours apart)

Carbonic anhydrase inhibitors
(osteopenia induced by hydantoin anticonvulsants may be enhanced; it is recommended that patients receiving concurrent therapy be monitored for early signs of osteopenia and that the carbonic anhydrase inhibitor be discontinued and appropriate treatment initiated if necessary)

» Diazoxide, oral
(concurrent use with hydantoin anticonvulsants may decrease the efficacy of phenytoin and the hyperglycemic effect of diazoxide and is not recommended)

Dopamine
(use of intravenous phenytoin in patients maintained on dopamine may produce sudden hypotension and bradycardia; this reaction is considered to be dose-rate dependent; if anticonvulsant therapy is necessary during administration of dopamine, an alternative to phenytoin should be considered)

Enflurane or
Halothane or
Methoxyflurane
(chronic use of hydantoin anticonvulsants prior to anesthesia may increase metabolism of anesthetic, leading to increased risk of hepatotoxicity, nephrotoxicity [with methoxyflurane only], and hydantoin toxicity)

Enteral feeding solutions
(concurrent use with phenytoin may decrease phenytoin absorption, possibly necessitating an increase in dosage; some clinicians

recommend that at least 2 hours should elapse between feeding and phenytoin administration; if phenytoin suspension or capsule contents are administered via nasogastric tubing, flushing the tube with 2 to 4 ounces of water before and after administration has been suggested; phenytoin serum concentrations should be carefully monitored during concurrent therapy)

» Fluconazole or
  Ketoconazole or
  Miconazole
  (concurrent use of fluconazole with phenytoin may decrease the metabolism of phenytoin, resulting in increased plasma phenytoin concentrations; a 75% increase in the area under the curve [AUC] of phenytoin was found in volunteers given 200 mg of fluconazole per day; phenytoin concentrations must be carefully monitored)

  (concurrent use of ketoconazole with phenytoin may result in altered metabolism of either ketoconazole, phenytoin, or both; in addition, time to peak serum concentration of ketoconazole may be delayed; response to both medications should be closely monitored)

  (serum concentrations of phenytoin have been reported to be increased by miconazole, another imidazole derivative, resulting in phenytoin toxicity; dosage adjustments may be necessary before and after miconazole therapy)

» Fluoxetine
  (concurrent use of fluoxetine with phenytoin has been reported to cause elevated plasma phenytoin concentrations, resulting in symptoms of toxicity; caution and close monitoring are suggested)

  Folic acid
  (although hydantoin anticonvulsants deplete the body of folate stores, supplementation with folic acid may result in lowered serum hydantoin concentrations and possible loss of seizure control; therefore, an increase in hydantoin dosage may be necessary in patients who receive folate supplementation)

  Leucovorin
  (large doses of leucovorin may counteract the anticonvulsant effects of hydantoin anticonvulsants)

  Levothyroxine
  (concurrent use with phenytoin may reduce serum protein binding of levothyroxine and reduce total serum thyroxine [$T_4$] by 15 to 25%; however, most patients remain euthyroid, and dosage of thyroid hormone does not need to be altered)

» Lidocaine or
  Propranolol and probably other beta-adrenergic blocking agents
  (concurrent use with intravenous phenytoin may produce additive cardiac depressant effects; hydantoin anticonvulsants may also increase hepatic enzyme metabolism of lidocaine, reducing its intravenous concentration)

» Methadone
  (chronic use of phenytoin may increase methadone metabolism, probably by induction of hepatic microsomal enzyme activity, and may precipitate withdrawal symptoms in patients being treated for opioid dependence; methadone dosage adjustments may be necessary when phenytoin therapy is initiated or discontinued)

  Nifedipine or
  Verapamil
  (caution is advised when nifedipine or verapamil is used concurrently with hydantoin anticonvulsants, which are highly protein–bound medications, since changes in serum concentrations of the free, unbound medications may occur)

  Omeprazole
  (inhibition of the cytochrome P-450 enzyme system by omeprazole, especially at higher doses, may cause a decrease in the hepatic metabolism of phenytoin; delayed elimination and increased serum concentrations may result, with considerable interpatient variability)

» Phenacemide
  (risk of additive toxicity when phenacemide is used concurrently with hydantoin anticonvulsants; concurrent use of phenacemide with ethotoin has been reported to cause paranoid symptoms; extreme caution is recommended during concurrent use of these medications)

  Praziquantel
  (one small, single-dose, controlled study found that epileptic patients taking phenytoin had significantly lower plasma concentrations of praziquantel [24% of the control group]; this effect is thought to be due to induction of the cytochrome P-450 microsomal enzyme system by phenytoin; patients on phenytoin may require a larger dose of praziquantel)

» Rifampin
  (concurrent use with phenytoin may stimulate the hepatic metabolism of phenytoin, increasing its elimination and thus counteracting its anticonvulsant effect; careful monitoring of serum hydantoin concentrations and dosage adjustments may be necessary)

» Streptozocin
  (phenytoin may protect pancreatic beta cells from the toxic effects of streptozocin, thus reducing streptozocin's therapeutic effects; concurrent use is not recommended)

» Sucralfate
  (concurrent use of sucralfate may decrease the absorption of hydantoin anticonvulsants)

  Sulfinpyrazone
  (sulfinpyrazone may displace hydantoin anticonvulsants from plasma protein-binding sites and decrease their metabolism, possibly leading to increased plasma concentrations and elimination half-life; although plasma hydantoin concentration is not consistently increased, it is recommended that patients be monitored for signs of hydantoin toxicity)

  Trazodone
  (increased plasma hydantoin concentrations have been reported when hydantoin anticonvulsants are used concurrently with trazodone; caution and close monitoring are suggested)

» Valproic acid
  (valproic acid may displace phenytoin from protein-binding sites and may inhibit the metabolism of phenytoin; phenytoin, through enzyme induction, may lower valproate levels; there may be an increased risk of liver toxicity, especially in infants; close monitoring of the patient is required since variable serum phenytoin concentrations have resulted; monitoring of free phenytoin concentrations is advised by some clinicians; dosage of phenytoin should be adjusted as required by clinical situation; caution is advised also for use with other hydantoin anticonvulsants)

  Vitamin D
  (hydantoin anticonvulsants may reduce effect of vitamin D by accelerating metabolism through hepatic microsomal enzyme induction; patients on long-term anticonvulsant therapy may require vitamin D supplementation to prevent osteomalacia, although rickets is rare)

» Xanthines, such as:
  Aminophylline
  Caffeine
  Oxtriphylline
  Theophylline
  (concurrent use may stimulate hepatic metabolism of the xanthines [except dyphylline], resulting in increased theophylline clearance, especially if plasma phenytoin concentrations are in the usual therapeutic range for at least 5 days; also, simultaneous use with the xanthines may inhibit phenytoin absorption, resulting in decreased serum phenytoin concentrations; serum concentrations of phenytoin and theophylline should be monitored during concurrent therapy; dosage adjustments of both phenytoin and theophylline may be necessary)

**Laboratory value alterations**

The following have been selected on the basis of their potential clinical significance (possible effect in parentheses where appropriate)—not necessarily inclusive (» = major clinical significance):

With diagnostic test results
  Dexamethasone test or
  Metyrapone test
  (results may be inaccurate because of increased dexamethasone or metyrapone metabolism resulting from enzyme induction; dexamethasone or metyrapone doses may need to be increased)

  Gallium citrate Ga 67 imaging
  (phenytoin may stimulate a benign alteration in lymphoid tissue, which may result in a Ga 67 scintigram similar to that seen in patients with malignant melanoma)

  Schilling test
  (phenytoin in combination with other anticonvulsant medications may cause a reversible malabsorption of vitamin $B_{12}$)

  Thyroid function tests
  (free, circulating thyroxine [$FT_4$] and total thyroxine [$T_4$] concentrations are decreased by phenytoin therapy, mainly due to enhanced conversion to triiodothyronine [$T_3$]; however, $T_3$ and thyroid stimulating hormone [TSH] concentrations generally remain unchanged, and most patients remain euthyroid)

With physiology/laboratory test values
  Alkaline phosphatase, serum and
  Gamma glutamyl transpeptidase (GGT), serum and
  Glucose, serum
      (concentrations may be increased)

**Medical considerations/Contraindications**
The medical considerations/contraindications included here have been selected on the basis of their potential clinical significance (reasons given
in parentheses where appropriate)—not necessarily inclusive (» =
major clinical significance).

*Except under special circumstances, this medication should not be used
when the following medical problems exist:*

» Cardiac function impairment, such as Adams-Stokes syndrome, second
      and third degree AV block, sino-atrial block, and sinus bradycardia
      (parenteral phenytoin administration may affect ventricular auto-
      maticity and result in ventricular arrhythmias)

*Risk-benefit should be considered when the following medical problems
exist:*
  Alcoholism, active
      (serum phenytoin concentrations may be decreased)

» Blood dyscrasias
      (risk of serious infections may be increased)
  Cardiovascular disease
      (parenteral phenytoin administration may result in atrial and ven-
      tricular conduction depression, ventricular fibrillation, or reduced
      cardiac output, especially in the elderly or gravely ill patients;
      phenytoin should be administered at a rate of no more than 25 mg
      per minute, and if necessary, at a slow rate of 5 to 10 mg per
      minute)
  Diabetes mellitus
      (hyperglycemia may be potentiated)
  Fever or febrile illness—temperature >101 °F for more than 24 hours
      (serum concentrations of hydantoin anticonvulsants may be de-
      creased because of induction of hepatic oxidative enzymes during
      fever)

» Hepatic function impairment
      (metabolism of hydantoin anticonvulsants may be reduced, thereby
      increasing the possibility of toxic serum concentrations; protein-
      binding alterations are also likely, due to a secondary decrease in
      albumin concentrations)

» Porphyria
      (risk of exacerbation)

» Renal function impairment
      (excretion and protein binding may be altered)

» Sensitivity to hydantoin anticonvulsants
  Systemic lupus erythematosus
      (risk of exacerbation)
  Thyroid function impairment
      (free, circulating thyroxine [$FT_4$] and total thyroxine [$T_4$] con-
      centrations are decreased by phenytoin therapy; patients usually
      remain euthyroid)

**Patient monitoring**
The following may be especially important in patient monitoring (other
tests may be warranted in some patients, depending on condition;
» = major clinical significance):

  Albumin concentrations, serum and
  Calcium concentrations, serum and
» Complete blood cell and platelet counts and
» Hepatic function determinations
      (some or all may be required at periodic intervals during therapy
      depending on individual needs of the patient; however, these de-
      terminations may be necessary only during early weeks or months
      of treatment)

» Dental examinations
      (recommended at 3-month intervals for teeth cleaning and rein-
      forcement of patient's plaque control for inhibition of gingival
      hyperplasia)

» Electroencephalograms (EEGs) and
» Hydantoin concentrations, serum
      (frequent monitoring, possibly with video recording of seizures,
      and medical and physical reassessment may prevent neurotoxicity;
      all blood samples should be drawn at standardized times within
      the dosing schedule, preferably just before a dose is administered;
      since the hepatic metabolism of phenytoin is saturable, a small
      increment in dose, at higher doses, will produce a disproportionate
      and unpredictable increase in serum concentrations to the upper
      therapeutic ranges, and can lead to clinical toxicity)

(in patients with altered protein binding of phenytoin [e.g., neonates, and patients with renal failure, hypoalbuminemia, or acute
trauma], free hydantoin serum concentrations should be monitored)
(because of altered metabolism and protein binding, and/or increased metabolic clearance of hydantoin anticonvulsants during
pregnancy, monthly measurements of serum hydantoin concentrations are recommended to assess need for increase in dosage;
weekly measurements are recommended during postpartum period
to ascertain adequate reduction of dosage; some patients may have
a significant decrease in hydantoin metabolism at time of delivery;
therefore, serum hydantoin concentrations should be followed
closely during the immediate postpartum period [within 12 hours])

Folate concentrations, serum
    (recommended periodically because of increased folate require-
    ments of patients on long-term phenytoin therapy)

Physical examination, with special attention to lymph glands and skin
    (all cases of lymphadenopathy or skin rash should be monitored
    for an extended period because of possible phenytoin hypersensi-
    tivity syndrome with lymphadenopathy or pseudolymphoma;
    should these problems occur, every effort should be made to
    achieve seizure control using alternative anticonvulsants)

Thyroid function determinations
    (recommended during the first few months of therapy to detect
    symptoms of hypothyroidism, which may be unmasked by hydan-
    toins; when a patient receiving phenytoin is suspected of having
    hypothyroidism, $T_3$ and thyroid-stimulating hormone [TSH] con-
    centrations should be measured, not $T_4$ and free $T_4$ index [FTI],
    since the latter are both typically depressed in patients receiving
    phenytoin)

Even after patients have been stabilized on a maintenance dose, it is
    important that they have periodic examinations during therapy
    since phenytoin (and possibly other hydantoins) may deplete body
    stores of folic acid and vitamin D, possibly resulting in megalo-
    blastic anemia or osteomalacia.

## Side/Adverse Effects

Note: Although not all of these side effects have been attributed specifi-
        cally to each hydantoin anticonvulsant, a potential exists for their
        occurrence during the use of any hydantoin.

The following side/adverse effects have been selected on the basis of their
potential clinical significance (possible signs and symptoms in parentheses where appropriate)—not necessarily inclusive:

**Those indicating need for medical attention**
Incidence more frequent
    *CNS toxicity* (nystagmus [uncontrolled back-and-forth and/or rolling
    eye movements]; ataxia [clumsiness or unsteadiness]; confusion; mood
    or mental changes; muscle weakness; increased frequency of seizures;
    slurred speech or stuttering; trembling of hands; unusual excitement;
    nervousness; irritability)—usually with long-term use, but may be
    dose-related; *gingival hyperplasia* (bleeding, tender, or enlarged
    gums)—higher incidence in children and young adults; incidence in
    all age groups rare with ethotoin; *lupus erythematosus, phenytoin hy-
    persensitivity syndrome, Stevens-Johnson syndrome, or toxic epider-
    mal necrolysis* (fever; muscle pain; skin rash; or sore throat)

Note: *Phenytoin hypersensitivity syndrome* may be manifested in
        many ways. Fever, rash, and lymphadenopathy frequently occur
        together, and may be part of more than one hypersensitivity
        syndrome. Skin rash is the most frequent hypersensitivity re-
        action; licheniform or maculopapular or morbilliform rash, of-
        ten pruritic, may present simply or may be prodromal of more
        serious dermatological reactions such as *Stevens-Johnson syn-
        drome* or *toxic epidermal necrolysis.* Lymphoid syndromes (in-
        cluding lymphoid hyperplasia, pseudolymphomas, and pseudo-
        pseudolymphomas) occur less commonly and are generally
        reversible upon discontinuation of phenytoin. Phenytoin-in-
        duced hepatitis and hepatic necrosis are other major hypersen-
        sitivity reactions, as is eosinophilia, which occurs commonly.
        Less commonly occurring syndromes include polyarteritis, po-
        lymyositis, or systemic *lupus erythematosus;* disseminated in-
        travascular coagulopathy, serum sickness, and renal failure may
        also occur.

        Rash usually appears in the first two weeks of treatment; *hy-
        persensitivity syndrome* usually occurs 3 to 8 weeks after, but
        may occur as long as 12 weeks after initiation of phenytoin
        therapy. Syndrome may be life-threatening, but early interven-
        tion may prevent renal failure, severe rhabdomyolysis, or he-
        patic necrosis. Other factors, such as a positive family history
        for phenytoin hypersensitivity reactions or concomitant admin-

istration of cranial radiation therapy, may increase the risk of hypersensitivity syndrome occurring.

Incidence rare
  *Blood dyscrasias, including agranulocytosis* (chills; fever; sore throat; unusual tiredness or weakness); *leukopenia* (fever; chills; sore throat); *pancytopenia* (nosebleeds or other unusual bleeding or bruising); *thrombocytopenia* (fever; sore throat; unusual bleeding or bruising); *cholestatic jaundice or hepatitis* (dark urine; light gray–colored stools; loss of appetite and weight; severe stomach pain; yellow eyes or skin; skin rash or itching; dizziness; nausea or vomiting; joint pain; unusual tiredness or weakness); *choreoathetoid movements, transient* (restlessness or agitation; uncontrolled jerking or twisting movements of hands, arms, or legs; uncontrolled movements of lips, tongue, or cheeks); *cognitive impairment* (defects in intelligence, short-term memory, learning ability, and attention); *periarteritis nodosa* (abdominal pain; soreness of muscles; unusual tiredness or weakness; fever with or without chills; headache; loss of appetite and weight); *Peyronie's disease* (pain of penis on erection); *pulmonary infiltrates or fibrosis* (fever; troubled or quick, shallow breathing; unusual tiredness or weakness; loss of appetite and weight; chest discomfort); *vitamin D and/or calcium imbalance* (frequent bone fractures; bone malformations; slowed growth)

  Note: Many cases of mephenytoin-induced *blood dyscrasias* occur in patients given mephenytoin for a second time after a period of abstinence.

  *Choreoathetoid movements* may be due to sudden administration of intravenous phenytoin for status epilepticus; effect usually lasts 24 to 48 hours after discontinuation of phenytoin and may resolve spontaneously; effect is unrelated to serum hydantoin toxicity or duration of use.

With chronic use
  *Peripheral polyneuropathy, predominantly sensory* (numbness, tingling, or pain in hands or feet)—with phenytoin

With parenteral use only
  *Burning pain at injection site*—rarely with necrosis and sloughing

**Those indicating need for medical attention only if they continue or are bothersome**
Incidence more frequent
  *Constipation; mild dizziness; mild drowsiness; nausea and vomiting*
Incidence less frequent
  *Diarrhea*—with ethotoin; *enlargement of facial features, including thickening of lips, widening of nasal tip, and protrusion of jaw; gynecomastia* (swelling of breasts)—in males; *headache; hypertrichosis* (unusual and excessive hair growth on body and face)—primarily with phenytoin; *insomnia* (trouble in sleeping); *muscle twitching*

# Overdose

For specific information on the agents used in the management of hydantoin anticonvulsant overdose, see *Charcoal, Activated (Oral-Local)* monograph.

For more information on the management of overdose or unintentional ingestion, **contact a Poison Control Center** (see *Poison Control Center Listing*).

**Clinical effects of overdose**
The following effects have been selected on the basis of their potential clinical significance (possible signs and symptoms in parentheses where appropriate)—not necessarily inclusive:
  *Ataxia* (clumsiness or unsteadiness); *or staggering walk; blurred or double vision; severe confusion; severe dizziness or drowsiness; dysarthria* (stuttering); *or slurred speech; hyperreflexia; nausea and vomiting; nystagmus* (continuous, uncontrolled back-and-forth and/or rolling eye movements); *tremor; unusual tiredness or weakness*

  Note: The lethal dose of phenytoin in adults is estimated to be 2 to 5 grams. The lethal dose in children is unknown.

**Treatment of overdose**
Since there is no specific antidote for overdose with hydantoin anticonvulsants, treatment is symptomatic and supportive and may include the following:

To decrease absorption—Induction of emesis or gastric lavage. Multiple oral doses of charcoal and cathartic may shorten the duration of symptoms.

Supportive care—Oxygen, vasopressors, and assisted ventilation may be necessary for CNS, respiratory, or cardiovascular depression. Patients in whom intentional overdose is confirmed or suspected should be referred for psychiatric consultation.

Following recovery, careful evaluation of blood-forming organs is advisable.

# Patient Consultation

As an aid to patient consultation, refer to *Advice for the Patient, Anticonvulsants, Hydantoin (Systemic)*.

In providing consultation, consider emphasizing the following selected information (» = major clinical significance):

**Before using this medication**
» Conditions affecting use, especially:
  Sensitivity to hydantoin anticonvulsants
  Pregnancy—Hydantoin anticonvulsants cross placenta; risk-benefit should be considered because of possibility of increased birth defects; seizures may increase during pregnancy with need for dose increase; bleeding problems may occur in mother during delivery and in baby immediately after delivery
  Breast-feeding—Ethotoin and phenytoin distributed into breast milk
  Use in children—Bleeding, tender, and enlarged gums more common in children; unusual and excessive hair growth, more noticeable in young girls; decreased performance in school (cognitive impairment) may occur with long-term use of high doses
  Use in the elderly—Side effects more likely to occur in the elderly; hydantoin anticonvulsants metabolized more slowly in elderly, possibly leading to toxicity
  Dental—Gingival hyperplasia may appear; good dental hygiene and visits to dentist every 3 months for cleaning recommended; agranulocytosis or thrombocytopenia may cause gingival bleeding, slowed healing, and infections
  Other medications, especially estrogen-containing oral contraceptives, estrogens, aminophylline, amiodarone, antacids, anticoagulants, caffeine, CNS depressants, alcohol, chloramphenicol, cimetidine, corticosteroids, diazoxide, disulfiram, isoniazid, calcium-containing medicine, fluconazole, fluoxetine, lidocaine, methadone, oxtriphylline, phenacemide, phenylbutazone, rifampin, streptozocin, sucralfate, sulfonamides, theophylline, or valproic acid
  Other medical problems, especially blood dyscrasias, cardiac function impairment, hepatic function impairment, history of hydantoin hypersensitivity, porphyria, or renal function impairment

**Proper use of this medication**
*Proper administration*
  For liquid dosage forms—Shaking well; using an accurate measuring device, such as a specially marked measuring spoon, a plastic syringe, or a small graduated cup
  For chewable tablet dosage form—Chewing or crushing tablets or swallowing them whole
  For capsule dosage form—Swallowing capsule whole
  Taking with food to reduce gastrointestinal irritation
» Compliance with therapy; taking every day exactly as directed
» Proper dosing
» Missed dose: If dosing schedule is—
  One dose a day: Taking as soon as possible unless next day, then continuing on schedule; not doubling doses
  Several doses a day: Taking as soon as possible unless within 4 hours of next scheduled dose, then continuing on regular schedule; not doubling doses
  Checking with doctor if doses are missed for 2 or more days in a row
» Proper storage

**Precautions while using this medication**
» Regular visits to physician to check progress of therapy
» Not taking other medication without physician's advice
» Avoiding the use of alcoholic beverages and other CNS depressants while taking this medicine
  Not taking within 2 to 3 hours of taking antacids or medication for diarrhea
  Not changing brands or dosage forms of phenytoin without checking with physician or pharmacist
» Checking with physician before discontinuing medication; gradual dosage reduction is usually needed to maintain seizure control
  Carrying medical identification card or bracelet during therapy
  Diabetic patients: Checking blood or urine sugar concentrations
  Caution if any laboratory tests required; possible interference with test results of dexamethasone, metyrapone, or Schilling tests, thyroid function tests, or gallium citrate Ga 67 imaging
» Caution if any kind of surgery, dental treatment, or emergency treatment is required
» Caution when driving, using machines, or doing other jobs requiring alertness
» Using different or additional means of birth control than estrogen-containing oral contraceptives

*For phenytoin or mephenytoin only*
» Maintaining good dental hygiene and seeing dentist every 3 months for teeth cleaning, to prevent tenderness, bleeding, and enlargement of gums

### Side/adverse effects
Increased incidence of gingival hyperplasia in children and young adults taking phenytoin or mephenytoin

Unusual and excessive hair growth more noticeable in young girls

Signs of potential side effects, especially blood dyscrasias, CNS toxicity, cholestatic jaundice, cognitive impairment, hepatitis, an increase in seizures, lupus erythematosus, phenytoin hypersensitivity syndrome, periarteritis nodosa, Peyronie's disease, pulmonary infiltrates or fibrosis, Stevens-Johnson syndrome, toxic epidermal necrolysis, transient choreoathetoid movements, or vitamin D and/or calcium imbalance

## General Dosing Information

Dosage must be individualized. Monitoring of serum phenytoin concentrations is recommended because of the great variation of response among patients to the hydantoin anticonvulsants and because of the relatively narrow therapeutic serum concentration range.

Geriatric patients, seriously ill patients, or patients with impaired hepatic function may require lower initial dosage with subsequent adjustments, because of slow hydantoin metabolism or decreased protein binding. If phenytoin is administered intravenously, the rate must be slowed to not more than 25 mg a minute, and possibly to as low as 5 to 10 mg a minute.

When patients are transferred from hydantoins to other anticonvulsant medication or vice versa, there should be a gradual increase in the dosage of the added medication and a gradual decrease in the dosage of the discontinued medication over a period of a few weeks. When an enzyme-inducing medication is added to or removed from a regimen, the metabolism of the remaining medications will be altered. In most patients, changes in enzyme induction may occur over a period of weeks.

When single-drug anticonvulsant therapy is to be discontinued in patients with seizure disorders, dosage should be reduced gradually over a period of 6 to 12 months, to prevent possible recurrence of seizures. Abrupt withdrawal may lead to status epilepticus.

### Diet/Nutrition
Oral hydantoin anticonvulsants may be taken with or immediately after meals to lessen gastric irritation. However, the medication should always be taken at the same time in relation to meals to ensure consistent absorption.

Patients on long-term hydantoin therapy may have increased folic acid requirements. However, increased hydantoin dosages may be necessary in patients who receive folate supplementation because such supplementation may result in decreased serum hydantoin concentrations and possible loss of seizure control.

### For treatment of adverse effects
Intolerance or allergic reactions—Hydantoin anticonvulsants should be discontinued immediately. Effects are usually observed within 9 to 14 days after start of therapy. If rash is morbilliform (measles-like) or scarlatiniform (scarlet fever–like), therapy may be restarted after the rash has completely disappeared, but should be discontinued if the rash reappears. If rash is exfoliative, purpuric, bullous, or if lupus erythematosus or Stevens-Johnson syndrome is suspected, hydantoin therapy should not be resumed. Attempts should be made to differentiate lymph gland enlargement from other lymph node pathology. The patient should be monitored closely for an extended length of time, and alternative anticonvulsant therapy initiated.

CNS or cerebellar toxicity—Dosage reduction or discontinuation of hydantoin anticonvulsant may improve or reverse effects. Cerebellar toxicity may occur after long-term administration, usually at serum concentrations above 30 mcg. However, CNS toxicity has also been reported at lower serum concentrations, due to free fraction variability.

Gingival or gum enlargement—Consultation with dentist; following recommendations for care to reduce effects.

---

### *ETHOTOIN*

## Summary of Differences

Pharmacology/pharmacokinetics:
  Half-life—
    3 to 9 hours.
Side/adverse effects:
  Diarrhea has been reported.

Drowsiness and sedation are dose related and quite common.

Gum hyperplasia is rare; ethotoin is sometimes substituted for phenytoin therapy when gingival hyperplasia is a problem.

Incidence of ataxia is rare.

Incidence of hypertrichosis is lower than with other hydantoin anticonvulsants.

## Additional Dosing Information

See also *General Dosing Information.*

Ethotoin may be substituted for phenytoin without loss of seizure control for improvement of gum hyperplasia, or other side effects, during anticonvulsant therapy. Ethotoin doses are usually 4 to 6 times greater than those of phenytoin.

## Oral Dosage Forms
### ETHOTOIN TABLETS USP

#### Usual adult and adolescent dose
Anticonvulsant—
  Oral, 500 mg to 1 gram the first day, usually divided into four to six doses, the dosage being gradually increased over several days until seizure control is obtained.

Note: Maintenance dosage of less than 2 grams a day has been found to be ineffective in most adults.
  Geriatric and debilitated patients may require a lower initial dosage.

#### Usual adult prescribing limits
Up to 3 grams a day.

#### Usual pediatric dose
Anticonvulsant—
  Oral, up to 750 mg a day initially, on the basis of age and weight, the dosage being adjusted as needed and tolerated until seizure control is obtained.

Note: A total daily dose of 3 grams may be required for some patients.

#### Strength(s) usually available
U.S.—
  250 mg (Rx) [*Peganone* (scored; lactose)].
  500 mg (Rx) [*Peganone* (scored; lactose)].
Canada—
  Not commercially available.

#### Packaging and storage
Store below 40 °C (104 °F), preferably between 15 and 30 °C (59 and 86 °F), unless otherwise specified by manufacturer. Store in a tight container.

#### Auxiliary labeling
• May cause drowsiness.
• Avoid alcoholic beverages.

---

### *MEPHENYTOIN*

## Summary of Differences

Pharmacology/pharmacokinetics: Half-life averages 95 to 144 hours (including active metabolite, nirvanol).

Side/adverse effects: Drowsiness and sedation are dose related and quite common.

## Additional Dosing Information

See also *General Dosing Information.*

Mephenytoin is usually used only after safer anticonvulsants have been tried and have proven unsatisfactory.

## Oral Dosage Forms
### MEPHENYTOIN TABLETS USP

#### Usual adult and adolescent dose
Anticonvulsant—
  Oral, 50 to 100 mg once a day, the dosage being increased by an additional 50 to 100 mg a day at one-week intervals until seizure control is obtained up to a maximum of 1.2 grams a day.

Note: Geriatric patients and debilitated patients may require a lower initial dosage.

#### Usual pediatric dose
Anticonvulsant—
  Oral, 25 to 50 mg a day, the dosage being increased by an additional 25 to 50 mg a day at one-week intervals until seizure control is obtained.

**Usual pediatric prescribing limits**
Up to 400 mg a day.
Note: Dose may be divided and should be based on severity of seizures, age, and serum concentrations.

**Strength(s) usually available**
U.S.—
    100 mg (Rx) [*Mesantoin* (scored; lactose; sucrose)].
Canada—
    100 mg (Rx) [*Mesantoin* (scored; lactose)].

**Packaging and storage**
Store below 40 °C (104 °F), preferably between 15 and 30 °C (59 and 86 °F), unless otherwise specified by manufacturer. Store in a well-closed container.

**Auxiliary labeling**
• May cause drowsiness.
• Avoid alcoholic beverages.

---

## PHENYTOIN

# Summary of Differences

Category: Also used as an antiarrhythmic, for ventricular arrhythmias, especially when arrhythmia is digitalis-induced or caused by tricyclic antidepressant toxicity; as an antineuralgic in trigeminal neuralgia; and as a muscle relaxant in certain movement disorders.
Pharmacology/pharmacokinetics: Because phenytoin exhibits saturable or dose-dependent pharmacokinetics, the apparent half-life of phenytoin changes with dose and serum concentration.
Side/adverse effects: Incidence of hypertrichosis is more frequent than with other hydantoin anticonvulsants.

# Additional Dosing Information

See also *General Dosing Information.*

**For oral dosage forms**
Extended Phenytoin Sodium Capsules USP is the only dosage form used for once-a-day dosing, and then, only after patients have been stabilized on a divided dosage, generally 300 to 400 mg a day.
Phenytoin oral suspension is generally not recommended for once-a-day dosing because it is not an extended-release dosage form. The suspension may be adequate for more frequent dosing, if vigorously shaken to avoid inadequate dispersal of phenytoin throughout the vehicle.

**For parenteral dosage forms**
Intravenous phenytoin sodium should be administered by direct intravenous injection into a large vein through a large-gauge needle or intravenous catheter at a rate not to exceed 50 mg a minute. Faster rates of administration may result in hypotension, cardiovascular collapse, or CNS depression, related to the propylene glycol diluent.
Intravenous administration should be monitored by cardiac function and blood pressure readings.
To minimize local venous irritation from intravenous injection of phenytoin, each dose must be followed by 0.9% sodium chloride injection through the same in-place needle or catheter. Extravasation should be avoided, as phenytoin injection is caustic to tissues because of its high alkalinity (pH=12), and possibly also because of the propylene glycol in the vehicle. Soft tissue injury ranging from irritation to extensive necrosis and sloughing has been reported even when extravasation has not occurred.
Some clinicians suggest that, to prevent serious local inflammatory reactions, intermittent phenytoin infusion may be desirable and that such an infusion can be made feasible if all of the following criteria are met:
    • Phenytoin injection is admixed only with no more than 50 mL of 0.9% sodium chloride injection.
    • The final concentration of phenytoin is between 1 and 10 mg per mL.
    • Admixture is done *immediately* before beginning the infusion.
    • Infusion is completed within 1 hour.
    • All tubing is flushed with 0.9% sodium chloride injection before and after infusion.
    • A 0.45 to 0.22 micron filter is placed on the line.

When phenytoin injection is administered by infusion, the maximum rate of infusion is 50 mg a minute. However, for patients who may develop hypotension, who are on a sympathomimetic medication, who have cardiovascular disease, or who are older than 65 years of age, the maximum rate of infusion should be 25 mg a minute and possibly as low as 5 to 10 mg a minute. Vigilant ECG monitoring of cardio-

vascular status throughout the duration of infusion is required.
For rapid control of seizures, concomitant administration of an intravenous benzodiazepine or a short-acting barbiturate may be necessary because of the slow rate of administration necessary for phenytoin injection.
Because of the delayed absorption of intramuscularly administered phenytoin and the high degree of local irritation from the alkaline solution, the intramuscular route of administration is not recommended when the intravenous or oral route is available.
Intramuscular administration is not recommended for treatment of status epilepticus since serum concentrations in the therapeutic range cannot be readily achieved for up to 24 hours. Erratic absorption is partly caused by tissue precipitation of phenytoin. Muscle necrosis has also been reported.
Intramuscular administration during neurosurgery, for patients stabilized on oral phenytoin, requires a dose 50% greater than the oral dosage used to maintain serum concentrations. When a patient is returned to the oral route, dosage should be reduced by 50% of the original oral dosage for 1 week to compensate for the sustained release of medication from prior intramuscular injections.
If the need for intramuscular administration continues for more than 1 week, alternative routes such as gastric intubation should be considered.

**Bioequivalence information**
For oral dosage forms only—
    The prescribing physician should be consulted before a prescription is changed from one phenytoin dosage form to another because of possible differences in bioavailability, due to varying amounts of calcium sulfate excipient or amount of phenytoin acid contained in the product. Phenytoin dosage forms based on phenytoin acid (oral suspension and chewable tablets) contain 8% more drug on an mg-per-mg basis than those based on phenytoin sodium. Phenytoin intoxication has been reported following weight-for-weight substitution of phenytoin acid for phenytoin sodium.
    The prescribing physician should be consulted before a product is dispensed that is different from that currently taken by the patient, or from that originally prescribed. Bioavailability may vary enough among oral phenytoin sodium products of different manufacturers to result in either a loss of seizure control or a toxic blood concentration.

# Oral Dosage Forms

Note: Bracketed uses in the *Dosage Forms* section refer to categories of use and/or indications that are not included in U.S. product labeling.

## PHENYTOIN ORAL SUSPENSION USP

Note: Phenytoin Oral Suspension USP is not an extended phenytoin product and is not intended for once-a-day dosage.

**Usual adult and adolescent dose**
Anticonvulsant—
    Oral, initially, 125 mg three times a day, the dosage being adjusted at seven- to ten-day intervals as needed and tolerated.
Note: For seriously ill or debilitated patients, or patients with impaired hepatic function, the total dose is often reduced.

**Usual pediatric dose**
Anticonvulsant—
    Initial: Oral, 5 mg per kg of body weight a day, divided into two or three doses, the dosage being adjusted as needed and tolerated but not to exceed 300 mg a day.
    Maintenance: Oral, 4 to 8 mg per kg of body weight or 250 mg per square meter of body surface a day, divided into two or three doses.

**Usual geriatric dose**
Anticonvulsant—
    Oral, initially 3 mg per kg of body weight a day, in divided doses, the dosage being adjusted according to serum hydantoin concentrations and the patient's response.

**Strength(s) usually available**
U.S.—
    125 mg per 5 mL (Rx) [*Dilantin-125* (sucrose); GENERIC].
Canada—
    30 mg per 5 mL (Rx) [*Dilantin-30*].
    125 mg per 5 mL (Rx) [*Dilantin-125*].

**Packaging and storage**
Store below 40 °C (104 °F), preferably between 15 and 30 °C (59 and 86 °F), unless otherwise specified by manufacturer. Store in a tight container. Protect from freezing.

**Auxiliary labeling**
- Shake well.
- Protect from freezing.
- Avoid alcoholic beverages.

**Note**

Remind patient to shake bottle well before removing each dose.

Advise patient to use an accurate measuring spoon, plastic syringe, or graduated measuring cup.

**Additional information**

May contain 0.6% alcohol.

## PHENYTOIN TABLETS (CHEWABLE) USP

Note: Phenytoin chewable tablets are not intended for once-a-day dosage as they may be too promptly bioavailable. Once-a-day use of phenytoin chewable tablets may result in toxic serum concentrations of phenytoin.

**Usual adult and adolescent dose**

Anticonvulsant—

Oral, initially, 100 to 125 mg three times a day, the dosage being adjusted at seven- to ten-day intervals as needed and tolerated.

Note: For seriously ill or debilitated patients, or patients with impaired hepatic function, the total dose is often reduced.

**Usual pediatric dose**

Anticonvulsant—

Initial: Oral, 5 mg per kg of body weight a day, divided into two or three doses, the dosage being adjusted as needed and tolerated but not to exceed 300 mg a day.

Maintenance: Oral, 4 to 8 mg per kg of body weight or 250 mg per square meter of body surface a day, divided into two or three doses.

**Usual geriatric dose**

Anticonvulsant—

Oral, initially 3 mg per kg of body weight a day, in divided doses, the dosage being adjusted according to serum hydantoin concentrations and the patient's response.

**Strength(s) usually available**

U.S.—

50 mg (Rx) [*Dilantin Infatabs* (saccharin; sucrose)].

Canada—

50 mg (Rx) [*Dilantin Infatabs*].

Note: One 100-mg capsule of phenytoin sodium contains 92% phenytoin and is therefore not equivalent to two 50-mg phenytoin chewable tablets containing 100% phenytoin.

**Packaging and storage**

Store below 40 °C (104 °F), preferably between 15 and 30 °C (59 and 86 °F), unless otherwise specified by manufacturer. Store in a well-closed container.

**Auxiliary labeling**
- May be chewed or crushed.
- Avoid alcoholic beverages.

## EXTENDED PHENYTOIN SODIUM CAPSULES USP

Note: Only phenytoin sodium capsules labeled "Extended" are to be used for once-a-day dosage. Once-a-day use of capsules labeled "Prompt" may result in toxic serum phenytoin concentrations.

**Usual adult and adolescent dose**

Anticonvulsant—

Oral, initially, 100 mg three times a day, the dosage being adjusted at seven- to ten-day intervals as needed and tolerated. When established, the daily maintenance dosage may be given on a once-a-day basis in accordance with patient tolerance.

Note: An oral loading dose of 1 gram may be given, the dose being divided as follows: Initially 400 mg, then 300 mg after two hours, followed by an additional 300 mg in two hours; normal maintenance dosing is started twenty-four hours after the loading dose. Alternatively, some clinicians recommend an oral loading dose of 20 mg per kg of body weight, divided into three to four doses and administered at two-hour intervals.

Patients with a history of renal or liver disease should not receive a loading dose. Use of this regimen should be limited to patients in a clinic or hospital setting where phenytoin serum concentrations can be closely monitored.

Once-a-day dosage should be considered only for adult patients whose condition has been stabilized by divided doses of extended phenytoin sodium capsules given as 100 mg three times a day. This single 300-mg daily dosage has the advantage of convenience and improved compliance.

For geriatric or seriously ill patients or for debilitated patients or patients with impaired hepatic function, the total dose is often reduced.

[Antineuralgic][1]—

Oral, 200 to 600 mg a day, in divided doses, the dose being adjusted as needed and tolerated.

[Skeletal muscle relaxant][1]—

Oral, up to 300 to 600 mg a day, as needed and tolerated.

**Usual pediatric dose**

Anticonvulsant—

Initial: Oral, 5 mg per kg of body weight a day, divided into two or three doses, the dosage then being adjusted as needed and tolerated but not to exceed 300 mg a day.

Maintenance: Oral, 4 to 8 mg per kg of body weight or 250 mg per square meter of body surface a day, divided into two or three doses.

**Usual geriatric dose**

Anticonvulsant—

Oral, initially, 3 mg per kg of body weight a day, in divided doses, the dosage being adjusted according to serum hydantoin concentrations and the patient's response.

**Strength(s) usually available**

U.S.—

30 mg (Rx) [*Dilantin Kapseals* (lactose; sucrose); GENERIC].

100 mg (Rx) [*Dilantin Kapseals* (lactose; sucrose); *Phenytex*; GENERIC].

Canada—

30 mg (Rx) [*Dilantin* (lactose)].

100 mg (Rx) [*Dilantin* (lactose)].

Note: One 100-mg capsule of phenytoin sodium contains 92% phenytoin and is therefore not equivalent to two 50-mg phenytoin chewable tablets containing 100% phenytoin.

**Packaging and storage**

Store below 40 °C (104 °F), preferably between 15 and 30 °C (59 and 86 °F), unless otherwise specified by manufacturer. Store in a tight container.

**Auxiliary labeling**
- Avoid alcoholic beverages.

**Additional information**

The sodium content of phenytoin sodium is 0.35 mEq (8 mg) per 100-mg capsule.

## PROMPT PHENYTOIN SODIUM CAPSULES USP

Note: Phenytoin sodium capsules labeled "Prompt" are not intended for once-a-day dosage because the phenytoin may be too promptly bioavailable and may cause toxic serum concentrations of phenytoin.

**Usual adult and adolescent dose**

Anticonvulsant—

Oral, 100 mg three times a day, the dosage being adjusted at seven- to ten-day intervals as needed and tolerated.

Note: For geriatric or seriously ill patients or for debilitated patients or patients with impaired hepatic function, the total dose is often reduced.

**Usual pediatric dose**

Anticonvulsant—

Initial: Oral, 5 mg per kg of body weight a day, divided into two or three doses, the dosage then being adjusted as needed and tolerated but not to exceed 300 mg a day.

Maintenance: Oral, 4 to 8 mg per kg of body weight or 250 mg per square meter of body surface a day, divided into two or three doses in accordance with patient tolerance.

**Usual geriatric dose**

Anticonvulsant—

Oral, initial, 3 mg per kg of body weight a day, in divided doses, the dosage being adjusted according to serum hydantoin concentrations and the patient's response.

**Strength(s) usually available**

U.S.—

30 mg (Rx) [*Diphenylan*; GENERIC].

100 mg (Rx) [*Diphenylan*; GENERIC].

Canada—

Not commercially available.

Note: One 100-mg capsule of phenytoin sodium contains 92% phenytoin and is therefore not equivalent to two 50-mg phenytoin chewable tablets containing 100% phenytoin.

## Packaging and storage

Store below 40 °C (104 °F), preferably between 15 and 30 °C (59 and 86 °F), unless otherwise specified by manufacturer. Store in a tight container.

## Auxiliary labeling

• Avoid alcoholic beverages.

## Additional information

The sodium content of phenytoin sodium is 0.35 mEq (8 mg) per 100-mg capsule.

## Parenteral Dosage Forms

Note: Bracketed uses in the *Dosage Forms* section refer to categories of use and/or indictions that are not included in U.S. product labeling.

### PHENYTOIN SODIUM INJECTION USP

**Usual adult and adolescent dose**
Anticonvulsant in status epilepticus—
Initial:
Intravenous, direct, 15 to 20 mg per kg of body weight administered at a rate not to exceed 50 mg a minute.
Note: For obese patients, the loading dose should be calculated on the basis of ideal body weight plus 1.33 times the excess weight over ideal weight, since phenytoin preferentially distributes into fat.
Maintenance:
Intravenous, direct, 100 mg every six to eight hours, at a rate not exceeding 50 mg a minute.
Note: Maintenance therapy, intravenously, 100 mg every six to eight hours, or orally, 5 mg per kg of body weight a day, divided into two to four doses, should begin about twelve to twenty-four hours after a loading dose is given.
[Antiarrhythmic][1]—
Intravenous, direct, 50 to 100 mg every ten to fifteen minutes as needed and tolerated to stop arrhythmia, but not to exceed a total dose of 15 mg per kg of body weight, administered slowly at a rate not exceeding 50 mg a minute.
Note: For geriatric or seriously ill patients or for debilitated patients or patients with impaired hepatic function, the total dose is often reduced and the rate of intravenous administration slowed to 25 mg a minute, possibly as low as 5 to 10 mg a minute, to lessen the possibility of side effects.

Although the manufacturers recommend that phenytoin not be added to intravenous infusions, some clinicians routinely use such infusions. If phenytoin is administered by infusion, the rate of administration should not exceed 50 mg per minute; some investigators have suggested rates of 20 to 40 mg per minute.

**Usual pediatric dose**
Anticonvulsant in status epilepticus—
Intravenous, direct, 15 to 20 mg per kg of body weight, or 250 mg per square meter of body surface area, administered at a rate of 1 to 3 mg per kg of body weight per minute, not exceeding 50 mg a minute.

**Strength(s) usually available**
U.S.—
50 mg per mL (Rx) [*Dilantin* (alcohol 10%); GENERIC].
Canada—
50 mg per mL (Rx) [*Dilantin* (alcohol 10%); GENERIC].

**Packaging and storage**
Store between 15 and 30 °C (59 and 86 °F), unless otherwise specified by manufacturer. Protect from freezing.

**Stability**
A slight yellowing of the solution will not affect its potency. After being refrigerated, solution may form a precipitate which usually dissolves after being warmed to room temperature; however, do not use if the solution is not clear.

**Incompatibilities**
The manufacturers recommend that parenteral phenytoin sodium not be added to intravenous infusions or mixed with other medication because precipitation of phenytoin may occur. However, some clinicians routinely use infusion solutions of phenytoin in 0.9% sodium chloride in concentrations of 1 to 10 mg of phenytoin per mL, provided the infusion is started immediately after preparation and is completed within 1 hour; the admixture must be carefully observed for signs of precipitation, and use of a 0.45 to 0.22 micron in-line filter is recommended; in addition, flushing of all tubing with 0.9% sodium chloride injection before and after infusion of phenytoin is recommended.

**Additional information**
The sodium content of phenytoin sodium injection is approximately 0.2 mEq (4.5 mg) per mL.

[1]Not included in Canadian product labeling.

Revised: 03/09/93
Interim revision: 03/24/94; 04/29/94; 05/13/94

# ANTICONVULSANTS, SUCCINIMIDE    Systemic

This monograph includes information on the following: Ethosuximide; Methsuximide; Phensuximide†.
INN:
Methsuximide—Methsuximide
VA CLASSIFICATION (Primary): CN400
Note: For a listing of dosage forms and brand names by country availability, see *Dosage Forms* section(s). For a listing of brand names for the articles in this monograph, refer to the General Index.

†Not commercially available in Canada.

## Category

Anticonvulsant.

## Indications

Note: Bracketed information in the *Indications* section refers to uses that are not included in U.S. product labeling.

### Accepted

Epilepsy, absence seizure pattern (treatment)—Ethosuximide, the drug of choice, and phensuximide are indicated for the control of seizures in absence (petit mal) epilepsy. Methsuximide is indicated for the management of absence seizures refractory to other medication.

[Epilepsy, complex partial seizure pattern (treatment)][1]—Methsuximide may be used in the treatment of complex partial seizures.

[1]Not included in Canadian product labeling.

## Pharmacology/Pharmacokinetics

### Physicochemical characteristics

Molecular weight—
Ethosuximide: 141.17.
Methsuximide: 203.24.
Phensuximide: 189.21.

### Mechanism of action/Effect

Poorly defined; succinimide anticonvulsants are thought to increase the seizure threshold and suppress the paroxysmal three-cycle-per-second spike-and-wave pattern seen with absence (petit mal) seizures. The frequency of attacks is reduced by depression of nerve transmission in the motor cortex. These effects may be due to direct modification of membrane function in excitable cells and/or alteration of chemically mediated neurotransmission. The specific effect of ethosuximide against absence seizures appears to be due to its ability to block T-type calcium channels at concentrations that do not affect other ion channels.

### Absorption

Generally rapid and complete.

### Distribution

Freely distributed to all body tissues, except fat. Concentrations of ethosuximide in saliva and tears are equivalent to plasma concentrations. Concentrations of ethosuximide in breast milk may approach 94% of plasma concentrations.

### Protein binding

Not significant.

**Biotransformation**
Hepatic. Methsuximide metabolized to the active metabolite *N*-desmethylmethsuximide.

**Half-life**
Ethosuximide—
    Adults: 56 to 60 hours.
    Children: 30 to 36 hours.
Methsuximide—
    1 to 3 hours.
*N*-desmethylmethsuximide—
    34 to 80 hours.
Phensuximide—
    5 to 12 hours.

**Time to peak concentration**
Ethosuximide—
    Adults: 2 to 4 hours.
    Children: 3 to 7 hours.
Methsuximide—
    1 to 4 hours.
Phensuximide—
    1 to 4 hours.

**Therapeutic serum concentration**
Ethosuximide—40 to 100 mcg/mL (283.4 to 708.4 micromoles per L).
*N*-desmethylmethsuximide—10 to 40 mcg/mL (49.2 to 196.8 micromoles per L).

**Elimination**
Renal (ethosuximide, up to 20% unchanged).

## Precautions to Consider

### Cross-sensitivity and/or related problems
Patients sensitive to one succinimide anticonvulsant may be sensitive to the others also.

### Pregnancy/Reproduction
Pregnancy—Problems in humans have not been documented; however, teratogenic effects have been associated with other anticonvulsant medications.

### Breast-feeding
Ethosuximide is distributed into breast milk. It is not known whether methsuximide or phensuximide is distributed into breast milk. Problems in humans have not been documented.

### Pediatrics
Appropriate studies performed to date have not demonstrated pediatrics-specific problems that would limit the usefulness of succinimide anticonvulsants in children.

### Geriatrics
Appropriate studies on the relationship of age to the effects of succinimide anticonvulsants have not been performed in the geriatric population. However, no geriatrics-specific problems have been documented to date.

### Dental
The blood dyscrasia–causing effects of succinimide anticonvulsants may result in an increased incidence of microbial infection, delayed healing, and gingival bleeding. If leukopenia or thrombocytopenia occurs, dental work should be deferred until blood counts have returned to normal. Patients should be instructed in proper oral hygiene during treatment, including caution in use of regular toothbrushes, dental floss, and toothpicks.

### Drug interactions and/or related problems
The following drug interactions and/or related problems have been selected on the basis of their potential clinical significance (possible mechanism in parentheses where appropriate)—not necessarily inclusive (» = major clinical significance):

Note: Combinations containing any of the following medications, depending on the amount present, may also interact with this medication.

Alcohol or
» Central nervous system (CNS) depression–producing medications, other (See *Appendix II*)
    (CNS depression may be enhanced)
Antidepressants, tricyclic, or
Loxapine or
Maprotiline or

Molindone or
Monoamine oxidase (MAO) inhibitors or
Phenothiazines or
Pimozide or
Thioxanthenes
    (concurrent use may lower the convulsive threshold, enhance CNS depression, and decrease the effects of the anticonvulsant medication)
Carbamazepine or
Phenobarbital or
Phenytoin or
Primidone
    (induction of hepatic microsomal enzyme activity resulting in increased metabolism and decreased serum concentrations and elimination half-lives of succinimide anticonvulsants and/or these medications may occur during concurrent therapy; monitoring of serum concentrations as a guide to dosage is recommended, especially when any anticonvulsant is added to or withdrawn from an existing regimen)
Folic acid
    (requirements for folic acid may be increased in patients receiving anticonvulsant therapy)
» Haloperidol
    (concurrent use may cause a change in the pattern and/or the frequency of epileptiform seizures; dosage adjustments of the anticonvulsant may be necessary; serum concentrations of haloperidol may be significantly reduced)
Phenacemide
    (concurrent use may result in additive toxicity)
Valproic acid
    (concurrent use of valproic acid has been reported to both increase and decrease ethosuximide concentrations due to changes in metabolism; monitoring of serum concentrations as a guide to dosage is recommended)

### Medical considerations/Contraindications
The medical considerations/contraindications included here have been selected on the basis of their potential clinical significance (reasons given in parentheses where appropriate)—not necessarily inclusive (» = major clinical significance).

### Risk-benefit should be considered when the following medical problems exist:
Blood dyscrasias
    (condition may be exacerbated)
Hepatic function impairment or
Renal function impairment, severe
    (morphological and functional changes may occur in liver or kidneys)
Intermittent porphyria
    (condition may be exacerbated)
Sensitivity to succinimide anticonvulsants

### Patient monitoring
The following may be especially important in patient monitoring (other tests may be warranted in some patients, depending on condition; » = major clinical significance):
» Blood cell counts, including platelets, and
    Hepatic function determinations and
    Renal function determinations and
    Urinalysis
        (recommended at periodic intervals for patients on prolonged therapy)

## Side/Adverse Effects

The following side/adverse effects have been selected on the basis of their potential clinical significance (possible signs and symptoms in parentheses where appropriate)—not necessarily inclusive:

**Those indicating need for medical attention**
Incidence more frequent
    *Stevens-Johnson syndrome or systemic lupus erythematosus* (skin rash and itching; swollen glands; sore throat and fever; muscle pain)

Incidence less frequent
  *Aggressiveness; difficulty in concentration; mental depression; nightmares*
Incidence rare
  *Blood dyscrasias, including agranulocytosis* (chills; fever; sore throat; unusual tiredness or weakness); *aplastic anemia* (shortness of breath, troubled breathing, wheezing, or tightness in chest; sores, ulcers, or white spots on lips or in mouth; swollen or painful glands; unusual bleeding or bruising); *eosinophilia* (fever); *leukopenia* (fever; chills; sore throat); *pancytopenia* (nosebleeds or other unusual bleeding or bruising); *precipitation of tonic-clonic convulsions; paranoid psychosis* (mood or mental changes); *pruritic erythematous rash* (skin rash and itching)

**Those indicating need for medical attention only if they continue or are bothersome**
Incidence more frequent
  *Anorexia* (loss of appetite); *ataxia* (clumsiness or unsteadiness); *dizziness; drowsiness; headache; hiccups; nausea or vomiting; stomach cramps*
Incidence less frequent
  *Irritability; unusual tiredness or weakness*

**Those not indicating need for medical attention**
  *Discoloration of urine* (pink, red, or red-brown urine)—for phensuximide only

## Overdose

For specific information on the agents used in the management of succinimide anticonvulsants, see: *Charcoal, Activated (Oral-Local)* monograph.

For more information on the management of overdose or unintentional ingestion, **contact a Poison Control Center** (see *Poison Control Center Listing*).

**Clinical effects of overdose**
The following effects have been selected on the basis of their potential clinical significance (possible signs and symptoms in parentheses where appropriate)—not necessarily inclusive:

  *Central nervous system (CNS) depression* (severe drowsiness); *severe nausea and vomiting; respiratory depression* (shortness of breath; slow or irregular breathing; troubled breathing)

  Note: Methsuximide poisoning may have a biphasic profile due to the *N*-desmethyl metabolite; therefore it is important to monitor serum concentrations of *N*-desmethylmethsuximide.

**Treatment of overdose**
Because no specific antidote is available, treatment is essentially symptomatic and supportive.

crease absorption—
  Induction of emesis (unless the patient is or could rapidly become obtunded, comatose, or convulsing) or gastric lavage.
  Instillation of activated charcoal.
  Use of cathartics.
To enhance elimination—
  Hemodialysis may be useful in treating ethosuximide overdoses.
  Charcoal hemoperfusion may be useful to remove the *N*-desmethyl metabolite of methsuximide.
  Forced diuresis and exchange transfusions are ineffective in the treatment of succinimide anticonvulsant overdoses.
Supportive care—
  Patients in whom intentional overdose is confirmed or suspected should be referred for psychiatric consultation.

## Patient Consultation

As an aid to patient consultation, refer to *Advice for the Patient, Anticonvulsants, Succinimide (Systemic)*.

In providing consultation, consider emphasizing the following selected information (» = major clinical significance):

**Before using this medication**
» Conditions affecting use, especially:
    Sensitivity to succinimide anticonvulsants
    Pregnancy—Possible birth defects
    Other medications, especially CNS depressants or haloperidol
    Other medical problems, especially blood dyscrasias, hepatic function impairment, severe renal function impairment, or intermittent porphyria

**Proper use of this medication**
» Compliance with therapy; taking daily in regularly spaced doses as ordered
    Taking with food or milk to reduce gastric irritation

» Proper dosing
    Missed dose: Taking as soon as possible; if remembered within 4 hours of next dose, skipping missed dose and continuing on regular dosing schedule; not doubling doses
» Proper storage

**Precautions while using this medication**
» Regular visits to physician to check progress of therapy
» Checking with physician before discontinuing this medication; gradual dosage reduction may be necessary
» Not starting or stopping other medication without physician's advice
» Avoiding the use of alcoholic beverages and other CNS depressants while taking this medication
» Possibility of drowsiness; caution if driving or doing jobs requiring alertness
» Caution if any kind of surgery, dental treatment, or emergency treatment is required
    Carrying medical identification card or bracelet
*For methsuximide*
    Not taking capsules that are melted or not full; effectiveness may be reduced

**Side/adverse effects**
Signs of potential side effects, especially Stevens-Johnson syndrome, systemic lupus erythematosus, aggressiveness, difficulty in concentration, mental depression, nightmares, blood dyscrasias, tonic-clonic convulsions, paranoid psychosis, or pruritic erythematous rash
Phensuximide may cause harmless discoloration of urine (pink, red, or red-brown)

## General Dosing Information

When succinimide anticonvulsants are to be discontinued, dosage should be reduced gradually to prevent possible occurrence of petit mal status.

When used to replace other anticonvulsant therapy, the dosage of the succinimide anticonvulsant should be increased gradually while that of the other medication is gradually decreased, to maintain seizure control.

If succinimide anticonvulsants are used to supplement an existing anticonvulsant regimen, their dosage should be gradually increased to the required level.

When succinimide anticonvulsants are used alone in mixed types of epilepsy, the frequency of primary generalized tonic-clonic seizures may be increased in some patients.

---

### *ETHOSUXIMIDE*

## Summary of Differences

Pharmacology/pharmacokinetics:
  Half-life—56 to 60 hours in adults; 30 to 36 hours in children.
  Peak effect—3 to 7 hours.
  Serum concentrations, therapeutic—40 to 100 mcg/mL.

## Additional Dosing Information

See also *General Dosing Information*.

Strict supervision by the physician is required if total daily dosage of ethosuximide exceeds 1.5 grams for adults or 1 gram for children up to 6 years of age.

Ethosuximide dosage may be initiated at maintenance level. When this medication is used concurrently with intravenous diazepam in management of absence status epilepticus (petit mal status), higher-than-usual starting doses may be required to rapidly achieve a therapeutic serum level.

## Oral Dosage Forms

### ETHOSUXIMIDE CAPSULES USP

**Usual adult and adolescent dose**
Anticonvulsant—
  Oral, 15 to 30 mg per kg of body weight a day; or initially 250 mg two times a day, the dosage being increased by an additional 250 mg a day at four- to seven-day intervals until seizure control is obtained or until the total daily dose reaches 1.5 grams.

**Usual pediatric dose**
Anticonvulsant—
  Children up to 6 years of age: Oral, 15 to 40 mg per kg of body weight a day; or initially 250 mg once a day, the dosage being increased by an additional 250 mg a day at four- to seven-day

intervals until seizure control is obtained or until the total daily dose reaches 1 gram.

Children 6 years of age and over: See *Usual adult and adolescent dose.*

Note: The optimal dosage for most children is 20 mg per kg of body weight a day.

**Strength(s) usually available**

U.S.—

250 mg (Rx) [*Zarontin*].

Canada—

250 mg (Rx) [*Zarontin*].

**Packaging and storage**

Store below 30 °C (86 °F), preferably between 15 and 30 °C (59 and 86 °F), unless otherwise specified by manufacturer. Store in a tight container.

**Auxiliary labeling**

• May cause drowsiness.
• Keep container tightly closed.

## ETHOSUXIMIDE SYRUP

**Usual adult and adolescent dose**

See *Ethosuximide Capsules USP.*

**Usual pediatric dose**

See *Ethosuximide Capsules USP.*

**Strength(s) usually available**

U.S.—

250 mg per 5 mL (Rx) [*Zarontin* (sucrose); GENERIC].

Canada—

250 mg per 5 mL (Rx) [*Zarontin*].

**Packaging and storage**

Store between 15 and 30 °C (59 and 86 °F), in a tight, light-resistant container, unless otherwise specified by manufacturer. Protect from freezing.

**Auxiliary labeling**

• May cause drowsiness.

### *METHSUXIMIDE*

## Summary of Differences

Category:

Indicated in absence seizures refractory to other medication.

Pharmacology/pharmacokinetics:

Half-life—1 to 3 hours (36 to 45 hours for active metabolites).

Serum concentration, therapeutic—10 to 40 mcg/mL.

## Oral Dosage Forms

### METHSUXIMIDE CAPSULES USP

**Usual adult and adolescent dose**

Anticonvulsant—

Oral, initially 300 mg once a day, the dosage being increased by 300 mg a day at one-week intervals until seizure control is obtained or until the total daily dose reaches 1.2 grams. Alternatively, some clinicians advocate making dosage increases of 150 to 300 mg at intervals of no less than 14 days to allow plasma concentrations to reach steady-state levels.

**Usual pediatric dose**

See *Usual adult and adolescent dose.* (Small children may require dosage adjustments utilizing the 150-mg capsules.)

**Strength(s) usually available**

U.S.—

150 mg (Rx) [*Celontin*].

300 mg (Rx) [*Celontin*].

Canada—

300 mg (Rx) [*Celontin*].

**Packaging and storage**

Store below 30 °C (86 °F), preferably between 15 and 30 °C (59 and 86 °F), unless otherwise specified by manufacturer. Store in a tight container. Avoid exposure to excessive heat.

**Stability**

Methsuximide has a relatively low melting range (50 to 56 °C [122 to 133 °F]). Improper storage may result in melting and subsequent impaired absorption of the capsule contents.

**Auxiliary labeling**

• May cause drowsiness.

**Note**

Do not dispense or use capsules that are not full or in which contents have melted. Protect from excessive heat (40 °C [104 °F]).

### *PHENSUXIMIDE*

## Summary of Differences

Pharmacology/pharmacokinetics:

Half-life—5 to 12 hours.

Peak effect—1 to 4 hours.

Precautions:

Medical considerations/contraindications—

Should be used with caution in patients with intermittent porphyria.

Side/adverse effects:

Causes harmless pink, red, or red-brown discoloration of urine.

## Oral Dosage Forms

### PHENSUXIMIDE CAPSULES USP

**Usual adult and adolescent dose**

Anticonvulsant—

Oral, initially 500 mg two or three times a day, the dosage being increased by an additional 500 mg a day at one-week intervals until seizure control is obtained or until the total daily dose reaches 3 grams.

**Usual pediatric dose**

See *Usual adult and adolescent dose.*

**Strength(s) usually available**

U.S.—

500 mg (Rx) [*Milontin*].

Canada—

Not commercially available.

**Packaging and storage**

Store below 30 °C (86 °F), preferably between 15 and 30 °C (59 and 86 °F), unless otherwise specified by manufacturer. Store in a tight container.

**Auxiliary labeling**

• May cause drowsiness.
• May discolor urine.

Revised: 05/23/94

# ANTIDEPRESSANTS, MONOAMINE OXIDASE (MAO) INHIBITOR    Systemic

This monograph includes information on the following: Isocarboxazid; Phenelzine; Tranylcypromine.

VA CLASSIFICATION (Primary): CN602

Note: This monograph does not cover other MAO inhibitors, such as furazolidone and procarbazine, which are not used as antidepressants, and selegiline, which has its own monograph.

Note: For a listing of dosage forms and brand names by country availability, see *Dosage Forms* section(s). For a listing of brand names for the articles in this monograph, refer to the General Index.

## Category

Category

Antidepressant; antipanic agent; headache (vascular; tension) prophylactic

## Indications

Note: Bracketed information in the *Indications* section refers to uses that are not included in U.S. product labeling.

### Accepted

Depression, mental (treatment)—Phenelzine is effective in the treatment of patients with major depression with or without melancholia, or with atypical, nonendogenous depression, or depressive neurosis. These patients often have mixed anxiety and depression with phobic or hypo-chondriacal features. Phenelzine is more often used as a second-line antidepressant in patients who have failed to respond to other antide-pressants. Nevertheless, many clinicians may consider phenelzine the first choice for treatment of certain dysphorias and minor periodic or chronic depressions (dysthymic disorders).

Tranylcypromine is indicated for treatment of major depression [with or] without melancholia in closely supervised adult patients not re-sponding to or unable to tolerate other antidepressants. [It is also used to treat the depressed phase of bipolar disorder and depressive neurosis of moderate to severe intensity.]

Isocarboxazid is classified by the Food and Drug Administration (FDA) as being "probably" effective for the treatment of depressed patients who are refractory to tricyclic antidepressants or electrocon-vulsive therapy or in whom tricyclic antidepressants are contraindi-cated. This classification requires the submission of adequate and well-controlled studies in order to provide substantial evidence of effectiveness.

[Panic disorder (treatment)][1]—Phenelzine and, to a lesser extent, tranyl-cypromine are used in conjunction with psychotherapy and behavioral therapy in the treatment of panic disorder, with or without agoraphobia.

[Headache, vascular (prophylaxis)][1] or
[Headache, tension (prophylaxis)][1]—Monoamine oxidase inhibitors are used in the prophylaxis of vascular headaches (including migraine), tension-type headaches, and mixed headache syndrome. However, due to potentially severe side effects, these agents are not considered first-line therapy.

---

[1]Not included in Canadian product labeling.

## Pharmacology/Pharmacokinetics

### Physicochemical characteristics
Molecular weight—
  Isocarboxazid: 231.25.
  Phenelzine sulfate: 234.27.
  Tranylcypromine sulfate: 364.46.

### Mechanism of action/Effect
The exact mechanism of antidepressant effect is unknown; however, it is established that the activity of the enzyme monoamine oxidase (MAO) is inhibited. MAO subtypes A and B are involved in the metabolism of serotonin and catecholamine neurotransmitters such as epinephrine, norepinephrine, and dopamine. Isocarboxazid, phenelzine, and tran-ylcypromine, as nonselective MAO inhibitors, bind irreversibly to monoamine oxidase–A (MAO-A) and monoamine oxidase–B (MAO-B). The reduced MAO activity results in an increased concentration of these neurotransmitters in storage sites throughout the central nerv-ous system (CNS) and sympathetic nervous system. This increased availability of one or more monoamines has been thought to be the basis for the antidepressant activity of MAO inhibitors. The nonselec-tive MAO inhibitors, phenelzine, tranylcypromine, and isocarboxazid, result in downregulation (desensitization) of alpha$_2$- or beta-adrenergic and serotonin receptors. It is thought that changes in receptor char-acteristics produced by chronic administration of MAO inhibitors cor-relate better with antidepressant action than does the increased activity of the neuron secondary to increased neurotransmitter concentrations, and may also account for the delay of 2 to 4 weeks in therapeutic response.

### Other actions/effects
MAO inhibitors exhibit a hypotensive effect, which varies with the spe-cific agent; the hypotensive mechanism of action is probably mediated through central inhibition of vasomotor centers, or it may be due to chronic accumulation of the false neurotransmitter octopamine in ad-renergic terminals.

MAO inhibitors prevent the inactivation of tyramine by hepatic and gas-trointestinal monoamine oxidase. Circulating tyramine releases nor-epinephrine from the sympathetic nerve terminals and produces a sud-den increase in blood pressure.

### Absorption
Well absorbed from the gastrointestinal tract.

### Biotransformation
Hepatic; rapid; by oxidation; possible active metabolites.

### Onset of action
As early as 7 to 10 days with appropriate dosage in some patients, but may take up to 4 to 8 weeks to achieve full therapeutic effect.

### Time to peak plasma concentration
Isocarboxazid—3 to 5 hours after oral dose.
Phenelzine—2 to 4 hours after oral dose.
Tranylcypromine—1 to 3.5 hours.

### Duration of action
At least 10 days for MAO activity to be recovered because of irreversible binding.

### Elimination
Renal, as metabolites.

## Precautions to Consider

### Tumorigenicity
Phenelzine and isocarboxazid, like other hydrazine derivatives, have been reported in an uncontrolled lifetime study to induce pulmonary and vascular tumors in mice.

### Pregnancy/Reproduction
Pregnancy—Tranylcypromine (and probably isocarboxazid and phenel-zine) crosses the placenta. A limited study in humans reported an increased risk of fetal malformations when these medications were administered in the first trimester.

Animal studies have shown that MAO inhibitors, in doses much higher than the maximum recommended human dose (MRHD), cause hyper-excitability and a reduced rate of growth in the neonate.

For phenelzine: FDA Pregnancy Category C.

For isocarboxazid and tranylcypromine: FDA pregnancy category not cur-rently included in product labeling.

### Breast-feeding
Tranylcypromine is distributed into human breast milk; it is not known whether isocarboxazid or phenelzine is distributed into human breast milk. Problems in humans have not been documented.

### Pediatrics
Appropriate studies on the relationship of age to the effects of MAO inhibitors have not been performed in children up to 16 years of age. Safety and efficacy have not been established. Animal studies have shown that these medications may cause growth retardation in the young.

### Geriatrics
Experience with the use of MAO inhibitors in the elderly is relatively limited. However, there have been reports that phenelzine is safe and effective in the treatment of elderly depressed patients with a history of atypical depression or depressive neurosis. MAO inhibitors may also be useful for anergic or apathetic retarded depressions. The po-tential for increased vascular accidents (especially in the event of sud-den hypertensive episodes), increased sensitivity to hypotensive ef-fects, and reduced metabolic capacity discourages the first-time use of MAO inhibitors in patients over 60 years of age. When an MAO inhibitor is prescribed for an elderly patient, the patient's history of depression, ability to comply with prescribing instructions, and any potential drug interactions must also be considered.

### Drug interactions and/or related problems
The following drug interactions and/or related problems have been se-lected on the basis of their potential clinical significance (possible mechanism in parentheses where appropriate)—not necessarily inclu-sive (» = major clinical significance):

Note: Combinations containing any of the following medications, de-pending on the amount present, may also interact with this medication.

» Alcohol or
» CNS depression–producing medications, other, (See *Appendix II*)
    (concurrent use with MAO inhibitors may increase CNS depressant effects)

    (also, possible tyramine content in some alcoholic beverages, es-pecially beer, wine, or ale, may induce hypertensive reactions)

    (in addition to additive CNS depressant effects caused by some antihypertensives such as clonidine, guanabenz, methyldopa, me-tyrosine, and pargyline, postural hypotension may be aggravated)

» Anesthetics, local, with epinephrine or levonordefrin or
» Cocaine
    (concurrent use with MAO inhibitors may cause severe hyperten-sion due to sympathomimetic effects)

    (cocaine should not be administered during or within 14 days fol-lowing administration of an MAO inhibitor; phenelzine also inhib-its cholinesterase activity and may reduce or slow cocaine metab-olism, thereby increasing the risk of cocaine toxicity)

Anesthetics, spinal
(use of MAO inhibitors in patients receiving local anesthetics via subarachnoid block may increase the risk of hypotension; discontinuation of MAO inhibitors 10 days before elective surgery may be advisable; however, to avoid interruption of antidepressant therapy, patients receiving long-term MAO inhibition may undergo surgery without discontinuation of the MAO inhibitor; dosages of the anesthetic must be adjusted carefully)

Anticholinergics or other medications with anticholinergic activity (See *Appendix II*) or
Antidyskinetic agents or
Antihistamines
(concurrent use with MAO inhibitors may intensify the anticholinergic effects of these medications because of secondary anticholinergic activities of MAO inhibitors)

(also, concurrent use with MAO inhibitors may block detoxification of anticholinergics, thus potentiating their action; patients should be advised to report occurrence of gastrointestinal problems promptly since paralytic ileus may occur with concurrent therapy)

(concurrent use with MAO inhibitors may also prolong and intensify the CNS depressant and anticholinergic effects of antihistamines; concurrent use is not recommended)

Anticoagulants, coumarin- or indandione-derivative
(concurrent use may increase anticoagulant activity; although the mechanism of action and clinical significance are unknown, caution is recommended)

Anticonvulsants
(in addition to increasing CNS depressant effects, concurrent use with MAO inhibitors may cause a change in the pattern of epileptiform seizures; dosage adjustment of anticonvulsant may be necessary)

» Antidepressants, tricyclic or
» Fluoxetine or
» Paroxetine or
» Sertraline or
» Trazodone
(a potentially lethal hyperserotonergic state known as the serotonin syndrome may occur as the result of combining serotonergic agents [such as amitriptyline, clomipramine, doxepin, or imipramine; fluoxetine, paroxetine, or sertraline; or trazodone] with MAO inhibitors. The syndrome may be manifested by mental status changes [confusion, hypomania], restlessness, myoclonus, hyperreflexia, diaphoresis, shivering, tremor, diarrhea, incoordination, and/or fever. If recognized early, the syndrome usually resolves quickly upon withdrawal of the offending agents)

(in addition to increased anticholinergic effects, concurrent use of tricyclic antidepressants with MAO inhibitors has resulted in an increased risk of hyperpyretic episodes, hypertensive crises, severe convulsions, and death; however, recent studies have shown that some tricyclic antidepressants can be used concurrently with MAO inhibitors for refractory depression with no adverse effects if both medications are initiated simultaneously at lower than usual doses and the doses raised gradually, or if the MAO inhibitor is gradually added to the tricyclic, also at low doses; tricyclics should not be added to an established MAO inhibitor regimen; clomipramine, desipramine, imipramine, nortriptyline, and protriptyline are not recommended for use in such a regimen; careful monitoring for side effects of either medication is necessary)

(concurrent use of fluoxetine with MAO inhibitors may result in confusion, agitation, restlessness, and gastrointestinal symptoms, or possibly hyperpyretic episodes, severe convulsions, and hypertensive crises. Based on experience with tricyclic antidepressants, at least 14 days should elapse between discontinuation of an MAO inhibitor and initiation of fluoxetine. However, because of the long half-lives of fluoxetine and its active metabolite, at least 5 weeks [approximately 5 half-lives of norfluoxetine] should elapse between discontinuation of fluoxetine and initiation of therapy with an MAO inhibitor. Administration of an MAO inhibitor within 5 weeks of discontinuation of fluoxetine may increase the risk of serious events. While a causal relationship to fluoxetine has not been established, death has been reported following the initiation of an MAO inhibitor shortly after fluoxetine administration was stopped)

» Antidiabetic agents, oral or
» Insulin
(hypoglycemic effects may be enhanced by MAO inhibitors; reduction in dosage of hypoglycemic medication may be necessary during and after concurrent therapy)

Beta-adrenergic blocking agents
(a few cases of significant bradycardia have been reported in elderly patients receiving a beta-adrenergic blocking agent concurrently with phenelzine; monitoring of pulse rate during concurrent administration has been recommended)

Bromocriptine
(concurrent use may increase serum prolactin concentrations and interfere with effects of bromocriptine; dosage adjustment of bromocriptine may be necessary)

» Bupropion
(concurrent use of MAO inhibitors with bupropion may increase the risk of acute bupropion toxicity and is contraindicated; a medication-free interval of at least 2 weeks should elapse between discontinuation of the MAO inhibitor and initiation of bupropion therapy)

» Buspirone
(concurrent use with MAO inhibitors is not recommended because elevation of blood pressure may occur; at least 10 days should elapse between discontinuation of one medication and initiation of the other)

» Caffeine-containing medications
(concurrent use of excessive amounts of caffeine, consumed in coffee, tea, cola, chocolate, or "stay awake" products, with MAO inhibitors may produce dangerous cardiac arrhythmias or severe hypertension because of sympathomimetic side effects of caffeine)

» Carbamazepine or
» Cyclobenzaprine or
» Maprotiline or
» Monoamine oxidase (MAO) inhibitors, other, including furazolidone, procarbazine, or selegiline
(concurrent use with MAO inhibitors has resulted in hyperpyretic crises, hypertensive crises, severe convulsions, and death; a medication-free interval of at least 2 weeks should elapse between discontinuation of one medication and initiation of another; for patients switching from one MAO inhibitor to another, an interval of 2 weeks is recommended)

(in addition, MAO inhibitors cause a change in the pattern of epileptiform seizures in patients receiving carbamazepine as an anticonvulsant)

» Dextromethorphan
(concurrent use with MAO inhibitors may cause excitation, hypertension, and hyperpyrexia)

Diuretics
(concurrent use with MAO inhibitors may result in an increased hypotensive effect)

» Doxapram
(concurrent use may increase the pressor effects of either doxapram or the MAO inhibitor)

» Guanadrel or
» Guanethidine or
» Rauwolfia alkaloids
(concurrent use with these agents may result in moderate to severe hypertension due to release of catecholamines; withdrawal of MAO inhibitor at least 1 week prior to initiation of therapy with these agents is recommended)

(when an MAO inhibitor is added to existing therapy with a rauwolfia alkaloid, serious potentiation of CNS depressant effects may result; however, if a rauwolfia alkaloid is added to an MAO inhibitor regimen, CNS excitation and hypertension may result from release of excessive amounts of accumulated norepinephrine and serotonin)

Haloperidol or
Loxapine or
Molindone or
Phenothiazines or
Pimozide or
Thioxanthenes
(concurrent use may prolong and intensify the sedative, hypotensive, and anticholinergic effects of either these medications or MAO inhibitors)

» Levodopa
(concurrent use with MAO inhibitors is not recommended, as the combination may result in sudden moderate to severe hypertensive crisis; it is recommended that MAO inhibitors be discontinued for 2 to 4 weeks prior to initiation of levodopa therapy)

» Meperidine, and possibly other opioid (narcotic) analgesics
(concurrent use with MAO inhibitors may produce immediate excitation, sweating, rigidity, and severe hypertension; in some pa-

tients, hypotension, severe respiratory depression, coma, convulsions, hyperpyrexia, vascular collapse, and death may occur; reactions may be due to accumulation of serotonin resulting from MAO inhibition; avoidance of meperidine use within 2 to 3 weeks following MAO inhibition is recommended; other opioid analgesics such as morphine are not likely to cause such severe reactions and may be used cautiously in reduced dosage in patients receiving MAO inhibitors; however, it is recommended that a small test dose [$^1/_4$ of the usual dose] or several small incremental test doses over a period of several hours should first be administered to permit observation of any adverse effects; caution is also recommended in the use of alfentanil, fentanyl, or sufentanil as an adjunct to anesthesia if the patient has received an MAO inhibitor within 14 days; although the risk of a significant interaction has been questioned, the use of a small test dose is advised to detect any possible interaction)

» Methyldopa
(may cause hyperexcitability in patients receiving an MAO inhibitor; also headache, severe hypertension, and hallucinations have been reported with concurrent use)

» Methylphenidate
(concurrent use with MAO inhibitors may potentiate the CNS stimulant effects of methylphenidate, possibly resulting in a hypertensive crisis; methylphenidate should not be administered during or within 14 days following the administration of MAO inhibitors)

Metrizamide
(concurrent use with MAO inhibitors may lower the seizure threshold and increase the risk of seizures; MAO inhibitors should be discontinued at least 48 hours before myelography and should not be resumed for at least 24 hours after procedure)

Phenylephrine, nasal or ophthalmic
(if significant systemic absorption of nasal or ophthalmic phenylephrine occurs, concurrent use with MAO inhibitors may potentiate the pressor effect of phenylephrine; nasal or ophthalmic phenylephrine should not be administered during or within 14 days following the administration of an MAO inhibitor)

Succinylcholine
(concurrent use with phenelzine may decrease plasma concentrations or activity of pseudocholinesterase, the enzyme that metabolizes succinylcholine, thereby enhancing the neuromuscular blockade of succinylcholine and possibly resulting in prolonged respiratory depression or apnea)

» Sympathomimetics
(concurrent use with MAO inhibitors may prolong and intensify cardiac stimulant and vasopressor effects [including headache, cardiac arrhythmias, vomiting, sudden and severe hypertensive and hyperpyretic crises] of these medications because of release of catecholamines that accumulate in intraneuronal storage sites during MAO inhibitor therapy; these medications should not be administered during or within 14 days following the administration of an MAO inhibitor)

» Tryptophan
(concurrent use with MAO inhibitors may cause hyperreflexia, shivering, hyperventilation, hyperthermia, mania or hypomania, and disorientation or confusion; if tryptophan is added to an MAO inhibitor regimen, especially tranylcypromine, it should be started in low dosages and the dose titrated upwards gradually with close monitoring of mental status and blood pressure)

» Tyramine- or other high pressor amine–containing foods and beverages, such as aged cheese; fava or broad bean pods; yeast/protein extracts; smoked or pickled meats, poultry, or fish; fermented sausage (bologna, pepperoni, salami, summer sausage) or other fermented meat; sauerkraut; any overripe fruit; beer; reduced-alcohol and alcohol-free beer and wine; red and white wines; sherry; and liqueurs
(concurrent use with MAO inhibitors may cause sudden and severe hypertensive reactions; reactions are usually limited to a few hours and easily treated with rapidly acting hypotensive agents [such as labetolol, nifedipine, or if necessary in severe cases refractory to other agents, phentolamine]; severity depends on amount of tyramine ingested, rate of gastric emptying, and length of interval between dose of MAO inhibitor and ingestion of tyramine; when MAO inhibitors are discontinued, dietary restrictions must continue for at least 2 weeks; other tyramine- or high pressor amine–containing foods, such as yogurt, sour cream, cream cheese, cottage cheese, chocolate, and soy sauce, if eaten when fresh and in moderation, are considered unlikely to cause serious problems)

**Medical considerations/Contraindications**
The medical considerations/contraindications included here have been selected on the basis of their potential clinical significance (reasons given in parentheses where appropriate)—not necessarily inclusive (» = major clinical significance).

*Except under special circumstances, this medication should not be used when the following medical problems exist:*
» Alcoholism, active
» Congestive heart failure
» Hepatic function impairment, severe
(hepatic precoma may be precipitated in patients with cirrhosis, who are extremely sensitive to effects of MAO inhibitors)
» Pheochromocytoma
(pressor substances secreted by such tumors may alter blood pressure during therapy with MAO inhibitors)
» Renal function impairment, severe
(cumulative effects of MAO inhibitors may occur because of reduced renal excretion)
Sensitivity to any MAO inhibitor, including furazolidone, procarbazine, or selegiline

*Risk-benefit should be considered when the following medical problems exist:*
Asthma or bronchitis
(medications used in the treatment of these conditions may interact with MAO inhibitors)
Bipolar disorder
(switch from depressive to manic phase may occur)
» Cardiac arrhythmias
» Cardiovascular disease or coronary insufficiency or
Cerebrovascular disease
(ischemia may be aggravated as a result of reduced blood pressure; however, in patients with serious heart block or a conduction disturbance, an MAO inhibitor may be preferred to a tricyclic antidepressant because of significant slowing of resting pulse [heart rate] or shortening of the PR and QT intervals, and a significant decrease in blood pressure)
Diabetes mellitus
(insulin or oral hypoglycemic requirements may be altered)
Epilepsy
(pattern of epileptiform seizures may be changed)
» Headaches, severe or frequent
(headache as a first sign of hypertensive reaction during therapy may be masked)
» Hepatic function impairment
(hepatic precoma may be precipitated in patients with cirrhosis, who are extremely sensitive to effects of MAO inhibitors)
» Hypertension
(use of MAO inhibitors is not recommended in patients on multiple-drug therapy since hypotensive effects may be potentiated; hypertensive crises resulting from dietary lapses may be more severe in hypertensive patients)
Hyperthyroidism
(sensitivity to pressor amines may be increased)
Parkinson's disease
(may be aggravated)
» Renal function impairment
(cumulative effects may occur)
» Schizophrenia
(MAO inhibitors may aggravate psychosis and/or cause excessive stimulation in schizophrenic patients)
» Suicidal tendencies
(patients may continue to exhibit suicidal tendencies because significant improvement may not occur for several weeks after initiation of therapy with MAO inhibitors)
» Caution is required also in patients who have undergone sympathectomy; these patients may be more sensitive to the hypotensive effects of MAO inhibitors.

**Patient monitoring**
The following may be especially important in patient monitoring (other tests may be warranted in some patients, depending on condition; » = major clinical significance):
» Blood pressure measurements
(careful and frequent monitoring is recommended because of the variety of factors that may produce dangerous alterations in pressure during therapy)

Hepatic function determinations
(although rare, drug-induced hepatitis has occurred with MAO inhibitor therapy)

## Side/Adverse Effects

The following side/adverse effects have been selected on the basis of their potential clinical significance (possible signs and symptoms in parentheses where appropriate)—not necessarily inclusive:

**Those indicating need for medical attention**
Incidence more frequent
*Orthostatic hypotension, severe* (dizziness or lightheadedness, especially when getting up from a lying or sitting position)
Note: Falling or fainting may result. *Orthostatic hypotension* occurs in hypertensive as well as normal and hypotensive patients. Reduction in the dosage of MAO inhibitor may be required to bring blood pressure up to pretreatment levels.

Incidence less frequent
*Diarrhea; peripheral edema* (swelling of feet and lower legs); *sympathetic stimulation* (fast or pounding heartbeat; unusual excitement or nervousness)
Note: *Edema* may subside spontaneously within a week. However, if edema persists, electrolytes should be monitored to rule out syndrome of inappropriate antidiuretic hormone secretion (SIADH).

Incidence rare
*Hepatitis* (dark urine; skin rash; yellow eyes or skin); *leukopenia* (fever; sore throat); *parkinsonian syndrome* (slurred speech; staggering gait)
Note: A potentially lethal hyperserotonergic state known as the serotonin syndrome may occur, typically as the result of combining serotonergic agents (such as amitriptyline, clomipramine, doxepin, or imipramine; fluoxetine, paroxetine, or sertraline; or trazodone) with MAO inhibitors. The syndrome may be manifested by mental status changes (confusion, hypomania), restlessness, myoclonus, hyperreflexia, diaphoresis, shivering, tremor, diarrhea, incoordination, and fever. If recognized early, the syndrome usually resolves quickly upon withdrawal of the offending agents.

Symptoms of hypertensive crisis
*Severe chest pain; enlarged pupils; fast or slow heartbeat; severe headache; increased sensitivity of eyes to light; increased sweating, possibly with fever or cold, clammy skin; nausea or vomiting; stiff or sore neck*
Note: Intracranial bleeding (sometimes fatal in outcome) has occurred in association with *hypertensive crisis*.
*Palpitation or frequent headaches* may be prodromal signs of a hypertensive reaction.

**Those indicating need for medical attention only if they continue or are bothersome**
Incidence more frequent
*Anticholinergic effect or syndrome of inappropriate antidiuretic hormone secretion [SIADH]* (decreased urine output); *blurred vision; CNS stimulation* (muscle twitching during sleep; restlessness or agitation; trouble in sleeping)—more likely with tranylcypromine; *decreased sexual ability; drowsiness*—more likely with phenelzine and isocarboxazid; *mild headache without increase in blood pressure; increased appetite and weight gain, related to carbohydrate craving; increased sweating; orthostatic hypotension, mild* (dizziness or lightheadedness; tiredness and weakness); *shakiness or trembling; weakness*
Note: *Decreased sexual ability* may include anorgasmia in males and females; ejaculatory disorders; and, less commonly, impotence in males.

Incidence less frequent or rare
*Anorexia* (decreased appetite); *chills; constipation; dryness of mouth*

## Overdose

For specific information on the agents used in the management of monoamine oxidase (MAO) inhibitor antidepressant overdose, see:
• *Charcoal, Activated (Oral-Local)* monograph;
• *Dantrolene (Systemic)* monograph; and/or
• *Diazepam* in *Benzodiazepines (Systemic)* monograph.

For more information on the management of overdose or unintentional ingestion, **contact a Poison Control Center** (see *Poison Control Center Listing*).

**Clinical effects of overdose**
The following effects have been selected on the basis of their potential clinical significance (possible signs and symptoms in parentheses where appropriate)—not necessarily inclusive:
*Severe anxiety; confusion; convulsions; cool, clammy skin; severe dizziness; severe drowsiness; fast and irregular pulse; fever; hallucinations; severe headache; high or low blood pressure; hyperactive reflexes; muscle stiffness; respiratory depression or failure* (troubled breathing); *slowed reflexes; sweating; severe trouble in sleeping; unusual irritability*

Note: *Symptoms of overdose* may be absent or minimal for nearly 12 hours after ingestion, and develop slowly thereafter, reaching a maximum in 24 to 48 hours. Immediate hospitalization and close monitoring of patient is essential during this period. Death has resulted.
Treatment may include the following:
**Treatment of overdose**
To decrease absorption—
Induction of vomiting or gastric lavage with protected airway followed by instillation of charcoal slurry in early overdose.
To enhance elimination—
In tranylcypromine overdose, acidification of urine to pH of 5.
Hemodialysis may be beneficial but is of unproven value.
Specific treatment—
Treatment of signs and symptoms of CNS stimulation with diazepam, administered intravenously and slowly. Phenothiazines should not be used because of additive hypotensive effects.
Treatment of hypotension and vascular collapse with intravenous fluids and a dilute pressor agent.
Close monitoring of body temperature, and vigorous treatment of hyperpyrexia with antipyretics and a cooling blanket. Maintenance of fluid and electrolyte balance is essential.
Reduction of symptoms of hypermetabolic state (coma, respiratory failure, hyperpyrexia, tachycardia, muscular rigidity, tremor, and hyperreflexia) with intravenous dantrolene sodium at 2.5 mg per kg of body weight (mg/kg) a day in divided doses, with careful monitoring for signs of hepatotoxicity and pleural or pericardial effusions.
Monitoring—
Close monitoring of body temperature.
Supportive care—
Support of respiration by management of the airway, and mechanical ventilation with the use of supplemental oxygen, as required.
Patients in whom intentional overdose is known or suspected should be referred for psychiatric consultation.
Note: Pathophysiologic effects of massive overdose may persist for several days; recovery from mild overdose may take 3 to 4 days.

## Patient Consultation

As an aid to patient consultation, refer to *Advice for the Patient, Antidepressants, Monoamine Oxidase (MAO) Inhibitor (Systemic)*.
In providing consultation, consider emphasizing the following selected information (» = major clinical significance):
**Before using this medication**
» Conditions affecting use, especially:
Sensitivity to any MAO inhibitor, including furazolidone or procarbazine
Pregnancy—MAO inhibitors cross placenta; no appropriate human studies done; animal studies have shown hyperexcitability and reduced growth rate in neonates
Breast-feeding—Not known if distributed into human breast milk; animal studies have shown distribution into milk
Use in the elderly—Increased sensitivity to hypotensive effects
Other medications, especially CNS depressants, tricyclic antidepressants, oral antidiabetic agents, insulin, bupropion, buspirone, caffeine in high doses, carbamazepine, cyclobenzaprine, cocaine, maprotiline, dextromethorphan, fluoxetine, paroxetine, or sertraline, trazodone, guanadrel, guanethidine, rauwolfia alkaloids, levodopa, meperidine, methyldopa, methylphenidate, sympathomimetics, tryptophan, or foods and beverages containing tyramine
Other medical problems, especially alcoholism (active), congestive heart failure, hepatic function impairment, pheochromocytoma, renal function impairment, cardiac arrhythmias, cardiovascular disease, coronary insufficiency, severe or frequent headaches, hypertension, schizophrenia, or suicidal tendencies

**Proper use of this medication**
» May require up to 3 or 4 weeks of therapy to obtain signs of improvement; regular visits to physician, especially during first few months

of therapy, to check progress of therapy and to check for unwanted effects
» Taking exactly as directed by physician
» Importance of not taking more medication than the amount prescribed
» Proper dosing
Missed dose: Taking as soon as possible within 2 hours of next dose; going back to regular dosing schedule; not doubling doses
» Proper storage

**Precautions while using this medication**
» Avoiding tyramine-containing foods, alcoholic beverages, and large quantities of caffeine-containing beverages, over-the-counter cold and cough medicines, and other medications, unless prescribed; having list of such for reference
» Checking with hospital emergency room or physician if symptoms of hypertensive crisis develop
» Checking with physician before discontinuing medication; gradual reduction may be needed to prevent withdrawal effects
» Dizziness may occur; caution when getting up suddenly from a lying or sitting position
» Drowsiness and blurred vision may occur; caution when driving or doing things requiring alertness or clear vision
» Caution if any kind of surgery, dental treatment, or emergency treatment is required
Carrying medical identification card
» Patients with angina: Not increasing physical activities without consulting physician
Diabetic patients: Carefully checking urine or blood sugar; results may be lowered by this medication
» Obeying rules of caution for 14 days after discontinuing medication

**Side/adverse effects**
» Signs of potential side effects, especially symptoms of hypertensive crisis, severe orthostatic hypotension, diarrhea, peripheral edema, sympathetic stimulation, hepatitis, leukopenia, or parkinsonian syndrome

## General Dosing Information

This medication is usually used for closely supervised patients who have not responded to other antidepressant therapy.

Patient response to these agents is variable, and patients not responsive to one MAO inhibitor may be treated successfully with another.

Potentially suicidal patients should not have access to large quantities of this medication since depressed patients, particularly those who use alcohol excessively, may continue to exhibit suicidal tendencies until significant improvement occurs.

It has been recommended that therapy with an MAO inhibitor be withdrawn gradually at least 10 to 14 days prior to surgery; however, to avoid interruption of antidepressant therapy, patients receiving long-term MAO inhibition may undergo surgery without discontinuation of the MAO inhibitor. Reduction of opioid (narcotic) analgesic or other premedication dosage to 1/4 of the usual dose is recommended, along with careful adjustment of anesthetic dosage. Avoidance of meperidine or cocaine use within 2 to 3 weeks following MAO inhibition is recommended.

Because insomnia or other sleep disturbances may be produced by their psychomotor-stimulating effect, these medications are usually not given in the evening.

After dosage is stopped, the effects of these medications may persist for up to 2 weeks (time required for regeneration of monoamine oxidase). During this period, food and drug contraindications must be observed.

### Diet/Nutrition

Foods and beverages containing tyramine or other high pressor amines, such as aged cheese; fava or broad bean pods; yeast/protein extracts; smoked or pickled meats, poultry, or fish; fermented sausage (bologna, pepperoni, salami, summer sausage) or other fermented meat; sauerkraut; any overripe fruit; beer; reduced-alcohol and alcohol-free beer and wine; red and white wines; sherry; and liqueurs, when used concurrently with MAO inhibitors, may cause sudden and severe hypertensive reactions. The reactions are usually limited to a few hours and are easily treated with rapidly acting hypotensive agents (such as labetalol, nifedipine, or if necessary in severe cases refractory to other agents, phentolamine). The severity depends on the amount of tyramine ingested, rate of gastric emptying, and length of the interval between the dose of MAO inhibitor and ingestion of tyramine. When MAO inhibitors are discontinued, dietary restrictions must continue for at least 2 weeks. Other foods, such as yogurt, sour cream, cream cheese, cottage cheese, chocolate, and soy sauce, if eaten when fresh and in moderation, are considered unlikely to cause serious problems.

**For treatment of hypertensive crisis**
Recommended treatment includes:
• Discontinuing MAO inhibitor.
• Lowering blood pressure immediately with intravenous administration of 5 mg of phentolamine, with care being taken to inject slowly, to prevent excessive hypotensive effect. Alternatively, some clinicians prefer to use labetalol (intravenously or orally), reserving phentolamine for severe or non-responding cases.
• Reducing fever by external cooling.

---

## *ISOCARBOXAZID*

## Additional Dosing Information

See also *General Dosing Information*.

Isocarboxazid has a cumulative effect; therefore, as soon as clinical improvement is observed, dosage should be stabilized and the patient closely followed for clinical effects.

Daily doses greater than 60 mg are not recommended since the frequency and intensity of side effects become greater as the dosage is increased.

If improvement is not seen within 6 weeks, continued administration is unlikely to be beneficial.

## Oral Dosage Forms

### ISOCARBOXAZID TABLETS USP

**Usual adult dose**
Antidepressant—
Initial: Oral, 30 mg a day as a single dose or in divided doses until clinical improvement is evident, the dosage then being reduced to maintenance dose.
Maintenance: Oral, 10 to 20 mg a day, the dosage being adjusted as needed and tolerated.

**Usual adult prescribing limits**
Up to 60 mg a day.

**Usual pediatric dose**
Children up to 16 years of age—Safety and efficacy have not been established.

**Strength(s) usually available**
U.S.—
10 mg (Rx) [*Marplan* (gelatin; lactose; magnesium stearate; corn starch; talc; FD&C Red No. 3; FD&C Yellow No. 6)].
Canada—
10 mg (Rx) [*Marplan* (lactose)].

**Packaging and storage**
Store below 40 °C (104 °F), preferably between 15 and 30 °C (59 and 86 °F), unless otherwise specified by manufacturer. Store in a well-closed, light-resistant container.

**Auxiliary labeling**
• Avoid alcoholic beverages.
• May cause drowsiness.

**Note**
Depressed patients with suicidal tendencies, particularly those who use alcohol excessively, should not have access to large quantities of MAO inhibitors.

---

## *PHENELZINE*

## Additional Dosing Information

See also *General Dosing Information*.

The initial dosage should be increased gradually, depending on patient tolerance. Rapid dosage increases can cause early hypotensive effects and may result in patient noncompliance. A more conservative increase usually avoids this. At least 4 weeks at a given dosage may be necessary for some patients to achieve improvement and significant MAO inhibition.

## Oral Dosage Forms

Note: Bracketed uses in the *Dosage Forms* section refer to categories of use and/or indications that are not included in U.S. product labeling.

## PHENELZINE SULFATE TABLETS USP

### Usual adult dose

Antidepressant—
Initial: Oral, 1 mg per kg of body weight a day.
Maintenance: Oral, 45 mg a day.

[Antipanic agent][1]—
Oral, initially 15 mg every morning for the first four days, the dosage being increased gradually over two weeks as needed and tolerated, up to 15 mg three or four times a day.

### Usual adult prescribing limits

Up to 90 mg a day.

### Usual pediatric dose

Children up to 16 years of age—Safety and efficacy have not been established.

### Usual geriatric dose

Antidepressant—
Oral, initially 0.8 to 1 mg per kg of body weight a day in divided doses, the dosage being gradually increased as needed and tolerated, up to a maximum of 60 mg a day.

Note: Elderly patients are often started on 15 mg in the morning and require a more gradual titration of dose than other adults, to minimize the adverse effects, especially hypotension.

### Strength(s) usually available

U.S.—
15 mg (Rx) [*Nardil* (acacia; calcium carbonate; carnauba wax; corn starch; FD&C Yellow No. 6; gelatin; kaolin; magnesium stearate; mannitol; pharmaceutical glaze; povidone; sucrose; talc; white wax; white wheat flour)].

Canada—
15 mg (Rx) [*Nardil*].

### Packaging and storage

Store between 15 and 30 °C (59 and 86 °F). Store in a tight container. Protect from heat and light.

### Auxiliary labeling

• Avoid alcoholic beverages.
• May cause drowsiness.

### Note

Depressed patients with suicidal tendencies, particularly those who use alcohol excessively, should not have access to large quantities of MAO inhibitors.

[1]Not included in Canadian product labeling.

---

## *TRANYLCYPROMINE*

## Summary of Differences

Side/adverse effects: May produce more CNS stimulation than other MAO inhibitors.

## Additional Dosing Information

See also *General Dosing Information.*

Dosage should be individualized. If there are no signs of improvement after up to 2 weeks on the usual effective dosage of 30 mg a day, the

dosage may be increased by 10 mg a day at intervals of 1 to 3 weeks, up to a maximum of 60 mg a day.

When electroconvulsive therapy is being administered concurrently, 10 mg twice a day can usually be given during the series, the dose being reduced to 10 mg a day for maintenance therapy.

Gradual withdrawal from tranylcypromine is recommended, to avoid recurrence of original symptoms, which may reappear if medication is withdrawn prematurely.

## Oral Dosage Forms

Note: Bracketed uses in the *Dosage Forms* section refer to categories of use and/or indications that are not included in U.S. product labeling.

### TRANYLCYPROMINE SULFATE TABLETS

#### Usual adult dose

Antidepressant—
Initial: Oral, 30 mg a day in divided doses. If there are no signs of improvement after two weeks, the dosage may be increased by 10 mg a day at intervals of one to three weeks, up to a maximum of 60 mg a day.
Maintenance: Oral, 10 to 40 mg a day.

[Antipanic agent][1]—
Oral, initially 10 mg in the morning for the first four days, the dosage being increased gradually over two weeks as needed and tolerated, up to 20 to 30 mg a day.

#### Usual adult prescribing limits

Up to 60 mg a day.

#### Usual pediatric dose

Children up to 16 years of age—Safety and efficacy have not been established.

#### Usual geriatric dose

Antidepressant—
Oral, initially 2.5 to 5 mg a day, the dosage being increased gradually in increments of 2.5 to 5 mg every three to four days, up to a maximum of 45 mg a day.

#### Strength(s) usually available

U.S.—
10 mg (Rx) [*Parnate* (acacia; calcium sulfate; cellulose; ethylcellulose; FD&C Red No. 3; FD&C Yellow No. 6; gelatin; iron oxide; magnesium stearate; starch; sucrose)].

Canada—
10 mg (Rx) [*Parnate* (gluten; sodium <1 mmol [0.003 mg]; sucrose)].

#### Packaging and storage

Store below 40 °C (104 °F), preferably between 15 and 30 °C (59 and 86 °F), unless otherwise specified by manufacturer. Store in a well-closed, light-resistant container.

#### Auxiliary labeling

• Avoid alcoholic beverages.
• May cause drowsiness.

#### Note

Depressed patients with suicidal tendencies, particularly those who use alcohol excessively, should not have access to large quantities of MAO inhibitors.

[1]Not included in Canadian product labeling.

Revised: 05/23/94

---

# ANTIDEPRESSANTS, TRICYCLIC  Systemic

---

This monograph includes information on the following: Amitriptyline; Amoxapine; Clomipramine; Desipramine; Doxepin; Imipramine; Nortriptyline; Protriptyline; Trimipramine.

VA CLASSIFICATION (Primary/Secondary):
Amitriptyline—CN601/GU900; CN103; GA900
Amoxapine—CN601
Clomipramine—CN601/CN900; CN809
Desipramine—CN601/CN103; CN900; CN809; GA900
Doxepin—CN601/CN900; DE890; CN103; GA900
Imipramine—CN601/GU900; CN809; CN103; GA900
Nortriptyline—CN601/CN103
Protriptyline—CN601/CN809
Trimipramine—CN601/GA900

Note: For a listing of dosage forms and brand names by country availability, see *Dosage Forms* section(s). For a listing of brand names for the articles in this monograph, refer to the General Index.

## Category

Note: All of the tricyclic antidepressants have similar pharmacologic actions; however, clinical uses among specific agents may vary because of actual pharmacokinetic differences, availability of specific testing, differences in side effects, and/or availability of clinical-use data.

Antidepressant—Amitriptyline; Amoxapine; Clomipramine; Desipramine; Doxepin; Imipramine; Nortriptyline; Protriptyline; Trimipramine.
Antienuretic—Amitriptyline; Imipramine Hydrochloride.

Antiobsessive-compulsive agent—Clomipramine.
Antipanic agent—Clomipramine; Desipramine; Doxepin; Imipramine; Nortriptyline.
Antineuralgic—Amitriptyline; Clomipramine; Desipramine; Doxepin; Imipramine; Nortriptyline; Trimipramine.
Antiulcer agent—Amitriptyline; Doxepin; Trimipramine.
Antinarcolepsy adjunct—Imipramine; Protriptyline.
Anticataplectic—Clomipramine; Desipramine; Imipramine; Protriptyline.
Antibulimic—Amitriptyline; Clomipramine; Desipramine; Imipramine.
Antipruritic—Doxepin.

## Indications

Note: Bracketed information in the *Indications* section refers to uses that are not included in U.S. product labeling.

### Accepted

Depression, mental (treatment)—Amitriptyline, amoxapine, [clomipramine], desipramine, doxepin, imipramine, nortriptyline, protriptyline, and trimipramine are indicated for the relief of symptoms of major depressive episodes; bipolar disorder, depressed type; dysthymia; and atypical depressions. Some conditions associated with or accompanied by depression that are treated with tricyclic antidepressants include alcoholism, organic disease such as stroke or Parkinson's disease, and agitation or anxiety.

Enuresis (treatment adjunct)—Imipramine hydrochloride, but not pamoate, and [amitriptyline] are indicated as an aid in the temporary treatment of nocturnal enuresis in children 6 years of age or older, after possible organic causes have been excluded by appropriate tests.

Obsessive-compulsive disorder (treatment)—Clomipramine is used to relieve symptoms of obsessive-compulsive disorders, independent of concomitant depression.

[Panic disorder (treatment)][1]—Tricyclic antidepressants, especially clomipramine, desipramine, doxepin, imipramine, and nortriptyline are used in conjunction with psychotherapy and behavior therapy to block the recurrence of panic attacks, with or without phobias. Imipramine's antipanic effect does not appear to be correlated with presence of depressive symptoms.

[Pain, neurogenic (treatment)][1]—Tricyclic antidepressants, especially amitriptyline, clomipramine, desipramine, doxepin, imipramine, nortriptyline, and trimipramine are used in patients with normal or depressed mood for the management of chronic, severe pain as in cancer; migraine and chronic, daily muscle-contraction headaches; rheumatic disorders; atypical facial pain; post-herpetic neuralgia; post-traumatic neuropathy; and diabetic or other peripheral neuropathy.

[Attention deficit hyperactivity disorder (treatment)][1]—Desipramine, imipramine, and protriptyline are used to relieve the symptoms of attention deficit hyperactivity disorder in some children over 6 years of age and in young adults. Tricyclic antidepressants may be more useful than stimulants when the patient has become withdrawn and depressed.

[Headache (prophylaxis)][1]—Tricyclic antidepressants are used in the prophylaxis of vascular headache (including migraine) and mixed headache syndrome.

[Ulcer, peptic (treatment)][1]—Although amitriptyline, doxepin, and trimipramine are effective in the treatment of peptic ulcer disease and in relieving nocturnal ulcer pain, their use has been largely supplanted by histamine H$_2$-receptor antagonists, omeprazole, and sucralfate.

[Narcolepsy/cataplexy syndrome (treatment)][1] or
[Narcolepsy/cataplexy syndrome (treatment adjunct)][1]—Tricyclic antidepressants, especially clomipramine, desipramine, imipramine, and protriptyline, are used to treat cataplexy associated with narcolepsy, with little or no effect on narcoleptic sleep attacks. Imipramine may be used in combination with amphetamines or methylphenidate when a patient requires treatment for both cataplexy and sleep attacks. Patients with sleep disorders such as hypersomnia or impaired morning arousal may benefit by the use of protriptyline.

[Bulimia nervosa (treatment)][1]—Amitriptyline, clomipramine, desipramine, and imipramine have been shown to be effective in controlling the binge eating and subsequent purging of bulimia nervosa.

[Cocaine withdrawal (treatment)][1]—Desipramine and imipramine are used to reduce craving and/or prevent depression upon withdrawal of cocaine.

[Urinary incontinence (treatment)][1]—Imipramine is used for the treatment of stress and urge incontinence.

[Pruritus (treatment)][1]—Doxepin is used in treatment of pruritus in idiopathic cold urticaria.

---

[1]Not included in Canadian product labeling.

## Pharmacology/Pharmacokinetics

See also *Table 1*, page 276.

### Physicochemical characteristics

Molecular weight—
  Amitriptyline hydrochloride: 313.87.
  Amoxapine: 313.79.
  Clomipramine hydrochloride: 351.32.
  Desipramine hydrochloride: 302.85.
  Doxepin hydrochloride: 315.84.
  Imipramine hydrochloride: 316.87.
  Imipramine pamoate: 949.2.
  Nortriptyline hydrochloride: 299.84.
  Protriptyline hydrochloride: 299.84.
  Trimipramine maleate: 410.51.

pKa—
  Amitriptyline: 9.4.
  Amoxapine: 7.6.
  Clomipramine: 9.5.
  Desipramine: 1.5 and 10.2.
  Doxepin: 9.0.
  Imipramine: 9.5.
  Nortriptyline: 9.7.
  Trimipramine: 8.0.

### Mechanism of action/Effect

Antidepressant—
Although the exact mechanism of action in the treatment of depression is unclear, tricyclic antidepressants have been thought to increase the synaptic concentration of norepinephrine (levarterenol; NE) and/or serotonin (5-hydroxytryptamine; 5-HT) in the central nervous system (CNS). One theory suggests that these neurotransmitters are increased through inhibition of their reuptake by the presynaptic neuronal membrane.

Amoxapine, desipramine, trimipramine, nortriptyline, and probably protriptyline mainly inhibit the reuptake of norepinephrine. Amitriptyline and clomipramine appear to be more potent than other tricyclics in blocking serotonin, although, through their metabolites, they become powerful inhibitors of norepinephrine reuptake also. Clomipramine's effectiveness in the treatment of obsessive-compulsive disorder may be related to the inhibition of serotonin reuptake. Imipramine inhibits reuptake of norepinephrine and serotonin equally. Doxepin is a moderate inhibitor of norepinephrine and a weak inhibitor of serotonin.

Recent research has shown that after long-term treatment with antidepressants, changes in postsynaptic beta-adrenergic receptor sensitivity and increased responsiveness of the adrenergic and serotonergic systems to physiologic and environmental stimuli contribute to the mechanism of action. Antidepressants may produce a downregulation (desensitization) of alpha$_2$- or beta-adrenergic and serotonin receptors, equilibrating the noradrenergic system, and thus correcting the dysregulated monoamine output of depressed patients. Receptor changes resulting from chronic administration of tricyclic antidepressants appear to correlate better with antidepressant action than does the synaptic reuptake blockade of neurotransmitters, and may also account for the delay of 2 to 4 weeks in therapeutic response.

Amoxapine, as a metabolite of the neuroleptic, loxapine, also has a potent postsynaptic dopamine-blocking effect. This may account for the extrapyramidal side effects and increases in serum prolactin concentrations seen with amoxapine. Amoxapine is metabolized to 7-hydroxyamoxapine, also a potent dopamine-blocking agent.

Antienuretic—
The exact antienuretic action of imipramine hydrochloride has not been established. It is thought to be associated with the anticholinergic effects of imipramine.

Antiobsessional agent—
The exact antiobsessional action of clomipramine has not been established. It is thought to be associated with clomipramine's inhibition of serotonin reuptake and compensatory down regulation of serotonin receptor subtypes.

Antianxiety agent—
In panic disorders, studies suggest an impaired function of the autonomic nervous system that causes an excessive release of norepinephrine from the locus ceruleus. Tricyclic antidepressants are thought to decrease the firing rate of the locus ceruleus by regulating the alpha$_2$- and beta-adrenergic receptor functions and norepinephrine turnover.

Antineuralgic—
The exact mechanism by which tricyclic antidepressants relieve chronic pain is also unknown. Some studies support the theory that pain relief results when depression is relieved. However, other

studies have found that pain may be ameliorated without a significant change in depression. Analgesic activity may be effected by the changing concentrations of central monoamines, especially serotonin, and by the direct or indirect effect of tricyclic antidepressants on the endogenous opioid systems.

Antiulcer agent—

In peptic ulcer disease, tricyclic antidepressants are effective in relieving pain and aid in complete healing because of their histamine₂-receptor blocking property on the parietal cells, and their sedative and anticholinergic effects.

Antibulimic—

In bulimia nervosa, the mechanism of action is unclear, although it may be similar to that in depression. Evidence shows there is a distinct antibulimic effect in patients without depression and in depressed patients whose bulimia was relieved without a concomitant relief of depression.

Urinary incontinence—

The exact mechanism by which imipramine enhances urinary continence has not been established but may include anticholinergic activity, resulting in increased bladder capacity; direct beta-adrenergic stimulation; alpha-adrenergic agonist activity, resulting in increased sphincter tone; and central blockade of serotonin uptake.

## Other actions/effects

Tricyclic antidepressants also produce prominent peripheral and central anticholinergic effects due to their potent and high binding affinity for muscarinic receptors; sedative effects due to strong binding affinity for histamine H₁-receptors (although the central actions of histamine are poorly understood, increased cholinoceptive activity in the brain has been associated with clinical depression); and orthostatic hypotension due to alpha blockade. In addition, tricyclic antidepressants are Class 1A antiarrhythmic agents which, like quinidine, moderately slow ventricular conduction in therapeutic doses, and in overdose may cause severe conduction block and occasional ventricular arrhythmia.

## Absorption

Rapidly and well absorbed after oral administration.

## Protein binding

Very highly protein bound (90% or more) in plasma and tissues.

## Biotransformation

Exclusively hepatic, with first-pass effect.

## Onset of action

Antidepressant—2 to 3 weeks.

## Elimination

As metabolites, primarily renal, over several days; poorly dialyzable because of high protein binding.

# Precautions to Consider

## Cross-sensitivity and/or related problems

Patients sensitive to one tricyclic antidepressant may be sensitive to other tricyclic antidepressants, and possibly to carbamazepine, maprotiline, and trazodone, also.

## Carcinogenicity/Mutagenicity

Amitriptyline—In one study with rats, no evidence of increase in incidence of any tumor was found. However, amitriptyline has not been adequately studied in animals to permit an evaluation of its carcinogenic potential. No evidence of mutagenicity was found in rats tested with the Ames salmonella test.

Amoxapine—Pancreatic islet cell hyperplasia occurred in rats, with slightly increased incidence at doses 5 to 10 times the human dose.

## Pregnancy/Reproduction

Pregnancy—

*For amitriptyline—*
Adequate and well-controlled studies in pregnant women have not been done.
Animal studies have shown amitriptyline to cause teratogenic effects when used in doses many times the human dose.
FDA Pregnancy Category C.

*For amoxapine—*
Adequate and well-controlled studies in pregnant women have not been done.
Animal studies have shown amoxapine to cause embryotoxic effects in doses approximating the human dose and fetotoxic effects such as intrauterine death, stillbirth, decreased birth weight, and decreased postnatal (0 to 4 days) survival at doses many times the human dose.
FDA Pregnancy Category C.

*For clomipramine, desipramine, and nortriptyline—*
Adequate and well-controlled studies in pregnant women have not been done.
Animal reproduction studies have been inconclusive.
FDA Pregnancy Category C.

*For doxepin—*
Adequate and well-controlled studies in pregnant women have not been done.
Animal studies have shown no evidence of teratogenic effects at doses up to 25 mg per kg of body weight (mg/kg) per day for 8 to 9 months and no changes in litter size, number of live births, or lactation. However, a decreased rate of conception was observed when male rats were given 25 mg/kg per day for prolonged periods.

*For imipramine—*
Adequate and well-controlled studies in pregnant women have not been done. However, there have been clinical reports of congenital malformations associated with the use of imipramine.
Animal reproduction studies have been inconclusive.

*For protriptyline—*
Adequate and well-controlled studies in pregnant women have not been done.
Animal reproduction studies have shown that protriptyline causes no apparent adverse effects at doses 10 times greater than recommended human doses.

*For trimipramine—*
Adequate and well-controlled studies in pregnant women have not been done.
Animal studies have shown trimipramine to cause embryotoxicity and major anomalies at 20 times the human dose.
FDA Pregnancy Category C.

Delivery—For all tricyclic antidepressants: There have been reports of cardiac problems, irritability, respiratory distress, muscle spasms, seizures, and urinary retention in infants whose mothers received tricyclic antidepressants immediately prior to delivery.

## Breast-feeding

Tricyclic antidepressants have been found in small amounts in breast milk in an approximate milk to plasma ratio of 0.4:1.5. Doxepin has been reported to cause sedation and respiratory depression in the nursing infant.

## Pediatrics

Although tricyclic antidepressants are generally not recommended for depression in children under 12 years of age, some, especially amitriptyline, desipramine, imipramine, and nortriptyline, are used in children over the age of 6 years for recognized major depressive illness. However, the effectiveness of tricyclic antidepressants in the treatment of depression in children and adolescents has not been definitively established. Amitriptyline and imipramine are also used for treatment of enuresis in children 6 years of age or older. Clomipramine is used for the treatment of obsessive-compulsive disorder in children 10 years of age or older. Imipramine, desipramine, and protriptyline are being used in the treatment of attention deficit hyperactivity disorder in children over 6 years of age and adolescents. However, deaths have been reported in children treated with desipramine for hyperactivity.

Children are more sensitive than adults to acute overdosage, which should be considered serious and potentially fatal. Increasing the dose in children increases the risk of adverse effects, such as alterations in electrocardiogram (ECG) patterns, nervousness, sleep disorders, tiredness, hypertension in some children, or mild gastrointestinal problems, without necessarily enhancing the therapeutic effect. Adolescent patients may require reduced dosage because they are also prone to exhibit increased dose sensitivity.

## Geriatrics

Elderly patients often require lower dosage and more gradual dose increases to avoid toxicity, because of slower metabolic rates and/or excretion and an increased ratio of fat to lean tissue. The elderly also exhibit increased sensitivity to anticholinergic effects, such as urinary retention (especially in older men with prostatic hypertrophy), anticholinergic delirium, and increased sedative and hypotensive effects. Increased anxiety may result from these adverse effects, possibly leading to unnecessary dose increases. If cardiovascular disease is present, the risk of conduction defects, arrhythmias, tachycardia, stroke, congestive heart failure, or myocardial infarction is increased.

## Dental

The peripheral anticholinergic effects of tricyclic antidepressants may decrease or inhibit salivary flow, especially in middle-aged or elderly patients, thus contributing to the development of caries, periodontal disease, oral candidiasis, and discomfort.

The blood dyscrasia–causing effects of tricyclic antidepressants, although rare, may be life-threatening. The result may be an increased incidence of microbial infection, delayed healing, and gingival bleeding. If agranulocytosis, leukopenia, or thrombocytopenia occurs, dental work should be deferred until blood counts have returned to normal. Patient instruction in proper oral hygiene should include caution in use of regular toothbrushes, dental floss, and toothpicks.

Extrapyramidal reactions that may be induced by amoxapine will result in increased motor activity of the head, face, and neck. Occlusal adjustments, bite registrations, and treatment for bruxism may be made less reliable.

## Drug interactions and/or related problems

The following drug interactions and/or related problems have been selected on the basis of their potential clinical significance (possible mechanism in parentheses where appropriate)—not necessarily inclusive (» = major clinical significance):

Note: Combinations containing any of the following medications, depending on the amount present, may also interact with this medication.

Although not all of the following interactions have been reported for every tricyclic antidepressant, the potential for their occurrence exists and should be considered.

» Alcohol or
» CNS depression–producing medications, other (See *Appendix II*)
  (concurrent use with tricyclic antidepressants may result in serious potentiation of CNS depression, respiratory depression, and hypotensive effects; caution is recommended, and dosage of one or both agents should be reduced)

  (in addition, tricyclics may increase the effects of alcohol, especially during first few days of tricyclic antidepressant treatment; in patients who use alcohol excessively, tricyclics may increase the danger inherent in any suicide attempt)

Amantadine or
Anticholinergics or other medications with anticholinergic activity
  (See *Appendix II*) or
Antidyskinetics or
Antihistamines
  (concurrent use with tricyclic antidepressants may intensify anticholinergic effects, especially mental confusion, hallucinations, and nightmares, because of secondary anticholinergic activities of tricyclic antidepressants)

  (concurrent use may potentiate the CNS depressant effects of either antihistamines or tricyclic antidepressants)

  (concurrent use with tricyclic antidepressants may block detoxification of atropine and related compounds; patients should be advised to report occurrence of gastrointestinal problems promptly since paralytic ileus may occur with concurrent therapy)

Anticoagulants, coumarin- or indandione-derivative
  (concurrent use with tricyclic antidepressants, especially amitriptyline or nortriptyline, may increase anticoagulant activity, possibly by inhibiting enzymatic metabolism of the anticoagulant)

Anticonvulsants
  (tricyclic antidepressants may enhance CNS depression, lower the seizure threshold when taken in high doses, and decrease the effects of the anticonvulsant medication; dosage adjustment of the anticonvulsant may be necessary to control seizures; monitoring of serum concentrations of both medications may be necessary to detect possible interaction; concurrent use of phenytoin with desipramine may lower serum concentrations of desipramine; dosage increases of desipramine above maximum recommended doses may be required to produce clinical improvement in depression)

» Antithyroid agents
  (concurrent use with tricyclic antidepressants may increase the risk of agranulocytosis)

Barbiturates or
Carbamazepine
  (plasma concentrations and therapeutic effects of tricyclic antidepressants may be decreased during concurrent use with barbiturates, especially phenobarbital, or carbamazepine because of increased metabolism resulting from induction of hepatic microsomal enzymes)

Bupropion or
Clozapine or
Cyclobenzaprine or
Haloperidol or
Loxapine or
Maprotiline or
Molindone or

» Phenothiazines or
Thioxanthenes
  (the sedative and anticholinergic effects of either these medications or tricyclic antidepressants may be prolonged and intensified; these medications may increase the risk of seizures by lowering the seizure threshold and should be added or withdrawn with caution; psychotic depressions respond well to a combination of tricyclic antidepressant and antipsychotic agent, but both medications must be initially administered at lower doses and are increased only as clinically indicated)

  (concurrent use of phenothiazines may increase serum concentrations of tricyclic antidepressants, especially desipramine and imipramine, due to inhibition of metabolism; conversely, tricyclics may inhibit phenothiazine metabolism; also, the risk of neuroleptic malignant syndrome [NMS] may be increased)

» Cimetidine
  (cimetidine may inhibit tricyclic metabolism and increase plasma concentrations, leading to toxicity; lowering the dose of the tricyclic antidepressant by 20 to 30% may be necessary when cimetidine is given concurrently; patient should be closely observed for sedation, anticholinergic effects, and orthostatic hypotension)

» Clonidine or
» Guanadrel or
» Guanethidine
  (concurrent use may decrease the hypotensive effects of these medications)

  (concurrent use of clonidine with tricyclic antidepressants may result in potentiation of CNS depressant effects)

Cocaine
  (concurrent use with tricyclic antidepressants may increase the risk of cardiac arrhythmias; if use of cocaine is necessary in patients receiving tricyclics, it is recommended that the cocaine be administered with caution, in reduced dosage, and in conjunction with electrocardiographic monitoring)

Contraceptives, oral, estrogen-containing or
Estramustine or
Estrogens
  (concurrent use of imipramine and possibly other tricyclic antidepressants by chronic long-term users of oral contraceptives or estrogens may increase the bioavailability of imipramine because of inhibition of hepatic enzyme metabolism; this may result in toxicity, obscuring therapeutic effects and worsening depression; may be dose-related, with lower doses of estrogens having less effect on enzyme inhibition than larger doses; dosage adjustments of the tricyclic may be necessary)

Corticosteroids, glucocorticoid
  (tricyclic antidepressants do not relieve, and may exacerbate, corticosteroid-induced mental depression)

Disulfiram or
Ethchlorvynol
  (concurrent use with tricyclics, especially amitriptyline, may result in transient delirium)

  (also, CNS depressant effects may be increased when ethchlorvynol is used concurrently with tricyclic antidepressants)

Electroconvulsive therapy
  (although electroconvulsive therapy may be used in conjunction with tricyclic antidepressants, caution should be used as hazards may be increased)

» Extrapyramidal reaction–causing medications, other (See *Appendix II*)
  (concurrent use with amoxapine and possibly other tricyclic antidepressants may increase the severity and frequency of extrapyramidal effects)

Fluoxetine
  (concurrent use with tricyclic antidepressants has produced increased plasma concentrations of the tricyclic antidepressant, possibly due to inhibition of tricyclic antidepressant metabolism; some clinicians recommend dosage reductions for tricyclic antidepressants of about 50% if used concurrently with fluoxetine)

Methylphenidate
  (serum concentrations of tricyclic antidepressants, especially desipramine and imipramine, may be increased due to inhibition of metabolism when methylphenidate is used concurrently; also, concurrent use may antagonize the effects of methylphenidate)

» Metrizamide
  (administration of intrathecal metrizamide may lower the seizure threshold and increase the risk of seizures in patients taking tricyclic antidepressants; it is recommended that tricyclic antidepres-

sants be discontinued for at least 48 hours before and at least 24 hours after myelography)

» Monoamine oxidase (MAO) inhibitors, including furazolidone, procarbazine, and selegiline

(concurrent use with tricyclic antidepressants has resulted in an increased incidence of hyperpyretic episodes, severe convulsions, hypertensive crises, and death; however, recent studies have shown that concurrent use of some tricyclic antidepressants with MAO inhibitors can be used for refractory depression with no adverse effects if both medications are initiated simultaneously at lower than usual doses, with doses being raised gradually thereafter, or if the MAO inhibitor is gradually added to the tricyclic, also at low doses; a tricyclic should not be added to an existing MAO inhibitor regimen; the tricyclic antidepressants most commonly used in this combined therapy are amitriptyline, doxepin, and trimipramine; imipramine, desipramine, nortriptyline, protriptyline, and clomipramine are not recommended for use in such a regimen because of potential excessive stimulation)

Naphazoline, ophthalmic or
Oxymetazoline, nasal or ophthalmic or
Phenylephrine, nasal or ophthalmic or
Xylometazoline, nasal

(if significant systemic absorption occurs, concurrent use with tricyclic antidepressants may potentiate pressor effects of these medications)

Pimozide

(concurrent use with tricyclic antidepressants may potentiate cardiac arrhythmias, which are seen on ECG as prolongation of the QT interval)

Probucol

(additive QT interval prolongation may increase risk of ventricular tachycardia)

» Sympathomimetics

(concurrent use with tricyclic antidepressants may potentiate cardiovascular effects possibly resulting in arrhythmias, tachycardia, or severe hypertension or hyperpyrexia; phentolamine can control the adverse reaction)

(significant systemic absorption of ophthalmic epinephrine may also potentiate cardiovascular effects; also, local anesthetics with vasoconstrictors should be avoided or a minimal amount of the vasoconstrictor should be used with the local anesthetic)

(concurrent use with tricyclic antidepressants may decrease the pressor effect of ephedrine and mephentermine)

Thyroid hormones

(concurrent use with tricyclic antidepressants may increase the therapeutic and toxic effects of both medications, possibly due to increased receptor sensitivity to catecholamines; toxic effects include cardiac arrhythmias and CNS stimulation)

## Laboratory value alterations

The following have been selected on the basis of their potential clinical significance (possible effect in parentheses where appropriate)—not necessarily inclusive (» = major clinical significance):

With diagnostic test results
ECG

(changes include prolonged PR intervals, widened QRS complexes, and inverted or flattened T-waves)

Metyrapone test

(amitriptyline may decrease the response to metyrapone)

With physiology/laboratory test values
Blood sugar concentrations

(may be increased or decreased)

## Medical considerations/Contraindications

The medical considerations/contraindications included here have been selected on the basis of their potential clinical significance (reasons given in parentheses where appropriate)—not necessarily inclusive (» = major clinical significance).

Note: This medication should *not* be used during the acute recovery period following a myocardial infarction.

***Risk-benefit should be considered when the following medical problems exist:***

» Alcoholism, active
(CNS depression may be potentiated)

» Asthma
(may be aggravated)

» Bipolar disorder
(swing to hypomanic or manic phase may be accelerated and reversible rapid cycling between mania and depression may be in-

duced by antidepressants in some patients; tricyclic antidepressant may have to be discontinued and lithium considered for a sustained remission)

» Blood disorders
(may be potentiated)

» Cardiovascular disorders, especially in children and the elderly
(increased risk of arrhythmias, heart block, congestive heart failure, myocardial infarction, or stroke)

» Gastrointestinal disorders
(risk of paralytic ileus)

Genitourinary disease
(may be masked by the use of imipramine for enuresis in children)

» Glaucoma, narrow-angle, predisposition to or
» Increased intraocular pressure
(may be aggravated)

» Hepatic function impairment
(metabolism of tricyclic may be altered)

» Hyperthyroidism
(risk of cardiovascular toxicity)

» Prostatic hypertrophy
(risk of urinary retention)

» Renal function impairment
(excretion of tricyclic may be altered)

» Schizophrenia
(psychosis may be activated)

» Seizure disorders
(seizure threshold may be lowered)

» Sensitivity to tricyclic antidepressants, carbamazepine, maprotiline, or trazodone

» Urinary retention
(may be aggravated)

## Patient monitoring

The following may be especially important in patient monitoring (other tests may be warranted in some patients, depending on condition; » = major clinical significance):

Blood cell counts (usually during extended therapy and in patients with sore throat or fever) and

Blood pressure and pulse measurements and

Glaucoma tests and

Hepatic function determinations and

Renal function determinations

(may be required at periodic intervals during therapy to detect development of adverse effects that may not be evident to the patient)

Cardiac function monitoring

(ECG may be required in the elderly, in children, and in patients with existing cardiac disease, or in patients receiving antiarrhythmics such as quinidine, procainamide, or disopyramide, before initiation of therapy as a baseline and at periodic intervals thereafter)

(for children taking imipramine for enuresis who are not responding to standard doses, ECG may be required before dosage is increased)

Careful supervision of depressed patients with suicidal tendencies

(recommended especially during early weeks of treatment; hospitalization may be required as a protective measure)

Dental examination

(recommended at least twice yearly)

Plasma tricyclic determinations

(recommended for patients who fail to respond to treatment, when there are increased side effects, when patient is at high risk, when there is doubt about patient compliance, or as a means of maximizing the response; optimum sampling time is immediately before the first morning dose or a minimum of 8 hours after a dose; See *Table 1* for therapeutic plasma concentration ranges)

*For amoxapine (in addition to the above)*

Careful observation for early signs of tardive dyskinesia

(recommended at periodic intervals, especially in the elderly; if early symptoms of tardive dyskinesia appear, amoxapine should be discontinued)

# Side/Adverse Effects

Note: Although not all of these side effects have been attributed specifically to each tricyclic antidepressant, a potential exists for their occurrence during the use of any tricyclic antidepressant.

The following side/adverse effects have been selected on the basis of their potential clinical significance (possible signs and symptoms in parentheses where appropriate)—not necessarily inclusive:

**Those indicating need for medical attention**

Incidence less frequent

*For all tricyclic antidepressants*

*Anticholinergic effects* (blurred vision; confusion; delirium or hallucinations; constipation, especially in the elderly, possibly resulting in paralytic ileus; difficult urination; eye pain due to aggravation of glaucoma); *fast, slow, or irregular heartbeat; fine-muscle tremors, especially in arms, hands, head, and tongue* (shakiness); *hypotension* (fainting); *nervousness or restlessness; Parkinsonian syndrome* (difficulty in speaking or swallowing; loss of balance control; mask-like face; shuffling walk; slowed movements; stiffness of arms and legs; trembling and shaking of fingers and hands); *sexual function impairment*—more common with amoxapine and clomipramine

*For amoxapine only (in addition to the above)*

*Tardive dyskinesia* (lip smacking or puckering; puffing of cheeks; rapid or worm-like movements of tongue; uncontrolled chewing movements; uncontrolled movements of the arms or legs)

Incidence rare

*For all tricyclic antidepressants*

*Agranulocytosis or other blood dyscrasias* (red or brownish spots on skin; sore throat and fever; unusual bleeding or bruising); *allergic reaction* (increased sensitivity to sunlight; skin rash and itching; swelling of face and tongue); *alopecia* (hair loss); *anxiety; breast enlargement in both males and females*—more common with amoxapine; *cholestatic jaundice* (yellow eyes or skin); *galactorrhea* (inappropriate secretion of milk)—in females; *seizures*—more common with clomipramine; *syndrome of inappropriate secretion of antidiuretic hormone [SIADH]* (irritability; muscle twitching; weakness); *testicular swelling*—more common with amoxapine; *tinnitus* (ringing, buzzing, or other unexplained noises in the ears); *trouble with teeth or gums*—more common with clomipramine

*For amoxapine only (in addition to the above)*

*Neuroleptic malignant syndrome (NMS)* (convulsions; difficult or fast breathing; fast heartbeat or irregular pulse; fever; high or low [irregular] blood pressure; increased sweating; loss of bladder control; severe muscle stiffness; unusually pale skin; unusual tiredness or weakness)

Note: May occur after prolonged treatment or after combined treatment with *tricyclic antidepressants* and *neuroleptics*.

**Those indicating need for medical attention only if they continue or are bothersome**

Incidence more frequent

*Drowsiness; dryness of mouth; headache; increased appetite*—may include craving for sweets; *nausea; orthostatic hypotension* (dizziness); *tiredness or weakness, mild; unpleasant taste; weight gain*

Incidence less frequent

*Diarrhea; excessive sweating; heartburn; trouble in sleeping*—more common with protriptyline, especially when taken late in the day; *vomiting*

**Those indicating possible withdrawal and the need for medical attention if they occur after medication is discontinued**

Occurring upon abrupt withdrawal, due to cholinergic rebound

*For all tricyclic antidepressants*

*Headache; nausea, vomiting, or diarrhea; trouble in sleeping, with vivid dreams; unusual excitement*

Occurring with gradual withdrawal after long-term treatment

*For all tricyclic antidepressants*

*Irritability; restlessness; trouble in sleeping, with vivid dreams*

*For amoxapine only (in addition to the above)*

*Tardive dyskinesia, withdrawal-emergent* (lip smacking or puckering; puffing of cheeks; rapid or worm-like movements of tongue; uncontrolled chewing movements; uncontrolled movements of the arms and legs)

## Overdose

For specific information on the agents used in the management of tricyclic antidepressant overdose, see:

- *Anesthetics, Inhalation (Systemic)* monograph;
- *Charcoal, Activated (Oral-Local)* monograph;
- *Diazepam* in *Benzodiazepines (Systemic)* monograph;
- *Digitalis Glycosides (Systemic)* monograph;
- *Lidocaine (Systemic)* monograph;
- *Paraldehyde (Systemic)* monograph;
- *Phenytoin* in *Anticonvulsants, Hydantoin (Systemic)* monograph;

- *Physostigmine (Systemic)* monograph;
- *Propranolol* in *Beta-adrenergic Blocking Agents (Systemic)* monograph; and/or
- *Sodium Bicarbonate (Systemic)* monograph.

For more information on the management of overdose or unintentional ingestion, **contact a Poison Control Center** (see *Poison Control Center Listing*).

**Clinical effects of overdose**

The following effects have been selected on the basis of their potential clinical significance (possible signs and symptoms in parentheses where appropriate)—not necessarily inclusive:

Acute

*Confusion; convulsions*—more severe and refractory with amoxapine; *disturbed concentration; drowsiness, severe; enlarged pupils; fast, slow, or irregular heartbeat; fever; hallucinations; restlessness and agitation; shortness of breath or troubled breathing; unusual tiredness or weakness, severe; vomiting*

**Treatment of overdose**

Treatment is essentially symptomatic and supportive, possibly including:

To decrease absorption—

Emptying stomach with gastric lavage.

To enhance elimination—

Administering activated charcoal slurry repeatedly, followed by a stimulant cathartic.

Specific treatment—

Digitalizing cautiously for congestive heart failure.

Controlling cardiac arrhythmias with lidocaine or by alkalinizing blood to pH 7.4 to 7.5 with intravenous sodium bicarbonate. Arrhythmias refractory to lidocaine and sodium bicarbonate may be managed with slow intravenous infusion of phenytoin while monitoring ECG. Propranolol is also effective but should be used with caution because of its negative inotropic and hypotensive effects. Quinidine and procainamide should be avoided.

For all tricyclics except amoxapine: Although routine use is not recommended, administering physostigmine salicylate, 1 to 3 mg (adults) by slow intravenous infusion over 2 to 3 minutes, may help reverse severe anticholinergic effects (myoclonic seizures, severe hallucinations, hypertension, and ventricular arrhythmias). For children, start with 0.5 mg and repeat dosage at 5 minute intervals to determine the minimum effective dose, not exceeding 2 mg per dose. Because of the short duration of action of physostigmine, dosage may need to be repeated at 30- to 60-minute intervals, especially if life-threatening symptoms occur. Routine administration of physostigmine is not recommended because of its toxicity. When used in tricyclic antidepressant overdose, it may cause bronchospasm, increased respiratory secretions, muscle weakness, bradycardia, hypotension, and may itself cause seizures. Physostigmine should be reserved for patients in coma with respiratory depression, uncontrollable seizures, severe hypertension, or serious cardiac arrhythmias. Physostigmine is contraindicated in amoxapine overdose because it may increase seizure activity.

Administering anticonvulsants such as diazepam, paraldehyde, phenytoin, or an inhalation anesthetic to control convulsions. Seizures may be especially severe and refractory with amoxapine overdose and may lead to acute tubular necrosis and rhabdomyolysis.

Monitoring—

Monitoring cardiovascular function (ECG) for not less than 5 days.

Supportive care—

Maintaining respiratory and cardiac function.

Maintaining body temperature.

Using standard measures to manage circulatory shock and metabolic acidosis.

Patients in whom intentional overdose is known or suspected should be referred for psychiatric consultation.

Note: Hemodialysis, peritoneal dialysis, exchange transfusions, and forced diuresis of tricyclic antidepressants have not been successful because of their high protein binding and rapid fixation in tissues.

## Patient Consultation

As an aid to patient consultation, refer to *Advice for the Patient, Antidepressants, Tricyclic (Systemic)*.

In providing consultation, consider emphasizing the following selected information (» = major clinical significance):

**Before using this medication**

» Conditions affecting use, especially:

Sensitivity to tricyclic antidepressants, maprotiline, or trazodone

Pregnancy—Clinical reports of fetal malformations with imipramine; animal studies have shown some tricyclics to cause embryotoxic or fetotoxic effects, and decreased rate of conception;

when tricyclics taken by mother immediately before delivery, clinical reports of newborns suffering from muscle spasms, and heart, breathing, and urinary problems

Breast-feeding—Pass into breast milk and may cause drowsiness in nursing baby

Use in children—Children and adolescents more sensitive to effects, requiring lower doses; may cause nervousness, sleeping problems, tiredness, mild stomach upset; generally not recommended for depression in children

Use in the elderly—Elderly more sensitive to effects; lower doses and more gradual increases required

Dental—Decreased salivary flow contributes to caries, periodontal disease, candidiasis, and discomfort; blood dyscrasias may cause increased infections, delayed healing, and gingival bleeding; increased extrapyramidal motor activity of head, face, and neck with amoxapine may cause difficulty with occlusal and other procedures

Other medications, especially CNS depressants, antithyroid agents, cimetidine, clonidine, guanadrel, guanethidine, phenothiazines, extrapyramidal reaction–causing medications, MAO inhibitors, metrizamide, or sympathomimetics

Other medical problems, especially alcoholism (active), asthma, bipolar disorder, blood disorders, cardiovascular disorders, gastrointestinal disorders, glaucoma or increased intraocular pressure, hepatic function impairment, hyperthyroidism, prostatic hypertrophy, renal function impairment, schizophrenia, seizure disorders, or urinary retention

### Proper use of this medication

Taking with food to reduce gastrointestinal irritation

» Compliance with therapy; not taking more or less medicine than prescribed

» May require from 1 to 6 weeks of therapy to obtain antidepressant effects

*Proper administration of doxepin oral solution*

Using dropper provided by manufacturer for accurate measurement

Diluting medication in one-half glass of recommended beverage (water, milk, or fruit juice, but not grape juice or carbonated beverages) immediately before use

Not preparing or storing bulk solutions

» Proper dosing

Missed dose: If dosing schedule is—

More than one dose a day: Taking as soon as possible unless almost time for next dose; not doubling dose

One dose at bedtime: Not taking in morning because of side effects; checking with physician

» Proper storage

### Precautions while using this medication

Regular visits to physician to check progress of therapy

» Avoiding the use of alcoholic beverages; not taking other medication unless prescribed by physician

» Possible drowsiness; caution when driving or doing things requiring alertness

» Possible dizziness or lightheadedness; caution when getting up suddenly from a lying or sitting position

» Possible dryness of mouth; using sugarless gum or candy, ice, or saliva substitute for relief; checking with physician or dentist if dry mouth continues for more than 2 weeks

» Possible skin photosensitivity; avoiding unprotected exposure to sun; using protective clothing; using a sun block product that includes protection against both UVA-caused photosensitivity reactions and UVB-caused sunburn reactions; avoiding use of sunlamp, tanning bed, or tanning booth

Caution if any laboratory tests required; possible interference with results of metyrapone test.

» Caution if any kind of surgery, dental treatment, or emergency treatment is required

» Checking with physician before discontinuing medicine; gradual dosage reduction may be needed to avoid worsening of condition or withdrawal symptoms

» Observing precautions for 3 to 7 days after stopping medication

*For protriptyline*

Possibility of sleep interference if taken late in the day

### Side/adverse effects

Signs of potential side effects, especially anticholinergic effects; hypotension; fast, slow, or irregular heartbeat; Parkinsonian syndrome; nervousness or restlessness; sexual function impairment; shakiness or tremors; neuroleptic malignant syndrome (NMS) or tardive dyskinesia (with amoxapine only); anxiety; breast enlargement in males and females; galactorrhea; testicular swelling; alopecia; allergic reactions; blood dyscrasias; cholestatic jaundice; seizures; SIADH; tinnitus; or trouble with teeth or gums

## General Dosing Information

Dosage of tricyclic antidepressants must be individualized for each patient by titration.

Plasma concentrations of tricyclic antidepressants, in general, vary greatly among patients. However, nortriptyline appears to have a well-defined "therapeutic window" at 50 to 150 nanograms per mL of plasma. Other therapeutic plasma concentration ranges that are generally accepted include desipramine, 150 to 250 nanograms per mL, and imipramine, 200 to 250 nanograms per mL. See *Table 1*.

Although a sedative action may occur following the initial dose (with the possible exception of protriptyline), 1 to 6 weeks of therapy may be required before the desired antidepressant response is obtained.

Maintenance therapy of the sedating tricyclic antidepressants is usually given as a single dose at bedtime. A divided dose may be preferred, however, for protriptyline, and for all tricyclic antidepressants in geriatric or cardiovascular patients, or in adolescents or children. Maintenance is often continued for 6 months to 1 year. Recent data suggest that some patients with recurrent depression may benefit from prolonged maintenance treatment at the full (acute treatment) daily dose.

A trial of four to six weeks at the upper therapeutic dose range may be considered an adequate antidepressant trial, after which alternate therapy should be considered.

The single daily dose at bedtime is useful when side effects such as excessive drowsiness or dizziness might be bothersome or dangerous during working hours. An exception to bedtime dosage is protriptyline, which if taken late in the day may cause insomnia or nightmares in some patients. Therefore, protriptyline is often given in divided doses with the last daily dose in the afternoon.

Withdrawal symptoms, such as headache, malaise, nausea or vomiting, and vivid dreams, may occur if high or prolonged dosage is abruptly discontinued. Also, patients with a history of only unipolar depression may experience a fast-cycling bipolar disorder (manic-depressive illness) with mania or hypomania. Although this has not been reported with all of the tricyclics, a gradual reduction in dosage over a 1- to 2-month period is recommended when any of these medications is to be discontinued.

Potentially suicidal patients should not have access to large quantities of these medications since depressed patients, particularly those who may use alcohol excessively, may continue to exhibit suicidal tendencies until significant improvement occurs. Some clinicians recommend that not more than the equivalent of 1 gram of amitriptyline be dispensed to such patients at any one time. However, most clinicians agree that the judgment must be made according to each patient's individual condition.

The condition of depressed patients with bipolar disorder may sometimes change to the manic phase during tricyclic antidepressant therapy, although such change has not been reported with every tricyclic antidepressant.

### Diet/Nutrition

Oral doses may be taken with or immediately after food to lessen gastric irritation.

The requirements for riboflavin may be increased in patients receiving amitriptyline or imipramine.

### For treatment of adverse effects

Neuroleptic malignant syndrome (NMS) (for amoxapine only)—

Treatment is essentially symptomatic and supportive and includes

• *Discontinuing amoxapine immediately.*

• Hyperthermia: Administering antipyretics (aspirin or acetaminophen); using cooling blanket.

• Dehydration: Restoring fluids and electrolytes.

• Cardiovascular instability: Monitoring blood pressure and cardiac rhythm closely.

• Hypoxia: Administering oxygen; considering airway insertion and assisted ventilation.

• Muscle rigidity: Dantrolene sodium may be administered (100 to 300 mg a day in divided doses; 0.75 to 1 mg per kg, intravenously, every 6 hours, increased up to 3 mg per kg every 6 hours as needed).

Parkinsonism—

In most cases, mild effects may be reversed by dosage reduction. Administration of antiparkinsonism drugs such as benztropine, diphenhydramine, or trihexyphenidyl may reverse severe reactions.

Secretion of inappropriate antidiuretic hormone syndrome (SIADH)—
Recommended treatment includes
  • *Discontinuing tricyclic antidepressant.*
  • If urgent treatment is required, administering several hundred milliliters of 5% sodium chloride intravenously over several hours while monitoring serum sodium concentration and the symptoms, and watching for fluid overload.
  • After initial phase, or for less urgent treatment, restricting water intake to 1000 mL a day.
  • Monitoring serum electrolytes for several days.
Tardive dyskinesia (for amoxapine only)—
No known effective treatment. Dosage of the tricyclic should be lowered or medication gradually discontinued at earliest signs of tardive dyskinesia, to prevent irreversible effects.

---

## *AMITRIPTYLINE*

## Summary of Differences

Indications:
  Also used to manage some types of chronic, severe, neurogenic pain, and to treat bulimia and peptic ulcer disease.
Pharmacology/pharmacokinetics:
  Effects—
    Anticholinergic: High.
    Sedative: High.
    Orthostatic hypotension: Moderate to high.

## Oral Dosage Forms

Note: Bracketed uses in the *Dosage Forms* section refer to categories of use and/or indications that are not included in U.S. product labeling.

### AMITRIPTYLINE HYDROCHLORIDE TABLETS USP

**Usual adult dose**
Antidepressant—
  Oral, initially 25 mg two to four times a day, the dosage being adjusted gradually as needed and tolerated.

**Usual adult prescribing limits**
Outpatients—Up to 150 mg a day.
Hospitalized patients—Up to 300 mg a day.
Geriatric patients—Up to 100 mg a day.

**Usual pediatric dose**
Antidepressant—
  Children 6 to 12 years of age: Oral, 10 to 30 mg, or 1 to 5 mg per kg of body weight, a day in two divided doses.
  Adolescents: Oral, initially 10 mg three times a day and 20 mg at bedtime, the dosage being adjusted as needed and tolerated, up to a maximum of 100 mg a day in divided doses or as a single dose at bedtime.
[Enuresis]—
  Children up to 6 years of age: Oral, 10 mg a day as a single dose at bedtime.
  Children over 6 years of age: Oral, initially 10 mg a day as a single dose at bedtime, the dose being increased as needed and tolerated up to a maximum of 25 mg.

**Usual geriatric dose**
Antidepressant—
  Oral, initially 25 mg at bedtime, the dosage being adjusted as needed and tolerated, up to 10 mg three times a day and 20 mg at bedtime.

**Strength(s) usually available**
U.S.—
  10 mg (Rx) [*Elavil; Endep* (scored); GENERIC].
  25 mg (Rx) [*Elavil; Endep* (scored); GENERIC].
  50 mg (Rx) [*Elavil; Endep* (scored); GENERIC].
  75 mg (Rx) [*Elavil; Endep* (scored); GENERIC].
  100 mg (Rx) [*Elavil; Endep* (scored); GENERIC].
  150 mg (Rx) [*Elavil; Endep* (scored); GENERIC].
Canada—
  10 mg (Rx) [*Apo-Amitriptyline; Elavil; Novotriptyn*].
  25 mg (Rx) [*Apo-Amitriptyline; Elavil; Novotriptyn;* GENERIC].
  50 mg (Rx) [*Apo-Amitriptyline; Elavil; Novotriptyn*].
  75 mg (Rx) [*Apo-Amitriptyline; Elavil; Levate*].

**Packaging and storage**
Store below 40 °C (104 °F), preferably between 15 and 30 °C (59 and 86 °F), unless otherwise specified by manufacturer. Store in a well-closed container.

**Auxiliary labeling**
• May cause drowsiness.
• Avoid alcoholic beverages.

### AMITRIPTYLINE PAMOATE SYRUP

**Usual adult dose**
Antidepressant—
  Oral, initially 25 mg (base) two to four times a day, the dosage being adjusted gradually as needed and tolerated.

**Usual pediatric dose**
Antidepressant—
  Children 6 to 12 years of age: Oral, 10 to 30 mg (base), or 1 to 5 mg per kg of body weight, a day in two divided doses.
  Adolescents: Oral, initially 10 mg (base) three times a day and 20 mg at bedtime, the dosage being adjusted as needed and tolerated, up to a maximum of 100 mg a day, in divided doses or as a single dose at bedtime.
[Enuresis]—
  Children up to 6 years of age: Oral, 10 mg (base) a day as a single dose at bedtime.
  Children over 6 years of age: Oral, initially 10 mg (base) a day as a single dose at bedtime, the dose being increased as needed and tolerated up to a maximum of 25 mg.

**Usual geriatric dose**
Antidepressant—
  Oral, initially 10 mg (base) three times a day and 20 mg at bedtime, the dosage being adjusted as needed and tolerated, up to a maximum of 100 mg a day, in divided doses or as a single dose at bedtime.

**Strength(s) usually available**
U.S.—
  Not commercially available.
Canada—
  10 mg (base) per 5 mL (Rx) [*Elavil* (methyl- and propylparaben)].

**Packaging and storage**
Store below 40 °C (104 °F), preferably between 15 and 30 °C (59 and 86 °F), in a well-closed container, unless otherwise specified by manufacturer.

**Auxiliary labeling**
• May cause drowsiness.
• Avoid alcoholic beverages.

## Parenteral Dosage Forms

### AMITRIPTYLINE HYDROCHLORIDE INJECTION USP

**Usual adult dose**
Antidepressant—
  Intramuscular, 20 to 30 mg four times a day.

**Usual pediatric dose**
Antidepressant—
  Children up to 12 years of age: Dosage has not been established.

**Strength(s) usually available**
U.S.—
  10 mg per mL (Rx) [*Elavil* (dextrose; methylparaben; propylparaben); *Enovil* (dextrose; parabens); GENERIC].
Canada—
  Not commercially available.

**Packaging and storage**
Store below 40 °C (104 °F), preferably between 15 and 30 °C (59 and 86 °F), unless otherwise specified by manufacturer. Protect from freezing.

---

### *AMOXAPINE*

## Summary of Differences

Pharmacology/pharmacokinetics:
  Effects—
    Anticholinergic: Moderate.
    Sedative: Low to moderate.
    Orthostatic hypotension: Low.
  Onset of action—
    Antidepressant: Within 1 to 2 weeks.
Side/adverse effects:
  Neuroleptic malignant syndrome, parkinsonian reactions and tardive dyskinesia may occur. Sexual function impairment, breast enlargement in both males and females, testicular swelling, and severe, refractory seizures on acute overdose are all more frequent with amoxapine than with other tricyclic antidepressants.

## Oral Dosage Forms

### AMOXAPINE TABLETS USP

**Usual adult dose**
Antidepressant—
Oral, initially 50 mg two or three times a day, the dosage being increased to 100 mg two or three times a day within the first week of treatment as needed and tolerated.

Note: Increases above 300 mg a day should be made with caution and only if 300 mg a day has been ineffective during a trial period of at least two weeks.

**Usual adult prescribing limits**
Hospitalized patients—Up to 600 mg a day in divided doses.

**Usual pediatric dose**
Children up to 16 years of age—Dosage has not been established.

**Usual geriatric dose**
Antidepressant—
Oral, initially 25 mg two or three times a day, the dosage being increased, if tolerated, to 50 mg two or three times a day within the first week.

**Strength(s) usually available**
U.S.—
25 mg (Rx) [*Asendin* (scored); GENERIC].
50 mg (Rx) [*Asendin* (scored); GENERIC].
100 mg (Rx) [*Asendin* (scored); GENERIC].
150 mg (Rx) [*Asendin* (scored); GENERIC].
Canada—
25 mg (Rx) [*Asendin* (scored)].
50 mg (Rx) [*Asendin* (scored)].
100 mg (Rx) [*Asendin* (scored)].
150 mg (Rx) [*Asendin* (scored)].

**Packaging and storage**
Store below 40 °C (104 °F), preferably between 15 and 30 °C (59 and 86 °F), in a well-closed container, unless otherwise specified by manufacturer.

**Auxiliary labeling**
• May cause drowsiness.
• Avoid alcoholic beverages.

---

### CLOMIPRAMINE

## Summary of Differences

Indications:
Also used to treat obsessive-compulsive disorder, panic disorder, bulimia nervosa, cataplexy associated with narcolepsy, and to manage some types of chronic, severe, neurogenic pain.
Pharmacology/pharmacokinetics:
Effects—
Anticholinergic: High.
Sedative: Moderate.
Orthostatic hypotension: Moderate.
Precautions:
Drug interactions and/or related problems—
Not recommended for concurrent use with monoamine oxidase inhibitors.
Side/adverse effects:
Sexual function impairment, seizures, and nausea and vomiting may occur more frequently with clomipramine than with other tricyclic antidepressants.

## Additional Dosing Information

See also *General Dosing Information.*

Clomipramine should be given in divided doses with meals during initial titration to minimize gastrointestinal side effects; after titration, the total daily dose may be given at bedtime to minimize daytime sedation.

## Oral Dosage Forms

Note: Bracketed uses in the *Dosage Forms* section refer to categories of use and/or indications that are not included in U.S. product labeling.

### CLOMIPRAMINE HYDROCHLORIDE CAPSULES

**Usual adult dose**
[Antidepressant]—
Oral, initially 25 mg three times a day, the dosage being adjusted as needed and tolerated.

Antiobsessional agent—
Oral, initially 25 mg once a day, the dosage being gradually increased to 100 mg during the first two weeks. The dosage may be further increased over the next several weeks, up to a maximum of 250 mg a day.

**Usual adult prescribing limits**
Outpatients: Up to 250 mg a day.
Hospitalized patients: Up to 300 mg a day.

**Usual pediatric dose**
[Antidepressant]—
Children up to 12 years of age: Dosage has not been established.
Adolescents: Oral, 20 to 30 mg a day, the dosage being increased by 10 mg at 4 or 5 day intervals as needed and tolerated.
Antiobsessional agent—
Children up to 10 years of age: Dosage has not been established.
Children 10 years of age and over, and adolescents: Oral, initially 25 mg once a day, the dose being increased as needed and tolerated up to 100 mg a day or 3 mg per kg of body weight, whichever is less. The dosage may be further increased up to a maximum of 200 mg a day or 3 mg per kg of body weight, whichever is less.

Note: The strengths of the specific products may not conform to the recommended pediatric doses.

**Usual geriatric dose**
Oral, 20 to 30 mg a day, the dosage being increased as needed and tolerated.

Note: The strengths of the specific products may not conform to the recommended geriatric doses.

**Strength(s) usually available**
U.S.—
25 mg (Rx) [*Anafranil* (gelatin; methylparaben; propylparaben; silicon dioxide; sodium lauryl sulfate; starch; titanium dioxide; magnesium stearate; FD&C Yellow #6; D&C Red #33)].
50 mg (Rx) [*Anafranil* (gelatin; methylparaben; propylparaben; silicon dioxide; sodium lauryl sulfate; starch; titanium dioxide; magnesium stearate; FD&C Yellow #6; D&C Yellow #10; FD&C Blue #1)].
75 mg (Rx) [*Anafranil* (gelatin; methylparaben; propylparaben; silicon dioxide; sodium lauryl sulfate; starch; titanium dioxide; magnesium stearate; FD&C Yellow #6)].
Canada—
Not commercially available.

**Packaging and storage**
Store below 40 °C (104 °F), preferably between 15 and 30 °C (59 and 86 °F), in a tight, light-resistant container, unless otherwise specified by manufacturer.

**Auxiliary labeling**
• May cause drowsiness.
• Avoid alcoholic beverages.

### CLOMIPRAMINE HYDROCHLORIDE TABLETS

**Usual adult dose**
See *Clomipramine Hydrochloride Capsules.*

**Usual adult prescribing limits**
See *Clomipramine Hydrochloride Capsules.*

**Usual pediatric dose**
See *Clomipramine Hydrochloride Capsules.*

**Usual geriatric dose**
See *Clomipramine Hydrochloride Capsules.*

**Strength(s) usually available**
U.S.—
Not commercially available.
Canada—
10 mg (Rx) [*Anafranil* (lactose)].
25 mg (Rx) [*Anafranil* (lactose)].
50 mg (Rx) [*Anafranil* (lactose)].

**Packaging and storage**
Store below 40 °C (104 °F), preferably between 15 and 30 °C (59 and 86 °F), in a tight, light-resistant container, unless otherwise specified by manufacturer.

**Auxiliary labeling**
• May cause drowsiness.
• Avoid alcoholic beverages.

## DESIPRAMINE

## Summary of Differences

Indications:
Also used to manage some types of chronic, severe, neurogenic pain; to reduce craving and/or prevent depression upon withdrawal of cocaine; to control binge eating and purging in bulimia; and to treat cataplexy associated with narcolepsy and is being used to relieve the symptoms of attention deficit hyperactivity disorder in children over 6 years of age and in adolescents.

Pharmacology/pharmacokinetics:
Effects—
Anticholinergic: Low.
Sedative: Low.
Orthostatic hypotension: Moderate.

Precautions:
Drug interactions and/or related problems—
Not recommended for concurrent use with monoamine oxidase inhibitors.
Concurrent use of phenytoin with desipramine may lower serum concentrations of desipramine; dosage increases above maximum recommended doses of desipramine may be necessary for clinical improvement of depression.

## Oral Dosage Forms

### DESIPRAMINE HYDROCHLORIDE TABLETS USP

**Usual adult dose**
Antidepressant—
Oral, 100 to 200 mg a day in divided doses or as a single dose, the dosage being adjusted as needed and tolerated.

**Usual adult prescribing limits**
Up to 300 mg a day.
Note: Geriatric patients—Up to 150 mg a day.

**Usual pediatric dose**
Antidepressant—
Children 6 to 12 years of age: Oral, 10 to 30 mg, or 1 to 5 mg per kg of body weight, a day in divided doses.
Adolescents: Oral, 25 to 50 mg a day in divided doses, the dosage being adjusted as needed and tolerated, up to a maximum of 100 mg a day.

**Usual geriatric dose**
Antidepressant—
Oral, 25 to 50 mg a day in divided doses, the dosage being adjusted as needed and tolerated, up to a maximum of 150 mg a day.

**Strength(s) usually available**
U.S.—
10 mg (Rx) [Norpramin; GENERIC].
25 mg (Rx) [Norpramin; GENERIC].
50 mg (Rx) [Norpramin; GENERIC].
75 mg (Rx) [Norpramin; GENERIC].
100 mg (Rx) [Norpramin; GENERIC].
150 mg (Rx) [Norpramin; GENERIC].
Canada—
10 mg (Rx) [Norpramin (sucrose; mannitol; corn starch)].
25 mg (Rx) [Norpramin; Pertofrane; GENERIC].
50 mg (Rx) [Norpramin; Pertofrane; GENERIC].
75 mg (Rx) [Norpramin; GENERIC].
100 mg (Rx) [Norpramin].

**Packaging and storage**
Store below 40 °C (104 °F), preferably between 15 and 30 °C (59 and 86 °F), unless otherwise specified by manufacturer. Store in a tight container.

**Auxiliary labeling**
• May cause drowsiness.
• Avoid alcoholic beverages.

## DOXEPIN

## Summary of Differences

Indications:
Also used in treatment of some types of chronic, severe neurogenic pain; peptic ulcer disease; and pruritus in idiopathic cold urticaria.

Pharmacology/pharmacokinetics:
Effects—
Anticholinergic: High.
Sedative: High.
Orthostatic hypotension: High.

## Additional Dosing Information

See also General Dosing Information.

Patients with mild symptomology or emotional symptoms accompanying organic disease may be controlled on doses as low as 25 to 50 mg a day.

The once-a-day dosage maximum is 150 mg, which may be given at bedtime.

## Oral Dosage Forms

Note: Bracketed uses in the Dosage Forms section refer to categories of use and/or indications that are not included in U.S. product labeling.

### DOXEPIN HYDROCHLORIDE CAPSULES USP

**Usual adult dose**
Antidepressant—
Oral, initially 25 mg (base) three times a day, the dosage being adjusted gradually as needed and tolerated.
[Antipruritic][1]—
Oral, initially 10 mg (base) at bedtime, the dosage being increased gradually up to 25 mg, as needed and tolerated.

**Usual adult prescribing limits**
Outpatients: Up to 150 mg (base) a day.
Hospitalized patients: Up to 300 mg (base) a day.

**Usual pediatric dose**
Antidepressant—
Children up to 12 years of age: Dosage has not been established.

**Usual geriatric dose**
Antidepressant—
Oral, initially 25 to 50 mg (base) a day, the dosage being adjusted gradually as needed and tolerated.

**Strength(s) usually available**
U.S.—
10 mg (base) (Rx) [Sinequan; GENERIC].
25 mg (base) (Rx) [Sinequan; GENERIC].
50 mg (base) (Rx) [Sinequan; GENERIC].
75 mg (base) (Rx) [Sinequan; GENERIC].
100 mg (base) (Rx) [Sinequan; GENERIC].
150 mg (base) (Rx) [Sinequan; GENERIC].
Canada—
10 mg (base) (Rx) [Sinequan; Triadapin].
25 mg (base) (Rx) [Novo-Doxepin; Sinequan (sodium metabisulfite); Triadapin].
50 mg (base) (Rx) [Novo-Doxepin; Sinequan (sodium metabisulfite); Triadapin].
75 mg (base) (Rx) [Novo-Doxepin; Sinequan (sodium metabisulfite); Triadapin].
100 mg (base) (Rx) [Novo-Doxepin; Sinequan (sodium metabisulfite); Triadapin].
150 mg (base) (Rx) [Novo-Doxepin; Sinequan (sodium metabisulfite)].

**Packaging and storage**
Store between 15 and 30 °C (59 and 86 °F), unless otherwise specified by manufacturer. Store in a well-closed container.

**Auxiliary labeling**
• May cause drowsiness.
• Avoid alcoholic beverages.

**Note**
The 150-mg capsule is intended for maintenance therapy only, and not for initiation of therapy.

### DOXEPIN HYDROCHLORIDE ORAL SOLUTION USP

**Usual adult dose**
See Doxepin Hydrochloride Capsules USP.

**Usual adult prescribing limits**
See Doxepin Hydrochloride Capsules USP.

**Usual pediatric dose**
See Doxepin Hydrochloride Capsules USP.

**Strength(s) usually available**
U.S.—
10 mg (base) per mL (Rx) [Sinequan; GENERIC].
Canada—
Not commercially available.

**Packaging and storage**
Store between 15 and 30 °C (59 and 86 °F), unless otherwise specified by manufacturer. Store in a tight, light-resistant container.

**Incompatibilities**
Oral solution may be incompatible with many carbonated beverages and with grape juice.

**Auxiliary labeling**
• May cause drowsiness.
• Avoid alcoholic beverages.
• Must be diluted before taking.

**Note**
When dispensing, include the manufacturer-provided graduated dropper.

[1]Not included in Canadian product labeling.

---

### IMIPRAMINE

## Summary of Differences

Indications:
Imipramine hydrochloride (but not pamoate) is indicated in treatment of childhood enuresis.
Imipramine is also used to manage some types of chronic, severe, neurogenic pain; to reduce craving and/or prevent depression upon cocaine withdrawal; to relieve symptoms of attention deficit hyperactivity disorder in children over 6 years of age and in adolescents; as a treatment adjunct with amphetamines or methylphenidate in cataplexy associated with narcolepsy; to block the recurrence of panic attacks, with or without phobias; in the treatment of stress and urge incontinence; and to control binge eating and purging in bulimia.
Pharmacology/pharmacokinetics:
Effects:
Anticholinergic: Moderate.
Sedative: Moderate.
Orthostatic hypotension: High.
Precautions:
Drug interactions and/or related problems—
Not recommended for concurrent use with monoamine oxidase inhibitors.

## Additional Dosing Information

See also *General Dosing Information.*

**For oral dosage forms only**
In enuretic children, a daily dose exceeding 75 mg does not normally increase results. The usual pediatric prescribing limits are 2.5 mg per kg of body weight (mg/kg) a day.
For early-night bedwetters, the dosage may be more effective when one-half of the dose is given at mid-afternoon and one-half at bedtime.
A gradual decrease in dosage is less likely to cause relapse than an abrupt discontinuation.
Younger children should not be allowed to self-administer imipramine because of their increased sensitivity to side effects, especially cardiovascular effects and acute overdosage (plasma concentrations over 225 nanograms per mL), which are potentially fatal.
A medication-free interval after adequate therapeutic trial should be considered for children. However, dosage should be decreased gradually to prevent relapse. Children who have relapsed may not respond when treatment is reinitiated.

**For parenteral dosage forms only**
Used only for initiating therapy in patients who are not able or are unwilling to take oral medication. Oral dosage forms should replace the parenteral as soon as possible.

## Oral Dosage Forms

Note: Bracketed uses in the *Dosage Forms* section refer to categories of use and/or indications that are not included in U.S. product labeling.

### IMIPRAMINE HYDROCHLORIDE TABLETS USP

**Usual adult dose**
Antidepressant—
Oral, 25 to 50 mg three or four times a day, the dosage being adjusted as needed and tolerated.
[Urinary incontinence][1]—
Oral, 10 to 50 mg a day, the dosage being adjusted as needed and tolerated, to a maximum of 150 mg a day.

**Usual adult prescribing limits**
Outpatients: Up to 200 mg a day.
Hospitalized patients: Up to 300 mg a day.
Geriatric patients: Up to 100 mg a day.

**Usual pediatric dose**
Antidepressant—
Children up to 6 years of age: Use is not recommended.
Children 6 to 12 years of age: Oral, 10 to 30 mg a day in two divided doses.
Adolescents: Oral, 25 to 50 mg a day in divided doses, the dosage being adjusted as needed and tolerated, up to 100 mg a day.
Antienuretic—
Oral, 25 mg once a day, one hour before bedtime. If a satisfactory response is not obtained within one week, the dosage may be increased to 50 mg nightly in children under 12 years of age and to 75 mg nightly in children 12 or over.

**Usual geriatric dose**
Antidepressant—
Oral, initially 25 mg at bedtime, the dosage being adjusted as needed and tolerated, up to 100 mg a day in divided doses.

**Strength(s) usually available**
U.S.—
10 mg (Rx) [*Tipramine; Tofranil;* GENERIC].
25 mg (Rx) [*Norfranil; Tipramine; Tofranil;* GENERIC].
50 mg (Rx) [*Norfranil; Tipramine; Tofranil;* GENERIC].
Canada—
10 mg (Rx) [*Apo-Imipramine; Novopramine; Tofranil*].
25 mg (Rx) [*Apo-Imipramine; Novopramine; Tofranil*].
50 mg (Rx) [*Apo-Imipramine; Novopramine; Tofranil*].
75 mg (Rx) [*Apo-Imipramine* (scored); *Impril; Tofranil*].

**Packaging and storage**
Store between 15 and 30 °C (59 and 86 °F), unless otherwise specified by manufacturer. Store in a tight container.

**Auxiliary labeling**
• May cause drowsiness.
• Avoid alcoholic beverages.

### IMIPRAMINE PAMOATE CAPSULES

**Usual adult dose**
Antidepressant—
Oral, initially 75 mg a day, usually given at bedtime, the dosage being adjusted as needed and tolerated.

Note: The dose level at which optimum response is usually obtained is 150 mg a day, usually given at bedtime.

**Usual adult prescribing limits**
Outpatients: Up to 200 mg a day.
Hospitalized patients: Up to 300 mg a day.

**Usual pediatric dose**
Antidepressant—
Children up to 12 years of age: Use is not recommended.

**Strength(s) usually available**
U.S.—
75 mg (Rx) [*Tofranil-PM*].
100 mg (Rx) [*Tofranil-PM*].
125 mg (Rx) [*Tofranil-PM*].
150 mg (Rx) [*Tofranil-PM*].

Note: The above strengths of imipramine pamoate are equivalent to the same strengths of imipramine hydrochloride.
Canada—
Not commercially available.

**Packaging and storage**
Store between 15 and 30 °C (59 and 86 °F), in a tight container, unless otherwise specified by manufacturer.

**Auxiliary labeling**
• May cause drowsiness.
• Avoid alcoholic beverages.

## Parenteral Dosage Forms

### IMIPRAMINE HYDROCHLORIDE INJECTION USP

**Usual adult dose**
Antidepressant—
Intramuscular, up to 100 mg a day in divided doses.

**Usual adult prescribing limits**
Up to 300 mg a day.

**Usual pediatric dose**

Antidepressant—

Children up to 12 years of age: Use is not recommended.

**Strength(s) usually available**

U.S.—

12.5 mg per mL (Rx) [*Tofranil* (ascorbic acid 1 mg; sodium bisulfite 0.5 mg; anhydrous sodium sulfite 0.5 mg)].

Canada—

Not commercially available.

**Packaging and storage**

Store below 40 °C (104 °F), preferably between 15 and 30 °C (59 and 86 °F), unless otherwise specified by manufacturer. Protect from freezing.

**Auxiliary labeling**

• For intramuscular use only.

---

[1]Not included in Canadian product labeling.

---

## NORTRIPTYLINE

## Summary of Differences

Indications:

Also used to manage some types of chronic, severe, neurogenic pain and in the treatment of panic disorder.

Pharmacology/pharmacokinetics:

Effects—

Anticholinergic: Low.

Sedative: Moderate.

Orthostatic hypotension: Low.

## Oral Dosage Forms

### NORTRIPTYLINE HYDROCHLORIDE CAPSULES USP

**Usual adult dose**

Antidepressant—

Oral, 25 mg (base) three or four times a day, the dosage being adjusted as needed and tolerated.

**Usual adult prescribing limits**

Up to 150 mg (base) a day.

**Usual pediatric dose**

Antidepressant—

Children 6 to 12 years of age: Oral, 10 to 20 mg (base), or 1 to 3 mg per kg of body weight, a day in divided doses.

Adolescents: Oral, 25 to 50 mg, or 1 to 3 mg per kg of body weight, a day in divided doses, the dosage being adjusted as needed and tolerated.

**Usual geriatric dose**

Oral, 30 to 50 mg a day in divided doses, the dosage being adjusted as needed and tolerated.

**Strength(s) usually available**

U.S.—

10 mg (base) (Rx) [*Aventyl; Pamelor;* GENERIC].

25 mg (base) (Rx) [*Aventyl; Pamelor;* GENERIC].

50 mg (base) (Rx) [*Pamelor;* GENERIC].

75 mg (base) (Rx) [*Pamelor;* GENERIC].

Canada—

10 mg (base) (Rx) [*Aventyl*].

25 mg (base) (Rx) [*Aventyl*].

**Packaging and storage**

Store between 15 and 30 °C (59 and 86 °F), unless otherwise specified by manufacturer. Store in a tight container.

**Auxiliary labeling**

• May cause drowsiness.

• Avoid alcoholic beverages.

### NORTRIPTYLINE HYDROCHLORIDE ORAL SOLUTION USP

**Usual adult dose**

See *Nortriptyline Hydrochloride Capsules USP.*

**Usual pediatric dose**

See *Nortriptyline Hydrochloride Capsules USP.*

**Strength(s) usually available**

U.S.—

10 mg (base) per 5 mL (Rx) [*Aventyl* (alcohol 4%); *Pamelor* (alcohol 4%)].

Canada—

Not commercially available.

**Packaging and storage**

Store below 40 °C (104 °F), preferably between 15 and 30 °C (59 and 86 °F), unless otherwise specified by manufacturer. Store in a tight, light-resistant container. Protect from freezing.

**Auxiliary labeling**

• May cause drowsiness.

• Avoid alcoholic beverages.

---

## PROTRIPTYLINE

## Summary of Differences

Indications:

Also used in the treatment of narcolepsy, as an adjunct with amphetamines or methylphenidate in the treatment of cataplexy associated with narcolepsy, in sleep disorders such as hypersomnia or impaired morning arousal, and may be used to relieve symptoms of attention deficit hyperactivity disorder in some children over 6 years of age and in adolescents.

Pharmacology/pharmacokinetics:

Effects—

Anticholinergic: Moderate.

Sedative: Very low.

Orthostatic hypotension: Low.

## Additional Dosing Information

See also *General Dosing Information.*

When dosage increases of protriptyline are indicated, the increase should be made in the morning. This drug often has a psychic-energizing action and usually not the sedative action exhibited by other tricyclics, although it may intensify the sedative effect of other medications.

Protriptyline is often given in divided doses with the last daily dose in the afternoon to avoid insomnia or nightmares when given to some patients before bedtime.

When protriptyline is used in narcolepsy, 15 to 20 mg given in a single daily dose at bedtime may relieve symptoms of arousal difficulty and daytime sleepiness.

## Oral Dosage Forms

Note: Bracketed uses in the *Dosage Forms* section refer to categories of use and/or indications that are not included in U.S. product labeling.

### PROTRIPTYLINE HYDROCHLORIDE TABLETS USP

**Usual adult dose**

Antidepressant—

Oral, initially 5 to 10 mg three or four times a day, the dosage being adjusted as needed and tolerated.

[Anticataplectic][1]—

Oral, 15 to 20 mg a day at bedtime.

**Usual adult prescribing limits**

Up to 60 mg a day.

**Usual pediatric dose**

Antidepressant—

Children up to 12 years of age: Dosage has not been established.

Adolescents: Oral, initially 5 mg three times a day, the dosage being adjusted as needed and tolerated.

**Usual geriatric dose**

Antidepressant—

Oral, initially 5 mg three times a day, the dosage being adjusted as needed and tolerated.

Note: When the daily dose for geriatric patients exceeds 20 mg, the cardiovascular response should be closely monitored.

**Strength(s) usually available**

U.S.—

5 mg (Rx) [*Vivactil* (lactose; calcium phosphate; cellulose; guar gum; hydroxypropyl cellulose; hydroxypropyl methylcellulose; magnesium stearate; starch; talc; titanium dioxide; FD&C Yellow No. 6)].

10 mg (Rx) [*Vivactil* (lactose; calcium phosphate; cellulose; guar gum; hydroxypropyl cellulose; hydroxypropyl methylcellulose; magnesium stearate; starch; talc; titanium dioxide; FD&C Yellow No. 6; D&C Yellow No. 10)].

Canada—

10 mg (Rx) [*Triptil*].

**Packaging and storage**

Store between 15 and 30 °C (59 and 86 °F), unless otherwise specified by manufacturer. Store in a tight container.

**Auxiliary labeling**
- May cause drowsiness.
- Avoid alcoholic beverages.

[1]Not included in Canadian product labeling.

---

### TRIMIPRAMINE

## Summary of Differences

Indications:
Also used in treatment of peptic ulcer disease and in the management of some types of chronic, severe, neurogenic pain.
Pharmacology/pharmacokinetics:
Effects—
Anticholinergic: High.
Sedative: High.
Orthostatic hypotension: Moderate.

## Additional Dosing Information

See also *General Dosing Information*.

For patient compliance and convenience of therapy for outpatients, the total daily dosage may be given at bedtime.

Following remission, maintenance therapy should continue for about 3 months at the lowest dose necessary to maintain remission.

In resistant cases of depression in adults in which dosage exceeds 2.5 mg per kg of body weight (mg/kg) a day, the ECG should be monitored during initiation of therapy and at appropriate intervals during stabilization of dose.

## Oral Dosage Forms

Note: The dosing and strengths of the dosage forms available are expressed in terms of trimipramine base (not the maleate).

### TRIMIPRAMINE MALEATE CAPSULES

**Usual adult dose**
Antidepressant—
Outpatients:
Initial—Oral, 75 mg (base) a day in divided doses, the dosage being adjusted gradually to 150 mg a day as needed and tolerated, up to a maximum of 200 mg a day.
Maintenance—Oral, 50 to 150 mg (base) a day.
Hospitalized patients:
Oral, initially 100 mg (base) a day in divided doses, the dosage being increased gradually in a few days to 200 mg a day, up to 250 to 300 mg a day in two to three weeks.

**Usual pediatric dose**
Antidepressant—
Children up to 12 years of age: Dosage has not been established.

Adolescents: Oral, initially 50 mg (base) a day in divided doses, the dosage being adjusted as needed and tolerated, up to a maximum of 100 mg a day.

**Usual geriatric dose**
Oral, initially 50 mg (base) a day in divided doses, the dosage being adjusted as needed and tolerated, up to a maximum of 100 mg a day.

**Strength(s) usually available**
U.S.—
25 mg (base) (Rx) [*Surmontil;* GENERIC].
50 mg (base) (Rx) [*Surmontil;* GENERIC].
100 mg (base) (Rx) [*Surmontil;* GENERIC].
Canada—
75 mg (base) (Rx) [*Rhotrimine; Surmontil*].

**Packaging and storage**
Store between 15 and 30 °C (59 and 86 °F), in a tight container, unless otherwise specified by manufacturer.

**Auxiliary labeling**
- May cause drowsiness.
- Avoid alcoholic beverages.

### TRIMIPRAMINE MALEATE TABLETS

**Usual adult dose**
See *Trimipramine Maleate Capsules.*

**Usual pediatric dose**
See *Trimipramine Maleate Capsules.*

**Usual geriatric dose**
Antidepressant—
Oral, initially 25 to 50 mg (base) a day in divided doses, the dosage being increased by 25 mg a week, up to a maximum of 150 mg a day.

**Strength(s) usually available**
U.S.—
Not commercially available.
Canada—
12.5 mg (base) (Rx) [*Apo-Trimip; Rhotrimine; Surmontil*].
25 mg (base) (Rx) [*Apo-Trimip; Novo-Tripramine; Rhotrimine; Surmontil*].
50 mg (base) (Rx) [*Apo-Trimip; Novo-Tripramine; Rhotrimine; Surmontil*].
100 mg (base) (Rx) [*Apo-Trimip; Novo-Tripramine; Rhotrimine; Surmontil*].

**Packaging and storage**
Store between 15 and 30 °C (59 and 86 °F), in a tight container, unless otherwise specified by manufacturer.

**Auxiliary labeling**
- May cause drowsiness.
- Avoid alcoholic beverages.

---

Revised: 05/22/92
Interim revision: 06/01/92; 03/01/93; 04/29/94

---

## Table 1. Pharmacology/Pharmacokinetics

| Drug | Anticholinergic Effects* | Sedation* | Orthostatic Hypotension* | Active Metabolites | Protein Binding (%) | Volume of Distribution (L/Kg) | Half-life (hours) | Therapeutic Plasma Concentration (ng/mL)† |
|---|---|---|---|---|---|---|---|---|
| Amitriptyline | High | High | Moderate to high | Nortriptyline 10-Hydroxyamitriptyline | 95 | 12–18 | 10–26 | |
| Amoxapine | Moderate | Low to moderate | Low | 7- and 8-Hydroxyamoxapine | 92 | N.A.‡ | 8–30 | |
| Clomipramine | High | Moderate | Moderate | Desmethylclomipramine | 96–97 | 12 | 21–31 | |
| Desipramine | Low | Low | Moderate | 2-Hydroxydesipramine | 90–92 | 17–42 | 12–27 | 125–300 |

## Table 1. Pharmacology/Pharmacokinetics (continued)

| Drug | Anticholiner- gic Effects* | Sedation* | Orthostatic Hypotension* | Active Metabolites | Protein Binding (%) | Volume of Distribu- tion (L/Kg) | Half-life (hours) | Therapeutic Plasma Con- centration (ng/mL)† |
|---|---|---|---|---|---|---|---|---|
| Doxepin | High | High | High | Desmethyldoxepin | N.A.‡ | 12–28 | 11–23 | |
| Imipramine | Moderate | Moderate | High | Desipramine 2-Hydroxydesipr- amine | 89–95 | 15–31 | 11–25 | 150–300§ |
| Nortriptyline | Low | Moderate | Low | 10-Hydroxynortript- yline | 92 | 14–22 | 18–44 | 50–150** |
| Protriptyline | Moderate | Very low | Low | N.A.‡ | 92 | 22 | 67–89 | |
| Trimipramine | High | High | Moderate | N.A.‡ | N.A.‡ | N.A.‡ | 9–11 | |

*Relative effects among tricyclic antidepressants only.

†Although various values have been reported, there is little consensus about therapeutic plasma concentrations, except for desipramine, imipramine, and nortriptyline. Steady-state plasma levels exhibit marked interindividual variations due to genetic factors (e.g., hepatic metabolism) and physiochemical properties of the medication (e.g., lipid solubility).

‡Not available.

§Includes metabolites.

**Denotes therapeutic window, outside of which effects are lessened.

# ANTIDIABETIC AGENTS, SULFONYLUREA  Systemic

This monograph includes information on the following: Acetohexamide; Chlorpropamide; Gliclazide*; Glipizide†; Glyburide; Tolazamide†; Tolbutamide.

INN:
  Glyburide—Glibenclamide

BAN:
  Glyburide—Glibenclamide

JAN:
  Glyburide—Glibenclamide

VA CLASSIFICATION (Primary/Secondary):
  Acetohexamide—HS502
  Chlorpropamide—HS502/CV900
  Gliclazide—HS502
  Glipizide—HS502
  Glyburide—HS502
  Tolazamide—HS502
  Tolbutamide—HS502

Another commonly used name for glyburide is glibenclamide.

Note: For a listing of dosage forms and brand names by country availability, see Dosage Forms section(s). For a listing of brand names for the articles in this monograph, refer to the General Index.

*Not commercially available in the U.S.

†Not commercially available in Canada.

## Category

Antidiabetic—Acetohexamide; Chlorpropamide; Gliclazide; Glipizide; Glyburide; Tolazamide; Tolbutamide.

Antidiuretic—Chlorpropamide.

## Indications

Note: Bracketed information in the Indications section refers to uses that are not included in U.S. product labeling.

**Accepted**

Diabetes mellitus (treatment), including:

Diabetes mellitus, non–insulin-dependent (NIDDM)—Sulfonylureas are indicated as adjunctive therapy to diet and exercise in the treatment and control of certain patients with NIDDM (Type II diabetes; previously known as adult-onset diabetes, maturity-onset diabetes, ketosis-resistant diabetes, or stable diabetes), which occurs in individuals who produce or secrete insufficient quantities of endogenous insulin or who have developed resistance to endogenous insulin. An attempt to control diabetes through changes in diet and level of physical activity is usually first-line management before beginning pharmacologic treatment. Those patients not responding adequately to diet alone or those patients requiring diet plus insulin, especially if they require 40 USP Units or less of insulin a day, may be candidates for therapy with a sulfonylurea as monotherapy or combination therapy.

Diabetes mellitus, other, associated with certain conditions or syndromes, such as:

• Endocrine disease, including endocrine overactivity due to Cushing's syndrome, hyperthyroidism, pheochromocytoma, somatostatinoma, or aldosteronoma; or endocrine underactivity due to hypoparathyroidism-hypocalcemia, type I isolated growth hormone deficiency, or multitropic pituitary deficiency or

• Genetic syndromes, including, inborn errors of metabolism, such as glycogen-storage disease type I, or insulin-resistant syndromes, such as muscular dystrophies, late onset proximal myopathy, or Huntington's chorea.

• Sulfonylureas may be used in conditions causing diabetes mellitus induced by hormones, medications, or chemicals in patients who have functioning pancreatic beta cells when the diabetes cannot be controlled by diet or exercise.

Combination use of insulin and sulfonylurea agents in insulin-dependent diabetes mellitus (IDDM) patients is controversial because many studies have indicated that sulfonylureas are not effective in the treatment of these patients.

Short-term administration of a sulfonylurea or insulin for transient loss of blood glucose control may be sufficient for NIDDM patients normally well-controlled with diet. Switching to another sulfonylurea agent may be beneficial if one particular sulfonylurea does not optimally control the diabetes mellitus; however, use of a sulfonylurea should be discontinued if satisfactory reduction of blood glucose concentration is not achieved.

The effectiveness of sulfonylureas in controlling blood glucose can decrease over time. If maximum doses of a sulfonylurea fail to control blood glucose, switching to another sulfonylurea or adding metformin to a sulfonylurea treatment regimen may be beneficial in increasing glycemic control and lipoprotein metabolism, and to help avoid initiation of insulin therapy. This is especially successful in NIDDM patients poorly controlled by insulin alone, in short-term diabetics, or in patients who are 120 to 160% over ideal baseline body weight but who are not excessively insulin-resistant. Alternatively, low-dose insulin in conjunction with sulfonylureas can help to avoid using large doses of insulin, especially for obese NIDDM patients; however, complications, such as weight gain, the effects of hyperinsulinemia, and an increased risk of hypoglycemia need to be considered. Some nonobese NIDDM patients experiencing secondary sulfonylurea failure may be best treated with insulin. A sulfonylurea should be discontinued anytime it fails to contribute to the lowering of plasma glucose in a patient for whom compliance with proper diet and sulfonylurea dosing has been determined to be adequate.

[Diabetes insipidus, central, partial (treatment)][1]—Chlorpropamide is also used as secondary therapy in selected patients to treat partial central diabetes insipidus. Used as an antidiuretic, chlorpropamide has successfully reduced polyuria in about 50% of such treated patients. Chlorpropamide may be used alone or in combination with another agent such as carbamazepine or clofibrate so that the dose of both can be reduced and side effects minimized. Nasal or subcutaneous desmopressin is considered the primary treatment for diabetes insipidus.

### Unaccepted

Sulfonylureas are not effective in the treatment of insulin-dependent diabetes mellitus (IDDM; Type I diabetes).

Chlorpropamide is not effective in the treatment of nephrogenic diabetes insipidus.

[1]Not included in Canadian product labeling.

## Pharmacology/Pharmacokinetics

See also *Table 1*, page 289.

### Physicochemical characteristics

Chemical group—
  Sulfonylurea.
    First generation: Acetohexamide, chlorpropamide, tolazamide, tolbutamide.
    Second generation: Gliclazide, glipizide, glyburide.
Molecular weight—
    Acetohexamide: 324.4.
    Chlorpropamide: 276.75.
    Gliclazide: 323.42.
    Glipizide: 445.55.
    Glyburide: 494.01.
    Tolazamide: 311.41.
    Tolbutamide: 270.35.
pKa—
    Chlorpropamide: 4.8.
    Gliclazide: 5.98.
    Glipizide: 5.9.
    Glyburide: 5.3.
    Tolazamide: 3.5, 5.7.
    Tolbutamide: 5.3.

### Mechanism of action/Effect

Antidiabetic—
  Sulfonylureas lower blood glucose in NIDDM by directly stimulating the acute release of insulin from functioning beta cells of pancreatic islet tissue by an unknown process that involves a sulfonylurea receptor on the beta cell. Sulfonylureas inhibit the ATP-potassium channels on the beta cell membrane and potassium efflux, which results in depolarization and calcium influx, calcium-calmodulin binding, kinase activation, and release of insulin-containing granules by exocytosis, an effect similar to that of glucose. Insulin is a hormone that lowers blood glucose and controls the storage and metabolism of carbohydrates, proteins, and fats. Therefore, sulfonylureas are effective only in patients whose pancreata are capable of producing insulin.
  With chronic sulfonylurea treatment, insulin production is not increased and may return to pretreatment values, but insulin efficacy continues and is thought to involve extrapancreatic mechanisms to increase insulin sensitivity in target tissues, such as liver, muscle, and fat as well as in other cells, such as monocytes and erythrocytes. This can result in a decrease in hepatic glycogenolysis and gluconeogenesis. It is unclear if the sulfonylurea's extrapancreatic actions that increase insulin's efficacy are direct or indirect effects, but it is clear that the mechanism of action is not due to a direct sulfonylurea action on the insulin receptor. Because this peripheral effect is not apparent in IDDM patients, it suggests that this may not be the clinically significant mechanism for NIDDM patients either. However, it is clear that tissues of sulfonylurea-treated NIDDM patients become more responsive to lower levels of endogenous insulin. Primary failure of sulfonylurea therapy may occur if the ability of beta cells to function is severely impaired. In addition to stimulating insulin secretion through the beta-cell sulfonylurea receptor, gliclazide may have a direct effect on intracellular calcium transport that specifically improves the biphasic response of the beta cell to a meal, that is, the immediate first phase of insulin release as well as the normally delayed second phase.
Antidiuretic—
  Chlorpropamide seems to potentiate the effect of minimal levels of antidiuretic hormone present in patients with partial central diabetes insipidus.

### Other actions/effects

Acetohexamide and its more potent major metabolite, hydroxyhexamide, have uricosuric properties. Gliclazide, at therapeutic doses, reduces platelet adhesiveness and aggregation by inhibition of arachidonic acid release and thromboxane synthesis, increased production of $PGI_2$, and release of plasminogen activator, which increases fibrinolysis. It is also thought that gliclazide and glyburide have protective activity against cardiac arrhythmias because they can stabilize potassium and calcium concentrations by inhibition of the sodium-potassium-ATPase pump transport system. Tolbutamide and chlorpropamide decrease free water clearance while glyburide, glipizide, and tolazamide produce a mild diuresis effect by enhancement of renal free water clearance. In contrast to glyburide, tolazamide and tolbutamide increase hexose uptake in adipocytes and myocytes. Sulfonylureas directly increase the secretion of pancreatic and gastric somatostatin and do not seem to have a direct effect on glucagon.

### Absorption

Rapidly and well absorbed but may have wide inter- and intra-individual variability. By impairing gastric motility and gastric emptying, hyperglycemia may significantly delay sulfonylurea absorption; glipizide plasma concentration has been shown to be reduced by 50% with plasma glucose concentrations over 198 mg/dL (11 millimoles/L).
*Chlorpropamide*—Food delays absorption of chlorpropamide.
*Gliclazide*—Food delays absorption of gliclazide up to 187 minutes; may be best taken 30 minutes before or with a meal.
*Glipizide*—Food delays absorption of immediate release glipizide by 40 minutes; therefore, it is recommended that glipizide be taken 30 minutes before a meal. While food had no effect on the lag time of absorption (3 to 4 hours) for extended release glipizide, administration of glipizide to normal males before a meal high in fat showed a 40% increase in the time to peak serum concentrations; area-under-the-time curve (AUC) was not affected.
*Glyburide*—Bioavailability of nonmicronized glyburide is lowest when given with a high fat diet compared to fasting or a high carbohydrate diet. Micronized glyburide is more consistent in its bioavailability and in its time to reach peak serum concentrations with regard to all meal types than is the nonmicronized formulation. Also, micronized glyburide is better absorbed and is effective at a lower dose than is nonmicronized glyburide.
*Tolbutamide*—Absorption is unaltered if taken with food but is increased with high pH.

## Precautions to Consider

### Cross-sensitivity and/or related problems

Patients sensitive to one of the sulfonylureas may be sensitive to the others also; cross-sensitivity to other sulfonamide- or thiazide-type medications may also occur.

### Carcinogenicity

*Acetohexamide*—Long-term studies in rats and mice showed no evidence of carcinogenicity.
*Chlorpropamide*—Chronic toxicity studies in dogs treated for 6, 13, and 20 months with doses of chlorpropamide greater than 20 times the human dose showed no histological or pathological abnormalities.
*Gliclazide*—Specific carcinogenicity studies have not been done in animals; however, long-term toxicity studies have not shown any evidence of drug-related carcinogenicity.
*Glipizide*—Large dose studies using up to 75 times the maximum human dose in rats and in mice for 20 and 18 months, respectively, showed no evidence of drug-related carcinogenicity.
*Glyburide*—An 18-month study in rats given doses of up to 300 mg per kg of body weight (mg/kg) a day and a 2-year oncogenicity study in mice showed no evidence of drug-related carcinogenicity.
*Tolazamide*—A 103-week study in rats and mice at both low and high doses showed no evidence of carcinogenicity.
*Tolbutamide*—A 78-week study in male and female rats and mice showed no evidence of carcinogenicity.

### Mutagenicity

*Acetohexamide*—Sister chromatid exchange testing showed no evidence of mutagenicity.
*Chlorpropamide*—The micronucleus test in one strain of Swiss mice given chlorpropamide doses of 200, 400, 800, and 1600 mg/kg (32 times greater than the therapeutic adult dose) showed no evidence of mutagenicity; however, 3 strains of mice showed positive results when evaluated using the *Salmonella*/microsome test. The results are questionable because negative results were also shown in rats and Chinese hamsters. Although an increase in chromosomal breakage has not been observed in treated mammals, Chinese hamsters, rats, or mice, the sister chromatin exchange showed a positive reaction with Chinese hamsters *in vivo* and *in vitro*; however, spontaneous breakage in this study was not even doubled in extremely high doses. It is difficult to

assign a cause-and-effect to the slightly positive results in these animal studies.

*Gliclazide*—The Ames test, human lymphocyte test, and micronucleus test did not reveal mutagenicity.

*Glipizide*—Bacterial and *in vivo* mutagenicity testing showed no evidence of mutagenicity.

*Glyburide*—Testing with the Ames test, DNA damage/alkaline elution assay, and the micronucleus test (at doses 60 to 240 times the average human therapeutic dose) showed no evidence of mutagenicity.

*Tolbutamide*—The Ames test and the micronucleus test in mice (at doses of 500 mg/kg) showed no evidence of mutagenicity.

## Pregnancy/Reproduction

Fertility—

*Acetohexamide, tolazamide, tolbutamide*—
 Studies in humans have not been done.
 Studies in animals have not been done.

*Chlorpropamide*—
 Studies in humans have not been done.
 Studies in rats treated with high doses of chlorpropamide (125 mg/kg) for 6 to 12 months showed varying degrees of spermatogenesis suppression.

*Gliclazide*—
 Studies in humans have not been done.
 Studies in female rats and the first generation offspring of treated male and female rats showed no evidence of impaired fertility.

*Glipizide*—
 Studies in humans have not been done.
 Studies in male and female rats given 75 times the maximum human dose showed no evidence of impaired fertility.

*Glyburide*—
 Studies in humans have not been done.
 Studies in rats and rabbits given 500 times the human dose have not shown evidence of impaired fertility.

Pregnancy—Chlorpropamide crosses the placenta; glyburide does not significantly cross the placenta, and it is not known whether other sulfonylureas cross the placenta. Use of insulin rather than sulfonylurea antidiabetic agents during pregnancy allows for the maintenance of blood glucose concentrations that are as close to normal as possible. Abnormal blood glucose levels have been associated with a higher incidence of congenital abnormalities during early pregnancy, and with increased perinatal morbidity and mortality later in pregnancy. Adequate and well-controlled studies in humans have not been done to determine whether sulfonylureas are teratogenic. It remains possible that sulfonylureas cause congenital malformations if they cross the placenta, but current data leave unresolved the issue of whether the abnormalities are due to poor glucose control or to sulfonylurea treatment. Generally, sulfonylureas are not recommended during pregnancy. In the rare case that sulfonylureas are used during pregnancy, they should be discontinued to allow an interval before delivery appropriate for the particular sulfonylurea being used because of the risk that they will cause insulin release and hypoglycemia in the neonate at delivery.

*Acetohexamide*—
 Adequate and well-controlled studies in humans have not been done.
 Acetohexamide has been shown to be teratogenic in animal studies when large doses were administered.
 FDA Pregnancy Category C.

*Chlorpropamide*—
 Chlorpropamide crosses the placenta. Adequate and well-controlled studies have not been done in humans. Low doses (250 mg a day or less) of chlorpropamide have been used in pregnant women without adverse effects. The manufacturer recommends discontinuing chlorpropamide at least one month before expected delivery date.
 Using an *in vitro* method and whole embryo mouse culture, one study compared the difference between growth in embryos bathed in hypoglycemic and euglycemic chlorpropamide-treated rat serums. The teratologic evaluation of the treated early somite mouse embryos showed malformations and growth retardation at doses similar to human therapeutic concentrations, which suggested that the teratogenicity was due to chlorpropamide and not to hypoglycemia; untreated mouse embryos showed normal development.
 FDA Pregnancy Category C.

*Gliclazide*—
 Studies in humans have not been done. Gliclazide is not recommended for use during pregnancy.
 No teratogenic effects were found in studies of mice and rabbits. Embryotoxicity was not seen in studies of rats. However, a significant decrease in offspring viability at 48 hours was seen

when pregnant females were treated up to delivery. It is unclear how this relates or if it applies to humans.

*Glipizide*—
 Studies in humans have not been done. Glipizide should be discontinued at least 1 month before the expected delivery date.
 Studies in rats have shown glipizide to be fetotoxic at all doses from 5 to 50 mg/kg; the fetotoxicity is thought to be due to the pharmacologic hypoglycemic effect during the perinatal period. No teratogenic effects were found in studies in rats and rabbits.
 FDA Pregnancy Category C.

*Glyburide*—
 Glyburide does not significantly cross the placenta according to an *in vitro* study using human placentas. Studies in humans have not been done. Use should be discontinued at least 2 weeks before the expected delivery date.
 Studies in rats and rabbits given up to 500 times the human dose have produced no evidence of teratogenicity.
 FDA Pregnancy Category B *(Micronase, Glynase)*.
 FDA Pregnancy Category C *(Diabeta)*.

*Tolazamide*—
 Studies in humans have not been done. Use should be discontinued at least 2 weeks before the expected delivery date.
 Studies in rats given 10 times the human dose have shown tolazamide to cause reduced litter sizes. No teratogenic effects were found. High doses of 100 mg/kg a day also produced reduced litter sizes and increased perinatal mortality in pups.
 FDA Pregnancy Category C.

*Tolbutamide*—
 Studies in humans have not been done. Use should be discontinued at least 2 weeks before the expected delivery date.
 Studies in rats given doses of tolbutamide that were 25 to 100 times greater than the human dose have shown teratogenic effects, such as ocular and bone abnormalities, and increased mortality in the offspring. Repeat studies in rabbits showed no teratogenic effects.
 FDA Pregnancy Category C.

Delivery—Prolonged severe hypoglycemia lasting from 4 to 10 days has been reported in neonates born to mothers who were receiving a sulfonylurea antidiabetic agent at the time of delivery. This effect has been reported more frequently with those agents with longer half-lives, such as chlorpropamide. If sulfonylureas are used during pregnancy, they should be discontinued according to the manufacturer's labeling.

## Breast-feeding

Chlorpropamide and tolbutamide are distributed into breast milk and potentially may cause hypoglycemia in the infant. It is not known if acetohexamide, gliclazide, glipizide, glyburide, or tolazamide is distributed into breast milk.

*Chlorpropamide*: Chlorpropamide has been found to be distributed into breast milk at a concentration of 5 mcg per mL after 5 hours for a single 500-mg dose (after 5 hours, blood concentration for a single dose of 250 mg chlorpropamide is 30 mcg per mL); therefore, its use during breast-feeding is not recommended. Its effect on the nursing infant is not known.

*Tolbutamide*: Tolbutamide was distributed into breast milk at a concentration averaging 3 and 18 mcg per mL in two patients taking 500 mg twice a day (milk:plasma ratio of 0.09 and 0.4, respectively). The effect on the nursing infants is not known. The American Academy of Pediatrics considers tolbutamide to be compatible with breast-feeding.

## Pediatrics

Oral antidiabetic agents are not effective in insulin-dependent (juvenile-onset; type I) diabetes. Because type II diabetes occurs rarely in this age group, very little or no published pediatrics-specific information is available. Safety and efficacy have not been established.

## Geriatrics

In general, no overall difference in safety or efficacy was apparent in persons over 65 years of age when compared to persons younger than 65 years of age taking sulfonylureas for diabetes mellitus. Lower doses are used initially because of possible increased sensitivity to these agents due to age-related metabolism and excretion changes; the steady state concentration of extended-release glipizide has been delayed for 1 or 2 days in elderly patients. The risk of adverse reactions is relatively low when other factors for toxicity, including liver and kidney disease and known drug interactions, are considered. Special counseling with emphasis on hydration, diet, and exercise may be necessary because of the greater risk of hypoglycemia in this age group. Special instruction to recognize hypoglycemia may be needed because early warning adrenergic symptoms of hypoglycemia (such as sweating, weakness, tachycardia, and nervousness) are absent in many patients. Hypoglycemia manifests as neurological symptoms (such as, headache, irritability, mental confusion, unusual tiredness, and drowsiness) and may be more prolonged and severe in the elderly. Combining antidiabetic agents (sulfonylureas with metformin or insulin) or using long-acting sulfonylureas, such as chlorpropamide and glyburide, is most often associated with hypoglycemia in elderly patients and is not generally recommended; shorter acting sulfonylureas cause fewer problems. Also, instructions may be needed to help the patient monitor urine or blood glucose if visual problems are present.

Geriatric patients may be more likely to develop a reversible SIADH (syndrome of inappropriate antidiuretic hormone) from the use of chlorpropamide. The incidence of SIADH is rare and occurs with greater incidence when thiazides are taken concurrently with chlorpropamide than when chlorpropamide is taken alone (10% versus 3%, respectively). In one study, women over 70 years of age were affected 10 times more often than women under 60 years of age when thiazides were used concurrently with chlorpropamide. It is not thought to be a gender-oriented effect. SIADH has been rarely reported with tolbutamide.

**Drug interactions and/or related problems**

The following drug interactions and/or related problems have been selected on the basis of their potential clinical significance (possible mechanism in parentheses where appropriate)—not necessarily inclusive (» = major clinical significance):

Note: Combinations containing any of the following medications, depending on the amount present, may also interact with this medication.

There is an increased chance of hypoglycemia occurring if more than one hypoglycemia-causing agent is used concurrently with sulfonylureas. If the need exists to administer any medications that may affect metabolic or glycemic control of diabetes mellitus, blood glucose concentrations should be monitored by the patient or health care professional. This is particularly important when any medication is added or removed from an established drug regimen. Subsequent adjustments in diet or antidiabetic agent dosage or both may be necessary; these adjustments may differ depending on the severity of the diabetes.

» Alcohol

(a disulfiram-like reaction, which is characterized primarily by flushing of the face, neck, and arms, may occur with any of the sulfonylureas when alcohol is ingested concurrently, but has not been reported with glipizide; risk is lowest with tolbutamide and glyburide, and highest with chlorpropamide for which it has occurred 12 hours after a single 250-mg dose of chlorpropamide and 40 mL of 18% alcohol)

(the risk of hypoglycemia may be increased or prolonged when moderate or large amounts of alcohol have been consumed concurrently with sulfonylurea antidiabetic agents use; small amounts of alcohol taken with meals do not usually result in hypoglycemia)

Allopurinol

(increased risk of hypoglycemia due to inhibition of renal tubular secretion of chlorpropamide; closer monitoring required)

Angiotensin-converting enzyme agents, such as:
  Captopril or
  Enalapril

(the mechanism of enhanced hypoglycemia that occurs rarely is unknown; concurrent use need not be avoided and may be used advantageously in the treatment of diabetes mellitus; however, the dosage of the sulfonylurea may need to be modified in some patients)

» Anticoagulants, coumarin- or indandione-derivative

(the mechanism is not completely known; however, mutual interactions of both agents have increased their anticoagulant and hypoglycemic effects. A hypoglycemic effect may be partially due to the decrease in hepatic metabolism of sulfonylureas caused by anticoagulants, which can prolong the half-life of the sulfonylureas two- to three-fold. An increased protein binding displacement of anticoagulants by sulfonylureas has increased prothrombin times, but because metabolism of dicumarol is increased and can result in up to a 50% reduced half-life, an increase, decrease, or no effect on coagulation may result. Although these effects have been reported specifically for chlorpropamide, tolbutamide, and dicumarol, concurrent use of all sulfonylurea antidiabetic agents with anticoagulants should be well-monitored and dosage adjustments of both agents may be required)

(glipizide and glyburide have lower plasma concentrations and exhibit only nonionic plasma protein binding; therefore, they may be less susceptible to displacement from plasma proteins by other medications that exhibit ionic binding to plasma proteins; studies have not been done and caution is still warranted)

» Antifungal, azoles, systemic, such as:
  Miconazole
  Fluconazole

(severe hypoglycemia has been reported shortly after concurrent use of tolbutamide, glyburide, and glipizide with these oral azole antifungal agents. In one study, glipizide and fluconazole increased the area-under-the-time curve [AUC] of glipizide 56.9% [range, 35–81%]. Also, hypoglycemia has been reported for gliclazide taken concurrently with miconazole, but not with fluconazole)

Appetite suppressants

(when appetite suppressants and a concurrent dietary regimen are used, blood glucose concentrations may be altered in diabetic patients; dosage adjustment of antidiabetic agent may be necessary during and after therapy)

» Asparaginase or
» Corticosteroids or
» Diuretics, thiazide or
» Lithium

(these medications have intrinisic hyperglycemic activity in both diabetics and nondiabetics; dosage of the sulfonylurea may need to be modified during and after treatment. Some studies of lithium have reported hypoglycemia)

(concurrent treatment using thiazides with chlorpropamide, and more rarely with tolbutamide, may increase the chance of hyponatremia and hypo-osmolality, especially in patients over 70 years of age)

Barbiturates

(chlorpropamide may prolong the effect of barbiturates and barbiturates may prolong the effect of gliclazide; other sulfonylureas may also exhibit these effects; dosage adjustment of the sulfonylurea or the barbiturate may be necessary)

» Beta-adrenergic blocking agents, including ophthalmics, if significant absorption occurs

(beta-adrenergic blocking agents may decrease the hypoglycemic effects of sulfonylureas to some extent by inhibition of insulin secretion, modification of carbohydrate metabolism, and increased peripheral insulin resistance, leading to hyperglycemia; an adjustment in dose may be required. Other mechanisms that control the normal physiological response to a fall in blood glucose may be affected also, such as a blocked catecholamine mediated response to hypoglycemia [glycogenolysis and mobilization of glucose], thereby prolonging the time it takes to achieve euglycemia and increasing the risk of a severe hypoglycemic reaction. Selective beta$_1$-adrenergic blocking agents [such as, acebutolol, atenolol, betaxolol, bisoprolol, and metoprolol] exhibit the above actions to a lesser extent; however, any of the agents can blunt some of the symptoms of developing hypoglycemia, such as increased heart rate or tremors [increased sweating and blood pressure may not be altered], making detection of this complication more difficult)

» Cimetidine or
» Ranitidine

(these agents, in therapeutic doses, can significantly decrease the postprandial rise in blood glucose and increase the hypoglycemic effects of glipizide, gliclazide, and glyburide in diabetics; also, cimetidine has decreased tolbutamide's elimination and increased absorption of tolbutamide and glyburide; ranitidine did not affect glyburide's area-under-the-time curve [AUC]; close monitoring for dose adjustments of sulfonylureas may be needed when these agents are added or withdrawn)

» Ciprofloxacin

(use of glyburide with ciprofloxacin has caused hypoglycemia; since the mechanism is not understood, similar effects with other sulfonylurea antidiabetic agents should be considered when these medications are used together)

» Cyclosporine

(glipizide may significantly increase the plasma concentration of cyclosporine by reducing its metabolism; dose reduction of cyclosporine may be necessary; similar effects may be possible with other sulfonylureas)

» Guanethidine or
» Monoamine oxidase (MAO) inhibitors, including furazolidone, procarbazine, and selegiline or
» Quinidine or
» Quinine or
» Salicylates, in large doses

(these medications have intrinsic hypoglycemic activity in both diabetics and nondiabetics, possibly severe with quinine, quinidine, or salicylates in high doses but is unlikely with low doses of salicylates. Also, salicylates may interfere with chlorpropamide's renal excretion. Salicylate dose may need to be reduced)

Hemolytics, other (See *Appendix II*)
(concurrent use may increase the incidence of sulfonylurea-induced hemolysis through a possible additive effect; reported cases of hemolysis effects have rarely occurred with chlorpropamide or tolbutamide and have not been reported with other sulfonylureas)

Hepatic enzyme inducers, such as:
Rifabutin
Rifampin
(metabolism of sulfonylureas may be increased due to stimulation of hepatic microsomal enzymes; dosage adjustments may be necessary during and after concurrent treatment)

(drug interaction data for rifabutin are not available; it is structurally related to rifampin but appears to be a less potent enzyme inducer of the hepatic cytochrome P-450 system than is rifampin. It is recommended that patients taking rifabutin concurrently with sulfonylurea antidiabetic agents be monitored since the significance of possible drug interactions is not known)

Hepatic enzyme inhibitors, such as:
» Chloramphenicol
(metabolism of sulfonylureas may be decreased due to inhibition of hepatic microsomal enzymes; dosage adjustments may be necessary during and after concurrent use).

(also, chlorpropamide's half-life has increased up to 146 hours; this may be partially due to interference by chloramphenicol with renal excretion of chlorpropamide)

Highly protein-bound medications such as:
Anti-inflammatory drugs, nonsteroidal (NSAIDs), such as phenylbutazone
Clofibrate
Probenecid
Sulfinpyrazone
Sulfonamides
(these medications enchance the hypoglycemic effects of sulfonylureas when given concurrently; the mechanism is unknown but may be due to displacement of sulfonylureas from protein binding sites and alterations in their renal excretion; concurrent use need not be avoided; however, the dosage of the sulfonylurea may need to be modified in some patients)

(clofibrate also shows intrinsic hypoglycemic effects by causing increased insulin sensitivity and has been used advantageously in the treatment of diabetes mellitus; also, clofibrate has intrinsic antidiuretic effects that have been used to treat diabetes insipidus; this effect may be lessened with concurrent use of glyburide or increased with concurrent use of chlorpropamide or tolbutamide)

(sulfinpyrazone and phenylbutazone have been shown to inhibit the hepatic metabolism of tolbutamide; they also inhibit the renal excretion of acetohexamide but not of glyburide; the effect on other sulfonylureas by NSAIDs [other than ibuprofen, naproxen, sulindac, and tolmetin, which do not affect sulfonylureas] is not known)

(NSAIDs inhibit synthesis of prostaglandin E, which inhibits endogenous insulin secretion; this increases basal insulin secretion, the response to a glucose load, and the hypoglycemic effect of insulin secretion; dosage adjustment of each medicine used may be necessary following chronic use of NSAIDs)

(glipizide and glyburide have lower plasma concentrations and exhibit nonionic plasma protein binding only; therefore, these sulfonylureas may be less susceptible to displacement from plasma proteins by other medications that exhibit ionic binding to plasma proteins)

Hyperglycemia-causing agents, such as:
Calcium channel blockers
Clonidine
Danazol
Dextrothyroxine
Diazoxide, parenteral
Estrogen
Estrogen–progestin-containing oral contraceptives
Furosemide
Glucagon
Growth hormone
Hydantoin anticonvulsants
Isoniazid
Morphine
Nicotinic acid
Phenothiazines, such as chlorpromazine

Sympathomimetics, such as beta-adrenergic agents or epinephrine
Thyroid hormones
(these medications may change many factors that affect the metabolic control of glucose concentrations and, unless the changes can be controlled with diet, may necessitate an increased sulfonylurea dose and regular monitoring)

(hyperglycemic effects have resulted with doses greater than 100 mg of chlorpromazine; other phenothiazines or lower doses of chlorpromazine have not had this effect. However, caution may be warranted for concurrent use of phenothiazines with sulfonylureas)

(isoniazid usually causes hyperglycemia, but hypoglycemia has occurred in some diabetics taking tolbutamide; a decrease in dose of tolbutamide is then warranted)

(beta-adrenergic agonists increase risk of hyperglycemia by increasing glycogenolysis. If given during pregnancy, these agents may cause hypoglycemia in the fetus, independent of maternal blood glucose concentrations, by causing a depletion of fetal glycogen stores; sulfonylurea dose adjustment may be necessary if these agents are given together during pregnancy)

Hypoglycemia-causing agents, such as:
Anabolic steroids
Androgens
Bromocriptine
Disopyramide
Pyridoxine
Tetracycline
Theophylline
(these medications may change metabolic control of glucose concentrations and, unless the changes can be controlled with diet, may necessitate a decreased sulfonylurea dose; patients susceptible to hypoglycemia should be closely monitored)

Insulin
(sulfonylurea agents chronically stimulate the pancreatic beta cell to release insulin and increase receptor and tissue sensitivity to insulin; although concurrent use of the medications with insulin may increase the hypoglycemic response, the effect may be unpredictable)

(although the combination has been used to treat a select group of diabetic patients whose condition is not well-controlled with either agent alone, many studies have shown there is generally no additional benefit from using oral agents for the treatment of IDDM)

» Octreotide
(octreotide suppresses pancreatic insulin and counterregulatory hormones, such as glucagon and growth hormone, and delays or lowers glucose absorption from the gastrointestinal tract; depending on the dose, concurrent use with sulfonylureas may cause hypo- or hyperglycemia so that dose adjustment of the sulfonylurea may be needed; octreotide has been used beneficially for sulfonylurea overdose or insulinomas)

» Pentamidine
(pentamidine has a toxic effect on pancreatic beta cells resulting in a biphasic effect on glucose concentration, i.e., initial insulin release and hypoglycemia followed by hypoinsulinemia and hyperglycemia with continued use of pentamidine; dose alterations and continued use of sulfonylureas should be considered)

**Laboratory value alterations**
The following have been selected on the basis of their potential clinical significance (possible effect in parentheses where appropriate)—not necessarily inclusive (» = major clinical significance):

With diagnostic test results
Blood urea nitrogen (BUN)
(acetohexamide produces a reaction with diacetyl and falsely elevates results of this test)

Creatinine, serum
(acetohexamide has significantly increased the creatinine concentration for some laboratory tests by as much as 2.2 or 3.3 mg/dL and as little as 0.3 mg/dL for others)

Protein, total, serum
(tolbutamide interferes with sulfosalicylic acid test by causing turbidity)

» Sodium iodide I 123 or
» Sodium iodide I 131
(tolbutamide may decrease thyroidal uptake of I 123 or I 131; withdrawal of tolbutamide 1 week or longer before reactive iodine uptake test is necessary to prevent interference)

With physiology/laboratory test values
Alanine aminotransferase, serum (ALT [SGPT]) or
Alkaline phosphatase, serum or

Aspartate aminotransferase (AST [SGOT]) or
Lactate dehydrogenase (LDH)
(values may be mildly increased, usually not associated with clinical symptoms, and may be due to the sulfonylurea or to the underlying diabetes; however, hepatitis or cholestatic jaundice is caused rarely by sulfonylureas and should be considered with high values)

Bile, urine or
Bilirubin, urine
(concentrations may be mildly increased and usually do not present with clinical symptoms; however, hepatitis or cholestatic jaundice is caused rarely by sulfonylureas and should be considered with high values)

C-peptide, serum
(increased concentration for the first three months of sulfonylurea treatment; can return to pretreatment values long-term [18 months in one study])

Osmolality, urine or
Sodium, serum
(may be decreased with acetohexamide, gliclazide, glipizide, glyburide, or tolazamide because of their slight diuretic effect)

(chlorpropamide increases osmolality because of its antidiuretic effect and has caused dilutional hyponatremia)

(sodium may also decrease in response to hyperglycemia; each 100 mg/dL (5.51 mmol/L) increase in blood glucose decreases serum sodium by 1.6 mEq/L)

Uric acid, serum
(serum concentrations are considerably reduced by use of acetohexamide due to its mild uricosuric effect)

Urine collection, 24-hour
(quantity is mildly increased due to normal slight diuretic response by acetohexamide, gliclazide, glipizide, glyburide, or tolazamide)

(decreased with chlorpropamide due to its antidiuretic effect)

*For gliclazide*
Factors VIII, XI
(concentrations may be decreased with gliclazide)

Tissue plasminogen activator
(concentrations may be increased with gliclazide)

## Medical considerations/Contraindications
The medical considerations/contraindications included here have been selected on the basis of their potential clinical significance (reasons given in parentheses where appropriate)—not necessarily inclusive (» = major clinical significance).

*Except under special circumstances, this medication should not be used when the following medical problems exist:*
*For all oral sulfonylurea antidiabetic agents*
» Acidosis, significant or
» Burns, severe or
» Diabetic coma or
» Diabetic ketoacidosis, with or without coma or
» Hyperosmolar nonketotic coma or
» Surgery, major or
» Trauma, severe or
» Any other condition that causes severe blood glucose fluctuations or
» Any other condition in which insulin needs change rapidly
(fluctuations in blood glucose levels associated with certain disease states are more closely controlled by titration of insulin dosing, possibly on a short-term basis, rather than with oral antidiabetic agents, such as sulfonylureas)

*Risk-benefit should be considered when the following medical problems exist:*
*For all oral sulfonylurea antidiabetic agents*
Allergy to oral antidiabetic agents, sulfonamides, or thiazide-type diuretics
» Diarrhea, severe or
» Gastroparesis or
» Intestinal obstruction or
» Vomiting, prolonged or
» Other conditions causing delayed food absorption
(delayed stomach emptying or intestinal movement or vomiting may require modification of a sulfonylurea dose or a change to insulin therapy)
» Hepatic disease
(sulfonylureas that are extensively metabolized in the liver should not be used when there is hepatic impairment; hypoglycemia that develops may be more severe when these sulfonylureas are being used)

» Hyperglycemia-causing conditions, such as:
Female hormone changes or
Fever, high or
Hyperadrenalism, not optimally controlled or
Infection, severe or
Psychological stress
(these conditions, by increasing blood glucose, may increase the need for more frequent glucose monitoring and for a permanent or temporary dose increase for sulfonylureas or a change to insulin if blood glucose is uncontrolled)

» Hyperthyroidism, not optimally controlled
(hyperthyroidism aggravates diabetes mellitus by increasing plasma glycogen concentrations and glucose absorption, and by impairing glucose tolerance; thyroid hormone has dose-dependent biphasic effects on glycogenolysis and glycogeneogenesis; hyperthyroidism can make glycemic control difficult until the patient is euthyroid; patients with this condition may require an increased dose of the sulfonylurea until euthyroidism is achieved)

» Hypoglycemia-causing conditions, such as:
Adrenal insufficiency, not optimally controlled or
Debilitated physical condition or
Malnourishment or
Pituitary insufficiency, not optimally controlled
(these conditions, which inherently predispose patients to the risk of developing hypoglycemia, increase the patient's risk of developing severe hypoglycemia with concurrent treatment of sulfonylurea antidiabetic agents; reduced sulfonylurea dose or more frequent monitoring may be required for patients with these conditions)

Hypothyroidism, not optimally controlled
(sulfonylurea metabolism may be reduced with hypothyroidism and may mildly aggravate this underlying condition, which already exhibits reduced glucose absorption and altered glucose and lipoprotein metabolism [tolbutamide has goitrogenic properties]; low doses of a sulfonylurea may be needed when hypothyroid conditions exist and an increase in sulfonylurea dosing may be required when initiating thyroid treatment; euglycemic control may be difficult until the patient is euthyroid)

» Renal function impairment
(use of sulfonylureas increases the risk of possibly prolonged hypoglycemia with renal function impairment)

(the elimination half-lives of all the sulfonylureas are increased with renal function impairment, especially where tubular involvement predominates or if azotemia is present, and less so if the glomerular filtration rate is mildly reduced; sulfonylureas with longer half-lives, such as acetohexamide and chlorpropamide, are not recommended since renal excretion is important in the elimination of chlorpropamide and the active metabolite of acetohexamide [hydroxyhexamide]; weakly active metabolites of tolazamide and glyburide may also accumulate, particularly in those patients with a creatinine clearance of less than 30 mL/min [0.5 mL/sec]; sulfonylureas with shorter half-lives, such as gliclazide, glipizide, or tolbutamide, should present fewer problems but should be used cautiously in renal impairment)

*For chlorpropamide or tolbutamide*
» Congestive heart failure
(fluid retention, caused rarely by chlorpropamide and even less often by tolbutamide, may result in hyponatremia and precipitate congestive heart failure in the elderly when other risk factors for congestive heart failure are present)

## Patient monitoring
The following may be especially important in patient monitoring (other tests may be warranted in some patients, depending on condition; » = major clinical significance):

» Blood glucose determinations
(blood or plasma glucose reflects the current degree of metabolic control and should be routinely self-monitored by the patient at home and by the physician [every 3 months or more often when patient is not stabilized] to confirm that blood glucose concentration is maintained within agreed upon targets by the selected diet and dosing regimen; this is particularly important during dosage adjustments. Self-monitoring of blood glucose by the patient may require testing multiple times during the day or once to several times a week)

(caution in interpreting blood glucose concentrations is needed because normal whole blood glucose values are approximately 15% lower than plasma glucose values; it is also laboratory and method specific. Normal fasting whole blood glucose for adults of all ages is 65 to 95 mg/dL [3.6 to 5.3 mmol/L]. Normal fasting serum glucose is 70 to 105 mg/dL [3.9 to 5.8 mmol/L] for adults younger than 60 years of age and 80 to 115 mg/dL [4.4 to 6.4 mmol/L] for adults 60 years of age and older. For pregnant diabetic women, a normal fasting serum glucose is less than 105 mg/dL [5.8 mmol/L] and a fasting whole blood glucose is less than 120 mg/dL [6.7 mmol/L]. Goals of conventional sulfonylurea antidiabetic therapy are based on the absence of symptoms of hyper- and hypoglycemia)

(capillary blood glucose measurement provides important information when done properly, but caution is warranted because of potential errors in technique and readings; it has been suggested that the values be relied upon only if the reported glucose concentration for stable diabetics is between 75 mg/dL and 325 mg/dL [4.12 mmol/L and 17.88 mmol/L, respectively])

» Complete blood count (CBC)
(leukopenia, agranulocytosis, thrombocytopenia, and hemolytic and aplastic anemias have rarely occurred with sulfonylureas)

Glucose, urine or
Ketones, urine
(if blood glucose concentrations exceed 200 mg/dL [11.1 mmol/L], monitoring of urine for the presence of glucose and ketones may be necessary; normalization of glucose in the urine generally lags quantitatively behind serum glucose concentrations; test methods are generally capable of detecting serum glucose concentrations greater than 180 mg/dL [10 mmol/L])

» Glycosylated hemoglobin (hemoglobin $A_{1c}$) determinations
(hemoglobin $A_{1c}$ values [normal whole blood hemoglobin $A_{1c}$ is approximately 4 to 6% of total hemoglobin; specific values are laboratory-dependent] reflect the metabolic control over the preceding 3 months, but assessment of this parameter does not eliminate the need for daily blood glucose monitoring. Hemoglobin $A_{1c}$ may be falsely elevated in unstable diabetics when the intermediate precursor is elevated [i.e., in alcoholism] and falsely lowered in conditions of shortened red blood cell lifespan [i.e., in anemia and acute or chronic blood loss] or in patients with hemoglobinopathies [i.e., sickle cell])

Osmolarity determinations, plasma or
Sodium concentrations, serum
(may be necessary with use of chlorpropamide or tolbutamide, especially for the elderly or when thiazides are being taken concurrently)

pH measurements, serum or
Potassium concentrations, serum
(determinations may be important if patient is hypoglycemic and ketoacidotic)

## Side/Adverse Effects

Note: It has been suggested by some studies, including the University Group Diabetes Program (UGDP), that certain sulfonylurea antidiabetic agents increased cardiovascular mortality in diabetic patients, a population that already has a greater risk of cardiovascular disease and mortality when blood glucose is not controlled. Other studies have not reached a similar conclusion and have in fact suggested that control of elevated blood glucose with sulfonylurea antidiabetic agents may lessen the danger of cardiovascular disease and mortality. Despite questions regarding the interpretation of the results and the adequacy of the experimental design, the findings of the UGDP study provide an adequate basis for caution, especially for certain high risk patients with coronary artery disease, congestive heart failure, or angina pectoris. If sulfonylurea treatment is necessary, glyburide or gliclazide may be the preferred sulfonylureas for use in patients at risk for conditions causing cardiac hypoxia. The patient should be informed of the potential risks and advantages of sulfonylurea antidiabetic agents and of alternative modes of therapy.

The following side/adverse effects have been selected on the basis of their potential clinical significance (possible signs and symptoms in parentheses where appropriate)—not necessarily inclusive:

**Those indicating need for medical attention**
Incidence more frequent
*Hypoglycemia—mild, including nocturnal hypoglycemia* (anxiety; behavior change, similar to drunkenness; blurred vision; cold sweats; confusion; cool pale skin; difficulty in concentrating; drowsiness; excessive hunger; fast heartbeat; headache; nausea; nervousness; nightmares; restless sleep; shakiness; slurred speech; unusual tiredness or weakness); *weight gain*

Note: Predisposing factors related to diet, exercise, age, or concurrent use of other hypoglycemia-causing drugs (including insulin) in-

crease the chances of hypoglycemic episodes occurring. The occurrence of a recent episode of *hypoglycemia* may lessen the symptoms of a second episode. In the elderly, *hypoglycemia* symptoms are variable and harder to identify. Furthermore, *nocturnal hypoglycemia* may be asymptomatic in 33% or more of affected patients. Hypoglycemic episodes are experienced by 20% of the patients taking sulfonylureas every 6 months (6% experiencing monthly episodes).

*Weight gain* is greater with combination use of insulin and sulfonylureas than with sulfonylurea therapy alone. Gliclazide alone, or metformin in combination with sulfonylureas, usually results in less weight gain than other sulfonylureas and has exhibited a weight loss effect.

Incidence less frequent
*Erythema multiforme or exfoliative dermatitis* (peeling of skin; skin redness, itching, or rash); *hypoglycemia—severe* (convulsions or coma
*For chlorpropamide or, rarely, tolbutamide*
*Dilutional hyponatremia, hypo-osmolality, or syndrome of inappropriate antidiuretic hormone (SIADH)* (depression; dizziness; headache; lethargy; nausea; swelling or puffiness of face, ankles, or hands with occasional progression to seizures, coma, or stupor)

Note: The incidence of *severe hypoglycemia* episodes is 0.22 episodes per 1000 patient-years. It occurs more often with long-acting sulfonylureas, such as chlorpropamide or glyburide, when other predisposing factors or conditions are present, and can be relapsing and prolonged; glyburide results in a higher fatality rate than does chlorpropamide.

Incidence rare
*Anemia, aplastic or hemolytic* (continuing and unexplained tiredness or weakness, headache, shortness of breath brought on by exercise); *blood dyscrasias, specifically, agranulocytosis, leukopenia, pancytopenia* (fever and sore throat; pale skin; unusual bleeding or bruising; unusual tiredness, or weakness); *cholestasis, cholestatic jaundice, hepatic function impairment, hepatic porphyria, hepatitis, or porphyria cutanea tarda* (dark urine; fluid-filled skin blisters; itching of the skin; light-colored stools; sensitivity to the sun; skin thinness; yellow eyes or skin); *eosinophilia* (chills; increased sweating; general feeling of ill health; increased production of sputum; shortness of breath; chest pain; blood in sputum); *thrombocytopenia* (unusual bleeding or bruising)

Note: Sulfonylurea-induced *blood dyscrasias and dermatologic conditions* generally occur within the initial six weeks of therapy and are thought to be hypersensitivity reactions.

**Those indicating need for medical attention only if they continue or are bothersome**
Incidence more frequent
*Changes in sensation of taste; dizziness; drowsiness; gastrointestinal disturbances* (constipation; diarrhea; flatulence; heartburn; loss of or increase in appetite; nausea; stomach fullness; vomiting); *headache; polyuria* (increased volume of urine and frequency of urination)
Incidence less frequent or rare
*Photosensitivity* (increased sensitivity of skin to sunlight)

## Patient Consultation

As an aid to patient consultation, refer to *Advice for the Patient, Antidiabetic Agents, Sulfonylurea (Systemic)*.

In providing consultation, consider emphasizing the following selected information (» = major clinical significance):

**Before using this medication**
» Conditions affecting use, especially:
Allergy to sulfonylurea antidiabetic agents, sulfonamides, or thiazides
Pregnancy—Chlorpropamide crosses the placenta. Should not be used during pregnancy, especially when insulin is available. In the rare cases that a sulfonylurea is used, chlorpropamide and glipizide should be discontinued at least 1 month before delivery date and other sulfonylureas stopped at least 2 weeks before delivery date. Importance of controlling and monitoring blood glucose concentrations before, during, and after pregnancy by adjusting antidiabetic agent dosing in order to help prevent maternal and fetal problems, including fetal macrosomnia, anomalies, and hyperglycemia
Breast-feeding—Chlorpropamide and tolbutamide are distributed into breast milk, and their effect on breast-fed infants is not known; some physicians believe that tolbutamide is compatible with breast-feeding; it is not known if other sulfonylureas are distributed into breast milk

Use in children—Safety and efficacy have not been established. Published information is not available for this age group as NIDDM rarely occurs

Use in the elderly—May be more susceptible to hypoglycemia, especially when treated with glyburide and chlorpropamide, or when other hypoglycemia-causing agents are concurrently being prescribed along with sulfonylureas; also, the elderly have higher risk of developing hyponatremia or a reversible syndrome of inappropriate antidiuretic hormone when treated with chlorpropamide

Other medications, especially alcohol; asparaginase; azole antifungals; beta-adrenergic blocking agents; chloramphenicol; cimetidine; ciprofloxacin; corticosteroids; coumarin- or indandione-derivative anticoagulants; cyclosporine; guanethidine; lithium; MAO inhibitors including furazolidone, procarbazine, and selegiline; octreotide; pentamidine; quinidine; quinine; ranitidine; salicylates, large doses; or thiazide diuretics

Other medical problems, especially conditions causing delayed food absorption including gastroparesis, intestinal obstruction, prolonged vomiting, or severe diarrhea; conditions that cause severe blood glucose fluctuations or rapidly change insulin needs including diabetic coma, diabetic ketoacidosis, hyperosmolar nonketotic coma, major surgery, severe burns, severe trauma, or significant acidosis; hyperglycemia-causing conditions including female hormone changes, high fever, not optimally controlled hyperadrenalism, psychological stress, or severe infection; hypoglycemia-causing conditions including hepatic disease, debilitated physical condition, malnourishment, not optimally controlled adrenal or pituitary insufficiency or hyperthyroidism; renal function impairment; in addition, for chlorpropamide or tolbutamide, congestive heart failure

### Proper use of this medication
» Compliance with therapy, including not taking more or less medication than directed; alternative dosing or therapy changes for modifications in diet, exercise, and sick day management
» Proper dosing
Missed dose: Taking as soon as possible; not taking if almost time for next dose; not doubling doses
» Proper storage

### Precautions while using this medication
Regular visits to physician to check progress
*Carefully following special instructions of health care team*
» Discussing use of alcohol and tobacco
Not taking other medications unless discussed with physician
Getting counseling for family to help assist diabetic; also, special counseling for pregnancy planning and contraception
Making travel plans to include preparedness for diabetic emergencies and keeping meal times near the usual times with changing time zones
Wearing sunscreen and protective clothing to protect against sunburn and photosensitivity
» Preparing for and understanding what to do in case of an emergency by carrying medical history and current drug list, wearing medical identification, keeping nonexpired glucagon kit and needles and quick-acting sugar close by
» Recognizing what brings on symptoms of hypoglycemia, such as delaying or missing a meal, exercising more than usual, drinking significant amounts of alcohol, taking certain medicines, using too much antidiabetic medication, such as insulin or sulfonylurea, being sick, including vomiting or diarrhea
» Knowing what to do if symptoms of hypoglycemia occur, such as using glucagon, eating glucose tablets or gel, corn syrup, honey, or sugar cubes, or drinking fruit juice, nondiet soft drink, or dissolved sugar in water; also, eating small snack, such as crackers or half sandwich, when scheduled meal is longer than 1 hour away; not eating foods high in fat, such as chocolate, since fat slows gastric emptying
» Recognizing symptoms of hyperglycemia and ketoacidosis: blurred vision; drowsiness; dry mouth; flushed, dry skin; fruit-like breath odor; increased urination (frequency and volume); ketones in urine; loss of appetite; somnolence (sleepiness); stomachache, nausea, or vomiting; tiredness; troubled breathing (rapid and deep); unconsciousness; unusual thirst
» Recognizing what brings on symptoms of hyperglycemia, such as fever or infection; not taking enough insulin; skipping an insulin dose; exercising less than usual; taking certain medicines; overeating or not following meal plan
» Knowing what to do if symptoms of hyperglycemia occur, such as checking blood glucose and contacting a member of the health care team

### Side/adverse effects
Signs of potential side effects, especially mild or severe hypoglycemia; weight gain; erythema multiforme or exfoliative dermatitis; aplastic or hemolytic anemia; blood dyscrasias; cholestasis; cholestatic jaundice; hepatic function impairment; hepatic porphyria; hepatitis; or porphyria cutanea tarda; eosinophilia; thrombocytopenia; in addition, for chlorpropamide only—dilutional hyponatremia, hypoosmolality, or syndrome of inappropriate antidiuretic hormone (SIADH)

## General Dosing Information

There is little evidence that one sulfonylurea is more effective in lowering blood glucose than another, especially between first and second generation sulfonylureas. Some pharmacokinetic differences between sulfonylureas may result in small qualitative and temporal differences that may make one medication more suitable in a certain situation. For instance, glyburide and gliclazide exert a better effect on fasting blood glucose than does glipizide (possibly due to glyburide's longer duration of action and effect on hepatic glucose suppression), which results in lowered nocturnal and morning blood glucose; glipizide has greater postprandial insulin release and lower postprandial blood glucose levels. Overall, the resulting blood glucose level reduction is similar between sulfonylureas.

Conservative initial and maintenance doses may be required in patients with medical problems that make them more sensitive to effects of sulfonylureas.

Secondary failure of oral antidiabetic therapy may occur in certain patients. This may be due to increasing severity of diabetes or to diminished responsiveness to the medication.

When adding a sulfonylurea to an insulin regimen that is poorly controlled with insulin alone, the insulin dose at times may be reduced 25 to 50%.

When adding a sulfonylurea to maximum doses of metformin or metformin to maximum doses of a sulfonylurea, even if primary or secondary failure of a sulfonylurea has occurred, the new medication should be added gradually and titrated to the lowest effective dose. Both agents should be discontinued and insulin should be initiated if the patient does not respond to maximum doses within 3 months (or less, depending on clinician's decision). No transition time is needed when transferring between sulfonylureas, metformin, or insulin, except with chlorpropamide, which may require a 2-week transition because of chlorpropamide's prolonged duration of action.

### Diet/Nutrition
Absorption of chlorpropamide or glipizide may be delayed if the medication is ingested with food, and should be taken 30 minutes before a meal. Gliclazide may be taken 30 minutes before a meal or with a meal but not after a meal. Furthermore, nonmicronized glyburide should not be taken with a diet high in fat; nonmicronized glyburide does not have any other dietary restrictions.

### For treatment of adverse effects and/or overdose
Recommended treatment consists of the following:
For mild to moderate hypoglycemia—
• Treating with immediate ingestion of a source of sugar, such as glucose gel, glucose tablets, fruit juice, corn syrup, non-diet soft drinks, honey, sugar cubes, or table sugar dissolved in water. A frequently used source of sugar is a glassful of orange juice.
• Documenting blood glucose and rechecking in 15 minutes.
• Counseling patient to seek medical assistance promptly.
• Closely monitoring for at least 3 to 5 days patients who develop hypoglycemia during use of chlorpropamide.
For severe hypoglycemia or acute overdose, including coma
Note: Glucose administration is the basis for treatment of hypoglycemia; however, an exposure to sudden or excessive hyperglycemia caused by an injection of hypertonic glucose solution may further stimulate the sulfonylurea-primed pancreas to release more insulin, worsening the hypoglycemia.
• Counseling patient to obtain emergency medical assistance immediately
• Immediately treating with 50 mL of 50% dextrose given intravenously to stabilize the patient. Then, administering a continuous infusion of 5 to 10% dextrose in water to maintain slight hyperglycemia (approximately 100 mg/dL blood glucose concentration) for up to 12 days. The intravenous glucose therapy should not be terminated suddenly. A central venous line for long-term use (24 to 48 hours) in cases of chlorpropamide overdose may be required. (Oral glucose cannot be relied upon to maintain euglycemia because 60% of an oral

glucose dose is stored as hepatic glycogen with only 15% left for brain utilization and 15% for insulin-dependent tissues even though 75% of oral glucose is absorbed after 150 to 180 minutes.)

• Glucagon, 1 to 2 mg administered intramuscularly, is useful for fast onset of action to mobilize hepatic glucose stores but may be ineffective or variable in its effect if glycogen stores are depleted and must follow the use of glucose.

• Diazoxide therapy (200 mg orally every 4 hours or 300 mg intravenously over a 30-minute period every 4 hours) can be used for nonresponders to glucose therapy or for patients in a coma as an aid to glucose infusion to reduce hypoglycemia; patient should be monitored for sodium concentration and for hypotension.

• Emesis can be induced with ipecac syrup if sulfonylurea overdose is recent (within the past 30 minutes) if patient is alert, has an intact gag reflex, and is not obtunded or convulsing. Otherwise, gastric lavage after endotracheal tube placement is required.

• Gastric removal by administration of repeated doses of oral activated charcoal with appropriate cathartic, although the usefulness of this has not been established.

• Alkalinization of urine with sodium bicarbonate to pH of 8 can eliminate 80% of chlorpropamide over 24 hours, but is not useful with other sulfonylureas. Caution with concurrent use with diazoxide treatment because of possible significant sodium retention.

• Monitoring vital signs, arterial blood gases, blood glucose, and serum electrolytes (especially calcium, potassium, and sodium) as required. Initially, blood glucose concentrations should be monitored as frequently as every 1 to 3 hours. Blood urea nitrogen and serum creatinine concentrations should also be obtained.

• Cerebral edema—Managing with mannitol and dexamethasone.

• Hypokalemia—Managing with potassium supplements.

• Hospitalization for 6 to 91 hours (mean, 24 hours), because the hypoglycemia may be recurrent and prolonged; for chlorpropamide this period may be extended to 3 to 5 days or longer.

• Other supportive measures should also be employed as needed.

## ACETOHEXAMIDE

## Summary of Differences

Pharmacology/pharmacokinetics:
Protein binding—Very high, ionic.
Serum half-life—Parent 1.3 hours; metabolite 6 hours.
Duration of action—8 to 24 hours.
Active metabolite.
Precautions:
Laboratory value alterations—Reduces serum uric acid concentration.
Medical considerations/contraindications—Not recommended for use in patients with renal function impairment.

## Additional Dosing Information

See also *General Dosing Information.*

When patients are transferred to acetohexamide from another oral antidiabetic medication (with the exception of chlorpropamide), no transition period is required. When transferring patients from chlorpropamide, caution should be exercised during the first 1 to 2 weeks because of the prolonged retention of chlorpropamide in the body.

During conversion from insulin therapy to acetohexamide therapy, no gradual dosage adjustment usually is required for patients using less than 20 USP Units of insulin daily. For patients using 20 or more USP Units daily, a 25 to 30% reduction in insulin every day or every second day with gradual dosage adjustment is advisable. Hospitalization for some patients on a higher insulin dosage may be required for uneventful conversion.

## Oral Dosage Forms
### ACETOHEXAMIDE TABLETS USP

**Usual adult dose**
Antidiabetic—
Initial: Oral, 250 mg once a day, the dosage being increased by 250 or 500 mg every 5 to 7 days as needed.
Maintenance: Oral, 250 to 1000 mg once a day before breakfast or 1000 to 1500 mg divided into two doses taken before breakfast and evening meals.

**Usual adult prescribing limits**
Up to 1.5 grams daily.

**Usual pediatric dose**
Safety and efficacy have not been established.

**Usual geriatric dose**
See *Usual adult dose.*

Note: If an elderly patient tends toward hypoglycemia during the first 24 hours after an initial dose of 250 mg at breakfast, the dose should be reduced or the medication discontinued.

**Strength(s) usually available**
U.S.—
250 mg (Rx) [*Dymelor* (scored); GENERIC].
500 mg (Rx) [*Dymelor* (scored); GENERIC].
Canada—
500 mg (Rx) [*Dimelor* (scored)].

**Packaging and storage**
Store below 40 °C (104 °F), preferably between 15 and 30 °C (59 and 86 °F), unless otherwise specified by manufacturer. Store in a well-closed container.

**Auxiliary labeling**
• Avoid alcoholic beverages.
• Do not take other medicines without advice from your doctor.
• Avoid too much sun.

## CHLORPROPAMIDE

## Summary of Differences

Indications:
Also used in the treatment of central diabetes insipidus.
Pharmacology/pharmacokinetics:
Other actions/effects—Antidiuretic effect.
Protein binding—Very high, ionic.
Half-life, serum—36 hours.
Precautions:
Pregnancy—Crosses the placenta.
Breast-feeding—Distributed into breast milk.
Geriatrics—Use is generally avoided.
Drug interactions and/or related problems—Risk of disulfiram-like reaction with alcohol is higher with chlorpropamide than with other sulfonylureas.
Medical considerations/contraindications—Not recommended for use in patients with renal function impairment or congestive heart failure.
Side/adverse effects:
Potential for serious adverse effects (e.g., prolonged hypoglycemia and severe hyponatremia) because of prolonged action of chlorpropamide, especially with predisposed individuals.

## Additional Dosing Information

See also *General Dosing Information.*

When patients are transferred to chlorpropamide from another sulfonylurea, no transition period is required. When transferring patients from chlorpropamide, caution should be exercised during the first 1 to 2 weeks because of the prolonged retention of chlorpropamide in the body.

During conversion from insulin therapy to chlorpropamide therapy, no gradual dosage adjustment usually is required for patients using less than 40 Units of insulin daily. For patients using 40 Units or more daily, a 50% reduction in insulin the first few days is advisable. Hospitalization for some patients on a higher insulin dosage may be required for uneventful conversion.

## Oral Dosage Forms

Note: Bracketed uses in the *Dosage Forms* section refer to categories of use and/or indications that are not included in U.S. product labeling.

### CHLORPROPAMIDE TABLETS USP

**Usual adult dose**
Antidiabetic—
Initial: Oral, 250 mg once a day, the dosage being changed by 50 to 125 mg every three to five days if needed.
Maintenance: Oral, 100 to 500 mg a day as a single dose.
[Antidiuretic][1]—
Oral, 100 to 250 mg as a single dose daily, the dosage being adjusted at two- or three-day intervals as needed and tolerated.

Note: Occasionally, divided doses are administered, usually twice a day before the morning and evening meals, to improve gastrointestinal tolerance.

**Usual adult prescribing limits**
Antidiabetic—
Oral, up to 750 mg per day.

[Antidiuretic][1]—
 Oral, up to 500 mg per day.

**Usual pediatric dose**
Safety and efficacy have not been established.

**Usual geriatric dose**
Antidiabetic—
 Oral, initially, 100 to 125 mg once a day, the dosage being increased by 50 to 125 mg at three- to five-day intervals as needed.

**Strength(s) usually available**
U.S.—
 100 mg (Rx) [*Diabinese* (scored); GENERIC (may be scored)].
 250 mg (Rx) [*Diabinese* (scored); GENERIC (may be scored)].
Canada—
 100 mg (Rx) [*Apo-Chlorpropamide* (scored); *Diabinese* (scored); GENERIC].
 250 mg (Rx) [*Apo-Chlorpropamide* (scored); *Diabinese* (scored); *Novo-Propamide* (scored); GENERIC].

**Packaging and storage**
Store below 40 °C (104 °F), preferably between 15 and 30 °C (59 and 86 °F), unless otherwise specified by manufacturer. Store in a well-closed container.

**Auxiliary labeling**
• Avoid alcoholic beverages.
• Do not take other medicines without advice from your doctor.
• Avoid too much sun.

[1]Not included in Canadian product labeling.

## GLICLAZIDE

## Summary of Differences

Pharmacology/pharmacokinetics:
 Other actions/effects—Protective activity for some cardiac arrhythmias; also, reduces platelet adhesiveness and aggregation and has fibrinolytic activity.
 Protein binding—Very high, non-ionic.
 Serum half-life—Approximately 10.4 hours.
 Duration of action—Approximately 24 hours.
Precautions:
 Drug interactions and/or related problems—Displacement from plasma proteins by other medications is less likely.
 Medical considerations/contraindications—May be preferred for those patients with moderate renal function impairment; should not be used with severe renal failure.
Side/adverse effects:
 Less weight gain when compared to other sulfonylureas.

## Additional Dosing Information

See also *General Dosing Information*.

When patients are transferred to gliclazide from another oral antidiabetic medication (with the exception of chlorpropamide), no transition period is required. When transferring patients from chlorpropamide, caution should be exercised during the first 1 to 2 weeks because of the prolonged retention of chlorpropamide in the body.

During conversion from insulin therapy to gliclazide therapy, no gradual dosage adjustment usually is required for patients using less than 20 USP Units of insulin daily. For patients using 20 or more USP Units daily, a 25 to 30% reduction in insulin every day or every second day with gradual dosage adjustment is advisable. Hospitalization for some patients on a higher insulin dosage may be required for uneventful conversion.

## Oral Dosage Forms
## GLICLAZIDE TABLETS

**Usual adult dose**
Antidiabetic—
 Initial: Oral, 160 mg two times a day with meals.
 Maintenance: Oral, 80 to 320 mg a day with meals.

**Usual adult prescribing limits**
Oral, up to 320 mg daily.

**Usual pediatric dose**
Safety and efficacy have not been established.

**Usual geriatric dose**
See *Usual adult dose*.

**Strength(s) usually available**
U.S.—
 Not commercially available.
Canada—
 80 mg (Rx) [*Diamicron* (quad-scored)].

**Packaging and storage**
Store below 40 °C (104 °F), preferably between 15 and 30 °C (59 and 86 °F), in a well-closed container, unless otherwise specified by manufacturer.

**Auxiliary labeling**
• Avoid alcoholic beverages.
• Do not take other medicines without advice from your doctor.
• Avoid too much sun.

## GLIPIZIDE

## Summary of Differences

Pharmacology/pharmacokinetics:
 Other actions/effects—Has mild diuretic effect.
 Protein binding—Very high, non-ionic.
 Serum half-life—2 to 4 hours.
 Duration of action—12 to 24 hours.
Precautions:
 Drug interactions and/or related problems—
 Displacement from plasma proteins by other medications is less likely than with ionic sulfonylureas.

## Additional Dosing Information

See also *General Dosing Information*.

When patients are transferred to glipizide from another oral antidiabetic medication (with the exception of chlorpropamide), no transition period is required. When transferring patients from chlorpropamide, caution should be exercised during the first 1 to 2 weeks because of the prolonged retention of chlorpropamide in the body.

During conversion from insulin therapy to glipizide therapy, no gradual dosage adjustment usually is required for patients using less than 20 USP Units of insulin daily. For patients using 20 or more USP Units daily, a 50% reduction of insulin the first day, with gradual dosage adjustments of glipizide as needed, is desirable. Hospitalization for some patients on a higher insulin dosage may be required for uneventful conversion.

## Oral Dosage Forms
## GLIPIZIDE EXTENDED-RELEASE TABLETS

**Usual adult dose**
Antidiabetic—
 Initial: Oral, 5 mg once daily with breakfast; dosage is increased by 5 mg based on resulting hemoglobin $A_{1c}$ measurements taken three months later or, less commonly, based on two or more consecutive fasting blood glucose measurements taken seven days apart.
 Maintenance: Oral, 5 to 10 mg once a day with breakfast.

Note: In most cases, if no improvement of hemoglobin $A_{1c}$ is noted after three months of use of a higher dose, the previous dose should be resumed.

**Usual adult prescribing limits**
Up to 20 mg once a day.

**Usual pediatric dose**
Safety and efficacy have not been established.

**Usual geriatric dose**
See *Usual adult dose*.

Note: When adjusting the dose in the elderly, consider that steady-state levels for glipizide extended-release may be delayed by approximately one or two days as compared to other age groups.

**Strength(s) usually available**
U.S.—
 5 mg (Rx) [*Glucotrol XL*].
 10 mg (Rx) [*Glucotrol XL*].

Note: Although similar in appearance to a conventional tablet, *Glucotrol XL* actually is a specially formulated gastrointestinal system (GITS) consisting of a semipermeable membrane surrounding an osmotically active drug core, which is designed to release glipizide at a constant rate over twenty-four hours; following drug release, the system is eliminated in the feces as an insoluble shell.

Canada—
    Not commercially available.

**Packaging and storage**
Store below 40 °C (104 °F), preferably between 15 and 30 °C (59 and 86 °F), in a tight container, unless otherwise specified by manufacturer.

**Auxiliary labeling**
- Avoid alcoholic beverages.
- Do not take other medicines without advice from your doctor.
- Avoid too much sun.

## GLIPIZIDE TABLETS USP

**Usual adult dose**
Antidiabetic—
    Initial: Oral, 5 mg once a day thirty minutes before breakfast, with dosage being changed by 2.5 to 5 mg every several days as needed.
    Maintenance: Oral, up to 40 mg a day thirty minutes before meals. Single daily doses are adequate with 15 mg or less but may be divided when necessary, while larger doses should be divided into two doses a day and taken thirty minutes before meals.

**Usual adult prescribing limits**
Oral, up to 40 mg daily.

**Usual pediatric dose**
Safety and efficacy have not been established.

**Usual geriatric dose**
Antidiabetic—
    Initial: Oral, 2.5 mg per day thirty minutes before breakfast, with dosage being changed by 2.5 to 5 mg every several days as needed.
    Maintenance: Oral, See *Usual adult dose*.

**Strength(s) usually available**
U.S.—
    5 mg (Rx) [*Glucotrol* (scored); GENERIC (may be scored)].
    10 mg (Rx) [*Glucotrol* (scored); GENERIC (may be scored)].
Canada—
    Not commercially available.

**Packaging and storage**
Store below 40 °C (104 °F), preferably between 15 and 30 °C (59 and 86 °F), unless otherwise specified by manufacturer. Store in a tight container.

**Auxiliary labeling**
- Avoid alcoholic beverages.
- Do not take other medicines without advice from your doctor.
- Avoid too much sun.
- Take this medication on an empty stomach, 30 minutes before meals.

---

### *GLYBURIDE*

## Summary of Differences

Pharmacology/pharmacokinetics:
    Other actions/effects—
        Protective activity for some cardiac arrhythmias; also, has mild diuretic activity.
    Protein binding—
        Very high, nonionic.
    Half-life—
        10 hours.
    Duration of action—
        24 hours.
    Elimination—
        Biliary: 50%.
        Renal: 50%.
Precautions:
    Geriatrics—
        Use is generally avoided.
    Drug interactions and/or related problems—
        Disulfiram-type reaction with concurrent alcohol use less likely with glyburide than with other antidiabetics. Also, displacement from plasma proteins by other medications is less likely.
Side/adverse effects:
    Fatal hypoglycemia occurs more often with glyburide than with chlorpropamide; potential for serious adverse effect because of prolonged action of glyburide, especially with predisposed individuals.

## Additional Dosing Information

See also *General Dosing Information*.

When patients are transferred to glyburide from another oral antidiabetic medication (with the exception of chlorpropamide), no transition period is required. When transferring patients from chlorpropamide, caution should be exercised during the first 1 to 2 weeks because of the prolonged retention of chlorpropamide in the body and subsequent overlapping of drug effects that could cause hypoglycemia.

During conversion from insulin therapy to glyburide therapy, no gradual dosage adjustment usually is required for patients using less than 40 USP Units of insulin daily. Patients requiring more than 40 USP Units should receive a 50% reduction of insulin the first day with initiation of 3 mg of micronized glyburide or 5 mg of nonmicronized glyburide as a single dose and gradual dosage adjustments of glyburide as needed. Hospitalization for some patients on a higher insulin dosage may be required for uneventful conversion.

**Bioequivalence information**

Micronized glyburide cannot be substituted for nonmicronized glyburide. Bioavailability studies have demonstrated that micronized glyburide is not bioequivalent to glyburide (nonmicronized); retitration is necessary if patients are transferred.

Micronized glyburide has an AB rating but may not be deemed bioequivalent according to some state formularies when the scored tablet is divided.

Glyburide (nonmicronized) has a BX rating and is not substitutable. However, some specific products are manufactured under the same new drug application (NDA) and may be deemed bioequivalent by some state formularies:
- Upjohn's product, *Micronase*, and Greenstone's generic glyburide (nonmicronized) are manufactured at Upjohn under the same NDA; Greenstone's generic product is distributed by Geneva and Greenstone.
- Hoescht-Roussel produces *DiaBeta* and its own generic, which is distributed by Copley, under the same NDA.
The products manufactured under one NDA cannot be substituted for those products produced under the other NDA; the products are not bioequivalent nor substitutable. The FDA Orange Book will list an NDA only once with the original manufacturer that applied for the product; hence, the Orange Book does not address multiple manufacturers under one NDA. Pharmacists should verify the regulations and formularies of their state or verify with the physician before substituting a BX-rated product under one NDA for a similar product under another.

## Oral Dosage Forms
### GLYBURIDE TABLETS

Note: Glyburide (nonmicronized) has an FDA BX rating denoting that data are insufficient to determine therapeutic equivalence. However, glyburide produced and distributed by the U.S. manufacturer Hoescht-Roussel and also distributed by Copley may be substitutable by some state pharmacy formularies because they use the same new drug application (NDA). Similarly, glyburide distributed by the U.S. manufacturers Greenstone and Upjohn share the same NDA. As long as glyburide holds a BX rating, substitution of products of different NDAs is not permissible without the physician's permission.

In contrast, glyburide (micronized) has an AB rating, denoting that bioequivalence for many state formularies has been resolved; however, some state formularies have deemed the AB-rated generic nonsubstitutable if a scored tablet is divided. State formularies should be checked before substitution is made with this type of product.

**Usual adult dose**
Antidiabetic—
    Initial: Oral, 2.5 to 5 mg once a day with breakfast or the first main meal, with dosage changes being made by no more than 2.5 mg at weekly intervals if needed. Patients more sensitive to hypoglycemia may need 1.25 mg a day.
    Maintenance: Oral, 1.25 to 20 mg a day, of which doses up to 10 mg are usually taken as a single dose with breakfast or the first main meal, while doses over 10 mg are usually divided into two daily doses with meals.

**Usual adult prescribing limits**
Oral, up to 20 mg daily.

**Usual pediatric dose**
Safety and efficacy have not been established.

**Usual geriatric dose**
Antidiabetic—
    Initial: Oral, 1.25 to 2.5 mg a day with breakfast, with dosage changes being made by no more than 2.5 mg at weekly intervals if needed.
    Maintenance: See *Usual adult dose*.

    Note: This dose should also be used in patients with medical problems that make them more sensitive to the effects of glyburide.

**Strength(s) usually available**
U.S.—
    1.25 mg (Rx) [*DiaBeta* (scored); *Micronase* (scored); GENERIC (may be scored)].
    2.5 mg (Rx) [*DiaBeta* (scored); *Micronase* (scored); GENERIC (may be scored)].
    5 mg (Rx) [*DiaBeta* (scored); *Micronase* (scored); GENERIC (may be scored)].
Canada—
    2.5 mg (Rx) [*Albert Glyburide* (scored); *Apo-Glyburide* (scored); *DiaBeta* (scored); *Euglucon* (scored); *Gen-Glybe* (scored); *Novo-Glyburide* (scored); *Nu-Glyburide* (scored)].
    5 mg (Rx) [*Albert Glyburide* (scored); *Apo-Glyburide* (scored); *DiaBeta* (scored); *Euglucon* (scored); *Gen-Glybe* (scored); *Novo-Glyburide* (scored); *Nu-Glyburide* (scored)].

**Packaging and storage**
Store below 40 °C (104 °F), preferably between 15 and 30 °C (59 and 86 °F), in a well-closed container, unless otherwise specified by manufacturer.

**Auxiliary labeling**
• Avoid alcoholic beverages.
• Do not take other medicines without advice from your doctor.
• Avoid too much sun.

### GLYBURIDE TABLETS (MICRONIZED)

Note: Micronized glyburide has an AB rating. However, some state formularies may not consider certain generic products bioequivalent when scored tablets are divided; state formularies should be checked before substituting one product for another.

    Micronized glyburide cannot be substituted for nonmicronized glyburide. Bioavailability studies have demonstrated that micronized glyburide is not bioequivalent to glyburide (nonmicronized); retitration is necessary if patients are transferred.

**Usual adult dose**
Antidiabetic—
    Initial: Oral, 1.5 to 3 mg once a day with breakfast or the first main meal. Some patients sensitive to glyburide's effects may need to be started on 0.75 mg a day. Dose titration should be made with changes of no more than 1.5 mg at weekly increments.
    Maintenance: Oral, 0.75 to 12 mg a day; doses up to 6 mg are usually taken as a single dose with breakfast or the first main meal, while doses over 6 mg are usually taken as divided doses with meals.

**Usual adult prescribing limits**
Oral, up to 12 mg daily.

**Usual pediatric dose**
Safety and efficacy have not been established.

**Usual geriatric dose**
Antidiabetic—
    Initial: Oral, 0.75 to 3 mg per day with breakfast or the first main meal, with dosage being changed by no more than 1.5 mg at weekly increments.
    Maintenance: See *Usual adult dose*.

**Strength(s) usually available**
U.S.—
    1.5 mg (Rx) [*Glynase PresTab* (scored); GENERIC (may be scored)].
    3 mg (Rx) [*Glynase PresTab* (scored); GENERIC (may be scored)].
    6 mg (Rx) [*Glynase PresTab* (scored)].
    Note: *Glynase PresTab* is formulated to divide easily in even halves by pressing gently on the scored area of the tablet.
Canada—
    Not commercially available.

**Packaging and storage**
Store below 40 °C (104 °F), preferably between 15 and 30 °C (59 and 86 °F), in a well-closed container, unless otherwise specified by manufacturer.

**Auxiliary labeling**
• Avoid alcoholic beverages.
• Do not take other medicines without advice from your doctor.
• Avoid too much sun.

## Summary of Differences

Pharmacology/pharmacokinetics:
    Other actions/effects—Has mild diuretic activity.
    Protein binding—Very high, ionic.
    Serum half-life—7 hours.
    Duration of action—10 or 20 hours.
Precautions:
    Drug interactions and/or related problems—Displacement from plasma proteins by other medications is more likely than with non-ionic sulfonylureas.
    Medical considerations/contraindications—Tolazamide may accumulate in patients with creatinine clearance less than 30 mL per minute (0.5 mL/sec).

## Additional Dosing Information

See also *General Dosing Information*.

When patients are transferred to tolazamide from another oral antidiabetic medication (with the exception of chlorpropamide), no transition period is required. When transferring patients from chlorpropamide, caution should be exercised during the first 1 to 2 weeks because of the prolonged retention of chlorpropamide in the body.

During conversion from insulin therapy to tolazamide therapy, no gradual dosage adjustment usually is required for patients using less than 40 USP Units of insulin daily. For patients requiring 40 or more USP Units daily, a 50% reduction of insulin the first few days with gradual dosage adjustment of tolazamide as needed is advisable. Hospitalization for some patients on a higher insulin dosage may be required for uneventful conversion.

## Oral Dosage Forms

### TOLAZAMIDE TABLETS USP

**Usual adult dose**
Antidiabetic—
    Initial: Oral, 100 to 250 mg once a day with breakfast or the first main meal, with dosage being changed by 100 to 250 mg at weekly intervals as needed.
    Maintenance: Oral, 250 to 500 mg a day with breakfast or the first main meal; some patients may need less (100 mg a day) or more (up to 1000 mg a day). Doses greater than 500 mg should be divided and given two times a day with meals.

**Usual adult prescribing limits**
Oral, up to 1 gram daily.

**Usual pediatric dose**
Safety and efficacy have not been established.

**Usual geriatric dose**
Antidiabetic—
    Initial: Oral, 100 mg once a day in the morning with breakfast or the first main meal, with the dose being changed by 100 to 250 mg at weekly intervals as needed.
    Maintenance: See *Usual adult dose*.

Note: Lower initial doses may also be required in patients with medical problems that make them more sensitive to the effects of tolazamide.

**Strength(s) usually available**
U.S.—
    100 mg (Rx) [*Tolinase* (scored); GENERIC (may be scored)].
    250 mg (Rx) [*Tolinase* (scored); GENERIC (may be scored)].
    500 mg (Rx) [*Tolinase* (scored); GENERIC (may be scored)].
Canada—
    Not commercially available.

**Packaging and storage**
Store below 40 °C (104 °F), preferably between 15 and 30 °C (59 and 86 °F), unless otherwise specified by manufacturer. Store in a tight container.

**Auxiliary labeling**
• Avoid alcoholic beverages.
• Do not take other medicines without advice from your doctor.
• Avoid too much sun.

## TOLBUTAMIDE

### Summary of Differences

Pharmacology/pharmacokinetics:
Other actions/effects—
Has mild antidiuretic activity.
Protein binding—
Very high, ionic.
Serum half-life—
4.5 to 6.5 hours.
Duration of action—
6 to 12 hours.
Precautions:
Drug interactions and/or related problems—
Disulfiram-type reaction with concurrent alcohol use less likely with tolbutamide than with other antidiabetics. Also, displacement from plasma proteins by other medications is more likely than with non-ionic sulfonylureas.
Metabolism of tolbutamide inhibited by sulfinpyrazone and phenylbutazone.
Laboratory value alterations—
Tolbutamide interferes with thyroidal uptake of I 123 and I 131.
Medical considerations/contraindications—
May be preferred for those patients with moderate renal function impairment, but should be discontinued with renal failure.

### Additional Dosing Information

See also *General Dosing Information*.

When patients are transferred to tolbutamide from another oral antidiabetic medication (with the exception of chlorpropamide), no transition period is required. When transferring patients from chlorpropamide, caution should be exercised during the first 1 to 2 weeks because of the prolonged retention of chlorpropamide in the body.

During conversion from insulin therapy to tolbutamide therapy, no gradual dosage adjustment usually is required for patients using less than 20 USP Units of insulin daily. Patients using 20 to 40 USP Units require a 30 to 50% reduction in insulin the first day with gradual dosage adjustment as needed. Patients requiring more than 40 USP Units should receive a 20% reduction of insulin the first day with gradual dosage adjustment of tolbutamide as needed. Hospitalization for some patients on a higher insulin dosage may be required for uneventful conversion.

### Oral Dosage Forms
### TOLBUTAMIDE TABLETS USP

**Usual adult dose**
Antidiabetic—
Initial: Oral, 1000 to 2000 mg a day as single morning or divided doses.
Maintenance: Oral, 250 to 2000 mg a day as single morning or divided doses.

Note: Lower initial doses may also be required in patients with medical problems that make them more sensitive to the effects of tolbutamide.

**Usual adult prescribing limits**
Oral, up to 3000 mg a day.

**Usual pediatric dose**
Safety and efficacy have not been established.

**Usual geriatric dose**
Lower initial dose may be required. See *Usual adult dose*.

Note: Lower initial doses may also be required in patients with medical problems that make them more sensitive to the effects of tolbutamide.

**Strength(s) usually available**
U.S.—
500 mg (Rx) [*Orinase* (scored); *Tol-Tab;* GENERIC (may be scored)].
Canada—
500 mg (Rx) [*Apo-Tolbutamide* (scored); *Mobenol* (scored); *Novo-Butamide* (scored); *Orinase* (scored); GENERIC].
1000 mg (Rx) [*Orinase* (scored)].

**Packaging and storage**
Store below 40 °C (104 °F), preferably between 15 and 30 °C (59 and 86 °F), unless otherwise specified by manufacturer. Store in a well-closed container.

**Auxiliary labeling**
• Avoid alcoholic beverages.
• Do not take other medicines without advice from your doctor.
• Avoid too much sun.

Revised: 08/03/95

## Table 1. Pharmacology/Pharmacokinetics

| Drug | $V_D$ (L/kg) | Protein* binding (%) | Biotransformation (%) | Elimination half-life (hrs) | Time to peak (hrs) | Peak serum concentration | | Duration of Action (hrs) | Elimination (%) |
|---|---|---|---|---|---|---|---|---|---|
| | | | | | | Concentration per mL | Dose (mg) | | |
| Acetohexamide Hydroxyhexamide‡ (metabolite) | 0.21 | Very high, 65–90; Ionic | Hepatic, mainly; erythrocytes | 1.3† 4.6–6 | 1.5–2 2–6 | 47 mcg 60 mcg | 1000 | 8–24 | Renal: 71 Fecal: 15 |
| Chlorpropamide | 0.09–0.27 | Very high, >90; Ionic | Hepatic | 36§ (range, 24–48) | 2–4 | N/A | N/A | 24–72 | Renal: In 96 hours: Unchanged— 6–20 Active and inactive metabolites |

* Primarily to albumin.
† Renal impairment prolongs acetohexamide half-life to 30 hours..
‡ A primary metabolite for acetohexamide, hydroxyhexamide, accounts for 47–60% of dose and is 2.5 times more potent than parent.
§ A randomized crossover study of five phases conducted over a 2 to 3 week period demonstrated that the half-life of chlorpropamide can be affected by the pH of the urine; half-life is $69 \pm 26$ hours with acidic urine (pH 4.7 to 5.5) and $13 \pm 3$ hours with basic urine (pH 7.1 to 8.2).
# Micronized glyburide allows greater solubility, faster absorption and, therefore, faster elimination; it is not bioequivalent to nonmicronized glyburide; micronized glyburide's area under the curve (AUC) is 568 ng.hr/mL and nonmicronized glyburide's AUC is 746 ng.hr/mL.
** Tolazamide is approximately 5–6.7 times more potent than tolbutamide and equal in its potency to chlorpropamide on a milligram per milligram basis.
†† The majority of a single dose of tolazamide is eliminated in urine within 24 hours and elimination is complete after 5 days. Less active metabolites include carboxytolazamide, hydroxytolazamide, and p-toulene sulfonamide.

## Table 1. Pharmacology/Pharmacokinetics (continued)

| Drug | $V_D$ (L/kg) | Protein* binding (%) | Biotransformation (%) | Elimination half-life (hrs) | Time to peak (hrs) | Peak serum concentration | | Duration of Action (hrs) | Elimination (%) |
|---|---|---|---|---|---|---|---|---|---|
| | | | | | | Concentration per mL | Dose (mg) | | |
| Gliclazide | 0.2 | Very high, 94; Nonionic | Hepatic | 10.4 | 4–6 | 5 mcg | 3 | 24 | Renal: Unchanged—<1 Metabolites, conjugates—60–70 Fecal: Metabolites, conjugates—10–20 |
| Glipizide | 0.14–0.16 | Very high, 99; Nonionic | Hepatic (no first-pass) | 2–4 | | N/A | N/A | | Renal: Unchanged—<10 Metabolites, inactive, and conjugates—80 Fecal: 10 |
| immediate release | | | | | 1–3 | | | 12–24 | |
| extended release | | | | | 6–12 | | | 24 | |
| Glyburide | 0.14–0.16 | Very high, 99; Nonionic | Hepatic | | | | | 24 | Renal: 50 Metabolites, active—2 weak, short-lived Biliary: 50 |
| Nonmicronized | | | | 6–10# | 3.4–4.5 | 87.5 nanograms | 5 | | |
| Micronized | | | | 4# | 2.3–3.5 | 97.2 nanograms | 3 | | |
| Tolazamide** | N/A | Very high, 94; Ionic | Hepatic | 7 | 3–4 | N/A | | 10–20 | Renal: 85†† Metabolites, major—5 metabolites (potency 0–70%) Fecal: 7 |
| Tolbutamide** | 0.10 | Very high, 96; Ionic | Hepatic | 4.5–6.5 | 3–4 | N/A | | 6–12 | Renal: 100 Metabolites, inactive—75% |

\* Primarily to albumin.

† Renal impairment prolongs acetohexamide half-life to 30 hours..

‡ A primary metabolite for acetohexamide, hydroxyhexamide, accounts for 47–60% of dose and is 2.5 times more potent than parent.

§ A randomized crossover study of five phases conducted over a 2 to 3 week period demonstrated that the half-life of chlorpropamide can be affected by the pH of the urine; half-life is 69 ± 26 hours with acidic urine (pH 4.7 to 5.5) and 13 ± 3 hours with basic urine (pH 7.1 to 8.2).

# Micronized glyburide allows greater solubility, faster absorption and, therefore, faster elimination; it is not bioequivalent to nonmicronized glyburide; micronized glyburide's area under the curve (AUC) is 568 ng.hr/mL and nonmicronized glyburide's AUC is 746 ng.hr/mL.

\*\* Tolazamide is approximately 5–6.7 times more potent than tolbutamide and equal in its potency to chlorpropamide on a milligram per milligram basis.

†† The majority of a single dose of tolazamide is eliminated in urine within 24 hours and elimination is complete after 5 days. Less active metabolites include carboxytolazamide, hydroxytolazamide, and p-toulene sulfonamide.

# ANTIDYSKINETICS Systemic

This monograph includes information on the following: Benztropine; Biperiden; Ethopropazine; Procyclidine; Trihexyphenidyl.

INN:
Benztropine—Benzatropine
Ethopropazine—Profenamine

BAN:
Benztropine—Benzatropine

Trihexyphenidyl—Benzhexol

VA CLASSIFICATION (Primary): AU350

Note: For a listing of dosage forms and brand names by country availability, see *Dosage Forms* section(s). For a listing of brand names for the articles in this monograph, refer to the General Index.

## Category

Antidyskinetic.

## Indications

Note: Bracketed information in the *Indications* section refers to uses that are not included in U.S. product labeling.

### Accepted

Parkinsonism (treatment)—Antidyskinetics are indicated in the treatment of mild cases of postencephalitic, arteriosclerotic, or idiopathic parkinsonism (paralysis agitans) in patients in whom anticholinergic therapy is not contraindicated. Antidyskinetics also are indicated as adjuncts to more potent medications to maximize improvement of symptoms. Procyclidine usually produces a more beneficial effect in conditions of rigidity than in those of tremor.

Extrapyramidal reactions, drug-induced (treatment)—Antidyskinetics are indicated in the control of extrapyramidal disorders (except tardive dyskinesia) due to central nervous system (CNS) drugs such as reserpine, phenothiazines, dibenzoxazepines, thioxanthenes, and butyrophenones. However, concomitant therapy with antipsychotics is not recommended beyond 3 months because extrapyramidal symptoms resulting from antipsychotic therapy usually resolve in 3 to 6 months and because prolonged, routine use of antidyskinetics with antipsychotics may predispose patients to the more serious neurological condition, tardive dyskinesia.

[Athetosis, congenital (treatment)][1] or
[Degeneration, hepatolenticular (treatment)][1]—Ethopropazine is used for the symptomatic treatment of hepatolenticular degeneration and congenital athetosis.

---

[1]Not included in Canadian product labeling.

## Pharmacology/Pharmacokinetics

### Physicochemical characteristics

Molecular weight—
   Benztropine mesylate: 403.54.
   Biperiden hydrochloride: 347.93.
   Biperiden lactate: 401.54.
   Ethopropazine hydrochloride: 348.93.
   Procyclidine hydrochloride: 323.91.
   Trihexyphenidyl hydrochloride: 337.93.

### Mechanism of action/Effect

Specific mode of action is unknown, but it is thought that these agents partially block central (striatal) cholinergic receptors, thereby helping to balance cholinergic and dopaminergic activity in the basal ganglia; salivation may be decreased, and smooth muscle may be relaxed. Drug-induced extrapyramidal symptoms and those due to parkinsonism may be relieved, but tardive dyskinesia is not alleviated and may be aggravated by anticholinergic effects.

### Other actions/effects

Benztropine and ethopropazine also have a slight antihistaminic and local anesthetic effect. Biperiden may have a slight effect on the cardiovascular and respiratory systems. Procyclidine and trihexyphenidyl have a direct antispasmodic effect on smooth muscle. In small doses trihexyphenidyl depresses the CNS, but larger doses may cause cerebral excitation.

### Absorption

Well-absorbed from gastrointestinal tract.

### Onset of action

Benztropine—
   Oral: 1 to 2 hours.
   Intramuscular or intravenous: Within a few minutes.
Biperiden—
   Intramuscular: Average of 10 to 30 minutes.
   Intravenous: Within a few minutes.
Trihexyphenidyl—
   Oral: 1 hour.

### Duration of action

Benztropine—Oral, intramuscular, or intravenous: 24 hours.
Biperiden—Intravenous: 1 to 8 hours.
Ethopropazine—Oral: 4 hours.
Procyclidine—Oral: 4 hours.
Trihexyphenidyl—Oral: 6 to 12 hours.

## Precautions to Consider

### Pregnancy/Reproduction

Pregnancy—Problems in humans have not been documented with benztropine, ethopropazine, procyclidine, or trihexyphenidyl.

For biperiden—Studies have not been done with biperiden in humans. Studies have not been done in animals.

FDA Pregnancy Category C.

### Breast-feeding

It is not known whether antidyskinetics are distributed into breast milk. However, antidyskinetics may inhibit lactation.

### Pediatrics

No information is available on the relationship of age to the effects of antidyskinetics in pediatric patients. However, it is known that pediatric patients exhibit increased sensitivity to other medications with anticholinergic properties.

### Geriatrics

Chronic use of antidyskinetics may predispose geriatric patients to glaucoma.

Geriatric patients, especially those with arteriosclerotic changes, may respond to the usual doses of antidyskinetics, ethopropazine and procyclidine in particular, with mental confusion, disorientation, agitation, hallucinations, and psychotic-like symptoms.

Memory may become severely impaired in geriatric patients, especially those who already have memory problems, with the continued use of antidyskinetics since these drugs block the action of acetylcholine, which is responsible for many functions of the brain, including memory functions.

### Dental

Prolonged use of antidyskinetics may decrease or inhibit salivary flow, thus contributing to the development of caries, periodontal disease, oral candidiasis, and discomfort.

### Drug interactions and/or related problems

The following drug interactions and/or related problems have been selected on the basis of their potential clinical significance (possible mechanism in parentheses where appropriate)—not necessarily inclusive (» = major clinical significance):

Note: Combinations containing any of the following medications, depending on the amount present, may also interact with this medication.

» Alcohol or
» CNS depression–producing medications (See *Appendix II* )
   (concurrent use with antidyskinetics may cause increased sedative effects)

Amantadine or
» Anticholinergics or other medications with anticholinergic action (See *Appendix II*) or
Monoamine oxidase (MAO) inhibitors, including furazolidone, procarbazine, and selegiline
   (concurrent use may intensify anticholinergic effects of antidyskinetics because of the secondary anticholinergic activities of these medications; patients should be advised to report occurrence of gastrointestinal problems, fever, or heat intolerance promptly since paralytic ileus, hyperthermia, or heat stroke may occur with concurrent therapy)

Antidiarrheals, adsorbent
   (simultaneous administration may reduce therapeutic effects of antidyskinetics because of particle adsorption; to avoid this effect, patients should be advised to allow at least 1 or 2 hours between doses of the different medications)

Carbidopa and levodopa or
Levodopa
   (concurrent use of these medications with benztropine, procyclidine, or trihexyphenidyl may result in increased efficacy of levodopa; however, concurrent use is not recommended if there is a history of psychosis)

Chlorpromazine
   (concurrent use of chlorpromazine with antidyskinetics may increase metabolism of chlorpromazine, resulting in decreased plasma concentration because of reduction in gastrointestinal motility)

### Medical considerations/Contraindications

The medical considerations/contraindications included here have been selected on the basis of their potential clinical significance (reasons given in parentheses where appropriate)—not necessarily inclusive (» = major clinical significance).

*Risk-benefit should be considered when the following medical problems exist:*

Cardiac arrhythmias
   (increased risk of tachycardia)
» Cardiovascular instability
   (increased risk of cardiac arrhythmias)

» Dyskinesia, tardive
(may be aggravated)

Extrapyramidal reactions, such as those resulting from phenothiazines or reserpine, in patients with mental disorders
(mental symptoms may be intensified, precipitating toxic psychosis)

» Glaucoma, angle-closure, or predisposition to
(mydriatic effect resulting in increased intraocular pressure may precipitate an acute attack of angle-closure glaucoma)

» Glaucoma, open-angle
(mydriatic effect may cause a slight increase in intraocular pressure; glaucoma therapy may need to be adjusted)

Hepatic function impairment
(metabolism may be altered)

Hypertension
(may be aggravated)

» Intestinal obstruction, complete, partial or history of
(decreased motility and tone may aggravate or precipitate obstruction)

» Myasthenia gravis
(condition may be aggravated because of inhibition of acetylcholine action)

Prostatic hypertrophy, moderate to severe or
» Urinary retention
(anticholinergic effect of antidyskinetics may precipitate or aggravate urinary retention)

Renal function impairment
(decreased elimination may increase risk of side effects)

Sensitivity to antidyskinetics (history of)

**Patient monitoring**
The following may be especially important in patient monitoring (other tests may be warranted in some patients, depending on condition; » = major clinical significance):

Intraocular pressure determinations
(recommended at periodic intervals during therapy, especially in patients with angle-closure and open-angle glaucoma)

## Side/Adverse Effects

Note: Anticholinergic side effects that may occur with antidyskinetics are rarely severe and either disappear as therapy is continued, or diminish when the dose is reduced.

Anhidrosis and subsequent hyperthermia may occur with antidyskinetics when patients, especially geriatric, chronically ill, and alcoholic, are exposed to high environmental temperatures.

Ethopropazine is a phenothiazine derivative. Although the likelihood of ethopropazine causing such side effects as changes in vision, jaundice, rare hematologic reactions, and electrocardiogram (ECG) abnormalities associated with phenothiazines seems to be minimal, the possibility exists.

The following side/adverse effects have been selected on the basis of their potential clinical significance (possible signs and symptoms in parentheses where appropriate)—not necessarily inclusive:

**Those indicating need for medical attention**
Incidence rare
*Allergic reaction* (skin rash); *confusion*—more frequent in the elderly or with high doses; *increased intraocular pressure* (eye pain)

**Those indicating need for medical attention only if they continue or are bothersome**
Incidence more frequent
*Anticholinergic effects, mild* (blurred vision; constipation; decreased sweating; difficult or painful urination, especially in older men; drowsiness; dryness of mouth, nose, or throat; increased sensitivity of eyes to light; nausea or vomiting)
Incidence less frequent or rare
*False sense of well-being*—especially in the elderly or with high doses; *headache; loss of memory*—especially in the elderly; *muscle cramps; nervousness; numbness or weakness in hands or feet; orthostatic hypotension* (dizziness or lightheadedness when getting up from a lying or sitting position); *soreness of mouth and tongue; stom-*

*ach upset or pain; unusual excitement*—more frequent with high doses of trihexyphenidyl

**Those indicating possible withdrawal symptoms and the need for medical attention if they occur after discontinuation of long-term therapy**
*Anxiety; extrapyramidal symptoms, recurrence or worsening of* (difficulty in speaking or swallowing; loss of balance control; mask-like face; muscle spasms, especially of face, neck, and back; restlessness or desire to keep moving; shuffling walk; stiffness of arms or legs; trembling and shaking of hands and fingers; twisting movements of body)—especially after abrupt withdrawal of antidyskinetic medication; may require reinstatement of the antidyskinetic; *fast heartbeat; orthostatic hypotension* (dizziness or lightheadedness when getting up from a lying or sitting position); *trouble in sleeping*

## Overdose

For specific information on the agents used in the management of antidyskinetics, see:
*Barbiturates (Systemic)* monograph;
*Diazepam* in *Benzodiazepines (Systemic)* monograph;
*Physostigmine Salicylate (Systemic)* monograph; and/or
*Pilocarpine (Ophthalmic)* monograph.

For more information on the management of overdose or unintentional ingestion, **contact a Poison Control Center** (see *Poison Control Center Listing*).

**Clinical effects of overdose**
The following effects have been selected on the basis of their potential clinical significance (possible signs and symptoms in parentheses where appropriate)—not necessarily inclusive:
*Anticholinergic effects, severe* (clumsiness or unsteadiness; severe drowsiness; severe dryness of mouth, nose, or throat; fast heartbeat; shortness of breath or troubled breathing; warmth, dryness, and flushing of skin); *CNS depression* (severe drowsiness); *CNS stimulation* (hallucinations, seizures, trouble in sleeping); *toxic psychoses* (mood or mental changes)—especially in patients with mental illness being treated with neuroleptic drugs

**Treatment of overdose**
Recommended treatment for overdose with antidyskinetics includes the following:
To decrease absorption—
Emesis or gastric lavage, except in precomatose, convulsive, or psychotic states.
Specific treatment—
Intramuscular or *slow* intravenous administration of 1 to 2 mg of physostigmine salicylate, repeated after 2 hours if needed (0.5 mg initially in children, repeated at five-minute intervals, up to a maximum of 2 mg), to reverse the cardiovascular and CNS toxic effects.
Administration of small doses of diazepam or a short-acting barbiturate to manage excitement.
Administration of pilocarpine 0.5%, to counteract mydriasis.
Supportive care—
Respiratory assistance and symptomatic support.
Patients in whom intentional overdose is confirmed or suspected should be referred for psychiatric consultation.

## Patient Consultation

As an aid to patient consultation, refer to *Advice for the Patient, Antidyskinetics (Systemic)*.

In providing consultation, consider emphasizing the following selected information (» = major clinical significance):

**Before using this medication**
» Conditions affecting use, especially:
Sensitivity to antidyskinetics (history of)
Breast-feeding—May inhibit lactation
Use in children—Increased susceptibility to anticholinergic effects
Use in the elderly—Predisposition to glaucoma with chronic use; increased risk of mental confusion and other psychotic-like symptoms; impairment of memory
Dental—Decrease or inhibition of salivary flow
Other medications, especially other anticholinergics and CNS depressants
Other medical problems, especially cardiovascular instability, tardive dyskinesia, glaucoma, intestinal obstruction, myasthenia gravis, or urinary retention

**Proper use of this medication**
» Importance of not taking more medication than the amount prescribed
Taking with food to relieve gastric irritation

» Proper dosing
    Missed dose: Taking as soon as possible; not taking if within 2 hours of next dose; not doubling doses
» Proper storage

**Precautions while using this medication**
    Regular visits to physician to check progress during prolonged therapy; eye examination may also be needed
» Checking with physician before discontinuing medication; gradual dosage reduction may be necessary
» Avoiding use of alcohol or other CNS depressants
    Avoiding use of antidiarrheal medications within 1 or 2 hours of taking this medication
    Suspected overdose: Getting emergency help at once
    Possible increased eye sensitivity to bright light
» Caution if drowsiness or blurred vision occurs
    Caution when getting up suddenly from a lying or sitting position
» Caution during exercise and hot weather
    Possible dryness of mouth; using sugarless gum or candy, ice, or saliva substitute for relief; checking with physician or dentist if dry mouth continues for more than 2 weeks

**Side/adverse effects**
    Signs of potential side effects, especially allergic reaction, confusion, increased intraocular pressure, anticholinergic effects, or CNS depression or stimulation

## General Dosing Information

**For oral dosage forms only**
Therapy should be initiated with a low dose because of cumulative action, and dosage should be increased gradually at 5- or 6-day intervals.

Titrated dosage is necessary to achieve the individual required therapeutic level, especially for geriatric patients, who tend to be more sensitive to anticholinergic effects, and patients receiving other medications.

During therapy, necessary dosage adjustments of antidyskinetic or other medication used concurrently should be made gradually to maintain proper control of the patient's condition.

Postencephalitic and younger parkinsonism patients often require and tolerate higher dosages than idiopathic, arteriosclerotic, or geriatric parkinsonism patients.

A drug-abuse potential exists with these medications as they may cause euphoria and hallucinations at higher dosages.

When an antidyskinetic is to be discontinued, dosage should be reduced gradually to prevent a sudden increase in adverse symptoms.

**Diet/Nutrition**
Antidyskinetics may be taken with or immediately after meals to lessen gastric irritation.

---

### *BENZTROPINE*

## Summary of Differences

Pharmacology/pharmacokinetics:
    Other actions/effects—
        Has slight antihistaminic and local anesthetic effect.
    Onset of action—
        Oral: 1 to 2 hours.
        Intramuscular or intravenous: Within a few minutes.
    Duration of action—
        Oral, intramuscular, or intravenous: 24 hours.
Precautions:
    Drug interactions and/or related problems—
        May increase efficacy of levodopa if used concurrently; however, concurrent use not recommended if there is history of psychosis.

## Additional Dosing Information

A single daily oral dose of benztropine at bedtime often provides maximum benefit for the patient because of the long duration of effect.

## Oral Dosage Forms

### BENZTROPINE MESYLATE TABLETS USP

**Usual adult and adolescent dose**
Parkinsonism—
    Oral, 1 to 2 mg a day, the dosage being adjusted as needed and tolerated.

Note: Idiopathic parkinsonism—Therapy may be initiated in some patients with a single oral daily dose of 500 mcg (0.5 mg) to 1 mg

at bedtime.
    Postencephalitic parkinsonism—Therapy may be initiated in most patients with 2 mg a day, given once a day or in divided doses.
Drug-induced extrapyramidal reactions—
    Oral, 1 to 4 mg one or two times a day. Or, 1 to 2 mg two or three times a day if drug-induced extrapyramidal reactions develop soon after initiation of treatment with neuroleptic drugs.

**Usual adult prescribing limits**
Up to 6 mg daily.

**Usual pediatric dose**
Parkinsonism or drug-induced extrapyramidal reactions—
    Children up to 3 years of age: Use is not recommended.
    Children 3 years of age and over: Dosage must be individualized by physician.

**Usual geriatric dose**
See *Usual adult and adolescent dose.*

Note: Geriatric patients may be more sensitive to the effects of the usual adult dose.

**Strength(s) usually available**
U.S.—
    500 mcg (0.5 mg) (Rx) [*Cogentin* (scored); GENERIC].
    1 mg (Rx) [*Cogentin* (scored); GENERIC].
    2 mg (Rx) [*Cogentin* (scored); GENERIC].
Canada—
    500 mcg (0.5 mg) (Rx) [*PMS Benztropine*].
    1 mg (Rx) [*PMS Benztropine* (scored)].
    2 mg (Rx) [*Apo-Benztropine* (double-scored); *Cogentin* (scored; lactose); *PMS Benztropine* (scored); GENERIC].

**Packaging and storage**
Store below 40 °C (104 °F), preferably between 15 and 30 °C (59 and 86 °F), in a well-closed container, unless otherwise specified by manufacturer.

**Auxiliary labeling**
• May cause drowsiness.
• Avoid alcoholic beverages.

## Parenteral Dosage Forms

### BENZTROPINE MESYLATE INJECTION USP

**Usual adult and adolescent dose**
Parkinsonism—
    Intramuscular or intravenous, 1 to 2 mg a day, the dosage being adjusted as needed and tolerated.
Drug-induced extrapyramidal reactions—
    Intramuscular or intravenous, 1 to 4 mg one or two times a day.

**Usual adult prescribing limits**
Up to 6 mg daily.

**Usual pediatric dose**
Parkinsonism or drug-induced extrapyramidal reactions—
    Children up to 3 years of age: Use is not recommended.
    Children 3 years of age and over: Dosage must be individualized by physician.

**Usual geriatric dose**
See *Usual adult and adolescent dose.*

Note: Geriatric patients may be more sensitive to the effects of the usual adult dose.

**Strength(s) usually available**
U.S.—
    1 mg per mL (Rx) [*Cogentin* (sodium chloride 9 mg/mL)].
Canada—
    1 mg per mL (Rx) [*Cogentin* (sodium chloride 9 mg/mL); GENERIC].

**Packaging and storage**
Store below 40 °C (104 °F), preferably between 15 and 30 °C (59 and 86 °F), unless otherwise specified by manufacturer. Protect from freezing.

---

### *BIPERIDEN*

## Summary of Differences

Pharmacology/pharmacokinetics:
    Other actions/effects—
        Slight cardiovascular and respiratory effects.
Side/adverse effects:
    Has slight effect on cardiovascular and respiratory systems.

# Oral Dosage Forms
## BIPERIDEN HYDROCHLORIDE TABLETS USP

### Usual adult and adolescent dose
Parkinsonism—
    Oral, 2 mg three or four times a day, the dosage being adjusted as needed and tolerated.
Drug-induced extrapyramidal reactions—
    Oral, 2 mg one to three times a day.

### Usual adult prescribing limits
Parkinsonism—
    Up to 16 mg daily.

### Usual pediatric dose
Safety and efficacy have not been established.

### Usual geriatric dose
See *Usual adult and adolescent dose.*

Note: Geriatric patients may be more sensitive to the effects of the usual adult dose.

### Strength(s) usually available
U.S.—
    2 mg (Rx) [*Akineton* (scored; corn syrup; lactose; magnesium stearate; potato starch; talc)].
Canada—
    2 mg (Rx) [*Akineton*].

### Packaging and storage
Store below 40 °C (104 °F), preferably between 15 and 30 °C (59 and 86 °F), unless otherwise specified by manufacturer. Store in a tight container.

### Auxiliary labeling
• May cause drowsiness.
• Avoid alcoholic beverages.
• Keep container tightly closed.

# Parenteral Dosage Forms
## BIPERIDEN LACTATE INJECTION USP

### Usual adult and adolescent dose
Drug-induced extrapyramidal reactions—
    Intramuscular or slow intravenous, 2 mg repeated at half-hour intervals as needed and tolerated up to a total of four doses a day.

### Usual pediatric dose
Drug-induced extrapyramidal reactions—
    Intramuscular, initially 40 mcg (0.04 mg) per kg of body weight, or 1.2 mg per square meter of body surface; dose may be repeated at half-hour intervals if necessary, up to four doses a day.

### Usual geriatric dose
See *Usual adult and adolescent dose.*

Note: Geriatric patients may be more sensitive to the effects of the usual adult dose.

### Strength(s) usually available
U.S.—
    5 mg per mL (Rx) [*Akineton* (1.4% sodium lactate)].
Canada—
    Not commercially available.

### Packaging and storage
Store below 40 °C (104 °F), preferably between 15 and 30 °C (59 and 86 °F), unless otherwise specified by manufacturer. Protect from light. Protect from freezing.

---

## *ETHOPROPAZINE*

## Summary of Differences
Indications:
    Also used for the symptomatic treatment of hepatolenticular degeneration and congenital athetosis.
Pharmacology/pharmacokinetics:
    Other actions/effects—
        Has slight antihistaminic and local anesthetic effect.
    Duration of action—
        Oral: 4 hours.
Side/adverse effects:
    May possess phenothiazine side effects, especially in high dosages.

# Oral Dosage Forms
## ETHOPROPAZINE HYDROCHLORIDE TABLETS USP

### Usual adult and adolescent dose
Parkinsonism and
Drug-induced extrapyramidal reactions—
    Oral, 50 mg one or two times a day, the dosage being increased as needed and tolerated. In severe cases, the dose may be increased gradually to a total of 500 to 600 mg a day.

### Usual pediatric dose
Dosage has not been established.

### Usual geriatric dose
See *Usual adult and adolescent dose.*

Note: Geriatric patients may be more sensitive to the effects of the usual adult dose.

### Strength(s) usually available
U.S.—
    10 mg (Rx) [*Parsidol*].
    50 mg (Rx) [*Parsidol* (scored)].
Canada—
    50 mg (Rx) [*Parsitan* (scored)].

### Packaging and storage
Store below 40 °C (104 °F), preferably between 15 and 30 °C (59 and 86 °F), in a well-closed container, unless otherwise specified by manufacturer. Protect from light.

### Auxiliary labeling
• May cause drowsiness.
• Avoid alcoholic beverages.

---

## *PROCYCLIDINE*

## Summary of Differences
Pharmacology/pharmacokinetics:
    Other actions/effects—
        Direct antispasmodic effect on smooth muscle.
    Duration of action—
        Oral: 4 hours.
Precautions:
    Drug interactions and/or related problems—
        May increase efficacy of levodopa if used concurrently; however, concurrent use not recommended if there is history of psychosis.
General dosing information:
    Provides more beneficial effect in conditions of rigidity than in those of tremor.

# Oral Dosage Forms
## PROCYCLIDINE HYDROCHLORIDE ELIXIR

### Usual adult and adolescent dose
Parkinsonism—
    Oral, initially 2.5 mg three times a day after meals. If tolerated, the dosage may be gradually increased to 5 mg three times a day and, occasionally, 5 mg at bedtime.
Note: For patients being transferred from other therapy, 2.5 mg three times a day may be substituted for all or part of the original medication. The dose of procyclidine may be increased while the original medication is decreased until a level of maximum benefit is reached.
Drug-induced extrapyramidal reactions—
    Oral, initially 2.5 mg three times a day, the dosage being increased in 2.5-mg increments per day as needed and tolerated.

### Usual pediatric dose
Dosage has not been established.

### Usual geriatric dose
See *Usual adult and adolescent dose.*

Note: Geriatric patients may be more sensitive to the effects of the usual adult dose.

### Strength(s) usually available
U.S.—
    Not commercially available.
Canada—
    2.5 mg per 5 mL (Rx) [*Kemadrin* (alcohol 10%); *PMS Procyclidine* (spearmint-flavored); *Procyclid*.].

**Packaging and storage**
Store below 40 °C (104 °F), preferably between 15 and 30 °C (59 and 86 °F), unless otherwise specified by manufacturer. Store in a tight container. Protect from freezing.

**Auxiliary labeling**
• May cause drowsiness.
• Avoid alcoholic beverages.
• Keep container tightly closed.

## PROCYCLIDINE HYDROCHLORIDE TABLETS USP

**Usual adult and adolescent dose**
See *Procyclidine Hydrochloride Elixir.*

**Usual pediatric dose**
See *Procyclidine Hydrochloride Elixir.*

**Usual geriatric dose**
See *Procyclidine Hydrochloride Elixir.*

**Strength(s) usually available**
U.S.—
    5 mg (Rx) [*Kemadrin* (scored)].
Canada—
    2.5 mg (Rx) [*PMS Procyclidine* (scored)].
    5 mg (Rx) [*Kemadrin* (scored); *PMS Procyclidine* (scored); *Procyclid* (scored)].

**Packaging and storage**
Store below 40 °C (104 °F), preferably between 15 and 30 °C (59 and 86 °F), unless otherwise specified by manufacturer. Store in a tight container.

**Auxiliary labeling**
• May cause drowsiness.
• Avoid alcoholic beverages.
• Keep container tightly closed.

---

### *TRIHEXYPHENIDYL*

## Summary of Differences

Pharmacology/pharmacokinetics:
    Other actions/effects—
        Direct antispasmodic effect on smooth muscle; small doses depress CNS; larger doses may cause cerebral excitation.
    Onset of action—
        Oral: 1 hour.
    Duration of action—
        Oral: 6 to 12 hours.
Precautions:
    Drug interactions and/or related problems—
        May increase efficacy of levodopa if used concurrently; however, concurrent use not recommended if there is history of psychosis.
Side/adverse effects:
    Unusual excitement (with high doses).

## Oral Dosage Forms

### TRIHEXYPHENIDYL HYDROCHLORIDE EXTENDED-RELEASE CAPSULES USP

**Usual adult and adolescent dose**
Parkinsonism—
    Oral, 5 mg a day after breakfast with an additional 5 mg taken twelve hours later as needed.
Note: This dosage form is usually utilized only after the patient has been stabilized on the conventional dosage forms.

**Usual adult prescribing limits**
Up to 15 mg daily.

**Usual pediatric dose**
Dosage has not been established.

**Usual geriatric dose**
See *Usual adult and adolescent dose.*
Note: Geriatric patients may be more sensitive to the effects of the usual adult dose.

**Strength(s) usually available**
U.S.—
    5 mg (Rx) [*Artane Sequels*].

Canada—
    5 mg (Rx) [*Artane Sequels*].

**Packaging and storage**
Store below 40 °C (104 °F), preferably between 15 and 30 °C (59 and 86 °F), in a tight container, unless otherwise specified by manufacturer.

**Auxiliary labeling**
• May cause drowsiness.
• Avoid alcoholic beverages.

## TRIHEXYPHENIDYL HYDROCHLORIDE ELIXIR USP

**Usual adult and adolescent dose**
Parkinsonism—
    Oral, 1 to 2 mg the first day, the dosage being increased by an additional 2 mg at three- to five-day intervals until the desired response is obtained or until the total dose per day reaches 6 to 10 mg, usually divided into three doses taken at mealtimes.
    Note: Postencephalitic parkinsonism—A total dose of 12 to 15 mg per day may be required.
Drug-induced extrapyramidal reactions—
    Oral, initially 1 mg a day, the dosage being increased as needed and tolerated or until the total daily dose reaches 5 to 15 mg.

**Usual adult prescribing limits**
Up to 15 mg daily.

**Usual pediatric dose**
Dosage has not been established.

**Usual geriatric dose**
See *Usual adult and adolescent dose.*
Note: Geriatric patients may be more sensitive to the effects of the usual adult dose.

**Strength(s) usually available**
U.S.—
    2 mg per 5 mL (Rx) [*Artane* (lime-mint flavored); GENERIC].
Canada—
    2 mg per 5 mL (Rx) [*Artane* (lime flavored); *PMS Trihexyphenidyl*].

**Packaging and storage**
Store below 40 °C (104 °F), preferably between 15 and 30 °C (59 and 86 °F), unless otherwise specified by manufacturer. Store in a tight container. Protect from freezing.

**Auxiliary labeling**
• May cause drowsiness.
• Avoid alcoholic beverages.
• Keep container tightly closed.

## TRIHEXYPHENIDYL HYDROCHLORIDE TABLETS USP

**Usual adult and adolescent dose**
See *Trihexyphenidyl Hydrochloride Elixir USP.*

**Usual adult prescribing limits**
See *Trihexyphenidyl Hydrochloride Elixir USP.*

**Usual pediatric dose**
See *Trihexyphenidyl Hydrochloride Elixir USP.*

**Usual geriatric dose**
See *Trihexyphenidyl Hydrochloride Elixir USP.*

**Strength(s) usually available**
U.S.—
    2 mg (Rx) [*Artane* (scored); *Trihexane; Trihexy;* GENERIC].
    5 mg (Rx) [*Artane* (scored); *Trihexane; Trihexy;* GENERIC].
Canada—
    2 mg (Rx) [*Apo-Trihex* (scored; sodium <1 mmol (0.113 mg)/2 mg); *Artane* (scored); *PMS Trihexyphenidyl* (sodium <1 mmol (0.113 mg)/2 mg)].
    5 mg (Rx) [*Apo-Trihex* (scored; sodium <1 mmol (0.188 mg)/5 mg); *Artane* (scored); *PMS Trihexyphenidyl* (sodium <1 mmol (0.188 mg)/5 mg)].

**Packaging and storage**
Store below 40 °C (104 °F), preferably between 15 and 30 °C (59 and 86 °F), unless otherwise specified by manufacturer. Store in a tight container.

**Auxiliary labeling**
• May cause drowsiness.
• Avoid alcoholic beverages.
• Keep container tightly closed.

---

Revised: 05/11/93

# ANTIFUNGALS, AZOLE   Systemic

This monograph includes information on the following: Fluconazole; Itraconazole; Ketoconazole; Miconazole†.

VA CLASSIFICATION (Primary/Secondary):
   Fluconazole—AM700
   Itraconazole—AM700
   Ketoconazole—AM700/HS900; AN900
   Miconazole—AM700

Note: For a listing of dosage forms and brand names by country availability, see *Dosage Forms* section(s). For a listing of brand names for the articles in this monograph, refer to the General Index.

†Not commercially available in Canada.

## Category

Antiadrenal; antineoplastic (systemic)—Ketoconazole.
Antifungal (systemic)—Fluconazole; Itraconazole; Ketoconazole; Miconazole.

## Indications

Note: Bracketed information in the *Indications* section refers to uses that are not included in U.S. product labeling.

### Accepted

Aspergillosis (treatment)—Itraconazole is indicated in the treatment of aspergillosis caused by *Aspergillus* species in patients who are intolerant of or refractory to amphotericin B therapy.

Blastomycosis (treatment)—Itraconazole is indicated for the treatment of pulmonary and extrapulmonary blastomycosis caused by *Blastomyces dermatiditis* in immunocompromised and nonimmunocompromised patients. Ketoconazole[1] is indicated in the treatment of pulmonary and disseminated blastomycosis.

Candidiasis (prophylaxis)[1]—Fluconazole is indicated for the prophylaxis of candidiasis in patients undergoing bone marrow transplant who receive cytotoxic chemotherapy and/or radiation therapy.

Candidiasis, esophageal (treatment) or
Candidiasis, oropharyngeal (treatment)—Fluconazole, [itraconazole], and ketoconazole are indicated for the treatment of esophageal and oropharyngeal candidiasis (thrush) caused by *Candida* species.

Candidiasis, disseminated (treatment)—Fluconazole, ketoconazole, and miconazole are indicated for the treatment of serious infections caused by *Candida* species, including peritonitis, pneumonia, and urinary tract infections.

Candidiasis, mucocutaneous, chronic (treatment)—[Fluconazole][1], [itraconazole][1], ketoconazole, and miconazole are indicated in the treatment of severe, chronic extensive mucocutaneous candidiasis caused by *Candida* species.

Candidiasis, vulvovaginal (treatment)[1]—Fluconazole, [itraconazole], and [ketoconazole] are indicated in the treatment of vulvovaginal candidiasis caused by *Candida* species.

Chromomycosis (treatment)—[Itraconazole] and ketoconazole are indicated as secondary agents in the treatment of chromomycosis caused by *Cladosporium carrioni, Exophiala dermatitidis, Fonsecaea pedrosi, F. compactum, Phialophora verrucosa, Rhinocladiella aquaspersa,* and *R. cerophilum.*

Coccidioidomycosis (treatment)—[Fluconazole][1] and [itraconazole][1] are used in the treatment of pulmonary and disseminated coccidioidomycosis caused by *Coccidioides immitis.* Ketoconazole and parenteral miconazole are indicated as secondary agents in the treatment of severe coccidioidomycosis.

Cryptococcosis (treatment)—[Fluconazole][1] and [itraconazole][1] are used in the treatment of extrameningeal cryptococcosis caused by *Cryptococcus neoformans.* Parenteral miconazole is indicated as a secondary agent in the treatment of severe cryptococcosis.

Histoplasmosis (treatment)—Itraconazole is indicated for the treatment of histoplasmosis, including chronic cavitary pulmonary disease and disseminated disease caused by *Histoplasma* species, in immunocompromised and nonimmunocompromised patients. Ketoconazole is also indicated in the treatment of pulmonary and disseminated histoplasmosis caused by *Histoplasma capsulatum.*

Meningitis, cryptococcal (treatment) or
Meningitis, cryptococcal, suppression—Fluconazole is indicated for the treatment and suppression of cryptococcal meningitis. [Itraconazole][1] is used as an alternative agent as suppressive, maintenance therapy for cryptococcal meningitis.

Preliminary studies indicate that amphotericin B plus flucytosine may be more efficacious than fluconazole in the primary treatment of cryptococcal meningitis in patients with acquired immunodeficiency syndrome (AIDS), although there was a greater incidence of toxicity with this combination. Another study found that amphotericin B alone was superior to fluconazole in the treatment of acute cryptococcal meningitis; however, fluconazole was superior for maintenance therapy.

Paracoccidioidomycosis (treatment)—[Itraconazole] and ketoconazole are indicated in the treatment of paracoccidioidomycosis caused by *Paracoccidioides brasiliensis.* Parenteral miconazole is indicated as a secondary agent in the treatment of severe paracoccidioidomycosis.

Pityriasis versicolor (treatment)
Tinea corporis (treatment)
Tinea cruris (treatment) or
Tinea pedis (treatment)—Ketoconazole is indicated in the treatment of recalcitrant or very severe disfiguring or disabling pityriasis versicolor, tinea corporis, tinea cruris, and tinea pedis infections unresponsive to griseofulvin, or in patients allergic to or unable to tolerate griseofulvin. [Fluconazole][1] and [itraconazole][1] are used in the treatment of tinea corporis (ringworm of the body), tinea cruris (ringworm of the groin; jock itch), and tinea pedis (ringworm of the foot; athlete's foot).

Pseudallescheriasis (treatment)—Parenteral miconazole is indicated as a secondary agent in the treatment of severe pseudallescheriasis (petriellidiosis or allescheriosis) caused by *Pseudallescheria boydii.*

[Carcinoma, prostatic (treatment)][1]—High dose ketoconazole is used as a secondary agent in the treatment of advanced prostatic carcinoma.

[Cushing's syndrome (treatment)][1]—High dose ketoconazole is used as a secondary agent in the treatment of Cushing's syndrome.

[Histoplasmosis (suppression)][1]—Itraconazole is used for the suppression of disseminated histoplasmosis caused by *Histoplasma* species, in immunocompromised patients.

[Leishmaniasis, cutaneous (treatment)][1]—Itraconazole and ketoconazole are used for the treatment of cutaneous leishmaniasis.

[Onychomycosis (treatment)][1]—Fluconazole, itraconazole, and ketoconazole are used in the treatment of onychomycosis caused by *Trichophyton* species and *Candida* species.

[Paronychia (treatment)][1]—Itraconazole and ketoconazole are used in the treatment of paronychia.

[Pneumonia, fungal (treatment)][1]—Fluconazole, itraconazole, and ketoconazole are used in the treatment of fungal pneumonia.

[Septicemia, fungal (treatment)][1]—Fluconazole, itraconazole, ketoconazole, and parenteral miconazole are used in the treatment of fungal septicemia.

[Sporotrichosis, disseminated (treatment)][1]—Itraconazole and ketoconazole[1] are used in the treatment of disseminated sporotrichosis.

[Tinea barbae (treatment)][1] or
[Tinea capitis (treatment)][1]—Systemic ketoconazole is used in combination with topical imidazoles in the treatment of griseofulvin-resistant tinea barbae (ringworm of the beard) and tinea capitis (ringworm of the scalp).

[Tinea manuum (treatment)][1]—Fluconazole and itraconazole are used in the treatment of tinea manuum (ringworm of the hand).

Fluconazole is approved for the treatment of systemic candidal infections, and, although some medical experts may consider the data to be preliminary at this time, fluconazole may be an appropriate, less toxic alternative to amphotericin B.

Fluconazole has been shown to be efficacious *in vivo* in the treatment of animals infected with candidiasis, cryptococcosis, histoplasmosis, coccidioidosis, blastomycosis, aspergillosis, and paracoccidioidosis. The *in vitro* susceptibility testing of fluconazole is affected by culture medium, pH, inoculum size, incubation temperature, and time. Because of this, published *in vitro* minimum inhibitory concentration (MIC) data vary widely and a correlation between this and *in vivo* clinical efficacy cannot reliably be made.

Miconazole is indicated in the treatment of severe systemic fungal infections only. However, in the opinion of medical experts, intravenous miconazole is a second-line drug. It has been replaced by systemic amphotericin B, fluconazole, itraconazole, and ketoconazole because of the number of treatment failures with miconazole, the greater efficacy of fluconazole, itraconazole, and ketoconazole in certain mycoses, the high incidence of toxicity with miconazole, and the limited number of studies on patients treated with miconazole.

### Unaccepted

Ketoconazole is not effective in the treatment of fungal meningitis because it penetrates poorly into the cerebrospinal fluid (CSF). Also, it is not effective against *Aspergillus* or *Zygomycetes* (agents of mucormycosis) or in mycetoma.

Miconazole I.V. is not recommended in the treatment of common trivial fungal infections.

---

[1]Not included in Canadian product labeling.

## Pharmacology/Pharmacokinetics

See also *Table 1,* page 303, and *Table 2,* page 304.

### Physicochemical characteristics

Molecular weight—
   Fluconazole: 306.27.
   Itraconazole: 705.65.
   Ketoconazole: 531.44.
   Miconazole: 416.14.
Chemical class—
   Fluconazole: Triazole derivative
   Itraconazole: Triazole derivative
   Ketoconazole: Imidazole derivative
   Miconazole: Imidazole derivative

### Mechanism of action/Effect

Fungistatic; may be fungicidal, depending on concentration; azole antifungals interfere with cytochrome P-450 activity, which is necessary for the demethylation of 14-alpha-methylsterols to ergosterol. Ergosterol, the principal sterol in the fungal cell membrane, becomes depleted. This damages the cell membrane, producing alterations in membrane functions and permeability. In *Candida albicans*, azole antifungals inhibit transformation of blastospores into invasive mycelial form.

### Other actions/effects

High-dose ketoconazole therapy can interfere with the conversion of lanosterol to cholesterol, a major precursor of several hormones. It has been shown to suppress corticosteroid secretion and lower serum testosterone concentrations, which return to baseline values when ketoconazole is discontinued. ACTH-induced serum corticosteroid concentrations and serum testosterone concentrations may be decreased by doses of 800 mg of ketoconazole daily; serum testosterone concentrations are abolished by doses of 1.6 grams of ketoconazole daily, leading to reduced libido and impotence, but return to baseline values when ketoconazole is discontinued.

Compared to ketoconazole, fluconazole and itraconazole have a very weak, noncompetitive inhibitory effect on the liver cytochrome P-450 system, while maintaining a high affinity for fungal P-450 activity.

Fluconazole and itraconazole have not been reported to have antiandrogenic activity at currently used doses. Itraconazole has not affected cortisol metabolism in patients treated with clinically recommended doses; however, a decrease in cortisol synthesis was observed in a patient receiving high-dose itraconazole therapy (600 mg a day).

### Distribution

Fluconazole—Fluconazole is widely distributed throughout the body, with good penetration into the cerebrospinal fluid (CSF) (ranging from 52 to 85% in patients with fungal meningitis), the eye, and peritoneal fluid.

Itraconazole—Highly lipophilic; extensively distributed to tissues, concentrating in fatty tissues, the omentum, the liver, and the kidneys. Aqueous fluids, such as the CSF, aqueous humor, and saliva, contain negligible concentrations of itraconazole. Itraconazole also does not distribute into peritoneal dialysate effluent. Exudates, such as pus, may have up to 3.5 times the simultaneous plasma concentration; tissues that are prone to fungal invasion, such as skin, lung tissue, and the female genital tract, have several times the plasma concentration.

Ketoconazole—Well distributed; distributed to inflamed joint fluid, saliva, bile, urine, breast milk, sebum, cerumen, feces, tendons, skin and soft tissues, and testes (small amounts); crosses the placenta; crosses the blood-brain barrier poorly; only negligible amounts reach the CSF. Although concentrations of 2.2 to 3 mcg per mL have been reported in the CSF with corresponding serum concentrations of 9 to 12 mcg per mL, most studies indicate that CSF concentrations > 1 mcg per mL are rare, regardless of dose.

Miconazole—Miconazole appears to be widely distributed in body tissues. It penetrates well into inflamed joints, the vitreous humor of the eye, and the peritoneal cavity, but poorly into the saliva and sputum. Urine concentrations are low. Miconazole crosses the blood-brain barrier, but to only a small extent. To achieve fungicidal concentrations in the cerebrospinal fluid, the intravenous infusion must be supplemented with intrathecal administration of the drug.

## Precautions to Consider

### Cross-sensitivity and/or related problems

Patients allergic to one azole antifungal agent (fluconazole, itraconazole, ketoconazole, miconazole) may also be allergic to the other antifungals in this family.

### Carcinogenicity/Tumorigenicity

*Fluconazole*—Studies in rats and mice treated with oral doses of 2.5 to 10 mg per kg of body weight (mg/kg) per day (2 to 7 times the recommended human dose) for 24 months showed no carcinogenic potential. Male rats treated with 5 to 10 mg/kg per day had an increased incidence of hepatocellular adenomas.

*Itraconazole*—No evidence of carcinogenicity was found in mice given oral doses of up to 80 mg/kg a day, or approximately 10 times the maximum recommended human dose (MRHD), for 23 months. Male rats given 3 times the MRHD had a slightly increased incidence of soft tissue sarcoma. These sarcomas may have been a consequence of hypercholesterolemia, which is caused by chronic itraconazole administration in rats, but did not occur in dogs or humans. Female rats who were given 6.25 times the MRHD had an increased incidence of squamous cell carcinoma in the lung, compared to the untreated group, although the increase in this study was not statistically significant.

*Ketoconazole*—Long-term feeding studies in Swiss albino mice and in Wistar rats have not shown evidence of oncogenesis.

### Mutagenicity

*Fluconazole*—Mutagenicity tests for fluconazole (with and without metabolic activation) in 4 strains of *S. typhimurium* and in the mouse lymphoma L5178Y system were negative. Cytogenic studies *in vivo* and *in vitro* showed no evidence of chromosomal mutations.

*Itraconazole*—Itraconazole produced no mutagenic effects when assayed in appropriate bacterial, non-mammalian and mammalian test systems.

*Ketoconazole* —Dominant lethal mutation tests have not shown mutation in any stage of germ cell development in male and female mice given single oral doses of ketoconazole as high as 80 mg/kg. In addition, the Ames/Salmonella microsomal activator assays have not shown evidence of mutagenicity.

### Pregnancy/Reproduction

Fertility—*Fluconazole:* Fertility was not affected in male or female rats treated with oral daily doses of 5 to 20 mg/kg or parenteral doses of 5, 25, or 75 mg/kg, although the onset of parturition was slightly delayed with oral doses of 20 mg/kg.

*Itraconazole:* Itraconazole did not affect the fertility of male or female rats treated with oral doses of up to 5 times the MRHD, although parental toxicity was present at this dosage level.

*Ketoconazole:* Ketoconazole has been shown to decrease or abolish serum testosterone concentrations when used in high doses (e.g., 800 mg to 1.6 grams daily). Ketoconazole has also been shown to cause menstrual irregularities, oligospermia, azoospermia, impotence, and decreased male libido.

*Miconazole:* Studies in rats given 40 mg/kg and rabbits given 20 mg/kg of intravenous miconazole have shown no evidence that miconazole impairs fertility.

Pregnancy—
*Fluconazole:* Studies in humans have not been done.

Maternal weight gain was impaired in pregnant rabbits administered oral fluconazole at doses ranging from 5 to 75 mg/kg per day. Abortions occurred at 75 mg/kg (20 to 60 times the recommended human dose); no adverse fetal effects were detected. Pregnant rats administered oral fluconazole showed impaired maternal weight gain and increased placental weight at 25 mg/kg. A slight increase in the number of stillborn pups and a decrease in neonatal survival were also seen at these doses. Supernumerary ribs, renal pelvis dilation, and delays in ossification were observed at doses of 25 mg/kg and higher. Embryolethality in rats and fetal abnormalities, including wavy ribs, cleft palate, and abnormal craniofacial ossification, occurred at doses ranging from 80 to 320 mg/kg (approximately 20 to 60 times the recommended human dose). These effects are consistent with the inhibition of estrogen synthesis in rats and may be a result of known effects of lowered estrogen on pregnancy, organogenesis, and parturition; this effect has not been observed in women treated with fluconazole.

FDA Pregnancy Category C.
*Itraconazole:* Adequate and well-controlled studies in humans have not been done.

Studies in rats found that itraconazole causes a dose-related increase in maternal toxicity, embryotoxicity, and teratogenicity, consisting of major skeletal defects, at doses approximately 5 to 20 times the MRHD. Studies in mice also found that itraconazole causes a dose-related increase in maternal toxicity, embryotoxicity, and teratogenicity, consisting of encephaloceles and/or macroglossia, at doses approximately 10 times the MRHD.

FDA Pregnancy Category C.

*Ketoconazole:* Ketoconazole crosses the placenta. Adequate and well-controlled studies in humans have not been done.

Studies in rats given doses of 80 mg/kg per day (10 times the MRHD) have shown ketoconazole to be teratogenic, causing syndactyly and oligodactyly. Ketoconazole has also been shown to be embryotoxic in rats given doses greater than 80 mg/kg during the first trimester.

FDA Pregnancy Category C.

*Miconazole:* Adequate and well-controlled studies in humans have not been done.

Studies in rats given 40 mg/kg and rabbits given 20 mg/kg of intravenous miconazole have shown no evidence of harm to the fetus.

FDA Pregnancy Category C.

Labor—*Fluconazole:* Dystocia and prolongation of parturition were observed in a few pregnant rats given 20 and 40 mg/kg of intravenous fluconazole.

*Ketoconazole:* Ketoconazole has also been shown to cause dystocia in rats given doses greater than 10 mg/kg (greater than 1.25 times the MRHD) during the third trimester.

### Breast-feeding

*Fluconazole*—Fluconazole is distributed into breast milk at concentrations similar to those in plasma.

*Itraconazole*—Itraconazole is distributed into breast milk.

*Ketoconazole*—Ketoconazole is distributed into breast milk.

*Miconazole*—It is not known whether miconazole is distributed into breast milk.

### Pediatrics

*Fluconazole*—Appropriate studies on the relationship of age to the effects of fluconazole have not been performed in the pediatric population. Efficacy has not been established. However, a small number of patients from 2 weeks to 14 years of age have been safely treated with doses of 3 to 6 mg/kg per day.

*Itraconazole*—Appropriate studies on the relationship of age to the effects of itraconazole have not been performed in the pediatric population. Safety and efficacy have not been established. However, a small number of patients ages 3 to 16 years have been treated with 100 mg per day of itraconazole for systemic fungal infections, and no serious adverse effects have been reported.

*Ketoconazole*—Several cases of hepatitis have been reported in children who have taken ketoconazole. Appropriate studies on the relationship of age to the effects of ketoconazole have not been performed in children up to 2 years of age. However, no pediatrics-specific problems have been documented to date in children over 2 years of age.

*Miconazole*—Appropriate studies on the relationship of age to the effects of miconazole have not been performed in children up to 1 year of age. No unanticipated adverse effects were reported in 21 neonates treated with 3 to 50 mg/kg per day of intravenous miconazole for 1 to 56 days. Seven of 11 evaluable neonates recovered or improved. No pediatrics-specific problems have been documented to date in children over one year of age.

### Geriatrics

No information is available on the relationship of age to the effects of azole antifungals in geriatric patients. However, elderly patients are more likely to have an age-related decrease in renal function, which may require an adjustment in dosage or dosing interval in patients receiving fluconazole.

### Drug interactions and/or related problems

The following drug interactions and/or related problems have been selected on the basis of their potential clinical significance (possible mechanism in parentheses where appropriate)—not necessarily inclusive (» = major clinical significance):

Note: Combinations containing any of the following medications, depending on the amount present, may also interact with this medication.

» Alcohol or
» Hepatotoxic medications, other (See *Appendix II*)

(concurrent use with ketoconazole may result in an increased incidence of hepatotoxicity; patients, especially those on prolonged administration or those with a history of liver disease, should be carefully monitored and should be advised to avoid alcoholic beverages and other hepatotoxins)

(concurrent ingestion of alcohol with ketoconazole has been reported to result in a disulfiram-like reaction, characterized by facial flushing; other symptoms may include difficult breathing, slight fever, and tightness of the chest; these effects subsided spontaneously within 24 hours with no lasting ill effects)

» Antacids or
» Anticholinergics/antispasmodics or
» Histamine H$_2$-receptor antagonists or
» Omeprazole or
» Sucralfate

(these medications increase gastrointestinal pH; this may result in a marked reduction in absorption of itraconazole and ketoconazole; ketoconazole depends on stomach acid for dissolution and subsequent absorption; patients should be advised to take these medications at least 2 hours after taking itraconazole or ketoconazole)

» Antidiabetic agents, oral

(concurrent use of fluconazole or itraconazole with tolbutamide, chlorpropamide, glyburide, or glipizide has increased the plasma concentration of these sulfonylurea agents; hypoglycemia has been noted; blood glucose concentrations should be monitored, and the dose of the oral hypoglycemic may need to be reduced)

» Astemizole or
» Terfenadine

(concurrent use of these medications with itraconazole or ketoconazole is contraindicated; concurrent use of these antihistamines with itraconazole or ketoconazole may result in elevated plasma concentrations of astemizole or terfenadine by inhibiting the P-450 metabolic pathways; this has led to cardiac arrhythmias, including ventricular tachycardia and torsades de pointes, and death; in a small study, fluconazole was given with terfenadine and a small pharmacokinetic interaction was found; however, no change in cardiac repolarization or accumulation of parent terfenadine was found)

» Carbamazepine

(concurrent use may decrease itraconazole plasma concentrations, leading to clinical failure or relapse)

» Cisapride

(concurrent use of cisapride with oral itraconazole, oral ketoconazole, or intravenous miconazole is contraindicated; concurrent use of cisapride with these antifungals may inhibit the cytochrome P-450 metabolic pathways, resulting in elevated plasma concentrations of cisapride; this has led to ventricular arrhythmias, including torsades de pointes, in patients taking cisapride and oral ketoconazole)

» Cyclosporine

(itraconazole, ketoconazole, miconazole, and high doses of fluconazole have been reported to inhibit the metabolism of cyclosporine; this may increase the plasma concentration of cyclosporine to potentially toxic levels; a few studies have not found a significant interaction between fluconazole and cyclosporine; however, plasma cyclosporine concentrations should be carefully monitored in patients receiving any of the azole antifungals; the dose of cyclosporine may need to be reduced; it is currently recommended that the dose of cyclosporine be reduced by 50% when itraconazole is started)

» Didanosine (ddI)

(didanosine contains a buffer that increases gastrointestinal pH in order to increase its absorption; itraconazole and ketoconazole require an acidic environment for their optimal absorption; concurrent administration may result in a marked reduction in absorption of any of these medications; itraconazole and ketoconazole should be administered at least 2 hours before or 2 hours after didanosine is given)

» Digoxin

(itraconazole may increase serum digoxin concentrations, leading to toxicity; digoxin concentrations should be monitored)

Hydrochlorothiazide

(concurrent use of fluconazole with hydrochlorothiazide 50 mg for 10 days in volunteers resulted in a 41% increase in peak plasma concentration, and a 43% increase in the area under the curve [AUC] of fluconazole; this is thought to be due to a mean decrease of approximately 20% in the renal clearance of fluconazole)

» Isoniazid or
» Rifampin

(concurrent use of rifampin may increase the metabolism of fluconazole, itraconazole, and ketoconazole, lowering their plasma concentrations; this may lead to clinical failure or relapse; concurrent use of isoniazid with ketoconazole has also been reported to decrease serum concentrations of ketoconazole; isoniazid or rifampin should be used with caution when given concurrently with azole antifungals)

» Phenytoin

(concurrent use with any azole antifungal may decrease the metabolism of phenytoin, resulting in increased plasma phenytoin concentrations; a 75% increase in the AUC of phenytoin was found in volunteers given 200 mg of fluconazole per day; concurrent use has also been reported to decrease the plasma concentration of azole antifungals, which may lead to clinical failure or relapse of the fungal infection; response to both medications should be closely monitored)

Rifabutin
(pharmacokinetic studies with fluconazole and rifabutin show that fluconazole appears to increase the serum concentration of rifabutin; however, this is not thought to have clinical significance, and rifabutin dosing does not need to be modified in patients receiving fluconazole)

Theophylline
(fluconazole has been found to increase serum theophylline concentrations by approximately 13%, which may lead to toxicity; theophylline concentrations should be monitored)

» Warfarin
(anticoagulant effects may be increased when warfarin is used concurrently with any azole antifungal, resulting in an increase in prothrombin time [PT]; PT must be carefully monitored in patients receiving warfarin and azole antifungals)

## Laboratory value alterations
The following have been selected on the basis of their potential clinical significance (possible effect in parentheses where appropriate)—not necessarily inclusive (» = major clinical significance):

With physiology/laboratory test values
» Alanine aminotransferase (ALT [SGPT]) and
» Alkaline phosphatase and
» Aspartate aminotransferase (AST [SGOT]) and
» Bilirubin, serum
(values may be elevated)

Lipid profile, serum
(hyperlipidemia has occurred in patients receiving intravenous miconazole; this is reportedly due to the vehicle in the miconazole solution, PEG 40 castor oil [chremophor EL])

» Potassium, serum
(hypokalemia has occurred in approximately 2 to 6% of patients treated with itraconazole, and has resulted in ventricular fibrillation, especially at higher doses)

» Corticosteroid concentrations, serum, ACTH-induced and
» Testosterone concentrations, serum
(ACTH-induced serum corticosteroid concentrations and serum testosterone concentrations may be decreased by doses of 800 mg of ketoconazole daily; serum testosterone concentrations are abolished by doses of 1.6 grams of ketoconazole daily, but return to baseline values when ketoconazole is discontinued)

## Medical considerations/Contraindications
The medical considerations/contraindications included here have been selected on the basis of their potential clinical significance (reasons given in parentheses where appropriate)—not necessarily inclusive (» = major clinical significance):

*Except under special circumstances, this medication should not be used when the following medical problem exists:*
» Hypersensitivity to azole antifungals

*Risk-benefit should be considered when the following medical problems exist:*
» Achlorhydria or
» Hypochlorhydria
(may cause marked reduction in absorption of itraconazole and ketoconazole; patients with acquired immunodeficiency syndrome [AIDS] may have reduced itraconazole and ketoconazole absorption due to hypochlorhydria)

» Alcoholism, active or in remission or
» Hepatic function impairment
(azole antifungals are metabolized in the liver and may, infrequently, be hepatotoxic; azole antifungals, especially ketoconazole, should be used with caution in patients with liver function impairment or a history of alcoholism)

(ketoconazole has also been reported to cause a disulfiram-like reaction to alcohol, characterized by flushing, rash, peripheral edema, nausea, and headache; symptoms resolved within a few hours)

» Renal function impairment
(because fluconazole is excreted through the kidneys, a reduction in dosage, or increase in dosing interval, is recommended in patients with renal function impairment)

## Patient monitoring
The following may be especially important in patient monitoring (other tests may be warranted in some patients, depending on condition; » = major clinical significance):
Blood urea nitrogen or
Creatinine concentration, serum
(blood urea nitrogen or serum creatinine concentrations should be monitored as clinically indicated in patients taking fluconazole since patients with renal function impairment will require an adjustment in dosage)

» Hepatic function determinations
(liver function tests are recommended prior to treatment, monthly for 3 to 4 months after treatment is started, and periodically thereafter during treatment in patients receiving ketoconazole; elevated serum enzyme values may occur without clinical hepatitis; however, ketoconazole should be discontinued if even minor abnormalities in enzyme values persist or worsen, or if they are accompanied by symptoms of hepatotoxicity; mild, transient increase in transaminases may occur with fluconazole and itraconazole therapy, and may, on rare occasion, progress to hepatotoxicity; liver function tests should be monitored periodically during treatment; fluconazole and itraconazole should be discontinued if abnormal enzyme values persist or worsen, or if they are accompanied by symptoms of hepatotoxicity)

» Potassium, serum
(hypokalemia has occurred in patients treated with itraconazole, and has been associated with ventricular fibrillation)

# Side/Adverse Effects

Note: In patients taking ketoconazole, hepatotoxicity, consisting primarily of hepatocellular damage or mixed hepatocellular and cholestatic changes, has been reported in approximately 1 in 10,000 exposed patients. It is usually, but not always, reversible upon discontinuation of ketoconazole, and fatalities have been reported rarely. It is considered to be an idiosyncratic reaction and can occur at any time during therapy. Females and patients over the age of 40 may be predisposed to hepatotoxicity. Several cases of hepatitis have also been reported in children.

High-dose ketoconazole therapy has also been shown to suppress corticosteroid secretion. In addition, ketoconazole has been shown to lower serum testosterone concentrations at doses of 800 mg per day, and abolish concentrations at 1600 mg per day; these concentrations return to baseline values when ketoconazole is discontinued.

The overall incidence of side effects with fluconazole has been reported to be higher in HIV-infected patients (21%) than in those being treated with fluconazole who were not infected with HIV (13%); however, many patients in these studies were also receiving other medications known to be hepatotoxic or associated with exfoliative skin disorders, making a direct causal association with fluconazole difficult.

The following side/adverse effects have been selected on the basis of their potential clinical significance (possible signs and symptoms in parentheses where appropriate)—not necessarily inclusive:

## Those indicating need for medical attention
Incidence more frequent
*Phlebitis* (redness, swelling, or pain at injection site)—for miconazole
Incidence less frequent
*Hypersensitivity* (fever and chills; skin rash or itching)
Incidence rare
*Agranulocytosis* (fever and sore throat)—for fluconazole; *anemia* (unusual tiredness or weakness)—for miconazole; *exfoliative skin disorders, including Stevens-Johnson syndrome* (reddening, blistering, peeling, or loosening of skin and mucous membranes)—for fluconazole; *hepatotoxicity* (dark or amber urine; loss of appetite; pale stools; stomach pain; unusual tiredness or weakness; yellow eyes or skin); *thrombocytopenia* (unusual bleeding or bruising)—for fluconazole and miconazole

## Those indicating need for medical attention only if they continue or are bothersome
Incidence less frequent
*CNS effects* (dizziness; drowsiness; headache); *flushing or redness of face or skin*—for miconazole; *gastrointestinal disturbances* (abdominal pain; constipation; diarrhea; loss of appetite; nausea; vomiting)
Incidence rare—for ketoconazole
*Gynecomastia* (enlargement of the breasts in males); *impotence* (decreased sexual ability in males); *menstrual irregularities; photophobia* (increased sensitivity of the eyes to light)

Note: *Gynecomastia* and *impotence* are due to inhibition of testosterone and adrenal steroid synthesis.

## Patient Consultation

As an aid to patient consultation, refer to *Advice for the Patient, Antifungals, Azole (Systemic).*

In providing consultation, consider emphasizing the following selected information (» = major clinical significance):

**Before using this medication**
» Conditions affecting use, especially:
  Hypersensitivity to azole antifungals
  Fertility—High doses of ketoconazole have been shown to cause menstrual irregularities, oligospermia, azoospermia, and impotence
  Pregnancy—High doses of azole antifungals may cause maternal toxicity, embryotoxicity, and teratogenicity in animals
  Other medications, especially alcohol, antacids, anticholinergics/antispasmodics, oral antidiabetic agents, astemizole, carbamazepine, cisapride, cyclosporine, didanosine, digoxin, hepatotoxic medications, histamine $H_2$-receptor antagonists, isoniazid, omeprazole, phenytoin, rifampin, sucralfate, terfenadine, or warfarin
  Other medical problems, especially achlorhydria, alcoholism, hepatic function impairment, hypochlorhydria, or renal function impairment

**Proper use of this medication**
» Taking itraconazole and ketoconazole with food to increase absorption
  Proper administration technique for oral liquids
  Proper administration technique in achlorhydria
» Compliance with full course of therapy
» Importance of not missing doses and taking at evenly spaced times
» Proper dosing
  Missed dose: Taking as soon as possible; not taking if almost time for next dose; not doubling doses
» Proper storage

**Precautions while using this medication**
  Checking with physician if no improvement within a few days
» Not taking oral itraconazole, oral ketoconazole, or miconazole injection with terfenadine, cisapride, or astemizole; concurrent use may cause cardiac arrhythmias
» Avoiding alcoholic beverages or other alcohol-containing preparations while taking ketoconazole because of increased risk of hepatotoxicity
» Avoiding antacids and other medications that increase gastrointestinal pH while taking itraconazole or ketoconazole; concurrent use may decrease the absorption of itraconazole or ketoconazole
  Possible photophobic reactions when taking ketoconazole; wearing sunglasses and avoiding bright light to minimize potential eye discomfort

**Side/adverse effects**
  Phlebitis, hypersensitivity, agranulocytosis, anemia, exfoliative skin disorders, hepatotoxicity and thrombocytopenia

---

### *FLUCONAZOLE*

## Summary of Differences

Indications:
  Also indicated for the treatment of vulvovaginal candidiasis.
Pharmacology/pharmacokinetics:
  Good penetration into the cerebrospinal fluid; 80% of an administered dose is eliminated as unchanged drug in the urine.
Precautions:
  Medical considerations/contraindications—Dose may need to be adjusted in patients with renal function impairment.
  Drug interactions and/or related problems—Use with oral antidiabetic agents has increased the plasma concentration of these sulfonylurea agents, leading to hypoglycemia.
Side/adverse effects:
  Increased risk of exfoliative skin disorders, including Stevens-Johnson syndrome, agranulocytosis, and thrombocytopenia.

## Additional Dosing Information

Because oral fluconazole is almost completely bioavailable, the daily oral dose is the same as the intravenous dose.

Intravenous fluconazole should be administered at a maximum rate of approximately 200 mg per hour by continuous infusion.

---

The dose of fluconazole and the length of treatment should be based on the site of infection and the individual response to therapy. Treatment should be continued until clinical parameters and laboratory tests indicate that active fungal infection has subsided. AIDS patients with cryptococcal meningitis or recurrent oropharyngeal candidiasis require maintenance therapy to prevent relapse.

Patients undergoing bone marrow transplantion in whom severe granulocytopenia is anticipated should start fluconazole prophylaxis several days before the anticipated onset of neutropenia, and continue treatment for seven days after the neutrophil count rises above 1000 cells per mm³.

Adults with impaired renal function require an adjustment in dose as follows:

| Creatinine Clearance (mL/min)/ (mL/sec) | Percent of Recommended Dose |
|---|---|
| >50/0.83 | 100 |
| 11–50/0.18–0.83 | 50 |
| Hemodialysis patients | 100 after each dialysis |

On dialysis days, the dose of fluconazole should be administered after hemodialysis has been performed since a single 3-hour dialysis period will reduce plasma fluconazole concentrations by approximately 50%.

## Oral Dosage Forms
### FLUCONAZOLE FOR ORAL SUSPENSION
**Usual adult and adolescent dose**
Antifungal—
  Candidiasis (prophylaxis)[1]: Oral, 400 mg once a day.
  Candidiasis, disseminated (treatment): Oral, 400 mg on the first day, then 200 mg once a day for at least four weeks and for at least two weeks following the resolution of symptoms.
  Candidiasis, esophageal (treatment): Oral, 200 mg on the first day, then 100 mg once a day for at least three weeks and for at least two weeks following the resolution of symptoms. Doses of up to 400 mg once a day may be used depending on clinical response.
  Candidiasis, oropharyngeal (treatment): Oral, 200 mg on the first day, then 100 mg once a day for at least two weeks.
  Candidiasis, vulvovaginal (treatment)[1]: Oral, 150 mg as a single dose.
  Cryptococcal meningitis (treatment): Oral, 400 mg once a day until a clear clinical response is seen, then 200 to 400 mg once a day for at least ten to twelve weeks after the cerebrospinal fluid becomes culture negative.
  Note: Some clinicians prefer a loading dose of 400 mg two times a day for two days, then 400 mg a day for at least ten to twelve weeks after the cerebrospinal fluid becomes culture negative.
  Cryptococcal meningitis (suppressive therapy): Oral, 200 mg once a day.

**Usual pediatric dose**
Dosage has not been established; however, a small number of children from 2 weeks to 14 years of age have been safely treated with doses of 3 to 6 mg per kg of body weight once a day.

**Strength(s) usually available**
U.S.—
  10 mg per mL (when reconstituted according to manufacturer's instructions) (Rx) [*Diflucan* (sucrose)].
  40 mg per mL (when reconstituted according to manufacturer's instructions) (Rx) [*Diflucan* (sucrose)].
Canada—
  Not commercially available.

**Packaging and storage**
Store between 5 and 30 °C (41 and 86 °F) in a well-closed container. Protect from freezing.

**Stability**
After reconstitution, suspensions retain their potency for 14 days.

**Auxiliary labeling**
• Shake well.
• Continue medicine for full time of treatment.
• Beyond-use date.

**Note**
When dispensing, include a calibrated liquid-measuring device.

### FLUCONAZOLE TABLETS
**Usual adult and adolescent dose**
See *Fluconazole for Oral Suspension.*

**Usual pediatric dose**
See *Fluconazole for Oral Suspension.*

## Strength(s) usually available
U.S.—
    50 mg (Rx) [*Diflucan*].
    100 mg (Rx) [*Diflucan*].
    200 mg (Rx) [*Diflucan*].
Canada—
    50 mg (Rx) [*Diflucan*].
    100 mg (Rx) [*Diflucan*].

## Packaging and storage
Store below 40 °C (104 °F), preferably between 15 and 30 °C (59 and 86 °F), in a well-closed container, unless otherwise specified by manufacturer.

## Auxiliary labeling
• Continue for full time of treatment.

# Parenteral Dosage Forms
## FLUCONAZOLE INJECTION
### Usual adult and adolescent dose
Antifungal—
    Candidiasis (prophylaxis): Intravenous, 400 mg once a day.
    Candidiasis, disseminated (treatment): Intravenous, 400 mg on the first day, then 200 mg once a day for at least four weeks and for at least two weeks following the resolution of symptoms.
    Candidiasis, esophageal (treatment): Intravenous, 200 mg on the first day, then 100 mg once a day for at least three weeks and for at least two weeks following the resolution of symptoms. Doses of up to 400 mg once a day may be used depending on clinical response.
    Candidiasis, oropharyngeal (treatment): Intravenous, 200 mg on the first day, then 100 mg once a day for at least two weeks.
    Cryptococcal meningitis (treatment): Intravenous, 400 mg once a day until a clear clinical response is seen, then 200 to 400 mg once a day for at least ten to twelve weeks after the cerebrospinal fluid becomes culture negative. The patient should be switched to fluconazole tablets when oral therapy can be administered.
    Note: Some clinicians prefer a loading dose of 400 mg two times a day for two days, then 400 mg a day for at least ten to twelve weeks after the cerebrospinal fluid becomes culture negative.
    Cryptococcal meningitis (suppressive therapy): Intravenous, 200 mg once a day.

### Usual pediatric dose
Dosage has not been established; however, a small number of children from 3 to 13 years old have been safely treated with doses of 3 to 6 mg per kg of body weight once a day.

### Strength(s) usually available
U.S.—
    200 mg in 100 mL (Rx) [*Diflucan*].
    400 mg in 200 mL (Rx) [*Diflucan*].
Canada—
    200 mg in 100 mL (Rx) [*Diflucan*].

### Packaging and storage
Store below 40 °C (104 °F), preferably between 15 and 30 °C (59 and 86 °F), unless otherwise specified by manufacturer. Protect from freezing.

### Incompatibilities
Intravenous admixtures of fluconazole and other medications are not recommended.

---

[1]Not included in Canadian product labeling.

---

## *ITRACONAZOLE*

# Summary of Differences
Precautions:
    Drug interactions and/or related problems—
        Antacids, anticholinergics/antispasmodics, histamine H₂-receptor antagonists, or omeprazole will increase the pH of the stomach and decrease the absorption of itraconazole.
        Use with astemizole, cisapride, or terfenadine is contraindicated and may increase the risk of cardiac arrhythmias, including torsades de pointes.
        Didanosine contains a buffer to increase its absorption; this will decrease the absorption of itraconazole since itraconazole needs an acidic environment.
        Use with oral antidiabetic agents has increased the plasma concentration of these sulfonylurea agents, leading to hypoglycemia.
        Use with carbamazepine may decrease itraconazole plasma concentrations, leading to clinical failure or relapse.
        Itraconazole may increase digoxin concentrations, leading to digoxin toxicity.
    Medical considerations/contraindications—
        Achlorhydria or hypochlorhydria will decrease the absorption of itraconazole.

# Additional Dosing Information
The dose of itraconazole and the length of treatment should be based on the site of infection and the individual response to therapy. Treatment may be continued for weeks or months until clinical parameters and laboratory tests indicate that active fungal infection has subsided.

Because patients with acquired immunodeficiency syndrome (AIDS) may have reduced absorption of itraconazole due to hypochlorhydria, they may require higher doses to achieve a clinical response.

Although studies did not provide for a loading dose, in life-threatening situations, a loading dose of 200 mg 3 times a day (600 mg per day) for the first 3 days is recommended, based on pharmacokinetic data.

Doses above 200 mg per day should be given in two divided doses.

## Diet/Nutrition
Itraconazole should be taken with food to increase absorption of the medication.

# Oral Dosage Forms
Note: Bracketed uses in the *Dosage Forms* section refer to categories of use and/or indications that are not included in U.S. product labeling.

## ITRACONAZOLE CAPSULES
### Usual adult and adolescent dose
Antifungal—
    Aspergillosis (treatment): Oral, 200 mg one or two times a day with meals for at least three months.
    Blastomycosis (treatment)[1]; or
    Histoplasmosis (treatment): Oral, 200 mg once a day with meals. The dose may be increased by 100 mg, up to a maximum of 400 mg a day, if there is no obvious improvement or if there is evidence of progressive fungal disease.
    [Candidiasis, esophageal (treatment)] or
    [Candidiasis, oropharyngeal (treatment)]: Oral, 100 to 200 mg once a day with a meal for fourteen days; the dose for AIDS and neutropenic patients is increased to 200 mg for four weeks.
    [Candidiasis, vulvovaginal (treatment)][1]: Oral, 200 mg once a day with a meal for three days.
    [Chromomycosis (treatment)]—Oral, 100 to 200 mg once a day with a meal for three to six months.
    [Coccidioidomycosis (treatment)][1]: Oral, 200 mg two times a day with meals for six weeks.
    [Cryptococcal meningitis (suppression)][1] or
    [Cryptococcosis (treatment)][1]: Oral, 200 mg two times a day with meals.
    [Histoplasmosis (suppression)][1]: Oral, 200 mg two times a day with meals.
    [Onychomycosis (treatment)][1]: Oral, 100 to 200 mg once a day with a meal for three to six months.
    [Paracoccidioidomycosis (treatment)]—Oral, 100 mg once a day with a meal for six months.
    [Sporotrichosis (treatment)]—Oral, 100 mg once a day with a meal for three months.
    [Tinea corporis (treatment)][1] or
    [Tinea cruris (treatment)][1]: Oral, 100 mg once a day with a meal for fifteen days.
    [Tinea manuum (treatment)][1] or
    [Tinea pedis (treatment)][1]: Oral, 100 mg once a day with a meal for thirty days.

### Usual pediatric dose
Safety and efficacy have not been established. A small number of patients 3 to 16 years of age have been treated with 100 mg per day of itraconazole for systemic fungal infections, and no serious adverse effects have been reported.

### Strength(s) usually available
U.S.—
    100 mg (Rx) [*Sporanox*].
Canada—
    100 mg (Rx) [*Sporanox*].

**Packaging and storage**
Store below 40 °C (104 °F), preferably between 15 and 30 °C (59 and 86 °F), in a well-closed container, unless otherwise specified by manufacturer.

**Auxiliary labeling**
• Take with food.
• Continue medicine for full time of treatment.

---

[1]Not included in Canadian product labeling.

---

### *KETOCONAZOLE*

## Summary of Differences

Pharmacology/pharmacokinetics:
Ketoconazole has been shown to suppress corticosteroid secretion and lower serum testosterone concentrations.
Ketoconazole penetrates poorly into the cerebrospinal fluid.
Precautions:
Pregnancy/reproduction—
Ketoconazole may cause menstrual irregularities, oligospermia, azoospermia, impotence, and decreased male libido.
Drug interactions and/or related problems—
Alcohol and hepatotoxic medications may increase the risk of hepatotoxicity.
Antacids, anticholinergics/antispasmodics, histamine $H_2$-receptor antagonists, or omeprazole will increase the pH of the stomach and decrease the absorption of ketoconazole.
Use with astemizole, cisapride, or terfenadine is contraindicated and may increase the risk of cardiac arrhythmias, including torsades de pointes.
Didanosine contains a buffer to increase its absorption, which will decrease the absorption of ketoconazole.
Medical considerations/contraindications—
Achlorhydria or hypochlorhydria will decrease the absorption of ketoconazole.
Side/adverse effects:
Increased risk of hepatotoxicity and of side effects due to inhibition of testosterone and corticosteroid synthesis, such as menstrual irregularities, oligospermia, azoospermia, impotence, and decreased male libido.

## Additional Dosing Information

In patients with achlorhydria or hypochlorhydria, higher serum concentrations may be achieved by taking the medication with an acidic drink. Ketoconazole may be dissolved in cola or seltzer water and swallowed, or the medication may be taken with a glass of cola or seltzer water. An alternative is to dissolve each tablet in 4 mL of 0.2 $N$ hydrochloric acid. Patients may further dilute the resulting mixture in a small amount of water and should be instructed to drink it through a plastic or glass straw to avoid contact with the teeth. This should be followed by ½ glass (120 mL) of water, which is swished around in the mouth and swallowed.

Therapy should be continued for at least 1 to 2 weeks in candidiasis (3 to 5 days in vaginal candidiasis); for 1 to 8 weeks in dermatomycoses caused by yeasts or dermatophytes, and mycoses of hair and scalp; for 3 months to 1 year in paracoccidioidomycosis; and for 6 months or longer in other systemic mycoses. Chronic mucocutaneous candidiasis usually requires indefinite maintenance treatment to prevent relapse.

### Diet/Nutrition
Ketoconazole may be taken with a meal or snack to minimize nausea or vomiting and to promote absorption.

## Oral Dosage Forms

Note: Bracketed uses in the *Dosage Forms* section refer to categories of use and/or indications that are not included in U.S. product labeling.

### KETOCONAZOLE ORAL SUSPENSION

**Usual adult and adolescent dose**
Antifungal—
Oral, 200 to 400 mg once a day.
Note: Pityriasis versicolor—Oral, 200 mg once a day for five to ten days.
[Candidiasis, vulvovaginal][1]—Oral, 200 to 400 mg once a day for five days.
[Paronychia][1]—Oral, 200 to 400 mg once a day.
[Pneumonia, fungal][1] or
[Septicemia, fungal][1]—Oral, 400 mg to 1 gram once a day.

Cushing's syndrome[1]:—
Oral, 600 mg to 1.2 grams a day.
Carcinoma, prostatic[1]:—
Oral, 400 mg three times a day.

**Usual adult prescribing limits**
Antifungal—
Up to 1 gram a day.
[Antiadrenal; antineoplastic][1]—
Up to 1.2 grams a day

**Usual pediatric dose**
Antifungal—
Children up to 2 years of age:
Dosage has not been established.
Children over 2 years of age:
Oral, 3.3 to 6.6 mg per kg of body weight once a day.
Note: [Candidiasis, vulvovaginal][1]—Oral, 5 to 10 mg per kg of body weight once a day for five days.
[Paronychia][1] or
[Pneumonia, fungal][1] or
[Septicemia, fungal][1]—Oral, 5 to 10 mg per kg of body weight once a day.

**Strength(s) usually available**
U.S.—
Not commercially available.
Canada—
100 mg per 5 mL (Rx) [*Nizoral*].

**Packaging and storage**
Store below 40 °C (104 °F), preferably between 15 and 30 °C (59 and 86 °F), in a well-closed container, unless otherwise specified by manufacturer. Protect from freezing.

**Auxiliary labeling**
• Shake well.
• Avoid alcoholic beverages.
• May cause dizziness or drowsiness.
• Continue medicine for full time of treatment (antifungal only).

### KETOCONAZOLE TABLETS USP

**Usual adult and adolescent dose**
See *Ketoconazole Oral Suspension*.

**Usual adult prescribing limits**
See *Ketoconazole Oral Suspension*.

**Usual pediatric dose**
See *Ketoconazole Oral Suspension*.

**Strength(s) usually available**
U.S.—
200 mg (Rx) [*Nizoral* (scored; lactose)].
Canada—
200 mg (Rx) [*Nizoral* (scored; lactose)].

**Packaging and storage**
Store below 40 °C (104 °F), preferably between 15 and 30 °C (59 and 86 °F), unless otherwise specified by manufacturer. Store in a well-closed container.

**Auxiliary labeling**
• Avoid alcoholic beverages.
• May cause dizziness or drowsiness.
• Continue medicine for full time of treatment (antifungal only).

---

[1]Not included in Canadian product labeling.

---

### *MICONAZOLE*

## Summary of Differences

Precautions: Drug interactions and/or related problems—Use with cisapride is contraindicated and may increase the risk of cardiac arrhythmias, including torsades de pointes.

## Additional Dosing Information

Rapid administration of undiluted miconazole injection may result in transient tachycardia or arrhythmias. There have been reports of cardiorespiratory arrest and/or anaphylaxis. The intravenous infusion should be administered slowly over a period of approximately 2 hours per 200-mg dose.

An initial dose of 200 mg should be administered by intravenous infusion under the supervision of a physician to determine if the patient is hypersensitive to the medication.

In fungal meningitis, intravenous infusion of miconazole must be supplemented with intrathecal administration of miconazole to achieve a therapeutic drug concentration. Intrathecal injections may be alternated among lumbar, cervical, and cisternal punctures every 3 to 7 days.

In mycoses of the bladder, intravenous infusion of miconazole must be supplemented with bladder irrigation with miconazole to achieve a therapeutic drug concentration.

Nausea or vomiting may be minimized by reducing the dose, slowing the rate of infusion, avoiding administration at mealtime, or administering antihistaminics or antiemetics prior to miconazole intravenous infusion.

## Parenteral Dosage Forms
### MICONAZOLE INJECTION USP

**Usual adult and adolescent dose**
Antifungal:
Intravenous infusion, 200 mg to 1.2 grams per infusion. The following daily doses may be divided over three intravenous infusions:

| | Dose Range per Day | Duration of Therapy (wks) |
|---|---|---|
| Candidiasis | 600 mg to 1.8 grams | 1 to >20 |
| Coccidioidomycosis | 1.8 to 3.6 grams | 3 to >20 |
| Cryptococcosis | 1.2 to 2.4 grams | 3 to >12 |
| Paracoccidioidomycosis | 200 mg to 1.2 grams | 2 to >16 |
| Pseudallescheriasis | 600 mg to 3 grams | 5 to >20 |

Note: For use as an adjunct to the intravenous infusion of miconazole in the treatment of fungal meningitis—Intrathecal, 20 mg of undiluted miconazole injection, as a single dose, every three to seven days.

For use as an adjunct to the intravenous infusion of miconazole in the treatment of mycoses of the bladder—Irrigation, 200 mg of

diluted injection; may be instilled into the bladder two to four times a day or as a continuous irrigation.

**Usual pediatric dose**
Antifungal—
Children up to 1 year of age: Dosage has not been established. However, there are reports of twenty-one neonates treated with doses of 3 to 50 mg per kg of body weight per day, divided into three or four doses. The majority were treated with 15 to 30 mg per kg of body weight a day.
Children 1 year of age and over: Intravenous infusion, 20 to 40 mg per kg of body weight per day; each dose should not exceed 15 mg per kg of body weight.

**Strength(s) usually available**
U.S.—
200 mg in 20 mL (Rx) [Monistat i.v. (methylparaben 0.5 mg; propylparaben 0.05 mg; PEG 40 castor oil)].
Canada—
Not commercially available.

**Packaging and storage**
Store between 15 and 30 °C (59 and 86 °F).

**Preparation of dosage form**
To prepare intravenous infusion, dilute each ampul of miconazole in at least 200 mL of 0.9% sodium chloride injection. As an alternative, 5% dextrose injection may be used as the diluent.

**Stability**
Following dilution, miconazole solution is stable at room temperature for 48 hours.
If the solution darkens in color, it should be discarded, since this is a sign of deterioration.

**Incompatibilities**
Miconazole injection should not be admixed with other medications.

Revised: 05/20/94
Interim revision: 11/14/94; 04/18/95

## Table 1. Pharmacology/Pharmacokinetics*

| Drug | Route of Administration | Bioavailability (%) | Vol$_D$ | CSF/Serum Concentrations (%) | Protein Binding (%) | Metabolism |
|---|---|---|---|---|---|---|
| Fluconazole | IV, PO | 90 (fasting) | 0.7–1.0 L/kg | 54–85 (patients with meningitis) | 11 | Hepatic† |
| Itraconazole | PO | 40–55 (fasting) 90–100 (with food) | 796 L | <10 | 99 | Hepatic# |
| Ketoconazole | PO | 75 (with food) | 0.36 L/kg | <10 | 99 | Hepatic |
| Miconazole | IV | | 1400 L | <10 | 99 | Hepatic |

*IV=intravenous; PO=oral; Vol$_D$=apparent volume of distribution; CSF=cerebrospinal fluid; L/kg=liters per kilogram.
†Fluconazole is primarily excreted by the kidneys; however, a small amount of the drug is hepatically metabolized.
#Itraconazole is extensively metabolized by the liver, with more than 30 identifiable inactive metabolites. The major metabolite, hydroxyitraconazole, has antifungal activity.

## Table 2. Pharmacology/Pharmacokinetics

| Drug | Half-life (hr) | | Time to Peak Serum Concentration (hr) | Peak Serum Concentration After Dose | | Renal Excretion (% unchanged) | Biliary Excretion |
| | Normal Renal Function | Impaired Renal Function | | mcg/mL | Dose | | |
| --- | --- | --- | --- | --- | --- | --- | --- |
| Fluconazole | 30 (adults) 14–20 (children) | 98–125 | 1–2 | 4.5–8 | 100 mg | >80 | Yes; small amount |
| Itraconazole | 21 (single dose) 64 (steady state) | | 3–4 | 0.132* 0.234* | 100 mg (with food) 200 mg (with food) | 0.03 | 3–18% |
| Ketoconazole | 8 | | 1–4 | 3.5 | 200 mg (with food) | 2–4 | Yes; primary route of elimination |
| Miconazole | 2.1 (elimination) 24 (terminal) | | | >1 | >9 mg/kg | <1 | |

*The plasma concentrations reported were measured by high performance liquid chromatography (HPLC), specific for itraconazole. When itraconazole in plasma is measured by a bioassay, values reported are approximately 3.3 times higher than those detected by HPLC due to the presence of the bioactive metabolite, hydroxyitraconazole.

---

# ANTIFUNGALS, AZOLE   Vaginal

This monograph includes information on the following: Butoconazole†; Clotrimazole; Econazole*; Miconazole; Terconazole; Tioconazole.

VA CLASSIFICATION (Primary/Secondary): GU300

Note: For a listing of dosage forms and brand names by country availability, see *Dosage Forms* section(s). For a listing of brand names for the articles in this monograph, refer to the General Index.

*Not commercially available in the U.S.
†Not commercially available in Canada.

## Category

Antifungal (vaginal).

## Indications

### Accepted

Candidiasis, vulvovaginal (treatment)—Vaginal azoles are indicated in the local treatment of vulvovaginal candidiasis caused by *Candida albicans* and other species of *Candida* in pregnant (second and third trimesters only) and nonpregnant women.

Not all species or strains of a particular organism may be susceptible to a specific vaginal azole.

### Unaccepted

Vaginal azoles are not effective in the treatment of vulvovaginitis caused by other common pathogens such as *Trichomonas vaginalis*.

The three-day regimen of clotrimazole vaginal tablets is not effective in pregnant women.

## Pharmacology/Pharmacokinetics

### Physicochemical characteristics

Chemical group—
  Imidazoles: Butoconazole, clotrimazole, econazole nitrate, miconazole nitrate, tioconazole.
  Triazole: Terconazole.
Molecular weight—
  Butoconazole nitrate: 474.79.
  Clotrimazole: 344.84.
  Econazole nitrate: 444.70.
  Miconazole nitrate: 479.15.
  Terconazole: 532.47.
  Tioconazole: 387.71.

### Mechanism of action/Effect

Fungistatic; may be fungicidal, depending on concentration; exact mechanism of action unknown. Azoles inhibit biosynthesis of ergosterol or other sterols, damaging the fungal cell membrane and altering its permeability. As a result, loss of essential intracellular elements may occur.

Azoles also inhibit biosynthesis of triglycerides and phospholipids by fungi. In addition, azoles inhibit oxidative and peroxidative enzyme activity, resulting in intracellular buildup of toxic concentrations of hydrogen peroxide, which may contribute to deterioration of subcellular organelles and cellular necrosis. In *Candida albicans*, azoles inhibit transformation of blastospores into invasive mycelial form.

For terconazole—Triazoles are more slowly metabolized than imidazoles. Triazoles also affect sterol synthesis to a lesser degree.

### Absorption

Butoconazole—Approximately 5.5% absorbed systemically following intravaginal administration.

Clotrimazole—3 to 10% estimated to be absorbed following intravaginal administration.

Econazole; miconazole; tioconazole—Small amounts absorbed systemically following intravaginal administration.

Terconazole—Approximately 5 to 8% absorbed in hysterectomized patients and approximately 12 to 16% absorbed in nonhysterectomized patients with tubal ligations.

### Biotransformation

Clotrimazole—Rapidly metabolized to inactive metabolites.

## Precautions to Consider

### Carcinogenicity

For butoconazole; miconazole; terconazole; tioconazole—Long-term studies in animals have not been done.

For clotrimazole—Long-term studies of intravaginal clotrimazole in animals have not been done. However, a long-term study of oral clotrimazole in Wistar strains of rats has not shown that clotrimazole is carcinogenic.

For terconazole—Studies have not been done.

### Mutagenicity

For butoconazole—Butoconazole has not been shown to be mutagenic in studies in appropriate indicator microorganisms.

For terconazole—Terconazole has not been shown to be mutagenic in studies for induction of microbial point mutations (Ames test), induction of cellular transformation, chromosomal breaks (micronucleus test), or in studies for dominant lethal mutations in mouse germ cells.

For tioconazole—No mutagenic or cytogenic effects were observed.

**Pregnancy/Reproduction**

Fertility—For butoconazole: Studies in rabbits or rats, given oral doses of up to 30 or 100 mg per kg of body weight (mg/kg) daily respectively, have not shown that butoconazole causes impaired fertility.

For terconazole: Terconazole has not been shown to cause impairment of fertility in female rats given terconazole orally in doses up to 40 mg/kg daily.

Pregnancy—

*For butoconazole—*

Adequate and well-controlled studies in humans have not been done during the first trimester. Clinical studies in over 200 pregnant women, given butoconazole intravaginally for 3 or 6 days during the second and third trimesters, have not shown that butoconazole causes adverse effects on the fetus. Follow-up reports on infants born to these women have not shown that butoconazole causes any adverse effects.

Studies in rats, given intravaginal doses of 6 mg/kg daily (3 to 7 times the usual human dose) during organogenesis, have shown that butoconazole causes an increase in resorption rate and a decrease in litter size. Butoconazole was not shown to be teratogenic.

Studies in rats, given oral doses of up to 50 mg/kg daily throughout organogenesis, have not shown that butoconazole causes adverse effects on the fetus. The administration of oral doses of 100, 300, or 750 mg/kg daily has resulted in adverse effects (abdominal wall defects, cleft palate) on the fetus, although maternal stress was evident at these higher dosages.

Studies in rabbits, given oral doses (e.g., 150 mg/kg) that caused maternal stress, have not shown that butoconazole causes adverse effects on the fetus.

FDA Pregnancy Category C.

*For clotrimazole—*

Adequate and well-controlled studies in humans have not been done during the first trimester. Reports in up to 177 pregnant women, given clotrimazole intravaginally during the second and third trimesters, have not shown that clotrimazole causes adverse effects on the fetus. Follow-up reports on 71 infants born to these women have not shown that clotrimazole causes any adverse effects.

Studies in rats, given repeated intravaginal doses of up to 100 mg/kg daily, have not shown that clotrimazole causes adverse effects on the fetus.

Studies in rats and mice, given repeated oral doses of 50 to 120 mg/kg, have shown that clotrimazole causes embryotoxicity (possibly secondary to maternal toxicity), impairment of mating, decreased litter size and number of viable young, and decreased survival to weaning. Studies in mice, rabbits, and rats, given oral doses of up to 200, 180, and 100 mg/kg, respectively, have not shown that clotrimazole is teratogenic.

FDA Pregnancy Category B.

*For econazole—*

Adequate and well-controlled studies have not been performed in humans.

*For miconazole—*

Clinical studies in over 500 pregnant women, given miconazole intravaginally for 14 days, have not shown that miconazole causes adverse effects on the fetus. Follow-up reports on infants born to these women have not shown that miconazole causes any adverse effects.

Miconazole crosses the placenta in animals. Studies in animals have shown that miconazole, given in oral doses of 80 mg/kg, causes embryotoxicity and fetotoxicity. Studies in rats have shown that miconazole, given orally, causes prolonged gestation, although this was not shown in studies using rabbits.

FDA Pregnancy Category B.

*For terconazole—*

At oral doses less than or equal to 10 mg/kg, no embryotoxicity was seen in rats. Studies in rats, given terconazole orally in doses of 10 mg/kg daily, have shown that terconazole causes delayed fetal ossification. In studies in rats, given 20 to 40 mg/kg orally during organogenesis, terconazole was shown to cause embryotoxicity (e.g., decreased litter size and number of viable young, reduced fetal weight, delayed ossification, and increased incidence of skeletal abnormalities). The skeletal changes observed (delayed ossification, short wavy ribs) were felt to be secondary to maternal toxicity or stress, which was evident from reduced body weight gain during most of the organogenesis period.

Terconazole has not been shown to be teratogenic in rats given oral doses of up to 40 mg per kg daily or given subcutaneous

doses of up to 20 mg per kg daily, or in rabbits given doses of 20 mg per kg daily.

FDA Pregnancy Category C.

*For tioconazole—*

. Adequate and well-controlled studies have not been performed in humans.

In limited and uncontrolled clinical use in about 20 patients, a single dose administered at varying stages of pregnancy did not appear to interfere with normal progress of the pregnancy and delivery.

In studies in rats, adverse effects on parturition and/or fetal development were observed during local and systemic use.

Labor—Vaginal azoles have been shown to cause dystocia in rats when given through parturition.

For butoconazole: Butoconazole has not been shown to cause dystocia in rabbits given oral doses of up to 100 mg/kg.

For terconazole: Terconazole has not been shown to adversely affect parturition in rats given up to 40 mg/kg orally per day during pregnancy, up through three weeks of lactation.

**Breast-feeding**

It is not known whether vaginal azoles are distributed into breast milk. However, problems in humans have not been documented.

**Pediatrics**

No information is available on the relationship of age to the effects of vaginal azoles.

**Geriatrics**

Appropriate studies on the relationship of age to the effects of vaginal azoles have not been performed in the geriatric population. However, no geriatrics-specific problems have been documented to date.

**Medical considerations/Contraindications**

The medical considerations/contraindications included here have been selected on the basis of their potential clinical significance (reasons given in parentheses where appropriate)—not necessarily inclusive (» = major clinical significance).

*Risk-benefit should be considered when the following medical problem exists:*

Allergy to azoles

## Side/Adverse Effects

The following side/adverse effects have been selected on the basis of their potential clinical significance (possible signs and symptoms in parentheses where appropriate)—not necessarily inclusive:

**Those indicating need for medical attention**

Incidence less frequent

*Vaginal burning, itching, discharge, or other irritation not present before therapy*

Incidence rare

*Hypersensitivity* (skin rash or hives)

**Those indicating need for medical attention only if they continue or are bothersome**

Incidence less frequent or rare

*Abdominal or stomach cramps or pain; burning or irritation of penis of sexual partner; headache*

## Patient Consultation

As an aid to patient consultation, refer to *Advice for the Patient, Antifungals, Azole (Vaginal).*

In providing consultation, consider emphasizing the following selected information (» = major clinical significance):

**Before using this medication**

» Conditions affecting use, especially:

Allergy to azoles

Pregnancy—Some animal studies have shown that vaginal azoles may be embryotoxic or fetotoxic, however, problems have not been documented in humans

Labor—Vaginal azoles have been shown to cause dystocia in some studies when given through labor

**Proper use of this medication**

Reading patient instructions before using medication

Using at bedtime, unless otherwise directed by physician; retaining miconazole vaginal tampons overnight and removing them the following morning

Checking with physician before using applicator if pregnant

Using cream, which is packaged with some of the vaginal suppositories or tablets, by applying it externally to genitalia to treat genital itching

» Compliance with full course of therapy, even if menstruation begins
» Proper dosing
    Missed dose: Inserting as soon as possible; not inserting if almost time
    for next dose
» Proper storage

**Precautions while using this medication**
Checking with physician if no improvement within a few days
Protecting clothing because of possible soiling with vaginal azoles;
    avoiding the use of unmedicated tampons
*Using hygienic measures to cure infection and prevent reinfection*
» Wearing cotton panties instead of synthetic underclothes
    Wearing only freshly washed underclothes

» Use of condom by partner to prevent reinfection; possible need for
    concurrent treatment of male partner; continuing medication if in-
    tercourse occurs during treatment

» Using douche prior to next dose; not overfilling vagina with douche
    solution; avoiding use of a douche during pregnancy

**Side/adverse effects**
Signs of potential side effects, especially hypersensitivity, and vaginal
    burning, itching, or other irritation not present before therapy

## General Dosing Information

If there is no response to therapy, the course of therapy may be repeated
after other pathogens have been ruled out by potassium hydroxide
(KOH) smears and cultures.

If sensitization or irritation occurs, treatment with vaginal azoles should
be discontinued.

The vehicles for some vaginal azole products contain lipid-based components. It is not known whether these products affect the performance
of latex contraceptive devices, such as cervical caps, condoms, or
diaphragms.

---

### BUTOCONAZOLE

## Vaginal Dosage Forms
**BUTOCONAZOLE NITRATE CREAM (VAGINAL) USP**

**Usual adult and adolescent dose**
Antifungal (vaginal)—
    Nonpregnant patients: Intravaginal, 100 mg (1 applicatorful of a 2%
        cream) once a day at bedtime for three days. May be repeated for
        an additional three days if needed.
    Pregnant patients (second and third trimesters only): Intravaginal, 100
        mg (1 applicatorful of a 2% cream) once a day at bedtime for six
        days.

**Usual pediatric dose**
Dosage has not been established.

**Strength(s) usually available**
U.S.—
    2% (100 mg per applicatorful) (OTC) [*Femstat*].
    Note: Packaging may include either 3 prefilled applicators or 3 card-
        board applicators plus tube of cream.
Canada—
    Not commercially available.

**Packaging and storage**
Store below 40 °C (104 °F), preferably between 15 and 30 °C (59 and 86
    °F), unless otherwise specified by manufacturer. Store in a tight con-
    tainer. Protect from freezing.

**Auxiliary labeling**
• For vaginal use only.
• Continue medicine for full time of treatment.

**Note**
Include patient instructions when dispensing.

**BUTOCONAZOLE NITRATE VAGINAL
    SUPPOSITORIES**

**Usual adult and adolescent dose**
Antifungal (vaginal)—
    Nonpregnant patients: Intravaginal, 100 mg once a day at bedtime for
        three days. May be repeated for an additional three days if needed.

**Strength(s) usually available**
U.S.—
    Not commercially available.
Canada—
    Not commercially available.

**Packaging and storage**
Store below 40 °C (104 °F), preferably between 15 and 30 °C (59 and 86
    °F), unless otherwise specified by manufacturer. Store in a well-closed
    container.

**Auxiliary labeling**
• For vaginal use only.
• Continue medicine for full time of treatment.

**Note**
Include patient instructions when dispensing.

---

### CLOTRIMAZOLE

## Vaginal Dosage Forms
**CLOTRIMAZOLE CREAM (VAGINAL) USP**

**Usual adult and adolescent dose**
Antifungal (vaginal)—
    Intravaginal, 50 mg (1 applicatorful of a 1% vaginal cream), once a
        day, preferably at bedtime, for six to fourteen consecutive days;
        or
    Intravaginal, 100 mg (1 applicatorful of a 2% vaginal cream), once a
        day, preferably at bedtime, for three days; or
    Intravaginal, 500 mg (1 applicatorful of a 10% vaginal cream), as a
        single dose, preferably at bedtime.

**Usual pediatric dose**
Dosage has not been established.

**Strength(s) usually available**
U.S.—
    1% (50 mg per applicatorful) (OTC) [*FemCare; Femizole-7; Gyne-
        Lotrimin; Mycelex-7*].
Canada—
    1% (50 mg per applicatorful) (OTC) [*Canesten; Clotrimaderm;
        Myclo-Gyne*].
    2% (100 mg per applicatorful) (OTC) [*Canesten 3; Clotrimaderm*].
    10% (500 mg per applicatorful) (OTC) [*Canesten 1*].
Note: Many of these products are packaged with one reusable vaginal
    applicator or more than one single-use vaginal applicator, or as
    prefilled vaginal applicators.

**Packaging and storage**
Store between 2 and 30 °C (36 and 86 °F). Store in a collapsible tube or
    in a tight container.

**Auxiliary labeling**
• For vaginal use only.
• Continue medicine for full time of treatment.

**Note**
Include patient instructions when dispensing.

**CLOTRIMAZOLE VAGINAL TABLETS USP**

**Usual adult and adolescent dose**
Antifungal (vaginal)—
    Nonpregnant patients: Intravaginal, 500 mg as a single dose, prefera-
        bly at bedtime; 200 mg once a day, preferably at bedtime, for three
        consecutive days; or 100 mg once a day, preferably at bedtime,
        for six or seven consecutive days.
    Pregnant patients: Intravaginal, 100 mg once a day, preferably at bed-
        time, for seven consecutive days.
Note: The three-day regimen is not effective in pregnant women.

    In severe vulvovaginal candidiasis, single-dose treatment with clo-
        trimazole 500-mg vaginal tablets may not be effective. Longer
        treatment with the 100- or 200-mg vaginal tablets or vaginal cream
        is recommended.

**Usual pediatric dose**
Dosage has not been established.

**Strength(s) usually available**
U.S.—
    100 mg (OTC) [*FemCare; Gyne-Lotrimin; Mycelex-7*].
    500 mg (OTC) [*Gyne-Lotrimin; Gyne-Lotrimin Combination Pack*].
    500 mg (Rx) [*Mycelex-G; Mycelex Twin Pack*].
Canada—
    100 mg (OTC) [*Canesten; Canesten Combi-Pak 6-Day Therapy; My-
        clo-Gyne*].
    200 mg (OTC) [*Canesten 3; Canesten Combi-Pak 3-Day Therapy*].
    500 mg (OTC) [*Canesten 1; Canesten Combi-Pak 1-Day Therapy*].
Note: Twin, combination, or combi-paks also contain a small tube of 1%
    clotrimazole cream for external application to genitals for treatment
    of itching.

**Packaging and storage**

Store below 40 °C (104 °F), preferably between 15 and 30 °C (59 and 86 °F), unless otherwise specified by manufacturer. Store in a well-closed container.

**Auxiliary labeling**

• For vaginal use only.
• Continue medicine for full time of treatment.

**Note**

Include patient instructions when dispensing.

---

## ECONAZOLE

# Vaginal Dosage Forms

## ECONAZOLE NITRATE VAGINAL SUPPOSITORIES

**Usual adult and adolescent dose**

Antifungal (vaginal)—
  Intravaginal, 150 mg once a day at bedtime for three days. May be repeated if needed.

**Usual pediatric dose**

Dosage has not been established.

**Strength(s) usually available**

U.S.—
  Not commercially available.
Canada—
  150 mg (Rx) [*Ecostatin*].

**Packaging and storage**

Store below 30 °C (86 °F), in a well-closed container, unless otherwise specified by manufacturer.

**Auxiliary labeling**

• For vaginal use only.
• Continue medicine for full time of treatment.

**Note**

Include patient instructions when dispensing.

---

## MICONAZOLE

# Vaginal Dosage Forms

## MICONAZOLE NITRATE VAGINAL CREAM

**Usual adult and adolescent dose**

Antifungal (vaginal)—
  Intravaginal, one applicatorful once a day at bedtime for seven or fourteen days. May be repeated if needed.

**Usual pediatric dose**

Dosage has not been established.

**Strength(s) usually available**

U.S.—
  2% (OTC) [*Miconazole-7; Monistat 7*].
Canada—
  2% (OTC) [*Monistat 7*].

Note: Many of these products are packaged with one reusable vaginal applicator or more than one single-use vaginal applicator, or as prefilled vaginal applicators.

**Packaging and storage**

Store below 40 °C (104 °F), preferably between 15 and 30 °C (59 and 86 °F), unless otherwise specified by manufacturer. Store in a tight container. Protect from freezing.

**Auxiliary labeling**

• For vaginal use only.
• Continue medicine for full time of treatment.

**Note**

Include patient instructions when dispensing.

## MICONAZOLE NITRATE VAGINAL SUPPOSITORIES USP

**Usual adult and adolescent dose**

Antifungal (vaginal)—
  Intravaginal, 100 mg once a day at bedtime for seven days. May be repeated for seven days if needed; or
  Intravaginal, 200 or 400 mg once a day at bedtime for three days. May be repeated if needed.

**Usual pediatric dose**

Dosage has not been established.

**Strength(s) usually available**

U.S.—
  100 mg (OTC) [*Monistat 7; Monistat 7 Combination Pack*].
  200 mg (Rx) [*Monistat 3*].
  200 mg (OTC) [*Monistat 3 Combination Pack*].
Canada—
  100 mg (OTC) [*Monistat 7; Monistat 7 Dual-Pak*].
  400 mg (OTC) [*Monistat 3; Monistat 3 Dual-Pak*].

Note: Dual packs or combination packs also contain a small tube of 2% miconazole cream for external application to genitals for treatment of itching.

**Packaging and storage**

Store between 15 and 30 °C (59 and 86 °F). Store in a tight container.

**Auxiliary labeling**

• For vaginal use only.
• Continue medicine for full time of treatment.

**Note**

Include patient instructions when dispensing.

## MICONAZOLE NITRATE VAGINAL TAMPONS

**Usual adult and adolescent dose**

Antifungal (vaginal)—
  Intravaginal, 100 mg (1 tampon) once a day at bedtime for five consecutive days; retain vaginally overnight and remove tampon the following morning.

**Usual pediatric dose**

Dosage has not been established.

**Strength(s) usually available**

U.S.—
  Not commercially available.
Canada—
  Not commercially available.

**Packaging and storage**

Store below 40 °C (104 °F), preferably between 15 and 30 °C (59 and 86 °F), in a well-closed container, unless otherwise specified by manufacturer.

**Auxiliary labeling**

• For vaginal use only.
• Continue medicine for full time of treatment.

**Note**

Include patient instructions when dispensing.

---

## TERCONAZOLE

# Vaginal Dosage Forms

## TERCONAZOLE VAGINAL CREAM

**Usual adult and adolescent dose**

Antifungal (vaginal)—
  Intravaginal, 20 mg (1 applicatorful of a 0.4% cream) once a day at bedtime for seven days; or
  Intravaginal, 40 mg (1 applicatorful of a 0.8% cream) once a day at bedtime for three days.

**Usual pediatric dose**

Dosage has not been established.

**Strength(s) usually available**

U.S.—
  0.4% (20 mg per applicatorful) (Rx) [*Terazol 7*].
  0.8% (40 mg per applicatorful) (Rx) [*Terazol 3*].
Canada—
  0.4% (20 mg per applicatorful) (Rx) [*Terazol 7*].
  0.8% (40 mg per applicatorful) (Rx) [*Terazol 3*].

**Packaging and storage**

Store below 40 °C (104 °F), preferably between 15 and 30 °C (59 and 86 °F), in a well-closed container, unless otherwise specified by manufacturer. Protect from freezing.

**Auxiliary labeling**

• For vaginal use only.
• Continue medicine for full time of treatment.

**Note**

Include patient instructions when dispensing.

## TERCONAZOLE VAGINAL SUPPOSITORIES

### Usual adult and adolescent dose
Antifungal (vaginal)—
    Intravaginal, 80 mg once a day at bedtime for three days.

### Usual pediatric dose
Dosage has not been established.

### Strength(s) usually available
U.S.—
    80 mg (Rx) [*Terazol 3*].
Canada—
    80 mg (Rx) [*Terazol 3*].

### Packaging and storage
Store below 40 °C (104 °F), preferably between 15 and 30 °C (59 and 86 °F), in a well-closed container, unless otherwise specified by manufacturer.

### Auxiliary labeling
• For vaginal use only.
• Continue medicine for full time of treatment.

### Note
Include patient instructions when dispensing.

---

## TIOCONAZOLE

## Vaginal Dosage Forms

### TIOCONAZOLE VAGINAL OINTMENT

#### Usual adult and adolescent dose
Antifungal (vaginal)—
    Intravaginal, 300 mg (1 applicatorful of a 6.5% vaginal ointment), as a single dose, preferably at bedtime.
Note: Limited data suggest that a second dose, 1 to 2 weeks later, may be effective for those patients with residual symptoms after one dose.

#### Usual pediatric dose
Dosage has not been established.

#### Strength(s) usually available
U.S.—
    6.5% (300 mg per applicatorful) (Rx) [*Vagistat-1*].

Canada—
    6.5% (300 mg per applicatorful) (Rx) [*Gyno-Trosyd*].

### Packaging and storage
Store below 40 °C (104 °F), preferably between 15 and 30 °C (59 and 86 °F), in a well-closed container, unless otherwise specified by manufacturer.

### Auxiliary labeling
• For vaginal use only.

### TIOCONAZOLE VAGINAL SUPPOSITORIES

#### Usual adult and adolescent dose
Antifungal (vaginal)—
    Intravaginal, 300 mg, as a single dose, preferably at bedtime.
Note: Limited data suggest that a second dose, 1 to 2 weeks later, may be effective for those patients with residual symptoms after one dose.

#### Usual pediatric dose
Dosage has not been established.

#### Strength(s) usually available
U.S.—
    Not commercially available.
Canada—
    Not commercially available.

### Packaging and storage
Store below 40 °C (104 °F), preferably between 15 and 30 °C (59 and 86 °F), in a well-closed container, unless otherwise specified by manufacturer.

### Auxiliary labeling
• For vaginal use only.

### Note
Include patient instructions when dispensing.

## Selected Bibliography

Doering PL, Santiago TM. Drugs for treatment of vulvovaginal candidiasis: comparative efficacy of agents and regimens [review]. Drug Intell Clin Pharm 1990; 24: 1078-83.

---

Revised: 04/21/92
Interim revision: 07/23/92; 07/12/94; 06/07/95; 7/15/96

---

# ANTIGLAUCOMA AGENTS, CHOLINERGIC, LONG-ACTING   Ophthalmic

This monograph includes information on the following: Demecarium; Echothiophate; Isoflurophate.
INN:
    Echothiophate—Ecothiopate Iodide
VA CLASSIFICATION (Primary/Secondary): OP102/OP900; DX900
Other commonly used names are: DFP [Isoflurophate], Difluorophate [Isoflurophate], Dyflos [Isoflurophate]
Note: For a listing of dosage forms and brand names by country availability, see *Dosage Forms* section(s). For a listing of brand names for the articles in this monograph, refer to the General Index.

## Category

Antiglaucoma agent (ophthalmic); cyclostimulant (accommodative esotropia); diagnostic aid (accommodative esotropia).

## Indications

### Accepted

Glaucoma (treatment)—Demecarium, echothiophate, and isoflurophate, which are long-acting cholinesterase inhibitors, are potent miotics. Because of their toxicity, they should be reserved for use in patients with open-angle glaucoma or other chronic glaucomas not satisfactorily controlled with the short-acting miotics and other agents.
    Glaucoma, open-angle (treatment): Demecarium, echothiophate, and isoflurophate are indicated in the treatment of chronic open-angle glaucoma.
    Glaucoma, angle-closure, *after* iridectomy (treatment): Demecarium, echothiophate, and isoflurophate are indicated in the treatment of subacute or chronic angle-closure glaucoma following iridectomy if continued drug therapy is required and short-acting miotics and other agents are inadequate. Long-acting cholinesterase inhibitors are usu-

ally not recommended for use in angle-closure glaucoma *prior* to iridectomy, because they may increase the pupillary block. However, echothiophate may be indicated in subacute or chronic angle-closure glaucoma when surgery is refused or contraindicated in the informed patient who understands the increased risk of pupillary block.
    Glaucoma, secondary (treatment): Echothiophate is indicated in the treatment of certain nonuveitic secondary types of glaucoma, especially glaucoma following cataract surgery.

Esotropia, accommodative (diagnosis) or
Esotropia, accommodative (treatment)—Demecarium, echothiophate, and isoflurophate are indicated in the diagnosis of accommodative esotropia. Demecarium and isoflurophate are indicated in the treatment of accommodative esotropia uncomplicated by anisometropia. Echothiophate may be indicated in the treatment of concomitant esotropias with a significant accommodative component.

## Pharmacology/Pharmacokinetics

### Physicochemical characteristics
Molecular weight—
    Demecarium bromide: 716.60.
    Echothiophate iodide: 383.22.
    Isoflurophate: 184.15.

### Mechanism of action/Effect
Demecarium, echothiophate, and isoflurophate are indirect-acting parasympathomimetic agents, which are also known as cholinesterase inhibitors and anticholinesterases. Cholinesterase inhibitors prolong the effect of acetylcholine, which is released at the neuroeffector junction of parasympathetic postganglion nerves, by inactivating the cholinesterases that break it down. Echothiophate and isoflurophate primarily inactivate pseudocholinesterase and incompletely inactivate acetylcholinesterase, whereas demecarium inactivates both pseudocholinesterase

and acetylcholinesterase. In the eye, this causes constriction of the iris sphincter muscle (causing miosis) and the ciliary muscle (affecting the accommodation reflex and causing a spasm of the focus to near vision). The outflow of the aqueous humor is facilitated, which leads to a reduction in intraocular pressure. Of the 2 actions, the effect on the accommodation reflex is the more transient and generally disappears before termination of the miosis.

Antiglaucoma agent (ophthalmic)—Cholinesterase inhibitors reduce intraocular pressure in both types of primary glaucoma (i.e., angle-closure glaucoma and open-angle glaucoma) primarily by lowering the resistance to the outflow of the aqueous humor. In angle-closure glaucoma, the abnormal contact between the peripheral iris and the peripheral cornea blocks the access of the anterior chamber of aqueous humor to the trabecular meshwork. In open-angle glaucoma, the block is between the trabecular meshwork and the canal of Schlemm. Effects on the volumes of the various intraocular vascular beds (e.g., those of the iris and the ciliary body) and on the rate of secretion of the aqueous humor into the posterior chamber may contribute secondarily to the lowering of pressure. Contraction of the ciliary muscle may act to increase tone and alignment of the trabecular meshwork, which improves outflow of aqueous humor through the meshwork to the canal of Schlemm. The longitudinal ciliary muscle is the major component; the iris sphincter is not relevant in open-angle glaucoma, but its contraction may improve (or worsen) angle-closure glaucoma. In angle-closure glaucoma, the outflow of the aqueous humor is facilitated by the drug-induced contraction of the iris sphincter muscle. This contraction prevents the iris from blocking the entrance to the trabecular space at the canal of Schlemm by lessening pupillary block. However, extreme miosis may actually increase pupillary block, thus worsening angle-closure glaucoma prior to iridectomy. In open-angle glaucoma, although there is no physical obstruction at the entrance to the trabecular space, the trabeculae, which are a meshwork of small-diameter pores, increase their resistance and lose their permeability.

Cyclostimulant (accommodative esotropia)—Cholinesterase inhibitors reduce the amount of convergence associated with a given amount of accommodation, thereby reducing the degree of esotropia.

Diagnostic aid (accommodative esotropia)—See *Cyclostimulant (accommodative esotropia)* above. An accommodative factor is demonstrated if the eyes become better aligned.

### Onset of action
Miosis—Less than 1 hour.
Reduction in intraocular pressure—Within 4 hours.

### Time to peak effect
Miosis—Within 2 hours.
Reduction in intraocular pressure—Within 24 hours.

### Duration of action
Miosis—Up to 1 month.
Reduction in intraocular pressure—Up to 1 month, but usually 24 to 48 hours.

## Precautions to Consider

### Carcinogenicity/Mutagenicity
Studies have not been done for demecarium, echothiophate, and isoflurophate.

### Pregnancy/Reproduction
Fertility—Studies have not been done for demecarium, echothiophate, and isoflurophate.

Pregnancy—
*Demecarium and isoflurophate*—
   Use of demecarium and isoflurophate is not recommended during pregnancy, because of the toxicity of cholinesterase inhibitors in general. If pregnancy occurs while one of these medications is being administered, the patients should be advised of the potential hazard to the fetus.
   FDA Pregnancy Category X.
*Echothiophate*—
   Studies have not been done in humans. However, this ophthalmic medication may be systemically absorbed and should be administered to pregnant women only if clearly needed.
   Studies have not been done in animals.
   FDA Pregnancy Category C.
Note: Although the FDA Pregnancy Categories are different for the above medications, some experts think that all three medications should be rated the same, namely, category X.

### Breast-feeding
Problems in humans have not been documented; however, these ophthalmic medications may be systemically absorbed. Because of the toxicity of cholinesterase inhibitors in general, and the potential for serious adverse reactions in the nursing infant, some clinicians believe that a decision should be made whether to discontinue nursing or discontinue the medication. Other clinicians believe that the concentration of medication in breast milk would be so minute that it would not present a problem.

### Pediatrics
The iris cysts at the pupil margins that may occur following prolonged use of these medications occur frequently in children. The most common systemic effects, especially in children, are *nausea, vomiting, diarrhea,* and *stomach cramps* or *pain*. No other information is available on whether the risk of adverse effects is increased in children, except that one drop of medication will result in a greater systemic dose per kg of body weight in a child than in an adult. Because of the toxicity of these medications, they should be used with caution, after less toxic alternatives have been considered and/or found ineffective. Recommended doses should not be exceeded, and the patient should be carefully monitored during therapy.

### Geriatrics
No information is available on whether the risk of adverse effects from long-acting cholinergic antiglaucoma agents is increased in the elderly. However, because of the toxicity of these medications, they should be used with caution, after less toxic alternatives have been considered and/or found ineffective. Recommended doses should not be exceeded, and the patient should be carefully monitored during therapy.

### Drug interactions and/or related problems
The following drug interactions and/or related problems have been selected on the basis of their potential clinical significance (possible mechanism in parentheses where appropriate)—not necessarily inclusive (» = major clinical significance):

Note: Combinations containing any of the following medications, depending on the amount present, may also interact with this medication.

*For echothiophate or isoflurophate only*
Physostigmine, ophthalmic
   (use of this medication prior to echothiophate or isoflurophate may partially block the effects of the latter medications and shorten their duration of action. Echothiophate and isoflurophate primarily inactivate pseudocholinesterase and incompletely inactivate acetylcholinesterase, whereas physostigmine and demecarium inactivate both pseudocholinesterase and acetylcholinesterase. Prior use of physostigmine inactivates the available acetylcholinesterase, thereby rendering it inaccessible to the incomplete inactivation by echothiophate or isoflurophate. This effect does not occur when physostigmine is given prior to demecarium, because both medications inactivate acetylcholinesterase, thereby producing an additive effect)

*For demecarium, echothiophate, or isoflurophate*
Anesthetics, mucosal-local, ester-derivative, such as benzocaine, butacaine, butamben, and tetracaine or
Anesthetics, parenteral-local, ester-derivative, such as chloroprocaine, procaine, propoxycaine, and tetracaine
   (concurrent use with demecarium, echothiophate, or isoflurophate may inhibit the metabolism of these anesthetics leading to prolonged anesthetic effect and increased risk of toxicity)
» Anticholinergics or other medications with anticholinergic activity (See *Appendix II*) or
» Antimyasthenics (See *Appendix II*) or
» Cholinesterase inhibitors, other, possibly including topical malathion
   (concurrent use of these medications with demecarium, echothiophate, or isoflurophate is not recommended except under strict medical supervision, because of the possibility of additive toxicity; caution may also be warranted with topical application of malathion if excessive quantities of it are used)
Belladonna alkaloids, ophthalmic or
Cyclopentolate or
Tropicamide
   (concurrent use of these parasympatholytics may antagonize the antiglaucoma and miotic actions of demecarium, echothiophate, or isoflurophate; however, tropicamide is expected to have little effect, since it is so short acting)
Carbamate- or organophosphate-type insecticides or pesticides
   (exposure of patients using demecarium, echothiophate, or isoflurophate to these preparations may increase the possibility of systemic effects due to absorption of the insecticide or pesticide through the respiratory tract or skin; patients should be advised to

protect themselves from contact with such insecticides or pesticides during therapy with demecarium, echothiophate, or isoflurophate)

Cocaine
(inhibition of cholinesterase activity by demecarium, echothiophate, or isoflurophate reduces or slows cocaine metabolism, thereby increasing and/or prolonging cocaine's effects and increasing the risk of toxicity; cholinesterase inhibition may persist for weeks or months after demecarium, echothiophate, or isoflurophate has been discontinued)

Corticosteroids, ophthalmic
(chronic or intensive use of ophthalmic corticosteroids may increase intraocular pressure and decrease the efficacy of the antiglaucoma agents)

Edrophonium
(caution is recommended in administering edrophonium to patients with symptoms of myasthenic weakness who are also using demecarium, echothiophate, or isoflurophate; symptoms of cholinergic crisis [overdosage] may be similar to those occurring with myasthenic crisis [underdosage] and the patient's condition may be worsened by use of edrophonium)

» Succinylcholine
(demecarium, echothiophate, or isoflurophate may decrease plasma concentrations or activity of pseudocholinesterase, the enzyme that metabolizes succinylcholine, thereby enhancing the neuromuscular blockade of succinylcholine when it is used concurrently; cardiovascular collapse may occur; in addition, increased or prolonged respiratory depression or paralysis [apnea] may occur, which is of minor clinical significance while the patient is being mechanically ventilated; however, caution and careful monitoring of the patient are recommended during and following concurrent or sequential use, especially if there is a possibility of incomplete reversal of neuromuscular blockade postoperatively; the effects of this interaction may persist for several weeks or months after demecarium, echothiophate, or isoflurophate has been discontinued)

### Medical considerations/Contraindications

The medical considerations/contraindications included here have been selected on the basis of their potential clinical significance (reasons given in parentheses where appropriate)—not necessarily inclusive (» = major clinical significance).

***Risk-benefit should be considered when the following medical problems exist:***

Asthma, bronchial
(systemic absorption of medication may precipitate an attack)

Bradycardia and hypotension, pronounced

Down's syndrome (mongolism)
(echothiophate, and possibly demecarium or isoflurophate, may cause hyperactivity in these children)

Epilepsy

Gastrointestinal disturbances, spastic

Glaucoma, angle-closure, or predisposition to
(medication may increase the narrowing of the angle)

» Glaucoma associated with iridocyclitis
(medication may aggravate the inflammatory process and lead to the development of posterior synechiae)

Hypertension, systemic

Hyperthyroidism

Iritis, quiescent or history of
(medication may aggravate the inflammatory process)

Myasthenia gravis

Myocardial infarction, recent

Parkinsonism

Peptic ulcer

» Retinal detachment, predisposition to or history of
(may result from drug-induced spasm of accommodation)

Sensitivity to the long-acting cholinergic antiglaucoma agent prescribed

Surgery, intraocular
(intraocular surgery performed during the action of these medications may be complicated by severe uveitis that is very difficult to manage; it is recommended that elective intraocular surgery not be performed until the full duration of action of these medications has elapsed)

Urinary tract obstruction

» Uveitis, active or

Uveitis, quiescent or history of
(medication may predispose the patient to the development of posterior synechiae)

Vagotonia, marked

### Patient monitoring

The following may be especially important in patient monitoring (other tests may be warranted in some patients, depending on condition; » = major clinical significance):

Gonioscopy
(recommended prior to, and soon after, initiation of therapy)

Intraocular pressure determinations
(recommended at periodic intervals during therapy)

Ophthalmologic examinations
(recommended at periodic intervals for patients on prolonged therapy, since formation of iris cysts [especially in children], conjunctival thickening, obstruction of nasolacrimal canals, retinal detachment, and lens opacities may occur; also, the condition of the optic nerve should be monitored in patients with glaucoma)

## Side/Adverse Effects

Note: Lens opacities and cataracts may occur following prolonged use of echothiophate, isoflurophate, and possibly demecarium. While there is strong evidence implicating the phosphorylating medications, echothiophate and isofluorophate, there is little or no similar evidence implicating the carbamylating medication, demecarium. If lens opacities occur, they may regress if therapy is discontinued early in their development; however, once cataracts are established, they often continue developing despite cessation of therapy. The incidence of cataracts appears to be directly related to the age of the patient and the concentration, frequency, and duration of the medication.

Retinal detachment has been reported in a few patients during the use of ophthalmic long-acting cholinergic antiglaucoma agents, such as demecarium, echothiophate, or isoflurophate.

Repeated administration of demecarium, echothiophate, or isoflurophate may cause depression of the concentration of cholinesterase in the serum and erythrocytes, resulting in systemic effects.

Iris cysts, conjunctival thickening, and obstruction of nasolacrimal canals may occur following prolonged use of demecarium, echothiophate, or isoflurophate. If iris cysts occur and treatment with demecarium, echothiophate, or isoflurophate is continued, the cysts may enlarge and obscure the vision. In addition, rarely, the cysts may rupture or break free of the iris into the aqueous humor. The cysts usually decrease in size following discontinuation of the medication.

Activation of latent iritis or uveitis may occur following use of demecarium, echothiophate, or isoflurophate.

A paradoxical increase in intraocular pressure may occur following use of demecarium, echothiophate, or isoflurophate. This may be alleviated by the use of a sympathomimetic, such as phenylephrine.

The following side/adverse effects have been selected on the basis of their potential clinical significance (possible signs and symptoms in parentheses where appropriate)—not necessarily inclusive:

### Those indicating need for medical attention

Incidence rare
***Burning, redness, stinging, or other irritation of eyes; eye pain; retinal detachment*** (veil or curtain appearing across part of vision)

Symptoms of systemic absorption
***Bradycardia*** (slow or irregular heartbeat); ***bronchospasm*** (shortness of breath, tightness in chest, or wheezing); ***hypotension, severe*** (unusual tiredness or weakness); ***increased sweating; loss of bladder control; muscle weakness; nausea, vomiting, diarrhea, or stomach cramps or pain; watering of mouth***

Note: The most common systemic effects, especially in children, are *nausea, vomiting, diarrhea,* and *stomach cramps* or *pain.*

Systemic absorption is rare with isoflurophate because systemic absorption from ointment bases is minimal and the isoflurophate that is absorbed is hydrolyzed in the circulation almost immediately.

### Those indicating need for medical attention only if they continue or are bothersome

***Accommodative myopia*** (blurred vision or change in near or distance vision); ***browache; headache; miosis*** (difficulty in seeing at night or in dim light); ***twitching of eyelids; watering of eyes***

# Overdose

For specific information on the agents used in the management of ophthalmic long-acting cholinergic antiglaucoma agents overdose, see:
- *Atropine* in *Anticholinergics/Antispasmodics (Systemic)* monograph; and/or
- *Diazepam* in *Benzodiazepines (Systemic)* monograph.

For more information on the management of overdose or unintentional ingestion, **contact a Poison Control Center** (see *Poison Control Center Listing*).

## Treatment of overdose

Atropine sulfate injection is used as an antidote to the systemic cholinergic effects of demecarium, echothiophate, or isoflurophate.

*For adults*—Intravenous, 2 to 4 mg initially, then 2 mg repeated every five to ten minutes until cholinergic symptoms disappear or signs of atropine toxicity appear.

*For children*—Intravenous or intramuscular, 1 mg initially, then 0.5 to 1 mg every five to ten minutes until cholinergic symptoms disappear or signs of atropine toxicity appear.

Intravenous pralidoxime chloride (dose of 25 mg per kg of body weight [mg/kg]) may be used as an adjunct to atropine therapy to reverse the muscle paralysis caused by nicotinic effects of demecarium, echothiophate, or isoflurophate.

A short-acting barbiturate or diazepam may be administered for convulsions not controlled by atropine; however, the dosage of the barbiturate should be adjusted to avoid central respiratory depression.

Artificial respiration and maintenance of a clear airway are indicated for severe weakness or paralysis of muscles of respiration.

# Patient Consultation

As an aid to patient consultation, refer to *Advice for the Patient, Antiglaucoma Agents, Cholinergic, Long-acting (Ophthalmic)*.

In providing consultation, consider emphasizing the following selected information (» = major clinical significance):

## Before using this medication
» Conditions affecting use, especially:
    Sensitivity to demecarium, echothiophate, or isoflurophate
    Pregnancy—Because of the toxicity of cholinesterase inhibitors in general, these medications are not recommended during pregnancy
    Breast-feeding—Medications may be absorbed into the body and are not recommended during breast-feeding, since they may cause adverse effects in nursing infants; a decision should be made whether to discontinue nursing or discontinue the medication
    Use in children—The iris cysts that may occur following prolonged use of these medications occur frequently in children
    Other medications, especially antimyasthenics; anticholinergics or other medications with anticholinergic activity; or other cholinesterase inhibitors, possibly including topical malathion
    Recent exposure to pesticides or insecticides
    Other medical problems, especially glaucoma associated with iridocyclitis, predisposition to or history of retinal detachment, or active uveitis

## Proper use of this medication
    Proper administration technique for ophthalmic solution; removing excess solution around eye with clean tissue, being careful not to touch eye; washing hands immediately after application to avoid possible systemic absorption; not touching applicator tip to any surface; keeping container tightly closed
    Proper administration technique for ophthalmic ointment; washing hands immediately after application to avoid possible systemic absorption; not washing tip of ointment tube or allowing it to touch moist surface, since medication loses efficacy when exposed to moisture; not touching applicator tip to any surface, wiping tip of ointment tube with clean tissue; keeping container tightly closed; applying at bedtime, since ointment causes blurred vision after administration
» Importance of not using more medication than the amount prescribed
» Proper dosing
    **Missed dose**
    If dosing schedule is—
      Every other day: Applying as soon as possible if remembered same day; if not remembered until the next day, applying it at that time, then skipping a day; not doubling doses
      Once a day: Applying as soon as possible; if not remembered until next day, skipping missed dose and going back to regular dosing schedule; not doubling doses

      More than once a day: Applying as soon as possible; if almost time for next dose, skipping missed dose and going back to regular dosing schedule; not doubling doses
» Proper storage

## Precautions while using this medication
    Regular visits to physician during therapy to check eye pressure and, for patients on prolonged therapy, to examine eyes
» Caution if any kind of surgery is required
» Caution in exposure to carbamate- or organophosphate-type insecticides or pesticides during therapy
» Making sure vision is clear before driving, using machines, or doing anything else that could be dangerous if not able to see well; caution because of possibility of decreased night vision, blurred vision or change in near or distance vision, or blurred vision for short time if using ointment

## Side/adverse effects
    Signs of potential side effects, especially burning, redness, stinging, or other symptoms of systemic absorption; irritation of the eyes; eye pain; and retinal detachment

# General Dosing Information

To reduce the inconvenience of post-medication miosis, the daily dose or one of the daily doses of the medication may be administered at bedtime.

A stronger concentration may be required to produce adequate miosis and reduction in intraocular pressure in eyes with hazel or brown irides than in eyes with blue or light-colored irides because miotics are less effective in heavily pigmented eyes.

To reduce the incidence of iris cyst formation, the frequency of administration should be minimal in all patients, especially in children. In addition, the simultaneous administration of 2.5 to 10% ophthalmic phenylephrine with demecarium, echothiophate, or isoflurophate may prevent iris cyst formation. However, phenylephrine will not prevent iris cysts if the phenylephrine is administered several hours before or after demecarium, echothiophate, or isoflurophate. The 2.5% concentration of phenylephrine appears to be as effective as the 10% concentration and causes less burning upon administration.

Concurrent use of demecarium, echothiophate, or isoflurophate with epinephrine, a beta-adrenergic blocking agent, and/or a carbonic anhydrase inhibitor results in additive effects, thereby providing better control of glaucoma. A reduced dose of demecarium, echothiophate, or isoflurophate may be possible. A dosage reduction of the miotic medication (i.e., demecarium, echothiophate, or isoflurophate) results in the patient experiencing less miosis and/or accommodative block. In addition, concomitant administration of 2.5 to 10% ophthalmic phenylephrine or 1 to 2% ophthalmic epinephrine may improve the visual acuity of some patients by dilating the miotic eye without increasing the intraocular pressure.

Tolerance to demecarium, echothiophate, or isoflurophate may develop with prolonged use. Effectiveness may be restored by changing to another miotic for a short time and then resuming the original medication.

Following long-term use of these medications, dilation of blood vessels and resulting greater permeability will increase postoperative inflammation and may increase the risk of hyphema during ophthalmic surgery; therefore, demecarium, echothiophate, or isoflurophate should be discontinued 2 to 3 weeks before eye surgery.

## For the solution dosage forms only
Although some manufacturers recommend a dose of 2 drops of an ophthalmic solution at appropriate intervals, the conjunctival sac will usually hold only 1 drop. In addition, because of the potency of these medications and the possibility of systemic absorption, the smallest dose possible should be administered.

To avoid excessive systemic absorption, patient should press finger to the lacrimal sac during and for 1 or 2 minutes following instillation of medication.

---

## DEMECARIUM

# Summary of Differences

Precautions: Drug interactions and/or related problems—Physostigmine not listed as a precaution.

# Ophthalmic Dosage Forms
## DEMECARIUM BROMIDE OPHTHALMIC SOLUTION USP

### Usual adult and adolescent dose
Antiglaucoma agent (ophthalmic)—
   Topical, to the conjunctiva, 1 drop of a 0.125 or 0.25% solution one or two times a day.
Cyclostimulant (accommodative esotropia)—
   Topical, to the conjunctiva, 1 drop of a 0.125 or 0.25% solution once a day for two to three weeks, then 1 drop every two days for three to four weeks, at which time the patient's status should be reevaluated. Thereafter, 1 drop one or two times a week to once every two days, depending on the patient's condition.
Note: In the treatment of esotropia uncomplicated by anisometropia, the patient's condition should be evaluated every four to twelve weeks. It is recommended that therapy be discontinued after four months if a dosage of 1 drop every two days is still required to control condition.
Diagnostic aid (accommodative esotropia)—
   Topical, to the conjunctiva, 1 drop of a 0.125 or 0.25% solution once a day for two weeks, then 1 drop every two days for two to three weeks.

### Usual pediatric dose
Antiglaucoma agent (ophthalmic)
Cyclostimulant (accommodative esotropia) or
Diagnostic aid (accommodative esotropia)—
   For infants and young children: Use is not recommended.
   Older children: See *Usual adult and adolescent dose.*
Note: Clinicians differ as to the age at which children may receive this medication, their recommendations ranging from 12 months to 15 years. Other clinicians feel that the lower end of the adult dose range, administered less frequently, may be used for infants and children.

### Strength(s) usually available
U.S.—
   0.125% (Rx) [*Humorsol* (benzalkonium chloride 1:5000; sodium chloride)].
   0.25% (Rx) [*Humorsol* (benzalkonium chloride 1:5000; sodium chloride)].

### Packaging and storage
Store below 40 °C (104 °F), preferably between 15 and 30 °C (59 and 86 °F), unless otherwise specified by manufacturer. Store in a tight, light-resistant container. Protect from freezing.

### Auxiliary labeling
• For the eye.
• Keep container tightly closed.

---

## *ECHOTHIOPHATE*

---

# Ophthalmic Dosage Forms
## ECHOTHIOPHATE IODIDE FOR OPHTHALMIC SOLUTION USP

### Usual adult and adolescent dose
Antiglaucoma agent (ophthalmic)—
   Topical, to the conjunctiva, 1 drop of a 0.03 to 0.25% solution one or two times a day.
Cyclostimulant (accommodative esotropia)—
   Topical, to the conjunctiva, 1 drop of a 0.03 to 0.125% solution once a day or every two days.
Diagnostic aid (accommodative esotropia)—
   Topical, to the conjunctiva, 1 drop of a 0.125% solution once a day at bedtime for two to three weeks.

### Usual pediatric dose
Antiglaucoma agent (ophthalmic)
Cyclostimulant (accommodative esotropia) or
Diagnostic aid (accommodative esotropia)—
   For infants and young children: Use is not recommended.
   Older children: See *Usual adult and adolescent dose.*
Note: Clinicians differ as to the age at which children may receive this medication, their recommendations ranging from 12 months to 15 years, with 2 years being the most recommended age. Other clinicians feel that the lower end of the adult dose range, administered less frequently, may be used for infants and children.

### Strength(s) usually available
U.S.—
   0.03% (equivalent to 1.5 mg per 5 mL of sterile diluent) (Rx) [*Phospholine Iodide* (in powder—potassium acetate; in powder—sodium hydroxide; in powder—acetic acid; in diluent—chlorobutanol 0.55%; in diluent—mannitol; in diluent—boric acid; in diluent—sodium phosphate)].
   0.06% (equivalent to 3 mg per 5 mL of sterile diluent) (Rx) [*Phospholine Iodide* (in powder—potassium acetate; in powder—sodium hydroxide; in powder—acetic acid; in diluent—chlorobutanol 0.55%; in diluent—mannitol; in diluent—boric acid; in diluent—sodium phosphate)].
   0.125% (equivalent to 6.25 mg per 5 mL of sterile diluent) (Rx) [*Phospholine Iodide* (in powder—potassium acetate; in powder—sodium hydroxide; in powder—acetic acid; in diluent—chlorobutanol 0.55%; in diluent—mannitol; in diluent—boric acid; in diluent—sodium phosphate)].
   0.25% (equivalent to 12.5 mg per 5 mL of sterile diluent) (Rx) [*Phospholine Iodide* (in powder—potassium acetate; in powder—sodium hydroxide; in powder—acetic acid; in diluent—chlorobutanol 0.55%; in diluent—mannitol; in diluent—boric acid; in diluent—sodium phosphate)].
Canada—
   0.06% (equivalent to 3 mg per 5 mL of sterile diluent) (Rx) [*Phospholine Iodide* (in powder—potassium acetate; in powder—sodium hydroxide; in powder—acetic acid; in diluent—chlorobutanol 0.5%; in diluent—mannitol; in diluent—hydrochloric acid; in diluent—sodium phosphate)].
   0.125% (equivalent to 6.25 mg per 5 mL of sterile diluent) (Rx) [*Phospholine Iodide* (in powder—potassium acetate; in powder—sodium hydroxide; in powder—acetic acid; in diluent—chlorobutanol 0.5%; in diluent—mannitol; in diluent—hydrochloric acid; in diluent—sodium phosphate)].
   0.25% (equivalent to 12.5 mg per 5 mL of sterile diluent) (Rx) [*Phospholine Iodide* (in powder—potassium acetate; in powder—sodium hydroxide; in powder—acetic acid; in diluent—chlorobutanol 0.5%; in diluent—mannitol; in diluent—hydrochloric acid; in diluent—sodium phosphate)].

### Packaging and storage
Prior to reconstitution, store between 15 and 30 °C (59 and 86 °F), in a tight container. Protect the reconstituted solution from freezing.

### Preparation of dosage form
For reconstitution of echothiophate iodide powder, use only the diluent supplied by the manufacturer to provide for optimum stability. Use aseptic technique.

### Stability
Reconstituted solution is stable for about 3 to 4 weeks at room temperature or for 3 to 6 months if refrigerated, depending on the manufacturer.

### Auxiliary labeling
• For the eye.
• Beyond-use date.
• Keep container tightly closed.

---

## *ISOFLUROPHATE*

---

# Ophthalmic Dosage Forms
## ISOFLUROPHATE OPHTHALMIC OINTMENT USP

### Usual adult and adolescent dose
Antiglaucoma agent (ophthalmic)—
   Topical, to the conjunctiva, a thin strip (approximately 0.5 cm) of a 0.025% ointment once every three days to three times a day.
Cyclostimulant (accommodative esotropia)—
   Topical, to the conjunctiva, a thin strip (approximately 0.5 cm) of a 0.025% ointment once a day at bedtime for two weeks, then once a week to once every two days, depending on the patient's condition, for two months.
Note: In the treatment of esotropia uncomplicated by anisometropia, it is recommended that therapy be discontinued if the patient's condition cannot be maintained on a dosage interval of at least every two days.
Diagnostic aid (accommodative esotropia)—
   Topical, to the conjunctiva, a thin strip (approximately 0.5 cm) of a 0.025% ointment once a day at bedtime for two weeks.

### Usual pediatric dose
Antiglaucoma agent (ophthalmic)
Cyclostimulant (accommodative esotropia) or

Diagnostic aid (accommodative esotropia)—
  For infants and young children: Use is not recommended.
  Older children: See *Usual adult and adolescent dose.*
Note: Clinicians differ as to the age at which children may receive this
  medication, their recommendations ranging from 12 months to 15
  years, with 2 years being the most recommended age. Other clinicians feel that the lower end of the adult dose range, administered
  less frequently, may be used for infants and children.

**Strength(s) usually available**
U.S.—
  0.025% (Rx) [*Floropryl* (polyethylene mineral oil gel)].

**Packaging and storage**
Store below 40 °C (104 °F), preferably between 15 and 30 °C (59 and 86
  °F), unless otherwise specified by manufacturer. Protect from freezing.

**Stability**
Isoflurophate hydrolyzes in the presence of water to form hydrofluoric
  acid and becomes inactivated.

**Auxiliary labeling**
• For the eye.
• Keep container tightly closed.

**Selected Bibliography**
Havener, WH. Ocular pharmacology. 5th ed. St. Louis: Mosby, 1983: 261-
  418, 635-72.
Pavan-Langston D, editor. Manual of ocular diagnosis and therapy. 2nd
  ed. Boston: Little, Brown, 1985: 201-29.

Revised: 06/21/94

---

# ANTIHEMOPHILIC FACTOR    Systemic

VA CLASSIFICATION (Primary): BL300
Other commonly used names are AHF and factor VIII.
Note: For a listing of dosage forms and brand names by country availability,
  see *Dosage Forms* section(s). For a listing of brand names for the
  articles in this monograph, refer to the General Index.

## Category
Antihemorrhagic.

## Indications
Note: Bracketed information in the *Indications* section refers to uses that are
  not included in U.S. product labeling.

**Accepted**
Hemophilia A, hemorrhagic complications of (prophylaxis) or
Hemophilia A, hemorrhagic complications of (treatment)—Antihemophilic
  factor (AHF) is indicated for the control and prevention of bleeding, including bleeding during and following surgical procedures, in patients with
  hemophilia A (classical hemophilia). Human AHF is not likely to be effective in patients with acquired inhibitor antibodies to human AHF when
  the antibody concentration exceeds 5 to 10 Bethesda Units (BU) per mL.
  Alternative treatment modalities available to these patients include anti-
  inhibitor coagulant complex concentrates, factor IX complex concentrates,
  and porcine AHF.

AHF (Porcine) is indicated for the control and prevention of bleeding,
  including bleeding during and following surgical procedures, in hemophiliacs with antibodies to human factor VIII, and in previously non-
  hemophilic patients with spontaneously acquired antibodies to human factor VIII. AHF (Porcine) is used in patients with anti–human factor VIII
  antibody concentrations between 10 and 50 BU per mL, or more than 50
  BU per mL if the anti–porcine factor VIII antibody concentration is less
  than 15 to 20 BU per mL, provided that *in vitro* testing has demonstrated
  lack of cross-reactivity with the factor VIII antibody. Patients with antibody concentrations beyond these ranges are not likely to receive any
  therapeutic benefit from this product.

von Willebrand disease (treatment)
Hypofibrinogenemia (treatment) or
Factor XIII deficiency (treatment)—Cryoprecipitated AHF is indicated in the
  treatment of type I, type II, and type III (severe) von Willebrand disease
  and for the replacement of fibrinogen and factor XIII.

[Coagulation, disseminated intravascular (treatment adjunct)][1] or
[Kasabach-Merritt syndrome (treatment adjunct)][1]—Cryoprecipitated AHF
  may be used as a source of fibrinogen in the treatment of disseminated
  intravascular coagulation. It may be given in conjunction with fresh frozen
  plasma and platelet concentrates, which replace other clotting factors and
  platelets, respectively. Heparin may be added to this regimen, although
  such use is controversial, to inhibit the formation of thrombin and mi-
  crothrombi and to reduce the inappropriate activation and consumption of
  clotting factors and platelets.

Cryoprecipitated AHF may be used as a source of fibrinogen in the treatment of Kasabach-Merritt syndrome. It may be used in conjunction with
  aminocaproic acid and thrombin, which inhibit fibrinolysis and promote
  thrombosis in, and subsequent shrinkage of, the tumor.

**Unaccepted**
AHF products other than the cryoprecipitated AHF do not contain sufficient
  quantities of von Willebrand factor, and therefore are not indicated, in the
  treatment of von Willebrand disease.

---

[1]Not included in Canadian product labeling.

## Pharmacology/Pharmacokinetics

**Physicochemical characteristics**
Source—Antihemophilic factor (AHF) is obtained from pooled human plasma
  or purified porcine plasma, or produced by recombinant DNA technology.
Almost all of the plasma-derived AHF products currently available are sterile,
  nonpyrogenic, high-purity concentrates purified by gel permeation chromatography, ion exchange chromatography, or immunoaffinity chromatography utilizing murine monoclonal antibodies to factor VIII or von
  Willebrand factor (vWf). The purified concentrates contain 25 to 150 times
  as much AHF as an equal volume of fresh plasma. Some products contain
  albumin as a stabilizer, and monoclonal purified products contain trace
  amounts of mouse protein. *Humate-P* is an intermediate-purity product
  and contains small amounts of foreign proteins, including vWf. However,
  this product is not indicated for use in the treatment of von Willebrand
  disease.
AHF (Porcine) is a sterile, high-purity, freeze-dried concentrate, that also contains platelet aggregating factor, the equivalent of porcine vWf, at a concentration of 1 porcine vWf unit for at least 5 units of porcine factor VIII.
Human recombinant AHF (rAHF) is a sterile, nonpyrogenic concentrate with
  biologic activity comparable to that of plasma-derived AHF. rAHF contains albumin as a stabilizer and trace amounts of mouse, hamster, and
  bovine proteins. vWf is co-expressed with rAHF in the production of
  *Recombinate*, and helps to stabilize it; however, it is present in such minute
  quantities that it offers no therapeutic benefit to patients with von Willebrand disease.
Cryoprecipitated AHF is a sterile, frozen concentrate of human AHF obtained
  from the plasma of 1 unit of whole blood or from 1 or more units of
  single-donor fresh frozen plasma.

**Mechanism of action/Effect**
Antihemophilic Factor (AHF), or factor VIII, is an endogenous glycoprotein
  necessary for blood clotting and hemostasis. It is a cofactor necessary for
  factor IX to activate factor X in the intrinsic pathway. In hemophilia A
  (classical hemophilia), there is a deficiency of this clotting factor. The
  average normal plasma activity of factor VIII is designated as 100%, and
  a factor VIII concentration of 25% of normal is required for hemostasis.
  Patients with severe hemophilia have a factor VIII concentration of less
  than 1% of normal and frequently experience bleeding even in the absence
  of trauma. Patients with a factor VIII concentration between 1 and 5%
  (moderate hemophilia) experience less bleeding, and patients with a factor
  VIII concentration greater than 5% (mild hemophilia) usually experience
  bleeding only after obvious trauma. The administration of AHF temporarily replaces the missing clotting factor to correct or prevent bleeding
  episodes.

**Half-life**
Distribution—2.4 to 8 hours.

Elimination—8.4 to 19.3 hours. However, the half-life may be significantly
  reduced in the presence of inhibitor antibodies, or during active consumption of clotting factors.

**Time to peak concentration**
There is conflicting information regarding the time to achieve peak concentration; values have ranged from 10 minutes to 2 hours after intravenous
  administration.

**Time to peak effect**
1 to 2 hours after intravenous administration.

## Precautions to Consider

### Cross-sensitivity and/or related problems

Patients with a history of allergies, especially those who are allergic to pork or pork products, may be allergic to this medication also.

### Carcinogenicity

The carcinogenic potential of antihemophilic factor has not been investigated.

### Mutagenicity

Recombinant antihemophilic factor (rAHF) does not induce reverse mutations, chromosomal aberrations, or an increase in micronuclei in bone marrow polychromatic erythrocytes at doses considerably exceeding plasma concentrations of rAHF *in vitro*, and at doses 10 to 40 times the maximum clinical dose *in vivo*.

### Pregnancy/Reproduction

Pregnancy—Studies have not been done in humans.
Studies have not been done in animals.
FDA Pregnancy Category C.

### Breast-feeding

It is not known whether antihemophilic factor is distributed into breast milk. However, problems in humans have not been documented.

### Pediatrics

Appropriate studies performed to date have not demonstrated pediatrics-specific problems that would limit the usefulness of antihemophilic factor in children.

### Geriatrics

Appropriate studies performed to date have not demonstrated geriatrics-specific problems that would limit the usefulness of antihemophilic factor in the elderly.

### Medical considerations/Contraindications

The medical considerations/contraindications included here have been selected on the basis of their potential clinical significance (reasons given in parentheses where appropriate)—not necessarily inclusive (» = major clinical significance).

*Risk-benefit should be considered when the following medical problems exist:*

Sensitivity to mouse, hamster, or bovine protein
(risk of allergic reaction to these proteins, which may be present in monoclonal antibody–derived and recombinant AHF products)

Sensitivity to antihemophilic factor

### Patient monitoring

The following may be especially important in patient monitoring (other tests may be warranted in some patients, depending on condition; » = major clinical significance):

» Antibody determinations
(recommended periodically to detect the development and concentration of antibodies to factor VIII, and to predict whether or not a patient is likely to respond to AHF therapy. Patients with antibody concentrations lower than 10 Bethesda Units [BU] per mL may be given larger amounts of AHF to complex with and thereby inactivate the antibodies. However, patients with antibody concentrations greater than 10 BU per mL are not likely to respond, even to very large amounts of AHF, and therefore must be treated with alternative modalities)

Direct Coombs' test and
Hematocrit determinations
(recommended when large volumes and/or frequent doses are administered, to detect the onset of progressive anemia; some products contain red blood cell anti-A and anti-B isoantibodies, which may precipitate intravascular hemolysis in patients with blood types A, B, or AB)

» Plasma factor VIII determinations
(recommended periodically to assure that adequate factor VIII concentrations have been achieved and are maintained)

Platelet count
(recommended during the administration of AHF [Porcine] to detect thrombocytopenia)

Pulse rate determinations
(recommended before and during administration; if a significant increase in pulse rate occurs, the infusion should be slowed or halted until the pulse rate returns to normal)

## Side/Adverse Effects

Note: To reduce the risk of transmission of viruses by blood and blood components, potential blood donors are screened, and donor blood is tested and must be found negative for antibodies to human immunodeficiency virus (HIV), hepatitis B surface antigen, antibody to hepatitis B core antigen, and antibody to hepatitis C (non-A, non-B) virus. The concentration of alanine aminotransferase (ALT) also must be within normal limits. However, these precautions are not totally effective in eliminating viral infectivity. To further reduce the risk, plasma-derived AHF concentrates, with the exception of the cryoprecipitated product, are either treated with an organic solvent/detergent combination (tri-*n*-butyl-phosphate [TNBP] and polysorbate-80 [Tween-80], sodium cholate, or Triton X-100) or pasteurized by heating at 60 °C for 10 hours in an aqueous solution. Both processes effectively inactivate lipid-enveloped viruses such as HIV; hepatitis B virus; and hepatitis C virus. Hepatitis A is a non-enveloped virus and has been reported in patients receiving solvent/detergent-treated AHF. However, it is not known if these cases were caused by the concentrate, the water used in processing, or by other sources. AHF (Porcine) is screened for porcine viruses; there have been no reports of transmission of hepatitis or HIV associated with its use. Recombinant AHF carries a very slight risk of transmission of viruses; however, there have been no cases of viral infection attributed to this product.

Unlike the intermediate-purity AHF concentrates, the high-purity concentrates currently available contain virtually no contaminating proteins. The many foreign proteins and alloantigens contained in the intermediate-purity concentrates have been reported to cause downmodulation of immune function, primarily by inhibiting phagocytic function of monocytes and macrophages and by inhibiting secretion of interleukin-2. Studies have not shown downmodulation of immune function with high-purity concentrates; there is minimal evidence that the highly purified concentrates may stabilize the immune function of HIV-positive hemophiliacs.

The development of inhibitor antibodies, which neutralize the procoagulant activity of factor VIII, is a complication associated with the use of AHF. Many studies have found the incidence of antibody development to be between 10 and 15%. However, some studies report occurrences as high as 50% with recombinant AHF products, and occurrences as high as 52% with plasma-derived products. The antibody concentration begins to increase 4 to 7 days after AHF exposure and peaks in 2 to 3 weeks. The risk of developing an antibody is greatest in patients younger than 5 years of age. Antibodies also may develop spontaneously in postpartum women, patients with autoimmune disorders or cancer, or otherwise healthy older adults.

The following side/adverse effects have been selected on the basis of their potential clinical significance (possible signs and symptoms in parentheses where appropriate)—not necessarily inclusive:

### Those indicating need for medical attention

Incidence less frequent
*Anaphylaxis or other allergic reaction to AHF, or to mouse, hamster, or bovine protein* (changes in facial skin color; fast or irregular breathing; puffiness or swelling of the eyelids or around the eyes; shortness of breath, troubled breathing, tightness in chest, and/or wheezing; skin rash, hives, and/or itching—may include anaphylactic shock with sudden, severe decrease in blood pressure and collapse; *hemolytic anemia* (unusual tiredness or weakness); *thrombosis* (tenderness, pain, swelling, warmth, skin discoloration, and prominent superficial veins over affected area)

Incidence rare
*Allergic reaction to albumin* (chills; fever; hives; nausea); *hyperfibrinogenemia; thrombocytopenia* (unusual bleeding or bruising)—for AHF (Porcine) only

Note: Chills and fever also may occur independently of an *allergic reaction to albumin* (incidence less frequent).

### Those indicating need for medical attention only if they continue or are bothersome

Incidence less frequent
*Burning, stinging, or inflammation at injection site* (swelling); *dizziness or lightheadedness; dry mouth; fatigue* (unusual tiredness or weakness); *flushing* (redness of face); *headache; nausea or vomiting; nosebleed; skin rash; unpleasant taste*

## Patient Consultation

As an aid to patient consultation, refer to *Advice for the Patient, Antihemophilic Factor (Systemic).*

In providing consultation, consider emphasizing the following selected information (» = major clinical significance):

**Before using this medication**
» Conditions affecting use, especially:
  Sensitivity to antihemophilic factor or to mouse, hamster, or bovine protein

**Proper use of this medication**
» Proper preparation of medication: bringing dry concentrate and diluent to room temperature before reconstitution; when reconstituting, directing stream of diluent against side of vial of concentrate to avoid foaming of contents; gently swirling vial to dissolve contents; not shaking hard
» Administering within 1 or 3 hours of reconstitution, according to the individual manufacturer's instructions
» Use of plastic disposable syringe and filter needle; safe handling and disposal of syringe and needle
  Proper dosing
  Missed dose: Contacting physician as soon as possible for instructions; if physician is unavailable, using usual dose as soon as it is remembered
» Proper storage

**Precautions while using this medication**
Need for patients newly diagnosed with hemophilia to receive hepatitis B vaccine
» Need to carry identification stating condition and treatment
» Notifying physician if medication seems less effective than usual; this may indicate the development of antibodies to factor VIII

**Side/adverse effects**
Signs of potential side effects, especially allergic reactions, hemolytic anemia, thrombosis, hyperfibrinogenemia, or thrombocytopenia

## General Dosing Information

It is important to verify the existence of a factor VIII deficiency before administering antihemophilic factor (AHF).

AHF is recommended for intravenous use only.

AHF should be administered via plastic disposable syringes because it tends to adhere to the ground-glass surface of all glass syringes.

AHF should be filtered before administration.

Hemophilic patients undergoing surgery, including tooth extractions or other dental surgical procedures, require concurrent antifibrinolytic therapy to prevent or decrease hemorrhaging during and following surgery. Aminocaproic acid may be given as an oral dose of 5 grams immediately after surgery, followed by 2 to 4 grams orally or intravenously every six hours for nine or ten days. Alternatively, an initial oral dose of 2 grams may be given thirty to sixty minutes prior to surgery followed, after surgery, by 2 grams three or four times a day for three to seven days. Or, tranexamic acid may be given as a single dose of 25 mg per kg of body weight orally or 10 mg per kg of body weight intravenously two hours before surgery, followed, after surgery, by 25 mg per kg of body weight orally three or four times a day for two to eight days.

## Parenteral Dosage Forms

### ANTIHEMOPHILIC FACTOR (HUMAN) USP

Note: Each vial of AHF is labeled with the AHF activity expressed in International Units (IU) per vial. This potency assignment is referenced to the World Health Organization International Standard. One IU of factor VIII activity is approximately equal to the AHF activity of 1 mL of fresh plasma, and increases the plasma concentration of factor VIII by 2%. The specific factor VIII activity ranges from 2 to 200 AHF IU per mg of total protein.

Although the dose of AHF must be individualized for each patient based on patient weight, circulating antibody concentration, type of hemorrhage, and desired plasma factor VIII concentration, the following formulas may be used as guides in determining dosage:

Desired AHF increase (% of normal) =
([Dose AHF (IU)]/[Body weight (kg)]) × 2

Dose AHF (IU) =
Body weight (kg) × Desired AHF increase × 0.5

*Hemofil M* and *Profilate OSD* may be administered at a rate not exceeding 10 mL per minute; *Monoclate P* and *Humate-P* may be administered at a rate of 2 or 4 mL per minute, respectively; and the entire dose of *Koate-HP* may be administered over five to ten minutes. However, the rate at which AHF is administered should be guided by the comfort of the patient.

**Usual adult and adolescent dose**
Prophylaxis of spontaneous hemorrhage—
  Intravenous, 25 to 40 IU per kg of body weight, administered three times per week.
Treatment of hemorrhage—
  Mild hemorrhage:
    Intravenous, 8 to 15 IU per kg of body weight, or a quantity sufficient to raise the plasma factor VIII concentration to 20 to 40% of normal. Most mild hemorrhages respond to a single dose. However, if there is further evidence of bleeding, the dose may be repeated every eight to ten hours for one to three days, as needed.
  Moderate hemorrhage:
    Intravenous, initially 15 to 20 IU per kg of body weight or a quantity sufficient to raise the plasma factor VIII concentration to 30 to 50% of normal, followed by 10 to 15 IU per kg of body weight, administered every eight to twelve hours, as needed.
  Severe hemorrhage, or hemorrhage involving vital structures (central nervous system, gastrointestinal tract, iliopsoas sheath, retroperitoneal and retropharyngeal spaces):
    Intravenous, initially 30 to 50 IU per kg of body weight, or a quantity sufficient to raise the plasma factor VIII concentration to 60 to 100% of normal, followed by 20 to 25 IU per kg of body weight, administered every eight to twelve hours.
Control of perisurgical hemostasis—
  Tooth extraction:
    Intravenous, a quantity sufficient to raise the plasma factor VIII concentration to 30 to 50% of normal, administered one hour prior to the procedure. The dose may be repeated if bleeding occurs.
  Minor surgery:
    Intravenous, initially 15 to 20 IU per kg of body weight or a quantity sufficient to raise the plasma factor VIII concentration to 30 to 50% of normal, followed by 10 to 15 IU per kg of body weight, administered every eight to twelve hours, as needed.
  Major surgery:
    Intravenous, a quantity sufficient to raise the plasma factor VIII concentration to 50 to 100% of normal, administered one hour prior to surgery. A second dose, one-half the size of the initial dose, should be given five hours after the first dose. A plasma concentration of at least 30% of normal should be maintained for ten to fourteen days.

**Usual pediatric dose**
See *Usual adult and adolescent dose.*

**Size(s) usually available**
U.S.—
  250 IU with 2.5 mL sterile water for injection provided as diluent (Rx) [*Humate-P* (sodium citrate 14 to 28 mg per 100 IU; sodium chloride 8 to 16 mg per 100 IU; albumin human 16 to 24 mg per 100 IU; other proteins 4 to 20 mg per 100 IU); *Monoclate-P* (sodium ion 300 to 450 mmol per liter; calcium chloride 2 to 5 mmol per liter; albumin human 1 to 2%; mouse protein <50 nanograms per 100 IU)].
  250 IU with 5 mL sterile water for injection provided as diluent (Rx) [*Koate-HP* (heparin ≤5 units per mL; calcium chloride ≤3 mmol; aluminum ≤1 part per million (ppm); albumin human ≤10 mg per mL)].
  250 IU with 10 mL sterile water for injection provided as diluent (Rx) [*Hemofil M* (albumin human 12.5 mg per mL; mouse protein ≤0.1 nanogram); *MelATE* (aluminum 0.1 mcg per IU; sodium ≤320 mmol; chloride ≤300 mmol; citrate ≤20 mmol; calcium ≤2 mmol; heparin ≤1 unit per mL); *Profilate OSD* (heparin ≤2 units per mL); GENERIC].
  500 IU with 5 mL sterile water for injection provided as diluent (Rx) [*Humate-P* (sodium citrate 14 to 28 mg per 100 IU; sodium chloride 8 to 16 mg per 100 IU; albumin human 16 to 24 mg per 100 IU; other proteins 4 to 20 mg per 100 IU); *Koate-HP* (heparin ≤5 units per mL; calcium chloride ≤3 mmol; aluminum ≤1 ppm; albumin human ≤10 mg per mL); *Monoclate-P* (sodium ion 300 to 450 mmol per liter; calcium chloride 2 to 5 mmol per liter; albumin human 1 to 2%; mouse protein <50 nanograms per 100 IU)].
  500 IU with 10 mL sterile water for injection provided as diluent (Rx) [*Hemofil M* (albumin human 12.5 mg per mL; mouse protein ≤0.1 nanogram); *MelATE* (aluminum 0.1 mcg per IU; sodium ≤320 mmol; chloride ≤300 mmol; citrate ≤20 mmol; calcium ≤2 mmol; heparin ≤1 unit per mL); *Profilate OSD* (heparin ≤2 units per mL); GENERIC].
  750 IU with 25 mL sterile water for injection provided as diluent (Rx) [*Profilate OSD* (heparin ≤2 units per mL)].

1000 IU with 10 mL sterile water for injection provided as diluent (Rx) [*Hemofil M* (albumin human 12.5 mg per mL; mouse protein ≤0.1 nanogram); *Humate-P* (sodium citrate 14 to 28 mg per 100 IU; sodium chloride 8 to 16 mg per 100 IU; albumin human 16 to 24 mg per 100 IU; other proteins 4 to 20 mg per 100 IU); *Koate-HP* (heparin ≤5 units per mL; calcium chloride ≤3 mmol; aluminum ≤1 ppm; albumin human ≤10 mg per mL); *MelATE* (aluminum 0.1 mcg per IU; sodium ≤320 mmol; chloride ≤300 mmol; citrate ≤20 mmol; calcium ≤2 mmol; heparin ≤1 unit per mL); *Monoclate-P* (sodium ion 300 to 450 mmol per liter; calcium chloride 2 to 5 mmol per liter; albumin human 1 to 2%; mouse protein <50 nanograms per 100 IU); GENERIC].

1000 IU with 25 mL sterile water for injection provided as diluent (Rx) [*Profilate OSD* (heparin ≤2 units per mL)].

1250 IU with 25 mL sterile water for injection provided as diluent (Rx) [*Profilate OSD* (heparin ≤2 units per mL)].

1500 IU with 10 mL sterile water for injection provided as diluent (Rx) [*Koate-HP* (heparin ≤5 units per mL; calcium chloride ≤3 mmol; aluminum ≤1 ppm; albumin human ≤10 mg per mL)].

1500 IU with 25 mL sterile water for injection provided as diluent (Rx) [*Profilate OSD* (heparin ≤2 units per mL)].

Canada—
250 IU with 5 mL sterile water for injection provided as diluent (Rx) [*Koate-HP* (heparin ≤5 units per mL; calcium chloride ≤3 mmol; aluminum ≤1 ppm; albumin human ≤10 mg per mL); GENERIC].

250 IU with 10 mL sterile water for injection provided as diluent (Rx) [*Hemofil M* (albumin human 12.5 mg per mL; mouse protein ≤0.1 nanogram)].

500 IU with 5 mL sterile water for injection provided as diluent (Rx) [*Koate-HP* (heparin ≤5 units per mL; calcium chloride ≤3 mmol; aluminum ≤1 ppm; albumin human ≤10 mg per mL); GENERIC].

500 IU with 10 mL sterile water for injection provided as diluent (Rx) [*Hemofil M* (albumin human 12.5 mg per mL; mouse protein ≤0.1 nanogram)].

1000 IU with 10 mL sterile water for injection provided as diluent (Rx) [*Hemofil M* (albumin human 12.5 mg per mL; mouse protein ≤0.1 nanogram); *Koate-HP* (heparin ≤5 units per mL; calcium chloride ≤3 mmol; aluminum ≤1 ppm; albumin human ≤10 mg per mL); GENERIC].

1500 IU with 10 mL sterile water for injection provided as diluent (Rx) [*Koate-HP* (heparin ≤5 units per mL; calcium chloride ≤3 mmol; aluminum ≤1 ppm; albumin human ≤10 mg per mL); GENERIC].

## Packaging and storage
The dry concentrates are preferably stored between 2 and 8 °C (36 and 46 °F). However, some products may be stored at temperatures not exceeding 25 °C (77 °F) for 3 months (*Profilate OSD*) or 6 months (*Koate-HP, Monoclate-P, Humate-P*), according to the individual manufacturer's instructions. The solutions should not be refrigerated after reconstitution. The diluent should be protected from freezing.

## Preparation of dosage form
The diluent and dry concentrate should be brought to room temperature, approximately 25 °C (77 °F), prior to reconstitution. They may be removed from the refrigerator and allowed to sit just until they reach room temperature, or in an urgent situation, they may be placed in a warm water bath, 30 to 37 °C (86 to 96 °F). The reconstituted solution should not be shaken, since excessive shaking will cause foaming. The reconstituted solution should be at approximately room temperature at the time of administration.

## Stability
Administration should begin within 1 or 3 hours after reconstitution, according to the individual manufacturer's instructions. Partially used vials should be discarded.

## Incompatibilities
It is recommended that AHF, after reconstitution with the provided diluent, be administered through a separate line, by itself, and without mixing with other intravenous fluids or medications.

# ANTIHEMOPHILIC FACTOR (PORCINE)
Note: The specific activity of AHF (Porcine) is more than 15 porcine units per mg of protein.

*Hyate:C* must be tested *in vitro*, prior to administration, to demonstrate that it will not cross-react with anti-human factor VIII antibodies.

The dose of AHF (Porcine) must be individualized for each patient based on patient weight, circulating antibody concentration, type of hemorrhage, and desired plasma factor VIII concentration.

## Usual adult and adolescent dose
Antihemorrhagic—
Intravenous, 100 to 150 porcine units per kg of body weight administered at a rate of 2 to 5 mL per minute. The dose may be increased if an adequate response is not achieved. Increasing the dose of AHF (Porcine) has been shown to improve the plasma factor VIII concentration, possibly by complexing with and thereby inactivating circulating antibodies.

## Usual pediatric dose
See *Usual adult and adolescent dose*.

## Size(s) usually available
U.S.—
400 to 700 Porcine Units (Rx) [*Hyate:C* (sodium ion ≤200 mmol per liter; citrate ion ≤55 mmol per liter)].
Canada—
400 to 700 Porcine Units (Rx) [*Hyate:C* (sodium ion ≤200 mmol per liter; citrate ion ≤55 mmol per liter)].

## Packaging and storage
The dry concentrate should be stored between −20 and −15 °C (−4 and +5 °F).

## Preparation of dosage form
The dry concentrate should be warmed to 20 to 37 °C (68 to 96 °F) prior to reconstitution. It may be removed from the refrigerator and allowed to sit just until it reaches room temperature, or in an urgent situation, it may be placed in a warm water bath, 20 to 37 °C (68 to 96 °F). The dry concentrate should then be dissolved with 20 mL of sterile water for injection. The vial should be shaken gently until the concentrate is dissolved, taking care to prevent foaming.

## Stability
Administration should begin within 3 hours after reconstitution. Partially used vials should be discarded.

## Incompatibilities
It is recommended that AHF (Porcine), after reconstitution, be administered through a separate line, by itself, and without mixing with other intravenous fluids or medications.

# ANTIHEMOPHILIC FACTOR (RECOMBINANT)
Note: Each vial of AHF is labeled with the AHF activity expressed in International Units (IU) per vial. This potency assignment is referenced to the World Health Organization International Standard. One IU of factor VIII activity is approximately equal to the AHF activity of 1 mL of fresh plasma, and increases the plasma concentration of factor VIII by 2%. The following formulas may be used as guides in determining dosage:

$$\text{Desired AHF increase (\% of normal)} = ([\text{Dose AHF (IU)}]/[\text{Body weight (kg)}]) \times 2$$

$$\text{Dose AHF (IU)} = \text{Body weight (kg)} \times \text{Desired AHF increase} \times 0.5$$

*Kogenate* may be administered over five to ten minutes, and *Recombinate* at a rate of up to 10 mL per minute. However, the rate at which recombinant AHF is administered should be guided by the comfort of the patient.

## Usual adult and adolescent dose
Prophylaxis of spontaneous hemorrhage—
Intravenous, 25 to 40 IU per kg of body weight, administered three times per week.
Treatment of hemorrhage—
Mild hemorrhage:
Intravenous, 10 IU per kg of body weight, or a quantity sufficient to raise the plasma factor VIII concentration to 20 to 40% of normal. Most mild hemorrhages respond to a single dose. However, if there is evidence of further bleeding, the dose may be repeated every eight to ten hours for one to three days, as needed.
Moderate hemorrhage:
Intravenous, 15 to 25 IU per kg of body weight, or a quantity sufficient to raise the factor VIII concentration to 30 to 60%

of normal. The dose may be repeated every eight to ten hours, as needed.

Severe hemorrhage:

Intravenous, initially 40 to 50 IU per kg of body weight, or a quantity sufficient to raise the plasma factor VIII concentration to 60 to 100% of normal, followed by 20 to 25 IU per kg of body weight, administered every eight to twelve hours, as needed.

Control of perisurgical hemostasis—

Tooth extraction:

Intravenous, a quantity sufficient to raise the plasma factor VIII concentration to 30 to 50% of normal, administered as a single dose.

Minor surgery:

Intravenous, 15 to 25 IU per kg of body weight, or a quantity sufficient to raise the factor VIII concentration to 30 to 60% of normal. The dose may be repeated every eight to ten hours, as needed.

Major surgery:

Intravenous, 50 IU per kg of body weight, or a quantity sufficient to raise the factor VIII concentration to 80 to 100% of normal, administered prior to surgery and repeated every six to twenty-four hours after surgery for ten to fourteen days, as needed.

**Usual pediatric dose**

See *Usual adult and adolescent dose.*

**Size(s) usually available**

U.S.—

250 IU with 2.5 mL sterile water for injection provided as diluent (Rx) [*Helixate; Kogenate* (calcium chloride 2 to 5 mmol; sodium 100 to 130 mEq per liter; chloride 100 to 130 mEq per liter; albumin human 4 to 10 mg per mL; mouse protein ≤0.03 nanogram per IU; hamster protein ≤0.04 nanogram per IU)].

250 IU with 10 mL sterile water for injection provided as diluent (Rx) [*Bioclate; Recombinate* (albumin human 12.5 mg per mL; sodium 180 mEq per liter; calcium 200 mcg per mL; von Willebrand factor ≤2 nanograms per IU; mouse protein ≤0.1 nanogram per IU; hamster and bovine proteins ≤1 nanogram per IU)].

500 IU with 5 mL sterile water for injection provided as diluent (Rx) [*Helixate; Kogenate* (calcium chloride 2 to 5 mmol; sodium 100 to 130 mEq per liter; chloride 100 to 130 mEq per liter; albumin human 4 to 10 mg per mL; mouse protein ≤0.03 nanogram per IU; hamster protein ≤0.04 nanogram per IU)].

500 IU with 10 mL sterile water for injection provided as diluent (Rx) [*Bioclate; Recombinate* (albumin human 12.5 mg per mL; sodium 180 mEq per liter; calcium 200 mcg per mL; von Willebrand factor ≤2 nanograms per IU; mouse protein ≤0.1 nanogram per IU; hamster and bovine proteins ≤1 nanogram per IU)].

1000 IU with 10 mL sterile water for injection provided as diluent (Rx) [*Helixate; Kogenate* (calcium chloride 2 to 5 mmol; sodium 100 to 130 mEq per liter; chloride 100 to 130 mEq per liter; albumin human 4 to 10 mg per mL; mouse protein ≤0.03 nanogram per IU; hamster protein ≤0.04 nanogram per IU); *Bioclate; Recombinate* (albumin human 12.5 mg per mL; sodium 180 mEq per liter; calcium 200 mcg per mL; von Willebrand factor ≤2 nanograms per IU; mouse protein ≤0.1 nanogram per IU; hamster and bovine proteins ≤1 nanogram per IU)].

Canada—

250 IU with 2.5 mL sterile water for injection provided as diluent (Rx) [*Kogenate* (calcium chloride 2 to 5 mmol; sodium 100 to 130 mEq per liter; chloride 100 to 130 mEq per liter; albumin human 4 to 10 mg per mL; mouse protein ≤0.03 nanogram per IU; hamster protein ≤0.04 nanogram per IU)].

250 IU with 10 mL sterile water for injection provided as diluent (Rx) [*Recombinate* (albumin human 12.5 mg per mL; sodium 180 mEq per liter; calcium 200 mcg per mL; von Willebrand factor ≤2 nanograms per IU; mouse protein ≤0.1 nanogram per IU; hamster and bovine proteins ≤1 nanogram per IU)].

500 IU with 5 mL sterile water for injection provided as diluent (Rx) [*Kogenate* (calcium chloride 2 to 5 mmol; sodium 100 to 130 mEq per liter; chloride 100 to 130 mEq per liter; albumin human 4 to 10 mg per mL; mouse protein ≤0.03 nanogram per IU; hamster protein ≤0.04 nanogram per IU)].

500 IU with 10 mL sterile water for injection provided as diluent (Rx) [*Recombinate* (albumin human 12.5 mg per mL; sodium 180 mEq per liter; calcium 200 mcg per mL; von Willebrand factor ≤2 nanograms per IU; mouse protein ≤0.1 nanogram per IU; hamster and bovine proteins ≤1 nanogram per IU)].

1000 IU with 10 mL sterile water for injection provided as diluent (Rx) [*Kogenate* (calcium chloride 2 to 5 mmol; sodium 100 to 130 mEq per liter; chloride 100 to 130 mEq per liter; albumin human 4 to 10 mg per mL; mouse protein ≤0.03 nanogram per IU; ham-

ster protein ≤0.04 nanogram per IU); *Recombinate* (albumin human 12.5 mg per mL; sodium 180 mEq per liter; calcium 200 mcg per mL; von Willebrand factor ≤2 nanograms per IU; mouse protein ≤0.1 nanogram per IU; hamster and bovine proteins ≤1 nanogram per IU)].

**Packaging and storage**

The dry concentrates are preferably stored between 2 and 8 °C (36 and 46 °F). However, *Kogenate* may be stored at temperatures not exceeding 25 °C (77 °F) for 3 months. The solution should not be refrigerated after reconstitution. The diluent should be protected from freezing.

**Preparation of dosage form**

The diluent and dry concentrate should be brought to room temperature, approximately 25 °C (77 °F), prior to reconstitution. They may be removed from the refrigerator and allowed to sit just until they reach room temperature, or in an urgent situation, they may be placed in a warm water bath, 30 to 37 °C (86 to 96 °F). The reconstituted solution should not be shaken, since excessive shaking will cause foaming. The reconstituted solution should be at approximately room temperature at the time of administration.

**Stability**

Administration should begin within 3 hours after reconstitution. Partially used vials should be discarded.

**Incompatibilities**

It is recommended that recombinant AHF, after reconstitution with the provided diluent, be administered through a separate line, by itself, and without mixing with other intravenous fluids or medications.

## CRYOPRECIPITATED ANTIHEMOPHILIC FACTOR USP

Note: Cryoprecipitated AHF is blood group–specific; ABO-compatible material is preferred when large amounts of this component are infused, to avoid hemolysis.

Each bag of cryoprecipitated AHF contains a minimum of 80 IU of factor VIII. The following formula may be used as a guide in determining dosage:

Number of bags required = [Body weight (kg) × Desired AHF increase (% normal) × 0.5]/[Average IU cryoprecipitate per bag (minimum 80)]

**Usual adult and adolescent dose**

Hemophilia A—

Intravenous, initially, a loading dose to achieve the desired plasma factor VIII concentration, administered at a rate of 10 mL per minute, followed by a smaller maintenance dose every eight to twelve hours. To maintain hemostasis after surgery, it may be necessary to continue therapy for ten days or more.

von Willebrand disease—

Intravenous, 1 bag per 10 kg of body weight, administered every eight to twelve hours for several days.

Hypofibrinogenemia—

Intravenous, a quantity sufficient to raise the plasma fibrinogen concentration to 50 mg per 100 mL for minor bleeding, or to 100 mg per 100 mL for surgery. Each bag of cryoprecipitated AHF can be expected to raise the fibrinogen concentration 4 to 7 mg per 100 mL.

Disseminated intravascular coagulation—

Intravenous, 1 to 2 bags of cryoprecipitate per liter of patient's plasma.

Kasabach-Merritt syndrome—

Intravenous, a quantity sufficient to raise the plasma fibrinogen concentration to 100 mg per 100 mL.

**Usual pediatric dose**

See *Usual adult and adolescent dose.*

**Strength(s) usually available**

U.S.—

80 IU (Rx) [GENERIC (Available only through approved blood banks; fibrinogen ≥ 150 mg per 15 mL plasma; von Willebrand factor; factor XIII; fibronectin)].

Canada—

80 IU (Rx) [GENERIC (Available only through approved blood banks; fibrinogen ≥ 150 mg; von Willebrand factor)].

**Packaging and storage**

The concentrate should be stored at −18 °C (−0.4 °F). It may be stored for up to 1 year from the date of collection of source material. The solution should not be refrozen after thawing.

**Preparation of dosage form**

The frozen concentrate should be thawed in a water bath at 30 to 37 °C (86 to 98.6 °F) for up to 15 minutes. The reconstituted solution should be maintained at room temperature and administered as soon as possible, but no more than 6 hours after thawing, or 4 hours after the container is entered. For pooling, the precipitate in each concentrate may be mixed with 10 to 15 mL of 0.9% sodium chloride injection. Cryoprecipitated AHF, Pooled, usually requires no extra diluent.

**Stability**

Should not be used if container shows evidence of breakage or if thawing occurred during storage.

**Incompatibilities**

It is recommended that cryoprecipitated AHF be administered through a separate line, by itself, and without mixing with other intravenous fluids (with the exception of 0.9% sodium chloride injection) or medications.

## Selected Bibliography

Bloom AL. Progress in the clinical management of haemophilia. Thromb Haemost 1991; 66: 166-77.

Gill JC. Therapy of factor VIII deficiency. Semin Thromb Hemost 1993; 19: 1-12.

Revised: 7/30/93
Interim revision: 10/10/95

# ANTIHISTAMINES   Systemic

This monograph includes information on the following: Acrivastine#†; Astemizole; Azatadine; Bromodiphenhydramine‡; Brompheniramine; Carbinoxamine‡; Cetirizine*; Chlorpheniramine; Clemastine; Cyproheptadine; Dexchlorpheniramine; Dimenhydrinate; Diphenhydramine; Diphenylpyraline§*; Doxylamine†; Hydroxyzine; Loratadine; Phenindamine; Pyrilamine†; Terfenadine; Tripelennamine; Triprolidine†.

Note: Products listed in this monograph contain single-entity antihistamines. For products containing antihistamines in combination with other medications, refer to *Antihistamines and Decongestants (Systemic)*, *Antihistamines, Decongestants, and Analgesics (Systemic)*, and *Cough/Cold Combinations (Systemic)*.

INN:
Bromodiphenhydramine—Bromazine
Chlorpheniramine—Chlorphenamine
Pyrilamine—Mepyramine

VA CLASSIFICATION (Primary/Secondary):
Acrivastine—AH900
Astemizole—AH900
Azatadine—AH700
Bromodiphenhydramine—AH200
Brompheniramine—AH400
Carbinoxamine—AH200
Cetirizine—AH900
Chlorpheniramine—AH400
Clemastine—AH200
Cyproheptadine—AH700
Dexchlorpheniramine—AH400
Dimenhydrinate—AH200/CN550
Diphenhydramine
    Oral—AH200/AU350; CN309; CN550; RE302
    Parenteral—CN204
Diphenylpyraline—AH700
Doxylamine—AH200/CN309
Hydroxyzine—AH500/CN309
Loratadine—AH900
Phenindamine—AH900
Pyrilamine—AH300
Terfenadine—AH600
Tripelennamine—AH300
Triprolidine—AH400

Note: For a listing of dosage forms and brand names by country availability, see *Dosage Forms* section(s). For a listing of brand names for the articles in this monograph, refer to the General Index.

*Not commercially available in the U.S.
†Not commercially available in Canada.
#Not available in the U.S. as a single entity; however, it is available in the U.S. in a combination product.
§Not available in the U.S. or Canada as a single entity; however, it is available in Canada in combination products.
‡Not available in the U.S. or Canada as a single entity; however, it is available in combination products.

## Category

Antihistaminic (H₁-receptor)—Acrivastine; Astemizole; Azatadine; Bromodiphenhydramine; Brompheniramine; Carbinoxamine; Cetirizine; Chlorpheniramine; Clemastine; Cyproheptadine; Dexchlorpheniramine; Dimenhydrinate; Diphenhydramine; Diphenylpyraline;

Doxylamine; Hydroxyzine; Loratadine; Phenindamine; Pyrilamine; Terfenadine; Tripelennamine; Triprolidine.
Antianxiety agent—Hydroxyzine.
Antidyskinetic—Diphenhydramine.
Antiemetic—Dimenhydrinate; Diphenhydramine; Hydroxyzine (parenteral).
Antitussive—Diphenhydramine Syrup.
Antivertigo agent—Dimenhydrinate; Diphenhydramine.
Sedative-hypnotic—Diphenhydramine; Doxylamine; Hydroxyzine.
Appetite stimulant—Cyproheptadine.
Vascular headache suppressant—Cyproheptadine.
Antiasthmatic—Astemizole; Cetirizine; Loratadine; Terfenadine.

## Indications

Note: Bracketed information in the *Indications* section refers to uses that are not included in U.S. product labeling.

**Accepted**

Rhinitis, perennial and seasonal allergic or vasomotor (prophylaxis and treatment) or

Conjunctivitis, allergic (prophylaxis and treatment)—Antihistamines are indicated in the prophylactic and symptomatic treatment of perennial and seasonal allergic rhinitis, vasomotor rhinitis, and allergic conjunctivitis due to inhalant allergens and foods.

Pruritus (treatment)

Urticaria (treatment)

Angioedema (treatment)

Dermatographism (treatment) or

Transfusion reactions, urticarial (treatment)—Antihistamines are indicated for the symptomatic treatment of pruritus associated with allergic reactions and of mild, uncomplicated allergic skin manifestations of urticaria and angioedema, in dermatographism, and in urticaria associated with transfusions. Cyproheptadine may be particularly useful for cold urticaria. [Antihistamines are also used in the treatment of pruritus associated with pityriasis rosea.][1]

Sneezing (treatment) or

Rhinorrhea (treatment)—Antihistamines are indicated for the relief of sneezing and rhinorrhea associated with the common cold. However, controlled clinical studies have not demonstrated that antihistamines are significantly more effective than placebo in relieving cold symptoms. Non-sedating (i.e., second-generation) antihistamines are unlikely to be useful in the treatment of the common cold symptoms since they do not have clinically significant anticholinergic effects (e.g., drying effects on nasal mucosa)

Anaphylactic or anaphylactoid reactions (treatment adjunct)—Antihistamines are indicated as adjunctive therapy to epinephrine and other standard measures for anaphylactic reactions after the acute manifestations have been controlled, and to ameliorate the allergic reactions to blood or plasma.

Anxiety (treatment) and

Tension, psychosis-related (treatment)—Hydroxyzine is indicated for the relief of anxiety and tension associated with psychoneurosis and as an adjunct in organic disease states in which anxiety is manifested. The effectiveness of hydroxyzine as an antianxiety agent for long-term use (for example, more than 4 months) has not been assessed by systematic clinical studies.

Alcohol withdrawal (treatment)—Parenteral hydroxyzine is indicated in the acute or chronic alcoholic with anxiety withdrawal symptoms.

Parkinsonism (treatment)[1] or

Extrapyramidal reactions, drug-induced (treatment)[1]—Diphenhydramine is indicated for the symptomatic treatment of parkinsonism and drug-induced extrapyramidal reactions in elderly patients unable to tolerate more potent antidyskinetic medications, for mild cases of parkinsonism in other age groups and, in combination with centrally acting anticholinergic agents, for other cases of parkinsonism.

Cough (treatment)—Diphenhydramine hydrochloride syrup is currently indicated as a non-narcotic cough suppressant for control of cough due to colds or allergy.

Motion sickness (prophylaxis and treatment) or

Vertigo (treatment)—Dimenhydrinate and diphenhydramine are indicated for the prevention and treatment of the nausea, vomiting, dizziness, or vertigo of motion sickness.

Nausea or vomiting (prophylaxis and treatment)—Parenteral hydroxyzine is indicated for the control of nausea and vomiting, excluding nausea and vomiting of pregnancy.

Sedation—Diphenhydramine and hydroxyzine are indicated for their sedative and hypnotic effects and as preoperative medications.

Insomnia (treatment)—Diphenhydramine and doxylamine are indicated as nighttime sleep aids to help reduce the time to fall asleep in patients having difficulty falling asleep.

Analgesia adjunct, during surgery

Anesthesia, general, adjunct or

Anesthesia, local, adjunct—Parenteral hydroxyzine is useful as pre- and postoperative, and pre- and postpartum adjunctive medication to allow reduction in narcotic dosage, and to control anxiety and emesis.

[Appetite, lack of (treatment)]—Cyproheptadine is used as an appetite stimulant, in adults and children.

[Headache, vascular (treatment)]—Cyproheptadine is used for treatment of vascular headaches, such as migraine and histamine cephalalgia.

[Asthma, bronchial (treatment adjunct)][1]—Astemizole, cetirizine, loratadine, and terfenadine are used as adjunctive treatment to asthma medications to reduce symptoms and improve bronchodilation in patients with mild atopic asthma.

## Unaccepted

Cyproheptadine has been used in the treatment of Cushing's disease because of its pronounced antiserotonin properties, which may decrease corticotropin release. Cyproheptadine may also provide antidiarrheal action against intestinal hypermotility associated with the excessive production of serotonin in patients with carcinoid tumors, and in some other conditions involving the release of serotonin. However, there is no conclusive evidence of effectiveness for these uses.

---

[1]Not included in Canadian product labeling.

# Pharmacology/Pharmacokinetics

## Physicochemical characteristics

Chemical group—

Ethanolamine derivatives: Bromodiphenhydramine; Carbinoxamine; Clemastine; Dimenhydrinate (chlorotheophylline salt of diphenhydramine); Diphenhydramine; Doxylamine

Ethylenediamine derivatives: Pyrilamine; Tripelennamine

Piperidine derivatives: Astemizole; Azatadine; Cyproheptadine; Diphenylpyraline; Loratadine; Phenindamine; Terfenadine

Piperazine derivative: Cetirizine (metabolite of hydroxyzine); Hydroxyzine

Propylamine derivatives (alkylamines): Acrivastine; Brompheniramine; Chlorpheniramine; Dexchlorpheniramine; Triprolidine

Molecular weight—

Astemizole: 458.58.

Azatadine maleate: 522.55.

Bromodiphenhydramine hydrochloride: 370.72.

Brompheniramine maleate: 435.32.

Carbinoxamine maleate: 406.87.

Cetirizine: 461.8.

Chlorpheniramine maleate: 390.87.

Clemastine fumarate: 459.97.

Cyproheptadine hydrochloride: 350.89.

Dexchlorpheniramine maleate: 390.87.

Dimenhydrinate: 469.97.

Diphenhydramine hydrochloride: 291.82.

Diphenylpyraline hydrochloride: 317.86.

Doxylamine succinate: 388.46.

Hydroxyzine hydrochloride: 447.83.

Hydroxyzine pamoate: 763.29.

Loratadine: 382.89.

Phenindamine tartrate: 411.45.

Pyrilamine maleate: 401.46.

Terfenadine: 471.68.

Tripelennamine citrate: 447.49.

Tripelennamine hydrochloride: 291.82.

Triprolidine hydrochloride: 332.87.

pKa—

Azatadine maleate: 9.3.

Brompheniramine maleate: 3.59 and 9.12.

Carbinoxamine maleate: 8.1.

Chlorpheniramine maleate: 9.2.

Cyproheptadine hydrochloride: 9.3.

Diphenhydramine hydrochloride: 9.

Doxylamine succinate: 5.8 and 9.3.

Hydroxyzine hydrochloride: 2.6 and 7.

Tripelennamine: 3.9 and 9.

Triprolidine hydrochloride: 3.6 and 9.3.

## Mechanism of action/Effect

Antihistaminic ($H_1$-receptor)—Antihistamines used in the treatment of allergy act by competing with histamine for $H_1$-receptor sites on effector cells. They thereby prevent, but do not reverse, responses mediated by histamine alone. Antihistamines antagonize, in varying degrees, most of the pharmacological effects of histamine, including urticaria and pruritus. Also, the anticholinergic actions of most antihistamines provide a drying effect on the nasal mucosa.

Antianxiety agent—Hydroxyzine's sedative action may be due to a suppression of activity in certain key regions of the subcortical area of the central nervous system (CNS). It is not a cortical depressant.

Antidyskinetic—The actions of diphenhydramine in parkinsonism and in drug-induced dyskinesias appear to be related to a central inhibition of the actions of acetylcholine, which are mediated via muscarinic receptors (anticholinergic action), and to its sedative effects.

Antiemetic; antivertigo agent—The mechanism by which some antihistamines exert their antiemetic, anti–motion sickness, and antivertigo effects is not precisely known but may be related to their central anticholinergic actions. They diminish vestibular stimulation and depress labyrinthine function. An action on the medullary chemoreceptive trigger zone may also be involved in the antiemetic effect.

Antitussive—Diphenhydramine suppresses the cough reflex by a direct effect on the cough center in the medulla of the brain.

Sedative-hypnotic—Most antihistamines cross the blood-brain barrier and produce sedation due to inhibition of histamine N-methyltransferase and blockage of central histaminergic receptors. Antagonism of other central nervous system receptor sites, such as those for serotonin, acetylcholine, and alpha-adrenergic stimulation, may also be involved. Central depression is not significant with astemizole, cetirizine (low doses), loratadine, or terfenadine because they do not readily cross the blood-brain barrier. Also, they bind preferentially to peripheral $H_1$-receptors rather than to central nervous system $H_1$-receptors.

Appetite stimulant—Cyproheptadine competes with serotonin for receptor sites, thus blocking the responses to serotonin in vascular, intestinal, and other smooth muscles. It is possible that by altering serotonin activity in the appetite center of the hypothalamus, cyproheptadine stimulates appetite.

Vascular headache suppressant—Cyproheptadine's vascular headache suppressant effect is probably due to its antiserotonin action.

Antiasthmatic—Astemizole, cetirizine, loratadine, and terfenadine have been shown to cause mild bronchodilation and also to block histamine-induced bronchoconstriction in asthmatic patients. Also, astemizole, loratadine, and terfenadine have been shown to diminish exercise-induced bronchospasm and hyperventilation-induced bronchospasm. Cetirizine has not been shown to be uniformly effective in preventing allergen- or exercise-induced bronchoconstriction; however, due to its inhibition of late-phase eosinophil recruitment after local allergen challenge, it has been shown to be more effective, in higher doses, than other antihistamines in reducing the symptoms of pollen-induced asthma.

## Other actions/effects

Anticholinergic—Antihistamines prevent responses to acetylcholine that are mediated via muscarinic receptors. The ethanolamine derivatives may show greater anticholinergic activity than the other classes of antihistamines. Astemizole, loratadine, and terfenadine have no significant anticholinergic activity; cetirizine has minimal anticholinergic activity.

Anesthetic, local, dental—Antihistamines are structurally related to local anesthetics and have local anesthetic activity. Local anesthetics prevent the initiation and transmission of nerve impulses by decreasing the permeability of the nerve cell membrane to sodium ions. This action decreases the rate of depolarization of the membrane and prevents the generation of the action potential.

**Absorption**

Well absorbed after oral administration.

Note: Ingestion of food may enhance the absorption of loratadine by 40% and of its active metabolite by 15%; however, it may decrease the absorption of astemizole by 60%.

Food may delay the rate, but not the extent of cetirizine absorption.

In one study involving patients 66 to 78 years of age the extent of absorption and peak plasma levels of loratadine and its metabolite were significantly higher (55%) than those in studies with younger patients.

**Protein binding**

Astemizole—96%.

Cetirizine—93%.

Chlorpheniramine—72%.

Diphenhydramine—98 to 99%.

Loratadine—97% (at concentrations of 2.5 to 100 ng/mL). Descarboethoxyloratadine (active metabolite): 73 to 77% (at concentrations of 0.5 to 100 ng/mL).

Terfenadine—97%.

**Biotransformation**

Hepatic (cytochrome P-450 system); some renal. Of the second-generation antihistamines, astemizole, loratadine, and terfenadine are metabolized by the hepatic cytochrome P-450 system and have active metabolites; however, cetirizine is minimally metabolized and excreted unchanged primarily thorough the kidneys.

**Half-life**

Elimination—

Acrivastine—1.5 to 3.5 hours.

Astemizole (plus hydroxylated metabolites)—Multiple doses, biphasic with an initial half-life of 7 to 9 days (with plasma concentrations being reduced by 75% within this phase) and a terminal half-life of about 19 days.

Azatadine—12 hours.

Brompheniramine—25 hours.

Carbinoxamine—10 to 20 hours.

Cetirizine—8 hours (range, 6.5 to 10 hours).

　In dialysis patients: 20 hours.

　In children: 4.1 to 6 hours.

Chlorpheniramine—14 to 25 hours.

Diphenhydramine—1 to 4 hours.

Hydroxyzine—20 to 25 hours.

Loratadine—3 to 20 hours (mean, 8.4 hours). Descarbethoxyloratadine (active metabolite): 8.8 to 92 hours (mean, 28 hours).

Terfenadine—8.5 hours. Acid metabolite of terfenadine: Biphasic with an initial mean plasma half-life of 3.5 hours followed by a mean plasma half-life of 6 hours.

Triprolidine—3 to 3.3 hours.

Note: In children, cetirizine, chlorpheniramine, hydroxyzine, and terfenadine have been found to have shorter elimination half-life values.

**Onset of action**

Oral—

Most first-generation antihistamines: 15 to 60 minutes.

Acrivastine: 0.5 hour.

Astemizole: < 24 hours (depending on initial severity of symptoms, the maximum effect may not occur until the second or third day).

Cetirizine: 0.58 hour (mean).

Loratadine: 1 hour.

Terfenadine: 1 to 2 hours (reaching maximum effect at 3 to 4 hours, and lasting over 12 hours).

Parenteral—

Dimenhydrinate: Intramuscular, 20 to 30 minutes.

Rectal—

Dimenhydrinate: 30 to 45 minutes.

**Time to peak concentration**

Oral—

Acrivastine—0.8 to 1.7 hours.

Astemizole—Within 1 hour.

Azatadine—4 hours.

Brompheniramine—2 to 5 hours.

Cetirizine—1 hour.

Chlorpheniramine—2 to 6 hours.

Clemastine—2 to 4 hours.

Diphenhydramine—1 to 4 hours.

Loratadine—1 to 2 hours.

Descarbethoxyloratadine (active metabolite)—3 to 4 hours.

Terfenadine—2 hours.

Triprolidine—2 hours.

**Time to peak effect**

Oral—

Astemizole: 9 to 12 days.

Brompheniramine: 3 to 9 hours.

Cetirizine: 4 to 8 hours.

Chlorpheniramine: 6 hours.

Clemastine: 5 to 7 hours.

Loratadine: 4 to 6 hours.

Terfenadine: 3 to 4 hours.

Triprolidine: 2 to 3 hours.

**Duration of action**

Ethanolamine derivatives—

6 to 8 hours.

Clemastine: 12 hours.

Dimenhydrinate: 3 to 6 hours.

Ethylenediamine derivatives—

Pyrilamine: 8 hours.

Tripelennamine: 4 to 6 hours.

Piperazine derivatives—

4 to 6 hours.

Cetirizine: Up to 24 hours.

Piperidine derivatives—

Astemizole: Depending on the length of therapy, skin test suppression may last for several weeks after discontinuation of astemizole.

Azatadine: 12 hours.

Cyproheptadine: 8 hours.

Diphenylpyraline: 12 hours.

Loratadine: At least 24 hours.

Phenindamine: 4 to 6 hours.

Terfenadine: Over 12 hours.

Propylamine derivatives—

4 to 8 hours.

Acrivastine: 6 to 8 hours.

**Elimination**

Renal (primarily fecal with astemizole and terfenadine). Most of the antihistamines studied (except cetirizine) are excreted as metabolites within 24 hours.

Cetirizine—

Approximately 60% of the total dose administered is excreted unchanged in urine within 24 hours; about 10% is excreted in feces.

Loratadine—

Approximately 80% of the total dose administered is excreted equally in urine and feces in the form of metabolic products after 10 days. Twenty-seven percent of the total dose is excreted in the urine in the conjugated form within 24 hours.

Terfenadine—

Sixty percent of the dose is eliminated in the feces (50% as acid metabolite, 2% unchanged terfenadine, and the remainder as unidentified metabolites). Approximately 40% of the total dose is excreted renally (40% as acid metabolite, 30% dealkyl metabolite, and 30% unidentified metabolites).

## Precautions to Consider

### Cross-sensitivity and/or related problems

Patients sensitive to one of the antihistamines may be sensitive to others.

### Carcinogenicity/Tumorigenicity/Mutagenicity

Long-term animal studies to evaluate carcinogenic, tumorigenic, or mutagenic potential of most antihistamines have not been performed.

*Loratadine—*

In carcinogenicity studies, AUC data demonstrated that the exposure of mice given loratadine 40 mg/kg was 3.6 (loratadine) and 18 (active metabolite) times higher than that for a human given 10 mg/day. Exposure of rats given 25 mg/kg was 28 (loratadine) and 67 (active metabolite) times higher than that for a human given 10 mg/day. Male mice given 40 mg/kg had a significantly higher incidence of hepatocellular tumors (combined adenomas and carcinomas) than concurrent controls. In rats, a significantly higher incidence of hepatocellular tumors (combined adenomas and carcinomas) was observed in males given 10 mg/kg and males and females given 25 mg/kg. The clinical significance of these findings during long-term use of loratadine is not known.

*Terfenadine—*

Studies in mice and rats have not shown evidence of tumorigenicity when terfenadine was given in oral doses 63 times the recommended human daily dose. Microbial and micronucleus test assays with terfenadine have not shown evidence of mutagenesis.

## Pregnancy/Reproduction

Pregnancy—Animal studies have suggested that meclizine and cyclizine, chemically related to antihistamines, might have a teratogenic potential.

*Astemizole—*

Adequate and well-controlled studies in humans have not been done. However, on the basis of 6 times the terminal half-life of astemizole, metabolites may remain in the body as long as 4 months after dosing has stopped.

Studies in rats showed embryocidal effects accompanied by maternal toxicity at doses 100 times the recommended human dose. However, at doses 50 times the recommended human dose, embryotoxicity or maternal toxicity has not been observed in rats or rabbits.

FDA Pregnancy Category C.

*Azatadine, brompheniramine, chlorpheniramine, clemastine, cyproheptadine, dexchlorpheniramine, dimenhydrinate, loratadine, and triprolidine—*

Studies with azatadine, brompheniramine, chlorpheniramine, clemastine, cyproheptadine, dexchlorpheniramine, dimenhydrinate, loratadine, or triprolidine in humans have not been done.

Studies in animals have not shown that these medicines cause adverse effects on the fetus.

FDA Pregnancy Category B.

*Cetirizine—*

Adequate and well-controlled studies in humans have not been done. However, cetirizine is not recommended for use in the early months of pregnancy since studies in mice, rats, and rabbits have shown that it causes fetal abnormalities when given in doses substantially above the human therapeutic range.

*Diphenhydramine—*

Adequate and well-controlled studies in humans have not been done.

Studies in rats and rabbits at doses up to 5 times the human dose have revealed no evidence of impaired fertility or harm to the fetus.

FDA Pregnancy Category B.

*Doxylamine—*

The Food and Drug Administration has stated that human epidemiologic data have not produced convincing evidence that the doxylamine and pyridoxine combination, a medication previously prescribed to treat nausea and vomiting during pregnancy, causes diaphragmatic hernias or other birth defects, as suggested by some animal studies in rats and monkeys. However, further studies in animals and humans are being done.

*Hydroxyzine—*

Adequate and well-controlled studies in humans have not been done. However, hydroxyzine is not recommended for use in the early months of pregnancy since studies in rats have shown that it causes fetal abnormalities when given in doses substantially above the human therapeutic range.

*Terfenadine—*

Adequate and well-controlled studies in humans have not been done.

Studies in rats given doses 63 and 125 times the daily human dose have shown that terfenadine decreased pup weight gain and survival.

FDA Pregnancy Category C.

*Tripelennamine—*

Adequate and well-controlled studies in humans have not been done.

Limited animal reproduction studies have not shown that tripelennamine causes adverse effects in the fetus.

## Breast-feeding

First-generation antihistamines may inhibit lactation because of their anticholinergic actions.

Small amounts of antihistamines are distributed into breast milk; use is not recommended in nursing mothers because of the risk of adverse effects, such as unusual excitement or irritability, in infants.

*Astemizole—*

It is not known whether astemizole is distributed into human breast milk. Astemizole is distributed into the milk of dogs. However, problems in humans have not been documented.

*Cetirizine—*

The extent of distribution into human breast milk is unknown. Studies in beagle dogs indicated that approximately 3% of the dose is distributed into milk.

*Loratadine—*

Loratadine and its metabolite descarboethoxyloratadine are distributed into breast milk, achieving concentrations equivalent to plasma levels. In one study, approximately 0.03% of the administered dose was distributed into breast milk over 48 hours after maternal ingestion of a single oral dose of 40 mg.

*Terfenadine—*

A small amount of terfenadine metabolite is distributed into breast milk.

## Pediatrics

Use is not recommended in newborn or premature infants because this age group has an increased susceptibility to anticholinergic side effects, such as central nervous system (CNS) excitation, and an increased tendency toward convulsions.

A paradoxical reaction characterized by hyperexcitability may occur in children taking antihistamines.

*Astemizole, cetirizine, loratadine, and terfenadine—*

Although adequate and well-controlled studies have not been done in the pediatric population, astemizole, loratadine, and terfenadine are not likely, and cetirizine is less likely than first-generation antihistamines, to cause anticholinergic or significant CNS effects in children.

## Geriatrics

Dizziness, sedation, confusion, and hypotension may be more likely to occur in geriatric patients taking antihistamines.

A paradoxical reaction characterized by hyperexcitability may occur in geriatric patients taking antihistamines.

Geriatric patients are especially susceptible to the anticholinergic side effects, such as dryness of mouth and urinary retention (especially in males), of the antihistamines. If these side effects occur and continue or are severe, medication should probably be discontinued.

*Astemizole, cetirizine, loratadine, and terfenadine—*

Although adequate and well-controlled studies have not been done in the geriatric population, astemizole, loratadine, and terfenadine are not likely, and cetirizine is less likely than first-generation antihistamines, to cause anticholinergic or significant CNS effects in geriatric patients. However, because elderly patients are more likely to have age-related renal function impairment, cetirizine and loratadine may accumulate and cause anticholinergic or CNS effects when given in such patients at the usual adult dose.

## Dental

Prolonged use of antihistamines (except astemizole, cetirizine, loratadine, or terfenadine) may decrease or inhibit salivary flow, thus contributing to the development of caries, periodontal disease, oral candidiasis, and discomfort.

## Drug interactions and/or related problems

The following drug interactions and/or related problems have been selected on the basis of their potential clinical significance (possible mechanism in parentheses where appropriate)—not necessarily inclusive (» = major clinical significance):

Note: It is not likely that astemizole, cetirizine, loratadine, or terfenadine will interact with most of the following medications because they lack significant anticholinergic and CNS actions. However, cetirizine and loratadine have been shown to cause dose-related CNS effects (e.g., sedation); and cetirizine has minimal anticholinergic effects.

Combinations containing any of the following medications, depending on the amount present, may also interact with this medication.

» Alcohol or
» CNS depression–producing medications, other (See *Appendix II*)
(concurrent use may potentiate the CNS depressant effects of either these medications or antihistamines; also, concurrent use of maprotiline or tricyclic antidepressants may potentiate the anticholinergic effects of either antihistamines or these medications)

» Anticholinergics or other medications with anticholinergic activity (See *Appendix II*)
(anticholinergic effects may be potentiated when these medications are used concurrently with antihistamines; patients should be advised to report occurrence of gastrointestinal problems promptly since paralytic ileus may occur with concurrent therapy)

Apomorphine
(prior administration of dimenhydrinate, diphenhydramine, doxylamine, or hydroxyzine may decrease the emetic response to apomorphine in the treatment of poisoning)

Azithromycin
» Clarithromycin
» Erythromycin or
» Troleandomycin

(concurrent use of erythromycin with astemizole and terfenadine has been reported to increase the risk of cardiotoxic effects [prolongation of the QT interval, torsades de pointes, and other ventricular arrhythmias])

(concurrent use of terfenadine with erythromycin, clarithromycin, or troleandomycin is contraindicated; pending further evaluation, concurrent use of terfenadine and azithromycin is not recommended)

(concurrent use of astemizole with erythromycin is contraindicated; pending further evaluation, concurrent use of astemizole with other macrolide antibiotics, such as azithromycin, clarithromycin, and trolenadomycin is not recommended)

Fluconazole
» Itraconazole
» Ketoconazole
Metronidazole or
Miconazole

(concurrent use with ketoconazole or itraconazole may increase plasma levels of astemizole, loratadine, and terfenadine, because of inhibition of the P-450 metabolic pathways by these antifungals; increased plasma levels of astemizole and terfenadine may result in cardiotoxic effects [prolongation of the QT interval, torsades de pointes, and other ventricular arrhythmias]; there are no reports to date of serious ventricular arrhythmias associated with increased plasma levels of loratadine; due to the chemical similarity of fluconazole, metronidazole, and miconazole to ketoconazole, caution is also recommended with concurrent use of these other imidazole antifungals and astemizole or terfenadine)

» Medications causing QT interval prolongation, such as:
Antidepressants, tricyclic
Calcium channel blocking agents, especially bepridil
Disopyramide
Maprotiline
Phenothiazines
Pimozide
Procainamide
Quinidine

(concurrent use of these medications with astemizole or terfenadine may increase risk of cardiac arrhythmias, which are seen on electrocardiogram [ECG] as prolongation of the QT interval)

» Monoamine oxidase (MAO) inhibitors, including furazolidone and procarbazine

(concurrent use of MAO inhibitors with antihistamines may prolong and intensify the anticholinergic and CNS depressant effects of antihistamines; concurrent use is not recommended)

Ototoxic medications (See *Appendix II*)

(concurrent use with antihistamines may mask the symptoms of ototoxicity such as tinnitus, dizziness, or vertigo)

Photosensitizing medications, other

(concurrent use of these medications with antihistamines may cause additive photosensitizing effects)

» Quinine

(concurrent use of a single 430–mg dose of quinine with astemizole has been reported to increase plasma concentrations of astemizole and its metabolite, desmethylastemizole, resulting in prolongation of the electrocardiographic QT interval)

**Laboratory value alterations**
The following have been selected on the basis of their potential clinical significance (possible effect in parentheses where appropriate)—not necessarily inclusive (» = major clinical significance):

With diagnostic test results

*For all antihistamines*
Skin tests using allergen extracts

(antihistamines may inhibit the cutaneous histamine response, thus producing false-negative results; it is recommended that antihistamines be discontinued at least 72 hours before testing begins [at least 4 weeks with astemizole and 1 week with loratadine and terfenadine])

*For hydroxyzine (in addition to those listed for all antihistamines)*
Urine 17-hydroxycorticosteroid determinations

(false increases have been reported with concurrent use of hydroxyzine)

With physiology/laboratory test values

*For cyproheptadine*
Amylase and
Prolactin

(serum concentrations may be increased when cyproheptadine is administered with thyrotropin-releasing hormone)

**Medical considerations/Contraindications**
The medical considerations/contraindications included here have been selected on the basis of their potential clinical significance (reasons given in parentheses where appropriate)—not necessarily inclusive (» = major clinical significance).

*Except under special circumstances, this medication should not be used when the following medical problems exist:*
» Hepatic function impairment

(increased plasma concentrations of astemizole or terfenadine may result, increasing the risk of cardiac arrhythmias or QT prolongation)

» QT interval prolongation, history of

(increased risk of astemizole- or terfenadine-induced arrhythmias)

*Risk-benefit should be considered when the following medical problems exist:*
» Bladder neck obstruction or
» Prostatic hypertrophy, symptomatic or
» Urinary retention, predisposition to

(anticholinergic effects may precipitate or aggravate urinary retention)

» Glaucoma, angle-closure, or predisposition to

(anticholinergic mydriatic effect resulting in increased intraocular pressure may precipitate an attack of angle-closure glaucoma)

Glaucoma, open-angle

(anticholinergic mydriatic effect may cause a slight increase in intraocular pressure; glaucoma therapy may need to be adjusted)

» Hypokalemia

(potassium deficiency, especially from use of diuretics, should be corrected before initiation of therapy with astemizole or terfenadine because of risk of ventricular arrhythmias)

Sensitivity to the antihistamine used

Caution is recommended when dimenhydrinate, diphenhydramine, or hydroxyzine is used, since their antiemetic action may impede diagnosis of such conditions as appendicitis and obscure signs of toxicity from overdosage of other drugs.

## Side/Adverse Effects

The following side/adverse effects have been selected on the basis of their potential clinical significance (possible signs and symptoms in parentheses where appropriate)—not necessarily inclusive:

**Those indicating need for medical attention**
Incidence less frequent or rare
*Blood dyscrasias* (sore throat and fever, unusual bleeding or bruising, unusual tiredness or weakness); *cardiac arrhythmias* (fast or irregular heartbeat)—with high doses of astemizole or terfenadine

Note: *Prolonged QT intervals* and *ventricular arrhythmias* (torsades de pointes or fibrillation), accompanied by syncope and cardiac arrest, have been reported in association with high doses and/or overdose of astemizole and terfenadine. Severe ventricular arrhythmias have been reported with ingestion of 360 mg or more of terfenadine, and with overdoses greater than 200 mg of astemizole. There have been rare cases of this effect occurring with doses as low as 20 to 30 mg of astemizole a day, and in some patients, with possible potentiating circumstances (e.g., concurrent use of medications that prolong the QT interval), taking 10 mg daily. Prolongation of the QT interval < 10 msec has occurred with doses of 60 mg twice daily; greater prolongation has occurred at a higher dose (300 mg twice daily).

**Those indicating need for medical attention only if they continue or are bothersome**
Incidence more frequent—less frequent with cetirizine; rare with astemizole, loratadine, and terfenadine
*Drowsiness; thickening of mucus*

Note: In general, sedative effects are more pronounced with the ethanolamine derivatives (except clemastine) and less pronounced with the propylamine (alkylamine) derivatives.

Tolerance to central effects may develop quickly with some antihistamines, so that sedation is no longer troublesome after a few days.

Incidence of sedation may increase when the recommended doses of astemizole, cetirizine, loratadine, or terfenadine are exceeded.

Incidence less frequent or rare
*Blurred vision or any change in vision; confusion; difficult or painful urination; dizziness; dryness of mouth, nose, or throat; tachycardia* (fast heartbeat); *increased appetite or weight gain*—with as-

temizole, cetirizine, cyproheptadine, loratadine, and terfenadine only; *increased sweating; loss of appetite*—except with astemizole, cetirizine, cyproheptadine, loratadine, and terfenadine; *paradoxical reaction* (nightmares; unusual excitement, nervousness, restlessness, or irritability); *photosensitivity* (increased sensitivity of skin to sun); *ringing or buzzing in ears; skin rash; stomach upset or pain*—more frequent with the ethylenediamine derivatives

Note: Confusion; difficult or painful urination; drowsiness; dizziness; and dryness of mouth, nose, or throat are more likely to occur in the elderly.

Nightmares, unusual excitement, nervousness, restlessness, or irritability are more likely to occur in children and elderly patients.

## Overdose

For more information on the management of overdose or unintentional ingestion, **contact a Poison Control Center** (see *Poison Control Center Listing*).

**Clinical effects of overdose**

Symptoms of overdose

*Anticholinergic effects* (clumsiness or unsteadiness; severe drowsiness; severe dryness of mouth, nose, or throat; flushing or redness of face; shortness of breath or troubled breathing); *cardiac arrhythmias* (fast or irregular heartbeat)—especially with astemizole or terfenadine; *CNS depression* (severe drowsiness); *CNS stimulation* (hallucinations, seizures, trouble in sleeping); *hypotension* (feeling faint)

Note: *Anticholinergic* and *CNS stimulant* effects are more likely to occur in children with overdose. *Hypotension* may also occur in the elderly at usual doses.

Anticholinergic and CNS effects may be less likely to occur with astemizole, cetirizine, loratadine, or terfenadine than with the first-generation antihistamines.

**Treatment of overdose**

Since there is no specific antidote for overdose with antihistamines, treatment is symptomatic and supportive.

To decrease absorption—

Induction of emesis (syrup of ipecac recommended); however, precaution against aspiration is necessary, especially in infants and children.

Gastric lavage (isotonic or 0.45% sodium chloride solution) if patient is unable to vomit within 3 hours of ingestion.

To enhance elimination—

Saline cathartics (milk of magnesia) are sometimes used.

Specific treatment—

Vasopressors to treat hypotension; however, epinephrine should not be used since it may further lower blood pressure.

Oxygen and intravenous fluids.

Precaution against use of stimulants (analeptic agents) because they may cause seizures.

## Patient Consultation

As an aid to patient consultation, refer to *Advice for the Patient, Antihistamines (Systemic)*.

In providing consultation, consider emphasizing the following selected information (» = major clinical significance):

**Before using this medication**

» Conditions affecting use, especially:

Sensitivity to any antihistamine

Pregnancy—Not taking during early months of pregnancy because of fetal abnormalities in studies in animals (for hydroxyzine only); risk-benefit should be considered because of fetal abnormalities in studies in animals with doses above the human therapeutic range (for astemizole and terfenadine only)

Breast-feeding—Use not recommended; may cause unusual excitement or irritability in nursing infant

Use in children—Increased susceptibility to anticholinergic side effects in newborn or premature infants; hyperexcitability (paradoxical reaction) may occur in children

Use in the elderly—Increased susceptibility to anticholinergic side effects; hyperexcitability (paradoxical reaction) may occur

Dental—Increased risk of dental problems because of decrease or inhibition of salivary flow

Other medications, especially alcohol or other CNS depressants; anticholinergics; calcium channel blocking agents, disopyramide, maprotiline, phenothiazines, pimozide, procainamide, quinidine, and tricyclic antidepressants (with astemizole and terfenadine); erythromycin and other macrolide antibiotics (with astemizole and terfenadine only); itraconazole and keto-

conazole (with astemizole and terfenadine); MAO inhibitors; or quinine (with astemizole)

Other medical problems, especially angle-closure glaucoma, hepatic function impairment (with astemizole or terfenadine only), hypokalemia (with astemizole or terfenadine only), prostatic hypertrophy, or urinary retention

**Proper use of this medication**

» Importance of not taking more medication than the amount recommended

» Proper dosing

Missed dose: If on scheduled dosing regimen—Using as soon as possible; not using if almost time for next dose; not doubling doses

» Proper storage

*For oral dosage forms*

Taking with food, water, or milk to minimize gastric irritation; taking astemizole on an empty stomach to minimize absorption problems

Swallowing extended-release dosage forms whole

*For injection dosage forms*

Knowing correct administration technique for self-administration; checking with physician if necessary

*For rectal dosage forms*

Proper administration technique

*For dimenhydrinate and diphenhydramine when used as antivertigo agent*

Taking at least 30 minutes (preferably 1 to 2 hours) before traveling

**Precautions while using this medication**

Possible interference with skin tests using allergens; need to inform physician if using medication

May mask ototoxic effects of large doses of salicylates

» Avoiding use of alcohol or other CNS depressants

» Caution if drowsiness occurs

Possible dryness of mouth; using sugarless gum or candy, ice, or saliva substitute for relief; checking with physician or dentist if dry mouth continues for more than 2 weeks

*For dimenhydrinate, diphenhydramine, or hydroxyzine*

Need to inform physician of use: Possible interference with diagnosis of appendicitis; may mask signs of toxicity from overdosage of other drugs

*For diphenhydramine and doxylamine when used in the treatment of insomnia*

» Not using concurrently with other sedatives or tranquilizers

**Side/adverse effects**

Signs of potential side effects, especially blood dyscrasias and cardiac arrhythmias (with astemizole and terfenadine only)

## General Dosing Information

**For oral dosage forms only**

Most antihistamines may be taken with food, water, or milk to lessen gastric irritation. Astemizole should be taken on an empty stomach since food may decrease absorption.

**Diet/Nutrition**

Although administration of a single 430-mg dose of quinine has been reported to elevate the plasma concentration of astemizole and desmethylastemizole, resulting in prolongation of the electrocardiographic QT interval, ingestion of small amounts of quinine, such as that found in beverages containing quinine (up to 80 mg per day or about 32 ounces of tonic water), has not been shown to have a clinically or statistically significant effect on the QT interval

**For parenteral dosage forms only**

Intramuscular injections should be administered deeply into the muscle.

Intravenous injections should be administered slowly, preferably with the patient in a recumbent position.

For hydroxyzine—

Administration should be by deep intramuscular injection into a large muscle mass, preferably the upper outer quadrant of the buttock or the mid-lateral thigh.

Intramuscular injections should not be made into the lower or mid-third of the upper arm.

When used preoperatively or prepartum, narcotic requirements may be decreased as much as 50%.

---

## *ASTEMIZOLE*

## Summary of Differences

Indications:

Used as treatment adjunct in asthma.

Pharmacology/pharmacokinetics:
Chemical group—Piperidine derivative.
Other actions/effects—No significant anticholinergic activity. Mild bronchodilator.
Absorption—Decreased absorption with ingestion of food.
Protein binding—96%.
Half-life—With multiple doses: 7 to 9 days (initial); 19 days (terminal).
Onset of action—< 24 hours; effect may not occur until day 2 or 3, depending on initial severity of symptoms.
Time to peak concentration—Within 1 hour.
Time to peak effect—9 to 12 days.
Duration of action—Up to several weeks.
Elimination—Primarily fecal.
Precautions:
Dental—No dental precaution.
Drug interactions and/or related problems—Possible cardiotoxic effects with erythromycin and other macrolide antibiotics, itraconazole, or ketoconazole, or with medications causing QT interval prolongation.
Medical considerations/contraindications—Possible cardiotoxic effects with hepatic function impairment, history of QT interval prolongation, or with hypokalemia.
Side/adverse effects:
Sedative and anticholinergic effects less likely. Cardiac arrhythmias with high doses or overdose. May cause increased appetite and weight gain.

## Oral Dosage Forms

Note: Bracketed uses in the *Dosage Forms* section refer to categories of use and/or indications that are not included in U.S. product labeling.

### ASTEMIZOLE ORAL SUSPENSION

**Usual adult and adolescent dose**
Antihistaminic (H₁-receptor)—
Oral, 10 mg once a day.

**Usual pediatric dose**
Antihistaminic (H₁-receptor)—
Children up to 6 years of age: Oral, 2 mg per 10 kg of body weight once a day.
Children 6 to 12 years of age: Oral, 5 mg once a day.
Children 12 years of age and over: See *Usual adult and adolescent dose*.

**Usual geriatric dose**
See *Usual adult and adolescent dose*.
Note: Geriatric patients may be more sensitive to the effects of the usual adult dose.

**Strength(s) usually available**
U.S.—
Not commercially available.
Canada—
2 mg per mL (OTC) [*Hismanal* (alcohol 5%)].

**Packaging and storage**
Store below 40 °C (104 °F), preferably between 15 and 30 °C (59 and 86 °F), in a well-closed container, unless otherwise specified by manufacturer. Protect from freezing.

**Auxiliary labeling**
• Shake well.
• Take on empty stomach.

### ASTEMIZOLE TABLETS

**Usual adult and adolescent dose**
See *Astemizole Oral Suspension*.

**Usual pediatric dose**
[Antihistaminic (H₁-receptor)]—
Children 6 to 12 years of age: Oral, 5 mg once a day.
Children 12 years of age and over: Oral, 10 mg once a day.

**Usual geriatric dose**
See *Astemizole Oral Suspension*.
Note: Geriatric patients may be more sensitive to the effects of the usual adult dose.

**Strength(s) usually available**
U.S.—
10 mg (Rx) [*Hismanal* (scored)].
Canada—
10 mg (OTC) [*Hismanal* (scored)].

**Packaging and storage**
Store below 40 °C (104 °F), preferably between 15 and 30 °C (59 and 86 °F), unless otherwise specified by manufacturer.

**Auxiliary labeling**
• Take on empty stomach.

---

## AZATADINE

## Summary of Differences

Pharmacology/pharmacokinetics:
Chemical group—Piperidine derivative.
pKa—9.3.
Half-life—12 hours.
Time to peak concentration—4 hours.
Duration of action—12 hours.

## Oral Dosage Forms

### AZATADINE MALEATE TABLETS USP

**Usual adult and adolescent dose**
Antihistaminic (H₁-receptor)—
Oral, 1 to 2 mg every eight to twelve hours as needed.

**Usual pediatric dose**
Antihistaminic (H₁-receptor)—
Children up to 12 years of age: Use is not recommended.
Children 12 years of age and over: Oral, 500 mcg (0.5 mg) to 1 mg two times a day as needed.

**Usual geriatric dose**
See *Usual adult and adolescent dose*.
Note: Geriatric patients may be more sensitive to the effects of the usual adult dose.

**Strength(s) usually available**
U.S.—
1 mg (Rx) [*Optimine* (scored)].
Canada—
1 mg (Rx) [*Optimine* (scored)].

**Packaging and storage**
Store below 40 °C (104 °F), preferably between 15 and 30 °C (59 and 86 °F), unless otherwise specified by manufacturer. Store in a well-closed container.

**Auxiliary labeling**
• May cause drowsiness.
• Avoid alcoholic beverages.

---

## BROMPHENIRAMINE

## Summary of Differences

Pharmacology/pharmacokinetics:
Chemical group—Propylamine derivative.
pKa—3.59 and 9.12.
Half-life—25 hours.
Time to peak concentration—2 to 5 hours.
Time to peak effect—3 to 9 hours.
Duration of action—4 to 8 hours.
Side/adverse effects:
Sedative effects less pronounced.

## Oral Dosage Forms

### BROMPHENIRAMINE MALEATE CAPSULES

**Usual adult and adolescent dose**
Antihistaminic (H₁-receptor)—
Oral, 4 mg every four to six hours as needed.

**Usual adult prescribing limits**
Up to 24 mg daily.

**Usual pediatric dose**
See *Brompheniramine Maleate Elixir USP*.
Note: The available strength of the tablet may not conform to some of the recommended pediatric dosages.

**Usual geriatric dose**
See *Usual adult and adolescent dose*.
Note: Geriatric patients may be more sensitive to the effects of the usual adult dose.

**Strength(s) usually available**
U.S.—
    4 mg (Rx) [*Dimetapp Allergy Liqui-Gels*].
Canada—
    Not commercially available.

**Packaging and storage**
Store between 15 and 30 °C (59 and 86 °F), unless otherwise specified by manufacturer. Protect from freezing.

**Auxiliary labeling**
• May cause drowsiness.
• Avoid alcoholic beverages.

## BROMPHENIRAMINE MALEATE ELIXIR USP

**Usual adult and adolescent dose**
See *Brompheniramine Maleate Capsules*.

**Usual adult prescribing limits**
See *Brompheniramine Maleate Capsules*.

**Usual pediatric dose**
Antihistaminic (H₁-receptor)—

$ $Oral, 500 mcg (0.5 mg) per kg of body weight or 15 mg per square meter of body surface per day, in three or four divided doses, as needed; or for
    Children 2 to 6 years of age: Oral, 1 mg every four to six hours as needed.
    Children 6 to 12 years of age: Oral, 2 mg every four to six hours as needed.
    Children 12 years of age and over: Oral, 4 mg every four to six hours as needed.

Note: Premature and full-term neonates—Use is not recommended.

**Usual geriatric dose**
See *Brompheniramine Maleate Capsules*.

Note: Geriatric patients may be more sensitive to the effects of the usual adult dose.

**Strength(s) usually available**
U.S.—
    2 mg per 5 mL (Rx) [*Bromphen;* GENERIC].
    2 mg per 5 mL (OTC) [*Dimetane* (alcohol 3%); GENERIC].
Canada—
    2 mg per 5 mL (OTC) [*Dimetane* (alcohol 3%)].

**Packaging and storage**
Store below 40 °C (104 °F), preferably between 15 and 30 °C (59 and 86 °F), unless otherwise specified by manufacturer. Store in a well-closed, light-resistant container. Protect from freezing.

**Auxiliary labeling**
• May cause drowsiness.
• Avoid alcoholic beverages.
• Keep container tightly closed.

## BROMPHENIRAMINE MALEATE TABLETS USP

**Usual adult and adolescent dose**
See *Brompheniramine Maleate Capsules*.

**Usual pediatric dose**
See *Brompheniramine Maleate Elixir USP*.

Note: The available strength of the tablet may not conform to some of the recommended pediatric dosages.

**Usual geriatric dose**
See *Brompheniramine Maleate Capsules*.

Note: Geriatric patients may be more sensitive to the effects of the usual adult dose.

**Strength(s) usually available**
U.S.—
    4 mg (Rx) [*Veltane* (scored); GENERIC].
    4 mg (OTC) [*Dimetapp Allergy* (scored); GENERIC].
    8 mg (Rx) [GENERIC].
Canada—
    4 mg (OTC) [*Dimetane*].

**Packaging and storage**
Store below 40 °C (104 °F), preferably between 15 and 30 °C (59 and 86 °F), unless otherwise specified by manufacturer. Store in a tight container.

**Auxiliary labeling**
• May cause drowsiness.
• Avoid alcoholic beverages.

## BROMPHENIRAMINE MALEATE EXTENDED-RELEASE TABLETS

**Usual adult and adolescent dose**
Antihistaminic (H₁-receptor)—
    Oral, 8 mg every eight or twelve hours or 12 mg every twelve hours as needed.

**Usual pediatric dose**
Antihistaminic (H₁-receptor)—
    Children up to 6 years of age: Use is not recommended.
    Children 6 years of age and over: Oral, 8 or 12 mg every twelve hours as needed.

**Usual geriatric dose**
See *Usual adult and adolescent dose*.

Note: Geriatric patients may be more sensitive to the effects of the usual adult dose.

**Strength(s) usually available**
U.S.—
    8 mg (Rx) [*Diamine T.D.;* GENERIC].
    8 mg (OTC) [*Dimetane Extentabs*].
    12 mg (Rx) [*Diamine T.D.;* GENERIC].
    12 mg (OTC) [*Dimetane Extentabs*].
Canada—
    12 mg (OTC) [*Dimetane Extentabs*].

**Packaging and storage**
Store below 40 °C (104 °F), preferably between 15 and 30 °C (59 and 86 °F), in a well-closed container, unless otherwise specified by manufacturer.

**Auxiliary labeling**
• Swallow tablets whole.
• May cause drowsiness.
• Avoid alcoholic beverages.

# Parenteral Dosage Forms
## BROMPHENIRAMINE MALEATE INJECTION USP

**Usual adult and adolescent dose**
Antihistaminic (H₁-receptor)—
    Intramuscular, intravenous, or subcutaneous, 10 mg every eight to twelve hours as needed.

**Usual adult prescribing limits**
Up to 40 mg daily.

**Usual pediatric dose**
Antihistaminic (H₁-receptor)—
    Children up to 12 years of age: Intramuscular, intravenous, or subcutaneous, 125 mcg (0.125 mg) per kg of body weight or 3.75 mg per square meter of body surface three or four times a day as needed.

Note: Premature and full-term neonates—Use is not recommended.

**Usual geriatric dose**
See *Usual adult and adolescent dose*.

Note: Geriatric patients may be more sensitive to the effects of the usual adult dose.

**Strength(s) usually available**
U.S.—
    10 mg per mL (Rx) [*Chlorphed; Codimal-A; Conjec-B; Cophene-B; Dehist; Histaject Modified; Nasahist B; ND-Stat Revised; Oraminic II*].
    100 mg per mL (Rx) [*Nasahist B*].
Canada—
    Not commercially available.

**Packaging and storage**
Store below 40 °C (104 °F), preferably between 15 and 30 °C (59 and 86 °F), unless otherwise specified by manufacturer. Protect from light. Protect from freezing.

**Stability**
Crystallization may occur if cooled below 0 °C (32 °F); but on warming to 30 °C (86 °F), the crystals will redissolve.

**Additional information**
The period of protection provided by a single dose ranges from three to twelve hours.

The concentrated solution (100 mg per mL) is not recommended for intravenous use.

## *CETIRIZINE*

### Summary of Differences

Indications:
Used as treatment adjunct in asthma.
Pharmacology/pharmacokinetics:
Chemical group—Hydroxyzine metabolite.
Absorption—Decreased absorption rate, but not extent, with food.
Protein binding—93%.
Half-life—8 hours.
Time to peak concentration—1 hour.
Time to peak effect—4 to 8 hours.
Duration of action—Up to 24 hours.
Precautions:
Dental—
No dental precaution.
Side/adverse effects:
Minimal anticholinergic effects; dose-related sedation.

## Oral Dosage Forms

### CETIRIZINE HYDROCHLORIDE TABLETS

**Usual adult and adolescent dose**
Antihistaminic (H₁-receptor)—
Oral, 5 to 10 mg once a day. Dosage may be increased to 20 mg a day, depending on severity of symptoms and patient response.

Note: In patients with reduced creatinine clearance, a starting dose of 5 mg is recommended.

**Usual adult prescribing limits**
Up to 20 mg daily.

**Usual pediatric dose**
Antihistaminic (H₁-receptor)[1]—
Children 2 to 6 years of age: Oral, 5 mg a day.
Children 6 to 11 years of age: Oral, 10 mg a day.

**Usual geriatric dose**
See *Usual adult and adolescent dose.*

Note: Geriatric patients may be more sensitive to the effects of the usual adult dose.

**Strength(s) usually available**
U.S.—
Not commercially available.
Canada—
10 mg (Rx) [*Reactine*].

**Packaging and storage**
Store between 15 and 30 °C (59 and 86 °F), in a well-closed container, unless otherwise specified by manufacturer.

**Auxiliary labeling**
• May cause drowsiness.
• Avoid alcoholic beverages.

[1]Not included in Canadian product labeling.

## *CHLORPHENIRAMINE*

### Summary of Differences

Pharmacology/pharmacokinetics:
Chemical group—Propylamine derivative.
pKa—9.2.
Protein binding—72%.
Half-life—14 to 25 hours.
Time to peak concentration—2 to 6 hours.
Time to peak effect—6 hours.
Duration of action—4 to 8 hours.
Side/adverse effects:
Sedative effects less pronounced.

## Oral Dosage Forms

### CHLORPHENIRAMINE MALEATE EXTENDED-RELEASE CAPSULES USP

**Usual adult and adolescent dose**
Antihistaminic (H₁-receptor)—
Oral, 8 or 12 mg every eight to twelve hours as needed.

**Usual pediatric dose**
Antihistaminic (H₁-receptor)—
Children up to 12 years of age: Use is not recommended.

Children 12 years of age and over: Oral, 8 mg every twelve hours as needed.

**Usual geriatric dose**
See *Usual adult and adolescent dose.*

Note: Geriatric patients may be more sensitive to the effects of the usual adult dose.

**Strength(s) usually available**
U.S.—
8 mg (Rx) [*Phenetron Lanacaps; Telachlor;* GENERIC].
8 mg (OTC) [GENERIC].
12 mg (Rx) [*Chlorspan-12; Telachlor;* GENERIC].
12 mg (OTC) [*Teldrin;* GENERIC].
Canada—
Not commercially available.

**Packaging and storage**
Store below 40 °C (104 °F), preferably between 15 and 30 °C (59 and 86 °F), unless otherwise specified by manufacturer. Store in a tight container.

**Auxiliary labeling**
• Swallow capsules whole.
• May cause drowsiness.
• Avoid alcoholic beverages.

### CHLORPHENIRAMINE MALEATE SYRUP USP

**Usual adult and adolescent dose**
Antihistaminic (H₁-receptor)—
Oral, 4 mg every four to six hours as needed.

**Usual adult prescribing limits**
Up to 24 mg daily.

**Usual pediatric dose**
Antihistaminic (H₁-receptor)—
Oral, 87.5 mcg (0.0875 mg) per kg of body weight or 2.5 mg per square meter of body surface every six hours as needed; or for
Children up to 6 years of age: Use is not recommended.
Children 6 to 12 years of age: Oral, 2 mg three or four times a day as needed, not to exceed 12 mg per day.

**Usual geriatric dose**
See *Usual adult and adolescent dose.*

Note: Geriatric patients may be more sensitive to the effects of the usual adult dose.

**Strength(s) usually available**
U.S.—
1 mg per 5 mL (OTC) [*PediaCare Allergy Formula*].
2 mg per 5 mL (Rx) [*Phenetron* (alcohol 7%); GENERIC].
2 mg per 5 mL (OTC) [*Aller-Chlor* (alcohol 7%); *Chlor-Trimeton* (alcohol 7%); GENERIC].
Canada—
2.5 mg per 5 mL (OTC) [*Chlor-Tripolon* (alcohol 7%)].

**Packaging and storage**
Store below 40 °C (104 °F), preferably between 15 and 30 °C (59 and 86 °F), unless otherwise specified by manufacturer. Store in a tight, light-resistant container. Protect from freezing.

**Auxiliary labeling**
• May cause drowsiness.
• Avoid alcoholic beverages.

### CHLORPHENIRAMINE MALEATE TABLETS USP

**Usual adult and adolescent dose**
See *Chlorpheniramine Maleate Syrup USP.*

**Usual pediatric dose**
See *Chlorpheniramine Maleate Syrup USP.*

**Usual geriatric dose**
See *Chlorpheniramine Maleate Syrup USP.*

Note: Geriatric patients may be more sensitive to the effects of the usual adult dose.

**Strength(s) usually available**
U.S.—
4 mg (Rx) [*Chlortab-4; Phenetron* (scored); *Trymegen;* GENERIC].
4 mg (OTC) [*Aller-Chlor; Chlorate; Chlor-Niramine; Chlor-Trimeton* (scored); *Chlor-Trimeton Allergy; Gen-Allerate; Pfeiffer's Allergy;* GENERIC].
Canada—
4 mg (OTC) [*Chlor-Tripolon* (scored); *Novo-Pheniram* (scored)].

**Packaging and storage**
Store below 40 °C (104 °F), preferably between 15 and 30 °C (59 and 86 °F), unless otherwise specified by manufacturer. Store in a tight container.

**Auxiliary labeling**
• May cause drowsiness.
• Avoid alcoholic beverages.

## CHLORPHENIRAMINE MALEATE TABLETS (CHEWABLE) USP

**Usual adult and adolescent dose**
See *Chlorpheniramine Maleate Syrup USP*.

**Usual pediatric dose**
See *Chlorpheniramine Maleate Syrup USP*.

**Usual geriatric dose**
See *Chlorpheniramine Maleate Syrup USP*.

Note: Geriatric patients may be more sensitive to the effects of the usual adult dose.

**Strength(s) usually available**
U.S.—
    2 mg (OTC) [*Chlo-Amine*].
Canada—
    Not commercially available.

**Packaging and storage**
Store below 40 °C (104 °F), preferably between 15 and 30 °C (59 and 86 °F), unless otherwise specified by manufacturer. Store in a tight container.

**Auxiliary labeling**
• Chew before swallowing.
• May cause drowsiness.
• Avoid alcoholic beverages.

## CHLORPHENIRAMINE MALEATE EXTENDED-RELEASE TABLETS

**Usual adult and adolescent dose**
See *Chlorpheniramine Maleate Extended-release Capsules USP*.

**Usual pediatric dose**
See *Chlorpheniramine Maleate Extended-release Capsules USP*.

**Usual geriatric dose**
See *Chlorpheniramine Maleate Extended-release Capsules USP*.

Note: Geriatric patients may be more sensitive to the effects of the usual adult dose.

**Strength(s) usually available**
U.S.—
    8 mg (Rx) [*Chlortab-8; Phenetron;* GENERIC].
    8 mg (OTC) [*Chlor-Trimeton Repetabs;* GENERIC].
    12 mg (Rx) [*Phenetron* (sugar-coated); GENERIC].
    12 mg (OTC) [*Chlor-Trimeton Repetabs* (sugar-coated); GENERIC].
Canada—
    8 mg (OTC) [*Chlor-Tripolon*].
    12 mg (OTC) [*Chlor-Tripolon*].

**Packaging and storage**
Store below 40 °C (104 °F), preferably between 15 and 30 °C (59 and 86 °F), in a well-closed container, unless otherwise specified by manufacturer.

**Auxiliary labeling**
• Swallow tablets whole.
• May cause drowsiness.
• Avoid alcoholic beverages.

# Parenteral Dosage Forms

## CHLORPHENIRAMINE MALEATE INJECTION USP

**Usual adult and adolescent dose**
Antihistaminic (H₁-receptor)—
    Intramuscular, intravenous, or subcutaneous, 5 to 40 mg administered as a single dose as needed.

**Usual adult prescribing limits**
Up to 40 mg daily.

**Usual pediatric dose**
Antihistaminic (H₁-receptor)—
    Subcutaneous, 87.5 mcg (0.0875 mg) per kg of body weight or 2.5 mg per square meter of body surface every six hours as needed.

Note: Premature and full-term neonates—Use is not recommended.

**Usual geriatric dose**
See *Usual adult and adolescent dose*.

Note: Geriatric patients may be more sensitive to the effects of the usual adult dose.

**Strength(s) usually available**
U.S.—
    10 mg per mL (Rx) [*Chlor-Pro 10; Chlor-Trimeton;* GENERIC].
    100 mg per mL (Rx) [*Chlor-100; Chlor-Pro*].
Canada—
    100 mg per mL (Rx) [*Chlor-Tripolon*].

**Packaging and storage**
Store below 40 °C (104 °F), preferably between 15 and 30 °C (59 and 86 °F), unless otherwise specified by manufacturer. Protect from light. Protect from freezing.

**Additional information**
The 10-mg-per-mL solution may be administered intravenously, intramuscularly, or subcutaneously. The 100-mg-per-mL solution is intended for intramuscular or subcutaneous administration only.

---

## *CLEMASTINE*

---

# Summary of Differences

Pharmacology/pharmacokinetics:
    Chemical group—Ethanolamine derivative.
    Other actions/effects—Greater anticholinergic activity.
    Time to peak concentration—2 to 4 hours.
    Time to peak effect—5 to 7 hours.
    Duration of action—12 hours.
Side/adverse effects:
    Sedative effects not as pronounced.

# Oral Dosage Forms

## CLEMASTINE FUMARATE SYRUP

**Usual adult and adolescent dose**
Antihistaminic (H₁-receptor)—
    Oral, 1.34 mg two times a day or 2.68 mg one to three times a day as needed.

Note: Clemastine is indicated for dermatologic conditions at the 2.68-mg dosage level only.

**Usual adult prescribing limits**
Up to 8.04 mg daily.

**Usual pediatric dose**
Antihistaminic (H₁-receptor)—
    Children up to 6 years of age: Dosage has not been established.
    Children 6 to 12 years of age: Oral, 670 mcg (0.67 mg) to 1.34 mg two times a day, not to exceed 4.02 mg per day.

Note: Clemastine is indicated for dermatologic conditions at the 1.34-mg dosage level only.

**Usual geriatric dose**
See *Usual adult and adolescent dose*.

Note: Geriatric patients may be more sensitive to the effects of the usual adult dose.

**Strength(s) usually available**
U.S.—
    0.67 mg per 5 mL (Rx) [*Tavist* (alcohol 5.5%)].
Canada—
    0.67 mg per 5 mL (OTC) [*Tavist* (alcohol 6.1%)].

**Packaging and storage**
Store below 25 °C (77 °F), preferably between 15 and 25 °C (59 and 77 °F), in a well-closed container, unless otherwise specified by manufacturer. Protect from freezing.

**Auxiliary labeling**
• May cause drowsiness.
• Avoid alcoholic beverages.
• Store in upright position.

## CLEMASTINE FUMARATE TABLETS USP

**Usual adult and adolescent dose**
See *Clemastine Fumarate Syrup*.

Note: Clemastine is indicated for dermatologic conditions at the 2.68-mg dosage level only.

## Usual pediatric dose

See *Clemastine Fumarate Syrup.*

Note: Clemastine is indicated for dermatologic conditions at the 1.34-mg dosage level only.

## Usual geriatric dose

See *Clemastine Fumarate Syrup.*

Note: Geriatric patients may be more sensitive to the effects of the usual adult dose.

## Strength(s) usually available

U.S.—

1.34 mg (OTC) [*Contac 12 Hour Allergy; Tavist-1* (scored); GENERIC].
2.68 mg (Rx) [*Tavist* (scored); GENERIC].

Canada—

1 mg (base) (OTC) [*Tavist* (scored)].

## Packaging and storage

Store between 15 and 30 °C (59 and 86 °F), unless otherwise specified by manufacturer. Store in a tight, light-resistant container.

## Auxiliary labeling

• May cause drowsiness.
• Avoid alcoholic beverages.

---

### *CYPROHEPTADINE*

## Summary of Differences

Indications:
     Also indicated in cold urticaria and used as an appetite stimulant in adults and children.
Pharmacology/pharmacokinetics:
     Chemical group—Piperidine derivative.
     pKa—9.3.
     Other actions/effects—Serotonin antagonist.
     Duration of action—8 hours.
Precautions:
     Laboratory value alterations—
          May increase serum amylase and serum prolactin concentrations when administered with thyrotropin-releasing hormone.
Side/adverse effects:
     May cause increased appetite and weight gain.

## Oral Dosage Forms

Note: Bracketed uses in the *Dosage Forms* section refer to categories of use and/or indications that are not included in U.S. product labeling.

### CYPROHEPTADINE HYDROCHLORIDE SYRUP USP

## Usual adult and adolescent dose

Antihistaminic ($H_1$-receptor)—
     Oral, initially 4 mg every eight hours, the dosage being increased as needed. For most patients the therapeutic range is 4 to 20 mg a day. However, doses up to 32 mg a day have been used occasionally.
[Appetite stimulant]—
     Oral, 4 mg three times a day with meals.
     Note: Treatment period to promote weight gain should not exceed six months.
[Vascular headache suppressant]—
     Initial: Oral, 4 mg at the start of the attack, repeated after thirty minutes if necessary.
     Maintenance: Oral, 4 mg every four to six hours.

## Usual adult prescribing limits

Up to 500 mcg (0.5 mg) per kg of body weight daily.

## Usual pediatric dose

Antihistaminic ($H_1$-receptor)—
     Oral, 125 mcg (0.125 mg) per kg of body weight or 4 mg per square meter of body surface, every eight to twelve hours as needed or for
     Children 2 to 6 years of age: Oral, 2 mg every eight to twelve hours as needed, not to exceed 12 mg per day.
     Children 6 to 14 years of age: Oral, 4 mg every eight to twelve hours as needed, not to exceed 16 mg per day.
[Appetite stimulant]—
     Children 2 to 6 years of age: Oral, initially 2 mg two or three times a day with meals. The dosage may be increased, if necessary, but not to exceed 8 mg a day.
     Children 6 to 14 years of age: Oral, initially 2 mg three or four times a day with meals. The usual maintenance dose is 4 mg two or three times a day. The dosage may be increased, if necessary, but not to exceed 16 mg a day.

---

Note: Premature and full-term neonates—Use is not recommended.
     Treatment period to promote weight gain should not exceed 3 months.

## Usual geriatric dose

See *Usual adult and adolescent dose.*

Note: Geriatric patients may be more sensitive to the effects of the usual adult dose.

## Strength(s) usually available

U.S.—

2 mg per 5 mL (Rx) [*Periactin* (alcohol 5%); GENERIC].

Canada—

2 mg per 5 mL (OTC) [*Periactin* (alcohol 5%)].

## Packaging and storage

Store below 40 °C (104 °F), preferably between 15 and 30 °C (59 and 86 °F), unless otherwise specified by manufacturer. Store in a tight container. Protect from freezing.

## Auxiliary labeling

• May cause drowsiness.
• Avoid alcoholic beverages.

### CYPROHEPTADINE HYDROCHLORIDE TABLETS USP

## Usual adult and adolescent dose

See *Cyproheptadine Hydrochloride Syrup USP.*

## Usual adult prescribing limits

See *Cyproheptadine Hydrochloride Syrup USP.*

## Usual pediatric dose

See *Cyproheptadine Hydrochloride Syrup USP.*

## Usual geriatric dose

See *Cyproheptadine Hydrochloride Syrup USP.*

Note: Geriatric patients may be more sensitive to the effects of the usual adult dose.

## Strength(s) usually available

U.S.—

4 mg (Rx) [*Periactin* (scored); GENERIC].

Canada—

4 mg (OTC) [*Periactin* (scored)].

## Packaging and storage

Store below 40 °C (104 °F), preferably between 15 and 30 °C (59 and 86 °F), unless otherwise specified by manufacturer. Store in a well-closed container.

## Auxiliary labeling

• May cause drowsiness.
• Avoid alcoholic beverages.

---

### *DEXCHLORPHENIRAMINE*

## Summary of Differences

Pharmacology/pharmacokinetics:
     Chemical group—Propylamine derivative.
     Duration of action—4 to 8 hours.
Side/adverse effects:
     Sedative effects less pronounced.

## Oral Dosage Forms

### DEXCHLORPHENIRAMINE MALEATE SYRUP USP

## Usual adult and adolescent dose

Antihistaminic ($H_1$-receptor)—
     Oral, 2 mg every four to six hours as needed.

## Usual pediatric dose

Antihistaminic ($H_1$-receptor)—
     Children up to 12 years of age: Oral, 150 mcg (0.15 mg) per kg of body weight or 4.5 mg per square meter of body surface per day, in four divided doses or for
          Children 2 to 5 years of age: Oral, 500 mcg (0.5 mg) every four to six hours as needed.
          Children 5 to 12 years of age: Oral, 1 mg every four to six hours as needed.

Note: Premature and full-term neonates—Use is not recommended.

## Usual geriatric dose

See *Usual adult and adolescent dose.*

Note: Geriatric patients may be more sensitive to the effects of the usual adult dose.

**Strength(s) usually available**
U.S.—
 2 mg per 5 mL (Rx) [*Polaramine* (alcohol 6%)].
Canada—
 2 mg per 5 mL (OTC) [*Polaramine* (alcohol 5%)].

**Packaging and storage**
Store below 40 °C (104 °F), preferably between 15 and 30 °C (59 and 86 °F), unless otherwise specified by manufacturer. Store in a tight container. Protect from light. Protect from freezing.

**Auxiliary labeling**
• May cause drowsiness.
• Avoid alcoholic beverages.

## DEXCHLORPHENIRAMINE MALEATE TABLETS USP

**Usual adult and adolescent dose**
See *Dexchlorpheniramine Maleate Syrup USP.*

**Usual pediatric dose**
See *Dexchlorpheniramine Maleate Syrup USP.*

**Usual geriatric dose**
See *Dexchlorpheniramine Maleate Syrup USP.*

Note: Geriatric patients may be more sensitive to the effects of the usual adult dose.

**Strength(s) usually available**
U.S.—
 2 mg (Rx) [*Polaramine*].
Canada—
 2 mg (OTC) [*Polaramine*].

**Packaging and storage**
Store below 40 °C (104 °F), preferably between 15 and 30 °C (59 and 86 °F), unless otherwise specified by manufacturer. Store in a tight container.

**Auxiliary labeling**
• May cause drowsiness.
• Avoid alcoholic beverages.

## DEXCHLORPHENIRAMINE MALEATE EXTENDED-RELEASE TABLETS

**Usual adult and adolescent dose**
Antihistaminic (H₁-receptor)—
 Oral, 4 or 6 mg every eight to twelve hours as needed.

**Usual pediatric dose**
Use is not recommended.

**Usual geriatric dose**
See *Usual adult and adolescent dose.*

Note: Geriatric patients may be more sensitive to the effects of the usual adult dose.

**Strength(s) usually available**
U.S.—
 4 mg (Rx) [*Dexchlor; Polaramine Repetabs* (sugar-coated); GENERIC].
 6 mg (Rx) [*Dexchlor; Poladex T.D.; Polaramine Repetabs* (sugar-coated); GENERIC].
Canada—
 6 mg (OTC) [*Polaramine Repetabs*].

**Packaging and storage**
Store below 40 °C (104 °F), preferably between 15 and 30 °C (59 and 86 °F), in a well-closed container, unless otherwise specified by manufacturer.

**Auxiliary labeling**
• Swallow tablets whole.
• May cause drowsiness.
• Avoid alcoholic beverages.

---

### *DIMENHYDRINATE*

## Summary of Differences

Category:
 Also indicated as an antiemetic and antivertigo agent.
Pharmacology/pharmacokinetics:
 Chemical group—Ethanolamine derivative.
 Other actions/effects—Greater anticholinergic activity.
 Duration of action—3 to 6 hours.
Precautions:
 Drug interactions and/or related problems—May decrease emetic response to apomorphine.

Medical considerations/contraindications—May impede diagnosis of appendicitis; may obscure signs of overdose.
Side/adverse effects:
 Sedative effects more pronounced.

## Additional Dosing Information

See also *General Dosing Information.*

When dimenhydrinate is used for prophylaxis of motion sickness, it should be taken at least 30 minutes, and preferably 1 or 2 hours, before exposure to conditions that may precipitate motion sickness.
For parenteral dosage form only
 • Do not administer intra-arterially.

## Oral Dosage Forms

### DIMENHYDRINATE CAPSULES

**Usual adult and adolescent dose**
Antiemetic or
Antivertigo agent—
 Oral, 50 to 100 mg every four hours as needed.

**Usual adult prescribing limits**
Up to 400 mg daily.

**Usual pediatric dose**
Antiemetic or
Antivertigo agent—
 Oral, 5 mg per kg of body weight or 150 mg per square meter of body surface per day, in four divided doses, as needed, not to exceed 300 mg per day; or for
 Children 6 to 12 years of age: Oral, 25 to 50 mg every six to eight hours as needed, not to exceed 150 mg per day.

**Usual geriatric dose**
See *Usual adult and adolescent dose.*

Note: Geriatric patients may be more sensitive to the effects of the usual adult dose.

**Strength(s) usually available**
U.S.—
 50 mg (Rx) [*Nico-Vert*].
 50 mg (OTC) [*Tega-Vert; Vertab*].
Canada—
 Not commercially available.

**Packaging and storage**
Store below 40 °C (104 °F), preferably between 15 and 30 °C (59 and 86 °F), in a well-closed container, unless otherwise specified by manufacturer.

**Auxiliary labeling**
• May cause drowsiness.
• Avoid alcoholic beverages.

### DIMENHYDRINATE EXTENDED-RELEASE CAPSULES

**Usual adult and adolescent dose**
Antiemetic or
Antivertigo agent—
 Oral, 1 capsule every twelve hours.

**Usual pediatric dose**
Use is not recommended.

**Usual geriatric dose**
See *Usual adult and adolescent dose.*

Note: Geriatric patients may be more sensitive to the effects of the usual adult dose.

**Strength(s) usually available**
U.S.—
 Not commercially available.
Canada—
 25 mg for immediate release and 50 mg for extended release (OTC) [*Gravol L/A*].

**Packaging and storage**
Store below 40 °C (104 °F), preferably between 15 and 30 °C (59 and 86 °F), in a well-closed container, unless otherwise specified by manufacturer.

**Auxiliary labeling**
• May cause drowsiness.
• Avoid alcoholic beverages.

### DIMENHYDRINATE ELIXIR

**Usual adult and adolescent dose**
See *Dimenhydrinate Capsules.*

**Usual adult prescribing limits**
See *Dimenhydrinate Capsules*.

**Usual pediatric dose**
Antiemetic or
Antivertigo agent—
Oral, 5 mg per kg of body weight or 150 mg per square meter of body surface per day, in four divided doses, as needed, not to exceed 300 mg per day or for
Children 2 to 6 years of age: Oral, 12.5 to 25 mg every six to eight hours as needed, not to exceed 75 mg per day.
Children 6 to 12 years of age: Oral, 25 to 50 mg every six to eight hours as needed, not to exceed 150 mg per day.

Note: Premature and full-term neonates—Use is not recommended.

**Usual geriatric dose**
See *Dimenhydrinate Capsules*.

Note: Geriatric patients may be more sensitive to the effects of the usual adult dose.

**Strength(s) usually available**
U.S.—
12.5 mg per 5 mL (OTC) [*Children's Dramamine* (alcohol 5%)].
Canada—
15 mg per 5 mL [*Gravol* (alcohol 4–6%)].

**Packaging and storage**
Store below 40 °C (104 °F), preferably between 15 and 30 °C (59 and 86 °F), in a tight container, unless otherwise specified by manufacturer. Protect from freezing.

**Auxiliary labeling**
• May cause drowsiness.
• Avoid alcoholic beverages.
• Keep container tightly closed.

## DIMENHYDRINATE SYRUP USP

**Usual adult and adolescent dose**
See *Dimenhydrinate Capsules*.

**Usual adult prescribing limits**
See *Dimenhydrinate Capsules*.

**Usual pediatric dose**
See *Dimenhydrinate Elixir*.

Note: Premature and full-term neonates—Use is not recommended.

**Usual geriatric dose**
See *Dimenhydrinate Capsules*.

Note: Geriatric patients may be more sensitive to the effects of the usual adult dose.

**Strength(s) usually available**
U.S.—
12.5 mg per 4 mL (OTC) [*Dramamine Liquid* (alcohol 5%); GENERIC].
15.62 mg per 5 mL (Rx) [*Dramamine Liquid*].
Canada—
Not commercially available.

**Packaging and storage**
Store below 40 °C (104 °F), preferably between 15 and 30 °C (59 and 86 °F), unless otherwise specified by manufacturer. Store in a tight container. Protect from freezing.

**Auxiliary labeling**
• May cause drowsiness.
• Avoid alcoholic beverages.

## DIMENHYDRINATE TABLETS USP

**Usual adult and adolescent dose**
See *Dimenhydrinate Capsules*.

**Usual adult prescribing limits**
See *Dimenhydrinate Capsules*.

**Usual pediatric dose**
See *Dimenhydrinate Elixir*.

Note: Premature and full-term neonates—Use is not recommended.

**Usual geriatric dose**
See *Dimenhydrinate Capsules*.

Note: Geriatric patients may be more sensitive to the effects of the usual adult dose.

**Strength(s) usually available**
U.S.—
50 mg (Rx) [*Dimetabs*].
50 mg (OTC) [*Calm X* (scored); *Dramamine* (scored); *Marmine; Triptone Caplets;* GENERIC].

Canada—
50 mg (OTC) [*Apo-Dimenhydrinate; Gravol; Nauseatol; Novo-Dimenate; PMS-Dimenhydrinate; Travamine; Traveltabs*].

**Packaging and storage**
Store below 40 °C (104 °F), preferably between 15 and 30 °C (59 and 86 °F), unless otherwise specified by manufacturer. Store in a well-closed container.

**Auxiliary labeling**
• May cause drowsiness.
• Avoid alcoholic beverages.

## DIMENHYDRINATE TABLETS (CHEWABLE) USP

**Usual adult and adolescent dose**
See *Dimenhydrinate Capsules*.

**Usual adult prescribing limits**
See *Dimenhydrinate Capsules*.

**Usual pediatric dose**
See *Dimenhydrinate Elixir*.

Note: Premature and full-term neonates—Use is not recommended.

**Usual geriatric dose**
See *Dimenhydrinate Capsules*.

Note: Geriatric patients may be more sensitive to the effects of the usual adult dose.

**Strength(s) usually available**
U.S.—
50 mg (OTC) [*Dramamine Chewable* (scored)].
Canada—
Not commercially available.

**Packaging and storage**
Store below 40 °C (104 °F), preferably between 15 and 30 °C (59 and 86 °F), unless otherwise specified by manufacturer. Store in a well-closed container.

**Auxiliary labeling**
• May cause drowsiness.
• Avoid alcoholic beverages.

# Parenteral Dosage Forms

## DIMENHYDRINATE INJECTION USP

**Usual adult and adolescent dose**
Antiemetic or
Antivertigo agent—
Intramuscular, 50 mg repeated every four hours as needed.
Intravenous, 50 mg in 10 mL of 0.9% sodium chloride injection, administered slowly over a period of at least two minutes, repeated every four hours as needed.

**Usual pediatric dose**
Antiemetic or
Antivertigo agent—
Intramuscular, 1.25 mg per kg of body weight or 37.5 mg per square meter of body surface, every six hours as needed, not to exceed 300 mg per day.
Intravenous, 1.25 mg per kg of body weight or 37.5 mg per square meter of body surface, in 10 mL of 0.9% sodium chloride injection, administered slowly over a period of at least two minutes, every six hours as needed, not to exceed 300 mg per day.

Note: Premature and full-term neonates—Use is not recommended.

**Usual geriatric dose**
See *Usual adult and adolescent dose*.

Note: Geriatric patients may be more sensitive to the effects of the usual adult dose.

**Strength(s) usually available**
U.S.—
50 mg per mL (Rx) [*Dinate; Dommanate; Dramamine; Dramanate; Dramocen; Dramoject; Dymenate; Hydrate; Marmine;* GENERIC].
Canada—
50 mg per mL (Rx) [*Gravol;* GENERIC].

**Packaging and storage**
Store below 40 °C (104 °F), preferably between 15 and 30 °C (59 and 86 °F), unless otherwise specified by manufacturer. Protect from freezing.

# Rectal Dosage Forms

## DIMENHYDRINATE SUPPOSITORIES

**Usual adult and adolescent dose**
Antiemetic or
Antivertigo agent—
Rectal, 50 to 100 mg every six to eight hours as needed.

**Usual pediatric dose**
Antiemetic or
Antivertigo agent—
Children up to 6 years of age: Dosage has not been established.
Children 6 to 8 years of age: Rectal, 12.5 to 25 mg every eight to twelve hours as needed.
Children 8 to 12 years of age: Rectal, 25 to 50 mg every eight to twelve hours as needed.
Children 12 years of age and over: Rectal, 50 mg every eight to twelve hours as needed.

**Usual geriatric dose**
See *Usual adult and adolescent dose.*
Note: Geriatric patients may be more sensitive to the effects of the usual adult dose.

**Strength(s) usually available**
U.S.—
Not commercially available.
Canada—
50 mg (OTC) [*Gravol; Nauseatol*].
100 mg (OTC) [*Gravol; Nauseatol*].

**Packaging and storage**
Store between 8 and 15 °C (46 and 59 °F), in a well-closed container, unless otherwise specified by manufacturer.

**Auxiliary labeling**
• May cause drowsiness.
• Avoid alcoholic beverages.

**Note**
When dispensing, include patient instructions.

---

## *DIPHENHYDRAMINE*

# Summary of Differences

Category:
Also indicated as an antidyskinetic, antiemetic, antitussive (syrup only), antivertigo agent, and a sedative-hypnotic.
Pharmacology/pharmacokinetics:
Chemical group—Ethanolamine derivative.
pKa—9.
Other actions/effects—Greater anticholinergic activity.
Protein binding—98 to 99%.
Half-life—1 to 4 hours.
Time to peak concentration—1 to 4 hours.
Duration of action—6 to 8 hours.
Precautions:
Drug interactions and/or related problems—May decrease emetic response to apomorphine.
Medical considerations/contraindications—May impede diagnosis of appendicitis; may obscure signs of overdose.
Side/adverse effects:
Sedative effects more pronounced.

# Additional Dosing Information

See also *General Dosing Information.*
When diphenhydramine is used for prophylaxis of motion sickness, it should be taken at least 30 minutes, and preferably 1 or 2 hours, before exposure to conditions that may precipitate motion sickness.

# Oral Dosage Forms

## DIPHENHYDRAMINE HYDROCHLORIDE CAPSULES USP

**Usual adult and adolescent dose**
Antihistaminic (H₁-receptor)—
Oral, 25 to 50 mg every four to six hours as needed.
Antidyskinetic[1]—
For idiopathic and postencephalitic parkinsonism: Oral, 25 mg three times a day initially, the dose then being gradually increased to 50 mg four times a day if needed.
Antiemetic or

Antivertigo agent—
Oral, 25 to 50 mg every four to six hours as needed.
Sedative-hypnotic—
Oral, 50 mg twenty to thirty minutes before bedtime if needed.

**Usual adult prescribing limits**
Up to 300 mg daily.

**Usual pediatric dose**
Antihistaminic (H₁-receptor)—
Children up to 6 years of age: Oral, 6.25 to 12.5 mg every four to six hours.
Children 6 to 12 years of age: Oral, 12.5 to 25 mg every four to six hours, not to exceed 150 mg per day.
Antiemetic or
Antivertigo agent—
Oral, 1 to 1.5 mg per kg of body weight every four to six hours as needed, not to exceed 300 mg per day.
Note: The available strength of the capsule may not conform to some of the recommended pediatric dosages.

**Usual geriatric dose**
See *Usual adult and adolescent dose.*
Note: Geriatric patients may be more sensitive to the effects of the usual adult dose.

**Strength(s) usually available**
U.S.—
25 mg (Rx) [*Benadryl; Genahist; Nordryl;* GENERIC].
25 mg (OTC) [*Banophen; Benadryl 25; Dormin;* GENERIC].
50 mg (Rx) [*Banophen; Benadryl Kapseals; Nordryl; Unisom SleepGels Maximum Strength;* GENERIC].
Canada—
25 mg (Rx) [*Allerdryl*].
25 mg (OTC) [*Benadryl; Insomnal*].
50 mg (Rx) [*Allerdryl*].
50 mg (OTC) [*Benadryl*].

**Packaging and storage**
Store below 40 °C (104 °F), preferably between 15 and 30 °C (59 and 86 °F), unless otherwise specified by manufacturer. Store in a tight container.

**Auxiliary labeling**
• May cause drowsiness.
• Avoid alcoholic beverages.

## DIPHENHYDRAMINE HYDROCHLORIDE ELIXIR USP

**Usual adult and adolescent dose**
See *Diphenhydramine Hydrochloride Capsules USP.*

**Usual adult prescribing limits**
See *Diphenhydramine Hydrochloride Capsules USP.*

**Usual pediatric dose**
Antihistaminic (H₁-receptor)—
Oral, 1.25 mg per kg of body weight or 37.5 mg per square meter of body surface, every four to six hours, not to exceed 300 mg a day
or for
Children weighing up to 9.1 kg: Oral, 6.25 to 12.5 mg every four to six hours.
Children weighing 9.1 kg and over: Oral, 12.5 to 25 mg every four to six hours.
Antiemetic or
Antivertigo agent—
Oral, 1 to 1.5 mg per kg of body weight every four to six hours as needed, not to exceed 300 mg per day.
Note: Premature and full-term neonates—Use is not recommended.

**Usual geriatric dose**
See *Usual adult and adolescent dose.*
Note: Geriatric patients may be more sensitive to the effects of the usual adult dose.

**Strength(s) usually available**
U.S.—
12.5 mg per 5 mL (Rx) [*Benadryl* (alcohol 14%); *Fynex; Hydramine* (alcohol 14%); *Hydril; Noradryl; Nordryl* (alcohol 14%); *Siladryl* (alcohol 5.6%); GENERIC].
12.5 mg per 5 mL (OTC) [*Belix* (alcohol 14%); *Diphenhist; Genahist* (alcohol 14%); *Nidryl* (alcohol 14%); *Phendry* (alcohol 14%); *Phendry Children's Allergy Medicine* (alcohol 14%); *Sominex Formula 2;* GENERIC].
Canada—
12.5 mg per 5 mL (OTC) [*Benadryl* (alcohol 14%)].

**Packaging and storage**
Store below 40 °C (104 °F), preferably between 15 and 30 °C (59 and 86 °F), unless otherwise specified by manufacturer. Store in a tight container. Protect from light. Protect from freezing.

**Auxiliary labeling**
• May cause drowsiness.
• Avoid alcoholic beverages.
• Keep container tightly closed.

## DIPHENHYDRAMINE HYDROCHLORIDE SYRUP

**Usual adult and adolescent dose**
Antihistaminic (H₁-receptor)
Antidyskinetic[1]
Antiemetic
Antivertigo agent or
Sedative-hypnotic—
    See *Diphenhydramine Hydrochloride Capsules USP.*
Antitussive—
    Oral, 25 mg every four to six hours.

**Usual adult prescribing limits**
See *Diphenhydramine Hydrochloride Capsules USP.*

**Usual pediatric dose**
Antihistaminic (H₁-receptor)
Antiemetic or
Antivertigo agent—
    See *Diphenhydramine Hydrochloride Elixir USP.*
Antitussive—
    Children up to 2 years of age: Dosage must be individualized by physician.
    Children 2 to 6 years of age: Oral, 6.25 mg every four to six hours, as needed, not to exceed 25 mg per day.
    Children 6 to 12 years of age: Oral, 12.5 mg every four to six hours, as needed, not to exceed 75 mg per day.

Note: Premature and full-term neonates—Use is not recommended.

**Usual geriatric dose**
See *Diphenhydramine Hydrochloride Capsules USP.*

Note: Geriatric patients may be more sensitive to the effects of the usual adult dose.

**Strength(s) usually available**
U.S.—
    12.5 mg per 5 mL (Rx) [*Beldin; Hydramyn* (alcohol 5%); *Noradryl; Tusstat* (alcohol 5%); GENERIC].
    12.5 mg per 5 mL (OTC) [*Benylin Cough* (alcohol 5%); *Bydramine Cough* (alcohol 5%); *Diphenadryl; Diphen Cough* (alcohol 5%); *Gen-D-phen* (alcohol 5%); *Hydramine Cough* (alcohol 5%); *Nordryl Cough; Silphen Cough Syrup; Uni-Bent Cough* (alcohol 5%); GENERIC].
Canada—
    Not commercially available.

**Packaging and storage**
Store below 40 °C (104 °F), preferably between 15 and 30 °C (59 and 86 °F), in a well-closed container, unless otherwise specified by manufacturer. Protect from freezing.

**Auxiliary labeling**
• May cause drowsiness.
• Avoid alcoholic beverages.

## DIPHENHYDRAMINE HYDROCHLORIDE TABLETS

**Usual adult and adolescent dose**
See *Diphenhydramine Hydrochloride Capsules USP.*

**Usual adult prescribing limits**
See *Diphenhydramine Hydrochloride Capsules USP.*

**Usual pediatric dose**
See *Diphenhydramine Hydrochloride Elixir USP.*

**Usual geriatric dose**
See *Diphenhydramine Hydrochloride Capsules USP.*

Note: Geriatric patients may be more sensitive to the effects of the usual adult dose.

**Strength(s) usually available**
U.S.—
    25 mg (Rx) [*Genahist;* GENERIC].
    25 mg (OTC) [*AllerMax Caplets; Aller-med; Banophen Caplets; Benadryl 25; Diphenhist Captabs; Nervine Nighttime Sleep-Aid; Nytol with DPH; Sleep-Eze 3; Sominex Formula 2*].
    50 mg (Rx) [GENERIC].
    50 mg (OTC) [*AllerMax Caplets; Compoz; Dormarex 2; Nytol Maximum Strength; Twilite Caplets*].

Canada—
    Not commercially available.

**Packaging and storage**
Store below 40 °C (104 °F), preferably between 15 and 30 °C (59 and 86 °F), in a well-closed container, unless otherwise specified by manufacturer.

**Auxiliary labeling**
• May cause drowsiness.
• Avoid alcoholic beverages.

# Parenteral Dosage Forms

## DIPHENHYDRAMINE HYDROCHLORIDE INJECTION USP

**Usual adult and adolescent dose**
Antihistaminic (H₁-receptor) or
Antidyskinetic[1]—
    Intramuscular or intravenous, 10 to 50 mg.
Antiemetic or
Antivertigo agent—
    Intramuscular or intravenous, 10 mg initially, may be increased to 20 to 50 mg every two to three hours.

**Usual adult prescribing limits**
Up to 100 mg per dose or 400 mg daily.

**Usual pediatric dose**
Antihistaminic (H₁-receptor) or
Antidyskinetic—
    Intramuscular, 1.25 mg per kg of body weight or 37.5 mg per square meter of body surface, four times a day, not to exceed 300 mg per day.
Antiemetic or
Antivertigo agent—
    Intramuscular, 1 to 1.5 mg per kg of body weight every six hours, not to exceed 300 mg per day.

Note: Premature and full-term neonates—Use is not recommended.

**Usual geriatric dose**
See *Usual adult and adolescent dose.*

Note: Geriatric patients may be more sensitive to the effects of the usual adult dose.

**Strength(s) usually available**
U.S.—
    10 mg per mL (Rx) [*Bena-D 10; Benadryl; Benahist 10; Benoject-10; Nordryl; Wehdryl-10;* GENERIC].
    50 mg per mL (Rx) [*Bena-D 50; Benadryl; Benahist 50; Ben-Allergin-50; Benoject-50; Diphenacen-50; Hyrexin-50; Nordryl; Wehdryl-50;* GENERIC].
Canada—
    10 mg per mL [*Benadryl*].
    50 mg per mL [*Benadryl;* GENERIC].

**Packaging and storage**
Store below 40 °C (104 °F), preferably between 15 and 30 °C (59 and 86 °F), unless otherwise specified by manufacturer. Protect from light. Protect from freezing.

---

[1]Not included in Canadian product labeling.

---

### DOXYLAMINE

# Summary of Differences

Category:
    Also indicated as a sedative-hypnotic.
Pharmacology/pharmacokinetics:
    Chemical group—Ethanolamine derivative.
    pKa—5.8 and 9.3.
    Other actions/effects—Greater anticholinergic activity.
    Duration of action—6 to 8 hours.
Precautions:
    Drug interactions and/or related problems—
        May decrease emetic response to apomorphine.
Side/adverse effects:
    Sedative effects more pronounced.

# Oral Dosage Forms

## DOXYLAMINE SUCCINATE TABLETS USP

**Usual adult and adolescent dose**
Antihistaminic (H₁-receptor)—
Oral, 12.5 to 25 mg every four to six hours as needed.
Sedative-hypnotic—
Oral, 25 mg thirty minutes before bedtime if needed.

**Usual adult prescribing limits**
Up to 150 mg daily.

**Usual pediatric dose**
Antihistaminic (H₁-receptor)—
Children up to 6 years of age: Use is not recommended.
Children 6 to 12 years of age: Oral, 6.25 to 12.5 mg every four to six hours as needed.
Sedative-hypnotic—
Use is not recommended.

**Usual geriatric dose**
See *Usual adult and adolescent dose.*

Note: Geriatric patients may be more sensitive to the effects of the usual adult dose.

**Strength(s) usually available**
U.S.—
25 mg (OTC) [*Unisom Nighttime Sleep Aid* (scored)].
Canada—
Not commercially available.

**Packaging and storage**
Store below 40 °C (104 °F), preferably between 15 and 30 °C (59 and 86 °F), unless otherwise specified by manufacturer. Store in a well-closed container. Protect from light.

**Auxiliary labeling**
• May cause drowsiness.
• Avoid alcoholic beverages.

---

## *HYDROXYZINE*

# Summary of Differences

Category:
Also indicated in the treatment of anxiety and psychosis-related tension; antiemetic agent and sedative-hypnotic.
Pharmacology/pharmacokinetics:
Chemical group—Piperazine derivative.
pKa—Hydroxyzine hydrochloride: 2.6 and 7.
Half-life (elimination)—20 to 25 hours.
Duration of action—4 to 6 hours.
Precautions:
Drug interactions and/or related problems—May decrease emetic response to apomorphine.
Laboratory value alterations—False increases in urine 17-hydroxycorticosteroid determinations.
Medical considerations/contraindications—May impede diagnosis of appendicitis; may obscure signs of overdose.

# Oral Dosage Forms

## HYDROXYZINE HYDROCHLORIDE CAPSULES

**Usual adult and adolescent dose**
Antianxiety agent or
Sedative-hypnotic—
Oral, 50 to 100 mg as a single dose.
Antihistaminic (H₁-receptor) or
Antiemetic—
Oral, 25 to 100 mg three or four times a day as needed.

**Usual pediatric dose**
Antianxiety agent or
Sedative-hypnotic—
Oral, 600 mcg (0.6 mg) per kg of body weight as a single dose.
Antihistaminic (H₁-receptor) or
Antiemetic—
Oral, 500 mcg (0.5 mg) per kg of body weight or 15 mg per square meter of body surface every six hours as needed; or for
Children up to 6 years of age: Oral, 30 to 50 mg a day in divided doses, or 12.5 mg every six hours as needed.
Children 6 to 12 years of age: Oral, 50 to 100 mg a day in divided doses, or 12.5 to 25 mg every six hours as needed.

**Usual geriatric dose**
See *Usual adult and adolescent dose.*

Note: Geriatric patients may be more sensitive to the effects of the usual adult dose.

**Strength(s) usually available**
U.S.—
Not commercially available.
Canada—
10 mg (Rx) [*Apo-Hydroxyzine; Atarax; Multipax; Novo-Hydroxyzin*].
25 mg (Rx) [*Apo-Hydroxyzine; Atarax; Multipax; Novo-Hydroxyzin*].
50 mg (Rx) [*Apo-Hydroxyzine; Atarax; Multipax; Novo-Hydroxyzin*].

**Packaging and storage**
Store below 40 °C (104 °F), preferably between 15 and 30 °C (59 and 86 °F), unless otherwise specified by manufacturer.

**Auxiliary labeling**
• May cause drowsiness.
• Avoid alcoholic beverages.

## HYDROXYZINE HYDROCHLORIDE SYRUP USP

**Usual adult and adolescent dose**
See *Hydroxyzine Hydrochloride Capsules.*

**Usual pediatric dose**
See *Hydroxyzine Hydrochloride Capsules.*

**Usual geriatric dose**
See *Hydroxyzine Hydrochloride Capsules.*

Note: Geriatric patients may be more sensitive to the effects of the usual adult dose.

**Strength(s) usually available**
U.S.—
10 mg per 5 mL (Rx) [*Atarax* (alcohol 0.5%); GENERIC].
Canada—
10 mg per 5 mL (Rx) [*Atarax*].

**Packaging and storage**
Store below 40 °C (104 °F), preferably between 15 and 30 °C (59 and 86 °F), unless otherwise specified by manufacturer. Store in a tight, light-resistant container. Protect from freezing.

**Auxiliary labeling**
• May cause drowsiness.
• Avoid alcoholic beverages.

## HYDROXYZINE HYDROCHLORIDE TABLETS USP

**Usual adult and adolescent dose**
See *Hydroxyzine Hydrochloride Capsules.*

**Usual pediatric dose**
See *Hydroxyzine Hydrochloride Capsules.*

**Usual geriatric dose**
See *Hydroxyzine Hydrochloride Capsules..*

Note: Geriatric patients may be more sensitive to the effects of the usual adult dose.

**Strength(s) usually available**
U.S.—
10 mg (Rx) [*Atarax;* GENERIC].
25 mg (Rx) [*Anxanil; Atarax;* GENERIC].
50 mg (Rx) [*Atarax;* GENERIC].
100 mg (Rx) [*Atarax;* GENERIC].
Canada—
Not commercially available.

**Packaging and storage**
Store below 40 °C (104 °F), preferably between 15 and 30 °C (59 and 86 °F), unless otherwise specified by manufacturer. Store in a tight container.

**Auxiliary labeling**
• May cause drowsiness.
• Avoid alcoholic beverages.

## HYDROXYZINE PAMOATE CAPSULES USP

**Usual adult and adolescent dose**
Antianxiety agent or
Sedative-hypnotic—
Oral, 50 to 100 mg as a single dose.
Antihistaminic (H₁-receptor) or
Antiemetic—
Oral, 25 to 100 mg three to four times a day as needed.

**Usual pediatric dose**

Antianxiety agent or

Sedative-hypnotic—

Oral, 600 mcg (0.6 mg) per kg of body weight as a single dose.

Antihistaminic (H₁-receptor) or

Antiemetic—

Oral, 500 mcg (0.5 mg) per kg of body weight or 15 mg per square meter of body surface every six hours as needed; or for

Children 6 years of age and over: Oral, 12.5 to 25 mg every six hours as needed.

**Usual geriatric dose**

See *Usual adult and adolescent dose.*

Note: Geriatric patients may be more sensitive to the effects of the usual adult dose.

**Strength(s) usually available**

U.S.—The equivalent of hydroxyzine hydrochloride:

25 mg (Rx) [*Vistaril;* GENERIC].

50 mg (Rx) [*Vistaril;* GENERIC].

100 mg (Rx) [*Vistaril;* GENERIC].

Canada—

Not commercially available.

**Packaging and storage**

Store below 40 °C (104 °F), preferably between 15 and 30 °C (59 and 86 °F), in a well-closed container, unless otherwise specified by manufacturer.

**Auxiliary labeling**

• May cause drowsiness.

• Avoid alcoholic beverages.

## HYDROXYZINE PAMOATE ORAL SUSPENSION USP

**Usual adult and adolescent dose**

See *Hydroxyzine Pamoate Capsules USP.*

**Usual pediatric dose**

Antianxiety agent or

Sedative-hypnotic—

Oral, 600 mcg (0.6 mg) per kg of body weight as a single dose.

Antihistaminic (H₁-receptor) or

Antiemetic—

Oral, 500 mcg (0.5 mg) per kg of body weight or 15 mg per square meter of body surface every six hours as needed; or for

Children up to 6 years of age: Oral, 12.5 mg every six hours as needed.

Children 6 years of age and over: Oral, 12.5 to 25 mg every six hours as needed.

**Usual geriatric dose**

See *Hydroxyzine Pamoate Capsules USP.*

Note: Geriatric patients may be more sensitive to the effects of the usual adult dose.

**Strength(s) usually available**

U.S.—The equivalent of hydroxyzine hydrochloride:

25 mg per 5 mL (Rx) [*Vistaril*].

Canada—

Not commercially available.

**Packaging and storage**

Store below 40 °C (104 °F), preferably between 15 and 30 °C (59 and 86 °F), unless otherwise specified by manufacturer. Store in a tight, light-resistant container. Protect from freezing.

**Auxiliary labeling**

• Shake well.

• May cause drowsiness.

• Avoid alcoholic beverages.

## Parenteral Dosage Forms

### HYDROXYZINE HYDROCHLORIDE INJECTION USP

**Usual adult and adolescent dose**

Antianxiety agent—

Intramuscular, 50 to 100 mg, repeated as needed every four to six hours.

Sedative-hypnotic—

Intramuscular, 50 mg as a single dose.

Adjunct to narcotic medication: Intramuscular, 25 to 100 mg.

Antiemetic—

Intramuscular, 25 to 100 mg.

**Usual pediatric dose**

Adjunct to narcotic medication or

Antiemetic—

Intramuscular, 1 mg per kg of body weight, or 30 mg per square meter of body surface, as a single dose.

**Usual geriatric dose**

See *Usual adult and adolescent dose.*

Note: Geriatric patients may be more sensitive to the effects of the usual adult dose.

**Strength(s) usually available**

U.S.—

25 mg per ml (Rx) [*Vistaject-25; Vistaril;* GENERIC].

50 mg per mL (Rx) [*E-Vista; Hydroxacen; Hyzine-50; Quiess; Vistaject-50; Vistaril; Vistazine 50;* GENERIC].

Canada—

50 mg per mL (Rx) [*Atarax;* GENERIC].

**Packaging and storage**

Store below 40 °C (104 °F), preferably between 15 and 30 °C (59 and 86 °F), unless otherwise specified by manufacturer. Protect from light. Protect from freezing.

---

### LORATADINE

## Summary of Differences

Indications:

Used as treatment adjunct in asthma.

Pharmacology/pharmacokinetics:

Chemical group—Piperidine derivative.

Other actions/effects—No significant anticholinergic activity. Mild bronchodilator.

Protein binding—97%.

Half-life—3 to 20 hours.

Onset of action—1 hour.

Time to peak concentration—1 to 2 hours.

Time to peak effect—4 to 6 hours.

Duration of action—At least 24 hours.

Precautions:

Dental—

No dental precaution.

Side/adverse effects:

Anticholinergic effects not likely; dose-related sedation.

## Oral Dosage Forms

### LORATADINE SYRUP

**Usual adult and adolescent dose**

Antihistaminic (H₁-receptor)—Oral, 10 mg once a day.

**Usual pediatric dose**

Antihistaminic (H₁-receptor)—

Children 2 to 9 years of age: Oral, 5 mg once a day.

Children 10 years of age and over: See *Usual adult and adolescent dose.*

**Usual geriatric dose**

See *Usual adult and adolescent dose.*

Note: Geriatric patients may be more sensitive to the effects of the usual adult dose.

**Strength(s) usually available**

U.S.—

Not commercially available.

Canada—

5 mg per 5 mL (OTC) [*Claritin*].

**Packaging and storage**

Store between 2 and 30 °C (36 and 86 °F), in a well-closed container, unless otherwise specified by manufacturer.

### LORATADINE TABLETS

**Usual adult and adolescent dose**

See *Loratadine Syrup.*

**Usual pediatric dose**

See *Loratadine Syrup.*

**Usual geriatric dose**

See *Loratadine Syrup.*

Note: Geriatric patients may be more sensitive to the effects of the usual adult dose.

**Strength(s) usually available**
U.S.—
   10 mg (Rx) [*Claritin* (scored)].
Canada—
   10 mg (OTC) [*Claritin* (scored)].

**Packaging and storage**
Store below 40 °C (104 °F), preferably between 15 and 30 °C (59 and 86 °F), in a well-closed container, unless otherwise specified by manufacturer.

---

### PHENINDAMINE

## Summary of Differences

Pharmacology/pharmacokinetics:
   Chemical group—Piperidine derivative.
   Duration of action—4 to 6 hours.

## Oral Dosage Forms

### PHENINDAMINE TARTRATE TABLETS

**Usual adult and adolescent dose**
Antihistaminic (H₁-receptor)—
   Oral, 25 mg every four to six hours as needed.

**Usual adult prescribing limits**
Up to 150 mg daily.

**Usual pediatric dose**
Antihistaminic (H₁-receptor)—
   Children up to 6 years of age: Dosage must be individualized by physician.
   Children 6 to 12 years of age: Oral, 12.5 mg every four to six hours as needed, not to exceed 75 mg per day.
   Children 12 years of age and over: See *Usual adult and adolescent dose.*

**Usual geriatric dose**
See *Usual adult and adolescent dose.*

Note: Geriatric patients may be more sensitive to the effects of the usual adult dose.

**Strength(s) usually available**
U.S.—
   25 mg (OTC) [*Nolahist* (scored)].
Canada—
   Not commercially available.

**Packaging and storage**
Store below 40 °C (104 °F), preferably between 15 and 30 °C (59 and 86 °F), in a well-closed container, unless otherwise specified by manufacturer.

**Auxiliary labeling**
• May cause drowsiness.
• Avoid alcoholic beverages.

---

### PYRILAMINE

## Summary of Differences

Pharmacology/pharmacokinetics:
   Chemical group—Ethylenediamine derivative.
   Duration of action—8 hours.
Side/adverse effects:
   Gastrointestinal effects more pronounced.

## Oral Dosage Forms

### PYRILAMINE MALEATE TABLETS USP

**Usual adult and adolescent dose**
Antihistaminic (H₁-receptor)—
   Oral, 25 to 50 mg every eight hours as needed.

**Usual adult prescribing limits**
Up to 200 mg daily.

**Usual pediatric dose**
Antihistaminic (H₁-receptor)—
   Children 2 to 6 years of age: Use is not recommended.
   Children 6 years of age and over: Oral, 12.5 to 25 mg every eight hours as needed.

**Usual geriatric dose**
See *Usual adult and adolescent dose.*

Note: Geriatric patients may be more sensitive to the effects of the usual adult dose.

**Strength(s) usually available**
U.S.—
   25 mg (Rx) [*Nisaval*].
   25 mg (OTC) [GENERIC].
Canada—
   Not commercially available.

**Packaging and storage**
Store below 40 °C (104 °F), preferably between 15 and 30 °C (59 and 86 °F), unless otherwise specified by manufacturer. Store in a well-closed container.

**Auxiliary labeling**
• May cause drowsiness.
• Avoid alcoholic beverages.

---

### TERFENADINE

## Summary of Differences

Indications:
   Used as treatment adjunct in asthma.
Pharmacology/pharmacokinetics:
   Chemical group—Piperidine derivative.
   Other actions/effects—No significant anticholinergic activity. Mild bronchodilator.
   Protein binding—97%.
   Half-life—8.5 hours.
   Onset of action—1 to 2 hours.
   Time to peak concentration—2 hours.
   Time to peak effect—3 to 4 hours.
   Duration of action—Over 12 hours.
   Elimination—Primarily fecal.
Precautions:
   Dental—No dental precaution.
   Drug interactions and/or related problems—Possible cardiotoxic effects with erythromycin and other macrolide antibiotics, itraconazole, ketoconazole, or with medications causing QT interval prolongation.
   Medical considerations/contraindications—Possible cardiotoxic effects with hepatic function impairment, history of QT interval prolongation, or with hypokalemia.
Side/adverse effects:
   Sedative and anticholinergic side effects less likely. Cardiac arrhythmias with high doses or overdose. May cause increased appetite and weight gain.

## Oral Dosage Forms

Note: Bracketed uses in the *Dosage Forms* section refer to categories of use and/or indications that are not included in U.S. product labeling.

### TERFENADINE ORAL SUSPENSION

**Usual adult and adolescent dose**
Antihistaminic (H₁-receptor)—
   Oral, 60 mg every twelve hours, [or 120 mg once a day], as needed.

**Usual pediatric dose**
Antihistaminic (H₁-receptor)—
   Children 3 to 6 years of age: Oral, 15 mg every twelve hours as needed.
   Children 7 to 12 years of age: Oral, 30 mg every twelve hours as needed.

Note: Premature and full-term neonates—Use is not recommended.

**Usual geriatric dose**
See *Usual adult and adolescent dose.*

Note: Geriatric patients may be more sensitive to the effects of the usual adult dose.

**Strength(s) usually available**
U.S.—
   Not commercially available.
Canada—
   6 mg per mL (OTC) [*Seldane*].

**Packaging and storage**
Store below 40 °C (104 °F), preferably between 15 and 30 °C (59 and 86 °F), unless otherwise specified by manufacturer. Store in a well-closed

container, unless otherwise specified by manufacturer. Protect from freezing.

**Auxiliary labeling**
• Shake well.

## TERFENADINE TABLETS USP

**Usual adult and adolescent dose**
See *Terfenadine Oral Suspension*.

**Usual pediatric dose**
The available strength of the tablet does not conform to the recommended pediatric dosages for this age group. See *Terfenadine Oral Suspension*.

**Usual geriatric dose**
See *Terfenadine Oral Suspension*.

Note: Geriatric patients may be more sensitive to the effects of the usual adult dose.

**Strength(s) usually available**
U.S.—
    60 mg (Rx) [*Seldane*].
Canada—
    60 mg (OTC) [*Novo-Terfenadine; Seldane*].
    120 mg (OTC) [*Seldane Caplets*].

**Packaging and storage**
Store below 40 °C (104 °F), preferably between 15 and 30 °C (59 and 86 °F), in a tight container, unless otherwise specified by manufacturer.

---

### *TRIPELENNAMINE*

## Summary of Differences

Pharmacology/pharmacokinetics:
    Chemical group—Ethylenediamine derivative.
    pKa—3.9 and 9.0.
    Duration of action—4 to 6 hours.
Side/adverse effects:
    Gastrointestinal effects more pronounced.

## Oral Dosage Forms

### TRIPELENNAMINE CITRATE ELIXIR USP

**Usual adult and adolescent dose**
Antihistaminic (H₁-receptor)—
    Oral, the equivalent of tripelennamine hydrochloride: 25 to 50 mg every four to six hours as needed.

**Usual adult prescribing limits**
Up to the equivalent of 600 mg of tripelennamine hydrochloride daily.

**Usual pediatric dose**
Antihistaminic (H₁-receptor)—
    Oral, the equivalent of tripelennamine hydrochloride, 1.25 mg per kg of body weight or 37.5 mg per square meter of body surface every six hours as needed, not to exceed 300 mg per day.

Note: Premature and full-term neonates—Use is not recommended.

**Usual geriatric dose**
See *Usual adult and adolescent dose*.

Note: Geriatric patients may be more sensitive to the effects of the usual adult dose.

**Strength(s) usually available**
U.S.—
    37.5 mg of tripelennamine citrate (25 mg of tripelennamine hydrochloride) per 5 mL (Rx) [*PBZ* (alcohol 12%)].
Canada—
    Not commercially available.

**Packaging and storage**
Store below 40 °C (104 °F), preferably between 15 and 30 °C (59 and 86 °F), unless otherwise specified by manufacturer. Store in a tight, light-resistant container. Protect from freezing.

**Auxiliary labeling**
• May cause drowsiness.
• Avoid alcoholic beverages.
• Keep container tightly closed.

### TRIPELENNAMINE HYDROCHLORIDE TABLETS USP

**Usual adult and adolescent dose**
Antihistaminic (H₁-receptor)—Oral, 25 to 50 mg every four to six hours as needed.

**Usual adult prescribing limits**
Up to 600 mg daily.

**Usual pediatric dose**
Antihistaminic (H₁-receptor)—Oral, 1.25 mg per kg of body weight or 37.5 mg per square meter of body surface every six hours as needed, not to exceed 300 mg per day.

Note: Premature and full-term neonates—Use is not recommended.

**Usual geriatric dose**
See *Usual adult and adolescent dose*.

Note: Geriatric patients may be more sensitive to the effects of the usual adult dose.

**Strength(s) usually available**
U.S.—
    25 mg (Rx) [*PBZ* (scored)].
    50 mg (Rx) [*PBZ* (scored); *Pelamine* (scored); GENERIC].
Canada—
    50 mg (OTC) [*Pyribenzamine* (scored)].

**Packaging and storage**
Store below 40 °C (104 °F), preferably between 15 and 30 °C (59 and 86 °F), unless otherwise specified by manufacturer. Store in a well-closed container.

**Auxiliary labeling**
• May cause drowsiness.
• Avoid alcoholic beverages.

### TRIPELENNAMINE HYDROCHLORIDE EXTENDED-RELEASE TABLETS

**Usual adult and adolescent dose**
Antihistaminic (H₁-receptor)—Oral, 100 mg every eight to twelve hours as needed.

**Usual adult prescribing limits**
Up to 600 mg daily.

**Usual pediatric dose**
Use is not recommended.

**Usual geriatric dose**
See *Usual adult and adolescent dose*.

Note: Geriatric patients may be more sensitive to the effects of the usual adult dose.

**Strength(s) usually available**
U.S.—
    100 mg (Rx) [*PBZ-SR*].
Canada—
    Not commercially available.

**Packaging and storage**
Store below 40 °C (104 °F), preferably between 15 and 30 °C (59 and 86 °F), in a well-closed container, unless otherwise specified by manufacturer. Protect from light.

**Auxiliary labeling**
• Swallow tablets whole.
• May cause drowsiness.
• Avoid alcoholic beverages.

---

### *TRIPROLIDINE*

## Summary of Differences

Pharmacology/pharmacokinetics:
    Chemical group—Propylamine derivative.
    pKa—3.6 and 9.3.
    Half-life—3 to 3.3 hours.
    Time to peak concentration—2 hours.
    Time to peak effect—2 to 3 hours.
    Duration of action—4 to 8 hours.
Side/adverse effects:
    Sedative effects less pronounced.

## Oral Dosage Forms

### TRIPROLIDINE HYDROCHLORIDE SYRUP USP

**Usual adult and adolescent dose**
Antihistaminic (H₁-receptor)—Oral, 2.5 mg every four to six hours as needed.

**Usual adult prescribing limits**
Up to 10 mg daily.

**Usual pediatric dose**

Antihistaminic (H₁-receptor)—

Children 4 months to 2 years of age: Oral, 312 mcg (0.312 mg) every six to eight hours as needed.

Children 2 to 4 years of age: Oral, 625 mcg (0.625 mg) every six to eight hours as needed.

Children 4 to 6 years of age: Oral, 937 mcg (0.937 mg) every six to eight hours as needed.

Children 6 to 12 years of age: Oral, 1.25 mg every six to eight hours as needed.

Note: Premature and full-term neonates—Use is not recommended.

**Usual geriatric dose**

See *Usual adult and adolescent dose.*

Note: Geriatric patients may be more sensitive to the effects of the usual adult dose.

**Strength(s) usually available**

U.S.—

1.25 mg per 5 mL (Rx) [*Myidil* (alcohol 4%); GENERIC].

Canada—

Not commercially available.

**Packaging and storage**

Store below 40 °C (104 °F), preferably between 15 and 30 °C (59 and 86 °F), unless otherwise specified by manufacturer. Store in a tight, light-resistant container. Protect from freezing.

**Auxiliary labeling**

• May cause drowsiness.
• Avoid alcoholic beverages.

## Selected Bibliography

Simons FE, et al. The comparative pharmacokinetics of H₁-receptor antagonists. Ann Allergy 1987 Dec; 59 (6 Pt 2): 20-4.

Simons FE, Simons KJ. Second-generation H₁-receptor antagonists. Review article. Ann Allergy 1991; 66: 5-15.

Wood-Baker R, Holgate ST. The comparative actions and adverse effect profile of single doses of H₁-receptor antihistamines in the airways and skin of subjects with asthma. J Allergy Clin Immunol 1993; 91: 1005-14.

Barnes CL, McKenzie CA, Webster KD. Cetirizine: a new, nonsedating antihistamine. Ann Pharmacother 1993; 27: 464-70.

Horak F. Seasonal allergic rhinitis—newer treatment approaches. Drugs 1993; 45: 518-27.

Simons FE, Simons KJ, Chung M, et al. The comparative pharmacokinetics of H₁-receptor antagonists. Ann Allergy 1987; 59: 20-4.

Revised: 07/26/94
Interim revision: 07/10/96

# ANTIHISTAMINES AND DECONGESTANTS   Systemic

This monograph includes information on the following: Acrivastine and Pseudoephedrine; Azatadine and Pseudoephedrine; Brompheniramine and Phenylephrine; Brompheniramine, Phenylephrine, and Phenylpropanolamine; Brompheniramine and Phenylpropanolamine; Brompheniramine and Pseudoephedrine; Carbinoxamine and Pseudoephedrine; Chlorpheniramine, Phenindamine, and Phenylpropanolamine; Chlorpheniramine and Phenylephrine; Chlorpheniramine, Phenylephrine, and Phenylpropanolamine; Chlorpheniramine and Phenylpropanolamine; Chlorpheniramine, Phenyltoloxamine, and Phenylephrine; Chlorpheniramine, Phenyltoloxamine, Phenylephrine, and Phenylpropanolamine; Chlorpheniramine and Pseudoephedrine; Chlorpheniramine, Pyrilamine, and Phenylephrine; Chlorpheniramine, Pyrilamine, Phenylephrine, and Phenylpropanolamine; Clemastine and Phenylpropanolamine; Dexbrompheniramine and Pseudoephedrine; Diphenhydramine and Pseudoephedrine; Loratadine and Pseudoephedrine; Pheniramine and Phenylephrine; Pheniramine, Phenyltoloxamine, Pyrilamine, and Phenylpropanolamine; Pheniramine, Pyrilamine, and Phenylpropanolamine; Promethazine and Phenylephrine; Terfenadine and Pseudoephedrine; Triprolidine and Pseudoephedrine.

INN:

Chlorpheniramine——Chlorphenamine

VA CLASSIFICATION (Primary): RE501

**NOTE:** The *Antihistamines and Decongestants (Systemic)* monograph is maintained on the USP DI electronic data base. For a printed copy of the most recent revision of the complete monograph, contact the USP Division of Information Development, 12601 Twinbrook Parkway, Rockville, MD 20852.

For information on the specific components of this combination, see the *USP DI* monographs for *Antihistamines (Systemic), Phenylephrine (Systemic), Phenylpropanolamine (Systemic),* and *Pseudoephedrine (Systemic),* and *Sympathomimetic Agents—Cardiovascular Use (Systemic).*

The information that follows is selectively abstracted from the complete monograph and is provided to facilitate drug use review and patient counseling.

Note: For a listing of dosage forms and brand names by country availability, see *Dosage Forms* section(s). For a listing of brand names for the articles in this monograph, refer to the General Index.

## Category

Antihistaminic (H₁-receptor)-decongestant.

## Indications

**Accepted**

Congestion, nasal (treatment)
Sneezing (treatment) and

Rhinorrhea (treatment)—Antihistamine and decongestant combinations are indicated for the temporary relief of nasal and sinus congestion, sneezing, and rhinorrhea associated with the common cold and allergic rhinitis.

The therapeutic effectiveness of oral phenylephrine as a nasal decongestant has been questioned, especially at the usual oral dose.

## Patient Consultation

As an aid to patient consultation, refer to *Advice for the Patient, Antihistamines and Decongestants (Systemic).*

In providing consultation, consider emphasizing the following selected information (» = major clinical significance):

**Before using this medication**

» Conditions affecting use, especially:

Sensitivity to any of the antihistamines or sympathomimetic amines

Pregnancy—Concern for the fetus and/or newborn infant only with high doses and long-term therapy; psychiatric disorders more likely with use of phenylpropanolamine in postpartum women

Breast-feeding—Antihistamines may cause excitement or irritability in nursing infants; high risk for infants from sympathomimetic amines

Use in children—Increased susceptibility to anticholinergic effects of antihistamines and to vasopressor effects of sympathomimetic amines; psychiatric disorders more likely with use of phenylpropanolamine in children under 6 years of age; hyperexcitability (paradoxical reaction) may occur

Use in the elderly—Anticholinergic and CNS stimulant effects more likely to occur

Other medications, especially anticholinergics; CNS depressants or stimulants; erythromycin and other macrolide antibiotics (with terfenadine-containing combination only); itraconazole and ketoconazole (with terfenadine-containing combination only); or medicine for high blood pressure or depression

Other medical problems, especially cardiovascular disease, diabetes, hepatic function impairment (with terfenadine-containing combination only), hypertension, hyperthyroidism, or prostatic hypertrophy

**Proper use of this medication**

» Importance of not taking more medication than the amount recommended

Taking with food, water, or milk to minimize gastric irritation

Swallowing extended-release dosage form whole

» Proper dosing

Missed dose: If on scheduled dosing regimen—Taking as soon as possible; not taking if almost time for next dose; not doubling doses

» Proper storage

**Precautions while using this medication**
    Caution if skin tests using allergens required; possible interference with test results
    May mask ototoxic effects of large doses of salicylates
» Avoiding use of alcohol or other CNS depressants
» Caution if drowsiness or dizziness occurs
» Caution if taking phenylpropanolamine-containing appetite suppressants
» Possible insomnia; taking the medication a few hours before bedtime
    Possible dryness of mouth; using sugarless gum or candy, ice, or saliva substitute for relief; checking with dentist if dry mouth continues for more than 2 weeks.

*For promethazine*
    Possible interference with diagnosis of intestinal obstruction, brain tumor, or overdosage of toxic drugs; need to inform physician of use

**Side/adverse effects**
    Signs of potential side effects, especially blood dyscrasias, cardiac arrhythmias, psychotic episodes, and tightness in chest

## Oral Dosage Forms
See *Table 1*, page 338.

Revised: 07/19/94
Interim revision: 07/25/95

### Table 1. Oral Dosage Forms
Note: Content per capsule, tablet, or 5 mL, unless otherwise stated.

| Brand or generic name [availability] | Antihistamines | Decongestants | Other content information as per product label | Usual adult and adolescent dose* prn | Usual pediatric dose prn | Packaging, storage, and auxiliary labeling† |
|---|---|---|---|---|---|---|
| *Actagen* Syrup USP (OTC) [U.S.] | Triprolidine HCl 1.25 mg | Pseudoephedrine HCl 30 mg | | 10 mL q 4–6 hr | 6–12 yrs: 5 mL q 4–6 hr | b, e, f, g |
| Tablets USP (OTC) [U.S.] | Triprolidine HCl 2.5 mg | Pseudoephedrine HCl 60 mg | | 1 tab q 4–6 hr | | b, f |
| *Actifed* Capsules (OTC) [U.S.] | Triprolidine HCl 2.5 mg | Pseudoephedrine HCl 60 mg | | 1 cap q 4–6 hr | | b, f, g |
| Syrup USP (OTC) [U.S./Canada] | Triprolidine HCl 1.25 mg | Pseudoephedrine HCl 30 mg | | 10 mL q 4–6 hr | 6–12 yrs: 5 mL q 4–6 hr | b, e, f, g |
| Tablets USP (OTC) [U.S./Canada] | Triprolidine HCl 2.5 mg | Pseudoephedrine HCl 60 mg | Scored | 1 tab q 4–6 hr | 6–12 yrs: ¹/₂ tab q 4–6 hr | b, f, g |
| *Actifed Allergy Nighttime Caplets* Tablets (OTC) [U.S.] | Diphenhydramine HCl 25 mg | Pseudoephedrine HCl 30 mg | Available in a dual package that also contains *Actifed Allergy Daytime Caplets* | 2 tabs hs, or 2 tabs q 4–6 hr | Not recommended | b, f, g |
| *Actifed Head Cold and Allergy Medicine* Syrup USP (OTC) [U.S.] | Triprolidine HCl 12.5 mg | Pseudoephedrine HCl 30 mg | Sorbitol | 10 mL q 4–6 hr | 6–12 yrs: 5 mL q 4–6 hr | b, e, f, g |
| *Alamine* Oral Solution (OTC) [U.S.] | Chlorpheniramine maleate 2 mg | Phenylpropanolamine HCl 5 mg | Alcohol 5% Sugar free | 10 mL q 4 hr | | a, e, g |
| *Alersule* Extended-release Capsules (Rx) [U.S.] | Chlorpheniramine maleate 8 mg | Phenylephrine HCl 20 mg | | 1 cap q 12 hr | | a, g |
| *Allent* Extended-release Capsules (Rx) [U.S.] | Brompheniramine maleate 12 mg | Pseudoephedrine HCl 120 mg | Dye free | 1 cap q 12 hr | | a, g |
| *Allercon* Tablets USP (OTC) [U.S.] | Triprolidine HCl 2.5 mg | Pseudoephedrine HCl 60 mg | | 1 tab q 4–6 hr (max 4 tabs daily) | | b, f, g |
| *Allerest, Children's* Chewable Tablets (OTC) [U.S.] | Chlorpheniramine maleate 1 mg | Phenylpropanolamine HCl 9.4 mg | Sorbitol | Intended for pediatric use | 6–12 yrs: 2 tabs q 4–6 hr (max 8 tabs daily) | b, g, h |
| *Allerest 12 Hour* Extended-release Tablets (OTC) [U.S.] | Chlorpheniramine maleate 12 mg | Phenylpropanolamine HCl 75 mg | | 1 tab q 12 hr | | a, g |

## Table 1. Oral Dosage Forms *(continued)*

Note: Content per capsule, tablet, or 5 mL, unless otherwise stated.

| Brand or generic name [availability] | Antihistamines | Decongestants | Other content information as per product label | Usual adult and adolescent dose* prn | Usual pediatric dose prn | Packaging, storage, and auxiliary labeling† |
|---|---|---|---|---|---|---|
| *Allerest Maximum Strength* Tablets (OTC) [U.S.] | Chlorpheniramine maleate 2 mg | Pseudoephedrine HCl 30 mg | | 2 tabs q 4–6 hr (max 8 tabs daily) | 6–12 yrs: 1 tab q 4–6 hr (max 4 tabs daily) | a, g |
| *Allerfrim* Syrup USP (OTC) [U.S.] | Triprolidine HCl 1.25 mg | Pseudoephedrine HCl 30 mg | | 10 mL q 4–6 hr (max 40 mL daily) | | b, e, f, g |
| Tablets USP (OTC) [U.S.] | Triprolidine HCl 2.5 mg | Pseudoephedrine HCl 60 mg | Scored | 1 tab q 4–6 hr (max 4 tabs daily) | | a, f, g |
| *Allerfrin* Syrup USP (OTC) [U.S.] | Triprolidine HCl 1.25 mg | Pseudoephedrine HCl 30 mg | | 10 mL q 4–6 hr | 6–12 yrs: 5 mL q 4–6 hr | b, e, f, g |
| Tablets USP (OTC) [U.S.] | Triprolidine HCl 2.5 mg | Pseudoephedrine HCl 60 mg | | 1 tab q 4–6 hr | | b, f, g |
| *Allergy Cold* Tablets USP (OTC) [U.S.] | Triprolidine HCl 2.5 mg | Pseudoephedrine HCl 60 mg | | 1 tab q 4–6 hr (max 4 tabs daily) | | b, f, g |
| *Allergy Formula Sinutab* Extended-release Tablets (OTC) [U.S.] | Dexbrompheniramine maleate 6 mg | Pseudoephedrine sulfate 120 mg | | 1 tab q 12 hr | | a, g |
| *Allergy Relief Medicine* Tablets (OTC) [U.S.] | Chlorpheniramine maleate 4 mg | Phenylpropanolamine HCl 37.5 mg | | 1 tab q 4 hr | | a, g |
| *Allerphed* Syrup USP (OTC) [U.S.] | Triprolidine HCl 1.25 mg | Pseudoephedrine HCl 30 mg | | 10 mL q 4–6 hr | 6–12 yrs: 5 mL q 4–6 hr | b, e, f, g |
| *Amaril D* Syrup (Rx) [U.S.] | Chlorpheniramine maleate 2.5 mg, Phenyltoloxamine citrate 7.5 mg | Phenylephrine HCl 5 mg, Phenylpropanolamine HCl 20 mg | | 5 mL q 4 hr | 6–12 yrs: 2.5 mL q 4 hr | a, e, g |
| *Amaril D Spantab* Extended-release Tablets (Rx) [U.S.] | Chlorpheniramine maleate 5 mg, Phenyltoloxamine citrate 15 mg | Phenylephrine HCl 10 mg, Phenylpropanolamine HCl 40 mg | | 1 tab q 8 hr | | a, g |
| *Ami-Drix* Extended-release Tablets (Rx) [U.S.] | Dexbrompheniramine maleate 6 mg | Pseudoephedrine sulfate 120 mg | Sugar coated | 1 tab q 8–12 hr | | a, g |
| *Anamine* Syrup (Rx) [U.S.] | Chlorpheniramine maleate 2 mg | Pseudoephedrine HCl 30 mg | Alcohol free Sugar free Dye free | 10 mL q 4–6 hr | | a, e, g |
| *Anamine T.D.* Extended-release Capsules (Rx) [U.S.] | Chlorpheniramine maleate 8 mg | Pseudoephedrine HCl 120 mg | | 1 cap q 8–12 hr | | a, g |

*Geriatric patients may be more sensitive to the effects of the usual adult dose.

†For appropriate *Packaging and storage* and *Auxiliary labeling* information refer to designated letters as follows:

    a—Store below 40 °C (104 °F), preferably between 15 and 30 °C (59 and 86 °F), in a tight container, unless otherwise specified by manufacturer.

    b—Store between 15 and 30 °C (59 and 86 °F), in a tight container, unless otherwise specified by manufacturer.

    c—Store between 2 and 30 °C (36 and 86 °F), in a tight container, unless otherwise specified by manufacturer.

    d—Store below 25 °C (77 °F), in a tight container, unless otherwise specified by manufacturer.

    e—Protect from freezing.

    f—Protect from light.

    g—Auxiliary labeling:
    • May cause drowsiness.
    • Avoid alcoholic beverages.

    h—Auxiliary labeling: • May be chewed.

    i—Auxiliary labeling: • Shake well.

## Table 1. Oral Dosage Forms *(continued)*

Note: Content per capsule, tablet, or 5 mL, unless otherwise stated.

| Brand or generic name [availability] | Antihistamines | Decongestants | Other content information as per product label | Usual adult and adolescent dose* prn | Usual pediatric dose prn | Packaging, storage, and auxiliary labeling† |
|---|---|---|---|---|---|---|
| *Aprodrine* Syrup USP (OTC) [U.S.] | Triprolidine HCl 1.25 mg | Pseudoephedrine HCl 30 mg | | 10 mL q 4–6 hr | 6–12 yrs: 5 mL q 4–6 hr | b, e, f, g |
| Tablets USP (OTC) [U.S.] | Triprolidine HCl 2.5 mg | Pseudoephedrine HCl 60 mg | Scored | 1 tab q 4–6 hr | 6–12 yrs: ¹/₂ tab q 4–6 hr | b, f, g |
| *A.R.M. Maximum Strength Caplets* Tablets (OTC) [U.S.] | Chlorpheniramine maleate 4 mg | Phenylpropanolamine HCl 25 mg | | 1 tab q 4 6 hr | 6–12 yrs: ¹/₂ tab q 4 6 hr | b, g |
| *Atrofed* Tablets USP (OTC) [U.S.] | Triprolidine HCl 2.5 mg | Pseudoephedrine HCl 60 mg | | 1 tab q 4–6 hr | 6–12 yrs: ¹/₂ tab q 4–6 hr | b, f, g |
| *Atrohist Pediatric* Extended-release Capsules (Rx) [U.S.] | Chlorpheniramine maleate 4 mg | Pseudoephedrine HCl 60 mg | | 2 caps q 12 hr | 6–12 yrs: 1 cap q 12 hr | b, g |
| Oral Suspension (Rx) [U.S.] | Chlorpheniramine tannate 2 mg, Pyrilamine tannate 12.5 mg | Phenylephrine tannate 5 mg | | Intended for pediatric use | 2–6 yrs: 2.5–5 mL, 6–12 yrs: 5–10 mL, q 12 hr | a, e, g, i |
| *Banophen* Capsules USP (OTC) [U.S.] | Diphenhydramine HCl 25 mg | Pseudoephedrine HCl 60 mg | | 1 tab q 4–6 hr (max 4 tabs daily) | | b, g |
| *Benadryl Allergy Decongestant* Oral Solution (OTC) [U.S.] | Diphenhydramine HCl 12.5 mg | Pseudoephedrine HCl 30 mg | Alcohol free Sugar free | 10 mL q 4–6 hr (max 40 mL daily) | >6 yrs: 5 mL q 4–6 hr (max 20 mL daily) | c, e, g |
| Tablets (OTC) [U.S./Canada] | Diphenhydramine HCl 25 mg | Pseudoephedrine HCl 60 mg | | 1 tab q 4–6 hr (max 4 tabs daily) | Not recommended | b, g |
| *Benylin Cold* Capsules (OTC) [Canada] | Chlorpheniramine maleate 4 mg | Pseudoephedrine HCl 60 mg | | 1 cap q 4–6 hr | | a, g |
| *Brexin L.A.* Extended-release Capsules (Rx) [U.S.] | Chlorpheniramine maleate 8 mg | Pseudoephedrine HCl 120 mg | | 1 cap q 12 hr | | b, g |
| *Brofed* Elixir (Rx) [U.S.] | Brompheniramine maleate 4 mg | Pseudoephedrine HCl 30 mg | | 10 mL q 8 hr | 2 6 yrs: 2.5 mL 6 12 yrs: 5 mL q 8 hr | a, e, g |
| *Bromaline* Elixir (OTC) [U.S.] | Brompheniramine maleate 2 mg | Phenylpropanolamine HCl 12.5 mg | Alcohol 2.3% | 10 mL q 4–6 hr | | a, e, g |
| *Bromanate* Elixir (OTC) [U.S.] | Brompheniramine maleate 2 mg | Phenylpropanolamine HCl 12.5 mg | Alcohol 2.3% Sugar free | 10 mL q 4–6 hr | | a, e, g |
| *Bromatap* Elixir (OTC) [U.S.] | Brompheniramine maleate 2 mg | Phenylpropanolamine HCl 12.5 mg | Alcohol 2.3% Sugar free | 10 mL q 4 hr | 6–12 yrs: 5 mL q 4 hr | b, e, g |
| *Bromatapp* Extended-release Tablets (Rx) [U.S.] | Brompheniramine maleate 12 mg | Phenylpropanolamine HCl 75 mg | | 1 tab q 12 hr | | a, g |

## Table 1. Oral Dosage Forms (continued)

Note: Content per capsule, tablet, or 5 mL, unless otherwise stated.

| Brand or generic name [availability] | Antihistamines | Decongestants | Other content information as per product label | Usual adult and adolescent dose* prn | Usual pediatric dose prn | Packaging, storage, and auxiliary labeling† |
|---|---|---|---|---|---|---|
| **Bromfed** Extended-release Capsules (Rx) [U.S.] | Brompheniramine maleate 12 mg | Pseudoephedrine HCl 120 mg | | 1 cap q 12 hr | | a, g |
| Syrup (OTC) [U.S.] | Brompheniramine maleate 2 mg | Pseudoephedrine HCl 30 mg | Alcohol free | 10 mL q 4–6 hr | 6–12 yrs: 5 mL q 4–6 hr | b, e, f, g |
| Tablets (Rx) [U.S.] | Brompheniramine maleate 4 mg | Pseudoephedrine HCl 60 mg | Scored | 1 tab q 4 hr | | a, g |
| **Bromfed-PD** Extended-release Capsules (Rx) [U.S.] | Brompheniramine maleate 6 mg | Pseudoephedrine HCl 60 mg | | 1–2 caps q 12 hr | 6–12 yrs: 1 cap q 12 hr | b, g |
| **Bromophen T.D.** Extended-release Tablets (Rx) [U.S.] | Brompheniramine maleate 12 mg | Phenylephrine HCl 15 mg, Phenylpropanolamine HCl 15 mg | Sugar coated | 1 tab q 8–12 hr | | b, f, g |
| **Bromphen** Elixir (OTC) [U.S.] | Brompheniramine maleate 2 mg | Phenylpropanolamine HCl 12.5 mg | Alcohol 2.3% Sugar free | 10 mL q 4 hr | | a, e, g |
| Extended-release Tablets (OTC) [U.S.] | Brompheniramine maleate 12 mg | Phenylpropanolamine HCl 75 mg | Lactose | 1 tab q 12 hr | | b, g |
| Brompheniramine Maleate, Phenylephrine HCl, and Phenylpropanolamine HCl Extended-release Tablets (Rx) [U.S./Canada] | Brompheniramine maleate 12 mg | Phenylephrine HCl 15 mg, Phenylpropanolamine HCl 15 mg | | 1 tab q 8–12 hr | | b, f, g |
| **Brompheril** Extended-release Tablets (OTC) [U.S.] | Dexbrompheniramine maleate 6 mg | Pseudoephedrine sulfate 120 mg | | 1 tab q 12 hr | | a, g |
| **Carbiset** Tablets (Rx) [U.S.] | Carbinoxamine maleate 4 mg | Pseudoephedrine HCl 60 mg | Dye free | 1 tab q 6 hr | 6–12 yrs: 1 tab q 6 hr | a, g |
| **Carbiset-TR** Extended-release Tablets (Rx) [U.S.] | Carbinoxamine maleate 8 mg | Pseudoephedrine HCl 120 mg | Dye free | 1 tab q 12 hr | | a, g |
| **Carbodec** Syrup (Rx) [U.S.] | Carbinoxamine maleate 4 mg | Pseudoephedrine HCl 60 mg | | 5 mL q 6 hr | 18 mos–6 yrs: 2.5 mL, 6–12 yrs: 5 mL, q 6 hr | a, e, g |
| Tablets (Rx) [U.S.] | Carbinoxamine maleate 4 mg | Pseudoephedrine HCl 60 mg | | 1 tab q 6 hr | | a, g |
| **Carbodec TR** Extended-release Tablets (Rx) [U.S.] | Carbinoxamine maleate 8 mg | Pseudoephedrine HCl 120 mg | | 1 tab q 12 hr | | a, g |
| **Cardec-S** Syrup (Rx) [U.S.] | Carbinoxamine maleate 4 mg | Pseudoephedrine HCl 60 mg | | 5 mL q 6 hr | 18 mos–6 yrs: 2.5 mL, 6–12 yrs: 5 mL, q 6 hr | a, e, g |

*Geriatric patients may be more sensitive to the effects of the usual adult dose.

†For appropriate *Packaging and storage* and *Auxiliary labeling* information refer to designated letters as follows:

　a—Store below 40 °C (104 °F), preferably between 15 and 30 °C (59 and 86 °F), in a tight container, unless otherwise specified by manufacturer.
　b—Store between 15 and 30 °C (59 and 86 °F), in a tight container, unless otherwise specified by manufacturer.
　c—Store between 2 and 30 °C (36 and 86 °F), in a tight container, unless otherwise specified by manufacturer.
　d—Store below 25 °C (77 °F), in a tight container, unless otherwise specified by manufacturer.
　e—Protect from freezing.
　f—Protect from light.

g—Auxiliary labeling:
　• May cause drowsiness.
　• Avoid alcoholic beverages.

h—Auxiliary labeling: • May be chewed.
i—Auxiliary labeling: • Shake well.

## Table 1. Oral Dosage Forms *(continued)*

Note: Content per capsule, tablet, or 5 mL, unless otherwise stated.

| Brand or generic name [availability] | Antihistamines | Decongestants | Other content information as per product label | Usual adult and adolescent dose* prn | Usual pediatric dose prn | Packaging, storage, and auxiliary labeling† |
|---|---|---|---|---|---|---|
| *Cenafed Plus* Tablets USP (OTC) [U.S.] | Triprolidine HCl 2.5 mg | Pseudoephedrine HCl 60 mg | | 1 tab q 4–6 hr | | b, f, g |
| *Cheracol Sinus* Extended-release Tablets (OTC) [U.S.] | Dexbrompheniramine maleate 6 mg | Pseudoephedrine sulfate 120 mg | | 1 tab q 12 hr | | a, g |
| *Chlorafed* Oral Solution (OTC) [U.S.] | Chlorpheniramine maleate 2 mg | Pseudoephedrine HCl 30 mg | Alcohol free Sugar free Dye free | 10 mL q 4–6 hr | | a, e, g |
| *Chlorafed H.S. Timecelles* Extended-release Capsules (Rx) [U.S.] | Chlorpheniramine maleate 4 mg | Pseudoephedrine HCl 60 mg | | 2 caps q 12 hr | | a, g |
| *Chlorafed Timecelles* Extended-release Capsules (Rx) [U.S.] | Chlorpheniramine maleate 8 mg | Pseudoephedrine HCl 120 mg | | 1 cap q 12 hr | | a, g |
| *Chlordrine S.R.* Extended-release Capsules (Rx) [U.S.] | Chlorpheniramine maleate 8 mg | Pseudoephedrine HCl 120 mg | | 1 cap q 12 hr | | a, g |
| *Chlorphedrine SR* Extended-release Capsules (Rx) [U.S.] | Chlorpheniramine maleate 8 mg | Pseudoephedrine HCl 120 mg | | 1 cap q 12 hr | | a, g |
| Chlorpheniramine Maleate and Phenyl-propanolamine HCl Extended-release Capsules (Rx) [U.S.] | Chlorpheniramine maleate 12 mg | Phenylpropanolamine HCl 75 mg | | 1 cap q 12 hr | | a, g |
| *Chlor-Rest* Tablets (OTC) [U.S.] | Chlorpheniramine maleate 2 mg | Phenylpropanolamine HCl 18.7 mg | | 2 tabs q 4 hr | | a, g |
| *Chlor-Trimeton 4 Hour Relief* Tablets (OTC) [U.S.] | Chlorpheniramine maleate 4 mg | Pseudoephedrine sulfate 60 mg | Lactose | 1 tab q 4–6 hr (max 4 tabs daily) | | c, g |
| *Chlor-Trimeton 12 Hour Relief* Extended-release Tablets (OTC) [U.S.] | Chlorpheniramine maleate 8 mg | Pseudoephedrine sulfate 120 mg | Lactose | 1 tab q 12 hr | | c, g |
| *Chlor-Tripolon Decongestant* Syrup (OTC) [Canada] | Chlorpheniramine maleate 2 mg | Phenylpropanolamine HCl 12.5 mg | Alcohol 7%, Tartrazine free | 5–10 mL q 6–8 hr | 1–6 yrs: 2.5 mL q 6–12 hr 6–12 yrs: 2.5–5 mL q 6–8 hr | a, e, g |
| *Chlor-Tripolon Decongestant Extra Strength* Extended-release Tablets (OTC) [Canada] | Chlorpheniramine maleate 12 mg | Pseudoephedrine sulfate 120 mg | Tartrazine free | 1 tab q 12 hr | | a, g |
| *Chlor-Tripolon N.D.* Tablets (OTC) [Canada] | Loratadine 5 mg | Pseudoephedrine sulfate 120 mg | | 1 tab q 12 hr | | d |
| *Claritin-D* Extended-release Tablets (Rx) [U.S.] | Loratadine 5 mg | Pseudoephedrine sulfate 120 mg | | 1 tab q 12 hr | | d |

## Table 1. Oral Dosage Forms (continued)

Note: Content per capsule, tablet, or 5 mL, unless otherwise stated.

| Brand or generic name [availability] | Antihistamines | Decongestants | Other content information as per product label | Usual adult and adolescent dose* prn | Usual pediatric dose prn | Packaging, storage, and auxiliary labeling† |
|---|---|---|---|---|---|---|
| *Claritin Extra* Extended-release Tablets (OTC) [Canada] | Loratadine 5 mg | Pseudoephedrine sulfate 120 mg | | 1 tab q 12 hr | | a |
| *Codimal–L.A.* Extended-release Capsules (Rx) [U.S.] | Chlorpheniramine maleate 8 mg | Pseudoephedrine HCl 120 mg | | 1 cap q 12 hr | | a, g |
| *Codimal–L.A. Half* Extended-release Capsules (Rx) [U.S.] | Chlorpheniramine maleate 4 mg | Pseudoephedrine HCl 60 mg | | 2 caps q 12 hr | 6–12 yrs: 1 cap q 12 hr | a, g |
| *Colfed-A* Extended-release Capsules (Rx) [U.S.] | Chlorpheniramine maleate 8 mg | Pseudoephedrine HCl 120 mg | | 1 cap q 12 hr | | a, g |
| *Coltab Children's* Chewable Tablets (OTC) [U.S.] | Chlorpheniramine maleate 1 mg | Phenylephrine HCl 2.5 mg | | Intended for pediatric use | 2–6 yrs: 1 tab, 6–12 yrs: 2 tabs, q 4 hr | a, g, h |
| *Comhist* Tablets (Rx) [U.S.] | Chlorpheniramine maleate 2 mg, Phenyltoloxamine citrate 25 mg | Phenylephrine HCl 10 mg | Scored | 1–2 tabs q 8 hr | | a, g |
| *Comhist LA* Extended-release ·Capsules (Rx) [U.S.] | Chlorpheniramine maleate 4 mg, Phenyltoloxamine citrate 50 mg | Phenylephrine HCl 20 mg | | 1 cap q 8–12 hr | | a, g |
| *Condrin–LA* Extended-release Capsules (Rx) [U.S.] | Chlorpheniramine maleate 12 mg | Phenylpropanolamine HCl 75 mg | | 1 cap q 12 hr | | a, g |
| *Conex`D.A.* Tablets (OTC) [U.S.] | Chlorpheniramine 4 mg | Phenylpropanolamine HCl 37.5 mg | | 1 tab q 4–6 hr | | a, g |
| *Contac 12-Hour* Extended-release Capsules (OTC) [U.S.] | Chlorpheniramine maleate 8 mg | Phenylpropanolamine HCl 75 mg | | 1 cap q 12 hr | | b, g |
| *Contac Maximum Strength 12-Hour Caplets* Extended-release Tablets (OTC) [U.S.] | Chlorpheniramine maleate 12 mg | Phenylpropanolamine HCl 75 mg | | 1 tab q 12 hr | | b, g |
| *Cophene No. 2* Extended-release Capsules (Rx) [U.S.] | Chlorpheniramine maleate 12 mg | Pseudoephedrine HCl 120 mg | | 1 cap q 12 hr | | a, g |
| *Co-Pyronil 2* Capsules (OTC) [U.S.] | Chlorpheniramine maleate 4 mg | Pseudoephedrine HCl 60 mg | | 1 cap q 6 hr | | a, g |
| *Coricidin D Long Acting* Extended-release Tablets (OTC) [Canada] | Chlorpheniramine maleate 8 mg | Phenylpropanolamine HCl 50 mg | | 1 tab q 12 hr | | a |

*Geriatric patients may be more sensitive to the effects of the usual adult dose.

†For appropriate *Packaging and storage* and *Auxiliary labeling* information refer to designated letters as follows:

   a—Store below 40 °C (104 °F), preferably between 15 and 30 °C (59 and 86 °F), in a tight container, unless otherwise specified by manufacturer.

   b—Store between 15 and 30 °C (59 and 86 °F), in a tight container, unless otherwise specified by manufacturer.

   c—Store between 2 and 30 °C (36 and 86 °F), in a tight container, unless otherwise specified by manufacturer.

   d—Store below 25 °C (77 °F), in a tight container, unless otherwise specified by manufacturer.

   e—Protect from freezing.

   f—Protect from light.

   g—Auxiliary labeling:
   • May cause drowsiness.
   • Avoid alcoholic beverages.

   h—Auxiliary labeling: • May be chewed.

   i—Auxiliary labeling: • Shake well.

## Table 1. Oral Dosage Forms *(continued)*

Note: Content per capsule, tablet, or 5 mL, unless otherwise stated.

| Brand or generic name [availability] | Antihistamines | Decongestants | Other content information as per product label | Usual adult and adolescent dose* prn | Usual pediatric dose prn | Packaging, storage, and auxiliary labeling† |
|---|---|---|---|---|---|---|
| *Corsym* Extended-release Oral Suspension (OTC) [Canada] | Equivalent of 4 mg of chlorpheniramine maleate (as polistirex) | Equivalent of 37.5 mg of phenylpropanolamine HCl (as polistirex) | Alcohol free Tartrazine free | 10 mL q 12 hr | 2–5 yrs: 2.5 mL, 6–12 yrs: 5 mL, q 12 hr | a, e, i |
| *Dallergy-D* Syrup (OTC) [U.S.] | Chlorpheniramine maleate 2 mg | Phenylephrine HCl 5 mg | Alcohol free | 10 mL q 4 hr | | a, g |
| *Dallergy Jr.* Extended-release Capsules (Rx) [U.S.] | Brompheniramine maleate 6 mg | Pseudoephedrine HCl 60 mg | | 1 cap q 12 hr | | a, g |
| *Deconamine* Syrup (Rx) [U.S.] | Chlorpheniramine maleate 2 mg | Pseudoephedrine HCl 30 mg | Alcohol free Dye free Sorbitol | 5–10 mL q 4–6 hr | 2–6 yrs: 2.5 mL, 6–12 yrs: 2.5–5 mL, q 4–6 hr | b, g |
| Tablets (Rx) [U.S.] | Chlorpheniramine maleate 4 mg | Pseudoephedrine HCl 60 mg | Dye free Scored | 1 tab q 4–6 hr | | b, g |
| *Deconamine SR* Extended-release Capsules (Rx) [U.S.] | Chlorpheniramine maleate 8 mg | Pseudoephedrine HCl 120 mg | | 1 cap q 12 hr | Not recommended See *Deconamine Syrup* | b, g |
| *Decongestabs* Extended-release Tablets (Rx) [U.S.] | Chlorpheniramine maleate 5 mg, Phenyltoloxamine citrate 15 mg | Phenylephrine HCl 10 mg, Phenylpropanolamine HCl 40 mg | | 1 tab q 12 hr | | a, g |
| *Demazin* Syrup (OTC) [U.S.] | Chlorpheniramine maleate 2 mg | Phenylpropanolamine HCl 12.5 mg | Alcohol 7.5% | 10 mL q 4–6 hr | 6–11 yrs: 5 mL q 4–6 hr | b, g |
| *Demazin Repetabs* Extended-release Tablets (OTC) [U.S.] | Chlorpheniramine maleate 4 mg | Phenylpropanolamine HCl 25 mg | Sugar coated | 2 tabs q 8 hr | 6–11 yrs: 1 tab q 8 hr | c, g |
| *Dexaphen SA* Extended-release Tablets (Rx) [U.S.] | Dexbrompheniramine maleate 6 mg | Pseudoephedrine sulfate 120 mg | | 1 tab q 12 hr | | a, g |
| Dexbrompheniramine Maleate and Pseudoephedrine Sulfate Extended-release Tablets (Rx) [U.S.] | Dexbrompheniramine maleate 6 mg | Pseudoephedrine sulfate 120 mg | Sugar coated | 1 tab q 12 hr | | a, g |
| *Dexophed* Extended-release Tablets (OTC) [U.S.] | Dexbrompheniramine maleate 6 mg | Pseudoephedrine sulfate 120 mg | | 1 tab q 12 hr | | a, g |
| *Dihistine* Elixir (OTC) [U.S.] | Chlorpheniramine maleate 2 mg | Phenylephrine HCl 5 mg | | 10 mL q 4 hr | | a, e, g |
| *Dimaphen* Elixir (OTC) [U.S.] | Brompheniramine maleate 2 mg | Phenylpropanolamine HCl 12.5 mg | Alcohol 2.3% | 10 mL q 4 hr | | a, e, g |
| Tablets (OTC) [U.S.] | Brompheniramine maleate 4 mg | Phenylpropanolamine HCl 25 mg | | 1 tab q 4 hr | | a, g |
| *Dimaphen S.A.* Extended-release Tablets (Rx) [U.S.] | Brompheniramine maleate 12 mg | Phenylephrine HCl 15 mg, Phenylpropanolamine HCl 15 mg | | 1 tab q 8–12 hr | | a, g |
| *Dimetane Decongestant* Elixir (OTC) [U.S.] | Brompheniramine maleate 2 mg | Phenylephrine HCl 5 mg | Alcohol 2.3% Sorbitol | 10 mL q 4 hr | 6–12 yrs: 5 mL q 4 hr | a, e, g |
| *Dimetane Decongestant Caplets* Tablets (OTC) [U.S.] | Brompheniramine maleate 4 mg | Phenylephrine HCl 10 mg | Scored | 1 tab q 4 hr | 6–12 yrs: tab q 4 hr | b, g |

## Table 1. Oral Dosage Forms *(continued)*

Note: Content per capsule, tablet, or 5 mL, unless otherwise stated.

| Brand or generic name [availability] | Antihistamines | Decongestants | Other content information as per product label | Usual adult and adolescent dose* prn | Usual pediatric dose prn | Packaging, storage, and auxiliary labeling† |
|---|---|---|---|---|---|---|
| *Dimetapp* Elixir (OTC) [U.S.] | Brompheniramine maleate 2 mg | Phenylpropanolamine HCl 12.5 mg | Alcohol 2.3% | 10 mL q 4 hr | 6–12 yrs: 5 mL q 4 hr | b, e, g |
| Elixir (OTC) [Canada] | Brompheniramine maleate 4 mg | Phenylephrine HCl 5 mg, Phenylpropanolamine HCl 5 mg | Alcohol 2.3% Sorbitol | 5–10 mL q 6–8 hr | 1–6 mos: 1.25 mL, 7–24 mos: 2.5 mL, 2–4 yrs: 3.75 mL, 4–12 yrs: 5 mL, q 6–8 hr | b, e, g |
| Tablets (OTC) [U.S.] | Brompheniramine maleate 4 mg | Phenylpropanolamine HCl 25 mg | Scored | 1 tab q 4 hr | 6–12 yrs: ¹/₂ tab q 4 hr | b, g |
| Tablets (OTC) [Canada] | Brompheniramine maleate 4 mg | Phenylephrine HCl 5 mg, Phenylpropanolamine HCl 5 mg | Scored | 1–2 tabs q 6–8 hr | 2–4 yrs: ¹/₂ tab, 4–12 yrs: 1 tab, q 6–8 hr | b, g |
| *Dimetapp Cold and Allergy* Chewable Tablets (OTC) [U.S.] | Brompheniramine maleate 1 mg | Phenylpropanolamine HCl 6.25 mg | Phenylalanine 8 mg Scored | Intended for pediatric use | 6–12 yrs: 2 tabs q 4 hr (max 12 tabs daily) | a, g, h |
| *Dimetapp Extentabs* Extended-release Tablets (OTC) [U.S.] | Brompheniramine maleate 12 mg | Phenylpropanolamine HCl 75 mg | Sugar coated | 1 tab q 12 hr | | b, g |
| Extended-release Tablets (OTC) [Canada] | Brompheniramine maleate 12 mg | Phenylephrine HCl 15 mg, Phenylpropanolamine HCl 15 mg | Sugar coated | 1 tab q 12 hr | | b, g |
| *Dimetapp 4-Hour Liqui-gels Maximum Strength* Capsules (OTC) [U.S.] | Brompheniramine maleate 4 mg | Phenylpropanolamine HCl 25 mg | | 1 cap q 4 hr (max 6 caps daily) | | a, g |
| *Dimetapp Oral Infant Drops* Oral Solution (OTC) [Canada] | Brompheniramine maleate 2 mg/mL | Phenylephrine HCl 2.5 mg/mL, Phenylpropanolamine HCl 2.5 mg/mL | Alcohol 2.3% | Intended for pediatric use | 5 kg: 0.5 mL, 7.5 kg: 0.75 mL, 10 kg: 1 mL, >10 kg: 1.5 mL, q 6–8 hr | b, e, g |
| *Disobrom* Extended-release Tablets (Rx) [U.S.] | Dexbrompheniramine maleate 6 mg | Pseudoephedrine sulfate 120 mg | | 1 tab q 12 hr | | a, g |
| *Disophrol* Tablets (OTC) [U.S.] | Dexbrompheniramine maleate 2 mg | Pseudoephedrine sulfate 60 mg | | 1 tab q 4–6 hr (max 4 tabs daily) | 6–11 yrs: ¹/₂ tab q 4–6 hr (max 4 doses daily) | b, g |
| *Disophrol Chronotabs* Extended-release Tablets (OTC) [U.S.] | Dexbrompheniramine maleate 6 mg | Pseudoephedrine sulfate 120 mg | Sugar coated | 1 tab q 12 hr | | c, g |

\*Geriatric patients may be more sensitive to the effects of the usual adult dose.

†For appropriate *Packaging and storage* and *Auxiliary labeling* information refer to designated letters as follows:

  a—Store below 40 °C (104 °F), preferably between 15 and 30 °C (59 and 86 °F), in a tight container, unless otherwise specified by manufacturer.

  b—Store between 15 and 30 °C (59 and 86 °F), in a tight container, unless otherwise specified by manufacturer.

  c—Store between 2 and 30 °C (36 and 86 °F), in a tight container, unless otherwise specified by manufacturer.

  d—Store below 25 °C (77 °F), in a tight container, unless otherwise specified by manufacturer.

  e—Protect from freezing.

  f—Protect from light.

  g—Auxiliary labeling:
    • May cause drowsiness.
    • Avoid alcoholic beverages.

  h—Auxiliary labeling: • May be chewed.

  i—Auxiliary labeling: • Shake well.

## Table 1. Oral Dosage Forms *(continued)*

Note: Content per capsule, tablet, or 5 mL, unless otherwise stated.

| Brand or generic name [availability] | Antihistamines | Decongestants | Other content information as per product label | Usual adult and adolescent dose* prn | Usual pediatric dose prn | Packaging, storage, and auxiliary labeling† |
|---|---|---|---|---|---|---|
| *Dorcol Children's Cold Formula* Oral Solution (OTC) [U.S.] | Chlorpheniramine maleate 1 mg | Pseudoephedrine HCl 15 mg | Sorbitol | Intended for pediatric use | 3–12 mos: 2 drops/kg of body weight, 1–2 yrs: 5 drops/kg of body weight, 2–6 yrs: 5 mL, 6–12 yrs: 10 mL, q 4–6 hr | a, e, g |
| *Dristan Allergy Caplets* Tablets (OTC) [U.S.] | Brompheniramine maleate 4 mg | Pseudoephedrine HCl 60 mg | | 1 tab q 4–6 hr (max 4 tabs daily) | | a, g |
| *Drixoral* Extended-release Capsules (OTC) [Canada] | Dexbrompheniramine maleate 6 mg | Pseudoephedrine sulfate 120 mg | | 1 cap q 8–12 hr | | c, g |
| Extended-release Tablets (OTC) [Canada] | Dexbrompheniramine maleate 6 mg | Pseudoephedrine sulfate 120 mg | Sugar coated | 1 tab q 12 hr | | c, g |
| *Drixoral Cold and Allergy* Extended-release Tablets (OTC) [U.S.] | Dexbrompheniramine maleate 6 mg | Pseudoephedrine sulfate 120 mg | Lactose | 1 tab q 12 hr | | c, g |
| *Drixtab Nighttime* Tablets (OTC) [Canada] | Dexbrompheniramine maleate 2 mg | Pseudoephedrine sulfate 60 mg | Tartrazine free Available in a dual package that also contains *Drixtab Day* | 1 tab hs | | a, g |
| *Drize* Extended-release Capsules (Rx) [U.S.] | Chlorpheniramine maleate 12 mg | Phenylpropanolamine HCl 75 mg | Dye free | 1 cap q 12 hr | | a, g |
| *Duralex* Extended-release Capsules (Rx) [U.S.] | Chlorpheniramine maleate 8 mg | Pseudoephedrine HCl 120 mg | | 1 cap q 12 hr | | a, g |
| *Dura-Tap PD* Capsules (Rx) [U.S.] | Chlorpheniramine maleate 4 mg | Pseudoephedrine HCl 60 mg | | 2 caps q 12 hr | 6–12 yrs: 1 cap q 12 hr | b, g |
| *Dura-Vent/A* Extended-release Capsules (Rx) [U.S.] | Chlorpheniramine maleate 10 mg | Phenylpropanolamine HCl 75 mg | | 1 cap q 12 hr | | b, g |
| *Ed A-Hist* Extended-release Capsules (Rx) [U.S.] | Chlorpheniramine maleate 8 mg | Phenylephrine HCl 20 mg | | 1 cap q 12 hr | | a, g |
| *Endafed* Extended-release Capsules (Rx) [U.S.] | Brompheniramine maleate 12 mg | Pseudoephedrine HCl 120 mg | | 1 cap q 12 hr | | a, g |
| *E.N.T* Extended-release Tablets (Rx) [U.S.] | Brompheniramine maleate 12 mg | Phenylpropanolamine HCl 75 mg | | 1 tab q 12 hr | | a, g |
| *Fedahist* Tablets (OTC) [U.S.] | Chlorpheniramine maleate 4 mg | Pseudoephedrine HCl 60 mg | Scored | 1 tab q 4–6 hr | 6–12 yrs: ½ tab q 4–6 hr | b, g |
| *Fedahist Gyrocaps* Extended-release Capsules (Rx) [U.S.] | Chlorpheniramine maleate 10 mg | Pseudoephedrine HCl 65 mg | | 1 cap q 12 hr | | b, g |

## Table 1. Oral Dosage Forms *(continued)*

Note: Content per capsule, tablet, or 5 mL, unless otherwise stated.

| Brand or generic name [availability] | Antihistamines | Decongestants | Other content information as per product label | Usual adult and adolescent dose* prn | Usual pediatric dose prn | Packaging, storage, and auxiliary labeling† |
|---|---|---|---|---|---|---|
| *Fedahist Timecaps* Extended-release Capsules (Rx) [U.S.] | Chlorpheniramine maleate 8 mg | Pseudoephedrine HCl 120 mg | | 1 cap q 12 hr | | b, f, g |
| *Genac* Tablets USP (OTC) [U.S.] | Triprolidine HCl 2.5 mg | Pseudoephedrine HCl 60 mg | | 1 tab q 4–6 hr | | b, f |
| *Genamin* Syrup (OTC) [U.S.] | Chlorpheniramine maleate 2 mg | Phenylpropanolamine HCl 12.5 mg | Alcohol free | 10 mL q 4–6 hr | 6–11 yrs: 5 mL q 4 hr | c, e, g |
| *Genatap* Elixir (OTC) [U.S.] | Brompheniramine maleate 2 mg | Phenylpropanolamine HCl 12.5 mg | Alcohol 2.3% Saccharin Sorbitol | 10 mL q 4 hr | | a, e, g |
| *Gencold* Extended-release Capsules (OTC) [U.S.] | Chlorpheniramine maleate 8 mg | Phenylpropanolamine HCl 75 mg | | 1 cap q 12 hr | | a, g |
| *Hayfebrol* Oral Solution (OTC) [U.S.] | Chlorpheniramine maleate 2 mg | Pseudoephedrine HCl 30 mg | Alcohol free Sugar free Dye free | 10 mL q 6 hr | | a, e, g |
| *Histalet* Syrup (Rx) [U.S.] | Chlorpheniramine maleate 3 mg | Pseudoephedrine HCl 45 mg | | 10 mL q 6 hr | | a, e, g |
| *Histalet Forte* Tablets (Rx) [U.S.] | Chlorpheniramine maleate 4 mg, Pyrilamine maleate 25 mg | Phenylephrine HCl 10 mg, Phenylpropanolamine HCl 50 mg | Scored | 1 tab q 8–12 hr | 6–12 yrs: ½ tab q 8–12 hr | b, f, g |
| *Histamic* Extended-release Capsules (Rx) [U.S.] | Chlorpheniramine maleate 12 mg, Phenyltoloxamine citrate 30 mg | Phenylephrine HCl 25 mg, Phenylpropanolamine HCl 50 mg | | 1 cap q 12 hr | | a, g |
| *Histatab Plus* Tablets (OTC) [U.S.] | Chlorpheniramine maleate 2 mg | Phenylephrine HCl 5 mg | | 2 tabs initially, then 1 tab q 4 hr | | a, g |
| *Histatan* Oral Suspension (Rx) [U.S.] | Chlorpheniramine tannate 2 mg, Pyrilamine tannate 12.5 mg | Phenylephrine tannate 5 mg | | Intended for pediatric use | 2–6 yrs: 2.5–5 mL, 6–12 yrs: 5–10 mL, q 12 hr | a, e, g, i |
| *Hista-Vadrin* Tablets (OTC) [U.S.] | Chlorpheniramine maleate 6 mg | Phenylephrine HCl 5 mg, Phenylpropanolamine HCl 40 mg | | 1 tab q 6 hr | | a, g |
| *Histor–D* Syrup (Rx) [U.S.] | Chlorpheniramine maleate 2 mg | Phenylephrine HCl 5 mg | Alcohol 2% | 5–10 mL q 4–6 hr | | a, e, g |
| *12-Hour Cold* Extended-release Capsules (OTC) [U.S.] | Chlorpheniramine maleate 4 mg | Phenylpropanolamine HCl 75 mg | | 1 cap q 12 hr | | a, g |

*Geriatric patients may be more sensitive to the effects of the usual adult dose.

†For appropriate *Packaging and storage* and *Auxiliary labeling* information refer to designated letters as follows:

    a—Store below 40 °C (104 °F), preferably between 15 and 30 °C (59 and 86 °F), in a tight container, unless otherwise specified by manufacturer.

    b—Store between 15 and 30 °C (59 and 86 °F), in a tight container, unless otherwise specified by manufacturer.

    c—Store between 2 and 30 °C (36 and 86 °F), in a tight container, unless otherwise specified by manufacturer.

    d—Store below 25 °C (77 °F), in a tight container, unless otherwise specified by manufacturer.

    e—Protect from freezing.

    f—Protect from light.

    g—Auxiliary labeling:
      • May cause drowsiness.
      • Avoid alcoholic beverages.

    h—Auxiliary labeling: • May be chewed.

    i—Auxiliary labeling: • Shake well.

## Table 1. Oral Dosage Forms *(continued)*

Note: Content per capsule, tablet, or 5 mL, unless otherwise stated.

| Brand or generic name [availability] | Antihistamines | Decongestants | Other content information as per product label | Usual adult and adolescent dose* prn | Usual pediatric dose prn | Packaging, storage, and auxiliary labeling† |
|---|---|---|---|---|---|---|
| *Isoclor* Oral Solution (OTC) [U.S.] | Chlorpheniramine maleate 2 mg | Pseudoephedrine HCl 30 mg | Sorbitol | 10 mL q 4–6 hr | 6–12 yrs: 5 mL q 4–6 hr | a, e, g |
| Tablets (OTC) [U.S.] | Chlorpheniramine maleate 4 mg | Pseudoephedrine HCl 60 mg | | 1 tab q 4–6 hr | 6–12 yrs: ¹/₂ tab q 4–6 hr | a, g |
| *Isoclor Timesules* Extended-release Capsules (OTC) [U.S.] | Chlorpheniramine maleate 8 mg | Pseudoephedrine HCl 120 mg | | 1 cap q 12 hr | | b, g |
| *Klerist-D* Extended-release Capsules (Rx) [U.S.] | Chlorpheniramine maleate 8 mg | Pseudoephedrine HCl 120 mg | Dye free | 1 cap q 12 hr | | a, g |
| Tablets (Rx) [U.S.] | Chlorpheniramine maleate 4 mg | Pseudoephedrine HCl 60 mg | Dye free | 1 tab q 6–8 hr | | b, g |
| *Kronofed-A Jr. Kronocaps* Extended-release Capsules (Rx) [U.S.] | Chlorpheniramine maleate 4 mg | Pseudoephedrine HCl 60 mg | Dye free | Intended for pediatric use | 6–12 yrs: 1 cap q 12 hr | a, g |
| *Kronofed-A Kronocaps* Extended-release Capsules (Rx) [U.S.] | Chlorpheniramine maleate 8 mg | Pseudoephedrine HCl 120 mg | Dye free | 1 cap q 12 hr | | a, g |
| *Lodrane LD* Extended-release capsules (Rx) (OTC) [U.S.] | Brompheniramine maleate 6 mg | Pseudoephedrine HCl 60 mg | Dye free | 1–2 caps q 12 hr | | a, g |
| *Lodrane Liquid* Oral Solution (Rx) [U.S.] | Brompheniramine maleate 4 mg | Pseudoephedrine HCl 60 mg | Dye free Sugar free Alcohol free | Intended for pediatric use | 2 6 yrs: 1.25 mL 6 12 yrs: 2.5 mL >12 yrs: 5 mL q 4 6 hr | b, e, g |
| *Myphetapp* Elixir (OTC) [U.S.] | Brompheniramine maleate 2 mg | Phenylpropanolamine HCl 12.5 mg | Alcohol 2.3% | 10 mL q 4 hr | | a, e, g |
| *Naldecon* Syrup (Rx) [U.S.] | Chlorpheniramine maleate 2.5 mg, Phenyltoloxamine citrate 7.5 mg | Phenylephrine HCl 5 mg, Phenylpropanolamine HCl 20 mg | Sorbitol | 5 mL q 3–4 hr | 6–12 yrs: 2.5 mL q 3–4 hr | a, e, g |
| Extended-release Tablets (Rx) [U.S.] | Chlorpheniramine maleate 5 mg, Phenyltoloxamine citrate 15 mg | Phenylephrine HCl 10 mg, Phenylpropanolamine HCl 40 mg | Scored | 1 tab q 6 hr | 6–12 yrs: ¹/₂ tab q 6 hr | a, g |
| *Naldecon Pediatric Drops* Oral Solution (Rx) [U.S.] | Chlorpheniramine maleate 0.5 mg/mL, Phenyltoloxamine citrate 2 mg/mL | Phenylephrine HCl 1.25 mg/mL, Phenylpropanolamine HCl 5 mg/mL | Sorbitol | Intended for pediatric use | 3–6 mos: mL, 6–12 mos: ¹/₂ mL, 1–6 yrs: 1 mL, q 3–4 hr | a, e, g |
| *Naldecon Pediatric Syrup* Syrup (Rx) [U.S.] | Chlorpheniramine maleate 0.5 mg, Phenyltoloxamine citrate 2 mg | Phenylephrine HCl 1.25 mg, Phenylpropanolamine HCl 5 mg | | Intended for pediatric use | 6–12 mos: 2.5 mL, 1–6 yrs: 5 mL, 6–12 yrs: 10 mL, q 3–4 hr | a, e, g |
| *Naldelate* Syrup (Rx) [U.S.] | Chlorpheniramine maleate 2.5 mg, Phenyltoloxamine citrate 7.5 mg | Phenylephrine HCl 5 mg, Phenylpropanolamine HCl 20 mg | | 5 mL q 4 hr | 6–12 yrs: 2.5 mL q 4 hr | a, e, g |

## Table 1. Oral Dosage Forms (continued)

Note: Content per capsule, tablet, or 5 mL, unless otherwise stated.

| Brand or generic name [availability] | Antihistamines | Decongestants | Other content information as per product label | Usual adult and adolescent dose* prn | Usual pediatric dose prn | Packaging, storage, and auxiliary labeling† |
|---|---|---|---|---|---|---|
| *Naldelate Pediatric Syrup*<br>Syrup (Rx) [U.S.] | Chlorpheniramine maleate 0.5 mg, Phenyltoloxamine citrate 2 mg | Phenylephrine HCl 1.25 mg, Phenylpropanolamine HCl 5 mg/mL | | Intended for pediatric use | 6–12 mos: 2.5 mL, 1–6 yrs: 5 mL, 6–12 yrs: 10 mL, q 3–4 hr | a, e, g |
| *Nalgest*<br>Extended-release Tablets (Rx) [U.S.] | Chlorpheniramine maleate 5 mg, Phenyltoloxamine citrate 15 mg | Phenylephrine HCl 10 mg, Phenylpropanolamine HCl 40 mg | | 1 tab q 8 hr | | a, g |
| *Nalgest Pediatric*<br>Oral Solution (Rx) [U.S.] | Chlorpheniramine maleate 0.5 mg, Phenyltoloxamine citrate 2 mg | Phenylephrine HCl 1.25 mg, Phenylpropanolamine HCl 5 mg | Sorbitol | Intended for pediatric use | 3–6 mos: 0.25 mL, 6–12 mos: 0.5 mL, 1–6 yrs: 1 mL, q 3–4 hr | a, e, g |
| Syrup (Rx) [U.S.] | Chlorpheniramine maleate 0.5 mg, Phenyltoloxamine citrate 2 mg | Phenylephrine HCl 1.25 mg, Phenylpropanolamine HCl 5 mg | Sorbitol | Intended for pediatric use | 6–12 mos: 2.5 mL q 3–4 hr (max 10 mL daily), 1–6 yrs: 5 mL q 3–4 hr (max 20 mL daily), 6–12 yrs: 10 mL q 3–4 hr (max 40 mL daily) | a, e, g |
| *ND Clear T.D.*<br>Extended-release Capsules (Rx) [U.S.] | Chlorpheniramine maleate 8 mg | Pseudoephedrine HCl 120 mg | | 1 cap q 12 hr | | a, g |
| *NeoCitran A for Oral Solution* (OTC) [Canada] | Pheniramine maleate 20 mg/packet | Phenylephrine HCl 10 mg/packet | Vitamin C 50 mg/packet | 1 packet dissolved in 225 mL of hot water q 3–4 hr | | a, g |
| *New-Decongestant Pediatric*<br>Oral Solution (Rx) [U.S.] | Chlorpheniramine maleate 0.5 mg, Phenyltoloxamine citrate 2 mg | Phenylephrine HCl 1.25 mg, Phenylpropanolamine HCl 5 mg | Alcohol free Sugar free | Intended for pediatric use | 3–6 mos: 0.25 mL, 6–12 mos: 0.5 mL, 1–6 yrs: 1 mL, q 3–4 hr | a, e, g |
| Extended-release Tablets (Rx) [U.S.] | Chlorpheniramine maleate 5 mg, Phenyltoloxamine citrate 5 mg | Phenylephrine HCl 10 mg, Phenylpropanolamine HCl 40 mg | | 1 tab q 8 hr | | a, g |
| *New-Decongest Pediatric Syrup*<br>Syrup (Rx) [U.S.] | Chlorpheniramine maleate 0.5 mg, Phenyltoloxamine citrate 2 mg | Phenylephrine HCl 1.25 mg, Phenylpropanolamine HCl 5 mg | | Intended for pediatric use | 6–12 mos: 2.5 mL, 1–6 yrs: 5 mL, 6–12 yrs: 10 mL, q 3–4 hr | a, e, g |

*Geriatric patients may be more sensitive to the effects of the usual adult dose.
†For appropriate *Packaging and storage* and *Auxiliary labeling* information refer to designated letters as follows:
  a—Store below 40 °C (104 °F), preferably between 15 and 30 °C (59 and 86 °F), in a tight container, unless otherwise specified by manufacturer.
  b—Store between 15 and 30 °C (59 and 86 °F), in a tight container, unless otherwise specified by manufacturer.
  c—Store between 2 and 30 °C (36 and 86 °F), in a tight container, unless otherwise specified by manufacturer.
  d—Store below 25 °C (77 °F), in a tight container, unless otherwise specified by manufacturer.
  e—Protect from freezing.     g—Auxiliary labeling:     h—Auxiliary labeling: • May be chewed.
  f—Protect from light.      • May cause drowsiness.     i—Auxiliary labeling: • Shake well.
                          • Avoid alcoholic beverages.

## Table 1. Oral Dosage Forms *(continued)*

Note: Content per capsule, tablet, or 5 mL, unless otherwise stated.

| Brand or generic name [availability] | Antihistamines | Decongestants | Other content information as per product label | Usual adult and adolescent dose* prn | Usual pediatric dose prn | Packaging, storage, and auxiliary labeling† |
|---|---|---|---|---|---|---|
| *Nolamine* Extended-release Tablets (Rx) [U.S.] | Chlorpheniramine maleate 4 mg, Phenindamine tartrate 24 mg | Phenylpropanolamine HCl 50 mg | | 1 tab q 8 hr | | b, f, g |
| *Noraminic* Syrup (OTC) [U.S.] | Chlorpheniramine maleate 2 mg | Phenylpropanolamine HCl 12.5 mg | | 10 mL q 4 hr | 6–11 yrs: 5 mL q 4 hr | c, e, g |
| *Normatane* Elixir (Rx) [U.S.] | Brompheniramine maleate 4 mg | Phenylephrine HCl 5 mg, Phenylpropanolamine HCl 5 mg | Alcohol 2.3% | 5–10 mL q 6–8 hr | | a, e, g |
| *Novafed A* Extended-release Capsules (Rx) [U.S.] | Chlorpheniramine maleate 8 mg | Pseudoephedrine HCl 120 mg | | 1 cap q 12 hr | | b, f, g |
| *Novahistex* Extended-release Capsules (OTC) [Canada] | Chlorpheniramine maleate 8 mg | Pseudoephedrine HCl 120 mg | | 1 cap q 12 hr | | a, g |
| *Novahistine* Elixir (OTC) [U.S.] | Chlorpheniramine maleate 2 mg | Phenylephrine HCl 5 mg | Alcohol 5% Sugar free Sorbitol | 10 mL q 4 hr | 2–6 yrs: 2.5 mL, 6–12 yrs: 5 mL, q 4 hr | a, e, g |
| *Oraminic Spancaps* Extended-release Capsules (Rx) [U.S.] | Chlorpheniramine maleate 12 mg | Phenylpropanolamine HCl 75 mg | | 1 cap q 10–12 hr | | a, g |
| *Ornade* Oral Solution (OTC) [Canada] | Chlorpheniramine maleate 1.5 mg | Phenylpropanolamine HCl 15 mg | Alcohol 3.8% Sugar free | 5–10 mL q 6–8 hr | 1–5 yrs: 2.5 mL, 6–12 yrs: 5 mL, q 6–8 hr | a, e, g |
| *Ornade-A.F.* Extended-release Capsules (OTC) [Canada] | Chlorpheniramine maleate 12 mg | Phenylpropanolamine HCl 75 mg | | 1 cap q 12 hr | Not recommended | a, g |
| Oral Solution (OTC) [Canada] | Chlorpheniramine maleate 2.5 mg | Phenylpropanolamine HCl 15 mg | Alcohol 3.8% Sugar free | 5–10 mL q 6–8 hr | 1–5 yrs: 2.5 mL, 6–12 yrs: 5 mL, q 6–8 hr | a, e, g |
| *Ornade Spansules* Extended-release Capsules (Rx) [U.S.] | Chlorpheniramine maleate 12 mg | Phenylpropanolamine HCl 75 mg | | 1 cap q 12 hr | Not recommended | b, f, g |
| Extended-release Capsules (OTC) [Canada] | Chlorpheniramine maleate 8 mg | Phenylpropanolamine HCl 75 mg | | 1 cap q 12 hr | | b, g |
| *Parhist SR* Extended-release Capsules (Rx) [U.S.] | Chlorpheniramine maleate 12 mg | Phenylpropanolamine HCl 75 mg | | 1 cap q 12 hr | | a, g |
| *Partapp TD* Extended-release Tablets (Rx) [U.S.] | Brompheniramine maleate 12 mg | Phenylephrine HCl 15 mg, Phenylpropanolamine HCl 15 mg | | 1 tab q 8–12 hr | | a, g |
| *PediaCare Cold Formula* Oral Solution (OTC) [U.S.] | Chlorpheniramine maleate 1 mg | Pseudoephedrine HCl 15 mg | Alcohol free Saccharin free | Intended for pediatric use | 6–11 yrs: 10 mL q 4–6 hr | b, e, g |
| *Phenergan VC* Syrup (Rx) [U.S.] | Promethazine HCl 6.25 mg | Phenylephrine HCl 5 mg | Alcohol 7% Saccharin | 5 mL q 4–6 hr | 2–6 yrs: 1.25–2.5 mL, 6–12 yrs: 2.5–5 mL, q 4–6 hr | d, e, f, g |

## Table 1. Oral Dosage Forms (continued)

Note: Content per capsule, tablet, or 5 mL, unless otherwise stated.

| Brand or generic name [availability] | Antihistamines | Decongestants | Other content information as per product label | Usual adult and adolescent dose* prn | Usual pediatric dose prn | Packaging, storage, and auxiliary labeling† |
|---|---|---|---|---|---|---|
| *Pherazine VC* Syrup (Rx) [U.S.] | Promethazine HCl 6.25 mg | Phenylephrine HCl 5 mg | Alcohol 7% | 5 mL q 4–6 hr | 2–6 yrs: 1.25–2.5 mL, 6–12 yrs: 2.5–5 mL, q 4–6 hr | d, e, f, g |
| *Poly-Histine-D* Extended-release Capsules (Rx) [U.S.] | Pheniramine maleate 16 mg, Phenyltoloxamine citrate 16 mg, Pyrilamine maleate 16 mg | Phenylpropanolamine HCl 50 mg | | 1 cap q 8–12 hr | | a, g |
| Elixir (Rx) [U.S.] | Pheniramine maleate 4 mg, Phenyltoloxamine citrate 4 mg, Pyrilamine maleate 4 mg | Phenylpropanolamine HCl 12.5 mg | Alcohol 4% | 10 mL q 4 hr | | a, e, g |
| *Poly-Histine-D Ped* Extended-release Capsules (Rx) [U.S.] | Pheniramine maleate 8 mg, Phenyltoloxamine citrate 8 mg, Pyrilamine maleate 8 mg | Phenylpropanolamine HCl 25 mg | | Intended for pediatric use | 6–12 yrs: 1 cap q 8–12 hr | a, g |
| *Prehist* Extended-release Capsules (Rx) [U.S.] | Chlorpheniramine maleate 8 mg | Phenylephrine HCl 20 mg | | 1 cap q 12 hr | | a, g |
| *Promethazine VC* Syrup (Rx) [U.S.] | Promethazine HCl 6.25 mg | Phenylephrine HCl 5 mg | | 5 mL q 4–6 hr | 2–6 yrs: 1.25–2.5 mL, 6–12 yrs: 2.5–5 mL, q 4–6 hr | d, e, f, g |
| *Prometh VC Plain* Syrup (Rx) [U.S.] | Promethazine HCl 6.25 mg | Phenylephrine HCl 5 mg | Alcohol 7% | 5 mL q 4–6 hr | 2–6 yrs: 1.25–2.5 mL, 6–12 yrs: 2.5–5 mL, q 4–6 hr | d, e, f, g |
| *Pseudo-Chlor* Extended-release Capsules (Rx) [U.S.] | Chlorpheniramine maleate 8 mg | Pseudoephedrine HCl 120 mg | | 1 cap q 12 hr | | a, g |
| *Pseudo-gest Plus* Tablets (OTC) [U.S.] | Chlorpheniramine maleate 4 mg | Pseudoephedrine HCl 60 mg | | 1 tab q 4–6 hr | | a, g |
| *Quadra-Hist* Extended-release Tablets (Rx) [U.S.] | Chlorpheniramine maleate 5 mg, Phenyltoloxamine citrate 15 mg | Phenylephrine HCl 10 mg, Phenylpropanolamine HCl 40 mg | | 1 tab q 8 hr | | a, g |

*Geriatric patients may be more sensitive to the effects of the usual adult dose.

†For appropriate *Packaging and storage* and *Auxiliary labeling* information refer to designated letters as follows:

a—Store below 40 °C (104 °F), preferably between 15 and 30 °C (59 and 86 °F), in a tight container, unless otherwise specified by manufacturer.

b—Store between 15 and 30 °C (59 and 86 °F), in a tight container, unless otherwise specified by manufacturer.

c—Store between 2 and 30 °C (36 and 86 °F), in a tight container, unless otherwise specified by manufacturer.

d—Store below 25 °C (77 °F), in a tight container, unless otherwise specified by manufacturer.

e—Protect from freezing.

f—Protect from light.

g—Auxiliary labeling:
• May cause drowsiness.
• Avoid alcoholic beverages.

h—Auxiliary labeling: • May be chewed.

i—Auxiliary labeling: • Shake well.

## Table 1. Oral Dosage Forms *(continued)*

Note: Content per capsule, tablet, or 5 mL, unless otherwise stated.

| Brand or generic name [availability] | Antihistamines | Decongestants | Other content information as per product label | Usual adult and adolescent dose* prn | Usual pediatric dose prn | Packaging, storage, and auxiliary labeling† |
|---|---|---|---|---|---|---|
| *Quadra-Hist Pediatric* Syrup (Rx) [U.S.] | Chlorpheniramine maleate 0.5 mg, Phenyltoloxamine citrate 2 mg | Phenylephrine HCl 1.25 mg Phenylpropanolamine HCl 5 mg | Sorbitol | Intended for pediatric use | 6–12 mos: 2.5 mL q 3–4 hr (max 10 mL daily), 1–6 yrs: 5 mL q 3–4 hr (max 20 mL daily), 6–12 yrs: 10 mL q 3–4 hr (max 40 mL daily) | a, e, g, i |
| *Resaid S.R.* Extended-release Capsules (Rx) [U.S.] | Chlorpheniramine maleate 12 mg | Phenylpropanolamine HCl 75 mg | | 1 cap q 12 hr | | b, f, g |
| *Rescon* Extended-release Capsules (Rx) [U.S.] | Chlorpheniramine maleate 12 mg | Pseudoephedrine HCl 120 mg | | 1 cap q 12 hr | | a, g |
| Oral Solution (OTC) [U.S.] | Chlorpheniramine maleate 2 mg | Phenylpropanolamine HCl 12.5 mg | | 10 mL q 4 hr (max 40 mL daily) | | a, e, g |
| *Rescon-ED* Extended-release Capsules (Rx) [U.S.] | Chlorpheniramine maleate 8 mg | Pseudoephedrine HCl 120 mg | | 1 cap q 12 hr | | a, g |
| *Rescon JR* Extended-release Capsules (Rx) [U.S.] | Chlorpheniramine maleate 4 mg | Pseudoephedrine HCl 60 mg | Dye free | Intended for pediatric use | 6–12 yrs: 1 cap q 12 hr | a, g |
| *Respahist* Extended-release Capsules (Rx) [U.S.] | Brompheniramine maleate 6 mg | Pseudoephedrine HCl 60 mg | Dye free | 1–2 caps q 12 hr | 6–12 yrs: 1 cap q 12 hr | a, f, g |
| *Rhinatate* Tablets (Rx) [U.S.] | Chlorpheniramine tannate 8 mg, Pyrilamine tannate 25 mg | Phenylephrine tannate 25 mg | | 1–2 tabs q 12 hr | | a, g |
| *Rhinolar-EX* Extended-release Capsules (Rx) [U.S.] | Chlorpheniramine maleate 8 mg | Phenylpropanolamine HCl 75 mg | Dye free | 1 cap q 12 hr | | a, g |
| *Rhinolar-EX 12* Extended-release Capsules (Rx) [U.S.] | Chlorpheniramine maleate 12 mg | Phenylpropanolamine HCl 75 mg | Dye free | 1 cap q 12 hr | | a, g |
| *Rhinosyn* Oral Solution (OTC) [U.S.] | Chlorpheniramine maleate 4 mg | Pseudoephedrine HCl 60 mg | Alcohol 0.45% | 5 mL q 4 hr | | a, e, g |
| *Rhinosyn-PD* Oral Solution (OTC) [U.S.] | Chlorpheniramine maleate 2 mg | Pseudoephedrine HCl 30 mg | Alcohol 1.2% | 10 mL q 4 hr | | a, e, g |
| *Rinade B.I.D.* Extended-release Capsules (Rx) [U.S.] | Chlorpheniramine maleate 8 mg | Pseudoephedrine HCl 120 mg | Dye free | 1 cap q 12 hr | | a, g |
| *Rolatuss Plain* Oral Solution (OTC) [U.S.] | Chlorpheniramine maleate 2 mg | Phenylephrine HCl 5 mg | Alcohol 5% | 10 mL q 4–6 hr | | a, e, g |

## Table 1. Oral Dosage Forms (continued)

Note: Content per capsule, tablet, or 5 mL, unless otherwise stated.

| Brand or generic name [availability] | Antihistamines | Decongestants | Other content information as per product label | Usual adult and adolescent dose* prn | Usual pediatric dose prn | Packaging, storage, and auxiliary labeling† |
|---|---|---|---|---|---|---|
| *Rondec* Syrup (Rx) [U.S.] | Carbinoxamine maleate 4 mg | Pseudoephedrine HCl 60 mg | | 5 mL q 6 hr | 18 mos–6 yrs: 2.5 mL, 6–12 yrs: 5 mL, q 6 hr | a, e, g |
| Tablets (Rx) [U.S.] | Carbinoxamine maleate 4 mg | Pseudoephedrine HCl 60 mg | Film coated | 1 tab q 6 hr | 6–12 yrs: 1 tab q 6 hr | a, g |
| *Rondec Drops* Oral Solution (Rx) [U.S.] | Carbinoxamine maleate 2 mg/mL | Pseudoephedrine HCl 25 mg/mL | | Intended for pediatric use | 1–3 mos: 1/4 mL, 3–6 mos: 1/2 mL, 6–9 mos: 3/4 mL, 9–18 mos: 1 mL, q 6 hr | a, e, g |
| *Rondec-TR* Extended-release Tablets (Rx) [U.S.] | Carbinoxamine maleate 8 mg | Pseudoephedrine HCl 120 mg | Film coated | 1 tab q 12 hr | | a, g |
| *R-Tannamine* Tablets (Rx) [U.S.] | Chlorpheniramine tannate 8 mg, Pyrilamine tannate 25 mg | Phenylephrine tannate 25 mg | | 1–2 tabs q 12 hr | | a, g |
| *R-Tannamine Pediatric* Oral Suspension (Rx) [U.S.] | Chlorpheniramine tannate 2 mg, Pyrilamine tannate 12.5 mg | Phenylephrine tannate 5 mg | | Intended for pediatric use | 2–6 yrs: 2.5–5 mL, 6–12 yrs: 5–10 mL, q 12 hr | a, e, g, i |
| *R-Tannate* Oral Suspension (Rx) [U.S.] | Chlorpheniramine tannate 2 mg, Pyrilamine tannate 12.5 mg | Phenylephrine tannate 5 mg | Saccharin | Intended for pediatric use | 2–6 yrs: 2.5–5 mL, 6–12 yrs: 5–10 mL, q 12 hrs | b, e, g |
| Tablets (Rx) [U.S.] | Chlorpheniramine tannate 8 mg, Pyrilamine tannate 25 mg | Phenylephrine tannate 25 mg | | 1–2 tabs q 12 hr | | a, g |
| *R-Tannate Pediatric* Oral Suspension (Rx) [U.S.] | Chlorpheniramine tannate 2 mg, Pyrilamine tannate 12.5 mg | Phenylephrine tannate 5 mg | | Intended for pediatric use | 2–6 yrs: 2.5–5 mL, 6–12 yrs: 5–10 mL, q 12 hr | a, e, g, i |
| *Ru-Tuss* Elixir (OTC) [U.S.] | Chlorpheniramine maleate 2 mg | Phenylephrine HCl 5 mg | Alcohol 5% | 10 mL q 4–6 hr | | a, e, g |
| *Ryna* Oral Solution (OTC) [U.S.] | Chlorpheniramine maleate 2 mg | Pseudoephedrine HCl 30 mg | Alcohol free Sugar free Sorbitol | 10 mL q 6 hr | 2–6 yrs: 2.5 mL, 6–12 yrs: 5 mL, q 6 hr | a, e, g |
| *Rynatan* Oral Suspension (Rx) [U.S.] | Chlorpheniramine tannate 2 mg, Pyrilamine tannate 12.5 mg | Phenylephrine tannate 5 mg | | Intended for pediatric use | 2–6 yrs: 2.5–5 mL, 6–12 yrs: 5–10 mL, q 12 hr | b, e, g |
| Tablets (Rx) [U.S.] | Chlorpheniramine tannate 8 mg, Pyrilamine tannate 25 mg | Phenylephrine tannate 25 mg | Scored | 1–2 tabs q 12 hr | | a, g |

*Geriatric patients may be more sensitive to the effects of the usual adult dose.

†For appropriate *Packaging and storage* and *Auxiliary labeling* information refer to designated letters as follows:

  a—Store below 40 °C (104 °F), preferably between 15 and 30 °C (59 and 86 °F), in a tight container, unless otherwise specified by manufacturer.

  b—Store between 15 and 30 °C (59 and 86 °F), in a tight container, unless otherwise specified by manufacturer.

  c—Store between 2 and 30 °C (36 and 86 °F), in a tight container, unless otherwise specified by manufacturer.

  d—Store below 25 °C (77 °F), in a tight container, unless otherwise specified by manufacturer.

| | | |
|---|---|---|
| e—Protect from freezing. | g—Auxiliary labeling: | h—Auxiliary labeling: • May be chewed. |
| f—Protect from light. | • May cause drowsiness. | i—Auxiliary labeling: • Shake well. |
| | • Avoid alcoholic beverages. | |

## Table 1. Oral Dosage Forms *(continued)*

Note: Content per capsule, tablet, or 5 mL, unless otherwise stated.

| Brand or generic name [availability] | Antihistamines | Decongestants | Other content information as per product label | Usual adult and adolescent dose* prn | Usual pediatric dose prn | Packaging, storage, and auxiliary labeling† |
|---|---|---|---|---|---|---|
| *Rynatan Pediatric* Oral Suspension (Rx) [U.S.] | Chlorpheniramine tannate 2 mg, Pyrilamine tannate 12.5 mg | Phenylephrine tannate 5 mg | | Intended for pediatric use | 2–6 yrs: 2.5–5 mL, 6–12 yrs: 5–10 mL, q 12 hr | a, e, g, i |
| *Rynatan-S Pediatric* Oral Suspension (Rx) [U.S.] | Chlorpheniramine tannate 2 mg, Pyrilamine tannate 12.5 mg | Phenylephrine tannate 5 mg | | Intended for pediatric use | 2–6 yrs: 2.5–5 mL, 6–12 yrs: 5–10 mL, q 12 hr | a, e, g, i |
| *Seldane-D* Extended-release Tablets (Rx) [U.S.] | Terfenadine 60 mg | Pseudoephedrine HCl 120 mg (10 mg immediate-release outer core; 110 mg extended-release core) | | 1 tab q 12 hr | | b |
| *Semprex-D* Capsules (Rx) [U.S.] | Acrivastine 8 mg | Pseudoephedrine HCl 60 mg | | 1 cap q 4–6 hr | | a, g |
| *Sinucon Pediatric Drops* Oral Solution (Rx) [U.S.] | Chlorpheniramine maleate 0.5 mg/mL, Phenyltoloxoamine citrate 2 mg/mL | Phenylephrine HCl 1.25 mg/mL, Phenylpropanolamine HCl 5 mg/mL | | Intended for pediatric use | 3–6 mos: ¼ mL, 6–12 mos: ½ mL, 1–6 yrs: 1 mL, q 3–4 hr | a, e, g |
| *Snaplets-D* Granules (OTC) [U.S.] | Chlorpheniramine maleate 1 mg/pack | Phenylpropanolamine HCl 6.25 mg/pack | | Intended for pediatric use | 2–6 yrs: 1 pack, 6–12 yrs: 2 packs, sprinkled on soft food q 4 hr | a, g |
| *Sudafed Plus* Oral Solution (OTC) [U.S.] | Chlorpheniramine maleate 2 mg | Pseudoephedrine HCl 30 mg | | 10 mL q 4–6 hr | 6–12 yrs: 5 mL q 4–6 hr | b, e, f, g |
| Tablets (OTC) [U.S.] | Chlorpheniramine maleate 4 mg | Pseudoephedrine HCl 60 mg | Scored | 1 tab q 4–6 hr | 6–12 yrs: ½ tab q 4–6 hr | b, f, g |
| *Tamine S.R.* Extended-release Tablets (Rx) [U.S.] | Brompheniramine maleate 12 mg | Phenylephrine HCl 15 mg, Phenylpropanolamine HCl 15 mg | Sugar coated | 1 tab q 8–12 hr | | b, f, g |
| *Tanoral* Tablets (Rx) [U.S.] | Chlorpheniramine tannate 8 mg, Pyrilamine tannate 25 mg | Phenylephrine tannate 25 mg | | 1–2 tabs q 12 hr | | a, g |
| *Tavist-D* Extended-release Tablets (OTC) [U.S.] | Clemastine fumarate 1.34 mg | Phenylpropanolamine HCl 75 mg | Film coated | 1 tab q 12 hr | | a, g |
| *T-Dry* Extended-release Capsules (OTC) [U.S.] | Chlorpheniramine maleate 12 mg | Pseudoephedrine HCl 120 mg | | 1 cap q 12 hr | | a, g |
| *T-Dry Junior* Extended-release Capsules (Rx) [U.S.] | Chlorpheniramine maleate 4 mg | Pseudoephedrine HCl 60 mg | | Intended for pediatric use | 6–12 yrs: 1 cap q 12 hr | a, g |
| *Temazin Cold* Syrup (OTC) [U.S.] | Chlorpheniramine maleate 2 mg | Phenylpropanolamine HCl 12.5 mg | | 10 mL q 4 hr (max 40 mL daily) | | a, e, g |

## Table 1. Oral Dosage Forms *(continued)*

Note: Content per capsule, tablet, or 5 mL, unless otherwise stated.

| Brand or generic name [availability] | Antihistamines | Decongestants | Other content information as per product label | Usual adult and adolescent dose* prn | Usual pediatric dose prn | Packaging, storage, and auxiliary labeling† |
|---|---|---|---|---|---|---|
| *Touro A&H* Extended-release Capsules (Rx) [U.S.] | Brompheniramine maleate 6 mg | Pseudoephedrine HCl 60 mg | | 1 cap q 12 hr | 6–12 yrs: 1 cap q 12 hr | a, g |
| *Triafed* Syrup USP (OTC) [U.S.] | Triprolidine HCl 1.25 mg | Pseudoephedrine HCl 30 mg | | 10 mL q 4–6 hr (max 40 mL daily) | | b, e, f, g |
| *Triaminic* Syrup (OTC) [Canada] | Chlorpheniramine maleate 2 mg | Phenylpropanolamine HCl 12.5 mg | Alcohol free Tartrazine free | 5–10 mL q 6–8 hr | 2–5 yrs: 2.5 mL 6–12 yrs: 5 mL, q 6–8 hr | a, e, g |
| Extended-release Tablets (OTC) [Canada] | Pheniramine maleate 25 mg, Pyrilamine maleate 25 mg | Phenylpropanolamine HCl 50 mg | Tartrazine free | 1 tab q 8 hr | | a, g |
| *Triaminic-12* Extended-release Tablets (OTC) [U.S.] | Chlorpheniramine maleate 12 mg | Phenylpropanolamine HCl 75 mg | | 1 tab q 12 hr | | a, g |
| *Triaminic Allergy* Tablets (OTC) [U.S.] | Chlorpheniramine maleate 4 mg | Phenylpropanolamine HCl 25 mg | Scored | 1 tab q 4 hr | 6–12 yrs: ½ tab q 4 hr | a, g |
| *Triaminic Chewables* Tablets (OTC) [U.S.] | Chlorpheniramine maleate 0.5 mg | Phenylpropanolamine HCl 6.25 mg | | Intended for pediatric use | 2–6 yrs: 1 tab, 6–12 yrs: 2 tabs, q 4 hr | a, g, h |
| *Triaminic Cold* Syrup (OTC) [U.S.] | Chlorpheniramine maleate 2 mg | Phenylpropanolamine HCl 12.5 mg | Alcohol free Sorbitol | 10 mL q 4 hr | 3–12 mos: 1 drop/kg of body weight, 1–2 yrs: 3 drops/kg of body weight, 2–6 yrs: 2.5 mL, 6–12 yrs: 5 mL, q 4 hr | b, e, g |
| Tablets (OTC) [U.S.] | Chlorpheniramine maleate 2 mg | Phenylpropanolamine HCl 12.5 mg | | 2 tabs q 4 hrs | 6–12 yrs: 1 tab q 4 hr | a, g |
| *Triaminic Oral Infant Drops* Oral Solution (Rx) [U.S./Canada] | Pheniramine maleate 10 mg/mL, Pyrilamine maleate 10 mg/mL | Phenylpropanolamine HCl 20 mg/mL | | Intended for pediatric use | 1.1 drop/kg (1 drop/2 lb) body weight q 6 hr | a, e, g |
| *Triaminic TR* Extended-release Tablets (Rx) [U.S.] | Pheniramine maleate 25 mg, Pyrilamine maleate 25 mg | Phenylpropanolamine HCl 50 mg | Film coated | 1 tab q 8–12 hr | | a, g |
| *Trifed* Tablets USP (Rx) [U.S.] | Triprolidine HCl 2.5 mg | Pseudoephedrine HCL 60 mg | | 1 tab q 6–8 hr | | b, f, g |
| *Trinalin Repetabs* Extended-release Tablets (Rx) [U.S./Canada] | Azatadine maleate 1 mg | Pseudoephedrine sulfate 120 mg | Sugar coated | 1 tab q 12 hr | | a, g |

*Geriatric patients may be more sensitive to the effects of the usual adult dose.

†For appropriate *Packaging and storage* and *Auxiliary labeling* information refer to designated letters as follows:

a—Store below 40 °C (104 °F), preferably between 15 and 30 °C (59 and 86 °F), in a tight container, unless otherwise specified by manufacturer.

b—Store between 15 and 30 °C (59 and 86 °F), in a tight container, unless otherwise specified by manufacturer.

c—Store between 2 and 30 °C (36 and 86 °F), in a tight container, unless otherwise specified by manufacturer.

d—Store below 25 °C (77 °F), in a tight container, unless otherwise specified by manufacturer.

e—Protect from freezing.

f—Protect from light.

g—Auxiliary labeling:
• May cause drowsiness.
• Avoid alcoholic beverages.

h—Auxiliary labeling: • May be chewed.

i—Auxiliary labeling: • Shake well.

## Table 1. Oral Dosage Forms *(continued)*

Note: Content per capsule, tablet, or 5 mL, unless otherwise stated.

| Brand or generic name [availability] | Antihistamines | Decongestants | Other content information as per product label | Usual adult and adolescent dose* prn | Usual pediatric dose prn | Packaging, storage, and auxiliary labeling† |
|---|---|---|---|---|---|---|
| *Tri-Nefrin Extra Strength* Tablets (OTC) [U.S.] | Chlorpheniramine maleate 4 mg | Phenylpropanolamine HCl 25 mg | | 1 tab q 4 hr | | a, g |
| *Triofed* Syrup USP (OTC) [U.S.] | Triprolidine HCl 1.25 mg | Pseudoephedrine HCl 30 mg | | 10 mL q 4–6 hr | 6–12 yrs: 5 mL q 4–6 hr | b, e, f, g |
| *Triotann* Extended-release Tablets (Rx) [U.S.] | Chlorpheniramine tannate 8 mg, Pyrilamine tannate 25 mg | Phenylephrine tannate 25 mg | | 1–2 tabs q 12 hr | | a, g |
| *Triotann Pediatric* Oral Suspension (Rx) [U.S.] | Chlorpheniramine tannate 2 mg, Pyrilamine tannate 12.5 mg | Phenylephrine tannate 5 mg | | Intended for pediatric use | 2–6 yrs: 2.5–5 mL, 6–12 yrs: 5–10 mL, q 12 hr | a, e, g, i |
| *Tripalgen Cold* Syrup (OTC) [U.S.] | Chlorpheniramine maleate 2 mg | Phenylpropanolamine HCl 12.5 mg | Alcohol free Sorbitol | 10 mL q 4–6 hr | | a, e, g |
| *Tri-Phen-Chlor* Syrup (Rx) [U.S.] | Chlorpheniramine maleate 2.5 mg, Phenyltoloxamine citrate 7.5 mg | Phenylephrine HCl 5 mg, Phenylpropanolamine HCl 20 mg | | 5 mL q 4 hr | 6–12 yrs: 2.5 mL q 4 hr | a, e, g |
| *Tri-Phen-Chlor Pediatric* Oral Solution (Rx) [U.S.] | Chlorpheniramine maleate 0.5 mg, Phenyltoloxamine citrate 2 mg | Phenylephrine HCl 1.25 mg, Phenylpropanolamine HCl 5 mg | | Intended for pediatric use | 3–6 mos: 0.25 mL, 6–12 mos: 0.5 mL, 1–6 yrs: 1 mL, q 3–4 hr | a, e, g |
| Syrup (Rx) [U.S.] | Chlorpheniramine maleate 0.5 mg Phenyltoloxamine citrate 2 mg | Phenylephrine HCl 1.25 mg, Phenylpropanolamine HCl 5 mg | Sorbitol | Intended for pediatric use | 6–12 mos: 2.5 mL q 3–4 hr (max 10 mL daily) 1–6 yrs: 5 mL q 3–4 hr (max 20 mL daily) 6–12 yrs: 10 mL q 3–4 hr (max 40 mL daily) | a, e, g, i |
| *Tri-Phen-Chlor T.R.* Extended-release Tablets (Rx) [U.S.] | Chlorpheniramine maleate 5 mg, Phenyltoloxamine citrate 15 mg | Phenylephrine HCl 10 mg, Phenylpropanolamine HCl 40 mg | | 1 tab q 8 hr | 6–12 yrs: ½ tab q 6 hr | a, g |
| *Triphenyl* Syrup (OTC) [U.S.] | Chlorpheniramine maleate 2 mg | Phenylpropanolamine HCl 12.5 mg | Alcohol free | 10 mL q 4 hr | | a, e, g |
| *Triphenyl T.D.* Extended-release Tablets (Rx) [U.S.] | Pheniramine maleate 25 mg, Pyrilamine maleate 25 mg | Phenylpropanolamine HCl 50 mg | | 1 tab q 8–12 hr | | a, g |
| *Triposed* Syrup USP (OTC) [U.S.] | Triprolidine HCl 1.25 mg | Pseudoephedrine HCl 30 mg | | 10 mL q 4–6 hr | 6–12 yrs: 5 mL q 4–6 hr | b, e, f, g |
| Tablets USP (OTC) [U.S.] | Triprolidine HCl 2.5 mg | Pseudoephedrine HCl 60 mg | Scored | 1 tab q 4–6 hr | 6–12 yrs: ½ tab q 4–6 hr | b, f, g |

## Table 1. Oral Dosage Forms *(continued)*

Note: Content per capsule, tablet, or 5 mL, unless otherwise stated.

| Brand or generic name [availability] | Antihistamines | Decongestants | Other content information as per product label | Usual adult and adolescent dose* prn | Usual pediatric dose prn | Packaging, storage, and auxiliary labeling† |
|---|---|---|---|---|---|---|
| Triprolidine HCl and Pseudoephedrine HCl Syrup USP (Rx) [U.S.] | Triprolidine HCl 1.25 mg | Pseudoephedrine HCl 30 mg | | 10 mL q 4–6 hr | 6–12 yrs: 5 mL q 4–6 hr | b, e, f, g |
| Tablets USP (Rx) [U.S.] | Triprolidine HCl 2.5 mg | Pseudoephedrine HCl 60 mg | | 1 tab q 6–8 hr | | b, e, f, g |
| *Tritann* Tablets (Rx) [U.S.] | Chlorpheniramine tannate 8 mg, Pyrilamine tannate 25 mg | Phenylephrine tannate 25 mg | Lactose Scored | 1–2 tabs q 12 hr | | a, g |
| *Tritann Pediatric* Oral Suspension (Rx) [U.S.] | Chlorpheniramine tannate 2 mg, Pyrilamine tannate 12.5 mg | Phenylephrine tannate 5 mg | | Intended for pediatric use | 2–6 yrs: 2.5–5 mL, 6–12 yrs: 5–10 mL, q 12 hr | a, e, g, i |
| *Tri-Tannate* Tablets (Rx) [U.S.] | Chlorpheniramine tannate 8 mg, Pyrilamine tannate 25 mg | Phenylephrine tannate 25 mg | | 1–2 tabs q 12 hr | | a, g |
| *Tri-Tannate Pediatric* Oral Suspension (Rx) [U.S.] | Chlorpheniramine tannate 2 mg, Pyrilamine tannate 12.5 mg | Phenylephrine tannate 5 mg | | Intended for pediatric use | 2–6 yrs: 2.5–5 mL, 6–12 yrs: 5–10 mL, q 12 hr | a, e, g, i |
| *Tussanil Plain* Syrup (Rx) [U.S.] | Chlorpheniramine maleate 4 mg | Phenylephrine HCl 10 mg | Alcohol 5% | 5 mL q 6–8 hr | | a, e, g |
| *ULTRAbrom PD* Extended-release Capsules (Rx) [U.S.] | Brompheniramine maleate 6 mg | Pseudoephedrine HCl 60 mg | | Intended for pediatric use | 6–12 yrs: 1 cap q 12 hr | a, g |
| *Uni-Decon* Extended-release Tablets (Rx) [U.S.] | Chlorpheniramine maleate 5 mg, Phenyltoloxamine citrate 15 mg | Phenylephrine HCl 10 mg, Phenylpropanolamine HCl 40 mg | | 1 tab q 8 hr | | a, g |
| *Vanex Forte Caplets* Tablets (Rx) [U.S.] | Chlorpheniramine maleate 4 mg, Pyrilamine maleate 25 mg | Phenylephrine HCl 10 mg, Phenylpropanolamine HCl 50 mg | Scored Film coated | 1 tab q 12 hr | 6–12 yrs: ¹/₂ tab q 12 hr | a, g |
| *Veltap* Elixir (Rx) [U.S.] | Brompheniramine maleate 4 mg | Phenylephrine HCl 5 mg, Phenylpropanolamine HCl 5 mg | Alcohol 3% | 5–10 mL q 6–8 hr | | a, e, g |
| *Vicks Children's NyQuil Allergy/ Head Cold* Oral Solution (OTC) [U.S.] | Chlorpheniramine maleate 0.67 mg | Pseudoephedrine HCl 10 mg | Alcohol free | Intended for pediatric use | 6–11 yrs: 15 mL hs or q 6 hr | a, e, g |
| *Vicks DayQuil 4 Hour Allergy Relief* Tablets (OTC) [U.S.] | Brompheniramine maleate 4 mg | Phenylpropanolamine HCl 25 mg | | 1 tab q 4 hr | 6–12 yrs: ¹/₂ tab q 4 hr | b, g |

*Geriatric patients may be more sensitive to the effects of the usual adult dose.

†For appropriate *Packaging and storage* and *Auxiliary labeling* information refer to designated letters as follows:
  a—Store below 40 °C (104 °F), preferably between 15 and 30 °C (59 and 86 °F), in a tight container, unless otherwise specified by manufacturer.
  b—Store between 15 and 30 °C (59 and 86 °F), in a tight container, unless otherwise specified by manufacturer.
  c—Store between 2 and 30 °C (36 and 86 °F), in a tight container, unless otherwise specified by manufacturer.
  d—Store below 25 °C (77 °F), in a tight container, unless otherwise specified by manufacturer.
  e—Protect from freezing.                    g—Auxiliary labeling:                    h—Auxiliary labeling: • May be chewed.
  f—Protect from light.                         • May cause drowsiness.                i—Auxiliary labeling: • Shake well.
                                                • Avoid alcoholic beverages.

## Table 1. Oral Dosage Forms (*continued*)

Note: Content per capsule, tablet, or 5 mL, unless otherwise stated.

| Brand or generic name [availability] | Antihistamines | Decongestants | Other content information as per product label | Usual adult and adolescent dose* prn | Usual pediatric dose prn | Packaging, storage, and auxiliary labeling† |
|---|---|---|---|---|---|---|
| *Vicks DayQuil 12 Hour Allergy Relief* Extended-release Tablets (OTC) [U.S.] | Brompheniramine maleate 12 mg | Phenylpropanolamine HCl 75 mg | | 1 tab q 12 hr | | b, g |

*Geriatric patients may be more sensitive to the effects of the usual adult dose.

†For appropriate *Packaging and storage* and *Auxiliary labeling* information refer to designated letters as follows:

  a—Store below 40 °C (104 °F), preferably between 15 and 30 °C (59 and 86 °F), in a tight container, unless otherwise specified by manufacturer.

  b—Store between 15 and 30 °C (59 and 86 °F), in a tight container, unless otherwise specified by manufacturer.

  c—Store between 2 and 30 °C (36 and 86 °F), in a tight container, unless otherwise specified by manufacturer.

  d—Store below 25 °C (77 °F), in a tight container, unless otherwise specified by manufacturer.

  e—Protect from freezing.

  f—Protect from light.

  g—Auxiliary labeling:
    • May cause drowsiness.
    • Avoid alcoholic beverages.

  h—Auxiliary labeling: • May be chewed.

  i—Auxiliary labeling: • Shake well.

---

# ANTIHISTAMINES, DECONGESTANTS, AND ANALGESICS   Systemic

This monograph includes information on the following: Brompheniramine, Phenylpropanolamine, and Acetaminophen; Brompheniramine, Pseudoephedrine, and Acetaminophen; Chlorpheniramine, Phenylephrine, and Acetaminophen; Chlorpheniramine, Phenylephrine, Acetaminophen, and Salicylamide; Chlorpheniramine, Phenylephrine, Acetaminophen, Salicylamide, and Caffeine; Chlorpheniramine, Phenylpropanolamine, and Acetaminophen; Chlorpheniramine, Phenylpropanolamine, and Aspirin; Chlorpheniramine, Phenylpropanolamine, Acetaminophen, and Caffeine; Chlorpheniramine, Phenylpropanolamine, Aspirin, and Caffeine; Chlorpheniramine, Phenyltoloxamine, Phenylpropanolamine, and Acetaminophen; Chlorpheniramine, Pseudoephedrine, and Acetaminophen; Chlorpheniramine, Pyrilamine, Phenylephrine, and Acetaminophen; Chlorpheniramine, Pyrilamine, Phenylephrine, Phenylpropanolamine, and Acetaminophen; Dexbrompheniramine, Pseudoephedrine, and Acetaminophen; Diphenhydramine, Phenylpropanolamine, and Aspirin; Diphenhydramine, Pseudoephedrine, and Acetaminophen; Diphenylpyraline, Phenylpropanolamine, Acetaminophen, and Caffeine; Pheniramine, Phenylephrine, and Acetaminophen; Pheniramine, Phenylephrine, Sodium Salicylate, and Caffeine; Phenyltoloxamine, Phenylpropanolamine, and Acetaminophen; Pyrilamine, Phenylephrine, Aspirin, and Caffeine; Pyrilamine, Phenylpropanolamine, Acetaminophen, and Caffeine; Triprolidine, Pseudoephedrine, and Acetaminophen.

VA CLASSIFICATION (Primary): RE599

**NOTE:** The *Antihistamines, Decongestants, and Analgesics (Systemic)* monograph is maintained on the USP DI electronic data base. For a printed copy of the most recent revision of the complete monograph, contact the USP Division of Information Development, 12601 Twinbrook Parkway, Rockville, MD 20852.

For information on the specific components of this combination, see the *USP DI* monographs for *Acetaminophen (Systemic), Antihistamines (Systemic), Caffeine (Systemic), Phenylpropanolamine (Systemic), Pseudoephedrine (Systemic), Salicylates (Systemic),* and *Sympathomimetic Agents—Cardiovascular Use (Parenteral-Systemic).*

The information that follows is selectively abstracted from the complete monograph and is provided to facilitate drug use review and patient counseling.

Note: For a listing of dosage forms and brand names by country availability, see *Dosage Forms* section(s). For a listing of brand names for the articles in this monograph, refer to the General Index.

## Category

Antihistaminic (H₁-receptor)-decongestant-analgesic.

## Indications

### Accepted

Cold symptoms (treatment)

Congestion, nasal (treatment) and

Congestion, sinus (treatment)—Antihistamine, decongestant, and analgesic combinations are indicated for the temporary relief of nasal and sinus congestion and headaches, pains, and general discomfort due to colds, flu, or allergies. The antihistamine in these combinations may provide added relief of nasal congestion, rhinorrhea, and sneezing. It may also serve as an adjunct because of its anticholinergic drying effects.

The therapeutic effectiveness of oral phenylephrine as a nasal decongestant has been questioned, especially at the usual oral dose.

## Patient Consultation

As an aid to patient consultation, refer to *Advice for the Patient, Antihistamines, Decongestants, and Analgesics (Systemic).*

In providing consultation, consider emphasizing the following selected information (» = major clinical significance):

### Before using this medication

» Conditions affecting use, especially:

  Sensitivity to any of the medications in the combination being taken

  Pregnancy—Concern for the fetus and/or newborn infant only with high doses and long-term therapy; psychiatric disorders more likely with use of phenylpropanolamine in postpartum women; use of aspirin-containing combinations not recommended during third trimester

  Breast-feeding—Antihistamines may cause excitement or irritability in nursing infant; high risk for infants from sympathomimetic amines; also, concern with high doses and chronic use because of high salicylate intake by infant

  Use in children—Increased susceptibility to anticholinergic effects of antihistamines and to vasopressor effects of sympathomimetic amines; psychiatric disorders more likely with use of phenylpropanolamine in children under 6 years of age; hyperexcitability (paradoxical reaction) may occur; also, increased susceptibility to toxic effects of salicylates, especially if fever and dehydration present; possible association between aspirin usage and Reye's syndrome

  Use in adolescents—Possible association between aspirin usage and Reye's syndrome

  Use in the elderly—Anticholinergic and CNS stimulant effects more likely to occur; increased susceptibility to toxic effects of salicylates

Other medications, especially anticholinergics, medicine for high blood pressure or depression, or CNS depressants or stimulants

Other medical problems, especially alcoholism, cardiovascular disease, diabetes, gastritis or peptic ulcer (with salicylate-containing), hypertension, hyperthyroidism, or prostatic hypertrophy

## Proper use of this medication

» Importance of not taking more medication than the amount recommended

Taking with food, water, or milk to minimize gastric irritation

Swallowing extended-release dosage form whole

» Not taking combinations containing aspirin if a strong vinegar-like odor is present

» Proper dosing

Missed dose: If on scheduled dosing regimen—Taking as soon as possible; not taking if almost time for next dose; not doubling doses

» Proper storage

## Precautions while using this medication

Caution if skin tests using allergens required; possible interference with test results

Checking with physician if symptoms persist or become worse, or if high fever is present

» Avoiding alcoholic beverages or other CNS depressants while taking these medications; also, alcohol consumption may increase risk of salicylate-induced gastrointestinal toxicity and acetaminophen-induced liver toxicity

» Caution if drowsiness or dizziness occurs

» Possible insomnia; taking the medication a few hours before bedtime

» Caution if taking phenylpropanolamine-containing appetite suppressants

Need to inform physician or dentist of use of medication if any kind of surgery (including dental surgery) or emergency treatment is required

Possible dryness of mouth; using sugarless gum or candy, ice, or saliva substitute for relief; checking with dentist if dry mouth continues for more than 2 weeks

» Caution if other medications containing acetaminophen, aspirin, or other salicylates (including diflunisal) are used

» Suspected overdose: Getting emergency help at once

Not taking products containing aspirin for 5 days prior to any kind of surgery, unless otherwise directed by physician

Diabetics: Aspirin present in some combination formulations may cause false urine sugar test results with prolonged use of 8 or more 325-mg (5-grain) doses per day

## Side/adverse effects

Signs of potential side effects, especially allergic reactions, anticholinergic effects, blood dyscrasias, jaundice (with acetaminophen-containing), and signs of gastrointestinal irritation or bleeding (with salicylate-containing)

## Oral Dosage Forms

See *Table 1*, page 359.

Revised: 08/30/94
Interim revision: 07/18/95

## Table 1. Oral Dosage Forms

Note: Content per capsule, tablet, or 5 mL, unless otherwise stated.

| Brand or generic name [availability] | Antihistamines | Decongestants | Analgesics | Other content information as per product label | Usual adult and adolescent dose* (prn) | Usual pediatric dose (prn) | Packaging, storage, and auxiliary labeling† |
|---|---|---|---|---|---|---|---|
| Aclophen Tablets (Rx) [U.S.] | Chlorpheniramine maleate 8 mg | Phenylephrine HCl 40 mg | Acetaminophen 500 mg | Dye-free | 1 tab q 4 hr | | a, d |
| Actifed-A Tablets (OTC) [Canada] | Triprolidine HCl 2.5 mg | Pseudoephedrine HCl 60 mg | Acetaminophen 325 mg | Scored | 1 tab q 4 hr | >10 yrs: ½ tab q 4 hr | a, d |
| Actifed Plus Tablets (OTC) [U.S.] | Triprolidine HCl 1.25 mg | Pseudoephedrine HCl 30 mg | Acetaminophen 500 mg | | 2 tabs q 6 hr | | a, d |
| Actifed Plus Caplets Tablets (OTC) [U.S.] | Triprolidine HCl 1.25 mg | Pseudoephedrine HCl 30 mg | Acetaminophen 500 mg | | 2 tabs q 6 hr | | a, d |
| Actified Sinus Nighttime Caplets Tablets (OTC) [U.S.] | Diphenhydramine HCl 25 mg | Pseudoephedrine HCl 30 mg | Acetaminophen 500 mg | In dual package that also contains *Actified Sinus Daytime* | 2 tabs hs or 2 tabs q 6 hr (max 8 tabs daily) | | a, d |
| Alka-Seltzer Plus Allergy Medicine Liqui-Gels Capsules (OTC) [U.S.] | Chlorpheniramine maleate 2 mg | Pseudoephedrine HCl 30 mg | Acetaminophen 250 mg | | 2 caps q 4 hr (max 8 caps daily) | 6–12 yrs: 1 cap q 4 hr (max 4 caps daily) | a, d |

*Geriatric patients may be more sensitive to the effects of usual adult dose.

†For appropriate *Packaging and storage* and *Auxiliary labeling* information refer to designated letters as follows:

a—Store below 40 °C (104 °F), preferably between 15 and 30 °C (59 and 86 °F), in a tight container, unless otherwise specified by manufacturer.

b—Store between 2 and 30 °C (36 and 86 °F), in a well-closed container, unless otherwise specified by manufacturer.

c—Protect from freezing.

d—Auxiliary labeling: • May cause drowsiness. • Avoid alcoholic beverages.

## Table 1. Oral Dosage Forms *(continued)*

Note: Content per capsule, tablet, or 5 mL, unless otherwise stated.

| Brand or generic name [availability] | Antihistamines | Decongestants | Analgesics | Other content information as per product label | Usual adult and adolescent dose* (prn) | Usual pediatric dose (prn) | Packaging, storage, and auxiliary labeling† |
|---|---|---|---|---|---|---|---|
| *Alka-Seltzer Plus Cold* Effervescent Tablets (OTC) [U.S.] | Chlorpheniramine maleate 2 mg | Phenylpropanol-amine bitartrate 24.08 mg | Aspirin 325 mg | Sodium 506 mg | 2 tabs q 4 hr dissolved in 120 mL water (max 8 tabs daily) | | a, d |
| *Alka-Seltzer Plus Cold Medicine Liqui-Gels* Capsules (OTC) [U.S.] | Chlorpheniramine maleate 2 mg | Pseudoephedrine HCL 30 mg | Acetaminophen 250 mg | | 2 caps q 4 hr (max 8 caps daily) | 6–12 yrs: 1 cap q 4 hr (max 4 caps daily) | a, d |
| *Allerest Headache Strength* Tablets (OTC) [U.S.] | Chlorpheniramine maleate 2 mg | Pseudoephedrine HCl 30 mg | Acetaminophen 325 mg | | 2 tabs q 4 hr (max 8 tabs daily) | 6–12 yrs: 1 tab q 4 hr | a, d |
| *Allerest Sinus Pain Formula* Tablets (OTC) [U.S.] | Chlorpheniramine maleate 2 mg | Pseudoephedrine HCl 30 mg | Acetaminophen 500 mg | | 2 tabs q 6 hr | | a, d |
| *Alumadrine* Tablets (Rx) [U.S.] | Chlorpheniramine maleate 4 mg | Phenylpropanol-amine HCl 25 mg | Acetaminophen 500 mg | Scored | 1 tab q 4 hr | 6-12 yrs: ½ tab q 4 hr | a, d |
| *BC Multi Symptom Cold Powder* for Oral Solution (OTC) [U.S.] | Chlorpheniramine maleate 4 mg per packet | Phenylpropanolam-ine HCl 25 mg per packet | Aspirin 650 mg per packet | Lactose | 1 packet dissolved in water q 4 hr | | a, d |
| *Benadryl Cold/Flu* Tablets (OTC) [U.S.] | Diphenhydramine HCl 12.5 mg | Pseudoephedrine HCl 30 mg | Acetaminophen 500 mg | | 2 tabs q 6 hr | | a, d |
| *Benadryl Cold Nighttime Liquid* Oral Solution (OTC) [U.S.] | Diphenhydramine HCl 8.3 mg | Pseudoephedrine HCl 10 mg | Acetaminophen 167 mg | Alcohol 10% | 30 mL q 6 hr | | a, c, d |
| *BQ Cold* Tablets (OTC) [U.S.] | Chlorpheniramine maleate 2 mg | Phenylpropanol-amine HCl 12.5 mg | Acetaminophen 325 mg | | 2 tabs q 4 hr | | a, d |
| *Bromaline Plus* Tablets (OTC) [U.S.] | Brompheniramine maleate 2 mg | Phenylpropanol-amine HCl 12.5 mg | Acetaminophen 500 mg | | 2 tabs q 6 hr | | a, d |
| *Children's Tylenol Cold* Oral Solution (OTC) [U.S.] | Chlorpheniramine maleate 1 mg | Pseudoephedrine HCl 15 mg | Acetaminophen 160 mg | Sorbitol; Alcohol-free | Intended for pediatric use | 2–5 yrs: 5 mL, 6–11 yrs: 10 mL, q 4–6 hr | a, c, d |
| Chewable Tablets (OTC) [U.S.] | Chlorpheniramine maleate 0.5 mg | Pseudoephedrine HCl 7.5 mg | Acetaminophen 80 mg | Phenylalanine 4 mg | Intended for pediatric use | 2–5 yrs: 2 tabs, 6–11 yrs: 4 tabs, q 4–6 hr | a, d |
| *Chlor-Trimeton Allergy-Sinus Caplets* Tablets (OTC) [U.S.] | Chlorpheniramine maleate 2 mg | Phenylpropanol-amine HCl 12.5 mg | Acetaminophen 500 mg | | 2 tabs q 6 hr | | b, d |

## Table 1. Oral Dosage Forms *(continued)*

Note: Content per capsule, tablet, or 5 mL, unless otherwise stated.

| Brand or generic name [availability] | Antihistamines | Decongestants | Analgesics | Other content information as per product label | Usual adult and adolescent dose* (prn) | Usual pediatric dose (prn) | Packaging, storage, and auxiliary labeling† |
|---|---|---|---|---|---|---|---|
| *Codimal* Capsules (OTC) [U.S.] | Chlorpheniramine maleate 2 mg | Pseudoephedrine HCl 30 mg | Acetaminophen 325 mg | | 2 caps or tabs q 4–6 hr | 6–12 yrs: 1 cap or tab q 4–6 hr | a, d |
| Tablets (OTC) [U.S.] | | | | Scored, coated | | | |
| *Comtrex Allergy-Sinus* Tablets (OTC) [U.S.] | Chlorpheniramine maleate 2 mg | Pseudoephedrine HCl 30 mg | Acetaminophen 500 mg | Coated | 2 tabs q 6 hr | | a, d |
| *Comtrex Allergy-Sinus Caplets* Tablets (OTC) [U.S.] | Chlorpheniramine maleate 2 mg | Pseudoephedrine HCl 30 mg | Acetaminophen 500 mg | Coated | 2 tabs q 6 hr | | a, d |
| *Congestant D* Tablets (OTC) [U.S.] | Chlorpheniramine maleate 2 mg | Phenylpropanol-amine HCl 12.5 mg | Acetaminophen 325 mg | | 2 tabs q 4 hr | | a, d |
| *Contac Allergy/ Sinus Night Caplets* Tablets (OTC) [U.S.] | Diphenhydramine HCl 50 mg | Pseudoephedrine HCl 60 mg | Acetaminophen 650 mg | In dual package that also contains *Contac Allergy/Sinus Day Caplets* | 1 tab q 6 hr (max 4 tabs daily) | | a, d |
| *Coricidin D* Tablets (OTC) [Canada] | Chlorpheniramine maleate 2 mg | Phenylpropanol-amine HCl 12.5 mg | Aspirin 325 mg | Coated | 2 tabs q 4 hr (max 8 tabs daily) | 10–14 yrs: 1 tab q 4 hr | b, d |
| Tablets (OTC) [U.S.] | | | | | 2 tabs q 4 hr | 6–11 yrs: 1 tab q 4 hr | b, d |
| *Covangesic* Tablets (OTC) [U.S.] | Chlorpheniramine maleate 2 mg, Pyrilamine maleate 12.5 mg | Phenylephrine HCl 7.5 mg, Phenylpropanol-amine HCl 12.5 mg | Acetaminophen 275 mg | Tartrazine | 1 tab q 4–6 hr | | a, d |
| *Dapacin Cold* Capsules (OTC) [U.S.] | Chlorpheniramine maleate 2 mg | Phenylpropanol-amine HCl 12.5 mg | Acetaminophen 325 mg | | 2 caps q 4 hr | | a, d |
| *Dimetapp Cold and Flu Caplets* Tablets (OTC) [U.S.] | Brompheniramine maleate 2 mg | Phenylpropanol-amine HCl 12.5 mg | Acetaminophen 500 mg | Coated | 2 tabs q 4 hr | | a, d |
| *Dristan* Capsules (OTC) [Canada] | Chlorpheniramine maleate 2 mg | Phenylpropanol-amine HCl 12.5 mg | Aspirin 325 mg, Caffeine 16 mg | | 2 caps or tabs q 4 hr | 10–14 yrs: 1 cap or tab q 4 hr | a, d |
| Tablets (OTC) [Canada] | | | | | | | |
| *Dristan Cold Maximum Strength Caplets* Tablets (OTC) [U.S.] | Brompheniramine maleate 2 mg | Pseudoephedrine HCl 30 mg | Acetaminophen 500 mg | | 2 tabs q 6 hr | | a, d |

*Geriatric patients may be more sensitive to the effects of usual adult dose.

†For appropriate *Packaging and storage* and *Auxiliary labeling* information refer to designated letters as follows:
   a—Store below 40 °C (104 °F), preferably between 15 and 30 °C (59 and 86 °F), in a tight container, unless otherwise specified by manufacturer.
   b—Store between 2 and 30 °C (36 and 86 °F), in a well-closed container, unless otherwise specified by manufacturer.
   c—Protect from freezing.
   d—Auxiliary labeling: • May cause drowsiness. • Avoid alcoholic beverages.

## Table 1. Oral Dosage Forms *(continued)*

Note: Content per capsule, tablet, or 5 mL, unless otherwise stated.

| Brand or generic name [availability] | Antihistamines | Decongestants | Analgesics | Other content information as per product label | Usual adult and adolescent dose* (prn) | Usual pediatric dose (prn) | Packaging, storage, and auxiliary labeling† |
|---|---|---|---|---|---|---|---|
| *Dristan Cold Multi-Symptom Formula* Tablets (OTC) [U.S.] | Chlorpheniramine maleate 2 mg | Phenylephrine HCl 5 mg | Acetaminophen 325 mg | | 2 tabs q 4 hr | | a, d |
| *Dristan Formula P* Tablets (OTC) [Canada] | Pyrilamine maleate 12.5 mg | Phenylephrine HCl 5 mg | Aspirin 325 mg, Caffeine 16 mg | Tartrazine-free | 2 tabs q 4 hr | 10–14 yrs: 1 tab q 4 hr | a, d |
| *Drixoral Allergy-Sinus* Extended-release Tablets (OTC) [U.S.] | Dexbrompheniramine maleate 3 mg | Pseudoephedrine sulfate 60 mg | Acetaminophen 500 mg | | 2 tabs q 12 hr | | b, d |
| *Drixoral Cold and Flu* Extended-release Tablets (OTC) [U.S.] | Dexbrompheniramine maleate 3 mg | Pseudoephedrine sulfate 60 mg | Acetaminophen 500 mg | | 2 tabs q 12 hr | | b, d |
| *Duadacin* Capsules (OTC) [U.S.] | Chlorpheniramine maleate 2 mg | Phenylpropanolamine HCl 12.5 mg | Acetaminophen 325 mg | | 2 caps q 4 hr | | a, d |
| *Gendecon* Tablets (OTC) [U.S.] | Chlorpheniramine maleate 2 mg | Phenylephrine HCl 5 mg | Acetaminophen 325 mg | | 2 tabs q 4 hr | | a, d |
| *Histagesic Modified* Tablets (OTC) [U.S.] | Chlorpheniramine maleate 4 mg | Phenylephrine HCl 10 mg | Acetaminophen 324 mg | | 1 tab q 4 hr | | a, d |
| *Histosal* Tablets (OTC) [U.S.] | Pyrilamine maleate 12.5 mg | Phenylpropanolamine HCl 20 mg | Acetaminophen 324 mg, Caffeine 30 mg | | 1–2 tabs q 4 hr | | a, d |
| *Kolephrin* Capsules (OTC) [U.S.] | Chlorpheniramine maleate 2 mg | Phenylephrine HCl 10 mg | Acetaminophen 195 mg, Salicylamide 130 mg, Caffeine 65 mg | | 1 cap before meals and at bedtime | | a, d |
| *Maximum Strength Tylenol Allergy Sinus Caplets* Tablets (OTC) [U.S.] | Chlorpheniramine maleate 2 mg | Pseudoephedrine HCl 30 mg | Acetaminophen 500 mg | | 2 tabs q 4–6 hr | 6–12 yrs: 1 tab q 4–6 hr | a, d |
| *ND-Gesic* Tablets (Rx) [U.S.] | Chlorpheniramine maleate 2 mg, Pyrilamine maleate 12.5 mg | Phenylephrine HCl 5 mg | Acetaminophen 300 mg | Sugar coated | 2 tabs q 4–6 hr | | a, d |
| *NeoCitran Colds and Flu Calorie Reduced* for Oral Solution (OTC) [Canada] | Pheniramine maleate 20 mg per packet | Phenylephrine HCl 10 mg per packet | Acetaminophen 325 mg per packet | Vitamin C 50 mg per packet | 1 packet dissolved in 8 oz of hot water q 3–4 hr | | a, d |
| *NeoCitran Extra Strength Colds and Flu* for Oral Solution (OTC) [Canada] | Pheniramine maleate 20 mg per packet | Phenylephrine HCl 10 mg per packet | Acetaminophen 325 mg per packet | Vitamin C 50 mg per packet | 1 packet dissolved in 8 oz of hot water q 3–4 hr | | a, d |

# Table 1. Oral Dosage Forms *(continued)*

Note: Content per capsule, tablet, or 5 mL, unless otherwise stated.

| Brand or generic name [availability] | Antihistamines | Decongestants | Analgesics | Other content information as per product label | Usual adult and adolescent dose* (prn) | Usual pediatric dose (prn) | Packaging, storage, and auxiliary labeling† |
|---|---|---|---|---|---|---|---|
| *Night-Time Effervescent Cold* Effervescent Tablets (OTC) [U.S.] | Diphenhydramine citrate 38.33 mg | Phenylpropanolamine HCl 15 mg | Aspirin 325 mg | | 2 tabs dissolved in water q 4–6 hr (max 8 tabs daily) | | a, d |
| *Norel Plus* Capsules (Rx) [U.S.] | Chlorpheniramine maleate 4 mg, Phenyltoloxamine dihydrogen citrate 25 mg | Phenylpropanolamine HCl 25 mg | Acetaminophen 325 mg | | 1 cap q 3–4 hr | | a, d |
| *Oradrine-2* Tablets (OTC) [Canada] | Diphenylpyraline HCl 2 mg | Phenylpropanolamine HCl 25 mg | Acetaminophen 325 mg | Caffeine 32.4 mg | 1 tab q 4 hr | | a, d |
| *Phenapap Sinus Headache & Congestion* Tablets (OTC) [U.S.] | Chlorpheniramine maleate 2 mg | Pseudoephedrine HCl 30 mg | Acetaminophen 325 mg | | 1 tab q 4 hr | | a, d |
| *Phenate T.D.* Extended-release Tablets (Rx) [U.S.] | Chlorpheniramine maleate 4 mg | Phenylpropanolamine HCl 40 mg | Acetaminophen 325 mg | | 1 tab q 6–8 hr | | a, d |
| *Pyrroxate Caplets* Tablets (OTC) [U.S.] | Chlorpheniramine maleate 4 mg | Phenylpropanolamine HCl 25 mg | Acetaminophen 650 mg | | 1 tab q 4 hr | | a, d |
| *Remcol Cold* Capsules (OTC) [U.S.] | Chlorpheniramine maleate 2 mg | Phenylpropanolamine HCl 25 mg | Acetaminophen 300 mg | | 1 cap q 4 hr | | a, d |
| *Rhinogesic* Tablets (OTC) [U.S.] | Chlorpheniramine maleate 2 mg | Phenylephrine HCl 5 mg | Acetaminophen 150 mg, Salicylamide 250 mg | | 1 tab q 3 hr | | a, d |
| *Salphenyl* Capsules (OTC) [U.S.] | Chlorpheniramine maleate 2 mg | Phenylephrine HCl 10 mg | Acetaminophen 130 mg, Salicylamide 200 mg | | 1 cap q 3–4 hr | | a, d |
| *Scot-tussin Original 5-Action Cold Formula* Syrup (OTC) [U.S.] | Pheniramine maleate 13.3 mg | Phenylephrine HCl 4.2 mg | Sodium salicylate 83.3 mg; Caffeine citrate 25 mg | Sodium citrate 83.3 mg; Alcohol-free | 5 mL q 3–4 hr | | a, c, d |
| *Scot-tussin Original 5-Action Cold Medicine* Oral Solution (OTC) [U.S.] | Pheniramine maleate 13.3 mg | Phenylephrine HCl 4.2 mg | Sodium salicylate 83.3 mg; Caffeine citrate 25 mg | Sodium citrate 83.3 mg; Alcohol-free; Sugar-free | 5 mL q 3–4 hr | | a, c, d |
| *Simplet* Tablets (OTC) [U.S.] | Chlorpheniramine maleate 4 mg | Pseudoephedrine HCl 60 mg | Acetaminophen 650 mg | | 1 tab q 4–6 hr (max 4 tabs daily) | | a, d |

*Geriatric patients may be more sensitive to the effects of usual adult dose.

†For appropriate *Packaging and storage* and *Auxiliary labeling* information refer to designated letters as follows:
    a—Store below 40 °C (104 °F), preferably between 15 and 30 °C (59 and 86 °F), in a tight container, unless otherwise specified by manufacturer.
    b—Store between 2 and 30 °C (36 and 86 °F), in a well-closed container, unless otherwise specified by manufacturer.
    c—Protect from freezing.
    d—Auxiliary labeling: • May cause drowsiness. • Avoid alcoholic beverages.

## Table 1. Oral Dosage Forms *(continued)*

Note: Content per capsule, tablet, or 5 mL, unless otherwise stated.

| Brand or generic name [availability] | Antihistamines | Decongestants | Analgesics | Other content information as per product label | Usual adult and adolescent dose* (prn) | Usual pediatric dose (prn) | Packaging, storage, and auxiliary labeling† |
|---|---|---|---|---|---|---|---|
| *Sinapils* Tablets (OTC) [U.S.] | Chlorpheniramine maleate 1 mg | Phenylpropanolamine HCl 12.5 mg | Acetaminophen 324 mg, Caffeine 32.5 mg | | 2 tabs q 4 hr | | a, d |
| *Sinarest* Tablets (OTC) [U.S.] | Chlorpheniramine maleate 2 mg | Pseudoephedrine HCl 30 mg | Acetaminophen 325 mg | | 2 tabs q 4 hr (max 8 tabs daily) | | a, d |
| *Sinarest Extra Strength* Tablets (OTC) [U.S.] | Chlorpheniramine maleate 2 mg | Pseudoephedrine HCl 30 mg | Acetaminophen 500 mg | | 2 tabs q 6 hr | | a, d |
| *Sine-Off Maximum Strength Allergy/ Sinus Formula Caplets* Tablets (OTC) [U.S.] | Chlorpheniramine maleate 2 mg | Pseudoephedrine HCl 30 mg | Acetaminophen 500 mg | | 2 tabs q 6 hr | | a, d |
| *Sine-Off Sinus Medicine* Tablets (OTC) [U.S.] | Chlorpheniramine maleate 2 mg | Phenylpropanolamine HCl 12.5 mg | Aspirin 325 mg | | 2 tabs q 4 hr | 6–12 yrs: 1 tab q 4 hr | a, d |
| *Singlet* Tablets (OTC) [U.S.] | Chlorpheniramine maleate 4 mg | Pseudoephedrine HCl 60 mg | Acetaminophen 650 mg | | 1 tab q 4 hr | | a, d |
| *Sinulin* Tablets (OTC) [U.S.] | Chlorpheniramine maleate 4 mg | Phenylpropanolamine HCl 25 mg | Acetaminophen 650 mg | Scored | 1 tab q 4–6 hr | | a, d |
| *Sinutab Extra Strength* Capsules (OTC) [Canada] | Chlorpheniramine maleate 2 mg | Pseudoephedrine HCl 30 mg | Acetaminophen 500 mg | | 1–2 caps q 4–6 hr | | a, d |
| *Sinutab Sinus Allergy Maximum Strength* Tablets (OTC) [U.S.] | Chlorpheniramine maleate 2 mg | Pseudoephedrine HCl 30 mg | Acetaminophen 500 mg | | 2 tabs q 6 hr | | a, d |
| *Sinutab Sinus Allergy Maximum Strength Caplets* Tablets (OTC) [U.S.] | Chlorpheniramine maleate 2 mg | Pseudoephedrine HCl 30 mg | Acetaminophen 500 mg | | 2 tabs q 6 hr | | a, d |
| *Sinutab Regular* Tablets (OTC) [Canada] | Chlorpheniramine maleate 2 mg | Pseudoephedrine HCl 30 mg | Acetaminophen 325 mg | Scored | 1–2 tab q 4–6 hr | 6–12 yrs: ¹/₂–1 tab q 4–6 hr | a, d |
| *Sinutab SA* Extended-release Tablets (OTC) [Canada] | Phenyltoloxamine citrate 66 mg | Phenylpropanolamine HCl 100 mg | Acetaminophen 600 mg | Scored | 1 tab q 12 hr | 10–14 yrs: ¹/₂ tab q 12 hr | a, d |
| *Sinutrex Extra Strength* Tablets (OTC) [U.S.] | Chlorpheniramine maleate 2 mg | Pseudoephedrine HCl 30 mg | Acetaminophen 500 mg | | 2 tabs q 6 hr | | a, d |
| *TheraFlu/Flu and Cold Medicine* for Oral Solution (OTC)[U.S.] | Chlorpheniramine maleate 4 mg per packet | Pseudoephedrine HCl 60 mg per packet | Acetaminophen 500 mg per packet | | 1 packet dissolved in 6-oz cup of hot water q 4 hr | | a, d |

## Table 1. Oral Dosage Forms *(continued)*

Note: Content per capsule, tablet, or 5 mL, unless otherwise stated.

| Brand or generic name [availability] | Antihistamines | Decongestants | Analgesics | Other content information as per product label | Usual adult and adolescent dose* (prn) | Usual pediatric dose (prn) | Packaging, storage, and auxiliary labeling† |
|---|---|---|---|---|---|---|---|
| *Triaminicin Cold, Allergy, Sinus* Tablets (OTC) [U.S.] | Chlorpheniramine maleate 4 mg | Phenylpropanol-amine HCl 25 mg | Acetaminophen 650 mg | | 1 tab q 4 hr | | a, d |
| *Tricom Caplets* Tablets (OTC) [U.S.] | Chlorpheniramine maleate 4 mg | Pseudoephedrine HCl 60 mg | Acetaminophen 650 mg | | 1 tab q 4–6 hr | | a, d |
| *Tylenol Allergy Sinus Night Time Maximum Strength Caplets* Tablets (OTC) [U.S.] | Diphenhydramine HCl 25 mg | Pseudoephedrine HCl 30 mg | Acetaminophen 500 mg | | 2 tabs hs | | a, d |
| *Tylenol Cold Medication* Effervescent Tablets (OTC) [U.S.] | Chlorpheniramine maleate 2 mg | Phenylpropanol-amine HCl 12.5 mg | Acetaminophen 325 mg | Sodium 525 mg | 2 tabs dissolved in water q 4 hr | 6–11 yrs: 1 tab dissolved in water q 4 hr | a, d |
| *Tylenol Cold Night Time* Oral Solution (OTC) [U.S.] | Diphenhydramine HCl 8.3 mg | Pseudoephedrine HCl 10 mg | Acetaminophen 108.3 mg | Alcohol 10% | 30 mL q 6 hr | | a, c, d |
| *4-Way Cold* Tablets (OTC) [U.S.] | Chlorpheniramine maleate 2 mg | Phenylpropanol-amine HCl 12.5 mg | Acetaminophen 325 mg | | 2 tabs q 4 hr | | a, d |

*Geriatric patients may be more sensitive to the effects of usual adult dose.

†For appropriate *Packaging and storage* and *Auxiliary labeling* information refer to designated letters as follows:
   a—Store below 40 °C (104 °F), preferably between 15 and 30 °C (59 and 86 °F), in a tight container, unless otherwise specified by manufacturer.
   b—Store between 2 and 30 °C (36 and 86 °F), in a well-closed container, unless otherwise specified by manufacturer.
   c—Protect from freezing.
   d—Auxiliary labeling: • May cause drowsiness. • Avoid alcoholic beverages.

# ANTIHISTAMINES, DECONGESTANTS, AND ANTICHOLINERGICS   Systemic

This monograph includes information on the following: .

VA CLASSIFICATION (Primary): RE599

**NOTE:** The *Antihistamines, Decongestants, and Anticholinergics (Systemic)* monograph is maintained on the USP DI electronic data base. For a printed copy of the most recent revision of the complete monograph, contact the USP Division of Information Development, 12601 Twinbrook Parkway, Rockville, MD 20852.

For information on the specific components of this combination, see the *USP DI* monographs for *Anticholinergics/Antispasmodics (Systemic), Antihistamines (Systemic), Phenylpropanolamine (Systemic), Pseudoephedrine (Systemic),* and *Sympathomimetic Agents—Cardiovascular Use (Systemic).*

The information that follows is selectively abstracted from the complete monograph and is provided to facilitate drug use review and patient counseling.

Note: For a listing of dosage forms and brand names by country availability, see *Dosage Forms* section(s). For a listing of brand names for the articles in this monograph, refer to the General Index.

## Category

Antihistaminic (H₁-receptor)-decongestant-anticholinergic.

## Indications

**Accepted**

Congestion, nasal (treatment)
Cold symptoms (treatment) and
Rhinitis, perennial and seasonal allergic or vasomotor (treatment)—Antihistamine, decongestant, and anticholinergic combinations are indicated in the symptomatic treatment of allergic rhinitis, sinusitis, and the common cold.

The therapeutic effectiveness of oral phenylephrine as a nasal decongestant has been questioned, especially at the usual oral dose.

## Patient Consultation

As an aid to patient consultation, refer to *Advice for the Patient, Antihistamines, Decongestants, and Anticholinergics (Systemic).*

In providing consultation, consider emphasizing the following selected information (» = major clinical significance):

**Before using this medication**
» Conditions affecting use, especially:

      Sensitivity to any of the medications in the combination being taken
      Pregnancy—Postpartum women are particularly susceptible to psychiatric disorders that may be caused by phenylpropanolamine

Breast-feeding—Antihistamines may cause excitement or irritability in nursing infant; high risk to infants from sympathomimetic amines; possible inhibition of lactation

Use in children—Increased susceptibility to anticholinergic effects and to vasopressor effects; children under 6 years of age may be particularly susceptible to psychiatric disorders that may be caused by phenylpropanolamine; hyperexcitability (paradoxical reaction) may occur; increased response to anticholinergics in infants and children with spastic paralysis or brain damage

Use in the elderly—Anticholinergic and CNS stimulant effects more likely to occur in older patients; danger of precipitating undiagnosed glaucoma; possible impairment of memory

Dental—Possible development of dental problems because of decreased salivary flow

Other medications, especially alcohol, other anticholinergics, beta-adrenergic blocking agents, medicine for high blood pressure or depression, CNS depressants or stimulants, digitalis glycosides, and potassium chloride

Other medical problems, especially cardiovascular disease, diabetes mellitus, hemorrhage, severe hypertension, hyperthyroidism, myasthenia gravis, obstruction in gastrointestinal or urinary tract, prostatic hypertrophy, tachycardia, urinary retention, and xerostomia

**Proper use of this medication**

» Importance of not taking more medication than the amount recommended

Taking with food, water, or milk to minimize gastric irritation

Swallowing extended-release dosage form whole

» Proper dosing

Missed dose: Taking as soon as possible; not taking if almost time for next dose; not doubling doses

» Proper storage

**Precautions while using this medication**

Checking with physician if symptoms persist or become worse, or if high fever is present

Caution if skin tests using allergens required; possible interference with test results

» Caution during exercise or hot weather; overheating may result in heat stroke

» Possible increased sensitivity of eyes to light

» Caution if blurred vision occurs

» Caution if drowsiness or dizziness occurs

» Possible insomnia; taking the medication a few hours before bedtime

» Caution if taking phenylpropanolamine-containing appetite suppressants

Need to inform physician or dentist of use of medication if any kind of surgery (including dental surgery or emergency treatment) is required

Possible dryness of mouth; using sugarless gum or candy, ice, or saliva substitute for relief; checking with dentist if dry mouth continues for more than 2 weeks

» Suspected overdose: Getting emergency help at once

**Side/adverse effects**

Signs of potential side effects, especially allergic reactions, severe anticholinergic effects, blood dyscrasias, CNS stimulation, severe drowsiness, hypertension, psychotic episodes, and tightness in chest

## Oral Dosage Forms

See *table 1,* page 366.

Revised: 07/19/94
Interim revision: 07/18/95

## Table 1. Oral Dosage Forms

Note: Content per capsule, tablet, or 5 mL, unless otherwise stated.

| Brand or generic name [availability] | Antihistamines | Decongestants | Anticholinergics | Other information | Usual adult and adolescent dose* (prn) | Usual pediatric dose (prn) | Packaging, storage, and auxiliary labeling† |
|---|---|---|---|---|---|---|---|
| *AH-chew* Chewable Tablets (Rx) [U.S.] | Chlorpheniramine maleate 2 mg | Phenylephrine HCl 10 mg | Methscopolamine nitrate 1.25 mg | Scored | 2 tabs q 4 hr | 6–12 yrs: 1 tab q 4 hr | a, c, d |
| *Atrohist Plus* Extended-release Tablets (Rx) [U.S.] | Chlorpheniramine maleate 8 mg | Phenylephrine HCl 25 mg, Phenylpropanolamine HCl 50 mg | Atropine sulfate 0.04 mg, Hyoscyamine sulfate 0.19 mg, Scopolamine HBr 0.01 mg | Scored | 1 tab q 12 hr | | a, d |
| *D.A. Chewable* Chewable Tablets (Rx) [U.S.] | Chlorpheniramine maleate 2 mg | Phenylephrine HCl 10 mg | Methscopolamine nitrate 1.25 mg | Scored | 1–2 tabs q 4 hr | 6–12 yrs: 1 tab q 4 hr | a, c, d |
| *Dallergy* Syrup (Rx) [U.S.] | Chlorpheniramine maleate 2 mg | Phenylephrine HCl 10 mg | Methscopolamine nitrate 0.625 mg | | 10 mL q 4–6 hr | 6–12 yrs: 5 mL q 4–6 hr | a, b, d |
| Tablets (Rx) [U.S.] | Chlorpheniramine maleate 4 mg | Phenylephrine HCl 10 mg | Methscopolamine nitrate 1.25 mg | Scored | 1 tab q 4–6 hr | 6–12 yrs: ½ tab q 4–6 hr | a, d |
| *Dallergy Caplets* Extended-release Tablets (Rx) [U.S.] | Chlorpheniramine maleate 8 mg | Phenylephrine HCl 20 mg | Methscopolamine nitrate 2.5 mg | Scored | 1 tab q 12 hr | 6–12 yrs: ½ tab q 12 hr | a, d |
| *Dura-Vent/DA* Extended-release Tablets (Rx) [U.S.] | Chlorpheniramine maleate 8 mg | Phenylephrine HCl 20 mg | Methscopolamine nitrate 2.5 mg | Scored | 1 tab q 12 hr | 6–12 yrs: ½ tab q 12 hr | a, d |

## Table 1. Oral Dosage Forms *(continued)*

Note: Content per capsule, tablet, or 5 mL, unless otherwise stated.

| Brand or generic name [availability] | Antihistamines | Decongestants | Anticholinergics | Other information | Usual adult and adolescent dose* (prn) | Usual pediatric dose (prn) | Packaging, storage, and auxiliary labeling† |
|---|---|---|---|---|---|---|---|
| *Extendryl* Syrup (Rx) [U.S.] | Chlorpheniramine maleate 2 mg | Phenylephrine HCl 10 mg | Methscopolamine nitrate 1.25 mg | | 10 mL q 4 hr | 6–12 yrs: 5 mL q 4 hr | a, b, d |
| Chewable Tablets (Rx) [U.S.] | Chlorpheniramine maleate 2 mg | Phenylephrine HCl 10 mg | Methscopolamine nitrate 1.25 mg | | 2 tabs q 4 hr | 6–12 yrs: 1 tab q 4 hr | a, c, d |
| *Extendryl JR* Extended-release Capsules (Rx) [U.S.] | Chlorpheniramine maleate 4 mg | Phenylephrine HCl 10 mg | Methscopolamine nitrate 1.25 mg | | Intended for pediatric patients | 6–12 yrs: 1 cap q 12 hr | a, d |
| *Extendryl SR* Extended-release Capsules (Rx) [U.S.] | Chlorpheniramine maleate 8 mg | Phenylephrine HCl 20 mg | Methscopolamine nitrate 2.5 mg | | 1 cap q 12 hr | | a, d |
| *Histor-D Timecelles* Extended-release Capsules (Rx) [U.S.] | Chlorpheniramine maleate 8 mg | Phenylephrine HCl 20 mg | Methscopolamine nitrate 2.5 mg | | 1 cap q 12 hr | | a, d |
| *OMNIhist L.A.* Extended-release Tablets (Rx) [U.S.] | Chlorpheniramine maleate 8 mg | Phenylephrine HCl 20 mg | Methscopolamine nitrate 2.5 mg | Scored | 1 tab q 12 hr | | a, d |
| *Phenahist-TR* Extended-release Tablets (Rx) [U.S.] | Chlorpheniramine maleate 8 mg | Phenylephrine HCl 25 mg, Phenylpropanol amine HCl 50 mg | Atropine sulfate 0.0362 mg, Hyoscyamine sulfate 0.1936 mg, Scopolamine HBr 0.0121 mg | | 1 tab q 8–12 hr | | a, d |
| *Phenchlor SHA* Extended-release Tablets (Rx) [U.S.] | Chlorpheniramine maleate 8 mg | Phenylephrine HCl 25 mg, Phenylpropanol amine HCl 50 mg | Atropine sulfate 0.04 mg, Hyoscyamine sulfate 0.19 mg, Scopolamine HBr 0.01 mg | | 1 tab q 12 hr | | a, d |
| *Prehist D* Extended-release Tablets (Rx) [U.S.] | Chlorpheniramine maleate 8 mg | Phenylephrine HCl 20 mg | Methscopolamine nitrate 2.5 mg | Scored | 1 cap q 12 hr | 6–12 yrs: ½ tab q 12 hr | a, d |
| *Rhinolar* Extended-release Capsules (Rx) [U.S.] | Chlorpheniramine maleate 8 mg | Phenylpropanolamine HCl 75 mg | Methscopolamine nitrate 2.5 mg | | 1 cap q 12 hr | | a, d |

*Geriatric patients may be more sensitive to the effects of usual adult dose.

†For appropriate *Packaging and storage* and *Auxiliary labeling* information refer to designated letters as follows:
    a—Store below 40 °C (104 °F), preferably between 15 and 30 °C (59 and 86 °F), in a tight container, unless otherwise specified by manufacturer.
    b—Protect from freezing.
    c—May be chewed.
    d—Auxiliary labeling: • May cause drowsiness. • Avoid alcoholic beverages.

## Table 1. Oral Dosage Forms (continued)

Note: Content per capsule, tablet, or 5 mL, unless otherwise stated.

| Brand or generic name [availability] | Antihistamines | Decongestants | Anticholinergics | Other information | Usual adult and adolescent dose* (prn) | Usual pediatric dose (prn) | Packaging, storage, and auxiliary labeling† |
|---|---|---|---|---|---|---|---|
| *Ru-Tuss* Extended-release Tablets (Rx) [U.S.] | Chlorpheniramine maleate 8 mg | Phenylephrine HCl 25 mg, Phenylpropanolamine HCl 50 mg | Atropine sulfate 0.04 mg, Hyoscyamine sulfate 0.19 mg, Scopolamine HBr 0.01 mg | Scored | 1 tab q 12 hr | | a, d |
| *Stahist* Extended-release Tablets (Rx) [U.S.] | Chlorpheniramine maleate 8 mg | Phenylephrine HCl 25 mg Phenylpropanolamine HCl 50 mg | Atropine sulfate 0.04 mg, Hyoscyamine sulfate 0.19 mg, Scopolamine HBr 0.01 mg | Scored | 1 tab q 12 hr | | a, d |

\*Geriatric patients may be more sensitive to the effects of usual adult dose.

†For appropriate *Packaging and storage* and *Auxiliary labeling* information refer to designated letters as follows:
    a—Store below 40 °C (104 °F), preferably between 15 and 30 °C (59 and 86 °F), in a tight container, unless otherwise specified by manufacturer.
    b—Protect from freezing.
    c—May be chewed.
    d—Auxiliary labeling: • May cause drowsiness. • Avoid alcoholic beverages.

# ANTIHISTAMINES, PHENOTHIAZINE-DERIVATIVE   Systemic

This monograph includes information on the following: Methdilazine†; Promethazine; Trimeprazine.

INN:
    Trimeprazine—Alimemazine

VA CLASSIFICATION (Primary/Secondary):
    Methdilazine—AH100
    Promethazine—AH100/CN309; GA700
    Trimeprazine—AH100

Note: For a listing of dosage forms and brand names by country availability, see *Dosage Forms* section(s). For a listing of brand names for the articles in this monograph, refer to the General Index.

    †Not commercially available in Canada.

## Category

Antihistaminic ($H_1$-receptor)—Methdilazine; Promethazine; Trimeprazine.
Antiemetic—Promethazine.
Antivertigo agent—Promethazine.
Sedative-hypnotic—Promethazine; Trimeprazine.

## Indications

Note: Bracketed information in the *Indications* section refers to uses that are not included in U.S. product labeling.

**Accepted**
Rhinitis, perennial and seasonal allergic or vasomotor (treatment) or
Conjunctivitis, allergic (treatment)—Antihistamines are indicated in the symptomatic treatment of perennial and seasonal allergic rhinitis, vasomotor rhinitis, and allergic conjunctivitis due to inhalant allergens and foods.

Pruritus (treatment)
Urticaria (treatment)
Angioedema (treatment)
Dermatographism (treatment) or
Transfusion reactions, urticarial (treatment)—Antihistamines are indicated for the symptomatic treatment of pruritus associated with allergic reactions and of mild, uncomplicated allergic skin manifestations of urticaria and angioedema, in dermatographism, and in urticaria associated with transfusions. Methdilazine is also indicated in the treatment of pruritus associated with pityriasis rosea.

Sneezing (treatment) or
Rhinorrhea (treatment)—Antihistamines are indicated for the relief of sneezing and rhinorrhea associated with the common cold. However, controlled clinical studies have not demonstrated that antihistamines are significantly more effective than placebo in relieving cold symptoms.

Anaphylactic or anaphylactoid reactions (treatment adjunct)—Antihistamines are indicated as adjunctive therapy to epinephrine and other standard measures for anaphylactic reactions after the acute manifestations have been controlled, and to ameliorate the allergic reactions to blood or plasma.

Motion sickness (prophylaxis and treatment) or
Vertigo (treatment)—Promethazine is indicated for the prevention and treatment of the nausea, vomiting, dizziness, or vertigo of motion sickness.

Nausea or vomiting (prophylaxis and treatment)—Promethazine is indicated in the control of nausea and vomiting associated with certain types of anesthesia and surgery.

Sedation—Promethazine and [trimeprazine][1] are indicated for their sedative and hypnotic effects and as adjuncts to preoperative and postoperative medication.

Pain, postoperative (treatment adjunct)—Promethazine is indicated as an adjunct to analgesics for control of postoperative pain.

Analgesia adjunct, during surgery
Anesthesia, general, adjunct or
Anesthesia, local, adjunct—Intravenous administration of promethazine is indicated in special surgical situations (such as repeated bronchoscopy, ophthalmic surgery, and poor-risk patients) in combination with reduced amounts of meperidine or other narcotic analgesics as an adjunct to anesthesia and analgesia.

    [1]Not included in Canadian product labeling.

## Pharmacology/Pharmacokinetics

**Physicochemical characteristics**
Chemical group—
    Phenothiazine derivatives
Molecular weight—
    Methdilazine hydrochloride: 332.89.
    Promethazine hydrochloride: 320.88.
    Trimeprazine tartrate: 746.98.

pKa—
    Promethazine: 9.1.

## Mechanism of action/Effect

Antihistaminic ($H_1$-receptor)—Antihistamines used in the treatment of allergy act by competing with histamine for $H_1$-receptor sites on effector cells. They thereby prevent, but do not reverse, responses mediated by histamine alone. Antihistamines antagonize, in varying degrees, most of the pharmacological effects of histamine, including urticaria and pruritus. In addition, the anticholinergic actions of most antihistamines provide a drying effect on the nasal and oral mucosa.

Antiemetic; antivertigo—The mechanism by which some antihistamines exert their antiemetic, anti-motion sickness, and antivertigo effects is not precisely known but may be related to their central anticholinergic actions. They diminish vestibular stimulation and depress labyrinthine function. Activity on the medullary chemoreceptive trigger zone may also be involved in the antiemetic effect.

Sedative-hypnotic—Most antihistamines cross the blood-brain barrier and produce sedation due to inhibition of histamine *N*-methyltransferase and blockage of central histaminergic receptors. Antagonism of other central nervous system receptor sites, such as those for serotonin, acetylcholine, and alpha-adrenergic stimulation, may also be involved. Phenothiazines are thought to cause indirect reduction of stimuli to the brain stem reticular system.

## Other actions/effects

Anticholinergic—Antihistamines prevent responses to acetylcholine that are mediated via muscarinic receptors.

Antiemetic—Methdilazine and trimeprazine also possess antiemetic properties. However, only promethazine is labeled for this indication.

## Absorption

Well absorbed after oral administration.

## Protein binding

Promethazine—High (65–90%).

## Biotransformation

Hepatic; some renal.

## Half-life

Elimination—Promethazine: 7 to 14 hours.

## Onset of action

Oral—
    15 to 60 minutes.
Parenteral—
    Promethazine:
        Intramuscular—20 minutes.
        Intravenous—3 to 5 minutes.
Rectal—
    Promethazine:
        20 minutes.

## Duration of action

Methdilazine—6 to 12 hours.
Promethazine—4 to 6 hours; may persist for up to 12 hours.
Trimeprazine—3 to 6 hours.

## Elimination

Renal. Most of the antihistamines studied are excreted as metabolites within 24 hours.

# Precautions to Consider

## Cross-sensitivity and/or related problems

Patients sensitive to other phenothiazines may be sensitive to methdilazine, promethazine, and trimeprazine also.

## Carcinogenicity/Tumorigenicity/Mutagenicity

Long-term animal studies to evaluate the carcinogenic, tumorigenic, or mutagenic potential of most antihistamines have not been performed.

## Pregnancy/Reproduction

Pregnancy—Phenothiazines have been reported to cause jaundice and extrapyramidal symptoms in infants whose mothers received these medications during pregnancy.

    *For promethazine—*
        Adequate and well-controlled studies in humans have not been done. However, promethazine taken within 2 weeks prior to delivery may inhibit platelet aggregation in the newborn.
        Studies in rats with doses 2.1 to 4.2 times the maximum recommended human daily dose have not shown that promethazine causes adverse effects on fetal development.

    FDA Pregnancy Category C.

## Breast-feeding

Small amounts of antihistamines may be distributed into breast milk; use is not recommended in nursing mothers because of the risk of adverse effects, such as unusual excitement or irritability, in infants.

Antihistamines may inhibit lactation because of their anticholinergic actions.

Some studies have indicated that the use of promethazine in children up to 2 years of age may be associated with the sudden infant death syndrome (SIDS) and an increase in sleep apnea, thus possibly increasing the risk to the nursing infant. Therefore, the use of phenothiazine-derivative antihistamines by nursing mothers should be discouraged until more studies have been performed to confirm the potential risk to the nursing infant.

## Pediatrics

Use is not recommended in newborn or premature infants because this age group has an increased susceptibility to anticholinergic side effects, such as central nervous system (CNS) excitation, and an increased tendency toward convulsions.

A paradoxical reaction characterized by hyperexcitability may occur in children taking antihistamines.

The use of phenothiazine-derivative antihistamines is not recommended in infants up to 3 months of age, because of the possible absence or deficiency of detoxifying enzyme and inefficient renal function usually noted in this age group. Also, increased susceptibility to dystonias has been reported in newborn or premature infants, acutely ill or dehydrated children, and children with acute infections who have received phenothiazine medication.

Some studies have associated the use of promethazine with sudden infant death syndrome (SIDS) and with an increase in infant sleep apnea. Until more studies have been performed to confirm this potential risk, phenothiazine derivatives should not be used in children up to 2 years of age.

In children with signs and symptoms suggestive of Reye's syndrome, phenothiazine-derivative antihistamines should not be used since the extrapyramidal symptoms that may occur, especially after parenteral administration of large doses, may be confused with the CNS signs of this syndrome, thus making diagnosis difficult.

## Adolescents

In adolescents with signs and symptoms suggestive of Reye's syndrome, phenothiazine-derivative antihistamines should not be used since the extrapyramidal symptoms that may occur, especially after parenteral administration of large doses, may be confused with the CNS signs of this syndrome, thus making diagnosis difficult.

## Geriatrics

Dizziness, sedation, confusion, and hypotension may be more likely to occur in geriatric patients taking antihistamines.

A paradoxical reaction characterized by hyperexcitability may occur in geriatric patients taking antihistamines.

Geriatric patients are especially susceptible to the anticholinergic side effects, such as dryness of the mouth and urinary retention (especially in males), of the antihistamines. If these side effects occur and continue or are severe, the medication should probably be discontinued.

Extrapyramidal signs, especially parkinsonism, akathisia, and persistent dyskinesia, may also be more likely to occur in geriatric patients, especially at the higher doses or with parenteral administration.

## Dental

Prolonged use of antihistamines may decrease or inhibit salivary flow, especially in middle-aged or elderly patients, thus contributing to the development of caries, periodontal disease, oral candidiasis, and discomfort.

Involuntary orofacial muscle movement may result from extrapyramidal effects. These involuntary movements may result in occlusal adjustments, bite registrations, and treatment for bruxism being less reliable.

## Drug interactions and/or related problems

The following drug interactions and/or related problems have been selected on the basis of their potential clinical significance (possible mechanism in parentheses where appropriate)—not necessarily inclusive ($»$ = major clinical significance):

Note: Combination products containing any of the following medications, depending on the amount present, may also interact with this medication.

$»$   Alcohol or

$»$   CNS depression–producing medications, other (See *Appendix II*) (concurrent use may potentiate the CNS depressant effects of either these medications or antihistamines; also, concurrent use of maprotiline or tricyclic antidepressants may potentiate the anticholinergic effects of either antihistamines or these medications)

Amphetamines
(concurrent use may decrease stimulant effects of amphetamines since phenothiazine derivatives produce alpha-adrenergic blockade)

» Anticholinergics or other medications with anticholinergic activity (See *Appendix II*)
(anticholinergic effects may be potentiated when these medications are used concurrently with antihistamines; patients should be advised to report occurrence of gastrointestinal problems promptly since paralytic ileus may occur with concurrent therapy)

Anticonvulsants, including barbiturates
(phenothiazine derivatives may lower the convulsion threshold; dosage adjustment of anticonvulsant medications may be necessary; potentiation of anticonvulsant effects does not occur)

Appetite suppressants
(concurrent use with phenothiazine derivatives may antagonize the anorectic effect of appetite suppressants)

Beta-adrenergic blocking agents, especially propranolol
(concurrent use with phenothiazine derivatives may result in increased plasma concentration of each medication because of inhibition of metabolism; this may result in additive hypotensive effects, irreversible retinopathy, cardiac arrhythmias, and tardive dyskinesia)

Bromocriptine
(concurrent use may increase serum prolactin concentrations and interfere with effects of bromocriptine; dosage adjustments of bromocriptine may be necessary)

Dopamine
(concurrent use may antagonize peripheral vasoconstriction produced by high doses of dopamine because of the alpha-adrenergic blocking action of phenothiazine derivatives)

Ephedrine or
Metaraminol or
Methoxamine
(alpha-adrenergic blocking action of phenothiazine derivatives may decrease the pressor response to these medications when used concurrently)

» Epinephrine
(alpha-adrenergic effects of epinephrine may be blocked when it is used concurrently with phenothiazine derivatives, possibly resulting in severe hypotension and tachycardia)

» Extrapyramidal reaction–causing medications, other (See *Appendix II*)
(concurrent use with phenothiazine derivatives may increase the severity and frequency of extrapyramidal effects)

Guanadrel or
Guanethidine
(neuronal uptake of these medications may be inhibited when they are used concurrently with phenothiazine derivatives, causing a decrease of their antihypertensive effect)

Hepatotoxic medications, other (See *Appendix II*)
(concurrent use of phenothiazine derivatives with other hepatotoxic medications may increase the potential for hepatotoxicity; patients, especially those on prolonged therapy or with a history of liver disease, should be carefully monitored)

Hypotension-producing medications, other (See *Appendix II*)
(concurrent use with phenothiazine derivatives may produce additive hypotensive effects)

» Levodopa
(antiparkinsonian effects of levodopa may be inhibited when used concurrently with phenothiazine derivatives because of blockade of dopamine receptors in the brain; levodopa has not been shown to be effective in phenothiazine-induced parkinsonism)

» Metrizamide, intrathecal
(concurrent use with phenothiazine derivatives may lower the seizure threshold; phenothiazine derivatives should be discontinued at least 48 hours before, and not resumed for at least 24 hours following, myelography)

» Monoamine oxidase (MAO) inhibitors, including furazolidone, procarbazine, and selegiline
(concurrent use of MAO inhibitors with antihistamines in general may prolong and intensify the anticholinergic and CNS depressant effects of antihistamines; concurrent use of MAO inhibitors with phenothiazine-derivative antihistamines may increase the risk of hypotension and extrapyramidal reactions; concurrent use is not recommended)

Ototoxic medications (See *Appendix II*)
(concurrent use with antihistamines may mask the symptoms of ototoxicity such as tinnitus, dizziness, or vertigo)

Quinidine
(concurrent use with phenothiazine-derivative antihistamines may result in additive cardiac effects)

Riboflavin
(requirements for riboflavin may be increased in patients receiving phenothiazine-derivative antihistamines)

**Laboratory value alterations**
The following have been selected on the basis of their potential clinical significance (possible effect in parentheses where appropriate)—not necessarily inclusive (» = major clinical significance):

With diagnostic test results
Glucose tolerance test
(an increase in glucose tolerance has been reported in patients receiving phenothiazine-derivative antihistamines)

Immunologic urine pregnancy tests
(may produce false-positive or false-negative results in patients receiving phenothiazine-derivative antihistamines, depending on the test used)

Skin tests using allergen extracts
(antihistamines may inhibit the cutaneous histamine response, thus producing false-negative results; it is recommended that antihistamines be discontinued at least 72 hours before testing begins)

**Medical considerations/Contraindications**
The medical considerations/contraindications included here have been selected on the basis of their potential clinical significance (reasons given in parentheses where appropriate)—not necessarily inclusive (» = major clinical significance).

*Risk-benefit should be considered when the following medical problems exist:*

» Bladder neck obstruction or
» Prostatic hypertrophy, symptomatic or
» Urinary retention, predisposition to
(anticholinergic effects may precipitate or aggravate urinary retention)

Bone marrow depression
(increased risk of leukopenia and agranulocytosis)

Cardiovascular disease
(increased risk of transient hypotension)

» Coma
(may be exacerbated)

Epilepsy
(parenteral administration of promethazine may increase severity of seizures)

» Glaucoma, angle-closure or predisposition to
(mydriatic effect resulting in increased intraocular pressure may precipitate an attack of angle-closure glaucoma)

Glaucoma, open-angle
(mydriatic effect may cause a slight increase in intraocular pressure; glaucoma therapy may need to be adjusted)

Hepatic function impairment
(metabolism may be decreased; higher serum concentrations may increase sensitivity to CNS effects)

» Jaundice
(may be exacerbated with parenteral administration of promethazine)

Reye's syndrome
(extrapyramidal symptoms that may be produced by parenteral administration of promethazine may be confused with CNS signs of Reye's syndrome)

Sensitivity to the antihistamine used

Caution is recommended when phenothiazine-derivative antihistamines are used, since their antiemetic action may impede diagnosis of such conditions as appendicitis and obscure signs of toxicity from overdosage of other drugs.

# Side/Adverse Effects

The following side/adverse effects have been selected on the basis of their potential clinical significance (possible signs and symptoms in parentheses where appropriate)—not necessarily inclusive:

**Those indicating need for medical attention**
Incidence less frequent or rare
*Blood dyscrasias* (sore throat; fever; unusual bleeding or bruising; unusual tiredness or weakness)

**Those indicating need for medical attention only if they continue or are bothersome**
Incidence more frequent
*Drowsiness; thickening of mucus*

Note: Sedative effects are more pronounced with promethazine and less pronounced with trimeprazine and methdilazine, in that order.

Incidence less frequent or rare

*Blurred vision or any change in vision; burning or stinging of rectum*—for promethazine rectal dosage form only; *confusion; difficult or painful urination; dizziness; dryness of mouth, nose, or throat; hypotension* (feeling faint); *increased sweating; loss of appetite; paradoxical reaction* (nightmares; unusual excitement, nervousness, restlessness, or irritability); *photosensitivity* (increased sensitivity of skin to sun); *ringing or buzzing in ears; skin rash; tachycardia* (fast heartbeat)

Note: *Confusion; difficult or painful urination; dizziness; drowsiness; and dryness of mouth, nose, or throat* are more likely to occur in the elderly.

*Nightmares, unusual excitement, nervousness, restlessness, or irritability* are more likely to occur in children and elderly patients.

## Overdose

For specific information on the agents used in the management of phenothiazine-derivative antihistamines overdose, see:

• *Antidyskinetics (Systemic)* monograph;
• *Antihistamines (Systemic)* monograph;
• *Barbiturates (Systemic)* monograph; and/or
• *Ipecac (Oral-local)* monograph.

For more information on the management of overdose or unintentional ingestion, **contact a Poison Control Center** (see *Poison Control Center Listing*).

### Clinical effects of overdose

The following effects have been selected on the basis of their potential clinical significance (possible signs and symptoms in parentheses where appropriate)—not necessarily inclusive:

Acute and chronic

*Anticholinergic effects* (clumsiness or unsteadiness; severe drowsiness; severe dryness of mouth, nose, or throat; flushing or redness of face; shortness of breath or troubled breathing); *CNS depression* (severe drowsiness); *CNS stimulation* (hallucinations; seizures; trouble in sleeping); *extrapyramidal effects* (muscle spasms, especially of neck and back; restlessness; shuffling walk; tic-like [jerky] movements of head and face; trembling and shaking of hands); *hypotension, severe* (feeling faint)

Note: *Anticholinergic* and *CNS stimulant* effects are more likely to occur in children with overdose. *Hypotension* may also occur in the elderly at usual doses.

### Treatment of overdose

Since there is no specific antidote for overdose with antihistamines, treatment is symptomatic and supportive with possible utilization of the following:

To decrease absorption—

Induction of emesis (syrup of ipecac recommended); however, precaution against aspiration is necessary, especially in infants and children.

Gastric lavage (isotonic or 0.45% sodium chloride solution) if patient is unable to vomit within 3 hours of ingestion.

To enhance elimination—

Saline cathartics (milk of magnesia) are sometimes used.

Specific treatment—

Vasopressors to treat hypotension; however, epinephrine should not be used since it may further lower blood pressure.

Anticholinergic antiparkinson agents, diphenhydramine, or barbiturates, to control extrapyramidal reactions.

Precaution against use of stimulants (analeptic agents) because they may cause seizures.

Supportive care—

Oxygen and intravenous fluids.

## Patient Consultation

As an aid to patient consultation, refer to *Advice for the Patient, Antihistamines, Phenothiazine-derivative (Systemic).*

In providing consultation, consider emphasizing the following selected information (» = major clinical significance):

### Before using this medication

» Conditions affecting use, especially:

Sensitivity to the antihistamine used or to phenothiazine medications

Pregnancy—Not taking during the 2 weeks before delivery, to avoid possible inhibition of platelet aggregation in newborn; also, jaundice and extrapyramidal effects may occur in infant

Breast-feeding—Use not recommended; may cause unusual excitement or irritability in nursing infant; possible association with sudden infant death syndrome (SIDS) and sleep apnea

Use in children—Increased susceptibility to anticholinergic side effects in newborn or premature infants; hyperexcitability (paradoxical reaction) may occur in children; possible association with sudden infant death syndrome (SIDS) and sleep apnea; diagnosis of Reye's syndrome may be obscured if extrapyramidal effects occur

Use in adolescents—Diagnosis of Reye's syndrome may be obscured if extrapyramidal effects occur

Use in the elderly—Increased susceptibility to CNS and anticholinergic side effects; hyperexcitability (paradoxical reaction) may occur; extrapyramidal symptoms more likely to occur

Dental—Increased risk of dental problems with prolonged use because of decrease or inhibition of salivary flow; involuntary orofacial muscle movements may result from extrapyramidal effects

Other medications, especially alcohol or other CNS depressants, anticholinergics, epinephrine, extrapyramidal reaction–causing medications, levodopa, MAO inhibitors, or metrizamide (intrathecal)

Other medical problems, especially angle-closure glaucoma (or predisposition to), bladder neck obstruction, prostatic hypertrophy, or urinary retention; jaundice (for parenteral promethazine)

### Proper use of this medication

» Importance of not taking more medication than the amount recommended

» Proper dosing

Missed dose: If on scheduled dosing regimen—Using as soon as possible; not using if almost time for next dose; not doubling doses

» Proper storage

*For oral dosage forms*

Taking with food, water, or milk to minimize gastric irritation

Swallowing extended-release dosage forms whole

*For injection dosage forms*

Knowing correct administration technique for self-administration; checking with physician if necessary

*For rectal dosage forms*

Proper administration technique

*For promethazine when used to prevent motion sickness*

Taking 30 minutes to 1 hour before traveling

### Precautions while using this medication

Possible interference with skin tests using allergens; need to inform physician of using medication

May mask ototoxic effects of large doses of salicylates

» Avoiding use of alcohol or other CNS depressants

» Caution if drowsiness occurs

Possible dryness of mouth; using sugarless gum or candy, ice, or saliva substitute for relief; checking with physician or dentist if dry mouth continues for more than 2 weeks

Need to inform physician of use: Possible interference with diagnosis of appendicitis; may mask signs of toxicity from overdosage of other drugs

### Side/adverse effects

Signs of potential side effects, especially blood dyscrasias

## General Dosing Information

### For oral dosage forms only

Most antihistamines may be taken with food, water, or milk to lessen gastric irritation.

### For parenteral dosage forms only

For promethazine—

The preferred route of administration is by deep intramuscular injection. Although intravenous administration is well tolerated, promethazine should not be administered in concentrations greater than 25 mg per mL and at a rate in excess of 25 mg per minute. Rapid intravenous administration of promethazine may produce a transient fall in blood pressure.

Intra-arterial administration is not recommended because of the possibility of severe arteriospasm and resultant gangrene; also, subcutaneous administration is not recommended, since chemical irritation has been noted and necrotic lesions have resulted on rare occasions.

## METHDILAZINE

## Summary of Differences

Indications: Used in the treatment of pruritus associated with pityriasis rosea.

Pharmacology/pharmacokinetics: Duration of action—6 to 12 hours.

Side/adverse effects: Least sedative effects.

## Oral Dosage Forms

### METHDILAZINE HYDROCHLORIDE SYRUP USP

**Usual adult and adolescent dose**
Antihistaminic (H₁-receptor)—
Oral, 8 mg every six to twelve hours as needed.

**Usual pediatric dose**
Antihistaminic (H₁-receptor)—
Children up to 3 years of age: Use is not recommended.
Children 3 to 12 years of age: Oral, 4 mg every six to twelve hours as needed.

**Usual geriatric dose**
See *Usual adult and adolescent dose.*

Note: Geriatric patients may be more sensitive to the effects of the usual adult dose.

**Strength(s) usually available**
U.S.—
4 mg per 5 mL (Rx) [*Tacaryl* (alcohol 7.37%)].
Canada—
Not commercially available.

**Packaging and storage**
Store below 40 °C (104 °F), preferably between 15 and 30 °C (59 and 86 °F), unless otherwise specified by manufacturer. Store in a tight, light-resistant container. Protect from freezing.

**Auxiliary labeling**
• May cause drowsiness.
• Avoid alcoholic beverages.

### METHDILAZINE HYDROCHLORIDE TABLETS USP

**Usual adult and adolescent dose**
See *Methdilazine Hydrochloride Syrup USP.*

**Usual pediatric dose**
See *Methdilazine Hydrochloride Syrup USP.*

**Usual geriatric dose**
See *Usual adult and adolescent dose.*

Note: Geriatric patients may be more sensitive to the effects of the usual adult dose.

**Strength(s) usually available**
U.S.—
8 mg (Rx) [*Tacaryl* (scored)].
Canada—
Not commercially available.

**Packaging and storage**
Store below 40 °C (104 °F), preferably between 15 and 30 °C (59 and 86 °F), unless otherwise specified by manufacturer. Store in a tight, light-resistant container.

**Auxiliary labeling**
• May cause drowsiness.
• Avoid alcoholic beverages.

### METHDILAZINE HYDROCHLORIDE TABLETS (CHEWABLE) USP

**Usual adult and adolescent dose**
See *Methdilazine Hydrochloride Syrup USP.*

**Usual pediatric dose**
See *Methdilazine Hydrochloride Syrup USP.*

**Usual geriatric dose**
See *Usual adult and adolescent dose.*

Note: Geriatric patients may be more sensitive to the effects of the usual adult dose.

**Strength(s) usually available**
U.S.—
4 mg (Rx) [*Tacaryl*].
Canada—
Not commercially available.

**Packaging and storage**
Store below 40 °C (104 °F), preferably between 15 and 30 °C (59 and 86 °F), unless otherwise specified by manufacturer. Store in a tight, light-resistant container.

**Auxiliary labeling**
• May cause drowsiness.
• Avoid alcoholic beverages.

## PROMETHAZINE

## Summary of Differences

Pharmacology/pharmacokinetics: Duration of action—Usually 4 to 6 hours.

Precautions: Medical considerations/contraindications—Caution needed in epilepsy, jaundice, and Reye's syndrome (with parenteral administration).

Side/adverse effects: Most pronounced sedative effects.

## Oral Dosage Forms

### PROMETHAZINE HYDROCHLORIDE SYRUP USP

**Usual adult and adolescent dose**
Antihistaminic (H₁-receptor)—
Oral, 10 to 12.5 mg four times a day before meals and at bedtime; or 25 mg at bedtime as needed.
Antiemetic—
Oral, 25 mg initially, then 10 to 25 mg every four to six hours as needed.
Antivertigo agent—
Oral, 25 mg two times a day as needed.

Note: For motion sickness, the initial 25-mg dose should be taken one-half to one hour before travel, and the dose repeated eight to twelve hours later, if necessary.

Sedative-hypnotic—
Oral, 25 to 50 mg for nighttime, presurgical, postsurgical, or obstetrical sedation.

Note: A 50-mg dose (with an equal amount of meperidine and an appropriate dose of an atropine-like drug) is used the night before surgery to relieve apprehension and produce sleep.

**Usual adult prescribing limits**
Up to 150 mg daily.

**Usual pediatric dose**
Children up to 2 years of age:
Use is not recommended.
Children 2 years of age and older:
Antihistaminic (H₁-receptor)—
Oral, 125 mcg (0.125 mg) per kg of body weight or 3.75 mg per square meter of body surface every four to six hours, or 500 mcg per kg of body weight or 15 mg per square meter of body surface at bedtime as needed; or 5 to 12.5 mg three times a day or 25 mg at bedtime as needed.
Antiemetic—
Oral, 250 to 500 mcg (0.25 to 0.5 mg) per kg of body weight or 7.5 to 15 mg per square meter of body surface every four to six hours as needed; or 10 to 25 mg every four to six hours as needed.
Antivertigo agent—
Oral, 500 mcg (0.5 mg) per kg of body weight or 15 mg per square meter of body surface every twelve hours as needed; or 10 to 25 mg two times a day as needed.
Sedative-hypnotic—
Oral, 500 mcg (0.5 mg) to 1 mg per kg of body weight or 15 to 30 mg per square meter of body surface as needed; or 10 to 25 mg as needed.

Note: For preoperative sedation, children require doses of 1.1 mg per kg of body weight in combination with an equal dose of meperidine and the appropriate dose of an atropine-like drug.

For postoperative sedation, 10 to 25 mg may be used.

**Usual geriatric dose**
See *Usual adult and adolescent dose.*

Note: Geriatric patients may be more sensitive to the effects of the usual adult dose.

---

**Packaging and storage**
Store below 40 °C (104 °F), preferably between 15 and 30 °C (59 and 86 °F), unless otherwise specified by manufacturer. Store in a tight, light-resistant container.

**Auxiliary labeling**
• May cause drowsiness.
• Avoid alcoholic beverages.

## Strength(s) usually available
U.S.—

6.25 mg per 5 mL (Rx) [*Pentazine; Phenergan Plain* (alcohol 7%); *Prothazine Plain* (alcohol 7%); GENERIC].

25 mg per 5 mL (Rx) [*Phenergan Fortis* (alcohol 1.5%); GENERIC].

Canada—

10 mg per 5 mL (OTC) [*Phenergan* (alcohol 3%)].

## Packaging and storage
Store below 40 °C (104 °F), preferably between 15 and 30 °C (59 and 86 °F), unless otherwise specified by manufacturer. Store in a tight, light-resistant container. Protect from freezing.

## Auxiliary labeling
• May cause drowsiness.
• Avoid alcoholic beverages.

# PROMETHAZINE HYDROCHLORIDE TABLETS USP

## Usual adult and adolescent dose
See *Promethazine Hydrochloride Syrup USP.*

## Usual adult prescribing limits
Up to 150 mg daily.

## Usual pediatric dose
See *Promethazine Hydrochloride Syrup USP.*

## Usual geriatric dose
See *Usual adult and adolescent dose.*

Note: Geriatric patients may be more sensitive to the effects of the usual adult dose.

## Strength(s) usually available
U.S.—

12.5 mg (Rx) [*Phenergan* (scored); GENERIC].

25 mg (Rx) [*Phenergan* (scored); *Promacot;* GENERIC].

50 mg (Rx) [*Phenergan;* GENERIC].

Canada—

10 mg (OTC) [*Phenergan* (scored)].

25 mg (OTC) [*Histantil* (film coated); *Phenergan* (film coated)].

50 mg (OTC) [*Histantil* (film coated); *Phenergan* (scored)].

## Packaging and storage
Store below 40 °C (104 °F), preferably between 15 and 30 °C (59 and 86 °F), unless otherwise specified by manufacturer. Store in a tight, light-resistant container.

## Auxiliary labeling
• May cause drowsiness.
• Avoid alcoholic beverages.

# Parenteral Dosage Forms
## PROMETHAZINE HYDROCHLORIDE INJECTION USP

## Usual adult and adolescent dose
Antihistaminic (H₁-receptor)—

Intramuscular or intravenous, 25 mg; may be repeated within two hours if necessary.

Antiemetic—

Intramuscular or intravenous, 12.5 to 25 mg every four hours as needed.

Sedative-hypnotic—

Intramuscular or intravenous, 25 to 50 mg for nighttime, presurgical, postsurgical, or obstetrical sedation.

Note: For preoperative and postoperative sedation, 25 to 50 mg of promethazine may be combined with appropriately reduced doses of analgesics and anticholinergics.

For obstetrical sedation, in the early stages of labor, 50 mg of promethazine will provide sedation and relief of apprehension. After labor is definitely established, 25 to 75 mg of promethazine may be administered with an appropriately reduced dose of an opioid analgesic, and may be repeated once or twice every four hours during the course of a normal labor.

## Usual adult prescribing limits
Up to 150 mg daily.

## Usual pediatric dose
Children up to 2 years of age:
Use is not recommended.
Children 2 years of age and older:
Antihistaminic (H₁-receptor)—

Intramuscular, 125 mcg (0.125 mg) per kg of body weight or 3.75 mg per square meter of body surface every four to six hours or 500 mcg (0.5 mg) per kg of body weight or 15 mg per square meter of body surface at bedtime as needed;

or 6.25 to 12.5 mg three times a day or 25 mg at bedtime as needed.

Antiemetic—

Intramuscular, 250 to 500 mcg (0.25 to 0.5 mg) per kg of body weight or 7.5 to 15 mg per square meter of body surface every four to six hours as needed; or 12.5 to 25 mg every four to six hours as needed.

Sedative-hypnotic—

Intramuscular, 500 mcg (0.5 mg) to 1 mg per kg of body weight as needed; or 12.5 to 25 mg as needed.

Note: For preoperative sedation, children require doses of 1.1 mg per kg of body weight in combination with an equal dose of meperidine and the appropriate dose of an atropine-like drug.

For postoperative sedation, 12.5 to 25 mg may be used.

## Usual geriatric dose
See *Usual adult and adolescent dose.*

Note: Geriatric patients may be more sensitive to the effects of the usual adult dose.

## Strength(s) usually available
U.S.—

25 mg per mL (Rx) [*Anergan 25; Phenazine 25; Phenergan; Prorex-25; Prothazine; Shogan; V-Gan-25;* GENERIC].

50 mg per mL (Rx) [*Anergan 50; Antinaus 50; Pentazine; Phenazine 50; Phencen-50; Phenergan; Phenerzine; Phenoject-50; Pro-50; Promacot; Pro-Med 50; Promet; Prorex-50; Prothazine; Shogan; V-Gan-50;* GENERIC].

Canada—

25 mg (base) per mL (Rx) [*Phenergan;* GENERIC].

## Packaging and storage
Store below 40 °C (104 °F), preferably between 15 and 30 °C (59 and 86 °F), unless otherwise specified by manufacturer. Protect from light. Protect from freezing.

## Stability
Do not use if discolored or if a precipitate is present.

# Rectal Dosage Forms
## PROMETHAZINE HYDROCHLORIDE SUPPOSITORIES USP

## Usual adult and adolescent dose
Antihistaminic (H₁-receptor)—

Rectal, 25 mg; may be repeated in two hours if necessary.

Antiemetic—

Rectal, 25 mg initially, then 12.5 to 25 mg every four to six hours as needed.

Antivertigo agent—

Rectal, 25 mg two times a day as needed.

Sedative-hypnotic—

Rectal, 25 to 50 mg for nighttime, presurgical, postsurgical, or obstetrical sedation.

Note: A 50-mg dose (with an equal amount of meperidine and an appropriate dose of an atropine-like drug) is used the night before surgery to relieve apprehension and produce sleep.

## Usual adult prescribing limits
Up to 150 mg daily.

## Usual pediatric dose
Children up to 2 years of age:
Use is not recommended.
Children 2 years of age and older:
Antihistaminic (H₁-receptor)—

Rectal, 125 mcg (0.125 mg) per kg of body weight or 3.75 mg per square meter of body surface every four to six hours, or 500 mcg (0.5 mg) per kg of body weight or 15 mg per square meter of body surface at bedtime as needed; or 6.25 to 12.5 mg three times a day or 25 mg at bedtime as needed.

Antiemetic—

Rectal, 250 to 500 mcg (0.25 to 0.5 mg) per kg of body weight or 7.5 to 15 mg per square meter of body surface every four to six hours as needed; or 12.5 to 25 mg every four to six hours as needed.

Antivertigo agent—

Rectal, 500 mcg (0.5 mg) per kg of body weight or 15 mg per square meter of body surface every twelve hours as needed; or 12.5 to 25 mg two times a day as needed.

Sedative-hypnotic—
Rectal, 500 mcg (0.5 mg) to 1 mg per kg of body weight or 15 to 30 mg per square meter of body surface as needed; or 12.5 to 25 mg as needed.

Note: For preoperative sedation, children require doses of 1.1 mg per kg of body weight in combination with an equal dose of meperidine and the appropriate dose of an atropine-like drug.

For postoperative sedation, 12.5 to 25 mg may be used.

### Usual geriatric dose
See *Usual adult and adolescent dose.*

Note: Geriatric patients may be more sensitive to the effects of the usual adult dose.

### Strength(s) usually available
U.S.—

12.5 mg (Rx) [*Phenergan*].

25 mg (Rx) [*Phenergan*].

50 mg (Rx) [*Phenergan*; GENERIC].

Canada—

Not commercially available.

### Packaging and storage
Store between 2 and 8 °C (36 and 46 °F), in a tight, light-resistant container, unless otherwise specified by manufacturer.

### Auxiliary labeling
• May cause drowsiness.
• Avoid alcoholic beverages.

### Note
Include patient instructions when dispensing.

Explain administration technique.

---

## *TRIMEPRAZINE*

## Summary of Differences

Pharmacology/pharmacokinetics: Duration of action—3 to 6 hours.

## Oral Dosage Forms

Note: The dosing and strengths of the dosage forms available are expressed in terms of trimeprazine base (not the tartrate salt).

### TRIMEPRAZINE TARTRATE EXTENDED-RELEASE CAPSULES

#### Usual adult and adolescent dose
Antihistaminic (H₁-receptor)—

Oral, 5 mg (base) every twelve hours as needed.

#### Usual pediatric dose
Antihistaminic (H₁-receptor)—

Children up to 6 years of age: Use is not recommended.

Children 6 years of age and over: Oral, 5 mg (base) once a day as needed.

#### Usual geriatric dose
See *Usual adult and adolescent dose.*

Note: Geriatric patients may be more sensitive to the effects of the usual adult dose.

#### Strength(s) usually available
U.S.—

5 mg (base) (Rx) [*Temaril*].

Canada—

Not commercially available.

#### Packaging and storage
Store below 40 °C (104 °F), preferably between 15 and 30 °C (59 and 86 °F), in a well-closed container, unless otherwise specified by manufacturer.

#### Auxiliary labeling
• May cause drowsiness.
• Avoid alcoholic beverages.

### TRIMEPRAZINE TARTRATE SYRUP USP

#### Usual adult and adolescent dose
Antihistaminic (H₁-receptor)—

Oral, 2.5 mg (base) four times a day as needed.

#### Usual pediatric dose
Antihistaminic (H₁-receptor)—

Children up to 2 years of age: Use is not recommended.

Children 2 to 3 years of age: Oral, 1.25 mg (base) at bedtime or three times a day as needed.

Children 3 years of age and over: Oral, 2.5 mg (base) at bedtime or three times a day as needed.

#### Usual geriatric dose
See *Usual adult and adolescent dose.*

Note: Geriatric patients may be more sensitive to the effects of the usual adult dose.

#### Strength(s) usually available
U.S.—

2.5 mg (base) per 5 mL (Rx) [*Temaril* (alcohol 5.7%); GENERIC].

Canada—

2.5 mg (base) per 5 mL (Rx) [*Panectyl* (alcohol 0.6%)].

#### Packaging and storage
Store below 40 °C (104 °F), preferably between 15 and 30 °C (59 and 86 °F), unless otherwise specified by manufacturer. Store in a tight, light-resistant container. Protect from freezing.

#### Auxiliary labeling
• May cause drowsiness.
• Avoid alcoholic beverages.

### TRIMEPRAZINE TARTRATE TABLETS USP

#### Usual adult and adolescent dose
Antihistaminic (H₁-receptor)—

Oral, 2.5 mg (base) four times a day as needed.

#### Usual pediatric dose
Antihistaminic (H₁-receptor)—

Children up to 2 years of age: Use is not recommended.

Children 2 to 3 years of age: The available strength of the tablet may not conform to the recommended pediatric dosage. See *Trimeprazine Tartrate Syrup USP.*

Children 3 years of age and over: Oral, 2.5 mg (base) at bedtime or three times a day as needed.

#### Usual geriatric dose
See *Usual adult and adolescent dose.*

Note: Geriatric patients may be more sensitive to the effects of the usual adult dose.

#### Strength(s) usually available
U.S.—

2.5 mg (base) (Rx) [*Temaril*].

Canada—

2.5 mg (base) (Rx) [*Panectyl*].

5 mg (base) (Rx) [*Panectyl*].

#### Packaging and storage
Store below 40 °C (104 °F), preferably between 15 and 30 °C (59 and 86 °F), unless otherwise specified by manufacturer. Store in a well-closed, light-resistant container.

#### Auxiliary labeling
• May cause drowsiness.
• Avoid alcoholic beverages.

## Selected Bibliography

Simons FE, Simons KJ: H₁-receptor antagonist treatment of chronic rhinitis. J Allergy Clin Immunol 1988; 81: 975-80.

Simons FE, Simons KJ, Chung M, Yeh J. The comparative pharmacokinetics of H₁-receptor antagonists. Ann Allergy 1987 Dec; 59: 20-4.

Revised: 07/26/94

# ANTI-INFLAMMATORY DRUGS, NONSTEROIDAL Ophthalmic

This monograph includes information on the following: Diclofenac; Flurbiprofen; Indomethacin**; Suprofen†.

INN:
Indomethacin—Indometacin

VA CLASSIFICATION (Primary/Secondary):
Diclofenac—OP300/OP900
Flurbiprofen—OP900/OP300
Indomethacin—OP900/OP300
Suprofen—OP900

Another commonly used name for indomethacin is indometacin.

Note: For a listing of dosage forms and brand names by country availability, see *Dosage Forms* section(s). For a listing of brand names for the articles in this monograph, refer to the General Index.

*Not commercially available in the U.S.
†Not commercially available in Canada.

## Category

Prostaglandin synthesis inhibitor, ophthalmic—Diclofenac; Flurbiprofen; Indomethacin; Suprofen.

Anti-inflammatory, nonsteroidal, ophthalmic—Diclofenac; Flurbiprofen; Indomethacin.

Miosis inhibitor, in ophthalmic surgery—Diclofenac; Flurbiprofen; Indomethacin; Suprofen.

## Indications

Note: Bracketed information in the *Indications* section refers to uses that are not included in U.S. product labeling.

### Accepted

Inflammation, ocular (treatment)—Diclofenac is indicated to reduce postoperative inflammation following cataract surgery. [Diclofenac is also indicated in the treatment of conjunctivitis, keratoconjunctivitis, corneal ulcers, and post-traumatic inflammation of the cornea and conjunctiva, provided that these conditions are not associated with an ocular infection.] [Flurbiprofen] and indomethacin[1] are indicated to reduce inflammation of the anterior segment of the eye following ocular surgery or laser trabeculoplasty. However, flurbiprofen and indomethacin have produced inconsistent results in clinical studies and may not produce clinically significant reductions in post-procedure inflammation. In one study, these nonsteroidal anti-inflammatory drugs (NSAIDs) reduced conjunctival injection, but not the anterior chamber reaction, following argon laser trabeculoplasty.

Ophthalmic NSAIDs may be administered concurrently with an ophthalmic corticosteroid, if necessary. There is some evidence of a synergistic or additive effect when the 2 types of medication are used together.

Miosis, during ophthalmic surgery (prophylaxis)—[Diclofenac], flurbiprofen, indomethacin, and suprofen are indicated to inhibit intraoperative miosis, which may occur in response to surgical trauma despite preoperative establishment of mydriasis. These NSAIDs may facilitate cataract extraction and lens implantation. However, published clinical studies have shown small and variable effects on pupil size, and some investigators have reported flurbiprofen to be ineffective. Also, studies demonstrating that ophthalmic NSAIDs produce clinically significant inhibition of miosis in surgical procedures other than cataract surgery have not been published.

Use of ophthalmic NSAIDs to inhibit miosis during surgery does not eliminate the need for mydriatic agents prior to and during surgery.

Edema, cystoid macular, following cataract surgery (prophylaxis and treatment)—[Diclofenac] and indomethacin are indicated to reduce the occurrence and severity of cystoid macular edema following cataract surgery. These agents are usually used concurrently with an ophthalmic corticosteroid; clinical studies indicate that concurrent use of both types of medication provides a synergistic effect.

There is insufficient evidence to determine whether flurbiprofen or suprofen is effective in reducing cystoid macular edema following cataract surgery.

[1]Not included in Canadian product labeling.

## Pharmacology/Pharmacokinetics

### Physicochemical characteristics

Chemical group—
Anti-inflammatory drug, nonsteroidal (NSAID)—
Indoleacetic acid derivative—Indomethacin.
Phenylacetic acid derivative—Diclofenac.
Propionic acid derivatives—Flurbiprofen, suprofen.

Molecular weight—
Diclofenac sodium: 318.13.
Flurbiprofen sodium: 302.28.
Indomethacin: 357.79.
Suprofen: 260.31.

### Mechanism of action/Effect

Ophthalmic NSAIDs inhibit the activity of the enzyme cyclo-oxygenase in ocular tissues, resulting in decreased formation of precursors of prostaglandins from arachidonic acid and subsequent inhibition of prostaglandin synthesis. These medications do not inhibit the actions of prostaglandins. Studies in animals have shown that trauma to the anterior segment of the eye, especially the iris, increases endogenous prostaglandin synthesis; that endogenous prostaglandins produce constriction of the iris sphincter independently of cholinergic mechanisms; and that endogenous prostaglandins may contribute to the development of intraocular inflammation by causing disruption of the blood–aqueous humor barrier, vasodilatation, increased vascular permeability, and leukocytosis. It is proposed that inhibition of prostaglandin synthesis in ocular tissues by ophthalmic NSAIDs decreases these effects, thereby reducing the severity of intraoperative miosis, signs and symptoms of postoperative inflammation, and postoperative cystoid macular edema (which may occur, independently of inflammation, because of prostaglandin-induced alterations in vascular permeability). Diclofenac and indomethacin have been shown to stabilize, or speed postoperative re-establishment of, the blood–aqueous humor barrier. However, the clinical consequences (benefit or harm) of this action in the treatment of postoperative inflammation have not been determined. Also, studies of flurbiprofen's or indomethacin's efficacy in reducing ocular inflammation following ophthalmic procedures have produced conflicting results. It is proposed that the anti-inflammatory activity of these medications may be limited, possibly because they do not inhibit the formation or activity of mediators of inflammation in the eye other than prostaglandins.

### Other actions/effects

Clinical studies indicate that perioperative use of ophthalmic NSAIDs does not significantly affect intraocular pressure.

Ophthalmic NSAIDs may increase the risk of bleeding in ocular tissues following ophthalmic procedures; postoperative bleeding, including hyphema, has been documented with flurbiprofen.

Studies in animals have shown that ophthalmic flurbiprofen may delay wound healing following certain types of surgery. Diclofenac may also slow or delay healing postoperatively. However, ophthalmic suprofen did not delay wound healing in a study in animals.

The anti-inflammatory activity of ophthalmic NSAIDs may mask the onset and/or progression of ocular infections.

### Absorption

Diclofenac—Studies suggest that limited, if any, systemic absorption occurs after a single application of up to 16 drops of a 0.1% solution.

Flurbiprofen—Flurbiprofen penetrates the cornea; significant systemic absorption may occur. In one study, 74% of the quantity of flurbiprofen applied to the conjunctiva appeared in the systemic circulation.

Indomethacin—The medication has not been detected in serum after ophthalmic administration. However, the possibility of significant systemic absorption must be considered, because a bronchospastic reaction has been reported in one asthmatic patient following ophthalmic administration of the medication.

Suprofen—No data regarding the extent of systemic absorption following ophthalmic application are available.

## Precautions to Consider

### Cross-sensitivity and/or related problems

Patients sensitive to aspirin or other systemically administered nonsteroidal anti-inflammatory drugs (NSAIDs) may be sensitive to ophthalmic NSAIDs also.

### Carcinogenicity

*Diclofenac*—No evidence of carcinogenicity was found in long-term studies in rats or mice receiving up to 2 mg per kg of body weight (mg/kg) per day orally.

*Flurbiprofen*—No evidence of carcinogenicity was found in a 24-month study in rats receiving up to 4 mg/kg per day, a second 24-month study in rats receiving 12 mg/kg per day for 32 weeks followed by 5 mg/kg per day thereafter, or an 80-week study in mice receiving up to 12 mg/kg per day orally.

*Indomethacin*—No evidence of carcinogenicity was found in long-term studies in rats or mice receiving up to 1.5 mg/kg per day orally.

*Suprofen*—No evidence of carcinogenicity was found in long-term studies in rats or mice receiving up to 40 mg/kg per day orally.

**Tumorigenicity**

*Diclofenac*—A slight increase in the occurrence of benign mammary fibroadenomas was found in female rats, but the increase was not significant for this common rat tumor. No other evidence of tumorigenicity was found in rats receiving up to 2 mg/kg per day orally.

*Flurbiprofen*—No evidence of tumorigenicity was found in a 2-year study in rats receiving up to 12 mg/kg per day for 32 weeks, followed by up to 5 mg/kg per day orally for the remainder of the study period.

*Indomethacin*—No evidence of tumorigenicity was found in an 81-week study in rats receiving up to 1 mg/kg per day orally.

*Suprofen*—An increased incidence of benign hepatomas occurred in female mice receiving 40 mg/kg per day and in male mice receiving 2 mg/kg per day or more orally.

**Mutagenicity**

*Diclofenac*—No mutagenic activity was found in *in vitro* tests using mammalian cells or bacteria (with or without microsomal activation) or in various *in vivo* tests.

*Flurbiprofen*—Long-term mutagenicity studies have not been performed.

*Indomethacin*—No mutagenic activity was found in *in vitro* tests (Ames test or *E. coli*, with or without metabolic activation) or in *in vivo* tests (host-mediated assay, sex-linked recessive lethals in *Drosophila*, and micronucleus test in mice).

*Suprofen*—No mutagenic activity was found in the Ames, micronucleus, and dominant lethal tests.

**Pregnancy/Reproduction**

Fertility—*Diclofenac*: No impairment of fertility was found in reproduction studies in rats receiving up to 4 mg/kg per day orally.

*Flurbiprofen*: No impairment of fertility was found in reproduction studies in rats receiving up to 4 mg/kg per day orally.

*Indomethacin*: No impairment of fertility was found in a 2-generation reproduction study in rats or in a 2-litter reproduction study in rats receiving up to 0.5 mg/kg per day orally.

*Suprofen*: No impairment of fertility was found in reproduction studies in rats receiving up to 40 mg/kg per day. However, a slight reduction in fertility was found in rats receiving 80 mg/kg per day orally. Testicular atrophy and hypoplasia occurred in a 6-month study in dogs receiving 80 mg/kg per day and a 12-month study in rats receiving 40 mg/kg per day orally.

Pregnancy—Adequate and well-controlled studies with ophthalmic NSAIDs have not been performed in pregnant women. However, use of ophthalmic NSAIDs late in pregnancy is not recommended, because oral NSAIDs caused premature closure of the ductus arteriosus in animal studies.

*First trimester*—

Diclofenac:

Diclofenac readily crosses the placenta.

No teratogenicity occurred in reproduction studies in mice receiving up to 20 mg/kg per day orally and in rats and rabbits receiving up to 10 mg/kg per day orally. However, maternal toxicity and embryotoxicity (reduced fetal weights and growth, reduced fetal survival) occurred in studies in rats receiving 2 or 4 mg/kg per day. Also, increases in resorption rates, decreased fetal weight, abnormal skeletal findings, and definite embryotoxicity occurred in studies in rabbits receiving 5 or 10 mg/kg per day orally.

FDA Pregnancy Category B.

Flurbiprofen:

Flurbiprofen crosses the placenta.

No teratogenicity occurred in reproduction studies in mice receiving up to 12 mg/kg per day, rats receiving up to 25 mg/kg per day, or rabbits receiving up to 7.5 mg/kg per day, orally. However, studies in rats have shown doses of 0.4 mg/kg per day or higher to be embryotoxic or embryocidal (causing reduced weight or slower fetal growth, increased stillbirths, and decreased pup survival). Also, stillbirths, retained fetuses, and/or fetal distress occurred in studies in rats receiving as little as 0.2 mg/kg per day. In addition, fetotoxicity related to maternal toxicity (gastrointestinal ulceration, retardation of weight gain, intrauterine hemorrhage, and maternal deaths) occurred in rats receiving 25 mg/kg per day from Days 1 through 20 of pregnancy.

With lower doses (0.2, 0.675, or 2.25 mg/kg per day), such effects did not occur when the medication was discontinued on Day 17 of pregnancy. Maternal deaths due to gastrointestinal ulceration also occurred in rabbits receiving the medication.

FDA Pregnancy Category C.

Indomethacin:

Indomethacin crosses the placenta.

Studies in rats and mice have shown that indomethacin in doses of 4 mg/kg per day orally causes retarded ossification secondary to decreased average fetal weight. In other studies in mice, higher doses (5 to 15 mg/kg per day orally) caused maternal toxicity and death, increased fetal resorptions, and fetal malformations. Doses lower than 4 mg/kg per day produced no adverse effects in these studies.

Suprofen:

Studies in rats receiving 40 mg/kg or more per day, and rabbits receiving 80 mg/kg or more per day, orally have shown that suprofen causes an increased incidence of fetal resorption associated with maternal toxicity. In rats receiving 2.5 mg/kg or more per day orally, there was an increase in stillbirths and a decrease in pup survival.

FDA Pregnancy Category C.

*Third trimester:*—

Diclofenac:

Studies in animals have shown that maternally toxic doses, administered orally, are associated with prolonged gestation and dystocia.

Flurbiprofen:

Studies in rats have shown that administration of 0.4 mg/kg or more per day orally causes prolonged gestation and delayed parturition.

Indomethacin:

Studies in rats and mice have shown that administration of 4 mg/kg per day orally during the last 3 days of gestation is associated with an increased incidence of neuronal necrosis in the diencephalon and some maternal and fetal deaths. Indomethacin also caused a slight delay in the onset of parturition in rats, but not in rabbits.

Suprofen:

Studies in rats have shown that suprofen causes a delay in parturition.

**Breast-feeding**

Although it is not known whether NSAIDs are distributed into breast milk after ophthalmic administration, it is known that orally administered diclofenac, indomethacin, and suprofen are distributed into human breast milk. It is not known whether orally administered flurbiprofen is distributed into breast milk. However, problems in humans have not been documented with any of these medications.

**Pediatrics**

Appropriate studies on the relationship of age to the effects of ophthalmic NSAIDs have not been performed in the pediatric population. Safety and efficacy have not been established.

**Geriatrics**

Studies performed to date have not demonstrated geriatrics-specific problems that would limit the usefulness of ophthalmic NSAIDs in the elderly.

**Drug interactions and/or related problems**

The following drug interactions and/or related problems have been selected on the basis of their potential clinical significance (possible mechanism in parentheses where appropriate)—not necessarily inclusive (» = major clinical significance):

Note: Combinations containing any of the following medications, depending on the amount present, may also interact with this medication.

Acetylcholine chloride or

Carbachol

(these medications may be less effective when administered after an ophthalmic NSAID has been used to inhibit miosis during ocular surgery; although the pharmacologic basis for the interaction has not been established, it has been suggested that NSAID-induced maintenance of a larger pupillary diameter during surgery, and the possibility that the duration of action of the NSAID may exceed that of acetylcholine chloride, may account for the apparent reduction in the ability of acetylcholine chloride to reverse mydriasis postoperatively)

Any medication that may interfere with blood clotting or prolong bleeding time, such as:

Anticoagulants, coumarin- or indandione-derivative or

Heparin or
Platelet aggregation inhibitors
(concurrent use with ophthalmic NSAIDs, which may also increase the bleeding tendency, may increase the risk of postoperative ocular bleeding)
Epinephrine (ophthalmic) and possibly other antiglaucoma agents
(the possibility should be considered that ophthalmic flurbiprofen may decrease the intraocular pressure–lowering effects of these medications; however, in one study, administration of ophthalmic flurbiprofen [1 drop every 10 minutes for 4 doses] had no effect on the intraocular pressure–lowering effect of 1% apraclonidine or 0.5% timolol)

## Medical considerations/Contraindications

The medical considerations/contraindications included here have been selected on the basis of their potential clinical significance (reasons given in parentheses where appropriate)—not necessarily inclusive (» = major clinical significance).

*Risk-benefit should be considered when the following medical problems exist:*

» Allergic reaction, such as anaphylaxis, bronchospasm, angioedema, allergic rhinitis, or urticaria, to aspirin or other systemic NSAIDs, history of
(possibility of cross-sensitivity)
Epithelial herpes simplex keratitis, active
(in one study in rabbits, ophthalmic flurbiprofen exacerbated herpes simplex keratitis [i.e., increased ulceration and conjunctivitis] and delayed healing; however, in another study in rabbits, neither flurbiprofen nor diclofenac exacerbated or prolonged acute herpes keratitis or prolonged viral shedding; although the risk of exacerbation or delayed healing of active epithelial herpes simplex keratitis in humans has not been determined, it is recommended that ophthalmic NSAIDs be administered with caution and in conjunction with an antiviral agent)
Epithelial herpes simplex keratitis, history of
(close monitoring of the patient following flurbiprofen administration is recommended because the risk of reactivation has not been determined)
Hemophilia or other bleeding problems or coagulation defects or
Prolonged bleeding time
(increased risk of bleeding)
» Sensitivity to the ophthalmic NSAID considered for use

## Side/Adverse Effects

Note: Oral administration of suprofen has caused acute flank pain and renal insufficiency, possibly manifestations of acute uric acid nephropathy. This reaction has occurred after ingestion of as few as 1 or 2 doses of 200 mg, > 25 times more than the total quantity of suprofen that would be administered over 2 days with recommended ophthalmic doses. The risk of such a reaction occurring after ophthalmic administration is unknown.

Keratitis, elevated intraocular pressure, corneal edema, chemosis, and anterior chamber reaction have also been reported with various ophthalmic nonsteroidal anti-inflammatory drugs (NSAIDs). Since these effects frequently occur following some types of ophthalmic procedures, a causal relationship has not been established.

The following side/adverse effects have been selected on the basis of their potential clinical significance (possible signs and symptoms in parentheses where appropriate)—not necessarily inclusive:

**Those indicating need for medical attention**
Incidence less frequent or rare
*For diclofenac*
**Allergic reaction** (itching; tearing)—in a patient hypersensitive to systemic NSAIDs
*For flurbiprofen*
**Bleeding in eye; redness in eye**—not resulting from surgery and not present before use
*For indomethacin*
**Bronchospastic allergic reaction** (shortness of breath; troubled breathing; tightness in chest; wheezing)—reported in an asthmatic patient; **corneal epithelial defects, including corneal abrasion and punctate keratitis; redness in eye**—not resulting from surgery and not present before use; **striate keratopathy**
*For suprofen*
**Iritis** (throbbing pain; tearing; sensitivity to light); **punctate epithelial staining**
Note: *Eye pain* and *photophobia* have also been reported independently of iritis.

**Those indicating need for medical attention only if they continue or are bothersome**
Incidence more frequent
**Irritation, ocular** (burning; stinging; itching; mild discomfort)

## Overdose

For more information on the management of overdose or unintentional ingestion, **contact a Poison Control Center** (see *Poison Control Center Listing*).

**Treatment of overdose**
Recommended treatment in case of accidental ingestion consists of drinking large quantities of fluids, to dilute the medication.

## Patient Consultation

As an aid to patient consultation, refer to *Advice for the Patient, Anti-inflammatory Drugs, Nonsteroidal (Ophthalmic)*.

In providing consultation, consider emphasizing the following selected information (» = major clinical significance):

**Before using this medication**
» Conditions affecting use, especially:
Sensitivity to aspirin or other systemic nonsteroidal anti-inflammatory drugs (NSAIDs), or to the ophthalmic NSAID considered for use
Pregnancy—Diclofenac, flurbiprofen, and indomethacin known to cross the placenta when administered systemically
Breast-feeding—Indomethacin and suprofen known to be distributed into breast milk after oral administration

**Proper use of this medication**
Proper administration technique
Preventing contamination: Not touching dropper or applicator tip to any surface and keeping container tightly closed.
» Importance of not using more medication than the amount prescribed
» Checking with physician before using medication for future eye problems
» Proper dosing
Missed dose: Using as soon as possible; not using if almost time for next dose
» Proper storage

**Precautions while using this medication**
» For diclofenac: Not wearing soft contact lenses during treatment

**Side/adverse effects**
Signs of potential side effects, especially bleeding or redness in the eye, iritis, allergic reaction

## General Dosing Information

When an ophthalmic nonsteroidal anti-inflammatory drug (NSAID) is used to prevent or reduce postoperative inflammation and/or cystoid macular edema, therapy should be started prior to the procedure. Ophthalmic NSAIDs are more effective in inhibiting the development of these complications than in treating them after they have fully developed.

---

### DICLOFENAC

## Additional Dosing Information

It is recommended that patients not wear hydrocel soft contact lenses during diclofenac therapy. Ocular irritation manifested by redness and burning has occurred in patients wearing this type of contact lens while using the medication.

## Ophthalmic Dosage Forms

Note: Bracketed uses in the *Dosage Forms* section refer to categories of use and/or indications that are not included in U.S. product labeling.

### DICLOFENAC SODIUM OPHTHALMIC SOLUTION

**Usual adult dose**
Anti-inflammatory, nonsteroidal, ophthalmic—
Treatment of inflammation following cataract surgery: Topical, to the conjunctiva, 1 drop in the affected eye four times a day, starting twenty-four hours postoperatively and continuing for the first two postoperative weeks. In some patients, treatment has been continued for six weeks or longer.
[Treatment of conjunctivitis, keratoconjunctivitis, corneal ulcers, or post-traumatic inflammation]: Topical, to the conjunctiva, 1 drop in the affected eye four to five times a day, depending on the severity of the disease.

[Miosis inhibitor, in ophthalmic surgery] and
[Prostaglandin synthesis inhibitor, ophthalmic]—
   Prevention or reduction of intraoperative miosis and postoperative cystoid macular edema: Topical, to the conjunctiva, 1 drop in the affected eye, applied up to five times during the three hours prior to surgery; fifteen minutes, thirty minutes, and forty-five minutes postoperatively; then three to five times a day for as long as needed.

**Usual pediatric dose**
Safety and efficacy have not been established.

**Strength(s) usually available**
U.S.—
   0.1% (1 mg per mL) (Rx) [*Voltaren Ophthalmic* (boric acid; edetate disodium 1 mg per mL; polyoxyl 35 castor oil; sorbic acid 2 mg per mL; tromethamine)].
Canada—
   0.1% (1 mg per mL) (Rx) [*Voltaren Ophtha* (boric acid; cremophor EL; tromethamine [TRIS]; thimerosal)].

**Packaging and storage**
Store between 15 and 30 °C (59 and 86 °F), protected from light and from freezing, unless otherwise directed by manufacturer.

**Auxiliary labeling**
• • For the eye.

**Note**
Dispense in original unopened container.

---

## FLURBIPROFEN

## Ophthalmic Dosage Forms

Note: Bracketed uses in the *Dosage Forms* section refer to categories of use and/or indications that are not included in U.S. product labeling.

### FLURBIPROFEN SODIUM OPHTHALMIC SOLUTION USP

**Usual adult dose**
Miosis inhibitor, in ophthalmic surgery—
   Topical, to the conjunctiva, 1 drop every thirty minutes, beginning two hours prior to surgery, for a total of 4 drops.
[Anti-inflammatory, nonsteroidal, ophthalmic]—
   Treatment of inflammation following ophthalmic surgery or laser trabeculoplasty: Topical, to the conjunctiva, 1 drop every four hours for one to three weeks.

**Usual pediatric dose**
Safety and efficacy have not been established.

**Strength(s) usually available**
U.S.—
   0.03% (Rx) [*Ocufen* (polyvinyl alcohol 1.4%; edetate disodium; thimerosal 0.005%; potassium chloride; sodium chloride; sodium citrate; citric acid; hydrochloric acid and/or sodium hydroxide)].
Canada—
   0.03% (Rx) [*Ocufen*].

**Packaging and storage**
Store below 40 °C (104 °F), preferably between 15 and 30 °C (59 and 86 °F), unless otherwise specified by manufacturer. Store in a tight container. Protect from freezing.

**Auxiliary labeling**
• • For the eye.

**Note**
Dispense in original unopened container.

---

## INDOMETHACIN

## Additional Dosing Information

Because an ophthalmic dosage form of indomethacin is not commercially available in the U.S., ophthalmic preparations are being compounded extemporaneously in some pharmacies. Eye injuries resulting from *Pseudomonas* contamination have occurred following use of such preparations. Pharmacists are advised **not** to use the contents of commercially available indomethacin capsules in the preparation of ophthalmic indomethacin solutions or suspensions, because of a lack of data on stability, concentration, and possible effects of excipients. Also, the sterility of compounded preparations must be assured.

## Ophthalmic Dosage Forms

### INDOMETHACIN OPHTHALMIC SUSPENSION

**Usual adult dose**
Prostaglandin synthesis inhibitor, ophthalmic and
Miosis inhibitor, in cataract surgery—
   Prevention or reduction of intraoperative miosis and postoperative cystoid macular edema: Topical, to the conjunctiva, 1 drop four times a day on the day prior to surgery, 1 drop forty-five minutes before surgery, then 1 drop four times a day for ten to twelve weeks postoperatively or as long as needed.

**Usual pediatric dose**
Safety and efficacy have not been established.

**Strength(s) usually available**
U.S.—
   Not commercially available.
Canada—
   1% (10 mg per mL) (Rx) [*Indocid* (lecithin; sodium bisulfite; sodium chloride; polysorbate 80; hydroxyethylcellulose; sorbitol; disodium edetate; benzalkonium chloride solution 0.02%; benzyl alcohol 0.25%; phenylethyl alcohol 0.25%)].

**Packaging and storage**
Store between 15 and 30 °C (59 and 86 °F), protected from light and from freezing, unless otherwise specified by manufacturer.

**Auxiliary labeling**
• • For the eye.
• • Shake well before using.

**Note**
Dispense in original unopened container.

---

## SUPROFEN

## Ophthalmic Dosage Forms

### SUPROFEN OPHTHALMIC SOLUTION USP

**Usual adult dose**
Miosis inhibitor, in ophthalmic surgery—
   Topical, to the conjunctiva, 2 drops three, two, and one hour prior to surgery. If desired, 2 drops may be applied every four hours while the patient is awake on the day prior to surgery.

**Usual pediatric dose**
Safety and efficacy have not been established.

**Strength(s) usually available**
U.S.—
   1% (10 mg per mL) (Rx) [*Profenal* (thimerosal 0.005%; caffeine 2%; edetate disodium; dibasic sodium phosphate; monobasic sodium phosphate; sodium chloride; sodium hydroxide and/or hydrochloric acid)].
Canada—
   Not commercially available.

**Packaging and storage**
Store below 40 °C (104 °F), preferably between 15 and 30 °C (59 and 86 °F), protected from freezing, unless otherwise directed by manufacturer.

**Auxiliary labeling**
• • For the eye.

**Note**
Dispense in original unopened container.

## Selected Bibliography

Keates RH, McGowan KA. Clinical trial of flurbiprofen to maintain pupillary dilation during cataract surgery. Ann Ophthalmol 1984; 16: 919-21.

Heinrichs DA, Leith AB. Effect of flurbiprofen on the maintenance of pupillary dilation during cataract surgery. Can J Ophthalmol 1990; 25: 239-42.

Stark WJ, Fagadau WR, Stewart RH, et al. Reduction of pupillary constriction during cataract surgery using suprofen. Arch Ophthalmol 1986; 104: 364-6.

Flach AJ. Cyclo-oxygenase inhibitors in ophthalmology. Surv Ophthalmol 1992; 36: 259-84.

---

Revised: 09/08/92
Interim revision: 01/24/95

# ANTI-INFLAMMATORY DRUGS, NONSTEROIDAL   Systemic

This monograph includes information on the following: Diclofenac; Diflunisal; Etodolac†; Fenoprofen; Floctafenine*; Flurbiprofen; Ibuprofen; Indomethacin; Ketoprofen; Meclofenamate†; Mefenamic Acid; Nabumetone; Naproxen; Oxaprozin†; Phenylbutazone; Piroxicam; Sulindac; Tenoxicam*; Tiaprofenic Acid*; Tolmetin.

Note: See also individual *Ketorolac (Systemic)* monograph.

See also *Indomethacin (Systemic—For Patent Ductus Arteriosus).*

See also *Anti-inflammatory Agents, Nonsteroidal (Ophthalmic)* for information on ophthalmic use of diclofenac, flurbiprofen, and indomethacin.

See also *Salicylates (Systemic)* for information on aspirin and other salicylates.

INN:
Etodolac—Etodolic acid.
Indomethacin—Indometacin.
Meclofenamate—Meclofenamic acid.

BAN:
Meclofenamate—Meclofenamic acid.

JAN:
Indomethacin—Indometacin.

VA CLASSIFICATION (Primary/Secondary):
Diclofenac—MS102/CN104; MS400; CN105
Diflunisal—MS102/CN104; MS400; CN105
Etodolac—MS102/CN104; MS400; CN105
Fenoprofen—MS102/CN104; MS400; CN105
Floctafenine—CN104/CN105; MS400
Flurbiprofen—MS102
Ibuprofen—MS102/CN104; CN850; MS400; CN105
Indomethacin—MS102/MS400; CN850; CN105; CV900
Ketoprofen—MS102/CN104; MS400; CN105
Meclofenamate—MS102/CN104; CN105
Mefenamic Acid—CN104/CN105
Nabumetone—MS102
Naproxen—MS102/CN104; CN850; MS400; CN105
Oxaprozin—MS102
Phenylbutazone—MS102/MS400
Piroxicam—MS102/MS400
Sulindac—MS102/MS400
Tenoxicam—MS102
Tiaprofenic Acid—MS102
Tolmetin—MS102

Other commonly used names are Etodolic acid [Etodolac] , Indometacin [Indomethacin] , Meclofenamic acid [Meclofenamate]

Note: For a listing of dosage forms and brand names by country availability, see *Dosage Forms* section(s). For a listing of brand names for the articles in this monograph, refer to the General Index.

*Not commercially available in the U.S.
†Not commercially available in Canada.

# Category

Note: All of these medications have analgesic, antipyretic, and anti-inflammatory actions; however, indications for specific agents may vary because of lack of specific testing and/or clinical-use data as well as the toxicity of the individual nonsteroidal anti-inflammatory drug (NSAID). **Clinically, most of these agents are used to treat a variety of painful and/or inflammatory conditions, both rheumatic and nonrheumatic, even though the specific uses are not listed in U.S. or Canadian product labeling.**

Antirheumatic (nonsteroidal anti-inflammatory)—Diclofenac; Diflunisal; Etodolac; Fenoprofen; Flurbiprofen; Ibuprofen; Indomethacin; Ketoprofen; Meclofenamate; Nabumetone; Naproxen; Oxaprozin; Phenylbutazone; Piroxicam; Sulindac; Tenoxicam; Tiaprofenic Acid; Tolmetin.

Analgesic—Diclofenac; Diflunisal; Etodolac; Fenoprofen; Floctafenine; Ibuprofen; Ketoprofen; Meclofenamate; Mefenamic Acid; Naproxen.

Antigout agent—Diclofenac; Diflunisal; Etodolac; Fenoprofen; Floctafenine; Ibuprofen; Indomethacin; Ketoprofen; Naproxen; Phenylbutazone; Piroxicam; Sulindac.

Anti-inflammatory (nonsteroidal)—Flurbiprofen; Indomethacin; Naproxen; Sulindac; Tenoxicam.

Antipyretic—Ibuprofen; Indomethacin; Naproxen.

Antidysmenorrheal—Diclofenac; Flurbiprofen; Ibuprofen; Indomethacin; Ketoprofen; Meclofenamate; Mefenamic Acid; Naproxen; Piroxicam.

Vascular headache prophylactic—Fenoprofen; Ibuprofen; Indomethacin; Mefenamic Acid; Naproxen.

Vascular headache suppressant—Diclofenac; Diflunisal; Etodolac; Fenoprofen; Floctafenine; Ibuprofen; Indomethacin; Ketoprofen; Meclofenamate; Mefenamic Acid; Naproxen.

Prostaglandin synthesis inhibitor, renal (Bartter's syndrome)—Indomethacin.

# Indications

Note: Bracketed information in the *Indications* section refers to uses that are not included in U.S. product labeling.

## Accepted

Rheumatic disease (treatment), such as:
Arthritis, rheumatoid—Diclofenac, diflunisal, fenoprofen, flurbiprofen, ibuprofen, indomethacin, ketoprofen, meclofenamate, nabumetone, naproxen, oxaprozin, phenylbutazone[1], piroxicam, sulindac, tenoxicam, tiaprofenic acid, and tolmetin are indicated for the treatment of acute or chronic rheumatoid arthritis.
Osteoarthritis—Diclofenac, diflunisal, etodolac, fenoprofen, flurbiprofen, ibuprofen, indomethacin, ketoprofen, meclofenamate, nabumetone, naproxen, oxaprozin, phenylbutazone[1], piroxicam, sulindac, tenoxicam, tiaprofenic acid, and tolmetin are indicated for relief of acute or chronic osteoarthritis.
Ankylosing spondylitis—Diclofenac[1], [diflunisal][1], [fenoprofen][1], [flurbiprofen], [ibuprofen][1], indomethacin, [ketoprofen], naproxen, phenylbutazone[1], [piroxicam], sulindac, tenoxicam, and [tolmetin] are indicated for relief of acute or chronic ankylosing spondylitis.
Arthritis, juvenile—Ibuprofen, indomethacin[1], naproxen, and tolmetin are indicated for relief of acute or chronic juvenile arthritis.
[Arthritis, psoriatic][1]—Diflunisal, fenoprofen, ibuprofen, indomethacin, ketoprofen, meclofenamate, phenylbutazone, and tolmetin are used in the treatment of psoriatic arthritis.
[Reiter's disease][1]—Indomethacin is used in the treatment of Reiter's disease.
[Rheumatic complications associated with Paget's disease of bone][1]—Indomethacin is used in the treatment of this condition.
Although NSAIDs may be required for relief of [rheumatic complications occurring in association with systemic lupus erythematosus (SLE)][1], extreme caution is recommended because patients with SLE may be predisposed toward NSAID-induced central nervous system (CNS) and/or renal toxicity. Several NSAIDs, including ibuprofen, sulindac, and tolmetin, have been shown to cause serious adverse effects, including aseptic meningitis, in patients with SLE. In addition, ibuprofen (although a causal relationship has not been established), meclofenamate, and phenylbutazone have rarely been reported to cause an SLE-like syndrome and/or to exacerbate pre-existing SLE.
NSAIDs do not affect the progressive course of some forms of rheumatic disease. Some patients with rheumatoid arthritis may need additional treatment.

Pain (treatment)—Diclofenac, diflunisal, etodolac, fenoprofen[1], floctafenine, ibuprofen, ketoprofen, meclofenamate, mefenamic acid, and naproxen are indicated for relief of mild to moderate pain, especially when anti-inflammatory actions may also be desired, e.g., following dental, obstetric, or orthopedic surgery, and for relief of musculoskeletal pain due to soft tissue athletic injuries (strains or sprains). Only immediate-release dosage forms are recommended for relief of acute pain because of their more rapid onset of action relative to delayed-release or extended-release dosage forms.
Mefenamic acid is indicated for relief of mild to moderate pain when therapy will not exceed 1 week.
Those NSAIDs indicated for relief of pain are also recommended for relief of mild to moderate bone pain caused by metastatic neoplastic disease. However, careful patient selection is necessary, especially in patients receiving chemotherapy, because of the potential gastrointestinal or renal toxicity and the platelet aggregation–inhibiting actions of these medications.

Gouty arthritis, acute (treatment) or
[Calcium pyrophosphate deposition disease, acute (treatment)][1]—[Diclofenac][1], [diflunisal][1], [etodolac], [fenoprofen][1], floctafenine[1], [ibuprofen][1], indomethacin, [ketoprofen][1], [meclofenamate], [mefenamic acid][1], naproxen[1], phenylbutazone, [piroxicam][1], and sulindac are indicated [or used ] for relief of the pain and inflammation of acute gouty arthritis and [acute calcium pyrophosphate deposition disease (pseudogout; chondrocalcinosis articularis; synovitis, crystal-induced)][1]. Only immediate-release dosage forms are recommended for

relief of acute attacks because of their more rapid onset of action relative to delayed-release or extended-release dosage forms.

[Long-term prophylactic use of an NSAID may decrease the incidence or severity of recurrent acute gout attacks, especially during the early months of antihyperuricemic therapy. The NSAIDs do not correct hyperuricemia (although diclofenac, diflunisal, etodolac, oxaprozin, and phenylbutazone have some uricosuric activity) and do not eliminate the need for administration of an antihyperuricemic agent for the long-term management of chronic gout. Colchicine is the recommended agent for preventing acute gout attacks because, in low (prophylactic) doses, it is less toxic for long-term use than NSAIDs. NSAIDs (other than phenylbutazone, which is *not recommended for long-term treatment*) should be used only for patients unable to tolerate even prophylactic doses of colchicine.]

Inflammation, nonrheumatic (treatment)—Most of the NSAIDs are indicated [or used] in the treatment of painful nonrheumatic inflammatory conditions, such as:

Athletic injuries
Bursitis
Capsulitis
Synovitis
Tendinitis or
Tenosynovitis—[Flurbiprofen is indicated for relief of bursitis, tendinitis, and soft tissue injuries.] Indomethacin[1] and sulindac are indicated for treatment of bursitis and/or tendinitis of the shoulder. Naproxen is indicated for treatment of bursitis and/or tendinitis of any joint. Tenoxicam is indicated for treatment of tendinitis, bursitis, and periarthritis of the shoulders or hips. [Other NSAIDs, especially those approved by U.S. and/or Canadian regulatory agencies for relief of pain, are also used in the treatment of these and other painful inflammatory conditions.][1]

Fever (treatment)—Ibuprofen and naproxen[1] are indicated for reduction of fever.

[Fever, due to malignancy (treatment)][1]—Indomethacin (rapidly acting dosage forms only) is used to reduce fever in patients with Hodgkin's disease, other lymphomas, and hepatic metastases of solid tumors. Indomethacin should be used only after aspirin and acetaminophen have proven ineffective. If antipyretic therapy at an adequate dosage is not effective within 48 hours, indomethacin should be discontinued.

Dysmenorrhea (treatment)—Diclofenac, [flurbiprofen], ibuprofen, [indomethacin][1], ketoprofen, meclofenamate, mefenamic acid, naproxen, and [piroxicam] are indicated for relief of the pain and other symptoms of primary dysmenorrhea. [Other NSAIDs that have been approved by U.S. and/or Canadian regulatory agencies for relief of pain are also used to relieve dysmenorrhea.][1] Only immediate-release dosage forms are recommended for relief of dysmenorrhea because of their more rapid onset of action relative to delayed-release or extended-release dosage forms.

[Because of the high incidence of adverse effects with effective doses of indomethacin, it is recommended that indomethacin be used only for severe primary dysmenorrhea unresponsive to other, less toxic, NSAIDs.]

Hypermenorrhea (treatment)—Meclofenamate is indicated for treatment of idiopathic excessive menstrual bleeding. The absence of an underlying pathologic condition should be verified before meclofenamate therapy is instituted. [NSAIDs that are used for relief of dysmenorrhea (see *Dysmenorrhea*, above) may also decrease excessive menstrual blood loss caused by an intrauterine device in addition to relieving other symptoms.][1]

[Headache, vascular (prophylaxis)][1] or
[Headache, vascular (treatment)][1]—Diclofenac, diflunisal, etodolac, fenoprofen, floctafenine, ibuprofen, indomethacin, ketoprofen, meclofenamate, mefenamic acid, and naproxen are used to relieve (when taken at the first sign of onset) migraine headache or other vascular headaches. Fenoprofen, ibuprofen, indomethacin, and naproxen are also used chronically to prevent recurrence of such headaches. Fenoprofen, ibuprofen, indomethacin, mefenamic acid, and naproxen may also be taken prior to and during menstruation to prevent migraine associated with menstruation.

[Bartter's syndrome (treatment)][1]—Indomethacin is used in the treatment of Bartter's syndrome. However, its use in this condition has been associated with adverse effects, including pseudotumor cerebri. Because long-term therapy is required, it has been suggested that other, less toxic, NSAIDs may be suitable alternatives to indomethacin.

[Pericarditis][1]—Indomethacin (rapidly acting dosage forms only) is used to relieve pain, fever, and inflammation associated with pericarditis.

**Unaccepted**
Except in the treatment of ankylosing spondylitis, for which it is a treatment of choice, and Bartter's syndrome, indomethacin is not recom-

mended as initial therapy because of its potential for causing severe side effects. Also, although indomethacin, like other NSAIDs, has analgesic and antipyretic activity, it should not be used indiscriminately (because of its toxicity) to relieve pain or reduce fever.

Phenylbutazone is not recommended as initial therapy for any indication. Because of its potential for causing severe side effects, including agranulocytosis and aplastic anemia, it should be used only after less toxic treatments (including other, less toxic, NSAIDs) have been found ineffective. In many countries, phenylbutazone is approved only for treatment of severe ankylosing spondylitis unresponsive to other NSAIDs. Use of phenylbutazone to relieve the pain and inflammation of acute painful shoulder (i.e., peritendinitis, capsulitis, or bursitis of that joint) is no longer FDA-approved. It is strongly recommended that use of phenylbutazone be restricted to short-term treatment of severe flares of rheumatic disease, gout, or calcium pyrophosphate deposition disease.

---

[1]Not included in Canadian product labeling.

## Pharmacology/Pharmacokinetics

See *Table 1*, page 411, and *Table 2*, page 415.

**Physicochemical characteristics**
Chemical group—
   Fenamate derivatives: Meclofenamate, mefenamic acid.
   Indoleacetic acid derivative: Indomethacin. Indomethacin is chemically related to the pyrroleacetic acid derivatives sulindac and tolmetin and to the pyranoindoleacetic acid derivative etodolac.
   Naphthylalkanone derivative: Nabumetone.
   Oxicam derivative: Piroxicam, tenoxicam.
   Phenylacetic acid derivative: Diclofenac.
   Propionic acid derivatives: Fenoprofen, flurbiprofen, ibuprofen, ketoprofen, naproxen, oxaprozin, tiaprofenic acid.
   Pyranoindoleacetic acid: Etodolac. This medication is chemically related to the indoleacetic acid derivative indomethacin and to the pyrroleacetic acid derivatives sulindac and tolmetin.
   Pyrazole derivative: Phenylbutazone.
   Pyrroleacetic acid derivatives: Sulindac, tolmetin. These medications are chemically related to the indoleacetic acid derivative indomethacin and to the pyranoindoleacetic acid derivative etodolac.
   Salicylic acid derivative: Diflunisal. However, diflunisal is not metabolized to salicylic acid *in vivo*
Molecular weight—
   Diclofenac potassium: 334.24.
   Diclofenac sodium: 318.13.
   Diflunisal: 250.2.
   Etodolac: 287.36.
   Fenoprofen calcium: 558.64.
   Floctafenine: 406.36.
   Flurbiprofen: 244.26.
   Ibuprofen: 206.28.
   Indomethacin: 357.79.
   Ketoprofen: 254.28.
   Meclofenamate sodium: 336.15.
   Mefenamic acid: 241.29.
   Nabumetone: 228.29
       Active nabumetone metabolite 6-methoxy-2-naphthylacetic acid (6-MNA)—216.25.
   Naproxen: 230.26.
   Naproxen sodium: 252.24.
   Oxaprozin: 293.32.
   Phenylbutazone: 308.38.
   Piroxicam: 331.35.
   Sulindac: 356.41.
   Tenoxicam: 337.32.
   Tiaprofenic acid: 260.31.
   Tolmetin sodium: 315.3.
Other characteristics—
   Ketoprofen: Highly lipophilic.
   Oxaprozin: Lipophilic.
pKa—
   Diclofenac potassium: 4.0.
   Diclofenac sodium: 4.0.
   Diflunisal: 3.3.
   Etodolac: 4.65.
   Fenoprofen calcium: 4.5 (25 °C).
   Flurbiprofen: 4.22.
   Ibuprofen: 4.43.
   Indomethacin: 4.5.
   Ketoprofen: 5.94 (in methanol:water [3:1]).
   Mefenamic acid: 4.2.
   Naproxen: 4.2.

Oxaprozin: 4.3.
Piroxicam: 1.8 and 5.1.
Tiaprofenic acid: 3.0.
Tolmetin sodium: 3.5.

Note: 6-MNA, the active metabolite of nabumetone, but not nabumetone itself, is acidic. Other NSAIDs not listed above are also acidic.

## Mechanism of action/Effect

Nonsteroidal anti-inflammatory drugs (NSAIDs) inhibit the activity of the enzyme cyclo-oxygenase, resulting in decreased formation of precursors of prostaglandins and thromboxanes from arachidonic acid. Also, meclofenamate and mefenamic acid have been shown to inhibit competitively the actions of prostaglandins. Although the resultant decrease in prostaglandin synthesis and activity in various tissues may be responsible for many of the therapeutic (and adverse) effects of NSAIDs, other actions may also contribute significantly to the therapeutic effects of these medications.

Antirheumatic (nonsteroidal anti-inflammatory)—
Act via analgesic and anti-inflammatory mechanisms; the therapeutic effects are not due to pituitary-adrenal stimulation. These medications do not affect the progressive course of rheumatoid arthritis.

Analgesic—
May block pain impulse generation via a peripheral action that may involve reduction of the activity of prostaglandins, and possibly inhibition of the synthesis or actions of other substances that sensitize pain receptors to mechanical or chemical stimulation. The antibradykinin activity of ketoprofen may also be involved in relief of pain, because bradykinin has been shown to act together with prostaglandins to cause pain.

Antigout agent—
Act via analgesic and anti-inflammatory mechanisms; do not correct hyperuricemia.

Anti-inflammatory (nonsteroidal)—
Exact mechanisms have not been determined. NSAIDs may act peripherally in inflamed tissue, probably by reducing prostaglandin activity in these tissues and possibly by inhibiting the synthesis and/or actions of other local mediators of the inflammatory response. Inhibition of leukocyte migration, inhibition of the release and/or actions of lysosomal enzymes, and actions on other cellular and immunological processes in mesenchymal and connective tissue may be involved. Indomethacin has been shown to inhibit phosphodiesterase, with a resultant increase in intracellular cyclic adenosine monophosphate (cAMP) concentration. Ketoprofen has been shown to inhibit leukotriene synthesis, inhibit bradykinin activity, and stabilize lysosomal membranes.

Antipyretic—
Probably produce antipyresis by acting centrally on the hypothalamic heat-regulating center to produce peripheral vasodilation, resulting in increased blood flow through the skin, sweating, and heat loss. The central action probably involves reduction of prostaglandin activity in the hypothalamus.

Antidysmenorrheal—
By inhibiting the synthesis and activity of intrauterine prostaglandins (which are thought to be responsible for the pain and other symptoms of primary dysmenorrhea), NSAIDs decrease uterine contractility and uterine pressure, increase uterine perfusion, and relieve ischemic as well as spasmodic pain. The antibradykinin activity of ketoprofen may also be involved in relief of dysmenorrhea, because bradykinin has been shown to induce uterine contractions and to act together with prostaglandins to cause pain. Also, NSAIDs may relieve to some extent extrauterine symptoms (such as headache, nausea, and vomiting) that may be associated with excessive prostaglandin production.

Vascular headache prophylactic and suppressant—
Analgesic actions may be involved in relief of headache. Also, by reducing prostaglandin activity, NSAIDs may directly prevent or relieve certain types of headache thought to be caused by prostaglandin-induced dilation or constriction of cerebral blood vessels.

Prostaglandin synthesis inhibitor, renal—
Inhibition of renal prostaglandin synthesis probably is responsible for indomethacin's beneficial effect in patients with Bartter's syndrome, which is thought to be caused by excessive production of renal prostaglandins.

## Other actions/effects

Most of the NSAIDs inhibit platelet aggregation. However, their antiplatelet effect, unlike that of aspirin, is reversible. Single doses of 4 to 10 mg of flurbiprofen inhibit platelet aggregation. Oxaprozin is as potent as aspirin in inhibiting platelet aggregation induced by epinephrine or collagen in vitro. With diflunisal, the effect is clinically significant only with greater-than-recommended daily doses. Also, usual doses of diclofenac, meclofenamate, mefenamic acid, or nabu-

metone (as determined after administration of 1000 mg per day for 7 to 10 days) may not significantly alter platelet aggregability. Recovery of platelet function may occur within 1 day after discontinuation of diclofenac, diflunisal, flurbiprofen, ibuprofen, indomethacin, or sulindac; 2 days after discontinuation of tolmetin; 4 days after discontinuation of naproxen; or 2 weeks following discontinuation of slowly eliminated agents such as oxaprozin or piroxicam.

Diclofenac, diflunisal, etodolac, oxaprozin, and phenylbutazone also have uricosuric activity.

Phenylbutazone also induces hepatic microsomal enzyme activity.

Studies have demonstrated that IgM rheumatoid factor production (which may be partially mediated by prostaglandins) may be decreased (but not totally inhibited) during NSAID therapy. However, because these medications do not affect the progressive course of rheumatoid arthritis, the clinical significance of this effect has not been determined.

It has been proposed that the gastrointestinal toxicity of NSAIDs may be caused primarily by reduction of the synthesis and activity of prostaglandins (which exert a protective effect on the gastrointestinal mucosa) because upper gastrointestinal toxicity has been reported following rectal or parenteral administration of some of these medications. However, when administered orally, some of these acidic medications probably also exert a direct irritant or erosive effect on the mucosa. Because nabumetone is a nonacidic prodrug, and the active metabolite 6-MNA is not formed until after absorption, the risk of serious upper gastrointestinal tract toxicity may be lower with nabumetone than with other NSAIDs. Also, in one study, gastric and duodenal prostaglandin concentrations were not altered by 4 weeks of administration of therapeutic doses of etodolac.

The renal toxicity associated with NSAIDs (i.e., decreased renal perfusion, sodium and fluid retention, and decreased renal function) may be caused by inhibition of renal prostaglandins, which are directly involved in the maintenance of renal hemodynamics and sodium and fluid balance. Renal prostaglandins are especially important in maintaining renal function in the presence of generalized vasoconstriction or volume depletion. Sulindac is a prodrug; its sulfide metabolite is the active substance. Because this active metabolite is not excreted via the kidneys, renal toxicity may be less likely with sulindac than with other NSAIDs. However, there have been reports of renal toxicity associated with sulindac therapy. Etodolac has been shown to decrease some measures of renal function, with maximum effects occurring within 1.5 to 2.5 hours after a dose. However, with administration of up to 500 mg every 12 hours, recovery of renal function occurred prior to administration of the next dose, even in patients with pre-existing mild to moderate renal function impairment (creatinine clearances ranging from 20 to 88 mL per minute). Whether more frequent administration of etodolac may cause cumulative effects on renal function has not been determined.

The analgesic, antipyretic, and anti-inflammatory effects of NSAIDs may mask symptoms of the onset and/or progression of an infection.

## Therapeutic effect

When these medications are used in the treatment of arthritis, their analgesic actions may produce some relief of pain within the first day or two. Significant relief of other symptoms of inflammation usually occurs within a few days to a week; however, in severe cases, 2 weeks or more of continuous use may be required.

| Drug and Indication | Onset of Action | Peak Effect | Duration of Action |
|---|---|---|---|
| Diclofenac Tablets Pain | 30 min | | Up to 8 hr |
| Diflunisal Pain | 1 hr | 2–3 hr | 8–12 hr |
| Etodolac Pain 200 mg 400 mg | 30 min | 1–2 hr | 4–5 hr 5–6 hr, but 8–12 hr in some patients |
| Ibuprofen Fever 5 mg/kg 10 mg/kg Pain | 0.5 hr | 2-4 hr | 6 hr 8 hr or more 4–6 hr |

| Drug and Indication | Onset of Action | Peak Effect | Duration of Action |
|---|---|---|---|
| Indomethacin Gout Heat, tenderness Swelling | 2–4 hr | 2–3 days 3–5 days | |
| Meclofenamate Pain | 1 hr | | 4–6 hr |
| Naproxen Gout Pain | 1 hr | 1–2 days 2–4 hr | Up to 7 hr |
| Piroxicam Gout | 2–4 hr | 3–5 days | 24 hr |

### Synovial fluid concentrations

Studies with several of the NSAIDs have shown that these medications enter the synovial fluid and that, several hours after administration of a single dose, synovial fluid concentrations equal or exceed the simultaneously measured plasma concentration. In addition, there is some evidence that ketoprofen, oxaprozin, and possibly other NSAIDs, may accumulate in synovial fluid when administered chronically.

| Drug and Dose | Concentration | | Half-life* (hr) |
|---|---|---|---|
| | Time to peak (hr) | Peak (mcg/mL) | |
| Diclofenac | 3 † | 0.28 † | Up to 6 |
| Etodolac ‡ | 2.7–3.7 | Total 2.6 Free (unbound) 44–84 nanograms/mL | 6.5–7 |
| Flurbiprofen 100 mg † | 5.2 | 4.4 | 4.6 |
| Indomethacin 50 mg | 2 | 0.69 | |
| Ketoprofen 50 mg 100 mg | 2 | 0.7–0.9 0.7–0.9 | |
| Nabumetone 1000 mg | ±8 | 20 §; 35 # | |
| Tenoxicam 40 mg | 10 | 1.82 | |
| Tiaprofenic Acid Tablets 200 mg † 300 mg † Extended-release Capsules | 4 4 8 | 5.3 7.7 | 8.6 |
| Tolmetin 400 mg † | 2 | 5.6 | 6.9 |

*Elimination.

†Determined at steady-state, after administration of a single dose in patients receiving chronic therapy (for diclofenac—50 mg 3 times a day; for flurbiprofen—100 mg twice a day; for tiaprofenic acid—200 mg 3 times a day for 7 days or 300 mg twice a day for 7 days; for tolmetin—400 mg 4 times a day for 7 days).

‡Determined at steady-state.

§Single dose; simultaneous plasma concentration 36 mcg/mL.

#Multiple doses (1000 mg every 12 hours on the first day, then 1000 mg per day for 3 days); simultaneous plasma concentration 41 mcg/mL.

## Precautions to Consider

### Cross-sensitivity and/or related problems

Patients sensitive to one of the nonsteroidal anti-inflammatory drugs (NSAIDs), including aspirin, ketorolac, and NSAIDs no longer commercially available (such as oxyphenbutazone, suprofen, and zomepirac) may be sensitive to any of the other NSAIDs also.

NSAIDs may cause bronchoconstriction or anaphylaxis in aspirin-sensitive asthmatics, especially those with aspirin-induced nasal polyps, asthma, and other allergic reactions (the "aspirin triad").

Patients with bronchospastic reactions to aspirin may be desensitized to this effect by administration of initially small and gradually increasing doses of aspirin. Desensitization must be carried out by physicians who are experienced with the technique, in a facility having personnel,

equipment, and medications immediately available for treatment of any adverse reaction to the medication (especially anaphylaxis or severe bronchospasm). Desensitization to aspirin also desensitizes the patient to other NSAIDs. However, unless aspirin or another NSAID is then administered on a daily basis, sensitivity to these medications redevelops within a few days.

### Carcinogenicity

*Diclofenac—*
No oncogenic potential was demonstrated with diclofenac sodium in a 2-year carcinogenicity study in male mice given up to 0.3 mg per kg of body weight (mg/kg) (0.9 mg per square meter of body surface area [mg/m²]) per day or in female mice given up to 1 mg/kg (3 mg/m²) per day.

*Diflunisal—*
No effect on the incidence or type of neoplasia was found in a 105-week study in rats given up to 40 mg/kg per day (approximately 1.3 times the maximum recommended human dose [MRHD]) or in long-term studies in mice given up to 80 mg/kg per day (approximately 2.7 times the MRHD).

*Etodolac—*
No carcinogenicity was demonstrated in mice or rats receiving up to 15 mg/kg per day (corresponding to 45 mg/m² for mice and 89 mg/m² for rats) for 2 years or 18 months, respectively.

*Floctafenine—*
No effect on the incidence of neoplasia was found in studies in CD-1 mice receiving up to 240 mg/kg per day.

*Flurbiprofen—*
No evidence of carcinogenicity was found in an 80-week study in mice receiving up to 14 mg/kg per day or in a 2-year study in rats receiving up to 12 mg/kg per day for 32 weeks, then up to 5 mg/kg per day thereafter.

*Indomethacin—*
No evidence of carcinogenicity was found in studies in mice receiving up to 1.5 mg/kg per day for 62 to 88 weeks or in studies in rats receiving up to 1.5 mg/kg per day for 73 to 110 weeks.
Leukemia has been reported in a few patients receiving indomethacin; however, a causal relationship has not been established.

*Ketoprofen—*
No evidence of carcinogenicity was found in studies in mice receiving up to 32 mg/kg (96 mg/m²) per day (approximately 0.5 times the MRHD based on body surface area).

*Meclofenamate—*
No evidence of carcinogenicity was found in an 18-month study in rats.

*Naproxen—*
No evidence of carcinogenicity was found in a 24-month study in rats.

*Oxaprozin—*
An increased incidence of hepatic adenomas and carcinomas occurred in 2-year studies in male CD mice, but not in female CD mice or in rats, given oxaprozin. The significance of this species-specific finding is not known.

*Phenylbutazone—*
Leukemia has been reported in a few patients receiving phenylbutazone; however, a causal relationship has not been established.
Long-term studies in animals have not been done to determine whether phenylbutazone has carcinogenic activity.

*Tenoxicam—*
No evidence of carcinogenicity was found in an 80-week study in mice receiving up to 5 mg/kg per day or in a 104-week study in rats receiving up to 6 mg/kg per day.

*Tiaprofenic acid—*
No evidence of carcinogenicity was found in an 80-week study in mice receiving up to 30 mg/kg per day or in a 104-week study in rats receiving up to 30 mg/kg per day.

*Tolmetin—*
No evidence of carcinogenicity was found in an 18-month study in mice receiving up to 50 mg/kg per day or in a 24-month study in rats receiving up to 75 mg/kg per day.

### Tumorigenicity

*Diclofenac—*
No tumorigenicity was demonstrated in studies in rats receiving up to 2 mg/kg per day (approximately the recommended human dose). Although there was a slight increase in benign mammary fibroadenomas in female rats given 0.5 mg/kg (3 mg/m²) per day, the increase was not significant.

*Flurbiprofen—*
No tumorigenicity was demonstrated in a 2-year study in rats receiving up to 12 mg/kg per day for 32 weeks, then up to 5 mg/kg per day.

*Indomethacin—*
No tumorigenicity was demonstrated in an 81-week study in rats receiving up to 1 mg/kg per day.

*Ketoprofen—*
No tumorigenicity was demonstrated in studies in rats receiving 6 mg/kg (36 mg/m$^2$) per day for 81 weeks or lower doses for 104 weeks.

*Nabumetone—*
No tumorigenicity was demonstrated in 2-year studies in mice and rats.

## Mutagenicity

*Diclofenac—*
No mutagenic activity was demonstrated in *in vitro* tests using mammalian cells or bacteria (with or without microsomal activation) or in *in vivo* tests, including dominant lethal and male germinal epithelial chromosomal studies in mice and nucleus anomaly and chromosomal aberration studies in Chinese hamsters.

*Diflunisal—*
No mutagenic activity was demonstrated in the dominant lethal assay, Ames microbial mutagen test, or V-79 Chinese hamster lung cell assay.

*Etodolac—*
No mutagenic activity was demonstrated in *in vitro* tests performed with *Salmonella typhimurium* and mouse lymphoma cells or in an *in vivo* mouse micronucleus test. However, in the *in vitro* human peripheral lymphocyte test, concentrations of 50 to 200 mcg per mL (mcg/mL) of etodolac produced an increase in the number of gaps (3 to 5.3% unstained regions in the chromatid without dislocation, compared with 2% in controls).

*Indomethacin—*
No mutagenic activity was demonstrated in *in vitro* tests (Ames test or *E. coli* , with or without metabolic activation) or in *in vivo* tests (host-mediated assay, sex-linked recessive lethals in *Drosophila*, and micronucleus test in mice).

*Ketoprofen—*
No mutagenic activity was demonstrated in the Ames test.

*Nabumetone—*
No mutagenic activity was demonstrated in the Ames test or in the mouse micronucleus test *in vivo*. However, chromosomal aberrations occurred in lymphocytes exposed *in vitro* to nabumetone or its active metabolite 6-methoxy-2-naphthylacetic acid (6-MNA) at concentrations of 80 mcg/mL (369.6 micromoles/L) or higher.

*Oxaprozin—*
No mutagenic activity was demonstrated in the Ames test, forward mutation testing in yeast and Chinese hamster ovary cells, DNA repair testing in Chinese hamster ovary cells, micronucleus testing in mouse bone marrow, chromosomal aberration testing in human lymphocytes, or cell transformation testing in mouse fibroblasts.

*Phenylbutazone—*
No mutagenic activity was demonstrated in tests in mice, Chinese hamsters, or rats given up to 33 times the maximum daily human dose, or in bacteria and fungi. However, *in vitro* tests using Chinese hamster fibroblast cells have shown that phenylbutazone concentrations exceeding 860 mg/L produce chromosome abnormalities. Although an increased incidence of chromosome anomalies has been reported in cultured leukocyte cells from patients receiving therapeutic doses of the medication, other similar studies in humans and in horses have yielded inconclusive or negative results.

*Piroxicam—*
No mutagenic activity was demonstrated (test systems used not specified).

*Tenoxicam—*
No mutagenic activity was demonstrated in studies in 3 bacterial systems and 4 eukaryotic test systems.

*Tiaprofenic acid—*
No mutagenic activity was demonstrated in the Ames test or in the micronucleus test in mice.

*Tolmetin—*
No mutagenic activity was demonstrated in the Ames test.

## Pregnancy/Reproduction

Fertility—

*Diclofenac—*
No impairment of fertility was demonstrated in reproduction studies in rats receiving up to 4 mg/kg (24 mg/m$^2$) per day.

*Diflunisal—*
No impairment of fertility was demonstrated in reproduction studies in rats receiving up to 50 mg/kg per day.

*Etodolac—*
A reduction in the implantation of fertilized eggs was demonstrated in reproduction studies in rats receiving 8 mg/kg per day, but no impairment of fertility was demonstrated in male or female rats receiving up to 16 mg/kg (94 mg/m$^2$) per day.

*Floctafenine—*
No impairment of fertility was demonstrated in reproduction studies in rats receiving up to 160 mg/kg per day.

*Flurbiprofen—*
No impairment of fertility was demonstrated in reproduction studies in rats receiving 2.25 mg/kg per day.

*Indomethacin—*
No impairment of fertility was demonstrated in a 2-generation reproduction study in mice or in a 2-litter reproduction study in rats receiving up to 0.5 mg/kg per day.

*Ketoprofen—*
No impairment of fertility was demonstrated in reproduction studies in male rats receiving up to 9 mg/kg (54 mg/m$^2$) per day. However, a decrease in the number of implantation sites was demonstrated in female rats receiving 6 or 9 mg/kg (36 or 54 mg/m$^2$) per day. In other studies, high doses of ketoprofen caused abnormal spermatogenesis or inhibition of spermatogenesis in rats and dogs, and decreased testicular weight in dogs and baboons.

*Mefenamic acid—*
Impairment of fertility was demonstrated in reproduction studies in rats receiving 10 times the human dose.

*Nabumetone—*
No impairment of fertility was demonstrated in male or female rats receiving 320 mg/kg (1888 mg/m$^2$) per day.

*Naproxen—*
No impairment of fertility was demonstrated in mice, rats, or rabbits receiving up to 6 times the human dose.

*Oxaprozin—*
No impairment of fertility was demonstrated in male or female rats receiving up to 200 mg/kg (1180 mg per square meter of body surface area [mg/m$^2$]) per day. For comparison, the usual human dose is about 17 mg/kg (629 mg/m$^2$) per day. However, testicular degeneration occurred in beagle dogs given 37.5 mg/kg (750 mg/m$^2$) or more per day for 42 days or longer. This finding did not occur in other species, and the clinical relevance to humans is unknown.

*Phenylbutazone—*
No impairment of fertility was demonstrated in reproduction studies in mice, Chinese hamsters, and rats receiving up to 33 times the maximum daily human dose.

*Piroxicam and tolmetin—*
No impairment of fertility was demonstrated in animal reproduction studies.

*Tenoxicam—*
No impairment of fertility was demonstrated in male rats receiving up to 8 mg per day for at least 63 days prior to mating. Administration of 8 mg per day, but not lower doses, to female rats from 14 days prior to, to 7 days after, mating resulted in a significant decrease in the number of corpora lutea and implantations, resulting in fewer live fetuses.

*Tiaprofenic—*
No impairment of fertility was demonstrated in reproduction studies in female or male rats receiving up to 20 mg/kg per day. However, an increased number of pre- and post-implantation losses was demonstrated in studies in female rats receiving 20 mg/kg per day, and a decrease in the number of implantation sites was demonstrated in studies in rabbits receiving 75 mg/kg per day.

Pregnancy—

*First trimester—*
Diclofenac:
Adequate and well-controlled studies in humans have not been done.

Diclofenac crosses the placenta in mice and rats. Studies in rats receiving 2 or 4 mg/kg per day have shown that diclofenac is embryotoxic (causing low birth weight, a slightly decreased growth rate, and failure to survive, especially with the higher dose). Also, in studies in rabbits receiving 5 or 10 mg/kg per day, diclofenac caused increases in the resorption rates, decreased fetal weights, abnormal skeletal findings, and definite embryotoxicity with the higher dose. However, no teratogenicity was demonstrated in reproduction studies in rabbits receiving up to 10 mg/kg (80 mg/m$^2$) per day, in mice receiving up to 20 mg/kg (60 mg/m$^2$) per day, or in rats receiving up to 10 mg/kg (60 mg/m$^2$) per day.

FDA Pregnancy Category B.

Diflunisal:
Adequate and well-controlled studies in humans have not been done.

Studies in animals have shown that diflunisal is teratogenic in rabbits (causing fetal vertebral and rib malformations at doses ranging from 40 to 50 mg/kg per day) but not in mice (in doses of 45 mg/kg per day) or rats (in doses of 100 mg/kg per day). Diflunisal also caused maternotoxicity and embryotoxicity (increased fetal resorptions) in rabbits receiving 60 mg/kg per day (2 times the maximum human dose).

FDA Pregnancy Category C.

Etodolac:

Adequate and well-controlled studies in humans have not been done.

Isolated alterations of limb development, including polydactyly (extra digits), oligodactyly (missing digits), syndactyly (digits attached by webbing), and unossified phalanges, occurred in rats receiving 2 to 14 mg/kg per day. Also, oligodactyly and synostosis of metatarsals occurred in rabbits receiving 2 to 14 mg/kg per day. However, the frequency and dosage group distribution in initial and repeated studies did not establish a clear drug- or dose-response relationship.

FDA Pregnancy Category C.

Fenoprofen, ibuprofen, naproxen, and tolmetin:

Adequate and well-controlled studies in humans have not been done.

Studies in animals have not shown that these agents cause adverse effects on fetal development. Naproxen was studied in mice, rats, and rabbits receiving up to 6 times the human dose. Tolmetin was studied in rats and rabbits receiving up to 50 mg/kg (1.5 times the maximum human dose).

Naproxen: FDA Pregnancy Category B.

Tolmetin: FDA Pregnancy Category C.

Floctafenine:

Studies in mice receiving up to 320 mg/kg per day, rats receiving up to 240 mg/kg per day, and rabbits receiving up to 160 mg/kg per day have not shown that floctafenine is teratogenic. However, embryotoxicity (increased fetal losses in mice, decreased fetal weight in rats, and increased fetal losses in rabbits) was demonstrated with these high doses (but not at lower dosage levels).

Flurbiprofen:

Although adequate and well-controlled studies in humans have not been done, it has been shown that flurbiprofen crosses the placenta.

Studies in mice receiving up to 12 mg/kg per day, rats receiving up to 25 mg/kg per day, and rabbits receiving up to 7.5 mg/kg per day have not shown evidence of teratogenicity. However, studies in rats have shown doses of 0.4 mg/kg per day or higher to be embryocidal (causing reduced weight or slower fetal growth, increased stillbirths, and decreased pup survival). Also, stillbirths, retained fetuses, and/or fetal distress occurred in studies in rats receiving as little as 0.2 mg/kg per day. In addition, fetotoxicity related to maternal toxicity (gastrointestinal ulceration, retardation of weight gain, intrauterine hemorrhage, and maternal deaths) occurred in rats receiving 25 mg/kg per day from Days 1 through 20 of pregnancy. With lower doses (0.2, 0.675, or 2.25 mg/kg per day), such effects did not occur when the medication was discontinued on Day 17 of pregnancy. Maternal deaths due to gastrointestinal ulceration also occurred in rabbits receiving the medication.

FDA Pregnancy Category B.

Indomethacin:

Although studies in humans have not been done, it has been shown that indomethacin crosses the placenta.

Studies in rats and mice have shown that indomethacin (at a dosage of 4 mg/kg per day) causes decreased average fetal weight and retarded ossification. In other studies in mice, higher doses (5 to 15 mg/kg per day) caused maternal toxicity and death, increased fetal resorptions, and fetal malformations.

Ketoprofen:

Adequate and well-controlled studies in humans have not been done.

Studies in animals have not shown evidence of teratogenicity or embryotoxicity in mice receiving up to 12 mg/kg (36 mg/m$^2$) per day or in rats receiving up to 9 mg/kg (54 mg/m$^2$) per day. In studies in rabbits, maternally toxic doses were embryotoxic but not teratogenic.

FDA Pregnancy Category B.

Meclofenamate:

Adequate and well-controlled studies in humans have not been done.

Animal studies have shown meclofenamate to cause fetotoxicity, minor skeletal malformations (e.g., supernumerary ribs), and delayed ossification, but no major teratogenicity.

Mefenamic acid:

Although adequate and well-controlled studies in humans have not been done, it has been demonstrated that mefenamic acid metabolites readily cross the placenta.

Mefenamic acid caused increases in the number of resorptions in rabbits receiving 2.5 times the human dose and decreases in survival to weaning (possibly due to maternal neglect) in rats receiving 10 times the human dose. Although no fetal abnormalities were reported in these studies or in studies in dogs receiving up to 10 times the human dose, it has been recommended that mefenamic acid not be used during pregnancy.

FDA Pregnancy Category C.

Nabumetone:

Adequate and well-controlled studies in humans have not been done.

Nabumetone did not cause teratogenicity in rats receiving up to 400 mg/kg (2360 mg/m$^2$) per day or in rabbits receiving up to 300 mg/kg (3540 mg/m$^2$) per day. However, fetotoxicity (post-implantation losses) occurred in rats receiving 100 mg/kg (590 mg/m$^2$) per day or more. These doses are equivalent to the maximum recommended human dose of nabumetone.

FDA Pregnancy Category C.

Oxaprozin:

Adequate and well-controlled studies in humans have not been done.

Fetal malformations occurred infrequently in rabbits receiving 7.5 to 30 mg/kg per day (doses within the usual human dose range). However, no teratogenicity occurred in mice or rats receiving 50 to 200 mg/kg (225 to 900 mg/m$^2$) per day.

FDA Pregnancy Category C.

Phenylbutazone:

Adequate and well-controlled studies in humans have not been done.

Although studies in rats and rabbits have not shown that phenylbutazone (in doses up to 16 times the maximum daily human dose) is teratogenic, slightly reduced litter sizes were demonstrated in both species.

FDA Pregnancy Category C.

Piroxicam:

Studies in humans have not been done.

Studies in animals have not shown that piroxicam causes teratogenic effects in doses up to 10 mg/kg per day.

Sulindac:

Studies in humans have not been done.

Animal studies have shown that sulindac (at dosage levels of 20 and 40 mg/kg per day—2.5 and 5 times the MRHD) causes decreased average fetal weight and an increased number of deaths (observed on the first day of the postpartum period). Also, some studies in rabbits have shown a low incidence of visceral and skeletal malformations with sulindac. However, these effects did not occur in repeat studies using the same or higher dosages.

Tenoxicam:

Studies in mice receiving up to 8 mg/kg per day from Day 6 to Day 15 of gestation did not show tenoxicam to adversely affect the fetuses or neonates. Teratogenic effects did not occur in offspring of rats receiving up to 12 mg/kg per day from Day 7 to Day 17 of gestation. However, a higher mortality rate associated with panperitonitis, gastric lesions characteristic of NSAIDs, and uterine hemorrhage occurred in dams receiving 8 or 12 mg/kg, but not 4 mg/kg or less, per day. Tenoxicam was embryotoxic (causing increased resorptions), but not teratogenic, in rabbits receiving 32 mg/kg, but not 16 mg/kg or less, per day from Day 6 to Day 18 of gestation.

Tiaprofenic acid:

Tiaprofenic acid crosses the placenta.

Studies in mice receiving up to 100 mg/kg per day have not shown that the medication is teratogenic. However, an increase in the fetal loss rate was demonstrated in studies in mice receiving 100 mg/kg per day, rats receiving 10 or 25 (but not 5) mg/kg per day, and rabbits receiving 75 (but not 25 or 50) mg/kg per day.

*Second and third trimesters—*
   All NSAIDs:
      Although studies in humans have not been done with NSAIDs
      other than indomethacin, use of NSAIDs during the second
      half of pregnancy is not recommended because of possible
      adverse effects on the fetus, such as premature closure of
      the ductus arteriosus, which may lead to persistent pul-
      monary hypertension in the newborn. Studies in full-term
      pregnant rats have shown that diclofenac, fenoprofen, flur-
      biprofen, ibuprofen, indomethacin, ketoprofen, mefenamic
      acid, naproxen, and tolmetin have a strong constrictive ef-
      fect on the fetal ductus arteriosus, whereas floctafenine,
      phenylbutazone, piroxicam, sulindac, and tiaprofenic acid
      have a moderate constrictive effect.
      Animal studies have also shown that administration of NSAIDs
      during late pregnancy may cause prolonged gestation, dys-
      tocia, and delayed parturition, possibly because of de-
      creased uterine contractility resulting from inhibition of
      uterine prostaglandins. Decreases in pup survival rates also
      have been reported. Studies with piroxicam and nabume-
      tone (at a dose of 320 mg/kg per day) have indicated that
      dystocia may cause an increased mortality rate in both off-
      spring and dams, and a study with tenoxicam showed a
      dose-dependent prolongation of gestation and decrease in
      neonatal viability with doses ranging between 0.5 and 2
      mg/kg per day. Also, delayed and prolonged parturition
      was associated with decreased pup survival in studies with
      etodolac and with an increased number of stillbirths in stud-
      ies with flurbiprofen and tiaprofenic acid. Administration
      of indomethacin to rats and mice during the last 3 days of
      gestation increased the incidence of neuronal necrosis in
      the diencephalon and caused maternal and fetal deaths. Ad-
      ministration of oxaprozin to rats during late pregnancy re-
      sulted in decreased pup survival, and administration of 3.5
      times the maximum human daily dose of phenylbutazone
      to rats during late pregnancy and lactation resulted in an
      increased number of stillbirths and reduced survival of off-
      spring. Studies in animals have also shown that adminis-
      tration of piroxicam during the third trimester may increase
      the risk of maternal gastrointestinal tract toxicity.
   Indomethacin:
      In addition to the adverse effects in animal studies described
      above, administration of indomethacin to pregnant women
      during the third trimester has caused closure of the ductus
      arteriosus, inhibition of platelet function resulting in bleed-
      ing, renal function impairment or failure with oligohydram-
      nios, gastrointestinal bleeding or perforation, and myocar-
      dial degenerative changes in the fetus.

**Breast-feeding**
Problems in humans have not been documented with most of the NSAIDs.
*Diclofenac—*
   Diclofenac is distributed into breast milk. In one study, long-term use
   of 150 mg per day produced concentrations of 100 nanograms per
   gram in the breast milk. An infant of 4 to 5 kg consuming one
   liter per day would therefore ingest approximately 0.03 mg/kg per
   day.
*Diflunisal—*
   Diflunisal is distributed into breast milk. Concentrations may reach 2
   to 7% of the maternal plasma concentration.
*Etodolac, floctafenine, and tiaprofenic acid—*
   It is not known whether these medications are distributed into breast
   milk.
*Fenoprofen and mefenamic acid—*
   Fenoprofen and mefenamic acid are distributed into breast milk in very
   small quantities.
*Flurbiprofen—*
   Flurbiprofen is distributed into breast milk in very small quantities. In
   one study, the peak concentration of 0.09 mcg/mL occurred 3
   hours following a single 100-mg dose. A maximum of 0.07% of
   the dose appeared in breast milk within 24 hours after administration. A nursing infant whose mother is taking 200 mg per day
   could receive approximately 0.1 mg of flurbiprofen per day.
*Ibuprofen—*
   Studies in humans have failed to detect ibuprofen in breast milk using
   methodology capable of detecting the medication in a concentration of 1 mcg/mL. The maternal dosage was 400 mg four times a
   day.
*Indomethacin—*
   Indomethacin is distributed into breast milk. Risk-benefit must be considered because convulsions were reported in one breast-fed infant

whose mother received 200 mg of indomethacin per day, of which
   0.5 to 2 mg per day was distributed into the breast milk.
*Ketoprofen—*
   It is not known whether ketoprofen is distributed into human breast
   milk; however, in animal studies, the concentration in the milk of
   lactating dogs was 4 to 5% of the maternal plasma concentration.
   In other studies, no adverse effect on perinatal development was
   observed in offspring of rats receiving 9 mg/kg (54 mg/m $^2$) per
   day, corresponding to 1.5 times the MRHD based on weight or 0.3
   times the MRHD based on body surface area.
*Meclofenamate—*
   Trace amounts of meclofenamate are distributed into breast milk. Use
   of meclofenamate in nursing mothers is not recommended because
   animal studies have shown meclofenamate to interfere with normal
   development of the young before weaning.
*Nabumetone—*
   It is not known whether nabumetone or its metabolites are distributed
   into human breast milk. Problems in humans have not been documented. However, 6-MNA is distributed into the milk of lactating
   rats in concentrations approximately equal to those in plasma.
*Naproxen—*
   Naproxen is distributed into breast milk; concentrations may reach 1%
   of the maternal plasma concentration. The peak concentration in
   breast milk occurs 4 hours after a dose.
*Oxaprozin—*
   It is not known whether oxaprozin is distributed into human breast
   milk. However, it is distributed into the milk of lactating rats.
*Phenylbutazone—*
   Phenylbutazone is distributed into breast milk; use by nursing mothers
   may cause severe adverse effects, including blood dyscrasias, in
   the infant.
*Piroxicam—*
   Piroxicam is distributed into breast milk; concentrations may reach 1
   to 3% of the maternal plasma concentration. Also, use of piroxicam
   by nursing mothers is not recommended because studies in rats
   have shown that piroxicam causes a dose-dependent inhibition of
   lactation.
*Sulindac—*
   It is not known whether sulindac is distributed into human breast milk,
   but it is distributed into the milk of lactating rats.
*Tolmetin—*
   Tolmetin is distributed into breast milk. In one study, an average concentration of 0.075 mcg/mL was measured, with the peak concentration occurring 1 hour following administration to the mother.
   The half-life in breast milk was 1.5 hours.

**Pediatrics**
*Ibuprofen—*
   Appropriate studies performed to date have not demonstrated pediatrics-specific problems that would limit the usefulness of ibuprofen
   in children 6 months of age or older. Safety and efficacy in infants
   younger than 6 months of age have not been established.
*Indomethacin—*
   Although appropriate studies have not been done in the pediatric population, no pediatrics-specific problems have been documented to
   date (with the immediate-release capsule or oral suspension dosage
   form; the extended-release dosage form is not recommended for
   pediatric patients). However, because of indomethacin's toxicity,
   it is recommended that its use be limited to patients unresponsive
   to (or intolerant of) other antirheumatic agents, that the patient be
   carefully monitored (especially for the presence of infection), and
   that the recommended pediatric doses not be exceeded.
*Naproxen—*
   Studies in children 2 years of age and older with juvenile arthritis have
   shown higher incidences of naproxen-induced skin rash and increased bleeding time as compared with adults. Studies in children
   younger than 2 years of age have not been done.
*Oxaprozin—*
   Although a study with oxaprozin has been conducted in patients 3 to
   16 years of age, controlled studies have not been published. Preliminary evidence indicates that, although the risk of overt hepatotoxicity appears to be minimal, elevated aspartate aminotransferase (AST [SGOT]) values during oxaprozin therapy may occur
   more often in patients treated for juvenile arthritis than in patients
   treated for other forms of arthritic disease. Safety and efficacy in
   pediatric patients have not been established.
*Phenylbutazone—*
   Because of phenylbutazone's toxicity, use in children younger than 15
   years of age is not recommended.
*Tolmetin—*
   Appropriate studies performed to date have not demonstrated pediatrics-specific problems that would limit the usefulness of tolmetin

in children 2 years of age or older. Studies in children younger than 2 years of age have not been done.

*Other NSAIDs—*

No information is available on the relationship of age to the effects of these medications in pediatric patients. Safety, efficacy, and appropriate dosages have not been established.

### Geriatrics

*All NSAIDs—*

Whether geriatric patients are at increased risk of serious gastrointestinal toxicity during NSAID therapy has not been established. However, NSAID-induced gastrointestinal ulceration and/or bleeding may be more likely to cause serious consequences, including fatalities, in geriatric patients than in younger adults. In addition, elderly patients are more likely to have age-related renal function impairment, which may increase the risk of NSAID-induced hepatic or renal toxicity and may also require dosage reduction to prevent accumulation of the medication. Some clinicians recommend that geriatric patients, especially those 70 years of age or older, be given one-half of the usual adult dose initially. Also, careful monitoring of the patient is recommended.

*Etodolac—*

Studies performed to date with 200 mg of etodolac twice a day have not shown differences in the pharmacokinetics of the medication in geriatric patients compared with younger adults. Also, studies with 600 mg of etodolac per day have not shown differences in the side effects profile of etodolac in geriatric patients compared with younger adults.

*Flurbiprofen—*

Studies have shown that the peak plasma concentration of flurbiprofen may be increased in females 74 to 94 years of age, but not in males 66 to 90 years of age.

*Indomethacin—*

In addition to the increased risks of therapy with any NSAID as described above, geriatric patients are more likely to develop adverse CNS effects, especially confusion, while taking indomethacin.

*Ketoprofen—*

Studies have shown that protein binding and clearance of ketoprofen may be reduced, leading to increased and prolonged serum concentration and elimination half-life.

*Nabumetone—*

Studies in geriatric patients have not shown differences in the efficacy or safety of nabumetone compared with younger adults. However, plasma concentrations of 6-MNA are higher in geriatric patients, and interpatient variability in the pharmacokinetic parameters for 6-MNA is greater in geriatric patients than in younger adults.

*Naproxen—*

Studies have shown that the unbound (free) fraction of naproxen, but not the total plasma concentration, may be increased in geriatric patients. The steady-state concentration of unbound naproxen may be almost doubled in geriatric patients as compared with younger adults.

*Oxaprozin—*

Studies have not demonstrated a need for adjustment of initial oxaprozin dosage in elderly patients on the basis of pharmacokinetic considerations.

The relationship of age to the risk of adverse effects in patients receiving oxaprozin has been examined using data from 3 studies in patients with rheumatoid arthritis and 1 study in patients with osteoarthritis. The data indicate that oxaprozin is more likely to cause a potentially significant decrease in renal function, adverse gastrointestinal effects, or a significant decrease in hemoglobin concentration in patients older than 60 years of age than in younger adults. Although it has also been reported, with other NSAIDs, that geriatric patients seem to be more susceptible to NSAID-induced hepatotoxicity, there were no significant age-related differences in measures of hepatic function in the 4 studies with oxaprozin.

*Phenylbutazone—*

In patients 60 years of age and over, therapy should be limited to short periods (not to exceed 1 week if possible) because of the high risk of severe, possibly fatal, toxic reactions. Specifically, the risk of aplastic anemia and agranulocytosis is increased in elderly patients.

*Piroxicam—*

Studies in geriatric patients have shown a tendency toward increased elimination half-life and steady-state plasma concentration in these patients, especially elderly females.

*Tenoxicam—*

The risk of hyperkalemia may be increased in elderly patients.

*Tiaprofenic acid—*

The risk of adverse renal effects reflected by hyperkalemia and/or an increase in blood urea nitrogen (BUN) may be increased in elderly

patients; an increase in BUN occurred in 11.8% of elderly patients, but only 2.5% of all patients, in clinical trials.

### Dental

NSAIDs may cause soreness, irritation, or ulceration of the oral mucosa. Most of the NSAIDs may rarely cause leukopenia and/or thrombocytopenia, which may result in an increased incidence of microbial infection, delayed healing, and gingival bleeding. If leukopenia or thrombocytopenia occurs, dental work should be deferred until blood counts have returned to normal, and patients should be instructed in proper oral hygiene, including caution in use of regular toothbrushes, dental floss, and toothpicks.

### Surgical

Caution is recommended in patients who require surgery. Most NSAIDs inhibit platelet aggregation and may prolong bleeding time, which may increase intra- and postoperative bleeding. The risk may be lower with usual doses of diclofenac, diflunisal, meclofenamate, mefenamic acid, or nabumetone, which may not significantly alter platelet aggregability (although mefenamic acid–induced hypoprothrombinemia, if present, could be hazardous to the patient). Recovery of platelet function may occur within 1 day after discontinuation of diclofenac, diflunisal, flurbiprofen, ibuprofen, indomethacin, or sulindac; 2 days after discontinuation of tolmetin; 4 days after discontinuation of naproxen; or 2 weeks following discontinuation of slowly eliminated agents such as oxaprozin or piroxicam. Consideration should be given to discontinuing NSAID treatment for an appropriate length of time prior to elective surgery, depending on the potency and duration of effect of the individual agent on platelet aggregability. In particular, it is recommended that treatment with oxaprozin, which is as potent as aspirin in inhibiting platelet aggregation, be discontinued 1 to 2 weeks prior to elective surgery.

### Drug interactions and/or related problems

The following drug interactions and/or related problems have been selected on the basis of their potential clinical significance (possible mechanism in parentheses where appropriate)—not necessarily inclusive (» = major clinical significance):

Note: Combinations containing any of the following medications, depending on the amount present, may also interact with this medication.

In addition to the interactions listed below, the possibility should be considered that additive or multiple effects leading to impaired blood clotting and/or increased risk of bleeding may occur if any NSAID is used concurrently with any medication having a significant potential for causing hypoprothrombinemia, thrombocytopenia, or gastrointestinal ulceration or hemorrhage.

*For all NSAIDs*

Note: All of the following interactions have not been documented with every NSAID. However, they have been reported with several of these medications and should be considered potential precautions to the use of any NSAID, especially with chronic administration.

Acetaminophen

(prolonged concurrent use of acetaminophen with an NSAID may increase the risk of adverse renal effects; it is recommended that patients be under close medical supervision while receiving such combined therapy)

(concurrent use with diflunisal may also increase the risk of acetaminophen-induced hepatotoxicity because diflunisal may increase the acetaminophen plasma concentration by 50%)

Alcohol or

Corticosteroids, glucocorticoid or

Corticotropin (chronic therapeutic use) or

Potassium supplements

(concurrent use with an NSAID may increase the risk of gastrointestinal side effects, including ulceration or hemorrhage; however, concurrent use with a glucocorticoid or corticotropin in the treatment of arthritis may provide additional therapeutic benefit and permit reduction of glucocorticoid or corticotropin dosage)

» Anticoagulants, coumarin- or indandione-derivative or

» Heparin or

» Thrombolytic agents, such as:

Alteplase

Anistreplase

Streptokinase

Urokinase

(inhibition of platelet aggregation by NSAIDs, and the possibility of NSAID-induced gastrointestinal ulceration or bleeding, may be hazardous to patients receiving anticoagulant or thrombolytic therapy; although nabumetone may be less likely than other NSAIDs to increase the risk of bleeding because it may be less likely to cause gastrointestinal ulceration or hemorrhage and because it has minimal, if any, platelet aggregation–inhibiting activity, caution is recommended; also, with usual doses, diclofenac, diflunisal, me- clofenamate, and mefenamic acid may be less likely than other NSAIDs to significantly alter platelet aggregability)

(diflunisal, etodolac, fenoprofen, floctafenine, flurbiprofen, indo- methacin, meclofenamate, mefenamic acid, phenylbutazone, pirox- icam, sulindac, tiaprofenic acid, and tolmetin have been reported to potentiate the effects of coumarin- or indandione-derivative an- ticoagulants; the effect of floctafenine on coagulation test results becomes apparent only after 2 weeks of concurrent use; potentia- tion may result from displacement of the anticoagulant from pro- tein-binding sites and, with phenylbutazone, from inhibition of the metabolism of the anticoagulant; concurrent use of phenylbutazone with an anticoagulant is not recommended; if another NSAID is used concurrently, coagulation tests should be monitored and an- ticoagulant dosage adjustments made, if necessary, when NSAID therapy is initiated or discontinued)

Antidiabetic agents, oral or
Insulin
(NSAIDs may increase the hypoglycemic effect of these medica- tions because prostaglandins are directly involved in regulatory mechanisms of glucose metabolism and possibly because of dis- placement of the oral antidiabetics from serum proteins; dosage adjustments of the antidiabetic agent may be necessary; glipizide and glyburide, due to their nonionic binding characteristics, may not be affected as much as the other oral antidiabetic agents; how- ever, caution with concurrent use is recommended)

(diclofenac has also been reported to decrease the effects of these medications, leading to hyperglycemia)

Antihypertensives or
Diuretics, especially
»   Triamterene
(increased monitoring of the response to an antihypertensive agent may be advisable when any NSAID is used concurrently because flurbiprofen, indomethacin, ibuprofen, naproxen, oxaprozin, and piroxicam have been shown to reduce or reverse the effects of antihypertensives, possibly by inhibiting renal prostaglandin syn- thesis and/or by causing sodium and fluid retention)

(NSAIDs may decrease the diuretic, natriuretic, and antihyperten- sive effects of diuretics, probably by inhibiting renal prostaglandin synthesis; flurbiprofen has also been shown to interfere with fu- rosemide-induced kaliuresis; however, diflunisal does not decrease the diuretic effect of furosemide)

(indomethacin may block the increase in plasma renin activity [PRA] induced by bumetanide, furosemide, or indapamide)

(concurrent use of an NSAID and a diuretic may increase the risk of renal failure secondary to a decrease in renal blood flow caused by inhibition of renal prostaglandin synthesis; specifically, con- current use of triamterene and indomethacin is not recommended because this combination has caused renal function impairment [azotemia and reduced creatinine clearance] and a few cases of renal failure requiring hemodialysis)

(concurrent use of a potassium-sparing diuretic with indomethacin or diclofenac, and possibly other NSAIDs, may increase the risk of hyperkalemia)

(diflunisal significantly increases the plasma concentration of hy- drochlorothiazide and decreases the hyperuricemic effect of hy- drochlorothiazide or furosemide)

» Aspirin or
NSAIDs, two or more concurrently, especially
»   Diflunisal and indomethacin concurrently or
Salicylates other than aspirin and diflunisal
(concurrent use of two or more NSAIDs, including aspirin, is not recommended; concurrent therapy may increase the risk of gastro- intestinal toxicity, including ulceration or hemorrhage, without providing additional symptomatic relief; specifically, concurrent use of diflunisal and indomethacin has resulted in fatal gastroin- testinal hemorrhage)

(concurrent use of aspirin with other NSAIDs may also increase the risk of bleeding at sites other than the gastrointestinal tract because of additive inhibition of platelet aggregation)

(concurrent administration of two or more NSAIDs may alter the pharmacokinetic profile of at least one of the medications, which may alter the therapeutic effect and/or increase the risk of adverse effects; specifically, aspirin decreases protein binding of ketopro- fen and etodolac [but does not alter etodolac clearance], increases plasma clearance of ketoprofen, interferes with the formation and excretion of ketoprofen conjugates, decreases concentrations of the

active sulfide metabolite of sulindac, and decreases the bioavaila- bility of diclofenac, diflunisal, fenoprofen, flurbiprofen [by 50%], ibuprofen [by 50% in multiple-dose studies], indomethacin [by 20%], meclofenamate, piroxicam [by 20%], a single dose of ten- oxicam [by 20%], and tolmetin. Also, diflunisal decreases the renal clearance of indomethacin, resulting in significantly increased in- domethacin plasma concentrations, and decreases the concentration of the active sulfide metabolite of sulindac by 33%. Although stud- ies to determine whether phenylbutazone alters etodolac clearance have not been done, phenylbutazone has been shown *in vitro* to decrease the protein binding of etodolac, leading to an 80% in- crease in the concentration of unbound etodolac))

Bone marrow depressants (See *Appendix II*)
(leukopenic and/or thrombocytopenic effects of these medications may be increased with concurrent or recent therapy if an NSAID causes the same effects; dosage adjustment of the bone marrow depressant, if necessary, should be based on blood counts)
» Cefamandole or
» Cefoperazone or
» Cefotetan or
» Plicamycin or
» Valproic acid
(these medications may cause hypoprothrombinemia; in addition, plicamycin or valproic acid may inhibit platelet aggregation; con- current use with an NSAID may increase the risk of bleeding be- cause of additive interferences with platelet function and/or the potential occurrence of NSAID-induced gastrointestinal ulceration or hemorrhage)

Colchicine
(concurrent use with an NSAID may increase the risk of gastro- intestinal ulceration or hemorrhage, and concurrent use with phen- ylbutazone may also increase the risk of adverse hematologic effects)

(inhibition of platelet aggregation by NSAIDs, added to colchi- cine's effects on blood clotting mechanisms [colchicine may cause thrombocytopenia with chronic use and clotting defects, including disseminated intravascular coagulation, with overdose], may in- crease the risk of bleeding at sites other than the gastrointestinal tract)

» Cyclosporine or
Gold compounds or
Nephrotoxic medications, other (See *Appendix II*)
(inhibition of renal prostaglandin activity by NSAIDs may increase the plasma concentration of cyclosporine and/or the risk of cy- closporine-induced nephrotoxicity; patients should be carefully monitored during concurrent use)

(the risk of adverse renal effects may also be increased when an NSAID is used concurrently with other nephrotoxic medications, possibly including gold compounds [although NSAIDs and gold compounds are commonly used concurrently in the treatment of arthritis])

Digitalis glycosides
(diclofenac and ibuprofen have been shown to increase serum di- goxin concentrations, and indomethacin has increased digitalis concentrations in neonates being treated for patent ductus arterio- sus; the possibility should be considered that some of the other NSAIDs may also increase digoxin concentrations, leading to an increased risk of digitalis toxicity; increased monitoring and dos- age adjustments of the digitalis glycoside may be necessary during and following concurrent NSAID therapy; however, studies have failed to show that flurbiprofen, ketoprofen, piroxicam, or tenoxi- cam increases digoxin concentrations, and phenylbutazone may de- crease digitalis concentrations [see individual *For phenylbutazone* listing, below])

» Lithium
(diclofenac, ibuprofen, indomethacin, naproxen, and piroxicam have been reported to increase the steady-state concentration of lithium, possibly by decreasing its renal clearance; with indometh- acin, the steady-state lithium concentration was increased by up to 50%; other NSAIDs may have a similar effect; increased moni- toring of lithium concentrations is recommended during and fol- lowing concurrent use)

» Methotrexate
(concurrent use with phenylbutazone may increase the risk of agranulocytosis or bone marrow depression and is not recommended)

(NSAIDs may decrease protein binding and/or renal elimination of methotrexate, resulting in increased and prolonged methotrexate plasma concentrations and an increased risk of toxicity, especially during high-dose methotrexate infusion therapy; indomethacin has caused toxicity with intermediate-dose methotrexate infusions; fatalities have been reported; it is recommended that NSAID therapy be withheld for varying periods of time, depending on the elimination half-life of the individual NSAID [12 to 24 hours for agents with a short elimination half-life to up to 10 or 12 days for agents with a very long elimination half-life] prior to administration of a high-dose methotrexate infusion [for indomethacin, an intermediate- or high-dose methotrexate infusion]; also, NSAID therapy should not be resumed following the infusion until the methotrexate plasma concentration has decreased to a nontoxic level, usually at least 12 hours)

(severe, sometimes fatal, methotrexate toxicity has also been reported when NSAIDs were used concurrently with low to moderate doses of methotrexate, including doses commonly used in the treatment of rheumatoid arthritis or psoriasis; caution in concurrent use is recommended, with dosage of methotrexate being adjusted as determined by monitoring the plasma methotrexate concentration and/or adequacy of the patient's renal function)

Photosensitizing medications, other
(concurrent use with photosensitizing NSAIDs may cause additive photosensitizing effects)

Platelet aggregation inhibitors, other (See *Appendix II*)
(concurrent use with an NSAID may increase the risk of bleeding because of additive inhibition of platelet aggregation, as well as the potential for NSAID-induced gastrointestinal ulceration or hemorrhage)

(concurrent use of sulfinpyrazone with NSAIDs may also increase the risk of gastrointestinal ulceration or hemorrhage)

» Probenecid
(concurrent use of probenecid with ketoprofen is not recommended; probenecid decreases ketoprofen's renal clearance [by approximately 66%] and protein binding [by 28%], and inhibits formation and renal clearance of ketoprofen conjugates, leading to greatly increased ketoprofen plasma concentration and risk of toxicity)

(probenecid has also been shown to decrease renal and biliary clearance of indomethacin, and to increase plasma concentrations of indomethacin and naproxen, leading to increased risk of toxicity and possibly to increased effectiveness of the NSAID; if concurrent use is necessary, it is recommended that these NSAIDs be administered in reduced dosage and that increases in dosage be made slowly and in small increments)

(probenecid may also decrease excretion and increase serum concentrations of other NSAIDs, possibly enhancing effectiveness and/or increasing the potential for toxicity; a decrease in dosage of the NSAID may be necessary if adverse effects occur)

(probenecid may increase the plasma concentration of sulindac and its sulfone metabolite, and slightly decrease the plasma concentration of the active sulfide metabolite)

*For diflunisal (in addition those listed for all NSAIDs)*
Antacids
(concurrent chronic use may significantly decrease the plasma concentration of diflunisal)

*For fenoprofen (in addition to those listed for all NSAIDs)*
Antacids
(concurrent chronic use may significantly decrease the plasma concentration of fenoprofen)

Phenobarbital
(phenobarbital may increase metabolism of fenoprofen by inducing hepatic microsomal enzymes, leading to a decrease in the elimination half-life of fenoprofen; fenoprofen dosage adjustment may be required)

*For indomethacin (in addition to those listed for all NSAIDs)*
Aminoglycosides
(administration of indomethacin to neonates being treated for a patent ductus has decreased the renal clearance and increased the plasma concentration of concurrently administered aminoglycoside antibiotics; although not documented, similar effects may occur in other patients, leading to increased risk of toxicity; adjustment of aminoglycoside dosage may be required)

» Zidovudine
(indomethacin may competitively inhibit hepatic glucuronidation and decrease the clearance of zidovudine, possibly leading to potentiation of zidovudine toxicity; indomethacin toxicity may also be increased; concurrent use of the two medications should be avoided)

*For phenylbutazone (in addition to those listed for all NSAIDs)*
Note: Phenylbutazone induces hepatic microsomal enzymes and is itself metabolized by the same enzymes. It has been reported to increase the metabolism of several medications metabolized by hepatic microsomal enzymes and to decrease the metabolism of others. Although not documented, it has been proposed that, in some cases, phenylbutazone may compete with other medications for the enzymes.

Alcohol
(concurrent use of alcohol with phenylbutazone may increase the potential for impairment of psychomotor skills)

Anticonvulsants, hydantoin, especially
» Phenytoin
(phenylbutazone may displace hydantoin anticonvulsants from their protein-binding sites and inhibit their metabolism, possibly leading to increased elimination half-life and toxicity; hydantoin dosage adjustment, based on monitoring of plasma concentrations and/or observed signs of toxicity, may be required)

Barbiturates or
Cortisone
(phenylbutazone may decrease the efficacy of these medications by inducing hepatic microsomal enzymes and increasing their metabolism; the possibility should be considered that corticosteroids other than cortisone may be similarly affected)

Cholestyramine
(cholestyramine may decrease absorption of phenylbutazone; administration of phenylbutazone 1 hour before or 4 to 6 hours after cholestyramine may decrease the risk of impaired absorption and of toxicity resulting from sudden increases in absorption and serum concentration of phenylbutazone if cholestyramine therapy is discontinued)

Contraceptives, estrogen-containing, oral
(concurrent long-term use with phenylbutazone may result in reduced contraceptive reliability and increased incidence of breakthrough bleeding)

Dermatitis-causing medications, especially
Chloroquine
Hydroxychloroquine
(concurrent use with phenylbutazone may increase the risk of severe dermatologic reactions)

» Digitalis glycosides, possibly excepting digoxin
(phenylbutazone may increase the hepatic metabolism of digitalis, leading to a decrease in digitalis serum concentration; digitalis glycoside dosage adjustment may be necessary during and following concurrent use)

Hepatic enzyme inducers, other (See *Appendix II*)
(hepatic enzyme inducers may increase phenylbutazone metabolism and decrease its half-life)

Methylphenidate
(methylphenidate may inhibit metabolism of phenylbutazone, leading to increased plasma concentrations and toxicity; dosage adjustments may be necessary)

» Penicillamine
(concurrent use with phenylbutazone may increase the risk of serious hematologic and/or renal adverse effects)

Sulfonamides
(sulfonamides may displace phenylbutazone from its protein binding sites and potentiate its effects; phenylbutazone has also been reported to potentiate the effects of sulfonamides)

Other medications, oral, especially:
» Ciprofloxacin
» Enoxacin
» Itraconazole
» Ketoconazole
» Lomefloxacin
» Norfloxacin
» Ofloxacin
» Tetracyclines, oral
(antacids present in buffered phenylbutazone formulations may decrease absorption of many other orally administered medications by forming nonabsorbable complexes and/or increasing intragastric pH; if used concurrently, buffered phenylbutazone should be taken at least 6 hours before or 2 hours after ciprofloxacin or lomefloxacin, 8 hours before or 2 hours after enoxacin, 2 hours after itraconazole, 3 hours before or after ketoconazole, 2 hours before or after norfloxacin or ofloxacin, 1 to 3 hours before or after tetracycline, and at least 1 to 2 hours before or after other orally administered medications)

*For sulindac (in addition to those listed for all NSAIDs)*
  Antacids
    (concurrent chronic use may significantly decrease the plasma concentration of sulindac)

  Dimethyl sulfoxide (DMSO)
    (topical application of DMSO to arthritic joints [not recommended because safety and efficacy are unproven] by patients receiving sulindac has been reported to cause peripheral neuropathy and to decrease the plasma concentration of sulindac's active metabolite, thereby decreasing its efficacy)

*For tenoxicam (in addition to those listed for all NSAIDs)*
  Cholestyramine
    (cholestyramine decreased the average half-life of an intravenous dose of tenoxicam from 67.4 to 31.9 hours and increased the apparent clearance of tenoxicam by 105%)

*For tiaprofenic acid (in addition to those listed for all NSAIDs)*
  Anticonvulsants, hydantoin, especially
 »  Phenytoin
    (tiaprofenic acid may displace hydantoin anticonvulsants from their protein-binding sites, which may lead to an increase in the concentration of the unbound fraction and to toxicity; hydantoin dosage adjustment, based on monitoring of plasma concentrations and/or observed signs of toxicity, may be required)

**Laboratory value alterations**
The following have been selected on the basis of their potential clinical significance (possible effect in parentheses where appropriate)—not necessarily inclusive (» = major clinical significance):

With diagnostic test results
*For diflunisal*
  Salicylate concentrations, serum
    (diflunisal may produce falsely elevated serum salicylate values determined via the Abbott TDx fluorescence polarization immunoassay, the Trinder colorimetric assay, or the Du Pont *aca* method, despite the fact that diflunisal is not metabolized to salicylate *in vivo*)

*For etodolac*
  Bilirubin, urine, determinations
    (phenolic metabolites of etodolac may cause false-positive test results)
  Ketones, urine, determinations
    (false-positive test results may occur with dipstick method of determination)

*For fenoprofen*
  Triiodothyronine ($T_3$) determinations
    (fenoprofen may interfere with total and free $T_3$ determinations in the Amerlex-M kit assay; thyroid stimulating hormone, total thyroxine, and thyrotropin releasing hormone test responses are not affected)

*For indomethacin*
  Dexamethasone suppression test for endogenous depression
    (indomethacin may produce false-negative test results [i.e., no indication of endogenous depression] because plasma cortisol concentration is reduced to a greater extent than with dexamethasone alone)
  5-Hydroxyindoleacetic acid (5-HIAA), urinary, determinations
    (false 5-HIAA concentration values may be measured via the Goldenberg modification of Undenfriend's method because indomethacin metabolites are structurally similar to 5-HIAA)

*For ketoprofen*
  Albumin, urine, determinations and
  Bile salts, urine, determinations and
  17-Ketosteroid (17-KS), urine, determinations and
  17-Hydroxycorticosteroid (17-OHCS), urine, determinations
    (ketoprofen metabolites in urine may interfere with test procedures that rely on acid precipitation as an end point or on color reactions of carbonyl groups; no interference occurs in tests for urinary protein using commercially available dye-impregnated test strips)

*For mefenamic acid*
  Bile, urinary, determinations
    (false-positive test results may occur when the diazo tablet test is used; the Harrison test is not affected)

*For naproxen*
  5-HIAA, urine, determinations
    (naproxen may interfere with some assays)

  Steroid, urine, determinations
    (17-ketogenic steroid concentrations may be falsely increased by naproxen when *m*-dinitrobenzene reagent is used; although 17-hydroxycorticosteroid measurements are not significantly altered when the Porter-Silber test is used, naproxen therapy should be discontinued 72 hours before adrenal function tests are performed)

*For phenylbutazone*
  Thyroid function tests
    (phenylbutazone may decrease 24-hour $^{131}$I thyroidal uptake [effect lasts about 14 days] or increase resin or red cell $T_3$ uptake)

*For tolmetin*
  Protein, urine, determinations
    (the metabolites of tolmetin in urine produce false-positive tests for urine protein when the sulfosalicylic acid method is used; no interference occurs in tests for urine protein when commercially available dye-impregnated reagent strips are used)

With physiology/laboratory test values
  Bleeding time
    (may be prolonged by most NSAIDs [with ketoprofen, by 3 to 4 minutes above baseline values] because of suppressed platelet aggregation; effects may persist for less than 1 day [flurbiprofen, ibuprofen, indomethacin, sulindac], 2 days [tolmetin], 4 days [naproxen], or 2 weeks [oxaprozin and piroxicam] following discontinuation of therapy)
    (effects on platelet aggregation and bleeding time appear minimal with usual doses of diclofenac, meclofenamate, or mefenamic acid, up to 1000 mg twice a day of diflunisal, or up to 1000 mg per day of nabumetone)

  Glucose concentrations
    (decrease in blood glucose concentration has been reported with ibuprofen, indomethacin, and piroxicam)
    (increase in blood glucose concentration has been reported with indomethacin, phenylbutazone, piroxicam, and sulindac)
    (increase in urine glucose concentration has also been reported with indomethacin)

  Hematocrit or
  Hemoglobin
    (values may be decreased, possibly because of gastrointestinal bleeding or microbleeding and/or hemodilution caused by fluid retention)

  Leukocyte count and
  Platelet count
    (may be decreased)

  Liver function tests, including:
  Alkaline phosphatase, serum and
  Lactate dehydrogenase (LDH), serum and
  Transaminases, serum
    (values may be increased; liver function test abnormalities may return to normal despite continued use; however, if significant abnormalities occur, clinical signs and symptoms consistent with liver disease develop, or systemic manifestations such as eosinophilia or rash occur, the medication should be discontinued)
    (the incidence of significantly increased transaminase values is higher with diclofenac than with other NSAIDs; in clinical trials with diclofenac, elevations to more than 3 times the upper limit of normal occurred with overall rates of 2% in patients treated for 2 months and 4% in patients treated for 2 to 6 months; values in excess of 8 times the upper limit of normal occurred in approximately 1% of the patients)

  Plasma renin activity (PRA)
    (indomethacin has been reported to decrease PRA and to block the increase in PRA usually produced by bumetanide, furosemide, or indapamide)

  Potassium, serum, concentrations
    (may be increased)

  Protein, urine (including albumin) concentrations
    (increases have been reported with diclofenac, diflunisal, indomethacin, phenylbutazone, piroxicam, sulindac, tenoxicam, and tolmetin)

  Renal function tests, including:
  Blood urea nitrogen (BUN)
  Creatinine, serum
  Electrolyte, blood and urine, concentrations
  Urine volume
    (NSAIDs may decrease renal function, resulting in increased BUN, serum creatinine, and serum electrolyte concentrations and in decreased urine volume and urine electrolyte concentrations; how-

ever, in some cases, water retention may exceed that of sodium, resulting in dilutional hyponatremia)

Uric acid concentrations
(serum concentrations may be decreased and urine concentrations increased by diclofenac, diflunisal, etodolac, oxaprozin, and phenylbutazone; in clinical trials with etodolac, the serum concentration was usually decreased by 1 to 2 mg per 100 mL [59 to 118 micromoles/L] after 4 weeks of therapy with 600 to 1000 mg per day and the reduction was maintained during the study period)

*For mefenamic acid only*
Prothrombin time
(may be prolonged)

## Medical considerations/Contraindications
The medical considerations/contraindications included here have been selected on the basis of their potential clinical significance (reasons given in parentheses where appropriate)—not necessarily inclusive (» = major clinical significance).

*Except under special circumstances, this medication should not be used when the following medical problems exist:*

*For all NSAIDs*
» Allergic reaction, severe, such as anaphylaxis or angioedema, induced by aspirin or other NSAIDs, history of or
» Nasal polyps associated with bronchospasm, aspirin-induced
(high risk of severe allergic reactions because of cross-sensitivity)

*For diclofenac (in addition to those listed for all NSAIDs)*
» Blood dyscrasias, active or history of or
» Bone marrow depression
(diclofenac may induce or exacerbate these conditions)

*For phenylbutazone (in addition to those listed for all NSAIDs)*
» Blood dyscrasias, active or history of or
» Bone marrow depression
(phenylbutazone may induce or exacerbate these conditions)

» Cardiac disease, severe or
» Cardiac failure, incipient or
» Cardiopulmonary disease, severe
(sodium and fluid retention caused by phenylbutazone may increase plasma volume and the risk of edema, acute pulmonary edema, and cardiac decompensation)

» Hepatic disease, severe or
» Renal disease, severe
(increased phenylbutazone blood concentrations and potential for toxicity may result from decreased clearance; also, potential for adverse renal effects may be increased in the presence of pre-existing severe hepatic or renal disease)

» Peptic ulcer disease, active
(may be exacerbated; increased risk of perforation and/or bleeding)

*Risk-benefit should be considered when the following medical problems exist:*

*For all NSAIDs*
Allergic reaction, mild, such as allergic rhinitis, urticaria, or skin rash, induced by aspirin or other NSAIDs, history of
(possibility of cross-sensitivity)

Anemia or
Asthma
(may be exacerbated)

Conditions predisposing to and/or exacerbated by fluid retention, such as:
Compromised cardiac function
Congestive heart disease
Edema, pre-existing
Hypertension
Renal function impairment or failure
(NSAIDs may cause fluid retention and edema)

Conditions predisposing to gastrointestinal toxicity, such as:
Alcoholism, active
» Inflammatory or ulcerative disease of the upper or lower gastrointestinal tract, including Crohn's disease, diverticulitis, peptic ulcer disease, or ulcerative colitis, active or history of
Tobacco use, or recent history of
(NSAIDs should preferably not be given to patients with active peptic ulcer disease or gastrointestinal bleeding; if NSAID administration is considered essential, an antiulcer regimen should be administered concurrently)

(caution and close supervision are also recommended for other patients in whom there is a significant risk of gastrointestinal toxicity; misoprostol or sucralfate should be considered as prophylaxis for those at high risk)

Congestive heart failure or
Diabetes mellitus or
Edema, pre-existing or
Extracellular volume depletion or
Sepsis
(increased risk of renal failure)

» Hemophilia or other bleeding problems including coagulation or platelet function disorders
(increased risk of bleeding because most NSAIDs inhibit platelet aggregation and may cause gastrointestinal ulceration or hemorrhage; although the risk of these problems is lower with nabumetone than with most other NSAIDs, caution is recommended)

Hepatic cirrhosis or
Hepatic function impairment
(risk of renal failure is increased in patients with hepatic function impairment)

(most NSAIDs are metabolized hepatically; impairment of metabolism may be particularly problematic for nabumetone, since metabolism to the active metabolite 6-MNA may be decreased sufficiently to reduce efficacy)

(although stable hepatic cirrhosis does not alter the clearance of etodolac, the possibility should be considered that unstable hepatic disease or severe hepatic function impairment may do so)

(hepatic function impairment, especially if associated with chronic alcoholic cirrhosis, produces variability in ketoprofen pharmacokinetics and reduces ketoprofen protein binding; the concentration of unbound ketoprofen may be doubled; caution and careful monitoring are recommended; also, only immediate-release ketoprofen dosage forms should be used if the patient's serum albumin is lower than 3.5 grams per deciliter)

(hepatic cirrhosis, especially if associated with chronic alcoholism, increases the concentration of unbound naproxen, even though the total plasma concentration may be decreased; the lowest effective dose should be administered and the patient carefully monitored)

(although the clearance of oxaprozin is not altered by well-compensated hepatic cirrhosis, caution is recommended in patients with severe hepatic function impairment)

(biotransformation of sulindac to the active sulfide metabolite is slowed; however, biliary elimination of the metabolite is greatly decreased, leading to increased and prolonged plasma concentrations and increased risk of toxicity; the patient should be carefully monitored and dosage adjusted as necessary)

Renal function impairment
(increased risk of hyperkalemia and of adverse renal effects, including acute renal failure; especially careful monitoring of the patient is recommended)

(NSAIDs and/or their metabolites are excreted primarily via the kidneys; a reduction in dosage may be required to prevent accumulation)

(etodolac has not been shown to increase the risk of renal toxicity, and the pharmacokinetic profile of etodolac is not altered, when up to 500 mg of etodolac is administered every 12 hours to patients with mild to moderate renal function impairment; however, the possibility of renal toxicity associated with a reduction of renal prostaglandin synthesis leading to a decrease in renal blood flow cannot be discounted; caution and monitoring of patients considered to be at risk are recommended)

(although less than 1% of the active 6-MNA metabolite of nabumetone is eliminated in the urine unchanged, and increased concentrations of 6-MNA were not measured after administration of a single dose, caution is recommended in patients with renal function impairment because the extent to which metabolites may accumulate and cause adverse effects has not been determined)

(in end-stage renal disease, conversion of sulindac to its active metabolite is decreased)

» Renal function impairment
(the risk of toxicity associated with accumulation of the NSAID and/or the risk of adverse renal effects may be higher with diflunisal, fenoprofen, indomethacin, and piroxicam than with other NSAIDs; individualization of dosage and especially careful monitoring of the patient are recommended)

» Stomatitis
(may be induced by NSAIDs; this symptom of possible NSAID-induced blood dyscrasias may be masked by pre-existing stomatitis)

Systemic lupus erythematosus (SLE)
(patient may be predisposed to NSAID-induced central nervous system and/or renal adverse effects)

» Caution is also recommended in geriatric patients, who may be more likely to develop adverse hepatic or renal effects with these medications and in whom gastrointestinal ulceration or bleeding is more likely to cause serious consequences, including fatalities.

Caution is also recommended when an NSAID, especially fenoprofen, is used in patients who developed genitourinary tract problems such as dysuria, cystitis, hematuria, nephritis, or nephrotic syndrome during treatment with another NSAID.

The sodium content of diclofenac sodium, meclofenamate sodium, naproxen sodium, naproxen oral suspension, and tolmetin sodium should be considered when selecting an NSAID for patients who must restrict their sodium intake.

*For diclofenac (in addition to those listed for all NSAIDs)*
Porphyria, hepatic
(diclofenac may precipitate an acute attack)

*For indomethacin (in addition to those listed for all NSAIDs)*
Epilepsy or
» Mental depression or other psychiatric disturbances or
Parkinsonism
(indomethacin may aggravate these conditions)

*For mefenamic acid (in addition to those listed for all NSAIDs)*
» Hypoprothrombinemia, when prothrombin activity is 10 to 20% of normal
(increased risk of bleeding, since mefenamic acid may further increase the prothrombin time)

*For phenylbutazone (in addition to those listed for all NSAIDs)*
» Polymyalgia rheumatica or
» Temporal arteritis
(phenylbutazone may aggravate these conditions)

*For sulindac (in addition to those listed for all NSAIDs)*
» Renal calculus or history of
(renal calculi containing sulindac metabolites have occurred, rarely, in patients receiving sulindac; it is recommended that the medication be used with caution, and in conjunction with adequate fluid intake, in patients who may be predisposed to calculus formation)

*For rectal administration (in addition to those listed as applying to oral use of the NSAIDs with rectal dosage forms)*
» Bleeding, rectal or anal, active or recent history of or
» Hemorrhoids or
» Lesions, inflammatory, of anus or rectum or
» Proctitis or recent history of
(may be exacerbated or reactivated)

**Patient monitoring**
The following may be especially important in patient monitoring (other tests may be warranted in some patients, depending on condition; » = major clinical significance):

Blood urea nitrogen (BUN) determinations or
Creatinine concentrations, serum and/or
Potassium concentrations, serum
(monitoring may be required at periodic intervals during therapy, especially in patients with documented hepatic or renal function impairment, other patients known or suspected to be at risk for renal function impairment, and/or those taking diuretics concurrently; also, may be required if signs of possible renal toxicity, such as substantial increases in blood pressure, fluid retention, or rapid weight gain occur)

Complete physical examinations, including urinalyses
(recommended prior to and at regular frequent intervals during phenylbutazone therapy)

Hematocrit determinations and/or
Hemoglobin determinations and/or
Stool tests for occult blood loss
(may be performed at one- to six-month intervals to detect blood loss during prolonged therapy, depending on the individual patient's risk of developing gastrointestinal toxicity; however, these tests [unlike endoscopy, which is not recommended on a routine basis] are not capable of detecting ulcerations that are developing asymptomatically or of predicting whether severe gastrointestinal bleeding is likely to occur)

» Hematologic determinations
(recommended prior to initiation of phenylbutazone therapy and at regular intervals of 3 to 4 weeks during therapy for patients receiving the medication for periods longer than 1 week)
(although routine monitoring is not necessary during therapy with other NSAIDs, appropriate testing should be performed if symptoms of blood dyscrasias occur)

Liver function tests, especially determination of transaminase (AST [SGOT]; ALT [SGPT]) values
(may be required at periodic intervals during indomethacin therapy; also, it is recommended that hepatic function tests be performed within eight weeks following initiation of diclofenac therapy and periodically thereafter)
(may also be required at periodic intervals during therapy with other NSAIDs if the patient is known or suspected to be at increased risk of developing hepatic adverse effects)
(although routine monitoring is not necessary for most patients during therapy with NSAIDs other than diclofenac or indomethacin, appropriate tests should be performed if signs and/or symptoms of hepatotoxicity occur)

Ophthalmologic examinations
(may be required if vision problems such as blurred vision occur during therapy)

Upper gastrointestinal diagnostic tests
(recommended for patients with persistent or severe dyspepsia or other signs of possible gastrointestinal toxicity)

## Side/Adverse Effects

See also *Table 3*, page 417.

Note: *Hypersensitivity reactions* with these medications may be similar to those reported for aspirin, i.e., *rhinosinusitis/asthma* or *angioedema/urticaria. Anaphylaxis* has also been reported, both in aspirin-sensitive patients and in those without known hypersensitivity to any of these agents. The risk of anaphylaxis, characterized by respiratory distress, circulatory collapse, and angioedema and/or urticaria with or without pruritus, may be increased when previously discontinued therapy with one of these medications is reinstituted. Although anaphylaxis occurs rarely with these agents, several reports have indicated a higher incidence of anaphylactic reactions with tolmetin than with the others.

Other *hypersensitivity reactions* affecting multiple body systems have also been reported with several of the NSAIDs. A hypersensitivity syndrome consisting of fever and chills, skin rashes or other cutaneous manifestations, hepatotoxicity, renal toxicity (including renal failure), leukopenia, thrombocytopenia, eosinophilia, inflamed glands or lymph nodes, and arthralgias has been reported rarely with diflunisal and with sulindac. Fever, skin rashes, and arthralgias have also preceded fenoprofen-induced renal toxicity. In addition, a syndrome of fever and chills, nausea, vomiting, and abdominal pain has been reported with ibuprofen, and a serum sickness– or influenza-like syndrome that may consist of troubled breathing, arthralgias, fever and chills, fatigue, pruritus, and/or skin rash or other cutaneous manifestations, has been reported with ibuprofen (although a positive causal relationship has not been established), meclofenamate, phenylbutazone, piroxicam, and tolmetin.

The antipyretic, analgesic, and anti-inflammatory actions of NSAIDs may mask symptoms of the occurrence or worsening of infections. *Reactivation of latent pulmonary tuberculosis* has been reported in a few patients receiving indomethacin.

Two cases of *biliary obstruction* associated with sulindac therapy have been reported. The obstruction was caused in each case by the presence in the common bile duct of a ''sludge'' of crystals containing a sulindac metabolite.

*Metabolic acidosis* and *respiratory alkalosis* have also been reported rarely (incidences < 1%) with phenylbutazone.

Patients 40 years of age and older may be more susceptible to the toxic effects of phenylbutazone. In patients 60 years of age and older, there is an increased risk of severe, possibly fatal, toxic reactions.

Phenylbutazone-induced *agranulocytosis* may occur with a rapid onset, especially in relatively young patients. *Aplastic anemia* may occur more frequently in patients receiving prolonged therapy, especially older female patients. Both *agranulocytosis* and *aplastic anemia* are more likely to occur in geriatric patients.

Because diflunisal is a salicylic acid derivative, the possibility that it may be associated with the development of *Reye's syndrome* in children, teenagers, or young adults with acute febrile illnesses, especially influenza or varicella, should be kept in mind.

The following side/adverse effects have been selected on the basis of their potential clinical significance (possible signs and symptoms in parentheses where appropriate)—not necessarily inclusive:

# Overdose

For specific information on the agents used in the mangement of anti-inflammatory agents, nonsteroidal overdose, see:

- *Diazepam* in *Benzodiazepines (Systemic)* monograph;
- *Dopamine* or *Dobutamine* in *Sympathomimetic Agents—Cardiovascular Use (Parenteral-Systemic)* monograph; and/or
- *Vitamin K₁—Phytonadione* in *Vitamin K (Systemic)* monograph.

For more information on the management of overdose or unintentional ingestion, **contact a Poison Control Center** (see *Poison Control Center Listing*).

## Clinical effects of overdose

The following effects have been selected on the basis of their potential clinical significance (possible signs and symptoms in parentheses where appropriate)—not necessarily inclusive:

Acute and chronic

For phenylbutazone

*Bluish color of fingernails, lips, or skin; convulsions, especially in children; difficulty in hearing or ringing or buzzing in the ears; dizziness or lightheadedness; hallucinations; headache, severe and continuing; increase or decrease in blood pressure; mood or mental changes; nausea, vomiting, or stomach pain, severe; periorbital edema* (swelling around the eyes); *shortness of breath, troubled breathing, or unusually slow, fast, or irregular breathing; swelling of face, hands, feet, or lower legs*

Note: The lowest fatal doses reported for phenylbutazone are 14 grams (in an adult) and 2 grams (in a 3-year-old child). The highest doses reported to have been survived are 40 grams (in a young adult) and 5 grams (in a 3-year-old child).

Laboratory findings in overdose may reveal respiratory or metabolic acidosis or alkalosis, other electrolyte disturbances, impaired hepatic or renal function, and abnormalities of formed blood elements.

Late manifestations of massive overdosage may occur 2 to 7 days following ingestion and may include hepatomegaly, jaundice, electrocardiographic abnormalities, blood dyscrasias, and ulceration of the buccal or gastrointestinal mucosa.

For other NSAIDs

Note: The symptoms of overdose of most of the other NSAIDs have not been described as completely as for phenylbutazone. Reported symptoms have generally reflected the gastrointestinal, renal, and CNS toxicities of these medications. Following overdosage with a propionic acid derivative or indomethacin, patients may remain asymptomatic or experience only relatively mild *CNS effects* (e.g., lethargy, drowsiness) or *gastrointestinal symptoms* (e.g., abdominal pain, nausea, vomiting). However, more serious effects, such as *gastrointestinal hemorrhage, acute renal failure, convulsions,* and *coma* have been reported with these, as well as other, NSAIDs. *Convulsions* may be especially likely to occur following mefenamic acid overdose. Also, *hypoprothrombinemia* has been reported following overdose of several NSAIDs.

## Treatment of overdose

To decrease absorption—Emptying the stomach via induction of emesis (in alert patients only) or gastric lavage. However, syrup of ipecac may induce symptoms similar to those of NSAID toxicity, which may complicate diagnosis, and is therefore not recommended for induction of emesis.

Administering activated charcoal. The efficacy of activated charcoal in decreasing absorption of these medications when given more than 2 hours (6 hours for piroxicam) following ingestion of the overdose has not been determined. However, there is some evidence that repeated administration of activated charcoal may interrupt enterohepatic circulation and/or bind any of the medication that has diffused from the circulation into the intestine, thereby increasing nonrenal excretion.

To enhance elimination—Administering antacids or other urinary alkalizers may increase diflunisal or sulindac excretion. Antacids may also relieve adverse gastrointestinal effects.

Instituting symptomatic and other supportive treatment as necessary. Certain adverse effects of NSAIDs, including nephritis or nephrotic syndrome, thrombocytopenia, hemolytic anemia, and severe cutaneous or other hypersensitivity reactions, may respond to glucocorticoid administration.

Inducing diuresis may be helpful in overdosage with fenoprofen, ibuprofen, or tolmetin; however, furosemide does not lower fenoprofen blood concentration.

Hemodialysis may be necessary to treat renal failure, but cannot be relied upon to decrease plasma concentrations of most NSAIDs because of their high degree of protein binding. Studies have shown that diclofenac and ketoprofen are dialyzable, but that diflunisal, etodolac, ibuprofen, indomethacin, and oxaprozin are not.

Specific treatment—

For severe hypotension plasma:

Use of volume expanders

For convulsions:

Diazepam or other appropriate benzodiazepine anticonvulsants. See the package insert or *Diazepam* in *Benzodiazepines (Systemic)* for specific dosing guidelines for use of this product.

For hypoprothrombinemia:

Vitamin K₁. See the package insert or *Vitamin K₁—Phytonadione* in *Vitamin K (Systemic)* for specific dosing guidelines for use of this product.

For prevention or reversal of early indications of, renal failure:

Use of dopamine plus dobutamine intravenously. See the package insert or *Dopamine* or *Dobutamine* in *Sympathomimetic Agents—Cardiovascular Use (Parenteral-Systemic)* for specific dosing guidelines for use of this product.

Monitoring—The possibility must be considered that gastrointestinal ulceration or hemorrhage, and phenylbutazone-induced blood dyscrasias, may occur several days after ingestion of an overdose. Patients being discharged after initial treatment should be informed of possible presenting symptoms and advised to seek immediate treatment if they occur.

Supportive care—Monitoring and supporting vital functions. If respiratory support is required following phenylbutazone overdose, respiratory stimulants should not be used. Patients in whom intentional overdose is known or suspected should be referred for psychiatric consultation.

# Patient Consultation

As an aid to patient consultation, refer to *Advice for the Patient, Anti-inflammatory Drugs, Nonsteroidal (Systemic)*.

In providing consultation, consider emphasizing the following selected information (» = major clinical significance):

**Before using this medication**

» Conditions affecting use, especially:

Allergies to aspirin or any of the nonsteroidal anti-inflammatory drugs (NSAIDs)

Pregnancy—Use of an NSAID during second half of pregnancy not recommended because of potential adverse effect on fetal blood flow and possible prolongation of pregnancy, dystocia, and difficult and/or delayed delivery

Breast-feeding—*For indomethacin:* Has caused convulsions in a nursing infant

*For meclofenamate and piroxicam:* These NSAIDs have caused adverse effects in animal studies

*For phenylbutazone:* May cause blood dyscrasias or other adverse effects in the infant

Use in children—*For indomethacin:* Because of toxicity, should be used with caution and only in patients unresponsive to less toxic NSAIDs

*For naproxen:* Skin rash more common in pediatric patients

*For phenylbutazone:* Because of toxicity, not recommended in children < 15 years of age

Use in the elderly—Increased risk of toxicity; initial dosage should be reduced and patients carefully monitored

Other medications, especially—

*For all NSAIDs:* Anticoagulants, aspirin, cephalosporins that may induce hypoprothrombinemia, cyclosporine, lithium, methotrexate, plicamycin, probenecid, triamterene, and valproic acid

*For indomethacin (in addition to those applying to all NSAIDs):* Zidovudine

*For phenylbutazone (in addition to those applying to all NSAIDs):* Digitalis, penicillamine, and phenytoin

*For buffered phenylbutazone (in addition to those applying to all NSAIDs and to phenylbutazone):* Ciprofloxacin, enoxacin, itraconazole, ketoconazole, lomefloxacin, norfloxacin, ofloxacin, and oral tetracyclines

*For tiaprofenic acid (in addition to those applying to all NSAIDs):* Phenytoin

Other medical problems, especially—

*For all NSAIDs:* Blood dyscrasias, bone marrow depression, cardiac or cardiopulmonary disease or predisposition to, clotting defects, hepatic disease, peptic ulcer or other inflammatory or ulcerative gastrointestinal tract disease or predisposition to, renal disease or predisposition to, and stomatitis

*For indomethacin (in addition to those applying to all NSAIDs):* Epilepsy, mental illness, and parkinsonism

*For phenylbutazone (in addition to those applying to all NSAIDs):* Polymyalgia rheumatica and temporal arteritis

*For sulindac (in addition to those applying to all NSAIDs):* Renal calculus or history of

*For rectal dosage forms (in addition to those applying to oral use of the NSAIDs with rectal dosage forms):* Anal or rectal bleeding, hemorrhoids, inflammatory lesions of anus or rectum, and proctitis or recent history of

## Proper use of this medication

*For all NSAIDs*

» Not taking more medication than prescribed or recommended on OTC package label

» For use in arthritis—Compliance with therapy; noticeable improvement in condition usually requires a few days to a week of treatment (but up to 2 weeks, and sometimes even longer, in severe cases) and maximum effectiveness may require several weeks of treatment

» Proper dosing

Missed dose (scheduled dosing): If dosing schedule is—

Once or twice a day: Taking as soon as possible if remembered within one or two hours after dose should have been taken; skipping dose if not remembered until later

More than twice a day: Taking as soon as possible; not taking if almost time for next dose; not doubling doses

» Proper storage

*For all capsule and tablet dosage forms*

Taking with a full glass of water and not lying down for 15 to 30 minutes after taking

*For indomethacin, mefenamic acid, phenylbutazone, and piroxicam*

» Taking oral dosage forms with meals or antacids (a magnesium– and aluminum-containing antacid may be preferred) to reduce gastrointestinal irritation

*For flurbiprofen extended-release tablets, nabumetone, and naproxen extended-release tablets*

Taking with food or antacids (a magnesium- and aluminum-containing antacid may be preferred) to reduce gastrointestinal irritation; taking with food also increases absorption

*For immediate-release and extended-release oral dosage forms of NSAIDs not listed above*

Taking with food or antacids (a magnesium- and aluminum-containing antacid may be preferred) to reduce gastrointestinal irritation, although when used for acute conditions (e.g., pain, gout, fever, or dysmenorrhea) the first 1 or 2 doses may be taken on an empty stomach to speed the onset of action

*For oral suspensions*

Not mixing suspension with an antacid or other liquid prior to use

*For delayed-release (enteric-coated) or extended-release dosage forms, diflunisal tablets, and all phenylbutazone tablet formulations*

Swallowing whole; not breaking, chewing or crushing before swallowing

*For all suppository dosage forms*

Proper administration technique

*For indomethacin suppositories*

Retaining in rectum for 1 full hour to ensure maximum absorption

*For nonprescription use of ibuprofen or naproxen*

» Reading patient information sheet provided in package

*For phenylbutazone*

» Taking for prescribed indications only; not taking to relieve other aches and pains

*For mefenamic acid*

» Not taking longer than 7 days at a time unless otherwise directed by physician

## Precautions while using this medication

» Regular visits to physician during prolonged therapy

» Possibility that use of alcohol may increase the risk of ulceration and, with phenylbutazone, depressant effects

Not taking 2 or more NSAIDs, including ketorolac, concurrently, and not taking acetaminophen or aspirin or other salicylates for more than a few days while receiving NSAID therapy, unless concurrent use is prescribed by, and patient remains under the care of, a physician or dentist

Caution if any surgery is required because of possible enhanced bleeding (although may be less of a problem with diclofenac, diflunisal, meclofenamate, mefenamic acid, and nabumetone)

Caution if confusion, dizziness or lightheadedness, drowsiness, or vision problems occur

» Possibility of photosensitivity

Possibility of gastrointestinal ulceration and bleeding

» Notifying physician immediately if influenza-like symptoms (chills, fever, or muscle aches and pains) occur shortly prior to or together with a skin rash; rarely, these symptoms may indicate a serious reaction to the medication

Possibility of anaphylaxis

*For buffered phenylbutazone*

» Not taking within:

—6 hours before or 2 hours after ciprofloxacin or lomefloxacin

—8 hours before or 2 hours after enoxacin

—2 hours after itraconazole

—3 hours before or after ketoconazole

—2 hours before or after norfloxacin or ofloxacin

—1 to 3 hours before or after an oral tetracycline

*For mefenamic acid*

Discontinuing use and checking with physician if severe diarrhea occurs

*For nonprescription use of ibuprofen or naproxen*

Checking with health care professional if symptoms do not improve or if they worsen, if using for fever and fever lasts more than 3 days or returns, or if painful area is red or swollen

## Side/adverse effects

» Stopping medication and obtaining emergency treatment if symptoms of any of the following occur

*For all NSAIDs*

Anaphylaxis, angioedema, or bronchospasm

» Stopping medication and checking with physician immediately if symptoms of the following occur

*For all NSAIDs*

Spitting up blood, unexplained nosebleeds, chest pain, convulsions, fainting, gastrointestinal ulceration or bleeding, and blood dyscrasias

*For mefenamic acid (in addition to those applying to all NSAIDs)*

Diarrhea

*For phenylbutazone (in addition to those applying to all NSAIDs)*

Edema

Signs and symptoms of other potential side effects, especially

*For all NSAIDs*

Dysarthria, hallucinations, aseptic meningitis, migraine, mood or mental changes, peripheral neuropathy, syncope, or other central nervous system effects; dermatitis (allergic or exfoliative), Stevens-Johnson syndrome, or other dermatologic effects; colitis, dysphagia, esophagitis, gastritis, gastroenteritis, or other digestive system effects; crystalluria, urinary tract irritation or infection, or other genitourinary effects; anemia or hypocoagulation; hepatitis; angiitis, fever, allergic rhinitis, or other hypersensitivity reactions not listed previously; loosening or splitting of fingernails; lymphadenopathy; vision problems, conjunctivitis, or other ocular effects; stomatitis, glossitis, or other oral/perioral effects; hearing problems or tinnitus; pancreatitis; and edema, hyperkalemia, polyuria, renal impairment or failure, or other renal effects

*For indomethacin (in addition to those applying to all NSAIDs)* Headache (severe), especially in the morning

Possibility that the following may occur many days or weeks after medication is discontinued

*For phenylbutazone*

Blood dyscrasias

## General Dosing Information

The sodium content of diclofenac sodium, meclofenamate sodium, naproxen sodium, naproxen oral suspension, and tolmetin sodium should be considered when selecting a nonsteroidal anti-inflammatory drug (NSAID) for patients who must restrict their sodium intake. Also, the sucrose content of ibuprofen and naproxen suspensions must be considered when selecting an NSAID for patients who must restrict their sucrose intake.

Patients who do not respond to one NSAID may respond to another. In responsive patients, partial symptomatic relief of arthritic symptoms usually occurs within 1 or 2 weeks, although maximum effectiveness may occur only after several weeks of therapy.

A reduction of initial dosage, possibly to as low as one-half the usual adult dose, is recommended for geriatric patients, especially those 70 years of age or older. However, if the reduced dose fails to produce an adequate clinical response and the medication is well tolerated, dosage may be increased as required and tolerated.

A reduction of dosage may also be required to prevent accumulation of NSAIDs and/or their metabolites (some of which may be unstable and may be hydrolyzed to the parent compound when their excretion is delayed) in patients with renal function impairment.

Long-term use of NSAIDs in doses that approach or exceed maximum dosage recommendations should be considered only if the clinical benefit is increased sufficiently to offset the higher risk of gastrointestinal toxicity or other adverse effects.

Indomethacin, mefenamic acid, phenylbutazone, and piroxicam should be administered immediately after meals or with food or antacids to reduce gastrointestinal irritation. Flurbiprofen extended-release capsules, nabumetone, or naproxen extended-release tablets should also be taken with food to increase absorption as well as reduce gastrointestinal irritation. The other NSAIDs (except for delayed-release [enteric-coated] and rectal dosage forms) are also preferably taken after meals or with food or antacids to reduce gastrointestinal irritation, especially during chronic use; however, for faster absorption when a rapid initial effect is required (as for analgesic or antipyretic use), the first 1 or 2 doses may be taken 30 minutes before meals or at least 2 hours after meals. If an antacid is taken concurrently, an aluminum and magnesium-containing formulation may be preferred, since studies have shown that this formulation does not adversely affect absorption of most NSAIDs (See *Table 1*, page 411.

It is recommended that solid oral dosage forms of NSAIDs be taken with a full glass (240 mL) of water and that the patient remain in an upright position for 15 to 30 minutes after administration. These measures may reduce the risk of tablets or capsules becoming lodged in the esophagus, which has been reported to cause prolonged esophageal irritation and difficulty in swallowing in some patients receiving these medications.

In the treatment of primary dysmenorrhea, maximum benefit is achieved by initiating NSAID therapy as rapidly as possible after the onset of menses. Prophylactic therapy (i.e., starting NSAID administration a few days prior to the expected onset of the menstrual period) has not been found to provide additional therapeutic benefit.

Concurrent use of an NSAID with an opioid analgesic provides additive analgesia and may permit lower doses of the opioid analgesic to be utilized.

The analgesic activity of non-opioid analgesics is subject to a ceiling effect. Therefore, administration of an NSAID in higher-than-recommended analgesic doses may not provide additional therapeutic benefit in the treatment of pain not associated with inflammation.

In the treatment of arthritis, most of these agents have been shown to provide additional symptomatic relief when administered concurrently with gold compounds or glucocorticoids. NSAIDs may permit reduction of glucocorticoid dosage; however, reductions of glucocorticoid dosage, especially following long-term use, should be gradual to avoid symptoms associated with adrenal insufficiency or other manifestations of too-sudden withdrawal.

---

## *DICLOFENAC*

## Summary of Differences

Indications:
Indicated for rheumatoid arthritis, osteoarthritis, and ankylosing spondylitis. Immediate-release tablets only indicated for pain and primary dysmenorrhea, and may also be used to relieve acute attacks of gout or calcium pyrophosphate deposition disease (pseudogout) and pain associated with nonrheumatic inflammatory conditions or vascular headaches.

Pharmacology/pharmacokinetics:
Physicochemical characteristics—Chemical group: A phenylacetic acid derivative.
Other actions/effects—
With usual doses, has lesser effect on platelet aggregation than most NSAIDs.
Also has uricosuric activity.
Biotransformation—Almost 50% of a dose eliminated via first-pass metabolism.
Half-life—Elimination: 1.2–2 hours.
Onset of action—Pain: Tablets—30 minutes.
Duration of action—Pain: Tablets—Up to 8 hours.
Precautions:
Pregnancy/reproduction—Embryotoxicity and other adverse effects, but not teratogenicity, demonstrated in animal studies.

Surgical—With recommended doses may be less likely than most other NSAIDs to increase perisurgical bleeding.
Drug interactions and/or related problems—
Also, reported to increase digoxin plasma concentrations.
Also, concurrent use with potassium-sparing diuretics may cause hyperkalemia.
Also, reported to decrease effects of antidiabetic agents or insulin.
Laboratory value alterations—
With usual doses is less likely than most other NSAIDs to increase bleeding time significantly.
Higher incidence of transaminase values being elevated to > 3 times the upper limit of normal than with other NSAIDs.
Also, may decrease plasma concentration and increase urine concentration of uric acid.
Medical considerations/contraindications—
Not recommended for patients with blood dyscrasias (or history of) or bone marrow depression.
Caution also required in patients with hepatic porphyria; may precipitate an acute attack.
Caution with diclofenac sodium–containing dosage forms in patients who must restrict their sodium intake.
Patient monitoring—Routine liver function tests recommended.

Side/adverse effects:
See *Table 3*, page 417.

## Additional Dosing Information

See also *General Dosing Information*.

Diclofenac therapy should be discontinued if gastrointestinal bleeding or ulceration occurs.

### For oral dosage forms only

The delayed-release tablets and the extended-release tablets are to be swallowed whole, not crushed or chewed.

## Oral Dosage Forms

### DICLOFENAC POTASSIUM TABLETS

**Usual adult dose**

Analgesic and
Antidysmenorrheal—
Oral, 50 mg three times a day as needed. If necessary, 100 mg may be administered for the first dose only.

Rheumatoid arthritis—
Oral, 150 to 200 mg per day in three or four divided doses, initially. After a satisfactory response has been obtained, dosage should be reduced to the minimum dose that provides continuing control of symptoms, usually 75 to 100 mg a day in three divided doses.

Osteoarthritis—
Oral, 100 to 150 mg per day in two or three divided doses, initially. After a satisfactory response has been obtained, dosage should be reduced to the minimum dose that provides continuing control of symptoms.

Ankylosing spondylitis[1]:—
Oral, 100 to 125 mg a day in four or five divided doses, initially. After a satisfactory response has been obtained, dosage should be reduced to the minimum dose that provides continuing control of symptoms.

**Usual adult prescribing limits**

Analgesic and
Antidysmenorrheal—
Up to 200 mg on the first day, then 150 mg per day thereafter.

Rheumatoid arthritis—
225 mg per day.

Osteoarthritis—
150 mg per day; higher doses have not been studied.

**Usual pediatric dose**

Safety and efficacy have not been established.

**Strength(s) usually available**

U.S.—
25 mg (Rx) [*Cataflam* (calcium phosphate; colloidal silicon dioxide; iron oxides; magnesium stearate; microcrystalline cellulose; polyethylene glycol; povidone; sodium starch glycolate; starch; sucrose; talc; titanium dioxide)].

50 mg (Rx) [*Cataflam* (calcium phosphate; colloidal silicon dioxide; iron oxides; magnesium stearate; microcrystalline cellulose; polyethylene glycol; povidone; sodium starch glycolate; starch; sucrose; talc; titanium dioxide)].

Canada—
50 mg [*Voltaren Rapide* (carnauba wax; cellulose; colloidal silicon dioxide; corn starch; ferric oxide; magnesium stearate; polyethyl-

ene glycol; povidone; sodium carboxymethyl starch; sucrose; talc; titanium dioxide; tribasic calcium phosphate; white ink)].

**Packaging and storage**
Store below 30 °C (86 °F), in a tight container, unless otherwise directed by manufacturer. Protect from moisture.

**Auxiliary labeling**
• Take with food.
• Take with a full glass of water.
• Avoid alcoholic beverages.

## DICLOFENAC SODIUM DELAYED-RELEASE TABLETS

**Usual adult dose**
Analgesic
and Antidysmenorrheal—
    The delayed-release formulation is not recommended. See *Diclofenac Potassium Tablets*, which should be used for these indications.
Antirheumatic (nonsteroidal anti-inflammatory)—
    See *Diclofenac Potassium Tablets*.

**Usual pediatric dose**
Safety and efficacy have not been established.

**Strength(s) usually available**
U.S.—
    25 mg (Rx) [*Voltaren* (hydroxypropyl methylcellulose; iron oxide; lactose; magnesium stearate; methacrylic acid copolymer; microcrystalline cellulose; polyethylene glycol; povidone; propylene glycol; sodium hydroxide; sodium starch glycolate; talc; titanium dioxide; D&C Yellow #10 Aluminum Lake)].
    50 mg (Rx) [*Voltaren* (hydroxypropyl methylcellulose; iron oxide; lactose; magnesium stearate; methacrylic acid copolymer; microcrystalline cellulose; polyethylene glycol; povidone; propylene glycol; sodium hydroxide; sodium starch glycolate; talc; titanium dioxide; FD&C Blue #1 Aluminum Lake)].
    75 mg (Rx) [*Voltaren* (hydroxypropyl methylcellulose; iron oxide; lactose; magnesium stearate; methacrylic acid copolymer; microcrystalline cellulose; polyethylene glycol; povidone; propylene glycol; sodium hydroxide; sodium starch glycolate; talc; titanium dioxide)].
Canada—
    25 mg (Rx) [*Apo-Diclo* (sodium <1 mmol [1.81 mg]); *Novo-Difenac; Nu-Diclo* (sodium <1 mmol); *Voltaren* (lactose; sodium < 1 mmol [2.03 mg])].
    50 mg (Rx) [*Apo-Diclo* (sodium <1 mmol [3.62 mg]); ; *Novo-Difenac; Nu-Diclo* (sodium <1 mmol); *Voltaren* (lactose; sodium < 1 mmol [4.06 mg])].

**Packaging and storage**
Store below 30 °C (86 °F), in a tight container, unless otherwise specified by manufacturer. Protect from moisture.

**Auxiliary labeling**
• Swallow tablets whole.
• Take with a full glass of water.
• Avoid alcoholic beverages.

## DICLOFENAC SODIUM EXTENDED-RELEASE TABLETS

**Usual adult dose**
Antirheumatic (nonsteroidal anti-inflammatory)—
    Oral, 75 or 100 mg once a day, in the morning or evening, or 75 mg two times a day, in the morning and evening.

Note:  The extended-release dosage form is not intended as initial therapy; the daily maintenance dose should be determined using an immediate- or delayed-release formulation. The extended-release dosage form may then be used, if desired, provided that the required dose can be achieved with the available strengths.

**Usual pediatric dose**
Safety and efficacy have not been established.

**Strength(s) usually available**
U.S.—
    Not commercially available.
Canada—
    75 mg (Rx) [*Voltaren SR* (sodium < 1 mmol [6.1 mg])].
    100 mg (Rx) [*Novo-Difenac SR; Voltaren SR* (sodium < 1 mmol [8.13 mg])].

**Packaging and storage**
Store below 40 °C (104 °F), preferably between 15 and 30 °C (59 and 86 °F), unless otherwise specified by manufacturer.

**Auxiliary labeling**
• Take with food.
• Swallow tablets whole.

• Take with a full glass of water.
• Avoid alcoholic beverages.

## Rectal Dosage Forms
### DICLOFENAC SODIUM SUPPOSITORIES

**Usual adult dose**
Antirheumatic (nonsteroidal anti-inflammatory)—
    Rectal, 50 or 100 mg, as a substitute for the last oral dose of the day.

**Usual adult prescribing limits**
Total daily dosage (oral and rectal) should not exceed 150 mg.

**Usual pediatric dose**
Safety and efficacy have not been established.

**Strength(s) usually available**
U.S.—
    Not commercially available.
Canada—
    50 mg (Rx) [*Voltaren* (sodium < 1 mmol [4.06 mg])].
    100 mg (Rx) [*Voltaren* (sodium < 1 mmol [8.13 mg])].

**Packaging and storage**
Store below 40 °C (104 °F), preferably between 15 and 30 °C (59 and 86 °F), unless otherwise specified by manufacturer.

**Auxiliary labeling**
• Avoid alcoholic beverages.
• For rectal use.

¹Not included in Canadian product labeling.

---

*DIFLUNISAL*

## Summary of Differences
Indications:
    Indicated for rheumatoid arthritis, osteoarthritis, ankylosing spondylitis, and psoriatic arthritis, and pain. May also be used to relieve acute attacks of gout or calcium pyrophosphate deposition disease (pseudogout), dysmenorrhea, and pain associated with nonrheumatic inflammatory conditions or vascular headaches.
Pharmacology/pharmacokinetics:
    Physicochemical characteristics—Chemical group: A salicylate derivative, although not metabolized to salicylate *in vivo*.
    Other actions/effects—
        Platelet aggregation inhibition significant only with greater-than-recommended doses.
        Also has uricosuric activity.
    Half-life—Elimination: 8–12 hours; greatly prolonged by renal function impairment.
    Onset of action—Pain: 1 hour.
    Duration of action—Pain: 8–12 hours.
Precautions:
    Pregnancy/reproduction—Embryotoxic and teratogenic effects demonstrated in rabbits, but not found to be teratogenic in mice.
    Surgical—With recommended doses may be less likely than most other NSAIDs to increase perisurgical bleeding.
    Drug interactions and/or medical problems—
        Also, may increase risk of acetaminophen-induced hepatotoxicity.
        Also, chronic concurrent use of antacids significantly decreases diflunisal plasma concentration.
        Diflunisal also increases plasma concentration of hydrochlorothiazide and decreases hyperuricemic effect of hydrochlorothiazide or furosemide, but has not been shown to decrease furosemide-induced diuresis.
    Laboratory value alterations—
        Interference with salicylate determinations; may cause falsely elevated salicylate values.
        With usual doses is less likely than most other NSAIDs to increase bleeding time significantly.
        May decrease plasma concentrations and increase urine concentrations of uric acid.
    Medical considerations/contraindications—Higher risk than with most other NSAIDs in patients with renal function impairment.
Side/adverse effects:
    Reported to cause a characteristic hypersensitivity syndrome.
    Possibility of Reye's syndrome in children and adolescents with acute febrile illness should be considered (as with other salicylates).
    See also *Table 3*, page 417.

## Additional Dosing Information

See also *General Dosing Information.*

Administration of a 1-gram initial loading dose is recommended to provide faster onset of analgesic action, shorter time to peak analgesic effect, and greater peak analgesic action. For long-term use, the initial loading dose decreases the time needed to reach steady-state plasma concentrations; if a loading dose is not administered, 2 to 3 days may be required to evaluate changes in treatment regimens.

In patients with impaired renal function, especially if renal function is decreased to ¹/₂ the normal value or below, a reduction in dosage and/ or an increase in the dosing interval may be necessary to prevent diflunisal accumulation.

Tablets are to be swallowed whole, not crushed or chewed.

Because diflunisal is not hydrolyzed to salicylic acid *in vivo*, serum salicylate concentration cannot be used as a guide to dosage or potential toxicity during therapy.

## Oral Dosage Forms
### DIFLUNISAL TABLETS USP

#### Usual adult dose
Rheumatoid arthritis or
Osteoarthritis—
    Oral, 250 to 500 mg two times a day; dosage may be increased or decreased according to patient response.
Analgesic—
    Oral, 1 gram initially, followed by 500 mg every eight to twelve hours as needed.
    Note: For some patients, 500 mg initially followed by 250 mg every eight to twelve hours may be appropriate, depending on the severity of pain or the age, weight, or response of the patient.

#### Usual adult prescribing limits
Up to 1.5 grams daily.

#### Usual pediatric dose
Dosage has not been established.

#### Strength(s) usually available
U.S.—
    250 mg (Rx) [*Dolobid;* GENERIC].
    500 mg (Rx) [*Dolobid;* GENERIC (talc; titanium dioxide)].
Canada—
    250 mg (Rx) [*Apo-Diflunisal; Dolobid; Novo-Diflunisal*].
    500 mg (Rx) [*Apo-Diflunisal; Dolobid; Novo-Diflunisal*].

#### Packaging and storage
Store below 40 °C (104 °F), preferably between 15 and 30 °C (59 and 86 °F). Store in a well-closed container.

#### Auxiliary labeling
• Take with food.
• Swallow tablets whole.
• Take with a full glass of water.
• Avoid alcoholic beverages.

---

### *ETODOLAC*

## Summary of Differences

Indications:
    Indicated for treatment of osteoarthritis and for pain. May also be used to relieve acute attacks of gout or calcium pyrophosphate deposition disease (pseudogout), dysmenorrhea, and pain associated with nonrheumatic inflammatory conditions or vascular headaches.
Pharmacology:
    Physicochemical characteristics—Chemical group: A pyranoindole-acetic acid derivative.
    Other actions/effects—Also has uricosuric activity.
        Decreases renal function, but with administration of up to 500 mg every 12 hours recovery occurs prior to administration of next dose.
    Half-life—Elimination:
        Single dose—6–7 hours.
        At steady-state—7.3 ± 4 hours.
    Onset of action—Pain: 30 minutes.
    Time to peak effect—Pain: 1–2 hours.
    Duration of action—Pain:
        200-mg single dose—4–5 hours.
        400-mg single dose—Generally 5–6 hours; up to 8–12 hours in some patients.

Precautions:
    Pregnancy/reproduction—Alterations of limb development demonstrated in animal studies, but drug- or dose-response relationship not established.
    Geriatrics—No differences relative to younger adults in pharmacokinetic profile with 200 mg twice a day or in side effects profile with 600 mg per day.
    Laboratory value alterations—May cause false-positive test results in urinary bilirubin and urinary ketone determinations.
    Decrease in serum uric acid concentration may be expected.
    Medical considerations/contraindications: Significant problems have not been demonstrated in patients with mild to moderate renal function impairment receiving up to 500 mg every 12 hours.
Side/adverse effects:
    See *Table 3,* page 417.

## Oral Dosage Forms
### ETODOLAC CAPSULES

#### Usual adult dose
Antirheumatic (nonsteroidal anti-inflammatory)—
    Oral, 400 mg two or three times a day or 300 mg three or four times a day, initially. After a satisfactory response has been obtained, dosage should be individualized according to patient tolerance and response. Most patients are maintained on 600 to 1200 mg per day. However, as little as 200 mg two times a day has been effective in some patients.
    Note: Although doses of up to 1 gram per day have been effective when administered in two divided doses (500 mg every twelve hours), administration on a three-dose-a-day schedule may provide greater benefit.
Analgesic—
    Oral, 400 mg initially, then 200 to 400 mg every six to eight hours as needed. If a 400-mg dose fails to provide eight hours of analgesia, a regimen of 300 mg every six hours may be effective.

#### Usual adult prescribing limits
Patients weighing less than 60 kg—20 mg per kg of body weight per day.
Patients weighing 60 kg or more—1.2 grams per day.

#### Usual pediatric dose
Safety and efficacy have not been established.

#### Usual geriatric dose
See *Usual adult dose.*

#### Strength(s) usually available
U.S.—
    200 mg (Rx) [*Lodine* (cellulose; gelatin; iron oxides; lactose; magnesium stearate; povidone; sodium lauryl sulfate; sodium starch glycolate; titanium dioxide)].
    300 mg (Rx) [*Lodine* (cellulose; gelatin; iron oxides; lactose; magnesium stearate; povidone; sodium lauryl sulfate; sodium starch glycolate; titanium dioxide)].
Canada—
    Not commercially available.

#### Packaging and storage
Store below 40 °C (104 °F), preferably between 15 and 30 °C (59 and 86 °F), unless otherwise specified by manufacturer.

#### Auxiliary labeling
• Take with food.
• Take with a full glass of water.
• Avoid alcoholic beverages.

### ETODOLAC TABLETS

#### Usual adult dose
See *Etodolac Capsules.*

#### Usual adult prescribing limits
See *Etodolac Capsules.*

#### Usual pediatric dose
Safety and efficacy have not been established.

#### Usual geriatric dose
See *Etodolac Capsules.*

#### Strength(s) usually available
U.S.—
    400 mg (Rx) [*Lodine* (cellulose; FD&C Yellow #10; FD&C Blue #2; FD&C Yellow #6; hydroxypropyl methylcellulose; lactose; magnesium stearate; polyethylene glycol; polysorbate 80; povidone; sodium starch glycolate; titanium dioxide)].
Canada—
    Not commercially available.

**Packaging and storage**
Store below 40 °C (104 °F), preferably between 15 and 30 °C (59 and 86 °F), unless otherwise specified by manufacturer.

**Auxiliary labeling**
• Take with food.
• Take with a full glass of water.
• Avoid alcoholic beverages.

---

## FENOPROFEN

## Summary of Differences

Indications:
Indicated for rheumatoid arthritis, osteoarthritis, ankylosing spondylitis, and psoriatic arthritis; pain; and acute attacks of gout or calcium pyrophosphate deposition disease (pseudogout). May also be used to relieve dysmenorrhea and pain associated with nonrheumatic inflammatory conditions or vascular headaches. Also used for vascular headache prophylaxis.
Pharmacology/pharmacokinetics:
Physicochemical characteristics—Chemical group: A propionic acid derivative.
Half-life—Elimination: 3 hours.
Precautions:
Pregnancy/reproduction—No teratogenic or other adverse effects demonstrated in animal studies.
Drug interactions and/or related problems—Concurrent chronic use with antacids significantly decreases fenoprofen plasma concentration.
Also, phenobarbital may increase metabolism and decrease half-life of fenoprofen.
Laboratory value alterations—Interference with triiodothyronine ($T_3$) determinations using the Amerlex-M kit assay.
Medical considerations/contraindications—Higher risk than with most other NSAIDs in patients with renal function impairment.
Side/adverse effects:
See *Table 3*, page 417.

## Additional Dosing Information

See also *General Dosing Information*.

In the treatment of arthritis, improvement in condition may occur within a few days, but 2 to 3 weeks of continuous use on a regular basis may be required for maximum effectiveness.

## Oral Dosage Forms

Note: Bracketed uses in the *Dosage Forms* section refer to categories of use and/or indications that are not included in U.S. product labeling. The dosing and strengths of the available dosage forms are expressed in terms of the free acid (not the calcium salt).

### FENOPROFEN CALCIUM CAPSULES USP

**Usual adult dose**
Antirheumatic (nonsteroidal anti-inflammatory)—
Oral, 300 to 600 mg (free acid), depending on the severity of the symptoms, three or four times a day, then adjusted as needed.
Note: Higher doses generally are required in rheumatoid arthritis than in osteoarthritis.
Analgesic[1] or
[Antidysmenorrheal][1]—
Oral, 200 mg (free acid) every four to six hours as needed.

**Usual adult prescribing limits**
Antirheumatic (nonsteroidal anti-inflammatory)—
Up to 3.2 grams (free acid) daily.

**Usual pediatric dose**
Safety and dosage have not been established.

**Strength(s) usually available**
U.S.—
200 mg (free acid) (Rx) [*Nalfon 200;* GENERIC].
300 mg (free acid) (Rx) [*Nalfon;* GENERIC].
Canada—
300 mg (free acid) (Rx) [*Nalfon*].

**Packaging and storage**
Store below 40 °C (104 °F), preferably between 15 and 30 °C (59 and 86 °F). Store in a well-closed container.

**Auxiliary labeling**
• Take with food.
• Take with a full glass of water.

• May cause drowsiness.
• Avoid alcoholic beverages.

### FENOPROFEN CALCIUM TABLETS USP

**Usual adult dose**
See *Fenoprofen Calcium Capsules USP*.

**Usual adult prescribing limits**
See *Fenoprofen Calcium Capsules USP*.

**Usual pediatric dose**
Safety and dosage have not been established.

**Strength(s) usually available**
U.S.—
600 mg (free acid) (Rx) [*Nalfon* (scored); GENERIC].
Canada—
600 mg (free acid) (Rx) [*Nalfon*].

**Packaging and storage**
Store below 40 °C (104 °F), preferably between 15 and 30 °C (59 and 86 °F). Store in a well-closed container.

**Auxiliary labeling**
• Take with food.
• Take with a full glass of water.
• May cause drowsiness.
• Avoid alcoholic beverages.

---

[1]Not included in Canadian product labeling.

---

## FLOCTAFENINE

## Summary of Differences

Indications:
Indicated for relief of pain. May also be used to relieve acute attacks of gout or calcium pyrophosphate deposition disease (pseudogout), dysmenorrhea, and pain associated with nonrheumatic inflammatory conditions or vascular headaches.
Precautions:
Pregnancy/reproduction—Embryotoxicity but not teratogenicity demonstrated in animal studies.
Drug interactions and/or related problems—Floctafenine-induced increase in effect of coumarin- or indandione-derivative anticoagulants may not become apparent until after 2 weeks of concurrent use.
Side/adverse effects:
See *Table 3*, page 417.

## Additional Dosing Information

See also *General Dosing Information*.

Because the safety and efficacy of floctafenine for long-term administration has not been established, this medication is recommended for short-term use only.

## Oral Dosage Forms

### FLOCTAFENINE TABLETS

**Usual adult dose**
Analgesic—
Oral, 200 to 400 mg every six to eight hours, as needed.

**Usual adult prescribing limits**
Dosage should not exceed 1.2 grams per day.

**Usual pediatric dose**
Use is not recommended.

**Strength(s) usually available**
U.S.—
Not commercially available.
Canada—
200 mg (Rx) [*Idarac* (corn starch)].
400 mg (Rx) [*Idarac* (corn starch)].

**Packaging and storage**
Store below 40 °C (104 °F), preferably between 15 and 30 °C (59 and 86 °F), unless otherwise specified by manufacturer. Protect from light.

**Auxiliary labeling**
• Take with food.
• Take with a full glass of water.
• May cause drowsiness.
• Avoid alcoholic beverages.

## *FLURBIPROFEN*

## Summary of Differences

Indications:

Indicated for rheumatoid arthritis, osteoarthritis, ankylosing spondylitis, bursitis, tendinitis, soft tissue injuries, and dysmenorrhea.

Pharmacology/pharmacokinetics:

Physicochemical characteristics—Chemical group: A propionic acid derivative.

Half-life—Elimination: 5.7 hours.

Peak plasma concentration—Extended-release capsules: Increased by food.

Precautions:

Pregnancy/reproduction—Embryocidal and fetotoxic, but not teratogenic, effects demonstrated in animal studies.

Geriatrics—Peak plasma concentrations increased in elderly females.

Drug interactions and/or related problems—Studies failed to show that flurbiprofen increases digoxin plasma concentrations.

Side/adverse effects:

See *Table 3*, page 417.

## Oral Dosage Forms

Note: Bracketed uses in the *Dosage Forms* section refer to categories of use and/or indications that are not included in U.S. product labeling.

### FLURBIPROFEN EXTENDED-RELEASE CAPSULES

**Usual adult dose**

Antirheumatic (nonsteroidal anti-inflammatory)—

Oral, 200 mg once a day in the evening.

Note: The extended-release dosage form is not intended as initial therapy; the daily maintenance dose should be determined using the immediate-release formulation. The extended-release dosage form may then be used, if desired, provided that the required dose can be achieved with the available strength.

**Usual pediatric dose**

Safety and efficacy have not been established.

**Strength(s) usually available**

U.S.—

Not commercially available.

Canada—

200 mg (Rx) [*Froben SR*].

**Packaging and storage**

Store below 40 °C (104 °F), preferably between 15 and 30 °C (59 and 86 °F), unless otherwise specified by manufacturer.

**Auxiliary labeling**

• Take with food.

• Swallow capsules whole.

• Take with a full glass of water.

• Avoid alcoholic beverages.

### FLURBIPROFEN TABLETS USP

**Usual adult dose**

Rheumatoid arthritis or

Osteoarthritis—

Oral, 200 to 300 mg a day in two to four divided doses, initially. Dosage may then be individualized according to the severity of the disease and patient response.

[Ankylosing spondylitis]—

Oral, 200 mg a day in four divided doses, initially, although some patients may require 250 to 300 mg a day.

Note: After a satisfactory response has been obtained, dosage should be decreased to the lowest dose that provides continuing control of symptoms.

[Antidysmenorrheal]—

Oral, 50 mg four times a day.

[Anti-inflammatory (nonsteroidal)]—

Oral, 50 mg every four to six hours as needed.

**Usual adult prescribing limits**

The maximum recommended single dose is 100 mg. Total daily dosage should not exceed 300 mg. This maximum dose is recommended for short-term use only, i.e., for initiation of therapy or for treating acute exacerbations of symptoms; it should not be used as a maintenance dose.

**Usual pediatric dose**

Safety and efficacy have not been established.

**Strength(s) usually available**

U.S.—

50 mg (Rx) [*Ansaid* (lactose); GENERIC].

100 mg (Rx) [*Ansaid* (lactose); GENERIC].

Canada—

50 mg (Rx) [*Ansaid; Apo-Flurbiprofen; Froben; Novo-Flurprofen; Nu-Flurbiprofen;* GENERIC].

100 mg (Rx) [*Ansaid; Apo-Flurbiprofen; Froben; Novo-Flurprofen; Nu-Flurbiprofen;* GENERIC].

**Packaging and storage**

Store below 40 °C (104 °F), preferably between 15 and 30 °C (59 and 86 °F), unless otherwise specified by manufacturer.

**Auxiliary labeling**

• Take with food.

• Take with a full glass of water.

• Avoid alcoholic beverages.

## *IBUPROFEN*

## Summary of Differences

Indications:

Indicated for rheumatoid arthritis, osteoarthritis, juvenile arthritis, and psoriatic arthritis; pain; gouty arthritis or calcium pyrophosphate deposition disease (pseudogout); fever; and dysmenorrhea. May also be used for prophylaxis and treatment of vascular headaches.

Pharmacology/pharmacokinetics:

Physicochemical characteristics—Chemical group: A propionic acid derivative.

Half-life—Elimination: 1.8–2 hours.

Onset of action—Pain: 0.5 hour.

Time to peak effect—Fever: 2–4 hours.

Duration of action—

Fever:

5-mg/kg dose—6 hours.

10-mg/kg dose—8 hours or more.

Pain: 4–6 hours.

Precautions:

Pregnancy/reproduction—Teratogenic effects in animals have not been shown.

Breast-feeding—Methodology capable of detecting 1 mcg/mL failed to show that ibuprofen is distributed in breast milk.

Pediatrics—Studied in children 6 months of age and older; pediatrics-specific problems have not been demonstrated.

Drug interactions and/or related problems—Also, reported to increase digoxin plasma concentrations.

Laboratory value alterations—Also, may decrease blood glucose concentrations.

Side/adverse effects:

Reported to cause a characteristic hypersensitivity syndrome.

Reported to cause a serum sickness– or influenza-like syndrome.

See also *Table 3*, page 417.

## Additional Dosing Information

See also *General Dosing Information*.

In the treatment of arthritis, improvement in condition may occur within 7 days, but 1 to 2 weeks of continuous use on a regular basis may be required for maximum effectiveness.

## Oral Dosage Forms

### IBUPROFEN ORAL SUSPENSION

**Usual adult and adolescent dose**

Antirheumatic (nonsteroidal anti-inflammatory)—

Oral, 1200 to 3200 mg a day in three or four divided doses. After a satisfactory response has been obtained, dosage should be reduced to the lowest maintenance dose that provides continuing control of symptoms.

Note: Higher doses generally are required in rheumatoid arthritis than in osteoarthritis.

Analgesic (mild to moderate pain)

Antipyretic or

Antidysmenorrheal—

Oral, 200 to 400 mg every four to six hours as needed.

**Usual adult prescribing limits**

Antirheumatic (nonsteroidal anti-inflammatory)—

Up to 3600 mg per day. The maximum dosage should be used only if the clinical benefit is increased sufficiently to offset the higher risk of adverse effects.

Analgesic
Antipyretic; or
Antidysmenorrheal—
　For patient self-medication (over-the-counter use): Not to exceed 1200
　　mg per day.

**Usual pediatric dose**
Antirheumatic (nonsteroidal anti-inflammatory)—
　Infants up to 6 months of age: Safety and efficacy have not been
　　established.
　Children 6 months to 12 years of age: Oral, initially 30 to 40 mg per
　　kg of body weight a day in three or four divided doses, although
　　20 mg per kg of body weight per day may be sufficient for patients
　　with mild disease. After a satisfactory response has been achieved,
　　dosage should be reduced to the lowest dose needed to control
　　disease activity.
Antipyretic—
　Infants up to 6 months of age: Safety and efficacy have not been
　　established.
　Children 6 months to 12 years of age: Oral, 5 mg per kg of body
　　weight for fevers less than 39.17 °C (102.5 °F) and 10 mg per kg
　　of body weight for higher fevers. Dosage may be repeated, if nec-
　　essary, at intervals of 4 to 6 hours or more.

**Usual pediatric prescribing limits**
Antirheumatic—
　Oral, 50 mg per kg of body weight per day.
Antipyretic—
　Oral, 40 mg per kg of body weight per day.

**Strength(s) usually available**
U.S.—
　40 mg per mL (OTC) [*Motrin, Children's Oral Drops*].
　40 mg per mL (Rx) [*Motrin, Children's Oral Drops*].
　100 mg per 5 mL (OTC) [*Advil, Children's* (sucrose; cellulose gum;
　　citric acid; disodium EDTA; FD&C Red #40; glycerin; microcrys-
　　talline cellulose; polysorbate 80; sodium benzoate; sorbitol; xan-
　　than gum)].
　100 mg per 5 mL (Rx) [*Advil, Children's* (sucrose; cellulose gum;
　　citric acid; disodium EDTA; FD&C Red #40; glycerin; microcrys-
　　talline cellulose; polysorbate 80; sodium benzoate; sorbitol; xan-
　　than gum)].
　100 mg per 5 mL (OTC) [*Motrin, Children's* (sucrose; citric acid;
　　glycerin; polysorbate 80; sodium benzoate; starch; xanthan gum;
　　yellow #10; red #40)].
　100 mg per 5 mL (Rx) [*Motrin, Children's* (sucrose; citric acid; glyc-
　　erin; polysorbate 80; sodium benzoate; starch; xanthan gum; yel-
　　low #10; red #40)].
Canada—
　Not commercially available.

**Packaging and storage**
Store between 15 and 30 °C (59 to 86 °F). Protect from freezing.

**Auxiliary labeling**
• Take with food or antacids.
• Shake well.
• Avoid alcoholic beverages.

## IBUPROFEN TABLETS USP

**Usual adult and adolescent dose**
See *Ibuprofen Oral Suspension.*

**Usual adult prescribing limits**
See *Ibuprofen Oral Suspension.*

**Usual pediatric dose**
See *Ibuprofen Oral Suspension.*

**Usual pediatric prescribing limits**
See *Ibuprofen Oral Suspension.*

**Strength(s) usually available**
U.S.—
　100 mg (Rx) [*Motrin, Junior Strength Caplets*].
　100 mg (OTC) [*Motrin, Junior Strength Caplets*].
　200 mg (OTC) [*Advil; Advil Caplets; Bayer Select Ibuprofen Pain
　　Relief Formula Caplets; Cramp End; Excedrin IB; Excedrin IB
　　Caplets; Genpril; Genpril Caplets; Haltran; Ibu-200; Ibuprin;
　　Ibuprohm; Ibuprohm Caplets; Ibu-Tab; Medipren; Medipren Ca-
　　plets; Midol IB; Motrin-IB; Motrin-IB Caplets; Nuprin; Nuprin
　　Caplets; Pamprin-IB; Q-Profen; Trendar; GENERIC*].
　300 mg (Rx) [*Motrin; GENERIC*].
　400 mg (Rx) [*Dolgesic; Ibu; Ibu-4; Ibuprohm; Ibu-Tab; Motrin; Ru-
　　fen; GENERIC*].

　600 mg (Rx) [*Ibifon 600 Caplets; Ibren; Ibu; Ibu-6; Ibu-Tab; Motrin;
　　Rufen; GENERIC*].
　800 mg (Rx) [*Ibu; Ibu-8; Ibu-Tab; Motrin; Rufen; GENERIC*].
Canada—
　200 mg (OTC) [*Actiprofen Caplets; Advil; Advil Caplets; Apo-Ibu-
　　profen; Medipren Caplets; Motrin-IB; Motrin-IB Caplets; Novo-
　　Profen; GENERIC*].
　300 mg (Rx) [*Apo-Ibuprofen; Motrin; Novo-Profen; Nu-Ibuprofen;
　　GENERIC*].
　400 mg (Rx) [*Apo-Ibuprofen; Motrin; Novo-Profen; Nu-Ibuprofen;
　　GENERIC*].
　600 mg (Rx) [*Apo-Ibuprofen; Motrin; Novo-Profen; Nu-Ibuprofen;
　　GENERIC*].

**Packaging and storage**
Store between 15 and 30 °C (59 and 86 °F), in a light-resistant container,
　unless otherwise specified by manufacturer. Store in a well-closed
　container.

**Auxiliary labeling**
• Take with food.
• Take with a full glass of water.
• May cause drowsiness.
• Avoid alcoholic beverages.

## IBUPROFEN TABLETS (CHEWABLE)

**Usual adult and adolescent dose**
See *Ibuprofen Oral Suspension.*

**Usual adult prescribing limits**
See *Ibuprofen Oral Suspension.*

**Usual pediatric dose**
See *Ibuprofen Oral Suspension.*

**Usual pediatric prescribing limits**
See *Ibuprofen Oral Suspension.*

**Strength(s) usually available**
U.S.—
　50 mg (Rx) [*Motrin Chewables*].
　100 mg (Rx) [*Motrin Chewables*].
Canada—
　Not commercially available.

**Packaging and storage**
Store between 15 and 30 °C (59 and 86 °F), in a well-closed, light-resistant
　container, unless otherwise specified by manufacturer.

**Auxiliary labeling**
• Take with food.
• Take with a full glass of water.
• May cause drowsiness.
• Avoid alcoholic beverages.

---

## *INDOMETHACIN*

## Summary of Differences

Indications:
　Indicated for rheumatoid arthritis, osteoarthritis, ankylosing spondyli-
　　tis, juvenile arthritis, psoriatic arthritis, Reiter's disease, and rheu-
　　matic complications associated with Paget's disease of bone; acute
　　gouty arthritis and calcium pyrophosphate deposition disease
　　(pseudogout); bursitis and tendinitis; fever associated with malig-
　　nancy; dysmenorrhea; prevention and treatment of vascular head-
　　aches; Bartter's disease; and pericarditis.
　Drug of first choice in ankylosing spondylitis; for other indications
　　(except Bartter's syndrome), recommended only for patients un-
　　responsive to less toxic NSAIDs or, in the case of fever, to other
　　antipyretic agents.
Pharmacology/pharmacokinetics:
　Physicochemical characteristics—Chemical group: An indoleacetic
　　acid derivative.
　Absorption—Oral: Capsules and oral suspension—90% of a dose ab-
　　sorbed within 4 hours.
　Extended-release capsules—90% of a dose absorbed within 12 hours.
　Rectal: 80 to 90% of a dose absorbed; incomplete absorption may
　　result from failure to retain suppository in rectum for a full hour.
　Half-life—Elimination: Average, about 4.5 hours; subject to substan-
　　tial intersubject variability, possibly because of differences in en-
　　terohepatic circulation and subsequent reabsorption.
　Onset of action—Gout: 2–4 hours.
　Time to peak effect—Gout (capsules or oral suspension): 2–3 days for
　　relief of heat and tenderness; 3–5 days for relief of swelling.

Precautions:

Pregnancy/reproduction—

First trimester: Crosses the placenta; fetotoxic, teratogenic, and other adverse effects demonstrated in animal studies.

Third trimester: Has caused closure of the ductus arteriosus, inhibition of platelet function resulting in bleeding, renal function impairment or failure with oligohydramnios, gastrointestinal bleeding or perforation, and myocardial degenerative changes in fetuses when given to pregnant women during the third trimester.

Breast-feeding—Distributed into breast milk; one report of convulsions in a breast-fed infant exposed to the medication.

Pediatrics—Recommended only for pediatric patients who are unresponsive to or intolerant of less toxic agents. Only immediate-release oral dosage forms should be used. Also, recommended doses should not be exceeded and the patient carefully monitored.

Geriatrics—Also, increased risk of adverse CNS effects, especially confusion.

Drug interactions and/or related problems—

Also, concurrent use with potassium-sparing diuretics may cause hyperkalemia.

Also, may block the increase in plasma renin activity induced by bumetanide, furosemide, or indapamide.

Also, concurrent use with zidovudine not recommended; toxicity of either or both of the medications may be increased.

Caution also recommended with aminoglycosides and digitalis glycosides; indomethacin has caused increased plasma concentrations of these medications in infants.

Laboratory value alterations—Also, may cause false-negative test results with dexamethasone suppression test for endogenous depression and one test for urinary 5-hydroxyindoleacetic acid (5-HIAA). Also, may increase or decrease blood glucose concentrations.

Medical considerations/contraindications—

Higher risk than with most other NSAIDs in patients with renal function impairment.

Also, may aggravate epilepsy, mental depression or other mental disturbances, or parkinsonism.

Patient monitoring—Routine monitoring of liver function recommended.

Side/adverse effects:

See *Table 3*, page 417.

## Additional Dosing Information

See also *General Dosing Information*.

Indomethacin should be administered in the lowest dose that provides symptomatic relief. Doses greater than 150 to 200 mg per day may increase the risk of adverse effects without providing additional clinical benefit. If therapy is to be continued after the acute phase of the disease has been controlled, periodic attempts should be made to reduce the dose to the lowest dose providing continuing control of symptoms.

If minor adverse effects occur, dosage should be reduced and the patient carefully monitored. If severe side effects occur, therapy should be discontinued.

### For oral dosage forms only

Oral dosage forms of indomethacin should always be administered after meals or with food or an antacid to reduce gastrointestinal irritation. However, the oral suspension should not be mixed with an antacid or other liquid prior to use.

To facilitate dosage adjustment and assessment of patient tolerance of the medication, it is recommended that an immediate-release, rather than the extended-release, dosage form be used for initiation of therapy or to increase the daily dose. If the extended-release dosage form is used for initial therapy, or to increase the daily dose, careful observation of the patient is recommended.

### For rectal dosage form only

To ensure maximum absorption, the suppository should be retained for at least one full hour after insertion.

## Oral Dosage Forms

Note: Bracketed uses in the *Dosage Forms* section refer to categories of use and/or indications that are not included in U.S. product labeling.

### INDOMETHACIN CAPSULES USP

#### Usual adult dose

Antirheumatic (nonsteroidal anti-inflammatory)—

Oral, initially 25 or 50 mg two to four times a day; if well tolerated, the dosage per day may be increased by 25 or 50 mg at weekly intervals until a satisfactory response is obtained or up to a maximum dose of 200 mg per day. After a satisfactory response has been achieved, dosage should be reduced to the lowest dose that provides continuing control of symptoms.

Note: In acute flare-ups of rheumatoid arthritis, dosage may be increased by 25 or 50 mg daily, as needed and tolerated.

For those arthritic patients who have persistent night pain and/or morning stiffness, up to 100 mg of the total daily dose may be given at bedtime. Lower bedtime doses may not provide adequate symptomatic relief.

A daily dose of less than 75 mg may not be effective in active inflammatory disease.

A daily dose of more than 150 to 200 mg may increase the risk of adverse effects without providing additional clinical benefit.

Antigout agent—

Oral, 100 mg initially, then 50 mg three times a day until pain is relieved, with the dosage then being reduced until medication is discontinued.

Anti-inflammatory (nonsteroidal)[1]—

75 to 150 mg per day in three or four divided doses.

Note: When used to treat conditions not requiring chronic therapy, such as acute bursitis or tendinitis of the shoulder, indomethacin should be discontinued when symptoms of inflammation have been controlled for several days. The usual length of treatment is 7 to 14 days.

[Antipyretic][1]—

Oral, 25 or 50 mg three or four times a day.

#### Usual adult prescribing limits

Oral, 200 mg a day.

#### Usual pediatric dose

Antirheumatic (nonsteroidal anti-inflammatory)—

Oral, 1.5 to 2.5 mg per kg of body weight per day, administered in three or four divided doses, up to a maximum of 4 mg per kg of body weight per day or 150 to 200 mg per day, whichever is less. After a satisfactory response has been obtained, dosage should be reduced to the lowest dose that provides continuing control of symptoms.

#### Strength(s) usually available

U.S.—

25 mg (Rx) [*Indocin* (lactose); GENERIC].

50 mg (Rx) [*Indocin* (lactose); GENERIC].

Canada—

25 mg (Rx) [*Apo-Indomethacin; Indocid* (lactose); *Novo-Methacin; Nu-Indo*].

50 mg (Rx) [*Apo-Indomethacin; Indocid* (lactose); *Novo-Methacin; Nu-Indo*].

#### Packaging and storage

Store below 40 °C (104 °F), preferably between 15 and 30 °C (59 and 86 °F). Store in a well-closed container.

#### Auxiliary labeling

• Take with food or antacids.

• Take with a full glass of water.

• Avoid alcoholic beverages.

### INDOMETHACIN EXTENDED-RELEASE CAPSULES USP

#### Usual adult dose

Antirheumatic (nonsteroidal anti-inflammatory)—

Oral, 75 mg once a day, in the morning or at bedtime; may be increased to 75 mg two times a day if necessary.

Note: It is generally recommended that the daily maintenance dose be determined using the immediate-release formulation. The extended-release dosage form may then be used, if desired, provided that the required dose can be achieved with the available strength.

Careful observation of the patient for signs of intolerance is recommended if the extended-release capsule is used for initiating indomethacin therapy or for increasing the daily dose. Initiation of therapy with one extended-release capsule daily provides the maximum initial dose recommended by the manufacturer. Use of the extended-release capsule to increase the dose provides a greater-than-recommended increase in daily dosage.

#### Usual pediatric dose

Dosage has not been established.

#### Strength(s) usually available

U.S.—

75 mg (Rx) [*Indocin SR* (sugar); GENERIC].

Canada—

75 mg (Rx) [*Indocid SR* (sucrose)].

**Packaging and storage**
Store below 40 °C (104 °F), preferably between 15 and 30 °C (59 and 86 °F), unless otherwise specified by manufacturer. Store in a well-closed container.

**Auxiliary labeling**
- Take with food or antacids.
- Take with a full glass of water.
- Avoid alcoholic beverages.

**Additional information**
The extended-release capsules are designed to release 25 mg of indomethacin immediately and the remaining 50 mg over a 12-hour period.

## INDOMETHACIN ORAL SUSPENSION USP

**Usual adult dose**
See *Indomethacin Capsules USP.*

**Usual adult prescribing limits**
See *Indomethacin Capsules USP.*

**Usual pediatric dose**
See *Indomethacin Capsules USP.*

**Strength(s) usually available**
U.S.—
25 mg per 5 mL (Rx) [*Indocin* (alcohol 1%); GENERIC].
Canada—
Not commercially available.

**Packaging and storage**
Store below 30 °C (86 °F). Store in a tight, light-resistant container. Protect from freezing.

**Incompatibilities**
Indomethacin is unstable in an alkaline medium and should not be mixed with antacids or other liquids having an alkaline pH.

**Auxiliary labeling**
- Take with food or antacids.
- Shake well.
- Avoid alcoholic beverages.

# Rectal Dosage Forms

## INDOMETHACIN SUPPOSITORIES USP

**Usual adult dose**
Antirheumatic (nonsteroidal anti-inflammatory)
Anti-inflammatory (nonsteroidal)[1]
Antigout agent or
[Antipyretic][1]—
Rectal, 50 mg up to four times a day.

Note: A daily dose of less than 75 mg may not be effective in active inflammatory disease.

For those arthritic patients who have persistent night pain and/or morning stiffness, up to 100 mg of the total daily dose may be given at bedtime. Lower bedtime doses may not provide adequate symptomatic relief.

A daily dose of more than 150 to 200 mg may increase the risk of adverse effects without providing additional clinical benefit.

**Usual adult prescribing limits**
Rectal or combined oral and rectal, 200 mg per day.

**Usual pediatric dose**
Antirheumatic (nonsteroidal anti-inflammatory)—
Rectal, 1.5 to 2.5 mg per kg of body weight per day, administered in 3 or 4 divided doses, up to a maximum of 4 mg per kg of body weight or 150 to 200 mg per day, whichever is less.

**Strength(s) usually available**
U.S.—
50 mg (Rx) [*Indocin* (butylated hydroxyanisole; butylated hydroxytoluene; edetic acid; glycerin; polyethylene glycol 3350; polyethylene glycol 8000; sodium chloride)].
Canada—
50 mg (Rx) [*Indocid*].
100 mg (Rx) [*Indocid*].

**Packaging and storage**
Store below 40 °C (104 °F), preferably between 15 and 30 °C (59 and 86 °F), unless otherwise specified by manufacturer. Store in a well-closed container. Protect from freezing.

**Auxiliary labeling**
- For rectal use.
- Avoid alcoholic beverages.

---

[1]Not included in Canadian product labeling.

---
### *KETOPROFEN*
---

## Summary of Differences

Indications:
Indicated for rheumatoid arthritis, osteoarthritis, ankylosing spondylitis, and psoriatic arthritis; pain; acute gouty arthritis and calcium pyrophosphate deposition disease (pseudogout); and dysmenorrhea. May also be used to relieve pain associated with nonrheumatic inflammatory disorders or vascular headaches.
Pharmacology/pharmacokinetics:
Physicochemical characteristics—Chemical group: A propionic acid derivative.
Half-life—Elimination:
Capsules—1.6 hours; increased by 26% in geriatric patients; also increased by renal function impairment.
Extended-release capsules—About 5.4 hours; higher value (relative to immediate-release capsules) represents prolonged absorption; increased by 54% in geriatric patients.
Extended-release tablets—About 3–4 hours; higher value (relative to immediate-release capsules) represents prolonged absorption.
Elimination—Dialyzable.
Precautions:
Pregnancy/reproduction—Fertility: Decreased number of implantation sites in female rats (but no effect on fertility in male rats); high doses caused abnormal spermatogenesis or impaired spermatogenesis in rats and dogs and decreased testicular weight in dogs and baboons.
First trimester: No teratogenicity demonstrated in animal studies; in rabbits, maternally toxic doses shown to be embryotoxic.
Geriatrics—Protein binding and clearance reduced in elderly people, leading to increased plasma concentration and prolonged half-life.
Drug interactions and/or related problems—
Probenecid may greatly increase ketoprofen plasma concentration and the risk of toxicity; concurrent use not recommended.
Studies failed to show that ketoprofen increases digoxin plasma concentration.
Laboratory value alterations—Interference with determinations of urinary albumin, bile salts, 17-ketosteroids, and 17-hydroxycorticosteroids via test procedures that rely on acid precipitation or on color reaction of carbonyl groups as an end point.
Side/adverse effects:
See *Table 3*, page 417.

## Oral Dosage Forms

### KETOPROFEN CAPSULES

**Usual adult dose**
Antirheumatic (nonsteroidal anti-inflammatory)—
Oral, 150 to 300 mg a day in three or four divided doses, usually 75 mg three times a day or 50 mg four times a day, initially, then adjusted according to patient response.
Analgesic or
Antidysmenorrheal—
Oral, 25 to 50 mg every six to eight hours as needed. Dosage may be increased if necessary, but single doses higher than 75 mg have not been shown to provide additional analgesia. In the treatment of dysmenorrhea, 75-mg doses may be more effective than lower doses.

Note: In patients with renal function impairment, a 33 to 50% reduction of dosage is recommended.

The analgesic dosage for self-medication with ketoprofen using the over-the-counter product is 12.5 mg every four to six hours.

**Usual adult prescribing limits**
Oral, 300 mg a day in three or four divided doses.

Note: Risk/benefit must be considered when the maximum dose is prescribed because the incidence of gastrointestinal effects and headache is increased with administration of 300 mg per day (as compared with 200 mg per day).

**Usual pediatric dose**
Safety and efficacy have not been established.

**Strength(s) usually available**
U.S.—
25 mg (Rx) [*Orudis* (lactose); GENERIC].
50 mg (Rx) [*Orudis* (lactose); GENERIC].
75 mg (Rx) [*Orudis* (lactose); GENERIC].
Canada—
50 mg (Rx) [*Apo-Keto; Orudis; Rhodis*].

**Packaging and storage**
Store below 40 °C (104 °F), preferably between 15 and 30 °C (59 and 86 °F), in a tight container, unless otherwise specified by manufacturer.

**Auxiliary labeling**
• Take with food.
• Take with a full glass of water.
• Avoid alcoholic beverages.

## KETOPROFEN EXTENDED-RELEASE CAPSULES

**Usual adult dose**
Antirheumatic (nonsteroidal anti-inflammatory)—
  Oral, 150 or 200 mg once a day, in the morning or evening. Elderly or debilitated patients may require lower doses.

Note: The extended-release dosage form is not intended as initial therapy; the daily maintenance dose should be determined using an immediate- or delayed-release formulation. The extended-release dosage form may then be used, if desired, provided that the required dose can be achieved with the available strength (s).

**Usual pediatric dose**
Safety and efficacy have not been established.

**Strength(s) usually available**
U.S.—
  100 mg (Rx) [*Oruvail*].
  150 mg (Rx) [*Oruvail*].
  200 mg (Rx) [*Oruvail*].
Canada—
  150 mg (Rx) [*Oruvail*].
  200 mg (Rx) [*Oruvail*].

**Packaging and storage**
Store below 40 °C (104 °F), preferably between 15 and 30 °C (59 and 86 °F), in a well-closed container, unless otherwise specified by manufacturer.

**Auxiliary labeling**
• Swallow capsule whole.
• Take with a full glass of water.
• Avoid alcoholic beverages.

**Note**
The extended-release capsule is formulated with delayed-release as well as extended-release characteristics. Dissolution of the contents of the capsules (coated pellets) does not occur until the medication reaches the alkaline pH of the small intestine.

## KETOPROFEN DELAYED-RELEASE TABLETS

**Usual adult dose**
See *Ketoprofen Capsules.*

**Usual adult prescribing limits**
See *Ketoprofen Capsules.*

**Usual pediatric dose**
Safety and efficacy have not been established.

**Strength(s) usually available**
U.S.—
  Not commercially available.
Canada—
  50 mg (Rx) [*Apo-Keto-E; Novo-Keto-EC; Orudis-E; Rhodis-EC*].
  100 mg (Rx) [*Apo-Keto-E; Novo-Keto-EC; Orudis-E; Rhodis-EC*].

**Packaging and storage**
Store below 40 °C (104 °F), preferably between 15 and 30 °C (59 and 86 °F), in a well-closed container, unless otherwise specified by manufacturer.

**Auxiliary labeling**
• Take with a full glass of water.
• Swallow tablets whole.
• Avoid alcoholic beverages.

## KETOPROFEN EXTENDED-RELEASE TABLETS

**Usual adult dose**
See *Ketoprofen Extended-release Capsules.*

**Usual pediatric dose**
Safety and efficacy have not been established.

**Strength(s) usually available**
U.S.—
  Not commercially available.
Canada—
  200 mg (Rx) [*Orudis-SR;* GENERIC].

**Packaging and storage**
Store below 40 °C (104 °F), preferably between 15 and 30 °C (59 and 86 °F), in a well-closed container, unless otherwise specified by manufacturer.

**Auxiliary labeling**
• Take with food.
• Take with a full glass of water.
• Swallow tablets whole.
• Avoid alcoholic beverages.

## KETOPROFEN TABLETS

**Usual adult dose**
See *Ketoprofen Capsules.*

**Usual adult prescribing limits**
See *Ketoprofen Capsules.*

**Usual pediatric dose**
Safety and efficacy have not been established.

**Strength(s) usually available**
U.S.—
  12.5 mg (OTC) [*Orudis KT* (tartrazine)].
  12.5 mg (OTC) [*Actron* (lactose)].
Canada—
  Not commercially available.

**Packaging and storage**
Store below 40 °C (104 °F), preferably between 15 and 30 °C (59 and 86 °F), in a well-closed container, unless otherwise specified by manufacturer.

**Auxiliary labeling**
• Take with a full glass of water.
• Avoid alcoholic beverages.

# Rectal Dosage Forms

## KETOPROFEN SUPPOSITORIES

**Usual adult dose**
Antirheumatic (nonsteroidal anti-inflammatory)—
  Rectal, 50 or 100 mg two times a day, in the morning and evening; or 50 or 100 mg in the evening in conjunction with oral administration during the day.

**Usual adult prescribing limits**
Rectal or combined oral and rectal, 300 mg a day.

**Usual pediatric dose**
Safety and efficacy have not been established.

**Strength(s) usually available**
U.S.—
  Not commercially available.
Canada—
  50 mg (Rx) [*Orudis*].
  100 mg (Rx) [*Orudis; Rhodis*].

**Packaging and storage**
Store below 30 °C (86 °F), in a well-closed container, unless otherwise specified by manufacturer. Protect from freezing.

**Auxiliary labeling**
• For rectal use.
• Avoid alcoholic beverages.

---

## *MECLOFENAMATE*

# Summary of Differences

Indications:
  Indicated for rheumatoid arthritis, osteoarthritis, psoriatic arthritis, pain, dysmenorrhea, and idiopathic hypermenorrhea. May also be used to relieve acute attacks of gout or calcium pyrophosphate deposition disease (pseudogout) and pain associated with nonrheumatic inflammatory conditions or vascular headaches.
Pharmacology/pharmacokinetics:
  Physicochemical characteristics—Chemical group: A fenamate derivative.
  Other actions/effects—With usual doses has lesser effect on platelet aggregation than most other NSAIDs.
  Biotransformation—Hydroxymethyl metabolite has anti-inflammatory activity.
  Half-life—Elimination:
  Single dose—2 hours.
  Multiple doses—3.3 hours.

Onset of action—Pain: 1 hour.
Duration of action—Pain: 4–6 hours.

Precautions:

Pregnancy/reproduction—Fetotoxicity and developmental abnormalities have been demonstrated in animals.

Breast-feeding—Use not recommended because animal studies have shown this agent to interfere with normal development of the young before weaning.

Surgical—With recommended doses may be less likely than most other NSAIDs to increase perisurgical bleeding.

Laboratory value alterations—With usual doses may be less likely than most other NSAIDs to increase bleeding time significantly.

Medical considerations/contraindications—Caution in patients on a sodium-restricted diet.

Side/adverse effects:

Reported to cause a serum sickness or influenza-like syndrome.

See also *Table 3*, page 417.

## Additional Dosing Information

See also *General Dosing Information.*

Improvement in condition may occur within a few days, but 2 to 3 weeks of continuous use on a regular basis may be required for maximum effectiveness.

Gastrointestinal side effects may respond to a reduction in dosage; however, if severe adverse reactions occur, therapy should be discontinued.

## Oral Dosage Forms

Note: The dosing and strengths of the available dosage form are expressed in terms of meclofenamic acid (not the sodium salt).

### MECLOFENAMATE SODIUM CAPSULES USP

**Usual adult dose**
Antirheumatic (nonsteroidal anti-inflammatory)—

Oral, 200 mg (meclofenamic acid) a day, in three or four divided doses, initially. Dosage may be increased to up to 400 mg a day if necessary. After a satisfactory response has been obtained, dosage should be reduced to the lowest maintenance dose that provides continuing control of symptoms.

Analgesic—

Oral, 50 mg (meclofenamic acid) every four to six hours. If necessary, dosage may be increased to 100 mg every four to six hours.

Antidysmenorrheal and
Antihypermenorrheal—

Oral, 100 mg (meclofenamic acid) three times a day for up to six days.

**Usual adult prescribing limits**
Antirheumatic (nonsteroidal anti-inflammatory)
and analgesic—
Up to 400 mg daily.

**Usual pediatric dose**
Children up to 14 years of age—Safety and efficacy have not been established.

**Strength(s) usually available**
U.S.—

50 mg (meclofenamic acid) (Rx) [*Meclomen* (lactose); GENERIC].
100 mg (meclofenamic acid) (Rx) [*Meclomen* (lactose); GENERIC].

Canada—
Not commercially available.

**Packaging and storage**
Store between 15 and 30 °C (59 and 86 °F), unless otherwise specified by manufacturer. Store in a tight, light-resistant container.

**Auxiliary labeling**
• Take with food.
• Take with a full glass of water.
• Avoid alcoholic beverages.

---

## MEFENAMIC ACID

## Summary of Differences

Indications:

Indicated for short-term use (7 days or less) to relieve pain and dysmenorrhea. May also be used for acute attacks of gout or calcium pyrophosphate deposition disease (pseudogout), for pain associated with nonrheumatic inflammatory conditions or vascular headaches, and to prevent migraines associated with menstruation.

Pharmacology/pharmacokinetics:

Physicochemical characteristics—Chemical group: A fenamate derivative.

Other actions/effects—With usual doses has lesser effect on platelet aggregation than most other NSAIDs.

Half-life—Elimination: 2 hours

Precautions:

Pregnancy/reproduction—

Fertility: Decreased fertility demonstrated in rodents.

Pregnancy: Increased number of resorptions and decreased survival to weaning demonstrated in rodents.

Surgical—With usual doses may be less likely than other NSAIDs to inhibit platelet aggregation significantly, but has been reported to cause hypoprothrombinemia, which may increase the risk of perisurgical bleeding.

Laboratory value alterations—

Interference with urinary bile determinations via the diazo tablet test.

With usual doses is less likely than most other NSAIDs to increase bleeding time significantly because of lesser effect on platelet aggregation; however, may prolong prothrombin time.

Medical considerations/contraindications—Also, may exacerbate pre-existing hypoprothrombinemia.

Side/adverse effects:

See *Table 3*, page 417.

## Additional Dosing Information

See also *General Dosing Information.*

It is recommended that mefenamic acid therapy be discontinued promptly if diarrhea or a skin rash develops. Patients who develop diarrhea during mefenamic acid therapy are usually unable to tolerate the drug thereafter.

Mefenamic acid should not be used for more than 7 days at a time.

## Oral Dosage Forms

### MEFENAMIC ACID CAPSULES USP

**Usual adult dose**
Analgesic or
Antidysmenorrheal—

Oral, 500 mg initially, followed by 250 mg every six hours as needed.

Note: It is recommended that mefenamic acid be used for no longer than 7 days at a time.

**Usual pediatric dose**
Children up to 14 years of age—Safety and efficacy have not been established.

**Strength(s) usually available**
U.S.—

250 mg (Rx) [*Ponstel* (lactose; sodium benzoate)].

Canada—

250 mg (Rx) [*Ponstan* (lactose)].

**Packaging and storage**
Store below 40 °C (104 °F), preferably between 15 and 30 °C (59 and 86 °F). Store in a tight container.

**Auxiliary labeling**
• Take with food.
• Take with a full glass of water.
• May cause drowsiness.
• Avoid alcoholic beverages.

---

## NABUMETONE

## Summary of Differences

Indications:

Indicated for rheumatoid arthritis and osteoarthritis.

Pharmacology/pharmacokinetics:

Physicochemical characteristics—

Chemical group: A naphthylalkanone derivative.

Other characteristics:

Nabumetone (prodrug)—Nonacidic.

6-MNA (active metabolite)—Acidic.

Other actions/effects—With usual doses has lesser effect on platelet aggregation than most other NSAIDs.

Absorption—Rate and extent increased by food or milk.

Biotransformation—Metabolite 6-MNA, not nabumetone itself, is active substance.

Half-life (plasma)—Elimination: 6-MNA—23 ± 3.7 hours; increased in geriatric patients to 30 ± 8.1 hours (although values as high as 74 hours have been reported) and to 39 hours in patients with renal function impairment (creatinine clearance < 30 mL/minute/1.73 cubic meters of body surface area).

Time to peak plasma concentration—6-MNA, at steady-state: Decreased by food; significantly delayed by hepatic cirrhosis.

Peak plasma concentration—6-MNA: Increased by food; may be increased in geriatric patients and substantially decreased in patients with hepatic cirrhosis.

Elimination—6-MNA: Significantly delayed by moderately severe renal function impairment (creatinine clearance < 30 mL/minute/1.73 cubic meters of body surface area).

Precautions:

Mutagenicity—Induced chromosomal aberrations in lymphocytes.

Pregnancy/reproduction—Fetotoxicity but not teratogenicity demonstrated in rats.

Geriatrics—Higher plasma concentrations and greater interpatient variability in pharmacokinetics of 6-MNA in geriatric patients.

Surgical—In doses up to 1000 mg per day may be less likely than most other NSAIDs to increase perisurgical bleeding.

Drug interactions and/or related problems—May be less likely than other NSAIDs to cause problems in patients receiving anticoagulant or thrombolytic therapy.

Medical considerations/contraindications—Hepatic function impairment may decrease biotransformation to active metabolite sufficiently to decrease efficacy.

Side/adverse effects:

Lower incidence of peptic ulceration and bleeding than with other NSAIDs.

See also *Table 3*, page 417.

## Oral Dosage Forms
### NABUMETONE TABLETS

**Usual adult dose**

Antirheumatic (nonsteroidal anti-inflammatory)—

Oral, initially 1000 mg a day, as a single dose (usually at night) or in two divided doses (in the morning and evening). Dosage may be increased, if necessary, to 1500 mg or 2000 mg a day in two divided doses. After a satisfactory response has been obtained, dosage should be individualized according to patient tolerance and response. The lowest dose that provides continuing control of symptoms should be used for maintenance.

**Usual adult prescribing limits**

Doses larger than 2000 mg a day have not been studied and are not recommended.

**Usual pediatric dose**

Safety and efficacy have not been established

**Usual geriatric dose**

See *Usual adult dose.*

**Strength(s) usually available**

U.S.—

500 mg (Rx) [*Relafen*].

750 mg (Rx) [*Relafen*].

Canada—

500 mg (Rx) [*Relafen*].

**Packaging and storage**

Store between 15 and 30 °C (59 and 86 °F), in a well-closed container, unless otherwise specified by manufacturer.

**Auxiliary labeling**

• Take with food.

• Take with a full glass of water.

• Avoid alcoholic beverages.

---

### *NAPROXEN*

## Summary of Differences

Indications:

Indicated for rheumatoid arthritis, osteoarthritis, ankylosing spondylitis, and juvenile arthritis; pain; acute attacks of gout and calcium pyrophosphate deposition disease (pseudogout); bursitis and tendinitis; fever; and dysmenorrhea; and for prophylaxis and treatment of vascular headaches.

Pharmacology/pharmacokinetics:

Physicochemical characteristics—Chemical group: A propionic acid derivative.

Absorption—May be increased by sodium bicarbonate.

Half-life—Elimination: 13 hours

Onset of action—Naproxen sodium: Pain—1 hour.

Time to peak plasma concentration—Extended-release tablets: Decreased by food.

Peak plasma concentration—Extended-release tablets: Increased by food.

Time to peak effect—Gout: 1–2 days.

Pain: 2–4 hours.

Duration of action—Pain: Up to 7 hours.

Precautions:

Pregnancy/reproduction—Teratogenic effects in animals have not been shown.

Pediatrics—Higher risk of skin rash and increases in bleeding time than in adults receiving the medication.

Laboratory value alterations—Interference with some assays for urinary 5-hydroxyindoleacetic acid (5-HIAA) and urinary 17-ketogenic steroids.

Medical considerations/contraindications—Caution with naproxen sodium and naproxen oral suspension for patients who must restrict their sodium intake.

Side/adverse effects:

See *Table 3*, page 417.

## Additional Dosing Information

See also *General Dosing Information.*

In arthritis, improvement in condition may occur within 2 weeks, but 2 to 4 weeks of continuous use on a regular basis may be required for maximum effectiveness.

Naproxen should be administered in the lowest effective dose to geriatric patients, patients with hepatic function impairment, or patients with renal function impairment (especially if creatinine clearance is < 20 mL per minute).

## Oral Dosage Forms
### NAPROXEN ORAL SUSPENSION

**Usual adult dose**

Antirheumatic (nonsteroidal anti-inflammatory)—

Oral, 250, 375, or 500 mg two times a day, morning and evening.

Note: During long-term administration, dosage may be adjusted according to patient response; lower doses may suffice.

For acute exacerbations of rheumatic disease, dosage may be increased to up to 1.5 grams per day for limited periods. Use of this high dose requires that the clinical benefit be increased sufficiently to offset the potential increased risk of adverse effects.

Anti-inflammatory (nonsteroidal)

Analgesic (mild to moderate pain) and

Antidysmenorrheal—

Oral, 500 mg initially, then 250 mg every six to eight hours as needed.

Antigout agent[1]—

Oral, 750 mg initially, then 250 mg every eight hours until the attack has subsided.

**Usual adult prescribing limits**

For mild to moderate pain and dysmenorrhea—

Up to a total dose of 1.25 grams daily.

**Usual pediatric dose**

Antirheumatic (nonsteroidal anti-inflammatory)—

Oral, 10 mg per kg of body weight per day, given in two divided doses.

**Strength(s) usually available**

U.S.—

125 mg per 5 mL (Rx) [*Naprosyn* (fumaric acid; imitation orange flavor; imitation pineapple flavor; magnesium aluminum silicate; methylparaben; sodium 8 mg [<1 mmol] per mL; sorbitol; sucrose)].

Canada—

125 mg per 5 mL (Rx) [*Naprosyn*].

**Packaging and storage**

Store below 40 °C (104 °F), preferably between 15 and 30 °C (59 and 86 °F), in a well-closed, light-resistant container, unless otherwise specified by manufacturer. Protect from freezing.

**Auxiliary labeling**

• Take with food.

• Shake well.

• Avoid alcoholic beverages.

### NAPROXEN TABLETS USP

**Usual adult dose**

See *Naproxen Oral Suspension.*

**Usual adult prescribing limits**
See *Naproxen Oral Suspension.*

**Usual pediatric dose**
See *Naproxen Oral Suspension.*

**Strength(s) usually available**
U.S.—

    250 mg (Rx) [*Naprosyn;* GENERIC].

    375 mg (Rx) [*Naprosyn;* GENERIC].

    500 mg (Rx) [*Naprosyn;* GENERIC].

Canada—

    125 mg (Rx) [*Apo-Naproxen; Naprosyn* (lactose); *Naxen* (lactose); *Novo-Naprox; Nu-Naprox*].

    250 mg (Rx) [*Apo-Naproxen; Naprosyn* (lactose); *Naxen* (lactose); *Novo-Naprox; Nu-Naprox*].

    375 mg (Rx) [*Apo-Naproxen* (scored); *Naprosyn* (scored; lactose); *Naxen* (scored; lactose); *Novo-Naprox* (scored); *Nu-Naprox* (scored)].

    500 mg (Rx) [*Apo-Naproxen* (scored); *Naprosyn* (scored; lactose); *Naxen* (scored; lactose); *Novo-Naprox* (scored); *Nu-Naprox* (scored)].

**Packaging and storage**
Store between 15 and 30 °C (59 and 86 °F). Store in a well-closed container.

**Auxiliary labeling**
- Take with food.
- Take with a full glass of water.
- May cause drowsiness.
- Avoid alcoholic beverages.

## NAPROXEN DELAYED-RELEASE TABLETS

**Usual adult dose**
See *Naproxen Oral Suspension.*

**Usual adult prescribing limits**
See *Naproxen Oral Suspension.*

**Usual pediatric dose**
See *Naproxen Oral Suspension.*

**Strength(s) usually available**
U.S.—

    375 mg (Rx) [*EC-Naprosyn* (croscarmellose sodium; povidone; magnesium stearate; methacrylic acid copolymer; talc; triethyl citrate; sodium hydroxide; simethicone emulsion)].

    500 mg (Rx) [*EC-Naprosyn* (croscarmellose sodium; povidone; magnesium stearate; methacrylic acid copolymer; talc; triethyl citrate; sodium hydroxide; simethicone emulsion)].

Canada—

    250 mg (Rx) [*Naprosyn-E*].

    375 mg (Rx) [*Naprosyn-E*].

    500 mg (Rx) [*Naprosyn-E*].

**Packaging and storage**
Store between 15 and 30 °C (59 and 86 °F), unless otherwise directed by manufacturer.

**Auxiliary labeling**
- Swallow tablets whole.
- Take with a full glass of water.
- Avoid alcoholic beverages.

## NAPROXEN EXTENDED-RELEASE TABLETS

**Usual adult dose**
Antirheumatic (nonsteroidal anti-inflammatory)—

    Oral, 750 mg once a day in the morning or evening.

Note: The extended-release dosage form is not intended as initial therapy; the daily maintenance dose should be determined using an immediate- or delayed-release formulation. The extended-release dosage form may then be used, if desired, provided that the required dose can be achieved with the available strength.

**Usual pediatric dose**
Pediatric strength not available.

**Strength(s) usually available**
U.S.—

    Not commercially available.

Canada—

    750 mg (Rx) [*Naprosyn-SR*].

**Packaging and storage**
Store between 15 and 30 °C (59 and 86 °F), in a well-closed container, unless otherwise specified by manufacturer.

**Auxiliary labeling**
- Take with food.
- Take with a full glass of water.
- Swallow tablets whole.
- May cause drowsiness.
- Avoid alcoholic beverages.

## NAPROXEN SODIUM TABLETS USP

**Usual adult dose**
Antirheumatic (nonsteroidal anti-inflammatory)—

    Oral, 275 or 550 mg two times a day, morning and evening; or 275 mg in the morning and 550 mg in the evening.

    Note: During long-term administration, dosage may be adjusted according to patient response; lower doses may suffice.

        If necessary, dosage may be increased to up to 1650 mg per day for short periods. The use of this higher dose requires that the clinical benefit be increased sufficiently to offset the potential increased risk.

Anti-inflammatory (nonsteroidal) or
Analgesic (mild to moderate pain)—

    Oral, 550 mg initially, then 275 mg every six to eight hours as needed.

Antigout agent[1]—

    Oral, 825 mg initially, then 275 mg every eight hours until the attack has subsided.

Antidysmenorrheal—

    Oral, 550 mg initially, then 275 mg every six to eight hours as needed.

Note: For patient self-medication (over-the-counter use) for pain, fever, or dysmenorrhea—Patients 12 years of age and older: Oral, 220 mg every eight to twelve hours while symptoms persist, or

    Oral, 440 mg for the first dose only, followed by 220 mg twelve hours later and every eight to twelve hours thereafter as needed.

**Usual adult prescribing limits**
For mild to moderate pain and
dysmenorrhea—

    Up to a total dose of 1375 mg daily.

Note: For patient self-medication (over-the-counter use) for pain, fever, or dysmenorrhea—Not to exceed 2 tablets (220 mg each) in twenty-four hours for patients 65 years of age or older or 3 tablets in twenty-four hours for patients 12 to 65 years of age.

**Usual pediatric dose**
Pediatric strength not available. It is recommended that naproxen oral suspension or tablets be administered instead.

**Strength(s) usually available**
U.S.—

    220 mg (equivalent to 200 mg of naproxen, with 20 mg of sodium) (OTC) [*Aleve* (magnesium stearate; microcrystalline cellulose; povidone; talc; Opadry YS-1-4215)].

    275 mg (equivalent to 250 mg of naproxen, with 25 mg [approximately 1.1 mmol] of sodium) (Rx) [*Anaprox* (lactose); GENERIC].

    550 mg (equivalent to 500 mg of naproxen, with 50 mg [approximately 2.2 mmol] of sodium) (Rx) [*Anaprox DS;* GENERIC].

Canada—

    275 mg (equivalent to 250 mg of naproxen, with 25 mg [approximately 1.1 mmol] of sodium) (Rx) [*Anaprox* (lactose); *Apo-Napro-Na; Novo-Naprox Sodium; Synflex*].

    550 mg (equivalent to 500 mg of naproxen, with 50 mg [approximately 2.2 mmol] of sodium) (Rx) [*Anaprox DS; Apo-Napro-Na DS; Novo-Naprox Sodium DS; Synflex DS*].

**Packaging and storage**
Store between 15 and 30 °C (59 and 86 °F). Store in a well-closed container.

**Auxiliary labeling**
- Take with food.
- Take with a full glass of water.
- May cause drowsiness.
- Avoid alcoholic beverages.

# Rectal Dosage Forms
## NAPROXEN SUPPOSITORIES

**Usual adult dose**
Antirheumatic (nonsteroidal anti-inflammatory)—

    Rectal, 500 mg at bedtime, administered in conjunction with oral administration during the day.

**Usual adult prescribing limits**
Total daily dose administered orally and rectally should not exceed 1.5 grams a day. The 1.5-gram daily dose is recommended only for short-term administration during acute exacerbations of rheumatic disease.

Also, use of this high dose requires that the additional clinical benefit be sufficient to offset the potential increased risk of adverse effects.

**Usual pediatric dose**
Dosage has not been established.

**Strength(s) usually available**
U.S.—
    Not commercially available.
Canada—
    500 mg (Rx) [*Naprosyn; Naxen*].

**Packaging and storage**
Store below 40 °C (104 °F), preferably between 15 and 30 °C (59 and 86 °F), unless otherwise specified by manufacturer. Protect from freezing.

**Auxiliary labeling**
• For rectal use.
• Avoid alcoholic beverages.

---

[1]Not included in Canadian product labeling.

---

## OXAPROZIN

## Summary of Differences

Indications:
    Indicated for rheumatoid arthritis and osteoarthritis.
Pharmacology/pharmacokinetics:
    Physicochemical characteristics—Chemical group: A proprionic acid derivative.
    Other actions/effects—
        Is as potent as aspirin as an inhibitor of platelet aggregation.
        Also has uricosuric activity.
    Half-life—Elimination
        600 mg per day—25 hours
        1200 mg per day—21 hours
    Peak plasma concentration—Accumulates with chronic dosing.
Precautions:
    Carcinogenicity—Increased hepatic adenomas and carcinomas in male CD mice, but not in female CD mice or in rats.
    Pregnancy/reproduction—Caused fetal malformations in rabbits with doses within the usual human therapeutic range, but not in mice or rats.
    Pediatrics—Preliminary studies done in patients 3 to 16 years of age; elevated aspartate aminotransferase values occurred more frequently in patients treated for juvenile arthritis than for other forms of arthritis.
    Geriatrics—Dosage adjustment not needed on basis of pharmacokinetic considerations. Studies showed increased occurrence of impaired renal function and of decreased hemoglobin concentration, but not of changes in hepatic function, in patients 60 years of age and older compared to younger adults.
    Surgical—Recommended that oxaprozin be discontinued 1 to 2 weeks before elective surgery; may be more likely than most other NSAIDs to increase risk of perisurgical bleeding because of potent and prolonged inhibitory effect on platelet aggregation.
    Laboratory value alterations—Also, may decrease plasma concentrations and increase urine concentrations of uric acid.
Side/adverse effects:
    See *Table 3*, page 417.

## Oral Dosage Forms

### OXAPROZIN TABLETS

**Usual adult dose**
Rheumatoid arthritis—
    Oral, 1200 mg per day, initially, then adjusted according to patient tolerance and response.
Osteoarthritis—
    Oral, 1200 mg per day, initially, although a lower dose of 600 mg per day may be sufficient for mild disease or for patients of low body weight.
Note: Initial dosage must be individualized according to the severity of disease and patient variables such as body weight and renal function.

    A single 1200-mg or 1800-mg loading dose may be administered to patients with normal renal function if necessary to speed the onset of action.

    An initial dose of 600 mg per day is recommended for patients with renal function impairment. If this dose is well tolerated, higher doses may be administered if needed.

Doses of up to 1200 mg per day are usually administered once a day, but patients who are unable to tolerate a single dose of this size may tolerate divided doses.

Very severe arthritis may require doses higher than 1200 mg per day, which should be administered in two or three divided doses. It is recommended that these higher doses be reserved for patients weighing more than 50 kg who have normal hepatic and renal function and a low risk of peptic ulceration and who have not experienced adverse effects with lower doses.

After a beneficial response has been achieved, dosage should be reduced to the lowest dose that provides continuing control of symptoms.

**Usual adult prescribing limits**
Oral, 1800 mg per day or 26 mg per kg of body weight per day, whichever is lower, in two or three divided doses.

**Usual pediatric dose**
Safety and efficacy in children have not been established. However, one preliminary study in children 3 to 16 years of age used a starting dose of 10 mg per kg of body weight. The dose was increased to 20 mg per kg of body weight if necessary.

**Strength(s) usually available**
U.S.—
    600 mg (Rx) [*Daypro* (scored)].
Canada—
    Not commercially available.

**Packaging and storage**
Store below 30 °C (86 °F), preferably between 15 and 30 °C (59 and 86 °F), in a tight, light-resistant container, unless otherwise specified by manufacturer.

Note: Protect unit-dose packages from light.

**Auxiliary labeling**
• Take with food.
• Take with a full glass of water.
• Avoid alcoholic beverages.

---

## PHENYLBUTAZONE

## Summary of Differences

Indications:
    Recommended only for short-term treatment of severe arthritic conditions, gout, or calcium pyrophosphate deposition disease (pseudogout) in patients unresponsive to less toxic NSAIDs. Not recommended as initial therapy for any indication.
Pharmacology/pharmacokinetics:
    Physicochemical characteristics—Chemical group: A pyrazole derivative.
    Other actions/effects—Also induces hepatic microsomal enzyme activity.
    Also has uricosuric activity.
    Biotransformation—Metabolized via hepatic microsomal enzymes. Metabolite oxyphenbutazone is active.
    Half-life—Elimination: 54–99 (average, 77) hours; increased to 105 hours in geriatric patients.
Precautions:
    Mutagenicity—High concentrations induced chromosome abnormalities in Chinese hamster fibroblast cells *in vitro* .
    Pregnancy/reproduction—Fetotoxicity, but not teratogenicity, demonstrated in animal studies.
    Breast-feeding—Distributed into breast milk; may cause blood dyscrasias or other adverse effects in nursing infants.
    Pediatrics—Use in children up to 15 years of age not recommended.
    Geriatrics—Also, increased risk of blood dyscrasias. Recommended that duration of treatment be limited to 1 week in patients 60 years of age and older.
    Drug interactions and/or related problems—
        Concurrent use with alcohol may also impair psychomotor skills.
        Higher risk of bleeding with coumarin- or indandione-derivative anticoagulants than with other NSAIDs because phenylbutazone inhibits the anticoagulant's metabolism; concurrent use not recommended.
        Also, increased risk of toxicity with hydantoin anticonvulsants because phenylbutazone may displace them from protein-binding sites and inhibit their metabolism.
        Also, by inducing hepatic microsomal enzymes, phenylbutazone may decrease effects of barbiturates, cortisone and possibly other coricosteroids, estrogen-containing oral contraceptives, and digitalis glycosides.

Also, increased risk of severe dermatologic reactions with other dermatitis-causing medications.

Also, cholestyramine may decrease absorption of phenylbutazone; recommend administering phenylbutazone 1 hour before or 4 to 6 hours after cholestyramine.

Also, increased risk of adverse hematologic effects if used concurrently with colchicine.

Also, other hepatic enzyme inducers may increase phenylbutazone metabolism and decrease its half-life.

Concurrent use with methotrexate may also increase risk of agranulocytosis or bone marrow depression.

Also, methylphenidate may inhibit phenylbutazone metabolism, leading to increased plasma concentration and risk of toxicity.

Also, concurrent use with penicillamine may increase risk of serious hematologic and/or renal adverse effects.

Also, concurrent use with sulfonamides may potentiate effects of either or both medications.

Also, antacids in buffered formulations may interfere with absorption of many other medications.

Laboratory value alterations—Interference with thyroid function tests, specifically, decreases 24-hour $^{131}$I thyroidal uptake and increases resin or red cell triiodothyronine ($T_3$) uptake.

Also, may decrease blood glucose concentrations.

Also, may decrease plasma concentrations and increase urine concentrations of uric acid.

Medical considerations/contraindications—Also, not recommended in patients with blood dyscrasias (or history of), bone marrow depression, severe cardiac or cardiopulmonary disease or cardiac failure, severe hepatic or renal disease, or active peptic ulcer disease.

Also, may aggravate polymyalgia rheumatica or temporal arteritis.

Patient monitoring—Complete physical examinations, including urinalyses, and hematologic examinations recommended at regular intervals.

Side/adverse effects:

Higher risk of blood dyscrasias than with other NSAIDs, especially in geriatric patients.

Reported to cause a serum sickness– or influenza-like syndrome.

Blood dyscrasias may occur days or weeks after medication is discontinued.

See also *Table 3*, page 417.

## Additional Dosing Information

See also *General Dosing Information*.

Because of its toxicity, phenylbutazone should be used in the minimum effective dosage and for the shortest possible time.

In geriatric patients, therapy should be limited to short periods, preferably not to exceed 1 week, because of the high risk of severe, possibly fatal, toxic reactions.

Phenylbutazone is generally better tolerated when administered with food to lessen gastric irritation.

If therapy is not effective within 1 week, the medication should be discontinued.

Edema may be dose-related and may be prevented in some patients by reducing the dosage.

## Oral Dosage Forms

Note: Bracketed uses in the *Dosage Forms* section refer to categories of use and/or indications that are not included in U.S. product labeling.

### PHENYLBUTAZONE CAPSULES USP

**Usual adult dose**
Rheumatoid arthritis[1] or
Osteoarthritis, acute attacks[1] or
Ankylosing spondylitis or
[Psoriatic arthritis]—
    Oral, 300 to 600 mg a day in three or four divided doses.
Antigout agent—
    Oral, initially 400 mg as a single dose; then 100 mg every four hours for approximately four days or until a satisfactory response is obtained, with the duration of therapy not exceeding one week.
    Note: Some clinicians use a dose of 200 mg every four hours for approximately four days or until a satisfactory response is obtained, with the duration of therapy not exceeding two weeks.

**Usual pediatric dose**
Children up to 15 years of age—Use is not recommended.

**Strength(s) usually available**
U.S.—
    100 mg (Rx) [*Cotylbutazone;* GENERIC].

Canada—
    Not commercially available.

**Packaging and storage**
Store below 40 °C (104 °F), preferably between 15 and 30 °C (59 and 86 °F), unless otherwise specified by manufacturer. Store in a tight container.

**Auxiliary labeling**
• Take with food.
• Take with a full glass of water.
• Avoid alcoholic beverages.

### PHENYLBUTAZONE TABLETS USP

**Usual adult dose**
See *Phenylbutazone Capsules USP*.

**Usual pediatric dose**
Children up to 15 years of age—Use is not recommended.

**Strength(s) usually available**
U.S.—
    100 mg (Rx) [GENERIC].
Canada—
    100 mg (Rx) [*Apo-Phenylbutazone; Butazolidin*].

**Packaging and storage**
Store below 40 °C (104 °F), preferably between 15 and 30 °C (59 and 86 °F), unless otherwise specified by manufacturer. Store in a tight container.

**Auxiliary labeling**
• Take with food.
• Swallow tablets whole.
• Take with a full glass of water.
• Avoid alcoholic beverages.

### PHENYLBUTAZONE TABLETS BUFFERED

**Usual adult dose**
See *Phenylbutazone Capsules USP*.

**Usual pediatric dose**
Children up to 15 years of age—Use is not recommended.

**Strength(s) usually available**
U.S.—
    Not commercially available.
Canada—
    100 mg of phenylbutazone, with 150 mg of magnesium trisilicate and 100 mg of dried aluminum hydroxide gel (Rx) [*Alka Butazolidin*].

**Packaging and storage**
Store below 40 °C (104 °F), preferably between 15 and 30 °C (59 and 86 °F), in a tight container, unless otherwise specified by manufacturer.

**Auxiliary labeling**
• Take with food.
• Swallow tablets whole.
• Take with a full glass of water.
• Avoid alcoholic beverages.

---

[1]Not included in Canadian product labeling.

---

## *PIROXICAM*

## Summary of Differences

Indications:
    Indicated for rheumatoid arthritis, osteoarthritis, ankylosing spondylitis, acute attacks of gout or calcium pyrophosphate deposition disease (pseudogout), and dysmenorrhea.
Pharmacology/pharmacokinetics:
    Physicochemical characteristics—Chemical group: An oxicam derivative.
    Half-life—Elimination: 50 hours, although values ranging from 14 to 158 hours have been reported. Increased in patients with renal function impairment. May also be increased in elderly patients, especially females.
    Onset of action—Gout: 2–4 hours.
    Peak effect time—Gout: 3–5 days.
    Duration of action—Gout: 24 hours.
Precautions:
    Pregnancy/reproduction—Teratogenic effects not demonstrated in animal studies.
    Breast-feeding—Distributed into breast milk; use by breast-feeding mothers not recommended because piroxicam inhibits lactation in animals.

Geriatrics—Tendency toward increased half-life and steady-state concentrations, especially in females.

Drug interactions and/or related problems—Studies failed to show that piroxicam increases digoxin plasma concentrations.

Laboratory value alterations—Also, may increase or decrease blood glucose concentrations.

Medical considerations/contraindications—Higher risk than with most other NSAIDs in patients with renal function impairment.

Side/adverse effects:

Reported to cause a serum sickness– or influenza-like syndrome. See also *Table 3*, page 417.

## Additional Dosing Information

See also *General Dosing Information.*

Because steady-state plasma concentrations are not reached for 7 to 12 days following initiation of therapy, the effectiveness of therapy with piroxicam should not be assessed for 2 weeks.

## Oral Dosage Forms

Note: Bracketed uses in the *Dosage Forms* section refer to categories of use and/or indications that are not included in U.S. product labeling.

### PIROXICAM CAPSULES USP

**Usual adult dose**
Antirheumatic (nonsteroidal anti-inflammatory)—
Oral, 20 mg once a day or 10 mg two times a day.
[Antidysmenorrheal]—
Oral, 40 mg at the onset of symptoms on the first day only, then 20 mg once a day thereafter if necessary.

**Usual pediatric dose**
Dosage has not been established.

**Strength(s) usually available**
U.S.—
10 mg (Rx) [*Feldene* (lactose); GENERIC].
20 mg (Rx) [*Feldene* (lactose); GENERIC].
Canada—
10 mg (Rx) [*Apo-Piroxicam; Feldene* (lactose); *Novo-Pirocam; Nu-Pirox; PMS-Piroxicam*].
20 mg (Rx) [*Apo-Piroxicam; Feldene* (lactose); *Novo-Pirocam; Nu-Pirox; PMS-Piroxicam*].

**Packaging and storage**
Store below 30 °C (86 °F). Store in a tight, light-resistant container.

**Auxiliary labeling**
• Take after meals.
• Take with a full glass of water.
• Avoid alcoholic beverages.

## Rectal Dosage Forms
### PIROXICAM SUPPOSITORIES

**Usual adult dose**
Antirheumatic (nonsteroidal anti-inflammatory)—
Rectal, 20 mg once a day or 10 mg two times a day.

**Usual adult prescribing limits**
Rectal or combined oral and rectal—20 mg a day.

**Usual pediatric dose**
Dosage has not been established.

**Strength(s) usually available**
U.S.—
Not commercially available.
Canada—
10 mg (Rx) [*Feldene*].
20 mg (Rx) [*Feldene*].

**Packaging and storage**
Store below 40 °C (104 °F), preferably between 15 and 30 °C (59 and 86 °F), unless otherwise specified by manufacturer. Protect from freezing.

**Auxiliary labeling**
• For rectal use.
• Avoid alcoholic beverages.

## Summary of Differences

Indications:
Indicated for rheumatoid arthritis, osteoarthritis, ankylosing spondylitis, acute attacks of gout or calcium pyrophosphate deposition disease (pseudogout), bursitis, and tendinitis.

Pharmacology/pharmacokinetics:
Physicochemical characteristics—Chemical group: A pyrroleacetic acid derivative.
Biotransformation—Hepatic; sulfide metabolite, not sulindac itself, is active substance.
Half-life—Elimination:
Sulindac—7.8 hours
Sulindac sulfide—16.4 hours
Time to peak plasma concentration—Sulindac sulfide: Substantially delayed in patients with alcoholic hepatic disease.
Elimination: Less than 1% of a sulindac dose excreted via the kidneys as the active sulfide metabolite.

Precautions:
Pregnancy/reproduction—Fetotoxicity, and, in some studies, a low incidence of teratogenicity, have been demonstrated in animals.
Drug interactions and/or related problems—
Concurrent chronic use of antacids significantly decreases sulindac plasma concentration.
Decreased concentration of active sulfide metabolite of sulindac and peripheral neuropathy reported with concurrent (topical) use of dimethyl sulfoxide.
Laboratory value alterations—Also, may increase blood glucose concentrations.
Medical considerations/contraindications—
Hepatic function impairment may slow metabolism to, but also decrease biliary elimination of, the active sulfide metabolite; net result is increased and prolonged plasma concentration and higher risk of toxicity.
Also, caution and adequate fluid intake recommended for patients with renal calculi (or history of) because renal calculi containing sulindac metabolites have occurred in a few patients.

Side/adverse effects:
May be less likely than most other NSAIDs to cause renal toxicity.
Reported to cause biliary obstruction.
Reported to cause a characteristic hypersensitivity syndrome.
See also *Table 3*, page 417.

## Additional Dosing Information

See also *General Dosing Information.*

In the treatment of arthritis, improvement in condition may occur within 7 days, but 2 to 3 weeks of continuous use on a regular basis may be required for maximum effectiveness.

Patients with impaired renal function may require lower doses.

Therapy for 7 days in acute gouty arthritis and for 7 to 14 days in acute painful shoulder is usually sufficient.

## Oral Dosage Forms
### SULINDAC TABLETS USP

**Usual adult dose**
Antirheumatic (nonsteroidal anti-inflammatory)—
Oral, 150 or 200 mg two times a day; may be increased or decreased, depending on patient response.
Note: Although some patients have received doses higher than 400 mg per day, such doses have not been fully evaluated and are not recommended.
Antigout agent—
Oral, 200 mg two times a day; dosage to be decreased according to patient response.
Anti-inflammatory (acute painful shoulder)—
Oral, 200 mg two times a day; dosage to be decreased according to patient response.

**Usual pediatric dose**
Safety and efficacy have not been established.

**Strength(s) usually available**
U.S.—
150 mg (Rx) [*Clinoril;* GENERIC].
200 mg (Rx) [*Clinoril* (scored); GENERIC (may be scored)].

Canada—
    150 mg (Rx) [*Apo-Sulin* (scored); *Clinoril; Novo-Sundac* (scored)].
    200 mg (Rx) [*Apo-Sulin* (scored); *Clinoril* (scored); *Novo-Sundac* (scored)].

**Packaging and storage**
Store below 40 °C (104 °F), preferably between 15 and 30 °C (59 and 86 °F). Store in a well-closed container.

**Auxiliary labeling**
• Take with food.
• Take with a full glass of water.
• Avoid alcoholic beverages.

---

### TENOXICAM

## Summary of Differences

Indications:
    Indicated for rheumatoid arthritis, osteoarthritis, ankylosing spondylitis, bursitis, tendinitis, and periarthritis.
Pharmacology/pharmacokinetics:
    Physicochemical characteristics—Chemical group: An oxicam derivative.
    Half-life—Elimination: $72 \pm 26$ (range, 32–110) hours.
Precautions:
    Pregnancy/reproduction—
        Fertility: Decreased number of corpora lutea and implantations in female rats, but no impairment of fertility in male rats, demonstrated in animal studies.
        First trimester: Maternotoxicity (panperitonitis, gastric lesions, and uterine hemorrhage) and embryotoxicity, but not teratogenicity, demonstrated in animal studies.
    Geriatrics—Also, risk of hyperkalemia may be increased in geriatric patients.
    Drug interactions and/or related problems—
        Studies failed to show that tenoxicam increases digoxin concentrations.
        Also, cholestyramine administered in conjunction with intravenously administered tenoxicam shown to decrease half-life of tenoxicam from 67.4 to 31.9 hours and increase tenoxicam clearance by 105%.
Side/adverse effects:
    See *Table 3*, page 417.

## Oral Dosage Forms
### TENOXICAM TABLETS

**Usual adult dose**
Antirheumatic (nonsteroidal anti-inflammatory)
and Anti-inflammatory (nonsteroidal)—
    Oral, 20 mg once a day, at the same time each day. For some patients, 10 mg once a day may be sufficient. The smallest effective dose should be used.

**Usual adult prescribing limits**
20 mg per day. Higher doses may increase the risk of adverse effects without providing a significantly greater therapeutic response.

**Usual pediatric dose**
Children up to 16 years of age—Dosage has not been established.

**Strength(s) usually available**
U.S.—
    Not commercially available.
Canada—
    20 mg (Rx) [*Mobiflex* (scored; corn starch; hydroxypropyl methylcellulose; iron oxide; lactose; magnesium stearate; talc; titanium dioxide)].

**Packaging and storage**
Store between 15 and 30 °C (59 and 86 °F), unless otherwise specified by manufacturer.

**Auxiliary labeling**
• Take with food.
• Take with a full glass of water.
• Avoid alcoholic beverages.

---

### TIAPROFENIC ACID

## Summary of Differences

Indications:
    Indicated for rheumatoid arthritis and osteoarthritis.

Pharmacology/pharmacokinetics:
Physicochemical characteristics—Chemical group: A propionic acid derivative.
Half-life—Elimination
Single dose—Tablets: 1.7 hours; increased to 2.5 hours in geriatric patients.
At steady-state—Extended-release capsules (600 mg once a day): 4.2 hours.
Precautions:
    Pregnancy/reproduction—
        Fertility: Decreased number of implantation sites in female rabbits, but no effect on fertility in male or female rats.
        First trimester:
            Crosses the placenta.
            Fetotoxicity, but not teratogenicity, demonstrated in animal studies.
    Geriatrics—Substantially higher frequency of hyperkalemia and/or increased blood urea nitrogen documented in studies.
    Drug interactions and/or related problems—Also, may displace hydantoin anticonvulsants from their protein-binding sites, possibly leading to increased hydantoin half-life and toxicity.
Side/adverse effects:
    See *Table 3*, page 417.

## Oral Dosage Forms
### TIAPROFENIC ACID EXTENDED-RELEASE CAPSULES

**Usual adult dose**
Antirheumatic (nonsteroidal anti-inflammatory)—
    Oral, 600 mg once a day, at the same time each day.

**Usual pediatric dose**
Safety and efficacy have not been established.

**Strength(s) usually available**
U.S.—
    Not commercially available.
Canada—
    300 mg (Rx) [*Surgam SR*].

**Packaging and storage**
Store below 40 °C (104 °F), preferably between 15 and 30 °C (59 and 86 °F), unless otherwise specified by manufacturer.

**Auxiliary labeling**
• Take with food.
• Swallow capsules whole.
• Take with a full glass of water.
• Avoid alcoholic beverages.

### TIAPROFENIC ACID TABLETS

**Usual adult dose**
Rheumatoid arthritis—
    Oral, 600 mg a day in two or three divided doses.
Osteoarthritis—
    Oral, 600 mg a day in two or three divided doses, initially. After a satisfactory response has been obtained, dosage may be reduced. Some patients may be maintained on 300 mg a day in divided doses.

**Usual adult prescribing limits**
600 mg a day.

**Usual pediatric dose**
Safety and efficacy have not been established.

**Strength(s) usually available**
U.S.—
    Not commercially available.
Canada—
    200 mg (Rx) [*Albert Tiafen* (scored); *Surgam* (scored)].
    300 mg (Rx) [*Albert Tiafen* (scored); *Surgam* (scored)].

**Packaging and storage**
Store below 40 °C (104 °F), preferably between 15 and 30 °C (59 and 86 °F), unless otherwise specified by manufacturer.

**Auxiliary labeling**
• Take with food.
• Take with a full glass of water.
• Avoid alcoholic beverages.

---
### *TOLMETIN*
---

## Summary of Differences

Indications:
Indicated for rheumatoid arthritis, osteoarthritis, ankylosing spondylitis, juvenile arthritis, and psoriatic arthritis.

Pharmacology/pharmacokinetics:
Physicochemical characteristics—Chemical group: A pyrroleacetic acid derivative.
Absorption—Extent decreased by food and milk.
Half-life—Elimination: 5 hours

Precautions:
Pregnancy/reproduction—No teratogenicity or other adverse effects on fetal development demonstrated in animal studies.
Pediatrics—Studied in pediatric patients 2 years of age and older; no pediatrics-specific problems documented.
Laboratory value alterations—Interference with sulfosalicylic acid test method for urinary protein.
Medical considerations/contraindications—Caution in patients who must restrict their sodium intake.

Side/adverse effects:
Higher incidence of anaphylactic reactions than with other NSAIDs.
Reported to cause a serum sickness– or influenza-like syndrome.
See also *Table 3*, page 417.

## Additional Dosing Information

See also *General Dosing Information.*

Improvement in condition may occur within 7 days, but 1 to 2 weeks of continuous use on a regular basis may be required for maximum effectiveness.

## Oral Dosage Forms

Note: The dosing and strengths of the available dosage forms are expressed in terms of the free acid (not the sodium salt).

### TOLMETIN SODIUM CAPSULES USP

**Usual adult dose**
Antirheumatic (nonsteroidal anti-inflammatory)—
Initial: Oral, 400 mg (free acid) three times a day, preferably including a dose in the morning and a dose at bedtime.
Maintenance: Rheumatoid arthritis—
Oral, 600 mg to 1.8 grams (free acid) a day in three or four divided doses.
Osteoarthritis—
Oral, 600 mg to 1.6 grams (free acid) a day in three or four divided doses.

**Usual adult prescribing limits**
Up to 2 grams (free acid) daily for rheumatoid arthritis or 1.6 grams (free acid) daily for osteoarthritis.

**Usual pediatric dose**
Antirheumatic (nonsteroidal anti-inflammatory)—
Children up to 2 years of age: Dosage has not been established.

Children 2 years of age and over: Initial—Oral, 20 mg (free acid) per kg of body weight a day in three or four divided doses.
Maintenance—Oral, 15 to 30 mg (free acid) per kg of body weight a day in divided doses.

Note: Doses higher than 30 mg (free acid) per kg of body weight per day have not been studied and therefore are not recommended.

**Strength(s) usually available**
U.S.—
400 mg (free acid, with 36 mg [1.568 mmol] of sodium) (Rx) [*Tolectin DS;* GENERIC].
Canada—
400 mg (free acid, with 36 mg [1.568 mmol] of sodium) (Rx) [*Novo-Tolmetin; Tolectin 400*].

**Packaging and storage**
Store below 40 °C (104 °F), preferably between 15 and 30 °C (59 and 86 °F). Store in a tight container.

**Auxiliary labeling**
• Take with food.
• Take with a full glass of water.
• Avoid alcoholic beverages.

### TOLMETIN SODIUM TABLETS USP

**Usual adult dose**
See *Tolmetin Sodium Capsules USP.*

**Usual adult prescribing limits**
See *Tolmetin Sodium Capsules USP.*

**Usual pediatric dose**
See *Tolmetin Sodium Capsules USP.*

**Strength(s) usually available**
U.S.—
200 mg (free acid, with 18 mg [0.784 mmol] of sodium) (Rx) [*Tolectin 200* (scored); GENERIC].
600 mg (free acid, with 54 mg [2.352 mmol] of sodium) (Rx) [*Tolectin 600;* GENERIC].
Canada—
200 mg (free acid, with 18 mg [0.784 mmol] of sodium) (Rx) [*Tolectin 200* (scored)].
600 mg (free acid, with 54 mg [2.352 mmol] of sodium) (Rx) [*Tolectin 600*].

**Packaging and storage**
Store between 15 and 30 °C (59 and 86 °F). Store in a well-closed container.

**Auxiliary labeling**
• Take with food.
• Take with a full glass of water.
• Avoid alcoholic beverages.

---
Revised: 09/13/94
Interim revision: 07/24/96

## Table 1. Pharmacology/Pharmacokinetics

| | Absorption | | | Plasma Concentration | | | |
|---|---|---|---|---|---|---|---|
| Drug and Route | Rate (Factors that decrease) | Extent (Factors that decrease) | % Protein-Binding* (Factors that decrease) | Time to Peak (hr) [dose in mg] | Peak (mcg/mL) [dose in mg] | Time to Steady-State (days) [dose in mg/ doses per day] | Steady-State (mcg/mL) [dose in mg/ doses per day] |
| Diclofenac | | | >99 | | | | |
| Oral | | | | | | | |
| Tablets | Rapid (food) | Complete | | 1, range 0.33–2†; up to 3.6‡ | | | |
| Delayed-release Tablets | Rapid (food) | Complete | | 2, range 0.25–4†; 6‡ | 0.7–1.1 [25] 1.5–1.6 [50]† 2 [75] Decreased 40% by food | | |
| Extended-release Tablets | | | | 4 | | | |
| Rectal | Rapid | | | 0.5–2 | | | |
| Diflunisal | | | >99 | | | | |
| Oral | Rapid (food) | Complete | | 2–3 | 41 [250] 87 [500] 124 [1000] | | 56 [250/2] 190 [500/2] |
| Etodolac | | | >99 | | | | |
| Oral | Rapid (food)§ | Extensive | | 1.3, range 0.8–1.8†; 2.2–5.6‡ [200–600]; Steady-state 1.7±1.3 | 10–46 [200–600] Decreased 50% by food and 15–20% by antacids | | 16.5–19 [200/2] |
| Fenoprofen | | | 99 | | | | |
| Oral | Rapid (food, milk)§ | | | 1–2 [600]† Increased by food | 50 [600]† Decreased by food | | |
| Floctafenine | | | | | | | |
| Oral | Rapid (food) | | | 1–2 | | Within 3 | |

*To albumin.

†Taken on an empty stomach.

‡Taken with food.

§Absorption not affected by antacids, specifically: For fenoprofen, ibuprofen, ketoprofen, meclofenamate, piroxicam, sulindac, tolmetin—Aluminum- and magnesium-containing; For tiaprofenic acid—Aluminum-containing

#May be increased in geriatric patients (For flurbiprofen, geriatric females only).

**Decreased by 40% in patients with end-stage renal disease undergoing continuous ambulatory peritoneal dialysis.

††Decrease to 37 mcg/mL demonstrated in obese patients, probably because volume of distribution increased.

‡‡Failure to retain suppository in rectum for one full hour may be responsible for incomplete absorption.

§§Bioavailability 73–93% of that achieved with oral administration.

##Mean 8 hours in patients with hepatic cirrhosis. Not significantly different in geriatric patients than in younger adults.

***Administration of a second 1000-mg dose 12 hours after an initial 1000-mg dose produced peak concentrations of ±71 mcg/mL. Peak concentrations are significantly decreased (to as low as 18 mcg/mL) in patients with hepatic cirrhosis.

†††May be increased by concurrent administration of sodium bicarbonate.

‡‡‡Similar values reported with administration of 500-mg tablets to adults and with administration of 5 mg/kg of oral suspension to children 5 to 16 years of age with juvenile arthritis.

§§§Increased to 70.7 mcg/mL by concurrent administration with antacid.

###May be increased to 2 to 3 weeks if elimination half-life is greatly prolonged.

****May be increased if elimination half-life is greatly prolonged and/or renal function is impaired.

††††May be increased to 4 to 7 hours in patients with alcoholic hepatic disease.

## Table 1. Pharmacology/Pharmacokinetics *(continued)*

| Drug and Route | Absorption | | % Protein-Binding* (Factors that decrease) | Plasma Concentration | | | |
|---|---|---|---|---|---|---|---|
| | Rate (Factors that decrease) | Extent (Factors that decrease) | | Time to Peak (hr) [dose in mg] | Peak (mcg/mL) [dose in mg] | Time to Steady-State (days) [dose in mg/ doses per day] | Steady-State (mcg/mL) [dose in mg/ doses per day] |
| Flurbiprofen Oral | | | 99 | | | | |
| Tablets | Rapid (food) | | | 1.5; range 0.5–4 | 5–6; 8.7# [50] 10–15 [100]** Decreased by food | | 5–6 [50/3] |
| Extended-release Capsules | | | | 5.5†; 8.3‡ | 8.56 Increased by food | 2–3 [200/1] | 10.78 [200/1] |
| Ibuprofen Oral | Rapid (food)§ | | 99 | 1.2–2.1 | 22–27 [200] 23–45 [400] 42–57 [600]†† 56–66 [800] Decreased up to 30% by food | | |
| Indomethacin Oral | | | 99 | | | | |
| Capsules; Oral Suspension | Rapid (food, antacids [Al- and/or Mg-containing]) | Complete; 90% in 4 hr | | 0.5–2 [25] | 0.8–2.5 [25] 2.5–4 [50] | | 1.4 [25/3] 2.8 [50/3] |
| Extended-release Capsules | | 90% in 12 hr | | 2–4.25 [75] | 1.5–3 [75] | | 1.4 [75/1] |
| Rectal | Rapid | 80–90‡‡ | | | | | |
| Ketoprofen | | | 99 (hepatic cirrhosis, advanced age) | | | <1 | |
| Oral Capsules | Rapid (food, milk)§ | Complete | | 0.5–2 [50] average 1.1† average 2‡ | 4.1 [50]†# 2.4 [50]‡# | | |
| Extended-release Capsules | Slow | Almost complete | | 6–7†; 8–9‡ | 3.1 ± 1.2†; 3.4 ± 1.3‡ [200] | | |
| Delayed-release Tablets | Delayed by ± 1.5 hr | | | 1.5–4 [50] | | | |
| Extended-release Tablets | | | | 5.5–8 | Decreased 20% by high-fat meal | | |
| Rectal§§ | | | | 0.5–2 | | | |
| Meclofenamate Oral | Rapid (food)§ | Complete (food) | >99 | 0.5–2 | 8–9 [100] | | 4.8, range 1.8-7.2 [100/3] Decreased by food |
| Mefenamic Acid Oral | Rapid | | | 2.5 [250] 1–2 [500] 2–4 [1000] | 3.6 [250] 3.5 [500] 10 [1000] | 2 [1000/4] | 20 [1000/4] |

Table 1. Pharmacology/Pharmacokinetics *(continued)*

| Drug and Route | Absorption | | % Protein-Binding* (Factors that decrease) | Plasma Concentration | | | |
|---|---|---|---|---|---|---|---|
| | Rate (Factors that decrease) | Extent (Factors that decrease) | | Time to Peak (hr) [dose in mg] | Peak (mcg/mL) [dose in mg] | Time to Steady-State (days) [dose in mg/ doses per day] | Steady-State (mcg/mL) [dose in mg/ doses per day] |
| Nabumetone (prodrug) Oral 6-methoxy-2-naph-thylacetic acid (6-MNA) (active substance) | Increased by food, milk§ | Increased by food, milk§ | >99 | Steady-state 3, range 1–12 [1000]##; 2.5, range 1–8 [2000] Decreased by food | 24 [500]‡ 22–23†; 36–38‡# [1000]***  64 [2000] | 3 [500/2 or 1000/1] | 18.5 [500/2]; trough 33, peak 52 [1000/1]# |
| Naproxen | | | >99 (hepatic cirrhosis, advanced age) | | | | |
| Oral Tablets; Oral Suspension | Rapid (food, antacids [Al- and Mg-contain-ing])††† | Complete | | Naproxen: 2–4 [750]  Sodium salt: 1–2 [825] | 46.6 [375] 63.1 [500]‡‡‡ 90 [750] | 2–2.5 (500/2) | 55 [500/2] |
| Delayed-release Tablets | | | | 4.2-4.5 Decreased by antacids Increased by high-fat meal | 47.9 [375] 58.2 [2×250] 60.7 [500]§§§ | | |
| Extended-release Tablets | | | | 9.7†; 7.7‡ [1000] | 63.1†; 86.1‡ [1000] | | |
| Oxaprozin | | | ±99.9 (renal impairment, congestive heart failure, hepatic cirrhosis | | | | |
| Oral | Relatively slow§ (food–slight effect) | | | 3-5 | 70-80 [1200] | 4-7 | 98-230 [600/1 or 1200/1] Accumulates with chronic dosing |

*To albumin.

†Taken on an empty stomach.

‡Taken with food.

§Absorption not affected by antacids, specifically: For fenoprofen, ibuprofen, ketoprofen, meclofenamate, piroxicam, sulindac, tolmetin—Aluminum- and magnesium-containing; For tiaprofenic acid—Aluminum-containing

#May be increased in geriatric patients (For flurbiprofen, geriatric females only).

**Decreased by 40% in patients with end-stage renal disease undergoing continuous ambulatory peritoneal dialysis.

††Decrease to 37 mcg/mL demonstrated in obese patients, probably because volume of distribution increased.

‡‡Failure to retain suppository in rectum for one full hour may be responsible for incomplete absorption.

§§Bioavailability 73–93% of that achieved with oral administration.

##Mean 8 hours in patients with hepatic cirrhosis. Not significantly different in geriatric patients than in younger adults.

***Administration of a second 1000-mg dose 12 hours after an initial 1000-mg dose produced peak concentrations of ±71 mcg/mL. Peak concentrations are significantly decreased (to as low as 18 mcg/mL) in patients with hepatic cirrhosis.

†††May be increased by concurrent administration of sodium bicarbonate.

‡‡‡Similar values reported with administration of 500-mg tablets to adults and with administration of 5 mg/kg of oral suspension to children 5 to 16 years of age with juvenile arthritis.

§§§Increased to 70.7 mcg/mL by concurrent administration with antacid.

###May be increased to 2 to 3 weeks if elimination half-life is greatly prolonged.

****May be increased if elimination half-life is greatly prolonged and/or renal function is impaired.

††††May be increased to 4 to 7 hours in patients with alcoholic hepatic disease.

## Table 1. Pharmacology/Pharmacokinetics *(continued)*

| Drug and Route | Absorption | | | Plasma Concentration | | | |
|---|---|---|---|---|---|---|---|
| | Rate (Factors that decrease) | Extent (Factors that decrease) | % Protein-Binding* (Factors that decrease) | Time to Peak (hr) [dose in mg] | Peak (mcg/mL) [dose in mg] | Time to Steady-State (days) [dose in mg/ doses per day] | Steady-State (mcg/mL) [dose in mg/ doses per day] |
| Phenylbutazone Oral | Rapid | | 98 | 2–2.5 | 43 [300] | | Phenylbuta-zone: up to 172 Oxyphenbuta-zone: up to 86 |
| Piroxicam Oral | (food)§ | | | 3–5 [20] | 1.5–2 [20] | 7–12 [20/1]### | 3–8 [20/1]**** |
| Rectal | | | | 10 [20] | | | |
| Sulindac (prodrug) Oral | (food)§ | 90% | | 2† 3–4‡ | 1–2 [200] | | |
| Sulindac sulfide (active substance) | | | | 1.7†††† | | 4–5 [200/2] | 4 [200/2] |
| Tenoxicam Oral | (food)§ | Extensive§ | 98–99 | 1.25, range 0.5–6† | 1.46–3.31† [20] | | |
| Tiaprofenic Acid Oral Tablets | Rapid (food)§ | | 98 | 0.5–1.5† Up to 2‡ | 26 [200] 50 [300] | Within 1 [200/3] | |
| Extended-release Capsules | | | | Steady-state 4–8 [600/1] | | | |
| Tolmetin Oral | Rapid (food)§ | Almost complete (food, milk) | >99 | 0.5–1 | 40 [400]† 20 [400]‡ | | |

*To albumin.

†Taken on an empty stomach.

‡Taken with food.

§Absorption not affected by antacids, specifically: For fenoprofen, ibuprofen, ketoprofen, meclofenamate, piroxicam, sulindac, tolmetin—Aluminum- and magnesium-containing; For tiaprofenic acid—Aluminum-containing

#May be increased in geriatric patients (For flurbiprofen, geriatric females only).

**Decreased by 40% in patients with end-stage renal disease undergoing continuous ambulatory peritoneal dialysis.

††Decrease to 37 mcg/mL demonstrated in obese patients, probably because volume of distribution increased.

‡‡Failure to retain suppository in rectum for one full hour may be responsible for incomplete absorption.

§§Bioavailability 73–93% of that achieved with oral administration.

##Mean 8 hours in patients with hepatic cirrhosis. Not significantly different in geriatric patients than in younger adults.

***Administration of a second 1000-mg dose 12 hours after an initial 1000-mg dose produced peak concentrations of ±71 mcg/mL. Peak concentrations are significantly decreased (to as low as 18 mcg/mL) in patients with hepatic cirrhosis.

†††May be increased by concurrent administration of sodium bicarbonate.

‡‡‡Similar values reported with administration of 500-mg tablets to adults and with administration of 5 mg/kg of oral suspension to children 5 to 16 years of age with juvenile arthritis.

§§§Increased to 70.7 mcg/mL by concurrent administration with antacid.

###May be increased to 2 to 3 weeks if elimination half-life is greatly prolonged.

****May be increased if elimination half-life is greatly prolonged and/or renal function is impaired.

††††May be increased to 4 to 7 hours in patients with alcoholic hepatic disease.

## Table 2. Pharmacology/Pharmacokinetics

| Drug | Biotransformation | Half-Life | | Renal Elimination | | Biliary/Fecal Elimination | |
|---|---|---|---|---|---|---|---|
| | | Distribution (hr) | Elimination (hr) | % of Dose | % Unchanged | % of Dose | % Unchanged |
| Diclofenac* | Hepatic; almost 50% eliminated via first-pass metabolism† | | 1.2–2 | 40–65 | Little or none | 35 | Little or none |
| Diflunisal‡ | | | 8–12<br><br>22<br>(GFR 10–50)§#<br>60<br>(GFR 2–10)§#<br>115<br>(GFR <2)§# | 80–95 in 72–96 hr<br>53 in 72 hr<br>(GFR 10–50)§<br>9.5 in 72 hr<br>(GFR 2–10)§<br>2.7 in 72 hr<br>(GFR <2)§ | <5 | Little or none | |
| Etodolac‡ | Hepatic, extensive. No significant first-pass metabolism | 0.71 ± 0.5, at steady-state | Single dose 6–7; Steady-state 7.3 ± 4 | 72; 60% in 24 h | <1 | 16 | |
| Fenoprofen | Hepatic | | 3 | 90 in 24 hr | | | |
| Floctafenine | Hepatic; rapid | 1 | 8 | 40** | | 60** | |
| Flurbiprofen | | 3 | 5.7, range 2–12 | 88–98; 73 within 48 hr | 20–25 | | |
| Ibuprofen‡ | Hepatic | | 1.8–2 | 100 in 24 hr | <1 | | |
| Indomethacin‡ | Hepatic | 1 | 2.6–11.2 (average 4.5)†† | 60 | 10–20 | 33‡‡ | 1.5 |
| Ketoprofen* | Primarily hepatic; glucuronide conjugation may also occur in other tissues | 0.33 | Capsules 1.6; Extended-release Capsules 5.4 ± 2.2; Extended-release Tablets 3–4## | 80 in 24 hr | Up to 10 | *** | |
| Meclofenamate | ††† | | 2 (single dose) 3.3 (multiple doses) | 66 | Little or none | 33 | |
| Mefenamic Acid | Hepatic | | 2 | 67 | | Up to 25 | |

*Dialyzable.

†Some metabolites may be active.

‡Not dialyzable.

§In patients with renal function impairment. GFR=glomerular filtration rate in mL per minute, when specified.

#Reason for prolonged half-life is unclear because only small amounts are excreted unchanged. It has been proposed that biliary excretion of metabolites with subsequent hydrolysis to, and reabsorption of, the parent compound may occur in renal failure. Alternatively, slower renal excretion may permit hydrolysis of an unstable metabolite to the parent compound.

**Excretion (renal plus biliary/fecal) complete within 24 hours.

††Subject to large interindividual variation, possibly because of differences in enterohepatic circulation and subsequent reabsorption.

‡‡Undergoes extensive enterohepatic circulation.

§§Acyl-glucuronide conjugate is unstable; in patients with renal function impairment, this conjugate may accumulate and be deconjugated to the parent compound.

##Higher values for the extended-release dosage forms reflect prolonged absorption. In geriatric patients, values for the capsules and the extended-release capsules are prolonged by 26% and 54%, respectively. Also, values for the capsules may be prolonged to 3 hours in patients with mild renal function impairment and to 5 to 9 hours in patients with moderate to severe renal function impairment.

***Enterohepatic recirculation has been proposed to account for elimination of the other 40% of the dose; however, studies to confirm this possibility have not been done.

†††Hydroxymethyl metabolite has anti-inflammatory activity approximately 20% of that of the parent compound.

‡‡‡In geriatric patients, in whom values are especially subject to substantial interpatient variability; values as high as 74 hours have been measured. Also, increased to about 39 hours in patients with creatinine clearances <30 mL/minute/1.73 cubic meters of body surface area), but not in patients with lesser degrees of renal function impairment or in patients receiving hemodialysis.

§§§In patients with moderately severe renal function impairment (creatinine clearances 10–30 mL/min/1.73 cubic meters of body surface area).

###Several studies reported terminal elimination half-life values of 50 to 60 hours. However, these lower "accumulation" half-life values are recommended for use in clinical practice, e.g., for estimating time to reach steady-state, determining appropriate dosing intervals, and determining intervals for dosage adjustment.

****In geriatric patients.

††††Average; usual range 30 to 60 hours, but values ranging from 14 to 158 hours have been reported. Half-life may be especially prolonged in patients with renal function impairment.

Table 2. Pharmacology/Pharmacokinetics *(continued)*

| Drug | Biotransformation | Half-Life Distribution (hr) | Half-Life Elimination (hr) | Renal Elimination % of Dose | Renal Elimination % Unchanged | Biliary/Fecal Elimination % of Dose | Biliary/Fecal Elimination % Unchanged |
|---|---|---|---|---|---|---|---|
| Nabumetone | Hepatic, with extensive first-pass metabolism. 35–38% of a 1000-mg dose metabolized to the active substance 6-MNA, which is further metabolized hepatically; bioavailability of 6-MNA decreased in patients with severe hepatic function impairment | | 6-MNA: 23 ± 3.7; 30 ± 8.1‡‡‡ | 6-MNA: 80; 75 in 48 hr; complete in 168 hr; 32.5 in 96 hr§§§ | 6-MNA: <1 | | |
| Naproxen | Hepatic | | 13 | 95 | | | |
| Oxaprozin‡ | Hepatic, 65% via microsomal oxidation followed by glucuronic acid conjugation and 35% via direct glucuronic acid conjugation | | Steady-state (mg/day) 25 (600) 21 (1200)### | 65%, as glucuronide metabolites | Very small amounts | 35%, as glucuronide metabolites | Very small amounts |
| Phenylbutazone | Slow, via hepatic microsomal enzymes | | 54–99 (average 77) 105**** | 61–75; may remain in body 7–10 days after last dose | Trace amounts | 25–27 | <5 |
| Oxyphenbutazone (active metabolite) | | | | 4 | | | |
| Piroxicam | Hepatic | | 50†††† | 66 | <5 | 33 | |
| Sulindac | Hepatic; sulfide metabolite, not sulindac itself, is active | | 7.8 | 50 | | ‡‡ | |
| Sulindac sulfide | | | 16.4 | <1 | | 25‡‡ | |
| Tenoxicam | | | 72 ± 28 (range, 32–110) | 66 | < 0.5 | 17 | |
| Tiaprofenic Acid | | | Tablets 1.7; 2.5**** Extended-release Capsules (at steady-state) 4.2 | 60 | 90 | 40 | |
| Tolmetin | Hepatic | 1–2 | 5 | 100 in 24 hr | Up to 17 | | |

*Dialyzable.

†Some metabolites may be active.

‡Not dialyzable.

§In patients with renal function impairment. GFR=glomerular filtration rate in mL per minute, when specified.

#Reason for prolonged half-life is unclear because only small amounts are excreted unchanged. It has been proposed that biliary excretion of metabolites with subsequent hydrolysis to, and reabsorption of, the parent compound may occur in renal failure. Alternatively, slower renal excretion may permit hydrolysis of an unstable metabolite to the parent compound.

**Excretion (renal plus biliary/fecal) complete within 24 hours.

††Subject to large interindividual variation, possibly because of differences in enterohepatic circulation and subsequent reabsorption.

‡‡Undergoes extensive enterohepatic circulation.

§§Acyl-glucuronide conjugate is unstable; in patients with renal function impairment, this conjugate may accumulate and be deconjugated to the parent compound.

##Higher values for the extended-release dosage forms reflect prolonged absorption. In geriatric patients, values for the capsules and the extended-release capsules are prolonged by 26% and 54%, respectively. Also, values for the capsules may be prolonged to 3 hours in patients with mild renal function impairment and to 5 to 9 hours in patients with moderate to severe renal function impairment.

***Enterohepatic recirculation has been proposed to account for elimination of the other 40% of the dose; however, studies to confirm this possibility have not been done.

†††Hydroxymethyl metabolite has anti-inflammatory activity approximately 20% of that of the parent compound.

‡‡‡In geriatric patients, in whom values are especially subject to substantial interpatient variability; values as high as 74 hours have been measured. Also, increased to about 39 hours in patients with creatinine clearances <30 mL/minute/1.73 cubic meters of body surface area), but not in patients with lesser degrees of renal function impairment or in patients receiving hemodialysis.

§§§In patients with moderately severe renal function impairment (creatinine clearances 10–30 mL/min/1.73 cubic meters of body surface area).

###Several studies reported terminal elimination half-life values of 50 to 60 hours. However, these lower "accumulation" half-life values are recommended for use in clinical practice, e.g., for estimating time to reach steady-state, determining appropriate dosing intervals, and determining intervals for dosage adjustment.

****In geriatric patients.

††††Average; usual range 30 to 60 hours, but values ranging from 14 to 158 hours have been reported. Half-life may be especially prolonged in patients with renal function impairment.

## Table 3. Side/Adverse Effects*

Legend:
I = Diclofenac
II = Diflunisal
III = Etodolac
IV = Fenoprofen
V = Floctafenine
VI = Flurbiprofen
VII = Ibuprofen
VIII = Indomethacin
IX = Ketoprofen
X = Meclofenamate
XI = Mefenamic Acid
XII = Nabumetone
XIII = Naproxen
XIV = Oxaprozin
XV = Phenylbutazone
XVI = Piroxicam
XVII = Sulindac
XVIII = Tenoxicam
XIX = Tiaprofenic Acid
XX = Tolmetin

| Side/Adverse effect | I | II | III | IV | V | VI | VII | VIII | IX | X | XI | XII | XIII | XIV | XV | XVI | XVII | XVIII | XIX | XX |
|---|---|---|---|---|---|---|---|---|---|---|---|---|---|---|---|---|---|---|---|---|
| **Medical attention needed** | | | | | | | | | | | | | | | | | | | | |
| *Cardiovascular effects* | | | | | | | | | | | | | | | | | | | | |
| Note: Many of these cardiovascular effects may occur secondary to NSAID-induced renal function impairment. | | | | | | | | | | | | | | | | | | | | |
| *Angina pectoris or exacerbation of* (chest pain) | L | | U | U | U | R† | U | U | U | U | U | R† | U | U | U | R | U | U | R | U |
| *Bleeding, other than gastrointestinal, including:* | | | | | | | | | | | | | | | | | | | | |
| Hemoptysis (spitting blood) | U | U | U | U | U | U | U | U | R | U | U | U | U | U | U | U | U | U | U | U |
| Nosebleeds, unexplained | R | U | U | U | U | R | R† | R | R | U | U | U | U | U | U | R | R | R | L | R |
| *Cardiac arrhythmias* | L | U | R† | R† | U | R† | R† | R | R† | U | U | R† | U | U | U | U | R† | U | U | U |
| *Chest pain* | R† | R† | U | U | U | R | U | R | U | R | R | R | U | U | U | U | U | U | R | L |
| *Congestive heart failure or exacerbation of* (chest pain; shortness of breath; troubled breathing, tightness in chest, and/or wheezing; decrease in amount of urine; swelling of face, fingers, feet, or lower legs; unusual tiredness; weight gain) | R | U | | U | U | R | R | R | R | U | U | U | R | U | U | U | R | U | R | R |
| *Edema, pulmonary* (shortness of breath, troubled breathing, tightness in chest, and/or wheezing) | U | U | U | R† | U | U | U | R | U | U | U | U | U | U | U | U | U | R | U | U |
| *Increased blood pressure*—may reach hypertensive levels | R | U | R | U | U | R | R | R | R | U | U | R† | U | R | U | R | R | R | U | M |
| *Pericarditis* (chest pain; fever with or without chills; shortness of breath, troubled breathing, and/or tightness in chest) | U | U | U | U | U | U | U | U | U | U | U | U | U | U | U | U | U | U | U | U |
| **Central nervous system effects** | | | | | | | | | | | | | | | | | | | | |
| Confusion | U | R | R† | L | U | R | R | R | R | R | R | R | R | L | R | R† | U | R | U | U |
| Convulsions | R† | U | U | R† | U | U | U | R | U | U | U | U | U | U | R | U | R | R | R | U |
| Dysarthria (trouble in speaking) | U | U | U | U | U | U | U | U | U | U | U | U | U | U | U | U | U | U | U | U |
| Forgetfulness | R† | U | U | U | L | U | L | R | R | U | U | U | U | U | U | U | U | U | U | U |
| Hallucinations | U | R | U | U | U | U | R† | R | R† | U | U | U | U | U | U | R† | U | U | U | U |
| Headache, severe, especially in the morning | U | U | U | U | U | U | U | M§ | U | U | U | U | U | U | U | U | U | U | U | U |

*Differences in frequency of occurrence may reflect either lack of clinical-use data or actual pharmacologic distinctions among agents (although their pharmacologic similarity suggests that side effects occurring with one may occur with the others). M=more frequent (3–9%); L=less frequent (1–3%); R=rare (<1%); U=unknown; unless otherwise specified.

†Has been reported, but a causal relationship has not been established.

‡Has been reported, but actual frequency of occurrence unknown.

§Frequency of occurrence 10% or higher.

#Serious gastrointestinal effects, including ulceration, perforation, and/or bleeding, may occur at any time, with or without warning signs and/or symptoms, during chronic therapy with nonsteroidal anti-inflammatory drugs (NSAIDs). The risk of NSAID-induced gastrointestinal toxicity may increase with the duration of therapy as well as with dosage. In clinical trials with nabumetone, peptic ulceration occurred in approximately 0.3%, 0.5%, and 0.8% of patients treated for 6 months, 1 year, and 2 years, respectively. In clinical trials with other NSAIDs, upper gastrointestinal tract ulceration, bleeding, or perforation occurred in approximately 1% of patients treated for 3 to 6 months and in approximately 2 to 4% of patients treated for 1 year. Risk factors that may increase the risk of NSAID-induced gastrointestinal toxicity, other than those associated with an increased risk of peptic ulcer disease in any patient, have not been identified.

**See also Dermatologic effects, Hematologic effects, Hepatic effects, and Renal effects for signs and symptoms of many of the reported components of this syndrome.

††Diarrhea occurring during mefenamic acid therapy requires medical attention.

Table 3. Side/Adverse Effects* (continued)

Legend:
I = Diclofenac
II = Diflunisal
III = Etodolac
IV = Fenoprofen
V = Floctafenine
VI = Flurbiprofen
VII = Ibuprofen
VIII = Indomethacin
IX = Ketoprofen
X = Meclofenamate
XI = Mefenamic Acid
XII = Nabumetone
XIII = Naproxen
XIV = Oxaprozin
XV = Phenylbutazone
XVI = Piroxicam
XVII = Sulindac
XVIII = Tenoxicam
XIX = Tiaprofenic Acid
XX = Tolmetin

| | I | II | III | IV | V | VI | VII | VIII | IX | X | XI | XII | XIII | XIV | XV | XVI | XVII | XVIII | XIX | XX |
|---|---|---|---|---|---|---|---|---|---|---|---|---|---|---|---|---|---|---|---|---|
| **Meningitis, aseptic** (severe headache, drowsiness, confusion, stiff neck and/or back, general feeling of illness, nausea) | R | U | U | U | U | R | R | U | U | U | U | U | R† | U | U | U | R | U | U | R |
| **Migraine** (headache, severe and throbbing, sometimes with nausea or vomiting) | U | U | U | U | U | U | U | U | U | U | U | U | U | U | U | U | U | U | U | U |
| **Mood or mental changes, including:** | | | | | | | | | | | | | | | | | | | | |
|   *Disorientation* | U | R | U | R | U | U | U | U | U | U | U | R | U | U | U | U | U | U | R | U |
|   *Feeling of depersonalization or muzziness* | U | U | U | U | U | U | U | R | U | U | U | U | U | U | U | U | U | U | R | U |
|   *Mental depression* | R | R | L | R† | U | L | R | L | R† | R† | ‡ | R | R | R | R | R | R | R | L | L |
|   *Psychotic reaction* | R† | U | U | U | U | U | U | R | U | U | U | U | U | U | U | U | R | U | M | L |
| **Neuropathy, peripheral** (numbness, tingling, pain, or weakness in hands or feet) | R† | R† | U | U | U | U | R† | R | R† | R† | U | R† | R† | U | R† | R† | R | U | R | U |
| **Syncope** (fainting) | U | R† | R | U | U | U | U | R | U | U | U | R† | U | U | U | U | R | U | U | U |
| **Dermatologic effects** | | | | | | | | | | | | | | | | | | | | |
|   *Dermatitis, allergic* | | | | | | | | | | | | | | | | | | | | |
|     (bullous eruption/blisters) | R | U | R | U | U | U | R | U | R | U | U | R | U | U | U | R | R | U | U | U |
|     (eczema) | U | U | U | U | R | R | U | U | U | U | U | U | U | U | U | U | U | U | R | U |
|     (hives) | R | R | R | R | R | R | R | R | R | L | ‡ | R | M | R | R | R | U | R | U | R |
|     (itching) | L | R | L | M | L | R | L | R | L | L | ‡ | M | R† | R | R | L | L | L | L | L |
|     (skin rash) | L | M | L | U | L | L | M | R | L | M | U | M | M | M | L | L | M | L | M | L |
| **Dermatitis, exfoliative** (fever with or without chills; red, thickened, or scaly skin; swollen and/or painful glands; unusual bruising) | R† | R | U | R† | U | U | U | R | R | U | U | U | R | U | U | R | R | U | U | U |
| **Desquamation** (peeling of skin) | U | U | R† | U | U | U | U | U | U | U | U | U | U | U | U | R | R | U | R | U |
| **Erythema** (reddening of skin) *or other skin discoloration* | U | U | U | U | U | U | U | U | R | U | U | R | U | U | U | R | U | U | R | R |
| **Erythema multiforme** (fever with or without chills; muscle cramps or pain; skin rash; sores, ulcers, or white spots on lips or in mouth) | R | R | U | U | U | U | R | R | U | R | U | U | R† | U | R | R | R | U | U | R |
| **Erythema nodosum** (fever with or without chills; skin rash) | U | U | U | U | U | U | U | R | U | R† | U | R† | U | R | R | U | U | U | U | U |
| **Photosensitivity reactions resembling porphyria cutanea tarda and epidermolysis bullosa** (blistering, scarring, darkening or lightening of skin color) | U | | | | | | | | U | | | | R† | | | U | U | | | U |
| **Stevens-Johnson syndrome** (bleeding or crusting sores on lips; chest pain; fever with or without chills; muscle cramps or pain; skin rash; sores, ulcers, or white spots in mouth; sore throat) | R | R | R | R† | R | R | R | R | R | U | R | R† | R† | U | R | R | R | U | U | R |
| **Toxic epidermal necrolysis** (redness, tenderness, itching, burning, or peeling of skin; sore throat; fever with or without chills) | U | R | R | R† | R | R | R† | R | U | U | U | R | U | U | R | R | R | U | U | R |

## Table 3. Side/Adverse Effects* (continued)

Legend:
I = Diclofenac
II = Diflunisal
III = Etodolac
IV = Fenoprofen
V = Floctafenine
VI = Flurbiprofen
VII = Ibuprofen
VIII = Indomethacin
IX = Ketoprofen
X = Meclofenamate
XI = Mefenamic Acid
XII = Nabumetone
XIII = Naproxen
XIV = Oxaprozin
XV = Phenylbutazone
XVI = Piroxicam
XVII = Sulindac
XVIII = Tenoxicam
XIX = Tiaprofenic Acid
XX = Tolmetin

| | I | II | III | IV | V | VI | VII | VIII | IX | X | XI | XII | XIII | XIV | XV | XVI | XVII | XVIII | XIX | XX |
|---|---|---|---|---|---|---|---|---|---|---|---|---|---|---|---|---|---|---|---|---|
| **Digestive system effects** | | | | | | | | | | | | | | | | | | | | |
| Abdominal distention (swelling of abdomen) | L | U | U | U | U | U | U | R | U | — | U | U | U | U | R | U | U | R | U | U |
| Bleeding from rectum—with rectal dosage forms | ‡ | — | — | — | — | — | — | R | M | — | — | — | R | — | — | L | — | — | — | — |
| Colitis or exacerbation of or | R | U | R† | U | U | U | U | R | R | R | U | U | R | U | R | U | R | U | U | U |
| Enterocolitis or | U | U | U | U | U | U | U | R | U | U | U | U | U | U | U | U | U | U | R | U |
| Regional enteritis or exacerbation of (abdominal pain, cramping, or discomfort; bloody stools; diarrhea) | U | U | U | U | U | U | U | R | U | U | U | U | U | U | R | U | U | U | U | U |
| Dysphagia (difficulty in swallowing) | U | U | U | U | U | U | U | U | U | U | U | R | U | U | U | U | R | U | U | U |
| Esophagitis (burning feeling in throat or chest, difficulty in swallowing) | U | U | R† | U | U | U | U | R | U | U | U | U | U | U | R | U | U | U | U | U |
| Gastritis (burning feeling in chest or stomach, indigestion, tenderness in stomach area) | U | R | L | R | M | R | R | R | R | U | U | L | U | R | R | U | R | U | U | L |
| Gastroenteritis (severe abdominal pain, diarrhea, loss of appetite, nausea, weakness) | U | U | U | U | U | U | R | R | R | U | U | R | U | U | R | U | R | R | L | U |
| Gastrointestinal bleeding or hemorrhage—reported independently of gastrointestinal ulceration or perforation, including *melena* (bloody stools) and *hematemesis* (vomiting blood or material that looks like coffee grounds)** | R | R | L | R | M | L | R | R | R | R | R | R | R | R | R | R | R | R | R | R |

*Differences in frequency of occurrence may reflect either lack of clinical-use data or actual pharmacologic distinctions among agents (although their pharmacologic similarity suggests that side effects occurring with one may occur with the others). M=more frequent (3–9%); L=less frequent (1–3%); R=rare (<1%); U=unknown; unless otherwise specified.

†Has been reported, but a causal relationship has not been established.

‡Has been reported, but actual frequency of occurrence unknown.

§Frequency of occurrence 10% or higher.

#Serious gastrointestinal effects, including ulceration, perforation, and/or bleeding, may occur at any time, with or without warning signs and/or symptoms, during chronic therapy with nonsteroidal anti-inflammatory drugs (NSAIDs). The risk of NSAID-induced gastrointestinal toxicity may increase with the duration of therapy as well as with dosage. In clinical trials with nabumetone, peptic ulceration occurred in approximately 0.3%, 0.5%, and 0.8% of patients treated for 6 months, 1 year, and 2 years, respectively. In clinical trials with other NSAIDs, upper gastrointestinal tract ulceration, bleeding, or perforation occurred in approximately 1% of patients treated for 3 to 6 months and in approximately 2 to 4% of patients treated for 1 year. Risk factors that may increase the risk of NSAID-induced gastrointestinal toxicity, other than those associated with an increased risk of peptic ulcer disease in any patient, have not been identified.

**See also Dermatologic effects, Hematologic effects, Hepatic effects, and Renal effects for signs and symptoms of many of the reported components of this syndrome.

††Diarrhea occurring during mefenamic acid therapy requires medical attention.

Table 3. Side/Adverse Effects* (continued)

Legend:
I = Diclofenac
II = Diflunisal
III = Etodolac
IV = Fenoprofen
V = Floctafenine
VI = Flurbiprofen
VII = Ibuprofen
VIII = Indomethacin
IX = Ketoprofen
X = Meclofenamate
XI = Mefenamic Acid
XII = Nabumetone
XIII = Naproxen
XIV = Oxaprozin
XV = Phenylbutazone
XVI = Piroxicam
XVII = Sulindac
XVIII = Tenoxicam
XIX = Tiaprofenic Acid
XX = Tolmetin

| Side/Adverse Effects | I | II | III | IV | V | VI | VII | VIII | IX | X | XI | XII | XIII | XIV | XV | XVI | XVII | XVIII | XIX | XX |
|---|---|---|---|---|---|---|---|---|---|---|---|---|---|---|---|---|---|---|---|---|
| *Gastrointestinal perforation# and/or* *Gastrointestinal ulceration#, including esophageal, gastric, or peptic ulceration, multiple gastrointestinal ulcerations, and perforation of pre-existing sigmoid lesions, e.g., diverticula, carcinoma* (severe pain, cramping, or burning; bloody or black, tarry stools; vomiting of blood or material that looks like coffee grounds; severe and continuing nausea, heartburn, and/or indigestion)# | U | R | U | R | U | U | R | R | R | R | U | U | R | U | U | R | R | U | U | R |
| | L | R | L | R | M | R | R | R | R | L | R | R | R | R | R | R | R | R | R | L |
| Note: *Intestinal ulceration may lead to stenosis and obstruction. Also, paralytic ileus has been reported with meclofenamate, but a causal relationship has not been established.* | | | | | | | | | | | | | | | | | | | | |
| *Genitourinary effects* *Bladder pain* | U | U | U | U | U | U | U | U | U | U | U | U | U | U | U | U | U | U | U | U |
| *Bleeding from vagina, unexplained, unexpected, and/or unusually heavy menstrual* | R† | U | R† | U | U | R† | R† | R | R | R | U | R | R | R | U | U | R | R | R | U |
| *Blood in urine* | R† | U | R† | R | M | R | R | R | R | U | ‡ | U | R | R | R | R | R | U | U | R |
| *Crystalluria, renal calculi, or ureteral obstruction* (blood in urine; difficult, burning, or painful urination; severe pain in lower back, side, or abdomen)—with phenylbutazone, may be composed of uric acid crystals and with sulindac, may be composed of sulindac metabolites | U | U | R† | U | U | U | U | R† | U | U | U | U | U | U | R | U | R | U | U | U |
| *Cystitis or* | R | R | R† | R | M | R | R | R† | L | U | R | U | R | R | U | R† | U | R | R | U |
| *Urethritis or* | U | U | U | U | M | U | U | U | U | U | U | U | U | U | U | U | U | U | U | U |
| *Urinary tract infection* (bloody or cloudy urine; difficult, burning, or painful urination; frequent urge to urinate) | U | U | U | U | U | M | U | U | U | U | U | U | U | U | U | U | L | U | U | U |
| *Dysuria* (burning, painful, or difficult urination) | U | R | L | L | M | U | U | U | U | U | U | U | U | U | U | R† | R | U | R | R |
| *Frequent urge to urinate* | R† | U | L | U | U | R | U | U | U | U | U | U | U | L | U | U | U | R | U | U |
| *Incontinence* (loss of bladder control) | U | U | U | U | U | R | U | U | U | U | U | U | U | U | R | U | U | U | R | U |
| *Proteinuria* (cloudy urine) | R | R | U | U | M | U | U | U | U | U | U | U | U | R | R | R | R | U | R | R |
| *Strong-smelling urine* | U | U | U | U | M | U | U | U | U | U | U | U | U | U | U | U | U | U | U | U |
| *Hematologic effects* *Agranulocytosis [granulocytopenia]* (fever with or without chills; sores, ulcers, or white spots on lips or in mouth; sore throat) | R | R | U | R | U | U | R | R | R | R | R | R | R | R | U | U | R | R | U | R |
| *Anemia* (unusual tiredness or weakness)—may be associated with gastrointestinal bleeding or microbleeding or with hemodilution caused by fluid retention | R | U | R | U | U | R | R | R | R | R | L | R | U | R | L | L | U | R | U | L |

Table 3. Side/Adverse Effects* *(continued)*

Legend:
I = Diclofenac
II = Diflunisal
III = Etodolac
IV = Fenoprofen
V = Floctafenine
VI = Flurbiprofen
VII = Ibuprofen
VIII = Indomethacin
IX = Ketoprofen
X = Meclofenamate
XI = Mefenamic Acid
XII = Nabumetone
XIII = Naproxen
XIV = Oxaprozin
XV = Phenylbutazone
XVI = Piroxicam
XVII = Sulindac
XVIII = Tenoxicam
XIX = Tiaprofenic Acid
XX = Tolmetin

| Side/Adverse Effect | I | II | III | IV | V | VI | VII | VIII | IX | X | XI | XII | XIII | XIV | XV | XVI | XVII | XVIII | XIX | XX |
|---|---|---|---|---|---|---|---|---|---|---|---|---|---|---|---|---|---|---|---|---|
| Aplastic anemia [pancytopenia] (shortness of breath, troubled breathing, tightness in chest, and/or wheezing; sores, ulcers, or white spots on lips or in mouth; sore throat) | R | U | U | R | U | R | R | R | U | U | R | R | R† | U | R | R | R | U | U | U |
| Bone marrow depression—signs and symptoms are listed under individual entries for *Aplastic anemia* and *Thrombocytopenia* | | | | | | | | | | | | | | | | | | | | |
| Disseminated intravascular coagulation | U | U | U | U | U | U | U | R | U | U | U | U | U | U | R | R | R | U | U | U |
| Ecchymosis/bruising | R† | U | R | R | U | R | R | U | R | R | U | U | L | R | U | R | U | R | R | R |
| Eosinophilia | U | U | U | U | R | R | R | R | R | R | ‡ | U | R | R | U | L | U | U | U | U |
| Hemolytic anemia (troubled breathing, exertional; unusual tiredness or weakness) | R | R | U | R | U | R | R | R | R | R | R | U | R† | U | R | R† | R | U | R | R |
| Hypocoagulability (bleeding from cuts or scratches that lasts longer than usual) | U | U | U | U | U | U | U | U | R | U | U | U | U | U | U | U | U | U | U | U |
| Leukopenia [neutropenia] (usually asymptomatic; rarely, fever or chills, cough or hoarseness, lower back or side pain, painful or difficult urination) | R | U | R† | U | U | R | R | R | R | R | R | R | R | R | R | L | R | R | R | R |
| Petechia (pinpoint red spots on skin) | U | U | U | U | U | U | U | R | U | U | U | U | U | U | R | R | U | R | U | U |
| Purpura (bruises and/or red spots on skin)—may be associated with thrombocytopenia | | | | | | | | | | | | | | | | | | | | |
| Thrombocytopenia with or without purpura (usually asymptomatic; rarely, unusual bleeding or bruising; black, tarry stools; blood in urine or stools; pinpoint red spots on skin) | | | | | | | | | | | | | | | | | | | | |
| Hepatic effects, including: Cholestatic hepatitis or jaundice (dark urine; fever; itching; light-colored stools; pain, tenderness, and/or swelling in upper abdominal area; skin rash; swollen glands) | U | R | R | R | U | R | U | R | U | R | R | R | R | R | R | U | R | U | R | R |
| Hepatitis or jaundice, toxic (loss of appetite, nausea, vomiting, yellow eyes or skin, swelling in upper abdominal area) | R | R | R | R | U | R | R | R | R | U | R | R | R | R | R | R | R | R | U | R |

*Differences in frequency of occurrence may reflect either lack of clinical-use data or actual pharmacologic distinctions among agents (although their pharmacologic similarity suggests that side effects occurring with one may occur with the others). M=more frequent (3–9%); L=less frequent (1–3%); R=rare (<1%); U=unknown; unless otherwise specified.

†Has been reported, but a causal relationship has not been established.

‡Has been reported, but actual frequency of occurrence unknown.

§Frequency of occurrence 10% or higher.

#Serious gastrointestinal effects, including ulceration, perforation, and/or bleeding, may occur at any time, with or without warning signs and/or symptoms, during chronic therapy with nonsteroidal anti-inflammatory drugs (NSAIDs). The risk of NSAID-induced gastrointestinal toxicity may increase with the duration of therapy as well as with dosage. In clinical trials with nabumetone, peptic ulceration occurred in approximately 0.3%, 0.5%, and 0.8% of patients treated for 6 months, 1 year, and 2 years, respectively. In clinical trials with other NSAIDs, upper gastrointestinal tract ulceration, bleeding, or perforation occurred in approximately 1% of patients treated for 3 to 6 months and in approximately 2 to 4% of patients treated for 1 year. Risk factors that may increase the risk of NSAID-induced gastrointestinal toxicity, other than those associated with an increased risk of peptic ulcer disease in any patient, have not been identified.

**See also Dermatologic effects, Hematologic effects, Hepatic effects, and Renal effects for signs and symptoms of many of the reported components of this syndrome.

††Diarrhea occurring during mefenamic acid therapy requires medical attention.

## Table 3. Side/Adverse Effects* (continued)

Legend:
I = Diclofenac
II = Diflunisal
III = Etodolac
IV = Fenoprofen
V = Floctafenine
VI = Flurbiprofen
VII = Ibuprofen
VIII = Indomethacin
IX = Ketoprofen
X = Meclofenamate
XI = Mefenamic Acid
XII = Nabumetone
XIII = Naproxen
XIV = Oxaprozin
XV = Phenylbutazone
XVI = Piroxicam
XVII = Sulindac
XVIII = Tenoxicam
XIX = Tiaprofenic Acid
XX = Tolmetin

| Side/Adverse Effect | I | II | III | IV | V | VI | VII | VIII | IX | X | XI | XII | XIII | XIV | XV | XVI | XVII | XVIII | XIX | XX |
|---|---|---|---|---|---|---|---|---|---|---|---|---|---|---|---|---|---|---|---|---|
| **Hypersensitivity reactions** *See also Dermatologic effects* | | | | | | | | | | | | | | | | | | | | |
| *Anaphylaxis or anaphylactoid reactions* (changes in facial skin color; skin rash, hives, and/or itching; fast or irregular breathing; puffiness or swelling of the eyelids or around the eyes; shortness of breath, troubled breathing, tightness in chest, and/or wheezing)—may include anaphylactic shock with sudden, severe decrease in blood pressure and collapse | R | R | U | R | R | R | R | R | R | U | R | R | R | R | R | R | R | U | R | R |
| *Angiitis [vasculitis]* (muscle pain, cramps, and/or weakness; shortness of breath, troubled breathing, tightness in chest, and/or wheezing; skin rash; spitting blood; unusual tiredness or weakness) | U | R | R | U | U | U | R† | R | R | U | U | R | R | R | R | R | R | U | U | U |
| *Angioedema* (large, hive-like swellings on face, eyelids, mouth, lips, and/or tongue) | R | R | R | R | R | U | R† | R | U | U | U | R | R† | U | R | R | R | R | U | U |
| *Bronchospastic allergic reactions* (shortness of breath, troubled breathing, tightness in chest, and/or wheezing) | R | R | R | R | R | R | R | R | R | U | U | R† | R† | U | R | R | R | R | U | U |
| *Fever with or without chills* | U | U | L | R† | U | U | U | R | R | U | U | R† | R | U | R | R | R | U | R | R |
| *Hypersensitivity syndrome, multisystemic, diflunisal-induced, including dermatologic reactions; hematologic effects including eosinophilia, leukopenia, thrombocytopenia, and disseminated intravascular coagulation; jaundice; renal impairment or failure; and nonspecific signs and symptoms* (disorientation, fever and chills, general feeling of illness or discomfort, loss of appetite, muscle and/or joint pain, swollen and/or painful glands)** | — | R | — | — | — | — | — | — | — | — | — | — | — | — | — | — | — | — | — | — |
| *Hypersensitivity syndrome, multisystemic, sulindac-induced, including dermatologic reactions; conjunctivitis; hepatic failure and jaundice; pancreatitis; pneumonitis with or without pleural effusions* (difficulty in breathing, coughing, tightness in chest, wheezing); *hematologic effects including leukopenia, leukocytosis, eosinophilia, disseminated intravascular coagulation, and anemia; renal impairment or failure; and nonspecific signs and symptoms* (chest pain, fast heartbeat, fever and chills, flushing, general feeling of illness or discomfort, low blood pressure, muscle and/or joint pain, sweating, tiredness)** | — | — | — | — | — | — | — | — | — | — | — | — | — | — | — | — | R | — | — | — |
| *Laryngeal edema* (shortness of breath or troubled breathing) | R | U | U | U | U | U | U | U | R | U | U | R | U | U | U | U | R | U | U | U |
| *Loeffler syndrome [eosinophilic pneumonitis]* (chest pain; fever with or without chills; shortness of breath, troubled breathing, tightness in chest, and/or wheezing; unusual weakness) | U | U | U | U | U | U | U | U | U | U | U | U | R | U | U | U | U | U | U | U |

## Table 3. Side/Adverse Effects* (continued)

Legend:
I = Diclofenac
II = Diflunisal
III = Etodolac
IV = Fenoprofen
V = Floctafenine
VI = Flurbiprofen
VII = Ibuprofen
VIII = Indomethacin
IX = Ketoprofen
X = Meclofenamate
XI = Mefenamic Acid
XII = Nabumetone
XIII = Naproxen
XIV = Oxaprozin
XV = Phenylbutazone
XVI = Piroxicam
XVII = Sulindac
XVIII = Tenoxicam
XIX = Tiaprofenic Acid
XX = Tolmetin

| Side/Adverse Effect | I | II | III | IV | V | VI | VII | VIII | IX | X | XI | XII | XIII | XIV | XV | XVI | XVII | XVIII | XIX | XX |
|---|---|---|---|---|---|---|---|---|---|---|---|---|---|---|---|---|---|---|---|---|
| **Rhinitis, allergic** (unexplained runny nose or sneezing) | U | U | U | U | U | L | R | U | R | U | U | U | U | U | U | U | U | U | R | U |
| **Serum sickness-like reaction** (fever with or without chills; muscle cramps, pain, and/or weakness; skin rash, hives, and/or itching; shortness of breath, troubled breathing, tightness in chest, and/or wheezing; swollen and/or painful glands) | U | U | | U | U | | R† | | U | | U | | U | R | R | R | | | U | R |
| **Systemic lupus erythematosus [SLE]-like syndrome** (bloody or cloudy urine; chest pain; fever with or without chills; shortness of breath, troubled breathing, tightness in chest, and/or wheezing; skin rash, hives, and/or itching; sudden decrease in amount of urine; swelling of face, fingers, feet, and/or lower legs; swollen and/or painful glands; unusual weakness; rapid weight gain) | U | U | | U | U | | R† | U | U | | U | | U | U | R | U | U | | U | U |
| **Loosening or splitting of fingernails or other nail disorder** | U | U | U | U | U | | U | U | R | R | U | | U | U | U | U | R | U | R | U |
| **Lymphadenopathy** (swollen and/or painful glands) | U | U | U | U | U | R† | U | U | R | U | U | U | U | U | U | R† | R | U | R | R |
| **Muscle cramps or pain**—not present before treatment and not related to condition being treated | U | R† | U | M | U | | U | R | R | U | U | R | R | U | R | U | U | U | U | M |
| **Ocular effects** | | | | | | | | | | | | | | | | | | | | |
| Amblyopia, toxic, or | R† | U | U | U | U | U | R | U | U | U | U | U | U | R | R† | U | U | U | U | U |
| Corneal opacity or | U | U | U | U | U | R | U | U | U | U | U | U | U | U | U | U | R | U | U | U |
| Retinal or macular disturbances (blurred vision or other vision change) | U | U | U | U | U | U | U | R | R† | R† | U | U | U | U | R† | U | R† | U | U | R† |
| **Blurred or double vision or any change in vision** | R | R | L | L | L | L | L | R | L | R† | ‡ | R | L | R | R† | R | R | L | R | R |
| **Conjunctivitis** (eye pain, redness, irritation, and/or swelling) | U | U | R† | U | U | R | R† | U | R† | R† | U | U | U | U | U | U | R | R | U | U |
| **Corneal deposits** | U | U | U | U | U | R | U | R | U | U | U | U | U | U | U | U | U | U | U | U |
| **Dry, irritated, or swollen eyes** | U | U | U | U | R | R | R | U | R† | R† | ‡ | U | U | U | R | U | R | U | R | U |
| **Eye pain** | U | U | U | U | U | R | R | R | U | U | U | U | R | U | U | U | U | U | U | U |
| **Palpebral edema** (swollen eyelids) | U | U | U | U | U | R | U | R | U | U | U | R | U | U | U | U | U | U | R | U |

*Differences in frequency of occurrence may reflect either lack of clinical-use data or actual pharmacologic distinctions among agents (although their pharmacologic similarity suggests that side effects occurring with one may occur with the others). M=more frequent (3–9%); L=less frequent (1–3%); R=rare (<1%); U=unknown; unless otherwise specified.
†Has been reported, but a causal relationship has not been established.
‡Has been reported, but actual frequency of occurrence unknown.
§Frequency of occurrence 10% or higher.
#Serious gastrointestinal effects, including ulceration, perforation, and/or bleeding, may occur at any time, with or without warning signs and/or symptoms, during chronic therapy with nonsteroidal anti-inflammatory drugs (NSAIDs). The risk of NSAID-induced gastrointestinal toxicity may increase with the duration of therapy as well as with dosage. In clinical trials with nabumetone, peptic ulceration occurred in approximately 0.3%, 0.5%, and 0.8% of patients treated for 6 months, 1 year, and 2 years, respectively. In clinical trials with other NSAIDs, upper gastrointestinal tract ulceration, bleeding, or perforation occurred in approximately 1% of patients treated for 3 to 6 months and in approximately 2 to 4% of patients treated for 1 year. Risk factors that may increase the risk of NSAID-induced gastrointestinal toxicity, other than those associated with an increased risk of peptic ulcer disease in any patient, have not been identified.
**See also Dermatologic effects, Hematologic effects, Hepatic effects, and Renal effects for signs and symptoms of many of the reported components of this syndrome.
††Diarrhea occurring during mefenamic acid therapy requires medical attention.

Table 3. Side/Adverse Effects* *(continued)*

Legend:
I = Diclofenac
II = Diflunisal
III = Etodolac
IV = Fenoprofen
V = Floctafenine
VI = Flurbiprofen
VII = Ibuprofen
VIII = Indomethacin
IX = Ketoprofen
X = Meclofenamate
XI = Mefenamic Acid
XII = Nabumetone
XIII = Naproxen
XIV = Oxaprozin
XV = Phenylbutazone
XVI = Piroxicam
XVII = Sulindac
XVIII = Tenoxicam
XIX = Tiaprofenic Acid
XX = Tolmetin

| | I | II | III | IV | V | VI | VII | VIII | IX | X | XI | XII | XIII | XIV | XV | XVI | XVII | XVIII | XIX | XX |
|---|---|---|---|---|---|---|---|---|---|---|---|---|---|---|---|---|---|---|---|---|
| *Retinal hemorrhage* (red eyes) | U | U | U | U | U | R† | U | U | R | U | U | U | U | U | R† | U | U | U | U | U |
| *Scotomata* (change in vision) | R | U | U | U | U | U | R | U | U | U | U | U | U | U | R† | U | U | U | U | U |
| ***Oral/perioral effects*** | | | | | | | | | | | | | | | | | | | | |
| *Gingival ulceration* or | U | U | U | U | U | U | R | U | U | U | U | U | U | U | R† | U | U | U | U | U |
| *Stomatitis, aphthous* (sores, ulcers, or white spots on lips or in mouth) | R | R | R | R† | U | R | R | R | L | L | L | L | L | R | R | L | R | R | L | R |
| *Glossitis* (irritated tongue) | U | U | U | U | U | U | U | U | U | U | R† | U | U | U | U | U | R | U | U | R |
| *Swelling of lips and tongue* | R | U | U | U | U | U | U | U | U | U | U | U | U | U | U | U | R | U | U | U |
| ***Otic effects*** | | | | | | | | | | | | | | | | | | | | |
| *Decreased hearing or any change in hearing* | R | U | R† | L | U | R† | R | R | R | U | U | U | L | R† | R | R† | R | R | U | R |
| *Ringing or buzzing in ears* | L | L | U | L | L | L | L | L | L | L | U | M | M | R | L | L | L | R | R | L |
| *Pancreatitis* (abdominal pain, fever with or without chills, swelling and/or tenderness in upper abdominal or stomach area) | R | U | U | R† | U | U | R | R | R† | U | R | R† | U | U | R† | R† | R | U | U | U |
| ***Renal effects*** | | | | | | | | | | | | | | | | | | | | |
| *Fluid retention/edema* (increased blood pressure; decrease in amount of urine; swelling of face, fingers, feet, and/or lower legs; rapid weight gain) | M | R | U | M | U | M | L | M | M | L | L | M | M | M | M | L | L | L | L | M |
| *Glomerulitis or glomerulonephritis* | U | U | U | U | U | U | U | U | U | U | R | U | U | U | R | R | U | U | U | U |
| *Hyperkalemia* (difficulty in speaking, low blood pressure, slow or irregular heartbeat, troubled breathing, severe weakness in arms or legs) | U | U | U | U | U | R† | U | R | U | U | U | R† | U | U | R† | R | U | U | L | U |
| *Interstitial nephritis* (bloody or cloudy urine; increased blood pressure; sudden decrease in amount of urine; swelling of face, fingers, feet, and/or lower legs; rapid weight gain)—may be hypersensitivity-mediated | R | R | R† | R | R | U | U | R | R | U | U | R | R | R | R | R | R | R | R | R |
| *Nephrosis* (sudden decrease in amount of urine; swelling of face, fingers, feet, and/or lower legs; rapid weight gain) | U | U | U | R | U | U | U | U | U | U | U | U | U | U | U | U | U | U | U | U |
| *Nephrotic syndrome* (cloudy urine, swelling of face) | R | R† | U | U | U | U | U | R | R | U | R | U | U | U | R | R | U | U | R | R |
| *Oliguria/anuria* (cessation of urination)—reported independently of renal impairment or failure | R | U | U | U | U | U | R† | U | R | R | R | U | R | U | R | U | U | R | U | R |
| *Polyuria* (sudden, large increase in frequency and quantity of urine) | U | U | U | U | U | U | U | U | U | U | U | U | U | U | U | U | U | U | U | U |
| *Renal impairment or failure* (increased blood pressure; shortness of breath, troubled breathing, tightness in chest, and/or wheezing; sudden decrease in amount of urine; swelling of face, fingers, feet, and/or lower legs; continuing thirst; unusual tiredness or weakness; weight gain) | R | R† | R | R | U | R† | R | R | R | R | R | U | R | R | R | R | R | R | R | R |
| *Renal papillary or tubular necrosis* | R | R† | R† | M | U | R† | R | R | R | R | ‡ | R | M | U | R | R† | R | U | U | R |
| *Shortness of breath or troubled breathing* | R | R† | R | U | L | R | R | R | R | R | R | R | M | U | R | U | R | U | U | R |
| *Thirst, continuing* | U | U | R | U | L | U | R | U | R | R | U | U | L | U | R | U | U | U | U | U |

Table 3. Side/Adverse Effects* (*continued*)

Legend:
I = Diclofenac
II = Diflunisal
III = Etodolac
IV = Fenoprofen
V = Floctafenine
VI = Flurbiprofen
VII = Ibuprofen
VIII = Indomethacin
IX = Ketoprofen
X = Meclofenamate
XI = Mefenamic Acid
XII = Nabumetone
XIII = Naproxen
XIV = Oxaprozin
XV = Phenylbutazone
XVI = Piroxicam
XVII = Sulindac
XVIII = Tenoxicam
XIX = Tiaprofenic Acid
XX = Tolmetin

| | I | II | III | IV | V | VI | VII | VIII | IX | X | XI | XII | XIII | XIV | XV | XVI | XVII | XVIII | XIX | XX |
|---|---|---|---|---|---|---|---|---|---|---|---|---|---|---|---|---|---|---|---|---|
| **Medical attention needed only if continuing or bothersome** | | | | | | | | | | | | | | | | | | | | |
| *Cardiovascular effects* | | | | | | | | | | | | | | | | | | | | |
| Fast heartbeat | R† | U | U | L | L | L | R† | R | R | U | U | U | U | U | U | U | U | R | U | U |
| Flushing or hot flashes | R† | U | R | U | L | L | R | R | U | U | U | U | U | U | U | U | U | R | L | U |
| Increased sweating | R† | R | U | L | L | R† | U | L | L | U | ‡ | L | L | L | U | R | U | R | R | U |
| Pounding heartbeat | R† | R† | R | M | U | R | R | R | R | R† | R† | R† | L | R† | U | R† | R | R | R | U |
| *Central nervous system effects* | | | | | | | | | | | | | | | | | | | | |
| Anxiety | U | U | U | U | U | L | U | U | U | U | R | R | U | U | U | U | U | U | R | U |
| Dizziness | L | L | M | M | M | L | M | M | L | M | M | M | M | U | U | L | M | M | M | M |
| Drowsiness | R | L | R | M | M | L | R | M | L | U | L | L | M | L | R | L | R | U | L | L |
| Headache, mild to moderate | M | M | M | M | M | M | L | M§ | M | M | ‡ | M | U | L | R | L | L | M | M | M |
| Lightheadedness/vertigo | U | R | U | U | U | U | U | L | R | M | U | R | L | U | R | L | R | U | R | U |
| Nervousness or irritability | R | R | L | M | M | L | L | R | M | U | ‡ | L | U | U | U | R | L | L | U | L |
| Trembling or twitching | R† | U | U | L | L | L | L | U | U | R† | U | R | U | U | L | U | U | U | L | U |
| Trouble in sleeping | R | L | R | L | M | L | R | R | L | R† | ‡ | L | R | L | R | R | R | R | R | R |
| Unusual weakness with no other signs or symptoms | R | L | M | M | L | M | U | R | U | R† | R | R | R | R | R | R† | R | | R | M |
| *Dermatologic effects* | | | | | | | | | | | | | | | | | | | | |
| Photosensitive or photoallergic dermatologic reaction (severe sunburn; skin rash, redness, itching, and/or discoloration after exposure to sunlight) | R | R | R† | U | U | R | R† | R | R | R | R | R | R | R | R | R | R | R | U | U |
| *Gastrointestinal effects* | | | | | | | | | | | | | | | | | | | | |
| Abdominal cramps, pain, or discomfort, mild to moderate | M | M | M | L | M | M | M | M | M | M | M§ | M | M | L | M | R | M§ | U | M | M |
| Bitter taste or other taste change | R | U | U | R† | L | R | U | U | R† | R† | U | R | U | R† | U | U | R | U | R | U |
| Bloated feeling or gas | L | L | M | L | L | L | L | R | M | M | M | L | L | L | R | L | L | L | L | M |
| Constipation | M | L | L | M | M | M | M | M | L | L | M | M | M | M | R | M | M | M | L | L |
| Decreased appetite or loss of appetite | R | L | R | L | M | L | L | R | L | L | L | U | U | U | R | L | L | L | R | R |
| Diarrhea | M | M | M | M | L | M | L | L | M | M§ | M†† | M§ | M | L | M | L | M | L | L | M |

*Differences in frequency of occurrence may reflect either lack of clinical-use data or actual pharmacologic distinctions among agents (although their pharmacologic similarity suggests that side effects occurring with one may occur with the others). M=more frequent (3–9%); L=less frequent (1–3%); R=rare (<1%); U=unknown; unless otherwise specified.

†Has been reported, but a causal relationship has not been established.

‡Has been reported, but actual frequency of occurrence unknown.

§Frequency of occurrence 10% or higher.

#Serious gastrointestinal effects, including ulceration, perforation, and/or bleeding, may occur at any time, with or without warning signs and/or symptoms, during chronic therapy with nonsteroidal anti-inflammatory drugs (NSAIDs). The risk of NSAID-induced gastrointestinal toxicity may increase with the duration of therapy as well as with dosage. In clinical trials with nabumetone, peptic ulceration occurred in approximately 0.3%, 0.5%, and 0.8% of patients treated for 6 months, 1 year, and 2 years, respectively. In clinical trials with other NSAIDs, upper gastrointestinal tract ulceration, bleeding, or perforation occurred in approximately 1% of patients treated for 3 to 6 months and in approximately 2 to 4% of patients treated for 1 year. Risk factors that may increase the risk of NSAID-induced gastrointestinal toxicity, other than those associated with an increased risk of peptic ulcer disease in any patient, have not been identified.

**See also Dermatologic effects, Hematologic effects, Hepatic effects, and Renal effects for signs and symptoms of many of the reported components of this syndrome.

††Diarrhea occurring during mefenamic acid therapy requires medical attention.

## Table 3. Side/Adverse Effects* (continued)

Legend:
I = Diclofenac
II = Diflunisal
III = Etodolac
IV = Fenoprofen
V = Floctafenine
VI = Flurbiprofen
VII = Ibuprofen
VIII = Indomethacin
IX = Ketoprofen
X = Meclofenamate
XI = Mefenamic Acid
XII = Nabumetone
XIII = Naproxen
XIV = Oxaprozin
XV = Phenylbutazone
XVI = Piroxicam
XVII = Sulindac
XVIII = Tenoxicam
XIX = Tiaprofenic Acid
XX = Tolmetin

| | I | II | III | IV | V | VI | VII | VIII | IX | X | XI | XII | XIII | XIV | XV | XVI | XVII | XVIII | XIX | XX |
|---|---|---|---|---|---|---|---|---|---|---|---|---|---|---|---|---|---|---|---|---|
| *Epigastric pain or discomfort* (stomach pain or discomfort, mild to moderate) | U | U | U | U | U | U | M | U | U | U | U | U | U | U | U | M | U | L | L | U |
| *Heartburn* | U | M | U | U | U | M | M | U | U | M | L | L | M | U | U | U | U | L | M | U |
| *Indigestion* | M | M | M | M§ | M | L | L | M | M§ | L | L | M§ | L | L | L | L | M | M | M§ | M |
| *Nausea* | M | M | M | M | M | M | M | R | M | M§ | M | M | M | M | M | M | M | L | M | M§ |
| *Rectal irritation*—with rectal dosage forms | ‡ | — | — | — | — | — | — | R | M | — | — | — | — | — | — | ‡ | — | — | — | — |
| *Vomiting* | R | L | R | L | U | L | L | L | L | L | U | L | R | R | R | R | L | R | M | M |
| *General feeling of discomfort or illness* | R | U | U | L | U | L | U | L | L | U | U | R | R | R | U | L | R | R | U | U |
| *Irritation, dryness, or soreness of mouth* | R | L | R | L | L | R† | R | R | R | R† | U | L | U | U | U | U | R | R | L | R |
| *Muscle weakness* | U | U | U | U | U | R† | U | R | U | U | U | U | R | U | U | U | R | U | U | U |
| *Photophobia* (increased sensitivity of eyes to light) | U | U | R | U | U | U | U | U | U | U | U | U | U | R | U | U | U | U | U | U |
| *Weight loss, unexplained* | R† | U | U | U | U | U | U | U | R | U | U | R | U | U | U | U | U | U | U | M |

*Differences in frequency of occurrence may reflect either lack of clinical-use data or actual pharmacologic distinctions among agents (although their pharmacologic similarity suggests that side effects occurring with one may occur with the others). M=more frequent (3–9%); L=less frequent (1–3%); R=rare (<1%); U=unknown; unless otherwise specified.

†Has been reported, but a causal relationship has not been established.

‡Has been reported, but actual frequency of occurrence unknown.

§Frequency of occurrence 10% or higher.

#Serious gastrointestinal effects, including ulceration, perforation, and/or bleeding, may occur at any time, with or without warning signs and/or symptoms, during chronic therapy with nonsteroidal anti-inflammatory drugs (NSAIDs). The risk of NSAID-induced gastrointestinal toxicity may increase with the duration of therapy as well as with dosage. In clinical trials with nabumetone, peptic ulceration occurred in approximately 0.3%, 0.5%, and 0.8% of patients treated for 6 months, 1 year, and 2 years, respectively. In clinical trials with other NSAIDs, upper gastrointestinal tract ulceration, bleeding, or perforation occurred in approximately 2 to 4% of patients treated for 1 year. Risk factors that may increase the risk of NSAID-induced gastrointestinal toxicity, other than those associated with an increased risk of peptic ulcer disease in any patient, have not been identified.

**See also Dermatologic effects, Hematologic effects, Hepatic effects, and Renal effects for signs and symptoms of many of the reported components of this syndrome.

††Diarrhea occurring during mefenamic acid therapy requires medical attention.

# ANTIMYASTHENICS Systemic

This monograph includes information on the following: Ambenonium†; Neostigmine; Pyridostigmine.

VA CLASSIFICATION (Primary): AU300

Note: For a listing of dosage forms and brand names by country availability, see *Dosage Forms* section(s). For a listing of brand names for the articles in this monograph, refer to the General Index.

†Not commercially available in Canada.

## Category

Note: Cholinergic (cholinesterase inhibitor) is the basic category; the other categories are specific categories of use.

Cholinergic (cholinesterase inhibitor)—Ambenonium; Neostigmine; Pyridostigmine;

Antimyasthenic—Ambenonium; Neostigmine; Pyridostigmine;

Antidote (to nondepolarizing neuromuscular block)—Neostigmine (parenteral only); Pyridostigmine (parenteral only);

Diagnostic aid (myasthenia gravis)—Neostigmine (parenteral only).

## Indications

Note: Bracketed information in the *Indications* section refers to uses that are not included in U.S. product labeling.

### Accepted

Myasthenia gravis (treatment)—Ambenonium, neostigmine, and pyridostigmine are indicated in the treatment of myasthenia gravis. Ambenonium is used less commonly than neostigmine or pyridostigmine but may be preferred in patients hypersensitive to the bromide ion. Oral neostigmine or pyridostigmine is most useful in prolonged therapy where no difficulty in swallowing is present. In acute myasthenic crisis where difficulty in breathing and swallowing is present, the parenteral dosage form should be used and the patient transferred to the oral dosage form as soon as tolerated.

In the treatment of myasthenia gravis, other treatment (such as respiratory therapy and control of secondary infection) must be administered concurrently with the antimyasthenic.

Ileus, gastrointestinal, postoperative (prophylaxis and treatment); or

Urinary retention, postoperative (prophylaxis and treatment)—Parenteral neostigmine is indicated in the treatment of postoperative nonobstructive urinary retention. Although it is not commonly used, parenteral neostigmine may also be indicated for the prevention and treatment of postoperative gastrointestinal ileus and prevention of postoperative urinary retention.

Neuromuscular blockade, nondepolarizing (treatment)—Parenteral neostigmine and pyridostigmine are indicated as antidotes to tubocurarine and other nondepolarizing neuromuscular blocking agents.

[Myasthenia gravis (diagnosis)][1]—Parenteral neostigmine has been used as a diagnostic test for myasthenia gravis. Although edrophonium is usually considered the agent of first choice because of its rapid onset and brief duration of action, neostigmine is sometimes used to confirm the edrophonium response.

### Unaccepted

Although parenteral neostigmine has been used as a screening test for pregnancy and in the treatment of delayed menstruation, these uses of neostigmine are obsolete.

[1]Not included in Canadian product labeling.

## Pharmacology/Pharmacokinetics

See also *Table 1*, page 432.

### Physicochemical characteristics

Molecular weight—
Neostigmine bromide: 303.20.
Neostigmine methylsulfate: 334.39.
Pyridostigmine bromide: 261.12.

Other characteristics—
Neostigmine methylsulfate injection: pH approximately 5.9.
Pyridostigmine bromide injection: pH approximately 5.0.

### Mechanism of action/Effect

Cholinergic (cholinesterase inhibitor)—
Antimyasthenics inhibit destruction of acetylcholine by acetylcholinesterase, thereby facilitating transmission of impulses across the myoneural junction. Cholinergic responses produced are miosis, bradycardia, increased tonus of intestinal and skeletal muscle, con-

striction of bronchi and ureters, and stimulation of secretion by salivary and sweat glands. In addition, these medications have a direct cholinomimetic effect on skeletal muscle. Neostigmine may also act on autonomic ganglion cells and neurons of the central nervous system (CNS).

Neostigmine prevents or relieves postoperative distention by stimulating gastric motility and increasing gastric tone, which probably represents a combination of actions at the ganglion cells of Auerbach's plexus and at the muscle fibers as a result of the preservation of acetylcholine released by the cholinergic preganglionic and postganglionic fibers, respectively.

Neostigmine prevents or relieves urinary retention by increasing the tone of the detrusor muscle of the urinary bladder to produce contractions strong enough to initiate micturition.

Antimyasthenic—
Muscle strength and response to repetitive nerve stimulation is increased as a result of these medications enhancing the peak effect and prolonging the duration of action of acetylcholine at the motor end plate.

Antidote (to nondepolarizing neuromuscular block)—
Since nondepolarizing neuromuscular blocking agents combine reversibly with the receptors, preventing access of acetylcholine, antagonism can be overcome by increasing the amount of agonist at the receptors; therefore, muscle paralysis induced by nondepolarizing neuromuscular blocking agents is reversed by neostigmine or pyridostigmine, which increases concentration of acetylcholine at the receptors.

Diagnostic aid (myasthenia gravis)—
By prolonging the duration of action of acetylcholine at the motor end plate, neostigmine increases muscle strength in patients with myasthenia gravis, whereas patients with other disorders develop either no increase in muscle strength or even a slight weakness and possibly fasciculations.

### Absorption

Oral—Poorly absorbed from the gastrointestinal tract.
Parenteral—Intramuscular: Neostigmine is rapidly absorbed.

## Precautions to Consider

### Cross-sensitivity and/or related problems

Patients sensitive to bromides may be sensitive to neostigmine (oral) or pyridostigmine also.

### Pregnancy/Reproduction

Pregnancy—Problems with cholinesterase inhibitors in the human fetus have not been documented; however, transient muscular weakness has occurred in about 20% of infants born to mothers who received these medications during pregnancy.
For neostigmine: Studies with neostigmine have not been done in either animals or humans.

FDA Pregnancy Category C.

Labor and delivery—Anticholinesterase agents may cause uterine irritability and induce premature labor when given intravenously to pregnant women near term.

### Breast-feeding

Pyridostigmine is distributed into breast milk in concentrations of 36 to 113% of maternal plasma concentrations. It is not known whether ambenonium and neostigmine are distributed into breast milk. However, problems in humans have not been documented.

### Pediatrics

Appropriate studies on the relationship of age to the effects of cholinesterase inhibitors have not been performed in the pediatric population. However, no pediatrics-specific problems have been documented to date.

### Geriatrics

Extensive studies with cholinesterase inhibitors have not been performed in the geriatric population. However, in one study in which 14 out of 32 adult patients were over 60 years of age, the duration of antagonism of neuromuscular blockade by neostigmine and pyridostigmine in the elderly group was prolonged compared to younger patients.

### Drug interactions and/or related problems

The following drug interactions and/or related problems have been selected on the basis of their potential clinical significance (possible mechanism in parentheses where appropriate)—not necessarily inclusive (» = major clinical significance):

Note: Combinations containing any of the following medications, depending on the amount present, may also interact with this medication.

Aminoglycosides, systemic or
Anesthetics, hydrocarbon inhalation, such as:
  Chloroform
  Cyclopropane
  Enflurane
  Halothane
  Methoxyflurane
  Trichloroethylene or
Anesthetics, parenteral-local, large doses or
Capreomycin or
Lidocaine, intravenous or
Lincomycins or
Polymyxins, such as colistimethate, colistin, and polymyxin B or
Quinine
  (neuromuscular blocking action of these medications may antagonize the effect of antimyasthenics on skeletal muscle; temporary dosage adjustments of antimyasthenics may be necessary to control symptoms of myasthenia gravis during and following concurrent use)
  (antimyasthenics, especially in large doses, may decrease the neuromuscular blocking activity of these medications)

Anesthetics, local, ester-derivative
  (antimyasthenic agent–induced inhibition of plasma cholinesterase activity reduces the metabolism of these anesthetics, leading to increased risk of toxicity; it is recommended that local anesthetics that are not ester derivatives be used instead)

Anticholinergic agents, especially atropine and related compounds
  (atropine may be used to reduce or prevent the muscarinic effects of antimyasthenics; however, routine concurrent use is not recommended since the muscarinic effects may be the first signs of overdose and masking them with atropine may prevent early recognition of cholinergic crisis)
  (concurrent use of anticholinergics with antimyasthenics may further reduce intestinal motility; therefore, caution is recommended)

» Cholinesterase inhibitors, other, including demecarium, echothiophate, and isoflurophate, and possibly topical malathion
  (concurrent use of other cholinesterase inhibitors with antimyasthenics is not recommended except under strict medical supervision because of the possibility of additive toxicity; caution may also be warranted with topical application of malathion if excessive quantities are used)

Edrophonium
  (caution is recommended in administering edrophonium to patients with symptoms of myasthenic weakness who are also receiving antimyasthenics, since symptoms of cholinergic crisis [overdosage] may be similar to those occurring with myasthenic crisis [underdosage] and the patient's condition may be worsened by use of edrophonium)

» Guanadrel or
» Guanethidine or
» Mecamylamine or
» Trimethaphan
  (these ganglionic-blocking medications may antagonize the effects of antimyasthenics when used concurrently, leading to increased muscle weakness, respiratory weakness, and/or difficulty in swallowing; the possibility should be considered that the antihypertensive effects of the ganglionic-blocking medication may also be decreased during concurrent use)

Neuromuscular blocking agents
  (phase I block of depolarizing neuromuscular blocking agents such as succinylcholine may be prolonged when used concurrently with neostigmine or pyridostigmine; however, if a depolarizing neuromuscular blocking agent has been used over a prolonged period of time and the depolarization block has changed to a nondepolarization block, neostigmine or pyridostigmine may reverse the nondepolarization block)
  (effects of nondepolarizing neuromuscular blocking agents are antagonized by parenteral neostigmine or pyridostigmine; this interaction may be used to therapeutic advantage to reverse muscle relaxation following surgery)
  (neuromuscular blockade antagonizes the effect of antimyasthenics on skeletal muscle; temporary dosage adjustments of antimyasthenics may be required to control symptoms of myasthenia gravis following use of a neuromuscular blocking agent)

» Procainamide or
  Quinidine
  (neuromuscular blocking activity and/or secondary anticholinergic effects of these medications may antagonize the action of antimyasthenics; caution is recommended during concurrent use in patients with myasthenia gravis)

**Medical considerations/Contraindications**
The medical considerations/contraindications included here have been selected on the basis of their potential clinical significance (reasons given in parentheses where appropriate)—not necessarily inclusive (» = major clinical significance).

*Risk-benefit should be considered when the following medical problems exist:*
  Asthma, bronchial
    (increase in bronchial secretions and other respiratory effects of antimyasthenics may aggravate condition)
  Atelectasis, postoperative, or
  Pneumonia
    (may be exacerbated)
  Cardiac dysrhythmias, especially bradycardia and atrioventricular (AV) block
    (increased risk of cardiac arrhythmias)
» Intestinal or urinary tract obstruction, mechanical
    (may be exacerbated)
  Sensitivity to any of these medications or to bromides
» Urinary tract infections
    (increase in urinary bladder muscle tone may aggravate symptoms)
» Caution is also recommended in the postsurgical patient because antimyasthenics may exacerbate respiratory problems caused by postoperative pain, sedation, retained secretions, or atelectasis. In the myasthenic patient, if a postoperative respiratory problem cannot be attributed to myasthenia gravis alone, mechanical ventilation is recommended.

## Side/Adverse Effects

Note: Most common adverse reactions to cholinesterase inhibitors are caused by excessive cholinergic stimulation. These include both muscarinic and nicotinic effects.
  Ambenonium produces fewer muscarinic side/adverse effects than neostigmine but more than pyridostigmine.
  Neostigmine produces more severe muscarinic side effects than ambenonium or pyridostigmine.
  Pyridostigmine may produce a significantly lower degree and incidence of bradycardia, salivation, and gastrointestinal stimulation than neostigmine.

The following side/adverse effects have been selected on the basis of their potential clinical significance (possible signs and symptoms in parentheses where appropriate)—not necessarily inclusive:

**Those indicating need for medical attention**
Incidence rare
  *Sensitivity to bromide ion of neostigmine or pyridostigmine* (skin rash); *thrombophlebitis* (redness, swelling, or pain at injection site)—for pyridostigmine injection only

**Those indicating need for medical attention only if they continue or are bothersome**
Incidence more frequent
  *Muscarinic effects* (diarrhea; increased sweating; increased watering of mouth; nausea or vomiting; stomach cramps or pain)
Incidence less frequent
  *Muscarinic effects* (frequent urge to urinate; increase in bronchial secretions; unusually small pupils; unusual watering of eyes)

## Overdose

For specific information on the agents used in the management of antimyasthenics overdose, see: *Atropine* in *Anticholinergics/Antispasmodics (Systemic)* monograph.

For more information on the management of overdose or unintentional ingestion, **contact a Poison Control Center** (see *Poison Control Center Listing.*

**Clinical effects of overdose**

The following effects have been selected on the basis of their potential clinical signifiance (possible signs and symptoms in parentheses where appropriate)—not necessarily inclusive:

Acute and chronic

*CNS effects* (clumsiness or unsteadiness; confusion; difficulty in breathing; seizures; slurred speech; unusual irritability, nervousness, restlessness, or fear); *muscarinic effects* (blurred vision; severe diarrhea; excessive increase in bronchial secretions or salivation; severe vomiting; shortness of breath; troubled breathing; wheezing, or tightness in chest; slow heartbeat; severe stomach cramps or pain; unusual tiredness or weakness); *nicotinic effects* (increasing muscle weakness or paralysis, especially in the arms, neck, shoulders, and tongue; muscle cramps or twitching)

Note: *Breathing problems* may also be caused by atelectasis.

*Unusual tiredness or weakness* may also be caused by hypokalemia resulting from severe diarrhea and vomiting.

In the myasthenic patient, *increased muscle weakness* may be caused by underdosage or resistance instead of by overdosage.

Note: Overdosage may induce cholinergic crisis, which is characterized by nicotinic effects in addition to intensified muscarinic effects.

In patients with myasthenia gravis or in the postoperative patient, cholinergic crisis may be difficult to distinguish from myasthenic crisis on a symptomatic basis because the principal symptom common to both is generalized muscle weakness. The time of onset of weakness may help determine whether the crisis is caused by overdosage or underdosage (or resistance). Weakness beginning about 1 hour after administration of antimyasthenic is probably overdosage while that occurring 3 or more hours after administration is probably underdosage or resistance.

If a differential diagnosis cannot be made on the basis of signs and symptoms, edrophonium may be used to distinguish cholinergic crisis from myasthenic crisis; however, caution is recommended because edrophonium will cause increased oropharyngeal secretions and further weakness in muscles of respiration in a cholinergic crisis. This may be especially critical in the postoperative patient.

**Treatment of overdose**

Recommended treatment for cholinergic crisis—

Prompt discontinuation of antimyasthenic.

Specific treatment—Use of intravenous atropine sulfate to counteract muscarinic effects.

Supportive care—May include establishment of endotracheal tube, if necessary.

## Patient Consultation

As an aid to patient consultation, refer to *Advice for the Patient, Antimyasthenics (Systemic)*.

In providing consultation, consider emphasizing the following selected information (» = major clinical significance):

**Before using this medication**

» Conditions affecting use, especially:

Sensitivity to antimyasthenics or to bromides

Pregnancy—Possible transient muscle weakness in newborns whose mothers received antimyasthenics during pregnancy

Use in the elderly—In one study in a limited number of patients, duration of antagonism of neuromuscular blockade by neostigmine and pyridostigmine was prolonged

Other medications, especially other cholinesterase inhibitors, guanadrel, guanethidine, mecamylamine, procainamide, or trimethaphan

Other medical problems, especially intestinal or urinary tract blockage or, urinary tract infection

**Proper use of this medication**

Taking with food or milk to decrease possibility of side effects

» Importance of not taking more medication than the amount prescribed

For use in myasthenia gravis: Keeping daily record of dosing and effects on condition during initial therapy

Missed dose: Taking as soon as possible; not taking if almost time for next dose; not doubling doses

» Proper dosing

» Proper storage

**Side/adverse effects**

Signs of potential side effects, especially thrombophlebitis at injection site (for pyridostigmine only), and sensitivity

## General Dosing Information

In myasthenia gravis, the dosage must be individualized according to the severity of the disease and the response of the patient.

To assist the physician in arranging an optimum therapeutic regimen in the treatment of myasthenia gravis, patients should keep a daily record of their condition.

Therapy in myasthenia gravis is frequently required day and night. Larger portions of the total daily dose may be taken at times of greater fatigue such as in the afternoons or at mealtimes.

Following prolonged therapy, myasthenic patients may become refractory to these medications. Responsiveness may be restored, especially when the resistance may have been caused by overdosage, by reducing the dosage or discontinuing the medication for a few days.

**For parenteral dosage forms only**

Patients should be closely observed for cholinergic reactions, especially when neostigmine or pyridostigmine is administered intravenously.

Atropine injection and antishock medication should always be readily available because of the possibility of hypersensitivity reactions.

When large doses of parenteral neostigmine or pyridostigmine are administered, as during reversal of muscle relaxants, prior or concurrent administration of atropine injection is recommended to counteract the muscarinic side effects.

**Diet/Nutrition**

Administration of oral forms of these medications with food or milk may decrease the muscarinic side effects by slowing down absorption of the medication and reducing serum peaks.

---

### *AMBENONIUM*

## Summary of Differences

Pharmacology/pharmacokinetics:

Has longer duration of action than neostigmine or pyridostigmine.

Side/adverse effects:

Produces fewer muscarinic side effects than neostigmine, but more than pyridostigmine.

## Oral Dosage Forms

### AMBENONIUM CHLORIDE TABLETS

**Usual adult and adolescent dose**

Antimyasthenic—

Oral, initially 5 mg three or four times a day, the dosage being adjusted as required at intervals of one to two days to avoid accumulation of medication and overdosage.

Note: When doses of more than 200 mg per day are administered, the patient should be closely observed for cholinergic reactions.

**Usual pediatric dose**

Antimyasthenic—

Oral, initially 300 mcg (0.3 mg) per kg of body weight or 10 mg per square meter of body surface per day (divided into three or four doses), the dosage being increased, if necessary, to 1.5 mg per kg of body weight or 50 mg per square meter of body surface per day (divided into three or four doses).

**Usual geriatric dose**

See *Usual adult and adolescent dose.*

**Strength(s) usually available**

U.S.—

10 mg (Rx) [*Mytelase Caplets* (scored; acacia; dibasic calcium phosphate; gelatin; lactose; magnesium stearate; starch; and sucrose)].

Canada—

Not commercially available.

**Packaging and storage**

Store below 40 °C (104 °F), preferably between 15 and 30 °C (59 and 86 °F), unless otherwise specified by manufacturer. Store in a tight container.

---

### *NEOSTIGMINE*

## Summary of Differences

Category: Parenteral neostigmine:

Also indicated as an antidote (to nondepolarizing neuromuscular block) and a diagnostic aid (myasthenia gravis).

Indications: Parenteral neostigmine:

Also indicated in the treatment of postoperative nonobstructive urinary retention.

May also be indicated for prevention and treatment of postoperative gastrointestinal ileus and prevention of postoperative urinary retention.

Pharmacology/pharmacokinetics:

Has shorter duration of action than ambenonium.

Precautions: Cross-sensitivity and/or related problems:

Oral neostigmine contains bromide ion to which some patients may be sensitive.

Side/adverse effects:

Produces more severe muscarinic side effects than ambenonium or pyridostigmine.

## Additional Dosing Information

See also *General Dosing Information*.

Generally, 15 mg of neostigmine bromide administered orally is equivalent to 500 mcg (0.5 mg) of neostigmine methylsulfate administered parenterally.

*For oral dosage forms only*

- Neostigmine is poorly absorbed from the gastrointestinal tract following oral administration; therefore, much larger doses are required for oral than for parenteral use.
- Large oral doses should be avoided in conditions where there may be an increased absorption rate from the intestinal tract, in order to avoid possible toxicity.

*For parenteral dosage forms only: When used as an antidote to nondepolarizing neuromuscular block*

- It is recommended that the exact dose required be titrated, using a peripheral nerve stimulator device.
- Unless tachycardia is present, atropine (0.6 to 1 mg) should be administered concomitantly or several minutes before neostigmine to prevent bradycardia.
- In the presence of bradycardia, the pulse rate should be increased to about 80 per minute with atropine prior to administration of neostigmine.

*When used as a diagnostic aid (myasthenia gravis)*

- Significant improvement of muscle weakness occurring within several minutes to 1 hour following administration of neostigmine usually indicates myasthenia gravis. However, diagnosis also should include clinical and electromyographic (EMG) evaluation.

## Oral Dosage Forms

### NEOSTIGMINE BROMIDE TABLETS USP

**Usual adult and adolescent dose**

Antimyasthenic—

Initial—Oral, 15 mg every three to four hours, the dose and frequency of administration being adjusted as necessary.

Maintenance—Oral, 150 mg administered over a twenty-four-hour period, the intervals between doses being determined by response of the patient.

Note: The twenty-four-hour maintenance dose is highly variable among individuals.

**Usual pediatric dose**

Antimyasthenic—

Oral, 2 mg per kg of body weight or 60 mg per square meter of body surface per day, divided into six to eight doses.

**Usual geriatric dose**

See *Usual adult and adolescent dose*.

**Strength(s) usually available**

U.S.—

15 mg (Rx) [*Prostigmin* (scored; lactose); GENERIC].

Canada—

15 mg (Rx) [*Prostigmin* (scored; lactose)].

**Packaging and storage**

Store below 40 °C (104 °F), preferably between 15 and 30 °C (59 and 86 °F), unless otherwise specified by manufacturer. Store in a tight container.

## Parenteral Dosage Forms

Note: Bracketed uses in the Dosage Forms section refer to categories of use and/or indications that are not included in U.S. product labeling.

## NEOSTIGMINE METHYLSULFATE INJECTION USP

**Usual adult and adolescent dose**

Antimyasthenic—

Intramuscular or subcutaneous, 500 mcg (0.5); subsequent doses should be based on the patient's response.

Antidote (to nondepolarizing neuromuscular block)—

Intravenous, 500 mcg (0.5) to 2 mg administered slowly, repeated as required up to a total dose of 5 mg.

Note: Subsequent doses may be less than 500 mcg (0.5mg).

When neostigmine is administered intravenously, it is recommended that 600 mcg (0.6) to 1.2 mg of atropine sulfate be administered intravenously prior to or concurrently with neostigmine to counteract its muscarinic side effects.

Diagnostic aid (myasthenia gravis)[1]—

Intramuscular or subcutaneous, 1.5 mg administered simultaneously with 600 mcg (0.6 mg) of atropine

Note: Significant improvement of muscle weakness occurring within several minutes to one hour indicates myasthenia gravis.

Prevention of postoperative distention or urinary retention—

Intramuscular or subcutaneous, 250 mcg (0.25 mg) immediately following surgery, repeated every four to six hours for two or three days.

Treatment of postoperative distention—

Intramuscular or subcutaneous, 500 mcg (0.5 mg) as needed.

Treatment of urinary retention—

Intramuscular or subcutaneous, 500 mcg (0.5 mg); dose repeated every three hours for at least five doses after patient has voided or the bladder has been emptied.

Note: If urination does not occur within one hour following the initial 500–mcg (0.5–mg) dose, the patient should be catheterized.

**Usual pediatric dose**

Antimyasthenic—

Intramuscular or subcutaneous, 10 to 40 mcg (0.01 to 0.04 mg) per kg of body weight every two to three hours.

Note: A dose of 10 mcg (0.01 mg) of atropine per kg of body weight may be administered intramuscularly or subcutaneously with each dose or with alternate doses of neostigmine to counteract the muscarinic side effects.

Antidote (to nondepolarizing neuromuscular block)—

Intravenous, 40 mcg (0.04 mg) per kg of body weight administered with 20 mcg (0.02 mg) of atropine per kg of body weight.

[Diagnostic aid (myasthenia gravis)][1]—

Intramuscular, 40 mcg (0.04 mg) per kg of body weight or 1 mg per square meter of body surface per dose.

Intravenous, 20 mcg (0.02 mg) per kg of body weight or 500 mcg (0.5 mg) per square meter of body surface.

**Usual geriatric dose**

See *Usual adult and adolescent dose*.

**Strength(s) usually available**

U.S.—

0.25 mg per mL (1:4000) (Rx) [*Prostigmin* (parabens 0.2% [methyl and propyl]; sodium hydroxide); GENERIC].

0.5 mg per mL (1:2000) (Rx) [*Prostigmin* (parabens 0.2% [methyl and propyl]; sodium hydroxide—in 1-ml ampuls; phenol 0.45%; sodium acetate 0.02%; acetic acid; sodium hydroxide—in 10-mL vials); GENERIC].

1 mg per mL (1:1000) (Rx) [*Prostigmin* (phenol 0.45%; sodium acetate 0.02%; acetic acid; sodium hydroxide); GENERIC].

Canada—

0.5 mg per mL (1:2000) (Rx) [*Prostigmin* (methylparaben 1.8 mg; propylparaben 0.2 mg; sodium <0.01 mmol/mL—in 1–mL ampuls; phenol 0.45%; sodium acetate; acetic acid; sodium <0.01 mmol/mL—in 10-mL vials)].

1 mg per mL (1:1000) (Rx) [*Prostigmin* (phenol 0.45%; sodium acetate; acetic acid; sodium hydroxide; sodium <0.01 mmol/mL)].

2.5 mg per mL (1:400) (Rx) [*Prostigmin* (phenol 0.4%,; sodium chloride; sodium hydroxide; sodium <0.01 mmol/mL)].

**Packaging and storage**

Store below 40 °C (104 °F), preferably between 15 and 30 °C (59 and 86 °F), unless otherwise specified by manufacturer. Protect from freezing. Protect from light.

---

[1]Not included in Canadian product labeling.

## PYRIDOSTIGMINE

## Summary of Differences

Category:
Parenteral pyridostigmine also indicated as an antidote (to nondepolarizing neuromuscular block).

Pharmacology/pharmacokinetics:
Generally has shorter duration of action than ambenonium and a slower onset and longer duration of action than neostigmine.

Precautions:
Cross-sensitivity and/or related problems—Contains bromide ion to which some patients may be sensitive.

Side/adverse effects:
May produce a significantly lower degree and incidence of bradycardia, salivation, and gastrointestinal stimulation than neostigmine.

## Additional Dosing Information

See also *General Dosing Information*.

For oral dosage forms only:

• The syrup dosage form may be preferred for use in children and "brittle" myasthenic patients who require fractions of 60-mg doses. Also, the syrup is more easily swallowed, especially in the morning, by patients with bulbar involvement.

• It has been reported that the extended-release dosage form may pass intact through the gastrointestinal tract in patients with increased gastrointestinal activity or diarrhea. Use of other oral dosage forms may be required temporarily for continued control of symptoms.

## Oral Dosage Forms

### PYRIDOSTIGMINE BROMIDE SYRUP USP

**Usual adult and adolescent dose**
Antimyasthenic—
Initial—Oral, 30 to 60 mg every three to four hours, the dosage being adjusted as required.
Maintenance—Oral, 600 mg (range 60 mg to 1.5 grams) per day.

**Usual pediatric dose**
Antimyasthenic—
Oral, 7 mg per kg of body weight or 200 mg per square meter of body surface per day, divided into five or six doses.

**Usual geriatric dose**
See *Usual adult and adolescent dose.*

**Strength(s) usually available**
U.S.—
60 mg per 5 mL (Rx) [*Mestinon* (alcohol 5%; glycerin; lactic acid; sodium benzoate; sorbitol; sucrose; FD&C Red No. 40; FD&C Blue No. 1; flavors; water)].
Canada—
Not commercially available.

**Packaging and storage**
Store below 40 °C (104 °F), preferably between 15 and 30 °C (59 and 86 °F), unless otherwise specified by manufacturer. Store in a tight, light-resistant container. Protect from freezing.

### PYRIDOSTIGMINE BROMIDE TABLETS USP

**Usual adult and adolescent dose**
See *Pyridostigmine Bromide Syrup USP.*

**Usual pediatric dose**
See *Pyridostigmine Bromide Syrup USP.*

**Usual geriatric dose**
See *Pyridostigmine Bromide Syrup USP.*

**Strength(s) usually available**
U.S.—
60 mg (Rx) [*Mestinon* (scored; lactose; silicon dioxide; stearic acid)].
Canada—
60 mg (Rx) [*Mestinon* (scored; lactose 272 mg)].

**Packaging and storage**
Store below 40 °C (104 °F), preferably between 15 and 30 °C (59 and 86 °F), unless otherwise specified by manufacturer. Store in a tight container.

### PYRIDOSTIGMINE BROMIDE EXTENDED-RELEASE TABLETS

**Usual adult and adolescent dose**
Antimyasthenic—
Oral, 180 to 540 mg one or two times a day, with at least six hours between doses.

Note: For optimum control of symptoms, it may be necessary to administer the more rapidly acting regular tablet or syrup dosage form concurrently with extended-release therapy.

Extended-release preparations may increase the risk of cholinergic crisis and, therefore, are usually not recommended.

**Usual pediatric dose**
Dosage has not been established.

**Usual geriatric dose**
See *Usual adult and adolescent dose.*

**Strength(s) usually available**
U.S.—
180 mg (Rx) [*Mestinon Timespans* (carnauba wax; corn-derived proteins; magnesium stearate; silica gel; tribasic calcium phosphate)].
Canada—
180 mg (Rx) [*Mestinon-SR* (scored)].

**Packaging and storage**
Store below 40 °C (104 °F), preferably between 15 and 30 °C (59 and 86 °F), in a well-closed container, unless otherwise specified by manufacturer.

**Auxiliary labeling**
• Swallow tablets whole.

## Parenteral Dosage Forms

### PYRIDOSTIGMINE BROMIDE INJECTION USP

**Usual adult and adolescent dose**
Antimyasthenic—
Intramuscular or intravenous, 2 mg (approximately one-thirtieth of the usual oral dose) every two to three hours.
Antidote (to nondepolarizing neuromuscular block)—
Intravenous, 10 to 20 mg.

Note: Prior to administration of pyridostigmine, it is recommended that 600 mcg (0.6 mg) to 1.2 mg of atropine sulfate be given intravenously to counteract the muscarinic effects.

**Usual pediatric dose**
Antimyasthenic—
Neonates of myasthenic mothers—Intramuscular, 50 to 150 mcg (0.05 to 0.15 mg) per kg of body weight every four to six hours.

**Usual geriatric dose**
See *Usual adult and adolescent dose.*

**Strength(s) usually available**
U.S.—
5 mg per mL (Rx) [*Mestinon* (parabens 0.2% [methyl and propyl]; sodium citrate 0.02%; citric acid; sodium hydroxide); *Regonol* (benzyl alcohol 1%)].
Canada—
5 mg per mL (Rx) [*Regonol* (parabens 0.2% [methyl and propyl]; sodium citrate 0.02%; citric acid; sodium hydroxide)].

**Packaging and storage**
Store below 40 °C (104 °F), preferably between 15 and 30 °C (59 and 86 °F), unless otherwise specified by manufacturer. Protect from light. Protect from freezing.

Revised: 09/30/91
Interim revision: 07/18/94

## Table 1. Pharmacology/Pharmacokinetics

| Drug | Oral Bioavailability | Volume of Distribution $V_D$ (L/kg) | Half-life Distribution (min) | Half-life Elimination (min) | Protein Binding | Biotransformation | Onset of Action (min) | Time to Peak Plasma Concentration (hr) | Peak Plasma Concentration (mcg/mL) | Peak Effect (min) | Duration of Action (hr) | Elimination (% excreted unchanged) | Clearance (L/hr/kg) |
|---|---|---|---|---|---|---|---|---|---|---|---|---|---|
| **Ambenonium** | | | | | | | 20–30 | | | | 3–8 | | |
| **Neostigmine** | | | | | | | | | | | | | |
|   Oral | 1–2% | | | | Low (15–25%) | Plasma; hepatic | 45–75* | 1–2 | 1–5† | 30 | 3–6 | Renal (about 50) | |
|   Parenteral | | | | | | | ‡ | | | | | | |
|   Intramuscular | | 0.74±0.2 | 3.6±1.2 | 77.4±48 | | | 20–30 | 0.5 | | | 2–4 | | 0.55±0.14 |
|   Intravenous | | 0.37–1.08 | 5.4 | 24–79.2 | | | 4–8 | | | | 2–4 | | 0.24–1.0 |
| **Pyridostigmine** | | | | | | | | | | | | | |
|   Oral | 10–20% | | | | Not bound | Plasma; hepatic | 30–45 | 1–2 | 40–60§ | 60–120 | 3–6 | Renal | |
|     Syrup, Tablets | | | | | | | | | | | | | |
|     Extended-release Tablets | | | | | | | 30–60 | | | | 6–12 | | |
|   Parenteral | | | | | | | | | | | | | |
|     Intramuscular | | | | | | | <15 | | | | 2–4 | | |
|     Intravenous | | 1.03–1.76 | 7.2–8.4 | 63–112 | | | 2–5 | | | | 2–4 | | 0.52–1.0 |

*Peristaltic activity begins in 2 to 4 hours.
†Following a single 30-mg oral dose.
‡Peristaltic activity begins in 10 to 30 minutes.
§Following a single 60-mg oral dose.

# ANTIPYRINE AND BENZOCAINE  Otic

INN: Antipyrine—Phenazone.
BAN: Antipyrine—Phenazone.
JAN: Benzocaine—Ethyl aminobenzoate.
VA CLASSIFICATION (Primary/Secondary): OT400/OT300

Note: For a listing of dosage forms and brand names by country availability, see *Dosage Forms* section(s). For a listing of brand names for the articles in this monograph, refer to the General Index.

## Category

Analgesic-anesthetic (otic); cerumen removal adjunct.

## Indications

### Unaccepted

Antipyrine and benzocaine otic combination has been used to relieve pain and inflammation in the congestive and serous stages of acute otitis media and to facilitate removal of cerumen from the wall of the ear canal. However, it is no longer recommended for these purposes, because of questionable effectiveness and because benzocaine frequently causes contact dermatitis.

## Pharmacology/Pharmacokinetics

### Physicochemical characteristics

Chemical group—
Antipyrine: A pyrazolone derivative.
Benzocaine: An aminobenzoic acid (para-aminobenzoic acid; PABA) derivative.
Molecular weight—
Antipyrine: 188.23.
Benzocaine: 165.19.
Glycerin: 92.09.

### Mechanism of action/Effect

Both antipyrine and benzocaine are employed for their analgesic/local anesthetic effects. The anhydrous glycerin vehicle is hygroscopic and may provide a decongestant action.

## Precautions to Consider

### Cross-sensitivity and/or related problems

Patients sensitive to benzocaine or other ester-derivative anesthetics may be sensitive to this medication also.

### Carcinogenicity/Mutagenicity

Studies have not been done.

### Pregnancy/Reproduction

Pregnancy—Studies in humans have not been done. However, problems have not been documented.
Studies in animals have not been done.
FDA Pregnancy Category C.

### Breast-feeding

It is not known whether this medication is distributed into breast milk. However, problems in humans have not been documented.

### Pediatrics

The risk of benzocaine-induced methemoglobinemia may be increased in infants, especially infants up to 3 months of age. However, pediatrics-specific problems that would limit the usefulness of antipyrine and benzocaine combination in older children are not expected.

### Geriatrics

Appropriate studies on the relationship of age to the effects of antipyrine and benzocaine combination have not been performed in the geriatric population. However, no geriatrics-specific problems have been documented to date.

### Medical considerations/Contraindications

The medical considerations/contraindications included here have been selected on the basis of their potential clinical significance (reasons given in parentheses where appropriate)—not necessarily inclusive (» = major clinical significance).

*Risk-benefit should be considered when the following medical problems exist:*
Sensitivity to antipyrine or benzocaine
Spontaneous perforation of or drainage through the eardrum membrane (increased risk of otorrhea and irritation)

## Side/Adverse Effects

The following side/adverse effects have been selected on the basis of their potential clinical significance (possible signs and symptoms in parentheses where appropriate)—not necessarily inclusive:

**Those indicating need for medical attention only if they continue or are bothersome**
*Allergic reaction, local* (itching, burning, redness, or oozing sores in the ear)

## Patient Consultation

As an aid to patient consultation, refer to *Advice for the Patient, Antipyrine and Benzocaine (Otic).*

In providing consultation, consider emphasizing the following selected information (» = major clinical significance):

**Before using this medication**
» Conditions affecting use, especially:
Sensitivity to benzocaine or antipyrine
Use in children—Risk of methemoglobinemia in infants

**Proper use of this medication**
*Proper administration technique*
May warm medication to body temperature (37 °C or 98.6 °F) by holding bottle in hand for a few minutes before using
Slowly fill ear canal while lying on side or tilting head with affected ear facing up
Keep ear facing up for 5 minutes or, for patients who cannot stay still that long, for at least 1 or 2 minutes
A cotton plug moistened with medication may be gently placed at the ear opening for no longer than 5 to 10 minutes to ensure retention
For cerumen removal, the ear canal should be irrigated with warm water after the medication has been used for 2 or 3 days
Preventing contamination of ear drops by not touching dropper to any surface including ear
» Not rinsing dropper after use; keeping container tightly closed
Missed dose: Using as soon as possible; not using if almost time for next dose
» Proper dosing
» Proper storage

**Side/adverse effects**
Discontinuing treatment if signs and symptoms of local allergic reaction occur

## General Dosing Information

This medication may be warmed to body temperature (37 °C or 98.6 °F) by holding the bottle in the hand for a few minutes prior to using.

The medication should be instilled with the affected ear facing up. Several minutes after the medication has been instilled the patient should gently place a cotton plug moistened with a little medication at the ear opening for no longer than 5 to 10 minutes to ensure retention.

When the medication is used to facilitate removal of cerumen, the ear canal should be irrigated with warm water, preferably by the physician, after the medication has been used for 2 or 3 days.

Treatment should be discontinued immediately if any sign of hypersensitivity or irritation occurs.

## Otic Dosage Forms

### ANTIPYRINE AND BENZOCAINE OTIC SOLUTION USP

**Usual adult and adolescent dose**
Analgesic-anesthetic, otic—
Topical, to the ear canal, a sufficient quantity to fill the ear canal every one to two hours until relief is obtained.
Cerumen removal adjunct[1]—
Topical, to the ear canal, a sufficient quantity to fill the ear canal three times a day for two or three days. After two or three days the ear canal should be irrigated with warm water.

**Usual pediatric dose**
See *Usual adult and adolescent dose.*

**Strength(s) usually available**
U.S.—
54 mg of antipyrine and 14 mg of benzocaine, dissolved in anhydrous glycerin to make 1 mL (Rx) [*A/B Otic; Allergen; Analgesic Otic* (oxyquinoline sulfate); *Antiben; Auralgan* (oxyquinoline sulfate);

*Aurodex; Auroto* (oxyquinoline sulfate); *Dolotic; Ear Drops* (oxyquinoline sulfate); *Otocalm;* GENERIC].

Canada—
- ·54 mg of antipyrine and 14 mg of benzocaine, dissolved in anhydrous glycerin to make 1 mL (OTC) [*Auralgan*].
- 90 mg of antipyrine and 14 mg of benzocaine, dissolved in anhydrous glycerin to make 1 mL (OTC) [*Earache Drops*].

**Packaging and storage**

Store below 40 °C (104 °F), preferably between 15 and 30 °C (59 and 86 °F), unless otherwise specified by manufacturer. Store in a tight, light-resistant container. Protect from freezing.

Note: The solution congeals at 0 °C (32 °F) but returns to liquid state at room temperature. Therapeutic qualities are not affected.

**Auxiliary labeling**
- For the ear.
- Keep container tightly closed.

†Not included in Canadian product labeling.

Revised: 07/14/95

---

# ANTIPYRINE-CONTAINING COMBINATIONS—

Antipyrine and Benzocaine (Otic)

---

# ANTITHROMBIN III    Systemic†

VA CLASSIFICATION (Primary): BL100

Other commonly used names are ATIII and heparin cofactor I.

Note: For a listing of dosage forms and brand names by country availability, see *Dosage Forms* section(s). For a listing of brand names for the articles in this monograph, refer to the General Index.

  †Not commercially available in Canada.

---

## Category

Anticoagulant; antithrombotic.

## Indications

Note: Bracketed information in the *Indications* section refers to uses that are not included in U.S. product labeling.

**Accepted**

Thromboembolism associated with hereditary antithrombin III deficiency (prophylaxis)—Antithrombin III is indicated as prophylaxis against the development of thrombotic complications in patients with hereditary antithrombin III deficiency in situations in which the risk of thromboembolism is increased, such as surgery, delivery (including spontaneous or induced abortion), [pregnancy], [trauma], and [prolonged (> 24 hours) immobilization]. Heparin enhances the effects of antithrombin III (and vice versa) and may be given concurrently, using a full-dose, adjusted-dose, or low-dose heparin regimen as determined by the clinical circumstances.

Although long-term prophylaxis may be required in patients with hereditary antithrombin III deficiency, antithrombin III is usually not used, whether or not a high-risk situation, such as those listed above, exists. A coumarin- or indandione-derivative anticoagulant is usually used for this purpose. However, these anticoagulants should not be administered during the first trimester of pregnancy, and some clinicians recommend that they not be used at all during pregnancy. Heparin is usually used instead, but may be ineffective when concentrations of endogenous antithrombin III are low. Long-term prophylactic use of antithrombin III may therefore be required if heparin alone fails to produce adequate anticoagulation.

Thromboembolism associated with hereditary antithrombin III deficiency (treatment adjunct)—Antithrombin III is indicated as an adjunct to heparin therapy for the treatment of thromboembolism in patients with hereditary antithrombin III deficiency.

[The safety and efficacy of antithrombin III as an adjunct to heparin for the treatment of thromboembolism associated with acquired antithrombin III deficiency have not been established. However, use of antithrombin III may be considered for individual patients in whom heparin alone is ineffective.]

## Pharmacology/Pharmacokinetics

**Physicochemical characteristics**

Source—Pooled human plasma.

Chemical group—An alpha-2-globulin.

Molecular weight—58,000 daltons.

Description—A glycoprotein consisting of 425 amino acids in a single polypeptide chain cross-linked by three disulfide bridges.

pH (after reconstitution with 10 mL of sterile water for injection)—6.5–7.5

**Mechanism of action/Effect**

Antithrombin III, which is synthesized in the liver and endothelial cells, is an endogenous inhibitor of blood coagulation, providing approxi-

mately 75% of the antithrombin activity of the blood. It combines in a 1:1 molar ratio with the activated serine proteases of the intrinsic coagulation pathway (primarily thrombin [factor IIa] and factor Xa, and, to a lesser extent, factors IXa, XIa, and XIIa) to form inactive complexes. The active binding center is at the $Arg_{384}$–$Ser_{385}$ peptide bond. Hereditary antithrombin III deficiency has been shown to increase the risk of thromboembolism in some individuals; initial episodes in these patients have occurred most often between 15 and 30 years of age. Administration of exogenous antithrombin III corrects the deficiency, thus normalizing the patient's coagulation-inhibiting capability and inhibiting formation of thromboemboli.

Note: Antithrombin III also has lysine binding sites to which heparin binds in a 1:1 molar ratio. Formation of the antithrombin III–heparin complex produces a conformational change in the antithrombin III molecule that results in more rapid binding with and inactivation of the clotting factors than can be achieved by antithrombin III alone. Because heparin produces its anticoagulant effect only through its cofactors (the primary cofactor being antithrombin III), the efficacy of heparin is substantially reduced in antithrombin III deficiency. A reduction in the plasma activity of antithrombin III to 70% of the normal value may decrease the efficacy of heparin to 45%, and a reduction to 50% of the normal antithrombin III value may decrease the efficacy of heparin to 20%, of that achieved in the presence of normal antithrombin III activity. Administration of antithrombin III augments or restores the efficacy of heparin.

**Other actions/effects**

Antithrombin III also inactivates the fibrinolytic enzyme plasmin, but to a lesser extent than it inactivates the clotting factors.

**Distribution**

Antithrombin III is removed from the blood by binding to the epithelium and by redistribution into the extravascular compartment.

Antithrombin III–clotting factor complexes are removed rapidly from the circulation by binding to a specific receptor present on hepatocytes.

**Half-life**

Elimination—2 to 3 days; may be decreased by concurrent use of heparin, following surgery, and in patients with disseminated intravascular coagulation.

**Therapeutic plasma concentration**

Therapeutic benefit requires an antithrombin III activity of 80% or more of the normal value, which ranges between 100 and 200 mcg per mL (100 to 200 mg per L) in individuals 3 months of age and older.

Note: Plasma antithrombin III activity in patients with a hereditary deficiency is generally 25 to 60% of that present in normal adult plasma.

Plasma antithrombin III activity is normally reduced in neonates. Healthy, full-term neonates exhibit 40 to 85% of the antithrombin III activity present in normal adults; gradual increases occur until adult values are reached, generally at about 3 months of age. Antithrombin III activity is even lower in premature neonates.

## Precautions to Consider

**Pregnancy/Reproduction**

Note: Transmission of hereditary antithrombin III deficiency is autosomal-dominant; a deficiency state may occur in the child if either parent is affected. Homozygous fetuses often do not survive (depending on the specific type of antithrombin III deficiency). Patients with hereditary antithrombin III deficiency should be counseled about the potential risk to a child. Also, female patients with diagnosed hereditary antithrombin III deficiency and their spouses should be informed of the very high risk of thrombosis in antithrombin III–deficient women during pregnancy and delivery.

Pregnancy—Antithrombin III is effective in preventing thrombotic complications during pregnancy in women with hereditary antithrombin III deficiency, including women with a prior history of thrombosis, and women who are heparin-resistant. Studies in pregnant women have not shown that antithrombin III increases the risk of fetal abnormalities when administered during the third trimester of pregnancy. Antithrombin III has also been administered to a few women during the first 2 trimesters of pregnancy. No adverse effects on the fetus attributable to antithrombin III were reported.

Studies have not been done in animals.

FDA Pregnancy Category C.

Labor and delivery—Administration of a coumarin- or indandione-derivative anticoagulant or heparin during pregnancy increases the risk of hemorrhage during and following delivery; heparin should be discontinued 12 hours, and coumarin- or indandione-derivative anticoagulants several days, prior to delivery or therapeutic abortion. Antithrombin III therapy, when instituted or continued after another anticoagulant has been discontinued, is effective in preventing thromboembolic complications during and following delivery or therapeutic abortion, even in women who had previously had such complications. Such use of antithrombin III has not been reported to cause problems in the neonate.

**Breast-feeding**

Problems in nursing infants have not been reported. Distribution of antithrombin III into breast milk is highly unlikely because of antithrombin III's large molecule size.

**Pediatrics**

Appropriate studies on the relationship of age to the effects of antithrombin III have not been performed in the pediatric population. However, the medication has been administered to a limited number of neonates and children.

Because hereditary antithrombin III deficiency is transmitted in an autosomal-dominant manner, neonates born to a parent with hereditary antithrombin III deficiency should be tested at birth. Fatal thromboemboli have occurred in these neonates. However, even healthy, full-term neonates normally have low antithrombin III activity (compared to adults), and antithrombin III activity is even further reduced in preterm infants (especially if they are ill with respiratory distress syndrome, necrotizing enterocolitis, sepsis, or disseminated intravascular coagulation). Therefore, identification of infants at risk for thrombotic complications associated with hereditary antithrombin III deficiency may be difficult, and the advice of an expert should be sought before any prophylactic measure, including antithrombin III administration, is instituted.

**Geriatrics**

Appropriate studies on the relationship of age to the effects of antithrombin III have not been performed in the geriatric population. However, no geriatrics-specific problems have been documented to date.

**Drug interactions and/or related problems**

The following drug interactions and/or related problems have been selected on the basis of their potential clinical significance (possible mechanism in parentheses where appropriate)—not necessarily inclusive (» = major clinical significance):

Heparin

   (concurrent administration of heparin and antithrombin III increases the anticoagulant effect of both medications, and usually decreases heparin dosage requirements, because antithrombin III is the primary cofactor required for heparin to exert an anticoagulant effect; in some patients [especially patients in whom disseminated intravascular coagulation caused by multiple trauma has produced an acquired antithrombin III deficiency] concurrent use may also increase the risk of bleeding, even with very low doses of heparin)

   (heparin decreases the half-life of antithrombin III)

**Patient monitoring**

The following may be especially important in patient monitoring (other tests may be warranted in some patients, depending on condition; » = major clinical significance):

Antithrombin III activity

   (monitoring is essential as a guide to dosage requirements and patient response; for patients with hereditary antithrombin III deficiency, it is recommended that determinations be performed twice a day until the dosage requirement has stabilized, after which determinations may be performed once daily, immediately prior to a dose; however, under certain circumstances, more frequent determinations may be needed)

Note: Antithrombin III may be measured quantitatively, using immunoassays, or qualitatively, using procedures that determine functional activity (e.g., measurement of the thrombin-inhibiting or factor Xa–inhibiting ability of the blood). Functional assays are preferred because, in some forms of antithrombin III deficiency, functional antithrombin III activity may be decreased despite normal immunologic (quantitative) test results.

## Side/Adverse Effects

Note: All products derived from human blood or plasma have the potential to transmit viral diseases, including acquired immunodeficiency syndrome (AIDS) and non-A, non-B hepatitis. Plasma used for preparation of antithrombin III for injection has been tested and found nonreactive for hepatitis B surface antigen and for antibody to the human immunodeficiency virus (HIV). In addition, prior to freeze-drying, the product is heat-treated (60 °C for not less than 10 hours). These measures may not be completely effective in eliminating the risk of viral transmission, but no documented cases of hepatitis resulting from administration of antithrombin III to patients with hereditary deficiencies have been reported to date.

Diuretic and vasodilatory effects leading to a fall in blood pressure were reported in 2 of 65 patients receiving antithrombin III for an acquired deficiency caused by severe disseminated intravascular coagulation. In addition, dyspnea and increased blood pressure occurred in one patient who received the medication at a too-rapid rate of administration (1500 IU in 5 minutes).

Chest pain or tightness, fever, hematoma, hives, oozing, and shortness of breath were also reported in a small number of patients. However, it was not clearly indicated that the symptoms were caused by the medication and were not related to the disease states of the patients. If these side/adverse effects should occur secondary to the infusion of antithrombin III, they may be abated by slowing or temporarily discontinuing the infusion.

## General Dosing Information

The potency of antithrombin III is expressed in international units (IU) and is determined using a standard calibrated against a World Health Organization (WHO) antithrombin III reference standard. One IU is equivalent to the quantity of endogenous antithrombin III present in 1 mL of normal human plasma.

## Parenteral Dosage Forms

### ANTITHROMBIN III (HUMAN) FOR INJECTION

**Usual adult and adolescent dose**

Thromboembolism associated with hereditary antithrombin III deficiency—

Intravenous, administered at a rate of 50 to 100 IU (not to exceed 100 IU) per minute:

Initial—A sufficient quantity to increase the antithrombin III activity, determined 30 minutes after administration, to 120% of the normal activity.

Maintenance—A sufficient quantity to increase the antithrombin III activity to 80% or more of the normal activity. Maintenance doses are generally administered at twenty-four-hour intervals.

Note: Initial dosage is calculated according to the following formula, based on an anticipated 1% increase in plasma antithrombin III (ATIII) activity for each 1 IU per kg of body weight:

Dose = [desired ATIII activity (as % of normal) − baseline ATIII activity (as % of normal)] × body weight (in kg) ÷ 1%.

Maintenance dosage is also calculated using the formula shown above for calculating initial dosage, but the actual increase in ATIII activity (in %) produced by 1 IU per kg of body weight, determined 30 minutes after administration of the initial dose, should be substituted for the 1% (the divisor) in the formula.

Increasing the antithrombin III activity to 120% (rather than 100%) of the normal value with the initial dose prolongs the interval before a second dose is required. However, dosage requirements may be increased in some patients. More frequent monitoring of antithrombin III activity may be required, with the dosage and frequency of administration being adjusted accordingly.

The duration of therapy depends on the indication for antithrombin III administration, the patient's condition and history, and the judgment of the physician. Treatment is usually continued for 2 to 8 days. In some circumstances (e.g., during pregnancy), more prolonged administration may be needed. Also, when treatment is given in conjunction with surgery or during prolonged immobilization, it is recommended that antithrombin III therapy be continued until the patient is fully mobilized.

**Usual pediatric dose**
See *Usual adult and adolescent dose.* The target percentage of normal human antithrombin III activity to be achieved for pediatric patients, is the same as for other patients.

**Size(s) usually available**
U.S.—
500 IU (Rx) [*ATnativ* (human albumin 100 mg; sodium chloride 90 mg); *Thrombate III* (sodium chloride 110 to 210 mEq per L; alanine 0.075 to 0.125M; heparin ≤0.004 USP units per IU antithrombin III)].
1000 IU (Rx) [*Thrombate III* (sodium chloride 110 to 210 mEq per L; alanine 0.075 to 0.125M; heparin ≤0.004 USP units per IU antithrombin III)].
Canada—
Not commercially available.

**Packaging and storage**
Store at 2 to 8 °C (36 and 46 °F), unless otherwise specified by manufacturer.

**Preparation of dosage form**
Antithrombin III for injection is reconstituted using 10 mL of sterile water for injection (provided by the manufacturer) or an alternate solution,

such as 0.9% sodium chloride injection or 5% dextrose injection. Do not shake the vial while reconstituting. The solution should then be brought to room temperature before administration. If desired, the reconstituted injection may be further diluted, using the same diluent.
Caution—Use of diluents containing benzyl alcohol is not recommended for preparation of medications for use in neonates. A fatal toxic syndrome consisting of metabolic acidosis, CNS depression, respiratory problems, renal failure, hypotension, and possibly seizures and intracranial hemorrhages has been associated with this use.

**Stability**
After reconstitution, the solution must be used within 3 hours.
Because antithrombin III for injection contains no preservative, any unused solution should be discarded.

**Selected Bibliography**

Vinazzer H. Clinical use of antithrombin III concentrates. Vox Sang 1987; 53: 193-8.
Rosenberg RD, editor. Role of antithrombin III in coagulation disorders: state-of-the-art review. Am J Med 1989; 87 (3B Suppl): 1S-67S.

Revised: 02/23/94

---

# ANTITHYROID AGENTS   Systemic

This monograph includes information on the following: Methimazole; Propylthiouracil.

INN:
Methimazole—Thiamazole

VA CLASSIFICATION (Primary): HS852

Note: For a listing of dosage forms and brand names by country availability, see *Dosage Forms* section(s). For a listing of brand names for the articles in this monograph, refer to the General Index.

## Category
Antihyperthyroid agent.

## Indications

**Accepted**
Hyperthyroidism (treatment)—Methimazole and propylthiouracil are indicated in the treatment of hyperthyroidism, including prior to surgery or radiotherapy, and as adjuncts in the treatment of thyrotoxicosis or thyroid storm. Propylthiouracil may be preferred over methimazole for use in thyroid storm, since propylthiouracil inhibits peripheral conversion of thyroxine [T₄] to triiodothyronine [T₃].

Further studies are needed to establish the safety and efficacy of using propylthiouracil for the treatment of alcoholic liver disease.

**Unaccepted**
Efficacy of antithyroid medications has been inconsistent in the treatment of angina pectoris. These agents are probably useful for this purpose only in hyperthyroid patients with angina pectoris.

Antithyroid medications are not effective in the treatment of thyrotoxicosis resulting from exogenous thyroid hormone overdosage.

## Pharmacology/Pharmacokinetics

**Physicochemical characteristics**
Chemical group—
Methimazole and propylthiouracil are thioamide derivatives.
Molecular weight—
Methimazole: 114.16.
Propylthiouracil: 170.23.
pKa—
Propylthiouracil: 7.8.

**Mechanism of action/Effect**
Inhibit synthesis of thyroid hormone within the thyroid gland by serving as substrates for thyroid peroxidase, which catalyzes the incorporation of oxidized iodide into tyrosine residues in thyroglobulin molecules and couples iodotyrosines. This diverts iodine from the synthesis of thyroid hormones. Antithyroid agents do not interfere with the actions of exogenous thyroid hormone or inhibit the release of thyroid hormones. Therefore, stores of thyroid hormones must be depleted before

clinical effects will be apparent. Antithyroid agents may also have moderating effects on the underlying immunologic abnormalities in hyperthyroidism due to Graves' disease (toxic diffuse goiter), but evidence on this point reported to date is inconclusive.
Propylthiouracil—
Additionally, inhibits peripheral conversion of T₄ to T₃, which may theoretically make it more effective in the treatment of thyroid storm.

**Absorption**
Rapid.
Methimazole—
Oral: Bioavailability 93%. Absorption may be unpredictably affected by food.
Rectal: In one study in healthy subjects, absorption of extemporaneously compounded 60-mg rectal suppositories was similar to that of oral tablets.
Propylthiouracil—
Oral: Bioavailability 65 to 75%.
Rectal: In one study in healthy subjects, absorption of extemporaneously compounded 100-mg rectal suppositories was slower and less extensive than that of oral tablets ($AUC_{0\ to\ 8h}$: 23.77 ± 1.24 mcg•hr/mL [oral], 6.16 ± 2.07 mcg•hr/mL [rectal]).

**Distribution**
Both methimazole and propylthiouracil are actively concentrated by the thyroid.
Methimazole—Volume of distribution is approximately 0.6 liter per kilogram (L/kg) of body weight.
Propylthiouracil—Volume of distribution is approximately 0.4 L/kg of body weight.

**Protein binding**
Methimazole—Not significant.
Propylthiouracil—High (80%), primarily to albumin.

**Biotransformation**
Primarily hepatic; active metabolites of either compound have not been demonstrated.
Propylthiouracil—Primarily undergoes glucuronidation. Approximately 33% of an orally administered dose is metabolized by a first-pass effect.

**Half-life**
Methimazole—5 to 6 hours.
Propylthiouracil—1 to 2 hours.

**Onset of action**
Methimazole—In one study, substantial reductions in mean serum thyroxine and triiodothyronine concentrations were seen after 5 days of methimazole therapy at 40 mg per day.

## Time to peak serum concentration
Methimazole—
Oral/Rectal:
Approximately 30 to 60 minutes (occurrence of peak blood concentrations, after administration of a 60-mg rectal suppository or a 60-mg oral dose to healthy subjects).

Propylthiouracil—
Oral:
1.99 ± 0.26 hours (after administration of a 100-mg dose to healthy subjects).
Rectal:
Solution—Approximately 3 hours (after administration of a 400-mg rectal dose of propylthiouracil in an aqueous solution of sodium phosphates to a patient with thyroid storm).
Suppository—4.72 ± 0.96 hours (after administration of a 100-mg suppository to healthy subjects).

## Peak serum concentration
Methimazole—
Oral:
1.184 ± 0.12 mcg/mL (blood concentrations, after administration of a 60-mg dose to healthy subjects).
Rectal:
1.163 ± 0.15 mcg/mL (blood concentrations, after administration of a 60-mg suppository to healthy subjects).

Propylthiouracil—
Oral:
7.12 ± 0.48 mcg/mL (after administration of a 100-mg dose to healthy subjects).
Rectal:
Solution—3.1 mcg/mL (approximate, after administration of a 400-mg rectal dose of propylthiouracil in an aqueous solution of sodium phosphates to a patient with thyroid storm).
Suppository—1.2 ± 0.31 mcg/mL (after administration of a 100-mg rectal suppository to healthy subjects).

## Time to peak effect
Methimazole—7 weeks (average) to normalize serum $T_3$ and $T_4$ concentrations with use of 30 mg per day. In one study, 4 weeks (approximate) to normalize serum $T_3$ and $T_4$ concentrations with use of 40 mg per day.

Propylthiouracil—17 weeks (average) to normalize serum $T_3$ and $T_4$ concentrations with use of 300 mg per day.

## Elimination
Methimazole—
Less than 10% is excreted in the urine unchanged. Total body clearance is approximately 10 L per hour.

Propylthiouracil—
Less than 1% is excreted in the urine unchanged. Total body clearance is approximately 7 L per hour.
In dialysis: Elimination and pharmacokinetics are not significantly altered in hemodialysis. In one patient undergoing hemodialysis, 5% of a 200-mg oral dose was removed by 3 hours of hemodialysis; elimination rate was not significantly altered. Peak serum concentration was decreased (from 7.9 to 4.9 mcg/mL), although it remained within an approximate therapeutic range.

# Precautions to Consider

## Cross-sensitivity and/or related problems
Cross-sensitivity may occur frequently (in about 50% of patients) between antithyroid thioamide medications.

If a persistent or severe reaction necessitates withdrawal of one agent, therapy may be switched to the other, although there is a risk of cross-reactivity occurring. However, if agranulocytosis, thrombocytopenia, or hepatic dysfunction occurs, substitution with another thioamide is not recommended.

## Carcinogenicity/Mutagenicity
Methimazole—Studies have not been done in either animals or humans.

Propylthiouracil—Thyroid hyperplasia and carcinoma have occurred in laboratory animals treated with propylthiouracil for longer than 1 year. Similar effects are seen with continuous thyroid suppression with various antithyroid agents, dietary iodine deficiency, subtotal thyroidectomy, and ectopic thyrotropin-secreting pituitary tumors. Pituitary adenomas have also occurred.

## Pregnancy/Reproduction
Pregnancy—Methimazole and propylthiouracil cross the placenta and can cause fetal hypothyroidism and goiter. However, the possible risks of adverse effects due to antithyroid agents must be weighed against the risks of possible adverse effects due to continuing hyperthyroidism during pregnancy. Propylthiouracil is considered by some clinicians as the agent of choice for women who require antithyroid medications

during pregnancy. Propylthiouracil crosses the placenta less readily than methimazole, and the use of methimazole during pregnancy has been associated with several cases of scalp defects (aplasia cutis) in the infant. The reduced placental transfer of propylthiouracil is presumably due to its high level of serum protein binding and high level of ionization at a pH of 7.4.

The actual risk of fetal death, goiter, hypothyroidism, or certain congenital abnormalities with administration of antithyroid agents appears to be low, especially if maternal doses are low (for example, less than 100 to 150 mg of propylthiouracil or an equivalent dose of methimazole per day). Fetal goiters induced by antithyroid agents are generally not as large as iodide-induced fetal goiters and have not usually been reported to be obstructive. Fetal hypothyroidism and goiter usually occur when the antithyroid agents are used close to term, since the fetal thyroid does not begin to produce thyroid hormones until the 11th or 12th week of gestation. In long-term follow-up of some children exposed in utero to maternal therapeutic doses of propylthiouracil, gross abnormalities in development or diminished intellectual performance have not been observed.

It is recommended that antithyroid medication be prescribed at the lowest effective dose to maintain maternal thyroid function within the upper-normal range for normal pregnant women, especially during the last trimester, to reduce the risk of fetal and maternal hypothyroidism and goiter. Thyroid hyperfunction may diminish as pregnancy progresses, allowing a reduction in antithyroid dosage and, in some cases, withdrawal of antithyroid therapy 2 to 3 months before delivery. However, thyroid function may vary and dosing should be based on frequent and careful monitoring. Hyperthyroidism may recur soon after delivery. Because radioactive iodine is absolutely contraindicated during pregnancy, thyroidectomy may be very rarely required in refractory cases of hyperthyroidism or in patients who are noncompliant with the use of antithyroid medications.

Thyroid hormones are minimally transferred across the placenta and therefore have little protective effect on the fetus. They may also mask signs of remission of hyperthyroidism, resulting in fetal and maternal exposure to unnecessarily high doses of antithyroid agents. For these reasons, adjunctive treatment with thyroid hormones is not recommended during pregnancy.

Several case reports have been published in which antithyroid agents were given to a euthyroid mother of a hyperthyroid fetus. Fetal heart rate monitoring and ultrasound examinations were used to monitor fetal response. Fetal tachycardia was reduced and the infants were euthyroid at delivery. However, further data are needed regarding this form of therapy for fetal hyperthyroidism.

FDA Pregnancy Category D.

## Breast-feeding
Small amounts of methimazole and propylthiouracil are distributed into breast milk. However, the use of average maintenance doses of these agents is not generally considered an absolute contraindication to breast-feeding, although serial monitoring of thyroid function (by measurement of serum thyrotropin and thyroxine concentrations) of the infant is advisable. Propylthiouracil is generally preferred over methimazole during lactation because methimazole is distributed into breast milk more readily (approximately ten-fold), presumably due to its insignificant level of protein binding and ionization. Maternal serum and breast milk concentrations of methimazole are nearly equal. However, some clinicians feel that small doses of methimazole (e.g., ≤ 10–15 mg per day) do not pose a significant risk to the infant if thyroid function is monitored frequently.

There is a theoretical risk of causing hypothyroidism and/or agranulocytosis in the infant with high maternal doses of antithyroid agents. Termination of breast-feeding may be necessary prior to initiation of high-dose therapy.

## Pediatrics
Antithyroid agents are frequently used to treat hyperthyroidism in children. Children seem to respond to antithyroid agents as well as do adults. Pharmacokinetic studies conducted in children also did not reveal any differences unique to the pediatric population.

Caution is necessary in interpreting results of thyroid function tests in neonates, because serum concentrations of thyroid hormones are higher at birth than those of healthy children or adults and begin to fall to normal in the first week of life.

## Adolescents
Antithyroid agents are frequently used to treat hyperthyroidism in adolescents. Adolescents seem to respond to antithyroid agents as well as do adults. Pharmacokinetic studies conducted in adolescents did not reveal any differences unique to the adolescent population.

## Geriatrics

One study showed that agranulocytosis is more likely to occur in patients older than 40 years of age or in patients taking more than 40 mg of methimazole per day.

In one pharmacokinetic study, no significant differences were found for geriatric patients in certain pharmacokinetic parameters (e.g., Vd, Vd beta, Vd at steady state, area under the curve, and clearance). Rate of absorption was decreased (approximately one-third that of younger subjects) though there are no data regarding the clinical significance of this finding.

Geriatric patients with severe cardiac disease should be given antithyroid agents and/or beta-adrenergic blocking agents, such as propranolol, for 4 to 6 weeks prior to treatment with radioiodine to help reduce possible exacerbation of heart disease by radiation-induced thyroiditis. Antithyroid drugs must be discontinued at least 3 to 4 days prior to radioiodine treatment and should not be readministered until 1 week after treatment. However, a beta-adrenergic blocking agent may be used throughout the treatment period if needed.

## Dental

The bone marrow depressant effects of antithyroid agents may result in an increased incidence of microbial infection, delayed healing, and gingival bleeding. If leukopenia or thrombocytopenia occurs, dental work should be deferred until blood counts have returned to normal, and patients should be instructed in proper oral hygiene, including caution in use of regular toothbrushes, dental floss, and toothpicks.

## Drug interactions and/or related problems

The following drug interactions and/or related problems have been selected on the basis of their potential clinical significance (possible mechanism in parentheses where appropriate)—not necessarily inclusive (» = major clinical significance):

Note: Combinations containing any of the following medications, depending on the amount present, may also interact with this medication.

Aminophylline or
Oxtriphylline or
Theophylline
    (hyperthyroid patients have exhibited increased metabolic clearance of aminophylline and theophylline, which returned to normal as the patients became euthyroid; decreased dose of aminophylline, oxtriphylline, or theophylline may be necessary as patients become euthyroid)

» Amiodarone or
» Iodinated glycerol or
» Iodine or
» Potassium iodide
    (iodide or iodine excess may decrease response to antithyroid agents, requiring an increase in dosage or longer duration of therapy with antithyroid agents; amiodarone contains 37% iodine by weight, and therefore its use significantly increases iodine intake; iodine deficiency may increase response to antithyroid agents, requiring a decrease in dosage or shorter duration of therapy with antithyroid agents)

» Anticoagulants, coumarin- or indandione-derivative
    (as thyroid and metabolic status of patient decreases toward normal, response to oral anticoagulants may decrease; however, if thioamide-induced hypoprothrombinemia occurs, anticoagulant effect may be enhanced; adjustment of oral anticoagulant dosage on the basis of prothrombin time is recommended)

» Digitalis glycosides
    (serum concentrations of digoxin and digitoxin have been reported to increase as the thyroid and metabolic status of patients taking antithyroid agents decreased; reduction in dosage of any digitalis glycoside may be necessary as patients become euthyroid)

» Sodium iodide I 131
    (antithyroid agents may decrease thyroidal uptake of I 131; a rebound increase in uptake may occur up to 5 days after sudden withdrawal of the antithyroid agent)

## Laboratory value alterations

The following have been selected on the basis of their potential clinical significance (possible effect in parentheses where appropriate)—not necessarily inclusive (» = major clinical significance):

With diagnostic test results
» Sodium iodide I 123 or
» Sodium iodide I 131 or
» Sodium pertechnetate Tc 99m
    (antithyroid agents may decrease thyroidal uptake of I 123, I 131, or pertechnetate; withdrawal of the antithyroid agent 5 days or more before radioactive iodine uptake tests is necessary to prevent interference)

With physiology/laboratory test values
    Alanine aminotransferase (ALT [SGPT]), serum concentrations and
    Alkaline phosphatase, serum concentrations and
    Aspartate aminotransferase (AST [SGOT]), serum concentrations and
    Bilirubin, serum concentrations and
    Lactate dehydrogenase (LDH), serum concentrations and
    Prothrombin time (PT)
        (may be increased; may indicate hepatotoxicity and be associated with splenomegaly)

## Medical considerations/Contraindications

The medical considerations/contraindications included here have been selected on the basis of their potential clinical significance (reasons given in parentheses where appropriate)—not necessarily inclusive (» = major clinical significance).

*Except under special circumstances, this medication should not be used when the following medical problem exists:*

» Severe adverse reaction or severe allergic reaction to either methimazole or propylthiouracil, or history of

*Risk-benefit should be considered when the following medical problem exists:*

» Hepatic function impairment
    (elimination half-life may be prolonged, in proportion to the degree of hepatic insufficiency)

## Patient monitoring

The following may be especially important in patient monitoring (other tests may be warranted in some patients, depending on condition; » = major clinical significance):

Leukocyte count, total and differential
    (determinations recommended prior to initiation of treatment and if infection occurs)

» Free thyroxine ($T_4$), by direct assay and/or
» Thyrotropin (TSH) by sensitive radioimmunoassay and/or

Total thyroxine ($T_4$), either by competitive protein-binding assay or by radioimmunoassay and/or

Total triiodothyronine ($T_3$) by radioimmunoassay
    (determination of serum concentrations is recommended prior to initiation of therapy, at monthly intervals during initial therapy, then every 2 to 3 months; some clinicians recommend at least yearly follow-up for life in patients successfully treated with antithyroid medications; in patients treated with these agents who do not undergo thyroid ablation with sodium iodide I 131 or surgery, the risk of subsequent hypothyroidism is related to immunogenic thyroid disease itself, and not the medication; recurrence of hyperthyroidism is common)

# Side/Adverse Effects

Note: Incidence of most adverse reactions is dose-related; most side effects occur within the first 4 to 8 weeks.

The following side/adverse effects have been selected on the basis of their potential clinical significance (possible signs and symptoms in parentheses where appropriate)—not necessarily inclusive:

## Those indicating need for medical attention

Incidence more frequent
    *Fever, mild and transient; leukopenia* (continuing or severe fever or chills, throat infection, cough, mouth sores, or hoarseness)—usually asymptomatic; *skin rash or itching*

    Note: Mild *leukopenias* occur more frequently in patients (12% of adults and 25% of children) treated with antithyroid agents. Also, approximately 10% of untreated hyperthyroid patients have leukocyte levels below 4000 per cubic millimeter.

        Incidence of *skin rash or itching* is 3 to 5%. Usually consists of maculopapular eruptions. An allergic reaction occurs less frequently and may disappear spontaneously with continued treatment; appears to be dose-related. Skin rash may also be a sign of vasculitis.

Incidence less frequent
    *Agranulocytosis* (continuing or severe fever or chills, throat infection, cough, mouth sores, or hoarseness); *arthralgias or arthritis or vasculitis* (pain, swelling, or redness in joints)—usually with propylthiouracil; *lupus-like syndrome* (fever or chills; general feeling of discomfort or illness or weakness)—usually with propylthiouracil; *peripheral neuropathy* (numbness or tingling of fingers, toes, or face)

    Note: *Agranulocytosis* (incidence 0.4%) usually occurs during the first 3 months of therapy. May occur less predictably and with lower doses of propylthiouracil. Deaths due to agranulocytosis have been reported.

Incidence rare

> *Aplastic anemia* (continuing or severe fever or chills, throat infection, cough, mouth sores, or hoarseness); *hypoprothrombinemia (for propylthiouracil); or thrombocytopenia* (rarely, increase in bleeding or bruising; black, tarry stools; blood in urine or stools; pinpoint red spots on skin)—usually asymptomatic; *cholestatic jaundice* (yellow eyes or skin)—for methimazole; *hepatic necrosis* (yellow eyes or skin)—primarily with propylthiouracil; *interstitial pneumonitis* (cough or shortness of breath)—with propylthiouracil; *lymphadenopathy* (swollen lymph nodes); *sialadenopathy* (swollen salivary glands); *nephritis (for methimazole) or renal vasculitis (usually with propylthiouracil)* (backache; increase or decrease in urination; swelling of feet or lower legs)

> Note: *Jaundice* may persist for up to 10 weeks after drug discontinuance. Fatal *hepatic necrosis* has been reported with both agents.

**Those indicating need for medical attention only if they continue or are bothersome**
Incidence less frequent

> *Dizziness; loss of taste*—for methimazole; *nausea or vomiting; stomach pain*

## Overdose

For more information on the management of overdose or unintentional ingestion, **contact a Poison Control Center** (see *Poison Control Center Listing*).

**Clinical effects of overdose (hypothyroidism)**
The following effects have been selected on the basis of their potential clinical significance (possible signs and symptoms in parentheses where appropriate)—not necessarily inclusive:

> *Changes in menstrual periods; coldness; constipation; dry, puffy skin; goiter* (swelling in the front of the neck); *headache; listlessness or sleepiness; muscle aches; nausea or vomiting, severe; unusual tiredness or weakness; weight gain, unusual*

> Note: *Hypothyroidism* may be an unavoidable long-term sequela to hyperthyroidism.

## Patient Consultation

As an aid to patient consultation, refer to *Advice for the Patient, Antithyroid Agents (Systemic)*.

In providing consultation, consider emphasizing the following selected information (» = major clinical significance):

**Before using this medication**
» Conditions affecting use, especially:
   Allergies to any thioamide
   Pregnancy—May be used but careful monitoring is necessary
   Breast-feeding—Distributed into breast milk, although propylthiouracil is distributed in much lesser amounts; may continue breast-feeding with low doses and monitoring of infant
   Other medications, especially iodides, coumarin- or indandione-derivative anticoagulants, amiodarone, digitalis glycosides, or radioiodide
   Other medical problems, especially hepatic function impairment

**Proper use of this medication**
» Importance of not taking more or less medication than the amount prescribed
» Importance of not missing doses and, if taking more than one dose per day, of taking at evenly spaced intervals
   Taking methimazole at same time in relation to meals every day
» Proper dosing
   Missed dose: Taking as soon as possible; taking both doses together if almost time for next dose; checking with physician if more than one dose is missed
» Proper storage

**Precautions while using this medication**
» Importance of close monitoring by the physician
» Checking with physician before discontinuing medication
» Caution if any kind of surgery (including dental surgery) or emergency treatment is required, because of the risk of thyroid storm
» Checking with physician immediately if injury, infection, or other illness occurs, because of the risk of thyroid storm
   Caution if any laboratory tests required; possible interference with test results

**Side/adverse effects**
   Signs of potential side effects, especially fever, skin rash or itching, bone marrow depression, hepatic dysfunction, lupus-like syndrome, arthralgias, arthritis, nephritis (for methimazole), vasculitis,

pneumonitis, lymphadenopathy, sialadenopathy, hypoprothrombinemia (for propylthiouracil), or peripheral neuropathy

## General Dosing Information

Dosage must be adjusted to meet the individual requirements of each patient, on the basis of clinical response and results of thyroid function tests.

In some patients, once- or twice-a-day therapy may be associated with a decreased incidence of side effects and improved compliance, although divided daily doses may be more effective. If divided daily doses are given, they should be administered at evenly spaced intervals throughout the day. Methimazole has a longer duration of action and therefore may frequently be more effective than propylthiouracil in once-daily dosing.

Confirmation of remission may be by sensitive TSH assay, trial withdrawal of the medication, protirelin test, thyroid suppression test, or thyroid-stimulating immunogloglubin (TSI) titer.

Duration of treatment necessary to produce a prolonged remission varies from 6 months to several years, with an average duration of 1 to 2 years. Control of hyperthyroidism with medication is sometimes followed by a spontaneous remission. Premature withdrawal may result in exacerbation of hyperthyroidism, although some clinicians feel that treatment may be withdrawn as soon as a euthyroid state is obtained (usually within 4 to 5 months), with no problems of rebound.

Iodide is usually added to thioamide antithyroid therapy for 7 to 10 days prior to surgery to reduce the vascularity of the thyroid gland, thereby decreasing subsequent blood loss during surgery.

If an antithyroid agent is being used in severely hyperthyroid patients to improve their thyroid state prior to radioactive iodine therapy, the antithyroid medication must be discontinued 2 to 4 days before treatment to prevent impairment of radioactive iodine uptake. Antithyroid treatment may be resumed, if desired, 3 to 7 days after radioactive iodine treatment to hasten return to euthyroidism, until effects of the iodine are apparent.

**Diet/Nutrition**
Food may inconsistently alter the bioavailability of methimazole. It is recommended that methimazole be taken at the same time in relation to meals every day.

**For treatment of adverse effects**
Reduction in dosage or temporary withdrawal of antithyroid medication may be recommended if signs and symptoms of hypothyroidism occur. Some clinicians recommend adjunctive thyroid therapy (except during pregnancy) to prevent development of hypothyroidism. However, hypothyroidism may be an unavoidable long-term sequela to hyperthyroidism.

It is recommended that antithyroid therapy be discontinued promptly and supportive measures initiated if signs and symptoms of agranulocytosis, aplastic anemia, hepatic dysfunction, lupus-like syndrome, severe skin rash, swelling of cervical lymph nodes, or vasculitis occur. If laboratory examinations show only a mild leukopenia, periodic blood count monitoring without withdrawal or reduction in dosage may be sufficient. Mild reactions may not require withdrawal, although they may precede more serious reactions. Leukocyte production usually returns to normal within 1 to 2 weeks after withdrawal.

---

### METHIMAZOLE

## Summary of Differences

General dosing information: May be more suitable for once-daily administration.

## Oral Dosage Forms

**METHIMAZOLE TABLETS USP**

**Usual adult and adolescent dose**
Hyperthyroidism—
   Initial:
      Mild hyperthyroidism—Oral, 15 mg a day as one daily dose or as two divided daily doses for six to eight weeks until the patient becomes euthyroid.
      Moderately severe hyperthyroidism—Oral, 30 to 40 mg a day as one daily dose or as two divided daily doses for six to eight weeks until the patient becomes euthyroid.
      Severe hyperthyroidism—Oral, 60 mg a day as one daily dose or as two divided daily doses for six to eight weeks until the patient becomes euthyroid.

Maintenance:
>    Oral, 5 to 30 mg a day in one daily dose or as two divided daily doses.

Thyrotoxic crisis:
>    Oral, 15 to 20 mg every four hours during the first day, as an adjunct to other measures.

### Usual pediatric dose
Hyperthyroidism—
>    Initial: Oral, 400 mcg (0.4 mg) per kg of body weight a day as one daily dose or as two divided daily doses.
>    Maintenance: Oral, 200 mcg (0.2 mg) per kg of body weight a day as one daily dose or as two divided daily doses.

### Strength(s) usually available
U.S.—
>    5 mg (Rx) [*Tapazole* (scored; lactose)].
>    10 mg (Rx) [*Tapazole* (scored; lactose)].

Canada—
>    5 mg (Rx) [*Tapazole* (scored)].

### Packaging and storage
Store below 40 °C (104 °F), preferably between 15 and 30 °C (59 and 86 °F), unless otherwise specified by manufacturer. Store in a well-closed, light-resistant container.

### Auxiliary labeling
• Take at the same time in relation to meals every day.

## Rectal Dosage Forms
### METHIMAZOLE SUPPOSITORIES

### Usual adult and adolescent dose
Hyperthyroidism—
>    Initial: Thyrotoxic crisis—Rectal, 15 to 20 mg every four hours during the first day, as an adjunct to other measures, with the dosage being adjusted according to patient response.

### Usual pediatric dose
Hyperthyroidism—
>    Initial: Thyrotoxic crisis—Rectal, 400 mcg (0.4 mg) per kg of body weight a day as one daily dose or as two divided daily doses.

### Strength(s) usually available
U.S.—
>    Not commercially available. Compounding required for prescription.

Canada—
>    Not commercially available. Compounding required for prescription.

### Packaging and storage
Store between 2 and 8 °C (36 and 46 °F). Store in a well-closed container. Protect from freezing.

### Preparation of dosage form
A formulation that has been used for the extemporaneous compounding of methimazole suppositories is as follows:
• 1200 mg methimazole dissolved in 12 mL of distilled water
• 2 drops of Span 80
• Cocoa butter (warmed to 37 °C [98.6 °F]) of sufficient quantity to make 20 suppositories containing 60 mg methimazole each.

### Auxiliary labeling
• Refrigerate.
• For rectal use only.

### Note
Use of methimazole suppositories is generally reserved for treatment of thyrotoxic emergencies, in patients who are unable to tolerate oral medications. The efficacy of chronic rectal dosing with extemporaneously compounded formulations has not been established.

---

## *PROPYLTHIOURACIL*

## Summary of Differences

Precautions:
>    Pregnancy—May be preferred to methimazole, due to lower rate of placental transfer.
>    Breast-feeding—May be preferred to methimazole, due to a lower rate of distribution into breast milk.

Side/adverse effects:
>    Agranulocytosis may be less predictable, because it is usually not dose-related.

## Oral Dosage Forms
### PROPYLTHIOURACIL TABLETS USP

### Usual adult and adolescent dose
Hyperthyroidism—
>    Initial:
>        Oral, 300 to 900 mg a day as one to four divided daily doses until the patient becomes euthyroid.
>        Note: Patients with severe hyperthyroidism may occasionally require up to 1.2 grams a day.
>    Maintenance:
>        Oral, 50 to 600 mg a day as one to four divided daily doses.

Thyrotoxic crisis:
>        Oral, 200 to 400 mg every four hours during the first day, as an adjunct to other measures, the dosage then being decreased as the crisis subsides.

### Usual pediatric dose
Hyperthyroidism—
>    Initial:
>        Children 6 to 10 years of age—Oral, 50 to 150 mg a day as one to four divided daily doses.
>        Children 10 years of age and over—Oral, 50 to 300 mg a day as one to four divided daily doses.
>    Maintenance:
>        Oral, determined by response.
>    Neonatal thyrotoxicosis:
>        Oral, 10 mg per kg of body weight a day in divided daily doses.

### Strength(s) usually available
U.S.—
>    50 mg (Rx) [GENERIC].

Canada—
>    50 mg (Rx) [*Propyl-Thyracil* (scored)].
>    100 mg (Rx) [*Propyl-Thyracil* (scored)].

### Packaging and storage
Store below 40 °C (104 °F), preferably between 15 and 30 °C (59 and 86 °F), unless otherwise specified by manufacturer. Store in a well-closed container.

### Auxiliary labeling
• Take at the same time in relation to meals every day.

## Rectal Dosage Forms
### PROPYLTHIOURACIL ENEMA

### Usual adult and adolescent dose
Hyperthyroidism—
>    Initial: Thyrotoxic crisis—Rectal, 200 to 400 mg every four hours during the first day, as an adjunct to other measures, with the dosage being adjusted according to patient response.

### Usual pediatric dose
Hyperthyroidism—Initial: Thyrotoxic crisis:
>    Children 6 to 10 years of age: Rectal, 50 to 150 mg a day as one to four divided daily doses, with the dosage being adjusted according to patient response.
>    Children 10 years of age and over: Rectal, 50 to 300 mg a day as one to four divided daily doses, with the dosage being adjusted according to patient response.
>    Neonatal thyrotoxicosis: Rectal, 10 mg per kg of body weight a day in divided daily doses, with the dosage being adjusted according to patient response.

### Strength(s) usually available
U.S.—
>    Not commercially available. Compounding required for prescription.

Canada—
>    Not commercially available. Compounding required for prescription.

### Packaging and storage
Store between 2 and 8 °C (36 and 46 °F). Store in a well-closed container. Protect from freezing.

### Preparation of dosage form
A formulation that has been used for the extemporaneous compounding of propylthiouracil enemas is as follows:
• 400 mg propylthiouracil (8-50 mg tablets)
• 60 mL aqueous sodium phosphates solution (*Fleet's Phospho-Soda*, pH 4.4 to 5.4).

### Auxiliary labeling
• For rectal use only.

**Note**

Use of propylthiouracil enema is generally reserved for treatment of thyrotoxic emergencies, in patients who are unable to tolerate oral medications. The efficacy of chronic rectal dosing with extemporaneously compounded formulations has not been established.

## PROPYLTHIOURACIL SUPPOSITORIES

**Usual adult and adolescent dose**

Hyperthyroidism—

Initial: Thyrotoxic crisis—Rectal, 200 to 400 mg every four hours during the first day, as an adjunct to other measures, with the dosage being adjusted according to patient response.

**Usual pediatric dose**

Hyperthyroidism—Initial: Thyrotoxic crisis—

Children 6 to 10 years of age: Rectal, 50 to 150 mg a day as one to four divided daily doses, with the dosage being adjusted according to patient response.

Children 10 years of age and over: Rectal, 50 to 300 mg a day as one to four divided daily doses, with the dosage being adjusted according to patient response.

Neonatal thyrotoxicosis: Rectal, 10 mg per kg of body weight a day in divided daily doses, with the dosage being adjusted according to patient response.

**Strength(s) usually available**

U.S.—

Not commercially available. Compounding required for prescription.

Canada—

Not commercially available. Compounding required for prescription.

**Packaging and storage**

Store between 2 and 8 °C (36 and 46 °F). Store in a well-closed container. Protect from freezing.

**Preparation of dosage form**

A formulation that has been used for the extemporaneous compounding of propylthiouracil suppositories is as follows:

• 400 mg propylthiouracil (8-50 mg tablets) in

• Hardfat (Witepsol H15), of sufficient quantity to make 4 suppositories containing 100 mg each.

**Auxiliary labeling**

• For rectal use only.

**Note**

Use of propylthiouracil suppositories is generally reserved for treatment of thyrotoxic emergencies, in patients who are unable to tolerate oral medications. The efficacy of chronic rectal dosing with extemporaneously compounded formulations has not been established.

## Selected Bibliography

Cooper DS. Antithyroid drugs. N Engl J Med 1984; 311 (21): 1353-62.
Cooper DS. Which antithyroid drug? Am J Med 1986; 80 (6): 1165-8.
Stockigt JR, Topliss DJ. Hyperthyroidism: current drug therapy. Drugs 1989; 37: 375-81.

Revised: 04/21/92
Interim revision: 06/03/94

---

# ANTIVENIN (CROTALIDAE) POLYVALENT    Systemic

VA CLASSIFICATION (Primary): IM300

Other commonly used names are: antivenin Crotalid serum and pit viper antivenin.

Note: For a listing of dosage forms and brand names by country availability, see *Dosage Forms* section(s). For a listing of brand names for the articles in this monograph, refer to the General Index.

## Category

Immunizing agent (passive).

## Indications

Note: If snakebite envenomation is known or suspected in a patient, it is very important that the attending physician contact a poison control center immediately, before treatment is attempted. Snake venoms are complex substances, and there may be multiple organ, system, or tissue effects. As an additional measure it is also very important to consult experts who have successfully treated snakebite poisoning. Physicians responsible for the treatment of such patients should be familiar with the signs and symptoms of crotalid envenomation and current methods of first aid and general supportive therapy for venomous snakebites.

**Accepted**

Envenomation, pit viper (treatment)—Antivenin (*Crotalidae*) polyvalent is indicated for the treatment of envenomation caused by bites of pit vipers (crotalids) native to Central, North, and South America, including rattlesnakes (*Crotalus* and *Sistrurus* species); copperhead and cottonmouth moccasins (*Agkistrodon* species, including *A. halys* of Korea and Japan); the fer-de-lance and other species of *Bothrops*; the tropical rattler (*Crotalus durissus* and similar species); the Cantil (*A. bilineatus*); and the bushmaster (*Lachesis mutus*) of Central and South America.

**Unaccepted**

Antivenin (*Crotalidae*) polyvalent is not effective against the venoms of coral snakes (family *Elapidae*) and should not be used to treat envenomation caused by the bites of these snakes.

## Pharmacology/Pharmacokinetics

**Physicochemical characteristics**

Source—Antivenin (*Crotalidae*) polyvalent is a sterile, non-pyrogenic, refined, and concentrated preparation of venom-neutralizing globulins obtained from the serum of healthy horses immunized with the venoms of Western diamond rattlesnake (*Crotalus atrox*); Eastern diamond rattlesnake (*C. adamanteus*); tropical rattlesnake, also known as Cascabel

(*C. durissus terrificus*); and fer-de-lance (*Bothrops atrox*). The antivenin is standardized by biological assay on mice, based on its ability to neutralize the lethal action of standard venoms. One dose of antivenin (*Crotalidae*) polyvalent neutralizes the venoms in not less than 180 mouse $LD_{50}$ of *C. atrox*, 1320 of *C. durissus terrificus*, and 780 of *B. atrox*.

**Mechanism of action/Effect**

Antivenin (*Crotalidae*) polyvalent specifically binds and neutralizes pit viper venom but does not reverse local injury. Early administration (ideally within 4 hours after envenomation) is necessary to prevent local and systemic injury.

**Half-life**

Mean half-life < 15 days.

**Onset of action**

Intravenous (preferred route)—Rapid.

Intramuscular—2 to 8 hours.

**Time to peak concentration**

Intravenous—2 hours or less.

Intramuscular—8 hours or longer.

## Precautions to Consider

**Pregnancy/Reproduction**

Fertility—Studies on the effects of antivenin (*Crotalidae*) polyvalent on fertility have not been done.

Pregnancy—Studies have not been done in humans. It is not known whether antivenin (*Crotalidae*) polyvalent can cause harm to the fetus when administered to a pregnant woman. However, the venom of pit vipers may precipitate spontaneous abortion. Before administering antivenin (*Crotalidae*) polyvalent to a pregnant woman, the risk of envenomation should be weighed against the risk of maternal and fetal toxicity from the antivenin.

Studies have not been done in animals.

**Breast-feeding**

Problems in humans have not been documented.

**Pediatrics**

A study shows that children have a lower incidence of adverse reactions to antivenin (*Crotalidae*) polyvalent and tolerate it better than do adults. However, children typically have more severe reactions to a given envenomation because of the greater amount of venom per body weight and may require larger doses of antivenin (*Crotalidae*) polyvalent than do adults. Pediatric doses should not be adjusted by the weight of the patient.

## Geriatrics

Appropriate studies on the relationship of age to the effects of antivenin (*Crotalidae*) polyvalent have not been performed in the geriatric population. However, no geriatrics-specific problems have been documented to date.

## Medical considerations/Contraindications

The medical considerations/contraindications included here have been selected on the basis of their potential clinical significance (reasons given in parentheses where appropriate)—not necessarily inclusive (» = major clinical significance).

*Risk-benefit should be considered when the following medical problems exist:*

» Hypersensitivity to antivenin (*Crotalidae*) polyvalent
» Hypersensitivity to horse serum
  (antivenin [*Crotalidae*] polyvalent is obtained from the serum of healthy horses immunized with the venoms of rattlesnakes; patients allergic to horse serum may be allergic to antivenin [*Crotalidae*] polyvalent; administration of antivenin [*Crotalidae*] polyvalent to these patients may result in severe systemic reactions)

## Side/Adverse Effects

Note: Antivenin (*Crotalidae*) polyvalent occasionally has caused immediate hypersensitivity reactions, such as anaphylaxis and shock. These reactions generally become evident within 30 minutes after antivenin administration; signs and symptoms of the reactions include apprehension; flushing; itching; urticaria; edema of the face, tongue, and throat; cough; dyspnea; cyanosis; vomiting; and collapse. In the event of a systemic reaction during antivenin administration, antivenin should be discontinued and appropriate treatment initiated.

The following side/adverse effects have been selected on the basis of their potential clinical significance (possible signs and symptoms in parentheses where appropriate)—not necessarily inclusive:

### Those indicating need for medical attention
Incidence more frequent
  *Anaphylactic reaction* (difficulty in breathing or swallowing; hives; itching, especially of feet or hands; reddening of skin, especially around ears; swelling of eyes, face, or inside of nose; unusual tiredness or weakness, sudden and severe); *serum sickness* (enlargement of the lymph glands; fever; generalized rash and itching; inflammation of joints)

## Patient Consultation

As an aid to patient consultation, refer to *Advice for the Patient, Antivenin, Pit Viper (Systemic)*.

In providing consultation, consider emphasizing the following selected information (» = major clinical significance):

### Before receiving this medication
» Conditions affecting use, especially:
  Hypersensitivity to antivenin (*Crotalidae*) polyvalent or horse serum

### Proper use of this medication
» Proper dosing

### Side/adverse effects
  Signs of potential side effects, especially anaphylactic reaction and serum sickness

## General Dosing Information

Note: In the management of poisonous snakebite, the following also should be considered. Cooling may predispose tissues already jeopardized by the snake venom enzymes to severe necrosis when rewarmed. Therefore, under no circumstances should the affected area be cooled, and so-called cryotherapy is contraindicated. A tourniquet should not be applied as a first-aid measure, and excisional therapy is not recommended. Fasciotomy also should not be considered unless there is objective evidence of true compartment syndrome, in which case a surgical consultation should be obtained.

Anaphylaxis may occur following antivenin (*Crotalidae*) polyvalent administration, even in individuals with no prior history of hypersensitivity to the antivenin or to horse serum. Before use of antivenin (*Crotalidae*) polyvalent, appropriate measures should be taken to detect the presence of a dangerous sensitivity. The patient's history (including any report of asthma, hay fever, urticaria, or other allergic manifestations; allergic reactions upon exposure to horses; and prior injections of horse serum) should be reviewed carefully. An intradermal skin test for serum sensitivity using normal horse serum or the antivenin and

sterile normal saline (0.9% sodium chloride injection) should be performed under close medical supervision in every patient, regardless of clinical history, prior to administration of the antivenin. A tourniquet and epinephrine injection (1:1000) should be at hand to combat any unexpected anaphylactic or other allergic reaction.

The skin test consists of an intradermal injection of 0.02 to 0.03 mL of a 1:10 dilution of normal horse serum, or of the reconstituted antivenin (*Crotalidae*) polyvalent, in 0.9% sodium chloride injection, and an injection of 0.9% sodium chloride in the opposite extremity to serve as a control. Use of larger amounts of diluted normal horse serum or of the antivenin for the skin test increases the likelihood of false-positive reactions, and, in extremely sensitive patients, increases the risk of a systemic reaction. When the patient has a history of sensitivity to horse serum, a 1:100 or greater dilution should be used for preliminary skin testing. A positive skin test result consists of a wheal, with or without pseudopods, and surrounding erythema, and occurs within 5 to 30 minutes after the injection. In general, the shorter the interval between the injection and the beginning of the skin reaction, the greater the sensitivity.

If the patient has no history of allergy and the skin test is negative, the antivenin may be administered. If the patient has a history of allergy and the skin test is strongly positive (especially if the positive sensitivity test is accompanied by systemic allergic manifestations), administration may be dangerous. In such instances, the risk of administering the crotaline antivenin must be weighed against the risk of withholding it, keeping in mind that severe envenomation can be fatal. If the patient does not have a history of allergy and the skin test is mildly or questionably positive, desensitization may be attempted to reduce the risk of a severe immediate systemic reaction. A negative allergic history and the absence of reaction to the skin test do not rule out the possibility of an immediate reaction to the antivenin.

The procedure of desensitization consists of subcutaneous injections of 0.1, 0.2, and 0.5 mL of a 1:100 dilution of antivenin (*Crotalidae*) polyvalent at 15-minute intervals; this process is repeated using the same amounts of a 1:10 dilution and then with undiluted antivenin. If there is any reaction after any of the injections, a tourniquet should be applied proximal to the sites of injection and epinephrine (1:1000) administered either proximal to the tourniquet or into another extremity. After 30 minutes, the procedure should be continued starting with the last dose of antivenin (*Crotalidae*) polyvalent that did not evoke a reaction. If no reaction occurs after administration of 0.5 mL of undiluted antivenin (*Crotalidae*) polyvalent, the usual therapeutic dose may be administered by intravenous infusion or, alternatively, by intramuscular injection by doubling the dose at 15-minute intervals until the entire dose has been injected.

The desensitization protocol may require 3 to 5 or more hours to administer the initial therapeutic dose. Since time is an important factor in neutralization of venom in critically ill patients, the following alternative procedure may be used for administering the antivenin in some severely envenomed patients who have positive sensitivity tests. Fifty to 100 mg of diphenhydramine hydrochloride should be given intravenously, followed by slow intravenous infusion of diluted antivenin (*Crotalidae*) polyvalent for 15 to 20 minutes, with close observation of the patient for symptoms and signs of anaphylaxis. If anaphylaxis does not occur, administration of antivenin (*Crotalidae*) polyvalent should be continued, with close observation of the patient.

For the treatment of patients who develop signs and symptoms of impending anaphylaxis in spite of desensitization or the alternative procedure, experts who have successfully treated snakebite poisoning or a poison control center should be consulted.

Pit viper (crotalid) venom varies widely between species in its systemic effects and local tissue destruction. The initial therapeutic dose of antivenin (*Crotalidae*) polyvalent is based on the severity of envenomation. An estimate of the severity of envenomation should be made as soon as possible, before any antivenin is administered, since, for example, in approximately 20% of rattlesnake bites, venom may not be injected.

The preferred route of administration is by intravenous infusion. However, antivenin (*Crotalidae*) polyvalent may be administered intramuscularly. If the intramuscular route is used, the antivenin should be administered into a large muscle mass, preferably into the gluteal area, with care to avoid nerve trunks. It should be kept in mind that maximum blood concentrations may not be attained for 8 or more hours after intramuscular administration.

Reconstituted antivenin (*Crotalidae*) polyvalent may be administered intravenously in a 1:1 to 1:10 dilution in 0.9% sodium chloride injection or 5% dextrose injection. Decisions concerning the dilution of antivenin to be used, the type of electrolyte solution used for dilution, and the rate of intravenous delivery of the diluted antivenin should take into account the age, weight, and cardiac status of the patient; the severity of the envenomation; the total amount and type of parenteral fluids one anticipates will be given; and the interval between the bite and the initiation of specific therapy.

The entire initial dose of antivenin (*Crotalidae*) polyvalent should be administered as soon as possible, preferably within 4 hours after the bite. Antivenin (*Crotalidae*) polyvalent is less effective when given 8 hours or more after envenomation and may be of questionable value when given after 12 hours. However, in severe poisonings, it is recommended that antivenin therapy be given even if 24 hours have elapsed since the bite.

The initial 5 to 10 mL of the diluted antivenin (*Crotalidae*) polyvalent should be infused over a 3- to 5-minute period, with careful observation of the patient for evidence of an untoward reaction. If no symptoms or signs of an immediate systemic reaction appear, infusion of the diluted antivenin may be continued at the maximum rate considered safe for intravenous fluid administration.

The decision to use additional antivenin (*Crotalidae*) polyvalent should be based on the clinical response to the initial dose and on continuing assessment of the severity of poisoning. If swelling continues to progress, if systemic symptoms or signs of envenomation increase in severity, or if new manifestations appear (for example, fall in hematocrit or hypotension), intravenous administration of an additional 10 to 50 mL (contents of 1 to 5 vials) or more may be necessary.

Pit viper bites on toes or fingers may require as much as 50% more antivenin (*Crotalidae*) polyvalent due to difficulties in achieving adequate antivenin (*Crotalidae*) polyvalent concentrations in the affected area. However, antivenin (*Crotalidae*) polyvalent should never be injected into a finger or toe.

Diluent is product specific. Only the diluent supplied by the manufacturer should be used.

The use of corticosteroids in the treatment of crotalid envenomation is controversial. Corticosteroids may mask the seriousness of hypovolemia in moderate or severe poisoning and have little, if any, effect on the local-tissue response to rattlesnake venoms. Corticosteroids should not be given simultaneously with antivenin (*Crotalidae*) polyvalent on a routine basis or during the acute state of envenomation. However, their use may be necessary for treatment of immediate allergic reactions to antivenin (*Crotalidae*) polyvalent, and corticosteroids are the agents of choice for treating serious delayed reactions to the antivenin.

Snakes' mouths do not harbor *Clostridium tetani*. However, appropriate tetanus prophylaxis is indicated, since tetanus spores may be carried into the fang puncture wounds by dirt present on the skin at the time of the bite or by nonsterile first-aid procedures. If local tissue damage is evident, a broad-spectrum antibiotic in adequate dosage is indicated. The bitten extremity should not be packed in ice, and cryotherapy is contraindicated.

The treatment of shock following crotalid envenomation is the same as treatment of hypovolemic shock of any cause. Aspirin, or preferably NSAIDs or codeine, is usually adequate for pain relief. Sedation with phenobarbital or mild tranquilizers may be used if indicated, but should not be used if respiratory failure is present.

Compartment syndromes may rarely complicate crotalid envenomations, especially those caused by bites on the lower extremities. Prompt surgical consultation is indicated whenever a closed-compartment syndrome is suspected. Defibrination and disseminated intravascular coagulation (DIC) syndromes have been associated with envenomation by some pit vipers native to the U.S.; appropriate therapy may be indicated.

Serum sickness occurs in 40 to 80% of patients. All patients should be observed for serum sickness for an average of 5 to 24 days following administration of antivenin (*Crotalidae*) polyvalent. In some patients, especially those who have received preparations containing horse serum in the past, the onset of serum sickness may be less than 5 days.

### For treatment of adverse effects

Recommended treatment consists of the following:
For anaphylaxis—
- Intravenous infusion:
  —Slowing or discontinuing administration.
  —Administering epinephrine.
- Intramuscular injection:
  —Applying tourniquet next to injection site.
  —Injecting epinephrine 1:1000 either next to tourniquet or into another extremity.
For serum sickness—Administering salicylates, antihistamines, or corticosteroids.

## Parenteral Dosage Forms

### ANTIVENIN ( (CROTALIDAE) POLYVALENT) USP

#### Usual adult and adolescent dose
Immunizing agent (passive)—Intravenous infusion:—
  Minimal envenomation—Initially, 20 to 40 mL (contents of 2 to 4 vials).
  Moderate envenomation—Initially, 50 to 90 mL (contents of 5 to 9 vials).
  Severe envenomation—Initially, 100 to 150 mL or more (contents of 10 to 15 vials or more).

Note: An estimate of the severity of envenomation should be made as soon as possible and before any antivenin is administered. The initial dose of antivenin (*Crotalidae*) polyvalent is based on the best estimate of the severity of envenomation at the beginning of treatment. The grades of severity of envenomation are: minimal envenomation (characterized by local swelling and other local changes; no systemic manifestations; normal laboratory findings), moderate envenomation (characterized by swelling progressing beyond the site of the bite and by one or more systemic manifestations; abnormal laboratory findings, for example, a fall in hematocrit or platelets), and severe envenomation (characterized by marked local response, severe systemic manifestations, and significant alteration in laboratory findings). The need for additional antivenin ( *Crotalidae*) polyvalent should be based on the clinical response to the initial dose and continuing assessment of the severity of poisoning. If swelling continues to progress, if systemic symptoms or signs of envenomation increase in severity, or if new manifestations appear (for example, fall in hematocrit or hypotension), an additional 10 to 50 mL (contents of 1 to 5 vials) or more should be administered intravenously. Envenomation by large snakes in small adults may require larger doses of antivenin (*Crotalidae*) polyvalent than average sized adults.

#### Usual pediatric dose
See *Usual adult and adolescent dose*.

Note: The amount of antivenin administered to children is not based on weight.

#### Strength(s) usually available
U.S.—
  One vial of antivenin neutralizes not less than 180 mouse $LD_{50}$ of *Crotalus atrox* (Western diamondback) venom; 1320 mouse $LD_{50}$ of *Crotalus durissus terrificus* (South American rattlesnake) venom; and 780 mouse $LD_{50}$ of *Bothrops atrox* (South American fer-de-lance) venom (Rx) [GENERIC (may contain phenol and thimerosal; diluent contains phenylmercuric nitrate)].
Canada—
  One vial of antivenin neutralizes not less than 180 mouse $LD_{50}$ of *Crotalus atrox* (Western diamondback) venom; 1320 mouse $LD_{50}$ of *Crotalus durissus terrificus* (South American rattlesnake) venom; and 780 mouse $LD_{50}$ of *Bothrops atrox* (South American fer-de-lance) venom (Rx) [GENERIC (may contain phenol and thimerosal)].

#### Packaging and storage
Store below 40 °C (104 °F), preferably between 15 and 30 °C (59 and 86 °F), unless otherwise specified by manufacturer.

#### Preparation of dosage form
To prepare the solution, 10 mL of the supplied diluent should be added to each vial. To avoid foaming, mix by gently swirling rather than shaking. The reconstituted solution is then prepared for intravenous injection by adding enough 0.9% sodium chloride or 5% dextrose injection to make a 1:1 to 1:10 dilution of reconstituted antivenin.

#### Stability
Reconstituted solutions of the antivenin should be used within 48 hours. Diluted solutions of the antivenin should be used within 12 hours.

### Selected Bibliography

Griffen D, Donovan JW. Significant envenomation from a preserved rattlesnake head (in a patient with a history of immediate hypersensitivity to antivenin). Ann Emerg Med 1986; 15: 955-8.

Smith TA II, Figge HL. Treatment of snakebite poisoning. Am J Hosp Pharm 1991; 48: 2190-6.

Durand LS, Hiebert JM, Rodeheaver GT, Edgerton MT, Edlich RF. Snake venom poisoning. Compr Ther 1981; 7: 51-7.

Developed: 07/20/95

# ANTIVENIN (LATRODECTUS MACTANS)   Systemic

VA CLASSIFICATION (Primary): IM300

Another commonly used name is black widow spider antivenin.

Note: For a listing of dosage forms and brand names by country availability, see *Dosage Forms* section(s). For a listing of brand names for the articles in this monograph, refer to the General Index.

## Category

Immunizing agent (passive).

## Indications

### Accepted

Envenomation, black widow spider (treatment)—Antivenin (*Latrodectus mactans*) is indicated in the treatment of serious or life-threatening symptoms resulting from the bites of the black widow spider (*Latrodectus mactans*). Early use of the antivenin is emphasized for prompt relief. The best effect occurs with antivenin administration within 4 hours after envenomation.

## Pharmacology/Pharmacokinetics

### Physicochemical characteristics

Source—Antivenin (*Latrodectus mactans*) is a sterile, non-pyrogenic preparation derived by drying a frozen solution of specific venom-neutralizing globulins obtained from the blood serum of healthy horses that have been immunized against venom of black widow spiders (*Latrodectus mactans*). One dose of antivenin neutralizes not less than 6000 mouse $LD_{50}$ of *Latrodectus mactans* venom

### Mechanism of action/Effect

The exact mechanism of action is unknown. However, the antivenin specifically binds with and neutralizes circulating venom.

### Half-life

Mean half-life < 15 days.

### Onset of action

Symptoms begin to subside in 1 to 3 hours following administration.

### Time to peak concentration

Intramuscular—2 to 3 days.
Intravenous—Almost immediately after end of infusion.

## Precautions to Consider

### Cross-sensitivity and/or related problems

Patients allergic to any product prepared from horse serum may be allergic to antivenin (*Latrodectus mactans*). A skin or conjunctival test for serum sensitivity should be performed under close medical supervision if antivenin administration is being considered. See *General Dosing Information*.

### Carcinogenicity/Mutagenicity

Long-term animal studies to evaluate carcinogenic or mutagenic potential of antivenin (*Latrodectus mactans*) have not been performed.

### Pregnancy/Reproduction

Fertility—Studies have not been performed.

Pregnancy—Studies have not been done in humans. It is not known whether antivenin (*Latrodectus mactans*) can cause harm to the fetus when administered to a pregnant woman. However, the venom of the black widow spider may precipitate spontaneous abortion.

Studies have not been done in animals.

FDA Pregnancy Category C.

### Breast-feeding

It is not known whether antivenin (*Latrodectus mactans*) is distributed into breast milk. However, problems in humans have not been documented.

### Pediatrics

Appropriate studies on the relationship of age to the effects of antivenin (*Latrodectus mactans*) have not been performed in the pediatric population. However, the toxicity of the bites themselves is more serious in children than in adults.

### Geriatrics

Appropriate studies on the relationship of age to the effects of antivenin (*Latrodectus mactans*) have not been performed in the geriatric population. However, the toxicity of the bites themselves is more serious in geriatric patients.

## Medical considerations/Contraindications

The medical considerations/contraindications included here have been selected on the basis of their potential clinical significance (reasons given in parentheses where appropriate)—not necessarily inclusive (» = major clinical significance).

*Risk-benefit should be considered when the following medical problem exists:*

» Hypersensitivity to antivenin (*Latrodectus mactans*) or horse serum

## Side/Adverse Effects

Note: Anaphylaxis may occur following antivenin (*Latrodectus mactans*) administration, even in individuals with no prior history of hypersensitivity to the antivenin or horse serum. Epinephrine hydrochloride injection (1:1000) should be readily available for use in case of an anaphylactic or acute hypersensitivity reaction. Serum sickness may occur following administration of antivenin (*Latrodectus mactans*); this lasts an average of 8 to 12 days. All patients should be observed, or followed for serum sickness.

The following side/adverse effects have been selected on the basis of their potential clinical significance (possible signs and symptoms in parentheses where appropriate)—not necessarily inclusive:

### Those indicating need for medical attention

Incidence more frequent

*Anaphylactic reaction* (difficulty in breathing or swallowing; hives; itching, especially of feet or hands; reddening of skin, especially around ears; swelling of eyes, face, or inside of nose; unusual tiredness or weakness, sudden and severe)

### Those indicating need for medical attention only if they continue or are bothersome

Incidence more frequent

*Serum sickness* (feeling of discomfort; fever; inflammation of joints; itching; muscle aches; rash; swollen lymph glands)

## Patient Consultation

As an aid to patient consultation, refer to *Advice for the Patient, Antivenin, Black Widow Spider (Systemic)*.

In providing consultation, consider emphasizing the following selected information (» = major clinical significance):

### Before using this medication

» Conditions affecting use, especially:
   Hypersensitivity to antivenin (*Latrodectus mactans*) or horse serum

### Side/adverse effects

Signs of potential side effects, especially anaphylactic reaction

## General Dosing Information

Anaphylaxis may occur following antivenin (*Latrodectus mactans*) administration, even in individuals with no prior history of hypersensitivity to the antivenin or horse serum. An intradermal skin test or conjunctival test with normal horse serum and sterile normal saline (0.9% sodium chloride injection) should be performed prior to use of the antivenin. However, intradermal skin tests have occasionally resulted in fatalities but conjunctival tests have not. Skin tests should not be performed unless epinephrine 1:1000 is within immediate reach to combat any unexpected anaphylactic or other allergic reactions.

The skin test consists of an intradermal injection of 0.02 mL of a 1:10 dilution of normal horse serum in 0.9% sodium chloride, and a 0.9% sodium chloride injection at a separate site to serve as a control. A positive skin test result consists of an urticarial wheal surrounded by an erythematous zone.

The conjunctival test consists of instillation of one drop of a 1:10 dilution (for adults) or a 1:100 dilution (for children) of normal horse serum into the conjunctival sac. One drop of 0.9% sodium chloride is instilled into the other conjunctival sac to serve as a control. A positive conjunctival test result consists of itching of the eye and reddening of the conjunctiva. Antivenin therapy should be avoided if the results of the sensitivity tests are positive.

Desensitization may be attempted if the results of the sensitivity tests are mildly or questionably positive, or if the administration of antivenin is considered necessary to save the patient's life. Epinephrine injection 1:1000 and a tourniquet should be immediately available during desensitization to combat anaphylactic or other allergic reactions.

The procedure of desensitization consists of subcutaneous injection of 0.1, then 0.2, and finally 0.5 mL of a 1:100 dilution of reconstituted antivenin in 0.9% sodium chloride at 15- or preferably 30-minute intervals; this process is repeated with a 1:10 dilution and finally with the undiluted reconstituted antivenin. If no reaction occurs after 0.5 mL of undiluted reconstituted antivenin has been given, it is probably safe to continue the dose at 15-minute intervals until the entire dose has been injected. However, if there is a reaction after any of the injections, a tourniquet should be applied next to the injection site and epinephrine 1:1000 administered either at a site next to the tourniquet or into another extremity.

Antivenin (*Latrodectus mactans*) may be given intramuscularly, preferably in the region of the anterolateral thigh so that a tourniquet may be applied in the event of a systemic reaction. However, when the patient is in shock, if the patient is under 12 years of age, or in severe cases of envenomation, the preferred route of administration is intravenous.

In otherwise healthy individuals between the ages of 16 and 60, the use of antivenin may be deferred and treatment with muscle relaxants considered.

Serum sickness may occur following administration of antivenin (*Latrodectus mactans*); this lasts an average of 8 to 12 days.

To help relieve symptoms of envenomation, it is also recommended that 10 mL of 10% calcium gluconate be administered by intravenous injection, as necessary, to control muscle pain. It may also be necessary to administer morphine to control pain and barbiturates to treat extreme restlessness. However, since black widow spider venom is a neurotoxin, the risk of respiratory paralysis must be weighed when the use of morphine or a barbiturate is considered.

### For treatment of adverse effects

Recommended treatment consists of the following:
- For anaphylaxis—Administering epinephrine 1:1000.
- For serum sickness—Administering salicylates, antihistamines, or corticosteroids.

## Parenteral Dosage Forms

### ANTIVENIN (LATRODECTUS MACTANS) USP

#### Usual adult and adolescent dose

Envenomation, black widow spider (treatment)—
Intravenous infusion, 2.5 mL (6000 antivenin units) administered over a fifteen-minute period, or intramuscular, 2.5 mL (6000 antivenin units), preferably in the region of the anterolateral thigh.

Note: A single dose of antivenin (*Latrodectus mactans*) usually is adequate. However, in some cases a second dose of 2.5 mL (6000 antivenin units) may be necessary.

#### Usual pediatric dose

See *Usual adult and adolescent dose.*

#### Strength(s) usually available

U.S.—

No less than 6000 antivenin units per 2.5 mL (Rx) [GENERIC (may contain thimerosal)].

Canada—

No less than 6000 antivenin units per 2.5 mL (Rx) [GENERIC (may contain thimerosal)].

Note: Antivenin is supplied with a 1-mL vial of normal horse serum (1:10 dilution) for sensitivity testing.

#### Packaging and storage

Store between 2 and 8 °C (36 and 46 °F).

#### Preparation of dosage form

Antivenin (*Latrodectus mactans*) is reconstituted by adding 2.5 mL of the diluent provided by the manufacturer to a vial labeled as containing at least 6000 antivenin units and shaking the vial to dissolve the contents completely. For intravenous administration, the reconstituted solution is further diluted in 10 to 50 mL of 0.9% sodium chloride injection.

#### Stability

The reconstituted solution should not be frozen.

## Selected Bibliography

Clark RF, Westhern-Kestner S, Vance MV, Gerkin R. Clinical presentation and treatment of black widow spider envenomation: a review of 163 cases. Ann Emerg Med 1992; 21: 782-7.

Moss HS, Binder LS. A retrospective review of black widow spider envenomation. Ann Emerg Med 1987; 16: 188-91.

Developed: 06/24/95

---

# ANTIVENIN (MICRURUS FULVIUS)     Systemic†

VA CLASSIFICATION (Primary): IM300

Another commonly used name is North American coral snake antivenin.

Note: For a listing of dosage forms and brand names by country availability, see *Dosage Forms* section(s). For a listing of brand names for the articles in this monograph, refer to the General Index.

†Not commercially available in Canada.

## Category

Immunizing agent (passive).

## Indications

Note: Coral snakebites are rare. If snakebite envenomation is known or suspected in a patient, it is very important that the attending physician contact a poison control center immediately, before treatment is attempted. Snake venoms are complex substances, and there may be multiple organ, system, or tissue effects. As an additional measure it is also very important to consult experts who have successfully treated snakebite poisoning. Physicians responsible for the treatment of such patients should be familiar with the signs and symptoms of coral snake envenomation and current methods of first aid and general supportive therapy for venomous snakebites.

### Accepted

Envenomation, North American coral snake (treatment)—Antivenin (*Micrurus fulvius*) is indicated for the treatment of envenomation caused by bites of the Eastern coral snake (*Micrurus fulvius fulvius*) and the Texas coral snake (*M. fulvius tenere*).

Antivenin (*Micrurus fulvius*) may partially neutralize the venom of *M. dumerilli carinicauda* and minimally neutralize that of *M. spixii*. It

may also provide some protection against the venom of *M. nigrocinctus.*

### Unaccepted

Antivenin (*Micrurus fulvius*) will not neutralize the venom of the Arizona or Sonoran coral snake (*Micruroides euryxanthus*), or the Brazilian giant coral snake (*Micrurus frontalis*). It is not effective against the venoms of pit vipers (family *Crotalidae*) and should not be used for the treatment of envenomation caused by the bites of these snakes.

## Pharmacology/Pharmacokinetics

### Physicochemical characteristics

Source—Antivenin (*Micrurus fulvius*) is a sterile, non-pyrogenic, refined, and concentrated preparation derived by drying a frozen solution of specific venom-neutralizing globulins obtained from the serum of healthy horses immunized against the venom of the Eastern coral snake (*Micrurus fulvius fulvius*). The antivenin is standardized by biological assay on mice by its ability to neutralize the lethal action of *M. fulvius fulvius* venom. The reconstituted contents of each vial (10 mL) will neutralize approximately 250 mouse $LD_{50}$ or approximately 2 mg of *M. fulvius fulvius* venom

### Mechanism of action/Effect

Antivenin (*Micrurus fulvius*) specifically binds and neutralizes coral snake venom. When indicated, antivenin should be administered as soon as possible, even before the onset of signs or symptoms of envenomation.

### Half-life

Mean half-life < 15 days.

### Onset of action
Effect is rapid after intravenous administration, which is the preferred route of administration, but 24 hours or more after intramuscular injection.

### Time to peak concentration
Concentration peaks rapidly after intravenous administration. Concentration may not peak until the next day after intramuscular injection.

## Precautions to Consider

### Pregnancy/Reproduction
Fertility—Studies on effects of antivenin (*Micrurus fulvius*) on fertility have not been done.

Pregnancy—Studies have not been done in humans. It is not known whether antivenin (*Micrurus fulvius*) can cause fetal harm when administered to a pregnant woman. However, the venom of coral snakes may precipitate spontaneous abortion.

Studies have not been done in animals.

### Breast-feeding
Problems in humans have not been documented.

### Pediatrics
Studies show that children have a lower incidence of adverse reaction to antivenin (*Micrurus fulvius*) and tolerate it better than do adults. However, children have more severe reactions to a given envenomation because of the greater amount of venom per body weight, and may require larger doses of antivenin (*Micrurus fulvius*) than adults do. Pediatric doses should not be adjusted by the weight of the patient.

### Geriatrics
Appropriate studies on the relationship of age to the effects of antivenin (*Micrurus fulvius*) have not been performed in the geriatric population. However, no geriatrics-specific problems have been documented to date.

### Medical considerations/Contraindications
The medical considerations/contraindications included here have been selected on the basis of their potential clinical significance (reasons given in parentheses where appropriate)—not necessarily inclusive (» = major clinical significance).

*Risk-benefit should be considered when the following medical problems exist:*
» Hypersensitivity to antivenin (*Micrurus fulvius*)
» Hypersensitivity to horse serum
     (Antivenin [*Micrurus fulvius*] is obtained from the serum of healthy horses immunized with the venom of the Eastern coral snake [*Micrurus fulvius fulvius*]. Patients allergic to horse serum may also be allergic to antivenin [*Micrurus fulvius*]; this may result in severe systemic reactions)

## Side/Adverse Effects

Note: Antivenin (*Micrurus fulvius*) occasionally has caused immediate hypersensitivity reactions, such as anaphylaxis and shock. These reactions generally become evident within 30 minutes after antivenin administration and include apprehension; flushing; itching; urticaria; edema of the face, tongue, and throat; cough; dyspnea; cyanosis; vomiting; and collapse. In the event of systemic reaction during antivenin administration, the antivenin should be discontinued and appropriate treatment should be initiated.

The following side/adverse effects have been selected on the basis of their potential clinical significance (possible signs and symptoms in parentheses where appropriate)—not necessarily inclusive:

**Those indicating need for medical attention**
Incidence more frequent
     *Anaphylactic reaction* (difficulty in breathing or swallowing; hives; itching, especially of feet or hands; reddening of skin, especially around ears; swelling of eyes, face, or inside nose; unusual tiredness or weakness, sudden and severe); *serum sickness* (fever; redness of joints; skin rash and itching; swollen glands)

## Patient Consultation

As an aid to patient consultation, refer to *Advice for the Patient, Antivenin, North American Coral Snake (Systemic)*.

In providing consultation, consider emphasizing the following selected information (» = major clinical significance):

**Before using this medication**
» Conditions affecting use, especially:
     Hypersensitivity to horse serum or antivenin (*Micrurus fulvius*)

**Proper use of this medication**
» Proper dosing

**Side/adverse effects**
     Signs of potential side effects, especially anaphylactic reaction and serum sickness

## General Dosing Information

Note: Coral snakebites, like bites by crotalids, are not always followed by envenomation. However, in contrast to crotalid bites, in which moderate-to-severe envenomation usually can be predicted by rapid onset of the local effects (e.g., pain, discoloration, edema), severe and even fatal envenomation from a coral snakebite can be present without any significant local tissue reaction. Systemic signs and symptoms of envenomation usually begin from 1 to 7 hours after the bite, but may be delayed for as long as 18 hours. Paralysis has been observed within 2.5 hours after envenomation and appears to be a bulbar type involving cranial motor nerves. Death from respiratory paralysis has occurred within 4 hours after envenomation. Systemic signs and symptoms of envenomation may include euphoria, lethargy, weakness, nausea, vomiting, excessive salivation, ptosis of the eyelids, dyspnea, abnormal reflexes, convulsions, and motor weakness or paralysis, including complete respiratory paralysis. Local signs and symptoms may include scratch marks or fang puncture wounds, edema, erythema, pain at the bite site, and paresthesia in the bitten extremity.

Anaphylaxis may occur following antivenin (*Micrurus fulvius*) administration, even in individuals with no prior history of hypersensitivity to the antivenin or horse serum. Prior to use of antivenin (*Micrurus fulvius*), appropriate measures should be taken in an effort to detect the presence of a dangerous sensitivity. A careful review of the patient's history should be made, including any report of asthma, hay fever, urticaria, or other allergic manifestations; allergic reactions upon exposure to horses; and prior injections of horse serum. An intradermal skin test for serum sensitivity using normal horse serum or the antivenin and 0.9% sodium chloride injection should be performed under close medical supervision in every patient prior to administration of the antivenin, regardless of clinical history. A tourniquet and epinephrine injection (1:1000) should be at hand to combat any unexpected anaphylactic or other allergic reaction.

The skin test consists of an intradermal injection of 0.02 to 0.03 mL of a 1:10 dilution of either normal horse serum or reconstituted antivenin (*Micrurus fulvius*) in 0.9% sodium chloride injection. A 0.9% sodium chloride injection should be administered in the opposite extremity to serve as a control. Use of larger amounts of diluted normal horse serum or diluted reconstituted antivenin for the skin test increases the likelihood of false-positive reactions, and, in extremely sensitive patients, increases the risk of a systemic reaction. When the patient has a history of sensitivity to horse serum, a 1:100 or greater dilution should be used for preliminary skin testing. A positive skin test result consists of a wheal with or without pseudopods and surrounding erythema, and occurs within 5 to 30 minutes. In general, the shorter the interval between injection and the beginning of the skin reaction, the greater the sensitivity. A negative allergic history and the absence of reaction to a skin test do not rule out the possibility of an immediate reaction.

If the patient has no history of allergy and the skin test is negative, or if the patient is not dangerously hypersensitive to horse serum, antivenin (*Micrurus fulvius*) may be administered as follows: An intravenous drip of 250 to 500 mL of sodium chloride injection USP should be started, and, depending on the nature and severity of the signs and symptoms of envenomation, the contents of 3 to 5 vials (30 to 50 mL) should be administered intravenously, either by slow injection directly into the intravenous tubing or by adding the contents of the vial to the reservoir bottle of the intravenous drip (if added to reservoir bottle, the contents should not be shaken but should be mixed by gentle swirling). In either case, the equivalent of the first 1 or 2 mL of the undiluted antivenin should be injected over a 3- to 5-minute period with careful observation of the patient for evidence of allergic reaction. If no signs or symptoms of anaphylaxis appear, the injection or intravenous infusion may be continued.

The rate of delivery should be regulated by the severity of signs and symptoms of envenomation and the tolerance of the patient to the antivenin. However, until the equivalent of 30 to 50 mL of undiluted antivenin has been given, the antivenin injection or intravenous infusion should be administered at the maximum safe rate for intravenous fluids, based on body weight and the general condition of the patient. For instance, if the antivenin is given by intravenous drip to a previously healthy adult, approximately 250 or 500 mL should be allowed to run in within 30 minutes. In small children, the first 100 mL should be allowed to run in rapidly but then should be decreased to a rate not to exceed 4 mL per minute.

If the history of sensitivity is positive and the skin test is strongly positive, administration of the antivenin may be dangerous, especially if the positive sensitivity test is accompanied by systemic allergic manifestations. In such instances, the risk of administering the antivenin must be weighed against the risk of withholding it, keeping in mind that severe envenomation can be fatal.

If the patient does not have a history of allergy and the skin test is mildly or questionably positive, desensitization may be attempted to reduce the risk of severe immediate systemic reaction.

The procedure of desensitization consists of subcutaneous injections of 0.1, 0.2, and 0.5 mL of a 1:100 dilution of reconstituted antivenin at 15 minute intervals; repeated with a 1:10 dilution and then with undiluted reconstituted antivenin. If there is any reaction after any of the injections, a tourniquet should be applied proximal to the sites of injection and epinephrine (1:1000) administered proximal to the tourniquet or into another extremity. After 30 minutes, the procedure should be continued, starting with the last dose of antivenin (*Micrurus fulvius*) that did not evoke a reaction. If no reaction occurs after 0.5 mL of undiluted antivenin (*Micrurus fulvius*) has been given, the usual therapeutic dose may be administered by intravenous infusion. Alternatively, antivenin (*Micrurus fulvius*) may be given by intramuscular injection by doubling the dose at 15 minute intervals until the entire therapeutic dose has been injected.

The desensitization protocol may require several hours to administer the initial therapeutic dose. Since time is an important factor in neutralization of venom in critically ill patients, the following alternative procedure may be used for administration of antivenin (*Micrurus fulvius*) in some severely envenomated patients who have positive sensitivity tests. Fifty to 100 mg of diphenhydramine hydrochloride should be given intravenously, followed by slow intravenous infusion of diluted antivenin (*Micrurus fulvius*) with close observation of the patient for symptoms and signs of anaphylaxis. If anaphylaxis does not occur, antivenin (*Micrurus fulvius*) administration should be continued with close observation of the patient.

For the treatment of patients who develop signs and symptoms of impending anaphylaxis in spite of desensitization or the alternative procedure, experts who have successfully treated snakebite poisoning or a poison control center should be consulted.

Additional antivenin (*Micrurus fulvius*) may be administered as required. Some envenomated patients may require administration of the contents of 10 or more vials of antivenin if the snake has injected its entire venom load into the patient.

Antivenin (*Micrurus fulvius*) should not be injected into a finger or toe.

Envenomation by large snakes in children or small adults requires larger doses of antivenin (*Micrurus fulvius*) than average size adults. The amount administered to a child or small adults is not based on weight.

Diluent is product specific. Only diluent supplied by the manufacturer should be used.

Snakes' mouths do not harbor *Clostridium tetani*. However, appropriate tetanus prophylaxis is indicated, since tetanus spores may be carried into the fang puncture wounds by dirt present on skin at time of bite or by nonsterile first-aid procedures.

Serum sickness occurs in 40 to 80% of patients. All patients should be observed for serum sickness for an average of 5 to 24 days following administration of antivenin (*Micrurus fulvius*). In some patients, especially those who have received preparations containing horse serum in the past, the onset of serum sickness may be less than 5 days.

### For treatment of adverse effects
Recommended treatment consists of the following:
   For anaphylaxis—
   • Intravenous infusion:
      —Slowing or discontinuing administration.
      —Administering epinephrine.
   • Intramuscular injection:
      —Applying tourniquet next to injection site.
      —Injecting epinephrine 1:1000 either next to tourniquet or into another extremity.
For serum sickness—Administering salicylates, antihistamines, or corticosteroids.

## Parenteral Dosage Forms

### ANTIVENIN (MICRURUS FULVIUS) USP

**Usual adult and adolescent dose**
Immunizing agent (passive)—
   Intravenous infusion, 3 to 5 vials (30 to 50 mL).

**Usual pediatric dose**
See *Usual adult and adolescent dose*.

**Strength(s) usually available**
U.S.—
   Each reconstituted vial (10 mL) neutralizes approximately 250 mouse median lethal doses or approximately 2 mg of *Micrurus fulvius fulvius* venom (Rx) [GENERIC (may contain phenol and thimerosal; diluent may contain phenylmercuric nitrate)].
Canada—
   Not commercially available.

**Packaging and storage**
Store between 2 and 8 °C (35 and 46 °F), unless otherwise specified by manufacturer.

**Preparation of dosage form**
To prepare solution, 10 mL of the supplied diluent should be added to each vial. Gentle agitation may be used to hasten complete dissolution of the lyophilized antivenin.

**Stability**
Reconstituted solutions of the antivenin should be used within 48 hours, and diluted solutions of the antivenin should be used within 12 hours.

## Selected Bibliography

Picchioni AL, Hardy DL, Russell FE, Kunkel DB. Management of poisonous snakebite. Vet Hum Toxicol 1984; 26 (2): 139-40.
Smith II TA, Figge HL. Treatment of snakebite poisoning. Am J Hosp Pharm 1991; 48: 2190-6.

Developed: 08/01/95

---

# APOMORPHINE   Systemic*

VA CLASSIFICATION (Primary): DX900

Note: For a listing of dosage forms and brand names by country availability, see *Dosage Forms* section(s). For a listing of brand names for the articles in this monograph, refer to the General Index.

*Not commercially available in the U.S.

## Category
Diagnostic aid (parkinsonism).

## Indications

### Accepted
Parkinsonism (diagnosis)—Apomorphine is used in the differential diagnosis of idiopathic parkinsonism syndrome and as a diagnostic test for dopaminergic responsiveness in parkinsonian syndromes to determine whether a patient will respond or is still responsive to levodopa therapy.

### Unaccepted
Apomorphine has been used as a centrally acting emetic in the treatment of acute oral drug overdose and accidental poisoning. However, this medication has been replaced by ipecac syrup, which is more convenient to use and does not produce central nervous system (CNS) or respiratory depression.

## Pharmacology/Pharmacokinetics

### Physicochemical characteristics
Molecular weight—312.80.

### Mechanism of action/Effect
Diagnostic aid (parkinsonism)—Apomorphine is a dopamine receptor agonist, whose clinical and pharmacological anti-parkinsonian effects resemble those of levodopa, but which is faster acting. Improvement of parkinsonian symptoms with apomorphine serves to predict responsiveness to levodopa.

**Other actions/effects**

Apomorphine induces vomiting by direct stimulation of the medullary chemoreceptor trigger zone (CTZ). Excitation of vestibular centers may also be involved since movement increases and recumbency decreases the emetic effect of apomorphine.

Apomorphine also depresses medullary centers that control respiration and vasomotor tone and stimulates salivation. It increases plasma concentrations of human growth hormone and decreases serum prolactin concentrations by stimulating dopamine receptors.

**Biotransformation**

Hepatic.

**Onset of action**

Adults: 5 to 10 minutes.
Children: 1 to 2 minutes.

**Elimination**

Renal. A very small percentage of a dose is excreted unchanged.

## Precautions to Consider

### Cross-sensitivity and/or related problems

Patients sensitive to morphine or its derivatives may be sensitive to this medication also.

### Pregnancy/Reproduction

Pregnancy—Studies have not been done in humans.
Studies have not been done in animals.

FDA Pregnancy Category C.

### Breast-feeding

It is not known whether apomorphine is distributed into breast milk. However, problems in humans have not been documented.

### Pediatrics

Apomorphine is not generally used in children.

### Geriatrics

No information is available on the relationship of age to the effects of apomorphine in geriatric patients. However, it is known that geriatric patients exhibit increased sensitivity to morphine-like medications and may be more susceptible to the respiratory depressant effects of apomorphine, especially with large or repeated doses.

In addition, the increase in blood pressure that may result from the vomiting action may place geriatric patients at greater risk of hemorrhage and vascular accidents because of possible pathologic changes of their blood vessels; therefore, caution is recommended.

### Drug interactions and/or related problems

The following drug interactions and/or related problems have been selected on the basis of their potential clinical significance (possible mechanism in parentheses where appropriate)—not necessarily inclusive (» = major clinical significance):

Note: Combinations containing any of the following medications, depending on the amount present, may also interact with this medication.

Dronabinol
(prior administration of dronabinol may decrease the emetic response to apomorphine; also, concurrent use may potentiate the central nervous system depressant effects of either apomorphine or dronabinol)

### Laboratory value alterations

The following have been selected on the basis of their potential clinical significance (possible effect in parentheses where appropriate)—not necessarily inclusive (» = major clinical significance):

With physiology/laboratory test values
Serum prolactin concentrations
(may be decreased)

### Medical considerations/Contraindications

The medical considerations/contraindications included here have been selected on the basis of their potential clinical significance (reasons given in parentheses where appropriate)—not necessarily inclusive (» = major clinical significance):

*Except under special circumstances, this medication should not be used when the following medical problems exist:*

» Any condition in which there is an increased risk of aspiration of vomitus, such as:
» Decreased patient alertness or
» Depressed gag reflex or
» Seizures or
» Unconsciousness
(risk of aspiration pneumonia)

» Narcosis due to opiates, barbiturates, or other CNS depressants or
» Shock
(increased risk of severe CNS, cardiovascular, and/or respiratory depression)

Sensitivity to apomorphine

*Risk-benefit should be considered when the following medical problems exist:*

Cardiac decompensation or
Cerebrovascular disease
(vomiting may cause an increase in blood pressure that may lead to hemorrhage and vascular accidents)

Caution is also recommended in debilitated patients, since they may show an increased susceptibility to apomorphine.

## Side/Adverse Effects

Note: Excessive doses of apomorphine may cause violent emesis, cardiac depression, and death.

Although the apomorphine test for parkinsonism is generally well tolerated, mild transient nausea and vomiting, moderate sedation, postural hypotension or vasovagal response, and yawning have been reported. These side effects usually resolve within thirty minutes. Apomorphine-induced side effects may be blocked by prior administration of domperidone, a peripheral dopamine antagonist.

The following side/adverse effects have been selected on the basis of their potential clinical significance (possible signs and symptoms in parentheses where appropriate)—not necessarily inclusive:

**Those indicating need for medical attention only if they continue or are bothersome**
Incidence more frequent
*CNS depression* (drowsiness; unusual tiredness or weakness); *increased salivation; increased sweating; nausea*
Incidence less frequent or rare
*CNS stimulation* (false sense of well-being; fast heartbeat; fast or irregular breathing; restlessness; trembling); *orthostatic hypotension* (dizziness or lightheadedness, especially when getting up from a lying or sitting position)—more frequent in patients with Parkinson's disease

## Overdose

For specific information on the agents used in the management of apomorphine overdose, see:
• *Atropine* in *Anticholinergics/Antispasmodics (Systemic)* monograph; and/or
• *Naloxone (Systemic)* monograph.

For more information on the management of overdose or unintentional ingestion, **contact a Poison Control Center** (See *Poison Control Center Listing*).

### Clinical effects of overdose

The following effects have been selected on the basis of their potential clinical significance (possible signs and symptoms in parentheses where appropriate)—not necessarily inclusive:
*Bradycardia* (slow heartbeat); *CNS depression, severe* (ranging from severe drowsiness to profound coma); *respiratory depression* (shortness of breath; troubled breathing); *vomiting, continuing*

Note: *CNS depression* may also occur at therapeutic doses.

### Treatment of overdose

Specific treatment—
Naloxone, to antagonize emetic effects and CNS and respiratory depression.
Atropine, to treat bradycardia.
Supportive care——
Patients in whom intentional overdose is known or suspected should be referred for psychiatric consultation.

## General Dosing Information

## Parenteral Dosage Forms

### APOMORPHINE HYDROCHLORIDE INJECTION

**Usual adult dose**

Diagnostic aid (parkinsonism)—
Subcutaneous, 1, 2, 4, and 5 mg of a solution containing 10 mg per mL, until a positive response is recorded (up to 10 mg), with thirty minutes between doses.

Note: The oral administration of domperidone, 20 mg three times a day for two to three days prior to the administration of apomorphine and 20 mg three times during the day of apomorphine administration beginning thirty to sixty minutes prior to the apomorphine dose, is recommended to reduce the incidence of side effects.

**Usual adult prescribing limits**
Up to 10 mg per twenty-four hours.

**Usual geriatric dose**
See *Usual adult dose.*

Note: Geriatric patients may be more sensitive to the effects of the usual adult dose.

**Strength(s) usually available**
U.S.—
Not commercially available.
Canada—
20 mg per 2 mL (Rx) [GENERIC].

**Packaging and storage**
Store between 2 and 8 °C (36 and 46 °F).

**Stability**
Solution should not be used if it turns green or brown or contains a precipitate.

**Incompatibilities**
Physically incompatible with alkalis, iodides, tannins, iron salts, and oxidizing agents.

## Selected Bibliography

Wheeler-Usher DH, Wanke LA, Bayer MJ. Gastric emptying—Risk versus benefit in the treatment of acute poisoning. Med Toxicol 1986; 1: 142-53.
Rodgers GC, Matyunas NJ. Gastrointestinal decontamination for acute poisoning. Pediatr Clin North Am 1986; 33: 261-85.

Revised: 03/02/94

---

# APPETITE SUPPRESSANTS   Systemic

This monograph includes information on the following: Benzphetamine†; Diethylpropion; Fenfluramine; Mazindol; Phendimetrazine†; Phentermine.
INN:
Benzphetamine—Benzfetamine
Diethylpropion—Amfepramone
VA CLASSIFICATION (Primary/Secondary):
Benzphetamine—GA751
Diethylpropion—GA751
Fenfluramine—GA751/CN900
Mazindol—GA751
Phendimetrazine—GA751
Phentermine—GA751

Note: Controlled substances in the U.S. and Canada as follows:

| Drug | U.S. | Canada |
|---|---|---|
| Benzphetamine | III | † |
| Diethylpropion | IV | C |
| Fenfluramine | IV | |
| Mazindol | IV | |
| Phendimetrazine | III | † |
| Phentermine | IV | C |

†Not commercially available in Canada.

Note: For a listing of dosage forms and brand names by country availability, see *Dosage Forms* section(s). For a listing of brand names for the articles in this monograph, refer to the General Index.

†Not commercially available in Canada.

## Category

Appetite suppressant.

## Indications

Note: Bracketed information in the *Indications* section refers to uses that are not included in U.S. product labeling.

**Accepted**
Obesity, exogenous (treatment)—Appetite suppressants are indicated in the management of exogenous obesity for short-term use (a few weeks) in conjunction with a regimen of weight reduction based on caloric restriction, exercise, and behavior modification. The limited usefulness of these agents should be measured against risk factors inherent in their use.

[Autism, infantile (treatment)][1]—Fenfluramine appears to be beneficial in treating some autistic children by decreasing motor activity, distractability and inattention, and mood disturbances. These changes may be accompanied by a decrease in serum serotonin concentration that is not necessarily related to initial serotonin concentrations, nor does it predict a clinical response.

---

[1]Not included in Canadian product labeling.

## Pharmacology/Pharmacokinetics

**Physicochemical characteristics**
Molecular weight—
Benzphetamine hydrochloride: 275.82.
Diethylpropion hydrochloride: 241.76.
Fenfluramine hydrochloride: 267.72.
Mazindol: 284.74.
Phendimetrazine tartrate: 341.36.
Phentermine: 149.24.
Phentermine hydrochloride: 185.70.

**Mechanism of action/Effect**
Although the mechanism of action of the appetite suppressants has not been completely established, they are sympathomimetic amines and have pharmacological effects similar to those of amphetamines, including central nervous system (CNS) stimulation and elevation of blood pressure. Tachyphylaxis or tolerance to appetite suppression has been shown to develop. It is believed that the main effect of these medications is on the appetite control center in the hypothalamus and that hunger is decreased by alteration of the chemical control of nerve impulse transmission.
Fenfluramine differs from the other appetite suppressants in that it is more likely to produce CNS depression instead of stimulation, and, often, a decrease in blood pressure. Its main CNS action is probably through serotonin metabolism instead of dopamine and norepinephrine metabolism.
Mazindol differs by lacking the phenethylamine structure of the other appetite suppressants. It appears to inhibit neuronal uptake of norepinephrine and synaptically released dopamine.
It has not been established that the action of these medications in treating obesity is primarily suppression of appetite. Other CNS actions and/or metabolic effects may be involved.

**Biotransformation**
Hepatic.

| Drug | Half-life (hr) | Duration of Action (hr) | Elimination |
|---|---|---|---|
| Benzphetamine | 6–12 | | |
| Diethylpropion | 4–6 | | Renal |
| Tablets | | 4 | |
| Extended-release Tablets | | 12 | |
| Fenfluramine | 11–30 | 4–6 | Renal |
| Mazindol | 10 | 8–15 | Renal |
| Phendimetrazine | 5–12.5 | 4 | |
| Phentermine | 19–24 | | Renal |
| Capsules, Tablets (8 mg) | | 4 | |
| Capsules (30 mg), Tablets (37.5 mg), or Resin Capsules | | 12–14 | |

## Precautions to Consider

**Cross-sensitivity and/or related problems**
Patients sensitive to other sympathomimetics (for example, amphetamines, ephedrine, epinephrine, isoproterenol, metaproterenol, norepinephrine,

phenylephrine, phenylpropanolamine, pseudoephedrine, terbutaline) may be sensitive to this medication also.

## Carcinogenicity/Mutagenicity
Studies have not been done.

## Pregnancy/Reproduction
Pregnancy—
*Benzphetamine*—
Benzphetamine is contraindicated during pregnancy because it may cause harm to the fetus. If pregnancy occurs during therapy, the patient should be informed of the risk to the fetus.
Studies in mammals have shown amphetamines to be teratogenic and embryotoxic when given in high multiples of the human dose.
FDA Pregnancy Category X.
*Diethylpropion*—
Adequate and well controlled studies in humans have not been done. Abuse of diethylpropion during pregnancy may result in withdrawal symptoms in the neonate since diethylpropion and its active metabolites are believed to cross the placenta.
Studies in rats given up to 9 times the human dose have shown no evidence of impaired fertility or harm to the fetus.
FDA Pregnancy Category B.
*Fenfluramine*—
Studies in humans have not been done.
Studies in animals have shown that fenfluramine is potentially embryotoxic and reduces conception rate when given in doses 20 times the human dose.
FDA Pregnancy Category C.
*Mazindol*—
Reproduction studies in animals have shown that mazindol increases neonatal mortality and possibly increases the incidence of rib anomalies when given in relatively high doses.
FDA pregnancy category not currently included in product labeling.
*Phendimetrazine*—
Problems with phendimetrazine in humans have not been documented.
FDA pregnancy category not currently included in product labeling.
*Phentermine*—
Problems with phentermine in humans have not been documented.
FDA pregnancy category not currently included in product labeling.

## Breast-feeding
Diethylpropion and its metabolites and benzphetamine are distributed into breast milk. It is not known if the other appetite suppressants are distributed into breast milk and problems in nursing infants have not been documented.

## Pediatrics
Appetite suppressants are not recommended for use in children up to 12 years of age, because appropriate studies have not been performed in the pediatric population.

## Geriatrics
No information is available on the relationship of age to the effects of the appetite suppressants in geriatric patients.

## Dental
Appetite suppressants may decrease or inhibit salivary flow, especially in middle-aged or elderly patients, thus contributing to the development of caries, periodontal disease, oral candidiasis, and discomfort.
The leukopenic and thrombocytopenic effects of diethylpropion, although rarely reported, may result in an increased incidence of microbial infection, delayed healing, and gingival bleeding. If leukopenia or thrombocytopenia occurs, dental work should be deferred until blood counts have returned to normal. Patient instruction in proper oral hygiene should include caution in use of regular toothbrushes, dental floss, and toothpicks.

## Drug interactions and/or related problems
See *Table 1*, page 454.

## Medical considerations/Contraindications
See *Table 2*, page 455.

## Side/Adverse Effects
Note: Although not all of these side effects have been attributed specifically to each appetite suppressant, a potential exists for their occurrence during the use of any appetite suppressant.

The following side/adverse effects have been selected on the basis of their potential clinical significance (possible signs and symptoms in parentheses where appropriate)—not necessarily inclusive:

**Those indicating need for medical attention**
Incidence more frequent
*Elevated blood pressure*—rare with fenfluramine
Incidence less frequent or rare
*Allergic reaction* (skin rash or hives); *blood dyscrasias* (sore throat and fever; unusual bleeding or bruising)—with diethylpropion; *confusion or mental depression; psychotic episodes; pulmonary hypertension* (difficult or troubled breathing brought on by physical effort)—with fenfluramine

**Those indicating need for medical attention only if they continue or are bothersome**
Incidence more frequent
*CNS stimulation* (false sense of well-being or mild euphoria; irritability; nervousness or restlessness; trouble in sleeping)
Note: Drowsiness, fatigue, or mental depression may follow the stimulant effects.

Incidence less frequent or rare
*Blurred vision; changes in libido* (changes in sexual desire); *constipation; clumsiness or unsteadiness*—with fenfluramine; *diarrhea; difficulty in talking*—with fenfluramine; *dizziness or lightheadedness; drowsiness; dryness of mouth; dysuria* (difficult or painful urination); *fast, pounding, or irregular heartbeat; headache; impotence* (decreased sexual ability); *increased sweating; nausea or vomiting; nightmares*—with fenfluramine; *polyuria or urinary frequency* (frequent urge to urinate or increased urination); *stomach cramps or pain; unpleasant taste; unusual tiredness or weakness*—with fenfluramine

**Those indicating possible withdrawal and/or the need for medical attention if they occur after medication is discontinued**
*Mental depression; nausea or vomiting; stomach cramps or pain; trembling; trouble in sleeping or nightmares; unusual tiredness or weakness*

## Overdose
For specific information on the agents used in the management of appetite suppressant overdose, see:
- *Barbiturates (Systemic)* monograph;
- *Beta-adrenergic Blocking Agents (Systemic)* monograph;
- *Charcoal, Activated (Oral-Local)* monograph;
- *Chlorpromazine* in *Phenothiazines (Systemic)* monograph;
- *Diazepam* in *Benzodiazepines (Systemic)* monograph;
- *Haloperidol (Systemic)* monograph;
- *Lidocaine (Systemic)* monograph;
- *Nitrates (Systemic)* monograph; and/or
- *Phentolamine (Systemic)* monograph.

For more information on the management of overdose or unintentional ingestion, **contact a Poison Control Center** (see *Poison Control Center Listing*).

### Clinical effects of overdose
The following effects have been selected on the basis of their potential clinical significance (possible signs and symptoms in parentheses where appropriate)—not necessarily inclusive:

*Abdominal or stomach cramps; arrhythmias* (irregular heartbeat); *confusion; diarrhea, severe; fast breathing; fever; hostility with assaultiveness; hallucinations* (seeing, hearing, or feeling things that are not there); *irregular blood pressure; nausea or vomiting, severe; panic state; restlessness; tremor*

Note: Hyperpyrexia, rhabdomyolysis, cardiovascular effects such as arrhythmias, hypertension or hypotension, and circulatory collapse may occur. Convulsions and coma usually precede death.
Diarrhea, hostility, hallucinations, irregular blood pressure, panic state, rhabdomyolysis, and cardiovascular effects have not been reported for fenfluramine.

### Treatment of overdose
Since there is no specific antidote for overdosage with appetite suppressants, treatment is symptomatic and supportive with possible utilization of the following:
To decrease absorption—
Induction of emesis and/or use of gastric lavage followed by the administration of activated charcoal is primary (fenfluramine overdose may produce early unconsciousness; drug-induced emesis is not recommended for fenfluramine).
To enhance elimination—
Acidification of urine and forced diuresis are recommended.

Specific treatment—
    Barbiturate sedatives or chlorpromazine (or haloperidol to lessen anticholinergic effects) are sometimes used to control excessive CNS stimulation. (Diazepam or phenobarbital may be used to control convulsions or muscular hyperactivity associated with fenfluramine overdosage. Caution necessary with use of CNS depressants and fenfluramine because of possible additive CNS depressant effects.)
    Intravenous phentolamine or nitrites to control hypertension.
    Intravenous lidocaine for cardiac arrhythmias.
    Beta-blocker for control of tachycardia.
Monitoring—
    Monitor cardiovascular and respiratory functions.
Supportive care—
    Intravenous fluids for hypotension control.
    Mechanical respirator, when necessary.
    Protect patient from self-injury by use of restraints if necessary.
    Patients in whom intentional overdose is known or suspected should be referred for psychiatric consultation.

## Patient Consultation

As an aid to patient consultation, refer to *Advice for the Patient, Appetite Suppressants (Systemic)* or *Fenfluramine (Systemic)*.

In providing consultation, consider emphasizing the following selected information (» = major clinical significance):

**Before using this medication**
» Conditions affecting use, especially:
    Sensitivity to appetite suppressants or other sympathomimetics
    Pregnancy—Benzphetamine is contraindicated in human pregnancy (FDA Category X); in animal studies, fenfluramine was shown to be embryotoxic and to reduce rate of conception; mazindol was shown to increase the incidence of neonatal mortality and possibly to increase the incidence of rib anomalies when given in relatively high doses
    Breast-feeding—Benzphetamine and diethylpropion are distributed into breast milk
    Use in children—Not recommended for appetite suppression in children up to 12 years of age
    Other medications, especially alcohol, MAO inhibitors, other CNS stimulants (with all appetite suppressants except fenfluramine), or CNS depressants (with fenfluramine)
    Other medical problems, especially agitated states, alcoholism, advanced arteriosclerosis, symptomatic cardiovascular disease including arrhythmias, cerebral ischemia, history of drug abuse or dependence, glaucoma, hypertension, hyperthyroidism, psychosis, or uremia

**Proper use of this medication**
    Taking the last dose of the regular dosage form for each day about 4 to 6 hours before bedtime (does not apply to fenfluramine)
» Importance of not taking more medication than the amount prescribed, because of habit-forming potential
» Not increasing dose if medication is not effective after a few weeks; checking with physician
» Proper dosing
» Proper storage
*For extended-release and long-acting dosage forms only*
    Proper administration: Swallowing whole; not breaking, crushing, or chewing
    Taking the daily dose about 10 to 14 hours before bedtime to minimize the possibility of insomnia (does not apply to fenfluramine)
*For mazindol*
    1-mg tablet—Taking last dose 4 to 6 hours before bedtime
    2-mg tablet—Taking once-a-day dose 10 to 14 hours before bedtime

**Precautions while using this medication**
    Regular visits to physician to check progress during therapy
    Possible dryness of mouth; using sugarless candy or gum, ice, or saliva substitute for relief; checking with physician or dentist if dry mouth continues for more than 2 weeks
» Caution if dizziness, drowsiness, lightheadedness, or elated mood or euphoria occurs; not driving or using machines or doing other things that require alertness
» Caution if any kind of surgery, dental treatment, or emergency treatment is required
» Suspected physical or psychological dependence: checking with physician
» Not increasing dosage if tolerance develops; checking with physician
    Diabetic patients: Insulin or oral antidiabetic–agent requirements may be altered

» Checking with physician before discontinuing medication after prolonged high-dose therapy; gradual dosage reduction may be necessary to avoid possibility of withdrawal symptoms
*For fenfluramine*
» Avoiding the use of alcoholic beverages or other CNS depressants

**Side/adverse effects**
    Symptoms of potential side effects, especially increased blood pressure, allergic reaction, blood dyscrasias (with diethylpropion), confusion or mental depression, psychotic episodes, or pulmonary hypertension (with fenfluramine)

## General Dosing Information

The dosage of appetite suppressants should be individualized to obtain an adequate response with the lowest effective dose.

To reduce the possibility of insomnia caused by appetite suppressants (except fenfluramine), the last dose of the regular dosage form for each day should be administered approximately 4 to 6 hours before bedtime and the daily dose of the extended-release or long-acting dosage form should be administered approximately 10 to 14 hours before bedtime.

Appetite suppressants are recommended for short-term use only, since tolerance to the anorectic effect may develop in a few weeks.

If tolerance to the anorectic effect develops, the medication should be discontinued. The dosage should not be increased in an attempt to increase the effect.

Prolonged use, especially of larger than usual therapeutic doses, may result in mental or physical dependence.

When the medication is to be discontinued following prolonged high-dose administration, the dosage should be reduced gradually in order to avoid the possibility of a rebound increase in appetite and to decrease withdrawal symptoms.

---

### *BENZPHETAMINE*

## Summary of Differences

Precautions:
    Pregnancy/reproduction—FDA Pregnancy Category X.
    Drug interactions and/or related problems—Caution is needed with concomitant use of urinary acidifiers and alkalizers with benzphetamine.

## Additional Dosing Information

See also *General Dosing Information*.

If a single daily dose is administered, it is preferably given either midmorning or mid-afternoon, depending on the patient's eating habits.

## Oral Dosage Forms

### BENZPHETAMINE HYDROCHLORIDE TABLETS

**Usual adult dose**
Appetite suppressant—
    Oral, initially 25 to 50 mg once a day in midmorning or midafternoon, the dosage being increased as needed and tolerated.

**Usual adult prescribing limits**
Up to 150 mg a day.

**Usual pediatric dose**
Children up to 12 years of age—Use is not recommended.

**Strength(s) usually available**
U.S.—
    50 mg (Rx) [*Didrex* (scored; lactose; sorbitol)].
Canada—
    Not commercially available.

**Packaging and storage**
Store between 15 and 30 °C (59 and 86 °F), in a tight container, unless otherwise specified by manufacturer.

**Note**
Controlled substance in the U.S.

---

### *DIETHYLPROPION*

## Summary of Differences

Precautions:
    Medical considerations/contraindications—Caution also needed in epilepsy.

## Oral Dosage Forms

### DIETHYLPROPION HYDROCHLORIDE TABLETS USP

**Usual adult dose**
Appetite suppressant—
Oral, 25 mg three times a day, one hour before meals. Alternatively, a dose may be taken in mid-evening, if desired, to overcome night hunger.

**Usual pediatric dose**
Children up to 12 years of age—Use is not recommended.

**Strength(s) usually available**
U.S.—
25 mg (Rx) [*Tenuate* (lactose); GENERIC].
Canada—
25 mg (Rx) [*Tenuate* (tartrazine)].

**Packaging and storage**
Store below 40 °C (104 °F), preferably between 15 and 30 °C (59 and 86 °F), unless otherwise specified by manufacturer. Store in a well-closed container.

**Note**
Controlled substance in both the U.S. and Canada.

### DIETHYLPROPION HYDROCHLORIDE EXTENDED-RELEASE TABLETS

**Usual adult dose**
Appetite suppressant—
Oral, 75 mg once a day at mid-morning.

**Usual pediatric dose**
Children up to 12 years of age—Use is not recommended.

**Strength(s) usually available**
U.S.—
75 mg (Rx) [*Tenuate Dospan; Tepanil Ten-Tab;* GENERIC].
Canada—
75 mg (Rx) [*Tenuate Dospan*].

**Packaging and storage**
Store below 40 °C (104 °F), preferably between 15 and 30 °C (59 and 86 °F), in a well-closed container, unless otherwise specified by manufacturer.

**Auxiliary labeling**
• Swallow tablets whole.

**Note**
Controlled substance in both the U.S. and Canada.

---

### FENFLURAMINE

## Summary of Differences

Indications:
Also used for treatment of infantile autism.
Pharmacology/pharmacokinetics:
More likely to produce CNS depression instead of CNS stimulation.
Precautions:
Pregnancy—
Animal reproduction studies have suggested an embryotoxic potential.
Drug interactions and/or related problems—
Hypotensive effects of antihypertensives may be increased with concurrent use of fenfluramine.
Enhanced CNS depressant effects may result from concurrent use of fenfluramine and CNS depression–producing medications.
No additive effects with CNS stimulation–producing medications or thyroid hormones.
No potential interaction with phenothiazines.
Medical considerations/contraindications—
Not contraindicated in agitated states, advanced arteriosclerosis, or hyperthyroidism.
Caution needed in patients with history of mental depression.
Side/adverse effects:
Elevated blood pressure is rare with fenfluramine.
Pulmonary hypertension may occur rarely.
CNS depressant side effects, such as drowsiness, occur more frequently than with other appetite suppressants.

## Additional Dosing Information

See also *General Dosing Information.*
Fenfluramine has an onset of action of 1 to 2 hours.

## Oral Dosage Forms

### FENFLURAMINE HYDROCHLORIDE EXTENDED-RELEASE CAPSULES

**Usual adult dose**
Appetite suppressant—
Oral, initially 60 mg once a day, the dosage being increased to 120 mg per day as needed and tolerated.

**Usual adult prescribing limits**
Up to 120 mg a day.

**Usual pediatric dose**
Appetite suppressant—
Children up to 12 years of age: Use is not recommended.

**Strength(s) usually available**
U.S.—
Not commercially available.
Canada—
60 mg (Rx) [*Ponderal Pacaps*].

**Packaging and storage**
Store below 40 °C (104 °F), preferably between 15 and 30 °C (59 and 86 °F), in a well-closed container, unless otherwise specified by manufacturer.

**Auxiliary labeling**
• Swallow capsules whole.

### FENFLURAMINE HYDROCHLORIDE TABLETS

**Usual adult dose**
Appetite suppressant—
Oral, initially 20 mg three times a day thirty minutes to one hour before meals, the dosage being increased by 20 mg per day at one-week intervals, if necessary, up to a maximum of 40 mg three times a day.
Note: If the initial dosage is not well tolerated, the dosage may be reduced to 20 mg twice daily and thereafter increased gradually in order to minimize side effects.

**Usual adult prescribing limits**
Up to 120 mg a day.

**Usual pediatric dose**
Appetite suppressant—
Children up to 12 years of age: Use is not recommended.

**Strength(s) usually available**
U.S.—
20 mg (Rx) [*Pondimin* (scored)].
Canada—
20 mg (Rx) [*Ponderal* (scored); *Pondimin* (scored; sodium < 1 mmol [0.10 mg])].

**Packaging and storage**
Store below 40 °C (104 °F), preferably between 15 and 30 °C (59 and 86 °F), in a well-closed container, unless otherwise specified by manufacturer.

**Note**
Controlled substance in the U.S.

---

### MAZINDOL

## Summary of Differences

Precautions:
Pregnancy—
Animal studies have suggested a teratogenic potential with high doses.
Drug interactions and/or related problems—
Effects of vasopressors may be potentiated when used concomitantly with mazindol.
Medical considerations/contraindications—
Contraindicated in cerebral ischemia, psychosis, and uremia.
Not contraindicated in advanced arteriosclerosis or hyperthyroidism.

## Oral Dosage Forms

### MAZINDOL TABLETS USP

**Usual adult dose**
Appetite suppressant—
Oral, initially, 1 mg once daily one hour before the first meal of the day, the dosage being increased to 1 mg three times a day one hour before meals; or 2 mg once a day one hour before lunch.

**Usual pediatric dose**
Children up to 12 years of age—Use is not recommended.

**Strength(s) usually available**
U.S.—
    1 mg (Rx) [*Mazanor* (scored; lactose); *Sanorex* (lactose)].
    2 mg (Rx) [*Sanorex* (scored; lactose)].
Canada—
    1 mg (Rx) [*Sanorex* (corn starch; lactose)].
    2 mg (Rx) [*Sanorex* (scored; corn starch; lactose; tartrazine)].

**Packaging and storage**
Store below 25 °C (77 °F), unless otherwise specified by manufacturer. Store in a tight container.

**Note**
Controlled substance in the U.S.

---

## *PHENDIMETRAZINE*

# Oral Dosage Forms

## PHENDIMETRAZINE TARTRATE CAPSULES USP

**Usual adult dose**
Appetite suppressant—
    Oral, 35 mg two or three times a day one hour before meals.

**Usual adult prescribing limits**
70 mg three times a day.

**Usual pediatric dose**
Children up to 12 years of age—Use is not recommended.

**Strength(s) usually available**
U.S.—
    35 mg (Rx) [*Obalan; Phendiet; Wehless;* GENERIC].
Canada—
    Not commercially available.

**Packaging and storage**
Store below 40 °C (104 °F), preferably between 15 and 30 °C (59 and 86 °F), unless otherwise specified by manufacturer. Store in a tight container.

**Note**
Controlled substance in the U.S.

## PHENDIMETRAZINE TARTRATE EXTENDED-RELEASE CAPSULES

**Usual adult dose**
Appetite suppressant—
    Oral, 105 mg once a day, thirty to sixty minutes before the morning meal.

**Usual pediatric dose**
Children up to 12 years of age—Use is not recommended.

**Strength(s) usually available**
U.S.—
    105 mg (Rx) [*Adipost; Anorex SR; Appecon; Bontril Slow-Release; Melfiat-105 Unicelles; Phendiet-105; Prelu-2; PT 105; Rexigen Forte; Wehless-105 Timecelles;* GENERIC].
Canada—
    Not commercially available.

**Packaging and storage**
Store below 40 °C (104 °F), preferably between 15 and 30 °C (59 and 86 °F), in a well-closed container, unless otherwise specified by manufacturer.

**Auxiliary labeling**
• Swallow capsules whole.

**Note**
Controlled substance in the U.S.

## PHENDIMETRAZINE TARTRATE TABLETS USP

**Usual adult dose**
Appetite suppressant—
    Oral, 17.5 to 35 mg two or three times a day one hour before meals.

**Usual adult prescribing limits**
70 mg three times a day.

**Usual pediatric dose**
Children up to 12 years of age—Use is not recommended.

**Strength(s) usually available**
U.S.—
    35 mg (Rx) [*Bontril PDM* (scored); *Obalan; Obezine; Parzine; Phendiet; Phendimet; Plegine* (scored); GENERIC].
Canada—
    Not commercially available.

**Packaging and storage**
Store below 40 °C (104 °F), preferably between 15 and 30 °C (59 and 86 °F), unless otherwise specified by manufacturer. Store in a well-closed container.

**Note**
Controlled substance in the U.S.

## PHENDIMETRAZINE TARTRATE EXTENDED-RELEASE TABLETS

**Usual adult dose**
See *Phendimetrazine Tartrate Extended-Release Capsules.*

**Usual pediatric dose**
See *Phendimetrazine Tartrate Extended-Release Capsules.*

**Strength(s) usually available**
U.S.—
    105 mg (Rx) [GENERIC].
Canada—
    Not commercially available.

**Packaging and storage**
Store below 40 °C (104 °F), preferably between 15 and 30 °C (59 and 86 °F), in a well-closed container, unless otherwise specified by manufacturer.

**Auxiliary labeling**
• Swallow capsules whole.

**Note**
Controlled substance in the U.S.

---

## *PHENTERMINE*

# Oral Dosage Forms

## PHENTERMINE HYDROCHLORIDE CAPSULES USP

**Usual adult dose**
Appetite suppressant—
    Oral, 15 to 37.5 mg (base) once a day before breakfast, or one to two hours after breakfast.

**Usual pediatric dose**
Children up to 12 years of age—Use is not recommended.

**Strength(s) usually available**
U.S.—
    15 mg (base) (Rx) [*Phentride;* GENERIC].
    18.75 mg (base) (Rx) [*Phentercot;* GENERIC].
    30 mg (base) (Rx) [*Fastin; Obe-Nix; OBY-CAP; Phentercot; Phentride; T-Diet; Teramine; Zantryl;* GENERIC].
    37.5 mg (base) (Rx) [*Adipex-P; Obe-Nix; Phentercot; Phentride;* GENERIC].
Canada—
    30 mg (base) (Rx) [*Fastin*].

**Packaging and storage**
Store below 40 °C (104 °F), preferably between 15 and 30 °C (59 and 86 °F), unless otherwise specified by manufacturer. Store in a tight container.

**Note**
Controlled substance in both the U.S. and Canada.

## PHENTERMINE HYDROCHLORIDE TABLETS USP

**Usual adult dose**
Appetite suppressant—
    Oral, 15 to 37.5 mg (base) a day, as a single dose before breakfast or one to two hours after breakfast, or in divided doses one half hour before meals.

**Usual pediatric dose**
Children up to 12 years of age—Use is not recommended.

**Strength(s) usually available**
U.S.—
    8 mg (base) (Rx) [*Phentercot; Phentride; Teramine;* GENERIC].
    30 mg (base) (Rx) [*Phentride;* GENERIC].

37.5 mg (base) (Rx) [*Adipex-P* (scored); *Panshape M; Phentercot;* GENERIC].

Canada—
Not commercially available.

### Packaging and storage
Store below 40 °C (104 °F), preferably between 15 and 30 °C (59 and 86 °F), unless otherwise specified by manufacturer. Store in a tight container.

### Note
Controlled substance in the U.S.

## PHENTERMINE RESIN CAPSULES

### Usual adult dose
Appetite suppressant—
Oral, 15 or 30 mg once a day before breakfast.

### Usual pediatric dose
Children up to 12 years of age—Use is not recommended.

### Strength(s) usually available
U.S.—
15 mg (Rx) [*Ionamin;* GENERIC].
30 mg (Rx) [*Ionamin;* GENERIC].
Canada—
15 mg (Rx) [*Ionamin*].
30 mg (Rx) [*Ionamin*].

### Packaging and storage
Store between 15 and 30 °C (59 and 86 °F), in a tight container, unless otherwise specified by manufacturer.

### Auxiliary labeling
• Swallow capsules whole.
• Take in the morning.

### Note
Controlled substance in both the U.S. and Canada.

Revised: 08/29/94
Interim revision: 06/30/95

## Table 1. Drug Interactions and/or Related Problems

The following drug interactions and/or related problems have been selected on the basis of their potential clinical significance (possible mechanism in parentheses where appropriate)—not necessarily inclusive (» = major clinical significance):

Note: Combinations containing any of the following medications, depending on the amount present, may also interact with this medication.

Legend:
I=Benzphetamine    IV=Mazindol
II=Diethylpropion   V=Phendimetrazine
III=Fenfluramine    VI=Phentermine

| | I | II | III | IV | V | VI |
|---|---|---|---|---|---|---|
| Acidifiers, urinary, such as:<br>Ammonium chloride<br>Ascorbic acid<br>Potassium or sodium phosphates<br>(concurrent use with benzphetamine may decrease serum concentrations and increase excretion of benzphetamine) | ✔ | | | | | |
| » Alcohol<br>(concurrent use with appetite suppressants is not recommended since this may increase the potential for CNS effects such as dizziness, lightheadedness, fainting, confusion, or drowsiness [with fenfluramine]) | ✔ | ✔ | ✔ | ✔ | ✔ | ✔ |
| Alkalizers, urinary, such as:<br>Antacids, calcium- and/or magnesium-containing<br>Carbonic anhydrase inhibitors<br>Citrates<br>Sodium bicarbonate<br>(concurrent use with benzphetamine may increase serum concentrations and decrease excretion of benzphetamine) | ✔ | | | | | |
| Anesthetics, hydrocarbon inhalation, especially halothane<br>(chronic use of appetite suppressants prior to anesthesia may result in cardiac arrhythmias because these anesthetics sensitize the myocardium to the effects of sympathomimetics) | ✔ | ✔ | ✔ | ✔ | ✔ | ✔ |
| Antidiabetic agents, oral, or<br>Insulin<br>(when appetite suppressants and the concurrent dietary regimen are used in the treatment of obesity, blood glucose concentrations may be altered in patients with diabetes mellitus; dosage adjustment of the hypoglycemic agent may be necessary during and after concurrent therapy) | ✔ | ✔ | ✔ | ✔ | ✔ | ✔ |
| Antihypertensives, especially clonidine, guanadrel, guanethidine, methyldopa, or rauwolfia alkaloids<br>(hypotensive effects may be increased when used concurrently with fenfluramine) | | | ✔ | | | |
| (hypotensive effects may be decreased when these medications are used concurrently with appetite suppressants because of displacement from and inhibition of uptake by adrenergic neurons) | ✔ | ✔ | | ✔ | ✔ | ✔ |
| » CNS depression–producing medications, other (See *Appendix II*)<br>(concurrent use may increase the CNS depressant effects of either these medications or fenfluramine) | | | ✔ | | | |
| » CNS stimulation–producing medications, other (See *Appendix II*), or<br>Thyroid hormones<br>(concurrent use may increase the CNS stimulant effects of either these medications or appetite suppressants) | ✔ | ✔ | | ✔ | ✔ | ✔ |
| » Monoamine oxidase (MAO) inhibitors, including furazolidone, procarbazine, and selegiline<br>(concurrent use may potentiate the sympathomimetic effects of appetite suppressants, possibly resulting in a hypertensive crisis; appetite suppressants should not be administered during or within 14 days following the administration of MAO inhibitors) | ✔ | ✔ | ✔ | ✔ | ✔ | ✔ |

## Table 1. Drug Interactions and/or Related Problems *(continued)*

| | Legend:<br>**I**=Benzphetamine<br>**II**=Diethylpropion<br>**III**=Fenfluramine | | | **IV**=Mazindol<br>**V**=Phendimetrazine<br>**VI**=Phentermine | | |
|---|---|---|---|---|---|---|
| | **I** | **II** | **III** | **IV** | **V** | **VI** |
| Phenothiazines, especially chlorpromazine<br>(concurrent use may antagonize the anorectic effect of appetite suppressants) | ✔ | ✔ | | ✔ | ✔ | ✔ |
| Vasopressors<br>(effects may be potentiated when vasopressors are used concurrently with mazindol; if necessary to administer a pressor amine agent to a patient who has recently received mazindol, initiating pressor therapy in reduced dosage and monitoring of blood pressure at frequent intervals are recommended) | | | | | | |

## Table 2. Medical considerations/Contraindications

| The medical considerations/contraindications included have been selected on the basis of their potential clinical significance (reasons given in parentheses where appropriate)—not necessarily inclusive (**»** = major clinical significance).* | Legend:<br>**I**=Benzphetamine<br>**II**=Diethylpropion<br>**III**=Fenfluramine | | | **IV**=Mazindol<br>**V**=Phendimetrazine<br>**VI**=Phentermine | | |
|---|---|---|---|---|---|---|
| | **I** | **II** | **III** | **IV** | **V** | **VI** |
| ***Except under special circumstances, this medicine should not be used when the following medical problems exist:*** | | | | | | |
| »    Agitated states or | ✔ | ✔ | | ✔ | ✔ | ✔ |
| »    Arteriosclerosis, advanced or | ✔ | ✔ | | ✔ | ✔ | ✔ |
| »    Cardiovascular disease, symptomatic, including arrhythmias or | ✔ | | ✔ | ✔ | ✔ | ✔ |
| »    Cerebral ischemia or | ✔ | | | ✔ | ✔ | ✔ |
| »    Glaucoma or | ✔ | ✔ | | ✔ | ✔ | ✔ |
| »    Hypertension, moderate to severe or | ✔ | ✔ | ✔ | ✔ | ✔ | ✔ |
| »    Hyperthyroidism or | ✔ | ✔ | | ✔ | ✔ | ✔ |
| »    Psychosis<br>(condition may be exacerbated) | | | | ✔ | ✔ | |
| »    Alcoholism, active or in remission, or | ✔ | ✔ | ✔ | ✔ | ✔ | ✔ |
| »    Drug abuse or dependence, history of<br>(dependence on appetite suppressants may develop) | ✔ | ✔ | ✔ | ✔ | ✔ | ✔ |
| »    Uremia<br>(excretion of appetite suppressants may be altered) | | | | ✔ | | |
| ***Risk-benefit should be considered when the following medical problems exist:*** | | | | | | |
| Cardiovascular disease, symptomatic, including arrhythmias or<br>Depression, mental, history of or<br>Hypertension, mild or<br>Psychosis, especially schizophrenia<br>(condition may be exacerbated) | ✔<br>✔ | ✔<br>✔<br>✔<br>✔ | ✔ | ✔<br>✔ | ✔<br>✔ | ✔<br>✔ |
| Diabetes mellitus<br>(use of appetite suppressants and concomitant dietary restrictions may change the amount of insulin or oral antidiabetic agents needed) | ✔ | ✔ | ✔ | ✔ | ✔ | ✔ |
| Epilepsy<br>(increased risk of seizures) | | ✔ | | | | |
| Sensitivity to appetite suppressants or other sympathomimetics | ✔ | ✔ | ✔ | ✔ | ✔ | ✔ |

*Fenfluramine differs from the other appetite suppressants in that it is more likely to produce CNS depression instead of CNS stimulation.

---

# APRACLONIDINE   Ophthalmic

VA CLASSIFICATION (Primary): OP100/OP900

Other commonly used names are aplonidine and p-aminoclonidine.

Note: For a listing of dosage forms and brand names by country availability, see *Dosage Forms* section(s). For a listing of brand names for the articles in this monograph, refer to the General Index.

## Category

Antiglaucoma agent (ophthalmic); antihypertensive, ocular.

## Indications

### Accepted

Glaucoma, open angle (treatment)—Apraclonidine 0.5% is indicated for short-term adjunctive therapy in patients who are on maximally tolerated doses of other medications intended to reduce intraocular pressure (IOP) and who need additional IOP reduction. Patients who already receive two aqueous suppressing medications (e.g., a beta-adrenergic blocking agent and a carbonic anhydrase inhibitor) may not derive additional IOP reduction from the addition of apraclonidine to their treatment regimen, since apraclonidine is also an aqueous-suppressing medication.

Hypertension, ocular (prophylaxis and treatment)—Apraclonidine 1% is indicated to control or prevent postsurgical elevations in intraocular pressure that occur in patients after argon laser trabeculoplasty, argon laser iridotomy, or Nd:YAG laser posterior capsulotomy.

## Pharmacology/Pharmacokinetics

### Physicochemical characteristics
Molecular weight—281.57.
pKa—9.22.
Other characteristics—The pH of apraclonidine hydrochloride ophthalmic solution is 4.4 to 7.8

### Mechanism of action/Effect
Apraclonidine is a relatively selective alpha$_2$ adrenergic agonist. When instilled into the eye, apraclonidine ophthalmic solution reduces elevated, as well as normal, intraocular pressure. Aqueous fluorophotometry studies demonstrate that the predominant mechanism of action of ophthalmic apraclonidine is the reduction of aqueous humor flow via stimulation of the alpha-adrenergic system.

### Other actions/effects
Apraclonidine does not have significant membrane stabilizing (local anesthetic) activity. In addition, ophthalmic apraclonidine has minimal effect on cardiovascular parameters.

### Half-life
For 0.5% apraclonidine—8 hours.

### Onset of action
Usually within one hour.

### Peak serum concentration
For 0.5% apraclonidine—0.9 nanograms per mL.

### Time to peak effect
Usually three to five hours after application of a single dose.

## Precautions to Consider

### Cross-sensitivity and/or related problems
Patients sensitive to clonidine may be sensitive to apraclonidine also.

### Carcinogenicity
Rats and mice administered oral apraclonidine for 2 years in doses of 1 and 0.6 mg per kg of body weight (mg/kg), respectively, did not have any significant change in tumor incidence or type.

### Mutagenicity
Apraclonidine was not shown to be mutagenic in an *in vivo* mouse micronucleus assay and a series of *in vitro* mutagenicity tests, including the Ames test, a mouse lymphoma forward mutation assay, a chromosome aberration assay in cultured Chinese hamster ovary (CHO) cells, a sister chromatid exchange assay in CHO cells, and a cell transformation assay.

### Pregnancy/Reproduction
Fertility—Studies on reproduction and fertility in male and female rats given 0.5 mg/kg of apraclonidine have not shown adverse effects on fertility.

Pregnancy—Adequate and well-controlled studies have not been done in humans.

Apraclonidine has been shown to have an embryocidal effect on rabbits that were given 3 mg/kg apraclonidine orally. Dose-related maternal toxicity was observed in pregnant rats given 0.3 mg/kg apraclonidine.

FDA Pregnancy Category C.

### Breast-feeding
It is not known whether ophthalmic apraclonidine is distributed into breast milk. However, problems in humans have not been documented. It is recommended that patients do not breast-feed on the day on which 1% apraclonidine is administered.

### Pediatrics
Appropriate studies on the relationship of age to the effects of apraclonidine have not been performed in the pediatric population. Safety and efficacy have not been established.

### Geriatrics
No information is available on the relationship of age to the effects of apraclonidine in geriatric patients.

## Drug interactions and/or related problems
The following drug interactions and/or related problems have been selected on the basis of their potential clinical significance (possible mechanism in parentheses where appropriate)—not necessarily inclusive (» = major clinical significance):

Note: Combinations containing any of the following medications, depending on the amount present, may also interact with this medication.

Monoamine oxidase (MAO) inhibitors, including furazolidone, procarbazine, and selegiline
(some clinicians believe that apraclonidine should not be used during or within 14 days following administration of MAO inhibitors, because the antihypertensive effects of either apraclonidine or the MAO inhibitor may be potentiated by concurrent use; however, this is controversial)

## Medical considerations/Contraindications
The medical considerations/contraindications included here have been selected on the basis of their potential clinical significance (reasons given in parentheses where appropriate)—not necessarily inclusive (» = major clinical significance).

*Risk-benefit should be considered when the following medical problems exist:*

» Cardiovascular disease, severe, including hypertension or
Cerebrovascular disease or
Coronary insufficiency or
Myocardial infarction, recent or
Raynaud's disease or
Thromboangiitis obliterans
(in clinical studies, the total usual adult dose of 2 drops of 1% and short-term three-times-a-day use of 0.5% ophthalmic apraclonidine had minimal effect on heart rate and blood pressure. However, since there is a possibility of systemic absorption and because apraclonidine is a potent medication, caution should be used when administering 0.5 or 1% apraclonidine to patients who have severe cardiovascular disease, including hypertension, and when administering 0.5% apraclonidine to patients with other cardiovascular diseases)

Depression
(use of apraclonidine 0.5% has been infrequently associated with depression; caution is recommended when apraclonidine is used in patients with depression)

Exaggerated response to medications that reduce intraocular pressure
(patients who exhibit an exaggerated response to medications that reduce intraocular pressure should be closely monitored during treatment with apraclonidine, since apraclonidine is a potent depressor of intraocular pressure)

Hepatic function impairment
(since a structurally related medication, clonidine, is partly metabolized in the liver, monitoring of cardiovascular parameters in patients with liver function impairment who are using apraclonidine 0.5% is recommended)

Renal function impairment
(since a structurally related medication, clonidine, undergoes a significant increase in half-life in patients with severe renal impairment, monitoring of cardiovascular parameters in patients with renal function impairment who are using apraclonidine 0.5% is recommended)

Sensitivity to apraclonidine

Vasovagal attack, history of
(the possibility of a vasovagal attack occurring during laser surgery should be considered; caution should be used when administering 1% apraclonidine to patients with a history of this medical problem)

## Patient monitoring
The following may be especially important in patient monitoring (other tests may be warranted in some patients, depending on condition; » = major clinical significance):

Ophthalmology examinations
(patients using 0.5% apraclonidine should have frequent followup examinations to check intraocular pressure, and their visual fields should be monitored periodically)

## Side/Adverse Effects

Note: Ophthalmic apraclonidine 0.5% used three times a day is systemically absorbed; the 2 drops of ophthalmic apraclonidine 1% used during laser surgery may also be systemically absorbed, but it may not be as likely to cause systemic side/adverse effects as is the 0.5% dosage.

The following side/adverse effects have been selected on the basis of their potential clinical significance (possible signs and symptoms in parentheses where appropriate)—not necessarily inclusive:

**Those indicating need for medical attention**
Incidence more frequent
　*For 0.5% ophthalmic apraclonidine*
　　*Allergic reaction* (redness of eye; itching of eye; tearing of eye)

Incidence less frequent or rare
　*For 0.5% ophthalmic apraclonidine*
　　*Abnormal coordination* (clumsiness or unsteadiness); *arrhythmia* (irregular heartbeat); *asthma* (wheezing or troubled breathing); *blepharitis; blepharoconjunctivitis; conjunctivitis* (redness of eye, eyelid, or inner lining of eyelid); *blurred vision or change in vision; chest pain; contact dermatitis* (rash around eyes); *corneal erosion; corneal infiltrate; foreign body sensation; keratitis; keratopathy* (eye redness, irritation, or pain); *depression; dizziness; dyspnea* (troubled breathing); *edema of eye, eyelid, or conjunctiva* (swelling of eye, eyelid, or inner lining of eyelid); *eye discharge; facial edema* (swelling of face); *lid retraction* (raising of upper eyelid); *paresthesia* (numbness or tingling in fingers or toes); *peripheral edema* (swelling of hands or feet)

　*For 1% ophthalmic apraclonidine*
　　*Allergic reaction* (redness of eye or inner lining of eyelid, swelling of eyelid, or watering of eye); *arrhythmia* (irregular heartbeat); *ocular inflammation or injection* (redness of eye)

**Those indicating need for medical attention only if they continue or are bothersome**
Incidence more frequent
　*For 0.5% ophthalmic apraclonidine*
　　*Dryness of mouth; eye discomfort*

　*For 1% ophthalmic apraclonidine*
　　*Conjunctival blanching* (paleness of eye or inner lining of eyelid); *lid retraction* (raising of upper eyelid); *mydriasis* (increase in size of pupil of eye)

Incidence less frequent or rare
　*For 0.5% ophthalmic apraclonidine*
　　*Asthenia* (tiredness or weakness); *conjunctival blanching* (paleness of eye or inner lining of eyelid); *constipation; corneal staining* (discoloration of white part of eye); *crusting or scales on eyelid or corner of eye; dry nose or eyes; headache; insomnia* (trouble in sleeping); *malaise* (general feeling of discomfort or illness); *myalgia* (muscle aches); *nausea; nervousness; parosmia or taste perversion* (change in taste or smell); *pharyngitis* (sore throat); *photophobia* (increased sensitivity of eyes to light); *rhinitis* (runny nose); *somnolence* (drowsiness or sleepiness)

　*For 1% ophthalmic apraclonidine*
　　*Nasal decongestion* (runny nose)

## Overdose

No information is available regarding overdosage of apraclonidine in humans.

## Patient Consultation

As an aid to patient consultation, refer to *Advice for the Patient, Apraclonidine (Ophthalmic).*

In providing consultation, consider emphasizing the following selected information (» = major clinical significance):

**Before using this medication**
» Conditions affecting use, especially:
　　Sensitivity to apraclonidine or clonidine
　　Pregnancy—Fetal death occurred after the administration of large oral doses of apraclonidine in rabbit studies
　　Breast-feeding—It may be necessary to stop breast-feeding during the day of surgery
　　Other medical problems, especially severe cardiovascular disease, including hypertension

**Proper use of this medication**
　　Waiting at least 10 minutes between instillation of two different ophthalmic solutions

Proper administration technique; using a second drop if necessary; not touching applicator tip to any surface; keeping container tightly closed
» Importance of not using more medication than the amount prescribed
» Regular visits to physician to check eye pressure during therapy
» Proper dosing
　　Missed dose: Using as soon as possible; not using if almost time for next dose; using next dose at regularly scheduled time; not doubling doses
» Proper storage

**Precautions while using this medication**
» Medication may cause dizziness or drowsiness; using caution when driving, using machines, or doing anything else requiring alertness
　　Possible photophobia; wearing sunglasses or avoiding bright light

**Side/adverse effects**
*Signs of potential side effects, especially*
　*For 0.5% ophthalmic apraclonidine*—Allergic reaction, abnormal coordination, arrhythmia, asthma, blepharitis, blepharoconjunctivitis, conjunctivitis, blurred vision or change in vision, chest pain, contact dermatitis, corneal erosion, corneal infiltrate, foreign body sensation, keratitis, keratopathy, depression, dizziness, dyspnea, edema of eye, eyelid, or conjunctiva, eye discharge, facial edema, lid retraction, paresthesia, or peripheral edema
　*For 1% ophthalmic apraclonidine*—Allergic reaction, arrhythmia, or ocular inflammation or injection

## General Dosing Information

The intraocular pressure (IOP) lowering efficacy of 0.5% ophthalmic apraclonidine diminishes over time and the benefit for most patients is less than one month.

When instilling two different ophthalmic solutions, patient should wait at least 10 minutes between instillations to avoid a "wash-out" effect.

If hypersensitivity develops, therapy with ophthalmic apraclonidine should be discontinued.

## Ophthalmic Dosage Forms
### APRACLONIDINE HYDROCHLORIDE OPHTHALMIC SOLUTION

**Usual adult and adolescent dose**
Open angle glaucoma—
　　Topical, to the conjunctiva, 1 drop of 0.5% solution in each eye two or three times a day.
Ocular hypertension—
　　Topical, to the conjunctiva, 1 drop of 1% solution in the affected eye one hour before initiating anterior segment laser surgery and 1 drop in the same eye immediately upon completion of the laser surgical procedure.

**Usual pediatric dose**
Safety and efficacy have not been established.

**Usual geriatric dose**
See *Usual adult and adolescent dose.*

**Strength(s) usually available**
U.S.—
　　0.5% (base) (Rx) [*Iopidine* (benzalkonium chloride 0.01%)].
　　1% (base) (Rx) [*Iopidine* (benzalkonium chloride 0.01%)].
Canada—
　　0.5% (base) (Rx) [*Iopidine* (benzalkonium chloride 0.01%)].
　　1% (base) (Rx) [*Iopidine* (benzalkonium chloride 0.01%)].
Note: Each mL of the 0.5% solution contains 5.75 mg of apraclonidine HCl equivalent to 5 mg of apraclonidine base.
　　Each mL of the 1% solution contains 11.5 mg of apraclonidine hydrochloride equivalent to 10 mg of apraclonidine base.

**Packaging and storage**
For the 0.5% solution—Store between 2 and 27 °C (36 and 80 °F), unless otherwise specified by manufacturer. Protect from freezing and light.
For the 1% solution—Store below 40 °C (104 °F), preferably between 15 and 30 °C (59 and 86 °F), unless otherwise specified by manufacturer. Protect from freezing and light.

**Auxiliary labeling**
- For the eye.
- Protect from light.
- Do not freeze.

## Selected Bibliography

Robin AL. Short-term effects of unilateral 1% apraclonidine therapy. Arch Ophthalmol 1988 Jul; 106 (7): 912-5.

Pollack IP, et al. Prevention of the rise in intraocular pressure following neodymium-YAG posterior capsulotomy using topical 1% apraclonidine. Arch Ophthalmol 1988 Jun; 106 (6): 754-7.

Revised: 06/21/94
Interim revision: 07/03/95

## APROBARBITAL—See *Barbiturates (Systemic)*

# APROTININ   Systemic

VA CLASSIFICATION (Primary): BL300
Note: For a listing of dosage forms and brand names by country availability, see *Dosage Forms* section(s). For a listing of brand names for the articles in this monograph, refer to the General Index.

## Category

Antifibrinolytic; antihemorrhagic; proteinase inhibitor.

## Indications

### Accepted

Hemorrhage, coronary artery bypass graft surgery–associated (prophylaxis)[1]—Aprotinin is indicated to reduce perioperative blood loss and the need for blood transfusion in patients undergoing cardiopulmonary bypass in the course of repeat coronary artery bypass graft (CABG) surgery. It is also indicated, in selected cases, in first CABG procedures when the risk of bleeding is especially high (e.g., impaired hemostasis due to platelet aggregation inhibitor therapy or other coagulopathy) or when transfusion is unavailable or unacceptable. However, when aprotinin is being considered for use in a first CABG procedure, the risk of renal function impairment and the risk of anaphylaxis should a second procedure be needed must be taken into account.

### Acceptance not established

Aprotinin has also been studied for use in the reduction of bleeding and transfusion requirements in other types of surgery including *orthotopic liver transplantation*, total hip replacement, colorectal surgery, peripheral vascular surgery, and *heart and heart-lung transplantation*. Study results evaluating the use of aprotinin for these indications are preliminary. Further studies are required to assess aprotinin's efficacy in these indications.

The use of aprotinin to control bleeding in *emergency cardiac surgery after thrombolysis* with alteplase, streptokinase, or urokinase has been reported. Although aprotinin may be effective in preventing severe hemorrhage in this setting, controlled studies to verify its efficacy and safety have not been done.

A few studies have evaluated the use of aprotinin in *pediatric patients* undergoing cardiac surgery. However, dosages and dosing regimens varied widely and the results have not been uniform. These studies have generally shown aprotinin to be less than beneficial in terms of reducing blood loss and the need for transfusions. Further studies are necessary to define the role of aprotinin in pediatric cardiac surgery.

### Unaccepted

Aprotinin was originally introduced for the treatment of acute pancreatitis because of its proteinase inhibiting property. However, most studies have failed to show any benefit from this use.

Use of aprotinin for the treatment of subcutaneous insulin resistance syndrome has been described in a limited number of case reports from the early 1980s. However, no recent reports are available supporting such use, possibly due to concern for its safety during long-term use.

[1]Not included in Canadian product labeling.

## Pharmacology/Pharmacokinetics

### Physicochemical characteristics

Source—Isolated from bovine lung
Molecular weight—6511.57.

### Mechanism of action/Effect

Aprotinin is a proteinase inhibitor. The exact mechanism by which it reduces bleeding is unclear; however, it has been shown to have a number of effects on the coagulation system.

Patients undergoing cardiopulmonary bypass (CPB) develop adverse changes in their blood components, blood cells, and specific proteins involved in coagulation, which increase the risk of serious postoperative bleeding. Platelet function impairment is considered to be the main hemostatic defect during CPB. There is evidence that aprotinin preserves platelet function; however, the mechanism by which this occurs is uncertain. In addition, aprotinin directly prevents fibrinolysis by inhibiting plasmin and kallikrein. It also inhibits the early phase of the intrinsic clotting cascade (contact phase) by inhibiting kallikrein, which in turn inhibits activation of factor XII.

### Distribution

Rapidly distributed into the total extracellular space following intravenous injection, leading to a rapid initial decrease in plasma aprotinin concentration. Aprotinin is actively reabsorbed and accumulated by the proximal tubules in the kidney.

### Biotransformation

Slowly degraded by lysosomal activity in the kidney.

### Half-life

Elimination—
Initial, following the distribution phase: Approximately 150 minutes.
Terminal, occuring beyond 5 hours after administration: Approximately 10 hours.

### Steady-state plasma concentration

Average steady-state intraoperative plasma concentrations were 250 Kallikrein Inhibitor Units per mL (KIU/mL) in cardiac surgery patients receiving a dosage regimen of 2 million KIU as an intravenous loading dose, 2 million KIU added to the pump prime fluid, and 500,000 KIU per hour as a continuous intravenous infusion during the procedure. Average steady-state intraoperative plasma concentrations were 137 KIU/mL after administration of half of the above regimen.

### Therapeutic plasma concentration

For plasma kallikrein inhibition—Approximately 200 KIU/mL.
For plasmin inhibition—Approximately 50 KIU/mL.

### Elimination

Renal: almost entirely as inactive metabolites.

## Precautions to Consider

### Carcinogenicity

Long-term animal studies to evaluate the carcinogenic potential of aprotinin have not been performed.

### Mutagenicity

Results of microbial *in vitro* tests using *Salmonella typhimurium* and *Bacillus subtilis* have shown no mutagenic effect of aprotinin.

### Pregnancy/Reproduction

Fertility—Studies in rats given intravenous doses up to 2.4 times the human dose on a mg per kg of body weight (mg/kg) basis (0.37 times the human dose on a mg per square meter of body surface area [mg/m² ] basis) for 11 days, and in rabbits given intravenous doses up to 1.2 times the human dose on a mg/kg basis (0.36 times the human dose on a mg/m² basis) for 13 days have revealed no evidence of impaired fertility.

Pregnancy—Adequate and well-controlled studies in pregnant women have not been done.

Studies in rats given intravenous doses up to 2.4 times the human dose on a mg/kg basis (0.37 times the human dose on a mg/m² basis) for 11 days, and in rabbits given intravenous doses up to 1.2 times the human dose on a mg/kg basis (0.36 times the human dose on a mg/m² basis) for 13 days have revealed no evidence of harm to the fetus.

FDA Pregnancy Category B.

**Breast-feeding**
There are no available studies on the distribution of aprotinin into breast milk. However, since aprotinin is not absorbed after oral administration, there would be no effect on a nursing infant even if the breast milk did contain any of the medication.

**Pediatrics**
Safety and efficacy have not been established.
A few studies have evaluated the use of aprotinin in pediatric patients undergoing cardiac surgery. Results of these studies have not been uniform, but they have generally shown aprotinin to be less than beneficial in terms of reducing blood loss and the need for transfusions. Further studies are necessary to define the role of aprotinin in pediatric cardiac surgery.

**Geriatrics**
Clinical trials of aprotinin in cardiac surgery have been conducted mainly in older patients, and geriatrics-specific problems that would limit the usefulness of this medication in the elderly have not been evident. However, retrospective data from patients undergoing surgery of the thoracic aorta, using deep hypothermic circulatory arrest, revealed an increase in renal function impairment and failure, and of myocardial infarction and death, in a subset of patients 65 years of age or older who received high-dose aprotinin. The incidence of these complications in the patients receiving aprotinin far exceeded that in a previous group of age-matched patients who underwent similar operations but did not receive aprotinin. The investigators suggest that profound hypothermia with low blood flow or circulatory arrest may be a predisposing factor for significant adverse effects, particularly in patients older than 65 years of age. However, no data to confirm these findings is available from prospective studies involving large numbers of patients. Caution should be used when administering aprotinin during deep hypothermic circulatory arrest, especially in patients over the age of 65.

**Drug interactions and/or related problems**
The following drug interactions and/or related problems have been selected on the basis of their potential clinical significance (possible mechanism in parentheses where appropriate)—not necessarily inclusive (» = major clinical significance):

Note: Combinations containing any of the following medications, depending on the amount present, may also interact with this medication.

   Angiotensin-converting enzyme (ACE) inhibitors
      (in a pharmacologic study evaluating the role of kinins in the antihypertensive effect of ACE inhibition, an intravenous infusion of aprotinin blocked the acute hypotensive effect of a 100-mg dose of captopril in 9 study patients with untreated hypertension; the clinical significance of this interaction is uncertain)

» Thrombolytic agents, such as:
   Alteplase
   Anistreplase
   Streptokinase
   Urokinase
      (the actions of antifibrinolytic agents and of thrombolytic agents are mutually antagonistic; although aprotinin may be effective in preventing severe hemorrhage in patients who have received a thrombolytic agent prior to cardiac surgery, controlled studies to verify its efficacy and safety for this use have not been done)

**Laboratory value alterations**
The following have been selected on the basis of their potential clinical significance (possible effect in parentheses where appropriate)—not necessarily inclusive (» = major clinical significance):

With diagnostic test results
» Activated clotting time (ACT) and
   Partial thromboplastin time (PTT)
      (aprotinin causes marked elevations in the ACT and PTT by inhibiting foreign surface contact–activation of the intrinsic clotting system, a method used in these tests; these elevations persist following surgery due to circulating concentrations of aprotinin)

      (aprotinin significantly prolongs the ACT as measured by the Hemochron® method, which utilizes a celite contact activator [used to monitor the adequacy of heparinization during cardiopulmonary bypass]; this is an artifactual prolongation of this particular test value and does not indicate excessive anticoagulation or a need to decrease heparin dosage)

With physiology/laboratory test values
   Creatine kinase (CK), serum
      (aprotinin may increase serum CK with increased MB fractions; however, the clinical significance of this effect is not known)

   Creatinine, serum
      (aprotinin may transiently increase serum creatinine concentrations, but this effect is generally not severe; during clinical use, aprotinin has had no clinically significant effect on serum creatinine or renal function)

   Transaminases, serum
      (may be increased; in controlled studies in the U.S., the percentage of subjects developing an elevation of alanine aminotransferase [ALT] greater than 1.8 times the upper limit of normal was higher in the aprotinin-treated group, but only in those patients undergoing repeat coronary artery bypass graft surgery, suggesting an indirect effect possibly related to the risk of repeated surgery; however, the etiology and clinical significance of this effect are uncertain)

**Medical considerations/Contraindications**
The medical considerations/contraindications included here have been selected on the basis of their potential clinical significance (reasons given in parentheses where appropriate)—not necessarily inclusive (» = major clinical significance).

*Except under special circumstances, this medication should not be used when the following medical problem exists:*
» Allergy to aprotinin

*Risk-benefit should be considered when the following medical problems exist:*
   Allergies, multiple, history of or
» Previous aprotinin therapy
      (there is an increased risk of allergic reactions; a case of fatal anaphylactic shock following re-exposure to aprotinin has been reported; it is important to verify any previous aprotinin exposure, and all patients should first receive a test dose to assess the potential for allergic reactions)

» Caution is also required in patients undergoing deep hypothermic circulatory arrest, especially those older than 65 years of age, as increases in renal failure and fatalities have been reported in patients receiving aprotinin in this setting in connection with surgery of the aortic arch.

**Patient monitoring**
The following may be especially important in patient monitoring (other tests may be warranted in some patients, depending on condition; » = major clinical significance):
» Observation for signs and symptoms of anaphylaxis

## Side/Adverse Effects

Note: Patients undergoing deep hypothermic circulatory arrest in connection with surgery of the aortic arch may be predisposed to significant adverse effects including renal failure and fatality, particularly patients older than 65 years of age. These effects appear to be attributable to *disseminated intravascular coagulation*, possibly caused by the combination of high-dose aprotinin and profound hypothermia with low blood flow or circulatory arrest.

A trend toward increased incidences of *vein graft closure* and *myocardial infarction* was found in pooled data of U.S. studies in aprotinin-treated patients undergoing cardiopulmonary bypass. However, the differences in the incidence rates were not statistically significant. Two studies that investigated graft occlusion rates showed no statistically significant difference in patency between treatment and placebo groups, although the number of patients was small. It has been suggested that the patients in the early studies were inadequately anticoagulated with heparin because the effect of aprotinin on the activated clotting time (ACT) in the presence of heparin was not fully taken into consideration. Current evidence suggests that aprotinin has no clinically significant effect on graft thrombosis.

The following side/adverse effects have been selected on the basis of their potential clinical significance (possible signs and symptoms in parentheses where appropriate)—not necessarily inclusive:

**Those indicating need for medical attention**
Incidence rare (1% or less)
   *Allergic reaction* (skin eruptions, itching, dyspnea, nausea, tachycardia, hypotension, and bronchospasm); *anaphylaxis, including shock with circulatory failure*

Note: A case of fatal *anaphylactic shock* following aprotinin re-exposure has been reported. It is important to verify any previous aprotinin exposure, and a test dose should be given to all patients to assess the potential for allergic reactions.

## General Dosing Information

Because of the increased risk of allergic reactions upon re-exposure to aprotinin, it is important to document the use of aprotinin in the patient's medical records and to ascertain any previous use of aprotinin.

Administration of aprotinin includes a 1-mL test dose, a loading dose, a dose to be added to the priming fluid of the cardiopulmonary bypass circuit ("pump prime" dose), and a constant infusion dose.

All intravenous doses of aprotinin should be administered through a central venous line. *No other medication should be administered through the same line.*

All patients should first receive a *test dose* to assess the potential for allergic reactions. The test dose (1 mL) should be administered intravenously at least 10 minutes prior to the loading dose.

Particular caution is needed when administering aprotinin (even test doses) to patients who have received it previously because of the risk of anaphylaxis. In *re-exposure cases*, after a successful test dose, prophylactic intravenous administration of an $H_1$-histamine antagonist (e.g., diphenhydramine) is recommended shortly before the loading dose of aprotinin.

Patients who experience any allergic reaction to the test dose of aprotinin should not receive further administration of the medication. Even after the uneventful administration of the test dose, the full therapeutic dose may cause anaphylaxis. In addition, anaphylaxis can occur in patients with no prior exposure to aprotinin. In the event of an anaphylactic reaction, the infusion should be stopped immediately and emergency treatment for anaphylaxis should begin. Patients with a history of allergies to medications or other agents may be at greater risk of developing an allergic reaction.

The loading dose of aprotinin should be given intravenously after induction of anesthesia but prior to sternotomy. The dose should be given with patients in the supine position and administered over a 20- to 30-minute period as rapid administration can cause a transient fall in blood pressure.

Either of 2 dosing regimens can be utilized, a high-dose regimen (Regimen A), or a low-dose regimen (Regimen B). The low-dose regimen is exactly one-half of the high-dose regimen. The high-dose regimen was used in the original studies in an effort to achieve plasma concentrations of aprotinin necessary to inhibit plasmin and plasma kallikrein. Interest in use of lower doses has arisen from a desire to find the most cost-effective regimen and, possibly, to reduce the potential for side effects. However, results of studies utilizing low-dose aprotinin have been equivocal, with variable effects on transfusion requirements.

No pharmacokinetic data is available from patients with pre-existing hepatic disease or renal insufficiency. Age and impaired renal function do not change aprotinin pharmacokinetics enough to warrant dosage adjustments.

### For treatment of adverse effects

Anaphylaxis or other severe allergic reactions require immediate emergency treatment, which consists of the following:
- Parenteral epinephrine.
- Oxygen.
- Parenteral antihistamines.
- Intravenous corticosteroids.
- Airway management (including intubation).

### During cardiopulmonary bypass (CPB) with heparin

Aprotinin prolongs the activated clotting time (ACT) as measured by the Hemochron® method, which utilizes a celite contact activator. Therefore, the standard method of monitoring heparinization by keeping the ACT above 400 to 450 seconds may lead to inadequate anticoagulation and the potential for coagulation through the extrinsic clotting system. Some investigators suggest maintaining the ACT above 750 seconds. Others propose utilizing tests not affected by aprotinin, such as high-dose thromboplastin time (HiPT) and high-dose thrombin time (HiTT), or kaolin-based activated coagulation time (AKT). However, the safety and efficacy of these alternative methods must be confirmed by further study. In any event, reduction of heparin dose is not recommended during CPB, as adequate heparin concentrations are needed to prevent clotting through the extrinsic system. Standard doses of heparin should be used during CPB; however, additional heparin may be administered based on the duration of CPB and patient weight, or the results of monitoring heparin concentrations using a heparin-protamine titration. Whole blood measurements of heparin are not affected by aprotinin and correlate well with plasma anti-Xa heparin measurements, making the automated protamine titration assay acceptable for monitoring of heparin concentrations in patients treated with aprotinin.

## Parenteral Dosage Forms

Note: The following doses are given in Kallikrein Inhibitor Units (KIU). The strength of commercially available aprotinin injection is labeled in KIU per mL.

### APROTININ INJECTION

#### Usual adult dose

Hemorrhage, coronary artery bypass graft surgery–associated (prophylaxis)[1]—

High-dose regimen:
  Test dose—Intravenous, 10,000 KIU (1 mL).
  Initial dose—Intravenous, 2,000,000 KIU (200 mL).
  Maintenance dose—Intravenous infusion, 500,000 KIU per hour (50 mL per hour).
  "Pump prime" dose—Added to the priming fluid, 2,000,000 KIU (200 mL).

Low-dose regimen:
  Test dose—Intravenous, 10,000 KIU (1 mL).
  Initial dose—Intravenous, 1,000,000 KIU (100 mL).
  Maintenance dose—Intravenous infusion, 250,000 KIU per hour (25 mL per hour).
  "Pump prime" dose—Added to the priming fluid, 1,000,000 KIU (100 mL).

Note: The test dose should be administered intravenously at least ten minutes prior to the initial dose. The initial dose is given slowly over twenty to thirty minutes with the patient in the supine position after induction of anesthesia but prior to sternotomy. Following the initial dose, the maintenance dose is given by constant infusion until surgery is complete and the patient leaves the operating room. The "pump prime" dose is added to the priming fluid of the cardiopulmonary bypass circuit, by replacement of an aliquot of the priming fluid, prior to initiation of cardiopulmonary bypass.

#### Usual adult prescribing limits

Total doses of more than 7,000,000 KIU have not been studied in controlled trials.

#### Usual pediatric dose

Safety and efficacy have not been established.

Note: A few studies have evaluated the use of aprotinin in pediatric patients undergoing cardiac surgery. However, dosages and dosing regimens varied widely and the results have not been uniform. These studies have generally shown aprotinin to be less than beneficial in terms of reducing blood loss and the need for transfusions. Further studies are necessary to define the role of aprotinin in pediatric cardiac surgery.

#### Strength(s) usually available

U.S.—
  10,000 KIU per mL (100- and 200-mL vials) (Rx) [*Trasylol*].

Canada—
  10,000 KIU per mL (50-mL vials) (Rx) [*Trasylol*].

#### Packaging and storage

Store between 2 and 25 °C (36 and 77 °F). Protect from freezing.

#### Stability

Aprotinin is stable when stored in sealed vials at room temperature. The medication should not be used if a precipitate or particulate matter is present or if the contents are cloudy. Once a vial has been opened, it should be used immediately. Any unused portion should be discarded.

#### Incompatibilities

Aprotinin is incompatible *in vitro* with corticosteroids, heparin, tetracyclines, and nutrient solutions containing amino acids or fat emulsions. If aprotinin is to be given concomitantly with another medication, each medication should be administered separately through a different venous line or catheter. **No other medication should be administered through the same intravenous line with aprotinin.**

---

[1]Not included in Canadian product labeling.

## Selected Bibliography

Royston D. High-dose aprotinin therapy: a review of the first five years' experience. J Cardiothorac Vasc Anesth 1992; 6: 76-100.

Lemmer JH, Stanford W, Bonney SL, et al. Aprotinin for coronary bypass operations: efficacy, safety, and influence on early saphenous vein graft patency. A multicenter, randomized, double-blind, placebo-controlled study. J Thorac Cardiovasc Surg 1994; 107: 543-53.

Davis R, Whittington R. Aprotinin: a review of its pharmacology and therapeutic efficacy in reducing blood loss associated with cardiac surgery. Drugs 1995; 49: 954-83.

Developed: 08/17/95

# ASCORBIC ACID    Systemic

This monograph includes information on the following: Ascorbic Acid; Sodium Ascorbate†.

VA CLASSIFICATION (Primary/Secondary):
    Ascorbic acid—VT400/AD900; DX900
    Sodium Ascorbate—VT400/AD900

Another commonly used name is vitamin C.

Note: For a listing of dosage forms and brand names by country availability, see *Dosage Forms* section(s). For a listing of brand names for the articles in this monograph, refer to the General Index.

    †Not commercially available in Canada.

## Category

Note: Ascorbic acid (vitamin C) is a water-soluble vitamin.

Nutritional supplement (vitamin)—Ascorbic Acid; Sodium Ascorbate.
Diagnostic aid adjunct (red blood cell disease)—Ascorbic Acid Injection.
Deferoxamine adjunct (chronic iron overdose)—Ascorbic Acid; Sodium Ascorbate.
Methemoglobinemia (idiopathic) therapy adjunct—Ascorbic Acid.

## Indications

Note: Bracketed information in the *Indications* section refers to uses that are not included in U.S. product labeling.

### Accepted

Vitamin C deficiency (prophylaxis and treatment)—Ascorbic acid and sodium ascorbate are indicated for prevention and treatment of ascorbic acid deficiency states. Ascorbic acid deficiency may occur as a result of inadequate nutrition but does not occur in healthy individuals receiving an adequate balanced diet. For prophylaxis of ascorbic acid deficiency, dietary improvement rather than supplementation is advisable. For treatment of vitamin C deficiency, supplementation is preferred.

Deficiency of ascorbic acid may lead to scurvy.

Requirements may be increased and/or supplementation may be necessary in the following persons or conditions (based on documented ascorbic acid deficiency):
AIDS (acquired immune deficiency syndrome)
Alcoholism
Burns
Cancer
Exposure to cold temperatures, prolonged
Fever, prolonged
Gastrectomy
Hemodialysis, chronic
Hyperthyroidism
Infants receiving unfortified formulas
Infection, continuing
Intestinal diseases—diarrhea, prolonged; ileal resection
Peptic ulcer
Smokers
Stress, continuing
Surgery
Trauma, continuing
Tuberculosis

Some unusual diets (e.g., reducing diets that drastically restrict food selection) may not supply minimum daily requirements for ascorbic acid. Supplementation is necessary in patients receiving total parenteral nutrition (TPN) or undergoing rapid weight loss or in those with malnutrition, because of inadequate dietary intake.

Recommended intakes for all vitamins and most minerals are increased during pregnancy. Many physicians recommend that pregnant women receive multivitamin and mineral supplements, especially those pregnant women who do not consume an adequate diet and those in high-risk categories (i.e., women carrying more than one fetus, heavy cigarette smokers, and alcohol and drug abusers). Taking excessive amounts of a multivitamin and mineral supplement may be harmful to the mother and/or fetus and should be avoided.

Recommended intakes for all vitamins and most minerals are increased during breast-feeding.

Red blood cells, labeling of, adjunct—Ascorbic acid injection is used as a reducing agent in the preparation of sodium chromate Cr 51 injection for the *in vitro* labeling of red blood cells.

[Toxicity, iron, chronic (treatment adjunct)][1]—Ascorbic acid or sodium ascorbate has been used to increase iron excretion by improving chelation during deferoxamine therapy.

Ascorbic acid has been used as treatment adjunct for idiopathic methemoglobinemia; however, its use has generally been replaced by more effective agents.

### Acceptance not established

There are insufficient data to show that ascorbic acid may reduce the risk of *cardiovascular disease* and certain types of *cancer*.

### Unaccepted

A potential role for ascorbic acid in the treatment of cancer has not been proven. Ascorbic acid is not useful for treatment of pyorrhea or gingival infections, hemorrhagic states, hematuria, retinal hemorrhages, immune system dysfunction, or mental depression not related to ascorbic acid deficiency. Ascorbic acid has not been proven effective for treatment of dental caries, anemia, acne, asthma, infertility, aging, atherosclerosis, peptic ulcer, tuberculosis, schizophrenia, dysentery, collagen disorders, fractures, skin ulcers, hay fever, or drug toxicity, nor for prevention of vascular thrombosis or the common cold.

[1]Not included in Canadian product labeling.

## Pharmacology/Pharmacokinetics

### Physicochemical characteristics

Molecular weight—
    Ascorbic acid: 176.13.
    Sodium ascorbate: 198.11.
pKa—
    4.2 and 11.6.

### Mechanism of action/Effect

Nutritional supplement (vitamin)—Ascorbic acid is necessary for collagen formation and tissue repair in the body and may be involved in some oxidation-reduction reactions. It is also involved in metabolism of phenylalanine, tyrosine, folic acid, norepinephrine, histamine, iron, and some drug enzyme systems; utilization of carbohydrates; synthesis of lipids, proteins, and carnitine; immune function; hydroxylation of serotonin; and preservation of blood vessel integrity. In addition, ascorbic acid enhances the absorption of nonheme iron.

Diagnostic aid adjunct (red blood cell disease)—Ascorbic acid reduces unbound dianionic chromium 51 to the anionic state, which does not penetrate red blood cells, thereby terminating the *in vitro* labeling of red blood cells.

Deferoxamine adjunct (chronic iron overdose)—Complex interaction; vitamin C given orally in small doses (150 to 250 mg per day) may improve the chelating action of deferoxamine and increase the amount of iron excreted.

### Absorption

Readily absorbed from gastrointestinal tract (jejunum); may be reduced with large doses.

### Protein binding

Low (25%).

### Storage

Ascorbic acid is taken up by all cells of the body. The highest concentrations are found in glandular tissues, leukocytes, the liver, and the lens of the eye. The body stores up to approximately 1500 mg of ascorbic acid with intake of the recommended daily amount, and 2500 mg with an intake of 200 mg a day.

### Biotransformation

Hepatic.

## Elimination

Renal, very little as unchanged vitamin and metabolites except with high doses; urinary excretion increases with plasma concentrations of greater than 1.4 mg per 100 mL.

In dialysis—Removable by hemodialysis.

## Precautions to Consider

### Pregnancy/Reproduction

Pregnancy—Studies have not been done in humans. Problems in humans have not been documented with intake of normal daily recommended amounts. Ascorbic acid crosses the placenta. Ingestion of large quantities of ascorbic acid daily throughout pregnancy may possibly harm the fetus.

Studies have not been done in animals.

FDA Pregnancy Category C (parenteral ascorbic acid).

### Breast-feeding

Problems in humans have not been documented with intake of normal daily recommended amounts. Ascorbic acid is distributed into breast milk.

### Pediatrics

Problems in pediatrics have not been documented with intake of normal daily recommended amounts.

### Geriatrics

Problems in geriatrics have not been documented with intake of normal daily recommended amounts.

### Dental

Excessive use of chewable ascorbic acid tablets has been reported to cause breakdown of tooth enamel.

### Drug interactions and/or related problems

The following drug interactions and/or related problems have been selected on the basis of their potential clinical significance (possible mechanism in parentheses where appropriate)—not necessarily inclusive (» = major clinical significance):

Note: Combinations containing any of the following medications, depending on the amount present, may also interact with this medication.

Large doses of ascorbic acid (but not sodium ascorbate) may lower urinary pH and cause renal tubular reabsorption of acidic medications with concurrent administration; alkaline medications may exhibit decreased reabsorption.

Anticoagulants, coumarin- or indandione-derivative
(doses of 10 grams or more a day of ascorbic acid have been reported to impair gastrointestinal absorption of the anticoagulant)

Cellulose sodium phosphate
(concurrent use may result in metabolism of ascorbic acid to oxalate)

» Deferoxamine
(concurrent use with ascorbic acid may enhance tissue iron toxicity, especially in the heart, causing cardiac decompensation; therefore, this regimen should be used with caution in older patients; the need for ascorbic acid supplementation should be completely documented by measurements of iron excretion before and after supplements, and the oral dose of ascorbic acid should be given an hour or two after the deferoxamine infusion has been initiated when adequate concentrations of deferoxamine have been achieved)

Disulfiram
(concurrent use with ascorbic acid, especially with chronic use or high doses, may interfere with the disulfiram-alcohol interaction)

### Laboratory value alterations

The following have been selected on the basis of their potential clinical significance (possible effect in parentheses where appropriate)—not necessarily inclusive (» = major clinical significance):

Note: Because ascorbic acid is a strong reducing agent, it interferes with laboratory tests based on oxidation-reduction reactions.

With diagnostic test results
Glucose determinations, urine, by cupric sulfate (Benedict's) reagent
(concentration may be falsely increased)

Glucose determinations, urine, by glucose oxidase (*Tes-Tape*) method
(concentration may be falsely decreased)

Lactate dehydrogenase (LDH) and
Transaminase, hepatic
(serum concentrations as measured by auto-analyzer may be decreased with doses of ascorbic acid greater than 200 mg a day)

Occult blood in stool
(large doses may cause false-negative results)

With physiology/laboratory test values
Bilirubin
(serum concentrations may be elevated)

pH, urine
(may be decreased by large doses of ascorbic acid, but not by sodium ascorbate)

Uric acid and
Oxalate, urine
(concentrations may be increased in patients receiving large doses of ascorbic acid)

### Medical considerations/Contraindications

The medical considerations/contraindications included here have been selected on the basis of their potential clinical significance (reasons given in parentheses where appropriate)—not necessarily inclusive (» = major clinical significance).

*Risk-benefit should be considered when the following medical problems exist:*

Diabetes mellitus
(possible interference with glucose determinations by very high doses of ascorbic acid)

Glucose-6-phosphate dehydrogenase (G6PD) deficiency
(high doses of ascorbic acid may cause hemolytic anemia)

Hemochromatosis or
Sideroblastic anemia or
Thalassemia
(high doses of ascorbic acid may increase iron absorption)

Hyperoxaluria or oxalosis or
Renal stones, history of
(risk of hyperoxaluria and possible precipitation of oxalate stones in urinary tract after high doses of ascorbic acid)

Sensitivity to ascorbic acid or sodium ascorbate

### Patient monitoring

The following may be especially important in patient monitoring (other tests may be warranted in some patients, depending on condition; » = major clinical significance):

Ascorbic acid determinations, buffy coat, plasma, or serum
(recommended to determine ascorbic acid deficiency; buffy coat levels are used to determine ascorbic acid stores)

## Side/Adverse Effects

Note: Withdrawal scurvy may occur after prolonged administration of 2 to 3 grams per day.

The following side/adverse effects have been selected on the basis of their potential clinical significance (possible signs and symptoms in parentheses where appropriate)—not necessarily inclusive:

### Those indicating need for medical attention
Incidence dose-related
*Kidney stones, oxalate* (side or lower back pain)

Note: Occasionally, prolonged doses of ascorbic acid in excess of 1 g per day have been reported to cause an increase in urinary oxalate, which may cause precipitation of oxalate stones in the urinary tract in patients with renal disease, especially those on hemodialysis, or in patients with a history of renal stones. However, studies have not found an increase in urinary oxalate formation with high doses of ascorbic acid.

### Those indicating need for medical attention only if they continue or are bothersome
Incidence less frequent or rare
*Dizziness or faintness*—with rapid intravenous administration

With high doses
*Diarrhea*—with oral doses greater than 1 gram per day; *flushing or redness of skin; headache; increase in urination, mild*—with doses greater than 600 mg per day; *nausea or vomiting; stomach cramps*

## Patient Consultation

As an aid to patient consultation, refer to *Advice for the Patient, Ascorbic Acid (Vitamin C) (Systemic)*.

In providing consultation, consider emphasizing the following selected information (» = major clinical significance):

### Description of use
Description should include function in the body, signs of deficiency, conditions that may cause deficiency, and unproven uses

### Importance of diet
Importance of proper nutrition; supplement may be needed because of inadequate dietary intake

Food sources of ascorbic acid; effects of processing
Not using vitamins as substitute for balanced diet
Recommended daily intake for ascorbic acid

### Before using this dietary supplement
» Conditions affecting use, especially:
   Pregnancy—Crosses placenta; large quantities during pregnancy
   may be harmful to the fetus
   Breast-feeding—Distributed into breast milk
   Dental—Breakdown of enamel has been reported with excessive
   use of chewable tablets
   Other medications, especially deferoxamine

### Proper use of this dietary supplement
» Proper dosing
   Missed dose: No cause for concern because of length of time necessary
   for depletion; remembering to take as directed
   Proper administration of oral solution:
   Taking by mouth even though it comes in dropper bottle
   May be dropped directly into the mouth or mixed with cereal, fruit
   juice, or other food
» Proper storage

### Precautions while using this dietary supplement
Ascorbic acid not stored; excessive amounts excreted in urine; very
high doses may interfere with glucose determinations and diagnostic tests for occult blood in stool

### Side/adverse effects
Signs of potential side effects, especially increase in urinary oxalate
and possible precipitation of oxalate kidney stones

## General Dosing Information

### For parenteral dosage forms
The intramuscular route is usually preferred because ascorbic acid is absorbed and utilized more efficiently with this method of administration.

### Diet/Nutrition
Recommended dietary intakes for ascorbic acid are defined differently
worldwide.
For U.S.—
   The Recommended Dietary Allowances (RDAs) for vitamins and min-
   erals are determined by the Food and Nutrition Board of the Na-
   tional Research Council and are intended to provide adequate nu-
   trition in most healthy persons under usual environmental stresses.
   In addition, a different designation may be used by the FDA for
   food and dietary supplement labeling purposes, as with Daily
   Value (DV). DVs replace the previous labeling terminology United
   States Recommended Daily Allowances (USRDAs).
For Canada—
   Recommended Nutrient Intakes (RNIs) for vitamins, minerals, and
   protein are determined by Health and Welfare in Canada and provide recommended amounts of a specific nutrient while minimizing
   the risk of chronic diseases.

Daily recommended intakes for ascorbic acid are generally defined as
follows:

| Persons | U.S. (mg) | Canada (mg) |
|---|---|---|
| Infants and children | | |
| Birth to 3 years of age | 30–40 | 20 |
| 4 to 6 years of age | 45 | 25 |
| 7 to 10 years of age | 45 | 25 |
| Adolescent and adult males | 50–60 | 25–40 |
| Adolescent and adult females | 50–60 | 25–30 |
| Pregnant females | 70 | 30–40 |
| Breast-feeding females | 90–95 | 55 |
| Smokers | 100 | 45–60 |

These are usually provided by nutritionally adequate diets.

Best dietary sources of ascorbic acid include citrus fruits (oranges, lemons,
grapefruit), green vegetables (peppers, broccoli, cabbage), tomatoes,
and potatoes. Gradual loss of ascorbic acid occurs in fresh foods with
storage, but not when frozen (except over prolonged periods). Ascorbic acid in foods is rapidly destroyed by exposure to air (oxygen),
drying, salting, and ordinary cooking (30 to 50%, especially in copper
pots). Mincing of fresh vegetables and mashing of potatoes also reduces the ascorbic acid content.

---

## Oral Dosage Forms
### ASCORBIC ACID EXTENDED-RELEASE CAPSULES
**Usual adult and adolescent dose**
Deficiency (prophylaxis)—
   Oral, amount based on normal daily recommended intakes:

| Persons | U.S. (mg) | Canada (mg) |
|---|---|---|
| Adolescent and adult males | 50–60 | 25–40 |
| Adolescent and adult females | 50–60 | 25–30 |
| Pregnant females | 70 | 30–40 |
| Breast-feeding females | 90–95 | 55 |
| Smokers | 100 | 45–60 |

Deficiency (treatment)—
   Treatment dose is individualized by prescriber based on severity of
   deficiency. The following dosage has been established: Scurvy—
   Oral, 500 mg a day for at least 2 weeks.

**Usual pediatric dose**
Dosage form not appropriate for pediatric patients.

**Strength(s) usually available**
U.S.—
   500 mg (OTC) [*Ascorbicap* (tartrazine); *Cebid Timecelles; Cetane;
   Cevi-Bid;* GENERIC].
Canada—
   Not commercially available.
Note: The strength of these ascorbic acid preparations may exceed the
   dosage range recommended by USP DI Advisory Panels based on
   the amount necessary to meet normal nutritional needs.

**Packaging and storage**
Store below 40 °C (104 °F), preferably between 15 and 30 °C (59 and 86
   °F), in a tight container, unless otherwise specified by manufacturer.
   Protect from light.

### ASCORBIC ACID ORAL SOLUTION USP
**Usual adult and adolescent dose**
See *Ascorbic Acid Extended-release Capsules.*

**Usual pediatric dose**
Deficiency (prophylaxis)—
   Oral, amount based on intake of normal daily recommended intakes:

| Persons | U.S. (mg) | Canada (mg) |
|---|---|---|
| Infants and children | | |
| Birth to 3 years of age | 30–40 | 20 |
| 4 to 6 years of age | 45 | 25 |
| 7 to 10 years of age | 45 | 25 |

Deficiency (treatment)—
   Treatment dose is individualized by prescriber based on severity of
   deficiency. The following dosage has been established: Scurvy—
   Oral, 100 to 300 mg a day for at least 2 weeks.

**Strength(s) usually available**
U.S.—
   50 mg per mL (OTC) [GENERIC].
   100 mg per mL (OTC) [*Cecon*].
Canada—
   Not commercially available.
Note: The strength of these ascorbic acid preparations may exceed the
   dosage range recommended by USP DI Advisory Panels based on
   the amount necessary to meet normal nutritional needs.

**Packaging and storage**
Store below 40 °C (104 °F), preferably between 15 and 30 °C (59 and 86
   °F), unless otherwise specified by manufacturer. Store in a tight, light-
   resistant container. Protect from freezing.

### ASCORBIC ACID SYRUP
**Usual adult and adolescent dose**
See *Ascorbic Acid Extended-release Capsules.*

**Usual pediatric dose**
See *Ascorbic Acid Oral Solution USP.*

**Strength(s) usually available**
U.S.—
   250 mg per 5 mL (OTC) [GENERIC].
   500 mg per 5 mL (OTC) [GENERIC].

Canada—
    Not commercially available.

Note: Some strengths of these ascorbic acid preparations may exceed the dosage range recommended by USP DI Advisory Panels based on the amount necessary to meet normal nutritional needs.

**Packaging and storage**
Store below 40 °C (104 °F), preferably between 15 and 30 °C (59 and 86 °F), in a tight container, unless otherwise specified by manufacturer. Protect from light. Protect from freezing.

## ASCORBIC ACID TABLETS USP

**Usual adult and adolescent dose**
See *Ascorbic Acid Extended-release Capsules.*

**Usual pediatric dose**
See *Ascorbic Acid Oral Solution USP.*

**Strength(s) usually available**
U.S.—
    25 mg (OTC) [GENERIC].
    50 mg (OTC) [GENERIC].
    100 mg (OTC) [GENERIC].
    125 mg (OTC) [GENERIC].
    250 mg (OTC) [GENERIC].
    500 mg (OTC) [*Sunkist;* GENERIC].
    1 gram (OTC) [GENERIC].
    1.5 grams (OTC) [GENERIC].
Canada—
    100 mg (OTC) [*Apo-C* (scored)].
    250 mg (OTC) [*Apo-C* (scored)].
    500 mg (OTC) [*Apo-C*].
    1 gram (OTC) [*Apo-C;* GENERIC].

Note: Some strengths of these ascorbic acid preparations may exceed the dosage range recommended by USP DI Advisory Panels based on the amount necessary to meet normal nutritional needs.

**Packaging and storage**
Store below 40 °C (104 °F), preferably between 15 and 30 °C (59 and 86 °F), unless otherwise specified by manufacturer. Store in a tight, light-resistant container.

## ASCORBIC ACID TABLETS (CHEWABLE) USP

**Usual adult and adolescent dose**
See *Ascorbic Acid Extended-release Capsules.*

**Usual pediatric dose**
See *Ascorbic Acid Oral Solution USP.*

**Strength(s) usually available**
U.S.—
    60 mg (OTC) [*Sunkist;* GENERIC].
    100 mg (OTC) [*Flavorcee;* GENERIC].
    250 mg (OTC) [*Flavorcee; Sunkist;* GENERIC].
    500 mg (OTC) [*Flavorcee; Sunkist;* GENERIC].
    1 gram (OTC) [GENERIC].
Canada—
    60 mg (OTC) [GENERIC].
    250 mg (OTC) [GENERIC].
    500 mg (OTC) [GENERIC].

Note: Some chewable ascorbic acid tablets may also contain sodium ascorbate.

Some strengths of these ascorbic acid preparations may exceed the dosage range recommended by USP DI Advisory Panels based on the amount necessary to meet normal nutritional needs.

**Packaging and storage**
Store below 40 °C (104 °F), preferably between 15 and 30 °C (59 and 86 °F), unless otherwise specified by manufacturer. Store in a tight, light-resistant container.

## ASCORBIC ACID TABLETS (EFFERVESCENT) USP

**Usual adult and adolescent dose**
See *Ascorbic Acid Extended-release Capsules.*

**Usual pediatric dose**
See *Ascorbic Acid Oral Solution USP.*

**Strength(s) usually available**
U.S.—
    1 gram (OTC) [GENERIC].
Canada—
    Not commercially available.

**Packaging and storage**
Store below 40 °C (104 °F), preferably between 15 and 30 °C (59 and 86 °F), unless otherwise specified by manufacturer. Store in a tight, light-resistant container.

**Preparation of dosage form**
Ascorbic acid effervescent tablets should be dissolved in a glass of water immediately prior to ingestion.

## ASCORBIC ACID EXTENDED-RELEASE TABLETS

**Usual adult and adolescent dose**
See *Ascorbic Acid Extended-release Capsules.*

**Usual pediatric dose**
Dosage form not appropriate for pediatric patients.

**Strength(s) usually available**
U.S.—
    500 mg (OTC) [*Cemill;* GENERIC].
    1 gram (OTC) [*Cemill;* GENERIC].
    1.5 gram (OTC) [GENERIC].
Canada—
    500 mg (OTC) [GENERIC].

Note: Some strengths of these ascorbic acid preparations may exceed the dosage range recommended by USP DI Advisory Panels based on the amount necessary to meet normal nutritional needs.

**Packaging and storage**
Store below 40 °C (104 °F), preferably between 15 and 30 °C (59 and 86 °F), in a tight container, unless otherwise specified by manufacturer. Protect from light.

# Parenteral Dosage Forms

## ASCORBIC ACID INJECTION USP

**Usual adult and adolescent dose**
Deficiency (prophylaxis)—
    Intravenous infusion, as part of total parenteral nutrition solutions, the specific amount determined by individual patient need.
Deficiency (treatment)—
    Intravenous infusion, as part of total parenteral nutrition solutions, the specific amount determined by individual patient need.
    Intramuscular, 100 to 500 mg a day for at least 2 weeks.
Diagnostic aid adjunct (red blood cell disease)—
    For use in labeling of red blood cells, 100 mg of ascorbic acid injection injected into the vial of sodium chromate Cr 51 injection.

**Usual pediatric dose**
Deficiency (prophylaxis)—
    Intravenous infusion, as part of total parenteral nutrition solutions, the specific amount determined by individual patient need.
Deficiency (treatment)—
    Intravenous infusion, as part of total parenteral nutrition solutions, the specific amount determined by individual patient need.
    Intramuscular, 100 to 300 mg a day for at least 2 weeks.

**Strength(s) usually available**
U.S.—
    222 mg per mL (Rx) [GENERIC].
    250 mg per mL (Rx) [GENERIC].
    500 mg per mL (Rx) [*Cecore 500; Cee-500; Mega-C/A Plus;* GENERIC].
Canada—
    Not commercially available.

**Packaging and storage**
Store below 40 °C (104 °F), preferably between 15 and 30 °C (59 and 86 °F), unless otherwise specified by manufacturer. Store in a light-resistant container. Protect from freezing.

**Stability**
Ascorbic acid is oxidized rapidly, especially in the presence of catalyzing metal ions such as copper. Loss of ascorbic acid is greatest from admixtures stored in plastic containers, especially for longer than 48 hours. Exposure to light causes degradation of ascorbic acid; however, the slight color that develops during storage does not impair therapeutic activity. Some clinicians recommend that total parenteral nutrition solutions that contain ascorbic acid should be protected from light.

**Incompatibilities**
Ascorbic acid injection is physically incompatible with aminophylline, bleomycin, cefazolin sodium, cephapirin, chlordiazepoxide, conjugated estrogen, dextran, doxapram hydrochloride, erythromycin lactobionate, methicillin sodium, nafcillin sodium, penicillin G potassium, phytonadione, sodium bicarbonate, and warfarin.

## SODIUM ASCORBATE

### SODIUM ASCORBATE INJECTION

**Usual adult and adolescent dose**
See *Ascorbic Acid Injection USP*.

**Usual pediatric dose**
See *Ascorbic Acid Injection USP*.

**Strength(s) usually available**
U.S.—
   250 mg (222 mg ascorbic acid) per mL (Rx) [*Ortho/CS;* GENERIC].
   562.5 mg (500 mg ascorbic acid) per mL (Rx) [*Cenolate* (0.5% sodium hydrosulfate)].
Canada—
   Not commercially available.

**Packaging and storage**
Store below 40 °C (104 °F), preferably between 15 and 30 °C (59 and 86 °F), protected from light, unless otherwise specified by manufacturer. Protect from freezing.

**Stability**
Ascorbic acid is oxidized rapidly, especially in the presence of catalyzing metal ions such as copper. Loss of ascorbic acid is greatest from admixtures stored in plastic containers, especially for longer than 48 hours. Exposure to light causes degradation of ascorbic acid; however, the slight color that develops during storage does not impair therapeutic activity. Some clinicians recommend that total parenteral nutrition solutions that contain ascorbic acid should be protected from light.

**Incompatibilities**
Ascorbic acid injection is physically incompatible with aminophylline, bleomycin, cefazolin sodium, cephapirin, chlordiazepoxide, conjugated estrogen, dextran, doxapram hydrochloride, erythromycin lactobionate, methicillin sodium, nafcillin sodium, penicillin G potassium, phytonadione, sodium bicarbonate, and warfarin.

**Additional information**
Each gram of sodium ascorbate contains approximately 5 mEq of sodium.

Revised: 05/01/95

## ASCORBIC ACID–CONTAINING COMBINATIONS—

Chlorpheniramine, Phenindamine, Phenylephrine, Dextromethorphan, Acetaminophen, Salicylamide, Caffeine, and Ascorbic Acid (Systemic)—See *Cough/Cold Combinations (Systemic)*
Chlorpheniramine, Pheniramine, Pyrilamine, Phenylephrine, Hydrocodone, Salicylamide, Caffeine, and Ascorbic Acid (Systemic)—See *Cough/Cold Combinations (Systemic)*
Pheniramine, Pyrilamine, Hydrocodone, Potassium Citrate, and Ascorbic Acid (Systemic)—See *Cough/Cold Combinations (Systemic)*

# ASPARAGINASE    Systemic

VA CLASSIFICATION (Primary): AN900
Another commonly used name is colaspase.
Note: For a listing of dosage forms and brand names by country availability, see *Dosage Forms* section(s). For a listing of brand names for the articles in this monograph, refer to the General Index.

## Category
Antineoplastic.

## Indications
Note: Bracketed information in the *Indications* section refers to uses that are not included in U.S. product labeling.

**Accepted**
Leukemia, acute lymphocytic (treatment)
[Leukemia, acute myelocytic (treatment)]
[Leukemia, acute myelomonocytic (treatment)] or
[Leukemia, chronic lymphocytic (treatment)]—Asparaginase is indicated, in combination with other agents, for induction of remissions in acute lymphocytic leukemia (primarily in children). It is recommended that asparaginase not be used as part of a maintenance regimen because of the rapid development of resistance (as cells develop the capability to synthesize asparagine) to the medication.

Asparaginase is also used for treatment of acute myelocytic leukemia, acute myelomonocytic leukemia, and chronic lymphocytic leukemia.

[Lymphomas, Hodgkin's (treatment)]—Asparaginase is used for treatment of Hodgkin's disease.

[Lymphomas, non-Hodgkin's (treatment)]—Asparaginase is used for treatment of lymphosarcoma and reticulum cell sarcoma (reticulosarcoma).

[Melanosarcoma (treatment)]—Asparaginase is used for treatment of melanosarcoma.

## Pharmacology/Pharmacokinetics

**Physicochemical characteristics**
Source—Asparaginase is a high molecular weight enzyme obtained commercially from *Escherichia coli*.

**Mechanism of action/Effect**
Asparaginase breaks down asparagine, which is required for cell survival, to aspartic acid and ammonia. Normal cells are capable of synthesizing their own asparagine but certain malignant cells are not. Asparaginase interferes with protein synthesis and also DNA and RNA synthesis, and appears to be cell cycle–specific for the $G_1$ phase of cell division.

**Other actions/effects**
Has immunosuppressant activity in animals.

**Distribution**
Crosses the blood-brain barrier to only a limited extent; cerebrospinal fluid concentrations are less than 1% of concurrent plasma concentrations.

**Protein binding**
Low (30%).

**Biotransformation**
Via slow sequestration by the reticuloendothelial system (wide individual variation); stimulates antibody response, which influences plasma clearance.

**Half-life**
Intramuscular—39 to 49 hours.
Intravenous—8 to 30 hours.

**Onset of action**
Blood concentrations of asparagine fall to undetectable levels almost immediately after administration of asparaginase.

**Time to peak plasma concentration**
After intramuscular administration—14 to 24 hours.

**Duration of action**
Asparagine reappears in the plasma within 23 to 33 days after withdrawal of therapy.

**Elimination**
Unknown, but appears to be biphasic; only trace amounts appear in the urine.

## Precautions to Consider

**Cross-sensitivity and/or related problems**
Cross-sensitivity between commercially available asparaginase and that for investigational use derived from *Erwinia carotovora* appears to be rare, although apparent cross-sensitivity has been reported in a few patients.

**Carcinogenicity**
Secondary malignancies are potential delayed effects of many antineoplastic agents, although it is not clear whether the effect is related to their mutagenic or immunosuppressive action. The effect of dose and duration of therapy is also unknown, although risk seems to increase with long-term use. Although information is limited, available data seem to indicate that the carcinogenic risk is greatest with the alkylating agents.
Intraperitoneal administration of 2500 Units of asparaginase per kg of body weight per day for 4 days reportedly caused a small increase in pulmonary adenomas in newborn Swiss mice.

**Mutagenicity**

Asparaginase was not found to be mutagenic at concentrations of 152–909 IU per plate in the Ames microbial mutagen test with or without metabolic activation.

**Pregnancy/Reproduction**

Pregnancy—Adequate and well-controlled studies in humans have not been done.

First trimester: It usually is recommended that use of antineoplastics, especially combination chemotherapy, be avoided whenever possible, especially during the first trimester. Although information is limited because of the relatively few instances of antineoplastic administration during pregnancy, the teratogenic and carcinogenic potential of these medications must be considered.

Other hazards to the fetus include adverse reactions seen in adults.

In general, use of a contraceptive is recommended during cytotoxic drug therapy.

Studies in mice and rats have shown that asparaginase, given in doses of greater than 1000 IU per kg of body weight (the recommended human dose), retards the weight gain of mothers and fetuses and causes resorptions, gross abnormalities, and skeletal abnormalities. Dose-dependent embryotoxicity and gross abnormalities also have been reported with intravenous administration of 50 or 100 IU of asparaginase per kg of body weight to pregnant rabbits on Days 8 and 9 of gestation.

FDA Pregnancy Category C.

**Breast-feeding**

It is not known whether asparaginase is distributed into breast milk. Although very little information is available regarding distribution of antineoplastic agents into breast milk, breast-feeding is not recommended while asparaginase is being administered because of the risks to the infant (adverse effects, carcinogenicity).

**Pediatrics**

Appropriate studies performed to date have not demonstrated pediatrics-specific problems that would limit the usefulness of asparaginase in children. In fact, incidence of toxicity appears to be lower in children than in adults.

**Geriatrics**

No information is available on the relationship of age to the effects of asparaginase in geriatric patients.

**Dental**

Asparaginase may cause stomatitis associated with considerable discomfort.

**Drug interactions and/or related problems**

The following drug interactions and/or related problems have been selected on the basis of their potential clinical significance (possible mechanism in parentheses where appropriate)—not necessarily inclusive (» = major clinical significance):

Note: Combinations containing any of the following medications, depending on the amount present, may also interact with this medication.

Allopurinol or
Colchicine or
» Probenecid or
» Sulfinpyrazone
(asparaginase may raise the concentration of blood uric acid; dosage adjustment of antigout agents may be necessary to control hyperuricemia and gout; allopurinol may be preferred to prevent or reverse asparaginase-induced hyperuricemia because of risk of uric acid nephropathy with uricosuric antigout agents)

Antidiabetic agents, oral or
Insulin
(asparaginase may alter blood glucose concentrations; for adult-onset diabetics, dosage adjustment of hypoglycemic medications may be necessary during and after asparaginase therapy)

Corticosteroids, glucocorticoid, especially prednisone or
Corticotropin (ACTH) or
» Vincristine
(concurrent use may enhance the hyperglycemic effect of asparaginase and may increase the risk of neuropathy and disturbances in erythropoiesis; toxicity appears to be less pronounced when asparaginase is administered after vincristine and prednisone rather than before or with these medications)

Immunosuppressant medications, other, such as:
Azathioprine
Chlorambucil
Cyclophosphamide
Cyclosporine

Mercaptopurine
Muromonab-CD3 or
Radiation therapy
(concurrent use with asparaginase may increase the total effects of these medications and radiation therapy; dosage reduction may be required)

» Methotrexate
(asparaginase may block the effects of methotrexate by inhibiting cell replication; this inhibition of methotrexate's action appears to correlate with suppression of asparagine concentrations. Some studies indicate that administration of asparaginase 9 to 10 days before or within 24 hours after methotrexate administration does not produce this inhibition of antineoplastic effect and may reduce the gastrointestinal and hematological effects of methotrexate)

Vaccines, killed virus
(because normal defense mechanisms may be suppressed by asparaginase therapy, the patient's antibody response to the vaccine may be decreased. The interval between discontinuation of medications that cause immunosuppression and restoration of the patient's ability to respond to the vaccine depends on the intensity and type of immunosuppression-causing medication used, the underlying disease, and other factors; estimates vary from 3 months to 1 year)

» Vaccines, live virus
(because normal defense mechanisms may be suppressed by asparaginase therapy, concurrent use with a live virus vaccine may potentiate the replication of the vaccine virus, may increase the side/adverse effects of the vaccine virus, and/or may decrease the patient's antibody response to the vaccine; immunization of these patients should be undertaken only with extreme caution after careful review of the patient's hematologic status and only with the knowledge and consent of the physician managing the asparaginase therapy. The interval between discontinuation of medications that cause immunosuppression and restoration of the patient's ability to respond to the vaccine depends on the intensity and type of immunosuppression-causing medication used, the underlying disease, and other factors; estimates vary from 3 months to 1 year. Patients with leukemia in remission should not receive live virus vaccine until at least 3 months after their last chemotherapy. In addition, immunization with oral poliovirus vaccine should be postponed in persons in close contact with the patient, especially family members)

**Laboratory value alterations**

The following have been selected on the basis of their potential clinical significance (possible effect in parentheses where appropriate)—not necessarily inclusive (» = major clinical significance):

With diagnostic test results
Thyroid function tests
(results may be altered because asparaginase decreases serum thyroxine-binding globulin concentrations within 2 days after the first dose; concentrations return to normal within 4 weeks of the last dose of asparaginase)

With physiology/laboratory test values
Alanine aminotransferase (ALT [SGPT]) and
Alkaline phosphatase and
Aspartate aminotransferase (AST [SGOT]) and
Bilirubin
(serum values may be increased; signs of hepatotoxicity)

Ammonia concentrations, blood and
Blood urea nitrogen (BUN) concentrations
(may be increased because of breakdown of asparagine)

Calcium
(serum concentrations may be decreased)

Cholesterol
(serum concentrations may be reversibly decreased; increases and decreases of total lipids have occurred)

Fibrinogen, antithrombin, and plasminogen concentrations, plasma and
Albumin concentrations, serum
(may be reversibly decreased in most patients due to inhibition of plasma protein synthesis by asparaginase)

Glucose
(blood concentrations may be increased)

Partial thromboplastin time (PTT) and
Platelet counts and
Prothrombin time (PT) and
Thrombin time (TT)
(may increase within the first 3 weeks of treatment)

Uric acid
(concentrations in blood and urine may be increased)

## Medical considerations/Contraindications

The medical considerations/contraindications included here have been selected on the basis of their potential clinical significance (reasons given
in parentheses where appropriate)—not necessarily inclusive (» =
major clinical significance).

*Except under special circumstances, this medication should not be used
when the following medical problems exist:*

» Pancreatitis, or history of
    (potentially fatal acute hemorrhagic pancreatitis has been associ-
    ated with asparaginase treatment)
» Previous allergic reaction to asparaginase

*Risk-benefit should be considered when the following medical problems
exist:*

» Chickenpox, existing or recent (including recent exposure) or
» Herpes zoster
    (risk of severe generalized disease)
  Diabetes mellitus
    (asparaginase may increase blood glucose concentrations)
  Gout, history of or
  Urate renal stones, history of
    (asparaginase may increase uric acid concentrations)
» Hepatic function impairment
    (may be increased by asparaginase)
» Infection
    (immunosuppressive effects)
» Caution should be used also in patients who have had previous cyto-
    toxic drug therapy and radiation therapy.

## Patient monitoring

The following are especially important in patient monitoring (other tests
may be warranted in some patients, depending on condition; » =
major clinical significance):

» Amylase concentrations, serum and
  Bone marrow aspiration studies and
  Calcium concentrations, serum and
» Central nervous system (CNS) function, clinical and
» Coagulation factor, plasma and
  Glucose concentrations, blood and
  Hepatic function and
  Peripheral blood count and
  Renal function and
  Uric acid concentrations, serum
    (recommended at the initiation of therapy and at frequent intervals
    during therapy)

# Side/Adverse Effects

Note: Incidence of toxicity appears to be greater in adults than in children.

The following side/adverse effects have been selected on the basis of their
potential clinical significance (possible signs and symptoms in parentheses where appropriate)—not necessarily inclusive:

**Those indicating need for medical attention**
Incidence more frequent
   *Allergic reaction* (trouble in breathing; joint pain; puffy face; skin rash
   or itching); *decrease in blood clotting factors* (usually asymptomatic;
   rarely, unusual bleeding or bruising); *hepatotoxicity, including fatty
   changes* (asymptomatic); *pancreatitis* (severe stomach pain with nausea and vomiting)
   Note: *Allergic reactions* occur frequently and may be severe or even
      fatal. The risk is increased with repeated doses, but may occur
      on initial administration, including during desensitization.
      An *allergic reaction* to a therapeutic dose may occur even after
      a negative reaction to the intradermal skin test. Rarely, an an-
      aphylactic reaction to the intradermal skin test itself may occur.
      *Anaphylaxis* may be less common after intramuscular than after
      intravenous administration in children with advanced leukemia
      (although incidence of mild allergic reactions may be in-
      creased), or when asparaginase is given in combination with
      immunosuppressive agents.
      The most common and most marked *decreases in blood clotting
      factors* occur in fibrinogen and factors V and VIII, with a var-
      iable decrease in factors VII and IX. Bleeding is rare, but in-
      tracranial hemorrhage and fatal bleeding have been reported. A
      compensatory increase in fibrinolytic activity has also occurred.
      *Hepatotoxicity* usually occurs within 2 weeks of start of
      treatment.

Incidence less frequent
   *CNS effects, reversible* (confusion; drowsiness; hallucinations; mental
   depression; nervousness; unusual tiredness); *hyperglycemia* (frequent
   urination; unusual thirst); *hyperuricemia or uric acid nephropathy*
   (lower back or side pain; swelling of feet or lower legs); *hypoalbuminemia or renal failure* (swelling of feet or lower legs); *stomatitis*
   (sores in mouth and on lips)
   Note: *CNS effects* occur mostly in adults, in whom incidence may be
      as high as 30 to 60%; they usually occur within the first day of
      treatment and subside 1 to 3 days after asparaginase is
      withdrawn.
      *Hyperglycemia* resembles hyperosmolar, nonketotic hypergly-
      cemia. It usually responds to withdrawal of asparaginase and
      appropriate treatment, but may occasionally be fatal.
      *Hyperuricemia or uric acid nephropathy* occurs most com-
      monly during initial treatment of patients with leukemia or lym-
      phoma, as a result of rapid cell breakdown leading to elevated
      serum uric acid concentrations.
      Azotemia, usually pre-renal, occurs frequently. Fatal *renal in-
      sufficiency* has been reported.

Incidence rare
   *Immunosuppression, leukopenia, infection, bacterial endotoxins in
   commercial preparation, or hyperthermia* (fever or chills); *intracranial hemorrhage or thrombosis* (severe headache; inability to move
   arm or leg); *leg vein thrombosis* (pain in lower legs); *seizures*
   Note: *Leukopenia* may be marked but bone marrow depression is
      transient.
      *Hyperthermia* may be fatal.

**Those indicating need for medical attention only if they continue
or are bothersome**
Incidence more frequent
   *Hyperammonemia* (mild headache; loss of appetite; nausea or vomiting; stomach cramps; weight loss)

**Those indicating the need for medical attention if they occur after
medication is discontinued**
   *Intracranial hemorrhage or thrombosis* (severe headache; inability to
   move arm or leg); *pancreatitis* (severe stomach pain with nausea and
   vomiting)

# Patient Consultation

As an aid to patient consultation, refer to *Advice for the Patient,
Asparaginase (Systemic).*

In providing consultation, consider emphasizing the following selected
information (» = major clinical significance):

**Before using this medication**
» Conditions affecting use, especially:
    Sensitivity to asparaginase
    Pregnancy—Embryotoxicity and abnormalities reported in ani-
      mals; advisability of using contraception; telling physician im-
      mediately if pregnancy is suspected
    Breast-feeding—Not recommended because of risk of serious side
      effects
    Other medications, especially probenecid, sulfinpyrazone, or pre-
      vious cytotoxic drug or radiation therapy
    Other medical problems, especially chickenpox, herpes zoster, pan-
      creatitis, hepatic function impairment, or infection

**Proper use of this medication**
   Caution with combination therapy; taking each medication at the right
     time
   Importance of ample fluid intake and subsequent increase in urine
     output to aid in excretion of uric acid
   Possible nausea, vomiting, and loss of appetite; importance of contin-
     uing medication despite stomach upset
» Proper dosing

**Precautions while using this medication**
» Importance of close monitoring by physician
» Avoiding immunizations unless approved by physician; other persons
    in patient's household should avoid immunizations with oral po-
    liovirus vaccine; avoiding persons who have taken oral poliovirus
    vaccine or wearing a protective mask that covers nose and mouth
   Caution if any laboratory tests required; possible interference with thy-
     roid function test results

**Side/adverse effects**
   Importance of discussing possible adverse effects, including cancer,
     with physician
   Signs of potential side effects, especially allergic reaction, decrease in
     blood clotting factors, pancreatitis, CNS effects, hyperglycemia,

hyperuricemia or uric acid nephropathy, hypoalbuminemia or renal failure, stomatitis, leukopenia, immunosuppression, infection, hyperthermia, intracranial hemorrhage or thrombosis, leg vein thrombosis, and seizures

Asymptomatic side effects, including hepatotoxicity

Physician or nurse can help in dealing with side effects

## General Dosing Information

It is recommended that asparaginase be administered to patients only in a hospital setting under the supervision of a physician experienced in cancer chemotherapy. It is also recommended that equipment and medications (including epinephrine, diphenhydramine, oxygen, and intravenous steroids) necessary for treatment of a possible anaphylactic reaction be immediately available during each administration of asparaginase.

A variety of dosage schedules and regimens of asparaginase, alone or in combination with other antitumor agents, are used. The prescriber may consult the medical literature as well as the manufacturer's literature in choosing a specific dosage.

Dosage must be adjusted to meet the individual requirements of each patient, on the basis of clinical response and appearance or severity of toxicity.

Although the intradermal skin test has not been found entirely reliable in predicting allergic reactions to asparaginase, it is recommended that this test be performed prior to the initial administration of asparaginase and when a week or more has passed between doses. The test solution is prepared by adding 5 mL of sterile water for injection or 0.9% sodium chloride injection to the 10,000–International Unit (IU) vial of asparaginase, shaking to dissolve, and withdrawing 0.1 mL of the resulting solution (2000 IU per mL) and injecting it into another vial containing 9.9 mL of diluent to produce a test solution containing approximately 20 IU per mL. An intradermal injection of 0.1 mL (about 2 IU) is administered and the site observed for 1 hour for the appearance of a wheal or erythema, which indicates a positive reaction.

It is recommended that a desensitization method of administration of the first dose be utilized in patients who have had a positive reaction to the intradermal skin test and on retreatment of a patient with asparaginase. A recommended schedule begins with the intravenous administration of 1 IU and doubles the dosage every 10 minutes, provided no allergic reaction has occurred, until the accumulated total dosage equals the dosage for that day.

It is recommended that when asparaginase is administered intravenously, it be given over a period of not less than 30 minutes through the side arm of an already running infusion of 0.9% sodium chloride injection or 5% dextrose injection. Asparaginase should not be infused through a filter. However, if gelatinous fiber-like particles develop on standing, reconstituted asparaginase may be filtered through a 5.0-micron filter during administration without loss in potency. Use of a 0.2-micron filter may result in a loss of potency.

No more than 2 mL of asparaginase solution should be injected at a single intramuscular injection site.

Development of uric acid nephropathy in patients with leukemia or lymphoma may be prevented by adequate oral hydration and, in some cases, administration of allopurinol. Alkalinization of urine may be necessary if serum uric acid concentrations are elevated.

If pancreatitis occurs, it is recommended that asparaginase therapy be permanently discontinued.

### Safety considerations for handling this medication

There is limited but increasing evidence and concern that personnel involved in preparation and administration of parenteral antineoplastics may be at some risk because of the potential mutagenicity, teratogenicity, and/or carcinogenicity of these agents, although the actual risk is unknown. USP advisory panels recommend cautious handling both in preparation and disposal of antineoplastic agents. Precautions that have been suggested include:

• Use of a biological containment cabinet during reconstitution and dilution of parenteral medications and wearing of disposable surgical gloves and masks.

• Use of proper technique to prevent contamination of the medication, work area, and operator during transfer between containers (including proper training of personnel in this technique).

• Cautious and proper disposal of needles, syringes, vials, ampuls, and unused medication.

A number of medical centers have developed detailed guidelines for handling of antineoplastic agents.

### Combination chemotherapy

Asparaginase may be used in combination with other agents in various regimens. As a result, incidence and/or severity of side effects may be altered and different dosages (usually reduced) may be used. For example, asparaginase is part of the following chemotherapeutic combination (a commonly used acronym is in parentheses):

—asparaginase, vincristine, and prednisone (VP-L-Asparaginase).

For specific dosages and schedules, consult the literature. For information regarding each agent, consult the individual monographs.

## Parenteral Dosage Forms

### ASPARAGINASE FOR INJECTION

#### Usual adult dose

Acute lymphocytic leukemia—

Induction: Intravenous, 200 IU per kg of body weight a day for twenty-eight days.

Note: Because use of asparaginase in adults is primarily investigational at this time, the prescriber should consult the medical literature in choosing a specific dosage.

#### Usual pediatric dose

Acute lymphocytic leukemia—

Intramuscular, 6000 IU per square meter of body surface on Days 4, 7, 10, 13, 16, 19, 22, 25, and 28 of the treatment period, in combination with vincristine and prednisone or

Intravenous, 1000 IU per kg of body weight per day for ten days beginning on Day 22 of the treatment period, in combination with vincristine and prednisone.

Note: Many dosage regimens of asparaginase are in use at this time. A review of all of them is impossible in this space. Consultation of current medical literature is recommended. Use of asparaginase as the sole induction agent generally is not recommended unless combination therapy is considered inappropriate.

#### Strength(s) usually available

U.S.—

10,000 IU (Rx) [*Elspar* (mannitol 80 mg)].

Canada—

10,000 IU (Rx) [*Kidrolase*].

#### Packaging and storage

Store below 8 °C (46 °F).

Note: Storage for several years at –20 °C (–4 °F) causes no apparent loss of activity.

#### Preparation of dosage form

Caution: Asparaginase is a contact irritant, and both the powder and solution should be handled with care to prevent inhalation of dust or vapors or contact with skin or mucous membranes (especially eyes). If accidental contact occurs, the affected area should be flushed with water for at least 15 minutes.

*Elspar* is reconstituted for intravenous use by adding 5 mL of sterile water for injection or 0.9% sodium chloride injection to a vial containing 10,000 IU of asparaginase and shaking to dissolve the medication. (Caution: Overly vigorous shaking may cause foaming and difficulty in withdrawing the contents of the vial.) Only a clear solution should be used. The resulting colorless solution, containing 2000 IU of asparaginase per mL, may be used for direct intravenous administration within 8 hours of reconstitution, provided the solution remains clear, or may be further diluted with 0.9% sodium chloride injection or 5% dextrose injection for administration by intravenous infusion. The infusion solution may also be used within 8 hours, provided it remains clear.

*Elspar* is reconstituted for intramuscular use by adding 2 mL of 0.9% sodium chloride injection to the 10,000-IU vial. The resulting solution should be used within 8 hours provided it remains clear.

If gelatinous fiber-like particles develop on standing, reconstituted *Elspar* may be filtered through a 5.0-micron filter during administration without loss in potency. Use of a 0.2-micron filter may result in a loss of potency.

*Kidrolase* is reconstituted for intramuscular or intravenous use by adding 4 mL of sterile water for injection to a vial containing 10,000 IU of asparaginase and rotating gently to dissolve the medication. (Caution: Vigorous shaking may cause foaming and difficulty in withdrawing the contents of the vial.) The resulting solution may be further diluted with 0.9% sodium chloride injection or isotonic glucose solution for administration by intravenous infusion.

**Stability**

*Elspar*—Contains no preservative. Unused, reconstituted solution should be stored at 2 to 8 °C (36 to 46 °F) and discarded after eight hours or sooner if it becomes cloudy.

*Kidrolase*—Unused, reconstituted solution may be stored at 2 to 8 °C (36 to 46 °F) for 14 days.

Revised: 04/09/93
Interim revision: 04/29/94

---

**ASPIRIN**—See *Salicylates (Systemic)*

---

**ASPIRIN, BUFFERED**—See *Salicylates (Systemic)*

---

**ASPIRIN-CONTAINING COMBINATIONS**—

Acetaminophen and Aspirin (Systemic)—See *Acetaminophen and Salicylates (Systemic)*

Acetaminophen, Aspirin, and Caffeine (Systemic)—See *Acetaminophen and Salicylates (Systemic)*

Acetaminophen, Aspirin, and Caffeine, Buffered (Systemic)—See *Acetaminophen and Salicylates (Systemic)*

Acetaminophen, Aspirin, and Salicylamide, Buffered (Systemic)—See *Acetaminophen and Salicylates (Systemic)*

Acetaminophen, Aspirin, Salicylamide, and Caffeine (Systemic)—See *Acetaminophen and Salicylates (Systemic)*

Aspirin, Buffered (Systemic)—See *Salicylates (Systemic)*

Aspirin and Caffeine (Systemic)—See *Salicylates (Systemic)*

Aspirin and Caffeine, Buffered (Systemic)—See *Salicylates (Systemic)*

Aspirin, Caffeine, and Dihydrocodeine (Systemic)—See *Opioid (Narcotic) Analgesics and Aspirin (Systemic)*

Aspirin and Codeine (Systemic)—See *Opioid (Narcotic) Analgesics and Aspirin (Systemic)*

Aspirin and Codeine, Buffered (Systemic)—See *Opioid (Narcotic) Analgesics and Aspirin (Systemic)*

Aspirin, Codeine, and Caffeine (Systemic)—See *Opioid (Narcotic) Analgesics and Aspirin (Systemic)*

Aspirin, Sodium Bicarbonate, and Citric Acid (Systemic)

Butalbital and Aspirin (Systemic)—See *Barbiturates and Analgesics (Systemic)*

Butalbital, Aspirin, and Caffeine (Systemic)—See *Barbiturates and Analgesics (Systemic)*

Butalbital, Aspirin, Caffeine, and Codeine (Systemic)—See *Barbiturates and Analgesics (Systemic)*

Chlorpheniramine, Phenylpropanolamine, and Aspirin (Systemic)—See *Antihistamines, Decongestants, and Analgesics (Systemic)*

Chlorpheniramine, Phenylpropanolamine, Aspirin, and Caffeine (Systemic)—See *Antihistamines, Decongestants, and Analgesics (Systemic)*

Chlorpheniramine, Phenylpropanolamine, Dextromethorphan, and Aspirin (Systemic)—See *Cough/Cold Combinations (Systemic)*

Diphenhydramine, Phenylpropanolamine, and Aspirin (Systemic)—See *Antihistamines, Decongestants, and Analgesics (Systemic)*

Doxylamine, Phenylpropanolamine, Dextromethorphan, and Aspirin (Systemic)—See *Cough/Cold Combinations (Systemic)*

Hydrocodone and Aspirin (Systemic)—See *Opioid (Narcotic) Analgesics and Aspirin (Systemic)*

Meprobamate and Aspirin (Systemic)

Orphenadrine, Aspirin, and Caffeine (Systemic)—See *Orphenadrine and Aspirin (Systemic)*

Oxycodone and Aspirin (Systemic)—See *Opioid (Narcotic) Analgesics and Aspirin (Systemic)*

Pentazocine and Aspirin (Systemic)—See *Opioid (Narcotic) Analgesics and Aspirin (Systemic)*

Phenobarbital, ASA, and Codeine (Systemic)—See *Barbiturates and Analgesics (Systemic)*

Phenylpropanolamine, Acetaminophen, and Aspirin (Systemic)—See *Decongestants and Analgesics (Systemic)*

Phenylpropanolamine, Acetaminophen, and Caffeine (Systemic)—See *Decongestants and Analgesics (Systemic)*

Phenylpropanolamine and Aspirin (Systemic)—See *Decongestants and Analgesics (Systemic)*

Propoxyphene and Aspirin (Systemic)—See *Opioid (Narcotic) Analgesics and Aspirin (Systemic)*

Propoxyphene, Aspirin, and Caffeine (Systemic)—See *Opioid (Narcotic) Analgesics and Aspirin (Systemic)*

Pseudoephedrine and Aspirin (Systemic)—See *Decongestants and Analgesics (Systemic)*

Pyrilamine, Phenylephrine, Aspirin, and Caffeine (Systemic)—See *Antihistamines, Decongestants, and Analgesics (Systemic)*

---

# ASPIRIN, SODIUM BICARBONATE, AND CITRIC ACID  Systemic

**VA CLASSIFICATION** (Primary/Secondary): CN103/BL700

**NOTE:** The *Aspirin, Sodium Bicarbonate, and Citric Acid (Systemic)* monograph is maintained on the USP DI electronic data base. For a printed copy of the most recent revision of the complete monograph, contact the USP DI Division of Information Development, 12601 Twinbrook Parkway, Rockville, MD 20852.

For information on the specific components of this combination, see the *USP DI* monographs for *Salicylates (Systemic), Sodium Bicarbonate (Systemic),* and *Citrates (Systemic).*

The information that follows is selectively abstracted from the complete monograph and is provided to facilitate drug use review and patient counseling.

Note: For a listing of dosage forms and brand names by country availability, see *Dosage Forms* section(s). For a listing of brand names for the articles in this monograph, refer to the General Index.

## Category

Analgesic-antacid; platelet aggregation inhibitor.

## Indications

Note: Bracketed information in the *Indications* section refers to uses that are not included in U.S. product labeling.

**Accepted**

Pain and upset stomach (treatment)—Aspirin, sodium bicarbonate, and citric acid combination is indicated to relieve pain, especially when an upset stomach is also present. However, this medication is not recommended for long-term, high-dose use because of the high sodium bicarbonate content.

Platelet aggregation (prophylaxis)[1]—Aspirin, sodium bicarbonate, and citric acid combination is indicated to provide the platelet aggregation-inhibiting action of aspirin in the following:

Ischemic attacks, transient, in males (prophylaxis);

Thromboembolism, cerebral (prophylaxis); or

[Thromboembolism, cerebral, recurrence (prophylaxis)]—Aspirin is indicated in the treatment of men who have had transient brain ischemia due to fibrin platelet emboli, to reduce the recurrence of transient ischemic attacks (TIAs) and the risk of stroke and death.

[Aspirin is also used in the treatment of women with transient brain ischemia due to fibrin platelet emboli. However, its efficacy in preventing stroke and death in female patients has not been established].

[Aspirin is also indicated in the treatment of patients with documented, unexplained TIAs associated with mitral valve prolapse. However, if TIAs continue to occur after an adequate trial of aspirin therapy, aspirin should be discontinued and an oral anticoagulant administered instead].

[Aspirin is also indicated to prevent initial or recurrent cerebrovascular embolism, TIAs, and stroke following carotid endarterectomy].

[Aspirin is indicated in the treatment of patients who have had a completed thrombotic stroke, to prevent a recurrence].

Myocardial infarction (prophylaxis); or

Myocardial reinfarction (prophylaxis)—Aspirin is indicated to prevent myocardial infarction in patients with unstable angina pectoris and to prevent recurrence of myocardial infarction in patients with a history of myocardial infarction.

In one study, aspirin significantly reduced the rate of reocclusion, reinfarction, stroke, and death when a single dose was administered within a few hours after the onset of symptoms of acute myocardial infarction and daily thereafter. The benefit of early treatment with aspirin was additive to that of streptokinase. Therefore, it is recommended that aspirin therapy be initiated as soon as possible after the onset of symptoms, even if the patient is receiving thrombolytic therapy.

[One study has shown that aspirin may also prevent myocardial infarction in individuals who have no history of unstable angina pectoris or myocardial infarction. However, an increased incidence of hemorrhagic stroke was reported in subjects receiving aspirin. Also, the incidence of myocardial infarction, although higher in the placebo group than in the aspirin group, was low in both groups. Therefore, use of aspirin for this purpose remains controversial; whether aspirin's benefit outweighs its risk in apparently healthy individuals has not been established. However, aspirin may be indicated for prevention of an initial myocardial infarction in selected patients, especially those who may be at risk because of the presence of chronic stable coronary artery disease (as shown by exertional or episodic angina pectoris, abnormal coronary arteriogram, or positive stress test) and/or other risk factors.]

[Thromboembolism (prophylaxis)]—Aspirin is used in low doses to decrease the risk of thromboembolism following orthopedic (hip) surgery (especially total hip replacement) and in patients with arteriovenous shunts.

Platelet aggregation inhibitors, although not as consistently effective as an anticoagulant or an anticoagulant plus dipyridamole, may provide some protection against the development of thromboembolic complications in patients with mechanical prosthetic heart valves. Therefore, administration of aspirin, alone or in combination with dipyridamole, may be considered if anticoagulant therapy is contraindicated for these patients. Patients with bioprosthetic cardiac valves who are in normal sinus rhythm generally do not require prolonged antithrombotic therapy, but long-term aspirin administration may be considered on an individual basis.

Aspirin is also indicated, alone or in combination with dipyridamole, to reduce the risk of thrombosis and/or reocclusion of saphenous vein aortocoronary bypass grafts following coronary bypass surgery.

Aspirin is also indicated, alone or in combination with dipyridamole, to reduce the risk of thrombosis and/or reocclusion of prosthetic or saphenous vein femoral popliteal bypass grafts.

Because the patient may be at risk for thromboembolic complications, including myocardial infarction and stroke, long-term aspirin therapy may also be indicated for maintaining patency following coronary or peripheral vascular angioplasty and for treating patients with peripheral vascular insufficiency caused by arteriosclerosis.

Prolonged antithrombotic therapy is generally not needed to maintain vessel patency following vascular reconstruction procedures in high-flow, low-resistance arteries larger than 6 mm in diameter. However, long-term aspirin therapy may be indicated, because patients requiring such procedures may be at risk for other thrombotic complications.

---

[1]Not included in Canadian product labeling.

## Patient Consultation

As an aid to patient consultation, refer to *Advice for the Patient, Aspirin, Sodium Bicarbonate, and Citric Acid (Systemic)*.

In providing consultation, consider emphasizing the following selected information (» = major clinical significance):

### Before using this medication
» Conditions affecting use, especially:

Sensitivity to aspirin, nonsteroidal anti-inflammatory drugs (NSAIDs), or sodium bicarbonate

Pregnancy—Not taking aspirin in third trimester unless prescribed by physician; high-dose, chronic use or abuse of aspirin in third trimester may be hazardous to the mother as well as the fetus and/or neonate, causing heart problems in fetus or neonate and/or bleeding in mother, fetus, or neonate; high-dose, chronic use or abuse may also prolong and complicate labor and delivery; sodium may cause edema and weight gain

Use in children—Checking with physician before giving to children with symptoms of acute febrile illness, especially influenza or varicella, because of the risk of Reye's syndrome; also, increased susceptibility to aspirin toxicity in children, especially with fever and dehydration

Use in teenagers—Checking with physician before giving to teenagers with symptoms of acute febrile illness, especially influenza or varicella, because of the risk of Reye's syndrome

Use in the elderly—Increased risk of aspirin toxicity; also, because of the very high sodium content, use should preferably be limited to 5 days at a time, unless more prolonged therapy is prescribed and monitored by a physician

Other medications, especially anticoagulants, oral antidiabetic agents, oral imidazole antifungals, mecamylamine, methenamine, methotrexate, NSAIDs, platelet aggregation inhibitors, those cephalosporins that may cause hypoprothrombinemia, probenecid, sulfinpyrazone, oral tetracyclines, and vancomycin

Other medical problems, especially symptoms of appendicitis, coagulation or platelet function disorders, conditions in which sodium may be detrimental, gastrointestinal problems such as ulceration or erosive gastritis (especially a bleeding ulcer) or gastrointestinal obstruction, and renal function impairment

### Proper use of this medication
» Importance of not taking more medication than recommended on package label, unless otherwise directed by physician, because of risk of aspirin- or sodium bicarbonate–induced adverse effects

Proper administration:

Taking in liquid form only; not ingesting tablets or tablet fragments

Preparing liquid: Placing 1 or 2 tablets in glass, then adding 1/2 glass (120 mL) cool water

Checking for complete tablet dissolution before drinking; drinking while solution is still effervescing, or after it has settled

Drinking entire amount, then rinsing glass with a little more water and drinking that, to ensure receiving full dosage

» Proper dosing

Missed dose (if on scheduled dosing): Taking as soon as possible; not taking if almost time for next dose; not doubling doses

» Proper storage

### Precautions while using this medication
» Regular visits to physician to check progress if long-term or high-dose therapy is prescribed

Checking with physician if symptoms persist for longer than 10 days for adults or 5 days for children, condition becomes worse, new symptoms occur, or the painful area is red or swollen

» Not taking this medication within:
—6 hours before or 2 hours after ciprofloxacin or lomefloxacin
—8 hours before or 2 hours after enoxacin
—2 hours after itraconazole
—3 hours before or after ketoconazole
—2 hours before or after norfloxacin or ofloxacin
—3 to 4 hours before or after an oral tetracycline
—1 or 2 hours before or after any other oral medication

Not taking a cellulose-containing laxative within 2 hours of taking aspirin

» Possibility of overdose if other medications containing aspirin or other salicylates (including diflunisal) or significant quantities of sodium are used

Not taking aspirin for 5 days prior to any kind of surgery, unless otherwise directed by physician

» If taking aspirin as a platelet aggregation inhibitor:

Taking only the amount prescribed; checking with physician to determine whether an alternative medication, rather than additional aspirin, should be used to relieve pain, fever, arthritis

Not discontinuing therapy without first checking with the prescriber

Not using an NSAID together with this medication for more than a few days, unless otherwise directed by physician

If taking more than an occasional 1 or 2 doses of this medication:

» Avoiding alcoholic beverages, because of the increased risk of aspirin-induced gastrointestinal toxicity

» Avoiding large amounts of milk or milk products

Possible need for sodium restriction

Caution if any laboratory tests required; possible interference with test results

Diabetics: Aspirin may cause false urine sugar test results with prolonged use of 8 or more 325-mg (5-grain) doses per day

» Suspected overdose: Getting emergency help at once

### Side/adverse effects

Signs of potential side effects, especially edema, hypercalcemia associated with milk-alkali syndrome, increased blood pressure, metabolic alkalosis, anaphylaxis, anemia, bronchospastic allergic reaction, allergic dermatitis, and gastrointestinal ulceration or bleeding

## Oral Dosage Forms

### ASPIRIN EFFERVESCENT TABLETS FOR ORAL SOLUTION USP

**Usual adult and adolescent dose**

Analgesic/antacid—
Oral, 325 to 500 mg of aspirin every three hours, 325 to 650 mg of aspirin every four hours, or 650 mg to 1 gram of aspirin every six hours as needed, while symptoms persist.

Note: It is recommended that the total daily dose of aspirin not exceed 4 grams, and that a physician be consulted if symptoms are not relieved within ten days.

Platelet aggregation inhibitor[1]—
Oral, 325 mg of aspirin a day.

Note: Optimal dosage has not been established. Doses lower than 325 mg of aspirin a day are often utilized, since there is evidence that 160 mg of aspirin every twenty-four hours may effectively inhibit platelet aggregation while minimizing the risk of aspirin-induced side effects. Doses higher than 325 mg of aspirin a day are also recommended for specific indications responsive to platelet aggregation inhibition. However, because of its high sodium bicarbonate content, this formulation is not recommended for long-term therapy with doses higher than 325 mg of aspirin a day.

**Usual adult prescribing limits**

Geriatric patients—Oral, up to 4 regular-strength or extra-strength tablets a day. Limiting the duration of treatment to five days may be advisable, unless longer treatment is prescribed and monitored by a physician.

Nongeriatric adults—Oral, up to 8 regular-strength unflavored tablets, 6 regular-strength flavored tablets, or 7 extra-strength tablets a day. A physician should be consulted if symptoms are not relieved within ten days.

Note: The lower maximum daily dosage recommended for the flavored regular-strength formulation, which contains more citric acid per tablet than the unflavored regular-strength formulation, is dictated by the FDA-mandated twenty-four-hour dosing limit for citric acid in OTC products.

**Usual pediatric dose**

Analgesic/antacid—
Children up to 3 years of age: Dosage must be individualized by physician.
Children 3 to 5 years of age: Oral, 167 mg of aspirin (one-half of a regular-strength tablet) every four to six hours as needed, while symptoms persist.
Children 6 to 12 years of age: Oral, 325 mg (one regular-strength tablet) every four to six hours as needed, while symptoms persist.

Note: It is recommended that children up to 12 years of age receive no more than five doses in each twenty-four-hour period, unless otherwise directed by a physician, and that a physician be consulted if symptoms are not relieved within five days.

**Strength(s) usually available**

Note: When dissolved in water, aspirin effervescent tablets for oral solution provide aspirin in the form of sodium acetylsalicylate.

U.S.—
Regular-strength:
325 mg of aspirin, with 1.916 grams of sodium bicarbonate and 1 gram of citric acid (OTC) [*Alka-Seltzer Effervescent Pain Reliever and Antacid* (sodium 567 mg [24.65 mmol] per tablet)].
325 mg of aspirin, with 1.71 grams of sodium bicarbonate and 1.22 grams of citric acid (OTC) [*Flavored Alka-Seltzer Effervescent Pain Reliever and Antacid* (sodium 506 mg [22 mmol] per tablet)].
Extra-strength:
500 mg of aspirin, with 1.985 grams of sodium bicarbonate and 1 gram of citric acid (OTC) [*Alka-Seltzer Effervescent Pain Reliever and Antacid* (sodium 588 mg [25.56 mmol] per tablet)].

Canada—
Regular strength:
325 mg of ASA, with 1.916 grams of sodium bicarbonate and 1 gram of citric acid (OTC) [*Alka-Seltzer Effervescent Pain Reliever and Antacid* (sodium 567 mg [24.65 mmol] per tablet)].
325 mg of ASA, with 1.71 grams of sodium bicarbonate and 1.22 grams of citric acid (OTC) [*Flavored Alka-Seltzer Effervescent Pain Reliever and Antacid* (sodium 506 mg [22 mmol] per tablet)].

Note: *Aspirin* is a brand name in Canada; acetylsalicylic acid is the generic name. ASA, a commonly used designation for aspirin (or acetylsalicylic acid) in both the U.S. and Canada, is the term used in Canadian product labeling.

**Auxiliary labeling**
• Keep container tightly closed.

[1]Not included in Canadian product labeling.

Revised: 08/29/94

---

## ASTEMIZOLE—See *Antihistamines (Systemic)*

---

## ATENOLOL—See *Beta-adrenergic Blocking Agents (Systemic)*

---

## ATENOLOL-CONTAINING COMBINATIONS—

Atenolol and Chlorthalidone (Systemic)—See *Beta-adrenergic Blocking Agents and Thiazide Diuretics (Systemic)*

---

# ATOVAQUONE   Systemic

---

**VA CLASSIFICATION (Primary): AP109**

Note: For a listing of dosage forms and brand names by country availability, see *Dosage Forms* section(s). For a listing of brand names for the articles in this monograph, refer to the General Index.

## Category

Antiprotozoal.

## Indications

**Accepted**

Pneumonia, *Pneumocystis carinii* (PCP) (treatment)—Atovaquone is indicated in the treatment of mild to moderate *Pneumocystis carinii* pneumonia (A-a gradient ≤ 45 mmHg and $pO_2$ ≥ 60 mmHg on room air) in patients who are intolerant of sulfamethoxazole and trimethoprim combination.

Atovaquone has not been evaluated for the treatment of more severe episodes of PCP, in patients who are failing sulfamethoxazole and trimethoprim combination therapy, or as a chronic suppressive agent for PCP prophylaxis.

**Unaccepted**

Atovaquone is not effective therapy against bacterial, viral, or fungal pneumonias or mycobacterial disease.

## Pharmacology/Pharmacokinetics

**Physicochemical characteristics**

Chemical group—1,4-Hydroxynaphthoquinone
Molecular weight—366.84.

**Mechanism of action/Effect**

Atovaquone has possible cidal activity against susceptible organisms. The action against *Pneumocystis carinii* is not fully understood. Atovaquone is structurally similar to ubiquinone, which inhibits the mitochondrial electron-transport chain at the site of the cytochrome $bc_1$ complex (complex III) in *Plasmodium* species. This may ultimately inhibit the synthesis of nucleic acid and ATP. Atovaquone also has been shown to have good *in vitro* activity against *Toxoplasma gondii*.

**Absorption**

The bioavailability of atovaquone is low and variable, and decreases significantly with single doses greater than 750 mg. A standard breakfast containing 23 grams of fat has been shown to enhance absorption significantly.

Oral suspension—The oral suspension provides a two-fold increase in bioavailability in fasting or fed conditions compared to the tablets. Bioavailability of the suspension increases two-fold when administered with meals; when administered with food, bioavailability is approximately 47%.

Tablets—Bioavailability increases three-fold when administered with meals; bioavailability of the tablets when administered with food is approximately 23%.

### Distribution

Atovaquone is highly lipophilic, with low aqueous solubility. The cerebrospinal fluid (CSF) to plasma ratio is very low (< 1%).

$Vol_D$ at steady state is approximately 0.6 liter per kg (L/kg).

### Protein binding

Very high (> 99.9%); primarily bound to albumin in serum.

### Biotransformation

There is indirect evidence that atovaquone may undergo limited metabolism; however, a specific metabolite has not been identified.

### Half-life

2.2 to 3.2 days in adult patients with acquired immunodeficiency syndrome (AIDS), adult healthy volunteers, and immunocompromised children (ages 5 months to 13 years).

### Time to peak concentration

A double peak has been observed. The first peak was 1 to 8 hours after dosing; the second peak was 24 to 96 hours after dosing. This is suggestive of enterohepatic recycling.

### Peak plasma concentration

Adults—
Oral suspension:
Approximately 24 mcg per mL (mcg/mL) in patients infected with human immunodeficiency virus (HIV) taking 750 mg two times a day with food.
Tablets:
Approximately 13 mcg/mL in AIDS patients taking 750 mg three times a day with food.
Children—
Oral suspension:
Ages 3 to 24 months (steady-state concentrations)—
Approximately 5.7 mcg/mL in HIV-infected children after administration of 10 mg per kg of body weight (mg/kg).
Approximately 8.9 mcg/mL in HIV-infected children after administration of 30 mg/kg.
Ages 2 to 13 years—
Approximately 16.8 mcg/mL in HIV-infected children after administration of 10 mg/kg.
Approximately 37.1 mcg/mL in HIV-infected children after administration of 30 mg/kg.
Tablets:
Ages 5 months to 13 years—
Steady-state average of 7.5 mcg/mL after administration of 10 mg per kg of body weight (mg/kg) once a day, and a steady-state average of 14 mcg/mL after administration of 40 mg/kg once a day.
There appears to be a correlation between plasma atovaquone concentrations and the likelihood of successful treatment and survival. Patients with atovaquone concentrations < 5 mcg/mL were more likely to die than those with concentrations ≥ 5 mcg/mL. In one study, 0 of 6 (0%) patients with a plasma atovaquone concentration of < 5 mcg/mL were successfully treated, compared to 30 of 38 (79%) patients with plasma concentrations of 10 to < 15 mcg/mL and 18 of 19 (95%) patients with plasma concentrations of 15 to < 20 mcg/mL.

Steady-state plasma concentrations in AIDS patients administered atovaquone tablets are about one-third to one-half of the levels achieved in asymptomatic HIV-infected patients; the reason for this is not yet known.

### Elimination

Fecal; > 94% of atovaquone was recovered in the feces over 21 days; <0.6% was excreted in the urine.

## Precautions to Consider

### Carcinogenicity

Studies in rats and mice have not been completed.

### Mutagenicity

Atovaquone was found to be negative with or without metabolic activation in the Ames *Salmonella* mutagenicity assay, the mouse lymphoma mutagenesis assay, and the cultured human lymphocyte cytogenic assay. No evidence of genotoxicity was seen in the *in vivo* mouse micronucleus assay.

### Pregnancy/Reproduction

Pregnancy—Studies have not been done in pregnant women.

Atovaquone was not teratogenic and did not cause reproductive toxicity in rats with plasma concentrations up to 2 to 3 times the estimated human exposure. It did cause maternal toxicity in rabbits with plasma

concentrations that were approximately equal to the estimated human exposure; mean fetal body lengths and weights were decreased and there were higher numbers of early resorption and post-implantation losses per dam. It is not clear whether these effects were caused by atovaquone or were secondary to maternal toxicity. Concentrations in rabbit fetuses averaged 30% of the concurrent maternal plasma concentrations. After a single $^{14}$C-radiolabeled dose, concentrations of radiocarbon in rat fetuses were 18% (middle gestation) and 60% (late gestation) of concurrent maternal plasma concentrations.

FDA Pregnancy Category C.

### Breast-feeding

It is not known whether atovaquone is distributed into human breast milk. A study done in rats found that the concentration of atovaquone in the milk was 30% of the concurrent concentration in the maternal plasma.

### Pediatrics

No information is available on the efficacy of atovaquone in pediatric patients. Clinical experience with atovaquone in children is limited to pharmacokinetic and safety data in immunocompromised children 1 month of age to 13 years of age. These data suggest that the pharmacokinetics of atovaquone are age dependent; also, no treatment-limiting adverse effects were seen.

### Geriatrics

No information is available on the relationship of age to the effects of atovaquone in geriatric patients.

### Drug interactions and/or related problems

The following drug interactions and/or related problems have been selected on the basis of their potential clinical significance (possible mechanism in parentheses where appropriate)—not necessarily inclusive (» = major clinical significance):

Note: Combinations containing any of the following medications, depending on the amount present, may also interact with this medication.

Highly plasma protein–bound medications
(because atovaquone is very highly plasma protein–bound, it could potentially displace other medications that are also very highly plasma protein–bound; this could increase the risk of toxicity from medications that have narrow therapeutic indexes; however, atovaquone protein binding has not been affected *in vitro* by therapeutic concentrations of phenytoin, and the binding of phenytoin has not been affected by atovaquone)

Rifabutin or
» Rifampin
(concurrent administration of oral rifampin with atovaquone suspension resulted in a 52% decrease in the average steady-state plasma concentration of atovaquone and a decrease in the elimination half-life of atovaquone from 82 hours to 50 hours; the average steady-state plasma concentration of rifampin increased by 37%; alternative agents to rifampin should be considered when treating patients with atovaquone. Although interaction trials have not been conducted with atovaquone and rifabutin, rifabutin is structurally similar to rifampin and it may have some of the same drug interactions as rifampin)

Sulfamethoxazole and trimethoprim combination
(concurrent administration of sulfamethoxazole and trimethoprim combination with atovaquone suspension resulted in an 8% and 17% decrease in the steady-state serum concentration of sulfamethoxazole and trimethoprim, respectively; this effect is thought to be minor and is not expected to produce clinically significant events)

Zidovudine
(concurrent administration of zidovudine with atovaquone tablets resulted in a decrease in zidovudine clearance by 24% and a 35% increase in the area under the plasma concentration-time curve [AUC] of zidovudine; the glucuronide metabolite:parent ratio of zidovudine decreased from a mean of 4.5 when zidovudine was administered alone to 3.1 when zidovudine was administered with atovaquone; this effect is thought to be minor and is not expected to produce clinically significant events; zidovudine has no effect on atovaquone pharmacokinetics)

### Laboratory value alterations

The following have been selected on the basis of their potential clinical significance (possible effect in parentheses where appropriate)—not necessarily inclusive (» = major clinical significance):

With physiology/laboratory test values
Alanine aminotransferase (ALT [SGPT]) and
Alkaline phosphatase and

Amylase, serum, and
Aspartate aminotransferase (AST [SGOT])
   (values may be increased)
Hemoglobin, serum, and
White blood cell count
   (hemoglobin concentrations and neutrophil counts may be mildly
   and transiently decreased)
Sodium, serum
   (concentrations may be decreased)

## Medical considerations/Contraindications

The medical considerations/contraindications included here have been selected on the basis of their potential clinical significance (reasons given
in parentheses where appropriate)—not necessarily inclusive (» =
major clinical significance).

*Except under special circumstances, this medication should not be used
when the following medical problem exists:*

» Allergic reaction to atovaquone

*Risk-benefit should be considered when the following medical problems
exist:*

» Gastrointestinal disorders that may inhibit absorption
   (patients with gastrointestinal disorders that may inhibit the absorption of atovaquone may not achieve therapeutic plasma concentrations; this may increase the risk of treatment failure and,
   possibly, death)

## Patient monitoring

The following may be especially important in patient monitoring (other
tests may be warranted in some patients, depending on condition;
» = major clinical significance):

Complete blood counts (CBCs)
   (because atovaquone may cause anemia and neutropenia, hemoglobin concentrations and neutrophil counts should be monitored
   periodically)
Liver function tests
   (liver function tests, including serum ALT [SGPT] and AST
   [SGOT] values, and serum amylase concentration, should be monitored periodically)

## Side/Adverse Effects

Note: Because many of the patients who participated in clinical trials with
   atovaquone had advanced HIV disease, it was often difficult to
   differentiate between the underlying medical condition and the adverse effects of atovaquone.

The following side/adverse effects have been selected on the basis of their
   potential clinical significance (possible signs and symptoms in parentheses where appropriate)—not necessarily inclusive:

**Those indicating need for medical attention**
Incidence more frequent
   *Fever; skin rash*

**Those indicating need for medical attention only if they continue
or are bothersome**
Incidence more frequent
   *Cough; diarrhea; headache; insomnia* (trouble in sleeping); *nausea;
   vomiting*

## Patient Consultation

As an aid to patient consultation, refer to *Advice for the Patient,
Atovaquone (Systemic).*

In providing consultation, consider emphasizing the following selected
information (» = major clinical significance):

**Before using this medication**
» Conditions affecting use, especially:
   Hypersensitivity to atovaquone
   Breast-feeding—Atovaquone is distributed into the milk of rats
   Other medications, especially rifampin
   Other medical problems, especially gastrointestinal disorders that
      may impair absorption

**Proper use of this medication**
» Taking with a meal
   Crushing tablets if necessary to ease administration
» Atovaquone oral suspension and tablets are not bioequivalent and can-
   not be interchanged or substituted for each other.
   Proper administration technique for oral liquid; not using after expi-
   ration date
» Compliance with full course of therapy
» Importance of not missing doses and taking at evenly spaced times

» Proper dosing
   Missed dose: Taking as soon as possible; not taking if almost time for
      next dose; not doubling doses
» Proper storage

**Precautions while using this medication**
   Checking with physician if no improvement within a few days

**Side/adverse effects**
   Signs of potential side effects, especially fever and skin rash

## General Dosing Information

Atovaquone tablets are uncoated and may be crushed if necessary to ease
   administration.

**Diet/Nutrition**
Atovaquone should be taken with a meal to enhance absorption. Failure
   to take with a meal may result in lower plasma concentrations of
   atovaquone, which may limit the response to therapy.

**Bioequivalence information**
Atovaquone oral suspension and tablets are not bioequivalent and cannot
   be interchanged or substituted for each other.

## Oral Dosage Forms

### ATOVAQUONE ORAL SUSPENSION

**Usual adult and adolescent dose**
Pneumonia, *Pneumocystis carinii*—
   Oral, 750 mg taken with a meal two times a day for twenty-one days.

**Usual pediatric dose**
Dosage has not been established; however, doses of 40 mg per kg of body
   weight per day have been used in children.

**Strength(s) usually available**
U.S.—
   750 mg per 5 mL (Rx) [*Mepron*].
Canada—
   Not commercially available.

**Packaging and storage**
Store between 15 and 25 °C (59 and 77 °F). Dispense in a tight container.
   Do not freeze.

**Auxiliary labeling**
• Take with food.
• Continue medicine for full time of treatment.
• Shake well.
• Beyond-use date.

**Note**
When dispensing, include a calibrated liquid-measuring device.

### ATOVAQUONE TABLETS

**Usual adult and adolescent dose**
Pneumonia, *Pneumocystis carinii*—
   Oral, 750 mg taken with a meal three times a day for twenty-one days.

**Usual pediatric dose**
Dose has not been established; however, doses of 40 mg per kg of body
   weight per day have been used in children.

**Strength(s) usually available**
U.S.—
   Not commercially available.
Canada—
   250 mg (Rx) [*Mepron*].

**Packaging and storage**
Store between 15 and 25 °C (59 and 77 °F). Dispense in a well-closed
   container.

**Auxiliary labeling**
• Take with food.
• Continue medicine for full time of treatment.

Revised: 08/14/95

---

**ATRACURIUM**—See *Neuromuscular Blocking Agents (Systemic)*

---

**ATROPINE**—See *Anticholinergics/Antispasmodics (Systemic)*; *Atropine (Ophthalmic)*

# ATROPINE   Ophthalmic

VA CLASSIFICATION (Primary): OP600

Note: For a listing of dosage forms and brand names by country availability, see *Dosage Forms* section(s). For a listing of brand names for the articles in this monograph, refer to the General Index.

## Category

Cycloplegic; mydriatic.

## Indications

Note: Bracketed information in the *Indications* section refers to uses that are not included in U.S. product labeling.

### Accepted

Refraction, cycloplegic—Atropine is indicated for measurement of refractive errors. Atropine is a commonly used cycloplegic for refraction in children up to 6 years of age and in children with convergent strabismus. It is not useful for refraction in adults, because of its long duration of action.

Uveitis (treatment)—Atropine is indicated for pupil dilation and ciliary muscle relaxation, which are desirable in acute inflammatory conditions of the iris and uveal tract.

[Synechiae, posterior (prophylaxis and treatment)]—Atropine may be used for pupil dilation to break posterior synechiae and decrease the possibility of serious complications resulting from synechiae. However, a more rapidly acting medication is usually used. Atropine may also be used to prevent formation of posterior synechiae.

[Mydriasis, preoperative and postoperative]—Atropine may be used for preoperative and postoperative mydriasis.

[Glaucoma, malignant (treatment)][1]—Atropine is used in the treatment of malignant (ciliary block) glaucoma, which may occur after inflammation, surgery, trauma, or use of miotics.

---

[1]Not included in Canadian product labeling.

## Pharmacology/Pharmacokinetics

### Mechanism of action/Effect

Atropine (a belladonna alkaloid) is an anticholinergic agent that blocks the responses of the sphincter muscle of the iris and the accommodative muscle of the ciliary body to stimulation by acetylcholine. Dilation of the pupil (mydriasis) and paralysis of accommodation (cycloplegia) result.

### Duration of action

Long-acting; effects on accommodation may last 6 days; mydriasis may persist for 12 days.

## Precautions to Consider

### Cross-sensitivity and/or related problems

Patients sensitive to any of the other belladonna alkaloids may be sensitive to atropine also.

### Carcinogenicity/Mutagenicity

Studies have not been done in either animals or humans to evaluate the carcinogenic or mutagenic potential of atropine.

### Pregnancy/Reproduction

Fertility—Studies have not been done in either animals or humans to evaluate the potential of atropine impairing fertility.

Pregnancy—Studies have not been done in humans; however, ophthalmic atropine may be systemically absorbed.

Studies have not been done in animals.

FDA Pregnancy Category C.

### Breast-feeding

Systemic atropine is distributed into breast milk in very small amounts. Ophthalmic atropine may be systemically absorbed and may possibly cause adverse effects, such as fast pulse, fever, or dry skin, in nursing infants of mothers using ophthalmic atropine.

### Pediatrics

Atropine should not be used in children who have previously had a severe systemic reaction to atropine.

An increased susceptibility to atropine has been reported in infants and young children and in children with blond hair, blue eyes, Down's syndrome, spastic paralysis, or brain damage; therefore, atropine should be used with great caution in these patients.

The ointment dosage form is generally preferred for use in children, since use of the solution presents a greater chance of systemic absorption.

### Geriatrics

Geriatric patients are more susceptible to the effects of atropine, thus increasing the potential for systemic side effects.

### Drug interactions and/or related problems

The following drug interactions and/or related problems have been selected on the basis of their potential clinical significance (possible mechanism in parentheses where appropriate)—not necessarily inclusive (» = major clinical significance):

Note: Combinations containing any of the following medications, depending on the amount present, may also interact with this medication.

Anticholinergics or medications with anticholinergic activity, other (See *Appendix II*)
(if significant systemic absorption of ophthalmic atropine occurs, concurrent use of other anticholinergics or medications with anticholinergic activity may result in potentiated anticholinergic effects)

Antiglaucoma agents, cholinergic, long-acting, ophthalmic
(concurrent use with atropine may antagonize the antiglaucoma and miotic actions of ophthalmic long-acting cholinergic antiglaucoma agents, such as demecarium, echothiophate, and isoflurophate; concurrent use with atropine may also antagonize the antiaccommodative convergence effects of these medications when they are used for the treatment of strabismus)

Antimyasthenics or
Potassium citrate or
Potassium supplements
(if significant systemic absorption of ophthalmic atropine occurs, concurrent use may increase the chance of toxicity and/or side effects of these systemic medications because of the anticholinergic-induced slowing of gastrointestinal motility)

Carbachol or
Physostigmine or
Pilocarpine
(concurrent use with atropine may interfere with the antiglaucoma action of carbachol, physostigmine, or pilocarpine. Also, concurrent use may counteract the mydriatic effect of atropine; this counteraction may be used to therapeutic advantage)

CNS depression–producing medications (See *Appendix II*)
(if significant systemic absorption of ophthalmic atropine occurs, concurrent use of medications having CNS effects, such as antiemetic agents, phenothiazines, or barbiturates, may result in opisthotonos, convulsions, coma, and extrapyramidal symptoms)

### Medical considerations/Contraindications

The medical considerations/contraindications included here have been selected on the basis of their potential clinical significance (reasons given in parentheses where appropriate)—not necessarily inclusive (» = major clinical significance).

*Except under special circumstances, this medication should not be used when the following medical problem exists:*

» Severe systemic reaction to atropine, especially in children, history of

*Risk-benefit should be considered when the following medical problems exist:*

Brain damage, in children

Down's syndrome (mongolism), in children and adults

» Glaucoma, primary, or predisposition to angle closure

Keratoconus
(atropine may produce fixed dilated pupil)

Sensitivity to atropine

Spastic paralysis, in children

Synechiae between the iris and lens

## Side/Adverse Effects

Note: An increased susceptibility to atropine has been reported in infants, young children, children with blond hair or blue eyes, adults and children with Down's syndrome, children with brain damage or spastic paralysis, and the elderly. This susceptibility increases the potential for systemic side effects.

Prolonged use of atropine may produce local irritation, resulting in follicular conjunctivitis, vascular congestion, edema, exudate, contact dermatitis, or an eczematoid dermatitis.

Severe reactions to atropine may occur and are evidenced by hypotension with progressive respiratory depression. Coma and death have been reported in the very young.

The following side/adverse effects have been selected on the basis of their potential clinical significance (possible signs and symptoms in parentheses where appropriate)—not necessarily inclusive:

**Those indicating need for medical attention**
Symptoms of systemic absorption
*Clumsiness or unsteadiness; confusion or unusual behavior; dizziness; dryness of skin; fever; flushing or redness of face; hallucinations; skin rash; slurred speech; swollen stomach in infants; tachycardia* (fast or irregular heartbeat); *unusual drowsiness; tiredness or weakness; xerostomia* (thirst or dryness of mouth)

**Those indicating need for medical attention only if they continue or are bothersome**
*Blurred vision; eye irritation not present before therapy; increased sensitivity of eyes to light; swelling of the eyelids*

## Overdose

For specific information on the agents used in the management of ophthalmic atropine overdose, see:
- *Atropine* in *Anticholinergics/Antispasmodics (Systemic)* monograph;
- *Diazepam* in *Benzodiazepines (Systemic)* monograph; and/or
- *Physostigmine (Systemic)* monograph.

For more information on the management of overdose or unintentional ingestion, **contact a Poison Control Center** (see *Poison Control Center Listing*).

**Treatment of overdose**
For accidental ingestion, emesis or gastric lavage with 4% tannic acid solution is recommended.

For systemic effects, 0.2 to 1 mg (0.2 mg in children) physostigmine should be administered intravenously, as a dilution containing 1 mg in 5 mL of normal saline. The solution should be injected over a period of not less than 2 minutes. Dosage may be repeated every 5 minutes up to a total dose of 2 mg in children and 6 mg in adults in each 30-minute period.

Physostigmine is contraindicated in hypertensive reactions.

ECG monitoring is recommended during physostigmine administration.

Excitement may be controlled by diazepam or a short-acting barbiturate.

It is recommended that 1 mg of atropine be available for immediate injection if the physostigmine causes bradycardia, convulsion, or bronchoconstriction.

Supportive therapy may require oxygen and assisted respiration; cool water baths for fever, especially in children; and catheterization for urinary retention. In infants and small children, the body surface should be kept moist.

## Patient Consultation

As an aid to patient consultation, refer to *Advice for the Patient, Atropine/Homatropine/Scopolamine (Ophthalmic)*.

In providing consultation, consider emphasizing the following selected information (» = major clinical significance):

**Before using this medication**
» Conditions affecting use, especially:
Sensitivity to atropine, homatropine, or scopolamine
Breast-feeding—Medication passes into the breast milk in very small amounts and may cause side effects, such as fast pulse, fever, or dry skin, in babies of nursing mothers using ophthalmic atropine
Use in children—Infants and young children and children with blond hair or blue eyes may be especially sensitive to the effects of atropine; this may increase the chance of side effects during treatment
Use in the elderly—Geriatric patients are more susceptible to the effects of atropine, thus increasing the potential for systemic side effects
Other medical problems, especially primary glaucoma or predisposition to angle closure

**Proper use of this medication**
Proper administration technique
Washing hands immediately after application to remove any medication that may be on them; if applying medication to infants or children, washing their hands immediately afterwards also, and not letting any medication get into their mouths; wiping

off any medication that may have accidentally gotten on the infant or child, including his or her face and eyelids
Preventing contamination: Not touching applicator tip to any surface; keeping container tightly closed
» Importance of not using more medication than the amount prescribed
» Proper dosing
Missed dose
If dosing schedule is—
Once a day: Applying as soon as possible if remembered same day; if remembered later, skipping missed dose and going back to regular dosing schedule; not doubling doses
More than once a day: Applying as soon as possible; if almost time for next dose, skipping missed dose and going back to regular dosing schedule; not doubling doses
» Proper storage

**Precautions while using this medication**
» Medication causes blurred vision and increased sensitivity of the eyes to light; checking with physician if these effects continue for longer than 14 days after discontinuation of atropine

**Side/adverse effects**
Signs of potential side effects, especially symptoms of systemic absorption

## General Dosing Information

A stronger concentration may be required to produce adequate cycloplegia in eyes with hazel or brown irides than in eyes with blue or light-colored irides.

The ointment dosage form is generally preferred for use in children, since use of the solution presents a greater chance of systemic absorption.

**For ointment dosage form only**
If the ointment is used for refraction, it should be applied several hours prior to the examination; otherwise it may impair the transparency of the cornea and alter the regularity of its refraction.

**For solution dosage form only**
Although some manufacturers recommend a dose of 2 drops of an ophthalmic solution at appropriate intervals, the conjunctival sac will usually hold only 1 drop.

To avoid excessive systemic absorption, patient should press finger to the lacrimal sac during, and for 2 or 3 minutes following, instillation of the solution.

## Ophthalmic Dosage Forms

Note: Bracketed uses in the *Dosage Forms* section refer to categories of use and/or indications that are not included in U.S. product labeling.

### ATROPINE SULFATE OPHTHALMIC OINTMENT USP

**Usual adult and adolescent dose**
Uveitis—
Topical, to the conjunctiva, 0.3 to 0.5 cm of a 1% ointment one or two times a day.

**Usual pediatric dose**
Cycloplegic refraction—
Topical, to the conjunctiva, 0.3 cm of the following concentrations three times a day for one to three days prior to refraction:
Children up to 2 years of age with blue irides:
0.5%.
Children up to 2 years of age with dark irides:
1%.
Children 2 years of age and over:
1%.
Uveitis
[Postoperative mydriasis]—
Topical, to the conjunctiva, 0.3 to 0.5 cm of a 0.5 or 1% ointment one to three times a day.

**Strength(s) usually available**
U.S.—
0.5% (Rx) [Atropine Sulfate S.O.P. (chlorobutanol 0.5%)].
1% (Rx) [Atropair; Atropine Sulfate S.O.P. (chlorobutanol 0.5%); Ocu-Tropine; GENERIC (may contain chlorobutanol)].
Canada—
1% (Rx) [GENERIC (may contain methylparaben, propylparaben)].

**Packaging and storage**
Store below 40 °C (104 °F), preferably between 15 and 30 °C (59 and 86 °F), in a tight container, unless otherwise specified by manufacturer. Protect from freezing.

**Auxiliary labeling**
- For the eye.
- Keep container tightly closed.

## ATROPINE SULFATE OPHTHALMIC SOLUTION USP

**Usual adult and adolescent dose**
Uveitis—
    Topical, to the conjunctiva, 1 drop of a 1% solution one or two times
        a day. In some cases, up to four doses a day may be required.
[To break posterior synechiae]—
    Topical, to the conjunctiva, 1 drop of a 1 to 3% solution alternated
        with 1 drop of a 2.5 or 10% phenylephrine solution every ten
        minutes for three applications of each. Extreme caution should be
        used if 10% phenylephrine is administered.
[Mydriasis]—
    Preoperative: Topical, to the conjunctiva, 1 drop of a 1% solution
        supplemented with 1 drop of a 2.5 or 10% phenylephrine solution,
        prior to surgery. Extreme caution should be used if 10% pheny-
        lephrine is administered.
    Postoperative: Topical, to the conjunctiva, 1 drop of a 1 to 3% solution
        one to three times a day.
[Malignant (ciliary block) glaucoma][1]—
    Initial: Topical, to the conjunctiva, 1 drop of a 1 to 3% solution ad-
        ministered concurrently with 1 drop of a 2.5 or 10% phenylephrine
        solution, three or four times a day. Extreme caution should be used
        if 10% phenylephrine is administered.
    Maintenance: Topical, to the conjunctiva, 1 drop of a 1 to 3% solution
        once every other day or once a day.

**Usual pediatric dose**
Cycloplegic refraction—
    Topical, to the conjunctiva, 1 drop of the following concentrations two
        times a day for one to three days prior to refraction:
        Infants up to 1 year of age:
            0.125%.
        Children 1 to 5 years of age:
            0.25%.
        Children 5 years of age and over with blue irides:
            0.25%.
        Children 5 years of age and over with dark irides:
            0.5 or 1%.
Uveitis—
    Topical, to the conjunctiva, 1 drop of a 0.125 to 1% solution one to
        three times a day.
[Postoperative mydriasis]—
    Topical, to the conjunctiva, 1 drop of a 0.5% solution one to three
        times a day or as determined by physician.

**Strength(s) usually available**
U.S.—
    0.5% (Rx) [*Atropisol; Isopto Atropine* (benzalkonium chloride
        0.01%)].
    1% (Rx) [*Atropair; Atropine Care; Atropisol; Atrosulf; Isopto Atro-
        pine* (benzalkonium chloride 0.01%); *I-Tropine; Ocu-Tropine;* GE-
        NERIC (may contain chlorobutanol)].
    2% (Rx) [*Atropisol;* GENERIC].
Canada—
    1% (Rx) [*Atropisol* (benzalkonium chloride); *Isopto Atropine* (benzal-
        konium chloride); *Minims Atropine;* GENERIC (may contain ben-
        zalkonium chloride)].
Note: The 0.125 and 0.25% strengths are no longer commercially avail-
    able; compounding required for prescriptions.

**Packaging and storage**
Store below 40 °C (104 °F), preferably between 15 and 30 °C (59 and 86
    °F), unless otherwise specified by manufacturer. Store in a tight con-
    tainer. Protect from freezing.

**Auxiliary labeling**
- For the eye.
- Keep container tightly closed.

---

[1]Not included in Canadian product labeling.

---

Revised: 06/21/94
Interim revision: 05/01/95

## ATROPINE-CONTAINING COMBINATIONS—

Atropine, Hyoscyamine, Methenamine, Methylene Blue, Phenyl Salicy-
    late, and Benzoic Acid (Systemic)
Atropine, Hyoscyamine, Scopolamine, and Phenobarbital (Systemic)—See
    *Belladonna Alkaloids and Barbiturates (Systemic)*
Atropine and Phenobarbital (Systemic)—See *Belladonna Alkaloids and
    Barbiturates (Systemic)*
Chlorpheniramine, Phenylephrine, Phenylpropanolamine, Atropine, Hyo-
    scyamine, and Scopolamine (Systemic)—See *Antihistamines, Decon-
    gestants, and Anticholinergics (Systemic)*
Difenoxin and Atropine (Systemic)
Diphenoxylate and Atropine (Systemic)
Kaolin, Pectin, Hyoscyamine, Atropine, and Scopolamine (Systemic)—
    See *Kaolin, Pectin, and Belladonna Alkaloids (Systemic)*
Magnesium Sulfate Tablets (Oral-Local)—See *Laxatives (Local)*

---

# ATROPINE, HYOSCYAMINE, METHENAMINE, METHYLENE BLUE, PHENYL SALICYLATE, AND BENZOIC ACID   Systemic†

VA CLASSIFICATION (Primary): GU200
Note: For a listing of dosage forms and brand names by country availa-
    bility, see *Dosage Forms* section(s). For a listing of brand names
    for the articles in this monograph, refer to the General Index.

    †Not commercially available in Canada.

## Category

Anticholinergic-antibacterial-analgesic (urinary tract).

## Indications

**Accepted**
Irritative voiding, symptoms of (treatment)—Indicated for the relief of
    local symptoms, such as inflammation, hypermotility, and pain, which
    accompany lower urinary tract infections.
Diagnostic procedure–induced symptoms, urinary (treatment)—Indicated
    for the relief of urinary tract symptoms caused by diagnostic
    procedures.

**Unaccepted**
This combination has a labeled indication for the treatment of cystitis,
    urethritis, and trigonitis caused by organisms that maintain or produce
    an acid urine and are susceptible to formaldehyde. In addition, it has
    a labeled indication for the prevention of recurring urinary tract infec-
    tions. However, the main value of this medication consists in the man-
    agement of the symptomatology of lower urinary tract infections and

it is best used when the acute infection has been destroyed by other
antibacterial agents. It is not intended as the primary drug for treatment
or as prophylactic therapy in these conditions.

## Pharmacology/Pharmacokinetics

**Mechanism of action/Effect**
Anticholinergic—
    Atropine; hyoscyamine: Relax smooth muscle spasm by inhibiting the
        muscarinic actions of acetylcholine on autonomic effectors inner-
        vated by postganglionic cholinergic nerves as well as on smooth
        muscle, which responds to endogenous acetylcholine but is not so
        innervated.
Antibacterial—
    Methenamine: Hydrolyzation of methenamine, in acidic urine, releases
        formaldehyde, which provides bactericidal or bacteriostatic action,
        depending on urine pH, volume, and flow rate.
    Methylene blue: Mild antiseptic activity may inhibit bacterial prolif-
        eration; relatively ineffective in the treatment of urinary tract
        infections.
    Benzoic acid: Mild antibacterial and antifungal action. It also helps
        maintain an acid pH in the urine necessary for the degradation of
        methenamine.
Analgesic—
    Phenyl salicylate: Produces analgesia through a peripheral action by
        blocking pain impulse generation and via a central action, possibly
        in the hypothalamus.

**Other actions/effects**
Phenyl salicylate—May produce antipyresis by acting centrally on the hypothalamic heat-regulating center to produce peripheral vasodilation, resulting in increased cutaneous blood flow, sweating, and heat loss.

**Absorption**
Well absorbed from gastrointestinal tract.

**Distribution**
Methenamine—Freely distributed to body tissues and fluids, but not clinically significant because methenamine does not hydrolyze at pH greater than 6.8

**Protein binding**
Atropine; hyoscyamine—Moderate.
Methenamine—Some formaldehyde is bound to substances in the urine and the surrounding tissues.

**Biotransformation**
Atropine; hyoscyamine—Hepatic.
Methenamine—Urine (70 to 90% of methenamine reaches the urine unchanged where it is hydrolyzed if the urine is acidic).

**Elimination**
Renal.
Atropine—30 to 50% excreted unchanged.
Hyoscyamine—Majority excreted unchanged.
Methenamine—Almost completely (90%) excreted within 24 hours; of this amount at pH 5, approximately 20% is formaldehyde.
Methylene blue—75% excreted unchanged.

# Precautions to Consider

**Cross-sensitivity and/or related problems**
Patients sensitive to other belladonna alkaloids or other salicylates may be sensitive to this medication also.

**Pregnancy/Reproduction**
Pregnancy—Atropine, hyoscyamine, and methenamine cross the placenta. Studies have not been done in humans.
Studies have not been done in animals.
FDA Pregnancy Category C.

**Breast-feeding**
Methenamine and traces of atropine and hyoscyamine are distributed into breast milk. However problems in humans have not been documented.

**Pediatrics**
No information is available on the relationship of age to the effects of this combination in pediatric patients. However, it is known that infants and young children are especially susceptible to the toxic effects of the belladonna alkaloids.
Close supervision is recommended for infants and children with spastic paralysis or brain damage since an increased response to anticholinergics has been reported in these patients and dosage adjustments are often required.
When anticholinergics are given to children where the environmental temperature is high, there is risk of a rapid increase in body temperature because of these medications' suppression of sweat gland activity.
A paradoxical reaction characterized by hyperexcitability may occur in children taking large doses of anticholinergics.

**Geriatrics**
No information is available on the relationship of age to the effects of this combination in geriatric patients. However, it is known that geriatric patients may respond to the usual doses of the belladonna alkaloids with excitement, agitation, drowsiness, or confusion. Also, geriatric patients are especially susceptible to anticholinergic side effects, such as constipation, dryness of mouth, and urinary retention (especially in males).
In addition, caution is recommended when anticholinergics are given to geriatric patients, because of the danger of precipitating undiagnosed glaucoma.
Memory may become severely impaired in geriatric patients, especially those who already have memory problems, with the continued use of atropine and hyoscyamine since these medications block the action of acetylcholine, which is responsible for many functions of the brain, including memory functions.

**Dental**
Prolonged use of belladonna alkaloids may decrease or inhibit salivary flow, thus contributing to the development of caries, periodontal disease, oral candidiasis, and discomfort.

**Drug interactions and/or related problems**
The following drug interactions and/or related problems have been selected on the basis of their potential clinical significance (possible mechanism in parentheses where appropriate)—not necessarily inclusive (» = major clinical significance):

Note: Combinations containing any of the following medications, depending on the amount present, may also interact with this medication.
Only specific interactions between this combination medication and other oral medications have been identified in this monograph. However, because of atropine's and hyoscyamine's effects on gastrointestinal motility and gastric emptying, absorption of other oral medications may be decreased during concurrent use with this combination medication.

» Alkalizers, urinary, such as:
Antacids, calcium- and/or magnesium-containing
Carbonic anhydrase inhibitors
Citrates
Sodium bicarbonate or
» Diuretics, thiazide
(may cause the urine to become alkaline, thereby reducing the effectiveness of methenamine by inhibiting its conversion to formaldehyde; concurrent use is not recommended)

» Anticholinergics, other, or other medications with anticholinergic action (See *Appendix II*)
(concurrent use of these medications may intensify anticholinergic effects of atropine and hyoscyamine; patients should be advised to report occurrence of gastrointestinal problems promptly since paralytic ileus may occur with concurrent therapy)

» Antacids or
» Antidiarrheals, adsorbent
(simultaneous use of these medications with this combination medication may reduce absorption of atropine and hyoscyamine, resulting in decreased therapeutic effectiveness; doses of these medications should be spaced 2 to 3 hours apart from doses of atropine and hyoscyamine)

(concurrent use of this combination medication with antacids, especially calcium carbonate–, magnesium-, or sodium bicarbonate–containing, may cause the urine to become alkaline, thereby reducing the effectiveness of methenamine by inhibiting its conversion to formaldehyde; simultaneous use may reduce absorption of atropine and hyoscyamine, resulting in decreased therapeutic effectiveness)

» Ketoconazole
(atropine and hyoscyamine may cause increased gastrointestinal pH; concurrent administration of ketoconazole with atropine and hyoscyamine may result in a marked reduction in absorption of ketoconazole; patients should be advised to take this combination at least 2 hours after ketoconazole)

Metoclopramide
(concurrent use of metoclopramide with atropine and hyoscyamine may antagonize the effects of metoclopramide on gastrointestinal motility)

Monoamine oxidase (MAO) inhibitors, including furazolidone, procarbazine, and selegiline
(concurrent use may result in intensified anticholinergic side effects because of these medications' secondary anticholinergic activities; also, concurrent use of MAO inhibitors may block detoxification of anticholinergics, thus potentiating their action)

Opioid (narcotic) analgesics
(concurrent use of opioids with atropine and hyoscyamine may result in increased risk of severe constipation, which may lead to paralytic ileus, and/or urinary retention)

» Potassium chloride, especially wax matrix preparations
(concurrent use with atropine and hyoscyamine may increase severity of potassium chloride–induced gastrointestinal lesions)

» Sulfonamides
(in acid urine, methenamine breaks down into formaldehyde, which may form an insoluble precipitate with certain sulfonamides and may also increase the danger of crystalluria; concurrent use is not recommended)

**Laboratory value alterations**
The following have been selected on the basis of their potential clinical significance (possible effect in parentheses where appropriate)—not necessarily inclusive (» = major clinical significance):

With diagnostic test results
Catecholamine determinations, urinary and
17-hydroxycorticosteroid (17-OHCS) determinations, urinary and
Vanillylmandelic acid (VMA), urinary
(methenamine may cause a false increase)

Estriol determinations, urinary and
5-Hydroxy indoleacetic acid (5-HIAA) determinations, urinary
(methenamine may cause a false decrease)

» Gastric acid secretion test
(atropine and hyoscyamine may antagonize the effect of pentagastrin and histamine in the evaluation of gastic acid secretory function; administration of this combination is not recommended during the 24 hours preceding the test)

» Phenolsulfonphthalein (PSP) excretion test
(methylene blue may cause a false positive)

Radionuclide gastric emptying studies
(atropine and hyoscyamine may result in delayed gastric emptying)

Urinary free formaldehyde and
Urine pH
(methylene blue may interfere with analysis)

## Medical considerations/Contraindications
The medical considerations/contraindications included here have been selected on the basis of their potential clinical significance (reasons given in parentheses where appropriate)—not necessarily inclusive (» = major clinical significance).

***Risk-benefit should be considered when the following medical problems exist:***

Brain damage, in children
(CNS effects may be exacerbated by atropine and hyoscyamine)

» Cardiac disease, especially cardiac arrhythmias, congestive heart failure, coronary heart disease, mitral stenosis or

» Hemorrhage, acute, with tachycardia or
Hyperthyroidism or
Tachycardia
(increase in heart rate caused by atropine and hyoscyamine may be undesirable)

Dehydration, severe or
Renal function impairment
(inadequate concentrations of this combination medicine may be achieved in urine; salts of methenamine may precipitate, causing crystalluria in patients with low urine output)

» Esophagitis, reflux
(decrease in esophageal and gastric motility and relaxation of lower esophageal sphincter caused by atropine and hyoscyamine may promote gastric retention by delaying gastric emptying and may increase gastroesophageal reflux through an incompetent sphincter)

Fever
(may be increased through suppression of sweat gland activity caused by atropine and hyoscyamine)

» Gastrointestinal tract obstructive disease
(decrease in motility and tone caused by atropine and hyoscyamine may result in obstruction and gastric retention)

» Glaucoma, angle-closure, or predisposition to
(mydriatic effect caused by atropine and hyoscyamine may result in increased intraocular pressure and may precipitate an acute attack of angle-closure glaucoma)

» Glaucoma, open-angle
(mydriatic effect of atropine and hyoscyamine may cause a slight increase in intraocular pressure; glaucoma therapy may need to be adjusted)

Glucose-6-phosphate dehydrogenase (G6PD) deficiency
(use of methylene blue may induce hemolysis)

Hepatic function impairment
(decreased metabolism of atropine and hyoscyamine; methenamine may facilitate ammonia production in the intestinal tract)

» Hernia, hiatal, associated with reflux esophagitis
(atropine and hyoscyamine may aggravate condition)

Hypertension
(atropine and hyoscyamine may aggravate condition)

» Intestinal atony in the elderly or debilitated patient or
» Paralytic ileus
(atropine and hyoscyamine may result in obstruction)

Lung disease, chronic, especially in infants, small children, and debilitated patients
(reduction in bronchial secretion caused by atropine and hyoscyamine can lead to inspissation and formation of bronchial plugs)

» Myasthenia gravis
(condition may be aggravated because of inhibition of acetylcholine action)

Neuropathy, autonomic
(urinary retention and cycloplegia may be aggravated by atropine and hyoscyamine)

» Prostatic hypertrophy, nonobstructive or
» Urinary retention or
» Uropathy, obstructive, such as bladder neck obstruction due to prostatic hypertrophy
(urinary retention may be precipitated or aggravated by atropine and hyoscyamine)

Sensitivity to any of the medications in this combination

Spastic paralysis, in children
(response to atropine and hyoscyamine may be increased)

Toxemia of pregnancy
(hypertension may be aggravated by atropine and hyoscyamine)

Ulcerative colitis
(large doses of atropine and hyoscyamine may suppress intestinal motility, possibly causing paralytic ileus; also, use may precipitate or aggravate toxic megacolon)

Xerostomia
(prolonged use of atropine and hyoscyamine may further reduce limited salivary flow)

Caution in use is also recommended in patients over 40 years of age because of the danger of precipitating undiagnosed glaucoma.

## Patient monitoring
The following may be especially important in patient monitoring (other tests may be warranted in some patients, depending on condition; » = major clinical significance):

Intraocular pressure determinations
(recommended at periodic intervals because atropine and hyoscyamine may increase the intraocular pressure by producing mydriasis)

Urine pH
(monitoring recommended before start of treatment and throughout therapy since the effectiveness of methenamine is increased if a pH of 5.5 or below is maintained. To check urine pH, phenaphthazine paper, which has a pH range of 4.5 to 7.5, may be used. However, the presence of methylene blue may interfere with urinary pH determination)

# Side/Adverse Effects

Note: This medication should be discontinued immediately if dizziness, increased pulse, or blurring of vision occurs.

Geriatric or debilitated patients may respond to usual doses of atropine and hyoscyamine with excitement, agitation, drowsiness, or confusion.

The following side/adverse effects have been selected on the basis of their potential clinical significance (possible signs and symptoms in parentheses where appropriate)—not necessarily inclusive:

## Those indicating need for medical attention
Incidence less frequent or rare
***Allergic reaction*** (skin rash or hives); ***difficulty in eye accommodation*** (blurred vision); ***increased intraocular pressure*** (eye pain)

## Those indicating need for medical attention only if they continue or are bothersome
Incidence less frequent
***Difficult urination***—more frequent with large doses over a prolonged period of time; ***dryness of mouth, nose, or throat; nausea or vomiting; stomach upset or pain***—more frequent with large doses over a prolonged period of time

## Those not indicating need for medical attention
Incidence more frequent
***Blue or blue-green urine and/or stools***—due to excretion of methylene blue

# Overdose
For specific information on the agents used in the management of this combination product overdose, see:
• *Physostigmine (Systemic)* monograph; and/or
• *Diazepam* in *Benzodiazepines (Systemic)* monograph.
For more information on the management of overdose or unintentional ingestion, **contact a Poison Control Center** (see *Poison Control Center Listing*).

**Clinical effects of overdose**

The following effects have been selected on the basis of their potential clinical significance (possible signs and symptoms in parentheses where appropriate)–not necessarily inclusive:

*Anticholinergic effects* (severe drowsiness; dizziness; fast heartbeat; flushing or redness of face; shortness of breath or troubled breathing); *hematuria; crystalluria* (blood in urine; lower back pain; pain or burning while urinating)—due to methenamine; *salicylate effects* (bloody stools; diarrhea; severe or continuing headache; dizziness; ringing or buzzing in ears; sweating; unusual tiredness or weakness)

**Treatment of overdose**

Recommended treatment for overdose includes:

To decrease absorption—
    Emesis or gastric lavage.

Specific treatment—
    Slow intravenous administration of physostigmine in doses of 1 to 4 mg (0.5 to 1 mg in children), repeated as needed in one to two hours, to reverse severe anticholinergic symptoms; use of physostigmine with caution and only with cardiac monitoring. Administration of small doses of diazepam to control excitement and seizures.

Supportive care—
    Artificial respiration with oxygen if needed for respiratory depression. Adequate hydration. Symptomatic treatment as necessary. Patients in whom intentional overdose is known or suspected should be referred for psychiatric consultation.

## Patient Consultation

As an aid to patient consultation, refer to *Advice for the Patient, Atropine, Hyoscyamine, Methenamine, Methylene Blue, Phenyl Salicylate, and Benzoic Acid (Systemic)*.

In providing consultation, consider emphasizing the following selected information (» = major clinical significance):

**Before using this medication**

» Conditions affecting use, especially:
    Sensitivity to any of the belladonna alkaloids or salicylates
    Pregnancy—Crosses the placenta
    Breast-feeding—Atropine, hyoscyamine, and methenamine distributed into breast milk
    Use in children—Increased susceptibility to toxic effects of belladonna alkaloids; increased response to anticholinergics in children with spastic paralysis or brain damage; suppression of sweat gland activity in children; possibility of paradoxical reaction characterized by hyperexcitability
    Use in the elderly—Increased susceptibility to CNS and anticholinergic effects of belladonna alkaloids; danger of precipitating undiagnosed glaucoma; possible impairment of memory
    Dental—Possible development of dental problems because of decreased salivary flow
    Other medications, especially antacids, other anticholinergics, antidiarrheals, ketoconazole, potassium chloride, sulfonamides, thiazide diuretics, or urinary alkalizers
    Other medical problems, especially cardiac disease, fever, glaucoma, hemorrhage, hiatal hernia, intestinal atony or paralytic ileus, lung disease, myasthenia gravis, obstruction in gastrointestinal or urinary tract, prostatic hypertrophy, reflux esophagitis, ulcerative colitis, or xerostomia

**Proper use of this medication**

» Importance of not taking more medication than the amount prescribed
    Maintaining fluid intake for adequate urinary output
» Compliance with full course of therapy
» Importance of maintaining acidic urine (pH 5.5 or below)
    Measuring urine pH with phenaphthazine paper; adjusting urine pH with appropriate diet
» Proper dosing
    Missed dose: Taking as soon as possible; if almost time for next dose, not taking at all; not doubling doses
» Proper storage

**Precautions while using this medication**

Checking with physician if no improvement within a few days
Caution during exercise or hot weather; overheating may result in heat stroke
» Caution if blurred vision occurs
    Possible dryness of mouth, nose, or throat; using sugarless gum or candy, ice, or saliva substitute for relief; checking with dentist if dry mouth continues for more than 2 weeks
    Avoid use of antacids and antidiarrheal medications within 2 or 3 hours of taking this medication

**Side/adverse effects**

Signs of potential side effects, especially allergic reaction, blurred vision, or eye pain
Blue or blue-green discoloration of urine and/or stools may be alarming to patient although medically insignificant

## General Dosing Information

An increase in the patient's fluid intake is not necessary; however, it is recommended that the patient drink enough liquids to satisfy normal fluid requirements and to maintain an adequate urine output.

In order to maintain a urine pH of 5.5 or below, most fruits (especially citrus fruits and juices), milk and other dairy products, and other alkalinizing foods should be avoided. A protein-rich diet with liberal amounts of cranberries (especially ascorbic acid–enriched cranberry juice), plums, or prunes may be helpful. If these measures do not produce a sufficiently acid urine, they may be supplemented with large doses of ascorbic acid (4 grams or more per day), arginine hydrochloride, or methionine. However, some brands of ascorbic acid may contain varying amounts of sodium ascorbate and may actually alkalinize the urine. Alternatively, ammonium chloride or sodium biphosphate may be given (caution—large doses of ammonium chloride may cause metabolic acidosis in patients with impaired renal function and may be contraindicated in patients with hepatic insufficiency).

Urea-splitting organisms (e.g., *Proteus mirabilis* and some strains of *Pseudomonas* and *Aerobacter*) may cause an increase in urine pH and thereby decrease the effectiveness of methenamine. Care should be taken to ensure urine acidification.

## Oral Dosage Forms

### ATROPINE SULFATE, HYOSCYAMINE, METHENAMINE, METHYLENE BLUE, PHENYL SALICYLATE, AND BENZOIC ACID TABLETS

**Usual adult and adolescent dose**

Oral, 1 or 2 tablets (depending on strength of product) four times a day.

**Usual pediatric dose**

Children up to 6 years of age—
    Use is not recommended.
Children 6 years of age and over—
    Dosage must be individualized by physician.

**Usual geriatric dose**

See *Usual adult and adolescent dose.*

Note: Geriatric patients may be more sensitive to the effects of the usual adult dose.

**Strength(s) usually available**

U.S.—
    30 mcg (0.03 mg) of atropine sulfate, 30 mcg (0.03 mg) of hyoscyamine, 40.8 mg of methenamine, 5.4 mg of methylene blue, 18.1 mg of phenyl salicylate, and 4.5 mg of benzoic acid, per tablet (Rx) [*Atrosept; Dolsed; Hexalol; UAA; Uridon Modified; Urimed; Urinary Antiseptic No. 2; Urised* (sugar-coated); *Uriseptic; Uritab; Uritin; Uro-Ves*].

    60 mcg (0.06 mg) of atropine sulfate, 30 mcg (0.03 mg) of hyoscyamine, 120 mg of methenamine, 6 mg of methylene blue, 30 mg of phenyl salicylate, and 7.5 mg of benzoic acid, per tablet (Rx) [*Trac Tabs 2X*].

    60 mcg (0.06 mg) of atropine sulfate, 60 mcg (0.06 mg) of hyoscyamine, 81.6 mg of methenamine, 10.8 mg of methylene blue, 36.2 mg of phenyl salicylate, and 9 mg of benzoic acid, per tablet (Rx) [*Prosed/DS*].

    Note: Exact strengths of specific products may vary slightly, depending on manufacturer.

Canada—
    Not commercially available.

**Packaging and storage**

Store below 40 °C (104 °F), preferably between 15 and 30 °C (59 and 86 °F), unless otherwise specified by manufacturer.

**Auxiliary labeling**

• Take with a full glass of water.
• May discolor urine and/or stools.

**Note**

Instruct patient on taking adequate amounts of fluids with each dose and during therapy.

Revised: 05/11/93

# ATTAPULGITE   Oral-Local

VA CLASSIFICATION (Primary): GA400

Note: For a listing of dosage forms and brand names by country availability, see *Dosage Forms* section(s). For a listing of brand names for the articles in this monograph, refer to the General Index.

## Category
Antidiarrheal (adsorbent).

## Indications
Note: The efficacy of any antidiarrheal medication for treatment of most cases of nonspecific diarrhea is questionable, especially in children. **Preferred treatment for acute, nonspecific diarrhea consists of fluid and electrolyte replacement, nutritional therapy, and, if possible, elimination of the underlying cause of the diarrhea.**

### Accepted
Diarrhea (treatment)—Attapulgite may be indicated as an adjunct to rest, fluids, and an appropriate diet in the symptomatic treatment of mild to moderately acute diarrhea. Use is recommended in chronic diarrhea only as temporary symptomatic treatment until the etiology is determined. Attapulgite should not be used if diarrhea is accompanied by fever, or if there is blood or mucus in the stool.

## Pharmacology/Pharmacokinetics

### Mechanism of action/Effect
Adsorbent and protectant. Attapulgite is a hydrated magnesium aluminum silicate that supposedly adsorbs large numbers of bacteria and toxins and reduces water loss. Activated attapulgite (contained in most of the products commercially available) is attapulgite that has been carefully heated to increase its adsorptive capacity. Results of animal studies with adsorbent antidiarrheals suggest that the fluidity of the stool is decreased but total water loss appears to be unchanged and sodium and potassium loss may be exacerbated.

### Absorption
Not absorbed.

## Precautions to Consider

### Pregnancy/Reproduction
Pregnancy—Problems in humans have not been documented. Attapulgite is not absorbed after oral administration.

### Breast-feeding
Problems in humans have not been documented. Attapulgite is not absorbed after oral administration.

### Pediatrics
In infants and children up to 3 years of age with diarrhea, use is not recommended unless directed by a physician because of the risk of fluid and electrolyte loss. Oral rehydration therapy is recommended in children with diarrhea to prevent loss of fluids and electrolytes.

### Geriatrics
In geriatric patients with diarrhea, caution is recommended because of the risk of fluid and electrolyte loss; these patients should be referred to a physician.

### Drug interactions and/or related problems
The following drug interactions and/or related problems have been selected on the basis of their potential clinical significance (possible mechanism in parentheses where appropriate)—not necessarily inclusive (» = major clinical significance):

Note: Combinations containing any of the following medications, depending on the amount present, may also interact with this medication.

Anticholinergics or other medications with anticholinergic activity (See *Appendix II*) or
Antidyskinetics or
Digitalis glycosides or
Lincomycins or
Loxapine or
Phenothiazines or
Thioxanthenes or
Xanthines, such as:
  Aminophylline
  Caffeine
  Dyphylline
  Oxtriphylline

Theophylline
(concurrent use with attapulgite may impair absorption of these medications when they are administered orally, resulting in decreased therapeutic effectiveness; it is recommended that attapulgite be administered not less than 2 hours before or 3 to 4 hours after oral lincomycins; patients on digitalis should be monitored closely for evidence of altered effect)

Oral medications, other
(prolonged use of adsorbents may interfere with absorption of other oral agents administered concurrently; it is recommended that attapulgite be administered at least 2 to 3 hours before or after other oral medications)

## Medical considerations/Contraindications
The medical considerations/contraindications included here have been selected on the basis of their potential clinical significance (reasons given in parentheses where appropriate)—not necessarily inclusive (» = major clinical significance):

*Risk-benefit should be considered when the following medical problems exist:*

» Dehydration
(although adsorbent antidiarrheals may increase the consistency of feces and decrease the frequency of evacuation, they do not reduce the amount of fluid loss, but only mask its extent; rehydration therapy is essential if symptoms of dehydration, such as dryness of mouth, excessive thirst, wrinkled skin, decreased urination, and dizziness or lightheadedness, are present; fluid loss may have serious consequences, such as circulatory collapse and renal failure, especially in young children and the elderly)

Diarrhea, parasite-associated, suspected
(use of adsorbent antidiarrheals may make recognition of parasitic causes of diarrhea more difficult; if parasitic agents are suspected pathogens, appropriate stool analyses should be performed prior to therapy with adsorbents)

» Dysentery, acute, characterized by bloody stools and elevated temperature
(sole treatment with adsorbent antidiarrheals may be inadequate; antibiotic therapy may be required)

Obstruction of the bowel, suspected
(condition may be aggravated)

## Side/Adverse Effects
The following side/adverse effects have been selected on the basis of their potential clinical significance (possible signs and symptoms in parentheses where appropriate)—not necessarily inclusive:

**Those indicating need for medical attention only if they continue or are bothersome**
Incidence dose-related
  *Constipation*—usually mild and transient, but may rarely lead to fecal impaction

## Patient Consultation
As an aid to patient consultation, refer to *Advice for the Patient, Attapulgite (Oral).*

In providing consultation, consider emphasizing the following selected information (» = major clinical significance):

### Before using this medication
» Conditions affecting use, especially:
  Use in children—Not using in infants and children up to 3 years of age unless prescribed by a physician because of risk of dehydration associated with diarrhea; oral rehydration therapy recommended in children with diarrhea
  Use in the elderly—Risk of dehydration associated with diarrhea
  Other medications; spacing doses of other oral medications 2 to 3 hours before or after doses of attapulgite is recommended
  Other medical problems, especially dehydration and acute dysentery

### Proper use of this medication
» Not using if diarrhea accompanied by fever or blood or mucus in the stool; contacting physician
  Taking after each loose bowel movement until diarrhea is controlled
» Importance of maintaining adequate hydration and proper diet
» Proper dosing
» Proper storage

**Precautions while using this medication**

» Checking with physician if diarrhea is not controlled within 48 hours and/or fever develops

## Oral-Local Dosage Forms
### ATTAPULGITE ORAL SUSPENSION

**Usual adult and adolescent dose**

Antidiarrheal—

Oral, 1.2 to 1.5 grams after each loose bowel movement, not to exceed 9 grams in twenty-four hours.

**Usual pediatric dose**

Antidiarrheal—

Children up to 3 years of age: Use is not recommended unless directed by a physician.

Children 3 to 6 years of age: Oral, 300 mg after each loose bowel movement, not to exceed 2.1 grams in twenty-four hours.

Children 6 to 12 years of age: Oral, 600 mg after each loose bowel movement, not to exceed 4.2 grams in twenty-four hours.

Children 12 years of age and over: See *Usual adult and adolescent dose*.

Note: In general, dietary treatment of diarrhea is preferred in children whenever possible.

**Strength(s) usually available**

U.S.—

600 mg per 15 mL (OTC) [*Donnagel; Kaopectate Advanced Formula; Kaopek; K-Pek; Parepectolin*].

750 mg per 5 mL (OTC) [*Diasorb*].

Canada—

600 mg per 15 mL (OTC) [*Kaopectate*].

750 mg per 15 mL (OTC) [*Kaopectate*].

900 mg per 15 mL (OTC) [*Fowler's*].

**Packaging and storage**

Store below 40 °C (104 °F), preferably between 15 and 30 °C (59 and 86 °F), in a well-closed container, unless otherwise specified by manufacturer. Protect from freezing.

**Auxiliary labeling**
• Shake well.

**Note**

Refer patients with recurrent or persistent diarrhea to a physician.

### ATTAPULGITE TABLETS

**Usual adult and adolescent dose**

Antidiarrheal—

Oral, 1.2 to 1.5 grams after each loose bowel movement, not to exceed 9 grams in twenty-four hours.

**Usual pediatric dose**

Antidiarrheal—

Children 3 to 6 years of age: The available strength of the tablet may not conform to the recommended dose for children 3 to 6 years of age; the oral suspension is the preferred dosage form for this age group.

Children 6 to 12 years of age: Oral, 750 mg after each loose bowel movement, not to exceed 4.5 grams in twenty-four hours.

Children 12 years of age and over: See *Usual adult and adolescent dose*.

Note: In general, dietary treatment of diarrhea is preferred in children whenever possible.

**Strength(s) usually available**

U.S.—

300 mg (OTC) [*Diarrest; Diatrol*].

750 mg (OTC) [*Diar-Aid* (pectin 150 mg); *Diasorb; Kaopectate Maximum Strength; Rheaban*].

Canada—

600 mg (OTC) [*Kaopectate*].

630 mg (OTC) [*Fowler's*].

750 mg (OTC) [*Kaopectate*].

**Packaging and storage**

Store below 40 °C (104 °F), preferably between 15 and 30 °C (59 and 86 °F), in a well-closed container, unless otherwise specified by manufacturer.

**Auxiliary labeling**
• Do not chew.

**Note**

Refer patients with recurrent or persistent diarrhea to a physician.

### ATTAPULGITE CHEWABLE TABLETS

**Usual adult and adolescent dose**

Antidiarrheal—

Oral, 1.2 grams after each loose bowel movement, not to exceed 8.4 grams in twenty-four hours.

**Usual pediatric dose**

Antidiarrheal—

Children up to 3 years of age: Use is not recommended unless directed by a physician.

Children 3 to 6 years of age: Oral, 300 mg after each loose bowel movement, not to exceed 2.1 grams in twenty-four hours.

Children 6 to 12 years of age: Oral, 600 mg after each loose bowel movement, not to exceed 4.2 grams in twenty-four hours.

Children 12 years of age and over: See *Usual adult and adolescent dose*.

Note: In general, dietary treatment of diarrhea is preferred in children whenever possible.

**Strength(s) usually available**

U.S.—

300 mg (OTC) [*Kaopectate*].

600 mg (OTC) [*Donnagel*].

Canada—

300 mg (OTC) [*Kaopectate*].

**Packaging and storage**

Store below 40 °C (104 °F), preferably between 15 and 30 °C (59 and 86 °F), in a well-closed container, unless otherwise specified by manufacturer.

**Auxiliary labeling**
• May be chewed.

**Note**

Refer patients with recurrent or persistent diarrhea to a physician.

## Selected Bibliography

DuPont HL. Using OTC drugs for acute diarrhea. Drug Ther 1983: 127-36.

Brownlee HJ. Family practitioner's guide to patient self-treatment of acute diarrhea. Am J Med 1990; 88 (6A Suppl): 27S-29S.

Revised: 08/12/94
Interim revision: 04/27/95

---

**AURANOFIN**—See *Gold Compounds (Systemic)*

---

**AUROTHIOGLUCOSE**—See *Gold Compounds (Systemic)*

---

**AVOBENZONE-CONTAINING COMBINATIONS**—

Avobenzone, Octocrylene, Octyl Salicylate, and Oxybenzone (Topical)—See *Sunscreen Agents (Topical)*

Avobenzone and Octyl Methoxycinnamate (Topical)—See *Sunscreen Agents (Topical)*

Avobenzone, Octyl Methoxycinnamate, Octyl Salicylate, and Oxybenzone (Topical)—See *Sunscreen Agents (Topical)*

Avobenzone, Octyl Methoxycinnamate, and Oxybenzone (Topical)—See *Sunscreen Agents (Topical)*

---

**AZATADINE**—See *Antihistamines (Systemic)*

---

**AZATADINE-CONTAINING COMBINATIONS**—

Azatadine and Pseudoephedrine (Systemic)—See *Antihistamines and Decongestants (Systemic)*

# AZATHIOPRINE   Systemic

VA CLASSIFICATION (Primary/Secondary): IM600/MS105; GA900

Note: For a listing of dosage forms and brand names by country availability, see *Dosage Forms* section(s). For a listing of brand names for the articles in this monograph, refer to the General Index.

## Category

Immunosuppressant; antirheumatic (disease-modifying); bowel disease (inflammatory) suppressant; lupus erythematosus suppressant.

## Indications

Note: Bracketed information in the *Indications* section refers to uses that are not included in U.S. product labeling.

### Accepted

Transplant rejection, organ (prophylaxis)—Azathioprine is indicated as an adjunct for prevention of rejection in renal homotransplantation. [It is also used in the prevention of rejection in cardiac, hepatic, and pancreatic transplantation.]

Arthritis, rheumatoid (treatment)—Azathioprine is indicated for the management of severe, active, and erosive rheumatoid arthritis unresponsive to rest or conventional medications.

[Bowel disease, inflammatory (treatment)][1]
[Hepatitis, chronic active (treatment)][1]
[Cirrhosis, biliary (treatment)][1]
[Lupus erythematosus, systemic (treatment)][1]
[Glomerulonephritis (treatment)][1]
[Nephrotic syndrome (treatment)][1]
[Myopathy, inflammatory (treatment)][1]
[Myasthenia gravis (treatment)][1]
[Dermatomyositis, systemic (treatment)][1]
[Pemphigoid (treatment)][1] or
[Pemphigus (treatment)][1]—Azathioprine is also used in the treatment of other immunologic diseases including regional and ulcerative colitis, chronic active hepatitis and biliary cirrhosis, systemic lupus erythematosus (SLE), glomerulonephritis, nephrotic syndrome, inflammatory myopathy, myasthenia gravis, systemic dermatomyositis (polymyositis), pemphigus, and pemphigoid.

[1]Not included in Canadian product labeling.

## Pharmacology/Pharmacokinetics

### Physicochemical characteristics

Molecular weight—277.26.

### Mechanism of action/Effect

The exact mechanism of immunosuppressive action is unknown since the exact mechanism of the immune response itself is complex and not completely understood. The immunosuppressive effects of azathioprine involve a greater suppression of delayed hypersensitivity and cellular cytotoxicity tests than of antibody responses. Azathioprine antagonizes purine metabolism and may inhibit synthesis of DNA, RNA, and proteins; it may also interfere with cellular metabolism and inhibit mitosis.

The mechanism of action of azathioprine in rheumatoid arthritis and other immunologic diseases is unknown but may be related to immunosuppression. Azathioprine has a steroid-sparing effect, which allows a reduction in steroid dose when the two are combined in chronic inflammatory diseases.

### Absorption

Well absorbed from the gastrointestinal tract.

### Protein binding

Low (30%).

### Biotransformation

Largely converted to 6-mercaptopurine and 6-thioinosinic acid (active metabolites). Further metabolism—Hepatic, largely by xanthine oxidase, and in erythrocytes. Proportions of metabolites vary among individual patients.

### Half-life

Approximately 5 hours (unchanged drug and metabolites).

### Onset of action

In rheumatoid arthritis—6 to 8 weeks.
In other inflammatory disorders—4 to 8 weeks.

### Time to peak concentration

Serum—1 to 2 hours.

### Duration of action

Immunosuppressant—Clinical effects may persist for long periods after the medication is eliminated.

### Elimination

Hepatic (biliary).
Renal (1 to 2% unchanged).
In dialysis—Partially (minimally) removable by hemodialysis.

## Precautions to Consider

### Carcinogenicity

Azathioprine has been shown to be carcinogenic in animals, and may be associated with an increased risk of development of carcinomas in humans, especially skin cancer and reticulum cell tumors or lymphomas in renal transplant patients and acute myelocytic leukemia and some solid tumors in rheumatoid arthritis patients. The risk of neoplastic toxicity appears to be lower in rheumatoid arthritis patients than in renal transplant patients; however, there is evidence that the risk is increased with prior use of alkylating agents.

### Mutagenicity

Mutagenic effects have been reported in animals, and chromosomal abnormalities (reversible when azathioprine is discontinued) have been noted in humans.

### Pregnancy/Reproduction

Fertility—Azathioprine has been reported to cause temporary depression in spermatogenesis and reduction in sperm viability and sperm count in mice at doses 10 times the human therapeutic dose; a reduced percentage of fertile matings occurred when animals received 5 mg per kg of body weight (mg/kg).

Pregnancy—Adequate and well-controlled studies in humans have not been done.

Azathioprine crosses the placenta.

Risk-benefit must be considered, especially during the first trimester, since azathioprine affects cell kinetics and can theoretically cause mutagenicity or teratogenicity.

There have been reports of limited immunologic abnormalities (lymphopenia, diminished IgG and IgM levels, cytomegalovirus [CMV] infection, and decreased thymic shadow; pancytopenia and severe immune deficiency) and other abnormalities (preaxial polydactyly in an infant whose mother received azathioprine and prednisone; meningomyelocele, bilateral dislocated hips, and bilateral talipes equinovarus in an infant whose father received azathioprine) in infants of renal homograft recipients treated with azathioprine.

Azathioprine is not recommended for use in pregnant women with rheumatoid arthritis.

Teratogenic effects (including skeletal malformations and visceral abnormalities) have been reported in rabbits and mice given doses equivalent to the human dose (5 mg/kg per day).

FDA Pregnancy Category D.

### Breast-feeding

Azathioprine is distributed, at low concentrations, into breast milk. Nursing mothers should be advised to contact physician, since use by nursing mothers is not recommended because of possible adverse effects (especially tumorigenicity) on the infant.

### Pediatrics

Appropriate studies performed to date have not demonstrated pediatrics-specific problems that would limit the usefulness of azathioprine in children.

### Geriatrics

Although appropriate studies on the relationship of age to the effects of azathioprine have not been performed in the geriatric population, geriatrics-specific problems are not expected to limit the usefulness of this medication in the elderly. However, elderly patients are more likely to have age-related renal function impairment, which may require reduced dosage in patients receiving azathioprine.

### Dental

The bone marrow depressant effects of azathioprine may result in an increased incidence of microbial infection, delayed healing, and gingival bleeding. Dental work, whenever possible, should be completed prior to initiation of therapy or deferred until blood counts have returned to normal. Patients should be instructed in proper oral hygiene during treatment, including caution in use of regular toothbrushes, dental floss, and toothpicks.

In addition, azathioprine rarely causes sores in the mouth and on the lips.

## Drug interactions and/or related problems

The following drug interactions and/or related problems have been selected on the basis of their potential clinical significance (possible mechanism in parentheses where appropriate)—not necessarily inclusive (» = major clinical significance):

Note: Combinations containing any of the following medications, depending on the amount present, may also interact with this medication.

» Allopurinol
(allopurinol-induced inhibition of xanthine oxidase–mediated metabolism may result in greatly increased azathioprine activity and toxicity; concurrent use should be avoided if possible, especially in renal transplant patients, because of the high risk of 6-mercaptopurine [azathioprine metabolite] accumulation and consequent azathioprine toxicity if the transplanted kidney is rejected; if concurrent use is essential, it is recommended that azathioprine dosage be reduced to one-quarter to one-third of the usual dosage, the patient be carefully monitored, and subsequent dosage adjustments be based on patient response and evidence of toxicity)

Blood dyscrasia–causing medications (See *Appendix II*)
(leukopenic and/or thrombocytopenic effects of azathioprine may be increased with concurrent or recent therapy if these medications cause the same effects; dosage adjustment of azathioprine, if necessary, should be based on blood counts)

Bone marrow depressants, other (See *Appendix II*) or
Radiation therapy
(concurrent use with azathioprine may increase the bone marrow depressant effects of these medications and radiation therapy; dosage reduction may be required; use prior to azathioprine therapy may be associated with an increased risk of development of neoplasms)

» Immunosuppressants, other, such as:
Chlorambucil
Corticosteroids, glucocorticoid
Cyclophosphamide
Cyclosporine
Mercaptopurine
Muromonab-CD3
(concurrent use with azathioprine may increase the risk of infection and development of neoplasms)

Vaccines, killed virus
(because normal defense mechanisms may be suppressed by azathioprine therapy, the patient's antibody response to the vaccine may be decreased. The interval between discontinuation of medications that cause immunosuppression and restoration of the patient's ability to respond to the vaccine depends on the intensity and type of immunosuppression-causing medication used, the underlying disease, and other factors; estimates vary from 3 months to 1 year)

» Vaccines, live virus
(because normal defense mechanisms may be suppressed by azathioprine therapy, concurrent use with a live virus vaccine may potentiate the replication of the vaccine virus, may increase the side/adverse effects of the vaccine virus, and/or may decrease the patient's antibody response to the vaccine; immunization of these patients should be undertaken only with extreme caution after careful review of the patient's hematologic status and only with the knowledge and consent of the physician managing the azathioprine therapy. The interval between discontinuation of medications that cause immunosuppression and restoration of the patient's ability to respond to the vaccine depends on the intensity and type of immunosuppression-causing medication used, the underlying disease, and other factors; estimates vary from 3 months to 1 year. Patients with leukemia in remission should not receive live virus vaccine until at least 3 months after their last chemotherapy. In addition, immunization with oral poliovirus vaccine should be postponed in persons in close contact with the patient, especially family members)

## Laboratory value alterations

The following have been selected on the basis of their potential clinical significance (possible effect in parentheses where appropriate)—not necessarily inclusive (» = major clinical significance):

With physiology/laboratory test values
Alanine aminotransferase (ALT [SGPT]) and
Alkaline phosphatase and
Amylase and

Aspartate aminotransferase (AST [SGOT]) and
Bilirubin
(serum values may be increased in association with toxic hepatitis and biliary stasis, primarily in allograft recipients; may also be increased as part of a gastrointestinal hypersensitivity reaction; uncommon in rheumatoid arthritis patients)

Albumin, plasma and
Hemoglobin and
Uric acid in blood and urine
(concentrations may be decreased)

Mean corpuscular volume (MCV)
(may be increased; occurs commonly, as a sign of macrocytosis)

## Medical considerations/Contraindications

The medical considerations/contraindications included here have been selected on the basis of their potential clinical significance (reasons given in parentheses where appropriate)—not necessarily inclusive (» = major clinical significance).

*Risk-benefit should be considered when the following medical problems exist:*

» Chickenpox, existing or recent (including recent exposure) or
» Herpes zoster
(risk of severe generalized disease)

» Gout
(because of interaction with allopurinol)

» Hepatic function impairment

» Infection
Pancreatitis

» Renal function impairment
(increased risk of hematologic toxicity; a lower dosage of azathioprine is recommended for patients with impaired renal function)

» Sensitivity to azathioprine

» Xanthine oxidase deficiency, severe
(reduced metabolism may result in increased azathioprine activity and toxicity)

» Caution should be used also in patients who have had previous cytotoxic drug therapy and radiation therapy.

## Patient monitoring

The following may be especially important in patient monitoring (other tests may be warranted in some patients, depending on condition; » = major clinical significance):

» Complete blood counts
(recommended at least weekly during the first 2 months of therapy; frequency may be reduced to monthly once the patient is stabilized)

# Side/Adverse Effects

Note: The risk of hematologic and neoplastic toxicity appears to be lower in rheumatoid arthritis patients because of the lower doses used. Bone marrow depression may be more severe in renal transplant patients whose hemografts are undergoing rejection.

The following side/adverse effects have been selected on the basis of their potential clinical significance (possible signs and symptoms in parentheses where appropriate)—not necessarily inclusive:

## Those indicating need for medical attention

Incidence more frequent
*Leukopenia or infection* (leukopenia is usually asymptomatic; less frequently, fever or chills; cough or hoarseness; lower back or side pain; painful or difficult urination); *megaloblastic anemia* (unusual tiredness or weakness)

Note: *Leukopenia* may be severe or delayed and is dose-related. Not correlated with therapeutic effect.

The incidence of *infection* in renal transplant patients is 30 to 60 times that in patients taking azathioprine for rheumatoid arthritis.

*Infections* may be fatal.

Incidence less frequent—dose-related
*Hepatitis or biliary stasis* (asymptomatic); *thrombocytopenia* (usually asymptomatic; rarely, unusual bleeding or bruising; black, tarry stools; blood in urine or stools; pinpoint red spots on skin)

Note: *Hepatotoxicity* usually occurs within 6 months of transplantation and is reversible on withdrawal of azathioprine. It is uncommon (incidence less than 1%) in rheumatoid arthritis patients. Hepatotoxicity occurs more frequently at dosages above 2.5 mg per kg of body weight (mg/kg) per day.

*Thrombocytopenia* may be severe or delayed and is dose-related.

Incidence rare
> *Gastrointestinal hypersensitivity reaction* (severe nausea and vomiting with diarrhea; sudden fever; joint pain; sudden unusual feeling of discomfort or illness); *hepatic veno-occlusive disease, potentially fatal* (stomach pain; swelling of feet or lower legs); *hypersensitivity* (fast heartbeat; sudden fever; muscle or joint pain; redness or blisters on skin); *pancreatitis, hypersensitivity* (severe stomach pain with nausea and vomiting); *pneumonitis* (cough; shortness of breath); *sores in mouth and on lips*

> Note: Symptoms of the *gastrointestinal hypersensitivity reaction* usually develop within the first several weeks of therapy and are reversible on withdrawal of azathioprine, although they will recur within hours after the first dose on rechallenge. Hypotension may occasionally occur. Hepatic enzymes may also be elevated.

> *Hypersensitivity* reactions usually occur after at least 1 week of therapy, and are reversible on withdrawal. The reaction may be more severe on rechallenge and can be fatal.

**Those indicating need for medical attention only if they continue or are bothersome**
Incidence more frequent
> *Loss of appetite; nausea or vomiting*

Incidence less frequent
> *Skin rash*

**Those indicating the need for medical attention if they occur after medication is discontinued**
> *Bone marrow depression, delayed* (black, tarry stools; blood in urine; cough or hoarseness; fever or chills; lower back or side pain; painful or difficult urination; pinpoint red spots on skin; unusual bleeding or bruising)

## Patient Consultation

As an aid to patient consultation, refer to *Advice for the Patient, Azathioprine (Systemic)*.

In providing consultation, consider emphasizing the following selected information (» = major clinical significance):

**Before using this medication**
» Conditions affecting use, especially:
> Sensitivity to azathioprine
> Pregnancy—Use not recommended because of mutagenic or teratogenic potential
> Breast-feeding—Not recommended because of risk of serious side effects
> Other medications, especially allopurinol, other immunosuppressants, or previous cytotoxic drug therapy or radiation therapy
> Other medical problems, especially chickenpox, herpes zoster, gout, hepatic function impairment, infection, or renal function impairment

**Proper use of this medication**
» Importance of not taking more or less medication than the amount prescribed
> Caution with combination therapy; taking each medication at the right time
» Checking with physician before discontinuing medication
> Possible nausea or vomiting; taking after meals or at bedtime to reduce stomach upset
> Checking with physician if vomiting occurs shortly after dose is taken
» Proper dosing
> Missed dose: If dosing schedule is—
>> Once a day: Not taking missed dose and not doubling next one
>> Several times a day: Taking as soon as possible or doubling next dose; checking with physician if more than one dose is missed
» Proper storage

**Precautions while using this medication**
» Importance of close monitoring by physician
» Avoiding immunizations unless approved by physician; other persons in patient's household should avoid immunizations with oral poliovirus vaccine; avoiding other persons who have taken oral poliovirus vaccine or wearing a protective mask that covers nose and mouth
*Caution if bone marrow depression occurs*
» Avoiding exposure to persons with bacterial or viral infections, especially during periods of low blood counts; checking with physician immediately if fever or chills, cough or hoarseness, lower back or side pain, or painful or difficult urination occurs

» Checking with physician immediately if unusual bleeding or bruising; black, tarry stools; blood in urine or stools; or pinpoint red spots on skin occur
> Caution in use of regular toothbrush, dental floss, or toothpick; physician, dentist, or nurse may suggest alternatives; checking with physician before having dental work done
> Not touching eyes or inside of nose unless hands washed immediately before
> Using caution to avoid accidental cuts with use of sharp objects such as safety razor or fingernail or toenail cutters
> Avoiding contact sports or other situations where bruising or injury could occur

**Side/adverse effects**
> Importance of discussing possible effects, including cancer, with physician
> Signs of potential side effects, especially leukopenia, infection, megaloblastic anemia, hepatitis, biliary stasis, thrombocytopenia, gastrointestinal hypersensitivity reaction, hepatic veno-occlusive disease, hypersensitivity, pancreatitis, pneumonitis, and sores in mouth and on lips
> Asymptomatic side effects, including hepatotoxicity

## General Dosing Information

Patients receiving azathioprine should be under supervision of a physician experienced in immunosuppressive therapy.

A variety of dosage schedules and regimens of azathioprine, alone or in combination with other immunosuppressive agents, are used. The prescriber may consult the medical literature as well as the manufacturer's literature in choosing a specific dosage.

Dosage must be adjusted to meet the individual requirements of each patient, on the basis of clinical response and appearance or severity of toxicity.

Cadaveric kidneys frequently develop a tubular necrosis with delayed onset of adequate function, necessitating a reduction in azathioprine dosage. If persistent negative nitrogen balance occurs, dosage should be reduced.

Because of the delayed action of azathioprine, dosage should be reduced or the medication withdrawn at the first sign of an abnormally large or persistent decrease in leukocyte count (to less than 3000 per cubic millimeter) or platelet count (to less than 100,000 per cubic millimeter) or other evidence of bone marrow depression. Therapy may be reinstituted at a lower dosage when leukocyte and platelet counts return to acceptable levels, usually after 7 to 10 days.

Special precautions are recommended in patients who develop thrombocytopenia as a result of administration of azathioprine. These may include extreme care in performing invasive procedures; regular inspection of intravenous sites, skin (including perirectal area), and mucous membrane surfaces for signs of bleeding or bruising; limiting frequency of venipuncture and avoiding intramuscular injections; testing urine, emesis, stool, and secretions for occult blood; care in use of regular toothbrushes, dental floss, toothpicks, safety razors, and fingernail and toenail cutters; avoiding constipation; and using caution to prevent falls and other injuries. Such patients should avoid alcohol and aspirin intake because of the risk of gastrointestinal bleeding. Platelet transfusions may be required.

Patients who develop leukopenia should be observed carefully for signs of infection. Antibiotic support may be required. In neutropenic patients who develop fever, broad-spectrum antibiotic coverage should be initiated empirically, pending bacterial cultures and appropriate diagnostic tests.

If an infection develops, it must be treated promptly; reduction of azathioprine dosage and/or use of other drugs may be necessary.

If symptoms of toxic hepatitis or biliary stasis appear, azathioprine therapy may have to be withdrawn. Patients with existing hepatic function impairment should be monitored carefully and treated with conservative doses (some clinicians recommend an initial dose of two-thirds the usual dose). If hepatic veno-occlusive disease is clinically suspected, it is recommended that azathioprine be permanently withdrawn.

If signs of homograft rejection occur, a larger dose may be necessary. Other therapy should be considered if signs persist.

**For parenteral dosage forms**
Azathioprine may be administered by intravenous push or infusion. Time for infusion is usually 30 to 60 minutes, but may range from 5 minutes to 8 hours.

**Diet/Nutrition**
Gastrointestinal upset may be reduced by giving oral azathioprine in divided doses or after meals.

## Safety considerations for handling this medication

There is limited but increasing evidence and concern that personnel involved in preparation and administration of parenteral antineoplastics and immunosuppressants may be at some risk because of the potential mutagenicity, teratogenicity, and/or carcinogenicity of these agents, although the actual risk is unknown. USP advisory panels recommend cautious handling both in preparation and disposal of antineoplastic and immunosuppressant agents. Precautions that have been suggested include:

• Use of a biological containment cabinet during reconstitution and dilution of parenteral medications and wearing of disposable surgical gloves and masks.

• Use of proper technique to prevent contamination of the medication, work area, and operator during transfer between containers (including proper training of personnel in this technique).

• Cautious and proper disposal of needles, syringes, vials, ampuls, and unused medication.

A number of medical centers have developed detailed guidelines for handling of antineoplastic and immunosuppressant agents.

## Oral Dosage Forms

Note: Bracketed uses in the *Dosage Forms* section refer to categories of use and/or indications that are not included in U.S. product labeling.

### AZATHIOPRINE TABLETS USP

#### Usual adult and adolescent dose

Transplant rejection, organ (prophylaxis)—
Initial: Oral, 3 to 5 mg per kg of body weight or 120 mg per square meter of body surface a day, one to three days before or at the time of surgery, the dosage being adjusted to maintain the homograft without causing toxicity.

Maintenance: Oral, 1 to 2 mg per kg of body weight or 45 mg per square meter of body surface a day.

[Bowel disease, inflammatory][1] or
[Hepatitis, chronic active][1] or
[Cirrhosis, biliary][1] or
[Glomerulonephritis][1] or
[Nephrotic syndrome][1] or
[Myopathy, inflammatory][1] or
[Myasthenia gravis][1] or
[Dermatomyositis, systemic][1] or
[Pemphigoid][1] or
[Pemphigus][1]—
Initial: Oral, 1 mg per kg of body weight per day, the dosage being increased in increments of 500 mcg (0.5 mg) per kg of body weight per day after six to eight weeks, then every four weeks as necessary up to a maximum dose of 2.5 mg per kg of body weight per day.

Maintenance: Oral, the dosage being reduced to the minimum effective dose in decrements of 500 mcg (0.5 mg) per kg of body weight per day every four to eight weeks.

Rheumatoid arthritis or
[Lupus erythematosus, systemic][1]—
Initial: Oral, 1 mg per kg of body weight per day, the dosage being increased in increments of 500 mcg (0.5 mg) per kg of body weight per day after six to eight weeks, then every four weeks as necessary up to a maximum dose of 2.5 mg per kg of body weight per day.

Maintenance: Oral, the dosage being reduced to the minimum effective dose in decrements of 500 mcg (0.5 mg) per kg of body weight per day every four to eight weeks.

#### Usual pediatric dose

See *Usual adult and adolescent dose.*

### Strength(s) usually available

U.S.—
50 mg (Rx) [*Imuran* (scored)].
Canada—
50 mg (Rx) [*Imuran* (scored)].

### Packaging and storage

Store below 40 °C (104 °F), preferably between 15 and 30 °C (59 and 86 °F), in a well-closed container, unless otherwise specified by manufacturer. Protect from light.

## Parenteral Dosage Forms

Note: The dosing and strengths of the dosage form available are expressed in terms of azathioprine base.

### AZATHIOPRINE SODIUM FOR INJECTION USP

#### Usual adult and adolescent dose

Transplant rejection, organ (prophylaxis)—
Initial: Intravenous 3 to 5 mg (base) per kg of body weight a day prior to, during, or soon after surgery, the dosage being adjusted to maintain the homograft without causing toxicity.

Maintenance: Intravenous, 1 to 2 mg (base) per kg of body weight a day.

#### Usual pediatric dose

See *Usual adult and adolescent dose.*

#### Size(s) usually available

U.S.—
100 mg (base) (Rx) [*Imuran;* GENERIC].
Canada—
100 mg (base) (Rx) [*Imuran*].

#### Packaging and storage

Store below 40 °C (104 °F), preferably between 15 and 30 °C (59 and 86 °F). Protect from light, unless otherwise specified by manufacturer.

#### Preparation of dosage form

Azathioprine Sodium for Injection USP is reconstituted for intravenous use by adding 10 mL of sterile water for injection to the vial and swirling to dissolve.

Reconstituted solutions may be further diluted for administration by intravenous infusion with 0.9% sodium chloride injection or 5% dextrose and 0.9% sodium chloride injection.

#### Stability

Reconstituted solutions of azathioprine are stable for 24 hours at room temperature. Although solutions may be stable for longer periods, because there is no preservative, use within 24 hours is recommended for reasons of sterility.

#### Incompatibilities

Mixing with alkaline solutions, especially on warming, may result in conversion to 6-mercaptopurine. Conversion to mercaptopurine also occurs in the presence of sulfhydryl compounds such as cysteine, glutathione, and hydrogen sulfide.

---

[1]Not included in Canadian product labeling.

## Selected Bibliography

Korman N. Pemphigus. J Am Acad Dermatol 1988 Jun; 18: 1219-38.
Pugh MC, Pugh CB. Current concepts in clinical therapeutics: disease-modifying drugs for rheumatoid arthritis. Clin Pharm 1987 Jun; 6: 475-91.

---

Revised: 05/06/93
Interim revision: 04/29/94

---

# AZELAIC ACID   Topical†

VA CLASSIFICATION (Primary/Secondary): DE752/DE900

Note: For a listing of dosage forms and brand names by country availability, see *Dosage Forms* section(s). For a listing of brand names for the articles in this monograph, refer to the General Index.

†Not commercially available in Canada.

## Category

Antiacne agent (topical); hypopigmentation agent (topical).

## Indications

Note: Bracketed information in the *Indications* section refers to uses that are not included in U.S. product labeling.

### Accepted

Acne vulgaris (treatment)—Azelaic acid is indicated in the treatment of mild to moderate acne vulgaris.

[Melasma (treatment)]—Azelaic acid has been used to treat melasma, caused by hyperfunctioning melanocytes. Azelaic acid will not similarly affect the function of normal melanocytes; thus, it will not lighten freckles.

# Pharmacology/Pharmacokinetics

### Physicochemical characteristics
Source—Dietary component (whole grain cereals and animal products).
Molecular weight—188.22.

### Mechanism of action/Effect
Antiacne agent—
The mechanism of action is not fully known but it is thought that azelaic acid causes antibacterial effects by inhibiting the synthesis of cellular protein in aerobic and anaerobic microorganisms, especially *Propionibacterium acnes* and *Staphylococcus epidermidis*. Within aerobic microorganisms, azelaic acid reversibly inhibits a variety of oxidoreductive enzymes including tyrosinase, mitochondrial enzymes of the respiratory chain, thioredoxin reductase, 5-alpha-reductase, and DNA polymerases. In anaerobic microorganisms, glycolysis is disrupted.

Also, azelaic acid improves acne vulgaris by decreasing microcomedo formation and normalizing the keratin process. Azelaic acid may be effective against both inflamed and noninflamed lesions. Specifically, azelaic acid reduces the thickness of the stratum corneum, shrinks keratohyalin granules by reducing the amount and distribution of filaggrin (a component of keratohyalin) in epidermal layers, and lowers the number of keratohyalin granules.

Hypopigmentation agent—
Azelaic acid's antityrosinase and antimitochondrial enzymatic activities may interrupt the hyperactivity of normal melanocytes and their resulting growth in melasma, a localized macular hyperpigmentation of facial or nuchal skin. Use of azelaic acid to treat hyperpigmentation disorders due to hyperactivity of abnormal melanocytes has not been consistently successful. The hypopigmentation action of azelaic acid may result, to a lesser extent, from its ability to scavenge free radicals that can cause hyperactivity of melanocytes. Free radicals are a metabolic product of peroxidation of cell membrane lipids, produced when cells are irradiated with ultraviolet light, including sunlight. There is no depigmenting effect on normal melanocytes.

### Other actions/effects
Azelaic acid is being studied for potential antimycotic and antiviral properties.

In time- and dose-dependent *in vitro* studies, azelaic acid has been shown to selectively penetrate rapidly growing human and murine tumor cells that are undifferentiated and possess chromosomal abnormalities while not affecting normal cells. The antiproliferative and cytotoxic effects are attributed to the antityrosinase and antimitochondrial activity of azelaic acid. Further *in vivo* studies are needed to fully characterize the clinical course of azelaic acid within these cell lines.

### Absorption
One study found the following levels of penetration after a single application to human skin *in vitro*—
Stratum corneum: Approximately 3 to 5%.
Dermis and epidermis: Up to 10%.
Plasma: Approximately 4%.

### Elimination
Renal, mainly unchanged.

# Precautions to Consider

### Carcinogenicity
Carcinogenic animal studies were deemed unnecessary because azelaic acid is normally found in the human diet and is not considered to be a carcinogenic substance.

### Mutagenicity
The Ames test, hypoxanthine-guanine phosphoribosyltransferase (HGPRT) test in Chinese hamster ovary cells, human lymphocyte test, and dominant lethal assay in mice suggest that azelaic acid is nonmutagenic.

### Pregnancy/Reproduction
Fertility—Adequate and well-controlled studies have not been done in humans.
Animal studies have shown no adverse effects.

Pregnancy—Systemically absorbed azelaic acid crosses the placenta; however, little systemic absorption of topical azelaic acid occurs. Adequate and well-controlled studies have not been done; problems in humans have not been documented.

In animal studies using toxic oral doses, embryotoxic effects occurred in Segment I and II studies of rats given doses of 2500 mg per kg of body weight (mg/kg) a day; similar effects were reported for Segment II studies in rabbits given doses of 150 to 500 mg/kg a day and mon-keys given doses of 500 mg/kg a day. No teratogenic effects occurred. Animal studies using topical administration have not been done.

FDA Pregnancy Category B.

### Breast-feeding
Azelaic acid may pass into breast milk, according to *in vitro* studies; however, the amount that is absorbed systemically from topical administration is insignificant and should not affect physiologic levels of azelaic acid. Problems in humans have not been documented.

### Pediatrics
No information is available on the relationship of age to the effects of azelaic acid in pediatric patients. Safety and efficacy have not been established.

### Geriatrics
No information is available on the relationship of age to the effects of azelaic acid in geriatric patients.

### Medical considerations/Contraindications
The medical considerations/contraindications included here have been selected on the basis of their potential clinical significance (reasons given in parentheses where appropriate)—not necessarily inclusive (» = major clinical significance).

*Risk-benefit should be considered when the following medical problem exists:*
Hypersensitivity to azelaic acid

# Side/Adverse Effects

The following side/adverse effects have been selected on the basis of their potential clinical significance (possible signs and symptoms in parentheses where appropriate)—not necessarily inclusive:

### Those indicating need for medical attention
Incidence rare
*Hypopigmentation* (white spots or lightening of treated areas of dark skin)—in patients with dark complexions
Note: Azelaic acid will consistently lighten hyperpigmented skin (skin that is darker than normal for a given individual) but will not typically lighten skin beyond its normal color. Rarely, patients with dark complexions may notice *hypopigmentation* of skin.

### Those indicating need for medical attention only if they continue or are bothersome
Incidence more frequent
*Desquamation* (peeling of skin); *dryness of skin; erythema* (redness of skin); *inflammatory reaction, mild* (burning, stinging, or tingling of skin, mild)—1 to 5% with continued use; *pruritus, mild* (itching of skin)—1 to 5% with continued use
Note: *Mild burning, stinging, or tingling of skin* and *pruritus* may occur at the start of each treatment and may last 5 to 20 minutes, especially if skin is inflamed or broken, but lessens with continued use. Dosage may be reduced until skin irritation lessens.

# Patient Consultation

As an aid to patient consultation, refer to *Advice for the Patient, Azelaic Acid (Topical)*.

In providing consultation, consider emphasizing the following selected information (» = major clinical significance):

### Before using this medication
» Conditions affecting use, especially:
Hypersensitivity to azelaic acid

### Proper use of this medication
Applying a small amount of medication as a thin film to clean, dry skin; gently and thoroughly rubbing into the affected area
Washing hands well after applying
» Not applying to mucous membranes and, if accidental contact occurs, washing affected area well with water immediately
» Compliance with full course of treatment
» Proper dosing
Missed dose: Applying as soon as possible; not applying if almost time for next dose; not doubling doses
» Proper storage

### Precautions while using this medication
Contacting health care professional if acne worsens or does not improve in the first 4 weeks or if medication causes too much redness, dryness, or peeling of skin
May take longer than 4 weeks before full improvement is noticed
Other topical medications may be used but recommend applying them at different times during the day

Conservative use of water-base cosmetics is permissible with use of azelaic acid

## General Dosing Information

Some skin irritation may be expected with first use of topical azelaic acid; however, if skin irritation persists, dosage may be reduced to one time a day until irritation lessens. If skin irritation continues, azelaic acid treatment should be discontinued.

Patient should apply azelaic acid as a thin film to clean dry skin and rub into skin thoroughly. Improvement of acne or hyperpigmentation condition may take 4 weeks or longer.

### Safety considerations for handling this medication

Wash hands thoroughly after handling topical azelaic acid.

Keep topical azelaic acid away from mouth, eyes, and other mucous membranes. If accidental contact occurs, large amounts of water should be used to wash affected area. If the eyes are involved and eye irritation persists after a thorough washing, contact a physician.

## Topical Dosage Form

Note: Bracketed uses in the *Dosage Forms* section refer to categories of use and/or indications that are not included in U.S. product labeling.

### AZELAIC ACID CREAM

**Usual adult and adolescent dose**
Antiacne agent or
[Hypopigmentation agent]—
Topical, to the affected area, two times a day (morning and evening).

Note: Initially, application once a day for a few days has been used for some patients sensitive to azelaic acid.

**Usual pediatric dose**
Safety and efficacy have not been established.

**Strength(s) usually available**
U.S.—
20% (Rx) [*Azelex*].
Canada—
Not commercially available.

**Packaging and storage**
Store below 40 °C (104 °F), preferably between 15 and 30 °C (59 and 86 °F), unless otherwise specified by manufacturer. Protect from freezing.

**Auxiliary labeling**
• External use only.

**Note**
Dermatologic use only; not for ophthalmic use.

## Selected Bibliography

Breathnach AS. Pharmacological properties of azelaic acid. Clin Drug Invest 1995; 10 (Suppl 2): 27-33.

Developed: 06/27/96

---

# AZITHROMYCIN   Systemic

VA CLASSIFICATION (Primary): AM200

Note: For a listing of dosage forms and brand names by country availability, see *Dosage Forms* section(s). For a listing of brand names for the articles in this monograph, refer to the General Index.

## Category

Antibacterial (systemic).

## Indications

Note: Bracketed information in the *Indications* section refers to uses that are not included in U.S. product labeling.

### General considerations

Azithromycin is the first of a new class of antibiotics called azalides. It has *in vitro* activity against many gram-positive and gram-negative aerobic and anaerobic bacteria. It also has greater stability than erythromycin in the presence of acid.

Azithromycin is active against staphylococci, including *Staphylococcus aureus* and *S. epidermidis*, as well as streptococci, such as *Streptococcus pyogenes* and *S. pneumoniae*. The minimum inhibitory concentration (MIC) of azithromycin is 2 to 4 times greater than that of erythromycin against staphylococcus and streptococcus; however, the clinical significance of this *in vitro* information is unclear since the concentrations attained in tissues are higher than the MIC for many pathogens. Most erythromycin-resistant strains of staphylococcus, enterococcus, and streptococcus, including methicillin-resistant *S. aureus*, are also resistant to azithromycin. Also, azithromycin is less potent than erythromycin and clarithromycin against erythromycin-sensitive enterococci.

Azithromycin has excellent activity against *Haemophilus influenzae*, being 2 to 8 times more active than erythromycin and 4 to 8 times more active than clarithromycin *in vitro*. MICs of 4 to 16 mcg per mL inhibit most *Escherichia coli*, *Salmonella*, *Shigella*, and *Aeromonas* species. *Pseudomonas aeruginosa*, *Klebsiella*, *Enterobacter*, *Citrobacter*, *Proteus*, *Providencia*, *Morganella*, and *Serratia* species are resistant to azithromycin.

Azithromycin is 2- to 4-fold more active than erythromycin against *Moraxella (Branhamella) catarrhalis*. Inhibition of anaerobes, such as *Clostridium perfringens*, is slightly better with azithromycin than with erythromycin, and azithromycin's inhibition of *Bacteroides fragilis* and other *Bacteroides* species is comparable to that of erythromycin. Azithromycin also has good *in vitro* activity against *Chlamydia trachomatis*, *C. pneumoniae*, *Mycoplasma pneumoniae*, *Legionella* species, *Borrelia burgdorferi*, *Ureaplasma urealyticum*, and *Gardnerella vaginalis*. Azithromycin has 8-fold more activity than erythromycin against *Neisseria gonorrhoeae* and 10-fold more activity against *Hae-*

*mophilus ducreyi*. It has also been shown to inhibit *Toxoplasma gondii in vitro* and in animal models. However, no potentiation against *Toxoplasma gondii* could be demonstrated when azithromycin was combined with pyrimethamine. Also, when azithromycin was administered as a single agent in the treatment of cerebral toxoplasmosis in 2 patients, it failed, although the patients responded to conventional treatment.

### Accepted

Bronchitis, bacterial exacerbations (treatment)
Cervicitis, chlamydial (treatment)
Pharyngitis, streptococcal (treatment)
Pneumonia, *Haemophilus influenzae* (treatment)
Pneumonia, *Streptococcus pneumoniae* (treatment)
Skin and soft tissue infections (treatment) or
Urethritis, chlamydial (treatment)—Azithroymycin is indicated in the treatment of these disease states when they are caused by susceptible organsims.

[Pneumonia, mycoplasmal (treatment)]—Azithromycin is used in the treatment of pneumonia caused by *Mycoplasma pneumoniae*.

## Pharmacology/Pharmacokinetics

### Physicochemical characteristics
Molecular weight—785.0.

### Mechanism of action/Effect
Azithromycin binds to the 50S ribosomal subunit of the 70S ribosome of susceptible organisms, thereby inhibiting RNA-dependent protein synthesis.

Azithromycin is bactericidal for *S. pyogenes*, *S. pneumoniae*, and *H. influenzae*; it is bacteriostatic for staphylococci and most aerobic gram-negative species.

### Absorption
Rapidly absorbed. Food decreases absorption of azithromycin, resulting in a decrease in the peak serum concentration ($C_{max}$) by approximately 52% and the area-under-the-concentration-time-curve (AUC) by approximately 43%. Oral bioavailability (F) is approximately 37%.

### Distribution
Rapidly and widely distributed throughout the body. Concentrates intracellularly, resulting in tissue concentrations 10 to 100 times those in plasma or serum. Azithromycin is highly concentrated in phagocytes and fibroblasts. Phagocytes transport the drug to the site of infection and inflammation. Release of azithromycin from phagocytes is gradual, but it is enhanced by exposure to the cell membrane of bacteria. Release of azithromycin from fibroblasts is not enhanced by bacteria, but fibroblasts may act as reservoirs of the antibiotic, releasing azith-

romycin to phagocytes. Very low concentrations ($< 0.01$ mcg per mL [mcg/mL]) were detected in the cerebrospinal fluid of human subjects with noninflamed meninges; however, higher concentrations were found in brain tissue in animal studies.

$Vol_D$ = Approximately 31 L per kg (steady-state).

**Protein binding**
Varies with concentration—Approximately 50% at 0.02 and 0.05 mcg/mL; approximately 7% at 1.0 mcg/mL.

**Biotransformation**
Hepatic; approximately 35% metabolized by demethylation. Up to 10 metabolites, which are thought to have no significant antimicrobial activity, may be found in the bile.

**Half-life**
Serum—11 to 14 hours when measured between 8 and 24 hours after a single dose; however, after several doses, the half-life is approximately the same as the half-life in tissues.

Tissue—2 to 4 days.

**Time to peak concentration**
Young subjects—2.5 to 3.2 hours.
Elderly subjects—3.8 to 4.4 hours.

**Peak serum concentration**
After a 500-mg loading dose on day 1, then 250 mg once a day on days 2 through 5—
    Day 1: Approximately 0.41 and 0.38 mcg/mL, respectively, for healthy and elderly adults.
    Day 5: Approximately 0.24 and 0.26 mcg/mL, respectively, for healthy and elderly adults.

**Elimination**
Over 50% of the dose is eliminated through biliary excretion as unchanged drug; approximately 4.5% of the dose is eliminated in the urine as unchanged drug within 72 hours.

## Precautions to Consider

**Cross-sensitivity and/or related problems**
Patients who are hypersensitive to erythromycin or other macrolides may also be hypersensitive to azithromycin.

**Carcinogenicity**
Long-term studies have not been done in animals to evaluate the carcinogenic potential of azithromycin.

**Mutagenicity**
Azithromycin was not found to be mutagenic in the mouse lymphoma assay, the human lymphoctye clastogenic assay, and the mouse bone marrow clastogenic assay.

**Pregnancy/Reproduction**
Fertility—Adequate and well-controlled studies in humans have not been done.
Reproduction studies done in rats and mice given azithromycin at doses up to moderately maternotoxic dose levels (i.e., 200 mg per kg of body weight [mg/kg] per day) have found no evidence of impaired fertility. On a mg per square meter of body surface (mg/m²) basis, these doses are estimated to be 4 times and 2 times the human daily dose of 500 mg in rats and mice, respectively.
Pregnancy—Adequate and well-controlled studies in humans have not been done.
Reproduction studies done in rats and mice given azithromycin at doses up to moderately maternotoxic dose levels (i.e., 200 mg/kg per day) have found no evidence of harm to the fetus. Based on a mg/m² basis, these doses are estimated to be 4 times and 2 times the human daily dose of 500 mg in rats and mice, respectively.

FDA Pregnancy Category B.

**Breast-feeding**
It is not known if azithromycin is distributed into human breast milk.

**Pediatrics**
Azithromycin is being studied in children. Although safety, efficacy, and dosage have not been established for children up to 16 years of age, pediatrics-specific problems that would limit the usefulness of this medication in children are not expected. One study found that doses of 10 mg/kg on day 1, followed by 5 mg/kg on days 2 through 5, produced serum concentrations that were similar to those reported in adults.

**Geriatrics**
Pharmacokinetic data in healthy elderly subjects (65 to 85 years old) were similar to those for younger volunteers (18 to 40 years old). A higher peak concentration (by 30 to 50%) was found in elderly women; however, no significant accumulation occurred. Dosage adjustment does

not appear to be necessary in older patients with normal renal and hepatic function.

**Drug interactions and/or related problems**
The following drug interactions and/or related problems have been selected on the basis of their potential clinical significance (possible mechanism in parentheses where appropriate)—not necessarily inclusive (» = major clinical significance):

Note: Combinations containing any of the following medications, depending on the amount present, may also interact with this medication.

» Antacids, aluminum- and magnesium-containing
    (concurrent use with antacids has decreased the peak serum concentration [$C_{max}$] of azithromycin by approximately 24%, but had no effect on the area-under-the-concentration-time-curve [AUC]; azithromycin should be administered at least 1 hour before or 2 hours after aluminum- and magnesium-containing antacids)

**Laboratory value alterations**
The following have been selected on the basis of their potential clinical significance (possible effect in parentheses where appropriate)—not necessarily inclusive (» = major clinical significance):
With physiology/laboratory test values
    Alanine aminotransferase (ALT [SGPT]) and
    Aspartate aminotransferase (AST [SGOT])
        (values may be increased)

**Medical considerations/Contraindications**
The medical considerations/contraindications included here have been selected on the basis of their potential clinical significance (reasons given in parentheses where appropriate)—not necessarily inclusive (» = major clinical significance).

*Except under special circumstances, this medication should not be used when the following medical problem exists:*

» Hypersensitivity to erythromycins or other macrolides

*Risk-benefit should be considered when the following medical problem exists:*

Hepatic function impairment, severe
    (because biliary excretion is the major route of elimination, caution should be used in patients with hepatic function impairment)

## Side/Adverse Effects

Note: Rarely, serious allergic reactions, such as anaphylaxis and angioedema, have been reported in patients taking azithromycin. Despite discontinuation of azithromycin and successful symptomatic treatment of the allergic reactions, allergic symptoms soon recurred in some patients when the symptomatic therapy was discontinued. These patients require prolonged periods of observation and symptomatic treatment.

The following side/adverse effects have been selected on the basis of their potential clinical significance (possible signs and symptoms in parentheses where appropriate)—not necessarily inclusive:

**Those indicating need for medical attention**
Incidence rare
    *Acute interstitial nephritis* (fever; joint pain; skin rash); *allergic reactions* (difficulty in breathing; swelling of face, mouth, neck, hands, and feet; skin rash)

**Those indicating need for medical attention only if they continue or are bothersome**
Incidence less frequent
    *Gastrointestinal disturbances* (abdominal pain; diarrhea; nausea; vomiting)

Incidence rare
    *Dizziness; headache*

## Patient Consultation

As an aid to patient consultation, refer to *Advice for the Patient, Azithromycin (Systemic)*.

In providing consultation, consider emphasizing the following selected information (» = major clinical significance):

**Before using this medication**
» Conditions affecting use, especially:
    Hypersensitivity to erythromycins or other macrolides
    Other medications, especially aluminum- and magnesium-containing antacids

**Proper use of this medication**
Azithromycin should be given at least 1 hour before or 2 hours after meals

Compliance with full course of therapy
» Importance of not taking more medication than prescribed; importance of not discontinuing medication without checking with physician
» Proper dosing
Missed dose: Taking as soon as possible; not taking if almost time for next dose; not doubling doses
» Proper storage

**Precautions while using this medication**
Checking with physician if no improvement within a few days or if condition becomes worse

**Side/adverse effects**
Signs of potential side effects, especially acute interstitial nephritis and allergic reactions

## General Dosing Information

No adjustment in dose is required in patients with mild renal function impairment (creatinine clearance ≥ 40 mL per minute [0.67 mL per second]). No data are available on the use of azithromycin in patients with more severe renal function impairment.

**Diet/Nutrition**
Azithromycin should be given at least 1 hour before or 2 hours after meals.

## Oral Dosage Forms

### AZITHROMYCIN CAPSULES USP

**Usual adult and adolescent dose**
Bronchitis, bacterial exacerbations and
Pharyngitis, streptococcal and
Pneumonia, due to *S. pneumoniae* or *H. influenzae*, and

Skin and soft tissue infections—
Oral, 500 mg as a single dose on day 1, then 250 mg once a day on days 2 through 5.
Cervicitis, chlamydial and
Urethritis, chlamydial—
Oral, 1000 mg as a single dose.

**Usual pediatric dose**
Safety, efficacy, and dosage have not been established in children up to 16 years of age; however, studies have been done in children 2 to 15 years of age using doses of 10 mg per kg of body weight on day 1, then 5 mg per kg of body weight once a day on days 2 through 5.

**Strength(s) usually available**
U.S.—
250 mg (Rx) [*Zithromax*].
Canada—
250 mg (Rx) [*Zithromax*].

**Packaging and storage**
Store below 40 °C (104 °F), preferably between 15 and 30 °C (59 and 86 °F) in a well-closed container, unless otherwise specified by manufacturer.

**Auxiliary labeling**
• Continue medicine for full time of treatment.

## Selected Bibliography

Drew RH, Gallis HA. Azithromycin—spectrum of activity, pharmacokinetics, and clinical applications. Pharmacotherapy 1992; 12 (3): 161-73.

Revised: 05/27/94
Interim revision: 06/28/94

# AZTREONAM   Systemic†

VA CLASSIFICATION (Primary): AM130
Note: For a listing of dosage forms and brand names by country availability, see *Dosage Forms* section(s). For a listing of brand names for the articles in this monograph, refer to the General Index.

†Not commercially available in Canada.

## Category

Antibacterial (systemic)
Note: Aztreonam is a narrow-spectrum antibacterial that is only active against aerobic, gram-negative organisms.

## Indications

Note: Bracketed information in the *Indications* section refers to uses that are not included in U.S. product labeling.

**Accepted**
Bronchitis (treatment) or
Pneumonia, gram-negative, bacterial (treatment)—Aztreonam is indicated as a secondary agent in the treatment of aerobic gram-negative bacterial bronchitis and pneumonia caused by *Enterobacter* species, *Escherichia coli*, *Haemophilus influenzae*, *Klebsiella pneumoniae*, *Proteus mirabilis*, *Pseudomonas aeruginosa*, and *Serratia marcescens*.

Skin and soft tissue infections (treatment)—Aztreonam is indicated as a secondary agent in the treatment of skin and soft tissue infections (including ulcers, burn wound infections, and postoperative wounds) caused by *Citrobacter* species, *Enterobacter* species, *E. coli*, *K. pneumoniae*, *P. mirabilis*, *Ps. aeruginosa*, and *S. marcescens*.

Cystitis (treatment) or
Urinary tract infections, bacterial (treatment)—Aztreonam is indicated as a secondary agent in the treatment of cystitis and complicated and uncomplicated urinary tract infections (including initial and recurrent pyelonephritis) caused by *Citrobacter* species, *E. cloacae*, *E. coli*, *K. oxytoca*, *K. pneumoniae*, *P. mirabilis*, *Ps. aeruginosa*, and *S. marcescens*.

Gynecologic infections (treatment)—Aztreonam is indicated as a secondary agent in the treatment of gynecologic infections (including endometritis and pelvic cellulitis) caused by *Enterobacter* species (including *E. cloacae*), *E. coli*, *K. pneumoniae*, and *P. mirabilis*.

Intra-abdominal infections (treatment)—Aztreonam is indicated as a secondary agent in the treatment of intra-abdominal infections (including peritonitis) caused by *Citrobacter* species (including *C. freundii*), *Enterobacter* species (including *E. cloacae*), *E. coli*, *Klebsiella* species (including *K. pneumoniae*), *Ps. aeruginosa*, and *Serratia* species (including *S. marcescens*).

Septicemia, bacterial (treatment)—Aztreonam is indicated as a secondary agent in the treatment of septicemia caused by *Enterobacter* species, *E. coli*, *K. pneumoniae*, *P. mirabilis*, *Ps. aeruginosa*, and *S. marcescens*.

[Bone and joint infections (treatment)]—Aztreonam is used as a secondary agent in the treatment of bone and joint infections caused by susceptible aerobic, gram-negative bacteria.

Aztreonam and aminoglycosides are synergistic *in vitro* against most strains of *Ps. aeruginosa*, many strains of Enterobacteriaceae, and other aerobic gram-negative bacilli.

Not all species or strains of a particular organism may be susceptible to aztreonam.

**Unaccepted**
Aztreonam is not effective against gram-positive organisms (e.g., *Staphylococcus aureus*, enterococci, *Streptococcus pneumoniae*) and anaerobes (e.g., *Bacteroides* species and *Clostridium* species).

## Pharmacology/Pharmacokinetics

**Physicochemical characteristics**
Molecular weight—435.43.

**Mechanism of action/Effect**
Bactericidal; binds to penicillin-binding protein-3 (PBP-3), which results in inhibition of bacterial cell wall synthesis, and often results ultimately in cell lysis and death; filamentation also occurs in Enterobacteriaceae and *Ps. aeruginosa*; does not induce beta-lactamase activity, but has a high degree of stability in the presence of bacterial beta-lactamases; does not bind appreciably to any essential PBPs in gram-positive or anaerobic organisms.

**Absorption**
Oral—Less than 1% absorbed from the gastrointestinal tract following oral administration.
Intramuscular—Completely absorbed following intramuscular administration.

## Distribution

Rapidly and widely distributed to body fluids and tissues; distributed to bile; breast milk; bronchial secretions; and blister, pericardial, pleural, synovial, amniotic, peritoneal, and cerebrospinal fluids (inflamed meninges); also distributed to atrial appendages, endometrium, fallopian tubes, fat, femurs, gallbladder, kidneys, large intestine, liver, lungs, myometrium, ovaries, prostate, skeletal muscles, skin, and sternum; also crosses the placenta and enters fetal circulation.

$Vol_D$ (steady state)—
  Adults:
    0.11 to 0.21 L per kg.
  Burn patients:
    Approximately 0.31 L per kg.
  Pediatric patients:
    Premature neonates—0.29 to 0.36 L per kg.
    Neonates (up to 1 month old)—0.26 to 0.30 L per kg.
    Infants and children (1 month to 12 years)—0.20 to 0.29 L per kg.
    Cystic fibrosis patients—Approximately 0.25 L per kg.

## Protein binding

Normal renal function—Moderate (56 to 60%).
Impaired renal function (creatinine clearance <30 mL per min [0.50 mL per sec])—36 to 43%.

## Biotransformation

Approximately 6 to 16% metabolized to inactive metabolites by hydrolysis of the beta-lactam bond, resulting in an open-ring compound.

## Half-life

Adults—
  Normal renal function:
    1.4 to 2.2 hours.
  Impaired renal function:
    4.7 to 6.0 hours.
  Impaired hepatic function:
    Primary biliary cirrhosis—Approximately 2.2 hours.
    Alcoholic cirrhosis—Approximately 3.4 hours.
  In elderly males (65 to 75 years of age):
    Slightly prolonged (2.1 hours).
Pediatric patients—
  Premature neonates:
    3.1 to 5.7 hours.
  Neonates (up to 1 month old):
    2.4 to 2.6 hours.
  Infants and children (1 month to 12 years):
    1.5 to 1.7 hours.
  Cystic fibrosis patients:
    1.0 to 1.3 hours.

## Time to peak serum concentration

Intramuscular—Approximately 0.6 to 1.3 hours.

## Time to peak bile concentration

Intravenous—Approximately 2.4 hours.

## Peak serum concentration

Linear kinetics—
  Adults:
    Intramuscular—1 gram: 40 to 46.5 mcg per mL.
    Intravenous injection—1 gram: Approximately 125 mcg per mL.
    Intravenous infusion—1 gram: 90 to 164 mcg per mL.
  Pediatric patients:
    Intravenous injection (over 3 to 5 minutes)—30 mg per kg of body weight (mg/kg).
    Premature neonates—Approximately 80 mcg per mL.
    Neonates and children up to 12 years of age—90 to 120 mcg per mL.

## Peak bile concentration

Approximately 43 mcg per mL following a 1-gram intravenous dose.

## Urine concentration

Intramuscular—Approximately 500 and 1200 mcg per mL 2 hours following intramuscular doses of 500 mg and 1 gram, respectively.
Intravenous—Approximately 1100, 3500, and 6600 mcg per mL 2 hours following 30-minute intravenous infusions of 500 mg, 1 gram, and 2 grams, respectively.

## Elimination

Renal—
  Approximately 60 to 75% excreted unchanged in urine within 8 hours by active tubular secretion and glomerular filtration (in approximately equal amounts); excretion essentially complete within 12 hours; inactive metabolites also excreted in urine.

Biliary/fecal—
  Excreted unchanged in feces following oral administration.
  Approximately 1.5 to 3.5% (up to 12%) excreted unchanged in feces following parenteral administration; inactive metabolites also excreted in feces.
In dialysis—
  Hemodialysis: A 4-hour period of hemodialysis reduces plasma aztreonam concentrations by 27 to 58%.
  Peritoneal dialysis: Reduces plasma aztreonam concentrations by approximately 10%.

# Precautions to Consider

## Cross-sensitivity and/or related problems

Studies in rabbits have shown negligible cross-reactivity between antiaztreonam, antibenzylpenicillin, and anticephalothin antibodies.

In studies in normal volunteers, aztreonam was shown to be only weakly immunogenic in humans. Of 41 patients with immunoglobulin E (IgE) antibodies to one or more penicillin moieties, none reacted to aztreonam. In a study of 36 patients receiving multiple doses of aztreonam over a 7-day period, there were no IgE antibody responses. Only one patient had an IgG response. In a study of 22 patients with positive skin tests to penicillin reagents, three had positive skin tests to aztreonam. Of those three, one was negative on rechallenge and one was confirmed as positive. Of the 20 patients with negative aztreonam skin tests who received aztreonam, none showed immediate hypersensitivity reactions.

Since cross-reactivity only rarely occurs between aztreonam and beta-lactam antibacterials, aztreonam may usually be given without incident to patients with ''rash-type'' beta-lactam allergy. However, patients who have had immediate hypersensitivity (e.g., anaphylactic or urticarial) reactions to beta-lactams should be closely monitored while receiving aztreonam.

## Carcinogenicity

Studies in animals have not been done.

## Mutagenicity

Studies with aztreonam in several standard in vivo and in vitro laboratory models have shown no evidence of mutagenic potential at the chromosome or gene level.

## Pregnancy/Reproduction

Fertility—Two-generation reproduction studies in rats given doses up to 20 times the maximum recommended human dose (MRHD) prior to and during gestation and lactation have not shown any evidence of impaired fertility.

Pregnancy—Aztreonam crosses the placenta and enters the fetal circulation. Adequate and well-controlled studies in humans have not been done.

Studies in rats and rabbits given daily doses up to 15 and 5 times the MRHD, respectively, have not shown that aztreonam is embryotoxic, fetotoxic, or teratogenic. Studies in rats given 15 times the MRHD during late gestation and lactation have not shown any aztreonam-induced changes.

FDA Pregnancy Category B.

## Breast-feeding

Aztreonam is excreted in breast milk in concentrations that are less than 1% of maternal serum concentrations. However, aztreonam is not absorbed from the gastrointestinal tract.

## Pediatrics

There is little information currently available on the use of aztreonam in children, especially those up to the age of 12. However, studies to date have shown aztreonam to be clinically effective in pediatric patients, and the side effects seen in children appear to be similar to those seen in adults.

## Geriatrics

Studies performed to date have not demonstrated geriatrics-specific problems that would limit the usefulness of aztreonam in the elderly. However, elderly patients are more likely to have an age-related decrease in renal function, which may require a decrease in dosage in patients receiving aztreonam.

## Laboratory value alterations

The following have been selected on the basis of their potential clinical significance (possible effect in parentheses where appropriate)—not necessarily inclusive (» = major clinical significance):

With diagnostic test results
  Coombs' (antiglobulin) tests
    (may become positive during therapy)

With physiology/laboratory test values
Alanine aminotransferase (ALT [SGPT]), serum and
Alkaline phosphatase, serum and
Aspartate aminotransferase (AST [SGOT]), serum and
Lactate dehydrogenase (LDH), serum
(values may be transiently increased during therapy)

Creatinine, serum
(concentration may be transiently increased during therapy)

Partial thromboplastin time (PTT) and
Prothrombin time (PT)
(may be prolonged during therapy)

## Medical considerations/Contraindications

The medical considerations/contraindications included here have been selected on the basis of their potential clinical significance (reasons given
in parentheses where appropriate)—not necessarily inclusive (» =
major clinical significance).

*Except under special circumstances, this medication should not be used
when the following medical problem exists:*
» Previous allergic reaction to aztreonam

*Risk-benefit should be considered when the following medical problems
exist:*
» Cirrhosis
(prolonged half-life; patients with cirrhosis may require a modest
reduction in dose [20-25%] when receiving high-dose, long-term
therapy with aztreonam)
» Renal function impairment
(it is recommended that aztreonam be administered in a reduced
dosage to patients with impaired renal function)

## Side/Adverse Effects

The following side/adverse effects have been selected on the basis of their
potential clinical significance (possible signs and symptoms in parentheses where appropriate)—not necessarily inclusive:

**Those indicating need for medical attention**
Incidence less frequent
*Hypersensitivity* (anaphylaxis; skin rash, redness, or itching); *throm-
bophlebitis* (inflammation or phlebitis at the injection site)

**Those indicating need for medical attention only if they continue
or are bothersome**
Incidence less frequent or rare
*Gastrointestinal upset* (abdominal or stomach cramps; diarrhea; nausea; vomiting)

## Overdose

For more information on the management of overdose or unintentional
ingestion, contact a **Poison Control Center** (see *Poison Control Center Listing*).

**Treatment of overdose**
Recommended treatment consists of the following:
Specific treatment—If necessary, hemodialysis to clear aztreonam from
the serum.
Supportive care—Patients in whom intentional overdose is known or sus-
pected should be referred for psychiatric consultation.

## Patient Consultation

As an aid to patient consultation, refer to *Advice for the Patient,
Aztreonam (Systemic)*.

In providing consultation, consider emphasizing the following selected
information (» = major clinical significance):

**Before receiving this medication**
» Conditions affecting use, especially:
Allergy to aztreonam or anaphylaxis to beta-lactam antibiotics
Pregnancy—Aztreonam crosses the placenta and enters the fetal
circulation
Breast-feeding—Aztreonam is excreted in breast milk
Other medical problems, especially cirrhosis or renal function
impairment

**Proper use of this medication**
» Importance of receiving medication for full course of therapy and on
regular schedule
» Proper dosing

**Side/adverse effects**
Signs of potential side effects, especially hypersensitivity or
thrombophlebitis

# General Dosing Information

Aztreonam may be administered intramuscularly or intravenously. In patients requiring single doses greater than 1 gram or in patients with
bacterial septicemia, localized parenchymal abscesses, peritonitis, or
other severe or life-threatening infections, the intravenous route is
recommended.

Aztreonam may be administered slowly over a 3- to 5-minute period either
by direct injection into a vein or by injection into the tubing of a
suitable intravenous administration set.

Aztreonam may also be administered by intermittent intravenous infusion
in 50 to 100 mL of a suitable fluid over a 20- to 60-minute period.

If aztreonam is administered via a volume-control administration set, the
final dilution should not exceed 2% (20 mg per mL).

Because of the serious nature of infections caused by *Pseudomonas aeruginosa*, the recommended dose in the treatment of such infections is
2 grams every 6 to 8 hours.

Patients with renal function impairment may need an adjustment in dosage, based on creatinine clearance. Creatinine clearance (in mL per
minute) may be calculated as follows:

Adult males: Creatinine clearance = [(140 − age) × (ideal body weight
in kg)]/[72 × serum creatinine (mg per dL)]
Adult females: Creatinine clearance = [(140 − age) × (ideal body weight
in kg)]/[72 × serum creatinine (mg per dL)] × 0.85

Creatinine clearance may also be calculated in SI units (as mL per second)
as follows:

Adult males: Creatinine clearance = [(140 − age) × (ideal body weight
in kg)]/[50 × serum creatinine (micromoles per L)]
Adult females: Creatinine clearance = [(140 − age) × (ideal body weight
in kg)]/[50 × serum creatinine (micromoles per L)] × 0.85

**For treatment of adverse effects**
Recommended treatment consists of the following:
• Discontinuation of aztreonam and institution of supportive treatment (e.g., maintenance of ventilation and administration of epinephrine, pressor amines, antihistamines, corticosteroids) if serious
hypersensitivity reactions or allergic reactions occur.

# Parenteral Dosage Forms

## AZTREONAM INJECTION

**Usual adult and adolescent dose**
Intravenous infusion over twenty to sixty minutes—
Moderately severe systemic infections: 1 to 2 grams every eight to twelve
hours.
Severe systemic or life-threatening infections: 2 grams every six to eight
hours.
Note: Urinary tract infections—Intravenous infusion over twenty to sixty
minutes, 500 mg to 1 gram every eight to twelve hours.

Adults with impaired renal function require a reduction in dose as
follows:

| Creatinine clearance (mL/min)(mL/sec) | Dose | | |
|---|---|---|---|
| | | Loading Dose | Maintenance dose (every 6-12 hours) |
| >30/0.50 | | | See *Usual adult and ado-lescent dose* |
| 10-30/0.17–0.50 | | 1–2 grams | ½ of the loading dose |
| <10/0.17 | | 500 mg–2 grams | ¼ of the loading dose; in serious or life-threatening infections, an additional ⅛ of the loading dose should be given after each hemodialysis period |

**Usual adult prescribing limits**
Up to a maximum of 8 grams daily.

**Usual pediatric dose**
Dosage has not been established.

**Strength(s) usually available**
U.S.—
1 gram in 50 mL (Rx) [*Azactam*].
2 grams in 50 mL (Rx) [*Azactam*].
Canada—
Not commercially available.

**Packaging and storage**
Do not store above −20 °C (−4 °F), unless otherwise specified by
manufacturer.

## Preparation of dosage form

Thaw container at room temperature or in a refrigerator before administration, making sure that all ice crystals have melted.

Do not use minibags in series connections. This may result in air embolism because of residual air being drawn from the primary container before administration of intravenous solution from the secondary container is complete.

## Stability

After thawing, solutions retain their potency for 48 hours at room temperature or for 14 days if refrigerated.

Once thawed, solutions should not be refrozen.

Do not use if the solution is cloudy or contains a precipitate.

## Incompatibilities

Additives or other medication should not be added to, or infused simultaneously through the same intravenous line.

## AZTREONAM FOR INJECTION USP

### Usual adult and adolescent dose

Intramuscular or intravenous

Moderately severe systemic infections: 1 to 2 grams every eight to twelve hours.

Severe systemic or life-threatening infections: 2 grams every six to eight hours.

Note: Urinary tract infections—Intramuscular or intravenous, 500 mg to 1 gram every eight to twelve hours.

Adults with impaired renal function require a reduction in dose as follows:

| Creatinine clearance (mL/min)(mL/sec) | Dose | |
| --- | --- | --- |
| | Loading Dose | Maintenance dose (every 6-12 hours) |
| >30/0.50 | See *Usual adult and adolescent dose* | |
| 10–30/0.17–0.50 | 1–2 grams | ¹/₂ of the loading dose |
| <10/0.17 | 500 mg–2 grams | ¹/₄ of the loading dose; in serious or life-threatening infections, an additional ¹/₈ of the loading dose should be given after each hemodialysis period |

### Usual adult prescribing limits

Up to a maximum of 8 grams daily.

### Usual pediatric dose

Antibacterial—

Dosage has not been established; however, the following doses have been reported in the literature:

Infants up to 7 days of age—30 mg per kg of body weight every twelve hours.

Infants 1 to 4 weeks of age—30 mg per kg of body weight every eight hours.

Infants over 4 weeks of age—30 mg per kg of body weight every six to eight hours.

Children with cystic fibrosis—50 mg per kg of body weight every six hours.

### Size(s) usually available

U.S.—

500 mg (Rx) [*Azactam* (L-arginine, 780 mg per gram)].

1 gram (Rx) [*Azactam* (L-arginine, 780 mg per gram)].

2 grams (Rx) [*Azactam* (L-arginine, 780 mg per gram)].

Canada—

Not commercially available.

### Packaging and storage

Prior to reconstitution, store below 40 °C (104 °F), preferably between 15 and 30 °C (59 and 86 °F), unless otherwise specified by manufacturer.

## Preparation of dosage form

To prepare initial dilution for intramuscular use (15-mL vial), for each gram of aztreonam add at least 3 mL of sterile water for injection, bacteriostatic water for injection (preserved with benzyl alcohol or methyl- and propylparabens), 0.9% sodium chloride injection, or bacteriostatic sodium chloride injection (preserved with benzyl alcohol or methyl- and propylparabens).

To prepare initial dilution for direct intravenous use, add 6 to 10 mL of sterile water for injection to each 15-mL vial.

To prepare initial dilution for intravenous infusion (15-mL vial), for each gram of aztreonam add at least 3 mL of sterile water for injection. The resulting solution may be further diluted in 0.9% sodium chloride injection, Ringer's injection, lactated Ringer's injection, dextrose injection (5 or 10%), dextrose and sodium chloride injection, sodium lactate injection (M/6), dextrose and lactated Ringer's injection, or other electrolyte-containing solutions (see manufacturer's package insert).

For reconstitution of piggyback infusion bottles (100-mL), add at least 50 mL of suitable diluent (see manufacturer's package insert) for each gram of aztreonam. The final concentration should not exceed 2% (20 mg per mL).

After addition of the diluent, contents of the vial should be shaken immediately and vigorously.

## Stability

Aztreonam vials are not intended for multiple-dose use. Unused solutions should be discarded.

Solutions range in color from colorless to light straw yellow, depending on the concentration and diluent.

Solutions may develop a slight pink tint on standing. This does not affect their potency.

After reconstitution for intramuscular use, solutions retain their potency for 48 hours at room temperature or for 7 days if refrigerated.

After reconstitution for intravenous use, solutions at concentrations not exceeding 2% (20 mg per mL) retain their potency for 48 hours at controlled room temperature (15 to 30 °C [59 to 86 °F]) or for 7 days if refrigerated at 2 to 8 °C (36 to 46 °F).

After reconstitution for intravenous use, solutions (except those reconstituted with sterile water for injection and sodium chloride injection) at concentrations exceeding 2% should be used promptly after reconstitution. Solutions reconstituted with sterile water for injection or sodium chloride injection retain their potency for 48 hours at controlled room temperature or for 7 days if refrigerated.

Frozen solutions (except those reconstituted with two untested diluents, 10% mannitol injection or dextrose and lactated Ringer's injection) retain their potency for up to 3 months at −20 °C (−4 °F). Frozen solutions may be thawed at controlled room temperature or by storage in a refrigerator overnight. Solutions that have been thawed and maintained at controlled room temperature or under refrigeration should be used within 24 or 72 hours, respectively. Once thawed, solutions should not be refrozen.

Admixtures of aztreonam and clindamycin phosphate, gentamicin sulfate, tobramycin sulfate, or cefazolin sodium in 0.9% sodium chloride injection or 5% dextrose injection retain their potency for 48 hours at room temperature or for 7 days if refrigerated.

Admixtures of aztreonam and ampicillin sodium in 0.9% sodium chloride injection retain their potency for 24 hours at room temperature (25 °C [77 °F]) or for 48 hours if refrigerated at 4 °C (39 °F). Admixtures containing aztreonam and ampicillin sodium in 5% dextrose injection retain their potency for 2 hours at room temperature (25 °C [77 °F]) or for 8 hours if refrigerated at 4 °C (39 °F).

Admixtures of aztreonam and cloxacillin sodium or aztreonam and vancomycin hydrochloride in peritoneal dialysis solution containing 4.25% dextrose retain their potency for 24 hours at room temperature.

## Incompatibilities

Admixtures of aztreonam and nafcillin sodium, cephradine, vancomycin, or metronidazole are incompatible.

In general, admixtures of aztreonam and other medications are not recommended. However, certain admixtures have been shown to be compatible (see *Stability*).

Revised: 02/23/93

**BACAMPICILLIN**—See *Penicillins (Systemic)*

# BACILLUS CALMETTE-GUÉRIN (BCG) LIVE    Mucosal-Local

VA CLASSIFICATION (Primary): AN900

Note:  For a listing of dosage forms and brand names by country availability, see *Dosage Forms* section(s). For a listing of brand names for the articles in this monograph, refer to the General Index.

## Category
Antineoplastic.

## Indications
Note:  Bracketed information in the *Indications* section refers to uses that are not included in U.S. product labeling.

### Accepted
Carcinoma, bladder (prophylaxis and treatment)—BCG is used intravesically for prophylaxis and treatment of primary (multifocal, high grade) and relapsed superficial transitional cell bladder carcinoma. It is used to reduce frequency of tumor recurrence after transurethral resection and to eliminate existing tumors, including [Ta and T1 tumors] and carcinoma in situ (CIS tumors) with or without associated papillary tumors. It is not indicated for treatment of papillary tumors occurring alone.

### Unaccepted
The product labeled for use only in treatment of bladder carcinoma is not intended to be used as an immunizing agent for the prevention of tuberculosis; the product labeled for use in both can be used for both. BCG is not a vaccine for the prevention of cancer.

## Pharmacology/Pharmacokinetics

### Physicochemical characteristics
Source—Is a live culture of the attenuated bacillus Calmette-Guérin strain of *Mycobacterium bovis*. Commercially available strains (which are substrains of the Pasteur Institute strain) include the Armand-Frappier, Connaught, Glaxo/Evans, and Tice substrains; of these, only the Connaught and Tice strains are approved for bladder carcinoma.

### Mechanism of action/Effect
The effect of BCG against carcinoma is not completely understood. It may be related to an inflammatory response and possibly also to an immune response.
Intravesical BCG suspension produces a granulomatous response locally and in regional lymph nodes; the inflammatory response stimulates production of macrophages that have tumoricidal effects. The presence of interleukin 2, which is a substance produced by activated helper T lymphocytes and which activates natural killer cells, has also been noted in the urine of patients who responded to BCG treatment. However, the relationship of these effects to the antineoplastic effect of BCG is unknown.

### Other actions/effects
Induces active immunity against tuberculosis by unknown mechanism; may involve stimulating the reticuloendothelial system (RES) to produce macrophages and other activated cells, which prevent multiplication of virulent *Mycobacterium tuberculosis*.
Viability and immunogenicity may vary between strains and viability varies between lots of any one strain. With intracavitary BCG, positive conversion of tuberculin (purified protein derivative [PPD]) skin test occurs in a majority of patients, usually after 3 to 12 weeks. Positive conversion of PPD skin test, when it occurs, is usually not permanent, although duration is variable and sometimes long.

## Precautions to Consider

### Tumorigenicity
Two cases of nephrogenic adenoma (adenomatous metaplasia of the bladder), which is usually benign and believed to result from chronic irritation or trauma, have been reported.

### Pregnancy/Reproduction
Pregnancy—Studies have not been done in humans.
Studies have not been done in animals.
FDA Pregnancy Category C.

### Breast-feeding
It is not known whether intravesical BCG is distributed into breast milk. However, problems in humans have not been documented.

### Pediatrics
No information is available on the relationship of age to the effects of BCG in pediatric patients. Safety and efficacy have not been established.

### Geriatrics
Studies performed to date have not demonstrated geriatrics-specific problems that would limit the usefulness of BCG as an antineoplastic in the elderly.

### Drug interactions and/or related problems
The following drug interactions and/or related problems have been selected on the basis of their potential clinical significance (possible mechanism in parentheses where appropriate)—not necessarily inclusive (» = major clinical significance):

Note:  Combinations containing any of the following medications, depending on the amount present, may also interact with this medication.

Antimicrobial therapy
(potential negative effect on actions of BCG)

» Bone marrow depressants or
» Immunosuppressants or
» Radiation
(may impair immune response to BCG. The interval between discontinuation of medications that cause immunosuppression and restoration of the patient's ability to respond to BCG depends on the intensity and type of immunosuppression-causing therapy used, the underlying disease, and other factors; estimates vary from 3 months to 1 year. Also, may increase the risk of osteomyelitis or disseminated BCG infection)

» Vaccines, killed or live virus
(concurrent administration with BCG is not recommended; it is recommended that live virus vaccines be given 6 to 8 weeks after BCG; it is recommended that killed virus vaccines be given 7 days before or 10 days after BCG)

### Laboratory value alterations
The following have been selected on the basis of their potential clinical significance (possible effect in parentheses where appropriate)—not necessarily inclusive (» = major clinical significance):

With physiology/laboratory test values
Hepatic function tests
(abnormalities have been reported rarely)

Tuberculin (purified protein derivative [PPD]) skin test
(positive conversion is produced in a majority of patients, usually after 3 to 12 weeks of intravesical BCG therapy; may complicate future interpretations of tuberculin skin test reactions in the diagnosis of suspected mycobacterial infections)

Microscopic examination of urine
(microscopic pyuria commonly seen; however, bacterial growth in urine is uncommon; returns to normal after completion of a course of BCG therapy)

### Medical considerations/Contraindications
The medical considerations/contraindications included here have been selected on the basis of their potential clinical significance (reasons given in parentheses where appropriate)—not necessarily inclusive (» = major clinical significance).

*Except under special circumstances, this medication should not be used when the following medical problems exist:*

» Fever
(BCG should not be administered until the cause has been determined; if fever is caused by infection, BCG should be withheld until the patient is afebrile and off all therapy)

» Urinary tract infection
(risk of disseminated BCG infection; increased severity of bladder irritation)

*Risk-benefit should be considered when the following medical problems exist:*

» Hematuria, gross, existing

    (risk of disseminated BCG infection; caution is necessary especially if the hematuria is induced by recent biopsy or resection, and it is recommended that intravesical BCG not be given until gross hematuria has cleared; if hematuria is from the tumor itself, BCG can still be given, but with caution because irritable bladder symptoms may be increased)

» Impaired immune response

    (decreased response to treatment; risk of osteomyelitis or disseminated BCG infection)

» Sensitivity to BCG live

Small bladder capacity

    (increased incidence and severity of local irritation; in addition, therapy with BCG may rarely cause bladder contracture, which further decreases capacity)

## Patient monitoring

The following may be especially important in patient monitoring (other tests may be warranted in some patients, depending on condition; » = major clinical significance):

» Bladder biopsy, cold cup

    (recommended at regular intervals to assess response; also recommended for any suspicious area found by cystoscopy or cytology studies)

» Cystoscopy and

» Urine cytology studies

    (recommended at regular intervals during and after treatment to assess response and confirm that the tumor is not progressing)

Hepatic function determinations

    (recommended if persistent [e.g., 101 °F for longer than 2 days] or severe [e.g., greater than 103 °F] fever or continuing malaise occurs)

Needle biopsy of prostate in males

    (recommended as indicated by presence of clinical signs of granulomatous prostatitis)

Tuberculin (PPD) skin test

    (recommended before treatment and at periodic intervals during treatment. However, although it may predict responsiveness to BCG treatment in general, this is controversial and it is unlikely to provide a prognosis for a specific individual patient, especially since positive conversion does not occur in all patients who respond to BCG therapy)

Urine cultures

    (recommended before and at periodic intervals during treatment; recommended if urinalysis or clinical symptoms suggest presence of urinary tract infection)

## Side/Adverse Effects

Note: Side/adverse effects are usually mild to moderate and transient, but may be cumulative.

The following side/adverse effects have been selected on the basis of their potential clinical significance (possible signs and symptoms in parentheses where appropriate)—not necessarily inclusive:

**Those indicating need for medical attention**

Incidence more frequent

    *Bladder infection, secondary to bladder irritation* (usually asymptomatic); *bladder irritation* (blood in urine; frequent urge to urinate; increased frequency of urination; painful urination, severe or continuing); *flu-like syndrome* (fever and chills; joint pain; nausea and vomiting; in a few patients, has progressed to a severe systemic reaction with high fever, malaise, and anorexia); *granulomatous prostatitis* (usually asymptomatic; appears as nodularity, enlargement, induration, and distortion of the prostate, which is clinically indistinguishable from prostatic carcinoma)

Note: *Bladder infection* responds rapidly to antibiotic treatment.

    *Bladder irritation* occurs in most patients, but is usually transient; may be severe in some patients. May predict antitumor response. Symptoms usually begin within 2 to 4 hours after a dose and last 24 to 72 hours. Granulomatous inflammation is seen on the histological examination; lesions that may be confused with tumors appear commonly within 4 weeks after BCG treatment; inflammation usually disappears within about 4 to 6 months after treatment.

    Symptoms of the *flu-like syndrome* usually begin within 4 hours after a dose and last 24 to 72 hours.

Incidence rare

    *Allergic reaction or erythema nodosum* (skin rash); *BCG infection, disseminated, with lung or liver involvement* (fever; cough); *bladder contracture; hepatic function impairment* (asymptomatic); *hypotension; leukopenia* (asymptomatic)

Note: Symptoms of *disseminated BCG infection* may be difficult to distinguish from those of gram negative sepsis or severe hypersensitivity reactions, or of progressing malignancy. Disseminated infection, with associated fever, may occur as late as 6 months or more after BCG therapy and may persist for 1 to 3 weeks after antituberculosis therapy is begun. It is usually diagnosed clinically based on the presence of fever (over 39 °C [103 °F] or persistently over 38 °C [101 °F] over 2 days) and chills, especially when associated with malaise and other systemic symptoms, negative blood and urine cultures, chest x-ray or computed tomography (CT) to exclude other pulmonary diseases, and hepatic function tests. Deaths have been reported.

    *Hepatic function impairment* is usually mild and transient; abnormalities peak by 20 days and may persist months after BCG administration.

**Those indicating need for medical attention only if they continue or are bothersome**

Incidence more frequent

    *Burning, slight, during first void after treatment*

**Those indicating the need for medical attention if they occur after medication is discontinued**

    *BCG infection, disseminated, with lung or liver involvement* (fever; cough)

## Patient Consultation

As an aid to patient consultation, refer to *Advice for the Patient, Bacillus Calmette-Guérin (BCG) Live (Mucosal-Local)*.

In providing consultation, consider emphasizing the following selected information (» = major clinical significance):

**Before using this medication**

» Conditions affecting use, especially:

    Sensitivity to BCG

    Other medications, especially bone marrow depressants or immunosuppressants

    Other medical problems, especially fever, gross hematuria, impaired immune response, or urinary tract infection

**Proper use of this medication**

Emptying bladder before instillation of each dose

» Following physician's instructions for holding solution in bladder; holding in bladder for 2 hours; telling physician if unable to retain solution for prescribed time; physician may recommend lying for 15 minutes each in prone and supine positions, and on each side, during first hour; sitting down while voiding

» Importance of ample fluid intake for several hours after instillation

    Bacteria will be present in urine; treating all urine voided within 6 hours after each instillation with an equal volume of 5% hypochlorite solution (undiluted household bleach; usually 6 to 8 ounces) and allowing to stand for 15 minutes before flushing

» Proper dosing

**Precautions while using this medication**

Avoiding persons with active tuberculosis for 6 to 12 weeks after treatment; telling physician about any exposure to active tuberculosis

Avoiding immunizations unless approved by physician

**Side/adverse effects**

Signs of potential side effects, especially bladder infection, bladder irritation, flu-like syndrome, allergic reaction, erythema nodosum, skin abscess, and disseminated BCG infection

## General Dosing Information

Patients receiving intravesical BCG should be under the supervision of a physician experienced in immunotherapy.

Prior to BCG administration, the bladder is emptied either by voiding or drainage through a urethral catheter inserted into the bladder under aseptic conditions. BCG is then instilled into the bladder by gravity flow via the catheter; the plunger should not be depressed to force the flow.

It is recommended that BCG instillation and equipment and materials used in preparation of the instillation be treated as biohazardous waste.

BCG should not be injected intravenously, subcutaneously, or intramuscularly.

Care and aseptic technique are necessary during administration of intravesical BCG therapy so as not to introduce contaminants into the urinary tract or to unduly traumatize the urinary mucosa.

If the physician believes that the bladder catheterization has been traumatic (e.g., associated with bleeding or possible false passage), instillation of BCG should be delayed by at least 1 week. However, beginning from the delayed dose, subsequent doses should be administered according to the original schedule (i.e., no doses should be omitted).

It is recommended that BCG therapy not be started until 7 to 14 days after bladder tumor resection or biopsy because fatalities from disseminated BCG infection have been reported with use of BCG after traumatic catheterization.

If development of systemic BCG infection is suspected, it is recommended that BCG be withheld and fast-acting antituberculosis therapy initiated.

Patients who do not respond after two 6-week courses of BCG therapy are unlikely to respond, and consideration of alternative therapy is recommended.

Most severe adverse effects can be prevented or reduced in severity with prophylactic isoniazid treatment given for 3 days beginning the morning of BCG treatment. Some clinicians also recommend use of antihistamines and nonsteroidal anti-inflammatory agents.

### Safety considerations for handling this medication

There is concern that personnel involved in preparation and administration of intravesical BCG may be at some risk because of the infectious potential of this agent, although the actual risk is unknown. USP advisory panels recommend cautious handling both in preparation and disposal of BCG for intravesical use. Precautions that have been suggested include:

• Use of a biological containment cabinet during reconstitution and dilution of parenteral medications and wearing of disposable surgical gloves and masks.

• Use of proper technique to prevent contamination of the medication, work area, and operator during transfer between containers (including proper training of personnel in this technique).

• Cautious and proper disposal of needles, syringes, vials, ampuls, and unused medication.

A number of medical centers have developed detailed guidelines for handling of antineoplastic and similar agents.

### For treatment of adverse effects

Most adverse effects respond to a reduction in BCG dose or temporary interruption of therapy; however, in some patients withdrawal of BCG therapy may be necessary.

Mild bladder irritation can usually be treated symptomatically with phenazopyridine hydrochloride and antispasmodics such as propantheline bromide or oxybutynin.

Recommended treatment of moderate to severe bladder irritation and flu-like syndrome may consist of the following:
• Isoniazid.
• Antihistamines, such as diphenhydramine hydrochloride.
• Nonsteroidal anti-inflammatory agents; parenteral narcotic analgesics may be necessary for severe bladder irritation.

Recommended treatment of disseminated BCG infection with liver and lung involvement consists of the following:
• Triple-drug antituberculosis therapy or
• A fast-acting antituberculosis medication such as cycloserine.

No specific treatment of granulomatous prostatitis secondary to BCG therapy is required.

## Topical Dosage Forms

### BCG LIVE (CONNAUGHT STRAIN)

**Usual adult dose**
Bladder carcinoma—
　Intracavitary, 3 vials (81 mg), reconstituted and then diluted with 50 mL of sterile, preservative-free 0.9% sodium chloride solution, to a final volume of 53 mL (less in patients with reduced bladder capacity), instilled into the empty bladder and retained for one to two hours (depending on irritative symptoms and the patient's ability to retain the solution). The procedure is repeated once a week for six weeks, followed by one treatment given at three, six, twelve, eighteen, and twenty-four months following the initial treatment or according to response.

Note: During the first hour after instillation, the patient may lie for 15 minutes in the prone position, supine position, and on each side, then may be up for the second hour the suspension is retained.
　The patient voids in a seated position.

**Usual pediatric dose**
Safety and efficacy have not been established.

### Size(s) usually available
U.S.—
　27 mg (dry weight) or $3.4 \pm 3.0 \times 10^8$ colony-forming units (CFU) per vial (3 vials per package) (Rx) [*TheraCys* (monosodium glutamate 5% w/v plus diluent)].
Canada—
　Approximately $3.0 \times 10^8$ colony-forming units (CFU) per vial (3 vials per package) (Rx) [*ImmuCyst* (monosodium glutamate 5% w/v plus diluent)].

### Packaging and storage
Store between 2 and 8 °C (36 and 46 °F). Protect from light.

### Preparation of dosage form
BCG live (Connaught strain) is reconstituted by adding 1.0 mL of diluent provided by manufacturer to the vial. The vial is then shaken gently until a fine, even suspension results. The suspension is then diluted in a suitable quantity of sterile, preservative-free 0.9% sodium chloride for administration.

Note: Aseptic technique must be used for reconstitution and dilution.
　　　The product should not be handled by persons with a known immunologic deficiency.

### Stability
Reconstituted suspension should be used immediately; otherwise, it should be refrigerated until use and should be discarded after 2 hours.

### Note
Commercially available BCG strains are not interchangeable. *One product should not be substituted for the other.* If patients are to be transferred from one to another, appropriate changes in dosage may be necessary.

### Additional information
After usage, all equipment and materials used for instillation of BCG into the bladder should be placed immediately into plastic bags labeled as infectious waste and disposed of properly as biohazardous waste.

Any unused portion of reconstituted BCG, and urine voided for 6 hours after instillation, should be disinfected with an equal volume of 5% hypochlorite solution (undiluted household bleach) and allowed to stand for 15 minutes before being flushed.

## BCG VACCINE (TICE STRAIN) USP

### Usual adult dose
Bladder carcinoma—
　Intracavitary, 1 vial ($1-8 \times 10^8$ colony-forming units [CFU]), reconstituted and then diluted to a total volume of 50 mL with sterile, preservative-free 0.9% sodium chloride injection (less in patients with reduced bladder capacity), instilled into the empty bladder and retained for one to two hours (depending on irritative symptoms and the patient's ability to retain the solution). The procedure is repeated once a week for six weeks; the schedule may be repeated once if circumstances warrant. This is followed by treatment at approximately monthly intervals for at least six to twelve months or according to response.

Note: During the first hour after instillation, the patient may lie for 15 minutes in the prone position, supine position, and on each side, then may be up for the second hour the suspension is retained.
　　　The patient voids in a seated position.

### Usual pediatric dose
Safety and efficacy have not been established.

### Size(s) usually available
U.S.—
　$1-8 \times 10^8$ CFU or approximately 50 mg (wet weight) per vial, (Rx) [*TICE BCG* (lactose)].
Canada—
　Not commercially available.

### Packaging and storage
Store between 2 and 8 °C (36 and 46 °F). Protect from light.

### Preparation of dosage form
BCG Vaccine USP (Tice Strain) is reconstituted by adding 1 mL of sterile, preservative-free 0.9% sodium chloride injection to ampul, drawing the mixture back into the syringe and expelling it into the ampul three times to mix it thoroughly (minimizes clumping of mycobacteria). The suspension is then diluted in a suitable quantity of sterile, preservative-free 0.9% sodium chloride injection for administration.

Note: Aseptic technique must be used for reconstitution and dilution.
　　　The product should not be handled by persons with a known immunologic deficiency.

### Stability
Reconstituted suspension should be used immediately and any unused portion discarded after 2 hours.

### Additional information

After usage, all equipment and materials used for instillation of BCG into the bladder should be placed immediately into plastic bags labeled as infectious waste and disposed of properly as biohazardous waste.

Any unused portion of reconstituted BCG, and urine voided for 6 hours after instillation, should be disinfected with an equal volume of 5% hypochlorite solution (undiluted household bleach) and allowed to stand for 15 minutes before being flushed.

## Selected Bibliography

Diagnostic and Therapeutic Technology Assessment (DATTA). BCG immunotherapy in bladder cancer: a reassessment. JAMA 1988 Apr 8; 259: 2153–5.

Debruyne FMJ, Denis L, van der Meijden APM (eds.). EORTC Genitourinary Group Monograph 6. BCG in superficial bladder cancer. Proceedings of an EORTC Genitourinary Group sponsored meeting held at Erenstein Castle, Kerkrade, The Netherlands, on September 7–8, 1988. New York: Alan R. Liss, Inc; 1989.

Revised: 07/11/94

---

# BACILLUS CALMETTE-GUÉRIN (BCG) LIVE    Systemic

This monograph is specific for the Bacillus Calmette-Guérin (BCG) live vaccine, intended for immunization of uninfected (tuberculin negative) persons to induce tuberculin sensitivity as a protection against tuberculosis infection. Only BCG live vaccine labeled for use against tuberculosis infection should be used for immunization, or where labeled for use both against tuberculosis infection and bladder cancer (for bladder cancer see *Bacillus Calmette-Guérin (BCG) Live, Mucosal-Local*). The efficacy of the BCG vaccines currently available has not been demonstrated directly and can only be inferred.

VA CLASSIFICATION (Primary): IM100

Note: For a listing of dosage forms and brand names by country availability, see *Dosage Forms* section(s). For a listing of brand names for the articles in this monograph, refer to the General Index.

## Category

Immunizing agent (active).

## Indications

### Accepted

Tuberculosis (prophylaxis)—BCG live vaccine is recommended for protection against tuberculosis in the following persons if tuberculin skin test (purified protein derivative [PPD]) result is negative.

• Infants and children who
—Are at high risk of intimate and prolonged exposure to persistently untreated or ineffectively treated patients with infectious pulmonary tuberculosis and who cannot be removed from the source of exposure, and cannot be placed on long-term preventive therapy;
—Are continuously exposed to persons with tuberculosis who have bacilli resistant to isoniazid and rifampin;
—Are in groups in which the rate of new infections exceeds 1% per year and for whom the usual surveillance and treatment programs have been attempted but are not operatively feasible.

• Household contacts of untreated or insufficiently treated tuberculosis patients, especially patients with a positive sputum culture, when the contacts cannot be effectively shielded from prolonged exposure to the patients.

Selective vaccination is indicated for international travelers with a negative or weakly positive PPD who may be in a high-risk environment for prolonged periods without access to tuberculin testing surveillance.

Health care workers who are likely to be exposed continuously to multidrug-resistant tuberculosis may benefit from vaccination with BCG live.

### Unaccepted

Routine BCG vaccination is no longer recommended in the U.S. since the risk of infection is very low. Also, routine vaccination of health care workers repeatedly exposed to tuberculosis infection is not recommended; tuberculin testing surveillance and prophylactic isoniazid are preferable.

BCG live vaccine labeled for use only as an immunizing agent for the prevention of tuberculosis is not intended for use in the treatment of bladder carcinoma. BCG live vaccine labeled for use against tuberculosis infection and bladder cancer can be used for both. BCG vaccine has no value in the treatment of tuberculosis disease.

## Pharmacology/Pharmacokinetics

### Physicochemical characteristics

Source—A live culture of attenuated organisms of bacillus Calmette-Guérin (BCG) strain of *Mycobacterium bovis*. The original attenuated strain was distributed by Calmette and Guérin widely throughout the world for preparation of BCG vaccine. Until the development of lyophilization techniques, by which the seed culture is preserved currently, the strain was continued by repeated subculturing. This has resulted in the appearance of a number of seed strains with differing characteristics in various countries.

In the U.S., approved BCG live vaccine is prepared from an acceptable seed lot shown to produce vaccines that meet all the prescribed requirements for the product and that have been evaluated in clinical trials for their ability to induce tuberculin sensitivity. No data are available concerning the clinical efficacy of this strain.

The efficacy of any of the currently available BCG vaccines has not been demonstrated directly and can only be inferred.

### Mechanism of action/Effect

BCG live vaccine induces cell-mediated immunity against tuberculosis. However, its mechanism of action is unknown, and it is unclear whether BCG induces antitubercular antibodies.

### Other actions/effects

BCG live vaccine induces antibodies that bind to *Mycobacterium leprae* and may be effective in providing protection against leprosy.

### Protective effect

BCG live vaccination induces tuberculin sensitivity in more than 90% of vaccinated individuals. The protection afforded by BCG live vaccination has been reported from different field trials ranging from 0 to 80%, 50% in meta-analysis. However, there is poor correlation between tuberculin skin test conversion rates or size of induration and protective immunity. Protection, while prolonged, has not been judged to be permanent. In some clinical trials, protection has been negligible. The level of protection against meningitis or miliary tuberculosis in children has been found to be 64 to 86% in clinical trials and 75 to 83% in case control studies.

## Precautions to Consider

### Pregnancy/Reproduction

Fertility—Studies have not been done.

Pregnancy—Studies have not been done in humans. It is not known whether BCG vaccine can cause harm to the fetus when administered to a pregnant woman. BCG vaccine should be given to a pregnant woman or a woman of childbearing age only if the potential benefits outweigh the possible risks.

Studies have not been done in animals.

FDA Pregnancy Category C.

### Breast-feeding

It is not known whether BCG vaccine is distributed into breast milk. However, problems in humans have not been documented.

### Pediatrics

Infants less than 1 month of age should be given one-half of the usual dose. If a vaccinated infant remains tuberculin negative and the vaccine is still indicated, the vaccination should be repeated at full dose after the infant reaches 1 year of age. The World Health Organization (WHO) does not recommend tuberculin skin testing prior to BCG vaccination for infants and children, who are the largest group of individuals receiving BCG in the world. The WHO has recommended that, in populations where the risk of tuberculosis is high, human immunodeficiency virus (HIV)-infected children who are asymptomatic should receive BCG vaccine at birth or as soon as possible thereafter. However, in populations where the incidence of tuberculosis is low, the risk of disseminated BCG infection outweighs the potential benefit from BCG live vaccination. For unvaccinated infants, the Expanded Programme on Immunization (EPI) at WHO recommends simultaneous administration of BCG, measles, DTP, and polio vaccines. EPI, however, does not recommend mixing different vaccines in one syringe, and if vaccines cannot be given on the same day, then live vaccines should be separated by at least 4 weeks. These recommendations of the WHO are based on the fact that the separate administration of live vaccines is not practical or feasible in many developing countries where BCG usage is greatest.

### Geriatrics
Appropriate studies on the relationship of age to the effects of BCG vaccine have not been performed in the geriatric population. However, no geriatrics-specific problems have been documented to date.

### Drug interactions and/or related problems
The following drug interactions and/or related problems have been selected on the basis of their potential clinical significance (possible mechanism in parentheses where appropriate)—not necessarily inclusive (» = major clinical significance):

Note: Combinations containing any of the following medications, depending on the amount present, may also interact with this medication.

» Antitubercular agents
(antitubercular agents, such as isoniazid, rifampin, and streptomycin, inhibit multiplication of BCG; therefore, BCG vaccine may not be effective if administered during treatment with these medications)

» Corticosteroids
(possibility of the vaccine establishing a systemic infection)

» Immunosuppressant agents
(immunosuppressant agents may interfere with the development of the immune response and should be used only under medical supervision)

» Vaccines, killed or live virus
(concurrent administration with BCG is not recommended; it is recommended that live virus vaccines be given 6 to 8 weeks after BCG; and that killed virus vaccines be given 7 days before or 10 days after BCG)

### Laboratory value alterations
The following have been selected on the basis of their potential clinical significance (possible effect in parentheses where appropriate)—not necessarily inclusive (» = major clinical significance):

With diagnostic test results
Tuberculin, purified protein derivative (PPD)
(a positive reaction is produced in most patients, usually 6 to 12 weeks after BCG vaccination; however, administration of a tuberculin test a few years after BCG vaccination may result in either positive or negative reaction)

### Medical considerations/Contraindications
The medical considerations/contraindications included here have been selected on the basis of their potential clinical significance (reasons given in parentheses where appropriate)—not necessarily inclusive (» = major clinical significance).

*Except under special circumstances, this medication should not be used when the following medical problems exist:*

» Fever
(BCG should not be administered until the cause of the fever has been determined; if the fever is caused by infection, BCG should be withheld until the patient is afebrile and off all therapy)

» Impaired immune response, including that associated with HIV infection
(BCG vaccine is less effective in patients with decreased natural immunity; in addition, the risk of disseminated BCG infection may be increased)

*Risk-benefit should be considered when the following medical problems exist:*

Extensive skin infections
Sensitivity to BCG live or any of its component substances

### Patient monitoring
The following may be especially important in patient monitoring (other tests may be warranted in some patients, depending on condition; » = major clinical significance):

Tuberculin, PPD skin test
(it is usually impossible to distinguish between tuberculin sensitivity caused by *M. tuberculosis* infection and tuberculin sensitivity resulting from the vaccine; therefore, caution should be exercised in interpreting tuberculin skin test reactions)

## Side/Adverse Effects

Note: The initial skin lesions, which are small red papules, appear in 10 to 14 days and reach a maximum diameter of 3 mm each after 4 to 6 weeks, which may scale and slowly subside. If not an abscess forms, which usually softens and tends to open spontaneously. The abscess heals within a few weeks, and, in such instances, a scar may form. The intensity and duration of the local reaction depend on the depth of penetration achieved in administration and the individual variation in tissue reaction.

The following side/adverse effects have been selected on the basis of their potential clinical significance (possible signs and symptoms in parentheses where appropriate)—not necessarily inclusive:

**Those indicating need for medical attention**
Incidence more frequent
*Abscesses* (accumulation of pus); *dermatologic reactions* (peeling or scaling of the skin); *granulomas* (aggregation of inflammatory cells); *lymphadenitis* (inflammation of 1 or more lymph nodes); *ulceration at site of injection* (sores at place of injection)

Incidence rare
*Allergic reaction or erythema nodosum* (skin rash); *BCG infection, disseminated* (fever; cough); *osteomyelitis* (increase in bone pain)

Note: Symptoms of disseminated BCG infection may be difficult to distinguish from those of gram-negative sepsis or severe hypersensitivity reactions. Disseminated BCG infection is usually diagnosed based on the presence of fever and chills. Disseminated infection following BCG administration has occurred in individuals with impaired immune responses, especially children. It has also occurred following administration of BCG vaccine in patients with acquired immune deficiency syndrome (AIDS) and symptomatic HIV infection, and, rarely, in patients with asymptomatic HIV infection. If disseminated BCG infection is suspected in an individual who has received BCG live, appropriate antitubercular therapy should be initiated.

## Patient Consultation

As an aid to patient consultation, refer to *Advice for the Patient, Bacillus Calmette-Guérin (BCG) Live (Systemic)*.

In providing consultation, consider emphasizing the following selected information (» = major clinical significance):

**Before receiving this vaccine**
» Conditions affecting use, especially:
Sensitivity to BCG live
Other medications, especially antitubercular agents, corticosteroids, immunosuppressant agents, or killed or live virus vaccines
Other medical problems, especially fever, or impaired immune response, including symptomatic HIV infection

**Proper use of this vaccine**
» Importance of telling the patient that the vaccine contains live organisms
» Proper dosing

**Side/adverse effects**
Signs of potential side effects, especially abscesses, allergic reaction or erythema nodosum, dermatologic reactions, disseminated BCG infection, granulomas, lymphadenitis, oseteomyelitis, and ulceration at site of injection.

## General Dosing Information

The potency of BCG vaccines varies markedly and is related to several factors. These factors include the intrinsic immunogenicity of the particular strain, as well as other properties conferred by the method of preparation of the vaccine. In each country, the use of a particular vaccine depends on what is permitted by the national control authority and is based on the results of controlled field trials, which may not have included the particular national vaccine. The results have shown considerable variations, depending on the particular vaccines included, and may also be related to the immunity status of the subject population.

BCG live vaccine for immunization against tuberculosis should be administered according to the manufacturer's instructions.

Before the vaccine is administered, the risks and benefits of the vaccination should be fully explained to the patient, parent, or guardian.

The patient should be advised that the vaccine contains live organisms.

BCG live vaccine should be used with caution in individuals with asymptomatic HIV infection and in individuals known to be at high risk for HIV infection.

BCG live vaccine should be administered only to individuals with a negative tuberculin skin test. The tuberculin skin test (preferably done by Mantoux method) should be performed within 6 weeks prior to administration of BCG live vaccine. In persons highly sensitive to tuberculosis antigens, severe reactions may occur. However, the WHO does not recommend tuberculin skin testing prior to BCG vaccination for infants and children, who are the largest group of individuals receiving BCG in the world.

### For BCG vaccine (Tice strain)

BCG vaccine (Tice strain) is administered percutaneously, using a sterile multiple-puncture disk. The multiple-puncture disk is a thin wafer-like stainless steel plate from which 36 points protrude. The disk is held by magnet type holder. In this method of administration a drop of vaccine is placed on the patient's arm and spread with the wide edge of the disk. The disk is placed gently over the vaccine and the magnet is centered. The arm is grasped firmly from underneath, tensing the skin appreciably. Downward pressure is applied on the magnet so the points of the disk are well buried in the skin. With pressure still exerted, the disk is rocked forward and backward and from side to side several times. Pressure underneath the arm is then released and the magnet is slid off the disk. In a successful procedure, the points of the disk remain in the skin. If the points are on top of the skin, the procedure must be repeated. After a successful puncture, the disk is removed and the vaccine is spread evenly over the puncture area with the wide edge of the disk. Each disk should be used only once and discarded after autoclaving. The magnet should be sterilized after each individual vaccination.

### For BCG vaccine (Connaught strain)

BCG vaccine (Connaught strain) is administered intracutaneously into the outer surface of the upper arm. Repeat vaccination is advisable for individuals remaining tuberculin negative to the Mantoux test more than 3 months after the initial vaccination.

### For BCG vaccine (Montreal strain)

BCG vaccine (Montreal strain) is administered intradermally into the deltoid region of the arm or the upper external part of the thigh. Any unused portion of BCG vaccine and all material used for reconstituting the vaccine must be sterilized prior to disposal.

### For treatment of adverse effects

Recommended treatment consists of the following:
- Triple-drug antituberculosis therapy or
- Appropriate 3- or 4-drug antitubercular therapy.

## Parenteral Dosage Forms

### BCG VACCINE (TICE STRAIN) USP

**Usual adult and adolescent dose**
Tuberculosis (prophylaxis)—
    Percutaneous, 0.02 to 0.03 mL of the reconstituted vaccine.

**Usual pediatric dose**
See *Usual adult and adolescent dose*.

Note: If BCG live is indicated in neonates younger than 1 month of age, the dosage should be decreased by 50%. If indications persist and the tuberculin skin test is negative, a full dose of BCG live should be given after 1 year of age.

**Size(s) usually available**
U.S.—
    1 to 8 × 10⁸ CFU, or approximately 50 mg (wet weight) per vial (Rx) [*TICE BCG*].
Canada—
    Not commercially available.

**Packaging and storage**
Store between 2 and 8 °C (35.6 and 46.4 °F). Protect from light.

**Preparation of dosage form**
Reconstituted by adding 1 mL (2 mL for neonates younger than 1 month of age) of sterile water for injection should be added to the vial using

a sterile syringe. The mixture should then be drawn back into the syringe, and expelled again into the vial 3 times to mix it thoroughly.

### BCG VACCINE ( (CONNAUGHT STRAIN))

**Usual adult and adolescent dose**
Tuberculosis (prophylaxis)—
    Intracutaneous, 0.1 mL of the reconstituted vaccine.

**Usual pediatric dose**
Tuberculosis (prophylaxis)—
    Children 1 year of age and over: See *Usual adult and adolescent dose*.
    Children up to 1 year of age: Intracutaneous, 0.05 mL of the reconstituted vaccine.

**Size(s) usually available**
U.S.—
    Not commercially available.
Canada—
    Multi-dose vial (Rx) [GENERIC].

**Packaging and storage**
Store between 2 and 8 °C (35.6 and 46.4 °F). Protect from light.

**Stability**
Reconstituted vaccine should be used immediately and any that is unused by the end of the day should be destroyed. The reconstituted vaccine should be stored at 4 °C during the day of reconstitution.

### BCG VACCINE ( (MONTREAL STRAIN))

**Usual adult and adolescent dose**
Tuberculosis (prophylaxis)—
    Intradermal, 0.1 mL (0.075 mg of BCG) of the reconstituted vaccine.

**Usual pediatric dose**
Tuberculosis (prophylaxis)—
    Children 2 years of age and over: See *Usual adult and adolescent dose*.
    Children up to 2 years of age: Intradermal, 0.1 mL (0.0375 mg of BCG) of the reconstituted vaccine.

**Size(s) usually available**
U.S.—
    Not commercially available.
Canada—
    0.75 mg of freeze-dried vaccine per ampule (Rx) [GENERIC].

**Packaging and storage**
Store between 2 and 8 °C (35.6 and 46.4 °F). Protect from light.

**Preparation of dosage form**
1 mL (2 mL for children under 2 years of age) of the diluent supplied with the vaccine is added to the ampule via a sterile syringe. The suspension is then drawn into the syringe, and expelled again into the ampule, 2 times to ensure homogenicity. The ampule should not be shaken, to avoid frothing of the solution. The reconstituted solution should be allowed to stand for one minute before use.

## Selected Bibliography

Colditz GA, Brewer TF, Berkey CS, Wilson ME, Burdick E, Fineberg HV, et al. Efficacy of BCG vaccine in the prevention of tuberculosis. Meta-analysis of the published literature. JAMA 1994; 271 (9): 698-702.

Centers for Disease Control. Use of BCG vaccines in the control of tuberculosis: a joint statement by the ACIP and the Advisory Committee for Elimination of Tuberculosis. MMWR. Morb Mortal Wkly Rep 1988; 37 (43): 663-75.

Developed: 07/20/95

## BACITRACIN-CONTAINING COMBINATIONS—

Neomycin, Polymyxin B, and Bacitracin (Ophthalmic)
Neomycin, Polymyxin B, and Bacitracin (Topical)

# BACLOFEN Systemic

VA CLASSIFICATION (Primary/Secondary): MS200/CN103

Note: For a listing of dosage forms and brand names by country availability, see *Dosage Forms* section(s). For a listing of brand names for the articles in this monograph, refer to the General Index.

## Category

Antispastic analgesic (in trigeminal neuralgia).

## Indications

Note: Bracketed information in the *Indications* section refers to uses that are not included in U.S. product labeling.

### Accepted

Spasticity (treatment)—Baclofen is indicated to relieve the signs and symptoms of spasticity caused by multiple sclerosis, spinal cord diseases, or spinal cord injury. It is especially useful in relieving flexor spasms and concomitant pain, clonus, and muscular rigidity. Baclofen may also improve bowel and bladder function in some patients with spinal lesions; however, it may not improve spastic stiff gait or manual dexterity.

[Neuralgia, trigeminal (treatment)][1]—Baclofen is used to reduce the number and severity of attacks of trigeminal neuralgia in patients who are not able to tolerate, or who have become refractory to the effects of, carbamazepine. In some patients, baclofen may provide additional benefit when used concurrently with carbamazepine.

### Unaccepted

Baclofen should not be used in patients who require spasticity to sustain upright posture or balance in locomotion, or to obtain increased function.

Baclofen may not be effective, and is not recommended, in the treatment of patients with cerebrovascular accident, parkinsonism, cerebral palsy, or trauma-induced cerebral lesions.

Baclofen is not indicated in the treatment of skeletal muscle spasm caused by rheumatic disorders.

[1]Not included in Canadian product labeling.

## Pharmacology/Pharmacokinetics

### Physicochemical characteristics
Molecular weight—213.66.

### Mechanism of action/Effect
The precise mechanism of action of baclofen has not been fully determined. It acts mainly at the spinal cord level to inhibit the transmission of both monosynaptic and polysynaptic reflexes, possibly by hyperpolarization of primary afferent fiber terminals resulting in antagonism of the release of putative excitatory transmitters (i.e., glutamic and aspartic acids). Actions at supraspinal sites may also be involved.

### Other actions/effects
Baclofen has general central nervous system (CNS)–depressant actions.

### Absorption
Rapid and extensive but subject to interpatient variation. Also, the rate and extent of absorption may decrease with increasing doses.

### Protein binding
Low.

### Biotransformation
Hepatic; only about 15% of a dose is metabolized.

### Half-life
2.5 to 4 hours.

### Onset of action
Highly variable; may range from hours to weeks.

### Time to peak concentration
2 to 3 hours.

### Peak serum concentration
500 to 600 nanograms per mL (ng/mL) (2.34 to 2.81 micromoles/L) following a 40-mg single dose; concentration remains above 200 ng/mL (0.94 micromoles/L) for 8 hours.

### Therapeutic serum concentration
80 to 400 ng/mL (0.37 to 1.87 micromoles/L).

### Elimination
Renal; 70 to 85% of a dose is excreted unchanged within 24 hours. Small amounts may also be excreted via the feces. About 40% of a dose is usually excreted within 6 hours, and excretion is usually complete within 3 days; however, with chronic use the rate of excretion is subject to interpatient variation.

## Precautions to Consider

### Pregnancy/Reproduction
Pregnancy—Studies have not been done in humans.

Some studies in rats have shown that baclofen increases the incidence of omphaloceles (ventral hernias) and incomplete sternebral ossification in the fetus when given in doses approximately 13 times the maximum recommended human dose (MRHD). However, these abnormalities did not occur in studies using mice or rabbits. Also, studies in rabbits have shown that baclofen causes an increased incidence of unossified phalangeal nuclei of forelimbs and hindlimbs in the fetus when given in doses approximately 7 times the MRHD. In addition, some studies in mice have shown that baclofen causes a reduction in fetal birth weight with consequent delays in skeletal ossification when given in doses 17 times or 34 times the MHRD.

### Breast-feeding
Baclofen is distributed into breast milk. However, problems in humans have not been documented.

### Pediatrics
No information is available on the relationship of age to the effects of baclofen in pediatric patients. Safety and efficacy in children up to 12 years of age have not been established.

### Geriatrics
Geriatric patients may be especially at risk for the development of CNS toxicity, leading to hallucinations, confusion or mental depression, other psychiatric disturbances, or incapacitating sedation, during baclofen therapy. Also, elderly patients are more likely to have age-related renal function impairment, which may require a reduction of dosage in patients receiving baclofen.

### Drug interactions and/or related problems
The following drug interactions and/or related problems have been selected on the basis of their potential clinical significance (possible mechanism in parentheses where appropriate)—not necessarily inclusive (» = major clinical significance):

Note: Combinations containing any of the following medications, depending on the amount present, may also interact with this medication.

Antidepressants, tricyclic
(concurrent use with baclofen may result in pronounced muscle hypotonia; caution is recommended)

Antidiabetic agents, oral or
Insulin
(baclofen may increase blood glucose concentrations; dosage adjustments of these medications and/or of baclofen may be necessary during and after concurrent therapy)

Antihypertensives or
Other hypotension-producing medications
(concurrent use with baclofen may increase the risk of hypotension; dosage adjustment of the antihypertensive agent may be needed)

» CNS depression–producing medications, other (See *Appendix II*) or
Monoamine oxidase (MAO) inhibitors, including furazolidone, procarbazine, and selegiline
(concurrent use may result in increased CNS-depressant and hypotensive effects; caution is recommended and dosage of one or both agents should be reduced)

### Laboratory value alterations
The following have been selected on the basis of their potential clinical significance (possible effect in parentheses where appropriate)—not necessarily inclusive (» = major clinical significance):

With physiology/laboratory test values
Alanine aminotransferase (ALT [SGPT]) and
Alkaline phosphatase and
Aspartate aminotransferase (AST [SGOT])
(values may be increased)

Glucose, blood
(concentration may be increased)

### Medical considerations/Contraindications
The medical considerations/contraindications included here have been selected on the basis of their potential clinical significance (reasons given

in parentheses where appropriate)—not necessarily inclusive (» = major clinical significance).

*Risk-benefit should be considered when the following medical problems exist:*

Cerebral lesions or
Cerebrovascular accident
(increased risk of CNS, respiratory, or cardiovascular depression; ataxia; and psychiatric disturbances such as hallucinations, euphoria, and mental excitation, confusion, or depression)

Diabetes mellitus
(baclofen may increase blood glucose concentrations)

Epilepsy
(baclofen may cause deterioration of seizure control, electroencephalographic [EEG] changes)

Psychiatric disorders, pre-existing
(increased risk of baclofen-induced psychiatric disturbances)

Renal function impairment
(baclofen may accumulate; reduction in dosage may be required)

Sensitivity to baclofen

Caution is also required in geriatric patients, who may be especially susceptible to baclofen-induced CNS toxicity and who are more likely than younger adults to have renal function impairment.

**Patient monitoring**

The following may be especially important in patient monitoring (other tests may be warranted in some patients, depending on condition; » = major clinical significance):

Electroencephalogram (EEG) and clinical state determinations
(increased or periodic monitoring recommended for epileptic patients because baclofen may cause deterioration of seizure control and EEG changes in these patients)

## Side/Adverse Effects

Note: Chronic administration of baclofen to female rats has caused a dose-related increase in the incidence of ovarian cysts and in enlarged and/or hemorrhagic adrenal glands. The clinical relevance of these findings to humans is not known.

Many of the CNS, visual, and genitourinary side effects listed below may be symptoms associated with the underlying spastic disease rather than baclofen-induced.

The following side/adverse effects have been selected on the basis of their potential clinical significance (possible signs and symptoms in parentheses where appropriate)—not necessarily inclusive:

**Those indicating need for medical attention**
Incidence rare
*Bloody or dark urine; chest pain; CNS toxicity* (visual and auditory hallucinations; mental depression or other mood changes; ringing or buzzing in ears); *dermatitis, allergic* (skin rash or itching); *syncope* (fainting)

**Those indicating need for medical attention only if they continue or are bothersome**
Incidence more frequent
*CNS effects* (drowsiness [up to 63%]; dizziness or lightheadedness [up to 15%]; weakness [up to 15%]; confusion [up to 11%]); *muscle weakness*—may be caused by CNS effect or become apparent if baclofen-induced reduction of muscle tone unmasks existing paresis; *nausea*—4 to 12%
Incidence less frequent or rare
*CNS effects* (clumsiness, unsteadiness, trembling, or other problems with muscle control; false sense of well-being; headache [up to 8%]; muscle pain; numbness or tingling in hands or feet; slurred speech or other speech problems; trouble in sleeping [up to 7%]; unexplained muscle stiffness; unusual excitement; unusual tiredness [up to 4%]); *constipation*—2 to 6%; *difficult or painful urination or decrease in amount of urine; fluid retention* (swelling of ankles; weight gain); *frequent urge to urinate; or uncontrolled urination*—2 to 6%; *gastrointestinal irritation* (abdominal or stomach pain or discomfort; diarrhea); *loss of appetite; low blood pressure*—up to 9%; *pounding heartbeat; sexual problems in males; stuffy nose*

**Those indicating need for medical attention and/or reinstitution of therapy if they occur after medication is abruptly discontinued**
*Convulsions; hallucinations, visual and auditory; increased spasticity; mood or mental changes such as paranoid ideation or manic psychosis; unusual nervousness or restlessness*

## Overdose

For specific information on the agents used in the management of baclofen overdose, see *Atropine* in *Anticholinergic/Antispasmodics (Systemic)* monograph.

For more information on the management of overdose or unintentional ingestion, **contact a Poison Control Center** (see *Poison Control Center Listing*).

**Clinical effects of overdose**

The following effects have been selected on the basis of their potential clinical significance (possible signs and symptoms in parentheses where appropriate)—not necessarily inclusive:

Acute and chronic
*CNS toxicity* (blurred or double vision; convulsions; myosis; mydriasis; severe muscle weakness; strabismus); *respiratory depression* (shortness of breath or unusually slow or troubled breathing); *vomiting*

**Treatment of overdose**

To decrease absorption—May include emptying the stomach by induction of emesis and/or gastric lavage.

Specific treatment—Administration of atropine has been recommended to increase ventilation, heart rate, blood pressure, and core body temperature.See the package insert or *Atropine* in *Anticholinergic/Antispasmodics (Systemic)* monograph.

Supportive care—May include maintaining adequate respiratory exchange. Respiratory stimulants should *not* be used. Patients in whom intentional overdose is known or suspected should be referred for psychiatric consultation.

## Patient Consultation

As an aid to patient consultation, refer to *Advice for the Patient, Baclofen (Systemic)*.

In providing consultation, consider emphasizing the following selected information (» = major clinical significance):

**Before using this medication**
» Conditions affecting use, especially:
Sensitivity to baclofen
Use in the elderly—Increased risk of adverse CNS effects
Other medications, especially other CNS depression–producing medications

**Proper use of this medication**
» Proper dosing
Missed dose: Taking if remembered within an hour or so; not taking if not remembered within an hour; not doubling doses
» Proper storage

**Precautions while using this medication**
» Checking with physician before discontinuing medication; gradual dosage reduction is necessary
» Avoiding alcohol or other CNS depressants
» Caution if drowsiness, dizziness, visual disturbances, or impaired coordination occur
Diabetics: May increase blood sugar concentrations

**Side/adverse effects**
» Convulsions, hallucinations, mood or mental changes, increased spasticity, or unusual nervousness or restlessness may occur following abrupt withdrawal
Signs and symptoms of potential side effects, especially bloody or dark urine, chest pain, CNS toxicity, allergic dermatitis, and syncope

## General Dosing Information

Side effects may be minimized by initiating therapy with low doses, which should be increased gradually until the desired response is obtained.

If the desired response is not achieved after a reasonable trial period, the medication should be slowly withdrawn.

Lower doses may be required in patients with renal function impairment.

Convulsions, hallucinations, other psychiatric disturbances, and exacerbation of spasticity have occurred following abrupt withdrawal of baclofen; gradual reduction of dosage over a period of 2 weeks or more is recommended before the medication is discontinued.

## Oral Dosage Forms

Note: Bracketed uses in the *Dosage Forms* section refer to categories of use and/or indications that are not included in U.S. product labeling.

## BACLOFEN TABLETS USP

### Usual adult and adolescent dose

Antispastic and

[Analgesic (in trigeminal neuralgia)][1]—

Oral, 5 mg three times a day initially, then increased by increments of 5 mg per dose every three days until the desired response is achieved.

Note: A smoother response may be achieved in some patients if the total daily dose is given in four divided doses.

### Usual adult prescribing limits

Up to 80 mg daily.

Note: Higher doses may be required in some patients.

### Usual pediatric dose

Safety and efficacy have not been established.

### Strength(s) usually available

U.S.—

10 mg (Rx) [*Lioresal* (scored); GENERIC].

20 mg (Rx) [*Lioresal* (scored); GENERIC].

Canada—

10 mg (Rx) [*Alpha-Baclofen; Lioresal* (scored); *PMS-Baclofen*].

20 mg (Rx) [*Alpha-Baclofen; Lioresal* (scored); *PMS-Baclofen*].

### Packaging and storage

Store below 40 °C (104 °F), preferably between 15 and 30 °C (59 and 86 °F). Store in a well-closed container.

### Auxiliary labeling

• May cause drowsiness.

• Avoid alcoholic beverages.

[1]Not included in Canadian product labeling.

Revised: 07/09/91

Interim revision: 06/13/95

---

# BARBITURATES  Systemic

This monograph includes information on the following: Amobarbital; Aprobarbital; Butabarbital; Mephobarbital; Metharbital\*†; Pentobarbital; Phenobarbital; Secobarbital; Secobarbital and Amobarbital.

VA CLASSIFICATION (Primary/Secondary):

Amobarbital

Oral—CN301

Parenteral—CN301/CN400

Aprobarbital

Oral—CN301

Butabarbital

Oral—CN301

Mephobarbital

Oral—CN400

Metharbital

Oral—CN400

Pentobarbital

Oral—CN301

Parenteral—CN301/CN400

Phenobarbital

Oral—CN301/CN400; GA900

Parenteral—CN301/CN400; GA900

Secobarbital

Oral—CN301

Parenteral—CN301/CN400

Note: Controlled substances in the U.S. and Canada as follows:

| Drug | U.S. | Canada |
|---|---|---|
| Amobarbital | II | C |
| Aprobarbital | III | |
| Butabarbital | III | C |
| Mephobarbital | IV | C |
| Pentobarbital | | |
|   Oral | II | C |
|   Parenteral | II | C |
|   Rectal | III | C |
| Phenobarbital | IV | C |
| Secobarbital | | |
|   Oral | II | C |
|   Parenteral | II | |
| Secobarbital and | | |
| Amobarbital | II | C |

Note: For a listing of dosage forms and brand names by country availability, see *Dosage Forms* section(s). For a listing of brand names for the articles in this monograph, refer to the General Index.

\*Not commercially available in the U.S.

†Not commercially available in Canada.

---

## Category

Sedative-hypnotic—Amobarbital; Aprobarbital; Butabarbital; Pentobarbital; Phenobarbital (parenteral only); Secobarbital.

Anticonvulsant—Amobarbital (parenteral only); Mephobarbital; Metharbital; Pentobarbital (parenteral only); Phenobarbital; Secobarbital (parenteral only).

Antihyperbilirubinemic—Phenobarbital.

## Indications

Note: Bracketed information in the *Indications* section refers to uses that are not included in U.S. product labeling.

### Accepted

Anesthesia, adjunct—Amobarbital, butabarbital, pentobarbital, phenobarbital (parenteral), and secobarbital are indicated for use as preoperative medication to help reduce anxiety and facilitate induction of anesthesia.

Narcoanalysis—Amobarbital (parenteral) may be indicated in narcoanalysis.

Epilepsy, tonic-clonic seizure pattern (treatment) or

Epilepsy, simple partial seizure pattern (treatment)—Phenobarbital, a long-acting barbiturate, is indicated as long-term anticonvulsant therapy for the treatment of generalized tonic-clonic and simple partial (cortical focal) seizures; mephobarbital and metharbital, also long-acting barbiturates, may be indicated as alternatives to phenobarbital.

Convulsions (treatment)

Seizures (prophylaxis and treatment)

Status epilepticus (treatment) or

Tetanus (treatment adjunct)—Parenteral barbiturates, especially phenobarbital, are indicated in the emergency treatment of certain acute convulsive episodes such as those associated with status epilepticus, eclampsia, meningitis, and toxic reactions to strychnine. They are also indicated as adjunctive treatment for acute convulsive episodes associated with tetanus.

Phenobarbital is used in the prophylaxis and treatment of febrile seizures.[1]

[Hyperbilirubinemia (prophylaxis and treatment)][1]—Phenobarbital (oral and parenteral) is used in the prevention and treatment of hyperbilirubinemia in neonates. It is used also to lower bilirubin concentrations in patients with congenital nonhemolytic unconjugated hyperbilirubinemia or chronic intrahepatic cholestasis.

[Ischemia, cerebral (treatment)][1] or

[Hypertension, cerebral (treatment)][1]—Pentobarbital (parenteral) is used for induction of coma to protect the brain from various states, including ischemia and increased intracranial pressure that follow stroke and head trauma; however, this use is controversial and further studies are needed.

Amobarbital, aprobarbital, butabarbital, pentobarbital, phenobarbital, secobarbital, and secobarbital and amobarbital have been used for the short-term treatment of insomnia; however, they generally *have been replaced* by benzodiazepines. If barbiturates are used, they are not recommended for long-term use since they appear to lose their effectiveness in sleep induction and maintenance after 2 weeks or less.

Amobarbital, aprobarbital, butabarbital, mephobarbital, pentobarbital, phenobarbital, and secobarbital have also been used for routine sedation to relieve anxiety, tension, and apprehension; however, barbiturates generally *have been replaced* by benzodiazepines for daytime sedation.

### Unaccepted

Amobarbital (parenteral) has been used as a diagnostic aid in schizophrenia but it generally has been replaced by other agents.

Amobarbital (parenteral) has also been used in the management of catatonic and negativistic reactions; however, phenothiazines generally are more appropriate therapy for catatonic reactions. It has also been used in the management of manic reactions, although benzodiazepines and lithium are usually preferred.

[Phenobarbital (oral and parenteral) has been used in the treatment of familial, senile, or essential action tremors; however, it generally has been replaced by other agents, such as benzodiazepines and beta-adrenergic blockers.]

¹Not included in Canadian product labeling.

## Pharmacology/Pharmacokinetics

See also *Table 1*, page 514.

### Physicochemical characteristics

Molecular weight—
Amobarbital: 226.27.
Amobarbital sodium: 248.26.
Aprobarbital: 210.23.
Butabarbital sodium: 234.23.
Mephobarbital: 246.27.
Metharbital: 198.22.
Pentobarbital: 226.27.
Pentobarbital sodium: 248.26.
Phenobarbital: 232.24.
Phenobarbital sodium: 254.22.
Secobarbital sodium: 260.27.

### Mechanism of action/Effect

Barbiturates act as nonselective depressants of the central nervous system (CNS), capable of producing all levels of CNS mood alteration from excitation to mild sedation, hypnosis, and deep coma. In sufficiently high therapeutic doses, barbiturates induce anesthesia. Recent studies have suggested that the sedative-hypnotic and anticonvulsant effects of barbiturates may be related to their ability to enhance and/or mimic the inhibitory synaptic action of gamma-aminobutyric acid (GABA).

Sedative-hypnotic—
Barbiturates depress the sensory cortex, decrease motor activity, alter cerebral function, and produce drowsiness, sedation, and hypnosis. Although the mechanism of action has not been completely established, the barbiturates appear to have a particular effect at the level of the thalamus where they inhibit ascending conduction in the reticular formation, thus interfering with the transmission of impulses to the cortex.

The mechanism of action of pentobarbital in protecting the brain from ischemia and intracranial pressure is not completely understood; however, it is related to pentobarbital's anesthetic action (produced by sufficiently high dosage) and possibly to the depression of neuronal activity and metabolism.

Anticonvulsant—
Barbiturates are believed to act by depressing monosynaptic and polysynaptic transmission in the CNS. They also increase the threshold for electrical stimulation of the motor cortex.

Antihyperbilirubinemic—
Phenobarbital lowers serum bilirubin concentrations probably by induction of glucuronyl transferase, the enzyme which conjugates bilirubin.

### Other actions/effects

Barbiturates have little analgesic action at subanesthetic doses and may increase reaction to painful stimuli.

Although phenobarbital, mephobarbital, and metharbital are the only barbiturates effective as anticonvulsants in subhypnotic doses, all of the barbiturates exhibit anticonvulsant activity in anesthetic doses.

Barbiturates are respiratory depressants; the degree of respiratory depression is dose-dependent.

Barbiturates have been shown to reduce the rapid eye movement (REM) phase of sleep or dreaming stage. Also, Stages III and IV sleep (slow-wave sleep, SWS) are decreased.

Animal studies have shown that barbiturates cause reduction in the tone and contractility of the uterus, ureters, and urinary bladder; however, concentrations required to produce this effect in humans are not attained with sedative-hypnotic doses.

Barbiturates have been shown to induce liver microsomal enzymes, thereby increasing and altering the metabolism of other medications or compounds.

### Absorption

Absorbed in varying degrees following oral, parenteral, or rectal administration.

Barbiturate sodium salts are absorbed more rapidly than the free acids because of rapid dissolution.

The rate of absorption is increased if barbiturates are taken well diluted or on an empty stomach.

### Distribution

Rapidly distributed to all tissues and fluids with high concentrations in the brain, liver, and kidneys.

Lipid solubility is the primary factor in distribution within the body. The more lipid soluble the barbiturate, the more rapidly it penetrates all tissues of the body; phenobarbital has the lowest lipid solubility and secobarbital the highest.

### Biotransformation

Hepatic, primarily by the hepatic microsomal enzyme system.

About 75% of a single oral dose of mephobarbital is metabolized to phenobarbital in 24 hours.

Metharbital is metabolized to barbital.

### Onset of action

Oral or rectal—Varies from 20 to 60 minutes.

Intramuscular—Slightly faster than for oral or rectal.

Intravenous—Ranges from almost immediately for pentobarbital sodium to 5 minutes for phenobarbital sodium.

### Therapeutic serum concentration

Anticonvulsant—Phenobarbital: 10 to 40 mcg per mL (43 to 172 micromoles/L).

Note: The optimal blood phenobarbital concentration should be determined by response in seizure control and the appearance of toxic effects.

To achieve blood concentrations considered therapeutic in children, higher-per-kg dosages of phenobarbital and most other anticonvulsants generally are required.

### Time to peak effect

Phenobarbital—Maximal CNS depression may not occur for 15 minutes or more after intravenous administration of phenobarbital sodium.

## Precautions to Consider

### Cross-sensitivity and/or related problems

Patients sensitive to one of the barbiturates may be sensitive to other barbiturates also.

### Carcinogenicity/Tumorigenicity/Mutagenicity

For butabarbital and secobarbital—No long-term studies in animals have been done to determine the carcinogenic and mutagenic potential of butabarbital or secobarbital.

For pentobarbital—Adequate studies have not been done in humans or animals to determine the carcinogenic potential of pentobarbital.

For phenobarbital—Studies in animals have shown that phenobarbital is carcinogenic in mice and rats following lifetime administration. It produced benign and malignant liver cell tumors in mice and benign liver cell tumors very late in life in rats. A study in humans did not provide sufficient evidence that phenobarbital is carcinogenic in humans.

### Pregnancy/Reproduction

Fertility—For butabarbital: No long-term studies in animals have been done to determine the effects of butabarbital on fertility.

Pregnancy—Barbiturates readily cross the placenta following oral or parenteral administration. They are distributed throughout fetal tissues, the highest concentrations being found in the placenta, fetal liver, and brain. Following parenteral administration, fetal blood concentration approaches maternal blood concentration.

Barbiturates have been shown to cause an increased incidence of fetal abnormalities. Risk-benefit must be carefully considered when the medication is required in life-threatening situations or in serious diseases for which other medications cannot be used or are ineffective.

Third trimester: Use of barbiturates throughout the last trimester of pregnancy may cause physical dependence with resulting withdrawal symptoms in the neonate. In infants suffering from long-term exposure in utero, the acute withdrawal syndrome of seizures and hyperirritability has been reported to occur from birth to a delayed onset of up to 14 days.

Use of long-acting barbiturates, especially phenobarbital, as anticonvulsants during pregnancy is reportedly associated with a neonatal coagulation defect that may cause bleeding during the early neonatal period (usually within 24 hours of birth). This coagulation defect is characterized by decreased concentrations of vitamin K–dependent clotting factors and prolongation of the prothrombin time and/or the partial thromboplastin time. Vitamin K should be given to the mother during delivery and to the infant (intramuscularly or subcutaneously) immediately after birth.

Also, one study in humans has suggested that prenatal exposure to barbiturates may be associated with an increased incidence of brain tumors.

**FDA Pregnancy Category D.**

Labor and delivery—Barbiturates in hypnotic doses do not appear to inhibit uterine activity; however, full anesthetic doses of barbiturates decrease the force and frequency of uterine contractions.

Use of barbiturates during labor may cause respiratory depression in the neonate, especially the premature neonate, because of immature hepatic function.

If barbiturates are used during labor and delivery, it is recommended that resuscitation equipment be readily available.

**Breast-feeding**

Barbiturates are distributed into breast milk; use by nursing mothers may cause CNS depression in the infant.

**Pediatrics**

Some children may react to barbiturates with paradoxical excitement.

**Geriatrics**

Geriatric patients may react to usual doses of barbiturates with excitement, confusion, or mental depression.

The risk of barbiturate-induced hypothermia may be increased in elderly patients, especially with high doses or in acute overdose of barbiturates.

In addition, elderly patients are more likely to have age-related hepatic or renal function impairment, which may require a reduction of dosage in patients receiving a barbiturate.

**Drug interactions and/or related problems**

The following drug interactions and/or related problems have been selected on the basis of their potential clinical significance (possible mechanism in parentheses where appropriate)—not necessarily inclusive (» = major clinical significance):

Note: Combinations containing any of the following medications, depending on the amount present, may also interact with this medication.

Acetaminophen
(therapeutic effects of acetaminophen may be decreased when the medication is used concurrently in patients receiving chronic barbiturate therapy because of increased metabolism resulting from induction of hepatic microsomal enzymes; also, risk of hepatotoxicity with single toxic doses or prolonged use of high doses of acetaminophen may be increased in alcoholics or in patients regularly using hepatic enzyme inducers such as barbiturates)

Addictive medications, other, especially CNS depressants with habituating potential
(prolonged concurrent use may increase the risk of habituation; caution is recommended)

» Adrenocorticoids, glucocorticoid and mineralocorticoid or
Chloramphenicol or
» Corticotropin or
Cyclosporine or
Dacarbazine or
Digitalis glycosides or
Metronidazole or
Quinidine
(effects may be decreased when these medications are used concurrently with barbiturates, especially phenobarbital, because of enhanced metabolism resulting from induction of hepatic microsomal enzymes; dosage adjustment of these medications, with the exception of digoxin, may be necessary)

» Alcohol or
» CNS depression–producing medications, other (See *Appendix II* )
(concurrent use may increase the CNS depressant effects of either these medications or barbiturates; caution is recommended and dosage of one or both agents should be reduced)

Amphetamines
(concurrent use may cause a delay in the intestinal absorption of phenobarbital)

Anesthetics, halogenated hydrocarbon
(chronic use of barbiturates prior to enflurane, halothane, or methoxyflurane anesthesia may increase anesthetic metabolism leading to increased risk of hepatotoxicity)
(chronic use of barbiturates prior to methoxyflurane anesthesia may increase formation of nephrotoxic metabolites leading to increased risk of nephrotoxicity)

» Anticoagulants, coumarin- or indandione-derivative
(effects may be decreased when these medications are used concurrently with barbiturates because of increased metabolism resulting from induction of hepatic microsomal enzymes; also, bleeding may result when the barbiturate is discontinued; periodic prothrombin-time determinations may be required to determine if dosage adjustments of anticoagulants are necessary)

Anticonvulsants, hydantoin
(concurrent use with barbiturates appears to produce variable and unpredictable effects on the metabolism of hydantoin anticonvulsants; blood concentrations of hydantoin anticonvulsants should be closely monitored when these medications are used concurrently)

Anticonvulsants, succinimide or
» Carbamazepine
(concurrent use with barbiturates may result in increased metabolism, leading to decreased serum concentrations and reduced elimination half-lives of carbamazepine or succinimide anticonvulsants because of induction of hepatic microsomal enzyme activity; monitoring of serum concentrations as a guide to dosage is recommended, especially when carbamazepine or a succinimide anticonvulsant is added to or withdrawn from an existing regimen)

Antidepressants, tricyclic
(effects of tricyclic antidepressants may be decreased when these medications are used concurrently with barbiturates, especially phenobarbital, because of increased metabolism resulting from induction of hepatic microsomal enzymes)

Calcium channel blocking agents
(caution is advised during titration of calcium channel blocker dosage for those patients taking medication known to promote hypotension, such as barbiturate preanesthetics, since the combination may result in excessive hypotension)

Carbonic anhydrase inhibitors
(osteopenia induced by barbiturates, especially phenobarbital, may be enhanced when carbonic anhydrase inhibitors are used concurrently; it is recommended that patients receiving concurrent therapy be monitored for early signs of osteopenia and that the carbonic anhydrase inhibitor be discontinued and appropriate treatment initiated if necessary)

» Contraceptives, estrogen-containing, oral
(concurrent use with barbiturates, especially phenobarbital, may result in reduced contraceptive reliability because of accelerated estrogen metabolism caused by induction of hepatic microsomal enzymes; use of a nonhormonal method of birth control or a progestin-only oral contraceptive may be necessary)

Cyclophosphamide
(concurrent use with barbiturates, especially phenobarbital, may induce microsomal metabolism to increase formation of alkylating metabolites of cyclophosphamide, thereby reducing the half-life and increasing the leukopenic activity of cyclophosphamide)

Disopyramide
(concurrent use with barbiturates, especially phenobarbital, may reduce serum disopyramide to ineffective concentrations; therefore, monitoring of its serum concentrations is necessary during concurrent therapy)

» Divalproex sodium or
» Valproic acid
(concurrent use may decrease the metabolism of barbiturates, resulting in increased serum concentrations, which may lead to increased CNS depression and neurological toxicity; barbiturate serum concentrations should be monitored to determine if dosage adjustment is necessary when these medications are used concurrently; also, the half-life of valproic acid may be decreased and dosage adjustment may be necessary)
(in addition, phenobarbital may enhance valproic acid hepatotoxicity, presumably through the formation of hepatotoxic valproate metabolites)

Doxycycline
(half-life of doxycycline may be shortened when this medication is used concurrently with barbiturates, especially phenobarbital, probably because of increased metabolism resulting from induction of hepatic microsomal enzymes; this effect may continue for up to 2 weeks after barbiturate therapy is discontinued; adjustment of doxycycline dosage during and after therapy or substitution of another tetracycline may be necessary)

Fenoprofen
(concurrent use with phenobarbital may decrease the elimination half-life of fenoprofen, possibly because of increased metabolism resulting from induction of hepatic microsomal enzyme activity; fenoprofen dosage adjustment may be required)

Griseofulvin
(absorption may be decreased when this medication is used concurrently with barbiturates, especially phenobarbital, resulting in decreased serum concentrations; although the effect of decreased serum concentrations on therapeutic response has not been established, concurrent use preferably should be avoided)

Guanadrel or
Guanethidine
(concurrent use with barbiturates may aggravate orthostatic hypotension)

Haloperidol
(concurrent use with barbiturate anticonvulsants may cause a change in the pattern and/or frequency of epileptiform seizures; dosage adjustments of anticonvulsants may be necessary; serum concentrations of haloperidol may be significantly reduced)

Hypothermia-producing medications, other (See *Appendix II*)
(concurrent use with barbiturates in high doses or acute overdose may increase the risk of hypothermia)

Ketamine
(concurrent use of ketamine, especially in high doses or when rapidly administered, with barbiturate preanesthetics may increase the risk of hypotension and/or respiratory depression)

Leucovorin
(large doses may counteract the anticonvulsant effects of barbiturate anticonvulsants)

Levothyroxine
(concurrent use of barbiturates may increase hepatic degradation of levothyroxine, which may result in increased requirements; dosage adjustment may be necessary)

Loxapine or
Phenothiazines or
Thioxanthenes
(may lower the seizure threshold; dosage adjustment of barbiturate anticonvulsants may be necessary)

(concurrent use of chlorpromazine with phenobarbital has been shown to increase the metabolism of chlorpromazine; therefore, phenobarbital may decrease serum concentrations of phenothiazines when used concurrently)

Maprotiline
(in addition to possibly enhancing CNS depressant effects, concurrent use of maprotiline may lower the convulsive threshold, at high doses, and decrease the effects of barbiturate anticonvulsants)

Methylphenidate
(concurrent use may increase serum concentrations of barbiturate anticonvulsants, especially phenobarbital, because of metabolism inhibition, possibly resulting in toxicity; dosage adjustment of the barbiturate anticonvulsant may be necessary)

Mexiletine
(concurrent use with barbiturates may accelerate metabolism and result in decreased plasma concentrations of mexiletine; plasma concentrations of mexiletine should be monitored during concurrent use to ensure efficacy is maintained)

Monoamine oxidase (MAO) inhibitors, including furazolidone, pargyline, and procarbazine
(concurrent use may prolong the CNS depressant effects of barbiturates, probably because metabolism of the barbiturate is inhibited)

(concurrent use with barbiturate anticonvulsants may cause a change in the pattern of epileptiform seizures; dosage adjustment of the barbiturate anticonvulsant may be necessary)

Phenylbutazone
(concurrent use may decrease the efficacy of barbiturates by inducing hepatic microsomal enzymes and increasing their metabolism; also, hepatic enzyme inducers such as barbiturates may increase phenylbutazone metabolism and decrease its half-life)

Posterior pituitary
(concurrent use with barbiturates may increase the risk of cardiac arrhythmias and coronary insufficiency)

Primidone
(although concurrent use with barbiturate anticonvulsants is rarely indicated, since primidone is metabolized to phenobarbital, it may cause a change in the pattern of epileptiform seizures because of altered medication metabolism and also increase the sedative effect of either primidone or the barbiturate anticonvulsant; decreases in primidone dosage may be necessary)

Rifampin
(concurrent use with rifampin may enhance the metabolism of hexobarbital by induction of hepatic microsomal enzymes, resulting in lower serum concentrations; there are conflicting data on rifampin's effect on phenobarbital; dosage adjustment may be required)

Vitamin D
(effects may be reduced by barbiturates, especially phenobarbital, because of accelerated metabolism by hepatic microsomal enzyme induction; vitamin D supplementation may be required in patients on long-term barbiturate anticonvulsant therapy to prevent osteomalacia, although rickets is rare)

Xanthines, such as:
 Aminophylline
 Caffeine
 Oxtriphylline
 Theophylline
(concurrent use with barbiturates, especially phenobarbital, may increase metabolism of the xanthines [except dyphylline] by induction of hepatic microsomal enzymes, resulting in increased theophylline clearance; also, concurrent use may antagonize hypnotic effects of barbiturates)

**Laboratory value alterations**
The following have been selected on the basis of their potential clinical significance (possible effect in parentheses where appropriate)—not necessarily inclusive (» = major clinical significance):

With diagnostic test results
Cyanocobalamin Co 57
(absorption of radioactive cyanocobalamin may be impaired by concurrent use of barbiturate anticonvulsants, especially phenobarbital)

Metyrapone test
(increased metabolism of metyrapone by an hepatic enzyme inducer such as a barbiturate may decrease the response to metyrapone)

Phentolamine test
(barbiturates may cause a false-positive phentolamine test; it is recommended that all medications be withdrawn at least 24 hours, preferably 48 to 72 hours, prior to a phentolamine test)

With physiology/laboratory test values
Bilirubin, serum
(concentrations may be decreased in neonates, in patients with congenital nonhemolytic unconjugated hyperbilirubinemia, and in epileptics; this effect is presumably due to induction of glucuronyl transferase, the enzyme responsible for the conjugation of bilirubin)

**Medical considerations/Contraindications**
The medical considerations/contraindications included here have been selected on the basis of their potential clinical significance (reasons given in parentheses where appropriate)—not necessarily inclusive (» = major clinical significance).

*Except under special circumstances, this medication should not be used when the following medical problem exists:*

» Porphyria, acute intermittent or variegata, or history of
(barbiturates may aggravate symptoms by inducing enzymes responsible for porphyrin synthesis)

*Risk-benefit should be considered when the following medical problems exist:*

Anemia, severe
(may be complicated by barbiturate-induced respiratory depression, especially with phenobarbital)

Asthma, history of
(hypersensitivity reactions such as bronchospasm more likely to occur in these patients)

Diabetes mellitus, especially with phenobarbital

» Drug abuse or dependence, history of
(predisposition of patient to habituation and dependence)

» Hepatic coma, premonitory signs of, or
Hepatic function impairment
(barbiturates metabolized in liver; medication should be administered with caution and, initially, in reduced dosage)

Hyperkinesis
(condition may be exacerbated)

Hyperthyroidism
(symptoms may be exacerbated because barbiturates displace thyroxine from plasma proteins)

Hypoadrenalism, borderline
(systemic effects of exogenous hydrocortisone and endogenous cortisol may be diminished by barbiturates)

Mental depression and/or
Suicidal tendencies
(condition may be exacerbated, especially in elderly patients)

» Pain, acute or chronic
(paradoxical excitement may be induced or important symptoms may be masked)

Renal function impairment, especially with intermediate- and long-acting barbiturates
  (barbiturates excreted primarily by kidneys; dosage reduction may be necessary)
» Respiratory disease involving dyspnea or obstruction, particularly status asthmaticus
  (serious ventilatory depression may occur)
» Sensitivity to barbiturate prescribed
  (in patients sensitive to barbiturates, severe hepatic damage can occur from ordinary doses and is usually associated with dermatitis and involvement of parenchymatous organs)
  Caution should be used also in debilitated patients because they may react to usual doses with marked excitement, mental depression, and confusion

*For parenteral dosage forms only*
Cardiac disease
  (adverse circulatory reactions may occur with intravenous administration, especially with too-rapid administration)
Hypertension
  (hypotension may occur with intravenous administration, especially in these patients; slow administration usually prevents this occurrence)

**Patient monitoring**
The following may be especially important in patient monitoring (other tests may be warranted in some patients, depending on condition; » = major clinical significance):
Folate concentrations, serum
  (determinations recommended periodically because of increased folate requirements of patients on long-term anticonvulsant therapy with phenobarbital and possibly mephobarbital)
Hematopoietic function and
Hepatic function and
Renal function
  (determinations recommended at periodic intervals during prolonged barbiturate therapy)
Barbital concentrations, serum
  (determinations recommended when clinically indicated during metharbital therapy)
Phenobarbital concentrations, serum
  (determinations recommended as clinically indicated when phenobarbital or mephobarbital is used as an anticonvulsant)

# Side/Adverse Effects

Note: Exfoliative dermatitis and Stevens-Johnson syndrome, possibly fatal, may occur rarely as hypersensitivity reactions to barbiturates. If dermatologic reactions occur, the barbiturate should be discontinued.
  Severe respiratory depression, apnea, laryngospasm, bronchospasm, or hypertension may occur with intravenous administration of barbiturates, especially if administered too rapidly.
  Prolonged barbiturate therapy may result in osteopenia or rickets.
  Barbiturate dependence may occur, especially following prolonged use of high doses. The characteristics of dependence include: a strong desire or need to continue taking the barbiturate; a tendency to increase the dose; a psychological dependence on the effects of the medication; and a physical dependence on the effects of the medication requiring its presence for maintenance of homeostasis and resulting in an abstinence syndrome when the barbiturate is discontinued. Symptoms of withdrawal are related to the pharmacokinetics of the specific barbiturate and can be severe and may even cause death.

The following side/adverse effects have been selected on the basis of their potential clinical significance (possible signs and symptoms in parentheses where appropriate)—not necessarily inclusive:

**Those indicating need for medical attention**
Incidence less frequent
  *Sensitivity to barbiturates* (confusion)—especially in geriatric or debilitated patients; *mental depression*—especially in geriatric or debilitated patients; *paradoxical reaction* (unusual excitement)—especially in children or geriatric or debilitated patients
Incidence rare
  *Agranulocytosis* (sore throat and/or fever); *allergic reaction* (skin rash or hives; swelling of eyelids, face, or lips; wheezing or tightness in chest)—especially in patients who have asthma, urticaria, angioedema, and similar conditions; *exfoliative dermatitis* (fever; red, thickened, or scaly skin); *hallucinations; hypotension or megaloblastic anemia* (-

unusual tiredness or weakness)—with chronic barbiturate use; *Stevens-Johnson syndrome* (bleeding sores on lips; chest pain; muscle or joint pain; painful sores, ulcers, or white spots in mouth; skin rash or hives; sore throat or fever); *thrombocytopenia* (unusual bleeding or bruising); *thrombophlebitis* (soreness, redness, swelling, or pain at injection site)—for parenteral dosage forms only
With prolonged or chronic use
  *Hepatic damage* (yellow eyes or skin); *osteopenia or rickets* (bone pain, tenderness, or aching; loss of appetite; muscle weakness; unusual weight loss)

**Those indicating need for medical attention only if they continue or are bothersome**
Incidence more frequent
  *Clumsiness or unsteadiness; dizziness or lightheadedness; drowsiness; "hangover" effect*
Incidence less frequent
  *Anxiety or nervousness; constipation; feeling faint; headache; irritability; nausea or vomiting; nightmares or trouble in sleeping*

**Those indicating possible barbiturate withdrawal and need for medical attention if they occur after medication is discontinued**
Minor symptoms—may occur within 8 to 12 hours and usually occur in the following sequence:
  *Anxiety or restlessness; muscle twitching; trembling of hands; weakness; dizziness; vision problems; nausea; vomiting; trouble in sleeping, increased dreaming, or nightmares; orthostatic hypotension* (feeling faint; lightheadedness)
Major symptoms—may occur within 16 hours and last up to 5 days
  *Convulsions; hallucinations*
  Note: Intensity of withdrawal symptoms gradually declines over a period of approximately 15 days.

# Overdose

For specific information on the agents used in the management of barbiturate overdose, see:
  • *Charcoal, Activated (Oral-Local)* monograph; and/or
  • *Ipecac (Oral-Local)* monograph.
For more information on the management of overdose or unintentional ingestion, **contact a Poison Control Center** (see *Poison Control Center Listing*).

**Clinical effects of overdose**
The following effects have been selected on the basis of their potential clinical significance (possible signs and symptoms in parentheses where appropriate)—not necessarily inclusive:
Acute
  *Confusion, severe; decrease in or loss of reflexes; drowsiness, severe; fever; hypothermia* (low body temperature); *shortness of breath or slow or troubled breathing; slow heartbeat; slurred speech; staggering; unusual movements of the eyes; weakness, severe*
  Note: In acute barbiturate overdosage, CNS and respiratory depression may progress to Cheyne-Stokes respiration, areflexia, slight constriction of the pupils (in severe toxicity, pupils may be dilated), oliguria, tachycardia, lowered body temperature, and coma. Typical shock syndrome (apnea, circulatory collapse, respiratory arrest, and death) may occur.
  In extreme barbiturate overdosage, all electrical activity in the brain may cease. In this case an electroencephalogram (EEG) may be "flat," but this does not necessarily indicate clinical death since, unless hypoxic damage occurs, this effect is fully reversible.
  Complications in barbiturate overdosage such as pneumonia, pulmonary edema, cardiac arrhythmias, congestive heart failure, and renal failure may occur.
  In acute overdosage, the blood barbiturate concentration for some of the barbiturates relative to the degree of CNS depression in nontolerant persons is as follows:
    See also *Table 2*, page 515.
Chronic
  *Confusion, severe; irritability, continuing; poor judgment; trouble in sleeping*

**Treatment of overdose**
Treatment of barbiturate overdose is primarily supportive and consists of the following:
To decrease absorption—
  If the patient is conscious and has not lost the gag reflex, emesis may be induced with ipecac syrup; care should be taken to prevent pulmonary aspiration of vomitus. After vomiting is completed, 30 to 60 grams of activated charcoal in a glass of

water or sorbitol may be administered to prevent absorption and increase excretion of the barbiturate.

If emesis is contraindicated, gastric lavage may be performed with a cuffed endotracheal tube in place with the patient face down. Activated charcoal should be left in the stomach and a saline cathartic may be administered.

To enhance elimination—

If renal function is normal, forced diuresis may help to eliminate the barbiturate.

Alkalinization of the urine increases renal excretion of some barbiturates, especially phenobarbital, also aprobarbital, and mephobarbital (which is metabolized to phenobarbital).

Although hemodialysis or hemoperfusion is not recommended as a routine procedure, it may be used in severe barbiturate poisoning or if the patient is anuric or in shock.

Monitoring—

Vital signs and fluid balance should be monitored.

Supportive care—

An adequate airway should be maintained, with assisted respiration and administration of oxygen as needed.

Blood pressure and body temperature should be maintained.

Fluid therapy and other standard treatment for shock should be administered, if necessary.

A vasopressor may be required if hypotension occurs.

Fluid or sodium overload should be avoided, especially if cardiovascular status is decreased.

Chest physiotherapy should be administered.

If pneumonia is suspected, appropriate cultures should be taken and antibiotics should be administered.

Also, appropriate care should be taken to prevent hypostatic pneumonia, decubiti, aspiration, and other complications that may occur with altered states of consciousness.

Patients in whom intentional overdose is known or suspected should be referred for psychiatric consultation.

## Patient Consultation

As an aid to patient consultation, refer to *Advice for the Patient, Barbiturates (Systemic)*.

In providing consultation, consider emphasizing the following selected information (» = major clinical significance):

### Before using this medication

» Conditions affecting use, especially:

Sensitivity to barbiturates

Pregnancy—Barbiturates readily cross placenta; increase in incidence of fetal abnormalities (FDA Pregnancy Category D); use during third trimester of pregnancy may cause physical dependence with resulting withdrawal symptoms in neonate; long-acting barbiturates associated with neonatal coagulation defect that may cause bleeding during early neonatal period; use during labor may cause respiratory depression in neonate

Breast-feeding—Barbiturates distributed into breast milk; use by nursing mothers may cause CNS depression in infant

Use in children—Children may react to barbiturates with paradoxical excitement

Use in the elderly—Elderly patients may react to usual doses of barbiturates with excitement, confusion, or mental depression; risk of barbiturate-induced hypothermia may be increased in elderly patients; elderly patients more likely to have age-related hepatic or renal function impairment, which may require a dosage reduction of barbiturates

Other medications, especially alcohol, adrenocorticoids, corticotropin, other CNS depression–producing medications, coumarin- or indandione-derivative anticoagulants, carbamazepine, divalproex sodium, estrogen-containing contraceptives, or valproic acid

Other medical problems, especially history of drug abuse or dependence, premonitory signs of hepatic coma, acute or chronic pain, or respiratory disease involving dyspnea or obstruction (particularly status asthmaticus)

Caution if any laboratory tests required; possible interference with results of metyrapone test.

### Proper use of this medication

» Importance of not using more medication than the amount prescribed because of habit-forming potential

» Not increasing dose if medication appears less effective after a few weeks; checking with physician

» For anticonvulsant use: Compliance with therapy; not missing any doses

» Proper dosing

Missed dose: If on scheduled dosing regimen—Taking as soon as possible; not taking if almost time for next dose; not doubling doses

*Proper administration*

*For extended-release dosage form*

Swallowing capsule or tablet whole

Not breaking, crushing, or chewing

*For suppository dosage form*

Proper administration technique

» Proper storage

### Precautions while using this medication

Regular visits to physician to check progress during prolonged therapy

Checking with physician before discontinuing medication after prolonged use; gradual dosage reduction may be necessary to avoid the possibility of withdrawal symptoms

» Avoiding use of alcohol or other CNS depressants

» Suspected psychological or physical dependence: Checking with physician

» Suspected overdose: Getting emergency help at once

» Caution if dizziness, lightheadedness, or drowsiness occurs

» Use of another or additional method of contraception if taking estrogen-containing oral contraceptives concurrently

### Side/adverse effects

Signs of potential side effects, especially allergic reaction or intolerance to barbiturate, blood dyscrasias, exfoliative dermatitis, hallucinations, hepatic damage (with prolonged or chronic use), mental depression, paradoxical reaction, osteopenia or rickets (with prolonged or chronic use), or Stevens-Johnson syndrome

Unusual excitement may be more likely to occur in children and in elderly or very ill patients

Confusion and mental depression may be more likely to occur in elderly or very ill patients

## General Dosing Information

See also *Table 2*, page 515.

Dosage of the barbiturates must be individualized, based on the patient's age, weight, and condition.

In patients with impaired hepatic function, lower doses should be used initially. Lower doses may be required also in patients with impaired renal function.

Patients on dialysis may require an increase in dosage.

Tolerance may occur with repeated administration of the barbiturates, especially of the long-acting ones and with large doses of the shorter-acting ones.

Prolonged administration of barbiturates as hypnotics generally is not recommended because they have not been shown to be effective for a period of more than 2 weeks.

Prolonged uninterrupted use of barbiturates, particularly the short-acting ones, may result in psychic or physical dependence.

Chronic use of barbiturates at doses 3 to 4 times the therapeutic concentration will usually produce physical dependence in about 75% of patients.

Daily administration in excess of 400 mg of pentobarbital or secobarbital for approximately 90 days is likely to produce some degree of physical dependence; a dosage of 600 to 800 mg taken for at least 35 days is sufficient to produce withdrawal seizures. The average daily dose for the barbiturate addict generally is about 1.5 grams.

Barbiturates should be withdrawn gradually in order to avoid the possibility of precipitating withdrawal symptoms.

To minimize the possibility of acute or chronic overdosage, the least possible quantity of a barbiturate should be prescribed and dispensed at any one time.

The toxic dose of barbiturates varies but generally an oral dose of 1 gram of most barbiturates produces serious poisoning in an adult. Death commonly occurs after 2 to 10 grams of ingested barbiturate.

### Diet/Nutrition

Patients on long-term anticonvulsant therapy with phenobarbital and possibly mephobarbital may have increased folic acid requirements. In addition, patients on long-term therapy may require supplements of vitamin D to prevent osteomalacia.

### For parenteral dosage forms only

Prior to administration, parenteral solutions should be inspected visually for particulate matter and discoloration, if possible.

For intravenous injections, it is preferable to use the larger veins to minimize the risk of irritation and the possibility of resulting thrombosis. Administration into varicose veins is not recommended because of poor circulation in these veins.

Intravenous injections should be administered slowly and patients should be carefully monitored during administration. This requires maintenance of blood pressure, respiration, and cardiac function and recording of vital signs. Equipment for resuscitation and artificial ventilation should be readily available.

Intramuscular injections should be administered deeply into large muscles, such as the gluteus maximus or vastus lateralis because superficial intramuscular injection may be painful and may produce sterile abscesses or sloughs.

No more than 5 mL, regardless of drug concentration, should be injected intramuscularly at any one site because of possible tissue irritation.

Parenteral solutions of barbiturate salts are highly alkaline; therefore, caution should be used to avoid perivascular extravasation or intra-arterial injection, since extravasation may cause local tissue damage with subsequent necrosis and intra-arterial injection may cause spasm, severe pain, and possibly gangrene.

**For rectal dosage forms only**

Barbiturates may be administered rectally when oral or parenteral administration may be undesirable. If the rectal dosage form is not available, the soluble sodium salt of the barbiturate may be incorporated in a retention enema.

To assure accuracy in dosage, suppositories should not be divided.

Rectal administration of barbiturates is not recommended for status epilepticus; intravenous injection is the preferred route of administration for this condition.

**For treatment of dependence**

Treatment of dependence consists of the following:
- Gradual withdrawal of the barbiturate.
- An example of the different withdrawal regimens used (all of which require an extended period of time) involves substituting a 30-mg dose of phenobarbital for each 100- to 200-mg dose of the barbiturate that the patient has been taking. The total daily amount of phenobarbital then is administered as a single dose or in 3 or 4 divided doses, not to exceed 600 mg per day. If signs of withdrawal occur on the first day of treatment, a loading dose of 100 to 200 mg of phenobarbital may be administered intramuscularly in addition to the oral dose. After stabilization on phenobarbital, the total daily dose is decreased by 30 mg a day as long as withdrawal is proceeding smoothly. This regimen may be modified by initiating treatment at the patient's regular dosage level and decreasing the daily dosage by 10% if tolerated by the patient.
- For infants physically dependent on barbiturates, initially a dose of 3 to 10 mg of phenobarbital per kg of body weight per day may be given. After withdrawal symptoms (hyperactivity, disturbed sleep, tremors, hyperreflexia) are relieved, the dosage of phenobarbital should be gradually decreased and completely withdrawn over a 2-week period.
- Also, barbiturate withdrawal may be accomplished with benzodiazepines, such as diazepam.

**For treatment of adverse effects**

For extravasation into subcutaneous tissues—Recommended treatment includes:
- Application of moist heat to affected area.
- Injection of a 0.5% procaine solution into the affected area.

For accidental intra-arterial injection—Recommended treatment includes:
- Release of tourniquet or restrictive garments to permit dilution of injected medication.
- Injection of 10 mL of a 1% procaine solution into the artery and, if necessary, brachial plexus block to relieve spasm.
- Anticoagulant therapy may prevent thrombosis.
- Supportive treatment.

---

## AMOBARBITAL

## Summary of Differences

Category:
  Parenteral amobarbital also may be indicated as an anticonvulsant.
Indications:
  Parenteral amobarbital also may be indicated in narcoanalysis; and has been used in diagnosis of schizophrenia and for catatonic, negativistic, and manic reactions, but generally has been replaced by other agents.
Pharmacology/pharmacokinetics:
  Long-acting barbiturate—
    Onset of action: 60 minutes or longer.
    Duration of action: 10 to 12 hours.
  Protein binding—
    Moderate.

## Additional Dosing Information

See also *General Dosing Information.*

**For parenteral dosage forms only**

The rate of intravenous injection should not exceed 100 mg per minute for adults or 60 mg per square meter of body surface per minute for children. Faster rates of administration may cause serious respiratory depression.

Superficial intramuscular or subcutaneous injections may be painful and may produce sterile abscesses or sloughs.

## Oral Dosage Forms

### AMOBARBITAL TABLETS USP

**Usual adult dose**

Sedative-hypnotic—
  Hypnotic:
    Oral, 65 to 200 mg at bedtime.
  Sedative:
    Daytime—Oral, 50 to 300 mg a day in divided doses.

Note: Geriatric and debilitated patients may react to usual doses with excitement, confusion, or mental depression. Lower doses may be required in these patients.

**Usual pediatric dose**

Sedative-hypnotic—
  Hypnotic:
    Dosage has not been established.
  Sedative:
    Daytime—Oral, 2 mg per kg of body weight or 60 mg per square meter of body surface three times a day.
    Preoperative—Oral, 2 to 6 mg per kg of body weight, up to a maximum of 100 mg per dose.

**Strength(s) usually available**

U.S.—
  Not commercially available.
Canada—
  30 mg (Rx) [*Amytal*].
  100 mg (Rx) [*Amytal*].

**Packaging and storage**

Store below 40 °C (104 °F), preferably between 15 and 30 °C (59 and 86 °F), unless otherwise specified by manufacturer. Store in a well-closed container.

**Auxiliary labeling**
- Avoid alcoholic beverages.
- May cause drowsiness.

**Note**

Controlled substance in the U.S. and Canada.

### AMOBARBITAL SODIUM CAPSULES USP

**Usual adult dose**

Sedative-hypnotic—
  Hypnotic:
    Oral, 65 to 200 mg at bedtime.
  Sedative:
    Daytime—Oral, 50 to 300 mg a day in divided doses.
    During labor—Oral, 200 to 400 mg, repeated every one to three hours, if necessary, up to a total dose of 1 gram.
    Preoperative—Oral, 200 mg one to two hours before surgery.

Note: Geriatric and debilitated patients may react to usual doses with excitement, confusion, or mental depression. Lower doses may be required in these patients.

**Usual pediatric dose**

Sedative-hypnotic—
  Hypnotic:
    Dosage has not been established.
  Sedative:
    Daytime—Oral, 2 mg per kg of body weight or 60 mg per square meter of body surface three times a day.
    Preoperative—Oral, 2 to 6 mg per kg of body weight, up to a maximum of 100 mg per dose.

**Strength(s) usually available**

U.S.—
  200 mg (Rx) [*Amytal;* GENERIC].
Canada—
  200 mg (Rx) [*Amytal*].

**Packaging and storage**
Store below 40 °C (104 °F), preferably between 15 and 30 °C (59 and 86 °F), unless otherwise specified by manufacturer. Store in a tight container.

**Auxiliary labeling**
• Avoid alcoholic beverages.
• May cause drowsiness.

**Note**
Controlled substance in the U.S. and Canada.

## Parenteral Dosage Forms
### AMOBARBITAL SODIUM STERILE USP

**Usual adult dose**
Sedative-hypnotic—
   Hypnotic:
      Intramuscular or intravenous, 65 to 200 mg.
   Sedative:
      Intramuscular or intravenous, 30 to 50 mg two or three times a day.
Anticonvulsant—
   Intravenous, 65 to 500 mg.

Note: Geriatric and debilitated patients may react to usual doses with excitement, confusion, or mental depression. Lower doses may be required in these patients.

**Usual adult prescribing limits**
Intramuscular, up to 500 mg per dose.
Intravenous, up to 1 gram per dose.

**Usual pediatric dose**
Sedative-hypnotic—
   Hypnotic:
      Children up to 6 years of age—
         Intramuscular, 2 to 3 mg per kg of body weight per dose.
      Children 6 years of age and over—
         Intramuscular, 2 to 3 mg per kg of body weight per dose.
         Intravenous, 65 to 500 mg per dose.
   Sedative:
      Preoperative—
         Intravenous, 65 to 500 mg or 3 to 5 mg per kg of body weight per dose.
Anticonvulsant—
   Children up to 6 years of age:
      Intramuscular or intravenous, 3 to 5 mg per kg of body weight or 125 mg per square meter of body surface per dose.
   Children 6 years of age and over:
      Intravenous, 65 to 500 mg per dose.

**Size(s) usually available**
U.S.—
   500 mg (Rx) [*Amytal*].
Canada—
   500 mg (Rx) [*Amytal*].

**Packaging and storage**
Prior to reconstitution, store below 40 °C (104 °F), preferably between 15 and 30 °C (59 and 86 °F), unless otherwise specified by manufacturer.

**Preparation of dosage form**
Solutions of amobarbital sodium should be prepared aseptically with sterile water for injection. For preparation of various concentrations of solutions for injection, see the manufacturer's package insert.

**Stability**
After reconstitution, solution should be used within 30 minutes since amobarbital sodium hydrolyzes in solution or upon exposure to air. Solution should not be used if it does not become absolutely clear within 5 minutes after reconstitution or if a precipitate forms after the solution clears.

**Note**
Controlled substance in the U.S. and Canada.

---

*APROBARBITAL*

## Summary of Differences
Pharmacology/pharmacokinetics:
   Intermediate-acting barbiturate—
      Onset of action: 45 to 60 minutes.
      Duration of action: 6 to 8 hours.
   Protein binding—
      Low.

## Oral Dosage Forms
### APROBARBITAL ELIXIR

**Usual adult dose**
Sedative-hypnotic—
   Hypnotic: Oral, 40 to 160 mg at bedtime.
   Sedative: Daytime—Oral, 40 mg three times a day.

Note: Geriatric and debilitated patients may react to usual doses with excitement, confusion, or mental depression. Lower doses may be required in these patients.

**Usual pediatric dose**
Dosage has not been established.

**Strength(s) usually available**
U.S.—
   40 mg per 5 mL (Rx) [*Alurate* (alcohol 20%; dextrose; saccharin; sorbitol; sucrose; FD&C Yellow No. 6; FD&C Red No. 40)].
Canada—
   Not commercially available.

**Packaging and storage**
Store below 40 °C (104 °F), preferably between 15 and 30 °C (59 and 86 °F), in a tight, light-resistant container, unless otherwise specified by manufacturer. Protect from freezing.

**Auxiliary labeling**
• Avoid alcoholic beverages.
• May cause drowsiness.
• Keep container tightly closed.

**Note**
Controlled substance in the U.S.

---

*BUTABARBITAL*

## Summary of Differences
Pharmacology/pharmacokinetics:
   Intermediate-acting barbiturate—
      Onset of action: 45 to 60 minutes.
      Duration of action: 6 to 8 hours.
   Protein binding—
      Low.

## Oral Dosage Forms
### BUTABARBITAL SODIUM ELIXIR USP

**Usual adult dose**
Sedative-hypnotic—
   Hypnotic:
      Oral, 50 to 100 mg at bedtime.
   Sedative:
      Daytime—Oral, 15 to 30 mg three or four times a day.
      Preoperative—Oral, 50 to 100 mg sixty to ninety minutes before surgery.

Note: Geriatric and debilitated patients may react to usual doses with excitement, confusion, or mental depression. Lower doses may be required in these patients.

**Usual pediatric dose**
Sedative-hypnotic—
   Hypnotic:
      Dosage must be individualized by physician.
   Sedative:
      Daytime—Oral, 2 mg per kg of body weight or 60 mg per square meter of body surface three times a day.
      Preoperative—Oral, 2 to 6 mg per kg of body weight, up to a maximum of 100 mg per dose.

**Strength(s) usually available**
U.S.—
   30 mg per 5 mL (Rx) [*Busodium; Butalan; Butisol* (alcohol [by volume] 7%; tartrazine); GENERIC].
Canada—
   Not commercially available.

**Packaging and storage**
Store below 40 °C (104 °F), preferably between 15 and 30 °C (59 and 86 °F), unless otherwise specified by manufacturer. Store in a tight container. Protect from freezing.

**Auxiliary labeling**
• Avoid alcoholic beverages.
• May cause drowsiness.
• Keep container tightly closed.

**Note**
Controlled substance in the U.S.

## BUTABARBITAL SODIUM TABLETS USP

**Usual adult dose**
See *Butabarbital Sodium Elixir USP.*

**Usual pediatric dose**
See *Butabarbital Sodium Elixir USP.*

**Strength(s) usually available**
U.S.—
    15 mg (Rx) [*Busodium; Butisol* (scored); GENERIC].
    30 mg (Rx) [*Busodium; Butisol* (scored; tartrazine); *Sarisol No. 2;*
      GENERIC].
    50 mg (Rx) [*Butisol* (scored; tartrazine)].
    100 mg (Rx) [*Busodium; Butisol* (scored); GENERIC].
Canada—
    15 mg (Rx) [*Butisol* (scored; sodium 2 mg)].
    30 mg (Rx) [*Butisol* (scored; sodium 3 mg; tartrazine)].
    100 mg (Rx) [*Butisol* (scored; sodium 10 mg)].

**Packaging and storage**
Store below 40 °C (104 °F), preferably between 15 and 30 °C (59 and 86 °F), unless otherwise specified by manufacturer. Store in a well-closed container.

**Auxiliary labeling**
• Avoid alcoholic beverages.
• May cause drowsiness.

**Note**
Controlled substance in the U.S. and Canada.

---

### *MEPHOBARBITAL*

## Summary of Differences

Category:
    Indicated only as an anticonvulsant.
Pharmacology/pharmacokinetics:
    Biotransformation—
        About 75% of a single dose metabolized to phenobarbital in 24 hours.
    Long-acting barbiturate—
        Onset of action: 60 minutes or longer.
        Duration of action: 10 to 12 hours.
Patient consultation:
    Compliance with therapy when used as an anticonvulsant.

## Additional Dosing Information

See also *General Dosing Information.*
In epilepsy
    • Therapy with mephobarbital should begin with small doses, the dosage being gradually increased over a period of 4 to 5 days until the optimum dosage is determined.
    • When used to replace another anticonvulsant, the dosage of mephobarbital should be gradually increased while the dosage of the other medication is maintained initially and then gradually decreased in order to maintain seizure control.
    • Mephobarbital may be alternated with phenobarbital therapy.
    • When used in conjunction with phenytoin, the dose of phenytoin may need to be reduced, but the full dose of mephobarbital may be given.
    • Mephobarbital should be withdrawn slowly in order to avoid precipitating seizures or status epilepticus. When the dosage is to be reduced to a maintenance level or discontinued, the amount should be reduced over a period of 4 to 5 days or possibly longer.

## Oral Dosage Forms

### MEPHOBARBITAL TABLETS USP

**Usual adult dose**
Anticonvulsant—
    Oral, 200 mg at bedtime to 600 mg a day in divided doses.
Sedative-hypnotic—
    Sedative: Daytime—Oral, 32 to 100 mg three or four times a day.
Note: Geriatric and debilitated patients may react to usual doses with excitement, confusion, or mental depression. Lower doses may be required in these patients.

**Usual pediatric dose**
Anticonvulsant—
    Children up to 5 years of age: Oral, 16 to 32 mg three or four times a day.
    Children 5 years of age and over: Oral, 32 to 64 mg three or four times a day.
Sedative-hypnotic—
    Sedative: Daytime—Oral, 16 to 32 mg three or four times a day.

**Strength(s) usually available**
U.S.—
    32 mg (Rx) [*Mebaral* (scored; lactose; starch; stearic acid; talc)].
    50 mg (Rx) [*Mebaral* (lactose; starch; stearic acid; talc)].
    100 mg (Rx) [*Mebaral* (lactose; starch; stearic acid; talc)].
Canada—
    30 mg (Rx) [*Mebaral* (lactose 65 mg)].
    100 mg (Rx) [*Mebaral* (lactose 59 mg)].

**Packaging and storage**
Store below 40 °C (104 °F), preferably between 15 and 30 °C (59 and 86 °F), unless otherwise specified by manufacturer. Store in a well-closed container.

**Auxiliary labeling**
• Avoid alcoholic beverages.
• May cause drowsiness.

**Note**
Controlled substance in the U.S. and Canada.

---

### *METHARBITAL*

## Summary of Differences

Category:
    Indicated only as an anticonvulsant.
Pharmacology/pharmacokinetics:
    Biotransformation—
        Metabolized to barbital.
    Long-acting barbiturate—
        Onset of action: 60 minutes or longer.
        Duration of action: 10 to 12 hours.
Patient consultation:
    Compliance with therapy.

## Additional Dosing Information

See also *General Dosing Information.*

Metharbital should be withdrawn gradually in order to avoid the possibility of precipitating seizures or status epilepticus.

When used to replace or supplement other anticonvulsant therapy, the dosage of metharbital should be gradually increased while the dosage of the other medication is maintained initially and then gradually decreased in order to maintain seizure control.

## Oral Dosage Forms

### METHARBITAL TABLETS

**Usual adult dose**
Anticonvulsant—
    Oral, initially 100 mg one to three times a day, the dosage being increased up to 800 mg per day, if necessary.
Note: Geriatric and debilitated patients may react to usual doses with excitement, confusion, or mental depression. Lower doses may be required in these patients.

**Usual pediatric dose**
Anticonvulsant—
    Oral, 50 mg one to three times a day; or 5 to 15 mg per kg of body weight per day in divided doses.

**Strength(s) usually available**
U.S.—
    Not commercially available.
Canada—
    Not commercially available.
In other countries—
    100 mg [*Gemonil* (scored; lactose)].

**Packaging and storage**
Store below 40 °C (104 °F), preferably between 15 and 30 °C (59 and 86 °F), unless otherwise specified by manufacturer. Store in a tight container.

**Auxiliary labeling**
• Avoid alcoholic beverages.
• May cause drowsiness.

---

## PENTOBARBITAL

## Summary of Differences

Category:
Parenteral pentobarbital also may be indicated as an anticonvulsant.
Indications:
Parenteral pentobarbital also used to protect brain from ischemia and increased intracranial pressure that follow stroke and head trauma.
Pharmacology/pharmacokinetics:
Short-acting barbiturate—
Onset of action: 10 to 15 minutes.
Duration of action: 3 to 4 hours.
Protein binding:
Moderate to high.

## Additional Dosing Information

See also *General Dosing Information*.

When administered during labor, doses greater than 200 mg may cause respiratory depression in the newborn.

**For parenteral dosage forms only**
The injection is for intramuscular or intravenous use only; it is not recommended for subcutaneous administration.
Intravenous injections should be made slowly, not to exceed 50 mg per minute, to avoid adverse respiratory and circulatory reactions.

## Oral Dosage Forms
### PENTOBARBITAL ELIXIR USP

**Usual adult dose**
Sedative-hypnotic—
Hypnotic:
Oral, 100 mg (pentobarbital sodium) at bedtime.
Sedative:
Daytime—Oral, 20 mg (pentobarbital sodium) three or four times a day.

Note: Geriatric and debilitated patients may react to usual doses with excitement, confusion, or mental depression. Lower doses may be required in these patients.

**Usual pediatric dose**
Sedative-hypnotic—
Hypnotic:
Dosage must be individualized by physician.
Sedative:
Daytime—Oral, 2 to 6 mg (pentobarbital sodium) per kg of body weight per day.
Preoperative—Oral, 2 to 6 mg (pentobarbital sodium) per kg of body weight, up to a maximum of 100 mg per dose.

**Strength(s) usually available**
U.S.—
20 mg of pentobarbital sodium (18.2 mg of pentobarbital) per 5 mL (Rx) [*Nembutal* (alcohol 18%)].
Canada—
Not commercially available.

**Packaging and storage**
Store below 40 °C (104 °F), preferably between 15 and 30 °C (59 and 86 °F), unless otherwise specified by manufacturer. Store in a tight container. Protect from freezing.

**Auxiliary labeling**
• Avoid alcoholic beverages.
• May cause drowsiness.
• Keep container tightly closed.

**Note**
Controlled substance in the U.S.

### PENTOBARBITAL SODIUM CAPSULES USP

**Usual adult dose**
Sedative-hypnotic—
Hypnotic: Oral, 100 mg at bedtime.
Sedative: Preoperative—Oral, 100 mg.

Note: Geriatric and debilitated patients may react to usual doses with excitement, confusion, or mental depression. Lower doses may be required in these patients.

**Usual pediatric dose**
Sedative-hypnotic—
Hypnotic: Dosage must be individualized by physician.
Sedative: Preoperative—Oral, 2 to 6 mg per kg of body weight, up to a maximum of 100 mg per dose.

**Strength(s) usually available**
U.S.—
50 mg (Rx) [*Nembutal;* GENERIC].
100 mg (Rx) [*Nembutal* (tartrazine); GENERIC].
Canada—
100 mg (Rx) [*Nembutal* (tartrazine); *Novopentobarb*].

**Packaging and storage**
Store below 40 °C (104 °F), preferably between 15 and 30 °C (59 and 86 °F), unless otherwise specified by manufacturer. Store in a tight container.

**Auxiliary labeling**
• Avoid alcoholic beverages.
• May cause drowsiness.

**Note**
Controlled substance in the U.S. and Canada.

## Parenteral Dosage Forms
### PENTOBARBITAL SODIUM INJECTION USP

**Usual adult dose**
Sedative-hypnotic—
Hypnotic:
Intramuscular, 150 to 200 mg.
Intravenous, 100 mg initially; after one minute, additional small doses may be administered at one-minute intervals, if necessary, up to a total of 500 mg.
Sedative:
Preoperative—Intramuscular, 150 to 200 mg.
Anticonvulsant—
Intravenous, 100 mg initially; after one minute, additional small doses may be administered at one-minute intervals, if necessary, up to a total of 500 mg.

Note: Geriatric and debilitated patients may react to usual doses with excitement, confusion, or mental depression. Lower doses may be required in these patients.

**Usual pediatric dose**
Sedative-hypnotic—
Hypnotic:
Intramuscular, 2 to 6 mg per kg of body weight, up to a maximum of 100 mg per dose.
Intravenous, 50 mg initially; after one minute, additional small doses may be administered at one-minute intervals, if necessary, until desired effect is obtained.
Sedative:
Preoperative—Intramuscular, 2 to 6 mg per kg of body weight, up to a maximum of 100 mg per dose.
Anticonvulsant—
Intramuscular or intravenous, 50 mg initially; after one minute, additional small doses may be administered at one-minute intervals, if necessary, until desired effect is obtained.

**Strength(s) usually available**
U.S.—
50 mg per mL (Rx) [*Nembutal* (alcohol 10%; propylene glycol 40% v/v); GENERIC].
Canada—
50 mg per mL (Rx) [*Nembutal* (alcohol 10%; propylene glycol 40%)].

**Packaging and storage**
Store below 40 °C (104 °F), preferably between 15 and 30 °C (59 and 86 °F), unless otherwise specified by manufacturer. Protect from freezing.

**Stability**
Do not use if solution is discolored or contains a precipitate.

**Note**
Controlled substance in the U.S. and Canada.

## Rectal Dosage Forms
### PENTOBARBITAL SODIUM SUPPOSITORIES

**Usual adult dose**
Sedative-hypnotic—
Hypnotic:
Rectal, 120 to 200 mg at bedtime.
Sedative:
Daytime—Rectal, 30 mg two to four times a day.

Note: Geriatric and debilitated patients may react to usual doses with excitement, confusion, or mental depression. Lower doses may be required in these patients.

**Usual pediatric dose**
Sedative-hypnotic—
Hypnotic:
Children up to 2 months of age: Dosage has not been established.
Children 2 months to 1 year of age (4.5 to 9 kg): Rectal, 30 mg.
Children 1 to 4 years of age (9 to 18 kg): Rectal, 30 or 60 mg.
Children 5 to 12 years of age (18 to 36 kg): Rectal, 60 mg.
Children 12 to 14 years of age (36 to 50 kg): Rectal, 60 or 120 mg.
Sedative:
Daytime—
Rectal, 2 mg per kg of body weight or 60 mg per square meter of body surface three times a day.
Preoperative—
Children up to 2 months of age: Dosage has not been established.
Children 2 months to 1 year of age: Rectal, 30 mg.
Children 1 to 4 years of age: Rectal, 30 or 60 mg.
Children 5 to 12 years of age: Rectal, 60 mg.
Children 12 to 14 years of age: Rectal, 60 or 120 mg.

**Strength(s) usually available**
U.S.—
30 mg (Rx) [*Nembutal* (semisynthetic glycerides)].
60 mg (Rx) [*Nembutal* (semisynthetic glycerides)].
120 mg (Rx) [*Nembutal* (semisynthetic glycerides)].
200 mg (Rx) [*Nembutal* (semisynthetic glycerides)].
Canada—
25 mg (Rx) [*Nova Rectal* (in a polyethylene glycol base)].
50 mg (Rx) [*Nova Rectal* (in a polyethylene glycol base)].

**Packaging and storage**
Store between 2 and 15 °C (36 and 59 °F), in a well-closed container, unless otherwise specified by manufacturer.

**Auxiliary labeling**
• For rectal use only.
• Avoid alcoholic beverages.
• May cause drowsiness.
• Refrigerate.

**Note**
Controlled substance in the U.S. and Canada.

---

## PHENOBARBITAL

## Summary of Differences

Category:
Also indicated as an anticonvulsant.
Oral and parenteral phenobarbital also used as an antihyperbilirubinemic; and has been used as an antitremor agent, although generally has been replaced by benzodiazepines and beta-adrenergic blockers.
Pharmacology/pharmacokinetics:
Distribution—
Distributed less rapidly than other barbiturates because it has lowest lipid solubility.
Time to peak effect—
Maximal CNS depression may not occur for 15 minutes or more after intravenous administration.
Long-acting barbiturate—
Onset of action: 60 minutes or longer.
Duration of action: 10 to 12 hours.
Protein binding—
Low to moderate.
Patient consultation:
Compliance with therapy when used as an anticonvulsant.

## Additional Dosing Information

See also *General Dosing Information*.
In epilepsy
• In children, higher-per-kg dosage of phenobarbital and most other anticonvulsants generally are required to achieve blood concentrations considered therapeutic.
• Several weeks of phenobarbital therapy may be required to achieve maximum antiepilepsy effects.
• Phenobarbital should be withdrawn slowly in order to avoid precipitating seizures or status epilepticus.

• When phenobarbital is replaced by another anticonvulsant, the dosage of phenobarbital should be maintained initially and then reduced gradually while, at the same time, the dosage of the replacement medication is increased gradually in order to maintain seizure control.
• When administered intravenously, phenobarbital sodium may require 15 minutes or more to attain peak concentrations in the brain; therefore, it is important to use the minimal dosage required and to wait for the anticonvulsant effect to develop before administering a second dose, in order to avoid the possibility of severe barbiturate-induced depression.

**For parenteral dosage forms only**
Sterile phenobarbital sodium may be administered subcutaneously after reconstitution, but phenobarbital sodium injection is not recommended for subcutaneous use.
The rate of the intravenous injection should not exceed 60 mg per minute. Faster rates of administration may cause serious respiratory depression.
Following intravenous administration, up to 30 minutes may be required for maximum effect.

**Bioequivalence information**
For phenobarbital tablets—
Bioavailability differences between generic products from different manufacturers have been reported in the past. However, no controlled studies systematically comparing the large number of tablets commercially available from different manufacturers have been conducted. In two studies published in 1979 and 1984 comparing phenobarbital tablets from different manufacturers in male volunteers, there were no significant differences in mean peak plasma concentrations ($C_{max}$) or relative area under the plasma concentration-time curve (AUC); however, statistically significant delays in reaching time of peak concentration ($t_{max}$) were demonstrated among products. In response to the potential problem of bio-inequivalence, official dissolution standards were changed, and problems have not been documented in the years following establishment of these standards. The current standard excludes slow-dissolving tablets.

## Oral Dosage Forms

Note: Bracketed uses in the *Dosage Forms* section refer to categories of use and/or indications that are not included in U.S. product labeling.

### PHENOBARBITAL CAPSULES

**Usual adult dose**
Anticonvulsant—
Oral, 60 to 250 mg (base) per day, as a single dose or in divided doses.
Sedative-hypnotic—
Hypnotic: Oral, 100 to 320 mg (base) at bedtime.
Sedative: Daytime—Oral, 30 to 120 mg (base) in two or three divided doses a day.
[Antihyperbilirubinemic][1]—
Oral, 30 to 60 mg (base) three times a day.
Note: Geriatric and debilitated patients may react to usual doses with excitement, confusion, or mental depression. Lower doses may be required in these patients.

**Usual pediatric dose**
Anticonvulsant—
Oral, 1 to 6 mg (base) per kg of body weight per day, as a single dose or in divided doses.
Sedative-hypnotic—
Hypnotic:
Dosage must be individualized by physician.
Sedative:
Daytime—Oral, 2 mg (base) per kg of body weight or 60 mg per square meter of body surface three times a day.
Preoperative—Oral, 1 to 3 mg (base) per kg of body weight.
[Antihyperbilirubinemic][1]—
Neonates: Oral, 5 to 10 mg (base) per kg of body weight per day for the first few days after birth.
Children up to 12 years of age: Oral, 1 to 4 mg (base) per kg of body weight three times a day.

**Strength(s) usually available**
U.S.—
15 mg (Rx) [*Solfoton*].
Canada—
Not commercially available.

**Packaging and storage**
Store below 40 °C (104 °F), preferably between 15 and 30 °C (59 and 86 °F), in a well-closed container, unless otherwise specified by manufacturer.

**Auxiliary labeling**
• Avoid alcoholic beverages.
• May cause drowsiness.

**Note**
Controlled substance in the U.S.

## PHENOBARBITAL ELIXIR USP

**Usual adult dose**
See *Phenobarbital Capsules.*

**Usual pediatric dose**
See *Phenobarbital Capsules.*

**Strength(s) usually available**
U.S.—
    20 mg per 5 mL (Rx) [GENERIC].
Canada—
    20 mg per 5 mL (Rx) [*Ancalixir*].

**Packaging and storage**
Store below 40 °C (104 °F), preferably between 15 and 30 °C (59 and 86 °F), unless otherwise specified by manufacturer. Store in a tight, light-resistant container. Protect from freezing.

**Auxiliary labeling**
• Avoid alcoholic beverages.
• May cause drowsiness.
• Keep container tightly closed.

**Note**
Controlled substance in the U.S. and Canada.

## PHENOBARBITAL TABLETS USP

Note: Bioavailability differences between products from different manufacturers have been reported in the past. However, no controlled studies systematically comparing the large number of tablets commercially available from different manufacturers have been conducted. In two studies published in 1979 and 1984 comparing phenobarbital tablets from different manufacturers in male volunteers, there were no significant differences in mean peak plasma concentrations ($C_{max}$) or relative area under the plasma concentration-time curve (AUC); however, statistically significant delays in reaching time of peak concentration ($T_{max}$) were demonstrated among products. In response to the potential problem of bio-inequivalence, official dissolution standards were changed, and problems have not been documented in the years following establishment of these standards. The current standard excludes slow-dissolving tablets.

**Usual adult dose**
See *Phenobarbital Capsules.*

**Usual pediatric dose**
See *Phenobarbital Capsules.*

**Strength(s) usually available**
U.S.—
    8 mg (Rx) [GENERIC].
    15 mg (Rx) [*Barbita; Solfoton;* GENERIC].
    30 mg (Rx) [GENERIC].
    60 mg (Rx) [GENERIC].
    100 mg (Rx) [GENERIC].
Canada—
    15 mg (Rx) [GENERIC].
    30 mg (Rx) [GENERIC].
    60 mg (Rx) [GENERIC].
    100 mg (Rx) [GENERIC].

**Packaging and storage**
Store below 40 °C (104 °F), preferably between 15 and 30 °C (59 and 86 °F), unless otherwise specified by manufacturer. Store in a well-closed container.

**Auxiliary labeling**
• Avoid alcoholic beverages.
• May cause drowsiness.

**Note**
Controlled substance in the U.S. and Canada.

## Parenteral Dosage Forms

Note: Bracketed uses in the *Dosage Forms* section refer to categories of use and/or indications that are not included in U.S. product labeling.

### PHENOBARBITAL SODIUM INJECTION USP

**Usual adult dose**
Anticonvulsant—
    Intravenous, 100 to 320 mg, repeated if necessary up to a total dose of 600 mg during a twenty-four-hour period.

Status epilepticus: Intravenous (slow), 10 to 20 mg per kg of body weight, repeated if necessary.
Sedative-hypnotic—
    Hypnotic:
        Intramuscular or intravenous, 100 to 325 mg.
    Sedative:
        Daytime—Intramuscular or intravenous, 30 to 120 mg a day in two or three divided doses.
        Preoperative—Intramuscular, 130 to 200 mg sixty to ninety minutes before surgery.
Note: Geriatric and debilitated patients may react to usual doses with excitement, confusion, or mental depression. Lower doses may be required in these patients.

**Usual pediatric dose**
Anticonvulsant—
    Initial: Intravenous, 10 to 20 mg per kg of body weight as a single loading dose.
    Maintenance: Intravenous, 1 to 6 mg per kg of body weight per day.
    Status epilepticus: Intravenous, 15 to 20 mg per kg of body weight, administered over a period of ten to fifteen minutes.
Sedative-hypnotic—
    Hypnotic: Dosage must be individualized.
    Sedative: Preoperative—Intramuscular or intravenous, 1 to 3 mg per kg of body weight, sixty to ninety minutes prior to surgery.
[Antihyperbilirubinemic][1]—
    Intramuscular, 5 to 10 mg per kg of body weight per day for the first few days after birth.

**Strength(s) usually available**
U.S.—
    30 mg per mL (Rx) [GENERIC].
    60 mg per mL (Rx) [GENERIC].
    65 mg per mL (Rx) [GENERIC].
    130 mg per mL (Rx) [*Luminal* (alcohol 10%; propylene glycol 67.8% by volume); GENERIC].
Canada—
    30 mg per mL (Rx) [GENERIC].
    120 mg per mL (Rx) [GENERIC].

**Packaging and storage**
Store below 40 °C (104 °F), preferably between 15 and 30 °C (59 and 86 °F), unless otherwise specified by manufacturer. Protect from freezing.

**Stability**
Do not use if solution is discolored or contains a precipitate.

**Note**
Controlled substance in the U.S. and Canada.

### PHENOBARBITAL SODIUM STERILE USP

**Usual adult dose**
Anticonvulsant—
    Intravenous, 100 to 320 mg, repeated if necessary up to a total dose of 600 mg during a twenty-four-hour period.
    Status epilepticus: Intravenous (slow), 10 to 20 mg per kg of body weight, repeated if necessary.
Sedative-hypnotic—
    Hypnotic:
        Intramuscular, intravenous, or subcutaneous, 100 to 325 mg.
    Sedative:
        Daytime—Intramuscular, intravenous, or subcutaneous, 30 to 120 mg a day in two or three divided doses.
        Preoperative—Intramuscular, 130 to 200 mg sixty to ninety minutes before surgery.
Note: Geriatric and debilitated patients may react to usual doses of barbiturates with excitement, confusion, or mental depression. Lower doses may be required in these patients.

**Usual pediatric dose**
Anticonvulsant—
    Initial: Intravenous, 10 to 20 mg per kg of body weight as a single loading dose.
    Maintenance: Intravenous, 1 to 6 mg per kg of body weight per day.
    Status epilepticus: Intravenous, 15 to 20 mg per kg of body weight, administered over a period of ten to fifteen minutes.
Sedative-hypnotic—
    Hypnotic: Dosage must be individualized.
    Sedative: Preoperative—Intramuscular, 1 to 3 mg per kg of body weight.
[Antihyperbilirubinemic][1]—
    Intramuscular, 5 to 10 mg per kg of body weight per day for the first few days after birth.

## Size(s) usually available
U.S.—
120 mg (Rx) [GENERIC].
Canada—
Not commercially available.

## Packaging and storage
Prior to reconstitution, store below 40 °C (104 °F), preferably between 15 and 30 °C (59 and 86 °F), unless otherwise specified by manufacturer.

## Preparation of dosage form
Solutions of phenobarbital sodium for subcutaneous or intramuscular injection may be prepared by dissolving 120 mg of anhydrous phenobarbital sodium powder in 1 mL of sterile water for injection. For intravenous use, 120 mg of anhydrous phenobarbital sodium powder should be dissolved in 3 mL of sterile water for injection. When solutions are prepared, the sterile water for injection should be introduced slowly into the vial by means of a sterile syringe. Several minutes may be required for the medication to dissolve completely; solution should not be injected if it has not become clear after 5 minutes.

## Stability
After reconstitution, solution should be used within thirty minutes since phenobarbital hydrolyzes in solution or upon exposure to air. Solution should not be used if it does not become absolutely clear within 5 minutes after reconstitution or if a precipitate forms after the solution clears.

## Note
Controlled substance in the U.S.

---

[1]Not included in Canadian product labeling.

---

## *SECOBARBITAL*

## Summary of Differences
Category:
Parenteral secobarbital also may be indicated as an anticonvulsant (in tetanus).
Pharmacology/pharmacokinetics:
Distribution:
Distributed more rapidly than other barbiturates because it has highest lipid solubility.
Short-acting barbiturate—
Onset of action: 10 to 15 minutes.
Duration of action: 3 to 4 hours.
Protein binding—
Moderate to high.

## Additional Dosing Information

See also *General Dosing Information.*

## For parenteral dosage forms only
The rate of the intravenous injection should not exceed 50 mg per 15-second period. Faster rates of administration may cause respiratory depression or apnea, laryngospasm, or vasodilation with fall in blood pressure.

## For rectal dosage forms only
To prepare a solution for rectal administration, dilute the commercially available 5% secobarbital sodium injection with lukewarm tap water to a concentration of 10 to 15 mg per mL (1 to 1.5%).

## Oral Dosage Forms
## SECOBARBITAL SODIUM CAPSULES USP

## Usual adult dose
Sedative-hypnotic—
Hypnotic:
Oral, 100 mg at bedtime.
Sedative:
Daytime—Oral, 30 to 50 mg three or four times a day.
Preoperative—Oral, 200 to 300 mg one to two hours before surgery.
Note: Geriatric and debilitated patients may react to usual doses with excitement, confusion, or mental depression. Lower doses may be required in these patients.

## Usual pediatric dose
Sedative-hypnotic—
Sedative:
Daytime—Oral, 2 mg per kg of body weight or 60 mg per square meter of body surface three times a day.

Preoperative—Oral, 2 to 6 mg per kg of body weight, up to a maximum of 100 mg per dose, one to two hours before surgery.

## Strength(s) usually available
U.S.—
100 mg (Rx) [*Seconal;* GENERIC].
Canada—
50 mg (Rx) [*Seconal*].
100 mg (Rx) [*Novosecobarb; Seconal*].

## Packaging and storage
Store below 40 °C (104 °F), preferably between 15 and 30 °C (59 and 86 °F), unless otherwise specified by manufacturer. Store in a tight container.

## Auxiliary labeling
• Avoid alcoholic beverages.
• May cause drowsiness.

## Note
Controlled substance in the U.S. and Canada.

## Parenteral Dosage Forms
## SECOBARBITAL SODIUM INJECTION USP

## Usual adult dose
Sedative-hypnotic—
Hypnotic:
Intramuscular, 100 to 200 mg.
Intravenous, 50 to 250 mg.
Sedative:
Dentistry—Intramuscular, 1.1 to 2.2 mg per kg of body weight ten to fifteen minutes before procedure.
Nerve block—Intravenous, 100 to 150 mg.
Anticonvulsant (in tetanus)—
Intramuscular or intravenous, 5.5 mg per kg of body weight, repeated every three to four hours as needed.
Note: Geriatric and debilitated patients may react to usual doses of barbiturates with excitement, confusion, or mental depression. Lower doses may be required in these patients.

## Usual pediatric dose
Sedative-hypnotic—
Hypnotic:
Intramuscular—
3 to 5 mg per kg of body weight or 125 mg per square meter of body surface, up to a maximum of 100 mg per dose.
Rectal, the following doses as a 1 to 1.5% solution—
Children weighing up to 40 kg: 5 mg per kg of body weight.
Children weighing 40 kg and over: 4 mg per kg of body weight.
Sedative:
Preoperative—
Intramuscular, 4 to 5 mg per kg of body weight.
Anticonvulsant (in tetanus)—
Intramuscular or intravenous, 3 to 5 mg per kg of body weight or 125 mg per square meter of body surface per dose.

## Strength(s) usually available
U.S.—
50 mg per mL (Rx) [GENERIC].
Canada—
Not commercially available.

## Packaging and storage
Store between 2 and 8 °C (36 and 46 °F). Protect from light.

## Preparation of dosage form
Secobarbital sodium injection may be administered in a concentration of 50 mg per mL or it may be diluted with sterile water for injection, 0.9% sodium chloride injection, or Ringer's injection.

## Stability
Do not use if solution is discolored or contains a precipitate.

## Note
Controlled substance in the U.S.

---

## *SECOBARBITAL AND AMOBARBITAL*

## Oral Dosage Forms
## SECOBARBITAL SODIUM AND AMOBARBITAL SODIUM CAPSULES USP

## Usual adult dose
Sedative-hypnotic—
Oral, 1 capsule at bedtime or one hour preoperatively.

Note: Geriatric and debilitated patients may react to usual doses with excitement, confusion, or mental depression. Lower doses may be required in these patients.

**Usual pediatric dose**
Dosage has not been established.

**Strength(s) usually available**
U.S.—
  50 mg of secobarbital and 50 mg of amobarbital (Rx) [*Tuinal*].
  100 mg of secobarbital and 100 mg of amobarbital (Rx) [*Tuinal*].
Canada—
  50 mg of secobarbital and 50 mg of amobarbital (Rx) [*Tuinal*].
  100 mg of secobarbital and 100 mg of amobarbital (Rx) [*Tuinal*].

**Packaging and storage**
Store below 40 °C (104 °F), preferably between 15 and 30 °C (59 and 86 °F), unless otherwise specified by manufacturer. Store in a well-closed container.

**Auxiliary labeling**
• Avoid alcoholic beverages.
• May cause drowsiness.

**Note**
Controlled substance in the U.S. and Canada.

Revised: 01/27/92
Interim revision: 08/29/94; 08/15/95

## Table 1. Pharmacology/Pharmacokinetics

| Drug | Protein Binding* (%) | Half-life (hr) | | Onset of Action† (min) | Duration of Action‡ (hr) | Elimination/ % Excreted Unchanged§ |
|------|------|------|------|------|------|------|
| | | Range | Mean | | | |
| Long-acting | | | | 60 or longer | 10–12 | |
| Mephobarbital# | | 11–67 | 34 | | | Renal |
| Metharbital | | | | | | Renal/2%; 20% excreted as barbital |
| Phenobarbital | Low to Moderate (20–45) | 53–118** | 79 | | | Renal/25–50% |
| Intermediate-acting | | | | 45–60 | 6–8 | |
| Amobarbital | Moderate (61) | 16–40 | 25 | | | Renal/<1% |
| Aprobarbital | Low (20) | 14–34 | 24 | | | Renal/25–50% |
| Butabarbital | Low (26) | 34–42 | †† | | | Renal/<1% |
| Short-acting | | | | 10–15 | 3–4 | |
| Pentobarbital | Moderate to High (60–70) | 15–50 | ‡‡ | | | Renal/<1% |
| Secobarbital | Moderate to High (46–70) | 15–40 | 28 | | | Renal/5% |

*Bound to plasma and tissue proteins to a varying degree; binding increases proportionate to lipid solubility.
†Following oral administration. Phenobarbital has the slowest, and secobarbital the fastest, onset of action.
‡Following oral administration. Duration of action is related to the rate at which the barbiturates are redistributed throughout the body and is variable among individuals and in the same individual from time to time. Phenobarbital has the longest, and secobarbital the shortest, duration of action.
§Metabolic products are excreted in the urine and, less commonly, in the feces. Inactive metabolites are excreted as conjugates of glucuronic acid.
  Peritoneal dialysis and hemodialysis remove phenobarbital from the body; serum phenobarbital concentrations should be determined during and after peritoneal dialysis and hemodialysis.
#Activity due mostly to accumulation of phenobarbital.
**Half-life is 60 to 180 hours in children (half-life 48 hours or less for newborns).
††One manufacturer states that the half-life of butabarbital is 100 hours.
‡‡Dose-dependent; the mean half-life of elimination is 50 and 22 hours following a 50- and 100-mg dose, respectively.

## Table 2. General Dosing Information

Note: In acute overdosage, the blood barbiturate concentration for some of the barbiturates relative to the degree of CNS depression in nontolerant persons is as follows:

| Drug | Onset/Duration of Action | Barbiturate Blood Concentrations (mcg/mL) | | | | |
|------|--------------------------|------|------|------|------|------|
| | | Categories of Degree of CNS Depression* | | | | |
| | | (1) | (2) | (3) | (4) | (5) |
| Pentobarbital | Fast/short | ≤2 | 0.5–3 | 10–15 | 12–25 | 15–40 |
| Secobarbital | Fast/short | ≤2 | 0.5–5 | 10–15 | 15–25 | 15–40 |
| Amobarbital | Intermediate/intermediate | ≤3 | 2–10 | 30–40 | 30–60 | 40–80 |
| Butabarbital | Intermediate/intermediate | ≤5 | 3–25 | 40–60 | 50–80 | 60–100 |
| Phenobarbital | Slow/long | ≤10 | 5–40 | 50–80 | 70–120 | 100–200 |

*Categories of degree of CNS depression in nontolerant persons:
(1) Under the influence and appreciably impaired for purposes of driving a motor vehicle or performing tasks requiring alertness and unimpaired judgment and reaction time.
(2) Sedated, therapeutic range, calm, relaxed, and easily aroused.
(3) Comatose, difficult to arouse, and significant respiratory depression.
(4) Comparable with death in aged or ill persons or in presence of obstructed airway, other toxic agents, or exposure to cold.
(5) Usual lethal concentration, the upper end of the range includes those who received some supportive treatment.

# BARBITURATES AND ANALGESICS   Systemic

This monograph includes information on the following: Butalbital and Acetaminophen; Butalbital and Aspirin; Butalbital, Aspirin‡, Caffeine, and Codeine; Phenobarbital, ASA‡, and Codeine.

PEN:
Butalbital, Acetaminophen, and Caffeine—Co-bucafAPAP

INN:
Acetaminophen—Paracetamol

VA CLASSIFICATION (Primary):
Butalbital and Acetaminophen—CN103
Butalbital and Aspirin—CN103
Butalbital, Aspirin, Caffeine, and Codeine—CN101
Phenobarbital, ASA‡, and Codeine—CN101

NOTE: The *Barbiturates and Analgesics (Systemic)* monograph is maintained in the USP DI electronic database. For a printed copy of the most recent revision of the complete monograph, contact the USP Division of Information Development, 12601 Twinbrook Parkway, Rockville, MD 20852.

The information that follows is selectively abstracted from the complete monograph and is provided to facilitate drug use review and patient counseling.

Note: For a listing of dosage forms and brand names by country availability, see *Dosage Forms* section(s). For a listing of brand names for the articles in this monograph, refer to the General Index.

‡In Canada, *Aspirin* is a brand name; acetylsalicylic acid is the generic name. ASA, a commonly used designation for aspirin (or acetylsalicylic acid) in both the U.S. and Canada, is the term used in Canadian product labeling.

## Category
Analgesic.

## Indications

Note: Bracketed information in the *Indications* section refers to uses that are not included in U.S. product labeling.

### Accepted
Headache, tension-type (treatment)—Barbiturate and analgesic combinations are indicated for relief of the symptoms of occasional tension-type (muscle contraction) headache.

[Headache, migraine (treatment)]—Barbiturate and analgesic combinations are indicated to relieve occasional migraine[1] and coexisting migraine and tension-type headaches ("mixed" headache syndrome).

Note: Because of the risk of habituation, barbiturate and analgesic combinations are not recommended for treatment of frequent, especially daily, headaches.

To reduce analgesic use, underlying problems that may contribute to tension-type headaches, such as inflammation or structural ab-

normalities in the cervical or temporomandibular areas, should be identified and treated. In some patients, application of heat, muscle relaxants, and/or physical therapy may be helpful. Other medications having the potential to cause habituation (e.g., benzodiazepines) should be used as infrequently as possible.

Chronic tension-type headaches and severe migraines that occur more frequently than twice a month may require additional prophylactic treatment to reduce the frequency, severity, and/or duration of the headaches. The prophylactic agents most commonly used for tension-type headaches are tricyclic antidepressants, especially amitriptyline, and/or beta-adrenergic blocking agents, especially propranolol. For migraines, beta-adrenergic blocking agents, calcium channel blocking agents, tricyclic antidepressants, monoamine oxidase inhibitors, methysergide, pizotyline (not commercially available in the U.S.), and sometimes cyproheptadine (especially in children) are used for prophylaxis. The combination of amitriptyline plus propranolol has been found superior to either agent used alone in preventing "mixed" headaches.

Identification and avoidance of precipitating factors is also important in the overall management of the patient with migraine headaches. Relaxation and/or biofeedback techniques may also be helpful in controlling migraine headaches, and may reduce the need for medication.

[Pain (treatment)]—Barbiturate and analgesic combinations are also indicated for relief of pain other than headache, especially when an antianxiety or relaxant effect is desired.

[1]Not included in Canadian product labeling.

## Pharmacology/Pharmacokinetics

Butalbital: 224.26
Phenobarbital: See *Barbiturates (Systemic)*.
Acetaminophen: See *Acetaminophen (Systemic)*.
Aspirin: See *Salicylates (Systemic)*.
Codeine phosphate: See *Opioid (Narcotic) Analgesics (Systemic)*.
Caffeine (anhydrous): See *Caffeine (Systemic)*.

Note: Gastric stasis that accompanies migraine headaches tends to inhibit absorption of orally administered medications, which may result in alteration of some of the pharmacokinetic values reported below. Consequently, the onset of action of these medications may be delayed and/or their efficacy decreased, especially if they are taken after a migraine is well established.

## Precautions to Consider

Butalbital: See *Barbiturates (Systemic)*. Although butalbital is not specifically mentioned in that monograph, general precautions applying to all barbiturates may apply to butalbital also.
Phenobarbital: See *Barbiturates (Systemic)*.
Acetaminophen: See *Acetaminophen (Systemic)*.
Aspirin: See *Salicylates (Systemic)*.

Codeine: See *Opioid (Narcotic) Analgesics (Systemic)*.
Caffeine: See *Caffeine (Systemic)*.

## Side/Adverse Effects

Butalbital: See *Barbiturates (Systemic)*. Although butalbital is not specifically mentioned in that monograph, butalbital may be expected to share general precautions that apply to, and side/adverse effects characteristics of, other barbiturates.

Phenobarbital: See *Barbiturates (Systemic)*.
Acetaminophen: See *Acetaminophen (Systemic)*.
Aspirin: See *Salicylates (Systemic)*.
Codeine: See *Opioid (Narcotic) Analgesics (Systemic)*.
Caffeine: See *Caffeine (Systemic)*.

## Patient Consultation

See *Table 1*, page 518.

## Overdose

Butalbital: See *Barbiturates (Systemic)*. Although butalbital is not specifically mentioned in that monograph, measures used to treat overdose of other barbiturates would be expected to be effective for treating butalbital overdose also.

Phenobarbital: See *Barbiturates (Systemic)*.
Acetaminophen: See *Acetaminophen (Systemic)*.
Aspirin: See *Salicylates (Systemic)*.
Codeine: See *Opioids (Narcotic) Analgesics (Systemic)*.
Caffeine: See *Caffeine (Systemic)*.

## General Dosing Information

When used for relief of headache, especially a migraine headache, a barbiturate and analgesic combination will be most effective if administered when the first symptoms appear (during the prodrome, for migraine with aura).

After the first dose has been administered, it is recommended that the patient lie down and relax in a quiet, darkened room, because this contributes to relief of headaches.

A reduction in dosage may be required for elderly or debilitated patients, who may react to usual doses of barbiturates with excitement, confusion, or depression. This is particularly important for the codeine-containing combinations, because these patients are also more sensitive to the respiratory depressant effects of codeine.

Tolerance may occur with repeated administration of large doses of barbiturates or codeine. Also, patients who are tolerant to the effects of other opioids may be at least partially cross-tolerant to the effects of codeine, and vice versa.

Prolonged uninterrupted use of codeine or barbiturates may result in psychic or physical dependence; in patients taking these medications for relief of pain other than headache pain, gradual withdrawal may be required to reduce the risk of precipitating withdrawal symptoms.

In headache-prone individuals, frequent use of analgesics may cause physical dependence, leading to both analgesic abuse and chronic (daily or near-daily) headaches. Chronic daily use of caffeine may also result in the development of physical dependence, leading to withdrawal (rebound) headaches when the medication is stopped and to further ingestion of caffeine-containing analgesics. Patients who experience frequent headaches may be dependent on a variety of medications, including opioid analgesics, nonopioid analgesics such as acetaminophen or aspirin, ergotamine-containing headache suppressants, and antianxiety agents or sedatives, as well as barbiturate and analgesic combinations.

Chronic headaches resulting from overmedication may be difficult to relieve, especially if the patient continues to take ergotamine-containing headache suppressants and/or analgesics. If such headaches occur, it is recommended that these medications be discontinued. In-patient treatment may be necessary during detoxification. Naproxen, alone or together with amitriptyline, may reduce the severity of the headaches. Repetitive intravenous administration of dihydroergotamine (in conjunction with metoclopramide [to control dihydroergotamine-induced nausea and vomiting]) is recommended by some headache specialists to relieve this type of headache. Appropriate treatment for symptoms of withdrawal from other substances frequently used or abused by chronic headache patients may also be needed. In addition, appropiate prophylactic treatment should be initiated or adjusted to reduce the frequency and severity of future headaches.

## Oral Dosage Forms

### BUTALBITAL AND ACETAMINOPHEN CAPSULES

**Usual adult and adolescent dose**
Analgesic—
Oral, 1 or 2 capsules containing 50 mg of butalbital and 325 mg of acetaminophen every four hours as needed, not to exceed 6 capsules a day; or
Oral, 1 capsule containing 50 mg of butalbital and 650 mg of acetaminophen every four hours as needed, not to exceed 4 capsules a day.

**Usual pediatric dose**
Dosage has not been established.

**Strength(s) usually available**
U.S.—
50 mg of butalbital and 325 mg of acetaminophen (Rx) [*Bancap; Triaprin*].
50 mg of butalbital and 650 mg of acetaminophen (Rx) [*Bucet; Conten; Phrenilin Forte; Tencon*].
Canada—
Not commercially available.

**Auxiliary labeling**
• May cause drowsiness.
• Avoid alcoholic beverages.
• May be habit-forming.

### BUTALBITAL AND ACETAMINOPHEN TABLETS

**Usual adult and adolescent dose**
Analgesic—
Oral, 1 or 2 tablets containing 50 mg of butalbital and 325 mg of acetaminophen every four hours as needed, not to exceed 6 tablets a day; or
Oral, 1 tablet containing 50 mg of butalbital and 650 mg of acetaminophen every four hours as needed, not to exceed 4 tablets a day.

**Usual pediatric dose**
Dosage has not been established.

**Strength(s) usually available**
U.S.—
50 mg of butalbital and 325 mg of acetaminophen (Rx) [*Phrenilin* (scored); GENERIC].
50 mg of butalbital and 650 mg of acetaminophen (Rx) [*Sedapap* (scored)].
Canada—
Not commercially available.

**Auxiliary labeling**
• May cause drowsiness.
• Avoid alcoholic beverages.
• May be habit-forming.

### BUTALBITAL, ACETAMINOPHEN, AND CAFFEINE CAPSULES USP

**Usual adult and adolescent dose**
Analgesic—Oral, 1 or 2 capsules every four hours as needed, not to exceed 6 capsules a day.

**Usual pediatric dose**
Dosage has not been established.

**Strength(s) usually available**
U.S.—
50 mg of butalbital, 325 mg of acetaminophen, and 40 mg of caffeine (Rx) [*Amaphen; Anolor-300; Anoquan; Butace; Dolmar; Endolor; Esgic; Ezol; Femcet; Isopap; Medigesic; Pacaps; Repan; Tencet; Triad; Two-Dyne*].
Canada—
Not commercially available.

**Auxiliary labeling**
• May cause drowsiness.
• Avoid alcoholic beverages.
• May be habit-forming.

## BUTALBITAL, ACETAMINOPHEN, AND CAFFEINE TABLETS USP

### Usual adult and adolescent dose
Analgesic—
Oral, 1 or 2 tablets containing 50 mg of butalbital and 325 mg of acetaminophen every four hours as needed, not to exceed 6 tablets a day; or
Oral, 1 tablet containing 50 mg of butalbital and 500 mg of acetaminophen every four hours as needed, not to exceed 6 tablets a day.

### Usual pediatric dose
Dosage has not been established.

### Strength(s) usually available
U.S.—
50 mg of butalbital, 325 mg of acetaminophen, and 40 mg of caffeine (Rx) [*Arcet; Dolmar; Esgic* (scored); *Fioricet; Isocet; Medigesic; Pharmagesic; Repan;* GENERIC].
50 mg of butalbital, 500 mg of acetaminophen, and 40 mg of caffeine (Rx) [*Esgic-Plus* (scored)].
Canada—
Not commercially available.

### Auxiliary labeling
• May cause drowsiness.
• Avoid alcoholic beverages.
• May be habit-forming.

---

### *BUTALBITAL AND ASPIRIN*

## Oral Dosage Forms

### BUTALBITAL AND ASPIRIN TABLETS USP

#### Usual adult and adolescent dose
Analgesic—
Oral, 1 tablet every four hours as needed, not to exceed 6 tablets a day.

#### Usual pediatric dose
Dosage has not been established.

#### Strength(s) usually available
U.S.—
50 mg of butalbital and 650 mg of aspirin (Rx) [*Axotal*].
Canada—
Not commercially available.

#### Auxiliary labeling
• Avoid alcoholic beverages.
• May cause drowsiness.
• Take with food or with a full glass of water.

#### Note
Not a federally controlled substance in the U.S.; however, state regulations may apply.

### BUTALBITAL, ASPIRIN, AND CAFFEINE CAPSULES USP

#### Usual adult and adolescent dose
Analgesic—
Oral, 1 or 2 capsules every four hours as needed, not to exceed 6 capsules a day.

#### Usual pediatric dose
Dosage has not been established.

#### Strength(s) usually available
U.S.—
50 mg of butalbital, 325 mg of aspirin, and 40 mg of caffeine (Rx) [*Butalgen; Fiorinal* (sodium bisulfite); *Isobutal; Isollyl; Laniroif; Lanorinal; Marnal;* GENERIC].
Canada—
50 mg of butalbital, 330 mg of ASA, and 40 mg of caffeine (Rx) [*Fiorinal; Tecnal*].
Note: Because *Aspirin* is a brand name in Canada, ASA is the term used in Canadian product labeling.

#### Auxiliary labeling
• Avoid alcoholic beverages.
• May cause drowsiness.
• Take with food or with a full glass of water.

#### Note
Controlled substance in both the U.S. and Canada.

## BUTALBITAL, ASPIRIN, AND CAFFEINE TABLETS USP

### Usual adult and adolescent dose
Analgesic—
Oral, 1 or 2 tablets containing 50 mg of butalbital, 325 mg of aspirin, and 40 mg of caffeine every four hours as needed, not to exceed 6 tablets a day.

### Usual pediatric dose
Dosage has not been established.

### Strength(s) usually available
U.S.—
50 mg of butalbital, 325 mg of aspirin, and 40 mg of caffeine (Rx) [*Butalgen; Fiorgen; Fiorinal* (lactose); *Fiormor; Fortabs; Isobutal; Isobutyl; Isolin; Isollyl; Laniroif; Lanorinal; Marnal; Vibutal;* GENERIC].
Canada—
50 mg of butalbital, 330 mg of ASA, and 40 mg of caffeine (Rx) [*Fiorinal; Tecnal*].
Note: Because *Aspirin* is a brand name in Canada, ASA is the term used in Canadian product labeling.

### Auxiliary labeling
• Avoid alcoholic beverages.
• May cause drowsiness.
• Take with food or with a full glass of water.

### Note
Products containing 325 mg of aspirin and 50 mg of butalbital per tablet are controlled substances in both the U.S. and Canada.

---

### *BUTALBITAL, ASPIRIN, CAFFEINE, AND CODEINE*

## Oral Dosage Forms

### BUTALBITAL, ASPIRIN, CAFFEINE, AND CODEINE PHOSPHATE CAPSULES USP

#### Usual adult and adolescent dose
Analgesic—
Oral, 1 or 2 capsules every four hours as needed, not to exceed 6 capsules a day.

#### Usual pediatric dose
Dosage has not been established.

#### Strength(s) usually available
U.S.—
50 mg of butalbital, 325 mg of aspirin, 40 mg of caffeine, and 30 mg of codeine phosphate (Rx) [*Ascomp with Codeine No.3; Butalbital Compound with Codeine; Butinal with Codeine No.3; Fiorinal with Codeine No.3; Idenal with Codeine; Isollyl with Codeine;* GENERIC].
Canada—
50 mg of butalbital, 330 mg of ASA, 40 mg of caffeine, and 15 mg of codeine phosphate (Rx) [*Fiorinal-C ¹/₄* (lactose); *Tecnal-C ¹/₄*].
50 mg of butalbital, 330 mg of ASA, 40 mg of caffeine, and 30 mg of codeine phosphate (Rx) [*Fiorinal-C ¹/₂* (lactose); *Tecnal-C ¹/₂*].
Note: Because *Aspirin* is a brand name in Canada, ASA is the term used in Canadian product labeling.

#### Auxiliary labeling
• Avoid alcoholic beverages.
• May cause drowsiness.
• Take with food or with a full glass of water.
• May be habit-forming.

#### Note
Controlled substance in both the U.S. and Canada.

### BUTALBITAL, ASPIRIN, CAFFEINE, AND CODEINE PHOSPHATE TABLETS

#### Usual adult and adolescent dose
See *Butalbital, Aspirin, Caffeine, and Codeine Phosphate Capsules USP.*

#### Usual pediatric dose
Dosage has not been established.

#### Strength(s) usually available
U.S.—
50 mg of butalbital, 325 mg of aspirin, 30 mg of codeine phosphate, and 40 mg of caffeine (Rx) [*Idenal with Codeine;* GENERIC].
Canada—
Not commercially available.

**Auxiliary labeling**
- Avoid alcoholic beverages.
- May cause drowsiness.
- Take with food or with a full glass of water.
- May be habit-forming.

**Note**
Controlled substance in the U.S.

---

### PHENOBARBITAL, ASA, AND CODEINE

## Oral Dosage Forms

### PHENOBARBITAL, ASA, AND CODEINE PHOSPHATE CAPSULES

**Usual adult and adolescent dose**
Analgesic—
Oral, 1 or 2 capsules containing 16.2 mg of phenobarbital, 325 mg of ASA, and 16.2 or 32.4 mg of codeine phosphate every three or four hours; or
Oral, 1 capsule containing 16.2 mg of phenobarbital, 325 mg of ASA, and 64.8 mg of codeine phosphate every three or four hours.

**Usual pediatric dose**
Dosage has not been established.

**Strength(s) usually available**
U.S.—
Not commercially available.
Canada—
16.2 mg of phenobarbital, 325 mg of ASA, and 16.2 mg of codeine phosphate (Rx) [*Phenaphen with Codeine No.2*].
16.2 mg of phenobarbital, 325 mg of ASA, and 32.4 mg of codeine phosphate (Rx) [*Phenaphen with Codeine No.3*].
16.2 mg of phenobarbital, 325 mg of ASA, and 64.8 mg of codeine phosphate (Rx) [*Phenaphen with Codeine No.4*].

Note: Because *Aspirin* is a brand name in Canada, ASA is the term used in Canadian product labeling.

**Auxiliary labeling**
- Avoid alcoholic beverages.
- May cause drowsiness.
- Take with food or with a full glass of water.

**Note**
Controlled substance in Canada.

---

Revised: 07/13/92
Interim revision: 07/19/94

---

## Table 1. Patient Consultation

As an aid to patient consultation, refer to *Advice for the Patient, Butalbital and Acetaminophen (Systemic); Butalbital and Aspirin (Systemic);* or *Barbiturates, Aspirin, and Codeine (Systemic).*

In providing consultation, consider emphasizing the following selected information (» = major clinical significance):

Legend:
I=Butalbital and Acetaminophen
II=Butalbital, Acetaminophen, and Caffeine
III=Butalbital and Aspirin
IV=Butalbital, Aspirin, and Caffeine
V=Butalbital, Aspirin, Caffeine, and Codeine
VI=Phenobarbital, Aspirin, and Codeine

| | I | II | III | IV | V | VI |
|---|---|---|---|---|---|---|
| **Before using this medication** | | | | | | |
| » Conditions affecting use, especially: | | | | | | |
| Sensitivity to— | | | | | | |
| Butalbital, phenobarbital, or other barbiturates | ✔ | ✔ | ✔ | ✔ | ✔ | ✔ |
| Acetaminophen | ✔ | ✔ | | | | |
| Aspirin or other nonsteroidal anti-inflammatory drugs (NSAIDs) | | | ✔ | ✔ | ✔ | ✔ |
| Codeine | | | | | ✔ | ✔ |
| Caffeine | | ✔ | | ✔ | ✔ | |
| Pregnancy— | | | | | | |
| Barbiturates cross the placenta; may cause fetal abnormalities and/or an increased risk of brain tumors in the neonate; may also cause breathing problems in the neonate if taken shortly before delivery | ✔ | ✔ | ✔ | ✔ | ✔ | ✔ |
| Aspirin crosses the placenta; should not be taken during third trimester unless prescribed by physician; chronic, high-dose use may cause adverse effects on the circulation in fetus or neonate, bleeding in fetus and/or mother, prolonged gestation, and complicated deliveries | | | ✔ | ✔ | ✔ | ✔ |
| Codeine crosses the placenta; may cause breathing problems in the neonate if taken just before delivery | | | | | ✔ | ✔ |
| Caffeine crosses the placenta; total daily intake should be limited because of risk of fetal arrhythmias | | ✔ | | ✔ | ✔ | |
| Breast-feeding— | | | | | | |
| Barbiturates distributed into breast milk; may cause CNS depression in the infant | ✔ | ✔ | ✔ | ✔ | ✔ | ✔ |
| Caffeine distributed into breast milk; total daily intake should be limited because of risk of CNS stimulation in the infant | | ✔ | | ✔ | ✔ | |
| Use in children— | | | | | | |
| Possibility of barbiturate-induced paradoxical excitement | ✔ | ✔ | ✔ | ✔ | ✔ | ✔ |
| Not giving aspirin to children with symptoms of viral illness (especially influenza or varicella) without physician's permission because of risk of Reye's syndrome; children without a viral illness are also more susceptible to aspirin-induced toxicity | | | ✔ | ✔ | ✔ | ✔ |
| Possibility of codeine-induced paradoxical excitement | | | | | ✔ | ✔ |

## Table 1. Patient Consultation (continued)

| | Legend:<br>I=Butalbital and Acetaminophen<br>II=Butalbital, Acetaminophen, and Caffeine<br>III=Butalbital and Aspirin | | | IV=Butalbital, Aspirin, and Caffeine<br>V=Butalbital, Aspirin, Caffeine, and Codeine<br>VI=Phenobarbital, Aspirin, and Codeine | | |
|---|---|---|---|---|---|---|
| | I | II | III | IV | V | VI |
| Use in teenagers—Checking with physician before giving to teenagers with symptoms of acute febrile illness, especially influenza or varicella, because of the risk of Reye's syndrome | | | ✔ | ✔ | ✔ | ✔ |
| Use in the elderly— | | | | | | |
|   Increased sensitivity to barbiturates; may react to usual doses with confusion, depression, or excitement | ✔ | ✔ | ✔ | ✔ | ✔ | ✔ |
|   Increased susceptibility to toxic effects of aspirin | | | ✔ | ✔ | ✔ | ✔ |
|   Increased susceptibility to respiratory depressant and other adverse effects of opioid analgesics | | | | | ✔ | ✔ |
| Other medications, especially: | | | | | | |
|   Alcohol | ✔ | ✔ | | ✔ | ✔ | ✔ |
|   Alkalizers, urinary | | | ✔ | ✔ | ✔ | ✔ |
|   Anticoagulants, coumarin- or indandione-derivative | ✔ | ✔ | ✔ | ✔ | ✔ | ✔ |
|   Carbamazepine | ✔ | ✔ | ✔ | ✔ | ✔ | ✔ |
|   Contraceptives, estrogen-containing, oral | ✔ | ✔ | ✔ | ✔ | ✔ | ✔ |
|   Corticosteroids, glucocorticoid and mineralocorticoid | ✔ | ✔ | ✔ | ✔ | ✔ | ✔ |
|   Corticotropin | ✔ | ✔ | ✔ | ✔ | ✔ | ✔ |
|   CNS depressants | ✔ | ✔ | ✔ | ✔ | ✔ | ✔ |
|   Divalproex sodium | ✔ | ✔ | ✔ | ✔ | ✔ | ✔ |
|   Heparin | | | ✔ | ✔ | ✔ | ✔ |
|   Methotrexate | | | ✔ | ✔ | ✔ | ✔ |
|   Naltrexone | | | | | ✔ | ✔ |
|   Probenecid | | | ✔ | ✔ | ✔ | ✔ |
|   Sulfinpyrazone | | | ✔ | ✔ | ✔ | ✔ |
|   Valproic acid | ✔ | ✔ | ✔ | ✔ | ✔ | ✔ |
|   Vancomycin | | | ✔ | ✔ | ✔ | ✔ |
| Other medical problems, especially: | | | | | | |
|   Alcohol abuse | ✔ | ✔ | | | ✔ | ✔ |
|   Asthma | ✔ | ✔ | ✔ | ✔ | ✔ | ✔ |
|   Bleeding ulcers, or other bleeding problems or coagulation defects | | | ✔ | ✔ | ✔ | ✔ |
|   Diarrhea caused by antibiotics or poisoning | | | | | ✔ | ✔ |
|   Drug abuse or history of | ✔ | ✔ | | | ✔ | ✔ |
|   Gastritis (erosive) or peptic ulcer, history of | | | ✔ | ✔ | ✔ | ✔ |
|   Inflammatory bowel disease, severe | | | ✔ | ✔ | ✔ | ✔ |
|   Liver disease | ✔ | ✔ | ✔ | ✔ | ✔ | ✔ |
|   Porphyria | ✔ | ✔ | ✔ | ✔ | ✔ | ✔ |
|   Respiratory disease | ✔ | ✔ | ✔ | ✔ | ✔ | ✔ |
|   Viral hepatitis | ✔ | ✔ | | | ✔ | ✔ |
| **Proper use of this medication** | | | | | | |
| » Taking with food or a full glass (240 mL) of water to minimize stomach irritation | | | ✔ | ✔ | ✔ | ✔ |
| » Not taking medication if it has a strong vinegar-like odor | | | ✔ | ✔ | ✔ | ✔ |
| » Importance of not taking more medication than the amount prescribed because of danger of: | | | | | | |
|   Habituation | ✔ | ✔ | ✔ | ✔ | ✔ | ✔ |
|   Hepatotoxicity | ✔ | ✔ | | | | |
|   Overdose | ✔ | ✔ | ✔ | ✔ | ✔ | ✔ |
| » For relief of headache: | | | | | | |
|   Most effective when taken as soon as headache appears or at first sign of migraine attack (prodromal stage) | ✔ | ✔ | ✔ | ✔ | ✔ | ✔ |
|   Lying down in a quiet, dark room for a while after taking | ✔ | ✔ | ✔ | ✔ | ✔ | ✔ |
|   Compliance with prophylactic therapy, if prescribed | ✔ | ✔ | ✔ | ✔ | ✔ | ✔ |
| » Proper dosing | ✔ | ✔ | ✔ | ✔ | ✔ | ✔ |
| » Missed dose (if on scheduled dosing regimen): Taking as soon as possible; not taking if almost time for next dose; not doubling doses | ✔ | ✔ | ✔ | ✔ | ✔ | ✔ |
| » Proper storage | ✔ | ✔ | ✔ | ✔ | ✔ | ✔ |

Table 1. Patient Consultation *(continued)*

| | Legend:<br>I=Butalbital and Acetaminophen<br>II=Butalbital, Acetaminophen, and Caffeine<br>III=Butalbital and Aspirin | | | IV=Butalbital, Aspirin, and Caffeine<br>V=Butalbital, Aspirin, Caffeine, and Codeine<br>VI=Phenobarbital, Aspirin, and Codeine | | |
|---|---|---|---|---|---|---|
| | I | II | III | IV | V | VI |
| **Precautions while using this medication** | | | | | | |
| » Checking with physician if effectiveness of medication decreases and/or frequency of headaches increases; possibility that tolerance to or physical dependence on the medication, leading to withdrawal headaches, has developed | ✔ | ✔ | ✔ | ✔ | ✔ | ✔ |
| » Risk of overdose if taking other medications containing: | | | | | | |
|     Barbiturates | ✔ | ✔ | ✔ | ✔ | ✔ | ✔ |
|     Acetaminophen | ✔ | ✔ | | | | |
|     Aspirin or other salicylates | | | ✔ | ✔ | ✔ | ✔ |
|     Codeine or other opioids | | | | | ✔ | ✔ |
| » Avoiding alcohol or other CNS depressants unless prescribed or otherwise approved by physician | ✔ | ✔ | ✔ | ✔ | ✔ | ✔ |
| Alcohol consumption may increase probability of stomach problems | | | ✔ | ✔ | ✔ | ✔ |
| Alcohol consumption may increase risk of hepatotoxicity, with high doses or prolonged use | ✔ | ✔ | | | | |
| » Caution if dizziness, lightheadedness, drowsiness, or a false sense of well-being occurs | ✔ | ✔ | ✔ | ✔ | ✔ | ✔ |
| Caution when getting up suddenly from a lying or sitting position | | | | | ✔ | ✔ |
| Lying down if nausea or vomiting, or dizziness or lightheadedness occurs | | | | | ✔ | ✔ |
| Need to inform physician or dentist of use of medication if any kind of surgery (including dental surgery) or emergency treatment is required | ✔ | ✔ | ✔ | ✔ | ✔ | ✔ |
| Caution if any kind of surgery is required; aspirin should be discontinued 5 days prior to surgery unless otherwise directed by physician | | | ✔ | ✔ | ✔ | ✔ |
| Diabetics: May cause false urine sugar test results with prolonged use of 8 or more capsules or tablets per day | | | ✔ | ✔ | ✔ | ✔ |
| Caution if any laboratory tests required | | | | | | |
|     Possible interference with laboratory test results | ✔ | ✔ | ✔ | ✔ | ✔ | ✔ |
|     Not taking caffeine for 8 to 12 hours prior to dipyridamole-assisted myocardial perfusion studies | | ✔ | | ✔ | ✔ | |
| » Checking with physician before discontinuing medication following prolonged use; gradual reduction in dosage may be required to reduce risk of withdrawal symptoms | ✔ | ✔ | ✔ | ✔ | ✔ | ✔ |
| » Suspected overdose: Getting emergency help at once | ✔ | ✔ | ✔ | ✔ | ✔ | ✔ |
| **Side/adverse effects** | | | | | | |
| Signs and symptoms of potential side effects, especially: | | | | | | |
|     Agranulocytosis | ✔ | ✔ | ✔ | ✔ | ✔ | ✔ |
|     Anaphylaxis | | | ✔ | ✔ | ✔ | ✔ |
|     Angioedema | ✔ | ✔ | ✔ | ✔ | ✔ | ✔ |
|     Bronchospastic allergic reaction | ✔ | ✔ | ✔ | ✔ | ✔ | ✔ |
|     CNS adverse effects | ✔ | ✔ | ✔ | ✔ | ✔ | ✔ |
|     CNS stimulation (paradoxical) | ✔ | ✔ | ✔ | ✔ | ✔ | ✔ |
|     Dermatitis, allergic | ✔ | ✔ | ✔ | ✔ | ✔ | ✔ |
|     Dermatitis, exfoliative | ✔ | ✔ | ✔ | ✔ | ✔ | ✔ |
|     Erythema multiforme | ✔ | ✔ | ✔ | ✔ | ✔ | ✔ |
|     Laryngeal edema, allergic | | | | | ✔ | ✔ |
|     Laryngospasm, allergic | | | | | ✔ | ✔ |
|     Stevens-Johnson syndrome | ✔ | ✔ | ✔ | ✔ | ✔ | ✔ |
|     Thrombocytopenia | ✔ | ✔ | ✔ | ✔ | ✔ | ✔ |
|     Toxic epidermal necrolysis | | | ✔ | ✔ | ✔ | ✔ |

# BARIUM SULFATE   Local

VA CLASSIFICATION (Primary): DX101

Note: For a listing of dosage forms and brand names by country availability, see *Dosage Forms* section(s). For a listing of brand names for the articles in this monograph, refer to the General Index.

## Category

Diagnostic aid, radiopaque (gastrointestinal disorders).

## Indications

### Accepted

**Radiography, gastrointestinal**—Oral or rectal barium sulfate suspension, and the oral tablet, are indicated for radiographic examination of the gastrointestinal tract. Barium sulfate suspension, when administered orally, provides contrast to help detect and evaluate abnormalities of the esophagus, the stomach, and/or the small intestine. The oral tablet form is used to detect minimal esophageal strictures. Rectal administration of barium sulfate helps detect and evaluate abnormalities of the colon and/or distal small intestine.

**Body imaging, computed tomographic**—Oral or rectal barium sulfate suspension, in low concentration, is indicated for enhancement of computed tomographic images (CT of the body) to delineate the gastrointestinal tract.

## Pharmacology/Pharmacokinetics

### Physicochemical characteristics

Molecular weight—233.39.

### Mechanism of action/Effect

Barium sulfate increases the absorption of x-rays as they pass through the body, thus delineating body structures, in which barium sulfate is localized.

### Absorption

No significant absorption from gastrointestinal tract (some of the additives are absorbed).

### Time to peak opacification:

**Esophagus, stomach, and duodenum**—Almost immediate after oral administration.

**Small intestine (anterograde examination)**—Dependent on gastric emptying rate and viscosity of the preparation; may be delayed 15 to 90 minutes.

**Small intestine (enteroclysis studies)**—Immediate, following direct instillation of preparation into small intestine.

**Colon and distal small intestine (retrograde examination)**—Patient positioning and hydrostatic pressure determines the rate and degree of opacification.

### Elimination

Fecal.

## Precautions to Consider

### Pregnancy/Reproduction

**Pregnancy**—Elective contrast radiography of the abdomen is usually not recommended during pregnancy because of the risks to the fetus from radiation exposure.

### Breast-feeding

Problems in humans have not been documented.

### Pediatrics

Two deaths of infants from barium aspiration have been reported; however, the volume of aspirated material rather than the nature of the material was probably the responsible factor.

### Geriatrics

Diagnostic studies performed to date have not demonstrated geriatrics-specific problems that would limit the usefulness of barium sulfate in the elderly. However, colon distention has caused electrocardiographic changes, especially in geriatric patients with a history of cardiac disease.

### Medical considerations/Contraindications

The medical considerations/contraindications included here have been selected on the basis of their potential clinical significance (reasons given in parentheses where appropriate)—not necessarily inclusive (» = major clinical significance).

*Except under special circumstances, this medication should not be used when the following medical problems exist:*

» Colon obstruction, known or suspected
  (oral administration of barium sulfate may increase risk of impaction)

» Gastrointestinal tract perforation
  (increased risk of intraperitoneal spread of barium sulfate with oral or rectal administration; prolonged exposure of peritoneum to barium sulfate may result in ascites, peritonitis, and adhesions)

*Risk-benefit should be considered when the following medical problems exist:*

  Allergies or asthma, history of, or
  Sensitivity to barium sulfate preparations
  (increased risk of anaphylactoid reaction to additives [e.g., suspending agents, flavoring agents] in the barium sulfate formulation)

  Cystic fibrosis
  (increased risk of obstruction of the small bowel)

» Dehydration
  (increased risk of impaction)

  Diverticulitis, acute, or
  Ulcerative colitis, acute
  (rectal administration of barium sulfate may increase risk of perforation of the colon)

» Gastrointestinal tract obstruction
  (condition may be aggravated)

## Side/Adverse Effects

Note: Perforation of the colon after rectal administration of barium sulfate suspension has occurred rarely due to hydrostatic pressure of the instilled suspension, trauma to the colon from the enema tip, or forceful or deep insertion of a firm enema tip. Perforation of the colon has led to peritonitis, adhesions, granulomas, and death.

The following side/adverse effects have been selected on the basis of their potential clinical significance (possible signs and symptoms in parentheses where appropriate)—not necessarily inclusive:

### Those indicating need for medical attention

Incidence rare

  *Anaphylactoid reaction* (wheezing, tightness in chest, or troubled breathing); *appendicitis* (stomach or lower abdominal pain, severe cramping, bloating, nausea, or vomiting); *fecal impaction* (severe continuing constipation)

  Note: Allergic-like reactions have been attributed to additives in the barium sulfate suspension, to other medications, such as glucagon, anticholinergic agents, or rectal lubricants, given at the time of the procedure, and, more recently, to the latex inflatable cuff on some enema tips.

### Those indicating need for medical attention only if they continue or are bothersome

Incidence more frequent

  *Constipation; intestinal cramping; diarrhea*

  Note: *Intestinal cramping* and *diarrhea* may be the result of intestinal distention produced by large volumes of barium sulfate enema.

## Patient Consultation

As an aid to patient consultation, refer to *Advice for the Patient, Barium Sulfate (Diagnostic)*.

In providing consultation, consider emphasizing the following selected information (» = major clinical significance):

### Description of use

  Action in the body: Oral/rectal administration; visualization of radiopacity in the gastrointestinal tract possible with x-rays

» Proper dosing

### Before having this test

» Conditions affecting use, especially:
  Sensitivity to barium sulfate formulations
  Pregnancy—Risk to the fetus from radiation exposure
  Other medical problems, especially dehydration, known or suspected obstruction of the colon, or gastrointestinal tract perforation or obstruction

**Preparation for this test**

Patient should inquire in advance regarding special instructions

For oral administration of barium sulfate: Not eating after 8 in the evening; not drinking liquids after midnight

For rectal administration of barium sulfate: Eating residue-free meals and using a laxative on day before examination

**Precautions after having this test**

Increased intake of liquids to prevent impaction after oral administration

**Side/adverse effects**

Signs of potential side effects, especially allergic-like reaction, appendicitis, and fecal impaction

# General Dosing Information

Barium sulfate should *not* be administered in its dry form since accidental inhalation, esophageal irritation or blockage, or intestinal blockage may occur. The powder must be reconstituted, and some of the commercially prepared suspensions require further dilution, prior to administration. The manufacturer's literature should be consulted for specific techniques and procedures for reconstitution and administration of the different barium sulfate preparations.

Increased intake of liquids is recommended after oral or rectal administration of barium sulfate to prevent severe constipation and the risk of impaction.

**For oral dosage forms**

On the evening before the examination, a residue-free dinner is recommended. Intake of food after 8 in the evening is not recommended; intake of clear liquids may continue up to midnight.

**For rectal dosage forms**

On the day prior to the examination, a residue-free diet and a laxative are usually recommended.

A bisacodyl suppository may be used the morning of the examination.

# Oral or Rectal Dosage Forms

## BARIUM SULFATE USP

**Usual adult and adolescent dose**

Gastrointestinal tract radiographic examination—

Oral:

Esophagus, single contrast—5 to 150 mL of a suspension containing 60 to 155% weight per volume (w/v) (40 to 75% weight in weight [w/w]) of barium sulfate.

Esophagus, double contrast—15 to 140 mL of a suspension containing 60 to 250% w/v (40 to 85% w/w) of barium sulfate.

Stomach and duodenum, single contrast—240 to 360 mL of a suspension containing 40 to 120% w/v (30 to 60% w/w) of barium sulfate.

Entire small intestine, single contrast—480 to 700 mL of a suspension containing 40 to 80% w/v (30 to 50% w/w) of barium sulfate.

Stomach, double contrast—Initially, 75 to 140 mL of a suspension containing 200 to 250% w/v (80 to 85% w/w) of barium sulfate for gastric coating. After gastric coating is observed and radiographs are taken, an additional 150 to 300 mL of a suspension containing 40 to 80% w/v (30 to 50% w/w) of barium sulfate is administered.

Single contrast enteroclysis studies (small intestine examination via oral tube into the duodenum)—500 to 2400 mL of a suspension containing 24 to 50% w/v (20 to 35% w/w) of barium sulfate.

Rectal:

Small intestine, retrograde examination—2 to 2.5 L of a suspension containing 20% w/v (17% w/w) of barium sulfate.

Colon, single contrast—1.5 to 2.5 L of a suspension containing 17 to 40% w/v (15 to 30% w/w) of barium sulfate.

Colon, double contrast—350 to 1000 mL of a suspension containing 85 to 125% w/v (50 to 65% w/w) of barium sulfate.

CT of the body—

Oral: 200 to 500 mL of a suspension containing 1 to 2% w/v (1 to 2% w/w) of barium sulfate.

**Usual pediatric dose**

Gastrointestinal tract radiographic examination—Dosage must be individualized by physician. In general, the following concentrations of barium sulfate suspensions are used—

Oral:

Upper GI, single contrast: 50 to 100% w/v (35 to 56% w/w).

Upper GI, double contrast: 200 to 250% w/v (80 to 85% w/w).

Small intestine follow-through studies: 50 to 100% w/v (35 to 56% w/w).

Enteroclysis studies: 20 to 30% w/v (17 to 20% w/w).

Rectal:

Colon, single contrast: 15 to 20% w/v (15 to 17% w/w).

Colon, double contrast: 80 to 120% w/v (50 to 60% w/w).

**Usual geriatric dose**

See *Usual adult and adolescent dose.*

**Size(s) usually available**

U.S.—

180 gram (Rx) [*Tonopaque*].

1 lb (Rx) [GENERIC].

5 lb (Rx) [GENERIC].

Canada—

25 kg (Rx) [GENERIC].

**Packaging and storage**

Store below 40 °C (104 °F), preferably between 15 and 30 °C (59 and 86 °F), unless otherwise specified by manufacturer. Store in a well-closed container.

**Preparation of dosage form**

Barium sulfate powder should not be taken in its dry form. To prepare suspension, water is added to the powder. Flavoring may be added, if needed.

See manufacturer's package insert for complete instructions on reconstitution.

**Note**

Suspension should be shaken vigorously just before administration.

## BARIUM SULFATE SUSPENSION

**Usual adult and adolescent dose**

See *Barium Sulfate USP.*

**Usual pediatric dose**

See *Barium Sulfate USP.*

**Usual geriatric dose**

See *Barium Sulfate USP.*

**Strength(s) usually available**

U.S.—

1.5% w/w (Rx) [*Prepcat*].

2.2% w/w (Rx) [*mede-SCAN*].

5% w/v (Rx) [*Tomocat*].

60% w/v (Rx) [*Liquid Barosperse*].

85% w/v (Rx) [*HD 85*].

100% w/v (Rx) [*Medebar Plus; Polibar Liquid*].

105% w/v (Rx) [*Polibar Plus*].

Canada—

1.2% w/v (Rx) [*Readi-CAT*].

100% w/v (Rx) [*Polibar*].

105% w/v (Rx) [*Polibar Plus; Polibar Rapide*].

**Packaging and storage**

Store below 40 °C (104 °F), preferably between 15 and 30 °C (59 and 86 °F), unless otherwise specified by manufacturer. Store in a well-closed container.

**Preparation of dosage form**

To achieve other desired concentrations, manufacturer's package insert should be consulted for dilution instructions.

**Note**

Suspension should be shaken vigorously just before administration.

# Oral Dosage Forms

## BARIUM SULFATE ORAL SUSPENSION

**Usual adult and adolescent dose**

Gastrointestinal tract radiographic examination—

Oral:

Esophagus, single contrast—5 to 150 mL of a suspension containing 60 to 155% weight per volume (w/v) (40 to 75% weight in weight [w/w]) of barium sulfate.

Esophagus, double contrast—15 to 140 mL of a suspension containing 60 to 250% w/v (40 to 85% w/w) of barium sulfate.

Stomach and duodenum, single contrast—240 to 360 mL of a suspension containing 40 to 120% w/v (30 to 60% w/w) of barium sulfate.

Entire small intestine, single contrast—480 to 700 mL of a suspension containing 40 to 80% w/v (30 to 50% w/w) of barium sulfate.

Stomach, double contrast—Initially, 75 to 120 mL of a suspension containing 200 to 250% w/v (80 to 85% w/w) of barium sulfate for gastric coating. After gastric coating is observed and radiographs are taken, an additional 150 to 300 mL of a suspension containing 40 to 80% w/v (30 to 50% w/w) of barium sulfate is administered.

Single contrast enteroclysis studies (small intestine examination via oral tube into the duodenum)—500 to 2400 mL of a suspension containing 24 to 50% w/v (20 to 35% w/w) of barium sulfate.
CT of the body—
Oral: 200 to 500 mL of a suspension containing 1 to 2% w/v (1 to 2% w/w) of barium sulfate.

### Usual pediatric dose
Gastrointestinal tract radiographic examination—Dosage must be individualized by physician. In general, the following concentrations of barium sulfate suspensions are used
Oral:Upper GI, single contrast: 50 to 100% w/v (35 to 56% w/w).Upper GI, double contrast: 200 to 250% w/v (80 to 85% w/w).Small intestine follow-through studies: 50 to 100% w/v (35 to 56% w/w).Enteroclysis studies: 20 to 30% w/v (17 to 20% w/w).

### Usual geriatric dose
See *Usual adult and adolescent dose.*

### Strength(s) usually available
U.S.—
1.2% w/w (Rx) [*Readi-CAT*].
1.5% w/w (Rx) [*Baro-cat*].
2.0% w/w (Rx) [*Readi-CAT 2*].
3.0% w/w (Rx) [*Esopho-CAT Esophageal Cream*].
4.9% w/v (Rx) [*E-Z-CAT; Tomocat; Tomocat 1000*].
50% w/v (Rx) [*Entrobar*].
60% w/v (Rx) [*E-Z-Paque Liquid; Gil-Paque*].
72% w/v (Rx) [*Sol-O-Pake Liquid*].
80% w/v (Rx) [*Entero-H*].
100% w/v (Rx) [*Esophotrast Esophageal Cream*].
120% w/v (Rx) [*E-Z-Paste Esophageal Cream*].
220% w/v (Rx) [*Liquid HD*].
Canada—
1.2% w/v (Rx) [*Readi-CAT*].
3.0% w/w (Rx) [*Esopho-CAT Esophageal Cream*].
4.6% w/w (Rx) [*E-Z-CAT*].
136% w/v (Rx) [*Esobar*].
210% w/v (Rx) [*Maxibar*].
100% w/v (Rx) [*Unibar-100*].

### Packaging and storage
Store below 40 °C (104 °F), preferably between 15 and 30 °C (59 and 86 °F), unless otherwise specified by manufacturer. Store in a well-closed container.

### Preparation of dosage form
To achieve other desired concentrations, manufacturer's package insert should be consulted for dilution instructions.

### Note
Suspension should be shaken vigorously just before administration.

## BARIUM SULFATE FOR SUSPENSION (ORAL) USP

### Usual adult and adolescent dose
See *Barium Sulfate Oral Suspension.*

### Usual pediatric dose
See *Barium Sulfate Oral Suspension.*

### Usual geriatric dose
See *Barium Sulfate Oral Suspension.*

### Strength(s) usually available
U.S.—
28% w/w (Rx) [*Liqui-Jug*].
28 to 56% w/w (Rx) [*Polibar Flavored*].
40% w/w (Rx) [*E-Z-Jug; Sol-O-Pake; Ultra-R*].
75% w/w (Rx) [*E-Z-Paque*].
85% w/w (Rx) [*Baricon; E-Z-HD*].
95% w/w (Rx) [*Barosperse*].
96% w/w (Rx) [*Tonojug 2000*].
98% w/w (Rx) [*Baricon; HD 200 Plus*].
Canada—
40% w/w (Rx) [*E-Z-Jug*].
40% w/w (Rx) [*Ultra-R*].
85% w/w [*E-Z-HD*].
Variable concentration (Rx) [*E-Z-Paque*].

### Packaging and storage
Store below 40 °C (104 °F), preferably between 15 and 30 °C (59 and 86 °F), unless otherwise specified by manufacturer. Store in a well-closed container.

### Preparation of dosage form
Barium sulfate powder should not be taken in its dry form. To prepare suspension, water is added to the powder. Flavoring may be added, if desired.

See manufacturer's package insert for complete instructions on reconstitution.

### Note
Suspension should be shaken vigorously just before administration.

## BARIUM SULFATE TABLETS

### Usual adult and adolescent dose
Esophageal stricture detection—
Oral, 1 tablet administered with one or two swallows of water just prior to esophagoscopy.

### Usual pediatric dose
Dosage has not been established.

### Usual geriatric dose
See *Usual adult and adolescent dose.*

### Strength(s) usually available
U.S.—
650 mg (Rx) [*E-Z-Disk*].
Canada—
Not commercially available.

### Packaging and storage
Store below 40 °C (104 °F), preferably between 15 and 30 °C (59 and 86 °F), unless otherwise specified by manufacturer. Store in a well-closed container.

# Rectal Dosage Forms
## BARIUM SULFATE RECTAL SUSPENSION

### Usual adult and adolescent dose
Gastrointestinal tract radiographic examination—
Rectal:
Small intestine, retrograde examination—2 to 2.5 L of a suspension containing 20% w/v (17% w/w) of barium sulfate.
Colon, single contrast—1.5 to 2.5 L of a suspension containing 17 to 40% w/v (15 to 30% w/w) of barium sulfate.
Colon, double contrast—350 to 1000 mL of a suspension containing 85 to 125% w/v (50 to 65% w/w) of barium sulfate.

### Usual pediatric dose
Gastrointestinal tract radiographic examination—Dosage must be individualized by physician. In general, the following concentrations of barium sulfate suspensions are used—
Rectal:
Colon, single contrast: 15 to 20% w/v (15 to 17% w/w).
Colon, double contrast: 80 to 120% w/v (50 to 60% w/w).

### Usual geriatric dose
See *Usual adult and adolescent dose.*

### Strength(s) usually available
U.S.—
1.2% w/w (Rx) [*Readi-CAT Unflavored*].
5% w/v (Rx) [*Enecat*].
43% w/w (Rx) [*EvacuPaste*].
85% w/v (Rx) [*Probar*].
100% w/v (Rx) [*Anatrast; E-Z-AC; Flo-Coat; Liquipake; Polibar Liquid*].
105% w/v (Rx) [*E-Z-Dose; Polibar Plus*].
150% w/v (Rx) [*Epi-C*].
Canada—
43% w/w (Rx) [*EvacuPaste*].
100% w/v (Rx) [*Polibar Liquid*].
105% w/v (Rx) [*Polibar Plus*].

### Packaging and storage
Store below 40 °C (104 °F), preferably between 15 and 30 °C (59 and 86 °F), unless otherwise specified by manufacturer. Store in a well-closed container.

### Preparation of dosage form
To achieve other desired concentrations, manufacturer's package insert should be consulted for dilution instructions.

### Note
Suspension should be shaken vigorously just before administration.

## BARIUM SULFATE FOR SUSPENSION (RECTAL) USP

### Usual adult and adolescent dose
See *Barium Sulfate Rectal Suspension.*

### Usual pediatric dose
See *Barium Sulfate Rectal Suspension.*

### Usual geriatric dose
See *Barium Sulfate Rectal Suspension.*

**Strength(s) usually available**

U.S.—

94% w/w (Rx) [*Polibar*].

95% w/w (Rx) [*Exacta I; Exacta II*].

95% w/w (Rx) [*Barosperse; E-Z-Paque Enema*].

96% w/w (Rx) [*Medebag*].

96.7% w/w (Rx) [*ACB*].

97% w/w (Rx) [*Barobag; Sol-O-Pake*].

Canada—

Variable strength (Rx) [*ACB; E-Z-Paque*].

Variable strength (Rx) [*Recto-Barium*].

**Packaging and storage**

Store below 40 °C (104 °F), preferably between 15 and 30 °C (59 and 86 °F), unless otherwise specified by manufacturer. Store in a well-closed container.

**Preparation of dosage form**

Barium sulfate powder should not be used in its dry form. To prepare suspension, water is added to the powder.

See manufacturer's package insert for complete instructions on reconstitution.

**Note**

Suspension should be shaken vigorously just before administration.

## Selected Bibliography

Cohen MD. Choosing contrast media for pediatric gastrointestinal examinations. Crit Rev Diagn Imaging 1990; 30 (4): 3174-80.

Foley MJ, Ghahremani GG, Rogers LF. Reappraisal of contrast media used to detect upper gastrointestinal perforations. Radiology 1982; 144: 231-7.

Revised: 07/26/94

---

**BECLOMETHASONE**—See *Corticosteroids (Inhalation-Local); Corticosteroids (Nasal); Corticosteroids (Topical)*

---

**BELLADONNA**—See *Anticholinergics/Antispasmodics (Systemic)*

---

## BELLADONNA ALKALOID–CONTAINING COMBINATIONS—

Atropine, Hyoscyamine, Methenamine, Methylene Blue, Phenyl Salicylate, and Benzoic Acid (Systemic)

Atropine, Hyoscyamine, Scopolamine, and Phenobarbital (Systemic)—See *Belladonna Alkaloids and Barbiturates (Systemic)*

Atropine and Phenobarbital (Systemic)—See *Belladonna Alkaloids and Barbiturates (Systemic)*

Belladonna and Butabarbital (Systemic)—See *Belladonna Alkaloids and Barbiturates (Systemic)*

Belladonna and Phenobarbital (Systemic)—See *Belladonna Alkaloids and Barbiturates (Systemic)*

Chlorpheniramine, Phenylephrine, Phenylpropanolamine, Atropine, Hyoscyamine, and Scopolamine (Systemic)—See *Antihistamines, Decongestants, and Anticholinergics (Systemic)*

Chlorpheniramine, Phenylpropanolamine, and Methscopolamine (Systemic)—See *Antihistamines, Decongestants, and Anticholinergics (Systemic)*

Difenoxin and Atropine (Systemic)

Diphenoxylate and Atropine (Systemic)

Ergotamine, Belladonna Alkaloids, and Phenobarbital (Systemic)

Ergotamine, Caffeine, and Belladonna Alkaloids (Systemic)—See *Vascular Headache Suppressants, Ergot Derivative–containing (Systemic)*

Ergotamine, Caffeine, Belladonna Alkaloids, and Pentobarbital (Systemic)—See *Vascular Headache Suppressants, Ergot Derivative–containing (Systemic)*

Hydrocodone and Homatropine (Systemic)—See *Cough/Cold Combinations (Systemic)*

Hyoscyamine and Phenobarbital (Systemic)—See *Belladonna Alkaloids and Barbiturates (Systemic)*

Kaolin, Pectin, Hyoscyamine, Atropine, and Scopolamine (Systemic)—See *Kaolin, Pectin, and Belladonna Alkaloids (Systemic)*

Magnesium Sulfate Tablets (Oral-Local)—See *Laxatives (Local)*

---

# BELLADONNA ALKALOIDS AND BARBITURATES   Systemic

This monograph includes information on the following: Atropine, Hyoscyamine, Scopolamine, and Phenobarbital; Atropine and Phenobarbital; Belladonna and Butabarbital; Belladonna and Phenobarbital; Hyoscyamine and Phenobarbital.

VA CLASSIFICATION (Primary): GA802

**NOTE:** The *Belladonna Alkaloids and Barbiturates (Systemic)* monograph is maintained on the USP DI electronic data base. For a printed copy of the most recent revision of the complete monograph, contact the USP Division of Information Development, 12601 Twinbrook Parkway, Rockville, MD 20852.

For information on the specific components of this combination, see the *USP DI* monographs for *Anticholinergics/Antispasmodics (Systemic)* and *Barbiturates (Systemic)*.

The information that follows is selectively abstracted from the complete monograph and is provided to facilitate drug use review and patient counseling.

Note: For a listing of dosage forms and brand names by country availability, see *Dosage Forms* section(s). For a listing of brand names for the articles in this monograph, refer to the General Index.

## Category

Anticholinergic-sedative.

## Indications

**Accepted**

Ulcer, peptic (treatment adjunct) or

Bowel syndrome, irritable (treatment adjunct)—FDA has classified these medications as possibly effective for use as adjunctive therapy in the treatment of peptic ulcer and irritable bowel syndrome (irritable colon, spastic colon, mucous colitis).

Note: Less than effective classification requires the submission of adequate and well-controlled studies in order to provide substantial evidence of effectiveness. In the past, FDA has notified manufac-

turers of the possible withdrawal from the market of products containing a combination of an anticholinergic and a sedative because their efficacy as fixed combinations had not been proven in adequately designed clinical trials. To date, no final action has been taken.

**Unaccepted**

Anticholinergic and sedative combinations have been used as adjuncts in the treatment of acute enterocolitis; however, their use for this condition is controversial since they cause a reduction in gastrointestinal motility resulting in retention of the causative organism or toxin and the consequent prolongation of symptoms.

## Patient Consultation

As an aid to patient consultation, refer to *Advice for the Patient, Belladonna Alkaloids and Barbiturates (Systemic)*.

In providing consultation, consider emphasizing the following selected information (» = major clinical significance):

**Before using this medication**

» Conditions affecting use, especially:

Sensitivity to any of the belladonna alkaloids or barbiturates

Pregnancy—Use not recommended because belladonna alkaloids and barbiturates cross placenta; barbiturates may cause fetal abnormalities; phenobarbital may cause neonatal hemorrhage

Breast-feeding—Distributed into breast milk; possible inhibition of lactation

Use in children—Increased susceptibility to toxic effects of anticholinergics; increased response in infants and children with spastic paralysis or brain damage; risk of increased body temperature in hot weather; hyperexcitability (paradoxical reaction); hyperkinesis may be induced in hypersensitive children

Use in the elderly—Increased susceptibility to mental and other toxic effects of anticholinergics and barbiturates; danger of precipitating undiagnosed glaucoma; possible impairment of memory

Dental—Possible development of dental problems because of decreased salivary flow

Other medications, especially adrenocorticoids or corticotropin, other anticholinergics, antacids, anticoagulants, antidiarrheals, ketoconazole, CNS depressants, MAO inhibitors, or potassium chloride

Other medical problems, especially gastrointestinal obstructive disease, glaucoma, hepatic function impairment, renal function impairment, or urinary retention

**Proper use of this medication**

Taking dose 30 to 60 minutes before meals unless otherwise directed by physician

» Importance of not taking more medication than the amount prescribed

» Proper dosing

Missed dose: Taking as soon as possible; not taking if almost time for next dose; not doubling doses

» Proper storage

**Precautions while using this medication**

» Avoiding use of alcohol or other CNS depressants

Not taking antacids and antidiarrheal medications within 1 hour of taking this medication

» Caution during exercise and hot weather; overheating may result in heat stroke

Possible increased sensitivity of eyes to light

» Caution if drowsiness or blurred vision occurs

Possible dryness of mouth, nose, and throat; using sugarless candy or gum, ice, or saliva substitute for relief; checking with physician or dentist if dry mouth continues for more than 2 weeks

**Side/adverse effects**

Signs of potential side effects, especially agranulocytosis, allergic reaction, hepatitis, increased intraocular pressure, and thrombocytopenia

---

### *ATROPINE, HYOSCYAMINE, SCOPOLAMINE, AND PHENOBARBITAL*

---

## Oral Dosage Forms

### ATROPINE SULFATE, HYOSCYAMINE SULFATE (or HYOSCYAMINE HYDROBROMIDE), SCOPOLAMINE HYDROBROMIDE, AND PHENOBARBITAL CAPSULES

**Usual adult and adolescent dose**

Anticholinergic-sedative—

Oral, 1 or 2 capsules two to four times a day, the dosage being adjusted as needed and tolerated.

**Usual pediatric dose**

Dosage must be individualized by physician.

**Usual geriatric dose**

See *Usual adult and adolescent dose.*

Note: Geriatric patients may be more sensitive to the effects of the usual adult dose.

**Strength(s) usually available**

U.S.—

19.4 mcg (0.0194 mg) of atropine sulfate, 104 mcg (0.104 mg) of hyoscyamine sulfate (or hydrobromide), 6.5 mcg (0.0065 mg) of scopolamine hydrobromide, and 16 mg of phenobarbital (Rx) [*Donnatal* (lactose); *Hyosophen*].

Note: Strengths of individual components may vary slightly among products of different manufacturers.

Canada—

Not commercially available.

**Auxiliary labeling**

• May cause drowsiness.

• Avoid alcoholic beverages.

### ATROPINE SULFATE, HYOSCYAMINE SULFATE (or HYOSCYAMINE HYDROBROMIDE), SCOPOLAMINE HYDROBROMIDE, AND PHENOBARBITAL ELIXIR

**Usual adult and adolescent dose**

Anticholinergic-sedative—

Oral, 5 to 10 mL three or four times a day, the dosage being adjusted as needed and tolerated.

**Usual pediatric dose**

Anticholinergic-sedative—

Children 4.5 to 9 kg of body weight: Oral, 0.5 to 0.75 mL every four to six hours.

Children 9 to 13.5 kg of body weight: Oral, 1.0 to 1.5 mL every four to six hours.

Children 13.5 to 22.5 kg of body weight: Oral, 1.5 to 2 mL every four to six hours.

Children 22.5 to 36.5 kg of body weight: Oral, 2.5 to 3.75 mL every four to six hours.

Children 36.5 to 45.4 kg of body weight: Oral, 3.75 to 5 mL every four to six hours.

Children 45.4 kg of body weight and over: Oral, 5 to 7.5 mL every four to six hours.

Note: Dosage must be adjusted for each patient as needed and tolerated.

**Usual geriatric dose**

See *Usual adult and adolescent dose.*

Note: Geriatric patients may be more sensitive to the effects of the usual adult dose.

**Strength(s) usually available**

U.S.—

19.4 mcg (0.0194 mg) of atropine sulfate, 103.7 mcg (0.1037 mg) of hyoscyamine sulfate (or hydrobromide), 6.5 mcg (0.0065 mg) of scopolamine hydrobromide, and 16 mg of phenobarbital, per 5 ml (Rx) [*Barophen; Donnamor; Donnapine; Donnatal; Hyosophen; Spasmophen; Spasquid; Susano*].

Note: Contain 23% alcohol.

34 mcg (0.034 mg) of atropine sulfate, 174 mcg (0.174 mg) of hyoscyamine sulfate (or hydrobromide), 10 mcg (0.01 mg) of scopolamine hydrobromide, and 21.6 mg of phenobarbital, per 5 mL (Rx) [*Barbidonna* (alcohol 15%)].

Canada—

19 mcg (0.019 mg) of atropine sulfate, 104 mcg (0.104 mg) of hyoscyamine sulfate, 7 mcg (0.007 mg) of scopolamine hydrobromide, and 16.2 mg of phenobarbital, per 5 ml (Rx) [*Donnatal* (alcohol 23%)].

Note: Strengths of individual components may vary slightly among products of different manufacturers.

**Auxiliary labeling**

• May cause drowsiness.

• Avoid alcoholic beverages.

• Keep container tightly closed.

### ATROPINE SULFATE, HYOSCYAMINE SULFATE (or HYOSCYAMINE HYDROBROMIDE), SCOPOLAMINE HYDROBROMIDE, AND PHENOBARBITAL TABLETS

**Usual adult and adolescent dose**

Anticholinergic-sedative—

Oral, 1 or 2 tablets two to four times a day, the dosage being adjusted as needed and tolerated.

**Usual pediatric dose**

Dosage must be individualized by physician.

**Usual geriatric dose**

See *Usual adult and adolescent dose.*

Note: Geriatric patients may be more sensitive to the effects of the usual adult dose.

**Strength(s) usually available**

U.S.—

19.4 mcg (0.0194 mg) of atropine sulfate, 104 mcg (0.104 mg) of hyoscyamine sulfate (or hydrobromide), 6.5 mcg (0.0065 mg) of scopolamine hydrobromide, and 16 mg of phenobarbital (Rx) [*Bellalphen; Donnapine; Donnatal; Malatal; Relaxadon; Spaslin; Spasmolin; Susano;* GENERIC].

19.4 mcg (0.0194) of atropine sulfate, 104 mcg (0.104 mg) of hyoscyamine sulfate, 6.5 mcg (0.0065 mg) of scopolamine hydrobromide, and 32 mg of phenobarbital (Rx) [*Donnatal No. 2*].

20 mcg (0.02 mg) of atropine sulfate, 100 mcg (0.1 mg) of hyoscyamine sulfate (or hydrobromide), 6.0 mcg (0.006 mg) of scopolamine hydrobromide, and 15 mg of phenobarbital (Rx) [*Donphen; Spasmophen*].

25 mcg (0.025 mg) of atropine sulfate, 128.6 mcg (0.1286 mg) of hyoscyamine sulfate (or hydrobromide), 7.4 mcg (0.0074 mg) of scopolamine hydrobromide, and 16 mg of phenobarbital (Rx) [*Barbidonna*].

25 mcg (0.025 mg) of atropine sulfate, 128.6 mcg (0.1286 mg) of hyoscyamine sulfate (or hydrobromide), 7.4 mcg (0.0074 mg) of scopolamine hydrobromide, and 32 mg of phenobarbital (Rx) [*Barbidonna No. 2*].

scopolamine hydrobromide, and 32 mg of phenobarbital (Rx) [*Barbidonna No. 2*].

Canada—

19 mcg (0.019 mg) of atropine sulfate, 104 mcg (0.104 mg) of hyoscyamine sulfate, 7 mcg (0.007 mg) of scopolamine hydrobromide, and 16.2 mg of phenobarbital (Rx) [*Donnatal*].

Note: Strengths of individual components may vary slightly among products of different manufacturers.

**Auxiliary labeling**
• May cause drowsiness.
• Avoid alcoholic beverages.

## ATROPINE SULFATE, HYOSCYAMINE SULFATE, SCOPOLAMINE HYDROBROMIDE, AND PHENOBARBITAL CHEWABLE TABLETS

**Usual adult and adolescent dose**
Anticholinergic-sedative—
Oral, 1 or 2 tablets three or four times a day, the dosage being adjusted as needed and tolerated.

**Usual pediatric dose**
Anticholinergic-sedative—
Children up to 2 years of age: Use is not recommended.
Children 2 to 12 years of age: Oral, 1/2 to 1 tablet three or four times a day, the dosage being adjusted as needed and tolerated.

**Usual geriatric dose**
See *Usual adult and adolescent dose*.
Note: Geriatric patients may be more sensitive to the effects of the usual adult dose.

**Strength(s) usually available**
U.S.—
120 mcg (0.12 mg) of atropine sulfate, 120 mcg (0.12 mg) of hyoscyamine sulfate, 7 mcg (0.007 mg) of scopolamine hydrobromide, and 16 mg of phenobarbital (Rx) [*Kinesed*].
Canada—
Not commercially available.

**Auxiliary labeling**
• May be chewed or swallowed with liquids.
• May cause drowsiness.
• Avoid alcoholic beverages.

## ATROPINE SULFATE, HYOSCYAMINE SULFATE, SCOPOLAMINE HYDROBROMIDE, AND PHENOBARBITAL EXTENDED-RELEASE TABLETS

**Usual adult and adolescent dose**
Anticholinergic-sedative—
Oral, 1 tablet every eight to twelve hours, the dosage being adjusted as needed and tolerated.

**Usual pediatric dose**
Use is not recommended.

**Usual geriatric dose**
See *Usual adult and adolescent dose*.
Note: Geriatric patients may be more sensitive to the effects of the usual adult dose.

**Strength(s) usually available**
U.S.—
58.2 mcg (0.0582 mg) of atropine sulfate, 311.1 mcg (0.3111 mg) of hyoscyamine sulfate, 19.5 mcg (0.0195 mg) of scopolamine hydrobromide, and 48.6 mg of phenobarbital (Rx) [*Donnatal Extentabs*].
Canada—
58.2 mcg (0.0582 mg) of atropine sulfate, 311.1 mcg (0.3111 mg) of hyoscyamine sulfate, 19.5 mcg (0.0195 mg) of scopolamine hydrobromide, and 48.6 mg of phenobarbital (Rx) [*Donnatal Extentabs*].

**Auxiliary labeling**
• Swallow tablets whole.
• May cause drowsiness.
• Avoid alcoholic beverages.

---

### ATROPINE AND PHENOBARBITAL

## Oral Dosage Forms
### ATROPINE SULFATE AND PHENOBARBITAL CAPSULES

**Usual adult and adolescent dose**
Anticholinergic-sedative—
Oral, 1 or 2 capsules two to four times a day, the dosage being adjusted as needed and tolerated.

**Usual pediatric dose**
Dosage must be individualized by physician.

**Usual geriatric dose**
See *Usual adult and adolescent dose*.
Note: Geriatric patients may be more sensitive to the effects of the usual adult dose.

**Strength(s) usually available**
U.S.—
195 mcg (0.195 mg) of atropine sulfate and 16 mg of phenobarbital (Rx) [*Antrocol*].
Canada—
Not commercially available.

**Auxiliary labeling**
• May cause drowsiness.
• Avoid alcoholic beverages.

## ATROPINE SULFATE AND PHENOBARBITAL ELIXIR

**Usual adult and adolescent dose**
Anticholinergic-sedative—
Oral, 5 to 10 mL three or four times a day, the dosage being adjusted as needed and tolerated.

**Usual pediatric dose**
Anticholinergic-sedative—
Children 7 to 14 kg of body weight: Oral, 0.5 to 1 mL every four to six hours.
Children 14 to 21 kg of body weight: Oral, 1 to 1.5 mL every four to six hours.
Children 21 to 28 kg of body weight: Oral, 1.5 to 2 mL every four to six hours.
Children 28 to 35 kg of body weight: Oral, 2 to 2.5 mL every four to six hours.
Children 41 kg of body weight and over: Oral, 3 mL every four to six hours.

Note: Dosage must be adjusted for each patient as needed and tolerated.

**Usual geriatric dose**
See *Usual adult and adolescent dose*.
Note: Geriatric patients may be more sensitive to the effects of the usual adult dose.

**Strength(s) usually available**
U.S.—
195 mcg (0.195 mg) of atropine sulfate and 16 mg of phenobarbital, per 5 mL (Rx) [*Antrocol (alcohol 20%)*].
Canada—
Not commercially available.

**Auxiliary labeling**
• May cause drowsiness.
• Avoid alcoholic beverages.
• Keep container tightly closed.

## ATROPINE SULFATE AND PHENOBARBITAL TABLETS

**Usual adult and adolescent dose**
Anticholinergic-sedative—
Oral, 1 or 2 tablets three or four times a day, the dosage being adjusted as needed and tolerated.

**Usual pediatric dose**
Dosage must be individualized by physician.

**Usual geriatric dose**
See *Usual adult and adolescent dose*.
Note: Geriatric patients may be more sensitive to the effects of the usual adult dose.

**Strength(s) usually available**
U.S.—
195 mcg (0.195 mg) of atropine sulfate and 16 mg of phenobarbital (Rx) [*Antrocol*].
Canada—
Not commercially available.

**Auxiliary labeling**
• May cause drowsiness.
• Avoid alcoholic beverages.

## BELLADONNA AND BUTABARBITAL

# Oral Dosage Forms

## BELLADONNA EXTRACT AND BUTABARBITAL SODIUM ELIXIR

**Usual adult and adolescent dose**
Anticholinergic-sedative—
  Oral, 5 to 10 mL three or four times a day, the dosage being adjusted as needed and tolerated.

**Usual pediatric dose**
Anticholinergic-sedative—
  Children up to 6 years of age: Oral, 1.25 to 2.5 mL three or four times a day, the dosage being adjusted as needed and tolerated.
  Children 6 to 12 years of age: Oral, 2.5 to 5 mL three or four times a day, the dosage being adjusted as needed and tolerated.

**Usual geriatric dose**
See *Usual adult and adolescent dose.*

Note: Geriatric patients may be more sensitive to the effects of the usual adult dose.

**Strength(s) usually available**
U.S.—
  15 mg of belladonna extract and 15 mg of butabarbital sodium, per 5 mL (Rx) [*Butibel* (alcohol 7%)].
Canada—
  Not commercially available.

**Auxiliary labeling**
• May cause drowsiness.
• Avoid alcoholic beverages.
• Keep container tightly closed.

## BELLADONNA EXTRACT AND BUTABARBITAL SODIUM TABLETS

**Usual adult and adolescent dose**
Anticholinergic-sedative—
  Oral, 1 or 2 tablets three or four times a day, the dosage being adjusted as needed and tolerated.

**Usual pediatric dose**
Dosage must be individualized by physician.

**Usual geriatric dose**
See *Usual adult and adolescent dose.*

Note: Geriatric patients may be more sensitive to the effects of the usual adult dose.

**Strength(s) usually available**
U.S.—
  15 mg of belladonna extract and 15 mg of butabarbital sodium (Rx) [*Butibel*].
Canada—
  Not commercially available.

**Auxiliary labeling**
• May cause drowsiness.
• Avoid alcoholic beverages.

## BELLADONNA AND PHENOBARBITAL

# Oral Dosage Forms

## BELLADONNA EXTRACT AND PHENOBARBITAL TABLETS

**Usual adult and adolescent dose**
Anticholinergic-sedative—
  Oral, 1 or 2 tablets two to four times a day, the dosage being adjusted as needed and tolerated.

**Usual pediatric dose**
Dosage must be individualized by physician.

**Usual geriatric dose**
See *Usual adult and adolescent dose.*

Note: Geriatric patients may be more sensitive to the effects of the usual adult dose.

**Strength(s) usually available**
U.S.—
  15 mg of belladonna extract and 15 mg of phenobarbital (Rx) [*Chardonna-2*].

Canada—
  Not commercially available.

Note: Strengths of individual components may vary slightly among products of different manufacturers.

**Auxiliary labeling**
• May cause drowsiness.
• Avoid alcoholic beverages.

## HYOSCYAMINE AND PHENOBARBITAL

# Oral Dosage Forms

## HYOSCYAMINE SULFATE AND PHENOBARBITAL ELIXIR

**Usual adult and adolescent dose**
Anticholinergic-sedative—
  Oral, 5 to 10 mL every four hours, the dosage being adjusted as needed and tolerated.

**Usual pediatric dose**
Anticholinergic-sedative—
  Children up to 2 years of age: Oral, 1.25 to 2.5 mL every four hours.
  Children 2 to 10 years of age: Oral, 2.5 to 5 mL every four hours.
  Children 10 years of age and over: See *Usual adult and adolescent dose.*

Note: Dosage must be adjusted for each patient as needed and tolerated.

**Usual geriatric dose**
See *Usual adult and adolescent dose.*

Note: Geriatric patients may be more sensitive to the effects of the usual adult dose.

**Strength(s) usually available**
U.S.—
  125 mcg (0.125 mg) of hyoscyamine sulfate and 15 mg of phenobarbital, per 5 mL (Rx) [*Levsin with Phenobarbital* (alcohol 20%)].
Canada—
  Not commercially available.

**Auxiliary labeling**
• May cause drowsiness.
• Avoid alcoholic beverages.

## HYOSCYAMINE SULFATE AND PHENOBARBITAL ORAL SOLUTION

**Usual adult and adolescent dose**
Anticholinergic-sedative—
  Oral, 1 to 2 mL every four hours, the dosage being adjusted as needed and tolerated.

**Usual pediatric dose**
Anticholinergic-sedative—
  Children up to 1 year of age: Oral, 0.1 to 0.5 mL every four hours.
  Children 1 to 10 years of age: Oral, 0.5 to 1 mL every four hours.
  Children 10 years of age and over: See *Usual adult and adolescent dose.*

Note: Dosage must be adjusted for each patient as needed and tolerated.

**Usual geriatric dose**
See *Usual adult and adolescent dose.*

Note: Geriatric patients may be more sensitive to the effects of the usual adult dose.

**Strength(s) usually available**
U.S.—
  125 mcg (0.125 mg) of hyoscyamine sulfate and 15 mg of phenobarbital, per mL (Rx) [*Levsin-PB* (alcohol 5%)].
Canada—
  Not commercially available.

**Auxiliary labeling**
• May cause drowsiness.
• Avoid alcoholic beverages.

## HYOSCYAMINE SULFATE AND PHENOBARBITAL TABLETS

**Usual adult and adolescent dose**
Anticholinergic-sedative—
  Oral, 1 to 2 tablets three or four times a day, the dosage being adjusted as needed and tolerated.

**Usual pediatric dose**
Dosage must be individualized by physician.

**Usual geriatric dose**
See *Usual adult and adolescent dose.*

Note: Geriatric patients may be more sensitive to the effects of the usual adult dose.

**Strength(s) usually available**
U.S.—
   125 mcg (0.125 mg) of hyoscyamine sulfate and 15 mg of phenobarbital (Rx) [*Levsin with Phenobarbital*].
Canada—
   Not commercially available.

**Auxiliary labeling**
• May cause drowsiness.
• Avoid alcoholic beverages.

Revised: 01/13/92
Interim revision: 08/29/94

---

**BELLADONNA–CONTAINING COMBINATIONS—**
Chlorpheniramine, Phenylephrine, and Methscopolamine (Systemic)—See *Antihistamines, Decongestants, and Anticholinergics (Systemic)*

---

**BENAZEPRIL**—See *Angiotensin-converting Enzyme (ACE) Inhibitors (Systemic)*

---

**BENDROFLUMETHIAZIDE**—See    *Diuretics,    Thiazide (Systemic)*

---

**BENDROFLUMETHIAZIDE-CONTAINING COMBINATIONS—**
Nadolol and Bendroflumethiazide (Systemic)—See *Beta-adrenergic Blocking Agents and Thiazide Diuretics (Systemic)*
Rauwolfia Serpentina and Bendroflumethiazide (Systemic)—See *Rauwolfia Alkaloids and Thiazide Diuretics (Systemic)*

---

# BENTIROMIDE    Systemic†

VA CLASSIFICATION (Primary): DX900
Note: For a listing of dosage forms and brand names by country availability, see *Dosage Forms* section(s). For a listing of brand names for the articles in this monograph, refer to the General Index.

   †Not commercially available in Canada.

---

## Category
Diagnostic aid (pancreatic function).

## Indications
**Accepted**
Pancreatic insufficiency (diagnosis)—Bentiromide is indicated as a screening test for pancreatic exocrine insufficiency. It is also indicated to monitor therapy with pancreatic supplements.

   A negative result with the bentiromide test does not rule out pancreatic disease. However, a positive test is a strong indication of pancreatic exocrine insufficiency, although it may require confirmatory studies.

## Pharmacology/Pharmacokinetics
**Physicochemical characteristics**
Molecular weight—404.42.
pKa—5.4.

**Mechanism of action/Effect**
Based on the ability of the patient to secrete chymotrypsin by the exocrine pancreas. When bentiromide is administered orally, it is cleaved by pancreatic chymotrypsin, thereby liberating most of the para-aminobenzoic acid (PABA), which is absorbed by the intestine, partially conjugated in the liver, and excreted in the urine, where it can be measured.

**Biotransformation**
Primarily hepatic. Enzymatic activity capable of hydrolyzing bentiromide has also been found in normal small intestine.

**Elimination**
Renal. Urinary arylamine metabolites consist of *N*-acetyl and glycine conjugates of PABA.

## Precautions to Consider
**Carcinogenicity**
Long-term studies to evaluate carcinogenic potential of bentiromide have not been performed.

**Pregnancy/Reproduction**
Pregnancy—It is not known whether bentiromide or PABA crosses the placenta. Studies in humans have not been done.

Studies in rabbits and rats with doses up to 50 and 100 times the recommended human dose, respectively, have not shown that bentiromide causes adverse effects in the fetus.

FDA Pregnancy Category B.

**Breast-feeding**
It is not known whether bentiromide is distributed into breast milk. However, problems in humans have not been documented.

**Pediatrics**
Appropriate studies on the relationship of age to the effects of bentiromide have not been performed in children up to 6 years of age.

**Geriatrics**
No information is available on the relationship of age to the effects of bentiromide in geriatric patients. However, elderly patients are more likely to have age-related renal function impairment, which may cause false-positive test results in patients receiving bentiromide.

**Drug interactions and/or related problems**
The following drug interactions and/or related problems have been selected on the basis of their potential clinical significance (possible mechanism in parentheses where appropriate)—not necessarily inclusive (» = major clinical significance):
See also *Laboratory value alterations.*

Note: Combinations containing any of the following medications, depending on the amount present, may also interact with this medication.

   Methotrexate
      (may be displaced from binding sites by PABA when given concurrently with bentiromide)

**Laboratory value alterations**
The following have been selected on the basis of their potential clinical significance (possible effect in parentheses where appropriate)—not necessarily inclusive (» = major clinical significance):

With results of *this* test
 *Due to other medications/foods*
   Acetaminophen or
   Benzocaine or
   Chloramphenicol or
   Diuretics, thiazide, or
   Lidocaine or
   PABA-containing medications, such as sunscreens and multivitamin preparations, or
   Procainamide or
   Procaine or
   Sulfonamides
      (concurrent administration of these medications during a bentiromide test period will invalidate test results since they are also metabolized to arylamines and will thus increase the percent of PABA recovered; discontinuation of these medications at least 3 days prior to the administration of bentiromide is recommended)

Arylamine-containing foods, such as prunes and cranberries (concurrent ingestion of these foods during a bentiromide test period will invalidate test results since their arylamine content will increase the percent of PABA recovered; these foods should be avoided for 3 days prior to the test)

» Pancreatic enzyme supplements, oral
(concurrent administration of pancreatic enzyme supplements with bentiromide may give false-negative results; discontinuation of these supplements at least 5 days in adults [1 day in children with cystic fibrosis] prior to the administration of bentiromide is recommended)

*Due to medical problems or conditions*
Gastrointestinal diseases or
Hepatic function impairment, severe or
» Renal function impairment
(may cause false-positive test results)

Steatorrhea secondary to small bowel disease
(occasionally may cause false-positive test results; D-xylose urinary excretion test may be used to exclude the possibility of small bowel disease as the cause of steatorrhea)

### Medical considerations/Contraindications

The medical considerations/contraindications included here have been selected on the basis of their potential clinical significance (reasons given in parentheses where appropriate)—not necessarily inclusive (» = major clinical significance).

See also *Laboratory value alterations.*

*Risk-benefit must be considered when the following medical problem exists:*

Sensitivity to bentiromide

## Side/Adverse Effects

The following side/adverse effects have been selected on the basis of their potential clinical significance (possible signs and symptoms in parentheses where appropriate)—not necessarily inclusive:

**Those indicating need for medical attention**
Incidence rare
*Allergic reaction* (shortness of breath or troubled breathing)

**Those indicating need for medical attention only if they continue or are bothersome**
Incidence more frequent
*Diarrhea; headache*

Incidence less frequent or rare
*Gas; nausea and vomiting; weakness*

## Patient Consultation

As an aid to patient consultation, refer to *Advice for the Patient, Bentiromide (Diagnostic).*

In providing consultation, consider emphasizing the following selected information (» = major clinical significance):

**Description of use**
Test procedure: Bentiromide given orally as single dose; total collection of urine obtained during first 6 hours after dosing; volume of the collection measured and 10 mL sample retained for analysis; test may be repeated after seven days

**Before having this test**
» Conditions affecting use, especially:
Sensitivity to bentiromide
Other medications, especially pancreatic enzyme supplements
Other medical problems, especially renal function impairment

**Preparation for this test**
» Not taking medications and/or foods that may increase arylamine content of urine for 72 hours before test is administered
Not eating after midnight before test is administered, unless otherwise directed by physician; test results may be affected
Voiding before taking bentiromide for best test results

Following dose with large glass of water (250 mL) and drinking additional glasses of water during the six hours after ingestion of dose to provide an adequate amount of urine for testing

**Side/adverse effects**
Signs of possible side effects, especially allergic reaction

## General Dosing Information

Fasting from food after midnight before having this test is usually recommended since some studies have shown that foods, such as complex starches or olive oil, may decrease the excretion of bentiromide. However, bentiromide is sometimes given with a test meal, such as a defined breakfast, to stimulate pancreatic secretion. Clinical experience has found no significant differences in test results when bentiromide was administered in the fasting state or with a meal.

Analysis of a pretest urine sample should be considered to detect background dietary PABA excretion or drug interference.

Voiding is recommended prior to the administration of bentiromide as a precaution to ensure the excretion of dietary PABA, or PABA from other sources, that may still be present in the urine.

Administration of bentiromide should be followed immediately by 250 mL of water. Two hours after dosing, the patient should take another 250 mL of water; an additional 500 mL of water should be taken during the two- to six-hour period after dosing, to promote diuresis.

A total collection of urine is obtained during the six hours after the administration of bentiromide. The volume of the collection is measured and a 10 mL sample is retained for analysis. Analysis of urinary arylamines is done using the Smith modification of the Bratton-Marshall test.

A recovery of less than 50% of PABA from the urine within 6 hours of administration of bentiromide may indicate pancreatic disease.

## Oral Dosage Forms

### BENTIROMIDE ORAL SOLUTION

**Usual adult and adolescent dose**
Pancreatic insufficiency (diagnosis)—
Oral, 500 mg as a single dose.

Note: Test may be repeated if needed after a period of at least 7 days. This waiting period will ensure the complete metabolism and excretion of prior doses of bentiromide.

**Usual pediatric dose**
Pancreatic insufficiency (diagnosis)—
Children up to 6 years of age: Dosage has not been established.
Children 6 years of age and over: Oral, 14 mg of bentiromide per kg of body weight, as a single dose.

**Usual geriatric dose**
See *Usual adult and adolescent dose.*

**Strength(s) usually available**
U.S.—
500 mg (containing 170 mg of PABA) per 7.5 mL (Rx) [*Chymex*].
Canada—
Not commercially available.

Note: In a 40% propylene glycol solution.

**Packaging and storage**
Store between 15 and 30 °C (59 and 86 °F), in a well-closed container, unless otherwise specified by manufacturer. Protect from freezing.

## Selected Bibliography

Toskes P. The bentiromide test for pancreatic exocrine insufficiency. Pharmacotherapy 1984; 4: 74-80.

Revised: 12/02/92
Interim revision: 06/16/94

## BENZALKONIUM CHLORIDE—See *Spermicides (Vaginal)*

# BENZNIDAZOLE   Systemic*†

VA CLASSIFICATION (Primary): AP100
Note: For a listing of dosage forms and brand names by country availability, see *Dosage Forms* section(s). For a listing of brand names
for the articles in this monograph, refer to the General Index.

*Not commercially available in the U.S.
†Not commercially available in Canada.

## Category
Antiprotozoal (systemic).

## Indications
Note: Because benznidazole is not commercially available in the U.S. or
Canada, the bracketed information and the use of the superscript 1
in this monograph reflect the lack of labeled (approved) indications
for this medication in these countries.

**Accepted**
[Trypanosomiasis, American (treatment)][1]—Benznidazole is used as an
alternative agent in the treatment of American trypanosomiasis (Chagas' disease) caused by *Trypanosoma cruzi*. However, nifurtimox is
considered the primary agent in the treatment of American
trypanosomiasis.

[1]Not included in Canadian product labeling.

## Pharmacology/Pharmacokinetics

**Physicochemical characteristics**
Source—Nitroimidazole derivative.
Molecular weight—260.25.

**Mechanism of action/Effect**
Trypanocidal; although the mode of action has not been studied in detail,
benznidazole appears to inhibit protein and ribonucleic acid (RNA)
synthesis in the trypanosome parasite.

**Absorption**
Rapidly absorbed from the gastrointestinal tract of healthy volunteers following a single oral 100-mg dose.

**Distribution**
Rapidly and evenly distributed between the plasma and the red blood cells
in humans.
Relative volume of distribution—Average 0.56 L per kg (L/kg).

**Protein binding**
About 44%.

**Half-life**
Elimination—Approximately 10.5 to 13.6 hours with an average of 12
hours.

**Time to peak concentration**
About 3 to 4 hours in healthy volunteers following a single oral 100-mg
dose.

**Peak plasma concentration**
About 2.2 to 2.8 mcg per mL (mcg/mL) with an average of 2.54 mcg/mL
in healthy volunteers following a single oral 100-mg dose.

**Elimination**
Renal—60 to 67% of the medication was eliminated in the urine within
4 days in healthy volunteers given a dose of 14 mg per kg of body
weight (mg/kg) of $^{14}$C-tagged benznidazole.
Fecal—About 22 to 28%.

## Precautions to Consider

**Carcinogenicity/Tumorigenicity**
Carcinogenicity bioassays of mice given 8 mg per kg of body weight (mg/
kg) per day of benznidazole for 60 days have shown an increase in
lymphomas.

**Mutagenicity**
A small study assessing the cytogenetic effect of benznidazole in 14 patients (aged 11 months to 11 years) with Chagas' disease has shown
a two-fold increase in chromosomal aberrations (CA).
Benznidazole has been shown to be mutagenic for *Klebsiella pneumoniae*
and *Salmonella typhimurium*.

**Pregnancy/Reproduction**
Pregnancy—Studies have not been done in humans. The World Health
Organization (WHO) prescribing information does not recommend the
use of benznidazole during the first trimester of pregnancy.
Studies done in female rats given benznidazole in oral doses of 25 to 75
mg/kg a day from the seventh to the sixteenth day of pregnancy and
in rabbits given oral doses of 25 mg/kg a day from the seventh to the
nineteenth day of pregnancy, have not shown benznidazole to be embryotoxic or teratogenic.

**Breast-feeding**
It is not known whether benznidazole is distributed into breast milk. However, problems in humans have not been documented.

**Pediatrics**
Appropriate studies on the relationship of age to the effects of benznidazole have not been performed in the pediatric population. No pediatrics-specific problems have been documented to date.

**Geriatrics**
Appropriate studies on the relationship of age to the effects of benznidazole have not been performed in the geriatric population. However,
no geriatrics-specific problems have been documented to date.

**Drug interactions and/or related problems**
The following drug interactions and/or related problems have been selected on the basis of their potential clinical significance (possible
mechanism in parentheses where appropriate)—not necessarily inclusive (» = major clinical significance):
Note: Combinations containing any of the following medications, depending on the amount present, may also interact with this
medication.

» Alcohol
(benznidazole should not be used concurrently with alcohol; accumulation of acetaldehyde may occur due to interference of benznidazole with the oxidation of alcohol, resulting in disulfiram-like
effects causing extreme discomfort such as abdominal cramps,
nausea, vomiting, headache, or flushing)

» Aspirin
(concurrent use with benznidazole may increase the chance of
bleeding)

» Anticoagulants, coumarin-derivative, such as warfarin
(effects may be potentiated when these agents are used concurrently with benznidazole, due to inhibition of enzymatic metabolism of anticoagulants)

**Laboratory value alterations**
The following have been selected on the basis of their potential clinical
significance (possible effect in parentheses where appropriate)—not
necessarily inclusive (» = major clinical significance):
With physiology/laboratory test values
» Complete blood count (CBC)
(benznidazole may decrease the concentration of leukocytes and
platelets on rare occasion)

**Medical considerations/Contraindications**
The medical considerations/contraindications included here have been selected on the basis of their potential clinical significance (reasons given
in parentheses where appropriate)—not necessarily inclusive (» =
major clinical significance).

***Risk-benefit should be considered when the following medical problems
exist:***
» Hematological impairment or
» Hepatic function impairment or
» Renal function impairment
(patients with these conditions may have an increased risk of side
effects)

Hypersensitivity to benznidazole

**Patient monitoring**
The following may be especially important in patient monitoring (other
tests may be warranted in some patients, depending on condition;
» = major clinical significance):
» Complete blood count (CBC)
(should be monitored throughout treatment since benznidazole may
cause leukopenia or thrombocytopenia on rare occasion; treatment
may have to be interrupted if these blood changes occur)

## Side/Adverse Effects

The following side/adverse effects have been selected on the basis of their potential clinical significance (possible signs and symptoms in parentheses where appropriate)—not necessarily inclusive:

**Those indicating need for medical attention**
Incidence more frequent
    *Peripheral neuropathy* (numbness; tingling pain; weakness in hands or feet); *progressive purpuric dermatitis* (reddish spots on skin or reddish discoloration of skin); *seizures*
Incidence rare
    *Blood dyscrasias, specifically leukopenia* (fever or chills; sore throat); *and thrombocytopenia* (pinpoint red spots on skin; unusual bleeding or bruising); *skin rash*

**Those indicating need for medical attention only if they continue or are bothersome**
Incidence more frequent
    *Gastrointestinal disturbances* (abdominal or stomach pain; diarrhea; nausea; vomiting)
Incidence rare
    *Fatigue* (unusual tiredness or weakness); *headache; psychic disturbances such as: disorientation* (confusion); *insomnia* (trouble in sleeping); *inability to concentrate; restlessness; amnesia, transient* (temporary loss of memory); *vertigo* (dizziness)

## Patient Consultation

As an aid to patient consultation, refer to *Advice for the Patient, Benznidazole (Systemic)*.

In providing consultation, consider emphasizing the following selected information (» = major clinical significance):

**Before using this medication**
» Conditions affecting use, especially:
    Hypersensitivity to benznidazole
    Mutagenicity—A small study of 14 pediatric patients has shown a two-fold increase in chromosomal aberrations
    Pregnancy—WHO does not recommend use during the first trimester of pregnancy
    Other medications, especially aspirin, alcohol, and coumarin-derivative anticoagulants
    Other medical problems, especially hematological conditions, hepatic function impairment, or renal function impairment

**Proper use of this medication**
    Taking with meals to minimize gastrointestinal irritation
» Compliance with full course of therapy
» Proper dosing
» Missed dose
» Proper storage

**Precautions while using this medication**
    Regular visits to physician to check progress
» Checking with physicians if symptoms get worse
    Caution if leukopenia or thrombocytopenia occurs:
» Checking with physician immediately if fever or chills occur or if you think you are getting an infection
» Checking with physician immediately if unusual bleeding or bruising; black, tarry stools; blood in urine or stools; or pinpoint red spots on skin occur
» Avoiding use of alcoholic beverages or other alcohol-containing preparations while taking this medication

**Side/adverse effects**
    Signs of potential side effects, especially peripheral neuropathy; seizures; blood dyscrasias; progressive purpuric dermatitis; and skin rash

## General Dosing Information

Nausea and mild rashes may occur during the initial phase (generally within the first 2 weeks) of therapy with benznidazole. Reduction of dose may not be necessary since these side/adverse effects may disappear spontaneously with continuous treatment. However, if rashes become severe or are accompanied by fever or purpura, treatment should be discontinued.

Symptoms of peripheral neuropathy are dose-related effects. If these symptoms occur, treatment should be discontinued immediately.

The daily dose of benznidazole should be taken after meals, in 2 divided doses, with a 12-hour interval between doses.

## Oral Dosage Forms

Note: Because benznidazole is not commercially available in the U.S. or Canada, the bracketed uses and the use of superscript 1 in the *Dosage Forms* section reflect the lack of labeled (approved) indications for this product in these countries.

### BENZNIDAZOLE TABLETS

**Usual adult and adolescent dose**
[Trypanosomiasis, American][1]—
    Oral, 5 to 7 mg per kg of body weight per day taken after meals, in two doses with an interval of twelve hours between doses. Therapy should continue for thirty to sixty days.

Note: Some medical authorities recommend treatment for up to one hundred and twenty days.

**Usual pediatric dose**
[Trypanosomiasis, American][1]—
    Children up to 12 years of age: Oral, 10 mg per kg of body weight per day taken after meals, in two doses with an interval of twelve hours between doses. Therapy should continue for thirty to sixty days.
    Children 12 years of age and over: See *Usual adult and adolescent dose.*

Note: Some medical authorities recommend treatment for up to one hundred and twenty days.

**Usual pediatric prescribing limits**
Up to a maximum of 10 mg per kg of body weight per day.

**Strength(s) usually available**
U.S.—
    Not commercially available.
Canada—
    Not commercially available.
Other (Brazil)—
    100 mg (Rx) [*Rochagan; Radanil; Ro7–1051*].

**Packaging and storage**
Store in a well-closed container below 40 °C (104 °F), preferably between 15 and 30 °C (59 and 86 °F), unless otherwise specified by manufacturer. Protect from light.

**Auxiliary labeling**
• Avoid alcoholic beverages.
• Continue medication for the full time of treatment.

---

[1]Not included in Canadian product labeling.

## Selected Bibliography

Cerisola JA. Chemotherapy of Chagas infection in man. In: Proceedings of an international symposium held in conjunction with the fifth international congress on protozoology; 1977 June 27; New York (NY): 35-47. (PAHO Scientific Publication No. 347).

Viotti R, Vigliano C, Armenti H, et al. Treatment of chronic Chagas' disease with benznidazole: clinical and serologic evolution of patients with long-term follow-up. Am Heart J 1994; 127 (1): 151-62.

---

Developed: 08/31/94

---

**BENZOCAINE**—See *Anesthetics (Mucosal-Local)*; *Anesthetics (Topical)*

---

**BENZOCAINE-CONTAINING COMBINATIONS**—

Antipyrine and Benzocaine (Otic)
Benzocaine, Butamben, and Tetracaine (Mucosal-Local)—See *Anesthetics (Mucosal-Local)*

---

**BENZOCAINE AND MENTHOL**—See *Anesthetics (Topical)*

# BENZODIAZEPINES   Systemic

This monograph includes information on the following: Alprazolam; Bromazepam*; Chlordiazepoxide; Clonazepam; Clorazepate; Diazepam; Estazolam†; Flurazepam; Halazepam†; Ketazolam*; Lorazepam; Nitrazepam*; Oxazepam; Prazepam†; Quazepam†; Temazepam; Triazolam.

VA CLASSIFICATION (Primary/Secondary):

Alprazolam
    Oral—CN302
Bromazepam
    Oral—CN302
Chlordiazepoxide
    Oral—CN302
    Parenteral—CN302
Clonazepam
    Oral—CN400
Clorazepate
    Oral—CN302/CN400
Diazepam
    Oral—CN302/CN400; MS200
    Parenteral—CN302/CN400; MS200
Estazolam
    Oral—CN302
Flurazepam
    Oral—CN302
Halazepam
    Oral—CN302
Ketazolam
    Oral—CN302
Lorazepam
    Oral—CN302/MS200
    Parenteral—CN302/CN400; MS200
Nitrazepam
    Oral—CN302/CN400
Oxazepam
    Oral—CN302
Prazepam
    Oral—CN302
Quazepam
    Oral—CN302
Temazepam
    Oral—CN302
Triazolam
    Oral—CN302

Note: All of the benzodiazepines in this monograph are controlled substances in the U.S.—Schedule IV.

Note: For a listing of dosage forms and brand names by country availability, see *Dosage Forms* section(s). For a listing of brand names for the articles in this monograph, refer to the General Index.

*Not commercially available in the U.S.
†Not commercially available in Canada.

## Category

Note: **All of the benzodiazepines have similar pharmacologic actions; however, clinical uses among specific agents may vary because of actual pharmacokinetic differences, availability of specific testing, and/or availability of clinical-use data.**

Antianxiety agent—Alprazolam; Bromazepam; Chlordiazepoxide; Clorazepate; Diazepam; Halazepam; Ketazolam; Lorazepam; Oxazepam; Prazepam.

Sedative-hypnotic—Alprazolam; Bromazepam; Chlordiazepoxide; Clorazepate; Diazepam; Estazolam; Flurazepam; Halazepam; Ketazolam; Lorazepam; Nitrazepam; Oxazepam; Prazepam; Quazepam; Temazepam; Triazolam.

Amnestic—Diazepam (parenteral only); Lorazepam (parenteral only).

Anticonvulsant—Clonazepam; Clorazepate; Diazepam; Lorazepam (parenteral only); Nitrazepam.

Antipanic agent—Alprazolam; Chlordiazepoxide (parenteral only); Clonazepam; Diazepam; Lorazepam.

Skeletal muscle relaxant adjunct—Diazepam; Lorazepam.

Antitremor agent—Chlordiazepoxide (oral only); Diazepam (oral only); Lorazepam (oral only).

Antiemetic, in cancer chemotherapy—Lorazepam (parenteral only).

## Indications

Note: Bracketed information in the *Indications* section refers to uses that are not included in U.S. product labeling.

**Accepted**

Anxiety (treatment)—Alprazolam, bromazepam, chlordiazepoxide, clorazepate, diazepam, halazepam, ketazolam, lorazepam, oxazepam, and prazepam are indicated for the management of anxiety disorders or for the short-term relief of the symptoms of anxiety. Oral chlordiazepoxide, [oral diazepam][1], and sublingual or intramuscular lorazepam are indicated for treatment of preoperative apprehension and anxiety.

Benzodiazepines are not indicated for the treatment of anxiety or tension associated with the stress of everyday life. Effectiveness of these medications for long-term management of anxiety has not been assessed by systematic clinical studies. The medication's efficacy should be reassessed at periodic intervals.

Anxiety associated with mental depression (treatment adjunct)[1]—Alprazolam, lorazepam (oral), and oxazepam are also indicated for the adjunctive management of anxiety associated with mental depression.

Alcohol withdrawal (treatment)—Chlordiazepoxide, clorazepate, diazepam (except the extended-release dosage form), [lorazepam][1], and oxazepam are indicated for the relief of acute alcohol withdrawal symptoms such as acute agitation, tremor, impending or acute delirium tremens, and hallucinosis.

Anesthesia, adjunct—Parenteral chlordiazepoxide and parenteral diazepam are indicated for preoperative procedures to relieve anxiety and tension. Also, parenteral lorazepam is indicated in adults as preanesthetic medication to produce sedation, relief of anxiety, and anterograde amnesia.

Amnesia, in cardioversion
Amnesia, in endoscopic procedures
Anxiety, in cardioversion (treatment) or
Anxiety, in endoscopic procedures (treatment adjunct)—Parenteral diazepam and [parenteral lorazepam][1] are indicated as adjuncts prior to endoscopic procedures if apprehension, anxiety, or acute stress reactions are present and to diminish patient's recall of the procedure.

Parenteral diazepam is also indicated for intravenous administration prior to cardioversion to relieve anxiety and tension and to produce anterograde amnesia.

[Sedation, conscious][1]—Parenteral diazepam is used in dentistry to relieve anxiety and produce amnesia in prolonged or difficult dental procedures. It is used frequently with a local anesthetic.

Insomnia (treatment)—Estazolam, flurazepam, nitrazepam, quazepam, temazepam, and triazolam are indicated for the short-term treatment of insomnia characterized by difficulty in falling asleep, frequent nocturnal awakenings, and/or early morning awakenings. Lorazepam[1] is indicated for insomnia due to anxiety or transient situational stress. Other benzodiazepines, such as [alprazolam][1], bromazepam[1], diazepam, ketazolam[1], [halazepam], and [prazepam], are also used in the treatment of insomnia. Failure of insomnia to remit after 7 to 10 days of treatment may indicate the presence of a primary psychiatric or medical illness. Worsening of insomnia or the emergence of new abnormalities of thinking or behavior may be the consequence of an unrecognized psychiatric or physical disorder.

[Short- and intermediate-acting benzodiazepine hypnotics may be useful in the prevention or treatment (short-term) of transient insomnia associated with a sudden sleep schedule change, such as occurs in trans-meridian travel and shift-work rotation.][1]

Seizures (treatment) or
Status epilepticus (treatment)—Diazepam injection (not the sterile emulsion) or [diazepam for rectal solution] is indicated as an adjunct in status epilepticus and severe recurrent convulsive seizures. It is not recommended for maintenance anticonvulsant therapy; therefore, once seizures are controlled, appropriate maintenance anticonvulsant therapy should be instituted. [Parenteral lorazepam also is used for the treatment of status epilepticus.]

Convulsions (treatment adjunct) or
Seizures (treatment adjunct)—Oral diazepam[1] (except the extended-release dosage form) is indicated as short-term (7 to 14 days) adjunctive therapy in convulsive disorders. It is not useful as sole therapy in convulsive disorders. [Clonazepam may be effective as an adjunct in convulsive disorders such as eclamptic convulsions, infantile spasms, reading epilepsy, and startle-induced seizures.][1]

Epilepsy, Lennox-Gastaut syndrome (treatment)
Epilepsy, akinetic seizure pattern (treatment) or

Epilepsy, myoclonic seizure pattern (treatment)—Clonazepam is indicated for use alone or, more frequently, as an adjunct in the treatment of the Lennox-Gastaut syndrome (petit mal variant), akinetic, and myoclonic seizures.

Nitrazepam also is indicated for the treatment of myoclonic seizures.

[Epilepsy, myoclonic seizure pattern (treatment adjunct)][1]—Oral diazepam is used as adjunctive therapy in myoclonus. It is not useful as sole therapy in this condition.

Epilepsy, absence seizure pattern (treatment)—Clonazepam may be useful in the treatment of absence (petit mal) seizures refractory to the succinimide anticonvulsants or valproic acid.

Epilepsy, simple partial seizure pattern (treatment adjunct)[1] or

Epilepsy, complex partial seizure pattern (treatment adjunct)[1]—Clorazepate may be indicated as adjunctive therapy in the management of partial seizures.

[Epilepsy, simple partial seizure pattern (treatment)][1] or

[Epilepsy, complex partial seizure pattern (treatment)][1]—Clonazepam may be effective in refractory seizures such as complex partial (psychomotor, temporal lobe) or elementary partial (focal) seizures.

[Epilepsy, tonic-clonic seizure pattern (treatment)][1]—Clonazepam may be effective in tonic-clonic (grand mal) seizures. However, when clonazepam is used in patients in whom several types of seizure disorders coexist, it may increase the incidence or rarely precipitate the onset of generalized tonic-clonic (grand mal) seizures; addition of another anticonvulsant and/or an increase in dosage may be required.

Panic disorders (treatment)—Alprazolam, [chlordiazepoxide (parenteral)], [clonazepam][1], [diazepam][1], and [lorazepam][1] are used in the treatment of panic disorders.

Spasm, skeletal muscle (treatment adjunct)—Diazepam and [lorazepam][1] are indicated as adjunctive therapy for the relief of skeletal muscle spasm due to reflex spasm of local pathology (such as inflammation of the muscles or joints, or secondary to trauma); spasticity caused by upper motor neuron disorders (such as cerebral palsy and paraplegia); athetosis; stiff-man syndrome; and tetanus. [Diazepam is also used to relieve spasms of facial muscles associated with problems of occlusion and temporomandibular joint disorders.][1]

[Nausea and vomiting, cancer chemotherapy–induced (prophylaxis)][1]—Lorazepam injection, alone or in combination with other agents, reduces the severity and duration of nausea and vomiting associated with emetogenic cancer chemotherapy. In addition, lorazepam-induced amnesia can reduce anticipatory anxiety, nausea, and vomiting.

[Headache, tension (treatment)]—Chlordiazepoxide, diazepam[1], lorazepam[1], and possibly other benzodiazepines[1] are used in the treatment of tension headache.

[Tremors (treatment)][1]—Oral alprazolam, chlordiazepoxide, diazepam, and lorazepam are also used in the treatment of familial, senile, or essential action tremors.

---

[1]Not included in Canadian product labeling.

## Pharmacology/Pharmacokinetics

See also *Table 1,* page 551.

### Physicochemical characteristics
Molecular weight—
Alprazolam: 308.77.
Bromazepam: 316.16.
Chlordiazepoxide: 299.76.
Chlordiazepoxide hydrochloride: 336.22.
Clonazepam: 315.72.
Clorazepate dipotassium: 408.92.
Diazepam: 284.74.
Estazolam: 294.74.
Flurazepam hydrochloride: 460.81.
Halazepam: 352.74.
Ketazolam: 368.82.
Lorazepam: 321.16.
Nitrazepam: 281.27.
Oxazepam: 286.72.
Prazepam: 324.81.
Quazepam: 386.79.
Temazepam: 300.74.
Triazolam: 343.21.

### Mechanism of action/Effect
In general, benzodiazepines act as depressants of the central nervous system (CNS), producing all levels of CNS depression from mild sedation to hypnosis to coma depending on dose.

The precise sites and mechanisms of action have not been completely established. Although various mechanisms of action have been pro-

posed, it is believed that benzodiazepines enhance or facilitate the inhibitory neurotransmitter action of gamma-aminobutyric acid (GABA), which is one of the major inhibitory neurotransmitters in the brain and mediates both pre- and post-synaptic inhibition in all regions of the CNS, following interaction between the benzodiazepine and a specific neuronal membrane receptor.

Benzodiazepines reportedly act as agonists at the benzodiazepine receptors, which have been shown to form a component of a functional supramolecular unit known as the benzodiazepine-GABA receptor-chloride ionophore complex. The receptor complex, believed to reside on neuronal membranes that regulate cell firing, functions mainly in the gating of the chloride channel. Activation of the GABA receptor results in the opening of the chloride channel, allowing the flow of chloride ions through the neuronal membrane. Usually this results in hyperpolarization of the post-synaptic neuron, which inhibits firing of that neuron. That inhibition translates into decreased neuronal excitability, thus attenuating subsequent depolarizing excitatory transmitters. Benzodiazepines reportedly increase the frequency of the chloride channel opening, probably by enhancing the binding of GABA to its receptor or by facilitating the link of the GABA receptors to the chloride ion channels. Benzodiazepines also appear to act at GABA-independent receptors.

Antianxiety agent; sedative-hypnotic—Believed to stimulate GABA receptors in the ascending reticular activating system. Since GABA is inhibitory, receptor stimulation increases inhibition and blocks both cortical and limbic arousal following stimulation of the brain stem reticular formation.

Amnestic—Mechanism of action has not been determined. However, as may occur with all sedative-hypnotic medications, preanesthetic doses of diazepam and lorazepam impair recent memory and interfere with the establishment of the memory trace, thus producing anterograde amnesia for events occurring while therapeutic concentrations of the benzodiazepine are present.

Anticonvulsant—Appear to act, at least partially, by enhancing presynaptic inhibition. Suppress the spread of seizure activity produced by epileptogenic foci in the cortex, thalamus, and limbic structures but do not abolish the abnormal discharge of the focus.

Skeletal muscle relaxant adjunct—The exact mechanism of action of benzodiazepines has not been completely established but these medications appear to produce skeletal muscle relaxation primarily by inhibiting spinal polysynaptic afferent pathways; however, monosynaptic afferent pathways may also be inhibited. Benzodiazepines may also directly depress motor nerve and muscle function.

### Absorption
Following oral administration—Benzodiazepines are well absorbed from the gastrointestinal tract, usually within 1 to 2 hours. Diazepam and clorazepate are among the most rapidly absorbed, and prazepam and oxazepam are the least rapidly absorbed.

Following intramuscular administration—Lorazepam absorption is rapid and complete, whereas chlordiazepoxide and diazepam absorption may be slow and erratic depending upon the site of administration. When diazepam is injected into the deltoid muscle, absorption is usually rapid and complete.

Following rectal administration—Absorption of diazepam rectal solution is rapid.

### Biotransformation
Hepatic.
Long half-life benzodiazepines—
Chlordiazepoxide, diazepam, flurazepam, halazepam, ketazolam, and quazepam are metabolized by oxidation to active, as well as inactive, metabolites before final inactivation as glucuronide conjugates.
Clorazepate and prazepam are metabolized in the stomach and liver, respectively, to desmethyldiazepam as a result of first-pass biotransformation prior to entering systemic circulation.
Short to intermediate half-life benzodiazepines—
Alprazolam undergoes oxidative metabolism to metabolites with little or no activity and is eliminated as glucuronide conjugates.
Bromazepam undergoes hepatic microsomal oxidation and is eliminated primarily as glucuronide conjugates.
Clonazepam and nitrazepam undergo nitro-reduction to inactive metabolites.
Estazolam undergoes oxidative metabolism and hydroxylation to metabolites with little or no activity.
Lorazepam, oxazepam, and temazepam are metabolized by direct conjugation with glucuronic acid.
Triazolam undergoes first-pass hepatic extraction; inactive metabolites are principally conjugated glucuronides.

### Accumulation
During repeated dosing with long half-life benzodiazepines, there is accumulation of the parent compound and/or any pharmacologically ac-

tive metabolites. Accumulation continues until a steady-state plasma concentration is reached, which usually takes 5 days to 2 weeks after initiation of therapy. Following termination of treatment, drug elimination is slow since active metabolites may remain in the blood for several days or even weeks, possibly resulting in persistent effects.

During repeated dosing with short to intermediate half-life benzodiazepines, accumulation is minimal, and a steady-state plasma concentration is usually attained within a few days after initiation of therapy. Following termination of treatment, blood concentrations are subclinical in 24 hours and return rapidly to zero (in about 4 days or less).

### Onset of action

After single oral doses, onset of action depends largely upon absorption rate. After multiple doses, effects depend partly upon rate and extent of drug accumulation, which in turn relate to elimination half-life and clearance.

### Duration of action

After single oral doses, duration of action depends upon rate and extent of drug distribution, as well as rate of elimination once distribution is complete. After multiple doses, effects depend partly upon rate and extent of drug accumulation, which in turn relate to elimination half-life and clearance. The duration of clinical effects of the benzodiazepines is not always predictable from the elimination half-life.

## Precautions to Consider

### Cross-sensitivity and/or related problems

Patients sensitive to one of the benzodiazepines may be sensitive to the other benzodiazepines also.

### Carcinogenicity/Tumorigenicity

For alprazolam—In a 24-month study in rats, alprazolam at doses up to 150 times the maximum recommended daily human dose showed no evidence of carcinogenic potential.

For estazolam—A 24-month study in mice and rats showed no evidence of tumorigenicity. Mice given 3 and 10 mg of estazolam per kg of body weight per day over the 2-year period showed an increase in hyperplastic liver nodules; however, the significance of this finding is unknown.

For halazepam—In oral oncogenicity studies in rats and mice, halazepam at doses 5 to 50 times the usual daily human dose of 120 mg showed no evidence of carcinogenicity.

For lorazepam—In an 18-month study in rats, lorazepam showed no evidence of carcinogenic potential.

For oxazepam—A 24-month study in rats given oxazepam at doses 30 times the maximum human dose showed an increase in benign thyroid follicular cell tumors, testicular interstitial cell adenomas, and prostatic adenomas. In a 9-month study in rats, oxazepam in doses 35 to 100 times the usual daily human dose caused dose-related increases in liver adenomas.

For quazepam—Oral oncogenicity studies in mice and hamsters showed no evidence of carcinogenicity.

For temazepam—Long-term studies in mice and rats showed temazepam to have no carcinogenic potential.

For triazolam—In a 24-month study in mice, triazolam in doses up to 4000 times the human dose showed no evidence of carcinogenic potential.

### Mutagenicity

For alprazolam—Mutagenicity was not demonstrated in appropriate tests on mice or bacteria.

For estazolam—Mutagenicity was not demonstrated in appropriate tests on mice, rats, and bacteria.

For halazepam—Halazepam demonstrated no mutagenic activity in the Ames test.

For lorazepam and oxazepam—Studies on the mutagenic potential of lorazepam or oxazepam have not been done

For quazepam—Mutagenicity was not demonstrated in tests on mice or bacteria.

### Pregnancy/Reproduction

Pregnancy—
*For all benzodiazepines—*
Chlordiazepoxide, clonazepam, diazepam, estazolam, flurazepam, lorazepam, nitrazepam, temazepam, and triazolam cross the placenta. Alprazolam, bromazepam, clorazepate, halazepam, ketazolam, oxazepam, prazepam, and quazepam may cross the placenta.
First trimester—Chlordiazepoxide and diazepam have been reported to increase the risk of congenital malformations when used during the first trimester of pregnancy. The other benzodiazepines may be associated with this increased risk also. Risk-benefit must be carefully considered. However, since the use of benzodiazepines (with the possible exception of anti-

convulsant use) is rarely a matter of urgency, it should be avoided during pregnancy, especially during the first trimester.
When benzodiazepines, such as clonazepam, clorazepate, diazepam, parenteral lorazepam, and nitrazepam, are used as anticonvulsants, risk-benefit must be considered since recent reports suggest an increased incidence of congenital abnormalities in children whose mothers used anticonvulsants during pregnancy; however, a definite cause and effect relationship has not been established.
Chronic usage of benzodiazepines during pregnancy may cause physical dependence with resulting withdrawal symptoms in the neonate.
Use of benzodiazepine hypnotics during the last weeks of pregnancy may result in neonatal CNS depression.
*For chlordiazepoxide—*
Reproduction studies in rats showed that chlordiazepoxide, at doses of 10, 20, and 80 mg per kg of body weight (mg/kg) per day, caused no congenital anomalies or adverse effects on the growth of the newborn animal. However, another study with chlordiazepoxide at doses of 100 mg/kg per day showed a significant decrease in the fertilization rate and a decrease in the viability and body weight of offspring, which may have been due to the sedative effect; also, one neonate in each of the first and second matings in this last study showed skeletal deformities.
*For clonazepam—*
Studies in rabbits have shown that clonazepam in oral doses of 0.2 and 5.0 mg/kg per day caused a non-dose-related incidence of cleft palates, open eyelids, fused sternebrae, and limb defects.
Withdrawal of clonazepam prior to or during pregnancy should be considered only when seizures are mild and infrequent in the absence of the medication and where the possibility of status epilepticus and withdrawal symptoms is considered low.
*For lorazepam—*
Studies in rabbits have shown that lorazepam causes fetal resorption and increased fetal loss at oral doses of 40 mg/kg and intravenous doses of 4 mg/kg and higher; however, lorazepam was also shown to cause anomalies in rabbits without relationship to dosage.
*For quazepam—*
Reproduction studies in mice given 66 to 400 times the human dose of quazepam showed minor developmental variations including delayed ossification of the sternum, vertebrae, distal phalanges, and supraoccipital bones. Studies in mice given 60 to 180 times the human dose produced slight reductions in the pregnancy rate.
*For temazepam—*
Studies in rats have shown that temazepam causes increased nursling mortality at oral doses of 60 mg/kg per day, increased incidence of fetal resorption at doses of 30 and 120 mg/kg, and increased occurrence of rudimentary ribs (considered skeletal variants) at doses of 240 mg/kg or higher. Also, studies in rabbits have shown that temazepam causes an increased incidence of the 13th rib variant at doses of 40 mg/kg or higher, and abnormalities such as exencephaly and fusion or asymmetry of ribs without relationship to dosage.

Alprazolam; Halazepam; Lorazepam [parenteral]—FDA Pregnancy Category D.
Estazolam; Quazepam; Temazepam; Triazolam—FDA Pregnancy Category X.
Other benzodiazepines—FDA pregnancy categories not presently included in product labeling.

Labor—For all benzodiazepines: Use of benzodiazepines just prior to or during labor may cause neonatal flaccidity.

Delivery—For diazepam: When diazepam is administered in doses of more than 30 mg (especially intramuscularly or intravenously) to women within 15 hours before delivery, the neonate may develop apnea, hypotonia, hypothermia, a reluctance to feed, and impaired metabolic response to cold stress.

### Breast-feeding

Chlordiazepoxide, diazepam, halazepam, and quazepam and their metabolites, including desmethyldiazepam (also the metabolite of clorazepate and prazepam), and nitrazepam are distributed into breast milk; alprazolam, bromazepam, clonazepam, flurazepam, lorazepam, oxazepam, and temazepam and/or their metabolites may be distributed into breast milk. Although studies with estazolam, ketazolam, and triazolam in humans have not been done, studies in rats have shown that estazolam, ketazolam, and triazolam and their metabolites are distributed into the milk of rats.

Since neonates metabolize benzodiazepines more slowly than adults and accumulation of the benzodiazepine and/or its metabolites may occur, use by nursing mothers may cause sedation, and possibly feeding difficulties and weight loss in the infant.

## Pediatrics
For all benzodiazepines—Children, especially the very young, are usually more sensitive to the CNS effects of benzodiazepines. Prolonged CNS depression may be produced in the neonate because of inability to biotransform the benzodiazepine into inactive metabolites.

For clonazepam—Risk-benefit must be considered in the long-term use of clonazepam in pediatric patients because of possible adverse effects on physical or mental development, which may not become apparent for many years.

## Geriatrics
Geriatric patients are usually more sensitive to the CNS effects of benzodiazepines. It is recommended that dosage be limited to the smallest effective dose and increased gradually, if necessary, to decrease the possibility of development of ataxia, dizziness, and oversedation. A retrospective case-control study has shown that elderly patients receiving long-acting benzodiazepines are more likely than those receiving short-acting benzodiazepines to suffer falls and fall-related fractures. However, both groups had an increased risk of these sequelae as compared to older patients who did not receive benzodiazepines or who received other short-acting sedative-hypnotics.

Parenteral administration of benzodiazepines may be more likely to cause apnea, hypotension, bradycardia, or cardiac arrest in geriatric patients.

## Drug interactions and/or related problems
The following drug interactions and/or related problems have been selected on the basis of their potential clinical significance (possible mechanism in parentheses where appropriate)—not necessarily inclusive (» = major clinical significance):

Note:   Combinations containing any of the following medications, depending on the amount present, may also interact with this medication.

Addictive medications, other, especially CNS depressants with habituating potential
(prolonged concurrent use may increase the risk of habituation; caution is recommended)

» Alcohol or
» CNS depression–producing medications, other (See *Appendix II*)
(concurrent use may increase the CNS depressant effects of either these medications or benzodiazepines; caution is recommended and dosage of one or both agents should be reduced; when a benzodiazepine is used concurrently with an opioid analgesic, the dosage of the opioid analgesic should be reduced by at least one-third and administered in small increments)

Antacids
(concurrent use may delay, but not reduce, the absorption of chlordiazepoxide and diazepam; whether this effect applies to other benzodiazepines has not been determined)

(concurrent use with clorazepate may decrease the rate of conversion of clorazepate to desmethyldiazepam, but does not affect the degree of absorption)

Antidepressants, tricyclic
(in addition to possibly increasing CNS depressant effects, concurrent use with alprazolam in doses of up to 4 mg per day has been reported to increase steady-state plasma concentrations of imipramine and desipramine by an average of 31% and 20%, respectively; however, the clinical significance of these changes is unknown)

Carbamazepine
(concurrent use with benzodiazepines metabolized via the hepatic enzyme system, especially clonazepam, may result in increased metabolism, leading to decreased serum concentrations and reduced elimination half-lives of benzodiazepines because of induction of hepatic microsomal enzyme activity; monitoring of carbamazepine blood concentrations as a guide to dosage is recommended, especially when carbamazepine is added to or withdrawn from existing benzodiazepine therapy)

Cimetidine or
Contraceptives, estrogen-containing, oral or
Disulfiram or
Erythromycin
(concurrent use may inhibit the hepatic metabolism of benzodiazepines that are metabolized by oxidation, especially chlordiazepoxide and diazepam, resulting in delayed elimination and increased plasma concentrations; however, the hepatic metabolism of benzodiazepines such as lorazepam, oxazepam, and temazepam is probably not affected, possibly because these medications do

not appear to affect glucuronide conjugation of these benzodiazepines)

(concurrent use of cimetidine or oral estrogen-containing contraceptives may inhibit the hepatic metabolism of benzodiazepines, such as nitrazepam, that are metabolized primarily by nitro-reduction, possibly resulting in delayed elimination and prolonged elimination half-life; also, during long-term use, serum concentrations may be increased)

(concurrent use of cimetidine or erythromycin may inhibit the hepatic metabolism of triazolam, resulting in increased plasma concentrations and delayed clearance of triazolam; dosage reductions may be necessary)

Clozapine
(collapse, sometimes accompanied by respiratory depression or arrest, has been reported in a few patients receiving clozapine concurrently with benzodiazepines. Caution is advised when clozapine is administered concomitantly with any agent that may depress respiration, and the dosage of clozapine should be titrated upwards slowly. Some clinicians have recommended that benzodiazepines be discontinued at least 1 week prior to initiation of therapy with clozapine)

Fentanyl derivatives
(premedication with diazepam or lorazepam may decrease the dose of a fentanyl derivative required for induction of anesthesia and decrease the time to loss of consciousness with induction doses; also, administration of diazepam or lorazepam prior to or during surgery may decrease risk of patient recall of surgical events postoperatively; however, these potential benefits must be weighed against the potential risks of concurrent use, such as an increased risk of severe hypotension associated with decreases in systemic vascular resistance, increased risk of respiratory depression, and delayed recovery time, especially when the benzodiazepine is administered intravenously)

Hypotension-producing medications, other (See *Appendix II*)
(concurrent use may potentiate the hypotensive effects of benzodiazepine preanesthetics used in surgery; dosage adjustments may be necessary)

(concurrent use of mecamylamine or trimethaphan with benzodiazepine preanesthetics used in surgery may potentiate the hypotensive response, with increased risk of severe hypotension, shock, and cardiovascular collapse during surgery)

(caution is advised during titration of calcium channel blocker dosage for those patients taking medication known to promote hypotension, such as benzodiazepine preanesthetics, since the combination may result in excessive hypotension)

Isoniazid
(concurrent use may inhibit the elimination of diazepam and triazolam, resulting in increased plasma concentrations; whether this effect applies to other benzodiazepines has not been determined; dosage adjustment may be necessary)

Levodopa
(concurrent use with benzodiazepines may decrease the therapeutic effects of levodopa)

Omeprazole
(concurrent use of omeprazole may prolong the elimination of diazepam)

Probenecid
(concurrent use may impair glucuronide conjugation of lorazepam, oxazepam, or temazepam, resulting in increased effects and possibly excessive sedation)

Rifampin
(concurrent use may enhance the elimination of diazepam, resulting in decreased plasma concentrations; whether this effect applies to other benzodiazepines has not been determined; dosage adjustment may be necessary)

Scopolamine, systemic
(concurrent use of scopolamine with parenteral lorazepam is reported to have no added beneficial effect and their combined effect may increase the incidence of sedation, hallucination, and irrational behavior)

Zidovudine
(concurrent use with benzodiazepines may, in theory, competitively inhibit hepatic glucuronidation and decrease the clearance of zidovudine; the toxicity of zidovudine potentially could be increased)

## Laboratory value alterations

The following have been selected on the basis of their potential clinical significance (possible effect in parentheses where appropriate)—not necessarily inclusive (» = major clinical significance):

With diagnostic test results

Metyrapone test

(chlordiazepoxide may interfere with the assay for urine 17-ketosteroids or 17-ketogenic steroids; in addition, the response to metyrapone may be decreased)

Sodium iodide I 123 and
Sodium iodide I 131

(benzodiazepines may decrease thyroidal uptake of I 123 and I 131)

## Medical considerations/Contraindications

The medical considerations/contraindications included here have been selected on the basis of their potential clinical significance (reasons given in parentheses where appropriate)—not necessarily inclusive (» = major clinical significance).

*Risk-benefit should be considered when the following medical problems exist:*

Alcohol intoxication, acute, with depressed vital signs
(additive CNS depression)

Coma or
Shock
(hypnotic or hypotensive effects may be prolonged or intensified by benzodiazepines administered parenterally)

Drug abuse or dependence, history of
(patients predisposed to habituation and dependence)

Epilepsy or
Seizures, history of
(initiation or abrupt withdrawal of clonazepam or diazepam therapy may increase frequency and/or severity of tonic-clonic [grand mal] seizures; use of intravenous diazepam for absence [petit mal] status or Lennox-Gastaut syndrome [petit mal variant] status may precipitate tonic status epilepticus)

(abrupt withdrawal of clonazepam or diazepam used to treat these disorders may precipitate seizures or status epilepticus)

» Glaucoma, angle-closure, acute or predisposition to
(benzodiazepines may have anticholinergic effect)

Hepatic function impairment
(elimination half-life may be prolonged; minimal effect with oxazepam, lorazepam, and temazepam)

Hyperkinesis
(paradoxical reactions may occur)

Hypoalbuminemia
(may predispose patient to higher incidence of sedative side effects, especially with chlordiazepoxide and diazepam)

Mental depression, severe
(suicidal tendencies may be present; protective measures may be necessary; also benzodiazepines, when used alone, may increase depression; episodes of hypomania and mania reported with use of alprazolam in patients with mental depression)

» Myasthenia gravis
(condition may be exacerbated)

Organic brain disorders
(patients may be more prone to disinhibition and CNS depressant effects of benzodiazepines)

Porphyria
(condition may be exacerbated with the use of chlordiazepoxide)

Psychoses
(benzodiazepines are rarely effective as primary treatment for psychosis; also, paradoxical reactions may occur)

» Pulmonary disease, severe chronic obstructive
(ventilatory failure may be exacerbated)

Renal function impairment
(elimination may be prolonged)

Sensitivity to benzodiazepines

Sleep apnea, established or suspected
(condition may be exacerbated)

Swallowing abnormality, in children
(condition may be exacerbated because drooling and aspiration induced by benzodiazepines, such as nitrazepam, may delay cricopharyngeal relaxation; patient should be closely monitored)

Caution should also be used in surgical or nonambulatory patients because of the cough-suppressant effects of clonazepam.

## Patient monitoring

The following may be especially important in patient monitoring (other tests may be warranted in some patients, depending on condition; » = major clinical significance):

Reassessment of medication's efficacy as an antianxiety agent or a sedative-hypnotic
(recommended at periodic intervals during therapy; see *Indications*)

# Side/Adverse Effects

Note: Although not all of these side effects have been attributed specifically to each benzodiazepine, a potential exists for their occurrence during the use of any benzodiazepine.

Geriatric and debilitated patients, children (especially the very young), and patients with liver disease or low serum albumin are usually more sensitive to the CNS effects of benzodiazepines.

Parenteral administration of benzodiazepines may cause apnea, hypotension, bradycardia, or cardiac arrest, especially in geriatric or severely ill patients and in patients with limited pulmonary reserve or unstable cardiovascular status or if intravenous administration of medication is too rapid.

Parenteral benzodiazepines have produced hypotension or muscular weakness in some patients, especially when used concurrently with narcotics, barbiturates, or alcohol.

Coughing, depressed respiration, dyspnea, hyperventilation, laryngospasm, and pain in throat and chest have been reported when parenteral diazepam was administered in peroral endoscopic procedures.

The following side/adverse effects have been selected on the basis of their potential clinical significance (possible signs and symptoms in parentheses where appropriate)—not necessarily inclusive:

### Those indicating need for medical attention

Incidence less frequent

*Intolerance to benzodiazepines* (confusion); *mental depression*

Incidence rare

*Allergic reaction* (skin rash or itching); *behavior problems* (including difficulty in concentrating and outbursts of anger); *blood dyscrasias, including agranulocytosis* (chills, fever, sore throat; unusual tiredness or weakness); *anemia* (unusual tiredness or weakness); *leukopenia* (chills, fever, sore throat); *neutropenia* (chills, fever, and/or sore throat; ulcers or sores in mouth or throat, continuing; unusual tiredness or weakness); *thrombocytopenia* (unusual bleeding or bruising); *extrapyramidal effects, dystonic* (uncontrolled movements of body, including the eyes); *hepatic dysfunction* (yellow eyes or skin); *hypotension* (low blood pressure); *memory impairment; muscle weakness; paradoxical reactions* (including hallucinations; insomnia; unusual excitement, nervousness, or irritability); *phlebitis or venous thrombosis* (redness, swelling, or pain at injection site)—for parenteral dosage forms only; *seizures*

Note: *Behavioral disturbances* associated with clonazepam are more likely to occur in children or in patients with pre-existing brain damage and/or mental retardation or a history of behavioral or psychiatric disturbances; if these effects occur, the medication should be discontinued.

*Anterograde amnesia* may occur at a higher rate with triazolam.

An increase in daytime *anxiety* has been reported for triazolam after as few as 10 days of continuous use. If this effect occurs, the medications should be discontinued.

Incidence of *phlebitis* or *venous thrombosis* is more common with diazepam, less common with lorazepam, and rare with chlordiazepoxide.

There may be an increased incidence and severity of *seizures*, especially on initiation or abrupt withdrawal of clonazepam and diazepam in patients with epilepsy or history of seizures.

### Those indicating need for medical attention only if they continue or are bothersome

Incidence more frequent

*Ataxia* (clumsiness or unsteadiness)—especially in elderly or debilitated patients; *dizziness or lightheadedness; drowsiness, including residual daytime drowsiness when used as a hypnotic*—especially in elderly or debilitated patients; *slurred speech*

Note: *Ataxia* and *drowsiness* are dose-related and are most severe during initial therapy. They may decrease in severity or disappear with continued or long-term therapy.

Daytime drowsiness may be dose-related.

Incidence less frequent or rare

*Abdominal or stomach cramps or pain; blurred vision or other changes in vision; changes in libido* (changes in sexual drive or performance); *constipation; diarrhea; dryness of mouth or increased thirst; euphoria* (false sense of well-being); *headache; increased bronchial secretions or watering of mouth; muscle spasm; nausea or vomiting; problems with urination; tachycardia/palpitations* (fast or pounding heartbeat); *trembling; unusual tiredness or weakness*

**Those indicating possible withdrawal and the need for medical attention if they occur (usually within 2 to 3 days with short to intermediate half-life benzodiazepines and 10 to 20 days with long half-life benzodiazepines) after medication is abruptly discontinued**

Incidence more frequent

*Irritability; nervousness; trouble in sleeping*

Incidence less frequent

*abdominal or stomach cramps; confusion; depersonalization* (loss of sense of reality); *increased sweating; mental depression; muscle cramps; nausea or vomiting; perceptual disturbances, including hyperacusis* (increased sense of hearing); *hypersensitivity to touch and pain; parasthesias* (tingling, burning, or prickly sensations); *or photophobia* (sensitivity of eyes to light); *tachycardia* (fast or pounding heartbeat); *trembling*

Incidence rare

*Convulsions; delirium* (confusion as to time, place, or person); *hallucinations; paranoid symptoms* (feelings of suspicion and distrust)

Note: *Withdrawal symptoms,* especially the more serious ones, are usually more common in patients who have received excessive doses over a prolonged period of time. However, symptoms have occurred following abrupt discontinuation of benzodiazepines that have been taken continuously, at therapeutic concentrations, for as few as 1 to 2 weeks. In some patients, withdrawal symptoms have occurred during gradual discontinuation or tapering of benzodiazepines. Withdrawal symptoms may be more likely to occur following the use of short-acting benzodiazepines than with long-acting benzodiazepines. There is no apparent correlation between the severity of withdrawal symptoms and previous benzodiazepine dose or plasma concentrations at the time the benzodiazepine was discontinued.

Rebound insomnia has occurred following withdrawal of single nightly doses of most benzodiazepines. It may occur sooner and be more frequent and severe following withdrawal of short half-life benzodiazepines. Since desmethyldiazepam (an active metabolite of chlordiazepoxide, clorazepate, diazepam, halazepam, ketazolam, and prazepam) and desalkylflurazepam (an active metabolite of flurazepam and quazepam) may persist in the blood for days or weeks, rebound insomnia may not occur for 10 to 20 days, if at all, after withdrawal of these long half-life benzodiazepines.

## Overdose

For specific information on the agents used in the management of benzodiazepine overdose, see:

- *Charcoal, Activated (Oral-Local)* monograph;
- *Dopamine* and/or *Metaraminol* and/or *Norepinephrine* in *Sympathomimetic Agents—Cardiovascular Use (Parenteral-Systemic)* monograph; and/or
- *Flumazenil (Systemic)* monograph.

For more information on the management of overdose or unintentional ingestion, **contact a Poison Control Center** (see *Poison Control Center Listing*).

### Clinical effects of overdose

The following effects have been selected on the basis of their potential clinical significance (possible signs and symptoms in parentheses where appropriate)—not necessarily inclusive:

*Confusion, continuing; decreased reflexes; drowsiness, severe; shakiness; slow heartbeat, shortness of breath, or troubled breathing; slurred speech, continuing; staggering; weakness, severe*

### Treatment of overdose

For benzodiazepine intoxication, treatment consists of general supportive therapy and includes the following:

To decrease absorption—

If the patient is conscious (and not at risk of becoming obtunded, comatose, or convulsing based on ingestion), emesis should be induced mechanically or with emetics; also, activated charcoal may be administered orally to increase clearance as well as decrease absorption of the benzodiazepine.

If the patient is unconscious, gastric lavage may be performed with a cuffed endotracheal tube in place to prevent aspiration of vomitus.

To enhance elimination—

Intravenous fluids may be administered to promote diuresis.

Specific treatment—

Oxygen should be administered if respiration is depressed.

Hypotension may be controlled, if necessary, by intravenous administration of vasopressors such as dopamine, norepinephrine, or metaraminol.

Flumazenil is now available, and other agents are currently under investigation to determine their usefulness as antagonists to reverse the effects of the benzodiazepines.

Monitoring—

Respiration, pulse, and blood pressure should be monitored.

Supportive care—

An adequate airway should be maintained.

Patients in whom intentional overdose is known or suspected should be referred for psychiatric consultation.

Note: If excitation occurs, barbiturates should *not* be used since they may exacerbate excitation and/or prolong CNS depression.

Dialysis is of limited value in the treatment of overdose.

## Patient Consultation

As an aid to patient consultation, refer to *Advice for the Patient, Benzodiazepines (Systemic).*

In providing consultation, consider emphasizing the following selected information (» = major clinical significance):

**Before using this medication**

» Conditions affecting use, especially:

Sensitivity to benzodiazepines

Pregnancy—Benzodiazepines reported to increase risk of congenital malformations when used during first trimester of pregnancy; chronic use may cause physical dependence in the neonate with resulting withdrawal symptoms; use during last weeks of pregnancy may cause neonatal CNS depression; use just prior to or during labor may cause neonatal flaccidity

Breast-feeding—Some benzodiazepines and their metabolites distributed into breast milk and others may be distributed into breast milk; use by nursing mothers may cause sedation, and possibly feeding difficulties and weight loss in the infant

Use in children—Children, especially the very young, usually more sensitive to CNS effects of benzodiazepines

Use in the elderly—Elderly patients usually more sensitive to CNS effects of benzodiazepines

Other medications, especially other CNS depression–producing medications

Other medical problems, especially acute angle-closure glaucoma, myasthenia gravis, or severe chronic obstructive pulmonary disease

**Proper use of this medication**

*Proper administration*

*For extended-release dosage form of diazepam*

Swallowing capsule whole

Not crushing, breaking, or chewing

*For oral solution dosage form of lorazepam*

Dose may be diluted with liquid or semisolid food such as water, soda or soda-like beverages, applesauce, or pudding

*For sublingual tablet dosage form of lorazepam*

Not chewing or swallowing tablet whole

Dissolving slowly under tongue; not swallowing for at least 2 minutes to allow sufficient absorption

» Importance of not taking more medication than the amount prescribed because of habit-forming potential

» Not increasing dose if medication is less effective after a few weeks; checking with physician

» Proper dosing

Missed dose: If on scheduled dosing regimen (e.g., for epilepsy)—Taking right away if remembered within an hour or so; if remembered later, not taking at all; not doubling doses

» Proper storage

*For anticonvulsant use of clonazepam, clorazepate, diazepam, or nitrazepam*

» Compliance with therapy; not missing any doses

*For flurazepam only*

» Maximum effectiveness of medication may not occur for 2 or 3 nights after initiation of therapy

## Precautions while using this medication

Regular visits to physician to check progress during prolonged therapy (and during initial therapy with clonazepam)

Checking with physician before discontinuing medication after prolonged use; gradual dosage reduction may be necessary to avoid the possibility of withdrawal symptoms and, in patients with epilepsy or history of seizures, the possibility of precipitating seizures

» Avoiding use of alcohol or other CNS depressants during therapy

» Suspected overdose: Getting emergency help at once

Caution if any laboratory tests required; possible interference with results of metyrapone test

» Caution if drowsiness, dizziness, lightheadedness, or clumsiness or unsteadiness occurs, especially in the elderly

*For anticonvulsant use of clonazepam, clorazepate, diazepam, or nitrazepam*

Carrying medical identification card or bracelet during therapy

## Side/adverse effects

Signs of potential side effects, especially allergic reaction, blood dyscrasias, CNS effects, extrapyramidal symptoms, hepatic dysfunction, muscle weakness, and paradoxical reaction

Most of side/adverse effects more likely to occur in children, especially the very young, and in elderly patients; these patients are usually more sensitive to effects of benzodiazepines

For patients receiving chlordiazepoxide, diazepam, or lorazepam injection: Checking with physician if redness, swelling, or pain at injection site occurs

## General Dosing Information

Geriatric or debilitated patients, children, or patients with hepatic or renal function impairment or low serum albumin should receive decreased initial dosage since elimination of benzodiazepines, especially those with long half-lives, may be decreased in these patients, resulting in increased CNS side effects such as oversedation, dizziness, or impaired coordination.

Benzodiazepines may suppress respiration, especially in the elderly, the very ill, the very young, and patients with limited pulmonary reserve. Lower doses may be required for these patients.

Optimal dosage of benzodiazepines varies with diagnosis and patient response. Individual dosage adjustments are important. The minimum effective dose should be used for the shortest period, with the need for continuing therapy with benzodiazepines reviewed regularly.

Prolonged use and/or larger than usual therapeutic doses of benzodiazepines may result in psychological or physical dependence. The risk of dependence among panic disorder patients taking higher doses of alprazolam (> 4 mg a day) may be greater than among patients taking lower doses for less severe anxiety. Similarly, rebound and withdrawal symptoms may also be more likely to occur in patients taking alprazolam at higher doses and for longer periods (> 8 to 12 weeks).

Following prolonged administration, benzodiazepines should be withdrawn gradually to lessen the possibility of precipitating withdrawal symptoms.

Depressed patients with suicidal tendencies, particularly those who use alcohol excessively, should not have access to large quantities of benzodiazepines.

## For parenteral dosage forms only

Following administration of parenteral dosage forms, patients should be kept under observation for a period of 3 to 8 hours or longer, based on the patient's clinical response and rate of recovery.

Too rapid intravenous administration may result in apnea, hypotension, bradycardia, or cardiac or respiratory arrest.

Inadvertent intra-arterial injection of benzodiazepines may produce arteriospasm, resulting in gangrene.

**When parenteral benzodiazepines are to be administered intravenously, equipment necessary to maintain a patent airway should be immediately available.**

## For treatment of dependence

There are no comparative studies to date documenting superiority of any one withdrawal schedule. Some clinicians substitute a long-acting benzodiazepine for short-acting agents before withdrawal is attempted.

Benzodiazepines should be tapered gradually. Withdrawal schedules ranging from 4 to 16 weeks are usually suggested; however, some practitioners believe withdrawal should be completed within 2 weeks, thus exposing patients to withdrawal symptoms for a shorter length of time.

---

## *ALPRAZOLAM*

## Summary of Differences

Category:
In addition to being indicated as an antianxiety agent, used as an antipanic agent.

Indications:
Also indicated for adjunctive management of anxiety associated with mental depression.

Pharmacology/pharmacokinetics:
Short to intermediate half-life benzodiazepine.
Accumulation is minimal during repeated dosing.
Steady-state plasma concentration usually attained within a few (2 to 3) days.
Elimination rapid following discontinuation of therapy.

Precautions:
Drug interactions and/or related problems—Elevation of steady-state plasma concentrations of imipramine and desipramine reported with concurrent use of alprazolam.
Medical considerations/contraindications—Episodes of hypomania and mania reported with use of alprazolam in patients with mental depression.

## Additional Dosing Information

See also *General Dosing Information.*

Dosage should be reduced gradually when therapy is discontinued or the daily dosage is decreased. It is suggested that the daily dosage be decreased by no more than 500 mcg (0.5 mg) every 3 days. However, some patients may need a slower reduction in dosage.

The occurrence of early morning anxiety or the emergence of anxiety symptoms between doses of alprazolam in panic disorder patients may reflect the development of tolerance, or a time interval between doses that exceeds the duration of clinical action of the administered dose. The manufacturer states that when these effects occur, the prescribed dose is presumed to be insufficient to maintain plasma levels above those needed to prevent relapse, rebound, or withdrawal symptoms over the course of the interdosing interval; they recommend that the same total daily dose be administered in more frequently divided doses.

## Oral Dosage Forms

### ALPRAZOLAM ORAL SOLUTION

**Usual adult dose**
Antianxiety agent—
Oral, initially 250 to 500 mcg (0.25 to 0.5 mg) three times a day, the dosage being titrated to the needs of the patient up to a maximum total dose of 4 mg per day.
Note: Debilitated patients—Oral, initially 250 mcg (0.25 mg) two or three times a day, the dosage being increased as needed and tolerated
Antipanic agent—
Oral, 500 mcg (0.5 mg) three times a day initially, the dosage being increased as needed and tolerated up to a maximum of 10 mg per day.

**Usual pediatric dose**
Antianxiety or antipanic agent—
Children up to 18 years of age: Safety and efficacy have not been established.

**Usual geriatric dose**
Antianxiety agent—
Oral, initially 250 mcg (0.25 mg) two or three times a day, the dosage being increased as needed and tolerated.

**Strength(s) usually available**
U.S.—
0.1 mg/1 mL (Rx) [GENERIC].
1 mg/mL (Rx) [*Alprazolam Intensol*].
Canada—
Not commercially available.

**Packaging and storage**
Store between 15 and 30 °C (59 and 86 °F), unless otherwise specified by manufacturer. Store in a tight, light-resistant container.

**Auxiliary labeling**
• Avoid alcoholic beverages.
• May cause drowsiness.

**Note**
Controlled substance in the U.S.

## ALPRAZOLAM TABLETS USP

**Usual adult dose**
See *Alprazolam Oral Solution*.

**Usual pediatric dose**
See *Alprazolam Oral Solution*.

**Usual geriatric dose**
See *Alprazolam Oral Solution*.

**Strength(s) usually available**
U.S.—

0.25 mg (Rx) [*Xanax* (scored; cellulose; corn starch; docusate sodium; lactose; magnesium stearate; silicon dioxide; sodium benzoate); GENERIC].

0.5 mg (Rx) [*Xanax* (scored; cellulose; corn starch; docusate sodium; lactose; magnesium stearate; silicon dioxide; sodium benzoate; FD&C Yellow No. 6); GENERIC].

1 mg (Rx) [*Xanax* (scored; cellulose; corn starch; docusate sodium; lactose; magnesium stearate; silicon dioxide; sodium benzoate; FD&C Blue No. 2); GENERIC].

2 mg (Rx) [*Xanax* (multi-scored; cellulose; corn starch; docusate sodium; lactose; magnesium stearate; silicon dioxide; sodium benzoate); GENERIC].

Canada—

0.25 mg (Rx) [*Apo-Alpraz* (scored); *Novo-Alprazol* (scored); *Nu-Alpraz* (scored); *Xanax* (scored)].

0.5 mg (Rx) [*Apo-Alpraz* (scored); *Novo-Alprazol* (scored); *Nu-Alpraz* (scored); *Xanax* (scored); GENERIC].

1 mg (Rx) [*Xanax* (scored)].

2 mg (Rx) [*Xanax TS* (triscored)].

**Packaging and storage**
Store between 15 and 30 °C (59 and 86 °F), unless otherwise specified by manufacturer. Store in a tight, light-resistant container.

**Auxiliary labeling**
• Avoid alcoholic beverages.
• May cause drowsiness.

**Note**
Controlled substance in the U.S.

---

### BROMAZEPAM

## Summary of Differences

Category:
Indicated only as an antianxiety agent.
Pharmacology/pharmacokinetics:
Short to intermediate half-life benzodiazepine.
Accumulation is minimal during repeated dosing.
Steady-state plasma concentration usually attained within a few (2 to 3) days.
Elimination rapid following discontinuation of therapy.

## Oral Dosage Forms
### BROMAZEPAM TABLETS

**Usual adult dose**
Antianxiety agent—
Oral, 6 to 30 mg per day in divided doses.
Note: Doses up to 60 mg may be used in severe cases.
Debilitated patients—Initial daily dose should not exceed 3 mg in divided doses, the dosage being carefully adjusted as needed and tolerated.

**Usual pediatric dose**
Antianxiety agent—
Children up to 18 years of age: Safety and efficacy have not been established.

**Usual geriatric dose**
Antianxiety agent—
Oral, up to 3 mg initially, the dosage being carefully adjusted as needed and tolerated.

**Strength(s) usually available**
U.S.—
Not commercially available.
Canada—
1.5 mg (Rx) [*Lectopam* (scored; lactose 96 mg)].
3 mg (Rx) [*Lectopam* (scored; lactose 94 mg)].
6 mg (Rx) [*Lectopam* (scored; lactose 91 mg)].

**Packaging and storage**
Store below 40 °C (104 °F), preferably between 15 and 30 °C (59 and 86 °F), in a well-closed container, unless otherwise specified by manufacturer.

**Auxiliary labeling**
• Avoid alcoholic beverages.
• May cause drowsiness.

---

### CHLORDIAZEPOXIDE

## Summary of Differences

Category:
In addition to being indicated as an antianxiety agent and a sedative-hypnotic, oral chlordiazepoxide is used as an antitremor agent and parenteral chlordiazepoxide is used as an antipanic agent.
Indications:
Also indicated for relief of acute alcohol withdrawal symptoms and as a preoperative medication.
Also used in treatment of tension headache.
Pharmacology/pharmacokinetics:
Absorption of intramuscular chlordiazepoxide may be slow and erratic.
Long half-life benzodiazepine.
Accumulation of chlordiazepoxide and its active metabolites is significant during repeated dosing.
Steady-state plasma concentration usually attained in 5 days to 2 weeks.
Elimination slow since metabolites remain in blood for several days or even weeks.
Precautions:
Drug interactions and/or related problems—
Antacids may delay the rate of but not reduce the extent of absorption of chlordiazepoxide.
Medical considerations/contraindications—
Hypoalbuminemia may predispose patient to an increased incidence of sedative side effects.
Porphyria may be exacerbated by use of chlordiazepoxide.
Side/adverse effects:
Intravenous chlordiazepoxide less likely to cause phlebitis or venous thrombosis than diazepam or lorazepam.

## Additional Dosing Information

See also *General Dosing Information*.

**For parenteral dosage forms only**
Intravenous administration of chlordiazepoxide is usually preferred, since absorption may be slow and erratic following intramuscular administration.
If intramuscular injections are used, they should be administered deeply into the muscle.
Intravenous administration of the intramuscular preparation is not recommended by the manufacturer because of the air bubbles that may form when the intramuscular diluent is added to the chlordiazepoxide hydrochloride powder.
Intravenous injections should be administered slowly over a 1-minute period.
The chlordiazepoxide hydrochloride solution prepared with 0.9% sodium chloride injection or sterile water for injection should not be administered intramuscularly because of pain on injection.

## Oral Dosage Forms
### CHLORDIAZEPOXIDE TABLETS USP

**Usual adult dose**
Antianxiety agent—
Oral, 5 to 25 mg three or four times a day.
Note: Debilitated patients—Oral, 5 mg two to four times a day, the dosage being increased gradually as needed and tolerated.
Sedative-hypnotic
Alcohol withdrawal—
Oral, 50 to 100 mg initially, repeated as needed, up to 400 mg per day, the dosage then reduced to maintenance levels.

**Usual pediatric dose**
Antianxiety agent—
Children up to 6 years of age: Safety and efficacy have not been established.
Children 6 years of age and over: Oral, 5 mg two to four times a day, the dosage being increased, if necessary, to 10 mg two or three times a day.

**Usual geriatric dose**
Antianxiety agent—
    Oral, 5 mg two to four times a day, the dosage being increased gradually as needed and tolerated.

**Strength(s) usually available**
U.S.—
    5 mg (Rx) [*Libritabs* (scored; lactose)].
    10 mg (Rx) [*Libritabs* (scored; lactose)].
    25 mg (Rx) [*Libritabs* (scored; lactose)].
Canada—
    Not commercially available.

**Packaging and storage**
Store below 40 °C (104 °F), preferably between 15 and 30 °C (59 and 86 °F), unless otherwise specified by manufacturer. Store in a tight, light-resistant container.

**Auxiliary labeling**
• Avoid alcoholic beverages.
• May cause drowsiness.

**Note**
Controlled substance in the U.S.

## CHLORDIAZEPOXIDE HYDROCHLORIDE CAPSULES USP

**Usual adult dose**
See *Chlordiazepoxide Tablets USP*.

**Usual pediatric dose**
See *Chlordiazepoxide Tablets USP*.

**Usual geriatric dose**
See *Chlordiazepoxide Tablets USP*.

**Strength(s) usually available**
U.S.—
    5 mg (Rx) [*Librium*; GENERIC].
    10 mg (Rx) [*Librium; Poxi;* GENERIC].
    25 mg (Rx) [*Librium*; GENERIC].
Canada—
    5 mg (Rx) [*Apo-Chlordiazepoxide; Librium; Novopoxide*].
    10 mg (Rx) [*Apo-Chlordiazepoxide; Librium; Novopoxide; Solium* (tartrazine)].
    25 mg (Rx) [*Apo-Chlordiazepoxide; Librium; Novopoxide; Solium*].

**Packaging and storage**
Store below 40 °C (104 °F), preferably between 15 and 30 °C (59 and 86 °F), unless otherwise specified by manufacturer. Store in a tight, light-resistant container.

**Auxiliary labeling**
• Avoid alcoholic beverages.
• May cause drowsiness.

**Note**
Controlled substance in the U.S.

# Parenteral Dosage Forms

Note: Bracketed uses in the *Dosage Forms* section refer to categories of use and/or indications that are not included in U.S. product labeling.

## CHLORDIAZEPOXIDE HYDROCHLORIDE STERILE USP

**Usual adult dose**
Antianxiety agent—
    Intramuscular or intravenous, 50 to 100 mg initially, then 25 to 50 mg three or four times a day, if necessary.
    Preoperative: Intramuscular, 50 to 100 mg one hour prior to surgery.
Sedative-hypnotic—
    Alcohol withdrawal: Intramuscular or intravenous, 50 to 100 mg initially, repeated in two to four hours, if necessary.
[Antipanic agent]—
    Intramuscular or intravenous, 50 to 100 mg initially, repeated in four to six hours if necessary.
Note: Debilitated patients—Intramuscular or intravenous, 25 to 50 mg per dose.

**Usual adult prescribing limits**
Up to 300 mg daily.

**Usual pediatric dose**
Antianxiety agent or
    sedative-hypnotic—
    Children up to 12 years of age: Safety and efficacy have not been established.

Children 12 years of age and over: Intramuscular or intravenous, 25 to 50 mg per dose.

**Usual geriatric dose**
Antianxiety agent or
    sedative-hypnotic—
    Intramuscular or intravenous, 25 to 50 mg per dose.

**Size(s) usually available**
U.S.—
    100 mg, with 2 mL of special intramuscular diluent (Rx) [*Librium* (benzyl alcohol 1.5%; polysorbate 80 4%; propylene glycol 20%; maleic acid 1.6%; sodium hydroxide)].
Canada—
    100 mg, with 2 mL of special intramuscular diluent (Rx) [*Librium* (benzyl alcohol 15 mg; propylene glycol 207 mg; sodium <1 mmol [3.0 mg], per mL)].

**Packaging and storage**
Prior to reconstitution, store below 40 °C (104 °F), preferably between 15 and 30 °C (59 and 86 °F), unless otherwise specified by manufacturer. Protect from light.
Note: Chlordiazepoxide injectable diluent should be stored between 2 and 8 °C (36 and 46 °F).

**Preparation of dosage form**
Solutions of chlordiazepoxide hydrochloride for intramuscular or intravenous use should be prepared immediately before administration.
To prepare solution for intramuscular use, add 2 mL of the special intramuscular diluent (supplied by manufacturer) to the ampul containing 100 mg of chlordiazepoxide hydrochloride. The diluent solution should not be used if it is opalescent or hazy. The diluent should be added carefully to the ampul of powder to avoid bubble formation. Agitate the ampul gently until the powder is completely dissolved. Caution—Use of diluents containing benzyl alcohol is not recommended for preparation of medications for use in neonates. A fatal toxic syndrome consisting of metabolic acidosis, CNS depression, respiratory problems, renal failure, hypotension, and possibly seizures and intracranial hemorrhages has been associated with this use.
To prepare solution for intravenous use, add 5 mL of 0.9% sodium chloride injection or sterile water for injection to the ampul containing 100 mg of chlordiazepoxide hydrochloride. Agitate the ampul gently until the powder is completely dissolved.

**Stability**
After reconstitution, solution should be used immediately.
Any unused portion of the solution should be discarded.
Sterilization by heating should not be done.

**Note**
Controlled substance in the U.S.

---

## *CLONAZEPAM*

# Summary of Differences

Category:
    In addition to being indicated as an anticonvulsant, used as an antipanic agent.
Pharmacology/pharmacokinetics:
    Intermediate half-life benzodiazepine.
Precautions:
    Pregnancy—
        Increased incidence of congenital abnormalities in children whose mothers used anticonvulsants during pregnancy; studies in animals have shown that clonazepam caused a non–dose-related incidence of cleft palates, open eyelids, fused sternebrae, and limb defects; withdrawal of clonazepam prior to or during pregnancy should be considered only when seizures mild and infrequent in absence of medication and the possibility of status epilepticus and withdrawal symptoms considered low.
    Pediatrics—
        Long-term use of clonazepam may cause possible adverse effects on physical or mental development which may not become apparent for many years.
    Medical considerations/contraindications—
        Initiation or abrupt withdrawal of clonazepam in patients with epilepsy or a history of seizures may precipitate seizures or status epilepticus.
        Caution should be used in surgical or non-ambulatory patients because of cough suppressant effects of clonazepam.

# Additional Dosing Information

See also *General Dosing Information*.

Dosage must be adjusted to meet the individual requirements of each patient, based on clinical response.

Since tolerance to clonazepam may develop after a few (often within 3) months of therapy, dosage adjustment may be necessary to restore efficacy of clonazepam.

In order to maintain seizure control, when clonazepam is used to replace other anticonvulsant therapy, the dosage of clonazepam should be gradually increased while the dosage of the other medication is gradually decreased; when clonazepam is used to supplement other anticonvulsant therapy, the dosage of clonazepam should be gradually increased until seizure activity is adequately controlled and then the dosage of the other medication may be gradually decreased if necessary.

Also, clonazepam should be withdrawn gradually, especially in those patients on long-term, high-dose therapy, since abrupt withdrawal may precipitate seizures or status epilepticus. During withdrawal of clonazepam, the simultaneous administration of another anticonvulsant may be indicated..

# Oral Dosage Forms

## CLONAZEPAM TABLETS USP

### Usual adult dose

Anticonvulsant—
Oral, initially 500 mcg (0.5 mg) three times a day, the dosage being increased in increments of 500 mcg (0.5 mg) to 1 mg every three days until seizures are controlled or until side effects prevent any further increase.

Note: Maintenance dose must be individualized, depending on patient's response.

### Usual adult prescribing limits

Up to 20 mg daily.

### Usual pediatric dose

Anticonvulsant—
Infants and children up to 10 years of age or 30 kg of body weight: Oral, initially 10 to 30 mcg (0.01 to 0.03 mg), not to exceed 50 mcg (0.05 mg), per kg of body weight per day (in two or three divided doses), the dosage being increased by no more than 250 to 500 mcg (0.25 to 0.5 mg) every third day until a maintenance dose of 100 to 200 mcg (0.1 to 0.2 mg) per kg of body weight per day is reached or until seizures are controlled or side effects prevent a further increase.

Note: The daily dose should be divided into three equal doses, if possible. If doses are not equally divided, the largest dose should be given before retiring.

### Strength(s) usually available

U.S.—
0.5 mg (Rx) [*Klonopin* (scored; lactose)].
1 mg (Rx) [*Klonopin* (scored; lactose)].
2 mg (Rx) [*Klonopin* (scored; lactose)].

Canada—
0.5 mg (Rx) [*Rivotril* (scored; lactose 122 mg); *Syn-Clonazepam*].
2 mg (Rx) [*Rivotril* (scored; lactose 122 mg); *Syn-Clonazepam*].

### Packaging and storage

Store between 15 and 30 °C (59 and 86 °F). Store in a tight, light-resistant container.

### Auxiliary labeling

• Avoid alcoholic beverages.
• May cause drowsiness.

### Note

Controlled substance in the U.S.

---

## *CLORAZEPATE*

# Summary of Differences

Category:
In addition to being indicated as an antianxiety agent and a sedative-hypnotic, indicated as an anticonvulsant.

Indications:
Also indicated for relief of acute alcohol withdrawal symptoms.

Pharmacology/pharmacokinetics:
Orally, one of most rapidly absorbed benzodiazepines.
Long half-life benzodiazepine.

Accumulation of active metabolites is significant during repeated dosing.

Steady-state plasma concentration usually attained in 5 days to 2 weeks.

Elimination slow since metabolites remain in blood for several days or even weeks.

Precautions:
Drug interactions and/or related problems—
Antacids may decrease rate of conversion to desmethyldiazepam but do not affect degree of absorption.

# Additional Dosing Information

See also *General Dosing Information*.

When used for alcohol withdrawal, excessive reductions in the total amount of medication administered on successive days should be avoided.

# Oral Dosage Forms

## CLORAZEPATE DIPOTASSIUM CAPSULES

### Usual adult and adolescent dose

Antianxiety agent—
Oral, 7.5 to 15 mg two to four times a day; or 15 mg initially, as a single dose at bedtime, the dosage being adjusted as needed and tolerated.

Note: Debilitated patients—Oral, initially, 3.75 to 15 mg per day, the dosage being increased gradually as needed and tolerated.

Sedative-hypnotic—
Alcohol withdrawal: Oral, 30 mg initially, followed by 15 mg two to four times a day the first day; 15 mg three to six times a day the second day; 7.5 to 15 mg three times a day the third day; 7.5 mg two to four times a day the fourth day; and thereafter, 3.75 mg two to four times a day.

Anticonvulsant[1]—
Oral, initially up to 7.5 mg three times a day, the dosage being increased by no more than 7.5 mg per week, not to exceed 90 mg per day.

### Usual adult prescribing limits

Up to 90 mg daily.

### Usual pediatric dose

Children up to 9 years of age: Safety and efficacy have not been established.
Anticonvulsant[1]—
Children 9 to 12 years of age: Oral, initially up to 7.5 mg two times a day, the dosage being increased by no more than 7.5 mg per week, not to exceed 60 mg per day.
Children 12 years of age and over: See *Usual adult and adolescent dose*.

### Usual geriatric dose

Antianxiety agent—
Oral, initially, 3.75 to 15 mg per day, the dosage being increased gradually as needed and tolerated.

### Strength(s) usually available

U.S.—
3.75 mg (Rx) [GENERIC].
7.5 mg (Rx) [GENERIC].
15 mg (Rx) [GENERIC].

Canada—
3.75 mg (Rx) [*Apo-Clorazepate; Novo-Clopate; Tranxene*].
7.5 mg (Rx) [*Apo-Clorazepate; Novo-Clopate; Tranxene*].
15 mg (Rx) [*Apo-Clorazepate; Novo-Clopate; Tranxene*].

### Packaging and storage

Store below 40 °C (104 °F), preferably between 15 and 30 °C (59 and 86 °F), in a tight, light-resistant container, unless otherwise specified by manufacturer.

### Auxiliary labeling

• Avoid alcoholic beverages.
• May cause drowsiness.

### Note

Controlled substance in the U.S.

## CLORAZEPATE DIPOTASSIUM TABLETS

### Usual adult and adolescent dose

See *Clorazepate Dipotassium Capsules*.

### Usual adult prescribing limits

See *Clorazepate Dipotassium Capsules*.

**Usual pediatric dose**
See *Clorazepate Dipotassium Capsules.*

**Usual geriatric dose**
See *Clorazepate Dipotassium Capsules.*

**Strength(s) usually available**
U.S.—
  3.75 mg (Rx) [*Gen-XENE* (scored); *Tranxene T-Tab* (scored); GENERIC].
  7.5 mg (Rx) [*Gen-XENE* (scored); *Tranxene T-Tab* (scored); GENERIC].
  11.25 mg (Rx) [*Tranxene-SD* (lactose; potassium carbonate; potassium chloride; castor oil wax; magnesium stearate; magnesium oxide; talc; FD&C Blue #2)].
  15 mg (Rx) [*Gen-XENE* (scored); *Tranxene T-Tab* (scored); GENERIC].
  22.5 mg (Rx) [*Tranxene-SD* (iron oxide; lactose; potassium carbonate; potassium chloride; castor oil wax; magnesium stearate; magnesium oxide; talc)].
Canada—
  Not commercially available.

**Packaging and storage**
Store between 15 and 30 °C (59 and 86 °F), in a tight, light-resistant container, unless otherwise specified by manufacturer.

**Stability**
Clorazepate dipotassium degrades in the presence of moisture. One of the degradation products is carbon dioxide gas, which tends to cause the tablets to "blow apart" and disintegrate very rapidly. The drug is also sensitive to heat and light. Pharmacists are advised to retain the desiccant when opening a new stock bottle of the product. If it is necessary to repackage the drug into unit doses, it is recommended that pharmacists be certain that the packaging materials used for unit-dose containers will produce a Class A package as defined in the USP. Multiple-dose containers should meet USP "tight" and "light-resistant" specifications. Pharmacists should consider using desiccant packets when dispensing a large number of tablets in a multiple-dose container. If shipping or mailing prescriptions, pharmacists should take into account these instability problems. Patients should be warned not to expose the product to moisture, light, or heat, and when possible to keep the tablets in the original containers.

**Auxiliary labeling**
• Avoid alcoholic beverages.
• May cause drowsiness.

**Note**
Controlled substance in the U.S.

---

[1]Not included in Canadian product labeling.

---

## DIAZEPAM

## Summary of Differences

Category:
  In addition to being indicated as an antianxiety agent and a sedative-hypnotic, indicated as an anticonvulsant and a skeletal muscle relaxant adjunct and used as an antipanic agent.
  Parenteral diazepam also indicated as an amnestic.
  Oral diazepam also used as an antitremor agent.
Indications:
  Also indicated for relief of acute alcohol withdrawal symptoms, for the treatment of status epilepticus, and as a preoperative medication.
  Parenteral diazepam also indicated as an adjunct prior to endoscopic procedures; indicated prior to cardioversion; and used in dentistry to produce conscious sedation.
  Also used to relieve spasms of facial muscles associated with problems of occlusion and temporomandibular joint disorders, and for the treatment of tension headache.
Pharmacology/pharmacokinetics:
  Orally, the most rapidly absorbed benzodiazepine.
  Absorption of intramuscular diazepam may be slow and erratic, depending upon administration site; usually rapid and complete when injected into the deltoid muscle.
  Absorption of rectal diazepam solution is rapid.
  Long half-life benzodiazepine.
  Accumulation of diazepam and its active metabolites is significant during repeated dosing.
  Steady-state plasma concentration usually attained in 5 days to 2 weeks.
  Elimination slow since metabolites remain in blood for several days or even weeks.

Precautions:
  Pregnancy—
    Administration (especially intramuscular or intravenous) in doses of more than 30 mg within 15 hours before delivery may cause apnea, hypotonia, hypothermia, a reluctance to feed, and impaired metabolic response to cold stress in the neonate.
  Drug interactions and/or related problems—
    Antacids may delay but not reduce the absorption of diazepam.
    Premedication with diazepam may decrease dose of a fentanyl derivative required for induction of anesthesia and decrease time to loss of consciousness with induction doses.
    Isoniazid may inhibit elimination of diazepam, resulting in increased plasma concentrations.
    Rifampin may enhance elimination of diazepam, resulting in decreased plasma concentrations.
  Medical considerations/contraindications—
    Initiation or abrupt withdrawal of diazepam in patients with epilepsy or a history of seizures may precipitate seizures or status epilepticus. Use of intravenous diazepam for absence status or Lennox-Gastaut syndrome status may precipitate tonic status epilepticus.
    Hypoalbuminemia may predispose patient to increased incidence of sedative side effects.
Side/adverse effects:
  Intravenous diazepam more likely to cause phlebitis or venous thrombosis than chlordiazepoxide and lorazepam.

## Additional Dosing Information

See also *General Dosing Information.*

**For oral dosage forms only**
When diazepam is used as an adjunct in treating convulsive disorders, the possibility of an increase in the frequency and/or severity of generalized tonic-clonic (grand mal) seizures may require an increase in dosage of standard anticonvulsant medication. Also, abrupt withdrawal of diazepam may result in a temporary increase in the frequency and/or severity of seizures.

**For parenteral dosage forms only**
Intravenous administration of diazepam is usually preferred, since absorption may be slow and erratic following intramuscular administration depending upon site of injection.
If intramuscular injections of diazepam (with the exception of sterile diazepam emulsion) are used, they should be administered deeply into the deltoid muscle.
For intravenous injections of diazepam (with the exception of sterile diazepam emulsion), small veins such as those on the back of the hand or wrist should not be used. Care should be taken with all parenteral forms of diazepam to avoid intra-arterial administration or extravasation in order to reduce the possibility of venous thrombosis, phlebitis, local irritation, swelling, and, rarely, vascular impairment.
For intravenous injections, the solutions should be injected slowly, into a large vein, at least one minute being taken for each 5 mg (1 mL) of medication given.
When subsequent doses are administered within 1 to 4 hours, consideration should be given to the possibility that active metabolites may still be present from the initial dose.
Continuous intravenous infusion of diazepam is not recommended because of the possibility of precipitation of diazepam in intravenous fluids and adsorption of the medication to the plastic of infusion bags and tubing.
If diazepam cannot be administered by direct intravenous injection, it may be injected slowly through an infusion tubing as close as possible to the insertion point.
When parenteral diazepam is used for peroral endoscopic procedures, the use of a topical anesthetic and availability of necessary countermeasures are recommended since an increase in cough reflex and laryngospasm may occur.

## Oral Dosage Forms

### DIAZEPAM EXTENDED-RELEASE CAPSULES USP

**Usual adult dose**
Antianxiety agent—
  Oral, 15 or 30 mg once a day.
Skeletal muscle relaxant adjunct—
  Oral, 15 or 30 mg once a day.

Note: Geriatric or debilitated patients—Use is recommended only when it has been determined that 5 mg of diazepam three times a day is the optimal daily dose; then, one 15–mg capsule per day may be used.

**Usual pediatric dose**
Antianxiety agent or
Skeletal muscle relaxant adjunct—
    Children up to 6 months of age: Use is not recommended.
    Children 6 months of age and over: Use is recommended only when
        it has been determined that 5 mg of diazepam three times a day is
        the optimal daily dose; then, one 15-mg capsule per day may be
        used.

**Strength(s) usually available**
U.S.—
    15 mg (Rx) [*Valrelease*].
Canada—
    Not commercially available.

**Packaging and storage**
Store below 40 °C (104 °F), preferably between 15 and 30 °C (59 and 86
°F), unless otherwise specified by manufacturer. Store in a tight, light-
resistant container.

**Auxiliary labeling**
• Swallow capsules whole.
• Avoid alcoholic beverages.
• May cause drowsiness.

**Note**
Controlled substance in the U.S.

# DIAZEPAM ORAL SOLUTION

**Usual adult dose**
Antianxiety agent—
    Oral, 2 to 10 mg two to four times a day.
Sedative-hypnotic—
    Alcohol withdrawal: Oral, 10 mg three or four times a day during the
        first twenty-four hours, the dosage being decreased to 5 mg three
        or four times a day as needed.
Anticonvulsant—
    Oral, 2 to 10 mg two to four times a day.
Skeletal muscle relaxant adjunct—
    Oral, 2 to 10 mg three or four times a day.
Note: Debilitated patients—Oral, 2 to 2.5 mg one or two times a day, the
    dosage being increased gradually as needed and tolerated.

**Usual pediatric dose**
Antianxiety agent or
Anticonvulsant or
Skeletal muscle relaxant adjunct—
    Children up to 6 months of age: Use is not recommended.
    Children 6 months of age and over: Oral, 1 to 2.5 mg, 40 to 200 mcg
        (0.04 to 0.2 mg) per kg of body weight, or 1.17 to 6 mg per square
        meter of body surface, three or four times a day, the dosage being
        increased gradually as needed and tolerated.

**Usual geriatric dose**
Antianxiety agent or
Sedative-hypnotic or
Anticonvulsant or
Skeletal muscle relaxant adjunct—
    Oral, 2 to 2.5 mg one or two times a day, the dosage being increased
        gradually as needed and tolerated.

**Strength(s) usually available**
U.S.—
    5 mg per mL (Rx) [*Diazepam Intensol*].
    5 mg per 5 mL (Rx) [GENERIC].
Canada—
    1 mg per mL (Rx) [*PMS-Diazepam*].

**Packaging and storage**
Store below 40 °C (104 °F), preferably between 15 and 30 °C (59 and 86
°F), in a well-closed container, unless otherwise specified by manu-
facturer. Protect from freezing.

**Auxiliary labeling**
• Avoid alcoholic beverages.
• May cause drowsiness.

**Note**
Controlled substance in the U.S.

# DIAZEPAM TABLETS USP

**Usual adult dose**
See *Diazepam Oral Solution*.

**Usual pediatric dose**
See *Diazepam Oral Solution*.

**Usual geriatric dose**
See *Diazepam Oral Solution*.

**Strength(s) usually available**
U.S.—
    2 mg (Rx) [*Valium* (scored); GENERIC].
    5 mg (Rx) [*Valium* (scored); GENERIC].
    10 mg (Rx) [*Valium* (scored); GENERIC].
Canada—
    2 mg (Rx) [*Apo-Diazepam* (scored); *Novodipam* (scored); *Valium*
        (scored); *Vivol* (scored; tartrazine)].
    5 mg (Rx) [*Apo-Diazepam* (scored); *Novodipam* (scored); *Valium*
        (scored); *Vivol* (scored; tartrazine)].
    10 mg (Rx) [*Apo-Diazepam* (scored); *Novodipam* (scored); *Valium*
        (scored); *Vivol* (scored; tartrazine)].

**Packaging and storage**
Store below 40 °C (104 °F), preferably between 15 and 30 °C (59 and 86
°F), unless otherwise specified by manufacturer. Store in a tight, light-
resistant container.

**Auxiliary labeling**
• Avoid alcoholic beverages.
• May cause drowsiness.

**Note**
Controlled substance in the U.S.

# Parenteral Dosage Forms

## DIAZEPAM INJECTION USP

**Usual adult dose**
Antianxiety agent—
    Preoperative medication: Dosage must be individualized; however, as
        a general guideline—Intramuscular or intravenous, 5 to 10 mg
        prior to surgery.
    Psychoneurotic reactions: Intramuscular or intravenous, 2 to 10 mg,
        the dosage being repeated in three or four hours, if necessary.
Sedative-hypnotic—
    Alcohol withdrawal: Intramuscular or intravenous, 10 mg initially, fol-
        lowed by 5 to 10 mg in three or four hours, if necessary.
Amnestic—
    Cardioversion:
        Intravenous, 5 to 15 mg five to ten minutes prior to the procedure.
    Endoscopic procedures:
        Intravenous (preferred route), up to 20 mg, the dosage being ti-
            trated to give the desired sedative response and administered
            immediately prior to the procedure.
        Intramuscular, 5 to 10 mg approximately thirty minutes prior to
            the procedure.
Anticonvulsant—
    Status epilepticus and severe recurrent convulsive seizures: Intrave-
        nous, 5 to 10 mg initially, the dosage being repeated, if necessary,
        at ten- to fifteen-minute intervals up to a maximum dose of 30 mg.
        If necessary, therapy may be repeated in two to four hours.
    Note: The intravenous route of administration is preferred; however,
        if intravenous administration is impossible, the intramuscular
        route of administration may be used.

        Some clinicians have used continuous intravenous infusions of
        diazepam in the treatment of selected patients with status epi-
        lepticus refractory to initial treatment. However, this method of
        administration is problematic due to inherent adsorption prob-
        lems with plastic infusion bags and tubing.
Skeletal muscle relaxant adjunct—
    Muscle spasm: Intramuscular or intravenous, 5 to 10 mg initially, the
        dosage being repeated in three or four hours, if necessary. For
        tetanus, larger doses may be required.
Note: Debilitated patients—Intramuscular or intravenous, initially 2 to 5
    mg per dose, the dosage being increased gradually as needed and
    tolerated.

**Usual pediatric dose**
Neonates up to and 30 days of age: Dosage has not been established.
    Anticonvulsant—
        Status epilepticus and severe recurrent convulsive seizures:
            Infants over 30 days of age and children up to 5 years of age—
                Intravenous (slow), 200 to 500 mcg (0.2 to 0.5 mg) every
                two to five minutes up to a maximum of 5 mg. If necessary,
                therapy may be repeated in two to four hours.
            Children 5 years of age and over—Intravenous (slow), 1 mg
                every two to five minutes up to a maximum of 10 mg. If
                necessary, therapy may be repeated in two to four hours.
            Note: The intravenous route of administration is preferred;
                however, if intravenous administration is impossible, the
                intramuscular route of administration may be used.

Skeletal muscle relaxant adjunct—
  Tetanus:
    Infants over 30 days of age and children up to 5 years of age—
      Intramuscular or intravenous, 1 to 2 mg, the dosage being re-
      peated every three or four hours as needed.
    Children 5 years of age and over—Intramuscular or intravenous,
      5 to 10 mg, the dosage being repeated every three or four hours
      as needed.
Note: When the intravenous route is used in infants and children, it is
      recommended that the medication be administered slowly over a
      three-minute period in a dosage not to exceed 250 mcg (0.25 mg)
      per kg of body weight. After an interval of fifteen to thirty minutes,
      the dosage may be repeated.
    Caution—Medications containing benzyl alcohol are not recom-
      mended for use in neonates. A fatal toxic syndrome consisting of
      metabolic acidosis, CNS depression, respiratory problems, renal
      failure, hypotension, and possibly seizures and intracranial hemor-
      rhages has been associated with this use.

**Usual geriatric dose**
Antianxiety agent or
Sedative-hypnotic or
Amnestic or
Anticonvulsant or
Skeletal muscle relaxant adjunct—
  Intramuscular or intravenous, initially 2 to 5 mg per dose, the dosage
  being increased gradually as needed and tolerated.

**Strength(s) usually available**
U.S.—
  5 mg per mL (Rx) [*D-Val; Valium* (benzoic acid; benzyl alcohol 1.5%;
    ethyl alcohol 10%; propylene glycol 40%; sodium benzoate 5%);
    *Zetran;* GENERIC].
Canada—
  5 mg per mL (Rx) [*Valium* (benzyl alcohol 16 mg; ethyl alcohol 80
    mg; propylene glycol 414 mg; sodium <1 mmol; sodium benzoate
    and benzoic acid 50 mg, per mL)].

**Packaging and storage**
Store below 40 °C (104 °F), preferably between 15 and 30 °C (59 and 86
  °F), unless otherwise specified by manufacturer. Protect from light.
  Protect from freezing.

**Stability**
Do not mix or dilute this medication with other solutions, intravenous
  fluids, or medications, because the resulting admixtures are unstable.
Diazepam is adsorbed to the plastic of intravenous infusion bags and
  tubing.

**Incompatibilities**
Diazepam injection is physically incompatible with aqueous solutions.

**Note**
Controlled substance in the U.S.

## STERILE DIAZEPAM EMULSION

**Usual adult dose**
Antianxiety agent—
  Preoperative medication: Dosage must be individualized; however, as
    a general guideline—Intramuscular or intravenous, 10 mg one to
    two hours prior to surgery.
  Psychoneurotic reactions: Intramuscular or intravenous, 2 to 10 mg,
    the dosage being repeated in three or four hours, if necessary.
Sedative-hypnotic—
  Alcohol withdrawal: Intramuscular or intravenous, 10 mg initially, fol-
    lowed by 5 to 10 mg in three or four hours, if necessary.
Amnestic—
  Cardioversion: Intravenous, 5 to 15 mg ten to twenty minutes prior to
    the procedure.
  Endoscopic procedures: Intramuscular or intravenous, 5 to 10 mg
    about thirty minutes prior to procedure.
Skeletal muscle relaxant adjunct—
  Muscle spasm: Intramuscular or intravenous, 5 to 10 mg initially, the
    dosage being repeated in three or four hours, if necessary.
Note: Debilitated patients—Intramuscular or intravenous, initially 2 to 5
      mg per dose, the dosage being increased gradually as needed and
      tolerated.

**Usual pediatric dose**
Antianxiety agent or
Amnestic or
Skeletal muscle relaxant adjunct—
  Neonates up to and 30 days of age: Dosage has not been established.
  Children over 30 days of age: Dosage must be individualized.

Note: When the intravenous route is used in infants and children, it is
      recommended that the medication be administered slowly over a
      three-minute period in a dosage not to exceed 250 mcg (0.25 mg)
      per kg of body weight. After an interval of fifteen to thirty minutes,
      the dosage may be repeated.

**Usual geriatric dose**
Antianxiety agent or
Sedative-hypnotic or
Amnestic or
Skeletal muscle relaxant adjunct—
  Intramuscular or intravenous, initially 2 to 5 mg per dose, the dosage
  being increased gradually as needed and tolerated.

**Strength(s) usually available**
U.S.—
  Not commercially available.
Canada—
  5 mg per mL (Rx) [*Diazemuls* (acetylated monoglycerides 50 mg;
    fractionated egg phospholipids 12 mg; fractionated soybean oil 150
    mg; glycerol 22.5 mg; sodium hydroxide, per mL)].
Note: Sterile diazepam emulsion is an oil/water emulsion.

**Packaging and storage**
Store below 25 °C (77 °F), unless otherwise specified by manufacturer.
  Protect from freezing.

**Preparation of dosage form**
Sterile diazepam emulsion may be administered without prior dilution or
  mixing with other products or solutions. However, it may be mixed
  or diluted with its emulsion base (*Intralipid* or *Nutralipid*) but the
  admixture should be used within 6 hours.

**Stability**
Sterile diazepam emulsion contains no preservatives.
Mixing or diluting sterile diazepam emulsion with products or solutions
  other than its own emulsion base (*Intralipid* or *Nutralipid*) may desta-
  bilize the emulsion. Although such an effect may not be recognized
  on visual inspection, it may result in potentially serious adverse
  reactions.

**Incompatibilities**
Sterile diazepam emulsion is incompatible with morphine and
  glycopyrrolate.
Infusion sets containing polyvinyl chloride should not be used for administration of sterile diazepam emulsion.

**Additional information**
For administration of sterile diazepam emulsion, polyethylene-lined or
  glass infusion sets and polyethylene/polypropylene plastic syringes are
  recommended; infusion sets containing polyvinyl chloride should not
  be used.

# Rectal Dosage Forms
## DIAZEPAM FOR RECTAL SOLUTION

**Usual adult and adolescent dose**
Anticonvulsant—
  Status epilepticus and severe recurrent convulsive seizures: Rectal, 150
    to 500 mcg (0.15 to 0.5 mg) of diazepam per kg of body weight,
    up to a maximum of 20 mg per dose.

**Usual pediatric dose**
Anticonvulsant—
  Status epilepticus and severe recurrent convulsive seizures: Rectal, 200
    to 500 mcg (0.2 to 0.5 mg) of diazepam per kg of body weight.

**Usual geriatric dose**
Rectal, 200 to 300 mcg (0.2 to 0.3 mg) of diazepam per kg of body weight.

**Strength(s) usually available**
U.S.—
  Not commercially available.
Canada—
  Not commercially available.

**Packaging and storage**
Store below 40 °C (104 °F), preferably between 15 and 30 °C (59 and 86
  °F), unless otherwise specified by manufacturer. Protect from light.
  Protect from freezing.

**Preparation of dosage form**
For rectal administration, Diazepam Injection USP has been used. The
  parenteral preparation may be instilled via a cannula or catheter fitted
  to the syringe or directly from a needleless 1-mL syringe inserted 4
  to 5 centimeters into the rectum to allow for optimum absorption.
  Alternatively, a dilution of Diazepam Injection USP with propylene
  glycol to make a solution containing 1 mg of diazepam per mL has
  been used.

## Stability

Do not mix or dilute this medication with other solutions, intravenous fluids, or medications, because the resulting admixtures are unstable. Diazepam is adsorbed to the plastic of intravenous infusion bags and tubing.

## Incompatibilities

Diazepam injection is physically incompatible with aqueous solutions.

---

## ESTAZOLAM

# Summary of Differences

Category:
Indicated only as a sedative-hypnotic.
Indications:
May be useful in prevention or treatment of transient insomnia associated with sudden sleep schedule changes.
Pharmacology/pharmacokinetics:
Intermediate half-life benzodiazepine.
Small degree of accumulation during repeated dosing.
Steady-state plasma concentration usually attained within a few days.
Intermediate rate of elimination following discontinuation of therapy.

# Oral Dosage Forms

## ESTAZOLAM TABLETS

### Usual adult dose

Sedative-hypnotic—
Oral, 1 mg.

Note: A dose of 2 mg may be necessary in some patients.

### Usual pediatric dose

Sedative-hypnotic—
Children up to 18 years of age: Safety and efficacy have not been established.

### Usual geriatric dose

Sedative-hypnotic—
Oral, 1 mg.

Note: Small or debilitated older patients may be started at 0.5 mg initially.

### Strength(s) usually available

U.S.—
1 mg (Rx) [*ProSom* (scored; lactose)].
2 mg (Rx) [*ProSom* (scored; lactose)].
Canada—
Not commercially available.

### Packaging and storage

Store below 30 °C (86 °F), in a well-closed container, unless otherwise specified by manufacturer.

### Auxiliary labeling

• Avoid alcoholic beverages.
• May cause daytime drowsiness.

### Note

Controlled substance in the U.S.

---

## FLURAZEPAM

# Summary of Differences

Category:
Indicated only as a sedative-hypnotic.
Pharmacology/pharmacokinetics:
Long half-life benzodiazepine.
Accumulation of active metabolites is significant during repeated dosing.
Steady-state plasma concentration usually attained in 7 to 10 days.
Elimination slow since metabolites remain in blood for several days.

# Additional Dosing Information

Flurazepam is increasingly effective on the second or third night of consecutive use, and for one or two nights after medication is discontinued both sleep latency and total wake time may still be decreased.

# Oral Dosage Forms

## FLURAZEPAM HYDROCHLORIDE CAPSULES USP

### Usual adult dose

Sedative-hypnotic—
Oral, 15 or 30 mg.

Note: Debilitated patients—Oral, 15 mg initially, the dosage being increased to 30 mg as needed and tolerated.

### Usual pediatric dose

Sedative-hypnotic—
Children up to 15 years of age: Safety and efficacy have not been established.

### Usual geriatric dose

Sedative-hypnotic—
Oral, 15 mg initially, the dosage being increased to 30 mg as needed and tolerated.

### Strength(s) usually available

U.S.—
15 mg (Rx) [*Dalmane;* GENERIC].
30 mg (Rx) [*Dalmane;* GENERIC].
Canada—
15 mg (Rx) [*Apo-Flurazepam; Dalmane; Novoflupam*].
30 mg (Rx) [*Apo-Flurazepam; Dalmane; Novoflupam*].

### Packaging and storage

Store below 40 °C (104 °F), preferably between 15 and 30 °C (59 and 86 °F), unless otherwise specified by manufacturer. Store in a tight, light-resistant container.

### Auxiliary labeling

• Avoid alcoholic beverages.
• May cause daytime drowsiness.

### Note

Controlled substance in the U.S.

## FLURAZEPAM MONOHYDROCHLORIDE TABLETS

### Usual adult dose

Sedative-hypnotic—
Oral, 15 or 30 mg (dihydrochloride).

Note: Debilitated patients—Oral, 15 mg (dihydrochloride) initially, the dosage being increased as needed and tolerated.

### Usual pediatric dose

Sedative-hypnotic—
Children up to 15 years of age: Safety and efficacy have not been established.

### Usual geriatric dose

Sedative-hypnotic—
Oral, 15 mg (dihydrochloride) initially, the dosage being increased as needed and tolerated.

### Strength(s) usually available

U.S.—
Not commercially available.
Canada—
15 mg (dihydrochloride) (Rx) [*Somnol* (scored; lactose)].
30 mg (dihydrochloride) (Rx) [*Somnol* (scored; lactose)].

### Packaging and storage

Store below 40 °C (104 °F), preferably between 15 and 30 °C, in a well-closed container, unless otherwise specified by manufacturer.

### Auxiliary labeling

• Avoid alcoholic beverages.
• May cause daytime drowsiness.

---

## HALAZEPAM

# Summary of Differences

Category:
Indicated only as an antianxiety agent.
Pharmacology/pharmacokinetics:
Long half-life benzodiazepine.
Accumulation of active metabolite is significant during repeated dosing.
Steady-state plasma concentration usually attained in 5 days to 2 weeks.
Elimination slow since metabolite remains in blood for several days or even weeks.

# Oral Dosage Forms

## HALAZEPAM TABLETS USP

### Usual adult dose

Antianxiety agent—
Oral, 20 to 40 mg three or four times a day.

Note: Debilitated patients—Oral, 20 mg one or two times a day, the dosage being adjusted as needed and tolerated.

### Usual pediatric dose
Antianxiety agent—
Children up to 18 years of age: Safety and efficacy have not been established.

### Usual geriatric dose
Antianxiety agent—
Oral, 20 mg one or two times a day, the dosage being adjusted as needed and tolerated.

### Strength(s) usually available
U.S.—
20 mg (Rx) [*Paxipam* (scored; lactose)].
40 mg (Rx) [*Paxipam* (scored; lactose)].
Canada—
Not commercially available.

### Packaging and storage
Store between 2 and 30 °C (36 and 86 °F), in a well-closed container, unless otherwise specified by manufacturer.

### Auxiliary labeling
• Avoid alcoholic beverages.
• May cause drowsiness.

### Note
Controlled substance in the U.S.

---

## KETAZOLAM

## Summary of Differences

Category:
Indicated only as an antianxiety agent.
Pharmacology/pharmacokinetics:
Long half-life benzodiazepine.
Accumulation of active metabolites is significant during repeated dosing.
Steady-state plasma concentration usually attained in 7 to 10 days.
Elimination slow since metabolites remain in blood for several days.

## Oral Dosage Forms
### KETAZOLAM CAPSULES

#### Usual adult dose
Antianxiety agent—
Oral, 15 mg one or two times a day, the dosage being increased in 15-mg increments as needed and tolerated.
Note: Debilitated patients—The recommended initial dose is one-half the lowest recommended initial adult dosage.

#### Usual pediatric dose
Antianxiety agent—
Children up to 18 years of age: Safety and efficacy have not been established.
Note: Use in infants is not recommended.

#### Usual geriatric dose
Antianxiety agent—
Oral, 15 mg once a day, the dosage being increased in 15-mg increments as needed and tolerated.

#### Strength(s) usually available
U.S.—
Not commercially available.
Canada—
15 mg (Rx) [*Loftran*].
30 mg (Rx) [*Loftran*].

#### Packaging and storage
Store below 40 °C (104 °F), preferably between 15 and 30 °C (59 and 86 °F), in a well-closed container, unless otherwise specified by manufacturer.

#### Auxiliary labeling
• Avoid alcoholic beverages.
• May cause drowsiness.

---

## LORAZEPAM

## Summary of Differences

Category:
In addition to being indicated as an antianxiety agent and a sedative-hypnotic, lorazepam is indicated as an amnestic and used as an anticonvulsant (parenteral only), an antiemetic in cancer chemotherapy (parenteral only), an antitremor agent (oral only), and a skeletal muscle relaxant adjunct.
Indications:
Oral lorazepam also indicated for adjunctive management of anxiety associated with mental depression.
Parenteral lorazepam also indicated as a preanesthetic medication; and used as an adjunct prior to endoscopic procedures, and for the treatment of status epilepticus.
Oral and parenteral lorazepam also used for relief of acute alcohol withdrawal symptoms and for treatment of tension headache.
Pharmacology/pharmacokinetics:
Absorption of intramuscular lorazepam is rapid and complete.
Short to intermediate half-life benzodiazepine.
Accumulation is minimal during repeated dosing.
Steady-state plasma concentration usually attained within a few (2 to 3) days.
Elimination rapid following discontinuation of therapy.
Precautions:
Drug interactions and/or related problems—
Cimetidine, oral estrogen-containing contraceptives, disulfiram, and erythromycin, which inhibit the oxidative metabolism of benzodiazepines, are less likely to affect lorazepam, which undergoes glucuronide conjugation.
Premedication with lorazepam may decrease dose of a fentanyl derivative required for induction of anesthesia and reduce time to loss of consciousness with induction doses.
Probenecid may impair glucuronide conjugation of lorazepam, resulting in increased effects and possibly excessive sedation.
Medical considerations/contraindications—
Prolongation of elimination half-life due to hepatic function impairment may be minimal with lorazepam.
Side/adverse effects:
Intravenous lorazepam more likely than chlordiazepoxide but less likely than diazepam to cause phlebitis or venous thrombosis.

## Additional Dosing Information

See also *General Dosing Information*.

#### For sublingual tablets only
Do not swallow for at least 2 minutes to allow sufficient time for absorption.

#### For parenteral dosage forms only
Immediately prior to intravenous use, lorazepam must be diluted with an equal amount of a compatible diluent such as sterile water for injection, 0.9% sodium chloride injection, or 5% dextrose injection.
Following proper dilution, the medication may be injected directly into the vein or into the tubing of an intravenous infusion.
Intravenous injection should be made slowly and with repeated aspiration.
The rate of the intravenous injection should not exceed 2 mg per minute.
Intra-arterial injection and perivascular extravasation should be avoided. Intra-arterial injection may produce arteriospasm, possibly resulting in gangrene.
When administered intramuscularly, the injection (undiluted) should be injected deeply into the muscle mass.
When parenteral lorazepam is used for peroral endoscopic procedures, the use of topical or regional anesthesia is recommended to minimize the reflex activity associated with such procedures.
When lorazepam is administered intravenously as premedication prior to regional or local anesthesia, potential excessive sleepiness or drowsiness may interfere with patient cooperation in determining levels of anesthesia. This is more likely to occur when doses greater than 0.05 mg per kg of body weight (mg/kg) are given and narcotic analgesics are used concomitantly with recommended doses.

## Oral Dosage Forms
### LORAZEPAM ORAL SOLUTION

#### Usual adult and adolescent dose
Antianxiety agent—
Oral, 1 to 3 mg two or three times a day.
Sedative-hypnotic—
Oral, 2 to 4 mg as a single dose at bedtime.

Note: Debilitated patients—Oral, initially 1 to 2 mg per day in divided doses, the dosage being increased gradually as needed and tolerated.

### Usual adult prescribing limits
Up to 10 mg per day.

### Usual pediatric dose
Antianxiety agent or
Sedative-hypnotic[1]—
   Children up to 12 years of age: Safety and efficacy have not been established.

### Strength(s) usually available
U.S.—
   2 mg per mL (Rx) [Lorazepam Intensol].
Canada—
   Not commercially available.

### Packaging and storage
Store between 2 and 8 °C (36 and 46 °F), unless otherwise specified by manufacturer. Store in a well-closed container.

### Preparation of dosage form
Each dose may be diluted with water, soda or soda-like beverages, or semisolid food, such as applesauce or pudding.

### Auxiliary labeling
• Avoid alcoholic beverages.
• May cause drowsiness.

### Note
Controlled substance in the U.S.

When preparing the label, directions should clearly explain the use of the dropper supplied with the product, which is calibrated in mL, not in mg.

## LORAZEPAM TABLETS USP

### Usual adult and adolescent dose
Antianxiety agent—
   Oral, 1 to 3 mg two or three times a day.
Sedative-hypnotic[1]—
   Oral, 2 to 4 mg as a single dose at bedtime.
Note: Debilitated patients—Oral, initially 500 mcg (0.5 mg) to 2 mg per day in divided doses, the dosage being increased gradually as needed and tolerated.

### Usual pediatric dose
Antianxiety agent or
Sedative-hypnotic[1]—
   Children up to 12 years of age: Safety and efficacy have not been established.

### Usual geriatric dose
Antianxiety agent or
Sedative-hypnotic[1]—
   Oral, initially 500 mcg (0.5 mg) to 2 mg per day in divided doses, the dosage being increased gradually as needed and tolerated.

### Strength(s) usually available
U.S.—
   0.5 mg (Rx) [Ativan; GENERIC].
   1 mg (Rx) [Ativan (scored); GENERIC].
   2 mg (Rx) [Ativan (scored); GENERIC].
Canada—
   0.5 mg (Rx) [Apo-Lorazepam; Ativan; Novo-Lorazem; Nu-Loraz].
   1 mg (Rx) [Apo-Lorazepam (scored); Ativan (scored); Novo-Lorazem (scored); Nu-Loraz (scored)].
   2 mg (Rx) [Apo-Lorazepam (scored); Ativan (scored); Novo-Lorazem (scored); Nu-Loraz (scored)].

### Packaging and storage
Store between 15 and 30 °C (59 and 86 °F), unless otherwise specified by manufacturer. Store in a tight, light-resistant container.

### Auxiliary labeling
• Avoid alcoholic beverages.
• May cause drowsiness.

### Note
Controlled substance in the U.S.

## LORAZEPAM SUBLINGUAL TABLETS

### Usual adult dose
Antianxiety agent—
   Sublingual, 2 to 3 mg per day in divided doses, the dosage being adjusted as needed, usually not exceeding 6 mg per day.
   Note: Debilitated patients—Sublingual, initially 500 mcg (0.5 mg) per day, the dosage being gradually adjusted as necessary.

Preoperative: Sublingual, 50 mcg (0.05 mg) per kg of body weight, up to a maximum of 4 mg, one to two hours before surgery.

### Usual pediatric dose
Antianxiety agent—
   Children up to 6 years of age: Use is not recommended.
   Children 6 to 18 years of age: Dosage has not been established.

### Usual geriatric dose
Antianxiety agent—
   Sublingual, initially 500 mcg (0.5 mg) per day, the dosage being gradually adjusted as necessary.

### Strength(s) usually available
U.S.—
   Not commercially available.
Canada—
   0.5 mg (Rx) [Ativan (lactose)].
   1 mg (Rx) [Ativan (lactose)].
   2 mg (Rx) [Ativan (lactose)].

### Packaging and storage
Store below 40 °C (104 °F), preferably between 15 and 30 °C (59 and 86 °F), in a well-closed container, unless otherwise specified by manufacturer.

### Auxiliary labeling
• Dissolve tablets under tongue.
• Avoid alcoholic beverages.
• May cause drowsiness.

## Parenteral Dosage Forms

Note: Bracketed uses in the Dosage Forms section refer to categories of use and/or indications that are not included in U.S. product labeling.

## LORAZEPAM INJECTION USP

### Usual adult dose
Antianxiety agent or
Sedative-hypnotic or
Amnestic—
   Intramuscular, 50 mcg (0.05 mg) per kg of body weight, up to a maximum of 4 mg. Dose should be administered at least two hours prior to surgery for optimum amnestic effect.
   Intravenous, initially 44 mcg (0.044 mg) per kg of body weight or a total dose of 2 mg, whichever is less. For greater amnestic effect, up to 50 mcg (0.05 mg) per kg of body weight, not to exceed a maximum of 4 mg, may be administered. Dose should be administered fifteen to twenty minutes prior to surgery for optimum amnestic effect.
[Antiemetic, in cancer chemotherapy][1]—
   Intravenous, initially 2 mg thirty minutes before initiation of chemotherapy, followed by 2 mg every four hours as needed.
[Status epilepticus]—
   Intravenous, initially 0.05 mg per kg of body weight up to a maximum of 4 mg, administered slowly. If seizures continue or recur after a ten- to fifteen-minute observation period, an additional dose of 0.05 mg per kg may be administered. If seizure control is not evident after another ten to fifteen minutes, other measures to control status epilepticus should be used. The total maximum dose should not exceed 8 mg of lorazepam in a twelve-hour period.

### Usual pediatric dose
Antianxiety agent or
Sedative-hypnotic or
Amnestic—
   Children up to 18 years of age: Safety and efficacy have not been established.
Caution—
   Use of medications containing benzyl alcohol is not recommended for use in neonates. A fatal toxic syndrome consisting of metabolic acidosis, CNS depression, respiratory problems, renal failure, hypotension, and possibly seizures and intracranial hemorrhages has been associated with this use.

### Strength(s) usually available
U.S.—
   2 mg per mL (Rx) [Ativan (benzyl alcohol 2%; polyethylene glycol 400 0.18 mL in propylene glycol); GENERIC].
   4 mg per mL (Rx) [Ativan (benzyl alcohol 2%; polyethylene glycol 400 0.18 mL in propylene glycol); GENERIC].
Canada—
   4 mg per mL (Rx) [Ativan (benzyl alcohol 2%; polyethylene glycol 18%; propylene glycol 80%)].

## Packaging and storage
Store between 2 and 8 °C (36 and 46 °F), unless otherwise specified by manufacturer. Protect from light. Protect from freezing.

## Preparation of dosage form
Immediately prior to use, lorazepam injection must be diluted with an equal volume of a compatible diluent, such as sterile water for injection, 0.9% sodium chloride injection, or 5% dextrose injection.

## Stability
Do not use if solution is discolored or contains a precipitate.

## Incompatibilities
Lorazepam injection is physically incompatible with buprenorphine injection.

## Note
Controlled substance in the U.S.

---

[1]Not included in Canadian product labeling.

---

### *NITRAZEPAM*

## Summary of Differences
Category:
> Also indicated as an anticonvulsant.

Pharmacology/pharmacokinetics:
> Absorption of nitrazepam is rapid.
> Short to intermediate half-life benzodiazepine.
> Accumulation is minimal during repeated dosing.
> Steady-state plasma concentration usually attained within a few (2 to 3) days.
> Elimination rapid following discontinuation of therapy.

Precautions:
> Drug interactions and/or related problems—Cimetidine or oral estrogen-containing contraceptives may inhibit the nitro-reduction of nitrazepam, resulting in delayed elimination and prolonged elimination half-life; serum concentrations may also be increased during long-term use.
> Medical considerations/contraindications—Nitrazepam may delay cricopharyngeal relaxation, exacerbating swallowing abnormalities in children.

## Oral Dosage Forms
### NITRAZEPAM TABLETS

**Usual adult dose**
Sedative-hypnotic—
> Oral, 5 or 10 mg before retiring.

Note: Debilitated patients—Oral, initially 2.5 mg, the dosage being increased as needed and tolerated up to 5 mg.

**Usual pediatric dose**
Sedative-hypnotic—
> Dosage has not been established.

Anticonvulsant—
> Children up to 30 kg: Oral, 300 mcg (0.3 mg) to 1 mg per kg of body weight per day given in three divided doses, the dosage being increased gradually as needed and tolerated.
> Note: If doses are not equally divided, the larger dose should be given before retiring.

**Usual geriatric dose**
Sedative-hypnotic—
> Oral, initially 2.5 mg, the dosage being increased as needed and tolerated up to 5 mg.

**Strength(s) usually available**
U.S.—
> Not commercially available.
Canada—
> 5 mg (Rx) [*Mogadon* (scored; lactose 53 mg)].
> 10 mg (Rx) [*Mogadon* (scored; lactose 105 mg)].

## Packaging and storage
Store below 40 °C (104 °F), preferably between 15 and 30 °C (59 and 86 °F), in a well-closed container, unless otherwise specified by manufacturer.

## Auxiliary labeling
• Avoid alcoholic beverages.
• May cause drowsiness.

---

### *OXAZEPAM*

## Summary of Differences
Indications:
> Also indicated for adjunctive management of anxiety associated with mental depression and relief of acute alcohol withdrawal symptoms.

Pharmacology/pharmacokinetics:
> Orally, one of least rapidly absorbed benzodiazepines.
> Short to intermediate half-life benzodiazepine.
> Accumulation is minimal during repeated dosing.
> Steady-state plasma concentration usually attained within a few days.
> Elimination rapid following discontinuation of therapy.

Precautions:
> Drug interactions and/or related problems—
> > Cimetidine, oral estrogen-containing contraceptives, disulfiram, and erythromycin, which inhibit the oxidative metabolism of benzodiazepines, are less likely to affect oxazepam, which undergoes glucuronide conjugation.
> > Probenecid may impair glucuronide conjugation of oxazepam, resulting in increased effects and possibly excessive sedation.
> Medical considerations/contraindications—
> > Prolongation of elimination half-life due to hepatic function impairment may be minimal with oxazepam.

## Oral Dosage Forms
### OXAZEPAM CAPSULES USP

**Usual adult dose**
Antianxiety agent—
> Oral, 10 to 30 mg three or four times a day.
Sedative-hypnotic—
> Alcohol withdrawal: Oral, 15 or 30 mg three or four times a day.

**Usual pediatric dose**
Antianxiety agent or
Sedative-hypnotic—
> Children up to 6 years of age: Use is not recommended.
> Children 6 to 12 years of age: Dosage has not been established.

**Usual geriatric dose**
Antianxiety agent—
> Oral, initially 10 mg three times a day, the dosage being increased as needed and tolerated to 15 mg three or four times a day. Alternatively, a dose of 5 mg one or two times a day has been recommended.

**Strength(s) usually available**
U.S.—
> 10 mg (Rx) [*Serax;* GENERIC].
> 15 mg (Rx) [*Serax;* GENERIC].
> 30 mg (Rx) [*Serax;* GENERIC].
Canada—
> Not commercially available.

Note: The strengths of specific products may not conform to some of the recommended geriatric dosages.

## Packaging and storage
Store below 40 °C (104 °F), preferably between 15 and 30 °C (59 and 86 °F), in a well-closed container, unless otherwise specified by manufacturer.

## Auxiliary labeling
• Avoid alcoholic beverages.
• May cause drowsiness.

## Note
Controlled substance in the U.S.

### OXAZEPAM TABLETS USP

**Usual adult dose**
See *Oxazepam Capsules USP.*

**Usual pediatric dose**
See *Oxazepam Capsules USP.*

**Usual geriatric dose**
See *Oxazepam Capsules USP.*

**Strength(s) usually available**
U.S.—
> 10 mg (Rx) [GENERIC].
> 15 mg (Rx) [*Serax* (tartrazine); GENERIC].
> 30 mg (Rx) [GENERIC].

Canada—
   10 mg (Rx) [*Apo-Oxazepam* (scored); *Novoxapam* (scored); *Serax* (scored)].
   15 mg (Rx) [*Apo-Oxazepam* (scored); *Novoxapam* (scored); *Serax* (scored)].
   30 mg (Rx) [*Apo-Oxazepam* (scored); *Novoxapam* (scored); *Serax* (scored)].

### Packaging and storage
Store below 40 °C (104 °F), preferably between 15 and 30 °C (59 and 86 °F), in a well-closed container, unless otherwise specified by manufacturer.

### Auxiliary labeling
• Avoid alcoholic beverages.
• May cause drowsiness.

### Note
Controlled substance in the U.S.

---

## PRAZEPAM

## Summary of Differences
Category:
   Indicated only as an antianxiety agent.
Pharmacology/pharmacokinetics:
   Orally, one of least rapidly absorbed benzodiazepines.
   Long half-life benzodiazepine.
   Accumulation of active metabolites is significant during repeated dosing.
   Steady-state plasma concentration usually attained in 5 days to 2 weeks.
   Elimination slow since metabolites remain in blood for several days.

## Oral Dosage Forms
### PRAZEPAM CAPSULES USP

### Usual adult dose
Antianxiety agent—
   Oral, 10 mg three times a day (range, 20 to 60 mg per day); or 20 to 40 mg at bedtime.
Note: Debilitated patients—Oral, initially 10 to 15 mg per day in divided doses, the dosage being increased gradually as needed and tolerated.

### Usual pediatric dose
Antianxiety agent—
   Children up to 18 years of age: Safety and efficacy have not been established.

### Usual geriatric dose
Antianxiety agent—
   Oral, initially 10 to 15 mg per day in divided doses, the dosage being increased gradually as needed and tolerated.

### Strength(s) usually available
U.S.—
   5 mg (Rx) [*Centrax;* GENERIC].
   10 mg (Rx) [*Centrax;* GENERIC].
   20 mg (Rx) [*Centrax*].
Canada—
   Not commercially available.

### Packaging and storage
Store between 15 and 30 °C (59 and 86 °F), unless otherwise specified by manufacturer. Store in a tight, light-resistant container.

### Auxiliary labeling
• Avoid alcoholic beverages.
• May cause drowsiness.

### Note
Controlled substance in the U.S.

### PRAZEPAM TABLETS USP

### Usual adult dose
See *Prazepam Capsules USP.*

### Usual pediatric dose
See *Prazepam Capsules USP.*

### Usual geriatric dose
See *Prazepam Capsules USP.*

### Strength(s) usually available
U.S.—
   5 mg (Rx) [GENERIC].
   10 mg (Rx) [*Centrax* (scored); GENERIC].
Canada—
   Not commercially available.

### Packaging and storage
Store between 15 and 30 °C (59 and 86 °F), unless otherwise specified by manufacturer. Store in a tight, light-resistant container.

### Auxiliary labeling
• Avoid alcoholic beverages.
• May cause drowsiness.

### Note
Controlled substance in the U.S.

---

## QUAZEPAM

## Summary of Differences
Category:
   Indicated only as a sedative-hypnotic.
Pharmacology/pharmacokinetics:
   Long half-life benzodiazepine.
   Accumulation of active metabolites may occur during repeated dosing.
   Steady-state plasma concentrations usually attained within 7 to 13 days.
   Elimination slow since metabolites remain in blood for several days.

## Oral Dosage Forms
### QUAZEPAM TABLETS

### Usual adult dose
Sedative-hypnotic—
   Oral, 15 mg initially, the dose being reduced to 7.5 mg as needed.
Note: Debilitated patients—Because of increased sensitivity to benzodiazepines, it is suggested that the nightly dose be reduced after 1 or 2 nights of treatment.

### Usual pediatric dose
Sedative-hypnotic—
   Children up to 18 years of age: Safety and efficacy have not been established.

### Usual geriatric dose
Sedative-hypnotic—
   Oral, 15 mg initially, the dose being reduced to 7.5 mg after one or two nights.

### Strength(s) usually available
U.S.—
   7.5 mg (Rx) [*Doral*].
   15 mg (Rx) [*Doral*].
Canada—
   Not commercially available.

### Packaging and storage
Store between 15 and 30 °C (59 and 86 °F), in a tight container, unless otherwise specified by manufacturer.

### Auxiliary labeling
• Avoid alcoholic beverages.
• May cause daytime drowsiness.

### Note
Controlled substance in the U.S.

---

## TEMAZEPAM

## Summary of Differences
Category:
   Indicated only as a sedative-hypnotic.
Indications:
   May be useful in prevention or treatment of transient insomnia associated with sudden sleep schedule changes.
Pharmacology/pharmacokinetics:
   Short to intermediate half-life benzodiazepine.
   Accumulation is minimal during repeated dosing.
   Steady-state plasma concentration usually attained within a few (about 3) days.
   Elimination rapid following discontinuation of therapy.

Precautions:
Drug interactions and/or related problems—
Cimetidine, oral estrogen-containing contraceptives, disulfiram, and erythromycin, which inhibit the oxidative metabolism of the benzodiazepines, are less likely to affect temazepam, which undergoes glucuronide conjugation.
Probenecid may impair glucuronide conjugation of temazepam, resulting in increased effects and possibly excessive sedation.
Medical considerations/contraindications—
Prolongation of elimination half-life due to hepatic function impairment may be minimal with temazepam.

# Oral Dosage Forms
## TEMAZEPAM CAPSULES USP

### Usual adult dose
Sedative-hypnotic—
Oral, 15 mg.

Note: In transient insomnia, 7.5 mg may be sufficient to improve sleep latency.
Debilitated patients—Oral, 7.5 mg initially, the dosage being adjusted as needed and tolerated.

### Usual pediatric dose
Sedative-hypnotic—
Children up to 18 years of age: Safety and efficacy have not been established.

### Usual geriatric dose
Sedative-hypnotic—
Oral, 7.5 mg initially, the dosage being adjusted as needed and tolerated.

### Strength(s) usually available
U.S.—
7.5 mg (Rx) [Restoril].
15 mg (Rx) [Restoril; GENERIC].
30 mg (Rx) [Restoril; GENERIC].
Canada—
15 mg (Rx) [Restoril (lactose)].
30 mg (Rx) [Restoril (lactose)].

### Packaging and storage
Store between 15 and 30 °C (59 and 86 °F), in a tight container, unless otherwise specified by manufacturer.

### Auxiliary labeling
• Avoid alcoholic beverages.
• May cause daytime drowsiness.

### Note
Controlled substance in the U.S.

## TEMAZEPAM TABLETS

### Usual adult dose
See Temazepam Capsules USP.

### Usual pediatric dose
See Temazepam Capsules USP.

### Usual geriatric dose
See Temazepam Capsules USP.

### Strength(s) usually available
U.S.—
15 mg (Rx) [GENERIC].
30 mg (Rx) [GENERIC].
Canada—
Not commercially available.

### Packaging and storage
Store below 40 °C (104 °F), preferably between 15 and 30 °C (59 and 86 °F), in a well-closed container, unless otherwise specified by manufacturer.

### Auxiliary labeling
• Avoid alcoholic beverages.
• May cause daytime drowsiness.

### Note
Controlled substance in the U.S.

---

## TRIAZOLAM

# Summary of Differences
Category:
Indicated only as a sedative-hypnotic.
Indications:
May be useful in prevention or treatment of transient insomnia associated with sudden sleep schedule change.
Pharmacology/pharmacokinetics:
Short half-life benzodiazepine.
Accumulation is minimal during repeated dosing.
Elimination rapid following discontinuation of therapy.
Precautions:
Drug interactions and/or related problems—
Cimetidine and erythromycin may inhibit the hepatic metabolism of triazolam, resulting in increased plasma concentrations and delayed clearance of triazolam; dosage reductions may be necessary.
Isoniazid may inhibit the elimination of triazolam, resulting in increased plasma concentrations.
Side/adverse effects:
Anterograde amnesia may be more likely to occur with triazolam than with most other benzodiazepines.

# Oral Dosage Forms
## TRIAZOLAM TABLETS USP

### Usual adult dose
Sedative-hypnotic—
Oral, 125 to 250 mcg (0.125 to 0.25 mg).

Note: A dose of 500 mcg (0.5 mg) may be necessary in some patients. However, this dose should be reserved for patients who do not respond adequately to lower doses, since the risk of side effects increases with dosage increases.
Debilitated patients—Oral, 125 mcg (0.125 mg) initially, the dosage being increased as needed and tolerated.

### Usual pediatric dose
Sedative-hypnotic—
Children up to 18 years of age: Safety and efficacy have not been established.

### Usual geriatric dose
Sedative-hypnotic—
Oral, 125 mcg (0.125 mg) initially, the dosage being increased as needed and tolerated.

### Strength(s) usually available
U.S.—
125 mcg (0.125 mg) (Rx) [Halcion (cellulose; corn starch; docusate sodium; lactose; magnesium stearate; silicon dioxide; sodium benzoate)].
250 mcg (0.25 mg) (Rx) [Halcion (scored; cellulose; corn starch; docusate sodium; lactose; magnesium stearate; silicon dioxide; sodium benzoate; FD&C Blue No. 2)].
Canada—
125 mcg (0.125 mg) (Rx) [Apo-Triazo (scored); Gen-Triazolam (scored); Halcion (scored); Novo-Triolam (scored); Nu-Triazo (scored); GENERIC].
250 mcg (0.25 mg) (Rx) [Apo-Triazo (scored); Gen-Triazolam (scored); Halcion (scored); Novo-Triolam (scored); Nu-Triazo (scored); GENERIC].

### Packaging and storage
Store between 15 and 30° C (59 and 86° F), unless otherwise specified by manufacturer. Store in a tight, light-resistant container.

### Auxiliary labeling
• Avoid alcoholic beverages.
• May cause daytime drowsiness.

### Note
Controlled substance in the U.S.

---

Revised: 08/04/92
Interim revision: 08/18/92; 08/17/94

## Table 1. Pharmacology/Pharmacokinetics

| Drug | Protein Binding (%) | Half-life* (hr) | Major Active Metabolites (half-life in hr) | Time to Peak Plasma Concentration† (oral dose) (hr) | Elimination‡ (% excreted unchanged) |
|---|---|---|---|---|---|
| *Long half-life* | | | | | |
| Chlordiazepoxide | Very high (96) | 5–30 | Desmethylchlordiazepoxide (18) Demoxepam (14–95) Desmethyldiazepam (30–100) Oxazepam (5–15) | 0.5–4 | Renal (1–2); 3–6% as conjugate |
| Clorazepate§ | Very high (97) | — | Desmethyldiazepam (30–100) Oxazepam (5–15) | 0.5–2 | Renal |
| Diazepam | Very high (98) | 20–70 | Desmethyldiazepam (30–100) Temazepam (9.5–12.4) Oxazepam (5–15) | 0.5–2 (IM, 0.5–1.5; IV, within 0.25) | Renal |
| Flurazepam§# | Very high (97) | 2.3 | Desalkylflurazepam (30–100) N-1-hydroxyethylflurazepam (2–4) | 0.5–1 | Renal |
| Halazepam | Very high (97) | 14 | Desmethyldiazepam (30–100) | 1–3 | Renal (< 1) |
| Ketazolam | Very high (93) | 2 | Desmethyldiazepam (30–100) N-methylketazolam (34–52) Diazepam (20–70) | 3 | Renal; fecal <1% |
| Prazepam§ | Very high (97) | — | Desmethyldiazepam (30–100) Oxazepam (5–15) | 2.5–6 for metabolite desmethyldiazepam with single dose | Renal |
| Quazepam | Very high (>95) | 39.3 | Desalkylflurazepam (30–100) 2-oxoquazepam (39) | 2 | Renal |
| *Short to intermediate half-life* | | | | | |
| Alprazolam | High (80) | 11–16 | None | 1–2 | Renal |
| Bromazepam | High (70) | 20–32 | None | 1–4 | Renal |
| Clonazepam | High (85) | 18–50 | None | 1–2** | Renal (<0.5 of 2-mg dose); fecal |
| Estazolam | Very high (93) | 10–24 | None | 2 (range, 0.5–6) | Renal (<5) |
| Lorazepam†† | High (85) | 10–20 | None | 1–6 (IM, 1–1.5) | Renal |
| Nitrazepam | High (87) | 16–48 | None | 2–3 | Renal (about 5) |
| Oxazepam | Very high (97) | 5–15 | None | 1–4 | Renal; fecal |
| Temazepam | Very high (96) | 8–15 | None | 1–2 | Renal |
| Triazolam | High (89) | 1.5–5.5 | None | Within 2 | Renal (small amount)‡‡; fecal |

*Elimination half-lives may be prolonged in children, especially premature and newborn infants, geriatric patients, and patients with hepatic disease; however, metabolic clearance of short to intermediate half-life benzodiazepines, especially lorazepam, oxazepam, temazepam, and triazolam, is affected less by age and hepatic disease than that of the long half-life benzodiazepines. The elimination half-life does not alway predict the duration of clinical effects.

†With multiple dosing, steady-state plasma concentrations of long half-life benzodiazepines are usually achieved within 5 days to 2 weeks and those of short to intermediate half-life benzodiazepines within a few days.

‡Benzodiazepines are not significantly removed from body by hemodialysis.

§Prodrugs or drug precursors; do not reach circulation in clinically significant amounts.

#Maximum effectiveness as a hypnotic may not be achieved for 2 to 3 days.

**Following a single dose; in some patients peak concentrations may not be achieved for 4 to 8 hours.

††Peak amnestic effect: IM, within 2 hours; IV, 15 to 20 minutes.

‡‡Appears to be biphasic in its time course.

# BENZONATATE Systemic

VA CLASSIFICATION (Primary): RE302

Note: For a listing of dosage forms and brand names by country availability, see *Dosage Forms* section(s). For a listing of brand names for the articles in this monograph, refer to the General Index.

## Category
Antitussive.

## Indications

**Accepted**

Cough (treatment)—Benzonatate is indicated for the symptomatic relief of nonproductive cough. It is used to provide relief of acute cough due to minor throat and bronchial irritation occurring with colds or inhaled irritants.

## Pharmacology/Pharmacokinetics

**Mechanism of action/Effect**

Suppresses cough through a peripheral action, anesthetizing the stretch or cough receptors of vagal afferent fibers, which are located in the respiratory passages, lungs, and pleura; also, may suppress transmission of the cough reflex by a central mechanism, at the level of the medulla.

**Other actions**

Local anesthetic activity when applied topically to the mucosa.

**Onset of action**

Usually within 15 to 20 minutes.

**Duration of action**

Up to 8 hours.

**Elimination**

As with other ester-type local anesthetics (e.g., tetracaine) to which benzonatate is chemically related, excretion may be primarily via metabolism, followed by renal excretion of metabolites.

## Precautions to Consider

**Cross-sensitivity and/or related problems**

Patients sensitive to tetracaine or other ester-type local anesthetics may also be sensitive to benzonatate.

**Pregnancy/Reproduction**

Pregnancy—Studies have not been done in humans.
Studies have not been done in animals.

FDA Pregnancy Category C.

**Breast-feeding**

It is not known whether benzonatate is distributed into breast milk. However, problems in humans have not been documented.

**Pediatrics**

Appropriate studies have not been performed in children up to 10 years of age. However, benzonatate should not be used in infants and young children since numbness of the mouth, tongue, and pharynx may occur, which may cause swallowing difficulty and aspiration.

**Geriatrics**

No information is available on the relationship of age to the effects of benzonatate in geriatric patients.

**Drug interactions and/or related problems**

The following drug interactions and/or related problems have been selected on the basis of their potential clinical significance (possible mechanism in parentheses where appropriate)—not necessarily inclusive (» = major clinical significance):

Note: Combinations containing any of the following medications, depending on the amount present, may also interact with this medication.

Central nervous system (CNS) depression–producing medications, other (see *Appendix II*)
(concurrent use may potentiate the CNS depressant effects of these medications or benzonatate)

**Medical considerations/Contraindications**

The medical considerations/contraindications included here have been selected on the basis of their potential clinical significance (reasons given in parentheses where appropriate)—not necessarily inclusive (» = major clinical significance).

*Risk-benefit should be considered when the following medical problems exist:*

» Cough, productive
(inhibition of cough reflex may lead to retention of secretions)
Sensitivity to benzonatate or topical anesthetics

## Side/Adverse Effects

The following side/adverse effects have been selected on the basis of their potential clinical significance (possible signs and symptoms in parentheses where appropriate)—not necessarily inclusive:

**Those indicating need for medical attention only if they continue or are bothersome**

Incidence less frequent or rare
*Constipation; dizziness, mild; drowsiness, mild; nausea or vomiting; skin rash; stuffy nose*

## Overdose

For more information on the management of overdose or unintentional ingestion, **contact a Poison Control Center** (see *Poison Control Center Listing*).

**Clinical effects of overdose**

The following effects have been selected on the basis of their potential clinical significance (possible signs and symptoms in parentheses where appropriate)–not necessarily inclusive:

*CNS stimulation* (convulsions; restlessness; trembling)

Note: *CNS stimulation* may be followed by profound CNS depression.

## Patient Consultation

As an aid to patient consultation, refer to *Advice for the Patient, Benzonatate (Systemic).*

In providing consultation, consider emphasizing the following selected information (» = major clinical significance):

**Before using this medication**

» Conditions affecting use, especially:
Sensitivity to benzonatate or topical anesthetics
Use in children—Children may chew capsule resulting in numbness of mouth, tongue, and pharynx, and choking may occur
Other medical problems, especially a productive cough

**Proper use of this medication**

Not chewing capsules; swallowing whole to avoid local anesthetic effect and choking

» Proper dosing
Missed dose: Taking as soon as possible; not taking if almost time for next dose; not doubling doses

» Proper storage

**Precautions while using this medication**

Checking with physician if cough persists after medication has been used for 7 days or if high fever, skin rash, or continuing headache is present with cough

## General Dosing Information

It is recommended that the capsules not be chewed before they are swallowed. Release of benzonatate from the capsule may produce temporary local anesthesia of the oral mucosa and choking may occur.

## Oral Dosage Forms

### BENZONATATE CAPSULES USP

**Usual adult and adolescent dose**

Antitussive—
Oral, 100 mg three times a day, as needed.

**Usual adult prescribing limits**

Up to 600 mg per day.

**Usual pediatric dose**

Antitussive—
Children up to 10 years of age: Dosage has not been established.
Children 10 years of age and older: See *Usual adult and adolescent dose.*

**Usual geriatric dose**

See *Usual adult and adolescent dose.*

**Strength(s) usually available**

U.S.—

   100 mg (Rx) [*Tessalon;* GENERIC].

Canada—

   100 mg (OTC) [*Tessalon*].

**Packaging and storage**

Store below 40 °C (104 °F), preferably between 15 and 30 °C (59 and 86 °F), in a tight, light-resistant container.

**Auxiliary labeling**

• Do not chew.

**Selected Bibliography**

Irwin RS, Curley FJ, Pratter MR. The effects of drugs on cough. Eur J Respir Dis Suppl 1987; 153: 173-81.

Irwin RS, Curley FJ, Bennett FM. Appropriate use of antitussives and protussives. Drugs 1993; 46 (1): 80-91.

Revised: 02/23/94

---

# BENZOYL PEROXIDE   Topical

VA CLASSIFICATION (Primary/Secondary): DE752/DE500

Note: For a listing of dosage forms and brand names by country availability, see *Dosage Forms* section(s). For a listing of brand names for the articles in this monograph, refer to the General Index.

## Category

Antiacne agent (topical); keratolytic (topical).

## Indications

Note: Bracketed information in the *Indications* section refers to uses that are not included in U.S. product labeling.

### Accepted

Acne vulgaris (treatment)—Indicated for the topical treatment of mild to moderate acne vulgaris. In more severe acne, benzoyl peroxide may be indicated as an adjunct in therapeutic regimens including antibiotics, retinoic acid preparations, and sulfur/salicylic acid–containing preparations.

[Ulcer, decubital (treatment)] or

[Ulcer, stasis (treatment)]—Benzoyl peroxide, usually in a 20% strength, is used as an oxidizing agent and to stimulate epithelial cell proliferation and the production of granulation tissue in the treatment of decubital or stasis ulcers.

## Pharmacology/Pharmacokinetics

### Physicochemical characteristics

Molecular weight—242.23 (anhydrous).

### Mechanism of action/Effect

Benzoyl peroxide slowly releases active oxygen, resulting in an antibacterial action against *Propionibacterium acnes*. The medication also has some keratolytic effect, which produces comedolysis as well as drying and desquamative actions that contribute to its efficacy.

### Absorption

Absorbed by the skin.

### Biotransformation

Metabolized in skin to benzoic acid. About 5% of the metabolized medication is systemically absorbed and eliminated unchanged in the urine.

### Onset of action

Improvement in condition is usually noticeable within 4 to 6 weeks.

### Elimination

Renal; excreted as benzoic acid in urine.

## Precautions to Consider

### Carcinogenicity/Tumorigenicity

Benzoyl peroxide is not considered to be a carcinogen; however, data from a study using mice known to be highly susceptible to cancer suggest that benzoyl peroxide acts as a tumor promoter.

### Pregnancy/Reproduction

Pregnancy—This medicine may be systemically absorbed. Studies have not been done in humans or animals.

FDA Pregnancy Category C.

### Breast-feeding

It is not known whether benzoyl peroxide is distributed into breast milk. Problems in humans have not been documented; however, benzoyl peroxide may be systemically absorbed.

### Pediatrics

Children up to 12 years of age—Appropriate studies on the relationship of age to the effects of benzoyl peroxide have not been performed in this age group. Safety and efficacy have not been established.

Children 12 years of age and over—Pediatrics-specific problems that would limit the usefulness of this medication in this age group are not expected.

### Geriatrics

Appropriate studies on the relationship of age to the effects of benzoyl peroxide have not been performed in the geriatric population. However, geriatrics-specific problems that would limit the usefulness of this medication in the elderly are not expected.

### Drug interactions and/or related problems

The following drug interactions and/or related problems have been selected on the basis of their potential clinical significance (possible mechanism in parentheses where appropriate)—not necessarily inclusive (» = major clinical significance):

Note: Combinations containing any of the following medications, depending on the amount present, may also interact with this medication.

   Abrasive or medicated soaps or cleansers or

   Acne preparations or preparations containing a peeling agent, such as
      Resorcinol
      Salicylic acid
      Sulfur
      Tretinoin or

   Acne preparations, topical, other or

   Alcohol-containing preparations, topical, such as
      After-shave lotions
      Astringents
      Perfumed toiletries
      Shaving creams or lotions or

   Cosmetics or soaps with a strong drying effect or

   Isotretinoin or

   Medicated cosmetics or "cover-ups"

      (concurrent use with benzoyl peroxide may cause a cumulative irritant or drying effect, especially with the application of peeling, desquamating, or abrasive agents, resulting in excessive irritation of the skin; in addition, concurrent use of benzoyl peroxide with tretinoin may inactivate the tretinoin)

### Medical considerations/Contraindications

The medical considerations/contraindications included here have been selected on the basis of their potential clinical significance (reasons given in parentheses where appropriate)—not necessarily inclusive (» = major clinical significance).

*Risk-benefit should be considered when the following medical problems exist:*

» Inflammation of skin, acute, or denuded skin

   Sensitivity to benzoyl peroxide

## Side/Adverse Effects

The following side/adverse effects have been selected on the basis of their potential clinical significance (possible signs and symptoms in parentheses where appropriate)—not necessarily inclusive:

**Those indicating need for medical attention**
Incidence less frequent or rare
  *Allergic contact dermatitis* (burning, blistering, crusting, itching, severe redness, or swelling of skin); *irritant effect* (painful irritation of skin); *skin rash*

**Those indicating need for medical attention only if they continue or are bothersome**
Incidence less frequent
  *Dryness or peeling of skin*—may occur after a few days; *feeling of warmth, mild stinging, or redness of skin*

## Overdose

For specific information on the agents used in the management of benzoyl peroxide overdose, see:
  • *Corticosteroids (Topical)* monograph.

For more information on the management of overdose or unintentional ingestion, **contact a Poison Control Center** (see *Poison Control Center Listing*).

**Clinical effects of overdose**
The following effects have been selected on the basis of their potential clinical significance (possible signs and symptoms in parentheses where appropriate)—not necessarily inclusive:
  *Burning, itching, scaling, redness, or swelling of skin, severe*

**Treatment of overdose**
Medication should be discontinued. After symptoms and signs of overdosage subside, a reduced dosage schedule may be cautiously reinstated.
Specific treatment—Emollients, cool compresses, and/or topical corticosteroid preparations may be used to hasten resolution of overdosage.

## Patient Consultation

As an aid to patient consultation, refer to *Advice for the Patient, Benzoyl Peroxide (Topical)*.

In providing consultation, consider emphasizing the following selected information (» = major clinical significance):

**Before using this medication**
» Conditions affecting use, especially:
    Sensitivity to benzoyl peroxide
    Other medical problems, especially acute inflammation of skin or denuded skin

**Proper use of this medication**
*Proper administration*
*For cream, gel, lotion, or stick dosage form*
    Before applying—Washing affected area with nonmedicated soap and water or with a degreasing cleanser; gently patting dry
    Applying enough medication to cover affected area and rubbing in gently
*For shave cream dosage form*
    Wetting area to be shaved; applying a small amount and gently rubbing over entire area; shaving; rinsing area and patting dry; not using after-shave lotions or other drying face products without checking with physician
*For cleansing bar or lotion or soap dosage form*
    Using to wash affected areas
*For facial mask dosage form*
    Before applying—Washing affected area with nonmedicated cleanser; rinsing and patting skin dry
    Using circular motion, applying thin layer of mask evenly over affected area
    Allowing mask to dry for 15 to 25 minutes
    Rinsing thoroughly with warm water and patting dry
» Importance of not using more medication than the amount recommended
» Avoiding contact with the eyes, other mucous membranes, and sensitive areas of the neck
» Not applying medication to raw or irritated skin
» Proper dosing
    Missed dose: Applying as soon as possible
» Proper storage

**Precautions while using this medication**
    Checking with physician if skin problem has not improved within 4 to 6 weeks

If medication causes excessive redness, peeling, or dryness, checking with physician; may be necessary to reduce the frequency of use or reduce its strength
» Avoiding simultaneous use with other topical acne preparations or preparations containing peeling agents, alcohol-containing preparations, abrasive soaps or cleansers, cosmetics or soaps with drying effect, medicated cosmetics, or other topical skin medication, unless otherwise directed by physician
» Medication may bleach hair or colored fabrics

**Side/adverse effects**
    Signs of potential side effects, especially allergic contact dermatitis, irritant effect, or skin rash

## General Dosing Information

This medication contains an oxidizing agent that may bleach hair and colored fabrics.

**For treatment of acne**
    • Benzoyl peroxide should not be applied to acutely inflamed, denuded, or highly sensitive skin, unless otherwise directed by physician as in treating an ulceration.
    • Therapy may be initiated with the 2.5 or 5% cream, gel, or lotion, then changed to the 10% strength after 3 to 4 weeks or sooner if tolerance to the lower strengths has been determined.
    • After treatment with benzoyl peroxide for approximately 8 to 12 weeks, maximum lesion reduction may be expected. Continued prophylactic use of benzoyl peroxide is usually required to maintain optimal therapeutic response.
    • In fair-skinned patients or under excessively dry atmospheric conditions, it is recommended that therapy be initiated with one application daily and gradually increased up to 2 to 4 times a day (depending on the dosage form) as tolerated.

**For treatment of decubital or stasis ulcers**
• A protective ointment should be applied to a wide area bordering the ulcer to decrease the possibility of irritant dermatosis of the surrounding skin.
• Ulcers should be treated by applying a sterile dressing of terry cloth moistened with normal saline and saturated with 20% lotion to the clean and surgically debrided ulcer. Occlude the dressed area with a plastic film and apply an abdominal dressing pad overall and tape firmly in place. Change the dressing every 8 hours in large ulcers and every 12 hours in small ulcers.
• For maximal therapeutic efficacy, the lotion dressing should be kept moist and as close to 37 °C (98.6 °F) as possible: the plastic film is used to retain moisture and the abdominal dressing pad is used to increase the local temperature through its insulating effect.
• Exuberant granulation tissue may be kept below the epidermal level with cauterization by a silver nitrate stick to facilitate ingrowth of epithelium.
• Severe ulcers may be treated by packing with surgical gauze saturated with 20% lotion to facilitate good contact with the walls of the cavity and then occluding.
• Large amounts of serous exudate appearing on the ulcer surface is a normal response to benzoyl peroxide therapy.
• Two weeks may pass before progress is visible in large chronic ulcers.

## Topical Dosage Forms

Note: Bracketed uses in the *Dosage Forms* section refer to categories of use and/or indications that are not included in U.S. product labeling.

### BENZOYL PEROXIDE CLEANSING BAR

**Usual adult and adolescent dose**
Acne vulgaris—
    Topical, to the skin, as a 5 or 10% cleansing bar two or three times a day or as directed.

**Usual pediatric dose**
Acne vulgaris—
    Children up to 12 years of age: Safety and efficacy have not been established.
    Children 12 years of age and over: See *Usual adult and adolescent dose*.

**Strength(s) usually available**
U.S.—
    5% (OTC) [*PanOxyl 5 Bar*].
    10% (OTC) [*Desquam-X 10 Bar; Fostex 10 Bar; PanOxyl 10 Bar*].
Canada—
    5% (OTC) [*Desquam-X 5 Bar; PanOxyl 5 Bar*].
    10% (Rx) [*PanOxyl 10 Bar*].

**Packaging and storage**

Store below 40 °C (104 °F), preferably between 15 and 30 °C (59 and 86 °F), in a well-closed container, unless otherwise specified by manufacturer.

**Auxiliary labeling**
• For external use only.

## BENZOYL PEROXIDE CREAM

**Usual adult and adolescent dose**

Acne vulgaris—
　　Topical, to the skin, as a 5 to 10% cream one or two times a day.

**Usual pediatric dose**

Acne vulgaris—
　　Children up to 12 years of age: Safety and efficacy have not been established.
　　Children 12 years of age and over: See *Usual adult and adolescent dose.*

**Strength(s) usually available**

U.S.—
　　5% [*BenzaShave 5 Cream* (Rx); *Cuticura Acne 5 Cream* (OTC)].
　　10% [*Acne Aid 10 Cream* (OTC) (methylparaben; propylparaben); *BenzaShave 10 Cream* (Rx); *Clearasil Maximum Strength Medicated Anti-Acne 10 Tinted Cream* (OTC) (methylparaben; propylparaben); *Clearasil Maximum Strength Medicated Anti-Acne 10 Vanishing Cream* (OTC); *Dry and Clear Double Strength 10 Cream* (OTC); *Fostex 10 Cream* (OTC); *pHisoAc BP 10 Cream* (OTC); *Stri-Dex Maximum Strength Treatment 10 Cream* (OTC)].

Canada—
　　5% (OTC) [*Clearasil BP Plus 5 Cream*].

**Packaging and storage**

Store between 15 and 30 °C (59 and 86 °F), in a well-closed container, unless otherwise specified by manufacturer. Protect from freezing.

**Auxiliary labeling**
• For external use only.

## BENZOYL PEROXIDE GEL USP

**Usual adult and adolescent dose**

Acne vulgaris—
　　Topical, to the skin, as a 2.5 to 20% gel one or two times a day.

**Usual pediatric dose**

Acne vulgaris—
　　Children up to 12 years of age: Safety and efficacy have not been established.
　　Children 12 years of age and over: See *Usual adult and adolescent dose.*

**Strength(s) usually available**

U.S.—
　　2.5% (Rx) [*Ben-Aqua-2½ Gel; Benzac Ac 2½ Gel; Benzac W 2½ Gel; Clear By Design 2.5 Gel; Desquam-E 2.5 Gel; Desquam-X 2.5 Gel; PanOxyl AQ 2½ Gel* (methylparaben)].
　　4% (Rx) [*Brevoxyl 4 Gel* (cetyl alcohol; stearyl alcohol)].
　　5% (Rx) [*Ben-Aqua-5 Gel; Benzac Ac 5 Gel; Benzac 5 Gel* (alcohol 12%); *Benzac W 5 Gel; Del-Aqua-5 Gel; Desquam-E 5 Gel; Desquam-X 5 Gel; Dryox 5 Gel* (methylparaben); *Fostex 5 Gel; PanOxyl AQ 5 Gel* (methylparaben); *PanOxyl 5 Gel* (alcohol 20%); *Persa-Gel 5* (acetone); *Persa-Gel W 5; Xerac BP 5 Gel; Zeroxin-5 Gel* (acetone); GENERIC].
　　10% (Rx) [*Ben-Aqua-10 Gel; Benzac Ac 10 Gel; Benzac 10 Gel* (alcohol 12%); *Benzac W 10 Gel; Del-Aqua-10 Gel; Desquam-E 10 Gel; Desquam-X 10 Gel; Dryox 10 Gel* (methyl paraben); *Fostex 10 Gel; PanOxyl AQ 10 Gel* (methylparaben); *PanOxyl 10 Gel* (alcohol 20%); *Persa-Gel 10* (acetone); *Persa-Gel W 10; Xerac BP 10 Gel; Zeroxin-10 Gel* (acetone); GENERIC].
　　20% (Rx) [*Dryox 20 Gel* (methylparaben)].

Canada—
　　2.5% (OTC) [*Acetoxyl 2.5 Gel* (acetone); *Dermoxyl 2.5 Gel* (acetone); *H₂ Oxyl 2.5 Gel*].
　　5% (OTC) [*Acetoxyl 5 Gel* (acetone); *Benzac W 5 Gel; Benzagel 5 Gel* (alcohol 15%); *Dermoxyl Aqua 5 Gel; Dermoxyl 5 Gel* (acetone); *Desquam-X 5 Gel; H₂ Oxyl 5 Gel; PanOxyl 5 Gel* (alcohol)].
　　10% (Rx) [*Acetoxyl 10 Gel* (acetone); *Benzac W 10 Gel; Benzagel 10 Gel* (alcohol 15%); *Dermoxyl 10 Gel* (acetone); *Desquam-X 10 Gel; H₂Oxyl 10 Gel; PanOxyl 10 Gel* (alcohol)].
　　15% (Rx) [*PanOxyl 15 Gel* (alcohol)].
　　20% (Rx) [*Acetoxyl 20 Gel* (acetone); *Dermoxyl 20 Gel* (acetone); *H₂Oxyl 20 Gel; PanOxyl 20 Gel* (alcohol)].

**Packaging and storage**

Store below 40 °C (104 °F), preferably between 15 and 30 °C (59 and 86 °F), unless otherwise specified by manufacturer. Store in a tight container. Protect from freezing.

**Auxiliary labeling**
• For external use only.

## BENZOYL PEROXIDE LOTION USP

**Usual adult and adolescent dose**

Acne vulgaris—
　　Topical, to the skin, as a 5 to 10% lotion one to four times a day.
[Decubital ulcer] or
[Stasis ulcer]—
　　Topical, to the ulcer, as a 20% lotion every 8 hours for large ulcers and every 12 hours for small ulcers.

**Usual pediatric dose**

Acne vulgaris—
　　Children up to 12 years of age: Safety and efficacy have not been established.
　　Children 12 years of age and over: See *Usual adult and adolescent dose.*

**Strength(s) usually available**

U.S.—
　　5% (OTC) [*Acne-5 Lotion; Ben-Aqua-5 Lotion; Benoxyl 5 Lotion; Dry and Clear 5 Lotion; Oxy 5 Tinted Lotion* (cetyl alcohol; stearyl alcohol; parabens); *Oxy 5 Vanishing Lotion* (cetyl alcohol; stearyl alcohol; parabens); *Theroxide 5 Lotion; Vanoxide 5 Lotion;* GENERIC].
　　5.5% (OTC) [*Loroxide 5.5 Lotion*].
　　10% (OTC) [*Acne-10 Lotion; Ben-Aqua-10 Lotion; Benoxyl 10 Lotion; Clearasil Maximum Strength Medicated Anti-Acne 10 Vanishing Lotion; Noxzema Clear-ups Maximum Strength 10 Lotion* (methylparaben; propylparaben); *Noxzema Clear-ups On-The-Spot 10 Lotion* (methylparaben; propylparaben); *Oxy 10 Tinted Lotion* (cetyl alcohol); *Oxy 10 Vanishing Lotion* (cetyl alcohol); *Theroxide 10 Lotion; Topex 10 Lotion;* GENERIC].

Canada—
　　5% (OTC) [*Acnomel B.P. 5 Lotion; Benoxyl 5 Lotion; Benzagel 5 Acne Lotion; Clearasil BP Plus 5 Lotion; Loroxide 5 Lotion with Flesh-Tinted Base; Oxyderm 5 Lotion; Oxy 5 Vanishing Formula Lotion; Topex 5 Lotion*].
　　10% (Rx) [*Benoxyl 10 Lotion; Oxyderm 10 Lotion*].
　　20% (Rx) [*Benoxyl 20 Lotion; Oxyderm 20 Lotion*].

**Packaging and storage**

Store below 40 °C (104 °F), preferably between 15 and 30 °C (59 and 86 °F), unless otherwise specified by manufacturer. Store in a tight container. Protect from freezing.

**Preparation of dosage form**

In some products, benzoyl peroxide powder is packaged separately and must be added to the lotion before dispensing.

**Auxiliary labeling**
• Shake well.
• For external use only.

## BENZOYL PEROXIDE CLEANSING LOTION

**Usual adult and adolescent dose**

Acne vulgaris—
　　Topical, to the skin, as a 5 to 10% cleansing lotion one or two times a day.

**Usual pediatric dose**

Acne vulgaris—
　　Children up to 12 years of age: Safety and efficacy have not been established.
　　Children 12 years of age and over: See *Usual adult and adolescent dose.*

**Strength(s) usually available**

U.S.—
　　5% (OTC) [*Benzac W Wash 5; Desquam-X 5 Wash; Dryox Wash 5*].
　　10% (OTC) [*Benzac W Wash 10; Desquam-X 10 Wash; Dryox Wash 10; Fostex 10 Wash; Oxy 10 Daily Face Wash* (methylparaben; propylparaben); *Propa P.H. 10 Liquid Acne Soap; Theroxide 10 Wash*].

Canada—
　　5% (OTC) [*Benoxyl 5 Wash; Benzagel 5 Acne Wash; Desquam-X 5 Wash*].
　　10% (Rx) [*Benoxyl 10 Wash; Desquam-X 10 Wash*].

**Packaging and storage**
Store between 15 and 30 °C (59 and 86 °F), in a well-closed container, unless otherwise specified by manufacturer. Protect from freezing.

**Auxiliary labeling**
- Shake well.
- For external use only.

Note: *Benzac W* does not require shaking.

## BENZOYL PEROXIDE FACIAL MASK

**Usual adult and adolescent dose**
Acne vulgaris—
Topical, to the skin, as a 5% facial mask once a week to once a day, or as directed.

**Usual pediatric dose**
Acne vulgaris—
Children up to 12 years of age: Safety and efficacy have not been established.
Children 12 years of age and over: See *Usual adult and adolescent dose*.

**Strength(s) usually available**
U.S.—
5% (OTC) [*Ben-Aqua Masque 5; Neutrogena Acne Mask 5*].
Canada—
Not commercially available.

**Packaging and storage**
Store below 40 °C (104 °F), preferably between 15 and 30 °C (59 and 86 °F), in a well-closed container, unless otherwise specified by manufacturer. Protect from freezing.

**Auxiliary labeling**
- For external use only.

## BENZOYL PEROXIDE STICK

**Usual adult and adolescent dose**
Acne vulgaris—
Topical, to the skin, as a 10% stick one to three times a day.

**Usual pediatric dose**
Acne vulgaris—
Children up to 12 years of age: Safety and efficacy have not been established.
Children 12 years of age and over: See *Usual adult and adolescent dose*.

**Strength(s) usually available**
U.S.—
10% (OTC) [*Propa P.H. 10 Acne Cover Stick*].
Canada—
Not commercially available.

**Packaging and storage**
Store below 40 °C (104 °F), preferably between 15 and 30 °C (59 and 86 °F), in a well-closed container, unless otherwise specified by manufacturer.

**Auxiliary labeling**
- For external use only.

Revised: 01/15/92
Interim revision: 05/20/94

## BENZOYL PEROXIDE–CONTAINING COMBINATIONS—
Erythromycin and Benzoyl Peroxide (Topical)

## BENZPHETAMINE—See *Appetite Suppressants (Systemic)*

## BENZTHIAZIDE—See *Diuretics, Thiazide (Systemic)*

## BENZTROPINE—See *Antidyskinetics (Systemic)*

# BENZYL BENZOATE   Topical*†

VA CLASSIFICATION (Primary/Secondary): AP300/AP900
Note: For a listing of dosage forms and brand names by country availability, see *Dosage Forms* section(s). For a listing of brand names for the articles in this monograph, refer to the General Index.

*Not commercially available in the U.S.
†Not commercially available in Canada.

## Category
Pediculicide; scabicide.

## Indications
Note: Because benzyl benzoate is not commercially available in the U.S. or Canada, the bracketed information and the use of the superscript 1 in this monograph reflect the lack of labeled (approved) indications for this medication.

**Accepted**
[Pediculosis (treatment)][1]—Benzyl benzoate is used in the topical treatment of pediculosis caused by *Pediculus capitis* (head louse) and *Phthirus pubis* (pubic or crab louse).

[Scabies (treatment)][1]—Benzyl benzoate is used in the topical treatment of scabies caused by the *Sarcoptes scabiei* mite.

[1]Not included in Canadian product labeling.

## Pharmacology/Pharmacokinetics

**Physicochemical characteristics**
Source—Prepared synthetically by the esterification of benzoic acid with benzyl alcohol.
Molecular weight—212.2.

**Mechanism of action/Effect**
Unknown, but in view of the medication's effects on vertebrates, it is thought that benzyl benzoate may act on the nervous system of the parasite, resulting in its death.
*In vitro*, benzyl benzoate has been found to kill the *Sarcoptes* mite within 5 minutes.

**Absorption**
No data are available on percutaneous absorption of benzyl benzoate. Older reports suggested some percutaneous absorption, but the amount was not quantified.

**Biotransformation**
If topical benzyl benzoate is systemically absorbed, it is rapidly hydrolyzed to benzoic acid and benzyl alcohol, which is further oxidized to benzoic acid. The benzoic acid is conjugated with glycine to form hippuric acid.

**Elimination**
Excreted in the urine primarily as hippuric acid.

## Precautions to Consider

**Mutagenicity**
Benzyl benzoate has not been shown to cause mutagenic effects.

**Pregnancy/Reproduction**
Problems in humans have not been documented. However, the manufacturer recommends that benzyl benzoate not be used in pregnant women unless considered essential.

**Breast-feeding**
Problems in humans have not been documented. However, the manufacturer recommends that breast-feeding be suspended during treatment and reinstated only after the medication has been discontinued.

**Pediatrics**
Appropriate studies on the relationship of age to the effects of benzyl benzoate have not been performed in the pediatric population. However, no pediatrics-specific problems have been documented to date.

### Geriatrics

Although appropriate studies on the relationship of age to the effects of benzyl benzoate have not been performed in the geriatric population, no geriatrics-specific problems have been documented to date. However, elderly patients are more likely to have age-related xerosis of the skin, which may make their skin more susceptible to the drying effects of benzyl benzoate, and irritation may be worse in this age group. An alternative medication may need to be considered.

### Medical considerations/Contraindications

The medical considerations/contraindications included here have been selected on the basis of their potential clinical significance (reasons given in parentheses where appropriate)—not necessarily inclusive (» = major clinical significance).

*Risk-benefit should be considered when the following medical problems exist:*
» Hypersensitivity to benzyl benzoate, history of
» Inflammation of skin, acute, or with raw, weeping surfaces
    (condition may be exacerbated because more benzyl benzoate may be absorbed, therefore causing more irritation of the skin)

## Side/Adverse Effects

Note: Benzyl benzoate applied topically at recommended doses appears to have a low order of toxicity.

The following side/adverse effects have been selected on the basis of their potential clinical significance (possible signs and symptoms in parentheses where appropriate)—not necessarily inclusive:

**Those indicating need for medical attention only if they continue or are bothersome**
Incidence less frequent or rare
    *Irritation of skin, slight* (burning sensation; itching)

## Overdose

For more information on the management of overdose or unintentional ingestion, contact a Poison Control Center (See *Poison Control Center Listing*).

The following effects have been selected on the basis of their potential clinical significance (possible signs and symptoms in parentheses where appropriate)—not necessarily inclusive:

**Acute and chronic effects**
*CNS convulsions or excitations* (muscle spasm or jerking of all extremities; sudden loss of consciousness); *contact dermatitis with repeated use* (blister formation, crusting, itching, oozing, reddening, or scaling of skin); *urinary retention* (difficulty in passing urine [dribbling])

**Treatment of overdose**
Recommended treatment consists of the following:
To decrease absorption—
    For accidental ingestion, emesis or gastric lavage should be induced.
Specific treatment—
    The body should be washed with soap and warm water to remove excess benzyl benzoate.
    Anticonvulsants may be given to control convulsions.
Supportive care—
    Symptomatic treatment.

## Patient Consultation

As an aid to patient consultation, refer to *Advice for the Patient, Benzyl Benzoate (Topical)*.

In providing consultation, consider emphasizing the following selected information (» = major clinical significance):

**Before using this medication**
» Conditions affecting use, especially:
    Sensitivity to benzyl benzoate
    Pregnancy—Not recommended for use in pregnant women unless considered essential
    Breast-feeding—Suspension of breast-feeding recommended during treatment
    Use in the elderly—Skin of older people may be more susceptible to the drying and irritating effects of benzyl benzoate
    Other medical problems, especially severe inflammation of skin

**Proper use of this medication**
Reading patient directions carefully before using
» Importance of using the medication only as directed
» Avoiding contact with the eyes and mucous membranes

» Not using on open wounds, such as cuts or sores on skin or scalp, to minimize systemic absorption
    If necessary, treating other members of household and close contacts, especially sexual partner or partners, since infestation may spread to persons in close contact; checking with doctor if these persons have not been examined or if there are any questions

*For lice—Proper administration*
    Shampooing, rinsing, and drying hair and scalp well before using benzyl benzoate if hair or scalp has any cream, lotion, ointment, or oil-based product on it
    Applying enough benzyl benzoate to thoroughly wet the dry hair and scalp or skin
    Leaving benzyl benzoate on affected areas for 24 hours
    Removing benzyl benzoate by washing thoroughly with soap or with regular shampoo and warm water
    Rinsing thoroughly; drying with clean towel
    When hair is dry, combing with a fine-toothed comb (less than 0.3 mm between the teeth) to remove any remaining nits or nit shells, or using tweezers or fingernails to pick out nits for persons with fine hair

*For scabies—Proper administration*
    Washing, rinsing, and drying skin well before using benzyl benzoate if skin has any cream, lotion, ointment, or oil on it
    Drying skin well if bath or shower is taken before use of benzyl benzoate
    Applying enough benzyl benzoate to dry skin to cover entire skin surface from neck down, including soles of feet; rubbing in well
    Leaving benzyl benzoate on skin for 24 hours
    Removing benzyl benzoate by washing thoroughly with soap and warm water
    Rinsing thoroughly; drying with clean towel
    Washing hands immediately after using to remove any benzyl benzoate that may be on them
    Repeating treatment for severe infestation
» Proper dosing
» Proper storage

**Precautions while using this medication**
*To help prevent reinfestation or spread of infestation to other persons*
*For lice*
    Disinfecting or washing combs, curlers, and brushes in very hot water for about 10 minutes immediately after using
    Washing all recently worn clothing and used bed linens and towels in very hot water or dry-cleaning
    Sealing stuffed toys and other non-washable articles in a plastic bag for 2 weeks, or placing these items in the freezer (in sealed plastic bags) for 12 to 24 hours
    Vacuuming all rugs, mattresses, pillows, furniture, and car seats to remove fallen hairs with lice
*For scabies*
    Washing all recently worn clothing such as underwear and pajamas, and used sheets, pillowcases, and towels in very hot water or dry-cleaning

## General Dosing Information

To minimize systemic absorption, benzyl benzoate should not be used on open wounds, such as cuts or sores on skin or scalp.

Sexual partners and other persons in close contact or living in the same household should be checked for infestation and treated if necessary, since the infestation may spread to persons in close contact.

To help prevent reinfestation or spreading of the infestation, all recently worn clothing such as underwear and pajamas, and used sheets, pillowcases, and towels should be washed in very hot water or dry-cleaned.

Itching due to circulating antigens from scabies may persist for up to 2 weeks after successful treatment. Further treatment with benzyl benzoate is not advisable; use of a topical corticosteroid is recommended.

Treatment may be repeated for severe infestation.

A follow-up examination one week after the last treatment is recommended to confirm disinfestation of lice.

**For treatment of adverse effects**
Recommended treatment consists of the following
    • For severe skin reaction, the medication should be washed off with soap and warm water.

## Topical Dosage Form

Note: Because benzyl benzoate is not commercially available in the U.S. or Canada, the bracketed information and the use of superscript 1 in the Dosage Forms section reflect the lack of labeled (approved) indications for this product.

## BENZYL BENZOATE EMULSION

### Usual adult and adolescent dose
[Pediculosis][1]—
Topical, one application to the affected areas as a 25% emulsion; emulsion should remain on the affected areas for twenty-four hours. Treatment may be repeated two or three times, if necessary, for severe infestation.

[Scabies][1]—
Topical, one application to the entire body except the head and face as a 25% emulsion, which should remain for twenty-four hours. Treatment may be repeated anytime within five days if necessary. Alternatively, the emulsion may be applied three times at twelve-hour intervals.

### Usual adult prescribing limits
No more than three applications within five days.

### Usual pediatric dose
See *Usual adult and adolescent dose.*

Note: To minimize the risk of irritation, dilute with water as follows—

For infants: Dilute with 3 parts water.

For older children: Dilute with an equal quantity of water.

### Strength(s) usually available
U.S.—
Not commercially available.

Canada—
Not commercially available.
Other (United Kingdom)—
25% (OTC) [*Ascabiol*].

### Packaging and storage
Store below 25 °C (77 °F), in a well-closed container. Protect from light. Protect from freezing.

### Auxiliary labeling
• For external use only.
• Shake the bottle before use.
• Keep out of reach of children.
• When dispensing, include patient instructions.

---

[1]Not included in Canadian product labeling.

## Selected Bibliography
Landegren J, Borglund E, Storgards K. Treatment of scabies with disulfiram and benzyl benzoate emulsion: a controlled study. Acta Derm Venereol (Stockh) 1979; 59 (3): 274-6.

---

Developed: 01/21/94

---

**BEPRIDIL**—See *Calcium Channel Blocking Agents (Systemic)*

---

# BERACTANT    Intratracheal-Local

VA CLASSIFICATION (Primary): RE900

Another commonly used name is modified bovine surfactant extract.

Note: For a listing of dosage forms and brand names by country availability, see *Dosage Forms* section(s). For a listing of brand names for the articles in this monograph, refer to the General Index.

## Category
Pulmonary surfactant.

## Indications

### Accepted
Respiratory distress syndrome, neonatal (prophylaxis and treatment)—
Beractant intratracheal suspension is indicated for the prophylaxis (prevention strategy) and treatment (rescue strategy) of respiratory distress syndrome (RDS), also known as hyaline membrane disease, in premature infants.

Beractant is used to prevent RDS in infants with birth weights of less than 1250 grams who are at risk of developing RDS or who show evidence of surfactant deficiency. For prevention of RDS, beractant should be given as soon as possible after the infant's birth, preferably within 15 minutes after birth.

Beractant is used in the rescue treatment of RDS in infants who have developed RDS, confirmed by chest radiography, and who require mechanical ventilation. For rescue treatment, beractant should be given as soon as possible after diagnosis of RDS is confirmed and the infant is placed on a respirator, preferably within 8 hours after the infant's birth.

## Pharmacology/Pharmacokinetics

### Mechanism of action/Effect
Beractant is a natural bovine lung extract containing phospholipids, neutral lipids, fatty acids, and the two hydrophobic, low-molecular-weight surfactant-associated proteins, SP-B and SP-C (beractant does not contain the hydrophilic, large-molecular-weight protein, SP-A). Colfosceril palmitate, palmitic acid, and tripalmitin are added to standardize the composition of beractant and make it similar to natural lung surfactant by optimizing surface tension–lowering properties. When beractant is used as a replacement for deficient endogenous lung surfactant, it is effective in lowering surface tension on alveolar surfaces during respiration and stabilizing the alveoli against collapse at resting transpulmonary pressures. Therefore, beractant reduces the incidence of RDS, mortality due to RDS, and air-leak complications.

Neonatal RDS develops primarily in premature infants because of pulmonary immaturity, including a deficiency of endogenous lung surfactant that results in higher alveolar surface tension and lower compliance properties. Without sufficient endogenous lung surfactant, progressive alveolar collapse occurs and both oxygen and carbon dioxide exchange are impaired. Also, RDS appears to be characterized by high pulmonary vascular permeability and increased lung tissue water. Fluid and protein that leak into alveoli inactivate both endogenous and exogenous surfactant, worsening lung function.

Natural lung surfactant is a mixture of lipids and apoproteins secreted by the alveolar cells into the alveoli and respiratory air passages. Surfactant reduces the surface tension of pulmonary fluids and thereby increases lung compliance. It exhibits not only surface tension–reducing properties (contributed by the lipids) but also rapid spreading and adsorption (contributed by the apoproteins). The major fraction of the lipid component of natural lung surfactant is dipalmitoylphosphatidylcholine (DPPC, colfosceril palmitate); this comprises up to 70% of the natural surfactant by weight.

### Absorption
Biophysical activity occurs locally at alveolar surface with no systemic absorption.

### Onset of action
Marked improvements in oxygenation may occur within minutes of administration.

### Duration of action
Significant improvements in arterial-alveolar oxygen ratio ($PaO_2$ /$PA\ O_2$), inspired oxygen fraction ($FI\ O_2$), and mean airway pressure (MAP) were sustained for 48 to 72 hours in several studies of beractant-treated infants who had RDS.

## Precautions to Consider

### Cross-sensitivity and/or related problems
Circulating antibodies to bovine surfactant proteins, SP-B and SP-C, as analyzed by Western blot immunoassay, were not detected in blood specimens taken from infants 7 and 28 days of age who had been treated previously with beractant after development of severe respiratory distress syndrome. Also, serum samples taken from infants 6 and 12 months of age who had been previously treated with beractant were negative for circulating antibodies to surfactant-associated proteins. However, the potential for an allergic response to foreign protein still exists with beractant.

### Carcinogenicity
Long-term studies have not been performed in animals to evaluate the carcinogenic potential of beractant.

### Mutagenicity
Ames mutagenicity studies with beractant were negative.

**Pregnancy/Reproduction**

Fertility—No adverse effect on fertility was observed in rats given beractant.

Pregnancy—No information is available on the use of beractant during pregnancy.

**Breast-feeding**

No information is available on the use of beractant during breast-feeding.

**Pediatrics**

Appropriate studies on the relationship of age to the effects of beractant have not been performed in the pediatric population. No information is available on administration more than 48 hours after birth.

**Geriatrics**

No information is available on the relationship of age to the effects of beractant.

**Patient monitoring**

The following may be especially important in patient monitoring (other tests may be warranted in some patients, depending on condition; » = major clinical significance):

» Arterial blood gases

(after both prophylactic and rescue dosing, frequent arterial and transcutaneous measurements of systemic oxygen and carbon dioxide are recommended to prevent hyperoxia and hypercarbia, which may occur within minutes of administration of beractant; if hyperoxia develops and transcutaneous oxygen saturation is in excess of 95%, Fi O$_2$ should be reduced until saturation is 90 to 95%; failure to reduce inspiratory ventilator pressures rapidly can result in lung overdistention and pulmonary air leaks)

Heart rate and
Oxygen saturation

(continuous monitoring is recommended during dosing procedure; if transient episodes of bradycardia and decreased oxygen saturation occur, procedure must be stopped and appropriate measures taken to relieve condition; dosing procedure may be resumed after stabilization of the infant)

## Side/Adverse Effects

Note: In controlled clinical studies, infants treated with beractant were at no greater risk than control infants for developing patent ductus arteriosus, intracranial hemorrhage, necrotizing enterocolitis, apnea, post-treatment infections, and pulmonary hemorrhage. Infants treated with beractant were at less risk for developing pulmonary air leaks and pulmonary interstitial emphysema. No particular surfactant or method of surfactant delivery was related to an increased incidence of intracranial hemorrhage. Surfactant therapy, in itself, may initiate hemodynamic changes that could predispose an infant to intracranial hemorrhage in certain circumstances. Such changes can probably be compensated for by careful management of oxygenation and ventilation.

Beractant-treated infants were at significantly greater risk for post-treatment nosocomial sepsis than were premature infants in control groups. However, the increased risk of sepsis was not associated with increased mortality.

The most commonly reported adverse effects in clinical trials were associated with particular dosing procedures or methods of administration. These effects include endotracheal tube reflux (noted in single-dose studies) and transient bradycardia and decreased oxygenation (noted in multidose studies).

The following side/adverse effects have been selected on the basis of their potential clinical significance (possible signs and symptoms in parentheses where appropriate)—not necessarily inclusive:

**Those indicating need for medical attention**

Incidence more frequent

*Bradycardia, transient (<60 beats per minute); carbon dioxide tension, increased; oxygen desaturation; reflux, endotracheal tube*

Incidence less frequent (<1%)

*Apnea; blockage, endotracheal tube; hypercarbia or hypocarbia; hypertension or hypotension; pallor; vasoconstriction*

## General Dosing Information

Beractant should be used only by neonatologists and other clinicians who are experienced in neonatal intubation and ventilatory management. Also, instillation of this medication should be performed only by trained medical personnel experienced in airway and clinical management of unstable premature infants. Adequate personnel, facilities, equipment, and medications are required to optimize the perinatal outcome in these premature infants. In addition, continuous clinical attention should be given to all infants prior to, during, and after administration of this medication.

Review of audiovisual materials provided by the manufacturer is recommended before using beractant to obtain a description of its dosing and administration procedures.

Prior to administration of beractant, proper placement of the endotracheal tube tip in the trachea (not in the esophagus or the right or left mainstream bronchus) should be confirmed. The endotracheal tube may be suctioned at the discretion of the clinician to ensure patency before administration of beractant.

Beractant intratracheal suspension is administered only by instillation into the trachea through a No. 5 end-hole French catheter. The length of the catheter should be shortened so that the tip of the catheter protrudes just beyond the endotracheal tube above the infant's carina. The catheter can be inserted into the endotracheal tube without interrupting ventilation by passing the catheter through a neonatal suction valve attached to the endotracheal tube. The neonatal suction valve maintains a closed airway circuit system by sealing the valve around the catheter. The catheter must be rigid enough to pass through the endotracheal tube without twisting or curling within the suction valve. Alternatively, beractant can be instilled through the catheter by briefly disconnecting the endotracheal tube from the ventilator. The infant should be allowed to stabilize before the dosing proceeds.

Prior to administration, the suspension should be warmed by allowing the vial to stand at room temperature for at least 20 minutes or by warming it in the hand for at least 8 minutes. No artificial warming methods should be used. For prophylactic doses, warming must begin before the infant's birth.

Four doses of four aliquots each can be administered in the infant's first 48 hours of life; doses should be given at least 6 hours apart, as follows:

**FIRST DOSE**

The total dose for both prevention and rescue strategies is determined from the dosing chart provided by the manufacturer and is dependent on the infant's birth weight.

To ensure homogeneous distribution of beractant throughout the lungs, the total dose (100 mg of phospholipids [4 mL of suspension] per kg of birth weight) is divided into 4 aliquots (25 mg [1 mL] per kg of birth weight). The infant is supine during the dosing procedure. The respective aliquots are administered with the infant held in the following positions: infant's head and body inclined slightly downward with head turned to the right; infant's head and body inclined downward with head turned to the left; infant's head and body inclined upward with head turned to the right; infant's head and body inclined upward with head turned to the left.

The entire contents of the vial are slowly drawn into a plastic syringe through a 20-gauge or larger needle without filtering or shaking. The catheter is attached to the syringe and filled with beractant suspension. Any excess suspension beyond the total dose is discarded through the catheter so that only the total dose remains in the syringe. With the infant positioned appropriately, the first aliquot is injected gently through the catheter into the endotracheal tube over 2 to 3 seconds.

Prevention strategy—The catheter is removed from the endotracheal tube after the first quarter-dose, and the infant is ventilated manually, by means of a hand-bag with sufficient oxygen to prevent cyanosis at a ventilation rate of 60 breaths per minute and with enough positive pressure to provide adequate air exchange and chest wall excursion.

Rescue strategy—The catheter is removed from the endotracheal tube after the first quarter-dose and the infant is placed on the mechanical ventilator.

Both strategies—The infant is then repositioned for administration of each of the next quarter-doses. Between aliquots, the catheter is removed and the infant is ventilated for at least 30 seconds or until the infant is stabilized. Immediately after the ventilation period, the next aliquot is instilled and the same procedure is followed until the entire dose is administered. After the final instillation, the catheter is removed without being flushed with air or liquid. The infant is not suctioned for at least 1 hour after dosing unless signs of significant airway obstruction appear.

After completion of the dosing procedure, usual ventilator management and clinical care are resumed.

**ADDITIONAL DOSES**

The need for subsequent doses is determined based on evidence of continuing respiratory distress in the infant. The following criteria for redosing are used

• Dose no sooner than 6 hours after the preceding dose if the infant remains intubated and requires at least 30% inspired oxygen to maintain a PaO$_2$ not less than 80 torr.

• For infants who received beractant as a prevention dose initially, radiographic confirmation of RDS is required before any additional doses are administered.

• Repeat doses are also 100 mg of phospholipids (or 4 mL suspension) per kg of birth weight, administered in four aliquots. The infant should not be reweighed.

Manual hand-bag ventilation should not be used for repeat doses. The infant is ventilated mechanically with ventilator settings adjusted to maintain appropriate oxygenation and ventilation.

## Intratracheal Dosage Forms

### BERACTANT INTRATRACHEAL SUSPENSION

**Usual pediatric dose**
Pulmonary surfactant (prophylaxis)—
Intratracheal, the equivalent of 100 mg of phospholipids (4 mL of suspension) per kg of birth weight for the first dose (administered as four quarter-doses) as soon as possible within 15 minutes after infant's birth; additional doses should be administered no sooner than 6 hours later to infants who remain intubated and require at least 30% inspired oxygen.
Pulmonary surfactant (treatment)—
Intratracheal, the equivalent of 100 mg of phospholipids (4 mL of suspension) per kg of birth weight for the first dose (administered as four quarter-doses) as soon as possible after diagnosis of respiratory distress syndrome (RDS) is confirmed and infant is placed on a respirator, preferably within 8 hours after birth; additional doses should be administered no sooner than 6 hours later to infants who remain intubated and require at least 30% inspired oxygen.

Note: Each dose is administered in four quarter-doses, with each quarter-dose being equivalent to 25 mg of beractant (1 mL of suspension) per kg of birth weight. Each quarter-dose is instilled slowly over 2 to 3 seconds through the catheter.

**Strength(s) usually available**
U.S.—
25 mg of phospholipids per mL (200 mg per 8-mL vial) (Rx) [*Survanta* (sodium chloride, 0.09%)].

Canada—
25 mg of phospholipids per mL (200 mg per 8-mL vial) (Rx) [*Survanta* (sodium chloride, 0.09%)].

**Packaging and storage**
Store unopened vials between 2 and 8 °C (35 and 46 °F). Protect from light.

**Preparation of dosage form**
The suspension should be warmed by allowing the vial to stand at room temperature for at least 20 minutes or by warming it in the hand for at least 8 minutes. No artificial warming methods should be used. For prevention doses, warming must begin before the infant's birth.

**Stability**
The optimum color of the suspension is off-white to light brown. Visual inspection before use is necessary to detect any discoloration of the product.
If the suspension appears to have separated, the vial should be swirled gently (not shaken) to resuspend any particles that may have settled during storage.

**Additional information**
Unopened, unused vials of the suspension that have been warmed to room temperature may be returned to the refrigerator within 8 hours of warming and stored for future use. However, warmed, unopened vials should not be returned to the refrigerator more than once.
Each single-use vial should be entered with a needle only once. Any unused suspension must be discarded.

## Selected Bibliography

Liechty EA, Donovan E, Purohit D, et al. Reduction of neonatal mortality after multiple doses of bovine surfactant in low birth weight neonates with respiratory distress syndrome. Pediatrics 1991 July; 88 (1): 19-28.

Reynolds MS, Wallander KA. Surfactant for neonatal respiratory distress syndrome. J Pediatr Health Care 1990 Jul-Aug; 4 (4): 209-15.

Yee WFH, Scarpelli EM. Surfactant replacement therapy. Pediatr Pulmonol 1991; 11: 65-80.

Developed: 8/15/95

---

# BETA-ADRENERGIC BLOCKING AGENTS   Ophthalmic

This monograph includes information on the following: Betaxolol; Carteolol; Levobunolol; Metipranolol†; Timolol.

VA CLASSIFICATION (Primary): OP101

Note: For a listing of dosage forms and brand names by country availability, see *Dosage Forms* section(s). For a listing of brand names for the articles in this monograph, refer to the General Index.

†Not commercially available in Canada.

## Category
Antiglaucoma agent (ophthalmic).

## Indications

Note: Bracketed information in the *Indications* section refers to uses that are not included in U.S. product labeling.

**Accepted**
Glaucoma, open-angle (treatment) or
Hypertension, ocular (treatment)—Ophthalmic beta-adrenergic blocking agents are indicated in the treatment of chronic open-angle glaucoma. They also may be used in the treatment of ocular hypertension. They may be used alone or in combination with other antiglaucoma agents.

Glaucoma, in aphakic eyes (treatment) or
Glaucoma, secondary (treatment)—[Betaxolol][1], [carteolol][1], [levobunolol][1], [metipranolol][1], and timolol are indicated in the treatment of glaucoma in aphakic eyes and in some cases of secondary glaucoma.

[Glaucoma, angle-closure (treatment adjunct)]—Betaxolol[1], carteolol[1], levobunolol[1], metipranolol[1], and timolol may be used in conjunction with miotics to reduce intraocular pressure in acute and chronic angle-closure glaucoma. However, the ophthalmic beta-adrenergic blocking agent's action alone is unlikely to terminate an acute attack of angle-closure glaucoma, because the agent produces little or no constriction of the pupil. Constriction of the pupil is necessary to pull the iris away from the trabeculum to relieve blockage of the trabecular meshwork.

[Glaucoma, angle-closure, *during* or *after* iridectomy (treatment)][1] or
[Glaucoma, malignant (treatment)][1]—Ophthalmic beta-adrenergic blocking agents may be used to lower intraocular pressure in the treatment of angle-closure glaucoma *during* or *after* iridectomy and in the treatment of malignant glaucoma.

Ophthalmic betaxolol may be especially useful in the treatment of glaucoma in patients with pulmonary disease because it is a relatively selective beta-1-adrenergic antagonist. Although ophthalmic betaxolol can have significant effects on pulmonary function in persons with pulmonary disease, it appears to do so much less frequently than nonselective beta-antagonists.

[1]Not included in Canadian product labeling.

## Pharmacology/Pharmacokinetics

**Physicochemical characteristics**
Molecular weight—
Betaxolol: 343.89.
Carteolol: 328.84.
Levobunolol: 327.85.
Metipranolol: 309.40.
Timolol: 432.49.

**Mechanism of action/Effect**
Betaxolol is a cardioselective (beta-1-adrenergic) receptor blocking agent. Carteolol, levobunolol, metipranolol, and timolol are beta-1 and beta-2 (nonselective) adrenergic blocking agents. The exact mechanism of the ocular hypotensive action of ophthalmic beta-adrenergic blocking agents has not been established. However, it appears that the ophthalmic beta-adrenergic blocking agents reduce aqueous humor production, as demonstrated by tonography and fluorophotometry. A slight increase in aqueous humor outflow may be an additional mechanism.

**Other actions/effects**
Ophthalmic beta-adrenergic blocking agents, if systemically absorbed, are capable of producing beta-adrenergic receptor blockade in the bronchi

and bronchioles. (This is less likely to occur with ophthalmic betaxolol because it is a relatively selective beta-1-adrenergic blocking agent.) This action results in an increase in airway resistance because of unopposed parasympathetic activity. This effect is in keeping with the beta-2-adrenergic blocking action of these medications. It is possible that carteolol, because of its partial beta-agonist activity, may have less of a beta-blockade effect than the other ophthalmic beta-2-adrenergic blocking agents; however, the possible protection conferred by the beta-agonist effect has not been clinically evaluated. Betaxolol 1% solution, when compared to a placebo, was not shown to have a significant effect on pulmonary function as measured by forced expiratory volume in 1 second (FEV$_1$), forced vital capacity (FVC), and FEV$_1$ / VC. However, in clinical use, ophthalmic betaxolol has caused a worsening of respiratory symptoms in some patients with pulmonary disease.

Ophthalmic beta-adrenergic blocking agents, if systemically absorbed, are also capable of reducing heart rate, myocardial contractility, and cardiac output, resulting in bradycardia and hypotension, in both healthy individuals and patients with heart disease. This is in keeping with the beta-1-adrenergic blocking action of these medications.

The ophthalmic beta-adrenergic blocking agents do not have significant membrane-stabilizing (local anesthetic) activity.

Ophthalmic beta-adrenergic blocking agents reduce normal as well as elevated intraocular pressure (IOP), whether or not it is accompanied by glaucoma.

Ophthalmic beta-adrenergic blocking agents have little or no effect on pupil size or accommodation compared with miosis produced by cholinergic agents.

### Absorption
Ophthalmic beta-adrenergic blocking agents may be systemically absorbed.

### Onset of action
Betaxolol, metipranolol, and timolol—Within 30 minutes following a single dose.

Levobunolol—Within 1 hour following a single dose.

### Time to peak effect
Betaxolol, carteolol, and metipranolol—Approximately 2 hours following a single dose. This applies to both betaxolol ophthalmic solution and suspension.

Levobunolol—Between 2 and 6 hours following a single dose.

Timolol—Within 1 to 2 hours following a single dose.

### Duration of action
Betaxolol—12 hours, following a single dose of either the ophthalmic solution or suspension.

Carteolol—More than 6 to 8 hours.

Levobunolol and timolol—A significant lowering of intraocular pressure may be maintained for up to 24 hours following a single dose.

Metipranolol—A reduction in intraocular pressure can be demonstrated 24 hours following a single dose.

## Precautions to Consider

### Cross-sensitivity and/or related problems
Patients sensitive to any of the ophthalmic or systemic beta-adrenergic blocking agents, such as acebutolol, atenolol, betaxolol, bisoprolol, carteolol, labetalol, levobunolol, metipranolol, metoprolol, nadolol, oxprenolol, penbutolol, pindolol, propranolol, sotalol, or timolol, may be sensitive to any other beta-adrenergic blocking agent also.

### Carcinogenicity
*Betaxolol*—In lifetime studies in mice and rats, betaxolol has not been shown to be carcinogenic when administered orally at doses of 6, 20, or 60 mg per kg of body weight (mg/kg) per day (mice) and at doses of 3, 12, or 48 mg/kg per day (rats).

*Carteolol*—In 2-year studies in mice and rats, carteolol has not been shown to be carcinogenic when administered orally at doses of up to 40 mg/kg per day.

*Metipranolol*—In lifetime studies, metipranolol has not been shown to be carcinogenic when administered orally to mice at doses of 5, 50, and 100 mg/kg per day and to rats at doses of up to 70 mg/kg per day.

*Timolol*—In a lifetime study in mice, timolol increased the incidence of malignant pulmonary tumors and mammary adenocarcinomas in female mice when administered orally at doses of 500 mg/kg per day, but not at 5 or 50 mg/kg per day.

### Tumorigenicity
*Betaxolol and carteolol*—Unknown.

*Levobunolol*—In a lifetime study, levobunolol increased the incidence of benign leiomyomas in female mice when administered orally at doses of 200 mg/kg per day (14,000 times the recommended human dose for glaucoma), but did not produce this effect at doses of 12 or 50 mg/kg per day (850 and 3500 times the human dose). In a 2-year

study in rats, levobunolol increased the incidence of benign hepatomas in male rats when administered orally at doses 12,800 times the recommended human dose for glaucoma. Similar differences were not observed in rats when levobunolol was administered at oral doses equivalent to 350 to 2000 times the recommended human dose for glaucoma.

*Metipranolol*—In lifetime studies, female mice had an increased number of pulmonary adenomas when they were given metipranolol at an oral dose of 5 mg/kg per day. However, doses of 50 and 100 mg/kg per day did not produce this effect.

*Timolol*—In a 2-year study in rats, timolol increased the incidence of adrenal pheochromocytomas in male rats when administered orally at doses of 300 mg/kg per day (which are 250 times the maximum recommended human oral dose of 30 mg [1 drop of ophthalmic timolol contains about 1/150th of this dose or about 0.2 mg of timolol]). However, similar effects were not observed in rats when timolol was administered at oral doses equivalent to 20 or 80 times the maximum recommended human oral dose. In a lifetime study in mice, timolol increased the incidence of benign pulmonary tumors and benign uterine polyps in female mice when administered orally at doses of 500 mg/kg per day. However, doses of 5 and 50 mg/kg per day did not produce this effect. In addition, timolol increased the overall incidence of neoplasms in female mice at oral doses of 500 mg/kg per day.

### Mutagenicity
*Betaxolol*—In vitro and in vivo bacterial and mammalian cell assays have not shown betaxolol to be mutagenic.

*Carteolol*—Carteolol was not shown to be mutagenic in the Ames test and recombinant (rec)-assay and in the *in vivo* cytogenetic and dominant lethal assays.

*Levobunolol*—In microbiological and mammalian *in vitro* and *in vivo* assays, levobunolol was not shown to be mutagenic.

*Metipranolol*—Metipranolol was nonmutagenic in *in vivo* and *in vitro* bacterial and mammalian cell assays.

*Timolol*—Timolol was not shown to be mutagenic when tested *in vivo* (mouse) in the micronucleus test and cytogenetic assay (at doses up to 800 mg/kg) and *in vitro* in a neoplastic cell transformation assay (up to 0.1 mg per mL).

### Pregnancy/Reproduction
Fertility—*Betaxolol*: Studies in rabbits and rats have shown that betaxolol, administered at oral doses above 12 mg/kg and 128 mg/kg, respectively, causes drug-related postimplantation loss.

*Carteolol*: Studies in rats and mice have not shown that carteolol causes any adverse effects on male and female fertility when administered at doses of up to 150 mg/kg per day.

*Levobunolol*: Reproduction and fertility studies in rats showed no adverse effects on male or female fertility when levobunolol was administered at doses of up to 1800 times the recommended human dose for glaucoma.

*Metipranolol*: Reproduction and fertility studies on metipranolol in rats and mice showed no adverse effect on female or male fertility at oral doses of up to 25 mg/kg per day and 50 mg/kg per day, respectively.

*Timolol*: Reproduction and fertility studies in rats have not shown that timolol causes any adverse effects on male and female fertility when administered at doses of up to 125 times the maximum recommended human oral dose.

Pregnancy—
  *Betaxolol*—
    Adequate and well-controlled studies in humans have not been done.

    In animal studies, betaxolol was not shown to cause teratogenic effects or other adverse effects on reproduction at subtoxic doses.

    FDA Pregnancy Category C.

  *Carteolol*—
    Although adequate and well-controlled studies in humans have not been done, carteolol may be absorbed systemically.

    In rabbits and rats, carteolol, administered in doses approximately 1052 and 5264 times the maximum recommended human oral dose of 10 mg per 70 kg of body weight per day, respectively, resulted in maternotoxicity, increased incidence of fetal resorptions, and decreased fetal weights. In rats, carteolol, administered in doses approximately 212 times the maximum recommended human oral dose, resulted in a dose-related increase in wavy ribs in the developing rat fetus. However, in mice, carteolol, administered in doses up to approximately 1052 times the maximum recommended human oral dose, did not result in wavy ribs.

    FDA Pregnancy Category C.

*Levobunolol—*
Adequate and well-controlled studies in humans have not been done.

Although levobunolol has been shown to cause fetotoxicity in rabbits when administered at doses equivalent to 200 and 700 times the recommended dose for the treatment of glaucoma, similar studies in rats have not shown levobunolol to cause fetotoxic effects when administered at doses of up to 1800 times the human dose for glaucoma. Moreover, in teratogenicity studies in rats, levobunolol was not shown to cause fetal malformations when administered at doses of up to 25 mg/kg per day (1800 times the recommended human dose for glaucoma). Also, levobunolol was not shown to have adverse effects on the postnatal development of animal offspring.

FDA Pregnancy Category C.

*Metipranolol—*
Adequate and well-controlled studies in humans have not been done.

No metipranolol-related effects were reported for the segment II teratology study in fetal rats when metipranolol was administered orally to pregnant rats in doses of up to 50 mg/kg per day during organogenesis. However, metipranolol has been shown to increase fetal resorption, fetal death, and delayed development when administered orally to pregnant rabbits at 50 mg/kg during organogenesis.

FDA Pregnancy Category C.

*Timolol—*
Although adequate and well-controlled studies in humans have not been done, timolol may be absorbed systemically.

Studies in rats have shown that timolol at doses of up to 50 mg/kg per day (50 times the maximum recommended human oral dose) causes delayed fetal ossification; however, there were no adverse effects on postnatal development of offspring. Teratogenic studies in mice and rabbits have not shown that timolol at doses of up to 50 mg/kg per day causes fetal malformations. In mice, timolol at doses of 1 gram per kg per day (1000 times the maximum recommended human oral dose) was maternotoxic and resulted in increased incidence of fetal resorptions. In rabbits, timolol at doses 100 times the maximum recommended human oral dose caused increased incidence of fetal resorptions but not maternotoxicity.

FDA Pregnancy Category C.

## Breast-feeding

*Betaxolol—*Systemic betaxolol is distributed into breast milk in large enough quantities to have pharmacological effects. However, it is not known whether ophthalmic betaxolol is distributed into breast milk and problems in humans have not been documented.

*Carteolol—*It is not known whether systemic or ophthalmic carteolol is distributed into human breast milk; however, carteolol has been shown to be distributed into animal milk.

*Levobunolol—*It is not known whether ophthalmic levobunolol is distributed into breast milk. However, problems in humans have not been documented.

*Metipranolol—*It is not known whether ophthalmic metipranolol is distributed into breast milk. However, problems in humans have not been documented.

*Timolol—*Systemic timolol is distributed into breast milk. Problems in humans have not been documented for ophthalmic timolol; however, ophthalmic timolol may be systemically absorbed and distributed into the breast milk, possibly causing serious adverse reactions in the infants of nursing mothers.

## Pediatrics

Although appropriate studies on the relationship of age to the effects of beta-adrenergic blocking agents, including the ophthalmic blocking agents, have not been performed in the pediatric population, infants should be treated cautiously and monitored for signs of dyspnea. In addition, the use of nasolacrimal occlusion should be emphasized for both infants and children.

## Geriatrics

Although appropriate studies on the relationship of age to the effects of ophthalmic beta-adrenergic blocking agents have not been performed in the geriatric population, no geriatrics-specific problems have been documented to date. However, if significant systemic absorption of ophthalmic beta-adrenergic blocking agents occurs, the same geriatrics-related problems may occur that are possible with the systemic beta-adrenergic blocking agents. These include bradycardia, increased myocardial depression because of reduced metabolic and excretory capabilities in many elderly patients, and the increased risk of beta-adrenergic blocking agent–induced hypothermia in elderly patients.

In addition, elderly patients are more likely to have age-related peripheral vascular disease, which may require caution in patients receiving beta-adrenergic blocking agents.

## Drug interactions and/or related problems

The following drug interactions and/or related problems have been selected on the basis of their potential clinical significance (possible mechanism in parentheses where appropriate)—not necessarily inclusive (» = major clinical significance):

Note: Combinations containing any of the following medications, depending on the amount present, may also interact with this medication.

Information concerning interactions between ophthalmic beta-adrenergic blocking agents and other medications is still limited. Some of the following potential interactions apply to beta-adrenergic blocking agents in general and are stated for cautionary reference until additional information specific to the ophthalmic beta-adrenergic blocking agents is available.

Allergen immunotherapy or
Allergenic extracts for skin testing
(if significant systemic absorption of ophthalmic beta-adrenergic blocking agents occurs, concurrent use of these agents in patients using ophthalmic beta-adrenergic blocking agents may increase the potential for serious systemic reaction or anaphylaxis)

Amiodarone
(if significant systemic absorption of ophthalmic beta-adrenergic blocking agents occurs, concurrent use may potentiate bradycardia, sinus arrest, and atrioventricular [AV] block, especially in patients with underlying sinus function impairment)

Anesthetics, hydrocarbon inhalation, such as:
Chloroform
Cyclopropane
Enflurane
Halothane
Isoflurane
Methoxyflurane
Trichloroethylene
(if significant systemic absorption of ophthalmic beta-adrenergic blocking agents occurs, concurrent use of hydrocarbon inhalation anesthetics may increase the risk of myocardial depression and hypotension because the beta-adrenergic blockade reduces the ability of the heart to respond to beta-adrenergically mediated sympathetic reflex stimuli; if it is necessary to reverse the effects of beta-adrenergic blocking agents during surgery, agonists, such as dobutamine, dopamine, isoproterenol, or norepinephrine, may be used but should be administered with caution, especially in patients receiving halothane. Some clinicians recommend gradual withdrawal of beta-adrenergic blocking agents 48 hours prior to elective surgery; however, this recommendation is controversial)

Antidiabetic agents, oral or
Insulin
(systemic beta-adrenergic blocking agents may affect diabetes mellitus therapy. This may also occur with ophthalmic beta-adrenergic blocking agents if there is significant systemic absorption. Nonselective beta-adrenergic blocking agents impair glycogenolysis and the hyperglycemic response to endogenous epinephrine, leading to persistence of hypoglycemia. Also, beta-adrenergic blocking agents, especially nonselective agents, decrease the release of insulin in response to hyperglycemia. Dosage adjustment of the antidiabetic agent may be required to avoid a severe hypoglycemic reaction. In addition, beta-adrenergic blocking agents may complicate patient monitoring by masking symptoms of hypoglycemia caused by epinephrine, such as increased heart rate and increased blood pressure, but not dizziness and sweating. Although selective or relatively selective beta-adrenergic blocking agents usually cause fewer problems with blood glucose levels, they may still mask symptoms of hypoglycemia)

Beta-adrenergic blocking agents, systemic
(if significant systemic absorption of ophthalmic beta-adrenergic blocking agents occurs, concurrent use of these medications may result in an additive effect on intraocular pressure or in additive systemic effects of beta-adrenergic blockade)

Calcium channel blocking agents
(if significant systemic absorption of ophthalmic beta-adrenergic blocking agents occurs, concurrent use of calcium channel blocking agents, such as bepridil, diltiazem, flunarizine, isradipine, nicardipine, nifedipine, nimodipine, and verapamil, may result in atrioventricular conduction disturbances, left ventricular failure, and hypotension; in some patients, if a calcium antagonist is necessary, nicardipine or nifedipine may be preferred because they

have less effect on heart rate and conduction, although they may also cause greater hypotension; concurrent use of calcium channel blockers and ophthalmic beta-adrenergic blocking agents should be used with care in patients with impaired cardiac function)

Catecholamine-depleting medications, such as the rauwolfia alkaloids:
Alseroxylon
Deserpidine
Rauwolfia serpentina
Reserpine
(if significant systemic absorption of ophthalmic beta-adrenergic blocking agents occurs, concurrent use of catecholamine-depleting medications may result in additive and possibly excessive beta-adrenergic blockade; although this effect is largely theoretical, close observation is recommended, since bradycardia and marked hypotension may occur)

Cimetidine
(if significant systemic absorption of ophthalmic beta-adrenergic blocking agents occurs, concurrent use with cimetidine may reduce the clearance of hepatically metabolized beta-adrenergic blocking agents, resulting in elevations of plasma concentrations)

Clonidine
(if significant systemic absorption of ophthalmic beta-adrenergic blocking agents occurs during concurrent use, discontinuation of clonidine therapy may increase the risk of clonidine-withdrawal hypertensive crisis; ideally, beta-adrenergic blocking agents should be discontinued several days before clonidine is discontinued; blood pressure control may also be impaired when the 2 are combined)

Cocaine
(cocaine may inhibit the therapeutic effects of systemic beta-adrenergic blocking agents, and may also have this effect on ophthalmic beta-adrenergic blocking agents)

(concurrent use of cocaine with systemic beta-adrenergic blocking agents may increase the risk of hypertension, excessive bradycardia, and possibly heart block because beta-adrenergic blockade may leave cocaine's alpha-adrenergic activity unopposed. This may also occur with ophthalmic beta-adrenergic blocking agents if significant systemic absorption of the ophthalmic beta-adrenergic blocking agent occurs)

Contrast media, iodinated
(if significant systemic absorption of ophthalmic beta-adrenergic blocking agents occurs, concurrent use with intravenous contrast media may increase the risk of moderate to severe anaphylaxis; these reactions may be refractory to treatment. There was no consensus among USP experts as to whether or not this interaction was clinically significant)

Fentanyl and derivatives
(preoperative chronic use of ophthalmic beta-adrenergic blocking agents [with the possible exception of betaxolol] may increase the risk of initial bradycardia following induction doses of fentanyl or any of its derivatives)

Flecainide
(if significant systemic absorption of ophthalmic beta-adrenergic blocking agents occurs, concurrent use may result in additive negative cardiac inotropic effects, especially, or perhaps only, in patients with cardiac problems)

Hypotension-producing medications, other (See *Appendix II*)
(if significant systemic absorption of ophthalmic beta-adrenergic blocking agents [with the possible exception of betaxolol] occurs, concurrent use may potentiate the hypotensive effects of these medications)

Methacholine
(if significant systemic absorption of ophthalmic beta-adrenergic blocking agents occurs, methacholine inhalation challenge should not be performed, since the reaction to methacholine may be exaggerated or prolonged and may not respond as rapidly to treatment with bronchodilators)

Nicotine
(nicotine increases the metabolism of beta-adrenergic blocking agents; if significant systemic absorption of ophthalmic beta-adrenergic blocking agents occurs, patients undergoing smoking cessation may experience an increase in the frequency of side/adverse effects caused by the blocking agents because of the subsequent decrease in the blocking agents' metabolism. There was no consensus among USP experts as to whether or not this interaction was clinically significant)

Phenothiazines
(if significant systemic absorption of ophthalmic beta-adrenergic blocking agents occurs, concurrent use may result in an increased plasma concentration of either the phenothiazine or the ophthalmic beta-adrenergic blocking agent because of inhibition of metabolism. This may result in additive hypotensive effects, irreversible retinopathy, cardiac arrhythmias, or tardive dyskinesia. There was no consensus among USP experts as to whether or not this interaction was clinically significant)

Phenytoin, intravenous
(if significant systemic absorption of ophthalmic beta-adrenergic blocking agents occurs, concurrent use may cause additive cardiac depressant effects. There was no consensus among USP experts as to whether or not this interaction was clinically significant)

Sympathomimetics, systemic
(if significant systemic absorption of ophthalmic beta-adrenergic blocking agents occurs, concurrent use may result in inhibition of the beta-adrenergic effects of sympathomimetics; depending on the type of sympathomimetic, this inhibition will occur with the beta-1-adrenergic cardiac effects and/or the beta-2-adrenergic bronchodilating effect; betaxolol will block primarily the beta-1-adrenergic effects)

(concurrent use of norepinephrine may result in mutual inhibition of therapeutic effects)

Xanthines, such as:
Aminophylline
Caffeine
Dyphylline
Oxtriphylline
Theophylline
(if significant systemic absorption of ophthalmic beta-adrenergic blocking agents [with the possible exception of betaxolol] occurs, concurrent use may result in inhibition of therapeutic effects of xanthines; in addition, concurrent use of xanthines [except dyphylline] with the ophthalmic beta-adrenergic blocking agents [with the possible exception of betaxolol] may decrease theophylline clearance, especially in patients with increased theophylline clearance induced by smoking; concurrent use requires careful monitoring)

(concurrent use with caffeine may result in inhibition of caffeine's therapeutic effect)

## Medical considerations/Contraindications

The medical considerations/contraindications included here have been selected on the basis of their potential clinical significance (reasons given in parentheses where appropriate)—not necessarily inclusive (» = major clinical significance).

*Except under special circumstances, this medication should not be used when the following medical problems exist:*

» Asthma, bronchial (or history of) or
» Pulmonary disease, obstructive, severe chronic
(severe respiratory reactions, including death due to bronchospasm, have been reported in patients with asthma, following administration of the ophthalmic beta-adrenergic blocking agents. Although betaxolol appears to have a minimal effect on pulmonary function, caution should be used in patients with severe restriction of pulmonary function)

» Cardiac failure, overt or
» Cardiogenic shock or
» Heart block, 2nd- or 3rd-degree atrioventricular (AV) or
» Sinus bradycardia
(risk of further myocardial depression may occur with the use of the ophthalmic beta-adrenergic blocking agents)

» Previous allergic reaction to the ophthalmic beta-adrenergic blocking agent prescribed

*Risk-benefit should be considered when the following medical problems exist:*

» Bronchitis, nonallergic or chronic or
» Emphysema or
» Pulmonary function impairment, other
(use of the ophthalmic beta-adrenergic blocking agents may promote bronchospasm and block bronchodilation produced by endogenous and exogenous catecholamine stimulation of beta-2-receptors. Although the effects of betaxolol on pulmonary function have been shown in some studies to be minimal in patients with reactive airway disease, there have been reports of asthmatic attacks and pulmonary distress during betaxolol treatment)

Cerebrovascular insufficiency
(potential effects on blood pressure and pulse; if signs of reduced cerebral blood flow occur following initiation of therapy, alternative therapy should be considered)

» Congestive heart failure
(risk of further depression of myocardial contractility)

» Cardiac failure, history of or
Heart block, history of
(possible risk of myocardial depression; treatment should be discontinued at first signs of cardiac failure)

» Diabetes mellitus, especially labile diabetes or
» Hypoglycemia
(ophthalmic beta-adrenergic blocking agents may mask some signs and symptoms of hypoglycemia, such as tachycardia and tremor, although they do not mask dizziness and sweating)

» Hyperthyroidism
(ophthalmic beta-adrenergic blocking agents may mask certain signs and symptoms of hyperthyroidism; abrupt withdrawal may precipitate a thyroid storm)

Myasthenia gravis
(beta-adrenergic blockade may potentiate muscle weakness related to certain myasthenic symptoms, such as diplopia, ptosis, and generalized weakness)

**Patient monitoring**
The following may be especially important in patient monitoring (other tests may be warranted in some patients, depending on condition; » = major clinical significance):

Intraocular pressure determination
(recommended during, and following, the first month of therapy during which stabilization of the pressure-lowering response to the ophthalmic beta-adrenergic blocking agent usually occurs; thereafter, intraocular pressure should be determined as necessary)

## Side/Adverse Effects

Note: Even in patients *without* a history of cardiac failure, continued depression of the myocardium with beta-blockers, including ophthalmic beta-adrenergic blocking agents, over a period of time can lead to cardiac failure, if significant systemic absorption occurs. However, betaxolol and metipranolol may be less likely to cause myocardial depression. At the first sign or symptom of cardiac failure, the ophthalmic beta-adrenergic blocking agent should be discontinued.

Although ophthalmic beta-adrenergic blocking agents have minimal membrane-stabilizing (local anesthetic) action, decreased corneal sensitivity may occur following prolonged use, and has been reported rarely with the use of betaxolol, levobunolol, and timolol, but not with the use of metipranolol. In contrast, carteolol has been reported to occasionally cause increased corneal sensitivity.

Because of betaxolol's relatively selective beta-1-adrenergic receptor inhibition, betaxolol may have less potential for systemic side/adverse effects than have the other ophthalmic beta-adrenergic blocking agents, which are nonselective beta-1 and beta-2 adrenergic receptor inhibitors. This may be especially important for patients for whom beta-2 adrenergic blockade could be harmful.

The ophthalmic suspension dosage form of betaxolol appears to be less irritating to the eye than the ophthalmic solution dosage form, although eye irritation occurs more frequently than other side effects with both dosage forms.

The side effects listed below have been reported for one or more of the ophthalmic beta-adrenergic blocking agents. However, all of these side effects are possible with any of the ophthalmic beta-adrenergic blocking agents. In addition, since the ophthalmic beta-adrenergic blocking agents may be systemically absorbed, any of the side effects that are possible for the systemic beta-adrenergic blocking agents are also theoretically possible for the ophthalmic beta-adrenergic blocking agents.

The following side/adverse effects have been selected on the basis of their potential clinical significance (possible signs and symptoms in parentheses where appropriate)—not necessarily inclusive:

**Those indicating need for medical attention**
Incidence more frequent
*Conjunctival hyperemia* (redness of eyes or inside of eyelids)—reported for carteolol, frequency 25%
Incidence less frequent or rare
*Anisocoria* (different size pupils of the eyes)—reported for betaxolol; *blepharitis*—reported for metipranolol and timolol; *blepharoconjunctivitis*—reported for carteolol and levobunolol; *conjunctivitis*—reported for metipranolol and timolol; *corneal punctate keratitis*—reported for betaxolol; *dermatitis of eyelid*—reported for metipranolol; *edema*—reported for carteolol and metipranolol; *iridocyclitis*—reported for levobunolol; *keratitis*—reported for betaxolol and timolol (-

severe swelling, irritation, or inflammation of eye or eyelid); *blepharoptosis* (droopy upper eyelid)—reported for carteolol and timolol; *corneal staining* (discoloration of the eyeball)—reported for betaxolol and carteolol; *decreased corneal sensitivity*—reported for betaxolol, levobunolol, and timolol; *diplopia* (seeing double)—reported for timolol; *eye pain*—reported for betaxolol suspension; *glossitis* (redness or irritation of the tongue)—reported for betaxolol; *vision disturbances* (blurred vision or other change in vision)—reported for betaxolol suspension, carteolol, metipranolol, and timolol

Symptoms of systemic absorption
*Allergic reaction* (skin rash, hives, or itching)—reported for all except levobunolol; *alopecia* (hair loss)—reported for betaxolol and timolol; *anxiety or nervousness*—reported for metipranolol only; *arthritis or myalgia* (muscle or joint aches or pain)—reported for metipranolol only; *ataxia* (clumsiness or unsteadiness)—reported for levobunolol only; *change in taste*—reported for carteolol only; *chest pain*—reported for timolol only; *confusion or mental depression*—reported for betaxolol, metipranolol, and timolol; *congestive heart failure* (swelling of feet, ankles, or lower legs)—reported for betaxolol and timolol; *coughing, wheezing, or troubled breathing, especially in patients with predisposition to bronchoconstriction*—reported for all; *diarrhea*—reported for timolol only; *dizziness or feeling faint*—reported for all; *drowsiness*—reported for metipranolol and timolol; *epistaxis* (bleeding nose)—reported for metipranolol and timolol; *hallucinations*—reported for timolol only; *headache*—reported for all; *heartblock*—reported for betaxolol and timolol; *hypertension*—reported for metipranolol and timolol; *impotence* (decreased sexual ability)—reported for timolol only; *insomnia* (trouble in sleeping)—reported for betaxolol and carteolol; *irregular, slow, or pounding heartbeat*—reported for all; *nasal congestion* (stuffy nose)—reported for timolol only; *nausea or vomiting*—reported for metipranolol and timolol; *paresthesia* (burning or prickling feeling on body)—reported for timolol only; *rhinitis or sinusitis* (runny nose)—reported for carteolol, metipranolol, and timolol; *systemic lupus erythematosus*—reported for timolol only; *toxic epidermal necrolysis* (raw or red areas of the skin)—reported for betaxolol; *unusual tiredness or weakness*—reported for all

**Those indicating need for medical attention only if they continue or are bothersome**
Incidence more frequent
*Decreased night vision*—reported for carteolol; *stinging of eye or other eye irritation, transient upon administration of medication*—reported for betaxolol, levobunolol, and metipranolol
Incidence less frequent or rare
*Browache*—reported with carteolol and metipranolol; *corneal sensitivity*—reported for carteolol; *crusting of eyelashes*—reported with betaxolol suspension; *dryness of eye*—reported with betaxolol suspension; *increased sensitivity of eye to light*—reported for betaxolol, carteolol, and metipranolol; *redness, itching, stinging, burning, or watering of eye or other eye irritation*—reported for all; more frequent for carteolol and levobunolol

## Overdose

For specific information on the agents used in the management of ophthalmic beta-adrenergic blocking agents overdose, see:
• *Aminophylline* in *Bronchodilators, Theophylline-derivative (Systemic)* monograph;
• *Atropine* in *Anticholinergics/Antispasmodics (Systemic)* monograph;
• *Charcoal, Activated (Oral-Local)* monograph;
• *Digitalis Glycosides (Systemic)* monograph;
• *Dobutamine* in *Sympathomimetic Agents-Cardiovascular Use (Parenteral-Systemic)* monograph;
• *Dopamine* in *Sympathomimetic Agents-Cardiovascular Use (Parenteral-Systemic)* monograph;
• *Glucagon (Systemic)* monograph;
• *Isoproterenol* in *Sympathomimetic Agents-Cardiovascular Use (Parenteral-Systemic)* monograph;
• *Norepinephrine* in *Sympathomimetic Agents-Cardiovascular Use (Parenteral-Systemic)* monograph; and/or
• *Theophylline* in *Bronchodilators, Theophylline-derivative (Systemic)* monograph.

For more information on the management of overdose or unintentional ingestion, **contact a Poison Control Center** (see *Poison Control Center Listing*).

**Treatment of overdose**
If an ophthalmic overdose occurs, immediately flush the eyes with warm tap water.

If an ophthalmic beta-adrenergic blocking agent is accidentally ingested, activated charcoal or gastric lavage may be appropriate to decrease further absorption.

For symptoms of systemic toxicity, the medication should be discontinued. Depending on severity of toxicity, the following supportive and symptomatic treatments should be utilized if necessary:

For bradycardia: Atropine (0.25 to 2 mg) should be administered intravenously to induce vagal blockade. If bradycardia persists, intravenous isoproterenol hydrochloride may be administered with caution. A transvenous cardiac pacemaker may be used, if necessary.

For hypotension: Glucagon and sympathomimetic pressor agents, such as dobutamine, dopamine, or norepinephrine, may be used. (See *Drug interactions and/or related problems* for precautions in use of sympathomimetic vasopressors.)

For bronchospasm: Isoproterenol hydrochloride should be administered. Additional therapy with a beta-2-agonist or a theophylline derivative may be used, if necessary.

For cardiac failure, acute: Digitalis, diuretics, and oxygen should be administered immediately. Intravenous aminophylline may be used in refractory cases. Also, glucagon hydrochloride may be used, if necessary.

For heart block, second or third degree: Isoproterenol hydrochloride or a transvenous cardiac pacemaker should be used.

## Patient Consultation

As an aid to patient consultation, refer to *Advice for the Patient, Beta-adrenergic Blocking Agents (Ophthalmic)*.

In providing consultation, consider emphasizing the following selected information (» = major clinical significance):

**Before using this medication**
» Conditions affecting use, especially:
  Allergy to any of the beta-adrenergic blocking agents, either ophthalmic or systemic, such as acebutolol, atenolol, betaxolol, bisoprolol, carteolol, labetalol, levobunolol, metipranolol, metoprolol, nadolol, oxprenolol, penbutolol, pindolol, propranolol, sotalol, or timolol
  Pregnancy—Ophthalmic beta-adrenergic blocking agents may be absorbed into the body. Studies in animals have not shown that betaxolol, levobunolol, metipranolol, or timolol causes birth defects. However, very large doses of carteolol given by mouth to pregnant rats have been shown to cause wavy ribs in rat babies. In addition, some studies in animals have shown that beta-adrenergic blocking agents increase the chance of death in the animal fetus
  Use in children—Infants may be especially sensitive to the effects of ophthalmic beta-adrenergic blocking agents, thus increasing the risk of side effects
  Use in the elderly—If significant systemic absorption of ophthalmic beta-adrenergic blocking agents occurs, the chance of side effects during treatment may be increased, since elderly people are especially sensitive to the effects of these medications
  Other medical problems, especially bronchial asthma, or history of, severe chronic obstructive pulmonary disease, overt cardiac failure, 2nd- or 3rd-degree atrioventricular (AV) heart block, cardiogenic shock, sinus bradycardia, nonallergenic or chronic bronchitis, emphysema or other pulmonary function impairment, congestive heart failure, history of cardiac failure, diabetes mellitus, spontaneous hypoglycemia, or hyperthyroidism

**Proper use of this medication**
» Proper administration technique; using nasolacrimal occlusion is especially important in infants and children
  Preventing contamination: Not touching applicator tip to any surface; keeping container tightly closed
  Proper use of medication having compliance cap
» Importance of not using more medication than the amount prescribed
» Proper dosing
  Missed dose: If dosing schedule is—
    Once a day: Applying as soon as possible; not applying if not remembered until next day; applying regularly scheduled dose
    More than once a day: Applying as soon as possible; not applying if almost time for next dose; applying next dose at regularly scheduled time
» Proper storage

**Precautions while using this medication**
  Regular visits to physician to check eye pressure during therapy
» Caution if any kind of surgery (including dental surgery) or emergency treatment is required
» Diabetics: May mask some signs of hypoglycemia, such as increased pulse rate and trembling, but not dizziness and sweating; also, may cause decreased or sometimes increased blood glucose concentrations
  Possible photophobia: Wearing sunglasses and avoiding too much exposure to bright light

**Side/adverse effects**
  Signs of potential side effects, especially conjunctival hyperemia, anisocoria, blepharitis, blepharoconjunctivitis, conjunctivitis, corneal punctate keratitis, dermatitis of eyelid, edema, iridocyclitis, keratitis, blepharoptosis, corneal staining, decreased corneal sensitivity, diplopia, eye pain, glossitis, vision disturbances, or symptoms of systemic absorption

## General Dosing Information

Although some manufacturers recommend a dose of 2 drops of an ophthalmic solution at appropriate intervals, the conjunctival sac will usually hold 1 drop or less.

When one ophthalmic beta-adrenergic blocking agent is used to replace another, the original beta-blocker may be discontinued simultaneously with initiation of therapy with the new one.

When an ophthalmic beta-adrenergic blocking agent is used to replace a single antiglaucoma agent other than another beta-blocker, the other antiglaucoma agent may be continued on the first day that the new beta-blocker is used but can be discontinued on the second day.

When an ophthalmic beta-adrenergic blocking agent is used to replace several concomitantly administered antiglaucoma agents, the patient's dosage should be individualized as required. If any of the other antiglaucoma agents used is a beta-blocker, it can be discontinued before the new ophthalmic beta-adrenergic blocking agent is added to the regimen. The other antiglaucoma agents being used may be continued on the first day that the new beta-blocker is used but one of the agents should be discontinued on the second day. Then the remaining antiglaucoma agents may be decreased or discontinued according to the patient's response. Additional adjustments usually should involve only one agent at a time and should be made at intervals of not less than one week.

Ophthalmic beta-adrenergic blocking agents may be used concurrently with direct and indirect cholinergic agonists (e.g., pilocarpine, echothiophate, carbachol), beta-agonists (e.g., ophthalmic epinephrine or dipivefrin), or systemic carbonic anhydrase inhibitors (such as acetazolamide), if necessary to control intraocular pressure.

In patients scheduled for major surgery, some practitioners recommend that beta-adrenergic blocking agents be gradually withdrawn 48 hours prior to surgery because beta-adrenergic receptor blockade impairs the ability of the heart to respond to beta-adrenergically mediated reflex stimuli. This recommendation is controversial. However, since ophthalmic beta-adrenergic blocking agents may be absorbed systemically, gradual withdrawal of the medication should be considered for patients undergoing elective surgery because prolonged severe hypotension during anesthesia has occurred in some patients receiving systemic beta-adrenergic blocking agents. If necessary during surgery, the effects of beta-adrenergic blocking agents may be reversed by sufficient doses of agonists, such as isoproterenol, dopamine, dobutamine, or norepinephrine.

To help reduce systemic side effects, the patient can be instructed to close the eyes gently and apply pressure to the inner canthus of each eye in order to block lacrimal drainage through the tear ducts after instillation of the ophthalmic drops.

---

### BETAXOLOL

## Summary of Differences

Indications:
  Betaxolol may be especially useful in the treatment of glaucoma in patients with pulmonary disease.
Pharmacology/pharmacokinetics:
  Mechanism of action/effect—Betaxolol is a cardioselective (beta-1-adrenergic) receptor blocking agent.
  Other actions/effects—Betaxolol is less likely to produce significant beta-adrenergic receptor blockade in the bronchi and bronchioles.
  Duration of action—12 hours.
Fertility:
  Studies in rabbits and rats have shown that betaxolol, at oral doses above 12 mg/kg and 128 mg/kg, respectively, causes drug-related postimplantation loss.
Breast-feeding:
  Systemic betaxolol is distributed into breast milk in large enough quantities to have pharmacological effects. However, it is not known whether ophthalmic betaxolol is distributed into breast milk and problems in humans have not been documented.

## Ophthalmic Dosage Forms
### BETAXOLOL HYDROCHLORIDE OPHTHALMIC SOLUTION USP

Note: The dosing and strength usually available are expressed in terms of betaxolol base.

**Usual adult and adolescent dose**
Ophthalmic antiglaucoma agent—
   Topical, to the conjunctiva, 1 drop of a 0.5% solution of betaxolol (base) two times a day.

**Usual pediatric dose**
Safety and efficacy have not been established.

**Strength(s) usually available**
U.S.—
   0.5% (5 mg base; 5.6 mg as hydrochloride) (Rx) [*Betoptic* (benzalkonium chloride 0.01%; edetate disodium; sodium chloride; hydrochloric acid; sodium hydroxide)].
Canada—
   0.5% (5 mg base; 5.6 mg as hydrochloride) (Rx) [*Betoptic* (benzalkonium chloride 0.01%; edetate disodium; sodium chloride; hydrochloric acid; sodium hydroxide)].

**Packaging and storage**
Store below 40 °C (104 °F), preferably between 15 and 30 °C (59 and 86 °F), in a tight container, unless otherwise specified by manufacturer. Protect from freezing.

**Auxiliary labeling**
• For the eye.
• Keep container tightly closed.

### BETAXOLOL HYDROCHLORIDE OPHTHALMIC SUSPENSION

**Usual adult and adolescent dose**
Ophthalmic antiglaucoma agent—
   Topical, to the conjunctiva, 1 drop of a 0.25% suspension of betaxolol (base) two times a day.

**Usual pediatric dose**
Safety and efficacy have not been established.

**Strength(s) usually available**
U.S.—
   0.25% (2.5 mg base; 2.8 mg as hydrochloride) (Rx) [*Betoptic S* (benzalkonium chloride 0.01%; mannitol; poly (styrene-divinyl benzene) sulfonic acid; Carbomer 934P; edetate disodium; hydrochloric acid; sodium hydroxide)].
Canada—
   Not commercially available.

**Packaging and storage**
Store below 40 °C (104 °F), preferably between 15 and 30 °C (59 and 86 °F), in a well-closed container, unless otherwise specified by manufacturer. Protect from freezing.

**Auxiliary labeling**
• Shake well.
• For the eye.
• Keep container tightly closed.

---

### *CARTEOLOL*

## Summary of Differences

Pharmacology/pharmacokinetics:
   Other actions/effects—Carteolol has intrinsic sympathomimetic activity.
   Duration of action—More than 6 to 8 hours.
Pregnancy:
   In rabbits and rats, carteolol, administered in doses approximately 1052 and 5264 times the maximum recommended human oral dose of 10 mg per 70 kg of body weight per day, respectively, resulted in maternotoxicity, increased incidence of fetal resorptions, and decreased fetal weights. In rats, carteolol, administered in doses approximately 212 times the maximum recommended human oral dose, resulted in a dose-related increase in wavy ribs in the developing rat fetus. However, in mice, carteolol, administered in doses up to approximately 1052 times the maximum recommended human oral dose, did not result in wavy ribs.
Breast-feeding:
   It is not known whether systemic or ophthalmic carteolol is distributed into human breast milk; however, carteolol has been shown to be distributed into animal milk.

## Ophthalmic Dosage Forms
### CARTEOLOL HYDROCHLORIDE OPHTHALMIC SOLUTION

**Usual adult and adolescent dose**
Ophthalmic antiglaucoma agent—
   Topical, to the conjunctiva, 1 drop two times a day.

**Usual pediatric dose**
Safety and efficacy have not been established.

**Strength(s) usually available**
U.S.—
   1% (10 mg carteolol hydrochloride per mL) (Rx) [*Ocupress* (benzalkonium chloride 0.005%; sodium chloride; monobasic sodium phosphate; dibasic sodium phosphate)].
Canada—
   Not commercially available.

**Packaging and storage**
Store between 15 and 25 °C (59 and 77 °F), in a well-closed container, unless otherwise specified by manufacturer. Protect from light. Protect from freezing.

**Auxiliary labeling**
• For the eye.
• Keep container tightly closed.

---

### *LEVOBUNOLOL*

## Summary of Differences

Pharmacology/pharmacokinetics:
   Onset of action—Within 1 hour.
   Time to peak effect—Between 2 and 6 hours.
   Duration of action—Up to 24 hours.
Pregnancy:
   Although levobunolol has been shown to cause fetotoxicity in rabbits when administered at doses equivalent to 200 and 700 times the recommended dose for the treatment of glaucoma, similar studies in rats have not shown levobunolol to cause fetotoxic effects when administered at doses of up to 1800 times the human dose for glaucoma. Moreover, in teratogenicity studies in rats, levobunolol was not shown to cause fetal malformations when administered at doses of up to 25 mg/kg per day (1800 times the recommended human dose for glaucoma). Also, levobunolol was not shown to have adverse effects on the postnatal development of animal offspring.

## Ophthalmic Dosage Forms
### LEVOBUNOLOL HYDROCHLORIDE OPHTHALMIC SOLUTION USP

**Usual adult and adolescent dose**
Ophthalmic antiglaucoma agent—
   Topical, to the conjunctiva, 1 drop of a 0.25% solution one or two times a day or 1 drop of a 0.5% solution once a day.

**Usual adult prescribing limits**
Dosages above 1 drop of a 0.5% solution two times a day are generally not more effective.

**Usual pediatric dose**
Safety and efficacy have not been established.

**Strength(s) usually available**
U.S.—
   0.25% (Rx) [*Betagan C Cap B.I.D.* (polyvinyl alcohol 1.4%; benzalkonium chloride 0.004%; sodium metabisulfite; edetate disodium; dibasic sodium phosphate; monobasic potassium phosphate; sodium chloride; hydrochloric acid; sodium hydroxide)].
   0.5% (Rx) [*Betagan C Cap B.I.D.* (polyvinyl alcohol 1.4%; benzalkonium chloride 0.004%; sodium metabisulfite; edetate disodium; dibasic sodium phosphate; monobasic potassium phosphate; sodium chloride; hydrochloric acid; sodium hydroxide); *Betagan C Cap Q.D.* (polyvinyl alcohol 1.4%; benzalkonium chloride 0.004%; sodium metabisulfite; edetate disodium; dibasic sodium phosphate; monobasic potassium phosphate; sodium chloride; hydrochloric acid; sodium hydroxide); *Betagan Standard Cap* (polyvinyl alcohol 1.4%; benzalkonium chloride 0.004%; sodium metabisulfite; edetate disodium; dibasic sodium phosphate; monobasic potassium phosphate; sodium chloride; hydrochloric acid; sodium hydroxide)].

Canada—

0.25% (Rx) [*Betagan C Cap B.I.D.* (polyvinyl alcohol 1.4%; benzalkonium chloride 0.004%; sodium metabisulfite; edetate disodium; dibasic sodium phosphate; monobasic potassium phosphate; sodium chloride; hydrochloric acid; sodium hydroxide)].

0.5% (Rx) [*Betagan C Cap B.I.D.* (polyvinyl alcohol 1.4%; benzalkonium chloride 0.004%; sodium metabisulfite; edetate disodium; dibasic sodium phosphate; monobasic potassium phosphate; sodium chloride; hydrochloric acid; sodium hydroxide); *Betagan Standard Cap* (polyvinyl alcohol 1.4%; benzalkonium chloride 0.004%; sodium metabisulfite; edetate disodium; dibasic sodium phosphate; monobasic potassium phosphate; sodium chloride; hydrochloric acid; sodium hydroxide)].

**Packaging and storage**
Store below 40 °C (104 °F), preferably between 15 and 30 °C (59 and 86 °F), in a tight container, unless otherwise specified by manufacturer. Protect from light. Protect from freezing.

**Auxiliary labeling**
• For the eye.
• Keep container tightly closed.

---

### METIPRANOLOL

## Summary of Differences

Pharmacology/pharmacokinetics: Duration of action—More than 24 hours.

Pregnancy: No metipranolol-related effects were reported for the segment II teratology study in fetal rats when metipranolol was administered orally in doses of up to 50 mg/kg per day during organogenesis. However, metipranolol has been shown to increase fetal resorption, fetal death, and delayed development when administered orally to pregnant rabbits at 50 mg/kg during organogenesis.

## Ophthalmic Dosage Forms

### METIPRANOLOL HYDROCHLORIDE OPHTHALMIC SOLUTION

Note: The dosing and strengths usually available are expressed in terms of metipranolol base.

**Usual adult and adolescent dose**
Ophthalmic antiglaucoma agent—
Topical, to the conjunctiva, 1 drop of a 0.3% solution of metipranolol (base) two times a day.

**Usual adult prescribing limits**
Dosages above 1 drop of a 0.3% solution two times a day are not known to be of benefit.

**Usual pediatric dose**
Safety and efficacy have not been established.

**Strength(s) usually available**
U.S.—

0.3% (3 mg base per mL) (Rx) [*OptiPranolol* (benzalkonium chloride 0.004%; glycerol; sodium chloride; edetate disodium; povidone; hydrochloric acid; sodium hydroxide)].

Canada—
Not commercially available.

**Packaging and storage**
Store below 40 °C (104 °F), preferably between 15 and 30 °C (59 and 86 °F), in a well-closed container, unless otherwise specified by manufacturer. Protect from freezing.

**Auxiliary labeling**
• For the eye.
• Keep container tightly closed.

---

### TIMOLOL

## Summary of Differences

Pharmacology/pharmacokinetics: Duration of action—Up to 24 hours.

Carcinogenicity: In a lifetime study in mice, timolol increased the incidence of malignant pulmonary tumors and mammary adenocarcinomas in female mice when administered orally at doses of 500 mg/kg per day, but not at 5 or 50 mg/kg per day.

Pregnancy: Studies in rats have shown that timolol at doses of up to 50 mg/kg per day (50 times the maximum recommended human oral dose) causes delayed fetal ossification; however, there were no adverse effects on postnatal development of offspring. Teratogenic studies in

mice and rabbits have not shown that timolol at doses of up to 50 mg/kg per day causes fetal malformations. In mice, timolol at doses of 1 gram per kg per day (1000 times the maximum recommended human oral dose) was maternotoxic and resulted in increased incidence of fetal resorptions. In rabbits, timolol at doses 100 times the maximum recommended human oral dose caused increased incidence of fetal resorptions but not maternotoxicity.

Breast-feeding: Systemic timolol is distributed into breast milk. Problems in humans have not been documented for ophthalmic timolol; however, ophthalmic timolol may be systemically absorbed and distributed into the breast milk, possibly causing serious adverse reactions in the infants of nursing mothers.

## Ophthalmic Dosage Forms

### TIMOLOL MALEATE OPHTHALMIC SOLUTION USP

Note: The dosing and strengths usually available are expressed in terms of timolol base.

**Usual adult and adolescent dose**
Ophthalmic antiglaucoma agent—
Topical, to the conjunctiva, 1 drop of a 0.25 or 0.5% solution of timolol (base) one or two times a day.

**Usual pediatric dose**
Ophthalmic antiglaucoma agent—
Infants and children up to 10 years of age: Topical, to the conjunctiva, 1 drop of a 0.25% solution of timolol (base) one or two times a day.
Children 10 years of age and older: See *Usual adult and adolescent dose*.

Note: Nasolacrimal occlusion should be emphasized to patient.

**Strength(s) usually available**
U.S.—

0.25% (2.5 mg base; 3.4 mg as maleate) (Rx) [*Timoptic* (benzalkonium chloride 0.01%; monobasic sodium phosphate; dibasic sodium phosphate; sodium hydroxide); *Timoptic in Ocudose* (monobasic sodium phosphate; dibasic sodium phosphate; sodium hydroxide)].

0.5% (5 mg base; 6.8 mg as maleate) (Rx) [*Timoptic* (benzalkonium chloride 0.01%; monobasic sodium phosphate; dibasic sodium phosphate; sodium hydroxide); *Timoptic in Ocudose* (monobasic sodium phosphate; dibasic sodium phosphate; sodium hydroxide)].

Canada—

0.25% (2.5 mg base; 3.4 mg as maleate) (Rx) [*Apo-Timop* (benzalkonium chloride 0.1%; monobasic sodium phosphate; dibasic sodium phosphate; sodium hydroxide); *Gen-Timolol* (benzalkonium chloride 0.01%; monobasic sodium phosphate; dibasic sodium phosphate; *Timoptic* (benzalkonium chloride 0.01%; ; monobasic sodium phosphate; dibasic sodium phosphate; sodium hydroxide)].

0.5% (5 mg base; 6.8 mg as maleate) (Rx) [*Apo-Timop* (benzalkonium chloride 0.1%; monobasic sodium phosphate; dibasic sodium phosphate; sodium hydroxide); *Gen-Timolol* (benzalkonium chloride 0.01%; monobasic sodium phosphate; dibasic sodium phosphate); *Timoptic* (benzalkonium chloride 0.01%; monobasic sodium phosphate; dibasic sodium phosphate; sodium hydroxide)].

**Packaging and storage**
Store between 15 and 30 °C (59 and 86 °F), in a tight container, unless otherwise specified by manufacturer. Protect from freezing. Protect from light.

**Auxiliary labeling**
• For the eye.
• Keep container tightly closed.

## Selected Bibliography

Gonzalez JP, Clissold SP. Ocular levobunolol. A review of its pharmacodynamic and pharmacokinetic properties, and therapeutic efficacy. Drugs 1987 Dec; 34 (60): 648-61.

Novack GD. Ophthalmic beta-blockers since timolol. Surv Ophthalmol 1987 Mar-Apr; 31 (5): 307-27.

Buckley MMT, et al. Ocular betaxolol. A review of its pharmacological properties, and therapeutic efficacy in glaucoma and ocular hypertension. Drugs 40. Auckland, New Zealand: ADIS Drug Information Services, 1990.

Battershill PE, Sorkin EM. Ocular metipranolol. A preliminary review of its pharmacodynamic and pharmacokinetic properties, and therapeutic efficacy in glaucoma and ocular hypertension. Drugs 1988 Nov; 36 (5): 601-15.

Bauer K, et al. Assessment of systemic effects of different ophthalmic beta-blockers in healthy volunteers. Clin Pharmacol Ther 1991 Jun; 49 (6): 658-64.

Brooks AM, Gillies WE. Ocular beta-blockers in glaucoma management. Clinical pharmacological aspects. Drugs Aging 1992 May-Jun; 2 (3): 208-21.

Chrisp P, Sorkin EM. Ocular carteolol. A review of its pharmacological properties, and therapeutic use in glaucoma and ocular hypertension. Drugs Aging 1992 Jan-Feb; 2 (1): 58-77.

Revised: 05/12/93

# BETA-ADRENERGIC BLOCKING AGENTS    Systemic

This monograph includes information on the following: Acebutolol; Atenolol; Betaxolol†; Bisoprolol†; Carteolol†; Labetalol; Metoprolol; Nadolol; Oxprenolol*; Penbutolol†; Pindolol; Propranolol; Sotalol; Timolol.

VA CLASSIFICATION (Primary/Secondary):
Acebutolol—CV100/CV250; CV300; CV490; CV900; CN900
Atenolol—CV100/CV250; CV300; CV490; CV900; CN105; CN900
Betaxolol—CV100/CV490
Bisoprolol—CV100/CV490
Carteolol—CV100/CV490
Labetalol—CV100/CV250; CV490
Metoprolol—CV100/CV250; CV300; CV490; CV900; CN105; CN900
Nadolol—CV100/CV250; CV300; CV490; CV900; CN105; CN900
Oxprenolol—CV100/CV250; CV300; CV490; CV900; CN900
Penbutolol—CV100/CV490
Pindolol—CV100/CV250; CV490; CN900
Propranolol—CV100/CV250; CV300; CV490; CV900; CN105; CN900
Sotalol—CV100/CV250; CV300; CV490; CV900; CN900
Timolol—CV100/CV250; CV300; CV490; CV900; CN105; CN900; OP107

Note: For a listing of dosage forms and brand names by country availability, see *Dosage Forms* section(s). For a listing of brand names for the articles in this monograph, refer to the General Index.

*Not commercially available in the U.S.
†Not commercially available in Canada.

## Category

Note: All of the beta-adrenergic blocking agents have similar pharmacologic actions; however, clinical uses among specific agents may vary because of pharmacologic or pharmacokinetic differences, availability of specific testing, and/or availability of clinical-use data.

Antiadrenergic—Acebutolol; Atenolol; Betaxolol; Carteolol; Labetalol; Metoprolol; Nadolol; Oxprenolol; Penbutolol; Pindolol; Propranolol; Sotalol; Timolol.
Antianginal—Acebutolol; Atenolol; Carteolol; Labetalol; Metoprolol; Nadolol; Oxprenolol; Penbutolol; Pindolol; Propranolol; Sotalol; Timolol.
Antiarrhythmic—Acebutolol; Atenolol; Metoprolol; Nadolol; Oxprenolol; Propranolol; Sotalol; Timolol.
Antihypertensive—Acebutolol; Atenolol; Betaxolol; Bisoprolol; Carteolol; Labetalol; Metoprolol; Nadolol; Oxprenolol; Penbutolol; Pindolol; Propranolol; Sotalol; Timolol.
Hypertrophic cardiomyopathy therapy adjunct—Acebutolol; Atenolol; Metoprolol; Nadolol; Oxprenolol; Pindolol; Propranolol; Sotalol; Timolol.
Myocardial infarction prophylactic and therapy—Acebutolol; Atenolol; Metoprolol; Nadolol; Oxprenolol; Propranolol; Sotalol; Timolol.
Neuroleptic–induced akathisia therapy—Betaxolol; Metoprolol; Nadolol; Propranolol.
Pheochromocytoma therapy adjunct—Acebutolol; Atenolol; Labetalol; Metoprolol; Nadolol; Oxprenolol; Propranolol; Sotalol; Timolol.
Vascular headache prophylactic—Atenolol; Metoprolol; Nadolol; Propranolol; Timolol.
Antitremor agent—Acebutolol; Atenolol; Metoprolol; Nadolol; Oxprenolol; Pindolol; Propranolol; Sotalol; Timolol.
Antianxiety therapy adjunct—Acebutolol; Atenolol; Metoprolol; Oxprenolol; Propranolol; Sotalol; Timolol.
Thyrotoxicosis therapy adjunct—Acebutolol; Atenolol; Metoprolol; Nadolol; Oxprenolol; Propranolol; Sotalol; Timolol.
Antiglaucoma agent—Timolol.

## Indications

Note: Bracketed information in the *Indications* section refers to uses that are not included in U.S. product labeling.

### Accepted

Angina pectoris, chronic (treatment)—[Acebutolol], atenolol, [carteolol], [labetalol][1], metoprolol, nadolol, oxprenolol[1], [penbutolol], [pindolol], propranolol, [sotalol], and [timolol] are indicated in the treatment of classic angina pectoris, also referred to as "effort-associated angina."

Arrhythmias, cardiac (prophylaxis and treatment)—Propranolol is indicated in the control and correction of supraventricular arrhythmias, ventricular tachycardias, digitalis-induced tachyarrhythmias, and catecholamine-induced tachyarrhythmias during anesthesia (with extreme caution because of possible additive myocardial depression with general anesthesia). Propranolol by intravenous injection is recommended only in the treatment of cardiac arrhythmias that occur while the patient is unable to receive oral medication, or when a rapid and observable effect is desired. [Acebutolol][1], [atenolol][1], [metoprolol][1], [nadolol][1], oxprenolol[1], sotalol[1], and [timolol][1] are also used for their antiarrhythmic effects, especially in supraventricular arrhythmias and ventricular tachycardias. Acebutolol[1] is indicated in the control and correction of premature ventricular contractions.

Hypertension (treatment)—Acebutolol, atenolol, betaxolol, bisoprolol, carteolol, labetalol, metoprolol, nadolol, oxprenolol, penbutolol, pindolol, propranolol, [sotalol], and timolol are indicated in the treatment of hypertension when used alone or in combination with other antihypertensive medication.

For additional information on initial therapeutic guidelines related to the treatment of hypertension, see *Appendix III*.

Parenteral labetalol is indicated for treatment of severe hypertension. Intravenous metoprolol and propranolol are not recommended for the management of hypertensive emergencies. However, intravenous propranolol has proven useful in controlling hypertension during anesthesia and surgery.

Cardiomyopathy, hypertrophic (treatment)—[Acebutolol][1], [atenolol][1], [metoprolol][1], [nadolol][1], oxprenolol[1], [pindolol][1], propranolol, [sotalol][1], and [timolol][1] are indicated in the management of angina, palpitations, and syncope associated with hypertrophic subaortic stenosis.

Myocardial infarction (treatment and prophylaxis)—[Acebutolol][1], atenolol[1], metoprolol, [nadolol][1], oxprenolol[1], propranolol, [sotalol][1], and timolol are indicated in clinically stable patients recovering from an initial definite or suspected acute myocardial infarction in order to reduce cardiovascular mortality and to decrease the risk of reinfarction.

Pheochromocytoma (treatment adjunct)—Propranolol is indicated in the management of symptoms of tachycardia due to excessive beta-receptor stimulation in pheochromocytoma. However, it should be used only after primary treatment with an alpha-adrenergic blocking agent (since use without concomitant alpha-blockade could lead to serious blood pressure elevation). [Acebutolol][1], [atenolol][1], [labetalol (with caution)][1], [metoprolol][1], [nadolol][1], oxprenolol[1], [sotalol][1], and [timolol][1] also may be used.

Headache, vascular (prophylaxis)—Propranolol and timolol are indicated for reducing frequency and severity of migraine headaches but are not recommended for treatment of acute attacks. [Atenolol][1], [metoprolol][1], and [nadolol][1] are also useful for prophylaxis of migraine. A beta-adrenergic blocking agent is the drug of choice for vascular headache prophylaxis.

Tremors (treatment)—Propranolol is indicated in the treatment of essential, familial, and senile tremors. Propranolol also has been used to reduce the agitation and tremors of alcohol withdrawal. [Acebutolol][1], [atenolol][1], [metoprolol][1], [nadolol][1], oxprenolol[1], [pindolol][1], [sotalol][1], and [timolol][1] also may be used to treat tremors. Propranolol is the drug of choice for treatment of essential tremor.

Anxiety (treatment adjunct)—[Propranolol][1] is used to control the physical manifestations of anxiety such as tachycardia and tremor. It is not particularly useful for chronic anxiety or panic attacks but is most useful for reducing anxiety and improving performance in specific stressful situations. [Acebutolol][1], [metoprolol][1], oxprenolol[1], [sotalol][1], and [timolol][1] also have been used for this purpose.

Thyrotoxicosis (treatment adjunct)—[Propranolol][1] has been effective in the short-term preoperative management of thyrotoxic crises (until thioamide therapy is effective) by reducing symptoms such as fever, tachycardia, and hyperkinesia. There is no effect on the hormone production of the thyroid. Abrupt withdrawal of beta-blocker treatment may provoke "thyroid storm." [Acebutolol][1], [atenolol][1], [metoprolol][1], [nadolol][1], oxprenolol[1], [sotalol][1], and [timolol][1] are also used for thyrotoxicosis.

Mitral valve prolapse syndrome (treatment)—[Acebutolol][1], [atenolol][1], [metoprolol][1], [nadolol][1], oxprenolol[1], [pindolol][1], [propranolol][1], [sotalol][1], and [timolol][1] are used in the treatment of mitral valve prolapse syndrome.

[Hypotension, controlled (induction and maintenance)][1]—Parenteral labetalol is used to produce controlled hypotension during surgery to reduce bleeding into the surgical field.

[Glaucoma, open-angle (treatment)][1]—Timolol is used to lower intraocular pressure in the treatment of open-angle glaucoma.

[Neuroleptic-induced akathisia (treatment)][1]—Propranolol may be used to relieve the somatic and subjective symptoms associated with neuroleptic-induced akathisia (NIA). Betaxolol, metoprolol, and nadolol have also been used for NIA.

---

[1]Not included in Canadian product labeling.

## Pharmacology/Pharmacokinetics

See *Table 1*, page 583.

### Physicochemical characteristics

Molecular weight—
Acebutolol: 336.43.
Atenolol: 266.34.
Betaxolol hydrochloride: 343.89.
Bisoprolol fumarate: 766.97.
Carteolol hydrochloride: 328.84.
Labetalol hydrochloride: 364.87.
Metoprolol succinate: 652.83.
Metoprolol tartrate: 684.82.
Nadolol: 309.40.
Oxprenolol hydrochloride: 301.81.
Penbutolol sulfate: 680.94.
Pindolol: 248.32.
Propranolol hydrochloride: 295.81.
Sotalol hydrochloride: 308.82.
Timolol maleate: 432.49.

pKa—
Acebutolol: 9.20.
Carteolol: 9.74.
Labetalol: 9.45.
Metoprolol: 9.68.
Nadolol: 9.67.
Penbutolol: 9.3.
Timolol: Approximately 9 in water at 25 °C.

Lipid solubility—
Acebutolol: Low
Atenolol: Very low (log partition coefficient for octanol/water=0.23)
Bisoprolol: Moderate (equally hydrophilic and lipophilic)
Carteolol: Low
Labetalol: Low
Metoprolol: Moderate
Nadolol: Low
Oxprenolol: Moderate
Penbutolol: Moderate
Pindolol: Moderate
Propranolol: High
Sotalol: Low
Timolol: Moderate

### Mechanism of action/Effect

Beta-adrenergic blocking agents block the agonistic effect of the sympathetic neurotransmitters by competing for receptor binding sites. When they predominantly block the beta-1 receptors in cardiac tissue, they are said to be cardioselective. When they block both beta-1 receptors and beta-2 receptors (primarily located in tissues other than cardiac), they are said to be nonselective. In general, so-called cardioselective beta-adrenergic blocking agents are relatively cardioselective—at lower doses they block beta-1 receptors only but begin to block beta-2 receptors as the dose increases.

Some beta-adrenergic blocking agents also have intrinsic sympathomimetic activity (ISA or partial agonist activity), which is the ability to cause weak stimulation of beta-adrenergic receptors while simultaneously blocking the effect of endogenous catecholamines; however, the significance of this property has not been established. Possession of ISA theoretically may result in fewer adverse effects related to unopposed beta blockade (e.g., bradycardia, heart block, bronchoconstriction, peripheral vascular constriction), but studies have not proven

clinical benefit. Pindolol exhibits the most ISA of the beta-adrenergic blocking agents currently available; carteolol, oxprenolol, and penbutolol have moderate ISA; acebutolol has mild to moderate ISA; and the other members of the group have little, if any, such activity.

Propranolol possesses moderate membrane-stabilizing (quinidine-like) activity; acebutolol, betaxolol, metoprolol, and oxprenolol have slight activity. The other beta-adrenergic blocking agents of this group show little, if any, such activity. At one time membrane-stabilizing activity was thought to be related to the antiarrhythmic effect, but it is no longer considered to be significant because it occurs only at very high (much greater than therapeutic) doses.

Antianginal—
Reduction in myocardial oxygen demand through negative chronotropic and inotropic effects.

Antiarrhythmic—
May involve beta-blockade–induced reduction in the rate of spontaneous firing of sinus and ectopic pacemakers and slowing of atrioventricular (AV) nodal conduction. In the Vaughan Williams classification of antiarrhythmics, beta-adrenergic blocking agents are considered to be class II agents.

Antihypertensive—
The precise mechanism of antihypertensive effect is not known. Possible mechanisms include reduced cardiac output, decreased sympathetic outflow to peripheral vasculature, and inhibition of renin release by the kidneys; with labetalol, may also be related to reduced peripheral vascular resistance as a result of alpha-adrenergic blockade.

Hypertrophic cardiomyopathy therapy adjunct—
Reduction of elevated outflow pressure gradient, which is exacerbated by beta-receptor stimulation.

Myocardial infarction therapy and prophylactic—
Possible reduction in severity of myocardial ischemia by decrease of myocardial oxygen requirements; postinfarction mortality may also be reduced through an antiarrhythmic action.

Vascular headache prophylactic—
Involves several mechanisms, including prevention of arterial dilation through beta-blockade, blockade of catecholamine-induced platelet aggregation and lipolysis, reduction of platelet adhesiveness, prevention of coagulation factor elevation during epinephrine release, promotion of oxygen release to tissues, and inhibition of renin secretion.

Antitremor agent—
Precise mechanism not known, but antitremor effect may be mediated predominantly by peripheral beta-2 receptor mechanisms.

Antianxiety therapy adjunct—
Precise mechanism unknown; however, thought to involve improvement of somatic symptoms secondary to beta-blockade.

Thyrotoxicosis therapy adjunct—
Unknown, but probably related to reduction of symptoms such as tremor, tachycardia, and elevated blood pressure caused by increased sensitivity to catecholamines.

### Other actions/effects

Labetalol also has selective alpha-1-adrenergic blocking effects, which lead to vasodilation, reduced peripheral vascular resistance, and postural hypotension.

## Precautions to Consider

Note: In general, because of the similarity of effect and because the cardioselectivity of beta-1 blockers is relative, the same precautions, especially drug interactions and medical problems, apply to all beta-adrenergic blocking agents.

### Carcinogenicity/Tumorigenicity

*Acebutolol*—Studies in rats and mice given up to 300 mg per kg of body weight (mg/kg) per day (equivalent to 15 times the maximum recommended human dose) found no evidence of carcinogenicity. Diacetolol, the major metabolite, also did not produce evidence of carcinogenicity in rats given up to 1800 mg/kg per day.

*Atenolol*—Two 18- to 24-month studies in rats and one study for up to 18 months in mice given up to 150 times the maximum recommended human antihypertensive dose found no evidence of carcinogenicity. However, a 24-month study in rats given up to 750 times the maximum recommended human antihypertensive dose revealed increased incidences of benign adrenal medullary tumors in males and females, mammary fibroadenomas in females, and anterior pituitary adenomas and thyroid parafollicular cell carcinomas in males.

*Betaxolol*—Studies in mice given up to 60 mg/kg per day orally (up to 90 times the maximum recommended human dose based on 60-kg body weight) and in rats given up to 48 mg/kg per day orally (up to 72 times the maximum recommended human dose) found no evidence of carcinogenicity.

*Bisoprolol*—Studies in mice and rats given 625 and 312 times, respectively, the maximum recommended human dose by weight found no evidence of carcinogenicity.

*Carteolol*—A 2-year study in rats and mice given 280 times the maximum recommended human dose (10 mg per 70 kg of body weight per day) found no evidence of carcinogenicity.

*Labetalol*—Studies for 18 months in mice and 2 years in rats found no evidence of carcinogenicity.

*Metoprolol*—A 1-year study in dogs given up to 105 mg/kg per day orally, a 2-year study in rats given up to 800 mg/kg per day orally, and a 21-month study in mice given up to 750 mg/kg per day orally found no evidence of carcinogenicity, although the incidence of small benign adenomas of the lung was higher in the treated female mice. A repeat of the 21-month study in mice found no increased incidence of any type of tumor.

*Nadolol*—A 2-year study in rats and mice found no evidence of carcinogenicity.

*Oxprenolol*—Long-term studies in mice and rats found no evidence of carcinogenicity.

*Penbutolol*—A 21-month study in mice and a 2-year study in rats at doses up to 500 times the maximum recommended human dose found no evidence of carcinogenicity.

*Pindolol*—Two-year studies in rats and mice found no evidence of carcinogenicity at doses as high as 50 and 100 times, respectively, the maximum recommended human dose.

*Propranolol*—Eighteen-month studies in rats and mice given up to 150 mg/kg per day found no evidence of carcinogenicity.

*Timolol*—A 2-year study found an increased incidence of adrenal pheochromocytomas in male rats given 300 times (but not 25 or 80 times) the maximum recommended human dose. Another study found an increased incidence of benign and malignant pulmonary tumors and benign uterine polyps in female mice given 500 (but not 5 or 50) mg/kg per day and an increase in mammary adenocarcinomas associated with elevations in serum prolactin at 500 mg/kg per day.

## Mutagenicity

*Acebutolol*—Ames mutagenicity studies with acebutolol and diacetolol were negative.

*Atenolol*—Mutagenicity studies were negative.

*Betaxolol*—Betaxolol was not found to be mutagenic in a variety of *in vitro* and *in vivo* bacterial and mammalian cell assays.

*Bisoprolol*—Bisoprolol was not found to be mutagenic in a variety of *in vitro* and *in vivo* assays.

*Carteolol*—Carteolol was not found to be mutagenic in the Ames test, recombinant (rec)-assay, *in vivo* cytogenetics tests, and dominant lethal assay.

*Labetalol*—Labetalol was not found to be mutagenic in dominant lethal assays in rats and mice or in modified Ames tests.

*Metoprolol*—Metoprolol was not found to be mutagenic in several tests, including a dominant lethal study in mice, chromosome studies in somatic cells, a *Salmonella*/mammalian-microsome mutagenicity test, and a nucleus anomaly test in somatic interphase nuclei.

*Penbutolol*—Penbutolol was not found to be mutagenic in the *Salmonella* mutagenicity test (Ames test), the point mutation induction test (*Saccharomyces*), or the micronucleus test.

*Timolol*—*In vivo* (mouse) and *in vitro* mutagenicity studies were negative; in Ames tests, some changes were seen, but not enough to make the test positive.

## Pregnancy/Reproduction

*Fertility*—*Acebutolol:* No adverse effect on fertility was observed in male or female rats given up to 240 mg/kg per day of acebutolol and 1000 mg/kg per day of diacetolol.

*Atenolol:* No adverse effect on fertility was observed in male or female rats given 100 times the maximum recommended human dose.

*Betaxolol:* No adverse effect on fertility or mating performance was observed in male or female rats given 380 times the maximum recommended human dose.

*Bisoprolol:* No adverse effect on fertility was observed in rats given 375 times the maximum recommended human dose by weight.

*Carteolol:* No adverse effect on fertility was observed in male or female rats and mice given 1052 times the maximum recommended human dose.

*Metoprolol:* No adverse effect on fertility was observed in rats given up to 55.5 times the maximum human daily dose of 450 mg.

*Nadolol:* No adverse effect on fertility was observed in rats given nadolol.

*Pindolol:* Mortality and decreased weight gain were observed in male rats given 100 mg/kg per day. Decreased mating was associated with atrophy and/or decreased spermatogenesis at 30 mg/kg per day. Mating behavior decreased and offspring mortality increased in females given 100 mg/kg per day and 30 mg/kg per day. In addition, there was an increase in prenatal mortality at a dose of 10 mg/kg per day, although there was not a clear dose-response relationship. In females necropsied

on the 15th day of gestation, an increased resorption rate was observed at a dose of 100 mg/kg per day.

*Propranolol:* No adverse effect on fertility was observed in animal studies.

*Timolol:* No adverse effect on fertility was observed in male or female rats at doses up to 125 times the maximum recommended human dose.

*Pregnancy*—Beta-adrenergic blocking agents cross the placenta. The safety of these agents in pregnancy is not fully established. Fetal and neonatal bradycardia, hypotension, hypoglycemia, and respiratory depression have been reported with administration of a cardioselective or a noncardioselective beta-adrenergic blocking agent to pregnant women. In addition, intrauterine growth retardation has been reported rarely with atenolol and nadolol. However, other reports seem to indicate successful treatment of maternal hypertension during pregnancy with no apparent effects on the fetus or neonate.

*Acebutolol*—

Acebutolol was not teratogenic in rats or rabbits given up to 31.5 and 6.8 times, respectively, the maximum recommended therapeutic dose in a 60-kg human. However, slight fetal growth retardation occurred in rabbits given 135 mg/kg per day. An elevation in postimplantation loss was seen in rabbit dams given 450 mg/kg per day of diacetolol.

FDA Pregnancy Category B.

*Atenolol*—

Dose-related increases in embryo/fetal resorptions were observed in rats given atenolol in doses greater than or equal to 25 times the maximum recommended human antihypertensive dose. This effect was not seen in rabbits given 12.5 times the maximum recommended human antihypertensive dose.

FDA Pregnancy Category D.

*Betaxolol*—

Administration of betaxolol to pregnant rats in doses up to 600 times the maximum recommended human dose was associated with increased postimplantation loss, reduced litter size and weight, and increased incidence of skeletal and visceral abnormalities, which may or may not have resulted from maternal drug toxicity. In another study, betaxolol, given at doses of up to 300 times the maximum recommended human dose, was associated with an increase in resorptions, but no teratogenicity. Administration of 380 times the maximum recommended human dose caused a marked increase in total litter loss within 4 days postpartum. A marked increase in postimplantation loss, but no teratogenicity, was observed in pregnant rabbits given up to 54 times the maximum recommended human dose.

FDA Pregnancy Category C.

*Bisoprolol*—

Bisoprolol was not teratogenic in rats or rabbits given 375 and 31 times, respectively, the maximum recommended human dose by weight. However, there was an increase in late resorptions in rats given bisoprolol at doses 125 times the maximum recommended human dose by weight.

FDA Pregnancy Category C.

*Carteolol*—

Increased resorptions and decreased fetal weights occurred in rabbits and rats given maternally toxic doses 1052 and 5264 times, respectively, the maximum recommended human dose. A dose-related increase in fetal wavy ribs was seen in pregnant rats given 212 times the maximum recommended human dose. However, this was not observed in mice given up to 1052 times the maximum recommended human dose.

FDA Pregnancy Category C.

*Labetalol*—

Teratogenic effects were not seen in rats and rabbits given 6 and 4 times, respectively, the maximum recommended human dose. Administration of labetalol to rats during late gestation through weaning at doses up to 2 to 4 times the maximum recommended human dose resulted in decreased neonatal survival.

FDA Pregnancy Category C.

*Metoprolol*—

Increased postimplantation loss and decreased neonatal survival were observed in rats given up to 55.5 times the maximum human daily dose of 450 mg. No evidence of teratogenicity was seen in animal studies.

FDA Pregnancy Category C.

*Nadolol*—

Evidence of embryotoxicity and fetotoxicity was found in rabbits given up to 10 times the maximum indicated human dose. However, these effects were not seen in rats or hamsters. Teratogenic effects were not seen in any of these species.

FDA Pregnancy Category C.

*Pindolol—*
> No evidence of embryotoxicity or teratogenicity was found in rats and rabbits given doses exceeding 100 times the maximum recommended human dose.
>
> FDA Pregnancy Category B.

*Propranolol—*
> Embryotoxicity occurred in animals given 10 times the maximum recommended human dose.
>
> FDA Pregnancy Category C.

*Timolol—*
> No evidence of fetal malformations was observed in mice and rabbits given up to 50 times the maximum recommended human dose. In rats, at similar doses, delayed fetal ossification was observed, but there were no adverse effects on postnatal development of offspring. Increased fetal resorptions were seen in mice and rabbits given 1000 and 100 times, respectively, the maximum recommended human dose.
>
> FDA Pregnancy Category C.

## Breast-feeding

Acebutolol (and diacetolol), atenolol, betaxolol, labetalol, metoprolol, nadolol, oxprenolol, pindolol, propranolol, sotalol, and timolol are distributed into breast milk. It is not known whether bisoprolol, carteolol, and penbutolol are distributed into breast milk. Cyanosis and bradycardia resulted from maternal therapy with atenolol in one breast-fed neonate; hypotension, bradycardia, and transient tachypnea resulted from maternal acebutolol therapy in another. Adverse neonatal effects resulting from maternal ingestion of other beta-adrenergic blocking agents have not been reported. Although the risk appears to be small, breast-fed infants should be monitored for signs of beta-adrenergic blockade, especially bradycardia, hypotension, respiratory distress, and hypoglycemia.

## Pediatrics

Use of beta-adrenergic blocking agents in a limited number of neonates, infants, and children has not demonstrated pediatrics-specific problems that would limit the usefulness of these medications in children.

## Geriatrics

Beta-adrenergic blocking agents have been used safely and efficaciously in elderly patients. However, elderly patients may be more susceptible to some adverse effects of these agents. Beta-adrenergic blocking agents have been reported to cause or exacerbate mental impairment in the elderly. However, other evidence suggests that these agents do not produce significant lethargy or impairment in mental performance. It is possible that the likelihood of central nervous system (CNS) effects may be related to lipophilicity of the beta-adrenergic blocking agent. However, this relationship has not been conclusively established.

Elderly patients are more likely to have age-related peripheral vascular disease, which may require caution in patients receiving beta-adrenergic blocking agents. In addition, the risk of beta-blocker–induced hypothermia may be increased in elderly patients.

## Surgical

Recent evidence suggests that withdrawal of antihypertensive therapy prior to surgery may be undesirable. However, the anesthesiologist must be aware of such therapy.

## Drug interactions and/or related problems

The following drug interactions and/or related problems have been selected on the basis of their potential clinical significance (possible mechanism in parentheses where appropriate)—not necessarily inclusive (» = major clinical significance):

Note: Combinations containing any of the following medications, depending on the amount present, may also interact with this medication.

     Information concerning interactions between beta-adrenergic blocking agents and other medications is still limited. Therefore, some of the following potential interactions are stated for cautionary reference until additional information is available.

» Allergen immunotherapy or
» Allergenic extracts for skin testing
     (use of these agents in patients taking beta-adrenergic blocking agents may increase the potential for serious systemic reaction or anaphylaxis; if possible, another medication should be substituted for a beta-adrenergic blocking agent in patients on allergen immunotherapy; allergen immunotherapy for conditions that are not life-threatening should be avoided in patients who cannot discontinue beta-adrenergic blocking agent therapy)

   Amiodarone
     (concurrent administration with beta-adrenergic blocking agents may result in additive depressant effects on conduction and neg-

ative inotropic effects, especially in patients with underlying sinus node dysfunction or atrioventricular node dysfunction)

   Anesthetics, hydrocarbon inhalation, such as:
     Chloroform
     Cyclopropane
     Enflurane
»   Halothane
     Isoflurane
     Methoxyflurane
     Trichloroethylene
     (concurrent use with beta-adrenergic blocking agents may increase the risk of myocardial depression and hypotension because beta-blockade reduces the ability of the heart to respond to beta-adrenergically mediated sympathetic reflex stimuli; if necessary to reverse the effects of beta-adrenergic blocking agents during surgery, agonists such as dobutamine, dopamine, isoproterenol, or norepinephrine may be used but should be administered with caution. In patients scheduled for major surgery, most practitioners believe the risk of precipitating myocardial infarction following abrupt cessation of beta-adrenergic blocking agent therapy prior to surgery outweighs the risks of continuing therapy while compensating for medication effects by anesthetic techniques)

     (high concentrations of halothane [3% or above] or high concentrations of other halogenated hydrocarbon anesthetics should not be used when labetalol is used to produce controlled hypotension during anesthesia because of the risk of excessive hypotension, large reduction in cardiac output, and increase in central venous pressure)

» Antidiabetic agents, oral or
» Insulin
     (concurrent use with beta-adrenergic blocking agents may impair glycemic control; there may be an increased risk of hyperglycemia secondary to a slight deterioration in carbohydrate metabolism and peripheral insulin resistance; beta-adrenergic blocking agents may impair recovery from hypoglycemia in diabetics because they block the effects of catecholamines, which promote glycogenolysis and mobilize glucose in response to hypoglycemia; beta-adrenergic blocking agents also may mask certain symptoms of developing hypoglycemia such as increases in pulse rate and blood pressure, thus complicating patient monitoring; labetalol and selective or relatively selective beta-adrenergic blocking agents, such as acebutolol, atenolol, betaxolol, bisoprolol, or metoprolol, may cause fewer problems with blood glucose levels, especially at lower dosages, although they may still mask the symptoms of hypoglycemia)

   Anti-inflammatory drugs, nonsteroidal (NSAIDs), especially indomethacin
     (NSAIDs may reduce the antihypertensive effects of beta-adrenergic blocking agents, possibly by inhibiting renal prostaglandin synthesis and/or causing sodium and fluid retention)

   Beta-adrenergic blocking agents, ophthalmic
     (if significant systemic absorption of the ophthalmic beta-adrenergic blocking agent occurs, concurrent use may result in an additive effect either on intraocular pressure or on systemic effects of beta-blockade)

» Calcium channel blocking agents or
» Clonidine or
     Diazoxide or
» Guanabenz or
     Reserpine or
     Hypotension-producing medications, other, (See *Appendix II*) with the exception of monoamine oxidase (MAO) inhibitors
     (blood pressure control may be impaired when clonidine or guanabenz is used concurrently with a beta-adrenergic blocking agent; potentiation of antihypertensive effect should be anticipated when other hypotension-producing medications are used concurrently; although combinations of antihypertensive agents and/or diuretics are often used for therapeutic advantage, dosage adjustment may be needed when any hypotension-producing medication is added to or withdrawn from a regimen including a beta-adrenergic blocking agent)

     (symptomatic bradycardia, with or without serious hemodynamic effects, has been reported during concurrent use of diltiazem or verapamil with systemic beta-adrenergic blocking agents; although these effects may occur in the absence of overt pre-existing sinoatrial disease, older patients and patients with left ventricular dysfunction or sinoatrial or atrioventricular conduction abnormalities may be at increased risk; concurrent use of nifedipine with beta-adrenergic blocking agents, although usually well tolerated, may produce excessive hypotension and in rare cases may increase the possibility of congestive heart failure)

(calcium channel blocking agents may decrease the hepatic metabolism of propranolol, metoprolol, and possibly other beta-adrenergic blocking agents with substantial hepatic biotransformation; although the clinical significance of this effect appears to be minimal, caution is warranted given the potential for additive cardiodepressant effects during concurrent use)

(concurrent use of diazoxide with beta-adrenergic blocking agents prevents the tachycardia produced by diazoxide but may also increase the hypotensive effects)

(concurrent use of reserpine with beta-adrenergic blocking agents may result in additive and possibly excessive beta-adrenergic blockade; close observation is recommended since bradycardia and hypotension may occur)

Cimetidine
(cimetidine may reduce the clearance of hepatically metabolized beta-adrenergic blocking agents, resulting in elevations of plasma concentrations)

» Cocaine
(cocaine may inhibit the therapeutic effects of beta-adrenergic blocking agents)

(although beta-adrenergic blocking agents are recommended to reduce tachycardia, myocardial ischemia, and/or arrhythmias induced by cocaine, concurrent use of a beta-adrenergic blocking agent with cocaine may increase the risk of hypertension, excessive bradycardia, and possibly heart block, because beta-adrenergic blockade may leave cocaine's alpha-adrenergic activity unopposed; the risk of these adverse effects may be decreased with labetalol because labetalol also has some alpha-adrenergic blocking activity, although its beta-adrenergic blocking activity predominates)

Contrast media, iodinated
(concurrent use of beta-adrenergic blocking agents with intravenous contrast media may increase the risk of moderate to severe anaphylaxis; an anaphylactic event may be refractory to treatment)

Estrogens
(concurrent use may decrease the antihypertensive effect of beta-adrenergic blocking agents because estrogen-induced fluid retention may lead to increased blood pressure)

Fentanyl and derivatives
(preoperative chronic use of systemic beta-adrenergic blocking agents may decrease the frequency and/or severity of hypertensive responses to surgery, especially during sternotomy and sternal spread in cardiac or coronary artery surgery; however, chronic preoperative use of systemic beta-adrenergic blocking agents may also increase the risk of initial bradycardia following induction doses of fentanyl or any of its derivatives)

Flecainide
(although there have been no reports of adverse effects during concurrent administration of flecainide with the beta-adrenergic blocking agents, caution is recommended because of the potential for additive negative inotropic effects, especially in patients with compromised left ventricular function [ejection fraction < 30%])

Lidocaine
(concurrent use with beta-adrenergic blocking agents may reduce lidocaine elimination and increase the risk of lidocaine toxicity because of reduced hepatic blood flow; lidocaine dosage should be adjusted on the basis of serum lidocaine concentrations)

Monoamine oxidase (MAO) inhibitors, including furazolidone, procarbazine, and selegiline
(significant hypertension theoretically may occur up to 14 days following discontinuation of the MAO inhibitor; although sufficient clinical reports are lacking, concurrent use with beta-adrenergic blocking agents is not recommended)

Neuromuscular blocking agents, nondepolarizing
(beta-adrenergic blocking agents may potentiate and prolong the action of nondepolarizing neuromuscular blocking agents when used concurrently; careful postoperative monitoring of the patient may be necessary following concurrent or sequential use, especially if there is a possibility of incomplete reversal of neuromuscular blockade)

Nicotine chewing gum or
Smoking deterrents, other or
Smoking, tobacco, cessation of
(smoking cessation may increase therapeutic effects of propranolol by decreasing metabolism, thereby increasing serum concentrations; dosage adjustments may be necessary)

Nitroglycerin
(labetalol reduces the reflex tachycardia caused by nitroglycerin and may increase the antihypertensive effect)

Phenothiazines
(concurrent use with beta-adrenergic blocking agents results in an increased plasma concentration of each medication)

Phenytoin
(concurrent use of propranolol, and probably other beta-adrenergic blocking agents, with intravenous phenytoin may produce additive cardiac depressant effects)

Phenoxybenzamine or
Phentolamine
(concurrent use with labetalol may result in additive alpha-adrenergic blocking effects)

Propafenone
(concurrent use with metoprolol or propranolol may result in significant increases in plasma concentrations and half-life of propranolol and metoprolol, without affecting plasma propafenone concentrations; dosage reduction of the beta-adrenergic blocking agent may be necessary)

» Sympathomimetics
(concurrent use of beta-adrenergic blocking agents with sympathomimetic amines having beta-adrenergic stimulant activity may result in mutual inhibition of therapeutic effects; for sympathomimetic agents with beta-adrenergic effects, beta-blockade may antagonize beta-1-adrenergic cardiac effects [dobutamine, dopamine] or the beta-2-adrenergic bronchodilating effect [albuterol, ethylnorepinephrine, isoetharine, isoproterenol, metaproterenol, terbutaline] or both [isoproterenol]; use of a cardioselective beta-1-adrenergic blocker [atenolol, betaxolol, or metoprolol] or labetalol [because of its alpha-blocking activity] at low doses may prevent antagonism of the bronchodilating effect)

(sympathomimetic agents with both alpha- and beta-adrenergic effects [amphetamines, ephedrine, epinephrine, metaraminol, norepinephrine, phenylephrine, pseudoephedrine], beta-blockade may result in unopposed alpha-adrenergic activity with a risk of hypertension and excessive bradycardia and possible heart block; risk should be less with labetalol because of its alpha-blocking activity; beta-blockade also antagonizes the bronchodilating effect of ephedrine and epinephrine)

» Xanthines, especially aminophylline or theophylline
(concurrent use with beta-adrenergic blocking agents may result in mutual inhibition of therapeutic effects; in addition, concurrent use with the xanthines [except dyphylline] may decrease xanthine clearance, especially in patients with increased theophylline clearance induced by smoking; concurrent use requires careful monitoring)

**Laboratory value alterations**
The following have been selected on the basis of their potential clinical significance (possible effect in parentheses where appropriate)—not necessarily inclusive (» = major clinical significance):
With diagnostic test results
Amphetamine determinations, urinary
(labetalol may produce false-positive results when commercially available assay methods [thin-layer chromatographic assay or radioenzymatic assay] are used; during labetalol therapy, positive results should be confirmed with more specific methods, such as a gas chromatographic-mass spectrometer technique)

Catecholamine determinations
(urinary concentrations of catecholamines and/or their metabolites [metanephrine, normetanephrine, vanillylmandelic acid] may be falsely increased by labetalol when measured by fluorimetric or photometric methods; a specific method, such as high performance liquid chromatography assay with solid phase extraction, should be used instead)

Glaucoma screening test
(may be interfered with by systemic beta-blockade, which reduces intraocular pressure)

Radionuclide ventriculography
(beta-adrenergic blocking agents may blunt the exercise-induced changes in cardiac function in the evaluation of coronary artery disease by decreasing heart rate)

With physiology/laboratory test values
Alkaline phosphatase, serum and
Lactate dehydrogenase (LDH), serum and
Transaminases, serum
(may be increased by acebutolol, labetalol, or metoprolol; it is recommended that labetalol be withdrawn if jaundice or laboratory signs of hepatic function impairment occur)

Antinuclear antibody (ANA) titers
(may be increased by beta-adrenergic blocking agents; dose-related)

Blood glucose concentrations

(nonselective beta-adrenergic blocking agents impair glycogenolysis and the hyperglycemic response to endogenous epinephrine, leading to persistence of hypoglycemia and delayed recovery of blood glucose to normal levels, especially in diabetics; studies have shown no such effect in resting nondiabetics with therapeutic doses; beta-adrenergic blocking agents, especially nonselective agents, decrease the release of insulin in response to hyperglycemia; effects on blood glucose may be less likely with labetalol or cardioselective agents such as acebutolol, betaxolol, atenolol, and metoprolol, especially at lower doses)

Blood urea nitrogen (BUN) (usually in patients with severe heart disease) and

Potassium concentrations, serum and

Uric acid concentrations, serum

(may be increased)

Lipoproteins, serum and

Triglycerides, serum

(concentrations may be increased)

## Medical considerations/Contraindications

The medical considerations/contraindications included here have been selected on the basis of their potential clinical significance (reasons given in parentheses where appropriate)—not necessarily inclusive (» = major clinical significance).

Note: In general, because of the similarity of effect and because the cardioselectivity of beta-1 blockers is relative, the same precautions apply to all beta-adrenergic blocking agents.

*Except under special circumstances, this medication should not be used when the following medical problems exist:*

*For all indications*
» Cardiac failure, overt or
» Cardiogenic shock or
» Heart block, 2nd- or 3rd-degree atrioventricular (AV) block or
» Sinus bradycardia (heart rate less than 45 beats per minute)
(risk of further myocardial depression; risk may be less with carteolol, labetalol, oxprenolol, penbutolol, and pindolol; beta-adrenergic blocking agents may be used with extreme caution in some patients with cardiac failure [e.g., high output failure associated with thyrotoxicosis])

*For use in myocardial infarction*
» Hypotension
(patients dependent on sympathetic stimulation to maintain adequate cardiac output and blood pressure, such as patients with hypotension in the setting of myocardial infarction, may not benefit from beta-adrenergic blockade; studies of beta-adrenergic blockade in the treatment of myocardial infarction excluded patients with systolic pressures less than 100 mm Hg)

*Risk-benefit should be considered when the following medical problems exist:*

*For all beta-adrenergic blocking agents*
» Allergy, history of or
» Asthma, bronchial or
» Emphysema or nonallergenic bronchitis
(beta-adrenergic blocking agents may promote bronchospasm and block the bronchodilating effect of epinephrine; cardioselective agents such as acebutolol, atenolol, betaxolol, bisoprolol, and metoprolol, or agents with ISA such as carteolol, oxprenolol, penbutolol, or pindolol are theoretically less likely to cause such effects when used at lower doses; labetalol may also pose less risk of bronchoconstriction; however, caution is necessary with all beta-adrenergic blocking agents)

(severity and duration of anaphylactic reactions to allergens and allergen immunotherapy may be increased in some patients being treated with beta-adrenergic blocking agents; if possible, another medication should be substituted for a beta-adrenergic blocking agent in patients receiving allergen immunotherapy, or, for conditions that are not life-threatening, allergen immunotherapy should be avoided in patients who cannot discontinue beta-adrenergic blocking agent therapy; caution is also recommended during skin testing in patients on beta-adrenergic blocking agents)

» Congestive heart failure
(risk of further depression of myocardial contractility; labetalol and agents with ISA such as carteolol, oxprenolol, penbutolol, pindolol, and possibly acebutolol may theoretically be associated with less risk and may be used with caution in patients who are well-compensated)

» Diabetes mellitus
(beta-adrenergic blocking agents may mask tachycardia associated with hypoglycemia, but not dizziness and sweating; beta-adrenergic blocking agents may adversely affect recovery from hypoglycemia and impair peripheral circulation; these effects may theoretically be more likely with the noncardioselective agents and less likely with labetalol and cardioselective agents)

Hepatic function impairment
(metabolism of beta-adrenergic blocking agents that undergo hepatic metabolism may be decreased; patients with impaired hepatic function may require lower doses of beta-adrenergic blocking agents [exceptions are atenolol, betaxolol, carteolol, metoprolol (except in severe impairment), and nadolol, which require no dosage adjustment]; such reduction in dosage frequently applies to geriatric patients, many of whom have reduced hepatic function)

» Hyperthyroidism
(beta-adrenergic blocking agents may mask tachycardic symptoms; abrupt withdrawal may intensify symptoms)

» Mental depression, or history of
(although the association between beta-adrenergic blocking agents and depression is not fully established, these medications should be used cautiously in these patients)

Myasthenia gravis
(beta-adrenergic blocking agents may potentiate a myasthenic condition, including muscle weakness and double vision)

Pheochromocytoma
(although labetalol is used to lower blood pressure, higher-than-usual doses may be required; paradoxical hypertensive responses to labetalol have been reported in a few patients; with other beta-adrenergic blocking agents, there is a risk of hypertension if effective alpha-adrenergic blockade is not achieved first)

Psoriasis
(may be exacerbated)

Renal function impairment
(may impair beta-adrenergic blocking agent clearance; risk of reduced renal blood flow; patients with impaired renal function may require reduced doses of beta-adrenergic blocking agents [exceptions are labetalol, metoprolol, oxprenolol, penbutolol, pindolol (unless impairment is severe), propranolol, and timolol, which require no dosage adjustment]; such reduction in dosage frequently applies to geriatric patients, many of whom have reduced renal function; specific dosage recommendations, where available, are included in the *Dosage Forms* section for the particular agent)

Sensitivity to the beta-blocker prescribed

*For all beta-adrenergic blocking agents except labetalol*
Raynaud's syndrome and other peripheral vascular diseases
(beta-adrenergic blocking agents may reduce peripheral circulation and worsen these conditions; cardioselective agents such as acebutolol, atenolol, betaxolol, bisoprolol, metoprolol, or agents with ISA such as acebutolol, carteolol, oxprenolol, penbutolol, or pindolol are theoretically less likely to produce adverse effect)

## Patient monitoring

The following may be especially important in patient monitoring (other tests may be warranted in some patients, depending on condition; » = major clinical significance):

Blood cell counts and
Blood glucose concentrations (for diabetic patients) and
» Cardiac function monitoring and
Hepatic function determinations and
» Pulse rate determinations and
Renal function determinations
(may be required at periodic intervals)

» Blood pressure and
» Electrocardiogram (ECG) and
» Heart rate
(should be carefully monitored during intravenous administration)

» Blood pressure determinations
(recommended at periodic intervals to monitor efficacy and safety of therapy in patients being treated for hypertension; selected patients may be trained to perform blood pressure measurements at home and report the results at regular physician visits)

## Side/Adverse Effects

The following side/adverse effects have been selected on the basis of their potential clinical significance (possible signs and symptoms in parentheses where appropriate)—not necessarily inclusive:

**Those indicating need for medical attention**
Incidence less frequent
*Bradycardia, symptomatic* (dizziness); *bronchospasm* (difficulty breathing and/or wheezing); *congestive heart failure* (swelling of ankles, feet, and/or lower legs; shortness of breath); *mental depression; reduced peripheral circulation* (cold hands and feet)—except labetalol

Note: Risk of *bronchospasm or reduced peripheral circulation* is theoretically reduced with acebutolol, atenolol, betaxolol, bisoprolol, carteolol, metoprolol, oxprenolol, penbutolol, or pindolol.

*Mental depression* is usually reversible and mild, but may progress to catatonia.

Incidence rare
*Allergic reaction* (skin rash); *arrhythmias* (irregular heartbeat); *back pain or joint pain; chest pain; confusion*—especially in the elderly; *hallucinations; hepatotoxicity* (dark urine, yellow eyes or skin)—for acebutolol, bisoprolol, or labetalol; *leukopenia* (fever, sore throat); *orthostatic hypotension* (dizziness or lightheadedness when getting up from a lying or sitting position); *psoriasiform eruption* (red, scaling, or crusted skin); *thrombocytopenia* (unusual bleeding and bruising);

Note: *Hepatotoxicity* is usually reversible; however, hepatic necrosis and death have been reported with labetalol.

**Those indicating need for medical attention only if they continue or are bothersome**
Incidence more frequent
*Decreased sexual ability; drowsiness*—especially with higher doses; *trouble in sleeping; unusual tiredness or weakness*

Incidence less frequent
*Anxiety and/or nervousness; constipation; diarrhea; nasal congestion* (stuffy nose); *nausea or vomiting; stomach discomfort*

Incidence rare
*Changes in taste; dry, sore eyes; frequent urination*—for acebutolol or carteolol; *itching of skin; nightmares and vivid dreams; numbness and/or tingling of fingers, toes, or skin, especially the scalp*—for labetalol

**Those indicating the need for medical attention if they occur after medication is discontinued**
*Arrhythmias* (fast or irregular heartbeat); *chest pain; general feeling of discomfort, illness, or weakness; headache; shortness of breath, sudden; sweating; trembling*

## Overdose

For more information on the management of overdose or unintentional ingestion, **contact a Poison Control Center** (see *Poison Control Center Listing*).

**Clinical effects of overdose**
The following effects have been selected on the basis of their potential clinical significance (possible signs and symptoms in parentheses where appropriate)—not necessarily inclusive:

*Bradycardia; dizziness, severe, or fainting; hypotension; irregular heartbeat; difficulty breathing; bluish-colored fingernails or palms of hands; or seizures*

**Treatment of overdose**
Decreased absorption—Gastric lavage and administration of activated charcoal.
Specific treatment—
*Atropine:* May be administered for severe bradycardia in the presence of hypotension.
*Diazepam or lorazepam*: May be used intravenously to treat associated seizures.
*Dobutamine, dopamine, epinephrine, norepinephrine, or isoproterenol:* May be administered for chronotropic and inotropic support and treatment of severe hypotension. However, the effects of sympathomimetic agents may be inhibited by the presence of significant beta-blockade. Therefore, hypotension and ensuing pump failure may be refractory to treatment with catecholamines.
*Glucagon:* Glucagon has been used effectively in the treatment of bradycardia and hypotension in beta-adrenergic blocking agent overdose. Glucagon demonstrates major inotropic and less dramatic chronotropic effects. These effects appear to be independent of the beta-adrenergic receptor. Therefore, glucagon may be an advantageous alternative treatment to reverse the hemodynamic depression of beta-adrenergic blocking agent overdose.
*Transvenous pacing:* May be necessary for heart block.
*Other therapy:* May include furosemide or digitalis glycoside for pulmonary edema or cardiac failure; or a beta-2 agonist such as isoproterenol and/or a theophylline derivative for bronchospasm.

There is limited evidence that calcium chloride may be effective in improving myocardial contractility and hemodynamic status. It is speculated that hypocalcemia resulting from beta-adrenergic blocking agent overdose may contribute to a decline in myocardial contractility.

## Patient Consultation

As an aid to patient consultation, refer to *Advice for the Patient, Beta-adrenergic Blocking Agents (Systemic)*.

In providing consultation, consider emphasizing the following selected information (» = major clinical significance):

**Before using this medication**
» Conditions affecting use, especially:
   Sensitivity to the beta-blocker prescribed
   Pregnancy—Beta-adrenergic blocking agents cross the placenta; risk of hypoglycemia, respiratory depression, bradycardia, and hypotension in the fetus and neonate
   Breast-feeding—Beta-adrenergic blocking agents pass into breast milk; bradycardia, cyanosis, hypotension, and tachypnea have been reported in breast-fed infants whose mothers ingested atenolol or acebutolol
   Use in the elderly—Older patients may be more susceptible to some side/adverse effects; increased risk of beta-blocker–induced hypothermia
   Other medications, especially allergen immunotherapy and allergenic extracts used for skin testing, oral antidiabetic agents, insulin, calcium channel blocking agents, clonidine, guanabenz, cocaine, MAO inhibitors, sympathomimetics, or xanthines
   Other medical problems, especially overt cardiac failure, cardiogenic shock, 2nd or 3rd degree AV block, sinus bradycardia, hypotension (when used in myocardial infarction), history of allergy, bronchial asthma, emphysema or nonallergenic bronchitis, congestive heart failure, diabetes mellitus, hyperthyroidism, or mental depression

**Proper use of this medication**
   Proper administration of extended-release dosage forms: Swallowing whole without crushing, breaking (except with metoprolol succinate), or chewing
   Proper use of concentrated oral propranolol solution:
   Measuring with calibrated dropper
   Mixing with liquid or semi-solid food such as water, juices, soda or soda-like beverages, applesauce, and puddings; making sure entire dose is taken
   Not storing after mixing
   Checking pulse as directed (checking with physician if less than 50 beats per minute)
   Getting into habit of taking at same time each day to help increase compliance
» Importance of not missing doses, especially with schedules of one dose per day
» Proper dosing
   Missed dose: Taking as soon as possible; not taking at all if within 4 hours of next scheduled dose (8 hours for atenolol, betaxolol, carteolol, labetalol, nadolol, penbutolol, sotalol, or extended-release oxprenolol or propranolol); not doubling doses
» Proper storage
*For use as an antihypertensive*
   Possible need for control of weight and diet, especially sodium intake
» Compliance with therapy; patient may not experience symptoms of hypertension; importance of taking medication only as directed and keeping appointments with physician, even if feeling well
» Does not cure, but helps control hypertension; possible need for lifelong therapy; checking with physician before discontinuing medication; serious consequences of untreated hypertension

**Precautions while using this medication**
   Regular visits to physician to check progress
» Checking with physician before discontinuing medication; gradual dosage reduction may be necessary
   Having enough medication on hand to get through weekends, holidays, and vacations; possibly carrying second written prescription for emergency use
   Carrying medical identification card during therapy

» Caution if any kind of surgery (including dental surgery) or emergency treatment is required

» Diabetics: May mask signs and symptoms of hypoglycemia or may cause increased blood glucose concentrations or prolong hypoglycemia

» Caution when driving or doing things requiring alertness, because of possible drowsiness, dizziness, or lightheadedness

Caution during exposure to cold weather because of possible increased sensitivity to cold

» Caution against overexertion in response to decreased chest pain

Caution if any laboratory tests required; possible interference with test results

Patients with allergies to foods, medications, or stinging insect venom: Possible increase in severity of allergic reactions; checking with physician immediately if severe allergic reaction occurs

*For use as an antihypertensive*

» Not taking other medications, especially nonprescription sympathomimetics, unless discussed with physician

*For oral labetalol only*

» Caution when getting up suddenly from a lying or sitting position, especially during initiation of therapy or when dosage is increased

» Caution in using alcohol, while standing for long periods or exercising, and during hot weather because of enhanced orthostatic hypotensive effects

*For parenteral labetalol only*

» Lying down during injection and for up to 3 hours after getting injection, then getting up gradually

**Side/adverse effects**

Signs of potential side effects, especially bradycardia, breathing difficulty and/or wheezing, congestive heart failure, mental depression, reduced peripheral circulation, allergic reaction, arrhythmias, back pain or joint pain, chest pain, confusion, hallucinations, hepatotoxicity, leukopenia, psoriasiform eruption, thrombocytopenia, and withdrawal reaction

For labetalol: Transient scalp tingling may occur, usually at beginning of treatment

# General Dosing Information

Although plasma concentrations of beta-adrenergic blocking agents can be ascertained, there is not always a predictable relationship between plasma concentration and pharmacological effects. Pharmacological effects have been observed when plasma concentrations were not discernible. Therefore, titration of dosage with measurement of heart rate and blood pressure is used to guide therapy.

In some patients, once-daily dosing is effective.

When beta-adrenergic blocking agent therapy is discontinued in patients concurrently receiving clonidine or guanabenz, the beta-adrenergic blocking agent should be gradually discontinued several days before the clonidine or guanabenz is gradually discontinued in order to avoid clonidine- or guanabenz-withdrawal hypertensive crisis.

**For oral dosage forms only**

When a beta-adrenergic blocking agent must be withdrawn from established therapy *(especially in patients with ischemic heart disease)*, it is recommended that the dosage be reduced gradually to minimize risk of exacerbation of angina or development of myocardial infarction. Dosage reduction should occur over a period of approximately 2 weeks. During this time the patient should avoid vigorous physical activity in order to minimize the danger of infarction or arrhythmias. If signs of withdrawal (e.g., angina) occur, beta-adrenergic blocking agent therapy should be reinstated temporarily and then carefully withdrawn after the patient has stabilized.

It is recommended that beta-adrenergic blocking agent therapy be withdrawn if drug-induced mental depression occurs.

**Diet/Nutrition**

Oral beta-adrenergic blocking agents may be taken either with food or on an empty stomach. Studies indicate that bioavailability of labetalol, propranolol, and possibly metoprolol may be enhanced by administration with food, which may slow the hepatic metabolism of the medication. Bioavailability of acebutolol, atenolol, nadolol, oxprenolol, penbutolol, and pindolol are not affected by food intake. Concurrent food intake may slow carteolol absorption, but does not affect bioavailability. Sotalol does not undergo significant first-pass metabolism. Food, especially milk and milk products, may reduce the bioavailability of sotalol.

---

## ACEBUTOLOL

# Summary of Differences

Pharmacology/pharmacokinetics:

Mechanism of action/Effect—Mild to moderate intrinsic sympathomimetic activity (ISA); relatively cardioselective; low lipid solubility.

Absorption—Bioavailability significantly reduced by first-pass metabolism but effect not reduced because of active metabolite.

Protein binding—Low.

Elimination—Removable by hemodialysis.

Precautions:

Medical considerations/contraindications—Dosage reduction necessary in hepatic function and renal function impairment.

Side/adverse effects:

Theoretical reduced risk of bronchospasm, hypoglycemia, and peripheral vasoconstriction because of cardioselectivity.

# Oral Dosage Forms

## ACEBUTOLOL HYDROCHLORIDE CAPSULES

**Usual adult dose**

Antiarrhythmic—

Oral, 200 mg two times a day, the dosage being adjusted according to response, generally in the range of 600 to 1200 mg per day.

Antihypertensive—

Oral, initially 400 mg per day as a single dose or in two divided daily doses, the dosage being adjusted according to response, with maintenance doses usually in the range of 400 to 800 mg per day.

Note: Geriatric patients may have increased or decreased sensitivity to the effects of the usual adult dose.

It is recommended that the dosage of acebutolol be reduced in patients with renal function impairment as follows:

| Creatinine clearance (mL/min/1.73m) | % of normal dose to be given |
|---|---|
| <50 | 50 |
| <25 | 25 |

**Usual geriatric prescribing limits**

In geriatric patients, daily doses should not exceed a total of 800 mg.

**Usual pediatric dose**

Dosage has not been established.

**Strength(s) usually available**

U.S.—

200 mg (Rx) [*Sectral*].

400 mg (Rx) [*Sectral*].

Canada—

Not commercially available.

**Packaging and storage**

Store below 40 °C (104 °F), preferably between 15 and 30 °C (59 and 86 °F), in a well-closed container, unless otherwise specified by manufacturer.

**Auxiliary labeling**

• Do not take other medicine without your doctor's advice.

**Note**

Check refill frequency to determine compliance in hypertensive patients.

## ACEBUTOLOL HYDROCHLORIDE TABLETS

**Usual adult dose**

Antianginal—

Oral, initially 200 mg two times a day, the dosage being adjusted according to response, generally in the range of 600 to 1200 mg per day.

Antihypertensive—

Oral, initially 100 mg two times a day, the dosage being adjusted weekly according to response, up to a maximum of 400 mg two times a day.

Antiarrhythmic[1]—

Oral, 200 mg two times a day, the dosage being adjusted according to response.

**Usual pediatric dose**

Dosage has not been established.

**Strength(s) usually available**

U.S.—

Not commercially available.

Canada—

100 mg (Rx) [*Monitan; Sectral* (scored)].

200 mg (Rx) [*Monitan* (scored); *Sectral* (scored)].
400 mg (Rx) [*Monitan* (scored); *Sectral* (scored)].

**Packaging and storage**
Store below 40 °C (104 °F), preferably between 15 and 30 °C (59 and 86 °F), in a well-closed container, unless otherwise specified by manufacturer.

**Auxiliary labeling**
• Do not take other medicines without your doctor's advice.

**Note**
Check refill frequency to determine compliance in hypertensive patients.

---

[1]Not included in Canadian product labeling.

---

### *ATENOLOL*

## Summary of Differences

Pharmacology/pharmacokinetics:
  Mechanism of action/Effect—Relatively cardioselective (beta-1); very low lipid solubility.
  Biotransformation—Minimal hepatic metabolism.
  Protein binding—Very low to low.
  Elimination—Removable by hemodialysis.
Precautions:
  Medical considerations/contraindications—Dosage reduction necessary in renal function impairment but not necessary in hepatic function impairment.
Side/adverse effects:
  Theoretical reduced risk of bronchospasm, hypoglycemia, and peripheral vasoconstriction when daily dosage is in the lower range, because of cardioselectivity.

## Oral Dosage Forms
### ATENOLOL TABLETS

**Usual adult dose**
Antianginal—
  Oral, initially 50 mg once a day, the dosage being increased gradually to 100 mg a day after one week if necessary and tolerated. Some patients may require up to 200 mg a day.
Antihypertensive—
  Oral, initially 25 to 50 mg once a day, the dosage being increased to 50 to 100 mg a day after two weeks if necessary and tolerated.
Myocardial infarction—
  In patients who tolerate the full intravenous dose: Oral, initially 50 mg ten minutes after the last intravenous dose, followed by another 50 mg twelve hours later. A dose of 100 mg once a day or 50 mg two times a day may then be given for six to nine days or until discharge from the hospital.
Note: Geriatric patients may have increased or decreased sensitivity to the effects of the usual adult dose.

  For patients with severe renal function impairment, the following maximum doses are recommended:

| Creatinine clearance (mL/min/1.73m) | Maximum dose |
|---|---|
| 15–35 | 50 mg per day |
| <15 | 50 mg every second day |

**Usual pediatric dose**
Dosage has not been established.

**Strength(s) usually available**
U.S.—
  25 mg (Rx) [*Tenormin*].
  50 mg (Rx) [*Tenormin* (scored); GENERIC].
  100 mg (Rx) [*Tenormin;* GENERIC].
Canada—
  50 mg (Rx) [*Apo-Atenolol; Novo-Atenol; Tenormin* (scored)].
  100 mg (Rx) [*Apo-Atenolol; Novo-Atenol; Tenormin* (scored)].

**Packaging and storage**
Store below 40 °C (104 °F), preferably between 15 and 30 °C (59 and 86 °F), in a well-closed container, unless otherwise specified by manufacturer. Protect from light.

**Auxiliary labeling**
• Do not take other medicine without your doctor's advice.

**Note**
Check refill frequency to determine compliance in hypertensive patients.

## Parenteral Dosage Forms
### ATENOLOL INJECTION

**Usual adult dose**
Myocardial infarction—
  Early treatment: Intravenous, 5 mg (over five minutes), the dose being repeated ten minutes later.
Note: Geriatric patients may have increased or decreased sensitivity to the effects of the usual adult dose.

  In patients who tolerate the full intravenous dose (10 mg), oral atenolol treatment should be initiated ten minutes after the last intravenous dose.

  For patients with severe renal function impairment, the following maximum doses are recommended:

| Creatinine clearance (mL/min/1.73m) | Maximum dose |
|---|---|
| 15–35 | 50 mg per day |
| <15 | 50 mg every second day |

**Usual pediatric dose**
Dosage has not been established.

**Strength(s) usually available**
U.S.—
  500 mcg (0.5 mg) per mL (Rx) [*Tenormin*].
Canada—
  Not commercially available.

**Packaging and storage**
Store between 2 and 30 °C (36 and 86 °F), unless otherwise specified by manufacturer. Protect from light. Protect from freezing.

---

### *BETAXOLOL*

## Summary of Differences

Pharmacology/pharmacokinetics:
  Mechanism of action/Effect—Relatively cardioselective; moderate lipid solubility.
  Protein binding—Moderate.
  Elimination—Not removable by hemodialysis.
Precautions:
  Medical considerations/contraindications—Dosage reduction may be recommended in renal function impairment; dosage reduction not necessary in hepatic function impairment.

## Oral Dosage Forms
### BETAXOLOL TABLETS

**Usual adult dose**
Antihypertensive—
  Oral, 10 mg once a day initially, the dosage being doubled, if necessary, after seven to fourteen days.
Note: Geriatric patients may have increased or decreased sensitivity to the effects of the usual adult dose. An initial dose of 5 mg should be considered for elderly patients.

  For patients with renal function impairment who are undergoing hemodialysis, an initial dose of 5 mg once a day is recommended, increased by 5 mg a day every fourteen days, as necessary, up to a maximum daily dose of 20 mg.

**Usual pediatric dose**
Dosage has not been established.

**Strength(s) usually available**
U.S.—
  10 mg (Rx) [*Kerlone* (scored)].
  20 mg (Rx) [*Kerlone*].
Canada—
  Not commercially available.

**Packaging and storage**
Store below 40 °C (104 °F), preferably between 15 and 30 °C (59 and 86 °F), unless otherwise specified by manufacturer.

**Auxiliary labeling**
• Do not take other medicine without your doctor's advice.

**Note**
Check refill frequency to determine compliance in hypertensive patients.

## BISOPROLOL

## Summary of Differences

Pharmacology/pharmacokinetics:
　Mechanism of action/Effect—Relatively cardioselective (beta-1).
　Protein binding—Low.
Precautions:
　Breast-feeding—Not known if distributed into breast milk.

## Oral Dosage Forms
### BISOPROLOL FUMARATE TABLETS

**Usual adult dose**
Antihypertensive—
　Oral, initially 5 mg once a day, the dosage being increased to 10 mg once a day if hypertension is not adequately controlled.

Note: An initial dose of 2.5 mg once a day may be appropriate for some patients, especially patients with bronchospastic disease.

**Usual adult prescribing limits**
20 mg once a day.

**Usual pediatric dose**
Dosage has not been established.

**Strength(s) usually available**
U.S.—
　5 mg (Rx) [*Zebeta* (scored)].
　10 mg (Rx) [*Zebeta*].
Canada—
　Not commercially available.

**Packaging and storage**
Store below 40 °C (104 °F), preferably between 15 and 30 °C (59 and 86 °F), in a tight container, unless otherwise specified by manufacturer.

**Auxiliary labeling**
• Do not take other medicine without your doctor's advice.

**Note**
Check refill frequency to determine compliance in hypertensive patients.

## CARTEOLOL

## Summary of Differences

Pharmacology/pharmacokinetics:
　Mechanism of action/Effect—Moderate intrinsic sympathomimetic activity (ISA); nonselective; low lipid solubility.
　Biotransformation—Minimal hepatic metabolism (one active metabolite).
　Protein binding—Low.
Precautions:
　Breast-feeding—Not known if distributed into breast milk.
　Medical considerations/contraindications—Dosage reduction necessary in renal function impairment but not necessary in hepatic function impairment.
Side/adverse effects:
　Theoretical reduced risk of bronchospasm, heart failure, and peripheral vasoconstriction because of ISA.

## Oral Dosage Forms
### CARTEOLOL HYDROCHLORIDE TABLETS

**Usual adult dose**
Antihypertensive—
　Oral, initially 2.5 mg once a day, the dosage being adjusted according to response, up to a maximum of 10 mg once a day.

Note: Geriatric patients may have increased or decreased sensitivity to the effects of the usual adult dose.

　It is recommended that the dosage interval be increased in patients with renal function impairment as follows:

| Creatinine clearance (mL/min) | Dosage interval (hrs) |
| --- | --- |
| >60 | 24 |
| 20–60 | 48 |
| <20 | 72 |

**Usual adult prescribing limits**
10 mg per day.

**Usual pediatric dose**
Dosage has not been established.

**Strength(s) usually available**
U.S.—
　2.5 mg (Rx) [*Cartrol* (lactose)].
　5 mg (Rx) [*Cartrol* (lactose)].
Canada—
　Not commercially available.

**Packaging and storage**
Store below 40 °C (104 °F), preferably between 15 and 30 °C (59 and 86 °F), in a well-closed container, unless otherwise specified by manufacturer.

**Auxiliary labeling**
• Do not take other medicine without your doctor's advice.

**Note**
Check refill frequency to determine compliance in hypertensive patients.

## LABETALOL

## Summary of Differences

Pharmacology/pharmacokinetics:
　Mechanism of action/Effect—Also has selective alpha-1-adrenergic blocking effects; nonselective beta-blocker; low lipid solubility.
　Absorption—Bioavailability significantly reduced by first-pass metabolism and enhanced by concurrent administration with food.
　Protein binding—Moderate.
　Elimination—Not removable by hemodialysis.
Precautions:
　Medical considerations/contraindications—May not exacerbate Raynaud's phenomenon or other peripheral vascular diseases; dosage reduction necessary in hepatic function impairment but not necessary in renal function impairment.
Side/adverse effects:
　Possible reduced risk of bradycardia, bronchoconstriction, cardiac failure, hypoglycemia, and peripheral vasoconstriction, and increased incidence of postural hypotension.

## Additional Dosing Information

See also *General Dosing Information*.

The hypotensive effect of labetalol may be especially pronounced when the patient is standing. If feasible, blood pressure should be taken in the supine position, after standing for 10 minutes, and immediately after exercise. Dosage increases should be made only if there has been no decrease in the standing blood pressure from previous levels.

Hospitalized patients should not be discharged until the effect of labetalol on their standing blood pressure has been determined.

Dosage reduction is indicated if the patient has excessive orthostatic fall in pressure and/or normal supine pressure.

Appropriate laboratory testing is recommended at the first sign and/or symptom of hepatotoxicity; if there is laboratory evidence of hepatotoxicity, it is recommended that labetalol be permanently withdrawn.

*For parenteral dosage form*

Labetalol hydrochloride injection may be administered as a direct intravenous injection (over a 2-minute period) or by continuous intravenous infusion.

When labetalol is administered by continuous intravenous infusion, it is recommended that it be administered by means of an infusion pump, a micro-drip regulator, or a similar device to allow precise adjustment of the flow rate.

To reduce the chance of postural hypotension, patients should remain supine for up to 3 hours after receiving parenteral labetalol. Ambulation should not be permitted until the ability of the patient to tolerate the upright position has been determined.

## Oral Dosage Forms
### LABETALOL HYDROCHLORIDE TABLETS USP

**Usual adult dose**
Antihypertensive—
　Initial: Oral, 100 mg two times a day, the dosage being adjusted in increments of 100 mg two times a day every two or three days until the desired response is achieved.
　Maintenance: Oral, 200 to 400 mg two times a day.

Note: Labetalol may be administered in three divided daily doses if necessary because of side effects such as nausea or dizziness.

　In severe hypertension, doses of 1.2 to 2.4 grams per day, in two or three divided doses, may be needed.

Geriatric patients may have increased or decreased sensitivity to the effects of the usual adult dose.

**Usual pediatric dose**
Dosage has not been established.

**Strength(s) usually available**
U.S.—
100 mg (Rx) [*Normodyne* (scored); *Trandate* (scored)].
200 mg (Rx) [*Normodyne* (scored); *Trandate* (scored)].
300 mg (Rx) [*Normodyne; Trandate* (scored)].
Canada—
100 mg (Rx) [*Trandate* (scored)].
200 mg (Rx) [*Trandate* (scored)].

**Packaging and storage**
Store between 2 and 30 °C (36 and 86 °F), unless otherwise specified by manufacturer. Store in a tight, light-resistant container.

**Auxiliary labeling**
• Do not take other medicines without your doctor's advice.

**Note**
Check refill frequency to determine compliance in hypertensive patients.

# Parenteral Dosage Forms
## LABETALOL HYDROCHLORIDE INJECTION USP

**Usual adult dose**
Antihypertensive—
Intravenous, 20 mg (0.25 mg per kg of body weight for an 80-kg patient) injected slowly over a two-minute period; additional injections of 40 mg and 80 mg may be given at ten-minute intervals until the desired blood pressure is achieved or a total of 300 mg has been given; or
Intravenous infusion, administered at a rate of 2 mg per minute, the dosage being adjusted according to response; the total dose necessary may range from 50 to 300 mg.

Note: Geriatric patients may have increased or decreased sensitivity to the effects of the usual adult dose.

**Usual pediatric dose**
Dosage has not been established.

**Strength(s) usually available**
U.S.—
5 mg per mL (Rx) [*Normodyne; Trandate*].
Canada—
5 mg per mL (Rx) [*Trandate*].

**Packaging and storage**
Store between 2 and 30 °C (36 and 86 °F), unless otherwise specified by manufacturer. Protect from light. Protect from freezing.

**Preparation of dosage form**
Labetalol hydrochloride may be prepared for administration by continuous intravenous infusion by either of the following methods—
Adding 200 mg to 160 mL of a commonly used intravenous fluid to produce 200 mL of solution containing 1 mg of labetalol hydrochloride per mL; or
Adding 200 mg to 250 mL of intravenous fluid to produce about 300 mL of solution containing approximately 2 mg of labetalol hydrochloride per 3 mL.

---

## *METOPROLOL*

---

# Summary of Differences

Pharmacology/pharmacokinetics:
Mechanism of action/Effect—Relatively cardioselective (beta-1); moderate lipid solubility.
Absorption—Bioavailability significantly reduced by first-pass metabolism.
Protein binding—Low.
Elimination—Not removable by hemodialysis.
Precautions:
Medical considerations/contraindications—No dosage reduction necessary in hepatic function impairment (unless severe) or renal function impairment.
Side/adverse effects:
Theoretical reduced risk of bronchospasm, hypoglycemia, and peripheral vasoconstriction when daily dosage does not exceed 200 mg, because of cardioselectivity; increased risk of central nervous system (CNS) side effects because of lipid solubility and relative ease of penetration into CNS.

# Oral Dosage Forms
Note: Bracketed uses in the *Dosage Forms* section refer to categories of use and/or indications that are not included in U.S. product labeling.

## METOPROLOL SUCCINATE EXTENDED-RELEASE TABLETS

**Usual adult dose**
Antihypertensive—
Oral, 50 to 100 mg once a day, the dosage being increased at weekly (or longer) intervals as needed and tolerated up to a total of 400 mg a day.
Antianginal—
Oral, 100 mg once a day, the dosage being increased gradually at weekly intervals as needed and tolerated up to a maximum of 400 mg a day.
[Vascular headache prophylactic][1]—
Oral, 200 mg once a day.

Note: Geriatric patients may have increased or decreased sensitivity to the effects of the usual adult dose.

**Usual pediatric dose**
Dosage has not been established.

**Strength(s) usually available**
U.S.—
50 mg (Rx) [*Toprol-XL* (scored)].
100 mg (Rx) [*Toprol-XL* (scored)].
200 mg (Rx) [*Toprol-XL* (scored)].
Canada—
Not commercially available.

**Packaging and storage**
Store between 15 and 30 °C (59 and 86 °F), unless otherwise specified by manufacturer. Store in a tight container.

**Auxiliary labeling**
• Do not take other medicine without your doctor's advice.

**Note**
Check refill frequency to determine compliance in hypertensive patients.

## METOPROLOL TARTRATE TABLETS USP

**Usual adult dose**
Antianginal
Antihypertensive—
Oral, initially 100 mg a day in single (hypertension) or divided (angina or hypertension) doses, the dosage being increased at one-week intervals as needed and tolerated up to a total of 450 mg a day if necessary.

Note: To maintain satisfactory blood pressure control, some patients may require division of the total daily dose into three separate doses.

Myocardial infarction—
Early treatment: Oral, 50 mg (for patients who tolerate the full intravenous dose) or 25 to 50 mg (for patients who do not tolerate the full intravenous dose) every six hours starting fifteen minutes after the last intravenous dose or as soon as clinical condition allows. This dosage is continued for forty-eight hours, followed by
Late treatment: Oral, 100 mg two times a day for at least three months and possibly for as long as one to three years.
[Vascular headache prophylactic][1]—
Oral, 50 to 100 mg two to four times a day.

Note: Geriatric patients may have increased or decreased sensitivity to the effects of the usual adult dose.

**Usual pediatric dose**
Dosage has not been established.

**Strength(s) usually available**
U.S.—
50 mg (Rx) [*Lopressor* (scored)].
100 mg (Rx) [*Lopressor* (scored)].
Canada—
50 mg (Rx) [*Apo-Metoprolol* (scored); *Apo-Metoprolol (Type L); Betaloc* (scored); *Lopresor* (scored); *Novometoprol* (scored); GENERIC].
100 mg (Rx) [*Apo-Metoprolol* (scored); *Apo-Metoprolol (Type L); Betaloc* (scored); *Lopresor* (scored); *Novometoprol* (scored); GENERIC].

**Packaging and storage**
Store between 15 and 30 °C (59 and 86 °F), unless otherwise specified by manufacturer. Store in a tight, light-resistant container.

**Auxiliary labeling**
• Do not take other medicine without your doctor's advice.

**Note**

Check refill frequency to determine compliance in hypertensive patients.

## METOPROLOL TARTRATE EXTENDED-RELEASE TABLETS

**Usual adult dose**

Antianginal

Antihypertensive—

Oral, 100 to 400 mg administered once a day for maintenance of established dosage requirements.

Note: Geriatric patients may have increased or decreased sensitivity to the effects of the usual adult dose.

**Usual pediatric dose**

Dosage has not been established.

**Strength(s) usually available**

U.S.—

Not commercially available.

Canada—

100 mg (Rx) [*Lopresor SR*].

200 mg (Rx) [*Betaloc Durules; Lopresor SR*].

**Packaging and storage**

Store below 40 °C (104 °F), preferably between 15 and 30 °C (59 and 86 °F), unless otherwise specified by manufacturer. Store in a light-resistant container.

**Auxiliary labeling**

• Do not take other medicine without your doctor's advice.

**Note**

Check refill frequency to determine compliance in hypertensive patients.

## Parenteral Dosage Forms

### METOPROLOL TARTRATE INJECTION USP

**Usual adult dose**

Myocardial infarction—

Early treatment: Intravenous (rapid), 5 mg every two minutes for three doses.

Note: Geriatric patients may have increased or decreased sensitivity to the effects of the usual adult dose.

**Usual pediatric dose**

Dosage has not been established.

**Strength(s) usually available**

U.S.—

1 mg per mL (Rx) [*Lopressor*].

Canada—

1 mg per mL (Rx) [*Betaloc* (sodium chloride 45 mg per mL); *Lopresor* (sodium chloride 45 mg per mL)].

**Packaging and storage**

Store below 40 °C (104 °F), preferably between 15 and 30 °C (59 and 86 °F), unless otherwise specified by manufacturer. Protect from light. Protect from freezing.

---

[1]Not included in Canadian product labeling.

---

### *NADOLOL*

## Summary of Differences

Pharmacology/pharmacokinetics:

Mechanism of action/Effect—Nonselective; low lipid solubility.

Biotransformation—Not hepatically metabolized.

Protein binding—Very low to low.

Elimination—Removable by hemodialysis.

Precautions:

Medical considerations/contraindications—Dosage reduction or increased dosing intervals recommended in renal function impairment; dosage reduction not necessary in hepatic function impairment.

## Oral Dosage Forms

Note: Bracketed uses in the *Dosage Forms* section refer to categories of use and/or indications that are not included in U.S. product labeling.

### NADOLOL TABLETS USP

**Usual adult dose**

Antianginal—

Oral, 40 mg once a day initially, the dosage being increased by 40 to 80 mg at three- to seven-day intervals as needed and tolerated up to a total of 240 mg a day if necessary.

Antihypertensive—

Oral, initially 40 mg once a day, the dosage being increased in increments of 40 to 80 mg at one-week intervals as needed and tolerated up to a total of 320 mg a day if necessary.

[Vascular headache prophylactic][1]—

Oral, 20 to 40 mg once a day initially, the dosage being gradually increased as tolerated up to 120 mg per day if necessary.

Note: Geriatric patients may have increased or decreased sensitivity to the effects of the usual adult dose.

Because of the long half-life, once-a-day dosage is sufficient to provide stable plasma concentrations; however, such steady-state concentrations may not be achieved for up to 5 days following initiation of therapy or change of dose.

For patients with renal function impairment, the following dosage adjustments are recommended:

| Creatinine clearance (mL/min/1.73m) | Dosage interval (hours) |
|---|---|
| >50 | 24 |
| 31–50 | 24–36 |
| 10–30 | 24–48 |
| <10 | 40–60 |

**Usual pediatric dose**

Dosage has not been established.

**Strength(s) usually available**

U.S.—

20 mg (Rx) [*Corgard* (scored)].

40 mg (Rx) [*Corgard* (scored)].

80 mg (Rx) [*Corgard* (scored)].

120 mg (Rx) [*Corgard* (scored)].

160 mg (Rx) [*Corgard* (scored)].

Canada—

40 mg (Rx) [*Corgard* (scored); *Syn-Nadolol* (scored); GENERIC].

80 mg (Rx) [*Corgard* (partially scored); *Syn-Nadolol* (partially scored); GENERIC].

160 mg (Rx) [*Corgard* (scored); *Syn-Nadolol* (scored); GENERIC].

**Packaging and storage**

Store between 15 and 30 °C (59 and 86 °F), unless otherwise specified by manufacturer. Store in a tight, light-resistant container.

**Auxiliary labeling**

• Do not take other medicine without your doctor's advice.

**Note**

Check refill frequency to determine compliance in hypertensive patients.

---

[1]Not included in Canadian product labeling.

---

### *OXPRENOLOL*

## Summary of Differences

Pharmacology/pharmacokinetics:

Mechanism of action/Effect—Moderate intrinsic sympathomimetic activity (ISA); nonselective; moderate lipid solubility.

Absorption—Bioavailability significantly reduced by first-pass metabolism.

Protein binding—High.

Precautions:

Medical considerations/contraindications—Dosage reduction necessary in hepatic function impairment but not necessary in renal function impairment.

Side/adverse effects:

Theoretical reduced risk of bronchospasm, heart failure, and peripheral vasoconstriction because of ISA.

## Oral Dosage Forms

Note: Dosage and strengths of the dosage forms available are expressed in terms of the hydrochloride salt.

## OXPRENOLOL TABLETS USP

**Usual adult dose**
Antihypertensive—
Oral, 20 mg three times a day initially, the dosage being increased in increments of 60 mg per day every one to two weeks until the desired response is achieved, usually in the range of 120 to 320 mg a day.
Note: Once the optimal daily dose has been reached, twice-daily dosing may be used.

Geriatric patients may have increased or decreased sensitivity to the effects of the usual adult dose.

**Usual adult prescribing limits**
480 mg per day.

**Usual pediatric dose**
Dosage has not been established.

**Strength(s) usually available**
U.S.—
Not commercially available.
Canada—
20 mg (hydrochloride) (Rx) [*Trasicor*].
40 mg (hydrochloride) (Rx) [*Trasicor* (scored)].
80 mg (hydrochloride) (Rx) [*Trasicor* (scored)].

**Packaging and storage**
Store below 40 °C (104 °F), preferably between 15 and 30 °C (59 and 86 °F), in a well-closed container, unless otherwise specified by manufacturer. Protect from light.

**Auxiliary labeling**
• Do not take other medicine without your doctor's advice.

**Note**
Check refill frequency to determine compliance in hypertensive patients.

## OXPRENOLOL EXTENDED-RELEASE TABLETS USP

**Usual adult dose**
Antihypertensive—
Oral, usually 120 to 320 mg a day administered once a day in the morning for maintenance of established dosage requirements.
Note: Geriatric patients may have increased or decreased sensitivity to the effects of the usual adult dose.

**Usual pediatric dose**
Dosage has not been established.

**Strength(s) usually available**
U.S.—
Not commercially available.
Canada—
80 mg (hydrochloride) (Rx) [*Slow-Trasicor* (lactose)].
160 mg (hydrochloride) (Rx) [*Slow-Trasicor* (lactose)].

**Packaging and storage**
Store below 40 °C (104 °F), preferably between 15 and 30 °C (59 and 86 °F), in a well-closed container, unless otherwise specified by manufacturer. Protect from light.

**Auxiliary labeling**
• Do not take other medicine without your doctor's advice.

**Note**
Check refill frequency to determine compliance in hypertensive patients.

---

### *PENBUTOLOL*

## Summary of Differences

Pharmacology/pharmacokinetics:
Mechanism of action/Effect—Moderate intrinsic sympathomimetic activity (ISA); high lipid solubility; nonselective.
Biotransformation—Although hepatically metabolized, penbutolol undergoes no significant first-pass effect.
Protein binding—High to very high.
Elimination—Not removable by hemodialysis.
Precautions:
Breast-feeding—Not known whether distributed into breast milk.
Medical considerations/contraindications—Dosage reduction necessary in hepatic function impairment but not necessary in renal function impairment.
Side/adverse effects:
Theoretical reduced risk of bronchospasm, heart failure, and peripheral vasoconstriction because of ISA.

## PENBUTOLOL SULFATE TABLETS

**Usual adult dose**
Antihypertensive—
Oral, 20 mg once a day.
Note: Geriatric patients may have increased or decreased sensitivity to the effects of the usual adult dose.

**Usual pediatric dose**
Dosage has not been established.

**Strength(s) usually available**
U.S.—
20 mg (Rx) [*Levatol* (scored; lactose)].
Canada—
Not commercially available.

**Packaging and storage**
Store below 40 °C (104 °F), preferably between 15 and 30 °C (59 and 86 °F), in a well-closed container, unless otherwise specified by manufacturer. Protect from light.

**Auxiliary labeling**
• Do not take other medicine without your doctor's advice.

**Note**
Check refill frequency to determine compliance in hypertensive patients.

---

### *PINDOLOL*

## Summary of Differences

Pharmacology/pharmacokinetics:
Mechanism of action/Effect—Exhibits the most intrinsic sympathomimetic activity (ISA) of beta-blockers currently available; moderate lipid solubility; nonselective.
Biotransformation—Although hepatically metabolized, pindolol undergoes no significant first-pass effect.
Protein binding—Moderate.
Precautions:
Medical considerations/contraindications—Dosage reduction necessary in hepatic function and severe renal function impairment.
Side/adverse effects:
Theoretical reduced risk of bronchospasm, heart failure, and peripheral vasoconstriction because of ISA; overdose may produce tachycardia and hypertension.

## Oral Dosage Forms

Note: Bracketed uses in the *Dosage Forms* section refer to categories of use and/or indications that are not included in U.S. product labeling.

## PINDOLOL TABLETS USP

**Usual adult dose**
Antihypertensive—
Oral, initially 5 mg two times a day, the dosage being increased in increments of 10 mg per day at two- or three-week intervals as needed and tolerated up to a maximum of 45 mg a day (Canada) or 60 mg a day (U.S.).
Note: Many hypertensive patients require a maintenance dose of only 5 mg of pindolol two times a day to provide an adequate reduction in blood pressure.

Once the optimal daily dose has been reached, once-daily dosing may be used.

Geriatric patients may have increased or decreased sensitivity to the effects of the usual adult dose.
[Antianginal]—
Oral, 5 mg three times a day, the dosage being increased at one to two week intervals up to a maximum of 40 mg per day.

**Usual adult prescribing limits**
45 mg a day (Canada) or 60 mg a day (U.S.).

**Usual pediatric dose**
Dosage has not been established.

**Strength(s) usually available**
U.S.—
5 mg (Rx) [*Visken* (scored)].
10 mg (Rx) [*Visken* (scored)].
Canada—
5 mg (Rx) [*Novo-Pindol; Syn-Pindolol; Visken* (scored)].
10 mg (Rx) [*Novo-Pindol; Syn-Pindolol; Visken* (scored)].
15 mg (Rx) [*Novo-Pindol; Syn-Pindolol; Visken* (scored)].

**Packaging and storage**

Store below 40 °C (104 °F), preferably between 15 and 30 °C (59 and 86 °F), in a well-closed container, unless otherwise specified by manufacturer. Protect from light.

**Auxiliary labeling**

• Do not take any other medicine without your doctor's advice.

**Note**

Check refill frequency to determine compliance in hypertensive patients.

---

## *PROPRANOLOL*

## Summary of Differences

Pharmacology/pharmacokinetics:

Mechanism of action/Effect—Nonselective; high lipid solubility.

Absorption—Bioavailability significantly reduced by first-pass metabolism.

Protein binding—Very high.

Elimination—Not removable by hemodialysis.

Precautions:

Medical considerations/contraindications—Dosage reduction necessary in hepatic function impairment but not necessary in renal function impairment.

Side/adverse effects:

Increased risk of CNS side effects because of high lipid solubility and ease of penetration into CNS.

## Oral Dosage Forms

Note: Bracketed uses in the *Dosage Forms* section refer to categories of use and/or indications that are not included in U.S. product labeling.

### PROPRANOLOL HYDROCHLORIDE EXTENDED-RELEASE CAPSULES USP

**Usual adult dose**

Antihypertensive—

Oral, 80 mg once a day, the dosage being increased gradually up to 160 mg once a day. Doses up to 640 mg per day may be needed in some patients.

Antianginal—

Oral, 80 mg once a day, the dosage being increased gradually at three- to seven-day intervals as needed up to 320 mg per day.

Vascular headache prophylaxis—

Oral, 80 mg once a day, the dosage being increased gradually as needed up to 240 mg once a day.

Note: Geriatric patients may have increased or decreased sensitivity to the effects of the usual adult dose.

**Usual pediatric dose**

Dosage has not been established.

**Strength(s) usually available**

U.S.—

60 mg (Rx) [*Inderal LA;* GENERIC].

80 mg (Rx) [*Inderal LA;* GENERIC].

120 mg (Rx) [*Inderal LA;* GENERIC].

160 mg (Rx) [*Inderal LA;* GENERIC].

Canada—

60 mg (Rx) [*Inderal LA* (sulfites)].

80 mg (Rx) [*Inderal LA* (sulfites)].

120 mg (Rx) [*Inderal LA* (sulfites)].

160 mg (Rx) [*Inderal LA* (sulfites)].

**Packaging and storage**

Store below 40 °C (104 °F), preferably between 15 and 30 °C (59 and 86 °F), unless otherwise specified by manufacturer. Protect from light.

**Auxiliary labeling**

• Do not take other medicine without your doctor's advice.

**Note**

Check refill frequency to determine compliance in hypertensive patients.

### PROPRANOLOL HYDROCHLORIDE ORAL SOLUTION

**Usual adult dose**

Antianginal—

Oral, 80 to 320 mg per day given in two, three, or four divided doses.

Antiarrhythmic—

Oral, 10 to 30 mg three or four times a day, the dosage being adjusted as needed and tolerated.

Antihypertensive—

Oral, 40 mg two times a day, the dosage being increased gradually as needed and tolerated, usually 120 to 240 mg a day; doses up to a total of 640 mg a day may be necessary (a total daily dose of 1 gram has been used by some clinicians).

Hypertrophic cardiomyopathy therapy adjunct—

Oral, 20 to 40 mg three or four times a day, the dosage being adjusted as needed and tolerated.

Myocardial infarction—

Oral, 180 to 240 mg a day in divided doses.

Pheochromocytoma therapy adjunct—

Oral, 20 mg three times a day to 40 mg three or four times a day (as necessary for sufficient beta-blockade) for three days prior to surgery, concomitantly with alpha-adrenergic blocking medication (should *never* be started until alpha-adrenergic blockade is at least partially established). Doses of 30 to 160 mg per day in divided doses have been used for management of inoperable tumor.

Vascular headache prophylactic—

Oral, 20 mg four times a day initially, the dosage being increased gradually as needed and tolerated up to a total of 240 mg a day if necessary.

Antitremor agent—

Oral, 40 mg two times a day, the dosage being adjusted as needed and tolerated, up to 120 mg a day; occasionally, doses up to 320 mg a day may be needed.

[Antianxiety therapy adjunct][1]—

Oral, 10 to 80 mg thirty to ninety minutes prior to the anxiety-provoking activity.

[Thyrotoxicosis therapy adjunct][1]—

Oral, 10 to 40 mg three or four times a day, the dosage being adjusted as needed and tolerated.

Note: Twice-daily or, in some patients, once-daily dosing may be effective for use as an antianginal, antihypertensive, or for myocardial infarction.

Geriatric patients may have increased or decreased sensitivity to the effects of the usual adult dose.

**Usual pediatric dose**

Antiarrhythmic

Antihypertensive—

Initial: Oral, 500 mcg (0.5 mg) to 1 mg per kg of body weight per day in two to four divided doses has been used as an initial dose, the dosage being adjusted as necessary to treat hypertension and prevent supraventricular tachycardia.

Maintenance: Oral, 2 to 4 mg per kg per day in two divided doses.

**Strength(s) usually available**

U.S.—

4 mg per mL (Rx) [GENERIC].

8 mg per mL (Rx) [GENERIC].

80 mg per mL (concentrated; must be diluted) (Rx) [GENERIC].

Canada—

Not commercially available.

**Packaging and storage**

Store below 40 °C (104 °F), preferably between 15 and 30 °C (59 and 86 °F), in a well-closed container, unless otherwise specified by manufacturer. Protect from light. Protect from freezing.

**Preparation of dosage form**

Propranolol concentrated oral solution is prepared for administration by mixing it with a liquid such as water, juice, or soda or soda-like beverage. After the patient drinks the mixture, the glass should be rinsed with more liquid to make sure all the medication is taken. Propranolol concentrated oral solution may also be mixed with semi-solid food such as applesauce or pudding.

**Auxiliary labeling**

• Do not take other medicine without your doctor's advice.

**Note**

Check refill frequency to determine compliance in hypertensive patients.

### PROPRANOLOL HYDROCHLORIDE TABLETS USP

**Usual adult dose**

See *Propranolol Hydrochloride Oral Solution.*

**Usual pediatric dose**

See *Propranolol Hydrochloride Oral Solution.*

**Strength(s) usually available**

U.S.—

10 mg (Rx) [*Inderal* (scored); GENERIC].

20 mg (Rx) [*Inderal* (scored); GENERIC (may be scored)].

40 mg (Rx) [*Inderal* (scored); GENERIC (may be scored)].

60 mg (Rx) [*Inderal* (scored); GENERIC (may be scored)].

80 mg (Rx) [*Inderal* (scored); GENERIC (may be scored)].

90 mg (Rx) [*Inderal* (scored); GENERIC (may be scored)].

Canada—
   10 mg (Rx) [*Apo-Propranolol* (scored); *Detensol* (scored); *Inderal* (scored); *Novopranol* (scored); *pms Propranolol* (scored)].
   20 mg (Rx) [*Apo-Propranolol* (scored); *Novopranol* (scored); *Inderal* (scored)].
   40 mg (Rx) [*Apo-Propranolol* (scored); *Detensol* (scored); *Inderal* (scored); *Novopranol* (scored); *pms Propranolol* (scored)].
   80 mg (Rx) [*Apo-Propranolol* (scored); *Detensol* (scored); *Inderal* (scored); *Novopranol* (scored); *pms Propranolol* (scored)].
   120 mg (Rx) [*Apo-Propranolol* (scored); *Inderal* (scored); *Novopranol* (scored); *pms Propranolol* (scored)].

### Packaging and storage
Store below 40 °C (104 °F), preferably between 15 and 30 °C (59 and 86 °F), unless otherwise specified by manufacturer. Store in a well-closed, light-resistant container.

### Auxiliary labeling
• Do not take other medicine without your doctor's advice.

### Note
Check refill frequency to determine compliance in hypertensive patients.

## Parenteral Dosage Forms
### PROPRANOLOL HYDROCHLORIDE INJECTION USP

### Usual adult dose
Antiarrhythmic—
   Intravenous, 1 to 3 mg administered at a rate not to exceed 1 mg per minute, repeated after two minutes and again after four hours if necessary.
Note: An intravenous dose of one-tenth the oral dose may be used to temporarily replace oral dosing in patients undergoing surgery.
   Geriatric patients may have increased or decreased sensitivity to the effects of the usual adult dose.

### Usual pediatric dose
Antiarrhythmic—
   Slow intravenous, 10 to 100 mcg (0.01 to 0.1 mg) per kg of body weight (up to a maximum of 1 mg per dose), repeated every six to eight hours if necessary.

### Strength(s) usually available
U.S.—
   1 mg per mL (Rx) [*Inderal;* GENERIC].
Canada—
   1 mg per mL (Rx) [*Inderal*].

### Packaging and storage
Store below 40 °C (104 °F), preferably between 15 and 30 °C (59 and 86 °F), unless otherwise specified by manufacturer. Store in a light-resistant container. Protect from freezing.

---

[1]Not included in Canadian product labeling.

---

## SOTALOL

## Summary of Differences
Pharmacology/pharmacokinetics:
   Mechanism of action/Effect—Nonselective; no intrinsic sympathomimetic activity (ISA) or membrane-stabilizing activity; low lipid solubility.
   Protein binding—Not protein bound.
   Elimination—Removable by hemodialysis.

## Oral Dosage Forms
Note: Bracketed uses in the *Dosage Forms* section refer to categories of use and/or indications that are not included in U.S. product labeling.

### SOTALOL HYDROCHLORIDE TABLETS

### Usual adult dose
[Antianginal]
[Antihypertensive]—
   Initial: Oral, 80 mg two times a day, the dosage being increased in increments of 80 mg two times a day at weekly intervals as needed and tolerated.
   Maintenance: Oral, 160 mg two times a day.
Note: Once-daily dosing may be effective in patients taking a total daily maintenance dose of 320 mg or less.
   Geriatric patients may have increased or decreased sensitivity to the effects of the usual adult dose.

Antiarrhythmic[1]—
   Initial: Oral, 80 mg two times a day, the dosage being increased gradually.
   Maintenance: Oral, 160 to 320 mg per day, given in two or three divided doses.
Note: It is recommended that the dosage interval be increased in patients with renal function impairment as follows:

| Creatinine clearance (mL/min) | Dosage interval (hrs) |
| --- | --- |
| >60 | 12 |
| 30–60 | 24 |
| 10–30 | 36–48 |
| <10 | Dosage and dosing interval must be individualized |

### Usual adult prescribing limits
For life-threatening arrhythmias—640 mg per day.
For other indications—480 mg per day.

### Usual pediatric dose
Dosage has not been established.

### Strength(s) usually available
U.S.—
   80 mg (Rx) [*Betapace* (scored)].
   160 mg (Rx) [*Betapace* (scored)].
   240 mg (Rx) [*Betapace* (scored)].
Canada—
   160 mg (Rx) [*Sotacor* (scored)].

### Packaging and storage
Store below 40 °C (104 °F), preferably between 15 and 30 °C (59 and 86 °F), in a well-closed container, unless otherwise specified by manufacturer.

### Auxiliary labeling
• Do not take other medicines without your doctor's advice.

### Note
Check refill frequency to determine compliance in hypertensive patients.

---

[1]Not included in Canadian product labeling.

---

## TIMOLOL

## Summary of Differences
Pharmacology/pharmacokinetics:
   Mechanism of action/Effect—Nonselective; no significant intrinsic sympathomimetic activity (ISA); moderate lipid solubility.
   Absorption—Bioavailability significantly reduced by first-pass metabolism.
   Protein binding—Very low.
   Elimination—Not removable by hemodialysis.
Precautions:
   Medical considerations/contraindications—Dosage reduction necessary in hepatic function impairment but not necessary in renal function impairment.

## Oral Dosage Forms
Note: Bracketed uses in the *Dosage Forms* section refer to categories of use and/or indications that are not included in U.S. product labeling.

### TIMOLOL MALEATE TABLETS USP

### Usual adult dose
Antihypertensive
[Antianginal]—
   Initial: Oral, 10 mg two times a day initially, the dosage being increased at one-week intervals as needed and tolerated.
   Maintenance: Oral, usually 20 to 40 mg per day; doses up to 60 mg per day divided into two doses may be necessary.
Myocardial infarction[1]—
   Oral, 10 mg two times a day prophylactically against reinfarction in clinically stable patients. Treatment is initiated one to four weeks following initial infarction.
Vascular headache prophylactic—
   Oral, 10 mg two times a day initially; maintenance, 20 mg a day (may be given as a single daily dose); maximum dose is 30 mg per day (10 mg in the morning and 20 mg at night).
Note: Geriatric patients may have increased or decreased sensitivity to the effects of the usual adult dose.

**Usual pediatric dose**

Dosage has not been established.

**Strength(s) usually available**

U.S.—

5 mg (Rx) [*Blocadren;* GENERIC].
10 mg (Rx) [*Blocadren* (scored); GENERIC].
20 mg (Rx) [*Blocadren* (scored); GENERIC].

Canada—

5 mg (Rx) [*Apo-Timol* (scored); *Blocadren* (scored); *Novo-Timol*].
10 mg (Rx) [*Apo-Timol* (scored); *Blocadren* (scored); *Novo-Timol*].
20 mg (Rx) [*Apo-Timol; Blocadren* (scored); *Novo-Timol*].

**Packaging and storage**

Store below 40 °C (104 °F), preferably between 15 and 30 °C (59 and 86 °F), unless otherwise specified by manufacturer. Store in a well-closed, light-resistant container.

**Auxiliary labeling**

• Do not take other medicine without your doctor's advice.

**Note**

Check refill frequency to determine compliance in hypertensive patients.

¹Not included in Canadian product labeling.

# Selected Bibliography

**General**

Gerber JG, Nies AS. Beta-adrenergic blocking drugs. Ann Rev Med 1985; 36: 145-64.

Prichard BN, Tomlinson B. The additional properties of beta adrenoreceptor blocking drugs. J Cardiovasc Pharmacol 1986; 8 (Suppl 4): S1-S15.

Drayer DE. Lipophilicity, hydrophilicity, and the central nervous system side effects of beta blockers. Pharmacother 1987; 7 (4): 87-91.

**For acebutolol**

Singh BN, Thoden WR, Wahl J. Acebutolol: a review of its pharmacology, pharmacokinetics, clinical uses, and adverse effects. Pharmacother 1986 Mar/Apr; 6: 45-63.

Anonymous. Acebutolol. Med Lett Drugs Ther 1985 Jul 5; 27: 58-9.

De Bono G, Kaye CM, Roland E, Summers AJH. Acebutolol: ten years of experience. Am Heart J 1985 May; 109: 1211-23.

**For betaxolol**

Beresford R, Heel RC. Betaxolol. A review of its pharmacodynamic and pharmacokinetic properties, and therapeutic efficacy in hypertension. Drugs 1986; 31: 6-28.

**For bisoprolol**

Lancaster SG, Sorkin EM. Bisoprolol. A preliminary review of its pharmacodynamic and pharmacokinetic properties, and therapeutic efficacy in hypertension and angina pectoris. Drugs 1988; 36: 256-85.

**For carteolol**

Luther RR, Glassman HN, Jordan DC, et al. Long-term treatment of angina pectoris with carteolol. J Int Med Res 1986; 14: 167-74.

Luther RR, Maurath CJ, Klepper MJ, et al. Carteolol treatment of essential hypertension. J Int Med Res 1986; 14: 175-84.

**For labetalol**

Blakey B, Williams LL, Lopez LM, Stein GH. Labetalol HCl: alpha- and beta-blocking properties may offer advantages over pure beta-blockers. Hosp Form 1987 Oct; 22: 864-9.

Weintraub M, Evans P. Labetalol: an alpha-blocker for treatment of hypertension. Hosp Form 1984 Apr; 19: 295-305.

MacCarthy EP, Bloomfield SS. Labetalol: a review of its pharmacology, pharmacokinetics, clinical uses, and adverse effects. Pharmacother 1983 Jul/Aug; 3: 193-219.

**For oxprenolol**

Weintraub M, Standish R. Oxprenolol: a nonselective beta blocking agent with intrinsic sympathomimetic activity. Hosp Form 1984 May; 19: 359-65.

**For penbutolol**

Marone C, Perisic M, Borer M. Antihypertensive efficacy and tolerance of penbutolol. Results of a cooperative study in 227 patients. Curr Med Res Opin 1985; 9: 417-25.

**For sotalol**

Singh BN, Deedwania P, Nademanee K, Ward A, Sorkin EM. Sotalol. A review of its pharmacodynamic and pharmacokinetic properties, and therapeutic use. Drugs 1987; 34: 311-49.

Revised: 05/13/93

## Table 1. Pharmacology/Pharmacokinetics

| Drug | Site of Effect | Oral Absorption (%) | Protein Binding | Biotransformation | Half-life (hr) | Time to Peak Effect— Single dose (hr) | Elimination (% unchanged) | Removable by Hemodialysis |
|---|---|---|---|---|---|---|---|---|
| Acebutolol | Beta-1* | 70† | Low (26%) | Hepatic‡ | 3–4‡ | 2.5‡ | 30–40% Renal; 50–60% Biliary/fecal | Yes |
| Atenolol | Beta-1* | 50–60 | Very low to low (6–16%) | Hepatic (minimal) | 6–7§ | 2–4 | 85–100% Renal | Yes** |

*Cardioselectivity tends to diminish with increased dosage.

†First-pass metabolism results in a decrease (usually significant) in bioavailability.

  Acebutolol—The effect is not reduced because of the active metabolite. Bioavailability of acebutolol may be increased 2-fold in the elderly because of reduced first-pass metabolism and renal function.

  Betaxolol—First-pass effect is small.

‡Acebutolol—Major metabolite (diacetolol) is pharmacologically active and even more cardioselective than acebutolol; time to peak effect is 3.5 hours; the half-life of diacetolol is 8 to 13 hours.

§Atenolol—Increased to 16–27 hours or more in patients with renal function impairment (up to 144 hours when severe).

  Betaxolol—Increased by approximately 33% in hepatic function impairment, but clearance unchanged.

     —Approximately doubled in renal function impairment; dosage reduction necessary.

  Carteolol—Prolonged in renal failure.

  Metoprolol—No change in renal failure.

  Nadolol—Increased in renal failure.

  Penbutolol—Increased in renal failure.

  Pindolol—Varies from 2.5 to more than 30 hours in patients with hepatic function impairment.

     —Increased to 3 to 11.5 hours in patients with renal function impairment.

     —Increased to an average of 7 hours (and as high as 15 hours) in the elderly.

  Sotalol—Increased in renal failure.

**Atenolol—Patients should receive 50 mg of atenolol after each dialysis and remain under supervision since marked hypotension may occur.

## Table 1. Pharmacology/Pharmacokinetics (continued)

| Drug | Site of Effect | Oral Absorption (%) | Protein Binding | Biotransforma-tion | Half-life (hr) | Time to Peak Effect— Single dose (hr) | Elimination (% un-changed) | Removable by Hemodialysis |
|---|---|---|---|---|---|---|---|---|
| Betaxolol | Beta-1* | 80–89† | Moderate (50–55%) | Hepatic | 14–22§ | 3–4 | >80% (15) Renal | No |
| Bisoprolol | Beta-1 | 80–90 | Low (26–33%) | Hepatic | 9–12 | | Renal (50) <2% Fecal | No |
| Carteolol | Beta-1; Beta-2 | 85 | Low (23–30%) | Hepatic (minimal) | 6§ | 1–3 | Renal (50–70) | ? |
| Labetalol | Beta-1; Beta-2 | 100† | Moderate (50%) | Hepatic | 6–8 (oral); ~5.5 (IV) | 2–4 (oral); 5 min (IV) | 55–60% (<5) Renal; Biliary/fecal | No |
| Metoprolol | Beta-1* | 95† | Low (12%) | Hepatic | 3–7§ | 1–2 (oral— regular); 6–12 (oral— long-acting); 20 min (IV) | Renal (3–10) | No |
| Nadolol | Beta-1; Beta-2 | 30 | Very low to low (4 to 30%) | None | 20–24§ | 4 | Renal (70) | Yes |
| Oxprenolol | Beta-1; Beta-2 | 90† | High (80%) | Hepatic | 1.3–1.5 | ? | Renal (<5) | ? |
| Penbutolol | Beta-1; Beta-2 | 100 | High to very high (80–98%) | Hepatic | 5§ | 1.5–3 | 90% (0) Renal | No |
| Pindolol | Beta-1; Beta-2 | 90–100 | Moderate (40%) | Hepatic | 3–4§ | 1–2 | Renal (40) | ? |
| Propranolol | Beta-1; Beta-2 | 90† | Very high (93%) | Hepatic | 3–5 | 1–1.5 | Renal (<1) | No |
| Sotalol | Beta-1; Beta-2 | > 80 | None | Hepatic | 7–18§ | 2–3 | Renal (75) | Yes |
| Timolol | Beta-1; Beta-2 | 90† | Very low (<10%) | Hepatic | 4 | 1–2 | Renal (20); Fecal | No |

*Cardioselectivity tends to diminish with increased dosage.

†First-pass metabolism results in a decrease (usually significant) in bioavailability.
    Acebutolol—The effect is not reduced because of the active metabolite. Bioavailability of acebutolol may be increased 2-fold in the elderly because of reduced first-pass metabolism and renal function.
    Betaxolol—First-pass effect is small.

‡Acebutolol—Major metabolite (diacetolol) is pharmacologically active and even more cardioselective than acebutolol; time to peak effect is 3.5 hours; the half-life of diacetolol is 8 to 13 hours.

§Atenolol—Increased to 16–27 hours or more in patients with renal function impairment (up to 144 hours when severe).
    Betaxolol—Increased by approximately 33% in hepatic function impairment, but clearance unchanged.
    —Approximately doubled in renal function impairment; dosage reduction necessary.
    Carteolol—Prolonged in renal failure.
    Metoprolol—No change in renal failure.
    Nadolol—Increased in renal failure.
    Penbutolol—Increased in renal failure.
    Pindolol—Varies from 2.5 to more than 30 hours in patients with hepatic function impairment.
    —Increased to 3 to 11.5 hours in patients with renal function impairment.
    —Increased to an average of 7 hours (and as high as 15 hours) in the elderly.
    Sotalol—Increased in renal failure.

**Atenolol—Patients should receive 50 mg of atenolol after each dialysis and remain under supervision since marked hypotension may occur.

# BETA-ADRENERGIC BLOCKING AGENTS AND THIAZIDE DIURETICS   Systemic

This monograph includes information on the following: Atenolol and Chlorthalidone; Bisoprolol and Hydrochlorothiazide; Metoprolol and Hydrochlorothiazide; Nadolol and Bendroflumethiazide; Pindolol and Hydrochlorothiazide; Propranolol and Hydrochlorothiazide; Timolol and Hydrochlorothiazide.

VA CLASSIFICATION (Primary/Secondary): CV400/CV490

**NOTE:** The *Beta-adrenergic Blocking Agents and Thiazide Diuretics (Systemic)* monograph is maintained on the USP DI electronic data base. For a printed copy of the most recent revision of the complete monograph, contact the USP Division of Information Development, 12601 Twinbrook Parkway, Rockville, MD 20852.

For information on the specific components of this combination, see the *USP DI* monographs for *Beta-adrenergic Blocking Agents (Systemic)* and *Diuretics, Thiazide (Systemic)*.

The information that follows is selectively abstracted from the complete monograph and is provided to facilitate drug use review and patient counseling.

Note: For a listing of dosage forms and brand names by country availability, see *Dosage Forms* section(s). For a listing of brand names for the articles in this monograph, refer to the General Index.

## Category
Antihypertensive.

## Indications

**Accepted**

Hypertension (treatment)—Beta-adrenergic blocking agent (beta-blocker) and thiazide diuretic combinations are indicated in the management of hypertension.

Fixed-dosage combinations generally are not recommended for initial therapy, but are utilized in maintenance therapy after the required dose is established, in order to increase convenience, economy, and patient compliance.

For additional information on initial therapeutic guidelines related to the treatment of hypertension, see *Appendix III*.

## Patient Consultation

As an aid to patient consultation, refer to *Advice for the Patient, Beta-adrenergic Blocking Agents and Thiazide Diuretics (Systemic)*.

In providing consultation, consider emphasizing the following selected information (» = major clinical significance):

**Before using this medication**
» Conditions affecting use, especially:
   Sensitivity to the beta-adrenergic blocking agent prescribed, or to any thiazide diuretic or other sulfonamide-type medications
   Pregnancy—Risk of hypoglycemia, respiratory depression, bradycardia, and hypotension with beta-adrenergic blocking agents; thiazide diuretics may cause jaundice, thrombocytopenia, hypokalemia in infant
   Breast-feeding—Distributed into breast milk; not known for bisoprolol
   Use in the elderly—Increased sensitivity to effects; increased risk of beta-blocker–induced hypothermia
   Other medications, especially allergen immunotherapy or skin testing, oral antidiabetic agents, calcium channel blocking agents, clonidine, cocaine, digitalis glycosides, guanabenz, insulin, lithium, MAO inhibitors, sympathomimetics, or xanthines
   Other medical problems, especially anuria or severe renal function impairment, bronchial asthma, cardiogenic shock, congestive heart failure, diabetes mellitus, emphysema or nonallergenic bronchitis, history of allergy, hyperthyroidism, hypotension, mental depression, overt cardiac failure, second or third degree AV block, or sinus bradycardia

**Proper use of this medication**
   Possible need for control of weight and diet, especially sodium intake
» Compliance with therapy; patient may not experience symptoms of hypertension; importance of taking medication only as directed and keeping appointments with physician, even if feeling well
» Does not cure, but helps control hypertension; possible need for life-long therapy; serious consequences of untreated hypertension

   Proper administration of extended-release dosage forms: Swallowing whole without crushing, breaking, or chewing
   Getting into habit of taking at same time each day to help increase compliance
   Checking pulse as directed (checking with physician if less than 50 beats per minute)
   Diuretic effects of the medication and timing of doses to minimize inconvenience of diuresis
» Importance of not missing doses, especially with schedules of one dose per day
» Proper dosing
   Missed dose: Taking as soon as possible; not taking at all if within 4 hours of next scheduled dose (8 hours for atenolol and chlorthalidone, nadolol and bendroflumethiazide, or extended-release propranolol and hydrochlorothiazide); not doubling doses
» Proper storage

**Precautions while using this medication**
   Regular visits to physician to check progress
» Checking with physician before discontinuing medication; gradual dosage reduction may be necessary
   Having enough medication on hand to get through weekends, holidays, and vacations; possibly carrying second written prescription for emergency use
   Carrying medical identification during therapy
» Not taking other medications, especially nonprescription sympathomimetics, unless discussed with physician
» Caution if any kind of surgery (including dental surgery) or emergency treatment is required
» Diabetics: May mask signs and symptoms of hypoglycemia or cause increased blood glucose concentrations
» Possibility of hypokalemia; possible need for additional potassium in diet; not changing diet without first checking with physician
   To prevent dehydration, checking with physician if severe nausea, vomiting, or diarrhea occurs and continues
» Caution when driving or doing things requiring alertness, because of possible drowsiness, dizziness, or lightheadedness
   Caution during exposure to cold weather because of possible increased sensitivity to cold
   Possible skin photosensitivity; avoiding unprotected exposure to sun; using protective clothing and sun block product; avoiding use of sunlamp, tanning bed, or tanning booth
   Caution if any laboratory tests required; possible interference with test results
   Patients with allergies to foods, medications, or stinging insect venom: Possible increase in severity of allergic reactions; checking with physician immediately if severe allergic reaction occurs

**Side/adverse effects**
Signs of potential side effects, especially electrolyte imbalance, bradycardia, bronchospasm, congestive heart failure, mental depression, reduced peripheral circulation, allergic reaction, arrhythmias, agranulocytosis, back pain, joint pain, chest pain, cholecystitis, pancreatitis, confusion (especially in elderly), hallucinations, hepatotoxicity, hyperuricemia, gout, leukopenia, psoriasiform eruption, and thrombocytopenia

---

### *ATENOLOL AND CHLORTHALIDONE*

## Oral Dosage Forms

### ATENOLOL AND CHLORTHALIDONE TABLETS

**Usual adult dose**
Antihypertensive—
   Oral, 1 or 2 tablets once a day, as determined by individual titration with the component agents.

Note: Geriatric patients may have increased or decreased sensitivity to the effects of the usual adult dose.

**Usual pediatric dose**
Dosage has not been established.

**Strength(s) usually available**
U.S.—
   50 mg of atenolol and 25 mg of chlorthalidone (Rx) [*Tenoretic* (scored); GENERIC].

100 mg of atenolol and 25 mg of chlorthalidone (Rx) [*Tenoretic;* GENERIC].

Canada—
    50 mg of atenolol and 25 mg of chlorthalidone (Rx) [*Tenoretic* (scored)].
    100 mg of atenolol and 25 mg of chlorthalidone (Rx) [*Tenoretic* (scored)].

**Auxiliary labeling**
• Do not take other medicines without your doctor's advice.

---

### BISOPROLOL AND HYDROCHLOROTHIAZIDE

## Oral Dosage Forms
### BISOPROLOL FUMARATE AND HYDROCHLOROTHIAZIDE TABLETS

**Usual adult dose**
Antihypertensive—
    Oral, 1 or 2 tablets once a day, as determined by individual titration with the component agents.

Note: Geriatric patients may have increased or decreased sensitivity to the effects of the usual adult dose.

**Usual pediatric dose**
Dosage has not been established.

**Strength(s) usually available**
U.S.—
    2.5 mg of bisoprolol and 6.25 mg of hydrochlorothiazide (Rx) [*Ziac*].
    5 mg of bisoprolol and 6.25 mg of hydrochlorothiazide (Rx) [*Ziac*].
    10 mg of bisoprolol and 6.25 mg of hydrochlorothiazide (Rx) [*Ziac*].
Canada—
    Not commercially available.

**Auxiliary labeling**
• Do not take other medicine without your doctor's advice.

---

### METOPROLOL AND HYDROCHLOROTHIAZIDE

## Oral Dosage Forms
### METOPROLOL TARTRATE AND HYDROCHLOROTHIAZIDE TABLETS USP

**Usual adult dose**
Antihypertensive—
    Oral, 1 or 2 tablets a day, as a single dose or in divided doses, as determined by individual titration with the component agents.

Note: Geriatric patients may have increased or decreased sensitivity to the effects of the usual adult dose.

**Usual pediatric dose**
Dosage has not been established.

**Strength(s) usually available**
U.S.—
    50 mg of metoprolol tartrate and 25 mg of hydrochlorothiazide (Rx) [*Lopressor HCT* (scored; lactose)].
    100 mg of metoprolol tartrate and 25 mg of hydrochlorothiazide (Rx) [*Lopressor HCT* (scored; lactose)].
    100 mg of metoprolol tartrate and 50 mg of hydrochlorothiazide (Rx) [*Lopressor HCT* (scored; lactose)].
Canada—
    Not commercially available.

**Auxiliary labeling**
• Do not take other medicines without your doctor's advice.

---

### NADOLOL AND BENDROFLUMETHIAZIDE

## Oral Dosage Forms
### NADOLOL AND BENDROFLUMETHIAZIDE TABLETS USP

**Usual adult dose**
Antihypertensive—
    Oral, 1 tablet once a day, as determined by individual titration with the component agents.

Note: Geriatric patients may have increased or decreased sensitivity to the effects of the usual adult dose.

**Usual pediatric dose**
Dosage has not been established.

**Strength(s) usually available**
U.S.—
    40 mg of nadolol and 5 mg of bendroflumethiazide (Rx) [*Corzide* (scored; lactose)].
    80 mg of nadolol and 5 mg of bendroflumethiazide (Rx) [*Corzide* (scored; lactose)].
Canada—
    40 mg of nadolol and 5 mg of bendroflumethiazide (Rx) [*Corzide* (scored)].
    80 mg of nadolol and 5 mg of bendroflumethiazide (Rx) [*Corzide* (scored)].

**Auxiliary labeling**
• Do not take other medicines without your doctor's advice.

---

### PINDOLOL AND HYDROCHLOROTHIAZIDE

## Oral Dosage Forms
### PINDOLOL AND HYDROCHLOROTHIAZIDE TABLETS

**Usual adult dose**
Antihypertensive—
    Oral, 1 or 2 tablets once a day, as determined by individual titration with the component agents.

Note: Geriatric patients may have increased or decreased sensitivity to the effects of the usual adult dose.

**Usual pediatric dose**
Dosage has not been established.

**Strength(s) usually available**
U.S.—
    Not commercially available.
Canada—
    10 mg of pindolol and 25 mg of hydrochlorothiazide (Rx) [*Viskazide*].
    10 mg of pindolol and 50 mg of hydrochlorothiazide (Rx) [*Viskazide*].

**Auxiliary labeling**
• Do not take other medicines without your doctor's advice.

---

### PROPRANOLOL AND HYDROCHLOROTHIAZIDE

## Oral Dosage Forms
### PROPRANOLOL HYDROCHLORIDE AND HYDROCHLOROTHIAZIDE EXTENDED-RELEASE CAPSULES USP

**Usual adult dose**
Antihypertensive—
    Oral, 1 capsule a day, as determined by individual titration with the component agents.

Note: Geriatric patients may have increased or decreased sensitivity to the effects of the usual adult dose.

**Usual pediatric dose**
Dosage has not been established.

**Strength(s) usually available**
U.S.—
    80 mg of propranolol hydrochloride and 50 mg of hydrochlorothiazide (Rx) [*Inderide LA* (lactose)].
    120 mg of propranolol hydrochloride and 50 mg of hydrochlorothiazide (Rx) [*Inderide LA* (lactose)].
    160 mg of propranolol hydrochloride and 50 mg of hydrochlorothiazide (Rx) [*Inderide LA* (lactose)].
Canada—
    Not commercially available.

**Auxiliary labeling**
• Do not take other medicines without your doctor's advice.

### PROPRANOLOL HYDROCHLORIDE AND HYDROCHLOROTHIAZIDE TABLETS USP

**Usual adult dose**
Antihypertensive—
    Oral, 1 or 2 tablets two times a day, as determined by individual titration with the component agents.

Note: Geriatric patients may have increased or decreased sensitivity to the effects of the usual adult dose.

**Usual pediatric dose**
Dosage has not been established.

**Strength(s) usually available**
U.S.—

40 mg of propranolol hydrochloride and 25 mg of hydrochlorothiazide (Rx) [*Inderide* (scored); GENERIC (may be scored)].

80 mg of propranolol hydrochloride and 25 mg of hydrochlorothiazide (Rx) [*Inderide* (scored); GENERIC (may be scored)].

Canada—

40 mg of propranolol hydrochloride and 25 mg of hydrochlorothiazide (Rx) [*Inderide* (scored)].

80 mg of propranolol hydrochloride and 25 mg of hydrochlorothiazide (Rx) [*Inderide* (scored)].

**Auxiliary labeling**
• Do not take other medicines without your doctor's advice.

---

### TIMOLOL AND HYDROCHLOROTHIAZIDE

## Oral Dosage Forms

### TIMOLOL MALEATE AND HYDROCHLOROTHIAZIDE TABLETS USP

**Usual adult dose**
Antihypertensive—
Oral, 1 tablet two times a day or 2 tablets once a day, as determined by individual titration with the component agents.

Note: Geriatric patients may have increased or decreased sensitivity to the effects of the usual adult dose.

**Usual pediatric dose**
Dosage has not been established.

**Strength(s) usually available**
U.S.—

10 mg of timolol maleate and 25 mg of hydrochlorothiazide (Rx) [*Timolide*].

Canada—

10 mg of timolol maleate and 25 mg of hydrochlorothiazide (Rx) [*Timolide*].

**Auxiliary labeling**
• Do not take other medicine without your doctor's advice.

Revised: 08/23/94

---

# BETA-CAROTENE   Systemic

VA CLASSIFICATION (Primary/Secondary): VT050/DE890

Note: For a listing of dosage forms and brand names by country availability, see *Dosage Forms* section(s). For a listing of brand names for the articles in this monograph, refer to the General Index.

---

## Category

Nutritional supplement (vitamin); photosensitivity reaction suppressant in erythropoietic protoporphyria; polymorphous light eruption suppressant.

Note: Beta-carotene is a precursor to a fat-soluble vitamin.

## Indications

Note: Bracketed information in the *Indications* section refers to uses that are not included in U.S. product labeling.

**Accepted**
Vitamin deficiency (prophylaxis and treatment)—Beta-carotene is indicated for prevention or treatment of vitamin A deficiency states. Vitamin A deficiency may occur as a result of inadequate nutrition or intestinal malabsorption but does not occur in healthy individuals receiving an adequate balanced diet. For prophylaxis of beta-carotene or vitamin A deficiency, dietary improvement, rather than supplementation, is advisable. For treatment of beta-carotene or vitamin A deficiency, supplementation is preferred.

Deficiency of vitamin A may lead to keratomalacia, xerophthalmia, and nyctalopia (night blindness).

Recommended intakes may be increased and/or supplementation may be necessary in the following conditions (based on documented beta-carotene or vitamin A deficiency):
Fat malabsorption (steatorrhea)
Fever, chronic
Hepatic-biliary tract disease—hepatic function impairment, cirrhosis, obstructive jaundice
Infection, prolonged
Malabsorption syndromes associated with pancreatic insufficiency—pancreatic disease, cystic fibrosis
Protein deficiency, severe

Some unusual diets (e.g., reducing diets that drastically restrict food selection) may not supply minimum daily requirements of vitamin A. Supplementation is necessary in patients receiving total parenteral nutrition (TPN) or undergoing rapid weight loss or in those with malnutrition, because of inadequate dietary intake.

Recommended intakes for all vitamins and most minerals are increased during pregnancy. Many physicians recommend that pregnant women receive multivitamin and mineral supplements, especially those pregnant women who do not consume an adequate diet and those in high-

risk categories (i.e., women carrying more than one fetus, heavy cigarette smokers, and alcohol and drug abusers). Taking excessive amounts of a multivitamin and mineral supplement may be harmful to the mother and/or fetus and should be avoided.

Recommended intakes for all vitamins and most minerals are increased during breast-feeding.

Recommended intakes may be increased by the following medications: Cholestyramine, colestipol, mineral oil, and neomycin.

Photosensitivity reactions in erythropoietic protoporphyria (prophylaxis and treatment)—Beta-carotene is indicated to reduce the severity of photosensitivity reactions in patients with erythropoietic protoporphyria (EPP).

[Polymorphous light eruption (prophylaxis and treatment)][1]—Beta-carotene is used in the prophylaxis and treatment of severe cases of polymorphous light eruption.

**Acceptance not established**
There are insufficient data to show that beta-carotene may reduce the occurrence of certain types of *cancer*.

**Unaccepted**
Beta-carotene has not been proven effective as a sunscreen.

---

[1]Not included in Canadian product labeling.

## Pharmacology/Pharmacokinetics

**Mechanism of action/Effect**
Nutritional supplement—Beta-carotene is a precursor to vitamin A which is essential for normal function of the retina; in the form of retinal, it combines with opsin (red pigment in the retina) to form rhodopsin (visual purple), which is necessary for visual adaptation to darkness. Other forms (retinol, retinoic acid) are necessary for growth of bone, testicular and ovarian function, and embryonic development, and for regulation of growth and differentiation of epithelial tissues; may act as a cofactor in biochemical reactions.

Photosensitivity reaction—Beta-carotene quenches singlet oxygen and free radicals that are generated when porphyrin is exposed to light and air.

**Absorption**
Absorption of beta-carotene depends on the presence of dietary fat and bile in the intestinal tract.

**Storage**
Unchanged beta-carotene is stored in various tissues, primarily fat tissues and adrenals. Small amounts are stored in the liver.

**Biotransformation**
Approximately 50 to 60% of beta-carotene is metabolized to retinaldehyde and then converted to retinol, primarily in the intestinal tract. A small amount of beta-carotene is converted to vitamin A in the liver. The

conversion of beta-carotene to vitamin A diminishes inversely to the intake of beta-carotene, as long as the dosages are higher than 1 to 2 times the daily requirements. High doses of beta-carotene do not lead to toxicity or abnormally high serum concentrations of vitamin A.

**Elimination**
Primarily fecal.

# Precautions to Consider

**Mutagenicity**
*In vitro* and *in vivo* mutagenicity studies were negative.

**Pregnancy/Reproduction**
Fertility—No problems with fertility have been documented in women taking up to 30 mg of beta-carotene a day. The effects of doses greater than 30 mg a day are not known.

Beta-carotene did not effect fertility in male rats at doses of up to 100 times the recommended human dose.

Pregnancy—Beta-carotene crosses the placenta. Adequate and well-controlled studies in humans have not been done. However, no problems with pregnancy have been documented in women taking up to 30 mg of beta-carotene a day. The effects of doses greater than 30 mg a day are not known.

Studies in rats at doses 300 to 400 times the recommended human dose have shown that beta-carotene causes an increase in resorption rate. No increase in resorption rate was noted in rats receiving 75 times the recommended human dose or less.

FDA Pregnancy Category C.

**Breast-feeding**
It is not known whether beta-carotene is distributed into breast milk. However, problems in humans have not been documented with intake of normal daily recommended amounts.

**Pediatrics**
Problems in pediatrics have not been documented with intake of normal daily recommended amounts.

**Geriatrics**
Problems in geriatrics have not been documented with intake of normal daily recommended amounts.

**Drug interactions and/or related problems**
The following drug interactions and/or related problems have been selected on the basis of their potential clinical significance (possible mechanism in parentheses where appropriate)—not necessarily inclusive (» = major clinical significance):

Note: Combinations containing any of the following, depending on the amount present, may also interact with beta-carotene.

Cholestyramine or
Colestipol or
Mineral oil or
Neomycin
(concurrent use may interfere with the absorption of beta-carotene; requirements for beta-carotene may be increased in patients receiving these medications)

Vitamin A
(for vitamin A deficiency, beta-carotene should fulfill normal vitamin A requirements; additional vitamin A supplementation may not be necessary)

Vitamin E
(concurrent use of vitamin E may facilitate absorption and utilization of beta-carotene and may reduce toxicity of vitamin A)

**Medical considerations/Contraindications**
The medical considerations/contraindications included here have been selected on the basis of their potential clinical significance (reasons given in parentheses where appropriate)—not necessarily inclusive (» = major clinical significance).

*Risk-benefit should be considered when the following medical problems exist:*
Hepatic function impairment or
Renal impairment
(may lead to an increase of serum beta-carotene concentrations)
Hypervitaminosis A
Sensitivity to beta-carotene

**Patient monitoring**
The following may be especially important in patient monitoring (other tests may be warranted in some patients, depending on condition; » = major clinical significance):

Beta-carotene concentrations, plasma and
Vitamin A concentrations, plasma
(determinations recommended to confirm deficiency; plasma vitamin A concentrations are not necessarily indicative of vitamin A nutritional status because of significant hepatic storage, although low concentrations correlate with deficiency)

# Side/Adverse Effects

The following side/adverse effects have been selected on the basis of their potential clinical significance (possible signs and symptoms in parentheses where appropriate)—not necessarily inclusive:

**Those indicating need for medical attention only if they continue or are bothersome**
Incidence more frequent
*Carotenodermia* (yellowing of palms, hands, or soles of feet, and to a lesser extent the face)—develops after 2 to 6 weeks of therapy
Incidence rare
*Arthralgia* (joint pain); *diarrhea; dizziness; ecchymoses* (unusual bleeding or bruising)

# Patient Consultation

As an aid to patient consultation, refer to *Advice for the Patient, Beta-carotene—For Dietary Supplement (Vitamin) (Systemic)* and *Beta-carotene—For Photosensitivity (Systemic)*.

In providing consultation, consider emphasizing the following selected information (» = major clinical significance):

**Description of use**
Description should include function in the body; indications for use; signs of deficiency; conditions that may cause deficiency; and unproven uses

**Importance of diet**
*For use as a dietary supplement*
Importance of proper nutrition; supplement may be needed because of inadequate dietary intake
Food sources of beta-carotene; effects of processing
Not using vitamins as substitute for balanced diet

**Before using this medication**
» Conditions affecting use, especially:
Sensitivity to beta-carotene

**Proper use of this medication**
*For use as a dietary supplement*
» Proper dosing
Function of beta-carotene in body
Missed dose: No cause for concern because of length of time necessary for depletion; remembering to take as directed

*For use in photosensitivity*
» Proper dosing
Missed dose: Taking as soon as possible; not taking if almost time for next dose; not doubling doses
» Proper storage

**Side/adverse effects**
Yellow discoloration of skin is to be expected; if taking as nutritional supplement, may be a sign that the dose is too high

# General Dosing Information

Because of the infrequency of beta-carotene or vitamin A deficiency alone, combinations of several vitamins are commonly administered. Many commercial vitamin complexes are available.

Therapy as a nutritional supplement may be discontinued when liver storage of vitamin A is determined to be adequate.

**Diet/Nutrition**
Although most manufacturers still label their beta-carotene products in terms of Units (U) of vitamin A activity, the preferred way of designating activity is in retinol equivalents (RE). Six micrograms of beta-carotene is equivalent to 1 RE and 10 Units of vitamin A activity.

The best dietary sources of beta-carotene include carrots; dark green leafy vegetables, such as spinach; green leafy lettuce; tomatoes; sweet potatoes; broccoli; cantaloupe; and winter squash. Ordinary cooking does not destroy beta-carotene.

# Oral Dosage Forms

Note: Bracketed uses in the *Dosage Forms* section refer to categories of use and/or indications that are not included in U.S. product labeling.

## BETA-CAROTENE CAPSULES USP

**Usual adults and adolescents dose**
Deficiency (prophylaxis)—
Oral, 1000 to 2500 RE (the equivalent of 10,000 to 25,000 Units of vitamin A activity or 6 to 15 mg of beta-carotene) per day.
Deficiency (treatment)—
Oral, 2500 to 10,000 RE (the equivalent of 25,000 to 100,000 Units of vitamin A activity or 15 to 60 mg of beta-carotene) per day.
Photosensitivity reaction suppressant—
Oral, 5000 to 50,000 RE (the equivalent of 50,000 to 500,000 Units of vitamin A activity or 30 to 300 mg of beta-carotene) per day.
[Polymorphous light eruption suppressant][1]—
Oral, 12,500 to 30,000 RE (the equivalent of 125,000 to 300,000 Units of vitamin A activity or 75 to 180 mg of beta-carotene) per day.

**Usual pediatric dose**
Deficiency (prophylaxis)—
Oral, 500 to 1000 RE (the equivalent of 5000 to 10,000 Units vitamin A activity or 3 to 6 mg of beta-carotene) per day.
Deficiency (treatment)—
Oral, 1000 to 2000 RE (the equivalent of 10,000 to 20,000 Units of vitamin A activity or 6 to 12 mg of beta-carotene) per day.
Photosensitivity reaction suppressant or
[Polymorphous light eruption suppressant][1]—
Oral, 5000 to 25,000 RE (the equivalent of 50,000 to 250,000 Units of vitamin A activity or 30 to 150 mg of beta-carotene) per day.

**Strength(s) usually available**
U.S.—
10,000 Units of vitamin A activity (6 mg of beta-carotene) (OTC) [GENERIC].
25,000 Units of vitamin A activity (15 mg of beta-carotene) (OTC) [*Max-Caro; Provatene;* GENERIC].
50,000 Units of vitamin A activity (30 mg of beta-carotene) (Rx) [*Solatene*].
Canada—
10,000 Units of vitamin A activity (6 mg of beta-carotene) (OTC) [GENERIC].
25,000 Units of vitamin A activity (15 mg of beta-carotene) (OTC) [GENERIC].
Note: Some strengths of these beta-carotene preparations may exceed the dosage range recommended by USP DI Advisory Panels based on the amount necessary to meet normal nutritional needs.

**Packaging and storage**
Store below 40 °C (104 °F), preferably between 15 and 30 °C (59 and 86 °F), unless otherwise specified by manufacturer.

## BETA-CAROTENE TABLETS

**Usual adult and adolescent dose**
See *Beta-carotene Capsules USP.*

**Usual pediatric dose**
See *Beta-carotene Capsules USP.*

**Strength(s) usually available**
U.S.—
10,000 Units of vitamin A activity (6 mg of beta-carotene) (OTC) [GENERIC].
25,000 Units of vitamin A activity (15 mg of beta-carotene) (OTC) [GENERIC].
Canada—
25,000 Units of vitamin A activity (15 mg of beta-carotene) (OTC) [GENERIC].
Note: Some strengths of these beta-carotene preparations may exceed the dosage range recommended by USP DI Advisory Panels based on the amount necessary to meet normal nutritional needs.

**Packaging and storage**
Store below 40 °C (104 °F), preferably between 15 and 30 °C (59 and 86 °F), unless otherwise specified by manufacturer.

## BETA-CAROTENE CHEWABLE TABLETS

**Usual adult and adolescent dose**
See *Beta-carotene Capsules USP.*

**Usual pediatric dose**
See *Beta-carotene Capsules USP.*

**Strength(s) usually available**
U.S.—
Not commercially available.
Canada—
5000 Units of vitamin A activity (3 mg of beta-carotene) (OTC) [GENERIC].

**Packaging and storage**
Store below 40 °C (104 °F), preferably between 15 and 30 °C (59 and 86 °F), unless otherwise specified by manufacturer.

[1]Not included in Canadian product labeling.

Revised: 11/27/91
Interim revision: 05/11/92; 08/15/94; 05/01/95

**BETAMETHASONE**—See *Corticosteroids—Glucocorticoid Effects (Systemic); Corticosteroids (Ophthalmic); Corticosteroids (Otic); Corticosteroids (Topical)*

**BETAMETHASONE-CONTAINING COMBINATIONS**—
Clotrimazole and Betamethasone (Topical)

**BETAXOLOL**—See *Beta-adrenergic Blocking Agents (Ophthalmic); Beta-adrenergic Blocking Agents (Systemic)*

# BETHANECHOL   Systemic

VA CLASSIFICATION (Primary): AU300
Note: For a listing of dosage forms and brand names by country availability, see *Dosage Forms* section(s). For a listing of brand names for the articles in this monograph, refer to the General Index.

## Category
Cholinergic.

## Indications
Note: Bracketed information in the *Indications* section refers to uses that are not included in U.S. product labeling.

**Accepted**
Urinary retention (treatment)—Although it generally has been replaced by more effective agents, bethanechol is indicated for the treatment of acute postoperative nonobstructive urinary retention and for neurogenic atony of the urinary bladder with retention.

[Atony, postoperative, gastric (treatment)][1] or
[Megacolon, congenital (treatment)][1]—Bethanechol is used in certain cases of gastric atony or stasis, and is also used in selected cases of congenital megacolon.

[Reflux, gastroesophageal (treatment)]—Oral bethanechol is used for treatment of gastroesophageal reflux associated with decreased pressure of the lower esophageal sphincter.

[1]Not included in Canadian product labeling.

## Pharmacology/Pharmacokinetics

**Physicochemical characteristics**
Molecular weight—196.68.

**Mechanism of action/Effect**

Bethanechol is a muscarinic cholinomimetic, which acts at cholinergic receptors in the smooth muscle of the urinary bladder and gastrointestinal tract. It increases the tone of the detrusor urinae muscle, producing an increase in the intravesical pressure. It may initiate micturition and empty the bladder; however, its clinical effectiveness in such conditions as voiding dysfunction has not been fully established. It also stimulates gastric and intestinal motility, and increases lower esophageal sphincter pressure.

**Other actions/effects**

Following oral or subcutaneous administration, cardiovascular effects and nicotinic activity are minimal.

**Onset of action**

Oral–Within 30 to 90 minutes.
Subcutaneous–Within 5 to 15 minutes.

**Time to peak effect**

Oral–About 1 hour.
Subcutaneous–Within 15 to 30 minutes.

**Duration of action**

Oral—Up to 6 hours, depending on dose.
Subcutaneous—About 2 hours.

## Precautions to Consider

### Pregnancy/Reproduction

Pregnancy—Adequate and well-controlled studies in humans have not been done.

Studies have not been done in animals.

FDA Pregnancy Category C.

### Breast-feeding

It is not known whether bethanechol is distributed into breast milk.

### Pediatrics

Appropriate studies on the relationship of age to the effects of bethanechol have not been performed in the pediatric population. However, no pediatrics-specific problems have been documented to date.

### Geriatrics

Appropriate studies on the relationship of age to the effects of bethanechol have not been performed in the geriatric population. However, geriatric-specific problems that would limit the usefulness of this medication in the elderly are not expected.

### Drug interactions and/or related problems

The following drug interactions and/or related problems have been selected on the basis of their potential clinical significance (possible mechanism in parentheses where appropriate)—not necessarily inclusive (» = major clinical significance):

Note: Combinations containing any of the following medications, depending on the amount present, may also interact with this medication.

Cholinergics, other, especially cholinesterase inhibitors
   (concurrent use may increase the effects of either these medications or bethanechol and increase the potential for toxicity)

Ganglionic blocking agents, such as mecamylamine, pentolinium, and trimethaphan
   (concurrent use with bethanechol may produce a critical fall in blood pressure, which is usually preceded by severe abdominal symptoms)

Procainamide or
Quinidine
   (concurrent use may antagonize the cholinergic effects of bethanechol)

### Laboratory value alterations

The following have been selected on the basis of their potential clinical significance (possible effect in parentheses where appropriate)—not necessarily inclusive (» = major clinical significance):

With physiology/laboratory test values
   Amylase, serum, and
   Lipase, serum
      (concentrations may be increased because bethanechol stimulates pancreatic secretion and constricts the sphincter of Oddi)

   Aspartate aminotransferase, serum (AST [SGOT])
      (concentrations may be increased because bethanechol impairs excretion by causing contractions in the sphincter of Oddi)

### Medical considerations/Contraindications

The medical considerations/contraindications included here have been selected on the basis of their potential clinical significance (reasons given in parentheses where appropriate)—not necessarily inclusive (» = major clinical significance).

***Risk-benefit should be considered when the following medical problems exist:***

» Asthma, bronchial, active or latent
   (bethanechol may cause bronchospasm and may precipitate asthmatic attack)

   Atrioventricular conduction defects
   (bethanechol may aggravate this condition by decreasing the rate of conduction)

» Bradycardia, pronounced
   (bethanechol slows heart rate and may exacerbate the condition)

» Hypotension
   (bethanechol may reduce blood pressure)

» Conditions in which increased muscular activity of the gastrointestinal tract or urinary bladder might be harmful, such as:
   Anastomosis
   Bladder surgery, recent
   Gastrointestinal resection

» Conditions in which strength or integrity of gastrointestinal or bladder wall is questionable or

» Gastrointestinal obstruction or
   Urinary tract obstruction
   (increased muscular activity of the gastrointestinal tract or urinary bladder may be harmful)

» Coronary artery disease, especially occlusion
   (bethanechol may decrease coronary blood flow)

   Epilepsy
   (although no causal relationship has been established, seizures have been reported in patients receiving bethanechol)

   Hypertension
   (bethanechol may cause sudden fall in blood pressure)

» Hyperthyroidism
   (risk of atrial fibrillation may be increased)

» Peptic ulcer
   (bethanechol may aggravate symptoms probably by increasing acid secretion and/or by increasing gastric motility)

   Parkinsonism or
   Vagotonia, marked
   (bethanechol may exacerbate these conditions)

» Peritonitis
   (bethanechol may increase cramping and exacerbate the condition and increase patient discomfort)

   Sensitivity to bethanechol

## Side/Adverse Effects

Note: In addition to those side/adverse effects needing medical attention listed below, other severe symptoms of cholinergic overstimulation such as circulatory collapse, hypotension, bloody diarrhea, shock, or sudden cardiac arrest are likely to occur in cases of hypersensitivity or overdosage, and may occur rarely after subcutaneous administration.

The following side/adverse effects have been selected on the basis of their potential clinical significance (possible signs and symptoms in parentheses where appropriate)—not necessarily inclusive:

**Those indicating need for medical attention**

Incidence rare—more frequent with subcutaneous injection
   *Shortness of breath, wheezing, or tightness in chest, especially in patients with predisposition to bronchoconstriction*

**Those indicating need for medical attention only if they continue or are bothersome**

Incidence less frequent or rare—more frequent with subcutaneous injection
   *Belching; blurred vision or change in near or distance vision; diarrhea; frequent urge to urinate*

With high doses
   *CNS stimulation* (sleeplessness, nervousness, or jitters); *orthostatic hypotension* (dizziness or lightheadedness; feeling faint); *parasympathetic stimulation* (headache; increased salivation or sweating; nausea or vomiting; redness or flushing of skin or feeling of warmth; stomach discomfort or pain); *seizures*

## Overdose

For specific information on the agents used in the management of bethanechol overdose, see:
   • *Atropine* in *Anticholinergics/Antispasmodics monograph.*

For more information on the management of overdose or unintentional ingestion, **contact a Poison Control Center** (see *Poison Contol Center Listing*).

### Treatment of overdose
Specific treatment—
Treatment consists of subcutaneous administration of atropine in doses of 500 mcg (0.5 mg) to 1 mg for adults and 10 mcg (0.01 mg) per kg of body weight for infants and children, repeated as needed every 2 hours. In emergencies, intravenous injection of atropine may be used to counteract severe toxic cardiovascular or bronchoconstrictor effects of bethanechol.

## Patient Consultation

As an aid to patient consultation, refer to *Advice for the Patient, Bethanechol (Systemic)*.

In providing consultation, consider emphasizing the following selected information (» = major clinical significance):

### Before using this medication
» Conditions affecting use, especially:
  Sensitivity to bethanechol
  Other medical problems, especially anastomosis, recent bladder surgery or gastrointestinal resection; asthma; pronounced bradycardia or hypotension; coronary artery disease; hyperthyroidism; peptic ulcer; peritonitis; or conditions in which the strength or integrity of the gastrointestinal or bladder wall is in question or in the presence of mechanical obstruction; or marked vagotonia

### Proper use of this medication
» Taking medication on an empty stomach to minimize the possibility of nausea and vomiting, unless otherwise directed by physician
» Importance of not taking more medication than the amount prescribed
» Proper dosing
  Missed dose: Taking if remembered within an hour or so; not taking if remembered after 2 or more hours; not doubling doses
» Proper storage

### Precautions while using this medication
Caution when getting up suddenly from a lying or sitting position

### Side/adverse effects
Signs of potential side effects, especially shortness of breath, wheezing, or tightness in chest

## General Dosing Information

### For oral dosage forms only
Preferably, bethanechol should be taken on an empty stomach to minimize the possibility of nausea and vomiting.

### For parenteral dosage forms only
Bethanechol injection is for subcutaneous use *only*. It should *not* be given intravenously or intramuscularly because severe symptoms of cholinergic overstimulation may occur, and the selectivity of bethanechol's action may be decreased.

After administration of bethanechol, the patient should be observed for 30 minutes to 1 hour for possible severe reactions, and a syringe containing a dose of atropine should be immediately available during this period.

## Oral Dosage Forms

Note: Bracketed uses in the *Dosage Forms* section refer to categories of use and/or indications that are not included in U.S. product labeling.

### BETHANECHOL CHLORIDE TABLETS USP

**Usual adult and adolescent dose**
Cholinergic—
Oral, 25 to 50 mg three or four times a day.

Note: The minimum effective dose may be determined by administering 5 or 10 mg initially and repeating the same dose at one- to two-

hour intervals until a satisfactory response is obtained or up to a maximum of 50 mg; or by administering 10 mg initially, and repeating with 25 mg and then 50 mg at six-hour intervals until the desired response is obtained.
[Treatment of gastroesophageal reflux]—
Oral, 10 to 25 mg four times a day, after meals and at bedtime.

**Usual pediatric dose**
Cholinergic—
Oral, 0.6 mg per kg of body weight a day in 3 or 4 divided doses.
[Treatment of gastroesophageal reflux]—
Oral, 0.4 mg per kg of body weight a day in 4 divided doses or 3 mg per square meter of body surface every eight hours.

**Usual geriatric dose**
See *Usual adult and adolescent dose.*

**Strength(s) usually available**
U.S.—
5 mg (Rx) [*Urabeth; Urecholine;* GENERIC (may be scored)].
10 mg (Rx) [*Duvoid* (scored); *Urabeth; Urecholine* (scored); GENERIC (may be scored)].
25 mg (Rx) [*Duvoid* (scored); *Urabeth; Urecholine* (scored); GENERIC (may be scored)].
50 mg (Rx) [*Duvoid* (scored); *Urabeth; Urecholine* (scored); GENERIC (may be scored)].
Canada—
10 mg (Rx) [*Duvoid* (scored); *Urecholine* (scored)].
25 mg (Rx) [*Duvoid* (scored); *Urecholine* (scored)].
50 mg (Rx) [*Duvoid* (scored)].

**Packaging and storage**
Store below 40 °C (104 °F), preferably between 15 and 30 °C (59 and 86 °F), unless otherwise specified by manufacturer. Store in a tight container.

## Parenteral Dosage Forms
### BETHANECHOL CHLORIDE INJECTION USP

**Usual adult and adolescent dose**
Cholinergic—
Subcutaneous, 5 mg three or four times a day as needed.
Note: The minimum effective dose may be determined by administering 2.5 mg initially and repeating the same dose at 15- to 30-minute intervals up to a maximum of four doses until a satisfactory response is obtained.
Single doses of 10 mg may be required. However, such a large dose may cause severe side effects and should be used only after single doses of 2.5 to 5 mg have proven to be ineffective.

**Usual pediatric dose**
Cholinergic—
Subcutaneous, 0.2 mg per kg of body weight a day in 3 or 4 divided doses.

**Usual geriatric dose**
See *Usual adult and adolescent dose.*

**Strength(s) usually available**
U.S.—
5 mg per mL (Rx) [*Urecholine*].
Canada—
5 mg per mL (Rx) [*Urecholine*].

**Packaging and storage**
Store below 40 °C (104 °F), preferably between 15 and 30 °C (59 and 86 °F), unless otherwise specified by manufacturer. Protect from freezing.

**Note**
For subcutaneous use only. Discard unused portion.

Revised: 05/12/93
Interim revision: 06/27/94

# BIOTIN Systemic

VA CLASSIFICATION (Primary): VT109

Other commonly used names are vitamin H, coenzyme R, or vitamin Bw.

Note: For a listing of dosage forms and brand names by country availability, see *Dosage Forms* section(s). For a listing of brand names for the articles in this monograph, refer to the General Index.

## Category

Nutritional supplement (vitamin)

Note: Biotin is a water-soluble B-complex vitamin.

# Indications

## Accepted

Biotin deficiency (prophylaxis and treatment)—The B vitamins are indicated for prevention and treatment of vitamin B deficiency. Vitamin B deficiency may occur as a result of inadequate nutrition or intestinal malabsorption but does not occur in healthy individuals receiving an adequate balanced diet. Simple nutritional deficiency of individual B vitamins is rare since dietary inadequacy usually results in multiple deficiencies. For prophylaxis of biotin deficiency, dietary improvement, rather than supplementation, is advisable. For treatment of biotin deficiency, supplementation is preferred.

Biotin deficiency may lead to dermatitis, alopecia, hypercholesterolemia, and cardiac abnormalities.

Requirements may be increased and/or supplementation may be necessary in the following conditions (based on documented biotin deficiency):
Biotinidase deficiency
Gastrectomy
Seborrheic dermatitis of infancy

Administration of large amounts of the biotin antagonist, avidin, which is found in raw egg whites, has also been found to cause biotin deficiency.

Some unusual diets (e.g., reducing diets that drastically restrict food selection) may not supply minimum daily requirements of biotin. Supplementation may be necessary in patients receiving total parenteral nutrition (TPN) or undergoing rapid weight loss or in those with malnutrition, because of inadequate dietary intake.

## Unaccepted

Biotin has not been proven effective in the treatment of acne, seborrheic eczema, or alopecia.

# Pharmacology/Pharmacokinetics

## Physicochemical characteristics

Molecular weight—244.31.

## Mechanism of action/Effect

Biotin is necessary for the proper functioning of enzymes that transport carboxyl units and fix carbon dioxide, and is required for various metabolic functions, including gluconeogenesis, lipogenesis, fatty acid biosynthesis, propionate metabolism, and catabolism of branched-chain amino acids.

## Absorption

Approximately 50%.

## Protein binding

Primarily to plasma proteins.

## Elimination

Primarily in urine.

# Precautions to Consider

## Pregnancy/Reproduction

Problems in humans have not been documented with intake of normal daily recommended amounts.

## Breast-feeding

Problems in humans have not been documented with intake of normal daily recommended amounts.

## Pediatrics

Problems in humans have not been documented with intake of normal daily recommended amounts.

## Geriatrics

Problems in humans have not been documented with intake of normal daily recommended amounts.

## Patient monitoring

The following may be especially important in patient monitoring (other tests may be warranted in some patients, depending on condition; » = major clinical significance):

Biotin, plasma or urine
(periodic determinations are recommended to assess biotin status)

# Side/Adverse Effects

No side effects have been reported with intakes of biotin as high as 10 mg daily.

# Patient Consultation

As an aid to patient consultation, refer to *Advice for the Patient, Biotin (Systemic).*

In providing consultation, consider emphasizing the following selected information (» = major clinical significance):

## Description of use

Description should include function in the body, signs of deficiency, and unproven uses

## Importance of diet

Importance of proper nutrition; supplement may be needed because of inadequate dietary intake
Food sources of biotin; effects of processing
Not using vitamins as substitute for balanced diet
Recommended daily intake for biotin

## Proper use of this dietary supplement

» Proper dosing
Missed dose: No cause for concern because of length of time necessary for depletion; remembering to take as directed
» Proper storage

# General Dosing Information

Because of the infrequency of single B vitamin deficiencies, combinations are commonly administered. Many commercial combinations of B vitamins are available.

## For parenteral dosage form only

Biotin is available as part of a multivitamin complex. Manufacturers recommend a dose of 60 mcg a day for adults and 20 mcg a day for children, added to a TPN solution.

## Diet/Nutrition

Recommended dietary intakes for biotin are defined differently worldwide.
For U.S.—
The Recommended Dietary Allowances (RDAs) for vitamins and minerals are determined by the Food and Nutrition Board of the National Research Council and are intended to provide adequate nutrition in most healthy persons under usual environmental stresses. In addition, a different designation may be used by the FDA for food and dietary supplement labeling purposes, as with Daily Value (DV), which replaces the previous labeling terminology United States Recommended Daily Allowances (USRDAs).
For Canada—
Recommended Nutrient Intakes (RNIs) for vitamins, minerals, and protein are determined by Health and Welfare in Canada and provide recommended amounts of a specific nutrient while minimizing the risk of chronic diseases.

There is no RDA or RNI established for biotin. Daily recommended intakes for biotin are generally defined as follows—
Infants and children:
Birth to 3 years of age: 10 to 20 mcg.
4 to 6 years of age: 25 mcg.
7 to 10 years of age: 30 mcg.
Adolescents and adults:
30 to 100 mcg.

The best sources of biotin include liver, cauliflower, salmon, carrots, bananas, soy flour cereals, and yeast. Additional biotin is added from synthesis by intestinal microorganisms. Processing and preservation of food reduces its biotin content.

# Oral Dosage Forms

## BIOTIN CAPSULES

### Usual adult and adolescent dose

Deficiency (prophylaxis)—
Oral, amount based on normal daily recommended intakes of 30 to 100 mcg.
Deficiency (treatment)—
Treatment dose is individualized by prescriber based on severity of deficiency.

### Usual pediatric dose

Deficiency (prophylaxis)—
Oral, amount based on normal daily recommended intakes:
Birth to 3 years of age—10 to 20 mcg.
4 to 6 years of age—25 mcg.
7 to 10 years of age—30 mcg.
Deficiency (treatment)—
Treatment dose is individualized by prescriber based on severity of deficiency.

### Strength(s) usually available

U.S.—
1000 mcg (1 mg) (OTC) [GENERIC].

Canada—
    Not commercially available.

Note: The strength of this preparation may exceed the dosage range recommended by USP DI Advisory Panels based on the amount necessary to meet normal nutritional needs.

**Packaging and storage**
Store below 40 °C (104 °F), preferably between 15 and 30 °C (59 and 86 °F), unless otherwise specified by manufacturer.

## BIOTIN TABLETS

**Usual adult and adolescent dose**
See *Biotin Capsules.*

**Usual pediatric dose**
See *Biotin Capsules.*

**Strength(s) usually available**
U.S.—
    300 mcg (0.3 mg) (OTC) [GENERIC].
    400 mcg (0.4 mg) (OTC) [GENERIC].
    600 mcg (0.6 mg) (OTC) [GENERIC].
    800 mcg (0.8 mg) (OTC) [GENERIC].
Canada—
    250 mcg (0.25 mg) (OTC) [GENERIC].

Note: The strength of these preparations may exceed the dosage range recommended by USP DI Advisory Panels based on the amount necessary to meet normal nutritional needs.

**Packaging and storage**
Store below 40 °C (104 °F), preferably between 15 and 30 °C (59 and 86 °F), unless otherwise specified by manufacturer.

Revised: 09/26/91
Interim revision: 06/02/92; 04/25/95

## BIPERIDEN—See *Antidyskinetics (Systemic)*

## BISACODYL—See *Laxatives (Local)*

## BISACODYL-CONTAINING COMBINATIONS—

Bisacodyl and Docusate (Oral-Local)—See *Laxatives (Local)*

# BISMUTH SUBSALICYLATE   Oral-Local

VA CLASSIFICATION (Primary): GA400
Note: For a listing of dosage forms and brand names by country availability, see *Dosage Forms* section(s). For a listing of brand names for the articles in this monograph, refer to the General Index.

## Category

Antidiarrheal (antisecretory); antacid; antiulcer agent.

## Indications

Note: Bracketed information in the *Indications* section refers to uses that are not included in U.S. product labeling.

**Accepted**
Diarrhea (treatment)—Bismuth subsalicylate is indicated for the symptomatic treatment of nonspecific diarrhea.

Gastric distress (treatment)—Bismuth subsalicylate is indicated for the symptomatic relief of upset stomach, including heartburn, acid indigestion, and nausea.

[Traveler's diarrhea (prophylaxis)][1]—Bismuth subsalicylate is used for the prevention of secretory diarrhea produced by enterotoxigenic *Escherichia coli* (traveler's diarrhea) and viral infections.

[Ulcer, duodenal, *Helicobacter pylori*–associated (treatment adjunct)][1] or [Gastritis, *Helicobacter pylori*–associated (treatment adjunct)][1]—Bismuth subsalicylate is used, in combination with oral antibiotic therapy, in the treatment of *Helicobacter pylori*–associated gastritis and duodenal ulcer.

---

[1]Not included in Canadian product labeling.

## Pharmacology/Pharmacokinetics

**Physicochemical characteristics**
Molecular weight—362.09.

**Mechanism of action/Effect**
Antidiarrheal—Exact mechanism has not been determined. Bismuth subsalicylate may exert its antidiarrheal action not only by stimulating absorption of fluid and electrolytes across the intestinal wall (antisecretory action) but also, when hydrolyzed to salicylic acid, by inhibiting synthesis of a prostaglandin responsible for intestinal inflammation and hypermotility. In addition, bismuth subsalicylate binds toxins produced by *Escherichia coli*. Both bismuth subsalicylate and the intestinal reaction products, bismuth oxychloride and bismuth hydroxide, are believed to have bactericidal action.

Antacid—Bismuth has weak antacid properties.

**Absorption**
Following oral administration, absorption of the salicylate component from the small intestine is generally rapid and complete (>90%). In contrast to the salicylate, the amount of bismuth absorbed is negligible (<0.005%).

**Protein binding**
Salicylate—High (to albumin).

**Biotransformation**
Based on *in vitro* dissociation data and *in vivo* animal data, bismuth subsalicylate is believed to be largely hydrolyzed in the stomach to bismuth oxychloride and salicylic acid. In the small intestine, nondissociated bismuth subsalicylate reacts with other anions (bicarbonate and phosphate) to form insoluble bismuth salts. In the colon, nondissociated bismuth subsalicylate and other bismuth salts react with hydrogen sulfide to produce bismuth sulfide, a highly insoluble black salt responsible for the darkening of the stools.

**Elimination**
Bismuth—Fecal (>99% of the bismuth present in an oral dose); renal.
Salicylate—Renal (primarily excreted as free salicylic acid and conjugated metabolites).

## Precautions to Consider

**Cross-sensitivity and/or related problems**
Patients sensitive to salicylates including methyl salicylate (oil of wintergreen), or to other nonsteroidal anti-inflammatory drugs (NSAIDs), may be sensitive to bismuth subsalicylate also.

**Pregnancy/Reproduction**
The occasional use of bismuth subsalicylate during pregnancy is not likely to result in adverse effects on the fetus or newborn; however, based on what is known about salicylates, the following information should be considered with higher doses and longer therapy.

Fertility—Salicylates have caused increased numbers of fetal resorptions in animal studies.

Pregnancy—First trimester: Salicylates readily cross the placenta. Studies in animals have shown that salicylates cause birth defects including fissure of the spine and skull; facial clefts; eye defects; and malformations of the central nervous system (CNS), viscera, and skeleton (especially the vertebrae and ribs). It has been reported that salicylate use during pregnancy may increase the risk of birth defects in humans.

Third trimester: Chronic, high-dose salicylate therapy may result in prolonged gestation, increased risk of postmaturity syndrome (fetal damage or death due to decreased placental function if pregnancy is greatly prolonged), and increased risk of maternal antenatal hemorrhage. Also, ingestion of salicylates during the last 2 weeks of pregnancy may increase the risk of fetal or neonatal hemorrhage. The possibility that regular use late in pregnancy may result in constriction or premature closure of the fetal ductus arteriosus, possibly leading to persistent pulmonary hypertension and heart failure in the neonate, must also be considered.

Labor and delivery—Chronic, high-dose salicylate therapy late in pregnancy may result in prolonged labor, complicated deliveries, and increased risk of maternal or fetal hemorrhage.

**Breast-feeding**
Problems in humans have not been documented. However, salicylate is
distributed into breast milk; with chronic, high-dose use, intake by the
infant may be high enough to cause adverse effects.

**Pediatrics**
In infants and children up to 3 years of age with diarrhea, caution is
recommended because of the risk of fluid and electrolyte loss; these
patients should be referred to a physician.

Pediatric patients, especially those with fever and dehydration, may be
more susceptible to the toxic effects of salicylates.

Although no cases have been documented with the use of bismuth subsalicylate, recent studies indicate that use of aspirin, a salicylate, may
be associated with the development of Reye's syndrome in children
with acute febrile illnesses, especially influenza and varicella. There
is insufficient data to establish an association between the use of non-
aspirin salicylates, such as bismuth subsalicylate, and the occurrence
of Reye's syndrome. However, it is recommended that children and
adolescents who have or are recovering from influenza or varicella not
be given bismuth subsalicylate to treat nausea or vomiting. Since nausea or vomiting could be an early sign of Reye's syndrome, these
patients should be referred to a physician.

Bismuth is more likely to cause impaction in children.

**Geriatrics**
In geriatric patients with diarrhea, caution is recommended because of the
risk of fluid and electrolyte loss; these patients should be referred to
a physician.

Also, elderly patients are more likely to have age-related renal function
impairment, which may increase the risk of salicylate toxicity. Dosage
reduction may be required to prevent accumulation of the medication.

Bismuth is more likely to cause impaction in elderly patients.

**Drug interactions and/or related problems**
The following drug interactions and/or related problems have been selected on the basis of their potential clinical significance (possible
mechanism in parentheses where appropriate)—not necessarily inclusive (» = major clinical significance):

Note: Although significant interactions are unlikely with usual doses of
bismuth subsalicylate in the treatment of diarrhea and for occasional
relief of gastric distress, the higher doses and the longer therapy
used in the prophylaxis of traveler's diarrhea increase the potential
for significant drug interactions.

Combinations containing any of the following medications, depending on the amount present, may also interact with this
medication.

» Anticoagulants, coumarin- or indandione-derivative or
» Heparin or
» Thrombolytic agents, such as:
   Alteplase (tissue-type plasminogen activator, recombinant)
   Anistreplase
   Streptokinase
   Urokinase
   (increased risk of bleeding may occur when these medications are
   used concurrently with salicylates)
» Antidiabetic agents, oral or
   Insulin
   (large doses of salicylate may enhance the hypoglycemic effect of
   these medications; dosage adjustment may be necessary)
» Probenecid or
» Sulfinpyrazone
   (concurrent use of salicylates is not recommended when these
   medications are used to treat hyperuricemia or gout because uricosuric effects of these medications may be decreased by doses of
   salicylates that produce serum salicylate concentrations above 50
   mcg per mL)
   (probenecid may decrease renal clearance and increase plasma
   concentrations and toxicity of salicylates)
» Salicylates, other
   (ingestion of large repeated doses of bismuth subsalicylate, as for
   traveler's diarrhea, may produce substantial plasma salicylate concentrations thus increasing the risk of salicylate toxicity during
   concurrent use with other salicylates)
» Tetracyclines, oral
   (calcium carbonate contained in the tablet dosage form may decrease gastrointestinal absorption and bioavailability of tetracyclines; patients should be advised not to take bismuth subsalicylate
   tablets within 1 to 3 hours of oral tetracyclines)

**Laboratory value alterations**
The following have been selected on the basis of their potential clinical
significance (possible effect in parentheses where appropriate)—not
necessarily inclusive (» = major clinical significance):

With diagnostic test results
Copper sulfate urine sugar tests
   (false-positive results may occur with chronic use of high doses of
   salicylate)

Gerhardt test for urine aceto-acetic acid
   (may be interfered with because reaction of salicylate with ferric
   chloride produces a reddish color that persists after boiling)

Glucose enzymatic urine sugar tests
   (false-negative results may occur with chronic use of high doses
   of salicylate)

Radiological examination of gastrointestinal tract
   (radiopacity of bismuth may interfere with radiologic examination
   of the gastrointestinal tract)

Serum uric acid determinations
   (falsely increased values may occur with colorimetric assay methods when plasma salicylate concentrations exceed 130 mcg per
   mL; the uricase assay method is not affected)

Thyroid imaging, radionuclide
   (chronic salicylate administration may decrease thyroidal uptake of
   iodide I 131 or of pertechnetate ion because of depressed thyroid
   function; salicylate therapy should be discontinued at least 1 week
   prior to administration of the radiopharmaceutical; however, a rebound effect may occur following discontinuation of salicylate
   therapy, resulting in a period of 3 to 10 days of increased thyroidal
   uptake)

Urine vanillylmandelic acid (VMA) concentrations
   (salicylate may falsely increase or decrease VMA concentrations,
   depending on method used)

With physiology/laboratory test values
Liver function tests, including:
   Serum alanine aminotransferase (ALT [SGPT]) and
   Serum alkaline phosphatase and
   Serum aspartate aminotransferase (AST [SGOT])
   (abnormalities may occur, especially in patients with juvenile rheumatoid arthritis, systemic lupus erythematosus, or history of liver
   disease, or when plasma salicylate concentrations exceed 250 mcg
   per mL)

Prothrombin time
   (may be prolonged with large doses of salicylates, especially if
   plasma concentrations exceed 300 mcg per mL)

Serum potassium concentrations
   (may be decreased because of increased potassium excretion
   caused by direct effect of salicylate on renal tubules)

Serum thyroxine (T$_4$) concentrations and
Serum triiodothyronine (T$_3$) concentrations
   (large doses of salicylate may decrease serum T$_4$ and T$_3$ concentrations when determined by radioimmunoassay)

Serum uric acid concentrations
   (may be increased or decreased, depending on salicylate dosage;
   plasma salicylate concentrations below 100 to 150 mcg per mL
   increase serum uric acid concentrations; salicylate concentrations
   above 100 to 150 mcg per mL decrease uric acid concentrations)

T$_3$ resin uptake
   (may be increased with large doses of salicylate)

Urine phenolsulfonphthalein (PSP) concentrations
   (may be decreased because of competition of salicylate with PSP
   for renal tubular secretion)

**Medical considerations/Contraindications**
The medical considerations/contraindications included here have been selected on the basis of their potential clinical significance (reasons given
in parentheses where appropriate)—not necessarily inclusive (» =
major clinical significance).

***Risk-benefit should be considered when the following medical problems
exist:***
» Bleeding ulcers or
» Hemorrhagic states, other active
   (may be exacerbated by the salicylate)
» Dehydration
   (rehydration therapy is essential if signs of dehydration, such as
   dry mouth, excessive thirst, wrinkled skin, decreased urination,
   dizziness or lightheadedness, are present with the diarrhea; fluid
   loss may have serious consequences, such as circulatory collapse
   and renal failure, especially in young children)

» Dysentery, acute, characterized by bloody stools and elevated temperature
(sole treatment with bismuth subsalicylate may be inadequate; antibiotic therapy may be required)

  Gout
(salicylates may have variable dose-dependent effects on serum uric acid concentrations; also, salicylates may interfere with efficacy of uricosuric antigout agents)

» Hemophilia
(salicylate may increase risk of hemorrhage)

  Renal function impairment
(increased risk of bismuth and salicylate toxicity because of decreased excretion)

  Sensitivity to bismuth subsalicylate

## Side/Adverse Effects

The following side/adverse effects have been selected on the basis of their potential clinical significance (possible signs and symptoms in parentheses where appropriate)—not necessarily inclusive:

**Those indicating need for medical attention**
Incidence rare—reported with higher-than-recommended doses and/or chronic dosing; may also be signs of overdose
*Bismuth encephalopathy* (anxiety; confusion; difficulty in speaking or slurred speech; severe and/or continuing headache; mental depression; muscle spasms, especially of face, neck, and back; muscle weakness; trembling; uncontrolled body movements); *constipation, severe; salicylism, symptoms of* (any loss of hearing; confusion; severe or continuing diarrhea; dizziness or lightheadedness; severe drowsiness; fast or deep breathing; severe or continuing headache; increased sweating; increased thirst; severe or continuing nausea or vomiting; continuing ringing or buzzing in ears; severe or continuing stomach pain; uncontrollable flapping movements of the hands, especially in elderly patients; vision problems)

**Those not indicating need for medical attention**
Incidence more frequent
*Discoloration produced by bismuth* (darkening of tongue or grayish black stools)

## Overdose

For specific information on the agents used in the management of bismuth subsalicylate overdose, see:
• *Charcoal, Activated (Oral-Local)* monograph;
• *Acetazolamide* in *Carbonic Anhydrase Inhibitors (Systemic)* monograph; and/or
• *Vitamin K (Systemic)* monograph.

For more information on the management of overdose or unintentional ingestion, **contact a Poison Control Center** (see *Poison Control Center Listing*).

**Clinical effects of overdose**
The following effects have been selected on the basis of their potential clinical significance (possible signs and symptoms in parentheses where appropriate)—not necessarily inclusive:
*Bismuth encephalopathy* (anxiety; confusion; difficulty in speaking or slurred speech; severe and/or continuing headache; mental depression; muscle spasms, especially of face, neck, and back; muscle weakness; trembling; uncontrolled body movements); *symptoms of salicylism* (any loss of hearing; confusion; severe or continuing diarrhea; dizziness or lightheadedness; severe drowsiness; fast or deep breathing; severe or continuing headache; increased sweating; increased thirst; severe or continuing nausea or vomiting; continuing ringing or buzzing in ears; severe or continuing stomach pain; uncontrollable flapping movements of the hands, especially in elderly patients; vision problems)

**Treatment of overdose**
Recommended treatment of overdose may include:
To decrease absorption—Emptying the stomach via induction of emesis or gastric lavage; administering activated charcoal.
To enhance elimination—Institution of exchange transfusion, hemodialysis, peritoneal dialysis, or hemoperfusion as needed in severe overdose.
Specific treatment—Monitoring serum salicylate concentration until it is apparent that the concentration is decreasing to the nontoxic range. Salicylate concentrations of 500 mcg per mL 2 hours after ingestion indicate serious toxicity; salicylate concentrations above 800 mcg per mL 2 hours after ingestion indicate possible fatality. In addition, prolonged monitoring may be necessary in massive overdosage because absorption may be delayed.

Inducing forced alkaline diuresis to increase salicylate excretion. However, bicarbonate should not be administered orally for this purpose because salicylate absorption may be increased. Also, if acetazolamide is used, the increased risk of severe metabolic acidosis and salicylate toxicity (caused by increased penetration of salicylate into the brain because of metabolic acidosis) must be considered. It is recommended that acetazolamide be given concurrently with an alkaline intravenous solution, e.g., one that contains sodium bicarbonate or sodium lactate. Administering blood or vitamin K₁ if necessary to treat hemorrhaging.
Monitoring—Monitoring and supporting vital functions; monitoring for pulmonary edema and convulsions and instituting appropriate therapy if required.
Supportive care—Correcting hyperthermia; fluid, electrolyte, and acid-base imbalances; ketosis; and plasma glucose concentration as needed. Patients in whom intentional overdose is confirmed or suspected should be referred for psychiatric consultation.

## Patient Consultation

As an aid to patient consultation, refer to *Advice for the Patient, Bismuth Subsalicylate (Oral)*.

In providing consultation, consider emphasizing the following selected information (» = major clinical significance):

**Before using this medication**
» Conditions affecting use, especially:
Allergies to salicylates or other nonsteroidal anti-inflammatory drugs
Pregnancy—Salicylates cross the placenta; concern only with high doses and long-term therapy because of salicylate effects
Breast-feeding—Concern only with high doses and chronic use because of salicylate intake by infant
Use in children—Risk of fluid and electrolyte loss due to diarrhea; increased susceptibility to toxic effects of salicylates if fever and dehydration present; risk of impaction due to bismuth
Use in the elderly—Risk of fluid and electrolyte loss due to diarrhea; increased susceptibility to toxic effects of salicylates possibly due to decreased renal function; risk of impaction due to bismuth
Other medications, especially anticoagulants, heparin, or thrombolytic agents; antidiabetic agents; probenecid or sulfinpyrazone; other salicylates; or oral tetracyclines (for tablet dosage form)
Other medical problems, especially bleeding ulcers or other active hemorrhagic states, acute dysentery, dehydration, or hemophilia

**Proper use of this medication**
Following physician's or manufacturer's instructions
» Not giving to children with symptoms of influenza or varicella without first checking with physician
Missed dose: If on a regular schedule—Taking as soon as possible; not taking if almost time for next dose; not doubling doses
» For use in treatment of diarrhea—Importance of maintaining adequate hydration and proper diet
» Proper dosing
» Proper storage

**Precautions while using this medication**
» Caution if other medications containing aspirin or other salicylates are used
Diabetics:
Possibility of false urine sugar test results with prolonged use
Checking with health care professional, if changes in urine sugar test results occur, or if any other questions, especially if diabetes is not well-controlled
» Suspected overdose: Getting emergency help immediately
*For antidiarrheal use*
Checking with physician if—
Symptoms do not improve within 2 days or become worse
Diarrhea is accompanied by high fever

**Side/adverse effects**
May cause encephalopathy, severe constipation, and/or salicylism with higher-than-recommended doses and/or chronic use
Dark tongue or grayish black stools may be alarming to patient although medically insignificant

## Oral Dosage Forms

Note: Bracketed uses in the *Dosage Forms* section refer to categories of use and/or indications that are not included in U.S. product labeling.

## BISMUTH SUBSALICYLATE ORAL SUSPENSION

### Usual adult and adolescent dose
Diarrhea (treatment); or
Gastric distress (treatment)—
    Oral, 524 or 528 mg every half-hour to one hour or 1048 or 1056 mg every hour if needed.
[Traveler's diarrhea (prophylaxis)][1]—
    Oral, 524 or 528 mg four times a day, starting one day prior to departure and continuing for two days after returning, but not to exceed three weeks of continued use.
[Ulcer, duodenal, *Helicobacter pylori*–associated (treatment adjunct)][1]; or
[Gastritis, *Helicobacter pylori*–associated (treatment adjunct)][1]—
    Dosage has not been established. However, in one study, 525 mg was administered orally three times a day one hour before meals, in conjunction with 500 mg of amoxicillin and 500 mg of metronidazole administered three times a day after meals, for one to two weeks.

### Usual adult prescribing limits
4.2 grams in twenty-four hours.

### Usual pediatric dose
Diarrhea (treatment); or
Gastric distress (treatment)—
    Children up to 3 years of age:
        According to weight as follows (may be repeated every four hours if needed, but not to exceed six doses in a day)——
        Children weighing 6.4 to 8 kg: Oral, 44 mg.
        Children weighing over 13 kg: Oral, 88 mg.
    Children 3 to 6 years of age:
        Oral, 88 mg every half-hour to one hour but not to exceed 704 mg in a day.
    Children 6 to 9 years of age:
        Oral, 174.6 or 176 mg every half-hour to one hour but not to exceed 1.4 grams in a day.
    Children 9 to 12 years of age:
        Oral, 262 or 264 mg every half-hour to one hour but not to exceed 2.1 grams in a day.

### Usual geriatric dose
See *Usual adult and adolescent dose.*
Note: Geriatric patients with reduced renal function may be more sensitive to the effects of the usual adult dose and may require lower doses.

### Strength(s) usually available
U.S.—
    262 mg per 15 mL (OTC) [*Pepto-Bismol* (salicylate 130 mg; sodium <3 mg); GENERIC].
    525 mg per 15 mL (OTC) [*Bismatrol Extra Strength; Pepto-Bismol Maximum Strength* (salicylate 236 mg; sodium <5 mg)].
Canada—
    264 mg per 15 mL (OTC) [*Bismed* (alcohol 2%; sodium <18 mg); *Pepto-Bismol* (sodium <1.3 mg)].
    525 mg per 15 mL (OTC) [*PMS-Bismuth Subsalicylate*].

### Packaging and storage
Store below 40 °C (104 °F), preferably between 15 and 30 °C (59 and 86 °F), unless otherwise specified by manufacturer. Protect from freezing.

### Auxiliary labeling
• Shake well.
• May cause darkening of tongue and/or stools.

## BISMUTH SUBSALICYLATE TABLETS

### Usual adult and adolescent dose
Diarrhea (treatment); or
Gastric distress (treatment)—
    Oral, 524 or 600 mg every half-hour to one hour or 1050 or 1200 mg every hour if needed.
[Traveler's diarrhea (prophylaxis)][1]—
    Oral, 524 or 600 mg four times a day, starting one day prior to departure and continuing for two days after returning, but not to exceed three weeks of continued use.
[Ulcer, duodenal, *Helicobacter pylori*–associated (treatment adjunct)][1]
[Gastritis, *Helicobacter pylori*–associated (treatment adjunct)][1]—
    Dosage has not been established. However, in one study, 525 mg was administered orally three times a day one hour before meals, in conjunction with 500 mg of amoxicillin and 500 mg of metronidazole administered three times a day after meals, for one to two weeks.

### Usual adult prescribing limits
4.8 grams in twenty-four hours.

### Usual pediatric dose
Diarrhea (treatment); or
Gastric distress (treatment)—
    Children up to 9 years of age: The available strength of the tablet may not conform to the recommended dose for children up to 9 years of age; the bismuth subsalicylate oral suspension is the preferred dosage form for this age group.
    Children 9 to 12 years of age: Oral, 262 or 300 mg every half-hour to one hour but not to exceed 2.4 grams in a day.

### Usual geriatric dose
See *Usual adult and adolescent dose.*
Note: Geriatric patients with reduced renal function may be more sensitive to the effects of the usual adult dose and may require lower doses.

### Strength(s) usually available
U.S.—
    262 mg (OTC) [*Pepto-Bismol Easy-to-Swallow Caplets* (salicylate 99 mg)].
Canada—
    Not commercially available.

### Packaging and storage
Store below 40 °C (104 °F), preferably between 15 and 30 °C (59 and 86 °F), unless otherwise specified by manufacturer.

### Auxiliary labeling
• Swallow with water. Do not chew.
• May cause darkening of tongue and/or stools.

## BISMUTH SUBSALICYLATE CHEWABLE TABLETS

### Usual adult and adolescent dose
See *Bismuth Subsalicylate Tablets.*

### Usual pediatric dose
See *Bismuth Subsalicylate Tablets.*

### Usual geriatric dose
See *Bismuth Subsalicylate Tablets.*

### Strength(s) usually available
U.S.—
    262 mg (OTC) [*Bismatrol; Pepto-Bismol* (salicylate 102 mg; sodium <2 mg; calcium carbonate 350 mg); GENERIC].
Canada—
    262 mg (OTC) [*Pepto-Bismol* (sodium <2 mg; calcium carbonate 350 mg)].
    300 mg (OTC) [*Bismed* (calcium carbonate 350 mg); *PMS-Bismuth Subsalicylate* (calcium carbonate 350 mg)].

### Packaging and storage
Store below 40 °C (104 °F), preferably between 15 and 30 °C (59 and 86 °F), unless otherwise specified by manufacturer.

### Auxiliary labeling
• Chew or allow to disintegrate in mouth before swallowing.
• May cause darkening of tongue and/or stools.

[1]Not included in Canadian product labeling.

## Selected Bibliography

Bierer DW. Bismuth subsalicylate: History, chemistry, and safety. Rev Infect Dis 1990; 12 (S1): S3-S7.
DuPont HL, Ericsson CD, Johnson PC, et al. Use of bismuth subsalicylate for the prevention of traveler's diarrhea. Rev Infect Dis 1990; 12: S64-S67.
Soriano-Brücher HE, Avendaõ P, O'Ryan M, et al. Use of bismuth subsalicylate in acute diarrhea in children. Rev Infect Dis 1990; 12: S51-S55.

Revised: 02/03/92
Interim revision: 09/01/94

**BISOPROLOL**—See *Beta-adrenergic Blocking Agents (Systemic)*

## BISOPROLOL-CONTAINING COMBINATIONS—

Bisoprolol and Hydrochlorothiazide (Systemic)—See *Beta-adrenergic Blocking Agents and Thiazide Diuretics (Systemic)*

**BITOLTEROL**—See *Bronchodilators, Adrenergic (Systemic)*

**BLENDERIZED ENTERAL NUTRITION FORMULAS**—See *Enteral Nutrition Formulas (Systemic)*

# BLEOMYCIN Systemic

VA CLASSIFICATION (Primary/Secondary): AN200/DE600

Note: For a listing of dosage forms and brand names by country availability, see *Dosage Forms* section(s). For a listing of brand names for the articles in this monograph, refer to the General Index.

## Category
Antineoplastic.

## Indications
Note: Bracketed information in the *Indications* section refers to uses that are not included in U.S. product labeling.

### Accepted
Carcinoma, head and neck (treatment)
Carcinoma, laryngeal (treatment)
[Carcinoma, paralaryngeal (treatment)]
Carcinoma, cervical (treatment)
Carcinoma, penile (treatment)
Carcinoma, skin (treatment)
Carcinoma, vulvar (treatment)
Carcinoma, testicular (treatment) or
[Carcinoma, renal (treatment)]—Bleomycin is indicated for treatment of squamous cell carcinomas of the head and neck (including the mouth, tongue, tonsil, nasopharynx, oropharynx, sinus, palate, lip, buccal mucosa, gingiva, epiglottis, and larynx and paralarynx), cervix, penis, skin and vulva. It is also indicated for treatment of testicular carcinoma (including embryonal cell carcinoma, choriocarcinoma, and teratocarcinoma) and has been used for treatment of renal carcinoma.

Lymphomas, Hodgkin's (treatment) or
Lymphomas, non-Hodgkin's (treatment)—Bleomycin is indicated for treatment of Hodgkin's and non-Hodgkin's lymphomas (including reticulum cell sarcoma and lymphosarcoma).

[Sarcomas, soft tissue (treatment)]—Bleomycin is indicated for treatment of some soft tissue sarcomas.

[Osteosarcoma (treatment)][1]—Bleomycin is used in the treatment of osteosarcoma.

[Malignant effusions, peritoneal (treatment)][1]
[Malignant effusions, pleural (prophylaxis)] or
[Malignant effusions, pleural (treatment)][1]—Bleomycin is used by intracavitary administration for treatment of peritoneal effusions and for prophylaxis and treatment of pleural effusions.

[Tumors, germ cell, ovarian (treatment)][1]—Bleomycin is used for treatment of germ cell ovarian tumors.

[Mycosis fungoides (treatment)][1]—Bleomycin is used, in combination with other agents, for treatment of advanced stage mycosis fungoides.

[Verruca vulgaris (treatment)][1]—Bleomycin is used by intralesional injection for treatment of severe, recalcitrant common warts (verrucae vulgaris) not responding to conventional treatment.

Extreme caution is recommended in use of bleomycin for non-neoplastic conditions because of potential carcinogenicity with long-term use of this agent.

[1]Not included in Canadian product labeling.

## Pharmacology/Pharmacokinetics

### Physicochemical characteristics
Hygroscopic; inactivated *in vitro* by agents containing sulfhydryl groups, hydrogen peroxide, and ascorbic acid.

### Mechanism of action/Effect
Bleomycin is classed as an antibiotic but is not used as an antimicrobial agent. Although bleomycin is effective against both cycling and non-cycling cells, it seems to be most effective in the $G_2$ phase of cell division. Its exact mechanism of antineoplastic action is unknown but may involve binding to DNA, inducing lability of the DNA structure, and reduced synthesis of DNA, and to a lesser extent, RNA and proteins.

### Absorption
Approximately 45% of a dose is absorbed into the systemic circulation following intrapleural or intraperitoneal administration.

### Protein binding
Very low (1%).

### Biotransformation
Unknown; probably by enzyme degradation in tissues (based on animal studies). Tissue enzyme activity varies, which may determine toxicity and antitumor effect of bleomycin; enzyme activity is high in the liver and kidneys, as well as in bone marrow and lymph nodes, but is low in the skin and lungs. It is not known if any metabolites are active.

### Half-life
Creatinine clearance greater than 35 mL per minute—115 minutes.

Creatinine clearance less than 35 mL per minute—Increased exponentially as creatinine clearance decreases.

### Elimination
Renal, 60 to 70%, largely as unchanged drug; markedly reduced in renal failure.

In dialysis—Probably not dialyzable.

## Precautions to Consider

### Carcinogenicity/Mutagenicity
Secondary malignancies are potential delayed effects of many antineoplastic agents, although it is not clear whether the effect is related to their mutagenic or immunosuppressive action. The effect of dose and duration of therapy is also unknown, although risk seems to increase with long-term use. Although information is limited, available data seem to indicate that the carcinogenic risk is greatest with the alkylating agents.

Carcinostatic antibiotics have been shown to be carcinogenic in animals, and have been associated with an increased risk of development of secondary carcinomas in humans.

Bleomycin has not been found to be mutagenic according to the Ames assay. However, chromosomal aberrations were reported in bone marrow cells and spermatogonia of mice given very high doses.

### Pregnancy/Reproduction
Fertility—Gonadal suppression, resulting in amenorrhea or azoospermia, may occur in patients taking antineoplastic therapy, especially with the alkylating agents. In general, these effects appear to be related to dose and length of therapy and may be irreversible. Prediction of the degree of testicular or ovarian function impairment is complicated by the common use of combinations of several antineoplastics, which makes it difficult to assess the effects of individual agents.

Pregnancy—First trimester: It is usually recommended that use of antineoplastics, especially combination chemotherapy, be avoided whenever possible, especially during the first trimester. Although information is limited because of the relatively few instances of antineoplastic administration during pregnancy, the mutagenic, teratogenic, and carcinogenic potential of these medications must be considered.

Other hazards to the fetus include adverse reactions seen in adults.

In general, use of a contraceptive is recommended during cytotoxic drug therapy.

Bleomycin has been found to be teratogenic in mice given intraperitoneal doses of 0.6 to 5 Units per kg of body weight on days 7 to 12 of gestation; increased fetal resorptions occurred at doses of 3 and 5 Units per kg of body weight.

### Breast-feeding
Although very little information is available regarding distribution of antineoplastic agents into breast milk, breast-feeding is not recommended while bleomycin is being administered because of the risks to the infant (adverse effects, mutagenicity, carcinogenicity).

### Pediatrics
Appropriate studies on the relationship of age to the effects of bleomycin have not been performed in the pediatric population. However, no pediatrics-specific problems have been documented to date.

### Geriatrics
Although appropriate studies on the relationship of age to the effects of bleomycin have not been performed in the geriatric population, there

may be an increased risk of pulmonary toxicity in the elderly (over 70 years of age). In addition, elderly patients are more likely to have age-related renal function impairment, which may require reduction of dosage in patients receiving bleomycin.

### Dental
Bleomycin may cause mild stomatitis.

### Drug interactions and/or related problems
The following drug interactions and/or related problems have been selected on the basis of their potential clinical significance (possible mechanism in parentheses where appropriate)—not necessarily inclusive (» = major clinical significance):

» Anesthetics, general
(use in patients previously treated with bleomycin may result in rapid pulmonary deterioration because bleomycin causes sensitization of lung tissue to oxygen; even with concentrations of inspired oxygen considered to be safe, pulmonary fibrosis may develop postoperatively)

Antineoplastics, other or
Radiation therapy
(concurrent use may result in increased bleomycin toxicity, including bone marrow depression, which is rarely caused by bleomycin alone, and mucosal and pulmonary toxicity; dosage adjustment may be necessary)

Cisplatin
(cisplatin-induced renal function impairment may result in delayed clearance and bleomycin toxicity even at low doses; caution is recommended because of the frequent combined use of these two agents)

Vincristine
(sequential administration prior to bleomycin arrests cells in mitosis so that they are more susceptible to bleomycin; frequently used to therapeutic advantage)

### Medical considerations/Contraindications
The medical considerations/contraindications included here have been selected on the basis of their potential clinical significance (reasons given in parentheses where appropriate)—not necessarily inclusive (» = major clinical significance).

*Risk-benefit should be considered when the following medical problems exist:*

Hepatic function impairment
(potential hepatotoxicity)

» Pulmonary function impairment

Raynaud's phenomenon or
Vascular disease, peripheral
(for intralesional use in treatment of warts; local Raynaud's phenomenon reported in fingers injected with bleomycin)

» Renal function impairment, severe —creatinine clearance less than 25 to 35 mL per minute
(toxicity of bleomycin may be increased; it is recommended that dosage of bleomycin be reduced in patients with renal function impairment)

Sensitivity to bleomycin

» Caution should be used also in patients who have had previous cytotoxic drug therapy and radiation therapy (especially chest irradiation), as well as in patients who smoke, because of the increased risk of pulmonary toxicity.

### Patient monitoring
The following are especially important in patient monitoring (other tests may be warranted in some patients, depending on condition; » = major clinical signfilcance):

» Auscultation of the lungs and
» Chest x-ray
(recommended prior to initiation of therapy and at periodic intervals during therapy)

Blood urea nitrogen (BUN) concentrations and
Creatinine concentrations, serum
(recommended prior to initiation of therapy and at periodic intervals during therapy; frequency varies according to clinical state, agent, dose, and other agents being used concurrently)

» Pulmonary function studies, including single-breath carbon monoxide diffusion capacity (DLco) and forced vital capacity
(recommended at frequent intervals during therapy to detect early asymptomatic interstitial damage; however, DLco results are sometimes difficult to interpret because of the effects of weakness and anemia or the presence of extensive lung tumor or effusion. Therapy with bleomycin should be discontinued at the first sign of pulmonary changes [for example, if forced vital capacity is reduced

to 75% or less or DLco to 40% or less of pretreatment level]; if the changes are determined to be drug-related, bleomycin therapy should not be resumed)

## Side/Adverse Effects

Note: There is some evidence that administration of bleomycin by continuous intravenous infusion over 24 hours rather than intermittently may be associated with less pulmonary and idiosyncratic toxicity, although mucocutaneous toxicity may be increased.

The main reported side effect with intralesional use is local burning or pain within 24 to 48 hours after injection. Blackening and eschar occur at the site of the lesion within 1 or 2 weeks and healing usually occurs within 2 to 3 weeks without scarring. Cases of urticaria, nail loss, and Raynaud's phenomenon have also been reported.

When bleomycin is used in combination with vinblastine for testicular carcinoma, vasospasm is a common vascular toxicity.

The following side/adverse effects have been selected on the basis of their potential clinical significance (possible signs and symptoms in parentheses where appropriate)—not necessarily inclusive:

### Those indicating need for medical attention
Incidence more frequent
*Fever and chills; pneumonitis, progressing to pulmonary fibrosis* (cough; shortness of breath); *stomatitis, mild, due to mucocutaneous toxicity* (sores in mouth and on lips)

Note: *Fever and chills* occur in approximately 20 to 60% of patients, usually 3 to 6 hours after administration, last 4 to 12 hours, and become less frequent with continued use.

*Pulmonary toxicity* occurs in 10 to 40% of treated patients, usually 4 to 10 weeks after initiation of treatment; approximately 1% of treated patients have died of pulmonary fibrosis. Pulmonary toxicity is age- and dose-related, occurring most frequently in patients over 70 years of age and/or receiving a total dose greater than 400 Units (although it has been reported with doses as low as 20 to 60 Units). It may be irreversible and fatal; however, there is some evidence that in patients who survive, symptoms and pulmonary function parameters return to normal in approximately 2 years. It occurs at lower doses in patients who have received other antineoplastics or thoracic radiation; mortality may be as high as 10% in patients who have received pulmonary irradiation. A low-dose allergic pneumonitis has also been reported.

The earliest signs of *pulmonary toxicity* are a decrease in diffusion capacity and fine rales. On chest x-ray, pneumonitis is seen as nonspecific patchy opacities, usually of the lower lung fields. Pulmonary function tests show a decrease in total lung volume and a decrease in vital capacity.

Incidence less frequent
*Idiosyncratic reaction* (confusion; faintness; fever and chills; wheezing)

Note: The *idiosyncratic reaction* occurs in approximately 1% of treated patients (1 to 6% of lymphoma patients). If not promptly treated, it may progress to sweating, dehydration, hypotension, and renal failure or cardiorespiratory collapse. It usually occurs at doses of 25 Units per square meter of body surface or greater, although it has occurred with a dose of 7.5 Units. May be immediate or delayed by several hours, and occurs after the first or second dose.

Incidence rare
*Hepatic toxicity* (seen as changes in hepatic function tests); *pleuropericarditis* (sudden severe chest pain); *renal toxicity* (seen as changes in renal function tests); *vascular toxicity, including cerebral arteritis, cerebrovascular accident, myocardial infarction, or thrombotic microangiopathy* (sudden weakness in arms or legs; sudden, severe chest pain)

### Those indicating need for medical attention only if they continue or are bothersome
Incidence more frequent
*Mucocutaneous toxicity* (darkening or thickening of skin; itching of skin; skin rash or colored bumps on fingertips, elbows, or palms; skin redness or tenderness; dark stripes on skin; swelling of fingers; less frequently, changes in fingernails or toenails); *vomiting and loss of appetite*

Note: *Skin toxicity* occurs in 25 to 50% of treated patients, usually 2 to 4 weeks after initiation of therapy; it appears to be related to cumulative dose and usually develops after 150 to 200 Units have been given.

*Vomiting and loss of appetite* occur in 15 to 30% of treated patients.

Incidence less frequent
*Weight loss*

**Those not indicating need for medical attention**
Incidence less frequent
*Loss of hair*
Note: *Loss of hair* begins after several weeks, with regrowth occurring several months later.

**Those indicating the need for medical attention if they occur after medication is discontinued**
*Pulmonary toxicity* (cough; shortness of breath)
Note: *Pulmonary toxicity* may occur up to 1 month after bleomycin is discontinued.

## Patient Consultation

As an aid to patient consultation, refer to *Advice for the Patient, Bleomycin (Systemic).*

In providing consultation, consider emphasizing the following selected information (» = major clinical significance):

**Before using this medication**
» Conditions affecting use, especially:
    Sensitivity to bleomycin
    Pregnancy—Use not recommended because of mutagenic, teratogenic, and carcinogenic potential; advisability of using contraception; telling physician immediately if pregnancy is suspected
    Breast-feeding—Not recommended because of risk of serious side effects
    Use in the elderly—Increased risk of pulmonary toxicity
    Other medical problems, especially pulmonary function impairment or severe renal function impairment
    Previous cytotoxic drug therapy or radiation therapy
    History of smoking

**Proper use of this medication**
    Caution in taking combination therapy; taking each medication at the proper time
    Frequency of nausea, vomiting, and loss of appetite; importance of continuing medication despite stomach upset
» Proper dosing

**Precautions while using this medication**
» Importance of close monitoring by physician
» Caution if any kind of surgery (including dental surgery) or emergency treatment is required

**Side/adverse effects**
    May cause adverse effects such as loss of hair and mucocutaneous and lung toxicity; importance of discussing possible effects with physician
    Signs of potential side effects, especially fever and chills, pneumonitis and pulmonary fibrosis, stomatitis, mucocutaneous toxicity, and idiosyncratic reaction
    Physician or nurse can help in dealing with side effects
    Possibility of hair loss; normal hair growth should return after treatment has ended (may take several months)
    Pulmonary toxicity more likely in smokers

## General Dosing Information

See also *Patient monitoring.*

It is recommended that bleomycin be administered to patients under supervision of a physician experienced in cancer chemotherapy. It is also recommended that equipment and medications (including epinephrine, oxygen, diphenhydramine, and intravenous corticosteroids) necessary for treatment of a possible anaphylactic reaction be readily available at each administration of bleomycin.

A variety of dosage schedules, routes, and regimens of bleomycin, alone or in combination with other antitumor agents, are used. The prescriber may consult the medical literature in choosing a specific dosage or route.

Because of the risk of an idiosyncratic reaction in lymphoma patients, one test dose of 1 or 2 Units or less of bleomycin (base) given 2 to 4 hours prior to initiation of therapy at regular dosage may be used, although the test dose does not always detect reactors.

Some clinicians recommend premedication of patients receiving bleomycin with acetaminophen, steroids, and diphenhydramine hydrochloride to reduce drug fever and the risk of anaphylaxis.

Bleomycin may be administered intravenously or intra-arterially slowly over a period of 10 minutes, or may be further diluted with 50 to 100 mL of the initial diluent for administration by regional infusion.

It is recommended that the dosage of bleomycin be reduced in patients with renal function impairment (creatinine clearance less than 25 to 35 mL per minute). For example, dosage may be adjusted as follows:

| Serum creatinine | | Fraction of normal dose to be given |
|---|---|---|
| (mg/dL) | (micromoles per liter) | |
| 1.5–2.0 | 130–180 | 1/2 |
| 2.5–4.0 | 180–350 | 1/4 |
| 4.0–6.0 | 350–530 | 1/5 |
| 6.0–10.0 | 530–900 | 1/10–1/20 |

**Safety considerations for handling this medication**
There is limited but increasing evidence and concern that personnel involved in preparation and administration of parenteral antineoplastics may be at some risk because of the potential mutagenicity, teratogenicity, and/or carcinogenicity of these agents, although the actual risk is unknown. USP advisory panels recommend cautious handling both in preparation and disposal of antineoplastic agents. Precautions that have been suggested include:

• Use of a biological containment cabinet during reconstitution and dilution of parenteral medications and wearing of disposable surgical gloves and masks.
• Use of proper technique to prevent contamination of the medication, work area, and operator during transfer between containers (including proper training of personnel in this technique).
• Cautious and proper disposal of needles, syringes, vials, ampuls, and unused medication.

A number of medical centers have developed detailed guidelines for handling of antineoplastic agents.

**Combination chemotherapy**
Bleomycin is usually used in combination with other agents in various regimens. As a result, incidence and/or severity of side effects may be altered and different dosages (usually reduced) may be used. For example, bleomycin is part of the following chemotherapeutic combinations (some commonly used acronyms are in parentheses):

—doxorubicin, bleomycin, vinblastine, and dacarbazine (ABVD).
—mechlorethamine, vincristine, procarbazine, prednisone, and bleomycin (MOPP-LO BLEO).
—vinblastine, cisplatin, and bleomycin (VBP).

For specific dosages and schedules, consult the literature. For information regarding each agent, consult the individual monographs.

**For treatment of adverse effects**
Treatment of the idiosyncratic reaction is symptomatic and may consist of volume expansion, pressor agents, antihistamines, and corticosteroids.

## Parenteral Dosage Forms

Note: Bracketed uses in the *Dosage Forms* section refer to categories of use and/or indications that are not included in U.S. product labeling.

A Unit of bleomycin is equal to the formerly used milligram activity. The term milligram activity is a misnomer and was changed to Units to be more precise.

### BLEOMYCIN SULFATE STERILE USP

**Usual adult and adolescent dose**
Antineoplastic—
    Initial:
        Hodgkin's disease, squamous cell carcinoma, lymphosarcoma, reticulum cell sarcoma, testicular carcinoma—
            Intramuscular, intravenous, or subcutaneous, 0.25 to 0.50 Units (base) per kg of body weight or 10 to 20 Units per square meter of body surface one or two times a week or
            Intravenous infusion, continuous, 0.25 Units (base) per kg of body weight or 15 Units per square meter of body surface per day (over 24 hours) for four to five days.
        Squamous cell carcinoma of the head, neck, or uterine cervix—
            Regional arterial infusion, 30 to 60 Units (base) a day over a period of one to twenty-four hours.
        [Malignant effusions][1]—
            Intrapleural, 15 to 120 Units (base) in 100 mL of sodium chloride injection, instilled, and after 24 hours, removed.
            Intraperitoneal, 60 to 120 Units (base) in 100 mL of sodium chloride injection, instilled, and after 24 hours, removed.

Maintenance
Hodgkin's disease—
Intramuscular or intravenous, after a 50% response occurs, 1 Unit (base) a day or 5 Units a week.
[Warts, common][1]—
Intralesional, 0.2 to 0.8 Units (base) (according to size) one or more times at intervals of two to four weeks, up to a maximum total dose of 2 Units, using a solution of 15 Units of Sterile Bleomycin Sulfate USP in 15 mL of 0.9% sodium chloride injection or water for injection.

**Usual adult prescribing limits**
Because of the risk of pulmonary toxicity, total doses exceeding 225 to 400 Units (base) (less in patients with renal or pulmonary function impairment) should be given with great caution. If bleomycin is administered intrapleurally or intraperitoneally, one-half of the administered dose should be counted towards this total.

**Usual pediatric dose**
See *Usual adult and adolescent dose.*

**Size(s) usually available**
U.S.—
15 Units (base) (Rx) [*Blenoxane*].
Canada—
15 Units (base) (Rx) [*Blenoxane*].

**Packaging and storage**
Store between 2 and 8 °C (36 and 46 °F).

**Preparation of dosage form**
U.S.—
Sterile Bleomycin Sulfate USP may be prepared for intravenous use by dissolving the contents of the ampul (15 Units [base]) in 5 mL or more of 0.9% sodium chloride injection or 5% dextrose injection.
Sterile Bleomycin Sulfate USP may be prepared for intramuscular or subcutaneous use by dissolving the contents of the ampul (15 Units [base]) in 1 to 5 mL of sterile water for injection, 0.9% sodium chloride injection, 5% dextrose injection, or bacteriostatic water for injection.
Canada—
Sterile bleomycin sulfate may be prepared for intramuscular or subcutaneous use by dissolving the contents of the vial (15 Units [base]) in 1 to 5 mL of sterile water for injection, sodium chloride injection, or dextrose in water.
Sterile bleomycin sulfate may be prepared for intravenous or intra-arterial use by dissolving the contents of the vial (15 Units [base]) in 5 to 20 mL of 5% dextrose in water, 10% invert sugar in normal saline, 20% mannitol in water (discard if a precipitate forms), or 10% dextrose in water.
Caution—
Use of diluents containing benzyl alcohol is not recommended for preparation of medications for use in neonates. A fatal toxic syndrome consisting of metabolic acidosis, central nervous system (CNS) depression, respiratory problems, renal failure, hypotension, and possibly seizures and intracranial hemorrhages has been associated with this use.

**Stability**
U.S.—Reconstituted solutions of Sterile Bleomycin Sulfate USP in 0.9% sodium chloride injection or 5% dextrose injection are stable for 24 hours at room temperature, or for at least 14 days if refrigerated.
Canada—Reconstituted solutions are stable for 8 hours at room temperature and at least 48 hours when refrigerated.

**Selected Bibliography**
Evans WE, Yee GC, Crom WR, et al. Clinical pharmacology of bleomycin and cisplatin. Drug Intell Clin Pharm 1982 Jun; 16: 448–58.
Dorr RT, Fritz WL. Cancer chemotherapy handbook. New York: Elsevier, 1980: 274-83.

Revised: 07/11/94

---

# BOTULINUM TOXIN TYPE A    Parenteral-Local

VA CLASSIFICATION (Primary): OP900
Note: For a listing of dosage forms and brand names by country availability, see *Dosage Forms* section(s). For a listing of brand names for the articles in this monograph, refer to the General Index.

## Category
Neuromuscular blocking agent (ophthalmic).

## Indications
Note: Bracketed information in the *Indications* section refers to uses that are not included in U.S. product labeling.

**Accepted**
Blepharospasm (treatment) or
Strabismus (treatment)—Botulinum toxin type A is indicated for the treatment of strabismus, including horizontal strabismus up to 50 prism diopters, vertical strabismus, and persistent VI nerve palsy of 1 month or longer duration, and for blepharospasm associated with dystonia, including benign essential blepharospasm or VII nerve disorders.

[Hemifacial spasm (treatment)]
[Facial spasm (treatment)]
[Spasmodic dysphonia (treatment)] or
[Spasmodic torticollis (treatment)]—Botulinum toxin type A is also used to treat the above listed dystonias or dysphonias.

Botulinum toxin type A is of doubtful efficacy for the following indications, or multiple injections over time may be required: deviations over 50 prism diopters, restrictive strabismus, Duane's syndrome with lateral rectus weakness, and secondary strabismus caused by prior surgical over-recession of the antagonist.

**Unaccepted**
Botulinum toxin type A is ineffective in chronic paralytic strabismus except to reduce antagonist contracture in conjunction with surgical repair.

## Pharmacology/Pharmacokinetics

**Physicochemical characteristics**
Botulinum toxin type A is a sterile, lyophilized form of purified botulinum toxin type A that is produced from a culture of the Hall strain of *Clostridium botulinum.*

**Mechanism of action/Effect**
Botulinum toxin type A blocks neuromuscular conduction by binding to receptor sites on motor nerve terminals, entering the nerve terminals, and inhibiting the release of acetylcholine. When injected intramuscularly in therapeutic doses, botulinum toxin type A produces a localized chemical denervation muscle paralysis. When the muscle is chemically denervated, it atrophies and may develop extrajunctional acetylcholine receptors. There is evidence that the nerve can sprout and reinnervate the muscle, thereby reversing the weakness. The paralytic effect on muscles injected with botulinum toxin type A reduces the excessive, abnormal contractions associated with blepharospasm. In the treatment of strabismus, it is postulated that the administration of botulinum toxin type A affects muscle pairs by inducing an atrophic lengthening of the injected muscle and a corresponding shortening of the muscle's antagonist. Following peri-ocular injection of botulinum toxin type A, distant muscles show electrophysiologic changes, but no clinical weakness or other clinical change, for a period of several weeks or months, corresponding to the duration of local clinical paralysis.

**Onset of action**
In the treatment of blepharospasm, the initial effect of the injections is seen within 3 days and the effect reaches a peak 1 to 2 weeks after treatment.
In the treatment of strabismus, the initial doses typically create paralysis of injected muscles beginning 1 or 2 days after injection and increasing in intensity during the first week.

**Duration of action**
In the treatment of blepharospasm, each treatment lasts approximately 3 months.
In the treatment of strabismus, the paralysis lasts for 2 to 6 weeks and gradually resolves over an additional 2 to 6 weeks.
In the treatment of hemifacial spasm, treatment may last 6 months.

# Precautions to Consider

## Carcinogenicity
Long term studies in animals have not been done to evaluate the carcinogenic potential of botulinum toxin type A.

## Pregnancy/Reproduction
Pregnancy—Studies have not been done in either animals or humans.

FDA Pregnancy Category C.

## Breast-feeding
It is not known whether botulinum toxin type A is excreted in breast milk. However, problems in humans have not been documented.

## Pediatrics
Appropriate studies on the relationship of age to the effect of botulinum toxin type A have not been performed in children up to 12 years of age. Safety and efficacy have not been established.

## Geriatrics
Appropriate studies on the relationship of age to the effects of botulinum toxin type A have not been performed in the geriatric population. However, no geriatrics-specific problems have been documented to date.

## Drug interactions and/or related problems
The following drug interactions and/or related problems have been selected on the basis of their potential clinical significance (possible mechanism in parentheses where appropriate)—not necessarily inclusive (» = major clinical significance):

Note: Combinations containing any of the following medications, depending on the amount present, may also interact with this medication.

Aminoglycoside antibiotics
(may potentiate the effects of botulinum toxin type A)

## Medical considerations/Contraindications
The medical considerations/contraindications included here have been selected on the basis of their potential clinical significance (reasons given in parentheses where appropriate)—not necessarily inclusive (» = major clinical significance).

*Risk-benefit should be considered when the following medical problems exist:*

Cardiac or other medical conditions that may worsen with rapidly increasing activity
(patients with blepharospasm may have been sedentary for a long time; sedentary patients should be cautioned to resume activity slowly and carefully following the administration of botulinum toxin type A)

Infection with *Clostridium botulinum* toxin, history of
(persons with a previous episode of botulism poisoning may have produced antibodies that may interfere with botulinum toxin type A therapy)

Sensitivity to botulinum toxin type A injection

# Side/Adverse Effects

Note: Treatment with botulinum toxin type A may cause the body to produce antibodies against the toxin. This may reduce the effectiveness of continued therapy. To forestall this, the dose of botulinum toxin type A should be kept as low as possible.

Two persons previously incapacitated by blepharospasm experienced cardiac collapse within 3 weeks following treatment with botulinum toxin type A. The collapse was attributed to physical overexertion. Sedentary patients should be cautioned to resume activity slowly and carefully following treatment with botulinum toxin type A.

During the treatment of strabismus, retrobulbar hemorrhages sufficient to compromise retinal circulation have occurred from needle penetrations into the orbit. It is recommended that appropriate instruments to decompress the orbit be accessible.

Ocular (globe) penetrations by needles have also occurred. An ophthalmoscope should be available to diagnose this condition.

The injection procedure for the treatment of strabismus has also caused scleral perforations, vitreous hemorrhage, and pupillary change consistent with ciliary ganglion damage (Adies pupil).

During the treatment of blepharospasm, reduced blinking as a result of injection of botulinum toxin type A into the orbicularis muscle can lead to corneal exposure, persistent epithelial defect, and corneal ulceration, especially in patients with VII nerve disorders. In one case, in an aphakic eye, reduced blinking resulted in corneal perforation that subsequently required corneal grafting. Careful test-

ing of corneal sensation in eyes previously operated upon, avoidance of injection into the lower lid area in order to avoid ectropion, and vigorous treatment of any epithelial defect should be employed. Treatment for the above problems may include protective drops, ointment, therapeutic soft contact lenses, or closure of the eye by patching or other means.

The following side/adverse effects have been selected on the basis of their potential clinical significance (possible signs and symptoms in parentheses where appropriate)—not necessarily inclusive:

## Those indicating need for medical attention
Incidence more frequent
*After treatment for blepharospasm*
**Keratoconjunctivitis sicca** (dryness of the eye); *lagophthalmos* (inability to close the eyelid completely)

Incidence less frequent or rare
*After treatment for blepharospasm*
**Decreased blinking; ectropion** (turning outward of the edge of the eyelid); **entropion** (turning inward of the edge of the eyelid); *keratitis* (irritation of the cornea [colored portion] of the eye)

## Those indicating need for medical attention only if they continue or are bothersome
Incidence more frequent
*After treatment for blepharospasm*
**Ecchymosis** (blue or purplish bruise on eyelid); *irritation or watering of the eye; photophobia* (sensitivity of the eye to light); *ptosis* (drooping of the upper eyelid)

*After treatment for horizontal strabismus*
**Ptosis** (drooping of the upper eyelid)—In trials, the average incidence was 10–20%; the incidence of ptosis was much less after inferior rectus injection (less than 1%) and much greater after superior rectus injection (30–40%); less than 1% of patients had ptosis lasting more than 180 days; **vertical deviation** (eye pointing upward or downward instead of straight ahead)—In trials, the incidence was 10–20%; 2% of patients had vertical deviation greater than 2 prism diopters lasting more than 180 days

Incidence less frequent
*After treatment for blepharospasm or strabismus*
**Skin rash, diffuse; swelling of the eyelid skin following injection into the eyelid**—may last several days

*After treatment for horizontal strabismus*
**Diplopia** (double vision); *past-pointing or spatial disorientation* (difficulty finding the location of objects)

Incidence rare (less than 1%)
*After treatment for blepharospasm*
**Diplopia** (double vision)

# Patient Consultation

As an aid to patient consultation, refer to *Advice for the Patient, Botulinum Toxin Type A (Parenteral-Local).*

In providing consultation, consider emphasizing the following selected information (» = major clinical significance):

## Before using this medication
» Conditions affecting use, especially:
Sensitivity to botulinum toxin type A
Use in children—No specific information about its use in children up to 12 years of age.

## Proper use of this medication
» Proper dosing

## Precautions while using this medication
Increasing activities slowly and carefully to allow the heart and body time to strengthen

## Side/adverse effects
Signs of potential side effects, especially lagophthalmos, keratoconjunctivitis sicca, decreased blinking, ectropion, entropion, and keratitis

# General Dosing Information

The cumulative dose of botulinum toxin type A in the treatment of either strabismus or blepharospasm should not exceed 200 units (U) in a 30-day period.

Physicians administering botulinum toxin type A should understand the standard electromyographic techniques as well as the relevant neuromuscular and orbital anatomy and any alterations to the anatomy because of prior surgical procedures.

### For treatment of blepharospasm

For blepharospasm, the diluted medication is injected using a sterile, 27 to 30 gauge needle without electromyographic guidance.

### For treatment of strabismus

For strabismus, botulinum toxin type A is intended for injection into extraocular muscles utilizing the electrical activity recorded from the tip of the injection needle as a guide to placement within the target muscle. Injection without surgical exposure or electromyographic guidance should not be attempted.

The injection should be prepared by drawing an amount of the properly diluted toxin that is slightly greater than the intended dose into a sterile 1.0 mL tuberculin syringe. Any air bubbles should be expelled from the syringe barrel and the syringe should be attached to the electromyographic injection needle, which is preferably a 1½ inch, 27 gauge needle. The injection volume that is in excess of the intended dose should be expelled through the needle; this assures patency of the needle and confirms that there is no syringe-needle leakage. A new, sterile needle and syringe should be used to enter the vial on each occasion for dilution or removal of the medication.

To prepare the eye for the injection, it is recommended that several drops of a local anesthetic and an ocular decongestant be administered several minutes prior to injection.

### For treatment of adverse effects

Recommended treatment consists of the following
  • Should accidental injection or oral ingestion occur, the person should be medically supervised for several days on an office or outpatient basis for signs or symptoms of systemic weakness or muscle paralysis.

A vial containing 100 U of lyophilized *Clostridium botulinum* toxin type A is considered to be below the estimated dose for systemic toxicity in humans weighing 6 kg (13.2 lb) or greater.

## Parenteral Dosage Forms

### BOTULINUM TOXIN TYPE A FOR INJECTION

#### Usual adult and adolescent dose

Strabismus—
  Vertical muscles; or horizontal strabismus of less than 20 prism diopters:
    Intramuscularly, initially, 1.25 to 2.5 units (U) into any one muscle.
  Horizontal strabismus of 20 to 50 prism diopters:
    Intramuscularly, initially, 2.5 to 5.0 U into any one muscle.
  Persistent VI nerve palsy of one month duration or longer:
    Intramuscularly, initially, 1.25 to 2.5 U into the medial rectus muscle.
  Note: The volume of botulinum toxin type A injected for treatment of strabismus should be between 0.05 to 0.15 mL per muscle.

    For initial treatment of strabismus—
    Use the lower of the initial doses for treatment of small deviations. Use the larger doses only for large deviations.

    The initial doses typically create paralysis of injected muscles beginning one or two days after injection and increasing in intensity during the first week. The paralysis usually lasts for two to six weeks and gradually resolves over an additional two to six weeks. Overcorrections lasting more than six months have been rare. About one-half of patients will require subsequent doses because of inadequate paralytic response of the muscle to the initial dose, or because of mechanical factors, such as large deviations or restrictions, or because of the lack of binocular motor fusion to stabilize the alignment.

    For subsequent treatment of residual or recurrent strabismus—
    It is recommended that patients be reexamined seven to fourteen days after each injection to assess the effect of that dose.

    Patients who experience adequate paralysis of the target muscle and who require subsequent injections should receive a dose comparable to the initial dose.

    Subsequent doses for patients experiencing incomplete paralysis of the target muscle may be increased up to twice the previously administered dose.

    Subsequent injections should not be administered until the effects of the previous dose have dissipated, as evidenced by substantial function in the injected and adjacent muscles.

    The maximum recommended dose as a single injection into any one muscle is 25 U.

Blepharospasm—
  Subcutaneously, initially, 1.25 to 2.5 U (using 0.05 to 0.1 mL volume at each site), injected into the medial and lateral pre-tarsal orbi-

cularis oculi of the upper lid and into the lateral pre-septal orbicularis oculi of the lower lid. An additional 2.5 to 5 U may be injected into the orbital portion of the orbicularis oculi at the zygomatic arch.

  Note: In general, the initial effect of the injections is seen within three days and the effect reaches a peak one to two weeks after treatment.

    Each treatment lasts approximately three months, following which the procedure can be repeated indefinitely.

    At subsequent treatment sessions, the dose may be increased up to two-fold if the response from the initial treatment is considered insufficient, which is usually defined as an effect that does not last longer than two months. There appears to be little benefit from injecting more than 5.0 U per site. In addition, some tolerance may occur when the medication is used in treating blepharospasm if the treatments are administered more frequently than every three months. Also, it is rare to have the effect be permanent.

#### Usual pediatric dose

Infants and children up to 12 years of age—Safety and efficacy have not been established.

Children 12 years of age and older—See *Usual adult and adolescent dose*.

#### Size(s) usually available

U.S.—
  100 units of lyophilized *Clostridium botulinum* toxin type A (Rx) [*Botox* (0.5 mg human albumin)].
Canada—
  100 units of lyophilized *Clostridium botulinum* toxin type A (Rx) [*Botox* (0.5 mg human albumin)].

Note: One unit corresponds to the calculated median lethal intraperitoneal dose (LD/50) in mice.

#### Packaging and storage

Lyophilized product—Store in a freezer at or below -5 °C (23 °F), unless otherwise specified by manufacturer.

Reconstituted product—Store in a refrigerator between 2 and 8 °C (36 and 46 °F), unless otherwise specified by manufacturer.

#### Preparation of dosage form

Botulinum toxin type A for injection should be reconstituted with sterile non–preserved normal saline, such as 0.9% sodium chloride injection. Dilution Table—

  Note: The dilutions and doses listed below are calculated for an injection volume of 0.1 mL. A decrease or increase in the dose is also possible by administering a smaller or larger injection volume; from 0.05 mL (50% decrease in dose) to 0.15 mL (50% increase in dose).

| Amount of Diluent Added | Resulting dose in Units per 0.1 mL |
|---|---|
| 1.0 mL | 10.0 U |
| 2.0 mL | 5.0 U |
| 4.0 mL | 2.5 U |
| 8.0 mL | 1.25 U |

#### Stability

Botulinum toxin type A is denatured by bubbling or similar violent agitation; the diluent should be injected into the vial gently.

Discard the vial if its vacuum does not pull the diluent into the vial.

The lyophilized medication and the diluent to be used contain no preservatives.

The medication should be administered within 4 hours after reconstitution and should be stored in a refrigerator during those 4 hours. The date and time of reconstitution should be recorded on the vial.

Reconstituted botulinum toxin type A is clear, colorless, and free of particulate matter. The solution should be discarded if it is discolored or contains particulate matter.

## Selected Bibliography

Biglan AW, et al. Management of strabismus with botulinum A toxin. Ophthalmology 1989 Jul;96 (7): 935-43.
Biglan, AW, et al. Management of facial spasm with Clostridium botulinum toxin, type A (Oculinum). Arch Otolaryngol Head Neck Surg 1988 Dec;114 (12): 1407-12.
Kalra, HK, et al. Side effects of the use of botulinum toxin for treatment of benign essential blepharospasm and hemifacial spasm. Ophthalmic Surg 1990 May; 21 (5): 335-8.

Revised: 01/09/92
Interim revision: 10/28/93

# BRETYLIUM   Systemic

INN: Bretylium tosilate

VA CLASSIFICATION (Primary): CV300

Note: For a listing of dosage forms and brand names by country availability, see *Dosage Forms* section(s). For a listing of brand names for the articles in this monograph, refer to the General Index.

## Category
Antiarrhythmic.

## Indications

### Accepted
Arrhythmias, ventricular (prophylaxis and treatment)—Bretylium is indicated in the prophylaxis and management of ventricular fibrillation.

    Bretylium is also indicated in the treatment of life-threatening ventricular arrhythmias (e.g., ventricular tachycardias) refractory to first-line treatment (lidocaine and cardioversion).

## Pharmacology/Pharmacokinetics

### Physicochemical characteristics
Molecular weight—Bretylium tosylate: 414.37.

### Mechanism of action/Effect
The exact mechanism of antiarrhythmic effects has not been fully determined. Bretylium is a quaternary ammonium compound that possesses both adrenergic and direct myocardial effects. Bretylium is selectively taken up into peripheral adrenergic nerve terminals where it produces an initial release of norepinephrine resulting in a sympathomimetic effect. After this initial release phase, bretylium inhibits norepinephrine release, producing adrenergic blockade. Finally, bretylium blocks the uptake of norepinephrine and epinephrine into adrenergic nerve endings. The importance of these effects in mediating bretylium's antiarrhythmic action is not clear.

Bretylium's direct myocardial effect includes prolongation of action potential duration and effective refractory period by inhibition of potassium conductance. However, it does not directly depress conduction velocity or automaticity. Bretylium elevates the ventricular fibrillation threshold. In infarcted canine hearts, bretylium reduces the disparity in action potential duration and refractory period between normal and infarcted regions and transiently improves conduction velocity in infarcted areas. In the Vaughan Williams classification of antiarrhythmics, bretylium is considered to be a class III agent.

### Other actions/effects
Bretylium produces a positive inotropic effect, which may or may not be related to the norepinephrine release.

### Biotransformation
Insignificant. No metabolites have been identified.

### Half-life
Mean, 10 hours (range 4 to 17 hours); this variability may result partially from differences in renal function or administration procedures; increased to 16 to 31.5 hours in renal function impairment.

### Onset of action

| | Onset of Effect after Administration | |
|---|---|---|
| | Ventricular Fibrillation (min) | Ventricular Tachycardia (min) |
| Intravenous | 5–10 | 20–120 |
| Intramuscular | 20–60 | 20–120 |

### Time to peak serum concentration
Intramuscular, 1 hour.

### Duration of action
6 to 24 hours.

### Elimination
Renal, 90% (unchanged).
In dialysis—Removable by hemodialysis.

## Precautions to Consider

### Carcinogenicity/Mutagenicity
No information is available on the carcinogenic or mutagenic potential of bretylium.

### Pregnancy/Reproduction
Pregnancy—Studies have not been done in humans.
Studies have not been done in animals.
FDA Pregnancy Category C.

### Breast-feeding
It is not known whether bretylium is distributed into breast milk.

### Pediatrics
Appropriate studies on the relationship of age to the effects of bretylium have not been performed in the pediatric population. Safety and efficacy have not been established.

### Geriatrics
No information is available on the relationship of age to the effects of bretylium in the geriatric population. However, elderly patients are more likely to have age-related renal function impairment, which may require reduction of dosage or increase of dosage intervals in patients receiving bretylium.

### Drug interactions and/or related problems
The following drug interactions and/or related problems have been selected on the basis of their potential clinical significance (possible mechanism in parentheses where appropriate)—not necessarily inclusive (» = major clinical significance):

» Digitalis glycosides
    (initial norepinephrine release caused by bretylium may aggravate digitalis toxicity; concurrent use is not recommended)

Procainamide or
Quinidine
    (concurrent administration may counteract inotropic effect of bretylium and potentiate hypotension)

Sympathomimetics, such as dopamine or norepinephrine
    (the pressor effects of these agents may be enhanced during concurrent administration with bretylium; blood pressure should be monitored closely during concurrent use and dilute solutions should be used)

### Medical considerations/Contraindications
The medical considerations/contraindications included here have been selected on the basis of their potential clinical significance (reasons given in parentheses where appropriate)—not necessarily inclusive (» = major clinical significance).

*Risk-benefit should be considered when the following medical problems exist:*
    Conditions with fixed cardiac output, such as:
      Aortic stenosis or
      Pulmonary hypertension, severe
      (severe hypotension may occur as a result of reduced peripheral resistance without a compensatory increase in cardiac output; bretylium may be used if necessary for survival, but vasoconstrictive catecholamines may be necessary if severe hypotension occurs)

    Renal function impairment
      (elimination reduced; dosage intervals should be increased)

    Sensitivity to bretylium

### Patient monitoring
The following may be especially important in patient monitoring (other tests may be warranted in some patients, depending on condition; » = major clinical significance):

Blood pressure determinations and
Electrocardiogram (ECG)
    (should be monitored continuously during administration)

## Side/Adverse Effects

Note: Hypotension (both postural and supine) occurs routinely, with an incidence of about 50% in supine patients, but is rarely symptomatic. Hypotension may occur at doses lower than those necessary to treat arrhythmias.

    An initial increase in frequency of arrhythmias and a transient hypertension may occur as a result of the initial release of norepinephrine, and may last a few minutes to an hour. This effect may be reduced by slowing the rate of administration of bretylium.

The following side/adverse effects have been selected on the basis of their potential clinical significance (possible signs and symptoms in parentheses where appropriate)—not necessarily inclusive:

### Those indicating need for medical attention
Incidence rare (less than 0.1%)
> *Hyperthermia; renal function impairment; respiratory depression from possible neuromuscular block*

Note: *Hyperthermia* has been reported in a small number of patients. Temperatures in excess of 106 °F have been observed. Temperature rise may begin within 1 hour or later after bretylium administration and may reach a peak within 1 to 3 days. If hyperthermia is suspected or diagnosed, bretylium should be discontinued and appropriate treatment instituted immediately.

### Those indicating need for medical attention only if they continue or are bothersome
Incidence less frequent (3%)
> *Nausea and vomiting*—especially following rapid (less than 8 minutes) intravenous administration

Incidence rare
> *Angina* (chest pain); *bradycardia* (slow heartbeat); *feeling of pressure in the chest; postural hypotension* (dizziness or lightheadedness when getting up from a lying or sitting position; sudden fainting)

## Overdose
For more information on the management of overdose or unintentional ingestion, **contact a poison control center** (see *Poison Control Center Listing*).

### Clinical effects of overdose
The following effects have been selected on the basis of their potential clinical significance (possible signs and symptoms in parentheses where appropriate)—not necessarily inclusive:
> *Hypertension; hypotension*

Note: Marked *hypertension* may be followed by marked refractory *hypotension*. This exaggerated hemodynamic response may be due to rapid injection of a very large dose of bretylium while some effective circulation is still present.

### Treatment of overdose
For hypertensive response—Administration of nitroprusside or other short-acting intravenous antihypertensive agent.
For hypotensive response—Appropriate fluid therapy and pressor agents such as dopamine or norepinephrine.

## General Dosing Information
Dosage must be adjusted to meet the individual requirements of each patient, on the basis of clinical response.

Bretylium injection is always diluted before intravenous administration, *except when used in life-threatening ventricular fibrillation* when it is administered undiluted and as rapidly as possible. Consult package insert for dilution information.

When administering bretylium by continuous intravenous infusion, an infusion pump or other suitable metering device should be used to control the rate of infusion.

Intramuscular administration should be limited to 5 mL, undiluted, at each injection site. The injection site should be rotated to avoid tissue destruction.

Bretylium is used clinically for short-term therapy only. It should be discontinued after 3 to 5 days by gradual dosage reduction and replaced with oral antiarrhythmic therapy if necessary.

Tolerance to the hypotensive effect of bretylium usually occurs within several days. Until that occurs, the patient should remain supine or be observed carefully for hypotension. No treatment is needed as long as the supine systolic blood pressure remains above 75 mm Hg, unless there are associated symptoms. If it falls to less than 75 mm Hg, treatment should consist of intravenous infusion of dobutamine, dopamine, or norepinephrine and volume replacement with blood or plasma and intravenous fluids if necessary. Hemodynamic monitoring is recommended in these unstable situations to help guide medication therapy.

## Parenteral Dosage Forms
### BRETYLIUM TOSYLATE INJECTION
**Usual adult and adolescent dose**
Ventricular fibrillation or
Ventricular tachycardia, hemodynamically unstable—
> Immediate suppression: Intravenous (rapid), 5 mg per kg of body weight administered *undiluted*. If the arrhythmia persists, the dosage may be increased to 10 mg per kg of body weight and repeated as necessary.
> Continuous suppression: Intravenous infusion, 1 to 2 mg per minute of the *diluted* solution. Alternatively, infuse the *diluted* solution at a dosage of 5 to 10 mg per kg of body weight over a period greater than eight minutes every six hours.

Note: For specific dilution information, see *Preparation of Dosage Form*.
Ventricular arrhythmias, other—
> Intravenous infusion, 5 to 10 mg per kg of body weight of the *diluted* solution infused over a period greater than eight minutes. If the arrhythmia persists, additional doses may be given at one- to two-hour intervals. This same dosage may be administered every six hours, or a constant infusion of 1 to 2 mg per minute may be used for maintenance therapy; or
> Intramuscular, 5 to 10 mg per kg of body weight administered *undiluted*. If the arrhythmia persists, subsequent doses may be given at one- to two-hour intervals and thereafter maintaining the same dosage every six to eight hours.

Note: The site of intramuscular injection should be rotated. No more than 5 mL should be injected intramuscularly into one site.

**Usual pediatric dose**
Safety and efficacy have not been established.

**Strength(s) usually available**
U.S.—
> 50 mg per mL (Rx) [*Bretylol* (preservative-free); GENERIC].
> 100 mg per mL (Rx) [GENERIC].
Canada—
> 50 mg per mL (Rx) [*Bretylate*].

**Packaging and storage**
Store between 15 and 30 °C (59 and 86 °F), unless otherwise specified by manufacturer. Protect from freezing.

**Preparation of dosage form**
For intravenous infusion—Using sterile environment and technique, dilute each 500 mg bretylium tosylate in at least 50 mL of 5% dextrose injection or 0.9% sodium chloride injection.

### BRETYLIUM TOSYLATE IN 5% DEXTROSE INJECTION
**Usual adult and adolescent dose**
Ventricular fibrillation or
Ventricular tachycardia, hemodynamically unstable—
> Intravenous infusion, 1 to 2 mg per minute; or 5 to 10 mg per kg of body weight infused over a period greater than eight minutes every six hours.

**Usual pediatric dose**
Safety and efficacy have not been established.

**Strength(s) usually available**
U.S.—
> 1 mg per mL (Rx) [GENERIC].
> 2 mg per mL (Rx) [GENERIC].
> 4 mg per mL (Rx) [GENERIC].
Canada—
> 2 mg per mL (Rx) [GENERIC].
> 4 mg per mL (Rx) [GENERIC].

**Packaging and storage**
Store below 40 °C (104 °F), preferably between 15 and 30 °C (59 and 86 °F), unless otherwise specified by manufacturer. Protect from freezing.

## Selected Bibliography
Anderson JL. Bretylium tosylate: profile of the only available class III antiarrhythmic agent. Clin Ther 1985; 7 (2): 205-24.

Revised: 06/28/96

## BROMAZEPAM—See *Benzodiazepines (Systemic)*

# BROMOCRIPTINE  Systemic

VA CLASSIFICATION (Primary/Secondary): AU900/HS900

Note: For a listing of dosage forms and brand names by country availability, see *Dosage Forms* section(s). For a listing of brand names for the articles in this monograph, refer to the General Index.

## Category

Dopamine agonist; antihyperprolactinemic; infertility therapy adjunct; lactation inhibitor; antidyskinetic; growth hormone suppressant (acromegaly); neuroleptic malignant syndrome therapy.

## Indications

Note: Bracketed information in the *Indications* section refers to uses that are not included in U.S. product labeling.

### Accepted

Prolactinomas, pituitary (treatment)—Bromocriptine is indicated in the treatment of prolactin–secreting pituitary tumors in men and women. Bromocriptine is usually considered to be the treatment of choice for microadenomas and for macroadenomas including those with visual defects. However, surgery may be required to treat macroadenomas in those patients who either cannot take bromocriptine or who exhibit a poor therapeutic response to bromocriptine. Bromocriptine may also be used as an adjunct to radiotherapy when the tumor is inoperable.

[Bromocriptine is used by some clinicians in the treatment of visual field defects that develop during pregnancy. Visual field defects that respond to bromocriptine are secondary to pituitary adenoma enlargement.][1]

Amenorrhea, secondary, due to hyperprolactinemia (treatment) or
Galactorrhea due to hyperprolactinemia (treatment) or
Hypogonadism, male, due to hyperprolactinemia (treatment) or
Infertility due to hyperprolactinemia (treatment)—Bromocriptine is indicated in the short-term symptomatic treatment of amenorrhea and/or galactorrhea or male or female infertility associated with hyperprolactinemia. Its usefulness in normoprolactinemic amenorrhea or anovulation is controversial.

[Lactation, after second- or third-trimester pregnancy loss (prophylaxis)][1]—Bromocriptine can be used in selected individuals for the prevention of physiological lactation and breast engorgement after stillbirth, neonatal death, or abortion. However, in many patients, breast engorgement is a benign, self-limited condition, which may respond to breast support and mild analgesics, such as acetaminophen and ibuprofen. Once bromocriptine has been discontinued, 18 to 40% of patients experience rebound symptoms of breast secretion, congestion, or engorgement. Also, the relative risk of all of bromocriptine's rare, severe, or life-threatening side effects, which have included strokes, seizures, and myocardial infarction, has yet to be determined.

Parkinsonism (treatment)—Bromocriptine is indicated, usually as an adjunct to levodopa/carbidopa therapy, in the treatment of the signs and symptoms of idiopathic or postencephalic parkinsonism.

Acromegaly (treatment)—Bromocriptine is indicated in the treatment of some cases of acromegaly, usually as an adjunct to surgery or radiotherapy. There are some reports that patients who respond may have elevated prolactin as well as elevated growth hormone concentrations.

[Neuroleptic malignant syndrome (treatment)][1]—Although controlled clinical trials have not been conducted, bromocriptine is sometimes used as adjunctive therapy in the treatment of neuroleptic malignant syndrome. Individual case reports and the known pharmacological activity of bromocriptine indicate that it may have some utility in the treatment of this disorder, as well as a lower incidence of side effects, as compared with other modes of therapy for this condition.

### Unaccepted

The routine use of bromocriptine for suppression of postpartum lactation is not recommended.

[1]Not included in Canadian product labeling.

## Pharmacology/Pharmacokinetics

### Physicochemical characteristics

Chemical group—Bromocriptine is an ergot alkaloid derivative.
Molecular weight—750.70.

### Mechanism of action/Effect

Dopamine agonist
Antihyperprolactinemic
Infertility therapy adjunct and

Lactation inhibitor—Reduction of serum prolactin concentrations by direct inhibition of release of prolactin from the anterior pituitary gland through binding to dopamine type 2 ($D_2$) receptors, resulting in restoration of testicular or ovarian function and suppression of lactation.

Antidyskinetic—In high doses, stimulation of post-synaptic dopamine type 2 ($D_2$) receptors in the neostriatum of the central nervous system (CNS); may also decrease dopamine turnover. At low doses, bromocriptine may worsen dyskinesia by stimulating pre-synaptic dopamine receptors. Is most effective when used concurrently with levodopa, as stimulation of $D_1$ receptors by levodopa enhances the antidyskinetic effects of postsynaptic $D_2$ receptor stimulation by bromocriptine.

Growth hormone suppressant (acromegaly)—Suppression of secretion and reduction of elevated growth hormone serum concentrations.

Neuroleptic malignant syndrome therapy—Some evidence exists that neuroleptic malignant syndrome may result from depletion of dopamine or blockade of dopamine receptors in the nigrostriatal, hypothalamic, and mesolimbic cortical pathways. Bromocriptine stimulates these dopamine receptors.

### Absorption

Approximately 28% of an oral dose is absorbed from the gastrointestinal tract, but because of first-pass metabolism, only 6% reaches the systemic circulation unchanged.

### Protein binding

Very high (90 to 96% to serum albumin).

### Biotransformation

Hepatic.

### Half-life

Biphasic—
    4 to 4.5 hours (alpha phase).
    15 hours (terminal).

### Onset of action

Single dose—
    Serum prolactin-lowering effect: 2 hours.
    Antiparkinsonism effect: 30 to 90 minutes.
    Growth hormone–lowering effect: 1 to 2 hours.

### Time to peak concentration

1 to 3 hours.

### Time to peak effect

Serum prolactin–lowering effect—8 hours (after a single dose).

Note: The maximum obtainable reduction in serum prolactin occurs after approximately 4 weeks of continuous therapy. The average duration of therapy required to reinitiate menses is 6 to 8 weeks. In the treatment of galactorrhea, a significant reduction in lactation usually occurs within 6 to 7 weeks, with cessation of lactation occurring by 12 to 13 weeks. Suppression of postpartum lactation requires 2 to 3 weeks of therapy; some clinicians believe that 3 weeks of therapy is necessary to prevent rebound lactation.

Antiparkinsonism effect—2 hours (after a single dose).
Growth hormone–lowering effect—A clinical response occurs within 4 to 8 weeks with continuous therapy.

### Duration of action

Serum prolactin–lowering effect—Approximately 24 hours (after a single dose).

Note: Serum prolactin concentrations usually return to pretreatment levels within 2 months after bromocriptine is discontinued.

Growth hormone–lowering effect—4 to 8 hours.

### Elimination

As metabolites—
    Biliary: Approximately 95%.
    Renal: 2.5 to 5.5%.

## Precautions to Consider

### Cross-sensitivity and/or related problems

Patients sensitive to other ergot derivatives may be sensitive to this medication also.

### Pregnancy/Reproduction

Fertility—Restoration of fertility may result in pregnancy with possible enlargement of a pituitary adenoma, leading to visual field defects, headaches, and excessive nausea and vomiting in the mother.

In general, use of a nonhormonal contraceptive is recommended in patients being treated for hyperprolactinemia until normal ovulatory menstrual cycles are established. At that time, contraception can be discontinued in patients desiring pregnancy, with careful monitoring to avoid inadvertent administration of bromocriptine after pregnancy is diagnosed.

*Pregnancy*—Bromocriptine is generally not recommended for use during pregnancy; however, in patients with a known pituitary tumor, some clinicians advocate use of bromocriptine to prevent or treat expansion of the tumor during pregnancy. Alternatively, surgery to remove a macroadenoma may be performed prior to conception.

Large and long-term studies performed in humans have found no increased incidence of birth defects. With clinical usage, successful pregnancies have occurred in humans with administration of bromocriptine both before conception and for periods ranging from the first 2 to 3 weeks to the full length of the pregnancy.

FDA Pregnancy Category B.

**Breast-feeding**
This medication should not be administered to mothers who intend to breast-feed, since bromocriptine interferes with lactation.

**Pediatrics**
Appropriate studies on the relationship of age to the effects of bromocriptine have not been performed in the pediatric population. Safety and efficacy have not been established.

**Adolescents**
Appropriate studies performed to date have not demonstrated adolescent-specific problems that would limit the use of bromocriptine in adolescents 15 years of age and older. However, appropriate studies to establish safety and efficacy in adolescents younger than 15 years of age have not been performed.

**Geriatrics**
Appropriate studies on the relationship of age to the effects of bromocriptine have not been performed in the geriatric population. However, clinical experience with the use of bromocriptine has shown that CNS effects may occur more frequently in the elderly.

**Dental**
Use of large doses of bromocriptine (for example, in the treatment of acromegaly or parkinsonism) may decrease or inhibit salivary flow, thus contributing to the development of caries, periodontal disease, oral candidiasis, and discomfort.

**Drug interactions and/or related problems**
The following drug interactions and/or related problems have been selected on the basis of their potential clinical significance (possible mechanism in parentheses where appropriate)—not necessarily inclusive (» = major clinical significance):

Note: Combinations containing any of the following medications, depending on the amount present, may also interact with this medication.

» Alcohol
  (disulfiram-like reaction may occur, including chest pain, confusion, fast or pounding heartbeat, flushing or redness of face, sweating, nausea, vomiting, throbbing headache, blurred vision, and severe weakness)

» Ergot alkaloids, other
  (although there is no conclusive evidence of a drug interaction, rarely occurring cases of hypertension associated with the use of bromocriptine may be aggravated with use of ergot alkaloids)

Haloperidol or
Loxapine or
Methyldopa or
Metoclopramide or
Molindone or
Monoamine oxidase (MAO) inhibitors, including furazolidone, procarbazine, and selegiline or
Phenothiazines or
Reserpine or
Thioxanthenes
  (may increase serum prolactin concentrations and interfere with effects of bromocriptine; dosage adjustment of bromocriptine may be necessary)

Hypotension-producing medications, other (See *Appendix II*)
  (concurrent use may result in additive hypotensive effects; antihypertensive dosage adjustment may be necessary)

Levodopa
  (bromocriptine may produce additive effects, allowing reduction in levodopa dosage)

**Laboratory value alterations**
The following have been selected on the basis of their potential clinical significance (possible effect in parentheses where appropriate)—not necessarily inclusive (» = major clinical significance):

With physiology/laboratory test values
  Growth hormone
    (plasma concentrations may be transiently increased in individuals with normal concentrations, paradoxically reduced in patients with acromegaly)

**Medical considerations/Contraindications**
The medical considerations/contraindications included here have been selected on the basis of their potential clinical significance (reasons given in parentheses where appropriate)—not necessarily inclusive (» = major clinical significance).

*Risk-benefit should be considered when the following medical problems exist:*
  Hepatic function impairment
    (metabolism may be reduced; dosage reduction may be required)

  Hypertension, or history of or
  Hypertension, pregnancy-induced, history of
    (may be aggravated; cautious use and monitoring of blood pressure are indicated with these conditions)

  Psychiatric disorders
    (may be exacerbated)

  Sensitivity to bromocriptine or other ergot alkaloids

**Patient monitoring**
The following may be especially important in patient monitoring (other tests may be warranted in some patients, depending on condition; » = major clinical significance):

» Blood pressure measurements
  (recommended especially when used for suppression of postpartum lactation; commonly decreases or rarely increases)

» Imaging studies of sella turcica
  (recommended prior to initiation of therapy for all patients with hyperprolactinemia, to rule out possible pituitary tumor, and once a year during therapy to detect enlargement of a tumor; after one or two years of therapy, this examination may be performed less frequently in asymptomatic patients)

» Pregnancy test
  (recommended in patients being treated for amenorrhea once menses resumes, whenever a menstrual period is missed)

» Prolactin, serum
  (measurement of serum concentrations is recommended monthly during initial treatment and twice yearly during maintenance treatment of hyperprolactinemia to assess effectiveness of bromocriptine)

  Visual field assessment
    (recommended if clinically indicated during pregnancy after treatment with bromocriptine in case of enlargement of a previously detected macroadenoma)

*For treatment of female infertility*
  Anterior pituitary function
    (complete evaluation may be warranted prior to initiation of treatment for infertility)

» Evaluation of ovulation, including:
  Daily basal body temperature and/or
  Progesterone, serum and/or
  Use of ovulation prediction test kits and
» Prolactin, serum
  (measurement of baseline serum prolactin concentration is recommended, with subsequent measurements as needed, along with other tests as may be appropriate for the evaluation and treatment of female infertility)

*For treatment of male infertility*
  FSH, serum and
  LH, serum and
  Prolactin, serum and
  Testosterone, serum
    (baseline serum concentration measurements recommended to rule out other causes of infertility and at 3- to 6-month intervals thereafter)

  Prolactin, serum
    (measurement of serum concentrations is recommended at 4- to 6-week intervals until normal levels are established, then at 3- to 6-month intervals)

Sperm counts
(recommended at periodic intervals beginning 3 months after initiation of treatment)

*For treatment of acromegaly*
» Growth hormone or
Insulin-like growth factor I concentrations (IGF-I), serum
(measurement of serum concentrations is recommended at periodic intervals to assess efficacy and aid in dosage adjustment)

Physical examination
(periodic examination, especially assessing changes in ring size, heel pad thickness, or soft-tissue volume)

## Side/Adverse Effects

Note: The most common side effects occur on initiation of therapy. Most side effects occurring with continuous therapy are dose-related.

Long-term treatment (6 to 36 months) with bromocriptine mesylate has rarely been associated with pulmonary infiltrates, pleural effusion, and thickening of the pleura. These occurred in a few patients taking doses ranging from 20 to 100 mg per day. When bromocriptine was discontinued, the changes slowly reversed toward normal.

The following side/adverse effects have been selected on the basis of their potential clinical significance (possible signs and symptoms in parentheses where appropriate)—not necessarily inclusive:

**Those indicating need for medical attention**
Incidence less frequent
*Confusion; dyskinesia* (uncontrolled movements of the body, such as the face, tongue, arms, hands, head, and upper body); *hallucinations*

Note: *Confusion, dyskinesia,* or *hallucinations* are usually associated with use of high doses but may occur in 20 to 25% of patients being treated for parkinsonism, even at low doses, and may persist for a week or more after bromocriptine is withdrawn.

Incidence rare
*Myocardial infarction* (severe chest pain,; fainting; fast heartbeat; increased sweating; continuing or severe nausea and vomiting; nervousness; unexplained shortness of breath; weakness); *seizures or strokes* (atypical headache; vision changes, such as blurred vision or temporary blindness; sudden weakness)

Note: There have been a few reports of *myocardial infarction* occurring in patients treated with bromocriptine, including patients that were treated with bromocriptine to suppress lactation, although a direct causal relationship has not been established.

There have been a number of reports of postpartum hypertension, *seizures,* and *strokes* as well as reports of fatalities occurring in patients treated with bromocriptine to suppress lactation; however, further studies are being conducted to determine if a causal relationship exists between the incidence of hypertension, strokes, and seizures and the use of bromocriptine for suppression of lactation. Mean onset of the reactions was 9 days postpartum. The cases of cerebrovascular accident were all associated with hypertension. Use of bromocriptine should be reevaluated in those patients who experience unexplained headaches and therapy discontinued if headache is severe and atypical.

*With high doses*
*Cerebrospinal fluid rhinorrhea* (continuing runny nose)—in patients treated for pituitary macroadenomas; *fainting*—has also occurred with low doses used in postpartum patients; *gastrointestinal hemorrhage or peptic ulcer* (black, tarry stools; blood in vomit; severe or continuing stomach pain); *retroperitoneal fibrosis* (continuing or severe abdominal or stomach pain; increased frequency of urination; continuing loss of appetite; lower back pain; continuing or severe nausea and vomiting; weakness)—with long-term use

**Those indicating need for medical attention only if they continue or are bothersome**
Incidence more frequent
*Hypotension* (dizziness or lightheadedness, especially when getting up from a lying or sitting position)—especially when getting up from a lying or sitting position; *nausea*

Note: *Hypotension* occurs frequently, but is symptomatic only in 1 to 5% of patients (8% of postpartum patients). Rarely, hypotension may be severe. A "first-dose phenomenon" has been reported.

Incidence less frequent—more frequent with high doses (for example, when used for acromegaly or parkinsonism)
*Constipation; diarrhea; drowsiness or tiredness; dry mouth; leg cramps at night; loss of appetite; mental depression; Raynaud's phenomenon* (tingling or pain in fingers or toes when exposed to cold); *stomach pain; stuffy nose; vomiting*

## Patient Consultation

As an aid to patient consultation, refer to *Advice for the Patient, Bromocriptine (Systemic)*.

In providing consultation, consider emphasizing the following selected information (» = major clinical significance):

**Before using this medication**
» Conditions affecting use, especially:
Sensitivity to bromocriptine or other ergot alkaloids
Pregnancy—Use is not generally recommended
Breast-feeding—Will prevent lactation in mothers who intend to breast-feed
Use in the elderly—CNS effects may occur more frequently
Dental—Reduced salivary flow caused by large doses may contribute to dental disorders
Other medications, especially alcohol or other ergot alkaloids

**Proper use of this medication**
Taking with meals or milk to reduce gastrointestinal irritation; taking dose at bedtime or the first doses vaginally to better tolerate nausea
» Proper dosing
Missed dose: Taking if remembered within 4 hours; otherwise not taking at all; not doubling doses
» Proper storage

**Precautions while using this medication**
Regular visits to physician to check progress
» Caution when driving or doing jobs requiring alertness because of possible drowsiness or dizziness
Dizziness may be more likely to occur after initial dose; taking first dose at bedtime or lying down; getting up slowly from sitting or lying position; taking first dose vaginally, if necessary
» Possible dryness of mouth; using sugarless gum or candy, ice, or saliva substitute for relief; checking with physician or dentist if dry mouth continues for more than 2 weeks
Checking with physician before reducing dosage or discontinuing medication
» Possibility of disulfiram-like reaction with alcohol
*For treatment of acromegaly, amenorrhea, infertility, galactorrhea, or pituitary prolactinomas in females of child-bearing potential*
Advisability of using nonhormonal contraception during therapy or, when using bromocriptine for female infertility, until normal menstrual cycle is established; patients desiring pregnancy should discuss with physician proper time to discontinue use of contraception; telling physician immediately if pregnancy is suspected
» Telling physician right away if symptoms of enlargement of pituitary tumor (blurred vision, sudden headache, severe nausea and vomiting) occur

**Side/adverse effects**
Signs of potential side effects, especially CNS effects, fainting, myocardial infarction, seizures, gastrointestinal hemorrhage, peptic ulcer, retroperitoneal fibrosis, rhinorrhea, and strokes

## General Dosing Information

Incidence and severity of side effects (especially nausea) may be reduced by initiating therapy at a low dose (for example, 1.25 mg at bedtime) and increasing gradually (increments of 2.5 mg every 14 to 28 days for parkinsonism and 3 to 7 days for other indications) to the minimum effective dose, and by administering bromocriptine with food. Also, dizziness and nausea may be better tolerated by administering some or all of the dose at bedtime or by administering one or more of the initial doses intravaginally. Since no first-pass effect occurs with a vaginal dose, a reduced first dose may be warranted in some cases and certainly with subsequent doses because higher serum concentrations may result.

Because of the risk of significant hypotension when bromocriptine is used rarely to treat postpartum lactation, it is recommended that the medication not be given until vital signs have stabilized, and not for at least 4 hours after delivery.

Treatment of hyperprolactinemia with bromocriptine may be symptomatic rather than curative. Following withdrawal, rebound amenorrhea usually occurs within 4 to 24 weeks and galactorrhea within 2 to 12 weeks. Pituitary adenoma regrowth and increase in serum prolactin concentrations may occur after withdrawal of bromocriptine. Elevated growth hormone concentrations will also return when the medication is withdrawn if the cause of acromegaly is not eliminated.

## Oral Dosage Forms

Note: Bracketed uses in the *Dosage Forms* section refer to categories of use and/or indications that are not included in U.S. product labeling.

### BROMOCRIPTINE MESYLATE CAPSULES USP

Note: For doses less than 5 mg, use *Bromocriptine Mesylate Tablets USP*.

#### Usual adult dose

Amenorrhea, secondary, due to hyperprolactinemia or
Galactorrhea due to hyperprolactinemia or
Hypogonadism, male, due to hyperprolactinemia or
Infertility due to hyperprolactinemia—
    Initial: Oral, 1.25 to 2.5 mg at bedtime with a snack. Dosage may be increased by 2.5 mg every three to seven days as needed to a total of 5 to 7.5 mg a day taken in divided doses with meals.
    Maintenance: Oral, 2.5 mg two or three times a day with meals. Doses of up to 15 mg have been used.
Prolactinomas, pituitary—
    Initial: Oral, 1.25 mg two or three times a day with meals. Dosage adjustment is gradual over several weeks to 10 to 20 mg a day taken in divided doses with meals. Occasionally, higher doses may be required.
    Maintenance: Oral, 2.5 to 20 mg a day taken in divided doses with meals.
Parkinsonism—
    Initial: Oral, 1.25 mg one or two times a day with meals; for single doses, at bedtime with a snack is preferred. Dosage may be increased by 2.5 mg increments every fourteen to twenty-eight days.
    Maintenance: Oral, 2.5 to 40 mg a day, taken in divided doses with meals. Although higher doses have been used, safety and efficacy have not been established with doses greater than 100 mg a day.
Acromegaly—
    Initial: Oral, 1.25 to 2.5 mg at bedtime with a snack for 3 days; dosage may be increased by 1.25 or 2.5 mg every three to seven days up to 30 mg a day taken in divided doses with meals or at bedtime with a snack.
    Maintenance: Oral, 10 to 30 mg a day taken in divided doses with meals or at bedtime with a snack. Up to 100 mg per day has been used.
[Lactation suppression][1]—
    Initial: Oral, 2.5 mg twice a day taken with meals. Patient may begin medication only after vital signs stabilize and no sooner than four hours after delivery.
    Maintenance: Oral, 2.5 to 7.5 mg a day taken in divided doses with meals or at bedtime with a snack for fourteen days. Has been used for up to twenty-one days if needed.
[Neuroleptic malignant syndrome][1]—
    Initial: Oral, 5 mg once a day taken at bedtime with a snack; dosage adjustment titrated according to patient response by 2.5 mg increments a day as needed, taken in divided doses with meals or at bedtime with a snack.
    Maintenance: Oral, up to 20 mg a day taken in divided doses with meals or at bedtime with a snack.

#### Usual adult prescribing limits

Parkinsonism—40 mg a day.
Other indications—20 mg a day.

Note: Although higher doses have been used, safety and efficacy have not been established with doses greater than 100 mg a day.

#### Usual pediatric dose

Children up to 15 years of age: Dosage has not been established.
Children 15 years of age and older: See *Usual adult dose*.

#### Strength(s) usually available

U.S.—
    5 mg (Rx) [*Parlodel* (lactose; sodium bisulfite)].
Canada—
    5 mg (Rx) [*Parlodel* (lactose)].

#### Packaging and storage

Store below 25 °C (77 °F), unless otherwise specified by manufacturer. Store in a tight, light-resistant container.

#### Auxiliary labeling

• Avoid alcoholic beverages.
• Take with meals or milk.
• May cause drowsiness.

#### Note

Unit-dose repackaging by any process involving heat is not recommended.

### BROMOCRIPTINE MESYLATE TABLETS USP

Note: For doses 5 mg or greater, consider using *Bromocriptine Mesylate Capsules USP*.

#### Usual adult dose

See *Bromocriptine Mesylate Capsules USP*..

#### Usual pediatric dose

See *Bromocriptine Mesylate Capsules USP*.

#### Strength(s) usually available

U.S.—
    2.5 mg (Rx) [*Parlodel SnapTabs* (scored; lactose)].
Canada—
    2.5 mg (Rx) [*Parlodel* (scored; lactose)].

#### Packaging and storage

Store below 25 °C (77 °F), unless otherwise specified by manufacturer. Store in a tight, light-resistant container.

#### Auxiliary labeling

• Avoid alcoholic beverages.
• Take with meals or milk.
• May cause drowsiness.

#### Note

Unit-dose repackaging by any process involving heat is not recommended.

[1]Not included in Canadian product labeling.

## Selected Bibliography

Ho Ky, Thorner Mo. Therapeutic applications of bromocriptine in endocrine and neurological diseases. Drugs 1988; 36: 67-82.

The American Fertility Society. Guideline for practice: The use of bromocriptine. Birmingham: American Fertility Society, 1991.

Revised: 08/09/95

**BROMODIPHENHYDRAMINE**—See *Antihistamines (Systemic)*

## BROMODIPHENHYDRAMINE-CONTAINING COMBINATIONS—

Bromodiphenhydramine and Codeine (Systemic)—See *Cough/Cold Combinations (Systemic)*
Bromodiphenhydramine, Diphenhydramine, Codeine, Ammonium Chloride, and Potassium Guaiacolsulfonate (Systemic)—See *Cough/Cold Combinations (Systemic)*

**BROMPHENIRAMINE**—See *Antihistamines (Systemic)*

## BROMPHENIRAMINE-CONTAINING COMBINATIONS—

Brompheniramine and Phenylephrine (Systemic)—See *Antihistamines and Decongestants (Systemic)*
Brompheniramine, Phenylephrine, and Phenylpropanolamine (Systemic)—See *Antihistamines and Decongestants (Systemic)*
Brompheniramine, Phenylephrine, Phenylpropanolamine, and Codeine (Systemic)—See *Cough/Cold Combinations (Systemic)*
Brompheniramine, Phenylephrine, Phenylpropanolamine, Codeine, and Guaifenesin (Systemic)—See *Cough/Cold Combinations (Systemic)*
Brompheniramine, Phenylephrine, Phenylpropanolamine, and Dextromethorphan (Systemic)—See *Cough/Cold Combinations (Systemic)*
Brompheniramine, Phenylephrine, Phenylpropanolamine, and Guaifenesin (Systemic)—See *Cough/Cold Combinations (Systemic)*
Brompheniramine, Phenylephrine, Phenylpropanolamine, Hydrocodone, and Guaifenesin (Systemic)—See *Cough/Cold Combinations (Systemic)*
Brompheniramine and Phenylpropanolamine (Systemic)—See *Antihistamines and Decongestants (Systemic)*

Brompheniramine, Phenylpropanolamine, and Acetaminophen (Systemic)—
    See *Antihistamines, Decongestants, and Analgesics (Systemic)*
Brompheniramine, Phenylpropanolamine, and Codeine (Systemic)—See
    *Cough/Cold Combinations (Systemic)*
Brompheniramine, Phenylpropanolamine, and Dextromethorphan (Sys-
    temic)—See *Cough/Cold Combinations (Systemic)*

Brompheniramine and Pseudoephedrine (Systemic)—See *Antihistamines
    and Decongestants (Systemic)*
Brompheniramine, Pseudoephedrine, and Acetaminophen (Systemic)—
    See *Antihistamines, Decongestants, and Analgesics (Systemic)*
Brompheniramine, Pseudoephedrine, and Dextromethorphan (Systemic)—
    See *Cough/Cold Combinations (Systemic)*

---

# BRONCHODILATORS, ADRENERGIC    Systemic

This monograph includes information on the following: Albuterol; Bitol-
terol†; Ephedrine; Epinephrine; Ethylnorepinephrine†; Fenoterol*; Is-
oetharine†; Isoproterenol; Metaproterenol; Pirbuterol†; Procaterol*;
Terbutaline.

INN:
    Albuterol—Salbutamol

VA CLASSIFICATION (Primary/Secondary):
    Albuterol
        Inhalation—RE102/RE109
        Oral—RE103
        Parenteral—RE103
    Bitolterol
        Inhalation—RE102/RE109
    Ephedrine
        Oral—RE103/RE200; CN809; DE890
        Parenteral—AU100/RE103; DE890
    Epinephrine
        Inhalation—RE102/RE109
        Parenteral—AU100/RE103; CN205; OP900; DE900; RE900
    Ethylnorepinephrine
        Parenteral—RE103
    Fenoterol
        Inhalation—RE102
        Oral—RE103
    Isoetharine
        Inhalation—RE102/RE109
    Isoproterenol
        Inhalation—RE102
        Oral—AU100/RE103
        Parenteral—AU100/RE103
    Metaproterenol
        Inhalation—RE102/RE109
        Oral—RE103
    Pirbuterol
        Inhalation—RE102/RE109
    Procaterol
        Inhalation—RE102/RE109
    Terbutaline
        Inhalation—RE102/RE109
        Oral—RE103/GU900
        Parenteral—AU100/RE103; GU900

Other commonly used names are: Orciprenaline [Metaproterenol], Sal-
butamol [Albuterol]

Note: For a listing of dosage forms and brand names by country availa-
    bility, see *Dosage Forms* section(s). For a listing of brand names
    for the articles in this monograph, refer to the General Index.

---

*Not commercially available in the U.S.
†Not commercially available in Canada.

---

## Category

Bronchodilator—Albuterol; Bitolterol; Ephedrine; Epinephrine; Ethylno-
    repinephrine; Fenoterol; Isoetharine; Isoproterenol; Metaproterenol;
    Pirbuterol; Procaterol; Terbutaline.
Asthma prophylactic—Albuterol Inhalation Aerosol; Albuterol Inhalation
    Solution; Bitolterol; Epinephrine (Inhalation); Isoetharine; Metaproter-
    enol (Inhalation); Pirbuterol; Procaterol; Terbutaline (Inhalation).
Anesthetic (local) adjunct—Epinephrine Injection.
Antiallergic (systemic)—Epinephrine Injection.
Surgical aid (antihemorrhagic; decongestant; mydriatic)—Epinephrine
    Injection.
Antihemorrhagic (topical)—Epinephrine Injection.
Decongestant, nasal (systemic)—Ephedrine (Oral).
Central nervous system (CNS) stimulant—Ephedrine (Oral).
Labor (premature) inhibitor—Terbutaline (Oral and Parenteral).
Urticaria therapy adjunct—Ephedrine.
Priapism reversal agent—Epinephrine Injection.

## Indications

Note: Bracketed information in the *Indications* section refers to uses that
    are not included in U.S. product labeling.

**Accepted**
Asthma, bronchial (treatment)
Bronchitis (treatment)
Bronchospasm (treatment)
Emphysema, pulmonary (treatment)
Bronchiectasis (treatment) or
Pulmonary disease, obstructive, other (treatment)—Albuterol, bitolterol,
    epinephrine, ethylnorepinephrine, fenoterol, isoetharine, isoproterenol
    inhalation, metaproterenol, pirbuterol, procaterol, and terbutaline are
    indicated for the symptomatic treatment of bronchial asthma. These
    medications are also indicated for the treatment of reversible bron-
    chospasm associated with bronchitis, pulmonary emphysema, bron-
    chiectasis, and other obstructive pulmonary diseases.

    Also, ephedrine may be indicated for the symptomatic treatment of
    bronchial asthma and reversible bronchospasm associated with other
    obstructive pulmonary diseases; however, agents with less beta-1-ad-
    renergic effects and more selective beta-2-adrenergic effects are gen-
    erally preferred. In the treatment of acute bronchospasm, parenteral
    ephedrine is usually less effective than epinephrine.

    Isoproterenol sublingual tablets may be used for the treatment of bron-
    chial asthma and in the management of obstructive pulmonary disease,
    but isoproterenol inhalation is preferred because absorption after sub-
    lingual administration may be erratic and unpredictable.

Asthma, bronchial (prophylaxis) or
Bronchospasm (prophylaxis)—Albuterol inhalation aerosol[1], bitolterol,
    and pirbuterol are indicated for the prophylaxis of bronchial asthma
    and reversible bronchospasm. [Other adrenergic bronchodilators, al-
    buterol inhalation solution, epinephrine inhalation, isoetharine, meta-
    proterenol inhalation, procaterol, and terbutaline inhalation, are also
    used for the prophylaxis of bronchial asthma and reversible
    bronchospasm.][1]

    Albuterol inhalation[1] and procaterol inhalation are indicated for the
    prevention of exercise-induced bronchospasm. [Other inhaled adre-
    nergic bronchodilators are also used in the prevention of exercise-
    induced bronchospasm.][1]

Bronchospasm, during anesthesia (treatment)—Parenteral isoproterenol
    may be indicated in the management of bronchospasm during anes-
    thesia. [Parenteral epinephrine and terbutaline may also be useful in
    the management of bronchospasm during anesthesia.]

Allergic reactions, drug-induced (treatment)
Anaphylactic reactions (treatment)
Angioedema (treatment)
Bites or stings, insect (treatment)
Laryngeal edema, acute noninfectious (treatment) or
Transfusion reactions, urticarial (treatment)—Epinephrine injection is in-
    dicated in the emergency treatment of severe allergic reactions to
    drugs, foods, sera, insect stings, or other allergens. It relieves symp-
    toms such as bronchospasm, urticaria, pruritus, hives, angioedema, and
    swelling of lips, eyelids, tongue, and nasal mucosa. Epinephrine in-
    jection is also used in the treatment of acute noninfectious laryngeal
    edema.

Croup (treatment)—Racepinephrine inhalation is indicated in the treatment
    of postintubation and infectious croup.

Anesthesia, local, adjunct—Epinephrine injection is indicated for concur-
    rent use with some local anesthetics to decrease the rate of vascular
    absorption and thereby localize anesthesia, prolong the duration of
    action, and decrease the risk of toxicity due to the local anesthetic.

Epinephrine injection should be used cautiously and in carefully circumscribed quantities, if at all, with local anesthetics for anesthetizing areas with end arteries (such as the fingers, toes, or penis) or otherwise compromised blood supply because ischemia leading to gangrene may result.

Hemorrhage, superficial, in ocular surgery (treatment)

Congestion, conjunctival, during surgery (treatment)

Mydriasis, during surgery or

Hypertension, ocular, during surgery (treatment)—Epinephrine may be injected intracamerally or subconjunctivally to control hemorrhage, produce conjunctival decongestion and mydriasis, and reduce intraocular pressure during ocular surgery.

Hemorrhage, superficial (treatment)—Epinephrine injection may be applied topically to control superficial bleeding from arterioles and capillaries in the skin, mucous membranes, or other tissues. However, only small doses should be used because topically applied epinephrine can be systemically absorbed.

Congestion, nasal (treatment) or

Congestion, sinus (treatment)—Oral ephedrine may be indicated for the local treatment of nasal congestion in acute coryza, vasomotor rhinitis, acute sinusitis, and hay fever. It may also be used in the treatment of sinus congestion.

Narcolepsy (treatment) or

Depression, mental (treatment)—Oral ephedrine may be indicated as a CNS stimulant in the treatment of narcolepsy and depressive states.

Status asthmaticus (treatment)—Parenteral albuterol is used for the treatment of status asthmaticus.

[Labor, premature (prophylaxis and treatment)][1]—Terbutaline (oral and parenteral) is used for prophylaxis and treatment of preterm labor.

[Urticaria (treatment adjunct)][1]—Ephedrine may be useful as an adjunct in the treatment of acute and chronic urticaria.

[Hemorrhage, gingival (treatment adjunct)][1] or

[Hemorrhage, pulpal (treatment)][1]—Epinephrine injection is used topically as an adjunct in the treatment of gingival hemorrhage. It is also used in the treatment of pulpal hemorrhage.

[Priapism (treatment)][1]—Epinephrine injection, administered intracavernosally, has been reported to be effective in the treatment of priapism resulting from use of intracavernosal papaverine or phentolamine or from other causes. However, epinephrine should be used with caution because hypertension and ischemic electrocardiographic changes can occur.

**Unaccepted**

Oral ephedrine has been used in the treatment of enuresis and myasthenia gravis but it has been replaced by more effective agents.

[1]Not included in Canadian product labeling.

# Pharmacology/Pharmacokinetics

See also *Table 1*, page 625.

### Physicochemical characteristics

Molecular weight—

Albuterol: 239.31.

Albuterol sulfate: 576.70.

Bitolterol mesylate: 557.66.

Ephedrine sulfate: 428.54.

Epinephrine: 183.21.

Epinephrine bitartrate: 333.29.

Ethylnorepinephrine hydrochloride: 233.69.

Fenoterol hydrobromide: 384.3.

Isoetharine hydrochloride: 275.77.

Isoetharine mesylate: 335.41.

Isoproterenol hydrochloride: 247.72.

Isoproterenol sulfate: 556.62.

Metaproterenol sulfate: 520.59.

Pirbuterol acetate: 300.3.

Procaterol hydrochloride hemihydrate: 335.83.

Racepinephrine: 183.21.

Terbutaline sulfate: 548.65.

### Mechanism of action/Effect

Bronchodilator—

Adrenergic bronchodilators act by stimulating beta-2-adrenergic receptors in the lungs to relax bronchial smooth muscle, thereby relieving bronchospasm, increasing vital capacity, decreasing residual volume, and reducing airway resistance. This action is believed to result from increased production of cyclic adenosine 3',5'-monophosphate (cyclic 3',5'-AMP or c-AMP) caused by activation of the enzyme adenyl cyclase, the enzyme that catalyzes the conversion of adenosine triphosphate (ATP) to c-AMP. Increased c-

AMP concentrations, in addition to relaxing bronchial smooth muscle, inhibit release of mediators of immediate hypersensitivity from cells, especially from mast cells. Also, epinephrine acts by stimulating alpha-adrenergic receptors to constrict bronchial arterioles.

Epinephrine also inhibits antigen-induced release of histamine and the slow-reacting substance of anaphylaxis and directly antagonizes histamine-induced bronchiolar constriction, vasodilation, and edema. Ephedrine, isoetharine, and metaproterenol may also inhibit antigen-induced release of histamine, and isoproterenol may inhibit antigen-induced release of histamine and the slow-reacting substance of anaphylaxis.

Anesthetic (local) adjunct—

Epinephrine acts on alpha-adrenergic receptors in the skin, mucous membranes, and viscera to produce vasoconstriction. This action decreases the rate of vascular absorption of the local anesthetic used with epinephrine, thereby localizing anesthesia, prolonging the duration of action, and decreasing the risk of toxicity due to the anesthetic.

Surgical aid (antihemorrhagic; decongestant; mydriatic)—

Epinephrine acts on alpha-adrenergic receptors in the conjunctiva to produce vasoconstriction and hemostasis in bleeding from small vessels; also, conjunctival congestion is decreased. Epinephrine contracts the dilator muscle of the pupil by acting on alpha-adrenergic receptors, resulting in dilation of the pupil (mydriasis).

Antihemorrhagic (topical)—

Epinephrine acts on alpha-adrenergic receptors in the skin, mucous membranes, and viscera to produce vasoconstriction and hemostasis in bleeding from small vessels.

Decongestant, nasal (systemic)—

Ephedrine acts on alpha-adrenergic receptors of blood vessels in the nasal mucosa, producing vasoconstriction, which may result in nasal decongestion.

CNS stimulant—

Ephedrine stimulates the cerebral cortex and subcortical centers to produce its effects in narcolepsy and depressive states.

Labor (premature) inhibitor—

Terbutaline acts primarily as a beta-adrenergic stimulant to relax the uterine muscle, thereby inhibiting uterine contractions.

Urticaria therapy adjunct—

Ephedrine acts on alpha-adrenergic receptors of blood vessels in the skin to produce vasoconstriction, which may help to reverse cutaneous vasodilation and thereby reduce the increased vascular permeability that results in localized edema in urticaria.

### Other actions/effects

Other adrenergic effects include alpha-receptor–mediated contraction of gastrointestinal and urinary sphincters; beta-1-receptor–mediated lipolysis; and beta-2-receptor–mediated decrease in gastrointestinal tone, and increases in uterine relaxation, renin secretion, hepatic glycogenolysis/gluconeogenesis, and pancreatic beta cell secretion.

### Absorption

Albuterol—

Inhalation: Albuterol is absorbed gradually from the bronchi, with a portion of the swallowed fraction being absorbed from the gastrointestinal tract. Systemic concentrations are low following inhalation of recommended doses because inhaled doses are only 5% of those required orally.

Oral: Rapidly and well absorbed from the gastrointestinal tract.

Ephedrine—

Rapidly absorbed after oral, intramuscular, or subcutaneous administration.

Epinephrine—

Inhalation: Absorption slight with usual doses, but increased with larger doses.

Intramuscular or subcutaneous: Well absorbed. Both rapid and prolonged following administration of the aqueous suspension.

Isoetharine—

Inhalation: Rapidly absorbed from respiratory tract.

Isoproterenol—

Inhalation or parenteral: Rapidly absorbed.

Sublingual or rectal: Variable and may be unreliable.

Metaproterenol—

Inhalation: Approximately 3% of the actuated dose absorbed intact through the lungs.

Oral: About 40% of an oral metaproterenol dose absorbed from gastrointestinal tract.

Pirbuterol—

Systemic blood concentrations of pirbuterol are below limit of assay sensitivity (2 to 5 nanograms per mL), following inhalation of doses up to 0.8 mg (two times the maximum recommended dose).

Terbutaline—
Oral: About 30 to 70% of an oral dose absorbed from gastrointestinal tract. Food reduces the bioavailability of terbutaline by one-third.
Subcutaneous: Well absorbed.

## Precautions to Consider

### Carcinogenicity/Tumorigenicity
For albuterol—In one 2-year study in rats, albuterol given orally in doses corresponding to 111, 555, and 2800 times the maximum human inhalation dose and 3, 16, and 78 times the maximum human oral dose caused a significant dose-related increase in the incidence of benign leiomyomas of the mesovarium. In another study, this effect was blocked by the coadministration of propranolol. Studies have shown that other beta agonists also induce mesovarium tumors in rats. An 18-month study with albuterol in mice and a lifetime study in hamsters showed no evidence of tumorigenicity. The relevance of these findings to humans is not known.

For bitolterol—In a 2-year study in Sprague-Dawley CD rats, bitolterol administered orally at doses corresponding to 23 or 114 times the maximal daily human inhalation dose was not shown to be tumorigenic (specifically, no increase in leiomyomas). In an 18-month study in Swiss-Webster mice, bitolterol administered orally at doses up to 568 times the maximum daily human inhalation dose was not shown to be tumorigenic.

For epinephrine, ethylnorepinephrine, isoetharine, isoproterenol, and metaproterenol—Long-term studies to evaluate carcinogenic potential in animals have not been done. There is no evidence from human data that epinephrine, ethylnorepinephrine, isoetharine, isoproterenol, or metaproterenol may be carcinogenic.

For pirbuterol—Pirbuterol hydrochloride showed no carcinogenicity when the medication was administered in the diet to rats for 24 months and to mice for 18 months at doses corresponding to 200 times the maximum human inhalation dose. Also, in a 12-month study in rats, pirbuterol was shown to cause no increase in tumors when the medication was administered via intragastric intubation at doses corresponding to 6250 times the maximum recommended human daily inhalation dose.

For terbutaline—An 18-month carcinogenicity study in NMRI strain mice showed that terbutaline administered orally in doses of 5, 50, and 200 mg per kg (500, 5000, and 20,000 times the clinical subcutaneous dose, respectively) caused no drug-related tumorigenicity. A 2-year carcinogenesis bioassay of terbutaline at oral doses of 50, 500, 1000, and 2000 mg per kg (corresponding to 167, 1667, 3333, and 6667 times the recommended daily adult oral dose, respectively) in Sprague-Dawley rats showed drug-related changes in the female genital system; female rats showed drug-related increases in leiomyomas of the mesovarium, which were significant at doses of 500, 1000, and 2000 mg per kg; the incidence of ovarian cysts was increased significantly at all dose levels except at 2000 mg per kg; and hyperplasia of the mesovarium was increased significantly at 500 and 2000 mg per kg. However, in a 21-month study in mice, terbutaline at oral doses of 5, 50, and 200 mg per kg (corresponding to 17, 167, and 667 times the recommended daily adult oral dose, respectively) showed no evidence of carcinogenicity.

### Mutagenicity
For albuterol—Studies with albuterol have not shown any evidence of mutagenesis.

For bitolterol—In Ames Salmonella and mouse lymphoma mutation assays *in vitro*, bitolterol was not shown to cause mutagenesis.

For epinephrine, ethylnorepinephrine, isoetharine, isoproterenol, metaproterenol, and terbutaline—Long-term mutagenicity studies in animals have not been done. There is no evidence from human data that epinephrine, ethylnorepinephrine, isoetharine, isoproterenol, metaproterenol, or terbutaline may be mutagenic.

For pirbuterol—Studies with pirbuterol have shown no evidence of mutagenesis.

### Pregnancy/Reproduction
Fertility—For albuterol: Animal (rat) reproduction studies with albuterol have shown no evidence of impaired fertility.

For bitolterol: Reproduction studies in male and female rats have shown no significant effects on fertility when bitolterol was administered at doses up to 364 times the maximum daily human inhalation dose.

For pirbuterol: Reproduction studies in rats have shown no evidence of impaired fertility.

For terbutaline: A reproduction study in rats with oral terbutaline at doses up to 50 mg per kg of body weight (mg/kg) (corresponding to 167 times the human oral dose) showed no adverse effects on fertility.

Pregnancy—
*For albuterol—*
Adequate and well-controlled studies in humans have not been done.

Some studies in CD-1 mice have shown that albuterol causes cleft palate formation when given subcutaneously in doses of 0.25 mg per kg (corresponding to 0.4 times the maximum human oral dose and 14 times the maximum human inhalation dose) and 2.5 mg per kg (corresponding to 140 times the maximum human inhalation dose). Another study in CD-1 mice has shown that albuterol causes malformations when given orally in doses of 25 and 50 mg per kg (corresponding to at least 32 times the maximum human oral daily dose). Also, a reproduction study in Stride Dutch rabbits has shown that albuterol causes cranioschisis when given in doses of 50 mg per kg (corresponding to 78 times the maximum human oral dose and 2800 times the maximum human inhalation dose).

FDA Pregnancy Category C.
*For bitolterol—*
Well-controlled studies in humans have not been done.
Studies in mice have shown that bitolterol mesylate, administered subcutaneously at doses of 2, 10, and 20 mg per kg (corresponding to 23, 114, and 227 times the maximum daily human inhalation dose), causes cleft palate formation. However, bitolterol caused no teratogenic effects when administered to rats and rabbits in oral doses up to 557 times the maximum daily human inhalation dose and to mice in oral doses up to 284 times the maximum daily human inhalation dose.

FDA Pregnancy Category C.
*For ephedrine—*
Studies have not been done in humans.
Studies have not been done in animals.

FDA Pregnancy Category C.
*For epinephrine—*
Epinephrine crosses the placenta. Adequate and well-controlled studies in humans have not been done. Use of epinephrine during pregnancy may cause anoxia in the fetus.
Studies in animals have shown that epinephrine causes teratogenic effects in rats when given in doses about 25 times the human dose.

FDA Pregnancy Category C.
*For ethylnorepinephrine, isoetharine, and isoproterenol—*
Studies have not been done in humans.
Studies have not been done in animals.

FDA Pregnancy Category C.
*For fenoterol—*
Problems in humans have not been documented.
*For metaproterenol—*
Adequate and well-controlled studies in humans have not been done.
Studies in rabbits have shown that metaproterenol was teratogenic (effects included skeletal abnormalities and hydrocephalus with bone separation) and embryocidal when given orally in doses 620 times the human inhalation dose and 62 times the human oral dose. Reproduction studies in mice, rats, and rabbits did not show metaproterenol to be teratogenic or embryocidal when given orally in doses up to 50 mg per kg or 310 times the human inhalation dose and 31 times the human oral dose. Studies in rabbits have shown metaproterenol to cause fetal loss and teratogenic effects when administered at and above oral doses of 50 and 100 mg/kg, respectively.

FDA Pregnancy Category C.
*For pirbuterol—*
Adequate and well-controlled studies in humans have not been done.
Reproduction studies with pirbuterol given by the inhalation route, at doses up to 12 times the maximum human inhalation dose in rats and 16 times the maximum human inhalation dose in rabbits, have shown no significant adverse effects. Also, animal reproduction studies in rats at oral doses up to 300 mg/kg and in rabbits at oral doses up to 100 mg/kg have shown no adverse effects on reproductive behavior, fertility, litter size, peri- and postnatal viability, or fetal development. However, studies in rabbits have shown that pirbuterol at the highest dose level, 300 mg/kg, causes abortions and fetal mortality.

FDA Pregnancy Category C.
*For procaterol—*
Studies have not been done in humans.
Studies have not been done in animals.
For terbutaline: Terbutaline crosses the placenta. Studies in humans have not been done. Parenteral administration of terbutaline during pregnancy has been reported to cause fetal tachycardia.
Studies in animals (mice and rats) have not shown that terbutaline, at doses up to 1000 times the human dose, causes adverse

effects on the fetus. Also, reproduction studies in mice with terbutaline at doses up to 1.1 mg/kg, administered subcutaneously (corresponding to 4 times the human oral dose and 110 times the human subcutaneous dose) and in rats and rabbits with terbutaline at doses up to 50 mg/kg orally (corresponding to 167 times the human oral dose and 5000 times the human subcutaneous dose) have shown no adverse effects on the fetus.

FDA Pregnancy Category B.

Labor—For albuterol: Albuterol administered intravenously or orally reportedly inhibits uterine contractions. Although albuterol administered orally has been reported to delay preterm labor, there are no well-controlled studies that show it will stop preterm labor or prevent labor at term.

For ephedrine: When ephedrine is administered just prior to or during labor, its effect on the neonate or on the child's later growth and development is not known.

For epinephrine: Epinephrine is not recommended for use during labor since its action in relaxing the muscles of the uterus may delay the second stage. Also, when administered in high dosage sufficient to reduce uterine contractions, epinephrine may cause prolonged uterine atony with hemorrhage.

For terbutaline: Terbutaline inhibits uterine activity during the second and third trimesters of pregnancy and may inhibit labor. When administered during labor, terbutaline has been reported to cause serious adverse reactions such as transient hypokalemia, pulmonary edema, and hypoglycemia in the mother and hypoglycemia in neonates of mothers treated with parenteral terbutaline.

Delivery—For ephedrine and epinephrine: Parenteral administration of ephedrine or epinephrine to maintain blood pressure during spinal anesthesia for delivery can cause acceleration of the fetal heart rate and should not be used when maternal blood pressure exceeds 130/80.

### Breast-feeding

For albuterol—Although it is not known whether albuterol is distributed into breast milk, problems in humans have not been documented. However, some animal studies have shown albuterol to be potentially tumorigenic.

For bitolterol, ethylnorepinephrine, isoetharine, isoproterenol, metaproterenol, pirbuterol, and procaterol—Although it is not known whether bitolterol (or colterol, the active compound), ethylnorepinephrine, isoetharine, isoproterenol, metaproterenol, pirbuterol, or procaterol is distributed into breast milk, problems in humans have not been documented.

For ephedrine—Ephedrine is distributed into breast milk. Use by nursing mothers is not recommended because of the higher than usual risks for infants.

For epinephrine—Epinephrine is distributed into breast milk; use by nursing mothers may cause serious adverse reactions in the infant.

For fenoterol—Problems in humans have not been documented.

For terbutaline—Problems in humans have not been documented. However, terbutaline is distributed into breast milk and some animal studies have shown this medication to be potentially tumorigenic.

### Pediatrics

For albuterol, bitolterol, ethylnorepinephrine, fenoterol, isoetharine, isoproterenol, metaproterenol, pirbuterol, procaterol, and terbutaline—Appropriate studies on the relationship of age to the effects of adrenergic bronchodilators have not been performed in the pediatric population. However, no pediatrics-specific problems have been documented to date.

For ephedrine—Caution should be used in infants because of the higher than usual risks with the use of ephedrine in these patients.

For epinephrine—Epinephrine should be used with caution in infants and children since syncope has occurred following administration of epinephrine to asthmatic children.

### Geriatrics

For albuterol, bitolterol, epinephrine, ethylnorepinephrine, fenoterol, isoproterenol, metaproterenol, pirbuterol, procaterol, and terbutaline—No information is available on the relationship of age to the effects of these medicines in geriatric patients.

For ephedrine—Although appropriate studies on the relationship of age to the effects of ephedrine have not been performed in the geriatric population, no geriatrics-specific problems have been documented to date. However, elderly patients are more likely to have age-related prostatic hypertrophy and caution should be used in patients receiving ephedrine.

### Dental

For epinephrine—Epinephrine is used in gingival retraction cords. Systemic absorption of epinephrine can occur from application of retraction cords, especially to abraded surfaces. Epinephrine retraction cords should be used with caution in patients with cardiovascular problems,

since the amount of epinephrine absorbed systemically cannot be predicted.

### Drug interactions and/or related problems

See *Table 2*, page 627.

### Laboratory value alterations

The following have been selected on the basis of their potential clinical significance (possible effect in parentheses where appropriate)—not necessarily inclusive (» = major clinical significance):

With physiology/laboratory test values

*For all adrenergic bronchodilators*

Potassium concentrations, serum
(may be decreased, possibly through intracellular shunting, when beta-agonists are given intravenously or by nebulization or in higher-than-recommended doses; decrease is usually transient, not requiring supplementation)

*For epinephrine*

Blood glucose concentrations and
Lactic acid concentrations, serum
(may be increased)

### Medical considerations/Contraindications

See *Table 3*, page 632.

## Side/Adverse Effects

Note: Supraventricular and ventricular ectopic beats have occurred with beta-adrenergic agonist inhalations.

Hypokalemia may be induced by higher-than-recommended doses of beta-agonists, especially in those patients receiving digitalis glycosides or diuretics or who are prone to cardiac dysrhythmias.

See also *Table 4*, page 633.

## Overdose

For more information on the management of overdose or unintentional ingestion, **contact a Poison Control Center** (see *Poison Control Center Listing*).

### Treatment of overdose

For all adrenergic bronchodilators—
Reducing dosage or discontinuing medication.
Supportive therapy.

For albuterol, bitolterol, ethylnorepinephrine, fenoterol, isoetharine, metaproterenol, and procaterol—
For oral overdose, performing gastric lavage.
Administering a cardioselective beta-adrenergic blocker (e.g., acebutolol, atenolol, metoprolol), if necessary for cardiac arrhythmias; however, the beta-adrenergic blocker should be used with caution because it could induce severe bronchospasm or an asthmatic attack.

For ephedrine—
Protecting patient's airway and supporting ventilation and perfusion.
Monitoring and maintaining, within acceptable limits, patient's vital signs, blood gases, and serum electrolytes. Also, monitoring electrocardiogram continuously.
In alert patients, removing ephedrine from the stomach by inducing emesis with ipecac, followed by activated charcoal (as long as ileus is not present); in depressed or hyperactive patients, removing ephedrine by airway-protected gastric lavage.
For supraventricular or ventricular tachycardias, administering a beta-adrenergic blocker, such as propranolol, by slow intravenous administration if necessary to control cardiac arrhythmias; however, in asthmatic patients, a cardioselective beta-adrenergic blocker (e.g., acebutolol, atenolol, metoprolol) may be more appropriate. The beta-blocker should be used with caution in asthmatic patients because it could induce severe bronchospasm or an asthmatic attack.
For marked hypertension, administering nitroprusside or phentolamine infusion, if necessary.
For "true" hypotension, administration of intravenous fluids, elevation of legs, or administration of inotropic vasopressors, such as norepinephrine, should be considered.
To control convulsions, administering diazepam. For refractory seizures, general anesthesia with thiopental or halothane and paralysis with a neuromuscular blocking agent may be necessary.
Controlling pyrexia by cool applications and by slow intravenous administration of 1 mg of dexamethasone per kg of body weight.

For epinephrine—
Treatment primarily supportive since epinephrine is rapidly inactivated in the body.
For anxiety, administering sedatives.

To counteract pressor effects, administering rapidly acting vasodilators or alpha-adrenergic blockers, if necessary; however, if prolonged hypotension follows such measures, it may be necessary to administer another pressor agent such as norepinephrine.

For epinephrine-induced pulmonary edema that interferes with respiration, administering a rapidly acting alpha-adrenergic blocker, such as phentolamine, and/or intermittent positive-pressure respiration.

For arrhythmias, administering a beta-adrenergic blocker, such as propranolol; however, in asthmatic patients, a cardioselective beta-adrenergic blocker, (e.g., acebutolol, atenolol, metoproterenol) may be more appropriate. The beta-blocker should be used with caution in asthmatic patients because it could induce severe bronchospasm or an asthmatic attack.

For isoproterenol—

For CNS stimulation, administering sedatives, such as barbiturates.

For tachycardia and arrhythmias induced by isoproterenol, administering a beta-adrenergic blocker, such as propranolol; however, in asthmatic patients, a cardioselective beta-adrenergic blocker (e.g., acebutolol, atenolol, metoprolol) may be more appropriate. The beta-blocker should be used with caution in asthmatic patients because it could induce severe bronchospasm or an asthmatic attack.

For terbutaline—

In the alert patient who has taken excessive oral terbutaline, inducing emesis followed by gastric lavage.

In the unconscious patient, performing gastric lavage after the airway is secured with a cuffed endotracheal tube; not inducing emesis.

Instilling activated charcoal slurry to help reduce absorption of terbutaline.

Maintaining an adequate respiratory exchange.

Providing cardiac and respiratory support as needed.

Monitoring patient until symptom-free.

## Patient Consultation
See also *Table 5*, page 635.

## General Dosing Information

Patients taking this medication for bronchial asthma, bronchitis, emphysema, or other obstructive pulmonary disease should be advised to contact their physician if they do not respond to the usual dose of this medication, since this may be a sign of seriously worsening asthma or bronchospasm that requires reassessment of therapy.

Following administration of an adrenergic bronchodilator, a sufficient interval of time should elapse before administration of another sympathomimetic agent.

**For inhalation aerosol dosage forms only**

When an adrenergic bronchodilator inhalation aerosol is used in conjunction with an adrenocorticoid or ipratropium oral inhalation aerosol, the adrenergic bronchodilator inhalation aerosol should be administered 5 minutes prior to the adrenocorticoid or ipratropium inhalation aerosol. This interval allows for bronchodilation to occur and increased deposition of the adrenocorticoid or ipratropium within the bronchi.

Repeated excessive use may result in paradoxical bronchospasm. If this occurs, the adrenergic bronchodilator should be discontinued immediately and alternative therapy instituted.

## *ALBUTEROL*

## Summary of Differences

Indications:
    Parenteral albuterol also used in treatment of status asthmaticus.
Pharmacology/pharmacokinetics:
    Half-life—
        Elimination: 3.8 hours.
        Plasma: 2.7 to 5 hours.
    Onset of action—
        Inhalation: 5 to 15 minutes.
        Oral: 15 to 30 minutes.
    Time to peak effect—
        Inhalation: 1 to 1.5 hours after 2 inhalations.
        Oral: 2 to 3 hours.
    Duration of action—
        Inhalation: 3 to 6 hours.
        Oral: 8 hours or more (12 hours for extended-release tablets).
    Elimination—
        Secondary route of elimination is fecal.
Precautions:
    Pregnancy/reproduction—Labor: Albuterol administered intravenously or orally reportedly inhibits uterine contractions.

Medical considerations/contraindications—Caution also needed in ketoacidosis when large parenteral doses of albuterol are administered.
Side/adverse effects:
    Difficult or painful urination, drowsiness, flushing or redness of face or skin, heartburn, loss of appetite, muscle cramps or twitching, unusual paleness, or unusual taste may occur.

## Additional Dosing Information

See also *General Dosing Information*.

**For parenteral dosage forms only**

Parenteral albuterol is preferably administered by continuous intravenous infusion. However, if a rapid response is required, it may be administered by direct intravenous injection, followed by a continuous intravenous infusion. Albuterol injection may also be administered by intramuscular injection, if necessary.

## Inhalation Dosage Forms

### ALBUTEROL INHALATION AEROSOL

**Usual adult and adolescent dose**

Bronchospasm in obstructive pulmonary disease (prophylaxis[1] and treatment)—

    Oral inhalation, 180 or 200 mcg (0.18 or 0.2 mg—2 inhalations) every four to six hours.

    Note: For some patients, a dose of 90 or 100 mcg (0.09 or 0.1 mg—1 inhalation) every four hours may be sufficient.

Bronchospasm, exercise-induced (prophylaxis)—

    Oral inhalation, 180 or 200 mcg (0.18 or 0.2 mg—2 inhalations) fifteen minutes prior to exercise.

**Usual pediatric dose**

Bronchodilator—

    Children up to 12 years of age: Dosage has not been established.
    Children 12 years of age and over: See *Usual adult and adolescent dose*.

**Strength(s) usually available**

U.S.—

    90 mcg (0.09 mg) per metered spray (Rx) [*Proventil* (dichlorodifluoromethane, trichloromonofluoromethane, oleic acid); *Ventolin* (dichlorodifluoromethane, trichloromonofluoromethane, oleic acid)].

Canada—

    100 mcg (0.1 mg) per metered spray (Rx) [*Novo-Salmol; Ventolin;* GENERIC].

Note: Each canister of the U.S. product provides at least 200 inhalations; each canister of the Canadian product provides 80 or 200 inhalations.

**Packaging and storage**

Store between 15 and 30 °C (59 and 86 °F), unless otherwise specified by manufacturer.

**Auxiliary labeling**
• For oral inhalation only.
• Shake well.
• Store away from heat and direct sunlight.

**Note**

Include patient instructions when dispensing.

### ALBUTEROL SULFATE INHALATION SOLUTION

**Usual adult and adolescent dose**

Bronchodilator—

    Oral inhalation, administered by nebulization or intermittent positive pressure breathing (IPPB), 1.25 to 5 mg (base) in 2 to 5 mL or more of sterile 0.9% sodium chloride solution or sterile water for inhalation, depending on product, repeated three or four times a day every four to six hours if necessary.

Note: When albuterol inhalation solution is administered through a nebulizer, a mouthpiece or face mask may be used. The nebulizer should be used with compressed air or oxygen and the gas flow should be about 6 to 10 liters per minute. With an average volume of 3 mL, a single treatment lasts about 10 (range, 5 to 15) minutes.

When administered through IPPB, the inspiratory pressure is usually 10 to 20 cm $H_2O$ and the duration of administration varies from 5 to 20 minutes, depending on the patient and the control of the apparatus.

**Usual pediatric dose**

Bronchodilator—

    Children up to 12 years of age: Dosage has not been established.

Children 12 years of age and over: See *Usual adult and adolescent dose.*

**Strength(s) usually available**
U.S.—
830 mcg (0.83 mg) (base) per mL (Rx) [*Airet; Proventil* (benzalkonium chloride); *Ventolin Nebules;* GENERIC].
5 mg (base) per mL (Rx) [*Proventil* (benzalkonium chloride); *Ventolin* (benzalkonium chloride); GENERIC].
Canada—
1 mg (base) per mL (Rx) [*Gen-Salbutamol; Ventolin Nebules P.F.* (benzalkonium chloride 0.01% [w/v])].
2 mg (base) per mL (Rx) [*Ventolin Nebules P.F.*].
5 mg (base) per mL (Rx) [*Ventolin* (benzalkonium chloride); GENERIC].

**Packaging and storage**
Store between 2 and 30 °C (36 and 86 °F), in a well-closed container, unless otherwise specified by manufacturer. Protect from freezing.

**Preparation of dosage form**
For preparation of the inhalation solution, diluents containing benzyl alcohol or preservatives other than benzalkonium chloride are not recommended since the safety of these preservatives has not been established for inhalation therapy.
The 0.83 mg-per-mL solution requires no dilution prior to administration. The 5 mg-per-mL solution is concentrated and must be diluted with 0.9% sterile sodium chloride solution or sterile water for inhalation, depending on product, prior to administration.

**Stability**
Diluted solutions should be used within 24 hours of dilution when stored at room temperature or within 48 hours when stored in the refrigerator.

**Auxiliary labeling**
• For oral inhalation only.
• Refrigerate.

## ALBUTEROL SULFATE FOR INHALATION

**Usual adult and adolescent dose**
Bronchospasm in obstructive pulmonary disease (treatment)—
Oral inhalation, 200 or 400 mcg (0.2 or 0.4 mg, respectively) every four to six hours.
Bronchospasm, exercise-induced (prophylaxis): Oral inhalation, 200 mcg (0.2 mg), fifteen minutes before exercise.

**Usual pediatric dose**
Bronchodilator—
Children up to 12 years of age: Dosage has not been established.
Children 12 years of age and over: See *Usual adult and adolescent dose.*

**Strength(s) usually available**
U.S.—
200 mcg (0.2 mg) per capsule (Rx) [*Ventolin Rotacaps* (lactose)].
Canada—
200 mcg (0.2 mg) per capsule or blister (Rx) [*Ventodisk; Ventolin Rotacaps* (lactose)].
400 mcg (0.4 mg) per capsule or blister (Rx) [*Ventodisk; Ventolin Rotacaps* (lactose)].

**Packaging and storage**
Store below 40 °C (104 °F), preferably between 15 and 30 °C (59 and 86 °F), in a well-closed container, unless otherwise specified by manufacturer.

**Auxiliary labeling**
• For oral inhalation only.

**Note**
Use of the capsule for inhalation requires a special device, which separates the capsule into halves and releases the medication.

## Oral Dosage Forms

### ALBUTEROL SULFATE ORAL SOLUTION

**Usual adult dose**
Bronchodilator—
Oral, 2 to 4 mg (base) three or four times a day.

**Usual pediatric dose**
Bronchodilator—
Children up to 2 years of age: Dosage has not been established.
Children 2 to 6 years of age: Oral, 100 mcg (0.1 mg) (base) per kg of body weight three or four times a day.
Children 6 to 12 years of age: Oral, 2 mg (base) three or four times a day.

**Strength(s) usually available**
U.S.—
Not commercially available.
Canada—
2 mg (base) per 5 mL (Rx) [*Ventolin*].

**Packaging and storage**
Store below 40 °C (104 °F), preferably between 15 and 30 °C (59 and 86 °F), unless otherwise specified by manufacturer. Protect from freezing.

## ALBUTEROL SULFATE SYRUP

**Usual adult and adolescent dose**
Bronchodilator—Bronchospasm in obstructive pulmonary disease (treatment): Oral, 2 to 6 mg (base) three or four times a day initially, the dosage being increased as needed and tolerated up to a maximum of 8 mg four times a day.
Note: Patients sensitive to beta-adrenergic stimulants—Oral, 2 mg (base) three or four times a day initially, the dosage being increased as needed and tolerated up to a maximum of 8 mg three or four times a day.

**Usual pediatric dose**
Bronchospasm in obstructive pulmonary disease (treatment)—
Children up to 2 years of age: Dosage has not been established.
Children 2 to 6 years of age: Oral, 100 mcg (0.1 mg) (base) per kg of body weight three times a day initially, the dosage being increased as needed and tolerated up to 200 mcg (0.2 mg) per kg of body weight, not to exceed 4 mg, three times a day.
Children 6 to 14 years of age: Oral, 2 mg (base) three or four times a day initially, the dosage being increased as needed and tolerated up to a maximum of 24 mg per day in divided doses.
Children 14 years of age and over: See *Usual adult and adolescent dose.*

**Usual geriatric dose**
Bronchodilator—
Oral, 2 mg (base) three or four times a day initially, the dosage being increased as needed and tolerated up to a maximum of 8 mg three or four times a day.

**Strength(s) usually available**
U.S.—
2 mg (base) per 5 mL (Rx) [*Proventil; Ventolin;* GENERIC].
Canada—
Not commercially available.

**Packaging and storage**
Store between 2 and 30 °C (36 and 86 °F), in a well-closed container, unless otherwise specified by manufacturer. Protect from light. Protect from freezing.

## ALBUTEROL TABLETS USP

**Usual adult and adolescent dose**
Bronchospasm in obstructive pulmonary disease (treatment)—
Oral, 2 to 6 mg (base) three or four times a day initially, the dosage being increased as needed and tolerated up to a maximum of 8 mg four times a day.
Note: Patients sensitive to beta-adrenergic stimulants—Oral, 2 mg (base) three or four times a day initially, the dosage being increased as needed and tolerated up to a maximum of 8 mg three or four times a day.

**Usual pediatric dose**
Bronchospasm in obstructive pulmonary disease (treatment)—
Children up to 6 years of age: Dosage has not been established.
Children 6 to 12 years of age: Oral, 2 mg (base) three or four times a day initially, the dosage being increased as needed and tolerated up to a maximum of 24 mg per day in divided doses.
Children 12 years of age and over: See *Usual adult and adolescent dose.*

**Usual geriatric dose**
Bronchodilator—
Oral, 2 mg (base) three or four times a day initially, the dosage being increased as needed and tolerated up to a maximum of 8 mg three or four times a day.

**Strength(s) usually available**
U.S.—
2 mg (base) (Rx) [*Proventil* (scored); *Ventolin* (scored); GENERIC].
4 mg (base) (Rx) [*Proventil* (scored); *Ventolin* (scored); GENERIC].
5 mg (base) (Rx) [GENERIC].
Canada—
2 mg (base) (Rx) [*Novo-Salmol* (scored); *Ventolin* (scored)].
4 mg (base) (Rx) [*Novo-Salmol* (scored); *Ventolin* (scored)].

**Packaging and storage**
Store between 2 and 30 °C (36 and 86 °F), in a tight container, unless otherwise specified by manufacturer.

## ALBUTEROL SULFATE EXTENDED-RELEASE TABLETS

**Usual adult and adolescent dose**
Bronchospasm in obstructive pulmonary disease (treatment)—
    Oral, 4 or 8 mg (base) every twelve hours.

**Usual adult prescribing limits**
Up to 32 mg (base) per day.

**Usual pediatric dose**
Bronchospasm in obstructive pulmonary disease (treatment)—
    Children up to 12 years of age: Dosage has not been established.
    Children 12 years of age and over: See *Usual adult and adolescent dose.*

**Strength(s) usually available**
U.S.—
    4 mg (base) (Rx) [*Proventil Repetabs; Volmax*].
    8 mg (base) (Rx) [*Volmax*].
Canada—
    4 mg (base) (Rx) [*Volmax*].
    8 mg (base) (Rx) [*Volmax*].

**Packaging and storage**
Store between 2 and 30 °C (36 and 86 °F), in a tight container, unless otherwise specified by manufacturer.

**Auxiliary labeling**
• Swallow tablets whole.

## Parenteral Dosage Forms

### ALBUTEROL SULFATE INJECTION

**Usual adult dose**
Bronchodilator—
    Intramuscular, 500 mcg (0.5 mg) (base), or 8 mcg (0.008 mg) per kg of body weight, repeated every four hours as required up to a maximum dose of 2 mg per day.
    Intravenous, 250 mcg (0.25 mg) (base), or 4 mcg (0.004 mg) per kg of body weight, administered over a period of two to five minutes, the dosage being repeated after fifteen minutes, if necessary, up to a maximum dose of 1 mg per day.
    Intravenous infusion, administered at a rate of 5 mcg (0.005 mg) (base) per minute, the dosage being increased to 10 mcg (0.01 mg) per minute and then 20 mcg (0.02 mg) per minute at fifteen-to-thirty minute intervals, if necessary.

**Usual pediatric dose**
Dosage has not been established.

**Strength(s) usually available**
U.S.—
    Not commercially available.
Canada—
    50 mcg (0.05 mg) (base) per mL (Rx) [*Ventolin* (sodium 3.5 mg per mL)].
    500 mcg (0.5 mg) (base) per mL (Rx) [*Ventolin* (sodium 3.5 mg per mL)].

**Packaging and storage**
Store below 30 °C (86 °F), unless otherwise specified by manufacturer. Protect from light. Protect from freezing.

**Preparation of dosage form**
For an intravenous infusion, albuterol injection may be diluted in water for injection, 0.9% sodium chloride injection, dextrose injection, or sodium chloride and dextrose injection.
An intravenous infusion may be prepared by diluting 10 mL of albuterol injection, 500 mcg (0.5 mg) (base) per mL, in 500 mL of an appropriate intravenous solution to provide an albuterol concentration of 10 mcg (0.01 mg) per mL.

**Stability**
Unused admixtures should be discarded 24 hours after preparation.

––––––––––––––––––––––––––––––––––
¹Not included in Canadian product labeling.

## BITOLTEROL

## Summary of Differences
Pharmacology/pharmacokinetics:
    Biotransformation—A prodrug hydrolyzed by esterases in tissue and blood to the active compound colterol.
    Onset of action—3 to 4 minutes.
    Time to peak effect—0.5 to 1 hour.
    Duration of action—5 to 8 hours.
Precautions:
    Medical considerations/contraindications—Caution also needed in convulsive disorders.
Side/adverse effects:
    Irregular heartbeat, flushing or redness of face or skin, or unpleasant taste may occur.

## Additional Dosing Information
See also *General Dosing Information.*

Although dosing studies showed bitolterol to be effective throughout a 3-month period of treatment in the majority of the patients, there was some decreased effectiveness in steroid-dependent asthmatic patients.

## Inhalation Dosage Forms

### BITOLTEROL MESYLATE INHALATION AEROSOL

**Usual adult and adolescent dose**
Prophylaxis—
    Oral inhalation, 740 mcg (0.74 mg—2 inhalations) every eight hours.
Treatment—
    Oral inhalation, 740 mcg (0.74 mg—2 inhalations), the 2 inhalations being separated by an interval of at least one to three minutes, followed by an additional 370 mcg (0.37 mg—1 inhalation) if needed. Dosage per day should not exceed 740 mcg (0.74 mg—2 inhalations) every four hours or 1.11 mg (3 inhalations) every six hours.

**Usual pediatric dose**
Bronchodilator—
    Children up to 12 years of age: Dosage has not been established.
    Children 12 years of age and over: See *Usual adult and adolescent dose.*

**Strength(s) usually available**
U.S.—
    370 mcg (0.37 mg) per metered spray (Rx) [*Tornalate* (alcohol 38% [w/w], dichlorodifluoromethane, dichlorotetrafluoroethane, saccharin)].
Canada—
    Not commercially available.
Note: Each container provides at least 300 metered sprays.

**Packaging and storage**
Store below 40 °C (104 °F), preferably between 15 and 30 °C (59 and 86 °F), unless otherwise specified by manufacturer. Protect from freezing.

**Auxiliary labeling**
• For oral inhalation only.
• Store away from heat and direct sunlight.

## EPHEDRINE

## Summary of Differences
Category:
    Oral ephedrine also indicated as a nasal decongestant and CNS stimulant.
    Oral and parenteral ephedrine also used as an urticaria therapy adjunct.
Indications:
    Oral ephedrine has been used in treatment of enuresis and myasthenia gravis, but has been replaced by more effective agents.
Pharmacology/pharmacokinetics:
    Ephedrine also has alpha- and beta-1-adrenergic receptor action.
    Half-life—
        Elimination:
            At urine pH 5—About 3 hours.
            At urine pH 6.3—About 6 hours.
    Onset of action—
        Oral: 15 to 60 minutes.
        Intramuscular: 10 to 20 minutes.
    Duration of action—
        Oral: 3 to 5 hours.

Intramuscular or subcutaneous: 0.5 to 1 hour after 25 to 50 mg dose.

Elimination—

Mostly excreted unchanged; dependent on urinary pH; increased in acidic urine.

Precautions:

Pregnancy/reproduction—

Delivery: Parenteral administration of ephedrine to maintain blood pressure during spinal anesthesia for delivery can cause acceleration of fetal heart rate and should not be used when maternal blood pressure exceeds 130/80.

Breast-feeding—

Ephedrine excreted in breast milk; use by nursing mothers not recommended because of higher than usual risks for infants.

Drug interactions and/or related problems—

Caution also needed with glucocorticoid adrenocorticoids, corticotropin, urinary alkalizers, alpha-adrenergic blocking agents, diatrizoates, iothalamate, ioxaglate, ergot alkaloids, methysergide, oxytocin, doxapram, guanadrel, guanethidine, mazindol, mecamylamine, methyldopa, trimethaphan, methylphenidate, and rauwolfia alkaloids.

Medical considerations/contraindications—

Caution also needed in angle-closure glaucoma (or predisposition to) and prostatic hypertrophy.

Side/adverse effects:

Hallucinations or mood or mental changes may occur rarely with high doses of ephedrine; also, difficult or painful urination, loss of appetite, or unusual paleness may occur.

## Additional Dosing Information

See also *General Dosing Information.*

Tolerance to ephedrine may develop with prolonged or excessive use. Discontinuation of the medication for a few days and subsequent readministration may restore its effectiveness.

### Bioequivalence information

For oral dosage forms only—

Bioavailability or bioequivalence problems among different brands of Ephedrine Sulfate Capsules have not been documented.

For oral dosage forms only:

To minimize the possibility of insomnia, the last dose of ephedrine for each day should be administered a few hours before bedtime.

### For parenteral dosage forms only

When ephedrine is administered intravenously, the injection should be given slowly.

## Oral Dosage Forms

### EPHEDRINE SULFATE CAPSULES USP

Note: Bioavailability or bioequivalence problems among different brands of Ephedrine Sulfate Capsules have not been documented.

**Usual adult dose**

Bronchodilator

Decongestant, nasal (systemic) or

CNS stimulant—

Oral, 25 to 50 mg every three or four hours, if necessary.

Note: Ephedrine has been used in the treatment of enuresis and myasthenia gravis. For enuresis, 25 to 50 mg once a day at bedtime; for myasthenia gravis, 25 mg three or four times a day.

**Usual pediatric dose**

Bronchodilator

Decongestant, nasal (systemic) or

CNS stimulant—

Oral, 3 mg per kg of body weight or 100 mg per square meter of body surface per day, in four to six divided doses.

**Strength(s) usually available**

U.S.—

25 mg (OTC) [GENERIC].

50 mg (OTC) [GENERIC].

Canada—

Not commercially available.

**Packaging and storage**

Store below 40 °C (104 °F), preferably between 15 and 30 °C (59 and 86 °F), unless otherwise specified by manufacturer. Store in a tight, light-resistant container.

## Parenteral Dosage Forms

### EPHEDRINE SULFATE INJECTION USP

**Usual adult dose**

Bronchodilator—Intramuscular, intravenous, or subcutaneous, 12.5 to 25 mg; subsequent dosage to be determined by patient response.

**Usual adult prescribing limits**

Up to 150 mg per twenty-four hours.

**Usual pediatric dose**

Bronchodilator—

Intravenous or subcutaneous, 3 mg per kg of body weight or 100 mg per square meter of body surface per day, in four to six divided doses.

**Strength(s) usually available**

U.S.—

25 mg per mL (Rx) [GENERIC].

50 mg per mL (Rx) [GENERIC].

Canada—

50 mg per mL (Rx) [GENERIC].

**Packaging and storage**

Store below 40 °C (104 °F), preferably between 15 and 30 °C (59 and 86 °F), unless otherwise specified by manufacturer. Store in a light-resistant container. Protect from freezing.

**Stability**

Ephedrine sulfate injection should not be used unless solution is clear. Unused portion should be discarded.

---

### *EPINEPHRINE*

## Summary of Differences

Category:

Epinephrine injection also indicated as a local anesthetic adjunct, surgical aid (antihemorrhagic; decongestant; mydriatic), and topical antihemorrhagic.

Indications:

Epinephrine injection also indicated in treatment of anaphylactic reactions; and may be used in management of bronchospasm during anesthesia.

Racepinephrine inhalation also indicated in treatment of postintubation and infectious croup.

Pharmacology/pharmacokinetics:

Epinephrine also has alpha- and beta-1-adrenergic receptor action.

Biotransformation—

Also metabolized in sympathetic nerve endings and other tissues.

Onset of action—

Inhalation: 3 to 5 minutes.

Intramuscular: Variable.

Subcutaneous: 6 to 15 minutes.

Time to peak effect—

Subcutaneous: 0.3 hours.

Duration of action—

Inhalation: 1 to 3 hours.

Intramuscular or subcutaneous: <1 to 4 hours.

Elimination—

Very small amount excreted unchanged.

Precautions:

Pregnancy/reproduction—

Epinephrine crosses placenta; use during pregnancy may cause anoxia in fetus; not recommended for use during labor since it may delay second stage; high doses, sufficient to reduce uterine contraction, may cause prolonged uterine atony with hemorrhage; parenteral administration of epinephrine to maintain blood pressure during spinal anesthesia for delivery can cause acceleration of fetal heart rate and should not be used when maternal blood pressure exceeds 130/80.

Breast-feeding—

Epinephrine excreted in breast milk; use by nursing mothers may cause serious adverse reactions in infant.

Pediatrics—

Syncope has occurred following administration of epinephrine to asthmatic children.

Drug interactions and/or related problems—

Caution also needed with alpha-adrenergic blocking agents, parenteral-local anesthetics, oral antidiabetic agents, insulin, diatrizoates, iothalamate, ioxaglate, ergot alkaloids, methysergide, oxytocin, doxapram, guanadrel, guanethidine, mazindol, mecamylamine, methyldopa, trimethaphan, methylphenidate, and rauwolfia alkaloids.

Medical considerations/contraindications—

Caution also needed in phenothiazine-induced circulatory collapse or hypotension; angle-closure glaucoma (or predisposition to); Parkinson's disease; prostatic hypertrophy; and cardiogenic, traumatic, or hemorrhagic shock.

Side/adverse effects:

Hallucinations may occur with high doses of epinephrine; also, flushing or redness of face or skin may occur.

## Additional Dosing Information

See also *General Dosing Information*.

Tolerance to epinephrine may develop with prolonged or excessive use. Discontinuation of the medication for a few days and subsequent readministration may restore its effectiveness.

**For inhalation dosage forms only**

When using epinephrine inhalation solution, approximately 10 drops of a 1% (base) solution should be placed in the reservoir of the nebulizer.

When racepinephrine inhalation solution is used for topical pulmonary chemotherapy in the combination nebulizer/respirator, the 2.25% solution must be diluted.

For epinephrine inhalation aerosol, epinephrine inhalation solution, or epinephrine bitartrate inhalation aerosol, an interval of 1 to 2 minutes should elapse between the first and second inhalations to make certain a second inhalation is necessary.

If difficulty in breathing persists or relief does not occur within 20 minutes of inhalation, or if condition becomes worse, the medication should be discontinued and physician contacted immediately.

Epinephrine, isoproterenol, and other beta-adrenergic agents may be used interchangeably, but not concurrently. An interval of 4 hours is recommended before changing from one medication to another.

**For parenteral dosage forms only**

The 1:1000 (1 mg/mL) concentration of epinephrine injection must be diluted before administering intracardially or intravenously.

If epinephrine injection is to be administered by intracardiac injection, it should be administered only by personnel well trained in the technique.

If the patient has been intubated, epinephrine can be injected via the endotracheal tube directly into the bronchial tree at the same dosage as for intravenous injection.

Intra-arterial administration of epinephrine injection is not recommended since marked vasoconstriction may result in gangrene.

It is recommended that sterile epinephrine suspension be administered with a tuberculin syringe and a 26-gauge, 1/2-inch needle.

After withdrawing a dose of sterile epinephrine suspension into the syringe, prompt injection is recommended to avoid settling of the suspension.

A single dose of sterile epinephrine suspension may be effective for up to 10 hours.

Repeated local injections may result in necrosis at the site of injection because of vascular constriction. Sites of injection should be rotated.

Intramuscular injection of epinephrine injection into the buttocks should be avoided since the vasoconstriction produced by the epinephrine reduces the oxygen tension of the tissues, enabling any anaerobic *Clostridium welchii* that may be present on the buttocks to multiply and possibly cause gas gangrene.

## Inhalation Dosage Forms

### EPINEPHRINE INHALATION AEROSOL USP

**Usual adult and adolescent dose**

Bronchodilator—

Oral inhalation, 200 to 275 mcg (0.2 to 0.275 mg—1 inhalation), repeated after one to two minutes, if necessary; subsequent dose (s) should not be administered for at least three hours.

**Usual pediatric dose**

Bronchodilator—

Children up to 4 years of age: Dosage must be individualized by physician.

Children 4 years of age and over: See *Usual adult and adolescent dose*.

**Strength(s) usually available**

U.S.—

0.125% (OTC) [GENERIC].

0.5% (200 mcg [0.2 mg] per metered spray) (OTC) [GENERIC].

0.5% (220 mcg [0.22 mg] per metered spray) (OTC) [*Primatene Mist* (alcohol 34%, fluorocarbon)].

0.5% (250 mcg [0.25 mg] per metered spray) (OTC) [*Bronkaid Mist* (alcohol 33%, dichlorodifluoromethane, dichlorotetrafluoroethane)].

Canada—

0.5% (275 mcg [0.275 mg] per metered spray) (OTC) [*Bronkaid Mistometer* (alcohol 33%)].

**Packaging and storage**

Store below 49 °C (120 °F), unless otherwise specified by manufacturer. Store in a light-resistant container.

**Auxiliary labeling**

• For oral inhalation only.
• Store away from heat and direct sunlight.

**Note**

Include patient instructions when dispensing.

### EPINEPHRINE INHALATION SOLUTION USP

**Usual adult and adolescent dose**

Bronchodilator—

Oral inhalation, 1 inhalation of a 1% solution of epinephrine (base), repeated if necessary after one or two minutes, as needed.

**Usual pediatric dose**

Bronchodilator—

Children up to 6 years of age: Dosage must be individualized by physician.

Children 6 years of age and over: See *Usual adult and adolescent dose*.

**Strength(s) usually available**

U.S.—

1% (base) (OTC) [*Adrenalin Chloride* (benzethonium chloride; sodium bisulfite)].

Canada—

Not commercially available.

**Packaging and storage**

Store below 40 °C (104 °F), preferably between 15 and 30 °C (59 and 86 °F), unless otherwise specified by manufacturer. Store in a tight, light-resistant container. Protect from freezing.

**Stability**

When exposed to air, the solution will turn pinkish to brownish in color because of oxidation. Also, light, heat, alkalies, and certain metals (for example, copper, iron, zinc) may promote deterioration. Do not use if solution is pinkish to brownish in color or contains a precipitate.

**Auxiliary labeling**

• For oral inhalation only.

### EPINEPHRINE BITARTRATE INHALATION AEROSOL USP

**Usual adult and adolescent dose**

Bronchodilator—

Oral inhalation, 160 mcg (0.16 mg—1 inhalation) (base), repeated after one minute, if necessary; subsequent dose(s) should not be administered for at least three hours.

**Usual pediatric dose**

Bronchodilator—

Children up to 4 years of age: Dosage must be individualized by physician.

Children 4 years of age and over: See *Usual adult and adolescent dose*.

**Strength(s) usually available**

U.S.—

300 mcg (0.3 mg) (160 mcg [0.16 mg] [base]) per metered spray (OTC) [*AsthmaHaler Mist* (dichlorodifluoromethane, dichlorotetrafluoroethane, trichloromonofluoromethane); *Bronitin Mist; Medihaler-Epi* (dichlorodifluoromethane, dichlorotetrafluoroethane, trichloromonofluoromethane); *Primatene Mist Suspension*].

Canada—

300 mcg (0.3 mg) (160 mcg [0.16 mg] [base]) per metered spray (OTC) [*Medihaler-Epi* (cetylpyridinium chloride, dichlorodifluoromethane, dichlorotetrafluoroethane, sorbitan trioleate, trichloromonofluoromethane)].

**Packaging and storage**

Store below 40 °C (104 °F), preferably between 15 and 30 °C (59 and 86 °F), unless otherwise specified by manufacturer. Store in a light-resistant container. Protect from freezing.

**Auxiliary labeling**

• For oral inhalation only.
• Shake well.
• Store away from heat and direct sunlight.

**Note**
Include patient instructions when dispensing.

## RACEPINEPHRINE INHALATION SOLUTION USP

**Usual adult and adolescent dose**
Bronchodilator—
Hand nebulizer: Oral inhalation, 2 or 3 inhalations of a 2.25% (epinephrine) solution, followed in five minutes by two or three additional inhalations if necessary, four to six times a day.
Nebulization via respirator: Oral inhalation, 5 mL of a 0.1% solution in a combination nebulizer/respirator for a period of fifteen minutes every three to four hours.

**Usual pediatric dose**
Bronchodilator—
Children up to 4 years of age: Dosage must be individualized by physician.
Children 4 years of age and over: See *Usual adult and adolescent dose*.

**Strength(s) usually available**
U.S.—
2% (OTC) [*Vaponefrin* (sodium metabisulfite 0.075%, chlorobutanol 0.5%, benzoic acid, glycerin)].
2.25% (epinephrine) (OTC) [*AsthmaNefrin* (sodium bisulfite); *microNefrin* (sodium bisulfite; potassium metabisulfite); *Nephron*; *S-2* (sodium bisulfite; potassium metabisulfite)].
Canada—
2.25% (epinephrine) (OTC) [*Vaponefrin* (sodium metabisulfite)].

**Packaging and storage**
Store below 40 °C (104 °F), preferably between 15 and 30 °C (59 and 86 °F), unless otherwise specified by manufacturer. Store in a tight, light-resistant container. Protect from freezing.

**Preparation of dosage form**
For dilution of 2.25% racepinephrine inhalation solution used for topical pulmonary chemotherapy in the combination nebulizer/respirator, see manufacturer's package insert for instructions.

**Stability**
When exposed to air, the solution will turn pinkish to brownish in color because of oxidation. Also, light, heat, alkalies, and certain metals (for example, copper, iron, zinc) may promote deterioration. Do not use if solution is pinkish to brownish in color or contains a precipitate.

**Auxiliary labeling**
• For oral inhalation only.

**Note**
Include patient instructions when dispensing.

# Parenteral Dosage Forms

## EPINEPHRINE INJECTION USP

**Usual adult and adolescent dose**
Bronchodilator—
Subcutaneous, initially 200 to 500 mcg (0.2 to 0.5 mg) (base), repeated every twenty minutes to four hours as needed, the dosage being increased up to a maximum of 1 mg per dose, if necessary.
Anaphylactic reactions—
Intramuscular or subcutaneous, initially 200 to 500 mcg (0.2 to 0.5 mg) (base), repeated every ten to fifteen minutes as needed, the dosage being increased up to a maximum of 1 mg per dose if necessary.
Anesthetic (local) adjunct—
For use with local anesthetics, 100 to 200 mcg (0.1 to 0.2 mg) (base) in a 1:200,000 to 1:20,000 solution.
For use with intraspinal anesthetics, 200 to 400 mcg (0.2 to 0.4 mg) (base) added to the anesthetic spinal fluid mixture.
Surgical aid (antihemorrhagic; decongestant; mydriatic)—
Intracameral or subconjunctival, a 0.01 to 0.1% (1:10,000 to 1:1000) (base) solution.
Antihemorrhagic (topical)—
Topical, a 0.002 to 0.1% (1:50,000 to 1:1000) (base) solution.

**Usual pediatric dose**
Bronchodilator
Anaphylactic reactions—
Subcutaneous, 10 mcg (0.01 mg) (base) per kg of body weight or 300 mcg (0.3 mg) per square meter of body surface up to a maximum of 500 mcg (0.5 mg) per dose, repeated every fifteen minutes for two doses, then every four hours as needed.
Anesthetic (local) adjunct—
See *Usual adult and adolescent dose*.
Surgical aid (antihemorrhagic; decongestant; mydriatic)—
See *Usual adult and adolescent dose*.

Antihemorrhagic (topical)—
See *Usual adult and adolescent dose*.

**Strength(s) usually available**
U.S.—
10 mcg (0.01 mg) (base) per mL (Rx) [GENERIC].
100 mcg (0.1 mg) (base) per mL (Rx) [GENERIC].
500 mcg (0.5 mg) (base) per mL (Rx) [*EpiPen Jr. Auto-Injector* (sodium metabisulfite 1.67 mg per mL)].
1 mg (base) per mL (Rx) [*Adrenalin Chloride Solution* (benzyl alcohol; chlorobutanol 0.5%; sodium bisulfite not more than 0.1% in ampuls and 0.15% in vials; sodium chloride); *Ana-Guard* (not more than 5 mg chlorobutanol and 1.5 mg sodium bisulfite per mL); *EpiPen Auto-Injector* (sodium chloride 6 mg per mL; sodium metabisulfite 1.67 mg per mL); GENERIC].
Canada—
100 mcg (0.1 mg) (base) per mL (Rx) [GENERIC].
500 mcg (0.5 mg) (base) per mL (Rx) [*EpiPen Jr. Auto-Injector* (sodium chloride 6 mg per mL; sodium metabisulfite 1.67 mg per mL)].
1 mg (base) per mL (Rx) [*Adrenalin* (sodium chloride; sulfites); *EpiPen Auto-Injector* (sodium chloride 6 mg per mL; sodium metabisulfite 1.67 mg per mL)].
Note: The auto-injector containing 500 mcg (0.5 mg) (base) per mL delivers a single dose of 150 mcg (0.15 mg); and the auto-injector containing 1 mg (base) per mL delivers a single dose of 300 mcg (0.3 mg).

**Packaging and storage**
Store below 40 °C (104 °F), preferably between 15 and 30 °C (59 and 86 °F), unless otherwise specified by manufacturer. Store in a tight, light-resistant container. Protect from freezing.

**Preparation of dosage form**
For intracardiac or intravenous administration of epinephrine injection, dilute 0.5 mL (0.5 mg) of a 1:1000 (1 mg/mL) solution to 10 mL with 0.9% sodium chloride injection.

**Stability**
Epinephrine is readily destroyed by alkalies and oxidizing agents (for example, oxygen, chlorine, bromine, iodine, permanganates, chromates, nitrites, and salts of easily reducible metals, especially iron). Do not use if solution is pinkish or brownish in color or contains a precipitate. Discard unused portion.

**Note**
For epinephrine auto-injector—Include patient instructions when dispensing.

## STERILE EPINEPHRINE SUSPENSION

**Usual adult dose**
Bronchodilator—
Subcutaneous, 500 mcg (0.5 mg) initially, then 500 mcg (0.5 mg) to 1.5 mg not more often than every six hours as needed.

**Usual pediatric dose**
Bronchodilator—
Subcutaneous, 25 mcg (0.025 mg) per kg of body weight or 625 mcg (0.625 mg) per square meter of body surface; dose may be repeated, if necessary, but not more often than every six hours.
Note: For children weighing 30 kg or less, the maximum single dose is 750 mcg (0.75 mg).

**Strength(s) usually available**
U.S.—
5 mg per mL (Rx) [*Sus-Phrine* (ascorbic acid 10 mg and thioglycolic acid 6.6 mg [as sodium salts]; glycerin 325 mg; phenol 5 mg; sodium hydroxide)].
Canada—
Not commercially available.

**Packaging and storage**
Store below 30 °C (86 °F), preferably between 2 and 8 °C (36 and 46 °F), unless otherwise specified by manufacturer. Store in a light-resistant container. Protect from freezing.

**Stability**
On removal of doses from the multiple dose vial, air is introduced which slowly oxidizes the epinephrine causing discoloration of the suspension and possible loss of potency. Do not use if suspension is pinkish or brownish in color.

**Auxiliary labeling**
• Shake well.
• Refrigerate.

## ETHYLNOREPINEPHRINE

## Summary of Differences

Pharmacology/pharmacokinetics:
Ethylnorepinephrine also has beta-1-adrenergic receptor action.
Onset of action—Intramuscular or subcutaneous: 6 to 12 minutes.
Duration of action—Intramuscular or subcutaneous: 1 to 2 hours.

## Additional Dosing Information

See also *General Dosing Information*.

Intraneural or intravascular injection of ethylnorepinephrine should be avoided.

## Parenteral Dosage Forms

### ETHYLNOREPINEPHRINE HYDROCHLORIDE INJECTION USP

**Usual adult dose**
Bronchodilator—
Intramuscular or subcutaneous, 1 to 2 mg.

Note: Smaller doses of 600 mcg (0.6 mg) to 1 mg may be sufficient, depending on the severity of the asthmatic attack.

**Usual pediatric dose**
Bronchodilator—
Intramuscular or subcutaneous, 200 mcg (0.2 mg) to 1 mg.

**Strength(s) usually available**
U.S.—
2 mg per mL (Rx) [*Bronkephrine* (acetone; sodium bisulfite 0.2%; sodium chloride 0.7%)].
Canada—
Not commercially available.

**Packaging and storage**
Store below 40 °C (104 °F), preferably between 15 and 30 °C (59 and 86 °F), unless otherwise specified by manufacturer. Store in a light-resistant container. Protect from freezing.

## FENOTEROL

## Summary of Differences

Pharmacology/pharmacokinetics:
Onset of action—
Inhalation: 5 minutes.
Oral: 30 to 60 minutes.
Time to peak effect—
Inhalation: 0.5 to 1 hour.
Oral: 2 to 3 hours.
Duration of action—
Inhalation: 2 to 3 hours.
Oral: 6 to 8 hours.
Precautions:
Medical considerations/contraindications—Caution also needed in angle-closure glaucoma (or predisposition to).
Side/adverse effects:
Heartburn, muscle cramps or twitching, or unpleasant taste (with inhalation dosage form only) may occur.

## Inhalation Dosage Forms

### FENOTEROL HYDROBROMIDE INHALATION AEROSOL

**Usual adult and adolescent dose**
Bronchodilator—
Oral inhalation, 200 or 400 mcg (0.2 or 0.4 mg—1 or 2 inhalations), repeated up to four times a day, if necessary, but not to be administered more often than every four hours.

**Usual pediatric dose**
Bronchodilator—
Children up to 12 years of age: Dosage has not been established.
Children 12 years of age and over: See *Usual adult and adolescent dose*.

**Strength(s) usually available**
U.S.—
Not commercially available.
Canada—
100 mcg (0.1 mg) per metered spray (Rx) [*Berotec*].

200 mcg (0.2 mg) per metered spray (Rx) [*Berotec* (dichlorodifluoromethane, dichlorotetrafluoroethane, trichloromonofluoromethane)].

**Packaging and storage**
Store below 40 °C (104 °F), preferably between 15 and 30 °C (59 and 86 °F), unless otherwise specified by manufacturer. Protect from freezing.

**Auxiliary labeling**
• For oral inhalation only.
• Store away from heat and direct sunlight.

### FENOTEROL HYDROBROMIDE INHALATION SOLUTION

**Usual adult and adolescent dose**
Bronchodilator—
Oral inhalation, administered via nebulization or intermittent positive-pressure breathing (IPPB), 500 mcg (0.5 mg) to 1 mg (up to 2.5 mg in some cases) as a 0.1% solution, diluted to 5 mL with 0.9% sodium chloride solution, the total volume nebulized over a period of ten to fifteen minutes. Dosage may be repeated every six hours, if necessary.

Note: When administered by IPPB, the inspiratory pressure should be set at 10 to 20 cm $H_2O$.
When administered by nebulization, motorized, compressed air, or ultrasonic nebulizers (which generate low pressure, low velocity aerosols) are recommended.

**Usual pediatric dose**
Bronchodilator—
Children up to 12 years of age: Dosage has not been established.
Children 12 years of age and over: See *Usual adult and adolescent dose*.

**Strength(s) usually available**
U.S.—
Not commercially available.
Canada—
1 mg per mL (Rx) [*Berotec*].

**Packaging and storage**
Store below 40 °C (104 °F), preferably between 15 and 30 °C (59 and 86 °F), in a well-closed container, unless otherwise specified by manufacturer. Protect from freezing.

**Auxiliary labeling**
• For oral inhalation only.

## Oral Dosage Forms

### FENOTEROL HYDROBROMIDE TABLETS

**Usual adult and adolescent dose**
Bronchodilator—
Oral, 2.5 mg two times a day initially, the dosage being increased up to a maximum of 5 mg three times a day, if necessary, but not to be administered more often than every six hours.

**Usual pediatric dose**
Bronchodilator—
Children up to 12 years of age: Dosage has not been established.
Children 12 years of age and over: See *Usual adult and adolescent dose*.

**Strength(s) usually available**
U.S.—
Not commercially available.
Canada—
2.5 mg (Rx) [*Berotec* (scored)].

**Packaging and storage**
Store below 40 °C (104 °F), preferably between 15 and 30 °C (59 and 86 °F), in a well-closed container, unless otherwise specified by manufacturer.

## ISOETHARINE

## Summary of Differences

Pharmacology/pharmacokinetics:
Biotransformation—Also metabolized in the lungs, gastrointestinal tract, and other tissues.
Onset of action—1 to 6 minutes.
Time to peak effect—0.25 to 1 hour.
Duration of action—1 to 4 hours.
Elimination—About 10% isoetharine excreted unchanged.

## Additional Dosing Information

See also *General Dosing Information*.

Excessive use may result in loss of effectiveness. If this occurs, discontinuation of the medication and use of alternative therapy such as epinephrine or another sympathomimetic are recommended.

## Inhalation Dosage Forms

### ISOETHARINE INHALATION SOLUTION USP

**Usual adult dose**
Bronchodilator—
Isoetharine inhalation solution may be administered by hand-bulb nebulizer, intermittent positive-pressure breathing (IPPB), or oxygen aerosolization, usually not more often than every four hours, as follows:

| Method of Administration | Strength (s) of Solution (%) | Usual Dose | Usual Dose Range | Usual Dilution |
|---|---|---|---|---|
| Hand-bulb nebulizer | 0.5 | 4 inhalations | | Undiluted |
| | 1 | 4 inhalations | 3–7 inhalations | Undiluted |
| IPPB | 0.062 | 4 mL | | Undiluted |
| | 0.08 | 3.0 mL | | Undiluted |
| | 0.1 | 2.5 mL | 2.5–10 mL | Undiluted |
| | 0.125 | 4 mL | 2–8 mL | Undiluted |
| | 0.14 | 3.5 mL | | Undiluted |
| | 0.167 | 3.0 mL | | Undiluted |
| | 0.2 | 2.5 mL | 1.25–5 mL | Undiluted |
| | 0.25 | 2 mL | | Undiluted |
| | 0.5 | 1 mL | | 1:3* |
| | 0.5 | 0.5 mL | | 1:3* |
| | 1 | 0.5 mL | 0.25–1 mL | 1:3* |
| Oxygen aerosolization | 0.062 | 4 mL | | Undiluted |
| | 0.08 | 3.0 mL | | Undiluted |
| | 0.1 | 2.5 mL | 2.5–5 mL | Undiluted |
| | 0.125 | 4 mL | 2–4 mL | Undiluted |
| | 0.14 | 3.5 mL | | Undiluted |
| | 0.167 | 3.0 mL | | Undiluted |
| | 0.2 | 2.5 mL | 1.25–2.5 mL | Undiluted |
| | 0.25 | 2 mL | | Undiluted |
| | 0.5 | 1 mL | | 1:3* |
| | 0.5 | 0.5 mL | | 1:3* |
| | 1 | 0.5 mL | 0.25–0.5 mL | 1:3* |

*With sterile purified water, sterile water, or 0.45 or 0.9% sodium chloride sterile solution.

Note: When administered by oxygen aerosolization, the oxygen flow is adjusted to 4 to 6 liters per minute over a period of 15 to 20 minutes.

When administered by IPPB, an inspiratory flow rate of 15 liters per minute at a cycling pressure of 15 cm of water is recommended. Depending on the patient and type of IPPB apparatus, it may be necessary to adjust the flow rate to 6 to 30 liters per minute and the cycling pressure to 10 to 15 cm of water, and to dilute further.

**Usual pediatric dose**
Bronchodilator—
Dosage has not been established.

**Strength(s) usually available**
U.S.—
0.062% (Rx) [*Arm-a-Med Isoetharine*].
0.08% (Rx) [*Dey-Lute Isoetharine S/F* (edetate disodium; sodium chloride; acetylcysteine); GENERIC].
0.1% (Rx) [*Dey-Lute Isoetharine S/F* (edetate disodium; sodium chloride; acetylcysteine); GENERIC].
0.125% (Rx) [*Arm-a-Med Isoetharine;* GENERIC].
0.167% (Rx) [*Arm-a-Med Isoetharine;* GENERIC].
0.17% (Rx) [*Dey-Lute Isoetharine S/F* (edetate disodium; sodium chloride; acetylcysteine); GENERIC].
0.2% (Rx) [*Arm-a-Med Isoetharine;* GENERIC].
0.25% (Rx) [*Arm-a-Med Isoetharine; Dey-Lute Isoetharine S/F* (edetate disodium; sodium chloride; acetylcysteine); GENERIC].
1% (Rx) [*Bronkosol* (acetone sodium bisulfite; glycerin; parabens; sodium chloride; sodium citrate); GENERIC].

Canada—
Not commercially available.

**Packaging and storage**
Store below 40 °C (104 °F), preferably between 15 and 30 °C (59 and 86 °F), unless otherwise specified by manufacturer. Store in a tight container. Protect from light. Protect from freezing.

**Stability**
Do not use if solution is brownish in color or contains a precipitate.

**Auxiliary labeling**
• For oral inhalation only.

### ISOETHARINE MESYLATE INHALATION AEROSOL USP

**Usual adult dose**
Bronchodilator—
Oral inhalation, 340 mcg (0.34 mg—1 inhalation), repeated after one to two minutes, if necessary. Dosage may be repeated every four hours as needed.

**Usual pediatric dose**
Bronchodilator—
Dosage has not been established.

**Strength(s) usually available**
U.S.—
0.61% (340 mcg [0.34 mg] [base] per metered spray) (Rx) [*Bronkometer* (alcohol 30%; acetone sodium bisulfite, ascorbic acid 0.1% w/w, dichlorodifluoromethane, dichlorotetrafluoroethane, menthol, saccharin); GENERIC].

Canada—
Not commercially available.

**Packaging and storage**
Store below 40 °C (104 °F), preferably between 15 and 30 °C (59 and 86 °F), unless otherwise specified by manufacturer. Store in a light-resistant container. Protect from freezing.

**Auxiliary labeling**
• For oral inhalation only.
• Store away from heat and direct sunlight.

**Note**
Include patient instructions when dispensing.

---

### *ISOPROTERENOL*

## Summary of Differences

Pharmacology/pharmacokinetics:
Isoproterenol also has beta-1-adrenergic receptor action.
Absorption of sublingual tablets may be erratic and unpredictable.
Biotransformation:
Also metabolized in the lungs and other tissues.
Onset of action:
Inhalation: 2 to 5 minutes.
Intravenous: Immediate.
Rectal: Within 30 minutes.
Sublingual: 15 to 30 minutes.
Duration of action:
Inhalation: 0.5 to 2 hours.
Intravenous: <1 hour.
Rectal: 2 to 4 hours.
Sublingual: 1 to 2 hours.
Elimination:
Intravenous: About 40 to 50% excreted unchanged.
Oral or inhalation: About 5 to 15% excreted unchanged.
Side/adverse effects:
Irregular heartbeat, pinkish to red coloration of saliva (for inhalation and sublingual dosage forms only), and flushing or redness of face or skin may occur.

## Additional Dosing Information

See also *General Dosing Information*.

**For inhalation dosage forms only**
Isoproterenol inhalation solution may be administered by hand-bulb nebulizer (all glass or plastic), nebulization by compressed air or oxygen, or intermittent positive-pressure breathing (IPPB). See manufacturer's package insert for instructions.

When used for bronchospasm in chronic obstructive lung disease, the treatment should not be repeated at less than 3- to 4-hour intervals.

When 0.25% isoproterenol inhalation solution is used and relief is not noticeable after 3 treatments of 6 to 12 inhalations at 15–minute intervals, the patient should immediately consult a physician.

Patients requiring more than 3 aerosol treatments within 24 hours should be under close medical supervision.

If 3 to 5 treatments within 6 to 12 hours provide minimal or no relief, further therapy with the aerosol alone is not recommended.

Excessive use may result in loss of effectiveness. If this occurs, discontinuation of the medication and use of alternative therapy are recommended.

# Inhalation Dosage Forms
## ISOPROTERENOL INHALATION SOLUTION USP

**Usual adult dose**
Bronchodilator—
Oral inhalation, 6 to 12 inhalations of a 0.25% nebulized solution, repeated at fifteen-minute intervals, if necessary, for three doses, not to exceed eight treatments per twenty-four hours or
Acute bronchial asthma:
Oral inhalation, 5 to 15 deep inhalations of a 0.5% nebulized solution or 3 to 7 deep inhalations of a 1% nebulized solution, repeated once, if necessary, after five to ten minutes; subsequent doses may be administered up to five times a day, if necessary.
Bronchospasm in chronic obstructive lung disease:
Hand-bulb nebulizer: Oral inhalation, 5 to 15 deep inhalations of a 0.5% solution or 3 to 7 deep inhalations of a 1% solution, not more often than every three to four hours.
Intermittent positive-pressure breathing (IPPB): Oral inhalation, 2 mL of a 0.125% solution or 2.5 mL of a 0.1% solution, administered over a period of ten to twenty minutes; treatment may be repeated up to five times a day, if necessary.
Nebulization by compressed air or oxygen: Oral inhalation, 2 mL of a 0.125% solution or 2.5 mL of a 0.1% solution, administered over a period of fifteen to twenty minutes; treatment may be repeated up to five times a day, if necessary.

**Usual pediatric dose**
Bronchodilator—
Oral inhalation, 6 to 12 inhalations of a 0.25% nebulized solution, repeated at fifteen-minute intervals, if necessary, for three doses, not to exceed eight treatments per twenty-four hours or
Acute bronchial asthma:
Oral inhalation, 5 to 15 deep inhalations of a 0.5% nebulized solution, repeated once, if necessary, after five to ten minutes; subsequent doses may be administered up to five times a day, if necessary.
Bronchospasm in chronic obstructive lung disease:
Hand-bulb nebulizer: Oral inhalation, 5 to 15 deep inhalations of a 0.5% solution, not more often than every three to four hours.
Intermittent positive-pressure breathing (IPPB) or nebulization by compressed air or oxygen: Oral inhalation, 2 mL of a 0.0625% solution or 2.5 mL of a 0.05% solution, administered over a period of ten to fifteen minutes; treatment may be repeated up to five times a day, if necessary.

**Strength(s) usually available**
U.S.—
0.25% (Rx) [GENERIC].
0.5% (Rx) [*Isuprel* (sodium metabisulfite 0.3%, chlorobutanol 0.5%, citric acid, glycerin, sodium chloride); GENERIC (may contain sodium bisulfite)].
1% (Rx) [*Isuprel* (sodium metabisulfite 0.3%, chlorobutanol 0.5%, saccharin sodium, sodium chloride, sodium citrate, citric acid)].
Canada—
0.5% (Rx) [*Isuprel*].

**Packaging and storage**
Store below 40 °C (104 °F), preferably between 15 and 30 °C (59 and 86 °F), unless otherwise specified by manfacturer. Store in a tight container. Protect from light. Protect from freezing.

**Stability**
When exposed to air, alkalies, or metals, isoproterenol solutions turn pinkish to brownish in color because of oxidation. Do not use if solution is pinkish to brownish in color or contains a precipitate.

**Auxiliary labeling**
• For oral inhalation only.

## ISOPROTERENOL HYDROCHLORIDE INHALATION AEROSOL USP

**Usual adult and adolescent dose**
Acute bronchial asthma—
Oral inhalation, 120 to 131 mcg (0.12 to 0.131 mg—1 inhalation), repeated after one to five minutes if necessary, four to six times a day.

Bronchospasm in chronic obstructive lung disease—
Oral inhalation, 120 to 131 mcg (0.12 to 0.131 mg—1 inhalation), not more often than every three to four hours.

**Usual pediatric dose**
Bronchodilator—
See *Usual adult and adolescent dose.*
Note: Administration of the aerosol solution to children is the same as for adults, since a child's smaller ventilatory exchange capacity automatically provides proportionally smaller aerosol intake.

**Strength(s) usually available**
U.S.—
0.25% (w/w) (120 mcg [0.12 mg] per metered spray) (Rx) [GENERIC].
0.25% (131 mcg [0.131 mg] per metered spray) (Rx) [*Isuprel Mistometer* (alcohol 33% [w/w], ascorbic acid 0.1% [w/w], dichlorodifluoromethane, dichlorotetrafluoroethane)].
Canada—
0.25% (w/w) (125 mcg [0.125 mg] per metered spray) (Rx) [*Isuprel Mistometer* (ethyl alcohol)].

**Packaging and storage**
Store below 49 °C (120 °F), preferably between 15 and 30 °C (59 and 86 °F), unless otherwise specified by manufacturer. Store in a light-resistant container.

**Auxiliary labeling**
• For oral inhalation only.
• Store away from heat and direct sunlight.

**Note**
Include patient instructions when dispensing.

## ISOPROTERENOL SULFATE INHALATION AEROSOL USP

**Usual adult and adolescent dose**
Bronchodilator—
Oral inhalation, 75 or 80 mcg (0.075 or 0.08 mg—1 inhalation), repeated after two to five minutes if necessary, four to six times a day.

**Usual pediatric dose**
See *Usual adult and adolescent dose.*
Note: Administration of the aerosol solution to children is the same as for adults, since a child's smaller ventilatory exchange capacity automatically provides proportionally smaller aerosol intake.

**Strength(s) usually available**
U.S.—
2 mg per mL (80 mcg [0.08 mg] per metered spray) (Rx) [*Medihaler-Iso* (dichlorodifluoromethane, dichlorotetrafluoroethane, trichloromonofluoromethane, sorbitan trioleate)].
Canada—
Not commercially available.

**Packaging and storage**
Store below 40 °C (104 °F), preferably between 15 and 30 °C (59 and 86 °F), unless otherwise specified by manufacturer. Store in a light-resistant container. Protect from freezing.

**Auxiliary labeling**
• For oral inhalation only.
• Shake well.
• Store away from heat and direct sunlight.

**Note**
Include patient instructions when dispensing.

# Oral Dosage Forms
## ISOPROTERENOL HYDROCHLORIDE TABLETS USP

**Usual adult dose**
Bronchodilator—
Sublingual, 10 to 15 mg three or four times a day.

**Usual pediatric dose**
Bronchodilator—
Sublingual, 5 to 10 mg three times a day.

**Strength(s) usually available**
U.S.—
10 mg (Rx) [*Isuprel Glossets* (lactose, saccharin sodium, sodium metabisulfite 2 mg)].
Canada—
Not commercially available.

## Packaging and storage

Store below 40 °C (104 °F), preferably between 15 and 30 °C (59 and 86 °F), unless otherwise specified by manufacturer. Store in a well-closed, light-resistant container.

## Auxiliary labeling

- Dissolve tablets under tongue.
- Keep container tightly closed.

# Parenteral Dosage Forms

## ISOPROTERENOL HYDROCHLORIDE INJECTION USP

### Usual adult dose

Bronchodilator (bronchospasm during anesthesia)—
    Intravenous, 10 to 20 mcg (0.01 to 0.02 mg), repeated as needed.

### Usual pediatric dose

Dosage must be individualized by physician.

### Strength(s) usually available

U.S.—
    20 mcg (0.02 mg) per mL (Rx) [GENERIC].
    200 mcg (0.2 mg) per mL (Rx) [*Isuprel* (sodium metabisulfite, sodium chloride 7 mg, sodium lactate 1.8 mg, lactic acid 0.2 mg); GENERIC].
Canada—
    200 mcg (0.2 mg) per mL (Rx) [*Isuprel* (sodium lactate, sodium metabisulfite)].

### Packaging and storage

Store below 40 °C (104 °F), preferably between 15 and 30 °C (59 and 86 °F), unless otherwise specified by manufacturer. Protect from light. Protect from freezing.

### Preparation of dosage form

For preparation of solutions for injection, see manufacturer's package insert.

### Stability

When exposed to air, alkalies, or metals, isoproterenol may turn pinkish to brownish in color because of oxidation. Do not use if solution is pinkish to brownish in color or contains a precipitate.

---

### *METAPROTERENOL*

---

## Summary of Differences

Pharmacology/pharmacokinetics:
    Onset of action—
        Inhalation aerosol: Within 1 minute.
        Inhalation by hand-bulb nebulizer or intermittent positive-pressure breathing (IPPB): 5 to 30 minutes.
        Oral: Within 15 to 30 minutes.
    Time to peak effect—
        Inhalation aerosol: About 1 hour.
        Oral: Within 1 hour.
    Duration of action—
        Inhalation aerosol: 1 to 5 hours after single dose; 1 to 2.5 hours after repeated doses.
        Inhalation by hand-bulb nebulizer or intermittent positive-pressure breathing (IPPB): 2 to 6 hours after single dose; 4 to 6 hours after repeated doses.
        Oral: Up to 4 hours.
    Elimination—
        Primarily excreted as glucuronic acid conjugates.
Precautions:
    Medical considerations/contraindications—Caution also needed in convulsive disorders.
Side/adverse effects:
    Muscle cramps or twitching or unpleasant taste may occur.

## Inhalation Dosage Forms

### METAPROTERENOL SULFATE INHALATION AEROSOL USP

#### Usual adult and adolescent dose

Bronchodilator—
    Oral inhalation, 1.3 to 2.25 mg (2 or 3 inhalations) every three to four hours, not to exceed 9 mg (12 inhalations) per day.

#### Usual pediatric dose

Bronchodilator—
    Children up to 12 years of age: Use is not recommended.

### Strength(s) usually available

U.S.—
    15 mg per mL (650 mcg [0.65 mg] per metered spray) (Rx) [*Alupent* (dichlorodifluoromethane, dichlorotetrafluoromethane, trichloromonofluoromethane, sorbitan trioleate); *Metaprel* (dichlorodifluoromethane, dichlorotetrafluoroethane, trichloromonofluoromethane, sorbitan trioleate)].
Canada—
    750 mcg (0.75 mg) per metered spray (Rx) [*Alupent*].

### Packaging and storage

Store below 49 °C (120 °F), unless otherwise specified by manufacturer. Store in a light-resistant container.

### Auxiliary labeling

- For oral inhalation only.
- Shake well.
- Store away from heat and direct sunlight.

### Note

Include patient instructions when dispensing.

## METAPROTERENOL SULFATE INHALATION SOLUTION USP

### Usual adult and adolescent dose

Bronchodilator—
    Oral inhalation, administered by using a hand-bulb nebulizer or intermittent positive-pressure breathing (IPPB), usually not more often than every four hours to relieve acute attacks of bronchospasm and three or four times a day in chronic bronchospastic pulmonary diseases, as follows:

| Method of Administration | Usual Dose | Usual Dose Range | Usual Dilution |
|---|---|---|---|
| Hand-bulb nebulizer | 10 inhalations | 5–15 inhalations | Undiluted |
| IPPB | 0.3 mL | 0.2–0.3 mL | * |

*Diluted in approximately 2.5 mL of saline solution or other diluent. The 0.4% unit dose vial contains the equivalent of 0.2 mL of a 5% solution diluted to 2.5 mL with normal saline. The 0.6% unit dose vial contains the equivalent of 0.3 mL of a 5% solution diluted to 2.5 mL with normal saline.

### Usual pediatric dose

Bronchodilator—
    Children up to 12 years of age: Dosage has not been established.

### Strength(s) usually available

U.S.—
    0.4% (Rx) [*Alupent* (edetate disodium, sodium chloride); *Arm-a-Med Metaproterenol* (edetate disodium, sodium chloride); *Dey-Lute Metaproterenol*; GENERIC].
    0.6% (Rx) [*Alupent* (edetate disodium, sodium chloride); *Arm-a-Med Metaproterenol* (edetate disodium, sodium chloride); *Dey-Lute Metaproterenol*; GENERIC].
    5% (Rx) [*Alupent* (edetate disodium, benzalkonium chloride); *Metaprel* (benzalkonium chloride, edetate disodium); GENERIC].
Canada—
    5% (Rx) [*Alupent*].

### Packaging and storage

Store below 40 °C (104 °F), preferably between 15 and 30 °C (59 and 86 °F), unless otherwise specified by manufacturer. Store in a tight container. Protect from light.

### Auxiliary labeling

- For oral inhalation only.

## Oral Dosage Forms

### METAPROTERENOL SULFATE SYRUP USP

#### Usual adult and adolescent dose

Bronchodilator—
    Oral, 20 mg three or four times a day.

#### Usual pediatric dose

Bronchodilator—
    Children up to 6 years of age: Dosage has not been established.
    Children 6 to 9 years of age and over or weighing up to 27 kg: Oral, 10 mg three or four times a day.
    Children 9 years of age and over or weighing 27 kg and over: See *Usual adult and adolescent dose.*

Note: Experience in children up to 6 years of age is limited; however, studies have shown a dose of 325 to 650 mcg (0.325 to 0.65 mg) per kg of body weight four times a day for this age group to be well tolerated.

**Strength(s) usually available**
U.S.—
    10 mg per 5 mL (Rx) [*Alupent; Metaprel; Prometa;* GENERIC].
Canada—
    10 mg per 5 mL (Rx) [*Alupent*].

**Packaging and storage**
Store below 40 °C (104 °F), preferably between 15 and 30 °C (59 and 86 °F), unless otherwise specified by manufacturer. Store in a tight, light-resistant container. Protect from freezing.

## METAPROTERENOL SULFATE TABLETS USP

**Usual adult and adolescent dose**
Bronchodilator—
    Oral, 20 mg three or four times a day.

**Usual pediatric dose**
Bronchodilator—
    Children up to 6 years of age: Dosage has not been established.
    Children 6 to 9 years of age and over; or
    Children weighing up to 27 kg: Oral, 10 mg three or four times a day.
    Children 9 years of age and over; or
    Children weighing 27 kg and over: See *Usual adult and adolescent dose*.

Note: Experience in children up to 6 years of age is limited; however, studies have shown a dose of 325 to 650 mcg (0.325 to 0.65 mg) per kg of body weight four times a day for this age group to be well tolerated.

**Strength(s) usually available**
U.S.—
    10 mg (Rx) [*Alupent* (scored); *Metaprel* (scored); GENERIC].
    20 mg (Rx) [*Alupent* (scored); *Metaprel* (scored); GENERIC].
Canada—
    20 mg (Rx) [*Alupent* (lactose)].

**Packaging and storage**
Store below 40 °C (104 °F), preferably between 15 and 30 °C (59 and 86 °F), unless otherwise specified by manufacturer. Store in a well-closed, light-resistant container.

---

### PIRBUTEROL

## Summary of Differences

Pharmacology/pharmacokinetics:
    Biotransformation—Metabolized primarily by sulfate conjugation; not metabolized by catechol-O-methyltransferase.
    Half-life—2 hours.
    Onset of action—Within 5 minutes.
    Time to peak effect—0.5 to 1 hour.
    Duration of action—5 hours.
    Elimination—51% of inhaled dose excreted as pirbuterol plus sulfate conjugate.
Side/adverse effects:
    Irregular heartbeat, mood or mental changes, numbness in hands or feet, unusual bruising, loss of appetite, or smell or taste changes may occur.

## Additional Dosing Information

See also *General Dosing Information*.

Pirbuterol may be administered concurrently with corticosteroid and/or theophylline therapy.

With chronic dosing of pirbuterol, tolerance to the bronchodilator effect has occurred in some patients.

## Inhalation Dosage Forms

### PIRBUTEROL ACETATE INHALATION AEROSOL

**Usual adult and adolescent dose**
Bronchodilator—
    Oral inhalation, 200 or 400 mcg (0.2 or 0.4 mg—1 or 2 inhalations) every four to six hours, not to exceed a total dose of 2.4 mg (12 inhalations) per day.

**Usual pediatric dose**
Bronchodilator—
    Children up to 12 years of age: Dosage has not been established.
    Children 12 years of age and over: See *Usual adult and adolescent dose*.

**Strength(s) usually available**
U.S.—
    200 mcg (0.2 mg) (base) per metered spray (Rx) [*Maxair* (dichloro-difluoromethane, trichloromonofluoromethane, sorbitan trioleate)].
Canada—
    Not commercially available.

**Packaging and storage**
Store below 40 °C (104 °F), preferably between 15 and 30 °C (59 and 86 °F), unless otherwise specified by manufacturer. Protect from freezing.

**Auxiliary labeling**
• For oral inhalation only.
• Shake well.
• Store away from heat and direct sunlight.

---

### PROCATEROL

## Summary of Differences

Pharmacology/pharmacokinetics:
    Onset of action—Within 5 minutes.
    Time to peak effect—About 1.5 hours.
    Duration of action—6 to 8 hours.

## Inhalation Dosage Forms

### PROCATEROL HYDROCHLORIDE HEMIHYDRATE INHALATION AEROSOL

**Usual adult and adolescent dose**
Bronchodilator—
    Oral inhalation, 20 mcg (0.02 mg—2 inhalations) three times a day.
    Bronchospasm, exercise-induced (prophylaxis): Oral inhalation, 20 mcg (0.02 mg—2 inhalations) at least fifteen minutes before exertion.

**Usual pediatric dose**
Bronchodilator—
    Children up to 12 years of age: Dosage has not been established.
    Children 12 years of age and over: See *Usual adult and adolescent dose*.

**Strength(s) usually available**
U.S.—
    Not commercially available.
Canada—
    10 mcg (0.01 mg) per metered spray (Rx) [*Pro-Air*].

**Packaging and storage**
Store below 40 °C (104 °F), preferably between 15 and 30 °C (59 and 86 °F), unless otherwise specified by manufacturer. Protect from freezing.

**Auxiliary labeling**
• For oral inhalation only.
• Shake well.
• Store away from heat and direct sunlight.

---

### TERBUTALINE

## Summary of Differences

Category:
    Oral and parenteral terbutaline also used as a labor (premature) inhibitor; and parenteral terbutaline may be used in management of bronchospasm during anesthesia.
Pharmacology/pharmacokinetics:
    Biotransformation:
        Metabolized primarily to inactive sulfate conjugate.
    Onset of action—
        Inhalation: 5 to 30 minutes.
        Oral: Within 60 to 120 minutes.
        Parenteral: Within 15 minutes.
    Time to peak effect—
        Inhalation: 1 to 2 hours.
        Oral: Within 2 to 3 hours.
        Parenteral: Within 0.5 to 1 hour.
    Duration of action—
        Inhalation: 3 to 6 hours.
        Oral: 4 to 8 hours.
        Parenteral: 1.5 to 4 hours.
Precautions:
    Pregnancy/reproduction—
        Pregnancy: Parenteral administration during pregnancy reported to cause fetal tachycardia.

Labor and delivery: Inhibits uterine activity during the second and third trimesters of pregnancy and may inhibit labor; when administered during labor, reported to cause serious adverse reactions such as transient hypokalemia, pulmonary edema, and hypoglycemia in the mother and hypoglycemia in neonates of mothers treated with parenteral terbutaline.

Medical considerations/contraindications—

Caution also needed in ketoacidosis when large parenteral doses of terbutaline are administered and in patients with history of seizures.

Side/adverse effects:

Irregular heartbeat, drowsiness, muscle cramps or twitching, or unusual taste may occur.

## Additional Dosing Information

See also *General Dosing Information*.

**For parenteral dosage forms only**
The subcutaneous injection is usually injected into the lateral deltoid area.

## Inhalation Dosage Forms

### TERBUTALINE SULFATE INHALATION AEROSOL

**Usual adult and adolescent dose**
Bronchodilator—

Oral inhalation, 200 to 500 mcg (0.2 to 0.5 mg—1 or 2 inhalations, 2 inhalations being separated by a sixty-second interval) every four to six hours.

**Usual pediatric dose**
Bronchodilator—

Children up to 12 years of age: Dosage has not been established.
Children 12 years of age and over: See *Usual adult and adolescent dose*.

**Strength(s) usually available**
U.S.—

200 mcg (0.2 mg) per metered spray (Rx) [*Brethaire* (dichlorodifluoromethane 5.16 grams, dichlorotetrafluoroethane 2.58 grams, and trichloromonofluoromethane 2.58 grams, per 7.5 mL [10.5 grams])].

Canada—

500 mcg (0.5 mg) per metered spray (Rx) [*Bricanyl*].

**Packaging and storage**
Store below 40 °C (104 °F), preferably between 15 and 30 °C (59 and 86 °F), unless otherwise specified by manufacturer. Protect from freezing.

**Auxiliary labeling**
• For oral inhalation only.
• Shake well.

**Note**
Include patient instructions when dispensing.

## Oral Dosage Forms

Note: Bracketed uses in the *Dosage Forms* section refer to categories of use and/or indications that are not included in U.S. product labeling.

### TERBUTALINE SULFATE TABLETS USP

**Usual adult dose**
Bronchodilator—

Oral, 2.5 to 5 mg three times a day, administered at approximately six-hour intervals.

[Labor (premature) inhibitor][1]—

Maintenance: Oral, 2.5 mg every four to six hours until term.

**Usual adult prescribing limits**
Up to 15 mg per twenty-four hours.

**Usual pediatric dose**
Bronchodilator—

Children up to 12 years of age: Dosage has not been established.
Children 12 to 15 years of age: Oral, 2.5 mg three times a day, administered at approximately six-hour intervals.

**Strength(s) usually available**
U.S.—

2.5 mg (Rx) [*Brethine* (scored); *Bricanyl*].
5 mg (Rx) [*Brethine* (scored); *Bricanyl* (scored; povidone)].

Canada—

2.5 mg (Rx) [*Bricanyl* (scored)].
5 mg (Rx) [*Bricanyl* (scored)].

**Packaging and storage**
Store between 15 and 30 °C (59 to 86 °F), in a tight container.

## Parenteral Dosage Forms

Note: Bracketed uses in the *Dosage Forms* section refer to categories of use and/or indications that are not included in U.S. product labeling.

### TERBUTALINE SULFATE INJECTION USP

**Usual adult dose**
Bronchodilator—

Subcutaneous, 250 mcg (0.25 mg), repeated after fifteen to thirty minutes if necessary; a total dose of 500 mcg (0.5 mg) should not be exceeded within a four-hour period.

[Labor (premature) inhibitor][1]—

Intravenous infusion, administered at a rate of 10 mcg (0.01 mg) per minute initially, the rate being increased by 5 mcg (0.005 mg) per minute every ten minutes until contractions cease or up to a maximum dose of 80 mcg (0.08 mg) per minute. After contractions cease for thirty minutes to one hour, the rate of administration is decreased by 5 mcg (0.005 mg) per minute to the lowest effective dose. The minimum effective dosage should be continued for four to eight hours after contractions cease.

Subcutaneous, 250 mcg (0.25 mg) every hour until contractions cease.

**Usual pediatric dose**
Bronchodilator—

Children up to 12 years of age: Dosage has not been established.

**Strength(s) usually available**
U.S.—

1 mg (820 mcg [0.82 mg] [base]) per mL (Rx) [*Brethine* (sodium chloride); *Bricanyl* (sodium chloride)].

Canada—

Not commercially available.

**Packaging and storage**
Store between 15 and 30 °C (59 and 86 °F). Protect from light.

**Stability**
Do not use if solution is discolored.

---

[1] Not included in Canadian product labeling.

Revised: July 1990
Interim revision: 09/12/94; 08/09/95

## Table 1. Pharmacology/Pharmacokinetics

| Drug | Adrenergic Receptor Action (Primary) | Biotransformation | Half-life (hr) | Onset of Action (min) | Time to Peak Effect (hr) | Duration of Action (hr) | Elimination Primary (% unchanged)/ Secondary |
|---|---|---|---|---|---|---|---|
| Albuterol* | Beta-2 | Hepatic† | | | | | Renal/Fecal‡ |
| Inhalation | | | Elimination: 3.8 | 5–15 | 1–1.5 after 2 inhalations | 3–6§ | |
| Oral | | | Plasma: 2.7–5 | 15–30 | 2–3 | 8 or more (12 for extended-release tablets) | |
| Bitolterol* Inhalation | Beta-2 | # | — | 3–4 | 0.5–1** | 5–8†† | ‡‡ |
| Ephedrine | Alpha; Beta-1; Beta-2 | Hepatic | Elimination: At urine pH 5— About 3 At urine pH 6.3—About 6 | | | | Renal (mostly unchanged); dependent on urinary pH; increased in acidic urine |
| Oral | | | | 15–60 | — | 3–5 | |
| Intramuscular | | | | 10–20 | — | 0.5–1 after 25–50 mg dose | |
| Subcutaneous | | | | — | — | 0.5–1 after 25–50 mg dose | |
| Epinephrine | Alpha; Beta-1; Beta-2 | Hepatic; also in sympathetic nerve endings and other tissues | | | | | Renal (very small amount) |
| Inhalation | | | — | 3–5 | — | 1–3 | |
| Intramuscular | | | — | Variable | — | <1–4 | |
| Subcutaneous | | | — | 6–15 | 0.3 | <1–4 | |
| Ethylnorepinephrine§§ | Beta-1; Beta-2 | — | | | | | — |
| Intramuscular | | | — | 6–12 | — | 1–2 | |
| Subcutaneous | | | — | 6–12 | — | 1–2 | |
| Fenoterol* | Beta-2 | — | | | | | Renal/Biliary/Fecal |
| Inhalation | | | — | 5 | 0.5–1 | 2–3 | |
| Oral | | | — | 30–60 | 2–3 | 6–8 | |
| Isoetharine* | Beta-2 | Hepatic; also in lungs, gastrointestinal tract, and other tissues | — | | | | Renal (about 10) |
| Inhalation | | | | 1–6 | 0.25–1 | 1–4 | |

*Has minor beta-1 activity.

†Primarily to albuterol 4'-0-sulfate, which has little or no beta-adrenergic stimulating effect and no beta-adrenergic blocking effect.

‡Inhalation—
    Renal: Approximately 72% of inhaled dose excreted within 24 hours in urine, consisting of 28% unchanged drug and 44% as metabolite.
    Fecal: About 10% of inhaled dose may be excreted in feces.
  Oral—
    Renal: Approximately 65 to 90% of oral dose excreted over 3 days in urine, the majority of dose being excreted within first 24 hours, consisting of 60% as metabolite.
    Fecal: About 4% of oral dose may be excreted in feces.

§Usually longer lasting than isoproterenol since albuterol is not a substrate for cellular uptake processes for catecholamines or for catechol-0-methyl transferase.

#A prodrug hydrolyzed by esterases in tissue and blood to the active compound colterol.

**Mean maximum increase in forced expiratory volume in 1 second ($FEV_1$) over baseline in most patients was 39 to 42%.

††Based on 15% or greater increase in $FEV_1$, at least 5 hours in most patients and 8 hours or more in 25 to 35% of patients; in steroid-dependent asthmatic patients, 3.5 to 5 hours. Based on mean maximal expiratory flow (MMEF) measurements, 6 to 7 hours.

‡‡Following oral administration of 5.9 mg of tritiated bitolterol mesylate, 83% of radioactivity of dose was excreted within first 24 hours. After 72 hours, 85.6% of tritium had been excreted in urine and 8.1% in feces. Majority of radioactivity was excreted as conjugated colterol; 2.1 to 3.7% of total radioactivity was excreted as free colterol; and no unchanged bitolterol was detected in urine.

§§Has minor alpha activity.

##Metabolized primarily by sulfate conjugation; not metabolized by catechol-O-methyltransferase.

***51% of inhaled dose excreted as pirbuterol plus sulfate conjugate.

## Table 1. Pharmacology/Pharmacokinetics *(continued)*

| Drug | Adrenergic Receptor Action (Primary) | Biotransformation | Half-life (hr) | Onset of Action (min) | Time to Peak Effect (hr) | Duration of Action (hr) | Elimination Primary (% unchanged)/ Secondary |
|---|---|---|---|---|---|---|---|
| Isoproterenol | Beta-1; Beta-2 | Hepatic; also in lungs and other tissues | | | | | Renal (IV, about 40–50; oral or inhalation, about 5–15) |
| Inhalation | | | — | 2–5 | — | 0.5–2 | |
| Intravenous | | | — | Immediate | — | <1 | |
| Rectal | | | — | Within 30 | — | 2–4 | |
| Sublingual | | | — | 15–30 | — | 1–2 | |
| Metaproterenol* | Beta-2 | Hepatic | | | | | Renal, primarily as glucuronic acid conjugates |
| Inhalation aerosol | | | — | Within 1 | About 1 | 1–5 after single dose 1–2.5 after repeated doses | |
| Inhalation by hand-bulb nebulizer or intermittent positive-pressure breathing (IPPB) | | | — | 5–30 | — | 2–6 after single dose; 4–6 after repeated doses | |
| Oral | | | — | Within 15–30 | Within 1 | Up to 4 | |
| Pirbuterol | Beta-2 | ## | 2 | | | | Renal*** |
| Inhalation | | | | Within 5 | 0.5–1 | 5 | |
| Procaterol | Beta-2 | — | — | | | | — |
| Inhalation | | | | Within 5 | About 1.5 | 6–8 | |
| Terbutaline* | Beta-2 | Hepatic, partially; primarily to inactive sulfate conjugate | | | | | Renal |
| Inhalation | | | — | 5–30 | 1–2 | 3–6 | |
| Oral | | | — | Within 60–120 | Within 2–3 | 4–8 | |
| Parenteral | | | — | Within 15 | Within 0.5–1 | 1.5–4 | |

*Has minor beta-1 activity.

†Primarily to albuterol 4'-0-sulfate, which has little or no beta-adrenergic stimulating effect and no beta-adrenergic blocking effect.

‡Inhalation—
   Renal: Approximately 72% of inhaled dose excreted within 24 hours in urine, consisting of 28% unchanged drug and 44% as metabolite.
   Fecal: About 10% of inhaled dose may be excreted in feces.

   Oral—
   Renal: Approximately 65 to 90% of oral dose excreted over 3 days in urine, the majority of dose being excreted within first 24 hours, consisting of 60% as metabolite.
   Fecal: About 4% of oral dose may be excreted in feces.

§Usually longer lasting than isoproterenol since albuterol is not a substrate for cellular uptake processes for catecholamines or for catechol-0-methyl transferase.

#A prodrug hydrolyzed by esterases in tissue and blood to the active compound colterol.

**Mean maximum increase in forced expiratory volume in 1 second (FEV₁) over baseline in most patients was 39 to 42%.

††Based on 15% or greater increase in FEV₁, at least 5 hours in most patients and 8 hours or more in 25 to 35% of patients; in steroid-dependent asthmatic patients, 3.5 to 5 hours. Based on mean maximal expiratory flow (MMEF) measurements, 6 to 7 hours.

‡‡Following oral administration of 5.9 mg of tritiated bitolterol mesylate, 83% of radioactivity of dose was excreted within first 24 hours. After 72 hours, 85.6% of tritium had been excreted in urine and 8.1% in feces. Majority of radioactivity was excreted as conjugated colterol; 2.1 to 3.7% of total radioactivity was excreted as free colterol; and no unchanged bitolterol was detected in urine.

§§Has minor alpha activity.

##Metabolized primarily by sulfate conjugation; not metabolized by catechol-O-methyltransferase.

***51% of inhaled dose excreted as pirbuterol plus sulfate conjugate.

## Table 2. Drug interactions and/or related problems

| The following drug interactions and/or related problems have been selected on the basis of their potential clinical significance (possible mechanism in parentheses where appropriate)—not necessarily inclusive (» = major clinical significance): | Legend:<br>**I**=Albuterol<br>**II**=Bitolterol<br>**III**=Ephedrine<br>**IV**=Epinephrine | | | | **V**=Ethylnorepinephrine<br>**VI**=Fenoterol<br>**VII**=Isoetharine<br>**VIII**=Isoproterenol | | | | **IX**=Metaproterenol<br>**X**=Pirbuterol<br>**XI**=Procaterol<br>**XII**=Terbutaline | | | |
|---|---|---|---|---|---|---|---|---|---|---|---|---|
| Note: Combinations containing any of the following medications, depending on the amount present, may also interact with this medication. | **I** | **II** | **III** | **IV** | **V** | **VI** | **VII** | **VIII** | **IX** | **X** | **XI** | **XII** |
| Alkalizers, urinary, such as:<br>  Antacids, calcium- and/or magnesium-containing<br>  Carbonic anhydrase inhibitors<br>  Citrates<br>  Sodium bicarbonate<br>    (urine alkalinization induced by these medications reduces urinary excretion of ephedrine and therefore may increase the half-life of ephedrine and prolong its duration of action, especially if the urine remains alkaline for several days or longer; patient should be monitored for ephedrine toxicity [e.g., nervousness, insomnia, excitability]; dosage adjustment of ephedrine may be necessary) | | | ✔ | | | | | | | | | |
| Alpha-adrenergic blocking agents, such as:<br>  Labetalol<br>  Phenoxybenzamine<br>  Phentolamine<br>  Prazosin<br>  Tolazoline, or<br>Other medications with alpha-adrenergic blocking action, such as:<br>  Haloperidol<br>  Loxapine<br>  Phenothiazines<br>  Thioxanthenes, or<br>Vasodilators, rapidly acting, such as nitrites<br>    (concurrent use may block the alpha-adrenergic effects of epinephrine, possibly resulting in severe hypotension and tachycardia) | | | | ✔ | | | | | | | | |
|     (concurrent use of ephedrine or epinephrine may reduce the antianginal effect of amyl nitrite) | | | ✔ | ✔ | | | | | | | | |
| »  Anesthetics, hydrocarbon inhalation, such as:<br>  Chloroform<br>  Cyclopropane<br>  Enflurane<br>  Halothane<br>  Isoflurane<br>  Methoxyflurane<br>  Trichloroethylene<br>    (concurrent use of chloroform, cyclopropane, halothane, or trichloroethylene with ephedrine, epinephrine, ethylnorepinephrine, or isoproterenol may increase the risk of severe ventricular arrhythmias because these anesthetics greatly sensitize the myocardium to the effects of sympathomimetics; these medications should be used with caution and in substantially reduced dosage in patients receiving hydrocarbon inhalation anesthetics) | | | ✔ | ✔ | ✔ | | | ✔ | | | | |
|     (administration of high doses of albuterol, bitolterol, fenoterol, isoetharine, metaproterenol, pirbuterol, procaterol, or terbutaline prior to or shortly after anesthesia with chloroform, cyclopropane, halothane, or trichloroethylene may increase the risk of severe ventricular arrhythmias, especially in patients with pre-existing heart disease, because these anesthetics greatly sensitize the myocardium to the effects of sympathomimetics) | ✔ | ✔ | | | | ✔ | ✔ | | ✔ | ✔ | ✔ | ✔ |
|     (enflurane, isoflurane, or methoxyflurane may also cause some sensitization of the myocardium to the effects of sympathomimetics; caution is recommended during concurrent use with the sympathomimetic) | ✔ | ✔ | ✔ | ✔ | ✔ | ✔ | ✔ | ✔ | ✔ | ✔ | ✔ | ✔ |

## Table 2. Drug interactions and/or related problems *(continued)*

Legend:
I=Albuterol  V=Ethylnorepinephrine  IX=Metaproterenol
II=Bitolterol  VI=Fenoterol  X=Pirbuterol
III=Ephedrine  VII=Isoetharine  XI=Procaterol
IV=Epinephrine  VIII=Isoproterenol  XII=Terbutaline

| | I | II | III | IV | V | VI | VII | VIII | IX | X | XI | XII |
|---|---|---|---|---|---|---|---|---|---|---|---|---|
| » Anesthetics, parenteral-local (epinephrine shoud be used cautiously and in carefully circumscribed quantities, if at all, with local anesthetics for anesthetizing areas with end arteries [such as the fingers, toes, or penis] or otherwise compromised blood supply; ischemia leading to gangrene may result) | | | | ✔ | | | | | | | | |
| » Antidepressants, tricyclic, or » Maprotiline (concurrent use may potentiate the cardiovascular effects of epinephrine or isoproterenol, possibly resulting in arrhythmias, tachycardia, or severe hypertension or hyperpyrexia) | | | | ✔ | | | | ✔ | | | | |
| (concurrent use of tricyclic antidepressants may potentiate the action of albuterol, metaproterenol, pirbuterol, procaterol, or terbutaline on the vascular system) | ✔ | | | | | | | | ✔ | ✔ | ✔ | ✔ |
| Antidiabetic agents, oral, or Insulin (effects may be decreased when these medications are used concurrently with epinephrine, since epinephrine increases blood glucose by inhibiting glucose uptake by peripheral tissues and by promoting glycogenolysis; dosage adjustments of oral antidiabetic agents or insulin may be necessary) | | | | ✔ | | | | | | | | |
| Antihypertensives or Diuretics used as antihypertensives (antihypertensive effects may be reduced when these medications are used concurrently with adrenergic bronchodilators; the patient should be carefully monitored to confirm that the desired effect is being obtained) | ✔ | ✔ | ✔ | ✔ | ✔ | ✔ | ✔ | ✔ | ✔ | ✔ | ✔ | ✔ |
| » Beta-adrenergic blocking agents, including ophthalmic agents (concurrent use with adrenergic bronchodilators may result in mutual inhibition of therapeutic effects) | ✔ | ✔ | ✔ | ✔ | ✔ | ✔ | ✔ | ✔ | ✔ | ✔ | ✔ | ✔ |
| (for adrenergic bronchodilators with both alpha- and beta-adrenergic effects [ephedrine, epinephrine], beta-adrenergic blockade may result in unopposed alpha-adrenergic activity with a risk of hypertension and excessive bradycardia with possible heart block; beta-blockade also antagonizes the beta-2-adrenergic bronchodilating effect of ephedrine and epinephrine) | | | ✔ | ✔ | | | | | | | | |
| (for adrenergic bronchodilators with beta-adrenergic effects, beta-blockade may antagonize the beta-2-adrenergic bronchodilating effect of albuterol, bitolterol, ethylnorepinephrine, fenoterol, isoetharine, metaproterenol, pirbuterol, procaterol, or terbutaline and the beta-1-adrenergic cardiac effect and the beta-2-adrenergic bronchodilating effect of isoproterenol; use of a cardioselective beta-1-adrenergic blocker, such as atenolol or metoprolol, at low doses may reduce antagonism of the bronchodilating effect) | ✔ | ✔ | | | ✔ | ✔ | ✔ | ✔ | ✔ | ✔ | ✔ | ✔ |
| CNS stimulation–producing medications, other (See *Appendix II*) (concurrent use with adrenergic bronchodilators may result in additive CNS stimulation to excessive levels, which may cause unwanted effects such as nervousness, irritability, insomnia, or possibly convulsions or cardiac arrhythmias; close observation is recommended) | ✔ | ✔ | ✔ | ✔ | ✔ | ✔ | ✔ | ✔ | ✔ | ✔ | ✔ | ✔ |

## Table 2. Drug interactions and/or related problems *(continued)*

| | Legend:<br>**I**=Albuterol<br>**II**=Bitolterol<br>**III**=Ephedrine<br>**IV**=Epinephrine | | | | **V**=Ethylnorepinephrine<br>**VI**=Fenoterol<br>**VII**=Isoetharine<br>**VIII**=Isoproterenol | | | | **IX**=Metaproterenol<br>**X**=Pirbuterol<br>**XI**=Procaterol<br>**XII**=Terbutaline | | | |
|---|---|---|---|---|---|---|---|---|---|---|---|---|
| | **I** | **II** | **III** | **IV** | **V** | **VI** | **VII** | **VIII** | **IX** | **X** | **XI** | **XII** |
| » Cocaine, mucosal-local<br>(in addition to increasing CNS stimulation, concurrent use of a sympathomimetic may increase the cardiovascular effects of either or both medications and the risk of adverse effects) | ✔ | ✔ | ✔ | ✔ | ✔ | ✔ | ✔ | ✔ | ✔ | ✔ | ✔ | ✔ |
| (concurrent use of epinephrine with cocaine [especially intranasal application of "cocaine mud," a potentially lethal substance obtained by moistening cocaine powder with an epinephrine solution] is not recommended because of the high risk of hypertensive episodes and cardiac arrhythmias; also, concurrent use of cocaine and epinephrine is unnecessary because epinephrine does not provide additional local vasoconstriction or slow absorption of cocaine from the mucosa) | | | | ✔ | | | | | | | | |
| Corticosteroids, glucocorticoid, or<br>Corticotropin, chronic therapeutic use of<br>(concurrent use of glucocorticoid corticosteroids or chronic therapeutic use of corticotropin with ephedrine may increase the metabolic clearance of corticosteroids or corticotropin; glucocorticoid dosage adjustment may be required) | | | ✔ | | | | | | | | | |
| Diatrizoates or<br>Iothalamate or<br>Ioxaglate<br>(neurologic effects of these medications, including paraplegia, may be increased during aortography when the medications are administered after hypertensive agents, such as parenteral ephedrine or epinephrine, used to increase contrast; increase of neurologic effects is due to contraction of vessels in the splanchnic circulation, forcing more of the contrast material into the vessels leading to the spine and spinal cord) | | | ✔ | ✔ | | | | | | | | |
| » Digitalis glycosides<br>(concurrent use with adrenergic bronchodilators may increase the risk of cardiac arrhythmias; caution and close electrocardiographic monitoring are very important if concurrent use is necessary) | ✔ | ✔ | ✔ | ✔ | ✔ | ✔ | ✔ | ✔ | ✔ | ✔ | ✔ | ✔ |
| Dihydroergotamine or<br>» Ergoloid mesylates or<br>Ergonovine or<br>» Ergotamine or<br>Methylergonovine or<br>Methysergide or<br>Oxytocin<br>(concurrent use of dihydroergotamine, ergonovine, methylergonovine, or methysergide with ephedrine or epinephrine may result in enhanced vasoconstriction; dosage adjustments may be necessary) | | | ✔ | ✔ | | | | | | | | |
| (concurrent use of ergoloid mesylates or ergotamine with ephedrine or epinephrine may produce peripheral vascular ischemia and gangrene and is not recommended) | | | ✔ | ✔ | | | | | | | | |
| (concurrent use of ergonovine, ergotamine, methylergonovine, or oxytocin may potentiate the pressor effect of ephedrine or epinephrine and result in severe hypertension; rarely, rupture of a cerebral blood vessel has occurred postpartum) | | | ✔ | ✔ | | | | | | | | |
| Doxapram<br>(in addition to possibly increasing CNS stimulation, concurrent use may increase the pressor effects of either doxapram or ephedrine or epinephrine) | | | ✔ | ✔ | | | | | | | | |

## Table 2. Drug interactions and/or related problems *(continued)*

| | Legend:<br>I=Albuterol<br>II=Bitolterol<br>III=Ephedrine<br>IV=Epinephrine | | | | V=Ethylnorepinephrine<br>VI=Fenoterol<br>VII=Isoetharine<br>VIII=Isoproterenol | | | | IX=Metaproterenol<br>X=Pirbuterol<br>XI=Procaterol<br>XII=Terbutaline | | | |
|---|---|---|---|---|---|---|---|---|---|---|---|---|
| | I | II | III | IV | V | VI | VII | VIII | IX | X | XI | XII |
| Guanadrel or<br>Guanethidine<br>(in addition to possibly decreasing the hypotensive effect of guanadrel or guanethidine, concurrent use may potentiate the pressor effect of ephedrine or epinephrine, as a result of inhibition of sympathomimetic uptake by adrenergic neurons, possibly resulting in hypertension and cardiac arrhythmias) | | | ✔ | ✔ | | | | | | | | |
| Levodopa<br>(concurrent use with adrenergic bronchodilators may increase the possibility of cardiac arrhythmias; dosage reduction of the sympathomimetic is recommended) | ✔ | ✔ | ✔ | ✔ | ✔ | ✔ | ✔ | ✔ | ✔ | ✔ | ✔ | ✔ |
| Mazindol<br>(in addition to possibly increasing CNS stimulation, concurrent use may potentiate the pressor effect of ephedrine or epinephrine; if necessary to administer a pressor amine agent to a patient who has recently received mazindol, initiating pressor therapy in reduced dosage and monitoring of blood pressure at frequent intervals are recommended) | | | ✔ | ✔ | | | | | | | | |
| Mecamylamine or<br>Methyldopa or<br>Trimethaphan<br>(in addition to possibly decreasing the hypotensive effects of these medications, concurrent use may enhance the pressor response to ephedrine or epinephrine) | | | ✔ | ✔ | | | | | | | | |
| Methylphenidate<br>(in addition to possibly increasing CNS stimulation, concurrent use may potentiate the pressor effects of ephedrine or epinephrine) | | | ✔ | ✔ | | | | | | | | |
| » Monoamine oxidase (MAO) inhibitors, including furazolidone and procarbazine<br>(concurrent use may potentiate the action of albuterol, fenoterol, metaproterenol, pirbuterol, procaterol, or terbutaline on the vascular system)<br>(concurrent use may prolong and intensify cardiac stimulant and vasopressor effects of ephedrine because of release of catecholamines, which accumulate in intraneuronal storage sites during MAO inhibitor therapy, resulting in headache, cardiac arrhythmias, vomiting, or sudden and severe hypertensive and/or hyperpyretic crises; ephedrine should not be administered during or within 14 days following the administration of an MAO inhibitor) | ✔ | | ✔ | | | ✔ | | | ✔ | ✔ | ✔ | ✔ |
| Nitrates<br>(concurrent use with adrenergic bronchodilators may reduce the antianginal effects of nitrates) | ✔ | ✔ | ✔ | ✔ | ✔ | ✔ | ✔ | ✔ | ✔ | ✔ | ✔ | ✔ |
| Papaverine, intracavernosal, or<br>Phentolamine, intracavernosal<br>(vasodilating effect of papaverine or phentolamine is reversed by epinephrine; epinephrine may be used to treat priapism or overdose due to these medications) | | | | ✔ | | | | | | | | |

## Table 2. Drug interactions and/or related problems *(continued)*

Legend:
I=Albuterol  V=Ethylnorepinephrine  IX=Metaproterenol
II=Bitolterol  VI=Fenoterol  X=Pirbuterol
III=Ephedrine  VII=Isoetharine  XI=Procaterol
IV=Epinephrine  VIII=Isoproterenol  XII=Terbutaline

| | I | II | III | IV | V | VI | VII | VIII | IX | X | XI | XII |
|---|---|---|---|---|---|---|---|---|---|---|---|---|
| Rauwolfia alkaloids (concurrent use with ephedrine may decrease the hypotensive effects of rauwolfia alkaloids) | | | ✔ | | | | | | | | | |
| (in addition to possibly decreasing the hypotensive effects of rauwolfia alkaloids, concurrent use may theoretically prolong the action of direct-acting sympathomimetics, such as epinephrine, by preventing uptake into storage granules; a "denervation supersensitivity" response is also possible; although concurrent use with epinephrine is not known to produce severe adverse effects, a significant increase in blood pressure has been documented when phenylephrine ophthalmic drops have been administered to patients taking reserpine, and caution and close observation are recommended) | | | | ✔ | | | | | | | | |
| Ritodrine (concurrent use may increase the effect of either these medications or ritodrine and the potential for side effects) | ✔ | ✔ | ✔ | ✔ | ✔ | ✔ | ✔ | ✔ | ✔ | ✔ | ✔ | ✔ |
| Sympathomimetics, other (in addition to possibly increasing CNS stimulation, concurrent use may increase the cardiovascular effects of either the other sympathomimetic or the adrenergic bronchodilator and the potential for side effects; however, an aerosol bronchodilator of the adrenergic stimulant type may be used to relieve acute bronchospasm in patients receiving chronic oral adrenergic bronchodilator therapy) | ✔ | ✔ | ✔ | ✔ | ✔ | ✔ | ✔ | ✔ | ✔ | ✔ | ✔ | ✔ |
| Thallous chloride Tl 201 (in animal studies, concurrent use of isoproterenol increased myocardial uptake of thallous chloride Tl 201; human data are not available) | | | | | | | | ✔ | | | | |
| Thyroid hormones (concurrent use may increase the effects of either these medications or adrenergic bronchodilators; thyroid hormones enhance risk of coronary insufficiency when sympathomimetic agents are administered to patients with coronary artery disease; dosage adjustment is recommended, although problem is reduced in euthyroid patients) | ✔ | ✔ | ✔ | ✔ | ✔ | ✔ | ✔ | ✔ | ✔ | ✔ | ✔ | ✔ |
| Xanthines, such as: Aminophylline Caffeine Dyphylline Oxtriphylline Theophylline (in addition to possibly increasing CNS stimulation, concurrent use with adrenergic bronchodilators may result in other additive toxic effects) | ✔ | ✔ | ✔ | ✔ | ✔ | ✔ | ✔ | ✔ | ✔ | ✔ | ✔ | ✔ |

## Table 3. Medical considerations/Contraindications

Note: A blank space usually signifies lack of information; it is not necessarily an indication that a given medical problem is of no concern. However, the pharmacologic similarity of these agents may suggest that if caution is required in particular medical problems for one agent, then it may be required for the others as well.

The medical considerations/contraindications included have been selected on the basis of their potential clinical significance (reasons given in parentheses where appropriate)—not necessarily inclusive (» = major clinical significance).

*Risk-benefit should be considered when the following medical problems exist:*

Legend:
I=Albuterol
II=Bitolterol
III=Ephedrine
IV=Epinephrine
V=Ethylnorepinephrine
VI=Fenoterol
VII=Isoetharine
VIII=Isoproterenol
IX=Metaproterenol
X=Pirbuterol
XI=Procaterol
XII=Terbutaline

| Medical problem | I | II | III | IV | V | VI | VII | VIII | IX | X | XI | XII |
|---|---|---|---|---|---|---|---|---|---|---|---|---|
| » Brain damage, organic | | | | ✔ | | | | | | | | |
| » Cardiovascular disease, including: Angina pectoris | | | ✔ | ✔ | | | | ✔ | | | | |
| Cardiac arrhythmias | ✔ | ✔ | ✔ | ✔ | | | | | ✔ | ✔ | ✔ | ✔ |
| Cardiac arrhythmias associated with tachycardia | | | | | | ✔ | | ✔ | ✔ | | ✔ | |
| Cardiac asthma | | | | | | | ✔ | | | | | |
| Cardiac dilatation | | | | ✔ | | | | | | | | |
| Cerebral arteriosclerosis | | | | ✔ | | | | | | | | |
| Congestive heart failure | | | | ✔ | | ✔ | | | ✔ | | ✔ | |
| Coronary artery disease | | | | ✔ | ✔ | ✔ | ✔ | ✔ | ✔ | | | |
| Coronary insufficiency | ✔ | | ✔ | ✔ | | | | ✔ | | | ✔ | ✔ |
| Degenerative heart disease | | | | ✔ | | | | ✔ | | | | |
| Hypertension | ✔ | ✔ | ✔ | ✔ | ✔ | ✔ | ✔ | ✔ | ✔ | ✔ | ✔ | ✔ |
| Idiopathic hypertrophic subvalvular aortic stenosis | | | | | | ✔ | | | | ✔ | | |
| Ischemic heart disease | ✔ | ✔ | | ✔ | | | | | ✔ | ✔ | | |
| Limited cardiac reserve | | | | | | | ✔ | | | | | |
| Organic heart disease | | | | ✔ | | | | ✔ | | | | |
| Stroke, history of | | | | | ✔ | | | | | | | |
| Tachycardia caused by digitalis intoxication (condition may be exacerbated due to drug-induced cardiovascular effects) | | | | | | | | ✔ | | | | |
| Circulatory collapse or hypotension, phenothiazine-induced (pressor effect of epinephrine may be reversed by the phenothiazine, resulting in further lowering of blood pressure) | | | | ✔ | | | | | | | | |
| Convulsive disorders | | ✔ | | | | | | | ✔ | ✔ | | |
| Diabetes mellitus (potential drug-induced hyperglycemia may result in loss of diabetic control; dosage of insulin or hypoglycemic agents may need to be increased, especially with epinephrine) | ✔ | ✔ | ✔ | ✔ | | ✔ | | ✔ | ✔ | ✔ | ✔ | ✔ |
| Glaucoma, angle-closure, or predisposition to | | | ✔ | ✔ | | ✔ | | | | | | |
| Hyperthyroidism (adverse reactions more likely to occur) | ✔ | ✔ | ✔ | ✔ | ✔ | ✔ | ✔ | ✔ | ✔ | ✔ | ✔ | ✔ |
| Ketoacidosis (large parenteral doses of albuterol or terbutaline may aggravate condition) | ✔ | | | | | | | | | | | ✔ |
| Parkinson's disease (rigidity and tremor may be increased temporarily) | | | | ✔ | | | | | | | | |
| Pheochromocytoma, diagnosed or suspected | ✔ | ✔ | ✔ | ✔ | ✔ | ✔ | ✔ | ✔ | | | | ✔ |
| Prostatic hypertrophy | | | ✔ | | | | | | | | | |
| Psychoneurotic disorders (worsening of symptoms) | | | | ✔ | | | | | | | | |
| Seizures, history of | | | | | | | | | | | | ✔ |

## Table 3. Medical considerations/Contraindications *(continued)*

Note: A blank space usually signifies lack of information; it is not necessarily an indication that a given medical problem is of no concern. However, the pharmacologic similarity of these agents may suggest that if caution is required in particular medical problems for one agent, then it may be required for the others as well.

Legend:
**I**=Albuterol   **V**=Ethylnorepinephrine   **IX**=Metaproterenol
**II**=Bitolterol   **VI**=Fenoterol   **X**=Pirbuterol
**III**=Ephedrine   **VII**=Isoetharine   **XI**=Procaterol
**IV**=Epinephrine   **VIII**=Isoproterenol   **XII**=Terbutaline

| | I | II | III | IV | V | VI | VII | VIII | IX | X | XI | XII |
|---|---|---|---|---|---|---|---|---|---|---|---|---|
| Sensitivity to sympathomimetics | ✓ | ✓ | ✓ | ✓ | ✓ | ✓ | ✓ | ✓ | ✓ | ✓ | ✓ | ✓ |
| » Shock, cardiogenic, traumatic, or hemorrhagic (increases myocardial oxygen demand in cardiogenic shock) | | | | ✓ | | | | | | | | |

## Table 4. Side/Adverse Effects*

Note: Fatalities have been reported in association with excessive use of inhaled sympathomimetics. The exact cause of death is unknown; however, cardiac arrest following unexpected development of a severe acute asthmatic crisis and subsequent hypoxia is suspected.

Parenteral albuterol may induce reversible metabolic changes, including hyperglycemia and hypokalemia, which are more pronounced during intravenous infusion.

If high arterial blood pressure is inadvertently induced by parenteral epinephrine, it may result in angina pectoris, aortic rupture, or cerebral hemorrhage.

The following side/adverse effects have been selected on the basis of their potential clinical significance (possible signs and symptoms in parentheses where appropriate)—not necessarily inclusive:

Legend:
**I**=Albuterol   **V**=Ethylnorepinephrine   **IX**=Metaproterenol
**II**=Bitolterol   **VI**=Fenoterol   **X**=Pirbuterol
**III**=Ephedrine   **VII**=Isoetharine   **XI**=Procaterol
**IV**=Epinephrine   **VIII**=Isoproterenol   **XII**=Terbutaline

| | I | II | III | IV | V | VI | VII | VIII | IX | X | XI | XII |
|---|---|---|---|---|---|---|---|---|---|---|---|---|
| **Medical attention needed** | | | | | | | | | | | | |
| *Chest discomfort or pain, continuing or severe, or* | ✓ | ✓ | ✓ | ✓ | ✓ | ✓ | ✓ | ✓ | ✓ | ✓ | ✓ | ✓ |
| *Chills or fever or* | | | ✓ | ✓ | ✓ | | | | | | | |
| *Convulsions or* | | | ✓ | ✓ | ✓ | | | | | | | |
| *Dizziness or lightheadedness, continuing or severe, or* | ✓ | ✓ | ✓ | ✓ | ✓ | ✓ | ✓ | ✓ | ✓ | ✓ | ✓ | ✓ |
| *Fast heartbeat, continuing, or* | ✓ | ✓ | ✓ | ✓ | ✓ | ✓ | ✓ | ✓ | ✓ | ✓ | ✓ | ✓ |
| *Hallucinations or* | | | ✓ | ✓ | | | | | | | | |
| *Headache, continuing or severe, or* | ✓ | ✓ | ✓ | ✓ | ✓ | ✓ | ✓ | ✓ | ✓ | ✓ | ✓ | ✓ |
| *Increase in blood pressure, severe, or* | ✓ | ✓ | ✓† | ✓† | ✓ | ✓ | ✓ | ✓ | ✓ | ✓ | ✓ | ✓ |
| *Irregular heartbeat, continuing or severe, or* | | | ✓ | ✓ | ✓ | | ✓ | | ✓ | ✓ | ✓ | ✓ |
| *Mood or mental changes or* | | | ✓ | | | | | | | | | |
| *Muscle cramps, severe, or* | | | | | | ✓ | | | | | ✓ | ✓ |
| *Nausea or vomiting, continuing or severe, or* | ✓ | | | ✓ | ✓ | ✓ | ✓ | ✓ | ✓ | ✓ | ✓ | ✓ |
| *Pounding heartbeat, continuing or severe, or* | ✓ | ✓ | | ✓ | ✓ | ✓ | ✓ | ✓ | ✓ | ✓ | ✓ | ✓ |
| *Shortness of breath or troubled breathing, severe, or* | | | ✓ | ✓ | | | | | | | | |
| *Slow heartbeat or* | | | | ✓ | ✓ | | | | | | | |
| *Trembling, severe, or* | ✓ | ✓ | ✓ | ✓ | ✓ | ✓ | ✓ | ✓ | ✓ | ✓ | ✓ | ✓ |
| *Unusual anxiety, nervousness, or restlessness or* | ✓ | ✓ | ✓ | ✓ | ✓ | ✓ | ✓ | ✓ | ✓ | ✓ | ✓ | ✓ |
| *Unusually large pupils or blurred vision or* | ✓ | | ✓ | ✓ | ✓ | | | | | | | |
| *Unusual paleness and coldness of skin or* | | | | ✓ | ✓ | | | | | | | |
| *Weakness, severe* (signs of overdose) | | | ✓ | ✓ | ✓ | ✓ | ✓ | ✓ | ✓ | ✓ | | ✓ |
| *Chest discomfort or pain* | R | R (1%) | R | R‡ | U | U | U | R | U | R | R§ | R |
| *Hallucinations* | U | U | § | § | U | U | U | U | U | U | U | U |
| *Irregular heartbeat* | U | R | R | R‡ | U | U | U | R | U | R | U | R |
| *Mood or mental changes* | U | U | § | U | U | U | U | U | U | R | U | U |
| *Numbness in hands or feet* | U | U | U | U | U | U | U | U | U | R | U | U |
| *Paradoxical bronchospasm* (increase in wheezing or difficulty in breathing) | R | R (<1%) | R | R | R | R | R | R | R | R | R | R |
| *Unusual bruising* | U | U | U | U | U | U | U | U | U | R | U | U |

## Table 4. Side/Adverse Effects* *(continued)*

| | I | II | III | IV | V | VI | VII | VIII | IX | X | XI | XII |
|---|---|---|---|---|---|---|---|---|---|---|---|---|
| Legend: I=Albuterol, II=Bitolterol, III=Ephedrine, IV=Epinephrine; V=Ethylnorepinephrine, VI=Fenoterol, VII=Isoetharine, VIII=Isoproterenol; IX=Metaproterenol, X=Pirbuterol, XI=Procaterol, XII=Terbutaline | | | | | | | | | | | | |
| **For preparations containing sulfites** | | | | | | | | | | | | |
| *Allergic reaction to sulfites* (bluish coloration of skin; dizziness, severe, or feeling faint; flushing or redness of skin, continuing; skin rash, hives, or itching; swelling of face, lips, or eyelids; wheezing or difficulty in breathing) | | | ✔ | ✔ | ✔ | ✔ | ✔ | ✔ | | | | |
| **Medical attention needed only if continuing or bothersome** | | | | | | | | | | | | |
| *Coughing or other bronchial irritation#* | L | L (4%) | — | § | — | L | U | L | L | L | U | U |
| *Difficult or painful urination* | L | U | L | U | U | U | U | U | U | U | U | U |
| *Dizziness or lightheadedness* | L | L (3%) | L | L** | L | L | L | L | L | L | L | L |
| *Drowsiness* | L | U | U | U | U | U | U | U | U | U | U | L |
| *Dryness or irritation of mouth or throat#* | L | L (5%) | L | R | — | L | L | M | U | R | R | L |
| *Fast heartbeat* | M | R (<1%) | L | M‡‡ | L | L | L | L | L | L | L | L |
| *Flushing or redness of face or skin* | L | L | U | L** | U | U | U | L | U | R | U | U |
| *Headache* | L | L (4%) | L | L** | L | L | L | L | L | L | M | L |
| *Heartburn* | L | U | U | U | — | L | U | U | U | U | U | U |
| *Increased sweating* | L | U | L | L** | U | L | U | L | L | U | U | L |
| *Increase in blood pressure* | L†† | L | L | L | L†† | U | L†† | L†† | L | R | U | L |
| *Loss of appetite* | R | U | L | U | U | U | U | U | U | U | R | U |
| *Muscle cramps or twitching* | L | U | U | U | U | L | U | U | L | U | U | L |
| *Nausea* | M | L (3%) | L | L** | L | L | L | L | L | L | L | L |
| *Nervousness or restlessness* | M | L (5%) | M | M‡‡ | U | M | L | M | M | M | L | M |
| *Pain or stinging at intramuscular injection site* | L | — | U | U | U | — | — | U | — | — | — | — |
| *Pounding heartbeat* | M | L (3%) | L | M‡‡ | L | L | L | L | L | L | L | L |
| *Trembling* | M | M (14%) | L | L** | L | M | L | L | L | M | M | M |
| *Trouble in sleeping* | L | R (<1%) | M | L** | U | L | L | M | U | R | U | L |
| *Unusual paleness* | R | U | L | L** | U | U | U | U | U | U | U | U |
| *Vomiting* | L | U | L | L** | U | L | L | L | L | L | U | L |
| *Weakness* | L | U | L | L** | L | L | L | L | L | R | U | L |
| **Medical attention *not* needed** | | | | | | | | | | | | |
| *Pinkish to red coloration of saliva* | — | — | — | — | — | — | — | M§§ | — | — | — | — |
| *Smell or taste changes* | U | U | U | U | — | U | U | U | U | L | U | U |
| *Unpleasant taste* | U | L | U | U | — | L# | U | U | L | U | U | U |
| *Unusual taste* | L | U | U | U | — | U | U | U | U | U | U | L |

*Differences in frequency of occurrence may reflect either lack of clinical-use data or actual pharmacologic distinctions among agents (although the agents' pharmacologic similarity suggests that side effects occurring with one may occur with the others). M=more frequent; L=less frequent; R=rare; U=unknown.

†Or possibly a severe decrease in blood pressure.

‡More frequent with high doses.

§With high doses.

#With inhalation dosage forms only.

**Less frequent with injection; rare with recommended doses of inhalation.

††Or possibly a decrease in blood pressure.

‡‡More frequent with injection; rare with recommended doses of inhalation.

§§For inhalation and sublingual dosage forms of isoproterenol only.

## Table 5. Patient Consultation

As an aid to patient consultation, refer to *Advice for the Patient, Bronchodilators, Adrenergic (Inhalation)* and *Bronchodilators, Adrenergic (Oral/Injection).*

In providing consultation, consider emphasizing the following selected information (» = major clinical signficance):

Legend:
I=Albuterol
II=Bitolterol
III=Ephedrine
IV=Epinephrine
V=Ethylnorepinephrine
VI=Fenoterol
VII=Isoetharine
VIII=Isoproterenol
IX=Metaproterenol
X=Pirbuterol
XI=Procaterol
XII=Terbutaline

| | I | II | III | IV | V | VI | VII | VIII | IX | X | XI | XII |
|---|---|---|---|---|---|---|---|---|---|---|---|---|
| **Before using this medication** | | | | | | | | | | | | |
| » Conditions affecting use, especially: | | | | | | | | | | | | |
| Sensitivity to sympathomimetics | ✔ | ✔ | ✔ | ✔ | ✔ | ✔ | ✔ | ✔ | ✔ | ✔ | ✔ | ✔ |
| Allergies to sulfites present in some preparations | | | ✔ | ✔ | ✔ | ✔ | ✔ | ✔ | | | | |
| Pregnancy— | | | | | | | | | | | | |
| Studies in animals have shown albuterol, bitolterol, epinephrine, and metaproterenol to cause teratogenic effects when medication given in doses many times human dose | ✔ | ✔ | | ✔ | | | | | ✔ | | | |
| Use of epinephrine during pregnancy may cause anoxia in fetus | | | | ✔ | | | | | | | | |
| Studies in animals have shown pirbuterol at high doses to cause abortions and fetal mortality | | | | | | | | | | ✔ | | |
| Parenteral administration of terbutaline during pregnancy reported to cause fetal tachycardia | | | | | | | | | | | | |
| Labor and/or delivery— | | | | | | | | | | | | |
| Albuterol given intravenously or orally reportedly inhibits uterine contractions | ✔ | | | | | | | | | | | |
| Epinephrine is not recommended for use during labor because it may delay second stage; also may cause prolonged uterine atony with hemorrhage when given in sufficient dosage to reduce uterine contractions | | | | ✔ | | | | | | | | |
| Terbutaline inhibits uterine activity during second and third trimesters of pregnancy and may inhibit labor: when administered during labor; terbutaline reported to cause serious adverse reactions (e.g., transient hypokalemia, pulmonary edema, hypoglycemia) in mother and hypoglycemia in neonates of mothers treated with parenteral terbutaline | | | | | | | | | | | | ✔ |
| Breast-feeding— | | | | | | | | | | | | |
| Not known if albuterol is distributed into breast milk; however, some animal studies have shown albuterol to be potentially tumorigenic | ✔ | | | | | | | | | | | |
| Epinephrine distributed into breast milk; use by nursing mothers may cause serious adverse reactions in infant | | | | ✔ | | | | | | | | |
| Terbutaline distributed into breast milk; some animal studies have shown terbutaline to be potentially tumorigenic | | | | | | | | | | | | ✔ |
| Use in children—Epinephrine should be used with caution in infants and children, since syncope has occurred following administration of epinephrine in asthmatic children | | | | ✔ | | | | | | | | |
| Dental—Epinephrine present in gingival retraction cords; systemic absorption of epinephrine from retraction cords may occur; epinephrine retraction cords should be used with caution in patients with cardiovascular problems | | | | ✔ | | | | | | | | |
| Other medications, especially— | | | | | | | | | | | | |
| Beta-adrenergic blocking agents | ✔ | ✔ | ✔ | ✔ | ✔ | ✔ | ✔ | ✔ | ✔ | ✔ | ✔ | ✔ |
| Cocaine, mucosal-local | ✔ | ✔ | ✔ | ✔ | ✔ | ✔ | ✔ | ✔ | ✔ | ✔ | ✔ | ✔ |
| Digitalis glycosides | ✔ | ✔ | ✔ | ✔ | ✔ | ✔ | ✔ | ✔ | ✔ | ✔ | ✔ | ✔ |
| Ergoloid mesylates | | | ✔ | ✔ | | | | | | | | |
| Ergotamine | | | ✔ | ✔ | | | | | | | | |
| Maprotiline | ✔ | | ✔ | | | | | | ✔ | ✔ | ✔ | ✔ |
| Monoamine oxidase (MAO) inhibitors | ✔ | | ✔ | | | ✔ | | | ✔ | ✔ | ✔ | ✔ |
| Tricyclic antidepressants | ✔ | | ✔ | | | | | | ✔ | ✔ | ✔ | ✔ |
| Other medical problems, especially— | | | | | | | | | | | | |
| Brain damage, organic | | | | ✔ | | | | | | | | |
| Cardiovascular disease | ✔ | ✔ | ✔ | ✔ | ✔ | ✔ | ✔ | ✔ | ✔ | ✔ | ✔ | ✔ |

*USOC permits use of inhalation beta-2 agonists.
†For inhalation dosage forms.
‡With high doses.

## Table 5. Patient Consultation (*continued*)

Legend:
I = Albuterol
II = Bitolterol
III = Ephedrine
IV = Epinephrine
V = Ethylnorepinephrine
VI = Fenoterol
VII = Isoetharine
VIII = Isoproterenol
IX = Metaproterenol
X = Pirbuterol
XI = Procaterol
XII = Terbutaline

| | I | II | III | IV | V | VI | VII | VIII | IX | X | XI | XII |
|---|---|---|---|---|---|---|---|---|---|---|---|---|
| **Proper use of this medication** | | | | | | | | | | | | |
| Not using if solution or suspension is pinkish to brownish in color or if solution contains a precipitate | | | | ✔ | | | ✔ | ✔ | | | | |
| » Not using inhalation dosage form of epinephrine without a physician's prescription unless medical problem is diagnosed as asthma | | | | ✔ | | | | | | | | |
| » Importance of not using more medication than the amount recommended | ✔ | ✔ | ✔ | ✔ | ✔ | ✔ | ✔ | ✔ | ✔ | ✔ | ✔ | ✔ |
| » Taking the medication a few hours before bedtime to minimize the possibility of insomnia | | | ✔ | | | | | | | | | |
| » Proper dosing | ✔ | ✔ | ✔ | ✔ | ✔ | ✔ | ✔ | ✔ | ✔ | ✔ | ✔ | ✔ |
| Missed dose: If on scheduled dosing regimen, using as soon as possible; using any remaining doses for the day at regularly spaced intervals; not doubling doses | ✔ | ✔ | ✔ | ✔ | | ✔ | ✔ | ✔ | ✔ | ✔ | ✔ | ✔ |
| *For all inhalation dosage forms* Proper administration: Reading patient instructions carefully before using | ✔ | ✔ | | ✔ | | | ✔ | ✔ | ✔ | ✔ | ✔ | ✔ |
| Knowing correct administration technique if using in a nebulizer or a combination nebulizer and respirator; checking with physician, nurse, or pharmacist if necessary | ✔ | | | ✔ | | ✔ | ✔ | ✔ | ✔ | | | |
| *For inhalation aerosols* » Avoiding contact with the eyes » Taking no more than 2 inhalations at one time with interval of 1 to 2 minutes between inhalations Saving applicator; refill units may be available | ✔ | ✔ | | ✔ | | ✔ | ✔ | ✔ | ✔ | ✔ | ✔ | ✔ |
| *For extended-release tablet dosage form* Swallowing tablet whole; not crushing, breaking, or chewing | ✔ | | | | | | | | | | | |
| *For sublingual tablet dosage form* Not chewing or swallowing tablet whole, but dissolving slowly under tongue; not swallowing until tablet completely dissolved | | | | | | | | ✔ | | | | |
| *For injection dosage forms* » Using only for conditions as prescribed by physician | | | | ✔ | ✔ | | | | | | | |
| Keeping ready for use at all times; also keeping telephone numbers for physician and nearest hospital emergency room readily available | | | | ✔ | ✔ | | | | | | | |
| Checking expiration date routinely; replacing medication before it expires | | | | ✔ | ✔ | | | | | | | |
| Knowing correct administration technique for self-administration; checking with physician if necessary | | | | ✔ | ✔ | | | | | | | |
| *For emergency use in allergic reaction—* » Using medication immediately | | | | ✔ | | | | | | | | |
| Notifying physician immediately or going to nearest hospital emergency room | | | | | | | | | | | | |
| If stung by an insect, removing insect's stinger; applying ice packs or sodium bicarbonate soaks, if available, to area stung | | | | | | | | | | | | |
| For auto-injector use: Importance of not removing safety cap on auto-injector before ready to use | | | | | | | | | | | | |
| Reading patient instructions carefully before need to use medication | | | | | | | | | | | | |
| Procedures for using— Removing gray safety cap Placing black tip on thigh at right angle to leg Pressing hard into thigh until auto-injector functions; holding in place several seconds; removing and properly discarding Massaging injection area for 10 seconds | | | | | | | | | | | | |

## Table 5. Patient Consultation (continued)

| | Legend:<br>I=Albuterol<br>II=Bitolterol<br>III=Ephedrine<br>IV=Epinephrine | | | | V=Ethylnorepinephrine<br>VI=Fenoterol<br>VII=Isoetharine<br>VIII=Isoproterenol | | | | IX=Metaproterenol<br>X=Pirbuterol<br>XI=Procaterol<br>XII=Terbutaline | | | |
|---|---|---|---|---|---|---|---|---|---|---|---|---|
| | I | II | III | IV | V | VI | VII | VIII | IX | X | XI | XII |
| » Proper storage | ✓ | ✓ | ✓ | ✓ | ✓ | ✓ | ✓ | ✓ | ✓ | ✓ | ✓ | ✓ |
| **Precautions while using this medication** | | | | | | | | | | | | |
| » Checking with physician immediately if difficulty in breathing persists after use of medication or if condition becomes worse | ✓ | ✓ | | ✓† | ✓ | ✓ | ✓ | ✓ | ✓ | ✓ | ✓ | ✓ |
| Diabetics: May increase blood glucose concentrations | | | | ✓ | | | | | | | | |
| » Possibility of allergic reaction to sulfites contained in some preparations; checking with physician immediately if signs of allergic reaction occur | | | | ✓ | ✓ | ✓ | ✓ | ✓ | | | | |
| *For inhalation dosage forms* | | | | | | | | | | | | |
| Possible dryness of mouth and throat; rinsing mouth with water after each dose to help prevent dryness | ✓ | ✓ | | | | ✓ | ✓ | | ✓ | ✓ | ✓ | ✓ |
| *For inhalation aerosol dosage forms* | | | | | | | | | | | | |
| » For patients also using an adrenocorticoid or ipratropium inhalation aerosol: Using adrenergic bronchodilator inhalation aerosol 5 minutes prior to the adrenocorticoid or ipratropium inhalation aerosol, unless otherwise directed by physician | ✓ | ✓ | | ✓ | | ✓ | ✓ | ✓ | ✓ | ✓ | ✓ | ✓ |
| Checking with physician if contents of one canister used in less than 2 weeks | ✓ | | | | | | | | | | | |
| **Side/adverse effects** | | | | | | | | | | | | |
| Signs of potential side effects, especially: | | | | | | | | | | | | |
|   Allergic reaction to sulfites present in some preparations | | | ✓ | ✓ | ✓ | ✓ | ✓ | ✓ | | | | |
|   Chest discomfort or pain | ✓ | ✓ | ✓ | ✓ | | | | ✓ | | ✓ | ✓‡ | ✓ |
|   Hallucinations, with high doses | | | ✓ | ✓ | | | | | | | | |
|   Irregular heartbeat | | | ✓ | ✓ | | | | ✓ | | ✓ | | ✓ |
|   Mood or mental changes | | | ✓ | | | | | | | | | |
|   Numbness in feet or hands | | | | | | | | | | ✓ | | |
|   Paradoxical bronchospasm | ✓ | ✓ | ✓ | ✓ | ✓ | ✓ | ✓ | ✓ | ✓ | ✓ | ✓ | ✓ |
|   Unusual bruising | | | | | | | | | | ✓ | | |
| In some animal studies, albuterol caused increased incidence of benign leiomyomas of mesovarium when administered at doses many times the maximum human inhalation or oral dose | ✓ | | | | | | | | | | | |
| Some studies in animals have shown that terbutaline caused increased incidence of leiomyomas of mesovarium, ovarian cysts, and hyperplasia of mesovarium when administered at oral doses many times the recommended daily adult dose | | | | | | | | | | | | ✓ |
| Pinkish to red coloration of saliva caused by oxidation of isoproterenol in mouth may be alarming to patient although medically insignificant | | | | | | | | ✓ | | | | |
| Unusual or bad taste may occur | ✓ | | | | | ✓ | | | ✓ | | | ✓ |
| Changes in smell or taste may occur | | | | | | | | | | ✓ | | |

*USOC permits use of inhalation beta-2 agonists.
†For inhalation dosage forms.
‡With high doses.

# BRONCHODILATORS, THEOPHYLLINE  Systemic

This monograph includes information on the following: Aminophylline; Oxtriphylline; Theophylline.

INN:
Oxtriphylline—Choline theophyllinate

BAN:
Oxtriphylline—Choline theophyllinate

JAN:
Oxtriphylline—Choline theophylline

VA CLASSIFICATION (Primary/Secondary):
Aminophylline
    Injection—RE104/RE900
    Oral solution—RE104/RE109; RE900
    Tablets—RE104/RE109
    Extended-release tablets—RE104/RE109
Oxtriphylline—RE104/RE109
Theophylline
    Capsules—RE104/RE109
    Extended-release capsules—RE104/RE109
    Elixir—RE104/RE109; RE900

Oral solution—RE104/RE109; RE900
Syrup—RE104/RE109; RE900
Tablets—RE104/RE109
Extended-release tablets—RE104/RE109
Theophylline in Dextrose—RE104/RE900

Note: For a listing of dosage forms and brand names by country availability, see *Dosage Forms* section(s). For a listing of brand names for the articles in this monograph, refer to the General Index.

## Category

Bronchodilator—Aminophylline; Oxtriphylline; Theophylline.

Asthma prophylactic—Aminophylline; Oxtriphylline; Theophylline.

Stimulant, respiratory—Aminophylline Injection USP; Aminophylline Oral Solution USP; Theophylline Elixir; Theophylline Oral Solution; Theophylline Syrup.

Antidote (to dipyridamole toxicity)—Aminophylline Injection USP.

## Indications

Note: Bracketed information in the *Indications* section refers to uses that are not included in U.S. product labeling.

### Accepted

Asthma, bronchial (prophylaxis and treatment)—Aminophylline, oxtriphylline, and theophylline are indicated for the prevention and treatment of bronchial asthma symptoms. They improve pulmonary function and reduce the frequency and severity of symptoms such as wheezing, cough, shortness of breath, or dyspnea.

Some studies have shown that theophylline does not provide additional benefit in the initial treatment of *acute* airway obstruction when optimal therapy is provided with inhaled or injected beta-2-adrenergic bronchodilators and systemic glucocorticoids in patients not already receiving a methylxanthine. Although patients hospitalized with asthma may benefit from administration of aminophylline or theophylline, these medications should not be relied upon to produce immediate bronchodilation, even if therapeutic theophylline concentrations are rapidly achieved.

Aminophylline, oxtriphylline, and theophylline may benefit those patients with an inadequate response to anti-inflammatory medications and beta-adrenergic bronchodilators; however, theophylline bronchodilators are not considered to be first-line therapy.

Bronchitis, chronic (treatment)
Emphysema, pulmonary (treatment) or
Pulmonary disease, chronic obstructive, other (treatment)—Aminophylline, oxtriphylline, and theophylline may be indicated in the treatment of reversible airway obstruction associated with chronic bronchitis, emphysema, or other chronic obstructive pulmonary disease.

[Apnea, neonatal (treatment adjunct)][1]—Aminophylline oral solution and injection and theophylline oral liquids are used in the treatment of idiopathic apnea in neonates, characterized by cessation of respiration that lasts 20 seconds or longer. Aminophylline or theophylline should be considered in addition to administration of oxygen, sensory stimulation, or low pressure nasal continuous positive airway pressure.

Toxicity, dipyridamole (treatment)[1]—Parenteral aminophylline is used to reverse the adenosine-mediated adverse effects of dipyridamole, such as angina pectoris, ventricular arrhythmias, bronchospasm, and severe hypotension.

### Unaccepted

Parenteral aminophylline and theophylline have been used in the treatment of Cheyne-Stokes respiration. However, there is insufficient evidence to establish the efficacy of these medications for this indication.

[1]Not included in Canadian product labeling.

## Pharmacology/Pharmacokinetics

### Physicochemical characteristics

Source—
Aminophylline: Theophylline compound with ethylenediamine
Oxtriphylline: The choline salt of theophylline
Molecular weight—
Aminophylline: 420.43.
Oxtriphylline: 283.33.
Theophylline: 198.18.

### Mechanism of action/Effect

The exact mechanism of action by which theophylline produces its pharmacologic effect is unknown; it is likely to involve multiple mechanisms.

Bronchodilator; asthma prophylactic—Theophylline directly relaxes smooth muscle in the bronchial airways and pulmonary blood vessels.

This action is believed to be mediated by selective inhibition of specific phosphodiesterases (PDEs), which in turn produces an increase in intracellular cyclic 3', 5'-adenosine monophosphate (cyclic AMP). *In vitro* study results demonstrate that the PDE isoenzyme types III and IV may play a primary role. Inhibition of these isoenzymes may also mediate certain theophylline side effects such as emesis, hypotension, and tachycardia. Theophylline also demonstrates adenosine receptor antagonism, which may contribute to its effect on bronchial airways.

Respiratory stimulant—Theophylline is believed to stimulate the medullary respiratory center, presumably by increasing sensitivity to the stimulatory actions of carbon dioxide.

Antidote (to dipyridamole toxicity)—Involves antagonism of the coronary vasodilatory effects of the increased concentrations of adenosine produced by intravenous administration of dipyridamole during myocardial perfusion studies.

### Other actions/effects

Theophylline may attenuate airway hyperreactivity associated with the late phase response that is induced by inhaled allergens by an undefined mechanism which is not attributable to PDE inhibition or adenosine antagonism. Theophylline also has been reported to increase the number and activity of suppressor T-cells in the peripheral blood. Whether these actions are clinically relevant is not clear.

Theophylline may produce other physiologic effects such as transient diuresis, stimulation of cardiac muscle, improved contractility of the diaphragm, reduction of systemic and pulmonary vascular resistance, increased gastric acid secretion, central nervous system stimulation, and cerebral vasoconstriction.

### Absorption

Immediate-release capsule, liquid, or tablet dosage forms—Rapidly and completely absorbed. The rate of absorption may be slowed by concurrent ingestion of food or magnesium-containing antacids; however, the effect on the extent of absorption is generally not clinically significant.

Delayed-release tablets—Enteric coating provides delayed and possibly incomplete absorption compared with immediate-release dosage forms.

Extended-release capsules or tablets—The rate of absorption varies among different formulations and is slower than with immediate-release products; the extent of absorption may also vary. Significant intra- and interindividual differences in absorption have been reported. Serum concentration fluctuations are most apparent in patients demonstrating increased theophylline clearance. Co-administration of antacids or food may only slow the rate of absorption from some extended-release formulations, while significantly altering the extent of absorption from others. Some formulations designed for once-a-day administration may be substantially affected by food.

Intramuscular—Slow absorption; medication may precipitate at the injection site.

Suppository—Slow and unreliable absorption.

### Distribution

Theophylline distributes rapidly into peripheral non-adipose tissues and body water, including breast milk and cerebrospinal fluid. It freely crosses the placenta. The apparent volume of distribution ($Vol_D$) for theophylline averages 0.45 L per kg of body weight (L/kg) and ranges from 0.3 to 0.7 L/kg (30 to 70% of ideal body weight) in both adults and children. The $Vol_D$ may be increased, probably due to altered protein binding, in premature neonates, adults with cirrhosis, patients with uncorrected acidemia, elderly patients, pregnant women during the third trimester, critically ill patients, mechanically ventilated adults, and children with protein-calorie malnutrition.

### Protein binding

Moderate (40%). Primarily to albumin. Patients with reduced protein binding may have low total serum theophylline concentrations when unbound theophylline is in the therapeutic range.

### Biotransformation

Aminophylline and oxtriphylline—
Release free theophylline at physiologic pH.

Theophylline—
Hepatic; no first-pass effect. Believed to occur over multiple parallel pathways, mediated by cytochrome P-450 isoenzymes P-4501A2, P-4503A3, and P-4502E1. In neonates, several of these pathways are undeveloped but mature slowly over the first year of life. Caffeine is a minor active metabolite, except in premature neonates and children less than 6 months of age, in whom caffeine's extremely long half-life results in significant accumulation. The half-life of caffeine shortens over the first 6 months of life because of maturation of its metabolic pathway. Thereafter, caffeine does not accumulate in older children and adults. Major inactive metabolites

in adults and children older than 6 months of age are 1,3-dimethyluric acid, 3-methylxanthine, and 1-methyluric acid.

Theophylline approximates first-order elimination kinetics, where serum concentrations follow a log-linear decay. However, zero-order kinetics, where elimination becomes dependent on the serum concentration, can be observed in patients at therapeutic concentrations. This is probably due to capacity limitations of the hepatic enzymes that metabolize theophylline, and is clinically relevant for some patients in that a small change in theophylline dosage may result in a disproportionately large change in serum concentration.

## Half-life

Elimination half-life and total body clearance values for theophylline in various patients are as follows—

| Patient characteristics | Half-life Mean (Range)* (hr) | Total body clearance Mean (Range)* (mL/kg/min) |
|---|---|---|
| **Age** | | |
| Premature neonates | | |
| 3–15 days† | 30 (17–43) | 0.29 (0.09–0.49) |
| 25–57 days† | 20 (9.4–30.6) | 0.64 (0.04–1.2) |
| Term infants | | |
| 1–2 days† | (25–26.5) | |
| 3–26 weeks† | 11 (6–29) | |
| Children | | |
| 1–4 yrs | 3.4 (1.2–5.6) | 1.7 (0.5–2.9) |
| 4–12 yrs | | 1.57 (0.83–2.31) |
| 13–15 yrs | | 0.88 (0.38–1.38) |
| 6–17 yrs‡ | 3.7 (1.5–5.9) | 1.4 (0.2–2.6) |
| Adults§ | 8.2 (6.1–12.8) | 0.65 (0.27–1.03) |
| Elderly# | 9.8 (1.6–18) | 0.41 (0.21–0.61) |
| **Concurrent illness or altered physiologic state** | | |
| Acute pulmonary edema | 19 (3.1–82)** | 0.33 (0.07–2.35)** |
| COPD†† | 11 (9.4–12.6) | 0.54 (0.44–0.64) |
| COPD and cor pulmonale | | 0.48 (0.08–0.88) |
| Cystic fibrosis‡‡ | 6 (1.8–10.2) | 1.25 (0.31–2.19) |
| Fever§§ | 7 (1–13) | |
| Hepatic disease | | |
| Acute hepatitis | 19.2 (16.6–21.8) | 0.35 (0.25–0.45) |
| Cholestasis | 14.4 (5.7–31.8) | 0.65 (0.25–1.45) |
| Cirrhosis | 32 (10–56)** | 0.31 (0.1–0.7)** |
| Hyperthyroidism | 4.5 (3.7–5.6) | 0.8 (0.68–0.97) |
| Hypothyroidism | 11.6 (8.2–25) | 0.38 (0.13–0.57) |
| Pregnancy | | |
| First trimester | 8.5 (3.1–13.9) | |
| Second trimester | 8.8 (3.9–13.8) | |
| Third trimester | 13.3 (8.4–17.6) | |
| Sepsis## | 18.8 (6.3–24.1) | 0.46 (0.19–1.9) |

*Reported or estimated range (mean ±2 SD) where actual range not reported.

†Postnatal age.

‡Elimination half-life and total body clearance gradually become slower until adult values are reached.

§Otherwise healthy, nonsmoking asthmatics.

#Nonsmokers with normal cardiac, liver, and renal function; 70 to 85 years of age.

**Median.

††Stable; older than 60 years of age; at least 1 year since stopped smoking.

‡‡Patients 14 to 28 years of age.

§§Associated with acute viral respiratory illness in children 9 to 15 years of age.

##With multi-organ failure.

## Time to peak concentration

Theophylline—

Immediate-release capsules, tablets, or oral solution: 1 to 2 hours.

Delayed-release tablets: Approximately 4 hours.

Extended-release capsules and tablets: 4 to 13 hours depending upon the specific product.

## Therapeutic serum concentration

Bronchodilator—

For most patients, a conservative goal of therapy would be to target peak steady-state serum concentrations in the range of 5 to 15 mcg/mL (27.5 to 82.5 micromoles/L). Although improved pulmonary function is evident over the range of 5 to 20 mcg/mL (27.5 to 110 micromoles/L), concentrations at the upper end of the therapeutic range may be associated with an increased potential for toxicity. When serum concentrations exceed 20 mcg/mL (110 micromoles/L), the probability of toxicity increases.

Respiratory stimulant—

Neonatal apnea: Steady-state peak serum concentrations of 5 to 12 mcg per mL (27.5 to 66 micromoles per L).

## Elimination

Theophylline—

Renal; approximately 10% excreted unchanged in the urine in adults; amount excreted unchanged may reach 50% in neonates.

In dialysis: Charcoal hemoperfusion increases theophylline clearance 2 to 4 times. Hemodialysis and peritoneal dialysis are estimated to increase theophylline clearance by approximately 50% and 30%, respectively.

# Precautions to Consider

## Carcinogenicity/Tumorigenicity

Long-term studies have not been done in humans. The results of long-term carcinogenicity studies performed in mice and rats are pending.

## Mutagenicity

Theophylline has not been shown to be mutagenic in Ames salmonella, *in vivo* and *in vitro* cytogenetics, micronucleus and Chinese hamster ovary test systems.

## Pregnancy/Reproduction

Fertility—Studies in rodents have shown that theophylline impairs fertility in mice given oral doses approximately 1 to 3 times the human dose on a mg per square meter of body surface area (mg/m²), and in rats given oral doses approximately 2 times the human dose on a mg/m² basis.

Pregnancy—Although adequate and well-controlled studies in pregnant women have not been done, these medications are used in pregnancy when the risk of treatment is preferable to the risk of placental hypoxemia from uncontrolled pulmonary disease. The Collaborative Perinatal Project monitored 193 mother-child pairs exposed to theophylline during the first trimester and found no evidence of association with teratogenicity.

Theophylline crosses the placenta; cord blood concentrations are approximately equal to the maternal serum concentration. Because of this, higher-than-recommended serum concentrations during pregnancy may result in potentially dangerous serum theophylline and caffeine concentrations in the neonate. Tachycardia, irritability, jitteriness, and vomiting have been reported; therefore, neonates of mothers taking these medications during pregnancy should be monitored for signs of theophylline toxicity.

Theophylline clearance is reported to be lower in the third trimester, which may necessitate more frequent theophylline serum concentration determinations and possible dosage reductions.

Theophylline was not teratogenic in mice or rats given oral doses approximately 2 and 3 times the recommended human dose on a mg/m² basis, respectively. Embryotoxicity was observed in rats given 220 mg per kg of body weight, in the absence of maternal toxicity.

FDA Pregnancy Category C.

Labor—Theophylline has been shown to slightly inhibit uterine contractions.

## Breast-feeding

Less than 1% of a maternal theophylline dose distributes into breast milk; this may cause irritability in the infant.

## Pediatrics

Caution is recommended in neonates and children less than 1 year of age, especially in premature neonates and in infants less than 3 months of age with renal function impairment, because theophylline clearance is reduced, resulting in lower dosage requirements. Clearance progressively increases over the first year of life, remains constant during the subsequent 9 years, and gradually declines to mean adult values by 16 years of age.

## Geriatrics

Caution is recommended when aminophylline, oxtriphylline, or theophylline is used in patients older than 60 years of age. Theophylline clearance in healthy adults older than 60 years of age is 30% lower than in healthy younger adults. These patients may require adjustment in dosage or dosing interval. Severe signs or symptoms of toxicity resulting from chronic overdose are more common in elderly patients, occurring in 65% of patients 60 years of age or older with serum theophylline concentrations > 30 mcg per mL (165 micromoles per L).

## Drug interactions and/or related problems

The following drug interactions and/or related problems have been selected on the basis of their potential clinical significance (possible mechanism in parentheses where appropriate)—not necessarily inclusive (» = major clinical significance):

Note: Combinations containing any of the following medications, depending on the amount present, may also interact with this medication.

*Pharmacokinetic interactions*

Medications that decrease theophylline clearance

(the medications listed in the table below probably decrease theophylline clearance by inhibition of one or more hepatic cytochrome P-450 isoenzyme; changes in clearance of approximately 25% or greater can have clinical significance; monitoring of serum theophylline concentrations and/or dosage adjustments are strongly recommended when concurrent use of these medications with aminophylline, oxtriphylline, or theophylline is initiated or discontinued

| Medication | Decrease in Clearance (avg. %) | Increase in Serum Concentration (avg. %)* |
|---|---|---|
| Alcohol† | 25 | 33 |
| Allopurinol‡ | 20 | 25 |
| » Cimetidine | 33 | 33–50 |
| Contraceptives, estrogen-containing, oral | 25–34 | 33–50 |
| Disulfiram§ | 21–33 | 25–50 |
| Fluoroquinolone antibiotics# | | |
| » Ciprofloxacin | 20–40 | 25–66 |
| » Enoxacin | 40–70 | 66–300 |
| » Fluvoxamine | 100 | >300 |
| » Interferon alpha, recombinant | 10–50 | 11–100 |
| Macrolide antibiotics** | | |
| » Clarithromycin | 20 | 25 |
| » Erythromycin | 5–35 | 5–50 |
| » Troleandomycin | 25–50†† | 33–100 |
| Methotrexate‡‡ | 15–25 | 18–33 |
| » Mexiletine | 43 | 75 |
| Propafenone | | 40§§ |
| » Pentoxifylline | | 30 (0–95) |
| » Propranolol | 30–50 | 40–100 |
| » Tacrine | 50 | 100 |
| » Thiabendazole | 66 | >200 |
| » Ticlopidine | 37 | 60 |
| Verapamil | 14–23 | 16–30 |

*Calculation based on reported change in clearance if actual change not reported.

†3 mL of whiskey per kg of body weight as a single dose decreased clearance up to 24 hrs.

‡≥600 mg per day.

§Dose-dependent, 250 and 500 mg.

#Norfloxacin, lomefloxacin, and ofloxacin are not considered to significantly decrease theophylline clearance.

**Azithromycin does not appear to alter theophylline clearance.

††Once-daily dose decreases clearance by average of 25%.

‡‡Low-dose intramuscular regimen of 15 mg per week.

§§Beta-2-antagonist effect may decrease effect of theophylline.

Medications that increase theophylline clearance

(the medications listed in the table below probably increase theophylline clearance by induction of one or more hepatic cytochrome P-450 isoenzyme; changes in clearance of approximately 25% or greater can have clinical significance; monitoring of serum theophylline concentrations and/or dosage adjustments are strongly recommended when concurrent use of these medications with aminophylline, oxtriphylline, or theophylline is initiated or discontinued

| Medication | Increase in Clearance (avg. %) | Decrease in Serum Concentration (avg. %)* |
|---|---|---|
| Aminoglutethimide | 18–43 | 15–30 |
| Carbamazepine | 33 | 25 |
| Isoproterenol, intravenous | 21 | 17 |
| » Moricizine | 44–66 | 30–40 |
| Phenobarbital | 33 | 25 |
| » Phenytoin | 35–75 | 25–43 |
| » Rifampin | 64–100 | 40–50 |

*Calculation based on reported change in clearance if actual change not reported.

*Pharmacodynamic or other drug interactions*

Adenosine

(concurrent use with theophylline may antagonize the cardiovascular effects of adenosine; larger doses of adenosine may be required or alternative therapy should be used)

Benzodiazepines

(theophylline may reverse benzodiazepine sedation; caution is recommended when starting or stopping either medication)

» Beta-adrenergic blocking agents, including ophthalmic agents

(concurrent use with theophylline may result in inhibition of its bronchodilator effect; although agents with beta-1-selectivity may be less antagonistic, extreme caution is recommended if beta-adrenergic blocking agents are used in patients with bronchospasm)

Ephedrine

(concurrent use with theophylline may result in increased frequency of nausea, nervousness, or insomnia)

» Halothane

(ventricular arrhythmias have been reported when halothane is used concurrently with theophylline)

» Ketamine

(concurrent use with theophylline may lower the seizure threshold)

Lithium

(concurrent use of lithium with theophylline may increase renal elimination of lithium, thus decreasing its therapeutic effect)

Neuromuscular blocking agents, nondepolarizing

(concurrent use with theophylline may antagonize neuromuscular blocking effects; a larger dose of neuromuscular blocking agent may be required)

» Smoking tobacco or marijuana

(induces the hepatic metabolism of theophylline, resulting in increased clearance and decreased serum concentrations. Passive smoking may also increase theophylline clearance. Induction is attributed to the polyaromatic hydrocarbons in smoke. Following cessation of cigarette smoking, theophylline clearance begins to decrease after 1 week; however, normalization may require 6 months to 2 years. Dosage adjustments and/or additional theophylline serum determinations may be necessary when smoking is started or stopped)

Sucralfate

(concurrent use with aminophylline, oxtriphylline, or theophylline may result in adsorption of the theophylline bronchodilator if medications are administered less than 2 hours apart)

## Laboratory value alterations

The following have been selected on the basis of their potential clinical significance (possible effect in parentheses where appropriate)—not necessarily inclusive (» = major clinical significance):

With diagnostic test results

» Dipyridamole-assisted myocardial perfusion studies

(the theophylline bronchodilators reverse the effects of dipyridamole on myocardial blood flow, thereby interfering with test results; dipyridamole-assisted myocardial perfusion studies should not be performed if therapy with aminophylline, oxtriphylline, or theophylline cannot be withheld for 36 hours prior to the test)

With physiology/laboratory test values

Cholesterol and

Free cortisol excretion, urinary and

Free fatty acids and

Glucose, plasma and

HDL and HDL/LDL ratio and

Uric acid, plasma

(concentrations may be increased by theophylline serum concentrations within the therapeutic range)

Triiodothyronine, serum
  (concentration may be transiently decreased by theophylline serum concentrations within the therapeutic range)

### Medical considerations/Contraindications

The medical considerations/contraindications included here have been selected on the basis of their potential clinical significance (reasons given in parentheses where appropriate)—not necessarily inclusive (» = major clinical significance).

*Risk-benefit should be considered when the following medical problems exist:*

» Acute pulmonary edema or
» Congestive heart failure or
  Fever, sustained or
» Hepatic disease or
» Hypothyroidism, not optimally controlled or
» Sepsis
  (theophylline clearance may be decreased, resulting in increased theophylline serum concentrations)

  (the extent to which fever, as opposed to other complicating factors such as acute viral illness, affects theophylline clearance is controversial; however, some practitioners recommend additional monitoring and/or dose reduction when the body temperature is 102 °F or greater for at least 24 hours, or when a lower temperature elevation persists for a longer period)

Gastritis, active or
Peptic ulcer disease, active
  (may be exacerbated because theophylline increases gastric acid secretion)

Gastroesophageal reflux
  (theophylline may decrease lower esophageal sphincter pressure, resulting in increased gastroesophageal reflux)

» Seizure disorder
  (aminophylline, oxtriphylline, or theophylline may lower the seizure threshold; caution is recommended unless the patient is receiving appropriate anticonvulsant therapy)

Tachyarrhythmias
  (condition may be exacerbated at higher theophylline serum concentrations)

» Sensitivity to a theophylline bronchodilator or ethylenediamine

### Patient monitoring

The following may be especially important in patient monitoring (other tests may be warranted in some patients, depending on condition; » = major clinical significance):

Caffeine concentrations, serum
  (determinations may be required in neonates; usually necessary only if adverse effects occur when the serum theophylline concentration is within the therapeutic range)

Pulmonary function tests
  (objective measures of lung function are essential for diagnosis and for guiding therapeutic decision making in asthma; measurement of forced expiratory airflow, using a spirometer or a peak expiratory flowmeter, is recommended at periodic intervals)

» Theophylline concentrations
  (dosage requirements are usually guided by measurement of the peak serum concentration obtained at the expected time of the peak, depending upon the specific product characteristics; the frequency of determinations should relate to the specific clinical situation)

  (theophylline determinations are recommended when initiating therapy, before increasing the dose when a patient fails to exhibit the expected results, at the appearance of any adverse reaction, whenever any change in physiologic state or medication known to alter theophylline elimination occurs, and upon the addition of any new medication with an unknown effect on theophylline elimination; also recommended at least every 6 to 12 months in stable patients)

  (blood samples obtained for guidance of therapy should be collected during steady-state conditions, which are generally reached after 48 to 72 hours of treatment, provided that the medication is taken at regular intervals, with no missed or extra doses. Steady-state conditions may not be reached for up to 5 days in patients with factors known to decrease theophylline clearance. On each occasion, blood samples should be obtained during the same dosing interval, due to the diurnal variation in the absorption of these medications)

  (for intravenous therapy, concentrations may be determined 30 to 60 minutes after an intravenous loading dose, approximately 8 to 12 hours after initiating continuous intravenous therapy, and at approximately 24-hour intervals during continuous intravenous therapy)

  (trough concentration may be useful when evaluating serum concentration–time profiles; determinations may be performed just before the next dose or, for once-daily evening administration of an extended-release product, the morning following a dose)

  (caution is recommended in interpreting serum theophylline concentrations in patients with low albumin; total serum theophylline concentrations may be low when unbound theophylline is in the therapeutic range; measurement of unbound serum theophylline concentration provides a more reliable basis for dosage adjustment)

  (caution is recommended in interpreting the results of rapid theophylline immunoassays for uremic patients, because falsely high values may occur. Also, when theophylline concentration is determined via high pressure liquid chromatography, sulfamethoxazole may cause inaccurate test results and large doses of ampicillin, cephalothin, or acetazolamide may cause falsely high concentrations. Determinations via specific immunoassay or high pressure liquid chromatography are not affected by caffeine or dyphylline. However, when theophylline is measured via spectrophotometry, caffeine [including caffeine-containing substances such as chocolate, coffee, tea, colas, or medications] or acetaminophen may cause falsely high concentrations)

Note: Concentrations in saliva are approximately 60% of serum concentrations; however, the saliva-to-serum concentration ratio may not remain constant within the same patient; caution is recommended in use and interpretation of the data without the use of special techniques.

## Side/Adverse Effects

Note: The less severe signs or symptoms of toxicity, such as continuing or severe abdominal pain, agitation, confusion or change in behavior, diarrhea, hematemesis, hypotension, trembling, and continued vomiting, do not always precede the more serious ones such as sinus tachycardia, ventricular arrhythmias, or seizures. Patients with chronic overdosage have a greater risk for serious toxicity at lower serum concentrations than patients with acute single overdosage. Severe signs or symptoms of toxicity resulting from chronic overdose are more common in elderly patients, occurring in 65% of patients 60 years of age or older with serum theophylline concentrations > 30 mcg/mL (165 micromoles/L). For additional information about acute or chronic overdose, refer to the *Overdose* section of this monograph.

Although some studies do not support the suggestion that theophylline has an adverse effect on behavioral and cognitive function in children, differences in individual response have been reported; monitoring for these effects may be advisable.

The following side/adverse effects have been selected on the basis of their potential clinical significance (possible signs and symptoms in parentheses where appropriate)—not necessarily inclusive:

### Those indicating need for medical attention
Incidence less frequent
  *Gastroesophageal reflux* (heartburn; vomiting)

Note: Aminophylline, oxtriphylline, or theophylline may relax the gastroesophageal sphincter; however, if *vomiting* occurs, theophylline toxicity should be considered.

Incidence rare
  *For aminophylline only*
    *Dermatitis, ethylenediamine hypersensitivity–induced* (hives; skin rash; sloughing of skin)

Note: *Ethylenediamine hypersensitivity–induced dermatitis* can appear up to 48 hours after administration of aminophylline.

### Those indicating need for medical attention only if they continue or are bothersome
Incidence less frequent
  *Headache; increased urination; insomnia* (trouble in sleeping); *nausea; nervousness; tachycardia* (fast heartbeat); *trembling*

Note: These caffeine-like side effects may occur at therapeutic theophylline serum concentrations, especially if the concentrations are rapidly attained. Tolerance generally develops within 1 or 2 weeks; however, the symptoms may persist in < 3% of children and < 10% of adults with chronic therapy despite therapeutic serum theophylline concentrations. Starting therapy at a low dose and slowly increasing the dose by no more than 25% at no less than 3-day intervals until the desired daily dose is reached may prevent the caffeine-like side effects.

*For parenteral aminophylline and theophylline—with too rapid intravenous administration*

**Anxiety; headache; nausea; vomiting**

Note: *Hypotension and cardiac arrest have been reported following rapid direct administration through a central venous catheter.*

## Overdose

For specific information on the agents used in the management of theophylline overdose, see:
- *Anesthetics, Inhalation (Systemic)* monograph;
- *Benzodiazepines (Systemic)* monograph;
- *Charcoal, Activated (Oral-Local)* monograph;
- *Metoclopramide (Systemic)* monograph;
- *Neuromuscular Blocking Agents (Systemic)* monograph;
- *Ondansetron (Systemic)* monograph;
- *Phenobarbital* in *Barbiturates (Systemic)* monograph;
- *Polyethylene Glycol and Electrolytes (Local)* monograph; and/or
- *Thiopental* in *Anesthetics, Barbiturate (Systemic)* monograph.

For more information on the management of overdose or unintentional ingestion, **contact a Poison Control Center** (see *Poison Control Center Listing*).

Theophylline is associated with a significant potential for toxicity because of its narrow therapeutic index. The upper limit of the therapeutic serum concentration range is considered to be 20 mcg per mL (mcg/mL) (110 micromoles per L [micromoles/L]). Clinical symptoms of toxicity become evident in some patients with serum concentrations above 15 mcg/mL (82.5 micromoles/L), and increase in frequency when 20 mcg/mL (110 micromoles/L) is exceeded. Less severe toxicities do not always precede major toxicities. Serum theophylline concentrations do not always predict who will experience life-threatening toxicity. Theophylline demonstrates concentration-dependent elimination kinetics as its metabolic pathways become saturated, resulting in prolonged elimination.

Theophylline overdose is associated with significant morbidity and mortality, primarily due to the development of arrhythmias or seizures. Patients who develop seizures are at the highest risk for further morbidity and mortality from associated hypoxia, acidosis, rhabdomyolysis, or myoglobinuric renal failure. The type of theophylline overdose has significant influence on clinical outcome. Chronic theophylline overdose appears to be associated with a greater frequency of seizures and arrhythmias at lower theophylline concentrations, when compared with acute overdose outcomes; this is especially true in patients older than 60 years of age. Although there is a lack of correlation between serum theophylline concentrations and clinical course of a chronic overdose, serum theophylline concentrations > 40 mcg/mL (220 micromoles/L) are considered potentially life-threatening. Following an acute overdose, serum theophylline concentrations of > 90 mcg/mL (495 micromoles/L) are associated with major toxicity, especially seizures. The onset and duration of theophylline toxicity vary and depend on the formulation used, the route of administration, the amount ingested, time since the ingestion, and the patient's theophylline elimination capacity.

### Clinical effects of overdose

The following effects have been selected on the basis of their potential clinical significance (possible signs and symptoms in parentheses where appropriate)—not necessarily inclusive:

Acute and chronic effects

*Abdominal pain, continuing or severe; agitation* (nervousness or restlessness, continuing); *confusion or change in behavior; diarrhea; hematemesis* (dark or bloody vomit); *hyperglycemia; hypokalemia; hypotension* (dizziness; lightheadedness); *metabolic acidosis; seizures* (convulsions); *tachyarrhythmias* (fast and irregular heartbeat); *tachycardia* (fast heartbeat); *trembling, continuing; vomiting*

### Treatment of overdose

There is no antidote for theophylline overdose. Treatment is symptomatic and supportive.

To decrease absorption—

Regardless of the route or mode of exposure resulting in toxicity, oral activated charcoal (OAC) should be administered. OAC binds medication remaining in the gastrointestinal tract and decreases serum concentrations by interrupting enteroenteric recirculation of theophylline. Use of an aqueous activated charcoal preparation is recommended. If the total dose of OAC is not tolerated, more frequent administration of smaller doses, slow instillation through a nasogastric tube, or concurrent use of an antiemetic may be tried.

The initial dose of charcoal may be followed by a single dose of sorbitol if the charcoal is not pre-mixed with sorbitol. Caution

is recommended when giving more than a single dose of sorbitol since frequent administration may result in dehydration and electrolyte imbalance secondary to diarrhea. Sorbitol is reported to be more effective than magnesium-containing cathartics and is not associated with hypermagnesemia; however, the role of cathartics is questionable.

**Ipecac syrup should generally be avoided** in the management of theophylline overdoses.

Gastric lavage is generally not necessary if the patient has vomited. Lavage may provide some benefit if performed via a large bore orogastric tube less than 1 hour after a large ingestion. This procedure may not be very effective for large, poorly soluble tablets.

Whole bowel irrigation with polyethylene glycol and electrolyte combination may be of some value if performed early in the treatment of large ingestions of extended-release dosage forms. Whole bowel irrigation with polyethylene glycol and electrolytes may also be useful when theophylline serum concentrations rapidly increase or when high concentrations persist despite other methods of removal.

To enhance elimination—

Repeated doses of OAC will at least double theophylline clearance and should be continued throughout the course of toxicity, until the patient is asymptomatic and serum concentration is below 20 mcg/mL (110 micromoles/L).

Extracorporeal elimination of theophylline by charcoal hemoperfusion is the most effective means of increasing theophylline clearance. Hemodialysis is less effective; however, it may be used if hemoperfusion is unavailable. Peritoneal dialysis is considered ineffective. Controversy exists about when to initiate extracorporeal elimination. It may be indicated when serum theophylline concentrations are approaching 90 mcg/mL (495 micromoles/L) in an acute overdose or when serum theophylline concentrations are greater than 40 mcg/mL (220 micromoles/L) in a chronic overdose or in certain patients with other significant risk factors, such as age greater than 60 years or presence of complicating illness. In addition, use of extracorporeal elimination is recommended in the presence of intractable seizures or life-threatening cardiovascular symptoms, regardless of serum concentration.

Nausea or vomiting—

The presence of nausea or vomiting should not cause postponement of OAC administration. Antiemetic therapy with metoclopramide or ondansetron, administered intravenously, may be useful. See the package insert or the *Metoclopramide (Systemic)* or *Ondansetron (Systemic)* monograph for specific dosing guidelines for use of these products. Phenothiazine antiemetics such as prochlorperazine or perphenazine should be avoided since they can lower the seizure threshold.

Seizures—

Seizures associated with serum concentrations > 30 mcg/mL (165 micromoles/L) are often resistant to anticonvulsant therapy and may produce a toxic encephalopathy and permanent brain damage if not rapidly controlled. An intravenous benzodiazepine is the drug of choice. See the package insert or the *Benzodiazepines (Systemic)* monograph for specific dosing guidelines for use of these products.

If seizures are repetitive or seizure prophylaxis is indicated in selected patients at high risk for theophylline-induced seizures, intravenous phenobarbital may be administered. In animal studies, the prophylactic use of phenobarbital in therapeutic doses has delayed the onset of theophylline-induced seizures and reduced mortality. There are no controlled studies in humans. See the package insert or the *Barbiturates (Systemic)* monograph for specific dosing guidelines for use of this product. Phenytoin is considered ineffective.

Should use of a benzodiazepine and phenobarbital fail to control seizure activity, the addition of the barbiturate anesthetic agent, thiopental, may be considered. Use of a neuromuscular blocking agent may also be considered to decrease the muscular manifestations of persistent seizures. General anesthesia should be used with caution because flourinated volatile anesthetics may sensitize the myocardium to endogenous catecholamines released by theophylline. Enflurane appears less likely to be associated with this effect than does halothane. See the package insert or the *Anesthetics, Inhalation (Systemic)*, *Anesthetics, Barbiturate (Systemic)*, and/or *Neuromuscular Blocking Agents (Systemic)* monographs for specific dosing guidelines for use of these products.

Ventricular tachyarrhythmias—

Ventricular tachyarrhythmias considered to be life-threatening require antiarrhythmic therapy specific for the type of arrhythmia.

Monitoring—
　　Serial theophylline serum concentrations should be obtained to guide and assess treatment decisions. Serial monitoring should continue at periodic intervals after treatment has been discontinued until it is clear that the serum concentration is no longer rising. Serious rebound theophylline toxicity has been reported, due to bezoar formation composed of undissolved extended-release tablets.
　　All monitoring interventions should be continued until the serum concentration remains below 20 mcg/mL (110 micromoles/L) and the patient is asymptomatic.
　　Abdominal physical examination should be performed to determine the presence of distention and/or the absence of bowel sounds when repeated doses of OAC are administered. Arterial blood gases, electrocardiograph, serum electrolytes and glucose, stool output, and vital signs should also be monitored as required.
Supportive care—
　　Respiration should be supported by airway management, oxygen administration, or mechanical ventilation as required, especially if higher doses of a benzodiazepine, phenobarbital, or a neuromuscular blocking agent are used.
　　Standard measures should be used to manage hypotension and metabolic complications.
　　Patients in whom intentional overdose is known or suspected should be referred for psychiatric consultation.

## Patient Consultation

As an aid to patient consultation, refer to *Advice for the Patient, Bronchodilators, Theophylline (Systemic)*.

In providing consultation, consider emphasizing the following selected information (» = major clinical significance):

**Before using this medication**
» Conditions affecting use, especially:
　　Sensitivity to theophylline bronchodilators or to ethylenediamine in aminophylline
　　Pregnancy—Crosses placenta; decreased elimination during third trimester may require more frequent serum concentration determinations
　　Breast-feeding—Distributes into breast milk; may result in irritability in infants
　　Use in children—Decreased theophylline clearance in children less than 1 year of age, especially neonates and infants less than 3 months of age with renal function impairment, results in lower dosage requirements; initially, use in children less than 1 year of age may require more frequent serum concentration determinations
　　Use in the elderly—Possible decreased theophylline clearance in patients 60 years of age or older may result in lower dosage requirements; severe signs or symptoms of toxicity are more common in these patients following chronic overdose that results in serum concentrations > 30 mcg per mL (165 micromoles per L)
　　Other medications, especially beta-adrenergic blocking agents; cimetidine; ciprofloxacin; clarithromycin; enoxacin; erythromycin; fluvoxamine; mexiletine; moricizine; pentoxifylline; phenytoin; rifampin; tacrine; thiabendazole; ticlopidine; or troleandomycin
　　Other medical problems, especially congestive heart failure, convulsions (seizures), hepatic disease, or hypothyroidism

**Proper use of this medication**
» Proper administration
　　For liquids and immediate-release capsules or tablets: Taking on an empty stomach with a glass of water for faster absorption or, if necessary, taking with meals or immediately after meals to lessen gastrointestinal irritation, unless otherwise directed
　　For once-a-day dosage forms: Taking the medication either in the morning at least 1 hour before eating or in the evening with or without food, depending on the specific product; taking consistently with or without food; taking at approximately the same time each day
　　For enteric-coated or delayed-release tablet dosage form: Swallowing tablets whole; not breaking (unless scored for breakage), crushing, or chewing
　　For extended-release dosage forms: Swallowing capsules whole or opening capsules and sprinkling contents on soft food, then swallowing without crushing or chewing; not breaking (unless scored for breakage), crushing, or chewing tablets; taking on an empty stomach with a glass of water for faster absorption or, if necessary, taking with meals or immediately after meals to lessen gastrointestinal irritation, unless otherwise directed
» Importance of not using more than amount prescribed

» Compliance with therapy; not missing doses
» Proper dosing
　　Missed dose: Taking as soon as possible; not taking if almost time for next dose; not doubling doses
» Proper storage

**Precautions while using this medication**
» Regular visits to physician required to check progress, including blood levels
» Not changing brands or dosage forms without first checking with physician
» Notifying physician of factors that may alter theophylline concentrations, such as:
　　—fever (≥102 °F ≥ 24 hours or a lower temperature elevation for a longer period)
　　—other medicines started or stopped
　　—smoking started or stopped
　　—an extended change in diet
　　Caution in eating or drinking large amounts of caffeine-containing foods or beverages during therapy with this medication

**Side/adverse effects**
　　Signs of potential side effects, especially heartburn and/or vomiting, hives, skin rash, and sloughing of skin
　　Signs of toxicity

## General Dosing Information

The bronchodilator action of aminophylline, oxtriphylline, and theophylline depends upon their theophylline content. The anhydrous theophylline content of various theophylline salts is as follows:
　　Aminophylline anhydrous—86%.
　　Aminophylline dihydrate—79%.
　　Oxtriphylline—64%.
　　Theophylline monohydrate—91%.

Theophylline does not distribute into fatty tissue; therefore, all dosages should be calculated on the basis of lean (ideal) body weight.

The recommended doses are given as a guideline for use in the average patient. Dosage of aminophylline, oxtriphylline, or theophylline must be adjusted to meet the individual requirements of each patient on the basis of product selected, patient characteristics, clinical response, and steady-state serum theophylline concentrations.

Administration of a single loading dose of theophylline is intended to produce a serum concentration in the therapeutic range as quickly as possible. A theophylline loading dose may be considered for all patient groups, including neonates. Although the intravenous route of administration provides the most rapid effect, immediate-release oral liquids, tablets, or capsules may also be used. Delayed- or extended-release dosage forms should not be used when rapid achievement of a therapeutic serum theophylline concentration is required.

Before a loading dose is administered, it is extremely important to determine the time, amount, dosage form, and route of administration of previous doses of aminophylline, oxytriphylline, or theophylline.

Once the desired theophylline serum concentration is obtained with a loading dose, it can be maintained with an oral or intravenous dosage form.

The goal of chronic therapy is to obtain maximum potential benefit with minimal risk of adverse effects. Transient caffeine-like side effects and excessively high serum concentrations can be avoided in most patients by starting with a lower dose and slowly increasing the dose by 25% at three-day intervals, approximately.

For final dosage adjustment in chronic therapy after serum theophylline measurement, the following dosage adjustments are recommended:

| Steady-state Peak Serum Theophylline Concentration (mcg/mL) | Recommended Dosage Adjustment |
| --- | --- |
| Below 9.9 | If *clinically indicated*, about 25% increase to nearest dose increment; recheck serum theophylline concentration after 3 days for further dosage adjustment |
| 10–14.9 | If *clinically indicated*, maintain dose and recheck serum theophylline concentration at 6- to 12-month intervals; if symptoms are not controlled, consider adding additional medication to treatment regimen |
| 15–19.9 | Consider 10% decrease in dose to increase margin of safety even if current dosage is tolerated |

| Steady-state Peak Serum Theophylline Concentration (mcg/mL) | Recommended Dosage Adjustment |
|---|---|
| 20–24.9 | Decrease dose by 25% even if no adverse effects are present; recheck serum theophylline concentration after 3 days |
| 25–30 | Omit next dose; 25% decrease in subsequent doses even if no adverse effects are present; recheck serum theophylline concentration after 3 days; if symptomatic, consider whether overdose treatment is indicated |
| > 30 | Treatment of overdose may be indicated; when theophylline is resumed, decrease subsequent dose by at least 50%; recheck serum theophylline concentration after 3 days |

Note: If asthma is well controlled and there are no side effects or intervening factors that would alter dose requirements, follow-up serum concentration measurements can be obtained at 6- to 12-month intervals. However, **whenever a patient develops nausea, vomiting, CNS stimulation or any other symptom of theophylline toxicity, even if another cause is suspected (e.g., viral gastroenteritis), the next dose should be withheld and a serum concentration measurement obtained.** In addition, various drug interactions and physiologic abnormalities can alter theophylline elimination and require serum concentration measurement and/or dose adjustment.

**For oral dosage forms only**
The dosing frequency should be individualized. When rapidly absorbed dosage forms such as liquids or immediate-release capsules or tablets are used, dosing to maintain therapeutic serum concentrations usually requires administration every 6 hours, especially in children and smoking adults. A dosing interval of up to 8 hours may be appropriate in some nonsmoking adults, elderly or debilitated patients, and neonates due to a slower clearance rate. In premature neonates and patients with hepatic disease, dosing every 12 hours or longer will usually provide relatively constant serum concentrations.

Patients requiring higher-than-usual doses (i.e., patients with rapid clearance rates) may be more effectively controlled during chronic therapy by being given extended-release dosage forms. These products have the potential to achieve relatively constant serum concentrations with 12-hour dosing intervals. Patients who metabolize theophylline rapidly may require an extended-release product every 8 hours. Patients who metabolize theophylline at a normal or slow rate (elimination half-life longer than 8 hours) are potential candidates for once-a-day formulations.

Alcohol-free liquid dosage forms are generally preferred.

For patients who have difficulty in swallowing, some extended-release capsules may be opened and the contents sprinkled on a spoonful of soft, cold food such as applesauce or pudding, then taken without chewing.

**For parenteral dosage forms only**
Therapy can be converted from an intravenous to an oral product by dividing the total daily dose that produced the desired steady-state peak serum concentration into equal parts, and giving in amounts and at intervals appropriate for the product. The intravenous infusion can usually be discontinued when the first oral dose of medication is administered. Extreme caution is recommended if intravenous and oral therapy are overlapped, since this practice may lead to inadvertent theophylline toxicity.

Use of intravenous aminophylline or theophylline should be reassessed after 24 to 72 hours. Oral therapy should be substituted for intravenous therapy as soon as the patient is able to take medication orally.

**Diet/Nutrition**
Dietary changes are of clinical importance only if a sustained and extreme change in the usual eating pattern occurs. High-carbohydrate, low-protein diets have been shown to decrease theophylline elimination. Low-carbohydrate, high-protein diets and daily ingestion of charcoal-broiled beef have been shown to increase theophylline elimination.

Large amounts of caffeine-containing foods or beverages should be avoided, since they may increase CNS stimulant effects of theophylline bronchodilators.

**Bioequivalence information**
For oral dosage forms only—
The formulation selected for maintenance therapy can have an important effect on the serum concentration–time profile. Selection of a theophylline product must be based upon the specific clinical indication, the absorption characteristics of the formulation, and the rate of theophylline elimination in the individual patient. Immediate-release oral formulations can generally be used interchangeably since they are not considered to have clinically important differences in rates of absorption. However, many brands of extended-release theophylline products have clinically important differences in their extent and/or rate of absorption. Different extended-release products having the same strength of active ingredient may not be equivalent due to formulation differences. Even with reliably absorbed extended-release formulations, a minority of patients can have marked day-to-day variations in absorption. When this occurs, alternative therapy should be considered.

Due to the significant variability in extended-release product characteristics, pharmacists should not substitute one brand for another without consulting the prescribing physician unless the product has proven bioequivalence, so that theophylline serum concentrations can be appropriately monitored.

---

### *AMINOPHYLLINE*

## Summary of Differences
Category:
 Aminophylline (injection, oral solution) is also used as a respiratory stimulant in neonatal apnea; aminophylline injection is used as an antidote to dipyridamole toxicity.
Pharmacology/pharmacokinetics:
 Aminophylline is a theophylline compound with ethylenediamine.
 Aminophylline releases free theophylline at physiologic pH.
Side/adverse effects:
 Ethylenediamine in aminophylline may cause hives, skin rash, or sloughing of skin.
General dosing information:
 Aminophylline anhydrous contains about 86% of anhydrous theophylline.
 Aminophylline dihydrate contains about 79% of anhydrous theophylline.

## Additional Dosing Information
See also *General Dosing Information.*

The recommended doses are given as a guideline for use in the average patient. Dosage of aminophylline must be adjusted to meet the individual requirements of each patient on the basis of product selected, patient characteristics, clinical response, and steady-state serum theophylline concentrations.

**For parenteral dosage forms only**
Intramuscular administration of aminophylline injection is not recommended since precipitation may occur at the site of injection, resulting in severe local pain and slow absorption.

Aminophylline may be administered by direct intravenous injection or by intravenous infusion; however, it is recommended that intravenous aminophylline be administered slowly, at a rate *not exceeding* 25 mg per minute.

**For rectal dosage forms only**
USP DI Advisory Panels do not recommend the use of aminophylline suppositories because of the potential for slow and unreliable absorption. The suppositories may also cause local irritation.

## Oral Dosage Forms
Note: Bracketed uses in the *Dosage Forms* section refer to categories of use and/or indications that are not included in U.S. product labeling.

### AMINOPHYLLINE ORAL SOLUTION USP

**Usual adult dose**
Bronchodilator—
 Loading dose:
  For patients *not* currently receiving theophylline preparations— Oral, the equivalent of 5 mg of anhydrous theophylline per kg of lean (ideal) body weight as a single dose to provide an average peak serum concentration of 10 mcg per mL (55 micromoles per L), range 5 to 15 mcg per mL (27.5 to 82.5 micromoles per L).

For patients currently receiving theophylline preparations—Obtaining a serum theophylline concentration prior to administering a partial loading dose is recommended. Once the theophylline concentration is known, the loading dose for theophylline is based on the principle that each 0.5 mg of theophylline per kg of lean (ideal) body weight will result in a 1 mcg per mL increase in serum theophylline concentration.

Maintenance:

Oral, the equivalent of anhydrous theophylline, initially, 300 mg per day. After three days, the dosage may be increased, if tolerated, to 400 mg per day. After three more days, the dosage may be increased, if tolerated, to 600 mg per day without measurement of serum concentration.

The total daily adult dose is administered in three or four divided doses given about six to eight hours apart. Patients with risk factors for impaired theophylline clearance may require a dosing interval of every twelve hours. Young adult smokers and patients with more rapid metabolism may require a dosing interval of every six hours.

Note:  **If the 600-mg-per-day dose is to be maintained or exceeded, monitoring of serum theophylline concentration and patient response is recommended to achieve the optimal therapeutic aminophylline dosage and minimize the risk of toxicity.**

**Usual pediatric dose**
Bronchodilator—

Loading dose:

For patients not currently receiving theophylline preparations—Infants and children up to 16 years of age: Oral, the equivalent of 5 mg of anhydrous theophylline per kg of lean (ideal) body weight as a single dose to provide an average peak serum concentration of 10 mcg per mL (55 micromoles per L), range 5 to 15 mcg per mL (27.5 to 82.5 micromoles per L).

For patients currently receiving theophylline preparations—Obtaining a serum theophylline concentration prior to administering a partial loading dose is recommended. Once the theophylline concentration is known, the loading dose for theophylline is based on the principle that each 0.5 mg of theophylline per kg of lean (ideal) body weight will result in a 1 mcg per mL increase in serum theophylline concentration.

Maintenance:

Premature infants, postnatal age less than 24 days—Oral, the equivalent of 1 mg of anhydrous theophylline per kg of body weight every twelve hours.

Premature infants, postnatal age 24 days and older—Oral, the equivalent of 1.5 mg of anhydrous theophylline per kg of body weight every twelve hours.

Full-term infants, postnatal age up to 52 weeks—Oral, the equivalent of anhydrous theophylline: total daily dose in mg per kg of body weight = (0.2) (postnatal age in weeks) + 5.

Note:  For full-term infants up to 26 weeks of age, divide the total daily dose into three equal amounts administered eight hours apart.

For full-term infants 26 to 52 weeks of age, divide the total daily dose into four equal amounts administered six hours apart.

Children 1 year of age and older, weighing less than 45 kg—Oral, the equivalent of anhydrous theophylline, 12 to 14 mg per kg of body weight, *up to a maximum of 300 mg,* per day in divided doses. The dosage may be increased, if tolerated, after three days to 16 mg per kg of body weight, *up to a maximum of 400 mg,* per day. After three more days, if tolerated, the dosage may be increased to 20 mg per kg of body weight, *up to a maximum of 600 mg,* per day. The total daily dose is administered in four to six divided doses and given every four to six hours.

Children weighing more than 45 kg—See *Usual adult dose.*

Note:  **If the above maintenance dose is to be maintained or exceeded, monitoring of serum theophylline concentration and patient response is recommended to achieve the optimal therapeutic aminophylline dosage and minimize the risk of toxicity.**

[Respiratory stimulant (neonatal apnea)][1]—

Loading dose:

For patients *not* currently receiving theophylline preparations—Oral, the equivalent of 5 mg of anhydrous theophylline per kg of lean (ideal) body weight as a single dose to provide an average peak serum concentration of 10 mcg per mL (55 micromoles per L), range 5 to 15 mcg per mL (27.5 to 82.5 micromoles per L).

For patients currently receiving theophylline preparations—Obtaining a serum theophylline concentration prior to administering a partial loading dose is recommended. Once the theophylline concentration is known, the loading dose for theophylline is based on the principle that each 0.5 mg of theophylline per kg of lean (ideal) body weight will result in a 1 mcg per mL increase in serum theophylline concentration.

Maintenance:

Premature infants, postnatal age less than 24 days—Oral, the equivalent of 1 mg of anhydrous theophylline per kg of body weight every twelve hours.

Premature infants, postnatal age 24 days and older—Oral, the equivalent of 1.5 mg of anhydrous theophylline per kg of body weight every twelve hours.

Note:  **If the above maintenance dose is to be maintained or exceeded, monitoring of serum theophylline concentration and patient response is recommended to achieve the optimal therapeutic aminophylline dosage and minimize the risk of toxicity.**

**Strength(s) usually available**
U.S.—

105 mg of anhydrous aminophylline (equivalent to 90 mg of anhydrous theophylline) per 5 mL (Rx) [GENERIC].

Canada—

Not commercially available.

**Packaging and storage**
Store between 15 and 30 °C (59 and 86 °F), unless otherwise specified by manufacturer. Store in a tight container.

## AMINOPHYLLINE TABLETS USP

**Usual adult dose**
See *Aminophylline Oral Solution USP.*

**Usual pediatric dose**
Bronchodilator—

Loading dose:

For patients not currently receiving theophylline preparations—Infants and children up to 16 years of age: Oral, the equivalent of 5 mg of anhydrous theophylline per kg of lean (ideal) body weight as a single dose to provide an average peak serum concentration of 10 mcg per mL (55 micromoles per L), range 5 to 15 mcg per mL (27.5 to 82.5 micromoles per L).

For patients currently receiving theophylline preparations—Obtaining a serum theophylline concentration prior to administering a partial loading dose is recommended. Once the theophylline concentration is known, the loading dose for theophylline is based on the principle that each 0.5 mg of theophylline per kg of lean (ideal) body weight will result in a 1 mcg per mL increase in serum theophylline concentration.

Maintenance:

Premature infants, postnatal age less than 24 days—Oral, the equivalent of 1 mg of anhydrous theophylline per kg of body weight every twelve hours.

Premature infants, postnatal age 24 days and older—Oral, the equivalent of 1.5 mg of anhydrous theophylline per kg of body weight every twelve hours.

Full-term infants, postnatal age up to 52 weeks—Oral, the equivalent of anhydrous theophylline: total daily dose in mg per kg of body weight = (0.2) (postnatal age in weeks) + 5.

Note:  For full-term infants up to 26 weeks of age, divide the total daily dose into three equal amounts administered eight hours apart.

For full-term infants 26 to 52 weeks of age, divide the total daily dose into four equal amounts administered six hours apart.

Children 1 year of age and older, weighing less than 45 kg—Oral, the equivalent of anhydrous theophylline, 12 to 14 mg per kg of body weight, *up to a maximum of 300 mg,* per day in divided doses. The dosage may be increased, if tolerated, after three days to 16 mg per kg of body weight, *up to a maximum of 400 mg,* per day. After three more days, if tolerated, the dosage may be increased to 20 mg per kg of body weight, *up to a maximum of 600 mg,* per day. The total daily dose is administered in four to six divided doses and given every four to six hours.

Children weighing more than 45 kg—See *Usual adult dose.*

Note:  **If the above maintenance dose is to be maintained or exceeded, monitoring of serum theophylline concentration and patient response is recommended to achieve the optimal therapeutic aminophylline dosage and minimize the risk of toxicity.**

**Strength(s) usually available**
U.S.—
    100 mg of hydrous aminophylline (equivalent to 79 mg of anhydrous theophylline) (Rx) [GENERIC (may be scored)].
    200 mg of hydrous aminophylline (equivalent to 158 mg of anhydrous theophylline) (Rx) [GENERIC (may be scored)].
Canada—
    100 mg of hydrous aminophylline (equivalent to 79 mg of anhydrous theophylline) (Rx) [GENERIC (may be scored)].
    200 mg of hydrous aminophylline (equivalent to 158 mg of anhydrous theophylline) (Rx) [GENERIC (may be scored)].

**Packaging and storage**
Store below 40 °C (104 °F), preferably between 15 and 30 °C (59 and 86 °F), unless otherwise specified by manufacturer. Store in a tight container.

## AMINOPHYLLINE EXTENDED-RELEASE TABLETS

**Usual adult dose**
Bronchodilator—
    Oral, the equivalent of anhydrous theophylline, initially, 300 mg per day. If tolerated, the dosage may be increased after three days, to 400 mg per day. After three more days, the dosage may be increased, if tolerated, to 600 mg per day without measurement of serum concentration. One-half of the daily dose may be given at twelve-hour intervals. However, certain patients metabolize theophylline more rapidly, especially the young and those who smoke, and may require dosing at eight-hour intervals.

Note: **If the 600-mg-per-day dose is to be maintained or exceeded, monitoring of serum theophylline concentration and patient response is recommended to achieve the optimal therapeutic aminophylline dosage and minimize the risk of toxicity.**

**Usual pediatric dose**
Bronchodilator—
    Children up to 6 years of age: Use is not recommended.
    Children 6 to 16 years of age: See *Usual adult dose.*

**Strength(s) usually available**
U.S.—
    225 mg of hydrous aminophylline (equivalent to 178 mg of anhydrous theophylline) (Rx) [*Phyllocontin* (scored)].
Canada—
    225 mg of hydrous aminophylline (equivalent to 182.25 mg of anhydrous theophylline) (Rx) [*Phyllocontin* (scored)].
    350 mg of hydrous aminophylline (equivalent to 283.5 mg of anhydrous theophylline (Rx) [*Phyllocontin-350* (scored)].

**Packaging and storage**
Store below 40 °C (104 °F), preferably between 15 and 30 °C (59 and 86 °F), in a well-closed container, unless otherwise specified by manufacturer.

# Parenteral Dosage Forms

Note: Bracketed uses in the *Dosage Forms* section refer to categories of use and/or indications that are not included in U.S. product labeling.

## AMINOPHYLLINE INJECTION USP

**Usual adult dose**
Bronchodilator—
    Loading dose:
        For patients *not* currently receiving theophylline preparations—Intravenous, the equivalent of 5 mg of anhydrous theophylline per kg of lean (ideal) body weight as a single dose, infused over twenty to thirty minutes, to provide an average peak serum concentration of 10 mcg per mL (55 micromoles per L), range 5 to 15 mcg per ml (27.5 to 82.5 micromoles per L).
        For patients currently receiving theophylline preparations—Obtaining a serum theophylline concentration prior to administering a partial loading dose is recommended. Once the theophylline concentration is known, the loading dose for theophylline is based on the principle that each 0.5 mg of theophylline per kg of lean (ideal) body weight will result in a 1 mcg per mL increase in serum theophylline concentration.
    Maintenance:
        Young adult smokers—Intravenous infusion, the equivalent of anhydrous theophylline, 700 mcg (0.7 mg) per kg of body weight per hour.
        Otherwise healthy nonsmoking adults—Intravenous infusion, the equivalent of anhydrous theophylline, 400 mcg (0.4 mg) per kg of body weight per hour.
        Older patients and patients with cardiac decompensation, cor pulmonale, or hepatic function impairment—Intravenous infusion,

the equivalent of anhydrous theophylline, 200 mcg (0.2 mg) per kg of body weight per hour.

Note: **If the above maintenance dose is to be maintained or exceeded, monitoring of serum theophylline concentration and patient response is recommended to achieve the optimal therapeutic aminophylline dosage and minimize the risk of toxicity.**

Antidote (to dipyridamole toxicity)[1]—
    Intravenous, the equivalent of 50 to 100 mg (range, 50 mg up to a maximum dose of 250 mg) administered over thirty to sixty seconds.

**Usual pediatric dose**
Bronchodilator—
    Loading dose:
        For patients not currently receiving theophylline preparations—Children up to 16 years of age: Intravenous, the equivalent of 5 mg of anhydrous theophylline per kg of lean (ideal) body weight as a single dose over twenty to thirty minutes to provide an average peak serum concentration of 10 mcg per mL (55 micromoles per L), range 5 to 15 mcg per mL (27.5 to 82.5 micromoles per L).
        For patients currently receiving theophylline preparations—Obtaining a serum theophylline concentration prior to administering a partial loading dose is recommended. Once the theophylline concentration is known, the loading dose for theophylline is based on the principle that each 0.5 mg of theophylline per kg of lean (ideal) body weight will result in a 1 mcg per mL increase in serum theophylline concentration.
    Maintenance:
        Premature infants, postnatal age less than 24 days—Intravenous, the equivalent of 1 mg of anhydrous theophylline per kg of body weight every twelve hours.
        Premature infants, postnatal age 24 days and older—Intravenous, the equivalent of 1.5 mg of anhydrous theophylline per kg of body weight every twelve hours.
        Full-term infants, postnatal age up to 52 weeks—Intravenous, the equivalent of anhydrous theophylline, total daily dose in mg per kg of body weight $= (0.2)$ (postnatal age in weeks) $+ 5$.
        For full-term infants up to 26 weeks of age, divide the total daily dose into three equal amounts administered eight hours apart. For full-term infants 26 to 52 weeks of age, divide the total daily dose into four equal amounts administered six hours apart.
        Note: May also be administered to infants less than 1 year as an intravenous infusion, the equivalent of anhydrous theophylline, dose in mg per kg of body weight per hour $= (0.008)$ (age in weeks) $+ 0.21$.
        Children 1 to 9 years of age—Intravenous infusion, the equivalent of anhydrous theophylline, 800 mcg (0.8 mg) per kg of body weight per hour.
        Children 9 to 16 years—Intravenous infusion, the equivalent of anhydrous theophylline, 700 mcg (0.7 mg) per kg of body weight per hour.

Note: **If the above maintenance dose is to be maintained or exceeded, monitoring of serum theophylline concentration and patient response is recommended to achieve the optimal therapeutic aminophylline dosage and minimize the risk of toxicity.**

[Respiratory stimulant (neonatal apnea)][1]—
    Loading dose:
        For patients *not* currently receiving theophylline preparations—Intravenous, the equivalent of 5 mg of anhydrous theophylline per kg of lean (ideal) body weight as a single dose over twenty to thirty minutes to provide an average peak serum concentration of 10 mcg per mL (55 micromoles per L), range 5 to 15 mcg per mL (27.5 to 82.5 micromoles per L).
        For patients currently receiving theophylline preparations: Obtaining a serum theophylline concentration prior to administering a partial loading dose is recommended. Once the theophylline concentration is known, the loading dose for theophylline is based on the principle that each 0.5 mg of theophylline per kg of lean (ideal) body weight will result in a 1 mcg per mL increase in serum theophylline concentration.
    Maintenance:
        Premature infants, postnatal age less than 24 days—Intravenous, the equivalent of 1 mg of anhydrous theophylline per kg of body weight every twelve hours.
        Premature infants, postnatal age 24 days and older—Intravenous, the equivalent of 1.5 mg of anhydrous theophylline per kg of body weight every twelve hours.

Note: **If the above maintenance dose is to be maintained or exceeded, monitoring of serum theophylline concentration and patient response is recommended to achieve the optimal therapeutic aminophylline dosage and minimize the risk of toxicity.**

**Strength(s) usually available**

U.S.—

25 mg of hydrous aminophylline (equivalent to 19.7 mg of anhydrous theophylline) per mL (Rx) [GENERIC].

Canada—

25 mg of hydrous aminophylline (equivalent to 19.7 mg of anhydrous theophylline) per mL (Rx) [GENERIC].

50 mg of hydrous aminophylline (equivalent to 39.4 mg of anhydrous theophylline) per mL (Rx) [GENERIC].

**Packaging and storage**

Store below 40 °C (104 °F), preferably between 15 and 30 °C (59 and 86 °F), unless otherwise specified by manufacturer. Protect from light. Protect from freezing.

**Preparation of dosage form**

To dilute the injection for intravenous administration, dextrose 5% in water, sodium chloride, or dextrose-sodium chloride combinations may be used.

**Stability**

A slight yellowing of the solution can occur when aminophylline is added to some dextrose-containing solutions. Because the aminophylline content remains constant, the discoloration is believed to result from the decomposition of dextrose.

Aminophylline solutions whose concentration does not exceed 40 mg/mL are reported to be stable for at least 48 hours at 77 °F (25 °C).

**Incompatibilities**

Although aminophylline has been reported to precipitate in acidic media, this generally does not apply to the dilute solutions for intravenous infusions.

No additives should be made directly to the same intravenous bag or bottle of aminophylline because dosages are titrated to response, and because admixture incompatibilities exist with a number of other medications.

Doxapram hydrochloride is reported to be incompatible with aminophylline when combined in the same syringe.

Medications that are incompatible when injected into Y-sites of administration sets with a continuous infusion of aminophylline include amiodarone hydrochloride, ciprofloxacin, diltiazem hydrochloride, dobutamine hydrochloride, hydralazine hydrochloride, and ondansetron hydrochloride.

## Rectal Dosage Forms

### AMINOPHYLLINE SUPPOSITORIES USP

Note: **USP DI Advisory Panels do not recommend the use of Aminophylline Suppositories USP because of the potential for slow and unreliable absorption.**

**Strength(s) usually available**

U.S.—

250 mg of hydrous aminophylline (equivalent to 197.5 mg of anhydrous theophylline) (Rx) [*Truphylline*; GENERIC].

500 mg of hydrous aminophylline (equivalent to 395 mg of anhydrous theophylline) (Rx) [*Truphylline*; GENERIC].

Canada—

Not commercially available.

---

¹Not included in Canadian product labeling.

---

## *OXTRIPHYLLINE*

## Summary of Differences

Pharmacology/pharmacokinetics:

Oxtriphylline is the choline salt of theophylline.

Oxtriphylline releases free theophylline at physiologic pH.

General dosing information:

Oxtriphylline contains about 64% of anhydrous theophylline.

## Additional Dosing Information

See also *General Dosing Information*.

The recommended doses are given as a guideline for use in the average patient. Dosage of oxtriphylline must be adjusted to meet the individual requirements of each patient on the basis of product selected, patient characteristics, clinical response, and steady-state serum theophylline concentrations.

## Oral Dosage Forms

### OXTRIPHYLLINE ORAL SOLUTION USP

**Usual adult dose**

Bronchodilator—

Loading dose:

For patients *not* currently receiving theophylline preparations—Oral, the equivalent of 5 mg of anhydrous theophylline per kg of lean (ideal) body weight as a single dose to provide an average peak serum concentration of 10 mcg per mL (55 micromoles per L), range 5 to 15 mcg per mL (27.5 to 82.5 micromoles per L).

For patients currently receiving theophylline preparations—Obtaining a serum theophylline concentration prior to administering a partial loading dose is recommended. Once the theophylline concentration is known, the loading dose for theophylline is based on the principle that each 0.5 mg of theophylline per kg of lean (ideal) body weight will result in a 1 mcg per mL increase in serum theophylline concentration.

Maintenance:

Oral, the equivalent of anhydrous theophylline, initially, 300 mg per day. After three days, the dosage may be increased, if tolerated, to 400 mg per day. After three more days, the dosage may be increased, if tolerated, to 600 mg per day without measurement of serum concentration.

The total daily adult dose is administered in three or four divided doses given about six to eight hours apart. Patients with risk factors for impaired theophylline clearance may require a dosing interval of every twelve hours. Young adult smokers and patients with more rapid metabolism may require a dosing interval of every six hours.

Note: **If the 600-mg-per-day dose is to be maintained or exceeded, monitoring of serum theophylline concentration and patient response is recommended to achieve the optimal therapeutic oxtriphylline dosage and minimize the risk of toxicity.**

**Usual pediatric dose**

Use is not recommended in children due to high alcohol content.

**Strength(s) usually available**

U.S.—

Not commercially available.

Canada—

100 mg (equivalent to 64 mg of anhydrous theophylline) per 5 mL (Rx) [*Choledyl* (alcohol 20%); *PMS-Oxtriphylline* (alcohol 20%)].

**Packaging and storage**

Store below 40 °C (104 °F), preferably between 15 and 30 °C (59 and 86 °F), unless otherwise specified by manufacturer. Store in a tight container. Protect from freezing.

### OXTRIPHYLLINE SYRUP

**Usual adult dose**

See *Oxtriphylline Oral Solution USP*.

**Usual pediatric dose**

Bronchodilator—

Loading dose:

For patients not currently receiving theophylline preparations—Infants and children up to 16 years of age: Oral, the equivalent of 5 mg of anhydrous theophylline per kg of lean (ideal) body weight as a single dose to provide an average peak serum concentration of 10 mcg/mL (55 micromoles per L), range 5 to 15 mcg per mL (27.5 to 82.5 micromoles per L).

For patients currently receiving theophylline preparations—Obtaining a serum theophylline concentration prior to administering a partial loading dose is recommended. Once the theophylline concentration is known, the loading dose for theophylline is based on the principle that each 0.5 mg of theophylline per kg of lean (ideal) body weight will result in a 1 mcg per mL increase in serum theophylline concentration.

Maintenance:

Premature infants, postnatal age less than 24 days—Oral, the equivalent of 1 mg of anhydrous theophylline per kg of body weight every twelve hours.

Premature infants, postnatal age 24 days and older—Oral, the equivalent of 1.5 mg of anhydrous theophylline per kg of body weight every twelve hours.

Full-term infants, postnatal age up to 52 weeks—Oral, the equivalent of anhydrous theophylline: Total daily dose in mg per kg of body weight = $(0.2)$ (postnatal age in weeks) + 5.

Note: For full-term infants up to 26 weeks of age, divide the total daily dose into three dosing intervals, eight hours apart.

For full-term infants 26 to 52 weeks of age, divide the total daily dose into four dosing intervals six hours apart.

Children 1 year of age and older, but weighing less than 45 kg— Oral, the equivalent of anhydrous theophylline, 12 to 14 mg per kg of body weight, *up to a maximum of 300 mg*, per day in divided doses. The dosage may be increased, if tolerated, after three days to 16 mg per kg of body weight, *up to a maximum of 400 mg per day*. After three more days, if tolerated, the dosage may be increased to 20 mg per kg of body weight *up to a maximum of 600 mg per day*. The total daily dose is administered in four to six divided doses given every four to six hours.

Children weighing more than 45 kg—See *Usual adult dose*.

Note: **If the above maintenance dose is to be maintained or exceeded, monitoring of serum theophylline concentration and patient response is recommended to achieve the optimal therapeutic oxtriphylline dosage and minimize the risk of toxicity.**

### Strength(s) usually available
U.S.—

Not commercially available.

Canada—

50 mg (equivalent to 32 mg of anhydrous theophylline) per 5 mL (Rx) [*Choledyl; PMS-Oxtriphylline*].

### Packaging and storage
Store below 40 °C (104 °F), preferably between 15 and 30 °C (59 and 86 °F), in a tight container, unless otherwise specified by manufacturer. Protect from freezing.

## OXTRIPHYLLINE TABLETS

### Usual adult dose
See *Oxtriphylline Oral Solution USP*.

### Usual pediatric dose
See *Oxtriphylline Syrup*.

### Strength(s) usually available
U.S.—

Not commercially available.

Canada—

100 mg (equivalent to 64 mg of anhydrous theophylline) (Rx) [*Apo-Oxtriphylline*].

200 mg (equivalent to 128 mg of anhydrous theophylline) (Rx) [*Apo-Oxtriphylline; Choledyl*].

300 mg (equivalent to 192 mg of anhydrous theophylline) (Rx) [*Apo-Oxtriphylline*].

### Packaging and storage
Store below 40 °C (104 °F), preferably between 15 and 30 °C (59 and 86 °F), unless otherwise specified by manufacturer. Store in a tight container.

## OXTRIPHYLLINE DELAYED-RELEASE TABLETS USP

### Usual adult dose
Bronchodilator—

Oral, the equivalent of anhydrous theophylline, initially, 300 mg per day. If tolerated, the dosage may be increased after three days to 400 mg per day. After three more days, the dosage may be increased, if tolerated, to 600 mg per day without measurement of serum concentration. The total daily adult dose is administered in three or four divided doses given about six to eight hours apart. Patients with risk factors for impaired theophylline clearance may require a dosing interval of every twelve hours. Young adult smokers and patients with more rapid metabolism may require a dosing interval of every six hours.

### Usual pediatric dose
Bronchodilator—

Children up to 6 years of age: Use is not recommended in children up to 6 years of age since this age group may not be capable of swallowing the tablets whole.

Children 6 to 16 years of age: See *Usual adult dose*.

### Strength(s) usually available
U.S.—

100 mg (equivalent to 64 mg of anhydrous theophylline) (Rx) [*Choledyl* (enteric, sugar-coated)].

200 mg (equivalent to 127 mg of anhydrous theophylline) (Rx) [*Choledyl* (enteric, sugar-coated)].

Canada—

Not commercially available.

### Packaging and storage
Store below 40 °C (104 °F), preferably between 15 and 30 °C (59 and 86 °F), unless otherwise specified by manufacturer. Store in a tight container.

### Auxiliary labeling
• Swallow tablets whole.

## OXTRIPHYLLINE EXTENDED-RELEASE TABLETS USP

### Usual adult dose
Bronchodilator—

Oral, the equivalent of anhydrous theophylline, initially, 300 mg per day. If tolerated, the dosage may be increased after three days to 400 mg per day. After three more days, the dosage may be increased, if tolerated, to 600 mg per day without measurement of serum concentration. One-half of the daily dose may be given at twelve-hour intervals. However, certain patients metabolize theophylline more rapidly, especially the young and those that smoke, and may require dosing at eight-hour intervals.

Note: **If the 600-mg-per-day dose is to be maintained or exceeded, monitoring of serum theophylline concentration and patient response is recommended to achieve the optimal therapeutic oxtriphylline dosage and minimize the risk of toxicity.**

### Usual pediatric dose
Bronchodilator—

Children up to 6 years of age: Use is not recommended. Children 6 to 16 years of age: See *Usual adult dose*.

### Strength(s) usually available
U.S.—

400 mg (equivalent to 254 mg of anhydrous theophylline) (Rx) [*Choledyl SA* (confectioner's sugar)].

600 mg (equivalent to 382 mg of anhydrous theophylline) (Rx) [*Choledyl SA* (confectioner's sugar)].

Canada—

400 mg (equivalent to 254 mg of anhydrous theophylline) (Rx) [*Choledyl SA* (scored)].

600 mg (equivalent to 382 mg of anhydrous theophylline) (Rx) [*Choledyl SA* (scored)].

### Packaging and storage
Store below 40 °C (104 °F), preferably between 15 and 30 °C (59 and 86 °F), unless otherwise specified by manufacturer. Store in a tight container.

---

## *THEOPHYLLINE*

## Summary of Differences

Category: Theophylline oral liquids are also used as a respiratory stimulant in neonatal apnea.

## Additional Dosing Information

See also *General Dosing Information*.

The recommended doses are given as a guideline for use in the average patient. Dosage of theophylline must be adjusted to meet the individual requirements of each patient on the basis of product selected, patient characteristics, clinical response, and steady-state serum theophylline concentrations.

### For parenteral dosage forms only
The rate of administration of theophylline and dextrose injection should *not exceed* 25 mg per minute.

## Oral Dosage Forms

Note: Bracketed uses in the *Dosage Forms* section refer to categories of use and/or indications that are not included in U.S. product labeling.

### THEOPHYLLINE CAPSULES USP

### Usual adult dose
Bronchodilator—

Loading dose:

For patients *not* currently receiving theophylline preparations— Oral, the equivalent of 5 mg of anhydrous theophylline per kg of lean (ideal) body weight as a single dose to provide an average peak serum concentration of 10 mcg per mL (55 micromoles per L), range 5 to 15 mcg per mL (27.5 to 82.5 micromoles per L.

For patients currently receiving theophylline preparations—Obtaining a serum theophylline concentration prior to administering a partial loading dose is recommended. Once the theophylline concentration is known, the loading dose for theophylline is based on the principle that each 0.5 mg of theophylline per kg of lean (ideal) body weight will result in a 1 mcg per mL increase in serum theophylline concentration.

Maintenance:
Oral, the equivalent of anhydrous theophylline, initially, 300 mg per day. After three days, the dosage may be increased, if tolerated, to 400 mg per day. After three more days, the dosage may be increased, if tolerated, to 600 mg per day without measurement of serum concentration.

The total daily adult dose is administered in three or four divided doses given about six to eight hours apart. Patients with risk factors for impaired theophylline clearance may require a dosing interval of every twelve hours. Young adult smokers and patients with more rapid metabolism may require a dosing interval of every six hours.

Note: **If the 600-mg-per-day dose is to be maintained or exceeded, monitoring of serum theophylline concentration and patient response is recommended to achieve the optimal therapeutic theophylline dosage and minimize the risk of toxicity.**

**Usual pediatric dose**
Bronchodilator—
Loading dose:
For patients *not* currently receiving theophylline preparations—Infants and children up to 16 years of age: Oral, the equivalent of 5 mg of anhydrous theophylline per kg of lean (ideal) body weight as a single dose to provide an average peak serum concentration of 10 mcg per mL (55 micromoles per L), range 5 to 15 mcg per mL (27.5 to 82.5 micromoles per L).

For patients currently receiving theophylline preparations—Obtaining a serum theophylline concentration prior to administering a partial loading dose is recommended. Once the theophylline concentration is known, the loading dose for theophylline is based on the principle that each 0.5 mg of theophylline per kg of lean (ideal) body weight will result in a 1 mcg per mL increase in serum theophylline concentration.

Maintenance:
Children 1 year of age and older, weighing less than 45 kg—Oral, the equivalent of anhydrous theophylline, 12 to 14 mg per kg of body weight, *up to a maximum of 300 mg*, per day in divided doses. The dosage may be increased, if tolerated, after three days to 16 mg per kg of body weight, *up to a maximum of 400 mg*, per day. After three more days, if tolerated, the dosage may be increased to 20 mg per kg of body weight *up to a maximum of 600 mg*, per day. The total daily dose is administered in four to six divided doses given every four to six hours.

Children weighing more than 45 kg—See *Usual adult dose.*

Note: **If the 600-mg-per-day dose is to be maintained or exceeded, monitoring of serum theophylline concentration and patient response is recommended to achieve the optimal therapeutic theophylline dosage and minimize the risk of toxicity.**

**Strength(s) usually available**
U.S.—
100 mg (equivalent of anhydrous theophylline) (Rx) [*Elixophyllin;* GENERIC].
200 mg (equivalent of anhydrous theophylline) (Rx) [*Elixophyllin;* GENERIC].
300 mg (equivalent of anhydrous theophylline) (Rx) [GENERIC].
Canada—
Not commercially available.

**Packaging and storage**
Store below 40 °C (104 °F), preferably between 15 and 30 °C (59 and 86 °F), unless otherwise specified by manufacturer. Store in a well-closed container.

## THEOPHYLLINE EXTENDED-RELEASE CAPSULES USP

Note: Due to the significant variability in extended-release product characteristics, pharmacists should not substitute one brand for another without consulting the prescribing physician unless the product has proven bioequivalence, so that theophylline serum concentrations can be appropriately monitored.

**Usual adult dose**
Bronchodilator—
Oral, the equivalent of anhydrous theophylline, initially, 300 mg per day. If tolerated, the dosage may be increased after three days to 400 mg per day. After three more days, the dosage may be increased, if tolerated, to 600 mg per day without measurement of

serum concentration. One-half of the daily theophylline dose may be given at twelve-hour intervals. However, certain patients metabolize theophylline more rapidly, especially the young and those that smoke, and may require dosing at eight-hour intervals.

Note: **If the 600-mg-per-day dose is to be maintained or exceeded, monitoring of serum theophylline concentration and patient response is recommended to achieve the optimal therapeutic theophylline dosage and minimize the risk of toxicity.**

**Usual pediatric dose**
Bronchodilator—
Children 1 year of age and older, weighing less than 45 kg: Oral, the equivalent of anhydrous theophylline, 12 to 14 mg per kg of body weight, *up to a maximum of 300 mg*, per day in divided doses. The dosage may be increased, if tolerated, after three days to 16 mg per kg of body weight, *up to a maximum of 400 mg*, per day. After three more days, if tolerated, the dosage may be increased to 20 mg per kg of body weight *up to a maximum of 600 mg*, per day. One-half of the daily theophylline dose may be given as aminophylline at twelve-hour intervals. However, younger patients may require dosing at eight-hour intervals.

Children weighing more than 45 kg: See *Usual adult dose.*

Note: **If the 600-mg-per-day dose is to be maintained or exceeded, monitoring of serum theophylline concentration and patient response is recommended to achieve the optimal therapeutic theophylline dosage and minimize the risk of toxicity.**

**Strength(s) usually available**
U.S.—
50 mg (equivalent of anhydrous theophylline) (Rx) [*Slo-Bid Gyrocaps*].
75 mg (equivalent of anhydrous theophylline) (Rx) [*Slo-Bid Gyrocaps*].
100 mg (equivalent of anhydrous theophylline) (Rx) [*Slo-Bid Gyrocaps; Theo-24*].
125 mg (equivalent of anhydrous theophylline) (Rx) [*Slo-Bid Gyrocaps; Theovent Long-Acting*].
200 mg (equivalent of anhydrous theophylline) (Rx) [*Slo-Bid Gyrocaps; Theo-24*].
250 mg (equivalent of anhydrous theophylline) (Rx) [*Theovent Long-Acting*].
260 mg (equivalent of anhydrous theophylline) (Rx) [*Aerolate Sr; Theobid Duracaps; Theoclear L.A.-260*].
300 mg (equivalent of anhydrous theophylline) (Rx) [*Slo-Bid Gyrocaps; Theo-24*].
400 mg (equivalent of anhydrous theophylline) (Rx) [*Theo-24*].
Canada—
50 mg (equivalent of anhydrous theophylline) (Rx) [*Slo-Bid Gyrocaps*].
100 mg (equivalent of anhydrous theophylline) (Rx) [*Slo-Bid Gyrocaps*].
200 mg (equivalent of anhydrous theophylline) (Rx) [*Slo-Bid Gyrocaps*].
300 mg (equivalent of anhydrous theophylline) (Rx) [*Slo-Bid Gyrocaps*].

**Packaging and storage**
Store below 40 °C (104 °F), preferably between 15 and 30 °C (59 and 86 °F), unless otherwise specified by manufacturer. Store in a well-closed container.

**Additional information**
Certain extended-release capsules may be opened and the contents sprinkled on soft food immediately prior to ingestion, then swallowed without crushing or chewing. Capsule contents should not be subdivided.

## THEOPHYLLINE ELIXIR

**Usual adult dose**
See *Theophylline Capsules USP.*

**Usual pediatric dose**
Use is not recommended in children due to the high alcohol content.

**Strength(s) usually available**
U.S.—
27 mg (equivalent of anhydrous theophylline) per 5 mL (Rx) [*Asmalix* (alcohol 20%); *Elixophyllin* (alcohol 20%); *Lanophyllin* (alcohol 20%); *Truxophyllin;* GENERIC].
Canada—
27 mg (equivalent of anhydrous theophylline) per 5 mL (Rx) [*PMS Theophylline* (alcohol 18%); *Pulmophylline* (alcohol 20% [v/v]); GENERIC].

**Packaging and storage**

Store below 40 °C (104 °F), preferably between 15 and 30 °C (59 and 86 °F), in a tight container, unless otherwise specified by manufacturer. Protect from freezing.

**Stability**

Exposure to cold temperatures may cause theophylline crystallization to occur. At room temperature the crystals redissolve and solution gradually clears.

**Auxiliary labeling**

• Do not refrigerate.

## THEOPHYLLINE ORAL SOLUTION

**Usual adult dose**

See *Theophylline Capsules USP*.

**Usual pediatric dose**

Bronchodilator—

Loading dose:

For patients not currently receiving theophylline preparations—Infants and children up to 16 years of age: Oral, the equivalent of 5 mg of anhydrous theophylline per kg of lean (ideal) body weight as a single dose to provide an average peak serum concentration of 10 mcg per mL (55 micromoles per L), range 5 to 15 mcg per mL (27.5 to 82.5 micromoles per L).

For patients currently receiving theophylline preparations—Obtaining a serum theophylline concentration prior to administering a partial loading dose is recommended. Once the theophylline concentration is known, the loading dose for theophylline is based on the principle that each 0.5 mg of theophylline per kg of lean (ideal) body weight will result in a 1 mcg per mL increase in serum theophylline concentration.

Maintenance:

Premature infants, postnatal age less than 24 days—Oral, the equivalent of 1 mg of anhydrous theophylline per kg of body weight every twelve hours.

Premature infants, postnatal age 24 days and older—Oral, the equivalent of 1.5 mg of anhydrous theophylline per kg of body weight every twelve hours.

Full-term infants, postnatal age up to 52 weeks—Oral, the equivalent of anhydrous theophylline: total daily dose in mg per kg of body weight = (0.2) (postnatal age in weeks) + 5.

Note: For full-term infants up to 26 weeks of age, divide the total daily dose into three equal amounts administered eight hours apart.

For full-term infants 26 to 52 weeks of age, divide the total daily dose into four equal amounts administered six hours apart.

Children 1 year of age and older, weighing less than 45 kg: Oral, the equivalent of anhydrous theophylline, 12 to 14 mg per kg of body weight, *up to a maximum of 300 mg*, per day in divided doses. The dosage may be increased, if tolerated, after three days to 16 mg per kg of body weight, *up to a maximum of 400 mg*, per day. After three more days, if tolerated, the dosage may be increased to 20 mg per kg of body weight *up to a maximum of 600 mg*, per day. The total daily dose is administered in four to six divided doses given every four to six hours.

Children weighing more than 45 kg: See *Usual adult dose*.

Note: **If the above maintenance dose is to be maintained or exceeded, monitoring of serum theophylline concentration and patient response is recommended to achieve the optimal therapeutic theophylline dosage and minimize the risk of toxicity.**

[Respiratory stimulant (neonatal apnea)][1]—

Loading dose:

For patients *not* currently receiving theophylline preparations—Infants and children up to 16 years of age: Oral, the equivalent of 5 mg of anhydrous theophylline per kg of lean (ideal) body weight as a single dose to provide an average peak serum concentration of 10 mcg per mL (55 micromoles per L), range 5 to 15 mcg per mL (27.5 to 82.5 micromoles per L).

For patients currently receiving theophylline preparations—Obtaining a serum theophylline concentration prior to administering a partial loading dose is recommended. Once the theophylline concentration is known, the loading dose for theophylline is based on the principle that each 0.5 mg of theophylline per kg of lean (ideal) body weight will result in a 1 mcg per mL increase in serum theophylline concentration.

Maintenance:

Premature infants, postnatal age less than 24 days—Oral, the equivalent of 1 mg of anhydrous theophylline per kg of body weight every twelve hours.

Premature infants, postnatal age 24 days and older—Oral, the equivalent of 1.5 mg of anhydrous theophylline per kg of body weight every twelve hours.

Note: **If the above maintenance dose is to be maintained or exceeded, monitoring of serum theophylline concentration and patient response is recommended to achieve the optimal therapeutic theophylline dosage and minimize the risk of toxicity.**

**Strength(s) usually available**

U.S.—

27 mg (equivalent of anhydrous theophylline) per 5 mL (Rx) [*Theolair;* GENERIC].

Canada—

27 mg (equivalent of anhydrous theophylline) per 5 mL (Rx) [*Theolair*].

**Packaging and storage**

Store below 40 °C (104 °F), preferably between 15 and 30 °C (59 and 86 °F), in a well-closed container, unless otherwise specified by manufacturer. Protect from freezing.

**Stability**

Exposure to cold temperatures may cause theophylline crystallization to occur. At room temperature the crystals redissolve and solution gradually clears.

**Auxiliary labeling**

• Do not refrigerate.

## THEOPHYLLINE SYRUP

**Usual adult dose**

See *Theophylline Capsules USP*.

**Usual pediatric dose**

See *Theophylline Oral Solution*.

**Strength(s) usually available**

U.S.—

27 mg (equivalent of anhydrous theophylline) per 5 mL (Rx) [*Slo-Phyllin; Theoclear-80*].

Canada—

Not commercially available.

**Packaging and storage**

Store below 40 °C (104 °F), preferably between 15 and 30 °C (59 and 86 °F), in a well-closed container, unless otherwise specified by manufacturer. Protect from freezing.

**Stability**

Exposure to cold temperatures may cause theophylline crystallization to occur. At room temperature the crystals redissolve and solution gradually clears.

**Auxiliary labeling**

• Do not refrigerate.

## THEOPHYLLINE TABLETS USP

**Usual adult dose**

See *Theophylline Capsules USP*.

**Usual pediatric dose**

See *Theophylline Capsules USP*.

**Strength(s) usually available**

U.S.—

100 mg (equivalent of anhydrous theophylline) (Rx) [*Slo-Phyllin* (scored); GENERIC].

125 mg (equivalent of anhydrous theophylline) (Rx) [*Theolair* (scored)].

200 mg (equivalent of anhydrous theophylline) (Rx) [*Slo-Phyllin* (scored); GENERIC].

250 mg (equivalent of anhydrous theophylline) (Rx) [*Theolair* (scored)].

300 mg (equivalent of anhydrous theophylline) (Rx) [*Quibron-T Dividose* (scored); GENERIC].

Canada—

125 mg (equivalent of anhydrous theophylline) (Rx) [*Theolair* (scored)].

250 mg (equivalent of anhydrous theophylline) (Rx) [*Theolair* (scored)].

## Packaging and storage

Store below 40 °C (104 °F), preferably between 15 and 30 °C (59 and 86 °F), unless otherwise specified by manufacturer. Store in a well-closed container.

## THEOPHYLLINE EXTENDED-RELEASE TABLETS

Note: Due to the significant variability in extended-release product characteristics, pharmacists should not substitute one brand for another without consulting the prescribing physician unless the product has proven bioequivalence, so that theophylline serum concentrations can be appropriately monitored.

### Usual adult dose

Bronchodilator—Oral, the equivalent of anhydrous theophylline, initially, 300 mg per day. If tolerated, the dosage may be increased after three days, to 400 mg per day. After three more days, the dosage may be increased, if tolerated, to 600 mg per day without measurement of serum concentration. One-half the daily theophylline dose may be given at twelve hour intervals. However, certain patients metabolize theophylline more rapidly, especially the young and those that smoke, and may require dosing at eight hour intervals.

Note: **If the 600-mg-per-day dose is to be maintained or exceeded, monitoring of serum theophylline concentration and patient response is recommended to achieve the optimal therapeutic theophylline dosage and minimize the risk of toxicity.**

### Usual pediatric dose

Bronchodilator—

Children 1 year of age and older, weighing less than 45 kg: Oral, the equivalent of anhydrous theophylline, 12 to 14 mg per kg of body weight, *up to a maximum of 300 mg*, per day in divided doses. The dosage may be increased, if tolerated, after three days to 16 mg per kg of body weight, *up to a maximum of 400 mg*, per day. After three more days, if tolerated, the dosage may be increased to 20 mg per kg of body weight *up to a maximum of 600 mg*, per day. One-half of the daily theophylline dose may be given at twelve-hour intervals. However, younger patients may require dosing at eight-hour intervals.

Children weighing more than 45 kg: See *Usual adult dose*.

Children 6 to 16 years of age: See *Usual adult dose*.

### Strength(s) usually available

U.S.—

100 mg (equivalent of anhydrous theophylline) (Rx) [*Theochron* (scored); *Theo-Dur* (scored); *Theo-Time; Theo-X;* GENERIC].

200 mg (equivalent of anhydrous theophylline) (Rx) [*Theochron* (scored); *Theo-Dur* (scored); *Theolair-SR* (scored); *Theo-Time; Theo-X; T-Phyl* (scored); GENERIC].

250 mg (equivalent of anhydrous theophylline) (Rx) [*Respbid* (scored); *Theolair-SR* (scored)].

300 mg (equivalent of anhydrous theophylline) (Rx) [*Quibron-T/SR Dividose* (scored); *Theochron* (scored); *Theo-Dur* (scored); *Theolair-SR* (scored); *Theo-Time; Theo-X;* GENERIC].

400 mg (equivalent of anhydrous theophylline) (Rx) [*Uni-Dur* (scored); *Uniphyl* (scored)].

450 mg (equivalent of anhydrous theophylline) (Rx) [*Theo-Dur* (scored); GENERIC (may be scored)].

500 mg (equivalent of anhydrous theophylline) (Rx) [*Respbid* (scored); *Theolair-SR* (scored)].

600 mg (equivalent of anhydrous theophylline) (Rx) [*Uni-Dur* (scored)].

Canada—

100 mg (equivalent of anhydrous theophylline) (Rx) [*Apo-Theo LA* (scored); *Theochron* (scored); *Theo-Dur* (scored)].

200 mg (equivalent of anhydrous theophylline) (Rx) [*Apo-Theo LA* (scored); *Theochron* (scored); *Theo-Dur* (scored); *Theolair-SR* (scored); *Theo-SR* (scored)].

250 mg (equivalent of anhydrous theophylline) (Rx) [*Theolair SR* (scored)].

300 mg (equivalent of anhydrous theophylline) (Rx) [*Apo-Theo LA* (scored); *Quibron-T/SR Dividose* (scored); *Theochron* (scored); *Theo-Dur* (scored); *Theolair-SR* (scored); *Theo-SR* (scored)].

400 mg (equivalent of anhydrous theophylline) (Rx) [*Uniphyl* (scored)].

450 mg (equivalent of anhydrous theophylline) (Rx) [*Theo-Dur* (scored)].

500 mg (equivalent of anhydrous theophylline) (Rx) [*Theolair-SR* (scored)].

600 mg (equivalent of anhydrous theophylline) (Rx) [*Uniphyl* (scored)].

## Packaging and storage

Store below 40 °C (104 °F), preferably between 15 and 30 °C (59 and 86 °F), in a well-closed container, unless otherwise specified by manufacturer.

### Auxiliary labeling

• Swallow tablets whole, unless otherwise directed.

# Parenteral Dosage Forms

Note: Bracketed uses in the *Dosage Forms* section refer to categories of use and/or indications that are not included in U.S. product labeling.

## THEOPHYLLINE IN DEXTROSE INJECTION USP

### Usual adult dose

Bronchodilator—

Loading dose:

For patients *not* currently receiving theophylline preparations—Intravenous, the equivalent of 5 mg of anhydrous theophylline per kg of lean (ideal) body weight as a single dose, infused over 20 to 30 minutes, to provide an average peak serum concentration of 10 mcg per mL (55 micromoles per L), range 5 to 15 mcg per mL (range 27.5 to 82.5 micromoles per L).

For patients currently receiving theophylline preparations—Obtaining a serum theophylline concentration prior to administering a partial loading dose is recommended. Once the theophylline concentration is known, the loading dose for theophylline is based on the principle that each 0.5 mg of theophylline per kg of lean (ideal) body weight will result in a 1 mcg per mL increase in serum theophylline concentration.

Maintenance:

Young adult smokers—Intravenous infusion, the equivalent of anhydrous theophylline: 700 mcg (0.7 mg) per kg of body weight per hour

Otherwise healthy nonsmoking adults—Intravenous infusion, the equivalent of anhydrous theophylline: 400 mcg (0.4 mg) per kg of body weight per hour.

Older patients and patients with cardiac decompensation, cor pulmonale, or hepatic function impairment—Intravenous infusion, the equivalent of anhydrous theophylline: 200 mcg (0.2 mg) per kg of body weight per hour.

Note: **If the above maintenance dose is to be maintained or exceeded, monitoring of serum theophylline concentration and patient response is recommended to achieve the optimal therapeutic theophylline dosage and minimize the risk of toxicity.**

### Usual pediatric dose

Bronchodilator—

Loading dose:

For patients *not* currently receiving theophylline preparations—Children 1 to 16 years of age: Intravenous, the equivalent of 5 mg of anhydrous theophylline per kg of lean (ideal) body weight as a single dose over twenty to thirty minutes to provide an average peak serum concentration of 10 mcg per mL (55 micromoles per L), range 5 to 15 mcg per mL (27.5 to 82.5 micromoles per L).

For patients currently receiving theophylline preparations—Obtaining a serum theophylline concentration prior to administering a partial loading dose is recommended. Once the theophylline concentration is known, the loading dose for theophylline is based on the principle that each 0.5 mg of theophylline per kg of lean (ideal) body weight will result in a 1 mcg per mL increase in serum theophylline concentration.

Maintenance:

Full-term infants, postnatal age up to 52 weeks—Intravenous infusion, the equivalent of anhydrous theophylline: Dose in mg per kg of body weight per hour = (0.008) (age in weeks) + 0.21.

Children 1 to 9 years of age—Intravenous infusion, the equivalent of anhydrous theophylline: 800 mcg (0.8 mg) per kg of body weight per hour.

Children 9 to 16 years—Intravenous infusion, the equivalent of anhydrous theophylline: 700 mcg (0.7 mg) per kg of body weight per hour.

Note: **If the above maintenance dose is to be maintained or exceeded, monitoring of serum theophylline concentration and patient response is recommended to achieve the optimal therapeutic theophylline dosage and minimize the risk of toxicity.**

**Strength(s) usually available**

U.S.—

Theophylline in 5% dextrose injection (Rx) [GENERIC ] contains the following amounts of anhydrous theophylline:

| Volume (approx.) mL | Theophylline Anhydrous | |
| --- | --- | --- |
| | Total mg | mg/mL |
| 50 | 200 | 4 |
| 100 | 200 | 2 |
| 100 | 400 | 4 |
| 250 | 400 | 1.6 |
| 250 | 800 | 3.2 |
| 500 | 400 | 0.8 |
| 500 | 800 | 1.6 |
| 1000 | 400 | 0.4 |
| 1000 | 800 | 0.8 |

Canada—

Theophylline in 5% dextrose injection (Rx) [GENERIC ] contains the following amounts of anhydrous theophylline:

| Volume (approx.) mL | Theophylline Anhydrous | |
| --- | --- | --- |
| | Total mg | mg/mL |
| 50 | 200 | 4 |
| 100 | 200 | 2 |
| 100 | 400 | 4 |
| 250 | 400 | 1.6 |
| 500 | 400 | 0.8 |
| 500 | 800 | 1.6 |
| 1000 | 400 | 0.4 |
| 1000 | 800 | 0.8 |

**Packaging and storage**

Store below 40 °C (104 °F), preferably between 15 and 30 °C (59 and 86 °F), unless otherwise specified by manufacturer. Protect from freezing.

**Stability**

Theophylline and dextrose solutions contain no bacteriostatic, antimicrobial agent, or added buffer; they are intended only for single-dose administration. When smaller doses are required, the unused portion should be discarded.

**Incompatibilities**

No additives should be made to theophylline and dextrose injection because dosages are titrated to response.

Hetastarch has been shown to be incompatible with theophylline in dextrose solution when injected into Y-sites of administration sets.

---

¹Not included in Canadian product labeling.

## Selected Bibliography

Edwards DJ, Zarowitz BJ, Slaughter RL. Theophylline. In: Evans WE, Schentag JJ, Jusko WJ, editors. Applied Pharmacokinetics: principles of therapeutic drug monitoring. Vancouver, WA: Applied Therapeutics, 1992: 13-1–13-38.

Weinberger MM. Methylxanthines. In: Weiss EB, Stein M, editors. Bronchial asthma—mechanisms and therapeutics. Boston: Little, Brown and Co, 1993: 746-83.

National Asthma Education Program. Expert Panel Report. Guidelines for the diagnosis and management of asthma. National Heart, Lung and Blood Institute, 1991.

---

Revised: 8/11/95

---

# BUCLIZINE   Systemic*†

VA CLASSIFICATION (Primary/Secondary): GA700

Note: For a listing of dosage forms and brand names by country availability, see *Dosage Forms* section(s). For a listing of brand names for the articles in this monograph, refer to the General Index.

---

*Not commercially available in the U.S.

†Not commercially available in Canada.

---

## Category

Antiemetic.

## Indications

**Accepted**

Motion sickness (prophylaxis)—Buclizine is indicated for the prophylaxis of nausea, vomiting, and dizziness associated with motion sickness.

## Pharmacology/Pharmacokinetics

**Physicochemical characteristics**

Molecular weight—505.96.

**Mechanism of action/Effect**

Antiemetic—The mechanism by which buclizine exerts its antiemetic and antimotion sickness effects is not precisely known but may be related to its central anticholinergic actions. It diminishes vestibular stimulation and depresses labyrinthine function. An action on the medullary chemoreceptive trigger zone may also be involved in the antiemetic effect.

**Other actions/effects**

Buclizine also has antihistaminic, anticholinergic, antivertigo, central nervous system (CNS) depressant, and local anesthetic effects.

**Duration of action**

4 to 6 hours.

## Precautions to Consider

**Pregnancy/Reproduction**

Pregnancy—Problems in humans have not been documented.

In studies in rats, buclizine has been shown to be teratogenic at doses above the human therapeutic range.

**Breast-feeding**

Buclizine may be distributed into breast milk. However, problems in humans have not been documented.

Because of its anticholinergic actions, buclizine may inhibit lactation.

**Pediatrics**

No information is available on the relationship of age to the effects of buclizine in pediatric patients. However, it is known that pediatric patients exhibit increased sensitivity to anticholinergics, which are related pharmacologically to buclizine.

**Geriatrics**

No information is available on the relationship of age to the effects of buclizine in geriatric patients. However, it is known that geriatric patients exhibit increased sensitivity to anticholinergics, which are related pharmacologically to buclizine. Therefore, constipation, dryness of mouth, and urinary retention (especially in males) are more likely to occur in the elderly.

**Drug interactions and/or related problems**

The following drug interactions and/or related problems have been selected on the basis of their potential clinical significance (possible mechanism in parentheses where appropriate)—not necessarily inclusive (» = major clinical significance):

Note: Combinations containing any of the following medications, depending on the amount present, may also interact with this medication.

» Alcohol or

» CNS depression–producing medications, other (See *Appendix II*)
    (concurrent use may potentiate the CNS depressant effects of either these medications or buclizine)

   Anticholinergics or other medications with anticholinergic activity (See *Appendix II*)
    (concurrent use with buclizine may potentiate anticholinergic effects)

   Apomorphine
    (prior administration of buclizine may decrease the emetic response to apomorphine)

**Laboratory value alterations**

The following have been selected on the basis of their potential clinical significance (possible effect in parentheses where appropriate)—not necessarily inclusive (» = major clinical significance):

With diagnostic test results
> Skin tests using allergen extracts
>> (use of buclizine may inhibit the cutaneous histamine response, thus producing false-negative results; it is recommended that buclizine be discontinued at least 72 hours before testing begins)

## Medical considerations/Contraindications

The medical considerations/contraindications included here have been selected on the basis of their potential clinical significance (reasons given in parentheses where appropriate)—not necessarily inclusive (» = major clinical significance).

*Risk-benefit should be considered when the following medical problems exist:*

Bladder neck obstruction or
Prostatic hyperplasia, symptomatic
> (anticholinergic effects of buclizine may precipitate urinary retention)

Gastroduodenal obstruction
> (decrease in motility and tone may occur, aggravating obstruction and gastric retention)

Glaucoma, angle-closure, or predisposition to
> (increased intraocular pressure may precipitate an attack of angle-closure glaucoma)

Sensitivity to buclizine

## Side/Adverse Effects

The following side/adverse effects have been selected on the basis of their potential clinical significance (possible signs and symptoms in parentheses where appropriate)—not necessarily inclusive:

**Those indicating need for medical attention only if they continue or are bothersome**
Incidence more frequent
> *Drowsiness*

Incidence less frequent
> *Blurred vision; dryness of mouth, nose, and throat; headache; nervousness, restlessness, or trouble in sleeping; upset stomach*

## Patient Consultation

As an aid to patient consultation, refer to *Advice for the Patient, Meclizine/Buclizine/Cyclizine (Systemic).*

In providing consultation, consider emphasizing the following selected information (» = major clinical significance):

**Before using this medication**
» Conditions affecting use, especially:
> Sensitivity to buclizine
> Pregnancy—Animal studies have shown buclizine to be teratogenic at doses above therapeutic range
> Breast-feeding—May be distributed into breast milk; may inhibit lactation due to anticholinergic effects
> Use in children—Possible increased susceptibility to anticholinergic side effects
> Use in the elderly—Possible increased susceptibility to anticholinergic side effects
> Other medications, especially other CNS depressants

**Proper use of this medication**
Not taking more medication than the amount recommended
» Proper dosing
> Missed dose (if on a regular dosing regimen): Taking as soon as possible; not taking if almost time for next dose; not doubling doses
» Proper storage

**Precautions while using this medication**
Possible interference with skin tests using allergens; need to inform physician of use of this medication
» Avoiding use of alcohol or other CNS depressants
» Caution if drowsiness occurs
> Possible dryness of mouth; using sugarless gum or candy, ice, or saliva substitute for relief

## General Dosing Information

For prophylaxis against motion sickness, this medication should be taken at least 30 minutes before exposure to conditions that may precipitate motion sickness.

## Oral Dosage Forms

### BUCLIZINE HYDROCHLORIDE CHEWABLE TABLETS

**Usual adult and adolescent dose**
Motion sickness (prophylaxis)—
> Oral, 50 mg thirty minutes before travel. Dose may be repeated every four to six hours as needed.

**Usual adult prescribing limits**
Up to 150 mg daily.

**Usual pediatric dose**
Dosage has not been established.

**Usual geriatric dose**
See *Usual adult and adolescent dose.*

Note: Geriatric patients may be more sensitive to the effects of the usual adult dose.

**Strength(s) usually available**
U.S.—
> Not commercially available.

Canada—
> Not commercially available.

**Packaging and storage**
Store below 40 °C (104 °F), preferably between 15 and 30 °C (59 and 86 °F), in a well-closed container, unless otherwise specified by manufacturer. Protect from light.

**Auxiliary labeling**
• May cause drowsiness.
• Avoid alcoholic beverages.
• May be chewed or allowed to dissolve in mouth.

Revised: 01/03/96

---

**BUDESONIDE**—See *Corticosteroids (Inhalation-Local); Corticosteroids (Nasal)*

---

**BUMETANIDE**—See *Diuretics, Loop (Systemic)*

---

**BUPIVACAINE**—See *Anesthetics (Parenteral-Local)*

---

**BUPIVACAINE-CONTAINING COMBINATIONS**—

Bupivacaine and Epinephrine (Parenteral-Local)—See *Anesthetics (Parenteral-Local)*

# BUPRENORPHINE  Systemic

**VA CLASSIFICATION** (Primary/Secondary): CN101/CN205

Note: Contolled substances in the U.S.—V.

Note: For a listing of dosage forms and brand names by country availability, see *Dosage Forms* section(s). For a listing of brand names for the articles in this monograph, refer to the General Index.

## Category

Analgesic; anesthesia adjunct.

Note: Buprenorphine is an opioid agonist/antagonist analgesic.

## Indications

Note: Bracketed information in the *Indications* section refers to uses that are not included in U.S. product labeling.

### Accepted

Pain (treatment)—Indicated for the treatment of moderate to severe pain.

[Anesthesia, general, adjunct]; or

[Anesthesia, local, adjunct]—Buprenorphine is used as an opioid analgesic adjunct to general and local anesthesia.

Prior to administration of buprenorphine, its antagonist activity and its high affinity for, and slow rate of dissociation from, receptor binding sites must be considered. Buprenorphine may precipitate withdrawal symptoms if administered to a patient physically dependent on an opioid analgesic. Also, buprenorphine may temporarily reduce or block the effects of subsequently administered opioid analgesics. In addition, buprenorphine-induced respiratory depression or other adverse effects may be difficult to reverse.

Buprenorphine (unlike pentazocine, which has cardiovascular effects that tend to increase cardiac work) may be administered to patients with angina pectoris or compromised cardiac function, following cardiac or cardiovascular surgery, and to relieve pain due to acute myocardial infarction.

## Pharmacology/Pharmacokinetics

### Physicochemical characteristics

Molecular weight—504.11.

pKa—8.42 and 9.92.

Other characteristics—Weakly acidic; highly lipophilic

### Mechanism of action/Effect

Analgesic—

Opioid analgesics bind with stereospecific receptors at many sites within the central nervous system (CNS) to alter processes affecting both the perception of pain and the emotional response to pain. Precise sites and mechanisms of action have not been fully determined, but may partially involve alterations in release of various neurotransmitters from afferent nerves sensitive to painful stimuli.

It has been proposed that there are multiple subtypes of opioid receptors, each mediating various therapeutic and/or side effects of opioid drugs. The actions of an opioid analgesic may therefore depend upon its binding affinity for each type of receptor and whether it acts as a full agonist or a partial agonist or is inactive at each type of receptor. At least two of these types of receptors (mu and kappa) mediate analgesia. Mu receptors are widely distributed throughout the CNS, especially in the limbic system (frontal cortex, temporal cortex, amygdala, and hippocampus), thalamus, striatum, hypothalamus, and midbrain as well as laminae I, II, IV, and V of the dorsal horn in the spinal cord. Kappa receptors are localized primarily in the spinal cord and in the cerebral cortex. A third type of receptor (sigma) may not mediate analgesia; actions at this receptor may produce the subjective and psychotomimetic effects characteristic of most opioids having mixed agonist/antagonist activity. Buprenorphine may act primarily as a partial agonist at the mu receptor; it may also have some agonist activity at the kappa receptor. Buprenorphine has little if any activity at the sigma receptor.

Antagonist—

Buprenorphine may displace mu-receptor opioid agonists from their receptor binding sites and competitively inhibit their actions. Because buprenorphine has high affinity for the mu receptor, but less intrinsic activity at this receptor than morphine or other potent mu-receptor agonists, it may precipitate withdrawal symptoms in physically dependent patients who are chronically receiving these agonists. However, because of its partial agonist activity, buprenorphine may attenuate spontaneous withdrawal symptoms caused by abrupt

discontinuation of opioid agonists. Also, buprenorphine dissociates from the mu receptor very slowly and may reduce or block the effects of subsequently administered mu-receptor agonists. In some animal studies, the antagonist activity of buprenorphine was comparable to that of naloxone. One study indicates that buprenorphine may also have some antagonist activity at the kappa receptor.

### Other actions/effects

Buprenorphine shares the CNS depressant, respiratory depressant, and hypotensive effects of opioid analgesics.

Buprenorphine may have less potential for causing habituation or abuse than other strong opioid analgesics. Studies in animals have indicated that it has less reinforcing efficacy than other opioids. Also, its slow rate of dissociation from the mu receptor reduces the risk that a severe abstinence syndrome will occur following abrupt withdrawal. Studies in opioid addicts have shown that withdrawal effects may not reach maximum intensity for up to 15 days following abrupt discontinuation. Withdrawal effects are morphine-like, mild to moderate, and may persist for 1 to 2 weeks. Despite the relatively low risk of habituation, abuse has been reported; further experience with this medication is necessary before its true abuse potential can be assessed.

Although studies in humans have not been done, animal studies have indicated that buprenorphine has potent, prolonged antitussive activity.

### Absorption

Intramuscular—Rapid; 5 to 10 minutes following intramuscular administration, plasma concentrations are equivalent to those measured 10 minutes following intravenous administration.

### Protein binding

Very high, primarily to alpha and beta globulin fractions; binding to albumin is not significant.

### Biotransformation

Hepatic; undergoes extensive enterohepatic circulation.

### Half-life

Triphasic—Following a dose of 0.3 mg intravenously—

Distribution—2 minutes

Redistribution—18 minutes

Elimination—1.2 to 7.2 hours; average 2 to 3 hours.

### Onset of action

Analgesic—

Intramuscular: About 15 minutes

Intravenous: More rapid than with intramuscular administration.

Antagonist—

When used to antagonize effects of fentanyl or sufentanil used in conjunction with nitrous oxide for anesthesia: 15 minutes.

Respiratory depressant—

1 to 3 hours following intramuscular administration.

Note: Pharmacokinetic studies have demonstrated no apparent relationship between the onset of buprenorphine's activity and its plasma concentration.

### Time to peak concentration

Intramuscular—2 to 5 minutes

Intravenous—2 minutes

### Peak plasma concentration

Intravenous—18 nanograms per mL following a 0.3-mg dose.

### Time to peak effect

Analgesic—

Intramuscular: 1 hour

Intravenous: Somewhat less than with intramuscular injection.

Antagonist—

When used to antagonize effects of fentanyl or sufentanil used in conjunction with nitrous oxide for anesthesia: 1.5 to 2 hours.

### Duration of action

Analgesia—

Adults:

Intramuscular or intravenous—Up to 6 hours in most patients, but 10 hours or longer in some studies.

Epidural—12 hours following a 0.3-mg dose; 6 hours following a 0.15-mg dose (when administered concurrently with a local anesthetic).

Children 2 to 12 years of age:

4 to 5 hours

Antagonist—

When used to antagonize effects of fentanyl or sufentanil used in conjunction with nitrous oxide for anesthesia: 4 hours.

Following chronic administration of large doses of buprenorphine: In one study in opioid addicts receiving chronic administration of 8 mg per day of buprenorphine subcutaneously, the effects of large doses (up to 120 mg) of subsequently administered morphine were blocked for more than 30 hours following the last dose of buprenorphine.

Respiratory depression—
May persist significantly longer than morphine-induced respiratory depression.

Note: Pharmacokinetic studies have demonstrated no apparent relationship between the duration of buprenorphine's activity and its plasma concentration. The medication's prolonged duration of action is more likely related to its slow rate of dissociation from receptor binding sites.

**Elimination**
Primarily biliary/fecal; about 68% (range 50 to 71%) of an intramuscular dose is eliminated in the feces as unchanged buprenorphine within 7 days. Up to 27% of an intramuscular dose may be excreted in the urine as conjugated buprenorphine and as a dealkylated metabolite; little if any unchanged buprenorphine appears in the urine. It has been proposed that the medication undergoes extensive enterohepatic circulation and is excreted into the bile as inactive conjugates, which are subsequently hydrolyzed in the gastrointestinal tract.

Note: A study in a limited number of pediatric patients 3 to 5 years of age showed that clearance of buprenorphine in children, although subject to high interpatient variability, may be more rapid than in adults.

# Precautions to Consider

### Carcinogenicity
Studies in animals have not shown that buprenorphine has carcinogenic potential.

### Mutagenicity
Studies utilizing *in vitro* and *in vivo* test systems have shown some evidence of mutagenicity with very high concentrations or doses in some test systems but not in others using similar concentrations or doses.

### Pregnancy/Reproduction
Fertility—Reproduction studies with rats have not shown evidence of impaired fertility with subcutaneous or intramuscular administration of 0.05, 0.5, or 5 mg per kg of body weight per day (up to 1000 times the human dose).

Pregnancy—Adequate and well-controlled studies in humans have not been done.

Studies in rats administered up to 1000 times the human dose intramuscularly or up to 160 times the human dose intravenously showed no evidence of teratogenicity. However, studies in rabbits showed a dose-related trend toward extra rib formation, which was statistically significant with intramuscular administration of 1000 times the human dose. Also, studies in rats showed an increased incidence of postimplantation losses and early fetal deaths with intramuscular administration of 10 or 100, but not 1000, times the human dose per day. A slight increase in postimplantation losses, possibly treatment-related, also occurred in rats receiving up to 160 times the human dose intravenously. In addition, intramuscular administration of 1000 times the human dose per day to rats throughout gestation caused dystocia, a high incidence of neonatal mortality, and a slow growth rate in surviving offspring.

FDA Pregnancy Category C.

Labor and delivery—Safe use of buprenorphine in labor and delivery has not been established. However, it has been recommended that the medication not be used during labor because of potential respiratory depressant effects in the neonate, which may be very difficult to reverse.

### Breast-feeding
Although it is not known whether buprenorphine is distributed into human breast milk, problems in humans have not been documented. Concentrations in the milk of lactating animals have been shown to equal or exceed maternal plasma concentrations; it is reasonable to assume that this highly lipophilic medication would be distributed into human breast milk also. In addition, animal studies have shown that administration of buprenorphine throughout the periods of gestation and lactation inhibits milk production.

### Pediatrics
Appropriate studies performed to date have not demonstrated pediatrics-specific problems that would limit the usefulness of buprenorphine in children 2 years of age and older.

### Geriatrics
Geriatric patients may be more sensitive to the effects, especially the respiratory depressant effects, of opioid analgesics, including buprenorphine. Also, elderly patients are more likely to have age-related renal function impairment, which may require caution and dosage adjustment in patients receiving buprenorphine. It is recommended that initial dosage for these patients be reduced by one-half. However, geriatric patients may also be more sensitive to the analgesic effects of the medication so that lower doses and/or a longer interval between doses may provide sufficient analgesia.

### Drug interactions and/or related problems
The following drug interactions and/or related problems have been selected on the basis of their potential clinical significance (possible mechanism in parentheses where appropriate)—not necessarily inclusive (» = major clinical significance):

Note: Combinations containing any of the following medications, depending on the amount present, may also interact with this medication.

Other interactions applying to opioid analgesics may apply to buprenorphine also, although documentation is currently not available.

» CNS depression–producing medications, other (See *Appendix II*) or
Monoamine oxidase (MAO) inhibitors, including furazolidone, procarbazine, and selegiline
(concurrent use may increase the CNS depressant, respiratory depressant, and hypotensive effects of these medications and/or buprenorphine; caution is recommended; it is recommended that dosage of buprenorphine be reduced by one-half; a reduction in dosage of the other agent may also be required)

Naltrexone
(although not documented, the possibility must be considered that usual doses of buprenorphine will be ineffective if administered to a patient receiving naltrexone therapy [because naltrexone blocks the therapeutic effects of other potent opioids] and that administration of increased doses of buprenorphine to override naltrexone-induced blockade of opioid receptors may increase the risk of adverse effects)

» Opioid analgesics, other
(if administered prior to another opioid analgesic, buprenorphine may reduce the therapeutic effects of the other opioid; in one study in opioid addicts receiving chronic administration of 8 mg per day of buprenorphine, the effects of large doses [up to 120 mg] of morphine were blocked during buprenorphine therapy and for at least 30 hours following the last dose of buprenorphine)
(buprenorphine antagonizes the respiratory depressant effects of large doses of previously administered opioids; however, additive respiratory depression may occur if buprenorphine is administered in conjunction with low doses of other opioids)
(when administered following fentanyl derivative–assisted anesthesia, buprenorphine may reverse the respiratory depressant effects of fentanyl or its derivatives [alfentanil and sufentanil] while providing adequate postoperative analgesia; however, in one study, administration of 0.3 or 0.45 mg of buprenorphine intramuscularly every 6 hours following opioid-assisted anesthesia with total doses of 0.2 or 0.3 mg of fentanyl or 1.75 or 4 mg of phenoperidine [not available in the U.S.] caused a higher incidence of hypotension, respiratory depression, and CNS depression than equianalgesic doses [10 or 15 mg] of morphine intramuscularly every 6 hours)
(buprenorphine may precipitate withdrawal symptoms in physically dependent patients who are chronically receiving potent mu-receptor agonists such as morphine; however, because of its partial agonist activity, buprenorphine may partially suppress spontaneous withdrawal symptoms caused by abrupt discontinuation of opioid agonists)

### Laboratory value alterations
The following have been selected on the basis of their potential clinical significance (possible effect in parentheses where appropriate)—not necessarily inclusive (» = major clinical significance):

With diagnostic test results
Gastric emptying studies
(buprenorphine may delay gastric emptying, thereby invalidating test results)

Hepatobiliary imaging using technetium Tc 99m disofenin
(delivery of technetium Tc 99m disofenin to the small bowel may be prevented because of buprenorphine-induced constriction of the sphincter of Oddi and increased biliary tract pressure; these actions result in delayed visualization and thus resemble obstruction of the common bile duct)

With physiology/laboratory test values
  Amylase, plasma and
  Lipase, plasma
      (values may be increased because buprenorphine can cause contrac-
      tions of the sphincter of Oddi and increased biliary tract pressure;
      the diagnostic utility of determinations of these enzymes may be
      compromised for up to 24 hours after medication has been given)
  Cerebrospinal fluid (CSF) pressure
      (may be increased; effect is secondary to respiratory depression–
      induced carbon dioxide retention)

**Medical considerations/Contraindications**
The medical considerations/contraindications included here have been selected on the basis of their potential clinical significance (reasons given
  in parentheses where appropriate)—not necessarily inclusive (» =
  major clinical significance).

*Except under special circumstances, this medication should not be used
when the following medical problems exist:*
» Diarrhea caused by poisoning, until toxic material has been eliminated
    from gastrointestinal tract
      (may slow elimination of toxic material)
» Respiratory depression, acute
      (may be exacerbated)

*Risk-benefit should be considered when the following medical problems
exist:*
  Abdominal conditions, acute
      (diagnosis or clinical course may be obscured)
» Asthma, acute attack or
» Respiratory impairment or disease, chronic
      (opioids may decrease respiratory drive and increase airway resis-
      tance in these patients; it is recommended that dosage be reduced
      by one-half, unless the patient is being mechanically ventilated)
  Cardiac arrhythmias or
  Seizures, history of
      (may be induced or exacerbated by opioids)
  Dependence on opioid analgesics, current
      (buprenorphine may precipitate withdrawal symptoms if patient is
      currently receiving other opioids)
  Drug abuse or dependence, history of, including acute alcoholism or
  Emotional instability or
  Suicidal ideation or attempts
      (increased risk of opioid abuse)
  Gallbladder disease or gallstones
      (opioids may cause biliary colic)
  Gastrointestinal tract surgery, recent
      (opioids may alter gastrointestinal motility)
  Head injury or
  Increased intracranial pressure, pre-existing or
  Intracranial lesions
      (risk of respiratory depression and further elevation of cerebrospinal
      fluid pressure is increased; also, opioids may cause sedation and
      pupillary changes that may obscure clinical course of head injury)
  Hepatic function impairment
      (opioids metabolized in liver)
  Hypothyroidism
      (risk of respiratory depression and prolonged CNS depression is
      greatly increased)
» Inflammatory bowel disease, severe
      (risk of toxic megacolon may be increased, especially with repeated
      dosing)
  Prostatic hypertrophy or obstruction or
  Urethral stricture or
  Urinary tract surgery, recent
      (opioids may cause urinary retention)
  Renal function impairment
      (buprenorphine metabolites excreted via kidneys; also, may cause
      urinary retention)
  Sensitivity to buprenorphine, history of
  Caution is also advised in administration to geriatric or very ill or
      debilitated patients, who may be more sensitive to the effects,
      especially the respiratory depressant effects, of buprenorphine.

## Side/Adverse Effects

Note: Buprenorphine appears less likely than other opioid agonist/antagonist
      analgesics to cause the subjective and psychotomimetic effects
      characteristic of this class of drugs. These effects may include

several or all of the following, occurring as a group: confusion,
delusions, feelings of depersonalization or unreality, hallucinations
(usually visual), dysphoria, nightmares, and nervousness or anxiety.
However, several of these effects have been reported individually
(incidence < 1%) in patients receiving buprenorphine.

Buprenorphine may have less dependence or abuse liability than
other potent opioid analgesics. However, abuse has been reported.

In some studies, the incidence and/or severity of nausea and vomiting
occurring with buprenorphine was greater than that induced by
meperidine or morphine.

Epidural administration of buprenorphine may be associated with a
lower incidence of adverse effects, such as late respiratory depression,
pruritus, and urinary retention, than has been reported with epidural
morphine. However, early respiratory depression resistant to naloxone
therapy has been reported. Also, signs of shock (pallor, cold skin,
low blood pressure, and tachycardia) have been reported in a few
patients following epidural buprenorphine. Although these signs
eventually abated spontaneously, naloxone and other treatments were
not effective in reversing them.

The following side/adverse effects have been selected on the basis of their
potential clinical significance (possible signs and symptoms in parentheses where appropriate)—not necessarily inclusive:

**Those indicating need for medical attention**
Incidence 1 to 5%
  *Decreased blood pressure; respiratory depression, mild* (unusually slow
  breathing)
  Note: Whether buprenorphine's respiratory depressant activity is subject
      to the same ceiling effect (i.e., the depth of respiratory depression
      is not increased with higher doses) reported for other opioid
      agonist/antagonist drugs has not been established in humans.
      Studies in animals indicate that such a ceiling effect may occur,
      but at higher dosage levels than with other opioid agonist/
      antagonist drugs.

Incidence <1%
  *CNS effects* (confusion, hallucinations, mental depression or other mood
  or mental changes; psychosis; ringing or buzzing in ears); *conjunctivitis*
  (red and/or irritated eyes); *dermatitis, allergic* (skin rash, hives, or
  itching); *increased blood presssure; increased or decreased heart rate;
  paresthesia* (pain, numbness, tingling, or burning feeling in hands or
  feet); *respiratory depression, severe* (blue color of face, lips, or
  fingernails; difficult or troubled breathing); *urinary retention* (decrease
  in amount of urine; swelling of face, fingers, hands, feet, or lower
  legs; weight gain); *Wenckebach block*

**Those indicating need for medical attention only if they continue
or are bothersome**
Incidence up to 66%
  *Drowsiness*

Incidence 5 to 10%
  *Dizziness or lightheadedness; nausea*—especially in ambulatory patients

Incidence 1 to 5%
  *Headache; increased sweating; vomiting*—especially in ambulatory
  patients

Incidence <1%
  *Blurred vision or any change in vision; false sense of well-being;
  general feeling of discomfort or illness; pain, redness, or swelling at
  place of injection; slurred speech; trembling; unusual nervousness;
  unusual tiredness; unusual weakness*

**Those indicating possible withdrawal and the need for medical
attention if they occur within 15 days after medication is
discontinued**
  *Body aches; diarrhea; fast heartbeat; gooseflesh; increased sweating;
  loss of appetite; nausea or vomiting; nervousness, restlessness, or
  irritability; runny nose; shivering or trembling; sneezing; stomach
  cramps; trouble in sleeping; unexplained fever; unusually large pupils
  of eyes; weakness; yawning*

## Overdose

For specific information on the agents used in the management of
buprenorphine overdose, see:
  • *Naloxone (Systemic)* monograph; and/or
  • *Doxapram (Systemic)* monograph.

For more information on the management of overdose or unintentional
ingestion, **contact a Poison Control Center** (see *Poison Control
Center Listing*).

### Clinical effects of overdose

The following effects have been selected on the basis of their potential clinical significance (possible signs and symptoms in parentheses where appropriate)—not necessarily inclusive:

Acute and chronic

*Cold, clammy skin; confusion; convulsions; dizziness, severe; drowsiness, severe; low blood pressure; nervousness or restlessness, severe; pinpoint pupils of eyes; slow heartbeat; slow or troubled breathing; unconsciousness; weakness, severe*

### Treatment of overdose

Specific treatment—Use of the opioid antagonist naloxone for buprenorphine-induced respiratory depression. However, even in doses as high as 16 mg, naloxone may not completely antagonize buprenorphine-induced respiratory depression or other adverse effects.

The respiratory stimulant doxapram may be administered if naloxone fails to reverse respiratory depression.

Assisted or controlled ventilation may be necessary despite administration of naloxone and/or doxapram.

Monitoring—May include monitoring the respiratory and cardiac status of the patient.

May include continual monitoring of the patient so that additional naloxone and/or doxapram may be administered as needed. Administration of these medications by continuous intravenous infusion, with the rate of infusion being adjusted according to patient response, may be preferable to intermittent administration.

Supportive care—May include establishing adequate respiratory exchange through provision of a patent airway and institution of assisted or controlled respiration using 100% oxygen if respiratory depression is severe; if respiratory depression is mild, i.e., a conscious and responsive patient is breathing unusually slowly (but without difficulty) and/or coaching the patient to breathe produces improvement, these measures may not be required.

May include administering intravenous fluids, vasopressors, and other supportive measures as needed.

## Patient Consultation

As an aid to patient consultation, refer to *Advice for the Patient, Narcotic Analgesics (Systemic—For Pain Relief)* and *Narcotic Analgesics (Systemic—For Surgery and Obstetrics).*

In providing consultation, consider emphasizing the following selected information (» = major clinical significance):

### Before using this medication

» Conditions affecting use, especially:

Allergic reaction to buprenorphine, history of

Breast-feeding—Buprenorphine has inhibited milk production in animal studies

Use in the elderly—Lower doses recommended because of increased sensitivity to opioids

Other medications, especially other CNS depression–producing medications and other opioids

Medical problems, especially diarrhea caused by poisoning, respiratory depression or disease (including asthma), and severe inflammatory bowel disease

### Proper use of this medication

Proper administration technique (if dispensed for home use)

» Importance of not taking more medication than the amount prescribed because of danger of overdose and habit-forming potential

» Not increasing dose if medication is less effective after a few weeks; checking with physician

» Missed dose (if on scheduled dosing): Using as soon as possible; not using if almost time for next dose; not doubling doses

» Proper dosing

» Proper storage

### Precautions while using this medication

Regular visits to physician to check progress during long-term therapy

» Avoiding alcohol or other CNS depressants during therapy

» Caution if dizziness, drowsiness, lightheadedness, or false sense of well-being occurs

Caution when getting up suddenly from a lying or sitting position

Lying down if nausea, vomiting, dizziness, or lightheadedness occurs

Caution if any kind of surgery (including dental surgery) or emergency treatment is required

» Checking with physician before discontinuing medication after prolonged use of high doses; gradual dosage reduction may be necessary to avoid withdrawal symptoms

» Suspected overdose: Getting emergency help at once

### Side/adverse effects

Signs and symptoms of potential side effects, especially respiratory and/or CNS depression, allergic dermatitis, hallucinations, and overdose

## General Dosing Information

Intramuscular administration of 300 mcg (0.3 mg) of buprenorphine provides analgesia equivalent to that produced by intramuscular administration of 10 mg of morphine.

Buprenorphine may suppress respiration, especially in geriatric, very ill, or debilitated patients and patients with respiratory problems. It is recommended that dosage for these patients be reduced by one-half initially, then adjusted as required and tolerated. However, geriatric patients may also be more sensitive to the analgesic effects of the medication so that lower doses and/or a longer interval between doses may be sufficient to provide effective analgesia.

Dosage and dosing intervals should be individualized on the basis of the severity of pain, the condition of the patient, other medications given concurrently, and patient response.

Some clinicians recommend that patients in chronic pain due to neoplastic disease receive opioid analgesics on a fixed dosage schedule in order that they remain free of pain rather than on an as needed basis after pain recurs.

Concurrent administration of a non-opioid analgesic (such as aspirin or other salicylates, other nonsteroidal anti-inflammatory analgesics, or acetaminophen) with opioid analgesics provides additive analgesia and may permit lower doses of the opioid analgesic to be utilized.

Although buprenorphine may have less potential for causing habituation or abuse than other opioid analgesics, psychological and physical dependence may occur with chronic administration. An abstinence syndrome may be precipitated when the medication is abruptly discontinued. Although withdrawal symptoms may not reach maximum intensity for up to 15 days following discontinuation, if they occur they may persist for 1 to 2 weeks. Also, abuse has been reported.

Rapid intravenous injection of most opioid analgesics has caused anaphylactoid reactions, severe respiratory depression, hypotension, peripheral circulatory collapse, and cardiac arrest. Although these effects have not been documented with buprenorphine, the same precautions applying to other opioid analgesics may apply, i.e., administering the medication slowly, with an opioid antagonist and equipment for artificial ventilation available. It is recommended that intravenous injections of buprenorphine be administered over at least 2 minutes.

Frequent monitoring of the patient's respiratory status is recommended during buprenorphine therapy because of the risk of respiratory depression.

When an opioid analgesic is administered parenterally, the patient usually should be lying down and should remain recumbent for a period of time to minimize side effects such as hypotension, dizziness, lightheadedness, nausea, and vomiting. If these side effects occur in an ambulatory patient, they may be relieved if the patient lies down.

In patients with shock, impaired perfusion may prevent complete absorption following intramuscular injection. Repeated administration may result in overdose due to an excessive amount suddenly being absorbed when circulation is restored.

Tolerance to buprenorphine requiring increased dosage to maintain adequate analgesia has not occurred in long-term studies in cancer patients. However, tolerance has been demonstrated in studies with opioid addicts.

## Parenteral Dosage Forms

Note: The dosing and strength of the available dosage form are expressed in terms of buprenorphine base (not the hydrochloride salt).

### BUPRENORPHINE HYDROCHLORIDE INJECTION

#### Usual adult and adolescent dose

Analgesic—

Intramuscular or slow intravenous, 300 mcg (0.3 mg) (base) every six or more hours as needed. An additional dose of up to 300 mcg (0.3 mg) may be administered thirty to sixty minutes following the initial dose, if necessary.

Note: Dosage may be increased to 600 mcg (0.6 mg), or the frequency of administration may be increased to every four hours if necessary, depending upon the severity of pain and patient response. This larger dose should be administered only via the intramuscular route and only to patients who are not at high risk for opioid toxicity. Although doses exceeding 600 mcg (0.6 mg) have been administered in some studies, long-term use of such doses is not recommended because of insufficient data.

**Usual pediatric dose**

Analgesic—

Children up to 2 years of age: Dosage has not been established.

Children 2 to 12 years of age: Intramuscular or slow intravenous, 2 to 6 mcg (0.002 to 0.006 mg) (base) per kg of body weight every four to six hours or as needed.

Note: Because of interpatient variability in buprenorphine clearance, it is recommended that the appropriate dosing interval for an individual pediatric patient be determined before a fixed-interval dosing regimen is scheduled.

**Strength(s) usually available**

U.S.—

Without preservative

300 mcg (0.3 mg) (base) per mL (Rx) [*Buprenex* (dextrose 5%)].

**Packaging and storage**

Store below 40 °C (104 °F), preferably between 15 and 30 °C (59 and 86 °F), unless otherwise specified by manufacturer. Protect from freezing. Avoid prolonged exposure to light.

**Incompatibilities**

Buprenorphine injection is chemically incompatible with diazepam and with lorazepam.

**Auxiliary labeling**

• May cause drowsiness.

• Avoid alcoholic beverages.

• May be habit-forming.

**Note**

Controlled substance in the U.S.

Revised: 07/29/94

---

# BUPROPION   Systemic†

INN: Amfebutamone

VA CLASSIFICATION (Primary): CN609

Note: For a listing of dosage forms and brand names by country availability, see *Dosage Forms* section(s). For a listing of brand names for the articles in this monograph, refer to the General Index.

†Not commercially available in Canada.

## Category

Antidepressant.

## Indications

**Accepted**

Depression, mental (treatment)—Bupropion is indicated for the treatment of major depression.

## Pharmacology/Pharmacokinetics

**Physicochemical characteristics**

Molecular weight—276.21.

**Mechanism of action/Effect**

Although the exact mechanism of antidepressant action is unclear, one *in vivo* effect of bupropion on biogenic amine systems appears to be its weak blockade of dopamine reuptake; however, this inhibition occurs at doses higher than those required for its antidepressant effects. Recent animal studies have suggested that bupropion's antidepressant activity may be mediated through noradrenergic pathways involving the locus ceruleus.

Bupropion is also a weak blocker of the neuronal reuptake of serotonin and norepinephrine, and it does *not* inhibit monoamine oxidase.

**Other actions/effects**

May be an inducer of hepatic microsomal enzymes.

May produce dose-related central nervous system (CNS) stimulation.

**Absorption**

Approximately 80%; rapidly absorbed from the gastrointestinal tract.

**Distribution**

Readily crosses the blood-brain barrier and placenta; a study of one subject demonstrated that bupropion and its metabolites pass into breast milk.

**Protein binding**

High (75 to 85%).

**Biotransformation**

Extensive presystemic or first-pass metabolism with metabolites of possible lesser therapeutic activity than parent drug. The major metabolites that have been identified are the *erythro-* and *threo-*amino alcohols of bupropion, the *erythro-*amino diol of bupropion, and a morpholinol metabolite.

**Half-life**

Distribution—

Approximately 1.5 hours.

Elimination—

Approximately 14 (range, 8 to 24) hours. Single-dose studies demonstrate a first-order elimination pattern with a mean total body clearance of 2 liters per hour per kilogram of body weight.

**Onset of action**

1 to 3 weeks.

**Time to peak concentration**

Within 1 to 3 hours, followed by biphasic decline.

**Elimination**

Renal—

Less than 1% excreted in urine unchanged. Over 60% excreted as metabolites within 24 hours, over 80% within 96 hours.

Hepatic—

Less than 10% (bupropion and metabolites) in feces.

## Precautions to Consider

**Carcinogenicity**

In a lifetime study of rats, there was an increase in nodular proliferative lesions of the liver at doses of 100 mg to 300 mg per kg of body weight (mg/kg) a day. However, whether such lesions may be precursors of neoplasms of the liver has not been resolved. Similar lesions were not seen in studies with mice given doses up to 150 mg/kg a day.

**Tumorigenicity**

Studies in rodents showed no increase in malignant tumors of the liver or other organs.

**Mutagenicity**

In studies in rats, bupropion produced a borderline positive response in some strains in the Ames bacterial mutagenicity test. Also, a high oral dose (300 mg/kg) produced a low incidence of chromosomal aberrations in rats.

**Pregnancy/Reproduction**

Fertility—Studies in rats and rabbits given doses up to 300 mg/kg a day have shown no evidence of impaired fertility.

Pregnancy—Adequate and well-controlled studies in humans have not been done. However, bupropion readily crosses the placenta.

Studies in rats and rabbits given doses up to 15 to 45 times the human daily dose have not shown that bupropion causes adverse effects in the fetus. In rabbits, two studies showed a slightly increased incidence of fetal abnormalities; however, there was no increase in any specific abnormality.

FDA Pregnancy Category B.

Labor and delivery—The effect of bupropion on labor and delivery in humans is unknown.

**Breast-feeding**

Bupropion is distributed into breast milk, and the potential exists for serious adverse reactions (such as seizures) in the infant.

**Pediatrics**

Appropriate studies on the relationship of age to the effects of bupropion have not been performed in children up to 18 years of age. Safety and efficacy have not been established.

**Geriatrics**

Studies performed in patients 60 years of age and older have not demonstrated geriatrics-specific problems that would limit the usefulness of bupropion in the elderly. However, older patients are known to be more sensitive to the anticholinergic, sedative, and cardiovascular side effects of antidepressants. In addition, elderly patients are more likely to have age-related renal or hepatic function impairment, which may require dosage adjustment in patients receiving bupropion.

### Drug interactions and/or related problems

The following drug interactions and/or related problems have been selected on the basis of their potential clinical significance (possible mechanism in parentheses where appropriate)—not necessarily inclusive ($\gg$ = major clinical significance):

Note: Combinations containing any of the following medications, depending on the amount present, may also interact with this medication.

$\gg$ Alcohol
(concurrent use or the cessation of chronic alcohol use during therapy may lower the seizure threshold and increase the risk of seizures; patients should be advised to minimize alcohol consumption or avoid the use of alcohol completely)

$\gg$ Antidepressants, tricyclic or
$\gg$ Clozapine or
$\gg$ Fluoxetine or
$\gg$ Haloperidol or
$\gg$ Lithium or
$\gg$ Loxapine or
$\gg$ Maprotiline or
$\gg$ Molindone or
$\gg$ Phenothiazines or
$\gg$ Thioxanthenes or
$\gg$ Trazodone
(concurrent use of these medications with bupropion may lower the seizure threshold and increase the risk of major motor seizures; in addition, changes in treatment regimen, such as abrupt discontinuation of a benzodiazepine, may precipitate a seizure)

Hepatic enzyme inducers, other (See *Appendix II*)
(concurrent use with bupropion may increase the metabolism of these agents or bupropion)

Hepatic enzyme inhibitors (See *Appendix II*)
(these medications may inhibit hepatic microsomal enzymes, thereby decreasing metabolism and increasing serum concentrations of bupropion, thus increasing the risk of seizures)

Levodopa
(concurrent use with bupropion may result in a greater incidence of adverse effects; small initial doses of bupropion and small gradual dose increases are recommended during concurrent therapy)

$\gg$ Monoamine oxidase (MAO) inhibitors, including furazolidone, procarbazine, and selegiline
(concurrent use of bupropion with these medications may increase the risk of acute toxicity of bupropion and is contraindicated; a medication-free interval of at least 2 weeks should elapse between discontinuation of the MAO inhibitor and initiation of bupropion therapy)

### Laboratory value alterations

The following have been selected on the basis of their potential clinical significance (possible effect in parentheses where appropriate)—not necessarily inclusive ($\gg$ = major clinical significance):

With diagnostic test results
Electrocardiogram (ECG) readings
(clinically symptomatic changes, such as premature beats and nonspecific ST-T changes, may occur with long-term treatment [up to a year])

With physiology/laboratory test values
White blood cell count
(decreased by 10 to 14% during the first 2 months of therapy in one study; unknown clinical significance)

### Medical considerations/Contraindications

The medical considerations/contraindications included here have been selected on the basis of their potential clinical significance (reasons given in parentheses where appropriate)—not necessarily inclusive ($\gg$ = major clinical significance).

*Except under special circumstances, this medication should not be used when the following medical problems exist:*

$\gg$ Anorexia nervosa or
$\gg$ Bulimia
(increased risk of seizures in patients with current or prior diagnosis of these conditions)

$\gg$ Seizure disorders
(increased risk of major motor seizures)

*Risk-benefit should be considered when the following medical problems exist:*

Bipolar disorder
(mania may be precipitated during the depressed phase in patients with manic-depressive illness)

$\gg$ CNS tumor or
$\gg$ Head trauma or
$\gg$ Spontaneous seizures, history of
(increased risk of major motor seizures)

Drug abuse
(patients with a history of amphetamine or stimulant abuse may be attracted to bupropion because of its mild amphetamine-like activity, especially at higher doses; however, risk of seizures has prevented adequate testing)

$\gg$ Hepatic function impairment or
$\gg$ Renal function impairment
(metabolism or excretion may be altered)

$\gg$ Myocardial infarction, recent history of or
Heart disease, unstable

Psychosis, especially schizoaffective disorder, depressed
(latent psychosis or mania may be activated in susceptible patients)
Sensitivity to bupropion

### Patient monitoring

The following may be especially important in patient monitoring (other tests may be warranted in some patients, depending on condition; $\gg$ = major clinical significance):

Careful supervision of depressed patients with suicidal tendencies
(recommended especially during early weeks of treatment; hospitalization may be required as a protective measure)

Hepatic function determinations or
Renal function determinations
(close monitoring is recommended in patients with kidney or liver function impairment to prevent excessive serum and tissue concentrations of bupropion or its metabolites; dosage adjustments may be necessary)

## Side/Adverse Effects

The following side/adverse effects have been selected on the basis of their potential clinical significance (possible signs and symptoms in parentheses where appropriate)—not necessarily inclusive:

**Those indicating need for medical attention**
Incidence more frequent
*CNS stimulation* (agitation or excitement; anxiety; restlessness; insomnia; confusion); *fast or irregular heartbeat; headache, severe*
Incidence less frequent
*Hallucinations; skin rash*
Incidence rare
*Fainting; seizures*—especially with higher doses
Note: The risk of *seizures* with bupropion may be greater than with other antidepressants, approximately 0.4% (4/1000 patients) at doses up to 450 mg of bupropion a day. At doses above 450 mg, the risk increases almost tenfold.

**Those indicating need for medical attention only if they continue or are bothersome**
Incidence more frequent
*Constipation; decrease in appetite; dizziness; dryness of mouth; increased sweating; nausea or vomiting; tremor; weight loss, unusual*
Incidence less frequent or rare
*Blurred vision; difficulty in concentration; drowsiness; fever or chills; hostility or anger; sleep disturbances; tiredness; unusual feeling of well-being*

## Overdose

For specific information on the agents used in the management of bupropion overdose, see:
• *Charcoal, Activated (Oral—Local)* monograph.

For more information on the management of overdose or unintentional ingestion, **contact a Poison Control Center** (see *Poison Control Center Listing*).

### Treatment of overdose

Recommended treatment consists of the following:
To decrease absorption—
Induction of emesis with syrup of ipecac.
In comatose, stuporous, or convulsing patients, initiation of airway intubation followed by gastric lavage within the first 12 hours of ingestion, when absorption is not yet complete.

Administration of activated charcoal every 6 hours within first 12 hours after ingestion.

Specific treatment—
Treatment of seizures with an intravenous benzodiazepine.

Monitoring—
Monitoring ECG and EEG for 48 hours.

Supportive care—
Maintenance of adequate fluid intake. Patients in whom intentional overdose is confirmed or suspected should be referred for psychiatric consultation.

## Patient Consultation

As an aid to patient consultation, refer to *Advice for the Patient, Bupropion (Systemic)*.

In providing consultation, consider emphasizing the following selected information (>> = major clinical significance):

### Before using this medication
>> Conditions affecting use, especially:
  Sensitivity to bupropion
  Pregnancy—Crosses placenta
  Breast-feeding—Distributed into breast milk; because of potential for serious adverse effects in the infant, use is not recommended
  Other medications, especially alcohol, antipsychotic medications, fluoxetine, lithium, MAO inhibitors, maprotiline, trazodone, or tricyclic antidepressants
  Other medical problems, especially anorexia nervosa, bulimia, CNS tumor, head trauma, hepatic or renal function impairment, recent myocardial infarction, or seizure disorders

### Proper use of this medication
>> Compliance with therapy; not taking more or less medication than prescribed
  Taking with food if needed to lessen gastrointestinal irritation
  May require up to 4 weeks or longer for optimal antidepressant effects
>> Proper dosing
  Missed dose: Taking as soon as possible; taking any remaining doses for that day at regularly spaced intervals of no less than 4 hours; not doubling doses
>> Proper storage

### Precautions while using this medication
  Regular visits to physician to check progress during therapy
>> Checking with physician before discontinuing medication; gradual dosage reduction may be necessary to prevent adverse effects
>> Minimizing consumption of or avoiding use of alcoholic beverages to prevent possible seizures
>> Possible dizziness, drowsiness, or euphoria; caution when driving, using machinery, or doing other things requiring alertness and judgment

### Side/adverse effects
  Signs of potential side effects, especially CNS stimulation, fast or irregular heartbeat, severe headache, hallucinations, skin rash, fainting, or seizures

## General Dosing Information

To reduce the risk of agitation, motor restlessness, or insomnia, which are more frequent at initiation of therapy, increases in dosage must be made gradually.

Seizures occur more frequently at higher doses, the incidence being approximately 0.4% (4/1000 patients) at doses up to 450 mg a day and increasing almost tenfold at doses between 450 mg and 600 mg a day.

Equally divided doses taken three or four times a day at 4- to 6-hour intervals will avoid high peak concentrations of bupropion or its metabolites.

Full antidepressant action may not be evident for 4 weeks or longer.

Potentially suicidal patients should not have access to large quantities of this medication since depressed patients, particularly those who use

alcohol excessively, may continue to exhibit suicidal tendencies until significant improvement occurs.

### Diet/Nutrition
Bupropion may be taken with food to lessen gastrointestinal irritation.

### For prevention of seizures
The risk of seizures may be reduced if:
  • The total daily dose does not exceed 450 mg and is administered in divided doses.
  • Each single dose does not exceed 150 mg.
  • The dosage is increased gradually.
  • Caution is used in patients with a history of seizures or cranial trauma; during concurrent use with other medications that may lower the seizure threshold; or when changes in treatment regimens occur.

### For treatment of adverse effects
Recommended treatment consists of the following:
• For agitation, excitement, or insomnia—Lowering dosage, and then increasing it gradually as needed and tolerated. Temporary sedative-hypnotic medication may be necessary, but is usually not required beyond the first week of treatment. If effects are severe, discontinuation of bupropion may be necessary.
• For nausea and vomiting—Taking with meals, or decreasing and then gradually increasing the dosage.

## Oral Dosage Forms
### BUPROPION HYDROCHLORIDE TABLETS

**Usual adult dose**
Antidepressant—
  Oral, initially 100 mg two times a day, the dosage being increased gradually, no sooner than three days after beginning therapy, to 100 mg three times a day as needed and tolerated.

Note: Dosing intervals must be at least every four hours.

**Usual adult prescribing limits**
450 mg a day, with no single dose exceeding 150 mg.

**Usual pediatric dose**
Safety and efficacy have not been established.

**Strength(s) usually available**
U.S.—
  75 mg (Rx) [*Wellbutrin* (D&C Yellow No. 10 Lake; FD&C Yellow No. 6 Lake; hydroxypropyl cellulose; hydroxypropyl methylcellulose; light mineral oil; microcrystalline cellulose; talc; titanium dioxide)].
  100 mg (Rx) [*Wellbutrin* (FD&C Red No. 40 Lake; FD&C Yellow No. 6 Lake; hydroxypropyl cellulose; hydroxypropyl methylcellulose; light mineral oil; microcrystalline cellulose; talc; titanium dioxide)].

Canada—
  Not commercially available.

**Packaging and storage**
Store below 40 °C (104 °F), preferably between 15 and 30 °C (59 and 86 °F), unless otherwise specified by manufacturer.

**Auxiliary labeling**
• May cause drowsiness.
• Avoid alcoholic beverages.

## Selected Bibliography

Dufresne RL, Weber SS, Becker RE. New drug evaluations: Bupropion hydrochloride. Drug Intell Clin Pharm 1984 Dec; 18: 957-64.
Preskorn SH, Othmer SC. Evaluation of bupropion hydrochloride: The first of a new class of atypical antidepressants. Pharmacotherapy 1984 Jan/Feb; 4 (1): 20-34.

Revised: 07/29/94

# BUSERELIN    Systemic*

VA CLASSIFICATION (Primary): AN500

Note: For a listing of dosage forms and brand names by country availability, see *Dosage Forms* section(s). For a listing of brand names for the articles in this monograph, refer to the General Index.

  *Not commercially available in the U.S.

## Category
Antineoplastic.

## Indications

### Accepted
Carcinoma, prostatic (treatment)—Buserelin is indicated for the palliative treatment of advanced prostatic carcinoma (stage D), especially as an alternative to orchiectomy or estrogen administration.

## Pharmacology/Pharmacokinetics

### Physicochemical characteristics
Molecular weight—1299.49.

### Mechanism of action/Effect
Buserelin is a synthetic luteinizing hormone–releasing hormone (LHRH) analog. Like naturally occurring LHRH that is produced by the hypothalamus, initial or intermittent administration of buserelin stimulates release of luteinizing hormone (LH) and follicle-stimulating hormone (FSH) from the anterior pituitary, which in turn transiently increases testosterone concentrations in males. However, continuous daily administration of buserelin in the treatment of prostatic carcinoma suppresses secretion of LH and FSH, with a resultant fall in testosterone concentrations and a "medical castration".

### Onset of action
Testosterone concentrations—Transient increase occurs within first week of therapy, but decline to castrate levels occurs within 2 to 4 weeks.

## Precautions to Consider

### Carcinogenicity
Studies in rats for two years at daily subcutaneous doses of 0.2 to 1.8 mcg per kg of body weight found no evidence of carcinogenicity.

### Mutagenicity
Mutagenicity studies in bacterial systems (Ames test in *Salmonella typhimurium* and *Escherichia coli*) and mammalian systems (micronuclei test in mice) found no evidence of mutagenic effects.

### Pregnancy/Reproduction
Fertility—Suppression of testosterone secretion results in impairment of fertility. Although it is not known whether fertility is restored after buserelin is withdrawn, reversal of fertility suppression does occur after withdrawal of similar analogs.

### Geriatrics
Appropriate studies on the relationship of age to the effects of buserelin have not been performed in the geriatric population. However, clinical trials were conducted mainly in older patients and geriatrics-specific problems that would limit the usefulness of this medication in the elderly are not expected.

### Laboratory value alterations
The following have been selected on the basis of their potential clinical significance (possible effect in parentheses where appropriate)—not necessarily inclusive (» = major clinical significance):

With physiology/laboratory test values
  Acid phosphatase
    (transient increases in serum values may occur early in treatment, but usually decrease to or near baseline by the fourth week; may decrease to below baseline levels if elevated concentrations were present before treatment)
  Testosterone
    (serum concentrations usually increase during the first week of therapy but then decrease; castrate levels are reached within 2 to 4 weeks)

### Medical considerations/Contraindications
The medical considerations/contraindications included here have been selected on the basis of their potential clinical significance (reasons given in parentheses where appropriate)—not necessarily inclusive (» = major clinical significance).

*Risk-benefit should be considered when the following medical problems exist:*
  Obstructive uropathy, history of
    (increased incidence of disease flare during initial buserelin treatment because of the initial increase in serum testosterone concentrations)
  Sensitivity to buserelin
  Vertebral metastases
    (risk of spinal cord compression as a result of disease flare during initial buserelin treatment)

### Patient monitoring
The following may be especially important in patient monitoring (other tests may be warranted in some patients, depending on condition; » = major clinical significance):

  Acid phosphatase concentrations, plasma prostatic or serum or
  Prostatic specific antigen concentrations, serum and
  Testosterone concentrations, serum
    (recommended at periodic intervals to monitor response)

## Side/Adverse Effects
The following side/adverse effects have been selected on the basis of their potential clinical significance (possible signs and symptoms in parentheses where appropriate)—not necessarily inclusive:

### Those indicating need for medical attention
Incidence less frequent—approximately 1%
  *Possible disease flare* (bone pain; numbness or tingling of hands or feet; trouble in urinating; weakness in legs)
  Note: *Possible disease flare* includes a transient (usually less than 10 days' duration), sometimes severe, increase in bone or tumor pain that may occur shortly after initiation of therapy, usually associated with the increase in serum testosterone, but that usually subsides with continued buserelin treatment. Analgesics may be required during this time. Other signs and symptoms of prostatic carcinoma, including difficult urination, may also worsen transiently. In addition, worsening of neurologic signs and symptoms in patients with vertebral metastases may result in temporary weakness and paresthesias of the lower extremities.

### Those indicating need for medical attention only if they continue or are bothersome
Incidence more frequent—incidence about 50%
  *Hot flashes* (sudden sweating and feelings of warmth)—incidence about 50%; *impotence or decrease in sexual desire*—incidence about 80 to 90%
Incidence less frequent
  *Burning, itching, redness, or swelling at site of injection; diarrhea; dry or sore nose*—with intranasal use only; *headache*—with intranasal use only; *increased sweating*—with intranasal use only; *loss of appetite; nausea or vomiting; swelling and increased tenderness of breasts; swelling of feet or lower legs*

## Patient Consultation
As an aid to patient consultation, refer to *Advice for the Patient, Buserelin (Systemic).*

In providing consultation, consider emphasizing the following selected information (» = major clinical significance):

### Before using this medication
» Conditions affecting use, especially:
  Sensitivity to buserelin
  Pregnancy—Pregnancy/reproduction—May cause sterility

### Proper use of this medication
» Carefully reading and following patient instruction sheet contained in package
  For patients using the injection:
    Using disposable syringes provided in kit
    Proper disposal of used syringes
  For patients using the nasal solution:
    Using nebulizer provided
» Importance of not using more or less medication than the amount prescribed
» Importance of continuing medication despite side effects
» Proper dosing
  Missed dose: Using as soon as remembered; not using if almost time for next dose; not doubling doses
» Proper storage

**Precautions while using this medication**

» Importance of close monitoring by the physician

**Side/adverse effects**

Signs of potential side effects, especially transient disease flare

## General Dosing Information

Patients receiving buserelin should be under supervision of a physician experienced in cancer therapy.

Buserelin has approximately 20 to 170 times the activity of naturally occurring luteinizing hormone–releasing hormone (LHRH) and a longer duration of action.

## Nasal Dosage Forms

### BUSERELIN ACETATE NASAL SOLUTION

**Usual adult dose**

Prostatic carcinoma—

    Maintenance: Intranasal, 400 mcg (0.4 mg) (base) (200 mcg in each nostril) every eight hours.

    Note: Initial treatment is by subcutaneous injection.

        Each pump action delivers 100 mcg (0.1 mL) of medication.

**Strength(s) usually available**

U.S.—

    Not commercially available.

Canada—

    1 mg (base) per mL (Rx) [*Suprefact* (benzyl alcohol 10 mg per mL; no propellants)].

**Packaging and storage**

Store below 25 °C (77 °F), unless otherwise specified by manufacturer. Protect from freezing.

**Auxiliary labeling**

• Do not freeze.

## Parenteral Dosage Forms

### BUSERELIN ACETATE INJECTION

**Usual adult dose**

Prostatic carcinoma—

    Initial: Subcutaneous, 500 mcg (0.5 mg) (base) every eight hours for seven days.

    Maintenance: Subcutaneous, 200 mcg (0.2 mg) (base) once a day.

    Note: Alternatively, the nasal solution may be used for maintenance dosing.

**Strength(s) usually available**

U.S.—

    Not commercially available.

Canada—

    1 mg (base) per mL (Rx) [*Suprefact* (benzyl alcohol 10 mg per mL)].

**Packaging and storage**

Store below 25 °C (77 °F), unless otherwise specified by manufacturer. Protect from freezing.

**Auxiliary labeling**

• Do not freeze.

## Selected Bibliography

Schroder FH (ed.). New treatment modalities in prostatic cancer: LHRH superagonists. Symposium held during World Congress of Oncology, Budapest, Hungary, August 26, 1986. Am J Clin Oncol 1988; 11 (Suppl 1): S1-46.

The management of clinically localized prostate cancer. National Institutes of Health Consensus Development Conference Statement 1987 June 15–17; 6 (10).

Korman LB. Treatment of prostate cancer. Clin Pharm 1989 Jun; 8: 412-24.

Furr BJA, Woodburn JR. Luteinizing hormone–releasing hormone and its analogues: a review of biological properties and clinical uses. J Endocrinol Invest 1988 Jul–Aug; 11: 535-57.

Revised: 07/11/94

---

# BUSPIRONE    Systemic

**VA CLASSIFICATION (Primary): CN309**

Note: For a listing of dosage forms and brand names by country availability, see *Dosage Forms* section(s). For a listing of brand names for the articles in this monograph, refer to the General Index.

## Category

Antianxiety agent.

## Indications

### Accepted

Anxiety (treatment)—Buspirone is indicated for the management of anxiety disorders or the short-term relief of the symptoms of anxiety. However, buspirone is usually not indicated for the treatment of anxiety or tension associated with the stress of everyday life.

    The efficacy of buspirone in the treatment of anxiety has been shown to be comparable to that of benzodiazepines, such as diazepam, clorazepate, alprazolam, and lorazepam.

    Buspirone has been shown to cause less sedation than other antianxiety agents, especially at lower doses. Therefore, it may be a useful alternative to other antianxiety agents in the treatment of generalized anxiety, particularly in patients hypersensitive to the sedative effects of the other agents.

    In controlled studies, buspirone has not been shown to be effective for long-term (more than 3 to 4 weeks) management of anxiety. However, buspirone has not been shown to cause adverse effects when used for several months. If buspirone is used for extended periods of time, efficacy of the medication should be reassessed at periodic intervals.

## Pharmacology/Pharmacokinetics

Note: Buspirone is not pharmacologically related to benzodiazepines, barbiturates, or other sedative/antianxiety agents.

**Physicochemical characteristics**

Molecular weight—421.97.

**Mechanism of action/Effect**

The site and mechanism of action of buspirone have not been determined. The medication is believed to have a unique anxioselective action, since it has no anticonvulsant or muscle relaxant activity and does not appear to cause physical dependence or significant sedation. Buspirone has been shown to have a high affinity for serotonin (5-HT$_{1A}$) receptors in the dorsal raphe neurons and a moderate affinity for brain D$_2$-dopamine receptors. It has no significant affinity for benzodiazepine receptors and does not affect gamma-aminobutyric acid (GABA) binding. Some studies have suggested that buspirone may have indirect effects on other neurotransmitter systems.

In contrast to the benzodiazepines, the spontaneous firing rate of noradrenergic cells in the locus ceruleus is increased rather than decreased by buspirone. Differences in dependence and tolerance between benzodiazepines and buspirone are due to these site-specific differences.

**Absorption**

Rapidly and completely absorbed from the gastrointestinal tract; however, extensive first-pass metabolism limits the bioavailability of buspirone.

Although concurrent administration of food slows the rate of absorption of buspirone, the presence of food increases the amount of unchanged buspirone reaching systemic circulation.

**Protein binding**

Plasma—Very high (95%). Although buspirone is highly protein-bound, it apparently does not displace other highly protein-bound medications, such as warfarin.

**Biotransformation**

Hepatic. Buspirone is rapidly metabolized and undergoes extensive first-pass metabolism. It is metabolized primarily by oxidation, producing several hydroxylated derivatives and a pharmacologically active metabolite, 1-pyrimidinylpiperazine (1-PP). In animal studies, 1-PP has been shown to have about one-fourth the activity of buspirone.

**Half-life**

Elimination (mean)—

    About 2 to 3 hours following single doses of 10 to 40 mg.

**Onset of therapeutic effect**
May require 1 to 2 weeks. Because buspirone does not cause muscle relaxation or significant sedation, patient may not immediately notice effects of medication.

**Time to peak plasma concentration**
40 to 90 minutes following single oral doses of 20 mg; and less than 1 hour following single oral doses of 10 mg.

**Peak plasma concentration**
Following oral administration, plasma concentrations of unchanged buspirone are very low and vary among individuals; 1 to 6 nanograms per mL 40 to 90 minutes following single oral doses of 20 mg.

Note: Dose increases and repeated dosing may result in higher blood concentrations of unchanged buspirone.

**Elimination**
In a single-dose study—
Renal: 29 to 63% of dose excreted in urine within 24 hours, primarily as metabolites.
Fecal: 18 to 38% of dose excreted in feces.
In dialysis—
Dialyzability of buspirone has not been determined.

## Precautions to Consider

**Carcinogenicity**
Buspirone was not shown to be potentially carcinogenic when it was administered to rats during a 24-month study at doses approximately 133 times the maximum recommended human oral dose or to mice during an 18-month study at doses approximately 167 times the maximum recommended human oral dose.

**Mutagenicity**
Buspirone was not shown to induce point mutations, with or without metabolic activation, in 5 strains of *Salmonella typhimurium* (Ames test) or mouse lymphoma L5178YTK+ cell cultures, nor was DNA damage observed with buspirone in Wi-38 human cells. Also, chromosomal abnormalities did not occur in bone marrow cells of mice given 1 or 5 daily doses of buspirone.

**Pregnancy/Reproduction**
Fertility—Reproduction studies in rats and rabbits showed no impairment of fertility when buspirone was administered at doses approximately 30 times the maximum recommended human dose (MRHD).

Pregnancy—Adequate and well-controlled studies in humans have not been done.

Reproduction studies in rats and mice have not shown buspirone to cause fetal damage when the medication was administered at doses approximately 30 times the MRHD.

FDA Pregnancy Category B.

Labor and delivery—Reproduction studies in rats have not shown buspirone to cause any adverse effects on labor and delivery.

**Breast-feeding**
Problems in humans have not been documented. However, buspirone and its metabolites are excreted in the milk of rats.

**Pediatrics**
Appropriate studies on the relationship of age to the effects of buspirone have not been performed in children up to 18 years of age. Safety and efficacy have not been established.

**Geriatrics**
Although buspirone has not been systematically evaluated in older patients, clinical studies performed in several hundred elderly patients have not demonstrated geriatrics-specific problems that would limit the usefulness of buspirone in the elderly. However, elderly patients are more likely to have age-related renal function impairment, which may require reduction of dosage in patients receiving buspirone.

**Drug interactions and/or related problems**
The following drug interactions and/or related problems have been selected on the basis of their potential clinical significance (possible mechanism in parentheses where appropriate)—not necessarily inclusive (» = major clinical significance):

Note: Combinations containing any of the following medications, depending on the amount present, may also interact with this medication.

Alcohol or
Central nervous system (CNS) depression–producing medications, other
(See *Appendix II*)
(although studies have shown that buspirone does not increase alcohol-induced impairment in mental and motor performance, caution is recommended with the concurrent use of buspirone and alcohol or other CNS depressants, since buspirone may cause

sedation, especially at doses greater than 30 mg per day, and its CNS effects in an individual patient may not be predictable)

Digoxin
(may be displaced from serum protein binding when used concurrently with buspirone)

» Monoamine oxidase (MAO) inhibitors, including furazolidone, procarbazine, and more than 10 mg a day of selegiline
(concurrent use with buspirone is not recommended because an elevation in blood pressure may occur)

**Medical considerations/Contraindications**
The medical considerations/contraindications included here have been selected on the basis of their potential clinical significance (reasons given in parentheses where appropriate)—not necessarily inclusive (» = major clinical significance).

*Risk-benefit should be considered when the following medical problems exist:*

Drug abuse or dependence, history of
(potential misuse or abuse of buspirone; patients should be observed closely for development of tolerance, incrementation of dose, and drug-seeking behavior)

Hepatic function impairment
(buspirone metabolized by liver)

Renal function impairment
(buspirone excreted via kidneys)

Sensitivity to buspirone

**Patient monitoring**
The following may be especially important in patient monitoring (other tests may be warranted in some patients, depending on condition; » = major clinical significance):

Hepatic function determinations and
Renal function determinations
(monitoring may be required; dosage adjustment may be necessary)

## Side/Adverse Effects

Note: Buspirone appears to have little potential for physical dependence or abuse. Although it does not produce euphoria and usually does not produce sedation at doses of 20 mg per day, buspirone has been shown to cause dysphoria and sedation at doses greater than 30 mg per day.

Studies have shown that buspirone causes less sedation than other antianxiety agents (about one-third of that occurring with benzodiazepines) and does not produce significant functional impairment. However, the CNS effects of buspirone in any individual patient may not be predictable.

If side/adverse effects occur, they usually appear at the beginning of buspirone therapy and subside during continued therapy, with or without dosage reduction.

Withdrawal symptoms or rebound anxiety has not been reported when the medication was abruptly discontinued.

The following side/adverse effects have been selected on the basis of their potential clinical significance (possible signs and symptoms in parentheses where appropriate)—not necessarily inclusive:

**Those indicating need for medical attention**
Incidence rare
*Chest pain; confusion or mental depression; fast or pounding heartbeat; neurological effects* (muscle weakness; numbness, tingling, pain, or weakness in hands or feet; uncontrolled movements of the body); *sore throat or fever*

**Those indicating need for medical attention only if they continue or are bothersome**
Incidence more frequent
*Dizziness or lightheadedness; headache; nausea; syndrome of restlessness* (restlessness, nervousness, or unusual excitement)

Note: May occur shortly after buspirone therapy is initiated; may be due to increased central noradrenergic activity or to dopaminergic effects.

Incidence less frequent or rare
*Blurred vision; decreased concentration; drowsiness*—more frequent with doses >20 mg per day; *dryness of mouth; musculoskeletal effects* (muscle pain, spasms, cramps, or stiffness); *ringing in the ears; stomach upset; trouble in sleeping; nightmares; or vivid dreams; unusual tiredness or weakness*

## Overdose

For more information on the management of overdose or unintentional ingestion, **contact a Poison Control Center** (see *Poison Control Center Listing*).

### Clinical effects of overdose

The following effects have been selected on the basis of their potential clinical significance (possible signs and symptoms in parentheses where appropriate)—not necessarily inclusive:

*Dizziness, severe; drowsiness, severe; stomach upset, including severe nausea or vomiting; unusually small pupils*

### Treatment of overdose

There is no known specific antidote to buspirone. Recommended treatment of buspirone overdose consists of the following:

To decrease absorption—
   Immediate gastric lavage.
Monitoring—
   Monitoring of respiration, pulse, and blood pressure.
Supportive care—
   General symptomatic and supportive measures. Patients in whom intentional overdose is known or suspected should be referred for psychiatric consultation.

## Patient Consultation

As an aid to patient consultation, refer to *Advice for the Patient, Buspirone (Systemic)*.

In providing consultation, consider emphasizing the following selected information (» = major clinical significance):

### Before using this medication

» Conditions affecting use, especially:
      Sensitivity to buspirone
      Other medications, especially monoamine oxidase (MAO) inhibitors

### Proper use of this medication

» Importance of not using more medication than the amount prescribed
   One to two weeks of therapy may be required before antianxiety effect is noticeable
» Proper dosing
   Missed dose: If on scheduled dosing regimen—Taking as soon as possible; not taking if almost time for next dose; not doubling doses
» Proper storage

### Precautions while using this medication

   Regular visits to physician to check progress during prolonged therapy
   Caution in taking alcohol or other CNS depressants during therapy
» Caution if dizziness or drowsiness occurs
» Suspected overdose: Getting emergency help at once

### Side/adverse effects

   Signs of potential side effects, especially chest pain, confusion, fast or pounding heartbeat, mental depression, neurological effects, and sore throat or fever

## General Dosing Information

Although buspirone does not appear to cause tolerance or physical or psychological dependence, patients with a history of drug abuse or dependence should be observed closely for development of tolerance to or dependence on the medication.

Since buspirone does not exhibit cross-tolerance with benzodiazepines and other common sedative/hypnotic agents, the medication will not block the withdrawal syndrome associated with discontinuation of therapy with these agents. Therefore, prior to initiating therapy with buspirone, these agents should be withdrawn gradually, especially in patients who have been chronically using these CNS depressants.

One to two weeks of therapy may be required before the antianxiety effect of buspirone is noticeable, as compared to the immediate effect of benzodiazepines.

## Oral Dosage Forms

### BUSPIRONE HYDROCHLORIDE TABLETS

#### Usual adult dose

Antianxiety—
   Oral, initially 5 mg three times a day, the dosage being increased by 5 mg per day at two- to three-day intervals until the desired response is obtained.

#### Usual adult prescribing limits

Up to 60 mg per day.

#### Usual pediatric dose

Antianxiety—
   Children up to 18 years of age: Safety and efficacy have not been established.

#### Strength(s) usually available

U.S.—
   5 mg (Rx) [*BuSpar* (scored; lactose; sodium starch glycolate)].
   10 mg (Rx) [*BuSpar* (scored; lactose; sodium starch glycolate)].
Canada—
   5 mg (Rx) [*BuSpar*].
   10 mg (Rx) [*BuSpar* (scored)].

#### Packaging and storage

Store between 15 and 30 °C (59 and 86 °F), in a tight, light-resistant container, unless otherwise specified by manufacturer.

#### Auxiliary labeling

• Avoid alcoholic beverages.
• May cause dizziness or drowsiness.

Revised: 03/09/93

---

# BUSULFAN   Systemic

VA CLASSIFICATION (Primary): AN100
Note: For a listing of dosage forms and brand names by country availability, see *Dosage Forms* section(s). For a listing of brand names for the articles in this monograph, refer to the General Index.

## Category

Antineoplastic.

## Indications

Note: Bracketed information in the *Indications* section refers to uses that are not included in U.S. product labeling.

### Accepted

Leukemia, chronic myelocytic (treatment)—Busulfan is indicated for palliative treatment of chronic myelocytic leukemia. It is not useful in the "blastic crisis" phase.

[Leukemia, acute myelocytic (treatment)][1]—Busulfan is used for treatment of acute myelocytic leukemia.

---

[1]Not included in Canadian product labeling.

## Pharmacology/Pharmacokinetics

### Physicochemical characteristics

Molecular weight—246.29.

### Mechanism of action/Effect

Busulfan is a bifunctional alkylating agent of the alkylsulfonate type and is cell cycle–phase nonspecific. Its mechanism of action is not clear but is thought to consist of alkylation and cross-linking of strands of DNA and myelosuppression.

### Absorption

Completely absorbed from the gastrointestinal tract. Radioactivity is detected in the blood $1/2$ to 2 hours after oral administration of radiolabeled busulfan.

### Biotransformation

Hepatic; rapid.

### Half-life

About 2.5 hours.

### Onset of action

A clinical response usually begins within 1 to 2 weeks after initiation of therapy.

## Elimination
Renal, slow, almost entirely as metabolites.

In dialysis—No information available; however, likely to have minimal effect because of poor water solubility of busulfan and prolonged retention of metabolites.

# Precautions to Consider

### Carcinogenicity
Secondary malignancies are potential delayed effects of many antineoplastic agents, although it is not clear whether the effect is related to their mutagenic or immunosuppressive action. The effect of dose and duration of therapy is also unknown, although risk seems to increase with long-term use. Although information is limited, available data seem to indicate that the carcinogenic risk is greatest with the alkylating agents.

Busulfan has been associated with development of acute leukemia in humans.

### Mutagenicity
Busulfan is mutagenic in mice. It has been reported to cause chromosome aberrations in human cells.

### Pregnancy/Reproduction
Fertility—Gonadal suppression, resulting in amenorrhea or azoospermia, may occur in patients taking antineoplastic therapy, especially with the alkylating agents. In general, these effects appear to be related to dose and length of therapy and may be irreversible. Prediction of the degree of testicular or ovarian function impairment is complicated by the common use of combinations of several antineoplastics, which makes it difficult to assess the effects of individual agents.

Busulfan produces sterility in the male and female offspring of rats due to germinal cell aplasia in testes and ovaries. It has also been associated with impairment of gonadal function in humans (ovarian suppression and amenorrhea with menopausal symptoms in premenopausal patients; sterility, azoospermia, and testicular atrophy in males).

Pregnancy—Adequate and well-controlled studies in humans have not been done. Although several successful pregnancies have been reported, one case of neonatal abnormalities has been reported in which the mother received radiation and combination chemotherapy including busulfan. In addition, there have been reports of small infants, especially after use of busulfan during the third trimester, and there is one report of mild anemia and neutropenia at birth after maternal administration of busulfan from the eighth week of pregnancy to term.

First trimester: It is usually recommended that use of antineoplastics, especially combination chemotherapy, be avoided whenever possible, especially during the first trimester. Although information is limited because of the relatively few instances of antineoplastic administration during pregnancy, the mutagenic, teratogenic, and carcinogenic potential of these medications must be considered.

Other hazards to the fetus include adverse reactions seen in adults.

In general, use of a contraceptive is recommended during cytotoxic drug therapy.

FDA Pregnancy Category D.

### Breast-feeding
Although very little information is available regarding distribution of antineoplastic agents into breast milk, breast-feeding is not recommended during chemotherapy because of the risks to the infant (adverse effects, mutagenicity, carcinogenicity). It is not known whether busulfan is distributed into breast milk.

### Pediatrics
Appropriate studies performed to date have not demonstrated pediatrics-specific problems that would limit the usefulness of busulfan in children.

### Geriatrics
Appropriate studies on the relationship of age to the effects of busulfan have not been performed in the geriatric population. However, geriatrics-specific problems that would limit the usefulness of this medication in the elderly are not expected.

### Dental
The bone marrow depressant effects of busulfan may result in an increased incidence of microbial infection, delayed healing, and gingival bleeding. Dental work, whenever possible, should be completed prior to initiation of therapy or deferred until blood counts have returned to normal. Patients should be instructed in proper oral hygiene during treatment, including caution in use of regular toothbrushes, dental floss, and toothpicks.

Busulfan may also cause stomatitis associated with considerable discomfort.

### Drug interactions and/or related problems
The following drug interactions and/or related problems have been selected on the basis of their potential clinical significance (possible mechanism in parentheses where appropriate)—not necessarily inclusive (» = major clinical significance):

Note: Combinations containing any of the following medications, depending on the amount present, may also interact with this medication.

Allopurinol or
Colchicine or
» Probenecid or
» Sulfinpyrazone
   (busulfan may raise the concentration of blood uric acid; dosage adjustment of antigout agents may be necessary to control hyperuricemia and gout; allopurinol may be preferred to prevent or reverse busulfan-induced hyperuricemia because of risk of uric acid nephropathy with uricosuric antigout agents)

Blood dyscrasia–causing medications (See *Appendix II*)
   (leukopenic and/or thrombocytopenic effects of busulfan may be increased with concurrent or recent therapy if these medications cause the same effects; dosage adjustment of busulfan, if necessary, should be based on blood counts)

» Bone marrow depressants, other (See *Appendix II*) or
» Radiation therapy
   (additive bone marrow depression may occur; dosage reduction may be required when two or more bone marrow depressants, including radiation, are used concurrently or consecutively)

Vaccines, killed virus
   (because normal defense mechanisms may be suppressed by busulfan therapy, the patient's antibody response to the vaccine may be decreased. The interval between discontinuation of medications that cause immunosuppression and restoration of the patient's ability to respond to the vaccine depends on the intensity and type of immunosuppression-causing medication used, the underlying disease, and other factors; estimates vary from 3 months to 1 year)

» Vaccines, live virus
   (because normal defense mechanisms may be suppressed by busulfan therapy, concurrent use with a live virus vaccine may potentiate the replication of the vaccine virus, may increase the side/adverse effects of the vaccine virus, and/or may decrease the patient's antibody response to the vaccine; immunization of these patients should be undertaken only with extreme caution after careful review of the patient's hematologic status and only with the knowledge and consent of the physician managing the busulfan therapy. The interval between discontinuation of medications that cause immunosuppression and restoration of the patient's ability to respond to the vaccine depends on the intensity and type of immunosuppression-causing medication used, the underlying disease, and other factors; estimates vary from 3 months to 1 year. Patients with leukemia in remission should not receive live virus vaccine until at least 3 months after their last chemotherapy. In addition, immunization with oral poliovirus vaccine should be postponed in persons in close contact with the patient, especially family members)

### Laboratory value alterations
The following have been selected on the basis of their potential clinical significance (possible effect in parentheses where appropriate)—not necessarily inclusive (» = major clinical significance):

With diagnostic test results
   Cytology studies of lung, bladder, breast, or uterine cervix tissue
   (cytologic dysplasia caused by busulfan may be severe enough to cause difficulty in interpretation)

With physiology/laboratory test values
   Uric acid in blood and urine
   (concentrations may be increased)

### Medical considerations/Contraindications
The medical considerations/contraindications included here have been selected on the basis of their potential clinical significance (reasons given in parentheses where appropriate)—not necessarily inclusive (» = major clinical significance).

*Risk-benefit should be considered when the following medical problems exist:*

» Bone marrow depression
» Chickenpox, existing or recent (including recent exposure) or
» Herpes zoster
   (risk of severe generalized disease)

Gout, history of or
Urate renal stones, history of
   (risk of hyperuricemia)

» Infection
Sensitivity to busulfan

Caution is necessary when using very high doses of busulfan in patients with head trauma or a history of seizure disorder; some clinicians use prophylactic anticonvulsant therapy.

» Caution should be used also in patients who have had previous cytotoxic drug therapy or radiation therapy or who have evidence of myelofibrosis.

### Patient monitoring

The following are especially important in patient monitoring (other tests may be warranted in some patients, depending on condition; » = major clinical significance):

Alanine aminotransferase values, serum and
Alkaline phosphatase values, serum and
Bilirubin concentrations, serum
    (recommended at periodic intervals to detect possible hepatotoxicity, including hepatic veno-occlusive disease)

» Hematocrit or hemoglobin and
» Leukocyte count, total and, if appropriate, differential and
    Platelet count
    (determinations recommended prior to initiation of therapy and at periodic intervals during therapy; frequency varies according to clinical state, agent, dose, and other agents being used concurrently; because of severe and delayed myelosuppression caused by busulfan, frequent monitoring is necessary so that therapy can be withdrawn promptly when indicated)

Uric acid concentrations, serum
    (recommended prior to initiation of therapy and at periodic intervals during therapy; frequency varies according to clinical state, agent, dose, and other agents being used concurrently)

## Side/Adverse Effects

Note: Many "side effects" of antineoplastic therapy are unavoidable and represent the medication's pharmacologic action. Some of these (for example, leukopenia and thrombocytopenia) are actually used as parameters to aid in individual dosage titration.

Busulfan can cause cellular dysplasia in many tissues, including lungs, lymph nodes, pancreas, thyroid, adrenal gland, liver, bone marrow, bladder, breast, and uterine cervix.

Seizures have been reported in 2 of 130 patients receiving very high investigational doses (1 mg per kg of body weight [mg/kg] four times a day for four days, total dose 16 mg/kg).

Hepatic veno-occlusive disease has been reported following investigational use of very high doses of busulfan in combination with other chemotherapy prior to bone marrow transplantation.

Continuous treatment with a combination of busulfan and thioguanine in approximately 330 patients was associated with esophageal varices along with abnormal hepatic function tests and evidence of nodular regenerative hyperplasia on liver biopsy in 12 patients after six to forty-five months of therapy. No hepatic toxicity was found in the busulfan alone arm of the study.

The following side/adverse effects have been selected on the basis of their potential clinical significance (possible signs and symptoms in parentheses where appropriate)—not necessarily inclusive:

### Those indicating need for medical attention
Incidence more frequent
    *Anemia; leukopenia or infection* (usually asymptomatic; less frequently, fever or chills; cough or hoarseness; lower back or side pain; painful or difficult urination); *thrombocytopenia* (unusual bleeding or bruising; black, tarry stools; blood in urine or stools; pinpoint red spots on skin)
    Note: Onset of *leukopenia* is usually 10 to 15 days after initiation of therapy (leukocyte counts usually increase transiently before this), with nadir of white cell count at 11 to 30 days; white cell counts may continue to fall for more than 1 month after withdrawal but usually recover within 12 to 20 weeks.
        *Bone marrow depression* may be severe and progressive, leading to pancytopenia. Recovery from pancytopenia after withdrawal of busulfan may take 1 month to 2 years.
        Symptoms of *bone marrow depression* may also indicate transformation of chronic myelocytic leukemia into the acute blastic form.

Incidence less frequent—occurring with long-term use or high dosage
    *Bronchopulmonary dysplasia with pulmonary fibrosis* (fever; cough; shortness of breath); *hyperuricemia or uric acid nephropathy* (joint pain; lower back or side pain; swelling of feet or lower legs); *stomatitis* (sores in mouth and on lips)
    Note: *Bronchopulmonary dysplasia with pulmonary fibrosis* usually occurs 8 months to 10 years (average 4 years) after initiation of

therapy and is usually fatal within 6 months after diagnosis. Associated with decreased diffusion capacity and pulmonary compliance. Histologically resembles changes following pulmonary irradiation. Lung biopsy may be necessary to establish the diagnosis.
    *Hyperuricemia or uric acid nephropathy* occurs most commonly during initial treatment of patients with leukemia or lymphoma, as a result of rapid cell breakdown which leads to elevated serum uric acid concentrations.

Incidence rare
    *Cataracts* (blurred vision)—occur after prolonged administration

### Those indicating need for medical attention only if they continue or are bothersome
Incidence more frequent
    *Amenorrhea and ovarian suppression* (missed or irregular menstrual periods); *darkening of skin*—5 to 10%
Incidence less frequent—occurring with long-term use
    *Confusion; diarrhea; hypotension* (dizziness); *loss of appetite; nausea and vomiting; unusual tiredness or weakness; sudden weight loss*
    Note: All of the above, as well as darkening of skin, may occur after prolonged therapy and may resemble adrenocortical insufficiency, although adrenocortical function is not suppressed in most patients. Symptoms are sometimes reversible on withdrawal of busulfan. Adrenal responsiveness to exogenous adrenocorticotropic hormone (ACTH) is usually normal, but pituitary function testing with metyrapone has shown blunted urinary 17-hydroxycorticosteroid excretion in some patients that returned to normal when busulfan was discontinued.

### Those indicating the need for medical attention if they occur after medication is discontinued
    *Bone marrow depression, thrombocytopenia, pancytopenia* (unusual bleeding or bruising; black, tarry stools; blood in urine or stools; pinpoint red spots on skin; fever or chills; cough or hoarseness; lower back or side pain; painful or difficult urination); *pulmonary fibrosis* (fever; cough; shortness of breath)

## Overdose

For more information on the management of overdose or unintentional ingestion, **contact a Poison Control Center** (see *Poison Control Center Listing*).

### Treatment of overdose
Induction of vomiting or gastric lavage followed by administration of charcoal if ingestion is recent.

Monitoring of hematologic status and supportive measures if necessary.

## Patient Consultation

As an aid to patient consultation, refer to *Advice for the Patient, Busulfan (Systemic)*.

In providing consultation, consider emphasizing the following selected information (» = major clinical significance):

### Before using this medication
» Conditions affecting use, especially:
    Sensitivity to busulfan
    Pregnancy—Use not recommended because of mutagenic, teratogenic, and carcinogenic potential; advisability of using contraception; telling physician immediately if pregnancy is suspected
    Breast-feeding—Not recommended because of risk of serious side effects
    Other medications, especially probenecid, sulfinpyrazone, other bone marrow depressants, or previous cytotoxic drug therapy or radiation therapy
    Other medical problems, especially chickenpox, herpes zoster, or infection

### Proper use of this medication
» Importance of not taking more or less medication than the amount prescribed
    Taking each dose at the same time each day to ensure uniform effect
    Importance of ample fluid intake and subsequent increase in urine output to aid in excretion of uric acid
» Possible nausea and vomiting; importance of continuing medication despite stomach upset
    Checking with physician if vomiting occurs shortly after dose is taken
» Proper dosing
    Missed dose: Not taking at all; not doubling doses
» Proper storage

### Precautions while using this medication
» Importance of close monitoring by the physician

» Avoiding immunizations unless approved by physician; other persons in patient's household should avoid immunizations with oral poliovirus vaccine; avoiding persons who have taken oral poliovirus vaccine or wearing a protective mask that covers nose and mouth

*Caution if bone marrow depression occurs*

» Avoiding exposure to persons with bacterial infections, especially during periods of low blood counts; checking with physician immediately if fever or chills, cough or hoarseness, lower back or side pain, or painful or difficult urination occurs

» Checking with physician immediately if unusual bleeding or bruising; black, tarry stools; blood in urine or stools; or pinpoint red spots on skin occur

Caution in use of regular toothbrush, dental floss, or toothpick; physician, dentist, or nurse may suggest alternatives; checking with physician before having dental work done

Not touching eyes or inside of nose unless hands washed immediately before

Using caution to avoid accidental cuts with use of sharp objects such as safety razor or fingernail or toenail cutters

Avoiding contact sports or other situations where bruising or injury might occur

Caution if any laboratory tests required; possible interference with tissue study results

### Side/adverse effects

May cause adverse effects such as lung or blood problems; importance of discussing possible effects with physician

Signs of potential side effects, especially anemia, leukopenia, infection, thrombocytopenia, bronchopulmonary dysplasia with pulmonary fibrosis, hyperuricemia, uric acid nephropathy, stomatitis, and cataracts

Physician or nurse can help in dealing with side effects

## General Dosing Information

Patients receiving busulfan should be under supervision of a physician experienced in cancer chemotherapy.

Dosage must be adjusted to meet the individual requirements of each patient, based on clinical response and degree of bone marrow depression.

Development of uric acid nephropathy in patients with leukemia or lymphoma may be prevented by adequate oral hydration and, in some cases, administration of allopurinol. Alkalinization of urine may be necessary if serum uric acid concentrations are elevated.

Busulfan therapy should be discontinued at the first sign of interstitial pulmonary fibrosis.

Because of the delayed effect, it is recommended that busulfan therapy be discontinued or dosage reduced at the first sign of a sudden large decrease in leukocyte (particularly granulocyte) count to prevent irreversible bone marrow depression.

Special precautions are recommended in patients who develop thrombocytopenia as a result of administration of busulfan. These may include extreme care in performing invasive procedures; regular inspection of intravenous sites, skin (including perirectal area), and mucous membrane surfaces for signs of bleeding or bruising; limiting frequency of venipuncture and avoiding intramuscular injections; testing urine, emesis, stool, and secretions for occult blood; care in use of regular toothbrushes, dental floss, toothpicks, safety razors, and fingernail and toenail cutters; avoiding constipation; and using caution to prevent falls and other injuries. Such patients should avoid alcohol and aspirin intake because of the risk of gastrointestinal bleeding. Platelet transfusions may be required.

Patients who develop leukopenia should be observed carefully for signs of infection. Antibiotic support may be required. In neutropenic patients who develop fever, broad-spectrum antibiotic coverage should be initiated empirically, pending bacterial cultures and appropriate diagnostic tests.

## Oral Dosage Forms

### BUSULFAN TABLETS USP

**Usual adult dose**
Chronic myelocytic leukemia—
Induction:
Oral, 1.8 mg per square meter of body surface or 60 mcg (0.06 mg) per kg of body weight a day until the white cell count falls below 15,000 cells per cubic millimeter. Usual dosage

range is 4 to 8 mg per day but may range from 1 to 12 mg per day. During remission, treatment is resumed when a monthly white cell count reaches 50,000 cells per cubic millimeter.

Note: Some patients may be unusually sensitive to busulfan and develop myelosuppression more rapidly than usual. Therefore, frequent and careful monitoring of blood counts is necessary. The total leukocyte count decreases exponentially at a constant busulfan dose, so a weekly plot of leukocyte count on semi-logarithmic paper can aid in predicting when leukocyte counts will reach 15,000 and busulfan should be discontinued.

Maintenance:
Oral, 1 to 3 mg per day.

Note: Maintenance therapy with busulfan is recommended only when a remission is shorter than 3 months.

**Usual pediatric dose**
Chronic myelocytic leukemia—
Induction: Oral, 60 to 120 mcg (0.06 to 0.12 mg) per kg of body weight or 1.8 to 4.6 mg per square meter of body surface per day.

Note: Dosage is titrated to reduce and maintain a leukocyte count of about 20,000 cells per cubic millimeter.

**Strength(s) usually available**
U.S.—
2 mg (Rx) [*Myleran* (scored)].
Canada—
2 mg (Rx) [*Myleran* (scored)].

**Packaging and storage**
Store below 40 °C (104 °F), preferably between 15 and 25 °C (59 and 77 °F), unless otherwise specified by manufacturer. Store in a well-closed container.

## Selected Bibliography

Rushing D et al. Hydroxyurea versus busulfan in the treatment of chronic myelogenous leukemia. Am J Clin Oncol 1982; 5: 307-13.

Revised: 06/12/92
Interim revision: 05/02/94

---

**BUTABARBITAL**—See *Barbiturates (Systemic)*

---

## BUTABARBITAL-CONTAINING COMBINATIONS—

Belladonna and Butabarbital (Systemic)—See *Belladonna Alkaloids and Barbiturates (Systemic)*

---

**BUTACAINE**—See *Anesthetics (Mucosal-Local)*

---

## BUTALBITAL-CONTAINING COMBINATIONS—

Butalbital and Acetaminophen (Systemic)—See *Barbiturates and Analgesics (Systemic)*

Butalbital, Acetaminophen, and Caffeine (Systemic)—See *Barbiturates and Analgesics (Systemic)*

Butalbital and Aspirin (Systemic)—See *Barbiturates and Analgesics (Systemic)*

Butalbital, Aspirin, and Caffeine (Systemic)—See *Barbiturates and Analgesics (Systemic)*

Butalbital, Aspirin, Caffeine, and Codeine (Systemic)—See *Barbiturates and Analgesics (Systemic)*

---

**BUTAMBEN**—See *Anesthetics (Topical)*

---

## BUTAMBEN-CONTAINING COMBINATIONS—

Benzocaine, Butamben, and Tetracaine (Mucosal-Local)—See *Anesthetics (Mucosal-Local)*

---

**BUTOCONAZOLE**—See *Antifungals, Azole (Vaginal)*

---

**BUTORPHANOL**—See *Opioid (Narcotic) Analgesics (Systemic)*

# CAFFEINE   Systemic

This monograph includes information on the following: Caffeine; Citrated Caffeine; Caffeine and Sodium Benzoate†.

VA CLASSIFICATION (Primary/Secondary):
Caffeine—CN809/RE900
Caffeine, Citrated—CN809/RE900
Caffeine and Sodium Benzoate—CN809

Note: For a listing of dosage forms and brand names by country availability, see *Dosage Forms* section(s). For a listing of brand names for the articles in this monograph, refer to the General Index.

---

†Not commercially available in Canada.

---

## Category

Central nervous system stimulant—Caffeine; Citrated Caffeine; Caffeine and Sodium Benzoate.
Analgesia adjunct—Caffeine.
Respiratory stimulant adjunct—Caffeine; Citrated Caffeine.

## Indications

Note: Bracketed information in the *Indications* section refers to uses that are not included in U.S. product labeling.

### Accepted

Fatigue or
Drowsiness (treatment)—Caffeine is used as a mild central nervous system stimulant to help restore mental alertness or wakefulness when fatigue or drowsiness is experienced.

[Apnea, neonatal (treatment adjunct)]—Caffeine or citrated caffeine (but not caffeine and sodium benzoate combination) is used in the management of neonatal apnea, especially primary apnea of prematurity, which is characterized by periodic breathing and apneic episodes of more than 15 seconds accompanied by cyanosis and bradycardia. However, caffeine should be considered only as an adjunct to nondrug measures such as decreased ambient temperature, oxygen, sensory stimulation, and mechanical support of ventilation. Caffeine may be considered a desirable alternative to theophylline when initiating therapy for premature neonatal apnea because some infants are unable to convert theophylline to caffeine, a major metabolite of theophylline in neonates. Caffeine also has a wider therapeutic index than theophylline. Caffeine therapy in the management of apnea is usually required for only a few weeks and rarely for more than a few months, the apnea usually resolving by about 34 to 36 weeks' gestational age.

[Apnea, infant, postoperative (prophylaxis)]—Caffeine or citrated caffeine has been used for the prevention of postoperative apnea in former preterm infants.

[Electroconvulsive therapy (ECT) (treatment adjunct)]—Caffeine pretreatment is used to augment ECT by increasing seizure duration and reducing the need for increases in stimulus intensity.

Caffeine is used in combination with ergotamine to treat vascular headaches such as migraine and cluster headaches (histaminic cephalalgia, migrainous neuralgia, Horton's headache).

Caffeine is also used, and has been shown to be effective, as an analgesic adjunct in combination with aspirin or acetaminophen and aspirin to enhance pain relief, although it has no analgesic activity of its own. However, caffeine's efficacy as an analgesic adjunct in combination with acetaminophen alone has been questioned.

### Unaccepted

Caffeine and sodium benzoate combination has been used in conjunction with other supportive measures to treat respiratory depression associated with overdose with central nervous system (CNS) depressants such as narcotic analgesics or alcohol; however, because of the availability of specific antagonists, such as flumazenil and naloxone, and caffeine's questionable benefit and transient effect, most authorities believe caffeine should not be used for these conditions and, therefore, recommend other supportive therapy.

Caffeine is used in combination with other agents such as analgesics and diuretics to relieve tension and fluid retention associated with menstruation; however, its usefulness for this purpose is in doubt because of its minimal diuretic action.

## Pharmacology/Pharmacokinetics

### Physicochemical characteristics

Source—
Coffee, tea, some soft drinks, and cocoa or chocolate. May also be synthesized from urea or dimethylurea.
Chemical group—
Methylated xanthine.
Molecular weight—
Caffeine (anhydrous): 194.19.
Citric acid: 192.12.
Sodium benzoate: 144.11.

### Mechanism of action/Effect

Central nervous system stimulant—Caffeine stimulates all levels of the CNS, although its cortical effects are milder and of shorter duration than those of amphetamines. In larger doses, caffeine stimulates medullary, vagal, vasomotor, and respiratory centers, promoting bradycardia, vasoconstriction, and increased respiratory rate. This action was previously believed to be primarily due to increased intracellular cyclic 3',5'-adenosine monophosphate (cyclic AMP) following inhibition of phosphodiesterase, the enzyme that degrades cyclic AMP. More recent studies indicate that caffeine exerts its physiological effects in large part through antagonism of central adenosine receptors.

Analgesia adjunct—Caffeine constricts cerebral vasculature with an accompanying decrease in cerebral blood flow and in the oxygen tension of the brain. It has been suggested that the addition of caffeine to aspirin or aspirin and acetaminophen combinations may help to relieve headache by providing a more rapid onset of action and/or enhanced pain relief with a lower dose of the analgesic. In some patients, caffeine may reduce headache pain by reversing caffeine withdrawal symptoms. Recent studies with ergotamine indicate that the enhancement of effect by the addition of caffeine may be due to improved gastrointestinal absorption of ergotamine when administered with caffeine.

Respiratory stimulant adjunct—Although the exact mechanism of action has not been completely established, caffeine, as other methylxanthines, is believed to act primarily through stimulation of the medullary respiratory center. This action is seen in certain pathophysiological states, such as in Cheyne-Stokes respiration and in apnea of preterm infants, and when respiration is depressed by certain drugs, such as barbiturates and opioids. Methylxanthines appear to increase the sensitivity of the respiratory center to the stimulatory actions of carbon dioxide, increasing alveolar ventilation, thereby reducing the severity and frequency of apneic episodes.

### Other actions/effects

Cardiac—Caffeine produces a positive inotropic effect on the myocardium and a positive chronotropic effect on the sinoatrial node, causing transient increases in heart rate, force of contraction, and cardiac output. Low concentrations of caffeine may produce small decreases in heart rate, possibly as a result of stimulation of the medullary vagal nuclei. At higher concentrations, caffeine produces definite tachycardia and sensitive persons may experience other arrhythmias, such as premature ventricular contractions.

Vascular—Caffeine causes constriction of cerebral vasculature with an accompanying decrease in cerebral blood flow and in the oxygen tension in the brain. Caffeine also causes an increase in systemic vascular resistance, resulting in an increase in blood pressure. These effects are believed to be mediated by blockade of adenosine-induced vasodilation and activation of the sympathetic nervous system.

Skeletal muscles—Caffeine stimulates voluntary skeletal muscle, possibly by inducing the release of acetylcholine, increasing the force of contraction and decreasing muscle fatigue. This stimulation of diaphragmatic muscles decreases the work of breathing.

Gastrointestinal secretions—Caffeine causes secretion of both pepsin and gastric acid from parietal cells.

Renal—Caffeine increases renal blood flow and glomerular filtration rate and decreases proximal tubular reabsorption of sodium and water, resulting in a mild diuresis.

Caffeine also inhibits uterine contractions, increases plasma and urinary catecholamine concentrations, and transiently increases plasma glucose by stimulating glycogenolysis and lipolysis.

### Absorption

Readily absorbed after oral or parenteral administration. Absorption of methylxanthines relates more to lipophilicity than to water solubility.

### Distribution

Rapidly distributed to all body compartments; readily crosses the placenta and blood-brain barrier. Volume of distribution ($Vol_D$) in adults ranges from 0.4 to 0.6 liter per kg of body weight (L/kg). Vol$_D$ in neonates averages between 0.78 and 0.92 L/kg.

**Protein binding**
Low (25–36%).

**Biotransformation**
Hepatic. In adults, about 80% of a dose of caffeine is metabolized to paraxanthine (1,7-dimethylxanthine), about 10% is metabolized to theobromine (3,7-dimethylxanthine), and about 4% is metabolized to theophylline (1,3-dimethylxanthine). These compounds are further demethylated to monomethylxanthines and then to methyl uric acids. In premature neonates, theophylline is converted to caffeine.

**Half-life**
Adults—3 to 7 hours.

Neonates—65 to 130 hours. Decreases to adult values by 4 to 7 months post-term.

Note: Half-life is increased in pregnant women and in patients with cirrhosis.

**Time to peak plasma concentration**
50 to 75 minutes following oral administration in adults.

**Therapeutic plasma concentration**
5 to 25 mcg per mL (25.8 to 128.8 micromoles per L).

**Elimination**
Adults—Renal; primarily as metabolites; about 1 to 2% excreted unchanged.
Neonates—Renal; about 85% excreted unchanged.

## Precautions to Consider

**Cross-sensitivity and/or related problems**
Patients sensitive to other xanthines (aminophylline, dyphylline, oxtriphylline, theobromine, theophylline) may be sensitive to caffeine also.

**Pregnancy/Reproduction**
Pregnancy—Caffeine crosses the placenta and achieves blood and tissue concentrations in the fetus that are similar to maternal concentrations. Studies in humans have shown that heavy caffeine consumption by pregnant women may increase the risk of spontaneous abortion and intrauterine growth retardation. Also, excessive intake of caffeine by pregnant women has resulted in fetal arrhythmias. It is therefore recommended that pregnant women limit their intake of caffeine to less than 300 mg (3 cups of coffee) per day.
Studies in animals have shown that caffeine causes skeletal abnormalities in the digits and phalanges when given in doses equivalent to the caffeine content of 12 to 24 cups of coffee daily throughout pregnancy or when given in very large single doses (i.e., 50 to 100 mg per kg of body weight), and causes retarded skeletal development when given in lower doses.

FDA Pregnancy Category C.

**Breast-feeding**
Caffeine is distributed into breast milk in very small amounts. Although the concentration of caffeine in breast milk is 1% of the mother's plasma concentration, caffeine can accumulate in the infant. The infant may show signs of caffeine stimulation such as hyperactivity and wakefulness when a breast-feeding mother drinks as much as 6 to 8 cups of caffeine-containing beverages. It is recommended that nursing mothers limit their intake of caffeine-containing beverages to 1 to 2 cups per day and avoid taking over-the-counter caffeine capsules or tablets. At recommended doses of caffeine-containing analgesic combinations, concentration in the infant is considered to be insignificant.

**Pediatrics**
With the exception of infants, appropriate studies on the relationship of age to the effects of caffeine have not been performed in children up to 12 years of age; however, no pediatrics-specific problems have been documented to date.
Caffeine and sodium benzoate injection is not recommended in neonatal apnea because the benzoate may interact competitively with bilirubin at the albumin binding site, which could cause or increase jaundice. In addition, elevated serum concentrations of benzyl alcohol and benzoate have been associated with neurological disturbances, hypotension, gasping respirations, and metabolic acidosis.

**Geriatrics**
No information is available on the relationship of age to the effects of caffeine in geriatric patients.

**Drug interactions and/or related problems**
The following drug interactions and/or related problems have been selected on the basis of their potential clinical significance (possible mechanism in parentheses where appropriate)—not necessarily inclusive (» = major clinical significance):

Note: Combinations containing any of the following medications, depending on the amount present, may also interact with this medication.

Adenosine
(effects of adenosine are antagonized by caffeine; larger doses of adenosine may be required, or adenosine may be ineffective)

Barbiturates or
Primidone
(concurrent use of barbiturates or primidone [because of the phenobarbital metabolite] with caffeine may increase the metabolism of caffeine by induction of hepatic microsomal enzymes, resulting in increased clearance of caffeine; in addition, concurrent use may antagonize the hypnotic or anticonvulsant effects of the barbiturates)

Beta-adrenergic blocking agents, systemic or
Beta-adrenergic blocking agents, ophthalmic
(concurrent use of beta-blocking agents, including ophthalmic agents [significant systemic absorption possible] with caffeine may result in mutual inhibition of therapeutic effects)

Bronchodilators, adrenergic
(concurrent use with caffeine may result in additive CNS stimulation and other additive toxic effects)

» Caffeine-containing beverages (coffee, tea, or soft drinks) or
» Caffeine-containing medications, other or
» CNS stimulation–producing medications, other (See *Appendix II*)
(excessive CNS stimulation causing nervousness, irritability, insomnia, or possibly convulsions or cardiac arrhythmias may occur; close observation is recommended)

Calcium supplements
(concurrent use with excessive amounts of caffeine may inhibit absorption of calcium)

Cimetidine
(decreased hepatic metabolism of caffeine results in delayed elimination and increased blood concentrations)

Ciprofloxacin or
Enoxacin or
Norfloxacin
(hepatic metabolism and clearance of caffeine may be reduced, increasing the risk of caffeine-related CNS stimulation)

Contraceptives, oral
(concurrent use may decrease caffeine metabolism)

Disulfiram
(concurrent use may reduce the elimination rate of caffeine by inhibiting its metabolism; recovering alcoholic patients on disulfiram therapy are best advised to avoid the use of caffeine to prevent the possibility of complicating alcohol withdrawal by caffeine-induced cardiovascular and cerebral excitation)

Erythromycin or
Troleandomycin
(concurrent use may reduce the hepatic clearance of caffeine)

Hydantoin anticonvulsants, especially phenytoin
(concurrent use of phenytoin may increase the clearance of caffeine)

Lithium
(concurrent use with caffeine increases urinary excretion of lithium, possibly reducing its therapeutic effect)

Mexiletine
(concurrent use with caffeine reduces the elimination of caffeine by up to 50% and may increase the potential for adverse effects)

» Monoamine oxidase (MAO) inhibitors, including furazolidone, procarbazine, and selegiline
(large amounts of caffeine may produce dangerous cardiac arrhythmias or severe hypertension because of the sympathomimetic side effects of caffeine; concurrent use with small amounts of caffeine may produce tachycardia and a mild increase in blood pressure)

Smoking, tobacco
(concurrent use of tobacco increases the elimination rate of caffeine)

Xanthines, other, such as:
Aminophylline
Dyphylline
Oxtriphylline
Theobromine
Theophylline

(caffeine may decrease the clearance of theophylline and possibly other xanthines, increasing the potential for additive pharmacodynamic and toxic effects)

**Laboratory value alterations**

The following have been selected on the basis of their potential clinical significance (possible effect in parentheses where appropriate)—not necessarily inclusive (» = major clinical significance):

With diagnostic test results

Dipyridamole- or adenosine-assisted cardiac diagnostic studies
(caffeine antagonizes the effects of dipyridamole and adenosine on myocardial blood flow, thereby interfering with test results; patients should be instructed to avoid ingesting caffeine [from a dietary or medicinal source] for 8 to 12 hours prior to the test)

Urate measurements, serum
(false-positive elevations when measured by the Bittner method)

Vanillylmandelic acid (VMA) and
Catecholamines, including norepinephrine and epinephrine and
5-hydroxyindoleacetic acid
(urine concentrations are slightly increased; high urinary concentrations of VMA or catecholamines may result in a false-positive diagnosis of pheochromocytoma or neuroblastoma; caffeine intake should be avoided during tests)

With physiology/laboratory test values

Glucose, blood
(concentrations may be increased; glucose tolerance may be impaired in diabetic patients)

**Medical considerations/Contraindications**

The medical considerations/contraindications included here have been selected on the basis of their potential clinical significance (reasons given in parentheses where appropriate)—not necessarily inclusive (» = major clinical significance).

*Risk-benefit should be considered when the following medical problems exist:*

» Anxiety disorders, including agoraphobia and panic attacks
(increased risk of anxiety, nervousness, fear, nausea, palpitations, rapid heartbeat, restlessness, and trembling)

» Cardiac disease, severe
(high doses not recommended because of increased risk of tachycardia or extrasystoles, which may lead to heart failure)

» Hepatic function impairment
(half-life of caffeine may be prolonged leading to toxic accumulation)

» Hypertension or
» Insomnia
(may be potentiated)

Sensitivity to caffeine or other xanthines

**Patient monitoring**

The following may be especially important in patient monitoring (other tests may be warranted in some patients, depending on condition; » = major clinical significance):

*For neonatal apnea*

Caffeine concentrations, plasma or serum
(determinations recommended 24 hours after loading dose, then 1 to 2 times a week; alternatively, some clinicians recommend checking caffeine concentrations every 2 weeks once the infant has been stabilized)

Theophylline concentrations, serum
(determinations may be indicated in the presence of adverse effects possibly caused by conversion of caffeine to theophylline in the neonate)

## Side/Adverse Effects

The following side/adverse effects have been selected on the basis of their potential clinical significance (possible signs and symptoms in parentheses where appropriate)—not necessarily inclusive:

**Those indicating need for medical attention**

Incidence more frequent
*CNS stimulation, excessive* (dizziness; fast heartbeat; irritability, nervousness, or severe jitters in neonates; tremors; trouble in sleeping); *gastrointestinal irritation* (diarrhea; nausea; vomiting)

**Those indicating need for medical attention only if they continue or are bothersome**

Incidence more frequent
*CNS stimulation, mild* (nervousness or jitters); *gastrointestinal irritation, mild* (nausea)

**Those indicating possible withdrawal if they occur after medication is abruptly discontinued after prolonged use**
*Anxiety; dizziness; headache; irritability; muscle tension; nausea; nervousness; stuffy nose; unusual tiredness*

## Overdose

For specific information on the agents used in the management of caffeine overdose, see:
- *Antacids (Oral-Local)* monograph;
- *Charcoal, Activated (Oral-Local)* monograph;
- *Diazepam* in *Benzodiazepines (Systemic)* monograph;
- *Ipecac (Oral-Local)* monograph;
- *Magnesium sulfate* in *Laxatives (Local)* monograph;
- *Phenobarbital* in *Barbiturates (Systemic)* monograph; and/or
- *Phenytoin* in *Anticonvulsants, Hydantoin (Systemic)* monograph.

For more information on the management of overdose or unintentional ingestion, **contact a Poison Control Center** (see *Poison Control Center Listing*).

**Clinical effects of overdose**

The following effects have been selected on the basis of their potential clinical significance (possible signs and symptoms in parentheses where appropriate)—not necessarily inclusive:
*Abdominal or stomach pain; agitation, anxiety, excitement, or restlessness; confusion or delirium; dehydration; fast or irregular heartbeat; fever; frequent urination; headache; increased sensitivity to touch or pain; irritability; muscle trembling or twitching; nausea and vomiting, sometimes with blood; painful, swollen abdomen or vomiting in neonates; ringing or other sounds in ears; seeing flashes of "zig-zag" lights; seizures, usually tonic-clonic seizures*—in acute overdose; *trouble in sleeping; whole body tremors in neonates*

**Treatment of acute overdose**

Acute caffeine toxicity has been reported rarely. Treatment is primarily symptomatic and supportive.

To decrease absorption—
Induction of emesis with ipecac syrup and/or gastric lavage if caffeine has been ingested within 4 hours in amounts over 15 mg per kg of body weight (mg/kg) and emesis has not been induced by caffeine.
Administration of activated charcoal may be useful within the first 4 hours if precautions are taken to minimize the risk of aspiration; magnesium sulfate cathartic may also be useful.

To enhance elimination—
Hemoperfusion is usually more effective than dialysis. Use of exchange transfusion in neonates, if necessary.

Specific treatment—
Control of CNS stimulation or seizures with intravenous diazepam, phenobarbital, or phenytoin.
Administration of antacids and iced saline lavage for hemorrhagic gastritis.

Supportive care—
Maintenance of fluid and electrolyte balance. Maintenance of ventilation and oxygenation. Patients in whom intentional overdose is confirmed or suspected should be referred for psychiatric consultation.

## Patient Consultation

As an aid to patient consultation, refer to *Advice for the Patient, Caffeine (Systemic)*.

In providing consultation, consider emphasizing the following selected information (» = major clinical significance):

**Before using this medication**

» Conditions affecting use, especially:
Sensitivity to caffeine or other xanthines (aminophylline, dyphylline, oxtriphylline, theobromine, theophylline)
Pregnancy—Crosses placenta; excessive use during pregnancy may result in spontaneous abortion, intrauterine growth retardation, or fetal arrhythmias; animal studies have shown skeletal

abnormalities with large doses and retarded skeletal development with lower doses

Breast-feeding—Distributed into breast milk in small amounts but accumulates in infant and may cause hyperactivity and wakefulness; nursing mothers should limit intake of caffeine from all sources

Use in children—Caffeine and sodium benzoate injection is not recommended in neonates because of the benzoate content. However, caffeine citrate may be used safely

Other medications, especially caffeine-containing medications or beverages, other CNS stimulation–producing medications, or monoamine oxidase (MAO) inhibitors

Other medical problems, especially anxiety disorders including agoraphobia and panic attacks, severe cardiac disease, hepatic function impairment, hypertension, or insomnia

## Proper use of this medication

» Importance of not taking more medication and not taking it more often than directed because of increased risk of side effects and habit-forming potential; should be used only occasionally

Proper administration of extended-release capsule: Swallowing whole; not breaking, crushing, or chewing

» Caution if tolerance develops; not increasing dose

» Proper dosing

» Proper storage

## Precautions while using this medication

» Checking with physician if fatigue or drowsiness persists or recurs often

Caution in concurrently drinking large amounts of coffee, tea, or colas or using other medications containing caffeine since amount of caffeine in medication is about the same as in a cup of coffee; importance of knowing amount of caffeine in common foods and beverages

» Discontinuing caffeine-containing medications or foods if fast pulse, dizziness, or pounding heartbeat occurs

Not taking too close to bedtime

## Side/adverse effects

Signs of potential side effects, especially excessive CNS stimulation or gastrointestinal irritation

# General Dosing Information

With prolonged use, habituation or psychological dependence and tolerance to cardiovascular, diuretic, and stimulant effects may occur.

Citrated caffeine injection or oral solution for use in neonatal apnea is not available commercially but must be prepared extemporaneously from citrated caffeine powder. Caffeine tablets may also be crushed and made into an oral suspension. Caffeine citrate powder may be combined with lactose to add to feedings.

Citrated caffeine injection should not be administered intramuscularly because of its acidic nature (pH 3 to 4). It may be administered intravenously.

Caffeine and sodium benzoate injection is not recommended in neonatal apnea because of the benzoate content.

## Diet/Nutrition

The amount of caffeine from dietary sources is as follows

Coffee, brewed—40 to 180 mg per cup.
Coffee, instant—30 to 120 mg per cup.
Coffee, decaffeinated—3 to 5 mg per cup.
Tea, brewed American—20 to 90 mg per cup.
Tea, brewed imported—25 to 110 mg per cup.
Tea, instant—28 mg per cup.
Tea, canned iced—22 to 36 mg per 12 ounces.
Cola and other soft drinks, caffeine-containing—36 to 90 mg per 12 ounces.
Cola and other soft drinks, decaffeinated—0 mg per 12 ounces.
Cocoa—4 mg per cup.
Chocolate, milk—3 to 6 mg per ounce.
Chocolate, bittersweet—25 mg per ounce.

---

## CAFFEINE

# Oral Dosage Forms

Note: Bracketed uses in the *Dosage Forms* section refer to categories of use and/or indications that are not included in U.S. product labeling.

## CAFFEINE EXTENDED-RELEASE CAPSULES

### Usual adult and adolescent dose

Fatigue; drowsiness—
Oral, 200 to 250 mg (anhydrous caffeine), the dosage to be repeated no sooner than three or four hours, as needed.

### Usual adult prescribing limits

Up to 1 gram a day.

### Usual pediatric dose

Fatigue; drowsiness—
Children up to 12 years of age: Use is not recommended.

### Strength(s) usually available

U.S.—
200 mg (anhydrous caffeine) (OTC) [*Caffedrine; Caffedrine Caplets;* GENERIC].
250 mg (anhydrous caffeine) (OTC) [*Dexitac;* GENERIC].

Canada—
Not commercially available.

### Packaging and storage

Store below 40 °C (104 °F), preferably between 15 and 30 °C (59 and 86 °F), in a well-closed container, unless otherwise specified by manufacturer.

### Auxiliary labeling

• Do not take at bedtime.

## CAFFEINE TABLETS

### Usual adult and adolescent dose

Fatigue; drowsiness—
Oral, 100 to 200 mg (anhydrous caffeine), the dosage to be repeated no sooner than three or four hours, as needed.

### Usual adult prescribing limits

Up to 1 gram a day.

### Usual pediatric dose

Fatigue; drowsiness—
Children up to 12 years of age: Use is not recommended.

[Neonatal apnea]—
Initial: Oral, 10 mg (anhydrous caffeine) per kg of body weight.
Maintenance: Oral, 2.5 mg (anhydrous caffeine) per kg of body weight a day, starting twenty-four hours after the initial dose, to maintain a serum concentration of 5 to 25 mcg per mL (25.8 to 128.8 micromoles per L).

Note: Caffeine tablets may be crushed and made into an oral suspension for use in neonatal apnea.

### Strength(s) usually available

U.S.—
75 mg (anhydrous caffeine) (OTC) [*Enerjets*].
100 mg (anhydrous caffeine) (OTC) [*NoDoz; Pep-Back;* GENERIC].
150 mg (anhydrous caffeine) (OTC) [*Quick Pep*].
200 mg (anhydrous caffeine) (OTC) [*Keep Alert; NoDoz Maximum Strength Caplets; Ultra Pep-Back; Vivarin*].

Canada—
100 mg (anhydrous caffeine) (OTC) [*Caffedrine*].
100 mg (caffeine alkaloid) (OTC) [*Wake-Up*].

### Packaging and storage

Store below 40 °C (104 °F), preferably between 15 and 30 °C (59 and 86 °F), in a well-closed container, unless otherwise specified by manufacturer.

### Auxiliary labeling

• Do not take at bedtime.

---

## CAFFEINE, CITRATED

# Oral Dosage Forms

Note: Bracketed uses in the *Dosage Forms* section refer to categories of use and/or indications that are not included in U.S. product labeling.

## CITRATED CAFFEINE SOLUTION

### Usual pediatric dose

[Neonatal apnea]—
Initial: Oral, 20 mg (10 mg of anhydrous caffeine and 10 mg of anhydrous citric acid) per kg of body weight.

Maintenance: Oral, 5 mg (2.5 mg of anhydrous caffeine and 2.5 mg of anhydrous citric acid) per kg of body weight a day, starting twenty-four hours after the initial dose, to maintain a serum concentration of 5 to 25 mcg per mL (25.8 to 128.8 micromoles per L).

Note: Premature neonates may require a smaller dose.

### Strength(s) usually available
U.S.—
Dosage form not commercially available. Compounding required.
Canada—
Dosage form not commercially available. Compounding required.

### Preparation of dosage form
Ten grams of citrated caffeine powder should be dissolved in 250 mL of sterile water for irrigation, and stirred until completely clear; then flavoring should be added (simple syrup and cherry syrup 2:1) to make 500 mL. The final concentration is 20 mg (10 mg of anhydrous caffeine and 10 mg of anhydrous citric acid) per mL.

### Stability
Compounded product as described above is stable for 3 months at room temperature.

### Note
Citrated caffeine powder may also be combined with lactose and added to infant feedings.

## CITRATED CAFFEINE TABLETS

### Usual adult and adolescent dose
Fatigue; drowsiness—
Oral, initially, 65 to 325 mg (32 to 162 mg of anhydrous caffeine and 32 to 162 mg of anhydrous citric acid) three times a day, as needed.

### Usual adult prescribing limits
Up to 1 gram of anhydrous caffeine a day.

### Usual pediatric dose
Children up to 12 years of age—
Use is not recommended.

### Strength(s) usually available
U.S.—
65 mg (32.5 mg of anhydrous caffeine and 32.5 mg of anhydrous citric acid) (OTC) [GENERIC].
Canada—
Not commercially available.

### Packaging and storage
Store below 40 °C (104 °F), preferably between 15 and 30 °C (59 and 86 °F), unless otherwise specified by manufacturer.

### Auxiliary labeling
• Do not take at bedtime.

## Parenteral Dosage Forms

Note: Bracketed uses in the *Dosage Forms* section refer to categories of use and/or indications that are not included in U.S. product labeling.

## CITRATED CAFFEINE INJECTION

### Usual pediatric dose
[Neonatal apnea]—
Initial: Intravenous, 20 mg (10 mg of anhydrous caffeine and 10 mg of anhydrous citric acid) per kg of body weight.
Maintenance: Intravenous, 5 mg (2.5 mg of anhydrous caffeine and 2.5 mg of anhydrous citric acid) per kg of body weight a day, starting twenty-four hours after the initial dose, to maintain a serum concentration of 5 to 25 mcg per mL (25.8 to 128.8 micromoles per L).

### Strength(s) usually available
U.S.—
Dosage form not commercially available. Compounding required.
Canada—
Dosage form not commercially available. Compounding required.

### Preparation of dosage form
Ten grams of citrated caffeine powder should be dissolved in 250 mL of sterile water for injection and transferred to a 500-mL empty evacuated container (EEC). The container should be filled with sterile water to the 500-mL mark and filtered through a 0.22-micron filter into another 500-mL EEC. Then the solution should be transferred to 10-mL vials and autoclaved at 121 °C for 15 minutes and allowed to cool. The resulting concentration is 20 mg (10 mg of anhydrous caffeine and 10 mg of anhydrous citric acid) per mL.

### Stability
Compounded product as described above is stable for 3 months at room temperature.

---

### *CAFFEINE AND SODIUM BENZOATE*

## Parenteral Dosage Forms
### CAFFEINE AND SODIUM BENZOATE INJECTION USP

### Usual adult and adolescent dose
CNS stimulant—
Intramuscular or intravenous, up to a maximum of 500 mg (250 mg of anhydrous caffeine and 250 mg of sodium benzoate), as needed and tolerated.

### Usual adult prescribing limits
2.5 grams (1.25 grams of anhydrous caffeine and 1.25 grams of sodium benzoate) a day.

### Usual pediatric dose
Dosage has not been established.

Note: Use not recommended in neonatal apnea because of benzoate content.

### Strength(s) usually available
U.S.—
250 mg (125 mg of anhydrous caffeine and 125 mg of sodium benzoate) per mL (Rx) [GENERIC].
Canada—
Not commercially available.

### Packaging and storage
Store below 40 °C (104 °F), preferably between 15 and 30 °C (59 and 86 °F), unless otherwise specified by manufacturer.

## Selected Bibliography

Nehlig A, Daval J-L, Debry G. Caffeine and the central nervous system: mechanisms of action, biochemical, metabolic and psychostimulant effects. Brain Res Rev 1992; 17: 139-70.

Revised: 07/12/94

---

## CAFFEINE, CITRATED—See *Caffeine (Systemic)*

---

## CAFFEINE-CONTAINING COMBINATIONS—
Acetaminophen, Aspirin, and Caffeine (Systemic)—See *Acetaminophen and Salicylates (Systemic)*
Acetaminophen, Aspirin, and Caffeine, Buffered (Systemic)—See *Acetaminophen and Salicylates (Systemic)*
Acetaminophen, Aspirin, Salicylamide, and Caffeine (Systemic)—See *Acetaminophen and Salicylates (Systemic)*
Acetaminophen and Caffeine (Systemic)—See *Acetaminophen (Systemic)*
Acetaminophen, Codeine, and Caffeine (Systemic)—See *Opioid (Narcotic) Analgesics and Acetaminophen (Systemic)*
Acetaminophen, Salicylamide, and Caffeine (Systemic)—See *Acetaminophen and Salicylates (Systemic)*
Aspirin and Caffeine (Systemic)—See *Salicylates (Systemic)*
Aspirin and Caffeine, Buffered (Systemic)—See *Salicylates (Systemic)*
Aspirin, Caffeine, and Dihydrocodeine (Systemic)—See *Opioid (Narcotic) Analgesics and Aspirin (Systemic)*
Aspirin and Codeine, Buffered (Systemic)—See *Opioid (Narcotic) Analgesics and Aspirin (Systemic)*
Aspirin, Codeine, and Caffeine (Systemic)—See *Opioid (Narcotic) Analgesics and Aspirin (Systemic)*
Butalbital, Acetaminophen, and Caffeine (Systemic)—See *Barbiturates and Analgesics (Systemic)*
Butalbital, Aspirin, and Caffeine (Systemic)—See *Barbiturates and Analgesics (Systemic)*
Butalbital, Aspirin, Caffeine, and Codeine (Systemic)—See *Barbiturates and Analgesics (Systemic)*
Caffeine and Sodium Benzoate (Systemic)—See *Caffeine (Systemic)*
Chlorpheniramine, Phenindamine, Phenylephrine, Dextromethorphan, Acetaminophen, Salicylamide, Caffeine, and Ascorbic Acid (Systemic)—See *Cough/Cold Combinations (Systemic)*
Chlorpheniramine, Pheniramine, Pyrilamine, Phenylephrine, Hydrocodone, Salicylamide, Caffeine, and Ascorbic Acid (Systemic)—See *Cough/Cold Combinations (Systemic)*

Chlorpheniramine, Phenylephrine, Acetaminophen, Salicylamide, and Caffeine (Systemic)—See *Antihistamines, Decongestants, and Analgesics (Systemic)*

Chlorpheniramine, Phenylephrine, Hydrocodone, Acetaminophen, and Caffeine (Systemic)—See *Cough/Cold Combinations (Systemic)*

Chlorpheniramine, Phenylpropanolamine, Acetaminophen, and Caffeine (Systemic)—See *Antihistamines, Decongestants, and Analgesics (Systemic)*

Chlorpheniramine, Phenylpropanolamine, Aspirin, and Caffeine (Systemic)—See *Antihistamines, Decongestants, and Analgesics (Systemic)*

Chlorpheniramine, Phenylpropanolamine, Dextromethorphan, Acetaminophen, and Caffeine (Systemic)—See *Cough/Cold Combinations (Systemic)*

Dihydrocodeine, Acetaminophen, and Caffeine (Systemic)—See *Opioid (Narcotic) Analgesics and Acetaminophen (Systemic)*

Diphenylpyraline, Phenylpropanolamine, Acetaminophen, and Caffeine (Systemic)—See *Antihistamines, Decongestants, and Analgesics (Systemic)*

Ergotamine and Caffeine (Systemic)—See *Vascular Headache Suppressants, Ergot Derivative-containing (Systemic)*

Ergotamine, Caffeine, and Belladonna Alkaloids (Systemic)—See *Vascular Headache Suppressants, Ergot Derivative-containing (Systemic)*

Ergotamine, Caffeine, Belladonna Alkaloids, and Pentobarbital (Systemic)—See *Vascular Headache Suppressants, Ergot Derivative-containing (Systemic)*

Ergotamine, Caffeine, and Cyclizine (Systemic)—See *Vascular Headache Suppressants, Ergot Derivative-containing (Systemic)*

Ergotamine, Caffeine, and Dimenhydrinate (Systemic)—See *Vascular Headache Suppressants, Ergot Derivative-containing (Systemic)*

Ergotamine, Caffeine, and Diphenhydramine (Systemic)—See *Vascular Headache Suppressants, Ergot Derivative-containing (Systemic)*

Orphenadrine, Aspirin, and Caffeine (Systemic)—See *Orphenadrine and Aspirin (Systemic)*

Pheniramine, Phenylephrine, Codeine, Sodium Citrate, Sodium Salicylate, and Caffeine (Systemic)—See *Cough/Cold Combinations (Systemic)*

Pheniramine, Phenylephrine, Sodium Salicylate, and Caffeine (Systemic)—See *Antihistamines, Decongestants, and Analgesics (Systemic)*

Pheniramine, Pyrilamine, Phenylpropanolamine, Codeine, Acetaminophen, and Caffeine (Systemic)—See *Cough/Cold Combinations (Systemic)*

Phenylephrine, Guaifenesin, Acetaminophen, Salicylamide, and Caffeine (Systemic)—See *Cough/Cold Combinations (Systemic)*

Phenylpropanolamine, Acetaminophen, and Caffeine (Systemic)—See *Decongestants and Analgesics (Systemic)*

Phenylpropanolamine, Acetaminophen, Salicylamide, and Caffeine (Systemic)—See *Decongestants and Analgesics (Systemic)*

Propoxyphene, Aspirin, and Caffeine (Systemic)—See *Opioid (Narcotic) Analgesics and Aspirin (Systemic)*

Pyrilamine, Phenylephrine, Aspirin, and Caffeine (Systemic)—See *Antihistamines, Decongestants, and Analgesics (Systemic)*

Pyrilamine, Phenylpropanolamine, Acetaminophen, and Caffeine (Systemic)—See *Antihistamines, Decongestants, and Analgesics (Systemic)*

# CALAMINE    Topical

VA CLASSIFICATION (Primary): DE900

Note: For a listing of dosage forms and brand names by country availability, see *Dosage Forms* section(s). For a listing of brand names for the articles in this monograph, refer to the General Index.

## Category

Skin protectant; antipruritic (topical).

## Indications

### Accepted

Skin irritations, minor (treatment)—Calamine is indicated for the topical relief of itching, pain, and discomfort of minor skin irritations, such as those caused by poison ivy, poison oak, and poison sumac.

Calamine also has a mild astringent action on the skin and dries oozing and weeping caused by poison ivy, poison oak, and poison sumac.

## Pharmacology/Pharmacokinetics

### Physicochemical characteristics

Calamine consists of a mixture of zinc oxide (not less than 98% and not more than 100.5%) and a small proportion of ferric oxide.

### Mechanism of action/Effect

Unknown.

### Absorption

Calamine applied topically is not absorbed through the skin.

## Precautions to Consider

### Pregnancy/Reproduction

Problems in humans have not been documented.

### Breast-feeding

Problems in humans have not been documented.

### Pediatrics

Appropriate studies on the relationship of age to the effects of calamine have not been performed in the pediatric population. However, no pediatrics-specific problems have been documented to date.

### Geriatrics

Appropriate studies on the relationship of age to the effects of calamine have not been performed in the geriatric population. However, no geriatrics-specific problems have been documented to date.

## Patient Consultation

As an aid to patient consultation, refer to *Advice for the Patient, Calamine (Topical)*.

In providing consultation, consider emphasizing the following selected information (» = major clinical significance):

**Proper use of this medication**

For external use only; keeping away from eyes and other mucous membranes such as the mouth, nose, and anogenital region

» To apply the lotion: shaking lotion well before use; using a pledget of cotton moistened with calamine and allowing to dry after application

» To apply the ointment: applying enough medication to cover affected area (s) of skin and rubbing in gently

» Proper dosing

» Proper storage

**Precautions while using this medication**

Discontinuing use and checking with physician if condition worsens, or does not improve within 7 days, or if rash, irritation, or sensitivity develops

## General Dosing Information

Calamine is for external use only; contact with the eyes and other mucous membranes should be avoided.

Calamine lotion should be applied to the affected area (s) of skin with a cotton pledget moistened with the lotion. Then the medication should be allowed to dry on the skin.

A sufficient amount of calamine ointment should be applied to cover the affected area (s) of skin and rubbed in gently.

Treatment should be discontinued and the physician consulted if the condition worsens or if it does not improve within 7 days, or if rash, irritation, or sensitivity develops.

Ingestion of calamine has been reported to cause adverse effects such as gastritis and vomiting due to irritation of gastric mucosa.

**For treatment of adverse effects**

Recommended treatment consists of the following
• For ingestion, milk or antacids may be used to allay gastritis.

Patients should seek medical help or **contact a Poison Control Center** (see *Poison Control Center Listing*) immediately. Patients in whom intentional ingestion is known or suspected should be referred for psychiatric consultation.

## Topical Dosage Forms

### CALAMINE LOTION USP

**Usual adult and adolescent dose**

Skin protectant or
Antipruritic (topical)—
Topical, to the affected area (s) of skin as often as necessary.

**Usual pediatric dose**
See *Usual adult and adolescent dose.*

**Strength(s) usually available**
U.S.—
  8% (OTC) [GENERIC].
Canada—
  8% (OTC) [GENERIC].

Note:
Calamine Lotion USP contains
    Calamine—80 grams
    Zinc oxide—80 grams
    Glycerin—20 mL
    Bentonite magma—250 mL
    Calcium hydroxide topical solution—A sufficient quantity to make
    1000 mL.
The quantity of Bentonite Magma may be increased to not more than 400
mL if a more viscous consistency is desired.

**Packaging and storage**
Store in a light-resistant container below 40 °C (104 °F), preferably be-
    tween 15 and 30 °C (59 and 86 °F), unless otherwise specified by
    manufacturer. Protect from freezing. Store in a tight container.

**Auxiliary labeling**
• For external use only.
• Shake well before using.

## CALAMINE OINTMENT

**Usual adult and adolescent dose**
See *Calamine Lotion USP.*

**Usual pediatric dose**
See *Calamine Lotion USP.*

**Strength(s) usually available**
U.S.—
  17 grams per 100 grams (OTC) [*Calamox*].
Canada—
  5% (OTC) [*Diaper Rash Ointment* (zinc oxide 5%)].
  16% (OTC) [*Onguent de Calamine*].

**Packaging and storage**
Store below 40 °C (104 °F), preferably between 15 and 30 °C (59 and 86
    °F), unless otherwise specified by manufacturer.

**Auxiliary labeling**
• For external use only.

## Selected Bibliography

Spilker B, Wilkins RD, Perkins JG. A novel double-blind method to eval-
    uate topically applied antipruritic drugs. Curr Ther Res Clin Exp 1984;
    35 (4): 593-605.

Developed: 05/26/95

**CALCIFEDIOL**—See *Vitamin D and Analogs (Systemic)*

---

# CALCIPOTRIENE    Topical

INN: Calcipotriol
BAN: Calcipotriol
VA CLASSIFICATION (Primary): DE802
Another commonly used name is MC 903.
Note: For a listing of dosage forms and brand names by country availa-
    bility, see *Dosage Forms* section(s). For a listing of brand names
    for the articles in this monograph, refer to the General Index.

## Category
Antipsoriatic (topical).

## Indications
Note: Bracketed information in the *Indications* section refers to uses that
    are not included in U.S. product labeling.

**Accepted**
Psoriasis (treatment)—Calcipotriene is indicated for the treatment of
    [mild] to moderate plaque psoriasis. [Calcipotriene also may be used
    in the treatment of extensive or severe chronic plaque psoriasis. How-
    ever, its use in this type of psoriasis is generally not recommended
    because of increased risk of hypercalcemia, secondary to excessive
    absorption of the medication when there is extensive skin involvement.
    If calcipotriene is to be used for severe extensive psoriasis, it is nec-
    essary to monitor the serum calcium levels at regular intervals.]

    [Calcipotriene is also used in combination with ultraviolet B light
    (UVB) phototherapy in the treatment of psoriasis.]

## Pharmacology/Pharmacokinetics

**Physicochemical characteristics**
Source—Synthetic vitamin $D_3$ derivative.
Molecular weight—412.6.

**Mechanism of action/Effect**
Unknown; however, calcipotriene inhibits keratinocyte proliferation (with-
    out any evidence of cytotoxic effect) and induces terminal differenti-
    ation of keratinocytes, thus reversing the abnormal keratinocyte
    change in psoriasis. Calcipotriene exhibits a vitamin D–like effect by
    competing for the cellular receptors for calcitriol $(1,25[OH]_2D_3)$, a bi-
    ologically active metabolite of vitamin D. These calcitriol receptors
    have been identified on keratinocytes of both normal and psoriatic
    skin.

**Other actions/effects**
Calcipotriene seems to have an immunoregulatory role that involves the
    skin immune system, and is associated with variable decreases in ker-
    atinocyte expression of markers of activation. Calcipotriene may re-
    duce the release of cytokines from different cell lineages; it may also
    govern a down-regulation of cell adhesion molecules (CAMs) that are
    known to mediate the passage of activated T-lymphocytes in the der-
    mis and in the epidermis, thereby producing a reduction of cellular
    infiltrate in psoriasis.

**Absorption**
Approximately 6% (± 3%, SD) of the applied dose of radiolabeled cal-
    cipotriene ointment is absorbed systemically when the ointment is ap-
    plied topically to psoriasis plaques; about 5% (± 2.6%, SD) is ab-
    sorbed when applied to normal skin.

**Protein binding**
*In vitro*, the affinity of calcipotriene for human serum vitamin D–binding
    protein is 30 times less than that of calcitriol.

**Biotransformation**
Clinical studies using radiolabeled calcipotriene ointment have shown that
    much of the active substance absorbed is converted to inactive metab-
    olites within 24 hours following topical application to psoriasis plaques
    and normal skin. In animal studies, calcipotriene is rapidly metabo-
    lized in the liver following systemic uptake and converted into inactive
    metabolites identified as MC 1046 and MC 1080.

**Elimination**
Only small amounts (< 1%) of radiolabeled calcipotriene were recovered
    in the urine and feces following topical application of this medication
    in 4 patients with psoriasis.

## Precautions to Consider

**Carcinogenicity**
Long-term animal studies have not been conducted to evaluate the carcin-
    ogenic potential of calcipotriene.

**Mutagenicity**
Calcipotriene did not show any mutagenic effects in the Ames mutagen-
    icity assay, the mouse lymphoma TK locus assay, the human lympho-
    cyte chromosome aberration test, or the mouse micronucleus test.

**Pregnancy/Reproduction**
Fertility—Studies in rats given calcipotriene in doses up to 54 mcg per
    kg of body weight (mcg/kg) per day (318 mcg per square meter of
    body surface [mcg/m²] per day) showed no impairment of fertility or
    general reproductive performance.

Pregnancy—Adequate and well-controlled studies in humans have not been done.

Studies in rabbits given doses of calcipotriene of up to 36 mcg/kg per day (396 mcg/m$^2$ per day) showed no teratogenic effects. However, increases in maternal and fetal toxicity were observed at doses of 12 mcg/kg per day (132 mcg/m$^2$ per day) and higher. Studies in rats given oral doses of 54 mcg/kg per day (318 mcg/m$^2$ per day) resulted in a significantly higher incidence of skeletal abnormalities consisting of enlarged fontanelles and extra ribs. The enlarged fontanelle is most likely due to the effect of calcipotriene on calcium metabolism.

FDA Pregnancy Category C.

### Breast-feeding
It is not known whether calcipotriene is distributed into breast milk. However, problems in humans have not been documented.

### Pediatrics
Appropriate studies on the relationship of age to the effects of calcipotriene have not been performed in the pediatric population. Safety and efficacy have not been established. Because of a higher ratio of skin surface area to body mass, children are at greater risk than adults of systemic adverse effects when they are treated with topical medication.

### Geriatrics
According to the manufacturer, about 12% of the total number of patients in the clinical studies of calcipotriene ointment were 65 years of age or older, while about 4% were 75 years of age and over. Skin-related adverse effects were more severe in those over 65 years of age than in those under 65 years of age.

### Laboratory value alterations
The following have been selected on the basis of their potential clinical significance (possible effect in parentheses where appropriate)—not necessarily inclusive (» = major clinical significance):

With physiology/laboratory test values
» Calcium concentrations, serum
(rapid, transient, and reversible increase may occur, which may or may not be dose-related; if increase in serum calcium is outside the normal range, treatment should be discontinued until normal calcium levels are restored)

» Calcium concentrations, urine
(transient, reversible increase may occur, usually with excessive dose; one study showed an increase in urine calcium level when calcipotriene was used within the recommended maximum dose of 100 grams per week; this increase was attributed to the following mechanisms: increased absorption of calcium by the gut, increased mobilization from bone, or altered renal handling; urine calcium levels may rise even in the absence of any apparent change in the serum calcium levels)

### Medical considerations/Contraindications
The medical considerations/contraindications included here have been selected on the basis of their potential clinical significance (reasons given in parentheses where appropriate)—not necessarily inclusive (» = major clinical significance).

*Risk-benefit should be considered when the following medical problems exist:*
» Hypercalcemia or
» Hypercalciuria, pre-existing or
» Hypervitaminosis D
(may result in renal impairment due to increased renal calculi formation secondary to precipitation of calcium salts in the renal parenchyma [nephrocalcinosis])

Hypersensitivity to calcipotriene or to other components of the preparation, history of
» Nephrolithiasis, history of
(may further aggravate condition due to increased renal calculi formation)

### Patient monitoring
The following may be especially important in patient monitoring (other tests may be warranted in some patients, depending on condition; » = major clinical significance):
» Calcium concentrations, serum
(transient, reversible increase may occur; generally, treatment with calcipotriene at recommended doses of up to 100 grams per week does not result in changes in laboratory values of serum calcium; however, it is recommended that baseline serum calcium levels be obtained prior to treatment and that monitoring be done at regular intervals, especially if calcipotriene is used at doses in excess of 100 grams per week or if it is used for severe psoriasis with extensive skin involvement; if serum calcium levels become elevated, treatment with calcipotriene should be discontinued and serum cal-

cium levels should be measured once a week until the levels return to normal; patients with marginally elevated serum calcium may be treated with calcipotriene, provided that the serum calcium is monitored at suitable intervals)

» Calcium concentrations, urine
(transient, reversible increase may occur; urine calcium is considered a more sensitive indicator of toxicity than serum calcium is; patients with extensive psoriasis who may require a dose approaching 100 grams per week should be screened for hypercalciuria by obtaining baseline urine calcium levels prior to treatment; urine calcium of these patients should be monitored if this dose is continued for more than a few weeks)

## Side/Adverse Effects

Note: According to the manufacturer, controlled clinical trials have reported side effects such as dermatitis, skin dryness, erythema, rash, and worsening of psoriasis, including development of psoriasis of the face and scalp, in 1 to 10% of patients. Atrophy of skin, folliculitis, hypercalcemia, and hyperpigmentation were reported in less than 1% of patients. One study reported transient burning, irritation, or itching of skin in 19.5% of patients. Another study reported nondermatologic symptoms such as fatigue, headache, hot flushes and flu-like symptoms, increasing bronchospasm, nausea and vomiting, and upper abdominal pain in about 2% of patients.

The following side/adverse effects have been selected on the basis of their potential clinical significance (possible signs and symptoms in parentheses where appropriate)—not necessarily inclusive:

### Those indicating need for medical attention
Incidence more frequent
*Dermatitis* (redness and swelling of skin with itching); *skin rash; worsening of psoriasis including development of psoriasis of the face and scalp*
Incidence rare
*Atrophy of skin* (thinning, weakness, or wasting away of skin); *folliculitis* (burning, itching, and pain in hairy areas; pus in the hair follicles); *hypercalcemia* (high blood levels of calcium usually asymptomatic in mild cases; in severe cases, abdominal pain, constipation, depression, easy fatigability, high blood pressure, loss of appetite, loss of weight, muscle weakness, nausea, thirst, and vomiting); *hypercalciuria* (high urine levels of calcium usually asymptomatic)
Note: Hypercalcemia and hypercalciuria are usually reversible upon withdrawal of the medication.

### Those indicating need for medical attention only if they continue or are bothersome
Incidence more frequent
*Burning, irritation, or itching of skin, transient*—about 10 to 15%; *dryness or peeling of skin; erythema* (redness of skin); *skin rash*
Incidence less frequent or rare
*Hyperpigmentation* (increased color of skin)

## Overdose
For specific information on the agents used in the management of calcipotriene overdose, see:
• *Corticosteroids/Corticotropin—Glucocorticoid Effects (Systemic)* monograph;
• *Diuretics, Loop (Systemic)* monograph; and/or
• *Potassium Supplements (Systemic)* monograph
For more information on the management of overdose or unintentional ingestion, **contact a Poison Control Center** (see *Poison Control Center Listing*).

### Clinical effects of overdose
The following effects have been selected on the basis of their potential clinical significance (possible signs and symptoms in parentheses where appropriate)—not necessarily inclusive:
Acute effects
*Hypercalcemia and/or hypercalciuria* (usually asymptomatic; however, in severe hypercalcemia, abdominal pain, constipation, depression, easy fatigability, high blood pressure, loss of appetite, loss of weight, muscle weakness, nausea, thirst, and vomiting)

### Treatment of overdose
To decrease absorption—For both mild and severe cases of hypercalcemia and/or hypercalciuria, treatment with calcipotriene should be discontinued. For mild cases, withdrawal of the medication should be sufficient treatment.

To enhance elimination—For severe hypercalcemia, intensive hydration to increase calcium excretion is necessary. Fluids should be given both orally and parenterally (sodium chloride given intravenously is most helpful).

Specific treatment—Diuretics such as furosemide may be given in conjunction with vigorous hydration. Prednisone may also be helpful. Sufficient potassium chloride with continuous cardiac monitoring may be given to prevent hypokalemia. For patients with impaired renal function, hemodialysis may be useful.

Monitoring—Fluid intake and output and serum and urine electrolytes should be monitored carefully.

Supportive care—Patients in whom intentional overdose is known or suspected should be referred for psychiatric consultation.

## Patient Consultation

As an aid to patient consultation, refer to *Advice for the Patient, Calcipotriene (Topical)*.

In providing consultation, consider emphasizing the following selected information (» = major clinical significance):

### Before using this medication
» Conditions affecting use, especially:
  Hypersensitivity to calcipotriene or to other components of the preparation
  Use in children—Safety and efficacy have not been established
  Use in the elderly—Skin-related side effects may be more severe when they occur in those over 65 years of age
  Other medical problems, especially hypercalcemia, hypercalciuria, hypervitaminosis D, or nephrolithiasis

### Proper use of this medication
» For external use only and not for ophthalmic, oral, or intravaginal use; using this medication only as directed by physician
  Compliance with full course of therapy
» Not using more than 100 grams per week
» Avoiding contact of medication with face or eyes; washing it off with water if medication accidentally gets onto face, into eyes, or onto normal skin surrounding the psoriatic area (s)
  Applying medication sparingly in folds of skin because of risk of irritation of skin where there is natural occlusion
» Applying enough medication to cover affected area (s) of skin and rubbing in gently and completely; avoiding use of occlusive dressing; washing hands after application to avoid inadvertently transferring medication onto face
» When used in combination with ultraviolet B light (UVB) phototherapy, applying medication after ultraviolet light exposure
  Not using medication for any skin disorder other than that for which it was prescribed
» Proper dosing
  Missed dose
» Proper storage

### Precautions while using this medication
  Medication may cause transient irritation of lesions and surrounding uninvolved skin after application; not scratching irritated skin
» Discontinuing use and checking with physician if irritation persists, or if facial rash or other problems develop
  While using this medication, visiting physician regularly for monitoring of serum and urine calcium levels
  Checking with physician if skin problem has not improved (usually within 2 to 8 weeks) or if skin condition becomes worse

### Side/adverse effects
  Signs of potential side effects, especially dermatitis, skin rash, worsening of psoriasis, atrophy of skin, folliculitis, hypercalcemia, and hypercalciuria

## General Dosing Information

Calcipotriene is for external use only and not for ophthalmic, oral, or intravaginal use.

In adequate controlled trials with patients treated with calcipotriene, improvement usually began after 2 weeks of therapy. This improvement

continued, with approximately 70% of patients showing marked improvement after 8 weeks of therapy but only approximately 10% showing complete clearing.

Calcipotriene should not be used on the face since it may cause itching and erythema of the facial skin. Patients should be instructed to wash their hands after using calcipotriene to avoid inadvertent transfer of this medication to the face or eyes. Should facial dermatitis develop, therapy should be discontinued.

Calcipotriene should be used cautiously in skin folds, such as the intertriginous areas, where the natural occlusion may give rise to an increase of the irritant effect of the medication.

Hypercalcemia generally does not occur with the use of calcipotriene at the usual dose of up to 100 grams per week. Excessive use may cause elevated serum calcium, which rapidly subsides when treatment is discontinued.

Treatment with calcipotriene may be combined with ultraviolet B light (UVB) phototherapy. With this form of treatment, patients are allowed to expose their skin to sunlight. Calcipotriene should be applied after exposure to ultraviolet (UV) light.

## Topical Dosage Forms
### CALCIPOTRIENE OINTMENT

**Usual adult dose**
Psoriasis—
  Topical, to the affected area (s) of skin, two times a day, in the morning and evening. Treatment may be continued for six to eight weeks.

  Note: Some clinicians would prescribe calcipotriene for more than eight weeks for maintenance therapy if initial treatment produces acceptable results.

**Usual adult prescribing limits**
The maximum recommended dose is 100 grams per week.

**Usual pediatric dose**
Safety and efficacy have not been established.

**Strength(s) usually available**
U.S.—
  50 mcg per gram (Rx) [*Dovonex* (dibasic sodium phosphate; edetate disodium; mineral oil; petrolatum; propylene glycol; tocopherol; steareth-2; water)].
Canada—
  50 mcg per gram (Rx) [*Dovonex* (disodium edetate; disodium phosphate dihydrate; DL-alpha-tocopherol; liquid paraffin; polyoxyethylene- (2)-stearyl ether; propylene glycol; purified water; white soft paraffin)].

**Packaging and storage**
Store between 15 and 25 °C (59 and 77 °F), unless otherwise specified by manufacturer. Protect from freezing.

**Auxiliary labeling**
• For external use only.

## Selected Bibliography

Bruce S, Epinette WW, Funicella T, et al. Comparative study of calcipotriene (MC 903) ointment and fluocinonide ointment in the treatment of psoriasis. J Am Acad Dermatol 1994; 31 (5 part 1): 755-9.

Cunliffe WJ, Berth-Jones J, Claudy A, et al. Comparative study of calcipotriol (MC 903) ointment and betamethasone 17-valerate ointment in patients with psoriasis vulgaris. J Am Acad Dermatol 1992; 26 (5 part 1): 736-43.

Highton A, Quell J, The Calcipotriene Study Group. Calcipotriene ointment 0.005% for psoriasis: A safety and efficacy study. J Am Acad Dermatol 1995; 32 (1): 67-72.

Developed: 04/25/95

# CALCITONIN   Systemic

This monograph includes information on the following: Calcitonin-Human; Calcitonin-Salmon.

VA CLASSIFICATION (Primary): HS900

Note: For a listing of dosage forms and brand names by country availability, see *Dosage Forms* section(s). For a listing of brand names for the articles in this monograph, refer to the General Index.

---

†Not commercially available in Canada.

---

## Category

Bone resorption inhibitor; osteoporosis therapy adjunct; antihypercalcemic therapy adjunct..

## Indications

Note: Bracketed information in the *Indications* section refers to uses that are not included in U.S. product labeling.

### Accepted

Paget's disease of bone (treatment)—Calcitonin-salmon and calcitonin-human are indicated in the treatment of moderate to severe symptomatic Paget's disease (osteitis deformans), characterized by abnormal and accelerated bone metabolism in one or more bones. Signs and symptoms may include bone pain, deformity, and/or fractures; increased concentrations of serum alkaline phosphatase and/or urinary hydroxyproline; neurologic disorders associated with skull lesions and spinal deformities; and elevated cardiac output and other vascular disorders associated with increased vascularity of bones. Calcitonin-human may be effective for treatment of patients who have developed resistance to calcitonin-salmon.

Osteoporosis, postmenopausal (treatment adjunct)—Calcitonin-salmon[1] is indicated [and calcitonin-human is used] for the treatment of osteoporosis in postmenopausal women in conjunction with an adequate intake of calcium (1.5 grams of elemental calcium per day) and vitamin D (400 IU per day) to aid in the prevention of the progressive loss of bone mass. An adequate diet is also essential.

Although calcitonin may increase bone mass or help slow the loss of bone mass in some patients, questions still remain as to whether treatment with calcitonin will actually decrease the incidence of compression fractures in postmenopausal women with osteoporosis.

Hypercalcemia (treatment adjunct)—Calcitonin-salmon is indicated [and calcitonin-human is used] with intravenous saline and other appropriate hypocalcemic agents in the treatment of hypercalcemic emergencies. Calcitonin has been shown to effectively lower serum calcium concentrations in patients with carcinoma, multiple myeloma, or, to a lesser degree, primary hyperparathyroidism. Calcitonin-salmon may be added to existing therapeutic regimens for the treatment of hypercalcemia, such as intravenous fluids, furosemide, oral phosphates, or adrenocorticoids.

[Osteoporosis, secondary (treatment adjunct)][1]—Calcitonin-human and calcitonin-salmon are used in conjunction with an adequate intake of calcium and vitamin D for the treatment of osteoporosis secondary to hormonal disturbances, drug therapy, immobilization, and other causes. Calcitonin therapy is initiated when treatment of the underlying etiology is not feasible.

---

[1]Not included in Canadian product labeling.

## Pharmacology/Pharmacokinetics

### Physicochemical characteristics

Molecular weight—
Calcitonin-human: 3527.20.
Calcitonin-salmon: 3431.88.

### Mechanism of action/Effect

Paget's disease—Calcitonin reduces the rate of bone turnover, possibly by an initial blocking of bone resorption, resulting in decreases in serum alkaline phosphatase (reflecting decreased bone formation) and decreases in urinary hydroxyproline excretion (reflecting decreased bone resorption, i.e., breakdown of collagen).

Osteoporosis or

Hypercalcemia—Calcitonin lowers serum calcium concentration primarily by a direct inhibition of bone resorption. The number and/or function of osteoclasts is reduced and a decrease in osteocytic resorption may also be involved. These effects may be mediated in part by a drug-induced increase in cyclic adenosine monophosphate concentration in bone cells and subsequent alteration of calcium and/or phosphate transport across the plasma membrane of the osteoclast.

### Other actions/effects

Calcitonin also has a direct effect on the kidneys, increasing the excretion of calcium, phosphate, and sodium by inhibiting their tubular reabsorption. These effects are also mediated in part by cyclic adenosine monophosphate. However, in some patients, calcitonin-induced inhibition of bone resorption has a greater effect on calcium excretion than does the drug's direct renal action, so that urinary calcium is decreased rather than increased.

Short-term administration of calcitonin results in decreases in the volume and acidity of gastric juice, and in trypsin and amylase content and volume of pancreatic juice.

### Duration of effect

Calcitonin-salmon—Hypercalcemia: 6 to 8 hours.

### Biotransformation

Calcitonin is rapidly metabolized, primarily in the kidneys but also in blood and peripheral tissues.

### Half-life

Calcitonin-human—60 minutes, after a single dose.

Calcitonin-salmon—70 to 90 minutes, after a single dose.

### Onset of therapeutic action

Calcitonin-human and calcitonin-salmon—Maximum reductions of serum alkaline phosphatase and urinary hydroxyproline excretion in Paget's disease may take 6 to 24 months of continuous treatment.

### Time to peak effect

Cacitonin-salmon—Hypercalcemia: 2 hours.

### Elimination

Renal; very small amounts are excreted unchanged.

## Precautions to Consider

### Cross-sensitivity and/or related problems

Patients who are allergic to proteins may be allergic to calcitonin, since calcitonin is a protein. Its use is not recommended in patients with suspected sensitivity who show a positive response to skin testing prior to initiating therapy. Since calcitonin-salmon is a foreign protein, it may induce antibodies with continued use. In short-term treatment (2 years or less), antibody titers appear in 30 to 60% of treated patients, but only 5 to 15% become resistant to treatment as a result. Long-term treatment may be possible in patients who are not limited by antibody formation. Because synthetic human calcitonin is identical to naturally occurring human calcitonin, antibody formation is rare, allowing longer term treatment that is not limited by antibody-mediated resistance.

### Carcinogenicity

No long-term studies have been done to evaluate carcinogenic potential of calcitonin. The incidence of osteogenic sarcoma is increased in Paget's disease with or without treatment. Pagetic lesions, with or without therapy, should be carefully evaluated to distinguish them from osteogenic sarcoma, since such lesions may show marked progression on x-ray, with possible loss of periosteal margins. Calcitonin does not appear to slow the progression of such sarcomas.

### Pregnancy/Reproduction

Pregnancy—No adequate and well-controlled studies in humans have been done. However, calcitonin does not cross the placenta.

In animal studies, calcitonin has been shown to decrease fetal birth weight, when given in doses 14 to 56 times the dose recommended for human use, possibly due to metabolic effects on the pregnant animal.

FDA Pregnancy Category C.

### Breast-feeding

Calcitonin is distributed into breast milk. However, problems in humans have not been documented. In animal studies, calcitonin has been shown to inhibit lactation.

### Pediatrics

Appropriate studies on the relationship of age to the effects of calcitonin have not been performed in the pediatric population.

### Geriatrics

Appropriate studies on the relationship of age to the effects of calcitonin have not been performed in the geriatric population. However, no geriatrics-specific problems have been documented to date.

**Drug interactions and/or related problems**
The following drug interactions and/or related problems have been selected on the basis of their potential clinical significance (possible mechanism in parentheses where appropriate)—not necessarily inclusive (» = major clinical significance):

Note: Combinations containing any of the following medications, depending on the amount present, may also interact with this medication.

Calcium-containing preparations or
Vitamin D, including calcifediol and calcitriol
(in the treatment of hypercalcemia, concurrent use may antagonize the effect of calcitonin; in the treatment of other conditions, calcium-containing preparations may be given 4 hours after calcitonin)

**Medical considerations/Contraindications**
The medical considerations/contraindications included here have been selected on the basis of their potential clinical significance (reasons given in parentheses where appropriate)—not necessarily inclusive (» = major clinical significance).

***Risk-benefit should be considered when the following medical problems exist:***
» Allergy to proteins (or history of) or
» Sensitivity to calcitonin
(possibility of systemic allergic reaction, especially in patients with a history of severe allergy, even with a negative skin test reaction to calcitonin, because of the protein nature of calcitonin; allergic reaction is more likely with calcitonin-salmon)

**Patient monitoring**
The following may be especially important in patient monitoring (other tests may be warranted in some patients, depending on condition; » = major clinical significance):

Alkaline phosphatase concentrations, serum and
Urinary hydroxyproline concentrations (24-hour)
(determinations recommended at periodic intervals during therapy with calcitonin-salmon in Paget's disease of bone; during therapy with calcitonin-human, biochemical determinations are recommended prior to initiation, and once during the first three months, and at approximately 3- to 6-month intervals during chronic treatment of Paget's bone disease to determine effectiveness and dosage of calcitonin; most clinicians prefer to measure serum alkaline phosphatase for routine use because urinary hydroxyproline concentrations are cumbersome to measure and expensive)

Calcium concentrations, serum
(determinations required at periodic intervals during therapy for hypercalcemia)

Skin testing for allergic reaction
(recommended prior to treatment for patients with suspected hypersensitivity to calcitonin or patients with a history of florid allergy to foreign proteins)

## Side/Adverse Effects

The following side/adverse effects have been selected on the basis of their potential clinical significance (possible signs and symptoms in parentheses where appropriate)—not necessarily inclusive:

**Those indicating need for medical attention**
Incidence rare
*Allergic reactions, specifically; skin rash; and urticaria* (hives)

**Those indicating need for medical attention only if they continue or are bothersome**
Incidence more frequent
*Flushing, redness, or tingling of face, ears, hands, or feet; gastrointestinal effects, specifically diarrhea; loss of appetite; nausea or vomiting; and stomach pain; redness, soreness, or swelling at injection site*

Incidence less frequent
*Increased frequency of urination*

Incidence rare
*Chills; dizziness; headache; pressure in chest; stuffy nose; tenderness or tingling of hands or feet; trouble in breathing; weakness*

## Patient Consultation

As an aid to patient consultation, refer to *Advice for the Patient, Calcitonin (Systemic).*

In providing consultation, consider emphasizing the following selected information (» = major clinical significance):

**Before using this medication**
» Conditions affecting use, especially:
Allergies (history of) or sensitivity to calcitonin or other proteins
Breast-feeding—Distributed into breast milk; lactation inhibited in animal studies

**Proper use of this medication**
Proper administration: Using aseptic technique; subcutaneous injection preferred for self-administration
Importance of using reconstituted solution of calcitonin-human within 6 hours
Importance of inspecting solution for particles or discoloration before administering
» Proper dosing
Missed dose: If dosage schedule is:
Two doses a day—Taking missed dose, if remembered within 2 hours, and continuing on schedule; if remembered later, skipping missed dose, not doubling doses, and continuing on schedule
One dose a day—Taking as soon as possible unless remembered the next day; then skipping missed dose and continuing on schedule, but not doubling doses
One dose every other day—Taking as soon as possible if on scheduled day; taking if remembered on alternate day, but skipping the following day and restarting schedule
One dose three times a week (Monday-Wednesday-Friday)—Taking missed dose the next day; setting each injection back a day and resuming regular schedule the following week
» Proper storage

**Precautions while using this medication**
Regular visits to physician to check progress during therapy
Possible need for calcium and vitamin D restriction, including calcifediol and calcitriol, in patients with hypercalcemia

**Side/adverse effects**
Signs of potential side effects, especially allergic reaction

## General Dosing Information

**For use in Paget's disease of bone**
Clinical or biochemical improvement (decreased serum alkaline phosphatase) usually occurs within the first few months of therapy if calcitonin is effective. A longer period of therapy, often more than a year, may be required for maximum improvement.

Dosage adjustments depend on clinical and radiologic evidence, changes in serum alkaline phosphatase and urinary hydroxyproline excretion, and severity of nausea or flushing.

Bedtime administration may help to reduce the severity of nausea or flushing. Reduction in dosage may also be helpful.

After at least 6 months of treatment for Paget's disease, if symptoms have been relieved, therapy may be reduced for 6 months, monitoring biochemical and clinical responses, before being discontinued. Since biochemical indexes will relapse after cessation of treatment, they cannot be relied on to indicate a need for restarting therapy.

---

### CALCITONIN-HUMAN

## Summary of Differences

Cross-sensitivity and/or related problems: May be used for longer term treatment with less antibody formation or protein hypersensitivity than calcitonin-salmon.

## Additional Dosing Information

See also *General Dosing Information.*

More severe cases of Paget's disease of bone (evidence of weak bones with osteolytic lesions) may require doses of up to 1 mg a day, given in divided doses.

## Parenteral Dosage Forms

### CALCITONIN-HUMAN FOR INJECTION

**Usual adult dose**
Paget's disease of bone—
Subcutaneous, initially 500 mcg (0.5 mg) a day, the dosage being reduced for some patients to 500 mcg (0.5 mg) two or three times a week, or 250 mcg (0.25 mg) a day.

Note: To diminish side effects, some clinicians recommend starting with a low dose and gradually increasing dosage over 2 weeks.

**Usual pediatric dose**
Dosage has not been established.

**Size(s) usually available**
U.S.—
  500 mcg (0.5 mg) (Rx) [*Cibacalcin*].
Canada—
  Not commercially available.

**Packaging and storage**
Store at a temperature not exceeding 25 °C (77 °F), unless otherwise specified by manufacturer. Protect from light. Do not refrigerate.

**Preparation of dosage form**
To reconstitute, push the barrel of the double-chambered syringe into the vial as far as possible, and press upward on the plunger to release the water into the dry powder. Shake gently to mix. Withdraw the reconstituted medication back into the syringe and inject.

**Stability**
The reconstituted solution should be used within 6 hours.

**Additional information**
One chamber of the dual syringe contains 0.5 mg of calcitonin-human for injection and mannitol (20 mg) in sterile, lyophilized form. The other chamber contains mannitol (30 mg) in 1 mL of water for injection.

---

## *CALCITONIN-SALMON*

## Summary of Differences

Cross-sensitivity and/or related problems: Risk of protein hypersensitivity and antibody-mediated resistance greater than with calcitonin-human.

## Additional Dosing Information

See also *General Dosing Information*.

This medicine is for intramuscular or subcutaneous injection. The subcutaneous route of administration is usually preferred for patient self-administration.

If the volume to be injected exceeds 2 mL, the intramuscular route of administration is usually preferred and multiple sites of injection should be used to minimize local inflammatory reactions.

Skin testing should be considered prior to treatment of patients with suspected sensitivity to calcitonin-salmon. The manufacturer's recommendation for preparing the solution for skin testing is as follows:
• Prepare a dilution of 10 IU per mL by withdrawing 0.05 mL into a tuberculin syringe (an insulin syringe with no "dead space" may be preferred for a more accurate dilution).
• Fill to 1 mL with 0.9% sodium chloride injection. Mix well.
• Discard 0.9 mL and inject 0.1 mL intracutaneously on the inner forearm.
• Observe injection site 15 minutes after injection.
• A positive response is considered to be the appearance of a more than mild erythema or wheal.

In any patient who has an acceptable initial response but later relapses, either clinically or biochemically, there is the possibility of antibody formation. Testing the patient for high antibody titer by an appropriate specialized test or by critical clinical evaluation should be considered. Alternatively, a trial of therapy with calcitonin-human may be considered. Patient compliance should also be assessed in the event of relapse.

In patients who have relapsed, a dosage increase above 100 IU per day does not appear to improve patient response.

## Parenteral Dosage Forms
### CALCITONIN-SALMON INJECTION

**Usual adult dose**
Paget's disease of bone—
  Intramuscular or subcutaneous, initially 100 IU a day, the dosage being decreased to 50 IU once a day, once every other day, or three times a week, in patients without serious deformity or bone involvement.
Hypercalcemia—
  Intramuscular or subcutaneous, initially 4 IU per kg of body weight every twelve hours, the dosage being increased, if necessary for a more satisfactory response, to 8 IU per kg of body weight every twelve hours, up to a maximum of 8 IU per kg of body weight every six hours.
Postmenopausal osteoporosis[1]—
  Intramuscular or subcutaneous, 100 IU once a day, once every other day, or three times a week.

Note: To diminish side effects, some clinicians recommend starting with a low dose and gradually increasing dosage over 2 weeks.

**Usual pediatric dose**
Dosage has not been established.

**Strength(s) usually available**
U.S.—
  200 IU per mL (Rx) [*Calcimar; Miacalcin*].
Canada—
  200 IU per mL (Rx) [*Calcimar*].

**Packaging and storage**
Store between 2 and 8 °C (36 and 46 °F), unless otherwise specified by manufacturer. Do not freeze.

**Auxiliary labeling**
• Refrigerate.

**Additional information**
May also contain 5 mg of phenol per mL, as a preservative.

The activity of calcitonin-salmon is stated in terms of International Units (IU), which are equal to Medical Research Council Units (MRC).

[1]Not included in Canadian product labeling.

Revised: 05/13/92
Interim revision: 06/27/94

---

## CALCITONIN-HUMAN—See *Calcitonin (Systemic)*

---

## CALCITONIN-SALMON—See *Calcitonin (Systemic)*

---

## CALCITRIOL—See *Vitamin D and Analogs (Systemic)*

---

## CALCIUM ACETATE—See *Calcium Supplements (Systemic)*

---

## CALCIUM CARBONATE—See *Antacids (Oral-Local)*; *Calcium Supplements (Systemic)*

---

## CALCIUM CARBONATE–CONTAINING COMBINATIONS—

Alumina, Magnesia, and Calcium Carbonate (Oral-Local)—See *Antacids (Oral-Local)*
Alumina, Magnesia, Calcium Carbonate, and Simethicone (Oral-Local)—See *Antacids (Oral-Local)*
Calcium Carbonate and Magnesia (Oral-Local)—See *Antacids (Oral-Local)*
Calcium Carbonate, Magnesia, and Simethicone (Oral-Local)—See *Antacids (Oral-Local)*
Calcium and Magnesium Carbonates (Oral-Local)—See *Antacids (Oral-Local)*
Calcium and Magnesium Carbonates and Magnesium Oxide (Oral-Local)—See *Antacids (Oral-Local)*
Calcium Carbonate and Simethicone (Oral-Local)—See *Antacids (Oral-Local)*

# CALCIUM CHANNEL BLOCKING AGENTS    Systemic

This monograph includes information on the following: Bepridil†; Diltiazem; Felodipine; Flunarizine*; Isradipine†; Nicardipine; Nifedipine; Nimodipine; Verapamil.

VA CLASSIFICATION (Primary/Secondary):
Bepridil—CV200/CV250
Diltiazem—CV200/CV250; CV300; CV490
Felodipine—CV200/CV490
Flunarizine—CV200/CN105
Isradipine—CV200/CV490
Nicardipine—CV200/CV250; CV490
Nifedipine—CV200/CV250; CV490
Nimodipine—CV200
Verapamil—CV200/CN105; CV250; CV300; CV490; CV900

Note: For a listing of dosage forms and brand names by country availability, see *Dosage Forms* section(s). For a listing of brand names for the articles in this monograph, refer to the General Index.

*Not commercially available in the U.S.
†Not commercially available in Canada.

## Category

Antianginal—Bepridil; Diltiazem; Felodipine; Isradipine; Nicardipine; Nifedipine; Verapamil.
Antiarrhythmic—Diltiazem; Verapamil.
Antihypertensive—Diltiazem; Felodipine; Isradipine; Nicardipine; Nifedipine; Verapamil.
Hypertrophic cardiomyopathy therapy adjunct—Verapamil.
Subarachnoid hemorrhage therapy—Flunarizine; Nicardipine; Nimodipine.
Vascular headache prophylactic—Flunarizine; Verapamil.

## Indications

Note: Bracketed information in the *Indications* section refers to uses that are not included in U.S. product labeling.

### Accepted

Angina pectoris, chronic (treatment)—Bepridil, diltiazem, [felodipine], [isradipine], nicardipine, nifedipine, and verapamil are indicated in the management of classic angina (chronic stable angina or effort-associated angina) with no evidence of vasospasm. Nicardipine [and other calcium channel blockers] may be used alone or in combination, with caution, with beta-adrenergic blocking agents.

Diltiazem, [felodipine] , [isradipine], [nicardipine], nifedipine, and verapamil are also indicated in the management of vasospastic angina (Prinzmetal's variant, or at-rest angina) or unstable angina in patients who are unable to tolerate or whose symptoms are not relieved by adequate doses of beta-adrenergic blocking agents or organic nitrates. They are generally indicated when vasospastic angina is confirmed by: (a) the classical pattern accompanied by elevation of ST segment; (b) ergonovine-induced angina or coronary artery spasm; or (c) coronary artery spasm demonstrated by angiography, although they may also be used when a vasospastic component is indicated but not confirmed (e.g., where pain has a variable threshold on exertion or in unstable angina where electrocardiographic findings are compatible with intermittent vasospasm).

Tachycardia, supraventricular (treatment and prophylaxis)—Verapamil and parenteral diltiazem are indicated in the treatment of supraventricular tachyarrhythmias. Diltiazem and verapamil produce rapid conversion to sinus rhythm of paroxysmal supraventricular tachycardia (including those associated with accessory bypass tracts, such as Wolff-Parkinson-White (W-P-W) or Lown-Ganong-Levine (L-G-L) syndrome) in patients who do not respond to vagal maneuvers when the atrioventricular (AV) node is required for reentry to sustain tachycardia. Parenteral diltiazem and verapamil also produce temporary control of rapid ventricular rate in atrial flutter or atrial fibrillation. Oral verapamil is indicated, alone or in association with digitalis, for control of ventricular rate at rest and during stress in patients with chronic atrial flutter and/or atrial fibrillation (not otherwise controllable with digitalis), and for prophylaxis of repetitive paroxysmal supraventricular tachycardia. Diltiazem and verapamil do not produce class I, II, or III antiarrhythmic effects.

Hypertension (treatment)—Diltiazem, felodipine, isradipine, nicardipine, nifedipine, and verapamil are indicated, alone or in combination with other agents, for treatment of hypertension.

For additional information on initial therapeutic guidelines related to the treatment of hypertension, see *Appendix III*.

[Cardiomyopathy, hypertrophic (treatment adjunct)]—Verapamil is used in the treatment of hypertrophic cardiomyopathy to relieve ventricular outflow obstruction. However, extreme caution is recommended when hypertrophic cardiomyopathy is complicated by left ventricular obstruction, high pulmonary wedge pressure, paroxysmal nocturnal dyspnea or orthopnea, sinoatrial (SA) nodal function impairment, or severe heart block.

Raynaud's phenomenon (treatment)—[Felodipine], [isradipine], [nicardipine], and [nifedipine][1] are used for symptomatic treatment of Raynaud's phenomenon.

Subarachnoid hemorrhage–associated neurologic deficits (treatment)—Nimodipine is indicated for improvement of neurological outcome by reducing the incidence and severity of ischemic deficits in patients with subarachnoid hemorrhage from ruptured congenital intracranial aneurysms who are in good neurological condition post-ictus (e.g., Hunt and Hess Grades I–III). [Flunarizine] and [nicardipine] are also used for this indication.

Headache, vascular (prophylaxis)—Flunarizine and [verapamil] are indicated for reducing frequency and severity of vascular headaches, but are not recommended for treatment of acute attacks.

### Unaccepted

Sublingual use of nifedipine capsules for hypertensive crisis is not recommended because it has been associated with severe hypotension, acute myocardial infarction, stroke, and death.

[1]Not included in Canadian product labeling.

## Pharmacology/Pharmacokinetics

### Physicochemical characteristics

Molecular weight—
Bepridil hydrochloride: 421.02.
Diltiazem hydrochloride: 450.98.
Felodipine: 384.26.
Flunarizine hydrochloride: 477.42.
Isradipine: 371.39.
Nicardipine hydrochloride: 515.99.
Nifedipine: 346.34.
Nimodipine: 418.45.
Verapamil hydrochloride: 491.07.

### Mechanism of action/Effect

These agents are calcium-ion influx inhibitors (slow-channel blocking agents). Although their mechanism is not completely understood, they are thought to inhibit calcium ion entry through select voltage-sensitive areas termed "slow channels" across cell membranes. By reducing intracellular calcium concentration in cardiac and vascular smooth muscle cells, they dilate coronary arteries and peripheral arteries and arterioles, and may reduce heart rate, decrease myocardial contractility (negative inotropic effect), and slow atrioventricular (AV) nodal conduction. Serum calcium concentrations are unchanged, although there is some evidence that elevated serum calcium concentrations may alter the therapeutic effect of verapamil.

Calcium channel blockers may be classified into subgroups according to structure—
Bepridil.
Benzothiazepine (diltiazem).
Diphenylpiperazine (flunarizine).
Dihydropyridine (felodipine, isradipine, nicardipine, nifedipine, nimodipine).
Diphenylalkylamine (verapamil).

Effects within each subgroup are generally the same—
Bepridil is a nonselective calcium channel blocker that affects both cardiac and smooth muscle. It also inhibits the fast sodium inward current in myocardial and vascular smooth muscle.
Piperazine derivatives act on vascular smooth muscle, with few or no direct myocardial effects.
Dihydropyridines are selective for vascular smooth muscle compared with myocardium and therefore act primarily as vasodilators. Hypotensive effects are accompanied by reflex tachycardia.
Diltiazem (a benzothiazepine) and verapamil (a diphenylalkylamine) are less selective vasodilators that also have direct effects on the myocardium, including depression of sinoatrial (SA) and atrioventricular (AV) nodal conduction.

See *Table 1*, page 692.
Antianginal—
Dilation of the peripheral vasculature reduces systemic pressure or cardiac afterload, which results in lessened myocardial wall tension and reduced oxygen requirements of the myocardial tissues. In

vasospastic angina, a relaxation of coronary arteries and arterioles and inhibition of coronary artery spasm improves blood flow and oxygen supply to myocardial tissues. May also be related to enhanced left ventricular diastolic relaxation and decreased wall stiffness (improved diastolic compliance).

Antiarrhythmic—

The inhibited influx of calcium ions in cardiac tissues prolongs the effective refractory period and results in slowed AV nodal conduction. Normal sinus rhythm is usually not affected, except in some elderly or patients with sick sinus syndrome, in whom calcium channel blockade may interfere with sinus-node impulse generation and may induce sinus or sinoatrial block. Normal atrial action potential or intraventricular conduction are not altered, but in depressed atrial fibers amplitude, velocity of depolarization, and conduction velocity are decreased. The antegrade effective refractory period of the accessory bypass tract may be shortened.

Antihypertensive—

Reduction of total peripheral vascular resistance as a result of vasodilation.

Hypertrophic cardiomyopathy therapy adjunct—

Improvement of left ventricular outflow. May also be related to enhanced left ventricular diastolic relaxation and decreased wall stiffness.

Subarachnoid hemorrhage therapy—

Theoretically, nimodipine may prevent cerebral arterial spasm following subarachnoid hemorrhage, but that has not been confirmed by arteriography. Its exact mechanism of action in treatment of neurologic deficits caused by subarachnoid hemorrhage is not known.

Vascular headache prophylactic—

By inhibiting the vasoconstriction that occurs in the prodrome phase, calcium channel blockade may relieve or prevent reactive vasodilation.

## Other actions/effects

Inhibition of platelet aggregation. Decrease in esophageal contraction amplitude. Diltiazem and verapamil may inhibit cytochrome P450 metabolism, thereby inhibiting the metabolism of other medications or compounds. Flunarizine has antihistaminic effects. Isradipine has diuretic effects. Verapamil decreases gastrointestinal transit time.

## Absorption

Bepridil—Rapid and complete; bioavailability 60 to 70% because of first-pass metabolism; rate, but not extent of absorption, is reduced in the presence of food.

Diltiazem—Well absorbed; bioavailability approximately 40% because of first-pass metabolism; bioavailability may increase with chronic use and increasing dose (i.e., bioavailability is nonlinear).

Felodipine—Almost completely absorbed; bioavailability approximately 20% because of first-pass metabolism. Bioavailability is not affected in the presence of food; however, bioavailability more than doubled when felodipine was taken with doubly concentrated grapefruit juice as compared to when it was taken with water or orange juice (a similar, but lesser, effect is also seen with other dihydropyridines).

Flunarizine—Well absorbed.

Isradipine—Absorption is 90 to 95%; bioavailability approximately 15 to 24% because of first-pass metabolism; rate, but not extent, of absorption is reduced in the presence of food.

Nicardipine—Completely absorbed; bioavailability approximately 35% because of first-pass metabolism.

Nifedipine—Rapidly and completely absorbed; bioavailability approximately 60 to 75% because of first-pass metabolism; bioavailability is increased with hepatic function impairment. Rate, but not extent, of absorption of *Procardia XL* may be reduced in the presence of food.

Nimodipine—Rapidly absorbed. Because of extensive first-pass metabolism, bioavailability is only about 13% (significantly increased [up to double the peak serum concentration] in patients with hepatic function impairment). The effect of food on absorption is unknown.

Verapamil—More than 90% of an oral dose is absorbed; bioavailability approximately 20 to 35% because of first-pass metabolism; bioavailability of oral verapamil may increase with chronic use and increasing dose (i.e., bioavailability is nonlinear).

## Distribution

Bepridil—In breast milk: Concentration is approximately one-third serum concentration.

## Protein binding

Bepridil—Very high (more than 99%).
Diltiazem—High (70 to 80%, 35 to 40% to albumin).
Felodipine—Very high (more than 99%).
Flunarizine—Very high (99%).
Isradipine—Very high (95%).
Nicardipine—Very high (more than 95%).
Nifedipine—Very high (92 to 98%).

Nimodipine—Very high (over 95%); independent of concentration.
Verapamil—Very high (approximately 90%).

## Biotransformation

Hepatic; extensive and rapid, with a prominent first-pass effect.

Bepridil—At least 17 metabolites, 1 or more of which may have cardiovascular activity.

Diltiazem—By cytochrome P450 mixed function oxidase. A major metabolite, detected following oral and continuous intravenous administration but not rapid intravenous administration, is desacetyl diltiazem, which has one-quarter to one-half the coronary dilatation activity of the parent compound.

Felodipine—Six metabolites, accounting for 23% of an oral dose, have been identified; none has significant vasodilating activity.

Isradipine—Completely metabolized; 6 metabolites identified.

Nifedipine—No known active metabolites.

Verapamil—Principal metabolite is norverapamil, which has approximately 20% of the hypotensive cardiovascular activity of verapamil; eleven other metabolites occur only in trace amounts.

## Half-life

Bepridil (biphasic)—
   Distribution:
      Approximately 2 hours.
   Elimination:
      Multiple doses: 42 hours (range, 26 to 64 hours); however, decline from peak plasma concentrations occurs rapidly, indicating a dosing interval half-life shorter than 24 hours.

Diltiazem—
   Oral (biphasic):
      Extended-release capsules—
         *Cardizem CD*—5 to 8 hours.
         *Cardizem SR*—5 to 7 hours.
      Tablets—
         Early—20 to 30 minutes.
         Terminal—Approximately 3.5 hours (5 to 8 hours with high and repetitive dosage).
   Intravenous:
      Approximately 3.4 hours.

Felodipine (polyphasic)—
   Terminal:
      11 to 16 hours.

Flunarizine—
   19 days.

Isradipine (biphasic)—
   Early—1.5 to 2 hours.
   Terminal—About 8 hours.

Nicardipine (biphasic)—
   Early—2 to 4 hours.
   Terminal—8.6 hours.

Nifedipine—
   Approximately 2 hours.

Nimodipine—
   Terminal—8 to 9 hours. Earlier, more rapid elimination rates (equivalent to a half-life of 1 to 2 hours) necessitate frequent dosing.

Verapamil—
   Oral:
      Single dose—Range, 2.8 to 7.4 hours.
      Repetitive dosage—Range, 4.5 to 12 hours (half-life is increased because of saturation of hepatic enzyme systems as plasma verapamil concentrations increase).
   Intravenous (biphasic):
      Early—About 4 minutes.
      Terminal—2 to 5 hours.

## Onset of action

Diltiazem—
   Oral:
      Extended-release capsules—2 to 3 hours.
      Tablets—30 to 60 minutes.
   Parenteral:
      Rapid intravenous injection—
         Reduction in heart rate or conversion of paroxysmal supraventricular tachycardia to sinus rhythm: Within 3 minutes.

Felodipine—
   Within 2 to 5 hours.

Isradipine—
   2 to 3 hours.

Nifedipine—
   Oral:
      Capsules and tablets—20 minutes.

Verapamil—
Oral:
1 to 2 hours.
Intravenous:
Antiarrhythmic—Within 1 to 5 minutes and usually less than 2 minutes.
Hemodynamic—Within 3 to 5 minutes.

**Time to peak concentration**
Bepridil—
2 to 3 hours.
Diltiazem—
Oral (wide individual variation in concentrations achieved):
Extended-release capsules—
*Cardizem CD:* 10 to 14 hours.
*Cardizem SR:* 6 to 11 hours.
Tablets—
2 to 3 hours.
Felodipine—
2.5 to 5 hours. Peak plasma concentrations at steady state are about 20% higher than after a single dose.
Flunarizine—
2 to 4 hours.
Isradipine—
About 1.5 hours.
Nicardipine—
30 minutes to 2 hours (mean, 1 hour).
Nifedipine—
Capsules:
About 30 to 60 minutes.
Tablets:
1 to 2 hours. Peak plasma concentrations achieved are 30% lower than those achieved with the same dosage of nifedipine capsules, although the antianginal effects are the same.
Extended-release tablets:
*Adalat P.A.*—4 hours.
*Procardia XL*—Approximately 6 hours.
Nimodipine—
Within 1 hour.
Verapamil—
Oral:
Extended-release capsules—7 to 9 hours.
Tablets—1 to 2 hours (wide individual variation in concentrations achieved).
Extended-release tablets—5 to 7 hours.

**Time to peak effect**
Bepridil—
Time to steady-state plasma concentration: 8 days.
Diltiazem—
Antihypertensive: Multiple doses—Within 2 weeks.
Antiarrhythmic: Rapid intravenous injection—Hypotension or reduction in heart rate: Within 2 to 7 minutes.
Flunarizine—
Multiple doses: Several weeks.
Isradipine—
Antihypertensive: Multiple doses—2 to 4 weeks.
Nicardipine—
Single dose: 1 to 2 hours.
Verapamil—
Oral: About 30 to 90 minutes. The maximum effects from oral dosage are usually evident sometime during the first 24 to 48 hours of therapy (for some patients the time may be slightly extended because the half-life of verapamil tends to increase during this period).
Intravenous: Within 3 to 5 minutes after completion of injection.

**Duration of action**
Bepridil—
24 hours.
Diltiazem—
Oral:
Extended-release capsules—
*Cardizem CD:* 24 hours.
*Cardizem SR:* 12 hours.
Tablets—
4 to 8 hours.
Parenteral:
Rapid intravenous injection—Hypotension or reduction in heart rate: 1 to 3 hours.
Continuous intravenous infusion—Hypotension or reduction in heart rate: 0.5 to more than 10 hours (median 7 hours).
Felodipine—
24 hours.

Isradipine—
More than 12 hours.
Nicardipine—
8 hours.
Nifedipine—
Capsules and tablets:
4 to 8 hours.
Extended-release tablets:
*Adalat P.A.*—12 hours.
*Procardia XL*—24 hours.
Verapamil—
Oral:
Extended-release capsules: 24 hours.
Tablets: 8 to 10 hours.
Extended-release tablets: 24 hours.
Intravenous:
Antiarrhythmic: About 2 hours.
Hemodynamic: 10 to 20 minutes.

**Elimination**
Bepridil—
Renal: 70% (none unchanged).
Biliary/fecal: 22% (none unchanged).
In dialysis: Not removable by hemodialysis.
Diltiazem—
Biliary and renal (2 to 4% unchanged).
In dialysis: Does not appear to be removable by hemodialysis or peritoneal dialysis.
Felodipine—
Renal: 70% (less than 0.5% unchanged).
Biliary/fecal: 10% (less than 0.5% unchanged).
Flunarizine—
Drug and metabolites: Very slow and prolonged.
Biliary/fecal: Less than 6% in the first 48 hours.
Renal: Less than 0.2% in the first 48 hours.
Isradipine—
Renal: 60 to 65% (none unchanged).
Biliary/fecal: 25 to 30% (none unchanged).
In dialysis: No information, but not likely to be removable by hemodialysis because of plasma protein binding.
Nicardipine—
Renal: 60% (less than 1% unchanged).
Biliary/fecal: 35%.
Nifedipine—
Renal: 80% (as metabolites), only traces unchanged.
Biliary/fecal: 20% (as metabolites).
In dialysis: Does not appear to be removed by hemodialysis or chronic ambulatory peritoneal dialysis; however, plasmapheresis may be beneficial.
Nimodipine—
Renal (less than 1% unchanged).
Biliary/fecal.
In dialysis: Because of extensive protein binding, unlikely to be significantly removed by hemodialysis or peritoneal dialysis.
Verapamil—
Renal:
As conjugated metabolites—70% as metabolites and 3 to 4% unchanged within 5 days.
Unmetabolized—3%.
Biliary/fecal:
9 to 16%.
In dialysis:
Not removable by hemodialysis.

# Precautions to Consider

## Carcinogenicity/Mutagenicity
*For bepridil—*
A lifetime study in mice at doses up to 60 times the maximum recommended human dose (MRHD) (based on a 60-kg subject) found no evidence of carcinogenicity. A lifetime study in rats at doses 20 times the usual recommended human dose found unilateral follicular adenomas of the thyroid.
Mutagenicity studies (micronucleus test for chromosomal effects, liver microsome activated bacterial assay for mutagenicity, Chinese hamster ovary cell assay for mutagenicity, sister chromatid exchange assay) were negative.
*For diltiazem—*
A 24-month study with diltiazem in rats and a 21-month study in mice found no evidence of carcinogenicity.
There was no mutagenic response in *in vitro* bacterial tests.

For felodipine—
A 2-year study in rats at doses of 7.7, 23.1, or 69.3 mg per kg of body weight (mg/kg) per day (up to 28 times the MRHD [based on a 50-kg subject]) found an increased incidence of benign interstitial cell tumors of the testes (Leydig cell tumors) in males, probably secondary to a reduction in testicular testosterone and corresponding increase in serum luteinizing hormone (which have not been observed in humans). In addition, a dose-related increase in the incidence of focal squamous cell hyperplasia in the esophageal groove of both males and females at all doses (humans have no anatomical structure comparable to the esophageal groove). Felodipine was not carcinogenic and did not increase the incidence of Leydig cell tumors in mice at doses up to 138.6 mg/kg per day (28 times the MRHD [based on a 50-kg subject]) for periods up to 80 and 99 weeks in males and females, respectively; no effect on the esophageal groove occurred.
Mutagenicity studies (Ames test, mouse lymphoma forward mutation assay, mouse micronucleus test, human lymphocyte chromosome aberration assay) were negative.

For flunarizine—
A 24-month study in 4 groups of 50 male and 50 female Wistar rats at doses of 0, 5, 20, or 40 mg/kg per day (the 40-mg/kg group received 80 mg/kg for the first 2 months) did not produce an effect on tumor rate or type; however, the validity of the study is questionable because of an extremely high mortality rate (more than 90% in the males and 80% in the females).
Mutagenicity studies (Ames test, sister chromatid exchange test in human lymphocytes, sex-linked recessive lethal test in Drosophila melanogaster, micronucleus test in male rats, dominant lethal test in male and female mice) were negative.

For isradipine—
A 2-year study in male rats at doses of 2.5, 12.5, or 62.5 mg/kg per day (approximately 6, 31, and 156 times the MRHD, respectively, based on a 50-kg subject) found a dose-dependent increase in the incidence of benign Leydig cell tumors and testicular hyperplasia relative to untreated control animals; these findings were replicated in a subsequent study. A 2-year study in mice at doses of 6, 38, and 200 times the MRHD found no evidence of oncogenicity.
Mutagenicity studies were negative.

For nicardipine—
A 2-year study in rats with nicardipine at dosage levels of 5, 15, or 45 mg/kg per day found a dose-dependent increase in thyroid hyperplasia and neoplasia (follicular adenoma/carcinoma). One- and three-month studies in the rat suggest that the mechanism for this effect is a nicardipine-induced reduction in plasma thyroxine ($T_4$) concentrations with a resulting increase in thyroid-stimulating hormone (TSH) concentrations, which is known to cause hyperstimulation of the thyroid; in rats on an iodine-deficient diet, one month of nicardipine administration produced thyroid hyperplasia that was prevented by $T_4$ supplementation. Studies in mice for up to 18 months at doses up to 100 mg/kg per day and in dogs for 1 year at doses up 25 mg/kg per day found no evidence of neoplasia of any tissue and no evidence of thyroid changes. No effects of nicardipine on thyroid function (plasma $T_4$ and TSH) have been reported in humans.
No evidence of mutagenicity was found in a battery of genotoxicity tests conducted on microbial indicator organisms, in micronucleus tests in mice and hamsters, or in a sister chromatid exchange study in hamsters.

For nifedipine—
Nifedipine was not shown to be carcinogenic when administered orally to rats for 2 years.
In vivo mutagenic tests were negative.

For nimodipine—
A 2-year study in rats found an increased incidence of adenocarcinoma of the uterus and Leydig-cell adenoma of the testes, but the increases were not significant. A 91-week study in mice found no evidence of carcinogenicity, although the life expectancy was shortened.
Mutagenicity studies, including the Ames, micronucleus, and dominant lethal tests, have been negative.

For verapamil—
A 2-year study in rats with verapamil at doses up to 12 times the MRHD found no evidence of carcinogenicity.
There was no mutagenic response in the Ames test in 5 test strains at 3 mg per plate with or without metabolic activation.

**Pregnancy/Reproduction**
Fertility—
For felodipine—
No significant effect on reproductive performance was found in male or female rats given doses of 3.8, 9.6, or 26.9 mg/kg per day.
For flunarizine—
In studies in male and female Wistar rats at doses of 0 and approximately 10, 40, and 160 mg/kg given for 60 days premating in the males or 14 days pre-mating and 21 days of gestation in the females, treated animals were mated with non-treated animals. In treated females at the highest dose, there were no pregnancies and a large number of deaths; at the 40-mg/kg dose, there was decreased weight gain during pregnancy, decreased rate of pregnancy, increase in the number of resorbed fetuses, decreased litter size, and decreased weight of pups at birth. In non-treated females mated with treated males, a slight increase in resorption was seen only at the highest dose.
For nifedipine—
Reduced fertility occurred in rats given 30 times the maximum recommended human dose (MRHD) prior to mating.
Pregnancy—
For bepridil—
Adequate and well-controlled studies in humans have not been done.
Studies in rats at maternal doses of 37 times the MRHD found reduced litter size at birth and decreased pup survival during lactation. No teratogenicity was observed in rats or rabbits at the same dose.
FDA Pregnancy Category C.
For diltiazem—
Well-controlled studies in humans have not been done.
Studies in mice, rats, and rabbits, using doses of diltiazem 5 to 10 times greater than the recommended daily dose on a mg/kg basis, resulted in embryo and fetal deaths, reduced neonatal survival rates, and skeletal abnormalities. In addition, there was an increased incidence of stillbirths at doses of 20 or more times the recommended human dose.
FDA Pregnancy Category C.
For felodipine—
Adequate and well-controlled studies in humans have not been done.
Studies in rabbits at doses of 0.46, 1.2, 2.3, and 4.6 mg/kg per day (from 0.4 to 4 times the MRHD [based on a 50-kg subject] on a mg per square meter of body surface basis) found digital anomalies consisting of reduction in size and degree of ossification of the terminal phalanges in the fetuses. Frequency and severity of the changes were dose-related and occurred even at the lowest dose. These changes are similar to those occurring with other dihydropyridines and may be the result of compromised uterine blood flow. The anomalies did not occur in rats; abnormal position of the distal phalanges (but not reduction in size of the terminal phalanges) occurred in about 40% of cynomolgus monkey fetuses.
Studies in rats at doses of 9.6 mg/kg per day (4 times the MRHD [based on a 50-kg subject] on a mg per square meter of body surface basis) produced a prolongation of parturition with a difficult labor and an increased frequency of fetal and early postnatal deaths.
Studies in rabbits at doses greater than or equal to 1.2 mg/kg per day (equal to the MRHD on a mg per square meter of body surface basis) found significant enlargement (in excess of normal) of the mammary glands during pregnancy, which regressed during lactation. These effects were not observed in rats or monkeys.
FDA Pregnancy Category C.
For flunarizine—
Studies in humans have not been done.
There was a slight increase in resorptions and decrease in number of live fetuses in female Wistar rats given 40 mg/kg, with no effects seen at doses of 0, 10, or 20 mg/kg; there was no evidence of teratogenicity. There was a dose-related increase in the number of resorptions in New Zealand rabbits given doses of 0, 2.5, or 10 mg/kg from day 6 to day 18 of pregnancy, with a corresponding decrease in number of live births; there was no evidence of teratogenicity.
For isradipine—
Studies in humans have not been done.
Studies in rats at doses of 6, 20, or 60 mg/kg per day produced a significant reduction in maternal weight gain at the highest dose (150 times the MRHD), but with no lasting effects on the

mother or offspring. Studies in rabbits at doses of 1, 3, or 10 mg/kg per day (2.5, 7.5, and 25 times the MRHD, respectively) found decreased maternal weight gain and increased fetal resorptions at the two highest doses. There was no evidence of embryotoxicity at doses that were not maternotoxic and no evidence of teratogenicity at any dose. With peri- and postnatal administration of doses of 20 and 60 mg/kg per day, reduced maternal weight gain during late pregnancy was associated with reduced birth weights and decreased peri- and postnatal pup survival.

FDA Pregnancy Category C.

*For nicardipine—*

Adequate and well-controlled studies in humans have not been done.

Studies in Japanese White rabbits at doses of 150 mg/kg per day during organogenesis (but not at doses of 50 mg/kg per day [25 times the MRHD]) found nicardipine to be embryocidal and to cause marked body weight gain suppression in the treated doe. Studies in rats with nicardipine at doses 50 times the MRHD found no evidence of embryolethality or teratogenicity, but dystocia, reduced birth weights, reduced neonatal survival, and reduced neonatal weight gain occurred.

FDA Pregnancy Category C.

*For nifedipine—*

Adequate and well-controlled studies in humans have not been done.

Nifedipine has been shown to be teratogenic in rodents and embryotoxic (increased fetal resorptions, reduced fetal weight, increase in stunted forms, increased fetal deaths, and decreased fetal survival) in rodents and rabbits at doses 30 times and 3 to 10 times the MRHD, respectively. In pregnant monkeys, small placentas and underdeveloped chorionic villi occurred at two-thirds and 2 times the MRHD. In rats, 3 times or more the MRHD caused prolongation of pregnancy.

FDA Pregnancy Category C.

*For nimodipine—*

Adequate and well-controlled studies in humans have not been done.

Two studies in Himalayan rabbits found an increased incidence of teratogenic malformations in the fetuses at doses of 1 and 10 (but not 3) mg/kg per day given on Days 6 through 18 of pregnancy; in these same studies, stunted fetuses were found at doses of 1 and 10 (but not 3) mg/kg per day in one study, and only at 1 mg/kg per day in the other. Studies in Long Evans rats at doses of 100 mg/kg per day given on Days 6 through 15 found embryotoxicity, including fetal resorption and stunted fetal growth. In other rat studies, doses of 30 mg/kg per day from Days 16 to 20 or 21 produced an increased incidence of skeletal variation, stunted fetuses, and stillbirths, but no malformations.

FDA Pregnancy Category C.

*For verapamil—*

Adequate and well-controlled studies in humans have not been done.

Verapamil crosses the placenta and can be detected in umbilical vein blood at delivery. Occasionally, rapid intravenous injection of verapamil in humans may cause maternal hypotension resulting in fetal distress.

Studies in rats, using doses of verapamil up to 6 times the recommended daily dose for humans, resulted in embryo deaths and slowed growth.

FDA Pregnancy Category C.

**Breast-feeding**

*For all calcium channel blockers—*

Although problems in humans have not been documented, bepridil, diltiazem, nifedipine, and verapamil, and possibly other calcium channel blockers, are distributed into breast milk.

*For felodipine only—*

It is not known whether felodipine is distributed into breast milk in humans.

*For flunarizine only—*

It is not known whether flunarizine is distributed into breast milk in humans; however, it is distributed into the milk of dogs, at concentrations much higher than in plasma.

*For nimodipine only—*

It is not known whether nimodipine is distributed into breast milk in humans; however, nimodipine and/or its metabolites have been found in the milk of treated rats, at concentrations much higher than maternal plasma concentrations.

**Pediatrics**

Although appropriate studies on the relationship of age to the effects of calcium channel blockers have not been performed in the pediatric population, pediatrics-specific problems that would limit the usefulness of calcium channel blockers in children are not expected. However, in rare instances, severe adverse hemodynamic effects have occurred after intravenous administration of verapamil in neonates and infants.

**Geriatrics**

*For diltiazem, nimodipine, verapamil, and possibly other calcium channel blockers—*

Half-life of calcium channel blockers may be increased in the elderly as a result of decreased clearance.

*For felodipine only—*

Plasma concentrations increase with age. Mean clearance at mean age of 76 was found to be only 45% of that at mean age of 26.

*For isradipine only—*

Bioavailability may be increased in patients over 65 years of age.

*For nicardipine only—*

Studies in patients 65 years of age and older found no difference in half-life or protein binding from that in young normal volunteers.

*For nimodipine only—*

Risk of hypotension may be increased.

*For all calcium channel blockers—*

Elderly patients are more likely to have age-related renal function impairment, which may require caution in patients receiving calcium channel blockers.

**Dental**

Gingival hyperplasia is a rare side effect that has been reported with diltiazem, felodipine, nifedipine, and verapamil. It usually starts as gingivitis or gum inflammation in the first 1 to 9 months of treatment. A strictly enforced program of teeth cleaning by a professional combined with plaque control by the patient will minimize growth rate and severity of gingival enlargement. Periodontal surgery may be indicated in some cases, and should be followed by careful plaque control to inhibit recurrence of gum enlargement.

**Drug interactions and/or related problems**

The following drug interactions and/or related problems have been selected on the basis of their potential clinical significance (possible mechanism in parentheses where appropriate)—not necessarily inclusive (» = major clinical significance):

Note: Information concerning interactions between calcium channel blockers and other medications is still limited. Therefore, some of the following potential interactions are stated for cautionary reference until additional information is available.

Combinations containing any of the following medications, depending on the amount present, may also interact with these medications.

Anesthetics, hydrocarbon inhalation
(concurrent use with calcium channel blockers may produce additive hypotension; although calcium channel blockers may be useful to prevent supraventricular tachycardias, hypertension, or coronary spasm during surgery, caution is recommended during use)

Anti-inflammatory drugs, nonsteroidal (NSAIDs), especially indomethacin
(indomethacin, and possibly other NSAIDs, may antagonize the antihypertensive effect of calcium channel blockers by inhibiting renal prostaglandin synthesis and/or by causing sodium and fluid retention; the patient should be carefully monitored to confirm that the desired effect is being obtained)

» Beta-adrenergic blocking agents, systemic or ophthalmic
(concurrent use of oral dosage forms with oral bepridil, diltiazem, or verapamil or intravenous verapamil usually results in no serious negative inotropic, chronotropic, or dromotropic effects. However, caution and careful monitoring are necessary since the additive effect may prolong sinoatrial [SA] and atrioventricular [AV] conduction [which may lead to severe hypotension, bradycardia, and cardiac failure], especially in patients with impaired ventricular function or abnormal cardiac conduction or sinus node depression. When verapamil and beta-adrenergic blocking agents are to be given intravenously, they should be administered at least a few hours apart since they may have additive depressant effects on myocardial contractility or SA or AV conduction, and asystole has been reported with concurrent use)

(in a single small study, diltiazem was reported to significantly increase the bioavailability of propranolol; in other studies, verapamil was found to decrease clearance of both metoprolol and propranolol, with a variable effect on atenolol)

(concurrent use with dihydropyridines, although usually well tolerated, may produce excessive hypotension, and in rare cases may increase the possibility of congestive heart failure. Occasionally, angina has occurred upon initiation of nicardipine or nifedipine therapy, especially after recent abrupt discontinuation of beta-adrenergic blocking agent therapy. If possible, it is recommended that beta-adrenergic blocking agent dosage be discontinued gradually, but especially before nicardipine or nifedipine therapy is begun. However, if concurrent use is necessary, nicardipine or nifedipine may be preferred over other calcium channel blockers in some patients because it has less effect on heart rate and conduction)

(if significant systemic absorption of an ophthalmic beta-blocker occurs, concurrent use of calcium channel blocking agents may result in atrioventricular conduction disturbances, left ventricular failure, and hypotension; in some patients, if a calcium antagonist is necessary, nicardipine or nifedipine may be preferred because it has less effect on heart rate and conduction, although it may also cause greater hypotension; concurrent use of calcium channel blockers and ophthalmic beta-blockers should be avoided in patients with impaired cardiac function)

Calcium supplements
(concurrent use in quantities sufficient to elevate serum calcium concentrations above normal may reduce the response to verapamil and probably other calcium channel blockers)

» Carbamazepine or
» Cyclosporine or
» Quinidine or
Theophylline or
Valproate
(diltiazem or verapamil may inhibit cytochrome P450 metabolism, resulting in increased concentrations and toxicity of these medications)

(an idiosyncratic reaction has been reported in which concurrent use of nifedipine and quinidine resulted in significantly reduced serum quinidine concentrations; caution is recommended when nifedipine therapy is initiated or discontinued in a patient stabilized on quinidine)

Cimetidine
(concurrent use may result in accumulation of calcium channel blockers as a result of inhibition of first-pass metabolism; caution and careful titration of calcium channel blocker dose is recommended on initiation of therapy in patients receiving cimetidine; ranitidine and famotidine do not appear to significantly affect calcium channel blocker metabolism)

» Digitalis glycosides
(concurrent use of digoxin with some calcium channel blocking agents [especially verapamil and, to a lesser extent, bepridil, diltiazem, and nifedipine] has been reported to increase the serum concentration of digoxin; the effect of verapamil on digoxin kinetics is enhanced in patients with hepatic function impairment; felodipine significantly increased peak plasma concentrations of digoxin, although there was no significant change in the area under the curve [AUC]; isradipine and nicardipine do not appear to have a significant effect. Digoxin serum concentrations should be monitored and dosage may need to be altered when concurrent dosage of the calcium channel blocking agent is initiated, changed, or discontinued. Concurrent use of oral digitalis preparations with oral diltiazem or verapamil or intravenous verapamil has resulted in no serious adverse effects when patients were closely monitored; however, both groups of medications slow AV conduction. Patients receiving them concurrently should be monitored for AV block or excessive bradycardia, especially during the first week of concurrent dosage. To avoid toxicity, dosage reduction of digitalis glycoside may be necessary)

» Disopyramide or
Flecainide
(disopyramide should not be administered within 48 hours before or 24 hours following verapamil administration since both medications possess negative inotropic properties; deaths have been reported; caution is also recommended when disopyramide is used concurrently with diltiazem, nicardipine, or nifedipine; caution is also recommended when flecainide is used concurrently with a calcium channel blocker)

Estrogens
(estrogen-induced fluid retention tends to increase blood pressure; the patient should be carefully monitored to confirm that the desired effect is being obtained)

Highly protein-bound medications, such as:
Anticoagulants, coumarin- and indandione-derivative
Anticonvulsants, hydantoin
Anti-inflammatory drugs, nonsteroidal
Quinine

Salicylates
Sulfinpyrazone
(caution is advised when these medications are used concurrently with nifedipine or verapamil since changes in serum concentrations of the free, unbound medications may occur)

» Hypokalemia-producing medications, such as:
Amphotericin B, parenteral
Carbonic anhydrase inhibitors
Corticosteroids, glucocorticoid, especially those with significant mineralocorticoid activity
Corticosteroids, mineralocorticoid
Corticotropin (ACTH)
Diuretics, potassium-depleting (such as bumetanide, ethacrynic acid, furosemide, indapamide, mannitol, or thiazides)
Sodium phosphates
(risk of bepridil-induced arrhythmias may be increased)

Hypotension-producing medications, other (See *Appendix II*)
(antihypertensive effects may be potentiated when these medications are used concurrently with hypotension-producing calcium channel blockers; although some antihypertensive and/or diuretic combinations are frequently used for therapeutic advantage, when any hypotension-producing medication is used concurrently dosage adjustments may be necessary)

Lithium
(concurrent use with calcium channel blockers may result in neurotoxicity in the form of nausea, vomiting, diarrhea, ataxia, tremors, and/or tinnitus; caution is recommended)

Neuromuscular blocking agents
(verapamil may potentiate the activity of curare-like and depolarizing neuromuscular blocking agents; dosage reduction of either or both medications may be necessary during concurrent use)

Phenobarbital
(may increase clearance of verapamil)

Prazosin, and possibly other alpha-adrenergic blocking agents
(concurrent use with calcium channel blockers may produce an increased hypotensive effect, possibly related to impairment of compensatory responses by alpha-blockade and/or inhibition of prazosin metabolism by calcium channel blockers; caution is recommended)

» Procainamide or
» Quinidine or
» Other medications causing QT interval prolongation
(risk of increased QT interval prolongation)
(caution is recommended when procainamide or quinidine is used with a calcium channel blocker since both groups of medications possess negative inotropic properties)

Rifampin, and possibly other hepatic enzyme inducers
(rifampin may reduce the bioavailability of oral verapamil by induction of first-pass metabolism; other calcium channel blockers may also be affected, depending on the extent of first-pass metabolism)

Sympathomimetics
(concurrent use may reduce antihypertensive effects of calcium channel blockers; the patient should be carefully monitored to confirm that the desired effect is being obtained)

## Laboratory value alterations
The following have been selected on the basis of their potential clinical significance (possible effect in parentheses where appropriate)—not necessarily inclusive (» = major clinical significance):

With physiology/laboratory test values
Antinuclear antibody (ANA) titers and
Direct Coombs test, with or without hemolytic anemia
(positive results have been reported during nifedipine therapy)

Arterial blood pressure
(may be reduced by calcium channel blockers [except bepridil and flunarizine])

*Electrocardiograph (ECG) effects*
PR interval
(may be increased by diltiazem and verapamil)
Note: Increase tends to be proportional to serum concentration.

QT interval
(may be increased by bepridil)

T-wave morphology
(may be altered by bepridil)

*Hepatic enzymes*
(may rarely be increased after several days of therapy; concentrations return to normal upon withdrawal of therapy)

*Prolactin*
(serum concentrations may be slightly increased by flunarizine)

Note: Total serum calcium concentrations are not affected by the calcium channel blocking agents.

### Medical considerations/Contraindications

The medical considerations/contraindications included here have been selected on the basis of their potential clinical significance (reasons given in parentheses where appropriate)—not necessarily inclusive (» = major clinical significance).

See *Table 2*, page 693.

### Patient monitoring

The following may be especially important in patient monitoring (other tests may be warranted in some patients, depending on condition; » = major clinical significance):

» Blood pressure determinations and
» ECG readings and
» Heart rate determinations
   (recommended primarily during dosage titration or when dosage is increased from established maintenance dosage level, or during addition of medications affecting cardiac conduction or blood pressure; also recommended during intravenous verapamil administration)

   (blood pressure determinations are recommended at periodic intervals in patients being treated for hypertension; selected patients may be trained to perform blood pressure measurements at home and report the results at regular physician visits)

Hepatic function determinations or
Renal function determinations
   (may be required at periodic intervals during long-term therapy)

*For bepridil*
Potassium concentrations, serum
   (recommended at periodic intervals during therapy to watch for hypokalemia)

*For nimodipine*
Neurological examinations
   (recommended at periodic intervals during treatment)

## Side/Adverse Effects

See *Table 3*, page 694.

## Patient Consultation

As an aid to patient consultation, refer to *Advice for the Patient, Calcium Channel Blocking Agents (Systemic).*

In providing consultation, consider emphasizing the following selected information (» = major clinical significance):

### Before using this medication
» Conditions affecting use, especially:
   Sensitivity to the calcium channel blocker prescribed
   Pregnancy—High doses in animals cause birth defects, prolonged pregnancy, poor bone development, and stillbirth
   Use in the elderly—Elderly patients may be more sensitive to effects
   Other medications, especially parenteral amphotericin B (for bepridil), beta-blockers, carbamazepine, carbonic anhydrase inhibitors, corticosteroids (for bepridil), cyclosporine, digitalis glycosides, disopyramide, potassium-depleting diuretics (for bepridil), procainamide, or quinidine
   Other medical problems, especially arrhythmias (for bepridil), other cardiovascular problems, or hypokalemia (for bepridil)

### Proper use of this medication
» Compliance with therapy; importance of not taking more medication than amount prescribed
» Proper dosing
   Missed dose: Taking as soon as possible; not taking if almost time for next scheduled dose; not doubling doses
» Proper storage
*For bepridil*
   If nausea occurs, may be taken with meals or at bedtime
*For extended-release diltiazem capsules*
   Swallowing capsules whole without crushing or chewing
» Caution if switching brands; one is for once-daily dosing and one is for twice-daily dosing
*For extended-release nifedipine or verapamil capsules*
   Swallowing capsules whole without crushing or chewing

*For regular nifedipine or extended-release felodipine or nifedipine tablets*
   Swallowing tablets whole, without breaking, crushing, or chewing
   For *Procardia XL*—Patient may notice empty shell in stool left over after medication is absorbed
*For extended-release verapamil tablets*
   Swallowing tablets whole, without crushing or chewing; may be broken in half on instructions from physician
   Taking with food or milk
*For use as an antihypertensive*
   Importance of diet; possible need for sodium restriction and/or weight reduction
» Patient may not experience symptoms of hypertension; importance of taking medication even if feeling well
» Does not cure, but helps control hypertension; possible need for lifelong therapy; serious consequences of untreated hypertension

### Precautions while using this medication

Regular visits to physician to check progress during therapy
Checking with physician before discontinuing medication; gradual dosage reduction may be necessary
» Discussing exercise or physical exertion limits with physician; reduced occurrence of chest pain may tempt patient to be overactive
Possible headache; checking with physician if continuing or severe
» Maintaining good dental hygiene and seeing dentist frequently for teeth cleaning to prevent tenderness, bleeding, and gum enlargement
*For use as an antihypertensive*
» Not taking other medications, especially nonprescription sympathomimetics, unless discussed with physician
*For patients taking bepridil, diltiazem, or verapamil*
» Checking pulse as directed; checking with physician if less than 50 beats per minute
*For patients taking flunarizine*
   Caution when driving or doing other things requiring alertness because of risk of drowsiness

### Side/adverse effects

Signs of potential side effects, especially angina, congestive heart failure or pulmonary edema, extrapyramidal effects (for flunarizine), galactorrhea (for flunarizine), peripheral edema, tachycardia, bradycardia, excessive hypotension, gingival hyperplasia, allergic reaction, mental depression (for flunarizine), arthritis (for nifedipine), and transient blindness (for nifedipine)

## General Dosing Information

### For oral dosage forms only
Oral dosage must be titrated for each patient as needed and tolerated.

Concurrent administration of nitroglycerin sublingually or long-acting nitrates with calcium channel blocking agents may produce an additive antianginal effect. Nitroglycerin may be used sublingually as required to abort acute angina attacks during calcium channel blocking agent therapy. Nitrate medication may be used during calcium channel blocking agent therapy for angina prophylaxis.

Although no "rebound effect" has been reported upon discontinuation of calcium channel blockers, a gradual decrease of dosage with physician supervision is recommended.

### For treatment of overdose or acute adverse effects
The following treatments have been proven effective for the indicated adverse effect:
   • Hypotension, symptomatic—Intravenous fluids. Intravenous dopamine or dobutamine, calcium chloride, isoproterenol, metaraminol, or norepinephrine. For parenteral verapamil, placement of patient in Trendelenburg position.
   • Tachycardia, rapid ventricular rate in patients with antegrade conduction in atrial flutter fibrillation, and accessory pathway with Wolff-Parkinson-White or Lown-Ganong-Levine syndrome—Direct-current cardioversion, intravenous lidocaine, or intravenous procainamide. Intravenous fluids given by slow-drip.
   • Bradycardia, rarely 2nd or 3rd degree atrioventricular (AV) block, with a few patients progressing to asystole—Intravenous atropine, isoproterenol, norepinephrine, or calcium chloride or use of electronic cardiac pacemaker.

## BEPRIDIL

### Summary of Differences

Pharmacology/pharmacokinetics:
  Nonselective calcium channel blocker; also affects fast sodium inward current.
  Depresses sinoatrial (SA) and atrioventricular (AV) nodes; negative inotropic effect; causes bradycardia.
Precautions:
  Laboratory value alterations—Increases QT interval and alters T-wave morphology.
  Medical considerations/contraindications—Contraindicated in patients with history of serious ventricular arrhythmias or QT interval prolongation. Also, contraindicated in patients with 2nd or 3rd degree atrioventricular (AV) block or sinoatrial (SA) nodal function impairment, except in patients with a functioning artificial ventricular pacemaker. Extreme caution necessary in patients with hypokalemia.
Side/adverse effects:
  Differences in frequencies are due to differences in pharmacological effects. Also causes agranulocytosis (rare); arrhythmias, including torsades de pointes (less common).

### Oral Dosage Forms

#### BEPRIDIL HYDROCHLORIDE TABLETS

**Usual adult dose**
Antianginal—
  Oral, initially 200 mg once a day, the dosage being increased after ten days, if necessary, to 300 mg once a day.

**Usual adult prescribing limits**
Up to 400 mg daily.

**Usual pediatric dose**
Safety and efficacy have not been established.

**Usual geriatric dose**
See *Usual adult dose.*

**Strength(s) usually available**
U.S.—
  200 mg (Rx) [*Bepadin; Vascor*].
  300 mg (Rx) [*Bepadin; Vascor*].
  400 mg (Rx) [*Bepadin; Vascor*].
Canada—
  Not commercially available.

**Packaging and storage**
Store below 40 °C (104 °F), preferably between 15 and 30 °C (59 and 86 °F), in a well-closed container, unless otherwise specified by manufacturer. Protect from light.

## DILTIAZEM

### Summary of Differences

Pharmacology/pharmacokinetics:
  Benzothiazepine structure.
  Depresses sinoatrial (SA) and atrioventricular (AV) nodes; little or no negative inotropic effect; usually does not significantly alter heart rate, but may cause slight bradycardia.
Precautions:
  Laboratory value alterations—Increases PR interval.
  Medical considerations/contraindications—Contraindicated in patients with 2nd or 3rd degree atrioventricular (AV) block, sinoatrial (SA) nodal function impairment, or Wolff-Parkinson-White or Lown-Ganong-Levine syndrome accompanied by atrial flutter or fibrillation, except in patients with a functioning artificial ventricular pacemaker.
Side/adverse effects:
  Differences in frequencies are due to differences in pharmacological effects.

### Additional Dosing Information

See also *General Dosing Information.*
Dermatologic side effects usually disappear even with continued use. However, if skin eruptions persist, it is recommended that diltiazem therapy be withdrawn, since progression to erythema multiforme and/or exfoliative dermatitis or Stevens-Johnson syndrome have been reported rarely.

### Oral Dosage Forms

Note: Bracketed uses in the *Dosage Forms* section refer to categories of use and/or indications that are not included in U.S. product labeling.

#### DILTIAZEM HYDROCHLORIDE EXTENDED-RELEASE CAPSULES

**Usual adult and adolescent dose**
Antihypertensive—
  *Cardizem CD* or *Dilacor-XR*: Oral, 180 to 240 mg once a day, the dosage being adjusted after fourteen days as needed and tolerated.
    Note: The total daily dose usually ranges from 240 to 360 mg.
  *Cardizem SR*: Oral, initially 60 to 120 mg two times a day, the dosage being adjusted after fourteen days as needed and tolerated.
Note: Geriatric patients may be more sensitive to the effects of the usual adult dose.

**Usual adult prescribing limits**
Up to 360 mg daily.

**Usual pediatric dose**
Dosage has not been established.

**Strength(s) usually available**
U.S.—
  60 mg (Rx) [*Cardizem SR* (sucrose); GENERIC].
  90 mg (Rx) [*Cardizem SR* (sucrose); GENERIC].
  120 mg (Rx) [*Cardizem SR* (sucrose); GENERIC].
  180 mg (Rx) [*Cardizem CD* (sucrose); *Dilacor-XR*].
  240 mg (Rx) [*Cardizem CD* (sucrose); *Dilacor-XR*].
  300 mg (Rx) [*Cardizem CD* (sucrose)].
Canada—
  90 mg (Rx) [*Cardizem SR*].
  120 mg (Rx) [*Cardizem SR*].

**Packaging and storage**
Store below 40 °C (104 °F), preferably between 15 and 30 °C (59 and 86 °F), in a well-closed container, unless otherwise specified by manufacturer.

**Auxiliary labeling**
• Do not take other medicines without physician's advice.

**Note**
Check refill frequency to determine compliance in hypertensive patients.
*Cardizem CD* and *Cardizem SR* can be used interchangeably on a total daily mg per mg dosing basis.

#### DILTIAZEM HYDROCHLORIDE TABLETS USP

**Usual adult and adolescent dose**
Antianginal or
[Antihypertensive][1]—
  Oral, initially 30 mg three or four times a day, the dosage being increased gradually at one- or two-day intervals as needed and tolerated.
Note: Geriatric patients may be more sensitive to the effects of the usual adult dose.

**Usual adult prescribing limits**
Up to 360 mg daily.

**Usual pediatric dose**
Dosage has not been established.

**Strength(s) usually available**
U.S.—
  30 mg (Rx) [*Cardizem*; GENERIC].
  60 mg (Rx) [*Cardizem* (scored); GENERIC].
  90 mg (Rx) [*Cardizem* (scored); GENERIC].
  120 mg (Rx) [*Cardizem* (scored); GENERIC].
Canada—
  30 mg (Rx) [*Apo-Diltiaz; Cardizem; Novo-Diltazem; Nu-Diltiaz; Syn-Diltiazem*; GENERIC].
  60 mg (Rx) [*Apo-Diltiaz; Cardizem* (scored); *Novo-Diltazem* (scored); *Nu-Diltiaz; Syn-Diltiazem* (scored); GENERIC].
  90 mg (Rx) [*Cardizem*].
  120 mg (Rx) [*Cardizem*].

**Packaging and storage**
Store below 40 °C (104 °F), preferably between 15 and 30 °C (59 and 86 °F), unless otherwise specified by manufacturer. Store in a tight container. Protect from light.

**Auxiliary labeling**
• Do not take other medicines without physician's advice.

**Note**
Check refill frequency to determine compliance in hypertensive patients.

## Parenteral Dosage Forms

### DILTIAZEM HYDROCHLORIDE INJECTION

#### Usual adult and adolescent dose
Antiarrhythmic—
- Intravenous (rapid), 250 mcg (0.25 mg) per kg of actual body weight administered slowly over a two-minute period with continuous ECG and blood pressure monitoring. If response is not adequate, 350 mcg (0.35 mg) per kg of actual body weight may be administered fifteen minutes after completion of initial dose. Subsequent doses should be individualized.
- Note: Some patients may respond to an initial dose of 150 mcg (0.15 mg) per kg of actual body weight, although the duration of action may be shorter.
- Intravenous infusion, continuous (for continued reduction of heart rate [up to twenty-four hours] in patients with atrial fibrillation or atrial flutter), initially 10 mg per hour beginning immediately after the last rapid intravenous dose. The rate of infusion may be increased in increments of 5 mg per hour as needed, up to a maximum rate of 15 mg per hour.
- Note: Some patients may respond to an initial rate of 5 mg per hour.

#### Usual pediatric dose
Safety and efficacy have not been established.

#### Strength(s) usually available
U.S.—
- 5 mg per mL (Rx) [*Cardizem* (citric acid; sodium citrate dihydrate; sorbitol solution; sodium hydroxide or hydrochloric acid)].

Canada—
- Not commercially available.

#### Packaging and storage
Store between 2 and 8 °C (36 and 46 °F), unless otherwise specified by manufacturer. May be stored at room temperature for 1 month; destroy after 1 month at room temperature. Protect from freezing.

#### Preparation of dosage form
Diltiazem hydrochloride injection may be prepared for administration by continuous intravenous infusion by diluting the appropriate quantity in the desired volume of 0.9% sodium chloride injection, 5% dextrose injection, or 5% dextrose in 0.45% sodium chloride injection, and mixing thoroughly, as follows:

| Diluent Volume | Quantity of Cardizem Injection | Final Concentrations | Administration | |
|---|---|---|---|---|
| | | | Dose* | Infusion Rate |
| 100 mL | 125 mg (25 mL) | 1.0 mg/mL | 10 mg/hr 15 mg/hr | 10 mL/hr 15 mL/hr |
| 250 mL | 250 mg (50 mL) | 0.83 mg/mL | 10 mg/hr 15 mg/hr | 12 mL/hr 18 mL/hr |
| 500 mL | 250 mg (50 mL) | 0.45 mg/mL | 10 mg/hr 15 mg/hr | 22 mL/hr 33 mL/hr |

*5 mg/hr may be appropriate for some patients.

#### Stability
After dilution for administration by intravenous infusion, diltiazem hydrochloride injection should be refrigerated until use and should be used within 24 hours.

#### Incompatibilities
Diltiazem hydrochloride injection is physically incompatible with furosemide solution.

---

¹Not included in Canadian product labeling.

---

### *FELODIPINE*

## Summary of Differences

Pharmacology/pharmacokinetics:
- Dihydropyridine structure.
- Potent peripheral vasodilator; does not depress sinoatrial (SA) or atrioventricular (AV) node; reflex increase in heart rate in response to vasodilation masks negative inotropic effect.

Precautions:
- Medical considerations/contraindications—No caution necessary in renal function impairment.

Side/adverse effects:
- Differences in frequencies are due to differences in pharmacological effects.

## Oral Dosage Forms

### FELODIPINE EXTENDED-RELEASE TABLETS

#### Usual adult dose
Antihypertensive—
- Initial: Oral, 5 mg once a day, the dosage being adjusted as needed, usually at intervals of not less than two weeks.
- Maintenance: Oral, 5 to 10 mg once a day.
Antianginal—
- Oral, 10 mg once a day.
- Note: Geriatric patients may be more sensitive to the effects of the usual adult dose.

#### Usual adult prescribing limits
Up to 20 mg once a day.

#### Usual pediatric dose
Safety and efficacy have not been established.

#### Strength(s) usually available
U.S.—
- 5 mg (Rx) [*Plendil*].
- 10 mg (Rx) [*Plendil*].
Canada—
- 5 mg (Rx) [*Plendil; Renedil*].
- 10 mg (Rx) [*Plendil; Renedil*].

#### Packaging and storage
Store below 30 °C (86 °F), unless otherwise specified by manufacturer. Store in a tight container. Protect from light.

#### Auxiliary labeling
- Do not take other medicines without physician's advice.

#### Note
Check refill frequency to determine compliance in hypertensive patients.

---

### *FLUNARIZINE*

## Summary of Differences

Indications:
- Indicated for prophylaxis of migraine.
Pharmacology/pharmacokinetics:
- Diphenylpiperazine structure.
- Does not depress sinoatrial (SA) or atrioventricular (AV) node; no negative inotropic effect; no reflex increase in heart rate; no antihypertensive effect.
- Cerebroselective.
Precautions:
- Medical considerations/contraindications—Caution required in patients with history of mental depression or with Parkinson's syndrome or other extrapyramidal disorders.
Side/adverse effects:
- Differences in frequencies are due to differences in pharmacological effects. Also causes parkinsonian extrapyramidal effects (less common), galactorrhea (rare), mental depression (less common), drowsiness (more common), dryness of mouth (less common), increased appetite and/or weight gain (more common).

## Oral Dosage Forms

### FLUNARIZINE HYDROCHLORIDE CAPSULES

#### Usual adult dose
Vascular headache prophylactic—
- Oral, 10 mg once a day in the evening.
- Note: Geriatric patients may be more sensitive to the effects of the usual adult dose.

#### Usual pediatric dose
Dosage has not been established.

#### Strength(s) usually available
U.S.—
- Not commercially available.
Canada—
- 5 mg (Rx) [*Sibelium*].

#### Packaging and storage
Store below 40 °C (104 °F), preferably between 15 and 30 °C (59 and 86 °F), in a well-closed container, unless otherwise specified by manufacturer. Protect from light.

## *ISRADIPINE*

## Summary of Differences

Pharmacology/pharmacokinetics:
    Dihydropyridine structure.
    Potent peripheral vasodilator; does not depress sinoatrial (SA) or atrioventricular (AV) node; reflex increase in heart rate in response to vasodilation masks negative inotropic effect.
Side/adverse effects:
    Differences in frequencies are due to differences in pharmacological effects.

## Oral Dosage Forms

### ISRADIPINE CAPSULES

**Usual adult dose**
Antihypertensive—
    Oral, initially 2.5 mg two times a day, alone or in combination with a thiazide diuretic, the dosage being increased, if necessary, in increments of 5 mg per day at two- to four-week intervals.
Note: Geriatric patients may be more sensitive to the effects of the usual adult dose.

**Usual adult prescribing limits**
Up to 10 mg two times a day.

**Usual pediatric dose**
Safety and efficacy have not been established.

**Strength(s) usually available**
U.S.—
    2.5 mg (Rx) [*DynaCirc*].
    5 mg (Rx) [*DynaCirc*].
Canada—
    Not commercially available.

**Packaging and storage**
Store below 40 °C (104 °F) between 15 and 30 °C (59 and 86 °F), unless otherwise specified by manufacturer. Store in a tight container. Protect from light.

**Auxiliary labeling**
• Do not take other medicines without physician's advice.

**Note**
Check refill frequency to determine compliance in hypertensive patients.

## *NICARDIPINE*

## Summary of Differences

Pharmacology/pharmacokinetics:
    Dihydropyridine structure.
    Potent peripheral vasodilator; does not depress sinoatrial (SA) or atrioventricular (AV) node; reflex increase in heart rate in response to vasodilation masks negative inotropic effect.
Precautions:
    Geriatrics—No change in half-life or protein binding.
    Medical considerations/contraindications—Caution necessary in patients with acute cerebral infarction or hemorrhage.
Side/adverse effects:
    Differences in frequencies are due to differences in pharmacological effects.

## Oral Dosage Forms

### NICARDIPINE HYDROCHLORIDE CAPSULES

**Usual adult and adolescent dose**
Antianginal or
Antihypertensive—
    Oral, initially 20 mg three times a day, the dosage being adjusted as needed and tolerated.

**Usual pediatric dose**
Dosage has not been established.

**Strength(s) usually available**
U.S.—
    20 mg (Rx) [*Cardene*].
    30 mg (Rx) [*Cardene*].

Canada—
    20 mg (Rx) [*Cardene*].
    30 mg (Rx) [*Cardene*].

**Packaging and storage**
Store between 15 and 25 °C (59 and 77 °F), in a well-closed, light-resistant container, unless otherwise specified by manufacturer.

**Auxiliary labeling**
• Do not take other medicines without physician's advice.

**Note**
Check refill frequency to determine compliance in hypertensive patients.

## *NIFEDIPINE*

## Summary of Differences

Pharmacology/pharmacokinetics:
    Dihydropyridine structure.
    Potent peripheral vasodilator; does not depress sinoatrial (SA) or atrioventricular (AV) node; reflex increase in heart rate in response to vasodilation masks negative inotropic effect.
Side/adverse effects:
    Differences in frequencies are due to differences in pharmacological effects. Also causes arthritis associated with elevated antinuclear antibody (ANA) titers (rare), transient blindness at peak plasma concentrations (rare).

## Additional Dosing Information

See also *General Dosing Information.*

In solution, degradation of nifedipine occurs more rapidly at 25 °C (77 °F) than at 4 °C (39 °F). However, when nifedipine solutions are protected from light and refrigerated, concentrations of nifedipine decline to approximately 90% of the original concentrations within 6 hours of preparation. It is recommended that extemporaneous preparations be made immediately before use.

## Oral Dosage Forms

Note: Bracketed uses in the *Dosage Forms* section refer to categories of use and/or indications that are not included in U.S. product labeling.

### NIFEDIPINE CAPSULES USP

**Usual adult and adolescent dose**
Antianginal or
[Antihypertensive][1]—
    Essential hypertension: Oral, initially 10 mg three times a day, the dosage being gradually increased over a seven- to fourteen-day period as needed and tolerated.
Note: For hospitalized patients under close supervision, dosage may be increased by 10-mg increments over four- to six-hour periods until symptoms are controlled.

    When justified by symptom frequency and/or severity, dosage titration may be accomplished over a three-day period (medication given three times a day and increased stepwise from 10 mg to 20 mg, then to 30 mg per dose as needed and tolerated), but only if the patient is monitored frequently.

    Geriatric patients may be more sensitive to the effects of the usual adult dose.

**Usual adult prescribing limits**
Single dose, up to 30 mg; total daily dose, up to 180 mg (a total daily dose greater than 120 mg is rarely required).

**Usual pediatric dose**
Dosage has not been established.

**Strength(s) usually available**
U.S.—
    10 mg (Rx) [*Adalat; Procardia;* GENERIC].
    20 mg (Rx) [*Adalat; Procardia;* GENERIC].
Canada—
    5 mg (Rx) [*Adalat*].
    10 mg (Rx) [*Adalat; Apo-Nifed; Novo-Nifedin; Nu-Nifed*].

**Packaging and storage**
Store between 15 and 25 °C (59 and 77 °F), unless otherwise specified by manufacturer. Store in a tight, light-resistant container.

**Auxiliary labeling**
• Do not take other medicines without physician's advice.

**Note**
Check refill frequency to determine compliance in hypertensive patients.

## NIFEDIPINE TABLETS

**Usual adult and adolescent dose**
Antianginal or
Antihypertensive[1]—
    Oral, initially 10 mg three times a day, the dosage being gradually increased over a seven- to fourteen-day period as needed and tolerated.
Note: For hospitalized patients under close supervision, dosage may be increased by 10-mg increments over four- to six-hour periods until symptoms are controlled.
    When justified by symptom frequency and/or severity, dosage titration may be accomplished over a three-day period (medication given three times a day and increased stepwise from 10 mg to 20 mg, then to 30 mg per dose as needed and tolerated), but only if the patient is monitored frequently.
    Geriatric patients may be more sensitive to the effects of the usual adult dose.

**Usual adult prescribing limits**
Single dose, up to 30 mg; total daily dose, up to 180 mg (a total daily dose greater than 120 mg is rarely required).

**Usual pediatric dose**
Dosage has not been established.

**Strength(s) usually available**
U.S.—
    Not commercially available.
Canada—
    10 mg (Rx) [*Adalat FT*].

**Packaging and storage**
Store between 15 and 25 °C (59 and 77 °F), unless otherwise specified by manufacturer. Store in a tight, light-resistant container.

**Auxiliary labeling**
• Do not take other medicines without physician's advice.

**Note**
Check refill frequency to determine compliance in hypertensive patients.

## NIFEDIPINE EXTENDED-RELEASE TABLETS

**Usual adult and adolescent dose**
Antianginal or
Antihypertensive—
    *Adalat CC* or *Procardia XL*:
        Oral, 30 or 60 mg once a day, the dosage being gradually adjusted over a seven- to fourteen-day period as needed and tolerated.
Antianginal[1] or
Antihypertensive—
    *Adalat P.A.*:
        Oral, initially 20 mg two times a day, the dosage being gradually increased as needed and tolerated.
Note: Geriatric patients may be more sensitive to the effects of the usual adult dose.

**Usual adult prescribing limits**
Up to 80 mg (*Adalat P.A.*), or 90 mg (antianginal) or 120 mg (antihypertensive) (*Procardia XL*) per day.

**Usual pediatric dose**
Dosage has not been established.

**Strength(s) usually available**
U.S.—
    30 mg (Rx) [*Adalat CC; Procardia XL*].
    60 mg (Rx) [*Adalat CC; Procardia XL*].
    90 mg (Rx) [*Adalat CC; Procardia XL*].
    Note: Although similar in appearance to a conventional tablet, *Procardia XL* actually is a specially formulated gastrointestinal system (GITS) consisting of a semipermeable membrane surrounding an osmotically active drug core, which is designed to release nifedipine at a constant rate over twenty-four hours; following drug release, the system is eliminated in the feces as an insoluble shell.

Canada—
    10 mg [*Adalat P.A.*].
    20 mg [*Adalat P.A.*].

**Packaging and storage**
Store below 40 °C (104 °F), preferably between 15 and 30 °C (59 and 86 °F), in a well-closed container, unless otherwise specified by manufacturer.

**Auxiliary labeling**
• Do not take other medicines without physician's advice.

**Note**
Check refill frequency to determine compliance in hypertensive patients.

[1]Not included in Canadian product labeling.

---

### NIMODIPINE

## Summary of Differences
Indications:
    Indicated for treatment of subarachnoid hemorrhage–associated neurologic deficits.
Pharmacology/pharmacokinetics:
    Dihydropyridine structure.
    Potent peripheral vasodilator; does not depress sinoatrial (SA) or atrioventricular (AV) node; no negative inotropic effect; reflex increase in heart rate in response to vasodilation occurs.
    Cerebroselective.
Side/adverse effects:
    Differences in frequencies are due to differences in pharmacological effects. Also causes thrombocytopenia (rare).

## Oral Dosage Forms
### NIMODIPINE CAPSULES

**Usual adult dose**
Oral, 60 mg every four hours, beginning within ninety-six hours after the subarachnoid hemorrhage and continuing for twenty-one days.
Note: In patients with hepatic function impairment, dosage should be reduced to 30 mg every four hours, with close monitoring of blood pressure and heart rate.
    Geriatric patients may be more sensitive to the effects of the usual adult dose.

**Usual pediatric dose**
Dosage has not been established.

**Strength(s) usually available**
U.S.—
    30 mg (Rx) [*Nimotop*].
Canada—
    30 mg (Rx) [*Nimotop*].

**Packaging and storage**
Store between 15 and 30 °C (59 and 86 °F), in a well-closed container, unless otherwise specified by manufacturer. Protect from light. Protect from freezing.

**Preparation of dosage form**
For patients who cannot take oral solids—
    For patients who cannot swallow, a hole may be made in both ends of the capsule with an 18 gauge needle and the contents of the capsule withdrawn into a syringe, and then emptied into the patient's nasogastric tube and washed down the tube with 30 mL of 0.9% sodium chloride solution.

---

### VERAPAMIL

## Summary of Differences
Indications:
    Indicated for treatment of supraventricular tachyarrhythmias; oral dosage form indicated for prophylaxis.
    Also used to treat hypertrophic cardiomyopathy.
Pharmacology/pharmacokinetics:
    Diphenylalkylamine structure.
    Depresses sinoatrial (SA) and atrioventricular (AV) nodes; usually does not significantly alter heart rate but may cause bradycardia; negative inotropic effect countered by reduction in afterload.

Precautions:

    Pediatrics—In rare instances, severe adverse hemodynamic effects have occurred after intravenous administration of verapamil in neonates and infants.

    Laboratory value alterations—Prolongs PR interval in serum concentrations greater than 30 nanograms per mL.

    Medical considerations/contraindications—Contraindicated in patients with 2nd or 3rd degree atrioventricular (AV) block, sinoatrial (SA) nodal function impairment, or Wolff-Parkinson-White or Lown-Ganong-Levine syndrome accompanied by atrial flutter or fibrillation, except in patients with a functioning artificial ventricular pacemaker. Caution necessary in patients with neuromuscular transmission deficiency, and wide-complex ventricular tachycardia (with intravenous use).

Side/adverse effects:

    Differences in frequencies are due to differences in pharmacological effects.

## Additional Dosing Information

See also *General Dosing Information.*

Dermatologic side effects usually disappear even with continued use. However, if skin eruptions persist, it is recommended that verapamil therapy be withdrawn, since progression to erythema multiforme has been reported rarely.

### For parenteral dosage forms only

Parenteral dosage is indicated in the management of cardiac arrhythmias with close monitoring. Emergency equipment and medications should be readily available.

## Oral Dosage Forms

Note: Bracketed uses in the *Dosage Forms* section refer to categories of use and/or indications that are not included in U.S. product labeling.

### VERAPAMIL TABLETS USP

Note: The dosing and strengths of verapamil are expressed in terms of hydrochloride salt.

#### Usual adult and adolescent dose

Antianginal
Antiarrhythmic
Antihypertensive or[1]
[Hypertrophic cardiomyopathy therapy adjunct]—

    Oral, initially 80 to 120 mg (HCl) three times a day, the dosage being increased at daily or weekly intervals as needed and tolerated.

Note: An initial dose of 40 mg (HCl) three times a day is recommended in patients who may have an increased response to verapamil (e.g., those with hepatic function impairment, elderly patients, patients with poor left ventricular function).

    The total daily dose usually ranges from 240 to 480 mg.

    Because of prolongation of the half-life with repeated dosing, decreased frequency of dosing may be possible; dosage should be individualized.

    Geriatric patients may be more sensitive to the effects of the usual adult dose.

#### Usual adult prescribing limits

Up to 480 mg (HCl) daily in divided doses; has been used in doses up to 720 mg per day in the treatment of hypertrophic cardiomyopathy.

#### Usual pediatric dose

For infants less than 1 year and children 1 to 15 years of age—Oral, 4 to 8 mg (HCl) per kg of body weight per day in divided doses.

#### Usual geriatric dose

Oral, initially 40 mg (HCl) three times a day, the dosage being adjusted as needed and tolerated.

#### Strength(s) usually available

U.S.—

    40 mg (HCl) (Rx) [*Calan; Isoptin* (scored); GENERIC].

    80 mg (HCl) (Rx) [*Calan* (scored); *Isoptin* (scored); GENERIC].

    120 mg (HCl) (Rx) [*Calan* (scored); *Isoptin* (scored); GENERIC].

Canada—

    80 mg (HCl) (Rx) [*Apo-Verap; Isoptin; Novo-Veramil; Nu-Verap;* GENERIC].

    120 mg (HCl) (Rx) [*Apo-Verap; Isoptin; Novo-Veramil; Nu-Verap;* GENERIC].

#### Packaging and storage

Store below 40 °C (104 °F), preferably between 15 and 30 °C (59 and 86 °F), unless otherwise specified by manufacturer. Store in a tight container. Protect from light.

### Auxiliary labeling

• Do not take other medicines without physician's advice.

### Note

Check refill frequency to determine compliance in hypertensive patients.

## VERAPAMIL HYDROCHLORIDE EXTENDED-RELEASE CAPSULES

### Usual adult and adolescent dose

Antihypertensive—

    Oral, initially 240 mg once a day, the dosage being increased in increments of 120 mg per day at daily or weekly intervals as needed and tolerated.

Note: An initial dose of 120 mg per day is recommended in patients who may have an increased response to verapamil (e.g., elderly, small people, etc.).

    The total daily dose usually ranges from 240 to 480 mg.

    Geriatric patients may be more sensitive to the effects of the usual adult dose.

### Usual pediatric dose

Dosage has not been established.

### Strength(s) usually available

U.S.—

    120 mg (Rx) [*Verelan*].

    180 mg (Rx) [*Verelan*].

    240 mg (Rx) [*Verelan*].

Canada—

    Not commercially available.

### Packaging and storage

Store below 40 °C (104 °F), preferably between 15 and 30 °C (59 and 86 °F), unless otherwise specified by manufacturer. Store in a tight container. Protect from light.

### Auxiliary labeling

• Do not take other medicines without physician's advice.

### Note

Check refill frequency to determine compliance in hypertensive patients.

## VERAPAMIL HYDROCHLORIDE EXTENDED-RELEASE TABLETS

### Usual adult and adolescent dose

Antihypertensive—

    Oral, initially 180 mg once a day in the morning with food, the dosage being increased at daily or weekly intervals as needed and tolerated in the following order: 240 mg once a day in the morning; 180 mg every twelve hours or 240 mg in the morning and 120 mg in the evening; 240 mg every twelve hours.

Note: Lower initial doses (e.g., 120 mg per day) may be necessary in patients with a potential increased response to verapamil.

    Tablets may be broken in half, but should not be crushed or chewed.

    Geriatric patients may be more sensitive to the effects of the usual adult dose.

### Usual pediatric dose

Dosage has not been established.

### Strength(s) usually available

U.S.—

    120 mg (Rx) [*Calan SR; Isoptin SR*].

    180 mg (Rx) [*Calan SR; Isoptin SR*].

    240 mg (Rx) [*Calan SR* (scored); *Isoptin SR* (scored)].

Canada—

    240 mg (Rx) [*Isoptin SR* (scored)].

### Packaging and storage

Store below 40 °C (104 °F), preferably between 15 and 30 °C (59 and 86 °F), unless otherwise specified by manufacturer. Store in a tight, light-resistant container.

### Auxiliary labeling

• Take with meals or milk.

• Do not take other medicines without physician's advice.

### Note

Check refill frequency to determine compliance in hypertensive patients.

## Parenteral Dosage Forms

### VERAPAMIL INJECTION USP

Note: The dosing and strengths of verapamil are expressed in terms of hydrochloride salt.

## Usual adult dose

Intravenous, initially 5 to 10 mg (HCl) (or 75 to 150 mcg [0.075 to 0.15 mg] per kg of body weight) administered slowly over a two-minute period with continuous ECG and blood pressure monitoring. If response is not adequate, 10 mg (or 150 mcg [0.15 mg] per kg of body weight) may be administered thirty minutes after completion of initial dose.

Note: In geriatric patients, the intravenous dose should be administered slowly over a three-minute period to minimize undesired effects.

## Usual pediatric dose

The following doses should be administered slowly over a two-minute period, with continuous ECG monitoring. If response is not adequate, a repeat dose may be administered thirty minutes after completion of initial dose.

Infants up to 1 year of age—Initially, 100 to 200 mcg (HCl) (0.1 to 0.2 mg) per kg of body weight (usual single dose range, 0.75 to 2 mg).

Children 1 to 15 years of age—Initially, 100 to 300 mcg (HCl) (0.1 to 0.3 mg) per kg of body weight (usual single dose range, 2 to 5 mg) not to exceed a total of 5 mg. For repeat dose, thirty minutes after initial dose, do not exceed 10 mg as a single dose.

## Strength(s) usually available

U.S.—

2.5 mg (HCl) per mL (Rx) [*Isoptin;* GENERIC (sodium chloride 8.5 mg per mL)].

Canada—

2.5 mg (HCl) per mL (Rx) [*Isoptin*].

## Packaging and storage

Store between 15 and 30 °C (59 and 86 °F), unless otherwise specified by manufacturer. Protect from light. Protect from freezing.

## Stability

Verapamil hydrochloride injection is physically and chemically compatible with Ringer's injection or 5% dextrose or 0.9% sodium chloride injection.

## Incompatibilities

Verapamil hydrochloride injection is physically incompatible with albumin, amphotericin B injection, hydralazine hydrochloride injection, and sulfamethoxazole and trimethoprim injection. Precipitation of verapamil hydrochloride will occur in any solution with a pH greater than 6.

¹Not included in Canadian product labeling.

## Selected Bibliography

Freedman DD, Waters DD. 'Second generation' dihydropyridine calcium antagonists. Greater vascular selectivity and some unique applications. Drugs 1987; 34: 578-98.

Flaim SF, Cummings DM. Bepridil hydrochloride: a review of its pharmacologic properties. Curr Ther Res 1986 Apr; 39: 568-97.

Tracy TS, Black CD. Calcium modulators: future agents, future uses. Drug Intell Clin Pharm 1987 Jul/Aug; 21: 575-83.

Hasegawa GR. Nicardipine, nitrendipine, and bepridil: new calcium antagonists for cardiovascular disorders. Clin Pharm 1988 Feb; 7: 97-108.

Pickard JD, Murray GD, Illingworth R, et al. Effect of oral nimodipine on cerebral infarction and outcome after subarachnoid hemorrhage: British aneurysm nimodipine trial. Br Med J 1989 Mar 11; 298: 636-42.

Lam YW. Calcium metabolism, calcium-channel blocking agents, and hypertension management. Drug Intell Clin Pharm 1988 Sep; 22: 659-71.

McAuley BJ, Schroeder JS. The use of diltiazem hydrochloride in cardiovascular disorders. Pharmacother 1982 May/Jun; 2: 121-33.

Chaffman M, Brogden RN. Diltiazem. A review of its pharmacological properties and therapeutic efficacy. Drugs 1985 May; 29: 387-454.

Yedinak KC, Lopez LM. Felodipine: a new dihydropyridine calcium-channel antagonist. DICP Ann Pharmacother 1991 Nov; 25: 1193-1206.

Holmes B, Brogden RN, Heel RC, et al. Flunarizine: a review of its pharmacodynamic and pharmacokinetic properties and therapeutic use. Drugs 1984; 27: 6-44.

Fitton A, Benfield P. Isradipine. A review of its pharmacodynamic and pharmacokinetic properties, and therapeutic use in cardiovascular disease. Drugs 1990; 40 (1): 31-74.

Sorkin EM, Clissold SP. Nicardipine. A review of its pharmacodynamic and pharmacokinetic properties, and therapeutic efficacy, in the treatment of angina pectoris, hypertension and related cardiovascular disorders. Drugs 1987; 33: 296-345.

Ferlinz J. Nifedipine in myocardial ischemia, systemic hypertension, and other cardiovascular disorders. Ann Intern Med 1986 Nov; 105: 714-29.

Allen GS, et al. A controlled trial of nimodipine in acute ischemic stroke. New Engl J Med 1988 Jan 28; 318: 203-7.

Petruk K, et al. Nimodipine treatment in poor-grade aneurysm patients. Results of a multicenter, double-blind, placebo-controlled trial. J Neurosurg 1988; 68: 505-17.

Baky SH, Singh BN. Verapamil hydrochloride: Pharmacological properties and role in cardiovascular therapeutics. Pharmacother 1982 Nov/Dec; 2: 328-53.

Revised: 08/21/92
Interim revision: 09/07/94; 04/13/95

## Table 1. Pharmacology/Pharmacokinetics

| Hemodynamic Effect | Legend*:<br>**I**=Bepridil<br>**II**=Diltiazem<br>**III**=Felodipine<br>**IV**=Flunarizine<br>**V**=Isradipine | | | | | **VI**=Nicardipine<br>**VII**=Nifedipine<br>**VIII**=Nimodipine<br>**IX**=Verapamil | | | |
|---|---|---|---|---|---|---|---|---|---|
| | **I** | **II** | **III** | **IV** | **V** | **VI** | **VII** | **VIII** | **IX** |
| Peripheral vasodilation | + | + | ++ | + | ++ | ++ | ++ | ++ | + |
| Heart rate | D | D | I† | N | I† | I† | I† | I† | D |
| Depression of sinoatrial (SA) or atrioventricular (AV) nodal conduction | + | + | − | − | − | − | − | − | + |
| Negative inotropic effect | +‡ | +/− | +/−‡ | − | +/−‡ | +/−‡ | +/−‡ | +/−‡ | +‡ |
| Antihypertensive effect | − | + | + | − | + | + | + | + | + |
| Cerebrovascular selectivity | | | | + | | + | | + | |

*Legend: I=Increase; D=Decrease; N=No effect; +=Some effect; ++=Significant effect; −=No effect.

†Reflex increase occurs in response to vasodilating action. Isradipine causes only a slight increase or no change.

‡Bepridil's negative inotropic effect is small and tends to occur at high doses.

For felodipine, isradipine, nicardipine, nifedipine, and nimodipine, the effect is masked by the reflex increase in heart rate.

The effect of verapamil is countered by a reduction in afterload.

## Table 2. Medical Considerations/Contraindications

| The medical considerations/contraindications included have been selected on the basis of their potential clinical significance (reasons given in parentheses where appropriate)—not necessarily inclusive (» = major clinical significance). | Legend: I=Bepridil II=Diltiazem III=Felodipine IV=Flunarizine V=Isradipine | | | | | VI=Nicardipine VII=Nifedipine VIII=Nimodipine IX=Verapamil | | | |
|---|---|---|---|---|---|---|---|---|---|
| | **I** | **II** | **III** | **IV** | **V** | **VI** | **VII** | **VIII** | **IX** |
| ***Except under special circumstances, this medication should not be used when the following medical problems exist:*** | | | | | | | | | |
| » Arrhythmias, ventricular, serious, history of or<br>» QT interval prolongation, history of<br>(increased risk of bepridil-induced arrhythmias) | ✔ | | | | | | | | |
| » Heart block—2nd or 3rd degree atrioventricular (AV) block, except in patients with a functioning artificial ventricular pacemaker<br>(use of calcium channel blocker may lead to excessive bradycardia) | ✔ | ✔ | | | | | | | ✔ |
| » Hypotension, severe | ✔ | ✔ | ✔ | | ✔ | ✔ | ✔ | ✔ | ✔ |
| » Sinoatrial (SA) nodal function impairment (sick sinus syndrome) except in patients with functioning artificial ventricular pacemaker<br>(use of calcium channel blocker may lead to severe hypotension, bradycardia, and asystole) | ✔ | ✔ | | | | | | | ✔ |
| » Wolff-Parkinson-White or Lown-Ganong-Levine syndrome accompanied by atrial flutter or fibrillation, except in patients with a functioning artificial ventricular pacemaker<br>(use of calcium channel blocker for treatment of atrial fibrillation or flutter may precipitate severe ventricular arrhythmias) | | ✔ | | | | | | | ✔ |
| ***Risk-benefit should be considered when the following medical problems exist:*** | | | | | | | | | |
| Aortic stenosis, severe<br>(increased risk of heart failure when calcium channel blocker initiated, because of fixed impedance to flow across aortic valve) | | ✔ | | | | ✔ | ✔ | | ✔ |
| » Bradycardia, extreme, or<br>» Heart failure<br>(reduced sinus node and AV node activity may be worsened)<br>Note: When not severe or rate-related, heart failure should be controlled with digitalization and diuretics before administration of a calcium channel blocker. Heart failure, severe or moderately severe (pulmonary wedge pressure above 20 mm of mercury, ejection fraction less than 30%), may be acutely worsened by administration of a calcium channel blocker. | ✔ | ✔ | | | | | | | ✔ |
| Bradycardia, extreme, or<br>Heart failure<br>(because these agents have a slight negative inotropic effect, caution is recommended) | | | ✔ | | ✔ | ✔ | ✔ | ✔ | |
| » Cardiogenic shock | ✔ | ✔ | ✔ | | ✔ | ✔ | ✔ | ✔ | ✔ |
| Cerebral infarction or hemorrhage, acute | | | | | | ✔ | | | |
| Hepatic function impairment<br>(clearance and duration of effect may be prolonged; clearance of felodipine is reduced to about 60%; half-life of nicardipine may be increased to 19 hours in patients with severe hepatic function impairment; half-life of verapamil may be increased to 14 to 16 hours and plasma clearance reduced to about 30% of normal; dosage reduction may be necessary) | ✔ | ✔ | ✔ | ✔ | ✔ | ✔ | ✔ | ✔ | ✔ |
| » Hypokalemia<br>(risk of bepridil-induced arrhythmias may be increased) | ✔ | | | | | | | | |
| Hypotension, mild to moderate<br>(tendency to hypotension is augmented by the peripheral vasodilating effect of the calcium channel blocker) | | ✔ | ✔ | | | ✔ | ✔ | ✔ | ✔ |
| Mental depression, history of<br>(flunarizine may precipitate mental depression) | | | | ✔ | | | | | |
| » Myocardial infarction, acute, with pulmonary congestion documented by x-ray on admission<br>(associated heart failure may be acutely worsened by administration of a calcium channel blocker) | ✔ | ✔ | | | | | | | ✔ |

## Table 2. Medical Considerations/Contraindications (continued)

| | Legend:<br>I=Bepridil<br>II=Diltiazem<br>III=Felodipine<br>IV=Flunarizine<br>V=Isradipine | | | | | VI=Nicardipine<br>VII=Nifedipine<br>VIII=Nimodipine<br>IX=Verapamil | | | |
|---|---|---|---|---|---|---|---|---|---|
| | **I** | **II** | **III** | **IV** | **V** | **VI** | **VII** | **VIII** | **IX** |
| Myocardial infarction, acute, with pulmonary congestion documented by x-ray on admission<br>(because these agents have a slight negative inotropic effect, there is a possibility that associated heart failure may be acutely worsened) | | | ✔ | | ✔ | ✔ | ✔ | ✔ | |
| Narrowing of the gastrointestinal tract, pathologic or iatrogenic, severe<br>(passage of the nondeformable extended-release nifedipine system [*Procardia XL*] may be impaired; obstructive symptoms may occur) | | | | | | | ✔ | | |
| Neuromuscular transmission deficiency<br>(verapamil has been reported to decrease neuromuscular transmission in patients with Duchenne's muscular dystrophy, and to prolong recovery from the neuromuscular blocking agent vecuronium; dosage reduction may be required) | | | | | | | | | ✔ |
| Parkinson's syndrome or<br>Extrapyramidal disorders, other<br>(flunarizine may produce parkinsonian extrapyramidal symptoms not responsive to parkinsonian medications) | | | | ✔ | | | | | |
| Renal function impairment<br>(possible reduced clearance of the calcium channel blocker or metabolites, although half-life is only slightly increased; dosage adjustment may be necessary)<br>(plasma concentrations of felodipine are unchanged; although reduced excretion results in increased concentrations of metabolites, they are inactive) | ✔ | ✔ | | | ✔ | ✔ | ✔ | | ✔ |
| » Sensitivity to the calcium channel blocker prescribed | ✔ | ✔ | ✔ | ✔ | ✔ | ✔ | ✔ | ✔ | ✔ |
| Ventricular tachycardia, wide-complex<br>(risk of ventricular fibrillation if intravenous diltiazem or verapamil administered) | | ✔ | | | | | | | ✔ |

## Table 3. Side/Adverse Effects

Note: Side/adverse effects tend to be dose-related and occur most frequently during periods of dosage titration.

Although not reported to occur in humans, lenticular changes and cataracts have developed during chronic dosage with verapamil in beagles. These effects resulted from daily dosage of 30 mg and more per kg of body weight and are considered likely to be species-specific.

A possible hyperglycemic effect has been reported with nicardipine (at a daily dose of 40 mg) and nifedipine therapy (when the daily dosage exceeds 60 mg). No significant effect on fasting serum glucose has been seen with felodipine.

Depression of atrioventricular (AV) and sinoatrial (SA) nodal conduction by bepridil, diltiazem, and verapamil may result in asymptomatic 1st degree block and transient sinus bradycardia, sometimes accompanied by nodal escape rhythms.

Use of verapamil for hypertrophic cardiomyopathy, especially in patients with pre-existing risk factors, has resulted in serious side effects (including pulmonary edema, sinus bradycardia, severe hypotension, 2nd degree AV block, and sudden death).

| The following side/adverse effects have been selected on the basis of their potential clinical significance (possible signs and symptoms in parentheses where appropriate)—not necessarily inclusive:* | Legend:<br>I=Bepridil<br>II=Diltiazem<br>III=Felodipine<br>IV=Flunarizine<br>V=Isradipine | | | | | VI=Nicardipine<br>VII=Nifedipine<br>VIII=Nimodipine<br>IX=Verapamil | | | |
|---|---|---|---|---|---|---|---|---|---|
| | **I** | **II** | **III** | **IV** | **V** | **VI** | **VII** | **VIII** | **IX** |
| **Medical attention needed**<br>*Agranulocytosis* (not symptomatic) | R | U | U | U | U | U | U | U | U |
| *Allergic reaction* (skin rash)<br>Note: May disappear, even with continued diltiazem use. Rarely, may progress to erythema multiform (diltiazem, verapamil), exfoliative dermatitis (diltiazem), or Stevens-Johnson syndrome (diltiazem, verapamil). | R | L | L | R | L | R | R | R | L |
| *Angina* (chest pain)—may occur about 30 minutes after administration<br>Note: Rarely, especially in patients with severe obstructive coronary artery disease, increased frequency, duration, and/or severity of angina or acute myocardial infarction have occurred when therapy is initiated or dosage increased. | U | R | L | U | L | L | R | U | R |

## Table 3. Side/Adverse Effects *(continued)*

| | Legend:<br>I=Bepridil<br>II=Diltiazem<br>III=Felodipine<br>IV=Flunarizine<br>V=Isradipine | | | | | VI=Nicardipine<br>VII=Nifedipine<br>VIII=Nimodipine<br>IX=Verapamil | | | |
|---|---|---|---|---|---|---|---|---|---|
| | **I** | **II** | **III** | **IV** | **V** | **VI** | **VII** | **VIII** | **IX** |
| *Arrhythmias, including torsades de pointes* (usually asymptomatic) | L | U | U | U | U | U | U | U | U |
| *Arthritis* (painful, swollen joints)—associated with elevated ANA titres | U | U | U | U | U | U | R | U | U |
| *Blindness, transient, at peak plasma concentration* | U | U | U | U | U | U | R | U | U |
| *Bradycardia less than 50 per minute; rarely, 2nd or 3rd degree AV block, with a few patients progressing to asystole* (slow heartbeat) | L | R | X | U | X | X | X | X | L |
| *Congestive heart failure or pulmonary edema, possible* (breathing difficulty, coughing, or wheezing) | L | L | U | U | R | R | L | R | L |
| *Extrapyramidal effects, parkinsonian* (loss of balance control, mask-like face, shuffling walk, stiffness of arms or legs, trembling and shaking of hands and fingers, trouble in speaking or swallowing)<br>Note: Symptoms are not responsive to antiparkinsonian medications, but are reversible on withdrawal of flunarizine. | U | R | U | L | U | U | U | U | U |
| *Galactorrhea* (unusual secretion of milk) | U | U | U | R | U | U | U | U | R |
| *Gingival hyperplasia* (bleeding, tender, or swollen gums) | U | R | R | U | U | U | R | U | R |
| *Hypotension* (usually not symptomatic; not orthostatic) | R | L | R | U | L | L | L | L | L |
| *Hypotension, excessive* (fainting) | R | R | R | U | R | R | R | R | R |
| *Mental depression* | U | R | R | L | U | U | U | U | U |
| *Peripheral edema* (swelling of ankles, feet, or lower legs) | R | L | M | U | L | L | M | L | L |
| *Tachycardia* (irregular or fast, pounding heartbeat)<br>Note: In patients receiving verapamil, rapid ventricular rate may occur in patients with atrial flutter/fibrillation and an accessory AV pathway as with Wolff-Parkinson-White, or Lown-Ganong-Levine syndrome; in patients receiving felodipine, isradipine, nicardipine, nifedipine, or nimodipine, reflex tachycardia may occur because of its hypotensive effect. | X | R | L | U | L | L | L | R | R |
| *Thrombocytopenia* (not symptomatic) | U | R | U | U | U | U | U | R | U |
| **Medical attention needed only if continuing or bothersome**<br>*Constipation* | L | L | L | U | R | R | L | U | L |
| *Diarrhea* | M | L | L | U | L | R | U | L | U |
| *Dizziness or lightheadedness* | M | L | L | L | L | L | L | M | L |
| *Drowsiness* | U | R | U | M | U | R | U | U | U |
| *Dryness of mouth* | U | R | R | L | U | R | U | U | U |
| *Flushing and feeling of warmth* | U | L | L | U | L | M | M | R | R |
| *Headache* | L | L | M | U | M | L | M | L | L |
| *Increased appetite and/or weight gain* | U | U | U | M | U | U | U | U | U |
| *Nausea* | M | L | L | L | L | L | M | L | L |
| *Unusual tiredness or weakness* | L | L | L | L | L | L | L | U | L |

\*Differences in frequency of occurrence may reflect either lack of clinical-use data or actual pharmacologic distinctions among agents (although their pharmacologic similarity suggests that side effects occurring with one may occur with the others). M = more frequent; L = less frequent; R = rare; U = unknown; X = does not occur.

---

**CALCIUM CHLORIDE**—See *Calcium Supplements (Systemic)*

**CALCIUM CITRATE**—See *Calcium Supplements (Systemic)*

**CALCIUM GLUBIONATE**—See *Calcium Supplements (Systemic)*

**CALCIUM GLUCEPTATE**—See *Calcium Supplements (Systemic)*

**CALCIUM GLUCEPTATE AND CALCIUM GLUCONATE**—See *Calcium Supplements (Systemic)*

**CALCIUM GLUCONATE**—See *Calcium Supplements (Systemic)*

**CALCIUM GLYCEROPHOSPHATE AND CALCIUM LACTATE**—See *Calcium Supplements (Systemic)*

**CALCIUM LACTATE**—See *Calcium Supplements (Systemic)*

**CALCIUM LACTATE-GLUCONATE AND CALCIUM CARBONATE**—See *Calcium Supplements (Systemic)*

**CALCIUM PANTOTHENATE**—See *Pantothenic Acid (Systemic)*

**CALCIUM PHOSPHATE, DIBASIC**—See *Calcium Supplements (Systemic)*

**CALCIUM PHOSPHATE, TRIBASIC**—See *Calcium Supplements (Systemic)*

# CALCIUM SUPPLEMENTS    Systemic

This monograph includes information on the following: Calcium Acetate†; Calcium Carbonate; Calcium Chloride; Calcium Citrate†; Calcium Glubionate‡§; Calcium Gluceptate†; Calcium Gluceptate and Calcium Gluconate*; Calcium Gluconate; Calcium Glycerophosphate and Calcium Lactate†; Calcium Lactate; Calcium Lactate-Gluconate and Calcium Carbonate*; Dibasic Calcium Phosphate†; Tribasic Calcium Phosphate†.

INN:
Calcium Gluceptate—Calcium Glucoheptonate

VA CLASSIFICATION (Primary/Secondary):
Calcium Acetate
     Parenteral—TN402
Calcium Carbonate
     Oral—TN402/GA105
Calcium Chloride
     Parenteral—TN402/CV900
Calcium Citrate
     Oral—TN402
Calcium Glubionate
     Oral—TN402
Calcium Gluceptate
     Parenteral—TN402
Calcium Gluceptate and Calcium Gluconate
     Oral—TN402
Calcium Gluconate
     Oral—TN402
     Parenteral—TN402/CV900
Calcium Glycerophosphate and Calcium Lactate
     Parenteral—TN402
Calcium Lactate
     Oral—TN402
Calcium Lactate-Gluconate and Calcium Carbonate
     Oral—TN402
Dibasic Calcium Phosphate
     Oral—TN402
Tribasic Calcium Phosphate
     Oral—TN402

Note: For a listing of dosage forms and brand names by country availability, see *Dosage Forms* section(s). For a listing of brand names for the articles in this monograph, refer to the General Index.

  *Not commercially available in the U.S.
  †Not commercially available in Canada.
  ‡Antacid product commonly recommended as calcium supplement.
  §In Canada, calcium glubionate is known as calcium glucono-galacto gluconate.

## Category

Antihypocalcemic—Calcium Acetate; Calcium Carbonate; Calcium Chloride; Calcium Citrate; Calcium Glubionate; Calcium Gluceptate; Calcium Gluconate; Calcium Glycerophosphate and Calcium Lactate; Calcium Lactate; Calcium Lactate-Gluconate and Calcium Carbonate; Dibasic Calcium Phosphate; Tribasic Calcium Phosphate.
Electrolyte replenisher—Calcium Acetate; Calcium Chloride; Calcium Gluceptate; Calcium Gluconate Injection.
Cardiotonic—Calcium Chloride; Calcium Gluconate Injection.

Antihyperkalemic—Calcium Chloride; Calcium Gluconate Injection.
Antihypermagnesemic—Calcium Chloride; Calcium Gluceptate; Calcium Gluconate Injection.
Antacid—Calcium Carbonate.
Nutritional supplement (mineral)—Calcium Carbonate; Calcium Citrate; Calcium Glubionate, Oral; Calcium Gluceptate and Calcium Gluconate; Calcium Gluconate, Oral; Calcium Lactate; Calcium Lactate-Gluconate and Calcium Carbonate; Dibasic Calcium Phosphate; Tribasic Calcium Phosphate.
Antihyperphosphatemic—Calcium Carbonate; Calcium Citrate.

## Indications

Note: Bracketed information in the *Indications* section refers to uses that are not included in U.S. product labeling.

### Accepted

Hypocalcemia, acute (treatment)—Parenteral calcium salts (i.e., acetate, chloride, gluceptate, and gluconate) are indicated in the treatment of hypocalcemia in conditions that require a rapid increase in serum calcium-ion concentration, such as in neonatal hypocalcemic tetany; tetany due to parathyroid deficiency; hypocalcemia due to ''hungry bones'' syndrome (remineralization hypocalcemia) following surgery for hyperparathyroidism; vitamin D deficiency; and alkalosis. Calcium salts have been used as adjunctive therapy for insect bites or stings, such as Black Widow Spider bites, and sensitivity reactions, especially when characterized by urticaria; and as an aid in the management of acute symptoms of lead colic. Parenteral calcium gluconate and calcium gluceptate are also used for the prevention of hypocalcemia during exchange transfusions.

Electrolyte depletion (treatment)—Calcium acetate, parenteral calcium chloride, calcium gluconate, and calcium gluceptate are used in conditions that require an increase in calcium ions for electrolyte adjustment.

Cardiac arrest (treatment adjunct)—Parenteral calcium chloride, [or calcium gluconate] may be used also as an adjunct in cardiac resuscitation, particularly after open heart surgery, to strengthen myocardial contractions, such as following defibrillation or when there is an inadequate response to catecholamines.

Hyperkalemia (treatment)—Calcium chloride and parenteral calcium gluconate, are used to decrease or reverse the cardiac depressant effects of hyperkalemia on electrocardiographic (ECG) function.

Hypermagnesemia (treatment adjunct)—Calcium chloride, [calcium gluceptate], and calcium gluconate injections have also been used as an aid in the treatment of central nervous system (CNS) depression due to overdosage of magnesium sulfate.

Hypocalcemia, chronic (treatment)—Oral calcium supplements provide a source of calcium ion for treating calcium depletion occurring in conditions such as chronic hypoparathyroidism, pseudohypoparathyroidism, osteomalacia, rickets, chronic renal failure, and hypocalcemia secondary to the administration of anticonvulsant medications. When chronic hypocalcemia is due to vitamin D deficiency, oral calcium salts may be administered concomitantly with vitamin D analogs. However, calcium phosphate should *not* be used in patients with hypoparathyroidism or renal failure, since phosphate levels may be too high and giving more phosphate would exacerbate the condition. Calcium supplements should not be used in hyperparathyroidism, unless the need for a calcium supplement is high and the patient is carefully monitored. For treatment of hypocalcemia, supplementation is preferred.

Calcium deficiency (prophylaxis)—Oral calcium salts are used as dietary supplemental therapy for persons who may not get enough calcium in their regular diet. However, for prophylaxis of calcium deficiency, dietary improvement, rather than supplementation, is preferred. Due to increased needs, children and pregnant women are at greatest risk. Pre- and postmenopausal women; adolescents, especially girls and the elderly may not receive adequate calcium in their diets. However, studies have shown that supplemental calcium in postmenopausal women without functioning ovaries does not lead to increases in bone density, even in the presence of supplemental vitamin D. Calcium supplements are used as part of the prevention and treatment of osteoporosis in patients with an inadequate calcium intake. The use of calcium citrate may reduce the risk of kidney stones in susceptible patients. The use of water-soluble salts of calcium (i.e., citrate, gluconate, and lactate) may be preferable to acid-soluble salts (i.e., carbonate and phosphate) for patients with reduced stomach acid or patients taking acid-inhibiting medication, such as the histamine $H_2$-receptor antagonists.

Some unusual diets (e.g., reducing diets that drastically restrict food selection) may not supply minimum daily requirements of calcium. Supplementation is necessary in patients receiving total parenteral nutrition (TPN) or undergoing rapid weight loss or in those with malnutrition, because of inadequate dietary intake.

Recommended intakes for all vitamins and most minerals are increased during pregnancy. Many physicians recommend that pregnant women receive multivitamin and mineral supplements, especially those pregnant women who do not consume an adequate diet and those in high-risk categories (i.e., women carrying more than one fetus, heavy cigarette smokers, and alcohol and drug abusers). Taking excessive amounts of a multivitamin and mineral supplement may be harmful to the mother and/or fetus and should be avoided.

Recommended intakes for all vitamins and most minerals are increased during breast-feeding.

Hyperacidity (treatment)—See Calcium Carbonate, *Antacids (Oral-Local)*.

[Hyperphosphatemia (treatment)]—Calcium carbonate is used in patients with end-stage renal failure (renal osteodystrophy) to lower serum phosphate concentrations. However, it should be used with caution in patients on chronic hemodialysis. See also *Patient monitoring*. Calcium citrate is also used in renal failure as a phosphate binder.

## Pharmacology/Pharmacokinetics

### Physicochemical characteristics
Molecular weight—
    Calcium acetate: 158.17.
    Calcium carbonate, precipitated: 100.09.
    Calcium chloride: 147.01.
    Calcium citrate: 570.50.
    Calcium glubionate: 610.53.
    Calcium gluceptate: 490.43.
    Calcium gluconate: 430.38.
    Calcium lactate: 218.22 (anhydrous).
    Calcium lactate-gluconate: 1551.5.
    Calcium phosphate, dibasic: 136.06.
    Calcium phosphate, tribasic: 503.31.

### Mechanism of action/Effect
Calcium is essential for the functional integrity of the nervous, muscular, and skeletal systems. It plays a role in normal cardiac function, renal function, respiration, blood coagulation, and cell membrane and capillary permeability. Also, calcium helps to regulate the release and storage of neurotransmitters and hormones, the uptake and binding of amino acids, absorption of vitamin $B_{12}$, and gastrin secretion. The major fraction (99%) of calcium is in the skeletal structure primarily as hydroxyapatite, $Ca_{10}(PO_4)_6(OH)_2$; small amounts of calcium carbonate and amorphous calcium phosphates are also present. The calcium of bone is in a constant exchange with the calcium of plasma. Since the metabolic functions of calcium are essential for life, when there is a disturbance in the calcium balance because of dietary deficiency or other causes, the stores of calcium in bone may be depleted to fill the body's more acute needs. Therefore, on a chronic basis, normal mineralization of bone depends on adequate amounts of total body calcium.

### Absorption
Approximately one-fifth to one-third of orally administered calcium is absorbed in the small intestine, depending on presence of vitamin D metabolites, pH in lumen, and on dietary factors, such as calcium binding to fiber or phytates. Calcium absorption is increased when a calcium deficiency is present or when a patient is on a low-calcium diet. In patients with achlorhydria or hypochlorhydria, calcium absorption, especially with the carbonate salt, may be reduced.

### Protein binding
Moderate, approximately 45% in plasma.

### Elimination
Renal (20%)—The amount excreted in the urine varies with degree of calcium absorption and whether there is excessive bone loss or failure of renal conservation.

Fecal (80%)—Consists mainly of nonabsorbed calcium, with only a small amount of endogenous fecal calcium excreted.

## Precautions to Consider

### Pregnancy/Reproduction
Pregnancy—Studies have not been done in humans. However, problems have not been documented with intake of normal daily recommended amounts.

Studies have not been done in animals.

Second and third trimesters: Some studies have shown that calcium supplementation begun in the second trimester may be effective in lowering blood pressure in pregnant women with pregnancy-induced hypertension or pre-eclampsia, both of which may possibly be associated with increased calcium demand of the fetus during the last trimester.

During pregnancy, there is an increased need for calcium to calcify fetal bones and to increase the maternal skeletal mass in preparation for lactation. This need is normally met by enhanced intestinal absorption of calcium, increased vitamin D production, and a concurrent increase in calcitonin secretion, which prevents unwanted bone resorption in the maternal skeleton. The maternal parathyroid glands undergo hyperplasia, producing greater amounts of parathyroid hormone, which acts indirectly to increase intestinal absorption of calcium, reabsorption at the distal renal tubules, and bone calcium mobilization. However, the prescribing of calcium supplements during pregnancy may be necessary since standard prenatal vitamins along with normal intake of dairy products may not provide sufficient elemental calcium for the average pregnant woman.

Calcium acetate, calcium chloride, calcium gluceptate, calcium gluconate injection—FDA Pregnancy Category C.

Other calcium salts—FDA pregnancy categories not currently included in product labeling.

Labor and delivery—The effect of calcium chloride, calcium gluceptate, and calcium gluconate on mother and fetus during labor and delivery is unknown.

### Breast-feeding
Problems in nursing babies have not been documented with intake of normal daily recommended amounts. Although some oral supplemental calcium may be distributed into breast milk, the concentration is not sufficient to produce an adverse effect in the neonate. It is not known whether calcium chloride or calcium gluconate is distributed into breast milk.

### Pediatrics
Problems in pediatrics have not been documented with intake of normal daily recommended amounts.
    *Parenteral calcium preparations, especially calcium chloride*—
        The extreme irritation and possibility of tissue necrosis and sloughing caused by intravenous injection of calcium preparations usually restricts its use in pediatric patients because of the small vasculature of this patient group.
    *For calcium gluceptate injection only*—
        It is not recommended that calcium gluceptate be administered intramuscularly to infants and children except in emergencies when the intravenous route is technically impossible, because of the possibility of severe tissue necrosis or sloughing.

### Geriatrics
Problems in geriatrics have not been documented with intake of normal daily recommended amounts. With advancing age, intestinal calcium absorption decreases. Therefore, calcium requirements are increased in the elderly, and dosages of oral supplements may need to be adjusted accordingly. Impaired absorption may be due to low levels of active vitamin D metabolites.

### Drug interactions and/or related problems
The following drug interactions and/or related problems have been selected on the basis of their potential clinical significance (possible mechanism in parentheses where appropriate)—not necessarily inclusive (» = major clinical significance):

Note: Combinations containing any of the following, depending on the amount present, may also interact with this medication.

Not all interactions between calcium supplements and other oral medications have been identified in this monograph. Because the rate and/or extent of absorption of other oral medications may vary when used concurrently with calcium supplements, especially calcium carbonate, patients should be advised not to take any other oral medications within 1 to 2 hours of calcium supplements.

Alcohol or
Caffeine, usually more than 8 cups of coffee a day or
Tobacco
 (concurrent use of excessive amounts of these substances has been reported to decrease calcium absorption)

Antacids containing aluminum
 (concurrent use with calcium citrate may enhance aluminum absorption)

Calcitonin
 (concurrent use with calcium supplements may antagonize the effect of calcitonin in the treatment of hypercalcemia; however, when calcitonin is prescribed for osteoporosis or Paget's disease of the bone, calcium intake should be generous to prevent hypocalcemia which might generate secondary hyperparathyroidism; calcium-containing preparations may be given 4 hours after calcitonin)

Calcium-channel blocking agents
 (concurrent use of these medications with calcium supplements in quantities sufficient to raise serum calcium concentrations above normal may reduce the response to verapamil and probably other calcium-channel blockers)

» Calcium-containing preparations, other or
Magnesium-containing preparations, oral
 (concurrent use with calcium supplements may increase serum calcium or magnesium concentrations in susceptible patients, mainly patients with impaired renal function, leading to hypercalcemia or hypermagnesemia, respectively)

» Cellulose sodium phosphate
 (concurrent use with calcium supplements may decrease effectiveness of cellulose sodium phosphate in preventing hypercalciuria)

Contraceptives, estrogen-containing, oral or
Estrogens
 (concurrent use with calcium supplements may increase calcium absorption, which is used to therapeutic advantage when estrogens are prescribed for the treatment of postmenopausal osteoporosis)

» Digitalis glycosides
 (concurrent use of parenteral calcium salts with digitalis glycosides may increase the risk of cardiac arrhythmias; therefore, when the parenteral administration of calcium salts to digitalized patients is deemed necessary, caution and close electrocardiographic [ECG] monitoring are recommended)

Diuretics, thiazide
 (concurrent use with large doses of calcium supplements may result in hypercalcemia because of reduced calcium excretion)

» Etidronate
 (concurrent use with calcium supplements may prevent absorption of etidronate; patients should be advised not to take etidronate within 2 hours of calcium supplements)

Fiber, found in bran, whole-grain breads and cereals or
Phytates, found in bran and whole-grain breads and cereals
 (concurrent use of large amounts of fiber or phytates, especially in patients being treated for hypocalcemia, with calcium supplements may reduce calcium absorption by formation of nonabsorbable complexes)

Fluoroquinolones
 (concurrent use with calcium carbonate may reduce absorption by chelation of fluoroquinolones, resulting in lower serum and urine concentrations of fluoroquinolones; therefore, concurrent use is not recommended)

» Gallium nitrate
 (concurrent use with calcium supplements may antagonize the effect of gallium nitrate)

Iron supplements
 (concurrent use with calcium carbonate and calcium phosphate will decrease the absorption of iron; iron supplements should not be taken within 1 or 2 hours of calcium carbonate or phosphate; however, when iron and calcium carbonate are present in multivitamin-with-minerals formulations, the absorption of iron is not significantly changed, possibly because the ascorbic acid in the formulation maintains the iron in the ferrous state, thus increasing its solubility and absorption)

» Magnesium sulfate, parenteral
 (parenteral calcium salts may neutralize effects of parenteral magnesium sulfate and should be readily available to counteract the potentially serious risk of magnesium intoxication; also, calcium sulfate may precipitate when a calcium salt is admixed with magnesium sulfate in the same intravenous solution, although commercial nutritional solutions are formulated to avoid precipitation; calcium and magnesium should be administered through separate intravenous lines if required in post-parathyroidectomy "hungry bones" syndrome or tetany associated with hypocalcemia and hypomagnesemia)

Milk or milk products
 (concurrent excessive and prolonged use with calcium supplements may result in the milk-alkali syndrome)

Neuromuscular blocking agents, except succinylcholine
 (concurrent use with parenteral calcium salts usually reverses the effects of nondepolarizing neuromuscular blocking agents; also, concurrent use with calcium salts has been reported to enhance or prolong the neuromuscular blocking action of tubocurarine)

» Phenytoin
 (concurrent use decreases the bioavailability of both phenytoin and calcium because of possible formation of a nonabsorbable complex; patients should be advised not to take calcium supplements within 1 to 3 hours of taking phenytoin; also, enteral feeding solutions containing calcium should not be administered through a nasogastric feeding tube together with phenytoin oral suspension; a 2-hour interval should elapse between the administration of the feeding solution and of the phenytoin)

Potassium phosphates or
Potassium and sodium phosphates
 (concurrent use with calcium supplements may increase potential for deposition of calcium in soft tissues if serum ionized calcium is high)

Sodium bicarbonate
 (concurrent and prolonged use with calcium supplements may result in milk-alkali syndrome)

Sodium fluoride
 (concurrent use with calcium supplements may cause the calcium ions to complex with fluoride and inhibit absorption of both fluoride and calcium; however, if sodium fluoride is used with calcium supplements to treat osteoporosis, a one- to two-hour interval should elapse between doses)

» Tetracyclines, oral
 (concurrent use with calcium supplements may decrease absorption of tetracyclines because of possible formation of nonabsorbable complexes and increase in intragastric pH; patients should be advised not to take calcium supplements within 1 to 3 hours of taking tetracyclines)

Vitamin A
 (excessive intake, more than 7500 RE or 25,000 Units per day, of vitamin A may stimulate bone loss and counteract the effects of calcium supplementation and may cause hypercalcemia)

Vitamin D, especially calcifediol and calcitriol
 (concurrent use of large doses of vitamin D with calcium supplements may excessively increase intestinal absorption of calcium, increasing risk of chronic hypercalcemia in susceptible patients; however, it may be therapeutically advantageous in elderly and high-risk groups when it is necessary to prescribe vitamin D or its derivatives with calcium; careful monitoring of serum calcium concentrations is essential during long-term therapy)

**Laboratory value alterations**
The following have been selected on the basis of their potential clinical significance (possible effect in parentheses where appropriate)—not necessarily inclusive (» = major clinical significance):

With physiology/laboratory test values
Phosphate, serum
 (concentrations may be decreased by excessive and prolonged calcium use)

**Medical considerations/Contraindications**
The medical considerations/contraindications included here have been selected on the basis of their potential clinical significance (reasons given in parentheses where appropriate)—not necessarily inclusive (» = major clinical significance).

*Except under special circumstances, these medications should not be used when the following medical problems exist:*

*For all calcium supplements*
- » Hypercalcemia, primary or secondary or
- » Hypercalciuria or
- » Renal calculi, calcium
  (risk of exacerbation)
- » Sarcoidosis
  (may potentiate hypercalcemia)

*For calcium phosphate, dibasic or tribasic, only*
- » Hypoparathyroidism or
- » Renal insufficiency
  (may increase risk of hyperphosphatemia)

*For parenteral calcium salts only*
- » Digitalis toxicity
  (increased risk of arrhythmias)

*Risk-benefit should be considered when the following medical problems exist:*

*For all calcium supplements*
- » Dehydration or
  Electrolyte imbalance, other
  (may increase risk of hypercalcemia)
- Diarrhea or
  Malabsorption, gastrointestinal, chronic
  (fecal excretion of calcium may be increased, although patients with chronic diarrhea or malabsorption commonly need calcium supplements)
- » Renal calculi, history of
  (risk of recurrent stone formation)
- » Renal function impairment, chronic
  (may increase risk of hypercalcemia; however, calcium carbonate or calcium citrate may be used as a phosphate binder in renal failure; also, some patients with renal failure have symptomatic hypocalcemia and need cautious treatment with calcium salts)

*For calcium carbonate and calcium phosphate only*
- Achlorhydria or hypochlorhydria
  (calcium absorption may be decreased unless the calcium carbonate or phosphate is taken with meals)

*For parenteral calcium salts only*
- » Cardiac function impairment
- » Ventricular fibrillation during cardiac resuscitation
  (increased risk of arrhythmias; however, calcium may increase strength of myocardial contraction, make fibrillation coarser, and help in electrical defibrillation, especially with concomitant hyperkalemia)

### Patient monitoring

The following may be especially important in patient monitoring (other tests may be warranted in some patients, depending on condition; » = major clinical significance):

*For hypocalcemia*
Blood pressure determinations and
Electrocardiographic monitoring and
Magnesium, concentrations, serum and
Parathyroid hormone (PTH) concentrations, serum and
Phosphate concentrations, serum and
Potassium concentrations, serum and
Renal function determinations
  (determinations recommended at initiation of therapy and at frequent intervals during treatment of hypocalcemia)
  Note: In elderly patients or patients with hypertension, blood pressure should be monitored during intravenous administration, since a transient increase in blood pressure may occur.
- » Calcium concentrations, serum or
- » Ionized calcium concentrations, serum
  (determinations recommended at frequent intervals during treatment of acute hypocalcemia to achieve normal serum calcium concentrations without exceeding them; at periodic intervals for patients on chronic hemodialysis to prevent hypercalcemia; for patients with chronic renal failure not yet on dialysis who are taking calcium as a phosphate binder; and during long-term therapy with oral calcium supplements. In patients with hypoparathyroidism, serum calcium concentrations should be kept in the low normal range, since significant hypercalciuria may occur intermittently or as a complication with higher concentrations, especially if vitamin D preparations are being used concurrently; serum ionized

calcium concentrations are preferable to determine free and bound calcium, but may not be readily available from a reliable lab)
Calcium concentrations, urine
  (urinary calcium excretion determinations are sometimes needed to avoid hypercalciuria)

## Side/Adverse Effects

Note: Side/adverse effects may be more likely to occur if oral calcium supplements are taken in much larger doses than recommended (greater than 2000 to 2500 mg a day), if they are taken for a longer period of time, or if they are taken by patients with renal function impairment or milk-alkali syndrome.

The following side/adverse effects have been selected on the basis of their potential clinical significance (possible signs and symptoms in parentheses where appropriate)—not necessarily inclusive:

### Those indicating need for medical attention
Incidence more frequent
  *With parenteral dosage forms only*
    Hypotension (dizziness); *flushing and/or sensation of warmth or heat; irregular heartbeat; nausea or vomiting; skin redness, rash, pain, or burning at injection site; sweating; tingling sensation; decrease in blood pressure, moderate*—with calcium chloride only
    Note: *Tingling sensation* may result when intravenous injection is too rapid; *skin redness, rash, pain,* or *burning* may indicate extravasation and can precede sloughing or necrosis of skin.
Incidence rare
    *Hypercalcemic syndrome, acute* (drowsiness; continuing nausea and vomiting; weakness); *renal calculi, calcific* (difficult or painful urination)—with oral dosage forms
Early symptoms of hypercalcemia
    *Constipation, severe; dryness of mouth; headache, continuing; increased thirst; irritability; loss of appetite; mental depression; metallic taste; unusual tiredness or weakness*
Late symptoms of hypercalcemia
    *Confusion; drowsiness; high blood pressure; increased sensitivity of eyes or skin to light, especially in hemodialysis patients; irregular, fast, or slow heartbeat; nausea and vomiting; unusually large amount of urine or increased frequency of urination*
    Note: In severe *hypercalcemia,* ECG changes consisting of shortened Q-T intervals are also seen.

## Patient Consultation

As an aid to patient consultation, refer to *Advice for the Patient, Calcium Supplements (Systemic).*

In providing consultation, consider emphasizing the following selected information (» = major clinical significance):

### Description of use
  Description should include function in the body, signs of deficiency, and conditions that may cause deficiency

### Importance of diet
  Importance of proper nutrition, supplement may be needed because of inadequate dietary intake
  Recommended daily intake for calcium
  Importance of adequate weight-bearing exercise, especially during younger years, for building and maintaining dense bones to prevent osteoporosis in later life
  Calcium content of selected foods
  Importance of adequate amounts of vitamin D or exposure to sunlight for enhancement of calcium absorption; avoiding too much vitamin D
  Importance of not using bonemeal or dolomite as a source of calcium because of potential lead contamination
  Calcium content per tablet of supplements

### Before using this dietary supplement
- » Conditions affecting use, especially:
    Use in children—Use of injectable calcium preparations may cause extreme irritation and possible tissue necrosis and sloughing
    Use in the elderly—Absorption is decreased; dosage adjustments may be necessary
    Other medications, especially cellulose sodium phosphate, digitalis glycosides (for parenteral calcium salts only), etidronate, gallium nitrate, parenteral magnesium sulfate (for parenteral calcium salts only), phenytoin, oral tetracyclines, or other calcium-containing preparations
    Other medical problems, especially hypercalcemia, hypercalciuria, calcium renal calculi, sarcoidosis, hypoparathyroidism (for cal-

cium phosphate only), dehydration, diarrhea or malabsorption, renal function impairment, or achlorhydria or hypochlorhydria (for calcium carbonate and calcium phosphates only)

## Proper use of this dietary supplement

» Proper dosing

Drinking full glass (8 ounces) of water or juice with all oral dosage forms, except when taking calcium carbonate as a phosphate binder in renal dialysis

» Proper administration of calcium carbonate or phosphate: Taking tablets 1 to 1½ hours after meals, unless otherwise directed by physician

Proper administration of chewable tablet: Chewing tablets well before swallowing

Proper administration of syrup: Taking calcium glubionate syrup *before* meals; diluting syrup in water or fruit juice, if desired, for infants or children

Missed dose: If on scheduled dosing regimen—Taking as soon as possible; then going back to regular schedule

» Proper storage

## Precautions while using this dietary supplement

Regular visits to physician to check progress if taking dietary supplement in large doses or if taking regularly for long period of time

» Not taking within 1 or 2 hours of other oral medication, if possible

» Avoiding concurrent use with other preparations containing significant amounts of calcium, phosphates, magnesium, or vitamin D, unless otherwise directed or approved by health care professional

» Avoiding concomitant use with certain fiber-containing foods such as bran and whole-grain breads and cereals; not eating these foods within 1 or 2 hours of taking calcium supplements

» Avoiding excessive use of alcoholic beverages, tobacco, or caffeine-containing beverages

» Importance of using calcium carbonate products labeled "USP," to avoid differences in bioavailability

## Side/adverse effects

Signs of potential side effects, especially calcium renal calculi or hypercalcemia

## General Dosing Information

The action of calcium supplements depends upon their content of calcium ion. The various calcium salts contain the following amounts of elemental calcium:

| Calcium salt | Calcium (mg/gram) | Calcium (mEq/gram) | % Calcium |
|---|---|---|---|
| Calcium acetate | 253 | 12.2 | 25.3 |
| Calcium carbonate | 400 | 20 | 40 |
| Calcium chloride | 272 | 13.6 | 27.2 |
| Calcium citrate | 211 | 10.5 | 21.1 |
| Calcium glubionate | 65 | 3.2 | 6.5 |
| Calcium gluceptate | 82 | 4.1 | 8.2 |
| Calcium gluconate | 90 | 4.5 | 9 |
| Calcium lactate | 130 | 6.5 | 13 |
| Calcium phosphate | | | |
| Dibasic | 230 | 11.5 | 23 |
| Tribasic | 380 | 19 | 38 |

The following table includes the number of tablets of each calcium salt required to provide 1000 mg of elemental calcium:

| Calcium supplement | Amount of salt in tablet (in milligrams) | Amount of calcium per tablet (in milligrams) | Number of tablets to provide 1000 milligrams of calcium |
|---|---|---|---|
| Calcium carbonate | 625 | 250 | 4 |
| | 650 | 260 | 4 |
| | 750 | 300 | 4 |
| | 835 | 334 | 3 |
| | 1250 | 500 | 2 |
| | 1500 | 600 | 2 |
| Calcium citrate | 950 | 200 | 5 |
| Calcium gluconate | 500 | 45 | 22 |
| | 650 | 58 | 17 |
| | 1000 | 90 | 11 |
| Calcium lactate | 325 | 42 | 24 |
| | 650 | 84 | 12 |

| Calcium supplement | Amount of salt in tablet (in milligrams) | Amount of calcium per tablet (in milligrams) | Number of tablets to provide 1000 milligrams of calcium |
|---|---|---|---|
| Calcium phosphate, dibasic | 500 | 115 | 9 |
| Calcium phosphate, tribasic | 800 | 304 | 4 |
| | 1600 | 608 | 2 |

Administration of calcium supplements should not preclude the use of other measures intended to correct the underlying cause of calcium depletion.

In the prevention of osteoporosis, postmenopausal women are sometimes also given estrogens to prevent bone resorption and/or small doses of vitamin D (usually 400 IU per day) to enhance calcium absorption. If estrogens are prescribed, either cyclically or continuously for women who have not undergone a hysterectomy, it is recommended that a progestin such as medroxyprogesterone acetate also be given to reduce or prevent the possibility of adverse endometrial changes from occurring.

The Food and Drug Administration has issued warnings that bonemeal and dolomite (sometimes used as sources of calcium) may contain lead in sufficient quantities to be dangerous.

### For parenteral dosage forms only

The injection should be warmed to body temperature prior to administration, unless precluded by an emergency situation. Following injection, the patient should remain recumbent for a short period of time to prevent dizziness.

Parenteral calcium salts are administered by *slow* intravenous injection (excepting calcium glycerophosphate and calcium lactate combination which is given by intramuscular injection) to prevent a high concentration of calcium from reaching the heart and causing cardiac syncope.

Side effects experienced by the conscious patient are often the result of too rapid a rate of intravenous administration of calcium salts. Administration should be temporarily discontinued with the appearance of abnormal electrocardiogram (ECG) readings or with patient complaints of discomfort; administration may be resumed when the abnormal reading or the discomfort has disappeared.

Severe necrosis, requiring skin grafting, and calcification can occur at the site of infiltration after intravenous injection, especially after push injection.

Transient increases in blood pressure, especially in the elderly or patients with hypertension, may occur during intravenous administration of calcium salts.

### Diet/Nutrition

Oral calcium supplements are best taken 1 to 1½ hours after meals in 3 to 4 daily doses. However, calcium glubionate syrup should be administered before meals to enhance absorption.

In the elderly, who may be more prone than younger patients to impaired stomach acid production, calcium absorption may be increased by the use of a more soluble calcium salt, such as calcium citrate, gluconate, or lactate. The poor solubility of carbonate and phosphate salts makes them less desirable as antihypocalcemic agents in patients with known achlorhydria or hypochlorhydria.

Recommended dietary intakes for calcium are defined differently worldwide.

For U.S.—

The Recommended Dietary Allowances (RDAs) for vitamins and minerals are determined by the Food and Nutrition Board of the National Research Council and are intended to provide adequate nutrition in most healthy persons under usual environmental stresses. In addition, a different designation may be used by the FDA for food and dietary supplement labeling purposes, as with Daily Value (DV). DVs replace the previous labeling terminology United States Recommended Daily Allowances (USRDAs).

For Canada—

Recommended Nutrient Intakes (RNIs) for vitamins, minerals, and protein are determined by Health and Welfare Canada and provide recommended amounts of a specific nutrient while minimizing the risk of chronic diseases.

Daily recommended intakes for calcium are generally defined as follows:

| Persons | U.S. (mg) | Canada (mg) |
|---|---|---|
| Infants and children | | |
| Birth to 3 years of age | 400–800 | 250–550 |
| 4 to 6 years of age | 800 | 600 |
| 7 to 10 years of age | 800 | 700–1100 |
| Adolescent and adult males | 800–1200 | 800–1100 |
| Adolescent and adult females | 800–1200 | 700–1100 |
| Pregnant females | 1200 | 1200–1500 |
| Breast-feeding females | 1200 | 1200–1500 |

The following table indicates the calcium content of selected foods:

| Food (amount) | Milligrams of calcium |
|---|---|
| Nonfat dry milk, reconstituted (1 cup) | 375 |
| Lowfat, skim, or whole milk (1 cup) | 290 to 300 |
| Yogurt (1 cup) | 275 to 400 |
| Sardines with bones (3 ounces) | 370 |
| Ricotta cheese, part skim (1/2 cup) | 340 |
| Salmon, canned, with bones (3 ounces) | 285 |
| Cheese, Swiss (1 ounce) | 272 |
| Cheese, cheddar (1 ounce) | 204 |
| Cheese, American (1 ounce) | 174 |
| Cottage cheese, lowfat (1 cup) | 154 |
| Tofu (4 ounces) | 154 |
| Shrimp (1 cup) | 147 |
| Ice milk (3/4 cup) | 132 |

### For treatment of adverse effects

Perivascular infiltration:Treatment may include the following—
- Immediate discontinuation of intravenous administration.
- Infusion of normal saline into the area by clysis.
- Local application of heat and elevation.

A serum calcium concentration exceeding 2.6 mmol per liter (10.5 mg per 100 mL) is considered a hypercalcemic condition. Withholding additional administration of calcium and any other medications that may cause hypercalcemia usually resolves mild hypercalcemia in asymptomatic patients, when patient renal function is adequate.

When serum calcium concentrations are greater than 2.9 mmol per liter (12 mg per 100 mL), immediate measures may be required with possible use of the following:
- Hydrating with intravenous 0.9% sodium chloride injection. Forcing diuresis with furosemide or ethacrynic acid may be used to rapidly increase calcium and sodium excretion when saline overload occurs.
- Monitoring of potassium and magnesium serum concentrations and starting replacement early to prevent complications of therapy.
- ECG monitoring and the possible use of beta-adrenergic blocking agents to protect the heart against serious arrhythmias.
- Possibly including hemodialysis, calcitonin, and corticosteroids in the treatment.
- Determining serum calcium concentrations at frequent intervals to guide therapy adjustments.

---

### *CALCIUM ACETATE*

## Summary of Differences

Category: Also used as an electrolyte replenisher.

## Additional Dosing Information

See also *General Dosing Information*.

For intravenous use only; subcutaneous or intramuscular injection may cause severe necrosis and sloughing.

Calcium acetate contains the equivalent of 253 mg of calcium ion per gram.

## Parenteral Dosage Forms

### CALCIUM ACETATE INJECTION

**Usual adult and adolescent dose**
Electrolyte replenisher or
Hypocalcemia (prophylaxis or treatment)—
    Intravenous infusion, as part of total parenteral nutrition solutions, the specific amount determined by individual patient need.

**Usual pediatric dose**
Electrolyte replenisher or
Hypocalcemia (prophylaxis or treatment)—
    Intravenous infusion, as part of total parenteral nutrition solutions, the specific amount determined by individual patient need.

**Strength(s) usually available**
U.S.—
    40 mg (10 mg [0.5 mEq] of calcium ion) per mL (Rx) [GENERIC].
Canada—
    Not commercially available.

**Packaging and storage**
Store below 40 °C (104 °F), preferably between 15 and 30 °C (59 and 86 °F), protected from light, unless otherwise specified by manufacturer. Protect from freezing.

**Incompatibilities**
Calcium acetate is precipitated by phosphates.

---

### *CALCIUM CARBONATE*

## Summary of Differences

Category:
    Also used as an antihyperphosphatemic and as an antacid (see *Calcium Carbonate, Antacids [Oral-Local]*).
Precautions:
    Drug interactions and/or related problems—Concurrent use with fluoroquinolones may decrease the absorption of fluoroquinolones, resulting in lower serum and urine concentrations of fluoroquinolones.
    Medical considerations/contraindications—Calcium absorption may be decreased in patients with achlorhydria or hypochlorhydria, unless the supplement is taken with meals.

## Additional Dosing Information

See also *General Dosing Information*.

Calcium carbonate contains the equivalent of 400 mg of calcium ion per gram.

## Oral Dosage Forms

Note: Bracketed uses in the *Dosage Forms* section refer to categories of use and/or indications that are not included in U.S. product labeling.

### CALCIUM CARBONATE CAPSULES

**Usual adult and adolescent dose**
Hypocalcemia (prophylaxis)—
    Oral, amount based on normal daily recommended intakes:

| Persons | U.S. (mg) | Canada (mg) |
|---|---|---|
| Adolescent and adult males | 800–1200 | 800–1100 |
| Adolescent and adult females | 800–1200 | 700–1100 |
| Pregnant females | 1200 | 1200–1500 |
| Breast-feeding females | 1200 | 1200–1500 |

Hypocalcemia (treatment)—
    Treatment dose is individualized by prescriber based on severity of deficiency.
Antacid—
    See *Calcium Carbonate, Antacids (Oral-Local)*.
[Antihyperphosphatemic]—
    Oral, 5 to 13 grams (2 to 5.2 grams of calcium ion) a day, in divided doses with meals.
    Note: Careful titration is recommended to prevent hypercalcemia, which has been reported with doses above 2 grams of calcium ion a day.

**Usual pediatric dose**
Dosage form not appropriate for use in children.

**Strength(s) usually available**
U.S.—
    1.25 grams (500 mg of calcium ion) (OTC) [*Calci-Mix*].
    1.5 grams (600 mg of calcium ion) (OTC) [*Liqui-Cal; Liquid Cal-600*].
Canada—
    1.25 grams (500 mg of calcium ion) (OTC) [*Calsan*].
Note: Some strengths of these calcium preparations may exceed the dosage range recommended by USP DI Advisory Panels based on the amount necessary to meet normal nutritional needs.

**Packaging and storage**
Store below 40 °C (104 °F), preferably between 15 and 30 °C (59 and 86 °F), in a well-closed container, unless otherwise specified by manufacturer.

**Auxiliary labeling**
• Drink a full glass of water.

Note: When taking as a phosphate binder in renal dialysis, patients should *not* be advised to take capsules with a glass of water.

## CALCIUM CARBONATE ORAL SUSPENSION USP

### Usual adult and adolescent dose
Hypocalcemia (prophylaxis or treatment)—
   See *Calcium Carbonate Capsules*.
Antacid—
   See *Calcium Carbonate, Antacids (Oral-Local)*.
[Antihyperphosphatemic]—
   Oral, 5 to 13 grams (2 to 5.2 grams of calcium ion) a day, in divided doses with meals.

   Note: Careful titration is recommended to prevent hypercalcemia, which has been reported with doses above 2 grams of calcium ion a day.

### Usual pediatric dose
Hypocalcemia (prophylaxis)—
   Oral, amount based on normal daily recommended intakes:

| Persons | U.S. (mg) | Canada (mg) |
|---|---|---|
| Infants and children | | |
| Birth to 3 years of age | 400–800 | 250–550 |
| 4 to 6 years of age | 800 | 600 |
| 7 to 10 years of age | 800 | 700–1100 |

Hypocalcemia (treatment)—
   Treatment dose is individualized by prescriber based on severity of deficiency.

### Strength(s) usually available
U.S.—
   1 gram (400 mg of calcium ion) per 5 mL (OTC) [*Titralac*].
   1.25 grams (500 mg of calcium ion) per 5 mL (OTC) [GENERIC].
Canada—
   Not commercially available.

Note: Some strengths of these calcium preparations may exceed the dosage range recommended by USP DI Advisory Panels based on the amount necessary to meet normal nutritional needs.

### Packaging and storage
Store below 40 °C (104 °F), preferably between 15 and 30 °C (59 and 86 °F), in a well-closed container, unless otherwise specified by manufacturer.

### Auxiliary labeling
• Shake well before using.
• Drink a full glass of water.

Note: When taking as a phosphate binder in renal dialysis, patients should *not* be advised to take suspension with a glass of water.

## CALCIUM CARBONATE TABLETS USP

### Usual adult and adolescent dose
Hypocalcemia (prophylaxis or treatment)—
   See *Calcium Carbonate Capsules*.
Antacid—
   See *Calcium Carbonate, Antacids (Oral-Local)*.
[Antihyperphosphatemic]—
   Oral, 5 to 13 grams (2 to 5.2 grams of calcium ion) a day, in divided doses with meals.

   Note: Careful titration is recommended to prevent hypercalcemia, which has been reported with doses above 2 grams of calcium ion a day.

### Usual pediatric dose
See *Calcium Carbonate Oral Suspension USP*.

### Strength(s) usually available
U.S.—
   650 mg (260 mg of calcium ion) (OTC) [GENERIC].
   667 mg (266.8 mg of calcium ion) (OTC) [*Calciday 667*].
   1 gram (OTC) [*Maalox Antacid Caplets*].
   1.25 grams (500 mg of calcium ion) (OTC) [*BioCal;* GENERIC].
   1.5 grams (600 mg of calcium ion) (OTC) [*Calcarb 600; Calcium 600; Cal-Plus; Caltrate 600; Gencalc 600; Nephro-Calci;* GENERIC].

Canada—
   625 mg (250 mg of calcium ion) (OTC) [*Apo-Cal*].
   1.25 grams (500 mg of calcium ion) (OTC) [*Apo-Cal*].
   1.5 grams (600 mg of calcium ion) (OTC) [*Caltrate 600;* GENERIC].

Note: Some strengths of these calcium preparations may exceed the dosage range recommended by USP DI Advisory Panels based on the amount necessary to meet normal nutritional needs.

### Packaging and storage
Store below 40 °C (104 °F), preferably between 15 and 30 °C (59 and 86 °F), unless otherwise specified by manufacturer. Store in a well-closed container.

### Auxiliary labeling
• Drink a full glass of water.

Note: When taking as a phosphate binder in renal dialysis, patients should *not* be advised to take tablets with a glass of water.

## CALCIUM CARBONATE TABLETS (CHEWABLE) USP

### Usual adult and adolescent dose
Hypocalcemia (prophylaxis or treatment)—
   See *Calcium Carbonate Capsules*.
Antacid—
   See *Calcium Carbonate, Antacids (Oral-Local)*.
[Antihyperphosphatemic]—
   Oral, 5 to 13 grams (2 to 5.2 grams of calcium ion) a day, in divided doses with meals.

   Note: Careful titration is recommended to prevent hypercalcemia, which has been reported with doses above 2 grams of calcium ion a day.

### Usual pediatric dose
See *Calcium Carbonate Oral Suspension USP*.

### Strength(s) usually available
U.S.—
   350 mg (140 mg calcium ion) (OTC) [*Amitone*].
   420 mg (168 mg of calcium ion) (OTC) [*Calcilac; Calglycine; Mallamint; Titralac*].
   500 mg (200 mg of calcium ion) (OTC) [*Chooz; Dicarbosil; Tums*].
   550 mg (220 mg of calcium ion) (OTC) [*Rolaids Calcium Rich*].
   750 mg (300 mg of calcium ion) (OTC) [*Caltrate Jr; Tums E-X*].
   850 mg (340 mg calcium ion) (OTC) [*Alka-Mints*].
   1.25 grams (500 mg of calcium ion) (OTC) [*Calci-Chew; OsCal 500 Chewable; Tums 500*].
   1.5 grams (600 mg calcium ion) (OTC) [*Calcium 600*].
Canada—
   500 mg (200 mg of calcium ion) (OTC) [*Tums Regular Strength*].
   750 mg (300 mg of calcium ion) (OTC) [*Tums Extra Strength*].
   1250 mg (500 mg of calcium ion) (OTC) [*Calsan*].

Note: Some strengths of these calcium preparations may exceed the dosage range recommended by USP DI Advisory Panels based on the amount necessary to meet normal nutritional needs.

### Packaging and storage
Store below 40 °C (104 °F), preferably between 15 and 30 °C (59 and 86 °F), unless otherwise specified by manufacturer. Store in a well-closed container.

### Auxiliary labeling
• Chew tablets before swallowing.
• Drink a full glass of water.

Note: When taking as a phosphate binder in renal dialysis, patients should *not* be advised to take tablets with a glass of water.

## CALCIUM CARBONATE (OYSTER-SHELL DERIVED) TABLETS

### Usual adult and adolescent dose
Hypocalcemia (prophylaxis or treatment)—
   See *Calcium Carbonate Capsules*.
Antacid—
   See *Calcium Carbonate, Antacids (Oral-Local)*.
[Antihyperphosphatemic]—
   Oral, 5 to 13 grams (2 to 5.2 grams of calcium ion) a day, in divided doses with meals.

   Note: Careful titration is recommended to prevent hypercalcemia, which has been reported with doses above 2 grams of calcium ion a day.

### Usual pediatric dose
Hypocalcemia (prophylaxis or treatment)—
   See *Calcium Carbonate Oral Suspension USP*.

## Strength(s) usually available

U.S.—

1.25 grams (500 mg of calcium ion) (OTC) [*Os-Cal 500; Oysco; Oyst-Cal 500; Oystercal 500;* GENERIC].

1.562 grams (625 mg of calcium ion) (OTC) [GENERIC].

Canada—

625 mg (250 mg of calcium ion) (OTC) [*Os-Cal*].

1.25 grams (500 mg of calcium ion) (OTC) [*Calcite 500; Nu-Cal; Os-Cal*].

Note: Some strengths of these calcium preparations may exceed the dosage range recommended by USP DI Advisory Panels based on the amount necessary to meet normal nutritional needs.

## Packaging and storage

Store below 40 °C (104 °F), preferably between 15 and 30 °C (59 and 86 °F), unless otherwise specified by manufacturer. Store in a well-closed container.

## Auxiliary labeling

• Drink a full glass of water.

Note: When taking as a phosphate binder in renal dialysis, patients should *not* be advised to take tablets with a glass of water.

## CALCIUM CARBONATE (OYSTER-SHELL DERIVED) TABLETS (CHEWABLE)

### Usual adult and adolescent dose

Antacid—

See *Calcium Carbonate, Antacids (Oral-Local)*.

Hypocalcemia (prophylaxis or treatment)—

See *Calcium Carbonate Capsules*.

[Antihyperphosphatemic]—

Oral, 5 to 13 grams (2 to 5.2 grams of calcium ion) a day, in divided doses with meals.

Note: Careful titration is recommended to prevent hypercalcemia, which has been reported with doses above 2 grams of calcium ion a day.

### Usual pediatric dose

See *Calcium Carbonate Oral Suspension USP*.

### Strength(s) usually available

U.S.—

1.25 grams (500 mg of calcium ion) (OTC) [*Oysco 500 Chewable;* GENERIC].

Canada—

1.25 grams (500 mg of calcium ion) (OTC) [*Os-Cal Chewable*].

1.875 grams (750 mg of calcium ion) (OTC) [*Os-Cal Chewable*].

Note: Some strengths of these calcium preparations may exceed the dosage range recommended by USP DI Advisory Panels based on the amount necessary to meet normal nutritional needs.

### Packaging and storage

Store below 40 °C (104 °F), preferably between 15 and 30 °C (59 and 86 °F), unless otherwise specified by manufacturer. Store in a well-closed container.

### Auxiliary labeling

• Chew tablets before swallowing.

• Drink a full glass of water.

Note: When taking as a phosphate binder in renal dialysis, patients should *not* be advised to take tablets with a glass of water.

---

### *CALCIUM CHLORIDE*

## Summary of Differences

Category: Also used as an electrolyte replenisher, a cardiotonic, an antihyperkalemic, and an antihypermagnesemic.

Precautions: Pediatrics—Parenteral calcium chloride use is usually restricted in pediatric patients due to possibility of irritation in small vasculature.

Side/adverse effects: Causes peripheral vasodilation with moderate decrease in blood pressure.

General dosing information: Has three times as much calcium per mL as calcium gluconate injection.

## Additional Dosing Information

See also *General Dosing Information*.

For intravenous use only; not to be administered intramuscularly, intramyocardially, subcutaneously, or permitted to extravasate into any body tissue; may cause severe tissue necrosis and/or sloughing and abscess formation.

Injected through a small-bore needle inserted into a large vein to minimize irritation.

Calcium chloride contains 272 mg of calcium ion per gram.

## Parenteral Dosage Forms

### CALCIUM CHLORIDE INJECTION USP

#### Usual adult dose

Hypocalcemia (prophylaxis)—

Intravenous infusion, as part of total parenteral nutrition solutions, the specific amount determined by individual patient need.

Hypocalcemia (treatment) or

Electrolyte replenisher—

Intravenous, 500 mg to 1 gram (136 to 272 mg of calcium ion) administered slowly at a rate not to exceed 0.5 mL (13.6 mg of calcium ion) to 1 mL (27.2 mg of calcium ion) a minute, the dosage being repeated at intervals of one to three days as indicated by patient response and serum calcium concentrations.

Note: For use in cases such as hungry bones syndrome, some clinicians recommend that calcium chloride be diluted in saline or dextrose and given by continuous intravenous infusion at a dosage of 0.5 to 1 mg per minute (up to 2 or more mg per minute). The rate and/or concentration can be adjusted until oral calcium supplements can be given.

Cardiotonic—

Intravenous, 500 mg to 1 gram (136 to 272 mg of calcium ion) administered at a rate not to exceed 1 mL (27.2 mg of calcium ion) a minute.

Intraventricular, 200 to 800 mg (54.4 to 217.6 mg of calcium ion) administered directly into cavity as a single dose.

Note: Injection into the cardiac muscle must be avoided.

Antihyperkalemic—

Dosage must be titrated by constant monitoring of ECG changes during administration.

Antihypermagnesemic—

Intravenous, initially 500 mg (136 mg of calcium ion) repeated as indicated by patient response.

#### Usual pediatric dose

Hypocalcemia (treatment) or

Electrolyte replenisher—

Intravenous, 25 mg (6.8 mg of calcium ion) per kg of body weight administered slowly.

Note: Calcium chloride injection is rarely used in pediatric patients, since a less irritating salt is preferred for use in the small vasculature.

#### Strength(s) usually available

U.S.—

100 mg (27.2 mg [1.36 mEq] of calcium ion) per mL (Rx) [GENERIC].

Canada—

100 mg (27.2 mg [1.36 mEq] of calcium ion) per mL (Rx) [*Calciject;* GENERIC].

#### Packaging and storage

Store below 40 °C (104 °F), preferably between 15 and 30 °C (59 and 86 °F), unless otherwise specified by manufacturer. Protect from freezing.

#### Incompatibilities

Calcium chloride is precipitated by carbonates or bicarbonates, phosphates, sulfates, and tartrates.

---

### *CALCIUM CITRATE*

## Summary of Differences

Indications:

May reduce risk of kidney stones in susceptible patients.

Also used to treat hyperphosphatenia in renal osteodystrophy.

## Additional Dosing Information

See also *General Dosing Information*.

Calcium citrate contains 211 mg of calcium ion per gram.

## Oral Dosage Forms

### CALCIUM CITRATE TABLETS

#### Usual adult and adolescent dose

Hypocalcemia (prophylaxis)—

Oral, amount based on normal daily recommended intakes:

| Persons | U.S. (mg) | Canada (mg) |
|---|---|---|
| Adolescent and adult males | 800–1200 | 800–1100 |
| Adolescent and adult females | 800–1200 | 700–1100 |
| Pregnant females | 1200 | 1200–1500 |
| Breast-feeding females | 1200 | 1200–1500 |

Hypocalcemia (treatment)—
  Treatment dose is individualized by prescriber based on severity of deficiency.

**Usual pediatric dose**
Dosage form not appropriate for use in children.

**Strength(s) usually available**
U.S.—
  950 mg (200 mg of calcium ion) (OTC) [*Citracal*].
Canada—
  Not commercially available.

Note: The strength of this calcium preparation may exceed the dosage range recommended by USP DI Advisory Panels based on the amount necessary to meet normal nutritional needs.

**Packaging and storage**
Store below 40 °C (104 °F), preferably between 15 and 30 °C (59 and 86 °F), in a well-closed container, unless otherwise specified by manufacturer.

**Auxiliary labeling**
• Drink a full glass of water.

## CALCIUM CITRATE EFFERVESCENT TABLETS

**Usual adult and adolescent dose**
See *Calcium Citrate Tablets*.

**Usual pediatric dose**
Hypocalcemia (prophylaxis)—
  Oral, amount based on normal daily recommended intakes:

| Persons | U.S. (mg) | Canada (mg) |
|---|---|---|
| Infants and children | | |
| Birth to 3 years of age | 400–800 | 250–550 |
| 4 to 6 years of age | 800 | 600 |
| 7 to 10 years | 800 | 700–1100 |

Hypocalcemia (treatment)—
  Treatment dose is individualized by prescriber based on severity of deficiency.

**Strength(s) usually available**
U.S.—
  2.38 grams (500 mg calcium ion) (OTC) [*Citracal Liquitabs*].
Canada—
  Not commercially available.

**Packaging and storage**
Store below 40°C (104°F), preferably between 15 and 30 °C (59 and 86 °F), unless otherwise specified by manufacturer. Store in a tight container or original foil packaging.

**Auxiliary labeling**
• Take dissolved in glass of water.

---

### *CALCIUM GLUBIONATE*

## Oral Dosage Forms
### CALCIUM GLUBIONATE SYRUP USP

**Usual adult and adolescent dose**
Hypocalcemia (prophylaxis)—
  Oral, amount based on normal daily recommended intakes:

| Persons | U.S. (mg) | Canada (mg) |
|---|---|---|
| Adolescent and adult males | 800–1200 | 800–1100 |
| Adolescent and adult females | 800–1200 | 700–1100 |
| Pregnant females | 1200 | 1200–1500 |
| Breast-feeding females | 1200 | 1200–1500 |

Hypocalcemia (treatment)—
  Treatment dose is individualized by prescriber based on severity of deficiency

**Usual pediatric dose**
Hypocalcemia (prophylaxis)—
  Oral, amount based on normal daily recommended intakes:

| Persons | U.S. (mg) | Canada (mg) |
|---|---|---|
| Infants and children | 400–800 | 250–550 |
| Birth to 3 years of age | | |
| 4 to 6 years of age | 800 | 600 |
| 7 to 10 years | 800 | 700–1100 |

Hypocalcemia (treatment)—
  Treatment dose is individualized by prescriber based on severity of deficiency.

**Strength(s) usually available**
U.S.—
  1.8 grams (115 mg of calcium ion) per 5 mL (OTC) [*Calcionate; Neo-Calglucon*].
Canada—
  1.2 grams calcium lactobionate, 530 mg calcium gluconate (110 mg of calcium ion) per 5 mL (OTC) [*Calcium-Sandoz*].

Note: Some strengths of these calcium preparations may exceed the dosage range recommended by USP DI Advisory Panels based on the amount necessary to meet normal nutritional needs.

**Packaging and storage**
Store below 30 °C (86 °F) preferably between 15 and 30 °C (59 and 86 °F), unless otherwise specified by manufacturer. Store in a tight container. Protect from freezing.

---

### *CALCIUM GLUCEPTATE*

## Summary of Differences

Category: Also used as an electrolyte replenisher and as an antihypermagnesemic.
Precautions: Pediatrics—Administered intramuscularly to infants and children only in emergencies when intravenous route is technically impossible.

## Additional Dosing Information

See also *General Dosing Information*.
Calcium gluceptate contains 82 mg of calcium ion per gram.
May also be administered intramuscularly to adults.

## Parenteral Dosage Forms

Note: Bracketed uses in the *Dosage Forms* section refer to categories of use and/or indications that are not included in U.S. product labeling.

### CALCIUM GLUCEPTATE INJECTION USP

**Usual adult and adolescent dose**
Hypocalcemia (prophylaxis)—
  Intravenous infusion, as part of total parenteral nutrition solutions, the specific amount determined by individual patient need.
Hypocalcemia (treatment) or
Electrolyte replenisher—
  Intramuscular, 440 mg to 1.1 gram (36 to 90 mg of calcium ion).
  Note: When a dose of 5 mL (90 mg of calcium ion) or more is administered, injection should be in the gluteal region.
  Intravenous, 1.1 to 4.4 grams (90 to 360 mg of calcium ion) administered slowly at a rate not to exceed 2 mL (36 mg of calcium ion) a minute.
[Antihypermagnesemic]—
  Intravenous, initially 1.2 to 2.4 grams (98 to 196 mg of calcium ion) administered slowly at a rate not to exceed 2 mL (36 mg of calcium ion) a minute.

**Usual pediatric dose**
Hypocalcemia (prophylaxis)—
  Intravenous infusion, part of total parenteral nutrition solutions, the specific amount determined by individual patient need.
Hypocalcemia (treatment)—
  Intramuscular, 440 mg to 1.1 gram (36 to 90 mg of calcium ion).
  Note: Calcium gluceptate may be administered intramuscularly to infants and children only in emergencies when intravenous administration is impossible.
    When a dose of 5 mL (90 mg of calcium ion) or more is administered to infants, injection should be administered in the lateral thigh.
  Intravenous, 440 mg to 1.1 gram (36 to 90 mg of calcium ion) as a single dose, administered at a rate not to exceed 2 mL (36 mg of calcium ion) a minute.
Exchange transfusions in newborns—
  Intravenous, 110 mg (9 mg of calcium ion) after every 100 mL of blood exchanged.

**Strength(s) usually available**
U.S.—
  220 mg (18 mg [0.9 mEq] of calcium ion) per mL (Rx) [GENERIC].
Canada—
  Not commercially available.

## Packaging and storage

Store below 38 °C (100 °F), preferably between 15 and 30 °C (59 and 86 °F), unless otherwise specified by manufacturer. Store in a tight container. Protect from freezing.

## Stability

Do not use if crystals are present.
Discard unused portion.

## Incompatibilities

Calcium glucaptate is precipitated by carbonates or bicarbonates, phosphates, sulfates, and tartrates.

---

## *CALCIUM GLUCEPTATE AND CALCIUM GLUCONATE*

# Oral Dosage Forms

## CALCIUM GLUCEPTATE AND CALCIUM GLUCONATE ORAL SOLUTION

### Usual adult and adolescent dose

Hypocalcemia (prophylaxis)—
Oral, amount based on normal daily recommended intakes:

| Persons | U.S. (mg) | Canada (mg) |
| --- | --- | --- |
| Adolescent and adult males | 800–1200 | 800–1100 |
| Adolescent and adult females | 800–1200 | 700–1100 |
| Pregnant females | 1200 | 1200–1500 |
| Breast-feeding females | 1200 | 1200–1500 |

Hypocalcemia (treatment)—
Treatment dose is individualized by prescriber based on severity of deficiency.

### Usual pediatric dose

Hypocalcemia (prophylaxis)—
Oral, amount based on normal daily recommended intakes:

| Persons | U.S. (mg) | Canada (mg) |
| --- | --- | --- |
| Infants and children | | |
| Birth to 3 years of age | 400–800 | 250–550 |
| 4 to 6 years of age | 800 | 600 |
| 7 to 10 years | 800 | 700–1100 |

Hypocalcemia (treatment)—
Treatment dose is individualized by prescriber based on severity of deficiency.

### Strength(s) usually available

U.S.—
Not commercially available.

Canada—
660 mg calcium glucaptate, and 560 mg calcium gluconate (total of 100 mg of calcium ion) per 5 mL (OTC) [*Calcium Stanley*].

Note: The strength of this calcium preparation may exceed the dosage range recommended by USP DI Advisory Panels based on the amount necessary to meet normal nutritional needs.

### Packaging and storage

Store below 40 °C (104 °F), preferably between 15 and 30 °C (59 and 86 °F), unless otherwise specified by manufacturer.

---

## *CALCIUM GLUCONATE*

# Summary of Differences

Category: Injection may also be used as an electrolyte replenisher, a cardiotonic, an antihyperkalemic, and an antihypermagnesemic.

# Additional Dosing Information

See also *General Dosing Information*.

Calcium gluconate injection is for intravenous use only; it is not to be administered intramuscularly, intramyocardially, subcutaneously, or permitted to extravasate into any body tissue; may cause severe tissue necrosis and/or sloughing, and abscess formation.

Calcium gluconate contains 90 mg of calcium ion per gram.

# Oral Dosage Forms

## CALCIUM GLUCONATE TABLETS USP

### Usual adult and adolescent dose

Hypocalcemia (prophylaxis)—
Oral, amount based on normal daily recommended intakes:

| Persons | U.S. (mg) | Canada (mg) |
| --- | --- | --- |
| Adolescent and adult males | 800–1200 | 800–1100 |
| Adolescent and adult females | 800–1200 | 700–1100 |
| Pregnant females | 1200 | 1200–1500 |
| Breast-feeding females | 1200 | 1200–1500 |

Hypocalcemia (treatment)—
Treatment dose is individualized by prescriber based on severity of deficiency.

### Usual pediatric dose

Dosage form not appropriate for use in children.

### Strength(s) usually available

U.S.—
325 mg (OTC) [GENERIC].
500 mg (45 mg of calcium ion) (OTC) [GENERIC].
650 mg (58.5 mg of calcium ion) (OTC) [GENERIC].
975 mg (87.75 mg of calcium ion) (OTC) [GENERIC].
1 gram (90 mg of calcium ion) (OTC) [GENERIC].

Canada—
650 mg (60 mg of calcium ion) (OTC) [GENERIC].

Note: Some strengths of these calcium preparations may exceed the dosage range recommended by USP DI Advisory Panels based on the amount necessary to meet normal nutritional needs.

## CALCIUM GLUCONATE TABLETS (CHEWABLE) USP

### Usual adult and adolescent dose

Hypocalcemia (prophylaxis)—
Oral, amount based on normal daily recommended intakes:

| Persons | U.S. (mg) | Canada (mg) |
| --- | --- | --- |
| Adolescent and adult males | 800–1200 | 800–1100 |
| Adolescent and adult females | 800–1200 | 700–1100 |
| Pregnant females | 1200 | 1200–1500 |
| Breast-feeding females | 1200 | 1200–1500 |

Hypocalcemia (treatment)—
Treatment dose is individualized by prescriber based on severity of deficiency.

### Usual pediatric dose

Hypocalcemia (prophylaxis)—
Oral, amount based on normal daily recommended intakes:

| Persons | U.S. (mg) | Canada (mg) |
| --- | --- | --- |
| Infants and children | | |
| Birth to 3 years of age | 400–800 | 250–550 |
| 4 to 6 years of age | 800 | 600 |
| 7 to 10 years | 800 | 700–1100 |

Hypocalcemia (treatment)—
Treatment dose is individualized by prescriber based on severity of deficiency.

### Strength(s) usually available

U.S.—
650 mg (58.5 mg of calcium ion) (OTC) [GENERIC].
1 gram (90 mg of calcium ion) (OTC) [GENERIC].

Canada—
Not commercially available.

Note: Some strengths of these calcium preparations may exceed the dosage range recommended by USP DI Advisory Panels based on the amount necessary to meet normal nutritional needs.

### Packaging and storage

Store below 40 °C (104 °F), preferably between 15 and 30 °C (59 and 86 °F), unless otherwise specified by manufacturer. Store in a well-closed container.

### Auxiliary labeling

• Chew tablets before swallowing.
• Drink a full glass of water.

## Parenteral Dosage Forms

Note: Bracketed uses in the *Dosage Forms* section refer to categories of use and/or indications that are not included in U.S. product labeling.

### CALCIUM GLUCONATE INJECTION USP

**Usual adult dose**

Hypocalemia (prophylaxis)—
   Intravenous infusion, as part of total parenteral nutrition solutions, the specific amount determined by individual patient need.
Hypocalcemia (treatment) or
Electrolyte replenisher—
   Intravenous, 970 mg (94.7 mg of calcium ion), administered slowly at a rate not to exceed 5 mL (47.5 mg of calcium ion) a minute. The dosage may be repeated, if necessary, until tetany is controlled.
   Note: For use in cases such as hungry bones syndrome, some clinicians recommend that calcium gluconate be diluted in isotonic solution and given by continuous intravenous infusion at a dosage of 0.5 to 1 mg per minute (up to 2 or more mg per minute). The rate and/or concentration can be adjusted until oral calcium supplements can be given.
Antihyperkalemic—
   Intravenous, 1 to 2 grams (94.7 to 189 mg of calcium ion), administered slowly at a rate not to exceed 5 mL (47.5 mg of calcium ion) a minute, the dosage being titrated and adjusted by constant monitoring of ECG changes during administration.
[Antihypermagnesemic]—
   Intravenous, 1 to 2 grams (94.7 to 189 mg of calcium ion), administered at a rate not to exceed 5 mL (47.5 mg of calcium ion) a minute.

**Usual adult prescribing limits**

15 grams (1.42 gram of calcium ion) a day.

**Usual pediatric dose**

Hypocalcemia (prophylaxis)—
   Intravenous infusion, as part of total parenteral nutrition solutions, the specific amount determined by individual patient need.
Hypocalcemia (treatment)—
   Intravenous, 200 to 500 mg (19.5 to 48.8 mg of calcium ion) as a single dose, administered slowly at a rate not to exceed 5 mL (47.5 mg of calcium ion) a minute, repeated if necessary until tetany is controlled.
Exchange transfusions in newborns—
   Intravenous, 97 mg (9.5 mg of calcium ion) administered after every 100 mL of citrated blood exchanged.

**Strength(s) usually available**

U.S.—
   100 mg (9.3 mg [0.465 mEq] of calcium ion) per mL (Rx) [GENERIC].
Canada—
   100 mg (9.3 mg [0.465 mEq] of calcium ion) per mL (Rx) [GENERIC].

**Packaging and storage**

Store below 40 °C (104 °F), preferably between 15 and 30 °C (59 and 86 °F), unless otherwise specified by manufacturer. Protect from freezing.

**Stability**

Only clear solutions should be administered. If any crystals form, they may be redissolved by warming to 30 to 40 °C (86 to 104 °F).

**Incompatibilities**

Calcium gluconate is precipitated by carbonates or bicarbonates, phosphates, sulfates, and tartrates.

**Additional information**

Injection also contains 3.5 mg of calcium d-saccharate tetrahydrate per mL for stabilization.

---

### CALCIUM GLYCEROPHOSPHATE AND CALCIUM LACTATE

## Additional Dosing Information

See also *General Dosing Information*.

Intramuscular administration does not produce inflammation or sloughing at site of injection.

## Parenteral Dosage Forms

### CALCIUM GLYCEROPHOSPHATE AND CALCIUM LACTATE INJECTION

**Usual adult and adolescent dose**

Hypocalcemia (prophylaxis)—
   Intravenous infusion, as part of total parenteral nutrition solutions, the specific amount determined by individual patient need.
Hypocalcemia (treatment)—
   Intramuscular, initially 10 mL one or two times a week for four to five weeks, the dosage being repeated as needed to raise serum calcium concentrations.

**Usual pediatric dose**

Dosage has not been established.

**Strength(s) usually available**

U.S.—
   5 mg of calcium glycerophosphate and 5 mg of calcium lactate (0.08 mEq of calcium ion) per mL (Rx) [*Calphosan* (in sodium chloride solution; 0.25% phenol)].
Canada—
   Not commercially available.

**Packaging and storage**

Store below 40 °C (104 °F), preferably between 15 and 30 °C (59 and 86 °F), unless otherwise specified by manufacturer. Protect from light. Protect from freezing.

**Note**

May also be administered intravenously or subcutaneously because of neutral pH (approximately 7).

**Additional information**

Contains phenol 0.25% as a preservative.

---

### CALCIUM LACTATE

## Additional Dosing Information

See also *General Dosing Information*.

Calcium lactate contains 130 mg of calcium ion per gram.

## Oral Dosage Forms

### CALCIUM LACTATE TABLETS USP

**Usual adult and adolescent dose**

Hypocalcemia (prophylaxis)—
   Oral, amount based on normal daily recommended intakes:

| Persons | U.S. (mg) | Canada (mg) |
|---|---|---|
| Adolescent and adult males | 800–1200 | 800–1100 |
| Adolescent and adult females | 800–1200 | 700–1100 |
| Pregnant females | 1200 | 1200–1500 |
| Breast-feeding females | 1200 | 1200–1500 |

Hypocalcemia (treatment)—
   Treatment dose is individualized by prescriber based on severity of deficiency.

**Usual pediatric dose**

Hypocalcemia (prophylaxis)—
   Oral, amount based on normal daily recommended intakes:

| Persons | U.S. (mg) | Canada (mg) |
|---|---|---|
| Infants and children | | |
|   Birth to 3 years of age | 400–800 | 250–550 |
|   4 to 6 years of age | 800 | 600 |
|   7 to 10 years | 800 | 700–1100 |

Hypocalcemia (treatment)—
   Treatment dose is individualized by prescriber based on severity of deficiency.

**Strength(s) usually available**

U.S.—
   325 mg (42.25 mg of calcium ion) (OTC) [GENERIC].
   650 mg (84.5 mg of calcium ion) (OTC) [GENERIC].
Canada—
   650 mg (84.5 mg of calcium ion) (OTC) [GENERIC].

Note: Some strengths of these calcium preparations may exceed the dosage range recommended by USP DI Advisory Panels based on the amont necessary to meet normal nutritional needs.

**Packaging and storage**
Store below 40 °C (104 °F), preferably between 15 and 30 °C (59 and 86 °F), unless otherwise specified by manufacturer. Store in a tight container.

**Auxiliary labeling**
• Drink a full glass of water.

---

### CALCIUM LACTATE-GLUCONATE AND CALCIUM CARBONATE

## Oral Dosage Forms

### CALCIUM LACTATE-GLUCONATE AND CALCIUM CARBONATE EFFERVESCENT TABLETS

**Usual adult and adolescent dose**
Hypocalcemia (prophylaxis)—
    Oral, amount based on normal daily recommended intakes:

| Persons | U.S. (mg) | Canada (mg) |
|---|---|---|
| Adolescent and adult males | 800–1200 | 800–1100 |
| Adolescent and adult females | 800–1200 | 700–1100 |
| Pregnant females | 1200 | 1200–1500 |
| Breast-feeding females | 1200 | 1200–1500 |

Hypocalcemia (treatment)—
    Treatment dose is individualized by prescriber based on severity of deficiency.

**Usual pediatric dose**
Hypocalcemia (prophylaxis)—
    Oral, amount based on normal daily recommended intakes:

| Persons | U.S. (mg) | Canada (mg) |
|---|---|---|
| Infants and children | | |
| Birth to 3 years of age | 400–800 | 250–550 |
| 4 to 6 years of age | 800 | 600 |
| 7 to 10 years | 800 | 700–1100 |

Hypocalcemia (treatment)—
    Treatment dose is individualized by prescriber based on severity of deficiency.

**Strength(s) usually available**
U.S.—
    Not commercially available.
Canada—
    2.37 grams calcium lactate-gluconate, and 1.75 grams calcium carbonate (total of 1000 mg of calcium ion) (OTC) [*Gramcal*].
    2.94 grams calcium lactate-gluconate, and 300 mg calcium carbonate (total of 500 mg of calcium ion) (OTC) [*Calcium-Sandoz Forte*].
Note: Some strengths of these calcium preparations may exceed the dosage range recommended by USP DI Advisory Panels based on the amount necessary to meet normal nutritional needs.

**Packaging and storage**
Store below 40 °C (104 °F), preferably between 15 and 30 °C (59 and 86 °F), in a well-closed container, unless otherwise specified by manufacturer.

---

### DIBASIC CALCIUM PHOSPHATE

## Summary of Differences

Medical considerations/contraindications:
    Calcium absorption may be decreased in patients with achlorhydria or hypochlorhydria, unless the supplement is taken with meals.
    Risk of hyperphosphatemia may be increased in patients with hypoparathyroidism or renal insufficiency.

## Additional Dosing Information

See also *General Dosing Information*.
Dibasic calcium phosphate contains 230 mg of calcium ion per gram.

## Oral Dosage Forms

### DIBASIC CALCIUM PHOSPHATE TABLETS USP

**Usual adult and adolescent dose**
Hypocalcemia (prophylaxis)—
    Oral, amount based on normal daily recommended intakes:

| Persons | U.S. (mg) | Canada (mg) |
|---|---|---|
| Adolescent and adult males | 800–1200 | 800–1100 |
| Adolescent and adult females | 800–1200 | 700–1100 |
| Pregnant females | 1200 | 1200–1500 |
| Breast-feeding females | 1200 | 1200–1500 |

Hypocalcemia (treatment)—
    Treatment dose is individualized by prescriber based on severity of deficiency.

**Usual pediatric dose**
Hypocalcemia (prophylaxis)—
    Oral, amount based on normal daily recommended intakes:

| Persons | U.S. (mg) | Canada (mg) |
|---|---|---|
| Infants and children | | |
| Birth to 3 years of age | 400–800 | 250–550 |
| 4 to 6 years of age | 800 | 600 |
| 7 to 10 years | 800 | 700–1100 |

Hypocalcemia (treatment)—
    Treatment dose is individualized by prescriber based on severity of deficiency.

**Strength(s) usually available**
U.S.—
    500 mg (115 mg of calcium ion) (OTC) [GENERIC].
Canada—
    Not commercially available.
Note: The strength of this calcium preparation may exceed the dosage range recommended by USP DI Advisory Panels based on the amount necessary to meet normal nutritional needs.

**Packaging and storage**
Store below 40 °C (104 °F), preferably between 15 and 30 °C (59 and 86 °F), unless otherwise specified by manufacturer. Store in a well-closed container.

**Auxiliary labeling**
• Drink a full glass of water.

---

### TRIBASIC CALCIUM PHOSPHATE

## Summary of Differences

Medical considerations/contraindications:
    Calcium absorption may be decreased in patients with achlorhydria or hypochlorhydria, unless the supplement is taken with meals.
    Risk of hyperphosphatemia may be increased in patients with hypoparathyroidism or renal insufficiency.

## Additional Dosing Information

See also *General Dosing Information*.
Tribasic calcium phosphate contains 380 mg of calcium ion per gram.

## Oral Dosage Forms

### TRIBASIC CALCIUM PHOSPHATE TABLETS

**Usual adult dose**
Hypocalcemia (prophylaxis)—
    Oral, amount based on normal daily recommended intakes:

| Persons | U.S. (mg) | Canada (mg) |
|---|---|---|
| Adolescent and adult males | 800–1200 | 800–1100 |
| Adolescent and adult females | 800–1200 | 700–1100 |
| Pregnant females | 1200 | 1200–1500 |
| Breast-feeding females | 1200 | 1200–1500 |

Hypocalcemia (treatment)—
    Treatment dose is individualized by prescriber based on severity of deficiency.

**Usual pediatric dose**
Hypocalcemia (prophylaxis)—
    Oral, amount based on normal daily recommended intakes:

| Persons | U.S. (mg) | Canada (mg) |
|---------|-----------|-------------|
| Infants and children | | |
| Birth to 3 years of age | 400–800 | 250–550 |
| 4 to 6 years of age | 800 | 600 |
| 7 to 10 years | 800 | 700–1100 |

**Hypocalcemia (treatment)—**
Treatment dose is individualized by prescriber based on severity of deficiency.

**Strength(s) usually available**
U.S.—
1.6 grams (600 mg of calcium ion) (OTC) [*Posture*].
Canada—
Not commercially available.

Note: The strength of this calcium preparation may exceed the dosage range recommended by USP DI Advisory Panels based on the amount necessary to meet normal nutritional needs.

**Packaging and storage**
Store below 40 °C (104 °F), preferably between 15 and 30 °C (59 and 86 °F), in a well-closed container, unless otherwise specified by manufacturer.

**Auxiliary labeling**
• Drink a full glass of water.

Revised: 06/10/92
Interim revision: 08/22/94; 07/18/95

# CAPREOMYCIN   Systemic

VA CLASSIFICATION (Primary): AM500

Note: For a listing of dosage forms and brand names by country availability, see *Dosage Forms* section(s). For a listing of brand names for the articles in this monograph, refer to the General Index.

## Category
Antibacterial (antimycobacterial).

## Indications

**Accepted**
Tuberculosis (treatment)—Capreomycin is indicated in combination with other antituberculosis medications in the treatment of pulmonary tuberculosis caused by *Mycobacterium tuberculosis* after failure with the primary medications (streptomycin, isoniazid, rifampin, pyrazinamide, and ethambutol) or when these cannot be used because of toxicity or development of resistant tubercle bacilli.

Since bacterial resistance may develop rapidly when capreomycin is administered alone, it should only be administered concurrently with other antituberculosis medications in the treatment of tuberculosis. Cross-resistance has been documented with kanamycin; however, no cross-resistance has been found between capreomycin and other available antimycobacterial agents.

Not all species or strains of a particular organism may be susceptible to capreomycin.

## Pharmacology/Pharmacokinetics

**Mechanism of action/Effect**
Unknown; polypeptide complex with toxicities similar to those of the aminoglycosides.

**Absorption**
Not absorbed from the gastrointestinal tract in sufficient quantities; must be given intramuscularly.

**Distribution**
Does not penetrate into the cerebrospinal fluid (CSF); high concentrations are achieved in the urine. Crosses the placenta.

**Half-life**
Normal renal function—
3 to 6 hours.
Impaired renal function—
Prolonged.

**Time to peak serum concentration**
1 to 2 hours following intramuscular administration.

**Peak serum concentration**
Mean, 28 to 32 mcg/mL (range, 20 to 47 mcg/mL) after a 1-gram dose.

**Urine concentration**
Mean, 1680 mcg/mL after a 1-gram dose.

**Elimination**
Renal—
50 to 60% excreted unchanged within 12 hours by glomerular filtration; capreomycin accumulates in the serum of patients with renal function impairment.
Biliary—
Small amounts may also be excreted in the bile.

## Precautions to Consider

**Carcinogenicity/Mutagenicity**
Studies have not been performed with capreomycin to determine its potential for carcinogenicity or mutagenicity.

**Pregnancy/Reproduction**
Pregnancy—Capreomycin crosses the placenta. Studies in pregnant women have not been done.
Studies in rats have shown that capreomycin is teratogenic, causing a low incidence of "wavy ribs" when it is given in daily doses of 50 mg per kg of body weight (mg/kg) (3½ times the human dose) or more.
FDA Pregnancy Category C.

**Breast-feeding**
It is not known whether capreomycin is distributed into breast milk. However, problems in humans have not been documented.

**Pediatrics**
No information is available on the relationship of age to the effects of capreomycin in pediatric patients. Safety and efficacy have not been established.

**Geriatrics**
No information is available on the relationship of age to the effects of capreomycin in geriatric patients. However, elderly patients are more likely to have an age-related decrease in renal function, which may require a decrease in dosage or an increased dosing interval in patients receiving capreomycin.

**Drug interactions and/or related problems**
The following drug interactions and/or related problems have been selected on the basis of their potential clinical significance (possible mechanism in parentheses where appropriate)—not necessarily inclusive (» = major clinical significance):

Note: Combinations containing any of the following medications, depending on the amount present, may also interact with this medication.

» Aminoglycosides, parenteral
(concurrent use of these medications with capreomycin should be avoided since the potential for ototoxicity, nephrotoxicity, and neuromuscular blockade may be increased; hearing loss may occur and may progress to deafness even after discontinuation of the drug and may be reversible, but usually is permanent; neuromuscular blockade may result in skeletal muscle weakness and respiratory depression or paralysis [apnea]; treatment with anticholinesterase agents or calcium salts may help reverse the blockade)

» Methoxyflurane or
» Polymyxins, parenteral
(concurrent and/or sequential use of these medications with capreomycin should be avoided since the potential for nephrotoxicity and/or neuromuscular blockade may be increased; neuromuscular blockade may result in skeletal muscle weakness and respiratory depression or paralysis [apnea]; caution is also recommended when these medications are used concurrently during surgery or in the postoperative period; treatment with anticholinesterase agents or calcium salts to help reverse the blockade)

» Nephrotoxic medications (See *Appendix II*) or
» Ototoxic medications (See *Appendix II*)
   (concurrent and/or sequential use of these medications with capreomycin may increase the potential for ototoxicity and/or nephrotoxicity; hearing loss may occur and may progress to deafness
   even after discontinuation of the drug; hearing loss may be reversible, but usually is permanent; serial audiometric function determinations may be required with concurrent or sequential use of
   other ototoxic antibacterials; renal function determinations may be
   required)
» Neuromuscular blocking agents or other medications with neuromuscular blocking activity
   (concurrent use of medications with neuromuscular blocking activity, including halogenated hydrocarbon inhalation anesthetics and
   massive transfusions with citrate anticoagulated blood, with capreomycin should be carefully monitored since neuromuscular
   blockade may be enhanced, resulting in skeletal muscle weakness
   and respiratory depression or paralysis [apnea]; caution is recommended when these medications and capreomycin are used concurrently during surgery or in the postoperative period, especially
   if there is a possibility of incomplete reversal of neuromuscular
   blockade postoperatively; treatment with anticholinesterase agents
   or calcium salts may help reverse the blockade)

## Laboratory value alterations
The following have been selected on the basis of their potential clinical
   significance (possible effect in parentheses where appropriate)—not
   necessarily inclusive (» = major clinical significance):

With physiology/laboratory test values
» Blood urea nitrogen (BUN) and
» Creatinine, serum
   (concentrations may be increased)

## Medical considerations/Contraindications
The medical considerations/contraindications included here have been selected on the basis of their potential clinical significance (reasons given
   in parentheses where appropriate)—not necessarily inclusive (» =
   major clinical significance).

*Risk-benefit should be considered when the following medical problems
exist:*
Dehydration
   (possible increased risk of toxicity because of elevated serum
   concentrations)
» Eighth-cranial-nerve impairment
   (capreomycin may cause auditory and vestibular toxicity)
» Hypersensitivity to capreomycin
» Myasthenia gravis or
» Parkinsonism
   (capreomycin has produced a partial neuromuscular blockade after
   being administered in large intravenous doses; use of capreomycin
   may result in further skeletal muscle weakness)
» Renal function impairment
   (capreomycin may cause nephrotoxicity; it is recommended that
   capreomycin be administered in a reduced dosage at fixed intervals, or in normal doses at prolonged intervals to patients with
   impaired renal function)

## Patient monitoring
The following may be especially important in patient monitoring (other
   tests may be warranted in some patients, depending on condition;
   » = major clinical significance):
» Audiograms and
» Vestibular function determinations
   (may be required prior to treatment, especially in patients with pre-
   existing renal or eighth-cranial-nerve impairment; twice-weekly or
   weekly audiometric testing to detect high-frequency hearing loss
   and periodic vestibular function determinations are recommended)
Potassium, serum
   (concentrations may be required prior to and monthly during therapy since hypokalemia may occur; however, hypokalemia is less
   likely to occur when capreomycin is given 2 or 3 times weekly)
» Renal function determinations
   (weekly renal function determinations may be required during therapy; patients with impaired renal function require a reduction in
   dose or withdrawal of the medication)

## Side/Adverse Effects
The following side/adverse effects have been selected on the basis of their
   potential clinical significance (possible signs and symptoms in parentheses where appropriate)—not necessarily inclusive:

**Those indicating need for medical attention**
Incidence more frequent
   *Nephrotoxicity* (greatly increased or decreased frequency of urination
   or amount of urine; increased thirst; loss of appetite; nausea; vomiting)
Incidence less frequent
   *Hypersensitivity* (skin rash; itching; redness; swelling; or fever); *hypokalemia* (irregular heartbeat; loss of appetite; nausea; muscle cramps
   or pain; unusual tiredness or weakness; vomiting); *neuromuscular
   blockade* (difficulty in breathing; drowsiness; unusual tiredness or
   weakness); *ototoxicity, auditory* (any loss of hearing; ringing or buzzing or a feeling of fullness in the ears); *ototoxicity, vestibular* (clumsiness or unsteadiness; dizziness; nausea or vomiting); *pain, hardness,
   unusual bleeding, or a sore at the place of injection*

## Patient Consultation
As an aid to patient consultation, refer to *Advice for the Patient,
Capreomycin (Systemic)*.

In providing consultation, consider emphasizing the following selected
   information (» = major clinical significance):

**Before using this medication**
» Conditions affecting use, especially:
   Hypersensitivity to capreomycin
   Pregnancy—Capreomycin crosses the placenta; studies in rats have
      found capreomycin to be teratogenic
   Use in the elderly—Geriatric patients may be at increased risk of
      renal toxicity because of an age-related decrease in renal
      function
   Other medications, especially parenteral aminoglycosides, other
      nephrotoxic or ototoxic medications, methoxyflurane, paren-
      teral polymyxins, or other agents with neuromuscular blocking
      activity
   Other medical problems, especially eighth-cranial-nerve impair-
      ment, myasthenia gravis, parkinsonism, or renal function
      impairment

**Proper use of this medicine**
» Compliance with full course of therapy; for tuberculosis, therapy may
   take months or years
» Proper dosing
   Missed dose: Using as soon as possible; not using if almost time for
      next dose; not doubling doses

**Side/adverse effects**
   Signs of potential side effects, especially nephrotoxicity; hypersensi-
      tivity; hypokalemia; neuromuscular blockade; auditory and vestib-
      ular ototoxicity; and pain, hardness, unusual bleeding, or a sore at
      the place of injection

## General Dosing Information
Sterile capreomycin sulfate should be administered only by deep intramuscular injection into a large muscle mass since superficial injections
   may be associated with increased pain and development of sterile
   abscesses.

Patients with renal function impairment may need an adjustment in dosage, based on creatinine clearance.

## Parenteral Dosage Forms
Note: The dosing and dosage forms available are expressed in terms of
   capreomycin base.

### CAPREOMYCIN SULFATE STERILE USP

**Usual adult and adolescent dose**
Tuberculosis—
   In combination with other antituberculosis medications: Intramuscular,
   1 gram (base) once a day for sixty to one hundred and twenty
   days, followed by 1 gram two or three times a week.

Note: Adults with impaired renal function require a reduction in dose as
   follows:

| Creatinine Clearance (mL/min)/ (mL/sec) | Dose (base) |
| --- | --- |
| >110/1.84 | See *Usual adult and adolescent dose* |
| 110/1.84 | 13.9 mg per kg every 24 hours |
| 100/1.67 | 12.7 mg per kg every 24 hours |
| 80/1.33 | 10.4 mg per kg every 24 hours |

| Creatinine Clearance (mL/min)/ (mL/sec) | Dose (base) |
|---|---|
| 60/1.00 | 8.2 mg per kg every 24 hours |
| 50/0.83 | 7 mg per kg every 24 hours; or 14 mg per kg every 48 hours |
| 40/0.67 | 5.9 mg per kg every 24 hours; or 11.7 mg per kg every 48 hours |
| 30/0.50 | 4.7 mg per kg every 24 hours; 9.5 mg per kg every 48 hours; or 14.2 mg per kg every 72 hours |
| 20/0.33 | 3.6 mg per kg every 24 hours; 7.2 mg per kg every 48 hours; or 10.7 mg per kg every 72 hours |
| 10/0.17 | 2.4 mg per kg every 24 hours; 4.9 mg per kg every 48 hours; or 7.3 mg per kg every 72 hours |
| 0/0 | 1.3 mg per kg every 24 hours; 2.6 mg per kg every 48 hours; or 3.9 mg per kg every 72 hours |

**Usual adult prescribing limits**
Up to a maximum of 20 mg (base) per kg of body weight daily.

**Usual pediatric dose**
Dosage has not been established.

# CAPSAICIN Topical

VA CLASSIFICATION (Primary): DE900

Note: For a listing of dosage forms and brand names by country availability, see *Dosage Forms* section(s). For a listing of brand names for the articles in this monograph, refer to the General Index.

## Category
Antineuralgic, specific pain syndromes (topical); analgesic, specific pain syndromes (topical).

## Indications
Note: Bracketed information in the *Indications* section refers to uses that are not included in U.S. product labeling.

**Accepted**
Neuralgia (treatment)—Capsaicin is indicated for the treatment of neuralgias, such as the pain following herpes zoster (shingles) and painful diabetic neuropathy.

Osteoarthritis (treatment); or
Rheumatoid arthritis (treatment)—Capsaicin is indicated for the treatment of pain from osteoarthritis and rheumatoid arthritis.

[Pain, neurogenic, other (treatment)]—Capsaicin is used to treat the pain associated with postmastectomy pain syndrome (PMPS) and reflex sympathetic dystrophy syndrome (RSDS, causalgia).

## Pharmacology/Pharmacokinetics

**Physicochemical characteristics**
Source—Capsaicin is a naturally occurring substance in plants of the Solanaceae family.
Molecular weight—305.4.

**Mechanism of action/Effect**
The precise mechanism of action has not been fully elucidated. Capsaicin is a neuropeptide-active agent that affects the synthesis, storage, transport, and release of substance P. Substance P is thought to be the principal chemical mediator of pain impulses from the periphery to the central nervous system. In addition, substance P has been shown to be released into joint tissues where it activates inflammatory intermediates that are involved with the development of rheumatoid arthritis. Capsaicin renders skin and joints insensitive to pain by depleting and preventing reaccumulation of substance P in peripheral sensory neurons. With the depletion of substance P in the nerve endings, local pain impulses cannot be transmitted to the brain.

Note: Capsaicin is not a local anesthetic, since it only blocks the conduction of painful impulses carried by the type-C fibers, whereas local anesthetics block the conduction of impulses in all afferent neurons, which impairs all sensations including touch, pressure, heat, and vibration.

Capsaicin is not a traditional counterirritant, since it does not produce vasodilation.

**Size(s) usually available**
U.S.—
1 gram (base) (Rx) [*Capastat*].
Canada—
Sterile capreomycin sulfate (*Capastat*) is available in Canada on a restricted basis from the manufacturer. For information on how to obtain this product, contact Eli Lilly and Company in Canada.

**Packaging and storage**
Prior to reconstitution, store below 40 °C (104 °F), preferably between 15 and 30 °C (59 and 86 °F), unless otherwise specified by manufacturer.

**Preparation of dosage form**
To prepare initial dilution for intramuscular use, add 2 mL of 0.9% sodium chloride injection or sterile water for injection to each 1-gram vial. Two to three minutes may be required for complete dissolution.

**Stability**
After reconstitution, solutions retain their potency for 48 hours at room temperature or for up to 14 days if refrigerated.
Reconstituted solutions may vary in color from almost colorless to pale straw-colored and may darken in time. This variation does not affect their potency.

Revised: 06/27/94

## Precautions to Consider

**Pregnancy/Reproduction**
Pregnancy—Problems in humans have not been documented.

**Breast-feeding**
Problems in humans have not been documented.

**Pediatrics**
Appropriate studies on the relationship of age to the effects of capsaicin have not been performed in infants and children up to 2 years of age.

**Geriatrics**
Appropriate studies on the relationship of age to the effects of capsaicin have not been performed in the geriatric population. However, geriatrics-specific problems that would limit the usefulness of this medication in the elderly are not expected.

**Medical considerations/Contraindications**
The medical considerations/contraindications included here have been selected on the basis of their potential clinical significance (reasons given in parentheses where appropriate)—not necessarily inclusive (» = major clinical significance).

*Except under special circumstances, this medication should not be used when the following medical problem exists:*
» Broken or irritated skin on area to be treated
(will cause pain and further irritation of skin)

*Risk-benefit should be considered when the following medical problem exists:*
Sensitivity to capsaicin or to the fruits of *capsicum* plants (e.g., hot peppers)

## Side/Adverse Effects
Note: Capsaicin has no known systemic side effects.

Patients may experience a warm, stinging, or burning sensation at the site of application, especially during the initial few days of use. Although this sensation frequently disappears after the first several days of treatment, it may persist for 2 to 4 weeks or longer. This effect is related to the initial excitatory effect of capsaicin on type-C fibers and their release of substance P. The burning usually decreases in frequency and intensity with continued administration of capsaicin. However, application schedules of capsaicin of less than 3 or 4 times daily may prolong the burning sensation while not providing optimum pain relief. Environmental factors, such as heat or humidity; wrappings, such as clothing or bandages; bathing in warm water; or sweating may intensify the sensation. The incidence of the burning sensation has been variable in different studies. This may be related to the etiology and pathogenesis of the pain syndrome in different persons. For example, patients with arthritis generally experience less intense burning than do patients with peripheral neuropathies.

Removal of clothing or bedsheets that have covered the area of topical capsaicin application has been associated rarely with respiratory irritation, such as coughing, in the patient and bystanders who were present at the time. This has been attributed to the inhalation of the residue of the dried cream.

There is some concern that capsaicin may be potentially neurotoxic, although animal and clinical studies with topical capsaicin have not shown this to occur. Capsaicin is thought to be capable of elevating the heat–pain threshold in the treated skin areas, especially in patients with diabetic neuropathy; these patients often already have an elevated threshold for heat and pain.

The following side/adverse effects have been selected on the basis of their potential clinical significance (possible signs and symptoms in parentheses where appropriate)—not necessarily inclusive:

**Those indicating need for medical attention only if they continue or are bothersome**
Incidence more frequent
  *Warm, stinging, or burning sensation at the site of application*

## Patient Consultation

As an aid to patient consultation, refer to *Advice for the Patient, Capsaicin (Topical)*.

In providing consultation, consider emphasizing the following selected information (» = major clinical significance):

**Before using this medication**
» Conditions affecting use, especially:
   Sensitivity to capsaicin or to the fruits of *capsicum* plants (e.g., hot peppers)
   Use in children—Not recommended in infants and children up to 2 years of age, except under the direction of a physician
   Other medical problems, especially broken or irritated skin on area to be treated

**Proper use of this medication**
   If using capsaicin for treatment of neuralgia due to herpes zoster, not applying medicine until after zoster sores have healed
   Washing areas to be treated will not cause harm, but is not necessary
   Rubbing cream into the affected area well so that little or no cream is left on surface of skin
   Washing hands with soap and water after applying capsaicin to avoid getting medicine in eyes or on other sensitive areas of body; however, if medication used on arthritic hands, not washing hands for at least 30 minutes after application
   If bandage is being used, not applying tightly
   Warm, stinging, or burning sensation may occur and is related to the action of capsaicin on the skin; usually disappears after first several days of treatment, however, may last 2 to 4 weeks or longer; heat, humidity, clothing, bathing in warm water, or sweating may increase sensation; sensation usually lessens in frequency and intensity the longer medication is used; reducing number of daily doses of capsaicin will not lessen sensation, and may prolong period of time that sensation occurs; reducing number of doses also will reduce amount of pain relief obtained
   Relief from pain may not occur right away; also, time it takes for capsaicin to work differs depending on type of pain; with arthritis, pain relief usually begins within 1 or 2 weeks; with neuralgia, pain relief usually begins within 2 to 4 weeks; with head and neck neuralgias, pain relief may take 4 to 6 weeks
   Using capsaicin 3 or 4 times a day or as directed by doctor; pain relief will last only as long as capsaicin is used regularly; if medicine is discontinued and pain recurs, capsaicin treatment may be restarted
» Proper dosage
   Missed dose: Using as soon as possible; if almost time for next dose, skipping missed dose and returning to regular dosing schedule; not doubling doses
» Proper storage

**Precautions while using this medication**
   If capsaicin gets into eyes, flushing with water; if capsaicin gets on other sensitive areas of body, washing with warm (not hot) soapy water
   If condition worsens, or does not improve after 1 month, discontinuing use and checking with physician

## General Dosing Information

The cream should be applied sparingly and rubbed well into the affected area so that little or no cream is left on the surface of the skin.

During the first 1 or 2 weeks of treatment, application of a topical lidocaine product before capsaicin application may reduce initial discomfort.

A therapeutic pain response is usually achieved within 14 to 28 days. Most patients with arthritis notice an initial response within 1 or 2 weeks. Most patients with neuralgia pain begin to respond within 2 to 4 weeks, although patients with pain from head and neck neuralgias may take 4 to 6 weeks to respond.

Continued application of capsaicin 3 or 4 times daily is necessary to sustain pain relief. If the medicine is discontinued and pain recurs, capsaicin treatment may be restarted.

Persons using capsaicin to treat arthritis in their hands should avoid washing their hands for at least 30 minutes after application.

When capsaicin is used for the treatment of neuralgia due to herpes zoster, it should not be applied to the skin until after the zoster lesions have healed.

If a bandage is being used on the treated area, it should not be applied tightly.

## Topical Dosage Forms
### CAPSAICIN CREAM

**Usual adult and adolescent dose**
Topical, to the affected area, three or four times a day.

**Usual pediatric dose**
Infants and children up to 2 years of age—Use is not recommended.
Children 2 years of age and older—See *Usual adult and adolescent dose*.

**Strength(s) usually available**
U.S.—
   0.025% (OTC) [*Zostrix* (benzyl alcohol, cetyl alcohol)].
   0.075% (OTC) [*Zostrix–HP* (benzyl alcohol, cetyl alcohol)].
Canada—
   0.025% (OTC) [*Zostrix*].
   0.075% (OTC) [*Axsain*].

**Packaging and storage**
Store below 40 °C (104 °F), preferably between 15 and 30 °C (59 and 86 °F), unless otherwise specified by manufacturer. Protect from freezing.

**Auxiliary labeling**
• For external use only.
• Avoid contact with eyes.

## Selected Bibliography

Zostrix Cream 0.025 and Zostrix-HP Cream 0.075% manufacturer's drug monograph, GenDerm (US). Received 2/92.
Rumsfield JA, West DP. Topical capsaicin in dermatologic and peripheral pain disorders. DICP 1991 Apr; 25: 381-387.
Watson CP, et al. Post-herpetic neuralgia: 208 cases [abstract]. Pain 1988 Dec; 35 (3): 289-297.

Revised: 07/14/92

---

## CAPTOPRIL—See *Angiotensin-converting Enzyme (ACE) Inhibitors (Systemic)*

---

## CAPTOPRIL-CONTAINING COMBINATIONS—

Captopril and Hydrochlorothiazide (Systemic)—See *Angiotensin-converting Enzyme (ACE) Inhibitors and Hydrochlorothiazide (Systemic)*

---

## CARAMIPHEN-CONTAINING COMBINATIONS—

Chlorpheniramine, Phenylpropanolamine, and Caramiphen (Systemic)—See *Cough/Cold Combinations (Systemic)*
Phenylpropanolamine and Caramiphen (Systemic)—See *Cough/Cold Combinations (Systemic)*

# CARBACHOL    Ophthalmic

**VA CLASSIFICATION (Primary/Secondary): OP102/OP109**
Another commonly used name is carbamylcholine.

Note: For a listing of dosage forms and brand names by country availability, see *Dosage Forms* section(s). For a listing of brand names for the articles in this monograph, refer to the General Index.

## Category

Antiglaucoma agent (ophthalmic)—Carbachol Ophthalmic Solution USP; Miotic—Carbachol Intraocular Solution USP; Carbachol Ophthalmic Solution USP.

## Indications

Note: Bracketed information in the *Indications* section refers to uses that are not included in U.S. product labeling.

**Accepted**

Miosis induction, during surgery—Carbachol intraocular solution is indicated to produce pupillary miosis during surgery.

Glaucoma, open-angle (treatment)—Carbachol ophthalmic solution is indicated for lowering intraocular pressure in the treatment of chronic open-angle glaucoma. It is especially useful as a replacement drug, particularly in eyes that have become intolerant of, or resistant to, pilocarpine.

[Glaucoma, angle-closure (treatment)][1]—Carbachol ophthalmic solution is used for emergency treatment of angle-closure glaucoma; however, pilocarpine is usually preferred.

[Glaucoma, angle-closure, *during* or *after* iridectomy (treatment)][1]—Carbachol ophthalmic solution is used in the treatment of angle-closure glaucoma during or after iridectomy.

[Glaucoma, secondary (treatment)][1]—Carbachol ophthalmic solution is used in the treatment of secondary glaucoma if there is no active intraocular inflammation present.

---

[1]Not included in Canadian product labeling.

## Pharmacology/Pharmacokinetics

**Physicochemical characteristics**
Molecular weight—182.65.

**Mechanism of action/Effect**
Carbachol is a parasympathomimetic that directly stimulates cholinergic receptors. It may also act indirectly by promoting release of acetylcholine and by a weak anticholinesterase action. Carbachol produces contraction of the iris sphincter muscle resulting in pupillary constriction (miosis), constriction of the ciliary muscle resulting in increased accommodation, and a reduction in intraocular pressure associated with decreased resistance to aqueous humor outflow.

In chronic open-angle glaucoma, the exact mechanism by which carbachol lowers intraocular pressure is not precisely known; however, contraction of the ciliary muscle apparently opens the intertrabecular spaces and facilitates aqueous humor outflow.

In angle-closure glaucoma, constriction of the pupil apparently pulls the iris away from the trabeculum, thereby relieving blockage of the trabecular meshwork.

**Onset of action**
Ophthalmic solution—Miosis: Within 10 to 20 minutes.

**Time to peak effect**
Intraocular solution—Miosis: Within 2 to 5 minutes.
Ophthalmic solution—Reduction in intraocular pressure: Within 4 hours.

**Duration of action**
Intraocular solution—
    Miosis: About 24 hours.
Ophthalmic solution—
    Miosis: About 4 to 8 hours.
    Reduction in intraocular pressure: About 8 hours.

## Precautions to Consider

**Carcinogenicity**
Long-term animal studies have not been done.

**Pregnancy/Reproduction**
Pregnancy—Studies have not been done in humans. However, carbachol may be systemically absorbed.

Studies have not been done in animals.
FDA Pregnancy Category C.

**Breast-feeding**
Carbachol may be systemically absorbed. It is not known whether carbachol is distributed into breast milk. However, problems in humans have not been documented.

**Pediatrics**
Appropriate studies on the relationship of age to the effects of carbachol have not been performed in the pediatric population. However, no pediatrics-specific problems have been documented to date.

**Geriatrics**
Appropriate studies on the relationship of age to the effects of carbachol have not been performed in the geriatric population. However, no geriatrics-specific problems have been documented to date.

**Drug interactions and/or related problems**
The following drug interactions and/or related problems have been selected on the basis of their potential clinical significance (possible mechanism in parentheses where appropriate)—not necessarily inclusive (» = major clinical significance):

Note: Combinations containing any of the following medications, depending on the amount present, may also interact with this medication.

    Belladonna alkaloids, ophthalmic or
    Cyclopentolate
      (concurrent use of these medications may interfere with the antiglaucoma action of carbachol. Also, concurrent use with carbachol counteracts the mydriatic effects of these medications; this counteraction may be used to therapeutic advantage)

    Flurbiprofen, ophthalmic
      (ophthalmic carbachol may be ineffective when administered following ophthalmic flurbiprofen; the pharmacologic basis for this interference is not known)

**Medical considerations/Contraindications**
The medical considerations/contraindications included here have been selected on the basis of their potential clinical significance (reasons given in parentheses where appropriate)—not necessarily inclusive (» = major clinical significance).

*Risk-benefit should be considered when the following medical problems exist:*
    Asthma, bronchial
    Cardiac failure, acute
    Corneal abrasion or injury
      (possible excessive absorption of medication, which can produce systemic toxicity)
    Gastrointestinal spasm
    Hyperthyroidism
»  Iritis, acute, or other conditions in which pupillary constriction is undesirable
    Parkinson's disease
    Peptic ulcer, active
    Sensitivity to carbachol
    Urinary tract obstruction

**Patient monitoring**
The following may be especially important in patient monitoring (other tests may be warranted in some patients, depending on condition; » = major clinical significance):

    Intraocular pressure determinations
      (recommended at periodic intervals during therapy when carbachol is used in the treatment of glaucoma)

## Side/Adverse Effects

Note: Corneal clouding, persistent bullous keratopathy, and post-operative iritis following cataract extraction have been reported occasionally when carbachol intraocular solution was used during cataract surgery.

With the exception of retinal detachment, the following side effects have not been reported following the use of carbachol intraocular solution.

The following side/adverse effects have been selected on the basis of their potential clinical significance (possible signs and symptoms in parentheses where appropriate)—not necessarily inclusive:

**Those indicating need for medical attention**
Incidence rare
  *Retinal detachment* (veil or curtain appearing across part of vision)
Symptoms of systemic absorption
  *Asthma* (shortness of breath, wheezing, or tightness in chest); *cardiac arrhythmia* (irregular heartbeat); *diarrhea, stomach cramps or pain, or vomiting; flushing or redness of face; frequent urge to urinate; hypotension* (unusual tiredness or weakness); *increased sweating; syncope* (fainting); *watering of mouth*

**Those indicating need for medical attention only if they continue or are bothersome**
Incidence more frequent
  *Blurred vision or change in near or distance vision; eye pain; stinging or burning of the eye*
Incidence less frequent
  *Headache; irritation or redness of eyes; twitching of eyelids*

## Overdose

For specific information on the agents used in the management of ophthalmic carbachol overdose, see:
  • Atropine in *Anticholinergics/Antispasmodics (Systemic)* monograph.

For more information on the management of overdose or unintentional ingestion, **contact a Poison Control Center** (see *Poison Control Center Listing*).

**Treatment of overdose**
Atropine sulfate injection is used as an antidote to the systemic effects of carbachol.

## Patient Consultation

As an aid to patient consultation, refer to *Advice for the Patient, Carbachol (Ophthalmic)*.

In providing consultation, consider emphasizing the following selected information (» = major clinical significance):

**Before using this medication**
» Conditions affecting use, especially:
    Sensitivity to carbachol
    Other medical problems, especially acute iritis or other conditions in which pupillary constriction is undesirable

**Proper use of this medication**
*For the ophthalmic solution*
» Importance of not using more medication than the amount prescribed
  Proper administration technique
  Washing hands immediately after applying eye drops
  Preventing contamination: Not touching applicator tip to any surface; keeping container tightly closed
» Proper dosing
  Missed dose: Applying as soon as possible; not applying if almost time for next dose; applying next dose at regularly scheduled time
» Proper storage

**Precautions while using this medication**
*For the ophthalmic solution*
  Regular visits to physician to check eye pressure during therapy
» Caution if driving or doing anything else at night or in dim light
» Caution if blurred vision or change in near or distance vision occurs

**Side/adverse effects**
  Signs of potential side effects, especially retinal detachment or symptoms of systemic absorption

## General Dosing Information

**For ophthalmic solution**
Although some manufacturers recommend a dose of 2 drops of an ophthalmic solution at appropriate intervals, the conjunctival sac will usually hold only 1 drop.

More frequent instillation or use of a stronger solution may be required to produce an adequate reduction in intraocular pressure in eyes with hazel or brown irides than is needed in eyes with blue or light-colored irides.

To avoid excessive systemic absorption, patient should press finger to the lacrimal sac during and for 1 or 2 minutes following instillation of medication.

Tolerance to carbachol may develop with prolonged use. Effectiveness may be restored by changing to another miotic for a short time and then resuming the original medication.

# Ophthalmic Dosage Forms

## CARBACHOL INTRAOCULAR SOLUTION USP

**Usual adult and adolescent dose**
Miotic—
    Intraocular irrigation, no more than 0.5 mL of a 0.01% solution instilled into the anterior chamber.

**Usual pediatric dose**
See *Usual adult and adolescent dose*.

**Usual geriatric dose**
See *Usual adult and adolescent dose*.

**Strength(s) usually available**
U.S.—
    0.01% (Rx) [*Miostat*].
Canada—
    0.01% (Rx) [*Miostat*].

**Packaging and storage**
Store between 15 and 30 °C (59 and 86 °F), in a tight container. Protect from freezing.

**Auxiliary labeling**
• For single-dose intraocular use only.
• Discard unused portion.

## CARBACHOL OPHTHALMIC SOLUTION USP

**Usual adult and adolescent dose**
Antiglaucoma agent (ophthalmic)—
    Topical, to the conjunctiva, 1 drop of a 0.75 to 3% solution one to three times a day.

**Usual pediatric dose**
See *Usual adult and adolescent dose*.

**Usual geriatric dose**
See *Usual adult and adolescent dose*.

**Strength(s) usually available**
U.S.—
    0.75% (Rx) [*Isopto Carbachol* (benzalkonium chloride 0.005%)].
    1.5% (Rx) [*Isopto Carbachol* (benzalkonium chloride 0.005%)].
    2.25% (Rx) [*Isopto Carbachol* (benzalkonium chloride 0.005%)].
    3% (Rx) [*Carboptic; Isopto Carbachol* (benzalkonium chloride 0.005%)].
Canada—
    1.5% (Rx) [*Isopto Carbachol* (benzalkonium chloride)].
    3% (Rx) [*Isopto Carbachol* (benzalkonium chloride)].

**Packaging and storage**
Store below 40 °C (104 °F), preferably between 15 and 30 °C (59 and 86 °F), unless otherwise specified by manufacturer. Store in a tight container. Protect from freezing.

**Auxiliary labeling**
• For the eye.
• Keep container tightly closed.

Revised: 06/21/94
Interim revision: 05/01/95

# CARBAMAZEPINE   Systemic

VA CLASSIFICATION (Primary/Secondary): CN400/CN103; CN900; HS900

Note: For a listing of dosage forms and brand names by country availability, see *Dosage Forms* section(s). For a listing of brand names for the articles in this monograph, refer to the General Index.

## Category

Anticonvulsant; antineuralgic (specific pain syndromes); antimanic; antidiuretic; antipsychotic.

## Indications

Note: Bracketed information in the *Indications* section refers to uses that are not included in U.S. product labeling.

**Accepted**

Epilepsy (treatment)—Carbamazepine is indicated for the treatment of partial seizures with simple or complex symptomatology (psychomotor, temporal lobe); generalized tonic-clonic seizures (grand mal); mixed seizure patterns that include the above; or other partial or generalized seizures.

Carbamazepine is a first-choice anticonvulsant because of its relatively low behavioral and psychological toxicity and the rarity of serious adverse effects.

Neuralgia, trigeminal (treatment)—Carbamazepine is indicated for relief of pain due to true trigeminal neuralgia (tic douloureux) and glossopharyngeal neuralgia.

[Pain, neurogenic, other (treatment)][1]—Carbamazepine may also be used in some patients to relieve the lightning pains of tabes dorsalis; neuralgic pain associated with multiple sclerosis, acute idiopathic neuritis (Guillain-Barré syndrome), peripheral diabetic neuropathy, phantom limb, restless leg syndrome (Ekbom's syndrome), and hemifacial spasm; post-traumatic neuropathy or neuralgia; and postherpetic neuralgia.

[Bipolar disorder (prophylaxis and treatment)][1]—Carbamazepine is used alone or in combination with lithium and/or antidepressants or antipsychotics to treat patients with manic-depressive illness who are unresponsive to, or cannot tolerate, lithium or neuroleptics alone.

[Diabetes insipidus, central partial (treatment)][1]—Carbamazepine is used alone or with other agents such as clofibrate or chlorpropamide in the treatment of partial central diabetes insipidus.

[Alcohol withdrawal (treatment)][1]—Carbamazepine is used for the detoxification of alcoholics. It has been found to be effective in rapidly relieving anxiety and distress of acute alcohol withdrawal and for such symptoms as seizures, hyperexcitability, and sleep disturbances.

[Psychotic disorders (treatment)][1]—Carbamazepine has been shown to be effective in certain psychiatric disorders including schizoaffective illness, resistant schizophrenia, and dyscontrol syndrome, associated with limbic system dysfunction.

**Unaccepted**

*Carbamazepine is not a simple analgesic and should not be used to relieve general aches or pains.*

Carbamazepine is *not* indicated for atypical or generalized absence seizures (petit mal) or myoclonic or atonic seizures.

Although carbamazepine has also been reported to relieve dystonic attacks in children, reduce migraine attacks, and relieve intractable hiccups in some patients, its therapeutic efficacy in such cases has not been established.

Carbamazepine should not be used prophylactically during long periods of remission in trigeminal neuralgia.

---

[1]Not included in Canadian product labeling.

## Pharmacology/Pharmacokinetics

**Physicochemical characteristics**

Chemical group—Tricyclic iminostilbene derivative. Structurally resembles the psychoactive agents imipramine, chlorpromazine, and maprotiline; shares some structural features with the anticonvulsant agents phenytoin, clonazepam, and phenobarbital.

Molecular weight—236.27.

pKa—7.

**Mechanism of action/Effect**

Anticonvulsant—Exact mechanism unknown; may act postsynaptically by limiting the ability of neurons to sustain high frequency repetitive firing of action potentials through enhancement of sodium channel inactivation; in addition to altering neuronal excitability, may act presynaptically to block the release of neurotransmitter by blocking presynaptic sodium channels and the firing of action potentials, which in turn decreases synaptic transmission.

Antineuralgic—Exact mechanism unknown; may involve gamma-aminobutyric acid (GABA$_B$) receptors, which may be linked to calcium channels.

Antidiuretic—Exact mechanism unknown; may exert a hypothalamic effect on the osmoreceptors mediated via secretion of antidiuretic hormone (ADH), or may have a direct effect on the renal tubule.

Antimanic; antipsychotic—Exact mechanism unknown; may be related to either the anticonvulsant or the antineuralgic effects of carbamazepine, or to its effects on neurotransmitter modulator systems.

**Other actions/effects**

Anticholinergic, antidepressant, neuromuscular transmission–inhibiting, and antiarrhythmic actions have been reported.

**Absorption**

Slow and variable, but almost completely absorbed from gastrointestinal tract.

**Distribution**

Apparent volume of distribution (vol$_D$)—
   Carbamazepine: Ranges from 0.8 to 2 L per kg.
   Carbamazepine-10,11-epoxide: Ranges from 0.59 to 1.5 L per kg.
In breast milk—
   May reach 60% of the maternal plasma concentration.

**Protein binding**

Carbamazepine—Moderate (55 to 59% in children, 76% in adults).
Carbamazepine-10,11-epoxide—Moderate (50%).

**Biotransformation**

Hepatic (97%); may induce its own metabolism. One metabolite, carbamazepine-10,11-epoxide, has anticonvulsant, antidepressant, and antineuralgic activity.

**Half-life**

Carbamazepine—
   Initial single dose: May range from 25 to 65 hours.
   Chronic dosing: May decrease to 8 to 29 hours (average 12 to 17 hours) because of autoinduction of metabolism.
Carbamazepine-10,11-epoxide—
   5 to 8 hours.

**Onset of action**

Anticonvulsant effect—Varies from hours to days, depending on individual patient. A stable therapeutic concentration may require a month to achieve due to autoinduction of metabolism.
Relief of pain of trigeminal neuralgia—8 to 72 hours.
Antimanic response—Usually 7 to 10 days.

**Time to peak concentration**

Suspension—1.5 hours following chronic administration.
Tablets—4 to 5 hours and possibly up to 12 hours after a 400-mg dose.

**Therapeutic plasma concentrations:**

4 to 12 mcg per mL (16.9 to 50.8 micromoles per L) (in adults); variations due to autoinduction of metabolism.

**Elimination**

Renal—72% (3% as unchanged drug).
Fecal—28%.
Clearance values ranged from 0.011 to 0.021 L per hour per kg following a single dose of carbamazepine in healthy volunteers, and from 0.025 to 0.540 L per hour per kg following multiple dosing in healthy volunteers and epilepsy patients.

Note: Large interindividual differences in apparent plasma half-life and total body clearance are related to the phenomenon of autoinduction, which reaches different levels in different individuals. Autoinduction may lead to time-dependent kinetics, in which clearance values increase with time and higher doses are required to maintain the same plasma concentrations. In healthy volunteers, it is estimated that a plateau for autoinduction is reached after 20 to 30 days; in epileptic patients, however, the time course may differ due to previous induction by other medications.

# Precautions to Consider

## Cross-sensitivity and/or related problems

Patients who are sensitive to tricyclic antidepressants may be sensitive to carbamazepine also. Carbamazepine should be given with caution, if at all, to such patients.

## Carcinogenicity/Tumorigenicity

Carbamazepine is considered carcinogenic in Sprague-Dawley rats because doses of 25, 75, and 250 mg per kg per day for 2 years caused a dose-related increase in the incidence of hepatocellular tumors in females and of benign interstitial cell adenomas in the testes of males. The significance of these findings for use of carbamazepine in humans is not known.

## Pregnancy/Reproduction

Pregnancy—Carbamazepine crosses the placenta. Although adequate and well-controlled studies in humans have not been done, there have been reports of babies prenatally exposed to carbamazepine having small head circumferences, low birth weights, craniofacial defects, fingernail hypoplasia, developmental delays, and spina bifida. When it is essential to continue carbamazepine therapy during pregnancy, serum carbamazepine concentrations must be monitored closely, since adverse effects in the fetus have been associated with high blood concentrations.

Studies in animals have shown that carbamazepine caused kinked ribs in 1.5% of the offspring of rats receiving 250 mg per kg. Also, carbamazepine caused cleft palate, deformities of the foot, or anophthalmos in about 3% of the offspring of rats receiving 650 mg per kg. These doses are 10 to 25 times the human daily dose.

FDA Pregnancy Category C.

Also, it must be kept in mind that other anticonvulsants used during pregnancy have been implicated in birth defects in infants born to epileptic mothers. In addition, retrospective studies have suggested that there may be a higher incidence of teratogenic effects with the use of combinations of anticonvulsants than with monotherapy.

## Breast-feeding

Carbamazepine is distributed into breast milk. Concentrations in breast milk and in the plasma of nursing infants have been reported to reach 60% of the maternal plasma concentration. Therefore, the possibility exists that carbamazepine may cause adverse effects in the nursing infant. In animal studies, nursing rats showed a lack of weight gain and an unkempt appearance with maternal doses of 200 mg per kg.

## Pediatrics

Appropriate studies have not been performed in children up to 6 years of age. However, behavioral changes are more likely to occur in children.

## Geriatrics

Geriatric patients may be more susceptible to carbamazepine-induced confusion or agitation, atrioventricular (AV) heart block, syndrome of inappropriate antidiuretic hormone (SIADH), and bradycardia than younger patients.

## Dental

The leukopenic and thrombocytopenic effects of carbamazepine may result in an increased incidence of microbial infection, delayed healing, and gingival bleeding. If leukopenia or thrombocytopenia occurs, dental work should be deferred until blood counts have returned to normal. Patient instruction in proper oral hygiene should include caution in use of regular toothbrushes, dental floss, and toothpicks.

## Drug interactions and/or related problems

The following drug interactions and/or related problems have been selected on the basis of their potential clinical significance (possible mechanism in parentheses where appropriate)—not necessarily inclusive (» = major clinical significance):

Note: Combinations containing any of the following medications, depending on the amount present, may also interact with this medication.

Acetaminophen
> (risk of hepatotoxicity with single toxic doses or prolonged use of high doses of acetaminophen may be increased, and therapeutic effects of acetaminophen may be decreased, in patients taking hepatic enzyme–inducing agents such as carbamazepine)

Aminophylline or
Oxtriphylline or
Theophylline
> (concurrent use with carbamazepine may stimulate hepatic metabolism of the xanthines [except dyphylline], resulting in increased theophylline clearance)

» Anticoagulants, coumarin- or indandione-derivative
> (anticoagulant effects may be decreased because of induction of hepatic microsomal enzyme activity, resulting in increased anticoagulant metabolism leading to decreased anticoagulant serum concentration and elimination half-life; dosage adjustments based on monitoring of prothrombin time may be necessary during and after carbamazepine therapy)

» Anticonvulsants, hydantoin or
» Anticonvulsants, succinimide or
» Barbiturates or
» Benzodiazepines metabolized via hepatic microsomal enzymes, especially clonazepam or
» Primidone or
» Valproic acid
> (concurrent use with carbamazepine may result in increased metabolism, leading to decreased serum concentrations and reduced elimination half-lives of these medications because of induction of hepatic microsomal enzyme activity; monitoring of blood concentrations as a guide to dosage is recommended, especially when any of these medications or carbamazepine is added to or withdrawn from an existing regimen)
> (valproic acid may prolong the half-life and reduce the protein-binding of carbamazepine; the concentration of the active 10,11-epoxide metabolite may be increased)
> (in addition, use of carbamazepine in combination with other anticonvulsants has been reported to be associated with an increased risk of congenital defects)

» Antidepressants, tricyclic or
Haloperidol or
Loxapine or
Maprotiline or
Molindone or
Phenothiazines or
Pimozide or
Thioxanthenes
> (concurrent use of these agents with carbamazepine may enhance the central nervous system [CNS] depressant effects of carbamazepine, lower the seizure threshold, and decrease the anticonvulsant effects of carbamazepine; dosage adjustments may be necessary to control seizures; anticholinergic effects may be potentiated, leading to confusion and delirium)
> (also, concurrent use of haloperidol, and possibly other neuroleptics, with carbamazepine may decrease plasma concentrations of the neuroleptic by about 60% with or without adverse clinical effects; close observation of patient for clinical signs of ineffectiveness of the neuroleptic is recommended; dosage adjustment may be necessary)

Carbonic anhydrase inhibitors
> (concurrent use may increase the risk of carbamazepine-induced osteopenia; it is recommended that patients receiving concurrent therapy be monitored for early signs of osteopenia and that the carbonic anhydrase inhibitor be discontinued and appropriate treatment initiated if necessary)

Chlorpropamide or
Desmopressin or
Lypressin or
Posterior pituitary or
Thiazide diuretics, when used for their paradoxical antidiuretic activity in the treatment of diabetes insipidus, or
Vasopressin
> (concurrent use with carbamazepine may potentiate the antidiuretic effect, leading to a lower sodium concentration and causing adverse effects that include increased seizure activity; a reduction in dosage of either or both medications may be necessary for optimal therapeutic effect in the treatment of diabetes insipidus)

» Cimetidine
> (concurrent use may result in increased plasma concentration of carbamazepine by delaying its clearance, leading to carbamazepine toxicity)

» Clarithromycin
> (administration of carbamazepine with clarithromycin has been shown to significantly increase the plasma concentration of carbamazepine; carbamazepine serum levels should be monitored)

» Contraceptives, estrogen-containing, oral or
Cyclosporine or
Dacarbazine or
Digitalis glycosides, with the possible exception of digoxin or
Disopyramide or

» Estrogens, including estramustine or
Levothyroxine or
Mexiletine or
» Quinidine
(concurrent use may decrease the effects of these medications because of increased metabolism resulting from induction of hepatic
microsomal enzyme activity; dosage adjustments may be
necessary)

(in addition, concurrent use of oral, estrogen-containing contraceptives with carbamazepine may result in breakthrough bleeding and
contraceptive failure due to the increased rate of hepatic enzyme
metabolism of steroids induced by carbamazepine; the dose of the
estrogenic substance in the oral contraceptive may be increased to
diminish bleeding and decrease the risk of conception; parenteral
medroxyprogesterone or nonhormonal methods of birth control
may be considered as alternatives)

» Corticosteroids
(concurrent use may decrease the corticosteroid effect because of
increased corticosteroid metabolism resulting from induction of hepatic microsomal enzymes)

Danazol or
» Diltiazem or
» Verapamil
(concurrent use of these agents with carbamazepine may inhibit
carbamazepine metabolism, resulting in increased plasma concentrations and toxicity)

(carbamazepine toxicity may be delayed for several weeks after
initiation of danazol therapy; carbamazepine dosage may need to
be reduced)

(it is recommended that nifedipine be used as an alternative to
verapamil or diltiazem)

Doxycycline
(concurrent use may decrease plasma concentration and elimination half-life of doxycycline because of induction of hepatic microsomal enzyme activity; if concurrent use cannot be avoided,
doxycycline plasma concentrations or the therapeutic response to
doxycycline should be closely monitored and dosage adjustments
made as necessary)

Enflurane or
Halothane or
Methoxyflurane
(chronic use of a hepatic enzyme–inducing agent such as carbamazepine prior to anesthesia may increase the metabolism of these
anesthetics, leading to an increased risk of hepatotoxicity)

(formation of nephrotoxic metabolites of methoxyflurane may be
increased by chronic use of a hepatic enzyme–inducing agent such
as carbamazepine prior to anesthesia, leading to increased risk of
nephrotoxicity)

(in addition, cardiac arrhythmias may occur, possibly due to sensitization of the myocardium resulting from increased concentrations of norepinephrine)

» Erythromycin or
Troleandomycin
(concurrent use of these agents with carbamazepine may inhibit
carbamazepine metabolism, resulting in increased plasma concentrations and toxicity; it is recommended that an alternate antibiotic
to erythromycin or troleandomycin be used)

» Felbamate
(concurrent use may decrease carbamazepine plasma concentrations by about 20 to 30% and increase carbamazepine-10,11–epox-
ide plasma concentrations by about 60%, leading to an increase in
adverse effects; enzyme induction by carbamazepine may lead to
decreased felbamate plasma concentrations; carbamazepine dosage
should be reduced by 20 to 33% when felbamate therapy is initiated, and plasma concentrations of carbamazepine should be monitored with further dosage adjustments made as clinically
necessary)

Folic acid
(requirements for folic acid may be increased in patients receiving
anticonvulsant therapy)

Influenza virus vaccine
(concurrent use with carbamazepine may inhibit carbamazepine
metabolism, resulting in increased plasma concentrations and toxicity; carbamazepine serum concentrations may be increased on
days 7 to 14 after influenza virus vaccination; dosage adjustments
of carbamazepine based on the patient's clinical status and serum
carbamazepine concentrations may be necessary)

» Isoniazid
(carbamazepine may induce microsomal metabolism of isoniazid,
increasing formation of a reactive intermediate and leading to hepatotoxicity; also, isoniazid administration may result in elevated
plasma concentrations of carbamazepine and possible toxicity)

Lithium
(concurrent use may decrease the antidiuretic effect of carbamazepine and increase the neurotoxic side effects even at nontoxic
blood concentrations of both lithium and carbamazepine; however,
the concurrent use of lithium with carbamazepine may be synergistic in the treatment of patients with manic-depressive illness
who fail to respond to either drug alone)

Mebendazole
(in patients receiving high oral doses of mebendazole for treatment
of tissue-dwelling organisms such as *Echinococcus multilocularis*
or *granulosus* [Hydatid disease], carbamazepine has been shown
to lower plasma mebendazole concentrations by induction of hepatic microsomal enzymes and to impair the therapeutic response;
if carbamazepine is being used for seizures, replacement with another anticonvulsant is recommended; treatment of intestinal helminths such as whipworms or hookworms does not appear to be
affected by the rate of hepatic metabolism of mebendazole)

» Monoamine oxidase (MAO) inhibitors, including furazolidone and
procarbazine
(concurrent use with carbamazepine has resulted in hyperpyretic
crises, hypertensive crises, severe convulsions, and death; a medication-free interval of at least 14 days is recommended between
discontinuation of MAO inhibitor therapy and initiation of carbamazepine therapy, or vice versa)

(MAO inhibitors may also cause a change in the pattern of epileptiform seizures in patients receiving carbamazepine as an
anticonvulsant)

Praziquantel
(one small, single-dose, controlled study found that epileptic patients taking carbamazepine had significantly lower plasma concentrations of praziquantel [7.9% of the control group]; this effect
is thought to be due to induction of the cytochrome P-450 microsomal enzyme system by carbamazepine; patients on carbamazepine may require a larger dose of praziquantel)

» Propoxyphene
(concurrent use with carbamazepine may inhibit carbamazepine
metabolism, resulting in increased plasma concentrations and toxicity; an analgesic other than propoxyphene should be used)

» Risperidone
(chronic administration of carbamazepine may increase the clearance of risperidone)

**Laboratory value alterations**
The following have been selected on the basis of their potential clinical
significance (possible effect in parentheses where appropriate)—not
necessarily inclusive (» = major clinical significance):

With diagnostic test results
» Metyrapone test
(increased metabolism of metyrapone by an hepatic enzyme inducer such as carbamazepine may decrease the response to
metyrapone)

Pregnancy test
(false negative results may occur with the use of tests that determine human chorionic gonadotropin [HCG])

With physiology/laboratory test values
Alanine aminotransferase (ALT [SGPT]), serum, and
Alkaline phosphatase, serum, and
Aspartate aminotransferase (AST [SGOT]), serum
(values may be increased)

Bilirubin, serum and
Blood urea nitrogen (BUN)
(concentrations may be increased)

Cholesterol, serum and
High-density lipoprotein cholesterol, serum and
Triglyceride, serum
(concentrations may occasionally be increased)

Free cortisol, urine
(may be increased)

Glucose, urine and
Protein (albumin), urine
(may be detected in the urine)

Ionized calcium, serum
(concentrations may be decreased)

Thyroid hormones
(serum concentrations of $T_3$, free $T_4$, and free $T_4$ index may be decreased due to increased hepatic metabolism of hormones during long-term therapy with carbamazepine; thyroid size may be increased as a compensatory mechanism)

## Medical considerations/Contraindications

The medical considerations/contraindications included here have been selected on the basis of their potential clinical significance (reasons given in parentheses where appropriate)—not necessarily inclusive (» = major clinical significance).

*Except under special circumstances, this medication should not be used when the following medical problems exist:*

» Absence seizures, atypical or generalized or
» Atonic seizures or
» Myoclonic seizures
(increased risk of generalized seizures)
» Atrioventricular (AV) heart block or
» Blood disorders characterized by serious abnormalities in blood count, platelets, or serum iron or
» Bone marrow depression, history of
(increased risk of exacerbation)

*Risk-benefit should be considered when the following medical problems exist:*

Alcoholism, active
(CNS depression may be potentiated; in addition, the metabolism of carbamazepine may be accelerated)

Behavioral disorders
(latent psychosis may be activated, or agitation or confusion may be produced in elderly patients, especially when carbamazepine is used concurrently with other medications)

Cardiac damage, including organic heart disease and congestive heart disease or
Coronary artery disease
(may be exacerbated)

Diabetes mellitus
(elevated urine glucose concentrations may occur)

Glaucoma or
Increased intraocular pressure
(may be exacerbated because of mild anticholinergic effects of carbamazepine)

Hematologic reactions, adverse, to other medications, history of
(patients may be especially at risk for carbamazepine-induced bone marrow depression)

Hepatic function impairment
(increased risk of liver damage)

Hyponatremia, dilutional, caused by syndrome of inappropriate antidiuretic hormone (SIADH) secretion or other conditions such as hypopituitarism, hypothyroidism, or adrenocortical insufficiency or
Urinary retention
(may be exacerbated)

Renal function impairment
(excretion of carbamazepine may be altered)

Sensitivity to carbamazepine or to tricyclic antidepressants

Caution is also advised in administration to patients who have had interrupted courses of therapy with carbamazepine.

## Patient monitoring

The following may be especially important in patient monitoring (other tests may be warranted in some patients, depending on condition; » = major clinical significance):

» Blood counts, complete (CBCs), including platelet and possibly reticulocyte counts and
» Iron concentrations, serum
(determinations recommended prior to initiation of therapy as a baseline. Patients who develop low or decreased white blood cell or platelet counts during the course of treatment should be monitored closely and carbamazepine discontinued if there is any evidence of significant bone marrow depression)

BUN determinations and
Ophthalmologic examinations, including slit-lamp funduscopy and tonometry, where indicated, and
Urinalysis, complete
(recommended prior to initiation of therapy and at periodic intervals during therapy)

» Carbamazepine concentrations, plasma
(determinations recommended periodically as a guide to efficacy and safety; plasma concentrations of 6 to 12 mcg per mL [25 to 51 micromoles per L] are optimal for anticonvulsant activity and,

in rare cases, concentrations may go up to 16 mcg per mL [68 micromoles per L]; when used to treat psychiatric disorders, carbamazepine plasma concentrations of 8 to 12 mcg per mL [34 to 51 micromoles per L] are optimal; taking sample prior to the morning dose to determine lowest daily concentration is suggested)

Electrocardiogram (ECG) readings and
Electrolyte concentrations, serum
(determinations recommended prior to therapy and periodically during therapy because of possibility of hyponatremia)

» Ionized calcium concentrations, serum
(recommended every 6 months or if seizure frequency increases after weeks or months of carbamazepine therapy, since hypocalcemia decreases seizure threshold)

Liver function tests
(recommended prior to initiation of therapy and at periodic intervals during therapy; discontinuation of carbamazepine should be considered immediately upon evidence of aggravated liver function impairment or new disease)

## Side/Adverse Effects

Note: Carbamazepine-induced stimulation of antidiuretic hormone (ADH) release may cause water retention resulting in significant volume expansion and dilutional hyponatremia (syndrome of inappropriate secretion of antidiuretic hormone). Patients reporting lethargy, weakness, nausea, vomiting, confusion or hostility, neurological abnormalities, stupor, or increased seizure frequency should be suspected of being hyponatremic, although many of these symptoms may also be associated with other carbamazepine-induced side effects.

A case of aseptic meningitis accompanied by myoclonus and peripheral eosinophilia has been reported in a patient taking carbamazepine in conjunction with other medications; rechallenge with carbamazepine resulted in recurrence of meningitits.

The following side/adverse effects have been selected on the basis of their potential clinical significance (possible signs and symptoms in parentheses where appropriate)—not necessarily inclusive:

### Those indicating need for medical attention
Incidence more frequent
*CNS toxicity, including blurred or double vision; or nystagmus* (continuous back-and-forth eye movements)

Incidence less frequent
*Allergic reaction; Stevens-Johnson syndrome; or toxic epidermal necrolysis* (skin rash, hives, or itching); *behavioral changes*—especially in children; *diarrhea, severe; hyponatremia, dilutional, or water intoxication (SIADH)* (confusion, agitation, or hostility, especially in the elderly; continuing headache; increase in seizure frequency; severe nausea and vomiting; unusual drowsiness; weakness); *systemic lupus erythematosus (SLE)-like syndrome* (skin rash, hives, or itching; fever; sore throat; bone or joint pain; unusual tiredness or weakness)

Note: The risk of *hyponatremia* and *SIADH* appears to increase with patient age and serum concentration of carbamazepine; *hyponatremia* seemingly does not occur in children.

Incidence rare
*Adenopathy or lymphadenopathy* (swollen glands); *blood dyscrasias, including aplastic anemia* (shortness of breath, troubled breathing, wheezing, or tightness in chest; sores, ulcers, or white spots on lips or in mouth; swollen or painful glands; unusual bleeding or bruising); *agranulocytosis* (chills; fever; sore throat; unusual tiredness or weakness); *eosinophilia* (fever); *leukopenia* (usually asymptomatic; rarely, fever or chills; cough or hoarseness; lower back or side pain; painful or difficult urination); *pancytopenia* (nosebleeds or other unusual bleeding or bruising); *and thrombocytopenia* (usually asymptomatic; rarely, unusual bleeding or bruising; black, tarry stools; blood in urine or stools; pinpoint red spots on skin); *bone marrow depression* (chills; fever; sore throat; unusual bleeding or bruising); *cardiovascular effects, including arrhythmias* (fast, slow, or irregular heartbeat); *atrioventricular (AV) heart block* (unusual weakness; pounding heartbeat; troubled breathing; fainting); *bradycardia* (slow heartbeat); *congestive heart failure* (chest pain; troubled breathing; swelling of feet or lower legs; rapid weight gain); *edema* (swelling of face, hands, feet, or lower legs); *hypertension, increased* (high blood pressure); *hypotension* (low blood pressure); *and syncope* (fainting); *CNS toxicity* (difficulty in speaking or slurred speech; mental depression with restlessness and nervousness; rigidity; ringing, buzzing, or other unexplained sounds in the ears; trembling; uncontrolled body movements; visual hallucinations); *hypersensitivity hepatitis* (darkening of urine; pale stools; yellow eyes or skin); *hypocalcemia* (increase in seizure frequency; mus-

cle or abdominal cramps); *renal toxicity, renal failure, acute, or water intoxication (SIADH)* (frequent urination; sudden decrease in amount of urine; swelling of feet or lower legs); *paresthesias or peripheral neuritis* (numbness, tingling, pain, or weakness in hands and feet); *porphyria, acute intermittent* (darkening of urine); *pulmonary hypersensitivity* (fever; troubled breathing; cough; shortness of breath; tightness in chest; wheezing); *thrombophlebitis* (pain, tenderness, bluish color, or swelling of leg or foot)

Note: Geriatric patients and those with a defective conduction system may be especially susceptible to *AV heart block* or *bradycardia* with carbamazepine.

*Hypocalcemia* may lead to osteopenia as a direct effect of carbamazepine on bone metabolism.

**Those indicating need for medical attention only if they continue or are bothersome**
Incidence more frequent, especially during initiation of therapy
*Clumsiness or unsteadiness; confusion; dizziness, mild, or lightheadedness; drowsiness, mild; nausea or vomiting, mild*

Incidence less frequent or rare
*Aching joints or muscles or leg cramps; alopecia* (loss of hair); *anorexia* (loss of appetite); *constipation; diaphoresis* (increased sweating); *diarrhea; dryness of mouth; glossitis or stomatitis* (irritation or soreness of tongue or mouth); *headache; increased sensitivity of skin to sunlight; sexual problems in males; stomach pain or discomfort; unusual tiredness or weakness*

## Overdose

Note: For specific information on the agents used in the management of carbamazepine overdose, see:
- *Barbiturates (Systemic)* monograph;
- *Benzodiazepines (Systemic)* monograph;
- *Charcoal, Activated (Oral-Local)* monograph; and/or
- *Laxatives (Local)* monograph.

For more information on the management of overdose or unintentional ingestion, **contact a Poison Control Center** (see *Poison Control Center Listing*).

**Clinical effects of overdose**
The following effects have been selected on the basis of their potential clinical significance (possible signs and symptoms in parentheses where appropriate)—not necessarily inclusive:

*Anuria, oliguria, or urinary retention* (sudden decrease in amount of urine); *cardiovascular effects, including conduction disorders or tachycardia* (fast or irregular heartbeat); *convulsions*—especially in small children; *dizziness, severe; drowsiness, severe; dysmetria* (poor control in body movements—for example, when reaching or stepping); *hyperreflexia, followed by hyporeflexia* (overactive reflexes, followed by underactive reflexes); *hypertension or hypotension* (high or low blood pressure); *motor restlessness; muscular twitching; mydriasis* (large pupils); *nausea or vomiting, severe; neurological effects, including ataxia* (clumsiness or unsteadiness); *athetoid movements or ballism* (abnormal body movements); *opisthotonus* (body spasm in which head and heels are bent backward and body bowed forward); *respiratory depression* (irregular, slow, or shallow breathing); *shock* (fainting); *tremor*

Note: Signs and symptoms of acute toxicity may occur 1 to 3 hours following ingestion of an overdose. Neurological and neuromuscular symptoms predominate, followed by cardiovascular toxicity. Symptoms resemble those observed following overdose with tricyclic antidepressants. Cardiotoxic effects are more likely to occur in elderly and cardiopathic patients.

Laboratory findings in overdosage may indicate leukocytosis, reduced leukocyte count, glycosuria, acetonuria, and electroencephalogram (EEG) dysrhythmias.

**Treatment of overdose**
Recommended treatment consists of the following:
To decrease absorption—Induction of emesis or gastric lavage, followed by administration of activated charcoal or laxatives to reduce further absorption.

To enhance elimination—Forced diuresis may accelerate elimination. Dialysis is indicated only in severe poisoning associated with renal failure. In small children, severe poisoning may require replacement transfusion.

Specific treatment—For hypotension and shock, elevation of patient's legs and administration of a plasma volume expander. Use of a vasopressor may be considered if other measures are insufficient. Administration of a benzodiazepine or a barbiturate as required for seizures. The fact that these agents may aggravate respiratory depression (especially in children), hypotension, and coma must be

considered. Also, barbiturates or benzodiazepines should not be used if the patient has taken a monoamine oxidase inhibitor within the previous 14 days.

Monitoring—Monitoring of respiration, cardiac function, blood pressure, body temperature, pupillary reflexes, and kidney and bladder function for several days.

Supportive care—Maintenance of a patent airway with tracheal intubation, artificial respiration, and/or administration of oxygen. Patients in whom intentional overdose is confirmed or suspected should be referred for psychiatric consultation.

## Patient Consultation

As an aid to patient consultation, refer to *Advice for the Patient, Carbamazepine (Systemic)*.

In providing consultation, consider emphasizing the following selected information (» = major clinical significance):

**Before using this medication**
» Conditions affecting use, especially:
    Sensitivity to tricyclic antidepressants or carbamazepine
    Pregnancy—Crosses placenta; babies reportedly born with small head circumference, low birth weight, craniofacial defects, fingernail hypoplasia, developmental delays, and spina bifida; animal studies have shown rib anomalies, cleft palate, foot deformities, or anophthalmos with doses 10 to 25 times the human dose
    Breast-feeding—Distributed into breast milk; animal studies have shown lack of weight gain and unkempt appearance of young at high doses
    Use in children—Appropriate studies have not been done in children up to 6 years of age; behavior changes more likely to occur in children
    Use in the elderly—Elderly more likely to have confusion or agitation, AV heart block, SIADH, or bradycardia than are younger people
    Dental—Increased incidence of blood dyscrasias that cause infection, delayed healing, or gingival bleeding; proper oral hygiene necessary
    Other medications, especially anticoagulants, other anticonvulsants, tricyclic antidepressants, barbiturates, benzodiazepines metabolized via hepatic microsomal enzymes (especially clonazepam), cimetidine, clarithromycin, oral estrogen-containing contraceptives, corticosteroids, diltiazem, erythromycin, estrogens, isoniazid, MAO inhibitors, propoxyphene, quinidine, risperidone, or verapamil
    Other medical problems, especially absence, atonic, or myoclonic seizures; AV heart block; blood disorders; or bone marrow depression

**Proper use of this medication**
» Taking with food to lessen gastrointestinal irritation
» Compliance with therapy; not taking more or less medication than prescribed
» Not using medication for minor aches and pains
» Proper dosing
    Missed dose: Taking as soon as possible; not taking if almost time for next dose; not doubling doses; calling physician if more than one dose a day is missed
» Proper storage; not storing tablet dosage forms in bathroom or other high-moisture areas due to loss of potency and effectiveness

*For use in epilepsy*
» Checking with physician before discontinuing medication; gradual dosage reduction may be necessary to prevent seizures or status epilepticus

**Precautions while using this medication**
» Regular visits to physician to check progress of therapy
» Avoiding the use of alcoholic beverages and other CNS depressants while taking this medicine
» Possible drowsiness, dizziness, lightheadedness, blurred or double vision, weakness, or muscular incoordination; caution when driving or using machinery, or doing jobs requiring alertness and coordination
» Possible skin photosensitivity; avoiding unprotected exposure to sun; using protective clothing; using a sun block product that includes protection against both UVA-caused photosensitivity reactions and UVB-caused sunburn reactions; avoiding use of sunlamp, tanning bed, or tanning booth
    Diabetic patients: May increase urine sugar concentrations
    Caution if any laboratory tests required; possible interference with results of metyrapone or pregnancy tests

» Caution if any kind of surgery, dental treatment, or emergency treatment is needed

Carrying medical identification card or bracelet during therapy

### Side/adverse effects

Signs of potential side effects, especially CNS toxicity, allergic reaction, Stevens-Johnson syndrome, toxic epidermal necrolysis, behavioral changes, severe diarrhea, dilutional hyponatremia or water intoxication (SIADH), SLE-like syndrome, adenopathy or lymphadenopathy, blood dyscrasias, bone marrow depression, cardiovascular effects, hypersensitivity hepatitis, hypocalcemia, renal toxicity or failure, paresthesias or peripheral neuritis, porphyria, pulmonary hypersensitivity, or thrombophlebitis

## General Dosing Information

Side effects may be minimized by initiating therapy with low doses, which should be increased gradually at weekly intervals until an adequate response is obtained; administering carbamazepine with meals, and giving the total daily dosage in 3 or 4 divided doses may also minimize side effects.

When carbamazepine is added to existing anticonvulsant therapy, it should be added gradually while the other anticonvulsants are maintained or gradually decreased, except for phenytoin, which may have to be increased.

The maintenance dosage of carbamazepine may need to be increased progressively over the first few weeks of treatment to avoid low plasma carbamazepine concentrations caused by autoinduction.

Abrupt discontinuation in a responsive epileptic patient may result in convulsions and possibly status epilepticus; gradual withdrawal is recommended.

Therapy should be discontinued if cardiovascular reactions or skin rashes occur.

When carbamazepine is used as an antineuralgic in specific pain syndromes, *an attempt should be made at least once every few months to reduce dosage or discontinue therapy* if the patient is totally free of pain.

If carbamazepine suspension is administered through a nasogastric feeding tube, it should be mixed with an equal volume of diluent before administration.

### Diet/Nutrition

Carbamazepine should be taken with food to lessen gastrointestinal irritation.

### Bioequivalence information

Administration of carbamazepine suspension results in higher peak serum concentrations than does the same dose administered as tablets. It is recommended that doses of the suspension be initially lower and be increased more slowly than doses of the tablets to avoid side effects.

### For treatment of adverse effects

Treatment of bone marrow depression includes the following:
- Discontinuing carbamazepine therapy.
- Daily CBC, platelet, and reticulocyte counts.
- Performing a bone marrow aspiration and trephine biopsy immediately and repeating with sufficient frequency to monitor recovery.
- Considering other studies that may be helpful, including white cell and platelet antibodies; $^{59}$Fe—ferrokinetic studies; peripheral blood cell typing; cytogenic studies on marrow and peripheral blood; bone marrow culture studies for colony-forming units; hemoglobin electrophoresis for $A^2$ and F hemoglobin; and serum folic acid and $B_{12}$ concentrations. If aplastic anemia develops, specialized consultation should be sought for appropriate monitoring and treatment.

## Oral Dosage Forms

Note: Bracketed uses in the *Dosage Forms* section refer to categories of use and/or indications that are not included in U.S. product labeling.

### CARBAMAZEPINE ORAL SUSPENSION USP

#### Usual adult and adolescent dose

Anticonvulsant—

Initial: Oral, 100 mg four times a day on the first day, the dosage being increased by up to 200 mg a day at weekly intervals. Some clinicians recommend initiating therapy at 100 mg a day and increasing to full therapeutic dosage slowly at weekly intervals to avoid side effects and potential noncompliance.

Maintenance: Oral, usually 800 mg to 1.2 grams a day.

Antineuralgic—

Initial: Oral, 50 mg four times a day on the first day, the dosage being increased by up to 200 mg a day, using increments of 50 mg four times a day only as needed until pain is relieved.

Maintenance: Oral, 200 mg to 1.2 grams a day (average 400 to 800 mg a day) in divided doses.

[Antidiuretic][1]—

Oral, 300 to 600 mg a day if used as sole therapy; or 200 to 400 mg a day if used concurrently with other antidiuretic agents.

[Antimanic][1] or

[Antipsychotic][1]—

Oral, initially 200 to 400 mg a day in divided doses, the dosage being gradually increased at weekly intervals up to a maximum of 1.6 grams a day as needed and tolerated according to clinical response.

Note: Whenever possible, total daily dosage should be given in 3 or 4 divided doses.

#### Usual adult and adolescent prescribing limits

Anticonvulsant—

Patients 12 to 15 years of age:

Dosage should generally not exceed 1 gram a day.

Patients 15 years of age and over:

Dosage should generally not exceed 1.2 grams a day. In rare instances, doses up to 1.6 grams a day have been used in adults.

Antineuralgic—

Dosage should not exceed 1.2 grams a day.

#### Usual pediatric dose

Anticonvulsant—

Children up to 6 years of age:

Initial—Oral, 10 to 20 mg per kg of body weight a day in two or three divided doses, the dosage being increased by up to 100 mg a day at weekly intervals as needed and tolerated.

Maintenance—Oral, adjusted to the minimum effective dosage, usually 250 to 350 mg a day, and generally not exceeding 400 mg or 35 mg per kg of body weight a day.

Children 6 to 12 years of age:

Initial—Oral, 50 mg four times a day on the first day, the dosage being increased by up to 100 mg a day at weekly intervals until the best response is obtained.

Maintenance—Oral, adjusted to the minimum effective dosage, usually 400 to 800 mg a day.

Note: Dosage generally should not exceed 1 gram a day.

Whenever possible, total daily dosage should be given in 3 or 4 divided doses.

#### Strength(s) usually available

U.S.—

100 mg per 5 mL (Rx) [*Tegretol* (sorbitol; sucrose)].

Canada—

Not commercially available.

#### Packaging and storage

Store below 30 °C (86 °F), in a tight, light-resistant container, unless otherwise specified by manufacturer. Protect from freezing.

#### Auxiliary labeling

- Shake well before using.
- May cause drowsiness.
- Take with meals.

### CARBAMAZEPINE TABLETS USP

#### Usual adult and adolescent dose

Anticonvulsant—

Initial: Oral, 200 mg two times a day on the first day, the dosage being increased by up to 200 mg a day at weekly intervals until the best response is obtained. Some clinicians recommend initiating therapy at 100 mg a day and increasing to full therapeutic dosage slowly at weekly intervals to avoid side effects and potential noncompliance.

Maintenance: Oral, adjusted to the minimum effective dosage, usually 600 mg to 1.6 grams a day.

Antineuralgic—

Initial: Oral, 100 mg two times a day on the first day, the dosage being increased by up to 200 mg a day, using increments of 100 mg every twelve hours only as needed until pain is relieved.

Maintenance: Oral, 200 mg to 1.2 grams a day (average 400 to 800 mg a day) in divided doses.

[Antidiuretic][1]—

Oral, 300 to 600 mg a day if used as sole therapy; or 200 to 400 mg a day if used concurrently with other antidiuretic agents.

[Antimanic][1] or

[Antipsychotic][1]—
> Oral, initially 200 to 400 mg a day in divided doses, the dosage being gradually increased at weekly intervals up to a maximum of 1.6 grams a day as needed and tolerated according to clinical response.

Note: Whenever possible, total daily dosage should be given in 3 or 4 divided doses.

**Usual adult and adolescent prescribing limits**

Anticonvulsant—
> Patients 12 to 15 years of age:
>> Dosage should generally not exceed 1 gram a day.
>
> Patients 15 years of age and over:
>> Dosage should generally not exceed 1.2 grams a day. In rare instances, doses up to 1.6 grams a day have been used in adults.

Antineuralgic—
> Dosage should not exceed 1.2 grams a day.

**Usual pediatric dose**

Anticonvulsant—
> Children up to 6 years of age:
>> Initial—Oral, 10 to 20 mg per kg of body weight a day in two or three divided doses, the dosage being increased by up to 100 mg a day at weekly intervals as needed and tolerated.
>> Maintenance—Oral, adjusted to the minimum effective dosage, usually 250 to 350 mg a day, and generally not exceeding 400 mg or 35 mg per kg of body weight a day.
>
> Children 6 to 12 years of age:
>> Initial—Oral, 100 mg two times a day on the first day, the dosage being increased by 100 mg a day at weekly intervals until the best response is obtained.
>> Maintenance—Oral, adjusted to the minimum effective dosage, usually 400 to 800 mg a day.

Note: Dosage generally should not exceed 1 gram a day.
> Whenever possible, total daily dosage should be given in 3 or 4 divided doses.

**Strength(s) usually available**

U.S.—
> 200 mg (Rx) [*Atretol* (scored); *Epitol* (scored); *Tegretol* (scored); GENERIC (scored)].

Canada—
> 200 mg (Rx) [*Apo-Carbamazepine* (double-scored); *Novo-Carbamaz* (scored); *Nu-Carbamazepine* (double-scored); *Tegretol* (double-scored)].

**Packaging and storage**

Store below 40 °C (104 °F), preferably between 15 and 30 °C (59 and 86 °F), unless otherwise specified by manufacturer. Store in a tight container.

**Auxiliary labeling**
- May cause drowsiness.
- Take with meals.
- Store in a dry place.
- Protect from moisture.

## CARBAMAZEPINE TABLETS (CHEWABLE) USP

**Usual adult and adolescent dose**

See *Carbamazepine Tablets USP.*

**Usual adult and adolescent prescribing limits**

See *Carbamazepine Tablets USP.*

**Usual pediatric dose**

See *Carbamazepine Tablets USP.*

**Strength(s) usually available**

U.S.—
> 100 mg (Rx) [*Epitol* (scored); *Tegretol* (scored; sucrose); GENERIC (scored)].

Canada—
> 100 mg (Rx) [*Tegretol Chewtabs* (scored)].
> 200 mg (Rx) [*Tegretol Chewtabs* (scored)].

**Packaging and storage**

Store below 40 °C (104 °F), preferably between 15 and 30 °C (59 and 86 °F), unless otherwise specified by manufacturer. Store in a tight container.

**Auxiliary labeling**
- May cause drowsiness.
- Take with meals.
- May be chewed.
- Store in a dry place.
- Protect from moisture.

## CARBAMAZEPINE EXTENDED-RELEASE TABLETS

**Usual adult and adolescent dose**

Anticonvulsant—
> Initial: Oral, 100 to 200 mg one or two times a day with meals, the dosage being increased gradually as needed and tolerated. Some clinicians recommend initiating therapy at 100 mg a day and increasing to full therapeutic dosage slowly at weekly intervals to avoid side effects and potential noncompliance.
> Maintenance: Oral, adjusted to the minimum effective dosage, usually 800 to 1200 mg a day.

Antineuralgic—
> Oral, initially 100 mg two times a day on the first day, the dosage being increased by 200 mg a day (in increments of 100 mg every twelve hours) only as needed and tolerated until pain is relieved.

Note: As soon as pain relief is maintained, the dosage should be reduced to the minimum effective dose.
> Attempts should be made at intervals of not more than 3 months to reduce or discontinue use.

**Usual adult and adolescent prescribing limits**

Anticonvulsant—
> Patients 12 to 15 years of age:
>> Dosage should generally not exceed 1 gram a day.
>
> Patients 15 years of age and over:
>> Dosage should not exceed 1.2 grams a day. In rare instances, doses up to 1.6 grams a day have been used in adults.

Antineuralgic—
> Dosage should not exceed 1.2 grams a day.

**Usual pediatric dose**

Anticonvulsant—
> Children 6 to 12 years of age:
>> Oral, initially 100 mg one to two times on the first day, the dosage being increased gradually by 100 mg a day as needed and tolerated until the best response is obtained.

Note: When seizure relief is maintained, the dosage should be reduced gradually to the lowest effective dose.
> Dosage generally should not exceed 1 gram a day.

**Strength(s) usually available**

U.S.—
> 100 mg (Rx) [*Tegretol-XR*].
> 200 mg (Rx) [*Tegretol-XR*].
> 400 mg (Rx) [*Tegretol-XR*].

Canada—
> 200 mg (Rx) [*Tegretol CR* (scored)].
> 400 mg (Rx) [*Tegretol CR* (scored)].

**Packaging and storage**

Store below 40 °C (104 °F), preferably between 15 and 30 °C (59 and 86 °F), in a tight container, unless otherwise specified by manufacturer.

**Auxiliary labeling**
- May cause drowsiness.
- Take with meals.
- Do not chew.

---

[1]Not included in Canadian product labeling.

---

Revised: 07/26/96

---

# CARBENICILLIN—See *Penicillins (Systemic)*

---

# CARBETAPENTANE-CONTAINING COMBINATIONS—

Chlorpheniramine, Ephedrine, Phenylephrine, and Carbetapentane (Systemic)—See *Cough/Cold Combinations (Systemic)*

Chlorpheniramine, Phenylephrine, Phenylpropanolamine, Carbetapentane, and Potassium Guaiacolsulfonate (Systemic)—See *Cough/Cold Combinations (Systemic)*

Phenylephrine, Phenylpropanolamine, Carbetapentane, and Potassium Guaiacolsulfonate (Systemic)—See *Cough/Cold Combinations (Systemic)*

---

# CARBIDOPA-CONTAINING COMBINATIONS—

Carbidopa and Levodopa (Systemic)

# CARBIDOPA AND LEVODOPA  Systemic

PEN: Co-Careldopa
VA CLASSIFICATION (Primary): CN500
Note: For a listing of dosage forms and brand names by country availability, see *Dosage Forms* section(s). For a listing of brand names for the articles in this monograph, refer to the General Index.

## Category
Antidyskinetic.

## Indications

### Accepted
Parkinsonism (treatment)—Carbidopa and levodopa combination is indicated in the treatment of idiopathic Parkinson's disease (paralysis agitans), postencephalitic parkinsonism, or symptomatic parkinsonism, which may follow injury to the nervous system by carbon monoxide intoxication or manganese intoxication, to permit achievement of symptomatic relief with a lower dosage of levodopa than with levodopa alone. Also, it permits a smoother and more rapid dosage titration, reduces nausea and vomiting, and allows concurrent administration of pyridoxine when necessary.

## Pharmacology/Pharmacokinetics

See also *Levodopa (Systemic)*.

### Physicochemical characteristics
Molecular weight—Carbidopa: 244.25.

### Mechanism of action/Effect
Carbidopa—Inhibits the peripheral decarboxylation of levodopa, thus slowing its conversion to dopamine in extracerebral tissues. This results in an increased availability of levodopa for transport to the brain where it undergoes decarboxylation to dopamine.

### Absorption
Carbidopa and levodopa combination—
Tablets: Absorption is rapid and virtually complete in 2 to 3 hours.
Extended-release tablets: Absorption is gradual and continuous for 4 to 6 hours, although the majority of the dose is absorbed in 2 to 3 hours.
Bioavailability of carbidopa and levodopa extended-release tablets—
Approximately 70 to 75% relative to the immediate-release tablets.
Increased somewhat in the presence of food.
Two half tablets approximately 20% more bioavailable than one intact tablet.

### Distribution
Carbidopa—Widely distributed in body tissues other than the central nervous system (CNS).

### Protein binding
Carbidopa—Moderate (approximately 36%).

### Biotransformation
Carbidopa—Not extensive. Inhibits metabolism of levodopa in the gastrointestinal tract, thus increasing its absorption from the gastrointestinal tract and its concentration in plasma.

### Half-life
Carbidopa—1 to 2 hours. When given in combination with levodopa, increases levodopa's plasma half-life from 1 hour to about 2 hours, and, in some cases to as long as 15 hours.

### Time to peak concentration
Peak levodopa concentrations at steady state—
Tablets:
0.7 hours.
Extended-release tablets:
2.4 hours.
Note: Peak plasma concentrations of levodopa are increased when the extended-release tablets are administered with food.

Plasma concentrations of levodopa fluctuate less with the extended-release tablets than with the immediate release tablets.

### Elimination
Carbidopa—Renal; 30% of dose of carbidopa excreted unchanged in urine within 24 hours. When given in combination with carbidopa, the amount of levodopa excreted unchanged in urine is increased by about 6%.

## Precautions to Consider

### Pregnancy/Reproduction
Pregnancy—Studies in humans have not been done.
Reproduction studies in rodents have shown that levodopa, when given in doses in excess of 200 mg per kg of body weight (mg/kg) per day, depresses fetal and postnatal growth and viability. Also, studies in rabbits have shown that levodopa alone or in combination with carbidopa causes visceral and skeletal malformations.
FDA Pregnancy Category C.

### Breast-feeding
Levodopa is distributed into breast milk. Although problems in humans have not been documented, breast-feeding is not recommended because of the potential for side effects in the infant.
Also, levodopa may inhibit lactation.

### Pediatrics
Appropriate studies on the relationship of age to the effects of carbidopa and levodopa have not been performed in children up to 18 years of age. Safety and efficacy have not been established.

### Geriatrics
Smaller doses may be required in geriatric patients since they may have reduced tolerance to the effects of levodopa. Also, peripheral dopa decarboxylase, the enzyme responsible for decarboxylation, decreases with age, thus making large doses unnecessary.
Geriatric patients, especially those with osteoporosis, responsive to antiparkinsonian therapy should resume normal activity gradually and with caution because increased mobility may increase risk of fractures.
Psychic side effects, such as anxiety, confusion, or nervousness, are more common in geriatric patients receiving other antiparkinsonian medications, especially anticholinergics.

### Dental
Involuntary movements of jaws may result in poor retention of full dentures; dosage reduction may be required.

### Drug interactions and/or related problems
The following drug interactions and/or related problems have been selected on the basis of their potential clinical significance (possible mechanism in parentheses where appropriate)—not necessarily inclusive (» = major clinical significance):
Note: Combinations containing any of the following medications, depending on the amount present, may also interact with this medication.

Amantadine or
Benztropine or
Procyclidine or
Trihexyphenidyl
(concurrent use may result in increased efficacy of levodopa; however, concurrent use is not recommended if there is a history of psychosis)
» Anesthetics, hydrocarbon inhalation
(administration prior to anesthesia with these agents may result in cardiac arrhythmias because of increased endogenous dopamine concentration; carbidopa and levodopa combination should be discontinued 6 to 8 hours before the administration of these anesthetics, especially halothane)
» Anticonvulsants, hydantoin or
Benzodiazepines or
Droperidol or
» Haloperidol or
Loxapine or
Metyrosine or
Papaverine or
» Phenothiazines or
Rauwolfia alkaloids or
Thioxanthenes
(concurrent use may decrease the therapeutic effects of levodopa; hydantoin anticonvulsants increase the metabolism of levodopa, thus decreasing its therapeutic effects; since droperidol, haloperidol, loxapine, papaverine, phenothiazines, and the thioxanthenes block the dopamine receptors in the brain, they may induce extrapyramidal symptoms, thus aggravating parkinsonism and antagonizing the effects of levodopa; the rauwolfia alkaloids cause dopamine depletion in the brain, thus opposing the effects of levodopa)

Bromocriptine
   (may produce additive effects, allowing reduction in levodopa dosage)

» Cocaine
   (concurrent use with levodopa may increase the risk of cardiac arrhythmias; if use of cocaine is necessary in patients receiving levodopa, it is recommended that cocaine be administered with caution, in reduced dosage, and in conjunction with electrocardiographic monitoring)

Foods, especially high-protein
   (concurrent or previous ingestion of food may decrease the absorption of levodopa from the gastrointestinal tract, consequently delaying its effect; in addition, proteins in food may be degraded into the amino acids that compete with levodopa for transport to the brain, thus decreasing and/or making erratic the response to levodopa; however, rather than cutting down on daily protein intake to avoid this effect on levodopa, it is recommended that the intake of proteins be distributed equally throughout the day)

Hypotension-producing medications, other (See *Appendix II*)
   (concurrent use with levodopa may result in an increased hypotensive effect)

Methyldopa
   (concurrent use with levodopa may alter the antiparkinsonian effects of levodopa and may also produce additive toxic CNS effects such as psychosis)

Metoclopramide
   (gastric emptying of levodopa may be accelerated with concurrent use of metoclopramide, thus possibly increasing levodopa's rate and extent of absorption from the small intestine; the clinical significance of this interaction has not been determined)

Molindone
   (concurrent use may inhibit antiparkinsonian effects of levodopa by blocking dopamine receptor in the brain; also, levodopa may counteract the antipsychotic effects of molindone)

» Monoamine oxidase (MAO) inhibitors, including furazolidone and procarbazine
   (although high doses [300 to 400 mg a day] of carbidopa in combination with levodopa may help suppress the hypertensive reactions caused by concurrent use with MAO inhibitors, it is recommended that MAO inhibitors be discontinued for 2 to 4 weeks prior to initiation of carbidopa and levodopa combination therapy)

» Selegiline
   (although sometimes used in conjunction with carbidopa and levodopa combination, selegiline may enhance levodopa-induced dyskinesias, nausea, orthostatic hypotension, confusion, and hallucinations; levodopa dosage should be reduced within 2 to 3 days after the initiation of selegiline therapy)

**Laboratory value alterations**
The following have been selected on the basis of their potential clinical significance (possible effect in parentheses where appropriate)—not necessarily inclusive (» = major clinical significance):

With diagnostic test results
   Coombs' (antiglobulin) test
      (occasionally becomes positive after long-term levodopa therapy)
   Gonadorelin test
      (levodopa may elevate serum gonadotropin concentrations)
   Glucose, urine
      (tests using copper reduction methods may cause false-positive results; tests using glucose oxidase methods may cause false-negative results)
   Ketones, urine
      (tests using dipstick or test tape methods may cause false-positive results)
   Norepinephrine, urine
      (test shows false-positive results)
   Protein, urine
      (use of the Lowery test may cause false-positive results)
   Thyroid function determinations
      (chronic use of levodopa may inhibit the TSH response to protirelin)
   Uric acid, serum and urine
      (tests may show high concentrations with colorimetric measurements, but not with uricase)

With physiology/laboratory values
   Alanine aminotransferase (ALT [SGPT]) and
   Alkaline phosphatase and
   Aspartate aminotransferase (AST [SGOT]) and

Bilirubin and
Lactate dehydrogenase (LDH) and
Protein-bound iodine (PBI)
   (serum concentrations may be increased)

Blood urea nitrogen (BUN)
   (concentrations may be increased)

   Note: Concentrations of BUN, creatinine, and uric acid, although elevated during carbidopa and levodopa therapy, are elevated to a lesser degree than when levodopa is used alone.

**Medical considerations/Contraindications**
The medical considerations/contraindications included here have been selected on the basis of their potential clinical significance (reasons given in parentheses where appropriate)—not necessarily inclusive (» = major clinical significance).

*Risk-benefit should be considered when the following medical problems exist:*

» Bronchial asthma, emphysema, and other severe pulmonary diseases
   (respiratory effects of levodopa may aggravate condition)

» Cardiovascular disease, severe
   (increased risk of cardiac arrhythmias)

Convulsive disorders, history of
   (use of levodopa may precipitate seizures)

Diabetes mellitus
   (use of levodopa may adversely affect control of glucose in blood)

Endocrine diseases
   (use of levodopa may adversely affect hypothalamus or pituitary function)

» Glaucoma, angle-closure, or predisposition to
   (mydriatic effect resulting in increased intraocular pressure may precipitate an acute attack of angle closure glaucoma)

Glaucoma, open-angle, chronic
   (mydriatic effect may cause a slight increase in intraocular pressure; glaucoma therapy may need to be adjusted)

Hepatic function impairment

» Melanoma, history of or suspected
   (use of levodopa may activate a malignant melanoma)

» Myocardial infarction, history of, with residual arrhythmias
   (use of levodopa may precipitate or aggravate condition)

» Peptic ulcer, history of
   (increased risk of upper gastrointestinal hemorrhage)

» Psychotic states
   (increased risk of developing depression and suicidal tendencies)

» Renal function impairment
   (use of levodopa may lead to urinary retention)

Sensitivity to carbidopa and/or levodopa

» Urinary retention
   (use of levodopa may precipitate or aggravate condition)

**Patient monitoring**
The following may be especially important in patient monitoring (other tests may be warranted in some patients, depending on condition; » = major clinical significance):

Blood cell counts and
Hemoglobin determinations and
Hepatic function determinations and
Ophthalmologic examinations for glaucoma and monitoring of intraocular pressure in patients with open angle glaucoma and
Renal function determinations
   (recommended at periodic intervals for patients on long-term levodopa therapy; also, blood cell counts and hepatic and renal function determinations are recommended after withdrawal of levodopa therapy as part of the evaluation of a patient with suspected neuroleptic malignant–like syndrome)

Cardiovascular monitoring for detection of arrhythmias or orthostatic hypotensive tendencies
   (recommended during the period of initial dosage adjustment)

Serum creatine phosphokinase concentrations
   (determinations recommended after discontinuation of levodopa therapy, especially if fever is present; an elevated serum creatine phosphokinase level may be an early indication of the presence of neuroleptic malignant–like syndrome)

# Side/Adverse Effects

Note: Carbidopa, in doses used to inhibit peripheral decarboxylation of levodopa, has no significant ability to produce side effects. However, it allows certain CNS side effects of levodopa, such as dyskinesias and mental effects, to develop sooner and at lower levodopa doses because of the resultant greater efficiency per dose of levodopa.

Patients receiving carbidopa and levodopa combination for one to several years may experience sudden, unexpected akinesia, tremor, and rigidity, such as the "on-off" phenomenon. Emotional stress may precipitate akinesia paradoxica or "start hesitation" in these patients.

A syndrome resembling neuroleptic malignant syndrome, which includes intermittent dystonia alternating with substantial agitation, hyperthermia and mental changes, has been reported after the abrupt discontinuation of levodopa therapy.

Convulsions have been reported but a causal relationship to the use of levodopa or carbidopa and levodopa combination has not been established.

The following side/adverse effects have been selected on the basis of their potential clinical significance (possible signs and symptoms in parentheses where appropriate)—not necessarily inclusive:

### Those indicating need for medical attention
Incidence more frequent
> *Mental depression; mood or mental changes, such as aggressive behavior; uncontrolled movements of the body, including the face, tongue, arms, hands, head, and upper body*—may indicate excessive concentration of dopamine in the corpus striatum

> Note: *Mental depression, mood or mental changes, and uncontrolled movements of the body* tend to appear earlier during therapy with carbidopa and levodopa than with levodopa alone.

> *Choreiform and other involuntary movements* occur in 50 to 80% of patients and are usually dose-related.

Incidence less frequent
> *Difficult urination; irregular heartbeat; nausea or vomiting, severe or continuing; orthostatic hypotension* (dizziness or lightheadedness when getting up from a lying or sitting position); *spasm or closing of eyelids*—possible early sign of overdose

> Note: *Nausea and vomiting* may occur frequently in early carbidopa and levodopa therapy with tolerance being gradually achieved during continued use. The concurrent use of carbidopa with levodopa often reduces the frequency and severity of nausea and vomiting, although approximately 15% of patients continue to experience these side effects.

Incidence rare
> *Duodenal ulcer* (stomach pain); *hemolytic anemia* (unusual tiredness or weakness); *hypertension* (high blood pressure)

### Those indicating need for medical attention only if they continue or are bothersome
Incidence more frequent
> *Anxiety, confusion, or nervousness*—especially in elderly patients receiving other antiparkinsonian medication

Incidence less frequent
> *Anorexia* (loss of appetite); *blurred vision; constipation; diarrhea; dryness of mouth; flushing of skin; headache; insomnia* (trouble in sleeping); *muscle twitching; nightmares; unusual tiredness or weakness*

### Those not indicating need for medical attention
Incidence less frequent
> *Darkening in color of urine or sweat*

## Overdose

For more information on the management of overdose or unintentional ingestion, **contact a Poison Control Center** (See *Poison Control Center Listing*).

### Clinical effects of overdose
*Spasm or closing of eyelids*—possible early sign of overdose

### Treatment of overdose
Since there is no specific antidote for acute overdose with carbidopa and levodopa, treatment is symptomatic and supportive, with possible utilization of the following
To decrease absorption—Immediate gastric lavage.
Specific treatment—
> Antiarrhythmic medication, if necessary.
> Pyridoxine is not effective in reversing the actions of carbidopa and levodopa combination.
> The value of dialysis in the treatment of overdose is not known.
Supportive care—Patients in whom intentional overdose is confirmed or suspected should be referred for psychiatric consultation.

## Patient Consultation

As an aid to patient consultation, refer to *Advice for the Patient, Levodopa (Systemic)*.

In providing consultation, consider emphasizing the following selected information (» = major clinical significance):

### Before using this medication
> Conditions affecting use, especially:
>> Sensitivity to carbidopa and/or levodopa
>> Pregnancy—No studies in humans; depressed growth and malformations in animal studies
>> Breast-feeding—Levodopa is distributed into breast milk; may inhibit lactation
>> Use in the elderly—Reduced tolerance to effects of levodopa; caution in resuming normal activity, especially in patients with osteoporosis; psychic effects more common with concurrent use of anticholinergics
>> Dental—Possible difficulty in retention of full dentures
>> Other medications, especially haloperidol, hydantoin anticonvulsants, hydrocarbon inhalation anesthetics, phenothiazines, cocaine, MAO inhibitors, and selegiline
>> Other medical problems, especially severe cardiovascular disease, severe pulmonary diseases, glaucoma, melanoma (history of or suspected), peptic ulcer (history of), psychosis, renal function impairment, or urinary retention

### Proper use of this medication
> Taking food shortly after taking medication to relieve gastric irritation; taking food before or concurrently may retard levodopa's effect
> Compliance with therapy; taking medication only as directed; not stopping medication unless ordered by physician
> Maximum effectiveness of medication may not occur for several weeks or months after therapy is initiated
> Missed dose: Taking as soon as possible; skipping dose if next scheduled dose is within 2 hours; not doubling doses
> Proper storage

### Precautions while using this medication
> Caution if any kind of surgery (including dental surgery) or emergency treatment is required
> For diabetic patients—May interfere with urine tests for sugar and ketones
> Caution if drowsiness occurs
> Caution when getting up suddenly from lying or sitting position; dizziness and fainting may occur
> Possibility of "on-off" phenomenon

### Side/adverse effects
> Occasional darkening of urine or sweat may be alarming to patient although medically insignificant
> Signs of potential side effects, especially difficult urination, duodenal ulcer, hemolytic anemia, hypertension, irregular heartbeat, mental depression, mood or mental changes, severe nausea or vomiting, orthostatic hypotension, spasm or closing of eyelids, or uncontrolled movements of body

## General Dosing Information

Titrated dosage is necessary to achieve the individual therapeutic blood concentration requirements and to avoid side effects. This is especially important for geriatric patients and patients receiving other medications.

Postencephalitic and geriatric patients often require and tolerate lower dosage levels than other parkinsonism patients.

Levodopa must be discontinued at least 8 hours before the carbidopa and levodopa combination dosage is begun. Levodopa may be discontinued in the evening and the carbidopa and levodopa combination started the following morning.

The concurrent administration of carbidopa may permit the dose of levodopa to be reduced by up to 75% with no decrease in therapeutic results. Carbidopa also reduces the adverse effect of pyridoxine on levodopa.

Because carbidopa and levodopa extended-release tablets are 25 to 30% less systemically bioavailable than Carbidopa and Levodopa Tablets USP, increased daily doses of the extended-release tablets may be required to achieve the same level of symptomatic relief.

Amantadine or anticholinergic medications are often used concurrently with carbidopa and levodopa in the more advanced cases of parkinsonism or when response to carbidopa and levodopa decreases. However, gradual dosage reduction of these medications is recommended during initiation of therapy with carbidopa and levodopa and after optimum dosage is reached to maintain proper control of patient's condition.

When carbidopa and levodopa combination is to be discontinued, dosage should be reduced gradually to prevent the occurrence of a syndrome that resembles the neuroleptic malignant syndrome. Careful patient monitoring after withdrawal of carbidopa and levodopa will allow early diagnosis and treatment of neuroleptic malignant–like syndrome.

### Diet/Nutrition

Food should be eaten shortly after carbidopa and levodopa combination is taken to relieve gastric irritation; taking food before or concurrently may retard levodopa's effects.

High protein diets should be avoided, because amino acid degradation products compete with levodopa for transport to the brain, resulting in a decreased or erratic response to levodopa. It is recommended that intake of normal amounts of protein be distributed equally throughout the day.

### For treatment of adverse effects

Immediate relief of nausea and vomiting may sometimes be obtained by reducing the daily dose, giving smaller individual doses at more frequent intervals, or having patient take food shortly after each dose; however, high-protein foods should be avoided since they may decrease levodopa's effect as well (see *Drug interactions and/or related problems*). Since the nausea results primarily from the CNS effects of levodopa, non-phenothiazine antiemetics are sometimes successfully used. Phenothiazine antiemetics may be more effective but should not be used because of their tendency to negate levodopa's therapeutic effect.

The appearance of choreiform and other involuntary movements may require a reduction in dosage since tolerance usually does not develop.

Serious psychiatric disturbances, such as severe mental depression, with or without suicidal tendencies, may require reduction in dosage or complete withdrawal of levodopa.

After discontinuation of levodopa therapy, dantrolene and/or bromocriptine may be used in patients with evidence of neuroleptic malignant–like syndrome, to help reduce fever and thus avoid a potentially lethal complication.

## Oral Dosage Forms

### CARBIDOPA AND LEVODOPA TABLETS USP

#### Usual adult dose

Antidyskinetic—
  For patients not being converted from levodopa therapy:
    Oral, initially, 10 mg of carbidopa and 100 mg of levodopa three or four times a day or 25 mg of carbidopa and 100 mg of levodopa three times a day, the dosage per day being increased gradually at one- or two-day intervals as needed and tolerated.
  For patients being converted from levodopa therapy (levodopa must be discontinued for at least eight hours prior to conversion to carbidopa and levodopa therapy)—
    Patients who require less than 1.5 grams of levodopa per day—Oral, 10 mg of carbidopa and 100 mg of levodopa or 25 mg of carbidopa and 100 mg of levodopa three or four times a day initially, the dosage per day being increased gradually at one- or two-day intervals as needed and tolerated.
    Patients who require more than 1.5 grams of levodopa per day—Oral, 25 mg of carbidopa and 250 mg of levodopa three or four times a day initially, the dosage per day being increased gradually at one- or two-day intervals as needed and tolerated.
  Note: Postencephalitic patients may be more sensitive to the effects of the usual adult dose.
    For patients being converted from levodopa therapy, the initial dose of carbidopa and levodopa per day should provide approximately 25% of the total dosage of levodopa per day previously required.

#### Usual adult prescribing limits

Up to 200 mg of carbidopa and 2 grams of levodopa in combination daily.

Note: Additional levodopa may be administered alone if it is required and tolerated.

#### Usual pediatric dose

Children up to 18 years of age—Safety and efficacy have not been established.

#### Usual geriatric dose

See *Usual adult dose*.

Note: Geriatric patients may be more sensitive to the effects of the usual adult dose.

### Strength(s) usually available

U.S.—
  10 mg of carbidopa and 100 mg of levodopa (Rx) [*Sinemet* (scored); GENERIC].
  25 mg of carbidopa and 100 mg of levodopa (Rx) [*Sinemet* (scored); GENERIC].
  25 mg of carbidopa and 250 mg of levodopa (Rx) [*Sinemet* (scored); GENERIC].

Canada—
  10 mg of carbidopa and 100 mg of levodopa (Rx) [*Sinemet* (scored)].
  25 mg of carbidopa and 100 mg of levodopa (Rx) [*Sinemet* (scored)].
  25 mg of carbidopa and 250 mg of levodopa (Rx) [*Sinemet* (scored)].

### Packaging and storage

Store below 40 °C (104 °F), preferably between 15 and 30 °C (59 and 86 °F), unless otherwise specified by manufacturer. Store in a well-closed, light-resistant container.

### Auxiliary labeling

• May darken urine or sweat.

## CARBIDOPA AND LEVODOPA EXTENDED-RELEASE TABLETS

### Usual adult dose

Antidyskinetic—
  Initial dosage:
    For patients not receiving levodopa therapy—
      Mild to moderate disease:
        Oral, initially, 50 mg of carbidopa and 200 mg of levodopa twice a day, at intervals of at least 6 hours.
    For patients currently treated with conventional carbidopa-levodopa preparations—
      Dosage with the extended-release tablets should be substituted at an amount that provides approximately 10% more levodopa per day, although this may need to be increased to 30% more levodopa per day based on clinical response. The interval between doses of the extended-release tablets should be 4 to 8 hours during the waking day, although a few patients may require more frequent dosing.
      Guidelines for initial conversion from Carbidopa and Levodopa Tablets USP to carbidopa and levodopa extended-release tablets:

| Total daily dose of levodopa (mg) | Suggested dosage regimen of carbidopa and levodopa extended-release tablets (based on levodopa content) |
|---|---|
| 300–400 | 200 mg twice a day |
| 500–600 | 300 mg twice a day or 200 mg three times a day |
| 700–800 | A total of 800 mg in 3 or more divided doses (e.g., 300 mg a.m., 300 mg early p.m., and 200 mg later p.m.) |
| 900–1000 | A total of 1000 mg in 3 or more divided doses (e.g., 400 mg a.m., 400 mg early p.m., and 200 mg later p.m.) |

  For patients currently treated with levodopa without a decarboxylase inhibitor—
    Levodopa must be discontinued at least 8 hours before initiating therapy with carbidopa and levodopa extended-release tablets. The extended-release tablets should be substituted at a dosage of approximately 25% of the previous levodopa dosage.
    Mild to moderate disease: Oral, initially, 50 mg of carbidopa and 200 mg of levodopa twice a day.
  Maintenance dosing:
    Depending upon therapeutic response, doses and dosing intervals may be increased or decreased following initiation of therapy. An interval of at least 3 days between dosage adjustments is recommended. Most patients have been adequately treated with 400 to 1600 mg of levodopa per day, administered as divided doses at intervals ranging from 4 to 8 hours. A few patients may require higher doses (12 or more tablets per day) and shorter intervals (less than 4 hours).
    When the extended-release tablets are given at less than 4-hour intervals, and/or if the divided doses are not equal, the smaller doses should be given at the end of the day.
    Carbidopa and Levodopa Tablets USP may be added to the dosage regimen in selected patients with advanced disease who need additional levodopa for a brief time during daytime hours. Usu-

ally one-half or one tablet of carbidopa 10 mg and levodopa 100 mg or carbidopa 25 mg and levodopa 100 mg is added.

**Usual pediatric dose**

Children up to 18 years of age—Safety and efficacy have not been established.

**Usual geriatric dose**

See *Usual adult dose*.

**Strength(s) usually available**

U.S.—

25 mg of carbidopa and 100 mg of levodopa (Rx) [*Sinemet CR 25-100*].

50 mg of carbidopa and 200 mg of levodopa (Rx) [*Sinemet CR 50-200* (scored)].

Canada—

25 mg of carbidopa and 100 mg of levodopa (Rx) [*Sinemet CR 25-100*].

50 mg of carbidopa and 200 mg of levodopa (Rx) [*Sinemet CR 50-200* (scored)].

**Packaging and storage**

Store below 40 °C (104 °F), preferably between 15 and 30 °C (59 and 86 °F), unless otherwise specified by manufacturer. Store in a well-closed, light-resistant container.

**Auxiliary labeling**

- May darken urine or sweat.
- Do not chew or crush tablets.

Revised: 08/18/92
Interim revision: 05/23/94

---

# CARBINOXAMINE—See *Antihistamines (Systemic)*

---

# CARBINOXAMINE-CONTAINING COMBINATIONS—

Carbinoxamine and Pseudoephedrine (Systemic)—See *Antihistamines and Decongestants (Systemic)*

Carbinoxamine, Pseudoephedrine, and Dextromethorphan (Systemic)—See *Cough/Cold Combinations (Systemic)*

---

# CARBOHYDRATES AND ELECTROLYTES   Systemic

This monograph includes information on the following: Dextrose and Electrolytes; Oral Rehydration Salts§*; Rice Syrup Solids and Electrolytes†.

VA CLASSIFICATION (Primary): TN490

Other commonly used names are oral rehydration salts, ORS-bicarbonate, and ORS-citrate.§

Note: For a listing of dosage forms and brand names by country availability, see *Dosage Forms* section(s). For a listing of brand names for the articles in this monograph, refer to the General Index.

*Not commercially available in the U.S.
†Not commercially available in Canada.
§Distributed by the World Health Organization (WHO).

## Category

Electrolyte replenisher.

## Indications

**Accepted**

Diarrhea (treatment) and

Electrolyte depletion (prophylaxis and treatment)—Carbohydrate and electrolytes solutions are indicated for oral replacement of fluids and electrolytes (especially sodium and potassium) in the treatment of clinically evident dehydration caused by diarrhea; to prevent severe dehydration by replacing losses early in the course of diarrhea; and to maintain hydration in the presence of continuing fluid loss. Oral rehydration therapy (ORT) consists of rehydration (the expansion of intravascular volume and deficit replacement); replacement of ongoing abnormal losses of fluids and electrolyte salts from continuing diarrhea and vomiting and normal water losses through skin and respiration; and the maintenance of fluids and electrolytes in the body until adequate nutrition can be restored. Acute diarrhea is not immediately terminated by oral rehydration therapy, but it is usually self-limiting. Some carbohydrate and electrolytes solutions are also used for maintenance of water and electrolytes when food and liquid intake has been discontinued after surgery, and some are indicated for maintenance of hydration only, rather than for rehydration.

ORT is recommended by the World Health Organization (WHO) Diarrheal Disease Control Program and United Nations Children's Fund (UNICEF) as a fundamental treatment for acute diarrheal disease in infants and children and provides the basis for all national programs of diarrhea control. The WHO formulations of ORS-bicarbonate or ORS-citrate rehydration salts, consisting of preweighed sodium chloride, potassium chloride, sodium citrate or sodium bicarbonate, and dextrose, are distributed in aluminum foil or polyethylene packets to be prepared at home and given at the onset of diarrhea. The solutions are simple to prepare (i.e., the contents of each packet are dissolved in one liter of potable water) and are very effective, inexpensive, and therapeutically appropriate for routine use in prevention and treatment

of dehydration from diarrhea of any cause in all age groups. These powders are not widely used or commercially available in the U.S.

Some commercial carbohydrate and electrolytes solutions available in the U.S. and Canada have a lower sodium content than the recommended WHO formulas. This reflects the concern that the higher sodium content of the WHO solution may cause hypernatremia, especially in developed countries, due to the use of high solute diets and the lower incidence of malnutrition in young children. However, there is no evidence that the WHO solution causes hypernatremia when used as directed. Carbohydrate and electrolytes solutions with a lower sodium content have been found to be as effective as the WHO formulas.

Intravenous replacement of fluids and electrolytes is not used routinely in treatment of diarrhea, but it may be necessary to treat severe dehydration (fluid loss of 10% or more of body weight) or impending shock.

## Pharmacology/Pharmacokinetics

**Physicochemical characteristics**

Molecular weight—

Calcium chloride: 147.02.
Citric acid: 192.12.
Dextrose (anhydrous): 180.16.
Dextrose (monohydrate): 198.17.
Dibasic sodium phosphate: 268.07.
Magnesium chloride: 203.30.
Potassium chloride: 74.55.
Potassium citrate: 324.41.
Sodium bicarbonate: 84.01.
Sodium chloride: 58.44.
Sodium citrate (anhydrous): 258.07.
Sodium citrate (dihydrate): 294.1.

**Mechanism of action/Effect**

During normal digestion, about 9 liters of fluid a day in adults and about 3 to 6 liters a day in infants and children pass through the duodenum where most of the dietary sugars, fats, and amino acids are absorbed. The fluid, containing ingested food and liquids and digestive secretions, reaches the ileum mainly as an isotonic salt solution that is similar to plasma in its ionic sodium and potassium content. The ileum absorbs most of this isotonic solution by various active transport mechanisms, but about 1 liter a day is emptied into the colon where all but about 100 mL is absorbed. The rest is excreted into the feces to prevent desiccation. In addition, cells in the small intestine both absorb and secrete water and electrolytes, but less secretion occurs than absorption, so that the net effect of small bowel transport is absorption. In acute diarrheal states, various infectious agents produce alterations in the intestinal mucosa, inhibiting absorption or stimulating secretion. The large volume of secretions thus produced cannot be fully absorbed by the colon and are expelled as watery diarrhea. Essential water and salts are lost in stools and vomitus, and dehydration results when blood volume is decreased because of fluid loss from the extracellular fluid compartment. Thirst is the first sign of dehydration when fluid loss is less than 5% of the body weight. Tachycardia, decreased skin elasticity, sunken eyes, hypotension, irritability, oliguria or anuria, severe thirst, and stupor or coma develop rapidly when fluid loss is greater than 5% of the body weight. Shock occurs when the deficit equals about 10% of body weight, and death is caused by greater losses of fluids.

Preservation of the facilitated glucose-sodium cotransport system in the small-bowel mucosa is the rationale of oral rehydration therapy. Glucose is actively absorbed in the normal intestine and carries sodium with it in about an equimolar ratio. Therefore, there is a greater net absorption of an isotonic salt solution with glucose than of one without it. During acute diarrhea, the absorption of sodium is impaired and an isotonic salt solution without glucose can increase stool volume by passing through the intestine unabsorbed. Since the glucose absorption system usually remains intact during diarrheal illnesses, the net absorption of water and electrolytes from an isotonic dextrose-salt or a hypotonic rice-salt solution can equal or exceed diarrheal stool volume, even if the loss is rapid. Sucrose (ordinary sugar) may be substituted for dextrose in the dextrose-based oral rehydration solutions, but twice the amount of sugar is needed for near equal efficacy. However, excessive use of dextrose or sucrose to increase palatability of the solution or to increase nutritive value for small children may exacerbate diarrhea, because of the osmotic effect of unabsorbed glucose. A solution with 2 to 2.5% dextrose in the dextrose-based oral rehydration solutions is optimal for promoting coupled absorption of sodium from the intestine.

Rice-based oral rehydration solutions use starch rather than dextrose as a base. The ingested starch gradually releases glucose which along with sodium preserves the glucose-sodium transport system in the manner described above. The rice-based formula has the advantage of a lower osmotic effect and provides a few more calories than the dextrose-based electrolytes solution. This formula has also been found to be more effective in reducing stool output and shortening the duration of diarrhea.

Potassium replacement during acute diarrhea prevents below-normal serum concentrations of potassium, especially in children, in whom stool potassium losses are higher than in adults.

When added to oral rehydration solutions, bicarbonate and citrate are equally effective in correcting the metabolic acidosis caused by diarrhea and dehydration. However, citrate is used instead of the bicarbonate in the WHO formulation, to prevent the occurrence of bicarbonate-induced discoloration and decomposition of the dextrose in the packets.

Treatment started early in the course of diarrhea minimizes vomiting, anorexia, lethargy, or coma, which interfere with continued feeding; allows the homeostatic mechanisms of thirst and renal function to remain intact; and avoids the risk of death from severe dehydration. Thirst determines the amount of rehydration required, and normal renal function allows the excretion of any excess water and salts.

**Time to peak effect:**
8 to 12 hours.

## Precautions to Consider

### Pregnancy/Reproduction
Pregnancy—Problems in humans have not been documented.

### Breast-feeding
Problems in humans have not been documented. Continued breast-feeding during the treatment and maintenance phases of oral rehydration therapy is vital for the management of diarrhea.

### Pediatrics
Although oral rehydration therapy appears to be safe and effective in neonates, it has not been evaluated in premature infants. The range of sodium concentrations recommended by the American Academy of Pediatrics/Committee on Nutrition is 40 to 60 mEq per liter for maintenance solutions and 75 to 90 mEq per liter for rehydration solutions. To allow adequate intake of free water in the prevention of hypernatremia with the use of WHO/ORS-bicarbonate or citrate solutions, feeding (including breast milk) may continue, and/or the infant may be given a separate feeding of plain water after every two doses of undiluted WHO solution.

### Geriatrics
Carbohydrate and electrolytes solutions are well tolerated by elderly patients.

### Medical considerations/Contraindications
The medical considerations/contraindications included here have been selected on the basis of their potential clinical significance (reasons given in parentheses where appropriate)—not necessarily inclusive (» = major clinical significance).

*Except under special circumstances, this medication should not be used when the following medical problems exist:*
» Anuria or
» Oliguria
(since normal renal function is required to allow the excretion of any excess water or salt, patients with prolonged anuria or oliguria usually require precise parenteral administration of water and electrolytes; however, transient oliguria is a feature of dehydration due to diarrhea and is not a contraindication for oral rehydration therapy)

» Dehydration, severe, with symptoms of shock
(oral rehydration is too slow; rapid intravenous therapy is necessary; symptoms of severe dehydration include severe thirst, rapid heartbeat, decreased skin turgor, hypotension, oliguria or anuria, sunken eyes, loss of body weight, convulsions, stupor, and coma; if symptoms of severe dehydration appear after oral therapy has been attempted, rehydration must be achieved with parenteral therapy)

» Diarrhea, severe
(when amounts of diarrhea exceed 30 mL per kg of body weight per hour, patient may be unable to drink enough fluids to replace continuing loss)

» Glucose malabsorption
(diarrhea is exacerbated and dehydration worsened when oral rehydration solutions are given to patients with this problem; volume of stool greatly increases and contains large amounts of glucose; rehydration therapy should be discontinued)

» Inability to drink or
» Vomiting, severe and sustained
(parenteral therapy is required for patients unable to drink because of extreme fatigue, stupor, coma, or uncontrollable vomiting)

» Intestinal obstruction or
» Paralytic ileus or
» Perforated bowel
(delayed passage of carbohydrate and electrolytes solutions through the gastrointestinal tract may increase risk of gastrointestinal irritation)

### Patient monitoring
The following may be especially important in patient monitoring (other tests may be warranted in some patients, depending on condition; » = major clinical significance):

Blood pressure measurements
(recommended to detect shock due to severe dehydration)

Body weight
(recommended periodically to determine the degree of rehydration or the recurrence of dehydration)

Electrolytes, serum and
pH, serum
(recommended to help determine status of individual ions and acid-base status)

Glucose malabsorption tests
(recommended when oral rehydration solution appears to exacerbate diarrhea; infant's feces should be monitored for reducing substances to detect transient monosaccharide malabsorption, which may occur during acute infectious diarrhea; sugar intake should be eliminated or decreased if glucose intolerance is present; intravenous fluid replacement may be required)

Observation for signs of rehydration
(observation of patients with frequent diarrhea is recommended every 3 to 6 hours for signs of rehydration, i.e., normal skin turgor, normal urine flow, normal pulse rate and volume, and a sense of well-being)

Stool volume measurements
(recommended periodically to determine the dose and continued need for maintenance therapy; the volume of ingested replacement solution should equal the volume of stool losses; if stool volume cannot be measured, an intake of 10 to 15 mL of rehydration solution per kilogram of body weight per hour is suggested)

## Side/Adverse Effects
The following side/adverse effects have been selected on the basis of their potential clinical significance (possible signs and symptoms in parentheses where appropriate)—not necessarily inclusive:

### Those indicating need for medical attention
Incidence rare
*Hypernatremia* (dizziness; fast heartbeat; high blood pressure; irritability; muscle twitching; restlessness; seizures; swelling of feet or lower legs; weakness)

Symptoms of overhydration
*Puffy eyelids*
Note: Therapy may need to be discontinued temporarily.

**Those indicating need for medical attention only if they continue or are bothersome**
Incidence more frequent
*Vomiting, mild*
Note: *Mild vomiting* may occur when oral therapy is begun, but therapy should be continued with frequent, small amounts of solution administered slowly.

## Patient Consultation

As an aid to patient consultation, refer to *Advice for the Patient, Carbohydrates and Electrolytes (Systemic)*.

In providing consultation, consider emphasizing the following selected information (» = major clinical significance):

**Before using this medication**
» Conditions affecting use, especially:
    Other medical problems, especially renal function impairment, severe dehydration, severe and continuing diarrhea, glucose malabsorption, inability to drink, severe and continuing vomiting, intestinal obstruction, paralytic ileus, or perforated bowel

**Proper use of this medication**
    Importance of helping infants and small children to drink solution slowly and frequently in small amounts, given with a spoon
    Importance of not taking for a longer time than recommended by physician
» Proper dosing
» Proper storage
*For patients using the commercial powder form*
    Adding recommended amount of boiled, cooled drinking water to contents of packet; stirring or shaking container for 2 or 3 minutes to dissolve completely
    Not adding more water to the solution after it is mixed
    Not boiling solution
    Making and using fresh solution each day
*For patients using the powder form distributed by the World Health Organization (WHO)*
    Adding powder to recommended amount of drinking water; shaking container for 2 or 3 minutes to dissolve completely
    Not adding more water to the solution after it is mixed
    Not boiling solution
    Making and using fresh solution each day

**Precautions while using this medication**
    Eating soft foods, such as cereals, bananas, cooked peas and beans, and potatoes, to maintain nutrition
    Giving breast milk to breast-fed infants between doses of solution
    Checking with physician if diarrhea does not improve in a day or 2 or becomes worse during treatment with this medication
    Checking with physician as soon as possible if signs of severe dehydration occur, including doughy skin (decreased skin turgor), sunken eyes, dizziness or lightheadedness, weakness or tiredness, irritability, and weight loss
*For patients taking ORS-citrate or ORS-bicarbonate*
    Drinking water between doses of rehydration solution (except breast-fed infants)
*For patients taking the premixed liquid form*
    Avoiding other electrolyte-containing foods or liquids, such as fruit juices or foods with added salt, until rehydration solutions are discontinued, to prevent excessive electrolyte ingestion or osmotic diarrhea

**Side/adverse effects**
    Signs of potential side effects, especially hypernatremia

## General Dosing Information

Infants and young children should be given small, frequent, and slowly administered amounts of oral rehydration fluid. Infants who finish 150 mL of solution per kg of body weight in less than 24 hours should be encouraged to drink plain water to prevent hypernatremia and to quench thirst.

The commercially prepared solutions do not require additional water intake because of the generally lower sodium content.

Rehydration solutions must not be diluted with water, because dilution decreases the absorptive properties of the glucose-sodium cotransport system.

Acute watery diarrhea, dysentery, and persistent diarrhea in children can also result in tissue catabolism, which may in turn lead to malnutrition. This can be further aggravated by the common practice of withholding fluids and nutrition during diarrhea. Although early feeding may result in slightly increased stool volume, nutrient absorption is increased and weight loss is lessened. Therefore, continued feeding (including breast milk) of infants and children and supplementation with plain drinking water during the maintenance phase of oral rehydration therapy are important for maintaining hydration and nutrition in the management of diarrhea.

The oral rehydration solution should be taken alternately with soft foods, such as rice cereal, bananas, cooked legumes, potatoes, or other non-lactose-containing, carbohydrate-rich food. Older children and adults should resume their normal diets as soon as the appetite returns. Other electrolyte-containing foods or liquids such as fruit juices or foods with added salt should be withheld until oral rehydration solutions are discontinued, to prevent excessive electrolyte ingestion or osmotic diarrhea.

Cow's milk should be discontinued only if diarrhea worsens considerably after feeding and the stool becomes acidic and contains reducing substances. This reflects a depression of lactase activity, which may occur when the brush borders of jejunal mucosal cells are damaged. Soy formulas without lactose are given alternately with carbohydrate and electrolytes solutions for the first 24 to 48 hours.

If the initial dehydration is severe, rehydration must be achieved by intravenous administration of an appropriate isotonic electrolyte solution, after which the oral solution may be used for maintenance when tolerance to oral intake has been established.

Parenteral rehydration therapy should be started if symptoms of dehydration reappear after aggressive oral replacement of fluids and electrolytes has been attempted.

---

## DEXTROSE AND ELECTROLYTES

## Oral Dosage Forms
### DEXTROSE AND ELECTROLYTES SOLUTION
**Usual adult and adolescent dose**
Rehydration—
    Mild dehydration: Oral, initially 50 mL of solution per kg of body weight over four to six hours, the amounts and rates being adjusted as needed and tolerated, depending on thirst and response to therapy.
    Moderate dehydration: Oral, initially 100 mL of solution per kg of body weight over six hours, the amounts and rates being adjusted as needed and tolerated, depending on thirst and response to therapy.
Note: Severe dehydration must be treated with intravenous electrolyte solutions.
Maintenance of hydration—
    Mild continuing diarrhea: Oral, 100 to 200 mL of solution per kg of body weight over twenty-four hours until diarrhea stops.
    Severe continuing diarrhea: Oral, 15 mL of solution per kg of body weight every hour until diarrhea stops.

**Usual adult prescribing limits**
Up to 1000 mL per hour.

**Usual pediatric dose**
Rehydration—
    Children up to 2 years of age: Oral, initially 150 mL of solution per kg of body weight over twenty-four hours (75 mL per kg of body weight during the first eight hours, and 75 mL per kg of body weight during the next sixteen hours), the amounts and rates being adjusted as needed and tolerated, depending on thirst and response to therapy.
    Children 2 to 10 years of age with moderate to severe dehydration: Oral, initially 50 mL of solution per kg of body weight over the first four to six hours, and 100 mL of solution per kg of body weight over the next eighteen to twenty-four hours, the amounts and rates being adjusted as needed and tolerated, depending on thirst and response to therapy.
Note: No more than 100 mL of fluid should be given during any 20-minute period.
Children over 10 years of age: See *Usual adult and adolescent dose.*

**Strength(s) usually available**

| Product | Electrolyte Content (mEq/liter) | | | | | | |
|---|---|---|---|---|---|---|---|
| | Na$^+$ | K$^+$ | Cl$^-$ | Citrate | Mg$^{++}$ | Ca$^{++}$ | Phosphate |
| **U.S.—** | | | | | | | |
| *Naturalyte\** (OTC) | 45 | 20 | 35 | 48 | | | |
| *Oralyte\** (OTC) | 45 | 20 | 35 | 48 | | | |
| *Pedialyte\** (OTC) | 45 | 20 | 35 | 30 | | | |
| *Rehydralyte\** (OTC) | 75 | 20 | 65 | 30 | | | |
| *Resol†* (OTC) | 50 | 20 | 50 | 34 | 4 | 4 | 5 |
| **Canada—** | | | | | | | |
| *Lytren†* (OTC) | 50 | 25 | 45 | 30 | | | |
| *Pedialyte\** (OTC) | 45 | 20 | 35 | 30 | | | |

\*Dextrose content=25 grams per liter.
†Dextrose content=20 grams per liter.

Note: *Resol* is available to hospitals only.

    Generic name product is available in the U.S.

**Packaging and storage**
Store below 40 °C (104 °F), preferably between 15 and 30 °C (59 and 86 °F), unless otherwise specified by manufacturer.

---

## *ORAL REHYDRATION SALTS*

# Oral Dosage Forms
## ORAL REHYDRATION SALTS (FOR ORAL SOLUTION)

**Usual adult and adolescent dose**
Rehydration—
    Mild dehydration: Oral, initially 50 mL of solution per kg of body weight over four to six hours, the amounts and rates being adjusted as needed and tolerated, depending on thirst and response to therapy.
    Moderate dehydration: Oral, initially 100 mL of solution per kg of body weight over six hours, the amounts and rates being adjusted as needed and tolerated, depending on thirst and response to therapy.
Note: Severe dehydration must be treated with intravenous electrolyte solutions.
Maintenance of hydration—
    Mild continuing diarrhea: Oral, 100 to 200 mL of solution per kg of body weight over twenty-four hours until diarrhea stops.
    Severe continuing diarrhea: Oral, 15 mL of solution per kg of body weight every hour until diarrhea stops.

**Usual adult prescribing limits**
Up to 1000 mL per hour.

**Usual pediatric dose**
Rehydration—
    Mild or moderate dehydration: Oral, initially 50 to 100 mL per kg of body weight during the first four hours, the dosage being adjusted to 100 mL per kg of body weight per day until diarrhea stops, the amounts and rates being adjusted as needed and tolerated, depending on thirst and response to therapy.

**Strength(s) usually available**

| Product | Electrolyte Content (mEq/liter) | | | | |
|---|---|---|---|---|---|
| | Na$^+$ | K$^+$ | Cl$^-$ | Bicarbonate | Citrate |
| **U.S.—** | | | | | |
| Not commercially available. | | | | | |
| **Canada—** | | | | | |
| *Gastrolyte†* (OTC) | 60 | 20 | 60 | 10 | |
| *Rapolyte\** (OTC) | 90 | 20 | 80 | 30 | |
| **Other—** | | | | | |
| ORS-bicarbonate\* | 90 | 20 | 80 | 30 | |
| ORS-citrate\* | 90 | 20 | 80 | | 30 |

\*Dextrose content=20 grams per liter.
†Dextrose content=17.8 grams per liter.

**Packaging and storage**
Store below 30 °C (86 °F), preferably between 15 and 30 °C (59 and 86 °F). Store in a tight container.

**Preparation of dosage form**
Packets distributed by WHO—To one quart or liter of drinking water, add contents of one packet containing sodium chloride, potassium chloride, sodium bicarbonate or citrate, and dextrose. Stir or shake well for 2 or 3 minutes to dissolve.
Packets available commercially—Add 200 mL (7 ounces) of boiled, cooled tap water to the contents of one packet containing sodium chloride, potassium chloride, sodium bicarbonate, and dextrose. Stir or shake well for 2 or 3 minutes to dissolve.
To prepare extemporaneous oral rehydration solution—Add 3.5 grams (0.5 teaspoonful) sodium chloride (table salt), 1.5 grams (1.2 teaspoonfuls) potassium chloride or potassium salt, 2.5 grams (0.5 teaspoonful) sodium bicarbonate (baking soda), and 40 grams (4 tablespoonfuls) sucrose (table sugar) to one liter of potable water.

**Stability**
The constituted solution may be stored in a refrigerator for up to a maximum of 24 hours after constitution, after which time the unused portion should be discarded.
ORS-bicarbonate can be stored up to 3 years if the product is dry, filled and sealed in a dry atmosphere in air-tight aluminum laminate, and stored at temperatures below 30 °C. In conditions other than these, the product may deteriorate (caramelize) and change color (yellow to brown).
ORS-citrate can be stored for at least 3 years. If moisture is absorbed, the product will lump or harden with no change in color and no effect on its dissolution in water.

**Additional information**
The WHO oral rehydration solution contains sodium chloride 3.5 grams, potassium chloride 1.5 grams, sodium bicarbonate 2.5 grams or sodium citrate (dihydrate) 2.9 grams, and dextrose 20.0 grams, per liter of water.

---

## *RICE SYRUP SOLIDS AND ELECTROLYTES*

# Oral Dosage Forms

## RICE SYRUP SOLIDS AND ELECTROLYTES SOLUTION

**Usual adult and adolescent dose**
See *Dextrose and Electrolytes Solution.*

**Usual pediatric dose**
See *Dextrose and Electrolytes Solution.*

**Strength(s) usually available**

| Product | Electrolyte Content (mEq/liter) | | | |
|---|---|---|---|---|
| | Na$^+$ | K$^+$ | Cl$^-$ | Citrate |
| **U.S.—** | | | | |
| *Infalyte\** (OTC) | 50 | 25 | 45 | 36 |
| **Canada—** | | | | |
| Not commercially available. | | | | |

\*Rice syrup solids content=30 grams per liter.

**Packaging and storage**
Store below 40 °C (104 °F), preferably between 15 and 30 °C (59 and 86 °F), unless otherwise specified by manufacturer.

**Stability**
The manufacturer of the rice-based oral electrolytes solution recommends that the product be refrigerated and used within 48 hours after opening.

---

Revised: 12/02/92
Interim revision: 08/09/94; 07/20/95

# CARBOL-FUCHSIN   Topical

VA CLASSIFICATION (Primary): DE102

Another commonly used name is Castellani Paint

Note: For a listing of dosage forms and brand names by country availability, see *Dosage Forms* section(s). For a listing of brand names for the articles in this monograph, refer to the General Index.

## Category

Antifungal (topical); drying agent (topical).

## Indications

Note: Bracketed information in the *Indications* section refers to uses that are not included in U.S. product labeling.

### Accepted

Skin and nail infections, fungal, minor (treatment)—Carbol-fuchsin is indicated in the topical treatment of minor fungal skin and nail infections, including tinea pedis (ringworm of the foot; athlete's foot) caused by *Trichophyton* species or *Epidermophyton floccosum* and onychomycosis (tinea unguium; ringworm of the nails) caused by *Trichophyton* species, *Epidermophyton floccosum*, or *Candida albicans*. Carbol-fuchsin is indicated only during the acute and chronic stages of dermatophytoses.

Macerations (treatment adjunct); or

Tinea pedis (treatment adjunct)—Carbol-fuchsin is indicated as a topical drying agent in the adjunctive treatment of macerations and tinea pedis (ringworm of the foot; athlete's foot).

[Tinea barbae (treatment)]; or

[Tinea capitis (treatment)]—Carbol-fuchsin is used in the topical treatment of tinea barbae and tinea capitis.

Not all species or strains of a particular organism may be susceptible to carbol-fuchsin.

## Pharmacology/Pharmacokinetics

### Physicochemical characteristics

Molecular weight—Phenol: 94.11.
Resorcinol: 110.11.
Acetone: 58.08.
Alcohol: 46.07.

### Mechanism of action/Effect

Antifungal (topical)—Has fungicidal properties. The dye, basic fuchsin, has been reported to stimulate granulation and epithelialization.

### Other actions/effects

Also has local anesthetic and bactericidal properties.

## Precautions to Consider

### Pregnancy/Reproduction

Problems in humans have not been documented.

### Breast-feeding

Problems in humans have not been documented.

### Pediatrics

Appropriate studies on the relationship of age to the effects of carbol-fuchsin topical solution have not been performed in the pediatric population. However, when used in the treatment of infantile eczema, carbol-fuchsin topical solution should not be applied more than once daily.

### Geriatrics

No information is available on the relationship of age to the effects of carbol-fuchsin topical solution in geriatric patients.

## Side/Adverse Effects

The following side/adverse effects have been selected on the basis of their potential clinical significance (possible signs and symptoms in parentheses where appropriate)—not necessarily inclusive:

**Those indicating need for medical attention**
*Skin irritation not present before therapy*

**Those indicating need for medical attention only if they continue or are bothersome**
*Mild, temporary stinging*

## Patient Consultation

As an aid to patient consultation, refer to *Advice for the Patient, Carbol-Fuchsin (Topical)*.

In providing consultation, consider emphasizing the following selected information (» = major clinical significance):

### Before using this medication
» Conditions affecting use, especially:
    Sensitivity to carbol-fuschin
    Use in children—Not using on infants and children with eczema more than once a day.

### Proper use of this medication
» Poison if swallowed; importance of using only on affected areas; not swallowing this medication
    Before applying, washing affected areas with soap and water and drying thoroughly
    Applying with an applicator or swab; not applying to large areas of the body
    Not bandaging if medication applied to fingers or toes
» Compliance with full course of therapy, which may take several months or more
» Proper dosing
    Missed dose: Applying as soon as possible; not applying if almost time for next dose
» Proper storage

### Precautions while using this medication
    Checking with physician if no improvement within 1 week
» Medication will stain skin and clothing; stain will slowly wear off from skin

### Side/adverse effects
    Signs of potential side effects, especially skin irritation not present before therapy

## General Dosing Information

Use of topical antifungals may lead to skin sensitization, resulting in hypersensitivity reactions with subsequent topical use of the medication.

Carbol-fuchsin topical solution should never be applied to large areas of the body, because the high concentration of the constituents (basic fuchsin, phenol, resorcinol, acetone) in the hydroalcoholic solution may cause irritation.

## Topical Dosage Forms

### CARBOL-FUCHSIN TOPICAL SOLUTION USP

**Usual adult and adolescent dose**
Antifungal; or
Drying agent—
    Topical, to the skin, one to three times a day.

**Usual pediatric dose**
Antifungal; or
Drying agent—
    See *Usual adult and adolescent dose*.
Note: For infantile eczema, topical carbol-fuchsin should be applied to the skin not more than once daily.

**Strength(s) usually available**
U.S.—
    0.3% basic fuchsin, 4.5% phenol, 10% resorcinol, 5% acetone, and 10% alcohol in an aqueous solution (OTC) [*Castel Plus;* GENERIC].

**Packaging and storage**
Store below 40 °C (104 °F), preferably between 15 and 30 °C (59 and 86 °F), unless otherwise specified by manufacturer. Store in a tight, light-resistant container. Protect from freezing.

**Auxiliary labeling**
• Poison if swallowed.
• For external use only.
• Keep container tightly closed.
• Continue medication for full time of treatment.
• Will stain clothing.

Revised: 02/10/92
Interim revision: 07/21/94

# CARBONIC ANHYDRASE INHIBITORS   Systemic

This monograph includes information on the following: Acetazolamide; Dichlorphenamide†; Methazolamide.

INN:
  Dichlorphenamide—Diclofenamide

VA CLASSIFICATION (Primary/Secondary):
  Acetazolamide—CV703/OP104; CN400; MS900; GU900
  Dichlorphenamide—CV703/OP104
  Methazolamide—CV703/OP104

Note: For a listing of dosage forms and brand names by country availability, see *Dosage Forms* section(s). For a listing of brand names for the articles in this monograph, refer to the General Index.

†Not commercially available in Canada.

## Category

Antiglaucoma agent (systemic)—Acetazolamide; Dichlorphenamide; Methazolamide.
Anticonvulsant—Acetazolamide (tablets and injection).
Altitude sickness (acute) prophylactic and therapeutic agent—Acetazolamide.
Antiparalytic (familial periodic paralysis)—Acetazolamide.
Diuretic, urinary alkalinizing—Acetazolamide (parenteral).
Antiurolithic (uric acid calculi; cystine calculi)—Acetazolamide Tablets USP.

## Indications

Note: Bracketed information in the *Indications* section refers to uses that are not included in U.S. product labeling.

**Accepted**

Glaucoma, open-angle (treatment)
Glaucoma, secondary (treatment)
Glaucoma, angle-closure (treatment) or
[Glaucoma, malignant (treatment)]—Carbonic anhydrase inhibitors are indicated primarily as adjuncts to other agents in the treatment of open-angle (chronic simple) glaucoma and secondary glaucoma, and to lower intraocular pressure prior to surgery for some types of glaucoma.

These medications should not be used for long-term therapy in non-congestive angle-closure (closed-angle) glaucoma; organic closure of the angle may occur while the worsening condition is masked by the lowered intraocular pressure.

[Acetazolamide is used to lower intraocular pressure in the treatment of malignant (ciliary block) glaucoma, which may occur after inflammation, surgery, trauma, or use of miotics.]

Epilepsy, absence seizure pattern (treatment)
Epilepsy, tonic-clonic seizure pattern (treatment)
Epilepsy, mixed seizure pattern (treatment)
Epilepsy, simple partial seizure pattern (treatment) or
Epilepsy, myoclonic seizure pattern (treatment)—Acetazolamide is indicated as an adjunct to other anticonvulsants in the management of absence seizures (petit mal), generalized tonic-clonic seizures (grand mal), mixed seizure patterns, simple partial seizure patterns, and myoclonic seizure patterns. It may be especially useful for intermittent therapy in females who experience increased seizure activity at the time of menstruation.

Altitude sickness (prophylaxis)[1] or
Altitude sickness (treatment)[1]—Oral acetazolamide is indicated to decrease the incidence and/or severity of symptoms (such as headache, nausea, shortness of breath, dizziness, drowsiness, and fatigue) associated with acute altitude sickness in mountain climbers who are attempting rapid ascent and in those who are very susceptible to altitude sickness despite gradual ascent. Gradual ascent is desirable for prevention of acute altitude sickness even when acetazolamide is used. However, prompt descent may still be necessary if severe manifestations of acute altitude sickness, such as pulmonary edema or cerebral edema, occur.

[Paralysis, familial periodic (treatment)][1]—Acetazolamide is used to treat both the hypokalemic and hyperkalemic forms of familial periodic paralysis. It terminates the acute attacks and, with chronic use, prevents their recurrence. It may be the drug of choice in the hypokalemic form of the condition.

[Toxicity, weakly acidic medications (treatment)]—Parenteral acetazolamide is used to produce a forced alkaline diuresis as a method of increasing the elimination of certain weakly acidic medications.

[Renal calculi, uric acid (prophylaxis)][1] or
[Renal calculi, cystine (prophylaxis)][1]—Oral acetazolamide is used to alkalinize the urine as a means of preventing the occurrence or recurrence of uric acid renal stones, especially in patients receiving uricosuric antigout agents, or of cystine renal stones.

**Unaccepted**

Acetazolamide has also been used to prevent or counteract metabolic alkalosis, including that which may occur following open-heart surgery; however, it is no longer used for these indications.

Acetazolamide has also been used as a diuretic in the treatment of edema due to congestive heart disease and drug-induced edema. However, it has been replaced by newer diuretics for these indications.

[1]Not included in Canadian product labeling.

## Pharmacology/Pharmacokinetics

**Physicochemical characteristics**

Molecular weight—
  Acetazolamide—222.24.
  Acetazolamide sodium—244.22.
  Dichlorphenamide—305.15.
  Methazolamide—236.26.

**Mechanism of action/Effect**

Nonbacteriostatic sulfonamide derivatives. Inhibition of the enzyme carbonic anhydrase decreases formation of hydrogen and bicarbonate ions from carbon dioxide and water and reduces the availability of these ions for active transport. These agents reduce plasma bicarbonate concentration and increase plasma chloride concentration, producing systemic metabolic acidosis. Although all of these medications may produce diuresis with acute or intermittent administration, loss of diuretic effect occurs with chronic administration. Therefore, dichlorphenamide and methazolamide are not used as diuretics, and acetazolamide is now being used only to produce alkaline diuresis in certain cases of drug overdose. Methazolamide has less diuretic effect and less influence on urinary bicarbonate than do other carbonic anhydrase inhibitors with doses used in glaucoma.

Antiglaucoma agent—
  Lowers intraocular pressure by decreasing the production of aqueous humor by 50 to 60%. The mechanism is not completely understood but probably involves a decrease of the bicarbonate ion concentration in ocular fluids. These agents have no effect on the facility of aqueous outflow. The ocular action is independent of any diuretic action.

Acetazolamide—
  Anticonvulsant:
    Mechanism of action has not been fully determined. Inhibition of carbonic anhydrase in the central nervous system (CNS) may increase carbon dioxide tension, resulting in a retardation of neuronal conduction. The production of systemic metabolic acidosis may also be involved. This action is independent of any diuretic action.
  Altitude sickness, acute, prophylactic and therapeutic agent:
    May act by producing metabolic acidosis resulting in increased respiratory drive and arterial oxygen tension and/or by causing diuresis.
    In clinical trials, pulmonary function, such as minute ventilation, expired vital capacity, and peak flow, was greater in climbers treated with acetazolamide, whether they had acute altitude sickness or were asymptomatic. Acetazolamide-treated climbers also had less difficulty sleeping.
  Antiparalytic (for familial periodic paralysis):
    May stabilize muscle membranes against abnormal fluxes of potassium ions. Alternatively, may produce metabolic acidosis resulting in prevention of the intracellular shift of potassium.
  Diuretic, urinary alkalinizing:
    Induces alkaline diuresis by lowering hydrogen ion concentration in the renal tubule and increasing excretion of bicarbonate, sodium, potassium, and water. This increases the solubility in urine of weakly acidic drugs and promotes their excretion.
  Antiurolithic:
    Alkalinization of the urine increases the solubility in urine of uric acid and cystine, thereby reducing the formation of uric acid- or cystine-containing renal stones.

**Absorption**

Well absorbed; methazolamide absorbed more slowly than acetazolamide or dichlorphenamide.

**Protein binding**
Acetazolamide—Very high (90%).
Methazolamide—Moderate.

**Half-life**
Acetazolamide (tablets)—10 to 15 hours.
Methazolamide—14 hours.

**Time to peak concentration**
Acetazolamide tablets—2 to 4 hours after a 500-mg dose.
Acetazolamide extended-release capsules—8 to 12 hours after a 500-mg dose.

**Peak serum concentration**
Acetazolamide tablets—12 to 27 mcg per mL with a 500-mg dose.
Acetazolamide extended-release capsules—6 mcg per mL with a 500-mg dose.

**Elimination**
Acetazolamide—Renal; as unchanged drug; 90 to 100% of a dose is excreted within 24 hours after administration of oral tablets or intravenous injection; 47% of a dose is excreted within 24 hours after administration of extended-release capsules.
Dichlorphenamide—Unknown.
Methazolamide—Renal; 15 to 30% excreted unchanged. Remainder unknown.

**Effects on intraocular pressure**

| Drug | Onset of Action | Peak Effect | Duration of Action (hr) |
|---|---|---|---|
| Acetazolamide | | | |
| Extended-release | | | |
| capsules | 2 hr | 8–12 hr | 18–24 |
| Tablets | 1–1.5 hr | 2–4 hr | 8–12 |
| Intravenous | 2 min | 15 min | 4–5 |
| Dichlorphenamide | | | |
| Tablets | 0.5–1 hr | 2–4 hr | 6–12 |
| Methazolamide | | | |
| Tablets | 2–4 hr | 6–8 hr | 10–18 |

# Precautions to Consider

**Cross-sensitivity and/or related problems**
Patients sensitive to antibacterial sulfonamides, thiazide diuretics, or other sulfonamide-derivative diuretics may be sensitive to carbonic anhydrase inhibitors also.

**Carcinogenicity**
Long-term studies in animals have not been conducted using carbonic anhydrase inhibitors.

**Mutagenicity**
*Acetazolamide*—In a bacterial mutagenicity assay, acetazolamide was not mutagenic when evaluated with and without metabolic activation.
*Methazolamide*—In the Ames bacterial test, methazolamide was not mutagenic.

**Pregnancy/Reproduction**
Fertility—*Acetazolamide:* Acetazolamide had no effect on fertility of male and female rats administered oral daily doses of up to 4 times the recommended human dose of 1000 mg in a 50 kg individual.
*Dichlorphenamide* and *methazolamide:* Long-term studies in animals have not been conducted.

Pregnancy—Adequate and well-controlled studies have not been done using carbonic anhydrase inhibitors in humans.
*Acetazolamide*—
Acetazolamide has been shown to cause limb defects in mice, rats, hamsters, and rabbits.

FDA Pregnancy Category C.
*Dichlorphenamide and methazolamide*—
Dichlorphenamide and methazolamide, when given in large doses, have been shown to cause skeletal anomalies in rats.

FDA Pregnancy Category C.

**Breast-feeding**
Because of the potential for serious adverse reactions, a decision should be made whether to discontinue nursing during therapy with carbonic anhydrase inhibitors.
*Acetazolamide*—Acetazolamide may be distributed into breast milk.
*Dichlorphenamide* and *methazolamide*—It is not known whether dichlorphenamide or methazolamide is distributed into breast milk.

**Pediatrics**
Appropriate studies on the relationship of age to the effects of carbonic anhydrase inhibitors have not been performed in the pediatric popu-

lation. However, no pediatrics-specific problems have been documented to date.

**Geriatrics**
No information is available on the relationship of age to the effects of carbonic anhydrase inhibitors in geriatric patients. However, elderly patients are more likely to have age-related renal function impairment, which may require caution in patients receiving these medications.

**Dental**
Acetazolamide may cause facial paresthesia, such as numbness, tingling, or burning feeling of the mouth, tongue, or lips. Other carbonic anhydrase inhibitors may cause similar side effects.

**Drug interactions and/or related problems**
The following drug interactions and/or related problems have been selected on the basis of their potential clinical significance (possible mechanism in parentheses where appropriate)—not necessarily inclusive (» = major clinical significance):

Note: Combinations containing any of the following medications, depending on the amount present, may also interact with this medication.

Corticosteroids, glucocorticoid, especially with significant mineralocorticoid activity or
Corticosteroids, mineralocorticoid or
Amphotericin B, parenteral or
Corticotropin, especially prolonged therapeutic use
(concurrent use with carbonic anhydrase inhibitors may result in severe hypokalemia and should be undertaken with caution; serum potassium concentrations and cardiac function should be monitored during concurrent use)
(concurrent use of corticosteroids or corticotropin with acetazolamide sodium may increase the risk of hypernatremia and/or edema because these medications cause sodium and fluid retention; the risk with corticosteroids or corticotropin may depend on the patient's sodium requirement as determined by the condition being treated)
(the possibility should be considered that concurrent chronic use of corticosteroids or corticotropin with carbonic anhydrase inhibitors may increase the risk of hypocalcemia and osteoporosis because these medications increase calcium excretion)

» Amphetamines or
Anticholinergics, especially atropine and related compounds or
» Mecamylamine or
» Quinidine
(therapeutic and/or side effects may be enhanced or prolonged when these medications are used concurrently with carbonic anhydrase inhibitors, especially acetazolamide, as a result of decreased excretion caused by alkalinization of urine; concurrent use with mecamylamine is not recommended; dosage adjustments of the other medications may be needed when carbonic anhydrase inhibitor therapy is initiated or discontinued or if the dosage is changed)

Antidiabetic agents, oral or
Insulin
(hypoglycemic response may be decreased during concurrent use because carbonic anhydrase inhibitors may cause hyperglycemia and glycosuria in diabetic patients; dosage adjustments may be required)

Barbiturates, especially phenobarbital or
Carbamazepine or
Phenytoin or other hydantoin anticonvulsants or
Primidone
(osteopenia induced by these agents may be enhanced; it is recommended that patients receiving concurrent therapy be monitored for early signs of osteopenia and that the carbonic anhydrase inhibitor be discontinued and appropriate treatment initiated if necessary)

Ciprofloxacin
(urinary alkalizers, such as carbonic anhydrase inhibitors, may reduce the solubility of ciprofloxacin in the urine; patients should be observed for signs of crystalluria and nephrotoxicity)

Digitalis glycosides
(concurrent use with carbonic anhydrase inhibitors may enhance the possibility of digitalis toxicity associated with hypokalemia)

Diuretics, other
(diuretic effects may be enhanced during concurrent therapy; however, the hypokalemic and hyperuricemic effects of many diuretics may also be enhanced during concurrent therapy)

Ephedrine
(urine alkalinization induced by carbonic anhydrase inhibitors may increase the half-life of ephedrine and prolong its duration of action, especially if the urine remains alkaline for several days or longer; dosage adjustment of ephedrine may be necessary)

Mannitol or
Urea
(concurrent use with carbonic anhydrase inhibitors may lead to increased reduction of intraocular pressure as well as increased diuresis)

» Methenamine
(efficacy may be reduced because alkaline urine produced by carbonic anhydrase inhibitors inhibits methenamine conversion to formaldehyde, which is the active bacteriostatic derivative of methenamine; concurrent use is not recommended)

Mexiletine
(marked alkalinization of urine by carbonic anhydrase inhibitors may retard renal excretion of mexiletine)

Neuromuscular blocking agents, nondepolarizing
(hypokalemia induced by carbonic anhydrase inhibitors may enhance the blockade of nondepolarizing neuromuscular blocking agents, possibly leading to increased or prolonged respiratory depression or paralysis [apnea]; serum potassium concentration determinations may be necessary prior to administration of a nondepolarizing neuromuscular blocking agent)

Salicylates
(the risk of salicylate intoxication in patients receiving large doses of salicylates may be increased during concurrent therapy because metabolic acidosis induced by carbonic anhydrase inhibitors may increase penetration of salicylate into the brain. Anorexia, tachypnea, lethargy, coma, and death have been reported with concurrent use of high-dose aspirin and carbonic anhydrase inhibitors. In addition, the increased risk of severe metabolic acidosis and salicylate toxicity should be considered if acetazolamide is used to produce forced alkaline diuresis in the treatment of salicylate overdose. With average doses of salicylates, alkalinization of the urine results in increased salicylate excretion and decreased salicylate plasma concentrations)

**Laboratory value alterations**
The following have been selected on the basis of their potential clinical significance (possible effect in parentheses where appropriate)—not necessarily inclusive (» = major clinical significance):

With diagnostic test results
Urine 17-hydroxysteroid (17-OHCS) determinations
(may produce false-positive results by interfering with absorbance in the modified Glenn-Nelson technique)

Urine protein determinations
(may produce false-positive results with bromophenol blue test reagent and with sulfosalicylic acid, heat and acetic acid, and nitric acid ring test methods because of alkalinization of urine)

With physiology/laboratory test values
Ammonia concentrations, blood and
Bilirubin concentrations, serum and
Urobilinogen concentrations, urine
(may be increased)

Bicarbonate concentrations, plasma
(usually are decreased)

Calcium concentrations, urine
(may be increased or unchanged)

Chloride concentrations, plasma
(may be increased, especially with acetazolamide)

Citrate concentrations, urine
(may be decreased; in combination with increased or unchanged urine calcium concentrations may result in renal calculi and ureteral colic)

Glucose concentrations, blood and
Glucose concentrations, urine
(may be increased, especially in diabetic or prediabetic patients receiving acetazolamide; patients not predisposed to diabetes are not significantly affected)

Iodine uptake by the thyroid gland
(may be decreased in hyperthyroid patients or those with normal thyroid function but not in hypothyroid patients)

Potassium concentrations, serum
(may be decreased, especially when therapy is initiated or with intermittent dosage; with continuous therapy, serum potassium concentrations usually return to normal)

Uric acid concentrations, serum
(may be increased; rarely, gout may be exacerbated)

**Medical considerations/Contraindications**
The medical considerations/contraindications included here have been selected on the basis of their potential clinical significance (reasons given in parentheses where appropriate)—not necessarily inclusive (» = major clinical significance).

*Risk-benefit should be considered when the following medical problems exist:*

» Adrenal gland failure or adrenocortical insufficiency (Addison's disease)
(patients more susceptible to electrolyte imbalances)

Diabetes mellitus
(may increase blood and urine sugar concentrations)

Gout, except when used to prevent uric acid calculi in patients receiving uricosuric antigout agents or

» Hyperchloremic acidosis or

» Hypokalemia, hyponatremia, or other electrolyte imbalance or
Respiratory acidosis
(may be exacerbated)

» Hepatic disease, including cirrhosis, or impairment
(patients more susceptible to electrolyte imbalances; increased risk of hepatic coma and hepatotoxicity)

Impaired alveolar ventilation due to pulmonary disease, edema, infection, or obstruction
(respiratory acidosis may be induced or increased)

» Renal failure, disease, or impairment
(excessively high plasma concentrations may result and the acidosis of renal failure may be aggravated)

» Renal calculi, calcium-containing, or history of
(may be exacerbated or induced during therapy)

Sensitivity to carbonic anhydrase inhibitors

**Patient monitoring**
The following may be especially important in patient monitoring (other tests may be warranted in some patients, depending on condition; » = major clinical significance):

Complete blood cell (CBC) count
Platelet count
(baseline CBC and platelet counts recommended prior to initiating therapy and at regular intervals during therapy. If significant changes occur, medication should be promptly discontinued and appropriate therapy instituted)

» Electrolyte concentrations, serum
(recommended prior to initiation of therapy and at periodic intervals during therapy, especially in patients for whom hypokalemia or other electrolyte imbalances would be detrimental, such as those with hepatic cirrhosis or those receiving potassium-wasting medications or digitalis)

Urologic examinations
(may be necessary to detect possible renal problems, especially crystalluria or renal calculi)

# Side/Adverse Effects

Note: Serious side/adverse effects occur infrequently; many of the serious adverse effects are those that are common to all sulfonamide derivatives, such as Stevens-Johnson syndrome, toxic epidermal necrolysis, fulminant hepatic necrosis, agranulocytosis, aplastic anemia, and other blood dyscrasias. Rarely, these serious adverse effects have caused fatalities. Many side effects are dose-related and may respond to a reduction of dosage.

Hypokalemia may occur if diuresis is brisk and may be especially likely to occur if hepatic cirrhosis is present, if potassium intake is inadequate, or if other potassium-wasting drugs are used concurrently. Potassium supplementation may be necessary in some patients.

Severe metabolic acidosis or acidotic coma may occur rarely during long-term carbonic anhydrase inhibitor therapy and may be corrected by administration of bicarbonate.

The following side/adverse effects have been selected on the basis of their potential clinical significance (possible signs and symptoms in parentheses where appropriate)—not necessarily inclusive:*

Legend:
**I** = Acetazolamide
**II** = Dichlorphenamide
**III** = Methazolamide

| | I | II | III |
|---|---|---|---|
| **Medical attention needed** | | | |
| *Acidosis* (shortness of breath, troubled breathing)# | R | R | R |
| *Blood dyscrasias* (fever and sore throat, unusual bruising or bleeding)† | R | R | R |
| *Bloody or black, tarry stools* | R | R | R |
| *Cholestatic jaundice* (darkening of urine, pale stools, yellow eyes or skin) | R | U | U |
| *Clumsiness or unsteadiness* | R | R | R |
| *Confusion* | R | R | R |
| *Convulsions* | R | R | R |
| *Crystalluria, renal calculus, or sulfonamide-like nephrotoxicity* (blood in urine, difficult urination, pain in lower back, pain or burning while urinating, sudden decrease in amount of urine)† | L | L | L |
| *Hypersensitivity* (fever, hives, itching, skin rash or sores) | R | R | R |
| *Hypokalemia* (dryness of mouth, increased thirst, irregular heartbeats, mood or mental changes, muscle cramps or pain, nausea or vomiting, unusual tiredness or weakness, weak pulse)‡ | R | R | R |
| *Mental depression* | L | L | L |
| *Nearsightedness*§ | R | R | R |
| *Ringing or buzzing in ears* | R | R | R |
| *Severe muscle weakness or trembling* | R | R | R |
| *Unusual tiredness or weakness*** | M | M | M |
| **Medical attention needed only if continuing or bothersome** | | | |
| *Constipation* | U | R | U |
| *Diarrhea* | M | M | M |
| *Dizziness or lightheadedness* | U | L | L |
| *Drowsiness* | L | L | L |
| *Feeling of choking or lump in throat* | U | R | U |
| *General feeling of discomfort or illness* | M | M | M |
| *Headache* | R | R | R |
| *Increase in frequency of urination or amount of urine* | M | M | R |
| *Increased sensitivity of eyes to sunlight* | R | U | R |
| *Loss of appetite* | M | M | M |
| *Loss of taste and smell* | R | R | R |
| *Metallic taste in mouth* | M | M | M |
| *Nausea or vomiting* | M | M | M |
| *Nervousness or irritability* | U | R | U |
| *Numbness, tingling, or burning in hands, fingers, feet, toes, mouth, tongue, lips, or anus*† | M | M | M |
| *Weight loss* | M | M | M |

*Acetazolamide is the most widely used carbonic anhydrase inhibitor; most of the data concerning side effects have been reported for that medication. The comparatively infrequent reports of side effects with other agents of this group may reflect their less frequent usage rather than actual reduced incidence. The pharmacologic similarity of these medications suggests that side effects occurring with one may potentially occur with the others. However, many side effects may not occur with the same severity or frequency with all carbonic anhydrase inhibitors, and patients unable to tolerate one of these medications may be able to tolerate another. Frequency of side effects (generalized): M = more frequent; L = less frequent; R = rare; U = unknown.

†May be more likely to occur with acetazolamide and least likely to occur with methazolamide.

‡May be more likely to occur with dichlorphenamide.

§Transient myopia may occur when therapy is initiated and usually responds to a reduction in dosage or withdrawal of therapy. Transient myopia may not recur if therapy is restarted.

#May be less likely to occur with dichlorphenamide.

**Usually part of a general feeling of malaise induced by these agents but should be evaluated because rarely may indicate acidosis, blood dyscrasias, or hypokalemia.

## Patient Consultation

As an aid to patient consultation, refer to *Advice for the Patient, Carbonic Anhydrase Inhibitors (Systemic)*.

In providing consultation, consider emphasizing the following selected information (» = major clinical significance):

**Before using this medication**
» Conditions affecting use, especially:
   Sensitivity to carbonic anhydrase inhibitors, antibacterial sulfonamides, thiazide diuretics, or other sulfonamide-derivative diuretics
   Pregnancy—Studies in animals have shown teratogenic (skeletal anomalies) and embryocidal effects
   Breast-feeding—Use is not recommended, because these medicines may be distributed into breast milk and have the potential for serious adverse reactions
   Other medications, especially amphetamines, mecamylamine, methenamine, or quinidine
   Other medical problems, especially adrenal gland failure or adrenocortical insufficiency; hepatic disease, including cirrhosis or impairment; hyperchloremic acidosis; hypokalemia, hyponatremia, or other electrolyte imbalance; renal calculi, calcium-containing, or history of; or renal failure, disease, or impairment

**Proper use of this medication**
» Importance of not taking more medication than the amount prescribed
   Taking medication with meals to lessen gastrointestinal upset
   How to minimize inconvenience of unwanted diuresis
» Proper dosing
   Missed dose: Taking as soon as possible; not taking if almost time for next dose; not doubling doses
» Proper storage

**Precautions while using this medication**
» Caution if drowsiness, dizziness, lightheadedness, or tiredness occurs
   Regular visits to physician to check progress during therapy
» Possibility of hypokalemia
   Diabetics: May increase blood and urine glucose concentrations
   Importance of adequate fluid intake during therapy to help prevent kidney stones
   Checking with physician before discontinuing acetazolamide (when used as anticonvulsant); gradual dosage reduction may be desirable

**Side/adverse effects**
   Signs of potential side effects, especially acidosis; blood dyscrasias; bloody or black, tarry stools; cholestatic jaundice; clumsiness or unsteadiness; confusion; convulsions; crystalluria, renal calculus, sulfonamide-like nephrotoxicity; hypersensitivity; hypokalemia; mental depression; nearsightedness; ringing or buzzing in ears; severe muscle weakness or trembling; or unusual tiredness or weakness

## General Dosing Information

Carbonic anhydrase inhibitors are usually used concurrently with other antiglaucoma agents including miotics, mydriatics, and osmotic agents.

Dosage should be adjusted according to the requirements and response of the individual patient as indicated by measurement of ocular tension and symptomatology.

Carbonic anhydrase inhibitors may be given with meals to minimize gastrointestinal upset.

Maintenance of a high fluid intake may be advisable, especially in patients with hypercalciuria or gout, to reduce the risk of renal calculi.

Patients unable to tolerate one carbonic anhydrase inhibitor because of side effects may be able to tolerate another.

If a satisfactory lowering of intraocular pressure is not achieved or maintained with one carbonic anhydrase inhibitor, one of the other agents in this group may provide a beneficial effect.

It is recommended that various brands of acetazolamide marketed by different manufacturers not be used interchangeably unless data indicating therapeutic equivalence are available; bioequivalence problems have been reported.

It is recommended that carbonic anhydrase inhibitor therapy be discontinued if hematopoietic reactions, fever, skin rash, or renal problems occur.

If potassium supplementation is needed in a patient receiving a carbonic anhydrase inhibitor, the fact that plasma chloride concentration may be elevated should be kept in mind and a potassium preparation chosen that does not contain chloride.

---

### *ACETAZOLAMIDE*

## Summary of Differences

Indications: Also indicated as an anticonvulsant, to prevent or reduce severity of symptoms of acute altitude sickness, to treat toxicity caused by weakly acidic medications, to treat familial periodic paralysis, and to prevent uric acid or cystine renal calculi.
Side effects: See *Side/Adverse Effects*.

## Additional Dosing Information

See also *General Dosing Information*.

When acetazolamide is added to existing anticonvulsant therapy, an initial daily dose of 4 to 5 mg per kg of body weight per day in addition to existing medication is recommended. Dosage may be increased as necessary. Changes from other anticonvulsants to acetazolamide or withdrawal of acetazolamide therapy should be gradual to prevent increased seizure activity and possible status epilepticus.

Tolerance to the anticonvulsant effect of acetazolamide develops rapidly, over weeks or months in some patients.

For oral dosage forms only:
• Both the acetazolamide tablets and extended-release capsules are indicated for use in glaucoma and for prophylaxis and treatment of acute altitude sickness. Although the extended release capsules may be better tolerated than the acetazolamide tablets or the tablets of the other carbonic anhydrase inhibitors, they may be less effective in some patients.
For parenteral dosage forms only:
• Direct intravenous administration is preferred; intramuscular injection is not recommended, because it is painful due to the alkaline pH of the solution.
• Parenteral administration is usually used when the patient cannot take oral medication or when a rapid initial intraocular pressure-lowering action is necessary. Therapy is usually continued with oral acetazolamide, depending on the patient's condition and response.

## Oral Dosage Forms

Note: Bracketed uses in the *Dosage Forms* section refer to categories of use and/or indications that are not included in U.S. product labeling.

### ACETAZOLAMIDE EXTENDED-RELEASE CAPSULES

**Usual adult and adolescent dose**
Antiglaucoma agent—
Oral, 500 mg two times a day, in the morning and evening.
Note: In the treatment of glaucoma, dosage greater than 1 gram per day usually does not produce an increased effect.
Altitude sickness, acute, prophylactic and therapeutic agent[1]—
Oral, 500 mg one or two times a day.
Note: During rapid ascent, such as in rescue or military operations, 1,000 mg a day is recommended. Therapy should preferably be initiated 24 to 48 hours before ascent and, while at high altitude, continued for 48 hours or longer as necessary to control symptoms.

The use of acetazolamide for rapid ascent does not obviate the need for prompt descent if severe forms of high altitude sickness, such as high altitude pulmonary edema (HAPE) or high altitude cerebral edema, occur.

**Usual pediatric dose**
Safety and efficacy have not been established.

### Strength(s) usually available
U.S.—
500 mg (Rx) [*Diamox Sequels*].
Canada—
500 mg (Rx) [*Diamox Sequels*].

### Packaging and storage
Store between 15 and 30 °C (59 and 86 °F), in a well-closed container, unless otherwise specified by manufacturer.

### Auxiliary labeling
• May cause drowsiness.

## ACETAZOLAMIDE TABLETS USP

### Usual adult and adolescent dose
Antiglaucoma agent—
Open-angle glaucoma:
Initial—Oral, 250 mg one to four times a day.
Maintenance—To be titrated according to patient response; lower doses may be sufficient.
Secondary glaucoma and preoperative lowering of intraocular pressure:
Oral, 250 mg every four hours. Some patients may respond to 250 mg two times a day. In some acute cases, an initial dose of 500 mg followed by 125 or 250 mg every four hours may be preferable.
Malignant (ciliary block) glaucoma:
Oral, 250 mg four times a day to reduce intraocular pressure.
Anticonvulsant—
Oral, 4 to 30 mg (usually 10 mg initially) per kg of body weight a day in up to 4 divided doses; usually 375 mg to 1 gram a day.
Altitude sickness, acute, prophylactic and therapeutic agent[1]—
Oral, 250 mg two to four times a day.
Note: During rapid ascent, such as in rescue or military operations, 1,000 mg a day is recommended. Therapy should preferably be initiated 24 to 48 hours before ascent and, while at high altitude, continued for 48 hours or longer as necessary to control symptoms.

The use of acetazolamide for rapid ascent does not obviate the need for prompt descent if severe forms of high altitude sickness, such as high altitude pulmonary edema (HAPE) or high altitude cerebral edema, occur.
[Antiparalytic][1]—
Oral, 250 mg to 1.5 grams a day in divided doses.
[Antiurolithic][1]—
Oral, 250 mg daily at bedtime.
Note: For use as an anticonvulsant or in open-angle glaucoma, dosage greater than 1 gram per day usually does not produce an increased effect.

### Usual pediatric dose
Glaucoma—
Oral, 8 to 30 mg per kg of body weight, usually 10 to 15 mg per kg, or 300 to 900 mg per square meter of body surface area a day in divided doses.
Anticonvulsant—
See *Usual adult and adolescent dose*.

### Strength(s) usually available
U.S.—
125 mg (Rx) [*Diamox* (scored); GENERIC].
250 mg (Rx) [*Ak-Zol; Dazamide; Diamox* (scored); *Storzolamide;* GENERIC].
Canada—
250 mg (Rx) [*Acetazolam; Apo-Acetazolamide; Diamox*].

### Packaging and storage
Store between 15 and 30 °C (59 and 86 °F), in a well-closed container, unless otherwise specified by manufacturer.

### Preparation of dosage form
For pediatric patients or adults unable to swallow tablets—An acetazolamide oral suspension may be prepared by crushing acetazolamide tablets and suspending the resultant powder in a highly flavored syrup (cherry, raspberry, chocolate, etc.). Up to 500 mg may be suspended in 5 mL of syrup, but a suspension containing 250 mg per 5 mL is

more palatable. Such a suspension is stable for 1 week. Refrigeration may improve the taste but does not increase or lengthen stability. Elixirs or other vehicles containing alcohol or glycerin will not provide a palatable suspension.

**Auxiliary labeling**
• May cause drowsiness.

## Parenteral Dosage Forms

Note: Bracketed uses in the *Dosage Forms* section refer to categories of use and/or indications that are not included in U.S. product labeling.

### ACETAZOLAMIDE SODIUM STERILE USP

**Usual adult and adolescent dose**
Antiglaucoma agent—
    For rapid initial lowering of intraocular pressure: Intravenous, the equivalent of acetazolamide—500 mg.
Note: Parenteral administration may be repeated in two to four hours in some acute cases, but therapy is usually continued with oral acetazolamide, depending on the patient's response.
[Diuretic (urinary alkalinizing)]—
    Intravenous, 5 mg per kg of body weight or as required to achieve and maintain a forced alkaline diuresis.
Note: For other uses or when the patient is unable to take oral medication, acetazolamide may be given parenterally in dosages equivalent to those recommended for the oral tablets. (See *Acetazolamide Tablets USP*.)

**Usual pediatric dose**
Antiglaucoma agent—
    Acute glaucoma: Intravenous, the equivalent of acetazolamide—5 to 10 mg per kg of body weight every six hours.
[Diuretic (urinary alkalinizing)]—
    Intravenous, the equivalent of acetazolamide: 5 mg per kg of body weight or 150 mg per square meter of body surface area once a day in the morning for one or two days alternated with a drug-free day.

**Strength(s) usually available**
U.S.—
    500 mg (Rx) [Diamox; GENERIC].
Canada—
    500 mg (Rx) [Diamox].

**Packaging and storage**
Prior to reconstitution, store below 40 °C (104 °F), preferably between 15 and 30 °C (59 and 86 °F), unless otherwise specified by manufacturer.

**Preparation of dosage form**
Sterile Acetazolamide Sodium USP is reconstituted for parenteral use by adding at least 5 mL of Sterile Water for Injection USP to the vial and shaking to dissolve. A solution prepared using 5 mL of diluent contains the equivalent of 100 mg of acetazolamide per mL.

**Stability**
After reconstitution, solutions retain their potency for 1 week if refrigerated. However, because they contain no preservative, use within 24 hours is strongly recommended.

¹Not included in Canadian product labeling.

## Summary of Differences
Side effects: See *Side/Adverse Effects*.

## Oral Dosage Forms
### DICHLORPHENAMIDE TABLETS USP

**Usual adult and adolescent dose**
Antiglaucoma agent—
    Initial: 100 to 200 mg for the first dose followed by 100 mg every twelve hours until the desired response is obtained.
    Maintenance: 25 to 50 mg one to three times a day.

**Usual pediatric dose**
Safety and efficacy have not been established.

**Strength(s) usually available**
U.S.—
    50 mg (Rx) [Daranide (scored)].
Canada—
    Not commercially available.

**Packaging and storage**
Store below 40 °C (104 °F), preferably between 15 and 30 °C (59 and 86 °F), in a well-closed container, unless otherwise specified by manufacturer.

**Auxiliary labeling**
• May cause drowsiness.

## Summary of Differences
Side effects: See *Side/Adverse Effects*.

## Oral Dosage Forms
### METHAZOLAMIDE TABLETS USP

**Usual adult and adolescent dose**
Antiglaucoma agent—
    Oral, 50 to 100 mg two or three times a day.

**Usual pediatric dose**
Safety and efficacy have not been established.

**Strength(s) usually available**
U.S.—
    25 mg (Rx) [MZM; Neptazane; GENERIC].
    50 mg (Rx) [MZM; Neptazane (scored); GENERIC].
Canada—
    50 mg (Rx) [Neptazane].

**Packaging and storage**
Store between 15 and 30 °C (59 and 86 °F), in a well-closed container, unless otherwise specified by manufacturer.

**Auxiliary labeling**
• May cause drowsiness.

Revised: 06/21/94
Interim revision: 01/24/95

# CARBOPLATIN    Systemic

VA CLASSIFICATION (Primary): AN900
Note: For a listing of dosage forms and brand names by country availability, see *Dosage Forms* section(s). For a listing of brand names for the articles in this monograph, refer to the General Index.

## Category
Antineoplastic.

## Indications
Note: Bracketed information in the *Indications* section refers to uses that are not included in U.S. product labeling.

### Accepted
Carcinoma, ovarian (treatment)—Carboplatin is indicated for palliative treatment of ovarian carcinoma refractory to standard chemotherapy that did or did not include cisplatin. It is also indicated for initial treatment of advanced ovarian carcinoma in established combination with other approved chemotherapeutic agents.

[Carcinoma, lung, small cell (treatment)][1]
[Carcinoma, lung, non–small cell (treatment)][1]
[Carcinoma, head and neck (treatment)][1]
[Carcinoma, testicular (treatment)][1] or
[Seminoma (treatment)][1]—Carboplatin is used for treatment of small cell and non–small cell lung carcinoma, head and neck tumors, nonseminomatous testicular carcinoma, and seminoma.

[1]Not included in Canadian product labeling.

## Pharmacology/Pharmacokinetics

### Physicochemical characteristics
Molecular weight—371.25.

### Mechanism of action/Effect
Carboplatin resembles an alkylating agent. Although the exact mechanism of action is unknown, action is thought to be similar to that of the bifunctional alkylating agents, that is, possible cross-linking and interference with the function of DNA. It is cell cycle–phase nonspecific.

### Protein binding
Very low; however, platinum from carboplatin is irreversibly bound to plasma proteins and is slowly eliminated with a minimum half-life of 5 days.

### Biotransformation
By hydrolysis in solution (aquation), at a rate slower than occurs with cisplatin, to the active species that reacts with DNA.

### Half-life
Alpha phase—1.1 to 2.0 hours.
Beta phase—2.6 to 5.9 hours.

### Elimination
Renal (71% within 24 hours at creatinine clearances of 60 mL per minute and greater).

## Precautions to Consider

### Cross-sensitivity and/or related problems
Patients sensitive to cisplatin or other platinum-containing compounds may be sensitive to carboplatin also.

### Carcinogenicity
Secondary malignancies are potential delayed effects of many antineoplastic agents, although it is not clear whether the effect is related to their mutagenic or immunosuppressive action. The effect of dose and duration of therapy is also unknown, although risk seems to increase with long-term use. Although information is limited, available data seem to indicate that the carcinogenic risk is greatest with the alkylating agents.

### Mutagenicity
Both *in vivo* and *in vitro* studies have shown carboplatin to be mutagenic.

### Pregnancy/Reproduction
Fertility—Gonadal suppression, resulting in amenorrhea or azoospermia, may occur in patients taking antineoplastic therapy, especially with the alkylating agents. In general, these effects appear to be related to dose and length of therapy and may be irreversible. Prediction of the degree of testicular or ovarian function impairment is complicated by the common use of combinations of several antineoplastics, which makes it difficult to assess the effects of individual agents.

Pregnancy—Carboplatin is embryotoxic and teratogenic in rats.
First trimester: It is usually recommended that use of antineoplastics, especially combination chemotherapy, be avoided whenever possible, especially during the first trimester. Although information is limited because of the relatively few instances of antineoplastic administration during pregnancy, the mutagenic, teratogenic, and carcinogenic potential of these medications must be considered.
Other hazards to the fetus include adverse reactions seen in adults.
In general, use of a contraceptive is recommended during cytotoxic drug therapy.
FDA Pregnancy Category D.

### Breast-feeding
Although very little information is available regarding distribution of antineoplastic agents into breast milk, breast-feeding is not recommended while carboplatin is being administered because of the risks to the infant (adverse effects, mutagenicity, carcinogenicity). It is not known whether carboplatin is distributed into breast milk.

### Pediatrics
No information is available on the relationship of age to the effects of carboplatin in pediatric patients.

### Geriatrics
Incidence of peripheral neurotoxicity is increased and myelotoxicity may be more severe in patients greater than 65 years of age. In addition, elderly patients are more likely to have age-related renal function impairment, which may require dosage reduction and careful monitoring of blood counts in patients receiving carboplatin.

### Dental
The bone marrow depressant effects of carboplatin may result in an increased incidence of microbial infection, delayed healing, and gingival bleeding. Dental work, whenever possible, should be completed prior to initiation of therapy or deferred until blood counts have returned to normal. Patients should be instructed in proper oral hygiene during treatment, including caution in use of regular toothbrushes, dental floss, and toothpicks.
Carboplatin may also rarely cause mucositis or stomatitis associated with considerable discomfort.

### Drug interactions and/or related problems
The following drug interactions and/or related problems have been selected on the basis of their potential clinical significance (possible mechanism in parentheses where appropriate)—not necessarily inclusive (» = major clinical significance):
Note: Combinations containing any of the following medications, depending on the amount present, may also interact with this medication.

Blood dyscrasia–causing medications (See *Appendix II*)
    (leukopenic and/or thrombocytopenic effects of carboplatin may be increased with concurrent or recent therapy if these medications cause the same effects; dosage adjustment of carboplatin, if necessary, should be based on blood counts)

» Bone marrow depressants, other (See *Appendix II*) or
Radiation therapy
    (concurrent use may increase the total effects of these medications and radiation therapy; dosage reduction is recommended)

Cisplatin
    (incidence of carboplatin-induced neurotoxicity or ototoxicity is increased in patients previously treated with cisplatin; use of carboplatin worsens pre-existing cisplatin-induced neurotoxicity [in about 30% of those patients] or ototoxicity; additive nephrotoxicity has not been reported)

Nephrotoxic medications, other (See *Appendix II*) or
Ototoxic medications, other (See *Appendix II*)
    (concurrent and/or sequential administration may increase the potential for ototoxicity and nephrotoxicity)

Vaccines, killed virus
    (because normal defense mechanisms may be suppressed by carboplatin therapy, the patient's antibody response to the vaccine may be decreased. The interval between discontinuation of medications that cause immunosuppression and restoration of the patient's ability to respond to the vaccine depends on the intensity and type of immunosuppression-causing medication used, the underlying disease, and other factors; estimates vary from 3 months to 1 year)

» Vaccines, live virus

(because normal defense mechanisms may be suppressed by carboplatin therapy, concurrent use with a live virus vaccine may potentiate the replication of the vaccine virus, may increase the side/adverse effects of the vaccine virus, and/or may decrease the patient's antibody response to the vaccine; immunization of these patients should be undertaken only with extreme caution after careful review of the patient's hematologic status and only with the knowledge and consent of the physician managing the carboplatin therapy. The interval between discontinuation of medications that cause immunosuppression and restoration of the patient's ability to respond to the vaccine depends on the intensity and type of immunosuppression-causing medication used, the underlying disease, and other factors; estimates vary from 3 months to 1 year. Patients with leukemia in remission should not receive live virus vaccine until at least 3 months after their last chemotherapy. In addition, immunization with oral poliovirus vaccine should be postponed in persons in close contact with the patient, especially family members)

**Laboratory value alterations**

The following have been selected on the basis of their potential clinical significance (possible effect in parentheses where appropriate)—not necessarily inclusive (» = major clinical significance):

With physiology/laboratory test values

Bilirubin concentrations, serum and
Alkaline phosphatase values, serum and
Aspartate aminotransferase (AST [SGOT]) values, serum

(may be increased; increases are usually mild and are reversible in 50% of cases; severe abnormalities occur at carboplatin doses of more than 4 times the recommended dose)

Blood urea nitrogen (BUN) concentrations and
Creatinine clearance and
Creatinine concentrations, serum

(may be increased, indicating nephrotoxicity; usually mild; reversible in about 50% of cases)

Calcium and
Magnesium and
Potassium and
Sodium

(serum concentrations may be decreased)

**Medical considerations/Contraindications**

The medical considerations/contraindications included here have been selected on the basis of their potential clinical significance (reasons given in parentheses where appropriate)—not necessarily inclusive (» = major clinical significance).

*Risk-benefit should be considered when the following medical problems exist:*

Ascites or
Pleural effusion

(increased risk of toxicity)

» Bleeding, significant
» Bone marrow depression
» Chickenpox, existing or recent (including recent exposure) or
» Herpes zoster

(risk of severe generalized disease)

Hearing impairment

» Infection
» Renal function impairment

(reduced elimination; increased bone marrow depression; incidence and severity of nephrotoxicity may be increased. A lower dosage of carboplatin is recommended in patients with impaired renal function and careful monitoring of blood counts between courses is recommended)

Sensitivity to carboplatin

» Caution should be used also in patients who have had previous cytotoxic drug therapy or radiation therapy.

**Patient monitoring**

The following are especially important in patient monitoring (other tests may be warranted in some patients, depending on condition; » = major clinical significance):

Audiometric testing

(recommended prior to initiation of therapy and if ototoxicity is suspected during therapy)

Blood urea nitrogen (BUN) concentrations and
» Creatinine clearance and
Creatinine concentrations, serum

(recommended prior to initiation of therapy and before each course of carboplatin to adjust dosage and detect renal toxicity)

Calcium concentrations, serum and
Magnesium concentrations, serum and
Potassium concentrations, serum and
Sodium concentrations, serum

(recommended at periodic intervals during therapy)

» Hematocrit or hemoglobin and
» Leukocyte count, total and, if appropriate, differential, and
» Platelet count

(determinations recommended prior to initiation of therapy and at periodic intervals during therapy; frequency varies according to clinical state, agent, dose, and other agents being used concurrently)

Neurologic function studies

(recommended prior to initiation of therapy and at periodic intervals during therapy)

## Side/Adverse Effects

Note: Many "side effects" of antineoplastic therapy are unavoidable and represent the medication's pharmacologic action. Some of these (for example, leukopenia and thrombocytopenia) are actually used as parameters to aid in individual dosage titration.

Carboplatin infrequently causes mild renal toxicity, which may be detected initially only by means of renal function tests.

The following side/adverse effects have been selected on the basis of their potential clinical significance (possible signs and symptoms in parentheses where appropriate)—not necessarily inclusive:

**Those indicating need for medical attention**

Incidence more frequent—dose-related

*Anemia* (usually not symptomatic; less frequently, unusual tiredness or weakness, which is usually related to asthenia); *leukopenia or neutropenia* (usually not symptomatic; less frequently, fever or chills; cough or hoarseness; lower back or side pain; painful or difficult urination); *pain at site of injection; thrombocytopenia* (usually not symptomatic; less frequently, unusual bleeding or bruising; black, tarry stools; blood in urine or stools; pinpoint red spots on skin)

Note: *Anemia* may be cumulative; transfusions are frequently necessary.

With *leukopenia* and *thrombocytopenia,* nadir of leukocyte and platelet counts occurs after 21 days and counts usually recover by 30 days after a dose. Nadir of granulocyte counts usually occurs after 21 to 28 days and counts usually recover by day 35.

*Leukopenia* and *thrombocytopenia* are dose-dependent and cumulative; in a small percentage of patients (less than 10%) they are unpredictable.

Incidence less frequent

*Allergic reaction* (skin rash or itching; rarely, wheezing); *peripheral neurotoxicity* (numbness or tingling in fingers or toes); *ototoxicity* (usually not symptomatic, but rarely may be associated with ringing in ears)

Note: *An allergic reaction* occurs within minutes of administration.

*Neurotoxicity* may be cumulative.

With *ototoxicity,* hearing loss usually occurs first with high frequencies (above speech tones) and may be unilateral or bilateral.

Incidence rare

*Blurred vision; mucositis or stomatitis* (sores in mouth and on lips)

**Those indicating need for medical attention only if they continue or are bothersome**

Incidence more frequent

*Asthenia* (unusual tiredness or weakness); *nausea and vomiting*

Note: Less frequently, *asthenia* may be related to anemia.

*Nausea and vomiting* occur in about 65% of patients; severe in about one-third of those. Nausea alone occurs in about 10-15% of patients. Usually begin 6 to 12 hours after a dose, and vomiting may persist for 24 hours. May be treated or prevented by antiemetic medication.

Incidence less frequent

*Constipation or diarrhea; loss of appetite*

**Those not indicating need for medical attention**

Incidence less frequent

*Loss of hair*

# Patient Consultation

As an aid to patient consultation, refer to *Advice for the Patient, Carboplatin (Systemic)*.

In providing consultation, consider emphasizing the following selected information (» = major clinical significance):

### Before using this medication
» Conditions affecting use, especially:

Sensitivity to cisplatin or other platinum-containing compounds, or to carboplatin

Pregnancy—Use not recommended because of mutagenic, teratogenic, and carcinogenic potential; advisability of using contraception; telling physician immediately if pregnancy is suspected

Breast-feeding—Not recommended because of risk of serious side effects

Use in the elderly—Increased incidence of peripheral neurotoxicity and severity of myelotoxicity

Other medications, especially other bone marrow depressants

Other medical problems, especially chickenpox, herpes zoster, infection, or renal function impairment

### Proper use of this medication
Caution if taking combination therapy; taking each medication at the right time

Frequency of nausea and vomiting; importance of continuing medication despite stomach upset
» Proper dosing

### Precautions while using this medication
» Importance of close monitoring by the physician
» Avoiding immunizations unless approved by physician; other persons in patient's household should avoid immunizations with oral poliovirus vaccine; avoiding persons who have taken oral poliovirus vaccine or wearing a protective mask that covers nose and mouth

*Caution if bone marrow depression occurs:*
» Avoiding exposure to persons with bacterial infections, especially during periods of low blood counts; checking with physician immediately if fever or chills, cough or hoarseness, lower back or side pain, or painful or difficult urination occur
» Checking with physician immediately if unusual bleeding or bruising; black, tarry stools; blood in urine or stools; or pinpoint red spots on skin occur

Caution in use of regular toothbrush, dental floss, or toothpick; physician, dentist, or nurse may suggest alternatives; checking with physician before having dental work done

Not touching eyes or inside of nose unless hands washed immediately before

Using caution to avoid accidental cuts with use of sharp objects such as safety razor or fingernail or toenail cutters

Avoiding contact sports or other situations where bruising or injury might occur

### Side/adverse effects
May cause adverse effects such as ear and kidney problems, blood problems, and cancer; importance of discussing possible effects with physician

Signs of potential side effects, especially anemia, leukopenia or neutropenia, thrombocytopenia, pain at site of injection, allergic reaction, peripheral neurotoxicity, ototoxicity, blurred vision, and mucositis or stomatitis

Physician or nurse can help in dealing with side effects

Possibility of hair loss; should return after treatment has ended

# General Dosing Information

It is recommended that carboplatin be administered to patients under supervision of a physician experienced in cancer chemotherapy. It is also recommended that equipment and medications (including epinephrine, oxygen, antihistamines, and intravenous adrenocorticoids) necessary for treatment of a possible anaphylactic reaction be readily available at each administration of carboplatin.

Dosage must be adjusted to meet the individual requirements of each patient, on the basis of clinical response and appearance or severity of toxicity.

Carboplatin may be used in combination with other agents in various regimens. As a result, incidence and/or severity of side effects may be altered and different dosages (usually reduced) may be used.

It is recommended that carboplatin be administered as an intravenous infusion, usually over 15 to 60 minutes. No pre- or post-treatment hydration or forced diuresis is required.

Carboplatin has also been administered as a continuous intravenous infusion over 24 hours or by dividing the total dose into 5 consecutive daily pulse doses; this method of administration appears to reduce nausea and vomiting but not nephrotoxicity or ototoxicity.

It is recommended that courses of carboplatin be administered no more frequently than every 4 weeks, to allow recovery of bone marrow.

Administration of subsequent doses of carboplatin is not recommended before platelet levels return to at least 100,000 per cubic millimeter and leukocyte levels to at least 2000 per cubic millimeter.

Special precautions are recommended in patients who develop thrombocytopenia as a result of administration of carboplatin. These may include extreme care in performing invasive procedures; regular inspection of intravenous sites, skin (including perirectal area), and mucous membrane surfaces for signs of bleeding or bruising; limiting frequency of venipuncture and avoiding intramuscular injections; testing urine, emesis, stool, and secretions for occult blood; care in use of regular toothbrushes, dental floss, toothpicks, safety razors, and fingernail and toenail cutters; avoiding constipation; and using caution to prevent falls and other injuries. Such patients should avoid alcohol and aspirin intake because of the risk of gastrointestinal bleeding. Platelet transfusions may be required.

Patients who develop leukopenia should be observed carefully for signs of infection. Antibiotic support may be required. In neutropenic patients who develop fever, broad-spectrum antibiotic coverage should be initiated empirically, pending bacterial cultures and appropriate diagnostic tests.

### Safety considerations for handling this medication
There is limited but increasing evidence and concern that personnel involved in preparation and administration of parenteral antineoplastics may be at some risk because of the potential mutagenicity, teratogenicity, and/or carcinogenicity of these agents, although the actual risk is unknown. USP advisory panels recommend cautious handling both in preparation and disposal of antineoplastic agents. Precautions that have been suggested include:
• Use of a biological containment cabinet during reconstitution and dilution of parenteral medications and wearing of disposable surgical gloves and masks.
• Use of proper technique to prevent contamination of the medication, work area, and operator during transfer between containers (including proper training of personnel in this technique).
• Cautious and proper disposal of needles, syringes, vials, ampuls, and unused medication.
A number of medical centers have developed detailed guidelines for handling of antineoplastic agents.

# Parenteral Dosage Forms
## CARBOPLATIN INJECTION

### Usual adult dose
Carcinoma, ovarian—

Intravenous, 360 mg per square meter of body surface once every four weeks (Day 1).

Note: An initial dose of 250 mg per square meter of body surface is recommended in patients with creatinine clearance of 41–59 mL per minute; an initial dose of 200 mg per square meter of body surface is recommended in patients with creatinine clearance of 16–40 mL per minute.

Geriatric patients may require lower doses.

A suggested dosage adjustment schedule for subsequent doses is:

| Nadir after Prior Dose (cells per cubic millimeter) | | % of Prior Dose to Be Given |
|---|---|---|
| Neutrophils | Platelets | |
| >2000 | >100,000 | 125 |
| 500–2000 | 50,000–100,000 | 100 |
| <500 | <50,000 | 75 |

Note: Only one dose escalation should be made.

### Usual pediatric dose
Dosage has not been established.

### Strength(s) usually available
U.S.—

Not commercially available.

Canada—

10 mg per mL (Rx) [*Paraplatin-AQ*].

### Packaging and storage
Store between 15 and 30 °C (59 and 86 °F), unless otherwise specified by manufacturer. Protect from light. Protect from freezing.

## Stability

Caution—A black platinum precipitate will form if carboplatin comes in contact with aluminum.

## Incompatibilities

Do not use needles, intravenous sets, or equipment containing aluminum for administration since carboplatin is incompatible with aluminum.

## CARBOPLATIN FOR INJECTION

### Usual adult dose

Carcinoma, ovarian—

Advanced, initial treatment: Intravenous, 300 mg per square meter of body surface once every four weeks (Day 1) for six cycles, in combination with cyclophosphamide 600 mg per square meter of body surface intravenously once every four weeks (Day 1) for six cycles.

Refractory to other chemotherapy: Intravenous, 360 mg per square meter of body surface once every four weeks (Day 1).

Note: An initial dose of 250 mg per square meter of body surface is recommended in patients with creatinine clearance of 41–59 mL per minute; an initial dose of 200 mg per square meter of body surface is recommended in patients with creatinine clearance of 16–40 mL per minute.

A suggested dosage adjustment schedule for subsequent doses is:

| Nadir after Prior Dose (cells per cubic millimeter) | | % of Prior Dose to Be Given |
|---|---|---|
| Neutrophils | Platelets | |
| >2000 | >100,000 | 125 |
| 500–2000 | 50,000–100,000 | 100 |
| <500 | <50,000 | 75 |

Note: Only one dose escalation should be made.

Geriatric patients may require lower doses.

### Usual pediatric dose

Dosage has not been established.

### Size(s) usually available

U.S.—

50 mg (Rx) [*Paraplatin* (mannitol, equal quantity by weight)].
150 mg (Rx) [*Paraplatin* (mannitol, equal quantity by weight)].
450 mg (Rx) [*Paraplatin* (mannitol, equal quantity by weight)].

Canada—

50 mg (Rx) [*Paraplatin* (mannitol, equal quantity by weight)].
150 mg (Rx) [*Paraplatin* (mannitol, equal quantity by weight)].
450 mg (Rx) [*Paraplatin* (mannitol, equal quantity by weight)].

### Packaging and storage

Store between 15 and 30 °C (59 and 86 °F), unless otherwise specified by manufacturer. Protect from light.

### Preparation of dosage form

Carboplatin for injection is reconstituted for intravenous use by adding 5, 15, or 45 mL of sterile water for injection, 5% dextrose injection, or 0.9% sodium chloride injection to the 50-mg, 150-mg, or 450-mg vial, respectively, producing a solution containing 10 mg of carboplatin per mL. The resulting solution may be further diluted to a concentration as low as 500 mcg (0.5 mg) per mL with 5% dextrose injection or 0.9% sodium chloride injection if further dilution for administration by intravenous infusion is required.

### Stability

Reconstituted solutions of carboplatin are stable for 8 hours at 25 °C (77 °F).

Caution—A black platinum precipitate will form if carboplatin comes in contact with aluminum.

### Incompatibilities

Do not use needles, intravenous sets, or equipment containing aluminum for administration since carboplatin is incompatible with aluminum.

## Selected Bibliography

Canetta R, Gragman K, Smaldone L, Rozencweig M. Carboplatin: current status and future prospects. Cancer Treat Rev 1988; 15 (Suppl B): 17-32.

Woloschuk DMM, Pruemer JM, Cluxton RJ. Carboplatin: a new cisplatin analog. Drug Intell Clin Pharm 1988 Nov; 22: 843-9.

Wagstaff AJ, Ward A, Benfield P, Heel RC. Carboplatin. A preliminary review of its pharmacodynamic and pharmacokinetic properties and therapeutic efficacy in the treatment of cancer. Drugs 1989; 37: 162-90.

Revised: 06/02/92
Interim revision: 05/02/94

---

# CARBOPROST Systemic

VA CLASSIFICATION (Primary/Secondary): HS875/GU600

Note: For a listing of dosage forms and brand names by country availability, see *Dosage Forms* section(s). For a listing of brand names for the articles in this monograph, refer to the General Index.

## Category

Oxytocic; abortifacient; antihemorrhagic (postpartum and postabortal uterine bleeding).

## Indications

Note: Bracketed information in the *Indications* section refers to uses that are not included in U.S. product labeling.

### Accepted

Abortion or

[Abortion, incomplete (treatment)][1]—Carboprost is used for aborting midtrimester pregnancy (between the thirteenth and twentieth weeks of gestation as calculated from the first day of the last normal menstrual period). Carboprost is also indicated for second trimester abortion when other methods lead to failure of expulsion of the fetus, premature rupture of membranes with insufficient or absent uterine activity, and requirement of a repeat intrauterine instillation of drug for expulsion of the fetus, or when rupture of membranes in the presence of a previable fetus occurs without adequate activity for expulsion. Carboprost can be used for abortion in the early weeks of pregnancy, but its use is associated with an increased incidence of side effects and failures. Carboprost is sometimes used in combination with hypertonic saline, urea, or oxytocin.

Carboprost is used for induction of labor in cases of intrauterine fetal death.

Postpartum hemorrhage (treatment)[1]—Carboprost is indicated to reduce blood loss and correct uterine atony during the postpartum period in patients unresponsive to conventional treatment such as oxytocin, ergonovine, or methylergonovine.

[Hydatidiform mole, benign (treatment)][1] or
[Induction of labor][1] or
[Cervical ripening][1]—Carboprost has been used in the treatment of benign hydatidiform mole, for medically indicated induction of labor at term, and to ripen the cervix prior to abortion procedures such as vacuum curettage. However, experience with the use of carboprost for these indications is limited.

[1]Not included in Canadian product labeling.

## Pharmacology/Pharmacokinetics

### Physicochemical characteristics

Chemical name—Prosta-5,13-dien-1-oic acid, 9,11,15-trihydroxy-15-methyl, (5Z,9 alpha,11 alpha,13E,15S)-, compound with 2-amino-2-(hydroxymethyl)-1,3-propanediol (1:1).

Chemical group—Carboprost tromethamine is the tromethamine salt of the (15S)-15 methyl analog of naturally occurring prostaglandin $F_{2\text{-alpha}}$.

Molecular weight—489.65.

### Mechanism of action/Effect

Carboprost appears to act directly on the myometrium, but this has not been completely established. Carboprost stimulates myometrial contractions in the gravid uterus similar to the contractions occurring in the term uterus during natural labor. These contractions are usually sufficient to cause abortion. Uterine response to prostaglandins increases gradually throughout pregnancy. Carboprost also facilitates cervical dilatation and softening.

### Other actions/effects

Carboprost stimulates the smooth muscle of the gastrointestinal tract, arterioles, and bronchioles.

## Biotransformation

Primarily hepatic oxidation and some enzymatic dehydrogenation in maternal lung tissues; occur more slowly than with prostaglandin $F_{2alpha}$, due to the presence of a 15-methyl group.

## Time to peak concentration

15 to 60 minutes.

## Peak serum concentration

2060 picograms of 15-methyl-prostaglandin $F_{2alpha}$ per mL at 30 minutes after a single intramuscular dose of 250 mcg, declining to 770 picograms per mL after 2 hours; slightly increased to 2663 picograms per mL at 30 minutes post-dosing with a second dose 2 hours later, declining to 1047 picograms per mL after 2 hours.

## Time to peak effect

The mean abortion time with carboprost is about 16 hours.

## Elimination

Primarily renal as metabolites; rapid and nearly complete at 24 hours after intravenous, subcutaneous, or intramuscular dosing.

# Precautions to Consider

## Carcinogenicity

Studies have not been done in either animals or humans.

## Mutagenicity

No evidence of mutagenicity was found in the micronucleus test or Ames assay.

## Pregnancy/Reproduction

Pregnancy—Although studies have not been done in humans, any pregnancy termination with carboprost that fails should be completed by another method.

Proliferation of bone has been reported with clinical use of prostaglandin $E_1$ during prolonged therapy. However, there is no evidence to date that the short-term use of carboprost causes proliferation of bone in the fetus.

Studies in rats and rabbits found that carboprost causes embryotoxicity. Carboprost did not cause teratogenicity in animal studies. Prostaglandins of the E and F series have caused proliferation of bone with high doses in other animal studies.

FDA Pregnancy Category C.

Labor and delivery—Use of high doses may result in excessive uterine tone, causing decreased uterine blood flow and fetal distress. Carboprost is not feticidal and may result in delivery of a live fetus.

## Drug interactions and/or related problems

The following drug interactions and/or related problems have been selected on the basis of their potential clinical significance (possible mechanism in parentheses where appropriate)—not necessarily inclusive (» = major clinical significance):

Oxytocin or other oxytocics
(concurrent use with carboprost may result in uterine hypertonus, possibly causing uterine rupture or cervical laceration, especially in the absence of adequate cervical dilatation; although combinations are sometimes used for therapeutic advantage, patient should be monitored closely when this combination is used)

## Laboratory value alterations

The following have been selected on the basis of their potential clinical significance (possible effect in parentheses where appropriate)—not necessarily inclusive (» = major clinical significance):

With physiology/laboratory test values
Blood pressure, maternal or
Heart rate, maternal
(may be decreased or increased, especially with large doses)

Body temperature
(a temperature increase of greater than 1.1 °C [2 °F] usually occurs within 1 to 16 hours after the first injection, and the temperature returns to normal within several hours after the last injection)

## Medical considerations/Contraindications

The medical considerations/contraindications included here have been selected on the basis of their potential clinical significance (reasons given in parentheses where appropriate)—not necessarily inclusive (» = major clinical significance):

*Except under special circumstances, this medication should not be used when the following medical problems exist:*

» Allergy or intolerance to carboprost or other oxytocics

» Asthma, or history of
(increased risk of bronchospasm)

» Pulmonary disease, active
(use of carboprost may decrease pulmonary blood flow and increase pulmonary arterial pressure)

*Risk-benefit should be considered when the following medical problems exist:*

Adrenal disease, history of
(carboprost stimulates steroid production)

Anemia
(increased incidence of excessive uterine bleeding may occur with the use of prostaglandins in performance of abortion)

» Cardiac disease, active
(decrease in blood pressure and bradycardia may result in cardiovascular collapse and angina pectoris)

Cardiovascular disease, history of or
Hypertension, or history of or
Hypotension, or history of or
Preeclampsia
(may be aggravated by possible vasoconstriction or decreased blood pressure)

Cervical stenosis or
Uterine fibroids or
Uterine surgery, history of
(increased risk of uterine rupture)

Diabetes mellitus, history of

Epilepsy, or history of
(rarely, seizures have occurred during the use of prostaglandins)

Glaucoma
(increase in intraocular pressure and miosis have occurred rarely during the use of prostaglandins)

» Hepatic disease, active, or
Hepatic disease, history of
(metabolism of carboprost may be impaired, resulting in prolonged half-life)

Hypersensitivity to carboprost or
Multiparity
(excessive dosage or use with oxytocin may cause uterine hypertonicity with spasm and tetanic contraction, which can lead to posterior cervical perforations, cervical lacerations, uterine rupture, and hemorrhage)

Jaundice, history of

» Pelvic inflammatory disease, acute
(induction of uterine contractions is not generally recommended)

» Renal disease, active
Renal disease, history of

## Patient monitoring

The following may be especially important in patient monitoring (other tests may be warranted in some patients, depending on condition; » = major clinical significance):

Contractions—frequency, duration and force of and
Temperature, pulse, and blood pressure, maternal and
Uterine tone, resting
(monitoring of these parameters is recommended at frequent intervals during abortion procedure or labor and delivery)

Vaginal examination
(recommended prior to each dose and postabortion or postdelivery to check for signs of cervical trauma)

# Side/Adverse Effects

The following side/adverse effects have been selected on the basis of their potential clinical significance (possible signs and symptoms in parentheses where appropriate)—not necessarily inclusive:

## Those indicating need for medical attention

Incidence less frequent or rare
*Anaphylaxis, generalized* (swelling of face, inside the nose, and eyelids; hives; shortness of breath; trouble in breathing; tightness in chest; wheezing); *bradycardia* (slow heartbeat); *bronchoconstriction* (wheezing; trouble in breathing; tightness in chest)—most likely in asthmatic patients; *hypertension* (severe and continuing headache)—with very large doses; *ileus, adynamic* (constipation; tender or mildly bloated abdomen); *increased uterine pain accompanying abortion*—correlates with efficacy; *inflammation and pain at injection site; peripheral vasoconstriction, possibly severe* (pale, cool, or blotchy skin on arms or legs; weak or absent pulse in arms or legs); *substernal*

*pressure or pain* (pressing or painful feeling in chest); *tachycardia* (fast heartbeat)

**Those indicating need for medical attention only if they continue or are bothersome**
Incidence more frequent
  *Diarrhea*—about 67%; *nausea*—about 33%; *vomiting*—about 67%
Incidence less frequent
  *Chills or shivering; dizziness; fever, transient*—about 12%; *flushing or redness of face*—about 7%; *headache; stomach cramps or pain*

**Those indicating possible postabortion complications and the need for medical attention if they occur after medication is discontinued**
  *Endometritis* (continuing chills; shivering; continuing fever—usually on third day after abortion; foul-smelling vaginal discharge; pain in lower abdomen); *unusual increase in uterine bleeding*

## Overdose

For more information on the management of overdose or unintentional ingestion, **contact a Poison Control Center** (see *Poison Control Center Listing*).

**Treatment of overdose**
Supportive therapy—Emphasis on intravenous fluid replacement.

## Patient Consultation

As an aid to patient consultation, refer to *Advice for the Patient, Carboprost (Systemic)*.

In providing consultation, consider emphasizing the following selected information (» = major clinical significance):

**Before using this medication**
» Conditions affecting use, especially:
    Allergies or intolerance to carboprost or other oxytocics
    Pregnancy—Because some prostaglandins are teratogenic in animals, any pregnancy termination with carboprost that fails should be completed by another method
    Other medical problems, especially lung disease, cardiac disease, liver disease, pelvic inflammatory disease, or renal disease

**Proper use of this medication**
» Proper dosing

**Side/adverse effects**
  Signs of potential side effects, especially adynamic ileus, anaphylaxis, bradycardia, bronchoconstriction, chest pain or pressure, endometritis, fever, hypertension, inflammation and pain at injection site, peripheral vasoconstriction, tachycardia, and uterine bleeding or pain

## General Dosing Information

Carboprost is sometimes used in combination with hypertonic saline or urea in the performance of abortion.

It is recommended that antiemetic and antidiarrheal medications be administered prior to or concurrently with carboprost to decrease the incidence and severity of gastrointestinal side effects. Narcotic analgesics may be given for uterine pain.

If carboprost is ineffective, it is recommended that alternative methods such as hypertonic saline not be used until the uterus has stopped contracting. Continuous administration of carboprost for more than two days is not recommended.

Caution should be taken to prevent exposure of skin to carboprost tromethamine. If carboprost injection is spilled on the skin, it should be washed off immediately with soap and water.

## Parenteral Dosage Forms

Note: Bracketed uses in the *Dosage Forms* section refer to indications and/or categories of use that are not included in U.S. product labeling.

**CARBOPROST TROMETHAMINE INJECTION USP**

**Usual adult and adolescent dose**
Abortifacient—
  [Intra-amniotic, 2.5 mg (base) administered over five minutes. An additional dose of 2.5 mg may be administered twenty-four hours after the initial dose if abortion has not occurred, provided the membranes are intact] or
  Deep intramuscular, initially 250 mcg (0.25 mg) (base), the dosage being repeated every one and one-half to three and one-half hours, depending on uterine response. Dose may be increased to 500 mcg (0.5 mg) if uterine contractility is inadequate after several doses of 250 mcg (0.25 mg).
  Note: An optional test dose of 100 mcg (0.1 mg) of carboprost (base) may be administered initially.
        Continuous administration for more than two days is not recommended.
Antihemorrhagic, postpartum and postabortal uterine bleeding[1]—
  Deep intramuscular, 250 mcg (0.25 mg) (base). If necessary, the dosage may be repeated at fifteen- to ninety-minute intervals on the basis of response.

**Usual adult prescribing limits**
Abortifacient—
  Intra-amniotic: 5 mg (base).
  Intramuscular: 6 to 12 mg (base), cumulative. Continuous administration for more than two days is not recommended.
Antihemorrhagic, postpartum and postabortal uterine bleeding[1]—
  2 mg (base), cumulative.

**Strength(s) usually available**
U.S.—
  250 mcg (0.25 mg) (base) per mL (Rx) [*Hemabate*].
Canada—
  250 mcg (0.25 mg) (base) per mL (Rx) [*Prostin/15M*].

**Packaging and storage**
Store between 2 and 8 °C (36 and 46 °F).

[1]Not included in Canadian product labeling.

Revised: 10/26/92
Interim revision: 06/08/94

---

**CARBOXYMETHYLCELLULOSE-CONTAINING COMBINATIONS—**

Psyllium Hydrophilic Mucilloid and Carboxymethylcellulose (Oral-Local)—See *Laxatives (Local)*

---

**CARISOPRODOL**—See *Skeletal Muscle Relaxants (Systemic)*

---

# CARMUSTINE   Systemic

VA CLASSIFICATION (Primary/Secondary): AN100/DE600
Another commonly used name is BCNU.
Note: For a listing of dosage forms and brand names by country availability, see *Dosage Forms* section(s). For a listing of brand names for the articles in this monograph, refer to the General Index.

---

## Category
Antineoplastic.

## Indications
Note: Bracketed information in the *Indications* section refers to uses that are not included in U.S. product labeling.

**Accepted**
Tumors, brain, primary (treatment)
[Carcinoma, hepatic (treatment)][1] or
[Carcinoma, gastrointestinal (treatment)]—Carmustine is indicated as palliative therapy as a single agent or in combination therapy for treatment of primary brain tumors (glioblastoma, brainstem glioma, medulloblastoma, astrocytoma, ependymoma, and metastatic brain tumors), for hepatic carcinoma (by intra-arterial injection), and for gastrointestinal carcinoma.

Lymphomas, Hodgkin's (treatment) or
Lymphomas, non-Hodgkin's (treatment)—Carmustine is indicated for treatment of Hodgkin's disease and non-Hodgkin's lymphomas, in-

cluding lymphosarcoma[1] and reticulum cell sarcoma[1]. Carmustine is indicated as secondary therapy in combination with other approved drugs in patients who relapse while being treated with primary therapy, or who fail to respond to primary therapy.

Multiple myeloma (treatment)—Carmustine is indicated for treatment of multiple myeloma, in combination with prednisone.

[Melanoma, malignant (treatment)]—Carmustine is used for treatment of disseminated malignant melanoma, in combination with vincristine sulfate.

[Mycosis fungoides (treatment)][1]—Carmustine is used topically for treatment of mycosis fungoides.

---

[1]Not included in Canadian product labeling.

## Pharmacology/Pharmacokinetics

### Physicochemical characteristics
Molecular weight—214.05.

### Mechanism of action/Effect
Carmustine is an alkylating agent of the nitrosourea type. Carmustine and/or its metabolites alkylate and interfere with the function of DNA and RNA and are also capable of cross-linking DNA. It is cell cycle–phase nonspecific. Carmustine may also act by protein modification.

### Distribution
Crosses the blood-brain barrier (because of high lipid solubility and relative lack of ionization at physiological pH).

### Biotransformation
Hepatic; rapid (active metabolites).

### Half-life
Biologic—Approximately 15 to 30 minutes.
Chemical—Approximately 5 minutes.
Metabolites may persist in the plasma for several days, which may explain the delayed hematologic toxicity.

### Elimination
Renal—60 to 70% (less than 1% unchanged); some enterohepatic circulation believed to occur.
Fecal—1%.
Respiratory—10% (as carbon dioxide).

## Precautions to Consider

### Carcinogenicity/Mutagenicity
Secondary malignancies are potential delayed effects of many antineoplastic agents, although it is not clear whether the effect is related to their mutagenic or immunosuppressive action. The effect of dose and duration of therapy is also unknown, although risk seems to increase with long-term use. Although information is limited, available data seem to indicate that the carcinogenic risk is greatest with the alkylating agents.

Carmustine is carcinogenic in rats and mice at doses approximating the clinical dose and has been associated with development of secondary malignancies, including acute leukemia, in humans.

### Pregnancy/Reproduction
Fertility—Gonadal suppression, resulting in amenorrhea or azoospermia, may occur in patients taking antineoplastic therapy, especially with the alkylating agents. In general, these effects appear to be related to dose and length of therapy and may be irreversible. Prediction of the degree of testicular or ovarian function impairment is complicated by the common use of combinations of several antineoplastics, which makes it difficult to assess the effects of individual agents.

Carmustine affects fertility in male rats at doses somewhat higher than the human dose.

Pregnancy—Adequate and well-controlled studies in humans have not been done.

First trimester: It is usually recommended that use of antineoplastics, especially combination chemotherapy, be avoided whenever possible, especially during the first trimester. Although information is limited because of the relatively few instances of antineoplastic administration during pregnancy, the mutagenic, teratogenic, and carcinogenic potential of these medications must be considered.

Other hazards to the fetus include adverse reactions seen in adults.

In general, use of a contraceptive is recommended during cytotoxic drug therapy.

Carmustine is embryotoxic and teratogenic in rats and embryotoxic in rats and rabbits at doses equivalent to the human dose.

FDA Pregnancy Category D.

### Breast-feeding
It is not known whether carmustine is distributed into milk. Although very little information is available regarding distribution of antineoplastic agents into breast milk, breast-feeding is not recommended while carmustine is being administered because of the risks to the infant (adverse effects, mutagenicity, carcinogenicity).

### Pediatrics
Appropriate studies on the relationship of age to the effects of carmustine have not been performed in the pediatric population. However, pediatrics-specific problems that would limit the usefulness of this medication in children are not expected.

Delayed, sometimes fatal, pulmonary fibrosis has been reported to occur up to 15 years after treatment with carmustine in childhood and early adolescence in cumulative doses ranging from 770 to 1800 mg per square meter of body surface in combination with cranial radiotherapy for intracranial tumors.

### Geriatrics
No information is available on the relationship of age to the effects of carmustine in geriatric patients. However, geriatric patients are more likely to have age-related renal function impairment, which may require caution in patients receiving carmustine.

### Dental
The bone marrow depressant effects of carmustine may result in an increased incidence of microbial infection, delayed healing, and gingival bleeding. Dental work, whenever possible, should be completed prior to initiation of therapy or deferred until blood counts have returned to normal. Patients should be instructed in proper oral hygiene during treatment, including caution in use of regular toothbrushes, dental floss, and toothpicks.

Carmustine may also cause stomatitis associated with considerable discomfort.

### Drug interactions and/or related problems
The following drug interactions and/or related problems have been selected on the basis of their potential clinical significance (possible mechanism in parentheses where appropriate)—not necessarily inclusive (» = major clinical significance):

Note: Combinations containing any of the following medications, depending on the amount present, may also interact with this medication.

Blood dyscrasia–causing medications (See *Appendix II*)
(leukopenic and/or thrombocytopenic effects of carmustine may be increased with concurrent or recent therapy if these medications cause the same effects; dosage adjustment of carmustine, if necessary, should be based on blood counts)

» Bone marrow depressants, other (See *Appendix II*) or
Radiation therapy
(additive bone marrow depression may occur; dosage reduction may be required when two or more bone marrow depressants, including radiation, are used concurrently or consecutively)

Hepatotoxic medications, other (See *Appendix II*) or
Nephrotoxic medications, other (See *Appendix II*)
(concurrent use with carmustine may result in enhanced hepatotoxicity or nephrotoxicity; either or both medications should be discontinued at the first sign of impairment)

Vaccines, killed virus
(because normal defense mechanisms may be suppressed by carmustine therapy, the patient's antibody response to the vaccine may be decreased. The interval between discontinuation of medications that cause immunosuppression and restoration of the patient's ability to respond to the vaccine depends on the intensity and type of immunosuppression-causing medication used, the underlying disease, and other factors; estimates vary from 3 months to 1 year)

» Vaccines, live virus
(because normal defense mechanisms may be suppressed by carmustine therapy, concurrent use with a live virus vaccine may potentiate the replication of the vaccine virus, may increase the side/adverse effects of the vaccine virus, and/or may decrease the patient's antibody response to the vaccine; immunization of these patients should be undertaken only with extreme caution after careful review of the patient's hematologic status and only with the knowledge and consent of the physician managing the carmustine therapy. The interval between discontinuation of medications that cause immunosuppression and restoration of the patient's ability to respond to the vaccine depends on the intensity and type of immunosuppression-causing medication used, the underlying disease, and other factors; estimates vary from 3 months to 1 year. Patients with leukemia in remission should not receive live virus

vaccine until at least 3 months after their last chemotherapy. Immunization with oral poliovirus vaccine should also be postponed in persons in close contact with the patient, especially family members)

**Laboratory value alterations**

The following have been selected on the basis of their potential clinical significance (possible effect in parentheses where appropriate)—not necessarily inclusive (» = major clinical significance):

With physiology/laboratory test values

Alkaline phosphatase values, serum and
Aspartate aminotransferase (AST [SGOT]) values, serum and
Bilirubin concentrations, serum
    (may be increased, indicating hepatotoxicity)

Blood urea nitrogen (BUN)
    (concentrations may be increased, indicating nephrotoxicity)

**Medical considerations/Contraindications**

The medical considerations/contraindications included here have been selected on the basis of their potential clinical significance (reasons given in parentheses where appropriate)—not necessarily inclusive (» = major clinical significance).

***Risk-benefit should be considered when the following medical problems exist:***

» Bone marrow depression
» Chickenpox, existing or recent (including recent exposure) or
» Herpes zoster
    (risk of severe generalized disease)
    Hepatic function impairment
    (carmustine may cause mild hepatotoxicity)
» Infection
» Pulmonary function impairment, existing or history of
» Renal function impairment
» Sensitivity to carmustine
» Caution should be used also in patients who have had previous cytotoxic drug therapy or radiation therapy, especially to the mediastinum, and in patients who smoke, because of the possible increased risk of pulmonary toxicity.

**Patient monitoring**

The following may be especially important in patient monitoring (other tests may be warranted in some patients, depending on condition; » = major clinical significance):

Alanine aminotransferase (ALT [SGPT]) values, serum and
Aspartate aminotransferase (AST [SGOT]) values, serum and
Bilirubin values, serum and
Lactate dehydrogenase (LDH) values, serum
    (recommended prior to initiation of therapy and at periodic intervals during therapy; frequency varies according to clinical state, agent, dose, and other agents being used concurrently)

Blood urea nitrogen (BUN) concentrations and
Creatinine concentrations, serum
    (recommended prior to initiation of therapy and at periodic intervals during therapy; frequency varies according to clinical state, agent, dose, and other agents being used concurrently)

» Hematocrit or hemoglobin and
» Leukocyte count, total and, if appropriate, differential and
» Platelet count
    (determinations recommended prior to initiation of therapy and at periodic intervals during therapy; frequency varies according to clinical state, agent, dose, and other agents being used concurrently)

» Pulmonary function studies
    (recommended prior to initiation of therapy and at frequent intervals during systemic therapy)

Uric acid concentrations, serum
    (recommended prior to initiation of therapy and at periodic intervals during therapy; frequency varies according to clinical state, agent, dose, and other agents being used concurrently)

# Side/Adverse Effects

Note: Many "side effects" of antineoplastic therapy are unavoidable and represent the medication's pharmacologic action. Some of these (for example, leukopenia and thrombocytopenia) are actually used as parameters to aid in individual dosage titration.

Encephalomyelopathy has been reported in patients who have received high-dose carmustine therapy.

Ocular toxicity has been associated with intra-arterial use.

The following side/adverse effects have been selected on the basis of their potential clinical significance (possible signs and symptoms in parentheses where appropriate)—not necessarily inclusive:

**Those indicating need for medical attention**
Incidence more frequent
    *Leukopenia or infection* (usually asymptomatic; less frequently, fever or chills; cough or hoarseness; lower back or side pain; painful or difficult urination); *phlebitis* (pain or redness at site of injection); *pneumonitis or pulmonary fibrosis* (cough; shortness of breath); *thrombocytopenia* (usually asymptomatic; less frequently, unusual bleeding or bruising; black, tarry stools; blood in urine or stools; pinpoint red spots on skin)

Note: Maximum *leukopenia* occurs about 5 to 6 weeks after a dose. Recovery usually occurs within 6 to 7 weeks but may take up to 10 to 12 weeks after prolonged therapy. Severity of bone marrow depression varies and determines subsequent dosage of carmustine.

*Burning at the injection site* is associated with rapid intravenous infusion; true thrombosis is rare.

*Pneumonitis or pulmonary fibrosis* is initially thought to occur after high cumulative doses (greater than 1200 to 1400 mg per square meter of body surface) or several courses (greater than 5) or months of therapy; however, there have been several reports of pulmonary toxicity after only 1 or 2 courses or low doses. Symptoms may be insidious or acute in onset, and damage may be reversible or irreversible. Fatalities have occurred. The relationship of pulmonary toxicity to dose is not yet clear and other factors (previous radiation to mediastinum, concurrent administration of cyclophosphamide or agents associated with pulmonary toxicity, history of lung disease or smoking) may be significant. Delayed pulmonary fibrosis has been reported to occur up to 15 years after treatment with carmustine in childhood and early adolescence in cumulative doses ranging from 770 to 1800 mg per square meter of body surface in combination with cranial radiotherapy for intracranial tumors. Chest x-rays demonstrated pulmonary hypoplasia with upper zone contraction, gallium scans were normal, and thoracic computed tomography (CT) scans demonstrated an unusual pattern of upper zone fibrosis. Late reduction of pulmonary function was noted in a substantial number of cases. This form of lung fibrosis may be slowly progressive and has been fatal in some cases.

Maximum *thrombocytopenia* occurs about 4 to 5 weeks after a dose. Recovery usually occurs within 6 to 7 weeks but may take up to 10 to 12 weeks after prolonged therapy. Severity of bone marrow depression varies and determines subsequent dosage of carmustine.

Incidence less frequent
    *Anemia* (unusual tiredness or weakness); *flushing of face; stomatitis* (sores in mouth and on lips)

Note: *Flushing of face* is caused by rapid intravenous infusion. Flushing occurs within 2 hours after a dose and persists approximately 4 hours.

Incidence rare
    *Hepatotoxicity* (asymptomatic); *renal toxicity and failure* (decrease in urination; swelling of feet or lower legs)

Note: *Renal toxicity and failure* usually occur in patients who have received large cumulative doses after prolonged therapy, but has occasionally been reported with lower cumulative doses.

**Those indicating need for medical attention only if they continue or are bothersome**
Incidence more frequent
    *Nausea and vomiting*

Note: *Nausea and vomiting* occur within 2 hours after a dose and usually last 4 to 6 hours; dose-related.

Incidence less frequent
    *Central nervous system (CNS) toxicity* (dizziness; trouble in walking); *diarrhea; discoloration of skin along vein of injection; loss of appetite; skin rash and itching; trouble in swallowing*

**Those not indicating need for medical attention**
Incidence less frequent
    *Loss of hair*

**Those indicating the need for medical attention if they occur after medication is discontinued**
    *Bone marrow depression* (fever or chills; cough or hoarseness; lower back or side pain; painful or difficult urination; unusual bleeding or bruising; black, tarry stools; blood in urine or stools; pinpoint red spots

on skin); *pneumonitis or pulmonary fibrosis* (cough or shortness of breath)

Note: Cumulative *myelosuppression* may occur with repeated doses.

## Patient Consultation

As an aid to patient consultation, refer to *Advice for the Patient, Carmustine (Systemic)*.

In providing consultation, consider emphasizing the following selected information (» = major clinical significance):

### Before using this medication
» Conditions affecting use, especially:
   Sensitivity to carmustine
   Pregnancy—Use not recommended because of mutagenic, teratogenic, and carcinogenic potential; advisability of using contraception; telling physician immediately if pregnancy is suspected
   Breast-feeding—Not recommended because of risk of serious side effects
   Other medications, especially other bone marrow depressants, or previous cytotoxic drug therapy or radiation therapy
   Other medical problems, especially chickenpox, herpes zoster, infection, pulmonary function impairment, or renal function impairment
   Smoking

### Proper use of this medication
   Caution in taking combination therapy; taking each medication at the right time
   Frequency of nausea and vomiting; importance of continuing medication despite stomach upset
» Proper dosing

### Precautions while using this medication
» Importance of close monitoring by the physician
» Avoiding immunizations unless approved by physician; other persons in patient's household should avoid immunizations with oral poliovirus vaccine; avoiding persons who have taken oral poliovirus vaccine or wearing a protective mask that covers nose and mouth
*Caution if bone marrow depression occurs:*
» Avoiding exposure to persons with bacterial infections, especially during periods of low blood counts; checking with physician immediately if fever or chills, cough or hoarseness, lower back or side pain, or painful or difficult urination occur
» Checking with physician immediately if unusual bleeding or bruising; black, tarry stools; blood in urine or stools; or pinpoint red spots on skin occur
   Caution in use of regular toothbrush, dental floss, or toothpick; physician, dentist, or nurse may suggest alternatives; checking with physician before having dental work done
   Not touching eyes or inside of nose unless hands washed immediately before
   Using caution to avoid accidental cuts with use of sharp objects such as safety razor or fingernail or toenail cutters
   Avoiding contact sports or other situations where bruising or injury could occur
» Possibility of local tissue injury and scarring if infiltration of intravenous solution occurs; telling doctor or nurse right away about redness, pain, or swelling at injection site

### Side/adverse effects
   Importance of discussing possible adverse effects, including cancer, with physician
   Signs of potential side effects, especially leukopenia, infection, phlebitis, pneumonitis, pulmonary fibrosis, thrombocytopenia, anemia, flushing of face, stomatitis, and renal toxicity and failure
   Asymptomatic side effects, including leukopenia, thrombocytopenia, hepatotoxicity, and pulmonary toxicity
   Physician or nurse can help in dealing with side effects
   Possibility of hair loss; should return after treatment has ended
   Pulmonary toxicity more likely to occur in smokers

## General Dosing Information

Patients receiving carmustine should be under supervision of a physician experienced in cancer chemotherapy.

A variety of dosage schedules and regimens of carmustine, alone or in combination with other antitumor agents, are used. The prescriber may consult the medical literature as well as the manufacturer's literature in choosing a specific dosage.

Dosage of carmustine subsequent to the initial course should be adjusted to meet the individual requirements of each patient, based on hema-

tologic response of the patient to the previous dose. An additional course of carmustine should be given only after circulating blood elements have returned to acceptable levels (leukocytes above 4000 per cubic millimeter and platelets above 100,000 per cubic millimeter).

Because of the delayed and cumulative bone marrow suppression caused by carmustine, the medication should be given no more frequently than every 6 weeks.

Some cross-resistance has been reported between carmustine and lomustine.

Frequency and duration of nausea and vomiting may be reduced in some patients by administration of antiemetics prior to dosing.

Intravenous infusion solutions should be administered over 1 to 2 hours to prevent irritation at the injection site. Some clinicians also recommend flushing the line with 5 to 10 mL of 0.9% sodium chloride injection or 5% dextrose injection both before and after administration of carmustine.

Special precautions are recommended in patients who develop thrombocytopenia as a result of administration of carmustine. These may include extreme care in performing invasive procedures; regular inspection of intravenous sites, skin (including perirectal area), and mucous membrane surfaces for signs of bleeding or bruising; limiting frequency of venipuncture and avoiding intramuscular injections; testing urine, emesis, stool, and secretions for occult blood; care in use of regular toothbrushes, dental floss, toothpicks, safety razors, and fingernail and toenail cutters; avoiding constipation; and using caution to prevent falls and other injuries. Such patients should avoid alcohol and aspirin intake because of the risk of gastrointestinal bleeding. Platelet transfusions may be required.

Patients who develop leukopenia should be observed carefully for signs of infection. Antibiotic support may be required. In neutropenic patients who develop fever, broad-spectrum antibiotic coverage should be initiated empirically, pending bacterial cultures and appropriate diagnostic tests.

Carmustine has been injected intra-arterially (hepatic artery) in the investigational treatment of hepatic tumors in a dose of 200 mg per square meter of body surface administered over 20 to 60 minutes.

### Safety considerations for handling this medication
There is limited but increasing evidence and concern that personnel involved in preparation and administration of parenteral antineoplastics may be at some risk because of the potential mutagenicity, teratogenicity, and/or carcinogenicity of these agents, although the actual risk is unknown. USP advisory panels recommend cautious handling both in preparation and disposal of antineoplastic agents. Precautions that have been suggested include:
• Use of a biological containment cabinet during reconstitution and dilution of parenteral medications and wearing of disposable surgical gloves and masks.
• Use of proper technique to prevent contamination of the medication, work area, and operator during transfer between containers (including proper training of personnel in this technique).
• Cautious and proper disposal of needles, syringes, vials, ampuls, and unused medication.
A number of medical centers have developed detailed guidelines for handling of antineoplastic agents.

### Combination chemotherapy
Carmustine may be used in combination with other agents in various regimens. As a result, incidence and/or severity of side effects may be altered and different dosages (usually reduced) may be used. For example, carmustine is part of the following chemotherapeutic combinations (some commonly used acronyms are in parentheses):
—doxorubicin and carmustine (Adria + BCNU).
—carmustine, cyclophosphamide, vinblastine, procarbazine, and prednisone (BCVPP).
—vincristine, carmustine, cyclophosphamide, melphalan, and prednisone (M-2 Protocol).
For specific dosages and schedules, consult the literature. For information regarding each agent, consult the individual monographs.

## Parenteral Dosage Forms

Note: Bracketed uses in the *Dosage Forms* section refer to categories of use and/or indications that are not included in U.S. product labeling.

### CARMUSTINE FOR INJECTION

#### Usual adult and adolescent dose
Tumors, brain, primary or
[Carcinoma, gastrointestinal] or
Lymphomas, Hodgkin's or
Lymphomas, non-Hodgkin's or
Multiple myeloma or

[Melanoma, malignant]—

Intravenous, 150 to 200 mg per square meter of body surface as a single dose every six to eight weeks, or 75 to 100 mg per square meter of body surface on two successive days every six weeks, or 40 mg per square meter of body surface on five successive days every six weeks.

A suggested dosage adjustment schedule for subsequent doses is:

| Nadir after Prior Dose (cells per cubic millimeter) | | % of Prior Dose to Be Given |
|---|---|---|
| Leukocytes | Platelets | |
| >4000 | >100,000 | 100 |
| 3000–3999 | 75,000–99,999 | 50 |
| 2000–2999 | 25,000–74,999 | 25 |
| <2000 | <25,000 | 0 |

**Usual pediatric dose**
See *Usual adult and adolescent dose.*

**Size(s) usually available**
U.S.—
100 mg (Rx) [*BiCNU*].
Canada—
100 mg (Rx) [*BiCNU*].

**Packaging and storage**
Store between 2 and 8 °C (36 and 46 °F), unless otherwise specified by manufacturer. Exposure of the dry material to temperatures of 30.5 to 32.0 °C (86.9 to 89.6 °F) or above will cause the drug to decompose and liquefy, appearing as an oily film in the bottom of the vial; if this occurs, the vial must be discarded.

**Preparation of dosage form**
Carmustine for injection is reconstituted for intravenous use by adding 3 mL of sterile diluent (dehydrated alcohol injection) supplied by the manufacturer to dissolve it, then adding 27 mL of sterile water for injection, producing a clear, colorless solution containing 3.3 mg of carmustine per mL.
Reconstituted solutions may be further diluted with 0.9% sodium chloride injection or 5% dextrose injection for administration by intravenous infusion.

**Stability**
Reconstituted solutions are stable for 8 hours at 25 °C (77 °F) or 24 hours at 4 °C (39 °F). Reconstituted solutions diluted further for administration by infusion are stable for 48 hours when refrigerated and an additional 8 hours at 25 °C (77 °F) under normal room fluorescent light. Freezing does not alter the potency. Because the product contains no preservative, it should not be used as a multiple-dose vial.

**Note**
Avoid contact of the reconstituted solution with skin and eyes; it will cause burning and brown staining of skin. If accidental contact with skin or mucosa occurs, the area should be washed immediately and thoroughly with soap and water.

## Selected Bibliography

Weiss RB, Issell BF. The nitrosoureas: carmustine (BCNU) and lomustine (CCNU). Cancer Treat Rev 1982; 9: 313-30.
Dorr RT, Fritz WL. Cancer chemotherapy handbook. New York: Elsevier, 1980: 295-302.

Revised: 07/15/94

**CARTEOLOL**—See *Beta-adrenergic Blocking Agents (Ophthalmic); Beta-adrenergic Blocking Agents (Systemic)*

**CASANTHRANOL**—See *Laxatives (Local)*

**CASANTHRANOL-CONTAINING COMBINATIONS**—

Casanthranol and Docusate (Oral-Local)—See *Laxatives (Local)*

**CASCARA SAGRADA**—See *Laxatives (Local)*

**CASCARA SAGRADA–CONTAINING COMBINATIONS**—
Cascara Sagrada and Aloe (Oral-Local)—See *Laxatives (Local)*
Cascara Sagrada and Phenolphthalein (Oral-Local)—See *Laxatives (Local)*
Magnesium Hydroxide and Cascara Sagrada (Oral-Local)—See *Laxatives (Local)*

**CASTOR OIL**—See *Laxatives (Local)*

**CEFACLOR**—See *Cephalosporins (Systemic)*

**CEFADROXIL**—See *Cephalosporins (Systemic)*

**CEFAMANDOLE**—See *Cephalosporins (Systemic)*

**CEFAZOLIN**—See *Cephalosporins (Systemic)*

**CEFIXIME**—See *Cephalosporins (Systemic)*

**CEFMETAZOLE**—See *Cephalosporins (Systemic)*

**CEFONICID**—See *Cephalosporins (Systemic)*

**CEFOPERAZONE**—See *Cephalosporins (Systemic)*

**CEFOTAXIME**—See *Cephalosporins (Systemic)*

**CEFOTETAN**—See *Cephalosporins (Systemic)*

**CEFOXITIN**—See *Cephalosporins (Systemic)*

**CEFPODOXIME**—See *Cephalosporins (Systemic)*

**CEFPROZIL**—See *Cephalosporins (Systemic)*

**CEFTAZIDIME**—See *Cephalosporins (Systemic)*

**CEFTIZOXIME**—See *Cephalosporins (Systemic)*

**CEFTRIAXONE**—See *Cephalosporins (Systemic)*

**CEFUROXIME**—See *Cephalosporins (Systemic)*

# CELLULOSE SODIUM PHOSPHATE   Systemic†

VA CLASSIFICATION (Primary): GU900

Note: For a listing of dosage forms and brand names by country availability, see *Dosage Forms* section(s). For a listing of brand names for the articles in this monograph, refer to the General Index.

†Not commercially available in Canada.

## Category

Antiurolithic (calcium calculi).

## Indications

### Accepted

Renal calculi, calcium (prophylaxis)—Cellulose sodium phosphate is indicated for reducing the incidence of new renal stone formation in patients with absorptive hypercalciuria Type I (characterized by recurrent formation or passage of calcium oxalate and/or calcium phosphate renal calculi; evidence of high intestinal calcium absorption, i.e., urinary calcium concentration >0.2 mg per mg creatinine after oral load of 1 gram of calcium; hypercalciuria, i.e., 24-hour urinary calcium >200 mg per day on a diet of 400 mg calcium and 100 mEq sodium per day; normal fasting urinary calcium; no evidence of bone disease; normal serum calcium and phosphorus; normal parathyroid function; and lack of excessive skeletal mobilization of calcium, or renal leak).

Although some clinicians recommend the use of cellulose sodium phosphate as the primary agent for treatment of absorptive hypercalciuria Type I, others prefer to use dietary restriction of calcium and oxalate, thiazide diuretics, and increased fluid intake as the primary method of treatment.

Minimal diagnostic tests for different causes of hypercalciuria include serum calcium, phosphorus, and parathyroid hormone (PTH) determinations obtained on an empty stomach; 24-hour urinary calcium on a diet restricted for at least 10 days in calcium and sodium; and a determination of urinary excretion of calcium while fasting for 12 hours.

### Unaccepted

Cellulose sodium phosphate is *not* indicated for causes of hypercalciuria other than hyperabsorption. This medication may be used on a temporary basis for absorptive hypercalciuria Type II (identical to Type I, but the hypercalciuria can usually be eliminated by a calcium-restricted diet alone). Cellulose sodium phosphate should not be used for absorptive hypophosphatemic hypercalciuria Type III because hypercalciuria may result, in part, from an increased skeletal mobilization of calcium.

## Pharmacology/Pharmacokinetics

### Physicochemical characteristics

Cellulose sodium phosphate exchanges sodium for calcium and other divalent cations. Inorganic phosphate content is approximately 34%; sodium content is approximately 11%.

### Mechanism of action/Effect

Binds dietary and secreted calcium, preventing intestinal calcium absorption. Thus, decreased urinary saturation of calcium, with only slightly increased urinary oxalate and phosphorus, may prevent the spontaneous nucleation of calcium oxalate and calcium phosphate to form stones.

### Other actions/effects

Also binds dietary magnesium and decreases urinary magnesium concentration. Increases urinary oxalate by binding divalent cations, making them unavailable to oxalate, thus increasing oxalate absorption. Increases urinary phosphorus, reflecting hydrolysis of 7 to 30% of cellulose sodium phosphate in the intestinal tract and absorption of released phosphorus.

### Absorption

None.

### Elimination

Fecal, as the complex of calcium and cellulose phosphate.

## Precautions to Consider

### Carcinogenicity

No long-term studies have been done.

### Pregnancy/Reproduction

Pregnancy—Studies have not been done in either humans or animals.

Because of the increased dietary calcium requirement during pregnancy, cellulose sodium phosphate should not be given to pregnant women unless clearly needed.

FDA Pregnancy Category C.

### Breast-feeding

It is not known whether cellulose sodium phosphate is distributed into breast milk. However, problems in humans have not been documented.

### Pediatrics

Because growing children have an increased dietary calcium requirement, the use of cellulose sodium phosphate is not recommended in children up to 16 years of age.

### Geriatrics

No information is available on the relationship of age to the effects of cellulose sodium phosphate in geriatric patients.

### Drug interactions and/or related problems

The following drug interactions and/or related problems have been selected on the basis of their potential clinical significance (possible mechanism in parentheses where appropriate)—not necessarily inclusive (» = major clinical significance):

Note: Combinations containing any of the following medications, depending on the amount present, may also interact with this medication.

Ascorbic acid
(concurrent use with cellulose sodium phosphate may result in metabolism of ascorbic acid to oxalate)

» Calcium-containing medications, including calcium supplements or
» Milk or other dairy products
(concurrent use may decrease effectiveness of cellulose sodium phosphate in preventing hypercalciuria)

Foods high in oxalate content, such as spinach (and similar dark greens), chocolate, brewed tea, and rhubarb
(concurrent use with cellulose sodium phosphate may lead to hyperoxaluria, negating the beneficial effect of hypocalciuria)

» Magnesium-containing medications, including magnesium supplements
(simultaneous use with cellulose sodium phosphate may result in binding of magnesium; patients should be advised not to take these medications within 1 hour of cellulose sodium phosphate)

### Medical considerations/Contraindications

The medical considerations/contraindications included here have been selected on the basis of their potential clinical significance (reasons given in parentheses where appropriate)—not necessarily inclusive (» = major clinical significance).

*Except under special circumstances, this medication should not be used when the following medical problems exist:*

» Bone disease, such as osteitis, osteomalacia, and osteoporosis
(may further deplete calcium needed to prevent loss of bone mass)

» High fasting urinary calcium, unless a high skeletal mobilization of calcium can be excluded or

» Hypophosphatemia
(may indicate presence of hyperparathyroidism or renal tubular defects; stimulation of parathyroid hormone [PTH] by drug-induced hypocalcemia may further deplete phosphorus and lead to muscle weakness and osteomalacia)

» Hyperoxaluria, enteric
(increases propensity of oxalate stone formation)

» Hyperparathyroidism, primary or secondary
(increases risk of parathyroid bone disease)

» Hypocalcemic states, such as hypoparathyroidism and intestinal malabsorption
(further depletion of calcium may lead to osteomalacia)

» Hypomagnesemic states—serum magnesium <1.5 mg per deciliter
(further depletion of magnesium may lead to generalized tonic-clonic seizures)

» Normal or low intestinal absorption and renal excretion of calcium
(may cause excessive PTH secretion and possible parathyroid bone disease)

*Risk-benefit should be considered when the following medical problems exist:*

Ascites or
Congestive heart failure or
Nephrotic syndrome
    (sodium content of cellulose sodium phosphate may increase fluid retention)
Sensitivity to cellulose sodium phosphate

### Patient monitoring

The following may be especially important in patient monitoring (other tests may be warranted in some patients, depending on condition; » = major clinical significance):

» Calcium concentrations, serum
    (determinations recommended every 3 to 6 months during therapy; if borderline values are obtained, determinations should be repeated promptly)

» Calcium concentrations, urinary
    (determinations recommended at periodic intervals during therapy; a reduction in urinary calcium of <30 mg per 5 grams of cellulose sodium phosphate is an inadequate hypocalciuric response to treatment)

Magnesium concentrations, serum
    (determinations recommended every 3 to 6 months during therapy)

» Oxalate concentrations, urinary
    (determinations recommended at periodic intervals during therapy; if urinary oxalate is more than 55 mg per day on moderate dietary oxalate restriction, cessation of treatment should be considered)

» PTH concentrations, serum
    (determinations recommended at least once between the first 2 weeks and 3 months of treatment; if borderline values are obtained, the determinations should be repeated promptly and treatment adjusted or stopped if serum PTH rises above normal)

## Side/Adverse Effects

The following side/adverse effects have been selected on the basis of their potential clinical significance (possible signs and symptoms in parentheses where appropriate)—not necessarily inclusive:

### Those indicating need for medical attention
With long-term use
*Hypomagnesemia* (drowsiness; loss of appetite; mood or mental changes; muscle spasms [tetany] or twitching; seizures; nausea or vomiting; trembling; unusual tiredness or weakness)

### Those indicating need for medical attention only if they continue or are bothersome
Incidence more frequent
*Abdominal or stomach discomfort; loose bowel movements or diarrhea*

## Patient Consultation

As an aid to patient consultation, refer to *Advice for the Patient, Cellulose Sodium Phosphate (Systemic).*

In providing consultation, consider emphasizing the following selected information (» = major clinical significance):

### Before using this medication
» Conditions affecting use, especially:
    Sensitivity to cellulose sodium phosphate
    Pregnancy—Use not recommended during pregnancy because of increased need for calcium in pregnant women, unless clearly needed
    Use in children—Use not recommended in children up to 16 years of age because of increased need for calcium in growing children
    Other medications, especially calcium- or magnesium-containing medications
    Other medical problems, especially bone disease, high fasting urinary calcium, hypophosphatemia, enteric hyperoxaluria, hypoparathyroidism, hypocalcemia, hypomagnesemia, or normal or low intestinal absorption and renal excretion of calcium

### Proper use of this medication
» Taking powder mixed with a full glass (240 mL) of water, soft drink, or fruit juice; rinsing glass and drinking all of liquid to get full dose
» Taking with a meal for optimum calcium binding
» Importance of not taking more medication than the amount prescribed
» Importance of high fluid intake (240 mL hourly while awake) during therapy to dilute urine and help prevent kidney stones

» Proper dosing
» Missed dose: Skipping missed dose; not doubling doses
» Proper storage

### Precautions while using this medication
» Regular visits to physician to check progress during therapy
    Avoiding simultaneous use of magnesium-containing medications; taking at least 1 hour before or after cellulose sodium phosphate
    Avoiding concurrent use with vitamin C or high oxalate foods such as spinach (and similar dark greens), chocolate, brewed tea, and rhubarb
    Avoiding concurrent use with milk or other dairy products
    Avoiding salty foods and use of extra salt to help achieve an intake of <150 mEq of sodium a day
    Patients on a sodium-restricted diet: Medication contains sodium

### Side/adverse effects
Signs of potential side effects, especially hypomagnesemia

## General Dosing Information

Both the initial and maintenance doses of cellulose sodium phosphate are based on measurements of 24-hour urinary calcium excretion.

If there is an inadequate hypocalciuric response (reduction of urinary calcium <30 mg per 5 grams of cellulose sodium phosphate) to treatment while patient is maintained on moderate calcium and sodium restriction, the treatment may be considered ineffective and should be stopped.

Cellulose sodium phosphate is usually administered concomitantly with magnesium supplements to replace dietary magnesium. However, supplemental magnesium should be taken at least 1 hour before or after cellulose sodium phosphate to avoid binding of magnesium.

The dose of oral magnesium supplements, given as magnesium gluconate, depends on the dose of cellulose sodium phosphate. Patients receiving 15 grams of cellulose sodium phosphate a day should take 1.5 grams of magnesium gluconate twice a day. Those taking 10 grams of cellulose sodium phosphate a day should take 1 gram of magnesium gluconate twice a day.

### Diet/Nutrition
Cellulose sodium phosphate should be taken with meals because the amount of calcium that is bound is reduced considerably when the medication is administered more than one hour after a meal. The amount of bound calcium depends on actual mixing of medication with food.

High fluid intake (240 mL hourly while awake) should be encouraged to achieve a urinary output of 2 liters a day. This keeps urine diluted and prevents stone formation.

Avoiding the use of salty foods or extra salt will help limit sodium intake to <150 mEq a day.

Ingestion of foods high in oxalate content, such as spinach or similar dark greens, chocolate, brewed tea, and rhubarb, may lead to hyperoxaluria, negating the beneficial effect of hypocalciuria.

Vitamin C supplementation may result in metabolism of ascorbic acid to oxalate.

Milk or other dairy products may decrease the effectiveness of cellulose sodium phosphate by adding more calcium to the diet.

## Oral Dosage Forms
### CELLULOSE SODIUM PHOSPHATE (FOR ORAL SUSPENSION)
#### Usual adult dose
Renal calculi—
    Patients with urinary calcium >300 mg a day:
        Oral, initially, 15 grams a day (5 grams three times a day with meals), the dosage being decreased to 10 grams a day (5 grams with main meal, 2.5 grams with each of other two meals) when urinary calcium concentration declines to <200 mg a day.
    Patients with controlled urinary calcium (<300 mg but >200 mg a day):
        Oral, initially, 10 grams a day with meals, the continuing dosage being determined by the physician.

#### Usual pediatric dose
Renal calculi—Children up to 16 years of age—
    Use is not recommended.

#### Size(s) usually available
U.S.—
    2.5 grams (Rx) [*Calcibind*].
    300 grams (Rx) [*Calcibind*].
Canada—
    Not commercially available.

**Packaging and storage**
Store below 40 °C (104 °F), preferably between 15 and 30 °C (59 and 86 °F), unless otherwise specified by manufacturer. Store in a well-closed container.

**Auxiliary labeling**
• Take with meals.
• Drink large amounts of fluids.

**Additional information**
Cellulose sodium phosphate contains 25 to 50 mEq of exchangeable sodium per 15 grams.

Revised: 12/02/92
Interim revision: 05/13/94

**CEPHALEXIN**—See *Cephalosporins (Systemic)*

# CEPHALOSPORINS   Systemic

This monograph includes information on the following: Cefaclor; Cefadroxil; Cefamandole; Cefazolin; Cefixime; Cefmetazole†; Cefonicid†; Cefoperazone; Cefotaxime; Cefotetan; Cefoxitin; Cefpodoxime†; Cefprozil†; Ceftazidime; Ceftizoxime; Ceftriaxone; Cefuroxime; Cephalexin; Cephalothin; Cephapirin†; Cephradine.

VA CLASSIFICATION (Primary):
Cefaclor—AM102
Cefadroxil—AM101
Cefamandole—AM102
Cefazolin—AM101
Cefixime—AM103
Cefmetazole—AM102
Cefonicid—AM102
Cefoperazone—AM103
Cefotaxime—AM103
Cefotetan—AM102
Cefoxitin—AM102
Cefpodoxime—AM103
Cefprozil—AM102
Ceftazidime—AM103
Ceftizoxime—AM103
Ceftriaxone—AM103
Cefuroxime—AM102
Cephalexin—AM101
Cephalothin—AM101
Cephapirin—AM101
Cephradine—AM101

Note: For a listing of dosage forms and brand names by country availability, see *Dosage Forms* section(s). For a listing of brand names for the articles in this monograph, refer to the General Index.

†Not commercially available in Canada.

## Category

Antibacterial (systemic).

## Indications

Note: Bracketed information in the *Indications* section refers to uses that are not included in U.S. product labeling.

**General considerations**
Cephalosporins have been classified by "generation" based on their spectrum of antibacterial activity, providing a useful, although somewhat arbitrary, means of grouping the many cephalosporins available. Several of the newer cephalosporins with an expanded spectrum of activity do not fit into any one generation, but overlap into others. These medications have been placed into the generation that most closely describes their antibacterial spectrum.
First-generation cephalosporins include cefadroxil, cefazolin, cephalexin, cephalothin, cephapirin, and cephradine.
Second-generation cephalosporins include cefaclor, cefamandole, cefmetazole, cefonicid, cefotetan, cefoxitin, cefprozil, and cefuroxime.
Third-generation cephalosporins include cefixime, cefoperazone, cefotaxime, cefpodoxime, ceftazidime, ceftizoxime, and ceftriaxone.
Cephalosporins are broad-spectrum, beta-lactam antibiotics indicated in the treatment of a wide range of infections. Cefamandole, cefazolin, cefmetazole, cefonicid, cefotaxime, cefotetan, cefoxitin, ceftriaxone, cefuroxime, cephalothin, and cephapirin are also indicated in the prophylaxis of perioperative infections. A few cephalosporins (e.g., cefazolin, cefotetan, cefoxitin) may be preferred agents in the prophylaxis of perioperative infections because of their pharmacokinetic properties and spectrum of antibacterial activity.
Selection of a cephalosporin is usually based on the organism(s) that are present or most likely to be present, site(s) of infection, resistance patterns, and the side effects, cost, and pharmacokinetic properties of the cephalosporin. (See also *Table 1*, page 771, and *Table 2*, page 774.)

First-generation cephalosporins have the highest degree of activity against most gram-positive bacteria, including beta-lactamase–producing *Staphylococcus aureus* and most streptococci; exceptions include methicillin-resistant staphylococci, and penicillin-resistant *Streptococcus pneumoniae*. No cephalosporin is effective against *Enterococcus faecalis* infections. Gram-negative bacteria coverage is generally limited to *Escherichia coli*, *Klebsiella* species, and *Proteus mirabilis*. Cephalothin and cefazolin have similar spectrums of activity *in vitro*, but cefazolin is more active against *E. coli* and *Klebsiella* species. Cefazolin may also be less stable against staphylococcal penicillinases than is cephalothin. Cephalexin, cefadroxil, and cephradine all have very similar activity *in vitro* and are available in an oral dosage form.
First-generation cephalosporins are used to treat septicemia, bone and joint infections, otitis media, pneumonia, skin and soft tissue infections, including burn wound infections, and urinary tract infections caused by susceptible bacterial organisms. They are not effective in treating meningitis. These medications are possible alternatives to the penicillins for staphylococcal and nonenterococcal streptococcal infections, including pneumonias, bone and joint infections, and bacterial endocarditis. Cefazolin is the preferred agent for use in perioperative prophylaxis because of its longer half-life. Because first-generation cephalosporins provide inconsistent coverage against gram-negative bacilli, their empiric use as monotherapy is not recommended.
Second-generation cephalosporins have enhanced activity against *Escherichia coli*, *Klebsiella* species, and *Proteus mirabilis*; in addition, they have greater activity *in vitro* against a larger number of gram-negative bacteria, including *Haemophilus influenzae*, indole-positive *Proteus*, *Neisseria meningitidis*, *N. gonorrhoeae*, and some strains of *Serratia* and *Enterobacter* species. *Serratia* and *Enterobacter* species may induce beta-lactamases that inactivate the drug after a period of exposure to the cephalosporin, producing a resistance that may be expressed late; this resistance may not be detectable by disc sensitivity techniques. These cephalosporins also have slightly less or variable activity against most gram-positive cocci. None of the second-generation cephalosporins have activity against *Pseudomonas aeruginosa*. Cefaclor and cephalexin have comparable activity *in vitro* against most gram-positive cocci; however, cefaclor has better activity than cephalexin against *H. influenzae*, *E. coli*, and *P. mirabilis*. Cefamandole, cefonicid, and cefuroxime all have similar activity *in vitro*. However, cefuroxime may be more stable against certain beta-lactamases (e.g., TEM-1) than is cefamandole, and cefonicid has less activity *in vitro* against *S. aureus*. Cefuroxime is the only second-generation cephalosporin to adequately penetrate into the cerebrospinal fluid (CSF). Cefmetazole is used to treat uncomplicated penicillinase and nonpenicillinase-producing strains of urethral, cervical, and rectal gonorrhea. Cefprozil has *in vitro* activity that covers a broader range of organisms, including many gram-positive and gram-negative organisms that are typically covered by first-generation cephalosporins. It also has good activity against *H. influenzae*, *Moraxella (Branhamella) catarrhalis*, *Citrobacter diversus*, and penicillinase-producing strains of *N. gonorrhoeae*.
Second-generation cephalosporins are used in the treatment of septicemia, bone and joint infections, gram-negative pneumonia, skin and soft tissue infections, including burn wound infections, and urinary tract infections caused by susceptible bacterial organisms. Cefuroxime is commonly used to treat community-acquired pneumonias because of its activity against *S. pneumoniae*, *S. aureus*, and *H. influenzae*. It has been used to treat meningitis caused by *S. pneumoniae*, *H. influenzae*, and *N. meningitidis*, although third-generation cephalosporins have better penetration into the CSF. Also, delayed sterilization of the CSF has been reported in children being treated with cefuroxime for bacterial meningitis. Because cefaclor has good activity against many

strains of *H. influenzae*, it is used in the treatment of amoxicillin-resistant otitis media and sinusitis. This is also true of cefuroxime axetil, an oral prodrug of cefuroxime that is hydrolyzed to cefuroxime after absorption. It has been used to treat mild to moderate bronchitis, otitis media, skin and soft tissue infections, uncomplicated gonococcal urethritis, and urinary tract infections. Cefprozil is also used to treat bronchitis, otitis media, and skin and soft tissue infections, as well as pharyngitis and tonsillitis.

Cefoxitin, cefotetan, and cefmetazole have the greatest activity of the cephalosporins against anaerobes, particularly the *Bacteroides fragilis* group. Cefoxitin has the greatest stability in the presence of beta-lactamases produced by the *Bacteroides fragilis* group. Cefotetan has similar activity against *B. fragilis*, but cefotetan has greater activity than cefmetazole, and cefmetazole has greater activity than cefoxitin, against aerobic gram-negative bacilli. Most strains of *Bacteroides distasonis*, *B. ovatus*, and *B. thetaiotaomicron* are resistant to cefotetan. Many of the second- and third-generation cephalosporins that are active against anaerobic organisms are not effective against resistant strains of the *Bacteroides fragilis* group.

Cefoxitin, cefotetan, and cefmetazole are used primarily in the treatment of mixed aerobic-anaerobic bacterial infections, including aspiration pneumonia, diabetic foot infections, intra-abdominal and female pelvic infections. They are also used prophylactically to help prevent perioperative infections that may result from colorectal surgery and appendectomies, and in the treatment of penicillin-resistant strains of gonorrhea.

Most third-generation cephalosporins have a high degree of stability in the presence of beta-lactamases (penicillinases and cephalosporinases), and, therefore, they have excellent activity against a wider spectrum of gram-negative bacteria, including penicillinase-producing strains of *N. gonorrhoeae* and most Enterobacteriaceae (*E. coli*, *Citrobacter*, *Enterobacter*, *Klebsiella*, *Morganella*, *Proteus*, *Providencia*, and *Serratia* species). Cefoperazone tends to have slightly less activity against Enterobacteriaceae than the other third-generation cephalosporins because of its greater susceptibility to certain beta-lactamases (e.g., TEM-1, TEM-2). Strains of *Pseudomonas aeruginosa*, *Serratia*, and *Enterobacter* species may induce beta-lactamases after a period of exposure to the cephalosporin, producing a resistance that may be expressed late. These medications are generally not as active against gram-positive cocci as are the first- and second-generation cephalosporins. Cefotaxime, ceftizoxime, and ceftriaxone all have similar activity *in vitro*. Cefixime, an oral third-generation cephalosporin, has the most activity of all oral cephalosporins against *S. pyogenes*, *S. pneumoniae*, and all gram-negative bacilli, including beta-lactamase–producing strains of *H. influenzae*, *Moraxella (Branhamella) catarrhalis*, and *N. gonorrhoeae*. Cefixime has little activity against staphylococci, and no activity against *Pseudomonas aeruginosa*. Cefpodoxime is also an oral third-generation cephalosporin; it is stable in the presence of many plasmid-mediated beta-lactamases. Cefpodoxime's spectrum is very similar to that of cefixime, except that cefpodoxime also has some activity against *S. aureus* and *S. saprophyticus*. Most species of *Enterobacter*, *Enterococcus*, *Pseudomonas*, *Morganella*, and *Serratia* are resistant to cefpodoxime.

Ceftazidime has the greatest activity of the third-generation cephalosporins against *Pseudomonas aeruginosa*. Cefoperazone also is somewhat effective against *P. aeruginosa*. The other third-generation cephalosporins tend to have variable activity against this pathogen. Cefoperazone achieves higher biliary concentrations than the other third-generation cephalosporins, but has poor CSF penetration.

Third-generation cephalosporins and aminoglycosides (amikacin, gentamicin, netilmicin, or tobramycin) are synergistic *in vitro* against certain susceptible and resistant strains of *P. aeruginosa*, *S. marcescens*, and other Enterobacteriaceae, including *Enterobacter cloacae*, *E. coli*, *K. pneumoniae*, and *P. mirabilis*.

Third-generation cephalosporins are used in the treatment of serious gram-negative bacterial infections, including septicemia, bone and joint infections, female pelvic infections, intra-abdominal infections, gram-negative pneumonia, skin and soft tissue infections, including burn wound infections, and complicated urinary tract infections caused by susceptible organisms. Cefotaxime, ceftriaxone, and ceftazidime are used to treat meningitis in both children and adults. Single-dose ceftriaxone, cefixime, cefotaxime, and cefpodoxime have been found to be effective in the treatment of uncomplicated gonorrhea; and [ceftriaxone and cefotaxime have also been used in the treatment of the later stages of Lyme disease][1].

## Accepted

Bone and joint infections (treatment)—[Cefaclor][1], [cefadroxil][1], cefamandole, cefazolin, [cefixime][1], [cefmetazole][1], cefonicid[1], [cefoperazone][1], cefotaxime, cefotetan, cefoxitin, [cefpodoxime][1], [cefprozil][1], ceftazidime, ceftizoxime, ceftriaxone, cefuroxime, cephalexin, cephalothin, cephapirin[1], and [cephradine][1] are indicated in the treatment of

bone and joint infections caused by susceptible organisms.

Bronchitis (treatment)—Cefixime, cefmetazole[1], cefpodoxime[1], cefprozil[1], cefuroxime axetil, and cephradine are indicated in the treatment of bronchitis caused by susceptible organisms.

Endocarditis, bacterial (treatment)—Cefazolin, cephalothin, cephapirin[1], and [cephradine][1] are indicated in the treatment of bacterial endocarditis caused by susceptible organisms.

Gonorrhea, endocervical and urethral, uncomplicated (treatment)—Cefixime, cefmetazole[1], cefotaxime, cefotetan, cefoxitin, cefpodoxime[1], ceftizoxime, ceftriaxone, and cefuroxime are indicated in the treatment of uncomplicated endocervical and urethral gonorrhea.

Impetigo (treatment)—Cefuroxime axetil is indicated in the treatment of impetigo.

Intra-abdominal infections (treatment)—Cefamandole, cefmetazole[1], cefoperazone, cefotaxime, cefotetan, cefoxitin, cefpodoxime[1], ceftazidime, ceftizoxime, and ceftriaxone are indicated in the treatment of intra-abdominal infections caused by susceptible organisms.

Meningitis (treatment)—Cefotaxime, ceftazidime, ceftizoxime, ceftriaxone, and cefuroxime are indicated in the treatment of meningitis caused by susceptible organisms.

Otitis media (treatment)—[Cefaclor][1], [cefadroxil][1], [cefazolin][1], cefixime, cefpodoxime[1], cefprozil[1], cefuroxime axetil, cephalexin, [cephalothin][1], [cephapirin][1], and cephradine are indicated in the treatment of otitis media caused by susceptible organisms.

Pelvic infections, female (treatment)—[Cefmetazole][1], cefoperazone, cefotaxime, cefotetan, cefoxitin, ceftazidime, ceftizoxime, and ceftriaxone are indicated in the treatment of female pelvic infections caused by susceptible organisms.

Perioperative infections (prophylaxis)—Cefamandole, cefazolin, cefmetazole[1], cefonicid[1], cefotaxime, cefotetan, cefoxitin, ceftriaxone, cefuroxime, cephalothin, and cephapirin[1] are indicated for the prophylaxis of perioperative infections caused by susceptible organisms.

Pharyngitis, bacterial (treatment)—Cefaclor, cefadroxil, cefixime, cefpodoxime[1], cefprozil[1], cefuroxime axetil, cephalexin, and cephradine are indicated in the treatment of bacterial pharyngitis caused by susceptible organisms.

Pneumonia, bacterial (treatment)—Cefaclor, [cefadroxil][1], cefamandole, cefazolin, [cefixime][1], cefmetazole[1], cefonicid[1], cefoperazone, cefotaxime, cefotetan, cefoxitin, cefpodoxime[1], [cefprozil][1], ceftazidime, ceftizoxime, ceftriaxone, cefuroxime, cephalexin, cephalothin, cephapirin[1], and cephradine are indicated in the treatment of bacterial pneumonia caused by susceptible organisms.

Septicemia, bacterial (treatment)—[Cefaclor][1], [cefadroxil][1], cefamandole, cefazolin, [cefixime][1], [cefmetazole][1], cefonicid[1], cefoperazone, cefotaxime, [cefotetan][1], cefoxitin, [cefpodoxime][1], [cefprozil][1], ceftazidime, ceftizoxime, ceftriaxone, cefuroxime, [cephalexin][1], cephalothin, cephapirin[1], [cephradine][1] are indicated in the treatment of bacterial septicemia caused by susceptible organisms.

Skin and soft tissue infections (treatment)—Cefaclor, cefadroxil, cefamandole, cefazolin, [cefixime][1], cefmetazole[1], cefonicid[1], cefoperazone, cefotaxime, cefotetan, cefoxitin, cefpodoxime[1], cefprozil[1], ceftazidime, ceftizoxime, ceftriaxone, cefuroxime, cephalexin, cephalothin, cephapirin[1], and cephradine are indicated in the treatment of skin and soft tissue infections caused by susceptible organisms.

Tonsillitis (treatment)—Cefaclor, cefadroxil, cefixime, cefpodoxime[1], cefprozil[1], cefuroxime axetil, cephalexin, and cephradine are indicated in the treatment of bacterial pharyngitis caused by susceptible organisms.

Urinary tract infections, bacterial (treatment)—Cefaclor, cefadroxil, cefamandole, cefazolin, cefixime, cefmetazole[1], cefonicid[1], cefoperazone, cefotaxime, cefotetan, cefoxitin, cefpodoxime[1], [cefprozil][1], ceftazidime, ceftizoxime, ceftriaxone, cefuroxime, cephalexin, cephalothin, cephapirin[1], and cephradine are indicated in the treatment of bacterial urinary tract infections caused by susceptible organisms.

[Lyme disease (treatment)][1]—Cefotaxime and ceftriaxone are used in the treatment of Lyme disease.

[Sinusitis (treatment)][1]—Cefaclor is used in the treatment of sinusitis resistant to amoxicillin.

## Unaccepted

None of the cephalosporins is considered to be effective against enterococci, *Listeria* species, chlamydia, *Clostridium difficile*, or methicillin-resistant *Staphylococcus epidermidis* or *S. aureus*.

---

[1]Not included in Canadian product labeling.

## Pharmacology/Pharmacokinetics

See also *Table 1*, page 771, and *Table 2*, page 774.

## Physicochemical characteristics

Molecular weight—
    Cefaclor: 385.83.
    Cefadroxil: 381.41.
    Cefamandole nafate: 512.51.
    Cefazolin sodium: 476.50.
    Cefixime: 507.51.
    Cefmetazole sodium: 493.53.
    Cefonicid sodium: 586.54.
    Cefoperazone sodium: 667.66.
    Cefotaxime sodium: 477.46.
    Cefotetan disodium: 619.60.
    Cefoxitin sodium: 449.44.
    Cefpodoxime proxetil: 557.61.
    Cefprozil: 407.45.
    Ceftazidime: 636.67.
    Ceftizoxime sodium: 405.39.
    Ceftriaxone sodium: 661.61.
    Cefuroxime axetil: 510.48.
    Cefuroxime sodium: 446.38.
    Cephalexin: 365.41.
    Cephalothin sodium: 418.43.
    Cephapirin sodium: 445.46.
    Cephradine: 349.41.

## Mechanism of action/Effect

Bactericidal; action depends on ability to reach and bind penicillin-binding proteins located in bacterial cytoplasmic membranes; cephalosporins inhibit bacterial septum and cell wall synthesis, probably by acylation of membrane-bound transpeptidase enzymes. This prevents cross-linkage of peptidoglycan chains, which is necessary for bacterial cell wall strength and rigidity. Also, cell division and growth are inhibited, and lysis and elongation of susceptible bacteria frequently occur. Rapidly dividing bacteria are those most susceptible to the action of cephalosporins.

## Distribution

Also distributed in bone, the myocardium, the gallbladder, and skin and soft tissue.

Cross the placenta and enter breast milk.

The only cephalosporins to achieve therapeutic concentrations in the cerebrospinal fluid (CSF) are cefuroxime, cefotaxime, ceftazidime, ceftizoxime, and ceftriaxone.

Cefoperazone and ceftriaxone reach the highest concentration in bile.

Cefuroxime, and ceftazidime reach the highest levels in the aqueous humor.

## Time to peak bile concentration

Cefoperazone—1 to 3 hours.

## Bile concentration

Cefixime—Approximately 56.9 mcg per mL following a single 200 mg oral dose.

Cefmetazole—Approximately 310 mcg per mL 2.8 hours following a 1 gram intravenous dose.

Cefoperazone—Approximately 65, 1940, and 6000 mcg per mL ½, 1, and 3 hours, respectively, following a 2-gram intravenous bolus dose.

# Precautions to Consider

## Cross-sensitivity and/or related problems

Patients allergic to one cephalosporin or cephamycin may be allergic to other cephalosporins or cephamycins also.

Patients allergic to penicillins, penicillin derivatives, or penicillamine may be allergic to cephalosporins or cephamycins also. Cephalosporin cross-reactivity is approximately 3 to 7% in patients with a documented history of penicillin allergy. Although cephalosporins have been administered without incident to some patients with rash-type penicillin allergy, caution is recommended when cephalosporins are administered to patients with a history of penicillin anaphylaxis since anaphylaxis may also occur after cephalosporin administration.

## Carcinogenicity

*Cefazolin, cefixime, cefmetazole, cefonicid, cefoperazone, cefotaxime, cefotetan, cefoxitin, cefpodoxime, cefprozil, ceftazidime, ceftriaxone, cefuroxime axetil, and cephradine*—Long-term studies in animals to evaluate the carcinogenic potential of these cephalosporins have not been done.

## Mutagenicity

*Cefazolin, cefoxitin, and cephradine*—Long-term studies in animals to evaluate the mutagenic potential of cefazolin, cefoxitin, and cephradine have not been done.

*Cefixime, cefmetazole, cefonicid, cefoperazone, cefotaxime, cefotetan, cefprozil, ceftazidime, ceftriaxone, and cefuroxime*—Studies have not shown that these cephalosporins are mutagenic.

## Pregnancy/Reproduction

Fertility—

*Cefamandole, cefmetazole, cefoperazone, and cefotetan*—
    Adequate and well-controlled studies in humans have not been done.

    Beta-lactam antibacterials containing the *N*-methyltetrazolethiol side chain have not been shown to cause adverse effects on fertility in rats exposed in utero, in neonatal rats (4 days of age or younger) that were treated prior to initiation of spermatogenesis, or in older rats (more than 40 days of age) after exposure for up to 6 months. Beta-lactam antibacterials containing the *N*-methyltetrazolethiol side chain have been shown to cause delayed maturation of the testicular germinal epithelium when given to neonatal rats during initial spermatogenic development (6 to 40 days of age), although the effect was slight in rats given 30 to 100 mg per kg of body weight (mg/kg) daily. However, in those neonatal rats given 1000 mg per kg daily (approximately 5 to 20 times the usual clinical dose), the delayed maturation was pronounced and was associated with decreased testicular weights, arrested spermatogenesis, a reduced number of germinal cells, and vacuolation of Sertoli cell cytoplasm. In addition, some neonatal rats given 1000 mg per kg daily from days 6 to 40 were infertile after reaching sexual maturity.

*Other cephalosporins*—
    Adequate and well-controlled studies in humans have not been done.

    However, studies in animals have not shown that these cephalosporins cause impaired fertility.

Pregnancy—

*Cefamandole, cefmetazole, cefoperazone, and cefotetan*—
    Cefamandole, cefoperazone, and cefotetan cross the placenta. Adequate and well-controlled studies in humans have not been done.

    Studies in mice, rats, and monkeys given doses up to 10 times the usual human dose have not shown that cefamandole, cefmetazole, cefoperazone, or cefotetan causes adverse effects on the fetus.

    FDA Pregnancy Category B.

*Cefoxitin*—
    Cefoxitin crosses the placenta. Adequate and well-controlled studies in humans have not been done.

    Studies in rats and mice given parenteral doses of approximately 1 to 7.5 times the maximum recommended human dose have not shown that cefoxitin is teratogenic or fetotoxic. However, a slight decrease in fetal weight was observed. Studies in rabbits have shown that cefoxitin, although not teratogenic, causes a high incidence of abortion and maternal death.

    FDA Pregnancy Category B.

*Other cephalosporins*—
    Cephalosporins cross the placenta. Adequate and well-controlled studies in humans have not been done.

    However, studies in animals have not shown that these cephalosporins cause adverse effects on the fetus.

    FDA Pregnancy Category B—Cefaclor, cefadroxil, cefazolin, cefixime, cefonicid, cefotaxime, cefpodoxime, cefprozil, ceftazidime, ceftizoxime, ceftriaxone, cefuroxime, cephalexin, cephalothin, cephapirin, and cephradine.

## Breast-feeding

*Cefixime*—It is not known whether cefixime is distributed into human breast milk. However, problems in humans have not been documented to date.

*Other cephalosporins*—Other cephalosporins are distributed into breast milk, usually in low concentrations. However, problems in humans have not been documented to date.

## Pediatrics

*All cephalosporins*—Lower metabolic and/or renal clearance of cephalosporins, with resulting prolonged half-life, has been reported in newborn infants. However, ceftriaxone has been found to have a shorter half-life in infants than it does in adults.

*Cefaclor, cefamandole, cefazolin*—Appropriate studies on the relationship of age to the effects of cefaclor, cefamandole, or cefazolin have not been performed in premature infants and infants up to 1 month of age. However, no pediatrics-specific problems have been documented to date in children 1 month of age and older.

*Cefixime, cefpodoxime, and cefprozil*—Appropriate studies on the relationship of age to the effects of cefixime, cefpodoxime, or cefprozil have not been performed in children up to 6 months of age.

*Cefmetazole, cefoperazone, cefotetan*—Appropriate studies on the relationship of age to the effects of cefmetazole, cefoperazone, or cefotetan have not been performed in the pediatric population.

*Cefonicid*—Cefonicid has been used in children 1 year of age and older, and no pediatrics-specific problems have been documented to date.

*Cefoxitin*—In children 3 months of age and older, higher doses of cefoxitin have been associated with an increased incidence of eosinophilia and elevated aspartate aminotransferase (AST [SGOT]).

*Ceftazidime L-arginine*—The safety of the arginine component of ceftazidime L-arginine has not been established in children. If treatment with ceftazidime is indicated for children under 12 years of age, the ceftazidime sodium product should be used.

*Ceftizoxime*—Although studies have been done in children up to 6 months of age, ceftizoxime is not indicated for this age group. In children 6 months of age and older, the use of ceftizoxime has been associated with transient elevated concentrations of eosinophils, alanine aminotransferase (ALT [SGPT]), aspartate aminotransferase (AST [SGOT]), and creatine kinase (CK).

*Ceftriaxone*—Because ceftriaxone is very highly bound to plasma proteins, it may be more likely than some other cephalosporins to displace bilirubin from serum albumin. Ceftriaxone should be used with caution in hyperbilirubinemic neonates, especially premature neonates.

*Cefuroxime, cephapirin*—Appropriate studies on the relationship of age to the effects of cefuroxime and cephapirin have not been performed in children up to 3 months of age. However, no pediatrics-specific problems have been documented to date in children 3 months of age and older.

*Cephradine*—Appropriate studies on the relationship of age to the effects of cephradine have not been performed in children up to 1 year of age. However, no pediatrics-specific problems have been documented to date in children 1 year of age and older.

*Other cephalosporins*—Appropriate studies on the relationship of age to the effects of these cephalosporins have not been performed in the pediatric population. However, no pediatrics-specific problems have been documented to date.

**Geriatrics**
Cephalosporins have been used in the geriatric population, and no geriatrics-specific problems have been documented to date. However, elderly patients are more likely to have an age-related decrease in renal function, which may require an adjustment of dosage and/or dosing interval in patients receiving cephalosporins.

**Dental**
Long-term therapy with cephalosporins may allow for the overgrowth of *Candida albicans*, resulting in oral candidiasis.

**Drug interactions and/or related problems**
The following drug interactions and/or related problems have been selected on the basis of their potential clinical significance (possible mechanism in parentheses where appropriate)—not necessarily inclusive (» = major clinical significance):

Note: Combinations containing any of the following medications, depending on the amount present, may also interact with this medication.

» Alcohol
(concurrent use of alcohol with cefamandole, cefmetazole, cefoperazone, or cefotetan is not recommended since these cephalosporins, due to their N-methylthiotetrazole side chain, may inhibit the enzyme acetaldehyde dehydrogenase, resulting in accumulation of acetaldehyde in the blood)

(disulfiram-like effects such as abdominal or stomach cramps, nausea, vomiting, headache, hypotension, palpitations, shortness of breath, tachycardia, sweating, or facial flushing may occur following ingestion of alcohol or administration of intravenous alcohol-containing solutions; these effects usually occur within 15 to 30 minutes following ingestion of alcohol and usually subside spontaneously over several hours)

(patients should be advised not to drink alcoholic beverages, take alcohol-containing medications, or receive intravenous alcohol-containing solutions while receiving these cephalosporins and for several days after discontinuing them)

Antacids or
Histamine H₂-receptor antagonists
(concurrent use of high doses of antacids or H₂-receptor antagonists with cefpodoxime decreases absorption of cefpodoxime by 27 to 32%, and decreases peak plasma levels by 24 to 42%)

» Anticoagulants, coumarin- or indandione-derivative, or
» Heparin or
» Thrombolytic agents
(concurrent use of these medications with cefamandole, cefmetazole, cefoperazone, or cefotetan may increase the risk of bleeding

because of the N-methylthiotetrazole [NMTT] side chain on these medications. However, critical illness, poor nutritional status, and the presence of liver disease may be more important risk factors for hypoprothrombinemia and bleeding. All cephalosporins can inhibit vitamin K synthesis by suppressing gut flora. Prophylactic vitamin K therapy is recommended when any of these medications is used for prolonged periods in malnourished or seriously ill patients. Dosage adjustments of anticoagulants may be necessary during and after therapy with cefamandole, cefmetazole, cefoperazone, or cefotetan; concurrent use of these 4 cephalosporins with thrombolytic agents may increase the risk of severe hemorrhage and is not recommended)

Nephrotoxic medications (See *Appendix II*)
(cephalothin has been associated with an increased incidence of nephrotoxicity when used concurrently with aminoglycosides; this effect has rarely been seen with other commercially available cephalosporins used at appropriate doses; the potential for increased nephrotoxicity exists when cephalosporins are used with other nephrotoxic medications, such as loop diuretics, especially in patients with pre-existing renal function impairment)

» Platelet aggregation inhibitors, other (See *Appendix II*)
(hypoprothrombinemia induced by large doses of salicylates and/or cephalosporins, and the gastrointestinal ulcerative or hemorrhagic potential of nonsteroidal anti-inflammatory drugs [NSAIDs], salicylates, or sulfinpyrazone may increase the risk of hemorrhage)

» Probenecid
(probenecid decreases renal tubular secretion of those cephalosporins excreted by this mechanism, resulting in increased and prolonged cephalosporin serum concentrations, prolonged elimination half-life, and increased risk of toxicity; probenecid has no effect on the excretion of cefoperazone, ceftazidime, or ceftriaxone; however, other cephalosporins and probenecid might be used concurrently in the treatment of infections, such as sexually transmitted diseases [STDs] or other infections, in which high and/or prolonged antibiotic serum and tissue concentrations are required)

**Laboratory value alterations**
The following have been selected on the basis of their potential clinical significance (possible effect in parentheses where appropriate)—not necessarily inclusive (» = major clinical significance):

With diagnostic test results
» Coombs' (antiglobulin) tests
(a positive Coombs' reaction frequently appears in patients who receive large doses of a cephalosporin; hemolysis rarely occurs, but has been reported; test may become positive in neonates whose mothers received cephalosporins before delivery)

Creatinine, serum and urine
(cefotetan, cefoxitin, and cephalothin may falsely elevate test values when the Jaffe reaction is used; serum samples should not be obtained within 2 hours after administration)

Glucose, blood
(cefuroxime may give false-negative test results with ferricyanide tests; glucose enzymatic or hexokinase tests are recommended to determine blood glucose concentrations)

» Glucose, urine
(some cephalosporins [cefaclor, cefamandole, cefazolin, cefotetan, cefoxitin, cefuroxime, cephalexin, cephalothin, cephapirin, cephradine] may produce false-positive or falsely elevated test results with copper sulfate tests [Benedict's, Fehling's, or *Clinitest* tablets]; glucose enzymatic tests, such as *Clinistix* and *Tes-Tape*, are not affected)

Protein, urine
(cefamandole may produce false-positive tests for proteinuria with acid and denaturization-precipitation tests)

» Prothrombin time (PT)
(may be prolonged; cephalosporins may inhibit vitamin K synthesis by suppressing gut flora; also, cephalosporins with the NMTT side chain [cefamandole, cefmetazole, cefoperazone, cefotetan] have been associated with an increased incidence of hypoprothrombinemia; patients who are critically ill, malnourished, or have liver function impairment may be at the highest risk of bleeding)

With physiology/laboratory test values
Alanine aminotransferase (ALT [SGPT]), serum, or
Alkaline phosphatase, serum, or
Aspartate aminotransferase (AST [SGOT]), serum, or
Bilirubin, serum, or
Lactate dehydrogenase (LDH), serum
(values may be increased)

Blood urea nitrogen (BUN) or
Creatinine, serum
    (concentrations may be increased)
Complete blood count (CBC) or
Platelet count
    (transient leukopenia, neutropenia, agranulocytosis, thrombocyto-
    penia, eosinophilia, lymphocytosis, and thrombocytosis have been
    seen on rare occasions)

## Medical considerations/Contraindications

The medical considerations/contraindications included here have been selected on the basis of their potential clinical significance (reasons given
in parentheses where appropriate)—not necessarily inclusive (» =
major clinical significance).

*Except under special circumstances, this medication should not be used
when the following medical problem exists:*

» Previous allergic reaction (anaphylaxis) to penicillins, penicillin deriv-
    atives, penicillamine, or cephalosporins

*Risk-benefit should be considered when the following medical problems
exist:*

» Bleeding disorders, history of
    (cefamandole, cefmetazole, cefoperazone, and cefotetan, which
    contain the NMTT side chain, have been associated with an in-
    creased risk of bleeding; however, all cephalosporins may cause
    hypoprothrombinemia and, potentially, bleeding)

» Gastrointestinal disease, history of, especially ulcerative colitis, re-
    gional enteritis, or antibiotic-associated colitis
    (cephalosporins may cause pseudomembranous colitis)

» Hepatic function impairment
    (cefoperazone is primarily excreted in bile; may also cause ele-
    vated AST [SGOT], ALT [SGPT], and alkaline phosphatase; it is
    recommended that patients with both severe liver disease and sig-
    nificant renal disease receive a reduced dosage of cefoperazone)

Phenylketonuria
    (cefprozil for oral suspension contains 28 mg of phenylalanine per
    5 mL)

» Renal function impairment
    (many cephalosporins are excreted renally; a reduced dosage is
    recommended in patients with renal function impairment receiving
    cefadroxil, cefamandole, cefazolin, cefixime, cefmetazole, cefoni-
    cid, cefotaxime, cefotetan, cefoxitin, cefpodoxime, cefprozil, cef-
    tazidime, ceftizoxime, cefuroxime, cephalexin, cephalothin, and
    cephradine)

## Patient monitoring

The following may be especially important in patient monitoring (other
tests may be warranted in some patients, depending on condition;
» = major clinical significance):

*For all cephalosporins*
Bleeding time and/or
» Prothrombin time (PT)
    (determinations may be required in selected patients prior to and
    during therapy since hypoprothrombinemia and decreased vitamin
    K–dependent clotting factors may occur, on rare occasion, result-
    ing in significant hemorrhage; administration of vitamin K
    promptly reverses the hypoprothrombinemia, which usually occurs
    in elderly, debilitated, malnourished, or other seriously ill patients
    with deficient vitamin K stores; prophylactic daily or periodic ad-
    ministration of vitamin K may be required, especially in such pa-
    tients receiving cefamandole, cefmetazole, cefoperazone, or
    cefotetan)

*For antibiotic-associated pseudomembranous colitis (AAPMC)*
Stool examinations
    (cytotoxin assays of stool samples for the presence of *Clostridium
    difficile* and its cytotoxin, neutralizable by *C. sordellii* antitoxin,
    may be required prior to treatment in patients with AAPMC to
    document the presence of *C. difficile* and/or its cytotoxin; however,
    *C. difficile* and its cytotoxin may persist following treatment with
    oral vancomycin, cholestyramine, bacitracin, or metronidazole de-
    spite clinical improvement; follow-up cytotoxin assays are gener-
    ally not recommended with complete clinical improvement)

## Side/Adverse Effects

The following side/adverse effects have been selected on the basis of their
potential clinical significance (possible signs and symptoms in parentheses where appropriate)—not necessarily inclusive:

### Those indicating need for medical attention

Incidence less frequent or rare
    *For all cephalosporins*
        ***Hypoprothrombinemia*** (unusual bleeding or bruising)—more fre-
        quent for cefamandole, cefmetazole, cefoperazone, and cefotetan;
        ***pseudomembranous colitis*** (severe abdominal or stomach cramps
        and pain; abdominal tenderness; watery and severe diarrhea, which
        may also be bloody; fever)

Incidence rare
    *For all cephalosporins*
        ***Allergic reactions, specifically anaphylaxis*** (bronchospasm; hy-
        potension); ***erythema multiforme, or Stevens-Johnson syndrome***
        (blistering, peeling, or loosening of skin and mucous membranes;
        may involve the eyes or other organ systems); ***hemolytic anemia,
        immune, drug-induced*** (unusual tiredness or weakness; yellowing
        of the eyes or skin)—has occurred with many cephalosporins, but
        has been reported more commonly with cefotetan; ***hypersensitivity***
        (fever; skin rash; itching; redness; swelling); ***renal dysfunction***
        (decrease in urine output or decrease in urine concentrating abil-
        ity); ***serum sickness–like reactions*** (skin rash; joint pain; fever)—
        may be more frequent with cefaclor; ***seizures***—especially with
        high doses and in patients with renal function impairment; ***throm-
        bophlebitis*** (pain, redness, and swelling at site of injection)

    *For ceftriaxone only*
        ***Biliary "sludge" or pseudolithiasis*** (epigastric pain; anorexia;
        nausea and vomiting)—more likely when administered by intra-
        venous bolus over 3 to 5 minutes

### Those indicating need for medical attention only if they continue or are bothersome

Incidence more frequent—less frequent with some cephalosporins
    ***Oral candidiasis*** (sore mouth or tongue); ***gastrointestinal reactions***
    (mild diarrhea; abdominal cramps; nausea or vomiting); ***vaginal can-
    didiasis*** (vaginal itching and discharge)

### Those indicating possible pseudomembranous colitis and the need for medical attention if they occur after medication is discontinued

    ***Severe abdominal or stomach cramps and pain; abdominal tender-
    ness; fever; watery and severe diarrhea, which may also be bloody***

## Patient Consultation

As an aid to patient consultation, refer to *Advice for the Patient,
Cephalosporins (Systemic).*

In providing consultation, consider emphasizing the following selected
information (» = major clinical significance):

### Before using this medication

» Conditions affecting use, especially:
    Allergies to penicillins, penicillin derivatives, penicillamine, or
        cephalosporins
    Pregnancy—Cephalosporins cross the placenta
    Breast-feeding—Most cephalosporins are distributed into breast-
        milk; however, it is not known if cefixime is distributed into
        breast-milk; no problems in humans have been documented
    Use in children—Accumulation of cephalosporins, with resulting
        prolonged half-life, has been reported in newborn infants. Ce-
        foxitin and ceftizoxime have been associated with an increased
        incidence of eosinophilia and elevated aspartate aminotransfer-
        ase (AST [SGOT]). Ceftizoxime has also been associated with
        elevated alanine aminotransferase (ALT [SGPT]) and creatine
        kinase (CK). Ceftriaxone should be used with caution in hy-
        perbilirubinemic neonates since it may be more likely than
        other cephalosporins to displace bilirubin from serum albumin
    Other medications, especially alcohol, anticoagulants, heparin,
        thrombolytic agents, platelet aggregation inhibitors, or
        probenecid
    Other medical problems, especially a history of bleeding disorders;
        a history of gastrointestinal disease, such as colitis; hepatic
        function impairment; or renal function impairment

### Proper use of this medication

    Taking on a full or empty stomach, or with food if gastrointestinal
        irritation occurs; absorption of cefuroxime axetil and cefpodoxime
        proxetil is enhanced when they are administered with food
    Proper administration technique for oral liquids and/or pediatric drops;
        not using after expiration date

» Compliance with full course of therapy, especially in streptococcal infections
» Importance of not missing doses and taking at evenly spaced times
» Proper dosing
  Missed dose: Taking as soon as possible; not taking if almost time for next dose; not doubling doses
» Proper storage
*For patients unable to swallow cefuroxime axetil tablets whole*
  Crushing tablets and mixing with food to mask the strong, persistent bitter taste

**Precautions while using this medication**

Checking with physician if no improvement within a few days
» Diabetics: False-positive reactions with copper sulfate urine glucose tests may occur
» For severe diarrhea, checking with physician before taking any anti-diarrheals; for mild diarrhea, kaolin- or attapulgite-containing, but not other, antidiarrheals may be tried; checking with physician or pharmacist if mild diarrhea continues or worsens
» Avoiding alcoholic beverages or other alcohol-containing preparations while receiving, and for several days after discontinuing, cefamandole, cefmetazole, cefoperazone, or cefotetan

**Side/adverse effects**

Signs of potential side effects, especially hypoprothrombinemia, pseudomembranous colitis, allergic reactions, hemolytic anemia, renal dysfunction, serum sickness–like reactions, hypersensitivity reactions, seizures, thrombophlebitis, or biliary ''sludge'' or pseudolithiasis

# General Dosing Information

Therapy should be continued for at least 10 days in group A beta-hemolytic streptococcal infections to help prevent the occurrence of acute rheumatic fever or glomerulonephritis.

**For oral dosage forms only**

Cephalosporins may be taken on a full or empty stomach. Taking them with food may help if gastrointestinal irritation occurs. Absorption of cefuroxime axetil and cefpodoxime proxetil is enhanced when they are administered with food.

**For parenteral dosage forms only**

Perioperative (preoperative, intraoperative, and postoperative) prophylactic administration of parenteral cephalosporins usually should be discontinued within 24 hours following surgery.

**For treatment of adverse effects and/or overdose**

Since there is no specific antidote, treatment of cephalosporin overdose should be symptomatic and supportive.

For antibiotic-associated pseudomembranous colitis (AAPMC)—

Some patients may develop AAPMC, caused by *Clostridium difficile* toxin, during or following administration of cephalosporins. Mild cases may respond to discontinuation of the drug alone. Moderate to severe cases may require fluid, electrolyte, and protein replacement.

In cases not responding to the above measures or in more severe cases, oral doses of metronidazole, bacitracin, cholestyramine, or vancomycin may be used. Oral vancomycin is effective in doses of 125 to 500 mg every 6 hours for 5 to 10 days. The dose of metronidazole is 250 to 500 mg every 8 hours; cholestyramine, 4 grams four times a day; and bacitracin, 25,000 units, orally, four times a day for 5 to 10 days. Recurrences are not uncommon, and may be treated with a second course of these medications.

Cholestyramine and colestipol resins have been shown to bind *C. difficile* toxin *in vitro*. If cholestyramine or colestipol resin is administered in conjunction with oral vancomycin, the medications should be administered several hours apart since the resins have been shown to bind oral vancomycin also.

In addition, AAPMC may result in severe watery diarrhea, which may occur during therapy or up to several weeks after therapy is discontinued. If diarrhea occurs, administration of antiperistaltic antidiarrheals (e.g., opiates, diphenoxylate and atropine combination, loperamide) is not recommended since they may delay the removal of toxins from the colon, thereby prolonging and/or worsening damage to the colon because of toxin retention.

If hypersensitivity reactions occur, cephalosporins should be discontinued and the patient should be treated with the usual agents (epinephrine or other pressor amines, antihistamines, or corticosteroids), oxygen, and airway management, including intubation.

If seizures occur, cephalosporins should be discontinued. Anticonvulsants may be administered if clinically indicated.

---

## CEFACLOR

# Summary of Differences

Category: Second-generation cephalosporin.
Indications: Good activity against *Haemophilus influenzae*.
Side/adverse effects: Serum sickness–like reactions more common.

# Oral Dosage Forms

## CEFACLOR CAPSULES USP

**Usual adult and adolescent dose**
Antibacterial—
  Oral, 250 to 500 mg every eight hours.

**Usual adult prescribing limits**
Up to 4 grams daily.

**Usual pediatric dose**
Antibacterial—
  Infants up to 1 month of age: Dosage has not been established.
  Infants 1 month of age and over: Oral, 6.7 to 13.4 mg per kg of body weight every eight hours, or 10 to 20 mg per kg of body weight every twelve hours.

Note: Doses up to 60 mg per kg of body weight daily have been used. However, in older children, the maximum daily dose should not exceed 1.5 grams.

**Strength(s) usually available**
U.S.—
  250 mg (Rx) [*Ceclor*].
  500 mg (Rx) [*Ceclor*].
Canada—
  250 mg (Rx) [*Ceclor*].
  500 mg (Rx) [*Ceclor*].

**Packaging and storage**
Store below 40 °C (104 °F), preferably between 15 and 30 °C (59 and 86 °F), unless otherwise specified by manufacturer. Store in a tight container.

**Auxiliary labeling**
• Continue medicine for full time of treatment.

## CEFACLOR FOR ORAL SUSPENSION USP

**Usual adult and adolescent dose**
See *Cefaclor Capsules USP*.

**Usual adult prescribing limits**
See *Cefaclor Capsules USP*.

**Usual pediatric dose**
See *Cefaclor Capsules USP*.

**Strength(s) usually available**
U.S.—
  125 mg per 5 mL (when reconstituted according to manufacturer's instructions) (Rx) [*Ceclor*].
  187 mg per 5 mL (when reconstituted according to manufacturer's instructions) (Rx) [*Ceclor*].
  250 mg per 5 mL (when reconstituted according to manufacturer's instructions) (Rx) [*Ceclor*].
  375 mg per 5 mL (when reconstituted according to manufacturer's instructions) (Rx) [*Ceclor*].
Canada—
  125 mg per 5 mL (when reconstituted according to manufacturer's instructions) (Rx) [*Ceclor*].
  250 mg per 5 mL (when reconstituted according to manufacturer's instructions) (Rx) [*Ceclor*].
  375 mg per 5 mL (when reconstituted according to manufacturer's instructions) (Rx) [*Ceclor*].

**Packaging and storage**
Prior to reconstitution, store below 40 °C (104 °F), preferably between 15 and 30 °C (59 and 86 °F), unless otherwise specified by manufacturer. Store in a tight container.

**Stability**
After reconstitution, suspensions retain their potency for 14 days if refrigerated.

**Auxiliary labeling**
• Refrigerate.
• Shake well.

• Continue medicine for full time of treatment.
• Beyond-use date.

**Note**

When dispensing, include a calibrated liquid-measuring device.

---

## *CEFADROXIL*

## Summary of Differences

Category: First-generation cephalosporin.

## Oral Dosage Forms
### CEFADROXIL CAPSULES USP

**Usual adult and adolescent dose**

Antibacterial—

Group A beta-hemolytic streptococcal pharyngitis (including tonsillitis): Oral, 500 mg every twelve hours; or 1 gram once a day for ten days.

Skin and soft tissue infections: Oral, 500 mg every twelve hours; or 1 gram once a day.

Urinary tract infections: Oral, 500 mg to 1 gram every twelve hours; or 1 to 2 grams once a day.

Note: After an initial loading dose of 1 gram, adults with impaired renal function may require a reduction in dose as follows:

| Creatinine Clearance (mL/min)/ (mL/sec) | Dose |
| --- | --- |
| >50/0.83 | See *Usual adult and adolescent dose* |
| 25–50/0.42–0.83 | 500 mg every 12 hours |
| 10–25/0.17–0.42 | 500 mg every 24 hours |
| 0–10/0–0.17 | 500 mg every 36 hours |

**Usual adult prescribing limits**

Up to 4 grams daily.

**Usual pediatric dose**

Antibacterial—

Group A beta-hemolytic streptococcal pharyngitis (including tonsillitis): Oral, 15 mg per kg of body weight every twelve hours; or 30 mg per kg of body weight once a day for ten days.

Skin and soft tissue infections: Oral, 15 mg per kg of body weight every twelve hours; or 30 mg per kg of body weight once a day.

Urinary tract infections: Oral, 15 mg per kg of body weight every twelve hours.

**Strength(s) usually available**

U.S.—

500 mg (Rx) [*Duricef; Ultracef;* GENERIC].

Canada—

500 mg (Rx) [*Duricef*].

**Packaging and storage**

Store below 40 °C (104 °F), preferably between 15 and 30 °C (59 and 86 °F), unless otherwise specified by manufacturer. Store in a tight container.

**Auxiliary labeling**

• Continue medicine for full time of treatment.

### CEFADROXIL FOR ORAL SUSPENSION USP

**Usual adult and adolescent dose**

See *Cefadroxil Capsules USP.*

**Usual adult prescribing limits**

See *Cefadroxil Capsules USP.*

**Usual pediatric dose**

See *Cefadroxil Capsules USP.*

**Strength(s) usually available**

U.S.—

125 mg per 5 mL (when reconstituted according to manufacturer's instructions) (Rx) [*Duricef; Ultracef;* GENERIC].

250 mg per 5 mL (when reconstituted according to manufacturer's instructions) (Rx) [*Duricef; Ultracef;* GENERIC].

500 mg per 5 mL (when reconstituted according to manufacturer's instructions) (Rx) [*Duricef;* GENERIC].

Canada—

Not commercially available.

**Packaging and storage**

Prior to reconstitution, store below 40 °C (104 °F), preferably between 15 and 30 °C (59 and 86 °F), unless otherwise specified by manufacturer. Store in a tight container.

**Stability**

After reconstitution, suspensions retain their potency for 14 days if refrigerated.

**Auxiliary labeling**

• Refrigerate.
• Shake well.
• Continue medicine for full time of treatment.
• Beyond-use date.

**Note**

When dispensing, include a calibrated liquid-measuring device.

### CEFADROXIL TABLETS USP

**Usual adult and adolescent dose**

See *Cefadroxil Capsules USP.*

**Usual adult prescribing limits**

See *Cefadroxil Capsules USP.*

**Usual pediatric dose**

See *Cefadroxil Capsules USP.*

**Strength(s) usually available**

U.S.—

1 gram (Rx) [*Duricef; Ultracef;* GENERIC].

Canada—

Not commercially available.

**Packaging and storage**

Store below 40 °C (104 °F), preferably between 15 and 30 °C (59 and 86 °F), unless otherwise specified by manufacturer. Store in a tight container.

**Auxiliary labeling**

• Continue medicine for full time of treatment.

---

## *CEFAMANDOLE*

## Summary of Differences

Category:
    Second-generation cephalosporin.
Pharmacology/pharmacokinetics:
    Contains *N*-methylthiotetrazole (NMTT) side chain.
Precautions:
    Drug interactions and/or related problems—Interacts with alcohol (disulfiram-like reaction), oral anticoagulants, and other medications that affect blood clotting.
    Laboratory value alterations—May produce false-positive tests for proteinuria with acid and denaturization-precipitation tests.
    Medical considerations/contraindications—Caution also required in patients with history of bleeding problems.
    Patient monitoring—PT determinations may be required.
Side/adverse effects:
    May also cause unusual bleeding or bruising.

## Parenteral Dosage Forms

Note: The dosing and strengths of the dosage forms available are expressed in terms of cefamandole base (not the nafate salt).

### CEFAMANDOLE NAFATE FOR INJECTION USP

**Usual adult and adolescent dose**

Antibacterial—

Pneumonia (uncomplicated) and skin and soft tissue infections—Intramuscular or intravenous, 500 mg (base) every six hours.

Urinary tract infections—Intramuscular or intravenous, 500 mg to 1 gram (base) every eight hours.

Other infections—Intramuscular or intravenous, 500 mg to 2 grams (base) every four to six hours.

Note: Perioperative prophylaxis[1] Intramuscular or intravenous, 1 to 2 grams (base) one-half to one hour prior to the start of surgery; and 1 to 2 grams every six hours following surgery for up to twenty-four hours.

After an initial loading dose of 1 to 2 grams (base), adults with impaired renal function may require a reduction in dose as follows:

| Creatinine Clearance (mL/min)/ (mL/sec) | Dose (base) | |
| | Severe Infections | Life-threatening Infections (maximum) |
| --- | --- | --- |
| >80/1.33 | 1–2 grams every 6 hours | 2 grams every 4 hours |
| 50–80/0.83–1.33 | 750 mg–1.5 grams every 6 hours | 1.5 grams every 4 hours; or 2 grams every 6 hours |
| 25–50/0.42–0.83 | 750 mg–1.5 grams every 8 hours | 1.5 grams every 6 hours; or 2 grams every 8 hours |
| 10–25/0.17–0.42 | 500 mg–1 gram every 8 hours | 1 gram every 6 hours; or 1.25 grams every 8 hours |
| 2–10/0.03–0.17 | 500–750 mg every 12 hours | 670 mg every 8 hours; or 1 gram every 12 hours |
| <2/0.03 | 250–500 mg every 12 hours | 500 mg every 8 hours; or 750 mg every 12 hours |

### Usual adult prescribing limits
Up to 12 grams (base) daily.

Note: Doses up to 16 grams (base) daily have been used.

### Usual pediatric dose
Antibacterial—
  Premature infants and infants up to 1 month of age: Dosage has not been established.
  Infants 1 month of age and over: Intramuscular or intravenous, 8.3 to 16.7 mg (base) per kg of body weight every four hours; 12.5 to 25 mg per kg of body weight every six hours; or 16.7 to 33.3 mg per kg of body weight every eight hours.

Note: Perioperative prophylaxis[1]—Children 3 months of age and over: Intramuscular or intravenous, 12.5 to 25 mg (base) per kg of body weight one-half to one hour prior to the start of surgery; and 12.5 to 25 mg per kg of body weight every six hours following surgery.
  The maximum daily dose should not exceed 150 mg (base) per kg of body weight or the maximum daily adult dose.

### Size(s) usually available
U.S.—
  1 gram (base) (Rx) [Mandol (sodium 3.3 mEq per gram)].
  2 grams (base) (Rx) [Mandol (sodium 3.3 mEq per gram)].
  10 grams (base) (Rx) [Mandol (sodium 3.3 mEq per gram)].
Canada—
  500 mg (base) (Rx) [Mandol (sodium 3.3 mEq per gram)].
  1 gram (base) (Rx) [Mandol (sodium 3.3 mEq per gram)].
  2 grams (base) (Rx) [Mandol (sodium 3.3 mEq per gram)].

### Packaging and storage
Prior to reconstitution, store below 40 °C (104 °F), preferably between 15 and 30 °C (59 and 86 °F), unless otherwise specified by manufacturer.

### Preparation of dosage form
To prepare initial dilution for intramuscular use, add 3 mL of sterile water for injection, bacteriostatic water for injection, 0.9% sodium chloride injection, or bacteriostatic sodium chloride injection to each 1-gram vial. Also, up to 10 mL of 0.5 to 2% lidocaine hydrochloride injection (without epinephrine) may be added to each 1-gram vial.

To prepare initial dilution for direct intermittent intravenous use, add 10 mL of sterile water for injection, 5% dextrose injection, or 0.9% sodium chloride injection to each 1-gram vial. The resulting solution may be administered over a 3- to 5-minute period.

To prepare initial dilution for continuous intravenous infusion, add 10 mL of sterile water for injection to each 1-gram vial. The resulting solution may be further diluted in suitable diluents (see manufacturer's package insert).

For reconstitution of piggyback infusion bottles or pharmacy bulk vials, see manufacturer's labeling for instructions.

### Stability
After reconstitution, solutions retain their potency for 24 hours at room temperature (25 °C [77 °F]) or for 96 hours if refrigerated (5 °C [41 °F]).

If frozen immediately after reconstitution with sterile water for injection, 5% dextrose injection, or 0.9% sodium chloride injection, solutions retain their potency in the original container for 6 months at –20 °C (–4 °F). After being warmed to a maximum of 37 °C (98.6 °F), the solution should not be heated after thawing is complete. Once thawed, solutions should not be refrozen.

Solutions range in color from light yellow to amber depending on the concentration and diluent used. Solutions should not be used if they are of a different color or if they contain a precipitate.

Caution: During storage at room temperature, carbon dioxide develops inside the vial after reconstitution. This is of little or no consequence if the solution is added to sufficient quantities of intravenous fluids. However, if reconstituted cefamandole nafate is repackaged into cer-

tain types of syringes, continued production of carbon dioxide may cause leakage, or the rubber closure may be forced out of the barrel of the syringe. Therefore, syringes should be filled immediately prior to use.

### Incompatibilities
The admixture of beta-lactam antibacterials (penicillins and cephalosporins) and aminoglycosides may result in substantial mutual inactivation. If they are administered concurrently, they should be administered in separate sites. Do not mix them in the same intravenous bag or bottle.

Since cefamandole nafate contains sodium carbonate, it may be incompatible with magnesium or calcium ions (including Ringer's injection and lactated Ringer's injection).

### Additional information
Cefamandole nafate is rapidly hydrolyzed to cefamandole after initial dilution.

A solution containing 1 gram in 22 mL of sterile water for injection is isotonic.

[1]Not included in Canadian product labeling.

---

## CEFAZOLIN

# Summary of Differences
Category: First-generation cephalosporin.

# Parenteral Dosage Forms
Note: The dosing and strengths of the dosage forms available are expressed in terms of cefazolin base (not the sodium salt).

## CEFAZOLIN SODIUM INJECTION USP
### Usual adult and adolescent dose
Antibacterial—
  Intravenous infusion, 250 mg to 1.5 grams (base) every six to eight hours.

Note: Perioperative prophylaxis—Intravenous infusion, 1 gram (base) one-half to one hour prior to the start of surgery; 500 mg to 1 gram during surgery; and 500 mg to 1 gram every eight hours following surgery for up to twenty-four hours.

  Pneumococcal pneumonia—Intravenous infusion, 500 mg (base) every eight to twelve hours.

  Urinary tract infections (acute, uncomplicated)—Intravenous infusion, 1 gram (base) every twelve hours.

  After an initial loading dose of 500 mg (base), adults with impaired renal function may require a reduction in dose as follows:

| Creatinine Clearance (mL/min)/ (mL/sec) | Dose (base) |
| --- | --- |
| ≥55/0.92 | See Usual adult and adolescent dose |
| 35–54/0.58–0.90 | Full dose every 8 hours or less frequently |
| 11–34/0.18–0.57 | ½ usual dose every 12 hours |
| ≤10/0.17 | ½ usual dose every 18–24 hours |

### Usual adult prescribing limits
Up to 6 grams (base) daily; however, doses up to 12 grams daily have been used in rare instances.

### Usual pediatric dose
Antibacterial—
  Premature infants and infants up to 1 month of age: Dosage form not appropriate for neonates.
  Infants and children 1 month of age and over: Intravenous infusion, 6.25 to 25 mg (base) per kg of body weight every six hours; or 8.3 to 33.3 mg per kg of body weight every eight hours.

Note: After an initial loading dose, children with impaired renal function may require a reduction in dose as follows:

| Creatinine Clearance (mL/min)/ (mL/sec) | Dose (base) |
| --- | --- |
| >70/1.17 | See Usual pediatric dose |
| 40–70/0.67–1.17 | 7.5–30 mg per kg of body weight every 12 hours |
| 20–40/0.33–0.67 | 3.1–12.5 mg per kg of body weight every 12 hours |
| 5–20/0.08–0.33 | 2.5–10 mg per kg of body weight every 24 hours |

**Strength(s) usually available**
U.S.—
    500 mg (base) per 50 mL (Rx)
        [*Ancef* (sodium 2 mEq per
        gram); GENERIC].
    500 mg (base) per 100 mL (Rx) [GENERIC].
    1 gram (base) per 50 mL (Rx) [*Ancef* (sodium 2 mEq per gram);
        GENERIC].
    1 gram (base) per 100 mL (Rx) [*Ancef* (sodium 2 mEq per gram);
        GENERIC].
Canada—
    Not commercially available.

**Packaging and storage**
Do not store above –10 °C (14 °F), unless otherwise specified by
    manufacturer.

**Preparation of dosage form**
Thaw container at room temperature before administration, making sure
    that all ice crystals have melted.
Do not use minibags in series connections. This may result in air embolism
    because of residual air being drawn from the primary container before
    administration of intravenous solution from the secondary container is
    complete.

**Stability**
After thawing, solutions retain their potency for 48 hours at room tem-
    perature or for 10 days if refrigerated at 5 °C (41 °F).
Once thawed, solutions should not be refrozen.
Do not use if the solution is cloudy or contains a precipitate.

**Incompatibilities**
The admixture of cefazolin sodium injection with other medications is not
    recommended.
The admixture of beta-lactam antibacterials (penicillins and cephalospo-
    rins) and aminoglycosides may result in substantial mutual inactiva-
    tion. If they are administered concurrently, they should be adminis-
    tered in separate sites. Do not mix them in the same intravenous bag
    or bottle.

### CEFAZOLIN SODIUM STERILE USP

**Usual adult and adolescent dose**
See *Cefazolin Sodium Injection USP*.

**Usual adult prescribing limits**
See *Cefazolin Sodium Injection USP*.

**Usual pediatric dose**
Antibacterial—
    Premature infants and infants up to 1 month of age:
        Less than 2000 grams of body weight, or more than 2000 grams
            of body weight and 7 days of age or less—Intravenous infu-
            sion, 20 mg (base) per kg of body weight every twelve hours.
        More than 2000 grams of body weight and over 7 days of age—
            Intravenous infusion, 20 mg (base) per kg of body weight every
            eight hours.
    Infants and children 1 month of age and over:
        See *Cefazolin Sodium Injection USP*.

**Size(s) usually available**
U.S.—
    500 mg (base) (Rx) [*Ancef* (sodium 46 mg per gram); *Kefzol* (sodium
        48.3 mg per gram); *Zolicef;* GENERIC].
    1 gram (base) (Rx) [*Ancef* (sodium 46 mg per gram); *Kefzol* (sodium
        48.3 mg per gram); *Zolicef;* GENERIC].
    5 grams (base) (Rx) [*Ancef* (sodium 46 mg per gram)].
    10 grams (base) (Rx) [*Ancef* (sodium 46 mg per gram); *Kefzol* (sodium
        48.3 mg per gram); GENERIC].
    20 grams (base) (Rx) [GENERIC].
Canada—
    500 mg (base) (Rx) [*Ancef* (sodium 46 mg per gram); *Gen-Cefazolin;*
        *Kefzol* (sodium 48.3 mg per gram)].
    1 gram (base) (Rx) [*Ancef* (sodium 46 mg per gram); *Gen-Cefazolin;*
        *Kefzol* (sodium 48.3 mg per gram)].
    10 grams (base) (Rx) [*Gen-Cefazolin; Kefzol* (sodium 48.3 mg per
        gram)].

**Packaging and storage**
Prior to reconstitution, store below 40 °C (104 °F), preferably between 15
    and 30 °C (59 and 86 °F), unless otherwise specified by manufacturer.

**Preparation of dosage form**
To prepare initial dilution for intramuscular use, add 2 mL of sterile water
    for injection, bacteriostatic water for injection, or 0.9% sodium chlo-
    ride injection to each 250- or 500-mg vial, or 2.5 mL of diluent to
    each 1-gram vial.

To prepare initial dilution for direct or intermittent intravenous use, add
    10 mL of sterile water for injection to each 500-mg or 1-gram vial.
    For direct intravenous use, the resulting solution may be administered
    over a 3- to 5-minute period. For intermittent intravenous use, the
    solution may be further diluted in 50 to 100 mL of suitable diluent
    (see manufacturer's package insert).
For reconstitution of piggyback infusion bottles, pharmacy bulk vials, and
    dual-compartment vials, see manufacturer's labeling for instructions.

**Stability**
After reconstitution, solutions retain their potency for 24 hours at room
    temperature or for 10 days if refrigerated.
If frozen immediately after reconstitution with sterile water for injection,
    5% dextrose injection, or 0.9% sodium chloride injection, solutions
    retain their potency in the original container up to 12 weeks at –20
    °C (–4 °F), depending on the manufacturer. Once thawed, solutions
    should not be refrozen.

**Incompatibilities**
The admixture of beta-lactam antibacterials (penicillins and cephalospo-
    rins) and aminoglycosides may result in substantial mutual inactiva-
    tion. If they are administered concurrently, they should be adminis-
    tered in separate sites. Do not mix them in the same intravenous bag
    or bottle.

---

### CEFIXIME

## Summary of Differences

Category: Third-generation cephalosporin. One of two oral third-generation cephalosporins.

## Additional Dosing Information

Patients with impaired renal function may require a reduction in dose as
follows:

| Creatinine Clearance (mL/min)/ (mL/sec) | Dose |
|---|---|
| >60/1.00 | See *Usual adult and adolescent dose* |
| 21–60/0.35–1.00 or hemodialysis patients | 75% of standard dosage at standard dosing interval |
| <20/0.33 or CAPD patients | 50% of standard dosage at standard dosing interval |

## Oral Dosage Forms
### CEFIXIME FOR ORAL SUSPENSION USP

**Usual adult and adolescent dose**
Antibacterial—
    Oral, 200 mg every twelve hours; or 400 mg once a day.
Note: Gonorrhea, uncomplicated urethral and cervical—Oral, 400 mg as
    a single dose.

**Usual pediatric dose**
Antibacterial—
    Infants up to 6 months of age: Dosage has not been established.
    Children 6 months of age and over: Oral, 4 mg per kg of body weight
        every twelve hours; or 8 mg per kg of body weight once a day.
    Children over 12 years of age or 50 kg of body weight: See *Usual
        adult and adolescent dose.*

**Strength(s) usually available**
U.S.—
    100 mg per 5 mL (when reconstituted according to manufacturer's
        instructions) (Rx) [*Suprax*].
Canada—
    100 mg per 5 mL (when reconstituted according to manufacturer's
        instructions) (Rx) [*Suprax*].

**Packaging and storage**
Prior to reconstitution, store below 40 °C (104 °F), preferably between 15
    and 30 °C (59 and 86 °F), unless otherwise specified by manufacturer.

**Stability**
After reconstitution, suspension retains its potency for 14 days at room
    temperature or if refrigerated.

**Auxiliary labeling**
• Does not require refrigeration.
• Shake well.
• Continue medicine for full time of treatment.
• Beyond-use date.

**Note**

When dispensing, include a calibrated liquid-measuring device.

## CEFIXIME TABLETS USP

**Usual adult and adolescent dose**

See *Cefixime for Oral Suspension USP.*

**Usual pediatric dose**

See *Cefixime for Oral Suspension USP.*

Note: Otitis media should be treated with cefixime suspension since the suspension results in higher peak blood levels than the tablet when administered at the same dose.

**Strength(s) usually available**

U.S.—

  200 mg (Rx) [*Suprax*].

  400 mg (Rx) [*Suprax*].

Canada—

  200 mg (Rx) [*Suprax* (scored)].

  400 mg (Rx) [*Suprax* (scored)].

**Packaging and storage**

Store below 40 °C (104 °F), preferably between 15 and 30 °C (59 and 86 °F), unless otherwise specified by manufacturer.

**Auxiliary labeling**

• Continue medicine for full time of treatment.

---

## CEFMETAZOLE

## Summary of Differences

Category:

  Cephamycin; second-generation cephalosporin.

Indications:

  Good activity against anaerobic organisms.

Pharmacology/pharmacokinetics:

  Contains *N*-methylthiotetrazole (NMTT) side chain.

Precautions:

  Drug interactions and/or related problems—Interacts with alcohol (disulfiram-like reaction), oral anticoagulants, and other medications that affect blood clotting.

  Medical considerations/contraindications—Caution also required in patients with history of bleeding problems.

  Patient monitoring—PT determinations may be required.

Side/adverse effects:

  May also cause unusual bleeding or bruising.

## Parenteral Dosage Forms

Note: The dosing and strengths of the dosage forms available are expressed in terms of cefmetazole base (not the sodium salt).

### CEFMETAZOLE SODIUM FOR INJECTION

**Usual adult and adolescent dose**

Antibacterial—

  Intravenous, 2 grams (base) every six to twelve hours for five to fourteen days.

Note: Gonorrhea, uncomplicated urethral, cervical, and rectal—Intramuscular, 1 gram (base) administered as a single dose, concurrently with, or one-half hour after, administration of a 1-gram oral dose of probenecid.

  Perioperative prophylaxis—Cesarean-section patients: Intravenous, 2 grams (base) as soon as the umbilical cord is clamped; or 1 gram as soon as the umbilical cord is clamped, and repeat in eight and sixteen hours.

  Perioperative prophylaxis—Other patients: Intravenous, 2 grams (base) thirty to ninety minutes prior to the start of surgery; or 1 to 2 grams thirty to ninety minutes prior to the start of surgery, and repeat in eight and sixteen hours.

  Adults with impaired renal function may require a reduction in dose as follows:

| Creatinine Clearance (mL/min)/ (mL/sec) | Dose (base) |
|---|---|
| >90/1.5 | See *Usual adult and adolescent dose* |
| 50–90/0.83–1.5 | 1 or 2 grams every 12 hours |
| 30–49/0.50–0.82 | 1 or 2 grams every 16 hours |
| 10–29/0.17–0.48 | 1 or 2 grams every 24 hours |
| <10/0.17 | 1 or 2 grams every 48 hours |

**Usual pediatric dose**

Dosage has not been established.

---

**Size(s) usually available**

U.S.—

  1 gram (base) (Rx) [*Zefazone*].

  2 grams (base) (Rx) [*Zefazone*].

Canada—

  Not commercially available.

**Packaging and storage**

Prior to reconstitution, do not store above 22 °C (72 °F), unless otherwise specified by manufacturer.

**Preparation of dosage form**

To prepare initial dilution for intravenous use, add sterile water for injection, bacteriostatic water for injection, or 0.9% sodium chloride injection to each vial.

**Stability**

After reconstitution for intravenous use, solutions retain their potency for 24 hours at room temperature (25 °C [77 °F]), 7 days if refrigerated at 8 °C (46 °F), or for 6 weeks if frozen. Once thawed, solutions should not be refrozen.

**Incompatibilities**

Cefmetazole inactivates heparin *in vitro*; therefore, these 2 medications should be administered at separate sites. The admixture of beta-lactam antibacterials (penicillins and cephalosporins) and aminoglycosides may result in substantial mutual inactivation. If they are administered concurrently, they should be administered in separate sites. Do not mix them in the same intravenous bag or bottle.

---

## CEFONICID

## Summary of Differences

Category: Second-generation cephalosporin.

## Additional Dosing Information

Intramuscular doses of 2 grams should be administered as divided doses in different sites.

## Parenteral Dosage Forms

Note: The dosing and strengths of the dosage forms available are expressed in terms of cefonicid base (not the sodium salt).

### CEFONICID SODIUM STERILE USP

**Usual adult and adolescent dose**

Antibacterial—

  Intramuscular or intravenous, 500 mg (base) to 1 gram every twenty-four hours.

Note: For severe or life-threatening infections—Intramuscular or intravenous, 2 grams (base) every twenty-four hours.

  Perioperative prophylaxis—Cesarean-section patients: Intravenous, 1 gram (base) as soon as the umbilical cord is clamped.

  Perioperative prophylaxis—Other surgical patients: Intravenous, 1 gram (base) one hour prior to the start of surgery.

  After an initial loading dose of 7.5 mg (base) per kg of body weight, adults with impaired renal function may require a reduction in dose as follows:

| Creatinine Clearance (mL/min)/(mL/sec) | Dose (base) | |
|---|---|---|
| | Mild to Moderate Infections | Severe Infections |
| ≥80/1.33 | See *Usual adult and adolescent dose* | See *Usual adult and adolescent dose* |
| 60–79/1.00–1.31 | 10 mg/kg every 24 hours | 25 mg/kg every 24 hours |
| 40–59/0.67–0.98 | 8 mg/kg every 24 hours | 20 mg/kg every 24 hours |
| 20–39/0.33–0.65 | 4 mg/kg every 24 hours | 15 mg/kg every 24 hours |
| 10–19/0.17–0.32 | 4 mg/kg every 48 hours | 15 mg/kg every 48 hours |
| 5–9/0.08–0.15 | 4 mg/kg every 3 to 5 days | 15 mg/kg every 3 to 5 days |
| <5/0.08 | 3 mg/kg every 3 to 5 days | 4 mg/kg every 3 to 5 days |

## Usual pediatric dose

Antibacterial—

Dosage has not been established; however, cefonicid has been used in children one year of age and older, and no pediatrics-specific problems have been reported.

## Size(s) usually available

U.S.—

500 mg (base) (Rx) [*Monocid* (sodium 3.7 mEq per gram)].

1 gram (base) (Rx) [*Monocid* (sodium 3.7 mEq per gram)].

10 grams (base) (Rx) [*Monocid* (sodium 3.7 mEq per gram)].

Canada—

Not commercially available.

## Packaging and storage

Prior to reconstitution, store below 8 °C (46 °F). Protect from light.

## Preparation of dosage form

To prepare initial dilution for intramuscular or intravenous use, add 2 mL of sterile water for injection to each 500-mg vial or 2.5 mL of diluent to each 1-gram vial. For direct intravenous use, the resulting solution may be administered over a 3- to 5-minute period. For intravenous infusions, the resulting solution may be further diluted in 50 to 100 mL of suitable fluids (see manufacturer's package insert).

For reconstitution of piggyback infusion bottles or pharmacy bulk vials, see manufacturer's labeling for instructions.

## Stability

After reconstitution for intramuscular or intravenous use, solutions retain their potency for 24 hours at room temperature or for 72 hours if refrigerated at 5 °C (41 °F).

Slight yellowing of cefonicid solutions does not affect their potency.

## Incompatibilities

The admixture of beta-lactam antibacterials (penicillins and cephalosporins) and aminoglycosides may result in substantial mutual inactivation. If they are administered concurrently, they should be administered in separate sites. Do not mix them in the same intravenous bag or bottle.

## Additional information

A solution containing 1 gram in 18 mL of sterile water for injection is isotonic.

---

## CEFOPERAZONE

## Summary of Differences

Category:

Third-generation cephalosporin.

Pharmacology/pharmacokinetics:

Achieves high biliary concentrations.

Contains *N*-methylthiotetrazole (NMTT) side chain.

Precautions:

Drug interactions and/or related problems—

Interacts with alcohol (disulfiram-like reaction), oral anticoagulants, and other medications that affect blood clotting.

Does not interact with probenecid.

Medical considerations/contraindications—

Caution required in patients with history of bleeding problems, and in patients with both severe hepatic function impairment and renal dysfunction.

Patient monitoring—

PT determinations may be required.

Side/adverse effects:

May also cause unusual bleeding or bruising.

## Additional Dosing Information

Cefoperazone should be administered intermittently by intravenous infusion over a 15- to 30-minute period or by continuous intravenous infusion. Rapid bolus injection is not recommended.

Patients with impaired renal function do not generally require a reduction in dose since cefoperazone is excreted primarily in the bile. Also, patients with impaired hepatic function or biliary obstruction who are not receiving maximum doses do not generally require a reduction in dose since a corresponding increase in renal excretion (up to 90% or more) usually compensates, to a large degree, for reduced biliary excretion.

Patients with combined renal and hepatic function impairment require a reduction in dose since cefoperazone is not significantly metabolized and toxic serum concentrations may occur.

## Parenteral Dosage Forms

Note: The dosing and strengths of the dosage forms available are expressed in terms of cefoperazone base (not the sodium salt).

## CEFOPERAZONE SODIUM INJECTION USP

## Usual adult dose

Antibacterial—

Mild to moderate infections—Intravenous infusion, 1 to 2 grams (base) every twelve hours.

Severe infections—Intravenous infusion, 2 to 4 grams (base) every eight hours; or 3 to 6 grams every twelve hours.

Note: Adults with impaired hepatic function and/or biliary obstruction should not receive more than 4 grams (base) daily.

Adults with combined hepatic and renal function impairment should not receive more than 1 to 2 grams (base) daily.

In patients who are receiving hemodialysis treatments, a dose should be scheduled to follow hemodialysis.

## Usual adult prescribing limits

Up to 12 grams (base) daily. However, up to 16 grams daily have been given by continuous infusion in severely immunocompromised patients without adverse effect.

## Usual pediatric dose

Dosage has not been established.

## Strength(s) usually available

U.S.—

1 gram in 50 mL (base) (Rx) [*Cefobid* (sodium 1.5 mEq per gram)].

2 grams in 50 mL (base) (Rx) [*Cefobid* (sodium 1.5 mEq per gram)].

Canada—

Not commercially available.

## Packaging and storage

Do not store above –20 °C (–4 °F), unless otherwise specified by manufacturer.

## Preparation of dosage form

Thaw container at room temperature before administration, making sure that all ice crystals have melted.

Do not use minibags in series connections. This may result in air embolism because of residual air being drawn from the primary container before administration of intravenous solution from the secondary container is complete.

## Stability

After thawing, solutions retain their potency for 48 hours at room temperature or for 10 days if refrigerated at 5 °C (41 °F).

Once thawed, solutions should not be refrozen.

Do not use if the solution is cloudy or contains a precipitate.

## Incompatibilities

The admixture of cefoperazone sodium injection with other medications is not recommended.

The admixture of beta-lactam antibacterials (penicillins and cephalosporins) and aminoglycosides may result in substantial mutual inactivation. If they are administered concurrently, they should be administered in separate sites. Do not mix them in the same intravenous bag or bottle.

## Additional information

Cefoperazone sodium injection is an iso-osmotic solution (approximately 300 mOsmol per L) containing approximately 3.6% dextrose hydrous USP (per 1 gram cefoperazone) or approximately 1.8% dextrose hydrous USP (per 2 grams cefoperazone).

## CEFOPERAZONE SODIUM STERILE USP

## Usual adult dose

See *Cefoperazone Sodium Injection USP*.

## Usual adult prescribing limits

See *Cefoperazone Sodium Injection USP*.

## Usual pediatric dose

See *Cefoperazone Sodium Injection USP*.

## Size(s) usually available

U.S.—

1 gram (base) (Rx) [*Cefobid* (sodium 1.5 mEq per gram)].

2 grams (base) (Rx) [*Cefobid* (sodium 1.5 mEq per gram)].

10 grams (base) (Rx) [*Cefobid* (sodium 1.5 mEq per gram)].

Canada—

1 gram (base) (Rx) [*Cefobid*].

2 grams (base) (Rx) [*Cefobid*].

## Packaging and storage

Prior to reconstitution, store below 40 °C (104 °F), preferably between 15 and 30 °C (59 and 86 °F), unless otherwise specified by manufacturer.

Reconstituted solutions may be stored in glass or plastic disposable syringes or in glass or plastic intravenous bags or bottles.

### Preparation of dosage form

To prepare initial dilution for intramuscular use resulting in final concentrations of less than 250 mg per mL, any suitable diluent (see manufacturer's package insert) may be used.

To prepare initial dilution for intramuscular use resulting in final concentrations of 250 mg per mL, add 2.8 mL of sterile water for injection to each 1-gram vial and shake well until dissolution is complete. Then add 1 mL of 2% lidocaine hydrochloride injection (without epinephrine) and mix well. Add 5.4 mL of sterile water for injection and 1.8 mL of 2% lidocaine hydrochloride injection to each 2-gram vial in the above manner.

To prepare initial dilution for intramuscular use resulting in final concentrations of 333 mg per mL, add 2 mL of sterile water for injection to each 1-gram vial and shake well until dissolution is complete. Then add 0.6 mL of 2% lidocaine hydrochloride injection (without epinephrine) and mix well. Add 3.8 mL of sterile water for injection and 1.2 mL of 2% lidocaine hydrochloride injection to each 2-gram vial in the above manner.

To prepare initial dilution for intravenous use, add a minimum of 2.8 mL (5 mL preferred) of a suitable diluent (see manufacturer's package insert) for each gram of cefoperazone. For intermittent infusion, the resulting solution should be further diluted in a suitable diluent (see manufacturer's package insert) and administered over a 15- to 30-minute period. For continuous infusion, the resulting solution should be further diluted to a final concentration of 2 to 25 mg per mL.

Solution should be allowed to stand following reconstitution. This allows the foam to dissipate, thus permitting visual inspection for complete dissolution. Vigorous and prolonged shaking may be required for complete dissolution, especially at higher concentrations (>333 mg per mL).

For reconstitution of piggyback infusion bottles, see manufacturer's labeling for instructions.

### Stability

After reconstitution, solutions stored in bacteriostatic water for injection, most dextrose-containing injections, dextrose and sodium chloride injection, lactated Ringer's injection, 0.5% lidocaine hydrochloride injection, 0.9% sodium chloride injection, and other electrolyte-containing injections (see manufacturer's package insert) at concentrations of 2 to 300 mg per mL retain their potency for 24 hours at controlled room temperature (15 to 25 °C [59 to 77 °F]) or for 5 days if refrigerated at 2 to 8 °C (36 to 46 °F).

Solutions stored in 5% dextrose injection and 5% dextrose and 0.2 or 0.9% sodium chloride injection at concentrations of 2 and 50 mg per mL retain their potency for 3 weeks if frozen at −20 to −10 °C (−4 to 14 °F).

Solutions stored in 0.9% sodium chloride injection or sterile water for injection at concentrations of 300 mg per mL retain their potency for 5 weeks if frozen at −20 to −10 °C (−4 to 14 °F).

Frozen solutions should be thawed at room temperature prior to use. Once thawed, solutions should not be refrozen.

Solutions may vary in color from colorless to straw yellow, depending on concentration.

### Incompatibilities

The admixture of beta-lactam antibacterials (penicillins and cephalosporins) and aminoglycosides may result in substantial mutual inactivation. If they are administered concurrently, they should be administered in separate sites. Do not mix them in the same intravenous bag or bottle.

---

## *CEFOTAXIME*

## Summary of Differences

Category: Third-generation cephalosporin.

## Additional Dosing Information

Intramuscular doses of 2 grams should be administered as divided doses in different sites.

## Parenteral Dosage Forms

Note: The dosing and strengths of the dosage forms available are expressed in terms of cefotaxime base (not the sodium salt).

### CEFOTAXIME SODIUM INJECTION USP

#### Usual adult and adolescent dose

Antibacterial—
    Intravenous infusion, 1 to 2 grams (base) every four to twelve hours.

Note: Uncomplicated infections—Intravenous infusion, 1 gram (base) every twelve hours.
      Moderate to severe infections—Intravenous infusion, 1 to 2 grams (base) every six to eight hours.
      Life-threatening infections—Intravenous infusion, 2 grams (base) every four hours.
      Adults with impaired renal function (creatinine clearance <20 mL/min or 0.33 mL/sec)—One-half the *Usual adult and adolescent dose.*

#### Usual adult prescribing limits

Up to 12 grams (base) daily.

#### Usual pediatric dose

Antibacterial—
    Neonates up to 1 week of age: Intravenous infusion, 50 mg (base) per kg of body weight every twelve hours.
    Neonates 1 to 4 weeks of age: Intravenous infusion, 50 mg (base) per kg of body weight every eight hours.
    Infants and children up to 50 kg of body weight: Intravenous infusion, 8.3 to 30 mg (base) per kg of body weight every four hours; or 12.5 to 45 mg per kg of body weight every six hours.
    Children over 50 kg of body weight: See *Usual adult and adolescent dose.*

Note: The maximum daily dose in infants and children less than 50 kg of body weight should not exceed 180 mg (base) per kg of body weight per day.

#### Strength(s) usually available

U.S.—
    1 gram (base) in 50 mL (Rx) [*Claforan* (sodium 2.2 mEq per gram)].
    2 grams (base) in 50 mL (Rx) [*Claforan* (sodium 2.2 mEq per gram)].
Canada—
    Not commercially available.

#### Packaging and storage

Do not store above −20 °C (−4 °F), unless otherwise specified by manufacturer.

#### Preparation of dosage form

Thaw container at room temperature before administration, making sure that all ice crystals have melted.

Do not use minibags in series connections. This may result in air embolism because of residual air being drawn from the primary container before administration of intravenous solution from the secondary container is complete.

#### Stability

After thawing, solutions retain their potency for 24 hours at room temperature or for 10 days if refrigerated at 5 °C (41 °F).

Once thawed, solutions should not be refrozen

Do not use if the solution is cloudy or contains a precipitate.

#### Incompatibilities

The admixture of beta-lactam antibacterials (penicillins and cephalosporins) and aminoglycosides may result in substantial mutual inactivation. If they are administered concurrently, they should be administered in separate sites. Do not mix them in the same intravenous bag or bottle.

### CEFOTAXIME SODIUM STERILE USP

#### Usual adult and adolescent dose

See *Cefotaxime Sodium Injection USP.*

Note: Gonococcal infections (uncomplicated cervical, urethral, rectal, and pharyngeal)—Intramuscular, 250 mg (base) as a single dose.

#### Usual adult prescribing limits

See *Cefotaxime Sodium Injection USP.*

#### Usual pediatric dose

See *Cefotaxime Sodium Injection USP.*

#### Size(s) usually available

U.S.—
    500 mg (base) (Rx) [*Claforan* (sodium 2.2 mEq per gram)].
    1 gram (base) (Rx) [*Claforan* (sodium 2.2 mEq per gram)].
    2 grams (base) (Rx) [*Claforan* (sodium 2.2 mEq per gram)].
    10 grams (base) (Rx) [*Claforan* (sodium 2.2 mEq per gram)].
Canada—
    500 mg (base) (Rx) [*Claforan*].
    1 gram (base) (Rx) [*Claforan*].
    2 grams (base) (Rx) [*Claforan*].

#### Packaging and storage

Prior to reconstitution, store below 30 °C (86 °F), preferably between 15 and 30 °C (59 and 86 °F), unless otherwise specified by manufacturer.

## Preparation of dosage form

To prepare initial dilution for intramuscular use, add 2, 3, or 5 mL of sterile water for injection or bacteriostatic water for injection to each 500-mg, 1-gram, or 2-gram vial, respectively.

To prepare initial dilution for intravenous use, add 10 mL of sterile water for injection to each 500-mg, 1-gram, or 2-gram vial. For direct intravenous use, the resulting solution should be administered over a 3- to 5-minute period.

For reconstitution of piggyback infusion bottles or pharmacy bulk vials, see manufacturer's labeling for instructions.

## Stability

After reconstitution, solutions retain their potency for 24 hours at room temperature (22 °C [72 °F]), for 10 days if refrigerated (below 5 °C [41 °F]), or for at least 13 weeks if frozen.

Reconstituted solutions retain their potency in disposable glass or plastic syringes or plastic bags for 24 hours at room temperature, for 5 days if refrigerated, or for 13 weeks if frozen

Reconstituted solutions further diluted to 50 to 1000 mL in suitable diluents (see manufacturer's package insert) retain their potency for 24 hours at room temperature or for at least 5 days if refrigerated.

Frozen solutions should be thawed at room temperature before use. They retain their potency for the time periods stated above. Once thawed, solutions should not be refrozen.

Reconstituted solutions exhibit maximum stability at pH 5 to 7. Therefore, sterile cefotaxime sodium should not be reconstituted with diluents having a pH above 7.5 (e.g., sodium bicarbonate injection)

Solutions range from light yellow to amber in color, depending on the concentration and diluent used. However, solutions tend to darken during storage. This does not affect their potency

## Incompatibilities

The admixture of beta-lactam antibacterials (penicillins and cephalosporins) and aminoglycosides may result in substantial mutual inactivation. If they are administered concurrently, they should be administered in separate sites. Do not mix them in the same intravenous bag or bottle.

## Additional information

A solution containing 1 gram in 14 mL of sterile water for injection is isotonic.

---

## *CEFOTETAN*

# Summary of Differences

Category:
  Cephamycin; second-generation cephalosporin.
Indications:
  Good activity against anaerobic organisms.
Pharmacology/pharmacokinetics:
  Contains *N*-methylthiotetrazole (NMTT) side chain.
Precautions:
  Drug interactions and/or related problems—Interacts with alcohol (disulfiram-like reaction), oral anticoagulants, and other medications that affect blood clotting.
  Laboratory value alterations—May falsely elevate serum and urine creatinine concentrations when the Jaffe method is used.
  Medical considerations/contraindications—Caution also required in patients with history of bleeding problems.
  Patient monitoring—PT determinations may be required.
Side/adverse effects:
  May also cause unusual bleeding or bruising.

# Parenteral Dosage Forms

Note: The dosing and strengths of the dosage forms available are expressed in terms of cefotetan base (not the disodium salt).

## CEFOTETAN DISODIUM STERILE USP

### Usual adult and adolescent dose

Antibacterial—
  Mild to moderate infections: Intramuscular or intravenous, 1 to 2 grams (base) every twelve hours for five to ten days.
  Severe infections: Intravenous, 2 grams (base) every twelve hours.
  Life-threatening infections: Intravenous, 3 grams (base) every twelve hours.

Note: Perioperative prophylaxis—Cesarean-section patients: Intravenous, 1 to 2 grams (base) as soon as the umbilical cord is clamped.
  Perioperative prophylaxis—Other patients: Intravenous, 1 to 2 grams (base) one-half to one hour prior to the start of surgery.

Urinary tract infections—Intramuscular or intravenous, 500 mg to 2 grams (base) every twelve hours; or 1 to 2 grams every twenty-four hours.

Adults with impaired renal function may require a reduction in dose as follows:

| Creatinine Clearance (mL/min)/ (mL/sec) | Dose (base) |
|---|---|
| >30/0.50 | See *Usual adult and adolescent dose* |
| 10–30/0.17–0.50 | Usual adult dose every 24 hours; or one-half the usual adult dose every 12 hours |
| <10/0.17 | Usual adult dose every 48 hours; or one-fourth the usual adult dose every 12 hours |
| Hemodialysis patients | One-fourth the usual adult dose every 24 hours on the days between hemodialysis sessions; and one-half the usual adult dose on the day of hemodialysis |

## Usual adult prescribing limits

Up to a maximum of 6 grams (base) daily.

## Usual pediatric dose

Dosage has not been established.

## Size(s) usually available

U.S.—
  1 gram (base) (Rx) [*Cefotan* (sodium 3.5 mEq per gram)].
  2 grams (base) (Rx) [*Cefotan* (sodium 3.5 mEq per gram)].
  10 grams (base) (Rx) [*Cefotan* (sodium 3.5 mEq per gram)].
Canada—
  1 gram (base) (Rx) [*Cefotan*].
  2 grams (base) (Rx) [*Cefotan*].

## Packaging and storage

Prior to reconstitution, do not store above 22 °C (72 °F), unless otherwise specified by manufacturer. Protect from light.

## Preparation of dosage form

To prepare initial dilution for intramuscular use, add 2 mL of sterile water for injection, bacteriostatic water for injection, 0.9% sodium chloride injection, or 0.5 or 1% lidocaine hydrochloride injection (without epinephrine) to each 1-gram vial to provide a concentration of approximately 400 mg per mL. Add 3 mL of diluent to each 2-gram vial to provide a concentration of approximately 500 mg per mL.

To prepare initial dilution for intravenous use, add 10 mL of sterile water for injection to each 1-gram vial to provide a concentration of approximately 95 mg per mL. Add 10 to 20 mL of diluent to each 2-gram vial to provide a concentration of approximately 95 to 182 mg per mL. For direct intermittent intravenous use, the resulting solution should be administered over a 3- to 5-minute period.

For reconstitution of piggyback infusion bottles, add 50 to 100 mL of 5% dextrose injection or 0.9% sodium chloride injection to each bottle. If the Y-type method of administration is used, the primary infusion should be temporarily discontinued during infusion of cefotetan.

## Stability

After reconstitution for intramuscular or intravenous use, solutions retain their potency for 24 hours at room temperature (25 °C [77 °F]), 96 hours if refrigerated at 5 °C (41 °F), or for at least 1 week if frozen. Frozen solutions should be thawed at room temperature prior to use and retain their potency for the time periods indicated above. Once thawed, solutions should not be refrozen.

After reconstitution as indicated above, solutions stored in disposable glass or plastic syringes retain their potency for 24 hours at room temperature or for 96 hours if refrigerated.

Solutions range from colorless to yellow in color, depending on the concentration.

## Incompatibilities

The admixture of beta-lactam antibacterials (penicillins and cephalosporins) and aminoglycosides may result in substantial mutual inactivation. If they are administered concurrently, they should be administered in separate sites. Do not mix them in the same intravenous bag or bottle.

---

## *CEFOXITIN*

# Summary of Differences

Category:
  Cephamycin; second-generation cephalosporin.
Indications:
  Good activity against anaerobic organisms.

Precautions:
   Pediatrics—Higher doses associated with increased incidence of eosinophilia and elevated AST (SGOT).
   Laboratory value alterations—May falsely elevate serum and urine creatinine concentrations when the Jaffe method is used.

## Parenteral Dosage Forms

Note: The dosage forms available contain cefoxitin sodium, but dosing and strengths are expressed in terms of cefoxitin base.

### CEFOXITIN INJECTION USP

**Usual adult and adolescent dose**
Antibacterial—
   Mild or uncomplicated infections: Intravenous, 1 gram every six to eight hours.
   Moderately severe or severe infections: Intravenous, 1 gram every four hours; or 2 grams every six to eight hours.
   Life-threatening infections: Intravenous, 2 grams every four hours; or 3 grams every six hours.

Note: Perioperative prophylaxis—Cesarean-section patients: Intravenous, 2 grams as soon as the umbilical cord is clamped; followed by 2 grams, intramuscularly or intravenously, four and eight hours after the first dose; or a single 2-gram dose as soon as the umbilical cord is clamped.

   Perioperative prophylaxis—Other surgical patients: Intravenous, 2 grams one-half to one hour prior to the start of surgery; and 2 grams every six hours following surgery for up to twenty-four hours.

   After an initial loading dose of 1 to 2 grams, adults with impaired renal function may require a reduction in dose as follows:

| Creatinine Clearance (mL/min)/ (mL/sec) | Dose |
|---|---|
| >50/0.83 | See *Usual adult and adolescent dose* |
| 30–50/0.50–0.83 | 1–2 grams every 8–12 hours |
| 10–29/0.17–0.48 | 1–2 grams every 12–24 hours |
| 5–9/0.08–0.15 | 500 mg–1 gram every 12–24 hours |
| <5/0.08 | 500 mg–1 gram every 24–48 hours |

**Usual adult prescribing limits**
Up to 12 grams daily.

**Usual pediatric dose**
Antibacterial—
   Infants and children up to 3 months of age: Dosage has not been established.
   Infants and children 3 months of age and over: Intravenous, 13.3 to 26.7 mg per kg of body weight every four hours; or 20 to 40 mg per kg of body weight every six hours.

Note: Perioperative prophylaxis—Infants and children 3 months of age and over: Intravenous, 30 to 40 mg per kg of body weight one-half to one hour prior to the start of surgery; and 30 to 40 mg per kg of body weight every six hours following surgery for up to twenty-four hours.

   The total daily dose in infants and children should not exceed 12 grams.

**Strength(s) usually available**
U.S.—
   1 gram in 50 mL (Rx) [*Mefoxin* (sodium 2.3 mEq per gram)].
   2 grams in 50 mL (Rx) [*Mefoxin* (sodium 2.3 mEq per gram)].
Canada—
   Not commercially available.

**Packaging and storage**
Do not store above –20 °C (–4 °F), unless otherwise specified by manufacturer.

**Preparation of dosage form**
Thaw container at room temperature before administration, making sure that all ice crystals have melted.
Do not use minibags in series connections. This may result in air embolism because of residual air being drawn from the primary container before administration of intravenous solution from the secondary container is complete.

**Stability**
After thawing, solutions retain their potency for 24 hours at room temperature or 5 days if refrigerated at 2 to 8 °C (36 to 46 °F).
Once thawed, solutions should not be refrozen.
Do not use if the solution is cloudy or contains a precipitate.

**Incompatibilities**
The admixture of other medications with cefoxitin injection is not recommended.

The admixture of beta-lactam antibacterials (penicillins and cephalosporins) and aminoglycosides may result in substantial mutual inactivation. If they are administered concurrently, they should be administered in separate sites. Do not mix them in the same intravenous bag or bottle.

### CEFOXITIN FOR INJECTION USP

**Usual adult and adolescent dose**
Antibacterial—
   Mild or uncomplicated infections: See *Cefoxitin Injection USP*.
   Moderately severe or severe infections: See *Cefoxitin Injection USP*.
   Life-threatening infections: See *Cefoxitin Injection USP*.

Note: Gonorrhea (uncomplicated)—Intramuscular, 2 grams and 1 gram of probenecid orally, administered approximately thirty minutes prior to cefoxitin or simultaneously as a single dose.

   Perioperative prophylaxis—Cesarean-section patients: See *Cefoxitin Injection USP*.

   Perioperative prophylaxis—Other surgical patients: See *Cefoxitin Injection USP*.

   After an initial loading dose of 1 to 2 grams, adults with impaired renal function may require a reduction in dose as follows:

| Creatinine Clearance (mL/min)/(mL/sec) | Dose |
|---|---|
| >50/0.83 | See *Usual adult and adolescent dose* |
| 30–50/0.50–0.83 | 1–2 grams every 8–12 hours |
| 10–29/0.17–0.48 | 1–2 grams every 12–24 hours |
| 5–9/0.08–0.15 | 500 mg–1 gram every 12–24 hours |
| <5/0.08 | 500 mg–1 gram every 24–48 hours |

**Usual adult prescribing limits**
See *Cefoxitin Injection USP*.

**Usual pediatric dose**
Antibacterial—
   Premature infants weighing 1500 grams or more to neonates up to 1 week of age: Intravenous, 20 to 40 mg per kg of body weight every twelve hours.
   Neonates 1 to 4 weeks of age: Intravenous, 20 to 40 mg per kg of body weight every eight hours.
   Infants 1 to 3 months of age: Intramuscular or intravenous, 20 to 40 mg per kg of body weight every six to eight hours.
   Infants and children 3 months of age and over—See *Cefoxitin Injection USP*.

**Size(s) usually available**
U.S.—
   1 gram (Rx) [*Mefoxin* (sodium 2.3 mEq per gram)].
   2 grams (Rx) [*Mefoxin* (sodium 2.3 mEq per gram)].
   10 grams (Rx) [*Mefoxin* (sodium 2.3 mEq per gram)].
Canada—
   1 gram (Rx) [*Mefoxin* (sodium 2.3 mEq per gram)].
   2 grams (Rx) [*Mefoxin* (sodium 2.3 mEq per gram)].
   10 grams (Rx) [*Mefoxin* (sodium 2.3 mEq per gram)].

**Packaging and storage**
Prior to reconstitution, store below 40 °C (104 °F), preferably between 15 and 30 °C (59 and 86 °F), unless otherwise specified by manufacturer.

**Preparation of dosage form**
To prepare initial dilution for intramuscular use, add 2 mL of sterile water for injection or 0.5 or 1% lidocaine hydrochloride injection (without epinephrine) to each 1-gram vial.
To prepare initial dilution for intravenous use, add at least 10 mL of sterile water for injection to each 1-gram vial or 10 to 20 mL of diluent to each 2-gram vial. For continuous intravenous infusion, the resulting solution may be further diluted in 5% dextrose injection, 0.9% sodium chloride injection, 5% dextrose and 0.9% sodium chloride injection, or 5% dextrose injection with 0.02% sodium bicarbonate added.
To prepare initial dilution for direct intermittent intravenous use, add 10 mL of sterile water for injection to each 1- or 2-gram vial. The resulting solution should be administered over a 3- to 5-minute period.
For reconstitution of piggyback infusion bottles or pharmacy bulk vials, see manufacturer's labeling for instructions.

**Stability**
After reconstitution for intramuscular use with sterile water for injection, bacteriostatic water for injection, or 0.5 or 1% lidocaine hydrochloride injection (without epinephrine), solutions retain their potency for 24 hours at room temperature, for 7 days if refrigerated (below 5 °C), and for at least 30 weeks if frozen. Once thawed, solutions should not be refrozen.
After reconstitution for intravenous use with sterile water for injection, bacteriostatic water for injection, 0.9% sodium chloride injection, or

5% dextrose injection, solutions retain their potency for 24 hours at room temperature, for 7 days if refrigerated (below 5 °C), and for at least 30 weeks if frozen. Once thawed, solutions should not be refrozen. Initial dilutions retain their potency for 24 hours at room temperature and for at least 48 hours if refrigerated when added to 50 to 1000 mL of suitable diluents (see manufacturer's package insert).

Intravenous solutions of cefoxitin in 0.9% sodium chloride injection, lactated Ringer's injection, and 5% dextrose injection retain their potency for 24 hours at room temperature, for 48 hours if refrigerated, or for 26 weeks if frozen when stored in certain commercially available intravenous plastic bags.

Intravenous solutions of cefoxitin in sterile water for injection retain their potency for 24 hours at room temperature or for 48 hours if refrigerated when stored in disposable plastic syringes.

Cefoxitin decomposes rapidly in alkaline or strongly acid solutions.

Solutions range from clear to light amber in color but tend to darken depending on storage conditions. This does not affect their potency.

### Incompatibilities

The admixture of beta-lactam antibacterials (penicillins and cephalosporins) and aminoglycosides may result in substantial mutual inactivation. If they are administered concurrently, they should be administered in separate sites. Do not mix them in the same intravenous bag or bottle. However, some studies indicate that cefoxitin may be compatible with certain aminoglycosides.

---

## CEFPODOXIME

## Summary of Differences

Category: Third-generation cephalosporin, with broad *in vitro* activity. One of two oral third-generation cephalosporins.

Precautions: Drug interactions and/or related problems—Interacts with antacids and histamine H$_2$-receptor antagonists.

## Oral Dosage Forms

Note: The dosing and strengths of the dosage forms available are expressed in terms of cefpodoxime base (not the proxetil salt).

### CEFPODOXIME PROXETIL FOR ORAL SUSPENSION

**Usual adult and adolescent dose**

Antibacterial—

Bronchitis, bacterial exacerbations: Oral, 200 mg (base) every twelve hours for ten days.

Gonorrhea (uncomplicated urethral, cervical, and rectal): Oral, 200 mg (base) once as a single dose.

Pharyngitis, bacterial: Oral, 100 mg (base) every twelve hours for ten days.

Pneumonia (uncomplicated): Oral, 200 mg (base) every twelve hours for fourteen days.

Skin and soft tissue infections: Oral, 400 mg (base) every twelve hours for seven to fourteen days.

Urinary tract infections, uncomplicated: Oral, 100 mg (base) every twelve hours for seven days.

Note: Patients with renal function impairment may require a reduction in dose as follows:

| Creatinine Clearance (mL/min)/(mL/sec) | Dosing Interval |
|---|---|
| ≥30/0.50 | Every 12 hours |
| 0–30/0–0.50 | Every 24 hours |
| Hemodialysis | 3 times a week after hemodialysis |

**Usual pediatric dose**

Antibacterial—

Infants up to 6 months of age: Dosage has not been established.

Infants and children 6 months to 12 years of age: Otitis media and pharyngitis—Oral, 5 mg (base) per kg of body weight every twelve hours for ten days.

**Strength(s) usually available**

U.S.—

50 mg (base) per 5 mL (when reconstituted according to manufacturer's instructions) (Rx) [*Vantin*].

100 mg (base) per 5 mL (when reconstituted according to manufacturer's instructions) (Rx) [*Vantin*].

Canada—

Not commercially available.

**Packaging and storage**

Prior to reconstitution, store between 15 and 30 °C (59 and 86 °F), unless otherwise specified by manufacturer. Store in a tight container.

**Stability**

After reconstitution, suspension retains its potency for 14 days if refrigerated.

**Auxiliary labeling**
- Refrigerate.
- Shake well.
- Continue medicine for full time of treatment.
- Beyond-use date.
- Take with food.

**Note**

When dispensing, include a calibrated liquid-measuring device.

### CEFPODOXIME PROXETIL TABLETS

**Usual adult and adolescent dose**

See *Cefpodoxime Proxetil for Oral Suspension.*

**Usual pediatric dose**

See *Cefpodoxime Proxetil for Oral Suspension.*

**Strength(s) usually available**

U.S.—

100 mg (base) (Rx) [*Vantin*].

200 mg (base) (Rx) [*Vantin*].

Canada—

Not commercially available.

**Packaging and storage**

Store between 15 and 30 °C (59 and 86 °F), unless otherwise specified by manufacturer. Store in a tight container.

**Auxiliary labeling**
- Continue medicine for full time of treatment.
- Take with food.

---

## CEFPROZIL

## Summary of Differences

Category: Second-generation cephalosporin, with broad *in vitro* activity.

Precautions: Medical considerations/contraindications—Patients with phenylketonuria should be aware that cefprozil for oral solution contains 28 mg of phenylalanine per 5 mL.

## Oral Dosage Forms

### CEFPROZIL FOR ORAL SUSPENSION USP

**Usual adult and adolescent dose**

Antibacterial—

Bronchitis, bacterial exacerbations: Oral, 500 mg every twelve hours for ten days.

Pharyngitis, bacterial: Oral, 500 mg every twenty-four hours for ten days.

Skin and soft tissue infections: Oral, 250 to 500 mg every twelve hours for ten days; or 500 mg every twenty-four hours for ten days.

Note: Patients with renal function impairment may require a reduction in dose as follows:

| Creatinine Clearance (mL/min)/(mL/sec) | Usual Dose (%) |
|---|---|
| ≥30/0.50 | 100 |
| 0–30/0–0.50 | 50 |
| Hemodialysis | 100, after hemodialysis |

**Usual pediatric dose**

Antibacterial—

Infants up to 6 month of age: Dosage has not been established.

Infants and children 6 months to 12 years of age: Otitis media—Oral, 15 mg per kg of body weight every twelve hours for ten days.

Children 2 to 12 years of age: Pharyngitis—Oral, 7.5 mg per kg of body weight every twelve hours for ten days.

**Strength(s) usually available**

U.S.—

125 mg per 5 mL (when reconstituted according to manufacturer's instructions) (Rx) [*Cefzil*].

250 mg per 5 mL (when reconstituted according to manufacturer's instructions) (Rx) [*Cefzil*].

Canada—

Not commercially available.

**Packaging and storage**

Prior to reconstitution, store between 15 and 30 °C (59 and 86 °F), unless otherwise specified by manufacturer. Store in a tight container.

**Stability**

After reconstitution, suspension retains its potency for 14 days if refrigerated.

**Auxiliary labeling**

• Refrigerate.
• Shake well.
• Continue medicine for full time of treatment.
• Beyond-use date.

**Note**

When dispensing, include a calibrated liquid-measuring device.

## CEFPROZIL TABLETS USP

**Usual adult and adolescent dose**

See *Cefprozil for Oral Suspension USP.*

**Usual pediatric dose**

See *Cefprozil for Oral Suspension USP.*

**Strength(s) usually available**

U.S.—

   250 mg (Rx) [*Cefzil*].

   500 mg (Rx) [*Cefzil*].

Canada—

   Not commercially available.

**Packaging and storage**

Store between 15 and 30 °C (59 and 86 °F), unless otherwise specified by manufacturer. Store in a tight container.

**Auxiliary labeling**

• Continue medicine for full time of treatment.

---

### CEFTAZIDIME

## Summary of Differences

Category: Third-generation cephalosporin.

Indications: Good activity against *Pseudomonas aeruginosa.*

Precautions: Drug interactions and/or related problems—Does not interact with probenecid.

## Additional Dosing Information

Patients with impaired hepatic function do not require a reduction in dose.

## Parenteral Dosage Forms

### CEFTAZIDIME INJECTION USP

**Usual adult and adolescent dose**

Antibacterial—

   Intramuscular or intravenous, 500 mg to 2 grams every eight to twelve hours.

Note: Urinary tract infections (uncomplicated)—Intramuscular or intravenous, 250 mg every twelve hours.

   Urinary tract infections (complicated)—Intramuscular or intravenous, 500 mg every eight to twelve hours.

   Pneumonia (uncomplicated), and skin structure infections—Intramuscular or intravenous, 500 mg to 1 gram every eight hours.

   Bone and joint infections—Intravenous, 2 grams every twelve hours.

   Severe or life-threatening infections—Intravenous, 2 grams every eight hours.

   After an initial loading dose of 1 gram, adults (including dialysis patients) with impaired renal function may require a reduction in dose as follows:

| Creatinine Clearance (mL/min)/(mL/sec) | Dose |
| --- | --- |
| >50/0.83 | See *Usual adult and adolescent dose* |
| 31–50/0.52–0.83 | 1 gram every 12 hours |
| 16–30/0.27–0.50 | 1 gram every 24 hours |
| 6–15/0.10–0.25 | 500 mg every 24 hours |
| <5/0.08 | 500 mg every 48 hours |
| Hemodialysis patients | 1 gram after each hemodialysis period |
| Peritoneal dialysis patients | 500 mg every 24 hours |

**Usual pediatric dose**

Antibacterial—

   Neonates up to 4 weeks of age: Intravenous infusion, 30 mg per kg of body weight every twelve hours.

   Infants and children 1 month to 12 years of age: Intravenous infusion, 30 to 50 mg per kg of body weight every eight hours.

Note: The maximum total daily dose in infants and children should not exceed 6 grams.

**Strength(s) usually available**

U.S.—

   1 gram in 50 mL (Rx) [*Fortaz* (sodium 2.3 mEq per gram)].

   2 grams in 50 mL (Rx) [*Fortaz* (sodium 2.3 mEq per gram)].

Canada—

   Not commercially available.

**Packaging and storage**

Do not store above –20 °C (–4 °F), unless otherwise specified by manufacturer.

**Preparation of dosage form**

Thaw container at room temperature before administration, making sure that all ice crystals have melted. Do not force thaw by immersion in water bath or by microwave irradiation.

Do not use minibags in series connections. This may result in air embolism because of residual air being drawn from the primary container before administration of intravenous solution from the secondary container is complete.

**Stability**

After thawing, solutions retain their potency for 24 hours at room temperature or for 7 days if refrigerated.

Once thawed, solutions should not be refrozen.

Do not use if the solution is cloudy or contains a precipitate.

**Incompatibilities**

The admixture of beta-lactam antibacterials (penicillins and cephalosporins) and aminoglycosides may result in substantial mutual inactivation. If they are administered concurrently, they should be administered in separate sites. Do not mix them in the same intravenous bag or bottle.

Vancomycin is physically incompatible with ceftazidime and a precipitate may form, depending on the concentration. Therefore, the intravenous lines should be flushed between the administration of these 2 medications if they are to be given through the same tubing.

### CEFTAZIDIME FOR INJECTION USP

**Usual adult and adolescent dose**

See *Ceftazidime Injection USP.*

**Usual pediatric dose**

Infants and children up to 12 years of age—The safety of the arginine component in the ceftazidime L-arginine formulation has not been established in children up to 12 years of age. If treatment with ceftazidime is indicated, the sodium formulation should be used. See *Ceftazidime Injection USP.*

**Size(s) usually available**

U.S.—

   500 mg (Rx) [*Fortaz* (sodium 2.3 mEq per gram); *Tazidime* (sodium 2.3 mEq per gram)].

   1 gram (Rx) [*Ceptaz* (L-arginine 349 mg per gram); *Fortaz* (sodium 2.3 mEq per gram); *Tazicef* (sodium 2.3 mEq per gram); *Tazidime* (sodium 2.3 mEq per gram)].

   2 grams (Rx) [*Ceptaz* (L-arginine 349 mg per gram); *Fortaz* (sodium 2.3 mEq per gram); *Tazicef* (sodium 2.3 mEq per gram); *Tazidime* (sodium 2.3 mEq per gram)].

   6 grams (Rx) [*Fortaz* (sodium 2.3 mEq per gram); *Tazicef* (sodium 2.3 mEq per gram); *Tazidime* (sodium 2.3 mEq per gram)].

   10 grams (Rx) [*Ceptaz* (L-arginine 349 mg per gram)].

Canada—

   500 mg (Rx) [*Fortaz; Tazidime* (sodium 2.3 mEq per gram)].

   1 gram (Rx) [*Ceptaz; Fortaz; Tazidime* (sodium 2.3 mEq per gram)].

   2 grams (Rx) [*Ceptaz; Fortaz; Tazidime* (sodium 2.3 mEq per gram)].

   6 grams (Rx) [*Fortaz; Tazidime* (sodium 2.3 mEq per gram)].

**Packaging and storage**

Prior to reconstitution, store between 15 and 30 °C (59 and 86 °F), unless otherwise specified by manufacturer. Protect from light.

**Preparation of dosage form**

To prepare initial dilution for intramuscular use, add 1.5 mL of sterile water for injection, bacteriostatic water for injection, or 0.5 or 1% lidocaine hydrochloride injection (without epinephrine) to each 500-mg vial or 3 mL of diluent to each 1-gram vial to provide a concentration of approximately 280 mg per mL.

To prepare initial dilution for intravenous use, add 5 mL of sterile water for injection to each 500-mg vial or 10 mL of diluent to each 1- or 2-gram vial. For direct intravenous use, the resulting solution should be administered slowly over a 3- to 5-minute period.

For reconstitution of piggyback infusion bottles and pharmacy bulk vials, see manufacturer's labeling for instructions. If the Y-type method of administration is used, the primary infusion should be temporarily discontinued during infusion of ceftazidime.

After reconstitution of the sodium carbonate formulation, carbon dioxide is formed, causing positive pressure inside the vial. This may require venting.

### Stability

After reconstitution with sterile water for injection, bacteriostatic water for injection, or lidocaine hydrochloride injection for intramuscular use, solutions retain their potency for 24 hours at room temperature or for 7 days if refrigerated. Solutions that are frozen immediately after reconstitution with sterile water for injection in the original container retain their potency for 3 months at –20 °C (–4 °F). Once thawed, solutions should not be refrozen. Thawed solutions retain their potency for up to 8 hours at room temperature or for 4 days if refrigerated.

After reconstitution with sterile water for injection for intravenous use, solutions retain their potency for 24 hours at room temperature or for 7 days if refrigerated. Solutions that are frozen immediately after reconstitution with sterile water for injection (in original containers) or with 0.9% sodium chloride injection (in polyvinyl chloride plastic small-volume containers) retain their potency for 6 months at –20 °C (–4 °F). Once thawed, solutions should not be refrozen. Thawed solutions retain their potency for up to 24 hours at room temperature or for 7 days if refrigerated.

Intravenous infusions at concentrations of 1 and 40 mg per mL retain their potency for up to 24 hours at room temperature or for 7 days if refrigerated, when stored in suitable fluids (see manufacturer's package insert). However, storage in sodium bicarbonate injection is not recommended since ceftazidime is less stable in sodium bicarbonate than in other fluids.

Solutions range in color from light yellow to amber, depending on the diluent and volume.

Ceftazidime powder and solutions tend to darken, depending on storage conditions. This does not affect their potency.

### Incompatibilities

The admixture of beta-lactam antibacterials (penicillins and cephalosporins) and aminoglycosides may result in substantial mutual inactivation. If they are administered concurrently, they should be administered in separate sites. Do not mix them in the same intravenous bag or bottle.

Vancomycin is physically incompatible with ceftazidime and a precipitate may form, depending on the concentration. Therefore, the intravenous lines should be flushed between the administration of these 2 medications if they are to be given through the same tubing.

---

### *CEFTIZOXIME*

## Summary of Differences

Category: Third-generation cephalosporin.
Precautions: Pediatrics—Associated with transient elevation in eosinophils, ALT (SGOT), AST (SGPT), and CK.

## Additional Dosing Information

Intramuscular doses of 2 grams should be administered as divided doses in different sites.

## Parenteral Dosage Forms

Note: The dosing and strengths of the dosage forms available are expressed in terms of ceftizoxime base (not the sodium salt).

### CEFTIZOXIME SODIUM INJECTION USP

#### Usual adult and adolescent dose

Antibacterial—
   Mild to moderate infections: Intravenous, 1 gram (base) every eight to twelve hours.
   Severe infections: Intravenous, 1 to 2 grams (base) every eight to twelve hours.
   Life-threatening infections: Intravenous, 3 to 4 grams (base) every eight hours.
Note: Pelvic inflammatory disease—Intravenous, 2 grams every eight hours.
   Urinary tract infections (uncomplicated)—Intravenous, 500 mg (base) every twelve hours.

After an initial loading dose of 500 mg (base) to 1 gram, adults with impaired renal function may require a reduction in dose as follows:

| Creatinine Clearance (mL/min)/(mL/sec) | Dose (base) | |
|---|---|---|
| | Less Severe Infections | Life-threatening Infections |
| ≥80/1.33 | See *Usual adult and adolescent dose* | See *Usual adult and adolescent dose* |
| 50–79/0.83–1.32 | 500 mg every 8 hours | 750 mg to 1.5 grams every 8 hours |
| 5–49/0.08–0.82 | 250 to 500 mg every 12 hours | 500 mg to 1 gram every 12 hours |
| 0–4 /0–0.07 | 500 mg every 48 hours; or 250 mg every 24 hours | 500 mg to 1 gram every 48 hours; or 500 mg every 24 hours |

#### Usual pediatric dose

Antibacterial—
   Infants and children up to 6 months of age: Dosage has not been established.
   Children 6 months of age and older: Intravenous, 50 mg (base) per kg of body weight every six to eight hours.
Note: The maximum total daily dose in children should not exceed 200 mg (base) per kg of body weight (not to exceed the maximum adult dose for serious infection).

#### Strength(s) usually available

U.S.—
   1 gram (base) per 50 mL (Rx) [*Cefizox* (sodium 2.6 mEq per gram)].
   1 gram (base) per 100 mL (Rx) [*Cefizox* (sodium 2.6 mEq per gram)].
   2 grams (base) per 50 mL (Rx) [*Cefizox* (sodium 2.6 mEq per gram)].
   2 grams (base) per 100 mL (Rx) [*Cefizox* (sodium 2.6 mEq per gram)].
Canada—
   Not commercially available.

#### Packaging and storage

Do not store above –20 °C (–4 °F), unless otherwise specified by manufacturer.

#### Preparation of dosage form

Thaw container at room temperature before administration, making sure that all ice crystals have melted.
Do not use minibags in series connections. This may result in air embolism because of residual air being drawn from the primary container before administration of intravenous solution from the secondary container is complete.

#### Stability

After thawing, solutions retain their potency for 24 hours at room temperature or for 10 days if refrigerated at 5 °C (41 °F).
Once thawed, solutions should not be refrozen.
Do not use if the solution is cloudy or contains a precipitate.

#### Incompatibilities

The admixture of beta-lactam antibacterials (penicillins and cephalosporins) and aminoglycosides may result in substantial mutual inactivation. If they are administered concurrently, they should be administered in separate sites. Do not mix them in the same intravenous bag or bottle.

### CEFTIZOXIME SODIUM STERILE USP

#### Usual adult and adolescent dose

Antibacterial—
   Mild to moderate infections: See *Ceftizoxime Sodium Injection USP*.
   Severe infections: See *Ceftizoxime Sodium Injection USP*.
   Life-threatening infections: See *Ceftizoxime Sodium Injection USP*.
Note: Gonorrhea (uncomplicated)—Intramuscular, 1 gram (base) as a single dose.
   Pelvic inflammatory disease—See *Ceftizoxime Sodium Injection USP*.
   Urinary tract infections (uncomplicated)—See *Ceftizoxime Sodium Injection USP*.
   After an initial loading dose of 500 mg to 1 gram (base), adults with impaired renal function may require a reduction in dose as follows:

| Creatinine Clearance (mL/min) | Dose (base) | |
|---|---|---|
| | Less Severe Infections | Life-threatening Infections |
| ≥80/1.33 | See *Usual adult and adolescent dose* | See *Usual adult and adolescent dose* |
| 50–79/0.83–1.32 | 500 mg every 8 hours | 750 mg to 1.5 grams every 8 hours |
| 5–49/0.08–0.82 | 250 to 500 mg every 12 hours | 500 mg to 1 gram every 12 hours |
| 0–4 /0–0.07 | 500 mg every 48 hours; or 250 mg every 24 hours | 500 mg to 1 gram every 48 hours; or 500 mg every 24 hours |

### Usual pediatric dose
See *Ceftizoxime Sodium Injection USP.*

### Size(s) usually available
U.S.—
500 mg (base) (Rx) [*Cefizox* (sodium 2.6 mEq per gram)].
1 gram (base) (Rx) [*Cefizox* (sodium 2.6 mEq per gram)].
2 grams (base) (Rx) [*Cefizox* (sodium 2.6 mEq per gram)].
10 grams (base) (Rx) [*Cefizox* (sodium 2.6 mEq per gram)].
Canada—
1 gram (base) (Rx) [*Cefizox*].
2 grams (base) (Rx) [*Cefizox*].

### Packaging and storage
Prior to reconstitution, store below 40 °C (104 °F), preferably between 15 and 30 °C (59 and 86 °F), unless otherwise specified by manufacturer. Protect from excess light.

### Preparation of dosage form
To prepare initial dilution for intramuscular use, add 3 mL of sterile water for injection to each 1-gram vial or 6 mL of diluent to each 2-gram vial to provide a concentration of approximately 270 mg per mL.

To prepare initial dilution for intravenous use, add 10 mL of sterile water for injection to each 1-gram vial or 20 mL of diluent to each 2-gram vial to provide a concentration of approximately 95 mg per mL. For direct intravenous use, the resulting solution should be administered slowly over a 3- to 5-minute period. For intermittent infusions, the resulting solution should be further diluted in 50 to 100 mL of suitable fluids (see manufacturer's package insert).

For reconstitution of piggyback infusion bottles and pharmacy bulk vials, see manufacturer's labeling for instructions.

### Stability
After reconstitution for intramuscular or intravenous use with suitable diluents (see manufacturer's package insert), solutions retain their potency for 24 hours at room temperature or for 96 hours if refrigerated at 5 °C (41 °F).

Solutions may vary in color from yellow to amber. This does not affect their potency.

### Incompatibilities
The admixture of beta-lactam antibacterials (penicillins and cephalosporins) and aminoglycosides may result in substantial mutual inactivation. If they are administered concurrently, they should be administered in separate sites. Do not mix them in the same intravenous bag or bottle.

### Additional information
A solution containing 1 gram in 13 mL of sterile water for injection is isotonic.

---

## CEFTRIAXONE

## Summary of Differences
Category: Third-generation cephalosporin.
Pharmacology/pharmacokinetics: Long half-life; may be dosed once a day.
Precautions: Drug interactions and/or related problems—Does not interact with probenecid.
Side/adverse effects: Associated with ''biliary sludge'' or pseudolithiasis.

## Additional Dosing Information
Patients with impaired hepatic function do not generally require a reduction in dose. However, in patients with both impaired hepatic and renal function, the daily dose should not exceed 2 grams.

## Parenteral Dosage Forms
Note: The dosing and strengths of the dosage forms available are expressed in terms of ceftriaxone base (not the sodium salt).

## CEFTRIAXONE SODIUM INJECTION USP
### Usual adult and adolescent dose
Antibacterial—
Intravenous, 1 to 2 grams (base) every twenty-four hours; or 500 mg to 1 gram every twelve hours.
Note: Perioperative prophylaxis—Intravenous, 1 gram administered one-half to two hours prior to the start of surgery.

### Usual adult and adolescent prescribing limits
Up to 4 grams (base) daily.

### Usual pediatric dose
Antibacterial—
Intravenous, 25 to 37.5 mg (base) per kg of body weight every twelve hours.
Note: Meningitis—Intravenous, 100 mg (base) per kg of body weight once a day, or 50 mg (base) per kg of body weight every twelve hours, with or without a loading dose of 100 mg per kg of body weight. This dose is usually given for seven to fourteen days.
Skin and soft tissue infections—Intravenous, 50 to 75 mg (base) per kg of body weight once a day.
The maximum total daily dose in children should not exceed 4 grams (base) for meningitis or 2 grams for other infections.

### Strength(s) usually available
U.S.—
1 gram (base) in 50 mL (Rx) [*Rocephin* (sodium 3.6 mEq per gram)].
2 grams (base) in 50 mL (Rx) [*Rocephin* (sodium 3.6 mEq per gram)].
Canada—
Not commercially available.

### Packaging and storage
Do not store above –20 °C (–4 °F), unless otherwise specified by manufacturer.

### Preparation of dosage form
Thaw container at room temperature before administration, making sure that all ice crystals have melted.
Do not use minibags in series connections. This may result in air embolism because of residual air being drawn from the primary container before administration of intravenous solution from the secondary container is complete.

### Stability
After thawing, solutions retain their potency for 72 hours at room temperature or for 10 days if refrigerated at 5 °C (41 °F).
Once thawed, solutions should not be refrozen.
Do not use if the solution is cloudy or contains a precipitate.

### Incompatibilities
The admixture of ceftriaxone sodium injection with other antibacterials is not recommended.
The admixture of beta-lactam antibacterials (penicillins and cephalosporins) and aminoglycosides may result in substantial mutual inactivation. If they are administered concurrently, they should be administered in separate sites. Do not mix them in the same intravenous bag or bottle.

## CEFTRIAXONE SODIUM STERILE USP
### Usual adult and adolescent dose
See *Ceftriaxone Sodium Injection USP.*
Note: Gonococcal infections (uncomplicated cervical, urethral, rectal, and pharyngeal)—Intramuscular, 250 mg (base) as a single dose.

### Usual adult prescribing limits
See *Ceftriaxone Sodium Injection USP.*

### Usual pediatric dose
See *Ceftriaxone Sodium Injection USP.*

### Size(s) usually available
U.S.—
250 mg (base) (Rx) [*Rocephin* (sodium 3.6 mEq per gram)].
500 mg (base) (Rx) [*Rocephin* (sodium 3.6 mEq per gram)].
1 gram (base) (Rx) [*Rocephin* (sodium 3.6 mEq per gram)].
2 grams (base) (Rx) [*Rocephin* (sodium 3.6 mEq per gram)].
10 grams (base) (Rx) [*Rocephin* (sodium 3.6 mEq per gram)].
Canada—
250 mg (base) (Rx) [*Rocephin* (sodium 3.6 mEq per gram)].
500 mg (base) (Rx) [*Rocephin* (sodium 3.6 mEq per gram)].
1 gram (base) (Rx) [*Rocephin* (sodium 3.6 mEq per gram)].
2 grams (base) (Rx) [*Rocephin* (sodium 3.6 mEq per gram)].
10 grams (base) (Rx) [*Rocephin* (sodium 3.6 mEq per gram)].
Note: Ceftriaxone disodium is the generic name of this product in Canada.

**Packaging and storage**

Prior to reconstitution, store below 25 °C (77 °F), preferably between 15 and 30 °C (59 and 86 °F), unless otherwise specified by manufacturer. Protect from light.

**Preparation of dosage form**

To prepare initial dilution for intramuscular use, add 0.9 mL of sterile water for injection, 0.9% sodium chloride injection, 5% dextrose injection, bacteriostatic water for injection (with benzyl alcohol), or 1% lidocaine hydrochloride injection (without epinephrine) to each 250-mg vial, 1.8 mL of diluent to each 500-mg vial, 3.6 mL of diluent to each 1-gram vial, or 7.2 mL of diluent to each 2-gram vial to provide a concentration of approximately 250 mg per mL.

Caution: Use of diluents containing benzyl alcohol is not recommended for preparation of medications for use in neonates. A fatal toxic syndrome consisting of metabolic acidosis, CNS depression, respiratory problems, renal failure, hypotension, and possibly seizures and intracranial hemorrhages has been associated with this use.

To prepare initial dilution for intravenous use, add 2.4 mL of diluent to each 250-mg vial, 4.8 mL of diluent to each 500-mg vial, 9.6 mL of diluent to each 1-gram vial, or 19.2 mL of diluent to each 2-gram vial to provide a concentration of approximately 100 mg per mL.

For reconstitution of piggyback infusion bottles and pharmacy bulk vials, see manufacturer's labeling for instructions.

**Stability**

After reconstitution for intramuscular use, solutions retain at least 90% of their potency for 1 to 3 days at room temperature (25 °C [77 °F]) or for 3 to 10 days if refrigerated at 4 °C (39 °F), depending on concentration.

After reconstitution for intravenous use, solutions retain at least 90% of their potency for 3 days at room temperature (25 °C [77 °F]) or for 10 days if refrigerated at 4 °C (39 °F), when stored in glass or polyvinyl chloride (PVC) containers in suitable diluents (see manufacturer's package insert).

After reconstitution for intravenous use with 5% dextrose injection or 0.9% sodium chloride injection, solutions in concentrations of 10 to 40 mg per mL retain their potency for 26 weeks at −20 °C (−4 °F) when stored in PVC or polyolefin containers. Solutions should be thawed at room temperature. Once thawed, solutions should not be refrozen.

Solutions may vary in color from light yellow to amber, depending on length of storage, concentration, and diluent.

**Incompatibilities**

The admixture of sterile ceftriaxone sodium with other antibacterials is not recommended.

The admixture of beta-lactam antibacterials (penicillins and cephalosporins) and aminoglycosides may result in substantial mutual inactivation. If they are administered concurrently, they should be administered in separate sites. Do not mix them in the same intravenous bag or bottle.

---

## CEFUROXIME

## Summary of Differences

Category:

Second-generation cephalosporin.

Pharmacology/pharmacokinetics:

Cefuroxime oral suspension reaches only 91% of the area under the concentration time curve (AUC) and 71% of the peak serum concentration that cefuroxime tablets reach.

Parenteral cefuroxime is the only second-generation cephalosporin to adequately penetrate into the CSF.

Precautions:

Laboratory value alteration—

May give false-negative test result with ferricyanide blood glucose test.

## Additional Dosing Information

For oral dosage forms only:

• Cefuroxime axetil may be given without regard to meals; however, absorption is enhanced when it is given with food.

• Cefuroxime axetil tablets and oral suspension are not bioequivalent and are not substitutable on a mg-per-mg basis.

• Cefuroxime axetil administered as a crushed tablet has a strong, persistent, bitter taste. Alternative therapy, such as the oral suspension, should be considered for children who cannot swallow tablets.

## Oral Dosage Forms

Note: The dosing and strengths of the dosage forms available are expressed in terms of cefuroxime base (not the axetil salt).

### CEFUROXIME AXETIL FOR ORAL SUSPENSION

**Usual adult and adolescent dose**

The oral suspension is usually used only in children. See *Cefuroxime Axetil Tablets USP.*

**Usual pediatric dose**

Antibacterial—

Impetigo or

Otitis media, acute: Oral, 15 mg per kg of body weight, up to 1000 mg, every twelve hours for ten days.

Pharyngitis or

Tonsillitis: Oral, 10 mg per kg of body weight, up to 500 mg, every twelve hours for ten days.

**Strength(s) usually available**

U.S.—

125 mg per 5 mL (when reconstituted according to manufacturer's instructions) (Rx) [*Ceftin*].

Canada—

Not commercially available.

**Packaging and storage**

Store between 2 and 30 °C (36 and 86 °F), in a well-closed container, unless otherwise specified by manufacturer.

**Stability**

After reconstitution, suspension retains its potency for ten days if refrigerated or stored at room temperature.

**Auxiliary labeling**

• Continue medicine for full time of treatment.

• Shake well.

• Beyond-use date.

**Note**

When dispensing, include a calibrated liquid-measuring device.

### CEFUROXIME AXETIL TABLETS USP

**Usual adult and adolescent dose**

Antibacterial—

Oral, 250 to 500 mg (base) every twelve hours.

Note: Urinary tract infections (uncomplicated)—Oral, 125 to 250 mg (base) every twelve hours.

Gonorrhea (uncomplicated cervical and urethral)—Oral, 1 gram (base) as a single dose.

**Usual pediatric dose**

Antibacterial—

Children up to 12 years of age: Oral, 125 mg (base) every twelve hours.

Children 12 years of age and over: See *Usual adult and adolescent dose.*

Note: Otitis media, acute—

Infants and children up to 2 years of age: Oral, 125 mg (base) every twelve hours.

Children 2 years of age and over: Oral, 250 mg (base) every twelve hours.

**Strength(s) usually available**

U.S.—

125 mg (base) (Rx) [*Ceftin*].

250 mg (base) (Rx) [*Ceftin*].

500 mg (base) (Rx) [*Ceftin*].

Canada—

125 mg (base) (Rx) [*Ceftin*].

250 mg (base) (Rx) [*Ceftin*].

500 mg (base) (Rx) [*Ceftin*].

**Packaging and storage**

Store between 15 and 30 °C (59 and 86 °F), in a well-closed container, unless otherwise specified by manufacturer.

**Preparation of dosage form**

For patients who cannot take oral solids—Cefuroxime axetil tablets may be crushed and mixed with food (e.g., applesauce, ice cream) or apple juice, orange juice, grape juice, or chocolate milk to mask the strong, persistent, bitter taste.

**Auxiliary labeling**

• Continue medicine for full time of treatment.

# Parenteral Dosage Forms

## CEFUROXIME SODIUM INJECTION USP

### Usual adult and adolescent dose

Antibacterial—

Intramuscular or intravenous, 750 mg to 1.5 grams every eight hours.

Note: Gonococcal infections (uncomplicated)—Intramuscular, 1.5 grams, divided into two doses and administered at two separate sites, and 1 gram of probenecid given orally, administered simultaneously as a single dose.

Meningitis, bacterial—Intravenous, up to 3 grams every eight hours.

Perioperative prophylaxis—Open-heart surgical patients: Intravenous, 1.5 grams at the induction of anesthesia and every twelve hours thereafter for a total of six grams.

Perioperative prophylaxis—Other surgical patients: Intravenous, 1.5 grams one-half to one hour prior to the start of surgery; and 750 mg intravenously or intramuscularly every eight hours if the surgical procedure is prolonged, for up to twenty-four hours.

Adults with impaired renal function may require a reduction in dose as follows:

| Creatinine Clearance (mL/min)/ (mL/sec) | Dose |
|---|---|
| >20/0.33 | 750 mg to 1.5 grams every 8 hours |
| 10–20/0.17–0.33 | 750 mg every 12 hours |
| <10/0.17 | 750 mg every 24 hours |
| Hemodialysis patients | 750 mg at the end of each dialysis period |

### Usual pediatric dose

Antibacterial—

Neonates: Intramuscular or intravenous, 10 to 33.3 mg per kg of body weight every eight hours; or 15 to 50 mg per kg of body weight every twelve hours.

Infants and children 3 months of age and over: Intramuscular or intravenous, 16.7 to 33.3 mg per kg of body weight every eight hours.

Note: Bone infections—Intravenous, 50 mg per kg of body weight every eight hours.

Meningitis, bacterial (neonates)—Intravenous, 33.3 mg per kg of body weight every eight hours, or 50 mg per kg of body weight every twelve hours.

Meningitis, bacterial (infants and children 3 months of age and older)—Intravenous, 50 to 60 mg per kg of body weight every six hours; or 66.7 to 80 mg per kg of body weight every eight hours.

Pediatric patients with impaired renal function may require a reduction in the frequency of dosage consistent with adult dosage recommendations in renal impairment.

### Strength(s) usually available

U.S.—

750 mg in 50 mL (Rx) [*Zinacef*].

1.5 grams in 50 mL (Rx) [*Zinacef*].

Canada—

Not commercially available.

### Packaging and storage

Do not store above −20 °C (−4 °F), unless otherwise specified by manufacturer.

### Preparation of dosage form

Thaw container at room temperature 25 °C (77 °F) or under refrigeration 5 °C (41 °F) before administration, making sure that all ice crystals have melted. Do not thaw by immersing in water baths or in a microwave oven.

Do not use minibags in series connections. This may result in air embolism because of residual air being drawn from the primary container before administration of intravenous solution from the secondary container is complete.

### Stability

Premixed frozen solutions are stable for 18 months when stored at −20 °C (−4 °F).

After thawing, solutions retain their potency for 24 hours at room temperature or for 28 days if refrigerated at 5 °C (41 °F).

Once thawed, solutions should not be refrozen.

Do not use if the solution is cloudy or contains a precipitate.

### Incompatibilities

The admixture of cefuroxime sodium injection with other antibacterials is not recommended.

The admixture of beta-lactam antibacterials (penicillins and cephalosporins) and aminoglycosides may result in substantial mutual inactivation. If they are administered concurrently, they should be administered in separate sites. Do not mix them in the same intravenous bag or bottle.

## CEFUROXIME SODIUM STERILE USP

### Usual adult and adolescent dose

See *Cefuroxime Sodium Injection USP*.

### Usual pediatric dose

See *Cefuroxime Sodium Injection USP*.

### Size(s) usually available

U.S.—

750 mg (Rx) [*Kefurox* (sodium 2.4 mEq per gram); *Zinacef* (sodium 2.4 mEq per gram)].

1.5 grams (Rx) [*Kefurox* (sodium 2.4 mEq per gram); *Zinacef* (sodium 2.4 mEq per gram)].

7.5 grams (Rx) [*Kefurox* (sodium 2.4 mEq per gram); *Zinacef* (sodium 2.4 mEq per gram)].

Canada—

750 mg (Rx) [*Kefurox; Zinacef*].

1.5 grams (Rx) [*Kefurox; Zinacef*].

7.5 grams (Rx) [*Kefurox; Zinacef*].

### Packaging and storage

Prior to reconstitution, store below 40 °C (104 °F), preferably between 15 and 30 °C (59 and 86 °F), unless otherwise specified by manufacturer.

### Preparation of dosage form

To prepare initial dilution for intramuscular use, add 3.0 mL of sterile water for injection to each 750-mg vial and withdraw the entire volume, which provides a suspension of cefuroxime.

To prepare initial dilution for intravenous use, add 8 mL of sterile water for injection to each 750-mg vial; withdraw the entire volume. Add 16 mL of diluent to each 1.5-gram vial; withdraw the entire volume for the 1.5-gram dose. For direct intermittent intravenous use, the resulting solution should be administered slowly over a 3- to 5-minute period.

For reconstitution of piggyback infusion bottles and pharmacy bulk vials, see manufacturer's labeling for instructions. If the Y-type method of administration is used, the primary infusion should be temporarily discontinued during infusion of cefuroxime.

### Stability

After reconstitution for intramuscular use, suspensions retain their potency for 24 hours at room temperature or for 48 hours if refrigerated at 5 °C (41 °F).

After reconstitution for intravenous use, solutions retain their potency for 24 hours at room temperature or for 48 hours if refrigerated at 5 °C (41 °F). Solutions stored in polyvinyl chloride (PVC) minibags in 50 or 100 mL of 5% dextrose injection or 0.9% sodium chloride injection retain their potency for 6 months at −20 °C (−4 °F). Solutions should be thawed at room temperature. Thawed solutions retain their potency for 24 hours at room temperature or for 7 days if refrigerated.

Intravenous infusions at concentrations of 7.5 and 15 mg per mL in sterile water for injection, 5% dextrose injection, or 0.9% sodium chloride injection retain their potency for 24 hours at room temperature or for 7 days if refrigerated. Use of sodium bicarbonate is not recommended for dilution.

Solutions may vary in color from light yellow to amber, depending on concentration and diluent. In addition, cefuroxime powder, suspensions, and solutions tend to darken, depending on storage conditions. This does not affect their potency.

### Incompatibilities

The admixture of beta-lactam antibacterials (penicillins and cephalosporins) and aminoglycosides may result in substantial mutual inactivation. If they are administered concurrently, they should be administered in separate sites. Do not mix them in the same intravenous bag or bottle.

---

## CEPHALEXIN

## Summary of Differences

Category: First-generation cephalosporin.

## Additional Dosing Information

When daily doses greater than 4 grams are required, parenteral cephalosporins should be considered.

# Oral Dosage Forms

## CEPHALEXIN CAPSULES USP

### Usual adult and adolescent dose
Antibacterial—
   Oral, 250 to 500 mg every six hours.

Note: Cystitis (uncomplicated), skin and soft tissue infections, and streptococcal pharyngitis: Oral, 500 mg every twelve hours.

### Usual adult prescribing limits
Up to 4 grams daily.

### Usual pediatric dose
Antibacterial—
   Oral, 6.25 to 25 mg per kg of body weight every six hours.

Note: Skin and soft tissue infections and streptococcal pharyngitis—Oral, 12.5 to 50 mg per kg of body weight every twelve hours.

### Strength(s) usually available
U.S.—
   250 mg (Rx) [*Cefanex; C-Lexin; Keflex;* GENERIC].
   500 mg (Rx) [*Cefanex; C-Lexin; Keflex;* GENERIC].
Canada—
   250 mg (Rx) [*Apo-Cephalex; Novo-Lexin*].
   500 mg (Rx) [*Apo-Cephalex; Novo-Lexin*].

### Packaging and storage
Store below 40 °C (104 °F), preferably between 15 and 30 °C (59 and 86 °F), unless otherwise specified by manufacturer. Store in a tight container.

### Auxiliary labeling
• Continue medicine for full time of treatment.

## CEPHALEXIN FOR ORAL SUSPENSION USP

### Usual adult and adolescent dose
See *Cephalexin Capsules USP*.

### Usual adult prescribing limits
See *Cephalexin Capsules USP*.

### Usual pediatric dose
See *Cephalexin Capsules USP*.

### Strength(s) usually available
U.S.—
   100 mg per mL (when reconstituted according to manufacturer's instructions) (Rx) [*Keflex*].
   125 mg per 5 mL (when reconstituted according to manufacturer's instructions) (Rx) [*C-Lexin; Keflex;* GENERIC].
   250 mg per 5 mL (when reconstituted according to manufacturer's instructions) (Rx) [*C-Lexin; Keflex;* GENERIC].
Canada—
   125 mg per 5 mL (when reconstituted according to manufacturer's instructions) (Rx) [*Keflex; Novo-Lexin*].
   250 mg per 5 mL (when reconstituted according to manufacturer's instructions) (Rx) [*Keflex; Novo-Lexin*].

### Packaging and storage
Prior to reconstitution, store below 40 °C (104 °F), preferably between 15 and 30 °C (59 and 86 °F), unless otherwise specified by manufacturer. Store in a tight container.

### Stability
After reconstitution, suspensions retain their potency for 14 days if refrigerated.

### Auxiliary labeling
• Refrigerate.
• Shake well.
• Continue medicine for full time of treatment.
• Beyond-use date.
• For oral use only (pediatric drops).

### Note
Explain administration technique for pediatric drops (100 mg per mL).

When dispensing, include a calibrated liquid-measuring device.

## CEPHALEXIN TABLETS USP

### Usual adult and adolescent dose
See *Cephalexin Capsules USP*.

### Usual adult prescribing limits
See *Cephalexin Capsules USP*.

### Usual pediatric dose
See *Cephalexin Capsules USP*.

### Strength(s) usually available
U.S.—
   250 mg (Rx) [GENERIC].
   500 mg (Rx) [GENERIC].
Canada—
   250 mg (Rx) [*Keflex; Novo-Lexin; Nu-Cephalex*].
   500 mg (Rx) [*Keflex; Novo-Lexin; Nu-Cephalex*].

### Packaging and storage
Store below 40 °C (104 °F), preferably between 15 and 30 °C (59 and 86 °F), unless otherwise specified by manufacturer. Store in a tight container.

### Auxiliary labeling
• Continue medicine for full time of treatment.

## CEPHALEXIN HYDROCHLORIDE TABLETS USP

### Usual adult dose
See *Cephalexin Capsules USP*.

### Usual adult prescribing limits
See *Cephalexin Capsules USP*.

### Usual pediatric dose
Dosage has not been established.

### Strength(s) usually available
U.S.—
   250 mg (Rx) [*Keftab*].
   500 mg (Rx) [*Keftab*].
Canada—
   Not commercially available.

### Packaging and storage
Store between 15 and 30 °C (59 and 86 °F), in a well-closed container, unless otherwise specified by manufacturer.

### Auxiliary labeling
• Continue medicine for full time of treatment.

---

## *CEPHALOTHIN*

# Summary of Differences
Category:
   First-generation cephalosporin.
Precautions:
   Drug interactions and/or related problems—May be more likely to interact with nephrotoxic medications.
   Laboratory value alterations—May falsely elevate serum and urine creatinine concentrations when the Jaffe method is used.

# Additional Dosing Information
Since pain, induration, tenderness, and elevated temperature may occur on intramuscular administration, cephalothin sodium for injection should be administered by deep intramuscular injection or by intravenous injection.

When intravenous doses greater than 6 grams daily are given for more than 3 days, thrombophlebitis may occur. To help minimize the incidence of thrombophlebitis, larger veins may be used, 10 to 25 mg of hydrocortisone may be added to intravenous infusions containing 4 to 6 grams, or more dilute solutions may be given.

# Parenteral Dosage Forms
Note: The dosing and strengths of the dosage forms available are expressed in terms of cephalothin base (not the sodium salt).

## CEPHALOTHIN SODIUM INJECTION USP

### Usual adult and adolescent dose
Antibacterial—
   Intravenous infusion, 500 mg to 2 grams (base) every four to six hours.

Note: Perioperative prophylaxis—Intravenous infusion, 1 to 2 grams (base) one-half to one hour prior to the start of surgery; 1 to 2 grams during surgery; and 1 to 2 grams every six hours following surgery for up to twenty-four hours.

   Pneumonia (uncomplicated), furunculosis (with cellulitis), and urinary tract infections—Intravenous infusion, 500 mg (base) every six hours.

   After an initial loading dose of 1 to 2 grams (base), adults with impaired renal function may require a reduction in dose as follows:

| Creatinine Clearance (mL/min)/ (mL/sec) | Dose (base) |
|---|---|
| >80/1.33 | See *Usual adult and adolescent dose* |
| 50–80/0.83–1.33 | Up to 2 grams every 6 hours |
| 25–50/0.42–0.83 | Up to 1.5 grams every 6 hours |
| 10–25/0.17–0.42 | Up to 1 gram every 6 hours |
| 2–10/0.03–0.17 | Up to 500 mg every 6 hours |
| <2/0.03 | Up to 500 mg every 8 hours |

**Usual adult prescribing limits**
Up to 12 grams (base) daily.

**Usual pediatric dose**
Antibacterial—
Intravenous infusion, 13.3 to 26.6 mg (base) per kg of body weight every four hours; or 20 to 40 mg per kg of body weight every six hours.

Note: Perioperative prophylaxis—Intravenous infusion, 20 to 30 mg (base) per kg of body weight one-half to one hour prior to the start of surgery; 20 to 30 mg per kg of body weight during surgery; and 20 to 30 mg per kg of body weight every six hours following surgery for up to twenty-four hours.

**Strength(s) usually available**
U.S.—
1 gram (base) in 50 mL (Rx) [*Keflin* (sodium 2.8 mEq per gram); GENERIC].
2 grams (base) in 50 mL (Rx) [*Keflin* (sodium 2.8 mEq per gram); GENERIC].
Canada—
Not commercially available.

**Packaging and storage**
Do not store above –20 °C (–4 °F), unless otherwise specified by manufacturer.

**Preparation of dosage form**
Thaw container at room temperature before administration, making sure that all ice crystals have melted.
Do not use minibags in series connections. This may result in air embolism because of residual air being drawn from the primary container before administration of intravenous solution from the secondary container is complete.

**Stability**
After thawing, solutions retain their potency for 12 hours at room temperature or for 96 hours if refrigerated at 5 °C (41 °F).
Once thawed, solutions should not be refrozen.
Do not use if the solution is cloudy or contains a precipitate.

**Incompatibilities**
The admixture of other medications with cephalothin sodium injection is not recommended.
The admixture of beta-lactam antibacterials (penicillins and cephalosporins) and aminoglycosides may result in substantial mutual inactivation. If they are administered concurrently, they should be administered in separate sites. Do not mix them in the same intravenous bag or bottle.

**Additional information**
The vehicles are 0.9% sodium chloride injection and 5% dextrose injection.

## CEPHALOTHIN SODIUM FOR INJECTION USP

**Usual adult and adolescent dose**
See *Cephalothin Sodium Injection USP.*

**Usual adult prescribing limits**
See *Cephalothin Sodium Injection USP.*

**Usual pediatric dose**
See *Cephalothin Sodium Injection USP.*

**Size(s) usually available**
U.S.—
1 gram (base) (Rx) [*Keflin* (sodium 2.8 mEq per gram); GENERIC].
2 grams (base) (Rx) [*Keflin* (sodium 2.8 mEq per gram); GENERIC].
Canada—
1 gram (base) (Rx) [*Keflin* (sodium 2.8 mEq per gram)].
2 grams (base) (Rx) [*Keflin* (sodium 2.8 mEq per gram)].
20 grams (base) (Rx) [*Keflin* (sodium 2.8 mEq per gram)].

**Packaging and storage**
Prior to reconstitution, store below 40 °C (104 °F), preferably between 15 and 30 °C (59 and 86 °F), unless otherwise specified by manufacturer.

**Preparation of dosage form**
To prepare initial dilution for intramuscular use, add 4 mL of sterile water for injection to each 1-gram vial. If necessary, additional small amounts of diluent (e.g., 0.2 to 0.4 mL) may be added and the contents warmed slightly to facilitate dissolution.
To prepare initial dilution for direct or intermittent intravenous use, add 10 mL of sterile water for injection, 5% dextrose injection, or 0.9% sodium chloride injection to each 1-gram vial. The resulting solution should be administered over a 3- to 5-minute period.
To prepare initial dilution for continuous intravenous infusion, add at least 20 mL of sterile water for injection to each 4-gram vial. The resulting solution should be further diluted in a suitable diluent (see manufacturer's package insert).
For reconstitution of pharmacy bulk vials or piggyback infusion bottles, see manufacturer's labeling for instructions.

**Stability**
After reconstitution, solutions retain their potency for 96 hours if refrigerated. Solutions for intramuscular use retain their potency for 12 hours at room temperature.
A precipitate may form in the solution. Upon being warmed to room temperature and shaken, this will redissolve.
Concentrated solutions will darken in color, especially at room temperature. However, slight discoloration does not affect potency.
If frozen immediately after reconstitution with sterile water for injection, 5% dextrose injection, or 0.9% sodium chloride injection, solutions retain their potency in the original container up to 12 weeks at –20 °C (–4 °F). Once thawed, solutions should not be refrozen.

**Incompatibilities**
The admixture of beta-lactam antibacterials (penicillins and cephalosporins) and aminoglycosides may result in substantial mutual inactivation. If they are administered concurrently, they should be administered in separate sites. Do not mix them in the same intravenous bag or bottle.

---

## *CEPHAPIRIN*

# Summary of Differences

Category: First-generation cephalosporin.

# Additional Dosing Information

Cephapirin sodium should be administered by deep intramuscular injection or by intravenous injection only.

# Parenteral Dosage Forms

Note: The dosing and strengths of the dosage forms available are expressed in terms of cephapirin base (not the sodium salt).

## CEPHAPIRIN SODIUM STERILE USP

**Usual adult and adolescent dose**
Antibacterial—
Intramuscular or intravenous, 500 mg to 1 gram (base) every four to six hours.

Note: Perioperative prophylaxis[1]—Intramuscular or intravenous, 1 to 2 grams (base) one-half to one hour prior to the start of surgery; 1 to 2 grams during surgery; and 1 to 2 grams every six hours following surgery for up to twenty-four hours.

Patients with impaired renal function (moderately severe oliguria or serum creatinine above 5 mg per 100 mL)—7.5 to 15 mg (base) per kg of body weight every twelve hours.

**Usual adult prescribing limits**
Up to 12 grams (base) daily.

**Usual pediatric dose**
Antibacterial—
Infants up to 3 months of age: Dosage has not been established.
Infants and children 3 months of age and over: Intramuscular or intravenous, 10 to 20 mg (base) per kg of body weight every six hours.

**Size(s) usually available**
U.S.—
500 mg (base) (Rx) [*Cefadyl* (sodium 2.36 mEq per gram)].
1 gram (base) (Rx) [*Cefadyl* (sodium 2.36 mEq per gram); GENERIC].
2 grams (base) (Rx) [*Cefadyl* (sodium 2.36 mEq per gram); GENERIC].
4 grams (base) (Rx) [*Cefadyl* (sodium 2.36 mEq per gram); GENERIC].
20 grams (base) (Rx) [*Cefadyl* (sodium 2.36 mEq per gram); GENERIC].
Canada—
Not commercially available.

**Packaging and storage**

Prior to reconstitution, store below 40 °C (104 °F), preferably between 15 and 30 °C (59 and 86 °F), unless otherwise specified by manufacturer.

**Preparation of dosage form**

To prepare initial dilution for intramuscular use, add 1 or 2 mL of sterile water for injection or bacteriostatic water for injection to each 500-mg or 1-gram vial, respectively.

To prepare initial dilution for direct or intermittent intravenous use, add 10 mL or more of bacteriostatic water for injection, dextrose injection, or 0.9% sodium chloride injection to each 500-mg or 1- or 2-gram vial. The resulting solution should be administered over a 3- to 5-minute period.

For reconstitution of pharmacy bulk vials or piggyback infusion bottles, see manufacturer's labeling for instructions.

**Stability**

After reconstitution, depending on the diluent, solutions retain their potency for 12 to 48 hours at room temperature or for 10 days if refrigerated at 4 °C (39 °F).

Color changes do not affect potency.

If frozen immediately after reconstitution with sterile water for injection, bacteriostatic water for injection, 0.9% sodium chloride injection, or 5% dextrose injection, solutions retain their potency up to 60 days at –15 °C (5 °F). After thawing at room temperature, solutions retain their potency for 12 hours at room temperature or for 10 days if refrigerated at 4 °C (39 °F).

Intravenous infusions of cephapirin sodium retain their potency for 24 hours at room temperature at concentrations of 2 to 30 mg per mL in suitable fluids (see manufacturer's package insert). Intravenous infusions of cephapirin sodium retain their potency for 10 days if refrigerated or for 14 days if frozen at –15 °C (5 °F) at a concentration of 4 mg per mL in suitable fluids (see manufacturer's package insert). After thawing at room temperature, these infusions retain their potency for 24 hours at room temperature.

**Incompatibilities**

The admixture of beta-lactam antibacterials (penicillins and cephalosporins) and aminoglycosides may result in substantial mutual inactivation. If they are administered concurrently, they should be administered in separate sites. Do not mix them in the same intravenous bag or bottle.

[1]Not included in Canadian product labeling.

---

## *CEPHRADINE*

## Summary of Differences

Category: First-generation cephalosporin.

## Additional Dosing Information

Adults with impaired renal function may require a reduction in dose as follows:

| Creatinine Clearance (mL/min)/ (mL/sec) | Dose |
|---|---|
| >20/0.33 | 500 mg every 6 hours |
| 5–20/0.08–0.33 | 250 mg every 6 hours |
| <5/0.08 | 250 mg every 12 hours |

For parenteral dosage forms only:
- A solution containing 30 mg per mL is approximately isotonic.
- Since sterile abscesses may occur following subcutaneous injection, cephradine for injection should be administered by deep intramuscular injection or by intravenous injection only.

## Oral Dosage Forms

### CEPHRADINE CAPSULES USP

**Usual adult and adolescent dose**

Antibacterial—

Oral, 250 to 500 mg every six hours; or 500 mg to 1 gram every twelve hours.

**Usual adult prescribing limits**

Up to 4 grams daily.

**Usual pediatric dose**

Antibacterial—

Oral, 6.25 to 25 mg per kg of body weight every six hours.

Note: The maximum daily dose should not exceed 4 grams.

Children over 9 months of age may receive the total daily dose in equally divided doses every twelve hours.

**Strength(s) usually available**

U.S.—

250 mg (Rx) [*Velosef;* GENERIC].

500 mg (Rx) [*Velosef;* GENERIC].

Canada—

250 mg (Rx) [*Velosef*].

500 mg (Rx) [*Velosef*].

**Packaging and storage**

Store below 30 °C (86 °F), preferably between 15 and 30 °C (59 and 86 °F), unless otherwise specified by manufacturer. Store in a tight container.

**Auxiliary labeling**

- Continue medicine for full time of treatment.

### CEPHRADINE FOR ORAL SUSPENSION USP

**Usual adult and adolescent dose**

See *Cephradine Capsules USP.*

**Usual adult prescribing limits**

See *Cephradine Capsules USP.*

**Usual pediatric dose**

See *Cephradine Capsules USP.*

**Strength(s) usually available**

U.S.—

125 mg per 5 mL (when reconstituted according to manufacturer's instructions) (Rx) [*Velosef;* GENERIC].

250 mg per 5 mL (when reconstituted according to manufacturer's instructions) (Rx) [*Velosef;* GENERIC].

Canada—

Not commercially available.

**Packaging and storage**

Prior to reconstitution, store below 40 °C (104 °F), preferably between 15 and 30 °C (59 and 86 °F), unless otherwise specified by manufacturer. Store in a tight container.

**Stability**

After reconstitution, suspensions retain their potency for 7 days at room temperature or for 14 days if refrigerated.

**Auxiliary labeling**

- Refrigerate.
- Shake well.
- Continue medicine for full time of treatment.
- Beyond-use date.

**Note**

When dispensing, include a calibrated liquid-measuring device.

## Parenteral Dosage Forms

### CEPHRADINE FOR INJECTION USP

**Usual adult and adolescent dose**

Antibacterial—

Intramuscular or intravenous, 500 mg to 1 gram every six hours.

Note: Perioperative prophylaxis—Cesarean-section patients: Intravenous, 1 gram as soon as the umbilical cord is clamped; and 1 gram intramuscularly or intravenously six and twelve hours after the first dose.

Perioperative prophylaxis—Other surgical patients: Intramuscular or intravenous, 1 gram one-half to one and one-half hours prior to the start of surgery; and 1 gram every four to six hours following surgery for up to twenty-four hours.

**Usual adult prescribing limits**

Up to 8 grams daily.

**Usual pediatric dose**

Antibacterial—

Premature infants and infants up to 1 year of age: Dosage has not been established.

Children 1 year of age and over: Intramuscular or intravenous, 12.5 to 25 mg per kg of body weight every six hours.

Note: Doses up to 300 mg per kg of body weight daily have been used in severely ill infants and children without apparent adverse effects.

The maximum daily dose should not exceed 8 grams.

**Size(s) usually available**

U.S.—

250 mg (Rx) [*Velosef* (sodium 6 mEq per gram)].

500 mg (Rx) [*Velosef* (sodium 6 mEq per gram)].

1 gram (Rx) [*Velosef* (sodium 6 mEq per gram)].

2 grams (Rx) [*Velosef* (sodium 6 mEq per gram)].

Canada—
Not commercially available.

**Packaging and storage**
Prior to reconstitution, store below 40 °C (104 °F), preferably between 15 and 30 °C (59 and 86 °F), unless otherwise specified by manufacturer.

**Preparation of dosage form**
To prepare initial dilution for intramuscular use, add 1.2 mL of sterile water for injection or bacteriostatic water for injection to each 250-mg vial, 2 mL of diluent to each 500-mg vial, or 4 mL of diluent to each 1-gram vial.

To prepare initial dilution for direct intravenous use, add 5 mL of sterile water for injection, 5% dextrose injection, or sodium chloride injection to each 250- or 500-mg vial, 10 mL of diluent to each 1-gram vial, or 20 mL of diluent to each 2-gram vial. The resulting solution should be administered over a 3- to 5-minute period.

To prepare initial dilution for intermittent intravenous use, add 10 mL of a suitable diluent (see manufacturer's package insert) to each 1-gram vial, 20 mL of diluent to each 2-gram vial, or 40 mL of diluent to each 4-gram vial. After initial dilution, solution may be further diluted to a concentration of 5% (50 mg per mL) or less.

For reconstitution of piggyback infusion bottles, see manufacturer's labeling for instructions.

**Stability**
After reconstitution for intramuscular or direct intravenous use, solutions retain their potency for 2 hours at room temperature or for 24 hours if refrigerated at 5 °C (41 °F).

Intravenous infusions of cephradine retain their potency for 10 hours at room temperature or 48 hours if refrigerated at 5 °C (41 °F). If frozen immediately after reconstitution with sterile water for injection, solutions retain their potency in the original container for up to 6 weeks at –20 °C (–4 °F).

Reconstituted solutions may vary in color from light straw to yellow; color changes do not affect the potency.

**Incompatibilities**
Cephradine for Injection USP contains sodium carbonate and therefore is not compatible with calcium-containing solutions (e.g., lactated Ringer's injection, Ringer's injection, dextrose and lactated Ringer's injection).

The admixture of beta-lactam antibacterials (penicillins and cephalosporins) and aminoglycosides may result in substantial mutual inactivation. If they are administered concurrently, they should be administered in separate sites. Do not mix them in the same intravenous bag or bottle.

The admixture of Cephradine for Injection USP with other antibiotics is not recommended.

Revised: 12/30/94
Interim revision: 04/26/95; 06/26/95

## Table 1. Pharmacology/Pharmacokinetics

| Drug | Bioavailability (%) | Half-life (hr) | | Time to Peak Serum Concentration (hr) | Peak Serum Concentration After Dose | | Peak Urine Concentration After Dose | |
| --- | --- | --- | --- | --- | --- | --- | --- | --- |
| | | Normal Renal Function | Impaired Renal Function | | mcg/mL | Dose | mcg/mL | Dose |
| **First-Generation** | | | | | | | | |
| Cefadroxil | 95 | 1.2–1.5 | 20–25 | | | | | |
| Oral | | | | 1.5–2 | 16 | 500 mg | 1800 | 500 mg |
| | | | | | 28 | 1 gram | | |
| Cefazolin | | 1.4–1.8* | 3–42 | | | | | |
| IM | | | | 1–2 | 17 | 250 mg | 1000 | 500 mg |
| | | | | | 38 | 500 mg | 4000 | 1 gram |
| | | | | | 64 | 1 gram | | |
| IV | | | | End of infusion | 188 | 1 gram | | |
| Cephalexin | 95 | 0.9–1.2 | 5–30 | | | | | |
| Oral | | | | 1 | 9 | 250 mg | 1000 | 250 mg |
| | | | | | 18 | 500 mg | 2200 | 500 mg |
| | | | | | 32 | 1 gram | 5000 | 1 gram |
| Cephalothin | | 0.5–1† | 3–18 | | | | | |
| IM | | | | 0.5 | 10 | 500 mg | 800 | 500 mg |
| | | | | | 20 | 1 gram | 2500 | 1 gram |
| IV | | | | 0.25–0.5 | 30 | 1 gram | | |
| | | | | | 80–100 | 2 grams | | |

*Half-life of cefazolin in neonates less than 1 week old is 4.5 to 5 hours.

†Half-life of cephalothin in neonates less than 1 week old is 1.5 to 2 hours.

‡Delayed in presence of food.

§In neonates, the half-life of cefuroxime can be 3 to 5 times longer than it is in adults.

#Bioavailability is increased when this medication is administered with food.

**In adults, not significantly different from normal values during hemodialysis; 2.8 to 4.2 hours between hemodialysis periods; 3 to 7 hours with impaired hepatic function and/or biliary obstruction. In pediatric patients, 6 to 10 hours in low-birth-weight neonates; 4 to 6 hours in infants approximately 1 month of age; 2.2 hours in infants and children 2 months to 11 years of age.

††Half-life of ceftriaxone in pediatric patients with meningitis after a 50- or 75-mg-per-kg dose.

## Table 1. Pharmacology/Pharmacokinetics *(continued)*

| Drug | Bioavailability (%) | Half-life (hr) Normal Renal Function | Half-life (hr) Impaired Renal Function | Time to Peak Serum Concentration (hr) | Peak Serum Concentration After Dose mcg/mL | Peak Serum Concentration After Dose Dose | Peak Urine Concentration After Dose mcg/mL | Peak Urine Concentration After Dose Dose |
|---|---|---|---|---|---|---|---|---|
| Cephapirin | | 0.5–0.8 | 1.5–2.7 | | | | | |
| IM | | | | 0.5–1 | 9 | 500 mg | 900 | 500 mg |
| | | | | | 16 | 1 gram | | |
| IV | | | | End of infusion | 35 | 500 mg | | |
| | | | | | 67 | 1 gram | | |
| Cephradine | 95 | 0.8–1.3 | 8–15 | | | | | |
| Oral | | | | 1‡ | 9 | 250 mg | 1600 | 250 mg |
| | | | | | 17 | 500 mg | 3200 | 500 mg |
| | | | | | 24 | 1 gram | 4000 | 1 gram |
| IM | | | | 0.8–2 | 6 | 500 mg | | |
| | | | | | 14 | 1 gram | | |
| IV | | | | End of infusion | 86 | 1 gram | | |
| **Second-Generation** | | | | | | | | |
| Cefaclor | 95 | 0.6–0.9 | 2.3–2.8 | | | | | |
| Oral | | | | 0.5–1‡ | 7 | 250 mg | 600 | 250 mg |
| | | | | | 13 | 500 mg | 900 | 500 mg |
| Cefamandole | | 0.5–1.2 | 3–18 | | | | | |
| IM | | | | 0.5–2 | 13 | 500 mg | 254 | 500 mg |
| | | | | | 25 | 1 gram | 1357 | 1 gram |
| IV | | | | End of infusion | 139 | 1 gram | 750 | 500 mg |
| | | | | | 240 | 2 grams | 1380 | 1 gram |
| Cefmetazole | | 0.8–1.8 | 3–29 | | | | | |
| IV | | | | End of infusion | 86 | 1 gram | | |
| | | | | | 290 | 2 grams | | |
| Cefonicid | | 4.5 | 17–56 | | | | | |
| IM | | | | 1 | 99 | 1 gram | 385 | 500 mg |
| IV | | | | End of infusion | 220 | 1 gram | | |
| Cefotetan | | 3–4.6 | Prolonged | | | | | |
| IM | | | | 1–3 | 71 | 1 gram | | |
| | | | | | 91 | 2 grams | | |
| IV | | | | End of infusion | 158 | 1 gram | 1700 | 1 gram |
| | | | | | 237 | 2 grams | 3500 | 2 grams |
| Cefoxitin | | 0.7–1.1 | 2–20 | | | | | |
| IM | | | | 0.3–0.5 | 24 | 1 gram | >3000 | 1 gram |
| IV | | | | End of infusion | 110 | 1 gram | | |
| Cefprozil | 95 | 1.3 | to 5.2 | | | | | |
| Oral | | | | 1.5 | 6.1 | 250 mg | 700 | 250 mg |
| | | | | | 10.5 | 500 mg | 1000 | 500 mg |
| Cefuroxime | | 1.2–1.9§ | 17 | | | | | |
| Oral suspension | | | | 2.7–3.6 | 3.3 | 10 mg/kg | | |
| | | | | | 5.1 | 15 mg/kg | | |
| Tablet | After food# (52); Fasting (37) | | | 2 | 2 | 125 mg | | |
| | | | | | 4 | 250 mg | | |
| | | | | | 7 | 500 mg | | |

## Table 1. Pharmacology/Pharmacokinetics *(continued)*

| Drug | Bioavailability (%) | Half-life (hr) Normal Renal Function | Half-life (hr) Impaired Renal Function | Time to Peak Serum Concentration (hr) | Peak Serum Concentration After Dose mcg/mL | Peak Serum Concentration After Dose Dose | Peak Urine Concentration After Dose mcg/mL | Peak Urine Concentration After Dose Dose |
|---|---|---|---|---|---|---|---|---|
| Cefuroxime *(continued)* | | | | | | | | |
| IM | | | | 0.75 | 27 | 750 mg | 1300 | 750 mg |
| IV | | | | End of infusion | 50 | 750 mg | 1150 | 750 mg |
| | | | | | 100 | 1.5 grams | 2500 | 1.5 grams |
| **Third-Generation** | | | | | | | | |
| Cefixime | 40–50 | 3–4 | 6.4–11.5 | | | | | |
| Oral | | | | 2–6 | 2–3 | 200 mg | 73 | 100 mg |
| | | | | | 3.7–4.6 | 400 mg | 107 | 200 mg |
| | | | | | | | 164 | 400 mg |
| Cefoperazone | | 1.6–2.6** | 2.8–4.2** | | | | | |
| IM | | | | 1–2 | 65–75 | 1 gram | 1000 | 2 grams |
| | | | | | 97 | 2 grams | | |
| IV | | | | End of infusion | 153 | 1 gram | >2200 | 2 grams |
| | | | | | 252 | 2 grams | | |
| | | | | | 340 | 3 grams | | |
| | | | | | 506 | 4 grams | | |
| Cefotaxime | | 1 | 3 | | | | | |
| IM | | | | 0.5 | 21 | 1 gram | | |
| IV | | | | | 102 | 1 gram | | |
| | | | | | 214 | 2 grams | | |
| Cefpodoxime | 50# | 2.1–2.8 | 3.5–9.8 | | | | | |
| Oral | | | | 2–3 | 1.4 | 100 mg | | |
| | | | | | 2.3 | 200 mg | | |
| | | | | | 3.9 | 400 mg | | |
| Ceftazidime | | 2 | 13 | | | | | |
| IM | | | | 1 | 17 | 500 mg | 2100 | 500 mg |
| | | | | | 39 | 1 gram | | |
| IV | | | | End of infusion | 42 | 500 mg | 12100 | 2 grams |
| | | | | | 69 | 1 gram | | |
| | | | | | 170 | 2 grams | | |
| Ceftizoxime | | 1.7 | 30 | | | | | |
| IM | | | | 1 | 14 | 500 mg | | |
| | | | | | 39 | 1 gram | | |
| IV | | | | End of infusion | 60 | 1 gram | >6000 | 1 gram |
| | | | | | 132 | 2 grams | | |
| | | | | | 220 | 3 grams | | |
| Ceftriaxone | | | | | | | | |
| IM | | 5.8–8.7 | 11.4–15.7 | 2–3 | 43 | 500 mg | 425 | 500 mg |
| | | | | | 76 | 1 gram | 628 | 1 gram |
| IV | | 4.3–4.6†† | | End of infusion | 82 | 500 mg | 526 | 500 mg |
| | | | | | 151 | 1 gram | 995 | 1 gram |
| | | | | | 257 | 2 grams | 2692 | 2 grams |

*Half-life of cefazolin in neonates less than 1 week old is 4.5 to 5 hours.

†Half-life of cephalothin in neonates less than 1 week old is 1.5 to 2 hours.

‡Delayed in presence of food.

§In neonates, the half-life of cefuroxime can be 3 to 5 times longer than it is in adults.

#Bioavailability is increased when this medication is administered with food.

**In adults, not significantly different from normal values during hemodialysis; 2.8 to 4.2 hours between hemodialysis periods; 3 to 7 hours with impaired hepatic function and/or biliary obstruction. In pediatric patients, 6 to 10 hours in low-birth-weight neonates; 4 to 6 hours in infants approximately 1 month of age; 2.2 hours in infants and children 2 months to 11 years of age.

††Half-life of ceftriaxone in pediatric patients with meningitis after a 50- or 75-mg-per-kg dose.

## Table 2. Pharmacology/Pharmacokinetics*

| Drug | Protein Binding (%) | Hepatic and Renal Biotransformation (%) | Renal Excretion (% unchanged/hr) | Vol$_D$ (liter/kg) | Removal by Dialysis | |
|------|------|------|------|------|------|------|
| | | | | | HD | PD |
| **First-Generation** | | | | | | |
| Cefadroxil | Low (15–20) | No | 93/24 (GF; TS) | 0.31 | Yes | |
| Cefazolin | High (85) | No | 56–89/6 80–100/24 (GF; TS) | 0.12 | Moderate | Yes |
| Cephalexin | Low (10–15) | No | 80/6 90/8 (TS; GF) | 0.26 | Moderate | Yes |
| Cephalothin | Moderate to high (70) | Yes; 20–30 | 60–70/6 (30 as metabolite/6) (TS) | 0.26 | Moderate | Yes |
| Cephapirin | Moderate (44–50) | Yes; 40 | 70/6 (TS; GF; TR) | 0.13 | Slight | |
| Cephradine | Low (8–17) | No | 60–80/6 (TS) | 0.25 | Signif | Yes |
| **Second-Generation** | | | | | | |
| Cefaclor | Low to moderate (25) | No | 60–85/8 | 0.35 | Moderate | |
| Cefamandole | Moderate to high (70–80) | No | 65–85/8 (GF; TS) | 0.16 | Moderate | Yes |
| Cefmetazole | Moderate to high (65–85) | No | 71/24 | 0.13 | Moderate | |
| Cefonicid | Very high (>90) | No | 99/24 | 0.11 | Slight | |
| Cefotetan | High (88) | No | 50–80/24 | 0.19 | Slight | NS |
| Cefoxitin | Moderate to high (70–80) | Slight; 0.2–5 (inactive metabolite) | 85/6 (GF; TS) | 0.16 | Moderate | NS |
| Cefprozil | Moderate (36) | No | 60/8 | | Moderate | |
| Cefuroxime Oral | Moderate (50) | No; prodrug rapidly hydrolyzed to cefuroxime | 32–48/12 (GF; TS) | | Moderate | NS |
| IM, IV | | | 89/8 | | | |
| **Third-Generation** | | | | | | |
| Cefixime | Moderate to high (65–70) | No | 50/24 | 0.11 | NS | No |
| Cefoperazone | High to very high (82–93) | No | 20–30/12† (GF) | 0.14–2.0 | Slight | |
| Cefotaxime | Moderate (38) | Yes; 30–50 (active and inactive metabolites) | 60/6 (15–25 as active metabolite) | 0.25–0.39 | Moderate | NS |
| Cefpodoxime | Moderate (40) | No; prodrug de-esterified to cefpodoxime | 29–33/12 | | Moderate | |
| Ceftazidime | Very low (<10) | No | 80–90/24 | 0.21–0.28 | Yes | Yes |
| Ceftizoxime | Low (30) | No | 85–95/24 | 0.35–0.40 | Moderate | |
| Ceftriaxone | High to very high (85–95) | No | 33–67/24 | 0.12–0.14 0.3‡ | No | No |

*Abbreviations: GF = glomerular filtration; HD = hemodialysis; PD = peritoneal dialysis; TR = tubular reabsorption; TS = tubular secretion; NS = not significant; Signif = significant.

†75% excreted unchanged in bile; 15 to 30% (range: 10 to 36%) excreted unchanged in urine within 6 to 12 hours, primarily by glomerular filtration; up to 90% or more excreted in urine in patients with severe hepatic function impairment or biliary obstruction.

‡In pediatric patients.

**CEPHALOTHIN**—See *Cephalosporins (Systemic)*

**CEPHAPIRIN**—See *Cephalosporins (Systemic)*

**CEPHRADINE**—See *Cephalosporins (Systemic)*

**CETIRIZINE**—See *Antihistamines (Systemic)*

# CHARCOAL, ACTIVATED   Oral-Local

This monograph includes information on the following: Activated Charcoal; Activated Charcoal and Sorbitol.

VA CLASSIFICATION (Primary): AD900

Note: For a listing of dosage forms and brand names by country availability, see *Dosage Forms* section(s). For a listing of brand names for the articles in this monograph, refer to the General Index.

## Category

Antidote (adsorbent)—Activated Charcoal USP; Activated Charcoal Oral Suspension.

Antidote (adsorbent)-laxative—Activated Charcoal and Sorbitol Oral Suspension.

Antidiarrheal (adsorbent)—Activated Charcoal Capsules.

Antiflatulent—Activated Charcoal Capsules; Activated Charcoal Tablets.

## Indications

### Accepted

Toxicity, nonspecific (treatment)—Activated charcoal powder (prepared as an aqueous slurry) and oral suspension and activated charcoal and sorbitol oral suspension are indicated for use as an emergency antidote in the treatment of poisoning by most drugs and chemicals. However, activated charcoal is relatively ineffective in adsorbing caustic alkalis, boric acid, lithium, petroleum distillates (e.g., kerosene, gasoline, coal oil, fuel oil, paint thinner, cleaning fluid), ethanol, methanol, iron salts, and mineral acids.

Diarrhea (treatment) or

Gas, intestinal (treatment)—Activated charcoal capsules and tablets are indicated in the treatment of diarrhea and as a temporary aid in the adsorption of intestinal gas causing flatulence; however, enough studies have not been done to confirm its efficacy for these uses.

## Pharmacology/Pharmacokinetics

### Mechanism of action/Effect

Activated charcoal—

Antidote (adsorbent): Adsorbs the toxic substance ingested, thus inhibiting gastrointestinal absorption.

Antidiarrheal (adsorbent): Adsorbs many toxic irritants that cause diarrhea and gastrointestinal discomfort.

Antiflatulent: Adsorbs intestinal gas to relieve discomfort.

Sorbitol—

Laxative, hyperosmotic: Hygroscopic action results in increased water in the large intestine and increased intraluminal pressure, thus stimulating catharsis.

Flavoring agent: Provides a sweet vehicle to enhance palatability.

### Absorption

Activated charcoal—Not absorbed from the gastrointestinal tract.

Sorbitol—Poorly absorbed from the gastrointestinal tract.

### Biotransformation

Activated charcoal—Not metabolized.

Sorbitol—Hepatic; slowly converted to fructose.

### Elimination

Activated charcoal—Intestinal.

## Precautions to Consider

### Pregnancy/Reproduction

Pregnancy—Problems in humans have not been documented.

### Breast-feeding

Problems in humans have not been documented.

### Pediatrics

*For use as an antidote—*

Preparations of activated charcoal with sorbitol are usually not recommended for use in children under 1 year of age because of the risk of excessive catharsis. In older children, the weight of the child must be taken into account to determine a safe dosage of sorbitol, which should not exceed 3 grams per kg of body weight.

Children should not receive preparations of activated charcoal with sorbitol unless they are under the direct supervision of a physician, so proper attention may be given to the patients' fluid and electrolyte needs.

*For antidiarrheal or antiflatulent use (preparations without sorbitol only)—*

When used as an antidiarrheal or antiflatulent, prolonged use of activated charcoal in infants and children under 3 years of age is not recommended since it may possibly interfere with nutrition.

In pediatric patients with diarrhea, caution is recommended because of the risk of fluid and electrolyte loss; these patients should be referred to a physician.

### Geriatrics

*For use as an antidote—*

Although adequate and well-controlled studies have not been done in the geriatric population, caution is recommended when using preparations of activated charcoal with sorbitol because of the increased risk of catharsis, which may result in fluid and electrolyte loss in geriatric patients.

*For antidiarrheal use (preparations without sorbitol only)—*

In geriatric patients with diarrhea, caution is recommended because of the risk of fluid and electrolyte loss; these patients should be referred to a physician.

### Drug interactions and/or related problems

The following drug interactions and/or related problems have been selected on the basis of their potential clinical significance (possible mechanism in parentheses where appropriate)—not necessarily inclusive (» = major clinical significance):

» Acetylcysteine, oral

(effectiveness of orally administered acetylcysteine as antidote in acetaminophen overdose may be decreased because of adsorption by activated charcoal; activated charcoal is recommended if ingestion of other substances [in addition to acetaminophen] is confirmed or suspected, but its removal by gastric lavage may be advisable prior to acetylcysteine administration)

Chocolate syrup or

Ice cream or sherbet

(should not be used as vehicles for the administration of activated charcoal since they will decrease the adsorptive capacity of the activated charcoal)

Ipecac

(if both ipecac and activated charcoal are to be used in the treatment for oral poisoning, it is generally recommended that the charcoal be administered only after vomiting has been induced and completed; however, in some clinical trials in which activated charcoal was administered pre-emesis 10 minutes after high doses of ipecac, the emetic properties of ipecac were not inhibited)

Oral medications, other

(the effectiveness of other concurrently used medications may be decreased because of adsorption and increased elimination by the activated charcoal; patients should be advised not to take any other medication within 2 hours of the activated charcoal)

### Medical considerations/Contraindications

The medical considerations/contraindications included here have been selected on the basis of their potential clinical significance (reasons given in parentheses where appropriate)—not necessarily inclusive (» = major clinical significance).

*Risk-benefit should be considered when the following medical problems exist:*

» Bowel sounds, absence of

(increased risk of gastrointestinal complications, such as gastrointestinal obstruction)

*For antidiarrheal use only (preparations without sorbitol only)*

» Dehydration

(rehydration therapy is essential if signs of dehydration, such as dry mouth, excessive thirst, wrinkled skin, decreased urination, dizziness or lightheadedness, are present; fluid loss may have serious consequences, such as circulatory collapse and renal failure, especially in young children and the elderly)

Diarrhea, parasite-associated, suspected

(use of adsorbent antidiarrheals may make recognition of parasitic causes of diarrhea more difficult; if parasitic agents are suspected pathogens, appropriate stool analyses should be performed prior to therapy with adsorbents)

» Dysentery, acute, characterized by bloody stools and elevated temperature

(sole treatment with adsorbent antidiarrheals may be inadequate; antibiotic therapy may be required)

## Side/Adverse Effects

The following side/adverse effects have been selected on the basis of their potential clinical significance (possible signs and symptoms in parentheses where appropriate)—not necessarily inclusive:

Note: Dehydration, cardiac arrest, and brain damage occurred as a result of sorbitol overdose in a 3-year-old child who was being treated with activated charcoal and sorbitol combination for an overdose of a drug used to treat asthma.

**Those indicating need for medical attention**
Incidence less frequent or rare
*Swelling of abdomen or pain*

**Those indicating need for medical attention only if they continue**
Incidence more frequent—with sorbitol-containing preparations
*Diarrhea or vomiting*

Note: *Diarrhea or vomiting* may persist for several hours; precautions should be taken against possible fluid and electrolyte loss.

**Those not indicating need for medical attention**
Incidence more frequent
*Black stools*

## Patient Consultation

As an aid to patient consultation, refer to *Advice for the Patient, Charcoal, Activated (Oral)*.

In providing consultation, consider emphasizing the following selected information (» = major clinical significance):

**Before using this medication**
» Conditions affecting use, especially:
   Use in children—Preparations with sorbitol are not recommended for children up to 1 year of age and should be used only under a physician's supervision in older children because of risk of excessive catharsis; prolonged use of activated charcoal as an antidiarrheal/antiflatulent in children under 3 years of age may interfere with nutrition; risk of dehydration associated with diarrhea (for antidiarrheal use)
   Use in the elderly—Risk of fluid and electrolyte loss with preparations containing sorbitol; risk of dehydration associated with diarrhea (for antidiarrheal use)
   Other medical problems, especially absence of bowel sounds (for antidote use); dehydration and acute dysentery (for antidiarrheal/antiflatulent use)

**Proper use of this medication**
» Importance of not taking medication mixed with chocolate syrup, ice cream, or sherbet
» Proper dosing
» Proper storage
*When used as an antidote only*
» Calling poison control center, physician, or emergency room before taking medication
» Importance of shaking the oral liquid dosage form well; taking full dose
» Taking medication only after vomiting has been induced and completed if ipecac syrup is used also
*When used as an antidiarrheal/antiflatulent only*
   Taking doses of other oral medications at least 2 hours before or after doses of activated charcoal

*When used as an antidiarrheal only*
» Importance of maintaining adequate hydration and proper diet

**Precautions while using this medication**
*When used as an antidiarrheal/antiflatulent only*
   Checking with physician if condition has not improved after 7 days (when used as an antiflatulent only)
   Checking with physician if diarrhea continues after medication has been used for 2 days or if fever is present with diarrhea

**Side/adverse effects**
   Signs of potential side effects, especially continuing diarrhea or vomiting (for sorbitol-containing preparations)
   Medication will color stools black, which may be alarming to patient although medically insignificant

## General Dosing Information

**For use as an antidote only**
Activated charcoal is most effective when it is administered early in acute poisoning, preferably within 30 minutes following ingestion of the poison.

When the amount of toxic substance ingested is known, the dose of activated charcoal recommended is usually 5 to 10 times the amount of toxic substance ingested; however, a dose of 50 grams is considered the minimum adult dose by many clinicians.

Tablets or granules of activated charcoal are less effective than the powder form of the medication and should not be used in the treatment of poisoning.

The administration of activated charcoal as an aqueous slurry is generally preferred. However, to improve the palatability of activated charcoal, it has been administered in combination with suspending agents such as bentonite or carboxymethylcellulose. Also, a flavoring agent such as chocolate syrup has been added to the combination at the time of administration. However, some studies have shown that these agents, especially the flavoring agents, decrease the adsorptive capacity of activated charcoal and should not be used.

Following administration of activated charcoal, it is recommended that a cathartic be administered to enhance removal of the drug/charcoal complex since failure to excrete the drug/charcoal complex promptly may result in enhanced toxicity. However, administration of a cathartic may not be necessary when an activated charcoal product containing sorbitol is used.

Multiple-dose activated charcoal therapy may be useful in severe poisonings to prevent desorption from the charcoal; to hasten elimination of chronically used medications by the gastrointestinal tract (gastrointestinal dialysis); also, to increase clearance of certain drugs or substances that undergo enterohepatic circulation, to prevent their reabsorption. Some substances for which multiple-dose activated charcoal therapy has been demonstrated to be effective are amitriptyline, carbamazepine, diazepam, digoxin, doxepin, meprobamate, methotrexate, nortriptyline, phenobarbital, piroxicam, salicylates, and theophylline.

When multiple doses of activated charcoal are required, preparations that contain sorbitol should not be used in each dose of the multiple-dose regimen since they may produce excessive catharsis, which may result in dehydration and hypotension. Instead, doses of activated charcoal preparations without sorbitol should be alternated with the sorbitol-containing products.

The presence of normal bowel sounds is necessary to determine whether to continue multiple-dose activated charcoal therapy. If bowel sounds are absent or hypoactive, continuing multiple dosing of activated charcoal with or without sorbitol is not recommended because of the possibility of constipation (or aggravation of) and the possibility of pooling of fluids in the colon if sorbitol continues to be administered with the activated charcoal.

If catharsis does not occur within four to eight hours after use of an activated charcoal preparation containing sorbitol, an additional dose of sorbitol (1.5 grams per kg of body weight) or a saline laxative, such as magnesium citrate, may be administered.

---

## ACTIVATED CHARCOAL

## Oral-Local Dosage Forms

### ACTIVATED CHARCOAL USP

**Usual adult and adolescent dose**
Antidote (adsorbent)—
   Oral, 25 to 100 grams, as a slurry in water.

**Usual pediatric dose**
Antidote (adsorbent)—
   Oral, 1 gram per kg of body weight, or 25 to 50 grams, as a slurry in water.

**Usual geriatric dose**
See *Usual adult and adolescent dose*.

**Size(s) usually available**
U.S.—
   15 grams (OTC) [GENERIC].
   30 grams (OTC) [GENERIC].
   40 grams (OTC) [GENERIC].
   120 grams (OTC) [GENERIC].
   125 grams (OTC) [GENERIC].
   240 grams (OTC) [GENERIC].
   500 grams (OTC) [GENERIC].
Canada—
   25 grams (OTC) [GENERIC].

**Packaging and storage**
Store below 40 °C (104 °F), preferably between 15 and 30 °C (59 and 86 °F), unless otherwise specified by manufacturer. Store in a well-closed container.

**Note**

If this medication is to be used as an antidote for emergency use in poisoning, consider providing on the label the telephone number for physician, poison control center, or emergency room.

## ACTIVATED CHARCOAL CAPSULES

Note: Activated charcoal capsules should not be used as an antidote for emergency use in poisoning.

### Usual adult and adolescent dose

Antidiarrheal (adsorbent)—
Oral, 520 mg, repeated every thirty minutes to one hour as needed up to 4.16 grams per day.

Antiflatulent—
Oral, 1.04 to 3.9 grams three times a day after meals.

### Usual pediatric dose

Antidiarrheal (adsorbent)—
Infants and children up to 3 years of age: Dosage must be individualized by physician.
Children 3 years of age and over: See *Usual adult and adolescent dose.*

Antiflatulent—
Dosage must be individualized by physician.

### Usual geriatric dose

See *Usual adult and adolescent dose.*

### Strength(s) usually available

U.S.—
250 mg (OTC) [*Charcocaps*].
260 mg (OTC) [*Charcocaps;* GENERIC].

Canada—
Content information not available (OTC) [GENERIC].

### Packaging and storage

Store below 40 °C (104 °F), preferably between 15 and 30 °C (59 and 86 °F), in a well-closed container, unless otherwise specified by manufacturer.

## ACTIVATED CHARCOAL ORAL SUSPENSION

### Usual adult and adolescent dose

Antidote (adsorbent)—
Oral, 25 to 100 grams as a single dose.

Note: For multiple-dose therapy—Oral, 25 to 50 grams every four to six hours.

### Usual pediatric dose

Antidote (adsorbent)—
Children up to 1 year of age: Oral, 1 gram per kg of body weight as a single dose.
Children 1 to 12 years of age: Oral, 25 to 50 grams as a single dose.

Note: For multiple-dose therapy, dose may be repeated every four to six hours.

### Usual geriatric dose

See *Usual adult and adolescent dose.*

### Strength(s) usually available

U.S.—
12.5 grams per 60 mL (OTC) [*Liqui-Char;* GENERIC].
15 grams per 72 mL (OTC) [*Actidose-Aqua;* GENERIC].
15 grams per 75 mL (OTC) [*Liqui-Char*].
15 grams per 120 mL (OTC) [*Pediatric Aqueous Insta-Char*].
25 grams per 120 mL (OTC) [*Actidose-Aqua; Liqui-Char; Pediatric Aqueous Insta-Char;* GENERIC].
30 grams per 120 mL (OTC) [*Liqui-Char*].
50 grams per 240 mL (OTC) [*Actidose-Aqua; CharcoAid 2000; Insta-Char Aqueous; Liqui-Char;* GENERIC].

Canada—
15 grams per 120 mL [*Insta-Char Aqueous*].
25 grams per 125 mL [*Pediatric Aqueous Charcodote*].
50 grams per 225 mL [*Charac-50*].
50 grams per 240 mL [*Insta-Char Aqueous*].
50 grams per 250 mL [*Aqueous Charcodote*].

Note: In Canada, this medication has not been assigned either Rx or OTC status. However, it may not be sold or dispensed directly to the patient.

### Packaging and storage

Store below 40 °C (104 °F), preferably between 15 and 30 °C (59 and 86 °F), in a well-closed container, unless otherwise specified by manufacturer. Protect from freezing.

### Auxiliary labeling

• Shake well.

**Note**

If this medication is to be used as an antidote for emergency use in poisoning, consider providing on the label the telephone number for poison control center, physician, or emergency room.

## ACTIVATED CHARCOAL TABLETS

Note: Activated charcoal tablets should not be used as an antidote for emergency use in poisoning.

### Usual adult and adolescent dose

Antiflatulent—
Oral, 975 mg to 3.9 grams three times a day after meals.

### Usual pediatric dose

Antiflatulent—
Dosage must be individualized by physician.

### Usual geriatric dose

See *Usual adult and adolescent dose.*

### Strength(s) usually available

U.S.—
260 mg (OTC) [*Charocaps*].
325 mg (OTC) [GENERIC].
650 mg (OTC) [GENERIC].

Canada—
Not commercially available.

### Packaging and storage

Store below 40 °C (104 °F), preferably between 15 and 30 °C (59 and 86 °F), in a well-closed container, unless otherwise specified by manufacturer.

---

### ACTIVATED CHARCOAL AND SORBITOL

## Oral-Local Dosage Forms

### ACTIVATED CHARCOAL AND SORBITOL ORAL SUSPENSION

### Usual adult and adolescent dose

Antidote (adsorbent)—
Oral, 50 grams of activated charcoal as a single dose.

Note: For multiple-dose therapy—Use is not recommended because of excessive catharsis, unless repeat doses are alternated with activated charcoal preparations that contain no sorbitol.

Sorbitol content is different among the different preparations available. Product label should be consulted to determine the amount of sorbitol. For adults, the usual dose of sorbitol 70% (70 grams per 100 mL) is 50 to 150 mL.

### Usual pediatric dose

Antidote (adsorbent)—
Children up to 1 year of age: Use is not recommended.
Children 1 to 12 years of age: Oral, 25 to 50 grams of activated charcoal as a single dose.

Note: For multiple-dose therapy—Use is not recommended because of excessive catharsis, unless repeat doses are alternated with activated charcoal preparations that contain no sorbitol.

Sorbitol content is different among the different preparations available. Product label should be consulted to determine the amount of sorbitol. For children, the usual dose of sorbitol 70% (70 grams per 100 mL) is 2 mL per kg of body weight, or a dose not to exceed 3 grams of sorbitol per kg of body weight.

### Usual geriatric dose

See *Usual adult and adolescent dose.*

### Strength(s) usually available

U.S.—
25 grams of activated charcoal and 25 grams of sorbitol per 120 mL (OTC) [*Insta-Char with Sorbitol*].
25 grams of activated charcoal and 27 grams of sorbitol per 120 mL (OTC) [*Liqui-Char with Sorbitol*].
25 grams of activated charcoal and 48 grams of sorbitol per 120 mL (OTC) [*Actidose with Sorbitol*].
30 grams of activated charcoal and 62 grams of sorbitol per 150 mL (OTC) [*Charcoaid*].
50 grams of activated charcoal and 50 grams of sorbitol per 240 mL (OTC) [*Insta-Char with Sorbitol*].
50 grams of activated charcoal and 54 grams of sorbitol per 240 mL (OTC) [*Liqui-Char with Sorbitol*].
50 grams of activated charcoal and 96 grams of sorbitol per 240 mL (OTC) [*Actidose with Sorbitol*].

Canada—

   25 grams of activated charcoal and 25 grams of sorbitol per 125 mL
   [*Charcodote TFS-25*].

   25 grams of activated charcoal and 90 grams (approximately) of sorbitol per 125 mL [*Pediatric Charcodote*].

   50 grams of activated charcoal and 50 grams of sorbitol per 250 mL
   [*Charac-tol 50; Charcodote TFS-50*].

   50 grams of activated charcoal and 180 grams (approximately) of sorbitol per 250 mL [*Charcodote*].

   Note: In Canada, this medication has not been assigned either Rx or
   OTC status. However, it may not be sold or dispensed directly
   to the patient.

### Packaging and storage

Store below 40 °C (104 °F), preferably between 15 and 30 °C (59 and 86
°F), in a well-closed container, unless otherwise specified by manufacturer. Protect from freezing.

### Auxiliary labeling

• Shake well.

### Note

If this medication is to be used as an antidote for emergency use in poisoning, consider providing on the label the telephone number for physician, poison control center, or emergency room.

### Selected Bibliography

Pond S. Role of repeated oral doses of activated charcoal in clinical toxicology. Med Toxicol 1986; 1: 3-11.

Albertson TE, et al. Superiority of activated charcoal alone compared with
ipecac and activated charcoal in the treatment of acute toxic ingestions.
Ann Emerg Med 1989; 18: 56-59.

---

Revised: 08/16/91
Interim revision: 06/14/95

### CHARCOAL-CONTAINING COMBINATIONS—

Activated Charcoal and Sorbitol (Oral-Local)—See *Charcoal, Activated
(Oral-Local)*

---

# CHENODIOL    Systemic*†

INN: Chenodeoxycholic acid

BAN: Chenodeoxycholic acid

JAN: Chenodeoxycholic acid

VA CLASSIFICATION (Primary): GA900

Note: For a listing of dosage forms and brand names by country availability, see *Dosage Forms* section(s). For a listing of brand names
for the articles in this monograph, refer to the General Index.

---

*Not commercially available in the U.S.
†Not commercially available in Canada.

## Category

Anticholelithic.

## Indications

### Accepted

Gallstone disease (treatment)—Chenodiol is indicated for dissolution of
cholesterol gallstones in selected patients with uncomplicated radiolucent gallstone disease and functioning gallbladder.

   Chenodiol therapy is more likely to be effective if the stones are small
   and of the floatable type.

   Body weight and dietary factors may influence gallstone formation
   and/or dissolution rate. A high-fiber and low-fat diet and maintenance
   of reduced body weight are recommended as adjunctive measures to
   increase response to therapy.

### Unaccepted

Chenodiol is *not* indicated when there is a confirmed nonvisualizing gallbladder, radiopaque stones (calcium-containing), or when surgery is
clearly indicated.

## Pharmacology/Pharmacokinetics

### Physicochemical characteristics

Molecular weight—392.58.

### Mechanism of action/Effect

Although the exact mechanism of chenodiol's anticholelithic action is not
completely understood, chenodiol given orally in pharmacological
doses contributes to desaturation of the bile by increasing the ratio of
bile acids to cholesterol. The reduced cholesterol saturation allows for
the gradual solubilization of cholesterol from gallstones, resulting in
their eventual dissolution.

### Other actions/effects

Chenodiol may increase secretion of bile acids. Chenodiol also increases
low-density lipoprotein (LDL) fraction of cholesterol (by about 10%),
inhibits colonic fluid absorption, and may induce fluid secretion.

### Absorption

Unconjugated chenodiol is well absorbed from the small intestine.

### Biotransformation

Hepatic (60 to 80% first-pass hepatic clearance). Exogenous chenodiol is
metabolized in the liver to its taurine and glycine conjugates.

### Time to peak concentration

50 to 120 minutes.

### Elimination

Fecal. Conjugated chenodiol is converted by bacteria in the colon to its
major metabolite, lithocholic acid; 80% of the lithocholate is excreted
in the feces and the remainder is reabsorbed and converted in the liver
to sulfolithocholyl conjugates.

## Precautions to Consider

### Cross-sensitivity and/or related problems

Patients sensitive to other bile acid products may be sensitive to chenodiol
also.

### Carcinogenicity/Tumorigenicity

Studies in rats have not shown that chenodiol has carcinogenic effects
when given orally in doses 1 to 4 times the maximum recommended
human dose (MRHD). In long-term studies in rats and mice administered oral doses 40 and 60 times the maximum recommended doses,
respectively, chenodiol caused benign and malignant liver cell tumors
in female rats and cholangiomata in female rats and male mice. Also,
epidemiologic studies suggest that bile acids may contribute to human
colon cancer; however, conclusive evidence is lacking.

### Pregnancy/Reproduction

Pregnancy—Chenodiol is not recommended for use during pregnancy.
Studies in animals have shown that chenodiol, when given in doses
several times the MRHD, causes hepatic, renal, and adrenal lesions in
the fetus. Risk-benefit must be carefully considered.

FDA Pregnancy Category X.

### Breast-feeding

It is not known whether chenodiol is distributed into breast milk. However,
problems in humans have not been documented.

### Pediatrics

Appropriate studies on the relationship of age to the effects of chenodiol
have not been performed in the pediatric population.

### Geriatrics

Appropriate studies on the relationship of age to the effects of chenodiol
have not been performed in the geriatric population. However, geriatrics-specific problems that would limit the usefulness of this medication in the elderly are not expected.

### Drug interactions and/or related problems

The following drug interactions and/or related problems have been selected on the basis of their potential clinical significance (possible
mechanism in parentheses where appropriate)—not necessarily inclusive (» = major clinical significance):

Note: Combinations containing any of the following medications, depending on the amount present, may also interact with this
medication.

Antacids, aluminum-containing or
Cholestyramine or
Colestipol
    (concurrent use may result in binding of chenodiol, thus decreasing
    its absorption)

Antihyperlipidemics, especially clofibrate or
Estrogens or
Neomycin or
Progestins
    (concurrent use of these medications with chenodiol may decrease
    the effect of chenodiol since they tend to increase cholesterol sat-
    uration of bile)

## Laboratory value alterations

The following have been selected on the basis of their potential clinical
significance (possible effect in parentheses where appropriate)—not
necessarily inclusive (» = major clinical significance):

With physiology/laboratory test values

Alanine aminotransferase (ALT [SGPT])
    (serum concentrations may be increased due to either a direct dose-
    related effect of chenodiol or to the inability of the patient to form
    sulfate conjugates of lithocholic acid)

Cholesterol
    (serum concentrations may be increased slightly)

## Medical considerations/Contraindications

The medical considerations/contraindications included here have been selected on the basis of their potential clinical significance (reasons given
in parentheses where appropriate)—not necessarily inclusive (» =
major clinical significance):

*Risk-benefit should be considered when the following medical problems
exist:*

Atherosclerosis
    (condition may be aggravated because of increase in the low-den-
    sity lipoprotein [LDL] fraction of cholesterol)

» Bile duct abnormalities, such as:
  Biliary cirrhosis, primary
  Cholangitis, sclerosing
  Cholestasis, intrahepatic or

» Gallstone complications, such as:
  Biliary gastrointestinal fistula
  Biliary obstruction
  Cholangitis
  Cholecystitis
  Pancreatitis
    (medical treatment with chenodiol would be too lengthy; surgery
    may be indicated)

» Hepatic function impairment
    (impaired bile acid metabolism may be further aggravated)

## Patient monitoring

The following may be especially important in patient monitoring (other
tests may be warranted in some patients, depending on condition;
» = major clinical significance):

Cholecystograms, oral or
Ultrasonograms
    (recommended prior to treatment to determine the presence of gall-
    bladder stones, and during treatment to monitor stone dissolution;
    also recommended annually after gallstone dissolution to monitor
    for possible recurrence)

Cholesterol concentrations, serum
    (determinations recommended at 6-month intervals during cheno-
    diol therapy; chenodiol therapy should be discontinued if choles-
    terol concentrations rise above patient's acceptable age-adjusted
    limit)

Hepatic function determinations
    (monitoring of serum transaminase concentrations is recommended
    before initiating treatment to rule out pre-existing liver disease and
    during treatment; optimal frequency of monitoring during treat-
    ment has not been established; however, it is suggested that de-
    terminations be done on a monthly basis for the first 3 months and
    every 3 months thereafter during chenodiol therapy; chenodiol
    must be discontinued if elevations over 3 times the upper normal
    limit occur)

## Side/Adverse Effects

Note: Although serious liver damage has not been observed in humans,
    hepatotoxicity has occurred in animal species unable to sulfate lith-
    ocholic acid. Also, mild, transient hypertransaminasemia has oc-
    curred in some patients.

The following side/adverse effects have been selected on the basis of their
    potential clinical significance (possible signs and symptoms in paren-
    theses where appropriate)—not necessarily inclusive:

**Those indicating need for medical attention**
Incidence less frequent or rare
    *Diarrhea, severe*—may indicate overdose

**Those indicating need for medical attention only if they continue
or are bothersome**
Incidence more frequent
    *Diarrhea, mild and transient*—dose related; may also occur at initi-
    ation of therapy
Incidence less frequent or rare
    *Constipation; frequent urge for bowel movement; gas or indiges-
    tion*—usually disappears within 2 to 4 weeks after initiation of treat-
    ment; *loss of appetite; nausea or vomiting; stomach cramps or pain*

## Overdose

For specific information on the agents used in the management of chenodiol overdose, see:
    • *Aluminum Hydroxide* in *Antacids (Oral-Local)* monograph;
    • *Charcoal, Activated (Oral-Local)* monograph; and/or
    • *Cholestyramine (Oral-Local)* monograph.

For more information on the management of overdose or unintentional
ingestion, **contact a Poison Control Center** (see *Poison Control Center Listing*).

### Clinical effects of overdose

The following effects have been selected on the basis of their potential
clinical significance (possible signs and symptoms in parentheses
where appropriate)–not necessarily inclusive:

    *Diarrhea, severe*—may indicate overdose

### Treatment of overdose

Recommended treatment for chenodiol overdose (no cases reported) includes:

To decrease absorption—Gastric lavage with at least 1 liter of a cholestyramine or charcoal suspension (concentration of 2 grams per 100
mL of water).

Specific treatment—Oral administration of 50 mL of aluminum hydroxide
suspension.

Supportive care—Patients in whom overdose in confirmed or suspected
should be referred for psychiatric consultation.

## Patient Consultation

As an aid to patient consultation, refer to *Advice for the Patient, Chenodiol
(Systemic)*.

In providing consultation, consider emphasizing the following selected
information (»= major clinical significance):

**Before using this medication**
» Conditions affecting use, especially:
    Sensitivity to bile acid products
    Pregnancy—Contraindicated in pregnancy because studies in ani-
      mals have shown hepatic, renal, and adrenal damage to fetus
    Other medical problems, especially bile duct abnormalities, gall-
      stone complications, or hepatic function impairment
    Diet—High-fiber diet may be recommended to help dissolve stones
      faster and keep new stones from forming; importance of going
      on a reducing diet, but checking with a physician before going
      on any diet

**Proper use of this medication**
    Taking with food or milk for optimal therapeutic effect
» Compliance with full course of therapy
» Proper dosing
    Missed dose: Taking as soon as possible; not taking if almost time for
      next dose; not doubling doses
» Proper storage

**Precautions while using this medication**
    Avoiding aluminum-containing antacids; may interfere with absorption
      of chenodiol
» Regular visits to physician to check progress; laboratory tests required
      during therapy
» Notifying physician immediately if symptoms of acute cholecystitis
      develop

**Side/adverse effects**
    Signs of potential side effects, especially severe diarrhea

## General Dosing Information

Chenodiol should be taken with food or milk since it dissolves more rapidly when bile and pancreatic juice are present in the intestinal chyme.

Gallstone dissolution may require 3 months to 2 years depending on the size and composition of the stone (s). Response should be monitored by oral cholecystograms or ultrasonograms performed at 6- to 9-month intervals. Therapy may be discontinued if dissolution has been confirmed by a second cholecystogram 1 to 3 months later.

Chenodiol therapy is unlikely to be effective if partial dissolution has not occurred after 9 to 12 months of treatment. If there are still no signs of response to therapy after 18 months, treatment with chenodiol should be discontinued.

Dosage of chenodiol should be reduced by one-half if diarrhea is persistent during dosage buildup or later in treatment. Antidiarrheal agents may also be used during this period. The dose may be increased gradually to the original level after diarrhea subsides.

Overweight patients are often less responsive to chenodiol therapy because of greater cholesterol secretion into bile and may require a higher dose based on body weight.

### Diet/Nutrition

Body weight and dietary factors may influence gallstone formation and/or dissolution rate. A high-fiber diet, including foods such as whole grain breads and cereals, bran, fruit, and green, leafy vegetables; and maintenance of reduced body weight are recommended as adjunctive measures to increase response to therapy.

## Oral Dosage Forms

### CHENODIOL TABLETS

#### Usual adult and adolescent dose

Gallstone disease—
> Oral, 13 to 16 mg per kg of body weight a day, divided into two doses, taken with food or milk in the morning and at night.

Note:  An initial dose of 250 mg per day is recommended for the first two weeks of treatment, the dose being increased thereafter by 250 mg a day until the recommended or maximum tolerated dose is reached.

> Overweight patients may require up to 20 mg per kg of body weight a day.

#### Usual pediatric dose

Dosage has not been established.

#### Usual geriatric dose

See *Usual adult and adolescent dose*.

#### Strength(s) usually available

U.S.—
> Not commercially available.

Canada—
> Not commercially available.

#### Packaging and storage

Store below 40 °C (104 °F), preferably between 15 and 30 °C (59 and 86 °F), in a well-closed container, unless otherwise specified by manufacturer.

#### Auxiliary labeling

• Continue medicine for full time of treatment.
• Take with food.

## Selected Bibliography

Abate MA. Medical management of cholesterol gallstones. Drug Intell Clin Pharm 1986; 20: 106-15.

Fromm H, Roat JW, Gonzalez V. Comparative efficacy and side effects of ursodeoxycholic acid and chenodeoxycholic acid in dissolving gallstones. Gastroenterology 1983; 85: 1257-64.

Revised: 04/27/94

---

# CHLOPHEDIANOL   Systemic*

VA CLASSIFICATION (Primary): RE302

Note:  For a listing of dosage forms and brand names by country availability, see *Dosage Forms* section(s). For a listing of brand names for the articles in this monograph, refer to the General Index.

*Not commercially available in the U.S.

## Category

Antitussive.

## Indications

### Accepted

Cough (treatment)—Indicated for the symptomatic relief of nonproductive cough. Chlophedianol is used to provide relief of acute cough due to minor throat and bronchial irritation occurring with colds or inhaled irritants.

## Pharmacology/Pharmacokinetics

### Physicochemical characteristics

Molecular weight—326.26.

### Mechanism of action/Effect

Suppresses the cough reflex by a direct effect on the cough center in the medulla of the brain.

### Other actions/effects

It may also possess moderate local anesthetic effect and some anticholinergic action.

### Biotransformation

Hepatic.

### Time to peak effect

Slower than narcotic antitussives.

### Duration of action

Longer than narcotic antitussives.

### Elimination

Renal.

## Precautions to Consider

### Pregnancy/Reproduction

Pregnancy—Studies have not been done in humans.
Studies have not been done in animals.

### Breast-feeding

It is not known whether chlophedianol is distributed into breast milk. However, problems in humans have not been documented.

### Pediatrics

Appropriate studies on the relationship of age to the effects of chlophedianol have not been performed in children up to 2 years of age.

### Geriatrics

No information is available on the relationship of age to the effects of chlophedianol in geriatric patients.

### Drug interactions and/or related problems

The following drug interactions and/or related problems have been selected on the basis of their potential clinical significance (possible mechanism in parentheses where appropriate)—not necessarily inclusive (» = major clinical significance):

Note:  Combinations containing any of the following medications, depending on the amount present, may also interact with this medication.

> Central nervous system (CNS) depression–producing medications (see *Appendix II*) or
> Monoamine oxidase (MAO) inhibitors, including furazolidone and procarbazine
> (concurrent use may potentiate CNS depressant effects of either these medications or chlophedianol)

> CNS stimulation–producing medications (see *Appendix II* )
> (concurrent use may potentiate CNS stimulant effects of chlophedianol)

### Medical considerations/Contraindications

The medical considerations/contraindications included here have been selected on the basis of their potential clinical significance (reasons given in parentheses where appropriate)—not necessarily inclusive (» = major clinical significance).

*Except under special circumstances, this medication should not be used when the following medical problems exist:*

» Cough, productive
   (inhibition of cough reflex may lead to retention of secretions)
   Sensitivity to chlophedianol

## Side/Adverse Effects

The following side/adverse effects have been selected on the basis of their potential clinical significance (possible signs and symptoms in parentheses where appropriate)—not necessarily inclusive:

**Those indicating need for medical attention**
Incidence rare
   *CNS stimulant effects* (hallucinations; nightmares; unusual excitement or irritability); *hypersensitivity* (skin rash; hives)

With large doses
   *Anticholinergic effects* (blurred vision; dizziness; drowsiness; dryness of the mouth; nausea; vomiting)

## Patient Consultation

As an aid to patient consultation, refer to *Advice for the Patient, Chlophedianol (Systemic)*.

In providing consultation, consider emphasizing the following selected information (» = major clinical significance):

**Before using this medication**
» Conditions affecting use, especially:
      Sensitivity to chlophedianol
      Other medical problems, especially a productive cough

**Proper use of this medication**
   Not taking liquids immediately after taking medication
» Importance of not taking more medication than the amount prescribed
» Proper dosing
   Missed dose (if on regular dosing schedule): Taking as soon as possible; not taking if almost time for next dose; not doubling doses
» Proper storage

**Precautions while using this medication**
   Checking with physician if cough persists after medication has been used for 7 days or if high fever, skin rash, or continuing headache is present with cough
» Avoiding use of alcohol or other CNS depressants
» Caution in taking appetite suppressants or drinking large amounts of xanthine-containing beverages during therapy
» Caution if drowsiness occurs

**Side/adverse effects**
   Signs of potential side effects, especially CNS stimulant effects, hypersensitivity, or anticholinergic effects (with large dose)

## General Dosing Information

Liquids should not be taken immediately after the syrup is taken because soothing effects will be decreased.

Reduced dosage may be necessary in sedated or debilitated patients since excessive depression of the cough reflex might be undesirable in these patients.

## Oral Dosage Forms

### CHLOPHEDIANOL HYDROCHLORIDE SYRUP

**Usual adult and adolescent dose**
Antitussive—
   Oral, 25 mg every six to eight hours as needed.

**Usual pediatric dose**
Antitussive—
   Children up to 2 years of age: Dosage has not been established.
   Children 2 to 6 years of age: Oral, 12.5 mg every six to eight hours as needed.
   Children 6 to 12 years of age: Oral, 12.5 to 25 mg every six to eight hours as needed.

**Usual geriatric dose**
See *Usual adult and adolescent dose*.

**Strength(s) usually available**
U.S.—
   Not commercially available.
Canada—
   25 mg per 5 mL (OTC) [*Ulone*].

**Packaging and storage**
Store below 40 °C (104 °F), preferably between 15 and 30 °C (59 and 86 °F), in a light-resistant container, unless otherwise specified by manufacturer. Protect from freezing.

**Auxiliary labeling**
• May cause drowsiness.
• Avoid alcoholic beverages.

## Selected Bibliography

Irwin RS, Curley FJ, Pratter MR. The effects of drugs on cough. Eur J Respir Dis Suppl 1987; 153: 173-81.
Irwin RS, Curley FJ, Bennett FM. Appropriate use of antitussives and protussives. Drugs 1993; 46 (1): 80-91.

Revised: 02/23/94

---

# CHLORAL HYDRATE   Systemic

VA CLASSIFICATION (Primary): CN309
Note: Controlled substance in the U.S.
Note: For a listing of dosage forms and brand names by country availability, see *Dosage Forms* section(s). For a listing of brand names for the articles in this monograph, refer to the General Index.

## Category

Sedative-hypnotic.

## Indications

Note: Bracketed information in the *Indications* section refers to uses that are not included in U.S. product labeling.

**Accepted**
Anesthesia, adjunct—Chloral hydrate is indicated preoperatively to relieve anxiety and produce sedation and/or sleep.

[Sedation for procedures in pediatric patients]—Chloral hydrate is used to produce sedation in pediatric patients for certain dental and medical procedures.

Chloral hydrate has been used for the treatment of insomnia. However, this medication is effective as a hypnotic only for short-term use; it has been shown to lose its effectiveness for both inducing and maintaining sleep after 2 weeks of administration. In addition, chloral hydrate generally *has been replaced* by agents with better pharmacokinetic and pharmacodynamic profiles.

Chloral hydrate has been used as a routine sedative. However, it generally *has been replaced* by safer and more effective agents.

Chloral hydrate also has been used as an adjunct to opiates and analgesics in postoperative care and control of pain. However, it generally *has been replaced* by agents with better pharmacokinetic and pharmacodynamic profiles.

**Unaccepted**
Chloral hydrate is not recommended for use in infants and children when repetitive dosing would be necessary. With repeated dosing, accumulation of the trichloroethanol and trichloroacetic acid metabolites may increase the potential for excessive CNS depression, predispose neonates to conjugated and nonconjugated hyperbilirubinemia, decrease albumin binding of bilirubin, and contribute to metabolic acidosis.

## Pharmacology/Pharmacokinetics

**Physicochemical characteristics**
Molecular weight—165.40.

**Mechanism of action/Effect**
The central nervous system (CNS) depressant effects of chloral hydrate are believed to be due to its active metabolite trichloroethanol. The mechanism of action is not known.

**Absorption**
Readily absorbed from the gastrointestinal tract, following oral administration.

**Protein binding**
Trichloroethanol (the active metabolite)—35 to 41%.

**Biotransformation**
Chloral hydrate is metabolized in the liver and erythrocytes to the active metabolite trichloroethanol, which may be further metabolized to inactive metabolites. It is also metabolized directly to inactive metabolites by the liver and kidneys.

**Half-life**
The plasma half-life of trichloroethanol, the active metabolite, is about 7 to 10 hours.

**Onset of action**
Oral—Within 30 minutes.

**Duration of action**
About 4 to 8 hours.

**Elimination**
Renal; approximately 40% of dose excreted in 24 hours.

## Precautions to Consider

**Carcinogenicity/Mutagenicity**
Long-term studies in animals have not been done.

**Pregnancy/Reproduction**
Pregnancy—Chloral hydrate crosses the placenta. Studies on teratogenicity have not been done in humans. Chronic use of chloral hydrate during pregnancy may cause withdrawal symptoms in the neonate.
Studies on teratogenicity have not been done in animals.
FDA Pregnancy Category C.

**Breast-feeding**
Chloral hydrate is distributed into breast milk; use by nursing mothers may cause sedation in the infant.

**Pediatrics**
Appropriate studies on the relationship of age to the effects of chloral hydrate have not been performed in the pediatric population. *Deaths have occurred prior to or following diagnostic or therapeutic procedures, particularly in pediatric patients, after chloral hydrate was administered to induce sedation before the procedure.* The current Guidelines for Monitoring and Management of Pediatric Patients During and After Sedation For Diagnostic and Therapeutic Procedures established by the American Academy of Pediatrics recommend that *sedatives be administered only at the health care facility,* where appropriate monitoring can be instituted. Monitoring must continue until the child's level of consciousness has returned to a state that meets appropriate approved discharge criteria. In addition, particular care must be taken in calculating and administering the proper dose appropriate to the age and weight of pediatric patients. Also, children with sleep apnea, especially obstructive sleep apnea with tonsillar hypertrophy, are particularly prone to respiratory compromise.
Chloral hydrate is not recommended for use in infants and children when repetitive dosing would be necessary. With repeated dosing, accumulation of the trichloroethanol and trichloroacetic acid metabolites may increase the potential for excessive CNS depression, predispose neonates to conjugated and nonconjugated hyperbilirubinemia, decrease albumin binding of bilirubin, and contribute to metabolic acidosis.

**Geriatrics**
No information is available on the relationship of age to the effects of chloral hydrate in geriatric patients. However, elderly patients are more likely to have age-related hepatic function impairment and renal function impairment, which may require reduction of dosage in patients receiving chloral hydrate.

**Drug interactions and/or related problems**
The following drug interactions and/or related problems have been selected on the basis of their potential clinical significance (possible mechanism in parentheses where appropriate)—not necessarily inclusive (» = major clinical significance):

Note: Combinations containing any of the following medications, depending on the amount present, may also interact with this medication.

Addictive medications, other, especially CNS depressants with habituating potential
(prolonged concurrent use may increase the risk of habituation; caution is recommended)

» Alcohol or
» CNS depression–producing medications, other (See *Appendix II*)
(concurrent use may increase the CNS depressant effects of either these medications or chloral hydrate; caution is recommended and dosage of one or both agents should be reduced)
» Anticoagulants, coumarin- or indandione-derivative
(hypoprothrombinemic effects may be increased when these medications are used concurrently with chloral hydrate, particularly during the first 2 weeks of concurrent therapy, because of displacement of the anticoagulant from its plasma protein binding sites; with continued concurrent use, anticoagulant activity may return to baseline level or be decreased; frequent prothrombin-time determinations may be required, especially during initiation of chloral hydrate therapy, to determine if dosage adjustment of the anticoagulant is necessary)

Furosemide, intravenous
(administration of chloral hydrate followed by intravenous furosemide within 24 hours may result in diaphoresis, hot flashes, and variable blood pressure, including hypertension, due to a hypermetabolic state caused by displacement of thyroxine from its bound state)

**Laboratory value alterations**
The following have been selected on the basis of their potential clinical significance (possible effect in parentheses where appropriate)—not necessarily inclusive (» = major clinical significance):

With diagnostic test results
Fluorometric tests for urine catecholamines
(it is recommended that chloral hydrate not be administered for 48 hours preceding the test)

Glucose, urine
(determinations may give false-positive test results with Benedict's solution, and possibly with cupric sulfate tablets, but not with glucose enzymatic tests)

Phentolamine test
(chloral hydrate may cause false-positive phentolamine test; it is recommended that all medications be withdrawn at least 24 hours, preferably 48 to 72 hours, prior to a phentolamine test)

Urinary 17-hydroxycorticosteroid determinations
(when using the Reddy, Jenkins, and Thorn procedure)

**Medical considerations/Contraindications**
The medical considerations/contraindications included here have been selected on the basis of their potential clinical significance (reasons given in parentheses where appropriate)—not necessarily inclusive (» = major clinical significance).

*Risk-benefit should be considered when the following medical problems exist:*
Cardiac disease, severe
(condition may be exacerbated by large doses of chloral hydrate)

Alcohol abuse or dependence, history of or
Drug abuse or dependence, history of
(dependence on chloral hydrate may develop)

» Esophagitis or
» Gastritis or
» Ulcers, gastric or duodenal
(condition may be exacerbated—for oral dosage forms only)

» Hepatic function impairment, severe
(chloral hydrate metabolized in liver)

Porphyria, intermittent
(acute attacks may be precipitated by chloral hydrate)

Proctitis or colitis
(condition may be exacerbated—for rectal dosage forms only)

» Renal function impairment, severe
(chloral hydrate excreted via kidneys)

» Sleep apnea in pediatric patients (especially with tonsillar hypertrophy)
(increased risk of respiratory compromise)

Sensitivity to chloral hydrate

## Side/Adverse Effects

The following side/adverse effects have been selected on the basis of their potential clinical significance (possible signs and symptoms in parentheses where appropriate)—not necessarily inclusive:

**Those indicating need for medical attention**
Incidence less frequent
*Allergic reaction* (skin rash or hives)

Incidence rare
   *Confusion; paradoxical reaction* (hallucinations; unusual excitement)
**Those indicating need for medical attention only if they continue or are bothersome**
Incidence more frequent
   *Nausea; stomach pain; vomiting*
Incidence less frequent
   *Clumsiness or unsteadiness; diarrhea; dizziness or lightheadedness; drowsiness; "hangover" effect*
**Those indicating possible withdrawal and the need for medical attention if they occur after medication is discontinued**
   *Confusion; hallucinations; nausea or vomiting; nervousness; restlessness; stomach pain; trembling; unusual excitement*

## Overdose

For more information on the management of overdose or unintentional ingestion, **contact a Poison Control Center** (see *Poison Control Center Listing*).

**Clinical effects of overdose**
The following have been selected on the basis of their potential clinical significance (possible signs and symptoms in parentheses where appropriate)—not necessarily inclusive:
   *Confusion, continuing; convulsions; difficulty in swallowing; drowsiness, severe; low body temperature; nausea, vomiting, or stomach pain, severe; shortness of breath or troubled breathing; slow or irregular heartbeat; slurred speech; staggering; weakness, severe*
   Note: Hepatic and renal function may be impaired, resulting in transient jaundice and albuminuria during recovery from chloral hydrate overdose.

**Treatment of overdose**
Treatment of chloral hydrate overdose consists of the following:
To decrease absorption—
   Gastric lavage following oral overdose (endotracheal tube with inflated cuff should be in place to prevent aspiration of vomitus).
To enhance elimination—
   Hemodialysis may be effective in promoting the clearance of trichloroethanol.
Monitoring—
   Continuous cardiac monitoring is important, especially in patients with predisposing cardiac disease.
Supportive care—
   Support of respiration and circulation.
   Maintenance of normal body temperature.
   Artificial respiration with oxygen may be required.
   Appropriate fluid and electrolyte therapy should be administered and an adequate urinary output maintained.
   Patients in whom intentional overdose is known or suspected should be referred for psychiatric consultation.

## Patient Consultation

As an aid to patient consultation, refer to *Advice for the Patient, Chloral Hydrate (Systemic)*.

In providing consultation, consider emphasizing the following selected information (» = major clinical significance):

**Before using this medication**
» Conditions affecting use, especially:
   Sensitivity to chloral hydrate
   Pregnancy—Chloral hydrate crosses placenta; chronic use during pregnancy may cause withdrawal symptoms in neonate
   Breast-feeding—Chloral hydrate is distributed into breast milk; use by nursing mothers may cause sedation in the infant
   Other medications, especially alcohol or other CNS depression–producing medications or coumarin- or indandione-derivative anticoagulants
   Other medical problems, especially esophagitis, gastritis, gastric or duodenal ulcers, hepatic function impairment, renal function impairment, or sleep apnea in children, especially with tonsillar hypertrophy

**Proper use of this medication**
» Importance of not using more medication than the amount prescribed because of habit-forming potential
*Proper administration*
For capsule dosage form
   Swallowing capsule whole; not chewing because of unpleasant taste
   Taking with a full glass (240 mL) of water, fruit juice, or ginger ale to reduce gastric irritation

For syrup dosage form
   Taking each dose mixed with clear liquid (e.g., water, apple juice, ginger ale) to improve flavor and reduce gastric irritation
For suppository dosage form
   Proper administration technique
   Chilling in refrigerator for 30 minutes or running cold water over suppository before removing foil wrapper if too soft for insertion
» Proper dosing
   Missed dose: Not taking missed dose; not doubling doses
» Proper storage

**Precautions while using this medication**
   Regular visits to physician to check progress during prolonged therapy
   Checking with physician before discontinuing medication after prolonged use; gradual dosage reduction may be necessary to avoid the possibility of withdrawal symptoms
» Avoiding use of alcohol or other CNS depressants
» Suspected overdose: Getting emergency help at once
» Caution if dizziness, lightheadedness, or drowsiness occurs

**Side/adverse effects**
   Signs of potential side effects, especially allergic reaction, confusion, and paradoxical reaction

## General Dosing Information

*Deaths have occurred prior to or following diagnostic or therapeutic procedures, particularly in pediatric patients, after chloral hydrate was administered to induce sedation before the procedure*. The current Guidelines for Monitoring and Management of Pediatric Patients During and After Sedation For Diagnostic and Therapeutic Procedures established by the American Academy of Pediatrics recommend that *sedatives be administered only at the health care facility,* where appropriate monitoring can be instituted. Monitoring must continue until the child's level of consciousness has returned to a state that meets appropriate approved discharge criteria. In addition, particular care must be taken in calculating and administering the proper dose appropriate to the age and weight of pediatric patients.

Use of chloral hydrate in infants and children is not recommended when repetitive dosing would be necessary.

Children with sleep apnea, especially obstructive sleep apnea with tonsillar hypertrophy, are particularly prone to respiratory compromise.

Tolerance may develop by the second week of continual administration.

Prolonged use of larger than usual therapeutic doses may result in psychic or physical dependence.

Following prolonged administration, chloral hydrate should be withdrawn gradually in order to avoid the possibility of precipitating withdrawal symptoms.

**For oral dosage forms only**
Chloral hydrate capsules should be administered with a full glass (240 mL) of water, fruit juice, or ginger ale to reduce gastric irritation.

Each dose of chloral hydrate syrup should be diluted in clear liquid (e.g., water, apple juice, ginger ale) to improve flavor and reduce gastric irritation.

In patients with gastritis, oral chloral hydrate preparations may be dissolved in olive oil or cottonseed oil and administered rectally.

## Oral Dosage Forms

### CHLORAL HYDRATE CAPSULES USP

**Usual adult dose**
Sedative-hypnotic—
   Hypnotic:
      Oral, 500 mg to 1 gram fifteen to thirty minutes before bedtime.
   Sedative:
      Daytime—Oral, 250 mg three times a day after meals.
      Preoperative—Oral, 500 mg to 1 gram thirty minutes before surgery.

**Usual adult prescribing limits**
Up to 2 grams daily.

**Usual pediatric dose**
Sedative-hypnotic—
   Premedication prior to dental or medical procedures: Oral, 50 mg per kg of body weight, up to a maximum of 1 gram per single dose. Doses of 25 to 100 mg per kg of body weight may be used in individual patients. The total dose should not exceed 100 mg per kg of body weight or 2 grams.
   Premedication prior to electroencephalographic evaluation: Oral, 25 mg per kg of body weight.

Note: *Deaths have occurred prior to or following diagnostic or therapeutic procedures, particularly in pediatric patients, after chloral hydrate was administered to induce sedation before the procedure.* The current Guidelines for Monitoring and Management of Pediatric Patients During and After Sedation For Diagnostic and Therapeutic Procedures established by the American Academy of Pediatrics recommend that *sedatives be administered only at the health care facility,* where appropriate monitoring can be instituted. Monitoring must continue until the child has returned to the presedation level of consciousness or meets appropriate approved discharge criteria. In addition, particular care must be taken in calculating and administering the proper dose appropriate to the age and weight of pediatric patients.

### Strength(s) usually available
U.S.—

250 mg (Rx) [GENERIC].
500 mg (Rx) [GENERIC].

Canada—

500 mg (Rx) [*Novo-Chlorhydrate*].

### Packaging and storage
Store between 15 and 30 °C (59 and 86 °F), in a tight container.

### Stability
Clarity of the capsules may vary without affecting the potency.

### Auxiliary labeling
• Swallow capsules whole.
• Avoid alcoholic beverages.
• May cause drowsiness.
• Keep container tightly closed.

### Note
Controlled substance in the U.S.

## CHLORAL HYDRATE SYRUP USP

### Usual adult dose
See *Chloral Hydrate Capsules USP.*

### Usual adult prescribing limits
See *Chloral Hydrate Capsules USP.*

### Usual pediatric dose
See *Chloral Hydrate Capsules USP.*

### Strength(s) usually available
U.S.—

250 mg per 5 mL (Rx) [GENERIC].
500 mg per 5 mL (Rx) [GENERIC].

Canada—

500 mg per 5 mL (Rx) [*PMS-Chloral Hydrate;* GENERIC].

### Packaging and storage
Store below 40 °C (104 °F), preferably between 15 and 30 °C (59 and 86 °F), unless otherwise specified by manufacturer. Store in a tight, light-resistant container. Protect from freezing.

### Auxiliary labeling
• Avoid alcoholic beverages.
• May cause drowsiness.

### Note
Controlled substance in the U.S.

## Rectal Dosage Forms
## CHLORAL HYDRATE SUPPOSITORIES

### Usual adult dose
Sedative-hypnotic—
Hypnotic: Rectal, 500 mg to 1 gram as a single dose at bedtime.
Sedative: Rectal, 325 mg three times a day.

### Usual adult prescribing limits
Up to 2 grams daily.

### Usual pediatric dose
Sedative-hypnotic—
Premedication prior to dental or medical procedures: Rectal, 50 mg per kg of body weight, up to a maximum of 1 gram per single dose. Doses of 25 to 100 mg per kg of body weight may be used in individual patients. The total dose should not exceed 100 mg per kg of body weight or 2 grams.
Premedication prior to electroencephalographic evaluation: Rectal, 25 mg per kg of body weight.

Note: *Deaths have occurred prior to or following diagnostic or therapeutic procedures, particularly in pediatric patients, after chloral hydrate was administered to induce sedation before the procedure.* The current Guidelines for Monitoring and Management of Pediatric Patients During and After Sedation For Diagnostic and Therapeutic Procedures established by the American Academy of Pediatrics recommend that *sedatives be administered only at the health care facility,* where appropriate monitoring can be instituted. Monitoring must continue until the child has returned to the presedation level of consciousness or meets appropriate approved discharge criteria. In addition, particular care must be taken in calculating and administering the proper dose appropriate to the age and weight of pediatric patients.

### Strength(s) usually available
U.S.—

325 mg (Rx) [*Aquachloral Supprettes* (tartrazine)].
500 mg (Rx) [GENERIC].
650 mg (Rx) [*Aquachloral Supprettes* (tartrazine)].

Canada—

Not commercially available.

### Packaging and storage
Store below 40 °C (104 °F), preferably between 15 and 30 °C (59 and 86 °F), in a well-closed container, unless otherwise specified by manufacturer.

### Auxiliary labeling
• For rectal use only.
• Avoid alcoholic beverages.
• May cause drowsiness.

### Note
Controlled substance in the U.S.

Revised: 08/02/94
Interim revision: 03/31/95

# CHLORAMBUCIL  Systemic

VA CLASSIFICATION (Primary/Secondary): AN100/IM600
Note: For a listing of dosage forms and brand names by country availability, see *Dosage Forms* section(s). For a listing of brand names for the articles in this monograph, refer to the General Index.

## Category
Antineoplastic; immunosuppressant.

## Indications
Note: Bracketed information in the *Indications* section refers to uses that are not included in U.S. product labeling.

### Accepted
Leukemia, chronic lymphocytic (treatment)—Chlorambucil is indicated for palliative treatment of chronic lymphocytic leukemia.

Lymphomas, Hodgkin's (treatment) or
Lymphomas, non-Hodgkin's (treatment)—Chlorambucil is indicated for palliative treatment of Hodgkin's disease and other malignant lymphomas including lymphosarcoma and giant follicular lymphoma.

[Carcinoma, ovarian (treatment)][1] or
[Carcinoma, testicular (treatment)][1]—Chlorambucil is used for treatment of ovarian and testicular carcinoma.

[Leukemia, hairy cell (treatment)][1]—Chlorambucil is used in the treatment of hairy cell leukemia.

[Polycythemia vera (treatment)][1]—Chlorambucil is used for treatment of polycythemia vera.

[Nephrotic syndrome (treatment)][1]—Chlorambucil has been used as an immunosuppressant, in combination with prednisone, in the treatment of steroid-resistant or frequently relapsing steroid-sensitive minimal-change nephrotic syndrome in children and adults, although there are significant risks associated with its use. The most common dose-limiting short-term toxicity is bone marrow depression. Because of potential long-term toxicity (male sterility, leukemia), use of chlorambucil is recommended only for patients unresponsive to or seriously intolerant of steroid treatment.

**Extreme caution is recommended in use of chlorambucil for non-neoplastic conditions because of potential carcinogenicity with long-term use of this agent.**

---

[1]Not included in Canadian product labeling.

## Pharmacology/Pharmacokinetics

### Physicochemical characteristics
Molecular weight—304.22.
pKa—1.3 and 5.8.

### Mechanism of action/Effect
Chlorambucil is a bifunctional alkylating agent of the nitrogen mustard type. Chlorambucil is cell cycle–phase nonspecific, although it is also cytotoxic to nonproliferating cells. Activity occurs as a result of formation of an unstable ethylenimmonium ion, which alkylates or binds with many intracellular molecular structures, including nucleic acids. Its cytotoxic action is primarily due to cross-linking of strands of DNA and RNA, as well as inhibition of protein synthesis.

### Other actions/effects
Also has immunosuppressant activity.

### Absorption
Rapidly and completely absorbed from the gastrointestinal tract.

### Protein binding
Very high (99%).

### Biotransformation
Hepatic, extensive and rapid. The primary metabolite, phenylacetic acid mustard (an aminophenyl acetic acid derivative), is active. Also undergoes spontaneous degradation.

### Half-life
Chlorambucil—Approximately 1.5 hours.
Aminophenyl acetic acid derivative metabolite—2.5 hours.

### Onset of action
Clinical effects usually occur within 3 to 4 weeks.

### Time to peak plasma concentration
1 hour.

### Elimination
Renal, less than 1% as chlorambucil or phenylacetic acid mustard.
In dialysis—Not dialyzable.

## Precautions to Consider

### Cross-sensitivity and/or related problems
Patients sensitive to other alkylating agents (i.e., those who experience skin rash) may also be sensitive to chlorambucil.

### Carcinogenicity
Secondary malignancies are potential delayed effects of many antineoplastic agents, although it is not clear whether the effect is related to their mutagenic or immunosuppressive action. The effect of dose and duration of therapy is also unknown, although risk seems to increase with long-term use. Although information is limited, available data seem to indicate that the carcinogenic risk is greatest with the alkylating agents.

Chlorambucil has been shown to be carcinogenic in mice. There are many reports of acute leukemia occurring in patients treated with chlorambucil for both malignant and nonmalignant diseases, often in combination with radiation or other chemotherapy. Risk appears to be related to cumulative dose and duration of therapy, but a threshold cumulative dose has not been defined.

### Mutagenicity
Chlorambucil has been shown to cause chromatid or chromosome damage in humans.

### Pregnancy/Reproduction
Fertility—Gonadal suppression, resulting in amenorrhea or azoospermia, may occur in patients taking antineoplastic therapy, especially with the alkylating agents. In general, these effects appear to be related to dose and length of therapy and may be irreversible. Prediction of the degree of testicular or ovarian function impairment is complicated by the common use of combinations of several antineoplastics, which makes it difficult to assess the effects of individual agents.

However, there have been numerous reports of prolonged or permanent azoospermia and permanent sterility with long-term use of chlorambucil, especially in prepubertal and pubertal males. Amenorrhea has

been reported in pubertal and adult females; autopsy studies of ovaries from women treated with combination therapy including chlorambucil have shown varying degrees of fibrosis, vasculitis, and depletion of primordial follicles.

Pregnancy—Adequate and well-controlled studies in humans have not been done. Although several successful pregnancies have been reported with chlorambucil use, two cases of an infant with an absent kidney and ureter have also been reported.

First trimester: It is usually recommended that use of antineoplastics, especially combination chemotherapy, be avoided whenever possible, especially during the first trimester. Although information is limited because of the relatively few instances of antineoplastic administration during pregnancy, the mutagenic, teratogenic, and carcinogenic potential of these medications must be considered.

Other hazards to the fetus include adverse reactions seen in adults.

In general, use of a contraceptive is recommended during cytotoxic drug therapy.

In rats, urogenital malformations including absence of a kidney have been reported.

FDA Pregnancy Category D.

### Breast-feeding
Although very little information is available regarding distribution of antineoplastic agents into breast milk, breast-feeding is not recommended during chemotherapy because of the risks to the infant (adverse effects, mutagenicity, carcinogenicity). It is not known whether chlorambucil is distributed into breast milk.

### Pediatrics
Appropriate studies performed to date generally have not demonstrated pediatrics-specific problems that would limit the usefulness of chlorambucil in children. However, children taking chlorambucil for nephrotic syndrome are reported to have an increased risk of seizures.

### Geriatrics
No information is available on the relationship of age to the effects of chlorambucil in geriatric patients.

### Dental
The bone marrow depressant effects of chlorambucil may result in an increased incidence of microbial infection, delayed healing, and gingival bleeding. Dental work, whenever possible, should be completed prior to initiation of therapy or deferred until blood counts have returned to normal. Patients should be instructed in proper oral hygiene during treatment, including caution in use of regular toothbrushes, dental floss, and toothpicks.

Chlorambucil may also cause stomatitis associated with considerable discomfort.

### Drug interactions and/or related problems
The following drug interactions and/or related problems have been selected on the basis of their potential clinical significance (possible mechanism in parentheses where appropriate)—not necessarily inclusive (» = major clinical significance):

Note: Combinations containing any of the following medications, depending on the amount present, may also interact with this medication.

Allopurinol or
Colchicine or
» Probenecid or
» Sulfinpyrazone
    (chlorambucil may raise the concentration of blood uric acid; dosage adjustment of antigout agents may be necessary to control hyperuricemia and gout; allopurinol may be preferred to prevent or reverse chlorambucil-induced hyperuricemia because of risk of uric acid nephropathy with uricosuric antigout agents)

Antidepressants, tricyclic and possibly, structurally related compounds such as cyclobenzaprine or
Haloperidol or
Loxapine or
Maprotiline or
Molindone or
Monoamine oxidase (MAO) inhibitors, including furazolidone, procarbazine, and selegiline or
Phenothiazines or
Pimozide or
Thioxanthenes
    (these medications may lower the seizure threshold and increase the risk of chlorambucil-induced seizures)

Blood dyscrasia–causing medications (See *Appendix II*)
    (leukopenic and/or thrombocytopenic effects of chlorambucil may be increased with concurrent or recent therapy if these medications

cause the same effects; dosage adjustment of chlorambucil, if necessary, should be based on blood counts)

» Bone marrow depressants, other (See *Appendix II*) or
» Radiation therapy
   (additive bone marrow depression may occur; dosage reduction may be required when two or more bone marrow depressants, including radiation, are used concurrently or consecutively)

» Immunosuppressants, other, such as:
   Azathioprine
   Corticosteroids, glucocorticoid
   Corticotropin (ACTH)
   Cyclophosphamide
   Cyclosporine
   Cytarabine
   Mercaptopurine
   Muromonab-CD3
   Tacrolimus
   (concurrent use with chlorambucil may increase the risk of infection and development of neoplasms)

   Lovastatin
   (concurrent use in cardiac transplant patients may be associated with an increased risk of rhabdomyolysis and acute renal failure)

   Vaccines, killed virus
   (because normal defense mechanisms may be suppressed by chlorambucil therapy, the patient's antibody response to the vaccine may be decreased. The interval between discontinuation of medications that cause immunosuppression and restoration of the patient's ability to respond to the vaccine depends on the intensity and type of immunosuppression-causing medication used, the underlying disease, and other factors; estimates vary from 3 months to 1 year)

» Vaccines, live virus
   (because normal defense mechanisms may be suppressed by chlorambucil therapy, concurrent use with a live virus vaccine may potentiate the replication of the vaccine virus, may increase the side/adverse effects of the vaccine virus, and/or may decrease the patient's antibody response to the vaccine; immunization of these patients should be undertaken only with extreme caution after careful review of the patient's hematologic status and only with the knowledge and consent of the physician managing the chlorambucil therapy. The interval between discontinuation of medications that cause immunosuppression and restoration of the patient's ability to respond to the vaccine depends on the intensity and type of immunosuppression-causing medication used, the underlying disease, and other factors; estimates vary from 3 months to 1 year. Patients with leukemia in remission should not receive live virus vaccine until at least 3 months after their last chemotherapy. In addition, immunization with oral poliovirus vaccine should be postponed in persons in close contact with the patient, especially family members)

**Laboratory value alterations**
The following have been selected on the basis of their potential clinical significance (possible effect in parentheses where appropriate)—not necessarily inclusive (» = major clinical significance):

With physiology/laboratory test values
   Alkaline phosphatase and
   Aspartate aminotransferase (AST [SGOT])
      (serum values may rarely be increased, indicating hepatotoxicity)
   Uric acid
      (concentrations in blood and urine may be increased)

**Medical considerations/Contraindications**
The medical considerations/contraindications included here have been selected on the basis of their potential clinical significance (reasons given in parentheses where appropriate)—not necessarily inclusive (» = major clinical significance).

***Risk-benefit should be considered when the following medical problems exist:***
» Bone marrow depression
» Chickenpox, existing or recent (including recent exposure) or
» Herpes zoster
   (risk of severe generalized disease)
   Gout, history of or
   Urate renal stones, history of
      (risk of hyperuricemia)
   Head trauma or
   Seizure disorder, history of
      (increased risk of seizures)
» Infection

Sensitivity to chlorambucil
» Tumor cell infiltration of bone marrow
» Caution should be used also in patients who have had previous cytotoxic drug therapy or radiation therapy.

**Patient monitoring**
The following are especially important in patient monitoring (other tests may be warranted in some patients, depending on condition; » = major clinical significance):

Alanine aminotransferase (ALT [SGPT]) values, serum and
Alkaline phosphatase values, serum and
Aspartate aminotransferase (AST [SGOT]) values, serum and
Lactate dehydrogenase (LDH) values, serum
   (recommended prior to initiation of therapy and at frequent intervals during therapy; frequency varies according to clinical state, agent, dose, and other agents being used concurrently)

» Hematocrit or hemoglobin and
» Leukocyte count, total and, if appropriate, differential and
» Platelet count
   (determinations recommended prior to initiation of therapy and at periodic intervals during therapy; frequency varies according to clinical state, agent, dose, and other agents being used concurrently)

Uric acid concentrations, serum
   (recommended prior to initiation of therapy and at periodic intervals during therapy; frequency varies according to clinical state, agent, dose, and other agents being used concurrently)

## Side/Adverse Effects

Note: Many "side effects" of antineoplastic therapy are unavoidable and represent the medication's pharmacologic action. Some of these (for example, leukopenia and thrombocytopenia) are actually used as parameters to aid in individual dosage titration.

The following side/adverse effects have been selected on the basis of their potential clinical significance (possible signs and symptoms in parentheses where appropriate)—not necessarily inclusive:

**Those indicating need for medical attention**
Incidence more frequent—dose-related
   *Lymphopenia, leukopenia, neutropenia, immunosuppression, or infection* (usually asymptomatic; less frequently, fever or chills; cough or hoarseness; lower back or side pain; painful or difficult urination); *thrombocytopenia* (usually asymptomatic; less frequently, unusual bleeding or bruising; black, tarry stools; blood in urine or stools; pinpoint red spots on skin)
   Note: With a short course of therapy, *leukopenia* and *thrombocytopenia* may not occur until the third week of treatment and usually persist for 1 to 2 weeks (or sometimes up to 3 to 4 weeks) after withdrawal of chlorambucil. The neutrophil count may continue to decrease for up to 10 days after the last dose. After a single high dose of chlorambucil, the nadir of the leukocyte and platelet counts occurs after 7 to 14 days, with recovery in 2 to 3 weeks.

   In general, short intermittent courses are thought to cause less risk of serious *bone marrow depression* than continuous therapy, by allowing bone marrow regeneration between courses. Excessive doses or prolonged therapy (a total dose of 6.5 mg per kg of body weight [mg/kg] in a single course) may result in pancytopenia and irreversible bone marrow damage.

Incidence less frequent
   *Allergic reaction* (skin rash); *hyperuricemia or uric acid nephropathy* (joint pain; lower back or side pain; swelling of feet or lower legs); *stomatitis* (sores in mouth and on lips)
   Note: *Skin rash* has been reported to progress rarely to erythema multiforme, toxic epidermal necrolysis, and Stevens-Johnson syndrome.

   *Hyperuricemia or uric acid nephropathy* occurs most commonly during initial treatment of patients with leukemia or lymphoma, as a result of rapid cell breakdown which leads to elevated serum uric acid concentrations.

   *Stomatitis* may be associated with neutropenia.

Incidence rare
   *Drug fever; hepatotoxicity, hepatic necrosis, or cirrhosis* (yellow eyes or skin); *neurotoxicity* (agitation; confusion; hallucinations; muscle twitching; seizures; severe weakness or paralysis; tremors; trouble in walking); *pulmonary fibrosis* (cough; shortness of breath)—occurs after long-term use; *skin reactions, severe, including erythema multiforme, epidermal necrolysis, and Stevens-Johnson syndrome* (blisters

on skin; severe skin rash; sores in mouth; fever may also be associated with Stevens-Johnson syndrome)

Note: Rare, focal and/or generalized seizures have been reported in both children and adults at therapeutic daily doses, and in pulse dosing regimens and acute overdose. However, the risk may be increased in children with nephrotic syndrome (seizures may occur 6 to 90 days after initiation of treatment) and in patients receiving high pulse doses. *Neurotoxicity* is usually reversible on withdrawal of chlorambucil.

*Pulmonary fibrosis* is usually reversible after chlorambucil is withdrawn, but fatalities have been reported.

**Those indicating need for medical attention only if they continue or are bothersome**

Incidence less frequent or rare

*Changes in menstrual period; dermatitis* (itching of skin); *nausea and vomiting*

Note: *Nausea and vomiting* are associated with single oral doses of 20 mg or more, usually last less than 24 hours, and become less frequent with continued therapy; may persist up to 7 days after a single high dose.

**Those indicating need for medical attention if they occur after medication is discontinued**

*Bone marrow damage, possibly irreversible* (fever or chills; cough or hoarseness; lower back or side pain; painful or difficult urination; unusual bleeding or bruising; black, tarry stools; blood in urine or stools; pinpoint red spots on skin); *pulmonary toxicity* (cough; shortness of breath)

## Overdose

For more information on the management of overdose or unintentional ingestion, **contact a Poison Control Center** (see *Poison Control Center Listing*).

**Clinical effects of overdose**

The following effects have been selected on the basis of their potential clinical significance (possible signs and symptoms in parentheses where appropriate)—not necessarily inclusive:

Symptoms of overdose, in order of frequency

*Pancytopenia, reversible* (fever or chills; cough or hoarseness; lower back or side pain; painful or difficult urination; unusual bleeding or bruising; black, tarry stools; blood in urine or stools; pinpoint red spots on skin); *neurotoxicity, including ataxia, agitation, and seizures* (agitation; seizures; trouble in walking)

**Treatment of overdose**

Recommended treatment consists of the following:
- Immediate evacuation of the stomach, followed by
- Supportive, symptomatic treatment and
- Monitoring of blood counts at least 3 times a week for at least 3 weeks or until bone marrow function has recovered.

## Patient Consultation

As an aid to patient consultation, refer to *Advice for the Patient, Chlorambucil (Systemic)*.

In providing consultation, consider emphasizing the following selected information (» = major clinical significance):

**Before using this medication**
» Conditions affecting use, especially:
  Sensitivity to chlorambucil or other alkylating agents
  Pregnancy—Use not recommended because of mutagenic, teratogenic, and carcinogenic potential; advisability of using contraception; telling physician immediately if pregnancy is suspected
  Breast-feeding—Not recommended because of risk of serious side effects
  Other medications, especially probenecid, sulfinpyrazone, other bone marrow depressants, other immunosuppressants, or previous cytotoxic drug or radiation therapy
  Other medical problems, especially chickenpox, herpes zoster, or infection

**Proper use of this medication**
» Importance of not taking more or less medication than the amount prescribed
  Caution in taking combination therapy; taking each medication at the right time
  Importance of ample fluid intake and subsequent increase in urine output to aid in excretion of uric acid
» Possible nausea and vomiting; importance of continuing medication despite stomach upset

Checking with physician if vomiting occurs shortly after dose is taken
» Proper dosing
  Missed dose: If dosing schedule is—
    Once a day: Taking as soon as possible if remembered same day; if not remembered until next day, skipping missed dose and taking next regularly scheduled dose
    Several times a day: Taking as soon as possible; however, if almost time for next dose, not taking missed dose; not doubling doses
» Proper storage

**Precautions while using this medication**
» Importance of close monitoring by the physician
» Avoiding immunizations unless approved by physician; other persons in patient's household should avoid immunizations with oral poliovirus vaccine; avoiding persons who have taken oral poliovirus vaccine or wearing a protective mask that covers nose and mouth

*Caution if bone marrow depression occurs:*
» Avoiding exposure to persons with bacterial infections, especially during periods of low blood counts; checking with physician immediately if fever or chills, cough or hoarseness, lower back or side pain, or painful or difficult urination occur
» Checking with physician immediately if unusual bleeding or bruising; black, tarry stools; blood in urine or stools; or pinpoint red spots on skin occur
  Caution in use of regular toothbrush, dental floss, or toothpick; physician, dentist, or nurse may suggest alternatives; checking with physician before having dental work done
  Not touching eyes or inside of nose unless hands washed immediately before
  Using caution to avoid accidental cuts with use of sharp objects such as safety razor or fingernail or toenail cutters
  Avoiding contact sports or other situations where bruising or injury might occur

**Side/adverse effects**
  May cause adverse effects such as blood problems and cancer
  Signs of potential side effects, especially lymphopenia, leukopenia, neutropenia, immunosuppression, infection, thrombocytopenia, allergic reaction, hyperuricemia, uric acid nephropathy, stomatitis, drug fever, hepatotoxicity, hepatic necrosis, cirrhosis, neurotoxicity, pulmonary fibrosis, and severe skin reactions
  Physician or nurse can help in dealing with side effects

## General Dosing Information

Patients receiving chlorambucil should be under supervision of a physician experienced in use of alkylating agents.

A variety of dosage schedules and regimens of chlorambucil, alone or in combination with other antitumor agents, are used. The prescriber may consult the medical literature as well as the manufacturer's literature in choosing a specific dosage.

Dosage must be adjusted to meet the individual requirements of each patient, based on clinical response and degree of bone marrow depression.

Development of uric acid nephropathy in patients with leukemia or lymphoma may be prevented by adequate oral hydration and, in some cases, administration of allopurinol. Alkalinization of urine may be necessary if serum uric acid concentrations are elevated.

It is recommended that chlorambucil be withdrawn if signs of pulmonary toxicity or a severe skin reaction occurs.

Because of the risk of enhanced bone marrow toxicity, use of chlorambucil is not recommended within 4 to 6 weeks of radiation therapy or chemotherapy with drugs that depress bone marrow function.

Because the decrease in neutrophil count may continue for 10 days after the last dose of chlorambucil, caution is necessary as the total dose approaches 65 mg per kg of body weight (mg/kg) because of the risk of pancytopenia.

If the white blood cell count (particularly granulocyte count) falls suddenly, a reduction in dosage or withdrawal of therapy plus continued monitoring is required until leukocyte and platelet levels become adequate. Persistence of low neutrophil and platelet counts or presence of peripheral lymphocytosis may indicate bone marrow infiltration; if that is confirmed by bone marrow examination, the daily dosage of chlorambucil should not exceed 100 mcg (0.1 mg) per kg of body weight.

Special precautions are recommended in patients who develop thrombocytopenia as a result of administration of chlorambucil. These may include extreme care in performing invasive procedures; regular inspection of intravenous sites, skin (including perirectal area), and mucous membrane surfaces for signs of bleeding or bruising; limiting frequency of venipuncture and avoiding intramuscular injections; testing urine, emesis, stool, and secretions for occult blood; care in use of regular toothbrushes, dental floss, toothpicks, safety razors, and fingernail and toenail cutters; avoiding constipation; and using caution to prevent falls and other injuries. Such patients should avoid alcohol and aspirin intake because of the risk of gastrointestinal bleeding. Platelet transfusions may be required.

Patients who develop leukopenia should be observed carefully for signs of infection. Antibiotic support may be required. In neutropenic patients who develop fever, broad-spectrum antibiotic coverage should be initiated empirically, pending bacterial cultures and appropriate diagnostic tests.

### Combination chemotherapy

Although chlorambucil is usually used alone, it may be used in combination with other agents in various regimens. As a result, incidence and/or severity of side effects may be altered and different dosages (usually reduced) may be used. For example, chlorambucil is part of the following chemotherapeutic combination (a commonly used acronym is in parentheses):

—chlorambucil and prednisone (CHL + PRED).

For specific dosages and schedules, consult the literature. For information regarding each agent, consult the individual monographs.

## Oral Dosage Forms

Note: Bracketed uses in the *Dosage Forms* section refer to categories of use and/or indications that are not included in U.S. product labeling.

### CHLORAMBUCIL TABLETS USP

#### Usual adult dose
Leukemia, chronic lymphocytic or
Lymphomas, Hodgkin's or
Lymphomas, non-Hodgkin's—
    Initiation or short course: Oral, 100 to 200 mcg (0.1 to 0.2 mg) per kg of body weight a day or 3 to 6 mg per square meter of body surface, usually 4 to 10 mg, a day, as a single dose or in divided doses.

    Note: An intermittent biweekly course of therapy may produce less hematologic toxicity; an initial dose of 400 mcg (0.4 mg) per kg of body weight or 12 mg per square meter of body surface

is increased by 100 mcg (0.1 mg) per kg or 3 mg per square meter of body surface every two weeks until an effective or toxic dose is reached, then adjusted as necessary.

[Nephrotic syndrome][1]—
    Oral, 100 to 200 mcg (0.1 to 0.2 mg) per kg of body weight per day, in a single dose, for 8 to 12 weeks.

    Note: The maximum recommended cumulative dose is 14 mg per kg of body weight or a maximum duration of treatment of 12 weeks; some clinicians recommend a maximum cumulative dose of 8.2 mg per kg of body weight or a maximum of 6 weeks of treatment.

#### Usual adult prescribing limits
Presence of lymphocytic infiltration of bone marrow or hypoplastic bone marrow—Up to 100 mcg (0.1 mg) per kg of body weight per day.

#### Usual pediatric dose
Leukemia, chronic lymphocytic or
Lymphomas, Hodgkin's or
Lymphomas, non-Hodgkin's—
    Oral, 100 to 200 mcg (0.1 to 0.2 mg) per kg of body weight or 4.5 mg per square meter of body surface a day, as a single dose or in divided daily doses.
[Nephrotic syndrome][1]—
    See *Usual adult dose.*

#### Strength(s) usually available
U.S.—
    2 mg (Rx) [*Leukeran* (lactose; sucrose)].
Canada—
    2 mg (Rx) [*Leukeran*].

#### Packaging and storage
Store below 40 °C (104 °F), preferably between 15 and 30 °C (59 and 86 °F), unless otherwise specified by manufacturer. Store in a well-closed, light-resistant container.

---

[1]Not included in Canadian product labeling.

Revised: 07/15/94

---

# CHLORAMPHENICOL   Ophthalmic

VA CLASSIFICATION (Primary): OP201
Note: For a listing of dosage forms and brand names by country availability, see *Dosage Forms* section(s). For a listing of brand names for the articles in this monograph, refer to the General Index.

## Category
Antibacterial (ophthalmic).

## Indications
Note: Bracketed information in the *Indications* section refers to uses that are not included in U.S. product labeling.

### Accepted
Ocular infections (treatment)—Chloramphenicol is indicated in the topical treatment of superficial ocular infections involving the conjunctiva and/or cornea caused by susceptible organisms, including *Escherichia coli*; *Haemophilus influenzae*; *Klebsiella* species; *Enterobacter (Aerobacter)* species; *Neisseria* species; *Staphylococcus aureus*; streptococci, including *Streptococcus hemolyticus* and *S. pneumoniae (Diplococcus pneumoniae)*; and *Moraxella lacunata* (Morax-Axenfeld bacillus). Chloramphenicol may also be effective against rickettsiae and the mycoplasma (PPLO) group of organisms. In serious ocular infections, topical chloramphenicol should be given concurrently with appropriate systemic antibacterials.

[Blepharitis, bacterial (treatment)]
[Blepharoconjunctivitis (treatment)]
[Conjunctivitis, bacterial (treatment)] or
[Keratitis, bacterial (treatment)]—Chloramphenicol is used in the topical treatment of bacterial blepharitis, blepharoconjunctivitis, bacterial conjunctivitis, and bacterial keratitis.

[Keratitis, exposure (treatment)] or
[Keratitis, neuroparalytic (treatment)]—Chloramphenicol is used in the topical treatment of exposure keratitis and neuroparalytic keratitis when a secondary bacterial infection is present.

[Keratoconjunctivitis, bacterial (treatment)]—Chloramphenicol is used in the topical treatment of bacterial keratoconjunctivitis.

Note: Not all species or strains of a particular organism may be susceptible to chloramphenicol.

    Although rare, bone marrow aplasia, resulting in aplastic anemia and death, has been reported with the use of chloramphenicol ophthalmic preparations. Because of reported systemic toxicity, some USP medical experts recommend that ophthalmic chloramphenicol be reserved for serious ocular infections in which the etiologic organisms are resistant to all other ophthalmic antibiotics or for infections in which less toxic antibiotics are ineffective. However, other USP experts still consider ophthalmic chloramphenicol valuable because of its lipid solubility and excellent corneal penetration, as well as its low ocular toxicity when compared with other antibacterials commonly used in the eye (e.g., neomycin).

### Unaccepted
Chloramphenicol is not effective against *Pseudomonas aeruginosa* or *Serratia marcescens*.

## Pharmacology/Pharmacokinetics

### Physicochemical characteristics
Molecular weight—323.13.

### Mechanism of action/Effect
Bacteriostatic; since chloramphenicol is lipid-soluble, it diffuses through the bacterial cell membrane and reversibly binds to the 50 S subunit of bacterial ribosomes where transfer of amino acids to growing peptide chains is prevented (perhaps by suppression of peptidyl transferase activity), thus inhibiting peptide bond formation and subsequent protein synthesis.
The mechanism for the irreversible aplastic anemia following ophthalmic use of chloramphenicol has not been established.

### Absorption
Intraocular and some systemic absorption occurs following topical application to the eye.

### Distribution

Aqueous humor—Measurable concentrations following topical application to the eye.

## Precautions to Consider

### Pregnancy/Reproduction

Problems in humans have not been documented.

### Breast-feeding

Problems in humans have not been documented.

### Pediatrics

Appropriate studies on the relationship of age to the effects of this medicine have not been performed in the pediatric population. However, no pediatrics-specific problems have been documented to date.

### Geriatrics

Appropriate studies on the relationship of age to the effects of this medicine have not been performed in the geriatric population. However, no geriatrics-specific problems have been documented to date.

### Medical considerations/Contraindications

The medical considerations/contraindications included here have been selected on the basis of their potential clinical significance (reasons given in parentheses where appropriate)—not necessarily inclusive (» = major clinical significance).

*Except under special circumstances, this medication should not be used when the following medical problem exists:*

» Previous allergy or toxic reaction to chloramphenicol

## Side/Adverse Effects

Note: Bone marrow hypoplasia, including aplastic anemia and death, has been reported following local application of chloramphenicol.

The following side/adverse effects have been selected on the basis of their potential clinical significance (possible signs and symptoms in parentheses where appropriate)—not necessarily inclusive:

### Those indicating need for medical attention

Incidence less frequent
*Hypersensitivity* (burning, itching, redness, skin rash, swelling, or other sign of irritation not present before therapy)

Incidence rare
*Blood dyscrasias* (pale skin, sore throat and fever, unusual bleeding or bruising, unusual tiredness or weakness)

### Those indicating need for medical attention only if they continue or are bothersome

Incidence less frequent
*Blurred vision*—for the ointment dosage form; *burning or stinging*

**Those indicating possible irreversible bone marrow depression, possibly leading to aplastic anemia, and the need for immediate medical attention if they occur after medication is discontinued**
*Pale skin; sore throat and fever; unusual bleeding or bruising; unusual tiredness or weakness*

## Patient Consultation

As an aid to patient consultation, refer to *Advice for the Patient, Chloramphenicol (Ophthalmic).*

In providing consultation, consider emphasizing the following selected information (» = major clinical significance):

### Before using this medication

» Conditions affecting use, especially:
   Allergy to chloramphenicol

### Proper use of this medication

Proper administration technique for ophthalmic solution and ointment
» Compliance with full course of therapy
» Proper dosing
   Missed dose: Applying as soon as possible; not applying if almost time for next dose
» Proper storage

### Precautions while using this medication

Checking with physician if no improvement within a few days

### Side/adverse effects

Blurred vision may occur for a few minutes after application of ophthalmic ointments
Signs of potential side effects, especially blood dyscrasias and hypersensitivity reactions

## General Dosing Information

At night the ophthalmic ointment may be used as an adjunct to the ophthalmic solution to provide prolonged contact with the medication.

Although some manufacturers recommend a dose of 2 drops of an ophthalmic solution at appropriate intervals, the conjunctival sac will usually hold only 1 drop.

## Ophthalmic Dosage Forms

### CHLORAMPHENICOL OPHTHALMIC OINTMENT USP

**Usual adult and adolescent dose**
Antibacterial (ophthalmic)—
   Topical, to the conjunctiva, a thin strip (approximately 1 cm) of ointment every three hours or more frequently.

**Usual pediatric dose**
See *Usual adult and adolescent dose.*

**Strength(s) usually available**
U.S.—
   1% (Rx) [*Ak-Chlor Ophthalmic Ointment; Chlorofair Ophthalmic Ointment; Chloromycetin Ophthalmic Ointment; Chloroptic S.O.P.* (chlorobutanol 0.5%); *Econochlor Ophthalmic Ointment; Ocu-Chlor Ophthalmic Ointment; Spectro-Chlor Ophthalmic Ointment;* GENERIC].
Canada—
   1% (Rx) [*Chloromycetin Ophthalmic Ointment; Chloroptic S.O.P.; Fenicol Ophthalmic Ointment; Pentamycetin Ophthalmic Ointment; Sopamycetin Ophthalmic Ointment*].

**Packaging and storage**
Store below 40 °C (104 °F), preferably between 15 and 30 °C (59 and 86 °F), unless otherwise specified by manufacturer. Protect from freezing.

**Auxiliary labeling**
• For the eye.
• Continue medicine for full time of treatment.

### CHLORAMPHENICOL OPHTHALMIC SOLUTION USP

**Usual adult and adolescent dose**
Antibacterial (ophthalmic)—
   Topical, to the conjunctiva, 1 drop every one to four hours.

**Usual pediatric dose**
See *Usual adult and adolescent dose.*

**Strength(s) usually available**
U.S.—
   0.5% (Rx) [*Ak-Chlor Ophthalmic Solution* (chlorobutanol 0.5%); *Chloracol Ophthalmic Solution* (chlorobutanol); *Chlorofair Ophthalmic Solution* (may contain chlorobutanol 0.5%); *Chloroptic Ophthalmic Solution* (chlorobutanol 0.5%); *Econochlor Ophthalmic Solution; I-Chlor Ophthalmic Solution; Ocu-Chlor Ophthalmic Solution; Ophthochlor Ophthalmic Solution; Spectro-Chlor Ophthalmic Solution;* GENERIC].
Canada—
   0.25% (Rx) [*Pentamycetin Ophthalmic Solution* (parabens); *Sopamycetin Ophthalmic Solution* (parabens 0.08%)].
   0.5% (Rx) [*Ak-Chlor Ophthalmic Solution* (chlorobutanol); *Chloroptic Ophthalmic Solution* (phenylmercuric nitrate 0.004%); *Ophtho-Chloram Ophthalmic Solution*].

**Packaging and storage**
Store below 40 °C (104 °F), preferably between 15 and 30 °C (59 and 86 °F), unless otherwise specified by manufacturer. Store in a tight container. Protect from freezing.

Note: Some manufacturers recommend storing between 2 and 8 °C (36 and 46 °F) until the medication is dispensed.

**Stability**
Some manufacturers recommend that the solution be discarded 20 or 21 days after date dispensed.

**Auxiliary labeling**
• For the eye.
• Continue medicine for full time of treatment.
• Beyond-use date.

**Note**
Dispense in original unopened container. Some manufacturers also recommend dispensing in original carton to protect the ophthalmic solution from light.

## CHLORAMPHENICOL FOR OPHTHALMIC SOLUTION USP

### Usual adult and adolescent dose
Antibacterial (ophthalmic)—
Topical, to the conjunctiva, 1 drop every three hours or more frequently.

### Usual pediatric dose
See *Usual adult and adolescent dose.*

### Size(s) usually available
U.S.—
25 mg with 15 mL of sterile distilled water (by varying the quantity of diluent, solutions ranging in strength from 0.16 to 0.5% may be prepared) (Rx) [*Chloromycetin for Ophthalmic Solution*].

Canada—
25 mg with 15 mL of sterile distilled water (by varying the quantity of diluent, solutions ranging in strength from 0.16 to 0.5% may be prepared) (Rx) [*Chloromycetin for Ophthalmic Solution*].

### Packaging and storage
Prior to reconstitution, store below 40 °C (104 °F), preferably between 15 and 30 °C (59 and 86 °F), unless otherwise specified by manufacturer. Store in a tight container. Protect diluent from freezing.

### Preparation of dosage form
To prepare a 0.5, 0.25, or 0.16% solution, add 5, 10, or 15 mL, respectively, of sterile distilled water to the 25-mg bottle.

### Stability
After reconstitution, solutions retain their potency for 10 days if stored at room temperature.

### Auxiliary labeling
• For the eye.
• Continue medicine for full time of treatment.
• Beyond-use date.

Revised: 01/15/92
Interim revision: 09/30/93

# CHLORAMPHENICOL  Otic

VA CLASSIFICATION (Primary): OT101

Note: For a listing of dosage forms and brand names by country availability, see *Dosage Forms* section(s). For a listing of brand names for the articles in this monograph, refer to the General Index.

## Category
Antibacterial (otic).

## Indications
Note: Bracketed information in the *Indications* section refers to uses that are not included in U.S. product labeling.

### Accepted
Ear canal infections, external (treatment)—Chloramphenicol is indicated in the topical treatment of superficial infections of the external ear canal caused by susceptible organisms, including *Staphylococcus aureus*, *Escherichia coli*, *Haemophilus influenzae*, *Pseudomonas aeruginosa*, *Enterobacter aerogenes (Aerobacter aerogenes)*, *Klebsiella pneumoniae*, and *Proteus* species.

In serious otic infections, topical chloramphenicol should be given concurrently with appropriate systemic antibacterials.

[Mastoidectomy cavity infections (treatment)] or

[Otitis media, chronic suppurative (treatment)]—Chloramphenicol is used in the topical treatment of mastoidectomy cavity infections and chronic suppurative otitis media.

Not all species or strains of a particular organism may be susceptible to chloramphenicol.

## Pharmacology/Pharmacokinetics

### Physicochemical characteristics
Molecular weight—323.13.

### Mechanism of action/Effect
Bacteriostatic; since it is lipid-soluble, it diffuses through the bacterial cell membrane and reversibly binds to the 50 S subunit of bacterial ribosomes where transfer of amino acids to growing peptide chains is prevented (perhaps by suppression of peptidyl transferase activity), thus inhibiting peptide bond formation and subsequent protein synthesis.

## Precautions to Consider

### Pregnancy/Reproduction
Pregnancy—Chloramphenicol crosses the placenta. However, studies in humans have not shown that this medicine causes adverse effects on the fetus.

### Breast-feeding
It is not known whether otic chloramphenicol is excreted in breast milk. However, problems in humans have not been documented.

### Pediatrics
Appropriate studies on the relationship of age to the effects of otic chloramphenicol have not been performed in the pediatric population. However, no pediatrics-specific problems have been documented to date.

### Geriatrics
No information is available on the relationship of age to the effects of this medicine in geriatric patients.

### Medical considerations/Contraindications
The medical considerations/contraindications included here have been selected on the basis of their potential clinical significance (reasons given in parentheses where appropriate)—not necessarily inclusive (» = major clinical significance).

*This medication should not be used when the following medical problems exist:*
» Perforated tympanic membrane
(ototoxicity may occur if medication enters the middle ear)

» Previous allergy or toxic reaction to chloramphenicol

## Side/Adverse Effects

Note: Bone marrow hypoplasia, including aplastic anemia and death, has been reported following local application of chloramphenicol.

The following side/adverse effects have been selected on the basis of their potential clinical significance (possible signs and symptoms in parentheses where appropriate)—not necessarily inclusive:

### Those indicating need for medical attention
Incidence less frequent
*Hypersensitivity* (burning, itching, redness, skin rash, swelling, or other sign of irritation not present before therapy)
Incidence rare
*Blood dyscrasias* (pale skin; sore throat and fever; unusual bleeding or bruising; unusual tiredness or weakness)

**Those indicating possible irreversible bone marrow depression, possibly leading to aplastic anemia, and the need for immediate medical attention if they occur after medication is discontinued**
*Pale skin; sore throat and fever; unusual bleeding or bruising; unusual tiredness or weakness*

## Patient Consultation
As an aid to patient consultation, refer to *Advice for the Patient, Chloramphenicol (Otic).*

In providing consultation, consider emphasizing the following selected information (» = major clinical significance):

### Before using this medication
» Conditions affecting use, especially:
Allergy to chloramphenicol
Other medical problems, especially perforated eardrum

### Proper use of this medication
Proper administration technique for otic solution
» Compliance with full course of therapy
» Proper dosing
Missed dose: Inserting as soon as possible; not inserting if almost time for next dose
» Proper storage

### Precautions while using this medication
Checking with physician if no improvement within a few days

**Side/adverse effects**
Signs of potential side effects, especially blood dyscrasias and hypersensitivity reactions

## Otic Dosage Forms

### CHLORAMPHENICOL OTIC SOLUTION USP

**Usual adult and adolescent dose**
Topical, to the ear canal, 2 or 3 drops every six to eight hours.

**Usual pediatric dose**
See *Usual adult and adolescent dose.*

**Strength(s) usually available**
U.S.—
0.5% (5 mg per mL) (Rx) [*Chloromycetin;* GENERIC].

Canada—
0.5% (5 mg per mL) (Rx) [*Chloromycetin*].
4.5% (45 mg per mL) (Rx) [*Sopamycetin*].

**Packaging and storage**
Store below 30 °C (86 °F), preferably between 15 and 30 °C (59 and 86 °F), unless otherwise specified by manufacturer. Store in a tight container. Protect from freezing.

**Auxiliary labeling**
• For the ear.
• Continue medicine for full time of treatment.

**Note**
Dispense in original unopened container.

Revised: 02/10/92
Interim revision: 02/17/94

---

# CHLORAMPHENICOL  Systemic

VA CLASSIFICATION (Primary): AM150

Note: For a listing of dosage forms and brand names by country availability, see *Dosage Forms* section(s). For a listing of brand names for the articles in this monograph, refer to the General Index.

## Category
Antibacterial (systemic).

## Indications

### General considerations
Chloramphenicol has *in vitro* activity against a large number of organisms, including various aerobic gram-positive and gram-negative bacteria, anaerobic bacteria, rickettsiae, spirochetes, and chlamydia. *Haemophilus influenzae*, *Streptococcus pneumoniae*, and *Neisseria meningitidis* are highly susceptible to chloramphenicol, which is considered to be bactericidal against these organisms. Chloramphenicol has bacteriostatic activity against *Staphylococcus aureus*, *Streptococcus pyogenes*, *S. viridans*, group B streptococcus, *Escherichia coli*, *Klebsiella pneumoniae*, *Proteus mirabilis*, *Salmonella typhi*, *S. paratyphi A*, *Shigella* species, *Pseudomonas pseudomallei*, and nearly all anaerobes, including *Bacteroides fragilis*. Bacteria that are generally considered to be resistant to chloramphenicol include *Pseudomonas aeruginosa*, *Acinetobacter* species, *Enterobacter* species, *Serratia marcescens*, indole positive *Proteus* species, methicillin-resistant staphylococcus, and *Enterococcus faecalis*.
Because of this drug's serious toxicities, chloramphenicol is indicated only for the treatment of serious infections in which less toxic antibacterials are ineffective or contraindicated. Other medications, such as the third-generation cephalosporins for the treatment of meningitis, and clindamycin or metronidazole for the treatment of anaerobic infections, have generally replaced chloramphenicol; however, under certain circumstances, chloramphenicol may still be the most appropriate drug to use.
Chloramphenicol is also used in the treatment of rickettsial infections that require parenteral treatment when other antibiotics are contraindicated.
**Chloramphenicol should be reserved for serious infections in which less toxic antibacterials are ineffective or contraindicated.**

### Accepted
Brain abscess (treatment)—Chloramphenicol is indicated in the treatment of brain abscess caused by *B. fragilis* or other susceptible organisms.
Ehrlichiosis (treatment)—Chloramphenicol is indicated in the treatment of ehrlichiosis caused by *Ehrlichia canis.*
Meningitis (treatment)—Chloramphenicol is indicated in the treatment of meningitis caused by *H. influenzae*, *S. pneumoniae*, and *N. meningitidis.*
Paratyphoid fever (treatment)—Chloramphenicol is indicated in the treatment of paratyphoid fever caused by *S. paratyphi A.*
Q fever (treatment)—Chloramphenicol is indicated in the treatment of Q fever caused by *Coxiella burnetii.*
Rocky Mountain spotted fever (treatment)—Chloramphenicol is indicated in the treatment of Rocky Mountain spotted fever caused by *Rickettsia* species.
Typhoid fever (treatment)—Chloramphenicol is indicated in the acute treatment of typhoid fever only, caused by *S. typhi.*

Typhus infections (treatment)—Chloramphenicol is indicated in the treatment of typhus infections caused by *Rickettsia* species.

Not all species or strains of a particular organism may be susceptible to chloramphenicol.

### Unaccepted
Chloramphenicol is not indicated in the routine treatment of typhoid carrier states; in the treatment of trivial infections, colds, influenza, or throat infections; or in the prophylaxis of infections.

## Pharmacology/Pharmacokinetics

### Physicochemical characteristics
Molecular weight—Chloramphenicol: 323.13.
Chloramphenicol palmitate: 561.54.
Chloramphenicol sodium succinate: 445.19.

### Mechanism of action/Effect
Chloramphenicol, a broad-spectrum antibiotic, is bacteriostatic. However, it may be bactericidal in high concentrations or when used against highly susceptible organisms.
Chloramphenicol, which is lipid soluble, diffuses through the bacterial cell membrane and reversibly binds to the 50 S subunit of bacterial ribosomes where transfer of amino acids to growing peptide chains is prevented (perhaps by suppression of peptidyl transferase activity), thus inhibiting peptide bond formation and subsequent protein synthesis.
The mechanism for the irreversible aplastic anemia following use of chloramphenicol has not been established.
The mechanism for the dose-related reversible bone-marrow depression during and following use of chloramphenicol is thought to be by inhibition of mitochondrial protein synthesis in bone-marrow cells.

### Absorption
Rapidly and completely absorbed from gastrointestinal tract.
Well absorbed after intramuscular administration; achieves serum concentrations comparable to intravenous administration.
Intravenous bioavailability—70%.
Oral bioavailability—80%.

### Distribution
Chloramphenicol diffuses rapidly and is widely, but not uniformly, distributed throughout the body to—
Liver and kidneys: Highest concentrations.
Urine: High concentrations.
Placenta: Fetal serum concentrations may be 30 to 80% of maternal serum concentrations.
Eye: Therapeutic concentrations in aqueous and vitreous humor.
Cerebrospinal fluid (CSF): Concentrations may be 21 to 50% of serum concentrations through uninflamed meninges and may be 45 to 89% of serum concentrations through inflamed meninges.
Other: Pleural fluid, ascitic fluid, synovial fluid, breast milk, and saliva (bitter aftertaste).
Vol$_D$ = 0.6–1.0 L/kg.

### Protein binding
Adults—Moderate (50–60%).
Premature neonates—Low (32%).

**Biotransformation**

Hepatic (free drug); 90% conjugated to inactive glucuronide.

Chloramphenicol palmitate is hydrolyzed to free drug in the gastrointestinal tract prior to absorption.

Chloramphenicol sodium succinate is hydrolyzed to free drug in the plasma, liver, lungs, and kidneys.

In the fetus and neonates, the immature liver cannot conjugate chloramphenicol, and toxic concentrations of active drug accumulate. In neonates and infants this may result in the "gray syndrome."

**Half-life**

Adults—
  Normal renal and hepatic function: 1.5 to 3.5 hours.
  Impaired renal function: 3 to 4 hours.
  Severely impaired hepatic function: Prolonged (4.6 to 11.6 hours).
Children (1 month to 16 years old)—
  3 to 6.5 hours.
Infants—
  1 to 2 days old: 24 hours or longer; highly variable, especially in low-birth-weight infants.
  10 to 16 days old: 10 hours.

**Time to peak serum concentration:**

Intravenous—1 to 1.5 hours.
Oral—1 to 3 hours.

**Peak serum concentration**

Adults—Oral, 12.5 mg per kg of body weight (mg/kg): 11.2 to 18.4 mcg/mL.

Children—Oral and intravenous: 25 mg/kg—19 to 28 mcg/mL.

**Elimination**

Renal, by glomerular filtration; 5 to 10% excreted unchanged within 24 hours; 80% rapidly excreted by tubular secretion as inactive metabolites. Inactive metabolites can accumulate in premature and newborn infants because of immaturity of renal tubular secretion mechanisms.

Fecal/biliary; small amounts excreted unchanged following oral administration.

Dialysis—Dialysis does not remove significant amounts of chloramphenicol from the blood. Charcoal hemoperfusion has been reported to lower blood concentrations in an infant.

# Precautions to Consider

## Pregnancy/Reproduction

Chloramphenicol readily crosses the placenta; fetal serum concentrations may be 30 to 80% of maternal serum concentrations. Although birth defects in humans have not been documented, use is not recommended in pregnancy at term or during labor because of potential toxicity ("gray syndrome" or bone marrow depression) in premature or full-term infants.

## Breast-feeding

Chloramphenicol is excreted in breast milk in concentrations up to 25 mcg per mL. Use is not recommended in nursing mothers because of the possibility of adverse effects, especially bone marrow depression, in the infant.

## Pediatrics

In the fetus and neonates, the immature liver cannot conjugate chloramphenicol, and toxic concentrations of active drug accumulate. In neonates and infants this may result in the "gray syndrome."

In infants 1 to 2 days old, the half-life is 24 hours or longer and may be highly variable, especially in low-birth-weight infants. In infants 10 to 16 days old, the half-life is 10 hours.

Inactive metabolites can accumulate in premature and newborn infants because of immaturity of renal tubular secretion mechanisms.

Serum concentrations must be performed in pediatric patients with impaired or immature metabolic functions or in patients who are receiving medications that are also metabolized by the liver (e.g., phenytoin, phenobarbital, acetaminophen, theophylline).

## Geriatrics

No information is available on the relationship of age to the effects of chloramphenicol in geriatric patients.

## Dental

The bone marrow–depressant effects of chloramphenicol may result in an increased incidence of microbial infection, delayed healing, and gingival bleeding. Dental work, whenever possible, should be completed prior to initiation of therapy or deferred until blood counts have returned to normal. Patients should be instructed in proper oral hygiene during treatment, including caution in use of regular toothbrushes, dental floss, and toothpicks.

**Drug interactions and/or related problems**

The following drug interactions and/or related problems have been selected on the basis of their potential clinical significance (possible mechanism in parentheses where appropriate)—not necessarily inclusive (» = major clinical significance):

Note: Combinations containing any of the following medications, depending on the amount present, may also interact with this medication.

» Alfentanil
(chronic preoperative or perioperative use of chloramphenicol, an hepatic enzyme inhibitor, may decrease the plasma clearance and prolong the duration of action of alfentanil)

» Anticonvulsants, hydantoin or
  Blood dyscrasia–causing medications (See *Appendix II*) or
» Bone marrow depressants, other (See *Appendix II* ) or
» Radiation therapy
(concurrent use with chloramphenicol may increase the bone marrow–depressant effects of these medications and radiation therapy; dosage reduction may be required)

» Antidiabetic agents, oral
(concurrent use of chloramphenicol with tolbutamide and chlorpropamide may enhance their hypoglycemic effect by inhibiting the hepatic metabolism of these medications and increasing their serum levels; dosage adjustments may be necessary; glipizide and glyburide, due to their non-ionic binding characteristics, may not be affected as much as the other oral antidiabetic agents; however, caution with concurrent use is recommended)

Contraceptives, estrogen-containing, oral
(concurrent long-term use of chloramphenicol may result in reduced contraceptive reliability and increased incidence of breakthrough bleeding)

» Clindamycin or
» Erythromycins or
» Lincomycin
(may be displaced from or prevented from binding to 50 S subunits of bacterial ribosomes by chloramphenicol, thus antagonizing the effects of erythromycins and lincomycins; concurrent use is not recommended)

Hepatic enzyme inducers
(concurrent use of chloramphenicol with hepatic microsomal enzyme inducing drugs, including phenobarbital and rifampin, can increase the metabolism of chloramphenicol, decreasing chloramphenicol serum concentrations)

Penicillins
(since bacteriostatic drugs may interfere with the bactericidal effects of penicillins in the treatment of meningitis or in other situations in which a rapid bactericidal effect is necessary, it is best to avoid concurrent therapy; however, chloramphenicol and ampicillin are sometimes administered concurrently in pediatric patients)

» Phenobarbital or
» Phenytoin or
» Warfarin or
» Other medications metabolized by mixed-function oxidase system
(inhibition of the cytochrome P-450 enzyme system by chloramphenicol may cause a decrease in the hepatic metabolism of these medications, resulting in delayed elimination and increased blood concentrations)

Vitamin B$_{12}$
(concurrent use may antagonize hematopoietic response to vitamin B$_{12}$; monitoring of hematologic status or use of an alternate antibiotic is recommended)

**Laboratory value alterations**

The following have been selected on the basis of their potential clinical significance (possible effect in parentheses where appropriate)—not necessarily inclusive (» = major clinical significance):

With diagnostic test results
  Bentiromide
  (concurrent administration of chloramphenicol during a bentiromide test period will invalidate test results since chloramphenicol is also metabolized to arylamines and will thus increase the percent of PABA recovered; discontinuation of chloramphenicol at least 3 days prior to the administration of bentiromide is recommended)

  Urine glucose determinations
  (chloramphenicol may give false-positive test results with copper sulfate urine glucose tests)

### Medical considerations/Contraindications

The medical considerations/contraindications included here have been selected on the basis of their potential clinical significance (reasons given in parentheses where appropriate)—not necessarily inclusive (» = major clinical significance).

*Except under special circumstances, this medication should not be used when the following medical problems exist:*

» Previous allergy or toxic reaction to chloramphenicol

*Risk-benefit should be considered when the following medical problems exist:*

» Bone marrow depression
    (chloramphenicol may cause a dose-related bone marrow depression, an idiosyncratic aplastic anemia, and other blood dyscrasias)

» Hepatic function impairment
    (chloramphenicol is metabolized in the liver; patients with impaired or immature hepatic or renal function, especially neonates and infants, or adults with both impaired hepatic and renal function, may require a reduction in dose; serum concentrations should be monitored)

» Risk-benefit should be considered in patients who have had previous cytotoxic drug therapy or radiation therapy also.

### Patient monitoring

The following may be especially important in patient monitoring (other tests may be warranted in some patients, depending on condition; » = major clinical significance):

» Chloramphenicol levels, serum
    (serum concentrations must be performed in low-birth-weight infants because the pharmacokinetics of chloramphenicol are so variable in this age group; serum concentrations should also be monitored in patients with impaired or immature metabolic functions or in patients who are receiving medications that are also metabolized by the liver; the desired serum concentration should fall within the range of 10 to 25 mcg/mL, the concentration to which most susceptible organisms respond; concentrations in excess of these increase the risk of reversible bone marrow depression and "gray syndrome")

» Complete blood counts (CBCs)
    (may be required frequently during therapy to detect dose-related reversible bone marrow depression; chloramphenicol should be discontinued if reticulocytopenia, leukopenia, thrombocytopenia, anemia, or other blood dyscrasias occur; however, CBCs are not useful in predicting aplastic anemia, which usually appears after treatment has been completed)
    (patients should be informed of the importance of having blood counts followed closely during therapy)

## Side/Adverse Effects

Note: The hematologic toxicity of chloramphenicol can manifest itself in 1 of 2 ways—either as a reversible bone marrow depression or an idiosyncratic aplastic anemia. Bone marrow depression is dose-related and most commonly seen when serum concentrations exceed 25 mcg/mL. Bone marrow changes are usually reversible when chloramphenicol is discontinued. Aplastic anemia is an idiosyncratic reaction that occurs in 1 of every 25,000 to 40,000 courses of treatment. It is not related to dose or duration of therapy. Most cases have been associated with oral chloramphenicol, and the onset of aplasia may not occur until weeks or months after treatment with chloramphenicol has been discontinued.

Gray syndrome (or "gray baby syndrome") almost always occurs in newborn infants treated with inappropriately high doses of chloramphenicol. Typically, the infant has been started on chloramphenicol within the first 48 hours of life; symptoms first appear after 3 to 4 days of continued treatment with high doses of chloramphenicol; and serum levels are high, often between 40 and 200 mcg/mL. If caught early and chloramphenicol is discontinued, the infant may have a complete recovery. On rare occasion, older patients, including adults with severe liver disease, have also had a gray syndrome–type reaction.

The following side/adverse effects have been selected on the basis of their potential clinical significance (possible signs and symptoms in parentheses where appropriate)—not necessarily inclusive:

### Those indicating need for medical attention
Incidence less frequent
    *Blood dyscrasias* (pale skin; sore throat and fever; unusual bleeding or bruising; unusual tiredness or weakness)

Incidence rare
    *Gray syndrome* (abdominal distension; blue-gray skin color; low body temperature; uneven breathing; unresponsiveness; cardiovascular collapse)—in neonates only; *hypersensitivity reactions* (skin rash; fever; shortness of breath); *neurotoxic reactions* (confusion; delirium; headache); *optic neuritis* (eye pain, blurred vision, or loss of vision); *peripheral neuritis* (numbness, tingling, burning pain, or weakness in the hands or feet)

### Those indicating need for medical attention only if they continue or are bothersome
Incidence less frequent
    *Gastrointestinal reaction* (diarrhea; nausea; vomiting)

### Those indicating possible fatal, irreversible bone marrow depression, leading to aplastic anemia, and the need for immediate medical attention if they occur weeks or months after medication is discontinued
    *Pale skin; sore throat and fever; unusual bleeding or bruising; unusual tiredness or weakness*

## Patient Consultation

As an aid to patient consultation, refer to *Advice for the Patient, Chloramphenicol (Systemic).*

In providing consultation, consider emphasizing the following selected information (» = major clinical significance):

### Before using this medication
» Conditions affecting use, especially:
    Allergies or toxic reactions to chloramphenicol
    Pregnancy—Chloramphenicol crosses the placenta; use at term or during labor may cause "gray syndrome" in infants
    Breast-feeding—Chloramphenicol is excreted in breast milk; may cause bone marrow depression in the infant
    Use in children—Because of possible accumulation and toxic reactions, serum concentrations must be measured in premature and newborn infants
    Dental—May result in an increased incidence of infection, delayed healing, and gingival bleeding
    Other medications, especially alfentanil, hydantoin anticonvulsants, bone marrow depressants, radiation therapy, oral antidiabetic agents, erythromycins, lincomycins, phenobarbital, phenytoin, warfarin, or other medicines metabolized by mixed-function oxidase system
    Other medical problems, especially bone marrow depression, liver dysfunction, previous cytotoxic drug therapy, or radiation therapy

### Proper use of this medication
    Taking on an empty stomach
    Proper administration technique for oral liquids
» Compliance with full course of therapy
» Proper dosing
    Missed dose: Taking as soon as possible; not taking if almost time for next dose; not doubling doses
» Proper storage

### Precautions while using this medication
    Checking with physician if no improvement within a few days
» Regular visits to physician to check for blood problems
    Using caution in use of regular toothbrushes, dental floss, and toothpicks; completing dental work prior to initiation of therapy or deferring dental work until blood counts have returned to normal; checking with physician or dentist concerning proper oral hygiene
» Diabetics: False-positive reactions with copper sulfate urine glucose tests may occur

### Side/adverse effects
    May also cause bone marrow aplasia and "gray syndrome"
    Signs of potential side effects, especially blood dyscrasias, gray syndrome, optic neuritis, peripheral neuritis, neurotoxic reactions, or hypersensitivity reactions

## General Dosing Information

Treatment should be continued no longer than required to produce a cure, yet long enough to provide little or no risk of relapse.

Repeated courses of the drug should be avoided if at all possible since reversible bone marrow depression may occur.

The serum chloramphenicol concentration should fall within the range of 10 to 25 mcg/mL, the concentration to which most susceptible organisms respond; concentrations higher than 30 mcg/mL increase the risk of bone marrow depression and "gray syndrome."

**For oral dosage forms only**

Chloramphenicol should preferably be taken with a full glass (240 mL) of water on an empty stomach (either 1 hour before or 2 hours after meals) to optimize absorption.

Chloramphenicol palmitate must be hydrolyzed in the gastrointestinal tract to chloramphenicol before being absorbed. The rate of absorption may be decreased in neonates or increased in older children, depending on the individual rate of hydrolysis. Serum concentrations are usually similar to those resulting from oral base administration of chloramphenicol.

## Oral Dosage Forms

### CHLORAMPHENICOL CAPSULES USP

**Usual adult and adolescent dose**

Antibacterial—
  Oral, 12.5 mg (base) per kg of body weight every six hours.

**Usual adult prescribing limits**

Up to a maximum of 4 grams (base) daily.

**Usual pediatric dose**

Antibacterial—
  Premature and full-term infants up to 2 weeks of age: Oral, 6.25 mg (base) per kg of body weight every six hours.
  Infants 2 weeks of age and over: Oral, 12.5 mg (base) per kg of body weight every six hours; or 25 mg per kg of body weight every twelve hours.

Note: In severe infections, such as bacteremia or meningitis, doses up to 75 to 100 mg (base) per kg of body weight daily may be used.
  Serum determinations are recommended in patients with impaired or immature metabolic functions.

**Strength(s) usually available**

U.S.—
  250 mg (base) (Rx) [*Chloromycetin;* GENERIC].

Canada—
  250 mg (base) (Rx) [*Novochlorocap*].

**Packaging and storage**

Store below 30 °C (86 °F), preferably between 15 and 30 °C (59 and 86 °F), unless otherwise specified by manufacturer. Store in a tight container.

**Auxiliary labeling**
• Continue medicine for full time of treatment.
• Take on empty stomach.

### CHLORAMPHENICOL PALMITATE ORAL SUSPENSION USP

**Usual adult and adolescent dose**

See *Chloramphenicol Capsules USP*.

**Usual adult prescribing limits**

See *Chloramphenicol Capsules USP*.

**Usual pediatric dose**

See *Chloramphenicol Capsules USP*.

**Strength(s) usually available**

U.S.—
  150 mg (base) per 5 mL (Rx) [*Chloromycetin* (sodium benzoate 2.5 mg per 5 mL)].

Canada—
  Not commercially available.

**Packaging and storage**

Store below 40 °C (104 °F), preferably between 15 and 30 °C (59 and 86 °F), unless otherwise specified by manufacturer. Store in a tight, light-resistant container. Protect from freezing.

**Auxiliary labeling**
• Shake well.
• Continue medicine for full time of treatment.
• Take on empty stomach.

**Note**

When dispensing, include a calibrated liquid-measuring device.

**Additional information**

The oral suspension is tasteless.

## Parenteral Dosage Forms

Note: The dosing and strengths of the dosage forms available are expressed in terms of chloramphenicol base.

### STERILE CHLORAMPHENICOL SODIUM SUCCINATE USP

**Usual adult and adolescent dose**

Antibacterial—
  Intravenous, 12.5 mg (base) per kg of body weight every six hours.

**Usual adult prescribing limits**

Up to a maximum of 4 grams (base) daily.

**Usual pediatric dose**

Antibacterial—
  Premature and full-term infants up to 2 weeks of age: Intravenous, 6.25 mg (base) per kg of body weight every six hours.
  Infants 2 weeks of age and over: Intravenous, 12.5 mg (base) per kg of body weight every six hours; or 25 mg per kg of body weight every twelve hours.

Note: In severe infections, such as bacteremia or meningitis, doses up to 75 to 100 mg (base) per kg of body weight daily may be used.
  Serum determinations are recommended in patients with impaired or immature metabolic functions.

**Size(s) usually available**

U.S.—
  1 gram (base) (Rx) [*Chloromycetin* (sodium 2.25 mEq per gram); GENERIC].

Canada—
  1 gram (base) (Rx) [*Chloromycetin*].

**Packaging and storage**

Prior to reconstitution, store below 40 °C (104 °F), preferably between 15 and 30 °C (59 and 86 °F), unless otherwise specified by manufacturer.

**Preparation of dosage form**

To prepare a 10% (100-mg-per-mL) solution, add 10 mL of an aqueous diluent such as sterile water for injection or 5% dextrose injection to each 1-gram vial.

**Stability**

After reconstitution, solutions (100-mg-per-mL) retain their potency for 2 to 30 days if stored at room temperature or if refrigerated, depending on the manufacturer.

Diluted solutions are stable for 24 to 48 hours if stored at room temperature or if refrigerated, depending on the manufacturer.

If frozen, solutions retain their potency for up to 6 months, depending on the manufacturer.

Do not use if solution is cloudy.

**Additional information**

Chloramphenicol sodium succinate must be hydrolyzed in the body to chloramphenicol; therefore, there may be a delay in achieving adequate serum concentrations of active drug.

May be given intravenously over at least a 1-minute period.

Chloramphenicol may also be given intramuscularly, achieving serum concentrations comparable to intravenous administration.

Revised: 05/13/92
Interim revision: 03/17/94; 06/20/95

# CHLORAMPHENICOL   Topical

VA CLASSIFICATION (Primary): DE101

Note: For a listing of dosage forms and brand names by country availability, see *Dosage Forms* section(s). For a listing of brand names for the articles in this monograph, refer to the General Index.

## Category
Antibacterial (topical).

## Indications
Note: Bracketed information in the *Indications* section refers to uses that are not included in U.S. product labeling.

**Accepted**
Skin infections, bacterial, minor (treatment)—Chloramphenicol is indicated in the topical treatment of minor bacterial skin infections caused by susceptible organisms.

In deeper skin infections, topical chloramphenicol should be given concurrently with appropriate systemic antibacterials.

[Skin infections, bacterial, minor (prophylaxis)]—Chloramphenicol is used in the topical prophylaxis of minor bacterial skin infections.

[Ulcer, dermal (treatment)]—Chloramphenicol is used in the topical treatment of dermal ulcer.

Not all species or strains of a particular organism may be susceptible to chloramphenicol.

## Pharmacology/Pharmacokinetics

**Physicochemical characteristics**
Molecular weight—323.13.

**Mechanism of action/Effect**
Bacteriostatic; since chloramphenicol is lipid-soluble, it diffuses through the bacterial cell membrane and reversibly binds to the 50 S subunit of bacterial ribosomes where transfer of amino acids to growing peptide chains is prevented (perhaps by suppression of peptidyl transferase activity), thus inhibiting peptide bond formation and subsequent protein synthesis.

**Absorption**
Extent of systemic absorption following topical application to skin, wounds, or mucous membranes unknown.

## Precautions to Consider

**Pregnancy/Reproduction**
Pregnancy—Chloramphenicol crosses the placenta. However, studies in humans have not shown that topical chloramphenicol causes adverse effects on the fetus.

**Breast-feeding**
It is not known whether topical chloramphenicol is distributed into breast milk. However, problems in humans have not been documented.

**Pediatrics**
Appropriate studies on the relationship of age to the effect of topical chloramphenicol have not been performed in the pediatric population. However, no pediatrics-specific problems have been documented to date.

**Geriatrics**
No information is available on the relationship of age to the effects of this medication in geriatric patients.

**Medical considerations/Contraindications**
The medical considerations/contraindications included here have been selected on the basis of their potential clinical significance (reasons given in parentheses where appropriate)—not necessarily inclusive (» = major clinical significance).

*Except under special circumstances, this medication should not be used when the following medical problem exists:*
» Previous allergy or toxic reaction to chloramphenicol

## Side/Adverse Effects
Note: Prolonged topical administration frequently results in contact sensitization.

Bone marrow hypoplasia, including aplastic anemia and death, has been reported following topical application of chloramphenicol.

The following side/adverse effects have been selected on the basis of their potential clinical significance (possible signs and symptoms in parentheses where appropriate)—not necessarily inclusive:

**Those indicating need for medical attention**
Incidence more frequent
    *Hypersensitivity* (burning, itching, redness, skin rash, swelling, or other signs of irritation not present before therapy)
Incidence rare
    *Blood dyscrasias* (pale skin; sore throat and fever; unusual bleeding or bruising; unusual tiredness or weakness)

**Those indicating possible irreversible bone marrow depression, possibly leading to aplastic anemia, and the need for immediate medical attention if they occur after medication is discontinued**
    *Pale skin; sore throat and fever; unusual bleeding or bruising; unusual tiredness or weakness*

## Patient Consultation
As an aid to patient consultation, refer to *Advice for the Patient, Chloramphenicol (Topical)*.

In providing consultation, consider emphasizing the following selected information (» = major clinical significance):

**Before using this medication**
» Conditions affecting use, especially:
    Allergy to chloramphenicol

**Proper use of this medication**
    Before applying, washing affected area with soap and water and drying thoroughly
» Compliance with full course of therapy; not using more often or for longer than prescribed
» Proper dosing
    Missed dose: Applying as soon as possible; not applying if almost time for next dose
» Proper storage

**Precautions while using this medication**
    Checking with physician if no improvement within 1 week

**Side/adverse effects**
    Signs of potential side effects, especially blood dyscrasias and hypersensitivity reactions

## General Dosing Information
Use of topical antibacterials may lead to skin sensitization, resulting in hypersensitivity reactions with subsequent topical or systemic use of the medication.

## Topical Dosage Forms

### CHLORAMPHENICOL CREAM USP

**Usual adult and adolescent dose**
Antibacterial—
    Topical, to the skin, three or four times a day.

**Usual pediatric dose**
Antibacterial—
    See *Usual adult and adolescent dose*.

**Strength(s) usually available**
U.S.—
    1% (10 mg per gram) (Rx) [*Chloromycetin* (propylparaben 0.1%)].
Canada—
    1% (10 mg per gram) (Rx) [*Chloromycetin* (parabens)].

**Packaging and storage**
Store below 30 °C (86 °F), preferably between 15 and 30 °C (59 and 86 °F), unless otherwise specified by manufacturer. Store in a collapsible tube or a tight container. Protect from freezing.

**Auxiliary labeling**
• For external use only.
• Continue medication for full time of treatment.

**Note**
Chloramphenicol cream is water-miscible.

Revised: 02/10/92
Interim revision: 06/13/94

**CHLORDIAZEPOXIDE**—See *Benzodiazepines (Systemic)*

---

# CHLORDIAZEPOXIDE AND AMITRIPTYLINE   Systemic

VA CLASSIFICATION (Primary): CN900

**NOTE:** The *Chlordiazepoxide and Amitriptyline (Systemic)* monograph is maintained on the USP DI electronic data base. For a printed copy of the most recent revision of the complete monograph, contact the USP Division of Information Development, 12601 Twinbrook Parkway, Rockville, MD 20852.

For information on the specific components of this combination, see the *USP DI* monographs for *Antidepressants, Tricyclic (Systemic)* and *Benzodiazepines (Systemic)*.

The information that follows is selectively abstracted from the complete monograph and is provided to facilitate drug use review and patient counseling.

Note: For a listing of dosage forms and brand names by country availability, see *Dosage Forms* section(s). For a listing of brand names for the articles in this monograph, refer to the General Index.

## Category
Antianxiety agent–antidepressant.

## Indications
**Accepted**
Anxiety associated with mental depression (treatment)—The combination of chlordiazepoxide and amitriptyline is indicated in the treatment of moderate to severe anxiety associated with moderate to severe depression.

The therapeutic response to chlordiazepoxide and amitriptyline combination may occur earlier than when either agent is used alone. Symptoms most likely to respond to therapy in the first week are feelings of guilt or worthlessness, insomnia, agitation, anxiety, suicidal thoughts, and anorexia.

## Patient Consultation
As an aid to patient consultation, refer to *Advice for the Patient, Chlordiazepoxide and Amitriptyline (Systemic)*.

In providing consultation, consider emphasizing the following selected information (» = major clinical significance):

**Before using this medication**
» Conditions affecting use, especially:
 Sensitivity to other benzodiazepines or tricyclic antidepressants
 Pregnancy—Chlordiazepoxide: Crosses placenta; chronic use may cause physical dependence in mother and withdrawal symptoms in neonate; reported to increase risk of congenital malformations when used during first trimester; during delivery, may cause neonatal flaccidity when used just prior to or during labor
 Amitriptyline: Animal studies have shown teratogenic effects when given in doses many times larger than the human dose; reports of cardiac problems, muscle spasms, respiratory distress, or urinary retention in neonates of mothers taking amitriptyline just prior to delivery
 Breast-feeding—Chlordiazepoxide excreted in breast milk; may cause sedation, feeding difficulties, or weight loss in infant
 Use in children—Adolescents are more likely to exhibit dose sensitivity to chlordiazepoxide and amitriptyline combination, requiring a lower initial dose
 Use in the elderly—Elderly tend to develop CNS and anticholinergic effects at lower doses; close supervision necessary for patients with cardiac problems, glaucoma, urinary retention, and/or gastrointestinal problems; elderly may better tolerate divided doses
 Dental—Dryness of mouth may contribute to development of caries, periodontal disease, oral candidiasis, and discomfort; pos-

sible dyscrasias caused by amitriptyline may increase incidence of microbial infection, delayed healing, and gingival bleeding
 Other medications, especially other addictive medications, antacids, antithyroid agents, cimetidine, clonidine, guanadrel, guanethidine, alcohol or other CNS depression-producing medications, monoamine oxidase (MAO) inhibitors, metrizamide, or sympathomimetics
 Other medical problems, especially alcoholism, active or in remission; seizure disorders; glaucoma; hepatic function impairment; latent psychosis; bipolar disorder; blood, cardiovascular, or gastrointestinal disorders; hyperthyroidism; prostatic hypertrophy; or urinary retention

**Proper use of this medication**
 Taking after meals or with food to reduce gastric irritation
» Several weeks of therapy may be required to produce optimal therapeutic effects.
» Importance of not taking more medication than the amount prescribed because of habit-forming potential
» Not increasing dose if medication is less effective after a few weeks; checking with physician
» Proper dosing
 Missed dose: Not taking dose at all; continuing on schedule; not doubling doses
» Proper storage

**Precautions while using this medication**
 Regular visits to physician to check progress of therapy
» Checking with physician before discontinuing medication; gradual dosage reduction may be needed to avoid the possibility of withdrawal symptoms
» Avoiding use of alcoholic beverages or other CNS depressants during therapy; not taking other medication unless discussed with physician
 Diabetics: May affect blood sugar determinations
 Caution if any laboratory tests required; possible interference with results of metyrapone test
» Caution if any kind of surgery, dental treatment, or emergency treatment is required
» Possible drowsiness; caution when driving or doing things requiring alertness
» Possible dizziness; caution when getting up suddenly from a lying or sitting position
 Possible dryness of mouth; using sugarless candy or gum, ice, or saliva substitute for relief; checking with dentist or physician if dry mouth continues for more than 2 weeks
 Possible skin photosensitivity; avoiding unprotected exposure to sun; using protective clothing; using a sun block product that includes protection against both UVA-caused photosensitivity reactions and UVB-caused sunburn reactions; avoiding use of sunlamp, tanning bed, or tanning booth

**Side/adverse effects**
 Signs of potential side effects, especially aggravation of glaucoma, agranulocytosis, allergic reactions, anticholinergic effects, convulsions, hallucinations, hypotension, irregular heartbeat, jaundice, mood or mental changes, muscle tremors, or paradoxical CNS stimulation

## Oral Dosage Forms
### CHLORDIAZEPOXIDE AND AMITRIPTYLINE HYDROCHLORIDE TABLETS USP

**Usual adult and adolescent dose**
Antianxiety agent–antidepressant—
 Oral, 5 mg of chlordiazepoxide and 12.5 mg of amitriptyline hydrochloride or 10 mg of chlordiazepoxide and 25 mg of amitriptyline

hydrochloride three or four times a day initially, the dosage being adjusted as needed and tolerated.

Note: The larger portion of the daily dose may be taken at bedtime. A single bedtime dose may be adequate for some patients.

**Usual adult prescribing limits**

10 mg of chlordiazepoxide and 25 mg of amitriptyline hydrochloride up to six times a day.

**Usual pediatric dose**

Antianxiety agent–antidepressant—
    Children up to 12 years of age: Dosage has not been established.
    Children 12 years of age and over: See *Usual adult and adolescent dose.*

**Strength(s) usually available**

U.S.—
    5 mg of chlordiazepoxide and 12.5 mg of amitriptyline hydrochloride (Rx) [*Limbitrol;* GENERIC].
    10 mg of chlordiazepoxide and 25 mg of amitriptyline hydrochloride (Rx) [*Limbitrol DS;* GENERIC].

Canada—
    Not commercially available.

**Auxiliary labeling**

• May cause drowsiness.
• Avoid alcoholic beverages.

Revised: 03/19/93

# CHLORDIAZEPOXIDE AND CLIDINIUM   Systemic

VA CLASSIFICATION (Primary): GA802

**NOTE:** The *Chlordiazepoxide and Clidinium (Systemic)* monograph is maintained on the USP DI electronic data base. For a printed copy of the most recent revision of the complete monograph, contact the USP Division of Information Development, 12601 Twinbrook Parkway, Rockville, MD 20852.

For information on the specific components of this combination, see the *USP DI* monographs for *Anticholinergics/Antispasmodics (Systemic)* and *Benzodiazepines (Systemic).*

The information that follows is selectively abstracted from the complete monograph and is provided to facilitate drug use review and patient counseling.

Note: For a listing of dosage forms and brand names by country availability, see *Dosage Forms* section(s). For a listing of brand names for the articles in this monograph, refer to the General Index.

## Category

Anticholinergic-sedative.

## Indications

**Accepted**

Ulcer, peptic (treatment adjunct) or
Bowel syndrome, irritable (treatment)—FDA has classified chlordiazepoxide and clidinium combination as possibly effective as adjunctive therapy in the treatment of peptic ulcer and irritable bowel syndrome.

Note: The less-than-effective classifications require submission of adequate and well-controlled studies to provide substantial evidence of effectiveness. FDA has notified manufacturers of the possible withdrawal from the market of products containing a combination of an anticholinergic and a sedative because their efficacy as fixed combinations has not been proven in adequately designed clinical trials. To date, no final action has been taken.

**Unaccepted**

Anticholinergic and sedative combinations have been used as adjuncts in the treatment of acute enterocolitis; however, their use for this condition is controversial since they cause a reduction in gastrointestinal motility, resulting in retention of the causative organism or toxin and the consequent prolongation of symptoms.

## Patient Consultation

As an aid to patient consultation, refer to *Advice for the Patient, Chlordiazepoxide and Clidinium (Systemic).*

In providing consultation, consider emphasizing the following selected information ( »= major clinical significance):

**Before using this medication**

» Conditions affecting use, especially:
    Sensitivity to clidinium and chlordiazepoxide or to other benzodiazepines or any of the belladonna alkaloids
    Pregnancy—Use is not recommended; chronic use of chlordiazepoxide may cause physical dependence and withdrawal symptoms in the neonate; chlordiazepoxide increases risk of congenital malformations in first trimester
    Breast-feeding—Chlordiazepoxide distributed into breast milk; clidinium may cause inhibition of lactation
    Use in children—Increased susceptibility to anticholinergic effects of clidinium and to CNS effects of chlordiazepoxide

Use in the elderly—Increased susceptibility to mental and other anticholinergic effects of clidinium and to CNS effects of chlordiazepoxide; danger of precipitating undiagnosed glaucoma; possible impairment of memory
Dental—Possible development of dental problems because of decreased salivary flow
Other medications, especially other anticholinergics, antacids, antidiarrheals, CNS depressants, ketoconazole, or potassium chloride
Other medical problems, especially cardiac disease, glaucoma, hepatic disease, hiatal hernia with reflux esophagitis, intestinal atony, myasthenia gravis, obstruction in gastrointestinal or urinary tract, ulcerative colitis, or urinary retention

**Proper use of this medication**

Taking dose 30 to 60 minutes before meals unless told otherwise by physician
» Taking medication only as directed
» Proper dosing
Missed dose: Taking as soon as possible; not taking if almost time for next dose; not doubling doses
» Proper storage

**Precautions while using this medication**

Regular visits to physician to check progress of therapy if used for extended period of time
Avoiding medicine for diarrhea within 1 to 2 hours of taking this medication
» Caution if dizziness, lightheadedness, drowsiness, or blurred vision occurs
» Avoiding use of alcohol or other CNS depressants during and for a few days following therapy
» Caution during exercise and hot weather; overheating may result in heat stroke
Possible dryness of mouth, nose, and throat; using sugarless gum or candy, ice, or saliva substitute for relief; checking with dentist if mouth continues to feel dry for more than 2 weeks
» Checking with physician if constipation occurs
Checking with physician before discontinuing medication after prolonged use; gradual dosage reduction may be necessary to avoid the possibility of withdrawal symptoms

**Side/adverse effects**

Signs of potential side effects, especially agranulocytosis, granulocytopenia, or leukopenia; allergic reaction; CNS depression; increased intraocular pressure; jaundice; and paradoxical reaction

## Oral Dosage Forms

### CHLORDIAZEPOXIDE HYDROCHLORIDE AND CLIDINIUM BROMIDE CAPSULES USP

**Usual adult dose**

Oral, 1 or 2 capsules one to four times a day, thirty to sixty minutes before meals or food, the dosage then being adjusted as needed and tolerated.

Note: Debilitated patients—See *Usual geriatric dose.*

**Usual adult prescribing limits**

Up to a total of 8 capsules daily (40 mg of chlordiazepoxide hydrochloride and 20 mg of clidinium bromide).

**Usual pediatric dose**

Dosage has not been established.

**Usual geriatric dose**
Oral, initially no more than 1 capsule two times a day, the dosage then
   being adjusted as needed and tolerated.

**Strength(s) usually available**
U.S.—
   5 mg of chlordiazepoxide hydrochloride and 2.5 mg of clidinium bro-
      mide per capsule (Rx) [*Clindex; Clinoxide; Clipoxide; Librax; Li-
      dox; Lidoxide; Zebrax;* GENERIC].
Canada—
   5 mg of chlordiazepoxide hydrochloride and 2.5 mg of clidinium bro-
      mide per capsule (Rx) [*Apo-Chlorax; Corium; Librax*].

**Auxiliary labeling**
• Take before meals.
• Avoid alcoholic beverages.
• May cause drowsiness.

Revised: 01/29/92
Interim revision: 08/10/94

## CHLORDIAZEPOXIDE-CONTAINING COMBINATIONS—

Chlordiazepoxide and Amitriptyline (Systemic)
Chlordiazepoxide and Clidinium (Systemic)

---

# CHLORHEXIDINE     Mucosal-Local†

VA CLASSIFICATION (Primary/Secondary): OR500/DE101
Note: For a listing of dosage forms and brand names by country availability, see *Dosage Forms* section(s). For a listing of brand names
   for the articles in this monograph, refer to the General Index.

   †Not commercially available in Canada.

## Category
Antibacterial (dental).

## Indications
Note: Bracketed information in the *Indications* section refers to uses that
   are not included in U.S. product labeling.

**Accepted**
Gingivitis (treatment)—Chlorhexidine is indicated for use between dental
   visits for the treatment of gingivitis that is characterized by redness
   and swelling of the gingivae or gingival bleeding upon probing.
[Gingivitis, necrotizing ulcerative, acute (treatment)]—Chlorhexidine is
   used along with other measures in the treatment of acute necrotizing
   ulcerative gingivitis (ANUG).
[Mouth infections (prophylaxis)] or
[Mouth infections (treatment)]—Chlorhexidine is used in the treatment of
   mouth infections in cancer patients who are being prepared for bone
   marrow transplants. Chlorhexidine is also used in the management of
   the oral complications that occur in leukemia patients.
   Chlorhexidine is also used following periodontal surgery to promote
   healing by minimizing mouth infections and plaque that may lead to
   increased inflammation and infection during the healing process.
[Stomatitis, denture (treatment)]—Chlorhexidine is used in the treatment
   of inflammation of the oral mucosa caused by bacterial or fungal actions associated with the wearing of dentures but should not be used
   when inflammation is caused by poor fit or other mechanical factors
   associated with dentures.
[Stomatitis, aphthous (treatment)]—Chlorhexidine is used in the management of minor aphthous ulcers.
[Plaque, dental (prophylaxis)]—Chlorhexidine is used for reduction of
   dental plaque.

Microorganisms with high susceptibility to chlorhexidine include some
   staphylococci, *Streptococcus mutans, Streptococcus salivarius, Candida albicans, Escherichia coli, Selenomonas,* and anaerobic propionic
   bacteria. *Streptococcus sanguis* has moderate susceptibility. Microorganisms with low susceptibility to chlorhexidine include *Proteus*
   strains, *Pseudomonas, Klebsiella,* and gram-negative cocci resembling
   *Veillonella.*
Samples of plaque taken during a 6-month period of use with chlorhexidine oral rinse showed a 54 to 97% reduction in certain aerobic and
   anaerobic bacteria. However, 3 months after chlorhexidine was discontinued, the number of bacteria in the plaque had returned to baseline levels.
A 6-month clinical study did not show any significant changes in bacterial
   resistance, overgrowth of potentially opportunistic organisms, or other
   adverse changes in the oral microbial ecosystem during the use of
   chlorhexidine. In addition, 3 months after chlorhexidine was discontinued, the resistance of plaque bacteria to the medication was found
   to be the same as before therapy was initiated.

## Pharmacology/Pharmacokinetics

**Physicochemical characteristics**
Molecular weight—Chlorhexidine gluconate: 897.77.

**Mechanism of action/Effect**
Because of its positive charge, chlorhexidine gluconate is adsorbed during
   oral rinsing onto the surfaces of teeth, plaque, and oral mucosa, which
   have a net negative charge. Subsequently, the adsorbed medication is
   gradually released from these sites by diffusion for up to 24 hours as
   the concentration of chlorhexidine gluconate in the saliva decreases.
   This release provides a continuing bacteriostatic effect.
Chlorhexidine gluconate is adsorbed onto the cell walls of microorganisms, which causes leakage of intracellular components. At low concentrations, chlorhexidine gluconate is bacteriostatic; at higher concentrations, chlorhexidine gluconate is bactericidal.

**Absorption**
Pharmacokinetic studies indicate that approximately 30% of chlorhexidine
   gluconate is retained in the oral cavity following rinsing and subsequently is slowly released into the oral fluids.
Studies using humans and animals have shown that chlorhexidine gluconate is poorly absorbed from the gastrointestinal tract. In humans, the
   mean plasma level of chlorhexidine gluconate reached a peak of 0.206
   mcg per gram 30 minutes following an oral dose of 300 mg.

**Elimination**
Following oral doses of 300 mg of chlorhexidine gluconate, excretion of
   chlorhexidine gluconate was primarily through the feces (approximately 90%); less than 1% of chlorhexidine gluconate was excreted
   in the urine. In addition, 12 hours after chlorhexidine gluconate was
   administered, it was not detectable in the plasma.

## Precautions to Consider

**Cross-sensitivity and/or related problems**
Patients sensitive to disinfectant skin cleansers containing chlorhexidine
   may be sensitive to chlorhexidine oral rinse also.

**Carcinogenicity**
Carcinogenesis was not observed in a drinking water study in rats where
   the highest dose of chlorhexidine used was 38 mg per kg of body
   weight (mg/kg) per day. This dose is at least 500 times the amount
   that would be ingested from the recommended human daily dose of
   chlorhexidine oral rinse.

**Mutagenicity**
Mutagenicity was not observed in 2 mammalian *in vivo* mutagenic studies
   with chlorhexidine.

**Pregnancy/Reproduction**
Fertility—Fertility studies have shown no evidence of impaired fertility in
   rats given chlorhexidine in doses of up to 100 mg/kg per day. This
   dose is approximately 100 times greater than the dose a person would
   receive if he/she ingested 30 mL (2 capfuls) of chlorhexidine oral rinse
   per day.
Pregnancy—Well-controlled studies in humans have not been done.
In animal studies, no evidence of harm to the fetus was observed in rats
   and rabbits given doses of chlorhexidine of up to 300 mg/kg per day
   and up to 40 mg/kg per day, respectively. These doses are approximately 300 and 40 times, respectively, greater than the dose a person
   would receive if she ingested 30 mL (2 capfuls) of chlorhexidine oral
   rinse per day.
FDA Pregnancy Category B.

**Breast-feeding**

Although it is not known whether chlorhexidine is distributed into breast milk, problems in humans have not been documented. In addition, studies in rats have shown no evidence of impaired parturition and no evidence of toxic effects to suckling pups when chlorhexidine was administered to dams at doses over 100 times greater than the dose a person would receive if she ingested 30 mL (2 capfuls) of chlorhexidine oral rinse per day.

**Pediatrics**

Appropriate studies on the relationship of age to the effects of this medicine have not been performed in the pediatric population. Safety and efficacy have not been established.

**Geriatrics**

Appropriate studies on the relationship of age to the effects of this medicine have not been performed in the geriatric population. However, no geriatrics-specific problems have been documented to date.

**Medical considerations/Contraindications**

The medical considerations/contraindications included here have been selected on the basis of their potential clinical significance (reasons given in parentheses where appropriate)—not necessarily inclusive (» = major clinical significance).

*Risk-benefit should be considered when the following medical problems exist:*

Anterior tooth restorations (front-tooth fillings)

(anterior tooth restorations having rough surfaces or margins may develop permanent discoloration from chlorhexidine, necessitating replacement for cosmetic reasons)

Periodontitis

(during clinical tests, an increase in supragingival calculus was noted in patients using chlorhexidine; it is not known whether use of chlorhexidine results in an increase in subgingival calculus)

(since gingival inflammation and bleeding may occur with both periodontitis and gingivitis and chlorhexidine oral rinse may reduce these signs, the presence or absence of these signs should not be used as indicators of periodontitis after the patient has been treated with chlorhexidine)

Sensitivity to chlorhexidine

**Patient monitoring**

The following may be especially important in patient monitoring (other tests may be warranted in some patients, depending on condition; » = major clinical significance):

Dental examination and prophylaxis

(tartar [calculus] deposits should be removed before therapy is initiated and during therapy at intervals of 6 months or less; the patient's condition should be reevaluated at intervals of 6 months or less, including monitoring of gingival pockets, because of the possible masking of coexisting periodontitis by chlorhexidine)

# Side/Adverse Effects

Note: Chlorhexidine causes staining of oral surfaces. Staining may be visible as early as 1 week after therapy; after 6 months of use, approximately 50% of patients may have a measurable increase in tooth stain and approximately 10% may have heavy staining. Staining is more pronounced in patients who have heavier accumulations of plaque. Tooth restorations having rough surfaces or margins may develop permanent staining. If this occurs on anterior surfaces, it may be necessary to replace the tooth restoration for cosmetic reasons.

Some patients develop an alteration in taste perception during treatment with chlorhexidine. This effect usually becomes less noticeable with continued treatment. No cases of permanent taste alteration have been reported.

No serious systemic side/adverse effects associated with the use of chlorhexidine oral rinse were reported during the clinical trials.

The following side/adverse effects have been selected on the basis of their potential clinical significance (possible signs and symptoms in parentheses where appropriate)—not necessarily inclusive:

**Those indicating need for medical attention**

Incidence rare

*Allergic reaction* (nasal congestion; shortness of breath or troubled breathing; skin rash, hives, or itching; swelling of face)

**Those indicating need for medical attention only if they continue or are bothersome**

Incidence more frequent

*Change in taste; increase in tartar (calculus) on teeth; staining of teeth, mouth, tooth restorations (fillings), and dentures or other mouth appliances*

Incidence less frequent or rare

*Parotid duct obstruction or parotitis* (swollen glands on side of face or neck); *superficial desquamative lesions* (mouth irritation)—reported mainly in children ages 10 to 18 years; the lesions are transient and may be painless; *tongue tip irritation*

# Overdose

For more information on the management of overdose or unintentional ingestion, **contact a Poison Control Center** (see *Poison Control Center Listing*).

**Treatment of overdose**

Medical attention and symptomatic treatment are recommended if signs of alcohol intoxication develop or if more than 4 ounces of chlorhexidine oral rinse is ingested by a child weighing approximately 10 kg (22 pounds) or less.

# Patient Consultation

As an aid to patient consultation, refer to *Advice for the Patient, Chlorhexidine (Dental)*.

In providing consultation, consider emphasizing the following selected information (» = major clinical significance):

**Before using this medication**

» Conditions affecting use, especially:

Allergy to chlorhexidine or to disinfectant skin cleansers containing chlorhexidine

**Proper use of this medication**

Using medication after brushing and flossing; rinsing toothpaste completely from mouth with water before using oral rinse; not eating or drinking for several hours after using oral rinse

Using the cap of the original container to measure the dose or acquiring another measuring device to use; asking your pharmacist for help

» Swishing medication around in mouth for 30 seconds and spitting out; using full strength; not swallowing

» Proper dosing

Missed dose: Using as soon as possible; not using if almost time for next dose; not doubling doses

» Proper storage

**Precautions while using this medication**

Not rinsing mouth with water immediately after using medication, since doing so will increase medication's bitter aftertaste and may decrease medication's effect

Medication causes change in taste; change may last up to 4 hours after dose; change in taste should be less noticeable as medication is continued; after medication is discontinued, taste should return to normal

Staining and increase in tartar (calculus) may occur; brushing with tartar-control toothpaste and flossing teeth daily to help reduce tartar build-up; visiting dentist at least every 6 months for teeth cleaning and gum examination

» Getting emergency help at once if a child weighing 22 pounds (10 kg) or less drinks more than 4 ounces of dental rinse or if any child experiences symptoms of alcohol intoxication, such as slurred speech, sleepiness, or staggering or stumbling walk, after drinking the dental rinse

**Side/adverse effects**

Signs of potential side effects, especially allergic reaction

# Dental Dosage Forms

Note: Bracketed uses in the *Dosage Forms* section refer to categories of use and/or indications that are not included in U.S. product labeling.

## CHLORHEXIDINE GLUCONATE ORAL RINSE

**Usual adult dose**

Gingivitis—

Topical, to the gingival membranes, 15 mL of a 0.12% oral rinse for 30 seconds two times a day after brushing and flossing teeth.

Note: Therapy with chlorhexidine oral rinse should start immediately following a dental prophylaxis.

[Denture stomatitis]—

Soak the dentures in chlorhexidine oral rinse 0.12% for 1 to 2 minutes two times a day. Rinsing the mouth for 30 seconds two times a day or brushing the gums or dentures two times a day with chlorhexidine oral rinse 0.12% may also be required.

**Usual pediatric dose**

Children up to 18 years of age—Safety and efficacy have not been established.

## Strength(s) usually available

U.S.—

0.12% (Rx) [*Peridex* (alcohol 11.6%); *PerioGard* (alcohol 11.6%)].

Canada—

Not commercially available; compounding is required.

## Packaging and storage

Store above freezing at a temperature not exceeding 25 °C (77 °F), unless otherwise specified by manufacturer. Protect from light.

## Preparation of dosage form

If the medication is not commercially available, it may be compounded as follows—3 mL chlorhexidine gluconate 20% should be added to approximately 200 mL distilled water. Separately, 5 mL essence of peppermint should be combined with 5 mL ethanol 95% and then 15 mL glycerin should be added. This mixture should be combined with the chlorhexidine and water solution and enough distilled water added to make 500 mL.

## Auxiliary labeling

• Do not swallow.
• Do not dilute.

## Note

Dispense with patient package insert.

Dispense in original container, which includes a measuring cap, or in an amber glass container and include a device for measuring 15 mL (¹/₂ fluid ounce).

Revised: 05/16/94
Interim revision: 08/22/94

# CHLORMEZANONE   Systemic†

VA CLASSIFICATION (Primary): CN309

Note: For a listing of dosage forms and brand names by country availability, see *Dosage Forms* section(s). For a listing of brand names for the articles in this monograph, refer to the General Index.

†Not commercially available in Canada.

## Category

Antianxiety agent.

## Indications

### Accepted

Anxiety (treatment)—Chlormezanone may be useful for the treatment of mild anxiety and tension states. However, this medication generally has been replaced by more effective antianxiety agents. Chlormezanone should not be used for the stress of everyday life.

Effectiveness of chlormezanone for long-term (more than 4 months) management of anxiety has not been assessed by systematic clinical studies. The medication's efficacy should be reassessed at periodic intervals.

## Pharmacology/Pharmacokinetics

### Physicochemical characteristics

Molecular weight—273.73.

### Mechanism of action/Effect

The exact mechanism of action of chlormezanone as an antianxiety agent is not known; however, studies in animals have shown that chlormezanone acts on subcortical levels of the central nervous system (CNS). The CNS depressant actions of chlormezanone are similar to those of meprobamate.

### Absorption

Rapidly absorbed from gastrointestinal tract.

### Protein binding

Plasma—Moderate (48%).

### Biotransformation

Hepatic; partially metabolized by oxidation and hydrolysis and conjugated with glucuronic acid in the liver.

### Half-life

Plasma—About 24 hours.

### Onset of action

15 to 30 minutes.

### Time to peak concentration

Within 1 to 2 hours.

### Duration of action

Up to 6 hours or longer.

### Elimination

Renal; fecal.

## Precautions to Consider

### Pregnancy/Reproduction

Pregnancy—Studies have not been done in either animals or humans.

### Breast-feeding

Problems in humans have not been documented.

### Pediatrics

Appropriate studies on the relationship of age to the effects of chlormezanone have not been performed in the pediatric population. However, no pediatrics-specific problems have been documented to date.

### Geriatrics

Although appropriate studies on the relationship of age to the effects of chlormezanone have not been performed in the geriatric population, no geriatrics-specific problems have been documented to date. However, elderly patients are more likely to have age-related hepatic function impairment and renal function impairment, which may require reduction of dosage in patients receiving chlormezanone.

### Drug interactions and/or related problems

The following drug interactions and/or related problems have been selected on the basis of their potential clinical significance (possible mechanism in parentheses where appropriate)—not necessarily inclusive (» = major clinical significance):

Note: Combinations containing any of the following medications, depending on the amount present, may also interact with this medication.

» Alcohol or
» CNS depression–producing medications (See *Appendix II*)
(concurrent use may increase the CNS depressant effects of either these medications or chlormezanone)

### Medical considerations/Contraindications

The medical considerations/contraindications included here have been selected on the basis of their potential clinical significance (reasons given in parentheses where appropriate)—not necessarily inclusive (» = major clinical significance).

*Risk-benefit should be considered when the following medical problems exist:*

Drug abuse or dependence, history of
(predisposition of patients to habituation and dependence)

Hepatic function impairment
(chlormezanone metabolized in liver)

Renal function impairment
(chlormezanone excreted via kidneys)

Sensitivity to chlormezanone

### Patient monitoring

The following may be especially important in patient monitoring (other tests may be warranted in some patients, depending on condition; » = major clinical significance):

Reassessment of medication's efficacy
(recommended at periodic intervals since the effectiveness of chlormezanone in long-term use [more than 4 months] has not been assessed by systematic clinical studies)

## Side/Adverse Effects

Note: Withdrawal symptoms have been reported rarely when chlormezanone was suddenly discontinued in patients who received the medication daily for weeks or months.

The following side/adverse effects have been selected on the basis of their potential clinical significance (possible signs and symptoms in parentheses where appropriate)—not necessarily inclusive:

**Those indicating need for medical attention**
Incidence less frequent
*Confusion; mental depression*

Incidence rare
*Allergic reaction* (skin rash); *cholestatic jaundice* (abdominal or stomach pains; aching muscles and joints; fever and chills; severe skin itching; skin rash; yellow eyes or skin)—reversible on discontinuation of medication; *swelling of the feet or lower legs; unusual excitement*

**Those indicating need for medical attention only if they continue or are bothersome**
Incidence more frequent
*Drowsiness*

Incidence less frequent
*Clumsiness or unsteadiness; difficult urination; dizziness; flushing or redness of skin; headache; nausea; trembling; weakness*

## Overdose

For specific information on the agents used in the management of chlormezanone overdose, see:
• *Charcoal, Activated (Oral-Local)* monograph.

For more information on the management of overdose or unintentional ingestion, **contact a Poison Control Center** (see *Poison Control Center Listing*).

**Clinical effects of overdose**
The following effects have been selected on the basis of their potential clinical significance (possible signs and symptoms in parentheses where appropriate)—not necessarily inclusive:

*Confusion, severe; drowsiness, severe; loss of reflexes; unusual tiredness or weakness, continuing*

**Treatment of overdose**
Recommended treatment consists of the following:
To decrease absorption—
If ingestion of drug is recent and patient is fully conscious, emesis should be induced.
If patient is comatose, gastric lavage may be performed if an endotracheal tube with cuff inflated is in place to prevent aspiration of gastric contents.
Administration of activated charcoal and a saline cathartic after gastric lavage and/or emesis to remove any remaining chlormezanone.
Supportive care—
General supportive therapy. Patients in whom intentional overdose is known or suspected should be referred for psychiatric consultation.

## Patient Consultation

As an aid to patient consultation, refer to *Advice for the Patient, Chlormezanone (Systemic).*

In providing consultation, consider emphasizing the following selected information (» = major clinical significance):

**Before using this medication**
» Conditions affecting use, especially:
Sensitivity to chlormezanone
Other medications, especially alcohol or other CNS depression–producing medications

**Proper use of this medication**
» Importance of not using more medication than the amount prescribed because of habit-forming potential and possible increase in side effects
» Proper dosing
Missed dose: Taking right away if remembered within an hour or so; not taking if remembered later; not doubling doses
» Proper storage

**Precautions while using this medication**
Regular visits to physician to check progress during prolonged therapy
Checking with physician before discontinuing medication after prolonged use; gradual dosage reduction may be necessary to avoid possibility of withdrawal symptoms
» Avoiding use of alcohol or other CNS depressants
» Suspected overdose: Getting emergency help at once
» Caution if dizziness or drowsiness occurs

**Side/adverse effects**
Signs of potential side effects, especially allergic reaction, cholestatic jaundice, confusion, edema, mental depression, and unusual excitement

## General Dosing Information

Dosage must be individualized. The smallest effective dosage should be used to avoid oversedation.

Following prolonged administration, chlormezanone should be withdrawn gradually to avoid the precipitation of withdrawal symptoms.

**For treatment of adverse effects**
Recommended treatment consists of the following:
• For drowsiness—Dosage should be reduced.

## Oral Dosage Forms
### CHLORMEZANONE TABLETS

**Usual adult and adolescent dose**
Antianxiety agent—
Oral, 100 to 200 mg three or four times a day.

**Usual pediatric dose**
Children up to 5 years of age: Dosage has not been established.
Children 5 to 12 years of age: Oral, 50 to 100 mg three or four times a day.

**Strength(s) usually available**
U.S.—
100 mg (Rx) [*Trancopal Caplets*].
200 mg (Rx) [*Trancopal Caplets*].
Canada—
Not commercially available.

**Packaging and storage**
Store below 40 °C (104 °F), preferably between 15 and 30 °C (59 and 86 °F), in a well-closed container, unless otherwise specified by manufacturer.

**Auxiliary labeling**
• Avoid alcoholic beverages.
• May cause drowsiness.

Revised: 03/09/93

---

**CHLOROPROCAINE**—See *Anesthetics (Parenteral-Local)*

---

# CHLOROQUINE  Systemic

VA CLASSIFICATION (Primary/Secondary): AP101/MS103; TN900
Note: For a listing of dosage forms and brand names by country availability, see *Dosage Forms* section(s). For a listing of brand names for the articles in this monograph, refer to the General Index.

## Category

Antiprotozoal—Chloroquine.
Antihypercalcemic—Chloroquine (Oral).
Antirheumatic (disease-modifying)—Chloroquine (Oral).
Lupus erythematosus suppressant—Chloroquine (Oral).
Polymorphous light eruption suppressant—Chloroquine (Oral).
Porphyria cutanea tarda suppressant—Chloroquine (Oral).

## Indications

Note: Bracketed information in the *Indications* section refers to uses that are not included in U.S. product labeling.

**General considerations**
Chloroquine-resistant strains of *Plasmodium falciparum*, originally seen only in Southeast Asia and South America, are now documented in all malarious areas except Central America west of the Canal Zone, the Middle East, and the Caribbean. Chloroquine is still the drug of choice for the treatment of susceptible strains of *P. falciparum* and the

other 3 malarial species; however, chloroquine-resistant *P. vivax* has recently been reported.

### Accepted

Malaria (prophylaxis and treatment)—Chloroquine is indicated in the suppressive treatment and the treatment of acute attacks of malaria caused by *P. vivax*, *P. malariae*, *P. ovale*, and chloroquine-susceptible strains of *P. falciparum*. The radical cure for *P. vivax* and *P. ovale* malaria requires the concurrent or subsequent administration of primaquine. However, there have been reports of chloroquine-resistant *P. vivax* in patients who have traveled to Papua New Guinea and Indonesia.

Liver abscess, amebic (treatment)—Chloroquine is indicated in the treatment of amebic liver abscess, usually in combination with an effective intestinal amebicide. However, it is not considered a primary drug.

[Hypercalcemia, sarcoid-associated (treatment)][1]—Chloroquine (oral) is used to reduce urinary calcium excretion and the levels of 1,25-dihydroxyvitamin D in the serum of sarcoid patients who are unable to take corticosteroids.

[Arthritis, juvenile (treatment)][1]—Chloroquine (oral) is used in the treatment of juvenile arthritis.

[Arthritis, rheumatoid (treatment)][1]—Chloroquine (oral) is indicated in the treatment of acute and chronic rheumatoid arthritis in patients who do not respond adequately to other less toxic antirheumatics. Chloroquine may be used in addition to nonsteroidal anti-inflammatory agents.

[Lupus erythematosus, discoid (treatment)][1] or

[Lupus erythematosus, systemic (treatment)][1]—Chloroquine (oral) is used as a suppressant for chronic discoid and systemic lupus erythematosus.

[Polymorphous light eruption (treatment)][1]—Chloroquine (oral) is used as a suppressant for polymorphous light eruption.

[Porphyria cutanea tarda (treatment)][1]—Chloroquine (oral) is used in the treatment of porphyria cutanea tarda.

[Urticaria, solar (treatment)][1] or

[Vasculitis, chronic cutaneous (treatment)][1]—Chloroquine is also used in the treatment of solar urticaria and chronic cutaneous vasculitis unresponsive to other therapy.

### Unaccepted

Chloroquine does not prevent relapses in patients with *P. vivax* or *P. ovale* malaria since it is not effective against exo-erythrocytic forms of the parasite. In these species, "hypnozoites," which remain dormant in the liver, are responsible for relapses.

Chloroquine is not indicated in the treatment of acute amebic dysentery or asymptomatic carriers.

---

[1]Not included in Canadian product labeling.

## Pharmacology/Pharmacokinetics

Note: Because chloroquine concentrates in the cellular fraction of blood, chloroquine concentrations measured in the blood are higher than those measured in the plasma, with concentration ratios between blood and plasma ranging from 1 to 25.

### Physicochemical characteristics

Molecular weight—Chloroquine: 319.88.
Chloroquine hydrochloride: 392.80.
Chloroquine phosphate: 515.87.

### Mechanism of action/Effect

Antiprotozoal—Malaria: Unknown, but may be based on ability of chloroquine to bind to and alter the properties of DNA. Chloroquine is also taken up into the acidic food vacuoles of the parasite in the erythrocyte. It increases the pH of the acid vesicles, interfering with vesicle functions and possibly inhibiting phospholipid metabolism. In suppressive treatment, chloroquine inhibits the erythrocytic stage of development of plasmodia. In acute attacks of malaria, chloroquine interrupts erythrocytic schizogony of the parasite. Its ability to concentrate in parasitized erythrocytes may account for its selective toxicity against the erythrocytic stages of plasmodial infection.

Antirheumatic—Chloroquine is thought to act as a mild immunosuppressant, inhibiting the production of rheumatoid factor and acute phase reactants. It also accumulates in white blood cells, stabilizing lysosomal membranes and inhibiting the activity of many enzymes, including collagenase and the proteases that cause cartilage breakdown.

### Absorption

Rate of absorption is variable; chloroquine is almost completely absorbed from the gastrointestinal tract. Bioavailability of tablets is approximately 89%.

### Distribution

Widely distributed in body tissues such as the eyes, heart, kidneys, liver, and lungs where retention is prolonged. Concentrations are 2 to 5 times higher in erythrocytes than in plasma. Very low concentrations are found in intestinal wall. Chloroquine crosses the placenta and is distributed into breast milk.

Apparent Vol$_D$ (in plasma)=204 L per kg (range, 116 to 285 L per kg); may be as large as 800 L per kg.

### Protein binding

Moderate (50 to 65%).

### Biotransformation

Hepatic (partially), to active de-ethylated metabolites. Principal metabolite is desethylchloroquine.

### Half-life

Terminal elimination half-life—1 to 2 months.

### Time to peak concentration

Adults (healthy, in plasma)—
  Oral: Approximately 3.5 hours.
  Parenteral (IV, IM, SQ): 30 minutes.
Children (with malaria, via nasogastric tube, in whole blood)—
  7.5 hours (range, 1 to 12 hours) after an initial dose of 10 mg [base] per kg of body weight and 5 mg [base] per kg of body weight six hours later.

### Peak concentrations

Adults (in plasma)—
  Oral:
    300 mg (base) in healthy patients—73 to 76 mcg per L.
  Parenteral:
    Intravenous infusion, 300 mg (base) over 24 minutes in healthy patients—Approximately 837 mcg per L.
    Intramuscular, 3 mg (base) per kg of body weight in malaria patients—236 to 256 mcg per L.
    Subcutaneous, 3 mg (base) per kg of body weight in malaria patients—Approximately 265 mcg per L.
Children (with malaria, in whole blood)—
  Oral (after an initial dose of 10 mg [base] per kg of body weight and 5 mg [base] per kg of body weight six hours later) via nasogastric tube: 897 mcg per L (491 to 1589 mcg per L).
  Parenteral (after first dose):
    Intravenous infusion, 5 mg (base) per kg of body weight over 4 hours—790 mcg per L (538 to 1249 mcg per L).
    Intramuscular, 3.5 mg (base) per kg of body weight—Approximately 718 mcg per L.
    Subcutaneous, 3.5 mg (base) per kg of body weight—Approximately 946 mcg per L.

### Elimination

Renal; 42 to 47% of chloroquine is excreted unchanged in the urine; 7 to 12% desethylchloroquine is excreted in urine. Chloroquine is excreted very slowly and may persist in urine for months or years after medication is discontinued. Urine acidification increases renal excretion by 20 to 90%.

Hemodialysis—Hemodialysis increases the clearance of chloroquine; however, due to chloroquine's large volume of distribution, hemodialysis may not remove appreciable amounts in an overdose.

## Precautions to Consider

### Cross-sensitivity and/or related problems

Patients hypersensitive to hydroxychloroquine may also be hypersensitive to chloroquine, a structurally similar 4-aminoquinoline compound.

### Pregnancy/Reproduction

Chloroquine crosses the placenta. Use is not recommended during pregnancy except in the suppression or treatment of malaria or hepatic amebiasis since malaria poses greater potential danger to the mother and fetus (i.e., abortion and death) than prophylactic administration of chloroquine. Chloroquine, given in weekly chemoprophylactic doses, has not been shown to cause adverse effects on the fetus. However, risk-benefit must be considered since chloroquine, given in therapeutic doses, has been shown to cause central nervous system (CNS) damage, including ototoxicity (auditory and vestibular); congenital deafness; retinal hemorrhages; and abnormal retinal pigmentation.

Chloroquine has been shown to accumulate selectively in melanin structures of fetal eyes of mice. It may be retained in ocular tissues for up to 5 months after elimination from the blood.

### Breast-feeding

Chloroquine is distributed into breast milk. Although problems in humans have not been documented, risk-benefit must be considered since infants and children are especially sensitive to the effects of chloroquine.

### Pediatrics

Infants and children are especially sensitive to the effects of chloroquine. Fatalities have been reported following the ingestion of as little as 300 mg of chloroquine base in a 12-month-old child. In addition, severe reactions and sudden death have been reported following parenteral administration of chloroquine in children. If chloroquine hydrochloride injection is given intravenously in pediatric patients, it should be diluted and administered very slowly.

### Geriatrics
No information is available on the relationship of age to the effects of chloroquine in geriatric patients.

### Drug interactions and/or related problems
The following drug interactions and/or related problems have been selected on the basis of their potential clinical significance (possible mechanism in parentheses where appropriate)—not necessarily inclusive (» = major clinical significance):

Note: Combinations containing any of the following medications, depending on the amount present, may also interact with this medication.

Penicillamine
(concurrent use of penicillamine with chloroquine may increase penicillamine plasma concentrations, increasing the potential for serious hematologic and/or renal adverse reactions, as well as the possibility of severe skin reactions)

### Medical considerations/Contraindications
The medical considerations/contraindications included here have been selected on the basis of their potential clinical significance (reasons given in parentheses where appropriate)—not necessarily inclusive (» = major clinical significance).

**Risk-benefit should be considered when the following medical problems exist:**
» Blood disorders, severe
(chloroquine may cause blood dyscrasias, including agranulocytosis, aplastic anemia, neutropenia, or thrombocytopenia)

Gastrointestinal disorders, severe
(chloroquine may cause gastrointestinal irritation)

Glucose-6-phosphate dehydrogenase (G6PD) deficiency
(chloroquine may cause hemolytic anemia in G6PD-deficient patients, although this is unlikely when chloroquine is given in therapeutic doses)

» Hepatic function impairment
(because chloroquine is metabolized in the liver, hepatic function impairment may increase blood concentrations of chloroquine, increasing the risk of side effects)

Hypersensitivity to chloroquine or hydroxychloroquine

» Neurological disorders, severe
(chloroquine may cause polyneuritis, ototoxicity, seizures, or neuromyopathy)

Porphyria
(chloroquine may cause exacerbation of porphyria)

Psoriasis
(chloroquine may precipitate severe attacks of psoriasis)

» Retinal or visual field changes, presence of
(chloroquine may cause corneal opacities, keratopathy, or retinopathy)

### Patient monitoring
The following may be especially important in patient monitoring (other tests may be warranted in some patients, depending on condition; » = major clinical significance):

» Complete blood counts (CBCs)
(recommended periodically during prolonged daily therapy with chloroquine; if severe blood dyscrasias occur that are not attributable to the disease being treated, discontinuation of chloroquine should be considered)

» Neuromuscular examinations, including knee and ankle reflexes
(recommended periodically during long-term therapy with chloroquine to detect muscle weakness; if muscle weakness occurs, chloroquine should be discontinued)

» Ophthalmologic examinations, including visual acuity, expert slit-lamp, funduscopic, and visual field tests
(recommended before and at least every 3 to 6 months during prolonged daily therapy since irreversible retinal damage has been reported with long-term or high-dosage therapy; serious ocular injury has been thought to be correlated with a total cumulative dose of greater than 100 grams [base] of chloroquine; however, a daily dose of greater than 150 mg [base], or 2.4 mg [base] per kg daily, of chloroquine may be a more important determinant; any retinal or visual abnormality that is not fully explainable by difficulties of accommodation or corneal opacities should be monitored fol-

lowing discontinuation of therapy, since retinal changes and visual disturbances may progress even after cessation of therapy)

## Side/Adverse Effects

Note: Side/adverse effects of chloroquine are usually dose-related. When chloroquine is used for the short-term treatment of malaria or other parasitic diseases, side/adverse effects are usually mild and reversible. However, following prolonged use and/or high-dose therapy such as in the treatment of rheumatoid arthritis, lupus erythematosus, or polymorphous light eruption, side/adverse effects may be serious and sometimes irreversible.

Irreversible retinal damage may be more likely to occur when the daily dosage equals or exceeds the equivalent of 150 mg (base), or 2.4 mg (base) per kg per day of chloroquine.

The following side/adverse effects have been selected on the basis of their potential clinical significance (possible signs and symptoms in parentheses where appropriate)—not necessarily inclusive:

### Those indicating need for medical attention
Incidence less frequent
*Ocular toxicity such as corneal opacities* (blurred vision or any other change in vision); *keratopathy* (blurred vision or any other change in vision); *or retinopathy* (blurred vision or any other change in vision)
Incidence rare
*Blood dyscrasias such as agranulocytosis* (sore throat and fever); *aplastic anemia* (weakness; fatigue); *neutropenia* (sore throat and fever); *or thrombocytopenia* (bleeding; bruising); *cardiovascular toxicity such as hypotension* (feeling faint or lightheaded); *or prolonged QRS interval; emotional changes or psychosis* (mood or other mental changes); *neuromyopathy* (increased muscle weakness); *ototoxicity* (any loss of hearing, ringing or buzzing in ears)—usually in patients with pre-existing auditory damage; *seizures*

### Those indicating need for medical attention only if they continue or are bothersome
Incidence more frequent
*Ciliary muscle dysfunction* (difficulty in reading); *gastrointestinal irritation* (diarrhea; loss of appetite; nausea; stomach cramps or pain; vomiting); *headache; itching*—especially in black patients, but not an indication for discontinuing their therapy
Incidence less frequent
*Bleaching of hair or increased hair loss; blue-black discoloration of skin, fingernails, or inside of mouth*—with prolonged oral therapy; *skin rash or itching*

### Those indicating possible retinal changes or visual disturbances and the need for medical attention if they occur or progress after medication is discontinued
*Blurred vision or any other change in vision*

## Overdose
For specific information on the agents used in the management of chloroquine overdose, see:
- *Charcoal, Activated (Oral-Local)* monograph;
- *Diazepam* in *Benzodiazepines (Systemic)* monograph; and/or
- *Sympathomimetic Agents—Cardiovascular Use (Parenteral-Systemic)* monograph.

For more information on the management of overdose or unintentional ingestion, **contact a Poison Control Center** (see *Poison Control Center Listing*).

After ingestion of an overdose of chloroquine, toxic symptoms may occur within 30 minutes, and death may occur as soon as 3 hours postingestion. Doses of chloroquine phosphate as small as 300 mg in children, and 2.25 to 3 grams in adults, may be fatal.

### Clinical effects of overdose
The following effects have been selected on the basis of their potential clinical significance (possible signs and symptoms in parentheses where appropriate)—not necessarily inclusive:
Acute
*Cardiovascular toxicities* (conduction disturbances; hypotension); *neurotoxicity* (drowsiness; headache; hyperexcitability; seizures; coma); *respiratory and cardiac arrest; visual disturbances* (blurred vision)

### Treatment of overdose
Since there is no specific antidote, treatment of chloroquine overdose should be symptomatic and supportive.
To decrease absorption—
Gastric lavage may be performed to empty the stomach. Activated charcoal should be administered with a cathartic. The dose of ac-

tivated charcoal should be 5 to 10 times the estimated dose of chloroquine ingested.

To enhance elimination—
Forcing diuresis and acidifying the urine, with ammonium chloride, for example, can help promote urinary excretion of chloroquine. The dose of the acidifying agent should be adjusted to maintain a urinary pH of 5.5 to 6.5. Monitoring of plasma potassium is recommended. Use with caution in patients with renal function impairment and/or metabolic acidosis.

Specific treatment—
For repetitive seizures or status epilepticus: Treat with intravenous diazepam (in 2.5 to 5.0 mg increments).
For life-threatening ventricular arrhythmias or cardiac arrest: Manage appropriately, as per Advanced Cardiac Life Support guidelines.
For hypotension and circulatory shock: Fluids should be administered at a sufficient rate to maintain urine output. Intravenous pressors and/or inotropic drugs, such as norepinephrine, dopamine, isoproterenol, or dobutamine, may be administered if required. High-dose diazepam infusion has been reported to improve hemodynamic function. Epinephrine has been shown to decrease the myocardial depressant and vasodilatory effects of chloroquine.

Supportive care—
Supportive measures such as securing and maintaining a patent airway, administering oxygen, and instituting assisted or controlled respiration may be required. In severe overdoses, early mechanical ventilation has been suggested to prevent hypoxemia. Patients in whom intentional overdose is confirmed or suspected should be referred for psychiatric consultation.

## Patient Consultation

As an aid to patient consultation, refer to *Advice for the Patient, Chloroquine (Systemic)*.

In providing consultation, consider emphasizing the following selected information (» = major clinical significance):

### Before using this medication
» Conditions affecting use, especially:
Hypersensitivity to chloroquine or hydroxychloroquine
Pregnancy—May cause toxicity to the fetus when given to mother in therapeutic doses; however, chloroquine has not been shown to cause adverse effects in the fetus when used as a prophylactic agent against malaria or hepatic amebiasis
Use in children—Infants and children are especially sensitive to effects of chloroquine
Other medical problems, especially impaired hepatic function, severe blood disorders, severe neurologic disorders, or presence of retinal or visual field changes

### Proper use of this medication
» Taking with meals or milk to minimize possible gastrointestinal irritation
» Keeping medication out of reach of children; fatalities reported with as little as 300 mg of chloroquine base (1 tablet) in a 12-month-old child
» Importance of not taking more medication than the amount prescribed
» Compliance with full course of therapy
» Importance of not missing doses and taking medication on regular schedule
» Proper dosing
Missed dose: If dosing schedule is—
Every 7 days: Taking as soon as possible
Once a day: Taking as soon as possible; not taking if not remembered until next day; not doubling doses
More than once a day: Taking right away if remembered within an hour or so; not taking if not remembered until later; not doubling doses
» Proper storage
*For prevention of malaria*
Starting medication 1 to 2 weeks before entering malarious area to ascertain patient response and allow time to substitute another medication if reactions occur
» Continuing medication while staying in area and for 4 weeks after leaving area; checking with physician immediately if fever develops while traveling or within 2 months after departure from endemic area

### Precautions while using this medication
» Regular visits to physician to check for blood problems, muscle weakness, and ophthalmologic examinations during or after long-term therapy
Checking with physician if no improvement within a few days (or a few weeks or months for arthritis)

» Caution if blurred vision, difficulty in reading, or other change in vision occurs
*Mosquito-control measures to reduce the chance of getting malaria:*
Avoiding exposure to mosquitoes, especially at peak feeding times (between dusk and dawn)
Sleeping in screened or air-conditioned room or under mosquito netting sprayed with insecticide
Wearing long-sleeved shirts or blouses and long trousers to protect arms and legs between dusk and dawn
Applying mosquito repellent to uncovered areas of skin between dusk and dawn
Using mosquito coils or spray

### Side/adverse effects
Signs of potential side effects, especially ocular toxicity such as corneal opacities, keratopathy, or retinopathy; blood dyscrasias such as agranulocytosis, aplastic anemia, or thrombocytopenia; cardiovascular toxicity such as hypotension or prolonged QRS interval; emotional changes or psychosis; neuromyopathy; ototoxicity; and seizures

## General Dosing Information

Long-term and/or high-dosage therapy may cause irreversible retinal damage and/or neurosensorial deafness.

Chloroquine should be discontinued if any of the following problems occur: any abnormality in visual acuity, visual fields, retinal macular changes, or any visual symptoms; muscle weakness; or severe blood disorders.

Malaria-suppressive therapy should be started 1 to 2 weeks before the patient enters a malarious area and should be continued for 4 weeks after patient leaves the area. Starting the medication in advance will help to determine the patient's tolerance to the medication and allow time to substitute other antimalarials if the patient develops allergies to the medication or other adverse effects.

### For oral dosage form only
Chloroquine should be taken with meals or milk to minimize the possibility of gastrointestinal irritation.

When chloroquine is used in the treatment of rheumatoid arthritis, up to 6 months of therapy may be required for it to reach its maximum effectiveness.

### For parenteral dosage forms only
If chloroquine hydrochloride injection is given intravenously in pediatric patients, it should be diluted and administered very slowly.

## Oral Dosage Forms

Note: Bracketed uses in the *Dosage Forms* section refer to categories of use and/or indications that are not included in U.S. product labeling.

### CHLOROQUINE PHOSPHATE TABLETS USP

**Usual adult and adolescent dose**
Malaria—
Suppressive: Oral, 500 mg (300 mg base) once every seven days.
Therapeutic: Oral, 1 gram (600 mg base) initially, followed by 500 mg (300 mg base) in six to eight hours, and 500 mg (300 mg base) once a day on the second and third days.
Liver abscess, amebic—
In combination with other "tissue-acting" antiprotozoals: Oral, 250 mg (150 mg base) four times a day for two days, followed by 250 mg (150 mg base) two times a day for at least two to three weeks.
Note: The dosage schedule may be revised up or down, if necessary, or the course of therapy may be repeated.
[Antirheumatic (disease-modifying)][1]—
Oral, up to 4 mg (2.4 mg base) per kg of lean body weight daily.
[Lupus erythematosus suppressant][1]—
Oral, up to 4 mg (2.4 mg base) per kg of lean body weight daily.
[Polymorphous light eruption suppressant][1]—
Oral, 250 mg (150 mg base) two times a day for two weeks; then 250 mg (150 mg base) once a day.

**Usual pediatric dose**
Malaria—
Suppressive: Oral, 8.3 mg (5 mg base) per kg of body weight, not to exceed the adult dose, once every seven days.
Therapeutic: Oral, 41.7 mg (25 mg base) per kg of body weight administered over a period of three days as follows: 16.7 mg (10 mg base) per kg of body weight, not to exceed a single dose of 1 gram (600 mg base); then 8.3 mg (5 mg base) per kg of body weight, not to exceed a single dose of 500 mg (300 mg base), six, twenty-four, and forty-eight hours after the first dose.

Liver abscess, amebic—
   Oral, 10 mg (6 mg base) per kg of body weight (up to a maximum of 500 mg [300 mg base]) per day for three weeks.

Note: Children are especially sensitive to the effects of chloroquine.

### Strength(s) usually available
U.S.—
   250 mg (equivalent to 150 mg base) (Rx) [GENERIC].
   500 mg (equivalent to 300 mg base) (Rx) [*Aralen;* GENERIC].
Canada—
   250 mg (equivalent to 150 mg base) (Rx) [*Aralen*].

### Packaging and storage
Store below 40 °C (104 °F), preferably between 15 and 30 °C (59 and 86 °F), unless otherwise specified by manufacturer. Store in a well-closed container.

### Auxiliary labeling
• Continue medication for full time of treatment.
• Keep out of reach of children.
• Take with food or milk.

### Note
Explain potential danger of accidental overdose in children.

Consider dispensing in unit-dose packaging in child-resistant containers ("double-barrier" packaging).

## Parenteral Dosage Forms
### CHLOROQUINE HYDROCHLORIDE INJECTION USP

#### Usual adult and adolescent dose
Malaria—
   Intramuscular, initially 200 to 250 mg (160 to 200 mg base), repeated in six hours if necessary, not to exceed 1 gram (800 mg base) in the first twenty-four hours.
Liver abscess, amebic—
   Intramuscular, 200 to 250 mg (160 to 200 mg base) per day for ten to twelve days.

Note: Slow intravenous infusion, over at least four hours, has not been associated with any increase in side effects compared with oral administration.

#### Usual pediatric dose
Malaria—
   Intramuscular or subcutaneous, 4.4 mg (3.5 mg base) per kg of body weight, repeated in six hours if necessary, not to exceed a total

dose of 12.5 mg (10 mg base) per kg of body weight per twenty-four hours.
   Intravenous infusion, initially 16.6 mg (13.3 mg base) per kg of body weight over eight hours, followed by 8.3 mg (6.6 mg base) per kg of body weight every six to eight hours over at least four hours.
Liver abscess, amebic—
   Intramuscular, 7.5 mg (6 mg base) per kg of body weight per day for ten to twelve days.

Note: In no instance should a single intramuscular or subcutaneous dose exceed 6.25 mg (5 mg base) per kg of body weight, since children are especially sensitive to the effects of the 4-aminoquinolines. Severe reactions and sudden death have been reported following parenteral administration in children.

### Strength(s) usually available
U.S.—
   50 mg (equivalent to 40 mg base) per mL (Rx) [*Aralen HCl*].
Canada—
   Not commercially available.

### Packaging and storage
Store below 40 °C (104 °F), preferably between 15 and 30 °C (59 and 86 °F), unless otherwise specified by manufacturer. Protect from freezing.

---

¹Not included in Canadian product labeling.

Revised: 8/11/95

---

## CHLOROTHIAZIDE—See *Diuretics, Thiazide (Systemic)*

---

## CHLOROTHIAZIDE-CONTAINING COMBINATIONS—
Methyldopa and Chlorothiazide (Systemic)—See *Methyldopa and Thiazide Diuretics (Systemic)*
Reserpine and Chlorothiazide (Systemic)—See *Rauwolfia Alkaloids and Thiazide Diuretics (Systemic)*

---

## CHLOROTRIANISENE—See *Estrogens (Systemic)*

---

# CHLOROXINE    Topical†

VA CLASSIFICATION (Primary): DE400
Note: For a listing of dosage forms and brand names by country availability, see *Dosage Forms* section(s). For a listing of brand names for the articles in this monograph, refer to the General Index.

---

†Not commercially available in Canada.

## Category
Antiseborrheic.

## Indications
### Accepted
Dandruff (treatment) or
Dermatitis, seborrheic, of scalp (treatment)—Chloroxine is indicated in the treatment of dandruff and mild to moderately severe seborrheic dermatitis of the scalp.

## Pharmacology/Pharmacokinetics
### Physicochemical characteristics
Molecular weight—214.05.

### Mechanism of action/Effect
Although the mechanism of action is not understood, chloroxine may slow down mitotic activity in the epidermis, thereby reducing excessive scaling associated with dandruff or seborrheic dermatitis of the scalp.

### Other actions/effects
Chloroxine has an antibacterial action, inhibiting the growth of gram-positive as well as some gram-negative organisms.

Also, chloroxine has shown some antifungal activity against certain dermatophytes and yeasts.

### Onset of action
Improvement in condition is usually noticeable after 14 days of therapy.

## Precautions to Consider
### Cross-sensitivity and/or related problems
Patients sensitive to hydroxyquinolines (for example, clioquinol [iodochlorhydroxyquin] or iodoquinol [diiodohydroxyquin]) or edetate disodium may be sensitive to this medication also.

### Carcinogenicity
No long-term studies in animals have been done to evaluate the carcinogenic potential of this medication.

### Mutagenicity
Results of the *in vitro* Ames Salmonella/Microsome Plate test indicate that this medication is non-mutagenic.

### Pregnancy/Reproduction
Pregnancy—Studies have not been done in humans.
Studies have not been done in animals.
FDA Pregnancy Category C.

### Breast-feeding
It is not known whether chloroxine is distributed into breast milk. However, problems in humans have not been documented.

### Pediatrics
Appropriate studies on the relationship of age to the effects of this medication have not been performed in the pediatric population.

### Geriatrics

Appropriate studies on the relationship of age to the effects of this medication have not been performed in the geriatric population. However, no geriatrics-specific problems have been documented to date.

### Medical considerations/Contraindications

The medical considerations/contraindications included here have been selected on the basis of their potential clinical significance (reasons given in parentheses where appropriate)—not necessarily inclusive (» = major clinical significance).

*Risk-benefit should be considered when the following medical problems exist:*
» Acutely inflamed or exudative lesions of scalp
   Sensitivity to chloroxine

## Side/Adverse Effects

The following side/adverse effects have been selected on the basis of their potential clinical significance (possible signs and symptoms in parentheses where appropriate)—not necessarily inclusive:

**Those indicating need for medical attention**
   *Allergic reaction* (skin rash); *scalp irritation or burning not present before therapy*

**Those indicating need for medical attention only if they continue or are bothersome**
   *Chemical conjunctivitis* (eye irritation)—may occur if this medication enters the eyes; *dryness or increased itching of scalp*

## Patient Consultation

As an aid to patient consultation, refer to *Advice for the Patient, Chloroxine (Topical)*.

In providing consultation, consider emphasizing the following selected information (» = major clinical significance):

**Before using this medication**
» Conditions affecting use, especially:
   Sensitivity to hydroxyquinolines, such as iodoquinol or clioquinol, or to edetate disodium or chloroxine
   Other medical problems, especially acutely inflamed or exudative lesions of scalp

**Proper use of this medication**
» Not using medication if blistered, raw, or oozing areas are present on scalp
» Avoiding contact with the eyes; if contact occurs, thoroughly flushing eyes with cool water
   Proper administration
      Wetting hair and scalp with lukewarm water
      Applying enough medication to scalp to work up lather; rubbing in well
      Allowing lather to remain on scalp for 3 minutes, then rinsing
      Applying medication again and rinsing thoroughly
      Using twice a week or as directed by physician
» Proper dosing
» Proper storage

**Precautions while using this medication**
   Medication may slightly discolor light-colored hair

**Side/adverse effects**
   Signs of potential side effects, especially allergic reaction and scalp irritation or burning not present before therapy

## General Dosing Information

Chloroxine should be massaged thoroughly onto the wet scalp. The lather should remain on the scalp for approximately 3 minutes; then the hair and scalp should be rinsed. The application should be repeated; then the hair and scalp should be rinsed thoroughly. Two treatments per week are usually sufficient.

## Topical Dosage Forms

### CHLOROXINE LOTION SHAMPOO

**Usual adult and adolescent dose**
Dandruff (treatment) or
Dermatitis, seborrheic, of scalp (treatment)—
   Topical, to the scalp, two times a week.

**Usual pediatric dose**
Dosage has not been established.

**Strength(s) usually available**
U.S.—
   2% (Rx) [*Capitrol* (benzyl alcohol 1%)].

Canada—
   Not commercially available.

**Packaging and storage**
Store below 40 °C (104 °F), preferably between 15 and 30 °C (59 and 86 °F), in a well-closed container, unless otherwise specified by manufacturer. Protect from freezing.

**Auxiliary labeling**
• For external use only.

Revised: 01/21/94

---

## CHLORPHENESIN—See *Skeletal Muscle Relaxants (Systemic)*

---

## CHLORPHENIRAMINE—See *Antihistamines (Systemic)*

---

## CHLORPHENIRAMINE-CONTAINING COMBINATIONS—

Chlorpheniramine and Dextromethorphan (Systemic)—See *Cough/Cold Combinations (Systemic)*
Chlorpheniramine, Dextromethorphan, and Acetaminophen (Systemic)—See *Cough/Cold Combinations (Systemic)*
Chlorpheniramine, Ephedrine, and Guaifenesin (Systemic)—See *Cough/Cold Combinations (Systemic)*
Chlorpheniramine, Ephedrine, Phenylephrine, and Carbetapentane (Systemic)—See *Cough/Cold Combinations (Systemic)*
Chlorpheniramine, Ephedrine, Phenylephrine, Dextromethorphan, Ammonium Chloride, and Ipecac (Systemic)—See *Cough/Cold Combinations (Systemic)*
Chlorpheniramine and Hydrocodone (Systemic)—See *Cough/Cold Combinations (Systemic)*
Chlorpheniramine, Phenindamine, Phenylephrine, Dextromethorphan, Acetaminophen, Salicylamide, Caffeine, and Ascorbic Acid (Systemic)—See *Cough/Cold Combinations (Systemic)*
Chlorpheniramine, Phenindamine, and Phenylpropanolamine (Systemic)—See *Antihistamines and Decongestants (Systemic)*
Chlorpheniramine, Pheniramine, Pyrilamine, Phenylephrine, Hydrocodone, Salicylamide, Caffeine, and Ascorbic Acid (Systemic)—See *Cough/Cold Combinations (Systemic)*
Chlorpheniramine and Phenylephrine (Systemic)—See *Antihistamines and Decongestants (Systemic)*
Chlorpheniramine, Phenylephrine, and Acetaminophen (Systemic)—See *Antihistamines, Decongestants, and Analgesics (Systemic)*
Chlorpheniramine, Phenylephrine, Acetaminophen, and Salicylamide (Systemic)—See *Antihistamines, Decongestants, and Analgesics (Systemic)*
Chlorpheniramine, Phenylephrine, Acetaminophen, Salicylamide, and Caffeine (Systemic)—See *Antihistamines, Decongestants, and Analgesics (Systemic)*
Chlorpheniramine, Phenylephrine, Codeine, and Ammonium Chloride (Systemic)—See *Cough/Cold Combinations (Systemic)*
Chlorpheniramine, Phenylephrine, Codeine, and Potassium Iodide (Systemic)—See *Cough/Cold Combinations (Systemic)*
Chlorpheniramine, Phenylephrine, and Dextromethorphan (Systemic)—See *Cough/Cold Combinations (Systemic)*
Chlorpheniramine, Phenylephrine, Dextromethorphan, Acetaminophen, and Salicylamide (Systemic)—See *Cough/Cold Combinations (Systemic)*
Chlorpheniramine, Phenylephrine, Dextromethorphan, and Guaifenesin (Systemic)—See *Cough/Cold Combinations (Systemic)*
Chlorpheniramine, Phenylephrine, Dextromethorphan, Guaifenesin, and Ammonium Chloride (Systemic)—See *Cough/Cold Combinations (Systemic)*
Chlorpheniramine, Phenylephrine, and Guaifenesin (Systemic)—See *Cough/Cold Combinations (Systemic)*
Chlorpheniramine, Phenylephrine, and Hydrocodone (Systemic)—See *Cough/Cold Combinations (Systemic)*
Chlorpheniramine, Phenylephrine, Hydrocodone, Acetaminophen, and Caffeine (Systemic)—See *Cough/Cold Combinations (Systemic)*
Chlorpheniramine, Phenylephrine, and Methscopolamine (Systemic)—See *Antihistamines, Decongestants, and Anticholinergics (Systemic)*
Chlorpheniramine, Phenylephrine, and Phenylpropanolamine (Systemic)—See *Antihistamines and Decongestants (Systemic)*
Chlorpheniramine, Phenylephrine, Phenylpropanolamine, Atropine, Hyoscyamine, and Scopolamine (Systemic)—See *Antihistamines, Decongestants, and Anticholinergics (Systemic)*

Chlorpheniramine, Phenylephrine, Phenylpropanolamine, Carbetapentane, and Potassium Guaiacolsulfonate (Systemic)—See *Cough/Cold Combinations (Systemic)*

Chlorpheniramine, Phenylephrine, Phenylpropanolamine, and Codeine (Systemic)—See *Cough/Cold Combinations (Systemic)*

Chlorpheniramine, Phenylephrine, Phenylpropanolamine, and Dextromethorphan (Systemic)—See *Cough/Cold Combinations (Systemic)*

Chlorpheniramine, Phenylephrine, Phenylpropanolamine, Dextromethorphan, Guaifenesin, and Acetaminophen (Systemic)—See *Cough/Cold Combinations (Systemic)*

Chlorpheniramine, Phenylephrine, Phenylpropanolamine, and Dihydrocodeine (Systemic)—See *Cough/Cold Combinations (Systemic)*

Chlorpheniramine and Phenylpropanolamine (Systemic)—See *Antihistamines and Decongestants (Systemic)*

Chlorpheniramine, Phenylpropanolamine, and Acetaminophen (Systemic)—See *Antihistamines, Decongestants, and Analgesics (Systemic)*

Chlorpheniramine, Phenylpropanolamine, Acetaminophen, and Caffeine (Systemic)—See *Antihistamines, Decongestants, and Analgesics (Systemic)*

Chlorpheniramine, Phenylpropanolamine, and Aspirin (Systemic)—See *Antihistamines, Decongestants, and Analgesics (Systemic)*

Chlorpheniramine, Phenylpropanolamine, Aspirin, and Caffeine (Systemic)—See *Antihistamines, Decongestants, and Analgesics (Systemic)*

Chlorpheniramine, Phenylpropanolamine, and Caramiphen (Systemic)—See *Cough/Cold Combinations (Systemic)*

Chlorpheniramine, Phenylpropanolamine, Codeine, Guaifenesin, and Acetaminophen (Systemic)—See *Cough/Cold Combinations (Systemic)*

Chlorpheniramine, Phenylpropanolamine, and Dextromethorphan (Systemic)—See *Cough/Cold Combinations (Systemic)*

Chlorpheniramine, Phenylpropanolamine, Dextromethorphan, and Acetaminophen (Systemic)—See *Cough/Cold Combinations (Systemic)*

Chlorpheniramine, Phenylpropanolamine, Dextromethorphan, and Ammonium Chloride (Systemic)—See *Cough/Cold Combinations (Systemic)*

Chlorpheniramine, Phenylpropanolamine, Dextromethorphan, and Aspirin (Systemic)—See *Cough/Cold Combinations (Systemic)*

Chlorpheniramine, Phenylpropanolamine, and Guaifenesin (Systemic)—See *Cough/Cold Combinations (Systemic)*

Chlorpheniramine, Phenylpropanolamine, Guaifenesin, Sodium Citrate, and Citric Acid (Systemic)—See *Cough/Cold Combinations (Systemic)*

Chlorpheniramine, Phenylpropanolamine, and Methscopolamine (Systemic)—See *Antihistamines, Decongestants, and Anticholinergics (Systemic)*

Chlorpheniramine, Phenyltoloxamine, Ephedrine, Codeine, and Guaiacol Carbonate (Systemic)—See *Cough/Cold Combinations (Systemic)*

Chlorpheniramine, Phenyltoloxamine, and Phenylephrine (Systemic)—See *Antihistamines and Decongestants (Systemic)*

Chlorpheniramine, Phenyltoloxamine, Phenylephrine, and Phenylpropanolamine (Systemic)—See *Antihistamines and Decongestants (Systemic)*

Chlorpheniramine, Phenyltoloxamine, Phenylpropanolamine, and Acetaminophen (Systemic)—See *Antihistamines, Decongestants, and Analgesics (Systemic)*

Chlorpheniramine and Pseudoephedrine (Systemic)—See *Antihistamines and Decongestants (Systemic)*

Chlorpheniramine, Pseudoephedrine, and Acetaminophen (Systemic)—See *Antihistamines, Decongestants, and Analgesics (Systemic)*

Chlorpheniramine, Pseudoephedrine, and Codeine (Systemic)—See *Cough/Cold Combinations (Systemic)*

Chlorpheniramine, Pseudoephedrine, and Dextromethorphan (Systemic)—See *Cough/Cold Combinations (Systemic)*

Chlorpheniramine, Pseudoephedrine, Dextromethorphan, and Acetaminophen (Systemic)—See *Cough/Cold Combinations (Systemic)*

Chlorpheniramine, Pseudoephedrine, Dextromethorphan, Acetaminophen, and Caffeine (Systemic)—See *Cough/Cold Combinations (Systemic)*

Chlorpheniramine, Pseudoephedrine, and Guaifenesin (Systemic)—See *Cough/Cold Combinations (Systemic)*

Chlorpheniramine, Pseudoephedrine, and Hydrocodone (Systemic)—See *Cough/Cold Combinations (Systemic)*

Chlorpheniramine, Pyrilamine, and Phenylephrine (Systemic)—See *Antihistamines and Decongestants (Systemic)*

Chlorpheniramine, Pyrilamine, Phenylephrine, and Acetaminophen (Systemic)—See *Antihistamines, Decongestants, and Analgesics (Systemic)*

Chlorpheniramine, Pyrilamine, Phenylephrine, and Phenylpropanolamine (Systemic)—See *Antihistamines and Decongestants (Systemic)*

Chlorpheniramine, Pyrilamine, Phenylephrine, Phenylpropanolamine, and Acetaminophen (Systemic)—See *Antihistamines, Decongestants, and Analgesics (Systemic)*

---

## CHLORPROMAZINE—See *Phenothiazines (Systemic)*

---

## CHLORPROPAMIDE—See *Antidiabetic Agents, Sulfonylurea (Systemic)*

---

## CHLORPROTHIXENE—See *Thioxanthenes (Systemic)*

---

## CHLORTETRACYCLINE—See *Tetracyclines (Ophthalmic); Tetracyclines (Topical)*

---

## CHLORTHALIDONE—See *Diuretics, Thiazide (Systemic)*

---

## CHLORTHALIDONE-CONTAINING COMBINATIONS—

Atenolol and Chlorthalidone (Systemic)—See *Beta-adrenergic Blocking Agents and Thiazide Diuretics (Systemic)*

Clonidine and Chlorthalidone (Systemic)

Reserpine and Chlorthalidone (Systemic)—See *Rauwolfia Alkaloids and Thiazide Diuretics (Systemic)*

---

## CHLORZOXAZONE—See *Skeletal Muscle Relaxants (Systemic)*

---

# CHLORZOXAZONE AND ACETAMINOPHEN   Systemic

**INN:** Acetaminophen—Paracetamol

**VA CLASSIFICATION (Primary):** MS200

**NOTE:** The *Chlorzoxazone and Acetaminophen (Systemic)* monograph is maintained on the USP DI electronic data base. For a printed copy of the most recent revision of the complete monograph, contact the USP Division of Information Development, 12601 Twinbrook Parkway, Rockville, MD 20852.

For information on the specific components of this combination, see the *USP DI* monographs for *Acetaminophen (Systemic)* and *Skeletal Muscle Relaxants (Systemic)*.

The information that follows is selectively abstracted from the complete monograph and is provided to facilitate drug use review and patient counseling.

Note: For a listing of dosage forms and brand names by country availability, see *Dosage Forms* section(s). For a listing of brand names for the articles in this monograph, refer to the General Index.

## Category

Analgesic–skeletal muscle relaxant.

## Indications

### Accepted

Spasm, skeletal muscle, accompanied by pain (treatment)—Chlorzoxazone and acetaminophen combination is indicated as an adjunct to other measures, such as rest and physical therapy, for relief of pain and muscle spasm associated with acute, painful musculoskeletal conditions.

## Patient Consultation

As an aid to patient consultation, refer to *Advice for the Patient, Chlorzoxazone and Acetaminophen (Systemic).*

In providing consultation, consider emphasizing the following selected information (» = major clinical significance):

**Before using this medication**
» Conditions affecting use, especially:
    Sensitivity to acetaminophen, aspirin, or chlorzoxazone
    Pregnancy—Acetaminophen crosses the placenta
    Breast-feeding—Acetaminophen is distributed into breast milk
    Other medications, especially alcohol or other CNS depression–producing medications
    Other medical problems, especially alcoholism (active), hepatic function impairment or other hepatic disease, and viral hepatitis

**Proper use of this medication**
» Importance of not taking more medication than the amount prescribed; acetaminophen may cause liver damage with long-term use or greater-than-recommended doses
» Proper dosing
    Missed dose: Taking as soon as possible; not taking if almost time for next dose; not doubling doses
» Proper storage

**Precautions while using this medication**
    Regular visits to physician if long-term therapy is prescribed
» Risk of overdose if other medications containing acetaminophen are used
» Avoiding alcohol or other CNS depressants during therapy unless prescribed or otherwise approved by physician
» Risk of hepatotoxicity may be increased if acetaminophen used with alcohol
    Not taking aspirin or other anti-inflammatory analgesics concurrently for more than a few days, unless directed by physician
» Caution if drowsiness, dizziness, or lightheadedness occurs
    Possible interference with some laboratory tests; preferably discussing use of the medication with physician in charge 3 to 4 days ahead of time; if this is not possible, informing physician in charge if acetaminophen taken within the past 3 or 4 days
    Diabetics: Possible false results with blood glucose tests; checking with physician, nurse, or pharmacist if changes in test results noted
» Suspected overdose: Getting emergency help at once even if no symptoms apparent; symptoms of severe acetaminophen overdosage may be delayed, but treatment must be begun as soon as possible; treatment started 24 hours or more after the overdose may be ineffective in preventing liver damage or fatality

**Side/adverse effects**
Medication may color the urine orange or reddish purple
Signs of potential side effects, especially agranulocytosis, anemia, angioedema, allergic dermatitis, gastrointestinal bleeding, hepatitis, renal colic, renal failure, sterile pyuria, and thrombocytopenia

## Oral Dosage Forms
### CHLORZOXAZONE AND ACETAMINOPHEN TABLETS

**Usual adult and adolescent dose**
Analgesic–skeletal muscle relaxant—
    Oral, 500 mg of chlorzoxazone and 600 mg of acetaminophen four times a day.

**Usual pediatric dose**
Administration of this combination medication to a child depends upon whether the appropriate dose of each ingredient, which must be individualized according to the child's age and weight, can be provided. Dosage of chlorzoxazone ranges between 125 and 500 mg, administered three or four times a day. The quantity of acetaminophen in one tablet of the chlorzoxazone and acetaminophen combination (300 mg) may be administered to children six years of age or older, but the quantity present in two tablets (600 mg) is higher than the maximum dose recommended for children younger than twelve years of age.

**Strength(s) usually available**
U.S.—
    Not commercially available.
Canada—
    250 mg of chlorzoxazone and 300 mg of acetaminophen (OTC) [*Parafon Forte* (scored; sodium bisulfite, tartrazine)].

**Auxiliary labeling**
• May cause drowsiness.
• Avoid alcoholic beverages.

Revised: 08/29/94

## CHLORZOXAZONE-CONTAINING COMBINATIONS—
Chlorzoxazone and Acetaminophen (Systemic)

---

# CHOLECYSTOGRAPHIC AGENTS, ORAL    Systemic

This monograph includes information on the following: Iocetamic Acid†; Iopanoic Acid; Ipodate†; Tyropanoate†.
INN:
    Tyropanoate—Sodium Tyropanoate
VA CLASSIFICATION (Primary/Secondary):
    Iocetamic Acid——DX102
    Iopanoic Acid——DX102
    Ipodate——DX102/HS852
    Tyropanoate——DX102
Note: For a listing of dosage forms and brand names by country availability, see *Dosage Forms* section(s). For a listing of brand names for the articles in this monograph, refer to the General Index.

---

†Not commercially available in Canada.

---

## Category
Note: Ipodate and tyropanoate are ionic radiopaque contrast media.
Diagnostic aid, radiopaque (gallbladder disorders)—Iocetamic Acid; Iopanoic Acid; Ipodate; Tyropanoate.
Antihyperthyroid agent—Ipodate.

## Indications
Note: Bracketed information in the *Indications* section refers to uses that are not included in U.S. product labeling.

**Accepted**
Cholecystography, oral—Oral cholecystographic agents are indicated for radiographic delineation of the gallbladder. However, oral cholecystography is no longer the primary test in the evaluation of gallbladder disease. Real-time ultrasonography is the procedure of choice in most patients suspected of having gallbladder disease. Oral cholecystography is being reserved for situations in which the diagnosis is uncertain

after ultrasonography, particularly in cases of chronic cholecystitis, or when there is a need to count or measure gallstones for extracorporeal shock wave lithotripsy (ESWL) or pharmacologic dissolution.

[Hyperthyroidism, in Graves' disease (treatment)]—Ipodate salts, and possibly iopanoic acid and tyropanoate, are used as an alternative treatment of Graves' hyperthyroidism, when conventional therapeutic agents are contraindicated or when rapid correction of thyrotoxicosis is needed. However, the efficacy of ipodate salts, and other cholecystographic agents, in other forms of hyperthyroidism, such as toxic multi-nodular goiter, has not been investigated.

Iopanoic acid and ipodate salts have been used for oral cholangiography to visualize the biliary ducts. However, cholescintigraphy performed after the intravenous injection of radioisotope-labeled substances that are rapidly excreted into the bile (e.g., technetium Tc 99m–labeled iminodiacetic acid derivatives) is the preferred method, especially in patients in whom acute cholecystitis is suspected.

## Pharmacology/Pharmacokinetics

**Physicochemical characteristics**
Molecular weight—
    Iocetamic acid: 613.96.
    Iopanoic acid: 570.93.
    Ipodate calcium: 1233.99.
    Ipodate sodium: 619.94.
    Tyropanoate sodium: 663.01.
pKa—
    Iocetamic acid: 4.1 and 4.25.
    Iopanoic acid: 4.8.

**Mechanism of action/Effect**
Diagnostic aid (gallbladder disorders; biliary tract disorders)—Organic iodine compounds block x-rays as they pass through the body, thereby allowing body structures containing iodine to be delineated in contrast

to those structures that do not contain iodine. The degree of opacity produced by these iodinated organic compounds is directly proportional to their iodine content. Radiopaque oral cholecystographic agents are concentrated in the functioning gallbladder and some may, upon contraction of the gallbladder, provide visualization of the extrahepatic ducts.

Antihyperthyroid agent—Ipodate inhibits peripheral conversion of thyroxine ($T_4$) to triiodothyronine ($T_3$). It also decreases the secretion of thyroid hormone in Graves' hyperthyroidism.

### Absorption
Generally well absorbed by passive diffusion across the gastrointestinal mucosa, primarily from the small intestine. However, iopanoic acid is poorly absorbed from the intestine in the absence of bile salts.

### Protein binding
High, to plasma albumin.

### Biotransformation
Hepatic (primarily converted to radiopaque glucuronic acid conjugates). Inorganic iodide is liberated during hepatic metabolism.

### Time to peak opacification:
Gallbladder—
  Iocetamic acid: 10 to 15 hours.
  Iopanoic acid: 14 to 19 hours.
  Ipodate: 10 to 12 hours.
  Tyropanoate: 4 to 10 hours.

### Elimination
Renal and fecal (primary route of excretion depends on the degree of binding to albumin and existing renal and/or hepatic disease). Most of administered dose is excreted within a week.
  Within 24 hours of administration, the following percentage of the dose is eliminated in the urine—
    Iocetamic acid: 62%.
    Iopanoic acid: 33%.
    Ipodate: 45%.
    Tyropanoate: 45%.

## Precautions to Consider

### Cross-sensitivity and/or related problems
Patients sensitive to iodine or other iodinated contrast media may be sensitive to these agents also.

### Carcinogenicity/Mutagenicity
Long-term animal studies to evaluate carcinogenic or mutagenic potential of cholecystographic agents have not been performed.

### Pregnancy/Reproduction
Pregnancy—Other organically bound iodine–containing preparations administered near term by intra-amniotic injection have caused hypothyroidism in some newborns. Also, elective contrast radiography of the abdomen is usually not recommended during pregnancy because of the risks to the fetus from radiation exposure.
*Iocetamic acid—*
  Studies in humans have not been done.
  Teratology studies in rats and rabbits have not shown that iocetamic acid causes adverse effects in the fetus.

  FDA Pregnancy Category B.
*Ipodate salts, iopanoic acid, and tyropanoate—*
  Studies with ipodate salts, iopanoic acid, and tyropanoate have not been done in either animals or humans.

  FDA Pregnancy Category C.

### Breast-feeding
Problems in humans have not been documented; however, risk-benefit must be considered since iocetamic acid, iopanoic acid, and tyropanoate are distributed into breast milk and the pharmacologic similarity of the oral cholecystographic agents suggests that the others may be distributed into breast milk also.

### Pediatrics
*Iocetamic acid and tyropanoate sodium—*
  Appropriate studies on the relationship of age to the effects of iocetamic acid or tyropanoate sodium have not been performed in the pediatric population. Safety and efficacy have not been established.
*Iopanoic acid and ipodate calcium—*
  Appropriate studies on the relationship of age to the effects of iopanoic acid or ipodate calcium have not been performed in the pediatric population. However, no pediatrics-specific problems have been documented to date.
*Ipodate sodium—*
  Studies performed to date using ipodate sodium in the treatment of neonatal hyperthyroidism due to Graves' disease, and in children up to 15 years of age with toxic ingestion of levothyroxine, have

not demonstrated pediatrics-specific problems that would limit the usefulness of ipodate sodium in children.

### Geriatrics
Elderly patients may be more sensitive to the toxic effects of oral cholecystographic agents; use of large or repeated doses over a period of several days is not recommended.

Dehydration in elderly patients receiving oral cholecystographic agents may lead to acute renal insufficiency; adequate hydration is recommended before and following administration of these agents.

The elderly may be more sensitive to the effects of cholecystographic agents on thyroid function. Iodine-induced thyrotoxicosis may occur 4 to 12 weeks following contrast radiography. Thyroid function monitoring may be needed in geriatric patients.

### Drug interactions and/or related problems
The following drug interactions and/or related problems have been selected on the basis of their potential clinical significance (possible mechanism in parentheses where appropriate)—not necessarily inclusive (» = major clinical significance):

See also *Diagnostic interference.*

Note: Combinations containing any of the following medications, depending on the amount present, may also interact with this medication.

Iodipamide meglumine, intravenous
  (hepatic excretion of iodipamide meglumine may be blocked after administration of oral cholecystographic agents, increasing the risk of adverse effects; administration of cholecystographic agents is not recommended within 24 hours before or after iodipamide meglumine)

Urographic agents, such as diatrizoate salts, iodamide, iothalamate salts, and ioxaglate salts
  (risk of renal toxicity may be increased when administration of oral cholecystographic agents is followed by urographic agents, especially in patients with hepatic or biliary function impairment)

### Diagnostic interference
The following have been selected on the basis of their potential clinical significance (possible effect in parentheses where appropriate)—not necessarily inclusive (» = major clinical significance):

With results of *this* test
*Due to other medications*
  Cholestyramine
    (concurrent use with cholecystographic agents may result in poor or non-visualization of gallbladder because of cholestyramine's high affinity for these agents; cholestyramine should be discontinued long enough [12 to 48 hours] to allow its complete evacuation from at least the small bowel prior to cholecystography)

*Due to medical problems or conditions*
  Gastrointestinal disorders, such as malabsorptive diseases, inflammatory small bowel disease, and short small intestines
    (absorption of cholecystographic agent may be decreased or impaired, resulting in nonvisualization)

  Hepatic or cystic duct obstruction
    (flow of cholecystographic agent to the gallbladder may be blocked, resulting in nonvisualization)

  Hepatic function impairment, severe, advanced
    (bilirubin concentration of more than 5 mg per 100 mL may result in nonvisualization)

With *other* diagnostic test results
  Hepatic function determinations
    (use of these agents may increase sulfobromophthalein [BSP] retention; BSP test should not be performed for at least 2 days following oral cholecystography)

  Thyroid function determinations and
  Thyroid imaging
    (cholecystographic agents may cause a decrease in radioactive iodine or pertechnetate ion uptake for a period varying from 1 week to several months; these agents may also depress total $T_3$ and elevate total $T_4$ and TSH values due to enzyme inhibition; other thyroid function tests not based on measurement of iodine are not affected)

  Urinalysis
    (use of these agents may produce false-positive results for up to 3 days following oral cholecystography. Pseudoalbuminuria may be present if sulfosalicylic acid and nitric acid ring tests are used; heat and acetic acid or colorimetric dip-strip method may be used to verify positive reactions)

With physiology/laboratory test values
Bilirubin, serum and
BSP, urine
(concentrations may be increased for a few days)
Uric acid, serum and urinary
(rate of excretion of uric acid may be increased, resulting in a decrease of uric acid serum concentration and an increase of urinary excretion values for a few days)

## Medical considerations/Contraindications

The medical considerations/contraindications included here have been selected on the basis of their potential clinical significance (reasons given in parentheses where appropriate)—not necessarily inclusive (» = major clinical significance).

See also *Diagnostic interference.*

*Except under special circumstances, this medication should not be used when the following medical problems exist:*

» Hepatorenal disease, advanced or
» Renal function impairment, severe
(use of cholecystographic agents may precipitate acute renal insufficiency)

*Risk-benefit should be considered when the following medical problems exist:*

Allergic reaction (anaphylaxis) to penicillins or to skin allergens, previous
(increased risk of anaphylactoid reaction in patients who have had a previous reaction to penicillins or to skin allergens)
Allergies or asthma, history of
(increased risk of hypersensitivity reactions)
Coronary artery disease
(increased risk of hypotension, bradycardia, and acute coronary insufficiency)
Dehydration, all patients, especially the elderly and/or those with pre-existing renal or hepatic disease
(increased risk of acute renal insufficiency)
» Hepatic function impairment, severe, advanced
(increased risk of renal toxicity and damage because of increased load of unchanged drug to the kidneys)
Hyperthyroidism
(thyroid storm may be precipitated)
Hyperuricemia
(administration of cholecystographic agents may increase risk of developing uric acid stones and decreased renal function; adequate hydration and alkalinization of the urine is recommended in these patients)
» Renal function impairment
(increased risk of acute renal insufficiency)
» Sensitivity to iodinated contrast media

## Patient monitoring

The following may be especially important in patient monitoring (other tests may be warranted in some patients, depending on condition; » = major clinical significance):

Blood pressure determinations
(recommended after administration of oral cholecystographic agent in patients with cardiovascular disease)
Blood urea nitrogen (BUN) determinations and
Creatinine determinations, serum and
Hepatic function monitoring and
Urinary output monitoring
(may be required after cholecystography in patients with liver disease)
Renal function determinations
(recommended before cholecystography in patients with liver disease, because of the possibility of acute renal insufficiency)
Thyroid function determinations
(iodine-induced thyrotoxicosis may occur 4 to 12 weeks following contrast radiography in geriatric patients; thyroid function monitoring may be needed)

## Side/Adverse Effects

Note: Acute renal insufficiency has been reported following oral administration of cholecystographic agents, especially when these agents were used in large doses or with other agents, or in dehydrated patients or those with hepatic disease.

The following side/adverse effects have been selected on the basis of their potential clinical significance (possible signs and symptoms in parentheses where appropriate)—not necessarily inclusive:

**Those indicating need for medical attention**
Incidence rare
*Pseudo-allergic reaction* (itching, skin rash or hives, swelling of skin); *unusual bleeding or bruising*—with iopanoic acid
Symptoms of overdose—reported only with iopanoic acid
*Severe diarrhea; severe nausea and vomiting; problems with urination*

**Those indicating need for medical attention only if they continue or are bothersome**
Incidence more frequent
*Mild diarrhea; mild to moderate nausea and vomiting*
Incidence less frequent or rare
*Abdominal or stomach spasms or cramps; severe diarrhea; difficult or painful urination; dizziness; frequent urge to urinate; headache; heartburn; severe or continuing nausea and vomiting*

## Overdose

### Treatment of overdose

Since there is no specific antidote for overdose with cholecystographic agents, treatment is symptomatic and supportive with possible utilization of the following:

To decrease absorption—Gastric lavage and administration of enema are recommended.

Specific treatment—

Administration of oral fluids to avoid concentration and possible precipitation or crystallization of the cholecystographic agent or uric acid in the kidneys.
Alkalinization of the urine to solubilize the glucoronide complex formed and the uric acid.
Use of cholestyramine to reduce absorption of the cholecystographic agent.

Monitoring—Frequent monitoring of blood pressure.

## Patient Consultation

As an aid to patient consultation, refer to *Advice for the Patient, Cholecystographic Agents, Oral (Diagnostic).*

In providing consultation, consider emphasizing the following selected information (» = major clinical significance):

### Description of use

Action in the body: Accumulation in gallbladder; visualization of radiopacity in gallbladder and extrahepatic ducts possible with x-rays

### Before having this test
» Conditions affecting use, especially:
Sensitivity to iodine or other iodinated contrast media
Pregnancy—Not recommended, because of possibility of hypothyroidism in newborn; risk to the fetus from radiation exposure
Breast-feeding—Distributed into breast milk
Use in the elderly—Increased sensitivity to toxic effects; importance of adequate hydration to prevent acute renal insufficiency; increased risk of thyrotoxicosis
Other medical problems, especially renal function impairment or severe hepatic function impairment

### Preparation for this test
Taking medication with water after dinner the evening(s) before test; also, adequate intake of fluids to prevent dehydration
Not eating or drinking anything, except water, after taking medication; not smoking or chewing gum
Special diet and/or preparatory instructions may apply; patient should inquire in advance

### Precautions after having this test
Possible interference with later thyroid tests

### Side/adverse effects
Signs of possible side effects, especially pseudo-allergic reaction (for all cholecystographic agents) or unusual bleeding or bruising (for iopanoic acid)

## General Dosing Information

The manufacturer's literature should be consulted for specific techniques and procedures for administration of contrast media.

Pretreatment with corticosteroids and/or antihistamines is recommended to minimize the incidence and severity of reactions in patients with a history of severe reactions to contrast media or with other high-risk conditions (e.g., asthma or history of allergies, positive allergy history to skin allergens or penicillin, dehydration).

As a preparatory measure for cholecystography, it is recommended that the patient ingest a fatty meal on the day prior to the initial oral dose of the cholecystographic agent, regardless of the nature of the agent. This will induce gallbladder contractions and elimination of the contents of the gallbladder. Whether or not the evening meal immediately prior to the administration of the cholecystographic agent should contain fat is dependent on the nature of the contrast medium used. When using iopanoic acid as the contrast agent, it has been shown that a reasonable amount of dietary fat enhances gastrointestinal absorption of the agent, and thus, better opacification of the gallbladder is obtained. Conversely, ingestion of a fatty meal with other cholecystographic agents decreases their absorption.

The fatty meal is being replaced, in some cases, by a commercially available oral fat emulsion, which is usually administered 20 minutes before diagnostic imaging of the gallbladder.

During the interval between ingestion of the cholecystographic agent and the time of the examination, the patient should not take anything by mouth except water. Also, smoking or chewing gum is not recommended since the resulting increase in gastric acidity may affect intestinal motility and absorption of the agent.

Adequate hydration is important in all patients, especially in those with renal or hepatic disease and in the elderly. Additional fluid intake is recommended after ingestion of the cholecystographic agent.

---

## IOCETAMIC ACID

## Oral Dosage Forms

Note: The dosing and strengths of the dosage forms available are expressed in terms of iocetamic acid (not the iodine content).

### IOCETAMIC ACID TABLETS USP

**Usual adult and adolescent dose**
Cholecystography—Oral, 3 to 4.5 grams.

Note: For repeat examination, on the same day as the initial cholecystography, the above dose may be given again.

In current practice, to avoid false positive diagnosis of gallbladder disease, the dose of the cholecystographic agent is administered on two consecutive evenings prior to cholecystography.

The use of large or repeated doses over several days is not recommended, especially in geriatric patients.

**Usual pediatric dose**
Safety and efficacy have not been established.

**Usual geriatric dose**
See *Usual adult and adolescent dose*.

**Strength(s) usually available**
U.S.—
750 mg with 62% of iodine (Rx) [*Cholebrine* (scored)].
Canada—
Not commercially available.

**Packaging and storage**
Store below 40 °C (104 °F), preferably between 15 and 30 °C (59 and 86 °F), unless otherwise specified by manufacturer. Store in a tight container.

---

## IOPANOIC ACID

## Oral Dosage Forms

Note: Bracketed uses in the *Dosage Forms* section refer to categories of use and/or indications that are not included in U.S. product labeling. The dosing and strengths of the dosage forms available are expressed in terms of iopanoic acid (not the iodine content).

### IOPANOIC ACID TABLETS USP

**Usual adult and adolescent dose**
Cholecystography—
Oral, 3 grams.

Note: For repeat examination, on the same day as the initial cholecystography, the above dose may be given again.

In current practice, to avoid false positive diagnosis of gallbladder disease, the dose of the cholecystographic agent is administered on two consecutive evenings prior to cholecystography.

The use of large or repeated doses over several days is not recommended, especially in geriatric patients.
[Antihyperthyroidism (Graves' disease)][1]—
Oral, 500 mg to 1 gram once a day.

**Usual adult prescribing limits**
Up to 6 grams in a twenty-four-hour period.

**Usual pediatric dose**
Cholecystography—
Children weighing up to 13 kg: Oral, 150 mg per kg of body weight.
Children weighing 13 to 23 kg: Oral, 2 grams.
Children weighing 23 kg or more: Oral, 3 grams.

**Usual geriatric dose**
See *Usual adult and adolescent dose*.

**Strength(s) usually available**
U.S.—
500 mg with 66.68% of iodine (Rx) [*Telepaque* (scored)].
Canada—
500 mg with 66.68% of iodine (Rx) [*Telepaque* (scored)].

**Packaging and storage**
Store below 40 °C (104 °F), preferably between 15 and 30 °C (59 and 86 °F), unless otherwise specified by manufacturer. Store in a tight, light-resistant container.

[1]Not included in Canadian product labeling.

---

## IPODATE

## Oral Dosage Forms

Note: Bracketed uses in the *Dosage Forms* section refer to categories of use and/or indications that are not included in U.S. product labeling. The dosing and strengths of the dosage forms available are expressed in terms of ipodate (not the iodine content).

### IPODATE CALCIUM FOR ORAL SUSPENSION USP

**Usual adult and adolescent dose**
Cholecystography—
Oral, 3 grams.

Note: For repeat examination, on the same day as the initial cholecystography, the above dose may be given again.

In current practice, to avoid false positive diagnosis of gallbladder disease, the dose of the cholecystographic agent is administered on two consecutive evenings prior to cholecystography.

The use of large or repeated doses over several days is not recommended, especially in geriatric patients.
[Antihyperthyroidism (Graves' disease)]—
Oral, 500 mg once a day.

**Usual adult prescribing limits**
Up to 6 grams in a twenty-four-hour period.

**Usual pediatric dose**
Cholecystography—Oral, 450 to 900 mg per kg of body weight.

Note: For infants, dose should be diluted in 50 mL of water and given in baby bottle.

**Usual geriatric dose**
See *Usual adult and adolescent dose*.

**Strength(s) usually available**
U.S.—
3 grams with 61.7% of iodine (Rx) [*Oragrafin Calcium*].
Canada—
Not commercially available.

**Packaging and storage**
Store below 40 °C (104 °F), preferably between 15 and 30 °C (59 and 86 °F), in a well-closed container, unless otherwise specified by manufacturer.

**Preparation of dosage form**
Granules should be mixed by vigorous stirring in about 60 mL of water.

**Stability**
Suspension should be ingested immediately after preparation.

### IPODATE SODIUM CAPSULES USP

**Usual adult and adolescent dose**
Cholecystography—
Oral, 3 grams, taken with as little water as possible (capsules may be swallowed in rapid succession or over a period of about 30 minutes).

Note: For repeat examination, on the same day as the initial chole-cystography, the above dose may be given again.

In current practice, to avoid false positive diagnosis of gall-bladder disease, the dose of the cholecystographic agent is ad-ministered on two consecutive evenings prior to cholecystography.

The use of large or repeated doses over several days is not recommended, especially in geriatric patients.

[Antihyperthyroidism (Graves' disease)]—
Oral, 500 mg to 1 gram once a day or 3 grams every third day.

**Usual adult prescribing limits**
Up to 6 grams in a twenty-four-hour period.

**Usual pediatric dose**
Safety and efficacy have not been established.

**Usual geriatric dose**
See *Usual adult and adolescent dose.*

**Strength(s) usually available**
U.S.—
500 mg with 61.4% of iodine (Rx) [*Bilivist; Oragrafin Sodium*].
Canada—
Not commercially available.

**Packaging and storage**
Store below 40 °C (104 °F), preferably between 15 and 30 °C (59 and 86 °F), unless otherwise specified by manufacturer. Store in a tight container.

---

## *TYROPANOATE*

## Oral Dosage Forms

Note: Bracketed uses in the *Dosage Forms* section refer to categories of use and/or indications that are not included in U.S. product labeling.

The dosing and strengths of the dosage forms available are ex-pressed in terms of tyropanoate (not the iodine content).

---

## TYROPANOATE SODIUM CAPSULES USP

**Usual adult and adolescent dose**
Cholecystography—
Oral, 3 grams.
Note: For repeat examination, on the day after the initial cholecystog-raphy, the above dose may be given again.

In current practice, to avoid false positive diagnosis of gall-bladder disease, the dose of the cholecystographic agent is ad-ministered on two consecutive evenings prior to cholecystography.

The use of large or repeated doses over several days is not recommended, especially in geriatric patients.

[Antihyperthyroidism (Graves' disease)]—
Oral, 1.5 grams once a day.

**Usual pediatric dose**
Safety and efficacy have not been established.

**Usual geriatric dose**
See *Usual adult and adolescent dose.*

**Strength(s) usually available**
U.S.—
750 mg with 57.4% of iodine (Rx) [*Bilopaque*].
Canada—
Not commercially available.

**Packaging and storage**
Store below 40 °C (104 °F), preferably between 15 and 30 °C (59 and 86 °F), unless otherwise specified by manufacturer. Store in a tight, light-resistant container.

## Selected Bibliography

Marton K, Doubilet P. How to image the gallbladder in suspected cho-lecystitis. Ann Intern Med 1988; 109: 722-9.

Revised: 06/29/95

---

# CHOLECYSTOKININ   Systemic*

BAN: Pancreozymin
VA CLASSIFICATION (Primary/Secondary): HS900/DX900
Other commonly used names are: CCK and pancreozymin.
Note: For a listing of dosage forms and brand names by country availa-bility, see *Dosage Forms* section(s). For a listing of brand names for the articles in this monograph, refer to the General Index.

---

*Not commercially available in the U.S.

---

## Category

Cholecystokinetic; diagnostic aid (gallbladder disorders; pancreatic dis-orders); peristaltic stimulant.

## Indications

**Accepted**
Cholecystography, oral, adjunct or
Cholangiography adjunct—Cholecystokinin is indicated as a diagnostic aid for evaluation of gallbladder disorders. It is used to stimulate gall-bladder contraction and emptying prior to, or during, cholecystography with contrast media to aid in visualization of the cystic duct and gall-bladder. As part of oral cholecystography or preoperative cholangi-ography, cholecystokinin facilitates the evaluation of the contractile patterns of the gallbladder, filling of the bile ducts, flow of contrast medium into the duodenum, and localization of gallstones in the lower common bile duct.

Although cholangiography is an acceptable procedure for visualizing the biliary ducts, it has generally been replaced by cholescintigraphy, in which a radioisotope-labeled substance that is rapidly excreted into the bile (e.g., a technetium Tc 99m–labeled iminodiacetic acid deriv-ative) is used. Cholescintigraphy is the preferred method rather than cholangiography, especially in patients in whom acute cholecystitis is suspected.

Small intestine studies—Cholecystokinin is indicated to accelerate small bowel transit time of contrast media, such as barium sulfate, thus de-creasing transit time and flocculation of the barium meal.

Pancreatic insufficiency (diagnosis adjunct)—In conjunction with secretin, cholecystokinin is indicated in the diagnosis of pancreatic insufficiency.

## Pharmacology/Pharmacokinetics

**Mechanism of action/Effect**
Cholecystokinetic and
Diagnostic aid (gallbladder disorders)—Cholecystokinin, a natural poly-peptide formed in the amine precursor uptake and decarboxylation (APUD) cells of the proximal mucosa of the small intestine, induces contraction of the gallbladder muscle, resulting in reduction of gall-bladder size and evacuation of bile.
Diagnostic aid (pancreatic disorders)—Cholecystokinin stimulates secre-tion of pancreatic digestive enzymes and secretion from the glands of Brunner.
Peristaltic stimulant—Cholecystokinin increases muscle contractions of the stomach and small intestine.

**Other actions**
Cholecystokinin inhibits contraction of the lower esophageal sphincter and the sphincter of Oddi.

**Onset of action**
Contraction of the gallbladder—Within 1 to 3 minutes.
Peristaltic stimulant—1 to 2 minutes.

**Time to peak effect**
Contraction of gallbladder—5 to 15 minutes after injection.

**Duration of action**
Contraction of gallbladder—Approximately 2 hours or more.

## Precautions to Consider

**Pregnancy/Reproduction**
Pregnancy—Although adequate studies in humans have not been done, cholecystokinin should not be administered to pregnant women near term because it is a smooth muscle stimulant and may induce spon-taneous abortion or premature labor.

**Breast-feeding**
It is not known whether cholecystokinin is distributed into breast milk. However, problems in humans have not been documented.

**Pediatrics**
Appropriate studies on the relationship of age to the effects of cholecystokinin have not been performed in the pediatric population.

**Geriatrics**
Appropriate studies performed to date have not demonstrated geriatrics-specific problems that would limit the usefulness of cholecystokinin in the elderly.

**Medical considerations/Contraindications**
The medical considerations/contraindications included here have been selected on the basis of their potential clinical significance (reasons given in parentheses where appropriate)—not necessarily inclusive (» = major clinical significance).

*Except under special circumstances, this medication should not be used when the following medical problem exists:*
» Intestinal obstruction
(stimulation of gastrointestinal motility may aggravate condition)

*Risk-benefit should be considered when the following medical problem exists:*
Sensitivity to the cholecystokinin preparation

## Side/Adverse Effects

The following side/adverse effects have been selected on the basis of their potential clinical significance (possible signs and symptoms in parentheses where appropriate)—not necessarily inclusive:

**Those indicating need for medical attention only if they continue or are bothersome**
Incidence more frequent
*Flushing or redness of skin*—with rapid administration; *gastrointestinal effects* (abdominal or stomach pain, cramps, or discomfort)

## Patient Consultation

As an aid to patient consultation, refer to *Advice for the Patient, Cholecystokinin (Diagnostic).*

In providing consultation, consider emphasizing the following selected information (» = major clinical significance):

**Description of use**
Procedure for cholecystokinin test: Dose of cholecystokinin is based on body weight and must be determined by physician; cholecystokinin is injected intravenously

**Before having this test**
» Conditions affecting use, especially:
Sensitivity to the cholecystokinin preparation
Pregnancy—Use not recommended; may induce spontaneous abortion or premature labor
Other medical problems, especially intestinal obstruction

**Preparation for this test**
Special preparatory instructions may be given; patient should inquire in advance

## Parenteral Dosage Forms

### CHOLECYSTOKININ FOR INJECTION

**Usual adult and adolescent dose**
Cholecystokinetic or
Diagnostic aid (gallbladder disorders)—
Cholecystography:
For prompt contraction of gallbladder—
Intravenous, 1 Ivy dog unit (IDU) (0.1 mL) per kg of body weight, administered slowly over 30 to 60 seconds.

Note: For oral cholecystography, the patient should be given the contrast medium on the evening before the examination. Fluoroscopy is recommended before the x-ray examination. If the gallbladder is visible, cholecystokinin may be injected.

For cholescintigraphy, prior administration of cholecystokinin is recommended for pre-emptying the gallbladder before the injection of the radiotracer (e.g., a technetium Tc 99m–labeled iminodiacetic acid derivative).
Cholangiography:
Preoperative—Intravenous, 40 Ivy dog units (IDU) (4 mL) administered approximately one minute prior to administration of contrast medium.
Secondary—Intravenous, 75 IDU administered daily for one week, if a concretion remains after surgery. Concurrent with the last injection, cholangiography may be performed.
Diagnostic aid (pancreatic disorders)—
Intravenous, 0.5 to 1 Ivy dog unit (IDU) per kg of body weight, administered slowly.
Peristaltic stimulant—
To accelerate small bowel transit time of barium sulfate: Intravenous, 0.5 to 1 Ivy dog unit (IDU) per kg of body weight, administered slowly after the barium meal has passed into the first part of the jejunum.
Note: After ingestion of 200 to 300 mL of barium mixture, patients should lie on their right side for 10 to 15 minutes; if fluoroscopy shows that most of the contrast medium has passed into the first part of the jejunum, cholecystokinin is injected.

**Usual pediatric dose**
Dosage has not been established.

**Usual geriatric dose**
See *Usual adult and adolescent dose.*

**Strength(s) usually available**
U.S.—
Not commercially available. However, sincalide (CCK-8), a synthetically prepared C-terminal octapeptide of cholecystokinin, is commercially available in the U.S.
Canada—
75 Ivy dog units (IDU) (Rx) [GENERIC (0.4 mg-cysteine, 0.1 mg-cysteine hydrochloride, 20 mg mannitol)].

**Packaging and storage**
Store at −20 °C (−4 °F), unless otherwise specified by manufacturer.

**Preparation of dosage form**
To prepare injection, 7.5 mL of an isotonic sodium chloride solution is added to the vial containing 75 Ivy dog units (IDU) of cholecystokinin, giving a final concentration of 10 IDU per mL.

**Stability**
Following reconstitution, cholecystokinin injection must be used immediately.
Any unused portion remaining in the container should be discarded.

## Selected Bibliography

Freeman LM, Sugarman LA, Weissmann HS. Role of cholecystokinetic agents in Tc 99m-IDA cholescintigraphy. Semin Nucl Med 1981; 11 (3): 186-93.

Developed: 05/27/96

# CHOLERA VACCINE   Systemic

VA CLASSIFICATION (Primary): IM100
Note: This monograph is specific for cholera vaccine prepared from equal parts of Ogawa and Inaba serotypes of killed *Vibrio cholerae* 01, and intended for parenteral use only.

Note: For a listing of dosage forms and brand names by country availability, see *Dosage Forms* section(s). For a listing of brand names for the articles in this monograph, refer to the General Index.

## Category

Immunizing agent (active).

## Indications

**General considerations**
Travelers to areas in which there is a recognized risk of exposure to *Vibrio cholerae* should take the necessary precautions. Risk is greatest for travelers to developing countries of Asia (especially South and South-

east Asia), Latin America, and Africa, who will have exposure to potentially contaminated food and drink.

Persons following the usual tourist itinerary who use standard accommodations in countries reporting cholera are at virtually no risk of infection. Travelers to cholera-infected areas are advised to avoid eating uncooked food, especially fish and shellfish, and to peel fruits themselves. Carbonated bottled water and carbonated soft drinks are safe. Travelers should be cautioned that cholera vaccination is not a substitute for careful selection of food and drink. Travelers should also be advised not to transport food from cholera-affected areas.

The World Health Organization (WHO) no longer recommends routine immunization with cholera vaccine for travel to or from cholera-infected areas and discourages countries from requiring cholera vaccination for visitors. Currently, no country or territory requires vaccination as a condition for entry. However, local authorities may continue to require documentation of vaccination against cholera. In such cases, a single dose of vaccine is sufficient to satisfy local requirements.

### Accepted

*Vibrio cholerae* (prophylaxis)—Cholera vaccine is indicated for immunization of adults and children 6 months of age and older against disease caused by *V. cholerae* 01.

The currently available killed cholera vaccine for parenteral use provides only limited and brief protection against *V. cholerae* 01, does not prevent asymptomatic infection, may not provide any protection against *V. cholerae* 0139, and has a high cost-benefit ratio; therefore, this vaccine is not recommended for travelers.

The complete primary series is suggested only for special high-risk groups who work and live in highly endemic areas under less than adequate sanitary conditions. The primary series does not need to be repeated for the booster doses to be effective.

## Pharmacology/Pharmacokinetics

### Physicochemical characteristics

Source—Cholera vaccine is a sterile suspension for intracutaneous (intradermal), subcutaneous, or intramuscular administration. The vaccine contains equal parts of Ogawa and Inaba serotypes of killed *V. cholerae* 01 in buffered sodium chloride injection. The Inaba and Ogawa strains of *V. cholerae* 01 are grown on trypticase soy agar medium, removed from the medium with buffered sodium chloride injection, and killed by addition of 0.5% phenol. The vaccine contains 8 units of each serotype antigen (Ogawa and Inaba) per mL.

### Mechanism of action/Effect

Inactivated *V. cholerae* 01 present in cholera vaccine promote the production of vibriocidal antibodies.

### Protective effect

Cholera vaccine confers protection against disease caused by *V. cholerae* 01 in only 25 to 50% of individuals who receive the vaccine, and may not provide any protection against *V. cholerae* 0139.

### Duration of protective effect

Immunity against cholera lasts only for a short duration (3 to 6 months), after vaccination, with the greatest protection occurring during the first 2 months. A booster dose is recommended every 6 months if there is continuing or repeated risk of exposure to *V. cholerae*.

## Precautions to Consider

### Pregnancy/Reproduction

Fertility—Studies on effects of cholera vaccine on fertility have not been done.

Pregnancy—Studies have not been done in humans.

Studies have not been done in animals.

FDA Pregnancy Category C.

### Breast-feeding

It is not known whether cholera vaccine is distributed into breast milk. However, problems in humans have not been documented.

### Pediatrics

Cholera vaccine is not recommended in infants up to 6 months of age. Breast-feeding is protective against cholera; careful preparation of formula and food from safe water and foodstuffs should protect non–breast-fed infants. Currently, no country or territory requires documentation of cholera vaccination for entry; local authorities, however, may still request documentation of vaccination. If a child less than 6 months of age is to travel to areas where documentation of cholera vaccination is likely to be requested, a medical waiver should be obtained before travel. For older infants and children, a single dose of vaccine is sufficient to satisfy local requirements.

### Geriatrics

Appropriate studies on the relationship of age to the effects of cholera vaccine have not been performed in the geriatric population. However, no geriatrics-specific problems have been documented to date.

### Drug interactions and/or related problems

The following drug interactions and/or related problems have been selected on the basis of their potential clinical significance (possible mechanism in parentheses where appropriate)—not necessarily inclusive (» = major clinical significance):

Note: Combinations containing any of the following medications, depending on the amount present, may also interact with this medication.

Plague vaccine or
Typhoid vaccine
   (concurrent use of cholera vaccine may increase the risk of local and systemic adverse effects)

Yellow fever vaccine
   (simultaneous administration has been reported to interfere with the immune response to each vaccine)

### Medical considerations/Contraindications

The medical considerations/contraindications included here have been selected on the basis of their potential clinical significance (reasons given in parentheses where appropriate)—not necessarily inclusive (» = major clinical significance).

*Except under special circumstances, this medication should not be used when the following medical problems exist:*

» Febrile illness, acute
   (administration of cholera vaccine should be postponed to avoid confusing manifestations of acute febrile illness with possible side/adverse effects of the vaccine; minor illness, such as upper respiratory infections, with or without low grade fever or mild diarrhea, does not preclude administration of the vaccine)

» Previous sensitivity reaction to cholera vaccine
   (cholera vaccine is contraindicated in patients with a history of severe systemic or allergic reaction to cholera vaccine)

## Side/Adverse Effects

The following side/adverse effects have been selected on the basis of their potential clinical significance (possible signs and symptoms in parentheses where appropriate)—not necessarily inclusive:

### Those indicating need for medical attention

Incidence rare
   *Anaphylactic reaction* (difficulty in breathing or swallowing; hives; itching, especially of soles or palms; reddening of skin, especially around ears; swelling of eyes, face, or inside of nose; unusual tiredness or weakness, sudden and severe)

### Those indicating need for medical attention only if they continue or are bothersome

Incidence more frequent
   *Fever; headache; malaise* (general feeling of discomfort or illness); *pain, redness, or swelling at injection site*

## Patient Consultation

As an aid to patient consultation, refer to *Advice for the Patient, Cholera Vaccine (Systemic).*

In providing consultation, consider emphasizing the following selected information (» = major clinical significance):

### Before using this medication

» Conditions affecting use, especially:
   Sensitivity to cholera vaccine
   Use in children—Use is not recommended in infants less than 6 months of age
   Other medical problems, especially acute febrile illness

### Proper use of this medication

» Proper dosing

### Side/adverse effects

   Signs of potential side effects, especially anaphylactic reaction

## General Dosing Information

Appropriate precautions should be taken prior to vaccine injection to prevent allergic or any other unwanted reactions. This should include review of the patient's history regarding possible sensitivity and the ready availability of epinephrine 1:1000 and other appropriate agents used for control of immediate allergic reactions.

Primary immunization with cholera vaccine consists of two doses administered at an interval of 1 week to 1 month or more.

Under conditions of continued or repeated exposure (in areas where cholera is epidemic or endemic), a single booster dose should be given every 6 months. It is not necessary to repeat the primary immunization series.

Even after immunization with cholera vaccine, not all recipients of the vaccine will be fully protected against cholera. Travelers should take all necessary precautions to avoid contact with, or ingestion of, potentially contaminated food or water.

Cholera vaccine does not prevent *V. cholerae* excretion. Therefore, it should not be used to manage contacts of imported cholera cases or to control the spread of infection, even during epidemics.

## Parenteral Dosage Forms

### CHOLERA VACCINE USP

**Usual adult and adolescent dose**
Immunizing agent (active)—
  Primary immunization:
    U.S.—
      Subcutaneous or intramuscular, two doses of 0.5 mL administered at intervals of one week to one month or more.
      Intradermal, two doses of 0.2 mL administered at intervals of one week to one month or more.
    Canada—
      First dose: Subcutaneous, 0.5 mL.
      Second dose: Subcutaneous, 1 mL three to four weeks after the first dose.
      Third dose: Subcutaneous, 1 mL three to four weeks after the second dose.
      Note: When time does not permit the above spacing of doses, the interval between doses may be shortened to seven days.
  Booster doses:
    U.S.—
      Subcutaneous or intramuscular, 0.5 mL every six months.
      Intradermal, 0.2 mL every six months.
    Canada—
      Subcutaneous, 1 mL every six months.

**Usual pediatric dose**
Immunizing agent (active)—
  Primary immunization:
    U.S.—
      Infants up to 6 months of age:
        Use is not recommended.
      Children 6 months to 5 years of age:
        Subcutaneous or intramuscular, two doses of 0.2 mL administered at intervals of one week to one month or more.

Children 5 to 10 years of age:
  Subcutaneous or intramuscular, two doses of 0.3 mL administered at intervals of one week to one month or more.
  Intradermal, two doses of 0.2 mL administered at intervals of one week to one month or more.
Children 10 years of age and older:
  See *Usual adult and adolescent dose*.
Canada—
  First dose:
    Children less than 5 years of age—Subcutaneous, 0.1 mL.
    Children 5 to 10 years of age—Subcutaneous, 0.3 mL.
    Children 10 years of age and older—See *Usual adult and adolescent dose*.
  Second dose:
    Children less than 5 years of age—Subcutaneous, 0.3 mL three to four weeks after the first dose.
    Children 5 to 10 years of age—Subcutaneous, 0.5 mL three to four weeks after the first dose.
    Children 10 years of age and older—See *Usual adult and adolescent dose*.
  Booster doses:
    U.S.—
      Children 6 months to 5 years of age:
        Subcutaneous or intramuscular, 0.2 mL every six months.
      Children 5 to 10 years of age:
        Subcutaneous or intramuscular, 0.3 mL every six months.
        Intradermal, 0.2 mL every six months.
      Children 10 years of age and older:
        See *Usual adult and adolescent dose*.
    Canada—
      Children less than 5 years of age:
        Subcutaneous, 0.3 mL every six months.
      Children 5 to 10 years of age:
        Subcutaneous, 0.5 mL every six months.
      Children 10 years of age and older:
        See *Usual adult and adolescent dose*.

Note: A booster dose may be repeated every six months as long as the likelihood of exposure continues.

**Strength(s) usually available**
U.S.—
  8 units of each serotype (Ogawa and Inaba) antigen per mL (Rx) [GENERIC].
Canada—
  Approximately 8 × 10⁹ killed *V. cholerae* per mL (Rx) [GENERIC].

**Packaging and storage**
Store between 2 and 8 °C (36 and 46 °F).

**Auxiliary labeling**
• Do not freeze.
• Shake well before using.

Developed: 02/05/96

---

# CHOLESTYRAMINE   Oral-Local

VA CLASSIFICATION (Primary/Secondary): CV350/AD400; DE890; GA400; GU900

Note: For a listing of dosage forms and brand names by country availability, see *Dosage Forms* section(s). For a listing of brand names for the articles in this monograph, refer to the General Index.

## Category

Antihyperlipidemic; antipruritic (cholestasis); antidiarrheal (postoperative colonic bile acids); antidote (anion-exchange resin); antihyperoxaluric.

## Indications

Note: Bracketed information in the *Indications* section refers to uses that are not included in U.S. product labeling.

**Accepted**
Hyperlipidemia (treatment)—Cholestyramine is indicated for use in patients with primary hypercholesterolemia (type IIa hyperlipidemia) and a significant risk of coronary artery disease who have not responded to diet or other measures alone. Cholestyramine reduces plasma total cholesterol and low density lipoprotein (LDL) concentrations, but

causes no change or a slight increase in serum triglyceride concentrations, and so is not useful in patients with elevated triglyceride concentrations alone. Its use is limited in other types of hyperlipidemia (including type IIb) because it may cause further elevation of triglycerides.

Studies have suggested that control of elevated cholesterol and triglycerides may not lessen the danger of cardiovascular disease and mortality, although incidence of nonfatal myocardial infarctions may be decreased.

For additional information on initial therapeutic guidelines related to the treatment of hyperlipidemia, see *Appendix III*.

Cholestyramine is indicated to reduce the risks of atherosclerotic heart disease and myocardial infarctions.

Pruritus, associated with partial biliary obstruction (treatment)—Cholestyramine is indicated for the relief of pruritus associated with partial biliary obstruction (including primary biliary cirrhosis and various other forms of bile stasis). It is not useful in patients with complete biliary obstruction or with pruritus due to other causes.

[Diarrhea, due to bile acids (treatment)]—Cholestyramine has also been used to treat diarrhea caused by increased bile acids in the colon after surgery, although the risk of steatorrhea is increased.

[Hyperoxaluria (treatment)][1]—Cholestyramine is also being used in the treatment of hyperoxaluria.

[Cholestyramine has been used in the treatment of digitalis glycoside overdose; however, it generally has been replaced by other agents such as digoxin immune fab.]

---

[1]Not included in Canadian product labeling.

## Pharmacology/Pharmacokinetics

### Physicochemical characteristics
Cholestyramine is an anion-exchange resin

### Mechanism of action/Effect
Cholestyramine binds with bile acids in the intestine, preventing their reabsorption and producing an insoluble complex, which is excreted in the feces.
Antihyperlipidemic—
   Cholestyramine binds with bile acids in the intestine, causing an increase in hepatic synthesis of bile acids from cholesterol. This depletion of hepatic cholesterol increases hepatic low-density lipoprotein (LDL) receptor activity, which removes LDL cholesterol from the plasma. Cholestyramine may also increase hepatic very–density lipoprotein (VLDL) production, thereby increasing the plasma concentration of triglycerides, especially in patients with hypertriglyceridemia.
Antipruritic (cholestasis)—
   Reduction of serum bile acids and subsequent reduction of excess bile acids, which are deposited in dermal tissue, may lead to reduced pruritus.
Antidiarrheal (postoperative colonic bile acids)—
   Cholestyramine binds with and removes bile acids.
Antidote (anion-exchange resin)—
   Because it is an anion-exchange resin, cholestyramine is capable of binding negatively charged medications as well as some others, causing a decreased effect or shortened half-life.

### Absorption
Not absorbed from the gastrointestinal tract.

### Onset of action
Reduction of plasma cholesterol concentrations—Generally reduced within 1 to 2 weeks after initiation of cholestyramine therapy, but may continue to fall for up to 1 year. In some patients, after the initial decrease, serum cholesterol concentrations return to or exceed baseline levels with continued therapy.
Relief of pruritus associated with biliary stasis—Usually occurs within 1 to 3 weeks after initiation of therapy.
Relief of diarrhea associated with bile acids—Within 24 hours.

### Duration of action
Reduction of plasma cholesterol concentrations—After withdrawal of cholestyramine, cholesterol concentrations return to baseline in about 2 to 4 weeks.
Relief of pruritus associated with biliary stasis—Pruritus returns within 1 to 2 weeks when the medication is withdrawn.

## Precautions to Consider

### Tumorigenicity
Cholestyramine was found to increase the incidence of intestinal tumors in rats receiving potent carcinogens.

### Pregnancy/Reproduction
Pregnancy—Problems in humans have not been documented. Cholestyramine is almost totally unabsorbed after oral administration; however, adverse effects on the fetus may potentially occur because of impaired maternal absorption of vitamins and nutrients.

### Breast-feeding
Problems in humans have not been documented. Cholestyramine is almost totally unabsorbed after oral administration. However, the possible impaired maternal vitamin and nutrient absorption may have an effect on nursing infants.

### Pediatrics
Several studies performed to date have not demonstrated pediatrics-specific problems that would limit the usefulness of cholestyramine in children. However, experience with cholestyramine in children younger than 10 years of age is limited. Therefore, caution is recommended since cholesterol is required for normal development.

### Geriatrics
Appropriate studies on the relationship of age to the effects of cholestyramine have not been performed in the geriatric population. However, patients over 60 years of age may be more likely to experience gastrointestinal side effects, as well as adverse nutritional effects.

### Drug interactions and/or related problems
The following drug interactions and/or related problems have been selected on the basis of their potential clinical significance (possible mechanism in parentheses where appropriate)—not necessarily inclusive (» = major clinical significance):

Note: Combinations containing any of the following medications, depending on the amount present, may also interact with this medication.

» Anticoagulants, coumarin- or indandione-derivative
   (concurrent use may significantly increase the anticoagulant effect as a result of depletion of vitamin K, but cholestyramine may also bind with oral anticoagulants in the gastrointestinal tract and reduce their effects; administration at least 6 hours before cholestyramine and adjustment of anticoagulant dosage based on frequent prothrombin-time determinations are recommended)

Chenodiol or
Ursodiol
   (effect may be decreased when chenodiol or ursodiol is used concurrently with cholestyramine, which binds these medications and decreases their absorption and also tends to increase cholesterol saturation of bile)

» Digitalis glycosides, especially digitoxin
   (cholestyramine may reduce the half-life of these medications by decreasing intestinal reabsorption and enterohepatic circulation; caution is recommended, especially when cholestyramine is withdrawn from a patient who was stabilized on the digitalis glycoside while receiving cholestyramine, because of the potential for serious toxicity; some clinicians recommend administration of cholestyramine approximately 8 hours after the digitalis glycoside)

» Diuretics, thiazide, oral or
» Penicillin G, oral or
» Phenylbutazone or
» Propranolol, oral or
» Tetracyclines, oral
   (concurrent use with cholestyramine may result in binding of these medications, thus decreasing their absorption; an interval of several hours between administration of cholestyramine and any of these medications is recommended)

Folic acid
   (concurrent use with cholestyramine may interfere with absorption of folic acid; folic acid supplementation recommended in patients receiving cholestyramine for prolonged periods)

» Thyroid hormones, including dextrothyroxine
   (concurrent use with cholestyramine may decrease the effects of thyroid hormones by binding and delaying or preventing absorption; an interval of 4 to 5 hours between administration of the two medications and regular monitoring of thyroid function tests are recommended)

» Vancomycin, oral
   (cholestyramine has been shown to bind oral vancomycin significantly when used concurrently, resulting in decreased stool concentrations and marked reduction in antibacterial activity of vancomycin; concurrent use is not recommended; patients should be advised to take oral vancomycin and cholestyramine several hours apart)

Vitamins, fat-soluble
   (cholestyramine may interfere with absorption of fat-soluble vitamins as a result of its interference with fat absorption; supplemental vitamins A and D in water-miscible or parenteral form are recommended in patients receiving cholestyramine for prolonged periods; supplemental vitamin K may be required in some patients who develop bleeding tendencies)

Medications, other
   (cholestyramine may delay or reduce absorption of other medications administered concurrently because of its anion-binding activity; administration of other medications 1 to 2 hours before or 4 to 6 hours after cholestyramine is recommended, although absorption of some medications is impaired even then; caution is recommended when cholestyramine is withdrawn because of the risk of toxicity when suddenly increased absorption of the other medication leads to higher serum concentrations)

**Laboratory value alterations**

The following have been selected on the basis of their potential clinical significance (possible effect in parentheses where appropriate)—not necessarily inclusive (» = major clinical significance):

With physiology/laboratory test values

Alkaline phosphatase (ALT [SGPT]) values and
Aspartate aminotransferase (AST [SGOT]) values and
Chloride concentrations, serum and
Phosphorus concentrations, serum
    (may be increased)

Calcium
    (serum concentrations may be decreased due to impaired absorption; may lead to osteoporosis, especially in patients with biliary cirrhosis who already have impaired calcium absorption)

Potassium and
Sodium
    (serum concentrations may be decreased)

Prothrombin time (PT)
    (may be prolonged)

Schilling test for absorption of vitamin $B_{12}$
    (test may be falsely abnormal due to drug binding with intrinsic factor, which prevents the formation of an intrinsic factor-vitamin $B_{12}$ complex needed for absorption)

**Medical considerations/Contraindications**

The medical considerations/contraindications included here have been selected on the basis of their potential clinical significance (reasons given in parentheses where appropriate)—not necessarily inclusive (» = major clinical significance).

*Risk-benefit should be considered when the following medical problems exist:*

Bleeding disorders or
Gallstones or
Gastrointestinal function impairment or
Hypothyroidism or
Malabsorption states, especially steatorrhea or
Peptic ulcer
    (these conditions may be exacerbated)

» Complete biliary obstruction or complete atresia
    (no bile acids in gastrointestinal tract for cholestyramine to bind)

» Constipation
    (risk of fecal impaction)

Coronary artery disease and
Hemorrhoids
    (exacerbation of these conditions may occur because of the risks associated with severe constipation)

» Phenylketonuria
    (sensitivity to phenylalanine in aspartame, which is included in sugar-free preparation)

Renal function impairment
    (increased risk of development of hyperchloremic acidosis)

Sensitivity to cholestyramine

**Patient monitoring**

The following may be especially important in patient monitoring (other tests may be warranted in some patients, depending on condition; » = major clinical significance):

Calcium concentrations, serum
    (recommended periodically because of decreased absorption of calcium associated with chronic use of cholestyramine)

Cholesterol concentrations, serum and
Triglyceride concentrations, serum
    (determinations recommended prior to initiation of therapy of hyperlipidemia and at periodic intervals during therapy to confirm efficacy and determine that a positive response is maintained)

Prothrombin-time (PT) determinations
    (recommended periodically because vitamin K deficiency associated with chronic use of cholestyramine may increase bleeding tendency)

## Side/Adverse Effects

Note: Side effects are more likely to occur with high doses and in patients over 60 years of age.

    Less frequently, osteoporosis has been reported as a result of chronic long-term cholestyramine use.

The following side/adverse effects have been selected on the basis of their potential clinical significance (possible signs and symptoms in parentheses where appropriate)—not necessarily inclusive:

**Those indicating need for medical attention**

Incidence more frequent
    *Constipation*—usually mild and transient, but may be severe and lead to fecal impaction

Incidence rare
    *Gallstones or pancreatitis* (severe stomach pain with nausea and vomiting); *gastrointestinal bleeding or peptic ulcer* (black, tarry stools); *steatorrhea or malabsorption syndrome* (sudden loss of weight)

**Those indicating need for medical attention only if they continue or are bothersome**

Incidence more frequent
    *Heartburn or indigestion; nausea or vomiting; stomach pain*

Incidence less frequent
    *Belching; bloating; diarrhea; dizziness; headache*

## Patient Consultation

As an aid to patient consultation, refer to *Advice for the Patient, Cholestyramine (Oral)*.

In providing consultation, consider emphasizing the following selected information (» = major clinical significance):

**Before using this medication**

» Conditions affecting use, especially:
    Sensitivity to cholestyramine
    Use in children—Caution with use in children less than 10 years of age since cholesterol is required for normal development
    Use in the elderly—Increased incidence of gastrointestinal side effects and potentially adverse nutritional effects in patients over 60 years of age
    Other oral medications, especially anticoagulants, digitalis glycosides, thiazide diuretics, penicillin G, phenylbutazone, propranolol, tetracyclines, thyroid hormones, or vancomycin
    Other medical problems, especially complete biliary obstruction or complete atresia, constipation, or phenylketonuria

**Proper use of this medication**

» Importance of not taking more or less medication than the amount prescribed

» Proper dosing
    Missed dose: Taking as soon as possible; not taking if almost time for next dose; not doubling doses

» Proper storage

» Importance of mixing with fluids before taking; instructions for measuring and mixing—Placing in 2 ounces of any beverage and stirring vigorously, then adding 2 to 4 ounces of beverage and shaking vigorously (does not dissolve); rinsing glass and drinking to make sure all medication is taken; may also be mixed with milk in cereals, thin soups, or pulpy fruits

*For use as an antihyperlipidemic*

» Diet as preferred therapy; importance of following prescribed diet
    This medication does not cure the condition but rather helps control it

**Precautions while using this medication**

» Importance of close monitoring by the physician

» Not taking any other medication unless discussed with physician
*For use as an antihyperlipidemic*

» Checking with physician before discontinuing medication; blood lipid concentrations may increase significantly

**Side/adverse effects**

    Signs of potential side effects, especially constipation, gallstones, pancreatitis, gastrointestinal bleeding, peptic ulcer, and steatorrhea or malabsorption syndrome

## General Dosing Information

To prevent accidental inhalation or esophageal distress with the dry form, it is recommended that cholestyramine for suspension be mixed with at least 120 to 180 mL of water or other fluids before being ingested. It may also be taken in soups or with cereals or pulpy fruits.

Reduction in cholestyramine dosage or withdrawal of the medication may be necessary in some patients if constipation occurs or worsens, to prevent impaction. Administration of a laxative or stool softener or increased fluid intake may be helpful.

**For use as an antihyperlipidemic**

If a paradoxical increase in plasma cholesterol concentrations occurs, it is recommended that cholestyramine therapy be withdrawn.

If response is inadequate after 1 to 3 months of treatment, cholestyramine therapy should be withdrawn, except in the case of xanthoma tuberosum, which may require up to 1 year of treatment as long as reduction in size and/or number of xanthomata occurs.

**For use as an antipruritic**
Dosage may be reduced when relief of pruritus occurs.

## Oral Dosage Forms

Bracketed uses in the *Dosage Forms* section refer to categories of use and/or indications that are not included in U.S. product labeling.

### CHOLESTYRAMINE FOR ORAL SUSPENSION USP

**Usual adult and adolescent dose**
Antihyperlipidemic; or
Antipruritic (cholestasis); or
[Antidiarrheal, postoperative colonic bile acids]—
    Initial: Oral, 4 grams (anhydrous cholestyramine) one or two times a day before meals, adjusted according to response.
    Maintenance: Oral, 8 to 24 grams (anhydrous cholestyramine) a day, in two to six divided doses.
Note: A single daily dose or two divided daily doses are equally effective, but up to six divided daily doses may be administered and may be more convenient for the patient, especially with the larger doses.

**Usual adult prescribing limits**
Antihyperlipidemic—24 grams (anhydrous cholestyramine) a day.
Antipruritic (cholestasis)—Up to 16 grams (anhydrous cholestyramine) a day.

**Usual pediatric dose**
Antihyperlipidemic—
    Initial: Oral, 4 grams (anhydrous cholestyramine) a day, in two divided doses.
    Maintenance: Oral, 8 to 24 grams (anhydrous cholestyramine) a day, in two or more divided doses.

**Size(s) usually available**
U.S.—
    5 grams (4 grams of anhydrous cholestyramine) per packet or level scoop (Rx) [*Questran Light* (aspartame; phenylalanine 16.8 mg per 5-gram dose)].
    9 grams (4 grams of anhydrous cholestyramine) per packet or level scoop (Rx) [*Questran* (sucrose)].
Canada—
    5 grams (4 grams of anhydrous cholestyramine) per packet or level scoop (Rx) [*Questran Light* (aspartame; phenylalanine 16.8 mg per 5-gram dose)].

9 grams (4 grams of anhydrous cholestyramine) per packet or level scoop (Rx) [*Questran*].

**Packaging and storage**
Store below 40 °C (104 °F), preferably between 15 and 30 °C (59 and 86 °F), unless otherwise specified by manufacturer. Store in a tight container.

**Preparation of dosage form**
Cholestyramine is prepared for administration by placing the measured powder in 2 ounces of any beverage and stirring vigorously. An additional 2 to 4 ounces of beverage should then be added, again shaking vigorously (does not dissolve). After the patient drinks the suspension, the glass should be rinsed with more liquid to make sure all the medication is taken. Cholestyramine may also be mixed with milk in hot or regular breakfast cereals, in thin soups (tomato or chicken noodle), or in pulpy fruits such as pineapple, pears, peaches, or fruit cocktail.

**Stability**
Variations in color do not reflect changes in potency of the product.

**Auxiliary labeling**
• Take mixed in cold water or juice.

## Selected Bibliography

The Expert Panel. Report of the National Cholesterol Education Program Expert Panel on Detection, Evaluation, and Treatment of High Blood Cholesterol in Adults. Arch Intern Med 1988; 148: 36-69.
NIH Consensus Conference. Lowering blood cholesterol to prevent heart disease. JAMA 1985; 253: 2080-6.
Knodel LC, Talbert RL. Adverse effects of hypolipidaemic drugs. Med Toxicol 1987; 2: 10-32.

Revised: 08/02/94

---

**CHOLINE SALICYLATE**—See *Salicylates (Systemic)*

---

### CHOLINE SALICYLATE–CONTAINING COMBINATIONS—

Choline and Magnesium Salicylates (Systemic)—See *Salicylates (Systemic)*

---

# CHORIONIC GONADOTROPIN   Systemic

VA CLASSIFICATION (Primary/Secondary): HS400/DX900; HS900
Note: Controlled substance in some states in the U.S.—Schedule IV.

Another commonly used name is human chorionic gonadotropin (hCG).
Note: For a listing of dosage forms and brand names by country availability, see *Dosage Forms* section(s). For a listing of brand names for the articles in this monograph, refer to the General Index.

## Category

Gonadotropin; cryptorchidism therapy adjunct; infertility therapy adjunct; diagnostic aid (hypogonadism).

## Indications

Note: Bracketed information in the *Indications* section refers to uses that are not included in U.S. product labeling.

**Accepted**
[Cryptorchidism (diagnosis)][1] or
Cryptorchidism (treatment)—Chorionic gonadotropin is indicated both as a diagnostic trial and for treatment of prepubertal cryptorchidism not due to anatomical obstruction. Treatment with chorionic gonadotropin usually begins at 4 to 9 years of age. If no signs of improvement occur during the initial course, surgery is indicated.

Infertility, male (treatment)—Chorionic gonadotropin is indicated, alone or in combination with menotropins or clomiphene, for treatment of male hypogonadism due to pituitary deficiency. Males who have been hypogonadotropic for prolonged periods may require treatment with

testosterone instead.

Infertility, female (treatment)—Chorionic gonadotropin is indicated in conjunction with menotropins, urofollitropin, or in some cases, clomiphene, to stimulate ovulation. In general, use of chorionic gonadotropin with menotropins or urofollitropin is the treatment of choice for induction of ovulation in patients who do not respond to clomiphene.

Reproductive technologies, assisted—Chorionic gonadotropin is indicated, in conjunction with menotropins or urofollitropin, to stimulate the development and maturation of multiple oocytes in ovulatory patients who are attempting to conceive by means of assisted reproductive technologies, such as gamete intrafallopian transfer (GIFT) or *in vitro* fertilization (IVF).

[Hypogonadism, male (diagnosis)][1]—Chorionic gonadotropin is also used to test the ability of the testes to respond to gonadotropin stimulation in males with delayed puberty.

[Corpus luteum insufficiency (treatment)][1]—Chorionic gonadotropin is used to treat corpus luteum dysfunction. Treatment should begin in the cycle of conception and not after the first missed menses. It is continued until hormone production is taken over by the placenta after 7 to 10 weeks of gestation.

**Unaccepted**
Chorionic gonadotropin has not been found effective and is not indicated for weight reduction.

---

[1]Not included in Canadian product labeling.

# Pharmacology/Pharmacokinetics

## Physicochemical characteristics

Source—Produced by the placenta; extracted from urine of pregnant women.

## Mechanism of action/Effect

The action of chorionic gonadotropin is almost identical to that of pituitary luteinizing hormone (LH). It is generally used as a substitute for LH.

Prepubertal cryptorchidism—
Stimulates androgen production by the testes, which may stimulate descent of the testes. The effect is usually permanent but may be temporary. In use as a diagnostic trial, chorionic gonadotropin administration should stimulate increased serum testosterone concentrations.

Hypogonadotropic hypogonadism—
Stimulates androgen production by the testes, which leads to the development of male secondary sexual characteristics.

For induction of ovulation and assisted reproductive technologies (ART)—
Clomiphene, menotropins, or urofollitropin prepare the ovarian follicle for ovulation. The combination of follicle-stimulating hormone (FSH) and LH stimulates follicular growth and maturation. Chorionic gonadotropin, whose actions are nearly identical to those of LH, is administered following administration of clomiphene, menotropins, or urofollitropin to mimic the naturally occurring surge of LH that triggers ovulation.

Diagnostic aid (hypogonadism)—
Should stimulate increased production of testosterone.

Corpus luteum insufficiency—
Promotes maintenance of the corpus luteum; stimulates ovarian production of progesterone.

## Half-life

Biphasic, 11 and 23 hours (serum).

## Time to peak effect

Females—Ovulation usually occurs within 32 to 36 hours after administration of chorionic gonadotropin.

## Elimination

Renal, unchanged; 10 to 12% within 24 hours.

# Precautions to Consider

## Carcinogenicity/Mutagenicity

Studies have not been done in either animals or humans.

## Pregnancy/Reproduction

Fertility—Use of chorionic gonadotropin in conjunction with menotropins or urofollitropin to induce ovulation is associated with a high incidence of multiple gestations and multiple births. As a result, this may increase the risk of neonatal prematurity, as well as other complications associated with multiple gestations.

Pregnancy—Appropriate studies have not been done in either animals or humans.

Ovarian hyperstimulation syndrome (OHS), which may occur during chorionic gonadotropin therapy, may be more common, more severe, and protracted in patients who conceive.

FDA Pregnancy Category C.

## Pediatrics

Precocious puberty has been reported in males treated with chorionic gonadotropin for cryptorchidism. Generally, therapy is withdrawn and the use of chorionic gonadotropin re-evaluated if signs of precocious puberty appear. Also, prolonged or high doses of chorionic gonadotropin may cause abnormally rapid advancement of skeletal maturation and lead to premature epiphyseal fusion. This could result in reduced final adult height.

## Laboratory value alterations

The following have been selected on the basis of their potential clinical significance (possible effect in parentheses where appropriate)—not necessarily inclusive (» = major clinical significance):

With diagnostic test results
Immunologic assay for endogenous chorionic gonadotropin
(pregnancy test should be performed at least 10 days or longer after administration of chorionic gonadotropin to avoid false-positive result)

With physiology/laboratory test values
17-Hydroxycorticosteroids and
17-Ketosteroids
(urine concentrations may be increased)

## Medical considerations/Contraindications

The medical considerations/contraindications included here have been selected on the basis of their potential clinical significance (reasons given in parentheses where appropriate)—not necessarily inclusive (» = major clinical significance).

***Except under special circumstances, this medication should not be used when the following medical problems exist:***

*For all indications*
» Pituitary hypertrophy or tumor
(pituitary enlargement may occur)

*For treatment of cryptorchidism*
» Precocious puberty

*For induction of ovulation*
» Abnormal vaginal bleeding, undiagnosed
(may indicate the presence of endometrial hyperplasia or carcinoma, which may be exacerbated by ovulation-induced increases in estrogen serum concentrations; other possible endocrinopathies should also be ruled out)

» Fibroid tumors of the uterus or
» Ovarian cyst or enlargement not associated with polycystic ovarian disease
(risk of further enlargement)

» Thrombophlebitis, active
(increased risk of arterial thromboembolism due to elevations in serum estrogen concentrations)

*For males only*
» Prostatic carcinoma or other androgen-dependent neoplasm
(may be exacerbated by hCG-induced increases in testosterone serum concentrations)

***Risk-benefit should be considered when the following medical problems exist:***

Sensitivity to chorionic gonadotropin or other gonadotropins

*For induction of ovulation*
» Polycystic ovarian disease
(an exaggerated response to hCG may occur; lower dosage may be required)

## Patient monitoring

The following may be especially important in patient monitoring (other tests may be warranted in some patients, depending on condition; » = major clinical significance):

*For induction of ovulation*
» Estradiol
(measurement of serum concentrations is recommended as needed, continuing through the day of chorionic gonadotropin administration; recommended to determine optimal dose and to lessen the risk of ovarian hyperstimulation)

» Ultrasound examination
(recommended prior to chorionic gonadotropin therapy to provide information on the number and size of mature follicles, to follow follicular development, and to lessen the risk of ovarian hyperstimulation syndrome and multiple gestation)

Daily basal body temperature
(can be used in ovulation induction to determine if ovulation has occurred; if basal body temperature following a treatment cycle is biphasic and is not followed by menses, a pregnancy test is recommended)

Progesterone
(measurement of serum concentrations can be performed after therapy to detect luteinized ovarian follicles)

*For treatment of male infertility (hypogonadism)*
Testosterone
(measurement of baseline serum concentrations recommended before and after chorionic gonadotropin administration to rule out other causes and evaluate success of treatment; should increase after chorionic gonadotropin therapy)

Sperm count and determinations of sperm motility
(to evaluate success of treatment)

*For diagnosis of male hypogonadism (delayed puberty)*
Testosterone
(measurement of baseline and post-treatment serum concentrations recommended prior to and 1 day following the course; should double if testes are normal)

## Side/Adverse Effects

Note: Use of chorionic gonadotropin in conjunction with other ovulation-inducing agents is associated with an increased risk of thromboembolic events, possibly due to increased serum estrogen concentrations.

The following side/adverse effects have been selected on the basis of their potential clinical significance (possible signs and symptoms in parentheses where appropriate)—not necessarily inclusive:

**Those indicating need for medical attention**
Incidence more frequent
*For induction of ovulation only*
 **Ovarian cysts or mild to moderate, uncomplicated ovarian enlargement** (mild bloating, stomach or pelvic pain)
  Note: Symptoms of *ovarian cysts or enlargement* are usually mild to moderate and abate within 2 or 3 weeks.

Incidence less frequent or rare
*For induction of ovulation only*
 **Severe ovarian hyperstimulation syndrome** (severe abdominal or stomach pain; feeling of indigestion; moderate to severe bloating; decreased amount of urine; continuing or severe nausea, vomiting, or diarrhea; severe pelvic pain; rapid weight gain; shortness of breath; swelling of lower legs); **peripheral edema** (swelling of feet or lower legs; rapid weight gain)
  Note: *Ovarian hyperstimulation syndrome (OHS)* may occur in patients treated with hCG for ovulation induction. OHS may often occur 7 to 10 days after ovulation or completion of therapy. OHS is usually avoided or short-lived in patients for whom chorionic gonadotropin is withheld. OHS differs from uncomplicated ovarian enlargement and can rapidly progress to cause serious medical problems. With OHS, a marked increase in vascular permeability results in rapid accumulation of fluid in the peritoneal, pleural, and pericardial cavities (third-spacing of fluids). Medical complications ultimately arising from this increased vascular permeability may include hypovolemia, hemoconcentration, electrolyte imbalance, ascites, hemoperitoneum, pleural effusions, hydrothorax, acute pulmonary distress, and thromboembolic events. OHS is more common, more severe, and protracted in patients who conceive.

Incidence less frequent
*In treatment of cryptorchidism only*
 **Precocious puberty** (acne; enlargement of penis or testes; growth of pubic hair; rapid increase in height)—generally requires discontinuance of chorionic gonadotropin and re-evaluation

**Those indicating need for medical attention only if they continue or are bothersome**
Incidence less frequent
 **Enlargement of breasts; headache; irritability; mental depression; pain at injection site; tiredness**

## Patient Consultation

As an aid to patient consultation, refer to *Advice for the Patient, Chorionic Gonadotropin (Systemic).*

In providing consultation, consider emphasizing the following selected information (» = major clinical significance):

**Before using this medication**
» Conditions affecting use, especially:
   Sensitivity to chorionic gonadotropin
   Use in children—Use of chorionic gonadotropin for treatment of cryptorchidism has resulted in precocious puberty
   Other medical problems, especially:
   For all indications—Pituitary hypertrophy or tumor
   For induction of ovulation—Abnormal vaginal bleeding, uterine fibroids, ovarian cyst or enlargement, polycystic ovarian disease, or thrombophlebitis
   For treatment of male hypogonadism—Prostatic carcinoma or other androgen-dependent neoplasm

**Proper use of this medication**
» Proper dosing

**Precautions while using this medication**
» Importance of close monitoring by physician
» May take a long time to work; importance of continuing treatment
*For induction of ovulation*
» Importance of following physician's instructions for recording of basal body temperature and timing of intercourse, when recommended by physician

**Side/adverse effects**
 Signs of potential side effects, especially peripheral edema, ovarian enlargement, cysts, or hyperstimulation syndrome (for ovulation induction), and precocious puberty (for treatment of cryptorchidism)

## General Dosing Information

Patients receiving chorionic gonadotropin should be under supervision of a physician experienced in the treatment of gynecologic or endocrine disorders.

**For induction of ovulation**
Dosage varies considerably and must be adjusted to meet the individual requirements of each patient, on the basis of clinical response.

Conception should be attempted within 48 hours of ovulation. It is recommended that the couple have intercourse or insemination performed daily or every other day beginning the day after chorionic gonadotropin is administered until ovulation is thought to have occurred.

If ovulation does not occur after any cycle of therapy, the therapeutic regimen employed should be re-evaluated. After 3 cycles of non-ovulatory menses, the appropriateness of continuing the use of chorionic gonadotropin for ovulation induction should be reconsidered.

**For corpus luteum insufficiency**
Treatment must begin in the cycle of conception and not after the first missed menses.

Administration of chorionic gonadotropin should continue until hormone production is taken over by the placenta after 7 to 10 weeks gestation.

**For treatment of adverse effects**
Ovarian enlargement or ovarian cyst formation
 • Discontinuing therapy until ovarian size has returned to baseline. Chorionic gonadotropin should also be withheld for that cycle.
 • Prohibiting intercourse until ovarian size has returned to baseline to prevent cyst rupture.
 • Reducing dosage in next course of therapy.
Ovarian hyperstimulation syndrome (OHS)
 Acute phase
 • Discontinuing therapy. Chorionic gonadotropin should also be withheld for that cycle.
 • Prohibiting intercourse until ovarian size has returned to baseline to prevent cyst rupture.
 • Most cases of OHS will spontaneously resolve when menses begins. In selected cases, hospitalization of the patient with bed rest may be necessary.
 • Utilizing therapy to prevent hemoconcentration and minimize risk of thromboembolism and renal injury.
 • Correcting (cautiously) electrolyte imbalance while maintaining acceptable intravascular volume; in the acute phase, intravascular volume deficit cannot be completely corrected without increasing third space fluid volume.
 • Monitoring fluid intake and output, body weight, hematocrit, serum and urine electrolytes, urine specific gravity, blood urea nitrogen (BUN), creatinine, and abdominal girth daily or as often as required.
 • Monitoring serum potassium concentrations for development of hyperkalemia.
 • Limiting performance of pelvic examinations since they may result in rupture of ovarian cysts and hemoperitoneum.
 • Administering intravenous fluids, electrolytes, and human serum albumin, as needed to maintain adequate urine output and to avoid hemoconcentration.
 • Administering analgesics as needed.
 • Avoiding diuretic use since it reduces intravascular volume further.
 • Removing ascitic, pleural, or pericardial fluid *only* if it is imperative for relief of symptoms such as respiratory distress or cardiac tamponade; to do so may increase risk of injury to the ovary.
 • In patients who require surgery to control bleeding from ovarian cyst rupture, employing surgical measures that also maximally conserve ovarian tissue.
 Intermediate phase
 • Once patient is stabilized, minimizing third spacing of fluids by cautiously replacing potassium, sodium, and fluids as required, based on monitoring of serum electrolyte concentrations.
 • Avoiding diuretic use.
 Resolution phase
 • The third space fluid shifts to intravascular compartment, resulting in decreased hematocrit value and increased urinary output.
 • Peripheral and/or pulmonary edema may result if third space fluid volume mobilized exceeds renal output.

   • Administering diuretics when required, to manage pulmonary edema.

## Parenteral Dosage Forms

Note: Bracketed uses in the *Dosage Forms* section refer to categories of use and/or indications that are not included in U.S. product labeling.

### CHORIONIC GONADOTROPIN FOR INJECTION USP

**Usual adult dose**
Hypogonadotropic hypogonadism in males—
   Intramuscular, 1000 to 4000 Units two to three times a week for several weeks to months; may be continued indefinitely as long as a response occurs.
   For induction of spermatogenesis in infertility, treatment is usually continued for 6 months or longer. If sperm counts are still not adequate (>5 million per mL), menotropins or urofollitropin may be added to the regimen. It may be necessary to continue a combined regimen for up to 12 additional months.
[Corpus luteum insufficiency][1]—
   Intramuscular, 1500 Units (average; dosage will vary depending upon patient) every other day from the day of ovulation until the time of expected menses or confirmed pregnancy. After pregnancy is confirmed, this dose may be continued for up to 10 weeks gestation.
Induction of ovulation or
Assisted reproductive technologies—
   Intramuscular, 5000 to 10,000 Units one day following the last dose of menotropins or urofollitropin or five to nine days following the last dose of clomiphene.
   Note: If the ovaries are abnormally enlarged or the serum estradiol concentration is excessively elevated on the last day of menotropins or urofollitropin therapy, chorionic gonadotropin should not be given for that cycle.
      Dosage varies considerably and must be adjusted to meet the individual requirements of each patient, on the basis of clinical response.

**Usual pediatric dose**
Prepubertal cryptorchidism—
   Intramuscular, 1000 to 5000 Units two to three times a week for a maximum of 10 doses, discontinuing when the desired response is achieved.
   Note: Treatment with more than 10 doses is not recommended if progressive descent does not occur.
      Several dosage schedules have been used; dosage will vary depending on the degree of sexual development already present.
[Diagnostic aid (hypogonadism) in males][1]—
   Intramuscular, 2000 Units once a day for three days.

**Size(s) usually available**
U.S.—
   5000 Units (Rx) [*A.P.L; Profasi;* GENERIC].
   10,000 Units (Rx) [*A.P.L; Pregnyl; Profasi;* GENERIC].
   20,000 Units (Rx) [*A.P.L;* GENERIC].
Canada—
   5000 Units (Rx) [GENERIC].
   10,000 Units (Rx) [*A.P.L; Profasi HP;* GENERIC].
   20,000 Units (Rx) [GENERIC].

**Packaging and storage**
Store below 40 °C (104 °F), preferably between 15 and 30 °C (59 and 86 °F), unless otherwise specified by manufacturer.

**Preparation of dosage form**
Using standard aseptic technique, add 1 to 10 mL of diluent provided to each vial, depending upon manufacturer labeling.

**Stability**
Reconstituted solution is stable in the refrigerator for 60 or 90 days, depending on manufacturer.

---

[1]Not included in Canadian product labeling.

---

Revised: 07/26/92
Interim revision: 06/03/94

---

## CHROMIC    CHLORIDE—See *Chromium Supplements (Systemic)*

---

# CHROMIC PHOSPHATE P 32   Parenteral-Local†

VA CLASSIFICATION (Primary): AN600

Note: For a listing of dosage forms and brand names by country availability, see *Dosage Forms* section(s). For a listing of brand names for the articles in this monograph, refer to the General Index.

---

†Not commercially available in Canada.

---

## Category
Antineoplastic.

## Indications

### Accepted
Malignant effusions, peritoneal (treatment) or
Malignant effusions, pleural (treatment)—Chromic phosphate P 32 is indicated by intracavity instillation for the treatment of peritoneal and pleural effusions caused by metastatic disease. In the presence of large tumor masses, other forms of treatment may be indicated; however, chromic phosphate P 32 may control the effusion when other treatment has failed. Bloody effusions may reduce the effectiveness of treatment.

Carcinoma, ovarian (treatment) or
Carcinoma, prostatic (treatment)—Chromic phosphate P 32 is indicated by interstitial injection for the treatment of cancer, such as cancer of the ovary (early-stage) and of the prostate.

## Physical Properties

### Nuclear data

| Radionuclide (half-life) | Mode of decay | Principal emissions (keV) | Mean number of emissions/ disintegration |
| --- | --- | --- | --- |
| P 32 (14.3 days) | Beta emission | 694.8 | 1 |

## Pharmacology/Pharmacokinetics

### Mechanism of action/Effect
Colloidal chromic phosphate P 32 introduced into a body cavity is phagocytized by free macrophages and fixed to the lining of the cavity wall, thus providing local irradiation to the affected area.

### Distribution
Chromic phosphate P 32 distributes from the pleural or peritoneal cavity, and from the site of interstitial injection depending on the particle size and on the instillation site. Thus, phosphate P 32 may locate in the lungs, adrenal glands, kidneys, lymph nodes, liver, spleen, bone marrow, plasma, erythrocytes, and leukocytes.

### Radiation dosimetry
Following a 740-megabequerel (20-millicurie) dose of chromic phosphate P 32—
Pleural and peritoneal surface areas: Assuming the pleural and peritoneal surface areas are 4000 and 5000 cm², respectively, the estimated radiation doses to the pleural and peritoneal cavities of an average 70-kg adult, with 90% retention of dose, at various tissue depths (0.004 to 0.2 cm) range from 230 to 21 Gy (23,000 to 2100 rads) and 180 to 17 Gy (18,000 to 1700 rads), respectively.
Prostate: Estimated absorbed radiation dose to the prostate of an average 70-kg adult is 9100 Gy (910,000 rads).

**Elimination**
Primarily renal.

## Precautions to Consider

### Pregnancy/Reproduction
Pregnancy—The possibility of pregnancy should be assessed in women of child-bearing potential. Clinical situations exist where the benefit to the patient and fetus from information derived from radiopharmaceutical use outweighs the risks from radiation exposure to the fetus. In this situation, the physician should use discretion and reduce the radiopharmaceutical dose to the lowest possible amount.

### Breast-feeding
Chromic phosphate P 32 is excreted in breast milk. Because of the potential risk of radiation exposure to the infant, temporary discontinuation of nursing is recommended for a length of time that may be assessed by measuring the activity of breast milk and estimating the radiation exposure to the infant. Also, it is possible that the dissociated radioactive phosphorus (P 32) may be incorporated into the normal phosphate metabolism of the newborn infant.

### Pediatrics
Appropriate studies on the relationship of age to the effects of chromic phosphate P 32 have not been performed in the pediatric population.

### Geriatrics
Appropriate studies on the relationship of age to the effects of chromic phosphate P 32 have not been performed in the geriatric population. However, no geriatrics-specific problems have been documented to date.

### Medical considerations/Contraindications
The medical considerations/contraindications included here have been selected on the basis of their potential clinical significance (reasons given in parentheses where appropriate)—not necessarily inclusive (» = major clinical significance).

*Except under special circumstances, this medication should not be used when the following medical problems exist:*
» Tumors, ulcerative
   (increased absorption into bloodstream)
» Extreme caution should be used to avoid administration into exposed cavities or in the presence of loculation, unless extent of loculation is determined, because of risk of radiation damage

## Side/Adverse Effects

Note: Intestinal fibrosis or necrosis and chronic fibrosis of the body wall have been reported as a result of inadvertent instillation into intrapleural or intraperitoneal loculations, bowel lumen, or the body wall.

   Radiation damage may result from accidental interstitial administration or injection into a loculation.

The following side/adverse effects have been selected on the basis of their potential clinical significance (possible signs and symptoms in parentheses where appropriate)—not necessarily inclusive:

**Those indicating need for medical attention**
Incidence less frequent or rare
   *Bone marrow depression, transitory* (sore throat and fever, unusual bleeding or bruising, unusual tiredness or weakness); *peritonitis* (severe abdominal or stomach pain, chills, severe nausea and vomiting); *pleuritis* (chest pain, chills and fever, dry cough, troubled breathing)

**Those indicating need for medical attention only if they continue or are bothersome**
Incidence more frequent
   *Radiation sickness* (abdominal or stomach cramps, diarrhea, feeling of discomfort, loss of appetite, nausea and vomiting, weakness)
   Note: *Radiation sickness* is usually self-limiting; onset within several hours after administration; may last 24 to 36 hours.

## Patient Consultation

As an aid to patient consultation, refer to *Advice for the Patient, Chromic Phosphate P 32 (Therapeutic)*.

In providing consultation, consider emphasizing the following selected information (» = major clinical significance):

**Description of use**
   Instillation into body cavity or injection into interspaces of affected tissue
   Local irradiation effect used for treatment of cancer or effusions caused by cancer

**Before using this medication**
» Conditions affecting use, especially:
      Pregnancy—Risk to fetus from radiation exposure as opposed to benefit derived from use should be considered
      Breast-feeding—Excreted in breast milk; discontinuation of nursing recommended because of risk of radiation exposure to infant

**Preparation for this treatment**
   Special preparatory instructions may be given; patient should inquire in advance

**Side/adverse effects**
   Signs of potential side effects, especially peritonitis, pleuritis, transitory bone marrow depression

## General Dosing Information

Radiopharmaceuticals are to be administered only by or under the supervision of physicians who have had extensive training in the safe use and handling of radionuclides and who are licensed by the Nuclear Regulatory Commission (NRC) or the appropriate Agreement State agency or, outside the U.S., the appropriate authority.

Chromic phosphate P 32 suspension should *not* be injected intravascularly.

Visual inspection of the injection is recommended to avoid accidental administration of sodium phosphate P 32. Chromic phosphate P 32 is a green, cloudy liquid, whereas sodium phosphate P 32 is a clear, colorless solution, intended for intravascular use only.

### Safety considerations for handling this radiopharmaceutical
Improper handling of this radiopharmaceutical may cause radioactive contamination. Guidelines for handling radioactive material have been prepared by scientific, professional, state, federal, and international bodies and are available to the specially qualified and authorized users who have access to radiopharmaceuticals.

## Parenteral Dosage Forms

### CHROMIC PHOSPHATE P 32 SUSPENSION USP

**Usual adult and adolescent dose**
Malignant effusions—
   Intraperitoneal instillation, 370 to 740 megabecquerels (10 to 20 millicuries).
   Intrapleural instillation, 222 to 444 megabecquerels (6 to 12 millicuries).
Carcinoma—
   Interstitial injection, 3.7 to 18.5 megabecquerels (0.1 to 0.5 millicurie) per gram of estimated tumor weight.

**Usual pediatric dose**
Dosage must be individualized by physician.

**Usual geriatric dose**
See *Usual adult and adolescent dose.*

**Strength(s) usually available**
U.S.—
   185 megabecquerels (5 millicuries) per mL, having a specific activity of up to 185 megabecquerels (5 millicuries) per milligram, at time of calibration (Rx) [*Phosphocol P 32*].
Canada—
   Not commercially available.

**Packaging and storage**
Store below 40 °C (104 °F), preferably between 15 and 30 °C (59 and 86 °F), unless otherwise specified by manufacturer. Protect from freezing.

**Note**
Caution—Radioactive material.

Shake well.

## Selected Bibliography

Powell JL, Burrell MO, Kirchner AB. Intraperitoneal radioactive chromic phosphate P 32 in the treatment of ovarian cancer. South Med J 1987 Dec; 80 (12): 1513-7.
Leichner PK, Cash SA, Backx C, et al. Effects of injection volume on the tissue dose, dose rate and therapeutic potential of intraperitoneal P 32. Radiology 1981; 141: 193.

Revised: 05/18/92
Interim revision: 08/02/94

**CHROMIUM**—See *Chromium Supplements (Systemic)*

# CHROMIUM SUPPLEMENTS   Systemic

This monograph includes information on the following: Chromic Chloride†; Chromium.

VA CLASSIFICATION (Primary): TN490

Note: For a listing of dosage forms and brand names by country availability, see *Dosage Forms* section(s). For a listing of brand names for the articles in this monograph, refer to the General Index.

---

†Not commercially available in Canada.

---

## Category

Nutritional supplement (mineral).

## Indications

### Accepted
Chromium deficiency (prophylaxis and treatment)—Chromium supplements are indicated in the prevention and treatment of chromium deficiency, which may result from inadequate nutrition, protein malnutrition, or intestinal malabsorption but does not occur in healthy individuals receiving an adequate balanced diet. For prophylaxis of chromium deficiency, dietary improvement, rather than supplementation, is advisable. For treatment of chromium deficiency, supplementation is preferred.

Deficiency of chromium may lead to glucose intolerance and peripheral or central neuropathy.

Some unusual diets (e.g., reducing diets that drastically restrict food selection) may not supply minimum daily requirements of chromium. Supplementation may be necessary in patients receiving total parenteral nutrition (TPN) or undergoing rapid weight loss or in those with malnutrition, because of inadequate dietary intake.

### Acceptance not established
There are insufficient data to show that chromium supplementation is beneficial in improving *glucose tolerance*.

## Pharmacology/Pharmacokinetics

### Physicochemical characteristics
Molecular weight—
    Chromic chloride: 266.45.
    Elemental chromium: 52.

### Mechanism of action/Effect
Chromium is part of the glucose tolerance factor (GTF), which is believed to potentiate the action of insulin at the cellular level. Chromium may also play a role in lipoprotein metabolism.

### Absorption
Oral chromium is poorly absorbed. Oral chromium products may be chelated to increase absorption. The absorption of inorganic chromic salts is 0.5 to 1%.

### Protein binding
10 to 17% bound to transferrin.

### Elimination
Primarily in urine, with small amounts excreted in bile.

## Precautions to Consider

### Pregnancy/Reproduction
Pregnancy—Problems in humans have not been documented with intake of normal daily recommended amounts. However, adequate and well-controlled studies in humans have not been done.

Adequate and well-controlled studies in animals have not been done.

FDA Pregnancy Category C (parenteral chromium).

### Breast-feeding
Problems in humans have not been documented with intake of normal daily recommended amounts.

### Pediatrics
Problems in pediatrics have not been documented with intake of normal daily recommended amounts.

Chromic chloride injection that contains benzyl alcohol as a preservative should not be used in newborn and immature infants. The use of benzyl alcohol in neonates has been associated with a fatal toxic syndrome consisting of metabolic acidosis and CNS, respiratory, circulatory, and renal function impairment.

### Geriatrics
Problems in geriatrics have not been documented with intake of normal daily recommended amounts.

### Drug interactions and/or related problems
The following drug interactions and/or related problems have been selected on the basis of their potential clinical significance (possible mechanism in parentheses where appropriate)—not necessarily inclusive (» = major clinical significance):

Note: Combinations containing any of the following medications, depending on the amount present, may also interact with chromium supplements.

  Insulin
    (some studies have found that administration of chromium supplements to a chromium deficient patient may improve glucose tolerance; this could decrease insulin requirements; careful monitoring of blood glucose may be necessary with chromium therapy to avoid hypoglycemia)

### Laboratory value alterations
The following have been selected on the basis of their potential clinical significance (possible effect in parentheses where appropriate)—not necessarily inclusive (» = major clinical significance):

With physiology/laboratory test values
  Glucose
    (serum concentrations may be decreased, as chromium has been reported to improve glucose tolerance and potentiate the action of insulin)

### Medical considerations/Contraindications
The medical considerations/contraindications included here have been selected on the basis of their potential clinical significance (reasons given in parentheses where appropriate)—not necessarily inclusive (» = major clinical significance).

*Risk-benefit should be considered when the following medical problem exists:*
  Diabetes mellitus
    (some studies have found that administration of chromium supplements to a chromium deficient patient may improve glucose tolerance; this could decrease insulin requirements; careful monitoring of blood glucose may be necessary with chromium therapy to avoid hypoglycemia)

### Patient monitoring
The following may be especially important in patient monitoring (other tests may be warranted in some patients, depending on condition; » = major clinical significance):

Glucose determinations, serum
    (determinations may be recommended at periodic intervals, especially in diabetes mellitus, to avoid hypoglycemia)

Hemoglobin A₁
    (some clinicians recommend that hemoglobin $A_1$ be monitored in patients receiving long-term TPN therapy because it is a more accurate method of assessing glucose tolerance)

Glucose tolerance
    (response to glucose tolerance tests or a change in insulin requirements during chromium supplementation may be useful in determining chromium status)

## Side/Adverse Effects

No side effects or overdoses have been reported with chromium supplements.

## Patient Consultation

As an aid to patient consultation, refer to *Advice for the Patient, Chromium Supplements (Systemic)*.

In providing consultation, consider emphasizing the following selected information (» = major clinical significance):

**Description of use**
  Description of use should include function in the body, signs of deficiency, conditions that may cause chromium deficiency

**Importance of diet**
  Importance of proper nutrition; supplement may be needed because of inadequate dietary intake
  Food sources of chromium
  Recommended daily intake for chromium

**Proper use of this dietary supplement**

» Proper dosing

Missed dose: No cause for concern because of length of time necessary for depletion; remembering to take as directed.

» Proper storage

## General Dosing Information

Because of the infrequency of chromium deficiency alone, combinations of several vitamins and/or minerals are commonly administered. Many commercial vitamin-mineral complexes are available.

**For parenteral dosage forms only**

In most cases, parenteral administration is indicated only when oral administration is not acceptable (for example, in nausea, vomiting, preoperative and postoperative conditions) or possible (for example, in malabsorption syndromes or following gastric resection).

**Diet/Nutrition**

Recommended dietary intakes for chromium are defined differently worldwide.

For U.S.—The Recommended Dietary Allowances (RDAs) for vitamins and minerals are determined by the Food and Nutrition Board of the National Research Council and are intended to provide adequate nutrition in most healthy persons under usual environmental stresses. In addition, a different designation may be used by the FDA for food and dietary supplement labeling purposes, as with Daily Value (DV). DVs replace the previous labeling terminology United States Recommended Daily Allowances (USRDAs).

For Canada—Recommended Nutrient Intakes (RNIs) for vitamins, minerals, and protein are determined by Health and Welfare Canada and provide recommended amounts of a specific nutrient while minimizing the risk of chronic diseases.

There is no RDA or RNI established for chromium. Normal daily recommended intakes for chromium are generally defined as follows:

Infants and children:

Birth to 3 years of age: 10 to 80 mcg.

4 to 6 years of age: 30 to 120 mcg.

7 to 10 years of age: 50 to 200 mcg.

Adolescents and adults:

50 to 200 mcg.

The best dietary sources of chromium include brewer's yeast, calf liver, American cheese, and wheat germ.

---

### *CHROMIC CHLORIDE*

## Parenteral Dosage Forms

### CHROMIC CHLORIDE INJECTION USP

**Usual adult and adolescent dose**

Deficiency (prophylaxis)—

Intravenous, 10 to 15 mcg (.01 to .015 mg) a day, added to total parenteral nutrition (TPN).

Deficiency (treatment)—

Intravenous, 20 mcg (.02 mg) a day, added to total parenteral nutrition (TPN).

**Usual pediatric dose**

Deficiency (prophylaxis or treatment)—

Intravenous, 0.14 to 0.2 mcg per kilogram of body weight a day, added to total parenteral nutrition (TPN).

Note: Chromic chloride injection that contains benzyl alcohol as a preservative should not be used in newborn and immature infants. The use of benzyl alcohol in neonates has been associated with a fatal toxic syndrome consisting of metabolic acidosis and CNS, respiratory, circulatory, and renal function impairment.

**Strength(s) usually available**

U.S.—

20.5 mcg (.0205 mg) (4 mcg elemental chromium) per mL (Rx) [*Chroma-Pak* (0.9% benzyl alcohol); GENERIC].

102.5 mcg (.1025 mg) (20 mcg elemental chromium) per mL (Rx) [*Chroma-Pak;* GENERIC].

Canada—

Not commercially available.

**Packaging and storage**

Store below 40 °C (104 °F), preferably between 15 and 30 °C (59 and 86 °F), unless otherwise specified by manufacturer.

**Preparation of dosage form**

Chromic chloride is compatible with amino acids, dextrose, electrolytes, and vitamins usually used for total parenteral nutrition (TPN).

---

### *CHROMIUM*

## CHROMIUM CAPSULES

**Usual adult and adolescent dose**

Deficiency (prophylaxis)—

Oral, amount based on normal daily recommended intakes: 50 to 200 mcg.

Deficiency (treatment)—

Treatment dose is individualized by prescriber based on severity of deficiency.

**Usual pediatric dose**

Deficiency (prophylaxis)—Oral, amount based on normal daily recommended amounts—

Birth to 3 years of age—10 to 80 mcg.

4 to 6 years of age—30 to 120 mcg.

7 to 10 years of age—50 to 200 mcg.

Deficiency (treatment)—

Treatment dose is individualized by prescriber based on severity of deficiency.

**Strength(s) usually available**

U.S.—

200 mcg (0.2 mg) elemental chromium (OTC) [GENERIC].

Canada—

Not commercially available.

Note: This chromium preparation may exceed the dosage range recommended by USP DI Advisory Panels based on the amount necessary to meet normal nutritional needs.

**Packaging and storage**

Store below 40 °C (104 °F), preferably between 15 and 30 °C (59 and 86 °F), unless otherwise specified by manufacturer.

## CHROMIUM TABLETS

**Usual adult and adolescent dose**

See *Chromium Capsules.*

**Usual pediatric dose**

See *Chromium Capsules.*

**Strength(s) usually available**

U.S.—

100 mcg (0.1 mg) elemental chromium (OTC) [GENERIC].

200 mcg (0.2 mg) elemental chromium (OTC) [GENERIC (yeast)].

1 mg elemental chromium (OTC) [GENERIC (amino acids)].

Canada—

200 mcg (0.2 mg) elemental chromium (OTC) [GENERIC (yeast)].

Note: Some strengths of these chromium preparations may exceed the dosage range recommended by USP DI Advisory Panels based on the amount necessary to meet normal nutritional needs.

**Packaging and storage**

Store below 40 °C (104 °F), preferably between 15 and 30 °C (59 and 86 °F), unless otherwise specified by manufacturer.

## Selected Bibliography

Mooradian A, Morely J. Micronutrient status in diabetes mellitus. Am J Clin Nutr 1987; 45: 877-95.

---

Revised: 03/24/92

Interim revision: 08/01/94; 05/26/95

# CHYMOPAPAIN   Parenteral-Local

VA CLASSIFICATION (Primary): MS900
Note: For a listing of dosage forms and brand names by country availability, see *Dosage Forms* section(s). For a listing of brand names
for the articles in this monograph, refer to the General Index.

## Category
Chemonucleolytic (herniated lumbar intervertebral disk therapy).

## Indications

### Accepted
Disk, herniated lumbar intervertebral (treatment)—Chymopapain is indicated in the treatment of patients with intractable sciatica and documented herniated intervertebral lumbar disks who have not responded
to conservative therapy. However, because chymopapain may cause
serious complications, especially if it is misused, it is recommended
that the medication be administered only by qualified and experienced
physicians, and only to carefully selected patients.

### Unaccepted
Chymopapain has not been studied, and is not recommended, in the treatment of herniated disks in areas other than the lumbar spine.

Chymopapain therapy is not recommended for treatment of a sequestrated
("migrated") disk, i.e., it should not be used when extruded nucleus
pulposus material has separated from, and is no longer contiguous
with, the disk.

## Pharmacology/Pharmacokinetics

### Physicochemical characteristics
Molecular weight—Approximately 27,000.

### Mechanism of action/Effect
Chymopapain is a proteolytic enzyme isolated from the crude latex of
*Carica papaya*. When injected into the nucleus pulposus, chymopapain hydrolyzes the polypeptides or proteins that maintain the structure
of the chondromucoprotein of the nucleus pulposus. Degradation of
the chondromucoprotein reduces intradiskal osmotic activity, thereby
decreasing fluid absorption and reducing intradiskal pressure. Chymopapain has no effect on collagen.

### Absorption
Chymopapain diffuses into the plasma, where it is inactivated by alpha$_2$-
macroglobulin, following injection into the central portion of the intervertebral disk. However, the medication acts directly at the site of
injection; absorption is not required for effectiveness.

## Precautions to Consider

### Cross-sensitivity and/or related problems
Patients hypersensitive to papaya or papaya derivatives (present in some
meat tenderizers, contact lens cleaners, and beers) may be hypersensitive to chymopapain also.

### Pregnancy/Reproduction
Pregnancy—Studies have not been done in humans.
Studies have not been done in animals.
FDA Pregnancy Category C.

### Breast-feeding
It is not known whether chymopapain is distributed into breast milk. However, problems in humans have not been documented.

### Pediatrics
No information is available on the relationship of age to the effects of
chymopapain in pediatric patients.

### Geriatrics
No information is available on the relationship of age to the effects of
chymopapain in geriatric patients.

### Drug interactions and/or related problems
The following drug interactions and/or related problems have been selected on the basis of their potential clinical significance (possible
mechanism in parentheses where appropriate)—not necessarily inclusive (» = major clinical significance):
Beta-adrenergic blocking agents, possibly including ophthalmic dosage forms
(gradual withdrawal of beta-adrenergic blocking agent therapy
prior to administration of chymopapain may be advisable because
beta-adrenergic blocking agents inhibit the actions of epinephrine,
which may be required to treat chymopapain-induced anaphylaxis)

» Contrast media, radiopaque
(concurrent use with chymopapain may increase the risk of toxicity, especially if either agent enters the subarachnoid space; it is
strongly recommended that diskography not be performed as part
of the chemonucleolysis procedure)

### Medical considerations/Contraindications
The medical considerations/contraindications included here have been selected on the basis of their potential clinical significance (reasons given
in parentheses where appropriate)—not necessarily inclusive (» =
major clinical significance).

*Except under special circumstances, this medication should not be used*
*when the following medical problems exist:*
» Allergic reaction to papaya or papaya derivatives, history of, or
» Previous chymopapain therapy
(increased risk of allergic reactions)
» Cauda equina lesion
» Paralysis, severe and progressing, as indicated by rapid deterioration
of neurologic function or increasing muscle weakness
» Spinal cord tumor
» Spinal stenosis, significant
» Spondylolisthesis, severe

*Risk-benefit should be considered when the following medical problems*
*exist:*
Allergies, multiple, history of
(increased risk of allergic reactions)
Cerebrovascular accident, history of in patient or strong history of in
patient's family, or
Cerebrovascular anomaly, known or suspected, or
Hypertension, history of
(increased risk of extensive or severe central nervous system
[CNS] hemorrhage and/or serious neurologic adverse effects)
Surgery, prior, of lumbar spine
(increased risk of serious neurologic adverse effects)
» Caution is also required for patients sensitive to iodine, who should
not receive absorbable iodine-containing contrast media if diskography is performed prior to injection of chymopapain.

### Patient monitoring
The following may be especially important in patient monitoring (other
tests may be warranted in some patients, depending on condition;
» = major clinical significance):
» Monitoring for signs and symptoms of anaphylaxis
(required during and for at least 2 hours after administration)

## Side/Adverse Effects
The following side/adverse effects have been selected on the basis of their
potential clinical significance (possible signs and symptoms in parentheses where appropriate)—not necessarily inclusive:

### Those indicating need for medical attention
Incidence rare (1% or less)
*Allergic reaction, which may include; angioedema; conjunctivitis;*
*pilomotor erection; vasomotor rhinitis* (runny nose); *and gastrointes-*
*tinal disturbances; as well as allergic dermatitis; and anaphylaxis*
(changes in facial skin color; fast or irregular breathing; hypotension;
puffiness or swelling of the eyelids or around the eyes; shortness of
breath, troubled breathing, tightness in chest, and/or wheezing; skin
rash, hives, and/or itching); *CNS hemorrhage, including intracerebral*
*or subarachnoid* (headache, sudden, severe, and continuing); *derma-*
*titis, allergic* (skin rash, hives, itching, or redness); *diskitis, aseptic or*
*bacterial; neurologic effects* (decreased or uncontrolled urination; paralysis or severe weakness of legs; uncontrolled bowel movements);
*paralytic ileus* (abdominal or stomach cramps or pain; severe constipation; swelling of abdomen or stomach; vomiting); *seizures; throm-*
*bophlebitis* (hot skin, pain, swelling, tenderness, and/or skin color
changes in leg or foot)—may lead to pulmonary embolism
Note: The incidence of *anaphylaxis* is approximately 0.6% in female
patients receiving local anesthesia, 0.9% in female patients receiving general anesthesia, and 0.3% in male patients receiving
either local or general anesthesia. The reaction may be immediate or delayed up to 2 hours following administration. The
severity of the reaction may be dose-dependent. Initial symptoms of bronchospasm and hypotension may progress to laryngeal edema, cardiac arrhythmia, shock, cardiac arrest, coma,
and death.

**Those indicating need for medical attention only if they continue or are bothersome**
Incidence more frequent
  *Back pain, stiffness, or soreness*—incidence 50%; *muscle spasm in lower back*—incidence 30%
  Note: *Back pain* and *muscle spasms in lower back* may persist for several days; residual *stiffness or soreness* may persist for several months.

Incidence less frequent or rare
  *Dizziness; headache; nausea; neurologic effects* (burning feeling in lower back or sacral area; cramps, pain, or mild weakness in legs; decreased sensitivity to pain; foot drop; numbness or tingling in legs or toes)

**Those indicating possible delayed reactions and the need for medical attention if they occur after the medication is discontinued**
  *Dermatitis, allergic* (skin rash, hives, or itching)—may occur up to 15 days after injection; *transverse myelitis/myelopathy, acute* (back pain, sudden and severe; muscle weakness, sudden and progressing)—may occur up to 2 to 4 weeks after injection

## Patient Consultation

As an aid to patient consultation, refer to *Advice for the Patient, Chymopapain (Parenteral-Local).*

In providing consultation, consider emphasizing the following selected information (»= major clinical significance):

**Before receiving this medication**
» Conditions affecting use, especially:
    Hypersensitivity to chymopapain, papaya, or papaya derivatives
    Prior chymopapain therapy
    Other medical problems, especially allergies, stroke, or hypertension

**Proper use of this medication**
» Proper dosing

**Side/adverse effects**
  Signs and symptoms of potential side effects, especially allergic reaction, CNS hemorrhage, allergic dermatitis, aseptic or bacterial diskitis, neurologic effects, paralytic ileus, seizures, thrombophlebitis, and acute transverse myelitis/myelopathy
  Possibility that back pain or muscle spasm may persist for several days, and stiffness or soreness may persist for several months, following administration of medication
  Notifying physician if symptoms of delayed reactions occur

## General Dosing Information

Chymopapain should be administered only by specially trained personnel in a hospital setting. Specifically, the medication should be administered only by surgeons who, by training and experience, can authoritatively perform, and advise patients about all accepted forms of treatment for herniated lumbar intervertebral disk disease, including surgery. In addition, these physicians and their support personnel should be capable of diagnosing and treating all potential chymopapain-induced complications.

*Equipment and medications needed to treat anaphylaxis should be immediately available whenever chymopapain is used.* At least 1 intravenous line must be in place to permit rapid management of anaphylaxis. Epinephrine hydrochloride is the drug of choice for treatment. The use of other agents such as antihistamines and/or glucocorticoids is generally reserved for cases in which use of epinephrine is ineffective.

Use of a preoperative screening test for chymopapain-specific IgE antibody may be considered to identify patients at risk of developing an anaphylactic reaction to the medication. However, the efficacy of such testing has not been demonstrated conclusively. Recent reports indicate that skin prick testing (using a 10-mg-per-mL concentration of chymopapain) is effective in identifying patients at risk of anaphylaxis, provided that the patient is not receiving a medication (such as $H_1$- or $H_2$-receptor antagonist antihistamines, cromolyn, or immunosuppressive doses of glucocorticoids) that will interfere with the test results.

Pretreatment of the patient with histamine ($H_1$ and $H_2$) receptor antagonists is recommended to decrease the severity of chymopapain-induced allergic reactions. A widely used regimen consists of cimetidine (300 mg orally) plus diphenhydramine (50 mg orally) every 6 hours for 24 hours prior to administration of chymopapain. Also, it is recommended that the patient be well hydrated, using oral or intravenous fluids, prior to the procedure because of the abrupt decrease in intravascular volume during anaphylaxis.

Patients receiving chymopapain injections at 2 or more disk spaces may be at increased risk of developing serious neurologic adverse effects. It is strongly recommended that chymopapain administration be limited to

one disk, unless specific clinical and/or diagnostic evidence clearly indicates that more than one disk is responsible for the patient's symptoms.

The patient should be anesthetized prior to insertion of the needle. General anesthesia may be administered if necessary. However, use of local anesthesia or supplemented local anesthesia may decrease the risk of anaphylaxis and/or serious neurologic adverse effects, and is therefore recommended. Also, because the awake patient is able to report early signs of these complications, appropriate countermeasures can be instituted more rapidly. In addition, use of epinephrine to counteract an anaphylactic reaction may produce cardiac arrhythmias in patients anesthetized with hydrocarbon inhalation anesthetics, especially halothane.

The needle should be inserted via the lateral approach to avoid puncture of the dura mater. *The transdural or posterior approach to needle placement must be avoided.* Because animal studies have shown intrathecal administration of chymopapain to be extremely toxic, especially when it is given in conjunction with radiopaque contrast media, *great caution must be exercised to prevent entry of chymopapain or contrast medium (if used) into the subarachnoid space. It is strongly recommended that diskography not be performed as part of the procedure.* Instead, examination of x-rays (obtained with an image intensifier) and, if desired, a saline or water acceptance test, may be used to ensure proper needle placement. However, if diskography is performed, at least 15 minutes should elapse following administration of the radiopaque contrast medium to permit diffusion and absorption of the medium prior to administration of chymopapain through the same needle. *It is recommended that the procedure be discontinued if there is any question regarding needle tip location within the nucleus of the disk, or if the contrast agent (if used) enters the subarachnoid space.*

Oxygen (100%) may be administered to the patient for 3 minutes prior to chymopapain injection to maximize oxygenation in case of anaphylaxis.

Administration of a 0.2-mL test dose of chymopapain is recommended to detect possible hypersensitivity. The remainder of the dose is injected if no adverse reaction occurs within 15 minutes.

## Parenteral Dosage Forms
### CHYMOPAPAIN FOR INJECTION

**Usual adult dose**
Chemonucleolytic—
    Intradiskal, 2000 to 4000 (usually 3000) picoKatal (pKat) units (2 to 4 [usually 3] nanoKatal [nKat] units) per disk.

**Usual adult prescribing limits**
For patients with multiple disk herniation—
    Up to 8000 pKat (8 nKat) units. However, it is strongly recommended that chymopapain administration be limited to one disk, unless clinical and/or diagnostic evidence clearly indicates that more than one disk is responsible for the patient's symptoms, because of the increased risk of neurological complications with multiple injections.

**Usual pediatric dose**
Dosage has not been established.

**Size(s) usually available**
U.S.—
    4000 pKat units (Rx) [*Chymodiactin*].
Canada—
    4 nKat units (Rx) [*Chymodiactin*].

**Packaging and storage**
Store between 2 and 8 °C (36 and 46 °F), unless otherwise specified by manufacturer.

**Preparation of dosage form**
Two mL of sterile water for injection should be added to each vial of chymopapain. Bacteriostatic water for injection should *not* be used because it may inactivate the enzyme. It is recommended that automatic filling syringes not be used for reconstitution because the manufacturing process results in a residual vacuum in the vial.

**Stability**
Alcohol used to cleanse the vial stopper prior to reconstitution must be allowed to air dry before proceeding with reconstitution because residual alcohol may inactivate the enzyme.
After chymopapain is reconstituted, the solution should be used within 2 hours.
Unused portions of the solution must be discarded.

Revised: 07/26/94

# CICLOPIROX    Topical

VA CLASSIFICATION (Primary): DE102
Note: For a listing of dosage forms and brand names by country availability, see *Dosage Forms* section(s). For a listing of brand names for the articles in this monograph, refer to the General Index.

## Category

Antifungal (topical).

Note: Ciclopirox is a broad-spectrum antifungal, which has an antifungal spectrum similar to that of the imidazoles.

## Indications

Note: Bracketed information in the *Indications* section refers to uses that are not included in U.S. product labeling.

### Accepted

Candidiasis, cutaneous (treatment)—Ciclopirox is indicated as a primary agent in the topical treatment of cutaneous candidiasis (moniliasis) caused by *Candida albicans (Monilia albicans)*.

Tinea corporis (treatment)
Tinea cruris (treatment) or
Tinea pedis (treatment)—Ciclopirox is indicated as a primary agent in the topical treatment of tinea corporis (ringworm of the body), tinea cruris (ringworm of the groin; jock itch), or tinea pedis (ringworm of the foot; athlete's foot) caused by *Trichophyton rubrum*, *T. mentagrophytes*, *Epidermophyton floccosum (Acrothesium floccosum)*, and *Microsporum canis*.

Tinea versicolor (treatment)—Ciclopirox is indicated as a primary agent in the topical treatment of tinea versicolor (pityriasis versicolor; "sun fungus") caused by *Pityrosporon orbiculare (Malassezia furfur)*.

[Onychomycosis (treatment)]—Ciclopirox is used as a secondary agent in the topical adjunctive treatment of onychomycosis (tinea unguium; ringworm of the nails).

Not all species or strains of a particular organism may be susceptible to ciclopirox.

## Pharmacology/Pharmacokinetics

### Physicochemical characteristics

Molecular weight—268.36.
pH——The 1% cream and 1% lotion have a pH of 7.

### Mechanism of action/Effect

Exact mechanism unknown; fungicidal *in vitro* against *Trichophyton rubrum*, *T. mentagrophytes*, *Epidermophyton floccosum (Acrothesium floccosum)*, *Microsporum canis*, and *Candida albicans (Monilia albicans)*; may inhibit transport of certain essential substrates into fungal cells; may also interfere with the synthesis of proteins, RNA, and DNA in growing fungal cells; alterations in cell permeability, osmotic fragility, and endogenous respiration are affected only at high concentrations of ciclopirox.

### Other actions/effects

Also has some activity against a wide variety of gram-positive and gram-negative bacteria.

### Absorption

1% Solution in polyethylene glycol 400—Rapid, but minimal; 1.3% of dose absorbed following topical application to 750 cm² of skin on the back, followed by occlusion for 6 hours.
1% Cream—In penetration studies of human cadaveric skin from the back, 0.8 to 1.6% of the dose was present in the stratum corneum 1.5 to 6 hours following application. In addition, the levels in the dermis were still 10 to 15 times the minimum inhibitory concentrations (MICs).
1% Lotion—Penetration studies have indicated that the penetration of the 1% cream and the 1% lotion are equivalent.
Ciclopirox olamine also penetrates into hair and through the epidermis and hair follicles into sebaceous glands and dermis.

### Protein binding

Very high (94–97%).

### Half-life

1% Solution in polyethylene glycol 400—1.7 hours.

### Elimination

1% Solution in polyethylene glycol 400——
Renal: Absorbed portion rapidly and almost completely excreted in urine; only 0.01% of dose remains in urine 2 days following topical application.
Fecal: Negligible.

## Precautions to Consider

### Carcinogenicity/Tumorigenicity

A study in female mice given cutaneous doses of ciclopirox twice a week for 50 weeks, followed by a six-month drug-free period, has shown that ciclopirox is not carcinogenic or tumorigenic at the application site.

### Mutagenicity

Several studies have shown that ciclopirox is not mutagenic.

### Pregnancy/Reproduction

Fertility—Studies in mice, rats, rabbits, and monkeys given ciclopirox by various routes at doses of 10 or more times the topical human dose have not shown that ciclopirox causes impaired fertility.

Pregnancy—Adequate and well-controlled studies in humans have not been done.

Studies in rats have shown that ciclopirox crosses the placenta in very small amounts. Studies in mice, rats, rabbits, and monkeys given ciclopirox by various routes at doses of 10 or more times the topical human dose have not shown that ciclopirox causes adverse effects in the fetus.

FDA Pregnancy Category B.

### Breast-feeding

It is not known whether ciclopirox is distributed into breast milk. However, problems in humans have not been documented.

### Pediatrics

Appropriate studies on the relationship of age to the effects of ciclopirox have not been performed in infants and children up to 10 years of age. Safety and efficacy have not been established.

### Geriatrics

Appropriate studies on the relationship of age to the effects of ciclopirox have not been performed in the geriatric population. However, no geriatrics-specific problems have been documented to date.

### Medical considerations/Contraindications

The medical considerations/contraindications included here have been selected on the basis of their potential clinical significance (reasons given in parentheses where appropriate)—not necessarily inclusive (» = major clinical significance).

*Risk-benefit should be considered when the following medical problem exists:*

Sensitivity to ciclopirox

## Side/Adverse Effects

The following side/adverse effects have been selected on the basis of their potential clinical significance (possible signs and symptoms in parentheses where appropriate)—not necessarily inclusive:

### Those indicating need for medical attention

Incidence rare
*Local irritation* (burning, itching, redness, swelling, or other signs of irritation not present before therapy)

## Patient Consultation

As an aid to patient consultation, refer to *Advice for the Patient, Ciclopirox (Topical)*.

In providing consultation, consider emphasizing the following selected information (» = major clinical significance):

### Before using this medication

» Conditions affecting use, especially:
Sensitivity to ciclopirox

### Proper use of this medication

Applying sufficient medication to cover affected and surrounding areas, and rubbing in gently
» Avoiding contact with the eyes
» Not applying occlusive dressing over this medication unless directed to do so by physician
» Compliance with full course of therapy; fungal infections may require prolonged therapy

» Proper dosing
   Missed dose: Applying as soon as possible; not applying if almost
   time for next dose
» Proper storage

## Precautions while using this medication

Checking with physician if no improvement within 2 to 4 weeks
» Using hygienic measures to cure infection and prevent reinfection:
*For tinea cruris*
   Avoiding underwear that is tight-fitting or made from synthetic ma-
   terials; wearing loose-fitting cotton underwear instead
   Using a bland, absorbent powder or an antifungal powder on the skin;
   using the powder between administration times for ciclopirox
*For tinea pedis*
   Carefully drying feet, especially between toes, after bathing
   Avoiding socks made from wool or synthetic materials; wearing clean,
   cotton socks and changing them daily or more often if feet perspire
   excessively
   Wearing sandals or well-ventilated shoes
   Using a bland, absorbent powder or an antifungal powder between
   toes, on feet, and in socks and shoes liberally once or twice daily;
   using the powder between administration times for ciclopirox

## Side/adverse effects

Signs of potential side effects, especially local irritation

## General Dosing Information

Use of topical antifungals may lead to skin sensitization, resulting in hypersensitivity reactions with subsequent topical use of the medication.

To reduce the possibility of recurrence, *Candida* infections, tinea cruris,
tinea corporis, and tinea versicolor should be treated for at least 2
weeks to 1 month; tinea pedis should be treated for at least 1 month
or longer.

When this medication is used in the treatment of candidiasis, occlusive
dressings should be avoided, since they provide conditions that favor
growth of yeast and release of its irritating endotoxin.

## Topical Dosage Forms

### CICLOPIROX OLAMINE CREAM USP

#### Usual adult and adolescent dose
Antifungal—
   Topical, to the skin and surrounding areas, two times a day, morning
   and evening.

#### Usual pediatric dose
Antifungal—
   Infants and children up to 10 years of age: Safety and efficacy have
   not been established.
   Children 10 years of age and over: See *Usual adult and adolescent
   dose*.

#### Strength(s) usually available
U.S.—
   1% (Rx) [*Loprox*].
Canada—
   1% (Rx) [*Loprox*].

#### Packaging and storage
Store between 15 and 30 °C (59 and 86 °F). Store in a collapsible tube.

#### Auxiliary labeling
• For external use only.
• Continue medicine for full time of treatment.

### CICLOPIROX OLAMINE LOTION

#### Usual adult and adolescent dose
See *Ciclopirox Olamine Cream USP*.

#### Usual pediatric dose
See *Ciclopirox Olamine Cream USP*.

#### Strength(s) usually available
U.S.—
   1% (Rx) [*Loprox*].
Canada—
   1% (Rx) [*Loprox*].

#### Packaging and storage
Store between 15 and 30 °C (59 and 86 °F). Protect from freezing.

#### Auxiliary labeling
• Shake well.
• For external use only.
• Continue medicine for full time of treatment.

Revised: 05/26/94

---

## CILASTATIN-CONTAINING COMBINATIONS—
Imipenem and Cilastatin (Systemic)

---

## CIMETIDINE—See *Histamine H₂-receptor Antagonists (Systemic)*

---

# CINOXACIN    Systemic†

VA CLASSIFICATION (Primary): AM900
Note: For a listing of dosage forms and brand names by country availability, see *Dosage Forms* section(s). For a listing of brand names
   for the articles in this monograph, refer to the General Index.

   †Not commercially available in Canada.

## Category

Antibacterial (systemic).
Note: Cinoxacin is a synthetic antibacterial similar in bacterial spectrum
   to nalidixic acid.

## Indications

### Accepted
Urinary tract infections, bacterial (prophylaxis)—Cinoxacin is indicated in
   the prophylaxis of urinary tract infections in women with a history of
   recurrent urinary tract infections.

Urinary tract infections, bacterial (treatment)—Cinoxacin is indicated in
   adults in the treatment of initial and recurrent urinary tract infections
   caused by susceptible gram-negative bacteria.

Not all species or strains of a particular organism may be susceptible to
   cinoxacin.

### Unaccepted
Cinoxacin is not effective against *Pseudomonas* species, *Enterococcus
faecalis*, or staphylococci.

## Pharmacology/Pharmacokinetics

### Physicochemical characteristics
Chemical group—A quinolone; similar in chemical structure to nalidixic
   acid and oxolinic acid.
Molecular weight—262.22.

### Mechanism of action/Effect
Bactericidal in the urine and acts by inhibition of bacterial DNA
   replication.

### Absorption
Rapidly and almost completely absorbed from the gastrointestinal tract.
   However, absorption delayed in the presence of food, although total
   absorption is unaffected.

### Distribution
High concentrations in the urine. Bladder tissue concentrations are approximately 60 to 70% of serum concentrations; prostatic tissue concentrations may range from < 1 to 6.3 mcg per gram of tissue (approximately 30 to 60% of serum concentrations), which may be below
   the minimum inhibitory concentrations (MICs) of many urinary
   pathogens.
Concentrated in renal tissue; concentrations somewhat higher than in the
   serum.
$Vol_D$=0.24 to 0.26 L per kg.

### Protein binding
High (60 to 80%).

**Biotransformation**

Probably hepatic; approximately 30 to 40% metabolized to inactive metabolites.

**Half-life**

Normal renal function—1.5 to 2 hours.

Normal renal function in patients receiving probenecid (2 grams daily) concurrently—3.5 hours.

Impaired renal function—May exceed 10 hours.

**Time to peak concentration**

2 to 3 hours.

**Peak serum concentration**

Up to approximately 15 mcg per mL following a 500-mg dose, but may be as low as 1 to 2 mcg per mL 6 hours following oral administration. Peak serum concentrations are reduced by 30% when cinoxacin is taken with food.

**Peak urine concentration**

May range up to approximately 900 mcg per mL. After a 500-mg dose, average urine concentrations are approximately 300 mcg per mL during the first 4 hours and may decline to approximately 100 mcg per mL during the second 4 hours.

**Elimination**

Renal, 97% excreted within 24 hours by glomerular filtration and tubular secretion; of this amount, 50 to 75% is excreted unchanged and the remainder is excreted as inactive metabolites.

In dialysis—Forced diuresis, peritoneal dialysis, hemodialysis, and charcoal hemoperfusion have not been shown to be beneficial in enhancing cinoxacin elimination.

## Precautions to Consider

**Cross-sensitivity and/or related problems**

Since cinoxacin is closely related chemically to other quinolone derivatives (e.g., nalidixic acid and the fluoroquinolones), patients allergic to other quinolones may be allergic to this medication also.

**Pregnancy/Reproduction**

Fertility—Studies in rats and rabbits given doses up to 10 times the daily human dose have not shown that cinoxacin causes impaired fertility.

Pregnancy—Adequate and well-controlled studies in humans have not been done. However, since cinoxacin has been shown to cause permanent lesions of the cartilage of weight-bearing joints and other signs of arthropathy in immature animals, use is not recommended during pregnancy.

Studies in rats and rabbits given doses up to 10 times the daily human dose have not shown that cinoxacin causes adverse effects on the fetus.

FDA Pregnancy Category C.

**Breast-feeding**

It is not known whether cinoxacin is distributed into breast milk. However, other quinolone derivatives are distributed into breast milk. Since cinoxacin has been shown to cause permanent lesions of the cartilage of weight-bearing joints and other signs of arthropathy in immature animals, use is not recommended in nursing mothers.

**Pediatrics**

Cinoxacin is not recommended for use in infants and children up to 18 years of age. Cinoxacin causes lameness in immature dogs given single doses of 250 mg per kg of body weight (mg/kg), due to permanent lesions of the cartilage of weight-bearing joints. In addition, related drugs (e.g., ciprofloxacin, nalidixic acid, norfloxacin, enoxacin, lomefloxacin, ofloxacin) have been reported to cause similar lesions, as well as other signs of arthropathy in immature animals of various species.

**Geriatrics**

No information is available on the relationship of age to the effects of cinoxacin in geriatric patients. However, elderly patients are more likely to have an age-related decrease in renal function, which may require an adjustment of dosage in patients receiving cinoxacin.

**Drug interactions and/or related problems**

The following drug interactions and/or related problems have been selected on the basis of their potential clinical significance (possible mechanism in parentheses where appropriate)—not necessarily inclusive (» = major clinical significance):

Note: Combinations containing any of the following medications, depending on the amount present, may also interact with this medication.

Aminophylline or
Caffeine or
Oxtriphylline or
Theophylline

(certain fluoroquinolones significantly reduce the hepatic metabolism and clearance of caffeine and theophylline, probably by competitive inhibition at the cytochrome P-450 binding sites; this may result in a prolonged elimination half-life of caffeine and theophylline, increased serum concentrations, and increased risk of caffeine- or theophylline-related toxicity; this possibility also exists with other xanthine derivatives, such as aminophylline and oxtriphylline; although this interaction has not been documented with cinoxacin, it should be considered in patients taking cinoxacin concurrently with any of these medications)

Antacids, aluminum-, calcium-, and/or magnesium-containing or
Sucralfate

(these antacids and sucralfate may chelate fluoroquinolones, reducing absorption, and consequently decreasing serum and urine concentrations, of the fluoroquinolones; although this interaction has not been documented with cinoxacin, it should be considered in patients taking cinoxacin concurrently with these medications)

Cyclosporine

(concurrent use with some fluoroquinolones has been reported to elevate serum creatinine and serum cyclosporine concentrations; other studies have not found fluoroquinolones to alter the pharmacokinetics of cyclosporine; although this interaction has not been documented with cinoxacin, it should be considered in patients taking cinoxacin concurrently with cyclosporine)

Probenecid

(probenecid decreases the renal tubular secretion of cinoxacin, resulting in decreased urinary excretion of the cinoxacin, prolonged elimination half-life [from 1.3 hours to 3.5 hours], and increased risk of toxicity)

Warfarin

(concurrent use of warfarin with ciprofloxacin or norfloxacin has been reported to increase the anticoagulant effect of warfarin, increasing the chance of bleeding; other studies have not found concurrent use of fluoroquinolones with warfarin to alter the prothrombin time [PT] significantly; although this interaction has not been documented with cinoxacin, it should be considered in patients taking cinoxacin concurrently with warfarin)

**Laboratory value alterations**

The following have been selected on the basis of their potential clinical significance (possible effect in parentheses where appropriate)—not necessarily inclusive (» = major clinical significance):

With physiology/laboratory test values

Alanine aminotransferase (ALT [SGPT]), serum and
Alkaline phosphatase, serum and
Aspartate aminotransferase (AST [SGOT]), serum
(values may be increased)

» Blood urea nitrogen (BUN) and

» Creatinine, serum
(concentrations may be increased)

**Medical considerations/Contraindications**

The medical considerations/contraindications included have been selected on the basis of their potential clinical significance (reasons given in parentheses where appropriate)—not necessarily inclusive (» = major clinical significance).

*Except under special circumstances, this medication should not be used when the following medical problem exists:*

» Previous allergic reaction to cinoxacin or other quinolones

*Risk-benefit should be considered when the following medical problem exists:*

» Renal function impairment
(cinoxacin is primarily excreted renally; it is recommended that cinoxacin be administered in a reduced dose in patients with impaired renal function)

## Side/Adverse Effects

The following side/adverse effects have been selected on the basis of their potential clinical significance (possible signs and symptoms in parentheses where appropriate)—not necessarily inclusive:

**Those indicating need for medical attention**

Incidence less frequent—3% or less
*Hypersensitivity* (skin rash, itching, redness, or swelling)

Incidence rare—1% or less
  *Central nervous system toxicity* (dizziness; headache); *photosensitivity* (increased sensitivity of skin to sunlight)

**Those indicating need for medical attention only if they continue or are bothersome**
Incidence less frequent—3% or less
  *Gastrointestinal reactions* (anorexia; diarrhea; nausea; stomach cramps; vomiting)

## Patient Consultation

As an aid to patient consultation, refer to *Advice for the Patient, Cinoxacin (Systemic)*.

In providing consultation, consider emphasizing the following selected information (» = major clinical significance):

**Before using this medication**
» Conditions affecting use, especially:
  Allergies to cinoxacin or other quinolone derivatives
  Pregnancy—Cinoxacin crosses the placenta. Cinoxacin is not recommended for use during pregnancy because it has been shown to cause arthropathy in immature animals
  Breast-feeding—Not recommended since cinoxacin has been shown to cause arthropathy in immature animals
  Use in children—Cinoxacin is not recommended for use in infants and children up to 18 years of age since it has been shown to cause arthropathy in immature animals
  Other medical problems, especially renal function impairment

**Proper use of this medication**
  Taking with food, unless otherwise directed by physician
» Not giving to infants or to children under 18 years of age; similar drugs have been reported to cause arthropathy in immature animals
» Compliance with full course of therapy
» Importance of not missing doses and taking at evenly spaced times
» Proper dosing
  Missed dose: Taking as soon as possible; not taking if almost time for next dose; not doubling doses
» Proper storage

**Precautions while using this medication**
  Checking with physician if no improvement within a few days
» Caution if dizziness occurs
» Possible photosensitivity reactions

**Side/adverse effects**
  Signs of potential side effects, especially hypersensitivity, central nervous system toxicity, and photosensitivity

## General Dosing Information

Cinoxacin may be taken with food.

Patients with impaired renal function may require a reduction in dosage based on creatinine clearance.

## Oral Dosage Forms
### CINOXACIN CAPSULES USP

**Usual adult dose**
Antibacterial—
  Prophylaxis: Oral, 250 mg at bedtime for up to five months.
  Treatment: Oral, 250 mg every six hours; or 500 mg every twelve hours for seven to fourteen days.

Note: After an initial loading dose of 500 mg, adults with impaired renal function may require a reduction in dose as follows:

| Creatinine Clearance (mL/min/1.73 M²)/ (mL/sec) | Dose |
|---|---|
| >80/ (1.33) | See *Usual adult dose* |
| 50–80/ (0.83–1.33) | 250 mg every eight hours |
| 20–50/ (0.33–0.83) | 250 mg every twelve to twenty-four hours |
| <20/ (0.33) | 250 mg every twenty-four hours |
| Anuria | Use is not recommended |

**Usual pediatric dose**
Use is not recommended in infants and children since cinoxacin causes arthropathy in immature animals.

**Strength(s) usually available**
U.S.—
  250 mg (Rx) [*Cinobac*].
  500 mg (Rx) [*Cinobac*; GENERIC].
Canada—
  Not commercially available.

**Packaging and storage**
Store below 30 °C (86 °F), preferably between 15 and 30 °C (59 and 86 °F), unless otherwise specified by manufacturer. Store in a well-closed container.

**Auxiliary labeling**
• Continue medicine for full time of treatment.
• May cause dizziness.

Revised: 07/19/95

---

## CIPROFLOXACIN—See *Fluoroquinolones (Systemic)*

---

# CIPROFLOXACIN   Ophthalmic

VA CLASSIFICATION (Primary): OP201
Note: For a listing of dosage forms and brand names by country availability, see *Dosage Forms* section(s). For a listing of brand names for the articles in this monograph, refer to the General Index.

## Category
Antibacterial (ophthalmic).

## Indications

**Accepted**
Corneal ulcers, bacterial (treatment)—Ophthalmic ciprofloxacin is indicated in the treatment of corneal ulcers caused by susceptible strains of bacteria, including *Pseudomonas aeruginosa, Serratia marcescens, Staphylococcus aureus, Staphylococcus epidermidis, Streptococcus pneumoniae,* and *Streptococcus (Viridans Group)*.

Conjunctivitis, bacterial (treatment)—Ophthalmic ciprofloxacin is indicated in the treatment of conjunctivitis caused by susceptible strains of *Staphylococcus aureus, Staphylococcus epidermidis,* and *Streptococcus pneumoniae*.

Note: Not all species or strains of a particular organism may be susceptible to ciprofloxacin. Streptococcal species are often less susceptible.

## Pharmacology/Pharmacokinetics

**Physicochemical characteristics**
Chemical group—Fluoroquinolone.
Molecular weight—385.82.

**Mechanism of action/Effect**
Ciprofloxacin's bactericidal action results from interference with the enzyme DNA gyrase, which is needed for the synthesis of bacterial DNA.

**Absorption**
During the patient's waking hours, ciprofloxacin was administered in each eye every 2 hours for 2 days followed by every 4 hours for an additional 5 days. The maximum reported plasma concentration of ciprofloxacin was less than 5 nanograms per mL. The mean concentration was usually less than 2.5 nanograms per mL.

## Precautions to Consider

**Cross-sensitivity and/or related problems**
Patients sensitive to other quinolones, such as cinoxacin, nalidixic acid, norfloxacin, or ofloxacin, may be sensitive to this medication also.

**Carcinogenicity**
Rats and mice administered ciprofloxacin orally for up to 2 years did not show carcinogenic effects.

## Mutagenicity

Ciprofloxacin was not found to be mutagenic in the following *in vitro* tests: *Salmonella* /Microsome test, *E. coli* DNA Repair assay, Chinese Hamster V₇₉ Cell HGPRT test, Syrian Hamster Embryo Cell Transformation assay, *Saccharomyces cerevisiae* Point Mutation assay, and *Saccharomyces cerevisiae* Mitotic Crossover and Gene Conversion assay. In addition, ciprofloxacin was not found to be mutagenic in the following *in vivo* tests: Rat Hepatocyte DNA Repair assay, Micronucleus test (mice), and Dominant Lethal test (mice). However, ciprofloxacin was found to be mutagenic in the *in vitro* Mouse Lymphoma Cell Forward Mutation assay and the *in vitro* Rat Hepatocyte DNA Repair assay.

## Pregnancy/Reproduction

Fertility—Studies performed in rats and mice administered ciprofloxacin in oral doses up to 6 times the usual daily human oral dose revealed no evidence of impaired fertility.

Pregnancy—Adequate and well-controlled studies in humans have not been done. However, problems in humans have not been documented.

Reproduction studies performed in rats and mice administered ciprofloxacin in oral doses up to 6 times the usual daily human oral dose revealed no evidence of harm to the fetus. In rabbits, ciprofloxacin, like most antimicrobial agents, when administered in oral doses of 30 and 100 mg per kg of body weight (mg/kg) per day produced gastrointestinal disturbances resulting in maternal weight loss and an increased incidence of abortion. However, no teratogenicity was observed at either dose. Ciprofloxacin administered intravenously in doses of up to 20 mg/kg, produced no embryotoxicity or teratogenicity.

FDA Pregnancy Category C.

## Breast-feeding

It is not known whether ophthalmic ciprofloxacin is distributed into breast milk. However, oral ciprofloxacin was shown to be distributed into breast milk after a single 500 mg dose.

## Pediatrics

Appropriate studies on the relationship of age to the effects of ciprofloxacin have not been performed in children up to 12 years of age. Safety and efficacy have not been established.

Although ciprofloxacin and other quinolones cause arthropathy in immature animals after oral administration, ophthalmic ciprofloxacin administered to immature animals did not cause any arthropathy. In addition, there is no evidence that the ophthalmic dosage form has any effect on the weight bearing joints.

## Geriatrics

No information is available on the relationship of age to the effects of ciprofloxacin in geriatric patients.

## Medical considerations/Contraindications

The medical considerations/contraindications included here have been selected on the basis of their potential clinical significance (reasons given in parentheses where appropriate)—not necessarily inclusive (» = major clinical significance).

*Risk-benefit should be considered when the following medical problem exists:*
Sensitivity to ciprofloxacin

## Side/Adverse Effects

Note: In corneal ulcer studies, frequent administration of ophthalmic ciprofloxacin resulted in white crystalline precipitates in the eyes of 17% of patients. This precipitate did not prevent the continued use of the medication and did not adversely affect treatment outcome.

The following side/adverse effects have been selected on the basis of their potential clinical significance (possible signs and symptoms in parentheses where appropriate)—not necessarily inclusive:

### Those indicating need for medical attention
Incidence rare
*Corneal infiltrates; corneal staining; decreased vision; keratopathy* (blurred vision or other change in vision); *keratitis* (severe irritation or redness of eye); *nausea; skin rash*

### Those indicating need for medical attention only if they continue or are bothersome
Incidence more frequent
*Burning or other discomfort of the eye; crusting or crystals in corner of eye*
Incidence less frequent
*Bad taste following instillation; foreign body sensation* (feeling of something in eye); *hyperemia, conjunctival* (redness of the lining of the eyelids); *itching of eye*

Rare
*Lid edema* (swelling of eyelid); *photophobia* (increased sensitivity of eyes to light); *tearing of eye*

## Patient Consultation

As an aid to patient consultation, refer to *Advice for the Patient, Ciprofloxacin (Ophthalmic).*

In providing consultation, consider emphasizing the following selected information (» = major clinical significance):

### Before using this medication
» Conditions affecting use, especially:
  Sensitivity to ciprofloxacin or other quinolones
  Breast-feeding—Oral ciprofloxacin is distributed into breast milk; it is not known whether ophthalmic ciprofloxacin is distributed into breast milk
  Use in children—Safety and efficacy have not been established in children up to 12 years of age

### Proper use of this medication
Proper administration technique
» Compliance with full course of therapy
» Proper dosing
  Missed dose: Applying as soon as possible; not applying if almost time for next dose
» Proper storage

### Precautions while using this medication
Checking with physician if no improvement within a few days
Possible photophobic reactions; wearing sunglasses and avoiding prolonged exposure to bright light

### Side/adverse effects
Signs of potential side effects, especially corneal infiltrates, corneal staining, decreased vision, keratopathy, keratitis, nausea, or skin rash

## General Dosing Information

Ciprofloxacin ophthalmic solution is not for injection into the eye.

Although some manufacturers recommend doses of 2 drops of ophthalmic solutions at appropriate intervals, the conjunctival sac usually holds less than 1 drop.

If hypersensitivity develops, therapy with ophthalmic ciprofloxacin should be discontinued.

### For treatment of adverse effects
Recommended treatment includes
  • For mild hypersensitivity reaction—Administering antihistamines and, if necessary, glucocorticoids.
  • For severe hypersensitivity or anaphylactic reaction—Administering epinephrine. Antihistamines and/or glucocorticoids may also be administered as required.

## Ophthalmic Dosage Forms

Note: The dosing and strengths of the dosage forms available are expressed in terms of ciprofloxacin base.

### CIPROFLOXACIN HYDROCHLORIDE OPHTHALMIC SOLUTION USP

**Usual adult and adolescent dose**
Bacterial conjunctivitis—
  Topical, to the conjunctiva, 1 drop in each eye every two hours, while patient is awake, for two days, then 1 drop every four hours, while patient is awake, for the next five days.
Corneal ulcers—
  Topical, to the conjunctiva, 1 drop into the affected eye every fifteen minutes for six hours, then 1 drop every thirty minutes, while patient is awake, for the rest of day one; 1 drop every hour, while patient is awake, on day two; and 1 drop every four hours, while patient is awake, on days three through fourteen. If corneal re-epithelialization has not occurred after fourteen days of treatment, treatment may be continued.

  Note: During the initial 24 to 48 hours, additional doses may be necessary during the night in some cases.

**Usual pediatric dose**
Bacterial conjunctivitis or
Corneal ulcers—
  Infants and children up to 12 years of age: Safety and efficacy have not been established.
  Children over 12 years of age: See *Usual adult and adolescent dose.*

## Strength(s) usually available
U.S.—
   3.5 mg (3 mg base) (Rx) [*Ciloxan* (benzalkonium chloride 0.006%)].
Canada—
   3.5 mg (3 mg base) (Rx) [*Ciloxan*].

## Packaging and storage
Store below 40 °C (104 °F), preferably between 15 and 30 °C (59 and 86 °F), unless otherwise specified by manufacturer. Store in a tight container. Protect from light.

## Auxiliary labeling
• For the eye.
• Continue medicine for full time of treatment.

## Selected Bibliography
Yolton DP. New antibacterial drugs for topical ophthalmic use. Optom Clin 1992; 2 (4): 59-72.

Revised: 07/29/93

---

# CISAPRIDE     Systemic

VA CLASSIFICATION (Primary): GA900

Note: For a listing of dosage forms and brand names by country availability, see *Dosage Forms* section(s). For a listing of brand names for the articles in this monograph, refer to the General Index.

## Category
Cholinergic enhancer; gastrointestinal emptying (delayed) adjunct.

## Indications
Note: Bracketed information in the *Indications* section refers to uses that are not included in U.S. product labeling.

### Accepted
Reflux, gastroesophageal (prophylaxis and treatment)—Cisapride is indicated for the symptomatic treatment of nocturnal [and daytime] heartburn, and of esophagitis due to reflux and delayed gastric emptying. Treatment may continue for up to 8 weeks; however, tolerance to cisapride may develop at some point in therapy.

[Gastroparesis (treatment)]—Cisapride is indicated in the treatment of gastroparesis, including idiopathic, diabetic, and intestinal pseudo-obstruction. Treatment may continue for up to 8 weeks; however, tolerance to cisapride may develop at some point in therapy.

## Pharmacology/Pharmacokinetics

### Physicochemical characteristics
Molecular weight—465.95.

### Mechanism of action/Effect
Cisapride exerts its effect by increasing the release of acetylcholine from the postganglionic nerve endings of the myenteric plexus. This release of acetylcholine increases esophageal activity and increases esophageal sphincter tone, thereby improving esophageal clearance and decreasing reflux of gastric contents into the esophagus. Cisapride enhances gastric and duodenal emptying as a result of increased gastric and duodenal contractivity and antroduodenal coordination. Duodenogastric reflux is also decreased. Cisapride improves transit in both small and large bowel.

### Absorption
Rapid and complete.

### Protein binding
97.5% bound to plasma proteins, primarily albumin.

### Biotransformation
Hepatic.

### Half-life
Elimination—7 to 10 hours after both single and multiple oral dosing regimens.

### Onset of action
30 to 60 minutes.

### Time to peak concentration
1 to 2 hours.

### Elimination
Renal and fecal.

## Precautions to Consider

### Carcinogenicity/Tumorigenicity
No tumorigenicity was demonstrated in rats receiving up to 80 mg of cisapride per kilogram of body weight (mg/kg) (50 times the maximum recommended human dose for a 50 kg person) a day for 25 months or in mice receiving up to 80 mg/kg (50 times the maximum recommended human dose) of cisapride a day for 19 months.

### Mutagenicity
No mutagenicity was demonstrated in the following *in vitro* and *in vivo* models: Ames test, chromosomal aberration assay on human lymphocytes, sex-linked recessive lethal test in *Drosophila melanogaster*, dominant lethal test in male and female mice germ cells, and micronucleus test in rats.

### Pregnancy/Reproduction
Fertility—At oral doses of up to 160 mg/kg a day (100 times the maximum recommended human dose), cisapride was found to have no effect on fertility in male rats. In female rats at oral doses of 40 mg/kg a day and higher, cisapride prolonged the breeding interval required for impregnation. These effects were also observed at maturity in the female offspring of female rats treated with oral doses of cisapride at 10 mg/kg a day or higher. At doses of 160 mg/kg a day, cisapride exerted contragestational/pregnancy disrupting effects in female rats.

Pregnancy—Adequate and well-controlled studies in humans have not been done.

Studies in rats (at doses of up to 160 mg/kg) and rabbits (at doses of up to 40 mg/kg) found no evidence of a teratogenic potential of cisapride. Studies in rats at doses of up to 160 mg/kg a day (100 times the maximum recommended human dose) and in rabbits at doses of 20 mg/kg (approximately 12 times the maximum recommended human dose) a day or higher found cisapride to be embryotoxic and fetotoxic. Doses of cisapride at 40 and 160 mg/kg a day reduced birth weights of pups in rats and adversely affected pup survival.

FDA Pregnancy Category C.

### Breast-feeding
Problems in humans have not been documented; however, risk-benefit must be considered since cisapride is distributed into breast milk at concentrations approximately one twentieth of those in plasma.

### Pediatrics
Studies performed in fewer than 50 patients for up to 8 weeks have not demonstrated pediatrics-specific problems that would limit the usefulness of cisapride in children.

### Geriatrics
Appropriate studies performed to date have not demonstrated geriatrics-specific problems that would limit the usefulness of cisapride in the elderly. However, the elimination half-life of cisapride has been found to be longer in some elderly patients, which may require adjustment of dosage in patients receiving cisapride.

### Drug interactions and/or related problems
The following drug interactions and/or related problems have been selected on the basis of their potential clinical significance (possible mechanism in parentheses where appropriate)—not necessarily inclusive (» = major clinical significance):

Note: Combinations containing any of the following medications, depending on the amount present, may also interact with this medication.

Only specific interactions between cisapride and other oral medications have been identified in this monograph. However, because of increased gastrointestinal motility and decreased gastric emptying time caused by cisapride, absorption of medications from the stomach may be decreased, while absorption from the small intestine may be enhanced.

Alcohol or
Benzodiazepines
   (cisapride has been reported to increase the rate of absorption of these agents)

» Anticholinergics or other medications with anticholinergic activity (See *Appendix II*)
   (concurrent use may antagonize the effects of cisapride on gastrointestinal motility)

Cimetidine or
Ranitidine
(cisapride accelerates the absorption of cimetidine and rantidine)

(cimetidine coadministration causes increased peak plasma concentration and area under the plasma concentration–time curve [AUC] of cisapride)

» Clarithromycin or
» Erythromycin or
» Troleandomycin
(concurrent use of clarithromycin, erythromycin, or troleandomycin with cisapride is contraindicated; concurrent use may result in elevated plasma concentrations of cisapride through inhibition of the cytochrome P450 3A4 enzyme; this has led to serious cardiac arrhythmias including ventricular tachycardia, ventricular fibrillation, torsades de pointes, and QT prolongation; some of these events have been fatal)

» Fluconazole or
» Itraconazole or
» Ketoconazole or
» Miconazole
(concurrent use of fluconazole, itraconazole, ketoconazole, or intravenous miconazole with cisapride is contraindicated; concurrent use may result in elevated plasma concentrations of cisapride through inhibition of the cytochrome P450 3A4 enzyme; this has led to serious cardiac arrhythmias including ventricular tachycardia, ventricular fibrillation, torsades de pointes, and QT prolongation; some of these events have been fatal)

### Medical considerations/Contraindications

The medical considerations/contraindications included here have been selected on the basis of their potential clinical significance (reasons given in parentheses where appropriate)—not necessarily inclusive (» = major clinical significance).

*Except under special circumstances, this medication should not be used when the following medical problem exists:*

» Gastrointestinal hemorrhage, mechanical obstruction or perforation (stimulation of gastrointestinal motility may aggravate these conditions)

*Risk-benefit should be considered when the following medical problems exist:*

Epilepsy or
Seizures, history of
(there have been isolated reports of seizures in patients with a history of seizures who are taking cisapride; however, a causal relationship to cisapride has not been established)

Hepatic insufficiency or
Renal insufficiency
(these conditions may cause a decrease in clearance of cisapride; reduced dosage may be recommended)

Predisposition to QT prolongation, including:
Congenital long QT syndrome
Intake of medications known to prolong the QT interval
Uncorrected electrolyte disturbances
(increased risk of serious cardiac arrhythmias with cisapride)

Sensitivity to cisapride

## Side/Adverse Effects

The following side/adverse effects have been selected on the basis of their potential clinical significance (possible signs and symptoms in parentheses where appropriate)—not necessarily inclusive:

### Those indicating need for medical attention

Incidence rare
*Seizures*
Note: *Seizures* have been reported only in patients with a history of seizures.

### Those indicating need for medical attention only if they continue or are bothersome

Incidence less frequent
*Abdominal cramping; constipation; diarrhea*—incidence 14.2%; *fatigue* (unusual tiredness or weakness); *headache; nausea; somnolence* (drowsiness)
Note: *Diarrhea* is dose-dependent.

## Overdose

For specific information on the agents used in the management of cisapride overdose, see *Charcoal, Activated (Oral-Local)* monograph.

For more information on the management of overdose or unintentional ingestion, **contact a Poison Control Center** (see *Poison Control Center Listing*).

### Treatment of overdose

Recommended treatment consists of the following:

Stopping administration of medication.

To decrease absorption—Use of gastric lavage and/or administration of activated charcoal.

Monitoring—Patients should be evaluated for possible QT prolongation and for factors that may predispose the patient to ventricular arrhythmias, including torsades de pointes.

Supportive care—Patients in whom intentional overdose is confirmed or suspected should be referred for psychiatric consultation.

## Patient Consultation

As an aid to patient consultation, refer to *Advice for the Patient, Cisapride (Systemic)*.

In providing consultation, consider emphasizing the following selected information (» = major clinical significance):

### Before using this medication

» Conditions affecting use, especially:
Sensitivity to cisapride
Pregnancy—High doses in animals shown to be embryotoxic and fetotoxic
Breast-feeding—Distributed into breast milk in small amounts
Other medications, especially anticholinergics, clarithromycin, erythromycin, fluconazole, itraconazole, ketoconazole, miconazole, and troleandomycin
Other medical problems, especially gastrointestinal bleeding, mechanical obstruction, or perforation

### Proper use of this medication

» Taking 15 minutes before meals and at bedtime with a beverage
» Proper dosing
Missed dose: Taking as soon as possible; not taking if almost time for next dose
» Proper storage

### Precautions while using this medication

» Checking with physician before using alcohol
» Caution if drowsiness occurs

### Side/adverse effects

Seizures

## General Dosing Information

Cisapride should be taken 15 minutes before meals and bedtime.

In patients with hepatic or renal function impairment, the initial daily dose should be reduced and adjusted depending on the therapeutic effect or possible side effects.

## Oral Dosage Forms

Note: Bracketed uses in the *Dosage Forms* section refer to categories of use and/or indications that are not included in U.S. product labeling.

### CISAPRIDE ORAL SUSPENSION

**Usual adult and adolescent dose**
Gastroesophageal reflux—
Prophylaxis:
Oral, 10 mg two times a day, before breakfast and at bedtime or 20 mg a day at bedtime.
Note: Dose used in prophylaxis may be increased to a maximum of 20 mg two times a day with severe disease.
Treatment:
Oral, 5 to 10 mg three to four times a day, fifteen minutes before meals and at bedtime.
Note: Some patients may require a dose of 20 mg four times a day, taken fifteen minutes before meals and at bedtime.
[Gastroparesis]—
Treatment:
Oral, 10 mg three to four times a day, fifteen minutes before meals and at bedtime.
Note: Dose may be increased to a maximum of 20 mg three times a day, fifteen minutes before meals.

**Usual pediatric dose**
Gastroesophageal reflux or
[Gastroparesis]—
Treatment: Oral, 0.15 to 0.3 mg per kg of body weight three or four times a day, before meals.

**Strength(s) usually available**
U.S.—
1 mg per mL (Rx) [*Propulsid*].
Canada—
1 mg per mL (Rx) [*Prepulsid*].

**Packaging and storage**
Store between 15 and 25 °C (59 and 77 °F), unless otherwise specified by manufacturer.

**Auxiliary labeling**
• Shake well.

## CISAPRIDE TABLETS

**Usual adult and adolescent dose**
See *Cisapride Oral Suspension*.

**Usual pediatric dose**
See *Cisapride Oral Suspension*.

**Strength(s) usually available**
U.S.—
10 mg (Rx) [*Propulsid* (scored)].
20 mg (Rx) [*Propulsid*].
Canada—
5 mg (Rx) [*Prepulsid*].
10 mg (Rx) [*Prepulsid*].
20 mg (Rx) [*Prepulsid*].

**Packaging and storage**
Store between 15 and 25 °C (59 and 77 °F), unless otherwise specified by manufacturer. Protect the 20 mg tablets from light.

## Selected Bibliography

McCallum R, Prakash C, Campoli-Richards D, Goa K. Cisapride: a preliminary review of its pharmacodynamic and pharmacokinetic properties, and therapeutic use as a prokinetic agent in gastrointestinal motility disorders. Drugs 1988; 36: 652-81.

Revised: 7/29/96

# CISPLATIN Systemic

VA CLASSIFICATION (Primary): AN900
Note: For a listing of dosage forms and brand names by country availability, see *Dosage Forms* section(s). For a listing of brand names for the articles in this monograph, refer to the General Index.

## Category

Antineoplastic.

## Indications

Note: Bracketed information in the *Indications* section refers to uses that are not included in U.S. product labeling.

**Accepted**
Carcinoma, bladder (treatment)—Cisplatin is indicated as a single agent for treatment of transitional cell bladder cancer that is no longer amenable to local treatments such as surgery and/or radiotherapy.

Carcinoma, ovarian (treatment)—Cisplatin is indicated in combination with other chemotherapeutic agents for treatment of metastatic ovarian tumors in patients who have already received appropriate surgical and/or radiotherapeutic procedures. It is indicated, as a single agent, as secondary therapy of metastatic ovarian tumors refractory to standard chemotherapy that did not include cisplatin.

Carcinoma, testicular (treatment)—Cisplatin is indicated in combination with other chemotherapeutic agents for treatment of metastatic testicular tumors in patients who have already received appropriate surgical and/or radiotherapeutic procedures.

[Carcinoma, adrenal cortex (treatment)][1]
[Carcinoma, breast (treatment)][1]
[Carcinoma, cervical (treatment)][1]
[Carcinoma, endometrial (treatment)][1]
[Carcinoma, gastric (treatment)][1]
[Carcinoma, lung (treatment)][1]
[Neuroblastoma (treatment)][1]
[Carcinoma, prostatic (treatment)][1] or
[Carcinoma, head and neck (treatment)]—Cisplatin is indicated for treatment of adrenocortical carcinoma, breast carcinoma, cervical carcinoma, endometrial carcinoma, gastric carcinoma, lung carcinoma, neuroblastoma in children, prostatic carcinoma, and squamous cell carcinoma of the head and neck.

[Tumors, germ cell, ovarian (treatment)][1] or
[Tumors, germ cell (treatment)][1]—Cisplatin is indicated for treatment of ovarian germ cell tumors and germ cell tumors in children.

[Osteosarcoma (treatment)][1]—Cisplatin is indicated for treatment of osteosarcoma in children.

[1]Not included in Canadian product labeling.

## Pharmacology/Pharmacokinetics

**Physicochemical characteristics**
Molecular weight—300.06.

**Mechanism of action/Effect**
Cisplatin resembles an alkylating agent. Although the exact mechanism of action is unknown, action is thought to be similar to that of the bifunctional alkylating agents, that is, possible cross-linking and interference with the function of DNA and a small effect on RNA. It is cell cycle–phase nonspecific. Stimulation of the host immune system is also possible.

**Distribution**
Does not readily cross the blood-brain barrier.

**Protein binding**
Metabolites—Very high (more than 90%) during excretory (beta) phase.

**Biotransformation**
By rapid nonenzymatic conversion to inactive metabolites.

**Half-life**
Alpha phase—
25 to 49 minutes.
Beta phase (in hours)—
Normal: 58 to 73.
Anuric: Up to 240.

**Duration of action**
Inhibition of DNA persists for several days following administration.

**Elimination**
Renal (27 to 43% after 5 days); platinum may be detected in tissues for 4 months or more after administration.
In dialysis—Cisplatin is removable by dialysis, but only within 3 hours after administration.

## Precautions to Consider

**Carcinogenicity**
Secondary malignancies are potential delayed effects of many antineoplastic agents, although it is not clear whether the effect is related to their mutagenic or immunosuppressive action. The effect of dose and duration of therapy is also unknown, although risk seems to increase with long-term use. Although information is limited, available data seem to indicate that the carcinogenic risk is greatest with the alkylating agents.

Development of acute leukemia has been reported to occur rarely in patients treated with cisplatin, usually in combination with other leukemogenic agents.

Studies in 50 BD IX rats at intraperitoneal doses of 3 times 1 mg per kg of body weight (mg/kg) for 3 weeks found that, 455 days after the first application, 33 animals had died. Thirteen of the deaths were related to malignancies (12 leukemias and 1 fibrosarcoma).

**Mutagenicity**
Cisplatin is mutagenic in bacteria and has been shown to cause chromosome aberrations in animal cells in tissue culture.

**Pregnancy/Reproduction**
Fertility—Gonadal suppression, resulting in amenorrhea or azoospermia, may occur in patients taking antineoplastic therapy, especially with the alkylating agents. In general, these effects appear to be related to dose and length of therapy and may be irreversible. Prediction of the degree

of testicular or ovarian function impairment is complicated by the common use of combinations of several antineoplastics, which makes it difficult to assess the effects of individual agents.

Pregnancy—Cisplatin may be toxic to the fetal urogenital tract.

First trimester: It is usually recommended that use of antineoplastics, especially combination chemotherapy, be avoided whenever possible, especially during the first trimester. Although information is limited because of the relatively few instances of antineoplastic administration during pregnancy, the mutagenic, teratogenic, and carcinogenic potential of these medications must be considered.

Other hazards to the fetus include adverse reactions seen in adults.

In general, use of a contraceptive is recommended during cytotoxic drug therapy.

Cisplatin is embryotoxic and teratogenic in mice.

FDA Pregnancy Category D.

**Breast-feeding**

Although very little information is available regarding distribution of antineoplastic agents into breast milk, breast-feeding is not recommended during chemotherapy because of the risks to the infant (adverse effects, mutagenicity, carcinogenicity).

**Pediatrics**

Ototoxic effects of cisplatin may be more severe in children.

**Geriatrics**

No information is available on the relationship of age to the effects of cisplatin in geriatric patients. However, elderly patients are more likely to have age-related renal function impairment, which may require reduction of dosage in patients receiving cisplatin.

**Dental**

The bone marrow depressant effects of cisplatin may result in an increased incidence of microbial infection, delayed healing, and gingival bleeding. Dental work, whenever possible, should be completed prior to initiation of therapy or deferred until blood counts have returned to normal. Patients should be instructed in proper oral hygiene during treatment, including caution in use of regular toothbrushes, dental floss, and toothpicks.

Cisplatin may also rarely cause stomatitis associated with considerable discomfort.

**Drug interactions and/or related problems**

The following drug interactions and/or related problems have been selected on the basis of their potential clinical significance (possible mechanism in parentheses where appropriate)—not necessarily inclusive (» = major clinical significance):

Note: Combinations containing any of the following medications, depending on the amount present, may also interact with this medication.

Allopurinol or
Colchicine or
» Probenecid or
» Sulfinpyrazone
(cisplatin may raise the concentration of blood uric acid; dosage adjustment of antigout agents may be necessary to control hyperuricemia and gout; allopurinol may be preferred to prevent or reverse cisplatin-induced hyperuricemia because of risk of uric acid nephropathy with uricosuric antigout agents)

Antihistamines or
Buclizine or
Cyclizine or
Loxapine or
Meclizine or
Phenothiazines or
Thioxanthenes or
Trimethobenzamide
(concurrent use with cisplatin may mask the symptoms of ototoxicity, such as tinnitus, dizziness, or vertigo)

Bleomycin
(cisplatin-induced renal function impairment may result in bleomycin toxicity even at low doses; caution is recommended because of the frequent combination of these two agents)

Blood dyscrasia–causing medications (See *Appendix II*)
(leukopenic and/or thrombocytopenic effects of cisplatin may be increased with concurrent or recent therapy if these medications cause the same effects; dosage adjustment of cisplatin, if necessary, should be based on blood counts)

» Bone marrow depressants, other (See *Appendix II*) or
Radiation therapy
(concurrent use may increase the total effects of these medications and radiation therapy; dosage reduction is recommended)

» Nephrotoxic medications, other (See *Appendix II*) or
» Ototoxic medications, other (See *Appendix II*)
(concurrent and/or sequential administration should be avoided since the potential for ototoxicity and nephrotoxicity may be increased, especially in the presence of renal function impairment)

Vaccines, killed virus
(because normal defense mechanisms may be suppressed by cisplatin therapy, the patient's antibody response to the vaccine may be decreased. The interval between discontinuation of medications that cause immunosuppression and restoration of the patient's ability to respond to the vaccine depends on the intensity and type of immunosuppression-causing medication used, the underlying disease, and other factors; estimates vary from 3 months to 1 year)

» Vaccines, live virus
(because normal defense mechanisms may be suppressed by cisplatin therapy, concurrent use with a live virus vaccine may potentiate the replication of the vaccine virus, may increase the side/adverse effects of the vaccine virus, and/or may decrease the patient's antibody response to the vaccine; immunization of these patients should be undertaken only with extreme caution after careful review of the patient's hematologic status and only with the knowledge and consent of the physician managing the cisplatin therapy. The interval between discontinuation of medications that cause immunosuppression and restoration of the patient's ability to respond to the vaccine depends on the intensity and type of immunosuppression-causing medication used, the underlying disease, and other factors; estimates vary from 3 months to 1 year. Patients with leukemia in remission should not receive live virus vaccine until at least 3 months after their last chemotherapy. In addition, immunization with oral poliovirus vaccine should be postponed in persons in close contact with the patient, especially family members)

**Laboratory value alterations**

The following have been selected on the basis of their potential clinical significance (possible effect in parentheses where appropriate)—not necessarily inclusive (» = major clinical significance):

With physiology/laboratory test values
Aspartate aminotransferase (ALT [SGOT]) values, serum and
Bilirubin concentrations, serum
(may be increased transiently)

Blood urea nitrogen (BUN) concentrations and
Creatinine concentrations, serum and
Uric acid concentrations, serum
(may be increased, indicating nephrotoxicity)

Calcium concentrations, serum and
Creatinine clearance and
Magnesium concentrations, serum and
Phosphate concentrations, serum and
Potassium concentrations, serum and
Sodium concentrations, serum
(may be decreased, probably as a result of renal toxicity; rarely, tetany associated with hypocalcemia and hypomagnesemia has occurred)

Coombs' test
(positive results, associated with hemolytic anemia, have been reported)

**Medical considerations/Contraindications**

The medical considerations/contraindications included here have been selected on the basis of their potential clinical significance (reasons given in parentheses where appropriate)—not necessarily inclusive (» = major clinical significance).

*Risk-benefit should be considered when the following medical problems exist:*

» Bone marrow depression
» Chickenpox, existing or recent (including recent exposure) or
» Herpes zoster
(risk of severe generalized disease)

Gout, history of or
Urate renal stones, history of
(risk of hyperuricemia)

» Hearing impairment
» Infection
» Renal function impairment
(reduced excretion; a lower dosage of cisplatin is recommended)

Sensitivity to cisplatin

» Caution should be used also in patients who have had previous cytotoxic drug therapy or radiation therapy.

## Patient monitoring

The following are especially important in patient monitoring (other tests may be warranted to some patients, depending on condition; » = major clinical significance):

» Audiometric testing and
» Neurologic function studies
   (recommended prior to initiation of therapy and at periodic intervals during therapy)

   Blood urea nitrogen (BUN) concentrations and
» Creatinine clearance and
   Creatinine concentrations, serum
   (recommended prior to initiation of therapy and before each course of cisplatin to detect renal toxicity)

   Calcium concentrations, serum and
   Magnesium concentrations, serum and
   Phosphate concentrations, serum and
   Potassium concentrations, serum
   (recommended at periodic intervals during therapy)

» Hematocrit or hemoglobin and
» Leukocyte count, total and, if appropriate, differential and
» Platelet count
   (determinations recommended prior to initiation of therapy and at periodic intervals during therapy; frequency varies according to clinical state, agent, dose, and other agents being used concurrently)

   Uric acid concentrations, serum
   (recommended prior to initiation of therapy and at periodic intervals during therapy; frequency varies according to clinical state, agent, dose, and other agents being used concurrently)

## Side/Adverse Effects

Note: Many "side effects" of antineoplastic therapy are unavoidable and represent the medication's pharmacologic action. Some of these (for example, leukopenia and thrombocytopenia) are actually used as parameters to aid in individual dosage titration.

Side effects are more pronounced at doses of cisplatin greater than 50 mg per square meter of body surface.

Vascular toxicities have been reported rarely when cisplatin is given in combination with other antineoplastic agents, although it is unknown whether the toxicity is related to cisplatin administration or to other factors. Vascular toxicities reported include myocardial infarction, cerebrovascular accident, thrombotic microangiopathy, cerebral arteritis, and Raynaud's phenomenon.

The following side/adverse effects have been selected on the basis of their potential clinical significance (possible signs and symptoms in parentheses where appropriate)—not necessarily inclusive:

### Those indicating need for medical attention
Incidence more frequent—severity increases with repeated doses
   *Anemia secondary to myelosuppression* (usually asymptomatic; unusual tiredness or weakness); *leukopenia* (usually asymptomatic; less frequently, fever or chills; cough or hoarseness; lower back or side pain; painful or difficult urination); *nephrotoxicity, hyperuricemia, or uric acid nephropathy* (joint pain; lower back or side pain; swelling of feet or lower legs); *ototoxicity* (loss of balance; ringing in ears; trouble in hearing); *thrombocytopenia* (usually asymptomatic; less frequently, unusual bleeding or bruising; black, tarry stools; blood in urine or stools; pinpoint red spots on skin)

Note: *Myelosuppression (leukopenia, thrombocytopenia, anemia)* is more pronounced at higher doses. Nadir of leukocyte and platelet counts occurs after 18 to 23 days and counts usually recover by 39 days after a dose.

Cisplatin frequently causes *nephrotoxicity* in the form of acute renal failure, which may be detected initially only by means of renal function tests. Laboratory abnormalities occur during the second week after a dose. Nephrotoxicity is dose-related and cumulative; it is usually reversible, but may become irreversible at high doses or with repeated treatments, and is occasionally fatal.

Hypocalcemia and hypomagnesemia may occur due to *nephrotoxicity*. Rarely, tetany associated with hypocalcemia may occur, and tremors or seizures may occur as a result of hypomagnesemia.

With *hyperuricemia*, peak uric acid concentrations occur 3 to 5 days after a dose.

*Ototoxicity* may be more severe in children and may not be reversible. Ototoxicity is cumulative; hearing loss usually occurs first with high frequencies (above speech tones) and may be unilateral or bilateral.

Incidence less frequent
   *Anaphylactic reaction, occurring within a few minutes after administration* (dizziness or fainting; fast heartbeat; swelling of face; wheezing); *extravasation* (pain or redness at site of injection); *neurotoxicity* (loss of reflexes; loss of taste; numbness or tingling in fingers or toes; seizures; trouble in walking; rarely, muscle cramps)

Note: *Extravasation* may rarely produce local soft tissue toxicity, the severity of which is related to the concentration of the solution. Infusion of solutions containing cisplatin in a concentration greater than 500 mcg (0.5 mg) per mL may result in tissue cellulitis, fibrosis, and necrosis.

*Neurotoxicity*, usually characterized by peripheral neuropathies, may occur after a single dose or prolonged therapy (4 to 7 months) and may be severe and irreversible. Signs and symptoms of neuropathy usually develop during treatment, but may rarely begin 3 to 8 weeks after the last dose, and may progress even after withdrawal of cisplatin. Muscle cramps (localized, painful, involuntary skeletal contractions of sudden onset and short duration) have been reported, usually in patients receiving a relatively high cumulative dose of cisplatin and in a relatively advanced symptomatic stage of peripheral neuropathy. Lhermitte's sign, dorsal column myelopathy, and autonomic neuropathy have also been reported.

Incidence rare
   *Hemolytic anemia* (usually asymptomatic; unusual tiredness or weakness); *optic neuritis, papilledema, or cerebral blindness* (blurred vision; change in ability to see colors, especially blue or yellow); *stomatitis* (sores in mouth and on lips); *syndrome of inappropriate antidiuretic hormone (SIADH) secretion* (dizziness, confusion, or agitation; unusual tiredness or weakness)

Note: A Coombs' positive *hemolytic anemia* has also been reported.

*Optic neuritis, papilledema, or cerebral blindness* is usually reversible after withdrawal. Fundoscopic examination usually finds only irregular retinal pigmentation of the macular area.

### Those indicating need for medical attention only if they continue or are bothersome
Incidence more frequent—occurs in most patients
   *Nausea and vomiting, severe*

Note: *Nausea and vomiting* usually begin 1 to 4 hours after a dose, and vomiting may persist for 24 hours. Nausea and anorexia may persist for up to 1 week. Serotonin antagonists (e.g., ondansetron), high-dose intravenous metoclopramide, or corticosteroids have been found to be useful in preventing severe nausea and vomiting; however, severe nausea and vomiting may require discontinuation of cisplatin.

Incidence less frequent
   *Loss of appetite*

### Those indicating need for medical attention if they occur after medication is discontinued
   *Myelosuppression* (black, tarry stools; blood in urine or stools; cough or hoarseness; fever or chills; lower back or side pain; painful or difficult urination; pinpoint red spots on skin; unusual bleeding or bruising); *nephrotoxicity* (decrease in urination; swelling of feet or lower legs); *neurotoxicity* (loss of reflexes; loss of taste; numbness or tingling in fingers or toes; seizures; trouble in walking); *ototoxicity* (loss of balance; ringing in ears; trouble in hearing)

## Patient Consultation

As an aid to patient consultation, refer to *Advice for the Patient, Cisplatin (Systemic)*.

In providing consultation, consider emphasizing the following selected information (» = major clinical significance):

### Before using this medication
» Conditions affecting use, especially:
   Sensitivity to cisplatin
   Pregnancy—Use not recommended because of mutagenic, teratogenic, and carcinogenic potential; advisability of using a contraceptive; telling physician immediately if pregnancy is suspected
   Breast-feeding—Not recommended because of serious side effects
   Use in children—Ototoxicity more severe
   Other medications, especially probenecid, sulfinpyrazone, other bone marrow depressants, other nephrotoxic medications, other

ototoxic medications, or previous cytotoxic drug therapy or radiation therapy

Other medical problems, especially chickenpox, herpes zoster, hearing impairment, infection, or renal function impairment

### Proper use of this medication

Caution if taking combination therapy; taking each medication at the right time

Importance of ample fluid intake and subsequent increase in urine output to aid in excretion of uric acid

Frequency of severe nausea and vomiting; importance of continuing medication despite stomach upset

» Proper dosing

### Precautions while using this medication

» Importance of close monitoring by the physician

» Avoiding immunizations unless approved by physician; other persons in patient's household should avoid immunizations with oral poliovirus vaccine; avoiding persons who have taken oral poliovirus vaccine or wearing a protective mask that covers nose and mouth

*Caution if bone marrow depression occurs:*

» Avoiding exposure to persons with bacterial infections, especially during periods of low blood counts; checking with physician immediately if fever or chills, cough or hoarseness, lower back or side pain, or painful or difficult urination occur

» Checking with physician immediately if unusual bleeding or bruising; black, tarry stools; blood in urine or stools; or pinpoint red spots on skin occur

Caution in use of regular toothbrush, dental floss, or toothpick; physician, dentist, or nurse may suggest alternatives; checking with physician before having dental work done

Not touching eyes or inside of nose unless hands washed immediately before

Using caution to avoid accidental cuts with use of sharp objects such as safety razor or fingernail or toenail cutters

Avoiding contact sports or other situations where bruising or injury could occur

» Possibility of local tissue injury and scarring if infiltration of intravenous solution occurs; telling doctor or nurse right away about redness, pain or swelling at injection site

### Side/adverse effects

Importance of discussing possible effects, including cancer, with physician

Signs of potential side effects, especially leukopenia, thrombocytopenia, anemia, hemolytic anemia, nephrotoxicity, hyperuricemia, uric acid nephropathy, ototoxicity, anaphylactic reaction, extravasation, neurotoxicity, optic neuritis, papilledema, cerebral blindness, stomatitis, and SIADH secretion

Physician or nurse can help in dealing with side effects

## General Dosing Information

It is recommended that cisplatin be administered to patients in an appropriate setting under supervision of a physician or nurse experienced in cancer chemotherapy. It is also recommended that equipment and medications (including epinephrine, oxygen, antihistamines, and intravenous corticosteroids) necessary for treatment of a possible anaphylactic reaction be readily available at each administration of cisplatin.

A variety of dosage schedules and regimens of cisplatin, alone or in combination with other antitumor agents, are used. The prescriber may consult the medical literature as well as the manufacturer's literature in choosing a specific dosage.

It is recommended that cisplatin be administered with vigorous parenteral infusion to increase hydration; this is intended to maintain urine output and reduce nephrotoxicity and ototoxicity, although it will not prevent them.

Vigorous pretreatment intravenous hydration, followed by adequate hydration and urinary output for 24 hours, are recommended. Mannitol or furosemide may also be used to produce acute diuresis, provided that salt and water depletion are avoided.

Cisplatin has also been administered as a continuous intravenous infusion over periods ranging from 24 hours to 5 days; this method of administration appears to reduce nausea and vomiting but not nephrotoxicity or ototoxicity. It is very important that orders for the total dose to be given over the entire course of the infusion *not* be misinterpreted as a daily dose, because of the risk of fatal overdose.

Development of uric acid nephropathy may be prevented by adequate oral hydration and, in some cases, administration of allopurinol. Alkalinization of urine may be necessary if serum uric acid concentrations are elevated.

It is recommended that courses of cisplatin be administered no more frequently than every 3 to 4 weeks, to reduce the risk of cumulative nephrotoxicity.

Subsequent doses of cisplatin must not be given before renal function approaches normal (measured by BUN, creatinine clearance, and serum creatinine). Administration of subsequent doses of cisplatin also is not recommended before platelet levels return to at least 100,000 per cubic millimeter and leukocyte levels to at least 4000 per cubic millimeter, or before auditory acuity is confirmed to be within normal limits.

Therapy with cisplatin should be discontinued at the first sign of significant neurotoxicity, which may be irreversible.

Special precautions are recommended in patients who develop thrombocytopenia as a result of administration of cisplatin. These may include extreme care in performing invasive procedures; regular inspection of intravenous sites, skin (including perirectal area), and mucous membrane surfaces for signs of bleeding or bruising; limiting frequency of venipuncture and avoiding intramuscular injections; testing urine, emesis, stool, and secretions for occult blood; care in use of regular toothbrushes, dental floss, toothpicks, safety razors, and fingernail and toenail cutters; avoiding constipation; and using caution to prevent falls and other injuries. Such patients should avoid alcohol and aspirin intake because of the risk of gastrointestinal bleeding. Platelet transfusions may be required.

Patients who develop leukopenia should be observed carefully for signs of infection. Antibiotic support may be required. In neutropenic patients who develop fever, broad-spectrum antibiotic coverage should be initiated empirically, pending bacterial cultures and appropriate diagnostic tests.

### Safety considerations for handling this medication

There is limited but increasing evidence and concern that personnel involved in preparation and administration of parenteral antineoplastics may be at some risk because of the potential mutagenicity, teratogenicity, and/or carcinogenicity of these agents, although the actual risk is unknown. USP advisory panels recommend cautious handling both in preparation and disposal of antineoplastic agents. Precautions that have been suggested include:

• Use of a biological containment cabinet during reconstitution and dilution of parenteral medications and wearing of disposable surgical gloves and masks.

• Use of proper technique to prevent contamination of the medication, work area, and operator during transfer between containers (including proper training of personnel in this technique).

• Cautious and proper disposal of needles, syringes, vials, ampuls, and unused medication.

A number of medical centers have developed detailed guidelines for handling of antineoplastic agents.

### Combination chemotherapy

Cisplatin may be used in combination with other agents in various regimens. As a result, incidence and/or severity of side effects may be altered and different dosages (usually reduced) may be used. For example, cisplatin is part of the following chemotherapeutic combinations (some commonly used acronyms are in parentheses):

—cyclophosphamide, doxorubicin, and cisplatin (CISCA or CAP).

—vinblastine, cisplatin, and bleomycin (VBP).

For specific dosages and schedules, consult the literature. For information regarding each agent, consult the individual monographs.

## Parenteral Dosage Forms

### CISPLATIN INJECTION

#### Usual adult and adolescent dose

Metastatic testicular tumors—

Intravenous, 20 mg per square meter of body surface a day for five days.

Metastatic ovarian tumors—

Intravenous, 50 mg per square meter of body surface once every three weeks (Day 1), in combination with 50 mg of doxorubicin hydrochloride per square meter of body surface intravenously every three weeks on Day 1 (administered sequentially), or

Intravenous, 100 mg per square meter of body surface once every four weeks (as a single agent).

Advanced bladder cancer—

Intravenous, 50 to 70 mg per square meter of body surface every three to four weeks (as a single agent). The lower end of the dosage range is recommended in patients heavily pretreated with radiation or chemotherapy.

**Usual adult prescribing limits**

Total dose for a single *course* of cisplatin (whether given as a single daily infusion or as a continuous infusion over several days, to be repeated every three to four weeks) should not exceed 120 mg per square meter of body surface. Administration of higher doses in a single course may lead to potentially fatal overdose. Exceptions should be made, and care of these patients should be handled, only by medical professionals who fully understand and are prepared to deal with the potential toxicities of such dosing.

**Usual pediatric dose**

See *Usual adult and adolescent dose.*

**Strength(s) usually available**

U.S.—

    1 mg per mL (50-, and 100-mL vials) (Rx) [*Platinol-AQ* (sodium chloride 9 mg per mL)].

Canada—

    500 mcg (0.5 mg) per mL (20- and 100-mL vials) (Rx) [*Platinol-AQ* (sodium chloride 9 mg per mL); GENERIC].

**Packaging and storage**

Store between 15 and 25 °C (59 and 77 °F), unless otherwise specified by manufacturer. Do not refrigerate.

**Stability**

Caution—A black platinum precipitate will form if cisplatin comes in contact with aluminum.

Solution remaining in amber vial following initial entry is stable for 28 days protected from light or for 7 days under fluorescent room light.

**Incompatibilities**

Do not use needles, intravenous sets, or equipment containing aluminum for administration since cisplatin is incompatible with aluminum.

**Note**

No more than 120 mg per square meter of body surface per course (with each course separated by three to four weeks) should be dispensed without verbal or written confirmation by the prescribing physician. To reduce the risk of fatal overdose, no more than the amount for one course should be dispensed at one time.

## CISPLATIN FOR INJECTION USP

**Usual adult and adolescent dose**

See *Cisplatin Injection.*

**Usual adult prescribing limits**

See *Cisplatin Injection.*

**Usual pediatric dose**

See *Cisplatin Injection.*

**Size(s) usually available**

U.S.—

    10 mg (Rx) [*Platinol*].

    50 mg (Rx) [*Platinol*].

Canada—

    10 mg (Rx) [*Platinol*].

    50 mg (Rx) [*Platinol*].

**Packaging and storage**

Store below 40 °C (104 °F), preferably between 15 and 30 °C (59 and 86 °F), unless otherwise specified by manufacturer. Protect from light.

**Preparation of dosage form**

Cisplatin for injection is reconstituted for intravenous use by adding 10 or 50 mL of sterile water for injection to the 10-mg or 50-mg vial, respectively, producing a clear, colorless solution containing 1 mg of cisplatin per mL. It is recommended that 5% dextrose injection in 0.3 or 0.45% sodium chloride injection be used if further dilution for administration by intravenous solution is required, in order to ensure stability.

**Stability**

Reconstituted solutions of cisplatin are stable for 20 hours at 27 °C (80 °F). Solution removed from the amber vial should be protected from light if it is not to be used within 6 hours.

Caution—

    A precipitate will form if reconstituted solutions are refrigerated.

    A black platinum precipitate will form if cisplatin comes in contact with aluminum.

**Incompatibilities**

Do not use needles, intravenous sets, or equipment containing aluminum for administration since cisplatin is incompatible with aluminum.

**Note**

No more than 120 mg per square meter of body surface per course (with each course separated by three to four weeks) should be dispensed without verbal or written confirmation by the prescribing physician. To reduce the risk of fatal overdose, no more than the amount for one course should be dispensed at one time.

## Selected Bibliography

Evans WE, et al. Clinical pharmacology of bleomycin and cisplatin. Drug Intell Clin Pharm 1982 Jun; 16: 448-58.

Loehrer PJ, Einhorn LH. Cisplatin. Ann Intern Med 1984 May; 100: 704-13.

Revised: 08/12/94

---

# CITRATES    Systemic

This monograph includes information on the following: Potassium Citrate; Potassium Citrate and Citric Acid; Potassium Citrate and Sodium Citrate; Sodium Citrate and Citric Acid; Tricitrates.

VA CLASSIFICATION (Primary/Secondary):

    Potassium Citrate—TN410/GU900

    Potassium Citrate and Citric Acid—TN410/GU900; TN900

    Potassium Citrate and Sodium Citrate—TN410/GU900

    Sodium Citrate and Citric Acid—TN410/GU900; TN900

    Tricitrates—TN410/GU900; TN900

Other commonly used names for sodium citrate and citric acid are Albright's solution and modified Shohl's solution.

Note: For a listing of dosage forms and brand names by country availability, see *Dosage Forms* section(s). For a listing of brand names for the articles in this monograph, refer to the General Index.

---

## Category

Antiurolithic, uric acid calculi—Potassium Citrate; Potassium Citrate and Citric Acid; Potassium Citrate and Sodium Citrate; Sodium Citrate and Citric Acid; Tricitrates.

Antiurolithic, cystine calculi—Potassium Citrate; Potassium Citrate and Citric Acid; Potassium Citrate and Sodium Citrate; Sodium Citrate and Citric Acid; Tricitrates.

Antiurolithic, calcium oxalate calculi—Potassium Citrate; Potassium Citrate and Citric Acid.

Antiurolithic, calcium phosphate calculi—Potassium Citrate; Potassium Citrate and Citric Acid.

Alkalizer, systemic—Potassium Citrate and Citric Acid; Sodium Citrate and Citric Acid; Tricitrates.

Alkalizer, urinary—Potassium Citrate; Potassium Citrate and Citric Acid; Potassium Citrate and Sodium Citrate; Sodium Citrate and Citric Acid; Tricitrates.

Buffer, neutralizing—Sodium Citrate and Citric Acid; Tricitrates.

## Indications

**Accepted**

Renal calculi, cystine (prophylaxis and treatment) or

Renal calculi, uric acid (prophylaxis and treatment)—Citrates are indicated as urinary alkalizers in the prevention and treatment of uric acid or cystine lithiasis. They are often used in gout therapy as urinary alkalizers to prevent crystallization of urates.

Renal calculi, calcium (prophylaxis and treatment) or

Hypocitraturia (prophylaxis and treatment)—Potassium citrate and potassium citrate and citric acid are also indicated to increase urinary citrate in the prevention and treatment of calcium phosphate, calcium oxalate, or uric acid kidney stones in such conditions as renal tubular acidosis with calcium stones, hypocitraturic calcium oxalate nephrolithiasis of any etiology, and uric acid or cystine lithiasis with or without calcium stones.

Acidosis, in renal tubular disorders (treatment)—Potassium citrate and citric acid, sodium citrate and citric acid, and tricitrates are also used in the treatment of chronic metabolic acidosis resulting from chronic renal insufficiency or the syndrome of renal tubular acidosis. Sodium citrate is especially useful when the administration of potassium salts is undesirable or contraindicated.

Pneumonitis, aspiration (prophylaxis)—Sodium citrate and citric acid and tricitrates are used in preanesthesia medication as nonparticulate acid-neutralizing buffers of gastric acid to lessen the danger from acid-aspiration pneumonitis in patients at risk. Citrates have generally been replaced by the equally or more effective $H_2$-receptor antagonists in the prevention of acid aspiration in elective surgery. However, citrates and other antacids have a more rapid onset of action than $H_2$-receptor antagonists and may be more useful in emergency situations.

# Pharmacology/Pharmacokinetics

## Physicochemical characteristics
Molecular weight—
> Potassium citrate: 324.41.
> Sodium citrate: 258.07 (anhydrous).
> Citric acid: 192.12.

## Mechanism of action/Effect
Alkalizer, urinary or
Antiurolithic, uric acid calculi or
Antiurolithic, cystine calculi—Sodium citrate and potassium citrate are metabolized to bicarbonates, which increase urinary pH by increasing the excretion of free bicarbonate ions, without producing systemic alkalosis when administered in recommended doses. A rise in urinary pH increases the solubility of cystine in the urine and the ionization of uric acid to more soluble urate ion. By maintaining an alkaline urine, the actual dissolution of uric acid stones may be accomplished.
Antiurolithic, calcium calculi—Metabolism of absorbed potassium citrate produces an alkaline load, raising urinary pH and increasing urinary citrate by augmenting citrate clearance. Thus, potassium citrate therapy appears to increase urinary citrate mainly by changing the renal handling of citrate, and, to a smaller extent, by increasing the filterable load of citrate. Increased urinary citrate and pH decreases calcium ion activity by increasing calcium complexation to dissociated anions and thus decreasing the saturation of calcium oxalate.
Potassium citrate also inhibits the crystallization and spontaneous nucleation of calcium oxalate and calcium phosphate in hypocitraturic calcium nephrolithiasis. However, potassium citrate does not alter the urinary saturation of calcium phosphate, because the effect of increased citrate complexation of calcium is antagonized by the rise in pH-dependent dissociation of phosphate. Calcium phosphate stones are more stable in alkaline urine.
Alkalizer, systemic—Increases the plasma bicarbonate, buffers excess hydrogen ion concentration, and raises blood pH, thereby reversing the clinical manifestations of acidosis.
Neutralizing buffer—Reacts chemically to neutralize or buffer existing quantities of gastric hydrochloric acid but has no direct effect on its output.

## Biotransformation
Oxidized in the body to form potassium bicarbonate or sodium bicarbonate. Effects are essentially those of chlorides before absorption and those of bicarbonates after absorption.

## Onset of action
Potassium citrate—Single dose: Within 1 hour.

## Duration of action
Potassium citrate tablets—
> Single dose: Up to 12 hours.
> Multiple doses: 3 days.
Potassium citrate and citric acid oral solution—Up to 24 hours at dosage of—
> 10 to 15 mL four times a day: Maintains a urine pH of 6.5 to 7.4.
> 15 to 20 mL four times a day: Maintains a urine pH of 7.0 to 7.6.
Tricitrates oral solution—Up to 24 hours at dosage of—
> 10 to 15 mL four times a day—Maintains a urine pH of 6.5 to 7.4.
> 15 to 20 mL four times a day—Maintains a urine pH of 7.0 to 7.6.

## Elimination
Urinary; less than 5% unchanged.

# Precautions to Consider

## Carcinogenicity
Long-term carcinogenicity studies in animals have not been performed.

## Pregnancy/Reproduction
Pregnancy—Studies have not been done in humans.
Studies have not been done in animals.

*Potassium citrate;* and *potassium citrate* and *sodium citrate*—FDA Pregnancy Category C.

## Breast-feeding
It is not known whether citrates are distributed into breast milk. However, problems in humans have not been documented.

## Pediatrics
Appropriate studies on the relationship of age to the effects of citrates have not been performed in the pediatric population. However, no pediatrics-specific problems have been documented to date.

## Geriatrics
No information is available on the relationship of age to the effects of citrates in geriatric patients.

## Drug interactions and/or related problems
The following drug interactions and/or related problems have been selected on the basis of their potential clinical significance (possible mechanism in parentheses where appropriate)—not necessarily inclusive (» = major clinical significance):

Note: Combinations containing any of the following medications, depending on the amount present, may also interact with this medication.

Amphetamines or
Ephedrine or
Pseudoephedrine or
» Quinidine
> (concurrent use with citrates may inhibit urinary excretion and prolong the duration of action of these medications)

» Antacids, especially those containing aluminum or sodium bicarbonate
> (concurrent use with citrates may result in systemic alkalosis)
> (concurrent use of sodium citrate with sodium bicarbonate may promote the development of calcium stones in patients with uric acid stones, due to sodium ion opposition to the hypocalciuric effect of the alkaline load; may also cause hypernatremia)
> (concurrent use of aluminum-containing antacids with citrate salts can increase aluminum absorption, possibly resulting in acute aluminum toxicity, especially in patients with renal insufficiency)

Anticholinergics or other medications with anticholinergic activity (See *Appendix II*)
> (concurrent use with potassium citrate may increase risk of gastrointestinal irritation because of slowed gastrointestinal transit time; patients should be carefully monitored endoscopically for evidence of lesions)

» Angiotensin-converting enzyme (ACE) inhibitors or
» Anti-inflammatory drugs, nonsteroidal (NSAIDs) or
Cyclosporine or
» Diuretics, potassium-sparing or
» Heparin or
» Low-salt milk or
» Potassium-containing medications, other or
» Salt substitutes
> (concurrent use with potassium citrate may increase serum potassium concentrations, which may cause severe hyperkalemia and lead to cardiac arrest, especially in renal insufficiency; low-salt milk may contain up to 60 mEq of potassium per liter and most salt substitutes contain substantial amounts of potassium)

Ciprofloxacin or
Norfloxacin or
Ofloxacin
> (citrates may reduce the solubility of ciprofloxacin, norfloxacin, or ofloxacin in the urine; patients should be observed for signs of crystalluria and nephrotoxicity)

» Digitalis glycosides
> (concurrent use with potassium citrate may increase risk of hyperkalemia in digitalized patients; careful monitoring of serum potassium concentrations during concurrent use is recommended)

Laxatives
> (concurrent administration with citrates may have an additive effect since sodium or potassium citrate may act as a saline laxative; however, these medications may be used concurrently as a preoperative for therapeutic advantage)

Lithium
> (concurrent use with sodium citrate may increase the urinary excretion of lithium and reduce its therapeutic effects, possibly due to the sodium content of the citrate and/or the effect of urinary alkalinization)

» Methenamine
> (concurrent use with citrates is not recommended because alkalinizing the urine may inhibit the effects of methenamine)

Salicylates
> (concurrent use with citrates may increase the urinary excretion and decrease the therapeutic effects of salicylates due to alkalinization of the urine)

Sodium-containing medications
(concurrent use with sodium citrate may increase the risk of hypernatremia, especially in patients with renal disease)

## Medical considerations/Contraindications

The medical considerations/contraindications included here have been selected on the basis of their potential clinical significance (reasons given in parentheses where appropriate)—not necessarily inclusive (» = major clinical significance).

*Except under special circumstances, this medication should not be used when the following medical problems exist:*

*For potassium citrate– and/or sodium citrate–containing*
» Aluminum toxicity
(citrate salts have been found to increase aluminum absorption and may exacerbate the condition, especially in renal insufficiency)

» Heart failure or
» Myocardial damage, severe
(because of impaired mechanisms for excreting potassium, potentially fatal asymptomatic hyperkalemia can develop, rapidly leading to cardiovascular failure and cardiac arrest)

(sodium retention may result when patients with congestive heart failure are administered sodium citrate)

» Renal impairment, severe, with azotemia or oliguria or
» Renal insufficiency, when glomerular filtration rate (GFR) is less than 0.7 mL per kg per minute
(danger of soft tissue calcification; increased risk of hyperkalemia or alkalosis)

(sodium retention may occur with use of sodium citrate)

» Urinary tract infection, active, with urea-splitting or other organisms, in association with calcium or struvite stones
(bacterial enzymatic degradation of citrate may occur, preventing it from increasing urinary citrate; also, the rise in urinary pH may promote further bacterial growth)

*For potassium citrate–containing only (in addition to those listed above)*
» Hyperkalemia, or conditions predisposing to hyperkalemia such as:
Adrenal insufficiency
Dehydration, acute
Diabetes mellitus, uncontrolled
Physical exercise, strenuous, in unconditioned persons
Renal failure, chronic
Tissue breakdown, extensive
(increased serum potassium concentrations leading to cardiac arrest may occur; exercise-induced hyperkalemia is transient and is a problem only in patients with renal insufficiency from dehydration or those taking medications that increase serum potassium)

» Peptic ulcer
(increased risk of gastrointestinal lesions with potassium citrate, especially with tablets)

*For potassium citrate tablets only (in addition to those listed above)*
» Gastric emptying, delayed or
» Esophageal compression or
» Intestinal obstruction or stricture
(delayed passage of tablets through gastrointestinal tract may increase risk of gastrointestinal irritation)

*Risk-benefit should be considered when the following medical problems exist:*

*For potassium citrate– and sodium citrate–containing*
» Acidosis, renal tubular, severe or
Diarrheal syndromes, chronic, such as ulcerative colitis, regional enteritis, or jejuno-ileal bypass surgery
(when urinary citrate in these conditions is very low [below 100 mg per day], citrates may be relatively ineffective in raising urinary citrate; higher doses may be required to produce the desired citraturic response; when urinary pH is high in renal tubular acidosis, citrates may produce only a small rise in pH; rapid transit time associated with diarrheal syndromes may prevent proper breakdown of tablets [especially wax matrix], liquid preparations should be used in diarrheal syndromes)

*For sodium citrate–containing only (in addition to those listed above)*
Edema, peripheral or pulmonary or
Hypertension or
Toxemia of pregnancy
(sodium salts should be used cautiously in patients with these conditions to prevent exacerbation; also, patients on sodium restricted diets should not take sodium citrate)

## Patient monitoring

The following may be especially important in patient monitoring (other tests may be warranted in some patients, depending on condition; » = major clinical significance):

Acid-base balance, serum, including pH and carbon dioxide and
Complete blood counts, including hematocrit and hemoglobin and
Creatinine concentrations, serum and
Electrolyte concentrations, serum, including sodium, potassium, chloride, and bicarbonate
(determinations recommended every 4 months during therapy, especially for patients with renal disease; treatment should be discontinued if there is a significant rise in serum potassium or in serum creatinine, or a significant fall in hematocrit or hemoglobin values)

Citrate, urinary, 24-hour, determinations and/or

pH determinations, urinary
(recommended at start of therapy, to determine adequacy of initial dosage, and every 4 months thereafter; patients taking citrate solutions should frequently check urinary pH to maintain alkalinity at all times)

Electrocardiogram (ECG)
(recommended periodically, especially in patients with cardiac disease; characteristic changes such as peaking of T-wave, loss of P-wave, depression of ST-segment, and prolongation of the QT-interval may indicate asymptomatic hyperkalemia)

# Side/Adverse Effects

The following side/adverse effects have been selected on the basis of their potential clinical significance (possible signs and symptoms in parentheses where appropriate)—not necessarily inclusive:

## Those indicating need for medical attention

Incidence rare
*For potassium citrate– and sodium citrate–containing*
*Metabolic alkalosis* (mood or mental changes; muscle pain or twitching; nervousness or restlessness; slow breathing; unpleasant taste; unusual tiredness or weakness)

*For potassium citrate–containing only (in addition to those listed above)*
*Bowel obstruction or bowel perforation* (abdominal or stomach cramps or pain; black, tarry stools; severe vomiting, sometimes with blood)—for tablet dosage form only; *hyperkalemia* (confusion; irregular heartbeat; numbness or tingling in hands, feet, or lips; shortness of breath or difficult breathing; unexplained anxiety; unusual tiredness or weakness; weakness or heaviness of legs)

Note: *Bowel obstruction* or *bowel perforation* caused by high concentration of potassium ions in region of dissolving tablets. Because the wax matrix is not an enteric coating, improper release of some of the potassium ions from the wax matrix into the stomach may cause upper gastrointestinal bleeding with the same frequency as other wax-matrix potassium products; if these adverse effects occur, potassium citrate should be discontinued immediately.

*Hyperkalemia* may often be asymptomatic or manifested only by characteristic ECG changes. Late signs may include muscle paralysis and cardiac arrest. When citrates are used at recommended doses, hyperkalemia is rare in patients without predisposing conditions.

*For sodium citrate–containing only (in addition to those listed for potassium citrate– or sodium citrate–containing)*
*Hypernatremia* (dizziness; fast heartbeat; high blood pressure; irritability; muscle twitching; restlessness; seizures; swelling of feet or lower legs; weakness)—occurs very rarely

## Those indicating need for medical attention only if they continue or are bothersome

Incidence less frequent
*For potassium citrate– and sodium citrate–containing*
*Laxative effect* (diarrhea or loose bowel movements)

*For potassium citrate only (in addition to those listed above)*
*Irritation, contact* (mild abdominal or stomach soreness or pain; nausea or vomiting)—for tablet dosage form only

Note: *Contact irritation* may be due to possible contact with ulcerous areas or high concentration of potassium ions in one area resulting from improper release of potassium ions from wax-matrix dosage form or delayed passage of dosage form through alimentary tract.

## Patient Consultation

As an aid to patient consultation, refer to *Advice for the Patient, Citrates (Systemic)*.

In providing consultation, consider emphasizing the following selected information (» = major clinical significance):

**Before using this medication**
» Conditions affecting use, especially:
    Other medications, especially—
*For all citrates:* Quinidine, calcium-containing medications, methenamine, antacids
*For potassium citrate–containing only:* Angiotensin-converting enzyme (ACE) inhibitors, digitalis glycosides, heparin, nonsteroidal anti-inflammatory drugs (NSAIDs), potassium-sparing diuretics, other potassium-containing medications

    Other medical problems, especially:
*For potassium citrate: and/or sodium citrate—containing:* Aluminum toxicity, heart failure, severe myocardial damage, severe renal function impairment with azotemia or oliguria, renal insufficiency, or urinary tract infection
*For potassium citrate—containing only:* Hyperkalemia or conditions predisposing to hyperkalemia, peptic ulcer, or severe renal tubular acidosis
*For potassium citrate tablets only:* Delayed gastric emptying, esophageal compression, or intestinal obstruction or stricture

**Proper use of this medication**
Proper administration:
*For tablet dosage form*
Swallowing tablet whole; not crushing, chewing, or sucking
Taking with a full glass (240 mL) of water or juice
» Checking with physician at once if trouble in swallowing tablets or if tablets seem to stick in the throat
*For oral liquid dosage form*
Diluting with 6 ounces of water or juice before swallowing; after swallowing, following with additional water, if desired
Chilling, but *not* freezing, before swallowing to enhance palatability
*For crystals dosage form*
Adding contents of one packet to at least 6 ounces of cool water or juice; stirring well to dissolve completely
Following with additional water after swallowing mixture, if desired
» Taking each dose immediately after a meal or within 30 minutes after a meal or bedtime snack to lessen gastrointestinal pain or saline laxative effect
» Importance of high fluid intake (at least 3 liters per day) to prevent supersaturation of urine and to assure a minimum urine volume of 2.5 liters per day
Compliance with therapy, especially when taking with diuretics and digitalis
» Proper dosing
Missed dose: Taking as soon as possible if remembered within 2 hours; not taking if almost time for next dose; not doubling doses
» Proper storage

**Precautions while using this medication**
Regular visits to physician to check progress of therapy
Checking with physician before starting strenuous physical exercise if out of condition, to prevent possible hyperkalemia
*For potassium citrate–containing only*
Not taking salt substitutes or drinking low-salt milk unless prescribed by physician
*For sodium citrate–containing only*
Avoiding salty foods and use of extra table salt
» Checking with physician at once if black, tarry stools or other signs of gastrointestinal bleeding are observed
Not being alarmed at appearance of "whole" tablet in stools; checking with physician

**Side/adverse effects**
Signs of potential side effects, especially:
*For potassium citrate–or sodium citrate–containing*—Metabolic alkalosis or diarrhea or loose bowel movements
*For potassium citrate–containing only*—Hyperkalemia
*For potassium citrate tablets only*—Bowel perforation or obstruction, or contact irritation resulting from improper release from wax matrix of tablets
*For sodium citrate–containing only*—Hypernatremia

## General Dosing Information

For patients on sodium-restricted diets, potassium citrate preparations may be preferable as urinary alkalizers; conversely, sodium citrate may be used when potassium citrate is contraindicated.

The goal of therapy with potassium citrate tablets or potassium citrate and citric acid solution is to increase the urinary citrate to normal (greater than 320 mg a day) and as close to the normal mean (640 mg a day) as possible, and to increase urinary pH to 6.0 to 7.0.

The rise in urinary citrate is directly dependent on the dosage of potassium citrate tablets or potassium citrate and citric acid oral solution. After long-term treatment, a dosage of 6.5 grams of potassium citrate (60 mEq of potassium ion) a day raises urinary citrate by approximately 400 mg a day and increases urinary pH by approximately 0.7 units. When treatment is withdrawn, urinary citrate begins to fall toward the pretreatment level of the first day.

Potassium citrate tablets and potassium citrate and citric acid oral solution are equally efficacious in raising urinary pH and citrate excretion.

**Diet/Nutrition**
Each dose should be taken immediately after a meal or within 30 minutes after a meal or bedtime snack, to lessen gastrointestinal pain or the saline laxative effect.

High fluid intake (at least 3 liters a day) is important to prevent supersaturation of urine and to assure a minimum urine volume of 2.5 liters a day.

Low-salt milk may contain up to 60 mEq of potassium per liter, and salt substitutes may contain substantial amounts of potassium. Both should be avoided if a patient is taking a potassium citrate–containing product, to prevent hyperkalemia.

**For treatment of adverse effects**
*For hyperkalemia*
Treatment includes:
• Discontinuing foods and medications containing potassium, including salt substitutes, ACE inhibitors, nonsteroidal anti-inflammatory drugs (NSAIDs), heparin, cyclosporine, and potassium-sparing diuretics.
• Administering 10% dextrose injection containing 10 to 20 units of insulin per liter at a rate of 300 to 500 mL of solution per hour. Monitoring for serial EKG and serum potassium concentration is recommended.
• Correcting acidosis with intravenous sodium bicarbonate.
• Using exchange resins, hemodialysis, or peritoneal dialysis.
• Observing caution when treating hyperkalemia in digitalized patients, since rapid reduction of serum potassium concentrations may induce digitalis toxicity.

*For hypernatremia*
Treatment includes:
• Discontinuing foods and medications containing sodium.
• If acute hypernatremia, administering hypotonic or isotonic saline solution intravenously to maintain fluid volume. In infants, to avoid a too rapid fall in serum sodium concentrations, use of a saline solution containing less than 70 mEq per liter is not recommended. Serum osmolality should be corrected over a 24- to 48-hour period.

*For metabolic alkalosis*
Treatment includes:
• Controlling symptoms by having patient rebreathe expired air into a paper bag or mask.
• Administering calcium gluconate injection if alkalosis is severe, to control tetany.

---

### *POTASSIUM CITRATE*

## Summary of Differences

Indications: Also used to prevent or treat hypocitraturia in patients with calcium renal calculi.
Precautions: Medical considerations/contraindications—May increase risk of gastrointestinal lesions in peptic ulcer disease; may increase risk of gastrointestinal irritation in delayed gastric emptying, esophageal compression, or intestinal obstruction.
Side/adverse effects: Tablets may cause severe abdominal or stomach pain; black, tarry stools; or severe vomiting, sometimes with blood.

## Additional Dosing Information

May be used as a urinary alkalizer when sodium citrate is contraindicated.

## Oral Dosage Forms

### POTASSIUM CITRATE TABLETS

**Usual adult dose**
Antiurolithic or
Alkalizer, urinary—
  Mild to moderate hypocitraturia (more than 150 mg of urinary citrate
  a day): Oral, initially 1.08 grams (10 mEq of potassium ion) three
  times a day with meals.
  Severe hypocitraturia (less than 150 mg of urinary citrate a day): Oral,
  initially, 2.16 grams (20 mEq of potassium ion) three times a day,
  with meals or within thirty minutes after a meal or bedtime snack;
  or 1.62 grams (15 mEq of potassium ion) four times a day, with
  meals or within thirty minutes after a meal or bedtime snack.
  Note: Dosage should be adjusted as determined by 24-hour fasting
  urinary citrate and/or urinary pH measurements.

**Usual adult prescribing limits**
10.8 grams of potassium citrate (100 mEq of potassium ion) a day.

**Usual pediatric dose**
Dosage has not been established.

**Strength(s) usually available**
U.S.—
  540 mg (5 mEq of potassium ion) (Rx) [*Urocit-K*].
  1080 mg (10 mEq of potassium ion) (Rx) [*Urocit-K*].

**Packaging and storage**
Store below 40 °C (104 °F), preferably between 15 and 30 °C (59 and 86
  °F), in a tight container, unless otherwise specified by manufacturer.

**Auxiliary labeling**
• Swallow tablets whole.
• Take with a full glass of water.
• Take with meals or snack.

**Note**
Dispense in original container.

**Additional information**
Intact wax matrix may appear in the feces.

---

### POTASSIUM CITRATE AND CITRIC ACID

## Summary of Differences

Indications: Also used to prevent or treat hypocitraturia in patients with
  calcium renal calculi.

## Additional Dosing Information

May be used as a urinary alkalizer when sodium citrate is contraindicated.

## Oral Dosage Forms

### POTASSIUM CITRATE AND CITRIC ACID ORAL SOLUTION USP

**Usual adult dose**
Antiurolithic or
Alkalizer, systemic or
Alkalizer, urinary—
  Oral, initially 10 to 15 mL (2.2 to 3.3 grams of potassium citrate [20
  to 30 mEq of potassium ion]) four times a day, after meals and at
  bedtime, the dosage being adjusted as needed and tolerated.
  Note: Dosage should be adjusted as determined by 24-hour fasting
  urinary citrate and/or urinary pH measurements.

**Usual pediatric dose**
Alkalizer, urinary—Oral, initially 5 to 15 mL (1.1 to 3.3 grams of potassium citrate [10 to 30 mEq of potassium ion]) four times a day, after
  meals and at bedtime, the dosage being adjusted as needed and
  tolerated.

**Strength(s) usually available**
U.S.—
  1.1 grams of potassium citrate (10 mEq of potassium ion) and 334 mg
  of citric acid per 5 mL (Rx) [*Polycitra-K*].

**Packaging and storage**
Store below 40 °C (104 °F), preferably between 15 and 30 °C (59 and 86
  °F), unless otherwise specified by manufacturer. Store in a tight con-
  tainer. Protect from freezing and excessive heat.

**Auxiliary labeling**
• Dilute with water or juice.
• Take with meals or snack.

**Additional information**
Citric acid is present as a temporary buffer with only a transient effect on
  the systemic acid-base balance.

### POTASSIUM CITRATE AND CITRIC ACID FOR ORAL SOLUTION

**Usual adult dose**
Antiurolithic or
Alkalizer, systemic or
Alkalizer, urinary—
  Oral, initially 3.3 grams of potassium citrate (30 mEq of potassium
  ion) four times a day, after meals and at bedtime, the dosage being
  adjusted as needed and tolerated.
  Note: Dosage should be adjusted as determined by 24-hour fasting
  urinary citrate and/or urinary pH measurements.

**Usual pediatric dose**
Use is not recommended.
Note: Because of the difficulty of regulating dosage with this dosage
  form, the oral solution is not recommended for pediatric patients.

**Size(s) usually available**
U.S.—
  3.3 grams of potassium citrate (30 mEq of potassium ion) and 1 gram
  of citric acid (Rx) [*Polycitra-K Crystals*].

**Packaging and storage**
Store below 40 °C (104 °F), preferably between 15 and 30 °C (59 and 86
  °F), in a tight container, unless otherwise specified by manufacturer.

**Preparation of dosage form**
Add contents of one packet to at least 6 ounces of cool water or juice.
  Stir well to dissolve.

**Auxiliary labeling**
• Dilute with water or juice.
• Take with meals or snack.

**Additional information**
Each packet provides the same amounts of potassium citrate and citric
  acid as 15 mL of potassium citrate and citric acid oral solution.
Citric acid is present as a temporary buffer with only a transient effect on
  the systemic acid-base balance.

---

### POTASSIUM CITRATE AND SODIUM CITRATE

## Summary of Differences

Indications: Used as a urinary alkalizing agent only, in patients with uric
  acid or cystine calculi.

## Oral Dosage Forms

### POTASSIUM CITRATE AND SODIUM CITRATE TABLETS

**Usual adult dose**
Antiurolithic or
Alkalizer, urinary—
  Oral, initially, 1 to 4 tablets (50 to 200 mg of potassium citrate [0.45
  to 1.8 mEq of potassium ion] and 950 mg to 3.8 grams of sodium
  citrate [9.5 to 38 mEq of sodium ion]) after meals and at bedtime.

**Usual pediatric dose**
Dosage has not been established.

**Strength(s) usually available**
U.S.—
  50 mg of potassium citrate (0.45 mEq of potassium ion) and 950 mg
  of sodium citrate (9.5 mEq of sodium ion) (Rx) [*Citrolith*].

**Packaging and storage**
Store below 40 °C (104 °F), preferably between 15 and 30 °C (59 and 86
  °F), in a well-closed container, unless otherwise specified by
  manufacturer.

**Auxiliary labeling**
• Swallow tablets whole.
• Take with a full glass of water.
• Take with meals or snack.

---

### SODIUM CITRATE AND CITRIC ACID

## Summary of Differences

Indications: Also used to prevent acid-aspiration pneumonitis.

## Additional Dosing Information

May be used when potassium citrate is contraindicated.

## Oral Dosage Forms
### SODIUM CITRATE AND CITRIC ACID ORAL SOLUTION USP

**Usual adult dose**
Antiurolithic or
Alkalizer, systemic or
Alkalizer, urinary—
> Oral, initially 10 to 30 mL (1 to 3 grams of sodium citrate [10 to 30 mEq of sodium ion]) four times a day, after meals and at bedtime, diluted in 30 to 90 mL of water, the dosage being adjusted as needed.
> Note: Dosage should be adjusted as determined by urinary pH measurements.

Neutralizing buffer—
> Oral, 15 to 30 mL (1.5 to 3 grams of sodium citrate [15 to 30 mEq of sodium ion]), as a single dose, or diluted in 15 to 30 mL of water.

**Usual adult prescribing limits**
Up to 150 mL (15 grams of sodium citrate [150 mEq of sodium ion]) a day.

**Usual pediatric dose**
Alkalizer, systemic—Oral, initially 5 to 15 mL (500 mg to 1.5 grams of sodium citrate [5 to 15 mEq of sodium ion]) four times a day, after meals and at bedtime, diluted in 30 to 90 mL of water, the dosage being adjusted as needed.

**Strength(s) usually available**
U.S.—
> 490 mg of sodium citrate (5 mEq of sodium ion) and 640 mg of citric acid per 5 mL (Rx) [*Oracit* (not USP)].
> 500 mg of sodium citrate (5 mEq of sodium ion) and 334 mg of citric acid per 5 mL (Rx) [*Bicitra*].

Canada—
> 490 mg of sodium citrate (5 mEq of sodium ion) and 640 mg of citric acid per 5 mL (OTC) [*Oracit*].

**Packaging and storage**
Store below 40 °C (104 °F), preferably between 15 and 30 °C (59 and 86 °F), unless otherwise specified by manufacturer. Store in a tight container. Protect from freezing.

**Auxiliary labeling**
• Dilute with water or juice.
• Take with meals or snack.

**Additional information**
Citric acid is a temporary buffer with only a transient effect on systemic acid-base balance.

---

### TRICITRATES

## Summary of Differences

Indications: Also used to treat chronic metabolic acidosis and to prevent acid-aspiration pneumonitis.

## Oral Dosage Forms
### TRICITRATES ORAL SOLUTION USP

**Usual adult dose**
Antiurolithic or
Alkalizer, systemic or
Alkalizer, urinary—
> Oral, initially 15 to 30 mL (1.6 to 3.3 grams of potassium citrate [15 to 30 mEq of potassium ion] and 1.5 to 3 grams of sodium citrate [15 to 30 mEq of sodium ion]) four times a day after meals and at bedtime, the dosage being adjusted as needed.
> Note: Dosage should be adjusted as determined by urinary pH measurements.

Neutralizing buffer—
> Oral, 15 mL (1.65 grams of potassium citrate [15 mEq of potassium ion] and 1.5 grams of sodium citrate [15 mEq of sodium ion]), as a single dose, diluted in 15 mL of water.

**Usual pediatric dose**
Alkalizer, systemic or
Alkalizer, urinary—
> Oral, initially 5 to 10 mL (550 mg to 1.10 grams of potassium citrate [5 to 10 mEq of potassium ion] and 500 mg to 1 gram of sodium citrate [5 to 10 mEq of sodium ion]) four times a day after meals and at bedtime, the dosage being adjusted as needed.

**Strength(s) usually available**
U.S.—
> 550 mg of potassium citrate (5 mEq of potassium ion), 500 mg of sodium citrate (5 mEq of sodium ion), and 334 mg of citric acid per 5 mL (Rx) [*Polycitra-LC; Polycitra Syrup* (sucrose)].

**Packaging and storage**
Store below 40 °C (104 °F), preferably between 15 and 30 °C (59 and 86 °F), unless otherwise specified by manufacturer. Store in a tight container. Protect from freezing.

**Auxiliary labeling**
• Dilute with water or juice.
• Take with meals or snack.

**Additional information**
Citric acid is a temporary buffer with only a transient effect on the systemic acid-base balance.

---

Revised: 01/18/93
Interim revision: 08/29/94

---

## CITRIC ACID–CONTAINING COMBINATIONS—

Acetaminophen, Sodium Bicarbonate, and Citric Acid (Systemic)
Aspirin, Sodium Bicarbonate, and Citric Acid (Systemic)
Chlorpheniramine, Phenylpropanolamine, Guaifenesin, Sodium Citrate, and Citric Acid (Systemic)—See *Cough/Cold Combinations (Systemic)*
Potassium Citrate and Citric Acid (Systemic)—See *Citrates (Systemic)*
Pyrilamine, Phenylpropanolamine, Dextromethorphan, Guaifenesin, Potassium Citrate, and Citric Acid (Systemic)—See *Cough/Cold Combinations (Systemic)*
Sodium Citrate and Citric Acid (Systemic)—See *Citrates (Systemic)*
Tricitrates (Systemic)—See *Citrates (Systemic)*

---

# CLADRIBINE   Systemic

VA CLASSIFICATION (Primary): AN300
Other commonly used names are 2-chlorodeoxyadenosine and 2-CdA.
Note: For a listing of dosage forms and brand names by country availability, see *Dosage Forms* section(s). For a listing of brand names for the articles in this monograph, refer to the General Index.

## Category
Antineoplastic.

## Indications

Note: Bracketed information in the *Indications* section refers to uses that are not included in U.S. product labeling.

**Accepted**
Leukemia, hairy cell (treatment)—Cladribine is indicated for active treatment of hairy cell leukemia as defined by clinically significant anemia, neutropenia, thrombocytopenia, or disease-related symptoms.

[Leukemia, chronic lymphocytic (treatment)][1]—Cladribine is accepted for treatment of B-cell chronic lymphocytic leukemia (CLL) in both previously untreated patients and patients refractory to previous treatment, based upon reports of objective tumor responses, most of which were partial, in noncomparative studies.

[Lymphomas, non-Hodgkin's (treatment)][1]—Cladribine is accepted for treatment of low-grade non-Hodgkin's lymphomas in patients refractory to previous treatment, based upon reports of objective tumor responses, most of which were partial, in two noncomparative studies.

[Waldenstrom macroglobulinemia (treatment)][1]—Cladribine is accepted for treatment of Waldenstrom macroglobulinemia, based upon reports of objective tumor responses in one noncomparative study.

---

[1]Not included in Canadian product labeling.

## Pharmacology/Pharmacokinetics

### Physicochemical characteristics
Source—Synthetic.
Chemical group—Cladribine is a halogenated purine nucleoside analog of deoxyadenosine.
Molecular weight—285.7.

### Mechanism of action/Effect
Cladribine is an antimetabolite. The exact mechanism of action in hairy cell leukemia is unknown. Cladribine is resistant to the action of adenosine deaminase (ADA), which deaminates deoxyadenosine to deoxyinosine. The phosphorylated metabolites of cladribine accumulate in cells with a high ratio of deoxycytidine kinase activity to 5' nucleotidase activity (lymphocytes, monocytes) and are converted to the active triphosphate deoxynucleotide. Intracellular accumulation of toxic deoxynucleotides selectively kills these cells, which become unable to properly repair single-strand DNA breaks, leading to disruption of cell metabolism. In addition, there is some evidence that deoxynucleotides are incorporated into the DNA of dividing cells and impair DNA synthesis. Cladribine also induces apoptosis (a form of programmed cell death in sensitive cells).
Cladribine's action is cell cycle–phase nonspecific; cladribine equally affects dividing and resting lymphocytes.

### Other actions/effects
Cladribine has immunosuppressant activity; restoration of lymphocyte subsets after treatment takes at least 6 to 12 months, although clinical immunocompetence is usually restored after about a month. Significant reductions in T and B lymphocytes occur during treatment (both CD4 and CD8 are affected) and CD4 counts recover more slowly after treatment.

### Distribution
Cladribine crosses the blood-brain barrier.

### Protein binding
Moderate (approximately 20%).

### Biotransformation
Metabolized in all cells with deoxycytidine kinase activity to 2-chloro-2'-deoxyadenosine-5'-triphosphate.

### Half-life
Distribution—With continuous intravenous infusion: Approximately 30 minutes.
Terminal—With continuous intravenous infusion: 7 hours.

### Onset of action
Time to achieve response—Median 4 months. (Response is defined as absence of hairy cells in bone marrow and peripheral blood together with normalization of peripheral blood parameters.)
Pharmacologic—Toxicity to lymphocytes: 7 days.

### Duration of action
Median duration of response—Greater than 8 months (range, up to and greater than 25 months).

### Elimination
Unknown.
In dialysis or hemofiltration—Unknown.

## Precautions to Consider

### Carcinogenicity
No studies have been done with cladribine in animals.
Secondary malignancies are potential delayed effects of many antineoplastic agents, although it is not clear whether the effect is related to their mutagenic or immunosuppressive action. The effect of dose and duration of therapy is also unknown, although risk seems to increase with long-term use. Although information is limited, available data seem to indicate that the carcinogenic risk is greatest with the alkylating agents.
Antimetabolites have been shown to be carcinogenic in animals and may be associated with an increased risk of development of secondary carcinomas in humans, although the risk appears to be less than with alkylating agents.

### Mutagenicity
In mammalian cells in culture, cladribine has been shown to cause an imbalance of intracellular deoxyribonucleotide triphosphate pools. This imbalance resulted in the inhibition of DNA synthesis and DNA repair, yielding DNA strand breaks and subsequently cell death. Inhibition of thymidine incorporation into human lymphoblastic cells was 90% at concentrations of 0.3 micromolar. Cladribine was also incorporated into DNA of these cells. Cladribine was not mutagenic to bacteria and did not induce unscheduled DNA synthesis in primary rat hepatocyte cultures.

### Pregnancy/Reproduction
Fertility—Gonadal suppression, resulting in amenorrhea or azoospermia, may occur in patients taking antineoplastic therapy, especially with the alkylating agents. In general, these effects appear to be related to dose and length of therapy and may be irreversible. Prediction of the degree of testicular or ovarian function impairment is complicated by the common use of combinations of several antineoplastics, which makes it difficult to assess the effects of individual agents.
Intravenous administration of cladribine to Cynomolgus monkeys has been shown to cause suppression of rapidly generating cells, including testicular cells.
Pregnancy—Adequate and well-controlled studies in women have not been done.
First trimester: It is usually recommended that use of antineoplastics, especially combination chemotherapy, be avoided whenever possible, especially during the first trimester. Although information is limited because of the relatively few instances of antineoplastic administration during pregnancy, the mutagenic, teratogenic, and carcinogenic potential of these medications must be considered.
Other hazards to the fetus include adverse reactions seen in adults.
In general, use of contraception is recommended during cytotoxic drug therapy.
Cladribine has been shown to cause a significant increase in fetal variations in mice at a dose of 1.5 mg per kg of body weight (mg/kg) (4.5 mg per square meter of body surface) per day, and to cause increased resorptions, reduced litter size, and increased fetal malformations in mice at a dose of 3 mg/kg (9 mg per square meter of body surface) per day. Cladribine was shown to cause fetal death and malformations in rabbits at a dose of 3 mg/kg (33 mg per square meter of body surface) per day. No fetal effects were produced in mice at a dose of 0.5 mg/kg (1.5 mg per square meter of body surface) per day or in rabbits at a dose of 1 mg/kg (11 mg per square meter of body surface) per day.
FDA Pregnancy Category D.

### Breast-feeding
Although very little information is available regarding distribution of antineoplastic agents into breast milk, breast-feeding is not recommended during chemotherapy because of the potential risks to the infant (adverse effects, mutagenicity, carcinogenicity). It is not known whether cladribine is distributed into breast milk.

### Pediatrics
No information is available on the relationship of age to the effects of cladribine in pediatric patients. However, phase I and phase II studies in children have been reported and some studies of cladribine for acute myelocytic leukemia and acute lymphocytic leukemia have included children.

### Geriatrics
Although appropriate studies on the relationship of age to the effects of cladribine have not been performed in the geriatric population, clinical trials have included patients over 65 years of age and geriatrics-specific problems that would limit the usefulness of this medication in the elderly are not expected.

### Dental
The bone marrow depressant effects of cladribine may result in an increased incidence of microbial infection, delayed healing, and gingival bleeding. Dental work, whenever possible should be completed prior to initiation of therapy or deferred until blood counts have returned to normal. Patients should be instructed in proper oral hygiene during treatment, including caution in use of regular toothbrushes, dental floss, and toothpicks.

### Drug interactions and/or related problems
The following drug interactions and/or related problems have been selected on the basis of their potential clinical significance (possible mechanism in parentheses where appropriate)—not necessarily inclusive (» = major clinical significance):
Note: Combinations containing any of the following medications, depending on the amount present, may also interact with this medication.

Allopurinol or
Colchicine or

» Probenecid or
» Sulfinpyrazone
   (cladribine may raise the concentration of blood uric acid; dosage adjustment of antigout agents may be necessary to control hyperuricemia and gout; allopurinol may be preferred to prevent or reverse cladribine-induced hyperuricemia because of risk of uric acid nephropathy with uricosuric antigout agents)

Blood dyscrasia–causing medications (See *Appendix II*)
   (leukopenic and/or thrombocytopenic effects of cladribine may be increased with concurrent or recent therapy if these medications cause the same effects; dosage adjustment of cladribine, if necessary, should be based on blood counts)

» Bone marrow depressants, other (See *Appendix II*) or
   Radiation therapy
   (additive bone marrow depression may occur; dosage reduction may be required when two or more bone marrow depressants, including radiation, are used concurrently or consecutively)

Vaccines, killed virus
   (because normal defense mechanisms may be suppressed by cladribine therapy, the patient's antibody response to the vaccine may be decreased. The interval between discontinuation of medications that cause immunosuppression and restoration of the patient's ability to respond to the vaccine depends on the intensity and type of immunosuppression-causing medication used, the underlying disease, and other factors)

» Vaccines, live virus
   (because normal defense mechanisms may be suppressed by cladribine therapy, concurrent use with a live virus vaccine may potentiate the replication of the vaccine virus, may increase the side/adverse effects of the vaccine virus, and/or may decrease the patient's antibody response to the vaccine; immunization of these patients should be undertaken only with extreme caution after careful review of the patient's hematologic status and only with the knowledge and consent of the physician managing the cladribine therapy. The interval between discontinuation of medications that cause immunosuppression and restoration of the patient's ability to respond to the vaccine depends on the intensity and type of immunosuppression-causing medication used, the underlying disease, and other factors. In addition, immunization with oral poliovirus vaccine should be postponed in persons in close contact with the patient, especially family members)

**Laboratory value alterations**
The following have been selected on the basis of their potential clinical significance (possible effect in parentheses where appropriate)—not necessarily inclusive (» = major clinical significance):

With physiology/laboratory test values
   Uric acid concentrations in blood and urine
   (may be increased as part of a tumor lysis syndrome, especially in patients with a large tumor burden)

**Medical considerations/Contraindications**
The medical considerations/contraindications included here have been selected on the basis of their potential clinical significance (reasons given in parentheses where appropriate)—not necessarily inclusive (» = major clinical significance).

*Risk-benefit should be considered when the following medical problems exist:*
» Bone marrow depression
» Chickenpox, existing or recent (including recent exposure) or
» Herpes zoster
   (risk of severe generalized disease)

Gout, history of or
Urate renal stones, history of
   (risk of hyperuricemia)
» Infection
» Sensitivity to cladribine
» Caution should be used also in patients who have had previous cytotoxic drug therapy or radiation therapy.

**Patient monitoring**
The following are especially important in patient monitoring (other tests may be warranted in some patients, depending on condition; » = major clinical significance):

CD4 T lymphocyte count and
CD8 T lymphocyte count
   (recommended prior to initiation of therapy and at periodic intervals during and after therapy)

» Hematocrit or hemoglobin and
» Leukocyte count, total and, if appropriate, differential and
» Platelet count
   (determinations recommended prior to initiation of therapy and at periodic intervals during therapy; frequency varies according to clinical state, agent, dose, and other agents being used concurrently)

Uric acid concentrations, serum
   (recommended prior to initiation of therapy and at periodic intervals during therapy; frequency varies according to clinical state, agent, dose, and other agents being used concurrently)

## Side/Adverse Effects

Note: Percentage figures for frequency of side/adverse effects listed below are based on a single study of patients with hairy cell leukemia and are included only as an indication of relative frequency of reported side/adverse effects.

   Cladribine has considerable hematopoietic stem cell toxicity.

   In patients with hairy cell leukemia, anemia, neutropenia, and thrombocytopenia may worsen during the first two weeks of cladribine therapy, before recovery begins.

   Prolonged bone marrow hypocellularity has been observed after treatment with cladribine.

   Administration of repeated courses for indications other than hairy cell leukemia has been associated with prolonged, dose-limiting thrombocytopenia, occasional pancytopenia, and prolonged erythroid macrocytosis.

   Neurotoxicity (paraparesis/quadraparesis of upper and/or lower extremities consistent with a demyelinating disease) and acute renal failure (possibly necessitating hemodialysis) occurred frequently in patients who received cladribine for indications other than hairy cell leukemia in doses above 0.26 mg per kg of body weight (mg/kg) per day for 10 to 14 days (4 to 9 times the recommended dose for hairy cell leukemia) in conjunction with alkylating agents, total body irradiation, and allogeneic bone marrow transplantation.

The following side/adverse effects have been selected on the basis of their potential clinical significance (possible signs and symptoms in parentheses where appropriate)—not necessarily inclusive:

**Those indicating need for medical attention**
Incidence more frequent
   *Anemia, severe* (usually asymptomatic)—37%; *fever*—40–70%; *infection* (fever or chills; cough or hoarseness; lower back or side pain; painful or difficult urination)—28%; *neutropenia, severe* (usually asymptomatic)—up to 70%; *skin rash*—27%; *thrombocytopenia* (unusual bleeding or bruising; black, tarry stools; blood in urine or stools; pinpoint red spots on skin)—12%

Note: *Anemia* may increase transfusion requirements during the first month of therapy; median time to normalization of hemoglobin has been reported to be 8 weeks.

   *Fever* (temperature above 100 °F [38 °C]) usually begins between the fifth and seventh day of therapy and lasts a few days. Severe fever (temperature of 104 °F [40 °C] or higher) occurs in about 10% of patients. In most patients, fever is associated with neutropenia, although non-neutropenic fever may also occur. Documented infections (including those related to central intravenous catheters) occur in fewer than one-third of patients who experience severe fever. Fever has generally not been reported when cladribine was used for indications other than hairy cell leukemia.

   *Infections* may be bacterial, viral, protozoal (e.g., *Pneumocystis*), or fungal, may occur even in the absence of neutropenia, and may be life-threatening. Cladribine causes prolonged depression of CD4 and CD8 lymphocyte subset counts; recovery of counts takes at least 6 to 12 months.

   The highest incidence of *severe neutropenia* is in patients with pre-existing neutropenia related to prior therapy. Median time to normalization of absolute neutrophil counts (ANC) has been reported to be 5 weeks.

   With *thrombocytopenia* occurring during cladribine therapy of hairy cell leukemia, median time to normalization of platelet counts has been reported to be 12 days. However, thrombocytopenia may become prolonged and dose-limiting with repeated courses (i.e., when cladribine is used for indications other than hairy cell leukemia).

Incidence less frequent—less than 10%
   *Cough; edema* (swelling of feet or lower legs); *injection site reaction* (pain or redness at site of injection)—9%; *phlebitis* (pain or redness

at site of injection)—2%; *shortness of breath; stomach pain; tachy-cardia* (unusually fast heartbeat)

**Those indicating need for medical attention only if they continue or are bothersome**
Incidence more frequent
*Anorexia* (loss of appetite)—17%; *headache*—22%; *nausea*—28%; *unusual tiredness*—45%; *vomiting*—13%

Note: *Nausea* is usually mild and does not usually require treatment with antiemetics.
*Skin rashes* are usually mild.

Incidence less frequent—less than 10%
*Constipation; diarrhea; dizziness; itching; malaise* (general feeling of discomfort or illness); *myalgia or arthralgia* (muscle or joint pain); *sweating; trouble in sleeping; weakness*

Note: *Dizziness* may be a neurologic effect.

## Overdose

For more information on the management of overdose or unintentional ingestion, **contact a Poison Control Center** (see *Poison Control Center Listing*).

**Treatment of overdose**
Treatment consists of:
Withdrawal of cladribine.
Observation.
Supportive therapy.

## Patient Consultation

As an aid to patient consultation, refer to *Advice for the Patient, Cladribine (Systemic)*.

In providing consultation, consider emphasizing the following selected information (» = major clinical significance):

**Before using this medication**
» Conditions affecting use, especially:
Sensitivity to cladribine
Pregnancy—Use not recommended because of mutagenic, terato-genic, and carcinogenic potential; advisability of using contra-ception; telling physician immediately if pregnancy is suspected
Breast-feeding—Not recommended because of risk of serious side effects
Other medications, especially probenecid, sulfinpyrazone, other bone marrow depressants, or other cytotoxic drug or radiation therapy
Other medical problems, especially chickenpox, herpes zoster, or infection

**Proper use of this medication**
Possibility of nausea and vomiting; importance of continuing medi-cation despite stomach upset
» Proper dosing

**Precautions while using this medication**
» Importance of close monitoring by the physician
» Avoiding immunizations unless approved by physician; other persons in patient's household should avoid immunizations with oral po-liovirus vaccine; avoiding other persons who have taken oral po-liovirus vaccine or wearing a protective mask that covers nose and mouth

*Caution if bone marrow depression occurs*
» Avoiding exposure to persons with bacterial infections, especially dur-ing periods of low blood counts; checking with physician imme-diately if fever or chills, cough or hoarseness, lower back or side pain, or painful or difficult urination occur
» Checking with physician immediately if unusual bleeding or bruising; black, tarry stools; blood in urine or stools; or pinpoint red spots on skin occur
Caution in use of regular toothbrush, dental floss, or toothpick; phy-sician, dentist, or nurse may suggest alternatives; checking with physician before having dental work done
Not touching eyes or inside of nose unless hands washed immediately before
Using caution to avoid accidental cuts with use of sharp objects such as safety razor or fingernail or toenail cutters
Avoiding contact sports or other situations where bruising or injury could occur

**Side/adverse effects**
May cause adverse effects such as blood problems; importance of dis-cussing possible effects with physician

Signs of potential side effects, especially anemia, fever, infection, neu-tropenia, thrombocytopenia, cough, edema, injection site reaction or phlebitis, shortness of breath, stomach pain, and tachycardia
Asymptomatic side effects including anemia and leukopenia
Physician or nurse can help in dealing with side effects

## General Dosing Information

Patients receiving cladribine should be under supervision of a physician experienced in cancer chemotherapy.

Cladribine injection must be diluted prior to administration by intravenous infusion.

If fever occurs, it is recommended that the patient be evaluated for pos-sible infection.

Development of uric acid nephropathy in patients with leukemia or lym-phoma may be prevented by adequate oral hydration and, in some cases, administration of allopurinol. Alkalinization of urine may be necessary if serum uric acid concentrations are elevated.

Special precautions are recommended in patients who develop thrombo-cytopenia as a result of administration of cladribine. These may in-clude extreme care in performing invasive procedures; regular inspec-tion of intravenous sites, skin (including perirectal area), and mucous membrane surfaces for signs of bleeding or bruising; limiting fre-quency of venipuncture and avoiding intramuscular injections; testing urine, emesis, stool, and secretions for occult blood; care in use of regular toothbrushes, dental floss, toothpicks, safety razors, and fin-gernail and toenail cutters; avoiding constipation; and using caution to prevent falls and other injuries. Such patients should avoid alcohol and aspirin intake because of the risk of gastrointestinal bleeding. Platelet transfusions may be required.

Subsequent courses of cladribine should not be administered until hema-tological effects from the previous course have subsided and then only with great caution.

Patients who develop leukopenia should be observed carefully for signs of infection. Antibiotic support may be required. In neutropenic pa-tients who develop fever, broad-spectrum antibiotic coverage should be initiated empirically, pending bacterial cultures and appropriate di-agnostic tests.

Red blood cell transfusions may be required for anemia.

If neurotoxicity occurs, it is recommended that withholding or discontin-uation of cladribine be considered.

**Safety considerations for handling this medication**

There is limited but increasing evidence and concern that personnel in-volved in preparation and administration of parenteral antineoplastics may be at some risk because of the potential mutagenicity, teratoge-nicity, and/or carcinogenicity of these agents, although the actual risk is unknown. USP advisory panels recommend cautious handling both in preparation and disposal of antineoplastic agents. Precautions that have been suggested include:
• Use of a biological containment cabinet during reconstitution and dilution of parenteral medications and wearing of disposable surgical gloves and masks.
• Use of proper technique to prevent contamination of the medication, work area, and operator during transfer between containers (including proper training of personnel in this technique).
• Cautious and proper disposal of needles, syringes, vials, ampuls, and unused medication.
A number of medical centers have developed detailed guidelines for handling of antineoplastic agents.

## Parenteral Dosage Forms

### CLADRIBINE INJECTION

**Usual adult dose**
Hairy cell leukemia—
Intravenous (by continuous infusion), 100 mcg (0.1 mg) per kg of body weight per day for seven days.

Note: Cladribine is usually given for only one course for treatment of hairy cell leukemia.

Early studies used an actual dose of 0.09 mg per kg of body weight per day as a result of a slight calculation error during formulation, but in most recent studies the patients received the 0.1 mg per kg dose.

**Usual adult prescribing limits**
A dose of 0.1 mg per kg of body weight per day by continuous infusion for seven days has been established as the maximum-tolerated dose (MTD) in phase I studies.

**Usual pediatric dose**

Dosage has not been established.

**Strength(s) usually available**

U.S.—

1 mg per mL (Rx) [*Leustatin* (sodium chloride 9 mg [0.15 mEq] per mL)].

Canada—

1 mg per mL (Rx) [*Leustatin* (sodium chloride 9 mg [0.15 mEq] per mL)].

**Packaging and storage**

Store between 2 and 8 °C (36 and 46 °F), unless otherwise specified by manufacturer. Protect from light. Not adversely affected by freezing; if freezing occurs, thawing naturally to room temperature is recommended (heat or microwave should not be used), and the solution should not be refrozen.

**Preparation of dosage form**

Cladribine injection must be diluted before administration. (Since the product contains no antimicrobial preservative or bacteriostatic agent, proper aseptic technique and environmental precautions are necessary.)

Cladribine injection is prepared for administration by a single 24-hour intravenous infusion (to be repeated daily for 7 days) by adding the calculated daily dose to an infusion bag containing 500 mL of 0.9% sodium chloride injection.

Cladribine injection is prepared for administration by a continuous 7-day intravenous infusion by adding the calculated 7-day dose to the infusion reservoir through a sterile 0.22 micron disposable hydrophilic syringe filter. Then bacteriostatic 0.9% sodium chloride injection

(0.9% benzyl alcohol preserved) is added through the filter, in an amount sufficient to make a total of 100 mL.

Caution—Use of diluents containing benzyl alcohol is not recommended for preparation of medications for use in neonates. A fatal toxic syndrome consisting of metabolic acidosis, CNS depression, respiratory problems, renal failure, hypotension, and possibly seizures and intracranial hemorrhages has been associated with this use.

**Stability**

Reconstituted solutions contain no preservative and should be used immediately or stored between 2 and 8 °C (36 and 46 °F) and used within 8 hours of reconstitution.

**Incompatibilities**

Use of 5% dextrose injection is not recommended for dilution of cladribine injection because increased degradation of cladribine will occur.

**Selected Bibliography**

Beutler E. Cladribine (2-chlorodeoxyadenosine). Lancet 1992 Oct 17; 340: 952-6.

Saven A, Piro LD. Treatment of hairy cell leukemia. Blood 1992 Mar 1; 79: 1111-20.

Bryson HM, Sorkin EM. Cladribine. A review of its pharmacodynamic and pharmacokinetic properties and therapeutic potential in haematological malignancies. Drugs 1993; 46 (5): 872-94.

Developed: 07/26/94
Interim revision: 08/15/94

# CLARITHROMYCIN   Systemic

VA CLASSIFICATION (Primary): AM200

Note: For a listing of dosage forms and brand names by country availability, see *Dosage Forms* section(s). For a listing of brand names for the articles in this monograph, refer to the General Index.

## Category

Antibacterial (systemic).

## Indications

Note: Bracketed information in the *Indications* section refers to uses that are not included in U.S. product labeling.

**General considerations**

Clarithromycin is a macrolide antibiotic with *in vitro* activity against many gram-positive and gram-negative aerobic and anaerobic organisms. The minimum inhibitory concentrations (MICs) of clarithromycin are generally 2- to 4-fold lower than those of erythromycin against gram-positive bacteria, such as methicillin-sensitive *Staphylococcus aureus* and most *Streptococcus* species. However, sensitivities vary and *S. aureus* strains that are resistant to erythromycin, methicillin, or oxacillin have also been found to be resistant to clarithromycin. Clarithromycin is bactericidal against *S. pyogenes* and *S. pneumoniae*; however, *Streptococcus* strains resistant to one macrolide antibiotic have demonstrated cross resistance to other macrolide antibiotics.

The activity of erythromycin is twice that of clarithromycin against *Haemophilus influenzae*; however, clarithromycin's active metabolite, 14-hydroxyclarithromycin, is as active as erythromycin. When clarithromycin and 14-hydroxyclarithromycin are combined, their MIC is 2- to 4-fold lower than that of erythromycin, suggesting additive or synergistic *in vitro* activity against *H. influenzae*.

Clarithromycin displays *in vitro* activity against *Mycobacterium avium* complex (MAC), being 8- to 32-fold more active than erythromycin. High intracellular concentrations are achieved with clarithromycin, and it has been found to be effective against MAC in human macrophages. Clarithromycin may act synergistically with other agents used to treat MAC. It is also very active against many different strains of mycobacteria. *In vitro* and *in vivo* activity against *M. leprae* has been demonstrated; and there has been good clinical response to the treatment of cutaneous disease, including disseminated disease, caused by *M. chelonae*.

Clarithromycin has been found to have greater *in vitro* activity than erythromycin against *Legionella pneumophila*, *Moraxella (Branhamella) catarrhalis*, *Chlamydia trachomatis*, and *Ureaplasma urealyticum*. Its activity is variable, and similar to that of erythromycin against *Neisseria gonorrhoeae*, anaerobic gram-positive cocci, and *Bacteroides* sp. Clarithromycin also has good *in vitro* activity against *Helicobacter*

*pylori* and has been clinically effective, when combined with omeprazole, in the treatment of duodenal ulcers.

**Accepted**

Clarithromycin is indicated to treat the following infections when caused by susceptible organisms:

Bronchitis, bacterial exacerbations of (treatment);

Otitis media, acute (treatment)[1];

Pharyngitis, streptococcal (treatment)

Pneumonia, mycoplasmal (treatment)

Pneumonia, streptococcal (treatment)

Sinusitis, acute maxillary (treatment) and

Skin and soft tissue infections (treatment)—Clarithromycin is indicated in the treatment of these disease states when caused by susceptible organisms.

*Mycobacterium avium* complex (MAC) (treatment)[1]—Clarithromycin is indicated, in combination with other antimycobacterials, in the treatment of disseminated *Mycobacterium avium* complex.

Acquired resistance of *Mycobacterium avium* complex to clarithromycin has been found to develop when clarithromycin is used as monotherapy. Clarithromycin should be used in combination with other antimycobacterials to prevent the development of resistance.

[Legionnaires' disease (treatment)][1]—Clarithromycin is used in the treatment of Legionnaires' disease, caused by *Legionella pneumophila*.

**Unaccepted**

Clarithromycin has not been found to have *in vitro* activity against *Mycobacterium tuberculosis*.

[1]Not included in Canadian product labeling.

## Pharmacology/Pharmacokinetics

**Physicochemical characteristics**

Molecular weight—747.96.

**Mechanism of action/Effect**

Clarithromycin binds to the 50S ribosomal subunit of the 70S ribosome of susceptible organisms, thereby inhibiting bacterial RNA-dependent protein synthesis.

**Absorption**

Well absorbed from the gastrointestinal tract; stable in gastric acid; food delays the rate, but not the extent, of absorption; bioavailability is approximately 55% in healthy volunteers. In adults, the bioavailability of the oral suspension was similar to that of the tablets.

## Distribution

Widely distributed into tissues and fluids; high concentrations found in nasal mucosa, tonsils, and lungs; concentrations in tissues are higher than those in serum because of high intracellular concentrations; readily enters leukocytes and macrophages.

$Vol_D$ =243 to 266 liters.

## Protein binding

65 to 75%.

## Biotransformation

Hepatically metabolized via 3 main pathways, demethylation, hydroxylation, and hydrolysis, to 8 metabolites. One metabolite, 14-hydroxyclarithromycin, has *in vitro* antimicrobial activity comparable to that of clarithromycin and may act synergistically with clarithromycin against *H. influenzae*. Saturation of metabolism involves the demethylation and hydroxylation pathways, and accounts for an increase in serum half-life.

## Half-life

Normal renal function—

Clarithromycin:

250 mg every 12 hours—3 to 4 hours.

500 mg every 12 hours—5 to 7 hours.

14-Hydroxyclarithromycin:

250 mg every 12 hours—5 to 6 hours.

500 mg every 12 hours—Approximately 7 hours.

Renal function impairment (creatinine clearance of <30 mL per minute [0.5 mL per second])—

Clarithromycin: Approximately 22 hours.

14-Hydroxyclarithromycin: Approximately 47 hours.

## Time to peak concentration

2 to 3 hours.

## Peak serum concentration

Adults—

Clarithromycin: Steady-state:

250 mg (suspension) every 12 hours: Approximately 2 mcg/mL.

250 mg (tablet) every 12 hours: Approximately 1 mcg/mL.

500 mg (tablet) every 12 hours: 2 to 3 mcg/mL.

14-Hydroxyclarithromycin: Steady-state:

250 mg (suspension) every 12 hours: Approximately 0.7 mcg/mL.

250 mg (tablet) every 12 hours: Approximately 0.6 mcg/mL.

500 mg (tablet) every 12 hours: Up to 1 mcg/mL.

Children—

Clarithromycin: Steady-state:

7.5 mg per kg of body weight (mg/kg) (suspension) every 12 hours: 3 to 7 mcg per mL.

15 mg/kg (suspension) every 12 hours: 6 to 15 mcg per mL.

14-Hydroxyclarithromycin: Steady-state:

7.5 mg/kg (suspension) every 12 hours: 1 to 2 mcg per mL.

## Elimination

Renal—Approximately 20 and 30%, respectively, of the dose of 250- and 500-mg tablets given twice-a-day is excreted in the urine as unchanged drug. Approximately 40% of the dose of 250-mg suspension given twice-a-day is excreted in the urine as clarithromycin. 14-Hydroxyclarithromycin accounts for 10 and 15%, respectively, of the dose excreted in the urine after a 250- and 500-mg twice-daily dose.

Fecal—Approximately 4% of a 250-mg dose is excreted in the feces.

# Precautions to Consider

## Cross-sensitivity and/or related problems

Patients who are hypersensitive to erythromycin or other macrolides may also be hypersensitive to clarithromycin.

## Carcinogenicity/Mutagenicity

Clarithromycin was not found to be mutagenic in the Salmonella/mammalian microsome test, the bacterial induced mutation frequency test, the rat hepatocyte DNA synthesis assay, the mouse lymphoma assay, the mouse dominant lethal study, and the mouse micronucleus test. However, the *in vitro* chromosome aberration test was weakly positive in one test and negative in another. The Ames test was negative when performed on clarithromycin metabolites.

## Pregnancy/Reproduction

Fertility—Adequate and well-controlled studies in humans have not been done.

Studies in male and female rats given 160 mg per kg of body weight (mg/kg) per day (plasma levels equivalent to approximately 2 times the human serum levels) showed no adverse effects on the estrous cycle, fertility, parturition, or the number and viability of offspring.

Pregnancy—Adequate and well-controlled studies in humans have not been done.

Monkeys administered oral doses of 150 mg/kg per day (plasma levels equivalent to 3 times the human serum levels) had embryonic loss, which was attributed to marked maternal toxicity at this dose. *In utero* fetal loss occurred in rabbits given intravenous doses of 33 mg per square meter of body surface (mg/m²), which is 17 times less than the maximum proposed human daily dose. Clarithromycin was not found to be teratogenic in 4 rat studies (3 with oral doses and 1 with intravenous doses of up to 160 mg/kg per day administered during the period of major organogenesis) and 2 rabbit studies (at oral doses of up to 125 mg/kg per day or intravenous doses of 30 mg/kg per day administered during gestation days 6 through 18). Two additional studies in a different rat strain demonstrated a low incidence of cardiovascular anomalies at oral doses of 150 mg/kg per day administered during gestation days 6 to 15. Cleft palate was seen at doses of 500 mg/kg per day. Fetal growth retardation was seen in monkeys given an oral dose of 70 mg/kg per day, which produced plasma levels that were 2 times the human serum levels.

FDA Pregnancy Category C.

## Breast-feeding

Clarithromycin and its active metabolite are distributed into human breast milk.

## Pediatrics

Appropriate studies on the relationship of age to the effects of clarithromycin have not been performed in children up to 6 months of age. Clarithromycin oral suspension has been studied in children 6 months to 12 years of age and appeared to be well tolerated.

## Geriatrics

One study performed in healthy elderly subjects found increased peak steady-state concentrations of clarithromycin and 14-hydroxyclarithromycin; this was thought to be due to an age-related decrease in renal function. There was no increase in side effects in elderly patients compared with younger subjects. Elderly patients with severe renal function impairment may require a decrease in dose.

## Drug interactions and/or related problems

The following drug interactions and/or related problems have been selected on the basis of their potential clinical significance (possible mechanism in parentheses where appropriate)—not necessarily inclusive (» = major clinical significance):

Note: Combinations containing any of the following medications, depending on the amount present, may also interact with this medication.

» Carbamazepine

(administration of carbamazepine with clarithromycin has been shown to increase significantly the plasma concentration of carbamazepine; carbamazepine serum levels should be monitored)

» Digoxin

(concurrent administration of digoxin with clarithromycin has been shown to increase serum digoxin concentrations; monitoring of digoxin serum levels is recommended in patients receiving digoxin and clarithromycin concurrently)

» Rifabutin or

» Rifampin

(concurrent use of clarithromycin and rifabutin or rifampin decreases the serum concentration of clarithromycin by > 50%)

» Terfenadine

(concurrent use of clarithromycin and terfenadine may increase the plasma concentration of terfenadine and its active metabolite by 2 to 3 times; concurrent use should be avoided)

» Theophylline

(concurrent administration with clarithromycin has been shown to increase the area under the plasma concentration time curve [AUC] of theophylline by 17%; monitoring of theophylline serum levels is recommended in patients receiving high doses of theophylline or patients with theophylline serum levels in the upper therapeutic range)

» Warfarin

(concurrent administration with clarithromycin has been shown to potentiate the effects of warfarin; prothrombin time should be closely monitored in patients receiving warfarin and clarithromycin concurrently)

» Zidovudine

(initial results of a dose escalation study in HIV-infected patients found that simultaneous oral administration of zidovudine and clarithromycin resulted in a lower peak serum concentration [$C_{max}$], lower AUC, and delayed time to peak concentration [$T_{max}$] of zidovudine; doses of clarithromycin and zidovudine should be taken at least 4 hours apart)

## Laboratory value alterations

The following have been selected on the basis of their potential clinical significance (possible effect in parentheses where appropriate)—not necessarily inclusive (» = major clinical significance):

With physiology/laboratory test values

Alanine aminotransferase (ALT [SGPT]) or
Aspartate aminotransferase (AST [SGOT])
(rarely, values may be elevated)

Blood urea nitrogen (BUN)
(rarely, concentration may be elevated)

## Medical considerations/Contraindications

The medical considerations/contraindications included here have been selected on the basis of their potential clinical significance (reasons given in parentheses where appropriate)—not necessarily inclusive (» = major clinical significance).

*Risk-benefit should be considered when the following medical problems exist:*

Hypersensitivity to erythromycins or other macrolides

» Renal function impairment, severe
(the elimination of clarithromycin is reduced in patients with renal function impairment, especially those with a creatinine clearance of < 30 mL/min [0.5 mL/second]; an adjustment in dose may be necessary in patients with a creatinine clearance of < 30 mL/min [0.5 mL/second])

(liver function impairment alters the pharmacokinetics of clarithromycin by decreasing the amount of metabolites formed and increasing the renal clearance of the parent drug; however, steady-state concentrations in patients with mild to severe hepatic function impairment do not differ from those in patients with normal hepatic function, unless there is also concurrent severe renal function impairment)

## Side/Adverse Effects

The following side/adverse effects have been selected on the basis of their potential clinical significance (possible signs and symptoms in parentheses where appropriate)—not necessarily inclusive:

**Those indicating need for medical attention**
Incidence rare
*Clostridium difficile colitis* (severe abdominal or stomach cramps and pain; abdominal tenderness; watery and severe diarrhea, which may also be bloody; fever); *hepatotoxicity* (fever; nausea and vomiting; yellow eyes or skin); *hypersensitivity* (shortness of breath; skin rash and itching); *thrombocytopenia* (unusual bleeding and bruising)

**Those indicating need for medical attention only if they continue or are bothersome**
Incidence less frequent
*Abnormal taste*—3%; *gastrointestinal disturbances* (abdominal discomfort or pain; diarrhea; nausea; vomiting)—2 to 3%; *headache*—2%

## Patient Consultation

As an aid to patient consultation, refer to *Advice for the Patient, Clarithromycin (Systemic).*

In providing consultation, consider emphasizing the following selected information (» = major clinical significance):

**Before using this medication**
» Conditions affecting use, especially:
Hypersensitivity to erythromycins or other macrolides
Pregnancy—Clarithromycin has produced embryotoxicity and fetal toxicity in animals
Breast-feeding—Passes into breast milk
Other medications, especially carbamazepine, digoxin, rifabutin, rifampin, terfenadine, theophylline, warfarin, and zidovudine
Other medical problems, especially severe renal function impairment

**Proper use of this medication**
May be taken with food or milk or on an empty stomach
» Compliance with full course of therapy
Proper administration technique for oral liquids
» Proper dosing
Missed dose: Taking as soon as possible; not taking if almost time for next dose; not doubling doses
» Proper storage

**Precautions while using this medication**
Checking with physician if no improvement within a few days

## Side/adverse effects
Signs of potential side effects, especially *Clostridium difficile* colitis, hepatotoxicity, hypersensitivity, and thrombocytopenia

## General Dosing Information

Clarithromycin tablets and suspension may be taken with meals or milk or on an empty stomach.

## Oral Dosage Forms

### CLARITHROMYCIN FOR ORAL SUSPENSION

**Usual adult and adolescent dose**
Antibacterial—
Bronchitis, bacterial exacerbations due to *H. influenzae*: Oral, 500 mg every twelve hours for seven to fourteen days.
Bronchitis, bacterial exacerbations due to other organisms: Oral, 250 mg every twelve hours for seven to fourteen days.
*Mycobacterium avium* complex, disseminated[1]: Oral, 500 mg every twelve hours.
Pharyngitis, streptococcal: Oral, 250 mg every twelve hours for ten days.
Pneumonia, due to *S. pneumoniae* or *M. pneumoniae*: Oral, 250 mg every twelve hours for seven to fourteen days.
Sinusitis, acute maxillary: Oral, 500 mg every twelve hours for fourteen days.
Skin and soft tissue infections: Oral, 250 mg every twelve hours for seven to fourteen days.
Note: The dose of clarithromycin should be adjusted in patients with severe renal function impairment (creatinine clearance [CrCl] < 30 mL/min or 0.50 mL/sec). The following dosing guidelines are suggested:

| Dose for CrCl of >30 mL/min (0.50 mL/sec) | Adjusted dose for CrCl of <30 mL/min (0.50 mL/sec) |
| --- | --- |
| 500 mg two times a day | 500 mg loading dose, then 250 mg two times a day |
| 250 mg two times a day | 250 mg once a day |

**Usual pediatric dose**
Antibacterial—
*Mycobacterium avium* complex, disseminated[1]:
Infants up to 6 months of age—Safety and efficacy have not been established.
Children 6 months of age and older—Oral, 7.5 mg per kg of body weight, up to 500 mg, every twelve hours for life if clinical and mycobacterial improvements are observed.
Otitis media, acute or
Pharyngitis, streptococcal or
Sinusitis, acute maxillary or
Skin and soft tissue infections:
Infants up to 6 months of age—Safety and efficacy have not been established.
Children 6 months of age and older—Oral, 7.5 mg per kg of body weight every twelve hours for ten days.

**Strength(s) usually available**
U.S.—
125 mg per 5 mL (when reconstituted according to manufacturer's instructions) (Rx) [*Biaxin* (sucrose)].
250 mg per 5 mL (when reconstituted according to manufacturer's instructions) (Rx) [*Biaxin* (sucrose)].
Canada—
Not commercially available.

**Packaging and storage**
Store between 15 and 30 °C (59 and 86 °F) in a well-closed container. Protect from light.

**Stability**
After reconstitution, suspension retains its potency for 14 days. Do not refrigerate.

**Auxiliary labeling**
• Shake well.
• Do not refrigerate.
• Continue for full time of treatment.
• Beyond-use date.

**Note**
When dispensing, include a calibrated liquid-measuring device.

## CLARITHROMYCIN TABLETS USP

**Usual adult and adolescent dose**
See *Clarithromycin for Oral Suspension*.

**Usual pediatric dose**
This product may not be suitable for young children. See *Clarithromycin for Oral Suspension*.

**Strength(s) usually available**
U.S.—
    250 mg (Rx) [*Biaxin*].
    500 mg (Rx) [*Biaxin*].
Canada—
    250 mg (Rx) [*Biaxin*].

**Packaging and storage**
Store below 40 °C (104 °F), preferably between 15 and 30 °C (59 and 86 °F), unless otherwise specified by manufacturer. Protect from light. Preserve in tight containers.

**Auxiliary labeling**
• Continue medicine for full time of treatment.

────────────

[1]Not included in Canadian product labeling.

## Selected Bibliography

Piscitelli SC, Danziger LH, Rodvold KA. Clarithromycin and azithromycin: new macrolide antibiotics. Clin Pharm 1992; 11: 137-52.
Peters DH, Clissold SP. Clarithromycin. Drugs 1992; 44 (1): 117-64.
Barradell LB, Plosker GL, McTavish D. Clarithromycin: a review of its pharmacological properties and therapeutic use in Mycobacterium av-

ium-intracellulare complex infection in patients with acquired immune deficiency syndrome. Drugs 1993; 46 (2): 289-312.

────────────

Revised: 07/24/95

## CLAVULANATE-CONTAINING COMBINATIONS—

Amoxicillin and Clavulanate (Systemic)—See *Penicillins and Beta-lactamase Inhibitors (Systemic)*
Ticarcillin and Clavulanate (Systemic)—See *Penicillins and Beta-lactamase Inhibitors (Systemic)*

## CLEMASTINE—See *Antihistamines (Systemic)*

## CLEMASTINE-CONTAINING COMBINATIONS—

Clemastine and Phenylpropanolamine (Systemic)—See *Antihistamines and Decongestants (Systemic)*

## CLIDINIUM—See *Anticholinergics/Antispasmodics (Systemic)*

## CLIDINIUM-CONTAINING COMBINATIONS—

Chlordiazepoxide and Clidinium (Systemic)

────────────────────────────────────────

# CLINDAMYCIN    Systemic

VA CLASSIFICATION (Primary/Secondary): AM350/AP101

Note: For a listing of dosage forms and brand names by country availability, see *Dosage Forms* section(s). For a listing of brand names for the articles in this monograph, refer to the General Index.

────────────

## Category

Antibacterial (systemic); antiprotozoal.

## Indications

Note: Bracketed information in the *Indications* section refers to uses that are not included in U.S. product labeling.

**Accepted**
Bone and joint infections (treatment)—Parenteral clindamycin is indicated in the adjunctive surgical treatment of chronic bone and joint infections, and acute hematogenous osteomyelitis caused by staphylococci.

Pelvic infections, female (treatment)—Clindamycin is indicated in the treatment of female pelvic infections, including endometritis, nongonococcal tubo-ovarian abscess, pelvic cellulitis, and postsurgical vaginal cuff infections caused by anaerobes.

Intra-abdominal infections (treatment)—Clindamycin is indicated in the treatment of intra-abdominal infections (such as peritonitis and abscesses) caused by anaerobes.

Pneumonia, anaerobic (treatment)
Pneumonia, pneumococcal (treatment)
Pneumonia, staphylococcal (treatment) or
Pneumonia, streptococcal (treatment)—Clindamycin is indicated as a primary agent in the treatment of pneumonia, including serious respiratory tract infections (such as empyema, pneumonitis, and lung abscess) caused by anaerobes. Clindamycin is indicated as a secondary agent in the treatment of pneumonia caused by susceptible strains of pneumococci, staphylococci, and streptococci.

Septicemia, bacterial (treatment)—Oral and parenteral clindamycin are indicated in the treatment of septicemia caused by anaerobes. In addition, parenteral clindamycin is indicated in the treatment of septicemia caused by streptococci and staphylococci.

Skin and soft tissue infections (treatment)—Clindamycin is indicated in the treatment of serious skin and soft tissue infections caused by anaerobes, streptococci, and staphylococci.

[Actinomycosis (treatment)][1]—Clindamycin is used in the treatment of actinomycosis.

[Babesiosis (treatment)][1]—Clindamycin is used concurrently with quinine in the treatment of severe babesiosis caused by *Babesia microti*.

[Erysipelas (treatment)][1]—Clindamycin is used in the treatment of erysipelas.

[Malaria (treatment)][1]—Clindamycin is used in combination with quinine in the treatment of chloroquine-resistant malaria caused by *Plasmodium falciparum* in patients for whom standard therapy is contraindicated (e.g., children, pregnant women, sulfa allergy).

[Otitis media, chronic suppurative (treatment)][1]—Clindamycin is used in the treatment of chronic suppurative otitis media.

[Pneumonia, *Pneumocystis carinii* (treatment)][1]—Clindamycin is used in combination with primaquine in the treatment of *Pneumocystis carinii* pneumonia (PCP) in patients unresponsive or intolerant to standard therapy.

[Sinusitis (treatment)][1]—Clindamycin is used in the treatment of sinusitis.

[Toxoplasmosis, central nervous system (CNS) (treatment)][1]—Clindamycin is used in combination with pyrimethamine in the treatment of CNS toxoplasmosis in patients who are unresponsive or intolerant to standard therapy.

Not all species or strains of a particular organism may be susceptible to clindamycin.

**Unaccepted**
Clindamycin is not indicated in the treatment of meningitis since it penetrates poorly into cerebrospinal fluid (CSF), even in the presence of inflamed meninges.

────────────

[1]Not included in Canadian product labeling.

## Pharmacology/Pharmacokinetics

**Physicochemical characteristics**
Molecular weight—Clindamycin hydrochloride: 461.44.
Clindamycin palmitate hydrochloride: 699.86.
Clindamycin phosphate: 504.96.

**Mechanism of action/Effect**
Antibacterial (systemic)—The lincomycins inhibit protein synthesis in susceptible bacteria by binding to the 50 S subunits of bacterial ribosomes and preventing peptide bond formation. They are usually considered bacteriostatic, but may be bactericidal in high concentrations or when used against highly susceptible organisms.

**Absorption**
Rapidly absorbed from the gastrointestinal tract following oral administration; not inactivated by gastric acid. Approximately 90% absorbed orally in fasting state; absorption unaffected by food.

**Distribution**
Widely and rapidly distributed to most fluids and tissues, except cerebrospinal fluid (CSF); high concentrations in bone, bile, and urine. Readily crosses the placenta. Also excreted in breast milk.
Vol$_D$—
     Adults: Approximately 0.66 liter per kg.
     Children: Approximately 0.86 liter per kg.

**Protein binding**
Very high (92–94%).

**Biotransformation**
Hepatic; some metabolites may possess antibacterial activity. Clindamycin palmitate and clindamycin phosphate are inactive; they are rapidly hydrolyzed *in vivo* to active clindamycin.

**Half-life**
Normal renal function—
     Adults: 2.4 to 3.0 hours.
     Infants and children: 2.5 to 3.4 hours.
     Premature infants: 6.3 to 8.6 hours.
End-stage renal failure or severe hepatic impairment—
     Slightly increased (3 to 5 hours in adults).

**Time to peak serum concentration**
Oral—0.75 to 1 hour.
Intramuscular—1 hour (children); 3 hours (adults).
Intravenous—End of infusion.

**Peak serum concentration**
Adults (steady-state)—
     300 mg intravenously over 10 minutes every 8 hours: Approximately 7 mcg/mL.
     600 mg intravenously over 20 minutes every 8 hours: Approximately 10 mcg/mL.
     900 mg intravenously over 30 minutes every 12 hours: Approximately 11 mcg/mL.
     1200 mg intravenously over 45 minutes every 12 hours: Approximately 14 mcg/mL.
     300 mg intramuscularly every 8 hours: Approximately 6 mcg/mL.
     600 mg intramuscularly every 12 hours: Approximately 9 mcg/mL.
Children (first dose)—
     5 to 7 mg per kg of body weight (mg/kg) intravenously over 1 hour: Approximately 10 mcg/mL.
     3 to 5 mg/kg intramuscularly: Approximately 4 mcg/mL.
     5 to 7 mg/kg intramuscularly: Approximately 8 mcg/mL.

**Elimination**
Approximately 10% of a total dose is eliminated in the urine and 3.6% in the feces as active drug. The remainder is excreted as inactive metabolites.
Dialysis—Not removed from the blood by hemodialysis or peritoneal dialysis.

# Precautions to Consider

**Cross-sensitivity and/or related problems**
Patients hypersensitive to lincomycin may be hypersensitive to clindamycin also. There is also a report of a possible cross-sensitivity between clindamycin and doxorubicin.

**Pregnancy/Reproduction**
Pregnancy—Clindamycin crosses the placenta and may be concentrated in the fetal liver. However, problems in humans have not been documented.

**Breast-feeding**
Clindamycin is excreted in breast milk. However, problems in humans have not been documented.

**Pediatrics**
Clindamycin should be used with caution in infants up to 1 month of age.
Clindamycin phosphate injection contains benzyl alcohol, which has been associated with a fatal gasping syndrome in infants.

**Geriatrics**
No information is available on the relationship of age to the effects of clindamycin in geriatric patients.

**Drug interactions and/or related problems**
The following drug interactions and/or related problems have been selected on the basis of their potential clinical significance (possible

mechanism in parentheses where appropriate)—not necessarily inclusive (» = major clinical significance):
Note: Combinations containing any of the following medications, depending on the amount present, may also interact with this medication.

» Anesthetics, hydrocarbon inhalation or
» Neuromuscular blocking agents
     (concurrent use of these medications with clindamycin, if necessary, should be carefully monitored since neuromuscular blockade may be enhanced, resulting in skeletal muscle weakness and respiratory depression or paralysis [apnea]; caution is also recommended when these medications are used concurrently with clindamycin during surgery or in the postoperative period; treatment with anticholinesterase agents or calcium salts may help reverse the blockade)

» Antidiarrheals, adsorbent
     (concurrent use of kaolin- or attapulgite-containing antidiarrheals with oral clindamycin may significantly delay the absorption of oral clindamycin; concurrent use should be avoided or patients should be advised to take adsorbent antidiarrheals not less than 2 hours before or 3 to 4 hours after oral lincomycins)

Antimyasthenics
     (concurrent use of medications with neuromuscular blocking action may antagonize the effect of antimyasthenics on skeletal muscle; temporary dosage adjustments of antimyasthenics may be necessary to control symptoms of myasthenia gravis during and following concurrent use)

» Chloramphenicol or
» Erythromycins
     (may displace clindamycin from or prevent its binding to 50 S subunits of bacterial ribosomes, thus antagonizing clindamycin's effects; concurrent use is not recommended)

Opioid (narcotic) analgesics
     (respiratory depressant effects of drugs with neuromuscular blocking activity may be additive to central respiratory depressant effects of opioid analgesics, possibly leading to increased or prolonged respiratory depression or paralysis [apnea]; caution and careful monitoring of the patient are recommended)

**Laboratory value alterations**
The following have been selected on the basis of their potential clinical significance (possible effect in parentheses where appropriate)—not necessarily inclusive (» = major clinical significance):
With diagnostic test results
     Alanine aminotransferase (ALT [SGPT]), serum and
     Alkaline phosphatase, serum and
     Aspartate aminotransferase (ALT [SGOT]), serum
     (concentrations may be increased)

**Medical considerations/Contraindications**
The medical considerations/contraindications included here have been selected on the basis of their potential clinical significance (reasons given in parentheses where appropriate)—not necessarily inclusive (» = major clinical significance).

*Risk-benefit should be considered when the following medical problems exist:*
» Gastrointestinal disease, history of, especially ulcerative colitis, regional enteritis, or antibiotic-associated colitis
     (clindamycin may cause pseudomembranous colitis)
» Hepatic function impairment, severe
     (the half-life of clindamycin is prolonged in patients with severe hepatic function impairment; this may require an adjustment in dosage)
Hypersensitivity to lincomycins or doxorubicin
Renal function impairment, severe
     (patients with impaired renal function do not generally require a reduction in dose unless the impairment is severe; however, patients receiving clindamycin with very severe renal impairment and/or very severe hepatic impairment accompanied by severe metabolic abnormalities may require a reduction in dosage)

**Patient monitoring**
The following may be especially important in patient monitoring (other tests may be warranted in some patients, depending on condition; » = major clinical significance):
*For antibiotic-associated pseudomembranous colitis (AAPMC)*
     Colonoscopy and/or
     Proctosigmoidoscopy
     (proctosigmoidoscopy and/or colonoscopy may be required in selected, severely ill patients with persistent symptoms of AAPMC

to document the presence of pseudomembranes; it is no longer recommended as a routine monitoring parameter)

Stool examinations
(cytotoxin assays of stool samples for the presence of *Clostridium difficile* and its cytotoxin, neutralizable by *C. sordellii* antitoxin, may be required prior to treatment in patients with AAPMC to document the presence of *C. difficile* and/or its cytotoxin; however, *C. difficile* and its cytotoxin may persist following treatment with oral vancomycin despite clinical improvement; follow-up cytotoxin assays are generally not recommended with complete clinical improvement)

## Side/Adverse Effects

The following side/adverse effects have been selected on the basis of their potential clinical significance (possible signs and symptoms in parentheses where appropriate)—not necessarily inclusive:

**Those indicating need for medical attention**
Incidence more frequent
  *Pseudomembranous colitis* (severe abdominal or stomach cramps and pain; abdominal tenderness; diarrhea, watery and severe, which may also be bloody; fever)
Incidence less frequent
  *Hypersensitivity* (skin rash, redness, and itching); *neutropenia* (sore throat and fever); *thrombocytopenia* (unusual bleeding or bruising)

**Those indicating need for medical attention only if they continue or are bothersome**
Incidence more frequent
  *Gastrointestinal disturbances* (abdominal pain; diarrhea; nausea and vomiting)
Incidence less frequent
  *Fungal overgrowth* (itching of rectal or genital areas)

**Those indicating possible pseudomembranous colitis and the need for medical attention if they occur after medication is discontinued**
  *Severe abdominal or stomach cramps and pain; abdominal tenderness; watery and severe diarrhea, which may also be bloody; fever*

## Patient Consultation

As an aid to patient consultation, refer to *Advice for the Patient, Clindamycin (Systemic)*.

In providing consultation, consider emphasizing the following selected information (» = major clinical significance):

**Before using this medication**
» Conditions affecting use, especially:
  Hypersensitivity to clindamycin, lincomycin, or doxorubicin
  Pregnancy—Clindamycin crosses the placenta
  Breast-feeding—Clindamycin is excreted in breast milk
  Use in children—Clindamycin should be used cautiously in infants up to 1 month of age; clindamycin injection contains benzyl alcohol, which has been associated with a fatal gasping syndrome in infants
  Other medications, especially hydrocarbon inhalation anesthetics, neuromuscular blocking agents, adsorbent antidiarrheals, chloramphenicol, or erythromycins
  Other medical problems, especially a history of gastrointestinal disease, particularly ulcerative colitis, or severe hepatic function impairment

**Proper use of this medication**
» Taking clindamycin capsules with a full glass of water or with meals to avoid esophageal ulceration
  Proper administration technique for clindamycin oral solution; not using after expiration date
» Compliance with full course of therapy, especially in streptococcal infections
» Importance of not missing doses and taking at evenly spaced times
» Proper dosing
  Missed dose: Taking as soon as possible; not taking if almost time for next dose; not doubling doses
» Proper storage

**Precautions while using this medication**
  Regular visits to physician to check progress
  Checking with physician if no improvement within a few days
» For severe diarrhea, checking with physician before taking any antidiarrheals; for mild diarrhea, taking attapulgite-containing antidiarrheals at least 2 hours before or 3 to 4 hours after taking oral clindamycin; other antidiarrheals may worsen or prolong the

diarrhea; checking with physician or pharmacist if mild diarrhea continues or worsens
  Caution if surgery with general anesthesia is required

**Side/adverse effects**
  Signs of potential side effects, especially pseudomembranous colitis, hypersensitivity, neutropenia, and thrombocytopenia

## General Dosing Information

Therapy should be continued for at least 10 days in group A beta-hemolytic streptococcal infections to help prevent the occurrence of acute rheumatic fever.

For oral dosage forms only:
• The capsule dosage form should be taken with food or a full glass (240 mL) of water to avoid esophageal irritation.

**For treatment of adverse effects**
  For antibiotic-associated pseudomembranous colitis (AAPMC)—
    • Some patients may develop antibiotic-associated pseudomembranous colitis (AAPMC), caused by *Clostridium difficile* toxin, during or following administration of lincomycins. Mild cases may respond to discontinuation of the drug alone. Moderate to severe cases may require fluid, electrolyte, and protein replacement.
    • In cases not responding to the above measures or in more severe cases, oral doses of metronidazole, bacitracin, cholestyramine, or vancomycin may be used. Oral vancomycin is effective in doses of 125 to 500 mg every 6 hours for 5 to 10 days. The dose of metronidazole is 250 to 500 mg every 8 hours; cholestyramine, 4 grams four times a day; and bacitracin, 25,000 units, orally, four times a day. Recurrences may be treated with a second course of these medications.
    • Cholestyramine and colestipol resins have been shown to bind *C. difficile* toxin *in vitro*. If cholestyramine or colestipol resin is administered in conjunction with oral vancomycin, the medications should be administered several hours apart since the resins have been shown to bind oral vancomycin also.
    • In addition, antibiotic-associated pseudomembranous colitis may result in severe watery diarrhea, which may occur during therapy or up to several weeks after therapy is discontinued. If diarrhea occurs, administration of antiperistaltic antidiarrheals (e.g., opiates, diphenoxylate and atropine combination, loperamide) is not recommended since they may delay the removal of toxins from the colon, thereby prolonging and/or worsening the condition.

## Oral Dosage Forms

Note: Bracketed uses in the *Dosage Forms* section refer to categories of use and/or indications that are not included in U.S. product labeling.

### CLINDAMYCIN HYDROCHLORIDE CAPSULES USP

**Usual adult and adolescent dose**
Antibacterial—
  Oral, 150 to 300 mg (base) every six hours.
[Malaria (treatment)][1]—
  Oral, 900 mg (base) three times a day for three days.
[Pneumonia, *Pneumocystis carinii* (treatment)][1]—
  Oral, 1200 to 1800 mg (base) per day in divided doses in combination with 15 to 30 mg of primaquine daily.
[Toxoplasmosis, central nervous system (CNS) (treatment)][1]—
  Oral, 1200 to 2400 mg (base) per day in divided doses in combination with 50 to 100 mg of pyrimethamine daily.

**Usual pediatric dose**
Antibacterial—
  Infants up to 1 month of age: Dosage must be individualized by physician. Use with caution.
  Infants 1 month of age and over: Oral, 2 to 5 mg (base) per kg of body weight every six hours; or 2.7 to 6.7 mg per kg of body weight every eight hours.
  Note: In children weighing 10 kg or less, the minimum recommended dose is 37.5 mg every eight hours.
[Malaria (treatment)][1]—
  Oral, 6.7 to 13.3 mg per kg of body weight three times a day for three days.

**Strength(s) usually available**
U.S.—
  75 mg (base) (Rx) [*Cleocin* (tartrazine); GENERIC].
  150 mg (base) (Rx) [*Cleocin* (tartrazine); GENERIC].
  300 mg (base) (Rx) [*Cleocin* (tartrazine)].
Canada—
  150 mg (base) (Rx) [*Dalacin C*].

**Packaging and storage**
Store below 40 °C (104 °F), preferably between 15 and 30 °C (59 and 86 °F), unless otherwise specified by manufacturer. Store in a tight container.

**Auxiliary labeling**
- Take with food or water.
- Continue medicine for full time of treatment.

## CLINDAMYCIN PALMITATE HYDROCHLORIDE FOR ORAL SOLUTION USP

**Usual adult and adolescent dose**
See *Clindamycin Hydrochloride Capsules USP*.

**Usual pediatric dose**
See *Clindamycin Hydrochloride Capsules USP*.

**Strength(s) usually available**
U.S.—
    75 mg per 5 mL (base) (when reconstituted according to manufacturer's instructions) (Rx) [*Cleocin Pediatric* (sucrose)].
Canada—
    75 mg per 5 mL (base) (when reconstituted according to manufacturer's instructions) (Rx) [*Dalacin C Palmitate*].

**Packaging and storage**
Prior to reconstitution, store below 40 °C (104 °F), preferably between 15 and 30 °C (59 and 86 °F), unless otherwise specified by manufacturer. Store in a tight container. Do not refrigerate the reconstituted solution since it may thicken and be difficult to pour when chilled.

**Stability**
After reconstitution, solutions retain their potency for 14 days at room temperature.

**Auxiliary labeling**
- Do not refrigerate.
- Shake well.
- Continue medicine for full time of treatment.
- Beyond-use date.

**Note**
When dispensing, include a calibrated liquid-measuring device.

## Parenteral Dosage Forms

Note: Bracketed uses in the *Dosage Forms* section refer to categories of use and/or indications that are not included in U.S. product labeling.

## CLINDAMYCIN PHOSPHATE INJECTION USP

**Usual adult and adolescent dose**
Antibacterial—
    Intramuscular or intravenous, 300 to 600 mg (base) every six to eight hours; or 900 mg every eight hours.
[Babesiosis (treatment)][1]—
    Intravenous, 300 to 600 mg clindamycin (base) four times a day with concurrent oral administration of 650 mg of quinine, three or four times a day for seven to ten days.
[Pneumonia, *Pneumocystis carinii* (treatment)][1]—
    Intravenous, 2400 to 2700 mg (base) per day in divided doses in combination with 15 to 30 mg of primaquine daily.
[Toxoplasmosis, central nervous system (CNS) (treatment)][1]—
    Intravenous, 1200 to 4800 mg (base) per day in divided doses in combination with 50 to 100 mg of pyrimethamine daily.

**Usual adult prescribing limits**
Up to 2.7 grams (base) daily.

Note: Doses up to 4.8 grams daily have been used. However, some medical experts recommend a maximum dose of 2.7 grams daily.

**Usual pediatric dose**
Antibacterial—
    Infants up to 1 month of age: Intramuscular or intravenous, 3.75 to 5 mg (base) per kg of body weight every six hours; or 5 to 6.7 mg per kg of body weight every eight hours.
    Infants 1 month of age and over: Intramuscular or intravenous, 3.75 to 10 mg (base) per kg of body weight or 87.5 to 112.5 mg per square meter of body surface every six hours; or 5 to 13.3 mg per kg of body weight or 116.7 to 150 mg per square meter of body surface every eight hours.

Note: In children, regardless of body weight, the minimum recommended dose is 300 mg (base) daily for severe infections.
    Bone infection—Intramuscular or intravenous, 7.5 mg per kg of body weight every six hours.
[Babesiosis (treatment)][1]—
    Dosage has not been established; however, based on one case report in an infant, the suggested dose is: Intravenous or intramuscular, 20 mg per kg of body weight per day of clindamycin with concurrent oral administration of 25 mg per kg of body weight per day of quinine for seven to ten days.

**Strength(s) usually available**
U.S.—
    300 mg (base) in 2 mL (Rx) [*Cleocin* (benzyl alcohol 9.45 mg); GENERIC].
    600 mg (base) in 4 mL (Rx) [*Cleocin* (benzyl alcohol 9.45 mg); GENERIC].
    900 mg (base) in 6 mL (Rx) [*Cleocin* (benzyl alcohol 9.45 mg); GENERIC].
    9000 mg (base) in 60 mL (Rx) [GENERIC].
Canada—
    300 mg (base) in 2 mL (Rx) [*Dalacin C Phosphate* (benzyl alcohol)].
    600 mg (base) in 4 mL (Rx) [*Dalacin C Phosphate* (benzyl alcohol)].
    900 mg (base) in 6 mL (Rx) [*Dalacin C Phosphate* (benzyl alcohol)].

**Packaging and storage**
Store below 40 °C (104 °F), preferably between 15 and 30 °C (59 and 86 °F), unless otherwise specified by manufacturer. Protect from freezing.

**Preparation of dosage form**
To prepare initial dilution for intravenous use, each dose must be diluted as follows (it must not be administered undiluted as a bolus):

| Dose (mg) | Diluent (mL) | Duration of Administration (min) |
|---|---|---|
| 300 | 50 | 10 |
| 600 | 100 | 20 |
| 900 | 100 | 30 |

Caution: Products containing benzyl alcohol are not recommended for use in neonates. A fatal toxic syndrome consisting of metabolic acidosis, CNS depression, respiratory problems, renal failure, hypotension, and possibly seizures and intracranial hemorrhages has been associated with this use.

**Stability**
Clindamycin phosphate retains its potency for 24 hours at room temperature in intravenous infusions containing sodium chloride, dextrose, potassium, vitamin B complex, cephalothin, kanamycin, gentamicin, penicillin, or carbenicillin.

**Incompatibilities**
Clindamycin phosphate is physically incompatible with ampicillin, phenytoin sodium, barbiturates, aminophylline, calcium gluconate, and magnesium sulfate.

**Additional information**
Clindamycin phosphate may also be administered as a single rapid infusion (initial dose) followed by continuous intravenous infusion as follows:

| Clindamycin Serum Concentrations (desired maintenance—mcg/mL) | Infusion Rate and Duration (initial) | | Infusion Rate (continuous— mg/min) |
|---|---|---|---|
| | Rate (mg/min) | Duration (min) | |
| >4 | 10 | 30 | 0.75 |
| >5 | 15 | 30 | 1.00 |
| >6 | 20 | 30 | 1.25 |

[1]Not included in Canadian product labeling.

Revised: 08/12/92
Interim revision: 03/18/94; 04/19/95

# CLINDAMYCIN   Topical

VA CLASSIFICATION (Primary/Secondary): DE752/DE101

Note: For a listing of dosage forms and brand names by country availability, see *Dosage Forms* section(s). For a listing of brand names for the articles in this monograph, refer to the General Index.

## Category

Antiacne agent (topical); antibacterial (topical).

## Indications

Note: Bracketed information in the *Indications* section refers to uses that are not included in U.S. product labeling.

### Accepted

Acne vulgaris (treatment)—Topical clindamycin is indicated in the treatment of acne vulgaris. It may be effective in grades II and III acne, which are characterized by inflammatory lesions such as papules and pustules. Topical antibacterials are not generally considered to be as effective as systemic antibacterials in the treatment of acne, especially more severe inflammatory acne. However, some studies have shown that clindamycin phosphate topical solution may be as effective as low-dose tetracycline for moderate cases of inflammatory acne.

[Skin infections, bacterial, minor (treatment)][1]—Topical clindamycin is used in the topical treatment of erythrasma caused by *Corynebacterium minutissimum*, rosacea, periorificial facial dermatitis, folliculitis, stasis, chronic lymphedema, and familial pemphigus.

[Ulcer, dermal (treatment)][1]—Clindamycin phosphate topical solution is used in the treatment of dermal ulcers.

Not all species or strains of a particular organism may be susceptible to clindamycin.

### Unaccepted

Topical clindamycin is not effective in the treatment of deep cystic lesions or noninflammatory lesions.

[1]Not included in Canadian product labeling.

## Pharmacology/Pharmacokinetics

### Physicochemical characteristics
Molecular weight—504.96.

### Mechanism of action/Effect
Antiacne agent (topical)—Probably due to its antibacterial activity. Topical clindamycin is thought to reduce free fatty acid concentrations on the skin and to suppress the growth of *Propionibacterium acnes* (*Corynebacterium acnes*), an anaerobe found in sebaceous glands and follicles. *P. acnes* produces proteases, hyaluronidases, lipases, and chemotactic factors, all of which can produce inflammatory components or inflammation directly.

### Absorption
Approximately 1.7% absorbed through the skin following topical application of the solution every 12 hours for 4 days to approximately 300 cm[2] of skin surface.

### Mean comedonal extract concentration
597 mcg per gram after 4 weeks of topical application.

### Biotransformation
Clindamycin phosphate is inactive *in vitro*, but is rapidly hydrolyzed *in vivo* by tissue phosphatases to active clindamycin.

### Peak serum concentration
<1 to 6 nanograms per mL following topical application of the solution every 12 hours for 4 days.

### Urine concentration
<1 to 53 nanograms per mL following topical application of the solution every 12 hours for 4 days.

### Elimination
Renal—0.15 to 0.25% of cumulative dose excreted in urine following topical application of the solution every 12 hours.

## Precautions to Consider

### Cross-sensitivity and/or related problems
Patients sensitive to one lincomycin may be sensitive to other lincomycins also.

### Pregnancy/Reproduction
Fertility—Studies in rats and mice receiving subcutaneous and oral doses of clindamycin ranging from 100 to 600 mg per kg per day have not shown that clindamycin causes impaired fertility.

Pregnancy—Adequate and well-controlled studies in humans have not been done.

Studies in rats and mice receiving subcutaneous and oral doses of clindamycin ranging from 100 to 600 mg per kg per day have not shown that clindamycin causes adverse effects on the fetus.

FDA Pregnancy Category B.

### Breast-feeding
It is not known whether topical clindamycin is distributed into breast milk. Since systemically administered clindamycin is distributed into breast milk, topical clindamycin may be also. However, clindamycin is unlikely to be distributed into breast milk in significant amounts following topical administration, since the total daily dose is small and only approximately 1.7% of the dose is absorbed through the skin.

### Pediatrics
Appropriate studies on the relationship of age to the effects of topical clindamycin have not been performed in children up to 12 years of age. Safety and efficacy have not been established.

### Geriatrics
No information is available on the relationship of age to the effects of topical clindamycin in geriatric patients.

### Drug interactions and/or related problems
The following drug interactions and/or related problems have been selected on the basis of their potential clinical significance (possible mechanism in parentheses where appropriate)—not necessarily inclusive (» = major clinical significance):

Note: Combinations containing any of the following medications, depending on the amount present, may also interact with this medication.

Abrasive or medicated soaps or cleansers or
Acne preparations or preparations containing a peeling agent, such as:

Resorcinol
Salicylic acid
Sulfur, or
Alcohol-containing preparations, topical, such as:
After-shave lotions
Astringents
Perfumed toiletries
Shaving creams or lotions, or
Cosmetics or soaps with a strong drying effect or
Isotretinoin or
Medicated cosmetics or "cover-ups"
(concurrent use with clindamycin phosphate topical solution may cause a cumulative irritant or drying effect, especially with the application of peeling, desquamating, or abrasive agents, resulting in excessive irritation of the skin)

### Medical considerations/Contraindications
The medical considerations/contraindications included here have been selected on the basis of their potential clinical significance (reasons given in parentheses where appropriate)—not necessarily inclusive (» = major clinical significance).

*Except under special circumstances, this medication should not be used when the following medical problem exists:*

» Sensitivity to clindamycin or lincomycin

*Risk-benefit should be considered when the following medical problems exist:*

» Antibiotic-associated colitis, ulcerative colitis, or regional enteritis, history of
(topical clindamycin may precipitate problems that may occur days, weeks, or months after start of therapy; also may occur up to several weeks after discontinuation of therapy)

Atopic reactions, history of

### Patient monitoring
The following may be especially important in patient monitoring (other tests may be warranted in some patients, depending on condition; » = major clinical significance):

Endoscopy, large bowel
(if severe diarrhea not controlled by administration of vancomycin occurs and persists during therapy, large bowel endoscopy may be required as an aid in the diagnosis of pseudomembranous colitis)

## Side/Adverse Effects

The following side/adverse effects have been selected on the basis of their potential clinical significance (possible signs and symptoms in parentheses where appropriate)—not necessarily inclusive:

**Those indicating need for medical attention**
Incidence less frequent
*Contact dermatitis or hypersensitivity* (skin rash, itching, redness, swelling, or other sign of irritation not present before therapy)
Incidence rare
*Pseudomembranous colitis* (abdominal or stomach cramps, pain, and bloating, severe; diarrhea, watery and severe, which may also be bloody; fever; increased thirst; nausea or vomiting; unusual tiredness or weakness; weight loss, unusual)

**Those indicating need for medical attention only if they continue or are bothersome**
Incidence more frequent
*Dryness, scaliness, or peeling of skin*—for the topical solution
Incidence less frequent
*Gastrointestinal disturbances* (abdominal pain; mild diarrhea); *irritation, sensitization or oiliness of skin; stinging or burning feeling of skin*—for the topical solution

**Those indicating possible pseudomembranous colitis and the need for medical attention if they occur after medication is discontinued**
*Abdominal or stomach cramps, pain, and bloating, severe; diarrhea, watery and severe, which may also be bloody; fever; increased thirst; nausea or vomiting; unusual tiredness or weakness; weight loss, unusual*

## Patient Consultation

As an aid to patient consultation, refer to *Advice for the Patient, Clindamycin (Topical)*.

In providing consultation, consider emphasizing the following selected information (» = major clinical significance):

**Before using this medication**
» Conditions affecting use, especially:
Sensitivity to clindamycin or lincomycin
Breast-feeding—May be distributed into breast milk in small quantities since systemic clindamycin is distributed into breast milk
Other medical problems, especially a history of antibiotic-associated colitis, ulcerative colitis, or regional enteritis

**Proper use of this medication**
Before applying, washing affected areas with warm water and soap, rinsing, and patting dry
» Importance of applying medication to entire affected area
Avoiding too frequent washing of affected areas
» Compliance with full course of therapy, which may take months or longer
» Proper dosing
Missed dose: Applying as soon as possible; not applying if almost time for next dose
» Proper storage
*For topical solution only*
Waiting 30 minutes after washing or shaving before applying
» Not using near heat, near open flame, or while smoking
Proper administration technique for applicator-tip bottle:
» Avoiding contact with eyes, nose, mouth, or other mucous membranes
Not using more often than prescribed
*For topical suspension only*
» Shaking well before using

**Precautions while using this medication**
Checking with physician or pharmacist if no improvement within about 6 weeks
Applying other medications at different times
Checking with physician if treated skin becomes excessively dry (for topical solution only)
» For severe diarrhea, checking with physician before taking any antidiarrheals; for mild diarrhea, taking attapulgite-containing, but not other, antidiarrheals; checking with physician or pharmacist if mild diarrhea continues or worsens
Using only "water-base" cosmetics; not applying too heavily or too often

**Side/adverse effects**
Signs of potential side effects, especially hypersensitivity reactions and pseudomembranous colitis

## General Dosing Information

Use of topical antibacterials may lead to skin sensitization, resulting in hypersensitivity reactions with subsequent topical or systemic use of the medication.

In the treatment of acne with topical clindamycin, noticeable improvement is usually seen after about 6 weeks in most patients. However, 8 to 12 weeks of treatment may be required before maximum benefit is seen.

**For treatment of adverse effects**
Some patients may develop antibiotic-associated pseudomembranous colitis (AAPMC), caused by *Clostridium difficile* toxin, during or following administration of topical clindamycin. Mild cases may respond to discontinuation of the drug alone. Moderate to severe cases may require fluid, electrolyte, and protein replacement.

In cases not responding to the above measures or in more severe cases, oral vancomycin, oral bacitracin, or oral metronidazole may be used. Oral vancomycin is effective in doses of 125 to 500 mg every 6 hours for 7 to 10 days. Recurrences may be treated with a second course of these medications.

Cholestyramine and colestipol resins have been shown to bind *C. difficile* toxin *in vitro*. If cholestyramine or colestipol resin is administered in conjunction with oral vancomycin, the medications should be administered several hours apart since the resins have been shown to bind oral vancomycin also.

In addition, AAPMC may result in severe watery diarrhea, which may occur during antibiotic therapy or up to several weeks after therapy is discontinued. If diarrhea occurs, administration of antiperistaltic antidiarrheals (e.g., opiates, diphenoxylate and atropine combination, loperamide) is *not* recommended since they may delay the removal of toxins from the colon, thereby prolonging and/or worsening the condition.

## Topical Dosage Forms

### CLINDAMYCIN PHOSPHATE GEL USP

**Usual adult and adolescent dose**
Antiacne agent (topical)—
Topical, to the skin, a thin film applied two times a day to the affected areas.

**Usual pediatric dose**
Children up to 12 years of age—Safety and efficacy have not been established.

**Strength(s) usually available**
U.S.—
1% (base) (Rx) [*Cleocin T Gel* (methylparaben; propylene glycol; sodium hydroxide)].
Canada—
Not commercially available.

**Packaging and storage**
Store below 40 °C (104 °F), preferably between 15 and 30 °C (59 and 86 °F), unless otherwise specified by manufacturer. Store in a tight container. Protect from freezing.

**Auxiliary labeling**
• For external use only.
• Continue medicine for full time of treatment.

**Additional information**
Clindamycin phosphate gel is an aqueous, nonalcoholic, nondrying formulation.

### CLINDAMYCIN PHOSPHATE TOPICAL SOLUTION USP

**Usual adult and adolescent dose**
Antiacne agent (topical)—
Topical, to the skin, two times a day to the affected areas.

Note: Solutions have been used one to four times a day.

**Usual pediatric dose**
See *Clindamycin Phosphate Gel USP*.

**Strength(s) usually available**
U.S.—
1% (base) (Rx) [*Cleocin T Topical Solution; Clinda-Derm* (isopropyl alcohol 50%; propylene glycol); GENERIC].
Canada—
1% (base) (Rx) [*Dalacin T Topical Solution* (isopropyl alcohol 50%; propylene glycol)].

**Packaging and storage**
Store below 40 °C (104 °F), preferably between 15 and 30 °C (59 and 86 °F), unless otherwise specified by manufacturer. Store in a tight container. Protect from freezing.

**Auxiliary labeling**
• For external use only.
• Continue medicine for full time of treatment.
• Keep container tightly closed.
• Flammable—Keep away from heat and flame.

## CLINDAMYCIN PHOSPHATE TOPICAL SUSPENSION USP

**Usual adult and adolescent dose**
Antiacne agent (topical)—
  See *Clindamycin Phosphate Topical Solution USP.*

**Usual pediatric dose**
See *Clindamycin Phosphate Topical Solution USP.*

**Strength(s) usually available**
U.S.—
  1% (base) (Rx) [*Cleocin T Lotion* (cetostearyl alcohol 2.5%; isostearyl alcohol 2.5%)].
Canada—
  Not commercially available.

**Packaging and storage**
Store below 40 °C (104 °F), preferably between 15 and 30 °C (59 and 86 °F), unless otherwise specified by manufacturer. Store in a tight container. Protect from freezing.

**Auxiliary labeling**
• Shake well.
• For external use only.
• Continue medicine for full time of treatment.

Revised: 02/22/94

---

# CLINDAMYCIN   Vaginal†

VA CLASSIFICATION (Primary): GU300

Note: For a listing of dosage forms and brand names by country availability, see *Dosage Forms* section(s). For a listing of brand names for the articles in this monograph, refer to the General Index.

  †Not commercially available in Canada.

## Category
Anti-infective (vaginal).

## Indications

**Accepted**
Vaginosis, bacterial (treatment)—Vaginal clindamycin is indicated in the local treatment of bacterial vaginosis (previously known as *Haemophilus* vaginitis, *Gardnerella* vaginitis, nonspecific vaginitis, *Corynebacterium* vaginitis, or anaerobic vaginosis).

  Because of the limited clinical data regarding vaginal clindamycin's efficacy in treating bacterial vaginosis, the Centers for Disease Control (CDC) recommend vaginal clindamycin only as alternative therapy to oral metronidazole.

Not all species or strains of a particular organism may be susceptible to clindamycin.

**Unaccepted**
Vaginal clindamycin is not effective in the treatment of vulvovaginitis caused by *Trichomonas vaginalis, Chlamydia trachomatis, Neisseria gonorrhoeae, Candida albicans,* or *Herpes simplex* virus.

## Pharmacology/Pharmacokinetics

**Physicochemical characteristics**
Molecular weight—Clindamycin phosphate: 504.96.

**Mechanism of action/Effect**
Clindamycin phosphate is hydrolyzed *in vivo* to clindamycin, which inhibits protein synthesis in susceptible bacteria by binding to the 50 S subunits of bacterial ribosomes and prevents peptide bond formation.

**Absorption**
Approximately 2 to 8% of the administered dose (100 mg) is absorbed systemically; little or no systemic accumulation has been produced with multiple dosing.

**Biotransformation**
Inactive clindamycin phosphate undergoes rapid hydrolysis *in vivo* to active clindamycin.

**Half-life**
Systemic—1.5 to 2.6 hours.

**Time to peak concentration**
Approximately 16 hours (range, 8 to 24 hours).

**Peak serum concentration**
Steady state—Approximately 16 mcg/L (0.032 micromoles/L).

## Precautions to Consider

**Cross-sensitivity and/or related problems**
Patients hypersensitive to lincomycin may be hypersensitive to clindamycin also.

**Carcinogenicity/Tumorigenicity**
Long-term studies in animals have not been done.

**Mutagenicity**
No evidence of mutagenicity was found in tests, including the Ames test and a rat micronucleus test.

**Pregnancy/Reproduction**
Fertility—No evidence of adverse effects on fertility was found in rats when they were treated with oral doses of 300 mg per kg of body weight (mg/kg) a day (31 times the human exposure based on mg per meter squared).

Pregnancy—Systemic clindamycin crosses the placenta. Adequate and well-controlled studies using vaginal clindamycin in humans have not been done. The Centers for Disease Control (CDC) recommend the use of vaginal clindamycin for bacterial vaginosis during the first trimester of pregnancy when treatment with vaginal metronidazole is not recommended (either medication may be used in the second and third trimesters). Vaginal administration is preferred over oral administration throughout all trimesters of pregnancy; however, studies have not determined whether treatment for bacterial vaginosis reduces the risk of adverse pregnancy outcomes, such as premature rupture of the membranes, preterm labor, or preterm delivery.

Reproduction studies in animals in which high systemic doses of clindamycin were used showed no evidence of fetal malformations, except one small study in which the fetuses of treated mice developed cleft palates. This result has not been duplicated in other animals or other mouse strains.

FDA Pregnancy Category B.

**Breast-feeding**
Systemic clindamycin is distributed into breast milk. Problems in humans have not been documented. It is not known if vaginally administered clindamycin phosphate is distributed into breast milk.

**Pediatrics**
No information is available on the relationship of age to the effects of vaginal clindamycin in pediatric patients. Safety and efficacy have not been established.

**Geriatrics**
No information is available on the relationship of age to the effects of clindamycin in geriatric patients.

**Medical considerations/Contraindications**
The medical considerations/contraindications included here have been selected on the basis of their potential clinical significance (reasons given in parentheses where appropriate)—not necessarily inclusive (» = major clinical significance).

*Risk-benefit should be considered when the following medical problems exist:*
» Gastrointestinal disease, history of, especially ulcerative colitis, regional enteritis, or antibiotic-associated colitis
(systemically and topically administered clindamycin may cause diarrhea and [although rarely with topical administration] colitis—including pseudomembranous colitis; although only up to 8% of the vaginal dose may be systemically absorbed, vaginal use may potentially worsen these conditions)
» Hypersensitivity to lincomycin or clindamycin

## Side/Adverse Effects

Note: The side effects listed below are those reported in studies with vaginal clindamycin administration. Systemic side effects may occur since up to 8% of the vaginal dose is absorbed systemically. Pseudomembranous colitis has occurred rarely with topical use of clindamycin but has not been reported with vaginal administration.

The following side/adverse effects have been selected on the basis of their potential clinical significance (possible signs and symptoms in parentheses where appropriate)—not necessarily inclusive:

**Those indicating need for medical attention**
Incidence more frequent
*Vaginitis or vulvovaginal pruritus, primarily due to Candida albicans* (itching of the vagina or genital area; pain during sexual intercourse; thick, white vaginal discharge with no odor or with a mild odor)
Incidence less frequent
*CNS effects* (dizziness; headache); *gastrointestinal disturbances* (diarrhea; nausea or vomiting; stomach pain or cramps)
Incidence rare
*Hypersensitivity* (burning, itching, redness, skin rash, swelling, or other signs of skin irritation not present before therapy)

**Those indicating possible need for medical attention if they occur after medication is discontinued**
*Vaginitis or vulvovaginal pruritus, primarily due to Candida albicans* (itching of the vagina or genital area; pain during sexual intercourse; thick, white vaginal discharge with no odor or with a mild odor)

## Patient Consultation

As an aid to patient consultation, refer to *Advice for the Patient, Clindamycin (Vaginal).*

In providing consultation, consider emphasizing the following selected information (» = major clinical significance):

**Before using this medication**
» Conditions affecting use, especially:
Hypersensitivity to clindamycin or lincomycin
Pregnancy—Systemic clindamycin crosses the placenta; up to 8% of vaginal clindamycin is systemically absorbed
Breast-feeding—Systemically administered clindamycin is distributed into breast milk. It is not known if vaginal clindamycin also distributes into breast milk
Other medical problems, especially history of gastrointestinal disease (particularly ulcerative colitis, regional enteritis, or antibiotic-associated colitis)

**Proper use of this medication**
Washing hands immediately before and after vaginal administration
Avoiding getting medication into the eyes; washing eyes out immediately with large amounts of cool tap water if medication does get into eyes; checking with physician if eyes continue to be painful
Reading patient directions carefully before use
*Proper administration technique*
Following directions regarding the filling of the applicator, insertion technique, and discarding the applicator after each use
» Compliance with full course of therapy, even during menstruation
» Not missing doses; using at evenly spaced times
» Proper dosing

Missed dose: Inserting as soon as possible; not inserting if almost time for next dose
» Proper storage

**Precautions while using this medication**
Checking with physician if no improvement within a few days
Follow-up visit to physician after treatment for bacterial vaginosis to ensure that infection has been properly treated
Caution if dizziness occurs
Protecting clothing because of possible soiling with vaginal clindamycin; avoiding use of tampons
» Using hygienic measures to help cure infection and prevent reinfection, e.g., wearing freshly washed cotton panties instead of synthetic panties
» Sexual abstinence is recommended during treatment to prevent a dilution of the dose, which may result in reduced efficacy of the medication and a relapse of the infection
» Not using latex contraceptives for up to 72 hours after vaginal clindamycin treatment as oils in the clindamycin weaken latex products and may affect efficacy

**Side/adverse effects**
Signs of potential side effects, especially vaginitis or cervicitis, and hypersensitivity

## General Dosing Information

Use of vaginal latex or rubber products, such as condoms, cervical caps, or diaphragms, is not recommended for up to 72 hours after completion of vaginal clindamycin treatment. Vaginal clindamycin cream contains mineral oil that can weaken or damage these products and reduce their efficacy.

Concurrent treatment of the male partner is generally unnecessary when treating bacterial vaginosis.

Vaginal applicators should be used with caution after the sixth month of pregnancy.

## Vaginal Dosage Form
### CLINDAMYCIN PHOSPHATE VAGINAL CREAM

**Usual adult and adolescent dose**
Anti-infective (vaginal)—
Intravaginal, 100 mg (one applicatorful) into vagina once a day, preferably at bedtime, for seven consecutive days.

**Usual pediatric dose**
Safety and efficacy have not been established.

**Strength(s) usually available**
U.S.—
2% (Rx) [*Cleocin*].
Canada—
Not commercially available.

**Packaging and storage**
Store below 40 °C (104 °F), preferably between 15 and 30 °C (59 and 86 °F), unless otherwise specified by manufacturer.

**Auxiliary labeling**
• May cause dizziness.
• Continue medicine for full time of treatment.
• For vaginal use only.

**Note**
Include patient package insert (PPI) when dispensing.

## Selected Bibliography

Fischbach F, Petersen EE, Weissenbacher ER, et al. Efficacy of clindamycin vaginal cream versus oral metronidazole in the treatment of bacterial vaginosis. Obstet Gynecol 1993 Sep; 82 (3): 405-10.
Livengood CH, Thomason JL, Hill GB. Bacterial vaginosis: diagnostic and pathogenetic findings during topical clindamycin therapy. Am J Obstet Gynecol 1990 Aug; 163 (2): 515-20.

Developed: 06/29/94

# CLIOQUINOL   Topical

VA CLASSIFICATION (Primary/Secondary): DE101/DE102

Another commonly used name is iodochlorhydroxyquin

Note: For a listing of dosage forms and brand names by country availability, see *Dosage Forms* section(s). For a listing of brand names for the articles in this monograph, refer to the General Index.

## Category

Antibacterial (topical); antifungal (topical).

## Indications

Note: Bracketed information in the *Indications* section refers to uses that are not included in U.S. product labeling.

### Accepted

Skin disorders, inflammatory (treatment)—Clioquinol is indicated in the topical treatment of inflammatory skin disorders.

Tinea pedis (treatment); or

Skin [and nail] infections, fungal, minor, other (treatment)—Clioquinol is indicated in the topical treatment of tinea pedis (ringworm of the foot; athlete's foot) and in the topical treatment of other minor fungal skin infections. Clioquinol is also used in the topical treatment of minor fungal nail infections.

[Skin infections, bacterial, minor (prophylaxis and treatment)];

[Tinea barbae (treatment)];

[Tinea capitis (treatment)]; or

[Ulcer, dermal (treatment)]—Clioquinol is used in the topical prophylaxis and treatment of minor bacterial skin infections and in the topical treatment of tinea barbae, tinea capitis, and dermal ulcer.

## Pharmacology/Pharmacokinetics

### Physicochemical characteristics

Molecular weight—305.50.

### Mechanism of action/Effect

Broad-spectrum antibacterial. Precise mechanism of action is unknown.

### Other actions/effects

Also possesses mild irritant properties.

### Absorption

Topical absorption is rapid and extensive, especially when the skin is covered with an occlusive dressing. Absorbed through the skin in sufficient amounts to affect thyroid function tests.

## Precautions to Consider

### Cross-sensitivity and/or related problems

Patients sensitive to chloroxine, iodine, or iodine-containing preparations may be sensitive to this medication also.

### Pregnancy/Reproduction

Pregnancy—Problems in humans have not been documented.

### Breast-feeding

It is not known whether clioquinol is distributed into breast milk. However, problems in humans have not been documented.

### Pediatrics

Use is not recommended in infants and children up to 2 years of age.

Clioquinol may produce false-positive ferric chloride test results for phenylketonuria (PKU) if clioquinol is present in the neonate's diaper or urine.

### Geriatrics

Appropriate studies on the relationship of age to the effects of this medicine have not been performed in the geriatric population. However, no geriatrics-specific problems have been documented to date.

### Laboratory value alterations

The following have been selected on the basis of their potential clinical significance (possible effect in parentheses where appropriate)—not necessarily inclusive (» = major clinical significance):

With diagnostic test results

Ferric chloride tests for phenylketonuria (PKU)
(may produce false-positive test results if clioquinol is present in neonate's diaper or urine)

» Thyroid function determinations
(may cause significant elevation of serum protein-bound iodine [PBI] or butanol-extractable iodine [BEI] and a decrease in radioactive iodine [RAI] uptake; at least 3 months should elapse between discontinuation of clioquinol and administration of these tests. Other thyroid function tests such as $T_3$ resin sponge tests or $T_4$ determinations are not affected)

### Medical considerations/Contraindications

The medical considerations/contraindications included here have been selected on the basis of their potential clinical significance (reasons given in parentheses where appropriate)—not necessarily inclusive (» = major clinical significance).

*Risk-benefit should be considered when the following medical problem exists:*

Sensitivity to clioquinol, chloroxine, iodine, or iodine-containing preparations

## Side/Adverse Effects

The following side/adverse effects have been selected on the basis of their potential clinical significance (possible signs and symptoms in parentheses where appropriate)—not necessarily inclusive:

### Those indicating need for medical attention

Incidence rare

*Skin sensitization* (itching, skin rash, redness, swelling, or other signs of irritation not present before therapy)

## Patient Consultation

As an aid to patient consultation, refer to *Advice for the Patient, Clioquinol (Topical)*.

In providing consultation, consider emphasizing the following selected information (» = major clinical significance):

### Before using this medication

» Conditions affecting use, especially:
Use in children—Not recommended in infants and children up to 2 years of age

### Proper use of this medication

Before applying, washing affected area with soap and water, and drying thoroughly

» Not for ophthalmic use or use in infants and children under 2 years of age

Proper administration technique for cream and ointment

» Compliance with full course of therapy

» Proper dosing
Missed dose: Applying as soon as possible; not applying if almost time for next dose

» Proper storage

### Precautions while using this medication

Checking with physician if no improvement within 1 to 2 weeks

May stain fabrics, skin, hair, and nails yellow

### Side/adverse effects

Signs of potential side effects, especially skin irritation

## General Dosing Information

Use of topical antibacterials may lead to skin sensitization, resulting in hypersensitivity reactions with subsequent topical or systemic use of the medication.

## Topical Dosage Forms

### CLIOQUINOL CREAM USP

#### Usual adult and adolescent dose

Antibacterial—
Topical, to the skin, two or three times a day.

Antifungal—
Topical, to the skin, two or three times a day.

#### Usual pediatric dose

Infants and children up to 2 years of age—Use is not recommended.

Children 2 years of age and over—See *Usual adult and adolescent dose*.

#### Strength(s) usually available

U.S.—
3% (OTC) [*Vioform*].

Canada—
3% (OTC) [*Vioform*].

### Packaging and storage
Store below 40 °C (104 °F), preferably between 15 and 30 °C (59 and 86 °F), unless otherwise specified by manufacturer. Store in a collapsible tube or tight, light-resistant container. Protect from freezing.

### Incompatibilities
Clioquinol is incompatible with oxidizing agents.

### Auxiliary labeling
- For external use only.
- Continue medication for full time of treatment.
- Do not use in or around the eyes.

## CLIOQUINOL OINTMENT USP

### Usual adult and adolescent dose
See *Clioquinol Cream USP*.

### Usual pediatric dose
See *Clioquinol Cream USP*.

### Strength(s) usually available
U.S.—
   3% (OTC) [*Vioform*].

---

Canada—
   3% (OTC) [*Vioform*].

### Packaging and storage
Store below 40 °C (104 °F), preferably between 15 and 30 °C (59 and 86 °F), unless otherwise specified by manufacturer. Store in a collapsible tube or tight, light-resistant container. Protect from freezing.

### Incompatibilities
Clioquinol is incompatible with oxidizing agents.

### Auxiliary labeling
- For external use only.
- Continue medication for full time of treatment.
- Do not use in or around the eyes.

Revised: 02/10/92
Interim revision: 06/03/94

---

## CLIOQUINOL-CONTAINING COMBINATIONS—
Clioquinol and Hydrocortisone (Topical)

---

# CLIOQUINOL AND HYDROCORTISONE    Topical

**VA CLASSIFICATION (Primary): DE250**

**NOTE:** The *Clioquinol and Hydrocortisone (Topical)* monograph is maintained on the USP DI electronic data base. For a printed copy of the most recent revision of the complete monograph, contact the USP Division of Information Development, 12601 Twinbrook Parkway, Rockville, MD 20852.

For information on the specific components of this combination, see the *USP DI* monographs for *Clioquinol (Topical)* and *Corticosteroids (Topical)*.

The information that follows is selectively abstracted from the complete monograph and is provided to facilitate drug use review and patient counseling.

Note: For a listing of dosage forms and brand names by country availability, see *Dosage Forms* section(s). For a listing of brand names for the articles in this monograph, refer to the General Index.

## Category
Antibacterial-antifungal-corticosteroid (topical)

Note: Therapeutic efficacy of the corticosteroid depends on drug release from the vehicle, solubilization of the drug at the skin surface, and its subsequent percutaneous absorption through the outer barrier layer of the epidermis (stratum corneum) so that it can reach the site of action in the living epidermis and/or the dermis.

Factors influencing product selection include skin hydration, site, severity, age, and whether the lesion is moist or dry, as well as potency and strength of the product, and the method of application.

## Indications
### Accepted
Dermatitis, atopic (treatment);
Dermatitis, contact (treatment);
Eczema (treatment);
Folliculitis (treatment);
Intertrigo (treatment);
Pruritus, anogenital (treatment); or
Skin infections, bacterial, minor (treatment)—Clioquinol and hydrocortisone combination is indicated in the topical treatment of atopic dermatitis, contact dermatitis, eczema, folliculitis, intertrigo, anogenital pruritus, and minor bacterial skin infections.

FDA has classified clioquinol and hydrocortisone combination as being possibly effective for its labeled indications. The less-than-effective classifications require the submission of adequate and well-controlled studies to provide substantial evidence of effectiveness.

## Patient Consultation
As an aid to patient consultation, refer to *Advice for the Patient, Clioquinol and Hydrocortisone (Topical).*

In providing consultation, consider emphasizing the following selected information (» = major clinical significance):

### Before using this medication
» Conditions affecting use, especially:
   Use in children—Use is not recommended in infants and children up to 2 years of age
   Other medical conditions, especially herpes simplex, vaccinia, eczema vaccinatum, varicella, or other viral infections of the skin

### Proper use of this medication
Before applying, washing affected area with soap and water, and drying thoroughly
» Not for ophthalmic use or use on infants and children under 2 years of age
   Proper administration technique for cream, lotion, and ointment
» Not bandaging or otherwise wrapping treated area unless directed by physician
» Checking with physician before using medication on other skin problems
» Compliance with full course of therapy
» Not using more often or longer or on thin skin areas unless directed by physician
» Proper dosing
   Missed dose: Applying as soon as possible; not applying if almost time for next dose
» Proper storage

### Precautions while using this medication
Checking with physician if no improvement within 1 to 2 weeks
» Taking special precautions when medication is used in children
   May stain fabrics, skin, hair, and nails yellow

### Side/adverse effects
Signs of potential side effects, especially skin sensitization, and thinning of skin with easy bruising

## Topical Dosage Forms

### CLIOQUINOL AND HYDROCORTISONE CREAM

### Usual adult and adolescent dose
Antibacterial—
   Topical, to the skin, three or four times a day.
Antifungal—
   Topical, to the skin, three or four times a day.

### Usual pediatric dose
Infants and children up to 2 years of age—Use is not recommended.
   Children 2 years of age and over—See *Usual adult and adolescent dose*.

### Strength(s) usually available
U.S.—
   3% of clioquinol and 0.5% of hydrocortisone (Rx) [*Vioform-Hydrocortisone Mild Cream*].
   3% of clioquinol and 1% of hydrocortisone (Rx) [*Vioform-Hydrocortisone Cream*].

Canada—
  3% of clioquinol and 0.5% of hydrocortisone (Rx) [*Vioform-Hydrocortisone Mild Cream*].
  3% of clioquinol and 1% of hydrocortisone (Rx) [*Vioform-Hydrocortisone Cream*].

**Auxiliary labeling**
• For external use only.
• Do not use in or around the eyes.
• Continue medication for full time of treatment.

## CLIOQUINOL AND HYDROCORTISONE LOTION

**Usual adult and adolescent dose**
See *Clioquinol and Hydrocortisone Cream.*

**Usual pediatric dose**
See *Clioquinol and Hydrocortisone Cream.*

**Strength(s) usually available**
U.S.—
  3% of clioquinol and 1% of hydrocortisone (Rx) [*Vioform-Hydrocortisone Lotion* (methylparaben; propylparaben)].
Canada—
  Not commercially available.

**Auxiliary labeling**
• Shake well.
• For external use only.
• Do not use in or around the eyes.
• Continue medication for full time of treatment.

## CLIOQUINOL AND HYDROCORTISONE OINTMENT

**Usual adult and adolescent dose**
See *Clioquinol and Hydrocortisone Cream.*

**Usual pediatric dose**
See *Clioquinol and Hydrocortisone Cream.*

**Strength(s) usually available**
U.S.—
  3% of clioquinol and 0.5% of hydrocortisone (Rx) [*Vioform-Hydrocortisone Mild Ointment*].
  3% of clioquinol and 1% of hydrocortisone (Rx) [*Vioform-Hydrocortisone Ointment*].
Canada—
  3% of clioquinol and 1% of hydrocortisone (Rx) [*Vioform-Hydrocortisone Ointment*].

**Auxiliary labeling**
• For external use only.
• Do not use in or around the eyes.
• Continue medication for full time of treatment.

Revised: 02/10/92
Interim revision: 4/13/92; 07/14/94

---

**CLOBETASOL**—See *Corticosteroids (Topical)*

---

**CLOBETASONE**—See *Corticosteroids (Topical)*

---

**CLOCORTOLONE**—See *Corticosteroids (Topical)*

---

# CLOFAZIMINE   Systemic†

VA CLASSIFICATION (Primary): AM900
Note: For a listing of dosage forms and brand names by country availability, see *Dosage Forms* section(s). For a listing of brand names for the articles in this monograph, refer to the General Index.

†Not commercially available in Canada.

## Category
Antibacterial (antimycobacterial).

## Indications
Note: Bracketed information in the *Indications* section refers to uses that are not included in U.S. product labeling.

**Accepted**
Leprosy (treatment)—Clofazimine is indicated as a secondary agent in the treatment of lepromatous leprosy (Hansen's disease), including dapsone-resistant lepromatous leprosy, caused by *Mycobacterium leprae* (Hansen's bacillus). In the initial treatment of multibacillary leprosy, clofazimine is recommended in combination with one or more other antileprosy agents to prevent the development of resistance.

Clofazimine is also indicated in the treatment of lepromatous leprosy complicated by erythema nodosum leprosum reactions. Corticosteroids may be given concurrently if nerve injury or skin ulceration shows signs of developing.

[Mycobacterial infections, atypical (treatment)]—Clofazimine is used in combination with up to 5 other antimycobacterial agents in the treatment of atypical mycobacterial infections caused by *Mycobacterium avium-intracellulare* (*Mycobacterium avium* complex; MAC) in patients with acquired immunodeficiency syndrome (AIDS). Despite clofazimine's high degree of *in vitro* activity, combination therapy has often been clinically ineffective.

**Unaccepted**
Clofazimine is not effective in the treatment of other leprosy-associated inflammatory reactions.

## Pharmacology/Pharmacokinetics

**Physicochemical characteristics**
Molecular weight—473.40.
Highly lipophilic; virtually insoluble in water.

**Mechanism of action/Effect**
Exact mechanism unknown; has a slowly bactericidal effect on *Mycobacterium leprae*; inhibits mycobacterial growth and binds preferentially to mycobacterial DNA.

**Other actions/effects**
Exerts anti-inflammatory effects in the control of erythema nodosum leprosum reactions.

**Absorption**
Variable (45 to 62%) following oral administration in leprosy patients; however, the bioavailability of the commercially available capsule is approximately 70%. Bioavailability and rate of absorption are increased when clofazimine is taken with food.

**Distribution**
Highly lipophilic; deposited primarily in fatty tissue and cells of the reticuloendothelial system; taken up by macrophages throughout the body; also distributed to breast milk, mesenteric lymph nodes, adrenal glands, subcutaneous fat, liver, bile, gallbladder, spleen, small intestine, muscles, bones, and skin. Does not appear to cross the blood-brain barrier.

**Biotransformation**
Three metabolites have been identified; two are conjugated and one is unconjugated. It is not known whether these metabolites have any pharmacologic activity.

**Half-life**
Approximately 10 days after a single dose.
Half-life of 2 to 3 months after long-term, high-dose therapy.

**Time to peak concentration**
1 to 6 hours, with chronic therapy.

**Mean serum concentration**
After 4 years of therapy—
  100 mg daily: 0.7 mcg per mL.
  300 mg daily: 1.0 mcg per mL.
  400 mg daily: 1.4 mcg per mL.

**Elimination**
Renal—Following daily administration of 300 mg in leprosy patients, approximately 0.6% of the 3 metabolites and 1% of unchanged clofazimine are excreted in the urine.
Fecal/biliary—Up to 50% of clofazimine is recovered unchanged from the feces.
Sputum, sebum, and sweat—Small amounts excreted.

# Precautions to Consider

### Carcinogenicity
Long-term carcinogenicity studies have not been done in animals.

### Mutagenicity
Mutagenicity studies (i.e., Ames tests) have not shown that clofazimine is mutagenic.

### Pregnancy/Reproduction
Fertility—One study in rats given doses of 25 times the usual human dose has shown that clofazimine causes a reduction in the number of offspring and a reduction in the proportion of implantations.

Pregnancy—Clofazimine crosses the human placenta. Adequate and well-controlled studies in humans have not been done. Although the skin of infants born to mothers who received clofazimine during pregnancy was deeply pigmented at birth, clofazimine has not been shown to be teratogenic in humans. A gradual fading of pigmentation over a 1-year period has been observed in neonates who were not breast fed.

Studies in rabbits given 8 times the usual human dose and studies in rats given 25 times the usual human dose have not shown that clofazimine is teratogenic. However, studies in mice given 12 to 25 times the human dose have shown that clofazimine causes retarded fetal skull ossification, increased incidence of abortions and stillbirths, and impaired neonatal survival.

FDA Pregnancy Category C.

### Breast-feeding
Clofazimine is excreted in breast milk. Use is not recommended in nursing mothers. The skin and fatty tissues of animal offspring become discolored approximately 3 days after birth. This has been attributed to the presence of clofazimine in the maternal milk. A gradual fading of pigmentation followed discontinuation of breast-feeding.

### Pediatrics
Appropriate studies on the relationship of age to the effects of clofazimine have not been performed in the pediatric population. However, there have been a few reports in the literature of children who have been treated with clofazimine.

### Geriatrics
No information is available on the relationship of age to the effects of clofazimine in geriatric patients.

### Dental
Clofazimine may cause discoloration of the sputum and changes in taste.

### Laboratory value alterations
The following have been selected on the basis of their potential clinical significance (possible effect in parentheses where appropriate)—not necessarily inclusive (» = major clinical significance):

With diagnostic test results
Erythrocyte sedimentation rate (ESR)
(may be increased)

With physiology/laboratory test values
Albumin, serum and
Aspartate aminotransferase (AST [SGOT]), serum and
Bilirubin, serum and
Blood glucose, serum
(concentrations may be increased)

Potassium, serum
(concentrations may be decreased)

### Medical considerations/Contraindications
The medical considerations/contraindications included here have been selected on the basis of their potential clinical significance (reasons given in parentheses where appropriate)—not necessarily inclusive (» = major clinical significance).

*Risk-benefit should be considered when the following medical problems exist:*

» Gastrointestinal problems, history of
(clofazimine may cause splenic infarction, bowel obstruction, gastrointestinal bleeding, colicky or burning pain in the abdomen, enteritis, and death following severe gastrointestinal symptoms)

Hepatic function impairment
(clofazimine may on rare occasion cause hepatitis and jaundice)

Sensitivity to clofazimine

# Side/Adverse Effects

Note: Clofazimine has rarely caused splenic infarction, bowel obstruction, gastrointestinal bleeding, eosinophilic enteritis, and death following severe abdominal symptoms. Crystalline deposits of clofazimine

have been recovered on autopsy in various tissues, including the intestinal mucosa, liver, spleen, and mesenteric lymph nodes.

Reversible pink or red to brownish-black discoloration of the skin may occur in 75 to 100% of patients within a few weeks of treatment. It may require several months or years to completely disappear after discontinuation of clofazimine. Also, 2 suicides have been reported as a result of mental depression secondary to skin discoloration.

The following side/adverse effects have been selected on the basis of their potential clinical significance (possible signs and symptoms in parentheses where appropriate)—not necessarily inclusive:

### Those indicating need for medical attention
Incidence rare
*Gastrointestinal bleeding* (bloody or black, tarry stools); *gastrointestinal toxicity* (colicky or burning abdominal or stomach pain); *hepatitis or jaundice* (yellow eyes or skin)—may be obscured due to pink to brownish-black discoloration of skin, cornea, and conjunctiva; *mental depression, secondary to skin discoloration*

### Those indicating need for medical attention only if they continue or are bothersome
Incidence more frequent
*Gastrointestinal disturbances* (anorexia; diarrhea; nausea or vomiting); *ichthyosis* (dry, rough, or scaly skin); *pink or red to brownish-black discoloration of skin; skin rash and itching*

Incidence less frequent or rare
*Changes in taste; dryness, burning, itching, or irritation of the eyes; photosensitivity* (increased sensitivity of skin to sunlight)

### Those not indicating need for medical attention
Incidence more frequent
*Discoloration of feces, lining of the eyelids, sputum, sweat, tears, and urine*

Note: Clofazimine may also cause bloody or black, tarry stools, a symptom of gastrointestinal bleeding, which does require medical attention.

# Overdose

For more information on the management of overdose or unintentional ingestion, **contact a Poison Control Center** (see *Poison Control Center Listing*).

### Treatment of overdose
Recommended treatment consists of the following:

To decrease absorption—Emptying the stomach by induction of vomiting or gastric lavage.

Supportive care—Giving supportive, symptomatic treatment as necessary. Patients in whom intentional overdose is known or suspected should be referred for psychiatric consultation.

# Patient Consultation

As an aid to patient consultation, refer to *Advice for the Patient, Clofazimine (Systemic)*.

In providing consultation, consider emphasizing the following selected information (» = major clinical significance):

### Before using this medication
» Conditions affecting use, especially:
Pregnancy—Clofazimine crosses the placenta; it can cause deeply pigmented skin in the infant; clofazimine has not been shown to be teratogenic in humans
Breast-feeding—Clofazimine is excreted in breast milk; it has caused skin discoloration in animals probably due to the presence of clofazimine in maternal milk
Dental—May cause discoloration of sputum and changes in taste
Other medical problems, especially a history of gastrointestinal problems

### Proper use of this medication
Taking with meals or milk
» Compliance with full course of therapy, which may take years
» Importance of not missing doses and taking at same time every day
» Proper dosing
Missed dose: Taking as soon as possible; not taking if almost time for next dose; not doubling doses
» Proper storage

### Precautions while using this medication
Checking with physician if no improvement within 1 to 3 months; may take up to 6 months before full therapeutic benefit is seen
» May cause mental depression, possibly leading to suicide, secondary to reversible skin discoloration; several months or years may be

required for skin discoloration to disappear; checking with physician immediately if mental depression or suicidal thoughts occur
» Possible skin photosensitivity; avoiding unprotected exposure to sun; using protective clothing and sun block product; avoiding use of sunlamp, tanning bed, or tanning booth
Using skin cream, lotion, or oil to treat dry, rough, or scaly skin

### Side/adverse effects
Signs of potential side effects, especially gastrointestinal bleeding, gastrointestinal toxicity, hepatitis or jaundice, and mental depression secondary to skin discoloration
Discoloration of feces, lining of the eyelids, sputum, sweat, tears, and urine may be alarming to patient, although medically insignificant; however, bloody or black, tarry stools may be due to gastrointestinal bleeding and requires medical attention

## General Dosing Information

Clofazimine should be taken with meals or milk.

Clofazimine should preferably be used in combination with one or more other antileprosy agents to prevent the development of resistance in the initial treatment of multibacillary leprosy.

Clofazimine may also be used in combination with corticosteroids in the treatment of lepromatous leprosy complicated by erythema nodosum leprosum reactions if nerve injury or skin ulceration appears likely to occur.

Depending on the drug regimen used, therapy may have to be continued for 2 years to life in multibacillary (borderline, borderline-lepromatous, and lepromatous) leprosy.

Doses of more than 100 mg daily should be given for as short a period of time as possible and only under close medical supervision.

## Oral Dosage Forms

Note: Bracketed uses in the *Dosage Forms* section refer to categories of use and/or indications that are not included in U.S. product labeling.

### CLOFAZIMINE CAPSULES USP

**Usual adult and adolescent dose**
Dapsone-resistant multibacillary leprosy—
  In combination with one or more other antileprosy agents: Oral, 50 to 100 mg of clofazimine once a day.
Multibacillary leprosy complicated by erythema nodosum leprosum reactions—
  Without threatened nerve injury or skin ulceration: See *Dapsone-resistant multibacillary leprosy*.
  With threatened nerve injury or skin ulceration: In combination with corticosteroids—Oral, 100 to 300 mg of clofazimine daily. This dosage of clofazimine may be useful in reducing or eliminating corticosteroid requirements (e.g., up to 40 to 80 mg of prednisone daily). Clofazimine dosage should be tapered to 100 mg daily as

soon as possible after control of the reaction is achieved. Since it may take approximately two months to reach adequate clofazimine tissue concentrations, corticosteroids should be tapered only after two months of clofazimine therapy. Both drugs may be tapered simultaneously.
[*Mycobacterium avium-intracellulare* infections]—
  In combination with up to five or six antitubercular agents: Oral, 100 mg of clofazimine every eight hours.
Note: In the treatment of dapsone-sensitive, multibacillary leprosy, combination therapy with two other antileprosy agents is recommended. This triple-drug regimen should be followed for at least two years and continued, if possible, until skin smears are negative. Following this, monotherapy with the appropriate antileprosy agent may be continued.

**Usual adult prescribing limits**
Leprosy—
  Doses above 300 mg daily are not recommended.
[Mycobacterial infections, atypical]—
  Up to 300 mg daily.

**Usual pediatric dose**
Dosage has not been established.

**Strength(s) usually available**
U.S.—
  50 mg (Rx) [*Lamprene* (parabens)].
  100 mg (Rx) [*Lamprene* (parabens)].
Canada—
  Not commercially available.

**Packaging and storage**
Store below 30 °C (86 °F), in a tight container, unless otherwise specified by manufacturer.

**Auxiliary labeling**
• Take with meals or milk.
• Avoid too much sun or use of sunlamp.
• May discolor skin and body fluids.
• Continue medicine for full time of treatment.

**Additional information**
*Lamprene* brand of clofazimine capsules contains micronized clofazimine suspended in an oil-wax base.

## Selected Bibliography

Holdiness MR. Clinical pharmacokinetics of clofazimine. Clin Pharmacokinetics 1989; 16: 74-85.
Garrelts JC. Clofazimine: a review of its use in leprosy and Mycobacterium avium complex infection. DICP Ann Pharmacother 5/91; 25: 525-31.

Revised: 02/23/93

---

# CLOFIBRATE   Systemic

VA CLASSIFICATION (Primary/Secondary): CV350/CV900
Note: For a listing of dosage forms and brand names by country availability, see *Dosage Forms* section(s). For a listing of brand names for the articles in this monograph, refer to the General Index.

## Category

Antihyperlipidemic; antidiuretic (central diabetes insipidus).

## Indications

Note: Bracketed information in the *Indications* section refers to uses that are not included in U.S. product labeling.

**Accepted**
Hyperlipidemia (treatment)—Clofibrate is indicated in the treatment of hyperlipidemia. Because of risks associated with its use (see *Side/Adverse Effects*), clofibrate is recommended for use as an adjunct only in patients with severe primary hyperlipidemia (type III hyperlipidemia) and a significant risk of coronary artery disease who have not responded to diet or other measures alone. Clofibrate reduces plasma triglyceride concentrations to a greater extent than plasma cholesterol concentrations, and so is not useful in patients with elevated cholesterol concentrations alone. Its use is limited in type II hyperlipidemia because of its variable effect on cholesterol concentrations. Clofibrate

is not recommended for community-wide prevention of ischemic heart disease.

Studies have suggested that control of elevated cholesterol and triglycerides may not lessen the danger of cardiovascular disease and mortality, although incidence of nonfatal myocardial infarctions may be decreased.

For additional information on initial therapeutic guidelines related to the treatment of hyperlipidemia, see *Appendix III*.

[Clofibrate has been used in the treatment of partial central diabetes insipidus in patients with some residual posterior pituitary function; however, it generally has been replaced by other agents.][1]

**Unaccepted**
Although clofibrate alters platelet function (decreases platelet adhesiveness), it has not shown significant efficacy as an antiplatelet drug.

---

[1]Not included in Canadian product labeling.

## Pharmacology/Pharmacokinetics

**Physicochemical characteristics**
Molecular weight—242.70.
pKa—2.95.

## Mechanism of action/Effect

Antihyperlipidemic—Not completely understood, but may involve inhibition of biosynthesis of cholesterol before mevalonate formation, increased secretion and fecal excretion of neutral sterols, enhanced catabolism of very low–density lipoproteins (VLDL) due to increased lipoprotein lipase activity in extrahepatic tissues, and/or increased clearance of triglycerides (VLDL) from the circulation.

Antidiuretic—May stimulate release of antidiuretic hormone (ADH) from the posterior pituitary.

## Absorption

Completely but slowly absorbed from the intestine.

## Protein binding

Very high (96%).

## Biotransformation

Hepatic and gastrointestinal; rapid de-esterification occurs in the gastrointestinal tract and/or on first-pass metabolism to produce the active form, clofibric acid (chlorophenoxy isobutyric acid [CPIB]).

## Half-life

Single dose—
Normal: 6 to 25 hours.
Anuria: 113 hours.
Steady state—
Normal: 54 hours.

## Onset of action

Plasma VLDL concentrations are reduced within 2 to 5 days.

## Time to peak plasma concentration

2 to 6 hours after a dose.

## Time to peak effect

3 weeks (with continued use).

## Duration of action

Return to pretreatment VLDL concentrations occurs within 3 weeks after clofibrate is withdrawn.

## Elimination

Renal; 10 to 20% of clofibric acid excreted unchanged; also as glucuronide conjugate (60%).

# Precautions to Consider

## Carcinogenicity

Clofibrate, in doses 5 to 8 times the human dose, has been found to increase the incidence of malignant hepatic tumors in rodents.

## Pregnancy/Reproduction

Pregnancy—Studies have not been done in humans. However, clofibrate may cross the placenta, and the fetus may not have developed the enzyme system required to excrete it; use is not recommended during pregnancy. If a pregnancy is planned, clofibrate therapy should be withdrawn several months before conception.

Studies in rabbits indicate that fetal serum concentrations of clofibrate may be higher than maternal serum concentrations.

FDA Pregnancy Category C.

## Breast-feeding

Clofibrate is distributed into breast milk. Use of clofibrate during breast-feeding is not recommended because of potentially serious adverse effects on nursing infants.

## Pediatrics

Appropriate studies on the relationship of age to the effects of clofibrate have not been performed in the pediatric population. However, use in children under 2 years of age is not recommended since cholesterol is required for normal development.

## Geriatrics

Although appropriate studies on the relationship of age to the effects of clofibrate have not been performed in the geriatric population, geriatrics-specific problems that would limit the usefulness of this medication in the elderly are not expected. However, elderly patients are more likely to have age-related renal function impairment, which may require dosage adjustment in patients receiving clofibrate.

## Drug interactions and/or related problems

The following drug interactions and/or related problems have been selected on the basis of their potential clinical significance (possible mechanism in parentheses where appropriate)—not necessarily inclusive (» = major clinical significance):

Note: Combinations containing any of the following medications, depending on the amount present, may also interact with this medication.

» Anticoagulants, coumarin- or indandione-derivative
(concurrent use with clofibrate may significantly increase the anticoagulant effect; adjustment of anticoagulant dosage based on frequent prothrombin-time determinations is recommended; some clinicians recommend reduction of the anticoagulant dosage by one-half)

Antidiabetic agents, oral, especially tolbutamide
(concurrent use of clofibrate with oral antidiabetic agents may enhance the hypoglycemic effect through displacement from serum proteins; dosage adjustments may be necessary. Glipizide and glyburide, due to their non-ionic binding characteristics, may not be affected as much as the other oral agents; however, caution with concurrent use is recommended)

Chenodiol or
Ursodiol
(effect may be decreased when chenodiol or ursodiol is used concurrently with clofibrate since clofibrate tends to increase cholesterol saturation of bile)

HMG-CoA reductase inhibitors
(concurrent use with clofibrate may increase the risk of rhabdomyolysis; cases of rhabdomyolysis have not been reported with concurrent use of clofibrate and HMG-CoA reductase inhibitors; however, there have been reported cases of rhadomyolysis with concurrent use of another fibrate, gemfibrozil, and lovastatin)

Oral contraceptives
(concurrent use may alter the effectiveness of clofibrate)

Probenecid
(concurrent use of probenecid may decrease renal and metabolic clearances and alter the protein binding of clofibrate, increasing the therapeutic and toxic effects of clofibrate)

Rifampin
(concurrent use with clofibrate may enhance the metabolism of clofibrate by induction of hepatic microsomal enzymes, resulting in significantly lower serum clofibrate concentrations)

## Laboratory value alterations

The following have been selected on the basis of their potential clinical significance (possible effect in parentheses where appropriate)—not necessarily inclusive (» = major clinical significance):

With physiology/laboratory test values
Alanine aminotransferase (ALT [SGPT]) and
Aspartate aminotransferase (AST [SGOT])
(serum concentrations may be increased, indicating hepatotoxicity)

Amylase
(serum concentrations may be increased)

Beta-lipoprotein, plasma
(low-density lipoprotein [LDL] or cholesterol concentrations may be increased as a paradoxical response to a large decrease in very low–density lipoprotein [VLDL] concentrations)

Creatine kinase (CK)
(concentrations may be increased, especially in patients with renal failure or hypoalbuminemia)

Fibrinogen
(plasma concentrations may be decreased)

## Medical considerations/Contraindications

The medical considerations/contraindications included here have been selected on the basis of their potential clinical significance (reasons given in parentheses where appropriate)—not necessarily inclusive (» = major clinical significance).

*Except under special circumstances, this medication should not be used when the following medical problem exists:*

» Primary biliary cirrhosis
(use of clofibrate may further raise the cholesterol)

*Risk-benefit should be considered when the following medical problems exist:*

Cardiovascular disease
(condition may be exacerbated)

Gallstones
(increased risk of biliary complications)

» Hepatic function impairment
(protein binding of clofibrate is reduced but half-life is not altered. It is recommended that patients with impaired hepatic function receive a reduced dose of clofibrate; some clinicians recommend reduction of dosage by one-half in patients with cirrhosis)

Hypothyroidism
(may predispose to clofibrate-induced myopathy)

Peptic ulcer
(reactivation has been reported)

» Renal function impairment
(reduced protein binding and clearance of clofibrate leads to increased incidence of side effects, especially myopathy and rhabdomyolysis. It is recommended that clofibrate be administered in reduced dosage to patients with impaired renal function. However, dosage reduction is not necessary in nephrotic syndrome when renal function is not impaired, since steady-state concentration of unbound drug is unchanged in spite of markedly reduced protein binding and half-life)

Sensitivity to clofibrate

## Patient monitoring

The following may be especially important in patient monitoring (other tests may be warranted in some patients, depending on condition; » = major clinical significance):

» Cholesterol, serum concentrations and

» Triglyceride, serum concentrations
(determinations recommended prior to initiation of therapy, at 2-week intervals during the first few months of therapy, at monthly intervals thereafter to detect a paradoxical rise in serum cholesterol or triglyceride concentrations as well as to confirm efficacy, then every few months when concentrations stabilize)

Complete blood counts
(recommended prior to initiation of therapy and at periodic intervals during therapy if signs of anemia or leukopenia occur)

Creatine kinase (CK) concentrations
(recommended at periodic intervals in uremic patients receiving clofibrate)

Liver function tests, including serum transaminase concentrations
(determinations recommended prior to initiation of therapy, every month for the first 2 months, then every 2 months until an effect is observed, and every 4 months thereafter)

## Side/Adverse Effects

Note: The suggestion that long-term use of clofibrate may increase the risk of death from noncardiovascular causes (malignancy, post-cholecystectomy complications, pancreatitis) was made after results first published in 1978 of a large prospective study (the WHO study). This suggestion has been controversial, in part because other studies (for example, the Coronary Drug Project report published in 1975) have not reached a similar conclusion, although both major studies agree that the risk of cholelithiasis and cholecystitis requiring surgery is greatly increased in clofibrate users. Clofibrate has been found to increase the risk of development of peripheral vascular disease, pulmonary embolism, thrombophlebitis, angina pectoris, arrhythmias, and intermittent claudication. Clofibrate, in doses 5 to 8 times the human dose, has been found to increase the incidence of malignant hepatic tumors in rodents.

Rhabdomyolysis and severe hyperkalemia have been reported in patients with pre-existing renal function impairment.

The following side/adverse effects have been selected on the basis of their potential clinical significance (possible signs and symptoms in parentheses where appropriate)—not necessarily inclusive:

### Those indicating need for medical attention
Incidence rare
*Anemia or leukopenia* (fever or chills; cough or hoarseness; lower back or side pain; painful or difficult urination); *angina* (chest pain; shortness of breath); *cardiac arrhythmias* (irregular heartbeat); *gallstones or pancreatitis* (severe stomach pain with nausea and vomiting); *renal toxicity* (blood in urine; decrease in urination; painful urination; swelling of feet and lower legs)

Note: Increased creatine kinase (CK) and serum transaminase concentrations may be caused by clofibrate rather than myocardial infarction.

### Those indicating need for medical attention only if they continue or are bothersome
Incidence more frequent
*Diarrhea; nausea*
Incidence less frequent or rare
*Decreased sexual ability; flu-like syndrome or myositis* (muscle aches or cramps; unusual tiredness or weakness); *headache; increased appetite or weight gain, slight; stomach pain, gas, or heartburn; stomatitis* (sores in mouth and on lips); *vomiting*

Note: *Flu-like syndrome* or *myositis* occurs more frequently in patients with existing renal disease, and usually is accompanied by increased CK and serum transaminases.

## Patient Consultation

As an aid to patient consultation, refer to *Advice for the Patient, Clofibrate (Systemic).*

In providing consultation, consider emphasizing the following selected information (» = major clinical significance):

### Before using this medication
Potential serious toxicity; WHO study controversy
Diet as preferred therapy
» Conditions affecting use, especially:
Sensitivity to clofibrate
Pregnancy—May cross placenta; enzyme system required for excretion may not be developed in fetus; withdrawal of clofibrate therapy several months before conception is recommended if pregnancy is planned
Breast-feeding—Use not recommended while nursing because of potentially serious adverse effects on nursing infants
Use in children—Not recommended in children less than 2 years of age since cholesterol is required for normal development
Other medications, especially anticoagulants
Other medical problems, especially primary biliary cirrhosis, hepatic function impairment, or renal function impairment

### Proper use of this medication
» Importance of not taking more or less medication than the amount prescribed
» Compliance with prescribed diet
Taking with meals to prevent possible gastric irritation
» Proper dosing
Missed dose: Taking as soon as possible; not taking if almost time for next dose; not doubling doses
» Proper storage

### Precautions while using this medication
» Importance of close monitoring by the physician
» Checking with physician before discontinuing medication; blood lipid concentrations may increase significantly

### Side/adverse effects
Signs of potential side effects, especially angina, cardiac arrhythmias, leukopenia, anemia, pancreatitis, gallstones, and renal toxicity

## General Dosing Information

If response is inadequate after 3 months of treatment, clofibrate therapy should be withdrawn, except in the case of xanthoma tuberosum, which may require up to 1 year of treatment as long as reduction in size and/or number of xanthomata occurs.

If results of hepatic function tests rise significantly or show significant abnormalities, it is recommended that clofibrate therapy be withdrawn and not resumed; laboratory abnormalities are usually reversible.

If an increase in serum amylase concentrations or a paradoxical increase in plasma cholesterol or plasma LDL concentrations occurs, it is recommended that clofibrate therapy be withdrawn.

When clofibrate is discontinued, an appropriate hypolipidemic diet and monitoring of serum lipids are recommended until the patient stabilizes, since a rise in serum cholesterol and triglyceride concentrations to or above the original base may occur.

### Diet/Nutrition
It is recommended that clofibrate be taken with food to minimize gastrointestinal upset.

## Oral Dosage Forms
### CLOFIBRATE CAPSULES USP

**Usual adult dose**
Antihyperlipidemic—
Oral, 1.5 to 2 grams per day in two to four divided doses.

Note: Clofibrate has been used in the treatment of diabetes insipidus at an oral dose of 6 to 8 grams per day in two or four divided doses.

**Usual adult prescribing limits**
Antihyperlipidemic—
2 grams daily.

**Usual pediatric dose**
Dosage has not been established.

**Strength(s) usually available**
U.S.—
500 mg (Rx) [*Abitrate; Atromid-S;* GENERIC].
Canada—
500 mg (Rx) [*Atromid-S; Claripex; Novofibrate*].
1 gram (Rx) [*Atromid-S*].

**Packaging and storage**
Store below 40 °C (104 °F), preferably between 15 and 30 °C (59 and 86 °F), unless otherwise specified by manufacturer. Store in a well-closed, light-resistant container.

**Auxiliary labeling**
• Take with meals.

## Selected Bibliography

The Expert Panel. Report of the National Cholesterol Education Program Expert Panel on Detection, Evaluation and Treatment of High Blood Cholesterol in Adults. Arch Intern Med 1988 Jan; 148: 36-69.

NIH Consensus Conference. Lowering blood cholesterol to prevent heart disease. JAMA 1985 Apr 12; 253: 2080-6.
Knodel LC, Talbert RL. Adverse effects of hypolipidaemic drugs. Med Toxicol 1987; 2: 10-32.

Revised: 11/24/92
Interim revision: 04/14/94

---

# CLOMIPHENE   Systemic

INN: Clomifene
JAN: Clomifene citrate
VA CLASSIFICATION (Primary/Secondary): HS400/DX900: HS900

Note: For a listing of dosage forms and brand names by country availability, see *Dosage Forms* section(s). For a listing of brand names for the articles in this monograph, refer to the General Index.

---

## Category

Antiestrogen; infertility therapy adjunct; diagnostic aid (ovarian function; hypothalamic-pituitary-gonadal axis function).

## Indications

Note: Bracketed information in the *Indications* section refers to uses that are not included in U.S. product labeling.

**Accepted**

Infertility, female (treatment)—Clomiphene is indicated in the treatment of anovulation or oligo-ovulation in patients desiring pregnancy, whose sexual partners have adequate sperm, and who have potentially functional hypothalamic-hypophyseal-ovarian systems and adequate endogenous estrogen.

[Corpus luteum insufficiency (treatment)][1]—Clomiphene may be used to treat corpus luteum dysfunction.

[Hypothalamic-pituitary-gonadal axis function, in males (diagnosis)][1]— Clomiphene is used to detect abnormalities of the hypothalamic-pituitary-gonadal axis in males.

[Infertility, male (treatment)][1]—Clomiphene is used to treat infertility in males with oligospermia.

[Ovarian function studies][1]—Clomiphene is sometimes given as a test dose to aid in predicting whether an ovulatory response might occur.

---

[1]Not included in Canadian product labeling.

## Pharmacology/Pharmacokinetics

**Physicochemical characteristics**
Source—Synthetic; nonsteroidal geometric isomer (30 to 50% is cis-clomiphene zuclomiphene and the remainder is trans-enclomiphene).
Molecular weight—598.10.

**Mechanism of action/Effect**
Clomiphene has mainly antiestrogenic effects and some estrogenic effects. The mechanism in stimulating ovulation is unknown but is believed to be related to its antiestrogenic properties. By clomiphene competing with estrogen for binding sites at the hypothalamic level, the gonadotropins, follicle-stimulating hormone (FSH) and luteinizing hormone (LH), secretion is increased, which results in ovarian follicle maturation, followed by the preovulatory LH surge, ovulation, and the subsequent development of the corpus luteum. Usefulness in male infertility is also likely related to the increases in FSH and LH secretion.

**Absorption**
Readily absorbed from gastrointestinal tract; undergoes enterohepatic recycling, especially with cis-zuclomiphene.

**Biotransformation**
Hepatic.

**Half-life**
Plasma—5 to 7 days.

**Time to peak effect**
Ovulation usually occurs 4 to 10 days (average 7 days) after the last day of treatment; this period of time may vary by patient and by cycle. In rare cases, ovulation may occur as late as 14 days after the last day of treatment.

**Elimination**
Biliary/fecal—Up to 42% of the oral dose; can be detectable in feces for up to 6 weeks.
Renal—Up to 8% of the oral dose.

## Precautions to Consider

**Carcinogenicity/Tumorigenicity/Mutagenicity**
Long-term carcinogenicity or mutagenicity studies have not been done. Studies are ongoing to determine the additional risk, if any, of developing ovarian cancer in women taking fertility medication beyond that contributed by infertility. Although a causal relationship between hyperstimulation of the ovaries and ovarian cancer has not been established, a correlation does exist for certain risk factors, including ovarian cancer, nulliparity, and increasing age. In addition, prolonged use of clomiphene may contribute to the risk of a borderline or invasive ovarian tumor, which should be considered whenever ovarian cysts do not regress with clomiphene therapy. Two cases of bilateral female breast carcinoma and one case of testicular carcinoma have occurred during clomiphene therapy.

**Pregnancy/Reproduction**
Fertility—Clomiphene may cause a decrease in quantity or change in quality of cervical mucus, which may interfere with sperm function, fertilization, and, subsequently, the occurrence of pregnancy.

Pregnancy—Clomiphene is not recommended during pregnancy. Controlled studies in humans have not been done. However, there have been reports of congenital malformations and fetal death occurring with clomiphene administration in humans. In clinical use, the cumulative rate of congenital abnormalities associated with ovulation induction therapy does not appear to be greater than that reported in the general population for spontaneous pregnancy. However, because a direct causal relationship has not been established, careful monitoring of the patient is recommended to prevent inadvertent administration of clomiphene during pregnancy.

Use of clomiphene is associated with an increased incidence of multiple pregnancies and, therefore, possible premature deliveries, as well as ectopic and heterotopic pregnancy. The incidence of reported multiple pregnancies was 7.98% (6.9% twins, 0.5% triplets, 0.3% quadruplets, and 0.1% quintuplets) with about an 83.3% survival rate, or a lower rate (73%) when including stillbirths, spontaneous abortions, or neonatal deaths. The ratio of monozygotic twins to dizygotic twins is 1 to 5.

Studies in rats and rabbits have shown clomiphene to be teratogenic. The observed malformations were similar to those produced by *in utero* exposure to diethylstilbestrol and may include vaginal adenosis and other defects in the vaginal, uterine, and Fallopian tube structures.

FDA Pregnancy Category X.

**Breast-feeding**
It is not known whether clomiphene is distributed into breast milk. However, clomiphene suppresses lactation.

**Laboratory value alterations**
The following have been selected on the basis of their potential clinical significance (possible effect in parentheses where appropriate)—not necessarily inclusive (» = major clinical significance):

With physiology/laboratory test values
    Desmosterol (only with long-term use, possibly indicating interference with cholesterol synthesis) and
    Sex hormone–binding globulin and
    Transcortin
      (plasma concentrations may be increased)

## Medical considerations/Contraindications

The medical considerations/contraindications included here have been selected on the basis of their potential clinical significance (reasons given in parentheses where appropriate)—not necessarily inclusive (» = major clinical significance).

*Except under special circumstances, this medication should not be used when the following medical problems exist:*

» Hepatic function impairment, active
   (potential for reduced clearance of clomiphene, leading to higher plasma concentrations or hepatoxicity)

» Mental depression
   (may be exacerbated)

» Ovarian cyst, not associated with polycystic ovary syndrome or
» Ovarian enlargement, not associated with polycystic ovary syndrome
   (risk of further enlargement)

» Thrombophlebitis, active
   (increased risk of thrombophlebitis in susceptible individuals can be caused by elevated estradiol levels associated with ovulation induction by clomiphene)

*Risk-benefit should be considered when the following medical problems exist:*

» Abnormal vaginal bleeding, undiagnosed
   (careful evaluation recommended; neoplastic lesions should be ruled out)

» Endometriosis
   (implants may be aggravated by elevated estradiol levels associated with ovulation induction)

» Fibroid tumors of the uterus
   (risk of further enlargement)

» Hepatic function impairment, history of
   (potential for reduced clearance of clomiphene, leading to higher plasma concentrations or hepatoxicity)

» Polycystic ovary syndrome or
   Sensitivity to pituitary gonadotropins
   (patient may have an exaggerated response to clomiphene; lower dose or shorter duration of therapy may be necessary)
   Sensitivity to clomiphene

## Patient monitoring

The following may be especially important in patient monitoring (other tests may be warranted in some patients, depending on condition; » = major clinical significance):

Immunologic assay for human chorionic gonadotropin (HCG)
   (recommended for detection of pregnancy if menses does not occur before start of next course of clomiphene; should be measured 10 days or later after exogenous HCG is administered)

Liver function tests
   (recommended in some patients prior to initiation of therapy with clomiphene, especially in patients with risk factors increasing their susceptibility to hepatic dysfunction)

Ophthalmologic, including slit-lamp, examination
   (recommended if treatment with clomiphene is continued for more than 1 year or if visual disturbances occur)

» Urinary luteinizing hormone surge testing
   (may be used as adjunctive therapy to predict ovulation)

## Side/Adverse Effects

Note: At the recommended dosage, adverse effects usually are rare. Incidence and severity of adverse effects tend to be related to dose and duration of treatment and are usually reversible after clomiphene therapy is discontinued. Doses over 100 mg a day for five days have been associated with a higher incidence of side effects; patients receiving these doses should be carefully monitored.

   Rare reports of ovarian cancer have been associated with fertility medications but a causal relationship has not been determined partly because it is not possible to predict beyond the risk that infertility brings to developing ovarian cancer.

The following side/adverse effects have been selected on the basis of their potential clinical significance (possible signs and symptoms in parentheses where appropriate)—not necessarily inclusive:

## Those indicating need for medical attention
Incidence more frequent—>5%

   *Ovarian cyst formation; ovarian enlargement; premenstrual syndrome; uterine fibroid enlargement* (abdominal bloating; stomach pain; pelvic pain)

   Note: Maximum *ovarian enlargement* occurs several days after clomiphene therapy is discontinued.

   A patient's report of *abdominal pain* during clomiphene therapy indicates the need for immediate pelvic examination. If ovarian enlargement or cyst formation has occurred, it is recommended that clomiphene therapy be withdrawn until the ovaries have returned to pretreatment size, usually within a few days or weeks. Dosage and duration of the next course of clomiphene should be reduced.

Incidence less frequent or rare

   *Hepatotoxicity* (yellow eyes or skin); *vision changes, especially afterimages* (persistence of visual images); *blurred vision*—especially with larger doses; *diplopia* (double vision); *floaters* (spots in visual field caused by protein deposits in the vitreous fluid of the eye); *phosphenes* (seeing flashes of light); *photophobia* (increased sensitivity of eyes to light); *scotoma* (area of decreased vision in visual field surrounded by normal or less-diminished vision)

   Note: If the patient receiving clomiphene experiences any *visual disturbances*, it is recommended that clomiphene therapy be withdrawn and a complete ophthalmologic examination performed. Ocular side effects usually disappear within a few days or weeks after the last dose of clomiphene.

## Those indicating need for medical attention only if they continue or are bothersome
Incidence more frequent—10%
   *Hot flashes*

Incidence less frequent or rare—1 to 2%
   *Breast discomfort in women; gynecomastia in men* (enlargement of breasts); *dizziness or lightheadedness; headache; menorrhagia* (increased amount of menstrual bleeding at regular monthly periods); *mental depression; nausea or vomiting; nervousness; restlessness; spotting* (light uterine bleeding between regular menstrual periods); *tiredness; trouble in sleeping*

# Patient Consultation

As an aid to patient consultation, refer to *Advice for the Patient, Clomiphene (Systemic)*.

In providing consultation, consider emphasizing the following selected information (» = major clinical significance):

## Before using this medication
» Conditions affecting use, especially:
   Sensitivity to clomiphene
   Pregnancy—Use during pregnancy is not recommended since animal studies have shown teratogenicity
   Breast-feeding—Suppresses lactation
   Other medical problems, especially hepatic function impairment, mental depression, ovarian cyst, ovarian enlargement, thrombophlebitis, undiagnosed abnormal vaginal bleeding, endometriosis, uterine fibroids, and polycystic ovary syndrome

## Proper use of this medication
» Compliance with therapy; clarification of schedule; taking at same time every day to aid in remembering each dose
» Proper dosing
   Missed dose: Taking as soon as possible; doubling dose if not remembered until time of next dose; checking with physician if more than one dose missed
» Proper storage

## Precautions while using this medication
» Importance of close monitoring by physician
» Importance of following physician's instructions for timing of intercourse
» Telling physician immediately if pregnancy is suspected; importance of not taking medication while pregnant
» Caution when driving or doing jobs requiring alertness because of visual disturbances, dizziness, or lightheadedness

## Side/adverse effects
   Signs of potential side effects, especially ovarian cyst formation, ovarian enlargement, uterine fibroid enlargement, premenstrual syndrome, hepatotoxicity, or vision changes

## General Dosing Information

Patients receiving clomiphene should be under supervision of a physician experienced in the treatment of gynecologic or endocrine disorders.

Patients who have been hypoestrogenic for prolonged periods may require pretreatment with estrogen to provide a more normal endometrium for ovum implantation. Estrogen therapy should be discontinued immediately before initiation of clomiphene therapy.

Properly timed coitus in relation to ovulation is important and may be predicted from ovulation test kits (the preferred method) or other appropriate tests for ovulation such as taking basal body temperature. Couples should be advised to have frequent intercourse at or around the time that ovulation is anticipated. Ovulation generally occurs 7 days (average) after the last dose of clomiphene (range is 5 to 10 days).

In some patients, a single injection of 5000 to 10,000 USP Units of human chorionic gonadotropin (HCG) given 5 to 9 days after the last dose of clomiphene to simulate the midcycle LH surge that results in ovulation may increase the efficacy of clomiphene.

If ovulation does not occur after 3 to 4 cycles of clomiphene therapy at the maximum dose, or if pregnancy does not result after a treatment interval of 3 to 6 months with documented ovulation, or if ovulatory menses does not occur, further treatment with clomiphene is not recommended and the diagnosis should be re-evaluated.

## Oral Dosage Forms

### CLOMIPHENE CITRATE TABLETS USP

**Usual adult dose**
Female infertility—
Oral, 50 mg a day for five days, starting on the fifth day of the menstrual cycle if bleeding occurs or at any time if the patient has had no recent uterine bleeding. If ovulation without conception occurs, this cycle is repeated until conception or for three or four cycles.

---

# CLONIDINE    Systemic

**VA CLASSIFICATION (Primary/Secondary):**
Oral—CV490/DX900; CN105; CN900
Transdermal—CV490

Note: For a listing of dosage forms and brand names by country availability, see *Dosage Forms* section(s). For a listing of brand names for the articles in this monograph, refer to the General Index.

## Category

Antihypertensive—Clonidine Hydrochloride Tablets; Clonidine Transdermal Systems.
Menopausal syndrome therapy adjunct—Clonidine Hydrochloride Tablets.
Vascular headache prophylactic—Clonidine Hydrochloride Tablets.
Antidysmenorrheal—Clonidine Hydrochloride Tablets.
Opioid withdrawal syndrome suppressant—Clonidine Hydrochloride Tablets.

## Indications

Note: Bracketed information in the *Indications* section refers to uses that are not included in U.S. product labeling.

**Accepted**
Hypertension (treatment)—Oral and transdermal dosage forms of clonidine are indicated in the treatment of hypertension. Because it causes only mild postural hypotension, clonidine may be useful as a substitute for guanethidine or other adrenergic blockers in patients who cannot tolerate these agents because of severe orthostatic hypotension.

For additional information on initial therapeutic guidelines related to the treatment of hypertension, see *Appendix III*.

[Oral clonidine is also used in the urgent treatment of hypertensive emergencies.][1]

[Pheochromocytoma (diagnosis)][1]—A clonidine suppression test is used in the diagnosis of pheochromocytoma.

[Headache, vascular (prophylaxis)][1]—Clonidine has been used orally in the prevention of migraine.

[Dysmenorrhea (treatment)][1] or
[Menopause, vasomotor symptoms of (treatment)]—Clonidine is used orally as an adjunct in the treatment of dysmenorrhea and menopausal flushing.

---

A smaller dose or shorter duration may be necessary for individuals unusually sensitive to clomiphene, such as women with polycystic ovary sydrome. If ovulation does not occur, the dose is increased to 75 to 100 mg a day for five days (the next course beginning as early as thirty days after the previous course), repeated if ovulation without conception occurs. Rarely, patients require up to 250 mg a day to induce ovulation.

Note: A physical exam prior to the first and each subsequent treatment is needed to exclude pregnancy, ovarian enlargement, or ovarian cysts (not due to polycystic ovary syndrome) and to ensure normal liver function and no abnormal uterine bleeding before next course of clomiphene may be initiated.

**Strength(s) usually available**
U.S.—
50 mg (Rx) [*Clomid* (scored; lactose; sucrose); *Milophene* (scored; lactose; sucrose); *Serophene* (scored); GENERIC]
Canada—
50 mg (Rx) [*Clomid* (scored; sucrose; lactose); *Serophene*].

**Packaging and storage**
Store below 40 °C (104 °F), preferably between 15 and 30 °C (59 and 86 °F), unless otherwise specified by manufacturer. Store in a well-closed container. Protect from light.

Revised: 08/08/95

---

**CLOMIPRAMINE**—See *Antidepressants, Tricyclic (Systemic)*

---

**CLONAZEPAM**—See *Benzodiazepines (Systemic)*

---

[Opioid (narcotic) abstinence syndrome (treatment)][1]—Clonidine is also used to control symptoms and aid in rapid detoxification in the treatment of opioid withdrawal.

[Nicotine dependence (treatment adjunct)][1]—Clonidine is used as an adjunct in the treatment of nicotine withdrawal.

[Gilles de la Tourette's syndrome (treatment)][1]—Clonidine is used in the treatment of Gilles de la Tourette's syndrome.

---

[1]Not included in Canadian product labeling.

## Pharmacology/Pharmacokinetics

**Physicochemical characteristics**
Molecular weight—Clonidine: 230.10.
Clonidine hydrochloride: 266.56.

**Mechanism of action/Effect**
Alpha-adrenergic agonist; also has some alpha-adrenergic antagonist effects.
Antihypertensive—
Thought to be due to central alpha$_2$-adrenergic stimulation, which results in a decreased sympathetic outflow to the heart, kidneys, and peripheral vasculature; this results in decreased peripheral vascular resistance, decreased systolic and diastolic blood pressure, and decreased heart rate.
Vascular headache prophylactic—
May block central vasomotor reflexes.
Dysmenorrhea therapy adjunct; or menopausal syndrome therapy adjunct—
Unknown, although may act as peripheral vascular stabilizer to reduce menopausal flushing.
Opioid withdrawal syndrome suppressant—
May be result of alpha-adrenergic inhibiting activity in areas of the brain such as the locus ceruleus.

**Other actions/effects**
Stimulates the release of growth hormone acutely, but not chronically.

**Absorption**
Oral—Well absorbed following oral administration. Bioavailability following chronic administration is approximately 65%.
Transdermal—Greatest from the chest and upper arm, and least from the thigh. Absorbed through the skin at a constant rate.

**Protein binding**
Low to moderate (20 to 40%).

**Biotransformation**
Hepatic (about 50% of the absorbed dose).

**Half-life**
Normal renal function—Range, 12 to 16 hours.

Renal function impairment—Up to 41 hours.

**Onset of effect**
Antihypertensive—
    Oral: 30 to 60 minutes.
    Transdermal: 2 to 3 days.

**Time to peak plasma concentration**
Oral—1.5 to 2.5 hours.
Transdermal—2 to 3 days.

**Time for peak effect**
Antihypertensive—Oral: 2 to 4 hours.

**Duration of action**
Antihypertensive—
    Oral—
        Up to 8 hours (24 to 36 hours in some patients).
    Transdermal—
        About 7 days with the system in place; about 8 hours after removal.

**Elimination**
Renal—40 to 60% (as unchanged drug) in 24 hours.
Biliary/fecal—20% (probably via enterohepatic circulation).
In dialysis—Very little (maximum 5%) removable by hemodialysis.

## Precautions to Consider

**Cross-sensitivity and/or related problems**
Patients sensitive to ophthalmic apraclonidine may be sensitive to clonidine.

**Carcinogenicity**
Studies in rats at doses 32 to 46 times the maximum recommended human dose for 132 weeks found no evidence of carcinogenicity.

**Pregnancy/Reproduction**
Fertility—Studies in male and female rats at doses up to 3 times the maximum recommended human dose found no impairment of fertility. However, fertility was affected in female rats given 10 to 40 times the maximum recommended human dose.

Pregnancy—Adequate and well-controlled studies in humans have not been done.

Studies in rats at doses as low as one-third the maximum recommended human dose given for 2 months prior to mating found an increased incidence of resorptions; this effect did not occur at doses of one-third to 3 times the maximum recommended human dose given on days 6 to 15 of gestation. Increased resorptions also occurred in rats and mice given doses up to 40 times the maximum recommended human dose on days 1 to 14 of gestation. No teratogenicity or embryotoxicity was observed in rabbits given up to 3 times the maximum recommended human dose.

FDA Pregnancy Category C.

**Breast-feeding**
Clonidine is distributed into breast milk. However, problems in humans have not been documented.

**Pediatrics**
Appropriate studies on the relationship of age to the effects of clonidine have not been performed in the pediatric population. However, there are numerous reports describing accidental clonidine overdose in the pediatric population. These reports seem to indicate that neonates, infants, and children are especially sensitive to the effects of clonidine. Caution is recommended.

**Geriatrics**
The elderly may be more sensitive than younger adults to clonidine's hypotensive effects. In addition, elderly patients are more likely to have age-related renal function impairment, which may require reduction of dosage in patients receiving clonidine.

**Dental**
Use of clonidine may decrease or inhibit salivary flow, thus contributing to the development of caries, periodontal disease, oral candidiasis, and discomfort.

**Drug interactions and/or related problems**
The following drug interactions and/or related problems have been selected on the basis of their potential clinical significance (possible mechanism in parentheses where appropriate)—not necessarily inclusive (» = major clinical significance):

Note: Combinations containing any of the following medications, depending on the amount present, may also interact with this medication.

Alcohol or
Central nervous system (CNS) depression–producing medications (See *Appendix II*)
    (concurrent use may enhance the CNS depressant effects of either these medications or clonidine)

» Antidepressants, tricyclic, or
Appetite suppressants, with the exception of fenfluramine
    (concurrent use may decrease the hypotensive effects of clonidine)

Anti-inflammatory drugs, nonsteroidal (NSAIDs), especially indomethacin
    (NSAIDs may reduce the antihypertensive effects of clonidine, possibly by inhibiting renal prostaglandin synthesis and/or causing sodium and fluid retention; the patient should be carefully monitored to confirm that the desired effect is being obtained)

» Beta-adrenergic blocking agents (systemic)
    (discontinuation of clonidine therapy during concurrent use of beta-adrenergic blocking agents may increase the risk of clonidine-withdrawal hypertensive crisis; ideally, beta-adrenergic blocking agents should be discontinued several days before clonidine is discontinued; blood pressure control may also be impaired when the 2 are combined)

Estrogens
    (estrogen-induced fluid retention may increase blood pressure)

Fenfluramine
    (concurrent use may increase the hypotensive effects of clonidine)

Hypotension-producing medications, other, (See *Appendix II*) with the exception of systemic beta-adrenergic blocking agents and tricyclic antidepressants
    (concurrent use may potentiate antihypertensive effects; although some antihypertensive and/or diuretic combinations are frequently used for therapeutic advantage, dosage adjustments may be necessary during concurrent use)

Sympathomimetics
    (concurrent use may reduce the antihypertensive effects of clonidine; the patient should be carefully monitored to confirm that the desired effect is being obtained)

**Laboratory value alterations**
The following have been selected on the basis of their potential clinical significance (possible effect in parentheses where appropriate)—not necessarily inclusive (» = major clinical significance):

With physiology/laboratory test values
Catecholamine concentrations, urinary, and
Vanillylmandelic acid (VMA) excretion, urinary
    (may be decreased but may increase on abrupt withdrawal)

Direct antiglobulin (Coombs') tests
    (may produce weakly positive results)

Growth hormone concentrations, plasma
    (may be increased transiently because of stimulation of growth hormone release, but are not elevated chronically with long-term use of clonidine)

**Medical considerations/Contraindications**
The medical considerations/contraindications included here have been selected on the basis of their potential clinical significance (reasons given in parentheses where appropriate)—not necessarily inclusive (» = major clinical significance).

*Risk-benefit should be considered when the following medical problems exist:*

Atrioventricular (AV) node function impairment
    (vagal effect of clonidine may exacerbate condition)

Cerebrovascular disease or
Coronary insufficiency or
Myocardial infarction, recent
    (lowered blood pressure may decrease perfusion and worsen ischemia)

Mental depression, history of or
Raynaud's syndrome
    (may be exacerbated by clonidine)

Renal function impairment, chronic
    (reduces the elimination of clonidine and may increase the risk of toxicity; dosage reduction may be necessary)

Sensitivity to clonidine

Sinus node function impairment
(function may be further impaired)

Thromboangiitis obliterans

*For transdermal dosage form only (in addition to above)*

Polyarteritis nodosa or

Scleroderma or

Systemic lupus erythematosus (SLE)
(absorption may be decreased; placement of patches on affected areas should be avoided)

Skin irritation or abrasion
(absorption may be increased; placement of patches on irritated or abraded areas should be avoided)

## Patient monitoring

The following may be especially important in patient monitoring (other tests may be warranted in some patients, depending on condition; » = major clinical significance):

» Blood pressure measurements
(recommended at periodic intervals in patients being treated for hypertension; selected patients may be taught to monitor their blood pressure at home and report the results at regular physician visits)

## Side/Adverse Effects

Note: Incidence and severity of adverse systemic effects may be reduced with the transdermal dosage form, possibly because this form of administration maintains lower peak blood concentrations than occur with oral administration and decreases fluctuation in blood concentration.

Administration of clonidine for 6 months or longer to albino rats has resulted in a dose-related increase in the incidence and severity of spontaneously occurring retinal degeneration. These effects have not been observed in humans.

The following side/adverse effects have been selected on the basis of their potential clinical significance (possible signs and symptoms in parentheses where appropriate)—not necessarily inclusive:

**Those indicating need for medical attention**

Incidence more frequent—about 15 to 20%, with transdermal systems only
*Itching or redness of skin*

Note: Patients who develop either a localized or an extended allergic reaction to the transdermal system may also experience a generalized allergic skin rash if oral clonidine is substituted.

Incidence less frequent
*Mental depression; sodium and water retention or edema* (swelling of feet and lower legs)

Incidence rare
*Raynaud's phenomenon* (paleness or cold feeling in fingertips and toes); *vivid dreams or nightmares*

**Those indicating need for medical attention only if they continue or are bothersome**

Incidence more frequent
*Constipation*—about 10%; *dizziness*—about 16% with oral use; *drowsiness*—about 33% with oral use; *dryness of mouth*—about 40% with oral use; *unusual tiredness or weakness*—about 10%

Incidence less frequent—1 to 5%
*Anorexia* (loss of appetite); *darkening of skin*—with transdermal systems only; *decreased sexual ability; dry, itching, or burning eyes; orthostatic hypotension* (dizziness, lightheadedness, or fainting, especially when getting up from a lying or sitting position); *nausea or vomiting; nervousness*

**Those indicating possible rebound hypertension and need for medical attention if they occur after medication is abruptly discontinued**

*Angina* (chest pain); *anxiety or tenseness; headache; increased salivation; nausea; nervousness; palpitations* (pounding heartbeat); *restlessness; shaking or trembling of hands and fingers; stomach cramps; sweating; tachycardia* (fast heartbeat); *trouble in sleeping; vomiting*

Note: *Rebound hypertension* may occur but is symptomatic in only 5 to 20% of patients. It is more likely to occur after abrupt withdrawal of clonidine in patients who had been receiving doses exceeding 1.2 mg per day or if clonidine therapy is discontinued before or at the same time as concurrent beta-adrenergic blocking agent therapy.

## Overdose

For more information on the management of overdose or unintentional ingestion, **contact a Poison Control Center** (see *Poison Control Center Listing*).

**Clinical effects of overdose**

The following effects have been selected on the basis of their potential clinical significance (possible signs and symptoms in parentheses where appropriate)—not necessarily inclusive:

*Apnea or respiratory depression* (difficulty in breathing); *bradycardia* (slow heartbeat); *hypotension* (dizziness or faintness); *hypothermia* (feeling cold); *lethargy* (unusual tiredness or weakness, extreme); *miosis* (pinpoint pupils of eyes)

Note: Overdose may result in hypertension, especially in pediatric patients.
Toxicity may occur with ingestion of 100 mcg (0.1 mg) in children.

**Treatment of overdose**

Specific treatment—

Recommended treatment for clonidine overdose is usually symptomatic and supportive and may include use of intravenous fluids.

For significant bradycardia: Atropine.

For hypotension: Dopamine infusion.

For hypertension: Intravenous furosemide, diazoxide, phentolamine, or nitroprusside.

Tolazoline infusion if necessary.

## Patient Consultation

As an aid to patient consultation, refer to *Advice for the Patient, Clonidine (Systemic)*.

In providing consultation, consider emphasizing the following selected information (» = major clinical significance):

**Before using this medication**

» Conditions affecting use, especially:
Sensitivity to clonidine or to ophthalmic apraclonidine
Pregnancy—Increased resorptions in rats and mice
Breast-feeding—Distributed into breast milk
Use in children—Caution recommended in children because accidental overdoses have been reported
Use in the elderly—Hypotensive effects may be more likely
Other medications, especially tricyclic antidepressants or beta-adrenergic blocking agents

**Proper use of this medication**

Proper administration of the transdermal dosage form:

» Compliance with therapy; reading patient instructions carefully
Not trimming or cutting patch
Applying to clean, dry skin area on upper arm or torso; area should be free of hair, scars, cuts, or irritation
Should remain in place even during showering, bathing, or swimming; applying adhesive overlay to loose systems; replacing systems that have loosened excessively or fallen off
Alternating application sites
Folding used patches in half with adhesive sides together; disposing of patch carefully, out of reach of children
Getting into the habit of taking or using at same time each day or week to help increase compliance

» Proper dosing

» Missed dose: Taking or using as soon as possible; checking with physician if miss two or more oral doses in a row or if are late in changing the transdermal system by 3 or more days; possible severe reaction if stopped abruptly

» Proper storage

*For use as an antihypertensive*

Possible need for control of weight and diet, especially sodium intake

» Patient may not experience symptoms of hypertension; importance of taking medication even if feeling well

» Does not cure, but helps control hypertension; possible need for lifelong therapy; serious consequences of untreated hypertension

**Precautions while using this medication**

Regular visits to physician to check progress

» Checking with physician before discontinuing medication; gradual dosage reduction may be necessary to avoid serious rebound hypertension

» Having enough medication on hand to get through weekends, holidays, and vacations; possibly carrying second prescription for emergency use

» Caution in taking alcohol or other CNS depressants

» Caution when driving or doing things requiring alertness, because of possible drowsiness

» Caution if any kind of surgery or emergency treatment is required

Caution when getting up suddenly from a lying or sitting position

Caution in using alcohol, while standing for long periods or exercising, and during hot weather, because of enhanced orthostatic hypotensive effects

Possible dryness of mouth; using sugarless candy or gum, ice, or saliva substitute for relief; checking with physician or dentist if dry mouth continues for more than 2 weeks

*For use as an antihypertensive*

» Not taking other medications, especially nonprescription sympathomimetics, unless discussed with physician

### Side/adverse effects

Signs of potential side effects, especially itching or redness of skin (transdermal), mental depression, sodium and water retention, edema, Raynaud's phenomenon, vivid dreams or nightmares, and withdrawal reaction

## General Dosing Information

With continued use, apparent tolerance to the antihypertensive effects of clonidine may develop as a result of fluid retention and expanded plasma volume. Concurrent administration of a diuretic may decrease this likelihood and will enhance the antihypertensive effects of clonidine. Other antihypertensives have also been used concurrently with clonidine. If combination therapy is indicated, individual titration is required to ensure the lowest possible therapeutic dose of each drug.

The abrupt interruption of clonidine therapy, including several consecutive missed doses, may result in rebound hypertension, which may be severe (acute post-treatment syndrome), or, in rare cases, overshoot hypertension, occurring within 12 to 48 hours of discontinuing therapy and lasting several days. Some patients may experience associated symptoms such as nervousness, agitation, and headache. At cessation of therapy, dosage should be gradually reduced (in the case of the transdermal system, by reducing patch strength and, if necessary, administering oral clonidine) over a 2- to 4-day period. Alternative therapy should be considered for unreliable or noncompliant patients. An excessive rise in blood pressure may be treated by resumption of oral clonidine therapy or by intravenous administration of diazoxide or an alpha-adrenergic blocking agent.

It is recommended that this medication be discontinued if mental depression occurs.

### For oral dosage form only

It is recommended that the last daily dose be taken at bedtime to ensure overnight control of blood pressure and reduce daytime drowsiness.

If clonidine therapy must be interrupted for surgery, it is recommended that the last dose be given no later than 4 to 6 hours prior to surgery, that parenteral hypotensive medication be administered throughout the procedure, and that clonidine therapy be reinstituted as soon as possible afterwards.

Clonidine has been used investigationally for rapid detoxification in the treatment of opioid withdrawal. One protocol used consists of a test dose of 5 to 6 mcg (0.005 to 0.006 mg) of clonidine hydrochloride per kg of body weight on the first day. Patients showing a positive response then receive 17 mcg (0.017 mg) of clonidine hydrochloride per kg of body weight in divided daily doses for 9 or 10 days (adjusted to avoid hypotension and oversedation), followed by a reduction to 50% of the dose on Days 11, 12, and 13, and no medication on Day 14. Dosage must be individualized according to each patient's tolerance.

### For transdermal dosage form only

Because the onset of action of transdermal clonidine is 2 to 3 days, when a patient is being switched from oral to transdermal therapy, the dose of oral clonidine should be gradually reduced over 2 to 3 days after transdermal therapy is begun, to avoid a withdrawal reaction.

Application should preferably be made at the same time of day each week to areas of clean, dry, hairless skin on the upper arm or torso. Skin areas with extensive scarring, calluses, or irritation should be avoided. Application sites should be alternated to avoid causing skin irritation.

The transdermal units *should not* be cut or trimmed in an attempt to adjust dosage.

If the transdermal system begins to loosen, the adhesive overlay provided by the manufacturer should be applied over the unit to hold it in place. A new dosage unit should be applied if the first becomes overly loosened or falls off.

If local skin irritation occurs before the system has been in place for 7 days, the system may be removed and a new one placed on a different

site. If contact sensitization persists, withdrawal of transdermal therapy may be necessary.

## Oral Dosage Forms

Note: Bracketed uses in the *Dosage Forms* section refer to categories of use and/or indications that are not included in U.S. product labeling.

### CLONIDINE HYDROCHLORIDE TABLETS USP

#### Usual adult dose

Antihypertensive—

Initial: Oral, 100 mcg (0.1 mg) two times a day, the dosage being increased by 100 or 200 mcg (0.1 or 0.2 mg, respectively) per day every two to four days if necessary for control of blood pressure.

Maintenance: Oral, 200 to 600 mcg (0.2 to 0.6 mg) per day, in divided doses.

Severe hypertension in the urgent but not emergency situation (loading dose): Oral, 200 mcg (0.2 mg), followed by 100 mcg (0.1 mg) every hour until diastolic blood pressure is controlled or a total of 800 mcg (0.8 mg) has been given; the patient is then controlled on a normal maintenance dose.

[Vascular headache prophylactic][1]—

Oral, 25 mcg (0.025 mg) two to four times a day up to 50 mcg (0.05 mg) three times a day.

[Antidysmenorrheal][1]—

Severe dysmenorrhea: Oral, 25 mcg (0.025 mg) two times a day for fourteen days before and during menses.

[Menopausal syndrome therapy adjunct]—

Oral, 25 to 75 mcg (0.025 to 0.075 mg) two times a day.

Note: Geriatric patients may be more sensitive to the effects of the usual adult dose.

#### Usual adult prescribing limits

Antihypertensive—Up to 2.4 mg daily.

#### Usual pediatric dose

Safety and efficacy have not been established.

#### Strength(s) usually available

U.S.—

100 mcg (0.1 mg) (Rx) [*Catapres* (scored; lactose); GENERIC (may be scored; may contain lactose)].

200 mcg (0.2 mg) (Rx) [*Catapres* (scored; lactose); GENERIC (may be scored; may contain lactose)].

300 mcg (0.3 mg) (Rx) [*Catapres* (scored; lactose); GENERIC (may be scored; may contain lactose)].

Note: Not commercially available in 25-mcg (0.025-mg) strength used for indications other than hypertension; extemporaneous compounding required.

Canada—

25 mcg (0.025 mg) (Rx) [*Dixarit* (lactose)].

100 mcg (0.1 mg) (Rx) [*Catapres* (scored)].

200 mcg (0.2 mg) (Rx) [*Catapres* (scored)].

Note: 100 mcg of the hydrochloride salt is equivalent to 87 mcg of the free base.

#### Packaging and storage

Store below 40 °C (104 °F), preferably between 15 and 30 °C (59 and 86 °F), unless otherwise specified by manufacturer. Store in a well-closed container.

#### Auxiliary labeling

• Avoid alcoholic beverages.

• Do not miss doses.

• Do not take other medicines without your doctor's advice.

#### Note

Check refill frequency to determine compliance in hypertensive patients.

## Topical Dosage Forms

### CLONIDINE TRANSDERMAL SYSTEM

#### Usual adult dose

Antihypertensive—

Topical, to the intact skin, 1 transdermal dosage system, beginning with the system delivering 100 mcg (0.1 mg) per day, once a week. Dosage adjustments may be made every one or two weeks by changing to the next larger dosage system or a combination of systems.

#### Usual pediatric dose

Dosage has not been established.

**Strength(s) usually available**

U.S.—

    2.5 mg (delivering 100 mcg [0.1 mg] per day) (Rx) [*Catapres-TTS*].

    5.0 mg (delivering 200 mcg [0.2 mg] per day) (Rx) [*Catapres-TTS*].

    7.5 mg (delivering 300 mcg [0.3 mg] per day) (Rx) [*Catapres-TTS*].

    Note: All systems are designed to release a constant, controlled dose of clonidine. The actual dose delivered will be as labeled and as intended, but less than the total content of each system.

Canada—

    Not commercially available.

**Packaging and storage**

Store below 30 °C (86 °F), unless otherwise specified by manufacturer.

**Auxiliary labeling**

• Avoid alcoholic beverages.

• For external use only.

• Do not miss doses.

• Do not take other medicines without your doctor's advice.

**Note**

Include patient instructions when dispensing.

Check refill frequency to determine compliance in hypertensive patients.

    [1]Not included in Canadian product labeling.

## Selected Bibliography

Transdermal clonidine for hypertension. Med Lett Drugs Ther 1985 Nov 8; 27: 95-6.

The fifth report of the Joint National Committee on Detection, Evaluation, and Treatment of High Blood Pressure (JNC V). Arch Intern Med 1993; 153 (2): 154-83.

Revised: 05/17/93

# CLONIDINE AND CHLORTHALIDONE  Systemic

VA CLASSIFICATION (Primary): CV400

Note: For a listing of dosage forms and brand names by country availability, see *Dosage Forms* section(s). For a listing of brand names for the articles in this monograph, refer to the General Index.

## Category

Antihypertensive.

## Indications

**Accepted**

Hypertension (treatment)—The combination of clonidine and chlorthalidone is indicated for treatment of hypertension.

    Fixed-dosage combinations are generally not recommended for initial therapy and are useful for subsequent therapy only when the proportion of the component agents corresponds to the dose of the individual agents, as determined by titration.

    For additional information on initial therapeutic guidelines related to the treatment of hypertension, see *Appendix III*.

## Pharmacology/Pharmacokinetics

**Physicochemical characteristics**

Molecular weight—Chlorthalidone: 338.77.

Clonidine: 230.10.

Clonidine hydrochloride: 266.56.

**Mechanism of action/Effect**

Chlorthalidone—Diuretics lower blood pressure initially by reducing plasma and extracellular fluid volume; cardiac output also decreases. Eventually, cardiac output returns to normal. Thiazide diuretics decrease peripheral resistance by a direct peripheral effect on blood vessels.

Clonidine—Antihypertensive effect is thought to be due to central alpha$_2$-adrenergic stimulation, which results in a decreased sympathetic outflow to the heart, kidneys, and peripheral vasculature; this results in decreased peripheral vascular resistance, decreased systolic and diastolic blood pressure, and decreased heart rate.

**Absorption**

Chlorthalidone—Thiazide diuretics are absorbed relatively rapidly after oral administration.

Clonidine—Well absorbed following oral administration. Bioavailability following chronic administration is approximately 65%.

**Protein binding**

Chlorthalidone—High (75% [58% to albumin]); increased affinity to carbonic anhydrase in red blood cells.

Clonidine—Low to moderate (20 to 40%).

**Biotransformation**

Clonidine—Hepatic (about 50% of the absorbed dose).

**Half-life**

Chlorthalidone—

    35 to 40 hours.

Clonidine—

    Normal renal function: Range, 12 to 16 hours.

    Renal function impairment: Up to 41 hours.

**Onset of action**

Clonidine—30 to 60 minutes.

**Time to peak plasma concentration**

Clonidine—1.5 to 2.5 hours.

**Time to peak effect**

Clonidine—2 to 4 hours.

**Elimination**

Chlorthalidone—

    Unchanged; almost totally via the kidneys, with minute quantities in the bile.

Clonidine—

    Renal: 40 to 60% (as unchanged drug) in 24 hours.

    Biliary/fecal: 20% (probably via enterohepatic circulation).

    In dialysis: Very little (maximum 5%) removable by hemodialysis.

## Precautions to Consider

**Cross-sensitivity and/or related problems**

Patients sensitive to ophthalmic apraclonidine or to sulfonamide-type medications, bumetanide, furosemide, or carbonic anhydrase inhibitors may be sensitive to this medication also.

**Carcinogenicity**

Studies in rats given doses 32 to 46 times the maximum recommended human dose for 132 weeks showed no evidence of carcinogenicity.

**Pregnancy/Reproduction**

Fertility—

    *Clonidine:*

        Studies in male and female rats given doses up to 3 times the maximum recommended human dose showed no impairment of fertility. However, fertility was affected in female rats given 10 to 40 times the maximum recommended human dose.

Pregnancy—

    *Chlorthalidone:*

        Thiazide diuretics cross the placenta and appear in cord blood. Although studies in humans have not been done, thiazide diuretics can cause fetal harm when given to pregnant women. Fetal or neonatal jaundice has been reported.

        Pregnant women should be advised to contact physician before taking this medication, since routine use of diuretics during normal pregnancy is inappropriate and exposes mother and fetus to unnecessary hazard. Thiazide diuretics do not prevent development of toxemia of pregnancy, and there is no satisfactory evidence that they are useful in the treatment of toxemia. Thiazide diuretics are indicated only in the treatment of edema due to pathologic causes or as a short course of treatment in patients with severe hypervolemia. Possible hazards include fetal or neonatal jaundice, thrombocytopenia, or other adverse reactions seen in adults.

        Studies in rats and rabbits at doses up to 420 times the human dose have not shown that chlorthalidone causes adverse effects in the fetus.

    FDA Pregnancy Category B.

    *Clonidine:*

        Adequate and well-controlled studies in humans have not been done.

Studies in rats given doses as low as one-third the maximum recommended human dose for 2 months prior to mating showed an increased incidence of resorptions; this effect did not occur at doses of one-third to 3 times the maximum recommended human dose given on days 6 to 15 of gestation. Increased resorptions also occurred in rats and mice given doses up to 40 times the maximum recommended human dose on days 1 to 14 of gestation. No teratogenicity or embryotoxicity was observed in rabbits given up to 3 times the maximum recommended human dose.

FDA Pregnancy Category C.

**Breast-feeding**
*Chlorthalidone*— Thiazide diuretics are distributed into breast milk. The American Academy of Pediatrics recommends that nursing mothers avoid thiazide diuretics during the first month of lactation because of reports of suppression of lactation.
*Clonidine*— Clonidine is distributed into breast milk.

**Pediatrics**
*Chlorthalidone*— Although appropriate studies on the relationship of age to the effects of thiazide diuretics have not been performed in the pediatric population, pediatrics-specific problems that would limit the usefulness of this medication in children are not expected. However, caution is required in jaundiced infants because of the risk of hyperbilirubinemia.
*Clonidine*— Appropriate studies on the relationship of age to the effects of clonidine have not been performed in the pediatric population. However, there are numerous reports describing accidental clonidine overdose in the pediatric population. These reports seem to indicate that neonates, infants, and children are especially sensitive to the effects of clonidine. Caution is recommended.

**Geriatrics**
The elderly may be more sensitive than younger adults to the hypotensive and electrolyte-depleting effects of clonidine and chlorthalidone combination. In addition, elderly patients are more likely to have age-related renal function impairment, which may require caution and/or reduction of dosage in patients receiving clonidine and chlorthalidone combination.

**Dental**
Use of clonidine may decrease or inhibit salivary flow, thus contributing to the development of caries, periodontal disease, oral candidiasis, and discomfort.

**Drug interactions and/or related problems**
The following drug interactions and/or related problems have been selected on the basis of their potential clinical significance (possible mechanism in parentheses where appropriate)—not necessarily inclusive (» = major clinical significance):

Note: Combinations containing any of the following medications, depending on the amount present, may also interact with this medication.

Alcohol or
Central nervous system (CNS) depression–producing medications (See *Appendix II*)
(concurrent use may enhance the CNS depressant effects of either these medications or clonidine)

Amiodarone
(concurrent use of thiazide diuretics with amiodarone may lead to an increased risk of arrhythmias associated with hypokalemia)

Anticoagulants, coumarin- or indandione-derivative
(effects may be decreased when used concurrently with thiazide diuretics as a result of reduction of plasma volume leading to concentration of procoagulant factors in the blood; in addition, diuretic-induced improvement of hepatic congestion may lead to improved hepatic function resulting in increased procoagulant factor synthesis; dosage adjustments may be necessary)

» Antidepressants, tricyclic or
Appetite suppressants, with the exception of fenfluramine
(concurrent use may decrease the hypotensive effects of clonidine)

Antidiabetic agents, oral or
Insulin
(thiazide diuretics may raise blood glucose concentrations; for adult-onset diabetics, dosage adjustment of hypoglycemic medications may be necessary during and after thiazide diuretic therapy; insulin requirements may be increased, decreased, or unchanged)

Anti-inflammatory drugs, nonsteroidal (NSAIDs), especially indomethacin
(NSAIDs may antagonize the natriuresis and increase in plasma renin activity [PRA] caused by thiazide diuretics; NSAIDs may also reduce the antihypertensive effects of clonidine and chlorthalidone combination, possibly by inhibiting renal prostaglandin synthesis and/or causing sodium and fluid retention; the patient should be carefully monitored to confirm that the desired effect is being obtained)
(in addition, concurrent use of NSAIDs with a diuretic may increase the risk of renal failure secondary to a decrease in renal blood flow caused by inhibition of renal prostaglandin synthesis)

» Beta-adrenergic blocking agents (systemic)
(discontinuation of clonidine therapy during concurrent use of beta-adrenergic blocking agents may increase the risk of clonidine-withdrawal hypertensive crisis; ideally, beta-adrenergic blocking agents should be discontinued several days before clonidine is discontinued; blood pressure control may also be impaired when the 2 are combined)

Calcium-containing medications
(concurrent use of thiazide diuretics with large doses of calcium may result in hypercalcemia because of reduced calcium excretion)

» Cholestyramine or
» Colestipol
(may inhibit gastrointestinal absorption of the thiazide diuretics; administration of thiazide diuretics 1 hour before or 4 hours after cholestyramine or colestipol is recommended)

Diazoxide
(concurrent use with thiazide diuretics may enhance hyperglycemic effects; monitoring of blood glucose levels and/or dosage adjustment of one or both agents may be necessary)
(in addition, concurrent use with thiazide diuretics may enhance hyperuricemic and antihypertensive effects)

» Digitalis glycosides
(concurrent use with thiazide diuretics may enhance the possibility of digitalis toxicity associated with hypokalemia or hypomagnesemia)

Dopamine
(concurrent use may increase the diuretic effect of either thiazide diuretics or dopamine, as a result of dopamine's direct effect on dopaminergic receptors to produce vasodilation of renal vasculature and increase renal blood flow; dopamine also has a direct natriuretic effect)

Estrogens
(estrogen-induced fluid retention may increase blood pressure)

Fenfluramine
(concurrent use may increase the hypotensive effects of clonidine)

Hypokalemia-causing medications, other (See *Appendix II*)
(risk of severe hypokalemia due to other hypokalemia-causing medications may be increased; monitoring of serum potassium concentrations and cardiac function and potassium supplementation may be necessary)

Hypotension-producing medications, other (See *Appendix II*), with the exception of systemic beta-adrenergic blocking agents and tricyclic antidepressants
(concurrent use may potentiate antihypertensive effects; although some antihypertensive and/or diuretic combinations are frequently used for therapeutic advantage, dosage adjustments may be necessary during concurrent use)

» Lithium
(concurrent use with thiazide diuretics is not recommended, as they may increase the risk of lithium toxicity because of reduced renal clearance; in addition, lithium has nephrotoxic effects)

Neuromuscular blocking agents, nondepolarizing
(thiazide diuretics may induce hypokalemia, which may enhance the blockade of nondepolarizing neuromuscular blocking agents; serum potassium determinations may be necessary prior to administration of nondepolarizing neuromuscular blocking agents; careful postoperative monitoring of the patient may be necessary following concurrent or sequential use, especially if there is a possibility of incomplete reversal of neuromuscular blockade)

Sympathomimetics
(concurrent use may reduce the antihypertensive effects of clonidine and chlorthalidone combination; the patient should be carefully monitored to confirm that the desired effect is being obtained)

**Laboratory value alterations**
The following have been selected on the basis of their potential clinical significance (possible effect in parentheses where appropriate)—not necessarily inclusive (» = major clinical significance):

With diagnostic test results
Bentiromide
(administration of thiazide diuretics during a bentiromide test period will invalidate test results since thiazide diuretics are also

metabolized to arylamines and will thus increase the percent of para-aminobenzoic acid [PABA] recovered; discontinuation of thiazide diuretics at least 3 days prior to the administration of bentiromide is recommended)

Direct antiglobulin (Coombs') tests
   (may produce weakly positive results)

With physiology/laboratory test values
Bilirubin
   (serum concentrations may be increased by displacement from albumin binding)

Calcium concentrations, serum
   (may be increased; thiazide diuretics should be discontinued before parathyroid function tests are carried out)

Calcium concentrations, urinary
   (may be decreased)

Catecholamine concentrations, urinary and
Vanillylmandelic acid (VMA) excretion, urinary
   (may be decreased but may increase on abrupt withdrawal of clonidine)

Cholesterol, low-density lipoprotein and
Triglyceride and
Creatinine
   (serum concentrations may be increased)

Glucose, blood and urine
   (concentrations may be increased, usually only in patients with a predisposition to glucose intolerance)

Growth hormone concentrations, plasma
   (may be increased transiently because of stimulation of growth hormone release, but are not elevated chronically with long-term use of clonidine)

Magnesium and
Potassium and
Sodium
   (serum concentrations may be decreased; serum magnesium concentrations may increase in uremic patients; a fall in sodium can be life-threatening)

Protein-bound iodine (PBI)
   (serum concentrations may be decreased)

Uric acid
   (serum concentrations may be increased)

## Medical considerations/Contraindications

The medical considerations/contraindications included here have been selected on the basis of their potential clinical significance (reasons given in parentheses where appropriate)—not necessarily inclusive (» = major clinical significance).

### Risk-benefit should be considered when the following medical problems exist:

» Anuria or severe renal function impairment
   (chlorthalidone ineffective and may precipitate azotemia; may produce cumulative effects)

Atrioventricular (AV) node function impairment
   (vagal effect of clonidine may exacerbate condition)

Cerebrovascular disease or
Coronary insufficiency or
Myocardial infarction, recent
   (lowered blood pressure may decrease perfusion and worsen ischemia)

Diabetes mellitus
   (hypoglycemic medication requirements may be altered)

Gout, history of or
Hyperuricemia
   (serum uric acid concentrations may be elevated by thiazide diuretics)

Hepatic function impairment
   (risk of dehydration, which may precipitate hepatic coma and death; plasma half-life is unaltered)

Hypercalcemia or
Hypercholesterolemia or
Hypertriglyceridemia or
Hyponatremia
   (conditions may be exacerbated by thiazide diuretics; onset of hyponatremia can be sudden and life-threatening)

Lupus erythematosus, history of
   (exacerbation or activation by thiazide diuretics has been reported)

Mental depression, history of or
Raynaud's syndrome
   (may be exacerbated by clonidine)

Pancreatitis

Renal function impairment, chronic
   (reduces the elimination of clonidine and may increase the risk of toxicity; dosage reduction may be necessary)

Sensitivity to clonidine or thiazide diuretics or other sulfonamide-derived medications

Sinus node function impairment
   (function may be further impaired by clonidine and chlorthalidone combination)

Sympathectomy
   (antihypertensive effects may be enhanced)

Thromboangiitis obliterans

» Caution is required also in jaundiced infants because of the risk of hyperbilirubinemia.

## Patient monitoring

The following may be especially important in patient monitoring (other tests may be warranted in some patients, depending on condition; » = major clinical significance):

Blood glucose and
Blood urea nitrogen (BUN) and
Creatinine, serum and
Uric acid, serum
   (determinations recommended prior to initiation of therapy and if clinical signs of a significant increase occur)

» Blood pressure measurements
   (recommended at periodic intervals; selected patients may be taught to monitor their blood pressure at home and report the results at regular physician visits)

Cholesterol, serum and
Triglycerides, serum
   (determinations recommended after 6 months of therapy and annually thereafter)

Electrolyte, serum, concentrations
   (determinations may be required for patients on long-term therapy, especially if they are also taking cardiac glycosides or systemic corticosteroids, or when severe cirrhosis is present)

# Side/Adverse Effects

Note: Administration of clonidine for 6 months or longer to albino rats has resulted in a dose-related increase in the incidence and severity of spontaneously occurring retinal degeneration. This effect has not been observed in humans.

## Those indicating need for medical attention

Incidence more frequent

**Electrolyte imbalance, such as hyponatremia, hypochloremic alkalosis, and hypokalemia** (confusion; convulsions; decreased mentation; dryness of mouth; fatigue; increased thirst; irregular heartbeat; irritability; mood or mental changes; muscle cramps or pain; nausea or vomiting; unusual tiredness or weakness; weak pulse)

Note: *Hyponatremia* as a complication is rare, but constitutes a medical emergency as onset may be rapid.

Incidence less frequent

**Mental depression; sodium and water retention or edema** (swelling of feet and lower legs)

Incidence rare

**Agranulocytosis** (fever or chills; cough or hoarseness); **allergic reaction** (skin rash or hives); **cholecystitis or pancreatitis** (severe stomach pain with nausea and vomiting); **gout or hyperuricemia** (joint pain, lower back or side pain); **hepatic function impairment** (yellow eyes or skin); **Raynaud's phenomenon** (paleness or cold feeling in fingertips and toes); **thrombocytopenia** (unusual bleeding or bruising; black, tarry stools; blood in urine or stools; pinpoint red spots on skin); **vivid dreams or nightmares**

## Those indicating need for medical attention only if they continue or are bothersome

Incidence more frequent

**Constipation**—about 10%; **dizziness**—about 16%; **drowsiness**—about 33%; **dryness of mouth**—about 40%; **unusual tiredness or weakness**

Incidence less frequent

**Anorexia** (loss of appetite); **decreased sexual ability; diarrhea; dry, itching, or burning eyes; orthostatic hypotension** (dizziness, lightheadedness, or fainting, especially when getting up from a lying or sitting position); *photosensitivity* (increased sensitivity of skin to sunlight); *nausea or vomiting; nervousness; upset stomach*

**Those indicating possible rebound hypertension and need for medical attention if they occur after medication is abruptly discontinued**

*Angina* (chest pain); *anxiety or tenseness; headache; increased salivation; nausea; nervousness; palpitations* (pounding heartbeat); *restlessness; shaking or trembling of hands and fingers; stomach cramps; sweating; tachycardia* (fast heartbeat); *trouble in sleeping; vomiting*

Note: *Rebound hypertension* may occur but is symptomatic in only 5 to 20% of patients. It is more likely to occur after abrupt withdrawal of clonidine in patients who had been receiving doses exceeding 1.2 mg per day or if clonidine therapy is discontinued before or at the same time as concurrent beta-adrenergic blocking agent therapy.

## Overdose

For specific information on the agents used in the management of clonidine and chlorthalidone overdose, see:
- *Atropine* in *Anticholinergics/Antispasmodics (Systemic)* monograph;
- *Diazoxide (Parenteral–Systemic)* monograph;
- *Dopamine* in *Sympathomimetic Agents (Parenteral-Systemic)* monograph;
- *Furosemide* in *Diuretics, Loop (Systemic)* monograph;
- *Nitroprusside (Systemic)* monograph;
- *Phentolamine Mesylate (Systemic)* monograph; and/or
- *Tolazoline (Parenteral–Systemic)* monograph.

For more information on the management of overdose or unintentional ingestion, **contact a Poison Control Center** (see *Poison Control Center Listing*).

**Clinical effects of overdose**

The following effects have been selected on the basis of their potential clinical significance (possible signs and symptoms in parentheses where appropriate)—not necessarily inclusive:

*Apnea or respiratory depression* (difficulty in breathing); *bradycardia* (slow heartbeat); *hypotension* (dizziness or faintness); *hypothermia* (feeling cold); *lethargy* (unusual tiredness or weakness, extreme); *miosis* (pinpoint pupils of eyes)

Note: Overdose may result in hypertension, especially in pediatric patients.

Toxicity may occur with ingestion of 100 mcg (0.1 mg) in children.

**Treatment of overdose**

Specific treatment—
Usually symptomatic and supportive and may include use of intravenous fluids.
For bradycardia—Atropine.
For hypotension—dopamine infusion.
For hypertension—Intravenous furosemide, diazoxide, phentolamine, or nitroprusside.
Tolazoline infusion if necessary.

Monitoring—
Monitoring of serum electrolyte concentrations and renal function.

Supportive care—
Patients in whom intentional overdose is confirmed or suspected should be referred for psychiatric consultation.

## Patient Consultation

As an aid to patient consultation, refer to *Advice for the Patient, Clonidine and Chlorthalidone (Systemic)*.

In providing consultation, consider emphasizing the following selected information (» = major clinical significance):

**Before using this medication**

» Conditions affecting use, especially:
  Sensitivity to clonidine or to ophthalmic apraclonidine, or to sulfonamide-type medications
  Pregnancy—Chlorthalidone: Risk of jaundice, thrombocytopenia, hypokalemia in infant
  Breast-feeding—Distributed into breast milk; may suppress lactation
  Use in children—Caution recommended in children because accidental overdoses have been reported
  Use in the elderly—Hypotensive and hypokalemic effects may be more likely

Other medications, especially tricyclic antidepressants, beta-adrenergic blocking agents, cholestyramine, colestipol, digitalis glycosides, or lithium
Other medical problems, especially severe renal function impairment

**Proper use of this medication**

Diuretic effects of the medication and timing of doses to minimize inconvenience of diuresis
Possible need for control of weight and diet, especially sodium intake
» Patient may not experience symptoms of hypertension; importance of taking medication even if feeling well
» Does not cure, but helps control hypertension; possible need for lifelong therapy; serious consequences of untreated hypertension
Getting into habit of taking at same time each day to help increase compliance
» Proper dosing
» Missed dose: Taking as soon as remembered; checking with physician if two or more doses in a row are missed
» Proper storage

**Precautions while using this medication**

Regular visits to physician to check progress
» Checking with physician before discontinuing medication; gradual dosage reduction may be necessary to avoid serious rebound hypertension
» Having enough medication on hand to get through weekends, holidays, and vacations; possibly carrying second prescription for emergency use
» Caution if any kind of surgery or emergency treatment is required
» Not taking other medications, especially nonprescription sympathomimetics, unless discussed with physician
» Caution in taking alcohol or other central nervous system (CNS) depressants
» Caution when driving or doing things requiring alertness, because of possible drowsiness
Caution when getting up suddenly from a lying or sitting position
Caution in using alcohol, while standing for long periods or exercising, and during hot weather because of enhanced orthostatic hypotensive effects
» Possibility of hypokalemia; possible need for additional potassium in diet; not changing diet without first checking with physician
To prevent dehydration, checking with physician if severe nausea, vomiting, or diarrhea occurs and continues
Diabetics: May increase blood sugar levels
Possible photosensitivity; avoiding unprotected exposure to sun; using protective clothing and sun block product; avoiding use of sunlamp, tanning bed, or tanning booth
Possible dryness of mouth; using sugarless candy or gum, ice, or saliva substitute for relief; checking with physician or dentist if dry mouth continues for more than 2 weeks

**Side/adverse effects**

Signs of potential side effects, especially electrolyte imbalance, mental depression, sodium and water retention or edema, agranulocytosis, allergic reaction, cholecystitis or pancreatitis, hyperuricemia or gout, hepatic function impairment, Raynaud's phenomenon, thrombocytopenia, and vivid dreams or nightmares

## General Dosing Information

Dosage must be adjusted to meet the individual requirements of each patient, on the basis of clinical response. The lowest effective dosage should be utilized to minimize potential electrolyte imbalance.

Fixed-dosage combinations are generally not recommended for initial therapy and are useful for subsequent therapy only when the proportion of the component agents corresponds to the dose of the individual agents, as determined by titration.

It is recommended that the last daily dose be taken at bedtime to ensure overnight control of blood pressure and reduce daytime drowsiness.

Concurrent administration of potassium supplements or potassium-sparing diuretics may be indicated in patients considered to be at higher risk for developing hypokalemia. Caution in administering potassium supplements is recommended, however, since loss of potassium is not clinically significant in most patients, and supplementation leads to a risk of development of hyperkalemia.

Because of the risk of sodium depletion due to chlorthalidone, severe dietary sodium restriction is not recommended.

The abrupt interruption of clonidine therapy, including several consecutive missed doses, may result in rebound hypertension, which may be severe (acute post-treatment syndrome) or, in rare cases, overshoot hypertension, occurring within 12 to 48 hours and lasting several days. Some patients may experience associated symptoms such as nervousness, agitation, and headache. At cessation of therapy, dosage should be gradually reduced over a 2- to 4-day period. Alternative therapy should be considered for unreliable or noncompliant patients. An excessive rise in blood pressure may be treated by resumption of clonidine therapy or by intravenous administration of diazoxide or an alpha-adrenergic blocking agent.

Recent evidence suggests that withdrawal of antihypertensive therapy prior to surgery may not be desirable. However, the anesthesiologist must be aware of such therapy.

If clonidine therapy must be interrupted for surgery, it is recommended that the last dose be given no later than 4 to 6 hours prior to surgery, that parenteral hypotensive medication be administered throughout the procedure, and that clonidine therapy be reinstituted as soon as possible afterwards.

It is recommended that therapy with clonidine and chlorthalidone be withdrawn if a significant rise in blood urea nitrogen (BUN) occurs.

It is recommended that this medication be discontinued if mental depression occurs.

## Oral Dosage Forms

### CLONIDINE HYDROCHLORIDE AND CHLORTHALIDONE TABLETS USP

**Usual adult dose**
Oral, 1 or 2 tablets two to four times a day, as determined by individual titration with the component agents.

Note: Geriatric patients may be more sensitive to the effects of the usual adult dose.

**Usual adult prescribing limits**
Up to 2.4 mg of clonidine hydrochloride daily.

**Usual pediatric dose**
Dosage has not been established.

**Strength(s) usually available**
U.S.—
  100 mcg (0.1 mg) clonidine hydrochloride and 15 mg chlorthalidone (Rx) [*Combipres* (scored; lactose); GENERIC].
  200 mcg (0.2 mg) clonidine hydrochloride and 15 mg chlorthalidone (Rx) [*Combipres* (scored; lactose); GENERIC].

  300 mcg (0.3 mg) clonidine hydrochloride and 15 mg chlorthalidone (Rx) [*Combipres* (scored; lactose); GENERIC].
Canada—
  100 mcg (0.1 mg) clonidine hydrochloride and 15 mg chlorthalidone (Rx) [*Combipres* (scored)].
Note: 100 mcg of clonidine hydrochloride is equivalent to 87 mcg of the free base.

**Packaging and storage**
Store below 40 °C (104 °F), preferably between 15 and 30 °C (59 and 86 °F), unless otherwise specified by manufacturer. Store in a well-closed container.

**Auxiliary labeling**
• Avoid alcoholic beverages.
• Do not miss doses.
• Do not take other medicines without your doctor's advice.

**Note**
Check refill frequency to determine compliance in hypertensive patients.

## Selected Bibliography
The fifth report of the Joint National Committee on Detection, Evaluation, and Treatment of High Blood Pressure (JNC V). Arch Intern Med 1993; 153 (2): 154-83.

Revised: 08/02/94

## CLONIDINE-CONTAINING COMBINATIONS—
Clonidine and Chlorthalidone (Systemic)

## CLORAZEPATE—See *Benzodiazepines (Systemic)*

## CLOTRIMAZOLE—See *Antifungals, Azole (Vaginal); Clotrimazole (Oral-Local); Clotrimazole (Topical)*

# CLOTRIMAZOLE   Oral-Local†

VA CLASSIFICATION (Primary): AM700
Note: For a listing of dosage forms and brand names by country availability, see *Dosage Forms* section(s). For a listing of brand names for the articles in this monograph, refer to the General Index.

  †Not commercially available in Canada.

## Category

Antifungal (oral-local)..
Note: Clotrimazole is a broad-spectrum antifungal.

## Indications

**Accepted**
Candidiasis, oropharyngeal (treatment)—Oral clotrimazole is indicated as a primary agent in nonimmunosuppressed and immunosuppressed patients in the local treatment of oropharyngeal candidiasis (thrush) caused by *Candida* species.

Candidiasis, oropharyngeal (prophylaxis)—Oral clotrimazole is indicated as a primary agent in immunosuppressed patients in the local prophylaxis of oropharyngeal candidiasis caused by *Candida* species.

Not all species or strains of a particular organism may be susceptible to clotrimazole.

**Unaccepted**
Clotrimazole lozenges are not indicated in the treatment of systemic mycoses.

## Pharmacology/Pharmacokinetics

**Physicochemical characteristics**
Molecular weight—344.84.

**Mechanism of action/Effect**
Fungistatic; may be fungicidal, depending on concentration; inhibits biosynthesis of ergosterol or other sterols, damaging the fungal cell wall membrane and altering its permeability; as a result, loss of essential intracellular elements may occur; also inhibits biosynthesis of triglycerides and phospholipids by fungi; in addition, inhibits oxidative and peroxidative enzyme activity, resulting in intracellular buildup of toxic concentrations of hydrogen peroxide, which may contribute to deterioration of subcellular organelles and cellular necrosis. In *Candida albicans*, inhibits transformation of blastospores into invasive mycelial form.

**Other actions/effects**
Also has some antibacterial activity.

**Absorption**
Poorly and erratically absorbed, even when swallowed.

**Binding**
Apparently bound to oral mucosa from which it is slowly released.

**Biotransformation**
When swallowed, absorbed clotrimazole is metabolized in the liver to inactive compounds; induces hepatic microsomal enzyme activity, resulting in acceleration of its own catabolism.

**Saliva concentration**
Sufficient to inhibit most species of *Candida* present in saliva (5.2 to 15 mcg per mL after dissolution of troche).

**Duration of action**
Up to 3 hours.

**Elimination**
Fecal.

# Precautions to Consider

## Carcinogenicity
An 18-month study in rats has not shown any carcinogenic effects.

## Pregnancy/Reproduction
Pregnancy—Adequate and well-controlled studies in humans have not been done.

Studies in rats and mice, given doses 100 times the usual adult human dose (in mg per kg), have shown that clotrimazole is embryotoxic. In addition, clotrimazole, given orally to mice in doses 120 times the usual human dose, has been shown to cause impairment of mating, decreased number of viable young, and decreased survival to weaning. No effects were seen at doses 60 times the usual human dose. When given to rats at doses 50 times the usual human dose, clotrimazole caused a slight decrease in the number of pups per litter and decreased pup viability. However, no teratogenic effects were seen in mice, rabbits, or rats given doses up to 200, 180, and 100 times the usual human dose, respectively.

FDA Pregnancy Category C.

## Breast-feeding
It is not known whether clotrimazole is excreted in breast milk; however, clotrimazole is poorly and erratically absorbed, even when swallowed.

## Pediatrics
Use of clotrimazole troches is not recommended in infants and children up to 5 years of age since this age group may not be capable of using the lozenge safely. No pediatrics-specific problems have been documented to date in children over 5 years old.

## Geriatrics
Appropriate studies on the relationship of age to the effects of clotrimazole have not been performed in the geriatric population. However, no geriatrics-specific problems have been documented to date.

## Laboratory value alterations
The following have been selected on the basis of their potential clinical significance (possible effect in parentheses where appropriate)—not necessarily inclusive (» = major clinical significance):

With physiology/laboratory test values
>   Aspartate aminotransferase (AST [SGOT]), serum
        (concentration may be minimally increased in up to 15% of patients)

## Medical considerations/Contraindications
The medical considerations/contraindications included here have been selected on the basis of their potential clinical significance (reasons given in parentheses where appropriate)—not necessarily inclusive (» = major clinical significance).

*Risk-benefit should be considered when the following medical problem exists:*

Hypersensitivity to clotrimazole

# Side/Adverse Effects

The following side/adverse effects have been selected on the basis of their potential clinical significance (possible signs and symptoms in parentheses where appropriate)—not necessarily inclusive:

**Those indicating need for medical attention only if they continue or are bothersome**
Incidence more frequent—when swallowed
   *Gastrointestinal disturbance* (abdominal or stomach cramping or pain; diarrhea; nausea or vomiting)

# Patient Consultation

As an aid to patient consultation, refer to *Advice for the Patient, Clotrimazole (Oral)*.

In providing consultation, consider emphasizing the following selected information (» = major clinical significance):

**Before using this medication**
>   Conditions affecting use, especially:
        Hypersensitivity to clotrimazole
        Use in children—Use is not recommended in children up to 5 years of age

**Proper use of this medication**
   Proper administration technique:
        Holding lozenge in mouth and allowing it to dissolve slowly and completely
        Swallowing saliva during this time
>   Not chewing or swallowing lozenge whole
>   Not giving to infants or children under 4 to 5 years of age
>   Compliance with full course of therapy; fungal infections may require prolonged therapy
>   Proper dosing
        Missed dose: Using as soon as possible; not using if almost time for next dose
>   Proper storage

**Precautions while using this medication**
   Checking with physician if no improvement within 1 week

# General Dosing Information

To provide prolonged oral contact with the medication and to achieve maximum effect, clotrimazole lozenges should be held in the mouth and allowed to dissolve slowly (and completely) over a 15- to 30-minute period. Saliva should be swallowed during this time. Clotrimazole lozenges should not be chewed or swallowed whole.

Since only limited data are available on the safety and efficacy of clotrimazole lozenges during prolonged administration, short-term administration is recommended whenever possible. However, clotrimazole lozenges have been used daily for approximately 3 months in renal transplant patients without apparent ill effects.

# Oral Dosage Forms
## CLOTRIMAZOLE LOZENGES

**Usual adult and adolescent dose**
Antifungal—
   Treatment: Oral, as a lozenge dissolved slowly and completely in the mouth, 10 mg five times a day for fourteen days or longer, especially in immunosuppressed patients.
   Prophylaxis: Oral, as a lozenge dissolved slowly and completely in the mouth, 10 mg three times a day in immunosuppressed patients.

**Usual pediatric dose**
Antifungal—
   Infants and children up to 5 years of age: Use is not recommended in infants and children up to 5 years of age since this age group may not be capable of using the lozenge safely.
   Children 5 years of age and over: See *Usual adult and adolescent dose*.

**Strength(s) usually available**
U.S.—
   10 mg (Rx) [*Mycelex Troches*].
Canada—
   Not commercially available.

**Packaging and storage**
Store below 30 °C (86 °F), in a tight container, unless otherwise specified by manufacturer.

**Auxiliary labeling**
• Dissolve slowly in mouth.
• Continue medicine for full time of treatment.

Revised: 02/23/93

# CLOTRIMAZOLE Topical

VA CLASSIFICATION (Primary): DE102

Note: For a listing of dosage forms and brand names by country availability, see *Dosage Forms* section(s). For a listing of brand names for the articles in this monograph, refer to the General Index.

## Category

Antifungal (topical).

## Indications

Note: Bracketed information in the *Indications* section refers to uses that are not included in U.S. product labeling.

**Accepted**

Candidiasis, cutaneous (treatment)—Topical clotrimazole is indicated in the treatment of cutaneous candidiasis (moniliasis) caused by *Candida albicans (Monilia albicans)*.

Tinea corporis (treatment)
Tinea cruris (treatment) or
Tinea pedis (treatment)—Topical clotrimazole is indicated in the treatment of tinea corporis (ringworm of the body), tinea cruris (ringworm of the groin; jock itch), and tinea pedis (ringworm of the foot; athlete's foot) caused by *Trichophyton rubrum*, *T. mentagrophytes*, *Epidermophyton floccosum (Acrothesium floccosum)*, and *Microsporum canis*.

Tinea versicolor (treatment)—Topical clotrimazole is indicated in the treatment of tinea versicolor (pityriasis versicolor; ''sun fungus'') caused by *Pityrosporon orbiculare (Malassezia furfur)*.

[Paronychia (treatment)][1]
[Tinea barbae (treatment)][1] or
[Tinea capitis (treatment)][1]—Topical clotrimazole is used in the treatment of paronychia, tinea barbae, and tinea capitis.

Not all species or strains of a particular organism may be susceptible to clotrimazole.

---

[1]Not included in Canadian product labeling.

## Pharmacology/Pharmacokinetics

**Physicochemical characteristics**
Molecular weight—344.84.

**Mechanism of action/Effect**
Fungistatic; may be fungicidal, depending on concentration; inhibits biosynthesis of ergosterol or other sterols, damaging the fungal cell wall membrane and altering its permeability; as a result, loss of essential intracellular elements may occur; also inhibits biosynthesis of triglycerides and phospholipids by fungi; in addition, inhibits oxidative and peroxidative enzyme activity, resulting in intracellular buildup of toxic concentrations of hydrogen peroxide, which may contribute to deterioration of subcellular organelles and cellular necrosis. In *Candida albicans*, inhibits transformation of blastospores into invasive mycelial form.

**Absorption**
Dermal penetration; minimal systemic absorption.

## Precautions to Consider

**Carcinogenicity**
Studies in rats given oral doses of clotrimazole for 18 months have not shown that clotrimazole is carcinogenic.

**Mutagenicity**
Studies in Chinese hamsters given clotrimazole in five oral doses of 100 mg per kg of body weight (mg/kg) prior to testing have shown no mutagenic effects in the spermatophore chromosomes.

**Pregnancy/Reproduction**
Fertility—Clotrimazole caused impairment of mating in studies in mice and rats given oral doses of 50 to 120 mg per kg (mg/kg).

Pregnancy—Adequate and well-controlled studies in humans have not been done during the first trimester. Studies in humans given intravaginal clotrimazole during the second and third trimesters have not shown that clotrimazole causes adverse effects on the fetus.

Studies in rats given intravaginal doses of up to 100 mg/kg have not shown that clotrimazole causes adverse effects on the fetus. However, clotrimazole caused embryotoxicity, decreased litter size and number of viable young, and decreased pup survival to weaning in studies in mice and rats given oral doses of 50 to 120 mg/kg. Clotrimazole was not shown to be teratogenic in studies in mice, rabbits, and rats given oral doses of up to 200, 180, and 100 mg/kg, respectively.

FDA Pregnancy Category B.

**Breast-feeding**
It is not known whether clotrimazole, applied topically, is distributed into breast milk. However, problems in humans have not been documented.

**Pediatrics**
Appropriate studies performed to date have not demonstrated pediatrics-specific problems that would limit the usefulness of topical clotrimazole in children.

**Geriatrics**
Appropriate studies on the relationship of age to the effects of topical clotrimazole have not been performed in the geriatric population. However, no geriatrics-specific problems have been documented to date.

**Medical considerations/Contraindications**
The medical considerations/contraindications included here have been selected on the basis of their potential clinical significance (reasons given in parentheses where appropriate)—not necessarily inclusive (» = major clinical significance).

*Risk-benefit should be considered when the following medical problem exists:*
Sensitivity to clotrimazole

## Side/Adverse Effects

The following side/adverse effects have been selected on the basis of their potential clinical significance (possible signs and symptoms in parentheses where appropriate)—not necessarily inclusive:

**Those indicating need for medical attention**
*Hypersensitivity* (skin rash, hives, blistering, burning, itching, peeling, redness, stinging, swelling, or other sign of skin irritation not present before therapy)

## Patient Consultation

As an aid to patient consultation, refer to *Advice for the Patient, Clotrimazole (Topical)*.

In providing consultation, consider emphasizing the following selected information (» = major clinical significance):

**Before using this medication**
» Conditions affecting use, especially:
   Sensitivity to clotrimazole

**Proper use of this medication**
   Proper administration technique
» Avoiding contact with the eyes
» Not applying occlusive dressing over this medication unless directed to do so by physician
» Compliance with full course of therapy
» Proper dosing
   Missed dose: Applying as soon as possible; not applying if almost time for next dose
» Proper storage

**Precautions while using this medication**
   Checking with physician if no improvement within 4 weeks

**Side/adverse effects**
   Signs of potential side effects, especially hypersensitivity reactions

## General Dosing Information

Use of topical antifungals may lead to skin sensitization, resulting in hypersensitivity reactions with subsequent topical use of the medication.

Improvement of condition, with relief of pruritus, usually occurs within the first week of therapy.

When this medication is used in the treatment of candidiasis, occlusive dressings should be avoided since they provide conditions that favor growth of yeast and release of its irritating endotoxin.

## Topical Dosage Forms

### CLOTRIMAZOLE CREAM USP

**Usual adult and adolescent dose**
Antifungal (topical)—
   Topical, to the affected area of skin and surrounding areas, two times a day, morning and evening.

**Usual pediatric dose**
Antifungal (topical)—
   See *Usual adult and adolescent dose.*

**Strength(s) usually available**
U.S.—
   1% (10 mg per gram) [*Lotrimin AF Cream* (OTC) (benzyl alcohol 1%); *Lotrimin Cream* (Rx) (benzyl alcohol 1%); *Mycelex Cream* (OTC) (benzyl alcohol 1%); GENERIC (Rx/OTC)].
Canada—
   1% (10 mg per gram) (Rx) [*Canesten Cream* (benzyl alcohol 1%); *Clotrimaderm Cream* (benzyl alcohol 1%); *Myclo Cream; Neo-Zol Cream*].

**Packaging and storage**
Store between 2 and 30 °C (36 and 86 °F). Store in a collapsible tube or in a tight container. Protect from freezing.

**Auxiliary labeling**
• For external use only.
• Continue medicine for full time of treatment.

## CLOTRIMAZOLE LOTION USP

**Usual adult and adolescent dose**
Antifungal (topical)—
   See *Clotrimazole Cream USP.*

**Usual pediatric dose**
Antifungal (topical)—
   See *Clotrimazole Cream USP.*

**Strength(s) usually available**
U.S.—
   1% (10 mg per gram) [*Lotrimin AF Lotion* (OTC) (benzyl alcohol; ceteryl alcohol); *Lotrimin Lotion* (Rx) (benzyl alcohol; ceteryl alcohol)].
Canada—
   Not commercially available.

**Packaging and storage**
Store between 2 and 30 °C (36 and 86 °F). Store in a tight container. Protect from freezing.

**Auxiliary labeling**
• Shake well.
• For external use only.
• Continue medicine for full time of treatment.

## CLOTRIMAZOLE TOPICAL SOLUTION USP

**Usual adult and adolescent dose**
Antifungal (topical)—
   See *Clotrimazole Cream USP.*

**Usual pediatric dose**
Antifungal (topical)—
   See *Clotrimazole Cream USP.*

**Strength(s) usually available**
U.S.—
   1% (10 mg per mL) [*Lotrimin AF Solution* (OTC) (polyethylene glycol); *Lotrimin Solution* (Rx) (polyethylene glycol); *Mycelex Solution* (OTC) (polyethylene glycol)].
Canada—
   1% (10 mg per mL) (Rx) [*Canesten Solution* (isopropyl alcohol); *Canesten Solution with Atomizer* (isopropyl alcohol); *Myclo Solution* (isopropyl alcohol); *Myclo Spray Solution* (isopropyl alcohol)].

**Packaging and storage**
Store between 2 and 30 °C (36 and 86 °F). Store in a tight container. Protect from freezing.

**Auxiliary labeling**
• For external use only.
• Keep container tightly closed.
• Continue medicine for full time of treatment.

Revised: 03/29/94

---

# CLOTRIMAZOLE AND BETAMETHASONE    Topical

**VA CLASSIFICATION (Primary): DE250**
**NOTE:** The *Clotrimazole and Betamethasone (Topical)* monograph is maintained on the USP DI electronic data base. For a printed copy of the most recent revision of the complete monograph, contact the USP Division of Information Development, 12601 Twinbrook Parkway, Rockville, MD 20852.

   For information on the specific components of this combination, see the *USP DI* monographs for *Clotrimazole (Topical)* and *Corticosteroids (Topical)*.

   The information that follows is selectively abstracted from the complete monograph and is provided to facilitate drug use review and patient counseling.

Note: For a listing of dosage forms and brand names by country availability, see *Dosage Forms* section(s). For a listing of brand names for the articles in this monograph, refer to the General Index.

## Category

Antifungal-corticosteroid (topical).
Note: Clotrimazole is a broad-spectrum antifungal agent.

## Indications

Note: Bracketed information in the *Indications* section refers to uses that are not included in U.S. product labeling.

**Accepted**
Tinea corporis (treatment)
Tinea cruris (treatment) or
Tinea pedis (treatment)—Clotrimazole and betamethasone dipropionate combination is indicated [as a secondary agent] in the topical treatment of tinea corporis (ringworm of the body), tinea cruris (jock itch; ringworm of the groin), and tinea pedis (athlete's foot; ringworm of the foot), [accompanied by inflammation], caused by *Epidermophyton floccosum (Acrothesium floccosum), Microsporum canis, Trichophyton rubrum*, and *T. mentagrophytes.*

   The use of clotrimazole and betamethasone dipropionate combination has been shown to provide greater benefit than either clotrimazole or betamethasone dipropionate alone [during the first few days of treatment or for as long as inflammation persists, except on the palms of

the hands and soles of the feet. After this time, USP medical experts recommend the use of plain clotrimazole or other topical antifungal agents].

[Candidiasis, cutaneous (treatment)][1]—Clotrimazole and betamethasone dipropionate combination is used as a secondary agent in the topical treatment of cutaneous candidiasis (moniliasis), accompanied by inflammation, caused by *Candida albicans (Monilia albicans).*

Not all species or strains of a particular organism may be susceptible to clotrimazole.

**Unaccepted**
Since corticosteroids may cause thinning of the skin and telangiectasias when used on the face or in intertriginous areas (e.g., axilla, genitals, perineum, groin, between the toes), clotrimazole and betamethasone dipropionate combination is not recommended for use in these areas for longer than a few days.

Clotrimazole is not effective against bacteria, protozoa, or viruses.

---

[1]Not included in Canadian product labeling.

## Patient Consultation

As an aid to patient consultation, refer to *Advice for the Patient, Clotrimazole and Betamethasone (Topical).*

In providing consultation, consider emphasizing the following selected information (» = major clinical significance):

**Before using this medication**
» Conditions affecting use, especially:
      Allergies to imidazoles or corticosteroids
      Pregnancy—Not recommended in pregnancy because of possibility of teratogenicity, especially when used on extensive surface areas, in large amounts, or for prolonged periods of time
      Breast-feeding—May cause systemic effects, such as growth suppression
      Use in children—May cause HPA axis suppression, Cushing's syndrome, intracranial hypertension, or growth suppression
      Other medical problems, especially eczema vaccinatum, herpes simplex, tubercular infections of the skin, vaccinia, varicella, or other viral infections of the skin

**Proper use of this medication**

Before applying, washing affected area with soap and water, and drying thoroughly

» Not for ophthalmic use

*To use*

» Checking with physician before using medication on other skin problems

Applying a thin layer of medication to affected area(s) and surrounding skin; rubbing in gently and thoroughly

» Not applying occlusive dressing over this medication unless directed to do so by physician; wearing loose-fitting clothing when using on inguinal area; avoiding tight-fitting diapers and plastic pants on diaper area of children

» Compliance with full course of therapy; not using more often or for longer than directed by physician; excessive use on thin skin areas may result in skin atrophy and stretch marks

» Proper dosing

Missed dose: Applying as soon as possible; not applying if almost time for next dose

» Proper storage

**Precautions while using this medication**

Checking with physician if no improvement within a few days

» Using hygienic measures to help cure infection and to help prevent reinfection:

*For tinea pedis*

Carefully drying feet, especially between toes, after bathing

Not wearing socks made from wool or synthetic materials; wearing clean, cotton socks and changing them daily or more often if feet perspire excessively

Wearing well-ventilated shoes or sandals

Using a bland, absorbent powder or an antifungal powder liberally between toes, on feet, and in socks and shoes once or twice daily; using the powder after cream has been applied and has disappeared into the skin; not using the powder as sole therapy for your fungal infection

*For tinea cruris*

Carefully drying inguinal area after bathing

Not wearing underwear that is tight-fitting or made from synthetic materials; wearing loose-fitting cotton underwear instead

Using a bland, absorbent powder or an antifungal powder liberally once or twice daily; using the powder after cream has been applied and has disappeared into the skin; not using the powder as sole therapy for your fungal infection

*For tinea corporis*

Carefully drying the body after bathing

Avoiding excess heat and humidity if possible; keeping moisture from accumulating on affected areas of the body

Wearing well-ventilated clothing

Using a bland, absorbent powder or an antifungal powder liberally once or twice daily; using the powder after cream has been applied and has disappeared into the skin; not using the powder as sole therapy for your fungal infection

» Diabetics: May rarely cause hyperglycemia and glucosuria, especially with severe diabetes and use of large amounts; checking with physician before changing diet or dosage of antidiabetic medication

**Side/adverse effects**

Signs of potential side effects, especially hypersensitivity and long-term effects, including skin atrophy

## Topical Dosage Forms

### CLOTRIMAZOLE AND BETAMETHASONE DIPROPIONATE CREAM USP

**Usual adult and adolescent dose**

Tinea corporis; or

Tinea cruris; or

Tinea pedis—

Topical, to the affected area(s) and surrounding skin, two times a day, morning and evening.

**Usual pediatric dose**

Infants and children up to 12 years of age—Safety and efficacy have not been established.

Children 12 years of age and over—See *Usual adult and adolescent dose.*

**Strength(s) usually available**

U.S.—

1% of clotrimazole and 0.05% of betamethasone (base) (Rx) [*Lotrisone* (propylene glycol; benzyl alcohol)].

Canada—

1% of clotrimazole and 0.05% of betamethasone (base) (Rx) [*Lotriderm* (propylene glycol; benzyl alcohol)].

**Auxiliary labeling**

• For external use only.

• Continue medication for full time of treatment.

• Do not use in the eyes.

Revised: 02/10/92

Interim revision: 07/01/94

---

## CLOTRIMAZOLE-CONTAINING COMBINATIONS—

Clotrimazole and Betamethasone (Topical)

---

**CLOXACILLIN—**See *Penicillins (Systemic)*

---

# CLOZAPINE   Systemic

VA CLASSIFICATION (Primary): CN709

Note: In the U.S. and Canada, *Clozaril* is available only through pharmacies that agree to participate with physicians in a program to monitor patients' weekly blood tests; a 7-day supply of medication may be dispensed if the results of the blood tests are within acceptable parameters.

Note: For a listing of dosage forms and brand names by country availability, see *Dosage Forms* section(s). For a listing of brand names for the articles in this monograph, refer to the General Index.

## Category

Antipsychotic.

Note: Clozapine is an atypical antipsychotic.

## Indications

**Accepted**

Schizophrenia (treatment)—Clozapine is indicated only in the management of severely ill schizophrenic patients who have failed to respond to other neuroleptic agents or who cannot tolerate the adverse effects produced by those agents. Clozapine may produce a significant improvement in both the positive and negative symptoms of schizophrenia.

Because of the significant risk of agranulocytosis and seizures with clozapine, the patient should be given an adequate trial with at least 2 different standard antipsychotic medications before clozapine therapy is initiated.

## Pharmacology/Pharmacokinetics

**Physicochemical characteristics**

Molecular weight—326.83.

**Mechanism of action/Effect**

The mechanism by which clozapine exerts its antipsychotic effect has not been defined. Clozapine is preferentially more active at limbic dopamine receptors in the brain, interfering with the binding of dopamine at both $D_1$ and $D_2$ receptors, although this effect is less pronounced and more balanced than that of typical neuroleptics. Clozapine binds primarily to nondopaminergic sites (e.g., alpha-adrenergic, serotonergic, histaminergic, and cholinergic receptors); it is unclear if a combination of these effects may contribute to clozapine's efficacy. Clozapine has little or no effect on serum prolactin concentrations, because it does not bind to the tuberoinfundibular dopamine tract.

**Absorption**
Rapid and nearly complete.

**Distribution**
Rapid and extensive; crosses the blood-brain barrier.

**Protein binding**
Very high (95%).

**Biotransformation**
Extensive first-pass hepatic metabolism to metabolites with limited or no activity.

**Half-life**
Elimination—
8 (range, 4 to 12) hours after a single 75-mg dose; 12 (range, 4 to 66) hours after reaching steady-state dosing of 100 mg twice a day.

**Time to peak concentration**
Average, 2.5 hours (range, 1 to 6 hours). Steady-state concentrations are attained in 8 to 10 days.

**Peak serum concentration**
Steady-state concentrations average 319 nanograms per mL (range, 102 to 771 nanograms per mL).

**Duration of action**
4 to 12 hours.

**Elimination**
Renal—
50%.
Fecal—
30%.

## Precautions to Consider

### Carcinogenicity
Long-term studies in mice and rats given clozapine in doses approximately 7 times the typical human dose (on a mg per kg basis) demonstrated no potential carcinogenicity.

### Tumorigenicity
Animal studies have shown no abnormalities.

### Mutagenicity
Clozapine was not found to be genotoxic or mutagenic when assayed in appropriate bacterial and mammalian tests.

### Pregnancy/Reproduction
Pregnancy—Clozapine crosses the placenta. Adequate and well-controlled studies in humans have not been done.
Studies in animals have not shown that clozapine causes adverse effects on the fetus.
FDA Pregnancy Category B.

### Breast-feeding
Animal studies have suggested that clozapine may be distributed into breast milk. Clozapine may cause sedation, decreased suckling, restlessness or irritability, seizures, and cardiovascular instability in the nursing infant.

### Pediatrics
Appropriate studies on the relationship of age to the effects of clozapine have not been performed in children up to 16 years of age. Safety and efficacy have not been established.

### Geriatrics
No information is available on the relationship of age to the effects of clozapine in geriatric patients. However, the elderly may be at greater risk for orthostatic hypotension, and for anticholinergic side effects such as confusion and excitement. Also, elderly males are more likely to have age-related prostatic hypertrophy, which requires caution in the use of clozapine.

### Dental
The peripheral anticholinergic effects of clozapine may decrease or inhibit salivary flow, thus contributing to the development of caries, periodontal disease, oral candidiasis, and discomfort. In contrast, hypersalivation may occur as a frequent consequence of clozapine administration.
The leukopenic and thrombocytopenic effects of clozapine may result in an increased incidence of microbial infection, delayed healing, and gingival bleeding. If leukopenia or thrombocytopenia occurs, dental work should be deferred until blood counts have returned to normal, and patients should be instructed in proper oral hygiene, including caution in the use of regular toothbrushes, dental floss, and toothpicks.

### Drug interactions and/or related problems
The following drug interactions and/or related problems have been selected on the basis of their potential clinical significance (possible mechanism in parentheses where appropriate)—not necessarily inclusive (» = major clinical significance):

Note: Combinations containing any of the following medications, depending on the amount present, may also interact with this medication.

» Alcohol or
» Central nervous system (CNS) depression–producing medications, other (See *Appendix II*)
(concurrent use with clozapine may increase the severity and frequency of CNS depressant effects)

Anticholinergics
(concurrent use with clozapine may potentiate the anticholinergic effects of these medications)

» Bone marrow depressants, other (See *Appendix II*)
(concurrent use with clozapine may potentiate the myelosuppressive effects of these medications)

Digoxin or
Highly protein-bound medications, such as:
  Heparin
  Phenytoin
  Warfarin
(concurrent use with clozapine may result in increased serum concentrations of these medications; also, clozapine may be displaced from its binding sites by these medications)

Hypotension-producing medications, other (See *Appendix II* )
(concurrent use with clozapine may cause additive hypotensive effects; epinephrine should not be used in the treatment of clozapine-induced hypotension because of a possible reverse epinephrine effect)

» Lithium
(concurrent use with clozapine may increase the risk of seizures, confusional states, neuroleptic malignant syndrome, and dyskinesias)

Smoking tobacco
(concurrent use may decrease the serum concentrations of clozapine)

### Medical considerations/Contraindications
The medical considerations/contraindications included here have been selected on the basis of their potential clinical significance (reasons given in parentheses where appropriate)—not necessarily inclusive (» = major clinical significance).

*Except under special circumstances, this medication should not be used when the following medical problems exist:*

» CNS depression, severe
    (may be potentiated)

» Myeloproliferative disorders, specifically:
    Blood dyscrasias, or history of
    Bone marrow depression
    (may be potentiated)

*Risk-benefit should be considered when the following medical problems exist:*

Cardiovascular disorders
    (increased risk of blood pressure alterations and arrhythmias)

Gastrointestinal disorders
    (condition may be exacerbated)

» Glaucoma, narrow-angle, predisposition to
    (may be aggravated)

Hepatic function impairment
    (metabolism of clozapine may be altered)

» Prostatic hypertrophy
    (condition may be exacerbated)

Renal function impairment
    (excretion of clozapine may be altered)

» Seizure disorders, or history of
    (risk of seizures may be increased)

### Patient monitoring
The following may be especially important in patient monitoring (other tests may be warranted in some patients, depending on condition; » = major clinical significance):

» White blood cell (WBC) and differential counts
(recommended prior to initiation of therapy and at weekly intervals during therapy and for 4 weeks after discontinuation of clozapine. If the baseline WBC count is less than 3500 per mm³, clozapine therapy should not be initiated. If treatment is started and the WBC count falls below 3500 per mm³, or if it drops substantially from baseline levels, or if immature forms are present, the WBC count

should be repeated and a differential count performed. If subsequent WBC and differential counts reveal a WBC count of 3000 to 3500 per mm³ and a granulocyte count greater than 1500 per mm³, WBC and differential counts should be done twice weekly. If the WBC count falls below 3000 per mm³ or the granulocyte count below 1500 per mm³, clozapine should be discontinued and the patient monitored for flu-like symptoms or symptoms suggesting infection. Clozapine may be resumed if the WBC count exceeds 3000 per mm³ and the granulocyte count exceeds 1500 per mm³; however, counts should be performed at least twice a week until the WBC count is greater than 3500 per mm³. If the WBC count falls below 2000 per mm³ or the granulocyte count below 1000 per mm³, discontinuation of clozapine is recommended; bone marrow aspiration may be considered to ascertain the patient's granulopoietic status; protective isolation and antibiotic therapy may be instituted if indicated. If the WBC count has fallen below 2000 per mm³ or the granulocyte count below 1000 per mm³, the patient should *not* be rechallenged with clozapine, as agranulocytosis may occur with a shorter latency period.)

## Side/Adverse Effects

The following side/adverse effects have been selected on the basis of their potential clinical significance (possible signs and symptoms in parentheses where appropriate)—not necessarily inclusive:

**Those indicating need for medical attention**
Incidence more frequent
   *Cardiovascular effects, specifically tachycardia* (fast or irregular heartbeat); *hypotension* (low blood pressure); *or orthostatic hypotension* (dizziness or fainting); *fever*
   Note: *Cardiovascular effects* can be minimized by gradually increasing dosage and tend to subside with continued use of clozapine.
      *Fever* usually occurs within the first 3 weeks of therapy and is benign and self-limiting; may be associated with an increase or decrease in white blood cell count. The patient should be evaluated to rule out underlying infectious processes or the development of agranulocytosis. If a high fever occurs in conjunction with severe muscle rigidity and autonomic changes, the possibility of neuroleptic malignant syndrome should be considered.

Incidence less frequent
   *Agitation* (unusual anxiety, nervousness, or irritability); *akathisia* (restlessness or need to keep moving); *confusion; difficulty in accommodation* (blurred vision); *electrocardiogram (ECG) changes; hypertension* (dizziness; severe or continuing headaches; increase in blood pressure); *syncope* (fainting)

Incidence rare
   *Blood dyscrasias, specifically agranulocytosis* (chills; fever; sore throat; unusual tiredness or weakness); *eosinophilia* (fever); *granulocytopenia* (chills; fever; sore throat; sores, ulcers, or white spots on lips or in mouth; unusual tiredness or weakness); *leukopenia* (chills; fever; sore throat); *or thrombocytopenia* (unusual bleeding or bruising); *difficulty in urinating; extrapyramidal effects, specifically akinesia or hypokinesia* (absence of or decrease in movement); *rigidity* (severe muscle stiffness); *tremor*—less frequent; *impotence* (decreased sexual ability); *insomnia or disturbed sleep* (trouble in sleeping); *mental depression; neuroleptic malignant syndrome (NMS)* (convulsions; difficult or fast breathing; fast heartbeat or irregular pulse; fever; high or low [irregular] blood pressure; increased sweating; loss of bladder control; severe muscle stiffness; unusually pale skin; unusual tiredness or weakness); *seizures; tardive dyskinesia* (lip smacking or puckering; puffing of cheeks; rapid or worm-like movements of tongue; uncontrolled chewing movements; uncontrolled movements of arms and legs)
   Note: Although no cases of *NMS* have been attributed to clozapine when used by itself, several cases have occurred in patients receiving clozapine concomitantly with lithium or other CNS-active agents.
      For *seizures,* a dose-dependent relationship has been suggested, with *seizures* occurring in 1 to 2% of patients receiving low doses (<300 mg per day), in 3 to 4% of patients receiving moderate doses (300 to 599 mg per day), and in 5% of patients receiving high doses (≥ 600 mg per day) of clozapine. Patients with a history of epilepsy or other predisposing factors may be at greater risk of developing seizures.
      Although no confirmed cases of *tardive dyskinesia* have been attributed to clozapine, the possibility of occurrence cannot be ruled out. The smallest dose and shortest duration of treatment should be used, with periodic reassessment of need for clozapine treatment.

**Those indicating need for medical attention only if they continue or are bothersome**
Incidence more frequent
   *Constipation; dizziness or lightheadedness; drowsiness; headache; hypersalivation* (increased watering of mouth); *nausea or vomiting; unusual weight gain*
   Note: *Salivation* may be profuse, very fluid and especially prevalent during sleep. It has been suggested by the manufacturer that this effect may be ameliorated in some cases by use of a peripherally acting anticholinergic medication; however, caution should be used since additive anticholinergic effects may lead to toxicity in some patients.

Incidence less frequent
   *Abdominal discomfort or heartburn; dryness of mouth; hyperhidrosis* (increased sweating)

## Overdose

For specific information on the agents used in the management of clozapine overdose, see:
   *Charcoal, Activated (Oral-Local)* monograph;
   *Dihydroergotamine* in *Vascular Headache Suppressants, Ergot Derivative–containing (Systemic)* monograph;
   *Norepinephrine* in *Sympathomimetic Agents—Cardiovascular Use (Parenteral-Systemic)* monograph;
   *Physostigmine (Systemic)* monograph.

For more information on the management of overdose or unintentional ingestion, **contact a Poison Control Center** (see *Poison Control Center Listing*).

### Clinical effects of overdose
The following effects have been selected on the basis of their potential clinical significance (possible signs and symptoms in parentheses where appropriate)—not necessarily inclusive:
   *Cardiac arrhythmias* (fast, slow, or irregular heartbeat); *delirium* (unusual excitement, nervousness, or restlessness; hallucinations); *drowsiness, severe; hypersalivation; hypotension* (dizziness or fainting); *respiratory depression* (slow, irregular, or troubled breathing); *tachycardia, severe* (fast or irregular heartbeat)

### Treatment of overdose
To decrease absorption—
   Induction of emesis or gastric lavage; administration of activated charcoal, which may be used with sorbitol.
To enhance elimination—
   Forced diuresis, dialysis, hemoperfusion, and exchange transfusions are not likely to be of benefit due to the high degree of protein binding.
Specific treatment—
   Considering use of physostigmine, dihydroergotamine, angiotensin, or norepinephrine to counteract anticholinergic symptoms; avoiding use of epinephrine and derivatives in treatment of hypotension; avoiding use of quinidine and procainamide in treatment of cardiac arrhythmias.
Monitoring—
   Monitoring of cardiac and vital signs; continued monitoring of patient for several days because of risk of delayed effects.
Supportive care—
   Establishment and maintenance of a patent airway, ensuring adequate oxygenation and ventilation.
   Patients in whom intentional overdose is confirmed or suspected should be referred for psychiatric consultation.

## Patient Consultation

As an aid to patient consultation, refer to *Advice for the Patient, Clozapine (Systemic)*.

In providing consultation, consider emphasizing the following selected information (» = major clinical significance):

**Before using this medication**
» Conditions affecting use, especially:
   Pregnancy—Crosses the placenta
   Breast-feeding—May cause sedation, decreased suckling, and restlessness or irritability in nursing infant
   Use in the elderly—Greater risk of orthostatic hypotension and anticholinergic side effects in these patients
   Dental—Clozapine-induced blood dyscrasias may result in infections, delayed healing, and bleeding; dry mouth may cause caries and candidiasis; hypersalivation occurs frequently
   Other medications, especially alcohol, other CNS depression-producing medications, other bone marrow depressants, or lithium

Other medical problems, especially severe CNS depression, myeloproliferative disorders, cardiovascular disorders, gastrointestinal disorders, predisposition to narrow-angle glaucoma, impairment of hepatic or renal function, prostatic hypertrophy,
and seizure disorders

**Proper use of this medication**
Compliance with therapy; not taking more or less medication than
prescribed
» Proper dosing
Missed dose: Taking as soon as possible; not taking if almost time for
next dose; not doubling doses
» Proper storage

**Precautions while using this medication**
Regular visits to physician to check progress of therapy and to laboratory for blood tests
Checking with physician before discontinuing medication; gradual
dosage reduction may be needed
Avoiding use of alcoholic beverages or other CNS depressants during
therapy
Possible drowsiness, blurred vision, or seizures; not driving, swimming, climbing, operating machinery, or doing other things that
require alertness or accurate vision
Possible orthostatic hypotension; caution when getting up from a lying
or sitting position
Possible dryness of mouth; using sugarless gum or candy, ice, or saliva
substitute for relief; checking with physician or dentist if dryness
of mouth continues for more than 2 weeks

**Side/adverse effects**
Signs of potential side effects, especially cardiovascular effects, fever,
difficulty in accommodation, agitation, akathisia, confusion, ECG
changes, extrapyramidal effects, insomnia, mental depression, syncope, blood dyscrasias, difficulty in urinating, impotence, neuroleptic malignant syndrome, tardive dyskinesia, and seizures

## General Dosing Information

Clozapine dosage must be individualized by cautious titration from the
lower dosage range. A divided dosage schedule should be used, the
need for clozapine periodically reassessed, and the patient maintained
at the lowest possible dosage level.

If clozapine is to be discontinued, the dosage should be tapered gradually
over 1 to 2 weeks. However, if abrupt termination is necessary, the
patient should be monitored for recurrence of psychotic symptoms, as
rapid decompensation has occurred after sudden withdrawal.

Caution should be exercised in restarting clozapine, as there may be an
increased risk in the occurrence and severity of agranulocytosis. Patients whose white blood cell (WBC) counts fall below 2000 per mm³
or granulocyte counts fall below 1000 per mm³ should *not* be restarted
on clozapine.

**For treatment of adverse effects**
Neuroleptic malignant syndrome (NMS)—
Treatment is essentially symptomatic and supportive and may in-
clude the following
• *Discontinuing clozapine immediately.*
• Hyperthermia—Administering antipyretics (aspirin or aceta-
minophen); using cooling blanket.
• Dehydration—Restoring fluids and electrolytes.
• Cardiovascular instability—Monitoring blood pressure and
cardiac rhythm closely. Use of sodium nitroprusside may allow
vasodilation with subsequent heat loss from the skin in patients
with less dominant muscle rigidity.
• Hypoxia—Administering oxygen; considering airway insertion and assisted ventilation.

• Muscle rigidity—Administering dantrolene sodium (100 to
300 mg a day orally in divided doses; or 1.25 to 1.5 mg per
kg of body weight [mg/kg], intravenously); or administering
amantadine (100 mg twice daily) or bromocriptine (5 mg three
times a day) to restore central balance of dopamine and acetylcholine at the receptor site.
Tardive dyskinesia—
No known effective treatment. Although no confirmed cases of tardive
dyskinesia have been attributed to clozapine, the dosage of clozapine should be lowered or medication discontinued at earliest
signs of tardive dyskinesia to prevent irreversible effects.
Agranulocytosis—
If the WBC count falls below 2000 per mm³ or the granulocyte count
falls below 1000 per mm³:
• *Discontinuing clozapine immediately.*
• Placing patient in protective isolation with close observation.
• Considering bone marrow aspiration to determine granulopoietic
status.
• Monitoring WBC and differential counts every 2 days until nor-
mal levels return.
• Performing appropriate cultures and instituting appropriate anti-
biotic therapy if signs of infection occur.
• *Not* rechallenging patient with clozapine.

## Oral Dosage Forms

### CLOZAPINE TABLETS

**Usual adult dose**
Antipsychotic—
Oral, initially 25 mg one to two times a day, the dosage being increased in increments of 25 to 50 mg a day, if tolerated, to achieve
a dose of 300 to 450 mg a day by the end of two weeks. Subsequent dosage increments should not exceed 100 mg one or two
times a week.
Note: For malnourished patients, or those with hepatic, renal, or cardiovascular disease, the initial dose should be decreased and the increases in dosage titrated more slowly.

**Usual adult prescribing limits**
Up to 900 mg a day.

**Usual pediatric dose**
Children up to 16 years of age—
Safety and efficacy have not been established.

**Strength(s) usually available**
U.S.—
25 mg (Rx) [*Clozaril* (lactose)].
100 mg (Rx) [*Clozaril* (lactose)].
Canada—
25 mg (Rx) [*Clozaril*].
100 mg (Rx) [*Clozaril*].

**Packaging and storage**
Store below 30 °C (86 °F), in a tight container, unless otherwise specified
by manufacturer.

**Auxiliary labeling**
• Avoid alcoholic beverages.

## Selected Bibliography

Bablenis E, Weber SS, Wagner RL. Clozapine: a novel antipsychotic
agent. DICP Ann Pharmacother 1989 Feb; 23: 109-15.
Ereshefsky L, Watanabe MD, Tran-Johnson TK. Clozapine: an atypical
antipsychotic. Clin Pharm 1989; 8: 691-709.

Revised: 07/17/91
Interim revision: 03/25/92; 06/08/94

# COAL TAR    Topical

VA CLASSIFICATION (Primary/Secondary): DE802/DE500; DE900
Note: For a listing of dosage forms and brand names by country availability, see *Dosage Forms* section(s). For a listing of brand names
for the articles in this monograph, refer to the General Index.

## Category
Keratolytic (topical); antipsoriatic (topical); antiseborrheic.

## Indications

### Accepted
Dandruff (treatment)
Dermatitis, seborrheic (treatment)
Dermatitis, atopic (treatment)
Eczema (treatment) or
Psoriasis (treatment)—Indicated for the relief of itching, burning, and
other symptoms associated with generalized persistent dermatoses,

such as psoriasis, eczema, atopic dermatitis, and seborrheic dermatitis, and for the control of dandruff.

Coal tar preparations are also used in conjunction with ultraviolet (UV) light or sunlight, under the supervision of a physician, in the treatment of psoriasis or other conditions responding to this combined therapy.

## Pharmacology/Pharmacokinetics

### Mechanism of action/Effect
Coal tar suppresses the hyperplastic skin in some proliferative disorders. Although there is no confirmed evidence as to its pharmacologic effects, its actions in humans have been reported as antiseptic, antipruritic, antiparasitic, antifungal, antibacterial, keratoplastic, and antiacantholic. Vasoconstrictive activity has also been reported.

## Precautions to Consider

### Cross-sensitivity and/or related problems
Patients sensitive to any of the tars may be sensitive to coal tar also.

### Carcinogenicity
In animal studies, coal tar has been shown to increase the incidence of epidermal carcinomas and self-limiting keratocanthomas. Studies of patients with psoriasis who are treated with coal tar do not indicate an increased incidence of skin cancer.

### Pregnancy/Reproduction
Pregnancy—Studies have not been done in humans. Studies have not been done in animals.

FDA Pregnancy Category C.

### Breast-feeding
It is not known whether coal tar is distributed into breast milk. Problems in humans have not been documented.

### Pediatrics
Infants—Coal tar products should not be used on infants, unless under close supervision of physician.

Children—Appropriate studies on the relationship of age to the effects of this medicine have not been performed in the pediatric population.

### Geriatrics
Appropriate studies on the relationship of age to the effects of this medicine have not been performed in the geriatric population. However, no geriatrics-specific problems have been documented to date.

### Drug interactions and/or related problems
The following drug interactions and/or related problems have been selected on the basis of their potential clinical significance (possible mechanism in parentheses where appropriate)—not necessarily inclusive (» = major clinical significance):

Note: Combinations containing any of the following medications, depending on the amount present, may also interact with this medication.

Photosensitizing medications, other
(concurrent use of coal tar with these medications may cause additive photosensitizing effects; concurrent use of coal tar with systemic or topical methoxsalen or trioxsalen is not recommended)

### Medical considerations/Contraindications
The medical considerations/contraindications included here have been selected on the basis of their potential clinical significance (reasons given in parentheses where appropriate)—not necessarily inclusive (» = major clinical significance).

***Risk-benefit should be considered when the following medical problems exist:***
» Acute inflammation, open wounds, or infection of skin
    Sensitivity to coal tar

## Side/Adverse Effects

The following side/adverse effects have been selected on the basis of their potential clinical significance (possible signs and symptoms in parentheses where appropriate)—not necessarily inclusive:

**Those indicating need for medical attention**
Incidence rare
   *Allergic or irritant contact dermatitis, folliculitis, or pustular or keratocystic response* (skin rash); *skin irritation not present before therapy*

**Those indicating need for medical attention only if they continue or are bothersome**
Incidence more frequent
   *Stinging, mild*—especially for gel and solution dosage forms

## Patient Consultation

As an aid to patient consultation, refer to *Advice for the Patient, Coal Tar (Topical)*.

In providing consultation, consider emphasizing the following selected information (» = major clinical significance):

### Before using this medication
» Conditions affecting use, especially:
    Allergy to coal tar or any of the other tars
    Use in children—Coal tar products should not be used on infants, unless under close supervision of physician
    Other medical problems, especially acute inflammation, open wounds, or infection of skin

### Proper use of this medication
» Importance of not using more medication than the amount recommended
» Protecting treated area from direct sunlight for 72 hours following application of medication, unless otherwise directed by physician
» Not applying medication to infected, blistered, raw, or oozing areas of skin
» Avoiding contact with the eyes
» Proper dosing
    Missed dose: Applying as soon as possible; not applying if almost time for next dose; not doubling doses
*Proper administration*
*For cream and ointment dosage forms*
    Applying enough to cover affected area and rubbing in gently
*For gel dosage form*
    Applying enough to cover affected area and rubbing in gently
    Allowing to remain on affected area for 5 minutes, then removing excess by patting with clean tissue
*For shampoo dosage form*
    Wetting scalp and hair with lukewarm water
    Applying generous amount and rubbing into scalp, then rinsing
    Applying again, working up lather, and allowing to remain on scalp for 5 minutes, then rinsing thoroughly
*For nonshampoo liquid dosage forms*
    Applying directly to dry or wet skin or adding to lukewarm bath water, depending on product
    If applying directly to skin, applying enough to cover affected area and rubbing in gently
    Possibly flammable; not using near heat, open flame, or while smoking
» Proper storage

### Precautions while using this medication
    Medication may temporarily discolor blond, bleached, or tinted hair
» Medication may stain skin or clothing

### Side/adverse effects
    Signs of potential side effects, especially folliculitis, allergic or irritant contact dermatitis, pustular or keratocystic response, or skin irritation not present before therapy

## General Dosing Information

After using this medication, patient should avoid exposure of treated areas to sunlamps or direct sunlight for 72 hours unless otherwise directed by physician, since a photosensitivity reaction may occur. Before subsequent exposure to direct sunlight or sunlamps, all coal tar should be removed from patient's skin.

If coal tar is used in conjunction with ultraviolet (UV) light or sunlight, exposure to light may be undertaken 2 to 72 hours after coal tar is applied. A determination of the minimal erythemal dosage (MED) should be made for each patient and the initial irradiation should not exceed the MED.

### For cleansing bar dosage form
For best results on hard scales, soak in a warm bath first, then lather with the cleansing bar.

### For gel dosage form
If dryness occurs, an emollient may be applied 1 hour after the gel is applied and between applications as needed.

### For lotion dosage form
This medication may be applied directly to dry or wet skin or added to lukewarm bath water, depending on the product.

### For shampoo dosage form
The scalp should be moistened with lukewarm water, and a liberal amount of shampoo massaged into the scalp, then rinsed. Application is to be repeated and the shampoo allowed to remain on the scalp for 5 minutes, then rinsed thoroughly. The shampoo may be reapplied as necessary or as directed by the physician.

**For solution dosage form**

The solution may be used full strength or diluted with 3 parts of water and applied to a cotton or gauze pad and then massaged gently on the affected area.

A coal tar solution bath may be prepared by adding 4 to 6 tablespoonfuls of the solution to a tubful of lukewarm water.

# Topical Dosage Forms

## COAL TAR CLEANSING BAR

**Usual adult and adolescent dose**

Topical, to the skin, one or two times a day or as directed.

**Usual pediatric dose**

Dosage has not been established.

**Strength(s) usually available**

U.S.—

2% (coal tar extract) (OTC) [*Tegrin Medicated Soap for Psoriasis*].

**Packaging and storage**

Store below 40 °C (104 °F), preferably between 15 and 30 °C (59 and 86 °F), unless otherwise specified by manufacturer.

**Auxiliary labeling**

• For external use only.

## COAL TAR CREAM

**Usual adult and adolescent dose**

Topical, to the skin, up to four times a day.

**Usual pediatric dose**

Dosage has not been established.

**Strength(s) usually available**

U.S.—

2% (coal tar) (OTC) [*Fototar* (methylparaben; propylparaben; stearyl alcohol)].

5% (coal tar extract) (OTC) [*Alphosyl* (allantoin 1.7%; cetyl alcohol; lanolin alcohol; methylparaben; oleyl alcohol; propylparaben); *Tarbonis; Tegrin Skin Cream for Psoriasis* (allantoin 1.7%; acetylated lanolin alcohol; alcohol SD-23A 4%; cetyl alcohol; lanolin alcohol; stearyl alcohol)].

Canada—

5% (coal tar extract) (OTC) [*Alphosyl* (2% allantoin; cetyl alcohol; methylparaben 0.1%; propylparaben 0.01%; oleyl alcohol)].

**Packaging and storage**

Store below 40 °C (104 °F), preferably between 15 and 30 °C (59 and 86 °F), in a well-closed container, unless otherwise specified by manufacturer. Protect from freezing.

**Auxiliary labeling**

• For external use only.

## COAL TAR GEL

**Usual adult and adolescent dose**

Topical, to the skin, one or two times a day.

**Usual pediatric dose**

Dosage has not been established.

**Strength(s) usually available**

U.S.—

2.5% (coal tar extract) (OTC) [*Aquatar*].

5% (coal tar) (OTC) [*Estar* (benzyl alcohol; SD alcohol 40 15%)].

7.5% (coal tar solution) (OTC) [*Psorigel* (alcohol 33%)].

Canada—

1.5% (crude coal tar) (OTC) [*Psorigel* (ethyl alcohol 33.3%)].

2% (coal tar extract) (OTC) [*Estar* (benzyl alcohol)].

**Packaging and storage**

Store below 40 °C (104 °F), preferably between 15 and 30 °C (59 and 86 °F), in a well-closed container, unless otherwise specified by manufacturer. Protect from freezing.

**Auxiliary labeling**

• For external use only.

## COAL TAR LOTION

**Usual adult and adolescent dose**

Topical, to the skin, as a direct application, as a bath, as a hand or foot soak, or as a hair rinse, depending on the product.

**Usual pediatric dose**

Dosage has not been established.

**Strength(s) usually available**

U.S.—

1.5% (coal tar) (OTC) [*Cutar Water Dispersible Emollient Tar* (lanolin alcohols extract)].

1.5% (coal tar extract) (OTC) [*T/Gel Therapeutic Conditioner*].

5% (coal tar extract) (OTC) [*Alphosyl* (allantoin 1.7%; cetyl alcohol; methylparaben; propylparaben; SD alcohol 23A 4%); *T/Derm Tar Emollient; Tegrin Lotion for Psoriasis* (allantoin 1.7%; alcohol SD-23A 4%; cetyl alcohol; methylparaben; propylparaben)].

5% (tar distillate) (OTC) [*Doak Tar Lotion* (acetylated lanolin alcohol; lanolin alcohol; methylparaben; propylparaben)].

Canada—

5% (crude coal tar extract) (OTC) [*Alphosyl* (cetyl alcohol; methylparaben 0.1%; propylparaben 0.01%)].

5% (tar distillate) (OTC) [*Tar Doak* (methylparaben; propylparaben)].

**Packaging and storage**

Store below 40 °C (104 °F), preferably between 15 and 30 °C (59 and 86 °F), in a well-closed container, unless otherwise specified by manufacturer. Protect from freezing.

**Auxiliary labeling**

• Shake well (depending on the product).

• For external use only.

## COAL TAR OINTMENT USP

**Usual adult and adolescent dose**

Topical, to the skin, two or three times a day.

**Usual pediatric dose**

Dosage has not been established.

**Strength(s) usually available**

U.S.—

1% (coal tar) (OTC) [*Medotar; Taraphilic* (stearyl alcohol; methylparaben; propylparaben)].

5% (tar distillate) (OTC) [*Tarpaste 'Doak'*].

Canada—

5% (tar distillate) (OTC) [*Tarpaste*].

**Packaging and storage**

Store below 40 °C (104 °F), preferably between 15 and 30 °C (59 and 86 °F), unless otherwise specified by manufacturer. Store in a tight container. Protect from freezing.

**Auxiliary labeling**

• For external use only.

## COAL TAR SHAMPOO

**Usual adult and adolescent dose**

Topical, to the scalp, once a week to once a day or as directed.

**Usual pediatric dose**

Dosage has not been established.

**Strength(s) usually available**

U.S.—

0.5% (coal tar) (OTC) [*DHS Tar Gel Shampoo; DHS Tar Shampoo*].

1% (whole coal tar) (OTC) [*Theraplex T Shampoo; Zetar Medicated Antiseborrheic Shampoo* (parachlorometaxylenol 0.5%)].

2% (crude coal tar) (OTC) [*Ionil T Plus*].

2% (coal tar extract) (OTC) [*Doctar Hair & Scalp Shampoo and Conditioner; Doctar Shampoo; Tegrin Medicated Shampoo Extra Conditioning Formula* (SD alcohol 23-A 2.8%, methylparaben; propylparaben); *T/Gel Therapeutic Shampoo*].

3% (tar distillate) (OTC) [*Doak Tar Shampoo* (isopropyl alcohol; methylparaben; propylparaben); *Tersa-Tar Soapless Tar Shampoo*].

4.3% (crude coal tar) (OTC) [*Pentrax Anti-Dandruff Tar Shampoo*].

5% (coal tar extract) (OTC) [*Tegrin Medicated Shampoo Concentrated Gel* (SD alcohol 23-A 4.6%; methylparaben; propylparaben); *Tegrin Medicated Shampoo Herbal Formula* (SD alcohol 23-A 4.6%; methylparaben; propylparaben); *Tegrin Medicated Shampoo Original Formula* (SD alcohol 23-A 4.6%; methylparaben; propylparaben)].

7% (coal tar solution) (OTC) [*Tegrin Medicated Cream Shampoo*].

9% (coal tar solution) (OTC) [*Denorex Medicated Shampoo* (menthol 1.5%; alcohol 7.5%); *Denorex Medicated Shampoo and Conditioner* (menthol 1.5%; alcohol 7.5%); *Denorex Mountain Fresh Herbal Scent Medicated Shampoo* (menthol 1.5%; alcohol 7.5%)].

12.5% (coal tar solution) (OTC) [*Denorex Extra Strength Medicated Shampoo* (menthol 1.5%; alcohol 10.4%); *Denorex Extra Strength Medicated Shampoo with Conditioners* (menthol 1.5%; alcohol 10.4%)].

Canada—

1% (colloidal whole tar) (OTC) [*Zetar Shampoo* (parachlorometaxylenol 0.5%)].

1% (tar distillate) (OTC) [*Tersa-Tar Mild Therapeutic Shampoo with Protein and Conditioner* (methylparaben; propylparaben)].

2% (coal tar extract) (OTC) [*T-Gel*].

3% (tar distillate) (OTC) [*Tersa-Tar Therapeutic Shampoo* (methylparabens; propylparabens)].

4.3% (coal tar) (OTC) [*Pentrax Extra-Strength Therapeutic Tar Shampoo*].

## Packaging and storage

Store between 15 and 30 °C (59 and 86 °F), in a well-closed container, unless otherwise specified by manufacturer.

## Auxiliary labeling

• Shake well (depending on the product).
• For external use only.

## COAL TAR TOPICAL SOLUTION USP

### Usual adult and adolescent dose

Topical, to the skin, as a direct application to wet skin or scalp or as a bath, depending on the product.

### Usual pediatric dose

Dosage has not been established.

### Strength(s) usually available

U.S.—

2% (tar distillate) (OTC) [*Doak Oil Therapeutic Bath Treatment For All-Over Body Care* (acetylated lanolin alcohol; lanolin alcohol)].

2.5% (coal tar) (OTC) [*Balnetar Therapeutic Tar Bath*].

2.5% (coal tar solution) (OTC) [*PsoriNail Topical Solution*].

10% (tar distillate) (OTC) [*Doak Oil Forte Therapeutic Bath Treatment* (acetylated lanolin alcohol; lanolin alcohol)].

25.5% (colloidal solution of tar distillate) (OTC) [*Lavatar*].

Canada—

2% (tar distillate) (OTC) [*Doak Oil*].

2.5% (coal tar) (OTC) [*Balnetar*].

7.5% (coal tar solution) (OTC) [*Denorex* (menthol 1.5%)].

10% (tar distillate) (OTC) [*Doak Oil Forte*].

20% (coal tar solution) (OTC) [*Liquor Carbonis Detergens*].

25.5% (tar distillate) (OTC) [*Lavatar*].

## Packaging and storage

Store below 40 °C (104 °F), preferably between 15 and 30 °C (59 and 86 °F), unless otherwise specified by manufacturer. Store in a tight container. Protect from freezing.

## Auxiliary labeling

• Shake well (depending on the product).
• For external use only.

## COAL TAR TOPICAL SUSPENSION

### Usual adult and adolescent dose

Topical, to the skin, as a bath.

### Usual pediatric dose

Dosage has not been established.

### Strength(s) usually available

U.S.—

300 mg per mL (whole coal tar) (Rx) [*Zetar Emulsion*].

Canada—

300 mg per mL (colloidal crude coal tar) (OTC) [*Zetar Emulsion*].

## Packaging and storage

Store below 40 °C (104 °F), preferably between 15 and 30 °C (59 and 86 °F), in a tight container, unless otherwise specified by manufacturer. Protect from freezing.

## Auxiliary labeling

• Shake well.
• For external use only.

Revised: 03/04/92
Interim revision: 06/03/94

## COAL TAR–CONTAINING COMBINATIONS—

Salicylic Acid, Sulfur, and Coal Tar (Topical)

# COCAINE    Mucosal-Local

VA CLASSIFICATION (Primary/Secondary): NT300/OR900

Note: Controlled substance classification—

     U.S.—Schedule II.

     Canada—N.

Note: For a listing of dosage forms and brand names by country availability, see *Dosage Forms* section(s). For a listing of brand names for the articles in this monograph, refer to the General Index.

## Category

Anesthetic-vasoconstrictor (mucosal-local).

## Indications

### Accepted

Anesthesia, local[1]—Cocaine hydrochloride is indicated to provide local anesthesia and vasoconstriction of accessible mucous membranes, especially in the oral, laryngeal, and nasal cavities, prior to instrumentation (e.g., bronchoscopy) or surgical procedures. Cocaine's toxicity must be considered prior to its use, especially when it is being applied to the tracheobronchial tree.

Although cocaine is an acceptable topical anesthetic for dental procedures, it is no longer extensively used in dentistry because of its toxicity.

### Unaccepted

Cocaine is not indicated for administration by injection and is not recommended for application to "closed" mucous surfaces, such as those of the urethra or bladder, because of the increased risk of severe toxic reactions.

[1]Not included in Canadian product labeling.

## Pharmacology/Pharmacokinetics

### Physicochemical characteristics

Molecular weight—339.82.

## Mechanism of action/Effect

Anesthetic, local—Acts primarily by blocking both the initiation and conduction of nerve impulses by decreasing the neuronal membrane's permeability to sodium ions. This reversibly stabilizes the membrane and inhibits depolarization, resulting in the failure of a propagated action potential and subsequent conduction blockade.

Vasoconstrictor—Cocaine is a potent indirect-acting sympathomimetic agent, i.e., it interferes with the uptake of norepinephrine by adrenergic nerve terminals and increases the concentration of this neurotransmitter at postsynaptic receptor sites. Norepinephrine acts on alpha-adrenergic receptors in blood vessels to produce vasoconstriction, which facilitates examination and surgery by reducing congestion, swelling, and bleeding at the site of application.

## Other actions/effects

Cocaine's indirect sympathetic nervous system–stimulating activity results in potentiation of the effects of endogenous catecholamines, i.e., epinephrine and dopamine as well as norepinephrine. This leads to systemic, as well as local, vasoconstriction; increased heart rate, arterial blood pressure, and blood glucose concentrations; mydriasis; and a risk of cardiac arrhythmias. Tachycardia and hypertension may increase myocardial work and oxygen demand; in some patients, especially those with predisposing cardiovascular disease, myocardial ischemia may result.

Cocaine is a potent central nervous system (CNS) stimulant.

Cocaine has pyrogenic activity that may result from CNS stimulation–induced increases in muscular activity (which increases heat production) as well as vasoconstriction (which decreases heat loss through the skin). There is some evidence that cocaine also produces pyresis via a direct effect on the heat-regulating centers in the CNS.

Cocaine has convulsant activity that may result from its pyrogenic activity as well as from its CNS effects.

Cocaine also blocks the uptake of dopamine, thereby increasing the concentration of dopamine at postsynaptic receptor sites and stimulating dopaminergic neurotransmission. However, repeated use of cocaine may cause dopamine depletion in the CNS. Studies have indicated that dopaminergic stimulation may be responsible for the development of cocaine-induced euphoria, whereas dopamine depletion may be responsible for the occurrence of dysphoria and/or mental depression following cessation of repeated cocaine use and may lead to psychological dependence on the drug. Cocaine abuse may also lead to physical dependence.

Topical application of cocaine to the oral or nasal mucosa decreases local sensory acuity; i.e., reduces or abolishes senses of taste and smell.

## Absorption

Cocaine is readily absorbed from all mucous membranes. Although cocaine's local vasoconstrictive effect may limit to some extent its rate of absorption (measurable quantities have been reported to remain in the nasal mucosa for 3 hours after application), the rate of absorption may exceed the rate of metabolism and/or excretion, leading to a significant risk of systemic toxicity. Entry of cocaine into the brain may be especially rapid following application to the nasal mucosa, particularly if the medication is applied as a fine-mist spray. Also, cocaine is more readily absorbed from inflamed or damaged tissue.

## Biotransformation

Cocaine is hydrolyzed by plasma and hepatic cholinesterases. The primary metabolites are benzoylecgonine and ecgonine methyl ester. Small quantities are also demethylated in the liver to an active metabolite, norcocaine, which has local anesthetic activity and, *in vitro*, inhibits norepinephrine uptake. Metabolism of cocaine is generally rapid, but may be significantly decreased or slowed in individuals with low levels of plasma or hepatic cholinesterase activity.

## Half-life

Elimination—1 to 1.5 hours; subject to wide inter- and intraindividual variability, but independent of the route of administration.

## Onset of action

Approximately 1 minute.

## Time to peak effect

Approximately 5 minutes.

## Duration of action

Approximately 30 minutes to 1 hour (average, 20 to 40 minutes), depending on the concentration.

## Elimination

Renal, primarily as metabolites. Approximately 10 to 20% of a dose may be excreted as unchanged cocaine, depending on the acidity of the urine (with larger quantities being excreted in acidic urine). The rate at which cocaine and its metabolites are cleared from the body is dose-dependent. Following intranasal administration of a single dose of about 100 mg, significant quantities of cocaine may appear in the urine for at least 10 hours, and significant quantities of its major metabolites may appear in the urine for 2 to 2.5 days.

In breast milk—Cocaine is excreted in breast milk.

# Precautions to Consider

## Carcinogenicity/Mutagenicity

Long-term studies have not been done.

## Pregnancy/Reproduction

Pregnancy—Cocaine has high water and lipid solubility and may therefore cross the placenta by simple diffusion. Although studies have not been done in pregnant women receiving cocaine clinically, the possibility should be considered that pregnant women may be especially sensitive to the effects of cocaine because of reduced plasma cholinesterase activity resulting in decreased or slower cocaine metabolism. Human fetuses and neonates also exhibit low cholinesterase activity. Use of cocaine by a pregnant woman 1 or 2 days prior to delivery may result in the appearance of measurable quantities of benzoylecgonine in the neonate's urine for up to 5 days after birth.

Studies in cocaine-abusing pregnant women have shown that cocaine may increase the risk of spontaneous abortion; premature labor and stillbirth associated with abruptio placentae, with onset of labor occurring shortly after use of cocaine during the third trimester; congenital malformations; decreased fetal growth (reduced neonatal birth weight, length, and head circumference); and neonatal neurobehavioral impairment. The congenital malformations reported in these studies include transposition of the great arteries, hypoplastic right heart syndrome, exencephaly, interparietal encephalocele, parietal bone defects, and, in one infant, major malformations of the urinary tract, with bilateral hydronephrosis and bilateral cryptorchidism. Also, one infant born to a mother who had used cocaine intranasally 15 hours prior to delivery displayed convulsions, right-sided muscle weakness, intermittent tachycardia, and hypertension at birth and was found to have had a cerebral infarction. It has been proposed that these effects result from cocaine-induced placental vasoconstriction as well as maternal hypertension, cardiac arrhythmias, and hyperpyrexia, which decrease the flow of blood and nutrients to the fetus and also increase the risk of spontaneous abortion or premature labor. Because of these adverse effects, and because less toxic local anesthetics are available, it is recommended that cocaine not be administered to pregnant women.

In animal studies, cocaine increased the fetal resorption rate in rats and mice, decreased fetal weight in rats, and caused edema in the rat fetus. In another study, administration of cocaine to CF-1 mice on one of Days 7 through 12 of gestation caused skeletal abnormalities (malformed sternebrae, fused sternebrae, and polysternebrae), exencephaly, cryptorchidism, hydronephrosis, butterfly xiphoid, ocular defects (including anophthalmia or malformed or missing lenses), and delayed ossification of the paws or skull. The occurrence of specific malformations or abnormalities was dependent on the day of administration and coincided with the period of ontogenesis for the structures involved. Also, in a study in pregnant ewes, cocaine increased maternal blood pressure and uterine vascular resistance, decreased uterine blood flow, and caused hypoxemia, hypertension, and tachycardia in the fetuses.

FDA Pregnancy Category C.

## Breast-feeding

Cocaine is distributed into human breast milk. Symptoms of cocaine intoxication, including tachycardia, tachypnea, hypertension, irritability, and tremulousness, occurred in a breast-fed infant whose mother used cocaine intranasally. The symptoms appeared within 3 hours after the mother first used cocaine and persisted for as long as significant quantities of the drug and/or its metabolites appeared in the infant's urine. Cocaine and benzoylecgonine were present in the breast milk for up to 36 hours, and in the infant's urine for up to 60 hours, after the mother's last dose of the drug. Another infant, whose mother applied cocaine to her nipples to relieve soreness prior to breast-feeding, developed convulsions. Neonates may be especially susceptible to cocaine-induced toxicity because of low levels of cholinesterase activity resulting in decreased and/or slowed inactivation of the drug. If clinical use of cocaine is unavoidable, temporary cessation of breast-feeding is recommended.

## Pediatrics

Because of cocaine's toxicity, it is recommended that the medication not be administered to children younger than 6 years of age. For children 6 years of age or older, it is recommended that cocaine be used with caution and in reduced dosage.

## Geriatrics

The risk of cocaine-induced adverse effects may be increased in geriatric patients, who are more likely to have cerebrovascular disease, and are therefore more likely to be adversely affected by sympathetic stimulation, than are younger adults. Also, elderly males may be especially sensitive to the effects of cocaine because of reduced plasma cholinesterase activity resulting in decreased or slower cocaine metabolism. A reduction in dosage is recommended.

## Drug interactions and/or related problems

The following drug interactions and/or related problems have been selected on the basis of their potential clinical significance (possible mechanism in parentheses where appropriate)—not necessarily inclusive (» = major clinical significance):

Note: Combinations containing any of the following medications, depending on the amount present, may also interact with this medication.

Anesthetics, hydrocarbon inhalation, such as:
» Chloroform
» Cyclopropane
   Enflurane
» Halothane
   Isoflurane
   Methoxyflurane
» Trichloroethylene
   (administration of cocaine prior to or shortly after anesthesia with chloroform, cyclopropane, halothane, or trichloroethylene may increase the risk of ventricular fibrillation or other severe ventricular arrhythmias, especially in patients with pre-existing heart disease, because these anesthetics greatly sensitize the myocardium to the effects of sympathomimetics; great caution and especially careful patient monitoring are recommended if concurrent use is necessary)

   (isoflurane, and, to a lesser extent, enflurane or methoxyflurane, may also sensitize the myocardium to the effects of sympathomimetics; caution in concurrent use is recommended)

   Antidepressants, tricyclic or
   Digitalis glycosides or
» Levodopa or
» Methyldopa
   (concurrent use with cocaine may increase the risk of cardiac arrhythmias; if use of cocaine is necessary in patients receiving these

medications, it is recommended that cocaine be administered with caution, in reduced dosage, and in conjunction with electrocardiographic monitoring)

Antihypertensives, especially:

» Postganglionic blocking antihypertensive agents, i.e., guanadrel or guanethidine
(cocaine may decrease the antihypertensive effects of these medications; careful monitoring of the patient is recommended)

(postganglionic blocking agents such as guanadrel or guanethidine may potentiate cocaine-induced sympathetic stimulation; concurrent use may increase the risk of hypertension and cardiac arrhythmias)

» Beta-adrenergic blocking agents, possibly including ophthalmic betaxolol, levobunolol, metipranolol or timolol
(cocaine may inhibit the therapeutic effects of systemic beta-adrenergic blocking agents)

(although systemic beta-adrenergic blocking agents are recommended to reduce tachycardia, myocardial ischemia, and/or arrhythmias induced by cocaine [see *Treatment of overdose* ], concurrent use of a systemic beta-adrenergic blocking agent with cocaine may increase the risk of hypertension, excessive bradycardia, and possibly heart block, because beta-blockade may leave cocaine's alpha-adrenergic activity unopposed; the risk of these adverse effects may be decreased with labetalol because labetalol also has some alpha-adrenergic blocking activity, although its beta-adrenergic blocking activity predominates; the possibility of adverse effects should also be considered if cocaine is administered to patients receiving ophthalmic beta-adrenergic blocking agents, which are extensively absorbed and cause significant systemic beta-adrenergic blockade)

» Cholinesterase inhibitors, such as:
  Antimyasthenics
  Cyclophosphamide
  Demecarium
  Echothiophate
  Insecticides, neurotoxic, possibly including large quantities of topical malathion
  Isoflurophate
  Thiotepa
(inhibition of cholinesterase activity by these agents reduces or slows cocaine metabolism, thereby increasing and/or prolonging its effects and increasing the risk of toxicity; cholinesterase inhibition caused by echothiophate, demecarium, or isoflurophate may persist for weeks or months after the medication has been discontinued)

» CNS stimulation–producing medications, other (See *Appendix II*)
(concurrent use with cocaine may result in excessive CNS stimulation, leading to nervousness, irritability, insomnia, or possibly convulsions or cardiac arrhythmias; close observation is recommended)

» Monoamine oxidase (MAO) inhibitors, including furazolidone, procarbazine, and selegiline
(MAO inhibitors may prolong and intensify the cardiac stimulant and vasopressor effects of cocaine because of release of catecholamines that accumulate in intraneuronal storage sites during MAO inhibitor therapy, resulting in headache, cardiac arrhythmias, vomiting, or sudden and severe hypertensive and/or hyperpyretic crises; cocaine should not be administered during, or within 14 days following, administration of an MAO inhibitor)

(phenelzine also inhibits cholinesterase activity and may reduce or slow cocaine metabolism, thereby increasing and/or prolonging its effects and increasing the risk of toxicity)

Nitrates
(cocaine may reduce the antianginal effects of these medications)

» Sympathomimetics, other, especially:
  Dobutamine or
  Dopamine or
  Epinephrine, topical
(in addition to increasing CNS stimulation, concurrent use may increase the cardiovascular effects of either or both medications and the risk of adverse effects)

(concurrent use of epinephrine with cocaine [especially intranasal application of ''cocaine mud'', a potentially lethal substance obtained by moistening cocaine crystals or flakes with an epinephrine solution] is not recommended because of the high risk of hypertensive episodes and cardiac arrhythmias; also, concurrent topical use of cocaine and epinephrine is unnecessary because epinephrine does not provide additional local vasoconstriction, slow absorption

of cocaine from the mucosa, or prolong cocaine's duration of action)

Thyroid hormones
(concurrent use may increase the effects of either these medications or cocaine; thyroid hormones enhance the risk of coronary insufficiency when sympathomimetic agents are administered to patients with coronary artery disease; dosage adjustment is recommended, although the risk is reduced in euthyroid patients)

**Laboratory value alterations**
The following have been selected on the basis of their potential clinical significance (possible effect in parentheses where appropriate)—not necessarily inclusive (» = major clinical significance):

With physiology/laboratory test values
  Blood pressure and
  Body temperature and
  Glucose, blood, concentrations and
  Heart rate
(may be increased; even low doses of cocaine may increase blood pressure by 15 to 20% and heart rate by 30 to 50%, although transient bradycardia may occur initially; the extent to which these values are increased may depend on patient predisposition as well as dosage)

**Medical considerations/Contraindications**
The medical considerations/contraindications included here have been selected on the basis of their potential clinical significance (reasons given in parentheses where appropriate)—not necessarily inclusive (» = major clinical significance).

*Risk-benefit should be considered when the following medical problems exist:*

» Cardiovascular disease, especially
»   Angina pectoris or
» Myocardial infarction, history of
(risk of severe hypertension, myocardial ischemia, angina, and/or myocardial infarction in patients with these predisposing conditions)

» Cardiac arrhythmias or history of or
» Convulsions, history of
(may be induced or exacerbated by cocaine)

» Cerebrovascular disease
(risk of cerebrovascular accident and subarachnoid hemorrhage)

» Decreased cholinesterase activity, genetic or induced by disease, including carcinoma or hepatic disease; administration of or exposure to cholinesterase inhibitors; or, to a lesser extent, pregnancy
(metabolism of cocaine is decreased or slowed, leading to increased and/or prolonged effects and increased risk of toxicity)

» Hypertension, not optimally controlled or
» Thyrotoxicosis
(cocaine-induced potentiation of endogenous catecholamines is detrimental to patients with these conditions; extreme caution is warranted)

Infection, local, at area of application
(may alter pH at area of application, leading to decrease or loss of local anesthetic effect)

Sensitivity to cocaine, history of

» Tourette's syndrome
(may be exacerbated, probably because of cocaine's dopaminergic activity)

» Traumatized mucosa, severe
(increased risk of systemic toxicity because of enhanced cocaine absorption)

» Caution is also required in elderly, debilitated, or acutely ill patients, who may be especially sensitive to the effects of the medication.

**Patient monitoring**
The following may be especially important in patient monitoring (other tests may be warranted in some patients, depending on condition; » = major clinical significance):

» Blood pressure and
» Cardiac rhythm and
  Core body temperature and
» Heart rate
(monitoring recommended because of the risk of hypertension, tachycardia, ventricular arrhythmias, and hyperpyrexia; when low doses are administered, tachycardia may initially be preceded by bradycardia caused by central vagal stimulation, although only tachycardia caused by central and peripheral sympathetic stimulation occurs following moderate or high doses)

## Side/Adverse Effects

Note: Many of cocaine's systemic adverse effects are due to excessive sympathetic activity and may be caused by rapid absorption, decreased patient tolerance, or, rarely, hypersensitivity. Toxic reactions are relatively uncommon with appropriate use of usual clinical doses.

The fatal dose of cocaine has been reported to be 1.2 grams. However, patient sensitivity to the effects of the medication is highly variable; adverse effects have been reported with as little as 20 mg.

Acute toxicity may occur very rapidly. Manifestations of systemic cocaine toxicity may occur in 3 stages (early stimulation, advanced stimulation, and depression). Although many of the signs and symptoms of early stimulation would not necessarily require medical intervention under other circumstances, their occurrence following use of cocaine indicates that prompt action is required, because progression from one stage of toxicity to the next may be very rapid.

The following side/adverse effects have been selected on the basis of their potential clinical significance (possible signs and symptoms in parentheses where appropriate)—not necessarily inclusive:

### Those indicating need for medical attention
Signs and symptoms of systemic toxicity
*Early stimulation*
*Cardiac/cardiovascular effects, including; increased blood pressure; increased heart rate; premature ventricular contractions* (irregular heartbeat); *vasoconstriction; chills and fever; CNS effects, including; agitation; excitement; nervousness; restlessness; apprehension; irritability; confusion; dizziness or lightheadedness; hallucinations; sudden headache; inability to remain still; mood or mental changes, including; elation or euphoria; dysphoria or dysphoric agitation; paranoid ideation or psychosis; preconvulsive movements; talkativeness; generalized tics or twitching of small muscles*—especially of the face, fingers, or feet; *gastrointestinal effects, including; abdominal pain; nausea or vomiting; grinding of teeth; increased sweating; rapid breathing; unusually large pupils,*—sometimes with bulging of eyes

Note: *Hallucinations* may be auditory, gustatory, olfactory, visual (e.g., "snow lights"), and/or tactile (e.g., formication ["cocaine bugs"], which may induce picking or stroking movements).

*Tachycardia* occurring after low doses of cocaine may initially be preceded by *bradycardia*.

*Advanced stimulation*
*Cardiac arrhythmias, including; ventricular arrhythmias such as; ventricular tachycardia and fibrillation* (blue discoloration of fingernails, lips, or skin; decreased blood pressure; rapid, irregular, or weak pulse); *CNS hemorrhage; congestive heart failure; convulsions, tonic-clonic*—may progress to status epilepticus; *decreased responsiveness to stimuli; delirium; hyperreflexia; loss of bladder or bowel control; malignant encephalopathy; myocardial ischemia; respiratory and/or cardiac weakness*

*Depression*
*Loss of reflexes; flaccid muscular paralysis; fixed, dilated pupils; loss of consciousness; ashen gray cyanosis; pulmonary edema; cardiac, circulatory, and/or respiratory failure*—may be fatal

### Those indicating need for medical attention only if continuing or bothersome
Incidence more frequent—following application to oral or nasal mucosa
*Loss of sense of smell and/or taste*
With repeated intranasal application
*Rebound hyperemia* (stuffy nose); *rhinitis, chronic* (sneezing or sniffling, continuing)—may lead to chronic sinusitis and increased risk of upper respiratory infections

Note: With repeated or prolonged intranasal use, *ischemic damage to the mucosa* may occur and may lead to *atrophy of the nasal mucosa, necrosis of septal tissue*, and *septal perforation*.

## Overdose

For specific information on the agents used in the management of cocaine overdose, see:
- *Benzodiazepines (Systemic)* monograph;
- *Beta-adrenergic Blocking Agents (Systemic)* monograph;
- *Calcium Channel Blocking Agents (Systemic)* monograph;
- *Lidocaine (Systemic)* monograph;
- *Nitrates (Systemic)* monograph;
- *Nitroprusside (Systemic)* monograph;
- *Phentolamine (Systemic)* monograph;
- *Sodium Bicarbonate (Systemic)* monograph; and/or
- *Thiopental* in *Anesthetics, Barbiturate (Systemic)* monograph.

For more information on the management of overdose or unintentional ingestion, **contact a Poison Control Center** (see *Poison Control Center Listing*).

### Clinical effects of overdose
The following effects have been selected on the basis of their potential clinical significance (possible signs and symptoms in parentheses where appropriate)—not necessarily inclusive:

Acute

*Cardiac arrhythmias; cardiovascular depression; convulsions; hypertension; hyperthermia; metabolic acidosis; myocardial ischemia*

### Treatment of overdose
To decrease absorption—
Measures to limit absorption in cases of overdosage (with recreational use of cocaine), such as administration of activated charcoal or gastric lavage (if the drug had been ingested orally) or application of a tourniquet (if the drug had been injected), may be of some value if they can be instituted rapidly. However, because severe cocaine toxicity may develop very quickly, *instituting the measures described below for treatment of cocaine-induced toxicity must always take precedence.*

Specific treatment—
For cardiac arrhythmias—Administering propranolol (1 mg intravenously, repeated at 1-minute intervals as needed up to a total of 6 mg) or other beta-adrenergic blocking agents is recommended to treat tachycardia or other cardiac arrhythmias. However, pure beta-adrenergic blocking agents such as propranolol do not reduce cocaine-induced hypertension and may actually increase the risk of hypertension, bradycardia, and possibly heart block by leaving unopposed cocaine's alpha-adrenergic stimulating activity. Labetalol, which also has some alpha-adrenergic blocking activity (although its beta-adrenergic blocking activity predominates) has been recommended instead. Administration of a pure alpha-adrenergic blocking agent such as phentolamine (5 mg intravenously, repeated every 15 to 20 minutes as needed) may also be required. Lidocaine hydrochloride (50 to 100 mg as a single intravenous injection, followed by infusion at a rate of 2 to 4 mg per minute as needed) or other antiarrhythmics may also be administered. In addition, cardiac massage and/or electrical defibrillation may be required for ventricular fibrillation.

For cardiovascular depression—Placing the patient in a 30-degree head down (Trendelenburg) position is recommended to increase venous return to the heart. Blood pressure should be maintained with intravenous fluids; administration of vasopressors is dangerous. For severe cardiovascular depression, cardiopulmonary resuscitation may be required, but inotropic agents should be given with great caution.

For convulsions—If convulsions do not respond to respiratory support, administration of a benzodiazepine such as diazepam (5 to 10 mg intravenously, repeated as needed) or an ultrashort-acting barbiturate such as thiopental or thiamylal (in 50- to 100-mg increments every 2 to 3 minutes, intravenously) is recommended. The fact that these agents, especially the barbiturates, may cause circulatory depression when administered intravenously must be kept in mind. A neuromuscular blocking agent has also been recommended to decrease the muscular manifestations of persistent convulsions; artificial respiration is mandatory if such an agent is used. However, succinylcholine may cause fasciculations and/or malignant hyperthermia, which may cause further problems in these patients. Other neuromuscular blocking agents may be less hazardous.

For hypertension—Administering phentolamine, labetalol, or a vasodilator such as nitroprusside.

For hyperthermia—Applying external cooling measures, such as a cooling blanket, sponging with ice water, and/or using fans.

For metabolic acidosis—Administering bicarbonate.

For myocardial ischemia—Administering nitrates, cardioselective beta-adrenergic blocking agents, and/or calcium-channel blocking agents.

Monitoring—
Monitoring vital signs and core body temperature continuously.

Supportive care—
Securing and maintaining a patent airway, administering 100% oxygen, and instituting assisted or controlled respiration as required. In some patients, endotracheal intubation may be necessary.

Establishing intravenous lines using an isotonic or hypotonic intravenous solution; hypertonic or hyperosmolar solutions should be avoided. All medications must be administered intravenously because cocaine-induced vasoconstriction may prevent absorption following intramuscular administration.

Minimizing all forms of sensory stimulation may be advisable, since these hyperstimulated patients may be agitated and/or paranoid and may become aggressive.

Patients in whom intentional overdose is known or suspected should be referred for psychiatric consultation.

## Patient Consultation

As an aid to patient consultation, refer to *Advice for the Patient, Cocaine (Mucosal-Local)*.

In providing consultation, consider emphasizing the following selected information (» = major clinical significance):

**Before receiving this medication**
» Conditions affecting use, especially:
Sensitivity to cocaine
Pregnancy—Cocaine crosses the placenta; spontaneous abortions, premature labor, and adverse effects on the fetus or neonate have resulted from cocaine abuse during pregnancy
Breast-feeding—Cocaine is distributed into breast milk and has caused convulsions, high blood presssure, fast heartbeat, breathing problems, trembling, and unusual irritability in nursing infants
Use in children—Caution required because of cocaine's toxicity
Use in the elderly—Increased risk of adverse effects
Other medications, especially beta-adrenergic blocking agents, guanadrel, guanethidine, levodopa, methyldopa, other CNS stimulants, cholinesterase inhibitors, monoamine oxidase inhibitors, and other sympathomimetics
Other medical problems, especially cardiovascular, cardiac, or cerebrovascular disease, conditions predisposing to decreased pseudocholinesterase activity, convulsions (history of), hypertension, thyrotoxicosis, and Tourette's syndrome

**Proper use of this medication**
Proper dosing

**Precautions after receiving this medication**
Caution if being tested for possible drug use because cocaine and/or its metabolites may be present in blood and/or urine for several days after administration

**Side/adverse effects**
Signs and symptoms of potential side effects, especially abdominal pain; chills; confusion; dizziness or lightheadedness; excitement, nervousness, or restlessness; fast or irregular heartbeat; general feeling of discomfort or illness; hallucinations; headache, sudden; increased sweating; mood or mental changes; and nausea

## General Dosing Information

Safe and effective clinical use of cocaine depends upon careful patient selection, proper dosage, correct administration technique, adequate precautions, and readiness for emergencies. *Resuscitative equipment, trained personnel, oxygen, and other required medications should be immediately available.*

The dosage of cocaine depends on the technique of anesthesia, the area to be anesthetized, the vascularity of the tissues at the application site, and the patient's tolerance. Because of cocaine's toxicity, the lowest dosage that provides adequate anesthesia should be used.

The recommended adult doses are given as a guideline for use in the average adult. *The actual dosage and maximum dosage must be individualized,* based on the age, size, and physical status of the patient and the expected rate of systemic absorption from the administration site. Lower concentrations and/or lower total dosage are recommended for pediatric, geriatric, acutely ill, or debilitated patients.

A standard textbook should be consulted for specific techniques and procedures applicable to the use of mucosal-local anesthetics for individual diagnostic procedures.

Premedication with a benzodiazepine such as diazepam, which has anxiolytic, anticonvulsant, and muscle relaxant properties, may reduce the incidence and/or severity of some cocaine-induced adverse effects.

Tolerance to the effects of cocaine may develop with repeated application.

Repeated use of cocaine may lead to the development of psychological and physical dependence.

**For treatment of adverse effects**
Recommended treatment consists of the following:
• Minimizing all forms of sensory stimulation may be advisable, since these hyperstimulated patients may be agitated and/or paranoid and may become aggressive.
• Treatment of CNS effects in patients who are not in immediate danger may include administering diazepam (2.5 to 5 mg) or a short-acting barbiturate (50 to 75 mg of amobarbital or secobar-

bital) for symptoms of CNS stimulation, such as hyperactivity or agitation; chlorpromazine or haloperidol for paranoia or psychosis; or tricyclic antidepressants (with great caution, because of the risk of cardiac arrhythmias) for mental depression associated with heavy cocaine abuse or withdrawal.

## Mucosal-Local Dosage Forms

### COCAINE HYDROCHLORIDE (CRYSTALS/FLAKES) USP

**Usual adult dose**
Anesthetic-vasoconstrictor (mucosal-local)[1]—
Topical, to the mucosa, a known (preweighed) quantity being applied via moistened cotton-tipped applicators.

**Usual adult prescribing limits**
400 mg, although the lowest effective dose should be used.

**Usual pediatric dose**
Dosage has not been established.

**Size(s) usually available**
U.S.—
Available as bulk chemical.
Canada—
Available as bulk chemical.

**Packaging and storage**
Store below 40 °C (104 °F), preferably between 15 and 30 °C (59 and 86 °F), unless otherwise specified by manufacturer. Store in a well-closed, light-resistant container.

**Note**
Controlled substance in both the U.S. and Canada.

### COCAINE HYDROCHLORIDE TABLETS FOR TOPICAL SOLUTION USP

**Usual adult dose**
Anesthetic-vasoconstrictor (mucosal-local)—
Topical, to the mucosa, as a 1 to 4% solution. The medication may be applied by means of cotton applicators, packs, or spray, or by instillation. Concentrations greater than 4% are generally not recommended because of difficulty in controlling dosage and the increased risk of toxic reactions.

**Usual adult prescribing limits**
400 mg, although the lowest effective dose should be used.

**Usual pediatric dose**
Children up to 6 years of age—Use is not recommended.
Children 6 years of age and older—Dosage must be individualized by the physician.

**Strength(s) usually available**
U.S.—
135 mg (Rx) [GENERIC].
Canada—
Not commercially available.

Note: This product is not to be dispensed directly to the patient.

**Packaging and storage**
Store below 40 °C (104 °F), preferably between 15 and 30 °C (59 and 86 °F), unless otherwise specified by manufacturer. Store in a well-closed, light-resistant container.

**Preparation of dosage form**
To prepare a 4% solution—Dissolve 1 tablet in 3.4 mL of distilled water.

**Incompatibilities**
Solutions of cocaine hydrochloride are incompatible with alkali and with alkaloidal precipitants.

**Note**
Controlled substance in the U.S.

### COCAINE HYDROCHLORIDE TOPICAL SOLUTION

**Usual adult dose**
Anesthetic-vasoconstrictor (mucosal-local)—
Topical, to the mucosa, as a 1 to 4% solution. The medication may be applied by means of cotton applicators, packs, or spray, or by instillation. Concentrations greater than 4% are generally not recommended because of the difficulty in controlling dosage and the increased risk of toxic reactions.

**Usual adult prescribing limits**
400 mg, although the lowest effective dose should be used.

**Usual pediatric dose**

Children up to 6 years of age—Use is not recommended.

Children 6 years of age and older—Dosage must be individualized by the physician.

**Strength(s) usually available**

U.S.—

4% (40 mg per mL) (Rx) [GENERIC].

10% (100 mg per mL) (Rx) [GENERIC].

Canada—

Not commercially available. Compounding (using cocaine hydrochloride crystals/flakes) is required for preparation of this dosage form.

Note: This product is not to be dispensed directly to the patient.

**Packaging and storage**

Store between 15 and 30 °C (59 and 86 °F), unless otherwise specified by manufacturer.

**Stability**

Ethylene oxide is recommended for sterilization of the external surface of glass bottles containing the solution. Do not steam autoclave.

**Incompatibilities**

Solutions of cocaine hydrochloride are incompatible with alkali and with alkaloidal precipitants.

**Note**

Controlled substance in the U.S.

## COCAINE HYDROCHLORIDE VISCOUS TOPICAL SOLUTION

**Usual adult dose**

Anesthetic-vasoconstrictor (mucosal-local)—

Topical, to the mucosa, as a 1 to 4% solution. The medication may be applied by means of cotton applicators or packs, or by instillation. Concentrations greater than 4% are generally not recommended because of the difficulty in controlling dosage and the increased risk of toxic reactions.

**Usual adult prescribing limits**

400 mg, although the lowest effective dose should be used.

**Usual pediatric dose**

Children up to 6 years of age—Use is not recommended.

Children 6 years of age and older—Dosage must be individualized by the physician.

**Strength(s) usually available**

U.S.—

4% (40 mg per mL) (Rx) [GENERIC].

10% (100 mg per mL) (Rx) [GENERIC].

Canada—

Not commercially available.

Note: This product is not to be dispensed directly to the patient.

**Packaging and storage**

Store between 15 and 30 °C (59 and 86 °F), unless otherwise specified by manufacturer.

**Stability**

Ethylene oxide is recommended for sterilization of the external surface of glass bottles containing the solution. Do not steam autoclave.

**Incompatibilities**

Solutions of cocaine hydrochloride are incompatible with alkali and with alkaloidal precipitants.

**Note**

Controlled substance in the U.S.

---

¹Not included in Canadian product labeling.

---

Revised: 08/08/92

Interim revision: 07/14/94

---

## CODEINE—See *Opioid (Narcotic) Analgesics (Systemic)*

---

## CODEINE-CONTAINING COMBINATIONS—

Acetaminophen and Codeine (Systemic)—See *Opioid (Narcotic) Analgesics and Acetaminophen (Systemic)*

Acetaminophen, Codeine, and Caffeine (Systemic)—See *Opioid (Narcotic) Analgesics and Acetaminophen (Systemic)*

Aspirin and Codeine (Systemic)—See *Opioid (Narcotic) Analgesics and Aspirin (Systemic)*

Aspirin and Codeine, Buffered (Systemic)—See *Opioid (Narcotic) Analgesics and Aspirin (Systemic)*

Aspirin, Codeine, and Caffeine (Systemic)—See *Opioid (Narcotic) Analgesics and Aspirin (Systemic)*

Bromodiphenhydramine and Codeine (Systemic)—See *Cough/Cold Combinations (Systemic)*

Bromodiphenhydramine, Diphenhydramine, Codeine, Ammonium Chloride, and Potassium Guaiacolsulfonate (Systemic)—See *Cough/Cold Combinations (Systemic)*

Brompheniramine, Phenylephrine, Phenylpropanolamine, and Codeine (Systemic)—See *Cough/Cold Combinations (Systemic)*

Brompheniramine, Phenylephrine, Phenylpropanolamine, Codeine, and Guaifenesin (Systemic)—See *Cough/Cold Combinations (Systemic)*

Brompheniramine, Phenylpropanolamine, and Codeine (Systemic)—See *Cough/Cold Combinations (Systemic)*

Butalbital, Aspirin, Caffeine, and Codeine (Systemic)—See *Barbiturates and Analgesics (Systemic)*

Chlorpheniramine, Phenylephrine, Codeine, and Ammonium Chloride (Systemic)—See *Cough/Cold Combinations (Systemic)*

Chlorpheniramine, Phenylephrine, Codeine, and Potassium Iodide (Systemic)—See *Cough/Cold Combinations (Systemic)*

Chlorpheniramine, Phenylephrine, Phenylpropanolamine, and Codeine (Systemic)—See *Cough/Cold Combinations (Systemic)*

Chlorpheniramine, Phenylpropanolamine, Codeine, Guaifenesin, and Acetaminophen (Systemic)—See *Cough/Cold Combinations (Systemic)*

Chlorpheniramine, Phenyltoloxamine, Ephedrine, Codeine, and Guaiacol Carbonate (Systemic)—See *Cough/Cold Combinations (Systemic)*

Chlorpheniramine, Pseudoephedrine, and Codeine (Systemic)—See *Cough/Cold Combinations (Systemic)*

Codeine, Ammonium Chloride, and Guaifenesin (Systemic)—See *Cough/Cold Combinations (Systemic)*

Codeine and Calcium Iodide (Systemic)—See *Cough/Cold Combinations (Systemic)*

Codeine and Guaifenesin (Systemic)—See *Cough/Cold Combinations (Systemic)*

Codeine and Iodinated Glycerol (Systemic)—See *Cough/Cold Combinations (Systemic)*

Diphenhydramine, Codeine, and Ammonium Chloride (Systemic)—See *Cough/Cold Combinations (Systemic)*

Pheniramine, Codeine, and Guaifenesin (Systemic)—See *Cough/Cold Combinations (Systemic)*

Pheniramine, Phenylephrine, Codeine, Sodium Citrate, Sodium Salicylate, and Caffeine (Systemic)—See *Cough/Cold Combinations (Systemic)*

Pheniramine, Pyrilamine, Phenylpropanolamine, and Codeine (Systemic)—See *Cough/Cold Combinations (Systemic)*

Pheniramine, Pyrilamine, Phenylpropanolamine, Codeine, Acetaminophen, and Caffeine (Systemic)—See *Cough/Cold Combinations (Systemic)*

Phenobarbital, ASA, and Codeine (Systemic)—See *Barbiturates and Analgesics (Systemic)*

Phenylephrine and Codeine (Systemic)—See *Cough/Cold Combinations (Systemic)*

Phenylpropanolamine, Codeine, and Guaifenesin (Systemic)—See *Cough/Cold Combinations (Systemic)*

Promethazine and Codeine (Systemic)—See *Cough/Cold Combinations (Systemic)*

Promethazine, Codeine, and Potassium Guaiacolsulfonate (Systemic)—See *Cough/Cold Combinations (Systemic)*

Promethazine, Phenylephrine, and Codeine (Systemic)—See *Cough/Cold Combinations (Systemic)*

Promethazine, Phenylephrine, Codeine, and Potassium Guaiacolsulfonate (Systemic)—See *Cough/Cold Combinations (Systemic)*

Pseudoephedrine and Codeine (Systemic)—See *Cough/Cold Combinations (Systemic)*

Pseudoephedrine, Codeine, and Guaifenesin (Systemic)—See *Cough/Cold Combinations (Systemic)*

Pyrilamine and Codeine (Systemic)—See *Cough/Cold Combinations (Systemic)*

Pyrilamine, Phenylephrine, and Codeine (Systemic)—See *Cough/Cold Combinations (Systemic)*

Triprolidine, Pseudoephedrine, and Codeine (Systemic)—See *Cough/Cold Combinations (Systemic)*

Triprolidine, Pseudoephedrine, Codeine, and Guaifenesin (Systemic)—See *Cough/Cold Combinations (Systemic)*

# COLCHICINE    Systemic

VA CLASSIFICATION (Primary): MS400

Note: For a listing of dosage forms and brand names by country availability, see *Dosage Forms* section(s). For a listing of brand names for the articles in this monograph, refer to the General Index.

## Category

Anti-inflammatory; antigout agent; familial Mediterranean fever suppressant; calcium pyrophosphate deposition disease suppressant; amyloidosis suppressant.

## Indications

Note: Bracketed information in the *Indications* section refers to uses that are not included in U.S. product labeling.

Note: The toxicity and narrow margin of safety of therapeutic doses of colchicine (e.g., doses required to relieve an acute attack of gout or calcium pyrophosphate deposition disease) must be carefully considered before treatment is initiated, especially when the medication is to be administered intravenously. However, long-term administration of prophylactic doses for chronic gout or other chronic conditions responsive to such treatment is relatively unlikely to cause serious toxicity in patients with normal renal and hepatic function.

### Accepted

Gouty arthritis, chronic (treatment) or

Gouty arthritis, acute (prophylaxis and treatment)—Colchicine is indicated to reduce the frequency and severity of acute attacks of gouty arthritis in patients with chronic gout. Complete remission of such attacks may occur in some patients. Prophylactic administration of colchicine may be especially important during the first several months of treatment with an antihyperuricemic agent (allopurinol, probenecid, or sulfinpyrazone) because the frequency of acute attacks may be increased when such therapy is initiated.

Although colchicine is also indicated to relieve the pain and inflammation of acute attacks of gouty arthritis, it has generally been replaced by less toxic medications for this purpose. Nonsteroidal anti-inflammatory drugs (NSAIDs) or corticosteroids (preferably via intrasynovial injection) are recommended for relief of an acute attack. Therapeutic doses of colchicine should be reserved for patients in whom these other agents are contraindicated or ineffective.

Intravenous administration of colchicine may be considered for treatment of acute attacks of gouty arthritis when oral administration is ineffective, gastrointestinal side effects limit administration of effective oral doses, or an especially rapid response is needed. Although the risk of gastrointestinal toxicity is considerably lower with intravenous administration than with oral administration, the risk of other forms of toxicity is very high, especially in patients with renal and/or hepatic function impairment; fatalities have been reported. It is recommended that the medication be administered intravenously with caution, in low doses, and only to carefully selected patients, if at all.

[Mediterranean fever, familial (prophylaxis and treatment)]—Colchicine is indicated to reduce the frequency and severity of acute attacks of familial Mediterranean fever (familial recurrent polyserositis). Complete remission of such attacks may occur in some patients.

Prophylactic use of colchicine prevents amyloidosis and amyloidosis-induced renal failure in patients with familial Mediterranean fever, including patients whose acute attacks are not suppressed by such treatment. Colchicine therapy must be started before nephrotic syndrome or uremia develops; initiation of treatment after either of these conditions is present will not prevent further deterioration of renal function. However, after renal transplantation, prophylactic colchicine prevents amyloid deposition and resultant tissue damage in the transplanted kidney. Prophylactic use of colchicine is therefore recommended for all patients with familial Mediterranean fever, even when frequent, severe attacks continue to occur despite colchicine administration.

Although colchicine may also be effective in aborting an acute attack of febrile polyserositis if taken at the earliest sign of an attack, it will not relieve or shorten a severe attack that is already in progress.

[Calcium pyrophosphate deposition disease, acute (prophylaxis and treatment)]—Colchicine is used for the symptomatic relief of acute attacks of calcium pyrophosphate deposition disease (chondrocalcinosis articularis; pseudogout; synovitis, crystal-induced). Intravenous administration of the medication is reported to be more consistently effective than oral administration for relief of an acute attack. However, the

high risk of toxicity associated with intravenous administration of colchicine must be considered. Prophylactic use of oral colchicine may prevent repeat acute attacks.

[Arthritis, sarcoid (treatment)][1]—Colchicine is used to relieve acute arthritic symptoms associated with sarcoidosis.

[Amyloidosis (treatment)][1]—Colchicine is indicated to decrease amyloid deposition and resultant tissue damage in patients with primary amyloidosis or amyloidosis secondary to conditions such as psoriatic arthritis, ankylosing spondylitis, or familial Mediterranean fever. Colchicine has been used together with melphalan and prednisone for the treatment of primary amyloidosis.

[Behçet's syndrome (treatment)][1]—Colchicine is used in the treatment of patients with Behçet's syndrome. It relieves or prevents erythema nodosum and arthralgias and may also reduce the frequency or severity of oral and/or genital ulcerations in some patients. However, colchicine does not reduce the frequency or severity of ocular lesions associated with this disease or improve visual acuity in affected patients.

[Cirrhosis, biliary (treatment)][1]—Colchicine is used in the treatment of primary biliary cirrhosis. Biochemical indicators of disease activity (serum albumin, bilirubin, alkaline phosphatase, cholesterol, and aminotransferases) improve during treatment. Although colchicine may retard the development of fibrosis and hepatic failure in patients with biliary cirrhosis, it does not relieve symptoms, prevent or reverse histological changes characteristic of the disease, or decrease the need for hepatic transplantation. In a few studies colchicine-treated patients survived significantly longer than control patients. Colchicine may provide additional benefit when used concurrently with ursodiol for this indication. However, colchicine clearance is substantially reduced in patients with alcoholic cirrhosis. Caution and careful attention to dosage are recommended to prevent accumulation and toxicity if colchicine is administered to these patients.

[Pericarditis, recurrent (treatment)][1]—Limited data indicate that colchicine may be useful for preventing acute attacks of pericarditis that recur despite treatment with NSAIDs and/or corticosteroids. Colchicine has permitted withdrawal of corticosteroid therapy in some patients with this condition.

---

[1]Not included in Canadian product labeling.

## Pharmacology/Pharmacokinetics

### Physicochemical characteristics

Source—Colchicine is the active alkaloidal principle derived from various species of *Colchicum*.

Molecular weight—399.44.

pKa—1.7 and 12.4.

### Mechanism of action/Effect

Anti-inflammatory and—

Antigout agent:

The precise mechanism of action has not been completely established. In patients with gout, colchicine apparently interrupts the cycle of monosodium urate crystal deposition in joint tissues and the resultant inflammatory response that initiates and sustains an acute attack. Colchicine decreases leukocyte chemotaxis and phagocytosis and inhibits the formation and release of a chemotactic glycoprotein that is produced during phagocytosis of urate crystals. Colchicine also inhibits urate crystal deposition, which is enhanced by a low pH in the tissues, probably by inhibiting oxidation of glucose and subsequent lactic acid production in leukocytes. Colchicine has no analgesic or antihyperuricemic activity.

Note: Colchicine inhibits microtubule assembly in various cells, including leukocytes, probably by binding to and interfering with polymerization of the microtubule subunit tubulin. Although some studies have found that this action probably does not contribute significantly to colchicine's antigout action, a recent *in vitro* study has shown that it may be at least partially involved.

Colchicine's effect on microtubule assembly and/or leukocyte function may be involved in the medication's efficacy in conditions other than gout. In patients with biliary cirrhosis, interference with microtubule formation may inhibit collagen production, thereby retarding the development of hepatic fibrosis. Colchicine may also increase degradation of collagen by stimulating production of collagenase. Also, colchicine corrects some of the abnormalities of lymphocyte and monocyte function that have been identified in patients with active biliary cirrhosis. In addition, colchicine has been found to reverse abnormalities in neutrophil activity that are present in patients with Behçet's disease, i.e., increased migration and reduced superoxide scavenging activity.

Familial Mediterranean fever suppressant and—
Amyloidosis suppressant:

The mechanism by which colchicine suppresses acute attacks of febrile polyserositis in patients with familial Mediterranean fever has not been determined, but it may differ from the mechanism responsible for suppression of amyloidosis in patients with this disease. Colchicine inhibits secretion of serum amyloid A in patients with familial Mediterranean fever. It has also been suggested that colchicine may interfere with polymerization of amyloid subunits into mature amyloid fibrils.

**Other actions/effects**

By inhibiting microtubule assembly, colchicine interferes with mitotic spindle formation, thereby arresting mitosis in metaphase.

Colchicine decreases body temperature, depresses the respiratory center, constricts blood vessels, and causes hypertension via central vasomotor stimulation.

**Absorption**

Colchicine is rapidly absorbed after oral administration, probably from the jejunum and ileum. However, the rate and extent of absorption are variable, depending on the tablet dissolution rate; variability in gastric emptying, intestinal motility, and pH at the absorption site; and the extent to which colchicine is bound to microtubules in gastrointestinal mucosal cells.

**Distribution**

Colchicine is rapidly distributed to peripheral leukocytes. Concentrations in these cells may exceed those in plasma. The medication can be detected in leukocytes for 9 to 10 days following administration of a single dose. Colchicine also concentrates in the kidneys, liver, and spleen. Accumulation in these tissues may lead to toxicity. Colchicine is distributed into breast milk; peak concentrations of 1.2 to 2.5 nanograms per mL (< 0.001 micromole per liter) have been measured 40 to 50 minutes after administration of a 0.6-mg dose to a patient receiving long-term therapy with 0.6 mg twice a day.

**Protein binding**

In plasma—Low to moderate (30 to 50%).

**Biotransformation**

Probably hepatic. Although colchicine metabolites have not been identified in humans, metabolism by mammalian hepatic microsomes has been demonstrated *in vitro*.

**Half-life**

Distribution—3 to 5 minutes

Elimination—Approximately 1 hour in healthy subjects, although a study with an extended sampling time reported mean terminal elimination half-life values of approximately 9 to 10.5 hours. Other studies have reported half-life values of approximately 2 hours in patients with alcoholic cirrhosis and approximately 2.5 hours in patients with familial Mediterranean fever.

**Onset of action**

Acute gouty arthritis (following first dose)—
Intravenous: Within 6 to 12 hours
Oral: Within 12 hours

**Time to peak concentration**

Oral—0.5 to 2 hours

**Time to peak effect**

Acute gouty arthritis—
Relief of pain and inflammation: 24 to 48 hours following the first oral dose.
Relief of swelling: May require several days.

**Elimination**

Primarily biliary, with enterohepatic recirculation; 10 to 20% renal. Renal elimination may be increased in patients with hepatic disease. Because of the high degree of tissue uptake, only 10% of a single dose is eliminated within 24 hours; elimination of colchicine from the body may continue for 10 days or more after cessation of administration. Also, elimination is slower in patients with biliary disease; in one study mean clearance rates of 10.65 mL per minute per kg of body weight (mL/min/kg) and 4.22 mL/min/kg were measured in healthy control subjects and in patients with alcoholic cirrhosis, respectively.

In dialysis—Because of the high degree of tissue binding, colchicine is not dialyzable.

# Precautions to Consider

## Pregnancy/Reproduction

Fertility—Colchicine arrests cell division in animals and plants. Although colchicine has been reported to cause reversible azoospermia and fertility problems in male patients receiving long-term treatment with prophylactic doses, several studies in patients receiving such treatment have shown no significant reproductive difficulties, abnormalities in sperm counts, or alterations in testosterone, prolactin, luteinizing hormone, or follicle-stimulating hormone concentrations. Administration of colchicine does not increase, and may actually reduce, the risk of serious fertility problems in women with familial Mediterranean fever, who are subject to formation of fibrous adhesions, ovulatory disturbances, and, consequently, sterility.

Pregnancy—Controlled studies in pregnant women have not been done, but colchicine has been used prior to and throughout pregnancy by patients receiving long-term prophylaxis for familial Mediterranean fever. Although several miscarriages have been reported, the miscarriage rate in untreated women with this disease is high. A large majority of the pregnancies in female patients and wives of male patients receiving colchicine produced healthy, normal, full-term infants. However, a group of investigators reported 2 cases of trisomy 21 (in 91 pregnancies) and recommend that amniocentesis be performed when either parent is receiving colchicine.

Colchicine has been shown to be teratogenic in mice given doses of 0.5 mg per kg of body weight (mg/kg) or more, causing microtia, exencephaly, microphthalmia, anophthalmia, skeletal malformations, gastrochisis, abnormalities of the liver and stomach, dextrocardia, missing pulmonary lobe, and cleft palate. Colchicine has also produced fetotoxic and teratogenic effects in hamsters given 10 mg/kg. Administration to hamsters on Day 8 of pregnancy resulted in fatalities in 50% of the fetuses and congenital malformations including microphthalmia, anophthalmia, exencephaly, rib fusions and other skeletal anomalies, and umbilical hernias in a large number of the surviving fetuses. In other studies, colchicine was embryotoxic in rabbits and cattle, but not monkeys. Studies in rats produced contradictory results.

FDA Pregnancy Category D.

## Breast-feeding

Colchicine is distributed into breast milk; peak concentrations of 1.2 to 2.5 nanograms per mL (< 0.001 micromole per liter) have been measured 40 to 50 minutes after administration of a 0.6-mg dose to a patient receiving long-term therapy with 0.6 mg twice a day. No adverse effects were apparent in the breast-fed infant during the first 6 months of life.

## Pediatrics

For gouty arthritis—Appropriate studies on the relationship of age to the effects of colchicine have not been performed in the pediatric population (in whom gouty arthritis rarely if ever occurs). Safety and efficacy for this indication have not been established.

For familial Mediterranean fever—Studies in pediatric patients 3 years of age and older receiving long-term prophylactic treatment have not demonstrated pediatrics-specific problems that would limit the usefulness of colchicine for this indication in children.

## Geriatrics

Geriatric patients, even those with normal renal and hepatic function, may be more susceptible to cumulative toxicity with colchicine. Also, elderly patients are more likely to have age-related renal function impairment, which increases the risk of myopathy and other toxic effects in patients receiving colchicine. Caution and careful attention to dosage are recommended.

## Dental

The leukopenic and thrombocytopenic effects of colchicine may result in an increased incidence of microbial infection, delayed healing, and gingival bleeding. If leukopenia or thrombocytopenia occurs, dental work should be deferred until blood counts have returned to normal and patients should be instructed in proper oral hygiene, including caution in use of regular toothbrushes, dental floss, and toothpicks.

## Drug interactions and/or related problems

The following drug interactions and/or related problems have been selected on the basis of their potential clinical significance (possible mechanism in parentheses where appropriate)—not necessarily inclusive (» = major clinical significance):

Note: Combinations containing any of the following medications, depending on the amount present, may also interact with this medication.

In addition to the interactions listed below, the possibility should be considered that colchicine, because of its potential for causing gastrointestinal hemorrhage, thrombocytopenia (with chronic use), and coagulation defects including disseminated intravascular coagulation (with an overdose), may cause increased risk to patients receiving other medications that may impair blood clotting or cause hemorrhage. Such medications may include anticoagulants (coumarin- or indandione-derivative) or other hypoprothrombinemia-inducing medications; heparin; thrombolytic agents; platelet aggregation inhibitors; other thrombocytopenia-inducing medications; and other medications having significant potential for causing gastrointestinal ulceration or hemorrhage.

Alcohol
(concurrent use with orally administered colchicine increases the risk of gastrointestinal toxicity, especially in alcoholics; also, alcohol increases blood uric acid concentrations and may decrease the efficacy of prophylactic gout therapy)

Anti-inflammatory drugs, nonsteroidal (NSAIDs), especially
» Phenylbutazone
(concurrent use of phenylbutazone with colchicine may increase the risk of leukopenia, thrombocytopenia, or bone marrow depression)

(concurrent use of any NSAID with colchicine may increase the risk of gastrointestinal ulceration or hemorrhage; also, NSAID-induced inhibition of platelet aggregation may increase the risk of bleeding in areas other than the gastrointestinal tract should colchicine-induced thrombocytopenia or clotting defects [with overdose] also occur)

Antineoplastic agents, rapidly cytolytic
(these medications may increase serum uric acid concentrations and decrease the efficacy of prophylactic gout therapy)

Blood dyscrasia–causing medications (See *Appendix II*)
(the leukopenic and/or thrombocytopenic effects of colchicine may be intensified with concurrent or recent therapy if these medications cause the same effects; blood counts should be monitored if concurrent or sequential use cannot be avoided)

» Bone marrow depressants, other (See *Appendix II*) or
Radiation therapy
(additive bone marrow depression may occur; dosage reductions may be required when 2 or more bone marrow depressants, including radiation, are used concurrently or consecutively)

Vitamin $B_{12}$
(absorption of this vitamin may be impaired by chronic administration or high doses of colchicine; requirement may be increased)

### Laboratory value alterations
The following have been selected on the basis of their potential clinical significance (possible effect in parentheses where appropriate)—not necessarily inclusive (» = major clinical significance):

With diagnostic test results
Hemoglobin, in urine, or
Red blood cells (RBC), in urine
(colchicine may cause false-positive test results)

17-Hydroxycorticosteroid determinations, in urine
(interference may occur when the Reddy, Jenkins, and Thorn procedure is used)

With physiology/laboratory test values
Alkaline phosphatase, serum and
Aspartate aminotransferase (AST [SGOT]), serum
(values may be increased)

Platelet count
(may be decreased)

### Medical considerations/Contraindications
The medical considerations/contraindications included here have been selected on the basis of their potential clinical significance (reasons given in parentheses where appropriate)—not necessarily inclusive (» = major clinical significance).

*Except under special circumstances, this medication should not be used when the following medical problems exist:*
» Hepatic and renal disease, concurrent
(risk of toxicity is very high, especially with intravenous administration)

» Renal function impairment, severe
(high risk of myopathy and other forms of toxicity; use in patients with severe renal function impairment [i.e., creatinine clearance 10 mL per minute (0.17 mL per second) or less] is not recommended)

*For intravenous administration only*
» Hepatic function impairment, severe
(intravenous administration is not recommended because of the high risk of impaired elimination and resultant toxicity)

» Leukopenia
(may be exacerbated; intravenous administration is not recommended)

*Risk-benefit should be considered when the following medical problems exist:*
Alcoholism, active
(increased risk of gastrointestinal toxicity with oral administration; parenteral administration is preferred; however, it is recommended that hepatic and renal function, which may be impaired in alcoholics, be assessed prior to initiation of therapy in these patients)

» Blood dyscrasias
(may be exacerbated)

» Cardiac disorders or
» Hepatic function impairment or
» Renal function impairment
(increased risk of cumulative toxicity, with the risk increasing as the severity of impairment increases; colchicine should be given with caution, with the dose being reduced and/or the intervals between doses being increased; it has been recommended that half of the usual dose be administered to patients with creatinine clearances of 50 mL per minute [0.83 mL per second] or less)

» Gastrointestinal disorders
(the risk of colchicine-induced damage to gastrointestinal tissues may be increased; also, colchicine's gastrointestinal toxicity may be particularly hazardous to patients with these conditions)

Sensitivity to colchicine, history of
Caution is also advised in administration to geriatric or debilitated patients, who may be more susceptible to cumulative toxicity.

### Patient monitoring
The following may be especially important in patient monitoring (other tests may be warranted in some patients, depending on condition; » = major clinical significance):

Complete blood counts
(recommended at periodic intervals during long-term treatment because bone marrow depression with agranulocytosis, thrombocytopenia, or aplastic anemia may occur)

## Side/Adverse Effects

Note: There is no clear separation of nontoxic, toxic, and lethal doses of colchicine. Various sources report lethal doses ranging between 20 and 65 mg, although considerably lower doses may be fatal, especially in patients with renal and/or hepatic function impairment and with intravenous administration. Fatalities have occurred after ingestion of single doses as low as 7 mg or intravenous administration of cumulative doses of only 5 mg.

The following side/adverse effects have been selected on the basis of their potential clinical significance (possible signs and symptoms in parentheses where appropriate)—not necessarily inclusive:

### Those indicating need for medical attention
Incidence rare
*Hypersensitivity reactions including dermatoses* (skin rash, hives); *and angioedema* (large, hive-like swellings on face, eyelids, mouth, lips, and/or tongue)

Note: *Skin rash* not associated with hypersensitivity may occur, especially with long-term treatment in patients with renal or hepatic function impairment.

*With intravenous administration*
*Cardiac arrhythmias*—with too-rapid administration; *localized reactions such as irritation, inflammation, or thrombophlebitis; median nerve neuritis in injected arm* (pain; tenderness; feeling of burning, "crawling," or tingling in the skin over the affected nerve); *or necrosis of the skin and soft tissues* (peeling of skin)—if extravasation occurs

*With prolonged or long-term use*
*Bone marrow depression with agranulocytosis* (fever with or without chills; sores, ulcers, or white spots on lips or in mouth; sore throat); *aplastic anemia* (unusual tiredness or weakness; headache; difficulty in breathing, exertional); *and thrombocytopenia* (usually asymptomatic; rarely, unusual bleeding or bruising; black, tarry stools; blood in urine or stools; pinpoint red spots on skin); *myopathy* (muscle weakness); *neuropathy* (mild numbness in fingers or toes)

Note: *Myopathy* is more likely to occur in patients with impaired renal or hepatic function who are receiving long-term treatment with prophylactic doses of colchicine. This condition is characterized by proximal muscle weakness, spontaneous activity in the electromyelogram, and elevated creatine kinase values. Because these findings are also present in patients with polymyositis, a muscle biopsy may be necessary to differentiate between the 2 conditions.

**Those indicating need for medical attention only if they continue or are bothersome**

Incidence more frequent (up to 80%) with therapeutic doses of oral colchicine; rare with intravenous administration
  *Gastrointestinal toxicity* (diarrhea; nausea or vomiting; stomach pain)—early symptoms

Incidence less frequent
  *Loss of appetite*

With long-term use or following recovery from severe toxicity
  *Loss of hair*

  Note: *Hair loss* may start to occur as soon as 2 to 3 weeks after initiation of long-term therapy; the risk is dose-dependent. Regrowth usually begins 3 to 12 weeks after discontinuation of the medication.

## Overdose

For specific information on the agents used in the management of colchicine overdose, see:
  • Atropine in *Anticholinergics/Antispasmodics (Systemic)* monograph;
  • *Benzodiazepines (Systemic)* monograph;
  • *Charcoal, Activated (Oral-Local)* monograph;
  • *Opioid (Narcotic) Analgesics (Systemic)* monograph; and/or
  • *Vitamin K (Systemic)* monograph.

For more information on the management of overdose or unintentional ingestion, **contact a Poison Control Center** (see *Poison Control Center Listing*).

**Clinical effects of overdose**

The following effects have been selected on the basis of their potential clinical significance (possible signs and symptoms in parentheses where appropriate)-not necessarily inclusive:

Acute

Acute—usually begins within 24 to 72 hours after an acute overdose

  *Fever*—may be the first sign of this stage and may be associated with septicemia; *cerebral edema; CNS toxicity* (ascending paralysis of the CNS; convulsions; delirium); *multiple organ failure caused by tissue damage, including bone marrow hypoplasia* (agranulocytosis or leukopenia; thrombocytopenia and disseminated intravascular coagulation or other coagulation abnormalities); *hepatocellular damage, possibly with necrosis; muscle damage, including rhabdomyolysis* (myoglobinuria; severe muscle weakness or paralysis); *or necrosis, possibly resulting in adult respiratory distress syndrome or other forms of respiratory distress* (fast, shallow breathing); *pulmonary edema, and hypoxia, and/or myocardial injury* (ST segment elevation in electrocardiogram; decreased cardiac contractility, creatine kinase elevation, hemorrhages and microinfarctions in the myocardium); *paralytic ileus; renal damage* (with hematuria; and oliguric renal failure)

  Note: After a cumulative overdose has been administered intravenously, symptoms associated with *bone marrow depression* may be the first indications of toxicity. In some patients, *disseminated intravascular coagulation* may be the first hematologic sign of toxicity, with the most severe coagulopathy occurring about 25 hours following administration of a large overdose.

  *Fluid and electrolyte disturbances* often occur in colchicine toxicity. *Hypovolemia* may lead to *hypokalemia, hyponatremia,* and *metabolic acidosis.* Also, *hypocalcemia, hypokalemia, hypophosphatemia,* and/or *metabolic acidosis* may occur in association with *renal damage.*

  Fatalities may result from *shock, respiratory or cardiac arrest,* or *rapidly progressive multiple organ failure.*

Chronic—may occur several hours after an acute overdose
  *Burning feeling in the throat or skin; gastrointestinal toxicity* (burning feeling in the stomach; severe abdominal pain; diarrhea; nausea, and/or vomiting); *sloughing of the gastrointestinal mucosa and/or; hemorrhagic gastroenteritis* (bloody diarrhea)—with oral ingestion only; *vascular damage*

  Note: Early *gastrointestinal symptoms* generally do not occur in overdosage caused by intravenous administration.

  *Vascular damage* may lead to *fluid extravasation* which, together with fluid losses caused by severe *diarrhea* and *vomiting,* may cause profound dehydration, hypotension, and shock. Also, *septicemia* secondary to severe intestinal damage may result in *septic shock.*

Chronic—generally begins about 10 days after an acute overdose
  *Alopecia* (hair loss)—reversible; *rebound leukocytosis; stomatitis* (sores, ulcers, or white spots on lips or in mouth)

**Treatment of overdose**

For early signs of overdose (gastrointestinal symptoms)—
  Immediate discontinuation of colchicine administration (when used for short-term relief of an acute attack) or reducing the dose (when used prophylactically).
  Specific treatment—Use of morphine or atropine for stomach pain.
  Use of an opioid or other antidiarrheal agents for diarrhea.
  For irritation caused by extravasation: Applying heat or cold to the affected area and administering analgesics.

For severe overdose—
  To decrease absorption—May include removing unabsorbed medication (if taken orally) via gastric lavage and/or administration of activated charcoal. Because of colchicine's extensive biliary elimination and enterohepatic recirculation, repeated doses of activated charcoal are recommended to bind absorbed colchicine that re-enters the intestinal tract, which interrupts enterohepatic recirculation and hastens elimination.
  To enhance elimination—Due to colchicine's high degree of uptake and binding in various tissues, forced diuresis, peritoneal dialysis, hemodialysis, charcoal hemoperfusion, or exchange transfusion cannot be expected to remove significant quantities of the medication from the body.

Specific treatment—
  For treatment of convulsions caused by overdose:
    Administering an anticonvulsant. A benzodiazepine, such as diazepam, may be administered. Since intravenously administered benzodiazepines may cause respiratory and circulatory depression, especially when administered rapidly, and respiratory distress and shock are also potential consequences of colchicine overdose, medications and equipment needed for support of respiration and for resuscitation must be immediately available.
  For bone marrow suppression and resultant coagulation defects:
    Vitamin $K_1$, fresh frozen plasma, platelets, and/or red blood cells may be administered as needed.
    Note: One patient with colchicine induced aplastic anemia has been successfully treated with a single 300–mg subcutaneous dose of granulocyte colony-stimulating factor
  For fever, leukopenia, and or sepsis:
    Use of broad-spectrum antibiotics.
  Monitoring— May include monitoring hemodynamic, cardiac, and respiratory status and blood electrolytes. Prolonged observation is recommended because the most severe toxic effects generally do not appear until 24 hours or more after ingestion of an acute overdose.
  Supportive care—
    May include correcting dehydration via fluid replacement and instituting other measures to prevent or treat shock, including administration of a vasopressor, if necessary.
    Correcting electrolyte imbalances and metabolic acidosis.
    For respiratory distress, securing and maintaining a patent airway, administering oxygen, and instituting assisted or controlled respiration as needed. Endotracheal intubation may be required.

## Patient Consultation

As an aid to patient consultation, refer to *Advice for the Patient, Colchicine (Systemic).*

In providing consultation, consider emphasizing the following selected information (» = major clinical significance):

**Before using this medication**
» Conditions affecting use, especially:
    Sensitivity to colchicine
    Use in the elderly—Increased susceptibility to cumulative toxicity
    Other medications, especially other bone marrow depressants or radiation therapy
    Other medical problems, especially blood dyscrasias, severe cardiac disorders, gastrointestinal disorders, renal function impairment, or hepatic function impairment

**Proper use of this medication**
» Importance of not taking more medication than prescribed
*For prophylactic use*
  Compliance with therapy
  Not using additional colchicine to relieve an acute gout attack that occurs during prophylactic therapy, unless otherwise directed by physician; using alternative treatment as prescribed
*For intermittent use to relieve acute attack*
  Starting medication at earliest sign of attack

&raquo; Stopping medication when pain is relieved; at first sign of diarrhea, nausea or vomiting, or stomach pain; or when maximum dosage is reached (even if symptoms are not relieved)

Noting total quantity of colchicine taken before gastrointestinal symptoms occur and, in subsequent attacks, stopping treatment before this cumulative dose has been reached

&raquo; Not taking additional colchicine for 3 days after using therapeutic oral doses to relieve an acute attack or for 7 days after receiving intravenous colchicine

&raquo; Continuing other gout medication (if applicable) while taking colchicine

&raquo; Proper dosing

Missed dose: If on fixed-dosage chronic therapy—Taking as soon as possible; not taking if almost time for next dose; not doubling doses

&raquo; Proper storage

**Precautions while using this medication**

Regular visits to physician to check progress and possibly to be tested for adverse effects during long-term therapy

&raquo; Possibility that large quantities of alcohol may increase the risk of gastrointestinal toxicity; also, alcohol may increase uric acid concentrations and thereby decrease the effectiveness of medication when used for gout

Not discontinuing prophylactic treatment without first consulting physician if acute attacks continue to occur

**Side/adverse effects**

&raquo; Checking with physician if diarrhea, nausea, vomiting, or stomach pain occurs and continues for more than 3 hours after medication is discontinued

&raquo; Checking with physician immediately if symptoms of angioedema, bone marrow depression, or overdose occur

Signs and symptoms of other potential side effects, especially skin rash or hives, localized reactions to extravasation after intravenous administration, myopathy, and neuropathy

# General Dosing Information

Colchicine's toxicity and narrow margin of safety must be considered before therapeutic doses of the medication are administered, especially intravenously. Fatalities have occurred after ingestion of single doses as low as 7 mg or intravenous administration of cumulative doses of 5 mg.

If colchicine is used to relieve an acute attack of gout or to abort an acute attack of familial Mediterranean fever, therapy should be instituted at the first sign of the attack. Delay in starting treatment reduces the medication's effectiveness.

A reduction in the size of individual doses, an increase in the interval between doses, or a reduction in the total daily dosage may be necessary in patients with renal or hepatic function impairment. Specifically, it is recommended that dosage be reduced by half (for prophylactic use, limited to no more than 600 mcg [0.6 mg] per day, orally) if the patient's creatinine clearance is 50 mL per minute (0.83 mL per second) or less and that the medication not be used at all if the patient's creatinine clearance is 10 mL per minute (0.17 mL per second) or less.

Oral administration of colchicine is preferable for prophylactic treatment of recurrent or chronic gout; intravenous administration should be reserved for patients who are temporarily unable to take medications orally.

**The risk of colchicine-induced toxicity depends on the total dose given over a period of time, as well as on the size of single doses, especially with intravenous administration.** The following measures are recommended to reduce the risk of cumulative toxicity:

When therapeutic doses of colchicine are given for relief of an acute attack, **the oral and intravenous routes of administration should not be used concurrently or sequentially. Additional colchicine should not be administered for at least 3 days after a course of oral treatment or for at least 7 days (21 days for geriatric patients) after a course of intravenous treatment.**

Patients who are receiving prophylactic doses of colchicine should not increase the dose to therapeutic levels if an acute attack of gout occurs. An alternative agent (e.g., a nonsteroidal anti-inflammatory drug [NSAID] or a corticosteroid, preferably via intrasynovial injection) should be used instead of additional colchicine.

Maximum dosage should be reduced if intravenous administration of colchicine cannot be avoided in geriatric patients and/or patients who are receiving prophylactic doses of colchicine.

Desensitization has been successfully accomplished in several patients with familial Mediterranean fever who were unable to tolerate pro-

phylactic doses of colchicine. The regimen used in a patient in whom adverse effects occurred with 1 mg per day of colchicine consisted of administering 1 mcg (0.001 mg) diluted in sodium chloride solution on the first day, doubling the dose each day until the tenth day, when 500 mcg (0.5 mg) was given, then increasing the dose to 750 mcg (0.75) mg per day after 3 months and to 1 mg per day after another 3 months.

**For oral dosage forms only**

Treatment with therapeutic doses of colchicine should be discontinued immediately, even if symptoms of the acute attack have not been relieved, when gastrointestinal symptoms (abdominal pain, diarrhea, nausea, or vomiting) occur. The patient should be instructed to note the total dose taken prior to the appearance of these symptoms and, during subsequent attacks, to discontinue treatment before this cumulative dose has been reached.

A reduction in prophylactic dosage is recommended if weakness, loss of appetite, nausea, vomiting, or diarrhea occurs.

**For parenteral dosage forms only**

Colchicine must be given intravenously because severe local irritation occurs if it is administered subcutaneously or intramuscularly. Also, care must be taken to ensure that the needle is properly positioned in the vein and to avoid extravasation because local irritation, inflammation, thrombophlebitis, and sloughing of the skin and subcutaneous tissues may occur.

It is recommended that the injection be diluted with 10 to 20 mL of 0.9% sodium chloride injection prior to administration. Alternatively, the medication may be injected into a large vein via an established intravenous line through which 0.9% sodium chloride injection is being infused.

The intravenous injection should be administered slowly, over a period of at least 2 to 5 minutes. Some clinicians recommend administering an intravenous dose over a period of 10 minutes.

Gastrointestinal symptoms occur rarely with intravenous administration and therefore cannot be used as an indicator of impending toxicity or guide to dosage. **The total dose administered and the duration of treatment should be limited and the patient carefully monitored.**

**Nutrition**

Colchicine impairs absorption of vitamin $B_{12}$ from the terminal ileum. Patients receiving long-term treatment may require supplementation with this vitamin.

# Oral Dosage Forms

Note: Bracketed uses in the *Dosage Forms* section refer to categories of use and/or indications that are not included in U.S. product labeling.

## COLCHICINE TABLETS USP

**Usual adult dose**

Antigout agent and

[Calcium pyrophosphate deposition disease suppressant][1]—
Prophylactic:

Oral, 500 or 600 mcg (0.5 or 0.6 mg) once a day, initially. If necessary, dosage may be increased to 500 or 600 mcg (0.5 or 0.6 mg) two or, rarely, three times a day. However, in mild cases, administration of a single dose one to four times a week may be sufficient.

In patients with gout who are undergoing surgery—Oral, 500 or 600 mcg (0.5 or 0.6 mg) three times a day for three days before and three days after surgery.

Therapeutic (relief of acute attack):

Oral, 1 or 2 tablets (500 or 600 mcg [0.5 or 0.6 mg] each), or a single 1-mg tablet, initially; then 500 or 600 mcg (0.5 or 0.6 mg) every one or two hours or 1 to 1.2 mg every two hours until pain is relieved; nausea, vomiting, or diarrhea occurs; or the maximum dose of 6 mg has been taken.

[Familial Mediterranean fever suppressant and]

[Amyloidosis suppressant][1]—
Prophylactic:

Oral, 500 or 600 mcg (0.5 or 0.6 mg) a day, initially. Dosage may be increased, if necessary and tolerated, up to a maximum of 2 mg a day in divided doses.

Note: Patients with familial Mediterranean fever who continue to experience frequent, severe acute attacks at a prophylactic dose of 2 mg a day are not likely to obtain relief with higher doses. However, prophylactic colchicine has been shown to prevent amyloidosis in these patients and therefore should not be discontinued.

Therapeutic (suppression of acute attack):

Oral, 600 mcg (0.6 mg) every hour for four doses, then every two hours for two additional doses on the first day; followed by 1.2

mg every twelve hours for two additional days. Administration may be discontinued at any time during this three-day regimen if it is apparent that the attack has been suppressed.

[Anti-inflammatory, in Behçet's disease][1]—

Oral, 1 to 1.8 mg a day in two or three divided doses.

[Anti-inflammatory, in biliary cirrhosis][1]—

Oral, 1 or 1.2 mg a day in two divided doses.

[Anti-inflammatory, in recurrent pericarditis][1]—

Oral, 1 mg a day in two divided doses. After a beneficial response has been attained, some patients may be maintained on 500 mcg (0.5 mg) a day.

**Usual adult prescribing limits**

Antigout agent—

Prophylactic:

Patients with renal function impairment (creatinine clearance between 10 and 50 mL per minute [0.17 and 0.83 mL per second])—600 mcg (0.6 mg) once a day.

Therapeutic (relief of acute attacks):

Patients with normal hepatic and renal function—6 mg.

Patients with renal function impairment (creatinine clearance between 10 and 50 mL per minute [0.17 and 0.83 mL per second])—3 mg.

**Usual pediatric dose**

[Familial Mediterranean fever suppressant]—

Children younger than 5 years of age: Oral, 500 mcg (0.5 mg) once a day.

Children 5 years of age and older: Oral, 500 mcg (0.5 mg) two times a day.

Other indications—Safety and efficacy have not been established.

Note: Dosage adjustment may be required as the child grows. One study found that children who were younger than 5 years of age when treatment was initiated often required an increase in dosage (to two 500–mcg [0.5–mg] doses a day) at about 7 years of age, and that children who were older than 5 years of age when treatment was initiated often required an increase in dosage (to three 500–mcg [0.5–mg] doses a day) at about 12.5 years of age.

**Strength(s) usually available**

U.S.—

500 mcg (0.5 mg) (Rx) [GENERIC].

600 mcg (0.6 mg) (Rx) [GENERIC].

Canada—

600 mcg (0.6 mg) (Rx) [GENERIC].

1 mg (Rx) [GENERIC].

**Packaging and storage**

Store below 40 °C (104 °F), preferably between 15 and 30 °C (59 and 86 °F). Store in a well-closed, light-resistant container.

## Parenteral Dosage Forms

Note: Bracketed uses in the *Dosage Forms* section refer to categories of use and/or indications that are not included in U.S. product labeling.

### COLCHICINE INJECTION USP

**Usual adult dose**

Antigout agent and

[Calcium pyrophosphate deposition disease suppressant][1]—

Prophylactic:

Intravenous, 500 mcg (0.5 mg) to 1 mg one or two times a day. Some clinicians recommend that single and total daily intravenous doses should be no larger than one-half of the doses recommended for oral administration if the intravenous route cannot be avoided.

Therapeutic (relief of acute attack):

Intravenous, 2 mg initially, then 500 mcg (0.5 mg) every six hours or 1 mg every six to twelve hours until the desired response is obtained or a maximum of 4 mg has been administered. However, some clinicians recommend administering an initial dose not higher than 1 mg, followed by 500 mcg (0.5 mg) one or two times a day. Other clinicians recommend that single and

cumulative intravenous doses should be no larger than one-half of the doses recommended for oral administration

Note: Administration of one-half of the above prophylactic and therapeutic doses is recommended for patients with renal function impairment (creatinine clearance between 10 and 50 mL per minute [0.17 and 0.83 mL per second]).

**Usual adult prescribing limits**

The cumulative dose administered over twenty-four hours or more is not to exceed—

For nongeriatric patients with normal renal and hepatic function: 4 mg. **After this quantity of colchicine has been administered, additional colchicine should not be administered by any route for at least seven days**.

For nongeriatric patients with renal function impairment (creatinine clearance between 10 and 50 mL per minute [0.17 and 0.83 mL per second]): 2 mg.

For geriatric patients: 2 mg. **After this quantity of colchicine has been administered, additional colchicine should not be administered by any route for at least twenty-one days**.

Note: It is recommended that patients who have been receiving oral prophylactic therapy receive total doses even lower than those recommended above. Specifically, a maximum dose of 1 or 2 mg is recommended for nongeriatric adults with normal hepatic and renal function.

**Usual pediatric dose**

Safety and efficacy have not been established.

**Strength(s) usually available**

U.S.—

1 mg per 2-mL ampul (500 mcg [0.5 mg] per mL) (Rx) [GENERIC].

Canada—

Not commercially available.

**Packaging and storage**

Store below 40 °C (104 °F), preferably between 15 and 30 °C (59 and 86 °F), unless otherwise specified by manufacturer. Protect from freezing. Protect from light.

**Preparation of dosage form**

To reduce the risk of sclerosis and other local reactions, it is recommended that the contents of 1 ampul (2 mL) be diluted to at least 10 to 20 mL with 0.9% sodium chloride injection. However, any solution that becomes turbid upon dilution should not be injected.

**Incompatibilities**

It is recommended that colchicine injection **not** be diluted with or injected into intravenous tubing containing 5% dextrose injection, solutions containing a bacteriostatic agent, or any other fluid that might change the pH of the colchicine solution, because precipitation may occur.

[1]Not included in Canadian product labeling.

## Selected Bibliography

Levy M, Spino M, Read SE. Colchicine: a state-of-the-art review. Pharmacotherapy 1991; 11: 196-211.

Star VL, Hochberg MC. Prevention and management of gout. Drugs 1993; 45: 212-22.

Zemer D, Livneh A, Danon YL, Pras M, Sohar E. Long-term colchicine treatment in children with familial Mediterranean fever. Arthritis Rheum 1991; 34: 973-7.

Henderson A, Emmerson BT, Bailey NL, Pond SM. Colchicine overdose in 6 patients. Prospects for prevention and therapy. Drug Invest 1993; 6: 114-7.

Revised: 01/31/94

## COLCHICINE-CONTAINING COMBINATIONS—

Probenecid and Colchicine (Systemic)

# COLESTIPOL    Oral-Local

VA CLASSIFICATION (Primary/Secondary): CV350/DE890; GA400

Note: For a listing of dosage forms and brand names by country availability, see *Dosage Forms* section(s). For a listing of brand names for the articles in this monograph, refer to the General Index.

## Category

Antihyperlipidemic; antipruritic (cholestasis); antidiarrheal (postoperative colonic bile acids).

## Indications

Note: Bracketed information in the *Indications* section refers to uses that are not included in U.S. product labeling.

### Accepted

Hyperlipidemia (treatment)—Colestipol is indicated for use as an adjunct only in patients with primary hypercholesterolemia (type IIa hyperlipidemia) and a significant risk of coronary artery disease who have not responded to diet or other measures alone. Colestipol reduces plasma cholesterol concentrations but causes no change or a slight increase in serum triglyceride concentrations, and so is not useful in patients with elevated triglyceride concentrations alone. Its use is limited in other types of hyperlipidemia (including type IIb) because it may cause further elevation of triglycerides.

Studies have suggested that control of elevated cholesterol and triglycerides may not lessen the danger of cardiovascular disease and mortality, although incidence of nonfatal myocardial infarctions may be decreased.

For additional information on initial therapeutic guidelines related to the treatment of hyperlipidemia, see *Appendix III.*

[Pruritus, associated with partial biliary obstruction (treatment)][1]—Colestipol is also used for the relief of pruritus associated with partial biliary obstruction (including primary biliary cirrhosis and various other forms of bile stasis). It is not useful in patients with complete biliary obstruction or with pruritus due to other causes.

[Diarrhea, due to bile acids (treatment)][1]—Colestipol may also be used to treat diarrhea caused by increased bile acids in the colon after surgery, although the risk of steatorrhea is increased.

[Colestipol has been used in the treatment of digitalis glycoside overdose and hyperoxaluria; however, it generally has been replaced by more effective agents.][1]

---

[1]Not included in Canadian product labeling.

## Pharmacology/Pharmacokinetics

### Physicochemical characteristics
Colestipol is an anion-exchange resin.

### Mechanism of action/Effect
Colestipol binds with bile acids in the intestine, preventing their reabsorption and producing an insoluble complex, which is excreted in the feces.

Antihyperlipidemic—
Colestipol binds with bile acids in the intestine, causing an increase in hepatic synthesis of bile acids from cholesterol. This depletion of hepatic cholesterol increases hepatic low-density lipoprotein (LDL) receptor activity, which removes LDL cholesterol from the plasma. Colestipol may also increase hepatic very low–density lipoprotein (VLDL) production, thereby increasing plasma concentration of triglycerides, especially in patients with hypertriglyceridemia.

Antipruritic (cholestasis)—
Reduction of serum bile acids and subsequent reduction of excess bile acids, which are deposited in dermal tissue, may lead to reduced pruritus.

Antidiarrheal (postoperative colonic bile acids)—
Colestipol binds with and removes bile acids.

### Other actions/effects
Because it is an anion-exchange resin, colestipol is capable of binding negatively charged medications as well as some others, causing a decreased effect or shortened half-life.

### Absorption
Not absorbed from the gastrointestinal tract.

### Onset of action
Plasma cholesterol concentrations are generally reduced within 24 to 48 hours after initiation of colestipol therapy.

### Time to peak effect
Within 1 month. In some patients, after the initial decrease, serum cholesterol concentrations return to or exceed baseline levels with continued therapy.

### Duration of action
After withdrawal of colestipol, cholesterol concentrations return to baseline in about 1 month.

## Precautions to Consider

### Tumorigenicity/Mutagenicity
In rats given colestipol for 18 months, no evidence of drug-related intestinal tumor formation was found. Colestipol was not mutagenic in the Ames assay.

### Pregnancy/Reproduction
Pregnancy—Studies have not been done in humans. Because colestipol is almost totally unabsorbed after oral administration, adverse effects on the fetus may potentially occur because of impaired maternal absorption of vitamins and nutrients.
Studies have not been done in animals.

### Breast-feeding
Problems in humans have not been documented.

### Pediatrics
Appropriate studies on the relationship of age to the effects of colestipol have not been performed in the pediatric population. However, use in children under 2 years of age is not recommended since cholesterol is required for normal development.

### Geriatrics
Appropriate studies on the relationship of age to the effects of colestipol have not been performed in the geriatric population. However, patients over 60 years of age may be more likely to experience gastrointestinal side effects, as well as adverse nutritional effects.

### Drug interactions and/or related problems
The following drug interactions and/or related problems have been selected on the basis of their potential clinical significance (possible mechanism in parentheses where appropriate)—not necessarily inclusive (» = major clinical significance):

Note: Combinations containing any of the following medications, depending on the amount present, may also interact with this medication.

» Anticoagulants, coumarin- or indandione-derivative
(concurrent use may significantly increase the anticoagulant effect as a result of depletion of vitamin K, but colestipol may also bind with oral anticoagulants in the gastrointestinal tract and reduce their effects; administration at least 6 hours before colestipol and adjustment of anticoagulant dosage based on frequent prothrombin-time determinations are recommended)

Chenodiol or
Ursodiol
(effect may be decreased when chenodiol or ursodiol is used concurrently with colestipol, which binds the medication and decreases its absorption and also tends to increase cholesterol saturation of bile)

» Digitalis glycosides
(colestipol may reduce the half-life of these medications by decreasing intestinal reabsorption and enterohepatic circulation; caution is recommended, especially when colestipol is withdrawn from a patient who was stabilized on the digitalis glycoside while receiving colestipol, because of the potential for serious toxicity; some clinicians recommend administration of colestipol approximately 8 hours after the digitalis glycoside)

» Diuretics, thiazide, oral or
» Penicillin G, oral or
» Propranolol, oral or
» Tetracyclines, oral
(concurrent administration with colestipol has been found to impair absorption of these medications; an interval of several hours between administration of colestipol and any of these medications is recommended; effects on absorption of other beta-blockers has not been determined)

» Thyroid hormones, including dextrothyroxine
   (concurrent use with colestipol may decrease the effects of thyroid hormones by binding and delaying or preventing absorption; an interval of 4 to 5 hours between administration of the 2 medications and regular monitoring of thyroid function tests are recommended)

» Vancomycin, oral
   (colestipol has been shown to bind oral vancomycin significantly when used concurrently, resulting in decreased stool concentrations and marked reduction in antibacterial activity of vancomycin; concurrent use is not recommended; patients should be advised to take oral vancomycin and colestipol several hours apart)

Vitamins, fat-soluble
   (colestipol may interfere with absorption of fat-soluble vitamins as a result of its interference with fat absorption; supplemental vitamin A and D in water-miscible or parenteral form are recommended in patients receiving colestipol for prolonged periods; supplemental vitamin K may be required in some patients who develop bleeding tendencies)

Medications, other
   (colestipol may delay or reduce absorption of other medications administered concurrently because of its anion-binding activity; administration of other medications 1 to 2 hours before or 4 hours after colestipol is recommended, although absorption of some medications is impaired even then; caution is recommended when colestipol is withdrawn because of the risk of toxicity when suddenly increased absorption of the other medication leads to higher serum concentrations)

**Laboratory value alterations**
The following have been selected on the basis of their potential clinical significance (possible effect in parentheses where appropriate)—not necessarily inclusive (» = major clinical significance):

With physiology/laboratory test values
Alkaline phosphatase and
Aspartate aminotransferase (AST [SGOT]), serum and
Chloride, serum and
Phosphorus, serum
   (concentrations may be increased)
Potassium and
Sodium
   (serum concentrations may be decreased)
Prothrombin time (PT)
   (may be prolonged)

**Medical considerations/Contraindications**
The medical considerations/contraindications included here have been selected on the basis of their potential clinical significance (reasons given in parentheses where appropriate)—not necessarily inclusive (» = major clinical significance):

*Except under special circumstances, this medication should not be used when the following medical problem exists:*
» Primary biliary cirrhosis
   (may further raise the cholesterol concentration)

*Risk-benefit should be considered when the following medical problems exist:*
Bleeding disorders and
Gallstones and
Gastrointestinal dysfunction and
Hypothyroidism and
Malabsorption states, especially steatorrhea and
Peptic ulcer
   (these conditions may be exacerbated)
» Complete biliary obstruction or complete atresia
   (no bile acids in gastrointestinal tract for colestipol to bind)
» Constipation
   (risk of fecal impaction)
Coronary artery disease and
Hemorrhoids
   (because of the risks associated with severe constipation)
Renal function impairment
   (increased risk of development of hyperchloremic acidosis)
Sensitivity to colestipol

**Patient monitoring**
The following may be especially important in patient monitoring (other tests may be warranted in some patients, depending on condition; » = major clinical significance):

Cholesterol and
Triglyceride
   (serum concentration determinations recommended prior to initiation of therapy for hyperlipidemia and every 2 months after stabilization to confirm efficacy and determine that a positive response is maintained)
Prothrombin-time (PT) determinations
   (recommended periodically because vitamin K deficiency associated with chronic use of colestipol may increase bleeding tendency)

## Side/Adverse Effects
The following side/adverse effects have been selected on the basis of their potential clinical significance (possible signs and symptoms in parentheses where appropriate)—not necessarily inclusive:

**Those indicating need for medical attention**
Incidence more frequent—about 10%
   *Constipation*—usually mild and transient, but may be severe and lead to fecal impaction
Incidence rare
   *Gallstones* (severe stomach pain with nausea and vomiting); *gastrointestinal bleeding or peptic ulcer* (black, tarry stools); *steatorrhea or malabsorption syndrome, especially with doses greater than 30 grams a day* (sudden loss of weight)

**Those indicating need for medical attention only if they continue or are bothersome**
Incidence less frequent
   *Belching; bloating; diarrhea; dizziness; headache; nausea or vomiting; stomach pain*

## Patient Consultation
As an aid to patient consultation, refer to *Advice for the Patient, Colestipol (Oral).*

In providing consultation, consider emphasizing the following selected information (» = major clinical significance):

**Before using this medication**
Diet as preferred therapy; importance of following prescribed diet
This medication does not cure the condition but rather helps control it
» Conditions affecting use, especially:
   Sensitivity to colestipol
   Use in children—Not recommended in children under 2 years of age since cholesterol is required for normal development
   Use in the elderly—Increased incidence of gastrointestinal side effects and adverse nutritional effects in patients over 60 years of age
   Other medications, especially anticoagulants, digitalis glycosides, oral penicillin G, oral tetracyclines, oral propranolol, thyroid hormones, thiazide diuretics, or oral vancomycin
   Other medical problems, especially primary biliary cirrhosis, complete biliary obstruction or complete atresia, or constipation

**Proper use of this medication**
» Importance of not taking more or less medication than the amount prescribed
» Compliance with prescribed diet
» Importance of mixing with fluids before taking; instructions for mixing: Stirring until completely mixed (does not dissolve); rinsing glass and drinking to make sure all medication is taken; may also be mixed with milk in cereals, thin soups, or pulpy fruits
» Proper dosing
   Missed dose: Taking as soon as possible; not taking if almost time for next dose; not doubling doses
» Proper storage

**Precautions while using this medication**
» Importance of close monitoring by the physician
» Checking with physician before discontinuing medication; blood lipid concentrations may increase significantly
» Not taking any other medication unless discussed with physician

**Side/adverse effects**
Signs of potential side effects, especially constipation, gallstones, gastrointestinal bleeding, peptic ulcer, and steatorrhea or malabsorption syndrome

## General Dosing Information
To prevent accidental inhalation or esophageal distress with the dry form, it is recommended that colestipol be mixed with at least 90 mL of water or other fluids (i.e., carbonated beverages, flavored drinks,

juices, or milk) before being ingested. It may also be taken in soups or with cereals or pulpy fruits.

Reduction in colestipol dosage or withdrawal of the medication may be necessary in some patients if constipation occurs or worsens, to prevent impaction. Administration of a laxative or stool softener or increased fluid intake may be helpful.

**For use as an antihyperlipidemic**

If a paradoxical increase in plasma cholesterol levels occurs, it is recommended that colestipol therapy be withdrawn.

If response is inadequate after 3 months of treatment, colestipol therapy should be withdrawn, except in the case of xanthoma tuberosum, which may require up to 1 year of treatment as long as reduction in size and/or number of xanthomata occurs.

## Oral Dosage Forms

### COLESTIPOL HYDROCHLORIDE FOR ORAL SUSPENSION USP

**Usual adult dose**
Antihyperlipidemic—
    Oral, 15 to 30 grams a day before meals in two to four divided doses.

Note: Colestipol has been used to treat digitalis glycoside toxicity at an oral dose of 10 grams, followed by 5 grams every six to eight hours.

**Usual pediatric dose**
Safety and efficacy have not been established.

**Size(s) usually available**
U.S.—
    5 grams per packet or level scoop (Rx) [*Colestid*].

Canada—
    5 grams per packet or level scoop (Rx) [*Colestid*].

**Packaging and storage**
Store below 40 °C (104 °F), preferably between 15 and 30 °C (59 and 86 °F), unless otherwise specified by manufacturer. Store in a tight container.

**Preparation of dosage form**
Colestipol is prepared for administration by adding the measured powder to the liquid and stirring to mix thoroughly (does not dissolve). After the patient drinks the suspension, the glass should be rinsed with more liquid to make sure all the medication is taken. Colestipol may also be mixed with milk in hot or regular breakfast cereals, in thin soups (tomato or chicken noodle), or with pulpy fruits such as pineapples, pears, peaches, or fruit cocktail.

**Auxiliary labeling**
• Take mixed in cold water or juice.

## Selected Bibliography

The Expert Panel. Report of the national cholesterol education program expert panel on detection, evaluation and treatment of high blood cholesterol in adults. Arch Intern Med 1988; 148: 36-69.

NIH Consensus Conference. Lowering blood cholesterol to prevent heart disease. JAMA 1985 Apr 12; 253: 2080-6.

Knodel LC, Talbert RL. Adverse effects of hypolipidaemic drugs. Med Toxicol 1987; 2: 10-32.

Revised: 10/21/92
Interim revision: 04/14/94

---

# COLFOSCERIL, CETYL ALCOHOL, AND TYLOXAPOL    Intratracheal-Local

VA CLASSIFICATION (Primary/Secondary): RE900

Other commonly used names for colfosceril are colfosceril palmitate, dipalmitoylphosphatidylcholine, DPPC, and synthetic lung surfactant.

Note: For a listing of dosage forms and brand names by country availability, see *Dosage Forms* section(s). For a listing of brand names for the articles in this monograph, refer to the General Index.

## Category
Pulmonary surfactant.

## Indications

### Accepted
Respiratory distress syndrome, neonatal (prophylaxis and treatment)—
    Colfosceril, cetyl alcohol, and tyloxapol combination is indicated for the prophylactic treatment of infants with birth weights of less than 1350 grams who are at risk of developing respiratory distress syndrome (RDS) and of infants with birth weights greater than 1350 grams who show evidence of pulmonary immaturity.

    Colfosceril, cetyl alcohol, and tyloxapol combination is also indicated for rescue treatment of infants who have developed RDS. Infants considered for rescue treatment with this medication should be on mechanical ventilation, and have a diagnosis of RDS based on the presence of respiratory distress that is not due to causes other than RDS (as shown by clinical and laboratory assessments) and on chest radiographic findings consistent with the diagnosis of RDS.

## Pharmacology/Pharmacokinetics

### Mechanism of action/Effect
Neonatal respiratory distress syndrome (RDS) develops primarily in premature infants because of pulmonary immaturity, including a deficiency of endogenous lung surfactant that results in higher alveolar surface tension and lower compliance properties. Without sufficient endogenous lung surfactant, progressive alveolar collapse occurs and both oxygen and carbon dioxide exchange are impaired. Also, RDS appears to be characterized by high pulmonary vascular permeability and increased lung tissue water. Fluid and protein that leak into alveoli inactivate both endogenous and exogenous surfactant, worsening lung function.

Natural lung surfactant is a mixture of lipids and apoproteins secreted by the alveolar cells into the alveoli and respiratory air passages. It reduces the surface tension of pulmonary fluids and thereby increases lung compliance. Surfactant exhibits not only surface tension–reducing properties (contributed by the lipids), but also rapid spreading and adsorption (contributed by the apoproteins). The major fraction of the lipid component of natural lung surfactant is dipalmitoylphosphatidylcholine (DPPC); this comprises up to 70% of the natural surfactant by weight.

Although the colfosceril (also known as DPPC) contained in the synthetic protein-free lung surfactant reduces surface tension, it alone is ineffective in RDS because it spreads and adsorbs poorly due to slow dispersion at air-fluid interfaces. Cetyl alcohol acts as the spreading agent for the colfosceril at the air-fluid interface, resulting in surface-tension effects that are similar to those of endogenous lung surfactant. Tyloxapol, a polymeric long-chain repeating alcohol, is a nonionic surfactant that acts to disperse both colfosceril and cetyl alcohol. Therefore, colfosceril, cetyl alcohol, and tyloxapol combination, when used as a replacement for deficient endogenous lung surfactant, is effective in reducing the surface tension of pulmonary fluids, thereby increasing lung compliance properties in RDS to prevent alveolar collapse and decrease work in breathing. The possibility exists that it may also improve ventilation/perfusion matching, independent of its direct effect on lung compliance.

### Absorption
In nonclinical studies, it has been shown that DPPC can be absorbed from the alveolus into lung tissue where it can be catabolized extensively and reutilized for further phospholipid synthesis and secretion. However, human pharmacokinetic studies on the absorption, biotransformation, and excretion of the components of colfosceril, cetyl alcohol, and tyloxapol combination have not been performed.

### Distribution
The lung surfactant administered endotracheally is distributed to the lung lobes, distal airways, and alveolar spaces. As the lung surfactant is distributed to the bronchi, bronchioles, and alveoli after administration in the upper airway, its concentration is highest at the alveolar air-fluid interface where it remains as a monolayer.

The lung surfactant does not enter systemic circulation from normal, healthy lungs; however, when the integrity of the alveolar lining is disrupted, as occurs in infants with RDS, the surfactant may be distributed outside the lungs into systemic circulation.

## Precautions to Consider

### Carcinogenicity
Long-term studies have not been performed in animals to evaluate the carcinogenic potential of colfosceril, cetyl alcohol, and tyloxapol combination.

**Mutagenicity**
Colfosceril, at concentrations up to 10,000 mcg per plate, was not mutagenic in the Ames Salmonella assay.

**Pregnancy/Reproduction**
Fertility—The effects of colfosceril, cetyl alcohol, and tyloxapol combination on fertility have not been studied.

Pregnancy—No information is available on the use of colfosceril, cetyl alcohol, and tyloxapol combination during pregnancy.

**Breast-feeding**
No information is available on the use of colfosceril, cetyl alcohol, and tyloxapol combination during breast-feeding.

**Pediatrics**
Appropriate studies performed to date have not demonstrated pediatrics-specific problems that would limit the usefulness of colfosceril, cetyl alcohol, and tyloxapol combination in children.

**Geriatrics**
No information is available on the relationship of age to the effects of colfosceril, cetyl alcohol, and tyloxapol combination.

**Patient monitoring**
The following may be especially important in patient monitoring (other tests may be warranted in some patients, depending on condition; » = major clinical significance):
Arterial blood gases
(after both prophylactic and rescue dosing, frequent arterial blood gas monitoring is recommended to prevent post-dosing hyperoxia and hypocarbia)
(if arterial or transcutaneous carbon dioxide [$CO_2$] measurements are < 30 torr, ventilation should be reduced at once; failure to reduce ventilator pressure or rate in such cases may result in severe hypocarbia, which can cause barotrauma and reduce brain blood flow)
(if the infant becomes pink and transcutaneous oxygen saturation is in excess of 95%, the fraction of inspired oxygen [$FiO_2$] should be reduced in small but repeated increments, until saturation is 90 to 95%, without waiting for confirmation of elevated arterial oxygen partial pressure [$PaO_2$] by blood gas assessment; failure to reduce $FiO_2$ in such cases may result in hyperoxia)
Arterial blood pressure and
Electrocardiogram (ECG)
(continuous monitoring of ECG during dosing is recommended; in most infants treated prophylactically, monitoring of ECG should be initiated prior to administration of the first dose of colfosceril, cetyl alcohol, and tyloxapol combination; for subsequent doses, arterial blood pressure monitoring during dosing is also recommended)
Chest expansion and
Color and
Endotracheal tube patency and position and
Heart rate and
Oxygen saturation, transcutaneous
(prior to dosing, it should be verified that the endotracheal tube tip is correctly positioned in mid-trachea; also, brisk and symmetrical chest movement with each mechanical inspiration and equal breath sounds in the two axillae should be confirmed)
(monitoring of chest expansion, color, endotracheal tube patency and position, heart rate, and transcutaneous oxygen saturation during dosing is recommended; if heart rate slows, the infant becomes dusky or agitated, or the medication backs up in the endotracheal tube, dosing should be slowed or stopped and, if necessary, the peak inspiratory pressure, ventilator rate, or $FiO_2$ should be increased; if transcutaneous oxygen saturation decreases during dosing, administration of the medication should be stopped and, if necessary, peak inspiratory pressure on the ventilator should be increased by 4 to 5 cm water for up to 15 to 20 minutes, depending on the infant's degree of tolerance versus oxygenation/ventilation compromise; increases of $FiO_2$ may also be required for 15 to 20 minutes; however, rapid improvement in lung function may require immediate reduction in peak inspiratory pressure, ventilator rate, or $FiO_2$)
(at the end of dosing, the proper position of the endotracheal tube should be confirmed by listening for equal breath sounds in the axillae; chest expansion, color, and transcutaneous oxygen saturation should also be checked; continuous monitoring of the patient for at least 30 minutes after dosing is recommended, since rapid lung function changes require immediate changes in peak inspiratory pressure, ventilator rate, or $FiO_2$)
(if chest expansion improves substantially after dosing, peak ventilator inspiratory pressure should be reduced immediately, without waiting for confirmation of respiratory improvement by blood gas assessment; failure to reduce inspiratory ventilator pressure rapidly in such cases may result in lung overdistention and pulmonary air leak)

## Side/Adverse Effects

Note: In controlled clinical studies of infants receiving colfosceril, cetyl alcohol, and tyloxapol combination, there was an increased incidence in some of the conditions associated with prematurity and RDS, including apnea and pulmonary hemorrhage. Hypoxia and bradycardia can occur during treatment and are directly related to the dosing procedure.

Infants treated with synthetic surfactant may develop apnea because they are taken off the ventilator sooner due to their improved respiratory status. Thus, apnea is not considered a direct side effect of this medication and is, in fact, associated with a favorable rather than an untoward outcome. Apneic infants, whether or not they received colfosceril, cetyl alcohol, and tyloxapol combination, had fewer episodes of grade III intraventricular hemorrhage or periventricular echodensities or both, fewer air leaks, and better survival rates than did nonapneic infants.

Pulmonary hemorrhage occurred more frequently in infants who were younger, smaller (< 700 grams at birth), or male, or in those who had a patent ductus arteriosus; it usually occurred in the first two days of life. Infants treated with colfosceril, cetyl alcohol, and tyloxapol combination who received steroids more than 24 hours prior to delivery or indomethacin postnatally had a lower rate of pulmonary hemorrhage than other infants treated with this medication.

Controlled clinical studies of infants receiving colfosceril, cetyl alcohol, and tyloxapol combination also showed a decreased incidence of pulmonary air leak and bronchopulmonary dysplasia, which are associated with mechanical ventilation in premature infants. Some studies have shown that, with rescue surfactant treatment, synthetic surfactant improved the chance of survival through 28 days without bronchopulmonary dysplasia.

During an open uncontrolled study, colfosceril, cetyl alcohol, and tyloxapol combination decreased oxygen ($O_2$) saturation ($\geq$ 20%) in 6% of infants on prophylactic treatment and in 22% of infants on rescue treatment; increased $O_2$ saturation ($\geq$ 10%) in 5% of infants on prophylactic treatment and in 6% of infants on rescue treatment; decreased transcutaneous oxygen partial pressure (Pa$O_2$) ($\geq$ 20 mm Hg) in 1% of infants on prophylactic treatment and in 8% of infants on rescue treatment; increased transcutaneous P$O_2$ ($\geq$ 20 mm Hg) in 2% of infants on prophylactic treatment and in 5% of infants on rescue treatment; decreased transcutaneous carbon dioxide partial pressure (Pa$CO_2$) ($\geq$ 20 mm Hg) in < 1% of infants on prophylactic treatment and in 1% of infants on rescue treatment; and increased transcutaneous P$CO_2$ ($\geq$ 20 mm Hg) in 1% of infants on prophylactic treatment and in 3% of infants on rescue treatment.

The following side/adverse effects have been selected on the basis of their potential clinical significance (possible signs and symptoms in parentheses where appropriate)—not necessarily inclusive:

**Those indicating need for medical attention**
Incidence rare
*Apnea; bradycardia (< 60 beats per minute); pulmonary air leak*—due to excess ventilation caused by rapid improvement in lung; *pulmonary hemorrhage; tachycardia (> 200 beats per minute)*

**Those indicating need for medical attention only if they continue or are bothersome**
Incidence less frequent or rare
*Gagging*

## General Dosing Information

Colfosceril, cetyl alcohol, and tyloxapol combination should be used only by neonatologists and other clinicians who are experienced at neonatal intubation and ventilatory management. Also, instillation of this medication should be performed only by trained medical personnel experienced in airway and clinical management of unstable premature infants. Adequate personnel, facilities, equipment, and medications are required to optimize the perinatal outcome in these premature infants. In addition, continuous clinical attention should be given to all infants prior to, during, and after administration of this medication.

Colfosceril, cetyl alcohol, and tyloxapol combination should be administered only by instillation into the trachea.

To ensure accurate dosing, the current weight of the infant should be accurately determined.

Colfosceril, cetyl alcohol, and tyloxapol combination for intratracheal suspension is to be used with one of the 5 special endotracheal tube adapters with a special right-angle Luer-lock sideport, supplied by the manufacturer. The adapters are used as follows:
- An adapter size should be selected that corresponds to the inside diameter of the endotracheal tube.
- The adapter is inserted into the endotracheal tube with a firm push-twist motion.
- The breathing circuit ''Y'' is connected to the adapter.
- The cap is removed from the sideport on the adapter and the syringe containing the medication is attached to the sideport.
- After completion of dosing, the syringe is removed and the sideport is capped.

Colfosceril, cetyl alcohol, and tyloxapol for intratracheal suspension is administered through the sideport on the special endotracheal tube adapter without interrupting mechanical ventilation.

Prior to dosing with colfosceril, cetyl alcohol, and tyloxapol combination, proper placement of the endotracheal tube tip in the trachea and not in the esophagus or right or left mainstem bronchus should be confirmed. Brisk and symmetrical chest movement with each mechanical inspiration and equal breath sounds in the two axillae should also be confirmed prior to dosing. In prophylactic treatment, dosing with colfosceril, cetyl alcohol, and tyloxapol combination should not be delayed pending radiographic confirmation of the endotracheal tube tip position. In rescue treatment, bedside confirmation of the endotracheal tube tip position is usually sufficient if at least one chest radiograph subsequent to the last intubation confirms proper position of the endotracheal tube tip. If the endotracheal tube tip is too low, some lung areas could remain undosed.

Infants whose ventilation becomes severely impaired during or shortly after dosing may have mucous plugging of the endotracheal tube, especially if pulmonary secretions were prominent prior to administration of the medication. Therefore, prior to administration of colfosceril, cetyl alcohol, and tyloxapol combination, the infant should be suctioned to lessen the chance of mucous plugs obstructing the endotracheal tube. If endotracheal tube obstruction is suspected, and suctioning is ineffective in removing the obstruction, the blocked endotracheal tube should be replaced immediately. Following administration of colfosceril, cetyl alcohol, and tyloxapol combination, the infant should not be suctioned for 2 hours except when it is clinically necessary.

In infants weighing 500 to 700 grams, a single prophylactic dose of colfosceril, cetyl alcohol, and tyloxapol combination has been shown to significantly improve the fraction of inspired oxygen ($FiO_2$) and ventilator settings, reduce pneumothorax, and reduce the incidence of death from respiratory distress syndrome (RDS), but it has also been shown to increase pulmonary hemorrhage. The effects of multiple doses of colfosceril, cetyl alcohol, and tyloxapol combination in infants in this weight group are not known; therefore, clinicians should carefully consider the potential risks and benefits of this medication in these infants.

Each dose is administered in two half-doses, with each half-dose being equivalent to 33.75 mg of colfosceril palmitate (2.5 mL of reconstituted suspension) per kg of body weight. Each half-dose is instilled slowly over a minimum of 1 to 2 minutes (30 to 50 mechanical breaths) in small bursts timed with inspiration. After the first half-dose (the equivalent of 33.75 mg of colfosceril palmitate [2.5 mL of reconstituted suspension] per kg of body weight) is administered in the midline position, the infant's head and torso are turned 45° to the right for 30 seconds while mechanical ventilation is continued. Then the infant is returned to the midline position, and the second half-dose (the equivalent of 33.75 mg of colfosceril palmitate [2.5 mL of reconstituted suspension] per kg of body weight) is given in an identical manner. The infant's head and torso are then turned 45° to the left for 30 seconds while mechanical ventilation is continued, after which the infant is turned back to the midline position. Using these maneuvers allows gravity to assist in the lung distribution of the colfosceril, cetyl alcohol, and tyloxapol combination.

The dosage volume of the equivalent of 67.5 mg of colfosceril palmitate (5 mL reconstituted suspension) per kg of body weight may cause transient impairment of gas exchange by physical blockage of the airway, especially in infants on low ventilator setting. This may result in a drop in oxygen saturation during dosing, especially if these infants are on low ventilator settings prior to dosing. These transient effects may be overcome by increasing peak inspiratory pressure on the ventilator during dosing. $FiO_2$ may also be increased if necessary. In infants who are especially fragile or reactive to external stimuli, increasing peak inspiratory pressure just prior to dosing may minimize any transient decrease in oxygenation. However, the infant should be returned to pre-dose settings within a very short time after dosing is completed.

Rapid administration of colfosceril, cetyl alcohol, and tyloxapol combination may cause reflux of the medication into the endotracheal tube during dosing. If reflux occurs, administration of the medication should be stopped and, if necessary, the peak inspiratory pressure on the ventilator should be increased until the endotracheal tube clears.

In controlled clinical studies with infants receiving colfosceril, cetyl alcohol, and tyloxapol combination, infants who received steroids more than 24 hours prior to delivery or indomethacin postnatally had a lower rate of pulmonary hemorrhage than did other infants treated with this medication. Careful attention should be given to early treatment (unless contraindicated) of patent ductus arteriosus during the first 2 days of life (while the ductus arteriosus is often clinically silent).

## Intratracheal Dosage Forms
### COLFOSCERIL PALMITATE, CETYL ALCOHOL, AND TYLOXAPOL FOR INTRATRACHEAL SUSPENSION

**Usual pediatric dose**
Pulmonary surfactant (prophylaxis)—
    Intratracheal, the equivalent of 67.5 mg of colfosceril palmitate (5 mL of reconstituted suspension) per kg of body weight for the first dose, administered (in two half-doses) as soon as possible after birth; second and third doses (each given in two half-doses) should be administered approximately twelve and twenty-four hours later to all infants remaining on mechanical ventilation at those times.
Pulmonary surfactant (rescue treatment)—
    Intratracheal, initially the equivalent of 67.5 mg of colfosceril palmitate (5 mL of reconstituted suspension) per kg of body weight administered (in two half-doses) as soon as possible after diagnosis of respiratory distress syndrome (RDS) is confirmed; a second dose (given in two half-doses) should be administered approximately twelve hours after the first dose, provided that the infant remains on mechanical ventilation. Administration of a third or fourth dose when signs of RDS persist or recur was not shown to be of overall clinical benefit.
Note: Each dose is administered in two half-doses, with each half-dose being equivalent to 33.75 mg of colfosceril palmitate (2.5 mL of reconstituted suspension) per kg of body weight. Each half-dose is instilled slowly over a minimum of one to two minutes (thirty to fifty mechanical breaths) in small bursts timed with inspiration.

**Strength(s) usually available**
U.S.—
    108 mg of colfosceril palmitate, 12 mg of cetyl alcohol, and 8 mg of tyloxapol per vial (13.5 mg of colfosceril palmitate, 1.5 mg of cetyl alcohol, and 1 mg of tyloxapol per mL, when reconstituted with 8 mL of Sterile Water for Injection supplied by manufacturer) (Rx) [Exosurf Neonatal (sodium chloride 47 mg per vial)].
Canada—
    108 mg of colfosceril palmitate, 12 mg of cetyl alcohol, and 8 mg of tyloxapol per vial (13.5 mg of colfosceril palmitate, 1.5 mg of cetyl alcohol, and 1 mg of tyloxapol per mL, when reconstituted with 8 mL of Sterile Water for Injection supplied by manufacturer) (Rx) [Exosurf Neonatal (sodium chloride 47 mg per vial)].

**Packaging and storage**
Store below 40 °C (104 °F), preferably between 15 and 30 °C (59 and 86 °F), unless otherwise specified by manufacturer.

**Preparation of dosage form**
Colfosceril, cetyl alcohol, and tyloxapol combination should be reconstituted immediately before use because it does not contain antibacterial preservatives.
Solutions containing buffers or preservatives should not be used for reconstitution; Bacteriostatic Water for Injection USP should also not be used.
Each vial of colfosceril, cetyl alcohol, and tyloxapol combination should be reconstituted only with 8 mL of the preservative-free Sterile Water for Injection provided by the manufacturer, as follows:
    A 10- or 12-mL syringe is filled with 8 mL of preservative-free Sterile Water for Injection, using an 18- or 19-gauge needle.
    The vacuum in the vial should be allowed to draw the sterile water into the vial.
    As much of the 8 mL as possible should be aspirated out of the vial into the syringe (while maintaining the vacuum), then the syringe plunger suddenly released; this step should be repeated three or four times to assure adequate mixing of the vial contents. If a vacuum is not present, the vial of colfosceril, cetyl alcohol, and tyloxapol combination should not be used.
    The appropriate dosage volume for the entire dose (5 mL [equivalent of 67.5 mg of colfosceril palmitate] per kg of body weight) should then be drawn into the syringe from below the froth in the vial (while maintaining the vacuum).

Following reconstitution, the colfosceril, cetyl alcohol, and tyloxapol combination preparation is a milky white suspension with a total volume of 8 mL per vial.

## Stability

The reconstituted suspension is chemically and physically stable and remains sterile for up to 24 hours following reconstitution (using aseptic technique) when stored at 2 to 30 °C (36 to 86 °F); however, the manufacturer's labeling states that it is best to reconstitute the colfosceril palmitate, cetyl alcohol, and tyloxapol combination immediately before use because the product does not contain antibacterial preservatives.

If the suspension appears to separate, the vial should be gently shaken or swirled to resuspend the preparation.

The reconstituted product should be inspected visually for homogeneity immediately before administration; if persistent large flakes or particulates are present, the vial should not be used.

## Selected Bibliography

Corbet A, Bucciarelli R, Goldman S, et al. Decreased mortality rate among small premature infants treated at birth with a single dose of synthetic surfactant: a multicenter controlled trial. J Pediatr 1991; 118: 277-84.

Jobe AH. Pulmonary surfactant therapy. N Engl J Med 1993; 32: 861-8.

Long W, Thompson T, Sundell H, et al. Effects of two rescue doses of a synthetic surfactant on mortality rate and survival without bronchopulmonary dysplasia in 700- to 1350-gram infants with respiratory distress syndrome. J Pediatr 1991; 118: 595-605.

Developed: 05/10/95

---

## COLISTIN-CONTAINING COMBINATIONS—
Colistin, Neomycin, and Hydrocortisone (Otic)

---

# COLISTIN, NEOMYCIN, AND HYDROCORTISONE    Otic

VA CLASSIFICATION (Primary): OT250

Note: For a listing of dosage forms and brand names by country availability, see *Dosage Forms* section(s). For a listing of brand names for the articles in this monograph, refer to the General Index.

---

## Category

Antibacterial-corticosteroid (otic).

## Indications

Note: Bracketed information in the *Indications* section refers to uses that are not included in U.S. product labeling.

### Accepted

Ear canal infections, external (treatment) or

Mastoidectomy cavity infections (treatment)[1]—Colistin, neomycin, and hydrocortisone otic combination is indicated in the treatment of superficial external ear canal infections and superficial mastoidectomy and fenestration cavity infections caused by susceptible organisms, including *Pseudomonas aeruginosa*, *Staphylococcus aureus*, *Klebsiella* species, *Enterobacter (Aerobacter)* species, and *Escherichia coli*.

[Otitis media, chronic suppurative (treatment)][1]—Colistin, neomycin, and hydrocortisone otic combination is used in the treatment of chronic suppurative otitis media.

Note: Not all species or strains of a particular organism may be susceptible to colistin and neomycin.

[1]Not included in Canadian product labeling.

## Pharmacology/Pharmacokinetics

### Physicochemical characteristics

Molecular weight—Hydrocortisone acetate: 404.50.
Family—Colistin sulfate: Polymyxins; also known as polymyxin E.
Neomycin sulfate: Aminoglycosides.
Hydrocortisone acetate: Corticosteroids.

### Mechanism of action/Effect

Colistin is bactericidal and active against *Pseudomonas aeruginosa* and other gram-negative bacteria. It is a surface-active basic polypeptide that binds to anionic phospholipid sites in bacterial cytoplasmic membranes, disrupts membrane structure, and alters membrane permeability to allow leakage of intracellular contents. Its action is antagonized by calcium and magnesium.

Neomycin is an aminoglycoside, bactericidal against most aerobic gram-negative bacilli and *Staphylococcus aureus*, but not effective against *Pseudomonas*. It is actively transported across the bacterial cell membrane, binds to a specific receptor protein on the 30 S subunit of bacterial ribosomes, and interferes with an initiation complex between mRNA (messenger RNA) and the 30 S subunit, thus inhibiting protein synthesis.

Hydrocortisone is a corticosteroid that diffuses across cell membranes and complexes with specific cytoplasmic receptors. These complexes then enter the cell nucleus, bind to DNA (chromatin), and stimulate transcription of mRNA and subsequent protein synthesis of various enzymes thought to be ultimately responsible for the anti-inflammatory effects of corticosteroids applied topically to the skin or ear.

### Absorption

Colistin and hydrocortisone—Not absorbed when applied to the ear.
Neomycin—May possibly be absorbed if the eardrum is perforated or the skin of the ear canal is abraded.

## Precautions to Consider

### Cross-sensitivity and/or related problems

Patients intolerant of one aminoglycoside or polymyxin may be intolerant of other aminoglycosides or polymyxins also.

### Pregnancy/Reproduction

Problems in humans have not been documented.

### Breast-feeding

Problems in humans have not been documented.

### Pediatrics

Appropriate studies on the relationship of age to the effects of this medicine have not been performed in the pediatric population. However, no pediatrics-specific problems have been documented to date.

### Geriatrics

Appropriate studies on the relationship of age to the effects of this medicine have not been performed in the geriatric population. However, no geriatrics-specific problems have been documented to date.

### Medical considerations/Contraindications

The medical considerations/contraindications included here have been selected on the basis of their potential clinical significance (reasons given in parentheses where appropriate)—not necessarily inclusive (» = major clinical significance).

**Risk-benefit should be considered when the following medical problems exist:**

Intolerance to colistin, neomycin, hydrocortisone, other aminoglycosides, polymyxins, or thimerosal

*For colistin and/or neomycin*
Otitis media, chronic or
Perforated eardrum
    (neomycin may cause ototoxicity)

*For hydrocortisone*
» Herpes simplex or
» Herpes zoster oticus or
» Tubercular or fungal infections of the ear or
» Vaccinia, varicella, or other viral disease of the ear
    (may be exacerbated)

## Side/Adverse Effects

The following side/adverse effects have been selected on the basis of their potential clinical significance (possible signs and symptoms in parentheses where appropriate)—not necessarily inclusive:

### Those indicating need for medical attention
Incidence more frequent
    *Hypersensitivity* (itching, skin rash, redness, swelling, or other sign of irritation not present before therapy)

## Patient Consultation

As an aid to patient consultation, refer to *Advice for the Patient, Colistin, Neomycin, and Hydrocortisone (Otic)*.

In providing consultation, consider emphasizing the following selected information (» = major clinical significance):

**Before using this medication**

» Conditions affecting use, especially:

    Intolerance to colistin, neomycin, hydrocortisone, other aminoglycosides, polymyxins, or thimerosal

    Other medical problems, especially herpes simplex, herpes zoster oticus, tubercular or fungal infections of the ear, vaccinia, varicella, or other viral disease of the ear

**Proper use of this medication**

Thoroughly cleaning and drying external auditory canal with sterile cotton applicator before inserting medication

Warming otic suspension to body temperature before inserting

Proper administration technique for otic suspension

Not touching dropper to any surface; keeping container tightly closed

» Not using longer than 10 days unless otherwise directed by physician

» Compliance with full course of therapy

» Proper dosing

Missed dose: Inserting as soon as possible; not inserting if almost time for next dose

» Proper storage

**Precautions while using this medication**

Checking with physician if no improvement within 1 week or immediately if symptoms become worse

**Side/adverse effects**

Signs of potential side effects, especially hypersensitivity reactions

## General Dosing Information

Prior to administration, the external auditory canal should be thoroughly cleaned and dried with a sterile cotton applicator.

This medication may be warmed prior to administration, but not above body temperature in order to avoid loss of potency.

A cotton wick may be placed in the ear canal and then saturated with the suspension. The wick should be kept moist by adding suspension every four to eight hours and it should be replaced at least once daily.

Therapy should not be continued for more than 10 days unless directed by physician.

## Otic Dosage Forms

### COLISTIN AND NEOMYCIN SULFATES AND HYDROCORTISONE ACETATE OTIC SUSPENSION USP

**Usual adult and adolescent dose**
Topical, to the ear canal, 4 drops every six to eight hours.

**Usual pediatric dose**
Topical, to the ear canal, up to 3 drops every six to eight hours.

**Strength(s) usually available**
U.S.—

    3 mg of colistin (base), 3.3 mg of neomycin (base), and 10 mg of hydrocortisone acetate per mL (Rx) [Coly-Mycin S Otic (thimerosal 0.002%)].

Canada—

    3 mg of colistin (base), 3.3 mg of neomycin (base), and 10 mg of hydrocortisone acetate per mL (Rx) [Coly-Mycin Otic].

**Packaging and storage**
Store below 40 °C (104 °F), preferably between 15 and 30 °C (59 and 86 °F), unless otherwise specified by manufacturer. Store in a tight container. Protect from freezing.

**Stability**
Stable for 18 months at room temperature.

**Auxiliary labeling**
• Shake well.
• For the ear.
• Continue medicine for full time of treatment.

Revised: 05/25/95

## COLLOIDAL GOLD PARTICLE IMMUNOASSAY PREGNANCY TEST KITS—See Pregnancy Test Kits for Home Use

---

# COLONY STIMULATING FACTORS    Systemic

This monograph includes information on the following: Filgrastim; Sargramostim†.

VA CLASSIFICATION (Primary): BL400

Other commonly used names are: Granulocyte colony stimulating factor, recombinant [Filgrastim], Granulocyte-macrophage colony stimulating factor, recombinant [Sargramostim], Recombinant human granulocyte-macrophage colony stimulating factor [Sargramostim], Recombinant methionyl human granulocyte colony stimulating factor [Filgrastim], rG-CSF [Filgrastim], rGM-CSF [Sargramostim], rHu GM-CSF [Sargramostim], r-met HuG-CSF [Filgrastim].

Note: For a listing of dosage forms and brand names by country availability, see Dosage Forms section(s). For a listing of brand names for the articles in this monograph, refer to the General Index.

†Not commercially available in Canada.

## Category

Hematopoietic stimulant; antineutropenic.

## Indications

Note: Bracketed information in the Indications section refers to uses that are not included in U.S. product labeling.

**Accepted**

Neutropenia, chemotherapy-related (treatment)—Filgrastim (rG-CSF) and [sargramostim (rGM-CSF)] are indicated to decrease the incidence of infection, as manifested by febrile neutropenia, in patients with non-myeloid malignancies receiving myelosuppressive anti-cancer drugs associated with a significant incidence of severe neutropenia with fever.

Caution is recommended in patients with myeloid malignancies such as acute myelocytic leukemia (AML) because of the potential of colony stimulating factors to stimulate leukemic blasts. Criteria to define

patients at increased risk (e.g., those with refractory anemia with excess blasts [RAEB] or refractory anemia with excess blasts in transformation [RAEBT], or cytogenetic abnormality) have been proposed but not established.

The theoretical risk that use of increased doses of chemotherapy permitted by administration of colony stimulating factors may result in an increase in other hematologic or nonhematologic toxicities not affected by colony stimulating factors has not been adequately studied, but caution is recommended.

Myeloid engraftment following bone marrow transplantation, promotion of—[Filgrastim][1] and sargramostim are indicated for acceleration of myeloid recovery in patients with non-Hodgkin's lymphoma, acute lymphoblastic leukemia, and Hodgkin's disease undergoing autologous bone marrow transplantation (BMT).

Myeloid engraftment following bone marrow transplantation, failure or delay of (treatment)—[Filgrastim][1] and sargramostim are indicated for prolonging survival in patients who have undergone allogeneic or autologous bone marrow transplantation (BMT) in whom engraftment is delayed or has failed, in the presence or absence of infection.

Note: Filgrastim and sargramostim are effective in patients receiving unpurged bone marrow or bone marrow purged with monoclonal (e.g., anti-B lymphocyte) antibodies; however, in vitro marrow purging with chemical agents may significantly reduce the number of responsive hematopoietic progenitors and prevent a response. The bone marrow purging process should preserve more than $1.2 \times 10^4$ progenitors per kg of body weight.

The effect may also be limited in patients who received extensive radiotherapy to hematopoietic sites for treatment of primary disease in the abdomen or chest or who have been exposed to multiple myelotoxic agents (alkylating agents, anthracycline antibiotics, and antimetabolites) before autologous BMT.

Peripheral progenitor cell yield, enhancement of—[Filgrastim][1] or [sargramostim] is used as an adjunct to enhance peripheral progenitor cell yield in autologous hematopoietic stem cell transplantation. However, the yield (quantity and quality) of peripheral progenitor cells is dependent on the extent of prior chemotherapy.

[Myeloid engraftment following hematopoietic stem cell transplantation, failure or delay of (treatment)]—Sargramostim is used for prolonging survival in patients who have undergone autologous hematopoietic stem cell transplantation in whom engraftment is delayed or has failed, in the presence or absence of infection.

Neutropenia, AIDS-associated (treatment)—[Filgrastim][1] and [sargramostim] are used to treat acquired immunodeficiency syndrome (AIDS) patients with neutropenia caused by the disease itself or infection of opportunistic organisms (such as cytomegalovirus), or antiretroviral agents (zidovudine, ganciclovir).

The effect on infections, hospitalization, or survival has not been established.

Because there is some evidence that sargramostim (but not filgrastim) may increase human immunodeficiency virus (HIV) replication, it is recommended that sargramostim only be given in combination with an antiretroviral agent.

Ganciclovir is toxic to stem cells. If neutrophil counts decrease despite use of colony stimulating factor, dose reduction or withdrawal of ganciclovir is recommended.

Myelodysplastic syndromes (treatment)—[Filgrastim][1] and [sargramostim] are used to enhance neutrophil function in patients with myelodysplastic syndromes and a history of infection.

Caution is necessary because of the risk that colony stimulating factors may precipitate transformation of myelodysplastic syndromes into acute myelocytic leukemia. Assessment of risk is complicated by the fact that progression to acute leukemia may occur in the natural course of the disease.

Colony stimulating factors do not have a consistent effect on erythrocytes or platelets in these conditions.

Neutropenia, severe chronic (treatment)—[Filgrastim][1] and [sargramostim] are used for treatment of severe chronic neutropenia, including congenital neutropenia (Kostmann's syndrome), idiopathic neutropenia, and cyclic neutropenia.

Neutropenia, drug-induced (treatment)—[Filgrastim][1] and [sargramostim] are used for treatment of drug-induced neutropenia.

---

[1]Not included in Canadian product labeling.

## Pharmacology/Pharmacokinetics

### Physicochemical characteristics
Source—
Filgrastim (rG-CSF): Synthetic. A protein chain of 175 amino acids produced by a recombinant DNA process involving genetically engineered *Escherichia coli* (the human granulocyte colony stimulating factor gene has been inserted into the bacteria). Has an amino acid sequence identical to the sequence in naturally occurring human granulocyte colony stimulating factor (G-CSF) predicted from human DNA sequence analysis, except for the addition of an N-terminal methionine necessary for expression in *E. coli*. In addition, unlike G-CSF isolated from a human cell, filgrastim is non-glycosylated. Purification is done by conventional means; prior to final purification, filgrastim is allowed to oxidize to its native state and final purity is achieved by sequential passage over a series of chromatography columns; the product is then formulated in an acetate buffer with mannitol and Tween 80.

Sargramostim (rGM-CSF): Synthetic. The commercially available form is a glycoprotein chain of 127 amino acids, characterized by 3 primary molecular species, produced by a recombinant DNA process involving a yeast (*S. cerevisiae*) expression system. The amino acid sequence differs from that of natural human granulocyte-macrophage colony stimulating factor (GM-CSF) by a substitution of leucine at position 23, and the carbohydrate moiety may be different. Sargramostim produced in a yeast system is glycosylated; rGM-CSF produced in other systems may not be.

Chemical group—
Related to naturally occurring colony stimulating factors, which are hormone-like glycoprotein growth factors also known as cytokines.

Molecular weight—
Filgrastim: 18,800 daltons.
Sargramostim: Contains 3 primary molecular species with molecular masses of 19,500, 16,800, and 15,500 daltons.

### Mechanism of action/Effect
In general, endogenous colony stimulating factors act on hematopoietic cells by binding to specific cell surface receptors and stimulating proliferation (clonal expansion), differentiation, and some end-cell functional activation. The recombinant colony stimulating factors have the same biological activity as the endogenous hormones. The actions of these growth factors promote differentiation of myeloid progenitor cells into granulocytes and monocytes; other pathways produce erythrocytes and platelets.

Filgrastim is a class II hematopoietic growth factor. It acts on progenitor cells capable of forming only one differentiated cell type—the neutrophil granulocyte; it is said to be lineage-specific. Sargramostim, a class I hematopoietic growth factor, stimulates formation of granulocytes (neutrophils, eosinophils) and macrophages and is therefore non–lineage specific.

Administration of colony stimulating factor to patients whose bone marrow has been depleted by myelotoxic agents or diseases such as acquired immunodeficiency syndrome (AIDS) results in an increased number of circulating hematopoietic progenitor cells. Filgrastim acts only on mature progenitor cells that are already committed to one pathway, the granulocyte pathway, and therefore increases only neutrophil concentrations. Sargramostim acts on progenitor cells at an earlier stage of development and can promote more than one lineage; it promotes formation of granulocyte, macrophage, and mixed granulocyte-macrophage colonies, resulting in increased concentrations of eosinophils and monocytes as well. Neither has a consistent effect on red cell or platelet counts.

### Other actions/effects
Colony stimulating factors may have a proliferative effect on myeloid and erythroid leukemic cells. Sargramostim has been reported in some studies to increase replication of human immunodeficiency virus. Sargramostim has been reported to reduce low-density lipoprotein (LDL) concentrations in blood, with a variable effect on high-density lipoproteins (HDL); it has also been reported to transiently decrease cholesterol concentrations. Filgrastim has been reported to decrease serum cholesterol with variable changes in triglycerides; these changes return to normal or near baseline within 1 to 2 weeks after it is withdrawn.

### Absorption
Filgrastim or sargramostim—Detected in serum within 5 minutes after subcutaneous administration.

### Half-life
Distribution—
Sargramostim:
Intravenous (2-hour infusion)—
12 to 17 minutes.
Elimination—
Filgrastim:
Approximately 3.5 hours.
Sargramostim:
Intravenous (2-hour infusion)—Approximately 2 hours.
Subcutaneous—Approximately 3 hours.

### Onset of action
Filgrastim—Decrease in circulating neutrophils occurs within the first 5 minutes of intravenous administration; after 4 hours, counts begin to rise, with an initial peak within 24 hours.
Sargramostim—Decrease in circulating neutrophils, eosinophils, and monocytes occurs, with a nadir at 30 minutes, and rebound to baseline or above by 2 hours. In addition, there is an apparent biphasic response over time; an initial plateau in leukocyte counts occurs after 3 to 7 days, which is followed by another increase and another plateau.

### Time to peak concentration
Filgrastim—After subcutaneous administration: 2 to 8 hours.
Sargramostim—After subcutaneous administration: 2 hours.

### Time to peak effect
Varies according to chemotherapy regimen, underlying disease and prior treatment history, and dose of colony stimulating factor.

## Precautions to Consider

### Cross-sensitivity and/or related problems
Patients sensitive to *Escherichia coli*–derived proteins may also be sensitive to filgrastim (rG-CSF).
Patients sensitive to yeast-derived products may also be sensitive to sargramostim (rGM-CSF).

### Carcinogenicity
Studies have not been done.

### Mutagenicity
Filgrastim did not induce bacterial gene mutations in either the presence or absence of a drug-metabolizing enzyme system.

### Pregnancy/Reproduction
Fertility—*For filgrastim:* No effect has been observed on the fertility of male or female rats or on gestation at doses up to 500 mcg per kg of body weight (mcg/kg).

*For sargramostim:* Studies in animals have not been done due to species specificity of the human protein.

Pregnancy—Adequate and well-controlled studies in humans have not been done.

*For filgrastim:* In pregnant rabbits, adverse effects have been observed at doses of 2 to 10 times the human dose. Studies in rabbits at doses of 80 mcg/kg per day found increased abortion and embryolethality. Studies in rabbits at doses of 100 mcg/kg per day during the period of organogenesis found increased fetal resorption, genitourinary bleeding, developmental abnormalities, and decreased body weight, live births, and food consumption; external abnormalities were not observed in the fetuses. Studies in rats at daily intravenous doses up to 575 mcg/kg per day during the period of organogenesis found no associated lethal, teratogenic, or behavioral effects on fetuses.

FDA Pregnancy Category C.

*For sargramostim:* Studies in animals have not been done due to species specificity of the human protein.

FDA Pregnancy Category C.

**Breast-feeding**

It is not known whether filgrastim or sargramostim is excreted in breast milk. However, problems in humans have not been documented.

**Pediatrics**

Appropriate studies on the relationship of age to the effects of colony stimulating factors have not been performed in the pediatric population. However, clinical trials have been conducted in infants and children; no differences in pharmacokinetics compared to studies in adults were found and no differences in type or incidence of adverse effects from those seen in adults have been documented to date. Subclinical increases in spleen size (seen during chronic use) detected by computed tomography (CT) or magnetic resonance imaging (MRI) studies were reported more often in children than in adults, but clinical significance of this is unknown.

**Geriatrics**

Appropriate studies on the relationship of age to the effects of colony stimulating factors have not been performed in the geriatric population. However, studies commonly include older patients and geriatrics-specific problems that would limit the usefulness of these medications in the elderly are not expected.

**Laboratory value alterations**

The following have been selected on the basis of their potential clinical significance (possible effect in parentheses where appropriate)—not necessarily inclusive (» = major clinical significance):

With physiology/laboratory test values

*For filgrastim and sargramostim*
Blood pressure
(transient decreases occur uncommonly; hypotension has been associated with a rare ''first-dose reaction'' to sargramostim)

*For filgrastim only (in addition to the above)*
Alkaline phosphatase, leukocyte (LAP scores) and serum values and
Lactic dehydrogenase (LDH), serum values and
Uric acid, serum concentrations
(commonly increased in patients receiving filgrastim; the increases coincide with the rise in neutrophil counts. Concentrations return to normal within 1 to 2 weeks after withdrawal of filgrastim)

*For sargramostim only (in addition to the above)*
Albumin, serum
(decreases have been reported during sargramostim therapy; possibly related to capillary leak syndrome)

Bilirubin, serum values and
Creatinine, serum concentrations and
Hepatic enzymes, serum values
(reportedly increased by sargramostim in some patients with renal or hepatic function impairment)

**Medical considerations/Contraindications**

The medical considerations/contraindications included here have been selected on the basis of their potential clinical significance (reasons given in parentheses where appropriate)—not necessarily inclusive (» = major clinical significance).

***Risk-benefit should be considered when the following medical problems exist:***

*For filgrastim and sargramostim*
Autoimmune disease, history of, e.g., autoimmune thrombocytopenia or
Inflammatory conditions, e.g., vaculitis
(may be exacerbated)

Cardiovascular disease, pre-existing
(supraventricular arrhythmia has been reported occasionally in patients receiving sargramostim, especially in patients with a history of cardiac arrhythmia; myocardial infarction and arrhythmias have been reported with filgrastim)

» Excessive leukemic myeloid blasts in the bone marrow or peripheral blood (10% or more)
(growth of leukemic blasts may be stimulated by colony stimulating factors, especially at high doses)

» Sensitivity to the colony stimulating factor prescribed

Sepsis
(theoretical potential of adult respiratory distress syndrome as a result of possible influx of neutrophils at the site of inflammation)

Caution should be used also in timing of colony stimulating factor administration to patients receiving chemotherapy or radiation therapy.

*For filgrastim only (in addition to the above)*
» Sensitivity to *E. coli*–derived proteins

*For sargramostim only (in addition to the above)*
Congestive heart failure or
Fluid retention, pre-existing (including peripheral edema, capillary leak syndrome, pleural and/or pericardial effusion) or
Pulmonary infiltrates
(sargramostim may aggravate fluid retention)

Hepatic function impairment or
Renal function impairment
(elevation of serum creatinine or bilirubin and hepatic enzymes by sargramostim has been reported; monitoring of function is recommended at least biweekly during treatment)

Pulmonary disease, including hypoxia
(caution is recommended because sargramostim causes sequestration of granulocytes in the pulmonary circulation; dyspnea has been reported)

» Sensitivity to yeast-derived proteins

**Patient monitoring**

The following may be especially important in patient monitoring (other tests may be warranted in some patients, depending on condition; » = major clinical significance):

*For filgrastim and sargramostim*
Cardiac monitoring
(recommended in patients with pre-existing cardiac conditions)

» Complete blood count (CBC) with differential (including examination for presence of blast cells) and
Platelet counts
(recommended twice weekly during treatment to monitor the neutrophil count to assess the hematopoietic response and avoid excessive leukocytosis)

Hepatic function and/or
Renal function
(monitoring recommended at least biweekly in patients with hepatic and/or renal function impairment)

*For sargramostim only (in addition to the above)*
Body weight and
Hydration status
(recommended during treatment with sargramostim)

# Side/Adverse Effects

Note: There are relatively few side/adverse effects directly associated with colony stimulating factor administration alone. Most side/adverse effects reported are due to the underlying malignancy or cytotoxic therapy. Neutropenic effects caused by cytotoxic therapy (fever, infection, mucositis) are decreased in frequency when colony stimulating factor is used. Only those side/adverse effects specifically caused by colony stimulating factor are listed below.

Development of antibodies to filgrastim (rG-CSF) has not been detected during treatment in 500 patients for up to almost 2 years and no blunting or diminishing of response has occurred. Neutralizing antibodies have been detected in 5 of 165 patients (3.0%) treated with sargramostim (rGM-CSF); because all 5 had impaired hematopoiesis prior to treatment, assessment of the effect of antibody development on normal hematopoiesis was not possible.

The following side/adverse effects have been selected on the basis of their potential clinical significance (possible signs and symptoms in parentheses where appropriate)—not necessarily inclusive:

**Those indicating need for medical attention**

*For filgrastim*

Incidence less frequent
*Excessive leukocytosis* (usually not symptomatic); *redness or pain at site of subcutaneous injection*

Incidence rare
*Allergic or anaphylactic reaction* (wheezing); *transient supraventricular arrhythmia* (rapid or irregular heartbeat); *splenomegaly* (not symptomatic); *Sweet's syndrome* (fever; sores on skin); *vasculitis* (sores on skin)

Note: *Splenomegaly* has been reported in patients receiving filgrastim for cyclic neutropenia. Subclinical splenomegaly occurs in approximately one-third of patients and clinical splenomegaly in about 3% of patients receiving chronic treatment with filgrastim.

*Sweet's syndrome* (also known as acute febrile neutrophilic dermatosis) appears to coincide with the increase in neutrophils.

*For sargramostim*

Incidence less frequent
*Capillary leak syndrome, including fluid retention, peripheral edema, or pleural and/or pericardial effusion* (swelling of feet or lower legs; sudden weight gain; shortness of breath); *fever; excessive leukocytosis* (usually not symptomatic); *redness or pain at site of subcutaneous injection; shortness of breath*

Note: *Capillary leak syndrome* is dose-related and dose-limiting; pleural and/or pericardial effusion usually occurs at doses above 32 mcg per kg of body weight per day. Fluid retention occurs at usual doses.

*Fever* is usually mild and dose-related. It occurs in about 50% of patients. It is not related to leukopenia, but may complicate assessment of fever associated with neutropenia. Fever resolves on withdrawal of sargramostim or administration of antipyretics such as acetaminophen.

*Shortness of breath* may be the result of sequestration of granulocytes in the pulmonary circulation. An adult respiratory distress syndrome has been reported.

Incidence rare
*Allergic or anaphylactic reaction* (wheezing); *transient supraventricular arrhythmia* (rapid or irregular heartbeat); *pericarditis* (chest pain; shortness of breath); *thrombophlebitis*—may occur during continuous infusion into small veins; *thromboses around tip of venous catheter; vasculitis* (sores on skin)

Note: *Pericarditis* is a dose-limiting effect.

Development of *thromboses* is a dose-limiting effect.

**Those indicating need for medical attention only if they continue or are bothersome**

*For filgrastim and sargramostim*

Incidence more frequent
*Arthralgias or myalgias* (pain in joints or muscles); *medullary bone pain* (pain in lower back or pelvis; less frequently, pain in arms or legs); *mild to moderate headache; skin rash or itching*

Note: *Arthralgias or myalgias* seem to occur when granulocyte counts are returning to normal. Pain usually occurs in the lower extremities.

*Bone pain* is usually mild to moderate and is alleviated by analgesics. It occurs in 20 to 50% of patients and is dose-related. It disappears within hours after withdrawal of colony stimulating factor, but usually resolves even with continued treatment. Bone pain is probably secondary to bone marrow expansion; it occurs over the 1- to 3-day period before myeloid recovery and the rise in peripheral blood neutrophils. It originates from sites containing bone marrow, including the sternum, spine, pelvis, and long bones.

*Skin rash* is usually generalized and mild.

*For sargramostim only (in addition to the above)*

Incidence less frequent or rare
*First-dose reaction, with flushing, hypotension, and syncope* (flushing of face; dizziness or faintness); *weakness*

Note: The *first-dose reaction* does not recur with the first dose of each course, although it may occur with the first dose of more than one course. The first-dose reaction has been described more consistently with bacterially-derived GM-CSF (molgramostim; not yet on the market), and included tachycardia, musculoskeletal pain, and dyspnea.

## Patient Consultation

As an aid to patient consultation, refer to *Advice for the Patient, Colony Stimulating Factors (Systemic)*.

In providing consultation, consider emphasizing the following selected information (» = major clinical significance):

**Before using this medication**
» Conditions affecting use, especially:
  Sensitivity to the colony stimulating factor prescribed
  Pregnancy—Adverse effects with filgrastim found in rabbits

**Proper use of this medication**

*For subcutaneous use*
» Compliance with therapy
» Reading patient directions carefully with regard to:
  —Preparation of the injection
  —Use of disposable syringes
  —Proper administration technique
  —Stability of the injection
» Proper dosing
  Missed dose: Checking with physician
» Proper storage

**Precautions while using this medication**
» Importance of close monitoring by physician
» Telling physician right away if signs or symptoms of infection (fever, chills) occur
  Possibility of mild bone pain as bone marrow begins to recover; usually relieved by mild analgesics; checking with physician if severe

**Side/adverse effects**
*Signs of potential side effects, especially—*
  For filgrastim: Redness or pain at site of subcutaneous injection, allergic or anaphylactic reaction, arrhythmias, and Sweet's syndrome and other dermatoses
  For sargramostim: Fluid retention, peripheral edema, pleural and/or pericardial effusion, fever, redness or pain at site of subcutaneous injection, shortness of breath, allergic or anaphylactic reaction, arrhythmias, pericarditis, and Sweet's syndrome and other dermatoses

## General Dosing Information

Patients receiving colony stimulating factor should be under supervision of a physician experienced in cytokine and/or cancer chemotherapy.

It is recommended that appropriate precautions be taken in the event that an allergic reaction occurs. If a serious allergic or anaphylactic reaction occurs, colony stimulating factor should be immediately discontinued and appropriate therapy initiated.

It is recommended that colony stimulating factor be discontinued when the absolute neutrophil count (ANC) reaches or exceeds 10,000 per cubic millimeter after the ANC nadir has occurred, to avoid excessive leukocytosis.

Colony stimulating factor should not be administered within 24 hours before or after administration of the last dose of chemotherapy or within 12 hours before or after radiotherapy, because of potential sensitivity of rapidly dividing hematopoietic progenitor cells to cytotoxic chemotherapy or radiologic therapies.

---

### *FILGRASTIM*

---

## Summary of Differences

Pharmacology/pharmacokinetics: Mechanism of action—Lineage-specific; stimulates production of neutrophil granulocytes.

Side/adverse effects: Causes splenomegaly with chronic use, Sweet's syndrome; development of antibodies not reported.

## Additional Dosing Information

Filgrastim may be administered subcutaneously (by rapid injection or as a continuous 24-hour infusion) or intravenously (as a short 30-minute or continuous 24-hour infusion). *Intravenous administration should be by infusion over at least 30 minutes*, because there is a decrease in efficacy when filgrastim is administered by rapid intravenous injection; in addition, it is preferable not to flush the intravenous line after administration is complete.

A variety of dosage schedules are used, depending on the indication and the individual patient, for indications not included in the official labeling. The prescriber may consult the medical literature in choosing a specific dosage.

The chemotherapy-induced nadir usually occurs 2 to 3 days earlier during cycles in which filgrastim is administered.

Bone pain usually responds to treatment with non-narcotic analgesics; infrequently, it may be severe enough to require narcotic analgesics.

## Parenteral Dosage Forms

Note: Bracketed uses in the *Dosage Forms* section refer to categories of use and/or indications that are not included in U.S. product labeling.

### FILGRASTIM INJECTION

#### Usual adult dose

Neutropenia, chemotherapy-related—

Intravenous or subcutaneous, 5 mcg per kg of body weight once a day, beginning no earlier than twenty-four hours after administration of the last dose of cytotoxic chemotherapy. This is continued for up to two weeks, until the absolute neutrophil count (ANC) reaches 10,000 per cubic millimeter following the nadir; in patients receiving dose intensified chemotherapy, filgrastim should be continued until two consecutive ANC's of at least 10,000 per cubic millimeter are documented. Dosage may be increased, if necessary, in increments of 5 mcg per kg of body weight for each chemotherapy cycle.

[Myeloid engraftment following bone marrow transplantation, promotion of][1]—

Intravenous or subcutaneous, 5 mcg per kg of body weight per day for twenty-one days beginning two to four hours after autologous bone marrow infusion, and not less than twenty-four hours after the last dose of chemotherapy and twelve hours after the last dose of radiotherapy.

[Myeloid engraftment following bone marrow transplantation, failure or delay (treatment)][1]—

Intravenous or subcutaneous, 5 mcg per kg of body weight per day for fourteen days; course of therapy may be repeated after seven days if engraftment has not occurred. If engraftment has not occurred within seven days after the second fourteen-day course of therapy, a course of 10 mcg per kg of body weight per day for fourteen days may be tried.

Note: The calculated dose may be rounded off, within reason, to the nearest vial size (300 or 480 mcg) to reduce wastage.

#### Usual adult prescribing limits

Not defined. Patients have received doses as high as 115 mcg per kg of body weight per day without toxic effects.

#### Usual pediatric dose

Dosage has not been established.

#### Strength(s) usually available

U.S.—

300 mcg (0.3 mg) per mL (300 mcg per 1-mL vial or 480 mcg per 1.6-mL vial) (Rx) [*Neupogen* (acetate; mannitol; Tween 80; sodium 0.035 mg per mL)].

Canada—

300 mcg (0.3 mg) per mL (300 mcg per 1-mL vial or 480 mcg per 1.6-mL vial) (Rx) [*Neupogen* (acetate; mannitol; Tween 80; sodium 0.035 mg per mL)].

Note: The specific activity is $1.0 \pm 0.6 \times 10^8$ Units per mg as measured by a cell mitogenesis assay.

#### Packaging and storage

Store between 2 and 8 °C (36 and 46 °F), unless otherwise specified by manufacturer. Protect from freezing. Avoid shaking.

#### Preparation of dosage form

Filgrastim injection may be diluted for administration by intravenous infusion in 5% dextrose injection to produce a concentration greater than or equal to 15 mcg of filgrastim per mL. If the final concentration is to be between 2 and 15 mcg per mL, addition of human albumin to the dextrose injection before addition of filgrastim injection is necessary to prevent adsorption to the components of the drug delivery system. The concentration of human albumin in the final solution should be 0.2% (2 mg per mL); this can be achieved with 2 mL of 5% human albumin in 50 mL of 5% dextrose injection.

#### Stability

Filgrastim injection contains no preservative. Before use, filgrastim injection may be allowed to reach room temperature for a maximum of 6 hours; after that period of time, the vial should be discarded.

#### Auxiliary labeling

• Do not shake.

---

[1]Not included in Canadian product labeling.

---

## Summary of Differences

Pharmacology/pharmacokinetics: Mechanism of action—Non–lineage specific; stimulates production of granulocytes, macrophages, and eosinophils.

Precautions: Medical considerations/contraindications—Pulmonary disease.

Side/adverse effects: Causes capillary leak syndrome and fluid retention, fever, shortness of breath, pericarditis, thrombophlebitis, thromboses, first-dose reaction, and weakness.

## Additional Dosing Information

Sargramostim is administered as a 2-hour intravenous infusion via a central venous line. An in-line membrane filter should not be used. Sargramostim may also be administered subcutaneously.

A variety of dosage schedules are used, depending on the indication and the individual patient, for indications not included in the official labeling. The prescriber may consult the medical literature in choosing a specific dosage.

Systemic adverse effects (bone pain, fever, asthenia, etc.) are usually prevented or reversed by administration of analgesics and antipyretics such as acetaminophen.

Fluid retention is reversible on withdrawal or dose reduction, with or without diuretic treatment.

If dyspnea occurs during sargramostim administration, the rate of administration should be reduced by half. The standard dosing schedule may be used, with careful monitoring, for subsequent infusions. If dyspnea persists following infusion rate reduction, the infusion should be discontinued.

If the absolute neutrophil count (ANC) exceeds 20,000 or the platelet count exceeds 500,000, sargramostim treatment should be discontinued or the dose reduced by half. Excessive blood counts usually return to normal or baseline levels within 3 to 7 days following withdrawal of sargramostim.

If progression of the underlying neoplastic disease (non-Hodgkin's lymphoma, acute lymphocytic leukemia, Hodgkin's disease) occurs during sargramostim therapy, it is recommended that sargramostim be discontinued.

If blast cells appear, it is recommended that sargramostim be discontinued.

## Parenteral Dosage Forms

Note: Bracketed uses in the *Dosage Forms* section refer to categories of use and/or indications that are not included in U.S. product labeling.

### SARGRAMOSTIM FOR INJECTION

#### Usual adult dose

Myeloid engraftment following bone marrow transplantation, promotion of—

Intravenous infusion (over two hours) or subcutaneous, 250 mcg per square meter of body surface per day for twenty-one days beginning two to four hours after autologous bone marrow infusion, and not less than twenty-four hours after the last dose of chemotherapy and twelve hours after the last dose of radiotherapy.

Myeloid engraftment following bone marrow transplantation, failure or delay (treatment)—

Intravenous infusion (over two hours) or subcutaneous, 250 mcg per square meter of body surface per day for fourteen days; course of therapy may be repeated after seven days if engraftment has not occurred. If engraftment has not occurred within seven days after the second fourteen-day course of therapy, a course of 500 mcg per square meter of body surface per day for fourteen days may be tried.

[Neutropenia, chemotherapy-related]—

Intravenous infusion (over two hours) or subcutaneous, 250 mcg per square meter of body surface per day beginning no earlier than twenty-four hours after administration of the last dose of cytotoxic chemotherapy. This is continued for up to two weeks, until the absolute neutrophil count (ANC) reaches 10,000 per cubic millimeter following the nadir; in patients receiving dose intensified chemotherapy, sargramostim should be continued until two consecutive ANC's of at least 10,000 per cubic millimeter are documented. Dosage may be increased, if necessary, in an increment of 250 mcg per square meter of body surface, up to 500 mcg per square meter of body surface.

Note: The calculated dose may be rounded off, within reason, to the nearest vial size (250 or 500 mcg) to reduce wastage.

### Usual pediatric dose
Dosage has not been established.

### Size(s) usually available
U.S.—
250 mcg (0.25 mg) (Rx) [*Leukine* (mannitol; sucrose; tromethamine)].
500 mcg (0.5 mg) (Rx) [*Leukine* (mannitol; sucrose; tromethamine)].
Canada—
Not commercially available.

Note: The specific activity is approximately $5 \times 10^7$ colony forming units per mg in a normal human bone marrow colony formation assay.

### Packaging and storage
Store between 2 and 8 °C (36 and 46 °F), unless otherwise specified by manufacturer. Protect reconstituted solution from freezing. Avoid shaking solution.

### Preparation of dosage form
Sargramostim for injection is reconstituted by adding 1.0 mL of sterile water for injection (without preservative) to the vial containing 250 or 500 mcg, producing a clear, colorless solution containing 250 or 500 mcg of sargramostim per mL, respectively. To avoid foaming during dissolution, the diluent should be directed at the side of the vial and the contents swirled gently; excessive or vigorous agitation should be avoided; the vial should not be shaken.

The reconstituted solution is diluted further for administration by intravenous infusion with 0.9% sodium chloride injection. If the final concentration of sargramostim is to be less than 10 mcg per mL, addition of human albumin to the saline before addition of sargramostim solution is necessary to prevent adsorption to the components of the drug delivery system. The concentration of human albumin in the final solution should be 0.1% (1 mg per mL); this can be achieved with 1 mL of 5% human albumin in 50 mL of 0.9% sodium chloride injection.

### Stability
Because sargramostim products contain no antibacterial preservative, reconstituted solutions should be used within 6 hours and any unused portion should be discarded.

### Auxiliary labeling
• Do not shake.

## Selected Bibliography

Mertelsmann R. Hematopoietins: biology, pathophysiology, and potential as therapeutic agents. Ann Oncol 1991; 2: 251-63.

Hollingshead LM, Goa KL. Recombinant granulocyte colony-stimulating factor (rG-CSF). A review of its pharmacological properties and prospective role in neutropenic conditions. Drugs 1991; 42 (2): 300-30.

Ruef C, Coleman DL. Granulocyte-macrophage colony-stimulating factor: pleiotropic cytokine with potential clinical usefulness. Rev Infect Dis 1990 Jan-Feb; 12: 41-62.

Metcalf D, Morstyn G. Colony-stimulating factors: general biology. In DeVita VT, Hellman S, Rosenberg SA (eds). Biologic therapy of cancer. New York: J.B. Lippincott, 1991: 417-44.

Gabrilove J. Colony-stimulating factors: clinical status. In DeVita VT, Hellman S, Rosenberg SA (eds). Biologic therapy of cancer. New York: J.B. Lippincott, 1991: 445-53.

Revised: 08/07/92
Interim revision: 04/22/93; 07/14/94

# CONDOMS

This monograph includes information on the following: Lamb Cecum Condoms; Lamb Cecum Condoms and Nonoxynol 9†; Latex Condoms; Latex Condoms and Nonoxynol 9.

VA CLASSIFICATION (Primary):
Lamb Cecum—XA900
Lamb and Nonoxynol 9—GU400
Latex—XA900
Latex and Nonoxynol 9—GU400

Note: For a listing of dosage forms and brand names by country availability, see *Dosage Forms* section(s). For a listing of brand names for the articles in this monograph, refer to the General Index.

†Not commercially available in Canada.

## Category
Contraceptive; sexually transmitted disease prophylactic.

## Indications
Note: Bracketed information in the *Indications* section refers to uses that are not included in U.S. product labeling.

### Accepted
Pregnancy (prophylaxis)—Condoms (both latex and lamb cecum) are used as a primary method of contraception. They are also used to prevent pregnancy at times when oral contraceptives or intrauterine devices may not be effective or are contraindicated or as an adjuvant to the periodic abstinence (rhythm) method of contraception. Concurrent use of a vaginal spermicide is also recommended since it may increase the efficacy of condoms by providing a back-up to the condom in case of leaking or spilling of ejaculate or rupture of the condom during coitus.

Sexually transmitted diseases (prophylaxis)—The use of latex or [lamb cecum] condoms is partially effective in reducing the risk of acquiring many sexually transmitted diseases (STDs). Latex condoms are preferred over lamb cecum condoms for the prevention of STDs. Lamb cecum condoms are generally recommended for use **only** by those individuals with a confirmed sensitivity to latex condoms.

Concurrent use of a spermicide is also recommended as a back-up to the condom in case of spilling of ejaculate or rupture of the condom during intercourse. However, the extent of this additional protection against acquiring STDs (especially viral) has not yet been determined.

Condoms may be recommended for use by patients in addition to nonbarrier contraceptives (such as the intrauterine device or oral contraceptives) or other barrier methods of contraception (such as the cervical cap, contraceptive sponge, or diaphragm) to reduce the risk of acquiring STDs. The use of latex condoms in combination with spermicides may also be considered for those patients at high risk of acquiring STDs (especially HIV infection) during pregnancy.

In *in vitro* studies, latex condoms have been shown to significantly reduce the passage of the following STD pathogens (approximate diameters in parentheses):
*Chlamydia trachomatis* (200 to 300 nanometers)
Cytomegalovirus (CMV) (200 to 300 nanometers)
Hepatitis B virus (HBV) (42 nanometers) and surface antigen
Herpes simplex virus II (HSV II) (120 to 150 nanometers)
Human immunodeficiency virus (HIV) (90 to 120 nanometers)
*Neisseria gonorrhoeae* (1000 to 2000 nanometers)

Epidemiologic studies have shown a reduction in the rate of occurrence of cervical human papillomavirus lesions or infections, chlamydia, cytomegalovirus infection, gonorrhea, hepatitis B infection, mycoplasma infection, syphilis, and ureaplasma infection with the use of condoms. Condoms are also recommended for the prevention of infections with the following pathogens: *Candida albicans*, group B streptococcus, *Trichomoniasis vaginalis*, *Haemophilus ducreyi*, and *Mycoplasma hominis*.

Lamb cecum condoms are not generally recommended for STD prophylaxis; latex condoms are preferred over lamb cecum condoms for the prevention of STDs. *In vitro* data concerning lamb cecum condoms are conflicting and some studies indicate that they may permit passage of HBV, HIV, CMV, and HSV. As compared with latex condoms, the surface layer of lamb cecum condoms shows large pores (up to 1500 nanometers) that may permit passage of smaller STD pathogens. Lamb cecum is composed of several layers of these porous membranes. Each pore on the surface layer membrane does not align directly with the porous membranes beneath to form a direct port of entry through the entire cecum. However, with prolonged contact or stretching of the cecum, it is theoretically possible for an infectious agent to traverse the entire cecum. Lamb cecum may also have naturally occurring thinner areas. When examined by scanning electron microscopy, the surface of a latex condom is irregular but exhibits no pores or breaks.

In small studies of heterosexual partners of HIV-positive patients, the lowest rates of HIV negative-to-positive seroconversion were associated with couples practicing sexual abstinence. Additionally, in the same studies and in others concerning female prostitutes, consistent users or partners of consistent users of latex condoms showed a reduced rate of seroconversion, as compared with never-users or inconsistent users of condoms. However, because a critical need exists for absolute protection from HIV infection, larger studies are needed to confirm these findings definitively, including information concerning anal, oral, and vaginal intercourse. Product-specific information is also needed regarding condom reliability during intercourse, since condoms may rupture or slip off the penis during intercourse. An especially high rate of condom rupture and slippage has been reported with their use during anal intercourse, which also carries the highest inherent risk of sexually transmitted HIV infection.

Although thicker latex condoms are less likely to deteriorate before use and rupture during intercourse, it has not been proven that they are more likely to provide greater protection against exposure to and infection with STDs.

[Pelvic inflammatory disease (prophylaxis)][1]—The use of condoms decreases the risk of development of pelvic inflammatory disease (PID) and subsequent tubal damage and infertility. Epidemiologic studies have shown a lower rate of hospitalization for pelvic inflammatory disease among women whose partners used condoms. One study showed a reduction in the incidence of tubal infertility among users of mechanical barrier contraceptives combined with a spermicide, which was greater than the reduction with either method alone. The use of latex condoms in combination with vaginal spermicides may also be considered for those patients at high risk of development of PID during pregnancy.

[Cervical neoplasia (prophylaxis and treatment)][1]—Use of condoms may provide some degree of protection against the development of cervical neoplasia. Epidemiologic studies have shown a lower rate of cervical neoplasia incidence among women whose partners used condoms. However, the extent of this protection has not yet been determined.

The use of condoms has been associated with regression of squamous cell cervical intraepithelial neoplasia in some patients. However, the use of condoms should not serve as a replacement for or to delay standard therapy for cervical neoplasia.

[Allergy, human seminal plasma (treatment)][1]—Condoms may be used rarely in the treatment of allergy to human seminal plasma. They may be used as interval therapy, prior to immunotherapy or other definitive therapies, to prevent the recurrence of symptoms upon re-exposure to seminal plasma, such as urticaria, pruritus, edema, bronchospasm, anaphylaxis, and pelvic pain.

Condoms have been used as adjunctive therapy in the treatment of female infertility resulting from the presence of antisperm antibodies. Theoretically, the use of condoms causes a decline in antisperm antibody titers after 3 to 6 months of use, due to reduction of female exposure to the sperm antigen. However, the effectiveness of condoms used in the treatment of this condition has not been demonstrated by well-controlled clinical trials.

[1]Not included in Canadian product labeling.

## Pharmacology/Pharmacokinetics

### Physicochemical characteristics
Nonoxynol 9—Chemical group: Nonionic surfactant

### Mechanism of action/Effect
Condoms—
For prevention of pregnancy:
Condoms are considered a mechanical form of barrier contraception because they block the passage of sperm (3000 nanometers in diameter) through the cervix by serving as a receptacle for ejaculate. There is also some minor evidence that latex condoms and other rubber products cause immobilization of spermatozoa. To be effective, condoms must be completely unrolled onto the penis before any genital contact occurs and remain intact throughout intercourse. The slight possibility exists that sufficient spermatozoa could be present in the pre-ejaculate fluid to result in conception.
Some latex condoms are designed with a pre-formed reservoir tip to hold semen. A reservoir helps to prevent spilling or leaking of sperm after ejaculation and before the penis is withdrawn and decreases the chance of condom rupture during intercourse. When condoms without this pre-formed reservoir tip are used, a reservoir is created by leaving approximately one-half inch of space at the tip of the condom and pressing out any trapped air. The condom should be completely unrolled onto the penis. After ejaculation and before the loss of erection, the base of the condom is grasped firmly and the penis withdrawn carefully to avoid spillage of the ejaculate and to prevent the condom from slipping off the penis. One type of condom has an adhesive which forms a seal around the base of the condom. Studies by the manufacturer have shown that this seal minimizes slippage and leaking of the condom during vaginal intercourse, regardless of whether the penis is erect. Lamb cecum condoms are more likely to slip off the penis because they are less elastic than latex condoms and therefore do not fit as tightly.

The following are the results of studies examining failure rates reported during the use of various contraceptive methods, as the percentage of women experiencing accidental pregnancy per year of use.

In the second column, interstudy variations in failure rates may be due to differences in study design or patient population characteristics, such as motivation, fecundity, or socioeconomic factors (including level of education). Studies reported also include failure rates beyond the first year, which generally decline with continued use of a specific method.

In the third column are failure rates expected among *typical* adult couples who start using the method listed (not necessarily for the first time) and do not stop use of this method in the first year for any reason other than accidental pregnancy. Failure rates among adolescents may be higher, due to poor compliance.

| Method used | Ranges seen in clinical studies (%) | Typical first year failure rates (%) |
|---|---|---|
| None | 78–94 | 89 |
| Spermicides* | 0.3–37 | 21 |
| Periodic abstinence | 13–35 | 20 |
| Withdrawal | 7–22 | 18 |
| Cervical cap with spermicide | 6–27 | 18 |
| Sponge | 5–>28 | 18 |
| Diaphragm with spermicide | | 2–23 |
| Condom without spermicide | 2–14 | 12 |
| IUD | 0.5–6 | 6 |
| Oral contraceptive | | |
| Combination | 0–6 | 3 |
| Progestin only | 1–10 | 5 |
| Progestin injection | 0–4 | |
| Medroxyprogesterone | | 0.3 |
| Norethisterone | | 2 |
| Implants | | |
| Capsules | 0.3–0.4 | 0.3 |
| Rods | 0–0.2 | 0.2 |
| Sterilization | | |
| Female | 0–8 | 0.4 |
| Male | 0–0.5 | 0.15 |

*Spermicides studied include creams, foams, gels, jellies, and suppositories.

For prevention of sexually transmitted diseases:
Condoms prevent sexual contact of infectious cervical, vaginal, vulvar, oral, or rectal secretions or lesions with the penis of the wearer. The partner is prevented from being exposed to any infectious agents present in semen and any lesions on the wearer's penis. Condoms may be less effective in the prevention of STDs acquired from lesions because the condom may not cover these infectious areas of skin or areas vulnerable to infection. To be most effective, condoms must be completely unrolled onto the penis before any genital contact occurs and remain intact throughout intercourse.

For prevention of pelvic inflammatory disease:
Condoms prevent the organisms causing pelvic inflammatory disease from reaching the cervix.

For prevention and treatment of cervical neoplasia:
Condoms may protect against cervical cancer and allow regression of cervical intraepithelial neoplasia, since there is some evidence that cervical neoplasia may result from sexual transmission of human papillomavirus.

Nonoxynol 9—
For prevention of pregnancy:
Vaginal spermicides are considered chemical forms of barrier contraceptives because they form a chemical barrier between the mucous membranes and ejaculate. The active chemicals in vaginal spermicides interact with the lipoproteins of the cell membrane to permanently disrupt the cell membranes of spermatozoa, resulting in severe damage to the acrosome (head), neck, midpiece, and tail of the sperm and rapid, irreversible loss of viability, function, and motility within the vagina. Cell permeability increases, and the leaking of cellular components occurs. Studies also indicate that carbohydrate-metabolizing enzymes and the mitochondriae are disturbed. The inactive vehicle itself may form a mechanical barrier to the cervical os, inhibiting the passage of sperm.

For prevention of sexually transmitted diseases:

*In vitro*, nonoxynol 9 has been shown to produce bactericidal and virucidal effects by disrupting the cell membrane and the viral envelope. The active chemicals in vaginal spermicides interact with the lipoproteins of the cell membrane to permanently disrupt the cell membranes. Nonoxynol 9 may also exert antimicrobial activity against *Chlamydia trachomatis* receptors on target cells. Low concentrations *in vitro* have been shown to block cellular attachment and/or penetration by *C. trachomatis* organisms. In one study, nonoxynol 9 caused significant chemorepulsion of *Trichomonas vaginalis in vitro*.

Any method covering the cervix may protect against gonorrhea and chlamydia because the causative organisms primarily infect cervical tissues. Therefore, spermicides alone or in combination with a mechanical barrier contraceptive may protect against transmission of these infections. Spermicidal preparations that are well-distributed within the vagina, such as foams or sponges, may be best for those organisms that reside mostly in the vagina, such as *T. vaginalis*.

Nonoxynol 9 has been shown to inhibit the *in vitro* growth of the following STD pathogens:

*Chlamydia trachomatis*
*Gardnerella vaginalis*
*Mycoplasma hominis*
*Neisseria gonorrhoeae*
*Trichomonas vaginalis*
*Ureaplasma urealyticum*

*In vitro*, nonoxynol 9 also decreases the infectivity of *Treponema pallidum*, the pathogenic agent of syphilis.

Clinical studies have shown a reduction in the rate of occurrence of chlamydia, gonorrhea, trichomoniasis, and bacterial vaginosis with the use of nonoxynol 9–containing preparations, especially in combination with mechanical barrier contraceptives.

*In vitro*, nonoxynol 9 has been shown to inactivate herpes simplex viruses (HSV) I and II and human immunodeficiency virus (HIV, AIDS virus).

## Absorption

Nonoxynol 9—Radiolabeled nonoxynol 9 has been shown to be rapidly and extensively absorbed into the systemic circulation from the vaginal mucosa of rats and rabbits. The rate of absorption is dependent upon the product vehicle. No direct information on the rate or extent of absorption of spermicides from human rectal or vaginal mucosa is available. However, disruption of the vaginal epithelial cells occurs, with increased thinning of the epithelium occurring with continuing exposure. Also, the vaginal mucosa is histologically similar to the buccal mucosa. Therefore, it is feasible that these agents could be absorbed into the systemic circulation in humans as well.

## Distribution

Nonoxynol 9 (systemic)—

Studies have not been published regarding systemic distribution in humans. However, in one study on the use of vaginal nonoxynol 9 in rabbits, the highest amounts of radiolabeled nonoxynol 9 were in the uterus and vaginal tissue. The liver also contained a greater amount than most other body tissues.

In one study of vaginally administered radiolabeled nonoxynol 9 in gravid rats, at 6 hours the medication in the uterus and placenta was in equilibrium with that of the maternal plasma. The concentration of nonoxynol 9 in the amniotic fluid was approximately one-third that of the maternal plasma.

## Biotransformation

Nonoxynol 9—In studies conducted in animals, there was little evidence that nonoxynol 9 is metabolized.

## Elimination

Nonoxynol 9—In one study in rabbits, a cumulative total of 40% of a dose of radiolabeled nonoxynol 9 was excreted in the urine and 10% in the feces in the 144 hours following vaginal administration. Within 24 hours, 20% was excreted in the urine, and the daily fecal excretion rate was approximately 1 to 2%. In rats, approximately 95% of the dose was excreted within 72 hours, 23% of which was present in the urine and 70% in the feces.

# Precautions to Consider

## Cross-sensitivity and/or related problems

Condoms—Patients with a confirmed latex sensitivity should notify the attending physician before undergoing medical and, especially, surgical procedures. Severe intraoperative anaphylaxis to latex surgical gloves and rubber anesthetic devices has been reported in patients who previously exhibited signs of contact dermatitis to latex rubber.

Nonoxynol 9—Because of close similarities in composition, activity, and structure, patients sensitive to octoxynol 9 are likely to be sensitive to nonoxynol 9 also and should avoid further use of either product if allergic reaction occurs.

## Pregnancy/Reproduction

Nonoxynol 9—The majority of evidence indicates that nonoxynol 9 does not increase the risk of occurrence of spontaneous abortion or major congenital anomalies when used at or near the time of conception or during pregnancy.

In a study of gravid rats, nonoxynol 9 appeared in the serum of the pups within 2 hours of vaginal administration of radiolabeled nonoxynol 9.

## Breast-feeding

Nonoxynol 9—

It is not known whether nonoxynol 9 is excreted in human breast milk. However, problems have not been documented.

In a study conducted in gravid rats, an amount of radiolabeled nonoxynol 9 corresponding to approximately 0.3% of the given dose was excreted in the milk in the 24 hours following vaginal administration.

## Adolescents

Consistent and careful use is critical in the employment of condoms to prevent pregnancy, and their use requires a considerable amount of interruption in sexual spontaneity. For this reason, typical first-year-usage failure rates associated with condom use by adolescents may be significantly higher than for adults. However, there are some advantages to the use of condoms in that they are a fairly effective, widely available, inexpensive, nonprescription contraceptive product. Thorough patient counseling and careful consideration of any psychosocial factors involved should be included in contraceptive choice.

## Medical considerations/Contraindications

The medical considerations/contraindications included here have been selected on the basis of their potential clinical significance (reasons given in parentheses where appropriate)—not necessarily inclusive (» = major clinical significance).

*Except under special circumstances, this medication should not be used when the following medical problems exist:*

*For latex condoms only*
» Sensitivity to latex

*For latex condoms and nonoxynol 9 only*
» Sensitivity to nonoxynol or octoxynol

*Risk-benefit should be considered when the following medical problems exist:*

*For contraceptive use only*
» Medical or psychosocial conditions where a critical need exists for highly effective contraception
   (patients must be sufficiently counseled regarding the need for consistent and correct use of condoms if they are to be effective in preventing pregnancy)

*For latex condoms and nonoxynol 9 only (in addition to the above)*
   Allergy, chronic, local or
   Contact dermatitis, genital
   (moderate to severe irritation may occur with the use of spermicides)

# Side/Adverse Effects

Note: The safety of the use of spermicides on the rectal mucosa is unknown. However, no serious adverse effects have been reported.

In one study in rats and rabbits given high doses of nonoxynol 9 peritoneally or vaginally, some evidence of hepatotoxicity and nephrotoxicity was seen. However, these effects or other serious systemic side effects have not been seen in humans.

The following side/adverse effects have been selected on the basis of their potential clinical significance (possible signs and symptoms in parentheses)—not necessarily inclusive:

## Those indicating need for medical attention

Incidence rare
   *For latex condoms and/or nonoxynol 9 only*
   ***Allergic vaginitis*** (recurring vaginal bleeding, redness, irritation, rash, dryness, or whitish discharge, associated with intercourse); ***contact dermatitis*** (recurring skin rash; local edema; redness; irritation; itching); ***anaphylaxis, generalized*** (rhinitis; conjunctivitis; hives; facial and laryngeal angioedema; bronchospasm); ***urinary tract infection, female*** (increased frequency of urination; pain on urination; bladder pain; cloudy or bloody urine)

Note: *Allergic vaginitis and contact dermatitis* may be due to exposure to latex, manufacturing contaminants from the latex, or the lubricant or spermicide applied to the condom. These symptoms may necessitate use of a different latex product or use of lamb cecum condoms.

*Anaphylaxis* has been reported very rarely with use of a latex condom during vaginal intercourse; use of latex gloves for vaginal examination, surgical procedures, or rectal manual disimpaction; inflation of rubber balloons; wearing of latex gloves; and use of latex dental dams.

An increased risk of *urinary tract infection* may occur with the use of nonoxynol 9 in females, possibly due to changes in vaginal flora.

**Those indicating need for medical attention only if they continue or are bothersome**
Incidence less frequent
> *For latex condoms and/or nonoxynol 9 only*
> > **Burning, stinging, warmth, itching, or other irritation of the skin, penis, rectum, or vagina; vaginal dryness or malodor**
> >
> > Note: *Local irritation* may be due to exposure to latex, manufacturing contaminants from the latex, or the lubricant or spermicide applied to the condom. These symptoms may necessitate use of a different product.

## Patient Consultation

As an aid to patient consultation, refer to *Advice for the Patient, Condoms.*

In providing consultation, consider emphasizing the following selected information (» = major clinical significance):

**Before using this product**
» Conditions affecting use, especially:
   Sensitivity to latex (latex condoms only)
   Sensitivity to nonoxynol 9 or octoxynol (latex condoms and nonoxynol 9 only)
   Medical problems, especially—
      For contraception only: Conditions where a critical need exists for contraception
      For latex condoms and nonoxynol 9 only: Local allergy or genital contact dermatitis

**Proper use of this product**
   To use: Reading package insert carefully and following manufacturer instructions
» Using correctly and consistently with every act of intercourse
» Proper use of lubricant or spermicide
» Proper storage

**Side/adverse effects**
   Signs of potential side effects, especially vaginitis, anaphylaxis, and dermatitis; in addition, for latex condoms and nonoxynol 9 only, urinary tract infection

## General Dosing Information

Some condom users find that they require the use of an additional lubricant. Condoms prevent the lubricating, pre-ejaculatory seminal fluid that leaks from the urethral meatus from coming in contact with the vaginal or rectal mucosa. They also prevent vaginal and cervical fluids from coming in contact with the penis. Some latex condoms have a pre-applied lubricant, which is a wet glycol jelly, a spermicidal jelly, or a silicone fluid. Lamb cecum condoms are packaged with a larger volume of a water-based lubricant that also serves as a preservative. The use of nonlubricated condoms may result in a sensation of dryness during intercourse. Use of additional lubrication or pre-lubricated condoms may decrease the risk of condom rupture or decrease frictional trauma to the rectal or vaginal mucosa or anus. The use of additional lubrication may be especially important during anal intercourse, since greater friction results in increased rates of condom rupture and slippage, as compared with vaginal intercourse. Only appropriate water-based lubricants should be used, such as sterile surgical lubricant, vaginal spermicides (especially gels and jellies), or a personal lubricant formulated for use with condoms or a latex diaphragm. Oil-based products such as hand, body, or face cream; petroleum jelly; cooking oils or shortenings; or mineral or baby oil will weaken latex and increase the risk of condom rupture during intercourse.

Although some brands of latex condoms are coated with a small quantity of spermicide, additional spermicide may be applied to ensure the maximum efficacy possible. Spermicide should be spread on the outside surface of the condom after it is unrolled onto the penis. It is especially important that a female partner also place spermicide in the vagina before coitus; such use is more likely to afford greater efficacy. If a condom ruptures after ejaculation, it has been suggested that im-

mediately applying a vaginal spermicide may provide some protection against pregnancy. It is not known if applying spermicide vaginally or rectally if a condom ruptures after ejaculation is effective in reducing the risk of STD transmission.

Condoms should not be opened until immediately before they are to be placed on the penis. Exposure to ultraviolet (UV) light, humidity, heat, or ozone will cause rapid deterioration of latex. This will result in an increased likelihood of condom rupture during use. Condoms should be purchased that are packaged in airtight, protective materials that also block UV light transmission. It is also recommended that condoms not be purchased well ahead of their time of use, since latex may deteriorate rapidly under less-than-ideal conditions. Condoms should be stored in a cool, dry location, out of direct sunlight.

Condoms should be inspected in a well-lighted area before they are placed on the penis and after they are completely unrolled onto the penis. The condom should not be used if it does not unroll easily; has tears, breaks, or holes after it is unrolled; or if the texture of the latex is sticky, brittle, discolored, or gummy. Condoms should not be reused; a new condom is necessary for each act of intercourse.

---

### LAMB CECUM CONDOMS

## Product Forms

### LAMB CECUM CONDOMS

**Product(s) usually available**
U.S.—
   Lubricated:
      (OTC) [*Fourex Natural Skins; Kling-Tite Naturalamb*].
Canada—
   Lubricated:
      (OTC) [*Fourex Natural Skins; Kling-Tite Naturalamb*].

**Packaging and storage**
Store below 40 °C (104 °F), preferably between 15 and 30 °C (59 and 86 °F), unless otherwise specified by manufacturer. Protect from light. Protect from freezing.

---

### LAMB CECUM CONDOMS AND NONOXYNOL 9

## Product Forms

### LAMB CECUM CONDOMS AND NONOXYNOL 9

**Product(s) usually available**
U.S.—
   (OTC) [*Fourex Natural Skins Spermicidally Lubricated; Kling-Tite Naturalamb with Spermicide Lubricant*].
Canada—
   Not commercially available.

**Packaging and storage**
Store below 40 °C (104 °F), preferably between 15 and 30 °C (59 and 86 °F), unless otherwise specified by manufacturer. Protect from light. Protect from freezing.

---

### LATEX CONDOMS

## Product Forms

### LATEX CONDOMS

**Product(s) usually available**
U.S.—
   Lubricated:
      (OTC) [*Beyond Seven; Class Act Ribbed & Sensitive; Class Act Ultra Thin & Sensitive; Crown; Embrace; Excita Fiesta; Excita Sensitrol; Gold Circle Coin; Gold Circle Rainbow Coin; Kimono; Kimono Microthins; Kimono Sensation; LifeStyles Assorted Colors; LifeStyles Form Fitting; LifeStyles Lubricated; LifeStyles Ultra Sensitive; LifeStyles Vibra-Ribbed; MAXX; Ramses Safe Play; Ramses Sensitol; Ramses Ultra Thin; Saxon Gold Ultra Sensitive; Sheik Classic Lubricated; Sheik Fiesta Colors; Sheik Super Thin Lubricated; Sheik Super Thin Ribbed Lubricated; Touch Lubricated; Touch Ribbed Lubricated; Touch Sunrise Colors; Touch Thins Lubricated; Trojan-Enz Large Lubricated; Trojan-Enz Lubricated; Trojan Extra Strength Lubricated; Trojan Magnum; Trojan Naturalube Ribbed; Trojan Plus; Trojan Ribbed; Trojans; Trojan Ultra Texture Lubricant; Trojan Very Sensitive with Lubricant; Trojan Very Thin with Lubricant;* GENERIC].

Non-Lubricated:
(OTC) [*LifeStyles Non-Lubricated; Ramses Non-Lubricated; Sheik Classic Non-Lubricated; Touch Non-Lubricated; Trojan-Enz Nonlubricated;* GENERIC].

Canada—
Lubricated:
(OTC) [*Embrace; Gold Circle Coin; LifeStyles Form Fitting; LifeStyles Lubricated; LifeStyles Ultra Sensitive; LifeStyles Vibra-Ribbed; Ortho Shields Lubricated; Ortho Shields X; Ortho Supreme; Ramses Sensitol; Ramses Thin Lub; Ramses Ultra; Sheik Denim; Sheik Sensi-Creme; Sheik Thin Lub; Titan Lubricated; Titan Ribbed; Trojan; Trojan-Enz Large Lubricated; Trojan-Enz Lubricated; Trojan Naturalube Ribbed; Trojan Plus; Trojan Ribbed*].

Non-Lubricated:
(OTC) [*Ortho Shields Non-Lubricated; Ramses Non-Lubricated; Sheik Non-Lubricated; Trojan-Enz*].

**Packaging and storage**
Store below 40 °C (104 °F), preferably between 15 and 30 °C (59 and 86 °F), unless otherwise specified by manufacturer. Protect from light. Protect from freezing.

---

### *LATEX CONDOMS AND NONOXYNOL 9*

## Product Forms

**LATEX CONDOMS AND NONOXYNOL 9**

**Product(s) usually available**
U.S.—
(OTC) [*Beyond Seven Plus; Class Act Ultra Thin & Sensitive Spermicidal Lubricated; Crown Plus; Kimono Microthins Plus; Kimono Plus; Kimono Sensation Plus; LifeStyles Extra Strength with Spermicide; LifeStyles Spermicidally Lubricated; LifeStyles Ultra Sensitive with Spermicide; LifeStyles Vibra-Ribbed with Spermicide; MAXX Plus; Ramses Extra Ribbed; Ramses Extra Strength; Ramses Ribbed; Ramses Ultra Thin Ribbed with Spermicide; Ramses Ultra Thin with Spermicide; Ramses with Spermicidal Lubricant; Saxon Gold Rainbow Ultra Spermicidal; Saxon Gold Ultra Spermicidal; Sheik Classic Spermicidally Lubricated; Sheik Excita Extra; Sheik Super Thin Ribbed Spermicidally Lubricated; Sheik Super Thin Spermicidally Lubricated; Touch Spermicidally Lubricated; Trojan-Enz Large with Spermicidal Lubricant; Trojan-Enz with Spermicidal Lubricant; Trojan Magnum Spermicidal Lubricant; Trojan Plus 2; Trojan Ribbed with Spermicidal Lubricant; Trojan Ultra Texture with Spermicidal Lubricant; Trojan Very Sensitive with Spermicidal Lubricant; Trojan Very Thin with Spermicidal Lubricant*].

Canada—
(OTC) [*LifeStyles Extra Strength with Spermicide; LifeStyles Lubricated with Spermicide; Ortho Shields Plus; Ramses Extra; Ramses*

*Extra-15; Ramses Ribbed; Ramses Thin Spermicidal Lub; Ramses Ultra-15; Sheik Elite; Sheik Excita; Sheik Thin Spermicidal Lub; Titan with Silicone Spermicidal Lubricant; Trojan-Enz Large with Spermicidal Lube; Trojan-Enz with Spermicidal Lubricant; Trojan Ribbed with Spermicidal Lube*].

**Packaging and storage**
Store below 40 °C (104 °F), preferably between 15 and 30 °C (59 and 86 °F), unless otherwise specified by manufacturer. Protect from light. Protect from freezing.

## Selected Bibliography

Stone KM, Grimes DA, Magder LS. Primary prevention of sexually transmitted diseases: a primer for clinicians. JAMA 1986; 255 (13): 1763-6.
Condoms for prevention of sexually transmitted diseases. MMWR 1988; 37 (9): 133-7.
Grimes DA. Reversible contraception for the 1980s. JAMA 1986; 255 (1): 69-75.

---

Revised: 03/04/93
Interim revision: 07/18/95

---

## CONDOMS, LAMB CECUM—See *Condoms*

---

## CONDOMS, LAMB CECUM, AND NONOXYNOL 9—
See *Condoms*

---

## CONDOMS, LATEX—See *Condoms*

---

## CONDOMS, LATEX, AND NONOXYNOL 9—See *Condoms*

---

## CONJUGATED ESTROGEN–CONTAINING COMBINATIONS—

Conjugated Estrogens and Methyltestosterone (Systemic)—See *Androgens and Estrogens (Systemic)*

---

## COPPER GLUCONATE—See *Copper Supplements (Systemic)*

---

# COPPER INTRAUTERINE DEVICES (IUDS)

This monograph includes information on the following: Copper-T 200*; Copper-T 200Ag*; Copper-T 380A†; Copper-T 380S*.

Note: Other copper devices that may be available worldwide include: Copper-7; Copper-T 200B; Copper-T 220C; Copper-T 380Ag; Multiload 250; Multiload 375; Shanghai V 200. Some of the following information may also apply to these devices.

VA CLASSIFICATION (Primary): GU900

Note: For a listing of dosage forms and brand names by country availability, see *Dosage Forms* section(s). For a listing of brand names for the articles in this monograph, refer to the General Index.

---

*Not commercially available in the U.S.
†Not commercially available in Canada.

---

## Category

Contraceptive (intrauterine-local).

## Indications

**Accepted**

Pregnancy (prophylaxis)—Copper intrauterine devices are recommended as a long-term contraceptive method, primarily for parous women who

are in a mutually monogamous relationship and have no history of pelvic inflammatory disease (PID).

An IUD may **not** be an appropriate choice for nulliparous or low parity women whose lifestyle (involvement in multiple relationships or in a nonmonogamous relationship) may expose them to sexually transmitted diseases (STDs) or for women at risk of developing PID. The IUD is **not** generally recommended for women whose uterine cavity measures less than 6.5 centimeters (cm).

IUDs do not protect against sexually transmitted diseases including human immunodeficiency virus (HIV) infection or acquired immunodeficiency syndrome (AIDS).

The following table presents the results of studies examining contraceptive failure rates calculated using the life-table method. The first column lists the contraceptive method used. The second column indicates the percentage of women experiencing an accidental pregnancy in the first year of use of a contraceptive method while using the method perfectly under clinical conditions. The range of failure rates in the clinical trials may be explained by interstudy variations in study design or patient population characteristics, such as motivation, fecundity, or socioeconomic factors (including education). The third column indicates contraceptive failure rates in the first year of contraceptive use under nonclinical conditions for typical couples who start using a method (not necessarily for the first time). Failure rates among adolescents may be higher due to poorer compliance than in other age groups.

| Method used | Failure rate range (over 12 months) in clinical studies (%) | Typical first year failure rate (%) |
|---|---|---|
| None | 78–94 | 85 |
| Spermicides[1] | 0.3–37 | 21 |
| Periodic abstinence[2] | 13–35 | 20 |
| Withdrawal | 7–22 | 18 |
| Cervical cap with spermicide | 6–27 | 18 |
| Sponge | 6–28 | |
| Parous women | 9->28 | 28 |
| Nonparous women | 6–18 | 18 |
| Diaphragm with spermicide | 2–23 | 18 |
| Condom without spermicide | 2–14 | 12 |
| IUD | | |
| Progesterone-releasing | 1.9–2.0 | |
| Copper-T 200 | 3.0–3.6 | |
| Copper-T 200Ag[3] | 0–1.2 | |
| Copper-T 220C[4] | 0.9–1.8 | |
| Copper-T 380A | 0.5–0.8 | |
| Copper-T 380S | 0.9 | |
| Oral contraceptive | | 3 |
| Combination | 0–6 | |
| Progestin only | 1–10 | |
| Progestin injection | | |
| Medroxyprogesterone (90-day) | 0–0.4 | 0.3 |
| Norethisterone (60-day) | 0–0.6 | 0.4 |
| Levonorgestrel (implants) | | |
| Six capsules | 0–0.4 | 0.4 |
| Two rods | 0–0.2 | 0.3 |
| Sterilization | | |
| Female[5] | 0–8 | 0.4 |
| Male | 0–0.5 | 0.15 |

[1] Spermicides studied include creams, foams, gels, jellies, and suppositories.
[2] Methods studied include calendar, ovulation method, symptothermal (cervical mucus method supplemented by basal body temperature in post-ovulatory phases, post-ovulation phases, post-ovulation).
[3] Life table method rate is unavailable for Copper-T 200Ag and the Pearl method rate at 12 months was reported; these methods at 12 months are considered comparable.
[4] Copper-T 220C is manufactured with copper sleeves instead of copper wire; often used as a control in clinical studies.
[5] Methods studied include culdotomy laparoscopy, minilaparotomy, electrocoagulation, laparotomy, tubal diathermy and/or use of rings or clips.

## Pharmacology/Pharmacokinetics

**Physicochemical characteristics**
Physical description—
In most cases, the number included in the name of the device refers to the surface area in square millimeters (mm²) of the copper on the device and the letter to the style. An exception is the *Copper-7* IUD, whose number refers to its shape.
Copper-T IUDs have certain common characteristics, including polyethylene T-shaped bodies containing radiopaque barium (to monitor location) and monofilament thread(s) (to monitor placement and aid in IUD removal). The devices differ in the amount and surface area of copper and style of copper covering; the bodies of the IUDs may vary in flexibility and size.
Copper-T 380A: Exposed surface area of copper is $380 \pm 23$ mm²; contains copper sleeves and wire; total copper weight is 309 mg.
Copper-T 380S: Exposed surface area of copper is 380 mm²; contains copper sleeves and wire; total copper weight is 320 mg.
Copper-T 200: Exposed surface area of copper is 208 mm²; contains copper wire; total copper weight is 120 mg.
Copper-T 200Ag: Exposed surface area of copper is 200 mm²; contains copper wire with an 11 to 29 mg silver core; total copper weight is 107 to 141 mg. The silver core of the copper wire may help prevent the copper coil from fragmenting.

**Mechanism of action/Effect**
Contraceptive, intrauterine-local—
The copper intrauterine device prevents pregnancy in 96 to 99% of users in the first year of use, depending on the specific device. The precise mechanism of action has not been fully elucidated; a number of mechanisms may contribute to the contraceptive effect.
IUDs produce cellular reactions that can lead to local superficial ulceration in adjacent uterine cells. This causes a foreign-body inflammatory response leading to biochemical and morphological changes in the endometrial tissue and uterine fluid, including increased vascular permeability, edema, and infiltration of leukocytes, especially macrophages. These actions result in interference with sperm migration, fertilization and, to a lesser extent, with implantation. Fertilization also may be hindered by an effect of the inflammatory response on the ovum and/or by an effect of copper ions on sperm and egg viability.
The copper released from the device increases the contraceptive effectiveness by enhancing the foreign body reaction and possibly by affecting several enzymes that decrease the number and activity of the viable sperm, retarding penetration and fertilization. The copper may exert an inhibitory effect on the ovum in the upper female reproductive tract before the ovum reaches the uterus. Copper may also increase the synthesis and decrease the metabolism of prostaglandins in the endometrium, which may increase uterine activity and alter the motility of ova within the fallopian tube.

**Other actions/effects**
Increased fibrinolytic activity may explain the presence of irregular bleeding.

**Absorption**
Copper IUDs release copper at an average rate of 38 mcg per day with the actual rate and extent of release subject to interindividual variability. Systemic absorption of copper occurs, but the quantity absorbed is well below the minimum daily requirement of 2 to 5 mg. However, enough copper may be absorbed to cause problems in women with Wilson's disease.

**Onset of action**
Local contraceptive action begins immediately after insertion.

**Duration of action**
Manufacturers recommend IUD replacement within the following time periods:
Copper-T 200—24 months.
Copper-T 200Ag—30 months.
Copper-T 380A—10 years.
Copper-T 380S—30 months.
Local contraceptive action terminates quickly on removal.

## Precautions to Consider

**Cross-sensitivity and/or related problems**
Women allergic to copper may also be allergic to copper-containing IUDs.

**Carcinogenicity**
One case-control study involving 481 women with invasive cervical cancer and 801 women from the general population used as controls reported no association between IUDs and increased risk of invasive cervical cancer. Carcinoma of the cervix was diagnosed in 8 of 8632 copper-T IUD users (6 being diagnosed within 6 months of insertion), a rate comparable to the incidence of cancer in women using other contraceptive methods, including oral contraceptives. One retrospective case-control study has reported a decreased incidence of endometrial carcinoma in IUD users.
Seven-year carcinogenicity studies using the copper-T IUD in the rhesus monkey have shown no evidence of uterine malignancy, although endometrial hyperplasia has been reported.

**Mutagenicity**
There is no evidence that copper IUDs cause DNA mutation in humans.

**Pregnancy/Reproduction**
Fertility—In most women, fertility resumes on removal of the IUD. Up to 94% of patients desiring pregnancy conceive successfully within 12 months after IUD removal, and 20.5% conceive within the first calendar month.
Monogamous women with monogamous partners have little risk of primary tubal infertility attributable to copper IUDs unless there are other risk factors. IUDs increase the risk of tubal infertility caused by obstruction in or damage to the fallopian tubes, which are problems associated with pelvic inflammatory disease (PID) or an infection in the uterus or fallopian tubes. This risk is highest within the first few months after IUD insertion.
Pregnancy—Use of a copper IUD is not recommended during pregnancy. A copper IUD *in utero* has resulted in maternal sepsis (usually, but not exclusively, in the second trimester, secondary to a septic abortion or chorioamnionitis) and, rarely, death. If pregnancy occurs with an IUD *in situ*, risk-benefit of leaving the IUD *in situ* versus IUD removal must be carefully considered. If an IUD remains *in utero*, possible

complications include a 50% risk of spontaneous abortion and an increased risk of premature rupture of membranes, labor, and delivery. In a study of 918 pregnant women who conceived while using a copper-T IUD, 157 viable births resulted.

If a pregnancy occurs with a copper IUD in place, the IUD should be removed if the string is visible and the removal is easy. However, manipulation of the IUD may stimulate spontaneous abortion. If the string is not visible, removal of the IUD may be attempted under ultrasound guidance, and/or the termination of the pregnancy should be considered.

When a pregnancy occurs with a copper IUD *in situ*, the possibility of an ectopic pregnancy should be considered. The total number of ectopic pregnancies is lower in women using IUDs compared to the general population. However, because the IUD protects against intrauterine pregnancy more than it protects against extrauterine pregnancy, the result is an increase in the relative number of ectopic pregnancies if a pregnancy occurs. Some studies indicate that about 3 to 9% of the pregnancies occurring with an IUD *in situ* will be ectopic. One study comparing 7 copper-containing devices found that, as the copper surface area was increased from 200 to 350 mm² or more, ectopic pregnancy rates decreased from 0.78 to 0.15 per 1000 woman-years over the first 2-year period. Similarly, total pregnancy rates decreased from 21.2 to 4.1 per 1000 woman-years with the devices of greater copper surface area.

Diagnosis of ectopic pregnancy may be difficult because early symptoms (enlarged and tender breasts, dizziness, faintness, nausea, unusual tiredness or weakness, lower abdominal pain, cramping or tenderness [possibly severe], vaginal bleeding [possibly heavy and/or unexpected], or absent or delayed menstrual cycle) are nonspecific and variable. Also, 83% of patients continue to have menses, and 53% do not suspect pregnancy.

Delivery—If an intrauterine pregnancy continues with an IUD *in situ*, the risk for premature delivery is increased along with the usual complications of premature infants.

Postpartum—It is recommended that postpartum IUD insertion be performed 8 weeks or more after delivery (interval insertion) or after complete involution of the uterus has occurred, although individual needs and desires should be taken into consideration by the physician. The risk of an IUD expulsion or uterine perforation caused by an IUD is lower for interval insertions than for postplacental insertions (insertions performed within 10 minutes after delivery). Immediate postpartum insertions (insertions performed within 48 hours after delivery) or immediate postabortion insertions may involve a similar risk of uterine perforation by the IUD as interval insertions, but the expulsion rate is higher. Higher expulsion rates in postpartum women may be due to the difficulty in placing the IUD sufficiently high in the fundus.

Modified IUDs for postpartum women have been designed with longer strings because missing strings are more prevalent in postpartum women.

**Breast-feeding**

Problems in humans have not been documented. Copper IUDs are recommended by the World Health Organization (WHO) for use as a contraceptive method because copper IUDs do not interfere with lactation.

**Adolescents**

Sexually active adolescents may be better served with a contraceptive method that also protects against sexually transmitted diseases (STDs). In general, young age and nulliparity in women appear to be associated with a higher expulsion rate, possibly due to a more reactive myometrium and irregular and heavy menses.

**Drug interactions and/or related problems**

The following drug interactions and/or related problems have been selected on the basis of their potential clinical significance (possible mechanism in parentheses where appropriate)—not necessarily inclusive (» = major clinical significance):

Note: Combinations containing the following medication, depending on the amount present, may also interact with this device.

Anticoagulants
  (administration of anticoagulants during IUD use may potentiate the risk of abnormal uterine bleeding and anemia secondary to menorrhagia and/or metrorrhagia)

**Medical considerations/Contraindications**

The medical considerations/contraindications included here have been selected on the basis of their potential clinical significance (reasons given in parentheses where appropriate)—not necessarily inclusive (» = major clinical significance).

*Except under special circumstances, this device should not be used when the following medical problems exist:*

» Acquired immunodeficiency syndrome (AIDS) or
» Autoimmune diseases or
» Immunosuppressive therapy or
» Malignancy treated with antineoplastic agents and/or radiation or
» Malignancy, uterine or cervical, known or suspected or
» Any other condition associated with or resulting in decreased immunity and/or increased susceptibility to infection
    (possible increased risk of infection with an IUD when a patient lacks an intact immune system)
» Bleeding, genital, of unknown etiology
    (use of an IUD may exacerbate bleeding or mask other serious underlying conditions, delaying the diagnosis of the condition)
» Ectopic pregnancy, history of
    (may increase risk of ectopic pregnancy with contraceptive failure, especially in nulliparous women)
» Infection or inflammation in female reproductive tract, including:
    Abortion, recent septic
    Cervicitis
    Endometritis
    Genital actinomyces-like infection
    PID, acute or history of
    Sexually transmitted diseases during last 12 months
    Vaginitis, excluding candidiasis but including bacterial vaginosis until controlled
    (use of an IUD when any of the above conditions is present may predispose the patient to upper genital tract infections that may range in severity from mild to life-threatening)
    (women with a history of PID may be at increased risk of developing acute, as opposed to chronic, PID; nulliparous women may be at greater risk than parous women)
    (significant risk of infection progressing to PID may be related to acquisition of or exposure to PID-associated sexually transmitted diseases)
    Sensitivity to copper
» Surgery involving the uterus or fallopian tubes
    (women currently using an IUD may have an increased risk of surgical complications)
» Uterine abnormalities or cavity distortion
    (possibility of decreased contraceptive effectiveness; increased risk of IUD expulsion or IUD perforation of the uterus)
    Wilson's disease
    (may be exacerbated by systemic absorption of copper from copper IUDs)

*Risk-benefit should be considered when the following medical problems exist:*

» Anemia
    (increased risk of hypochromic microcytic anemia because IUDs may increase and prolong menstrual and intermenstrual bleeding)
    Bradycardia, neurovascular, history of or
    Syncope, neurovascular, history of
    (short-term syncope or bradycardia may occur with IUD insertion; increased risk if these conditions are present)
    Cervical stenosis
    (may prevent ease of insertion of IUD; excessive force to overcome this resistance is not advised)
» Coagulopathy
    (increased vascularity and permeability, and decreased hemostatic response may increase risk of menorrhagia or metrorrhagia, possibly leading to anemia or increased risk of IUD expulsion)
    Diabetes, insulin-dependent
    (although one study suggests that IUDs may be a good short-term choice for diabetics, altered glucose metabolism has been reported to disrupt the normal release of copper and reduce the efficacy of a copper IUD; also, complications from infection, if infection occurs, are potentially greater)
    Heart defect, valvular or congenital
    (insertion of an IUD may represent a potential source of septic emboli, since these patients are prone to develop subacute bacterial endocarditis)
    Menorrhagia, history of or
    Metrorrhagia, history of
    (additive blood loss may occur and risk of IUD expulsion may be increased)

## Patient monitoring

The following may be especially important in patient monitoring (other tests may be warranted in some patients, depending on condition; » = major clinical significance):

Ferritin, serum
(recommended to assess possible hypochromic microcytic anemia in women with average blood loss at menses greater than 66 mL, or in women experiencing menorrhagia and/or metrorrhagia)

Papanicolaou (Pap) test
(recommended annually; examination for actinomycosis-like organisms and, if appropriate, gonococcal and chlamydial tests should be performed)

» Physical examination
(recommended once during the first 3 months and at 12 months after insertion, then annually thereafter to evaluate for expulsion or partial displacement of the IUD; special attention should be given to reports of delayed menses and/or pelvic pain because of the possibility of ectopic pregnancies with failed IUD contraception)

## Side/Adverse Effects

Note: Cervical laceration, cervical or uterine perforations, and/or abdominal displacement of the IUD may progress to peritonitis, sepsis, pelvic inflammatory disease (PID), abdominal adhesions, intestinal penetration, intestinal obstruction, cystic masses in the pelvis, and local inflammatory reaction with abscess formation, including tuboovarian abscess. Certain of these adverse effects of IUDs, although very rare, can lead to a loss of fertility, require partial or total removal of reproductive organs, and, in extremely rare circumstances, cause death. A copper IUD must be surgically removed as soon as feasible after IUD displacement has been diagnosed.

Vaginal bleeding and abdominal pain (cramping or dysmenorrhea) are the most common reasons for IUD removal, occurring in 4.4 to 13% of IUD users in the first year. Because many of the side effects listed below present with bleeding and pain, these symptoms should always be evaluated even though they may not signify a serious problem. Persistent or recurring abnormal vaginal bleeding and/or abdominal pain may lessen with continued IUD use. Other problems such as cervical or uterine perforation, IUD displacement, ectopic pregnancy, PID, and IUD embedment should be ruled out.

The following side/adverse effects have been selected on the basis of their potential clinical significance (possible signs and symptoms in parentheses where appropriate)—not necessarily inclusive:

### Those indicating need for medical attention

Incidence more frequent
*Menorrhagia* (increased amount of menstrual bleeding at regular monthly periods); *metrorrhagia* (normal menstrual bleeding occurring earlier, possibly lasting longer than expected); *neurovascular episodes* (dizziness; faintness)—at time of insertion

Note: Abdominal pain or vaginal bleeding may continue for several days after IUD insertion. However, increased dysmenorrhea and *metrorrhagia* can be expected for 3 to 4 menstrual periods after insertion; intermenstrual vaginal bleeding may stop within 3 months with a new higher level of menstrual blood loss occurring throughout IUD use.

Incidence less frequent
*Cervical perforation or laceration or endometritis* (abnormal vaginal bleeding not associated with period, possibly mild to moderate); *PID* (dull or aching abdominal pain, odorous vaginal discharge, pain on urination with increased urge to urinate, and unusual vaginal bleeding)

Note: Increased risk of *PID* occurs within the first 3 months of IUD insertion; ectopic pregnancy should be ruled out before treatment of PID because of similar presenting symptoms. Also, symptoms of PID and *actinomycosis-like infection* may be asymptomatic.

Incidence rare
*Actinomycosis-like infection* (abdominal pain or cramping, fever, nausea, and vomiting); *anemia, hypochromic* (unusual tiredness or weakness)—secondary to increased menstrual bleeding; *dyspareunia* (painful sexual intercourse); *embedment of IUD or perforation of the uterus* (severe abdominal pain or cramping; unexpected, heavy vaginal bleeding; sharp pain on insertion); *fragmentation or corrosion of copper*

### Those indicating need for medical attention only if they continue or are bothersome

Incidence more frequent
*Lower back pain; dysmenorrhea* (increased abdominal pain and cramping at menstrual periods)

## Patient Consultation

As an aid to patient consultation, refer to *Advice for the Patient, Copper Intrauterine Devices (IUDs)*.

In providing consultation, consider emphasizing the following selected information (» = major clinical significance):

### Before using this device

Note: In the U.S., the health care professional is required by U.S. federal regulation to provide a patient information brochure to the patient regarding the use of IUDs for contraception, discussing it and other methods of contraception.

» Conditions affecting use, especially:
Sensitivity to copper
Pregnancy—IUD use is not recommended for women during pregnancy, those planning to become pregnant shortly, or women who have had an ectopic pregnancy. If contraception fails with a copper IUD, complications to the mother or infant are possible whether the pregnancy continues with the IUD *in situ* or the device is removed; also, the risk of uterine perforation and expulsion of the IUD may be increased when an IUD is inserted before 8 weeks postpartum

Use in adolescents—Sexually active adolescents may be better served with a contraceptive method that also protects against sexually transmitted diseases (STDs); IUD use in adolescents of young age and nulliparous women appears to be associated with a higher expulsion rate

Other medical problems, especially acquired immunodeficiency syndrome (AIDS), autoimmune diseases, immunosuppressive therapy, malignancy of the cervix or uterus, or any other conditions of decreased immunity or increased risk of infection; genital bleeding of unknown etiology; history of ectopic pregnancy; infection or inflammation in reproductive tract; surgery involving the uterus or fallopian tubes; uterine abnormalities or cavity distortion; anemia; or coagulopathy

### Proper use of this device

» Reading a copy of the patient information brochure provided by the health care professional helps explain possible side effects, risks, and warning signs of trouble with the IUD
Spermicides are not needed with a properly placed IUD

» Checking for changes in the IUD thread length after the monthly menses, if not more often, as instructed by physician

» Proper dosing, including IUD removal or replacement times

### Precautions while using this device

» Visiting physician regularly to check progress, especially within the first 3 months and at 12 months during the first year after IUD insertion, and annually thereafter

» Alerting medical personnel before having diagnostic or therapeutic procedures such as short-wave or microwave radiation, or surgery involving the uterus or fallopian tubes

» Notifying physician immediately if a partial or complete expulsion is suspected; using another form of nonhormonal contraception until evaluated by a physician; patient should not try to remove the IUD or reinsert it

» Reporting missed or scanty menses to physician immediately and using other nonhormonal contraceptive methods

» Reporting symptoms of possible pregnancy, including ectopic pregnancy, to physician on the rare case when IUD contraceptive effects fail

» Notifying physician and using other nonhormonal contraceptive methods if any of the following occur:
—Abnormal vaginal bleeding
—Exposure to sexually transmitted diseases
—Feeling the tip of the IUD at the cervix or pain during sexual intercourse
—Change in length of IUD threads or disappearance of IUD threads on periodic observation after menses
—Lifestyle change from a mutually monogamous relationship
—Pelvic/lower abdominal pain or cramping, unusual or severe, possibly with fever
—Vaginal discharge or signs of genital lesions or sores
Copper-T IUDs should not interfere with the proper use of other vaginal products such as tampons or condoms

## Side/adverse effects

Signs of potential side effects, especially menorrhagia, metrorrhagia, neurovascular episodes on insertion cervical perforation or laceration, endometritis, pelvic inflammatory disease (PID), actinomycosis-like infection, hypochromic anemia, dyspareunia, embedment of IUD or perforation of the uterus, and fragmentation or corrosion of copper

## General Dosing Information

In the U.S., the health care professional is required by U.S. Federal Regulations (21 CFR 310.502) to give the patient a copy of the Patient Information for an Informed Decision to ensure complete understanding of the risks and benefits, safety, and efficacy of the copper-T IUD.

Copper IUD strength is measured by the copper surface area, which ranges from 200 to 380 mm² per device. Total pregnancy rates decreased from 21.2 to 4.1 per 1000 woman-years with the devices of greater copper surface area.

It is generally believed that perforations occur at the time of insertion, although they may not be detected until later. Adequate training of those health care professionals inserting the device may help prevent cervical or uterine perforation. A number of supervised insertions may be necessary before a solo attempt. The degree of training needed depends on the health care professional's skill and experience with IUD aseptic insertion techniques and uterus manipulation.

Insertion techniques differ for individual IUDs. The manufacturer's product information should be consulted for specific directions.

The IUD may be inserted at any time during the menstrual cycle. Many physicians prefer insertion at the end of or within 2 days after a menstrual period to reduce the possibility of inserting an IUD in the presence of an undiagnosed pregnancy. However, the optimal time for insertion appears to be the periovulatory period. Caution should be used to avoid inserting a second IUD, as patients may forget about a previously inserted IUD or may assume it to be expelled.

Using aseptic technique and removing the IUD from the sterile packaging no more than 5 minutes before the insertion procedure are recommended. Prophylactic treatment with antibiotics theoretically may reduce the risk of infection, which is 6 times higher within the first 20 days after insertion. Regimens include doxycycline 200 mg orally one hour before insertion, or erythromycin 500 mg orally one hour before insertion and 500 mg orally six hours after insertion. This may be of limited benefit and unnecessary for women at low risk of sexually transmitted disease (STDs).

It is recommended that an IUD be removed for the following medical reasons: anemia associated with excessive menstrual bleeding or intermenstrual bleeding, pelvic infection, genital actinomycosis, intractable pelvic pain, dyspareunia, pregnancy (when able to remove the IUD), endometrial or cervical malignancy, uterine or cervical perforation, or partial expulsion.

If the retrieval threads cannot be seen, they may have retracted into the uterus or have been broken, or the IUD may have been expelled. Pregnancy, both uterine and ectopic, should be considered before attempting to locate the IUD. Although ultrasound is the preferred method of locating a malpositioned IUD, high- or intermediate-strength magnetic resonance imaging (MRI), uterine probe, and x-rays may also be used.

Removing an intraperitoneal copper IUD as soon as medically feasible after the diagnosis is recommended because of the possibility of abdominal adhesion formation, intestinal penetration, and local inflammatory reaction with abscess formation and erosion of adjacent viscera, maternal sepsis, or, rarely, death.

The manufacturer's information should be consulted for the recommended removal procedure. If an IUD is difficult to remove, the procedure may need to be done in a hospital or operating room. Another type of contraception should begin immediately after IUD removal if contraception is desired.

### For treatment of adverse effects

Recommended treatment consists of the following
• For menorrhagia, or dysmenorrhea—Treating with nonsteroidal anti-inflammatory drugs (NSAIDs).
• For pain—Treating with mild analgesics for several hours after IUD insertion.
• For pelvic inflammatory disease (PID)—Removing the copper IUD and treating the patient with appropriate broad-spectrum antibiotics; the patient's partner may require treatment with broad-spectrum antibiotics as well.

Note: HIV-infected women with PID who are immunocompromised may be at increased risk of a complicated clinical course and should be hospitalized for intravenous therapy.

---

## COPPER-T 200

## Summary of Differences

Pharmacology/pharmacokinetics: Physicochemical characteristics—Exposed surface area of copper is 208 mm²; contains copper wire; total copper weight is 120 mg.

## Intrauterine Dosage Forms

### COPPER-T 200 INTRAUTERINE DEVICE

**Usual adult and adolescent dose**
Contraceptive—
Intrauterine, one device; the maximum duration of use is 24 months.

**Strength(s) usually available**
U.S.—
Not commercially available.
Canada—
Cu-T 200 (Rx) [*Gyne-T*].

**Packaging and storage**
Store below 40 °C (104 °F), preferably between 15 and 30 °C (59 and 86 °F), unless otherwise specified by manufacturer.

Note: Provide patient with patient package insert (PPI).

---

## COPPER-T 200Ag

## Summary of Differences

Pharmacology/pharmacokinetics: Physicochemical characteristics—Exposed surface area of copper is about 200 mm²; contains copper wire with an 11 to 29 mg silver core; total copper weight is 107 to 141 mg. The silver-cored wire was added to prevent the copper coil from fragmenting.

## Intrauterine Dosage Forms

### COPPER-T 200Ag INTRAUTERINE DEVICE

**Usual adult and adolescent dose**
Contraceptive—
Intrauterine, one device; the maximum duration of use is 30 months.

**Strength(s) usually available**
U.S.—
Not commercially available.
Canada—
Cu-T 200Ag (Rx) [*Nova-T*].

**Packaging and storage**
Store below 40 °C (104 °F), preferably between 15 and 30 °C (59 and 86 °F), unless otherwise specified by manufacturer.

Note: Provide patient with patient package insert (PPI).

---

## COPPER-T 380A

## Summary of Differences

Pharmacology/pharmacokinetics: Physicochemical characteristics—Exposed surface area of copper is 380 ± 23 mm²; contains copper sleeves and wire; total copper weight is 309 mg.

## Intrauterine Dosage Forms

### COPPER-T 380A INTRAUTERINE DEVICE

**Usual adult and adolescent dose**
Contraceptive—
Intrauterine, one device; the maximum duration of use is 10 years.

**Strength(s) usually available**
U.S.—
Cu-T 380A (Rx) [*ParaGard-T 380A*].
Canada—
Not commercially available.

**Packaging and storage**
Store between 15 and 30 °C (59 and 86 °F), unless otherwise specified by manufacturer.

Note: Provide patient with mandatory patient package insert (PPI).

## COPPER-T 380S

## Summary of Differences

Pharmacology/pharmacokinetics: Physicochemical characteristics—Exposed surface area of copper is 380 mm²; contains copper sleeves and wire; total copper weight is 320 mg.

## Intrauterine Dosage Forms

### COPPER-T 380S INTRAUTERINE DEVICE

**Usual adult and adolescent dose**
Contraceptive—
Intrauterine, one device; the maximum duration of use is 30 months.

**Strength(s) usually available**
U.S.—
Not commercially available.
Canada—
Cu-T 380S (Rx) [*Gyne-T 380 Slimline*].

## Packaging and storage

Store below 40 °C (104 °F), preferably between 15 and 30 °C (59 and 86 °F), unless otherwise specified by manufacturer.

Note: Provide patient with patient package insert (PPI).

## Selected Bibliography

Farley TM, Rosenberg MJ, Rowe PJ, Chen JH, Meirik O. Intrauterine devices and pelvic inflammatory disease: an international perspective. Lancet 1992 Mar 28; 339: 785-8.
Lisken L, Fox G. IUDs: An appropriate contraceptive for many women. Popul Reports [B]; Intrauterine Devices, (4), Washington, DC, 1982.
Trussell J, Hatcher RA, Cates W Jr, Stewart FH, Kost K. Contraceptive failure in the United States: an update. Stud Fam Plann 1990; 21 (1): 51-4.

Developed: 06/29/94

## COPPER REDUCTION URINE GLUCOSE TEST—See
*Urine Glucose and Ketone Test Kits for Home Use*

---

# COPPER SUPPLEMENTS   Systemic

This monograph includes information on the following: Copper Gluconate†; Cupric Sulfate†.

VA CLASSIFICATION (Primary): TN499

Note: For a listing of dosage forms and brand names by country availability, see *Dosage Forms* section(s). For a listing of brand names for the articles in this monograph, refer to the General Index.

†Not commercially available in Canada.

## Category

Nutritional supplement (mineral).

## Indications

### Accepted

Copper deficiency (prophylaxis and treatment)—Copper supplements are indicated in the prevention and treatment of copper deficiency, which may result from inadequate nutrition or intestinal malabsorption, but does not occur in healthy individuals receiving an adequate balanced diet. For prophylaxis of copper deficiency, dietary improvement, rather than supplementation, is advisable. For treatment of copper deficiency, supplementation is preferred.

Deficiency of copper may lead to hypochromic and microcytic anemias, neutropenia, and bone demineralization.

Recommended intakes may be increased and/or supplementation may be necessary in the following persons or conditions (based on documented copper deficiency):

Burns
Gastrectomy
Infants—premature
Intestinal diseases—celiac, diarrhea, sprue
Malabsorption syndromes associated with pancreatic insufficiency—cystic fibrosis
Malnutrition, especially protein
Renal disease—nephrotic syndrome
Stress, prolonged

Some unusual diets (e.g., reducing diets that drastically restrict food selection) may not supply minimum daily requirements of copper. Supplementation may be necessary in patients receiving total parenteral nutrition (TPN) or undergoing rapid weight loss or in those with malnutrition, because of inadequate dietary intake.

Recommended intakes may be increased by the following: penicillamine, trientine, oral zinc supplements.

### Unaccepted

Copper supplements should not be used as emetics, as death has been reported.

A potential role for copper supplements in the treatment of rheumatoid arthritis and psoriasis has not been proven.

## Pharmacology/Pharmacokinetics

### Physicochemical characteristics
Molecular weight—
Copper gluconate: 453.84.
Copper sulfate: 249.7.
Elemental copper: 63.54.

### Mechanism of action/Effect

Copper is necessary for the proper functioning of many metalloenzymes, including ceruloplasmin, monoamine oxidase, ferroxidase II, tyrosinase, dopamine beta-hydroxylase, and cytochrome-C-oxidase. Physiological functions that are copper dependent include oxidation of iron, erythro- and leukopoiesis, bone mineralization, elastin and collagen cross-linking, oxidative phosphorylation, catecholamine metabolism, melanin formation, myelin formation, glucose homeostasis, and antioxidant protection of the cell.

### Absorption

Approximately 40 to 60% of dietary copper is absorbed, primarily from the stomach and duodenum. Copper absorption increases in copper deficiency and decreases with adequate copper status. After absorption, copper is bound to the carrier protein, metallothionein.

### Protein binding

Copper is 90 to 95% bound to ceruloplasmin, 1 to 2% bound to amino acids or free, and the remaining is reversibly bound to albumin.

### Storage

Copper is stored primarily in the liver, with small amounts found in peripheral tissues.

### Biotransformation

Hepatic.

### Elimination

Primarily in bile, with small amounts eliminated in urine, sweat, and epidermal shedding.

## Precautions to Consider

### Pregnancy/Reproduction

Pregnancy—Problems in humans have not been documented with intake of normal daily recommended amounts. However, adequate and well-controlled studies in humans have not been done.

Studies have not been done in animals.

FDA Pregnancy Category C (parenteral copper).

### Breast-feeding

Problems in humans have not been documented with intake of normal daily recommended amounts.

### Pediatrics

Problems in pediatrics have not been documented with intake of normal daily recommended amounts.

Infusion of free amino acids of the total parenteral nutrition (TPN) solution has been reported to produce copper diuresis in infants.

Copper injection that contains benzyl alcohol as a preservative should not be used in newborn and immature infants. The use of benzyl alcohol in neonates has been associated with a fatal toxic syndrome consisting of metabolic acidosis and CNS, respiratory, circulatory, and renal function impairment.

**Geriatrics**
Problems in geriatrics have not been documented with intake of normal daily recommended amounts.

**Drug interactions and/or related problems**
The following drug interactions and/or related problems have been selected on the basis of their potential clinical significance (possible mechanism in parentheses where appropriate)—not necessarily inclusive (» = major clinical significance):

Note: Combinations containing any of the following, depending on the amount present, may also interact with copper supplements.

Copper-containing preparations, other
(concurrent use with copper supplements may increase serum copper concentrations)
» Penicillamine or
» Trientine
(copper chelation by penicillamine or trientine may lead to decreased serum copper concentrations; penicillamine or trientine should be given 2 hours before copper supplements)

» Zinc supplements, oral
(large doses of zinc supplements may inhibit copper absorption in the intestine; copper supplements should be taken 2 hours after zinc supplements)

**Medical considerations/Contraindications**
The medical considerations/contraindications included here have been selected on the basis of their potential clinical significance (reasons given in parentheses where appropriate)—not necessarily inclusive (» = major clinical significance).

*Except under special circumstances, this medication should not be used when the following medical problem exists:*
» Wilson's disease
(condition may be exacerbated)

*Risk-benefit should be considered when the following medical problems exist:*
» Biliary tract disease or
Hepatic disease
(may cause an accumulation of copper, since copper is normally eliminated in bile; a reduction in copper dosage may be necessary)

**Patient monitoring**
The following may be especially important in patient monitoring (other tests may be warranted in some patients, depending on condition; » = major clinical significance):
» Ceruloplasmin concentrations, serum or
» Copper concentrations, serum, plasma, or urinary
(determinations recommended monthly; however, these monitoring parameters are subject to many variables and may not be good indicators of copper overload)

## Overdose
For specific information on the agents used in the management of copper overdose, see:
• *Calcium Edetate Disodium (Systemic)* monograph;
• *Dimercaprol (Systemic)* monograph; and/or
• *Penicillamine (Systemic)*.

For more information on the management of overdose or unintentional ingestion, **contact a Poison Control Center** (see *Poison Control Center Listing*).

**Clinical effects of overdose**
The following effects have been selected on the basis of their potential clinical significance (possible signs and symptoms in parentheses where appropriate)—not necessarily inclusive:

*Coma; diarrhea; epigastric pain and discomfort* (heartburn); *hematuria* (blood in urine; lower back pain; pain or burning while urinating); *hepatotoxicity* (black or bloody vomit; severe or continuing headache; loss of appetite; severe or continuing nausea; pain in abdomen; yellow eyes or skin); *hypotension* (dizziness or fainting); *jaundice* (yellow eyes or skin); *metallic taste; vomiting*

**Treatment of overdose**
Dilution with milk or water
To decrease absorption—
Emptying stomach contents by emesis or gastric lavage if patient is not already vomiting

Specific treatment—
If patient is symptomatic, instituting chelation therapy with one of the following chelating agents:
Calcium edetate sodium—
Intravenous, 50 mg per kg of body weight (mg/kg) a day for 5 days; course may be repeated after a 2-day interval.
Intramuscular, 12.5 mg/kg every 4 to 6 hours for 5 days; course may be repeated after a 2-day interval.
Dimercaprol—
Intramuscular, 3 to 5 mg/kg every 4 hours for 2 days, then 3 mg/kg every 6 hours for 2 days, then 3 mg/kg every 12 hours for up to 7 days or until recovery is complete.
Penicillamine—Orally, 10 mg/kg in 4 divided doses a day (not to exceed 1 gram a day) for no longer than 1 week; if symptoms recur, allow 3 to 5 days before resuming therapy.

## Patient Consultation
As an aid to patient consultation, refer to *Advice for the Patient, Copper Supplements (Systemic)*.

In providing consultation, consider emphasizing the following selected information (» = major clinical significance):

**Description of use**
Description should include function in the body, signs of deficiency, conditions that may cause copper deficiency, unproven uses

**Importance of diet**
Importance of proper nutrition; supplement may be needed because of inadequate dietary intake
Food sources of copper; effects of processing
Recommended daily intake for copper

**Before using this dietary supplement**
» Conditions affecting use, especially:
Other medications or dietary supplements, especially penicillamine, trientine, or oral zinc supplements
Other medical problems, especially Wilson's disease and biliary tract disease

**Proper use of this dietary supplement**
» Proper dosing
Missed dose: No cause for concern because of length of time necessary for depletion; remembering to take as directed
» Proper storage

**Precautions while using this dietary supplement**
Not taking copper supplements within 2 hours of zinc supplements

## General Dosing Information
Because of the infrequency of copper deficiency alone, combinations of several vitamins and/or minerals are commonly administered. Many commercial vitamin/mineral complexes are available.

**For parenteral dosage forms only**
In most cases, parenteral administration is indicated only when oral administration is not acceptable (for example, in nausea, vomiting, and preoperative and postoperative conditions) or possible (for example, in malabsorption syndromes or following gastric resection).

**Diet/Nutrition**
Recommended dietary intakes for copper are defined differently worldwide.
For U.S.—
The Recommended Dietary Allowances (RDAs) for vitamins and minerals are determined by the Food and Nutrition Board of the National Research Council and are intended to provide adequate nutrition in most healthy persons under usual environmental stresses. In addition, a different designation may be used by the FDA for food and dietary supplement labeling purposes, as with Daily Value (DV). DVs replace the previous labeling terminology United States Recommended Daily Allowances (USRDAs).
For Canada—
Recommended Nutrient Intakes (RNIs) for vitamins, minerals, and protein are determined by Health and Welfare Canada and provide recommended amounts of a specific nutrient while minimizing the risk of chronic diseases.

There is no RDA or RNI established for copper. The following daily intakes are considered adequate for all individuals:
Infants and children:
Birth to 3 years of age: 0.4 to 1 mg.
4 to 6 years of age: 1 to 1.5 mg.
7 to 10 years of age: 1 to 2 mg.
Adolescent and adult males:
1.5 to 2.5 mg.

Adolescent and adult females:
　　1.5 to 3 mg.
The best sources of copper include organ meats (especially liver), seafoods, beans, nuts, and whole-grains. Additional copper can come from the interaction of drinking water with copper pipes, copper cookware, and copper-containing fungicides sprayed on agricultural products. The amount of copper in foods may be decreased as a result of prolonged storage in tin cans under acidic conditions.

---

## COPPER GLUCONATE

## Oral Dosage Forms

### COPPER GLUCONATE TABLETS

**Usual adult and adolescent dose**
Deficiency (prophylaxis)—Oral, amount based on normal daily recommended intakes:—
　　Adolescent and adult males—1.5 to 2.5 mg.
　　Adolescent and adult females—1.5 to 3 mg.
Deficiency (treatment)—
　　Treatment dose is individualized by prescriber based on severity of deficiency.

**Usual pediatric dose**
Deficiency (prophylaxis)—Oral, amount based on normal daily recommended intakes:—
　　Birth to 3 years of age—0.4 to 1 mg.
　　4 to 6 years of age—1 to 1.5 mg.
　　7 to 10 years of age—1 to 2 mg.
Deficiency (treatment)—
　　Treatment dose is individualized by prescriber based on severity of deficiency.

**Strength(s) usually available**
U.S.—
　　3 mg elemental copper (OTC) [GENERIC].
Canada—
　　Not commercially available.
Note: The strength of this preparation may exceed the dosage range recommended by USP DI Advisory Panels based on the amount necessary to meet normal nutritional needs.

**Packaging and storage**
Store below 40 °C (104 °F), preferably between 15 and 30 °C (59 and 86 °F), unless otherwise specified by manufacturer. Store in a tight container.

---

## CUPRIC SULFATE

## Parenteral Dosage Forms

Note: **Injectable copper products must be diluted prior to intravenous administration.**

### CUPRIC SULFATE INJECTION USP

**Usual adult and adolescent dose**
Deficiency (prophylaxis)—
　　Intravenous infusion, 0.5 to 1.5 mg of elemental copper a day added to TPN.

---

Deficiency (treatment)—
　　Intravenous infusion, 3 mg of elemental copper a day added to total parenteral nutrition (TPN).

**Usual pediatric dose**
Deficiency (prophylaxis)—For full-term infants and children:—
　　Intravenous infusion, 20 mcg elemental copper per kg of body weight per day added to TPN.
Deficiency (treatment)—For full-term infants and children:—
　　Intravenous infusion, 20 to 30 mcg elemental copper per kg of body weight per day added to TPN,
Note: Copper injection that contains benzyl alcohol as a preservative should not be used in newborn and immature infants. The use of benzyl alcohol in neonates has been associated with a fatal toxic syndrome consisting of metabolic acidosis and CNS, respiratory, circulatory, and renal function impairment.

**Strength(s) usually available**
U.S.—
　　0.4 mg elemental copper per mL (1.57 mg cupric sulfate) (Rx) [Cupri-Pak; GENERIC].
　　2 mg elemental copper per mL (7.85 mg cupric sulfate) (Rx) [GENERIC].
Canada—
　　Not commercially available.

**Packaging and storage**
Store below 40 °C (104 °F), preferably between 15 and 30 °C (59 and 86 °F), unless otherwise specified by manufacturer. Protect from freezing.

**Preparation of dosage form**
The manufacturer states that copper sulfate can be added to TPN solutions, and is physically compatible with amino acid solutions, dextrose solutions, and most vitamins with the exception of ascorbic acid.

**Incompatibilities**
Large doses of ascorbic acid are physically incompatible with copper. The manufacturer recommends that copper sulfate and other trace metal additives be added to TPN solutions immediately prior to infusion to avoid potential incompatibilities.

---

Revised: 09/01/91
Interim revision: 06/25/92; 08/17/94; 05/26/95

---

**COPPER-T 200AG INTRAUTERINE DEVICE**—See *Copper Intrauterine Devices (IUDs)*

---

**COPPER-T 380A INTRAUTERINE DEVICE**—See *Copper Intrauterine Devices (IUDs)*

---

**COPPER-T 200 INTRAUTERINE DEVICE**—See *Copper Intrauterine Devices (IUDs)*

---

**COPPER-T 380S INTRAUTERINE DEVICE**—See *Copper Intrauterine Devices (IUDs)*

---

# CORTICOSTEROIDS　Inhalation-Local

This monograph includes information on the following: Beclomethasone; Budesonide*; Dexamethasone†; Flunisolide; Triamcinolone.
INN:
　　Beclometasone—Beclomethasone
JAN:
　　Beclometasone dipropionate—Beclomethasone
VA CLASSIFICATION (Primary/Secondary): RE101/109
Other commonly used names for beclomethasone are beclomethasone dipropionate, beclometasone, and beclometasone dipropionate.
Note: For a listing of dosage forms and brand names by country availability, see *Dosage Forms* section(s). For a listing of brand names for the articles in this monograph, refer to the General Index.

---

*Not commercially available in the U.S.

†Not commercially available in Canada.

## Category

Anti-inflammatory (inhalation); antiasthmatic.

## Indications

### Accepted

Asthma, bronchial, chronic (treatment)—Beclomethasone, budesonide, flunisolide, and triamcinolone are indicated as primary maintenance treatment in patients with persistent symptoms of chronic bronchial asthma. Regular, continuous use controls chronic airway inflammation, decreases airway hyperresponsiveness, controls asthma symptoms, and reduces the frequency of asthma exacerbations. In clinical studies, inhaled corticosteroids appear to be effective in all types of asthma and in patients of all ages.

Initiation of therapy with daily doses of inhaled corticosteroids shortly after a diagnosis of chronic asthma (even if mild) may prevent irreversible structural changes in the airways resulting from uncontrolled inflammation, may decrease progression of severe disease, and may reduce the need for administration of systemic corticosteroids.

Information comparing dose-related systemic effects or the ratios of local to systemic activity of beclomethasone, budesonide, flunisolide, and triamcinolone is limited. However, since conclusive evidence is lacking and further studies are needed, the concept of using the lowest possible dose of an inhaled corticosteroid to achieve the desired clinical improvement in asthma seems prudent.

Because of the potent anti-inflammatory effects of inhaled corticosteroids and the potential morbidity and mortality associated with theophylline treatment, inhaled corticosteroids in conventional low doses are preferred to theophylline as first-line therapy for chronic asthma.

Guidelines for the treatment of children with asthma recommend that inhaled nonsteroidal anti-inflammatory medications, such as cromolyn and nedocromil, be considered as the first choice after beta-adrenergic bronchodilators. The use of beta-adrenergic bronchodilators more than three times a week suggests inadequate asthma control. An inhaled corticosteroid is then recommended to be substituted when asthma is not well controlled with cromolyn or nedocromil.

### Unaccepted

Corticosteroid inhalation therapy does not relieve acute bronchospasm and is not indicated for the primary treatment of status asthmaticus or other acute asthmatic episodes requiring more intensive or rapid treatment measures.

Corticosteroid inhalation therapy is not indicated in the treatment of non-asthmatic bronchitis.

Dexamethasone inhalation is not recommended for use in asthma because it has demonstrated a significantly higher incidence of systemic effects with no additional benefit over other inhaled corticosteroids. The high ratio of systemic glucocorticoid activity to local anti-inflammatory activity of inhaled dexamethasone may be due to its greater water solubility and longer metabolic half-life after absorption relative to the other inhaled corticosteroids.

## Pharmacology/Pharmacokinetics

### Physicochemical characteristics

Molecular weight—
    Beclomethasone dipropionate: 521.05.
    Budesonide: 430.54.
    Dexamethasone sodium phosphate: 516.41.
    Flunisolide: 443.51.
    Triamcinolone acetonide: 434.50.

### Mechanism of action/Effect

In the treatment of chronic bronchial asthma, orally inhaled corticosteroids have many probable sites of action. The net effect is to reduce the chronic inflammation in asthmatic airways.

The potent anti-inflammatory action may be due to an inhibition of the secretion of growth factors, endothelial activating and other cytokines from lymphocytes, eosinophils, macrophages, fibroblasts, and mast cells. The results are decreased influx of inflammatory cells into the bronchial walls, due in part to inhibition of expression of adhesion molecules on the endothelium and in the tissue. Decreased activation and survival of eosinophils in the lung tissue and a reduction in numbers of mast cells are further effects.

Corticosteroids may inhibit release of mediators from basophils and enzymes from macrophages. There is decreased permeability through vasoconstriction and direct inhibition of endothelial cell contraction.

Beta-adrenergic-receptor numbers may be increased, which results in an enhanced response to beta-adrenergic bronchodilators and reduced down-regulation of beta-receptors after prolonged beta-agonist exposure.

Inhaled corticosteroids also inhibit mucus secretion in airways, possibly by a direct action on submucosal gland cells and an indirect inhibitory effect caused by the reduction in inflammatory mediators that stimulate mucus secretion. The amount and viscosity of sputum are reduced.

The effect of inhaled corticosteroids on bronchial asthma is to block the late inflammatory response to inhaled allergens and reduce over time the response to nonspecific triggers such as exercise. Bronchial wall inflammation and edema are reduced, sputum production is diminished, and the airways become less hyperresponsive to direct and indirect challenges.

### Absorption

Beclomethasone, budesonide, and flunisolide are rapidly absorbed from the lungs and gastrointestinal tract. Triamcinolone is absorbed more slowly.

### Distribution

Without the use of a spacer, approximately 10 to 25% of an inhaled corticosteroid dose is deposited in the airways; the remainder is deposited in the mouth and throat, and swallowed. A greater percentage of the inhaled dose may reach the respiratory tract with the use of a spacer device.

### Biotransformation

For beclomethasone dipropionate—
    Rapidly transformed in the lungs to beclomethasone monopropionate, an active metabolite, which significantly increases the topical potency of beclomethasone.

For budesonide, flunisolide, and triamcinolone acetonide—
    Absorbed unchanged. Those portions of each drug absorbed through the lungs or absorbed after being swallowed are rapidly and extensively transformed to inactive metabolites in the liver.

### Half-life

For budesonide—120 minutes (plasma).

For flunisolide—90 to 120 minutes (plasma).

### Onset of action

Maximum improvement in pulmonary function and symptoms may take up to 4 weeks, while reduction in airway responsiveness occurs gradually over a period of weeks to months.

### Elimination

Fecal and renal.

## Precautions to Consider

### Pregnancy/Reproduction

Pregnancy—Chronic administration of systemic corticosteroids to pregnant women has shown decreased birth weight and a slight increase in the incidence of premature deliveries. In animal studies, decreases in fetal survival and weight have been demonstrated with systemic corticosteroids.

The use of conventional doses of inhaled corticosteroids by pregnant asthmatic women has not been reported to be associated with an increased incidence of congenital abnormalities in the newborn. Inhaled corticosteroids may be used during pregnancy when clinically necessary, since poorly controlled asthma and loss of pulmonary function and hypoxia present a greater risk to the mother and may cause fetal hypoxia. If inhaled corticosteroids are effective before pregnancy, it is advisable to continue regular maintenance dosing during pregnancy.

Beclomethasone is the preferred inhaled corticosteroid during pregnancy in the U.S. because of more extensive clinical experience with its use than with flunisolide or triamcinolone.

FDA Pregnancy Category C.

### Breast-feeding

It is not known whether inhaled corticosteroids are distributed into breast milk. However, problems in humans have not been documented. Although systemic corticosteroids are distributed into breast milk, it is unlikely that inhaled corticosteroids would reach significant quantities in maternal serum and the concentration in breast milk would probably be of minor clinical significance.

### Pediatrics

Inhaled corticosteroids in conventional low doses have been shown to be safe and effective in children with asthma. However, there have been reports that prolonged treatment and/or use of higher doses may, with great individual patient variation, result in systemic effects, such as decreased short-term growth rate and reduced cortisol secretion.

Studies have shown that high doses of inhaled corticosteroids may decrease short-term lower log linear growth but are not associated with long-term statural growth suppression. Minor degrees of growth suppression may be attributed to the transient drop in growth rate associated with delayed puberty in many asthmatic children, without the use of corticosteroids, suggesting that severity of asthma may influence growth. Monitoring of growth is advised in children who regularly require higher doses of inhaled corticosteroids.

Use of prolonged, high daily doses of inhaled corticosteroids may cause a reduction in secretion of endogenous cortisol, although there have been no reports of clinically significant adrenal insufficiency in children treated with inhaled corticosteroids only. However, monitoring for the possibility of some suppression of the hypothalamic-pituitary-adrenal axis may be advisable in children receiving prolonged treatment.

Using a spacer device, rinsing the mouth after inhalations, using the lowest possible doses, and reducing doses after favorable responses have been obtained appear to minimize the risk of adverse systemic and local side effects. A spacer device may enhance inhalation techniques and thus improve intrapulmonary delivery of inhaled corticosteroids and increase compliance in pediatric patients.

Children who are taking systemic corticosteroids in immunosuppressant doses may be more susceptible to infectious diseases, especially chickenpox and measles. Although it is highly unlikely that inhaled corticosteroids in usual doses would be associated with an increased risk of serious infection, some precautions are advisable for children who are taking larger than usual doses of inhaled corticosteroids and who have not had these diseases. Particular care should be taken to avoid exposure to chickenpox and measles and to immunize at an early age against infectious diseases for which there are vaccines, such as measles.

### Geriatrics

Appropriate studies on the relationship of age to the effects of inhaled corticosteroids have not been performed in the geriatric population. However, in studies that have included patients over 65 years of age, geriatrics-specific problems that would limit the usefulness of this medication in the elderly have not been documented.

### Drug interactions and/or related problems

Significant drug interactions are unlikely to occur with usual doses of inhaled corticosteroids. Although there are no defined drug interactions with inhaled corticosteroids, if these medications are used in high doses for a long time and systemic absorption occurs, some of the interactions seen with systemic corticosteroids have a potential to occur. (See *Corticosteroids/Corticotropin—Glucocorticoid Effects [Systemic]*.)

### Laboratory value alterations

The following have been selected on the basis of their potential clinical significance (possible effect in parentheses where appropriate)—not necessarily inclusive (» = major clinical significance):

With physiology/laboratory test values

Note: The following values may be affected with chronic use of larger-than-recommended doses of inhalation corticosteroids.

Adrenal function and
Hypothalamic-pituitary-adrenal (HPA) axis function as assessed by 24-hour urinary free cortisol, morning serum cortisol concentration, or short tetracosactrin cortisol test
   (may be decreased if significant absorption of inhaled corticosteroid occurs, especially in children)

Glucose, blood or urine
   (high-dose therapy may be associated with an increase in fasting insulin, peak glucose, and insulin to glucose ratios after glucose tolerance tests)

Hematologic status
   (neutrophils and total white blood cell count may be increased; eosinophils and lymphocytes may be decreased; clinical relevance of these systemic effects may be insignificant)

Osteocalcin, serum
   (may be decreased in children and adults taking inhaled corticosteroids; however, decrease may also be seen in asthma patients not taking corticosteroids)

### Medical considerations/Contraindications

The medical considerations/contraindications included here have been selected on the basis of their potential clinical significance (reasons given in parentheses where appropriate)—not necessarily inclusive (» = major clinical significance).

*Risk-benefit should be considered when the following medical problems exist:*

Osteoporosis
   (may be exacerbated in postmenopausal women taking high doses over a prolonged time and not receiving an estrogen supplement)

Tuberculosis
   (may be reactivated during prolonged inhaled corticosteroid therapy unless chemoprophylaxis is administered concurrently; asthmatic patients with a positive Mantoux test who are using inhaled corticosteroids should be carefully monitored for manifestation or reactivation, especially in countries with a high incidence of tuberculosis; inhaled corticosteroids should be avoided or used with great caution in patients with drug-resistant pulmonary tuberculosis or atypical tuberculosis)

### Patient monitoring

The following may be especially important in patient monitoring (other tests may be warranted in some patients, depending on condition; » = major clinical significance):

Adrenal function assessment

(may be advisable periodically during, and for several months following, transfer of a patient from systemic to inhalation corticosteroid therapy)

(may be advisable every year during treatment in both children and adults if dosing guidelines are exceeded, especially if systemic corticosteroids are used concurrently or prior to inhaled corticosteroids)

Growth and development in children
   (careful observation may be advisable periodically during prolonged therapy with inhaled corticosteroids)

Inhalation technique
   (frequent assessment of inhalation technique and patient education on the importance of continuous prophylactic treatment with inhaled corticosteroids is recommended to ensure compliance, enhance delivery of medication to lungs, and reduce local and systemic side effects)

Pulmonary function assessment
   (periodic assessment is advisable during, and for several months following, transfer of a patient from systemic to inhalation corticosteroid therapy; frequent pulmonary function monitoring may be necessary in some patients for as long as 4 to 8 months after discontinuation of oral corticosteroids; daily outpatient peak expiratory flow rate [PEFR] measurements are useful in following the course of asthma and the patient's response to therapy)

## Side/Adverse Effects

Note: Significant systemic absorption of inhaled corticosteroids has been reported to cause hypothalamic-pituitary-adrenal (HPA) axis suppression, growth inhibition in children, and possibly osteoporosis, glaucoma, and cataracts. However, most studies to date have been unable to correlate measurable effects on laboratory values with clinically important complications.

Generally, systemic adverse effects do not often occur with the use of conventional inhalation corticosteroid doses. However, the potential for systemic side effects increases with factors that affect absorption, such as high doses, prolonged therapy, the inspiratory technique used and the delivery system employed, patient variations in absorption in relation to lung anatomy and steroid pharmacokinetics, presence of bronchitis, and/or combination therapy with oral corticosteroids.

Side effects from usual doses of inhaled corticosteroids are generally limited to local effects on the upper airways caused by deposition of the inhaled corticosteroid in the oropharynx. Some of these effects may be prevented or alleviated with the use of a spacer and/or mouth rinsing after each treatment.

The following side/adverse effects have been selected on the basis of their potential clinical significance (possible signs and symptoms in parentheses where appropriate)—not necessarily inclusive:

### Those indicating need for medical attention
Incidence less frequent
   *Oropharyngeal candidiasis or thrush* (creamy white, curd-like patches in mouth or throat; pain when eating or swallowing)
Incidence rare
   *Bronchospasm, increased* (increased wheezing; tightness in chest; difficulty in breathing); *esophageal candidiasis* (pain or burning in chest); *psychic change* (nervousness; restlessness; mental depression; behavioral changes)—reported with budesonide only

### Those indicating need for medical attention only if they continue or are bothersome
Incidence more frequent
   *Cough; dry mouth; dysphonia* (hoarseness or other voice changes); *throat irritation*
Incidence less frequent
   *Dry throat; headache; nausea; skin bruising or thinning; unpleasant taste*

## Patient Consultation

As an aid to patient consultation, refer to *Advice for the Patient, Corticosteroids (Inhalation)*.

In providing consultation, consider emphasizing the following selected information (» = major clinical significance):

### Before using this medication
» Conditions affecting use, especially:
   Sensitivity to corticosteroids
   Use in children—Higher doses may result in retarded growth rate and reduced cortisol secretion; monitoring of growth and development and adrenal function is important with prolonged or

high-dose therapy. The use of a spacer is necessary for better compliance and improved airway delivery. Exposure to chickenpox or measles should be avoided

### Proper use of this medication

» Not using to relieve acute asthma attack; continuing use even if using other medication for asthma attack
» Importance of not using more medication than the amount prescribed
» Compliance with therapy by using every day in regularly spaced doses; patients who are not taking systemic corticosteroids when inhalation therapy started may require up to 4 weeks for initial improvement and several months for full benefits

  Gargling and rinsing mouth with water after each dose; not swallowing rinse water
» Reading patient instructions carefully; checking frequently with health care professional for proper use of inhaler
» Proper dosing

  Missed dose: Using as soon as possible; using any remaining doses for that day at regularly spaced intervals

  Checking with pharmacist to determine availability of refills for aerosol inhalers; saving inhaler if refills available
» Proper storage

  Proper dose may not be delivered if aerosol canister is cold

*For beclomethasone, flunisolide, or triamcinolone inhalation aerosol dosage form*

  Testing inhaler before using first time
  Proper administration technique
  Proper administration technique with use of spacer device
  Proper cleaning procedure for inhaler

*For beclomethasone capsule for inhalation dosage form*

» Not swallowing capsules; medication not effective if swallowed
  Proper loading technique for inhaler
  Proper administration technique
  Proper cleaning procedure for inhaler

*For beclomethasone powder for inhalation dosage form*

  Proper loading technique for inhaler
  Proper administration technique
  Proper cleaning procedure for inhaler

*For budesonide powder for inhalation dosage form*

  Proper loading technique for inhaler
  Proper administration technique

*For budesonide suspension for inhalation dosage form*

  Using in a power-operated nebulizer with an adequate flow rate and equipped with face mask or mouthpiece
  Preparation of medication for use in nebulizer
  Proper administration technique
  Proper cleaning procedure for nebulizer

### Precautions while using this medication

» Checking with physician if
    Unusual physical stress occurs, such as surgery, injury, or infections
    Asthma attack is not responsive to bronchodilator
    Any sign indicating possible mouth, throat, or lung infection occurs
    Symptoms do not improve or condition becomes worse
  Carrying medical identification card stating that supplemental systemic corticosteroid therapy may be required in emergency situations, periods of unusual stress, or acute asthma attack
» Caution if any kind of surgery or emergency treatment is required; informing physician or dentist in charge that inhalation corticosteroid is being used

*For patients receiving systemic corticosteroid therapy*

» Importance of not discontinuing systemic corticosteroid therapy without physician's advice; carefully reducing dose or discontinuing treatment if so directed
» Importance of regular visits to physician during time that systemic corticosteroid therapy is being withdrawn; obtaining physician's instructions to follow if severe asthma attack occurs, medical or surgical treatment is needed, or symptoms of corticosteroid withdrawal occur

### Side/adverse effects

  Signs of potential side effects, especially increased bronchospasm, oropharyngeal or esophageal candidiasis, and, with budesonide, psychic changes

## General Dosing Information

Pharmacologic doses of inhaled corticosteroids should be carefully titrated to minimum effective doses to control asthma symptoms and prevent systemic effects.

Gargling and rinsing the mouth with water after each dose are recommended to help prevent hoarseness, throat irritation, and oral candidiasis; the rinse water should not be swallowed. Rinsing the mouth without swallowing can also significantly reduce the amount of inhaled corticosteroid absorbed from the gastrointestinal tract.

The use of a spacer device with a metered dose inhaler may decrease the incidence of some adverse effects, especially oropharyngeal candidiasis and dysphonia. By reducing the need for proper coordination of timing of inhalation with activation of the inhaler and reducing the velocity and mean diameter of the aerosol particles, a spacer reduces the amount of medication deposited in the upper airways and increases the amount deposited in the lower respiratory tract. This enhances the local efficacy of the inhaled corticosteroid without significantly increasing systemic activity.

Some patients may require relatively high doses of inhaled corticosteroids to prevent severe asthma relapse. For this purpose, the highly concentrated beclomethasone aerosol inhalation product available outside the U.S. facilitates the clinical use of high doses. The risk of local side effects may be minimized by twice-daily dosing and the use of a spacer device. However, these measures do not eliminate the risk of systemic side effects associated with prolonged use of high doses.

Patients whose asthma is controlled by their usual dose of inhaled corticosteroids may require temporary emergency use of systemic corticosteroids, if their asthma control is rapidly deteriorating. The use of peak flow monitoring at home once or twice daily will provide objective information to the patient and the physician when this is necessary.

### For patients also receiving systemic corticosteroid therapy

Caution is required when transferring patients from systemic corticosteroids to inhaled corticosteroids. Deaths due to severe asthma relapse or possibly adrenal insufficiency have occurred in asthmatic patients during and after the transfer.

Systemic corticosteroids should be continued initially when inhalation therapy is instituted. After 1 to 2 weeks of inhalation therapy, systemic corticosteroid dosage may be reduced gradually at 1- or 2-week intervals, depending on patient response. *Dosage reductions must be made very slowly and in small decrements* when patient has been receiving prolonged systemic therapy or when systemic corticosteroid dose (prednisone or equivalent) is less than 10 to 15 mg daily.

Some patients may not be able to discontinue use of systemic corticosteroids. A minimal oral maintenance dose may be required along with the inhaled corticosteroid.

Continued monitoring of the patient for signs of adrenal insufficiency is recommended following complete withdrawal of systemic corticosteroid therapy. Recovery of adrenal function may require up to 12 months in some patients, depending on the dosage and duration of systemic therapy.

Supplementation with systemic corticosteroids may be advisable during periods of pronounced physical stress, such as during surgery or severe infections. Supplementation is usually recommended in any patient who has had systemic corticosteroid therapy in the past year and who needs general anesthesia.

Severe asthma relapse may occur upon withdrawal of the systemic corticosteroid. Reinstitution of systemic therapy may be required if a severe asthma attack occurs. Frequent pulmonary function monitoring (peak expiratory flow rate measurements) may be needed for some patients for as long as four to eight months after discontinuation of the systemic corticosteroid.

A syndrome of pseudo-rheumatism (consisting of joint or muscle pain, joint swelling, peripheral edema, lethargy, anorexia, and nausea) may occur when systemic corticosteroid is withdrawn. This syndrome can be avoided or minimized if the dosage of systemic corticosteroids is reduced slowly, using an alternate-day regimen. If the syndrome occurs, the symptoms may be alleviated by treatment with acetaminophen or nonsteroidal anti-inflammatory drugs (NSAIDs) in asthmatic patients who are not sensitive to NSAIDs. Resumption of systemic corticosteroid therapy may not be required.

### For treatment of adverse effects

For laryngeal or pharyngeal candidiasis—Recommended treatment includes
• Administration of an oral or systemic antifungal medication.
• Change in frequency of inhaled corticosteroid dosing from 4 to 2 times a day without decreasing the total daily dose. This may allow recovery and clearing of thrush or prevent its occurrence while maintaining therapeutic efficacy.
• Discontinuation of the inhaled corticosteroid is rarely necessary.

## BECLOMETHASONE

# Inhalation Dosage Forms

## BECLOMETHASONE DIPROPIONATE INHALATION AEROSOL

### Usual adult and adolescent dose
Antiasthmatic—
Oral inhalation, 84 or 100 mcg (0.084 or 0.1 mg—2 metered sprays) three or four times a day; or 168 or 200 mcg (0.168 or 0.2 mg—4 metered sprays) two times a day.

For severe asthma: Oral inhalation, initially, 504 to 800 mcg (0.504 to 0.8 mg—12 to 16 metered sprays) a day. Dosage should then be decreased according to patient response; or, 250 mcg (0.25 mg—1 metered spray) two to four times a day, or 500 mcg (0.5 mg—2 metered sprays) two times a day.

### Usual pediatric dose
Antiasthmatic—
Children up to 6 years of age: Dosage has not been established.
Children 6 to 12 years of age: Oral inhalation, 42 to 100 mcg (0.042 to 0.1 mg—1 or 2 metered sprays) three or four times a day; or 168 or 200 mcg (0.168 or 0.2 mg—4 metered sprays) two times a day.

### Usual pediatric prescribing limits
Up to 500 mcg (0.5 mg—10 metered sprays) per day.

### Strength(s) usually available
U.S.—
42 mcg (0.042 mg) per metered spray (Rx) [*Beclovent; Vanceril*].
Note: Each canister contains medication for about 200 inhalations.
Canada—
50 mcg (0.05 mg) per metered spray (Rx) [*Beclovent; Vanceril*].
Note: Each canister contains medication for about 200 inhalations.
250 mcg (0.25 mg) per metered spray (Rx) [*Becloforte*].
Note: The 250-mcg-per-metered-spray product is used only when the total daily dose equals or exceeds 500 mcg per day.
Each canister contains medication for about 80 or 200 inhalations.

### Packaging and storage
Store at temperature below 49 °C (120 °F) or between 2 and 30 °C (36 and 86 °F), depending on product, unless otherwise specified by manufacturer.

### Auxiliary labeling
• Shake well before using.
• For oral inhalation only.
• Store away from heat and direct sunlight.

### Note
Include patient instructions when dispensing.
Demonstrate administration technique.

### Additional information
In Canada, metered dose inhalers are labeled according to the amount of beclomethasone delivered at the valve; in the U.S., metered dose inhalers are labeled according to the amount of beclomethasone delivered at the mouthpiece or actuator. Thus, 50 mcg of beclomethasone delivered at the valve is equivalent to 42 mcg delivered at the mouthpiece.

This product contains dichlorodifluoromethane and trichloromonofluoromethane, substances that harm public health and the environment by destroying ozone in the upper atmosphere.

## BECLOMETHASONE DIPROPIONATE FOR INHALATION (CAPSULES)

### Usual adult dose
Antiasthmatic—
Oral inhalation, 200 mcg (0.2 mg) three or four times a day. Dosage should then be decreased according to patient response; many patients may be maintained on 400 mcg (0.4 mg) a day.

### Usual pediatric dose
Antiasthmatic—
Children up to 6 years of age: Dosage has not been established.
Children 6 to 14 years of age: Oral inhalation, 100 mcg (0.1 mg) two to four times a day. Dosage should then be decreased according to patient response.
Children over 14 years of age: See *Usual adult dose.*

### Usual pediatric prescribing limits
Up to 500 mcg (0.5 mg) per day.

### Strength(s) usually available
U.S.—
Not commercially available.
Canada—
100 mcg (0.1 mg) per capsule (Rx) [*Beclovent Rotacaps* (lactose)].
200 mcg (0.2 mg) per capsule (Rx) [*Beclovent Rotacaps* (lactose)].

### Packaging and storage
Store below 40 °C (104 °F), preferably between 15 and 30 °C (59 and 86 °F), in a well-closed container, unless otherwise specified by manufacturer.

### Auxiliary labeling
• Do not swallow capsule.

### Note
Include patient instructions when dispensing.
Demonstrate administration technique.
Use of beclomethasone for oral inhalation (capsules) requires a special device that separates the capsule into halves and releases the medication.

## BECLOMETHASONE DIPROPIONATE FOR INHALATION (POWDER)

### Usual adult dose
See *Beclomethasone Dipropionate for Inhalation (Capsules).*

### Usual pediatric dose
See *Beclomethasone Dipropionate for Inhalation (Capsules).*

### Usual pediatric prescribing limits
Up to 500 mcg (0.5 mg) per day.

### Strength(s) usually available
U.S.—
Not commercially available.
Canada—
100 mcg (0.1 mg) per blister (Rx) [*Beclodisk*].
200 mcg (0.2 mg) per blister (Rx) [*Beclodisk*].

### Packaging and storage
Store below 30 °C (86 °F), in a well-closed container, unless otherwise specified by manufacturer.

### Note
Include patient instructions when dispensing.
Demonstrate administration technique.
Use of beclomethasone for oral inhalation (powder) requires a special device that penetrates the blister and releases the medication.

## BUDESONIDE

# Inhalation Dosage Forms

## BUDESONIDE FOR INHALATION (POWDER)

### Usual adult and adolescent dose
Antiasthmatic—
Initial: Oral inhalation, 400 mcg (0.4 mg) to 2.4 mg a day, divided into two to four doses, during periods of severe asthma and/or while reducing or discontinuing systemic corticosteroids.
Maintenance: Oral inhalation, 200 to 400 mcg (0.2 to 0.4 mg) two times a day, the dosage being adjusted according to patient's response; or, for patients who require 400 mcg a day, 400 mcg (0.4 mg) once a day in the morning or evening.

### Usual pediatric dose
Antiasthmatic—
Children up to 6 years of age: Use is not recommended.
Children 6 to 12 years of age: Oral inhalation, 100 to 200 mcg (0.1 to 0.2 mg) two times a day during periods of severe asthma and/or while reducing or discontinuing systemic corticosteroids. Dosage should be decreased according to patient's response.

### Strength(s) usually available
U.S.—
Not commercially available.
Canada—
100 mcg (0.1 mg) (Rx) [*Pulmicort Turbuhaler*].
200 mcg (0.2 mg) (Rx) [*Pulmicort Turbuhaler*].
400 mcg (0.4 mg) (Rx) [*Pulmicort Turbuhaler*].

### Packaging and storage
Store between 15 and 30 °C (59 and 86 °F), unless otherwise specified by manufacturer. Protect from light.

### Auxiliary labeling
• For oral inhalation only.

# BUDESONIDE SUSPENSION FOR INHALATION

**Usual adult and adolescent dose**
Antiasthmatic—
Initial: Oral inhalation, 1 to 2 mg, diluted with sterile sodium chloride inhalation solution, if necessary, to a volume of two to four mL, and administered via nebulization over a period of ten to fifteen minutes two times a day.
Note: For severe asthma, dosage may be increased according to patient response.
Maintenance: Oral inhalation, 500 mcg (0.5 mg) to 1 mg, diluted with sterile sodium chloride inhalation solution, if necessary, to a volume of two to four mL, and administered via nebulization over a period of ten to fifteen minutes two times a day.

**Usual pediatric dose**
Antiasthmatic—
Children up to 3 months of age: Dosage has not been established.
Children 3 months to 12 years of age:
Initial—Oral inhalation, 500 mcg (0.5 mg) to 1 mg, diluted with sterile sodium chloride inhalation solution, if necessary, to a volume of two to four mL, and administered via nebulization over a period of ten to fifteen minutes two times a day.
Maintenance—Oral inhalation, 250 to 500 mcg (0.25 to 0.5 mg), diluted with sterile sodium chloride inhalation solution, if necessary, to a volume of two to four mL, and administered via nebulization over a period of ten to fifteen minutes two times a day.

**Strength(s) usually available**
U.S.—
Not commercially available.
Canada—
250 mcg (0.25 mg) per mL (500 mcg per 2-mL ampul) (Rx) [*Pulmicort Nebuamp*].
500 mcg (0.5 mg) per mL (1000 mcg per 2-mL ampul) (Rx) [*Pulmicort Nebuamp*].

**Packaging and storage**
Store between 15 and 30 °C (59 and 86 °F), unless otherwise specified by manufacturer. Protect from freezing. Protect from light.

**Stability**
Any unused suspension remaining in an opened ampul may be stored for later use as long as it is protected from light and is used within 12 hours after the ampul was opened. The entire contents of an ampul must be used within 12 hours after it is first opened.
Ampuls in an opened envelope should be used within 3 months.

**Auxiliary labeling**
• For oral inhalation only.
• Shake gently before using.

**Note**
When dispensing, include patient instructions for preparation of solution.

**Additional information**
For nebulization of budesonide inhalation suspension, a gas flow (oxygen or compressed air) of 6 to 10 liters per minute should be used. Nebulizers with either a facemask or mouthpiece have been used. Ultrasonic nebulizers are not recommended.

---

## *DEXAMETHASONE*

# Inhalation Dosage Forms

## DEXAMETHASONE SODIUM PHOSPHATE INHALATION AEROSOL USP

Note: **USP DI Advisory Panels do not recommend the use of Dexamethasone Sodium Phosphate Inhalation Aerosol USP, because of the potential for extensive systemic absorption and the long metabolic half-life after absorption resulting in an increased risk of adverse effects with usual inhalation doses.**

**Strength(s) usually available**
U.S.—
100 mcg (0.1 mg) dexamethasone phosphate per metered spray (Rx) [*Decadron Respihaler* (alcohol 2%)].

---

## *FLUNISOLIDE*

# Inhalation Dosage Forms

## FLUNISOLIDE INHALATION AEROSOL

**Usual adult and adolescent dose**
Antiasthmatic—
Oral inhalation, 500 mcg (0.5 mg—2 metered sprays) two times a day, morning and evening.

**Usual adult prescribing limits**
Oral inhalation, 2 mg per day (4 metered sprays twice a day).

**Usual pediatric dose**
Antiasthmatic—
Children up to 4 years of age: Dosage has not been established.
Children 4 years of age and older: See *Usual adult and adolescent dose.*
Note: Doses higher than 1 mg per day have not been studied in children 4 to 15 years of age. In the U.S., dosage has not been established for children under 6 years of age.

**Strength(s) usually available**
U.S.—
250 mcg (0.25 mg) per metered spray (Rx) [*AeroBid; AeroBid-M* (menthol)].
Canada—
250 mcg (0.25 mg) per metered spray (Rx) [*Bronalide*].
Note: Each canister delivers at least 100 inhalations.

**Packaging and storage**
Store below 49 °C (120 °F), preferably between 15 and 30 °C (59 and 86 °F), unless otherwise specified by manufacturer.

**Auxiliary labeling**
• Shake well before using.
• For oral inhalation only.

**Note**
Include patient instructions when dispensing.
Demonstrate administration technique.

**Additional information**
This product contains dichlorodifluoromethane, trichloromonomethane, and dichlorotetrafluoroethane, substances that harm public health and the environment by destroying ozone in the upper atmosphere.

---

## *TRIAMCINOLONE*

# Inhalation Dosage Forms

## TRIAMCINOLONE ACETONIDE INHALATION AEROSOL

**Usual adult and adolescent dose**
Antiasthmatic—
Initial: Oral inhalation, 200 mcg (0.2 mg—2 metered sprays) three or four times a day. For severe asthma–Oral inhalation, 1.2 to 1.6 mg (12 to 16 metered sprays) a day.
Maintenance: Dosage to be decreased according to patient response; maintenance may be achieved in some patients by administering the total daily dose in two divided doses.

**Usual pediatric dose**
Antiasthmatic—
Children up to 6 years of age: Dosage has not been established.
Children 6 to 12 years of age: Oral inhalation, 100 to 200 mcg (0.1 to 0.2 mg—1 or 2 metered sprays) three or four times a day. Dosage must be adjusted according to patient response.

**Usual pediatric prescribing limits**
Up to 1.2 mg (12 metered sprays) per day.

**Strength(s) usually available**
U.S.—
100 mcg (0.1 mg) per metered spray (Rx) [*Azmacort* (alcohol 1%)].
Canada—
100 mcg (0.1 mg) per metered spray (Rx) [*Azmacort* (alcohol 1%)].
Note: Each canister delivers at least 240 inhalations. Canister should not be used after 240 inhalations.

**Packaging and storage**
Store at temperatures below 49 °C (120 °F), preferably between 15 and 30 °C (59 and 86 °F), unless otherwise specified by manufacturer.

**Auxiliary labeling**
• Shake well before using.
• For oral inhalation only.

**Note**
Include patient instructions when dispensing.
Demonstrate administration technique.

**Additional information**
Each actuation releases approximately 200 mcg of triamcinolone acetonide, of which approximately 100 mcg are delivered from the unit.

This product contains dichlorodifluoromethane, a substance that harms public health and the environment by destroying ozone in the upper atmosphere.

Revised: 09/02/94
Interim revision: 10/13/94

# CORTICOSTEROIDS   Nasal

This monograph includes information on the following: Beclomethasone; Budesonide*; Dexamethasone†; Flunisolide; Triamcinolone.

INN:

Beclomethasone—Beclometasone

VA CLASSIFICATION (Primary): NT200

Note: For a listing of dosage forms and brand names by country availability, see *Dosage Forms* section(s). For a listing of brand names for the articles in this monograph, refer to the General Index.

*Not commercially available in the U.S.
†Not commercially available in Canada.

## Category

Anti-inflammatory (steroidal), nasal; corticosteroid (nasal).

## Indications

Note: Bracketed information in the *Indications* section refers to uses that are not included in U.S. product labeling.

**Accepted**

Rhinitis, perennial (treatment)

Rhinitis, seasonal (treatment) or

[Rhinitis, seasonal (prophylaxis)]—Nasal corticosteroids are indicated in the treatment of seasonal or perennial rhinitis in patients who have exhibited significant side effects from, or have exhibited poor response to, other therapies, such as antihistamines and decongestants. Antihistamines and decongestants are generally considered primary therapies for these disorders. However, some clinicians consider nasal corticosteroids primary therapy for perennial or seasonal rhinitis because they are more effective.

[Nasal corticosteroids are used in some patients for prophylaxis of seasonal rhinitis. This form of therapy is generally reserved for patients who have consistently demonstrated a need for nasal corticosteroids to control seasonal rhinitis symptoms. Antihistamines and decongestants are considered primary therapies for this disorder.]

Dexamethasone nasal aerosol is less frequently used because its use results in a significantly higher incidence of systemic adverse effects with no additional benefit over other nasal corticosteroids.

Allergic disorders, nasal (treatment)

Inflammatory conditions, noninfectious, nasal (treatment) or

Polyps, nasal (treatment)—Nasal corticosteroids are indicated in the treatment of allergic or inflammatory nasal conditions and nasal polyps.

Polyps, nasal, postsurgical recurrence of (prophylaxis)—Beclomethasone is indicated [and budesonide nasal solution, dexamethasone, flunisolide, and triamcinolone are used] to prevent recurrence of nasal polyps following their surgical removal and sufficient mucosal healing.

[Rhinitis, vasomotor (treatment)]—Budesonide is used in the treatment of vasomotor rhinitis in patients who are unresponsive to conventional therapy. Antihistamines are generally considered the primary therapy for this disorder.

## Pharmacology/Pharmacokinetics

**Physicochemical characteristics**

Molecular weight—
Beclomethasone dipropionate: 521.05 (anhydrous).
Beclomethasone dipropionate monohydrate: 539.07.
Budesonide: 430.54.
Dexamethasone sodium phosphate: 516.41.
Flunisolide: 443.51.
Triamcinolone acetonide: 434.5.

**Mechanism of action/Effect**

In the treatment of nasal symptoms, the primary action of nasally applied corticosteroids is anti-inflammatory. Nasal corticosteroids inhibit the IgE- and mast cell–mediated early-phase allergic reaction. They also inhibit the migration of inflammatory cells into the nasal tissue (the late-phase or late-onset allergic reaction), which may play a significant role in the pathology of chronic rhinitis.

During the late-phase allergic reaction, eosinophils, neutrophils, basophils, and mononuclear cells produce inflammatory mediators, which cause a reappearance of nasal symptoms.

**Absorption**

Beclomethasone dipropionate—Rapidly absorbed from the nasal mucosa; more slowly from the gastrointestinal tract.

Budesonide—Very little is absorbed from the nasal mucosa.

Flunisolide—50% of dose is absorbed from the nasal mucosa.

Dexamethasone sodium phosphate—Rapidly and extensively absorbed from the nasal mucosa; readily absorbed from the gastrointestinal mucosa.

**Distribution**

A portion of the drug administered nasally is swallowed.

**Protein binding**

Beclomethasone—87%, to albumin and transcortin.

Dexamethasone sodium phosphate—High (65–90%) to albumin and transcortin.

Flunisolide—Moderate, to albumin and transcortin.

**Biotransformation**

Beclomethasone—Hepatic to free beclomethasone and other inactive metabolites. The portion of the dose that is swallowed and absorbed from the gastrointestinal tract undergoes extensive first-pass metabolism to inactive compounds. Initially hydrolyzed to beclomethasone-17-propionate by fecal esterases.

Budesonide—Rapid; hepatic.

Flunisolide—Rapid; hepatic to less active 6-beta-hydroxy metabolites. The portion of the dose that is swallowed and absorbed from the gastrointestinal tract undergoes extensive first-pass metabolism to inactive compounds.

Triamcinolone acetonide—Hepatic to 3 less active metabolites, 6-beta-hydroxytriamcinolone acetonide, 21-carboxytriamcinolone acetonide, and 21-carboxy-6-beta-hydroxytriamcinolone acetonide.

**Half-life**

Beclomethasone dipropionate—
15 hours (plasma).

Budesonide—
Approximately 2 hours (plasma).

Dexamethasone sodium phosphate—
190 minutes (plasma).

Flunisolide—
1 to 2 hours (plasma).

Triamcinolone acetonide—
Intravenous: Approximately 90 minutes (plasma).
Intranasal: Apparent half-life is 4 hours (plasma) (range, 1 to 7 hours); however, this value probably reflects lingering absorption.

**Onset of action**

Beclomethasone and flunisolide—Usually 5 to 7 days; however, may rarely be as long as 2 to 3 weeks in some patients.

Triamcinolone acetonide—As early as 12 hours.

**Time to peak concentration**

Budesonide—
Oral, approximately 3 hours.
Inhalation, within 1 hour.

Flunisolide—
10 to 30 minutes.

Triamcinolone acetonide—
   Average of 3.4 hours (range, 0.5 to 8 hours).

**Peak plasma concentration**
Flunisolide—0.4 to 1.0 nanogram per mL.
Triamcinolone acetonide—Less than 1 nanogram per mL.

**Time to maximum benefit**
Beclomethasone and flunisolide—Up to 3 weeks in some patients.
Budesonide—Usually 2 or 3 days, but up to 3 weeks in some patients.
Triamcinolone acetonide—Usually 3 to 4 days.

**Elimination**
Beclomethasone—Fecal; renal, 12 to 15%.
Dexamethasone sodium phosphate—Renal.
Flunisolide—Renal, 50%; fecal, 40%.
Triamcinolone acetonide—Primarily fecal.

# Precautions to Consider

## Cross-sensitivity and/or related problems
Patients intolerant of benzalkonium chloride, disodium edetate, or phenylethanol may be intolerant of some nasal corticosteroid preparations, since they may contain these substances as preservatives.
Beclomethasone, dexamethasone, and triamcinolone aerosols also contain fluorocarbon propellants; beclomethasone monohydrate and flunisolide dosage forms contain no fluorocarbon propellants.
Flunisolide solution contains propylene glycol and polyethylene glycols.

## Carcinogenicity
*Beclomethasone*—No evidence of carcinogenicity was demonstrated in rats receiving beclomethasone for 95 weeks (13 weeks by inhalation and 82 weeks orally).
*Flunisolide*—In long-term studies, flunisolide given orally caused an increase in the incidence of pulmonary adenomas in mice but not in rats. Also, as reported for other corticosteroids, flunisolide caused an increased incidence of mammary adenocarcinoma in female rats receiving the highest oral doses.
*Triamcinolone*—No evidence of carcinogenicity was demonstrated in a 2-year study on male and female rats administered oral doses of 1 mcg per kg of body weight (mcg/kg) a day and male and female mice administered oral doses of 3 mcg/kg a day.

## Mutagenicity
*Beclomethasone*—Studies on mutagenicity have not been done.
*Triamcinolone*—Studies on mutagenicity have not been done.

## Pregnancy/Reproduction
*Fertility—Beclomethasone:* Female dogs administered beclomethasone orally showed impaired fertility (inhibition of the estrous cycle). However, this effect was not observed following administration of the medication via inhalation.
*Dexamethasone:* Dexamethasone may increase or decrease spermatozoa count or motility in some patients.
*Flunisolide:* Studies in female rats showed some evidence of impaired fertility.
*Triamcinolone:* Male and female rats administered triamcinolone acetonide orally at doses of up to 15 mcg/kg per day (maternally toxic doses are 2.5 to 15 mcg/kg per day) exhibited no evidence of impaired fertility. However, a few female rats administered 8 or 15 mcg/kg per day exhibited dystocia and prolonged delivery.

*Pregnancy*—Corticosteroids cross the placenta. Studies in humans have not been done with budesonide, dexamethasone, flunisolide, or triamcinolone nasal formulations.
Studies in animals have shown that corticosteroids are embryotoxic, fetotoxic, and/or teratogenic. However, teratogenic effects have not been confirmed in humans receiving systemic corticosteroids.
Infants born to mothers who have received substantial doses of corticosteroids during pregnancy should be carefully observed for signs of hypoadrenalism.
*Beclomethasone*—
   In one study of orally inhaled beclomethasone in humans, beclomethasone did not cause teratogenic or other adverse effects.
   Studies in rats, mice, and rabbits have shown that subcutaneously administered beclomethasone causes increased fetal resorptions and birth defects, including cleft palate, agnathia, microstomia, absence of tongue, delayed ossification, and partial agenesis of the thymus.
   FDA Pregnancy Category C.
*Budesonide*—
   Studies in rats, mice, and rabbits have shown that subcutaneously administered budesonide causes fetal malformations, primarily skeletal defects.

*Dexamethasone*—
   Although studies in humans have not been done with dexamethasone nasal aerosol, risk-benefit must be considered, since studies in animals have shown systemically administered dexamethasone to be teratogenic.
*Flunisolide*—
   Adequate and well-controlled studies in humans have not been done.
   Studies in rabbits and rats have shown that systemically administered flunisolide causes teratogenic and fetotoxic effects.
   FDA Pregnancy Category C.
*Trimacinolone*—
   Adequate and well-controlled studies in humans have not been done.
   Developmental toxicity, which included increases in fetal resorptions and stillbirths and decreases in pup body weight and survival, occurred at oral maternal doses of 2.5 to 15 mcg/kg per day. Studies in rats and rabbits administered systemic doses of 20 to 80 mcg/kg per day have shown teratogenic effects, including a low incidence of cleft palate and/or internal hydrocephaly and axial skeletal defects. Studies in non-human primates administered systemic doses of 500 mcg/kg per day have shown teratogenic effects, including CNS and cranial malformations. Administration of triamcinolone nasal aerosol to pregnant rats and rabbits resulted in embryotoxic and fetotoxic effects that were comparable to those produced by administration by other routes.
   FDA Pregnancy Category C.

## Breast-feeding
Distribution of significant quantities of corticosteroids into breast milk may suppress growth, interfere with endogenous corticosteroid production, or cause other adverse effects in the nursing infant.
*Beclomethasone, budesonide, flunisolide, and triamcinolone*—It is not known whether beclomethasone, budesonide, flunisolide, or triamcinolone is distributed into breast milk. However, systemic corticosteroids are distributed into breast milk.
*Dexamethasone*—Dexamethasone is distributed into breast milk. Nursing while receiving pharmacologic doses of dexamethasone is not recommended.

## Pediatrics
Significant suppression of growth has not been well documented with the use of usual doses of nasal beclomethasone and flunisolide. If significant systemic absorption of nasal corticosteroids occurs in pediatric patients, adrenal suppression and growth suppression may result. Prolonged or high-dose therapy with these medications, especially dexamethasone, requires careful attention to dosage and close monitoring of growth and development.

## Geriatrics
Appropriate studies with nasal corticosteroids have not been performed in the geriatric population. However, geriatrics-specific problems that would limit the usefulness of this medication in the elderly are not expected.

## Laboratory value alterations
The following have been selected on the basis of their potential clinical significance (possible effect in parentheses where appropriate)—not necessarily inclusive (» = major clinical significance):
With diagnostic test results
*For dexamethasone*
   Nitroblue tetrazolium test for bacterial infection
      (dexamethasone may produce false-negative results)
With physiology/laboratory test values
   Adrenal function as assessed by corticotropin (ACTH) stimulation or measurement of plasma cortisol and
   Hypothalamic-pituitary-adrenal (HPA) axis function
      (may be decreased if significant absorption occurs, especially in children; most likely with dexamethasone)

   Glucose concentration, blood and urine
      (may be increased if significant absorption occurs because of intrinsic hyperglycemic activity of glucocorticoids; most likely with dexamethasone)

   Hematologic status
      (should be monitored during long-term therapy)

## Medical considerations/Contraindications
The medical considerations/contraindications included here have been selected on the basis of their potential clinical significance (reasons given in parentheses where appropriate)—not necessarily inclusive (» = major clinical significance).

*Risk-benefit should be considered when the following medical problems exist:*

Amebiasis, latent or active
   (dexamethasone or other corticosteroids may activate latent amebiasis)

Glaucoma
   (may increase intraocular pressure)

Hepatic function impairment

Hypothyroidism

» Infections, fungal, bacterial, or systemic viral or
» Ocular herpes simplex
   (corticosteroids may mask infection)

Intolerance to corticosteroids

Nasal septal ulcers, recent or
Nasal surgery, recent or
Nasal trauma, recent
   (corticosteroids inhibit wound healing)

» Tuberculosis, latent or active, of respiratory tract

**Patient monitoring**

The following may be especially important in patient monitoring (other tests may be warranted in some patients, depending on condition; » = major clinical significance):

Adrenal function assessment
   (assessment of HPA axis function may be advisable at periodic intervals in patients receiving long-term nasal corticosteroid therapy; especially important in patients receiving usual doses of dexamethasone or greater-than-recommended doses of beclomethasone, flunisolide, or triamcinolone)

» Otolaryngologic examination
   (should be performed in patients on long-term therapy to monitor nasal mucosa and nasal passages for infection, nasal septal perforation, nasal membrane ulceration, or other histologic changes)

## Side/Adverse Effects

Note: The risk of systemic effects is minimal with usual doses of nasal beclomethasone and flunisolide. Side effects from usual doses of beclomethasone are generally limited to local effects.

Systemic effects including hypothalamic-pituitary-adrenal (HPA) axis suppression may occur with usual doses of nasal dexamethasone or greater-than-recommended doses of beclomethasone, flunisolide, or triamcinolone. (Doses of 440 mcg of triamcinolone acetonide administered daily for 42 days did not measurably affect adrenal response to a 6-hour cosyntropin test.) If the patient is particularly sensitive or has recently used systemic corticosteroids prior to using nasal corticosteroids, the patient may also be predisposed to hypercorticism.

The following side/adverse effects have been selected on the basis of their potential clinical significance (possible signs and symptoms in parentheses where appropriate)—not necessarily inclusive:

**Those indicating need for medical attention**

Incidence more frequent
   *For triamcinolone*
      *Headache*—incidence 18%

Incidence less frequent
   *For all nasal corticosteroids*
      *Crusting inside nose or epistaxis* (bloody mucus or unexplained nosebleeds)—especially if spray is improperly aimed toward nasal septum, rather than onto the turbinates; *sore throat; ulceration of nasal mucosa* (sores inside nose)

   *For dexamethasone*
      *Allergic reaction or bronchial asthma* (shortness of breath, troubled breathing, tightness in chest, hives, or wheezing)

   *For beclomethasone (monohydrate), budesonide, dexamethasone, and flunisolide*
      *Cough; dizziness or lightheadedness; headache; hoarseness*—not reported for budesonide; *lethargy* (unusual tiredness or weakness); *loss of sense of taste or smell*—reported for dexamethasone and flunisolide only; *nausea or vomiting; rhinorrhea, continuing* (runny nose); *stuffy nose, continuing; watery eyes, continuing*—not reported for budesonide; *stomach pains*—not reported for budesonide

Incidence rare
   *For all nasal corticosteroids*
      *Nasal candidiasis* (white patches inside nose); *nasal septal perforation* (bloody mucus or unexplained nosebleeds); *ocular hy-*

*pertension* (eye pain; nausea; vomiting; gradual loss of vision); *pharyngeal candidiasis* (white patches in throat)

   *For beclomethasone*
      *Hypersensitivity reaction, delayed or immediate* (hives; rash; shortness of breath or troubled breathing; swelling of eyelids, face, or lips); *rhinitis, atrophic* (bad smell; dry or stuffy nose; headache behind eye sockets)

   *For budesonide*
      *Dermatitis* (rash); *urticaria* (hives)

   *For triamcinolone*
      *Burning or stinging, continuing, after use of spray; irritation inside nose*

Symptoms of chronic overdose
   *Acneiform lesions* (acne); *Cushing's syndrome* (fullness or rounding of the face); *menstrual changes*

**Those indicating need for medical attention only if they continue or are bothersome**

Incidence more frequent
   *For all nasal corticosteroids*
      *Burning, dryness, or other irritation inside the nose, mild and transient*

   *For beclomethasone and flunisolide*
      *Irritation of throat*—possibly due to vehicle in nasal spray; *sneezing attacks*—may be more common in children using beclomethasone aerosol or flunisolide spray

Incidence less frequent
   *For all nasal corticosteroids*
      *Sneezing*

   *For budesonide*
      *Throat itching*

   *For triamcinolone*
      *Sinus congestion* (stuffy nose or headache); *stuffy nose; throat discomfort*

## Overdose

For more information on the management of overdose or unintentional ingestion, **contact a Poison Control Center** (see *Poison Control Center Listing*).

**Treatment of overdose**

For acute overdose—Adverse effects due to acute overdose are unlikely with the small quantities of corticosteroid contained in each canister.

For chronic overdose—If symptoms of chronic overdose occur, nasal corticosteroids should be discontinued slowly.

## Patient Consultation

As an aid to patient consultation, refer to *Advice for the Patient, Corticosteroids (Nasal)*.

In providing consultation, consider emphasizing the following selected information (» = major clinical significance):

**Before using this medication**

» Conditions affecting use, especially:
   Intolerance to corticosteroids
   Pregnancy—Risk-benefit must be considered, since systemic corticosteroids cross the placenta and have demonstrated embryotoxicity, fetotoxicity, and teratogenicity in animals; beclomethasone oral inhalation study in humans has shown no adverse effects on fetus; infants born to mothers who received substantial doses of corticosteroids during pregnancy should be observed for hypoadrenalism
   Breast-feeding—Use of dexamethasone is not recommended, since dexamethasone is distributed into breast milk
   Use in children—Significant effect on growth by beclomethasone or flunisolide has not been documented; importance of monitoring growth and development with prolonged or high-dose therapy
   Other medical problems, especially fungal, bacterial, or systemic viral infections, ocular herpes simplex, or latent or active tuberculosis of respiratory tract

**Proper use of this medication**

» Proper administration technique; reading patient directions carefully before use
   Blowing nose to clear nasal passages before administration; aiming spray away from nasal septum (aiming towards the inner corner of eye)

» Compliance with therapy; may require up to 3 weeks for full benefit

» Importance of not using more medication than the amount prescribed, because of potential enhanced absorption and increased severity of side effects
» Checking with physician before using medication for other nasal problems
   Saving special inhaler used for beclomethasone or dexamethasone; refills may be available
» Proper dosing
   Missed dose: Using as soon as possible if remembered within an hour or so; if remembered later, not using at all; not doubling doses
» Proper storage; not storing budesonide powder in damp places, especially if cap has not been tightly screwed on; decreased efficacy if aerosol canister is cold; not puncturing, breaking, or burning aerosol container; discarding unused portion of beclomethasone solution or flunisolide solution 3 months after opening package

**Precautions while using this medication**
Regular visits to physician to check progress during prolonged therapy
» Checking with physician if:
   —signs of infection of nose, throat, or sinuses occur
   —no improvement within 7 days (for dexamethasone)
   —no improvement within 3 weeks (for beclomethasone, budesonide, flunisolide, or triamcinolone)
   —condition becomes worse

**Side/adverse effects**
Signs of potential side effects, especially headache, crusting inside nose or epistaxis, sore throat, ulceration of nasal mucosa, allergic reaction or bronchial asthma, cough, dizziness or lightheadedness, hoarseness, lethargy, loss of sense of taste or smell, nausea or vomiting, continuing rhinorrhea, continuing stuffy nose, continuing watery eyes, stomach pains, nasal candidiasis, nasal septal perforation, ocular hypertension, pharyngeal candidiasis, delayed or immediate hypersensitivity reaction, atrophic rhinitis, dermatitis, urticaria, continuing burning or stinging after use of spray, or irritation inside nose

## General Dosing Information

In patients with blocked nasal passages, a topical decongestant may be used just prior to use of the nasal corticosteroid. However, because prolonged use of topical nasal decongestants may cause congestive rebound, they should preferably be used for a maximum of 3 to 5 days. An oral decongestant is recommended for chronic nasal congestion.

The smallest dose of a nasal corticosteroid required to control symptoms should be used as a maintenance dose after the desired clinical response is achieved.

The dosage of other corticosteroids being administered concurrently by other routes of administration, including oral inhalation, should be taken into account when determining the usual adult prescribing limits of nasal corticosteroids.

---

### *BECLOMETHASONE*

## Summary of Differences

Pharmacology/pharmacokinetics: See *Pharmacology/Pharmacokinetics*.
Precautions: Cross-sensitivity and/or related problems—Nasal spray dosage form contains no fluorocarbon propellants.
Side/adverse effects: See *Side/Adverse Effects*.

## Additional Dosing Information

Regular use is required to obtain full therapeutic benefit. Medication should be discontinued if improvement is not evident after 3 weeks.

See also *General Dosing Information*.

## Nasal Dosage Forms

### BECLOMETHASONE DIPROPIONATE NASAL AEROSOL

**Usual adult and adolescent dose**
Anti-inflammatory (steroidal), nasal—
   Nasal, 42 or 50 mcg (0.042 or 0.05 mg) (1 metered spray) in each nostril two to four times a day (total daily dose, 168 to 400 mcg [0.168 to 0.4 mg]).

**Usual adult prescribing limits**
Nasal, 1 mg per day.
Note: If orally inhaled beclomethasone is used concurrently, the combined total daily dose should not exceed 1 mg.

**Usual pediatric dose**
Anti-inflammatory (steroidal), nasal—
   Children up to 6 years of age: Safety and efficacy have not been established.
   Children 6 to 12 years of age: Nasal, 42 or 50 mcg (0.042 or 0.05 mg) (1 metered spray) in each nostril three or four times a day (total daily dose, 252 mcg [0.252 mg] to 400 mcg [0.4 mg]).
   Children 12 years of age and over: See *Usual adult and adolescent dose*.

**Usual pediatric prescribing limits**
Nasal, 500 mcg (0.5 mg) per day. If orally inhaled beclomethasone is used concurrently, the combined total daily dose should not exceed 500 mcg (0.5 mg).

**Strength(s) usually available**
U.S.—
   42 mcg (0.042 mg) per metered spray (Rx) [*Beconase* (fluorocarbons); *Vancenase* (fluorocarbons)].
Canada—
   50 mcg (0.05 mg) per metered spray (Rx) [*Beconase; Vancenase* (fluorocarbons); GENERIC].

**Packaging and storage**
Store between 2 and 30 °C (36 and 86 °F), unless otherwise specified by manufacturer.

**Auxiliary labeling**
• For the nose.
• Shake well.

**Note**
When dispensing, include patient instructions.

Explain administration technique.

### BECLOMETHASONE DIPROPIONATE MONOHYDRATE NASAL SOLUTION

**Usual adult and adolescent dose**
Anti-inflammatory (steroidal), nasal—
   Nasal, 42 to 100 mcg (0.042 to 0.1 mg) (1 or 2 metered sprays) in each nostril two times a day (total daily dose, 168 to 400 mcg [0.168 to 0.4 mg]).

**Usual adult prescribing limits**
Nasal, 600 mcg (0.6 mg) (12 metered sprays) per day.
Note: If orally inhaled beclomethasone is used concurrently, the combined total daily dose should not exceed 1 mg.

**Usual pediatric dose**
Anti-inflammatory (steroidal), nasal—
   Children up to 6 years of age: Safety and efficacy have not been established.
   Children 6 years of age and over: See *Usual adult and adolescent dose*.

**Usual pediatric prescribing limits**
Nasal, 400 mcg (0.4 mg) (8 metered sprays) per day. If orally inhaled beclomethasone is used concurrently, the combined total daily dose should not exceed 500 mcg (0.5 mg).

**Strength(s) usually available**
U.S.—
   42 mcg (0.042 mg) per metered spray (Rx) [*Beconase AQ* (benzalkonium chloride; phenylethanol 0.25%); *Vancenase AQ* (benzalkonium chloride; phenylethanol 0.25%)].
Canada—
   50 mcg (0.05 mg) per metered spray (Rx) [*Beconase AQ;* GENERIC].

**Packaging and storage**
Store between 15 and 30 °C (59 and 86 °F), unless otherwise specified by manufacturer.

**Auxiliary labeling**
• For the nose.
• Shake well.

**Note**
When dispensing, include patient instructions.

Explain administration technique.

---

### *BUDESONIDE*

## Summary of Differences

Pharmacology/pharmacokinetics: See *Pharmacology/Pharmacokinetics*.
Side/adverse effects: See *Side/Adverse Effects*.

## Additional Dosing Information

Regular use is required to obtain full therapeutic benefit. Treatment should not be continued beyond 3 weeks in the absence of significant symptomatic improvement.

See also *General Dosing Information.*

## Nasal Dosage Forms

### BUDESONIDE NASAL POWDER

#### Usual adult and adolescent dose

Anti-inflammatory (steroidal), nasal:

Nasal inhalation, initially 200 mcg (0.2 mg) (2 metered inhalations) in each nostril once a day in the morning (total daily dose, 400 mcg [0.4 mg]), the dosage then being decreased to the lowest effective dose according to patient response.

#### Usual adult prescribing limits

Nasal inhalation, 800 mcg (0.8 mg) (8 metered inhalations) per day.

#### Usual pediatric dose

Anti-inflammatory (steroidal), nasal inhalation—

Children up to 6 years of age: Safety and efficacy have not been established.

Children 6 years of age and older: See *Usual adult and adolescent dose.*

#### Usual pediatric prescribing limits

Nasal inhalation, 400 mcg (0.4 mg) (4 metered inhalations) per day.

#### Strength(s) usually available

U.S.—

Not commercially available.

Canada—

100 mcg (0.1 mg) per metered inhalation (Rx) [*Rhinocort Turbuhaler*].

#### Packaging and storage

Store below 40 °C (104 °F), preferably between 15 and 30 °C (59 and 86 °F), unless otherwise specified by manufacturer.

#### Auxiliary labeling

• For the nose.

#### Note

When dispensing, include patient instructions.

Explain administration technique.

### BUDESONIDE NASAL SOLUTION

#### Usual adult and adolescent dose

Anti-inflammatory (steroidal), nasal—

Initial: Nasal, 200 mcg (0.2 mg) (2 metered sprays) in each nostril once a day in the morning (total daily dose, 400 mcg [0.4 mg]).

Maintenance: Nasal, 100 mcg (0.1 mg) (1 metered spray) in each nostril once a day in the morning (total daily dose, 200 mcg [0.2 mg]).

#### Usual adult prescribing limits

Nasal, 800 mcg (0.8 mg) per day.

#### Usual pediatric dose

Anti-inflammatory (steroidal), nasal—

Children up to 6 years of age: Safety and efficacy have not been established.

Children 6 years of age and older: See *Usual adult and adolescent dose.*

#### Usual pediatric prescribing limits

Nasal, 400 mcg (0.4 mg) per day.

#### Strength(s) usually available

U.S.—

Not commercially available.

Canada—

100 mcg (0.1 mg) per metered spray (Rx) [*Rhinocort Aqua*].

#### Packaging and storage

Store below 40 °C (104 °F), preferably between 15 and 30 °C (59 and 86 °F), unless otherwise specified by manufacturer. Protect from freezing.

#### Auxiliary labeling

• For the nose.

• Shake well.

#### Note

When dispensing, include patient instructions.

Explain administration technique.

## Summary of Differences

Indications:

Less frequently used due to significantly increased incidence of adverse effects.

Pharmacology/pharmacokinetics:

See *Pharmacology/Pharmacokinetics.*

Precautions:

Laboratory value alterations—False-negative results may occur with nitroblue tetrazolium test for bacterial infections.

Side/adverse effects:

HPA axis suppression or other systemic corticosteroid effects may occur with usual nasal inhalation doses.

See also *Side/Adverse Effects.*

## Additional Dosing Information

When medication is to be discontinued, dosage usually should be reduced gradually according to the dose, frequency, and duration of therapy.

Patients whose conditions do not improve within 7 days should be reevaluated. Use of dexamethasone should be limited to a maximum of 2 weeks.

See also *General Dosing Information.*

## Nasal Dosage Forms

### DEXAMETHASONE SODIUM PHOSPHATE NASAL AEROSOL

#### Usual adult and adolescent dose

Anti-inflammatory (steroidal), nasal—

Nasal, initially 200 mcg (0.2 mg) (2 metered sprays) of dexamethasone phosphate in each nostril two or three times a day (total daily dose, 800 mcg [0.8 mg] to 1.2 mg of dexamethasone phosphate), the dosage then being decreased according to patient response.

Note: Some patients may be maintained on 100 mcg (0.1 mg) (1 metered spray) of dexamethasone phosphate in each nostril two times a day.

Therapy should be discontinued as soon as possible. If symptoms recur, therapy may be reinstituted.

#### Usual adult prescribing limits

Nasal, 1.2 mg (12 metered sprays) of dexamethasone phosphate per day.

#### Usual pediatric dose

Anti-inflammatory (steroidal), nasal—

Children up to 6 years of age: Use is not recommended.

Children 6 to 12 years of age: Nasal, 100 or 200 mcg (0.1 or 0.2 mg) (1 or 2 metered sprays) of dexamethasone phosphate in each nostril two times a day (total daily dose, 400 or 800 mcg [0.4 or 0.8 mg] of dexamethasone phosphate).

#### Usual pediatric prescribing limits

Nasal, 800 mcg (0.8 mg) (8 metered sprays) of dexamethasone phosphate per day.

#### Strength(s) usually available

U.S.—

100 mcg (0.1 mg) phosphate per metered spray (Rx) [*Decadron Turbinaire* (alcohol 2%; fluorocarbons)].

Canada—

Not commercially available.

#### Packaging and storage

Store below 49 °C (120 °F), preferably between 15 and 30 °C (59 and 86 °F), unless otherwise specified by manufacturer. Protect from freezing.

#### Auxiliary labeling

• For the nose.

• Shake well.

#### Note

When dispensing, include patient instructions.

Explain administration technique.

## Summary of Differences

Pharmacology/pharmacokinetics: See *Pharmacology/Pharmacokinetics.*

Precautions: Cross-sensitivity and/or related problems—Dosage form contains no fluorocarbon propellants.

Side/adverse effects: See *Side/Adverse Effects.*

## Additional Dosing Information

Regular use is required to obtain full therapeutic benefits. Medication should be discontinued if improvement is not evident after 3 weeks.

See also *General Dosing Information*.

## Nasal Dosage Forms

### FLUNISOLIDE NASAL SOLUTION USP

**Usual adult dose**

Anti-inflammatory (steroidal), nasal—

Initial: Nasal, 50 mcg (0.05 mg) (2 metered sprays) in each nostril two times a day (total daily dose, 200 mcg [0.2 mg]); if necessary, dosing frequency may be increased to three times a day (total daily dose, 300 mcg [0.3 mg]).

Maintenance: Nasal, as little as 25 mcg (0.025 mg) (1 metered spray) in each nostril once a day has been effective (total daily dose, 50 mcg [0.05 mg]).

**Usual adult prescribing limits**

Nasal, 400 mcg (0.4 mg) per day.

**Usual pediatric dose**

Anti-inflammatory (steroidal), nasal—

Children up to 6 years of age:

Safety and efficacy have not been established.

Children 6 to 14 years of age:

Initial—Nasal, 25 mcg (0.025 mg) (1 metered spray) in each nostril three times a day; or 50 mcg (0.05 mg) (2 metered sprays) in each nostril two times a day; (total daily dose, 150 or 200 mcg [0.15 or 0.2 mg]).

Maintenance—Nasal, as little as 25 mcg (0.025 mg) (1 metered spray) in each nostril once a day has been effective (total daily dose, 50 mcg [0.05 mg]).

Children 14 years of age and older:

See *Usual adult dose*.

**Usual pediatric prescribing limits**

Nasal, 200 mcg (0.2 mg) per day.

**Strength(s) usually available**

U.S.—

25 mcg (0.025 mg) per metered spray (Rx) [*Nasalide* (benzalkonium chloride; disodium edetate)].

Canada—

25 mcg (0.025 mg) per metered spray (Rx) [*Rhinalar* (benzalkonium chloride)].

**Packaging and storage**

Store between 15 and 30 °C (59 and 86 °F). Store in a tight container. Protect from light.

**Stability**

Opened container should be discarded after 3 months.

**Auxiliary labeling**

• For the nose.

**Note**

When dispensing, include patient instructions.

Explain administration technique.

---

### TRIAMCINOLONE

## Summary of Differences

Pharmacology/pharmacokinetics: See *Pharmacology/Pharmacokinetics*.

Side/adverse effects: See *Side/Adverse Effects*.

## Additional Dosing Information

Regular use is required to obtain full therapeutic benefit. Medication should be discontinued if improvement is not evident after 3 weeks.

See also *General Dosing Information*.

## Nasal Dosage Forms

### TRIAMCINOLONE ACETONIDE NASAL AEROSOL

**Usual adult and adolescent dose**

Anti-inflammatory (steroidal), nasal—

Nasal, 110 mcg (0.11 mg) (2 metered sprays) in each nostril once a day (total daily dose, 220 mcg [0.22 mg]).

**Usual adult prescribing limits**

Nasal, 440 mcg (0.44 mg) (8 metered sprays) per day.

**Usual pediatric dose**

Anti-inflammatory (steroidal), nasal—

Children up to 12 years of age: Safety and efficacy have not been established.

Children 12 years of age and older: See *Usual adult and adolescent dose*.

**Strength(s) usually available**

U.S.—

55 mcg (0.055 mg) per metered spray (Rx) [*Nasacort* (dehydrated alcohol 0.7% w/w; fluorocarbons)].

Canada—

55 mcg (0.055 mg) per metered spray (Rx) [*Nasacort* (dehydrated alcohol 0.7% w/w; fluorocarbons)].

**Packaging and storage**

Store between 15 and 30 °C (59 and 86 °F), unless otherwise specified by manufacturer.

**Auxiliary labeling**

• For the nose.

• Shake well.

**Note**

When dispensing, include patient instructions.

Explain administration technique.

---

Revised: 05/16/94

---

# CORTICOSTEROIDS    Ophthalmic

This monograph includes information on the following: Betamethasone*; Dexamethasone; Fluorometholone; Hydrocortisone*; Medrysone; Prednisolone.

VA CLASSIFICATION (Primary):

Betamethasone—OP300

Dexamethasone—OP300

Fluorometholone—OP300

Hydrocortisone—OP300

Medrysone—OP300

Prednisolone—OP300

Another commonly used name for hydrocortisone is cortisol.

Note: For a listing of dosage forms and brand names by country availability, see *Dosage Forms* section(s). For a listing of brand names for the articles in this monograph, refer to the General Index.

---

*Not commercially available in the U.S.

## Category

Corticosteroid (ophthalmic); anti-inflammatory (steroidal), ophthalmic.

Note: Ophthalmic dosage forms of betamethasone and hydrocortisone are not commercially available in the U.S.; therefore, there is no U.S. product labeling identifying approved indications.

## Indications

Note: Bracketed information in the *Indications* section refers to uses that are not included in U.S. product labeling.

**Accepted**

Ophthalmic disorders (treatment)—Ophthalmic corticosteroids are indicated in the treatment of corticosteroid-responsive allergic and inflammatory conditions of the palpebral and bulbar conjunctiva, cornea, and anterior segment of the globe.

Fluorometholone (0.1%), medrysone, or prednisolone (0.12 or 0.125%) may be preferred for long-term treatment because they are least likely to increase intraocular pressure.

Very severe ocular disorders that do not respond to topical corticosteroid therapy may require treatment with systemic corticosteroids. In some cases, concurrent topical and systemic corticosteroid therapy may be utilized.

See Table 1, page 935.

## Unaccepted

Topical corticosteroids for ophthalmic use are not indicated in the treatment of degenerative ocular disorders. Also, if corticosteroid therapy is required for the treatment of disorders involving deep ocular structures, the medication should be administered systemically because topical application will not be effective.

# Pharmacology/Pharmacokinetics

## Physicochemical characteristics

Molecular weight—
Betamethasone sodium phosphate: 516.41.
Dexamethasone: 392.47.
Dexamethasone sodium phosphate: 516.41.
Fluorometholone: 376.47.
Fluorometholone acetate: 418.51.
Hydrocortisone acetate: 404.50.
Medrysone: 344.49.
Prednisolone acetate: 402.49.
Prednisolone sodium phosphate: 484.39.

## Mechanism of action/Effect

Corticosteroids diffuse across cell membranes and complex with specific cytoplasmic receptors. These complexes then enter the cell nucleus, bind to DNA, and stimulate transcription of mRNA and subsequent protein synthesis of enzymes ultimately responsible for anti-inflammatory effects of topical application of corticosteroids to the eye. In high concentrations, which may be achieved after topical application, corticosteroids may exert direct membrane effects. Corticosteroids decrease cellular and fibrinous exudation and tissue infiltration, inhibit fibroblastic and collagen-forming activity, retard epithelial regeneration, diminish postinflammatory neovascularization, and reduce toward normal levels the excessive permeability of inflamed capillaries.

## Absorption

Absorbed into aqueous humor, cornea, iris, choroid, ciliary body, and retina. Systemic absorption occurs, but may be significant only at higher dosages or in extended pediatric therapy.

# Precautions to Consider

## Carcinogenicity/Mutagenicity

Dexamethasone—Long-term animal studies have not been conducted to evaluate the carcinogenicity of dexamethasone.

Fluorometholone, medrysone, and prednisolone—Studies in animals or humans have not been conducted to evaluate the carcinogenic or mutagenic potential of fluorometholone, medrysone, and prednisolone.

## Pregnancy/Reproduction

Pregnancy—Problems in humans have not been documented; however, adequate and well-controlled studies with these agents have not been done.

Infants born to mothers who have received substantial doses of corticosteroids during pregnancy should be carefully observed for signs of hypoadrenalism.

Studies in rabbits have shown that corticosteroids produce fetal resorptions and multiple abnormalities, including those of the head, ears, limbs, and palate.

Dexamethasone, hydrocortisone, and prednisolone—
Studies in pregnant mice have shown that these medications, when applied to both eyes 5 times a day on Days 10–13 of gestation, caused a significant increase in fetal cleft palate.

Dexamethasone and prednisolone—FDA Pregnancy Category C.

Fluorometholone—
Studies in pregnant rabbits have shown that fluorometholone is teratogenic and embryocidal when applied to the eyes at various dosage levels on Days 6–18 of gestation.

FDA Pregnancy Category C.

Medrysone—
Studies in pregnant rabbits have indicated that medrysone (doses 10 and 30 times the human dose or higher) is embryocidal. Also, application to the eyes (2 drops 4 times a day on Days

6–18 of gestation) of pregnant rabbits caused an increase in early resorptions.

FDA Pregnancy Category C.

## Breast-feeding

Problems in humans have not been documented.

## Pediatrics

Corticosteroids should be used with caution in children 2 years of age or younger because the different dose/weight ratio for children increases the risk of adrenal suppression. This risk increases with the length of therapy, which, therefore, should be limited to the shortest possible time (preferably less than 5 days).

## Geriatrics

Appropriate studies on the relationship of age to the effects of ophthalmic corticosteroids have not been performed in the geriatric population. However, no geriatrics-specific problems have been documented to date.

## Drug interactions and/or related problems

The following drug interactions and/or related problems have been selected on the basis of their potential clinical significance (possible mechanism in parentheses where appropriate)—not necessarily inclusive (» = major clinical significance):

Note: Combinations containing any of the following medications, depending on the amount present, may also interact with this medication.

Antiglaucoma agents
(chronic or intensive use of ophthalmic corticosteroids may increase intraocular pressure and decrease the efficacy of antiglaucoma agents)

Anticholinergics, especially atropine and related compounds
(risk of intraocular hypertension may be increased with prolonged corticosteroid therapy; may be more likely to occur during use of cycloplegic/mydriatic agents in patients predisposed to acute angle closure)

Contact lenses
(risk of infection increased)

## Medical considerations/Contraindications

The medical considerations/contraindications included here have been selected on the basis of their potential clinical significance (reasons given in parentheses where appropriate)—not necessarily inclusive (» = major clinical significance).

*Except under special circumstances, these medications should not be used when the following medical problems exist:*

» Fungal diseases, ocular, or
» Herpes simplex keratitis, acute superficial, or
» Tuberculosis, ocular, active or history of, or
» Viral disease, acute, infectious
(corticosteroids decrease human resistance to bacterial, fungal, and viral infections; application may exacerbate existing infections and encourage the development of new or secondary infections)

*Risk-benefit should be considered when the following medical problems exist:*

» Cataracts
(may be exacerbated)

Diabetes mellitus
(patient may be predisposed toward increases in intraocular pressure and/or cataract formation)

Diseases causing thinning of the cornea or sclera
(use may result in perforation)

» Glaucoma, chronic, open-angle, or family history of
(may be precipitated or exacerbated)

» Infections of the cornea or conjunctiva, other
(risk of exacerbation or development of secondary infections)

Sensitivity to corticosteroids

## Patient monitoring

The following may be especially important in patient monitoring (other tests may be warranted in some patients, depending on condition; » = major clinical significance):

Ophthalmologic examinations, especially tonometry and slit-lamp examination
(initial ophthalmologic examinations should be performed 2 to 3 weeks following onset of chronic therapy; subsequent examinations are performed at intervals as determined by patient status or risk factors)

## Side/Adverse Effects

Note: Frequent or intensive use of ophthalmic corticosteroids may retard corneal healing.

Systemic absorption occurs, but may be significant only at higher dosages or in extended pediatric therapy. The different dose/weight ratio for children increases the risk of adrenal suppression.

The following side/adverse effects have been selected on the basis of their potential clinical significance (possible signs and symptoms in parentheses where appropriate)—not necessarily inclusive:

### Those indicating need for medical attention
Incidence less frequent or rare
*Corneal thinning and/or globe perforation* (decreased vision; watering of the eyes); *glaucoma; ocular hypertension; optic nerve damage; posterior subcapsular cataract; visual acuity and field defects* (gradual blurring or loss of vision; eye pain; nausea; vomiting); *secondary ocular infection*

### Those indicating need for medical attention only if they continue or are bothersome
Incidence more frequent
*Temporary mild blurred vision*—may be expected to occur after use of ointments
Incidence less frequent or rare
*Burning, stinging, redness, or watering of the eyes*

## Overdose

For more information on the management of overdose or unintentional ingestion, **contact a Poison Control Center** (see *Poison Control Center Listing*).

### Treatment of overdose
Generally, acute oral overdose of ophthalmic corticosteroids does not result in serious adverse effects. Dilution with fluids is the mainstay of therapy.

## Patient Consultation

As an aid to patient consultation, refer to *Advice for the Patient, Corticosteroids (Ophthalmic).*

In providing consultation, consider emphasizing the following selected information (» = major clinical significance):

### Before using this medication
» Conditions affecting use, especially:
  Sensitivity to corticosteroids
  Use in children—Cautious and short-term use recommended
  Other medical problems, especially eye infections (other), cataracts, or glaucoma

### Proper use of this medication
For contact lens wearers: Checking with ophthalmologist prior to use; contact lenses should not be worn during, and possibly for a time following, application of these medications because of an increased risk of infection
Shaking suspensions vigorously before applying
Proper administration technique
Preventing contamination: Not touching applicator tip to any surface and keeping container tightly closed
» Importance of not using more medication than the amount prescribed (especially in children)
» Checking with physician before using medication for future eye problems
» Proper dosing
Missed dose: Using as soon as possible; not using if almost time for next dose
» Proper storage

### Precautions while using this medication
Need for ophthalmologic examinations during long-term therapy
Checking with physician if there is no improvement after 5 to 7 days of therapy or if condition worsens

### Side/adverse effects
Signs of potential side effects, especially corneal thinning and/or globe perforation, glaucoma, ocular hypertension, optic nerve damage, posterior subcapsular cataract, visual acuity and field defects, or secondary ocular infection

## General Dosing Information

The severity and location of ocular inflammation often requires dosage to be higher and/or more frequent than the usual adult dose initially, then gradually reduced to as little as necessary to maintain the therapeutic effect. If infections do not respond promptly, the ophthalmic corticosteroid should be discontinued until the infection has been controlled.

Increasing the frequency of administration is usually as effective as, or more effective than, using higher concentrations of the medication.

The duration of treatment may vary from a few days to several weeks or months in some cases, depending on the condition being treated. Daily or alternate-day therapy may be indicated for extended periods in certain situations, such as following penetrating keratoplasty.

Although ophthalmic corticosteroids should not be used longer than is medically necessary, it is recommended that treatment be continued after apparent response, with the dosage gradually tapered to avoid relapse.

At night, the ophthalmic ointment, where available, may be used as an adjunct to the ophthalmic solution or suspension to provide prolonged contact with the eye.

---

### BETAMETHASONE

## Ophthalmic Dosage Forms
### BETAMETHASONE SODIUM PHOSPHATE OPHTHALMIC/OTIC SOLUTION

Note: The dosing and strengths of the dosage form available are expressed in terms of betamethasone base.

**Usual adult and adolescent dose**
Ophthalmic disorders (treatment)—
Topical, to the conjunctiva, 1 or 2 drops of a 0.1% (base) solution every one or two hours initially, with dosage gradually being decreased as inflammation subsides.

**Usual pediatric dose**
See *Usual adult and adolescent dose.*

**Usual geriatric dose**
See *Usual adult and adolescent dose.*

**Strength(s) usually available**
U.S.—
Not commercially available.
Canada—
0.1% (base) (Rx) [*Betnesol*].

**Packaging and storage**
Store below 40 °C (104 °F), preferably between 15 and 30 °C (59 and 86 °F), unless otherwise specified by manufacturer. Protect from freezing.

**Auxiliary labeling**
• For the eye.

**Note**
Dispense in original unopened container.

---

### DEXAMETHASONE

## Ophthalmic Dosage Forms
### DEXAMETHASONE OPHTHALMIC OINTMENT

**Usual adult and adolescent dose**
Ophthalmic disorders (treatment)—
Topical, to the conjunctiva, a thin strip (approximately 1 cm) of a 0.1% ointment three or four times a day initially. After a favorable response is obtained, the number of applications per day may be gradually reduced prior to discontinuation.

**Usual pediatric dose**
See *Usual adult and adolescent dose.*

**Usual geriatric dose**
See *Usual adult and adolescent dose.*

**Strength(s) usually available**
U.S.—
Not commercially available.
Canada—
0.1% (Rx) [*Maxidex* (methylparaben; propylparaben)].

**Packaging and storage**
Store below 40 °C (104 °F), preferably between 15 and 30 °C (59 and 86 °F), unless otherwise specified by manufacturer. Store in a tight container. Protect from freezing.

**Auxiliary labeling**
• For the eye.

**Note**
Dispense in original unopened container.

## DEXAMETHASONE OPHTHALMIC SUSPENSION USP

### Usual adult and adolescent dose
Ophthalmic disorders (treatment)—
    Topical, to the conjunctiva, 1 or 2 drops of a 0.1% suspension four to
        six times a day.
Note: In severe conditions, treatment may be initiated with 1 or 2 drops
    every hour, with dosage gradually being decreased as inflammation
    subsides.

### Usual pediatric dose
See *Usual adult and adolescent dose.*

### Usual geriatric dose
See *Usual adult and adolescent dose.*

### Strength(s) usually available
U.S.—
    0.1% (Rx) [*Maxidex;* GENERIC].
Canada—
    0.1% (Rx) [*Maxidex* (benzalkonium chloride)].

### Packaging and storage
Store below 40 °C (104 °F), preferably between 15 and 30 °C (59 and 86
    °F), unless otherwise specified by manufacturer. Store in a tight con-
    tainer. Protect from freezing.

### Auxiliary labeling
• For the eye.
• Shake well.

### Note
Dispense in original unopened container.

## DEXAMETHASONE SODIUM PHOSPHATE OPHTHALMIC OINTMENT USP

Note: The dosing and strengths of the dosage form available are expressed
    in terms of dexamethasone phosphate not dexamethasone sodium
    phosphate.

### Usual adult and adolescent dose
Ophthalmic disorders (treatment)—
    Topical, to the conjunctiva, a thin strip (approximately 1 cm) of a
        0.05% (phosphate) ointment three or four times a day initially.
        After a favorable response is obtained, the number of applications
        per day may be gradually reduced prior to discontinuation.

### Usual pediatric dose
See *Usual adult and adolescent dose.*

### Usual geriatric dose
See *Usual adult and adolescent dose.*

### Strength(s) usually available
U.S.—
    0.05% (phosphate) (Rx) [*AK-Dex* (methylparaben, propylparaben);
        *Baldex* (methylparaben; propylparaben); *Decadron; Dexair* (meth-
        ylparaben; propylparaben); *Maxidex; Ocu-Dex;* GENERIC].
Canada—
    Not commercially available.

### Packaging and storage
Store below 40 °C (104 °F), preferably between 15 and 30 °C (59 and 86
    °F), unless otherwise specified by manufacturer. Protect from freezing.

### Auxiliary labeling
• For the eye.

### Note
Dispense in original unopened container.

## DEXAMETHASONE SODIUM PHOSPHATE OPHTHALMIC SOLUTION USP

Note: The dosing and strengths of the dosage form available are expressed
    in terms of dexamethasone phosphate not dexamethasone sodium
    phosphate.

### Usual adult and adolescent dose
Ophthalmic disorders (treatment)—
    Topical, to the conjunctiva, 1 or 2 drops of a 0.1% (phosphate) so-
        lution up to six times a day.
Note: In severe conditions, treatment may be initiated with 1 or 2 drops
    every hour, with dosage gradually being decreased as inflammation
    subsides.

### Usual pediatric dose
See *Usual adult and adolescent dose.*

### Usual geriatric dose
See *Usual adult and adolescent dose.*

### Strength(s) usually available
U.S.—
    0.1% (phosphate) (Rx) [*AK-Dex* (benzalkonium chloride); *Baldex* (so-
        dium bisulfite; benzalkonium chloride); *Decadron* (sodium bisul-
        fite 0.1%; benzalkonium chloride); *Dexair* (sodium bisulfite 0.1%;
        benzalkonium chloride); *Dexotic; Ocu-Dex; Storz-Dexa;* GENERIC].
Canada—
    0.1% (phosphate) (Rx) [*Decadron* (sodium bisulfite 0.1%; benzalkon-
        ium chloride); *Diodex* (disodium edetate; benzalkonium chloride);
        *PMS-Dexamethasone Sodium Phosphate; R.O.-Dexasone* (benzal-
        konium chloride); *Spersadex* (disodium edetate; benzalkonium
        chloride)].

### Packaging and storage
Store below 40 °C (104 °F), preferably between 15 and 30 °C (59 and 86
    °F), unless otherwise specified by manufacturer. Store in a tight, light-
    resistant container. Protect from freezing.

### Auxiliary labeling
• For the eye.

### Note
Dispense in original unopened container.

---

## *FLUOROMETHOLONE*

# Ophthalmic Dosage Forms
## FLUOROMETHOLONE OPHTHALMIC OINTMENT

### Usual adult and adolescent dose
Ophthalmic disorders (treatment)—
    Topical, to the conjunctiva, a thin strip (approximately 1 cm) of a
        0.1% ointment one to three times a day.
Note: In severe conditions, treatment may be initiated with application
    every four hours, with dosage gradually being decreased as inflam-
    mation subsides.

### Usual pediatric dose
See *Usual adult and adolescent dose.*

### Usual geriatric dose
See *Usual adult and adolescent dose.*

### Strength(s) usually available
U.S.—
    0.1% (Rx) [*FML S.O.P* (phenylmercuric acetate)].
Canada—
    Not commercially available.

### Packaging and storage
Store below 40 °C (104 °F), preferably between 15 and 30 °C (59 and 86
    °F), unless otherwise specified by manufacturer. Protect from freezing.

### Auxiliary labeling
• For the eye.

### Note
Dispense in original unopened container.

## FLUOROMETHOLONE OPHTHALMIC SUSPENSION USP

### Usual adult and adolescent dose
Ophthalmic disorders (treatment)—
    Topical, to the conjunctiva, 1 or 2 drops of a 0.1% or 0.25% suspen-
        sion two to four times a day.
Note: In severe conditions, treatment may be initiated with 1 or 2 drops
    every hour, with dosage gradually being decreased as inflammation
    subsides.

### Usual pediatric dose
See *Usual adult and adolescent dose.*

### Usual geriatric dose
See *Usual adult and adolescent dose.*

### Strength(s) usually available
U.S.—
    0.1% (Rx) [*Fluor-Op* (benzalkonium chloride); *FML Liquifilm* (ben-
        zalkonium chloride)].
    0.25% (Rx) [*FML Forte* (benzalkonium chloride)].
Canada—
    0.1% (Rx) [*FML Liquifilm* (benzalkonium chloride)].
    0.25% (Rx) [*FML Forte* (benzalkonium chloride)].

**Packaging and storage**
Store below 40 °C (104 °F), preferably between 15 and 30 °C (59 and 86 °F), unless otherwise specified by manufacturer. Store in a tight container. Protect from freezing.

**Auxiliary labeling**
• For the eye.
• Shake well.

**Note**
Dispense in original unopened container.

## FLUOROMETHOLONE ACETATE OPHTHALMIC SUSPENSION

**Usual adult and adolescent dose**
Ophthalmic disorders (treatment)—
Topical, to the conjunctiva, 1 or 2 drops of a 0.1% suspension two to four times a day.

Note: In severe conditions, treatment may be initiated with 2 drops every two hours during the initial twenty-four to forty-eight hours. Dosage should be gradually decreased as inflammation subsides.

**Usual pediatric dose**
See *Usual adult and adolescent dose.*

**Usual geriatric dose**
See *Usual adult and adolescent dose.*

**Strength(s) usually available**
U.S.—
0.1% (Rx) [*Eflone; Flarex* (benzalkonium chloride)].
Canada—
0.1% (Rx) [*Flarex* (benzalkonium chloride)].

**Packaging and storage**
Store below 40 °C (104 °F), preferably between 15 and 30 °C (59 and 86 °F), unless otherwise specified by manufacturer. Protect from freezing.

**Auxiliary labeling**
• For the eye.
• Shake well.

---

### *HYDROCORTISONE*

## Ophthalmic Dosage Forms
### HYDROCORTISONE ACETATE OPHTHALMIC OINTMENT USP

**Usual adult and adolescent dose**
Ophthalmic disorders (treatment)—
Topical, to the conjunctiva, a thin strip (approximately 1 cm) of a 2.5% ointment three or four times a day initially, with frequency of application gradually being decreased as inflammation subsides.

**Usual pediatric dose**
See *Usual adult and adolescent dose.*

**Usual geriatric dose**
See *Usual adult and adolescent dose.*

**Strength(s) usually available**
U.S.—
Not commercially available.
Canada—
2.5% (Rx) [*Cortamed*].

**Packaging and storage**
Store below 40 °C (104 °F), preferably between 15 and 30 °C (59 and 86 °F), unless otherwise specified by manufacturer. Protect from freezing.

**Auxiliary labeling**
• For the eye.

**Note**
Dispense in original unopened container.

---

### *MEDRYSONE*

## Ophthalmic Dosage Forms
### MEDRYSONE OPHTHALMIC SUSPENSION USP

**Usual adult and adolescent dose**
Ophthalmic disorders (treatment)—
Topical, to the conjunctiva, 1 drop of a 1% suspension up to every four hours.

**Usual pediatric dose**
See *Usual adult and adolescent dose.*

**Usual geriatric dose**
See *Usual adult and adolescent dose.*

**Strength(s) usually available**
U.S.—
1% (Rx) [*HMS Liquifilm* (benzalkonium chloride)].
Canada—
1% (Rx) [*HMS Liquifilm* (benzalkonium chloride)].

**Packaging and storage**
Store below 40 °C (104 °F), preferably between 15 and 30 °C (59 and 86 °F), unless otherwise specified by manufacturer. Store in a tight, light-resistant container. Protect from freezing.

**Auxiliary labeling**
• For the eye.
• Shake well.

**Note**
Dispense in original unopened container.

---

### *PREDNISOLONE*

## Ophthalmic Dosage Forms
### PREDNISOLONE ACETATE OPHTHALMIC SUSPENSION USP

**Usual adult and adolescent dose**
Ophthalmic disorders (treatment)—
Topical, to the conjunctiva, 1 or 2 drops of a 0.12 to 1% suspension two to four times a day.

Note: In severe conditions, treatment may be initiated with 1 or 2 drops every hour, with dosage gradually being decreased as inflammation subsides.

**Usual pediatric dose**
See *Usual adult and adolescent dose.*

**Usual geriatric dose**
See *Usual adult and adolescent dose.*

**Strength(s) usually available**
U.S.—
0.12% (Rx) [*Pred Mild* (sodium bisulfite; benzalkonium chloride)].
0.125% (Rx) [*Econopred* (benzalkonium chloride)].
1% (Rx) [*AK-Tate* (benzalkonium chloride); *Econopred Plus* (benzalkonium chloride); *Ocu-Pred-A; Predair A* (sodium bisulfite; benzalkonium chloride); *Pred Forte* (sodium bisulfite; benzalkonium chloride); *Ultra Pred;* GENERIC].
Canada—
0.12% (Rx) [*Pred Mild* (sodium bisulfite; benzalkonium chloride); GENERIC].
1% (Rx) [*AK-Tate* (sodium bisulfite); *Ophtho-Tate; Pred Forte* (sodium bisulfite; benzalkonium chloride); GENERIC].

**Packaging and storage**
Store between 8 and 24 °C (46 and 75 °F), unless otherwise specified by manufacturer. Store in a tight container. Protect from light. Protect from freezing.

**Auxiliary labeling**
• For the eye.
• Shake well.

**Note**
Dispense in original unopened container.

### PREDNISOLONE SODIUM PHOSPHATE OPHTHALMIC SOLUTION USP

**Usual adult and adolescent dose**
Ophthalmic disorders (treatment)—
Topical, to the conjunctiva, 1 or 2 drops of a 0.125 or 1% solution up to six times a day.

Note: In severe conditions, treatment may be initiated with 1 or 2 drops every hour, with dosage gradually being decreased as inflammation subsides.

**Usual pediatric dose**
See *Usual adult and adolescent dose.*

**Usual geriatric dose**
See *Usual adult and adolescent dose.*

**Strength(s) usually available**

U.S.—

0.125% (Rx) [*AK-Pred* (sodium bisulfite; benzalkonium chloride); *Inflamase Mild* (benzalkonium chloride); *I-Pred* (sodium metabisulfite; benzalkonium chloride); *Lite Pred; Ocu-Pred; Predair* (sodium bisulfite; benzalkonium chloride); GENERIC].

1% (Rx) [*AK-Pred* (sodium bisulfite; benzalkonium chloride); *Inflamase Forte* (benzalkonium chloride); *I-Pred* (sodium metabisulfite; benzalkonium chloride); *Ocu-Pred Forte; Predair Forte* (sodium bisulfite; benzalkonium chloride); GENERIC].

Canada—

0.125% (Rx) [*Inflamase Mild* (benzalkonium chloride)].

1% (Rx) [*Inflamase Forte* (benzalkonium chloride)].

**Packaging and storage**

Store below 40 °C (104 °F), preferably between 15 and 30 °C (59 and 86 °F), unless otherwise specified by manufacturer. Store in a tight, light-resistant container. Protect from freezing.

**Auxiliary labeling**
• For the eye.

**Note**

Dispense in original unopened container.

Revised: 01/05/94
Interim revision: 05/16/94; 01/27/95

## Table 1. Indications*

Note: Bracketed information refers to uses that are not included in U.S. product labeling.

Ophthalmic dosage forms of betamethasone and hydrocortisone are not commercially available in the U.S.; therefore, there is no U.S. product labeling identifying approved indications.

Legend:
I = Betamethasone  IV = Hydrocortisone
II = Dexamethasone  V = Medrysone
III = Fluorometholone  VI = Prednisolone

| | I | II | III | IV | V | VI |
|---|---|---|---|---|---|---|
| Indicated in the treatment of corticosteroid-responsive inflammatory conditions of the palpebral and bulbar conjunctiva, cornea, and anterior segment of the globe, such as: | | | | | | |
| Allergic disorders, ophthalmic (treatment) | ✔ | ✔ | ✔ | ✔ | | ✔ |
| Anterior segment disease, inflammatory (treatment) | ✔ | ✔ | ✔ | ✔ | | ✔ |
| Conjunctivitis, allergic (treatment) | ✔ | ✔ | ✔ | ✔ | ✔ | ✔ |
| Corneal injuries (treatment) | ✔ | ✔ | ✔ | ✔ | | ✔ |
| Cyclitis (treatment) | ✔ | ✔ | ✔ | ✔ | | ✔ |
| Episcleritis (treatment) | ✔ | ✔ | ✔ | ✔ | ✔ | ✔ |
| Iridocyclitis (treatment) | ✔ | ✔ | ✔ | ✔ | [✔]¹ | ✔ |
| Keratitis, herpes zoster (treatment) | ✔ | ✔ | ✔ | ✔ | [✔]¹ | ✔ |
| Keratitis not associated with herpes simplex or fungal infection (treatment) | ✔ | ✔ | ✔ | ✔ | [✔]¹ | ✔ |
| Keratitis, punctate, superficial (treatment) | ✔ | ✔ | ✔ | ✔ | [✔]¹ | ✔ |
| Keratitis, vernal (treatment) | ✔ | ✔ | ✔ | ✔ | [✔]¹ | ✔ |
| Keratoconjunctivitis, allergic (treatment) | ✔ | ✔ | ✔ | ✔ | [✔]¹ | ✔ |
| Keratoconjunctivitis, vernal (treatment) | ✔ | ✔ | ✔ | ✔ | ✔ | ✔ |
| Ocular infections, superficial (treatment adjunct)† | ✔ | ✔ | ✔ | ✔ | [✔]¹ | ✔ |
| Ocular sensitivity to epinephrine (treatment) | ✔ | ✔ | ✔ | ✔ | ✔ | ✔ |
| Ophthalmia sympathetic (treatment) | ✔ | ✔ | ✔ | ✔ | [✔]¹ | ✔ |
| Rosacea, ocular (treatment) | ✔ | ✔ | ✔ | ✔ | [✔]¹ | ✔ |

*Indications for specific agents may vary because of lack of specific testing and/or clinical-use data. Although all of these medications are used for all of the listed indications, medrysone may be less effective than the other ophthalmic corticosteroids for any condition other than conjunctivitis.

†Use in the treatment of ocular infection requires that the risk of corticosteroid-induced exacerbation of existing infection or development of secondary infections be weighed against the need for reducing inflammation and edema. Appropriate anti-infective therapy should also be administered as required.

¹Not included in Canadian product labeling.

# CORTICOSTEROIDS   Otic

This monograph includes information on the following: Betamethasone*; Dexamethasone; Hydrocortisone*.

**VA CLASSIFICATION (Primary): OT200**

Note: Otic corticosteroid formulations are identical to the corresponding ophthalmic formulations listed in *Corticosteroids (Ophthalmic)*. However, only the specific brand name products listed below are labeled for otic use.

Another commonly used name for hydrocortisone is cortisol.

Note: For a listing of dosage forms and brand names by country availability, see *Dosage Forms* section(s). For a listing of brand names for the articles in this monograph, refer to the General Index.

*Not commercially available in the U.S.

## Category

Corticosteroid (otic); anti-inflammatory (steroidal), otic.

# Indications

Note: Bracketed information in the *Indications* section refers to uses that are not included in U.S. product labeling.

## Accepted

Otic corticosteroids are indicated in the treatment of corticosteroid-responsive inflammatory disorders of the external auditory meatus such as:

Otitis externa, allergic (treatment)

Otitis, infective (treatment adjunct)

[Lichen simplex chronicus, localized (treatment)]

[Otitis externa, eczematoid, chronic (treatment)] or

[Otitis externa, seborrheic (treatment)]—Dexamethasone, betamethasone, and hydrocortisone are used in the treatment of these and other corticosteroid-responsive disorders of the external auditory meatus.

Use in the treatment of infective otitis requires that the risk of corticosteroid-induced exacerbation of existing infection or development of secondary infections be weighed against the need for reducing inflammation and edema. Appropriate anti-infective therapy should also be administered as required.

Dexamethasone is indicated in the treatment of lichen simplex chronicus of the external auditory meatus.

# Pharmacology/Pharmacokinetics

## Physicochemical characteristics

Molecular weight—

Betamethasone sodium phosphate: 516.41.

Dexamethasone sodium phosphate: 516.41.

Hydrocortisone acetate: 404.50.

## Mechanism of action/Effect

Corticosteroids diffuse across cell membranes and complex with specific cytoplasmic receptors. These complexes then enter the cell nucleus, bind to DNA, and stimulate transcription of messenger RNA and subsequent protein synthesis of enzymes responsible for anti-inflammatory effects of otic corticosteroids. In the high concentrations that may be achieved after otic use, corticosteroids may exert direct membrane effects. Corticosteroids decrease cellular and fibrinous exudation and tissue infiltration, inhibit fibroblastic and collagen-forming activity, retard epithelial regeneration, diminish postinflammatory neovascularization, and reduce toward normal levels the excessive permeability of inflamed capillaries.

# Precautions to Consider

## Carcinogenicity/Mutagenicity

For dexamethasone—Long-term animal studies have not been conducted to evaluate the carcinogenicity of dexamethasone ophthalmic/otic solution.

## Pregnancy/Reproduction

Problems in humans have not been documented.

## Breast-feeding

Problems in humans have not been documented.

## Pediatrics

Appropriate studies on the relationship of age to the effects of otic corticosteroids have not been performed in the pediatric population. However, pediatrics-specific problems that would limit the usefulness of these medications in children are not expected.

## Geriatrics

Appropriate studies on the relationship of age to the effects of otic corticosteroids have not been performed in the geriatric population. However, geriatrics-specific problems that would limit the usefulness of these medications in the elderly are not expected.

## Medical considerations/Contraindications

The medical considerations/contraindications included here have been selected on the basis of their potential clinical significance (reasons given in parentheses where appropriate)—not necessarily inclusive (» = major clinical significance).

*Except under special circumstances, these medications should not be used when the following medical problems exist:*

» Fungal diseases, aural or
» Tuberculosis, aural or
» Viral infection, acute, infectious
   (corticosteroids decrease human resistance to bacterial, fungal, and viral infections; application may mask or exacerbate existing infections and encourage the development of new or secondary infections)

» Otitis media, chronic, history of or

» Perforation of ear drum membrane
   (possibility of ototoxicity)

Sensitivity to corticosteroids

*Risk-benefit should be considered when the following medical problems exist:*

Infections, ear, acute or
Infections, ear, chronic or
Otitis media, especially in children
   (risk of exacerbation or development of secondary infections)

# Side/Adverse Effects

The following side/adverse effects have been selected on the basis of their potential clinical significance (possible signs and symptoms in parentheses where appropriate)—not necessarily inclusive:

**Those indicating need for medical attention only if they continue or are bothersome**

Incidence less frequent or rare

*Burning or stinging of the ear*

# Patient Consultation

As an aid to patient consultation, refer to *Advice for the Patient, Corticosteroids (Otic)*.

In providing consultation, consider emphasizing the following selected information (» = major clinical significance):

**Before using this medication**

» Conditions affecting use, especially:
   Sensitivity to corticosteroids
   Other medical problems, especially other ear infections, viral infections, or perforated ear drum

**Proper use of this medication**

Proper administration technique

Preventing contamination: Not touching applicator tip to any surface and keeping container tightly closed

» Importance of not using more medication than the amount prescribed
» Checking with physician before using medication for future ear problems
» Proper dosing
   Missed dose: Using as soon as possible; not using if almost time for next dose
» Proper storage

**Precautions while using this medication**

Checking with physician if no improvement after 5 to 7 days of therapy or if condition worsens

# General Dosing Information

To allow optimum contact between the medication and affected surfaces of the ear canal, all cerumen and debris should be carefully removed by a physician or a trained assistant prior to initiation of therapy.

Otic solutions may be instilled directly into the ear canal or administered by use of a saturated gauze or cotton wick gently placed into the canal. The wick should be kept moist with additional solution and replaced every 12 to 24 hours.

The duration of treatment may vary from a few days to several weeks or months in some cases, depending on the condition being treated. Daily or alternate-day therapy may be indicated for extended periods in certain situations.

Treatment should be continued after apparent response, with the dosage being gradually tapered to avoid relapse.

---

*BETAMETHASONE*

---

# Otic Dosage Forms

## BETAMETHASONE SODIUM PHOSPHATE OPHTHALMIC/OTIC SOLUTION

### Usual adult and adolescent dose

Topical, to the ear canal, 2 or 3 drops of a 0.1% (base) solution every 2 or 3 hours initially, with dosage gradually being decreased as inflammation subsides.

### Usual pediatric dose

See *Usual adult and adolescent dose*.

### Usual geriatric dose

See *Usual adult and adolescent dose*.

## Strength(s) usually available

U.S.—

Not commercially available.

Canada—

0.1% (base) (Rx) [*Betnesol*].

## Packaging and storage

Store below 40 °C (104 °F), preferably between 15 and 30 °C (59 and 86 °F), unless otherwise specified by manufacturer. Protect from freezing.

## Auxiliary labeling

• For the ear.

## Note

Dispense in original unopened container.

---

### *DEXAMETHASONE*

## Otic Dosage Forms

### DEXAMETHASONE SODIUM PHOSPHATE OPHTHALMIC SOLUTION (Otic use) USP

## Usual adult and adolescent dose

Topical, to the ear canal, 3 or 4 drops of a 0.1% (phosphate) solution two or three times a day. After a favorable response is obtained, dosage may be gradually reduced if required to provide continuing control of symptoms prior to discontinuation.

## Usual pediatric dose

See *Usual adult and adolescent dose.*

## Usual geriatric dose

See *Usual adult and adolescent dose.*

## Strength(s) usually available

U.S.—

0.1% (phosphate) (Rx) [*AK-Dex* (benzalkonium chloride 0.01%; sodium edetate); *Decadron* (sodium bisulfite 0.1%; benzalkonium chloride 0.02%; disodium edetate; phenylethanol 0.25%); *I-Methasone* (benzalkonium chloride 0.01%; disodium edetate)].

Canada—

0.1% (phosphate) (Rx) [*AK-Dex* (benzalkonium chloride 0.1%; sodium edetate); *Decadron* (sodium bisulfite 0.1%; benzalkonium chloride 0.02%; disodium edetate 0.05%; phenylethanol 0.25%,)].

## Packaging and storage

Store below 40 °C (104 °F), preferably between 15 and 30 °C (59 and 86 °F), unless otherwise specified by manufacturer. Store in a tight, light-resistant container. Protect from freezing.

## Auxiliary labeling

• For the ear.

## Note

Dispense in original unopened container.

---

### *HYDROCORTISONE*

## Otic Dosage Forms

### HYDROCORTISONE ACETATE OPHTHALMIC OINTMENT (Otic use) USP

## Usual adult and adolescent dose

Topical, to the external ear canal, a thin coating of a 2.5% ointment two or three times a day initially, with frequency of application gradually being decreased as inflammation subsides.

## Usual pediatric dose

Children up to 2 years of age—Dosage has not been established.
Children 2 years of age and older—See *Usual adult and adolescent dose.*

## Usual geriatric dose

See *Usual adult and adolescent dose.*

## Strength(s) usually available

U.S.—

Not commercially available.

Canada—

2.5% (Rx) [*Cortamed*].

## Packaging and storage

Store below 40 °C (104 °F), preferably between 15 and 30 °C (59 and 86 °F), unless otherwise specified by manufacturer. Protect from freezing.

## Auxiliary labeling

• For the ear.

## Note

Dispense in original unopened container.

Revised: 03/31/92
Interim revision: 02/17/94

---

# CORTICOSTEROIDS    Topical

This monograph includes information on the following: Alclometasone†; Amcinonide; Beclomethasone*; Betamethasone; Clobetasol; Clobetasone*; Clocortolone†; Desonide; Desoximetasone; Dexamethasone†; Diflorasone; Diflucortolone*; Flumethasone*; Fluocinolone; Fluocinonide; Flurandrenolide; Fluticasone†; Halcinonide; Halobetasol†; Hydrocortisone; Mometasone; Triamcinolone.

INN:

Beclomethasone—Beclometasone
Flumethasone—Flumetasone
Flurandrenolide—Fludroxycortide
Halobetasol—Ulobetasol
Hydrocortisone—Cortisol

VA CLASSIFICATION (Primary):

Alclometasone
   Topical—DE200
Amcinonide
   Topical—DE200
Beclomethasone
   Topical—DE200
Betamethasone
   Topical—DE200
Clobetasol
   Topical—DE200
Clobetasone
   Topical—DE200
Clocortolone
   Topical—DE200
Desonide
   Topical—DE200
Desoximetasone
   Topical—DE200

Dexamethasone
   Topical—DE200
Diflorasone
   Topical—DE200
Diflucortolone
   Topical—DE200
Flumethasone
   Topical—DE200
Fluocinolone
   Topical—DE200
Fluocinonide
   Topical—DE200
Flurandrenolide
   Topical—DE200
Fluticasone
   Topical—DE200
Halcinonide
   Topical—DE200
Halobetasol
   Topical—DE200
Hydrocortisone
   Dental—OR900
   Rectal—RS100
   Topical—DE200
Mometasone
   Topical—DE200
Triamcinolone
   Dental—OR900
   Topical—DE200

Other commonly used names are: Beclometasone [Beclomethasone], Cortisol [Hydrocortisone], Fludroxycortide [Flurandrenolide], Flumetasone [Flumethasone], Ulobetasol [Halobetasol].

Note: For a listing of dosage forms and brand names by country availability, see *Dosage Forms* section(s). For a listing of brand names for the articles in this monograph, refer to the General Index.

*Not commercially available in the U.S.
†Not commercially available in Canada.

## Category

Corticosteroid (topical); anti-inflammatory, steroidal (topical).

Note: Beclomethasone, Clobetasone, Diflucortolone, and Flumethasone are not commercially available in the U.S. Therefore, there is no U.S. product labeling identifying approved indications for these medications.

## Indications

Note: Bracketed information in the *Indications* section refers to uses that are not included in U.S. product labeling.

**Accepted**

Skin disorders (treatment):

Topical corticosteroids are indicated to provide symptomatic relief of inflammation and/or pruritus associated with acute and chronic corticosteroid-responsive disorders.

The location of the skin lesion to be treated should be considered in selecting a formulation. In areas with thinner skin, such as facial, eye, and intertriginous areas, low-potency corticosteroid preparations are preferred for long-term therapy. Low- to medium-potency products may be used on the ears, trunk, arms, legs, and scalp. Medium- to very high–potency formulations may be required for treatment of dermatologic disorders in areas with thicker skin, such as the palms and soles. Lotion, aerosol, and gel formulations are cosmetically better suited for hairy areas.

The type of lesion to be treated should also be considered in product selection. For dry, scaly, cracked, thickened, or hardened skin, ointments of medium potency are often used. Medium-potency lotions, aerosols, or creams are preferred in treating moister, weeping lesions or areas or in treating conditions with intense inflammation. High- to very high–potency ointments may be required to treat hyperkeratotic or thick skin lesions.

Topical corticosteroids of low to medium potency (See *Table 1, Pharmacology/Pharmacokinetics*) are used in the treatment of the following dermatologic disorders. Occlusive dressings may also be required for chronic or severe cases of lichen simplex chronicus, psoriasis, eczema, atopic dermatitis, or chronic hand eczema. The more potent topical corticosteroids and/or occlusive dressings may be required for conditions such as discoid lupus erythematosus, lichen planus, granuloma annulare, psoriatic plaques, and psoriasis affecting the palms, soles, elbows, or knees.

Dermatitis, atopic, mild to moderate
Dermatitis, contact
Dermatitis, nummular, mild
Dermatitis, seborrheic, facial and intertriginous areas
Dermatoses, inflammatory, other, mild to moderate
Dermatitis, other forms of, mild to moderate
Intertrigo
Lichen planus, facial and intertriginous areas
Lupus erythematosus, discoid, facial and intertriginous areas
Polymorphous light eruption
Pruritus, anogenital
Pruritus senilis
Psoriasis, facial and intertriginous areas or
Xerosis, inflammatory phase

Topical corticosteroids of medium to very high potency (See *Table 1, Pharmacology/Pharmacokinetics*) are used in the treatment of the following dermatologic disorders. Systemic therapy with, or intralesional injection of, a corticosteroid may be required for some of the disorders, as determined by the type and severity of the condition or inadequate response to topical therapy. Occlusive dressings may also be required for conditions such as discoid lupus erythematosus; bullous disorders; lichen planus; granuloma annulare; psoriatic plaques; and psoriasis affecting the palms, soles, elbows, or knees.

Alopecia areata
Dermatitis, atopic, moderate to severe
Dermatitis, exfoliative, generalized
Dermatitis, nummular, moderate to severe
Dermatoses, inflammatory, other, moderate to severe
Dermatitis, other forms of, moderate to severe
Granuloma annulare

Keloids, reduction of associated itching
Lichen planus
Lichen simplex chronicus
Lichen striatus
Lupus erythematosus, discoid and subacute cutaneous
Myxedema, pretibial
Necrobiosis lipoidica diabeticorum
Pemphigoid
Pemphigus
Pityriasis rosea
Psoriasis
Sarcoidosis or
Sunburn

Rectal disorders (treatment):

Hydrocortisone rectal suppositories are indicated as adjuvants in the treatment of ulcerative colitis of the rectum.

Hydrocortisone rectal ointment and suppositories are indicated in the treatment of inflammatory rectal disorders, such as cryptitis, inflamed hemorrhoids, and postirradiation or factitial proctitis.

Hydrocortisone rectal dosage forms are indicated in the treatment of anogenital pruritus.

Oral lesions, inflammatory or ulcerative (treatment):

Hydrocortisone acetate and triamcinolone acetonide dental pastes are indicated for adjunctive treatment and temporary relief of symptoms associated with nonherpetic oral inflammatory and ulcerative lesions, including recurrent aphthous stomatitis. [Formulations of high potency gels and very high potency ointments are also used in the treatment of aphthous stomatitis.][1]

[These agents are also used to treat other gingival disorders, such as desquamative gingivitis and oral lichen planus when the diagnosis has been confirmed by biopsy testing. Gel formulations of high potency corticosteroids and dental triamcinolone are used in the treatment of lichen planus of the mucous membranes.][1]

[Other topical corticosteroids are also used to treat gingival disorders.][1]

**Unaccepted**

Medium to very high potency topical corticosteroids should not be used in the treatment of rosacea and perioral dermatitis. Although topical corticosteroids may initially reduce the burning and pustulation associated with rosacea, a severe rebound flare-up may occur upon discontinuance of the steroid.

Topical corticosteroids should not be used in the treatment of acne.

Topical corticosteroids are not indicated for routine gingivitis, which should be treated by the removal of local causative factors and an improvement in oral hygiene.

---

[1]Not included in Canadian product labeling.

## Pharmacology/Pharmacokinetics

See *Table 1,* page 955.

**Physicochemical characteristics**

Molecular weight—

Alclometasone dipropionate: 521.05.
Amcinonide: 502.58.
Beclomethasone dipropionate: 521.05.
Betamethasone: 392.47.
Betamethasone benzoate: 496.57.
Betamethasone dipropionate: 504.59.
Betamethasone sodium phosphate: 516.41.
Betamethasone valerate: 476.58.
Clobetasol propionate: 466.99.
Clobetasone butyrate: 479.
Clocortolone pivalate: 495.03.
Desonide: 416.51.
Desoximetasone: 376.47.
Dexamethasone: 392.47.
Dexamethasone sodium phosphate: 516.41.
Diflorasone diacetate: 494.53.
Diflucortolone valerate: 478.6.
Flumethasone pivalate: 494.57.
Fluocinolone acetonide: 452.5.
Fluocinolone acetonide, dihydrate: 488.53.
Fluocinonide: 494.53.
Flurandrenolide: 436.52.
Fluticasone propionate: 500.57.
Halcinonide: 454.97.
Halobetasol propionate: 484.97.
Hydrocortisone: 362.47.
Hydrocortisone acetate: 404.5.
Hydrocortisone butyrate: 432.56.
Hydrocortisone valerate: 446.58.

Mometasone furoate: 521.44.
Triamcinolone acetonide: 434.5.

## Mechanism of action/Effect

Corticosteroids diffuse across cell membranes and complex with specific cytoplasmic receptors. These complexes then enter the cell nucleus, bind to DNA (chromatin), and stimulate transcription of messenger RNA (mRNA) and subsequent protein synthesis of various inhibitory enzymes responsible for anti-inflammatory effects of topical corticosteroids. These anti-inflammatory effects include inhibition of early processes such as edema, fibrin deposition, capillary dilatation, movement of phagocytes into the area, and phagocytic activities. Later processes, such as capillary production, collagen deposition, and keloid formation, are also inhibited by corticosteroids. The overall actions of topical corticosteroids are catabolic.

Factors that increase the clinical efficacy and potential for adverse effects of topical corticosteroids include enhancement of pharmacologic activity of the compound by altering molecular structure, increasing stratum corneum penetration of the compound, and increasing bioavailability of the compound from the vehicle.

The pharmacologic activity of topical corticosteroids is increased by several changes in molecular structure. Addition of a 9-alpha-fluorine atom increases the anti-inflammatory glucocorticoid activity, but simultaneously increases undesired mineralocorticoid activity. Mineralocorticoid activity is diminished by addition of a 16-hydroxy or 16-methyl group. Substitution or masking of 16- or 17-hydroxy groups with longer side chains such as acetonide, propionate, or valerate increases lipophilicity and subsequently stratum corneum penetration.

Dental paste in dental dosage forms acts as an adhesive vehicle for application of corticosteroids to oral mucosa. The vehicle also reduces pain by serving as a protective covering.

## Absorption

Absorbed systemically across the stratum corneum.

Stratum corneum penetration is primarily enhanced by increasing skin hydration and/or temperature, or by changes in molecular structure of the compound.

Hydrating the skin with occlusive dressings such as plastic wrap, a tight-fitting diaper or one covered with plastic pants, plastic tape, or dermatological patches can increase corticosteroid penetration by up to ten-fold. Ointment bases inhibit evaporation of moisture from skin. Intertriginous areas (axillae and groin) are self-occluding. Intertriginous areas and the face also have inherently thinner skin, are more macerated and therefore, allow for increased absorption.

Absorption of topical corticosteroids has been greatly increased by altering the product vehicle or the drug substance itself. Vehicles containing substances that solubilize the corticosteroid enhance absorption. Increasing the concentration of the drug increases skin penetration but may also increase wastage of the drug. Decreasing drug particle size has been shown to increase topical bioavailability.

Increased percutaneous absorption of corticosteroids also occurs when the skin or mucosa is abraded or inflamed, when body temperature is elevated, with prolonged use, or with extensive use.

There is some systemic absorption of topical corticosteroids through the oral mucosa; absorption increases with increased potency and prolonged use.

## Biotransformation

Primarily in skin; once absorbed systemically, in the liver. Corticosteroids that contain substituted 17-hydroxyl groups or that are fluorinated are resistant to local metabolism in the skin. Repeated application results in a cumulative depot effect in the skin, which may lead to a prolonged duration of action, increased side effects, and increased systemic absorption.

The following topical corticosteroids contain substituted 17-hydroxyl groups (S) and/or are fluorinated (F) compounds:

Alclometasone dipropionate—S
Amcinonide—S, F
Beclomethasone dipropionate—S
Betamethasone—F
Betamethasone benzoate—S, F
Betamethasone dipropionate—S, F
Betamethasone valerate—S, F
Clobetasol propionate—S, F
Clobetasone butyrate—S, F
Clocortolone pivalate—S, F
Desonide—S
Desoximetasone—S (17-hydrogen), F
Dexamethasone—F
Dexamethasone sodium phosphate—F
Diflorasone diacetate—S, F
Diflucortolone valerate—F
Flumethasone pivalate—F
Fluocinolone acetonide—S, F

Fluocinonide—S, F
Flurandrenolide—S, F
Fluticasone propionate—S, F
Halcinonide—S, F
Halobetasol propionate—S, F
Hydrocortisone butyrate—S
Hydrocortisone valerate—S
Mometasone furoate—S
Triamcinolone acetonide—S, F

# Precautions to Consider

## Carcinogenicity

Long-term animal studies have not been conducted on the carcinogenicity of topical corticosteroids.

## Mutagenicity

*Fluticasone*—No mutagenicity was shown with fluticasone propionate in the Ames test, *E. coli* fluctuation test, *S. cerevisiae* gene conversion test, or Chinese hamster ovarian cell assay. Fluticasone was not clastogenic in mouse micronucleus or cultured human lymphocyte tests.

*Halobetasol*—Halobetasol propionate was not found to be genotoxic in the Ames/*Salmonella* assay, sister chromatid exchange test in Chinese hamster somatic cells, chromosome aberration studies of germinal and somatic cells of rodents, and a mammalian spot test to determine point mutations. It was found to be mutagenic in a Chinese hamster micronucleus test, and in a mouse lymphoma gene mutation assay *in vitro*.

*Hydrocortisone* and *prednisolone*—Studies on mutagenicity with hydrocortisone and prednisolone yielded negative results.

*Mometasone*—No mutagenicity was shown with mometasone in the Ames test, mouse lymphoma assay, and a micronucleus test.

## Pregnancy/Reproduction

Pregnancy—Topical corticosteroids, especially the more potent ones, should not be used extensively, in large amounts, or for protracted periods in pregnant patients or in patients who are planning to become pregnant.

Appropriate studies in humans have not been done.

Studies in animals have shown that topical corticosteroids are systemically absorbed and may cause fetal abnormalities, especially when used in large amounts, with occlusive dressings, for prolonged periods of time, or if the more potent agents are used.

*Betamethasone*: A dose-related increase in fetal resorptions was observed in rabbits and mice given betamethasone dipropionate intramuscularly. This effect was not observed in rats. Teratogenic effects (umbilical hernia, cephalocele, cleft palate) were observed in rabbits when betamethasone dipropionate was administered intramuscularly.

*Desoximetasone*: In studies in mice, rats, and rabbits, desoximetasone has been shown to be teratogenic and embryotoxic with subcutaneous or dermal use.

*Fluticasone*: In studies in mice, fluticasone was found to be teratogenic (cleft palate) with subcutaneous usage of doses approximately 14 and 45 times the usual human topical dose.

*Halobetasol*: In studies in rats and rabbits, halobetasol propionate administered systemically was shown to be teratogenic at doses 3 to 33 times the usual human topical dose. Cleft palate was observed in both species. Omphalocele was seen in rats only. Halobetasol propionate was shown to be embryotoxic in rabbits but not in rats.

*Hydrocortisone dental dosage form*: Studies have not been done in animals.

FDA Pregnancy Category C.

## Breast-feeding

It is not known whether topical corticosteroids are distributed into breast milk. However, problems in humans have not been documented.

Systemic corticosteroids are distributed into breast milk and may cause unwanted effects in the infant such as growth suppression.

Topical corticosteroids should not be applied to the breasts prior to nursing.

## Pediatrics

Children and adolescents have a large skin surface area to body weight ratio and less developed, thinner skin, which may result in absorption of greater amounts of topical corticosteroids compared with older patients. Absorption is also greater in premature infants than in full term newborns, due to inadequate development of the stratum corneum.

Adrenal suppression, Cushing's syndrome, intracranial hypertension, and growth retardation due to the systemic absorption of topical corticosteroids have been documented in children. Therefore, special care must be exercised when these agents are used in children and growing adolescents, especially if factors that increase absorption are involved. It is recommended that only low-potency, unfluorinated topical corticosteroids that have a free 17-hydroxyl group be used in children or growing adolescents unless there is a demonstrated need for one of the other topical corticosteroids.

Generally, pediatric therapy continuing for longer than 2 weeks and consisting of doses in excess of one daily application (with medium- or high-potency corticosteroids) or two daily applications (with low-potency corticosteroids) should be evaluated carefully by the physician. This is especially important if medication is applied to more than 5 to 10% of the body surface or if an occlusive dressing is used. A tight-fitting diaper or one covered with plastic pants may constitute an occlusive dressing.

### Geriatrics

Although appropriate studies with topical corticosteroids have not been performed in the geriatric population, geriatrics-specific problems are not expected to limit the usefulness of topical corticosteroids in the elderly. However, elderly patients may be more likely to have pre-existing skin atrophy secondary to aging. Purpura and skin lacerations that may raise the skin and subcutaneous tissue from deep fascia may be more likely to occur with the use of topical corticosteroids in geriatric patients. Therefore, topical corticosteroids should be used infrequently, for brief periods, or under close medical supervision in patients with evidence of pre-existing skin atrophy. Use of lower potency topical corticosteroids may also be necessary in some patients.

### Laboratory value alterations

The following have been selected on the basis of their potential clinical significance (possible effect in parentheses where appropriate)—not necessarily inclusive (» = major clinical significance):

With physiology/laboratory test values

Adrenal function as assessed by corticotropin (ACTH) stimulation, measurement of 24-hour urine free cortisol or 17-hydroxycorticosteroids, or measurement of plasma cortisol and

Hypothalamic-pituitary-adrenal (HPA) axis function

(may be decreased if significant absorption of the corticosteroid occurs, especially in children)

Eosinophil count, total

(may be decreased as plasma cortisol concentration is decreased)

Glucose

(blood and urine concentrations may be increased if significant absorption of the corticosteroid occurs, because of intrinsic hyperglycemic activity of corticosteroids)

### Medical considerations/Contraindications

The medical considerations/contraindications included here have been selected on the basis of their potential clinical significance (reasons given in parentheses where appropriate)—not necessarily inclusive (» = major clinical significance).

*Risk-benefit should be considered when the following medical problems exist:*

Allergy to corticosteroids

Infection at treatment site

(may be exacerbated if no appropriate antimicrobial agent is used concurrently)

Skin atrophy, pre-existing

(may be exacerbated due to atrophigenic properties of corticosteroids)

*For use in the oral cavity*

Herpes simplex at treatment site

(may be transmitted to other sites, including the eye)

*With long-term use of more potent formulations or if substantial absorption occurs*

Cataracts

(corticosteroids may promote progression of cataracts, especially with the use of high- to very high–potency products in periorbital area)

Diabetes mellitus

(loss of control of diabetes may occur due to possible elevations in blood glucose)

Glaucoma

(intraocular pressure may be increased, especially with the use of high- to very high–potency products in periorbital area)

Tuberculosis

(may be exacerbated or reactivated; appropriate antitubercular chemotherapy or prophylaxis should be administered concurrently)

### Patient monitoring

The following may be especially important in patient monitoring (other tests may be warranted in some patients, depending on condition; » = major clinical significance):

Adrenal function assessment, such as urine or plasma cortisol concentration or ACTH stimulation test

(may be advisable during and following use if factors that increase percutaneous absorption are involved and treatment is prolonged)

## Side/Adverse Effects

Note: Generally, local or systemic adverse effects do not often occur with the use of low-potency topical corticosteroids. However, as with all topical corticosteroids, the incidence and severity of local or systemic side effects increase with factors that increase percutaneous absorption.

Percutaneous absorption of topical corticosteroids has resulted in systemic side effects such as hyperglycemia, glycosuria, and hypothalamic-pituitary-adrenal (HPA) axis suppression. HPA axis suppression has resulted from use of low doses of very high–potency products. HPA axis suppression has also resulted from use of less potent topical steroid preparations when occlusive dressings or excessive quantities were used. In all cases of HPA axis suppression, the effect was reversible upon discontinuation of therapy.

The following side/adverse effects have been selected on the basis of their potential clinical significance (possible signs and symptoms in parentheses where appropriate)—not necessarily inclusive:

### Those indicating the need for medical attention

Incidence less frequent or rare

*Allergic contact dermatitis* (burning and itching of skin; apparent chronic therapeutic failure)—may also be caused by vehicle ingredients; *folliculitis, furunculosis, pustules, pyoderma, or vesiculation* (painful, red or itchy, pus-containing blisters in hair follicles)—more frequent with occlusion or use of ointments in intertriginous areas; *hyperesthesia* (increased skin sensitivity); *numbness in fingers; purpura* (blood-containing blisters on skin); *rectal irritation* (rectal bleeding, pain, burning, itching, or blistering not present before therapy)—for rectal dosage forms; *skin atrophy* (thinning of skin with easy bruising, especially when used on facial or intertriginous areas); *skin infection, secondary*—more frequent with occlusion; *stripping of epidermal layer*—for tape dosage forms; *telangiectasia* (raised, dark red, wart-like spots on skin, especially when used on the face)

Incidence rare—with prolonged use or other factors that increase absorption

*Acneiform eruptions* (acne or oily skin, especially when used on the face); *cataracts, posterior subcapsular* (gradual blurring or loss of vision)—reported with use of systemic corticosteroids; caution advised with use of high- and very high–potency topical corticosteroids in periorbital area; *Cushing's syndrome* (filling or rounding out of the face; unusual tiredness or weakness; backache; irritability; mental depression; menstrual irregularities; in men—unusual decrease in sexual desire or ability); *dermatitis, perioral* (irritation of skin around mouth); *ecchymosis; edema* (increased blood pressure; swelling of feet or lower legs; rapid weight gain); *gastric ulcer* (loss of appetite; nausea; stomach bloating, pain, cramping, or burning; vomiting; weight loss); *glaucoma, secondary* (eye pain; gradual decrease in vision; nausea; vomiting)—with use of high- and very high–potency topical corticosteroids in periorbital area; *hirsutism or hypertrichosis* (unusual increase in hair growth, especially on the face); *hypertension; hypokalemic syndrome* (severe weakness of extremities and trunk; loss of appetite; nausea; vomiting; irregular heartbeat; muscle cramps or pain); *hypopigmentation* (lightened skin color); *or skin pigmentation changes, other; infection, aggravation of; miliaria rubra* (burning and itching of skin with pinhead-sized red blisters); *protein depletion* (muscle weakness); *skin laceration* (tearing of skin); *skin maceration* (softening of skin); *striae* (reddish purple lines on arms, face, legs, trunk, or groin); *subcutaneous tissue atrophy; unusual loss of hair*—especially on the scalp

### Those indicating need for medical attention only if they continue or are bothersome

Incidence less frequent or rare

*Burning, dryness, irritation, itching, or redness of skin, mild and transient; increased redness or scaling of skin lesions, mild and transient; skin rash, minor and transient*

## Overdose

For more information on the management of overdose or unintentional ingestion, **contact a Poison Control Center** (see *Poison Control Center Listing*).

### Treatment of overdose

For chronic topical overdose—Since there is no specific antidote available, treatment is symptomatic, supportive, and consists of discontinuance of topical corticosteroid therapy. Gradual withdrawal of the preparation may be necessary.

For acute oral overdose—Since there is no specific antidote available and serious adverse effects are unlikely, treatment consists of dilution with fluids.

## Patient Consultation

As an aid to patient consultation, refer to *Advice for the Patient, Corticosteroids (Dental)* or *Hydrocortisone (Rectal)*. For alclometasone, clocortolone, desonide, flumethasone, flurandrenolide (*Drenison-¹/₄* only), hydrocortisone, hydrocortisone acetate, and dexamethasone—*Corticosteroids—Low Potency (Topical)*. For amcinonide, betamethasone, clobetasol, clobetasone, desoximetasone, diflorasone, fluocinolone, fluocinonide, flurandrenolide (except *Drenison-¹/₄*), fluticasone, halcinonide, halobetasol, hydrocortisone butyrate, hydrocortisone valerate, mometasone, and triamcinolone—*Corticosteroids—Medium to Very High Potency (Topical)*.

In providing consultation, consider emphasizing the following selected information (» = major clinical significance):

### Before using this medication
» Conditions affecting use, especially:
    Allergies to corticosteroids
    Pregnancy—Use restricted because of possible fetal abnormalities
    Breast-feeding—Should not be applied to the breasts prior to nursing
    Use in children—Adrenal suppression, Cushing's syndrome, intracranial hypertension, growth retardation possible with improper use
    Use in the elderly—Caution recommended because purpura, skin lacerations may be more likely

### Proper use of this medication
    Proper administration technique:
*For all topical corticosteroids*
    Keeping away from eyes
» Not bandaging or otherwise wrapping the treated skin area unless directed to do so by physician
    Proper use of occlusive dressing, if prescribed
*For dental paste dosage forms*
    Applying with cotton applicator; pressing, not rubbing, paste on lesion
    Applying at bedtime and after meals for maximum effect
*For aerosol dosage forms*
    Reading and following patient directions carefully
    Avoiding breathing vapors of spray
    Avoiding getting vapors of spray in eyes
    Not smoking while using aerosols
    Not using aerosols near open flame
*For flurandrenolide tape*
    Reading and following patient directions carefully
*For rectal cream or ointment dosage forms*
    Reading and following patient directions carefully
*For rectal suppository dosage forms*
    Proper insertion technique
» Importance of not using more medication than the amount prescribed or recommended on package
» Checking with physician before using medication for other dental, skin, or rectal problems
    Missed dose: Using as soon as possible; not using if almost time for next dose
» Proper storage

### Precautions while using this medication
» Checking with physician or dentist if symptoms do not improve within 1 week or condition becomes worse
*For topical dosage forms*
    Not using tight-fitting diapers or plastic pants on a child if the diaper area is being treated with this medication

### Side/adverse effects
    Possible stinging when gel, lotion, solution, or aerosol form of medication is applied
    Signs of potential side effects, especially development of additional dermatologic problems, or rectal irritation (for rectal dosage forms)

## General Dosing Information

### For rectal and topical dosage forms
To minimize the possibility of significant systemic absorption of corticosteroids during long term therapy, treatment may be interrupted periodically, small amounts of the preparation may be applied, or one area of the body may be treated at a time.

Occlusion, whether by oleaginous ointment, a thin film of polyethylene, dermatological patch, or tape, promotes increased hydration of the stratum corneum and increased absorption. Rarely, body temperature may be elevated if large areas are covered with an occlusive dressing; occlusive dressings should not be used if body temperature is elevated. Use of intermittent, rather than continuous, occlusion may decrease the risk of side effects. Generally, occlusive dressings should be changed every 24 hours or more frequently. Very high–potency topical corticosteroid formulations should not be used with occlusive dressings.

Rarely, gradual withdrawal of therapy or supplemental systemic corticosteroid therapy may be required to avoid symptoms of steroid withdrawal. Gradual withdrawal of therapy by decreasing frequency of application or by using products of decreasing potency may be necessary also to avoid a rebound flare-up of certain conditions such as psoriasis. Tachyphylaxis may also result from continual usage.

Certain topical corticosteroids may be used as adjunctive therapy to antimicrobial agents for controlling inflammation, erythema, and pruritus associated with bacterial or fungal skin infections. If symptomatic relief is not noted within a few days to one week, the topical corticosteroid should be discontinued until the infection is controlled.

### For dental dosage forms only
Applying the paste with a cotton applicator will help to eliminate any possible absorption from contact with the skin.

The paste should be pressed, not rubbed, on the lesion. Rubbing the paste on the lesion will result in a granular, gritty sensation and cause the medication to crumble. A smooth, slippery film forms after application.

If significant repair or regeneration of oral tissues has not occurred in 7 days, the etiology of the lesion should be reinvestigated.

### For treatment of adverse effects
If a local infection develops at the site of application, discontinue occlusive dressings (if used) and institute appropriate antimicrobial therapy. Until the infection is controlled, discontinuance of the topical corticosteroid may be necessary.

If irritation or sensitization occurs at the site of application, discontinue use of the topical corticosteroid and institute appropriate symptomatic treatment.

---

### *ALCLOMETASONE*

## Summary of Differences

Pharmacology/pharmacokinetics:
    Substituted; non-fluorinated.
    Potency ranking—Low.

## Topical Dosage Forms

### ALCLOMETASONE DIPROPIONATE CREAM USP

**Usual adult dose**
Topical, to the skin, as a 0.05% cream two or three times a day.

**Usual pediatric dose**
Children and adolescents—Dosage has not been established.

**Strength(s) usually available**
U.S.—
    0.05% (Rx) [*Aclovate* (chlorocresol)].
Canada—
    Not commercially available.

**Packaging and storage**
Store below 40 °C (104 °F), preferably between 15 and 30 °C (59 and 86 °F), unless otherwise specified by manufacturer. Store in a tight container.

**Auxiliary labeling**
• For external use only.
• Do not use in or around the eye.

### ALCLOMETASONE DIPROPIONATE OINTMENT USP

**Usual adult dose**
Topical, to the skin, as a 0.05% ointment two or three times a day.

**Usual pediatric dose**
Children and adolescents—Dosage has not been established.

**Strength(s) usually available**
U.S.—
    0.05% (Rx) [*Aclovate*].
Canada—
    Not commercially available.

**Packaging and storage**
Store below 40 °C (104 °F), preferably between 15 and 30 °C (59 and 86 °F), unless otherwise specified by manufacturer. Store in a tight container.

**Auxiliary labeling**
- For external use only.
- Do not use in or around the eye.

---

## *AMCINONIDE*

## Summary of Differences

Pharmacology/pharmacokinetics:
    Substituted; fluorinated.
    Potency ranking—High.

## Topical Dosage Forms

### AMCINONIDE CREAM USP

**Usual adult dose**
Topical, to the skin, as a 0.1% cream two or three times a day.

**Usual pediatric dose**
Topical, to the skin, as a 0.1% cream once a day.

**Strength(s) usually available**
U.S.—
    0.1% (Rx) [*Cyclocort* (benzyl alcohol 2%)].
Canada—
    0.1% (Rx) [*Cyclocort* (benzyl alcohol 2%)].

**Packaging and storage**
Store below 40 °C (104 °F), preferably between 15 and 30 °C (59 and 86 °F), unless otherwise specified by manufacturer. Store in a tight container. Protect from freezing.

**Auxiliary labeling**
- For external use only.
- Do not use in or around the eye.

### AMCINONIDE LOTION

**Usual adult dose**
Topical, to the skin, as a 0.1% lotion two or three times a day.

**Usual pediatric dose**
Topical, to the skin, as a 0.1% lotion once a day.

**Strength(s) usually available**
U.S.—
    0.1% (Rx) [*Cyclocort* (benzyl alcohol 1%)].
Canada—
    0.1% (Rx) [*Cyclocort* (benzyl alcohol 1%)].

**Packaging and storage**
Store below 40 °C (104 °F), preferably between 15 and 30 °C (59 and 86 °F), in a well-closed container, unless otherwise specified by manufacturer. Protect from freezing.

**Auxiliary labeling**
- For external use only.
- Do not use in or around the eye.

### AMCINONIDE OINTMENT USP

**Usual adult dose**
Topical, to the skin, as a 0.1% ointment two times a day.

**Usual pediatric dose**
Topical, to the skin, as a 0.1% ointment once a day.

**Strength(s) usually available**
U.S.—
    0.1% (Rx) [*Cyclocort* (benzyl alcohol)].
Canada—
    0.1% (Rx) [*Cyclocort* (benzyl alcohol 2%)].

**Packaging and storage**
Store below 40 °C (104 °F), preferably between 15 and 30 °C (59 and 86 °F), unless otherwise specified by manufacturer. Store in a tight container. Protect from freezing.

**Auxiliary labeling**
- For external use only.
- Do not use in or around the eye.

---

## *BECLOMETHASONE*

## Summary of Differences

Pharmacology/pharmacokinetics:
    Substituted; non-fluorinated.
    Potency ranking—Medium.

## Topical Dosage Forms

### BECLOMETHASONE DIPROPIONATE CREAM

**Usual adult dose**
Topical, to the skin, as a 0.025% cream one or two times a day.

**Usual pediatric dose**
Dosage has not been established.

**Strength(s) usually available**
U.S.—
    Not commercially available.
Canada—
    0.025% (Rx) [*Propaderm*].

**Packaging and storage**
Store below 40 °C (104 °F), preferably between 15 and 30 °C (59 and 86 °F), unless otherwise specified by manufacturer.

**Auxiliary labeling**
- For external use only.
- Do not use in or around the eye.

### BECLOMETHASONE DIPROPIONATE LOTION

**Usual adult dose**
Topical, to the skin, as a 0.025% lotion one or two times a day.

**Usual pediatric dose**
Dosage has not been established.

**Strength(s) usually available**
U.S.—
    Not commercially available.
Canada—
    0.025% (Rx) [*Propaderm*].

**Packaging and storage**
Store below 40 °C (104 °F), preferably between 15 and 30 °C (59 and 86 °F), unless otherwise specified by manufacturer.

**Auxiliary labeling**
- For external use only.
- Do not use in or around the eye.

### BECLOMETHASONE DIPROPIONATE OINTMENT

**Usual adult dose**
Topical, to the skin, as a 0.025% ointment one or two times a day.

**Usual pediatric dose**
Dosage has not been established.

**Strength(s) usually available**
U.S.—
    Not commercially available.
Canada—
    0.025% (Rx) [*Propaderm*].

**Packaging and storage**
Store below 40 °C (104 °F), preferably between 15 and 30 °C (59 and 86 °F), unless otherwise specified by manufacturer.

**Auxiliary labeling**
- For external use only.
- Do not use in or around the eye.

---

## *BETAMETHASONE*

## Summary of Differences

Pharmacology/pharmacokinetics:
    Substituted (benzoate, dipropionate, valerate); fluorinated (base, benzoate, dipropionate, valerate).
        Potency ranking—
            Betamethasone benzoate, Medium.
            Betamethasone dipropionate (except for *Diprolene* and *Diprolene AF* products), High.
            *Diprolene* and *Diprolene AF* products, Very high.
            Betamethasone valerate, Medium.

# Topical Dosage Forms

## BETAMETHASONE BENZOATE CREAM

**Usual adult dose**
Topical, to the skin, as a 0.025% cream two to four times a day.

**Usual pediatric dose**
Topical, to the skin, as a 0.025% cream once a day.

**Strength(s) usually available**
U.S.—
   0.025% (Rx) [*Uticort*].

**Packaging and storage**
Store between 15 and 30 °C (59 and 86 °F), in a well-closed container, unless otherwise specified by manufacturer. Protect from freezing.

**Auxiliary labeling**
• For external use only.
• Do not use in or around the eye.

## BETAMETHASONE BENZOATE GEL USP

**Usual adult dose**
Topical, to the skin, as a 0.025% gel two to four times a day.

**Usual pediatric dose**
Topical, to the skin, as a 0.025% gel once a day.

**Strength(s) usually available**
U.S.—
   0.025% (Rx) [*Uticort* (alcohol 13.8%)].
Canada—
   0.025% (base) (Rx) [*Beben* (alcohol)].

**Packaging and storage**
Store below 40 °C (104 °F), preferably between 15 and 30 °C (59 and 86 °F), unless otherwise specified by manufacturer. Store in a tight container. Protect from freezing.

**Auxiliary labeling**
• For external use only.
• Do not use in or around the eye.

## BETAMETHASONE BENZOATE LOTION

**Usual adult dose**
Topical, to the skin, as a 0.025% lotion two to four times a day.

**Usual pediatric dose**
Topical, to the skin, as a 0.025% lotion once a day.

**Strength(s) usually available**
U.S.—
   0.025% (Rx) [*Uticort* (butylparaben; propylparaben; methylparaben)].

**Packaging and storage**
Store below 40 °C (104 °F), preferably between 15 and 30 °C (59 and 86 °F), in a well-closed container, unless otherwise specified by manufacturer. Protect from freezing.

**Auxiliary labeling**
• For external use only.
• Do not use in or around the eye.
• Shake well.

## BETAMETHASONE DIPROPIONATE CREAM (AUGMENTED)

Note: The dosing and strengths of betamethasone dipropionate cream (augmented) are expressed in terms of betamethasone base.

**Usual adult dose**
Topical, to the skin, as a 0.05% (base) cream one or two times a day. Augmented betamethasone dipropionate cream may be used for only a short duration of therapy and on small surface areas. Occlusive dressings should not be used.

**Usual pediatric dose**
Children up to 12 years of age—Use is not recommended.

**Strength(s) usually available**
U.S.—
   0.05% (base) (Rx) [*Diprolene AF*].
Canada—
   0.05% (base) (Rx) [*Diprolene*].

**Packaging and storage**
Store below 40 °C (104 °F), preferably between 15 and 30 °C (59 and 86 °F), unless otherwise specified by manufacturer. Store in a tight container. Protect from freezing.

**Auxiliary labeling**
• For external use only.
• Do not use in or around the eye.

## BETAMETHASONE DIPROPIONATE CREAM USP

Note: The dosing and strengths of betamethasone dipropionate cream are expressed in terms of betamethasone base.

**Usual adult dose**
Topical, to the skin, as a 0.05% (base) cream one or two times a day.

**Usual pediatric dose**
Topical, to the skin, as a 0.05% (base) cream once a day.

**Strength(s) usually available**
U.S.—
   0.05% (base) (Rx) [*Alphatrex; Diprosone; Maxivate; Teladar;* GENERIC].
Canada—
   0.05% (base) (Rx) [*Diprosone; Topilene; Topisone*].

**Packaging and storage**
Store below 40 °C (104 °F), preferably between 15 and 30 °C (59 and 86 °F), unless otherwise specified by manufacturer. Store in a tight container. Protect from freezing.

**Auxiliary labeling**
• For external use only.
• Do not use in or around the eye.

## BETAMETHASONE DIPROPIONATE GEL

Note: The dosing and strengths of betamethasone dipropionate gel are expressed in terms of betamethasone base.

**Usual adult dose**
Topical, to the skin, as a 0.05% (base) gel one or two times a day. Betamethasone dipropionate gel may be used for only a short duration of therapy and on small surface areas. Occlusive dressings should not be used.

**Usual pediatric dose**
Children up to 12 years of age—Use is not recommended.

**Strength(s) usually available**
U.S.—
   0.05% (base) (Rx) [*Diprolene*].
Canada—
   Not commercially available.

**Packaging and storage**
Store below 40 °C (104 °F), preferably between 15 and 30 °C (59 and 86 °F), unless otherwise specified by manufacturer. Store in a tight container. Protect from freezing.

**Auxiliary labeling**
• For external use only.
• Do not use in or around the eye.

## BETAMETHASONE DIPROPIONATE LOTION (AUGMENTED)

Note: The dosing and strengths of betamethasone dipropionate lotion (augmented) are expressed in terms of betamethasone base.

**Usual adult dose**
Topical, to the skin, as a 0.05% (base) lotion two times a day. Augmented betamethasone dipropionate lotion may be used for only a short duration of therapy and on small surface areas. Occlusive dressings should not be used.

**Usual pediatric dose**
Children up to 12 years of age—Dosage has not been established.

**Strength(s) usually available**
U.S.—
   0.05% (base) (Rx) [*Diprolene*].
Canada—
   Not commercially available.

**Packaging and storage**
Store below 40 °C (104 °F), preferably between 15 and 30 °C (59 and 86 °F), unless otherwise specified by manufacturer. Store in a tight container. Protect from light. Protect from freezing.

**Auxiliary labeling**
• For external use only.
• Do not use in or around the eye.
• Shake well.

## BETAMETHASONE DIPROPIONATE LOTION USP

Note: The dosing and strengths of betamethasone dipropionate lotion are expressed in terms of betamethasone base.

**Usual adult dose**
Topical, to the skin, as a 0.05% (base) lotion two times a day.

**Usual pediatric dose**

Topical, to the skin, as a 0.05% (base) lotion once a day.

**Strength(s) usually available**

U.S.—

0.05% (base) (Rx) [*Alphatrex; Diprosone; Maxivate;* GENERIC].

Canada—

0.05% (base) (Rx) [*Diprosone; Topisone*].

**Packaging and storage**

Store below 40 °C (104 °F), preferably between 15 and 30 °C (59 and 86 °F), unless otherwise specified by manufacturer. Store in a tight container. Protect from light. Protect from freezing.

**Auxiliary labeling**

• For external use only.
• Do not use in or around the eye.
• Shake well.

## BETAMETHASONE DIPROPIONATE OINTMENT (AUGMENTED)

Note: The dosing and strengths of betamethasone dipropionate ointment (augmented) are expressed in terms of betamethasone base.

**Usual adult dose**

Topical, to the skin, as a 0.05% (base) ointment one or two times a day. Augmented betametasone dipropionate ointment may be used for only a short duration of therapy and on small surface areas. Occlusive dressings should not be used.

**Usual pediatric dose**

Children up to 12 years of age—Use is not recommended.

**Strength(s) usually available**

U.S.—

0.05% (base) (Rx) [*Diprolene*].

Canada—

0.05% (base) (Rx) [*Diprolene*].

**Packaging and storage**

Store below 40 °C (104 °F), preferably between 15 and 30 °C (59 and 86 °F), unless otherwise specified by manufacturer. Store in a well-closed container. Protect from freezing.

**Auxiliary labeling**

• For external use only.
• Do not use in or around the eye.

## BETAMETHASONE DIPROPIONATE OINTMENT USP

Note: The dosing and strengths of betamethasone dipropionate ointment are expressed in terms of betamethasone base.

**Usual adult dose**

Topical, to the skin, as a 0.05% (base) ointment one or two times a day.

**Usual pediatric dose**

Topical, to the skin, as a 0.05% (base) ointment once a day.

**Strength(s) usually available**

U.S.—

0.05% (base) (Rx) [*Alphatrex; Diprosone; Maxivate;* GENERIC].

Canada—

0.05% (base) (Rx) [*Diprosone; Topilene; Topisone*].

**Packaging and storage**

Store below 40 °C (104 °F), preferably between 15 and 30 °C (59 and 86 °F), unless otherwise specified by manufacturer. Store in a well-closed container. Protect from freezing.

**Auxiliary labeling**

• For external use only.
• Do not use in or around the eye.

## BETAMETHASONE DIPROPIONATE TOPICAL AEROSOL

Note: The dosing and strengths of betamethasone dipropionate topical aerosol are expressed in terms of betamethasone base.

**Usual adult dose**

Topical, to the skin, a three-second spray of a 0.1% (base) aerosol three times a day.

**Usual pediatric dose**

Topical, to the skin, as a 0.1% (base) aerosol once a day.

**Strength(s) usually available**

U.S.—

0.1% (base) (Rx) [*Diprosone* (isobutane; isopropyl alcohol 10%; propane)].

Canada—

Not commercially available.

Note: A three-second spray delivers the equivalent of 60 mcg (0.06 mg) of betamethasone.

**Packaging and storage**

Store below 40 °C (104 °F), preferably between 2 and 30 °C (36 and 86 °F), unless otherwise specified by manufacturer. Protect from freezing.

**Auxiliary labeling**

• For external use only.
• Do not use in or around the eye.

**Note**

Explain administration technique.

When dispensing, include patient instructions.

## BETAMETHASONE VALERATE CREAM USP

Note: The dosing and strengths of betamethasone valerate cream are expressed in terms of betamethasone base.

**Usual adult dose**

Topical, to the skin, as a 0.01 or 0.1% (base) cream one to three times a day.

**Usual pediatric dose**

Topical, to the skin, as a 0.01% (base) cream one or two times a day; or a 0.1% (base) cream once a day.

**Strength(s) usually available**

U.S.—

0.01% (base) (Rx) [*Valisone Reduced Strength*].

0.1% (base) (Rx) [*Betatrex; Beta-Val; Dermabet; Valisone; Valnac;* GENERIC].

Canada—

0.05% (base) (Rx) [*Betaderm; Betnovate-¹/₂; Celestoderm-V/2; Ectosone Mild; Metaderm Mild; Novobetamet; Prevex B*].

0.1% (base) (Rx) [*Betaderm; Betnovate; Celestoderm-V; Ectosone Regular; Metaderm Regular; Novobetamet*].

**Packaging and storage**

Store below 40 °C (104 °F), preferably between 15 and 30 °C (59 and 86 °F), unless otherwise specified by manufacturer. Store in a tight container. Protect from freezing.

**Auxiliary labeling**

• For external use only.
• Do not use in or around the eye.

## BETAMETHASONE VALERATE LOTION USP

Note: The dosing and strengths of betamethasone valerate lotion are expressed in terms of betamethasone base.

**Usual adult dose**

Topical, to the skin, as a 0.1% (base) lotion one or two times a day.

**Usual pediatric dose**

Topical, to the skin, as a 0.1% (base) lotion once a day.

**Strength(s) usually available**

U.S.—

0.1% (base) (Rx) [*Betatrex; Beta-Val; Valisone;* GENERIC].

Canada—

0.05% (base) (Rx) [*Betnovate-¹/₂; Ectosone Mild*].

0.1% (base) (Rx) [*Betacort Scalp Lotion; Betaderm Scalp Lotion; Betnovate; Ectosone Regular; Ectosone Scalp Lotion; Valisone Scalp Lotion*].

**Packaging and storage**

Store between 15 and 30 °C (59 and 86 °F). Store in a tight, light-resistant container. Protect from freezing.

**Auxiliary labeling**

• For external use only.
• Do not use in or around the eye.
• Shake well.

## BETAMETHASONE VALERATE OINTMENT USP

Note: The dosing and strengths of betamethasone valerate ointment are expressed in terms of betamethasone base.

**Usual adult dose**

Topical, to the skin, as a 0.1% (base) ointment one to three times a day.

**Usual pediatric dose**

Topical, to the skin, as a 0.1% (base) ointment once a day.

**Strength(s) usually available**

U.S.—

0.1% (base) (Rx) [*Betatrex; Beta-Val; Valisone; Valnac;* GENERIC].

Canada—

0.05% (base) (Rx) [*Betaderm; Betnovate-¹/₂; Celestoderm-V/2; Metaderm Mild*].

0.1% (base) (Rx) [*Betaderm; Betnovate; Celestoderm-V; Metaderm Regular*].

**Packaging and storage**
Store below 40 °C (104 °F), preferably between 15 and 30 °C (59 and 86 °F). Store in a tight container. Protect from freezing.

**Auxiliary labeling**
• For external use only.
• Do not use in or around the eye.

---

### CLOBETASOL

## Summary of Differences
Pharmacology/pharmacokinetics:
   Substituted; fluorinated.
   Potency rating: Very high.

## Topical Dosage Forms
### CLOBETASOL PROPIONATE CREAM

**Usual adult dose**
Topical, to the skin, as a 0.05% cream two or three times a day. Clobetasol propionate cream may be used for only a short duration of therapy and on small surface areas. Occlusive dressings should not be used.

**Usual pediatric dose**
Children up to 12 years of age—Use is not recommended.

**Strength(s) usually available**
U.S.—
   0.05% (Rx) [*Temovate*].
Canada—
   0.05% (Rx) [*Dermovate*].

**Packaging and storage**
Store below 40 °C (104 °F), preferably between 15 and 30 °C (59 and 86 °F), in a well-closed container, unless otherwise specified by manufacturer. Do not refrigerate. Protect from freezing.

**Auxiliary labeling**
• For external use only.
• Do not use in or around the eye.

### CLOBETASOL PROPIONATE SOLUTION

**Usual adult dose**
Topical, to the scalp, as a 0.05% solution two times a day. Clobetasol propionate solution may be used for only a short duration of therapy and on small surface areas. Occlusive dressings should not be used.

**Usual pediatric dose**
Children up to 12 years of age—Use is not recommended.

**Strength(s) usually available**
U.S.—
   0.05% (Rx) [*Temovate Scalp Application* (isopropyl alcohol)].
Canada—
   0.05% (Rx) [*Dermovate Scalp Lotion* (alcohol)].

**Packaging and storage**
Store below 40 °C (104 °F), preferably between 15 and 30 °C (59 and 86 °F), in a well-closed container, unless otherwise specified by manufacturer. Protect from freezing.

**Auxiliary labeling**
• For external use only.
• Do not use in or around the eye.

### CLOBETASOL PROPIONATE OINTMENT

**Usual adult dose**
Topical, to the skin, as a 0.05% ointment two or three times a day. Clobetasol propionate ointment may be used for only a short duration of therapy and on small surface areas. Occlusive dressings should not be used.

**Usual pediatric dose**
Children up to 12 years of age—Use is not recommended.

**Strength(s) usually available**
U.S.—
   0.05% (Rx) [*Temovate*].
Canada—
   0.05% (Rx) [*Dermovate*].

**Packaging and storage**
Store below 40 °C (104 °F), preferably between 15 and 30 °C (59 and 86 °F), in a well-closed container, unless otherwise specified by manufacturer. Protect from freezing.

**Auxiliary labeling**
• For external use only.
• Do not use in or around the eye.

---

### CLOBETASONE

## Summary of Differences
Pharmacology/pharmacokinetics:
   Substituted; fluorinated.
   Potency rating—Medium.

## Topical Dosage Forms
### CLOBETASONE BUTYRATE CREAM

**Usual adult dose**
Topical, to the skin, as a 0.05% cream two or three times a day.

**Usual adult prescribing limits**
Topical, to the skin, up to 100 grams per week.

**Usual pediatric dose**
Dosage has not been established.

**Strength(s) usually available**
U.S.—
   Not commercially available.
Canada—
   0.05% (Rx) [*Eumovate*].

**Packaging and storage**
Store below 40 °C (104 °F), preferably between 15 and 30 °C (59 and 86 °F), unless otherwise specified by manufacturer.

**Auxiliary labeling**
• For external use only.
• Do not use in or around the eye.

### CLOBETASONE BUTYRATE OINTMENT

**Usual adult dose**
Topical, to the skin, as a 0.05% ointment two or three times a day.

**Usual adult prescribing limits**
Topical, to the skin, up to 100 grams per week.

**Usual pediatric dose**
Dosage has not been established.

**Strength(s) usually available**
U.S.—
   Not commercially available.
Canada—
   0.05% (Rx) [*Eumovate*].

**Packaging and storage**
Store below 40 °C (104 °F), preferably between 15 and 30 °C (59 and 86 °F), unless otherwise specified by manufacturer.

**Auxiliary labeling**
• For external use only.
• Do not use in or around the eye.

---

### CLOCORTOLONE

## Summary of Differences
Pharmacology/pharmacokinetics:
   Substituted; fluorinated.
   Potency rating—Low.

## Topical Dosage Forms
### CLOCORTOLONE PIVALATE CREAM USP

**Usual adult dose**
Topical, to the skin, as a 0.1% cream three times a day.

**Usual pediatric dose**
Dosage has not been established.

**Strength(s) usually available**
U.S.—
   0.1% (Rx) [*Cloderm* (methylparaben; propylparaben)].
Canada—
   Not commercially available.

**Packaging and storage**
Store below 40 °C (104 °F), preferably between 15 and 30 °C (59 and 86 °F), unless otherwise specified by manufacturer. Store in a tight, light-resistant container. Protect from freezing.

**Auxiliary labeling**
• For external use only.
• Do not use in or around the eye.

---

## *DESONIDE*

---

## Summary of Differences

Pharmacology/pharmacokinetics:
    Substituted; non-fluorinated.
    Potency rating—Low.

## Topical Dosage Forms

### DESONIDE CREAM

**Usual adult dose**
Topical, to the skin, as a 0.05% cream two to four times a day.

**Usual pediatric dose**
Topical, to the skin, as a 0.05% cream once a day.

**Strength(s) usually available**
U.S.—
    0.05% (Rx) [DesOwen; Tridesilon; GENERIC].
Canada—
    0.05% (Rx) [Tridesilon].

**Packaging and storage**
Store between 15 and 30 °C (59 and 86 °F), in a tight container, unless otherwise specified by manufacturer. Protect from freezing.

**Auxiliary labeling**
• For external use only.
• Do not use in or around the eye.

### DESONIDE LOTION

**Usual adult dose**
Topical, to the skin, as a 0.05% lotion two to four times a day.

**Strength(s) usually available**
U.S.—
    0.05% (Rx) [DesOwen].
Canada—
    Not commercially available.

**Packaging and storage**
Store between 15 and 30 °C (59 and 86 °F), in a tight container, unless otherwise specified by manufacturer. Protect from freezing.

**Auxiliary labeling**
• For external use only.
• Shake well before using.
• Do not use in or around the eye.

### DESONIDE OINTMENT

**Usual adult dose**
Topical, to the skin, as a 0.05% ointment two to four times a day.

**Usual pediatric dose**
Topical, to the skin, as a 0.05% ointment once a day.

**Strength(s) usually available**
U.S.—
    0.05% (Rx) [DesOwen; Tridesilon].
Canada—
    0.05% (Rx) [Tridesilon].

**Packaging and storage**
Store between 15 and 30 °C (59 and 86 °F), in a tight container, unless otherwise specified by manufacturer. Protect from freezing.

**Auxiliary labeling**
• For external use only.
• Do not use in or around the eye.

---

## *DESOXIMETASONE*

---

## Summary of Differences

Pharmacology/pharmacokinetics:
    Substituted (17-H); fluorinated.

Potency rating—
    High (except cream 0.05%).
    Cream 0.05%, Medium.

## Topical Dosage Forms

### DESOXIMETASONE CREAM USP

**Usual adult dose**
Topical, to the skin, as a 0.05 or 0.25% cream two times a day.

**Usual pediatric dose**
Topical, to the skin, as a 0.05 or 0.25% cream once a day.

**Strength(s) usually available**
U.S.—
    0.05% (Rx) [Topicort LP; GENERIC].
    0.25% (Rx) [Topicort; GENERIC].
Canada—
    0.05% (Rx) [Topicort Mild].
    0.25% (Rx) [Topicort].

**Packaging and storage**
Store between 15 and 30 °C (59 and 86 °F), in a well-closed container, unless otherwise specified by manufacturer. Protect from freezing.

**Auxiliary labeling**
• For external use only.
• Do not use in or around the eye.

### DESOXIMETASONE GEL USP

**Usual adult dose**
Topical, to the skin, as a 0.05% gel two times a day.

**Usual pediatric dose**
Topical, to the skin, as a 0.05% gel once a day.

**Strength(s) usually available**
U.S.—
    0.05% (Rx) [Topicort (alcohol 20%)].
Canada—
    0.05% (Rx) [Topicort (alcohol)].

**Packaging and storage**
Store between 15 and 30 °C (59 and 86 °F), in well-closed container, unless otherwise specified by manufacturer. Protect from freezing.

**Auxiliary labeling**
• For external use only.
• Do not use in or around the eye.

### DESOXIMETASONE OINTMENT USP

**Usual adult dose**
Topical, to the skin, as a 0.25% ointment two times a day.

**Usual pediatric dose**
Topical, to the skin, as a 0.25% ointment once a day.

**Strength(s) usually available**
U.S.—
    0.25% (Rx) [Topicort].
Canada—
    Not commercially available.

**Packaging and storage**
Store between 15 and 30 °C (59 and 86 °F), in well-closed container, unless otherwise specified by manufacturer. Protect from freezing.

**Auxiliary labeling**
• For external use only.
• Do not use in or around the eye.

---

## *DEXAMETHASONE*

---

## Summary of Differences

Pharmacology/pharmacokinetics:
    Unsubstituted; fluorinated.
    Potency rating—Low.

## Topical Dosage Forms

### DEXAMETHASONE GEL USP

**Usual adult dose**
Topical, to the skin, as a 0.1% gel three or four times a day.

**Usual pediatric dose**
Topical, to the skin, as a 0.1% gel one or two times a day.

**Strength(s) usually available**

U.S.—

0.1% (Rx) [*Decaderm*].

Canada—

Not commercially available.

**Packaging and storage**

Store below 30 °C (86 °F), in a tight container. Protect from freezing.

**Auxiliary labeling**

• For external use only.
• Do not use in or around the eye.

## DEXAMETHASONE TOPICAL AEROSOL USP (SOLUTION)

**Usual adult dose**

Topical, to the skin, as a 0.01 or 0.04% aerosol two to four times a day.

**Usual pediatric dose**

Topical, to the skin, as a 0.01 or 0.04% aerosol one or two times a day.

**Strength(s) usually available**

U.S.—

0.01% (Rx) [*Aeroseb-Dex* (alcohol 59%)].

0.04% (Rx) [*Decaspray*].

Note: Each one-second spray of 0.01% and 0.04% aerosols delivers 20 mcg (0.02 mg) and 75 mcg (0.075 mg) of dexamethasone, respectively.

Canada—

Not commercially available.

**Packaging and storage**

Store below 40 °C (104 °F). Protect from freezing.

**Auxiliary labeling**

• For external use only.
• Do not use in or around the eye.
• Shake gently.

**Note**

Explain administration technique.

When dispensing, include patient instructions.

This medication comes with a special applicator tube for use on the scalp.

## DEXAMETHASONE SODIUM PHOSPHATE CREAM USP

**Usual adult dose**

Topical, to the skin, as a 0.1% (phosphate) cream three or four times a day.

**Usual pediatric dose**

Topical, to the skin, as a 0.1% (phosphate) cream once a day.

**Strength(s) usually available**

U.S.—

0.1% (phosphate) (Rx) [*Decadron* (methylparaben)].

Canada—

Not commercially available.

**Packaging and storage**

Store below 40 °C (104 °F), preferably between 15 and 30 °C (59 and 86 °F), unless otherwise specified by manufacturer. Store in a tight container. Protect from freezing.

**Auxiliary labeling**

• For external use only.
• Do not use in or around the eye.

---

### DIFLORASONE

## Summary of Differences

Pharmacology/pharmacokinetics:

Substituted; fluorinated.

Potency rating—

High (except *Psorcon* ointment).

*Psorcon* ointment, Very high.

## Topical Dosage Forms

### DIFLORASONE DIACETATE CREAM USP

**Usual adult dose**

Topical, to the skin, as a 0.05% cream one to four times a day.

Note: Some patients may be maintained with once daily applications after the initial acute symptoms subside. Once daily dosage may also be used to taper therapy before discontinuance.

**Usual pediatric dose**

Topical, to the skin, as a 0.05% cream once a day.

**Strength(s) usually available**

U.S.—

0.05% (Rx) [*Florone; Florone E; Maxiflor*].

Canada—

0.05% (Rx) [*Florone*].

**Packaging and storage**

Store between 15 and 30 °C (59 and 86 °F), in a well-closed container, unless otherwise specified by manufacturer. Protect from freezing.

**Auxiliary labeling**

• For external use only.
• Do not use in or around the eye.

## DIFLORASONE DIACETATE OINTMENT USP

**Usual adult dose**

Topical, to the skin, as a 0.05% ointment one to four times a day.

Note: Some patients may be maintained with once daily applications after the initial acute symptoms subside. Once daily dosage may also be used to taper therapy before discontinuance.

*Psorcon* may be used for only a short duration of therapy and on small surface areas. Occlusive dressings should not be used with *Psorcon*.

**Usual pediatric dose**

Topical, to the skin, as a 0.05% ointment once a day.

Note: *Psorcon* should be used cautiously in patients up to 12 years of age.

**Strength(s) usually available**

U.S.—

0.05% (Rx) [*Florone; Maxiflor; Psorcon*].

Canada—

0.05% (Rx) [*Florone*].

**Packaging and storage**

Store between 15 and 30 °C (59 and 86 °F), in a well-closed container, unless otherwise specified by manufacturer. Protect from freezing.

**Auxiliary labeling**

• For external use only.
• Do not use in or around the eye.

---

### DIFLUCORTOLONE

## Summary of Differences

Pharmacology/pharmacokinetics:

Unsubstituted; fluorinated.

Potency rating—Medium.

## Topical Dosage Forms

### DIFLUCORTOLONE VALERATE CREAM

**Usual adult dose**

Topical, to the skin, as a 0.1% cream one to three times a day.

Note: Some patients may be maintained with once daily applications after the initial acute symptoms subside. Once daily dosage may also be used to taper therapy before discontinuance.

**Usual adult prescribing limits**

Topical, to the skin, up to 100 grams per week.

**Usual pediatric dose**

Dosage has not been established.

**Strength(s) usually available**

U.S.—

Not commercially available.

Canada—

0.1% (Rx) [*Nerisone; Nerisone Oily*].

**Packaging and storage**

Store below 40 °C (104 °F), preferably between 15 and 30 °C (59 and 86 °F), unless otherwise specified by manufacturer.

**Auxiliary labeling**

• For external use only.
• Do not use in or around the eye.

## DIFLUCORTOLONE VALERATE OINTMENT

**Usual adult dose**
Topical, to the skin, as a 0.1% ointment one to three times a day.

Note: Some patients may be maintained with once daily applications after the initial acute symptoms subside. Once daily dosage may also be used to taper therapy before discontinuance.

**Usual adult prescribing limits**
Topical, to the skin, up to 100 grams per week.

**Usual pediatric dose**
Dosage has not been established.

**Strength(s) usually available**
U.S.—
    Not commercially available.
Canada—
    0.1% (Rx) [*Nerisone*].

**Packaging and storage**
Store below 40 °C (104 °F), preferably between 15 and 30 °C (59 and 86 °F), unless otherwise specified by manufacturer.

**Auxiliary labeling**
• For external use only.
• Do not use in or around the eye.

---

### FLUMETHASONE

## Summary of Differences

Pharmacology/pharmacokinetics:
    Unsubstituted; fluorinated.
    Potency rating—Low.

## Topical Dosage Forms

### FLUMETHASONE PIVALATE CREAM USP

**Usual adult dose**
Topical, to the skin, as a 0.03% cream one to three times a day.

**Usual pediatric dose**
Topical, to the skin, as a 0.03% cream once a day.

**Strength(s) usually available**
U.S.—
    Not commercially available.
Canada—
    0.03% (Rx) [*Locacorten* (methylparaben; propylparaben)].

**Packaging and storage**
Store below 40 °C (104 °F), preferably between 15 and 30 °C (59 and 86 °F), in a well-closed container, unless otherwise specified by manufacturer. Protect from freezing.

**Auxiliary labeling**
• For external use only.
• Do not use in or around the eye.

### FLUMETHASONE PIVALATE OINTMENT

**Usual adult dose**
Topical, to the skin, as a 0.03% ointment one to three times a day.

**Usual pediatric dose**
Topical, to the skin, as a 0.03% ointment once a day.

**Strength(s) usually available**
U.S.—
    Not commercially available.
Canada—
    0.03% (Rx) [*Locacorten* (methylparaben; propylparaben)].

**Packaging and storage**
Store below 40 °C (104 °F), preferably between 15 and 30 °C (59 and 86 °F), in a well-closed container, unless otherwise specified by manufacturer. Protect from freezing.

**Auxiliary labeling**
• For external use only.
• Do not use in or around the eye.

---

### FLUOCINOLONE

## Summary of Differences

Pharmacology/pharmacokinetics:
    Substituted; fluorinated.

Potency rating—
    Medium (except cream 0.2%).
    Cream 0.2%, High.

## Topical Dosage Forms

### FLUOCINOLONE ACETONIDE CREAM USP

**Usual adult dose**
Topical, to the skin, as a 0.01 to 0.2% cream two to four times a day.

**Usual pediatric dose**
Topical, to the skin, as a 0.01% cream one or two times a day; or as a 0.025 or 0.2% cream once a day.

Note: The 0.2% strength is not recommended for use in children up to 2 years of age, should not be used for long periods, and should not be used in quantities greater than 2 grams per day.

**Strength(s) usually available**
U.S.—
    0.01% (Rx) [*Bio-Syn; Fluocet; Flurosyn; Synalar;* GENERIC].
    0.025% (Rx) [*Bio-Syn; Fluocet; Flurosyn; Synalar; Synemol*].
    0.2% (Rx) [*Synalar-HP*].
Canada—
    0.01% (Rx) [*Fluoderm; Fluolar; Fluonide; Synalar; Synamol*].
    0.025% (Rx) [*Fluoderm; Fluolar; Fluonide; Synalar; Synamol*].

**Packaging and storage**
Store below 40 °C (104 °F), preferably between 15 and 30 °C (59 and 86 °F), unless otherwise specified by manufacturer. Store in a tight container. Protect from freezing.

**Auxiliary labeling**
• For external use only.
• Do not use in or around the eye.

### FLUOCINOLONE ACETONIDE OINTMENT USP

**Usual adult dose**
Topical, to the skin, as a 0.025% ointment two to four times a day.

**Usual pediatric dose**
Topical, to the skin, as a 0.025% ointment once a day.

**Strength(s) usually available**
U.S.—
    0.025% (Rx) [*Flurosyn; Synalar;* GENERIC].
Canada—
    0.01% (Rx) [*Fluoderm*].
    0.025% (Rx) [*Fluoderm; Synalar*].

**Packaging and storage**
Store below 40 °C (104 °F), preferably between 15 and 30 °C (59 and 86 °F), unless otherwise specified by manufacturer. Store in a tight container. Protect from freezing.

**Auxiliary labeling**
• For external use only.
• Do not use in or around the eye.

### FLUOCINOLONE ACETONIDE TOPICAL SOLUTION USP

**Usual adult dose**
Topical, to the skin, as a 0.01% solution two to four times a day.

**Usual pediatric dose**
Topical, to the skin, as a 0.01% solution one or two times a day.

**Strength(s) usually available**
U.S.—
    0.01% (Rx) [*Fluonid; Synalar;* GENERIC].
Canada—
    0.01% (Rx) [*Synalar*].

**Packaging and storage**
Store below 40 °C (104 °F), preferably between 15 and 30 °C (59 and 86 °F), unless otherwise specified by manufacturer. Store in a tight container. Protect from freezing.

**Auxiliary labeling**
• For external use only.
• Do not use in or around the eye.

---

### FLUOCINONIDE

## Summary of Differences

Pharmacology/pharmacokinetics:
    Substituted; fluorinated.
    Potency rating—High.

# Topical Dosage Forms

## FLUOCINONIDE CREAM USP

**Usual adult dose**
Topical, to the skin, as a 0.05% cream two to four times a day.

**Usual pediatric dose**
Topical, to the skin, as a 0.05% cream once a day.

**Strength(s) usually available**
U.S.—
 0.05% (Rx) [*Fluocin; Licon; Lidex; Lidex-E;* GENERIC].
Canada—
 0.01% (Rx) [*Lidex*].
 0.05% (Rx) [*Lidemol; Lidex; Lyderm*].

**Packaging and storage**
Store below 40 °C (104 °F), preferably between 15 and 30 °C (59 and 86 °F), unless otherwise specified by manufacturer. Store in a tight container. Protect from freezing.

**Auxiliary labeling**
• For external use only.
• Do not use in or around the eye.

## FLUOCINONIDE GEL USP

**Usual adult dose**
Topical, to the skin, as a 0.05% gel two to four times a day.

**Usual pediatric dose**
Topical, to the skin, as a 0.05% gel once a day.

**Strength(s) usually available**
U.S.—
 0.05% (Rx) [*Lidex;* GENERIC].
Canada—
 0.05% (Rx) [*Topsyn*].

**Packaging and storage**
Store below 40 °C (104 °F), preferably between 15 and 30 °C (59 and 86 °F), unless otherwise specified by manufacturer. Protect from freezing. Store in a tight container.

**Auxiliary labeling**
• For external use only.
• Do not use in or around the eye.

## FLUOCINONIDE OINTMENT USP

**Usual adult dose**
Topical, to the skin, as a 0.05% ointment two to four times a day.

**Usual pediatric dose**
Topical, to the skin, as a 0.05% ointment once a day.

**Strength(s) usually available**
U.S.—
 0.05% (Rx) [*Lidex;* GENERIC].
Canada—
 0.01% (Rx) [*Lidex*].
 0.05% (Rx) [*Lidex*].

**Packaging and storage**
Store below 40 °C (104 °F), preferably between 15 and 30 °C (59 and 86 °F), unless otherwise specified by manufacturer. Store in a tight container. Protect from freezing.

**Auxiliary labeling**
• For external use only.
• Do not use in or around the eye.

## FLUOCINONIDE TOPICAL SOLUTION USP

**Usual adult dose**
Topical, to the skin, as a 0.05% solution two to four times a day.

**Usual pediatric dose**
Topical, to the skin, as a 0.05% solution once a day.

**Strength(s) usually available**
U.S.—
 0.05% (Rx) [*Lidex* (alcohol 35%); GENERIC].
Canada—
 0.05% (Rx) [*Lidex* (alcohol 35%)].

**Packaging and storage**
Store below 40 °C (104 °F), preferably between 15 and 30 °C (59 and 86 °F), unless otherwise specified by manufacturer. Store in a tight container. Protect from freezing.

**Auxiliary labeling**
• For external use only.
• Do not use in or around the eye.

# Summary of Differences

Pharmacology/pharmacokinetics:
 Substituted; fluorinated.
  Potency ranking—
   Medium (except cream and ointment 0.0125%).
   Cream and ointment 0.0125%, Low.

# Topical Dosage Forms

## FLURANDRENOLIDE CREAM USP

**Usual adult dose**
Topical, to the skin, as a 0.025 or 0.05% cream two or three times a day.

**Usual pediatric dose**
Topical, to the skin, as a 0.025% cream one or two times a day; or as a 0.05% cream once a day.

**Strength(s) usually available**
U.S.—
 0.025% (Rx) [*Cordran SP*].
 0.05% (Rx) [*Cordran SP*].
Canada—
 0.0125% (Rx) [*Drenison-¹/₄*].
 0.05% (Rx) [*Drenison*].

**Packaging and storage**
Store below 40 °C (104 °F), preferably between 15 and 30 °C (59 and 86 °F), unless otherwise specified by manufacturer. Store in a tight container. Protect from light. Protect from freezing.

**Auxiliary labeling**
• For external use only.
• Do not use in or around the eye.

## FLURANDRENOLIDE LOTION USP

**Usual adult dose**
Topical, to the skin, as a 0.05% lotion two or three times a day.

**Usual pediatric dose**
Topical, to the skin, as a 0.05% lotion once a day.

**Strength(s) usually available**
U.S.—
 0.05% (Rx) [*Cordran*].
Canada—
 Not commercially available.

**Packaging and storage**
Store below 40 °C (104 °F), preferably between 15 and 30 °C (59 and 86 °F). Store in a tight container. Protect from light. Protect from freezing.

**Auxiliary labeling**
• For external use only.
• Do not use in or around the eye.
• Shake well.

## FLURANDRENOLIDE OINTMENT USP

**Usual adult dose**
Topical, to the skin, as a 0.025 or 0.05% ointment two or three times a day.

**Usual pediatric dose**
Topical, to the skin, as a 0.025% ointment one or two times a day; or as a 0.05% ointment once a day.

**Strength(s) usually available**
U.S.—
 0.025% (Rx) [*Cordran*].
 0.05% (Rx) [*Cordran*].
Canada—
 0.0125% (Rx) [*Drenison-¹/₄*].
 0.05% (Rx) [*Drenison*].

**Packaging and storage**
Store below 40 °C (104 °F), preferably between 15 and 30 °C (59 and 86 °F), unless otherwise specified by manufacturer. Store in a tight container. Protect from light. Protect from freezing.

**Auxiliary labeling**
• For external use only.
• Do not use in or around the eye.

## FLURANDRENOLIDE TAPE USP

**Usual adult dose**
Topical, to the skin, as a tape containing 4 mcg (0.004 mg) of flurandrenolide per square centimeter, to be replaced every twelve to twenty-
four hours.

**Usual pediatric dose**
Topical, to the skin, as a tape containing 4 mcg (0.004 mg) of flurandrenolide per square centimeter; to be replaced once a day.

**Strength(s) usually available**
U.S.—
    4 mcg (0.004 mg) per square centimeter (Rx) [*Cordran*].
Canada—
    4 mcg (0.004 mg) per square centimeter (Rx) [*Drenison*].

**Packaging and storage**
Store between 15 and 30 °C (59 and 86 °F).

**Auxiliary labeling**
• For external use only.

**Note**
Explain administration technique.
When dispensing, include patient instructions.

**Additional information**
Tape of flexible polyethylene film impregnated with flurandrenolide in the
acrylic adhesive serves as an occlusive dressing, and should not be
used in intertriginous areas or applied to lesions exuding serum.

---

### *FLUTICASONE*

## Summary of Differences

Pharmacology/pharmacokinetics:
    Substituted; fluorinated.
    Potency ranking—Medium.

## Topical Dosage Forms

### FLUTICASONE PROPIONATE CREAM

**Usual adult dose**
Topical, to the skin, as a 0.05% cream two times a day.

**Usual pediatric dose**
Dosage has not been established.

**Strength(s) usually available**
U.S.—
    0.05% (Rx) [*Cutivate*].
Canada—
    Not commercially available.

**Packaging and storage**
Store below 40 °C (104 °F), preferably between 2 and 30 °C (36 and 86
°F), in a well-closed container, unless otherwise specified by
manufacturer.

**Auxiliary labeling**
• For external use only.
• Do not use in or around the eye.

### FLUTICASONE PROPIONATE OINTMENT

**Usual adult dose**
Topical, to the skin, as a 0.005% ointment two times a day.

**Usual pediatric dose**
Dosage has not been established.

**Strength(s) usually available**
U.S.—
    0.005% (Rx) [*Cutivate*].
Canada—
    Not commercially available.

**Packaging and storage**
Store below 40 °C (104 °F), preferably between 2 and 30 °C (36 and 86
°F), in a well-closed container, unless otherwise specified by
manufacturer.

**Auxiliary labeling**
• For external use only.
• Do not use in or around the eye.

---

### *HALCINONIDE*

## Summary of Differences

Pharmacology/pharmacokinetics:
    Substituted; fluorinated.
    Potency ranking—High.

## Topical Dosage Forms

### HALCINONIDE CREAM USP

**Usual adult dose**
Topical, to the skin, as a 0.025 or 0.1% cream one to three times a day.

**Usual pediatric dose**
Topical, to the skin, as a 0.025 or 0.1% cream once a day.

**Strength(s) usually available**
U.S.—
    0.025% (Rx) [*Halog*].
    0.1% (Rx) [*Halog; Halog-E*].
Canada—
    0.1% (Rx) [*Halog*].

**Packaging and storage**
Store between 15 and 30 °C (59 and 86 °F), unless otherwise specified by
manufacturer. Store in a well-closed container. Protect from freezing.

**Auxiliary labeling**
• For external use only.
• Do not use in or around the eye.

### HALCINONIDE OINTMENT USP

**Usual adult dose**
Topical, to the skin, as a 0.1% ointment two or three times a day.

**Usual pediatric dose**
Topical, to the skin, as a 0.1% ointment once a day.

**Strength(s) usually available**
U.S.—
    0.1% (Rx) [*Halog*].
Canada—
    0.1% (Rx) [*Halog*].

**Packaging and storage**
Store below 40 °C (104 °F), preferably between 15 and 30 °C (59 and 86
°F), unless otherwise specified by manufacturer. Store in a well-closed
container. Protect from freezing.

**Auxiliary labeling**
• For external use only.
• Do not use in or around the eye.

### HALCINONIDE TOPICAL SOLUTION USP

**Usual adult dose**
Topical, to the skin, as a 0.1% solution two or three times a day.

**Usual pediatric dose**
Topical, to the skin, as a 0.1% solution once a day.

**Strength(s) usually available**
U.S.—
    0.1% (Rx) [*Halog*].
Canada—
    0.1% (Rx) [*Halog*].

**Packaging and storage**
Store below 40 °C (104 °F), preferably between 15 and 30 °C (59 and 86
°F), unless otherwise specified by manufacturer. Store in a well-closed
container. Protect from freezing.

**Auxiliary labeling**
• For external use only.
• Do not use in or around the eye.

---

### *HALOBETASOL*

## Summary of Differences

Pharmacology/pharmacokinetics:
    Substituted; fluorinated.
    Potency ranking—Very high.

# Topical Dosage Forms

## HALOBETASOL PROPIONATE CREAM

### Usual adult dose
Topical, to the skin, as a 0.05% cream one or two times a day. Halobetasol propionate cream may be used for only a short duration of therapy and on small surface areas. Occlusive dressings should not be used.

### Usual pediatric dose
Dosage has not been established.

### Strength(s) usually available
U.S.—
    0.05% (Rx) [*Ultravate*].
Canada—
    Not commercially available.

### Packaging and storage
Store below 40 °C (104 °F), preferably between 2 and 30 °C (36 and 86 °F), in a well-closed container, unless otherwise specified by manufacturer.

### Auxiliary labeling
• For external use only.
• Do not use in or around the eye.

## HALOBETASOL PROPIONATE OINTMENT

### Usual adult dose
Topical, to the skin, as a 0.05% ointment one or two times a day. Halobetasol propionate ointment may be used for only a short duration of therapy and on small surface areas. Occlusive dressings should not be used.

### Usual pediatric dose
Dosage has not been established.

### Strength(s) usually available
U.S.—
    0.05% (Rx) [*Ultravate*].
Canada—
    Not commercially available.

### Packaging and storage
Store below 40 °C (104 °F), preferably between 2 and 30 °C (36 and 86 °F), in a well-closed container, unless otherwise specified by manufacturer.

### Auxiliary labeling
• For external use only.
• Do not use in or around the eye.

---

## *HYDROCORTISONE*

# Summary of Differences

Pharmacology/pharmacokinetics:
    Substituted (butyrate, valerate); non-fluorinated.
    Potency ranking—Low (acetate and base); Medium (butyrate and valerate).

# Dental Dosage Forms

## HYDROCORTISONE ACETATE DENTAL PASTE

### Usual adult dose
Topical, to the oral mucous membranes, as a 0.5% paste two or three times a day after meals and at bedtime.

### Usual pediatric dose
Dosage has not been established.

### Strength(s) usually available
U.S.—
    0.5% (Rx) [*Orabase-HCA*].
Canada—
    Not commercially available.

### Packaging and storage
Store between 4 and 30 °C (39 and 86 °F), unless otherwise specified by manufacturer. Protect from light. Protect from freezing.

### Auxiliary labeling
• For use in the mouth only.

# Rectal Dosage Forms

## HYDROCORTISONE CREAM USP

### Usual adult dose
Topical, to the anorectal area, as a 1% cream three or four times a day.

### Strength(s) usually available
U.S.—
    1% (Rx) [*Proctocort* (benzyl alcohol)].
Canada—
    Not commercially available.

### Packaging and storage
Store below 40 °C (104 °F), preferably between 15 and 30 °C (59 and 86 °F), unless otherwise specified by manufacturer. Store in a tight container. Protect from freezing.

### Auxiliary labeling
• For external use only.

## HYDROCORTISONE RECTAL OINTMENT

### Usual adult dose
Topical, to the anorectal area, as a 0.5 to 0.75% ointment one to four times a day.

### Usual pediatric dose
Children up to 2 years of age—Dosage has not been established.
Children 2 years of age and older—See *Usual adult dose*.

### Strength(s) usually available
U.S.—
    Not commercially available.
Canada—
    750 mg (0.75 grams) per 100 grams (Rx) [*Rectocort*].

### Packaging and storage
Store between 2 and 30 °C (36 and 86 °F), unless otherwise specified by manufacturer. Protect from freezing.

### Auxiliary labeling
• For external use only.

## HYDROCORTISONE SUPPOSITORIES

### Usual adult dose
Rectal, 20 to 30 mg a day.

### Usual pediatric dose
Dosage has not been established.

### Strength(s) usually available
U.S.—
    Not commercially available.
Canada—
    10 mg (Rx) [*Rectocort*].

### Packaging and storage
Store between 2 and 30 °C (36 and 86 °F), unless otherwise specified by manufacturer. Protect from freezing.

### Auxiliary labeling
• Store in a cool place.
• May be refrigerated.
• For rectal use only.

### Note
Explain administration technique.

## HYDROCORTISONE ACETATE CREAM USP

### Usual adult dose
Topical, to the anorectal area, as a 0.5 or 1% cream one to four times a day.

### Strength(s) usually available
U.S.—
    0.5% (OTC) [*Corticaine*].
    1% (OTC) [*Anusol-HC*].
Canada—
    Not commercially available.

### Packaging and storage
Store below 40 °C (104 °F), preferably between 15 and 30 °C (59 and 86 °F), unless otherwise specified by manufacturer. Store in a well-closed container. Protect from freezing.

### Auxiliary labeling
• For external use only.
• Do not use in or around the eye.

## HYDROCORTISONE ACETATE SUPPOSITORIES

### Usual adult dose
Rectal, up to 100 mg per day, in one to three divided doses.

### Usual pediatric dose
Dosage has not been established.

**Strength(s) usually available**

U.S.—

    25 mg (Rx) [*Anucort-HC; Anusol-HC; Cort-Dome High Potency; Hemril-HC;* GENERIC].

Canada—

    10 mg (Rx) [*Cortiment-10*].
    40 mg (Rx) [*Cortiment-40*].

**Packaging and storage**

Store between 2 and 15 °C (36 and 59 °F), in a well-closed container, unless otherwise specified by manufacturer. Protect from freezing.

**Auxiliary labeling**

• Store in a cool place.
• May be refrigerated.
• For rectal use only.

**Note**

Explain administration technique.

# Topical Dosage Forms

## HYDROCORTISONE CREAM USP

**Usual adult dose**

Topical, to the skin, as a 0.25 to 2.5% cream one to four times a day.

**Usual pediatric dose**

Children up to 2 years of age—Dosage has not been established.

Children 2 years of age and older—Topical, to the skin, as a 0.25 to 0.5% cream one to four times a day; or as a 1% cream one or two times a day.

**Strength(s) usually available**

U.S.—

    0.25% (OTC) [*Cort-Dome*].
    0.5% (OTC) [*Bactine; Cort-Dome; Cortifair; DermiCort; Dermtex HC; Hydro-Tex* (sodium bisulfite); *Hytone;* GENERIC].
    1% (Rx) [*Ala-Cort; Allercort; Alphaderm; Cort-Dome; Cortifair; Dermacort; Hi-Cor 1.0; Hydro-Tex* (sodium bisulfite); *Hytone; Lemoderm; Nutracort; Penecort; Synacort;* GENERIC].
    2.5% (Rx) [*Allercort; Anusol-HC; Hi-Cor 2.5; Hytone; Lemoderm; Penecort; Synacort;* GENERIC].

Canada—

    0.5% (OTC) [*Cortate; Unicort*].
    0.5% (Rx) [*Sential* (urea 4%)].
    1% (Rx) [*Barriere-HC; Emo-Cort; Prevex HC; Unicort*].
    2.5% (Rx) [*Emo-Cort*].

**Packaging and storage**

Store below 40 °C (104 °F), preferably between 15 and 30 °C (59 and 86 °F), unless otherwise specified by manufacturer. Store in a tight container. Protect from freezing.

**Auxiliary labeling**

• For external use only.
• Do not use in or around the eye.

## HYDROCORTISONE LOTION USP

**Usual adult dose**

Topical, to the skin, as a 0.25 to 2.5% lotion one to four times a day.

**Usual pediatric dose**

Children up to 2 years of age—Dosage has not been established.

Children 2 years of age and older—Topical, to the skin, as a 0.25 to 0.5% lotion one to four times a day; or as a 1% lotion one or two times a day; or as a 2.5% lotion once a day.

**Strength(s) usually available**

U.S.—

    0.25% (OTC) [*Cetacort; Cort-Dome*].
    0.5% (OTC) [*Cetacort; Delacort; MyCort; S-T Cort;* GENERIC].
    1% (Rx) [*Acticort 100; Ala-Cort; Allercort; Beta-HC; Cetacort; Dermacort; Gly-Cort; Hytone; LactiCare-HC; Lemoderm; Nutracort; Pentacort; Rederm;* GENERIC].
    2% (Rx) [*Ala-Scalp HP*].
    2.5% (Rx) [*Hytone; LactiCare-HC; Nutracort*].

Canada—

    0.5% (OTC) [*Cortate; Emo-Cort*].
    1% (Rx) [*Emo-Cort; Sarna HC 1.0%*].
    2.5% (Rx) [*Emo-Cort*].

**Packaging and storage**

Store below 40 °C (104 °F), preferably between 15 and 30 °C (59 and 86 °F), unless otherwise specified by manufacturer. Store in a tight container. Protect from freezing.

**Auxiliary labeling**

• For external use only.
• Do not use in or around the eye.
• Shake well.

## HYDROCORTISONE OINTMENT USP

**Usual adult dose**

Topical, to the skin, as a 0.5 to 2.5% ointment one to four times a day.

**Usual pediatric dose**

Children up to 2 years of age—Dosage has not been established.

Children 2 years of age and older—Topical, to the skin, as a 0.5% ointment one to four times a day; or as a 1% ointment one or two times a day; or as a 2.5% ointment once a day.

**Strength(s) usually available**

U.S.—

    0.5% (OTC) [GENERIC].
    1% [*Allercort; Cortril; Hytone; Lemoderm;* GENERIC].
    2.5% (Rx) [*Allercort; Hytone;* GENERIC].

Canada—

    0.5% (OTC) [*Cortate*].
    1% (Rx) [*Cortate; Cortef*].

**Packaging and storage**

Store below 40 °C (104 °F), preferably between 15 and 30 °C (59 and 86 °F), unless otherwise specified by manufacturer. Store in a well-closed container. Protect from freezing.

**Auxiliary labeling**

• For external use only.
• Do not use in or around the eye.

## HYDROCORTISONE TOPICAL SOLUTION

**Usual adult dose**

Topical, to the skin, as a 2.5% solution one to four times a day.

**Usual pediatric dose**

Topical, to the skin, as a 1% solution one or two times a day.

**Strength(s) usually available**

U.S.—

    0.5% (OTC) [*Aeroseb-HC* (alcohol 58%); *CaldeCORT Anti-Itch* (alcohol 89.5%); *Cortaid* (alcohol 46%; parabens); GENERIC].
    1% (OTC) [*Maximum Strength Cortaid* (alcohol 55%; parabens)].
    1% (Rx) [*Penecort* (alcohol 57%); *Texacort* (alcohol 33%)].
    2.5% (Rx) [*Texacort* (alcohol 49%)].

Canada—

    2.5% (Rx) [*Emo-Cort Scalp Solution* (alcohol)].

**Packaging and storage**

Store below 40 °C (104 °F), preferably between 15 and 30 °C (59 and 86 °F), in a well-closed container, unless otherwise specified by manufacturer. Protect from freezing.

**Auxiliary labeling**

• For external use only.
• Do not use in or around the eye.

## HYDROCORTISONE ACETATE CREAM USP

**Usual adult dose**

Topical, to the skin, as a 0.1 to 1% cream one to four times a day.

**Usual pediatric dose**

Children up to 2 years of age—Dosage has not been established.

Children 2 years of age and older—Topical, to the skin, as a 0.5 or 1% cream one to four times a day.

**Strength(s) usually available**

U.S.—

    0.5% (OTC) [*Corticaine; FoilleCort; Gynecort; Lanacort; 9-1-1; Pharma-Cort;* GENERIC].
    0.5% (base) (OTC) [*CaldeCORT Light; Cortaid; Cortef Feminine Itch;* GENERIC].
    1% (OTC) [*Anusol-HC; Gynecort 10; Lanacort 10*].
    1% (base) (OTC) [*Dermarest DriCort; Maximum Strength Cortaid*].
    1% (Rx) [*Carmol-HC* (sodium bisulfite); GENERIC].

Canada—

    0.1% (Rx) [*Corticreme*].
    0.5% (OTC) [*Cortacet; Hyderm; Novohydrocort*].
    1% (Rx) [*Corticreme; Hyderm; Novohydrocort*].

**Packaging and storage**

Store below 40 °C (104 °F), preferably between 15 and 30 °C (59 and 86 °F), unless otherwise specified by manufacturer. Store in a well-closed container. Protect from freezing.

**Auxiliary labeling**
- For external use only.
- Do not use in or around the eye.

## HYDROCORTISONE ACETATE TOPICAL AEROSOL FOAM

**Usual adult dose**
Topical, to the skin, as a 1% foam one to four times a day.

**Usual pediatric dose**
Topical, to the skin, as a 1% foam one or two times a day.

**Strength(s) usually available**
U.S.—
    1% (Rx) [*Epifoam* (butane; methylparaben; propane; propylparaben)].
Canada—
    Not commercially available.

**Packaging and storage**
Store below 49 °C (120 °F), unless otherwise specified by manufacturer.

**Auxiliary labeling**
- Shake well.
- For external use only.
- Do not use in or around the eye.

## HYDROCORTISONE ACETATE LOTION USP

**Usual adult dose**
Topical, to the skin, as a 0.5% lotion one to four times a day.

**Usual pediatric dose**
Children up to 2 years of age—Dosage has not been established.
Children 2 years of age and older—See *Usual adult dose*.

**Strength(s) usually available**
U.S.—
    0.5% (base) (OTC) [*Cortaid; Rhulicort*].
Canada—
    Not commercially available.

**Packaging and storage**
Store below 40 °C (104 °F), preferably between 15 and 30 °C (59 and 86 °F), unless otherwise specified by manufacturer. Store in a tight container. Protect from freezing.

**Auxiliary labeling**
- For external use only.
- Do not use in or around the eye.
- Shake well.

## HYDROCORTISONE ACETATE OINTMENT USP

**Usual adult dose**
Topical, to the skin, as a 0.5 to 2.5% ointment one to four times a day.

**Usual pediatric dose**
Children up to 2 years of age—Dosage has not been established.
Children 2 years of age and older—Topical, to the skin, as a 0.5% ointment one to four times a day; or as a 1% ointment one or two times a day; or as a 2.5% ointment once a day.

**Strength(s) usually available**
U.S.—
    0.5% (OTC) [*Lanacort*].
    0.5% (base) (OTC) [*Cortaid*].
    1% (Rx) [GENERIC].
    1% (base) (OTC) [*Maximum Strength Cortaid*].
Canada—
    0.5% (OTC) [*Cortoderm; Novohydrocort*].
    1% (Rx) [*Cortef; Cortoderm; Novohydrocort*].

**Packaging and storage**
Store below 40 °C (104 °F), preferably between 15 and 30 °C (59 and 86 °F), unless otherwise specified by manufacturer. Store in a well-closed container. Protect from freezing.

**Auxiliary labeling**
- For external use only.
- Do not use in or around the eye.

## HYDROCORTISONE BUTYRATE CREAM USP

**Usual adult dose**
Topical, to the skin, as a 0.1% cream two or three times a day.

**Usual pediatric dose**
Topical, to the skin, as a 0.1% cream one or two times a day.

**Strength(s) usually available**
U.S.—
    0.1% (Rx) [*Locoid* (methylparaben)].

Canada—
    Not commercially available.

**Packaging and storage**
Store below 40 °C (104 °F), preferably between 15 and 30 °C (59 and 86 °F), unless otherwise specified by manufacturer. Store in a well-closed container. Protect from freezing.

**Auxiliary labeling**
- For external use only.
- Do not use in or around the eye.

## HYDROCORTISONE BUTYRATE OINTMENT

**Usual adult dose**
Topical, to the skin, as a 0.1% ointment two or three times a day.

**Usual pediatric dose**
Topical, to the skin, as a 0.1% ointment one or two times a day.

**Strength(s) usually available**
U.S.—
    0.1% (Rx) [*Locoid*].
Canada—
    Not commercially available.

**Packaging and storage**
Store below 40 °C (104 °F), preferably between 15 and 30 °C (59 and 86 °F), unless otherwise specified by manufacturer. Protect from freezing.

**Auxiliary labeling**
- For external use only.
- Do not use in or around the eye.

## HYDROCORTISONE VALERATE CREAM USP

**Usual adult dose**
Topical, to the skin, as a 0.2% cream two or three times a day.

**Usual pediatric dose**
Topical, to the skin, as a 0.2% cream once a day.

**Strength(s) usually available**
U.S.—
    0.2% (Rx) [*Westcort*].
Canada—
    0.2% (Rx) [*Westcort*].

**Packaging and storage**
Store below 25 °C (77 °F), unless otherwise specified by manufacturer. Store in a well-closed container. Protect from freezing.

**Auxiliary labeling**
- For external use only.
- Do not use in or around the eye.

## HYDROCORTISONE VALERATE OINTMENT

**Usual adult dose**
Topical, to the skin, as a 0.2% ointment two or three times a day.

**Usual pediatric dose**
Topical, to the skin, as a 0.2% ointment once a day.

**Strength(s) usually available**
U.S.—
    0.2% (Rx) [*Westcort*].
Canada—
    0.2% (Rx) [*Westcort*].

**Packaging and storage**
Store below 26 °C (78 °F), in a well-closed container, unless otherwise specified by manufacturer. Protect from freezing.

**Auxiliary labeling**
- For external use only.
- Do not use in or around the eye.

---

## *MOMETASONE*

# Summary of Differences

Pharmacology/pharmacokinetics:
    Substituted; non-fluorinated.
    Potency ranking—Medium.

# Topical Dosage Forms

## MOMETASONE FUROATE CREAM

**Usual adult dose**
Topical, to the skin, as a 0.1% cream once a day.

**Usual pediatric dose**
Dosage has not been established.

**Strength(s) usually available**
U.S.—
  0.1% (Rx) [*Elocon*].
Canada—
  0.1% (Rx) [*Elocom*].

**Packaging and storage**
Store below 40 °C (104 °F), preferably between 2 and 30 °C (36 and 86 °F), in a well-closed container, unless otherwise specified by manufacturer.

**Auxiliary labeling**
• For external use only.
• Do not use in or around the eye.

## MOMETASONE FUROATE LOTION

**Usual adult dose**
Topical, to the skin, as a 0.1% lotion once a day.

**Usual pediatric dose**
Dosage has not been established.

**Strength(s) usually available**
U.S.—
  0.1% (Rx) [*Elocon* (isopropyl alcohol 40%)].
Canada—
  0.1% (Rx) [*Elocom*].

**Packaging and storage**
Store below 40 °C (104 °F), preferably between 2 and 30 °C (36 and 86 °F), in a well-closed container, unless otherwise specified by manufacturer.

**Auxiliary labeling**
• For external use only.
• Do not use in or around the eye.

## MOMETASONE FUROATE OINTMENT

**Usual adult dose**
Topical, to the skin, as a 0.1% ointment once a day.

**Usual pediatric dose**
Dosage has not been established.

**Strength(s) usually available**
U.S.—
  0.1% (Rx) [*Elocon*].
Canada—
  0.1% (Rx) [*Elocom*].

**Packaging and storage**
Store below 40 °C (104 °F), preferably between 2 and 30 °C (36 and 86 °F), in a well-closed container, unless otherwise specified by manufacturer.

**Auxiliary labeling**
• For external use only.
• Do not use in or around the eye.

---

### TRIAMCINOLONE

## Summary of Differences

Pharmacology/pharmacokinetics:
  Substituted; fluorinated.
    Potency ranking—
      Medium (except cream and ointment 0.5%).
      Cream and ointment 0.5%, High.

## Dental Dosage Forms

### TRIAMCINOLONE ACETONIDE DENTAL PASTE USP

**Usual adult dose**
Topical, to the oral mucous membranes, as a 0.1% paste two or three times a day after meals and at bedtime.

**Usual pediatric dose**
Dosage has not been established.

**Strength(s) usually available**
U.S.—
  0.1% (Rx) [*Kenalog in Orabase; Oracort; Oralone*].
Canada—
  0.1% (Rx) [*Kenalog in Orabase*].

**Packaging and storage**
Store below 40 °C (104 °F), preferably between 15 and 30 °C (59 and 86 °F), unless otherwise specified by manufacturer. Store in a tight container. Protect from freezing.

**Auxiliary labeling**
• For use in the mouth only.

## Topical Dosage Forms

### TRIAMCINOLONE ACETONIDE CREAM USP

**Usual adult dose**
Topical, to the skin, as a 0.025 to 0.5% cream two to four times a day.

**Usual pediatric dose**
Topical, to the skin, as a 0.025% cream one or two times a day; or as a 0.1 or 0.5% cream once a day.

**Strength(s) usually available**
U.S.—
  0.025% (Rx) [*Aristocort; Aristocort A; Flutex; Kenac; Kenalog; Kenonel; Triacet;* GENERIC].
  0.1% (Rx) [*Aristocort; Aristocort A; Delta-Tritex; Flutex; Kenac; Kenalog; Kenalog-H; Kenonel; Triacet; Triderm;* GENERIC].
  0.5% (Rx) [*Aristocort; Aristocort A; Flutex; Kenalog; Kenonel; Triacet;* GENERIC].
Canada—
  0.025% (Rx) [*Aristocort D; Triaderm; Trianide Mild*].
  0.1% (Rx) [*Aristocort R; Kenalog; Triaderm; Trianide Regular*].
  0.5% (Rx) [*Aristocort C*].

**Packaging and storage**
Store below 40 °C (104 °F), preferably between 15 and 30 °C (59 and 86 °F), unless otherwise specified by manufacturer. Store in a tight container. Protect from freezing.

**Auxiliary labeling**
• For external use only.
• Do not use in or around the eye.

### TRIAMCINOLONE ACETONIDE LOTION USP

**Usual adult dose**
Topical, to the skin, as a 0.025 or 0.1% lotion two to four times a day.

**Usual pediatric dose**
Topical, to the skin, as a 0.025% lotion one or two times a day; or as a 0.1% lotion once a day.

**Strength(s) usually available**
U.S.—
  0.025% (Rx) [*Kenalog;* GENERIC].
  0.1% (Rx) [*Kenalog; Kenonel;* GENERIC].
Canada—
  Not commercially available.

**Packaging and storage**
Store between 15 and 30 °C (59 and 86 °F), unless otherwise specified by manufacturer. Store in a tight container. Protect from freezing.

**Auxiliary labeling**
• For external use only.
• Do not use in or around the eye.
• Shake well.

### TRIAMCINOLONE ACETONIDE OINTMENT USP

**Usual adult dose**
Topical, to the skin, as a 0.025 to 0.5% ointment two to four times a day.

**Usual pediatric dose**
Topical, to the skin, as a 0.025% ointment one or two times a day; or as a 0.1 or 0.5% ointment once a day.

**Strength(s) usually available**
U.S.—
  0.025% (Rx) [*Flutex; Kenalog;* GENERIC].
  0.1% (Rx) [*Aristocort; Aristocort A; Flutex; Kenac; Kenalog; Kenonel;* GENERIC].
  0.5% (Rx) [*Aristocort; Flutex; Kenalog;* GENERIC].
Canada—
  0.025% (Rx) [*Aristocort D; Triaderm*].
  0.1% (Rx) [*Aristocort R; Kenalog; Triaderm*].

**Packaging and storage**
Store below 40 °C (104 °F), preferably between 15 and 30 °C (59 and 86 °F), unless otherwise specified by manufacturer. Store in a well-closed container. Protect from freezing.

**Auxiliary labeling**
• For external use only.
• Do not use in or around the eye.

## TRIAMCINOLONE ACETONIDE TOPICAL AEROSOL USP

**Usual adult dose**
Topical, to the skin, as a 0.015% aerosol spray three or four times a day.

**Usual pediatric dose**
Topical, to the skin, as a 0.015% aerosol spray one or two times a day.

**Strength(s) usually available**
U.S.—

0.015% (Rx) [*Kenalog* (alcohol 10.3%)].

Note: A 2-second spray delivers 0.2 mg of triamcinolone acetonide. Product applied to skin contains approximately 0.2% triamcinolone acetonide.

Canada—
Not commercially available.

**Packaging and storage**
Store below 40 °C (104 °F), preferably between 15 and 30 °C (59 and 86 °F). Protect from freezing.

**Auxiliary labeling**
• For external use only.
• Do not use in or around the eye.

**Note**
Explain administration technique.
When dispensing, include patient instructions.

Revised: 11/18/92

## Table 1. Pharmacology/Pharmacokinetics

Note: The following table lists topical corticosteroid products available in the U.S. and/or Canada. A potency rank is also listed for each preparation: Low, Medium, High, or Very High.

Products with a Low potency ranking have a modest anti-inflammatory effect and are safest for chronic application. These products are also the safest products for use on the face and intertriginous areas, with occlusion, and in infants and young children.

Products with a Medium potency ranking are used in moderate inflammatory dermatoses. Examples of conditions for which these products are frequently used include chronic eczematous dermatoses such as hand eczema and atopic eczema. Medium potency preparations may be used on the face and intertriginous areas for a limited duration.

High potency preparations are used in more severe inflammatory dermatoses. Examples of conditions for which these products are frequently used include more severe eczematous dermatoses, lichen simplex chronicus, and psoriasis. They may be used for an intermediate duration, or for longer periods in areas with thickened skin due to chronic conditions. High potency preparations may also be used on the face and intertriginous areas but only for a short treatment duration.

Very High potency products are used primarily as an alternative to systemic corticosteroid therapy when local areas are involved. Examples of conditions for which Very High potency products are frequently used include thick, chronic lesions caused by psoriasis, lichen simplex chronicus, and discoid lupus erythematosus. There is a high likelihood of skin atrophy with the use of Very High potency preparations. They may be used for only a short duration of therapy and on small surface areas. Occlusive dressings should not be used with these products.

| Generic drug name | Dosage Form(s) | Strength (%) | Potency Ranking |
|---|---|---|---|
| Alclometasone dipropionate | | | |
| | Cream | 0.05 | Low |
| | Ointment | 0.05 | Low |
| Amcinonide | | | |
| | Cream | 0.1 | High |
| | Lotion | 0.1 | High |
| | Ointment | 0.1 | High |
| Beclomethasone dipropionate | | | |
| | Cream | 0.025 | Medium |
| | Lotion | 0.025 | Medium |
| | Ointment | 0.025 | Medium |
| Betamethasone benzoate | | | |
| | Cream | 0.025 | Medium |
| | Gel | 0.025 | Medium |
| | Lotion | 0.025 | Medium |
| Betamethasone dipropionate | | | |
| | Cream | | |
| | *Diprolene AF* | 0.05 | Very high |
| | Others | 0.05 | High |
| | Gel | | |
| | *Diprolene* | 0.05 | Very high |
| | Lotion | | |
| | *Diprolene* | 0.05 | Very high |
| | Others | 0.05 | High |
| | Ointment | | |
| | *Diprolene* | 0.05 | Very high |
| | Others | 0.05 | High |
| | Topical aerosol | 0.1 | High |
| Betamethasone valerate | | | |
| | Cream | 0.01 | Medium |
| | Cream | 0.05 | Medium |
| | Cream | 0.1 | Medium |
| | Lotion | 0.05 | Medium |
| | Lotion | 0.1 | Medium |
| | Ointment | 0.05 | Medium |
| | Ointment | 0.1 | Medium |

| Generic drug name | Dosage Form(s) | Strength (%) | Potency Ranking |
|---|---|---|---|
| Clobetasol propionate | | | |
| | Cream | 0.05 | Very high |
| | Ointment | 0.05 | Very high |
| | Solution | 0.05 | Very high |
| Clobetasone butyrate | | | |
| | Cream | 0.05 | Medium |
| | Ointment | 0.05 | Medium |
| Clocortolone pivalate | | | |
| | Cream | 0.1 | Low |
| Desonide | | | |
| | Cream | 0.05 | Low |
| | Lotion | 0.05 | Low |
| | Ointment | 0.05 | Low |
| Desoximetasone | | | |
| | Cream | 0.05 | Medium |
| | Cream | 0.25 | High |
| | Gel | 0.05 | High |
| | Ointment | 0.25 | High |
| Dexamethasone | | | |
| | Gel | 0.1 | Low |
| | Topical aerosol | 0.01 | Low |
| | Topical aerosol | 0.04 | Low |
| Dexamethasone sodium phosphate | | | |
| | Cream | 0.1 (phosphate) | Low |
| Diflorasone diacetate | | | |
| | Cream | 0.05 | High |
| | Ointment | | |
| | *Psorcon* | 0.05 | Very high |
| | Others | 0.05 | High |

## Table 1. Pharmacology/Pharmacokinetics *(continued)*

| Diflucortolone valerate | | | |
|---|---|---|---|
| | Cream | 0.1 | Medium |
| | Ointment | 0.1 | Medium |

| Flumethasone pivalate | | | |
|---|---|---|---|
| | Cream | 0.03 | Low |
| | Ointment | 0.03 | Low |

| Fluocinolone acetonide | | | |
|---|---|---|---|
| | Cream | 0.01 | Medium |
| | Cream | 0.025 | Medium |
| | Cream | 0.2 | High |
| | Ointment | 0.01 | Medium |
| | Ointment | 0.025 | Medium |
| | Topical solution | 0.01 | Medium |
| | Ointment | 0.1 | Medium |

| Fluocinonide | | | |
|---|---|---|---|
| | Cream | 0.01 | High |
| | Cream | 0.05 | High |
| | Gel | 0.05 | High |
| | Ointment | 0.01 | High |
| | Ointment | 0.05 | High |
| | Topical solution | 0.05 | High |

| Flurandrenolide | | | |
|---|---|---|---|
| | Cream | 0.0125 | Low |
| | Cream | 0.025 | Medium |
| | Cream | 0.05 | Medium |
| | Lotion | 0.05 | Medium |
| | Ointment | 0.0125 | Low |
| | Ointment | 0.025 | Medium |
| | Ointment | 0.05 | Medium |
| | Tape | 4 mcg/cm² | Medium |

| Fluticasone propionate | | | |
|---|---|---|---|
| | Cream | 0.05 | Medium |
| | Ointment | 0.005 | Medium |

| Halcinonide | | | |
|---|---|---|---|
| | Cream | 0.025 | High |
| | Cream | 0.1 | High |
| | Ointment | 0.1 | High |
| | Topical solution | 0.1 | High |

| Halobetasol propionate | | | |
|---|---|---|---|
| | Cream | 0.05 | Very high |
| | Ointment | 0.05 | Very high |

| Hydrocortisone | | | |
|---|---|---|---|
| | Cream | 0.25 | Low |
| | Cream | 0.5 | Low |
| | Cream | 1 | Low |
| | Cream | 2.5 | Low |
| | Lotion | 0.25 | Low |
| | Lotion | 0.5 | Low |
| | Lotion | 1 | Low |
| | Lotion | 2 | Low |
| | Lotion | 2.5 | Low |
| | Ointment | 0.5 | Low |
| | Ointment | 1 | Low |
| | Ointment | 2.5 | Low |
| | Topical aerosol solution | 0.5 | Low |
| | Topical spray solution | 0.5 | Low |
| | Topical solution | 1 | Low |
| | Topical solution | 2.5 | Low |

| Hydrocortisone acetate | | | |
|---|---|---|---|
| | Ointment | 0.1 | Medium |
| | Cream | 0.1 | Low |
| | Cream | 0.5 | Low |
| | Cream | 1 | Low |
| | Lotion | 0.5 | Low |
| | Ointment | 0.5 | Low |
| | Ointment | 1 | Low |
| | Topical aerosol foam | 1 | Low |

| Hydrocortisone butyrate | | | |
|---|---|---|---|
| | Cream | 0.1 | Medium |
| | Ointment | 0.1 | Medium |

| Hydrocortisone valerate | | | |
|---|---|---|---|
| | Cream | 0.2 | Medium |
| | Ointment | 0.2 | Medium |

| Methylprednisolone acetate | | | |
|---|---|---|---|
| | Cream | 0.25 | Low |
| | Ointment | 0.25 | Low |
| | Ointment | 1 | Low |

| Mometasone furoate | | | |
|---|---|---|---|
| | Cream | 0.1 | Medium |
| | Lotion | 0.1 | Medium |
| | Ointment | 0.1 | Medium |

| Triamcinolone acetonide | | | |
|---|---|---|---|
| | Cream | 0.025 | Medium |
| | Cream | 0.1 | Medium |
| | Cream | 0.5 | High |
| | Lotion | 0.025 | Medium |
| | Lotion | 0.1 | Medium |
| | Ointment | 0.025 | Medium |
| | Ointment | 0.1 | Medium |
| | Ointment | 0.5 | High |
| | Topical aerosol | 0.015 | Medium |

# CORTICOSTEROIDS AND ACETIC ACID    Otic

This monograph includes information on the following: Desonide and Acetic Acid; Hydrocortisone and Acetic Acid.

VA CLASSIFICATION (Primary): OT250

Another commonly used name for hydrocortisone is cortisol.

Note: For a listing of dosage forms and brand names by country availability, see *Dosage Forms* section(s). For a listing of brand names for the articles in this monograph, refer to the General Index.

## Category

Corticosteroid-antiseptic (otic); anti-inflammatory (steroidal), otic.

## Indications

Note: Bracketed information in the *Indications* section refers to uses that are not included in U.S. product labeling.

**Accepted**

Ear canal infections, external (treatment)—Corticosteroid and acetic acid combinations are indicated in the treatment of superficial external ear canal infections that are accompanied by inflammation.

[Ear canal infections, external (prophylaxis)]—Hydrocortisone and acetic acid combination is indicated in the prophylaxis of external ear canal infections.

[Otitis externa, eczematoid, chronic (prophylaxis and treatment)]—Hydrocortisone and acetic acid combination is indicated in the prophylaxis and treatment of chronic eczematoid otitis externa.

[Otitis externa, seborrheic (prophylaxis and treatment)]—Hydrocortisone and acetic acid combination is indicated in the prophylaxis and treatment of seborrheic otitis externa.

## Pharmacology/Pharmacokinetics

**Physicochemical characteristics**

Molecular weight—
 Acetic acid: 60.05.
 Desonide: 416.51.
 Hydrocortisone: 362.47.

**Mechanism of action/Effect**

Corticosteroids—
 Otic corticosteroids possess anti-inflammatory, anti-allergic, and anti-pruritic actions.
 Corticosteroids diffuse across cell membranes and complex with specific cytoplasmic receptors. These complexes then enter the cell nucleus, bind to DNA, and stimulate transcription of messenger RNA (mRNA) and subsequent protein synthesis of enzymes ultimately responsible for anti-inflammatory effects of otic corticosteroids. In high concentrations, which may be achieved locally after topical application, corticosteroids may exert direct membrane effects. Corticosteroids decrease cellular and fibrinous exudation and tissue infiltration, inhibit fibroblastic and collagen-forming activity, retard epithelial regeneration, diminish post-inflammatory neovascularization, and reduce toward normal levels the excessive permeability of inflamed capillaries.

Acetic acid—
 Possesses antibacterial, astringent, and antifungal properties.

## Precautions to Consider

**Pregnancy/Reproduction**

Pregnancy—For desonide and acetic acid: Although problems in humans have not been documented, adequate and well-controlled studies have not been done.

FDA Pregnancy Category C.

For hydrocortisone and acetic acid: Problems in humans have not been documented.

**Breast-feeding**

Problems in humans have not been documented.

**Pediatrics**

Appropriate studies with these medications have not been performed in the pediatric population. However, pediatrics-specific problems that would limit the usefulness of these medications in children are not expected.

**Geriatrics**

Appropriate studies with these medications have not been performed in the geriatric population. However, geriatrics-specific problems that

would limit the usefulness of these medications in the elderly are not expected.

**Medical considerations/Contraindications**

The medical considerations/contraindications included here have been selected on the basis of their potential clinical significance (reasons given in parentheses where appropriate)—not necessarily inclusive (» = major clinical significance).

*Risk-benefit should be considered when the following medical problems exist:*

» Infection, aural, fungal or
» Infection, aural, acute untreated or
» Tuberculosis, aural or
 Viral infection, acute, infectious
  (infections may be exacerbated)
» Perforation of the ear drum membrane
  (possibility of ototoxicity)
 Sensitivity to acetic acid
 Sensitivity to corticosteroids

## Side/Adverse Effects

The following side/adverse effects have been selected on the basis of their potential clinical significance (possible signs and symptoms in parentheses where appropriate)—not necessarily inclusive:

**Those indicating need for medical attention only if they continue or are bothersome**
 *Stinging, itching, irritation, or burning in the ear*

## Patient Consultation

As an aid to patient consultation, refer to *Advice for the Patient, Corticosteroids and Acetic Acid (Otic).*

In providing consultation, consider emphasizing the following selected information (» = major clinical significance):

**Before using this medication**
» Conditions affecting use, especially:
  Sensitivity to acetic acid or corticosteroids
  Other medical problems, especially other untreated ear infections or perforated ear drum

**Proper use of this medication**
 Proper administration technique
 Preventing contamination: Avoid touching applicator tip to any surface; keeping container tightly closed
» Not washing dropper or applicator tip (to prevent dilution of medication with water)—applicable only to the hydrocortisone and acetic acid formulation; if necessary, wiping with clean tissue after use
 Importance of not using more medication than the amount prescribed
» Checking with physician before using medication for future ear problems
» Proper dosing
 Missed dose: Using as soon as possible; not using if almost time for next dose
» Proper storage

**Precautions while using this medication**
 Checking with physician if no improvement after 5 to 7 days of therapy or if ear condition becomes worse

## General Dosing Information

To allow optimum contact between the medication and infected surfaces of the ear canal, all cerumen and debris should be carefully removed by a physician or a trained assistant before initiation of therapy.

Otic solutions may be instilled directly into the ear canal or administered by use of a saturated gauze or cotton wick gently placed into the canal. The wick should be kept moist with additional solution and replaced every 12 to 24 hours.

The duration of treatment may vary from a few days to several weeks or months in some cases, depending on the condition being treated. Daily or alternate-day therapy may be indicated for extended periods in certain situations. In severe or persistent cases of external ear canal infections, more intensive anti-infective therapy may be required.

Treatment should be continued after apparent response, with the dosage being tapered gradually to avoid relapse.

## *DESONIDE AND ACETIC ACID*

## Otic Dosage Forms
### DESONIDE AND ACETIC ACID OTIC SOLUTION

**Usual adult and adolescent dose**
Topical, to the ear canal, 3 or 4 drops of the solution three or four times a day.

**Usual pediatric dose**
See *Usual adult and adolescent dose.*

**Usual geriatric dose**
See *Usual adult and adolescent dose.*

**Strength(s) usually available**
U.S.—
   0.05% desonide and 2% acetic acid (Rx) [*Otic Tridesilon Solution*].

**Packaging and storage**
Store below 30 °C (86 °F), unless otherwise specified by manufacturer. Protect from freezing.

**Auxiliary labeling**
• For the ear.
• Keep container tightly closed.

**Note**
Dispense in original unopened container.

---

## *HYDROCORTISONE AND ACETIC ACID*

## Otic Dosage Forms
Note: Bracketed uses in the *Dosage Forms* section refer to categories of use and/or indications that are not included in U.S. product labeling.

## HYDROCORTISONE AND ACETIC ACID OTIC SOLUTION USP

**Usual adult and adolescent dose**
[Prophylaxis]—Topical, to each ear canal, 2 drops of solution in the morning and evening.
Treatment—Topical, to the ear canal, 2 to 5 drops of the solution three or four times a day.
Note: To promote continuous contact for initial 24 to 48 hours, a saturated wick may be inserted into the ear canal. The wick should be moistened with 3 to 5 drops of solution every 4 to 6 hours.

**Usual pediatric dose**
See *Usual adult and adolescent dose.*

**Usual geriatric dose**
See *Usual adult and adolescent dose.*

**Strength(s) usually available**
U.S.—
   1% hydrocortisone and 2% acetic acid (Rx) [*VōSol HC* (benzethonium chloride 0.02%; propylene glycol diacetate 3%)].
Canada—
   1% hydrocortisone and 2% acetic acid (Rx) [*VōSol HC* (benzethonium chloride 0.02%; propylene glycol diacetate 3%)].

**Packaging and storage**
Store below 40 °C (104 °F), preferably between 15 and 30 °C (59 and 86 °F), unless otherwise specified by manufacturer. Store in a tight, light-resistant container. Protect from freezing.

**Auxiliary labeling**
• For the ear.
• Keep container tightly closed.

**Note**
Dispense in original unopened container.

---

Revised: 03/31/92
Interim revision: 04/01/94

---

# CORTICOSTEROIDS—GLUCOCORTICOID EFFECTS   Systemic

This monograph includes information on the following: Betamethasone; Cortisone; Dexamethasone; Hydrocortisone; Methylprednisolone; Prednisolone; Prednisone; Triamcinolone.

VA CLASSIFICATION (Primary/Secondary):
   Betamethasone—HS051/IM600
   Cortisone—HS051/IM600
   Dexamethasone—HS051/DX900; GA700; IM600
   Hydrocortisone—HS051/GA700; IM600
   Methylprednisolone—HS051/IM600
   Prednisolone—HS051/IM600
   Prednisone—HS051/GA700; IM600
   Triamcinolone—HS051/IM600

Another commonly used name for hydrocortisone is cortisol.

Note: For a listing of dosage forms and brand names by country availability, see *Dosage Forms* section(s). For a listing of brand names for the articles in this monograph, refer to the General Index.

## Category
Corticosteroid—Betamethasone; Cortisone; Dexamethasone; Hydrocortisone; Methylprednisolone; Prednisolone; Prednisone; Triamcinolone.
Anti-inflammatory (steroidal)—Betamethasone; Cortisone; Dexamethasone; Hydrocortisone; Methylprednisolone; Prednisolone; Prednisone; Triamcinolone.
Diagnostic aid (Cushing's syndrome)—Dexamethasone Elixir USP; Dexamethasone Oral Solution; Dexamethasone Tablets USP; Dexamethasone Sodium Phosphate Injection USP.
Immunosuppressant—Betamethasone; Cortisone; Dexamethasone; Hydrocortisone; Methylprednisolone; Prednisolone; Prednisone; Triamcinolone.
Antiemetic, in cancer chemotherapy—Dexamethasone Elixir USP; Dexamethasone Tablets USP; Dexamethasone Sodium Phosphate Injection USP; Hydrocortisone (oral and parenteral); Prednisone.
Diagnostic aid (endogenous depression)—Dexamethasone (oral dosage forms).

## Indications
See also *Table 1*, page 976.

**Accepted**
Corticosteroids are indicated (in physiologic doses) as replacement therapy in the treatment of adrenal insufficiency states.

In patients with known or suspected adrenal insufficiency, intravenous or intramuscular administration of a rapidly acting corticosteroid is indicated prior to surgery, including dental surgery, or if shock, severe trauma, illness, or other stress conditions occur. Patients already receiving replacement therapy require supplemental pharmacologic doses.

Glucocorticoids are indicated for their anti-inflammatory and immunosuppressant effects in the treatment of many disorders. Agents having minimal mineralocorticoid activity are preferred. For most indications, glucocorticoid administration provides symptomatic relief but has no effect on the underlying disease processes. Use of these medications does not eliminate the need for other therapies that may be required.

Corticosteroid therapy for conditions other than adrenocortical insufficiency, adrenogenital syndrome, or severe or life-threatening conditions is generally instituted only after less toxic therapies have proven ineffective.

## Pharmacology/Pharmacokinetics
See also *Table 2*, page 982, and *Table 3*, page 983.

**Physicochemical characteristics**
Molecular weight—
   Betamethasone—
      392.47
      Acetate:
         434.50
      Sodium phosphate:
         516.41
   Cortisone acetate—
      402.49
   Dexamethasone—
      392.47

Acetate:
452.52
Sodium phosphate:
516.41
Hydrocortisone—
362.47
Acetate:
404.50
Cypionate:
486.65
Sodium phosphate:
486.41
Sodium succinate:
484.52
Methylprednisolone—
374.48
Acetate:
416.51
Sodium succinate:
496.53
Prednisolone—
360.45 (anhydrous); 387.47 (sesquihydrate)
Acetate:
402.49
Sodium phosphate:
484.39
Tebutate:
458.59
Prednisone—
358.43
Triamcinolone—
394.44
Acetonide:
434.50
Diacetate:
478.51
Hexacetonide:
532.65

## Mechanism of action/Effect

Corticosteroids—Diffuse across cell membranes and complex with specific cytoplasmic receptors. These complexes then enter the cell nucleus, bind to DNA, and stimulate transcription of messenger RNA (mRNA) and subsequent protein synthesis of various enzymes thought to be ultimately responsible for two categories of effects of systemic corticosteroids. However, these agents may suppress transcription of mRNA in some cells (e.g., lymphocytes).

For glucocorticoid effects—

Anti-inflammatory (steroidal)—Glucocorticoids decrease or prevent tissue responses to inflammatory processes, thereby reducing development of symptoms of inflammation without affecting the underlying cause. Glucocorticoids inhibit accumulation of inflammatory cells, including macrophages and leukocytes, at sites of inflammation. They also inhibit phagocytosis, lysosomal enzyme release, and synthesis and/or release of several chemical mediators of inflammation. Although the exact mechanisms are not completely understood, actions that may contribute significantly to these effects include blockade of the action of macrophage inhibitory factor (MIF), leading to inhibition of macrophage localization; reduction of dilatation and permeability of inflamed capillaries and reduction of leukocyte adherence to the capillary endothelium, leading to inhibition of both leukocyte migration and edema formation; and increased synthesis of lipomodulin (macrocortin), an inhibitor of phospholipase $A_2$–mediated arachidonic acid release from membrane phospholipids, with subsequent inhibition of the synthesis of arachidonic acid–derived mediators of inflammation (prostaglandins, thromboxanes, and leukotrienes). Immunosuppressant actions may also contribute significantly to the anti-inflammatory effect.

Immunosuppressant—Mechanisms of immunosuppressant action are not completely understood but may involve prevention or suppression of cell-mediated (delayed hypersensitivity) immune reactions as well as more specific actions affecting the immune response. Glucocorticoids reduce the concentration of thymus-dependent lymphocytes (T-lymphocytes), monocytes, and eosinophils. They also decrease binding of immunoglobulin to cell surface receptors and inhibit the synthesis and/or release of interleukins, thereby decreasing T-lymphocyte blastogenesis and reducing expansion of the primary immune response. Glucocorticoids may also decrease passage of immune

complexes through basement membranes and decrease concentrations of complement components and immunoglobulins.

For mineralocorticoid effects—

Water and electrolyte balance—Sodium reabsorption, and potassium and hydrogen excretion, along with subsequent water retention, are mediated through an action of mineralocorticoids on the renal distal tubule that facilitates sodium transport. Cation transport in other secretory cells is similarly affected; excretion of water and electrolytes by the large intestine and by salivary and sweat glands is also altered, but to a lesser extent. Only cortisone and hydrocortisone have clinically useful mineralocorticoid activity.

For specific indications—

Adrenogenital syndrome—Glucocorticoids inhibit corticotropin (adrenocorticotropin or ACTH) secretion, leading to suppression of adrenal hypersecretion of androgens responsible for the androgenism associated with various enzyme deficiencies.

Hypercalcemia—Glucocorticoids reduce plasma calcium concentration by decreasing gastrointestinal absorption of calcium, probably by interfering with intestinal calcium transport (by decreasing the effect of vitamin D), and increasing calcium excretion.

Respiratory distress syndrome prophylaxis—Glucocorticoids may induce enzymes which accelerate or increase production of lung surfactant by type 2 pneumonocytes.

## Other actions/effects

Pharmacologic (supraphysiologic) doses of exogenous corticosteroids produce hypothalamic-pituitary-adrenal (HPA) axis suppression via a negative feedback mechanism, i.e., they inhibit pituitary ACTH secretion, thereby reducing ACTH-mediated production of corticosteroids and androgens in the adrenal cortex. The development of adrenocortical insufficiency and the time required for recovery of adrenal function depend primarily on the duration of corticosteroid therapy and, to a lesser extent, on dosage, timing, and frequency of administration, as well as on the potency and biologic (tissue) half-life of the specific agent. Adrenal insufficiency may occur in approximately 5 to 7 days with daily administration of doses equivalent to 20 to 30 mg of prednisone or in up to 30 days with lower doses. Following discontinuation of short-term (up to 5 days) high-dose use, adrenal recovery may occur within 1 week. Following prolonged high-dose use, complete recovery of adrenal function may require up to 1 year and, in some patients, may never occur.

Glucocorticoids stimulate protein catabolism and induce enzymes responsible for metabolism of amino acids. They decrease synthesis and increase degradation of protein in lymphoid tissue, connective tissue, muscle, and skin. With prolonged use, atrophy of these tissues may occur.

Glucocorticoids increase glucose availability by inducing hepatic enzymes involved in gluconeogenesis, stimulating protein catabolism (which increases hepatic concentrations of amino acids required for gluconeogenesis), and decreasing peripheral utilization of glucose. These actions lead to increased hepatic glycogen storage, increased blood glucose concentrations, and insulin resistance.

Glucocorticoids increase lipolysis and mobilize fatty acids from adipose tissues, leading to increased plasma fatty acid concentrations. With prolonged use, an abnormal redistribution of fat may occur.

Glucocorticoids decrease bone formation and increase bone resorption. They reduce plasma calcium concentration, leading to secondary hyperparathyroidism and subsequent stimulation of osteoclasts, and directly inhibit osteoblasts. These actions, together with a decrease in the protein matrix of bone secondary to increased protein catabolism, may lead to inhibition of bone growth in children and adolescents and the development of osteoporosis at any age.

## Absorption

Oral—
Rapidly and almost completely absorbed.

Parenteral—
Intramuscular:
Freely soluble esters (sodium phosphate, sodium succinate)—Rapidly absorbed.
Poorly soluble derivatives (acetate, acetonide, diacetate, hexacetonide, tebutate)—Slowly but completely absorbed.
Local:
Freely soluble esters—Less rapidly absorbed than with intramuscular injection.
Poorly soluble derivatives—Slowly but completely absorbed.

Rectal—
>20% of a dose is absorbed; may be increased to up to 50% if the mucosa is inflamed or damaged.

**Biotransformation**

Primarily hepatic (rapid); also renal and tissue; mostly to inactive metabolites. Cortisone and prednisone are inactive until metabolized to the active metabolites hydrocortisone and prednisolone, respectively. Fluorinated corticosteroids are metabolized more slowly than other members of the group.

**Duration of action**

Duration of action depends upon the route/site of administration, solubility of the dosage form, dose administered, and the condition being treated. Following oral or intravenous administration, the duration of action depends upon the biological (tissue) half-life. Following intramuscular administration, the duration of action depends upon the solubility of the dosage form as well as the biological (tissue) half-life. Following local injections, the duration of action depends upon the solubility of the dosage form and the specific route/site of administration.

**Elimination**

Primarily by renal excretion of inactive metabolites.

# Precautions to Consider

## Pregnancy/Reproduction

Fertility—Corticosteroids have been reported to increase or decrease the number or motility of spermatozoa. However, it is not known whether reproductive capacity in humans is adversely affected.

Pregnancy—

*For corticosteroids—*

Corticosteroids cross the placenta. Although adequate studies have not been done in humans, there is some evidence that pharmacologic doses of corticosteroids may increase the risk of placental insufficiency, decreased birthweight, or stillbirth. However, teratogenic effects in humans have not been confirmed.

Infants born to mothers who have received substantial doses of corticosteroids during pregnancy should be carefully observed for signs of hypoadrenalism and replacement therapy administered as required.

Prenatal administration of betamethasone or dexamethasone to the mother to prevent respiratory distress syndrome in the premature neonate has not been shown to affect the child's growth or development adversely. Physiologic replacement doses of corticosteroids administered for treatment of maternal adrenal insufficiency are also unlikely to adversely affect the fetus or neonate.

Studies in animals have shown that corticosteroids increase the incidence of cleft palate, placental insufficiency, spontaneous abortions, and intrauterine growth retardation.

FDA Pregnancy Category C.

## Breast-feeding

For corticosteroids—Problems in humans have not been documented. Administration of physiologic doses or low pharmacologic doses (the equivalent or less of 25 mg of cortisone or 5 mg of prednisone per day) is not considered likely to affect the infant adversely. Less than 1% of the administered dose of prednisolone is excreted in breast milk. However, breast-feeding during the use of higher pharmacologic doses is not recommended because corticosteroids are excreted in breast milk and may cause unwanted effects, such as growth suppression and inhibition of endogenous steroid production, in the infant.

## Pediatrics

Because infections such as chickenpox or measles may be more serious (or even fatal) in children receiving immunosuppressant doses of corticosteroids, extra care to avoid exposure to these infections is recommended. Prophylactic therapy with varicella zoster immune globulin (VCIG) or immune globulin intravenous (IGIV) or intramuscular (IGIM), as appropriate, may be indicated in exposed patients. Therapy with an antiviral agent may be indicated if chickenpox develops.

Chronic use of corticosteroids may suppress growth and development of the pediatric or adolescent patient and should be undertaken with caution. Use of long-acting glucocorticoids (betamethasone and dexamethasone) or daily doses of any corticosteroid that are larger than replacement therapy doses are especially likely to inhibit growth and are not recommended for any form of chronic therapy. For long-term therapy, a short-acting agent (cortisone or hydrocortisone) or an intermediate-acting agent (methylprednisolone, prednisolone, prednisone, or triamcinolone) is recommended. Alternate-day therapy with an oral intermediate-acting corticosteroid may decrease growth retardation effects. Some clinicians recommend that only cortisone, hydrocortisone, or prednisone be used for long-term replacement therapy. Also, pediatric patients may be at increased risk of developing osteoporosis, avascular necrosis of the femoral heads, glaucoma, or cataracts during

prolonged therapy. Children and adolescents receiving prolonged therapy should be closely monitored.

Pediatric dosage is determined more by the severity of the condition and the response of the patient than by age or body weight. Also, for treatment of adrenocortical insufficiency, pediatric dosage is preferably determined in terms of mg per square meter of body surface area. Determination of pediatric dosage in terms of mg per kg of body weight (mg/kg) increases the possibility of overdosage, especially in very young, short, or heavy children.

Caution should also be used in children and adolescents receiving rectal dosage forms because of possible systemic absorption that can affect growth.

## Geriatrics

Geriatric patients may be more likely to develop hypertension during corticosteroid therapy. Geriatric patients, especially postmenopausal women, may also be more likely to develop glucocorticoid-induced osteoporosis.

## Drug interactions and/or related problems

The following drug interactions and/or related problems have been selected on the basis of their potential clinical significance (possible mechanism in parentheses where appropriate)—not necessarily inclusive (» = major clinical significance):

See also *Laboratory value alterations.*

Note:   Combinations containing any of the following medications, depending on the amount present, may also interact with this medication.

Interactions listed below involving alterations in serum potassium concentration and/or changes in sodium or fluid balance are especially likely to occur with corticosteroids having significant mineralocorticoid activity. However, these interactions may also occur with other corticosteroids, depending on dosage and patient predisposition.

Acetaminophen

(induction of hepatic enzymes by corticosteroids may increase the formation of a hepatotoxic acetaminophen metabolite, thereby increasing the risk of hepatotoxicity, when they are used concurrently with chronic or high-dose acetaminophen therapy)

Alcohol or

Anti-inflammatory drugs, nonsteroidal (NSAIDs)

(risk of gastrointestinal ulceration or hemorrhage may be increased when these substances are used concurrently with glucocorticoids; however, concurrent use of NSAIDs in the treatment of arthritis may provide additive therapeutic benefit and permit glucocorticoid dosage reduction)

» Aminoglutethimide

(aminoglutethimide suppresses adrenal function so that glucocorticoid supplementation may be required; however, aminoglutethimide accelerates the metabolism of dexamethasone so that dexamethasone half-life may be reduced two-fold; hydrocortisone is recommended instead because its metabolism is not known to be altered by aminoglutethimide and because its mineralocorticoid activity may also be required)

» Amphotericin B, parenteral or

Carbonic anhydrase inhibitors

(concurrent use with corticosteroids may result in severe hypokalemia and should be undertaken with caution; serum potassium concentrations and cardiac function should be monitored during concurrent use)

(the use of hydrocortisone to control adverse reactions to amphotericin B has resulted in cases of cardiac enlargement and congestive heart failure)

(concurrent use of corticosteroids with acetazolamide sodium may increase the risk of hypernatremia and/or edema because corticosteroids cause sodium and fluid retention; the risk with corticosteroids may depend on the patient's sodium requirement as determined by the condition being treated)

(the possibility should be considered that concurrent chronic use of both carbonic anhydrase inhibitors and corticosteroids may increase the risk of hypocalcemia and osteoporosis because carbonic anhydrase inhibitors also increase calcium excretion)

Anabolic steroids or

Androgens

(concurrent use with glucocorticoids may increase the risk of edema; also, concurrent use may promote the development of severe acne)

» Antacids

(concurrent chronic use with prednisone or dexamethasone may decrease absorption of these glucocorticoids; efficacy may be decreased sufficiently to require dosage adjustment in patients receiving small doses, but probably not in those receiving large doses, of the corticosteroid)

Anticholinergics, especially atropine and related compounds
(concurrent long-term use with glucocorticoids may increase intraocular pressure)

Anticoagulants, coumarin- or indandione-derivative or
Heparin or
Streptokinase or
Urokinase
(effects of coumarin or indandione derivatives are usually decreased [but may be increased in some patients] when these medications are used concurrently with glucocorticoids; dosage adjustments based on prothrombin time determinations may be necessary during and after glucocorticoid therapy)

(the potential occurrence of gastrointestinal ulceration or hemorrhage during glucocorticoid therapy, and the effects of glucocorticoids on vascular integrity, may cause increased risk to patients receiving anticoagulant or thrombolytic therapy)

Antidepressants, tricyclic
(these medications do not relieve, and may exacerbate, corticosteroid-induced mental disturbances; they should not be used for treatment of these adverse effects)

» Antidiabetic agents, sulfonylurea or
» Insulin
(glucocorticoids may increase blood glucose concentration; dosage adjustment of one or both agents may be necessary during concurrent use; dosage readjustment of the hypoglycemic agent may also be required when glucocorticoid therapy is discontinued)

Antithyroid agents or
Thyroid hormones
(changes in the thyroid status of the patient that may occur as a result of administration, changes in dosage, or discontinuation of thyroid hormones or antithyroid agents may necessitate adjustment of corticosteroid dosage because metabolic clearance of corticosteroids is decreased in hypothyroid patients and increased in hyperthyroid patients. Dosage adjustment should be based on results of thyroid function tests)

Asparaginase
(glucocorticoids, especially prednisone, may increase the hyperglycemic effect of asparaginase and the risk of neuropathy and disturbances in erythropoiesis; the toxicity appears to be less pronounced when asparaginase is administered following, rather than before or with, these medications)

Contraceptives, oral, estrogen-containing or
Estrogens
(estrogens may alter the metabolism and protein binding of glucocorticoids, leading to decreased clearance, increased elimination half-life, and increased therapeutic and toxic effects of the glucocorticoid; glucocorticoid dosage adjustment may be required during and following concurrent use)

» Digitalis glycosides
(concurrent use with glucocorticoids may increase the possibility of arrhythmias or digitalis toxicity associated with hypokalemia)

» Diuretics
(natriuretic and diuretic effects of these medications may be decreased by sodium- and fluid-retaining actions of corticosteroids, and vice versa)

(concurrent use of potassium-depleting diuretics with corticosteroids may result in severe hypokalemia; monitoring of serum potassium concentration and cardiac function is recommended)

(effects of potassium-sparing diuretics and/or corticosteroids on serum potassium concentration may be decreased during concurrent use; monitoring of serum potassium concentration is recommended)

Ephedrine
(ephedrine may increase the metabolic clearance of corticosteroids; corticosteroid dosage adjustment may be required during and following concurrent use)

Folic acid
(requirements may be increased in patients receiving long-term corticosteroid therapy)

» Hepatic enzyme–inducing agents (See *Appendix II*)
(concurrent use may decrease the corticosteroid effect because of increased corticosteroid metabolism resulting from induction of hepatic microsomal enzymes)

Immunosuppressant agents, other
(concurrent use with immunosuppressant doses of glucocorticoids may increase the risk of infection and possibly the development of lymphomas or other lymphoproliferative disorders; these neoplasms may be associated with Epstein-Barr virus infections; a few studies in organ transplant patients receiving immunosuppressant therapy indicate that progression of the neoplasm may be reversed after immunosuppressant dosage is decreased or therapy is discontinued)

Iophendylate or
Metrizamide
(concurrent intrathecal administration of metrizamide or iophendylate with intrathecal administration of glucocorticoids may increase the risk of arachnoiditis)

Isoniazid
(glucocorticoids, especially prednisolone, may increase hepatic metabolism and/or excretion of isoniazid, leading to decreased plasma concentration and effectiveness of isoniazid, especially in patients who are rapid acetylators; isoniazid dosage adjustment may be required during and following concurrent use)

Mexiletine
(concurrent use with glucocorticoids may accelerate mexiletine metabolism, leading to decreased mexiletine plasma concentration)

» Mitotane
(mitotane suppresses adrenocortical function; glucocorticoid supplementation is usually required during mitotane administration, but higher doses than those generally used for replacement therapy may be required because mitotane alters glucocorticoid metabolism)

Neuromuscular blocking agents, nondepolarizing
(hypokalemia induced by glucocorticoids may enhance the blockade of nondepolarizing neuromuscular blocking agents, possibly leading to increased or prolonged respiratory depression or paralysis [apnea]; serum potassium determinations may be necessary prior to administration of these agents)

(hydrocortisone and prednisone have also been reported to decrease the efficacy of pancuronium by an unknown mechanism; increased dosage of pancuronium or use of an alternate neuromuscular blocking agent may be necessary)

» Potassium supplements
(effects of these medications and/or corticosteroids on serum potassium concentration may be decreased when these medications are used concurrently; monitoring of serum potassium concentration is recommended)

» Ritodrine
(concurrent use may cause pulmonary edema in the mother; maternal death has been reported; both medications should be discontinued at the first sign of pulmonary edema)

Salicylates
(although concurrent use with glucocorticoids in the treatment of arthritis may provide additive therapeutic benefit and permit glucocorticoid dosage reduction, glucocorticoids may increase salicylate excretion and reduce salicylate plasma concentrations so that the salicylate dosage requirement may be increased; salicylism may occur when glucocorticoid dosage is subsequently decreased or discontinued, especially in patients receiving large [antirheumatic] doses of salicylates; also, the risk of gastrointestinal ulceration or hemorrhage may be increased during concurrent use)

» Sodium-containing medications or foods
(concurrent use with pharmacologic doses of glucocorticoids may result in edema and increased blood pressure, possibly to hypertensive levels)

(although patients receiving replacement doses of glucocorticoids may require sodium supplementation, adjustment of dietary sodium intake may be required when a medication having a high sodium content is also administered concurrently)

» Somatrem or
» Somatropin
(inhibition of the growth response to somatrem or somatropin may occur with chronic therapeutic use of daily doses [per square meter of body surface] in excess of:

| | Oral | Parenteral |
| --- | --- | --- |
| Betamethasone | 300–450 mcg | 150–225 mcg |
| Cortisone | 12.5–18.8 mg | 6.25–9.4 mg |
| Dexamethasone | 375–563 mcg | 187.5–281.5 mcg |
| Hydrocortisone | 10–15 mg | 5–7.5 mg |
| Methylprednisolone | 2–3 mg | 1–1.5 mg |
| Prednisolone | 2.5–3.75 mg | 1.25–1.88 mg |
| Prednisone | 2.5–3.75 mg | |
| Triamcinolone | 2–3 mg | 1–1.5 mg |

It is recommended that these doses not be exceeded during somatrem or somatropin therapy; if larger doses are required, administration of somatrem or somatropin should be postponed

Streptozocin
(concurrent use with glucocorticoids may increase the risk of hyperglycemia)

Troleandomycin
(troleandomycin may decrease metabolism of methylprednisolone and possibly other glucocorticoids, leading to increased plasma concentration, elimination half-life, and therapeutic and toxic effects; glucocorticoid dosage adjustment may be required during and following concurrent use)

» Vaccines, live virus, or other immunizations
(administration of live virus vaccines to patients receiving pharmacologic [immunosuppressant] doses of glucocorticoids may potentiate replication of the vaccine virus, thereby increasing the risk of the patient's developing the viral disease, and/or decrease the patient's antibody response to the vaccine and is not recommended; the patient's immunologic status should be evaluated prior to administration of a live virus vaccine; also, immunization with oral poliovirus vaccine should be postponed in persons in close contact with the patient, especially family members)

(other immunizations are not recommended in patients receiving pharmacologic [immunosuppressant] doses of glucocorticoids because of the increased risk of neurological complications and the possibility of decreased or absent antibody response)

(immunizations may be administered to patients receiving glucocorticoids via routes or in quantities that are not likely to cause immunosuppression, for example, those receiving local injections, short-term [less than 2 weeks] therapy, or physiologic doses)

**Laboratory value alterations**
The following have been selected on the basis of their potential clinical significance (possible effect in parentheses where appropriate)—not necessarily inclusive (» = major clinical significance):

With results of dexamethasone suppression tests
*Due to other medications*
Alcohol (chronic abuse) or
Glutethimide or
Meprobamate or
Methaqualone or
Methyprylon
(may cause false-positive results in test for endogenous depression)

Benzodiazepines (high doses) or
Cyproheptadine (high doses) or
Glucocorticoid therapy, long-term or
Indomethacin
(may cause false-negative results in test for endogenous depression)

Ephedrine or
Estrogens (high doses) or
Hepatic enzyme–inducing agents (See *Appendix II*)
(may cause false-positive results in tests for Cushing's disease or endogenous depression)

*Due to medical problems or conditions*
Adrenal hyperfunction (Cushing's disease) or
Anorexia nervosa or malnutrition leading to extreme weight loss, recent or
Carcinoma, disseminated, with concurrent serious infection or
Cardiac failure or
Dehydration or
Diabetes mellitus, unstable or
Fever or
Hypertension or
Pregnancy or
Renal failure or
Temporal lobe disease
(may cause false-positive results in test for endogenous depression)

Adrenal insufficiency or
Hypopituitarism
(may cause false-negative results in test for endogenous depression)

Psychiatric disorders such as acute psychosis, mania, chronic schizophrenia, and primary degenerative dementia
(may interfere with results of test for endogenous depression)

With *other* diagnostic test results
Brain imaging using sodium pertechnetate Tc 99m, technetium Tc 99m gluceptate, or technetium Tc 99m pentetate
(uptake of these diagnostic aids into cerebral tumors may be decreased in patients receiving large doses of glucocorticoids because of glucocorticoid-induced reduction of peritumor edema)

Gonadorelin test for hypothalamic-pituitary-gonadal axis function
(glucocorticoids may alter the results of the gonadorelin test by affecting pituitary secretion of gonadotropins through a complicated feedback mechanism)

Nitroblue-tetrazolium test for bacterial infection
(false-negative test results may occur)

Protirelin test for thyroid function
(physiologic doses of corticosteroids have no effect, but pharmacologic doses may reduce the thyroid-stimulating hormone [TSH] response to protirelin; however, withdrawal of corticosteroids in patients with known hypopituitarism is generally not recommended)

Skeletal imaging using technetium Tc 99m medronate, technetium Tc 99m oxidronate, or technetium Tc 99m pyrophosphate
(long-term use of glucocorticoids may induce bone calcium depletion, thus causing decreased bone uptake of these diagnostic aids)

Skin tests, including tuberculin and histoplasmin skin tests and patch tests for allergy
(reactions may be suppressed, especially with daily administration of large doses of corticosteroids)

Thyroid $^{123}$I or $^{131}$I uptake
(may be decreased)

With physiology/laboratory test values
Adrenal function as assessed by ACTH stimulation or measurement of plasma or urinary free cortisol
(may be decreased with pharmacologic doses of glucocorticoids, especially in children)

Basophil count and
Eosinophil count and
Lymphocyte count and
Monocyte count
(may be decreased)

Calcium
(serum concentrations may be decreased)

Cholesterol and
Lipid (fatty acid)
(serum concentrations may be increased)

Glucose
(blood and urine concentrations may be increased because of intrinsic hyperglycemic activity)

17-Hydroxysteroid (17-OHCS) and
17-Ketosteroid (17-KS)
(urine concentrations may be decreased by potent corticosteroids)

Platelet count
(may be increased or decreased)

Polymorphonuclear leukocyte count
(may be increased)

Potassium
(serum concentrations may be decreased because of increased potassium excretion, especially with agents having significant mineralocorticoid activity)

Sodium
(serum concentrations may be increased because of sodium retention, especially with glucocorticoids having significant mineralocorticoid activity)

Uric acid
(serum concentrations may be increased in patients with acute leukemia; may be decreased in other patients because of weak uricosuric effect)

**Medical considerations/Contraindications**
The medical considerations/contraindications included here have been selected on the basis of their potential clinical significance (reasons given in parentheses where appropriate)—not necessarily inclusive (» = major clinical significance).

See also *Laboratory value alterations.*

Note: The medical problems listed below apply only to pharmacologic (supraphysiologic) doses of glucocorticoids, unless otherwise stated.

*Except under special circumstances, these medications should not be used when the following medical problems exist:*

*For intra-articular injection*

» Arthroplasty of joint, prior
   (increased risk of infection)

» Blood clotting disorders
   (risk of intra- and extra-articular hemorrhage)

» Fracture, intra-articular
   (healing may be retarded)

» Infection, periarticular, current or history of
   (may be exacerbated or reactivated)

» Osteoporosis, juxta-articular, non-arthritic
   (may be exacerbated)

» Unstable joint

*For rectal administration*

» Anastomoses, intestinal, recent

» Fistulas and sinus tracts, extensive

» Ileocolostomy, recent

» Infection, abdominal, including peritonitis and intestinal or rectal abscesses
   (may be exacerbated)

» Obstruction, intestinal

» Perforation, intestinal

*For neonatal respiratory distress syndrome prophylaxis*

» Amnionitis

» Bleeding, uterine

» Febrile illness or infection, especially tuberculosis, maternal or

» Herpes type II infection, active, maternal or

» Keratitis, viral, maternal
   (may be exacerbated; if corticosteroid administration is essential, appropriate antimicrobial therapy must be administered concurrently)

» Placental insufficiency

» Premature membrane rupture
   (increased risk of maternal infection; the glucocorticoid should be administered immediately if this occurs, since the risk of infection increases with time)

**Risk-benefit should be considered when the following medical problems exist:**

*For all indications*

» Acquired immunodeficiency syndrome (AIDS) or

» Human immunodeficiency virus (HIV) infection
   (although pharmacologic doses of corticosteroids can be effective in the treatment of certain HIV-related diseases, careful medical evaluation of the risks and benefits of this therapy must be done, due to the possible increased risk of severe uncontrollable infections and/or neoplasms; in one study in patients given tapering doses of intravenous methylprednisolone starting with 60 mg every 6 hours for 8 days as an adjunct to antipneumocystis therapy, an increase in frequency or severity of life-threatening opportunistic infections was observed; in a study of similar patients given tapering doses of prednisone starting at 40 mg two times a day for 21 days, no increase in the incidence of Kaposi's sarcoma or life-threatening opportunistic infections was observed, though the incidence of oral candidiasis and mucocutaneous herpes simplex infection did increase)

» Anastomoses, intestinal, recent

» Cardiac disease or

» Congestive heart failure or
   Hypertension or

» Renal function impairment or disease, severe
   (edema may be hazardous, especially with agents having significant mineralocorticoid activity)
   (patients undergoing dialysis may have increased risk of avascular necrosis with long-term corticosteroid use)

» Chickenpox, existing or recent (including recent exposure) or

» Measles, existing or recent (including recent exposure)
   (risk of severe, potentially fatal, generalized disease; extra care to avoid exposure to these infections is recommended; prophylactic therapy with varicella zoster immune globulin [VZIG] or immune globulin intravenous [IGIV] or intramuscular [IGIM], as appropriate, may be indicated in exposed patients; therapy with an antiviral agent may be indicated if chickenpox develops)

   Colitis, ulcerative nonspecific, with possibility of impending perforation, abscess, or other infection or

Diverticulitis or

» Esophagitis, gastritis, or peptic ulcer, active or latent
   (symptoms of progression or reactivation may be masked; hemorrhage and/or perforation may occur without warning)

» Diabetes mellitus or predisposition to
   (may be exacerbated or activated)

» Fungal infections, systemic
   (may be exacerbated; pharmacologic doses should not be given unless the patient is concurrently receiving an antifungal agent)

Glaucoma, open-angle
   (intraocular pressure may be increased)

Hepatic function impairment or disease
   (increased risk of glucocorticoid toxicity, especially if hypoalbuminemia present; possibility of impaired conversion of cortisone or prednisone to their active metabolites, although effect may be offset by decreased protein binding or clearance and/or conversion in other tissues)

» Herpes simplex, ocular
   (possible corneal perforation)

Herpetic lesions, oral

Hyperlipidemia
   (concentrations of fatty acids or cholesterol may be increased)

Hyperthyroidism
   (glucocorticoid effect may be impaired because of accelerated metabolism; may be especially important with physiologic doses or low pharmacologic doses)

Hypoalbuminemia or conditions predisposing to, including hepatic cirrhosis or nephrotic syndrome
   (increased risk of toxicity because reduced availability of albumin for glucocorticoid binding leads to increased serum concentration of unbound drug; reduction in initial dosage is recommended)

Hypothyroidism
   (decreased metabolism of corticosteroid may result)

Infections, viral or bacterial, uncontrolled, systemic or at site of local injection
   (may be exacerbated; concurrent antimicrobial therapy required)

Intolerance to corticosteroids

» Myasthenia gravis
   (muscle weakness may be increased initially, possibly leading to respiratory distress; patient should be hospitalized, and respiratory support should be immediately available, when glucocorticoid therapy is initiated)

Osteoporosis
   (may be exacerbated)

Renal function impairment, mild to moderate, or stones
   (fluid retention may exacerbate these conditions; increased risk of edema, especially with agents having mineralocorticoid activity)
   (patients receiving dialysis may have increased risk of avascular necrosis with long-term corticosteroid use)

Systemic lupus erythematosus (SLE)
   (cautious use is recommended because of an increased risk of aseptic necrosis)

» Tuberculosis—active, positive skin test, latent, or history of
   (may be exacerbated or reactivated; appropriate antitubercular chemotherapy or prophylaxis should be administered concurrently)

**Patient monitoring**

The following may be especially important in patient monitoring (other tests may be warranted in some patients, depending on condition; » = major clinical significance):

Glucose concentrations, blood or urine or

Glucose tolerance test
   (may be required for patients with diabetes mellitus or a predisposition to diabetes mellitus)

Growth and development determinations
   (recommended in children and adolescents receiving prolonged therapy)

Hypothalamic-pituitary-adrenal (HPA) axis function determination
   (may be required during and following withdrawal of, high-dose or long-term [more than 3 weeks] therapy to assess adrenal function; complete recovery of adrenal function may require up to 1 year following prolonged use, especially with high doses; in some patients receiving prolonged, high-dose therapy, complete recovery may never occur)

Ophthalmologic examinations
   (may be required at periodic intervals for adults or children receiving therapy for more than 6 weeks to detect the presence of

cataracts, increased intraocular pressure, glaucoma, or ocular infections)

Serum electrolyte determinations and
Stool tests for occult blood loss
   (may be required during long-term therapy)

## Side/Adverse Effects

Note:  The risk of adverse effects with pharmacologic doses of corticosteroids generally increases with the duration of therapy and frequency of administration and, to a lesser extent, with dosage.

Chronic administration of physiologic replacement doses of corticosteroids rarely causes adverse effects.

Administration of glucocorticoids rectally or via local injection reduces the risk of systemic effects. The risk of both systemic and local adverse effects is still present to a degree, however, and increases with the duration of rectal therapy and with the frequency of injections.

Pharmacologic doses of glucocorticoids lower resistance to infection; the patient may be predisposed to systemic infections during, and for a time following, therapy. Increased susceptibility to infection may occur with short-term high-dose use ("pulse" therapy) as well as with more prolonged use. Also, symptoms of onset or progression of infections may be masked.

The following side/adverse effects have been selected on the basis of their potential clinical significance (possible signs and symptoms in parentheses where appropriate)—not necessarily inclusive:

### Those indicating need for medical attention
Incidence less frequent
   *Local allergic reaction or rectal irritation* (rectal bleeding, blistering, burning, itching, or pain not present before therapy)—with rectal dosage forms; *cataracts* (decreased or blurred vision); *diabetes mellitus* (decreased or blurred vision; frequent urination; increased thirst)

Incidence rare
   *Generalized allergic reaction* (skin rash or hives); *local allergic reaction or infection at injection site* (redness, swelling, pain, or other signs of infection or allergic reaction); *sudden blindness; burning, numbness, pain, or tingling at or near place of injection; psychic disturbances such as delirium* (confusion; excitement; restlessness); *disorientation; euphoria* (false sense of well-being); *hallucinations* (seeing, hearing, or feeling things that are not there); *manic-depressive episodes* (sudden, wide mood swings); *mental depression, or paranoia* (mistaken feelings of self-importance or being mistreated)

   Note:  *Sudden blindness* following injection into sites in the head or neck area, such as nasal turbinates or scalp, due to possible entry of drug crystals into ocular blood vessels.

   *Psychic disturbances* are more likely in patients with chronic debilitating illnesses that predispose them to psychic disturbances and in patients receiving higher daily dosages. Psychic disturbances may be related to dose rather than duration of therapy; symptoms may appear within a few days to 2 weeks after initiation of therapy and are usually associated with doses equivalent to 40 mg or more of prednisone per day. Additionally, euphoria or fear of relapse may lead to psychological dependence or abuse of corticosteroids.

With rapid intravenous administration of high doses ("pulse" therapy)
   *Generalized anaphylaxis* (swelling of face, nasal membranes, and eyelids; hives; shortness of breath; tightness in chest; troubled breathing; wheezing); *flushing of face or cheeks; irregular or pounding heartbeat; seizures*

   Note:  *Rapid intravenous administration of high doses* of corticosteroids has been reported to cause convulsions, angioedema and/or anaphylactic reactions, and sudden death associated with cardiac arrhythmias. Monitoring of the electrocardiogram (ECG) is recommended. Equipment, medications, and trained personnel necessary for treating these complications should be immediately available.

### Those occurring principally during long-term use indicating need for medical attention
   *Acne or other skin problems; avascular necrosis* (hip or shoulder pain); *Cushing's syndrome* (filling or rounding out of the face); *edema* (swelling of feet or lower legs; rapid weight gain); *endocrine imbalance* (menstrual irregularities); *gastrointestinal irritation* (nausea; vomiting); *hypokalemic syndrome* (irregular heartbeat; muscle cramps or pain; unusual tiredness or weakness); *osteoporosis or bone fractures* (pain in back, ribs, arms, or legs)—includes vertebral compression and long bone pathologic fractures; *pancreatitis* (continuing ab-

dominal or stomach pain or burning; nausea; vomiting); *peptic ceration or intestinal perforation* (continuing abdominal or stomach pain or burning; bloody or black, tarry stools); *scarring at injection site; steroid myopathy* (muscle weakness); *striae* (reddish purple lines on arms, face, legs, trunk, or groin); *tendon rupture*—with local injection; *cutaneous or subcutaneous tissue atrophy* (thin, shiny skin; pitting or depression of skin at place of injection)—with frequent repository injections; *unusual bruising; wounds that will not heal*

### Those indicating need for medical attention only if they continue or are bothersome
Incidence more frequent
   *Increased appetite; indigestion; nervousness or restlessness; trouble in sleeping*

For triamcinolone
   *Loss of appetite*

Incidence less frequent or rare
   *Changes in skin color or hypopigmentation* (darkening or lightening of skin color); *dizziness or lightheadedness; flushing of face or cheeks; headache*—following intranasal injection; *increased joint pain*—following intra-articular injection; *increased sweating; nosebleeds*—following intranasal injection; *unusual increase in hair growth on body or face*

   Note:  *Hypopigmentation* is more likely at the injection site.

   *Flushing of face or cheeks* may persist for 24 to 48 hours.

   *Increased joint pain* may occur within a few hours postinjection and persist for up to 48 hours.

### Those occurring principally after medication is discontinued, indicating a corticosteroid withdrawal syndrome and the need for medical attention
   *Withdrawal syndrome* (abdominal or back pain; dizziness; fainting; frequent or continuing unexplained headaches; low-grade fever; muscle or joint pain; nausea; prolonged loss of appetite; rapid weight loss; reappearance of disease symptoms; shortness of breath; unusual tiredness or weakness; vomiting)

   Note:  Too-rapid *withdrawal of therapy*, especially after prolonged use, may cause acute, possibly life-threatening, adrenal insufficiency and/or a withdrawal syndrome not related to HPA axis suppression.

## Patient Consultation

As an aid to patient consultation, refer to *Advice for the Patient, Corticosteroids—Glucocorticoid Effects (Systemic)*.

In providing consultation, consider emphasizing the following selected information (» = major clinical significance):

### Before using this medication
» Conditions affecting use, especially:
   Allergies to corticosteroids
   Pregnancy—Pharmacologic doses in animals show some evidence of increased risk of placental insufficiency, decreased birthweight, or stillbirths; other animal studies show increased incidence of cleft palate, placental insufficiency, spontaneous abortions, or intrauterine growth retardation. Hypoadrenalism may occur in infants if mothers received substantial doses of corticosteroids prenatally
   Breast-feeding—Breast-feeding is not recommended during use of higher doses
   Use in children—Close monitoring required since chronic therapy may result in suppression of growth and development; possible increased severity of chickenpox or measles in children receiving immunosuppressant doses; discussing possible effects with physician
   Use in the elderly—Increased risk of osteoporosis (especially in postmenopausal females) or hypertension
   Other medications, especially aminoglutethimide, parenteral amphotericin B, antacids, sulfonylurea antidiabetic agents, insulin, digitalis glycosides, diuretics, hepatic enzyme–inducing agents, mitotane, potassium supplements, ritodrine, sodium-containing medications, human growth hormone, or immunizations
   Other medical problems, especially
      For all uses—AIDS, systemic or local infections, gastrointestinal disorders, cardiac disease, chickenpox, congestive heart failure, renal diseases, diabetes, measles, or myasthenia gravis
      For intra-articular injection only—Arthroplasty, clotting disorders, fracture, osteoporosis, or unstable joint
      For rectal use only—Recent ileocolostomy
      For neonatal respiratory distress syndrome prophylaxis only—Amnionitis, uterine bleeding, febrile illness, placental insufficiency, or premature membrane rupture

## Proper use of this medication

*For oral dosage forms*

» Taking with food to minimize gastrointestinal irritation
  Possibility that alcohol may enhance ulcerogenic effects of medication

*For rectal dosage forms*

  Proper administration technique; reading patient directions carefully
  Saving applicator for methylprednisolone acetate for enema; refill units may be available

» Importance of not using more medication than the amount prescribed
» Proper dosing
  Missed dose: If dosing schedule is—
    Every other day: Taking as soon as possible if remembered same morning; if remembered later, not taking until next morning, then skipping a day
    Once a day: Taking as soon as possible; not taking if almost time for next dose; not doubling doses
    Several times a day: Taking as soon as possible; doubling if time for next dose
» Proper storage

## Precautions while using this medication

» Regular visits to physician to check progress during and following therapy
» Checking with physician before discontinuing medication; gradual dosage reduction may be necessary
  Checking with physician if symptoms recur or worsen when dose decreased or therapy discontinued
» Possible need for calorie and/or sodium restriction or potassium supplementation during long-term therapy
  Possible need for increased protein intake during long-term therapy
  Ophthalmologic examinations during long-term therapy
  Carrying medical identification card indicating use of medication during long-term therapy
» Caution in receiving skin tests
» Caution if any kind of surgery or emergency treatment is required
» Avoiding exposure to chickenpox or measles (especially for children); telling physician right away if exposure occurs
» Caution in receiving vaccinations or other immunizations or coming in contact with persons receiving oral poliovirus vaccine
» Caution if serious infections or injuries occur
  Diabetics: May increase blood sugar concentrations

*For parenteral dosage forms*

  Restricting use of joint following intra-articular injection
  Checking with physician if redness or swelling occurs, and continues or becomes worse, following local injection

*For rectal dosage forms*

  Checking with physician if signs of rectal irritation or infection occur

## Side/adverse effects

  Signs of potential side effects, especially visual disturbances, diabetes mellitus, local irritation, allergic reactions, local or systemic infection, psychic disturbances, seizures, hypertension, tachycardia, musculoskeletal disorders, Cushing's syndrome, edema, endocrine imbalance, hypokalemic syndrome, gastrointestinal effects, myopathy, striae, tissue atrophy, scarring at injection site, bruising, or delayed wound healing

# General Dosing Information

See also *Table 4*, page 983.

For replacement therapy in chronic adrenocortical insufficiency states, corticosteroid therapy must be continued for the life of the patient. It is recommended that dosage of cortisone or hydrocortisone be timed to simulate endogenous corticosteroid secretion, with two-thirds of the daily dose administered in the morning and one-third in the evening. Other corticosteroids are usually given once a day.

For treatment of adrenogenital syndrome, suppression of corticotropin secretion is required to decrease hypersecretion of adrenal androgens. This is usually achieved by administering one-third of the daily dose of cortisone or hydrocortisone in the morning and two-thirds in the evening or giving one-third of the daily dose three times a day at evenly spaced intervals. Other corticosteroids are usually given once a day.

Except in severe conditions or emergency situations, it is recommended that therapy be instituted with low doses that should be increased as necessary to provide the desired effect. For most conditions, administration in the lowest effective dose for the shortest time possible is recommended. Dosage requirements are variable and should be individualized according to the disease being treated and patient response rather than by age or body weight. Whenever possible, local administration is recommended in order to concentrate the medication at the

affected site and reduce the risk of systemic effects. After a favorable response is obtained, the dosage should be decreased gradually to the lowest dose that will maintain an adequate clinical response.

Frequent monitoring of drug effect is required. Situations that may necessitate dosage adjustments include remissions or exacerbations of the disease process and the patient's response to the medication.

Clinically significant hypothalamic-pituitary-adrenal (HPA) axis suppression leading to adrenal insufficiency may occur more readily with multiple daily doses or evening administration than with single doses given every morning or every other morning. Administration of a single daily dose of a short- or intermediate-acting corticosteroid prior to 9 a.m. may reduce the risk of HPA axis suppression (because maximum endogenous corticosteroid secretion occurs in the morning) and is recommended for daily administration whenever possible. However, some disease conditions may require multiple daily doses.

Following discontinuation of short-term (up to 5 days) high-dose use, adrenal recovery may occur within 1 week; however, following prolonged high-dose administration, complete recovery of adrenal function may require up to 1 year. Following very prolonged suppression, complete recovery may never occur. During the recovery period, monitoring of adrenal function may be required to assess the patient's ability to respond to stress.

Patients with known or suspected adrenal insufficiency, including those already receiving replacement therapy, require an increase in dosage or reinstitution of therapy prior to, during, and for a time following, exposure to emotional stress or physical stress such as severe infection, surgery (including dental surgery), or injury. Administration of sodium and/or a mineralocorticoid may also be required. Dosage and duration of such therapy are dependent on the severity of the stress.

When medication is to be discontinued, dosage should be reduced gradually. The rate at which dosage can be decreased and the time required for complete withdrawal of therapy are variable, depending on the specific agent used; dose, frequency, and route of administration; duration of therapy; condition being treated; and patient response.

## For oral dosage forms only

If oral long-term use is required for disease therapy, an alternate-day regimen using an intermediate-acting corticosteroid is recommended to minimize HPA axis suppression and possibly other adverse effects. An intermediate-acting corticosteroid is one that suppresses HPA axis activity for 12 to 36 hours following a single dose. Administration of longer-acting corticosteroids on an alternate-day schedule does not reduce the risk of HPA axis suppression and is not recommended.

Alternate-day therapy utilizes a single dose administered every other morning, usually in a quantity equivalent to, or somewhat higher than, twice the usual or pre-established daily dose. The patient should have a normal or moderately responsive HPA axis.

If treatment has been initiated with daily administration, changes to alternate-day therapy should be made gradually, after the patient's condition has stabilized. However, for some diseases, such as childhood nephrosis, therapy may be initiated with alternate-day dosing.

Alternate-day therapy may not be effective in treating hematologic disorders, malignancies, ulcerative colitis, or severe conditions. Also, some patients, such as those with asthma or rheumatoid arthritis, may experience exacerbation of symptoms on the second day. Administration of (or increasing the dosage of) suitable supplemental therapy on the second day may provide sufficient symptomatic relief to permit alternate-day dosing in some patients.

## For parenteral dosage forms only

For acute adrenocortical insufficiency, initiation of corticosteroid therapy by intravenous injection followed by slow intravenous infusion or intramuscular administration is recommended. Certain other acute conditions may also require initiation of therapy with intravenous administration or intramuscular administration of a rapidly acting formulation.

In severe or life-threatening conditions, single-dose or short-term intravenous administration of a very high dose ("pulse" therapy) may produce the required therapeutic response with a minimum risk of prolonged HPA axis suppression or other adverse effects. Such therapy has been recommended for treating conditions such as organ transplant rejection reactions, acute nephritis associated with systemic lupus erythematosus, vasculitis, adult respiratory distress syndrome, and shock. However, rapid intravenous administration of high doses of corticosteroids has been reported to cause potentially life-threatening side effects and appropriate precautions should be observed.

When the suspension dosage forms are administered intramuscularly, they should be injected deeply into the gluteal muscle to prevent local tissue atrophy. It is recommended that the deltoid muscle not be used because of a higher incidence of local atrophy. In addition, do not inject repeatedly into the same site.

A standard textbook should be consulted for specific techniques and procedures applicable to local injection of corticosteroids for various indications.

It is recommended that intra-articular injections be repeated no more often than once every 3 weeks. Frequent repeated injections may cause joint damage.

Following intra-articular injection, the injected joint should not be over-used, even if pain is relieved, because of the increased risk of joint damage or deterioration. It is recommended that weight-bearing joints be rested for 24 to 48 hours postinjection.

Administration of a local anesthetic concurrently with intra-articular or soft tissue injection of a corticosteroid may reduce the pain of injection and provide immediate relief of symptoms. However, a post-injection flare of pain may occur when the local anesthetic effect subsides.

Dosages for local injections (e.g., intra-articular, intrabursal, intradermal, intralesional) are given as ranges only. The actual dosage depends upon the size of the joint or lesion and the severity of the condition being treated.

### Diet/Nutrition

Administration of oral dosage forms with food may relieve indigestion or mild gastrointestinal irritation that may occur.

Patients receiving prolonged therapy with pharmacologic doses of corticosteroids, especially those with significant mineralocorticoid activity, may require sodium restriction and/or potassium supplementation during therapy.

Because corticosteroids promote protein catabolism, increased protein intake may be necessary during prolonged therapy.

Administration of calcium and vitamin D and, if the patient's condition permits, exercise or physical therapy may reduce the risk of corticosteroid-induced osteoporosis during prolonged therapy.

### For treatment of adverse effects

Recommended treatment consists of the following

For gastrointestinal effects—Administration of antacids between meals may relieve indigestion or mild gastrointestinal irritation that may occur during parenteral, as well as oral, corticosteroid therapy. However, the efficacy of antacids or other antiulcer medications in preventing severe gastrointestinal problems, such as ulceration, hemorrhage, and/or bowel perforation, during corticosteroid therapy has not been established.

For mental depression or psychoses—If possible, decrease corticosteroid dosage or discontinue therapy. A phenothiazine may be administered if necessary; lithium has also been recommended. Some patients may require electroconvulsive therapy if severe depression persists. Tricyclic antidepressants should not be used since they do not relieve, and may exacerbate, corticosteroid-induced mental disturbances. Prophylactic administration of an antipsychotic agent may be indicated if additional courses of corticosteroid therapy are required by a patient with a history of corticosteroid-induced psychosis.

For withdrawal effects (non-HPA axis suppression)—Administration of aspirin or another nonsteroidal anti-inflammatory drug may alleviate some of the symptoms of this condition.

---

## *BETAMETHASONE*

## Summary of Differences

Indications: See *Table 1*.

Pharmacology/pharmacokinetics: See *Table 2* and *Table 3*.

Precautions: Pediatrics—Not recommended for chronic use; especially likely to inhibit growth.

General dosing information: See *Table 4*.

## Oral Dosage Forms

### BETAMETHASONE SYRUP USP

#### Usual adult and adolescent dose

Oral, 600 mcg (0.6 mg) to 7.2 mg a day as a single dose or in divided doses.

#### Usual pediatric dose

Adrenocortical insufficiency—
Oral, 17.5 mcg (0.0175 mg) per kg of body weight or 500 mcg (0.5 mg) per square meter of body surface a day in three divided doses.

Other indications—
Oral, 62.5 to 250 mcg (0.0625 to 0.25 mg) per kg of body weight or 1.875 to 7.5 mg per square meter of body surface a day in three or four divided doses.

#### Strength(s) usually available

U.S.—
600 mcg (0.6 mg) per 5 mL (Rx) [*Celestone* (alcohol <1%)].

#### Packaging and storage

Store between 2 and 30 °C (36 and 86 °F), protected from light. Store in a well-closed container. Protect from freezing.

### BETAMETHASONE TABLETS USP

#### Usual adult and adolescent dose

Oral, 600 mcg (0.6 mg) to 7.2 mg a day as a single dose or in divided doses.

#### Usual pediatric dose

Adrenocortical insufficiency—
Oral, 17.5 mcg (0.0175 mg) per kg of body weight or 500 mcg (0.5 mg) per square meter of body surface a day in three divided doses.

Other indications—
Oral, 62.5 to 250 mcg (0.0625 to 0.25 mg) per kg of body weight or 1.875 to 7.5 mg per square meter of body surface a day in three or four divided doses.

#### Strength(s) usually available

U.S.—
600 mcg (0.6 mg) (Rx) [*Celestone* (scored)].

Canada—
500 mcg (0.5 mg) (Rx) [*Betnelan* (scored); *Celestone* (scored)].

#### Packaging and storage

Store between 2 and 30 °C (36 and 86 °F). Store in a well-closed container.

Note: Protect the 21-tablet pack from excessive moisture.

### BETAMETHASONE EFFERVESCENT TABLETS

#### Usual adult and adolescent dose

Oral, 600 mcg (0.6 mg) to 7.2 mg a day as a single dose or in divided doses.

#### Usual pediatric dose

Adrenocortical insufficiency—
Oral, 17.5 mcg (0.0175 mg) per kg of body weight or 500 mcg (0.5 mg) per square meter of body surface a day in three divided doses.

Other indications—
Oral, 62.5 to 250 mcg (0.0625 to 0.25 mg) per kg of body weight or 1.875 to 7.5 mg per square meter of body surface a day in three or four divided doses.

#### Strength(s) usually available

U.S.—
Not commercially available.

Canada—
500 mcg (0.5 mg) (Rx) [*Betnesol* (scored)].

#### Packaging and storage

Store below 40 °C (104 °F), preferably between 15 and 30 °C (59 and 86 °F), in a well-closed container, unless otherwise specified by manufacturer. Protect from moisture.

#### Preparation of dosage form

Dissolve in water immediately prior to ingestion.

#### Note

When dispensing, explain dissolution requirement to patient.

### BETAMETHASONE SODIUM PHOSPHATE EXTENDED-RELEASE TABLETS

#### Usual adult and adolescent dose

Oral, 2 to 6 mg per day initially, then adjusted according to patient response.

#### Usual pediatric dose

Adrenocortical insufficiency—
Oral, 17.5 mcg (0.0175 mg) per kg of body weight or 500 mcg (0.5 mg) per square meter of body surface a day in three divided doses.

Other indications—
Oral, 62.5 to 250 mcg (0.0625 to 0.25 mg) per kg of body weight or 1.875 to 7.5 mg per square meter of body surface a day in three or four divided doses.

#### Strength(s) usually available

U.S.—
Not commercially available.

Canada—
1 mg (Rx) [*Celestone*].

#### Packaging and storage

Store below 40 °C (104 °F), preferably between 15 and 30 °C (59 and 86 °F), in a well-closed container, unless otherwise specified by manufacturer.

# Parenteral Dosage Forms

## BETAMETHASONE SODIUM PHOSPHATE INJECTION USP

### Usual adult and adolescent dose
Intra-articular, intralesional, or soft-tissue injection, up to 9 mg (base), repeated as needed.

Intramuscular or intravenous, up to 9 mg (base) a day.

### Usual pediatric dose
Adrenocortical insufficiency—
Intramuscular, 17.5 mcg (0.0175 mg) (base) per kg of body weight or 500 mcg (0.5 mg) (base) per square meter of body surface a day (in three divided doses) every third day; or 5.8 to 8.75 mcg (0.0058 to 0.00875 mg) (base) per kg of body weight or 166 to 250 mcg (0.166 to 0.25 mg) (base) per square meter of body surface once a day.

Other indications—
Intramuscular, 20.8 to 125 mcg (0.021 to 0.125 mg) (base) per kg of body weight or 625 mcg (0.625 mg) to 3.75 mg (base) per square meter of body surface every twelve to twenty-four hours.

### Strength(s) usually available
U.S.—
3 mg (base) (4 mg sodium phosphate) per mL (Rx) [*Celestone Phosphate* (sodium bisulfite 3.2 mg); *Selestoject* (sodium bisulfite); GENERIC].

### Packaging and storage
Store below 40 °C (104 °F), preferably between 15 and 30 °C (59 and 86 °F), protected from light, unless otherwise specified by manufacturer. Protect from freezing.

## STERILE BETAMETHASONE SODIUM PHOSPHATE AND BETAMETHASONE ACETATE SUSPENSION USP

### Usual adult and adolescent dose
Intra-articular, 1.5 to 12 mg, depending upon the size of the affected joint, repeated as needed.

Intrabursal, 6 mg, repeated as needed.

Intradermal or intralesional, 1.2 mg per square centimeter of affected skin up to a total amount of 6 mg, repeated at one-week intervals, if necessary.

Intramuscular, 500 mcg (0.5 mg) to 9 mg a day.

### Usual pediatric dose
Dosage has not been established.

### Strength(s) usually available
U.S.—
6 mg (3 mg of betamethasone acetate and 3 mg of betamethasone base) per mL (Rx) [*Celestone Soluspan*].

Canada—
6 mg (3 mg of betamethasone acetate and 3 mg of betamethasone base) per mL (Rx) [*Celestone Soluspan*].

### Packaging and storage
Store between 2 and 25 °C (36 and 77 °F), protected from light, unless otherwise specified by manufacturer. Protect from freezing.

### Incompatibilities
This medication should *not* be mixed with parenteral-local anesthetic formulations containing parabens, phenol, or other such preservatives, because flocculation of the corticosteroid may occur. Withdraw the required quantity of corticosteroid suspension into a syringe, then add the local anesthetic. *Do not introduce the local anesthetic directly into the multiple-dose vial.*

### Auxiliary labeling
• Shake well.

### Additional dosing information
For administration of injections, see manufacturer's labeling.

Do not administer this medication intravenously.

# Rectal Dosage Forms

## BETAMETHASONE DISODIUM PHOSPHATE ENEMA

### Usual adult and adolescent dose
Rectal, 5 mg (base) as a retention enema each night for fourteen to twenty-eight days initially, then as determined by patient response.

Note: It is recommended that the medication be discontinued, and alternate methods of treatment considered, if a favorable response is not obtained within 4 weeks.

### Usual pediatric dose
Dosage has not been established.

### Strength(s) usually available
U.S.—
Not commercially available.

Canada—
5 mg (base) per 100 mL (Rx) [*Betnesol*].

### Packaging and storage
Store below 40 °C (104 °F), preferably between 15 and 30 °C (59 and 86 °F), unless otherwise specified by manufacturer. Protect from freezing.

### Note
When dispensing, explain administration technique.

---

## CORTISONE

---

# Summary of Differences

Indications: See *Table 1*.
Pharmacology/pharmacokinetics: See *Table 2* and *Table 3*.
General dosing information: See *Table 4*.

# Oral Dosage Forms

## CORTISONE ACETATE TABLETS USP

### Usual adult and adolescent dose
Oral, 25 to 300 mg a day as a single dose or in divided doses.

### Usual pediatric dose
Adrenocortical insufficiency—
Oral, 700 mcg (0.7 mg) per kg of body weight or 20 to 25 mg per square meter of body surface a day in divided doses.

Other indications—
Oral, 2.5 to 10 mg per kg of body weight or 75 to 300 mg per square meter of body surface a day as a single dose or in divided doses.

### Strength(s) usually available
U.S.—
5 mg (Rx) [GENERIC (scored; lactose)].
10 mg (Rx) [GENERIC (scored)].
25 mg (Rx) [*Cortone Acetate* (scored); GENERIC (scored; sucrose)].

Canada—
5 mg (Rx) [*Cortone* (lactose)].
25 mg (Rx) [*Cortone* (scored; lactose); GENERIC].

### Packaging and storage
Store below 40 °C (104 °F), preferably between 15 and 30 °C (59 and 86 °F). Store in a well-closed container.

# Parenteral Dosage Forms

## STERILE CORTISONE ACETATE SUSPENSION USP

### Usual adult and adolescent dose
Intramuscular, 20 to 300 mg a day.

### Usual pediatric dose
Adrenocortical insufficiency—
Intramuscular, 700 mcg (0.7 mg) per kg of body weight or 37.5 mg per square meter of body surface a day every third day; or 233.33 to 350 mcg (0.23333 to 0.350 mg) per kg of body weight or 12.5 mg per square meter of body surface once a day.

Other indications—
Intramuscular, 833 mcg (0.833 mg) to 5 mg per kg of body weight or 25 to 150 mg per square meter of body surface every twelve to twenty-four hours.

### Strength(s) usually available
U.S.—
25 mg per mL (Rx) [GENERIC].
50 mg per mL (Rx) [*Cortone Acetate;* GENERIC].

Canada—
50 mg per mL (Rx) [*Cortone*].

### Packaging and storage
Store below 40 °C (104 °F), preferably between 15 and 30 °C (59 and 86 °F), unless otherwise specified by manufacturer. Protect from freezing.

### Stability
Dilutions or admixtures of this medication with other products are not recommended because the state of suspension or the rate of absorption may be affected.

This medication is heat-sensitive and should not be autoclaved.

### Auxiliary labeling
• Shake well.

### Additional information
Do not administer this medication intravenously.

---
### DEXAMETHASONE
---

## Summary of Differences

Category: Also, diagnostic aid (Cushing's syndrome and endogenous depression) and antiemetic (in cancer chemotherapy).

Indications: See *Table 1*.

Pharmacology/pharmacokinetics: See *Table 2* and *Table 3*.

Precautions: Pediatrics—Not recommended for chronic use; especially likely to inhibit growth.

General dosing information: See *Table 4*.

## Oral Dosage Forms

### DEXAMETHASONE ELIXIR USP

**Usual adult and adolescent dose**

Oral, 500 mcg (0.5 mg) to 9 mg a day as a single dose or in divided doses.

Dexamethasone suppression test—

Test for Cushing's syndrome: Oral, 1 mg as a single dose at 11:00 p.m. or 500 mcg (0.5 mg) every six hours for forty-eight hours.

Test to distinguish Cushing's syndrome due to pituitary ACTH excess from Cushing's syndrome due to other causes: Oral, 2 mg every six hours for forty-eight hours.

Depression diagnosis: Oral, 1 mg as a single dose at 11:00 p.m.

In cerebral edema associated with recurrent or inoperable brain tumor—

Oral, 2 mg two or three times a day, administered as maintenance therapy after cerebral edema has initially been controlled using parenteral dexamethasone sodium phosphate.

**Usual pediatric dose**

Adrenocortical insufficiency—

Oral, 23.3 mcg (0.0233 mg) per kg of body weight or 670 mcg (0.67 mg) per square meter of body surface a day in three divided doses.

Other indications—

Oral, 83.3 to 333.3 mcg (0.0833 to 0.3333 mg) per kg of body weight or 2.5 to 10 mg per square meter of body surface a day in three or four divided doses.

**Strength(s) usually available**

U.S.—

500 mcg (0.5 mg) per 5 mL (Rx) [*Decadron* (alcohol 5%); *Hexadrol* (alcohol 5%); *Mymethasone* (alcohol 5%); GENERIC].

**Packaging and storage**

Store below 40 °C (104 °F), preferably between 15 and 30 °C (59 and 86 °F), unless otherwise specified by manufacturer. Store in a tight container. Protect from freezing.

**Auxiliary labeling**

• Keep container tightly closed.

### DEXAMETHASONE ORAL SOLUTION

**Usual adult and adolescent dose**

Oral, 500 mcg (0.5 mg) to 9 mg a day as a single dose or in divided doses.

Dexamethasone suppression test—

Test for Cushing's syndrome: Oral, 1 mg as a single dose at 11:00 p.m. or 500 mcg (0.5 mg) every six hours for forty-eight hours.

Test to distinguish Cushing's syndrome due to pituitary ACTH excess from Cushing's syndrome due to other causes: Oral, 2 mg every six hours for forty-eight hours.

Depression diagnosis: Oral, 1 mg as a single dose at 11:00 p.m.

In cerebral edema associated with recurrent or inoperable brain tumor—

Oral, 2 mg two or three times a day, administered as maintenance therapy after cerebral edema has initially been controlled using parenteral dexamethasone sodium phosphate.

**Usual pediatric dose**

Adrenocortical insufficiency—

Oral, 23.3 mcg (0.0233 mg) per kg of body weight or 670 mcg (0.67 mg) per square meter of body surface a day in three divided doses.

Other indications—

Oral, 83.3 to 333.3 mcg (0.0833 to 0.3333 mg) per kg of body weight or 2.5 to 10 mg per square meter of body surface a day in three or four divided doses.

**Strength(s) usually available**

U.S.—

500 mcg (0.5 mg) per 5 mL (Rx) [GENERIC].

1 mg per mL (Rx) [*Dexamethasone Intensol* (alcohol 30%)].

**Packaging and storage**

Store below 40 °C (104 °F), preferably between 15 and 30 °C (59 and 86 °F), in a well-closed container, unless otherwise specified by manufacturer. Protect from freezing.

### DEXAMETHASONE TABLETS USP

**Usual adult and adolescent dose**

Oral, 500 mcg (0.5 mg) to 9 mg a day as a single dose or in divided doses.

Dexamethasone suppression test—

Test for Cushing's syndrome: Oral, 1 mg as a single dose at 11:00 p.m. or 500 mcg (0.5 mg) every six hours for forty-eight hours.

Test to distinguish Cushing's syndrome due to pituitary ACTH excess from Cushing's syndrome due to other causes: Oral, 2 mg every six hours for forty-eight hours.

Depression diagnosis: Oral, 1 mg as a single dose at 11:00 p.m.

In cerebral edema associated with recurrent or inoperable brain tumor—

Oral, 2 mg two or three times a day, administered as maintenance therapy after cerebral edema has initially been controlled using parenteral dexamethasone sodium phosphate.

**Usual pediatric dose**

Adrenocortical insufficiency—

Oral, 23.3 mcg (0.0233 mg) per kg of body weight or 670 mcg (0.67 mg) per square meter of body surface a day in three divided doses.

Other indications—

Oral, 83.3 to 333.3 mcg (0.0833 to 0.3333 mg) per kg of body weight or 2.5 to 10 mg per square meter of body surface a day in three or four divided doses.

**Strength(s) usually available**

U.S.—

250 mcg (0.25 mg) (Rx) [*Decadron* (scored); GENERIC].

500 mcg (0.5 mg) (Rx) [*Decadron* (scored); *Dexone 0.5* (scored); *Hexadrol* (scored); GENERIC].

750 mcg (0.75 mg) (Rx) [*Decadron* (scored); *Dexone 0.75* (scored); *Hexadrol* (scored); GENERIC].

1 mg (Rx) [GENERIC (scored)].

1.5 mg (Rx) [*Decadron* (scored); *Dexone 1.5* (scored); *Hexadrol* (scored); GENERIC].

2 mg (Rx) [GENERIC (scored)].

4 mg (Rx) [*Decadron* (scored); *Dexone 4* (scored); *Hexadrol* (scored); GENERIC].

6 mg (Rx) [*Decadron* (scored); GENERIC].

Canada—

500 mcg (0.5 mg) (Rx) [*Deronil* (scored); *Dexasone* (scored)].

750 mcg (0.75 mg) (Rx) [*Deronil* (scored); *Dexasone* (scored)].

4 mg (Rx) [*Deronil* (scored); *Dexasone* (scored); *Hexadrol* (scored); *Oradexon* (scored)].

**Packaging and storage**

Store below 40 °C (104 °F), preferably between 15 and 30 °C (59 and 86 °F). Store in a well-closed container.

## Parenteral Dosage Forms

### STERILE DEXAMETHASONE ACETATE SUSPENSION USP

**Usual adult and adolescent dose**

Intra-articular or soft-tissue injection, 4 to 16 mg of dexamethasone (base), repeated at one- to three-week intervals, if necessary.

Intralesional, 800 mcg (0.8 mg) to 1.6 mg of dexamethasone (base) per injection site, repeated as needed.

Intramuscular, 8 to 16 mg of dexamethasone (base), repeated at one- to three-week intervals, if necessary.

**Usual pediatric dose**

Dosage has not been established.

**Strength(s) usually available**

U.S.—

8 mg (base) per mL (Rx) [*Dalalone L.A* (sodium bisulfite); *Decadron-LA* (sodium bisulfite 1 mg); *Decaject-L.A.* (sodium bisulfite); *Dexacen LA-8* (benzyl alcohol; sodium bisulfite); *Dexasone-LA; Dexone LA* (sodium bisulfite); *Solurex-LA* (sodium bisulfite); GENERIC].

16 mg (base) per mL (Rx) [*Dalalone D.P.* (sodium bisulfite 1 mg)].

**Packaging and storage**

Store below 40 °C (104 °F), preferably between 15 and 30 °C (59 and 86 °F), unless otherwise specified by manufacturer. Protect from freezing.

**Stability**

This medication is heat-sensitive and should not be autoclaved.

**Auxiliary labeling**

• Shake well.

**Additional information**

For administration of injections, see manufacturer's labeling.

Do not administer this medication intravenously.

The suspension containing the equivalent of 16 mg of dexamethasone per mL is not for intralesional use.

## DEXAMETHASONE SODIUM PHOSPHATE INJECTION USP

### Usual adult and adolescent dose
Intra-articular, intralesional, or soft-tissue injection, 200 mcg (0.2 mg) to 6 mg of dexamethasone (phosphate), repeated at three-day to three-week intervals, if necessary.

Intramuscular or intravenous, 500 mcg (0.5 mg) to 9 mg of dexamethasone (phosphate) a day.

For cerebral edema—
Initial: Intravenous, 10 mg (phosphate), followed by 4 mg (phosphate) intramuscularly every six hours until symptoms subside. Dosage may be reduced after two to four days and gradually discontinued over a period of five to seven days, unless a brain tumor, which must be treated before dexamethasone can be discontinued, is present.

Maintenance (for recurrent or inoperable brain tumors): Intramuscular, 2 mg (phosphate) two or three times a day initially, then adjusted according to patient response.

For shock—
The following regimens have been utilized:
Intravenous, 20 mg (phosphate) as a single dose initially, followed by 3 mg (phosphate) per kg of body weight per 24 hours via continuous intravenous infusion, or

Intravenous, 2 to 6 mg (phosphate) per kg of body weight as a single injection, or

Intravenous, 40 mg (phosphate) as a single dose, administered every two to six hours as needed, or

Intravenous, 1 mg (phosphate) per kg of body weight as a single injection.

Note: Administration of high-dose therapy for shock should be discontinued after the patient's condition has stabilized and is usually continued for no longer than two to three days.

### Usual adult prescribing limits
Up to 80 mg daily.

### Usual pediatric dose
Adrenocortical insufficiency—
Intramuscular, 23.3 mcg (0.0233 mg) (phosphate) per kg of body weight or 670 mcg (0.67 mg) (phosphate) per square meter of body surface a day (in three divided doses) every third day; or 7.76 to 11.65 mcg (0.00776 to 0.01165 mg) (phosphate) per kg of body weight or 233 to 335 mcg (0.233 to 0.335 mg) (phosphate) per square meter of body surface once a day.

Other indications—
Intramuscular, 27.76 to 166.65 mcg (0.02776 to 0.16665 mg) (phosphate) per kg of body weight or 0.833 to 5 mg (phosphate) per square meter of body surface every twelve to twenty-four hours.

### Strength(s) usually available
U.S.—
4 mg (phosphate) per mL (Rx) [*AK-Dex; Dalalone* (sodium bisulfite); *Decadrol; Decadron Phosphate* (sodium bisulfite); *Decaject* (sodium bisulfite); *Dexacen-4* (sodium bisulfite); *Dexone* (sodium bisulfite); *Hexadrol Phosphate* (sodium sulfite); *Solurex* (sodium bisulfite); GENERIC (sodium metabisulfite)].

10 mg (phosphate) per mL (Rx) [*Hexadrol Phosphate* (sodium sulfite); GENERIC (sodium metabisulfite)].

20 mg (phosphate) per mL (Rx) [*Hexadrol Phosphate* (sodium sulfite); GENERIC (sodium metabisulfite)].

24 mg (phosphate) per mL (Rx) [*Decadron Phosphate* (sodium bisulfite); GENERIC (sodium metabisulfite)].

Canada—
4 mg (phosphate) per mL (Rx) [*Decadron* (sodium bisulfite 1 mg); GENERIC (sodium metabisulfite)].

10 mg (phosphate) per mL (Rx) [GENERIC (sodium metabisulfite)].

### Packaging and storage
Store below 40 °C (104 °F), preferably between 15 and 30 °C (59 and 86 °F), unless otherwise specified by manufacturer. Protect from light. Protect from freezing.

### Stability
This medication is heat-sensitive and should not be autoclaved.

### Additional information
For administration of injections, see manufacturer's labeling.

Dosage forms containing 24 mg (phosphate) per mL are for intravenous use only.

## HYDROCORTISONE

## Summary of Differences
Indications: See *Table 1*.
Pharmacology/pharmacokinetics: See *Table 2* and *Table 3*.
General dosing information: See *Table 4*.

## Oral Dosage Forms

### HYDROCORTISONE TABLETS USP

#### Usual adult and adolescent dose
Oral, 20 to 240 mg a day as a single dose or in divided doses.

#### Usual pediatric dose
Adrenocortical insufficiency—
Oral, 560 mcg (0.56 mg) per kg of body weight or 15 to 20 mg per square meter of body surface a day as a single dose or in divided doses.

Other indications—
Oral, 2 to 8 mg per kg of body weight or 60 to 240 mg per square meter of body surface a day as a single dose or in divided doses.

#### Strength(s) usually available
U.S.—
5 mg (Rx) [*Cortef* (scored)].
10 mg (Rx) [*Cortef* (scored); *Hydrocortone* (scored); GENERIC].
20 mg (Rx) [*Cortef* (scored); *Hydrocortone* (scored); GENERIC (scored)].

Canada—
10 mg (Rx) [*Cortef* (scored)].
20 mg (Rx) [*Cortef* (scored)].

#### Packaging and storage
Store below 40 °C (104 °F), preferably between 15 and 30 °C (59 and 86 °F). Store in a well-closed container.

### HYDROCORTISONE CYPIONATE ORAL SUSPENSION USP

#### Usual adult and adolescent dose
Oral, 20 to 240 mg (base) a day as a single dose or in divided doses.

#### Usual pediatric dose
Adrenocortical insufficiency—
Oral, 560 mcg (0.56 mg) (base) per kg of body weight or 15 to 20 mg per square meter of body surface a day as a single dose or in divided doses.

Other indications—
Oral, 2 to 8 mg (base) per kg of body weight or 60 to 240 mg per square meter of body surface a day as a single dose or in divided doses.

#### Strength(s) usually available
U.S.—
10 mg (base) per 5 mL (Rx) [*Cortef*].

#### Packaging and storage
Store below 40 °C (104 °F), preferably between 15 and 30 °C (59 and 86 °F), unless otherwise specified by manufacturer. Store in a tight, light-resistant container. Protect from freezing.

#### Auxiliary labeling
• Shake well.

## Parenteral Dosage Forms

### STERILE HYDROCORTISONE SUSPENSION USP

#### Usual adult and adolescent dose
Intramuscular, 15 to 240 mg a day.

#### Usual pediatric dose
Adrenocortical insufficiency—
Intramuscular, 560 mcg (0.56 mg) per kg of body weight or 30 to 37.5 mg per square meter of body surface a day every third day; or 186 to 280 mcg (0.186 to 0.28 mg) per kg of body weight or 10 to 12.5 mg per square meter of body surface once a day.

Other indications—
Intramuscular, 666 mcg (0.666 mg) to 4 mg per kg of body weight or 20 to 120 mg per square meter of body surface every twelve to twenty-four hours.

#### Strength(s) usually available
U.S.—
25 mg per mL (Rx) [GENERIC].
50 mg per mL (Rx) [GENERIC].

**Packaging and storage**
Store below 40 °C (104 °F), preferably between 15 and 30 °C (59 and 86 °F), unless otherwise specified by manufacturer. Protect from freezing.

**Auxiliary labeling**
• Shake well.

**Additional information**
Do not administer this medication intravenously.

## STERILE HYDROCORTISONE ACETATE SUSPENSION USP

**Usual adult and adolescent dose**
Intra-articular, intralesional, or soft-tissue injection, 5 to 75 mg, repeated at two- to three-week intervals.

Note: Severe conditions may require doses at one-week intervals.

**Usual pediatric dose**
Dosage has not been established.

**Strength(s) usually available**
U.S.—
25 mg per mL (Rx) [*Hydrocortone Acetate;* GENERIC].
50 mg per mL (Rx) [*Hydrocortone Acetate;* GENERIC].

**Packaging and storage**
Store below 40 °C (104 °F), preferably between 15 and 30 °C (59 and 86 °F), unless otherwise specified by manufacturer. Protect from freezing.

**Stability**
For concurrent use of a parenteral-local anesthetic, withdraw the required quantity of corticosteroid suspension into a syringe, then add the local anesthetic. *Do not introduce the local anesthetic directly into the multiple-dose vial.* Also, inject the mixture immediately and discard any unused portion.
This medication is heat-sensitive and should not be autoclaved.

**Auxiliary labeling**
• Shake well.

**Additional information**
For administration of injections, see manufacturer's labeling.
Do not administer this medication intravenously.

## HYDROCORTISONE SODIUM PHOSPHATE INJECTION USP

**Usual adult and adolescent dose**
Intramuscular, intravenous, or subcutaneous, 100 to 500 mg (base); may be repeated every two to six hours, depending upon patient condition and response.

**Usual pediatric dose**
Adrenocortical insufficiency—
Intramuscular or intravenous, 186 to 280 mcg (0.186 to 0.28 mg) (base) per kg of body weight or 10 to 12 mg (base) per square meter of body surface a day in three divided doses.
Other indications—
Intramuscular, 666 mcg (0.666 mg) to 4 mg (base) per kg of body weight or 20 to 120 mg (base) per square meter of body surface every twelve to twenty-four hours.

**Strength(s) usually available**
U.S.—
50 mg (base) per mL (Rx) [*Hydrocortone Phosphate* (sodium bisulfite 3.2 mg); GENERIC (sodium metabisulfite 2 mg)].

**Packaging and storage**
Store below 40 °C (104 °F), preferably between 15 and 30 °C (59 and 86 °F), unless otherwise specified by manufacturer. Protect from freezing.

**Stability**
This medication is heat-sensitive and should not be autoclaved.

**Additional information**
For administration of injections, see manufacturer's labeling.

## HYDROCORTISONE SODIUM SUCCINATE FOR INJECTION USP

**Usual adult and adolescent dose**
Intramuscular or intravenous, 100 to 500 mg (base); may be repeated every two to six hours, depending upon patient condition and response.

Note: Initial intravenous dosage should be administered over a period of thirty seconds (100-mg dose) to ten minutes (doses 500 mg or higher).
Maintenance dosage (if required) should be no less than 25 mg per day.

**Usual pediatric dose**
Adrenocortical insufficiency—
Intramuscular or intravenous, 186 to 280 mcg (0.186 to 0.28 mg) (base) per kg of body weight or 10 to 12 mg (base) per square meter of body surface a day in three divided doses.
Other indications—
Intramuscular, 666 mcg (0.666 mg) to 4 mg (base) per kg of body weight or 20 to 120 mg (base) per square meter of body surface every twelve to twenty-four hours.

**Size(s) usually available**
U.S.—
100 mg (base) (Rx) [*A-hydroCort; Solu-Cortef;* GENERIC].
250 mg (base) (Rx) [*A-hydroCort; Solu-Cortef;* GENERIC].
500 mg (base) (Rx) [*A-hydroCort; Solu-Cortef;* GENERIC].
1 gram (base) (Rx) [*A-hydroCort; Solu-Cortef;* GENERIC].
Canada—
100 mg (base) (Rx) [*Solu-Cortef*].
250 mg (base) (Rx) [*Solu-Cortef*].
500 mg (base) (Rx) [*Solu-Cortef*].
1 gram (base) (Rx) [*Solu-Cortef*].

**Packaging and storage**
Store below 40 °C (104 °F), preferably between 15 and 30 °C (59 and 86 °F), unless otherwise specified by manufacturer.

**Stability**
Reconstituted solution should be used only if it is clear and should be discarded after 3 days.
After reconstitution, protect the solution from light.

**Additional information**
For preparation and administration of injections, see manufacturer's labeling.

# Rectal Dosage Forms
## HYDROCORTISONE ENEMA USP

**Usual adult and adolescent dose**
Rectal, 100 mg as a retention enema each night for twenty-one days, or until clinical and proctological remission is obtained.

**Usual pediatric dose**
Dosage has not been established.

**Strength(s) usually available**
U.S.—
100 mg per 60 mL (Rx) [*Cortenema*].
Canada—
100 mg per 60 mL (Rx) [*Cortenema*].

**Packaging and storage**
Store below 40 °C (104 °F), preferably between 15 and 30 °C (59 and 86 °F), unless otherwise specified by manufacturer. Store in a tight container.

**Auxiliary labeling**
• Shake well.
• For rectal use only.

**Note**
Include patient instructions when dispensing.
Explain administration technique.

**Additional information**
If the hydrocortisone enema dosage form is to be discontinued after long-term (longer than 21 days) therapy, the dosage should be reduced gradually by decreasing the frequency to once every other night for 2 or 3 weeks.

## HYDROCORTISONE ACETATE RECTAL AEROSOL (FOAM)

**Usual adult and adolescent dose**
Rectal, 90 mg (one applicatorful) one or two times a day for two or three weeks, the frequency being decreased to every other day thereafter.

**Usual pediatric dose**
Dosage has not been established.

**Strength(s) usually available**
U.S.—
10% (90 mg hydrocortisone acetate [80 mg base] per applicatorful) (Rx) [*Cortifoam*].
Canada—
90 mg hydrocortisone acetate (80 mg base) per applicatorful (Rx) [*Cortifoam*].

Note: Each canister delivers a minimum of 14 applicatorfuls.

**Packaging and storage**
Store below 49 °C (120 °F), preferably between 15 and 30 °C (59 and 86 °F), unless otherwise specified by manufacturer.

**Auxiliary labeling**
- Shake well.
- For rectal use only.

**Note**
Include patient instructions when dispensing.
Explain administration technique.

---

## METHYLPREDNISOLONE

## Summary of Differences

Indications: See *Table 1*.
Pharmacology/pharmacokinetics: See *Table 2* and *Table 3*.
General dosing information: See *Table 4*.

## Oral Dosage Forms

### METHYLPREDNISOLONE TABLETS USP

**Usual adult and adolescent dose**
Oral, 4 to 48 mg a day as a single dose or in divided doses.
In multiple sclerosis—
Oral, 160 mg a day for one week, then 64 mg every other day for one month.

**Usual pediatric dose**
Adrenocortical insufficiency—
Oral, 117 mcg (0.117 mg) per kg of body weight or 3.33 mg per square meter of body surface a day in three divided doses.
Other indications—
Oral, 417 mcg (0.417 mg) to 1.67 mg per kg of body weight or 12.5 to 50 mg per square meter of body surface per day in three or four divided doses.

**Strength(s) usually available**
U.S.—
2 mg (Rx) [*Medrol* (scored)].
4 mg (Rx) [*Medrol* (scored); *Meprolone;* GENERIC].
8 mg (Rx) [*Medrol* (scored)].
16 mg (Rx) [*Medrol* (scored); GENERIC].
24 mg (Rx) [*Medrol* (scored; tartrazine); GENERIC].
32 mg (Rx) [*Medrol* (scored); GENERIC].
Canada—
2 mg (Rx) [*Medrol* (scored)].
4 mg (Rx) [*Medrol* (scored)].
16 mg (Rx) [*Medrol* (scored)].

**Packaging and storage**
Store below 40 °C (104 °F), preferably between 15 and 30 °C (59 and 86 °F), unless otherwise specified by manufacturer. Store in a tight container.

## Parenteral Dosage Forms

Note: Bracketed uses in the *Dosage Forms* section refer to categories of use and/or indications that are not included in U.S. product labeling.

### STERILE METHYLPREDNISOLONE ACETATE SUSPENSION USP

**Usual adult and adolescent dose**
Intra-articular, intralesional, or soft-tissue injection, 4 to 80 mg, repeated at one- to five-week intervals, if necessary.
Intramuscular, 40 to 120 mg, repeated at one-day to two-week intervals, if necessary.
For acute exacerbations of multiple sclerosis—
Intramuscular, 177.6 mg per day for one week, then 71 mg every other day for one month.

**Usual pediatric dose**
Adrenocortical insufficiency—
Intramuscular, 117 mcg (0.117 mg) per kg of body weight or 3.33 mg per square meter of body surface a day (in three divided doses) every third day; or 39 to 58.5 mcg (0.039 to 0.0585 mg) per kg of body weight or 1.11 to 1.66 mg per square meter of body surface once a day.
Other indications—
Intramuscular, 139 to 835 mcg (0.139 to 0.835 mg) per kg of body weight or 4.16 to 25 mg per square meter of body surface every twelve to twenty-four hours.

**Strength(s) usually available**
U.S.—
20 mg per mL (Rx) [*Depo-Medrol;* GENERIC].
40 mg per mL (Rx) [*depMedalone 40; Depoject-40; Depo-Medrol; Depopred-40; Depo-Predate 40; Duralone-40; Medralone-40; Rep-Pred 40;* GENERIC].
80 mg per mL (Rx) [*depMedalone 80; Depoject-80; Depo-Medrol; Depopred-80; Depo-Predate 80; Duralone-80; Medralone-80; Rep-Pred 80;* GENERIC].
Canada—
40 mg per mL (Rx) [*Depo-Medrol* (lidocaine 10 mg)].

**Packaging and storage**
Store below 40 °C (104 °F), preferably between 15 and 30 °C (59 and 86 °F), unless otherwise specified by manufacturer. Protect from freezing.

**Incompatibilities**
It is recommended that this medication not be diluted or mixed with other solutions because of possible physical incompatibility.

**Auxiliary labeling**
- Shake well.

**Additional information**
For preparation and administration of injections, see manufacturer's labeling.

Do not administer this medication intrathecally or intravenously.

### METHYLPREDNISOLONE SODIUM SUCCINATE FOR INJECTION USP

**Usual adult and adolescent dose**
Intramuscular or intravenous, 10 to 40 mg (base), repeated as needed.
For high-dose ("pulse" therapy)—Intravenous, 30 mg (base) per kg of body weight administered over at least thirty minutes. This dose may be repeated every four to six hours as needed.
For acute exacerbations of multiple sclerosis—
Intramuscular or intravenous, 160 mg (base) per day for one week, followed by 64 mg every other day for one month.
[For treatment of acute spinal cord injury][1]—
Intravenous, 30 mg (base) per kg of body weight administered over fifteen minutes, followed in forty-five minutes by a continuous infusion of 5.4 mg per kg of body weight per hour, for twenty-three hours.
[For adjunctive treatment in AIDS-associated *Pneumocystis carinii* pneumonia][1]—
Intravenous, 30 mg (base) two times a day on days one through five, 30 mg once a day on days six through ten, and 15 mg once a day on days eleven through twenty-one.

**Usual pediatric dose**
Adrenocortical insufficiency—
Intramuscular, 117 mcg (0.117 mg) (base) per kg of body weight or 3.33 mg (base) per square meter of body surface a day (in three divided doses) every third day; or 39 to 58.5 mcg (0.039 to 0.0585 mg) (base) per kg of body weight or 1.11 to 1.66 mg (base) per square meter of body surface once a day.
[For treatment of acute spinal cord injury][1]—
Intravenous, 30 mg (base) per kg of body weight administered over fifteen minutes, followed in forty-five minutes by a continuous infusion of 5.4 mg per kg of body weight per hour, for twenty-three hours.
Other indications—
Intramuscular, 139 to 835 mcg (0.139 to 0.835 mg) (base) per kg of body weight or 4.16 to 25 mg (base) per square meter of body surface every twelve to twenty-four hours.
[For adjunctive treatment in AIDS-associated *Pneumocystis carinii* pneumonia][1]—
Children 13 years of age and younger: Dosage has not been established.
Children over 13 years of age: See *Usual adult and adolescent dose*.

**Size(s) usually available**
U.S.—
40 mg (base) (Rx) [*A-methaPred; Solu-Medrol;* GENERIC].
125 mg (base) (Rx) [*A-methaPred; Solu-Medrol;* GENERIC].
500 mg (base) (Rx) [*A-methaPred; Solu-Medrol;* GENERIC].
1 gram (base) (Rx) [*A-methaPred; Solu-Medrol;* GENERIC].
2 grams (base) (Rx) [*Solu-Medrol*].
Canada—
40 mg (base) (Rx) [*Solu-Medrol*].
125 mg (base) (Rx) [*Solu-Medrol*].
500 mg (base) (Rx) [*Solu-Medrol*].
1 gram (base) (Rx) [*Solu-Medrol*].

**Packaging and storage**
Store below 40 °C (104 °F), preferably between 15 and 30 °C (59 and 86 °F), unless otherwise specified by manufacturer.

**Stability**
Use reconstituted solution within 48 hours. Do not use if solution is cloudy or contains a precipitate.

**Additional information**
For preparation and administration of injections, see manufacturer's labeling.

When used intravenously, Methylprednisolone Sodium Succinate for Injection USP should be administered over a period of 1 to several minutes.

## Rectal Dosage Forms

### METHYLPREDNISOLONE ACETATE FOR ENEMA USP

**Usual adult and adolescent dose**
Rectal, 40 mg three to seven times a week for two or more weeks.

**Usual pediatric dose**
Rectal, 500 mcg (0.5 mg) to 1 mg per kg of body weight or 15 to 30 mg per square meter of body surface, every one or two days for two or more weeks.

**Size(s) usually available**
U.S.—
    40 mg (Rx) [*Medrol Enpak*].

**Packaging and storage**
Store below 40 °C (104 °F), preferably between 15 and 30 °C (59 and 86 °F). Store in a well-closed container.

**Auxiliary labeling**
• For rectal use only.
• Shake well.

**Note**
Include patient instructions when dispensing.

Explain dilution and administration technique.

**Additional information**
The medication may be administered by continuous drip at a rate of 1 or 2 drops per second, or as a retention enema.

The constituted product is a suspension; when administered as continuous drip, shake bottle occasionally during administration.

---

¹Not included in Canadian product labeling.

---

### *PREDNISOLONE*

## Summary of Differences

Indications: See *Table 1*.
Pharmacology/pharmacokinetics: See *Table 2* and *Table 3*.
General dosing information: See *Table 4*.

## Oral Dosage Forms

### PREDNISOLONE SYRUP USP

**Usual adult and adolescent dose**
Oral, 5 to 60 mg a day as a single dose or in divided doses.
For acute exacerbations of multiple sclerosis—
    Oral, 200 mg per day for one week, followed by 80 mg every other day for one month.

**Usual adult prescribing limits**
Up to 250 mg daily.

**Usual pediatric dose**
Adrenocortical insufficiency—
    Oral, 140 mcg (0.14 mg) per kg of body weight or 4 mg per square meter of body surface a day in three divided doses.
Other indications—
    Oral, 500 mcg (0.5 mg) to 2 mg per kg of body weight or 15 to 60 mg per square meter of body surface a day in three or four divided doses.

**Strength(s) usually available**
U.S.—
    15 mg per 5 mL (Rx) [*Prelone* (alcohol 5%)].

**Packaging and storage**
Store below 40 °C (104 °F), preferably between 15 and 30 °C (59 and 86 °F), in a well-closed container, unless otherwise specified by manufacturer. Protect from freezing.

### PREDNISOLONE TABLETS USP

**Usual adult and adolescent dose**
Oral, 5 to 60 mg a day as a single dose or in divided doses.
For acute exacerbations of multiple sclerosis—
    Oral, 200 mg per day for one week, followed by 80 mg every other day for one month.

**Usual adult prescribing limits**
Oral, up to 250 mg a day.

**Usual pediatric dose**
Adrenocortical insufficiency—
    Oral, 140 mcg (0.14 mg) per kg of body weight or 4 mg per square meter of body surface a day in three divided doses.
Other indications—
    Oral, 500 mcg (0.5 mg) to 2 mg per kg of body weight or 15 to 60 mg per square meter of body surface a day in three or four divided doses.

**Strength(s) usually available**
U.S.—
    5 mg (Rx) [*Delta-Cortef* (scored); GENERIC (scored)].

**Packaging and storage**
Store below 40 °C (104 °F), preferably between 15 and 30 °C (59 and 86 °F). Store in a well-closed container.

### PREDNISOLONE SODIUM PHOSPHATE ORAL SOLUTION

**Usual adult and adolescent dose**
Oral, 5 to 60 mg (base) a day as a single dose or in divided doses.
For acute exacerbations of multiple sclerosis—
    Oral, 200 mg (base) per day for one week, followed by 80 mg every other day for one month.

**Usual adult prescribing limits**
Oral, up to 250 mg (base) a day.

**Usual pediatric dose**
Adrenocortical insufficiency—
    Oral, 140 mcg (0.14 mg) (base) per kg of body weight or 4 mg per square meter of body surface a day in three divided doses.
Other indications—
    Oral, 500 mcg (0.5 mg) (base) to 2 mg per kg of body weight or 15 to 60 mg per square meter of body surface a day in three or four divided doses.

**Strength(s) usually available**
U.S.—
    5 mg (base) per mL (Rx) [*Pediapred*].

**Packaging and storage**
Store below 40 °C (104 °F), preferably between 15 and 30 °C (59 and 86 °F). Protect from freezing.

**Auxiliary labeling**
• Keep container tightly closed.

## Parenteral Dosage Forms

### STERILE PREDNISOLONE ACETATE SUSPENSION USP

**Usual adult and adolescent dose**
Intra-articular, intralesional, or soft-tissue injection, 4 to 100 mg, repeated as needed.
Intramuscular, 4 to 60 mg a day.

**Usual pediatric dose**
Adrenocortical insufficiency—
    Intramuscular, 140 mcg (0.14 mg) per kg of body weight or 4 mg per square meter of body surface a day (in three divided doses) every third day; or 46 to 70 mcg (0.046 to 0.07 mg) per kg of body weight or 1.33 to 2 mg per square meter of body surface once a day.
Other indications—
    Intramuscular, 166 mcg (0.166 mg) to 1 mg per kg of body weight or 5 to 30 mg per square meter of body surface every twelve to twenty-four hours.

**Strength(s) usually available**
U.S.—
    25 mg per mL (Rx) [*Key-Pred 25*; *Predcor-25*; GENERIC].
    50 mg per mL (Rx) [*Articulose-50*; *Key-Pred 50*; *Predaject-50*; *Predalone 50*; *Predate 50*; *Predcor-50*; *Predicort-50*; GENERIC].

**Packaging and storage**
Store below 40 °C (104 °F), preferably between 15 and 30 °C (59 °F), unless otherwise specified by manufacturer. Protect from freezing.

### Auxiliary labeling
• Shake well.

### Additional information
Do not administer this medication intravenously.

## STERILE PREDNISOLONE ACETATE AND PREDNISOLONE SODIUM PHOSPHATE SUSPENSION

### Usual adult and adolescent dose
Intra-articular, intramuscular, or intrasynovial, 20 to 80 mg of prednisolone acetate and 5 to 20 mg of prednisolone sodium phosphate, repeated at three-day to four-week intervals, if necessary.

### Usual pediatric dose
Dosage has not been established.

### Strength(s) usually available
U.S.—
   80 mg of prednisolone acetate and 20 mg of prednisolone sodium phosphate per mL (Rx) [GENERIC].

### Packaging and storage
Store below 40 °C (104 °F), preferably between 15 and 30 °C (59 and 86 °F), unless otherwise specified by manufacturer. Protect from light. Protect from freezing.

### Auxiliary labeling
• Shake well.

### Additional information
Do not administer this medication intravenously.

## PREDNISOLONE SODIUM PHOSPHATE INJECTION USP

### Usual adult and adolescent dose
Intra-articular, intralesional, or soft-tissue injection, 2 to 30 mg of prednisolone phosphate, repeated at three-day to three-week intervals, if necessary.
Intramuscular or intravenous, 4 to 60 mg of prednisolone phosphate a day.

### Usual pediatric dose
Adrenocortical insufficiency—
   Intramuscular, 140 mcg (0.14 mg) (phosphate) per kg of body weight or 4 mg (phosphate) per square meter of body surface a day (in three divided doses) every third day; or 46 to 70 mcg (0.046 to 0.07 mg) (phosphate) per kg of body weight or 1.33 to 2 mg (phosphate) per square meter of body surface once a day.
Other indications—
   Intramuscular, 166 mcg (0.166 mg) to 1 mg (phosphate) per kg of body weight or 5 to 30 mg (phosphate) per square meter of body surface every twelve to twenty-four hours.

### Strength(s) usually available
U.S.—
   20 mg (phosphate) per mL (Rx) [Hydeltrasol (sodium bisulfite 1 mg); Key-Pred SP (sodium bisulfite); Predate S; Predicort-RP (sodium bisulfite); GENERIC].

### Packaging and storage
Store below 40 °C (104 °F), preferably between 15 and 30 °C (59 and 86 °F), unless otherwise specified by manufacturer. Protect from light. Protect from freezing.

### Stability
This medication is heat-sensitive and should not be autoclaved.

### Additional information
For preparation and administration of injections, see manufacturer's labeling.

## STERILE PREDNISOLONE TEBUTATE SUSPENSION USP

### Usual adult and adolescent dose
Intra-articular, intralesional, or soft-tissue injection, 4 to 40 mg, repeated at two- to three-week intervals, if necessary.
Note: Severe conditions may require doses at one-week intervals.

### Usual pediatric dose
Dosage has not been established.

### Strength(s) usually available
U.S.—
   20 mg per mL (Rx) [Hydeltra T.B.A.; Nor-Pred T.B.A.; Predalone T.B.A.; Predate TBA.; Predcor-TBA.; GENERIC].

### Packaging and storage
Store below 40 °C (104 °F), preferably between 15 and 30 °C (59 and 86 °F), protected from light, unless otherwise specified by manufacturer. Protect from freezing.

### Stability
For concurrent use of a parenteral-local anesthetic, withdraw the required quantity of corticosteroid suspension into a syringe, then add the local anesthetic. *Do not introduce the local anesthetic directly into the multiple-dose vial.* Also, inject the mixture immediately and discard any unused portion.
This medication is heat-sensitive and should not be autoclaved.

### Auxiliary labeling
• Shake well.

### Additional information
For preparation and administration of injections, see manufacturer's labeling.

Do not administer this medication intravenously.

---

## PREDNISONE

## Summary of Differences

Indications: See *Table 1*.
Pharmacology/pharmacokinetics: See *Table 2* and *Table 3*.
General dosing information: See *Table 4*.

## Oral Dosage Forms

Note: Bracketed uses in the *Dosage Forms* section refer to categories of use and/or indications that are not included in U.S. product labeling.

### PREDNISONE ORAL SOLUTION USP

### Usual adult and adolescent dose
Oral, 5 to 60 mg a day as a single dose or in divided doses.
For acute exacerbations of multiple sclerosis—
   Oral, 200 mg a day for one week followed by 80 mg every other day for one month.
For adrenogenital syndrome—
   Oral, 5 to 10 mg a day as a single dose.
[For adjunctive treatment in AIDS-associated *Pneumocystis carinii* pneumonia][1]—
   Oral, 40 mg two times a day on days one through five, 40 mg once a day on days six through ten, and 20 mg once a day on days eleven through twenty-one.

### Usual adult prescribing limits
Up to 250 mg daily.

### Usual pediatric dose
For nephrosis—
   Children up to 18 months of age: Dosage has not been established.
   Children 18 months to 4 years of age: Oral, initially 7.5 to 10 mg four times a day.
   Children 4 to 10 years of age: Oral, initially 15 mg four times a day.
   Children 10 years of age and older: Oral, initially 20 mg four times a day.
For rheumatic carditis, leukemia, tumors—
   Oral, 500 mcg (0.5 mg) per kg of body weight or 15 mg per square meter of body surface four times a day for two to three weeks; then 375 mcg (0.375 mg) per kg of body weight or 11.25 mg per square meter of body surface four times a day for four to six weeks.
For tuberculosis (with concurrent antitubercular therapy)—
   Oral, 500 mcg (0.5 mg) per kg of body weight or 15 mg per square meter of body surface four times a day for two months.
   Note: Medication should be gradually discontinued.
For adrenogenital syndrome—
   Oral, 5 mg per square meter of body surface area a day in two divided doses.
[For adjunctive treatment in AIDS-associated *Pneumocystis carinii* pneumonia][1]—
   Children 13 years of age and younger: Dosage has not been established.
   Children over 13 years of age: See *Usual adult and adolescent dose.*

### Strength(s) usually available
U.S.—
   5 mg per 5 mL (Rx) [GENERIC (alcohol 5%)].
   5 mg per mL (Rx) [Predisone Intensol (alcohol 30%)].

### Packaging and storage
Store below 40 °C (104 °F), preferably between 15 and 30 °C (59 and 86 °F), in a light-resistant container, unless otherwise specified by manufacturer. Store in a tight container. Protect from freezing.

## PREDNISONE SYRUP USP

**Usual adult and adolescent dose**
Oral, 5 to 60 mg a day as a single dose or in divided doses.
For acute exacerbations of multiple sclerosis—
Oral, 200 mg a day for one week followed by 80 mg every other day for one month.
For adrenogenital syndrome—
Oral, 5 to 10 mg a day as a single dose.
[For adjunctive treatment in AIDS-associated *Pneumocystis carinii* pneumonia][1]—
Oral, 40 mg two times a day on days one through five, 40 mg once a day on days six through ten, and 20 mg once a day on days eleven through twenty-one.

**Usual adult prescribing limits**
Up to 250 mg daily.

**Usual pediatric dose**
For nephrosis—
Children up to 18 months of age: Dosage has not been established.
Children 18 months to 4 years of age: Oral, initially 7.5 to 10 mg four times a day.
Children 4 to 10 years of age: Oral, initially 15 mg four times a day.
Children 10 years of age and older: Oral, initially 20 mg four times a day.
For rheumatic carditis, leukemia, tumors—
Oral, 500 mcg (0.5 mg) per kg of body weight or 15 mg per square meter of body surface four times a day for two to three weeks; then 375 mcg (0.375 mg) per kg of body weight or 11.25 mg per square meter of body surface four times a day for four to six weeks.
For tuberculosis (with concurrent antitubercular therapy)—
Oral, 500 mcg (0.5 mg) per kg of body weight or 15 mg per square meter of body surface four times a day for two months.
Note: Medication should be gradually discontinued.
For adrenogenital syndrome—
Oral, 5 mg per square meter of body surface area a day in two divided doses.
[For adjunctive treatment in AIDS-associated *Pneumocystis carinii* pneumonia][1]—
Children 13 years of age and younger: Dosage has not been established.
Children over 13 years of age: See *Usual adult and adolescent dose.*

**Strength(s) usually available**
U.S.—
5 mg per 5 mL (Rx) [*Liquid Pred* (alcohol 5%)].

**Packaging and storage**
Store below 40 °C (104 °F), preferably between 15 and 30 °C (59 and 86 °F), in a light-resistant container, unless otherwise specified by manufacturer. Store in a tight container. Protect from freezing.

## PREDNISONE TABLETS USP

**Usual adult and adolescent dose**
Oral, 5 to 60 mg a day as a single dose or in divided doses.
For acute exacerbations of multiple sclerosis—
Oral, 200 mg per day for one week followed by 80 mg every other day for one month.
For adrenogenital syndrome—
Oral, 5 to 10 mg a day as a single dose.
[For adjunctive treatment in AIDS-associated *Pneumocystis carinii* pneumonia][1]—
Oral, 40 mg two times a day on days one through five, 40 mg once a day on days six through ten, and 20 mg once a day on days eleven through twenty-one.

**Usual adult prescribing limits**
Up to 250 mg daily.

**Usual pediatric dose**
For nephrosis—
Children up to 18 months of age: Dosage has not been established.
Children 18 months to 4 years of age: Oral, initially 7.5 to 10 mg four times a day.
Children 4 to 10 years of age: Oral, initially 15 mg four times a day.
Children 10 years of age and older: Oral, initially 20 mg four times a day.
For rheumatic carditis, leukemia, tumors—
Oral, 500 mcg (0.5 mg) per kg of body weight or 15 mg per square meter of body surface four times a day for two to three weeks; then 375 mcg (0.375 mg) per kg of body weight or 11.25 mg per square meter of body surface four times a day for four to six weeks.

For tuberculosis (with concurrent antitubercular therapy)—
Oral, 500 mcg (0.5 mg) per kg of body weight or 15 mg per square meter of body surface four times a day for two months.
Note: Medication should be gradually discontinued.
For adrenogenital syndrome—
Oral, 5 mg per square meter of body surface area a day in two divided doses.
[For adjunctive treatment in AIDS-associated *Pneumocystis carinii* pneumonia][1]—
Children 13 years of age and younger: Dosage has not been established.
Children over 13 years of age: See *Usual adult and adolescent dose.*

**Strength(s) usually available**
U.S.—
1 mg (Rx) [*Meticorten; Orasone 1* (scored); GENERIC (scored)].
2.5 mg (Rx) [*Deltasone* (scored); GENERIC (scored)].
5 mg (Rx) [*Deltasone* (scored); *Orasone 5* (scored); *Prednicen-M* (scored); *Sterapred;* GENERIC (scored)].
10 mg (Rx) [*Deltasone* (scored); *Orasone 10* (scored); *Sterapred DS* (scored); GENERIC (scored)].
20 mg (Rx) [*Deltasone* (scored); *Orasone 20* (scored); GENERIC (scored)].
25 mg (Rx) [GENERIC].
50 mg (Rx) [*Deltasone* (scored); *Orasone 50* (scored); GENERIC (scored)].
Canada—
1 mg (Rx) [*Apo-Prednisone* (scored); *Winpred*].
5 mg (Rx) [*Apo-Prednisone* (scored); *Deltasone* (scored); *Winpred* (scored); GENERIC (scored)].
50 mg (Rx) [*Apo-Prednisone* (scored); *Deltasone* (scored)].

**Packaging and storage**
Store below 40 °C (104 °F), preferably between 15 and 30 °C (59 and 86 °F). Store in a well-closed container.

---

[1]Not included in Canadian product labeling.

---

*TRIAMCINOLONE*

## Summary of Differences

Indications: See *Table 1.*
Pharmacology/pharmacokinetics: See *Table 2* and *Table 3.*
General dosing information: See *Table 4.*

## Oral Dosage Forms

### TRIAMCINOLONE TABLETS USP

**Usual adult and adolescent dose**
Adrenocortical insufficiency—
Oral, 4 to 12 mg a day as a single dose or in divided doses.
Other indications—
Oral, 4 to 48 mg a day as a single dose or in divided doses.
Note: In some patients (e.g., those with systemic lupus erythematosus, acute rheumatic carditis, or certain hematologic disorders), initial doses as high as 60 mg per day may be required.

**Usual pediatric dose**
Adrenocortical insufficiency—
Oral, 117 mcg (0.117 mg) per kg of body weight or 3.3 mg per square meter of body surface a day as a single dose or in divided doses.
Other indications—
Oral, 416 mcg (0.416 mg) to 1.7 mg per kg of body weight or 12.5 to 50 mg per square meter of body surface a day as a single dose or in divided doses.
Note: Some pediatric patients with neoplastic disease (acute leukemia) may require initial doses as high as 2 mg per kg of body weight per day.

**Strength(s) usually available**
U.S.—
1 mg (Rx) [*Aristocort* (scored)].
2 mg (Rx) [*Aristocort* (scored)].
4 mg (Rx) [*Aristocort* (scored); *Kenacort;* GENERIC].
8 mg (Rx) [*Aristocort* (scored); *Kenacort* (scored; tartrazine)].
16 mg (Rx) [*Aristocort* (scored)].
Canada—
2 mg (Rx) [*Aristocort* (scored)].
4 mg (Rx) [*Aristocort* (scored); *Kenacort* (scored)].

**Packaging and storage**
Store below 40 °C (104 °F), preferably between 15 and 30 °C (59 and 86 °F). Store in a well-closed container.

## TRIAMCINOLONE DIACETATE SYRUP USP

**Usual adult and adolescent dose**
Adrenocortical insufficiency—
Oral, 4 to 12 mg (base) a day as a single dose or in divided doses.
Other indications—
Oral, 4 to 48 mg (base) a day as a single dose or in divided doses.

Note: After an initial response has been attained, this medication may be administered on an intermittent schedule. An example of this schedule is as follows: three or four days of medication followed by three medication-free days.

In some patients (e.g., those with systemic lupus erythematosus, acute rheumatic carditis, or certain hematologic disorders), initial doses as high as 60 mg (base) per day may be required.

**Usual pediatric dose**
Adrenocortical insufficiency—
Oral, 117 mcg (0.117 mg) (base) per kg of body weight or 3.3 mg per square meter of body surface a day as a single dose or in divided doses.
Other indications—
Oral, 416 mcg (0.416 mg) to 1.7 mg (base) per kg of body weight or 12.5 to 50 mg per square meter of body surface a day as a single dose or in divided doses.

Note: Some pediatric patients with neoplastic disease (acute leukemia) may require initial doses as high as 2 mg (base) per kg of body weight per day.

**Strength(s) usually available**
U.S.—
2 mg (diacetate) per 5 mL (Rx) [*Aristocort*].
4.85 mg anhydrous diacetate (4 mg base) per 5 mL (Rx) [*Kenacort Diacetate*].
Canada—
2 mg (diacetate) per 5 mL (Rx) [*Aristocort*].

**Packaging and storage**
Store below 40 °C (104 °F), preferably between 15 and 30 °C (59 and 86 °F), unless otherwise specified by manufacturer. Store in a tight, light-resistant container. Protect from freezing.

# Parenteral Dosage Forms

## STERILE TRIAMCINOLONE ACETONIDE SUSPENSION USP

**Usual adult and adolescent dose**
Intra-articular, intrabursal, or tendon-sheath injection, 2.5 to 15 mg.
Intradermal or intralesional, up to 1 mg per injection site, repeated at one-week or less frequent intervals, if necessary.
Intramuscular, 40 to 80 mg, repeated at four-week intervals, if necessary.

**Usual pediatric dose**
Children up to 6 years of age—Use is not recommended.
Children 6 to 12 years of age—
Intra-articular, intrabursal, or tendon-sheath injection, 2.5 to 15 mg, repeated as needed.
Intramuscular, 40 mg, repeated at four-week intervals if necessary; or 30 to 200 mcg (0.03 to 0.2 mg) per kg of body weight or 1 to 6.25 mg per square meter of body surface, repeated at one- to seven-day intervals.

**Strength(s) usually available**
U.S.—
3 mg per mL (Rx) [*Tac-3*].
10 mg per mL (Rx) [*Kenalog-10*].
40 mg per mL (Rx) [*Cenocort A-40; Cinonide 40; Kenaject-40; Kenalog-40; Triam-A; Triamonide 40; Tri-Kort; Trilog*; GENERIC].
Canada—
10 mg per mL (Rx) [*Kenalog-10*].
40 mg per mL (Rx) [*Kenalog-40*].

**Packaging and storage**
Store below 40 °C (104 °F), preferably between 15 and 30 °C (59 and 86 °F), unless otherwise specified by manufacturer. Protect from light. Protect from freezing.

**Auxiliary labeling**
• Shake well.

**Additional information**
For preparation and administration of injections, see manufacturer's labeling.
Do not administer this medication intravenously.
Do not administer the 40-mg-per-mL strength intradermally or intralesionally.
Do not administer the 10-mg-per-mL strength intramuscularly.

## STERILE TRIAMCINOLONE DIACETATE SUSPENSION USP

**Usual adult and adolescent dose**
Intra-articular, intrasynovial, intralesional, sublesional, or soft-tissue injection, 3 to 48 mg, repeated at one- to eight-week intervals, if necessary.
Intramuscular, 40 mg once a week. Alternatively, a dose equal to four to seven times the predetermined oral daily dose may be administered as a single injection and repeated at four-day to four-week intervals as required.

**Usual pediatric dose**
Children up to 6 years of age—Use is not recommended.
Children 6 to 12 years of age—Intramuscular, 40 mg once a week.

**Strength(s) usually available**
U.S.—
25 mg per mL (Rx) [*Aristocort Intralesional*].
40 mg per mL (Rx) [*Amcort; Aristocort Forte; Articulose-L.A; Cenocort Forte; Cinalone 40; Triam-Forte; Triamolone 40* (benzyl alcohol); *Trilone; Tristoject*; GENERIC].
Canada—
25 mg per mL (Rx) [*Aristocort Intralesional*].
40 mg per mL (Rx) [*Aristocort Forte*; GENERIC].

**Packaging and storage**
Store below 40 °C (104 °F), preferably between 15 and 30 °C (59 and 86 °F), unless otherwise specified by manufacturer. Protect from freezing.

**Stability**
Admixtures containing local anesthetics will retain their potency for one full week.

**Incompatibilities**
This medication should *not* be mixed with parenteral-local anesthetic formulations containing preservatives such as parabens or phenol because flocculation of the corticosteroid may occur.

**Auxiliary labeling**
• Shake well.

**Additional information**
For preparation and administration of injections, see manufacturer's labeling.
Do not administer this medication intravenously.

## STERILE TRIAMCINOLONE HEXACETONIDE SUSPENSION USP

**Usual adult and adolescent dose**
Intra-articular, 2 to 20 mg, repeated at three- or four-week intervals, if necessary.
Intralesional or sublesional, up to 500 mcg (0.5 mg) per square inch of affected skin, repeated as needed.

**Usual pediatric dose**
Dosage has not been established.

**Strength(s) usually available**
U.S.—
5 mg per mL (Rx) [*Aristospan Intralesional*].
20 mg per mL (Rx) [*Aristospan Intra-articular*].
Canada—
20 mg per mL (Rx) [*Aristospan Intra-articular*].

**Packaging and storage**
Store below 40 °C (104 °F), preferably between 15 and 30 °C (59 and 86 °F), unless otherwise specified by manufacturer. Protect from freezing.

**Stability**
Admixtures containing local anesthetics will retain their potency for one full week.

**Incompatibilities**

This medication should *not* be mixed with parenteral-local anesthetic formulations containing parabens, phenol, or other such preservatives because flocculation of the corticosteroid may occur.

**Auxiliary labeling**

• Shake well.

**Additional information**

For preparation and administration of injections, see manufacturer's labeling.

Do not administer this medication intravenously.

The 5-mg-per-mL strength is recommended for intralesional and sublesional injections only.

The 20-mg-per-mL strength is recommended for intra-articular injection only.

Revised: 04/14/92
Interim revision: 08/09/94; 04/01/96

## Table 1. Indications

Note: Bracketed information refers to uses or routes that are not included in U.S. product labeling.

| | Glucocorticoids* | | | |
|---|---|---|---|---|
| | Oral | IM; IV; SC† | Local‡ | Rectal§ |
| **Adrenocortical function abnormalities** | | | | |
| Adrenocortical insufficiency, acute (treatment)—Hydrocortisone and cortisone are preferred as replacement therapy because of their significant mineralocorticoid activity. Medication should be administered IV or by IM injection of a rapidly acting preparation initially. Replacement of sodium and fluids is also required. In some patients, additional mineralocorticoid replacement may also be necessary. | | ✔ | | |
| Adrenocortical insufficiency, chronic primary (Addison's disease) (treatment)—Hydrocortisone and cortisone are preferred as replacement therapy for most patients because of their significant mineralocorticoid activity. Administration of sodium (as dietary salt) is recommended; however, additional mineralocorticoid supplementation may also be required in some patients. If a glucocorticoid other than hydrocortisone or cortisone is administered, mineralocorticoid supplementation is usually mandatory. Rarely, however, a patient will have only a glucocorticoid deficiency and will not require mineralocorticoid or sodium supplementation. | ✔ | ✔ | | |
| Adrenocortical insufficiency, secondary (treatment)—Glucocorticoid replacement is usually sufficient; a mineralocorticoid is not always required. | ✔ | ✔ | | |
| Adrenogenital syndrome (adrenal hyperplasia, congenital) (treatment)—Indicated to reduce virilization caused by enzyme deficiency–induced adrenal androgen hypersecretion. Corticosteroid and supplemental therapy depends upon the enzyme deficiency involved and form of disease present. In salt-losing forms, hydrocortisone or cortisone, plus increased sodium intake, may be preferred. However, additional mineralocorticoid supplementation may be required. In salt-retaining or hypertensive forms, a glucocorticoid having minimal mineralocorticoid activity is preferred. However, long-acting glucocorticoids are best avoided because of the increased risk of growth retardation and difficulty in dosage adjustment. | ✔ | ✔ | | |
| Cushing's syndrome (diagnosis)—Dexamethasone is indicated in the diagnosis of Cushing's syndrome and to distinguish Cushing's syndrome caused by excessive corticotropin secretion from that due to other causes. | ✔ | ✔ | | |
| **Allergic disorders**—Indicated for the treatment of severe or incapacitating allergic disorders intractable to adequate trials of conventional treatment, such as: | | | | |
| Allergic reactions, drug-induced (treatment) | ✔ | ✔ | | |
| Anaphylactic or anaphylactoid reactions (treatment adjunct)—Use of glucocorticoids is generally reserved for prolonged reactions (those not responding to other forms of treatment within 1 hour), reactions requiring cardiovascular or respiratory resuscitation, or situations in which there is a significant risk of relapse. Medication should be administered IV or by IM injection of a rapidly acting preparation initially. | ✔ | ✔ | | |
| Angioedema (treatment adjunct)—Medication should be administered IV or by IM injection of a rapidly acting preparation initially. | ✔ | ✔ | | |
| Laryngeal edema, acute noninfectious (treatment adjunct)—If a corticosteroid is used, it should be administered IV or by IM injection of a rapidly acting preparation initially. (Epinephrine is the drug of first choice) | ✔ | ✔ | | |
| Rhinitis, allergic, perennial or seasonal, severe (treatment) | ✔ | ✔ | [✔]¹ | |
| Serum sickness (treatment) | ✔ | ✔ | | |
| Transfusion reactions, urticarial (treatment)—Medication should be administered IV or by IM injection of a rapidly acting preparation initially. | | ✔ | | |
| **Collagen disorders (treatment)**—Indicated during an acute exacerbation or as maintenance therapy in selected cases of: | | | | |
| Carditis, rheumatic [or nonrheumatic]¹, acute | ✔ | ✔ | | |
| Dermatomyositis, systemic (polymyositis)—Glucocorticoids may be the treatment of choice in children with this condition. | ✔ | ✔ | | |

## Table 1. Indications *(continued)*

| | Glucocorticoids* | | | |
|---|:---:|:---:|:---:|:---:|
| | Oral | IM; IV; SC† | Local‡ | Rectal§ |
| Lupus erythematosus, systemic | ✔ | ✔ | | |
| [Arteritis, giant-cell (temporal)]¹ | ✔ | ✔ | | |
| [Connective tissue disease, mixed]¹ | ✔ | ✔ | | |
| [Polyarteritis nodosa]¹ | ✔ | ✔ | | |
| [Polychondritis, relapsing]¹ | ✔ | ✔ | | |
| [Polymyalgia rheumatica]¹ | ✔ | ✔ | | |
| [Vasculitis]¹ | ✔ | ✔ | | |
| [Depression, mental, endogenous (diagnosis)]¹—Dexamethasone is used in diagnosing endogenous depression and in evaluating the efficacy of treatment. Dexamethasone reduces plasma cortisol to a greater extent in control subjects than in hospitalized patients with diagnosed depression; values return toward those of control subjects as the patient responds to therapy. However, the dexamethasone suppression test is less sensitive in patients with mild to moderate depression; also, many medications, medical problems, and other psychiatric disorders have been reported to interfere with the test results. The Health and Public Policy Committee of the American College of Physicians recommends that the dexamethasone suppression test not be used as a screening test for depression. | ✔ | | | |
| Dermatologic disorders (treatment)—Indicated in the treatment of dermatologic disorders, such as: | | | | |
| Alopecia areata | | | ✔ | |
| Dermatitis, atopic | ✔ | ✔ | | |
| Dermatitis, contact | ✔ | ✔ | | |
| Dermatitis, exfoliative | ✔ | ✔ | | |
| Dermatitis herpetiformis, bullous | ✔ | ✔ | | |
| Dermatitis, seborrheic, severe | ✔ | ✔ | | |
| Dermatoses, inflammatory, severe | ✔ | ✔ | ✔ | |
| Erythema multiforme, severe (Stevens-Johnson syndrome) | ✔ | ✔ | | |
| Granuloma annulare | | | ✔ | |
| Keloids | | | ✔ | |
| Lichen planus | | | ✔ | |
| Lichen simplex chronicus | | | ✔ | |
| Lupus erythematosus, discoid | | | ✔ | |
| Mycosis fungoides | ✔ | ✔ | | |
| Necrobiosis lipoidica diabeticorum | | | ✔ | |
| Pemphigus | ✔ | ✔ | | |
| Psoriasis, severe | ✔ | ✔ | ✔ | |
| [Eczema, severe] | ✔ | | | |
| [Pemphigoid]¹ | ✔ | ✔ | | |
| [Sarcoid, localized cutaneous]¹ | | | ✔ | |

*Unless otherwise specified in text, any glucocorticoid may be administered, subject to availability of a dosage form suitable for the recommended route of administration.

†IM=intramuscular; IV=intravenous; SC=subcutaneous. See *Table 4* for specific dosage forms.

‡Routes of local injection may include intra-articular, intrabursal, intralesional, intrasynovial, soft tissue, or [intranasal (intraturbinal)], depending on condition being treated. See *Table 4* for specific dosage forms.

§Rectal dosage forms include Betamethasone Sodium Phosphate Enema (Canada), Hydrocortisone Enema USP, Hydrocortisone Acetate Rectal Aerosol (Foam), and Methylprednisolone Acetate for Enema USP.

¹Not included in Canadian product labeling.

## Table 1. Indications *(continued)*

| | Glucocorticoids* | | | |
|---|---|---|---|---|
| | Oral | IM; IV; SC† | Local‡ | Rectal§ |
| **Gastrointestinal disorders (treatment)**—Indicated in the treatment of inflammatory bowel disease as listed below. Oral or parenteral dosage forms are indicated when systemic therapy is required during a critical period of the disease; long-term use is not recommended. | | | | |
| Bowel disease, inflammatory, including colitis, ulcerative: | ✔ | ✔ | | |
|  Enema dosage forms of [betamethasone], hydrocortisone, and methylprednisolone are also indicated in this condition. | | | | ✔ |
|  FDA has classified Methylprednisolone acetate for enema as being possibly effective in the treatment of ulcerative colitis; this classification requires submission of adequate and well-controlled studies to provide substantial evidence of effectiveness. | | | | |
| Colitis, ulcerative, of rectum: | | | | |
|  Rectal dosage forms of [betamethasone], hydrocortisone, and methylprednisolone are indicated in this condition. | | | | |
|  FDA has classified Methylprednisolone acetate for enema as being possibly effective in the treatment of ulcerative colitis; this classification requires submission of adequate and well-controlled studies to provide substantial evidence of effectiveness. | | | | |
| Enteritis, regional (Crohn's disease) | ✔ | ✔ | | |
| Proctitis, ulcerative: Hydrocortisone enema and, when only the distal portion of the rectum is affected, hydrocortisone acetate rectal aerosol (foam) are indicated. | | | | ✔ |
| Proctosigmoiditis, ulcerative: Hydrocortisone enema is indicated and [hydrocortisone acetate rectal aerosol (foam)] is used. | | | | ✔ |
| [Celiac disease, severe][1] | ✔ | ✔ | | |
| **Hematologic disorders (treatment)**—Indicated in the treatment of: | | | | |
| Anemia, hemolytic, acquired (autoimmune) | ✔ | ✔ | | |
| Anemia, hypoplastic, congenital (erythroid) | ✔ | ✔ | | |
| Anemia, red blood cell (erythroblastopenia) | ✔ | ✔ | | |
| Thrombocytopenia, secondary, in adults | ✔ | ✔ | | |
| Thrombocytopenic purpura, idiopathic, in adults: Oral or IV only; IM injections are contraindicated. | ✔ | ✔ | | |
| [Hemolysis][1] | ✔ | ✔ | | |
| **[Hepatic disease (treatment)][1]**—Although their use is controversial, methylprednisolone, prednisolone, and prednisone are used in the treatment of: | | | | |
| [Hepatitis, alcoholic, with encephalopathy][1] | ✔ | ✔ | | |
| [Hepatitis, chronic active][1] | ✔ | ✔ | | |
| [Hepatitis, nonalcoholic, in women][1] | ✔ | ✔ | | |
| [Necrosis, hepatic, subacute][1] | ✔ | ✔ | | |
| **Hypercalcemia associated with neoplasms [or sarcoidosis][1] (treatment)** | ✔ | ✔ | | |
| **Inflammation, nonrheumatic (treatment)**—Indicated during an acute episode or exacerbation of the disorders listed below. Local injections are preferred when only a few joints or areas are affected. | | | | |
| Bursitis, acute or subacute | ✔ | ✔ | ✔ | |
| Epicondylitis | ✔ | ✔ | ✔ | |
| Tenosynovitis, nonspecific acute | ✔ | ✔ | ✔ | |
| **[Nausea and vomiting, cancer chemotherapy–induced (prophylaxis)][1]**—Dexamethasone, hydrocortisone, and prednisone are used to prevent nausea and vomiting induced by antineoplastic agents. The medication is administered prior to and following each course of chemotherapy. However, the advisability of administering a potent glucocorticoid to a cancer patient, unless indicated for palliation of the disease has been questioned. Although an increased incidence of infection has not been reported in patients receiving such therapy, the possibility must be considered. | | ✔ | | |

## Table 1. Indications *(continued)*

| | Glucocorticoids* | | | |
|---|---|---|---|---|
| | Oral | IM; IV; SC† | Local‡ | Rectal§ |
| **Neoplastic disease (treatment adjunct)**—Indicated in conjunction with appropriate specific antineoplastic disease therapy for the palliative management of the following neoplastic diseases and related problems. | | | | |
|   Leukemia, acute or chronic lymphocytic | ✔ | ✔ | | |
|   Lymphomas, Hodgkin's or non-Hodgkin's | ✔ | ✔ | | |
|   [Carcinoma, breast][1] | ✔ | ✔ | | |
|   [Carcinoma, prostatic][1] | ✔ | ✔ | | |
|   [Fever, due to malignancy][1] | ✔ | ✔ | | |
|   [Multiple myeloma][1] | ✔ | ✔ | | |
| **Nephrotic syndrome (treatment)**—Indicated to induce diuresis or remission of proteinuria in idiopathic nephrotic syndrome (without uremia), and to improve renal function in patients with lupus erythematosus. In idiopathic nephrotic syndrome, long-term therapy may be required to prevent frequent relapses. | ✔ | ✔ | | |
| **Neurologic disease** | | | | |
|   Meningitis, tuberculous (treatment adjunct)—Indicated for administration concurrently with appropriate antitubercular chemotherapy in patients with concurrent or impending subarachnoid block. | ✔ | ✔ | | |
|   Multiple sclerosis (treatment)[1]—Indicated for treatment of acute exacerbations of the disease. | ✔ | ✔ | | |
|   [Myasthenia gravis (treatment)][1]—Used for treatment of severe cases not controlled by antimyasthenic agents alone. Glucocorticoid therapy may be more effective following thymectomy and in patients having disease onset after age 40. Long-term therapy may be required. | ✔ | | | |
| **Neurotrauma** | | | | |
| Note: Use in neurotrauma, except in conjunction with brain surgery and spinal cord injury, is controversial. Glucocorticoids are considered effective in preventing neurosurgery-associated cerebral edema and in treating edema caused by glioblastomas or metastatic brain tumors. They may be less effective in treating edema caused by astrocytomas or meningiomas. Beneficial effects in closed head injury or ischemic brain edema have not been established. Because very high doses are required, only those glucocorticoids having little or no mineralocorticoid activity should be used. | | | | |
|   Edema, cerebral, especially when associated with primary or metastatic brain tumor, craniotomy, or head injury ([prophylaxis and][1] treatment)—Dexamethasone (oral dosage forms and dexamethasone sodium phosphate injection) are indicated [and prednisone is used][1]. | ✔ | ✔ | | |
|   [Ischemia, cerebral (treatment)][1]—Dexamethasone is used. | ✔ | ✔ | | |
|   [Pseudotumor cerebri (treatment)][1]—Dexamethasone is used. | ✔ | ✔ | | |
|   [Spinal cord injury (treatment)][1]—Methylprednisolone is used. A large study concluded that patients receiving high-dose methylprednisolone therapy within 8 hours of acute spinal cord injury recover more motor and sensory function, as compared with those receiving placebo or naloxone. However, methylprednisolone did not improve patient prognosis when dosing was commenced more than 8 hours after spinal cord injury. | ✔ | ✔ | | |
| **Ophthalmic disorders (treatment)**—Indicated in the treatment of severe acute or chronic allergic and inflammatory ophthalmic conditions, such as: | | | | |
|   Chorioretinitis | ✔ | ✔ | | |
|   Choroiditis, posterior, diffuse | ✔ | ✔ | | |
|   Conjunctivitis, allergic (not controlled topically) | ✔ | ✔ | | |
|   Herpes zoster | ✔ | ✔ | | |
|   Iridocyclitis | ✔ | ✔ | | |
|   Keratitis not associated with herpes simplex or fungal infection | ✔ | ✔ | | |
|   Neuritis, optic | ✔ | ✔ | | |
|   Ophthalmia sympathetic | ✔ | ✔ | | |
|   Uveitis, posterior, diffuse | ✔ | ✔ | | |

\*Unless otherwise specified in text, any glucocorticoid may be administered, subject to availability of a dosage form suitable for the recommended route of administration.

†IM=intramuscular; IV=intravenous; SC=subcutaneous. See *Table 4* for specific dosage forms.

‡Routes of local injection may include intra-articular, intrabursal, intralesional, intrasynovial, soft tissue, or [intranasal (intraturbinal)], depending on condition being treated. See *Table 4* for specific dosage forms.

§Rectal dosage forms include Betamethasone Sodium Phosphate Enema (Canada), Hydrocortisone Enema USP, Hydrocortisone Acetate Rectal Aerosol (Foam), and Methylprednisolone Acetate for Enema USP.

[1]Not included in Canadian product labeling.

## Table 1. Indications *(continued)*

| | Glucocorticoids* | | | |
| --- | --- | --- | --- | --- |
| | Oral | IM; IV; SC† | Local‡ | Rectal§ |
| **[Oral disorders (treatment)][1]**—Systemic corticosteroids are indicated for treatment of oral lesions unresponsive to topical therapy. The presence of an oral herpetic lesion must be ruled out prior to initiation of glucocorticoid therapy. | | | | |
| [Gingivitis, desquamative (when the diagnosis is confirmed via immunofluorescent biopsy assay)][1] | ✔ | | | |
| [Lesions, oral, associated with corticosteroid-responsive disorders, such as systemic lupus erythematosus; discoid lupus erythematosus; pemphigus; pemphigoid; erythema multiforme, severe (Stevens-Johnson syndrome); and lichen planus][1] | ✔ | | | |
| [Stomatitis, aphthous, recurrent (recurrent aphthous ulcers)][1] | ✔ | | | |
| **[Pericarditis (treatment)][1]**—Used to relieve inflammation and fever | ✔ | ✔ | | |
| **Polyps, nasal (treatment)[1]** | ✔ | ✔ | | |
| **[Polyps, nasal, severe (treatment)][1]** | | | ✔ | |
| **Respiratory disorders (treatment [and prophylaxis][1])**— [Prophylactic uses include administration prior to or during extracorporeal circulation in heart surgery if the patient has a pre-existing pulmonary disorder, and administration prior to, during, and following oral, facial, or neck surgery to prevent edema that may threaten the airway.][1] Indicated in the treatment of respiratory disorders, such as: | | | | |
| Asthma, bronchial | ✔ | ✔ | | |
| Berylliosis | ✔ | ✔ | | |
| Loeffler syndrome (eosinophilic pneumonitis or hypereosinophilic syndrome) | ✔ | ✔ | | |
| Pneumonitis, aspiration | ✔ | ✔ | | |
| Sarcoidosis, symptomatic | ✔ | ✔ | | |
| Tuberculosis, pulmonary, disseminated or fulminating (treatment adjunct): Administered concurrently with appropriate antituberculosis chemotherapy | ✔ | ✔ | | |
| [Bronchitis, asthmatic, acute or chronic][1] | ✔ | ✔ | | |
| [Edema, pulmonary, noncardiogenic (protamine sensitivity–induced)][1]—Medication should be administered IV or by IM injection of a rapidly acting preparation initially. | ✔ | ✔ | | |
| [Hemangioma, airway-obstructing, in infants][1]—Medication should be administered IV or by IM injection of a rapidly acting preparation initially. | ✔ | ✔ | | |
| [Pneumonia, *Pneumocystis carinii*, associated with immunodeficiency syndrome, acquired (treatment adjunct)][1]—In a small number of studies, early use of corticosteroids (e.g., corticosteroid therapy begun within 24 to 72 hours of initial antipneumocystis therapy) as an adjunct to specific antipneumocystis therapy was shown to significantly reduce the risk of oxygenation deterioration, respiratory failure, and death in patients being treated for moderate-to-severe AIDS-associated pneumocystis pneumonia. The specific corticosteroids used in these studies were prednisone and intravenous methylprednisolone. No improvement in clinical outcome was shown in another study when adjunctive corticosteroid therapy was begun after the onset of respiratory failure and after the initiation of primary antipneumocystis therapy. Therefore, if adjunctive corticosteroid therapy is used, it should be started at the initiation of primary therapy for pneumocystis pneumonia in adults and children over 13 years of age who have documented or suspected HIV infection and documented or suspected pneumocystis pneumonia, accompanied by moderate-to-severe pulmonary dysfunction (PaO$_2$ < 70 mm Hg on room air or A-a gradient > 35 mm Hg). The diagnosis of HIV infection and pneumocystis pneumonia should be confirmed as soon as possible. | ✔ | ✔ | | |
| [Pulmonary disease, chronic obstructive (not controlled with theophylline and beta-adrenergic agonists)] | ✔ | ✔ | | |
| [Status asthmaticus]—Medication should be administered IV or by IM injection of a rapidly acting preparation initially. | | ✔ | | |
| **[Respiratory distress syndrome, neonatal (prophylaxis)][1]**—Betamethasone, dexamethasone, and hydrocortisone are used to reduce the incidence and severity of respiratory distress syndrome (hyaline membrane disease) in premature neonates. Long-acting agents (betamethasone or dexamethasone) are preferred. The medication is administered to the mother, preferably 24 to 48 hours prior to delivery to allow time for it to produce an effect. Glucocorticoids will not be effective when delivery is imminent. If necessary, ritodrine may be administered to delay delivery. If delivery does not occur within several days to 1 week following corticosteroid administration, but the risk of premature delivery persists, administration of a second course of corticosteroid therapy may be necessary. Glucocorticoids are not effective in the treatment of respiratory distress syndrome in the premature neonate. | | ✔ | | |

## Table 1. Indications (continued)

| | Glucocorticoids* | | | |
|---|---|---|---|---|
| | Oral | IM; IV; SC† | Local‡ | Rectal§ |
| **[Respiratory distress syndrome, adult (treatment)]**[1]—Dexamethasone is used in the treatment of respiratory distress syndrome in adults, especially those with post-traumatic pulmonary insufficiency or burns, and during or following massive blood transfusions. However, the benefits of such treatment have not been established. | | ✔ | | |
| **Rheumatic disorders (treatment)—** | | | | |
| Note: Local injections are preferred when only a few joints or areas are involved. | | | | |
| Indicated as adjunctive therapy during an acute episode or exacerbation of rheumatic disorders, such as: | | | | |
| Ankylosing spondylitis | ✔ | ✔ | | |
| Arthritis, psoriatic | ✔ | ✔ | ✔ | |
| Arthritis, rheumatoid (including juvenile arthritis): [Long-term use in the treatment of rheumatoid arthritis is controversial. It is recommended that such treatment be reserved for patients not responsive to other measures, such as aspirin or other nonsteroidal anti-inflammatory drugs, rest, and physical therapy.][1] | ✔ | ✔ | ✔ | |
| Gouty arthritis, acute | ✔ | ✔ | ✔ | |
| Osteoarthritis, post-traumatic | ✔ | ✔ | ✔ | |
| Synovitis of osteoarthritis | ✔ | ✔ | ✔ | |
| [Calcium pyrophosphate deposition disease, acute (pseudogout; chondrocalcinosis articularis; synovitis, crystal-induced)][1] | ✔ | ✔ | ✔ | |
| [Polymyalgia rheumatica][1] | ✔ | ✔ | | |
| [Reiter's disease][1] | ✔ | ✔ | | |
| [Rheumatic fever (especially if carditis is present)] | ✔ | ✔ | | |
| **Shock (treatment)**—Glucocorticoids are indicated in the treatment of shock caused by adrenocortical insufficiency (Addisonian shock) and as adjuncts in treating shock associated with anaphylactic or anaphylactoid reactions. Medication should be administered IV or by IM injection of a rapidly acting preparation initially. | ✔ | ✔ | | |
| [Intravenous glucocorticoids are also being used as adjuncts in the treatment of septic shock. Such use is very controversial because efficacy has not been established and superimposition of new infections has been reported. Specifically, methylprednisolone has been shown to be ineffective, and hazardous, in the treatment of septic shock and is not recommended.] | | ✔ | | |
| **Thyroiditis, nonsuppurative (treatment)** | ✔ | ✔ | | |
| **[Transplant rejection, organ (prophylaxis and treatment)]**[1]—Indicated concurrently with other immunosuppressants such as azathioprine or cyclosporine to reduce the risk of rejection of transplanted organs. | ✔ | ✔ | | |
| [High doses of rapidly acting corticosteroids are also indicated in the treatment of rejection reactions.][1] | | ✔ | | |
| **Trichinosis (treatment)**—Indicated for the treatment of trichinosis with neurological or myocardial involvement. | ✔ | ✔ | | |
| **Tumors, cystic, of a tendon or aponeurosis (treatment)** | | | ✔ | |

*Unless otherwise specified in text, any glucocorticoid may be administered, subject to availability of a dosage form suitable for the recommended route of administration.

†IM=intramuscular; IV=intravenous; SC=subcutaneous. See *Table 4* for specific dosage forms.

‡Routes of local injection may include intra-articular, intrabursal, intralesional, intrasynovial, soft tissue, or [intranasal (intraturbinal)], depending on condition being treated. See *Table 4* for specific dosage forms.

§Rectal dosage forms include Betamethasone Sodium Phosphate Enema (Canada), Hydrocortisone Enema USP, Hydrocortisone Acetate Rectal Aerosol (Foam), and Methylprednisolone Acetate for Enema USP.

[1]Not included in Canadian product labeling.

## Table 2. Pharmacology/Pharmacokinetics*

| Drug and Route | Onset of Action | Peak Effect | Duration of Action | Drug and Route | Onset of Action | Peak Effect | Duration of Action |
|---|---|---|---|---|---|---|---|
| **Betamethasone** | | | | **Methylprednisolone** | | | |
| Oral | | 1–2 hr | 3.25 days | Oral | | 1–2 hr | 1.25–1.5 days |
| Sodium phosphate | | | | Acetate | | | |
| IV | Rapid | | | IM | Slow | 4–8 days | 1–4 wk |
| IM | Rapid | | | | 6–48 hr | | |
| Acetate/Sodium phosphate | | | | IA, IL, ST | Very slow | 7 days | 1–5 wk |
| IM | 1–3 hr | | 1 wk | Sodium succinate | | | |
| IA, IS | | | 1–2 wk | IV | Rapid | | |
| IL, ST | | | 1 wk | IM | Rapid | | |
| **Cortisone acetate** | | | | **Prednisolone** | | | |
| Oral | Rapid | 2 hr | 1.25–1.5 days | Oral | | 1–2 hr | 1.25–1.5 days |
| IM | Slow | 20–48 hr | | Acetate | | | |
| **Dexamethasone** | | | | IM | Slow | | |
| Oral | | 1–2 hr | 2.75 days | Acetate/Sodium phosphate | | | |
| Acetate | | | | IM | | | Up to 4 wk |
| IM | | 8 hr | 6 days | IB, IS, IA, ST | | | 3 days–4 wk |
| IA, ST, IL | | | 1–3 wk | Sodium phosphate | | | |
| Sodium phosphate | | | | IV | Rapid | 1 hr | |
| IV | Rapid | | | IM | Rapid | 1 hr | |
| IM | Rapid | | | IA, IL, ST | | | 3 days–3 wk |
| IA, IS, IL, ST | | | 3 days–3 wk | Tebutate | | | |
| **Hydrocortisone** | | | | IA, IL, ST | Slow | | 1–3 wk |
| Oral | | 1 hr | 1.25–1.5 days | | 1–2 days | | |
| IM | | 4–8 hr | | **Prednisone** | | | |
| Rectal (retention enema) | 3–5 days | | | Oral | | 1–2 hr | 1.25–1.5 days |
| Acetate | | | | **Triamcinolone** | | | |
| IA, IS, IB, IL, ST | | 24–48 hr | 3 days–4 wk | Oral | | 1–2 hr | 2.25 days |
| Rectal (foam) | 5–7 days | | | Acetonide | | | |
| Cypionate | | | | IM | Slow | | 1–6 wk |
| Oral | Slower than tablet | 1–2 hr | | | 24–48 hr | | |
| | | | | IB, IA, IS, IL, ST | | | Several wk |
| Sodium phosphate | | | | Diacetate | | | |
| IV | Rapid | | | Oral | | 1–2 hr | |
| IM | Rapid | 1 hr | | IM | Slow | | 4 days–4 wk |
| Sodium succinate | | | | IL | | | 1–2 wk |
| IV | Rapid | | | IA, IS, ST | | | 1–8 wk |
| IM | Rapid | 1 hr | Variable | Hexacetonide | | | |
| | | | | IA, IL | | | 3–4 wk |

*Abbreviations: IA=intra-articular; IB=intrabursal; IL=intralesional; IM=intramuscular; IS=intrasynovial; ST=soft tissue.

## Table 3. Pharmacology/Pharmacokinetics

| | Relative Potency | | | | Half-life (hr) | |
|---|---|---|---|---|---|---|
| | Glucocorticoid Dose (mg)* | Glucocorticoid Activity† | Mineralocorticoid Activity‡ | Protein Binding§ | Plasma | Biological (Tissue) |
| **Corticosteroids** | | | | | | |
| *Short-acting* | | | | | | |
| Cortisone | 25 | 0.8 | 2+ | | 0.5 | 8–12 |
| Hydrocortisone | 20 | 1 | 2+ | Very high | 1.5–2 | 8–12 |
| *Intermediate-acting* | | | | | | |
| Methylprednisolone | 4 | 5 | 0# | | >3.5 | 18–36 |
| Prednisolone | 5 | 4 | 1+ | High | 2.1–3.5 | 18–36 |
| Prednisone | 5 | 4 | 1+ | High to very high | 3.4–3.8 | 18–36 |
| Triamcinolone | 4 | 5 | 0# | High | 2–>5 | 18–36 |
| *Long-acting* | | | | | | |
| Betamethasone | 0.6 | 20–30 | 0# | High | 3–5 | 36–54 |
| Dexamethasone | 0.5–0.75 | 20–30 | 0# | High | 3–4.5 | 36–54 |

*Approximate; applies to oral or intravenous administration only.

†Anti-inflammatory, immunosuppressant, metabolic effects.

‡Sodium and water retention, potassium depletion.

§Hydrocortisone binds to transcortin (corticosteroid binding globulin; CBG) and to albumin. Prednisone, but not betamethasone, dexamethasone, or triamcinolone, also binds to CBG.

#Although these glucocorticoids are considered not to have significant mineralocorticoid activity, hypokalemia and/or sodium and fluid retention may occur, depending on dosage and patient predisposition.

## Table 4. General Dosing Information*

| Drug | Parenteral Routes of Administration† | | | | | | | | |
|---|---|---|---|---|---|---|---|---|---|
| | Systemic | | | Local | | | | | |
| | IM | IV | SC | IA | IB | IL | IS | ST | [IT]¹ |
| **Betamethasone** | | | | | | | | | |
| Sodium phosphate | ✓ | ✓ | | ✓ | | ✓ | | ✓ | |
| Acetate/Sodium phosphate | ✓ | | | ✓ | | ✓ | ✓ | ✓ | |
| **Cortisone Acetate** | ✓ | | | | | | | | |
| **Dexamethasone** | | | | | | | | | |
| Acetate | ✓ | | | ✓ | | ✓ | | ✓ | |
| Sodium phosphate | ✓ | ✓ | | ✓ | | ✓ | ✓ | ✓ | |
| **Hydrocortisone** | | | | | | | | | |
| Sterile suspension | ✓ | | | | | | | | |
| Acetate | | | | ✓ | ✓ | ✓ | ✓ | ✓ | |
| Sodium phosphate | ✓ | ✓ | ✓ | | | | | | |
| Sodium succinate | ✓ | ✓ | | | | | | | |
| **Methylprednisolone** | | | | | | | | | |
| Acetate | ✓ | | | ✓ | | ✓ | | | |
| Sodium succinate | ✓ | ✓ | | | | | | | |
| **Prednisolone** | | | | | | | | | |
| Acetate | ✓ | | | ✓ | | ✓ | | | |
| Acetate/Sodium phosphate | ✓ | | | ✓ | ✓ | ✓ | ✓ | | |
| Sodium phosphate | ✓ | | | ✓ | | ✓ | ✓ | | |
| Tebutate | | | | ✓ | | ✓ | | ✓ | [✓]¹ |
| **Triamcinolone** | | | | | | | | | |
| Acetonide | ✓ | | | ✓ | ✓ | ✓ | | ✓ | [✓]¹ |
| Diacetate | ✓ | | | ✓ | | ✓ | ✓ | ✓ | [✓]¹ |
| Hexacetonide | | | | ✓ | | ✓ | | | [✓]¹ |

*Bracketed information refers to routes of administration that are not included in U.S. product labeling.

†Abbreviations: Systemic—IM=intramuscular; IV=intravenous; SC=subcutaneous. Local—IA=intra-articular; IB=intrabursal; IL=intralesional; IS=intrasynovial; ST=soft tissue; IT=intraturbinal.

¹Not included in Canadian product labeling.

# CORTICOTROPIN    Systemic

VA CLASSIFICATION (Primary):
    Corticotropin for Injection—DX900
    Repository Corticotropin—CN400

Another commonly used name is ACTH.

Note: For a listing of dosage forms and brand names by country availability, see *Dosage Forms* section(s). For a listing of brand names for the articles in this monograph, refer to the General Index.

## Category

Diagnostic aid (adrenocortical function)—Corticotropin for Injection USP.
Anticonvulsant (specific in infantile myoclonic seizures)—Repository Corticotropin Injection USP.

## Indications

Note: Bracketed information in the *Indications* section refers to uses that are not included in U.S. product labeling.

### Accepted

Adrenocortical insufficiency (diagnosis)—Corticotropin for injection is indicated as an aid in diagnosing adrenocortical insufficiency; however, the synthetic fragment of corticotropin, cosyntropin, is the preferred diagnostic aid because it is less antigenic. Additionally, corticotropin is purified from animal pituitary glands and can contain significant amounts of vasopressin and other peptides, which are not found in cosyntropin.

[Seizures, myoclonic, infantile (treatment)][1]—Repository corticotropin is used in the treatment of infantile myoclonic seizures (infantile spasms), although there are only limited data suggesting that it has greater efficacy than do glucocorticoids.

### Unaccepted

Corticotropin is no longer recommended for its anti-inflammatory and immunosuppressant properties. Although corticotropin is FDA-approved for the treatment of secondary adrenocortical insufficiency and many nonendocrine disorders that are responsive to glucocorticoid therapy, treatment with a corticosteroid is preferred.

---

[1]Not included in Canadian product labeling.

## Pharmacology/Pharmacokinetics

### Physicochemical characteristics
Hormone; obtained from porcine pituitary glands.

### Mechanism of action/Effect
Diagnostic aid (adrenocortical function)—Corticotropin combines with a specific receptor on the adrenal cell plasma membrane. In patients with normal adrenocortical function, it stimulates the initial reaction involved in the synthesis of adrenal steroids (including cortisol, cortisone, weak androgenic substances, and a limited quantity of aldosterone) from cholesterol by increasing the quantity of cholesterol within the mitochondria. Corticotropin does *not* significantly increase serum cortisol concentrations in patients with primary adrenocortical insufficiency (Addison's disease).

Anticonvulsant (specific in infantile myoclonic seizures)—The mechanism of action of corticotropin in the treatment of infantile myoclonic seizures is unknown.

### Other actions/effects
Corticotropin is not a corticosteroid. However, it shares many actions of the corticosteroids due to its ability to increase endogenous corticosteroid synthesis.

### Absorption
Corticotropin is rapidly absorbed following intramuscular administration; the repository dosage form is slowly absorbed over approximately 8 to 16 hours.

### Half-life
About 15 minutes following intravenous administration.

### Time to peak effect
Peak plasma cortisol concentrations are usually achieved within 1 hour after intramuscular or rapid intravenous administration of corticotropin for injection.

### Duration of action
Following intramuscular or rapid intravenous administration of corticotropin, peak plasma cortisol concentrations begin to decrease after 2 to 4 hours.
The effects of repository corticotropin may last up to 3 days.

## Precautions to Consider

### Cross-sensitivity and/or related problems
Patients allergic to proteins of porcine origin or cosyntropin may also be allergic to corticotropin.

### Carcinogenicity
Adequate and well-controlled animal studies have not been done in animals; however, use in humans has not shown an increase in malignant disease.

### Pregnancy/Reproduction
Fertility—Studies have not been done in humans or in animals.

Pregnancy—Adequate and well-controlled studies have not been done in humans.
Studies in animals have shown that corticotropin is embryocidal.
FDA Pregnancy Category C.

### Breast-feeding
It is not known whether corticotropin is distributed into breast milk. However, problems in humans have not been documented.

### Pediatrics
Appropriate studies performed to date using corticotropin have not demonstrated pediatrics-specific problems that would limit the usefulness of corticotropin in children. However, prolonged use of corticotropin in children will inhibit skeletal growth; therefore, close monitoring is recommended.

### Geriatrics
Appropriate studies performed to date using corticotropin have not demonstrated geriatrics-specific problems that would limit the usefulness of corticotropin in the elderly.

### Drug interactions and/or related problems
The following drug interactions and/or related problems have been selected on the basis of their potential clinical significance (possible mechanism in parentheses where appropriate)—not necessarily inclusive (» = major clinical significance):

Note: Combinations containing any of the following medications, depending on the amount present, may also interact with this medication.

Estrogens
    (estrogen may cause abnormally high plasma cortisol concentrations before and after corticotropin administration; however, a normal incremental response to corticotropin still occurs)

» Immunizations
    (during chronic therapy, patients should not be vaccinated against smallpox; extreme caution is recommended if other immunizations are to be given, because of the risk of neurological complications and lack of antibody response)

Verapamil
    (limited data show that chronic administration of oral verapamil may blunt the effect of corticotropin, resulting in a false negative diagnostic test result)

### Laboratory value alterations
The following have been selected on the basis of their potential clinical significance (possible effect in parentheses where appropriate)—not necessarily inclusive (» = major clinical significance):

With results of adrenocortical function testing
  *Due to other medications*
» Corticosteroids, glucocorticoid
    (if competitive protein binding assays or immunoassays showing cross-reactivity with prednisone or cortisone are used, a high baseline cortisol concentration with no response to corticotropin may be seen in patients taking these medications)

### Medical considerations/Contraindications
The medical considerations/contraindications included here have been selected on the basis of their potential clinical significance (reasons given in parentheses where appropriate)—not necessarily inclusive (» = major clinical significance).

*Except under special circumstances, this medication should not be used when the following medical problems exist:*

» Infections, serious bacterial or viral, especially varicella
    (possible immunosupression may lead to infectious complications with chronic use)

*Risk-benefit should be considered when the following medical problems exist:*
» Allergy to corticotropin, cosyntropin, or porcine derivatives
  (risk of allergic reaction)

**Patient monitoring**
The following may be especially important in patient monitoring (other tests may be warranted in some patients, depending on condition; » = major clinical significance):

*For treatment of infantile myoclonic seizures*
» Blood pressure and
» Calcium, serum and
» Electroencephalogram, waking and sleeping and
» Electrolytes, serum and
» Glucose, urine and
» Phosphorus, serum and
» Urinalysis and
» Weight
  (recommended at periodic intervals during therapy to assess therapeutic and/or adverse effects)
» Calcium, serum and
» Complete blood count and
» Electrolytes, serum and
» Endocrine profile and
» Glucose, serum, fasting and 2-hour postprandial and
» Phosphorus, serum, and
» Renal function tests and
» Urinalysis
  (recommended prior to initiation of therapy; caution in using corticotropin is recommended if any of these tests are abnormal)

## Side/Adverse Effects

Note: Except for rare allergic reactions, there are no side/adverse effects associated with the use of corticotropin as a diagnostic aid.

The following side/adverse effects have been selected on the basis of their potential clinical significance (possible signs and symptoms in parentheses where appropriate)—not necessarily inclusive:

**Those indicating need for medical attention**
Incidence less frequent—with chronic use only
  *Cerebral ventriculomegaly; congestive heart failure; hyperglycemia; hypertension; hypothalamic-pituitary suppression; metabolic abnormalities, such as; hypernatremia; hypokalemia; hypocalcemia; hypophosphatemia; sepsis*
Incidence rare
  *Allergic reaction* (dizziness; nausea and vomiting; shock; skin rash); *worsening of seizures*—with chronic use only

**Those indicating need for medical attention only if they continue or are bothersome**
Incidence more frequent—with chronic use only
  *Irritability, extreme*

**Those not indicating need for medical attention**
Incidence more frequent—with chronic use only
  *Cushingoid facies; cutaneous pigmentation; hirsutism; seborrheic dermatitis*

## General Dosing Information

Following administration of corticotropin as a diagnostic agent, adrenal insufficiency can be confirmed when a plasma, serum, or urinary free cortisol concentration does not increase above a baseline concentration.

During chronic therapy of infantile myoclonic seizures, patients should not be vaccinated against smallpox. Extreme caution is recommended if other immunizations are to be given, because of the risk of neurological complications and lack of antibody response.

**For treatment of adverse effects**
Recommended treatment for hypertension that may develop during treatment of infantile spasms consists of sodium restriction and diuretic therapy rather than discontinuation of corticotropin.

## Parenteral Dosage Forms

Note: Bracketed uses in the *Dosage Forms* section refer to categories of use and/or indications that are not included in U.S. product labeling.

## CORTICOTROPIN FOR INJECTION USP

**Usual adult and adolescent dose**
Adrenocortical insufficiency (diagnosis)—
  Intravenous infusion, 10 to 25 Units in 500 mL of 5% dextrose in water, infused over an eight-hour period.

**Usual pediatric dose**
Adrenocortical insufficiency (diagnosis)—
  Use is not recommended. The synthetic fragment of corticotropin, cosyntropin, is the recommended diagnostic agent.
[Seizures, myoclonic, infantile (treatment)][1]—
  Use is not recommended. Repository corticotropin injection USP is the preferred product.

**Size(s) usually available**
U.S.—
  25 USP Units per vial (Rx) [*Acthar*].
  40 USP Units per vial (Rx) [*ACTH; Acthar;* GENERIC].
Canada—
  40 IU per vial (Rx) [*Acthar Powder*].

**Packaging and storage**
Prior to reconstitution, store between 15 and 30 °C (59 and 86 °F), unless otherwise specified by manufacturer.

**Preparation of dosage form**
Corticotropin for injection should be reconstituted with sterile water or sodium chloride for injection, so that the individual dose is contained in 1 to 2 mL of solution.

**Stability**
After reconstitution, solution should be used immediately.

## REPOSITORY CORTICOTROPIN INJECTION USP

**Usual adult and adolescent dose**
Use is not recommended.

**Usual pediatric dose**
[Seizures, myoclonic, infantile (treatment)][1]—
  Intramuscular, 20 to 40 Units per day or 80 Units every other day.

  Note: The optimal dose of corticotropin for the treatment of infantile myoclonic seizures has not been established. Another recommended regimen for infantile myoclonic seizures is an initial dose of 150 Units per square meter of body surface area per day administered intramuscularly in two divided doses for one week, followed by 75 Units per square meter of body surface area per day for one week, then 75 Units per square meter of body surface area administered every other day for one week. Corticotropin dosage is then gradually tapered over the subsequent nine weeks.

  The optimal duration of therapy is not known.

  Dose should be tapered gradually when discontinuing corticotropin therapy.

**Strength(s) usually available**
U.S.—
  40 USP Units per mL (Rx) [*H.P. Acthar Gel;* GENERIC].
  80 USP Units per mL (Rx) [*H.P. Acthar Gel;* GENERIC].
Canada—
  40 IU per mL (Rx) [*Acthar Gel (H.P.)*].

**Packaging and storage**
Store between 2 and 8 °C (36 and 46 °F), unless otherwise specified by manufacturer.

---

[1]Not included in Canadian product labeling.

## Selected Bibliography

Snead OC. Other antiepileptic drugs: adrenocorticotropic hormone (ACTH). In: Levy R, Mattson R, Meldrum B, editors. Antiepileptic drugs. New York: Raven Press, 1995: 941-8.

Revised: 03/25/96

---

**CORTISONE**—See *Corticosteroids—Glucocorticoid Effects (Systemic)*

# COSYNTROPIN Systemic

INN: Tetracosactide

VA CLASSIFICATION (Primary/Secondary): DX900/HS701

Note: For a listing of dosage forms and brand names by country availability, see *Dosage Forms* section(s). For a listing of brand names for the articles in this monograph, refer to the General Index.

## Category

Diagnostic aid (adrenal-pituitary function).

## Indications

### Accepted

Adrenocortical insufficiency (diagnosis)—Cosyntropin is indicated as an aid for diagnosing adrenocortical insufficiency.

Cosyntropin is a synthetic subunit of corticotropin (adrenocorticotropic hormone; ACTH). Cosyntropin is preferable to ACTH for diagnosing primary adrenocortical insufficiency because it is less allergenic. Cosyntropin may be tolerated by most patients who have had an allergic reaction to ACTH or those with a history of allergies.

### Unaccepted

Cosyntropin is not indicated for the treatment of corticosteroid-responsive medical conditions.

## Pharmacology/Pharmacokinetics

### Physicochemical characteristics

Chemical group—Synthetic polypeptide identical to the first 24 of the 39 amino acids of corticotropin (ACTH).

Molecular weight—2933.46.

### Mechanism of action/Effect

Cosyntropin combines with a specific receptor in the adrenal cell plasma membrane and, in patients with normal adrenocortical function, stimulates the initial reaction involved in the synthesis of adrenal steroids (including cortisol, cortisone, weak androgenic substances, and a limited quantity of aldosterone) from cholesterol by increasing the quantity of the substrate within the mitochondria. Cosyntropin does not significantly increase plasma cortisol concentration in patients with primary or secondary adrenocortical insufficiency.

Cosyntropin has less immunogenic activity than ACTH because the amino acid sequence having most of the antigenic activity of ACTH (i.e., amino acids 25–39) is not present in cosyntropin.

### Time to peak effect

The maximal increase in plasma cortisol concentration usually occurs approximately 45 to 60 minutes following intravenous or subcutaneous administration of cosyntropin.

## Precautions to Consider

### Cross-sensitivity and/or related problems

Although most patients allergic to corticotropin do not exhibit allergy to cosyntropin, some of these patients may be allergic to cosyntropin also.

### Carcinogenicity/Mutagenicity

Long-term animal studies have not been conducted to evaluate the carcinogenic or mutagenic potential of cosyntropin.

### Pregnancy/Reproduction

Pregnancy—Studies have not been done in humans.
Studies have not been done animals.

FDA Pregnancy Category C.

### Breast-feeding

It is not known whether cosyntropin is distributed into breast milk. However, problems in humans have not been documented.

### Pediatrics

Appropriate studies on the relationship of age to the effects of cosyntropin have not been performed in the pediatric population. However, no pediatrics-specific problems have been documented to date.

### Geriatrics

No information is available on the relationship of age to the effects of cosyntropin in geriatric patients.

### Drug interactions and/or related problems

The following drug interactions and/or related problems have been selected on the basis of their potential clinical significance (possible mechanism in parentheses where appropriate)—not necessarily inclusive (» = major clinical significance):

Note: Combinations containing any of the following medications, depending on the amount present, may also interact with this medication.

Blood, whole, or
Plasma
(cosyntropin may be inactivated by enzymes)

### Laboratory value alterations

The following have been selected on the basis of their potential clinical significance (possible effect in parentheses where appropriate)—not necessarily inclusive (» = major clinical significance):

With results of *this* test

*Due to other medications*

Corticosteroids, glucocorticoid effects, especially cortisone or hydrocortisone
(baseline plasma cortisol concentration may be elevated in patients receiving cortisone or hydrocortisone on the test day and may decrease during the test period)
(with the exception of dexamethasone, other glucocorticoids may interfere with plasma cortisol determinations if radioligand assay tests used are not specific for cortisol)

Spironolactone
(because spironolactone metabolites also fluoresce, plasma cortisol concentrations following cosyntropin administration may be falsely elevated in patients receiving spironolactone when the fluorometric procedure is used but not when radioimmunoassay [RIA] or competitive protein-binding methods are used)

*Due to medical problems or conditions*

Elevated plasma bilirubin concentrations or
Free hemoglobin in plasma, presence of
(falsely elevated plasma cortisol concentrations may occur when the fluorometric method is used)

### Medical considerations/Contraindications

The medical considerations/contraindications included here have been selected on the basis of their potential clinical significance (reasons given in parentheses where appropriate)—not necessarily inclusive (» = major clinical significance).

***Risk-benefit should be considered when the following medical problems exist:***

Allergic disorders or history of
(increased risk of allergic reactions)

Allergy to ACTH or cosyntropin

## Side/Adverse Effects

The following side/adverse effects have been selected on the basis of their potential clinical significance (possible signs and symptoms in parentheses where appropriate)—not necessarily inclusive:

### Those indicating need for medical attention

Incidence rare
***Anaphylaxis, generalized*** (dizziness; lightheadedness; irritability; seizures; skin rash; hives; itching of skin; slow heartbeat; trouble in breathing; wheezing)

### Those indicating need for medical attention only if they continue or are bothersome

Incidence less frequent or rare
*Allergic reaction, mild* (mild fever; nausea; vomiting)

## General Dosing Information

A dose of 250 mcg (0.25 mg) of cosyntropin is equivalent to 25 USP Units of corticotropin.

When used as a diagnostic agent in the screening test for adrenocortical insufficiency, cosyntropin may be administered intramuscularly, subcutaneously, or by intravenous injection. If a greater stimulus is needed, cosyntropin may be administered as an intravenous infusion.

The following criteria may be used as guidelines to determine if the patient has a normal response to cosyntropin. Some interlaboratory variation may occur.

1. Morning control plasma cortisol concentration exceeds 5 mcg (0.005 mg) per 100 mL.

2. Thirty-minute cortisol concentration shows an increase of at least 7 mcg (0.007 mg) per 100 mL above the control level.

3. Thirty-minute cortisol concentration exceeds 18 mcg (0.018 mg) per 100 mL.

Patients who fail to respond to a single dose corticotropin stimulation test using a dose of 250 mcg (0.25 mg) of cosyntropin may be diagnosed as having primary or secondary adrenocortical insufficiency.

## Parenteral Dosage Forms

### COSYNTROPIN FOR INJECTION

**Usual adult and adolescent dose**
Diagnostic aid—
Intramuscular or subcutaneous, 250 mcg (0.25 mg).
Intravenous, 250 mcg (0.25 mg), administered over a two-minute period.
Intravenous infusion, 250 mcg (0.25 mg), administered at a rate of 40 mcg (0.04 mg) per hour over a six-hour period.

**Usual pediatric dose**
Diagnostic aid—
Children up to 2 years of age: Intramuscular, 125 mcg (0.125 mg).
Children 2 years of age and older: See *Usual adult and adolescent dose*.

**Size(s) usually available**
U.S.—
250 mcg (0.25 mg) per vial (Rx) [*Cortrosyn* (mannitol 10 mg)].
Canada—
250 mcg (0.25 mg) per vial (Rx) [*Cortrosyn* (mannitol 10 mg)].

**Packaging and storage**
Prior to reconstitution, store between 15 and 30 °C (59 and 86 °F), unless otherwise specified by manufacturer.

**Preparation of dosage form**
Add 1 mL of diluent provided (0.9% sodium chloride injection) to the vial containing 250 mcg (0.25 mg) of cosyntropin. The resultant solution contains 250 mcg (0.25 mg) of cosyntropin per mL.
For intravenous infusion, cosyntropin may be further diluted with 5% dextrose injection or 0.9% sodium chloride injection.

**Stability**
After reconstitution with 0.9% sodium chloride injection, 250 mcg (0.25 mg)-per-mL-solutions are stable for 24 hours at room temperature or for 21 days when refrigerated at 2 to 8 °C (36 to 46 °F). After further dilution, solutions are stable for 12 hours at room temperature.

Revised: 09/09/92

---

# COUGH/COLD COMBINATIONS  Systemic

**VA CLASSIFICATION (Primary):**
Bromodiphenhydramine and Codeine—RE301
Bromodiphenhydramine, Diphenhydramine, Codeine, Ammonium Chloride, and Potassium Guaiacolsulfonate—RE301
Brompheniramine, Phenylephrine, Phenylpropanolamine, and Codeine—RE301
Brompheniramine, Phenylephrine, Phenylpropanolamine, Codeine, and Guaifenesin—RE301
Brompheniramine, Phenylephrine, Phenylpropanolamine, and Dextromethorphan—RE502
Brompheniramine, Phenylephrine, Phenylpropanolamine, and Guaifenesin—RE503
Brompheniramine, Phenylephrine, Phenylpropanolamine, Hydrocodone, and Guaifenesin—RE301
Brompheniramine, Phenylpropanolamine, and Codeine—RE301
Brompheniramine, Phenylpropanolamine, and Dextromethorphan—RE502
Brompheniramine, Pseudoephedrine, and Dextromethorphan—RE502
Carbinoxamine, Pseudoephedrine, and Dextromethorphan—RE502
Chlorpheniramine and Dextromethorphan—RE507
Chlorpheniramine, Dextromethorphan, and Acetaminophen—RE509
Chlorpheniramine, Ephedrine, and Guaifenesin—RE503
Chlorpheniramine, Ephedrine, Phenylephrine, and Carbetapentane—RE502
Chlorpheniramine, Ephedrine, Phenylephrine, Dextromethorphan, Ammonium Chloride, and Ipecac—RE504
Chlorpheniramine and Hydrocodone—RE301
Chlorpheniramine, Phenindamine, Phenylephrine, Dextromethorphan, Acetaminophen, Salicylamide, Caffeine, and Ascorbic Acid—RE506
Chlorpheniramine, Pheniramine, Pyrilamine, Phenylephrine, Hydrocodone, Salicylamide, Caffeine, and Ascorbic Acid—RE301
Chlorpheniramine, Phenylephrine, Codeine, and Ammonium Chloride—RE301
Chlorpheniramine, Phenylephrine, Codeine, and Potassium Iodide—RE301
Chlorpheniramine, Phenylephrine, and Dextromethorphan—RE502
Chlorpheniramine, Phenylephrine, Dextromethorphan, Acetaminophen, and Salicylamide—RE506
Chlorpheniramine, Phenylephrine, Dextromethorphan, and Guaifenesin—RE504
Chlorpheniramine, Phenylephrine, Dextromethorphan, Guaifenesin, and Ammonium Chloride—RE504
Chlorpheniramine, Phenylephrine, and Guaifenesin—RE503
Chlorpheniramine, Phenylephrine, and Hydrocodone—RE301
Chlorpheniramine, Phenylephrine, Hydrocodone, Acetaminophen, and Caffeine—RE301
Chlorpheniramine, Phenylephrine, Phenylpropanolamine, Carbetapentane, and Potassium Guaiacolsulfonate—RE504
Chlorpheniramine, Phenylephrine, Phenylpropanolamine, and Codeine—RE301
Chlorpheniramine, Phenylephrine, Phenylpropanolamine, and Dextromethorphan—RE502
Chlorpheniramine, Phenylephrine, Phenylpropanolamine, Dextromethorphan, Guaifenesin, and Acetaminophen—RE505
Chlorpheniramine, Phenylephrine, Phenylpropanolamine, and Dihydrocodeine—RE301
Chlorpheniramine, Phenylpropanolamine, and Caramiphen—RE502
Chlorpheniramine, Phenylpropanolamine, Codeine, Guaifenesin, and Acetaminophen—RE301
Chlorpheniramine, Phenylpropanolamine, and Dextromethorphan—RE502
Chlorpheniramine, Phenylpropanolamine, Dextromethorphan, and Acetaminophen—RE506
Chlorpheniramine, Phenylpropanolamine, Dextromethorphan, and Ammonium Chloride—RE504
Chlorpheniramine, Phenylpropanolamine, Dextromethorphan, and Aspirin—RE506
Chlorpheniramine, Phenylpropanolamine, and Guaifenesin—RE503
Chlorpheniramine, Phenylpropanolamine, Guaifenesin, Sodium Citrate, and Citric Acid—RE503
Chlorpheniramine, Phenyltoloxamine, Ephedrine, Codeine, and Guaiacol Carbonate—RE301
Chlorpheniramine, Pseudoephedrine, and Codeine—RE301
Chlorpheniramine, Pseudoephedrine, and Dextromethorphan—RE502
Chlorpheniramine, Pseudoephedrine, Dextromethorphan, and Acetaminophen—RE506
Chlorpheniramine, Pseudoephedrine, Dextromethorphan, Acetaminophen, and Caffeine—RE506
Chlorpheniramine, Pseudoephedrine, and Guaifenesin—RE503
Chlorpheniramine, Pseudoephedrine, and Hydrocodone—RE301
Codeine, Ammonium Chloride, and Guaifenesin—RE301
Codeine and Calcium Iodide—RE301
Codeine and Guaifenesin—RE301
Codeine and Iodinated Glycerol—RE301
Dexchlorpheniramine, Pseudoephedrine, and Guaifenesin—RE503
Dextromethorphan and Acetaminophen—RE302
Dextromethorphan and Guaifenesin—RE302
Dextromethorphan and Iodinated Glycerol—RE302
Diphenhydramine, Codeine, and Ammonium Chloride—RE301
Diphenhydramine, Dextromethorphan, and Ammonium Chloride—RE502
Diphenhydramine, Pseudoephedrine, Dextromethorphan, and Acetaminophen—RE506
Doxylamine, Phenylpropanolamine, Dextromethorphan, and Aspirin—RE506
Doxylamine, Pseudoephedrine, Dextromethorphan, and Acetaminophen—RE506
Ephedrine and Guaifenesin—RE516
Ephedrine and Potassium Iodide—RE516
Hydrocodone and Guaifenesin—RE301
Hydrocodone and Homatropine—RE301
Hydrocodone and Potassium Guaiacolsulfonate—RE301
Hydromorphone and Guaifenesin—RE301
Pheniramine, Codeine, and Guaifenesin—RE301

Pheniramine, Phenylephrine, Codeine, Sodium Citrate, Sodium Salicylate, and Caffeine—RE301

Pheniramine, Phenylephrine, and Dextromethorphan—RE502

Pheniramine, Phenylephrine, Phenylpropanolamine, Hydrocodone, and Guaifenesin—RE301

Pheniramine, Pyrilamine, Hydrocodone, Potassium Citrate, and Ascorbic Acid—RE301

Pheniramine, Pyrilamine, Phenylephrine, Phenylpropanolamine, and Hydrocodone—RE301

Pheniramine, Pyrilamine, Phenylpropanolamine, and Codeine—RE301

Pheniramine, Pyrilamine, Phenylpropanolamine, Codeine, Acetaminophen, and Caffeine—RE301

Pheniramine, Pyrilamine, Phenylpropanolamine, and Dextromethorphan—RE502

Pheniramine, Pyrilamine, Phenylpropanolamine, Dextromethorphan, and Ammonium Chloride—RE504

Pheniramine, Pyrilamine, Phenylpropanolamine, Dextromethorphan, and Guaifenesin—RE504

Pheniramine, Pyrilamine, Phenylpropanolamine, and Guaifenesin—RE503

Pheniramine, Pyrilamine, Phenylpropanolamine, and Hydrocodone—RE301

Pheniramine, Pyrilamine, Phenylpropanolamine, Hydrocodone, and Guaifenesin—RE301

Phenylephrine and Codeine—RE512

Phenylephrine, Dextromethorphan, and Guaifenesin—RE513

Phenylephrine and Guaifenesin—RE516

Phenylephrine, Guaifenesin, Acetaminophen, Salicylamide, and Caffeine—RE599

Phenylephrine and Hydrocodone—RE512

Phenylephrine, Hydrocodone, and Guaifenesin—RE301

Phenylephrine, Phenylpropanolamine, Carbetapentane, and Potassium Guaiacolsulfonate—RE513

Phenylephrine, Phenylpropanolamine, and Guaifenesin—RE516

Phenylpropanolamine and Caramiphen—RE512

Phenylpropanolamine, Codeine, and Guaifenesin—RE301

Phenylpropanolamine and Dextromethorphan—RE512

Phenylpropanolamine, Dextromethorphan, and Acetaminophen—RE515

Phenylpropanolamine, Dextromethorphan, and Guaifenesin—RE513

Phenylpropanolamine and Guaifenesin—RE516

Phenylpropanolamine and Hydrocodone—RE301

Phenylpropanolamine, Hydrocodone, Guaifenesin, and Salicylamide—RE514

Phenyltoloxamine and Hydrocodone—RE301

Promethazine and Codeine—RE301

Promethazine, Codeine, and Potassium Guaiacolsulfonate—RE301

Promethazine and Dextromethorphan—RE507

Promethazine, Phenylephrine, and Codeine—RE301

Promethazine, Phenylephrine, Codeine, and Potassium Guaiacolsulfonate—RE301

Promethazine, Phenylephrine, and Potassium Guaiacolsulfonate—RE503

Pseudoephedrine and Codeine—RE301

Pseudoephedrine, Codeine, and Guaifenesin—RE301

Pseudoephedrine and Dextromethorphan—RE512

Pseudoephedrine, Dextromethorphan, and Acetaminophen—RE515

Pseudoephedrine, Dextromethorphan, and Guaifenesin—RE513

Pseudoephedrine, Dextromethorphan, Guaifenesin, and Acetaminophen—RE514

Pseudoephedrine and Guaifenesin—RE516

Pseudoephedrine and Hydrocodone—RE301

Pseudoephedrine, Hydrocodone, and Guaiacolsulfonate—RE301

Pseudoephedrine, Hydrocodone, and Guaifenesin—RE301

Pyrilamine and Codeine—RE301

Pyrilamine, Phenylephrine, and Codeine—RE301

Pyrilamine, Phenylephrine, and Dextromethorphan—RE502

Pyrilamine, Phenylephrine, and Hydrocodone—RE301

Pyrilamine, Phenylephrine, Hydrocodone, and Ammonium Chloride—RE301

Pyrilamine, Phenylpropanolamine, Dextromethorphan, Guaifenesin, Potassium Citrate, and Citric Acid—RE504

Pyrilamine, Phenylpropanolamine, Dextromethorphan, and Sodium Salicylate—RE506

Pyrilamine, Pseudoephedrine, Dextromethorphan, and Acetaminophen—RE506

Triprolidine, Pseudoephedrine, and Codeine—RE301

Triprolidine, Pseudoephedrine, Codeine, and Guaifenesin—RE301

Triprolidine, Pseudoephedrine, and Dextromethorphan—RE502

Note: For dosing information and appropriate controlled substances schedules or classification, see *Table 3*.

For other combination products that are used in the symptomatic treatment of colds, but which do not contain either an antitussive or an expectorant, see *Antihistamines and Decongestants (Systemic)*; *Antihistamines, Decongestants, and Analgesics (Systemic)*; *Antihistamines, Decongestants, and Anticholinergics (Systemic)*; and *Decongestants and Analgesics (Systemic)*.

Note: For a listing of dosage forms and brand names by country availability, see *Dosage Forms* section(s). For a listing of brand names for the articles in this monograph, refer to the General Index.

## Category

Antihistaminic (H$_1$-receptor)-decongestant-antitussive—Brompheniramine, Phenylephrine, Phenylpropanolamine, and Codeine; Brompheniramine, Phenylephrine, Phenylpropanolamine, and Dextromethorphan; Brompheniramine, Phenylpropanolamine, and Codeine; Brompheniramine, Phenylpropanolamine, and Dextromethorphan; Brompheniramine, Pseudoephedrine, and Dextromethorphan; Carbinoxamine, Pseudoephedrine, and Dextromethorphan; Chlorpheniramine, Ephedrine, Phenylephrine, and Carbetapentane; Chlorpheniramine, Phenylephrine, and Dextromethorphan; Chlorpheniramine, Phenylephrine, and Hydrocodone; Chlorpheniramine, Phenylephrine, Phenylpropanolamine, and Codeine; Chlorpheniramine, Phenylephrine, Phenylpropanolamine, and Dextromethorphan; Chlorpheniramine, Phenylephrine, Phenylpropanolamine, and Dihydrocodeine; Chlorpheniramine, Phenylpropanolamine, and Caramiphen; Chlorpheniramine, Phenylpropanolamine, and Dextromethorphan; Chlorpheniramine, Pseudoephedrine, and Codeine; Chlorpheniramine, Pseudoephedrine, and Dextromethorphan; Chlorpheniramine, Pseudoephedrine, and Hydrocodone; Pheniramine, Phenylephrine, and Dextromethorphan; Pheniramine, Pyrilamine, Phenylephrine, Phenylpropanolamine, and Hydrocodone; Pheniramine, Pyrilamine, Phenylpropanolamine, and Codeine; Pheniramine, Pyrilamine, Phenylpropanolamine, and Dextromethorphan; Pheniramine, Pyrilamine, Phenylpropanolamine, and Hydrocodone; Promethazine, Phenylephrine, and Codeine; Pyrilamine, Phenylephrine, and Codeine; Pyrilamine, Phenylephrine, and Dextromethorphan; Pyrilamine, Phenylephrine, and Hydrocodone; Triprolidine, Pseudoephedrine, and Codeine; Triprolidine, Pseudoephedrine, and Dextromethorphan.

Antihistaminic (H$_1$-receptor)-decongestant-expectorant—Brompheniramine, Phenylephrine, Phenylpropanolamine, and Guaifenesin; Chlorpheniramine, Ephedrine, and Guaifenesin; Chlorpheniramine, Phenylephrine, and Guaifenesin; Chlorpheniramine, Phenylpropanolamine, and Guaifenesin; Chlorpheniramine, Phenylpropanolamine, Guaifenesin, Sodium Citrate, and Citric Acid; Chlorpheniramine, Pseudoephedrine, and Guaifenesin; Dexchlorpheniramine, Pseudoephedrine, and Guaifenesin; Pheniramine, Pyrilamine, Phenylpropanolamine, and Guaifenesin; Promethazine, Phenylephrine, and Potassium Guaiacolsulfonate.

Antihistaminic (H$_1$-receptor)-decongestant-antitussive-expectorant—Brompheniramine, Phenylephrine, Phenylpropanolamine, Codeine, and Guaifenesin; Brompheniramine, Phenylephrine, Phenylpropanolamine, Hydrocodone, and Guaifenesin; Chlorpheniramine, Ephedrine, Phenylephrine, Dextromethorphan, Ammonium Chloride, and Ipecac; Chlorpheniramine, Phenylephrine, Codeine, and Ammonium Chloride; Chlorpheniramine, Phenylephrine, Codeine, and Potassium Iodide; Chlorpheniramine, Phenylephrine, Dextromethorphan, and Guaifenesin; Chlorpheniramine, Phenylephrine, Dextromethorphan, Guaifenesin, and Ammonium Chloride; Chlorpheniramine, Phenylephrine, Phenylpropanolamine, Carbetapentane, and Potassium Guaiacolsulfonate; Chlorpheniramine, Phenylpropanolamine, Dextromethorphan, and Ammonium Chloride; Chlorpheniramine, Phenyltoloxamine, Ephedrine, Codeine, and Guaiacol Carbonate; Pheniramine, Pyrilamine, Phenylpropanolamine, Dextromethorphan, and Ammonium Chloride; Pheniramine, Pyrilamine, Phenylpropanolamine, Dextromethorphan, and Guaifenesin; Pheniramine, Pyrilamine, Phenylpropanolamine, Hydrocodone, and Guaifenesin; Pheniramine, Phenylephrine, Phenylpropanolamine, Hydrocodone, and Guaifenesin; Promethazine, Phenylephrine, Codeine, and Potassium Guaiacolsulfonate; Pyrilamine, Phenylephrine, Hydrocodone, and Ammonium Chloride; Pyrilamine, Phenylpropanolamine, Dextromethorphan, Guaifenesin, Potassium Citrate, and Citric Acid; Triprolidine, Pseudoephedrine, Codeine, and Guaifenesin.

Antihistaminic (H$_1$-receptor)-decongestant-antitussive-expectorant-analgesic—Chlorpheniramine, Phenylephrine, Phenylpropanolamine, Dextromethorphan, Guaifenesin, and Acetaminophen; Chlorpheniramine, Phenylpropanolamine, Codeine, Guaifenesin, and Acetaminophen; Pheniramine, Phenylephrine, Codeine, Sodium Citrate, Sodium Salicylate, and Caffeine.

Antihistaminic (H$_1$-receptor)-decongestant-antitussive-analgesic—Chlorpheniramine, Phenindamine, Phenylephrine, Dextromethorphan, Acetaminophen, Salicylamide, Caffeine, and Ascorbic Acid; Chlorpheniramine, Pheniramine, Pyrilamine, Phenylephrine, Hydrocodone, Salicylamide, Caffeine, and Ascorbic Acid; Chlorpheniramine, Phenylephrine, Dextromethorphan, Acetaminophen, and Salicylamide; Chlorpheniramine, Phenylephrine, Hydrocodone, Acetaminophen, and Caffeine; Chlorpheniramine, Phenylpropanolamine, Dextromethorphan, and Acetaminophen; Chlorpheniramine, Phenylpropanolamine, Dextromethorphan, and Aspirin; Chlorpheniramine, Pseudoephedrine, Dextromethorphan, and Acetaminophen; Chlorpheniramine, Pseudoephedrine, Dextromethorphan, Acetaminophen, and Caffeine; Diphenhydramine, Pseudoephedrine, Dextromethorphan, and Acetaminophen; Doxylamine, Phenylpropanolamine, Dextromethorphan, and Aspirin; Doxylamine, Pseudoephedrine, Dextromethorphan, and Acetaminophen; Pheniramine, Pyrilamine, Phenylpropanolamine, Codeine, Acetaminophen, and Caffeine; Pyrilamine, Phenylpropanolamine, Dextromethorphan, and Sodium Salicylate; Pyrilamine, Pseudoephedrine, Dextromethorphan, and Acetaminophen.

Antihistaminic (H₁-receptor)-antitussive—Bromodiphenhydramine and Codeine; Chlorpheniramine and Dextromethorphan; Chlorpheniramine and Hydrocodone; Phenyltoloxamine and Hydrocodone; Promethazine and Codeine; Promethazine and Dextromethorphan; Pyrilamine and Codeine.

Antihistaminic (H₁-receptor)-antitussive-expectorant—Bromodiphenhydramine, Diphenhydramine, Codeine, Ammonium Chloride, and Potassium Guaiacolsulfonate; Diphenhydramine, Codeine, and Ammonium Chloride; Diphenhydramine, Dextromethorphan, and Ammonium Chloride; Pheniramine, Codeine, and Guaifenesin; Pheniramine, Pyrilamine, Hydrocodone, Potassium Citrate, and Ascorbic Acid; Promethazine, Codeine, and Potassium Guaiacolsulfonate.

Antihistaminic (H₁-receptor)-antitussive-analgesic—Chlorpheniramine, Dextromethorphan, and Acetaminophen.

Antitussive-expectorant—Codeine, Ammonium Chloride, and Guaifenesin; Codeine and Calcium Iodide; Codeine and Guaifenesin; Codeine and Iodinated Glycerol; Dextromethorphan and Guaifenesin; Dextromethorphan and Iodinated Glycerol; Hydrocodone and Guaifenesin; Hydrocodone and Potassium Guaiacolsulfonate; Hydromorphone and Guaifenesin.

Antitussive-analgesic—Dextromethorphan and Acetaminophen.

Antitussive-anticholinergic—Hydrocodone and Homatropine.

Decongestant-antitussive—Phenylephrine and Codeine; Phenylephrine and Hydrocodone; Phenylpropanolamine and Caramiphen; Phenylpropanolamine and Dextromethorphan; Phenylpropanolamine and Hydrocodone; Pseudoephedrine and Codeine; Pseudoephedrine and Dextromethorphan; Pseudoephedrine and Hydrocodone.

Decongestant-antitussive-expectorant—Phenylephrine, Dextromethorphan, and Guaifenesin; Phenylephrine, Phenylpropanolamine, Carbetapentane, and Potassium Guaiacolsulfonate; Phenylephrine, Hydrocodone, and Guaifenesin; Phenylpropanolamine, Codeine, and Guaifenesin; Phenylpropanolamine, Dextromethorphan, and Guaifenesin; Pseudoephedrine, Codeine, and Guaifenesin; Pseudoephedrine, Dextromethorphan, and Guaifenesin; Pseudoephedrine, Hydrocodone, and Guaiacolsulfonate; Pseudoephedrine, Hydrocodone, and Guaifenesin.

Decongestant-antitussive-expectorant-analgesic—Phenylpropanolamine, Hydrocodone, Guaifenesin, and Salicylamide; Pseudoephedrine, Dextromethorphan, Guaifenesin, and Acetaminophen.

Decongestant-antitussive-analgesic—Phenylpropanolamine, Dextromethorphan, and Acetaminophen; Pseudoephedrine, Dextromethorphan, and Acetaminophen.

Decongestant-expectorant—Ephedrine and Guaifenesin; Ephedrine and Potassium Iodide; Phenylephrine and Guaifenesin; Phenylephrine, Phenylpropanolamine, and Guaifenesin; Phenylpropanolamine and Guaifenesin; Pseudoephedrine and Guaifenesin.

Decongestant-expectorant-analgesic—Phenylephrine, Guaifenesin, Acetaminophen, Salicylamide, and Caffeine.

## Indications

### Accepted

Cough (treatment)—Combination products containing antitussives and/or expectorants may be indicated for the symptomatic relief of cough due to colds and minor upper respiratory infections.

Cough and nasal congestion (treatment)—Combination products containing antitussives and/or expectorants, and nasal decongestants may be indicated for the symptomatic relief of cough and nasal congestion due to the common cold and other respiratory infections. Also, products containing antihistamines may provide relief of the cough, nasal congestion, rhinorrhea, and sneezing associated with allergy and the common cold. However, controlled clinical studies have not demonstrated that antihistamines are significantly more effective than placebo in relieving cold symptoms.

Cold symptoms (treatment)—Combination products containing antihistamines, antitussives or expectorants, nasal decongestants, and analgesics may be indicated for the temporary relief of coughs, nasal congestion, and associated aches, pains, and general discomfort due to colds, flu, or allergy. The antihistamine in these cold combinations may provide relief of nasal congestion, rhinorrhea, and sneezing. It may also serve as an adjunct because of its anticholinergic drying effects. However, in many cough/cold combinations, the dosage level of the antihistamine is below that required to obtain a significant effect. Also, controlled clinical studies have not demonstrated that antihistamines are significantly more effective than placebo in relieving cold symptoms.

### Unaccepted

Cough/cold combination products that contain both an antitussive and an expectorant usually do not offer any advantage over products that contain only one of these agents. In some cases, their combination may be detrimental in the treatment of coughs, since antitussives should be used only in the treatment of dry coughs and not for productive coughs.

Some products containing an anticholinergic have been used to help dry excessive nasal secretions associated with the common cold and allergic rhinitis; however, the efficacy of anticholinergics for this use in these combination products has not been established. In most products, the anticholinergic is included in doses below the therapeutic level in an attempt to prevent abuse by deliberate overdosage (e.g., in combinations containing a narcotic antitussive).

Combination products that contain an analgesic are generally not recommended for regular use for the treatment of cold symptoms during the common cold or acute allergic rhinitis since they may mask fever, which may indicate a secondary bacterial infection.

Ammonium chloride, calcium iodide, citric acid, guaiacol carbonate, iodinated glycerol, ipecac, potassium citrate, potassium guaiacolsulfonate, potassium iodide, and sodium citrate are included as expectorants in these combinations; however, the Food and Drug Administration (FDA) has not found them to be useful for this indication. Therefore, FDA has requested manufacturers to reformulate their products to replace these ingredients with guaifenesin.

## Pharmacology/Pharmacokinetics

Antihistamine-containing—See *Antihistamines (Systemic)*.

Antihistamine- and decongestant-containing—See *Antihistamines and Decongestants (Systemic)*.

Decongestant-containing—See:

*Ephedrine* in *Bronchodilators, Adrenergic (Systemic)*.

*Phenylpropanolamine (Systemic)*.

*Pseudoephedrine (Systemic)*.

Dextromethorphan-containing—See *Dextromethorphan (Systemic)*.

Opioid (narcotic) antitussive–containing—See *Opioid (Narcotic) Analgesics (Systemic)*.

Expectorant-containing—See:

*Guaifenesin (Systemic)*.

*Iodinated Glycerol (Systemic)*.

Analgesic-containing—See:

*Acetaminophen (Systemic)*.

*Acetaminophen and Salicylates (Systemic)*.

*Salicylates (Systemic)*.

Homatropine-containing—See *Anticholinergics/Antispasmodics (Systemic)*.

## Precautions to Consider

Antihistamine-containing—See *Antihistamines (Systemic)*.

Antihistamine- and decongestant-containing—See *Antihistamines and Decongestants (Systemic)*.

Decongestant-containing—See: *Ephedrine* in *Bronchodilators, Adrenergic (Systemic)*; *Phenylpropanolamine (Systemic)*; *Pseudoephedrine (Systemic)*.

Dextromethorphan-containing—See *Dextromethorphan (Systemic)*.

Opioid (narcotic) antitussive–containing—See *Opioid (Narcotic) Analgesics (Systemic)*.

Expectorant-containing—See: *Guaifenesin (Systemic)*; *Iodinated Glycerol (Systemic)*.

Analgesic-containing—See: *Acetaminophen (Systemic)*; *Acetaminophen and Salicylates (Systemic)*; *Salicylates (Systemic)*.

Homatropine-containing—See *Anticholinergics/Antispasmodics (Systemic)*.

## Laboratory value alterations

See *Table 1*, page 990.

## Side/Adverse Effects

Antihistamine-containing—See *Antihistamines (Systemic)*.
Antihistamine- and decongestant-containing—See *Antihistamines and Decongestants (Systemic)*.
Decongestant-containing—See:
  *Ephedrine in Bronchodilators, Adrenergic (Systemic)*.
  *Phenylpropanolamine (Systemic)*.
  *Pseudoephedrine (Systemic)*.
Dextromethorphan-containing—See *Dextromethorphan (Systemic)*.
Opioid (narcotic) antitussive–containing—See *Opioid (Narcotic) Analgesics (Systemic)*.
Expectorant-containing—See:
  *Guaifenesin (Systemic)*.

*Iodinated Glycerol (Systemic)*.
Analgesic-containing—See:
  *Acetaminophen (Systemic)*.
  *Acetaminophen and Salicylates (Systemic)*.
  *Salicylates (Systemic)*.
Homatropine-containing—See *Anticholinergics/Antispasmodics (Systemic)*.

## Patient Consultation

See *Table 2*, page 992.

## Oral Dosage Forms

See *Table 3*, page 995.

Revised: 09/03/92
Interim revision: 08/11/95

## Table 1. Laboratory value alterations

| The following have been selected on the basis of their potential clinical significance (possible effect in parentheses where appropriate)—not necessarily inclusive (» = major clinical significance): | Legend:<br>**I**=Antihistamine-containing<br>**II**=Decongestant-containing<br>**III**=Antitussive-containing<br>**IV**=Expectorant-containing<br>**V**=Analgesic-containing | | | | |
|---|---|---|---|---|---|
| | **I** | **II** | **III** | **IV** | **V** |
| **With diagnostic test results** | | | | | |
| Copper sulfate urine sugar tests<br>(false-positive test results may occur with chronic use of salicylates in doses equivalent in salicylate content to 2.4 grams or more of aspirin a day) | | | | | ✔ |
| Gastric emptying studies<br>(opioids delay gastric emptying, thereby invalidating test results) | | | ✔ | | |
| Gerhardt test for urine aceto-acetic acid<br>(aspirin or sodium salicylate may cause interference because reaction with ferric chloride produces a reddish color that persists after boiling) | | | | | ✔ |
| Glucose, blood<br>(acetaminophen may cause falsely decreased blood glucose values when measured by the glucose oxidase/peroxidase method but probably not when measured by the hexokinase/glucose-6-phosphate dehydrogenase [G6PD] method)<br>(values may be falsely increased when certain instruments are used in glucose analysis if high acetaminophen concentrations are present; consult manufacturer's instruction manual) | | | | | ✔ |
| Glucose enzymatic urine sugar tests<br>(false-negative test results may occur with chronic use of salicylates in doses equivalent in salicylate content to 2.4 grams or more of aspirin a day) | | | | | ✔ |
| Hepatobiliary imaging using technetium Tc 99m disofenin, technetium Tc 99m lidofenin, technetium Tc 99m mebrofenin<br>(delivery of these technetium Tc 99m–labeled radiopharmaceuticals to the small bowel may be prevented because opioids may cause constriction of the sphincter of Oddi and increased biliary tract pressure; these actions result in delayed visualization and thus resemble obstruction of the common bile duct) | | | ✔ | | |
| 5-hydroxyindoleacetic acid (5-HIAA), urine<br>(urinary determinations may be falsely increased when nitrosonaphthol reagent is used because of color interference by guaifenesin metabolites)<br>(acetaminophen may cause false-positive results in qualitative screening tests using nitrosonaphthol reagent; the quantitative test is unaffected)<br>(aspirin may alter results when fluorescent method is used) | | | | | ✔ |
| Pancreatic function determinations using bentiromide<br>(administration of acetaminophen prior to the bentiromide test will invalidate test results because acetaminophen is also metabolized to an arylamine and will thus increase the apparent quantity of para-aminobenzoic acid [PABA] recovered; it is recommended that acetaminophen be discontinued at least 3 days prior to administration of bentiromide) | | | | | ✔ |
| Skin tests using allergen extracts<br>(antihistamines contained in these combinations may inhibit the cutaneous histamine response thus producing false-negative results; it is recommended that antihistamine-containing medication be discontinued at least 72 hours before testing begins) | ✔ | | | | |

# Table 1. Laboratory value alterations *(continued)*

|  | Legend:<br>**I** = Antihistamine-containing<br>**II** = Decongestant-containing<br>**III** = Antitussive-containing<br>**IV** = Expectorant-containing<br>**V** = Analgesic-containing | | | | |
|---|---|---|---|---|---|
|  | **I** | **II** | **III** | **IV** | **V** |
| Thyroid function tests<br>(iodides may alter the results of these tests, and a high intake of inorganic iodides has also been shown to interfere with determination of protein bound iodine [PBI]; these effects have not been reported with iodinated glycerol in usual recommended doses, but they should be kept in mind for patients receiving prolonged therapy) |  |  |  | ✔ |  |
| Uric acid, serum<br>(acetaminophen may cause falsely increased values when the phosphotungstate uric acid test method is used) |  |  |  |  | ✔ |
| Vanillylmandelic acid (VMA), urine<br>(guaifenesin or its metabolites may cause color interference with urinary determinations)<br>(values may be falsely increased or decreased by salicylates, depending on the method used) |  |  |  |  | ✔ |

## With physiology/laboratory test values

| Amylase activity, plasma, and<br>Lipase activity, plasma<br>(may be increased because opioids can cause contractions of the sphincter of Oddi and increased biliary tract pressure; the diagnostic utility of determinations of these enzymes may be compromised for up to 24 hours after the medication has been given) |  |  | ✔ |  |  |
|---|---|---|---|---|---|
| Bilirubin, serum, and<br>Lactate dehydrogenase (LDH), serum, and<br>Prothrombin time and<br>Transaminase, serum<br>(prothrombin time and concentrations of bilirubin, LDH, and transaminase may be increased indicating acetaminophen-induced hepatotoxicity, especially in alcoholics, patients taking hepatic enzyme–inducing agents, or those with pre-existing hepatic disease, when single toxic doses [>8–10 grams] are taken or with prolonged use of lower doses [>3–5 grams a day]) |  |  |  |  | ✔ |
| Bleeding time<br>(may be prolonged by aspirin for 4 to 7 days because of suppressed platelet aggregation; as little as 40 mg of aspirin affects platelet function for at least 96 hours following administration; however, clinical bleeding problems have not been reported with small doses [150 mg or less]) |  |  |  |  | ✔ |
| Platelet aggregation<br>(may be transiently decreased by guaifenesin; however, effects on bleeding time are unlikely) |  |  |  | ✔ |  |
| Potassium, serum<br>(concentrations may be decreased by aspirin or sodium salicylate because of increased potassium excretion caused by direct effect on renal tubules) |  |  |  |  | ✔ |
| Protirelin-induced thyroid-stimulating hormone (TSH) release<br>(TSH response to protirelin may be decreased by aspirin in doses of 2 to 3.6 grams daily; peak TSH concentrations occur at the same time after administration but are reduced) |  |  |  |  | ✔ |
| Uric acid, serum<br>(concentrations may be increased with doses of aspirin or sodium salicylate producing plasma salicylate concentrations below 100 to 150 mcg per mL or decreased with doses producing plasma salicylate concentrations above 100 to 150 mcg per mL) |  |  |  |  | ✔ |

## Table 2. Patient Consultation

As an aid to patient consultation, refer to *Advice for the Patient, Cough/Cold Combinations (Systemic)*.

In providing consultation, consider emphasizing the following selected information (» = major clinical significance):

**Legend**
I = Antihistamine-containing
II = Decongestant-containing
III = Opioid (Narcotic) Antitussive–containing
IV = Non-opioid Antitussive–containing
V = Expectorant-containing
VI = Analgesic-containing[1]
VII = Anticholinergic containing

| | I | II | III | IV | V | VI | VII |
|---|---|---|---|---|---|---|---|
| **Before using this medication** | | | | | | | |
| » Conditions affecting use, especially: | | | | | | | |
| Sensitivity to any of the medications in the combination being taken | ✓ | ✓ | ✓ | ✓ | ✓ | ✓ | ✓ |
| Pregnancy— | | | | | | | |
| Concern for the fetus or newborn infant, especially with high-dose and/or long-term usage | ✓ | ✓ | ✓ | ✓ | ✓ | ✓ | ✓ |
| Psychiatric disorders more likely with use of phenylpropanolamine in postpartum women | | ✓ | | | | | |
| Physical dependence in the neonate possible with regular use | | | ✓ | | | | |
| Iodinated glycerol not recommended, because may induce fetal goiter | | | | | ✓ | | |
| Breast-feeding— | | | | | | | |
| Antihistamines may cause excitement or irritability in nursing infant | ✓ | | | | | | |
| High risk for infants from sympathomimetic amines | | ✓ | | | | | |
| Concern with high doses and chronic use because of high salicylate intake by infant | | | | | | ✓[2] | |
| Iodinated glycerol not recommended, because may induce skin rash and thyroid suppression in nursing infant | | | | | ✓ | | |
| Use in children— | | | | | | | |
| Increased susceptibility to anticholinergic effects | ✓ | | | | | | ✓ |
| Increased susceptibility to vasopressor effects of sympathomimetic amines | | ✓ | | | | | |
| Psychiatric disorders more likely with use of phenylpropanolamine in children up to 6 years of age | | ✓ | | | | | |
| Paradoxical reaction (hyperexcitability) | ✓ | | | ✓ | | | ✓ |
| Increased susceptibility to toxic effects of salicylates, especially if fever and dehydration present | | | | | | ✓[2] | |
| Possible association between aspirin usage and Reye's syndrome | | | | | | ✓[2] | |
| Increased susceptibility to goitrogenic effects of iodides | | | | | ✓[3] | | |
| Increased susceptibility to respiratory depressant effects of opioids in children up to 2 years of age | | | | ✓ | | | |
| Use in the elderly— | | | | | | | |
| Anticholinergic effects more likely to occur | ✓ | | | | | | ✓ |
| Increased sensitivity to CNS and vasopressor effects of sympathomimetic amines | | ✓ | | | | | |
| Increased susceptibility to toxic effects of salicylates | | | | | | ✓[2] | |
| Increased susceptibility to respiratory depressant effects of opioids | | | | ✓ | | | |
| Other medications, especially: | | | | | | | |
| Alcohol | ✓ | | ✓ | ✓[4] | | ✓ | |
| Alkalizers, urinary | ✓ | | | | | ✓[2] | |
| Anticholinergics | ✓ | | | | | | ✓ |
| Anticoagulants | | | | | | ✓[2] | |
| Antidepressants, tricyclic | ✓ | ✓ | | | | | |
| Antidiabetic agents, oral | | | | | | ✓[2] | |
| Antihypertensives | | ✓ | | | | | |
| Anti-inflammatory drugs, nonsteroidal | | | | | | ✓[2] | |
| Antithyroid agents | | | | | ✓[3] | | |
| Beta-adrenergic blocking agents, oral | | ✓ | | | | | |
| CNS depressants | ✓ | ✓ | ✓ | ✓[4] | | | |
| CNS stimulants | | ✓ | | | | | |
| Heparin | | | | | | ✓[2] | |
| Lithium | | | | | ✓[3] | | |
| Methotrexate | | | | | | ✓[2] | |
| Monoamine oxidase (MAO) inhibitors | ✓ | ✓ | | ✓[4] | | | ✓ |
| Platelet aggregation inhibitors | | | | | | ✓[2] | |
| Probenecid | | | | | | ✓[2] | |
| Rauwolfia alkaloids | | ✓ | | | | | |
| Sulfinpyrazone | | | | | | ✓[2] | |
| Thrombolytic agents | | | | | | ✓[2] | |
| Vancomycin | | | | | | ✓ | |
| Zidovudine | | | | | | ✓ | |

## Table 3. Oral Dosage Forms

Note: Content per capsule, tablet, or 5 mL, unless otherwise stated.

| Brand or generic name [availability] | Antihistamines | Decongestants | Antitussives — Opioid | Antitussives — Non-opioid | Expectorants | Analgesics | Other content information as per product label | Usual Adult and Adolescent Dose prn‡ | Usual Pediatric Dose prn | Packaging, Storage, and Auxiliary labeling§ |
|---|---|---|---|---|---|---|---|---|---|---|
| *Actagen-C Cough* Syrup (Schedule V) [U.S.] | Triprolidine HCl 1.25 mg | Pseudoephedrine HCl 30 mg | Codeine PO$_4$ 10 mg | | | | Alcohol 4.3% | 10 mL q 4–6 hr | 2–6 yrs: 2.5 mL, 6–12 yrs: 5 mL, q 4–6 hr | b, c, d, e, f |
| *Actifed w/Codeine Cough* Syrup (Schedule V) [U.S.] | Triprolidine HCl 1.25 mg | Pseudoephedrine HCl 30 mg | Codeine PO$_4$ 10 mg | | | | Alcohol 4.3% | 10 mL q 4–6 hr | 2–6 yrs: 2.5 mL, 6–12 yrs: 5 mL, q 4–6 hr | b, c, d, e, f |
| *Actifed DM* Oral Solution (OTC) [Canada] | Triprolidine HCl 1.25 mg | Pseudoephedrine HCl 30 mg | | Dextromethorphan HBr 15 mg | | | Alcohol 5% | 10 mL q 8 hr | 6 mos 2 yrs: 1.25 mL 2 6 yrs: 2.5 mL q 8 hr | b, c, e |
| Tablets (OTC) [Canada] | Triprolidine HCl 2.5 mg | Pseudoephedrine HCl 60 mg | | Dextromethorphan HBr 30 mg | | | Scored | 1 tab q 4–6 hr (max 4 tabs daily) | 6–11 yrs: ½ tab q 4–6 hr | b, e |
| *Adatuss D.C.* Expectorant Oral Solution (Schedule III) [U.S.] | | | Hydrocodone bitartrate 5 mg | | Guaifenesin 100 mg | | Alcohol 5% | 5 mL q 4–6 hr | 2–6 yrs: 1.25 mL, 6–12 yrs: 2.5 mL, q 4–6 hr | b, c, d, e, f |

*Specific formulations may vary among the different manufacturers, check product labeling.

†Efficacy as expectorant has not been established.

‡Geriatric patients may be more sensitive to effects of usual adult dose.

§For appropriate *Packaging and storage* and *Auxiliary labeling* information refer to designated letters as follows:

a—Store below 40 °C (104 °F), preferably between 15 and 30 °C (59 and 86 °F), in a tight container, unless otherwise specified by manufacturer.

a¹—Store below 30 °C (86 °F), unless otherwise specified by manufacturer. Avoid exposure to excessive heat.

a²—Store below 25 °C (77 °F), unless otherwise specified by manufacturer.

b—Store below 40 °C (104 °F), preferably between 15 and 30 °C (59 and 86 °F), in a well-closed container, unless otherwise specified by manufacturer.

c—Protect from freezing.

d—Protect from light.

e—Auxiliary labeling: • May cause drowsiness. • Avoid alcoholic beverages.

f—Auxiliary labeling: • May be habit forming.

g—Auxiliary labeling: • Shake well.

h—Dispense in dropper bottle.

i—Chew well before swallowing.

**Included in subtherapeutic amount to discourage deliberate overdosage.

Table 3. Oral Dosage Forms (continued)

Note: Content per capsule, tablet, or 5 mL, unless otherwise stated.

| Brand or generic name [availability] | Antihistamines | Decongestants | Antitussives | | Expectorants | Analgesics | Other content information as per product label | Usual Adult and Adolescent Dose prn‡ | Usual Pediatric Dose prn | Packaging, Storage, and Auxiliary labeling§ |
|---|---|---|---|---|---|---|---|---|---|---|
| | | | Opioid | Non-opioid | | | | | | |
| Alamine-C Liquid Oral Solution (Schedule V) [U.S.] | Chlorpheniramine maleate 2 mg | Pseudoephedrine HCl 30 mg | Codeine PO$_4$ 10 mg | | | | Alcohol 5% | 10 mL q 4 hr | 2–6 yrs: 1.25–2.5 mL, 6–12 yrs: 2.5–5 mL, q 6 hr | a, c, e, f |
| Alamine Expectorant Oral Solution (Schedule V) [U.S.] | | Pseudoephedrine HCl 30 mg | Codeine PO$_4$ 10 mg | | Guaifenesin 100 mg | | Alcohol 7.5% | 10 mL q 4–6 hr | 2–6 yrs: 1.25–2.5 mL, 6–12 yrs: 2.5–5 mL, q 6 hr | a, c, e, f |
| Alka-Seltzer Plus Cold and Cough Effervescent Tablets (OTC) [U.S.] | Chlorpheniramine maleate 2 mg | Phenylpropanolamine bitartrate 20 mg | | Dextromethorphan HBr 10 mg | | Aspirin 325 mg | Phenylalanine 11.2 mg Sodium 507 mg | 2 tabs dissolved in 120 mL water q 4 hr (max 8 tabs daily) | | a, e |
| Alka-Seltzer Plus Cold & Cough Medicine Liqui-Gels Capsules (OTC) [U.S.] | Chlorpheniramine maleate 2 mg | Pseudoephedrine HCl 30 mg | | Dextromethorphan HBr 10 mg | | Acetaminophen 250 mg | | 2 caps q 4 hr (max 8 caps daily) | 6–12 yrs: 1 cap q 4 hr (max 4 caps daily) | a, e |
| Alka-Seltzer Plus Flu & Body Aches Effervescent Tablets (OTC) [U.S.] | Chlorpheniramine maleate 2 mg | Phenylpropanolamine bitartrate 20 mg | | Dextromethorphan HBr 10 mg | | Acetaminophen 325 mg | Sodium 111 mg Phenylalanine 11.2 mg | 2 tabs dissolved in 120 mL hot water q 4 hr (max 8 tabs daily) | | a, e |
| Alka-Seltzer Plus Flu & Body Aches Medicine Liqui-Gels Capsules (OTC) [U.S.] | | Pseudoephedrine HCl 30 mg | | Dextromethorphan HBr 10 mg | | Acetaminophen 250 mg | | 2 caps q 4 hr (max 8 caps daily) | 6–12 yrs: 1 cap q 4 hr (max 4 caps daily) | a, e |
| Alka-Seltzer Plus Night Time Cold Effervescent Tablets (OTC) [U.S.] | Doxylamine succinate 6.25 mg | Phenylpropanolamine bitartrate 20 mg | | Dextromethorphan HBR 15 mg | | Aspirin 500 mg | Sodium 506 mg Phenylalanine 16.2 mg | 2 tabs dissolved in 120 mL water q HS | | a, e |
| Alka-Seltzer Plus Night-Time Cold Liqui-Gels Capsules (OTC) [U.S.] | Doxylamine succinate 6.25 mg | Pseudoephedrine HCl 30 mg | | Dextromethorphan HBr 10 mg | | Acetaminophen 250 mg | Alcohol free | 2 caps hs | Not recommended | b, e |

Table 3. Oral Dosage Forms (continued)

Note: Content per capsule, tablet, or 5 mL, unless otherwise stated.

| Brand or generic name [availability] | Antihistamines | Decongestants | Antitussives Opioid | Antitussives Non-opioid | Expectorants | Analgesics | Other content information as per product label | Usual Adult and Adolescent Dose prn‡ | Usual Pediatric Dose prn | Packaging, Storage, and Auxiliary labeling§ |
|---|---|---|---|---|---|---|---|---|---|---|
| *Allerfrin w/Codeine* Syrup (Schedule V) [U.S.] | Triprolidine HCl 1.25 mg | Pseudoephedrine HCl 30 mg | Codeine PO$_4$ 10 mg | | | | Alcohol 4.3% | 10 mL q 4-6 hr | 2-6 yrs: 2.5 mL; 6-12 yrs: 5 mL, q 4-6 hr | b, c, d, e, f |
| *All-Nite Cold Formula* Oral Solution (OTC) [U.S.] | Doxylamine succinate 1.25 mg | Pseudoephedrine HCl 10 mg | | Dextromethorphan HBr 5 mg | | Acetaminophen 167 mg | Alcohol 25% | 30 mL hs or 30 mL q 6 hr | | a, c, e |
| *Ambay Cough* Syrup (Schedule V) [U.S.] | Bromodiphenhydramine HCl 12.5 mg | | Codeine PO$_4$ 10 mg | | | | Alcohol 5% | 5-10 mL q 4-6 hr | 2-6 yrs: 1.25-2.5 mL; 6-12 yrs: 2.5-5 mL, q 6 hr | a, c, d, e, f, g |
| *Ambenyl Cough* Syrup (Schedule V) [U.S.] | Bromodiphenhydramine HCl 12.5 mg | | Codeine PO$_4$ 10 mg | | | | Alcohol 5% | 5-10 mL q 4-6 hr | 6-12 yrs: 2.5-5 mL q 6 hr | a, c, d, e, f |
| Syrup (N) [Canada] | Bromodiphenhydramine HCl 3.75 mg, Diphenhydramine HCl 8.75 mg | | Codeine PO$_4$ 10 mg | | Ammonium Cl† 80 mg, Potassium guaiacolsulfonate† 80 mg | | Alcohol 5% | 5-10 mL q 4-6 hr (max 60 mL daily) | 2-6 yrs: 1.25-2.5 mL; 6-12 yrs: 2.5-5 mL, q 6 hr | a, c, d, e, f |
| *Ambenyl-D Decongestant Cough Formula* Oral Solution (OTC) [U.S.] | | Pseudoephedrine HCl 30 mg | | Dextromethorphan HBr 15 mg | Guaifenesin 100 mg | | Alcohol 9.5% | 10 mL q 6 hr | 2-6 yrs: 2.5 mL; 6-12 yrs: 5 mL, q 6 hr | b, c |

*Specific formulations may vary among the different manufacturers, check product labeling.

†Efficacy as expectorant has not been established.

‡Geriatric patients may be more sensitive to effects of usual adult dose.

§For appropriate *Packaging and storage* and *Auxiliary labeling* information refer to designated letters as follows:

a—Store below 40 °C (104 °F), preferably between 15 and 30 °C (59 and 86 °F), in a tight container, unless otherwise specified by manufacturer.

a¹—Store below 30 °C (86 °F), unless otherwise specified by manufacturer. Avoid exposure to excessive heat.

a²—Store below 25 °C (77 °F), unless otherwise specified by manufacturer.

b—Store below 40 °C (104 °F), preferably between 15 and 30 °C (59 and 86 °F), in a well-closed container, unless otherwise specified by manufacturer.

c—Protect from freezing.

d—Protect from light.

e—Auxiliary labeling: • May cause drowsiness. • Avoid alcoholic beverages.

f—Auxiliary labeling: • May be habit forming.

g—Auxiliary labeling: • Shake well.

h—Dispense in dropper bottle.

i—Chew well before swallowing.

**Included in subtherapeutic amount to discourage deliberate overdosage.

Table 3. Oral Dosage Forms (*continued*)

Note: Content per capsule, tablet, or 5 mL, unless otherwise stated.

| Brand or generic name [availability] | Antihistamines | Decongestants | Antitussives — Opioid | Antitussives — Non-opioid | Expectorants | Analgesics | Other content information as per product label | Usual Adult and Adolescent Dose prn‡ | Usual Pediatric Dose prn | Packaging, Storage, and Auxiliary labeling§ |
|---|---|---|---|---|---|---|---|---|---|---|
| *Ambophen Expectorant* Oral Solution (Schedule V) [U.S.] | Bromodiphenhydramine HCl 3.75 mg, Diphenhydramine HCl 8.75 mg | | Codeine PO$_4$ 10 mg | | Ammonium Cl† 80 mg, Potassium guaiacol-sulfonate† 80 mg | | Alcohol 5% | 5–10 mL q 4–6 hr | 2–6 yrs: 1.25–2.5 mL, 6–12 yrs: 2.5–5 mL, q 6 hr | b, c, d, e, f |
| *Amgenal Cough* Syrup (Schedule V) [U.S.] | Bromodiphenhydramine HCl 12.5 mg | | Codeine PO$_4$ 10 mg | | | | | 5–10 mL q 4–6 hr | | b, c, e, f |
| *Ami-Tex LA* Extended-release Tablets (Rx) [U.S.] | | Phenylpropanolamine HCl 75 mg | | | Guaifenesin 400 mg | | Scored | 1 tab q 12 hr | 6–12 yrs: ½ tab q 12 hr | b |
| *Anamine HD* Syrup (Schedule III) [U.S.] | Chlorpheniramine maleate 2 mg | Phenylephrine HCl 5 mg | Hydrocodone bitartrate 1.6 mg | | | | | 10 mL q 6–8 hr | 5 mL q 6–8 hr | b, c, e, f |
| *Anaplex HD* Syrup (Schedule III) [U.S.] | Chlorpheniramine maleate 2 mg | Phenylephrine HCl 5 mg | Hydrocodone bitartrate 1.7 mg | | | | Alcohol free Sugar free | 10 mL q 6–8 hr | | b, c, e, f |
| *Anatuss* Syrup (Rx) [U.S.] | Chlorpheniramine maleate 2 mg | Phenylephrine HCl 5 mg, Phenylpropanolamine HCl 12.5 mg | | Dextromethorphan HBr 5 mg | Guaifenesin 25 mg | Acetaminophen 130 mg | Alcohol 12% | 10 mL q 4–6 hr | Not recommended | b, c, e |
| Tablets (Rx) [U.S.] | Chlorpheniramine maleate 2 mg | Phenylephrine HCl 5 mg, Phenylpropanolamine HCl 25 mg | | Dextromethorphan HBr 10 mg | Guaifenesin 50 mg | Acetaminophen 300 mg | | 2 tabs q 4 hr | 6–12 yrs: 1–2 tabs q 4 hr | b, e |
| *Anatuss with Codeine* Syrup (Schedule V) [U.S.] | Chlorpheniramine maleate 2 mg | Phenylpropanolamine HCl 12.5 mg | Codeine PO$_4$ 10 mg | | Guaifenesin 25 mg | Acetaminophen 130 mg | Alcohol 12% | 10 mL q 4–6 hr | Not recommended | b, c, d, e, f |
| Tablets (Schedule III) [U.S.] | Chlorpheniramine maleate 2 mg | Phenylpropanolamine HCl 25 mg | Codeine PO$_4$ 10 mg | | Guaifenesin 100 mg | Acetaminophen 300 mg | | 1–2 tabs q 4–6 hr | 6–12 yrs: ½–1 q 6 hr | b, e, f |
| *Anatuss DM* Syrup (OTC) [U.S.] | | Pseudoephedrine HCl 30 mg | | Dextromethorphan HBr 10 mg | Guaifenesin 100 mg | | | 10 mL q 6 hr | 6–12 yrs: 5 mL q 6 hr | b, c |
| Tablets (OTC) [U.S.] | | Pseudoephedrine HCl 60 mg | | Dextromethorphan HBr 20 mg | Guaifenesin 400 mg | | | 1 tab q 6 hr | | b |

Table 3. Oral Dosage Forms (continued)

Note: Content per capsule, tablet, or 5 mL, unless otherwise stated.

| Brand or generic name [availability] | Antihistamines | Decongestants | Antitussives Opioid | Antitussives Non-opioid | Expectorants | Analgesics | Other content information as per product label | Usual Adult and Adolescent Dose prn‡ | Usual Pediatric Dose prn | Packaging, Storage, and Auxiliary labeling§ |
|---|---|---|---|---|---|---|---|---|---|---|
| Anatuss LA Extended-release Tablets (Rx) [U.S.] | | Pseudoephedrine HCl 120 mg | | | Guaifenesin 400 mg | | Scored | 1 q 12 hr | | b |
| Anti-Tuss DM Expectorant Oral Solution (OTC) [U.S.] | | | | Dextromethorphan HBr 15 mg | Guaifenesin 100 mg | | Alcohol 1.4% | 10 mL q 6–8 hr | 2–6 yrs: 2.5 mL; 6–12 yrs: 5 mL, q 6–8 hr | b, c |
| Aprodine with Codeine Syrup (Schedule V) [U.S.] | Triprolidine HCl 1.25 mg | Pseudoephedrine HCl 30 mg | Codeine PO₄ 10 mg | | | | | 10 mL q 4–6 hr | | b, c, e, f |
| Atuss DM Syrup (Rx) [U.S.] | Chlorpheniramine maleate 2 mg | Phenylephrine HCl 5 mg | | Dextromethorphan HBr 15 mg | | | Alcohol free | 10 mL q 6 hr | 6–12 yrs: 5 mL q 6 hr | a, d, e |
| Atuss EX Syrup (Schedule III) [U.S.] | | | Hydrocodone bitartrate 5 mg | | Guaifenesin 100 mg | | Alcohol free Sugar free | 5 mL q 4 hr (max 30 mL daily) | 2–12 yrs: 2.5 mL q 4 hr | a, f |
| Atuss HD Oral Solution (Schedule III) [U.S.] | Chlorpheniramine maleate 2 mg | Phenylephrine HCl 5 mg | Hydrocodone bitartrate 2.5 mg | | | | Alcohol free | 10 mL q 4 hr (max 40 mL daily) | 6–12 yrs: 5 mL q 4 hr (max 20 mL daily) | a, d, f |

*Specific formulations may vary among the different manufacturers, check product labeling.

†Efficacy as expectorant may has not been established.

‡Geriatric patients may be more sensitive to effects of usual adult dose.

§For appropriate Packaging and storage and Auxiliary labeling information refer to designated letters as follows:

a—Store below 40 °C (104 °F), preferably between 15 and 30 °C (59 and 86 °F), in a tight container, unless otherwise specified by manufacturer.

a¹—Store below 30 °C (86 °F), unless otherwise specified by manufacturer. Avoid exposure to excessive heat.

a²—Store below 25 °C (77 °F), unless otherwise specified by manufacturer.

b—Store below 40 °C (104 °F), preferably between 15 and 30 °C (59 and 86 °F), in a well-closed container, unless otherwise specified by manufacturer.

c—Protect from freezing.

d—Protect from light.

e—Auxiliary labeling: • May cause drowsiness. • Avoid alcoholic beverages.

f—Auxiliary labeling: • May be habit forming.

g—Auxiliary labeling: • Shake well.

h—Dispense in dropper bottle.

i—Chew well before swallowing.

**Included in subtherapeutic amount to discourage deliberate overdosage.

## Table 3. Oral Dosage Forms (*continued*)

Note: Content per capsule, tablet, or 5 mL, unless otherwise stated.

| Brand or generic name [availability] | Antihistamines | Decongestants | Antitussives Opioid | Antitussives Non-opioid | Expectorants | Analgesics | Other content information as per product label | Usual Adult and Adolescent Dose prn‡ | Usual Pediatric Dose prn | Packaging, Storage, and Auxiliary labeling§ |
|---|---|---|---|---|---|---|---|---|---|---|
| *Bunex* Capsules (Rx) [U.S.] | | Phenylephrine HCl 5 mg, Phenylpropanolamine HCl 45 mg | | | Guaifenesin 200 mg | | | 1 cap q 6 hr | Pediatric strength not available | b |
| *Banex-LA* Extended-release Tablets (Rx) [U.S.] | | Phenylpropanolamine HCL 75 mg | | | Guaifenesin 400 mg | | | 1 tab q 12 hr | 6-12 yrs: ½ tab q 12 hr | b |
| *Banex Liquid* Oral Solution (Rx) [U.S.] | | Phenylephrine HCl 5 mg, Phenylpropanolamine HCl 20 mg | | | Guaifenesin 100 mg | | Alcohol 5% | 10 mL q 6 hr | 2-4 yrs: 2.5 mL, 4-6 yrs: 5 mL, 6-12 yrs: 7.5 mL, q 6 hr | b, c |
| *Bayaminic Expectorant* Oral Solution (OTC) [U.S.] | | Phenylpropanolamine HCl 12.5 mg | | | Guaifenesin 100 mg | | Alcohol 5% Dye free | 10 mL q 4 hr | 2-6 yrs: 2.5 mL, 6-12 yrs: 5 mL, q 4 hr | b, c |
| *Bayaminicol* Oral Solution (OTC) [U.S.] | Chlorpheniramine maleate 2 mg | Phenylpropanolamine HCl 12.5 mg | | Dextromethorphan HBr 10 mg | | | | 10 mL q 4 hr | 2-6 yrs: 2.5 mL, 6-12 yrs: 5 mL, q 4 hr | b, c, e |
| *Baycodan* Syrup (Schedule III) [U.S.] | | | Hydrocodone bitartrate 5 mg | | | | Homatropine MBr 1.5 mg** | 5 mL q 4-6 hr | <2 yrs: 1.25 mL, 2-12 yrs: 2.5 mL, q 4-6 hr | b, c, d, e, f |
| *Baycomine* Syrup (Schedule III) [U.S.] | | Phenylpropanolamine HCl 25 mg | Hydrocodone bitartrate 5 mg | | | | | 5 mL q 4-6 hr | 6-12 yrs: 2.5 mL q 4-6 hr | a, c, d, e, f |
| *Baycomine Pediatric* Syrup (Schedule III) [U.S.] | | Phenylpropanolamine HCl 12.5 mg | Hydrocodone bitartrate 2.5 mg | | | | | Intended for pediatric use. See *Baycomine* Syrup | 2-6 yrs: 2.5 mL, 6-12 yrs: 5 mL, q 4-6 hr | b, c, d, e, f |

Table 3. Oral Dosage Forms (*continued*)

Note: Content per capsule, tablet, or 5 mL, unless otherwise stated.

| Brand or generic name [availability] | Antihistamines | Decongestants | Antitussives Opioid | Antitussives Non-opioid | Expectorants | Analgesics | Other content information as per product label | Usual Adult and Adolescent Dose prn‡ | Usual Pediatric Dose prn | Packaging, Storage, and Auxiliary labeling§ |
|---|---|---|---|---|---|---|---|---|---|---|
| *BayCotussend Liquid* Oral Solution (Schedule III) [U.S.] | | Pseudoephedrine HCl 60 mg | Hydrocodone bitartrate 5 mg | | | | Alcohol 5% | 5 mL q 4–6 hr | 2–6 yrs: 1.25 mL, 6–12 yrs: 2.5 mL, q 4–6 hr | a, c, d, e, f |
| *Baydec DM Drops* Oral Solution (Rx) [U.S.] | Carbinoxamine maleate 10 mg (2 mg/mL) | Pseudoephedrine HCl 125 mg (25 mg/mL) | | Dextromethorphan HBr 20 mg (4 mg/mL) | | | Alcohol <0.6% | Intended for pediatric use | 1–3 mos: 0.25 mL, 3–6 mos: 0.50 mL, 6–9 mos: 0.75 mL, 9–18 mos: 1 mL, q 4–6 hr | a, c, e, h |
| *Bayhistine DH* Oral Solution (Schedule V) [U.S.] | Chlorpheniramine maleate 2 mg | Pseudoephedrine HCl 30 mg | Codeine PO₄ 10 mg | | | | Alcohol 5% | 10 mL q 4 hr | 2–6 yrs: 2.5 mL, 6–12 yrs: 5 mL, q 4 hr | b, c, d, e, f |
| *Bayhistine Expectorant* Oral Solution (Schedule V) [U.S.] | | Pseudoephedrine HCl 30 mg | Codeine PO₄ 10 mg | | Guaifenesin 100 mg | | Alcohol 7.5% | 10 mL q 4 hr | 2–6 yrs: 2.5 mL, 6–12 yrs: 5 mL, q 4 hr | a, c, d, e, f |

*Specific formulations may vary among the different manufacturers, check product labeling.

†Efficacy as expectorant has not been established.

‡Geriatric patients may be more sensitive to effects of usual adult dose.

§For appropriate *Packaging and storage* and *Auxiliary labeling* information refer to designated letters as follows:

a—Store below 40 °C (104 °F), preferably between 15 and 30 °C (59 and 86 °F), in a tight container, unless otherwise specified by manufacturer.

a¹—Store below 30 °C (86 °F), unless otherwise specified by manufacturer. Avoid exposure to excessive heat.

a²—Store below 25 °C (77 °F), unless otherwise specified by manufacturer.

b—Store below 40 °C (104 °F), preferably between 15 and 30 °C (59 and 86 °F), in a well-closed container, unless otherwise specified by manufacturer.

c—Protect from freezing.

d—Protect from light.

e—Auxiliary labeling: • May cause drowsiness. • Avoid alcoholic beverages.

f—Auxiliary labeling: • May be habit forming.

g—Auxiliary labeling: • Shake well.

h—Dispense in dropper bottle.

i—Chew well before swallowing.

**Included in subtherapeutic amount to discourage deliberate overdosage.

Table 3. Oral Dosage Forms (*continued*)

Note: Content per capsule, tablet, or 5 mL, unless otherwise stated.

| Brand or generic name [availability] | Antihistamines | Decongestants | Antitussives Opioid | Antitussives Non-opioid | Expectorants | Analgesics | Other content information as per product label | Usual Adult and Adolescent Dose prn‡ | Usual Pediatric Dose prn | Packaging, Storage, and Auxiliary labeling§ |
|---|---|---|---|---|---|---|---|---|---|---|
| *Baytussin AC* Oral Solution (Schedule V) [U.S.] | | | Codeine PO$_4$ 10 mg | | Guaifenesin 100 mg | | Alcohol 3.5% | 10 mL q 4 hr | 2–6 yrs: 2.5 mL, 6–12 yrs: 5 mL, q 4 hr | b, c, e, f |
| *Baytussin DM* Syrup (OTC) [U.S.] | | | | Dextromethorphan HBr 15 mg | Guaifenesin 100 mg | | Alcohol 1.4% | 10 mL q 6–8 hr | 2–6 yrs: 2.5 mL, 6–12 yrs: 5 mL, q 6–8 hr | a, c, d, e, g |
| *Benylin Codeine D-E* Syrup (N) [Canada] | | Pseudoephedrine HCl 30 mg | Codeine PO$_4$ 3.3 mg | | Guaifenesin 100 mg | | Alcohol 5%, Sodium 25 mg, Sugar free | 10 mL q 4 hr (max 40 mL daily) | | b, c, e, f |
| *Benylin DM-D* Syrup (OTC) [Canada] | | Pseudoephedrine HCl 30 mg | | Dextromethorphan HBr 15 mg | | | Alcohol free Sodium 23.2 mg, Sugar free | 10 mL q 6 hr | 2–5 yrs: 2.5 mL, 6–11 yrs: 5 mL, q 6 hr | a |
| *Benylin DM-D for Children* Syrup [Canada] | | Pseudoephedrine HCl 15 mg | | Dextromethorphan HBr 7.5 mg | | | Alcohol free Sodium 11.04 mg, Sugar free | | 2–5 yrs: 5 mL, 6–12 yrs: 10 mL, q 6 hr | a |
| *Benylin DM-D-E* Syrup (OTC) [Canada] | | Pseudoephedrine HCl 30 mg | | Dextromethorphan HBr 15 mg | Guaifenesin 100 mg | | Alcohol 5%, Sodium 25 mg, Sugar free | 10 mL q 6 hr | 2–5 yrs: 2.5 mL, 6–11 yrs: 5 mL, q 6 hr | a |
| *Benylin DM-D-E Extra Strength* Syrup (OTC) [Canada] | | Pseudoephedrine HCl 30 mg | | Dextromethorphan HBr 15 mg | Guaifenesin 200 mg | | Alcohol 5%, Sodium 25 mg, Sugar free | 10 mL q 6 hr | Not recommended | a |
| *Benylin DM-E* Syrup (OTC) [Canada] | | | | Dextromethorphan HBr 15 mg | Guaifenesin 100 mg | | Alcohol 5%, Sodium 25 mg, Sugar free | 10 mL q 6 hr | 2–5 yrs: 2.5 mL, 6–11 yrs: 5 mL, q 6 hr | a |

## Table 3. Oral Dosage Forms (continued)

Note: Content per capsule, tablet, or 5 mL, unless otherwise stated.

| Brand or generic name [availability] | Antihistamines | Decongestants | Antitussives Opioid | Antitussives Non-opioid | Expectorants | Analgesics | Other content information as per product label | Usual Adult and Adolescent Dose prn‡ | Usual Pediatric Dose prn | Packaging, Storage, and Auxiliary labeling§ |
|---|---|---|---|---|---|---|---|---|---|---|
| *Benylin Expectorant* Syrup (OTC) [U.S.] | | | | Dextromethorphan HBr 5 mg | Guaifenesin 100 mg | | Alcohol free Sugar free | 20 mL q 4 hr | 2–6 yrs: 5 mL, 6–12 yrs: 10 mL, q 4 hr | b, c |
| *Benylin Multi-Symptom* Oral Solution (OTC) [U.S.] | | Pseudoephedrine HCl 15 mg | | Dextromethorphan HBr 5 mg | Guaifenesin 100 mg | | Alcohol free Sugar free | 20 mL q 4 hr (max 4 doses daily) | 2–6 yrs: 5 mL, 6–12 yrs: 10 mL, q 4 hr (max 4 doses daily) | b |
| *Biphetane DC Cough* Syrup (Schedule V) [U.S.] | Brompheniramine maleate 2 mg | Phenylpropanolamine HCl 12.5 mg | Codeine PO₄ 10 mg | | | | Alcohol 0.95% | 10 mL q 4 hr | 2–6 yrs: 2.5 mL, 6–12 yrs: 5 mL, q 4 hr | a, c, d, e, f |
| *Bromanate DC Cough* Syrup (Schedule V) [U.S.] | Brompheniramine maleate 2 mg | Phenylpropanolamine HCl 12.5 mg | Codeine PO₄ 10 mg | | | | Alcohol 0.95% | 10 mL q 4 hr | 2–6 yrs: 2.5 mL, 6–12 yrs: 5 mL, q 4 hr | a, c, d, e, f |
| *Bromanyl* Syrup (Schedule V) [U.S.] | Bromodiphenhydramine HCl 12.5 mg | | Codeine PO₄ 10 mg | | | | | 5–10 mL q 4–6 hr | | b, c, e, f |

*Specific formulations may vary among the different manufacturers, check product labeling.
†Efficacy as expectorant has not been established.
‡Geriatric patients may be more sensitive to effects of usual adult dose.
§For appropriate *Packaging and storage* and *Auxiliary labeling* information refer to designated letters as follows:
  a—Store below 40 °C (104 °F), preferably between 15 and 30 °C (59 and 86 °F), in a tight container, unless otherwise specified by manufacturer.
  a¹—Store below 30 °C (86 °F), unless otherwise specified by manufacturer. Avoid exposure to excessive heat.
  a²—Store below 25 °C (77 °F), unless otherwise specified by manufacturer.
  b—Store below 40 °C (104 °F), preferably between 15 and 30 °C (59 and 86 °F), in a well-closed container, unless otherwise specified by manufacturer.
  c—Protect from freezing.
  d—Protect from light.
  e—Auxiliary labeling: • May cause drowsiness. • Avoid alcoholic beverages.
  f—Auxiliary labeling: • May be habit forming.
  g—Auxiliary labeling: • Shake well.
  h—Dispense in dropper bottle.
  i—Chew well before swallowing.
**Included in subtherapeutic amount to discourage deliberate overdosage.

Table 3. Oral Dosage Forms (*continued*)

Note: Content per capsule, tablet, or 5 mL, unless otherwise stated.

| Brand or generic name [availability] | Antihistamines | Decongestants | Antitussives Opioid | Antitussives Non-opioid | Expectorants | Analgesics | Other content information as per product label | Usual Adult and Adolescent Dose prn‡ | Usual Pediatric Dose prn | Packaging, Storage, and Auxiliary labeling§ |
|---|---|---|---|---|---|---|---|---|---|---|
| *Bromarest DX Cough* Syrup (Rx) [U.S.] | Brompheniramine maleate 2 mg | Pseudoephedrine HCl 30 mg | | Dextromethorphan HBr 10 mg | | | Alcohol 0.95% | 10 mL q 4 hr | | b, c, e |
| *Bromatane DX Cough* Syrup (Rx) [U.S.] | Brompheniramine maleate 2 mg | Pseudoephedrine HCl 30 mg | | Dextromethorphan HBr 10 mg | | | | 10 mL q 4 hr | | b, c, e |
| *Bromfed-DM* Syrup (Rx) [U.S.] | Brompheniramine maleate 2 mg | Pseudoephedrine HCl 30 mg | | Dextromethorphan HBr 10 mg | | | | 10 mL q 4 hr | 2–6 yrs: 2.5 mL, 6–12 yrs: 5 mL, q 4 hr | a, c, d, e |
| *Bromotuss with Codeine* Syrup (Schedule V) [U.S.] | Bromodiphenhydramine HCl 12.5 mg | | Codeine PO₄ 10 mg | | | | | 5–10 mL q 4–6 hr | | b, c, e, f |
| *Bromphen DC w/Codeine Cough* Syrup (Schedule V) [U.S.] | Brompheniramine maleate 2 mg | Phenylpropanolamine HCl 12.5 mg | Codeine PO₄ 10 mg | | | | Alcohol 0.95% | 10 mL q 4 hr | 2–6 yrs: 2.5 mL, 6–12 yrs: 5 mL, q 4 hr | a, c, d, e, f |
| *Bromphen DX Cough* Syrup (Rx) [U.S.] | Brompheniramine maleate 2 mg | Pseudoephedrine HCl 30 mg | | Dextromethorphan HBr 10 mg | | | Alcohol 0.95% | 10 mL q 4 hr | | b, c, e |
| *Broncholate* Syrup (Rx) [U.S.] | | Ephedrine HCl 6.25 mg | | | Guaifenesin 100 mg | | | 10–20 mL q 4 hr | 2–6 yrs: 2.5–5 mL, 6–12 yrs: 5–10 mL, q 4 hr | a, c, d |
| *Bronkotuss Expectorant* Oral Solution (Rx) [U.S.] | Chlorpheniramine maleate 4 mg | Ephedrine sulfate 8.2 mg | | | Guaifenesin 100 mg | | Alcohol 5% | 5 mL q 3–4 hr | 6–12 yrs: 2.5 mL q 3–4 hr | b, c, e |
| *Brontex* Oral Solution (Schedule V) [U.S.] | | | Codeine PO₄ 2.5 mg | | Guaifenesin 75 mg | | | 20 mL q 4 hr (max 120 mL daily) | 6–12 yrs: 10 mL q 4 hr | b, e, f |
| Tablets (Schedule III) [U.S.] | | | Codeine PO₄ 10 mg | | Guaifenesin 300 mg | | | 1 tab q 4 hr | Not recommended | b, e, f |

## Table 3. Oral Dosage Forms (*continued*)

Note: Content per capsule, tablet, or 5 mL, unless otherwise stated.

| Brand or generic name [availability] | Antihistamines | Decongestants | Antitussives Opioid | Antitussives Non-opioid | Expectorants | Analgesics | Other content information as per product label | Usual Adult and Adolescent Dose prn‡ | Usual Pediatric Dose prn | Packaging, Storage, and Auxiliary labeling§ |
|---|---|---|---|---|---|---|---|---|---|---|
| *Brotane DX Cough Syrup* (Rx) [U.S.] | Brompheniramine maleate 2 mg | Pseudoephedrine HCl 30 mg | | Dextromethorphan HBr 10 mg | | | Alcohol 0.95% | 10 mL q 4 hr | 2–6 yrs: 2.5 mL, 6–12 yrs: 5 mL, q 4 hr | a, c, d, e |
| *Calcidrine Syrup* (Schedule V) [U.S.] | | | Codeine 8.4 mg | | Calcium iodide† 152 mg | | Alcohol 6% | 5–10 mL q 4 hr | 2–6 yrs: 2.5 mL, 6–10 yrs: 2.5–5 mL, q 4 hr | a, c, d, e, f |
| *Caldomine-DH Forte Oral Solution* (N) [Canada] | Pheniramine maleate 12.5 mg Pyrilamine maleate 12.5 mg | Phenylpropanolamine HCl 25 mg | Hydrocodone bitartrate 5 mg | | | | | 5 mL q 4 hr | 2–6 yrs: 1.25 mL, 6–12 yrs: 2.5 mL, q 4–6 hr See also *Caldomine-DH Pediatric Oral Solution* | b, c, e, f |
| *Caldomine-DH Pediatric Oral Solution* (N) [Canada] | Pheniramine maleate 6.25 mg Pyrilamine maleate 6.25 mg | Phenylpropanolamine HCl 12.5 mg | Hydrocodone bitartrate 1.66 mg | | | | | Intended for pediatric use. See *Caldomine-DH Forte Oral Solution* | 1–6 yrs: 2.5 mL, 6–12 yrs: 5 mL, q 4 hr | b, c, e, f |

*Specific formulations may vary among the different manufacturers, check product labeling.

†Efficacy as expectorant has not been established.

‡Geriatric patients may be more sensitive to effects of usual adult dose.

§For appropriate *Packaging and storage* and *Auxiliary labeling* information refer to designated letters as follows:

a—Store below 40 °C (104 °F), preferably between 15 and 30 °C (59 and 86 °F), in a tight container, unless otherwise specified by manufacturer.

a¹—Store below 30 °C (86 °F), unless otherwise specified by manufacturer. Avoid exposure to excessive heat.

a²—Store below 25 °C (77 °F), unless otherwise specified by manufacturer.

b—Store below 40 °C (104 °F), preferably between 15 and 30 °C (59 and 86 °F), in a well-closed container, unless otherwise specified by manufacturer.

c—Protect from freezing.

d—Protect from light.

e—Auxiliary labeling: • May cause drowsiness. • Avoid alcoholic beverages. • Avoid deliberate overdosage.

f—Auxiliary labeling: • May be habit forming.

g—Auxiliary labeling: • Shake well.

h—Dispense in dropper bottle.

i—Chew well before swallowing.

**Included in subtherapeutic amount to discourage deliberate overdosage.

## Table 3. Oral Dosage Forms (continued)

Note: Content per capsule, tablet, or 5 mL, unless otherwise stated.

| Brand or generic name [availability] | Antihistamines | Decongestants | Antitussives Opioid | Antitussives Non-opioid | Expectorants | Analgesics | Other content information as per product label | Usual Adult and Adolescent Dose prn‡ | Usual Pediatric Dose prn | Packaging, Storage, and Auxiliary labeling§ |
|---|---|---|---|---|---|---|---|---|---|---|
| *Calmylin #2* Syrup (OTC) [Canada] | | Pseudoephedrine HCl 30 mg | | Dextromethorphan HBr 15 mg | | | Alcohol free Sugar free | 5–10 mL q 6–8 hr | 2–5 yrs: 2.5 mL, 6–12 yrs: 5 mL, q 6–8 hr | a, c, e |
| *Calmylin #3* Syrup (OTC) [Canada] | | Pseudoephedrine HCl 30 mg | | Dextromethorphan HBr 15 mg | Guaifenesin 100 mg | | Alcohol 5% Sugar free | 10 mL q 6–8 hr | 2–5 yrs: 2.5 mL, 6–12 yrs: 5 mL, q 6–8 hr | a, c, e |
| *Calmylin #4* Syrup (OTC) [Canada] | Diphenhydramine HCl 12.5 mg | | | Dextromethorphan HBr 15 mg | Ammonium chloride† 125 mg | | Alcohol 5% | 5–10 mL q 6–8 hr | 2–3 yrs: 1.25 mL, 4–12 yrs: 2.5–5 mL, q 6–8 hr | a, c, e |
| *Calmylin Codeine* Oral Solution (N) [Canada] | | Pseudoephedrine HCl 30 mg | Codeine PO$_4$ 3.33 mg | | Guaifenesin 100 mg | | Sugar free | 10 mL q 4 hr (max 40 mL daily) | Not recommended | a, e |
| *Calmylin Cough & Flu* Oral Solution (OTC) [Canada] | | Pseudoephedrine HCl 30 mg/ 15 mL | | Dextromethorphan HBr 15 mg/15 mL | Guaifenesin 100 mg/ 15 mL | Acetaminophen 325 mg/ 15 mL | Alcohol free Sugar free | 15–30 mL q 6–8 hr (max 120 mL daily) | Not recommended | a, c, e |
| *Calmylin DM-D-E Extra Strength* Syrup (OTC) [Canada] | | Pseudoephedrine HCl 30 mg | | Dextromethorphan HBr 15 mg | Guaifenesin 200 mg | | Alcohol 5% Sugar free | 10 mL q 6 hr | Not recommended | a, c |
| *Calmylin DM-E* Syrup (OTC) [Canada] | | | | Dextromethorphan HBr 15 mg | Guaifenesin 100 mg | | Alcohol 5% Sugar free | 10 mL q 6 hr | 2–5 yrs: 2.5 mL, 6–11 yrs: 5 mL, q 6 hr | a, c |
| *Calmylin Pediatric* Syrup (OTC) [Canada] | | Pseudoephedrine HCl 15 mg | | Dextromethorphan HBr 7.5 mg | | | Alcohol free Sugar free | | 1–2 yrs: 2.5 mL, 2–6 yrs: 5 mL, 6–12 yrs: 10 mL, q 6–8 hr | a, c |

## Table 3. Oral Dosage Forms (continued)

Note: Content per capsule, tablet, or 5 mL, unless otherwise stated.

| Brand or generic name [availability] | Antihistamines | Decongestants | Antitussives Opioid | Antitussives Non-opioid | Expectorants | Analgesics | Other content information as per product label | Usual Adult and Adolescent Dose prn‡ | Usual Pediatric Dose prn | Packaging, Storage, and Auxiliary labeling§ |
|---|---|---|---|---|---|---|---|---|---|---|
| *Calmylin with Codeine Syrup* (N) [Canada] | Diphenhydramine HCl 12.5 mg | | Codeine PO$_4$ 3.33 mg | | Ammonium chloride† 125 mg | | Alcohol 5% | 5–10 mL q 3-4 hr | 6-12 yrs: 2.5-5 mL q 4 hr | b, c, e, f |
| *Carbinoxamine Compound Syrup* (Rx) [U.S.] | Carbinoxamine maleate 4 mg | Pseudoephedrine HCl 60 mg | | Dextromethorphan HBr 15 mg | | | Alcohol <0.2% | 5 mL q 4-6 hr | 18 mos–6 y.s.: 2.5 mL, > 6 yrs: 5 mL, q 4-6 hr | a, c, d, e |
| *Carbinoxamine Compound-Drops Oral Solution* (Rx) [U.S.] | Carbinoxamine maleate 2 mg/mL | Pseudoephedrine HCl 25 mg/mL | | Dextromethorphan HBr 4 mg/mL | | | Alcohol <0.2% | | 1–18 mos: 0.25–1 mL qid | b, c, e |
| *Carbodec DM Drops Oral Solution* (Rx) [U.S.] | Carbinoxamine maleate 10 mg (2 mg/mL) | Pseudoephedrine HCl 125 mg (25 mg/mL) | | Dextromethorphan HBr 20 mg (4 mg/mL) | | | Alcohol <0.6% | Intended for pediatric use. See *Carbodec DM Syrup* | 1–3 mos: 0.25 mL, 3–6 mos: 0.50 mL, 6–9 mos: 0.75 mL, 9–18 mos: 1 mL, q 4-6 hr | a, c, e, h |
| *Syrup* (Rx) [U.S.] | Carbinoxamine maleate 4 mg | Pseudoephedrine HCl 60 mg | | Dextromethorphan HBr 15 mg | | | Alcohol <0.6% | 5 mL q 4-6 hr | 18 mos–6 yrs: 2.5 mL, >6 yrs: 5 mL, q 4-6 hr | a, c, d, e |

*Specific formulations may vary among the different manufacturers, check product labeling.

†Efficacy as expectorant has not been established.

‡Geriatric patients may be more sensitive to effects of usual adult dose.

§For appropriate *Packaging and storage* and *Auxiliary labeling* information refer to designated letters as follows:

a—Store below 40 °C (104 °F), preferably between 15 and 30 °C (59 and 86 °F), in a tight container, unless otherwise specified by manufacturer.

a¹—Store below 30 °C (86 °F), unless otherwise specified by manufacturer. Avoid exposure to excessive heat.

a²—Store below 25 °C (77 °F), unless otherwise specified by manufacturer.

b—Store below 40 °C (104 °F), preferably between 15 and 30 °C (59 and 86 °F), in a well-closed container, unless otherwise specified by manufacturer.

c—Protect from freezing.

d—Protect from light.

e—Auxiliary labeling: • May cause drowsiness. • Avoid alcoholic beverages.

f—Auxiliary labeling: • May be habit forming.

g—Auxiliary labeling: • Shake well.

h—Dispense in dropper bottle.

i—Chew well before swallowing.

**Included in subtherapeutic amount to discourage deliberate overdosage.

**Table 3. Oral Dosage Forms** *(continued)*

Note: Content per capsule, tablet, or 5 mL, unless otherwise stated.

| Brand or generic name [availability] | Antihistamines | Decongestants | Antitussives Opioid | Antitussives Non-opioid | Expectorants | Analgesics | Other content information as per product label | Usual Adult and Adolescent Dose prn‡ | Usual Pediatric Dose prn | Packaging, Storage, and Auxiliary labeling§ |
|---|---|---|---|---|---|---|---|---|---|---|
| Cardec DM Syrup (Rx) [U.S.] | Carbinoxamine maleate 4 mg | Pseudoephedrine HCl 60 mg | | Dextromethorphan HBr 15 mg | | | | 5 mL q 6 hr | b, c, e | |
| Cardec DM Drops Oral Solution (Rx) [U.S.] | Carbinoxamine maleate 2 mg/mL | Pseudoephedrine HCl 25 mg/mL | | Dextromethorphan HBr 4 mg/mL | | | | Intended for pediatric use | 1–18 mos: 0.25–1 mL q 6 hr | b, c, e |
| Cardec DM Pediatric Syrup (Rx) [U.S.] | Carbinoxamine maleate 4 mg | Pseudoephedrine HCl 60 mg | | Dextromethorphan HBr 15 mg | | | Alcohol <0.6% | Intended for pediatric use | 2.5–5 mL q 6 hr | b, c |
| Cerose-DM Oral Solution (OTC) [U.S.] | Chlorpheniramine maleate 4 mg | Phenylephrine HCl 10 mg | | Dextromethorphan HBr 15 mg | | | Alcohol 2.4% Sugar free | 5 mL q 4 hr | 6–12 yrs: 2.5 mL q 4 hr | a, c, e |
| Cheracol Syrup USP (Schedule V) [U.S.] | | | Codeine PO₄ 10 mg | | Guaifenesin 100 mg | | Alcohol 4.75% | 5–10 mL q 4 hr | 2–6 yrs: 1.25–2.5 mL, 6–12 yrs: 2.5–5 mL, q 4–6 hr | a, d, e, f |
| Syrup (N) [Canada] | | | Codeine PO₄ 10 mg | | Ammonium Cl† 91 mg, Guaifenesin 100 mg | | Alcohol 3% | 5–15 mL q 4 hr (max 4 doses daily) | 1–6 yrs: 2.5 mL, 6–12 yrs: 2.5–5 mL, q 4 hr (max 4 doses daily) | b, c, e, f |
| Cheracol D Cough Syrup (OTC) [U.S.] | | | | Dextromethorphan HBr 10 mg | Guaifenesin 100 mg | | Alcohol 4.75% | 10 mL q 4 hr | 2–6 yrs: 2.5 mL, 6–12 yrs: 5 mL, q 4 hr | b, c |
| Cheracol Plus Oral Solution (OTC) [U.S.] | Chlorpheniramine maleate 4 mg | Phenylpropanolamine HCl 25 mg | | Dextromethorphan HBr 20 mg | | | Alcohol 8% | 15 mL q 4 hr | 6–12 yrs: 7.5 mL q 4 hr | b, c, e |
| Children's Formula Cough Syrup (OTC) [U.S.] | | | | Dextromethorphan HBr 5 mg | Guaifenesin 50 mg | | Alcohol free | | 2–<12 yrs: 5–10 mL q 6 hr | b, c |
| Children's Tylenol Cold Multi Symptom Plus Cough Oral Solution (OTC) [U.S.] | Chlorpheniramine maleate 1 mg | Pseudoephedrine HCl 15 mg | | Dextromethorphan HBr 5 mg | | Acetaminophen 160 mg | Alcohol free | | 6–11 yrs: 10 mL q 4–6 hr | b, c, e |

## Table 3. Oral Dosage Forms (continued)

Note: Content per capsule, tablet, or 5 mL, unless otherwise stated.

| Brand or generic name [availability] | Antihistamines | Decongestants | Antitussives — Opioid | Antitussives — Non-opioid | Expectorants | Analgesics | Other content information as per product label | Usual Adult and Adolescent Dose prn‡ | Usual Pediatric Dose prn | Packaging, Storage, and Auxiliary labeling§ |
|---|---|---|---|---|---|---|---|---|---|---|
| *Children's Vicks NyQuil Cold/Cough Relief* Oral Solution (OTC) [U.S.] | Chlorpheniramine maleate 2 mg/15 mL | Pseudoephedrine HCl 30 mg/15 mL | | Dextromethorphan HBr 15 mg/15 mL | | | Alcohol free | 30 mL q 4 hr (max 4 doses daily) | 6–11 yrs: 15 mL q 4 hr | b, c, e |
| *Chlorgest-HD* Oral Solution (Schedule III) [U.S.] | Chlorpheniramine maleate 2 mg | Phenylephrine HCl 5 mg | Hydrocodone bitartrate 1.67 mg | | | | Alcohol free Sugar free | 10 mL q 6–8 hr | | b, c, e, f |
| *Citra Forte* Capsules (Schedule III) [U.S.] | Chlorpheniramine maleate 1 mg, Pheniramine maleate 6.25 mg, Pyrilamine maleate 8.33 mg | Phenylephrine HCl 10 mg | Hydrocodone bitartrate 5 mg | | | Salicylamide 227 mg | Ascorbic acid 50 mg, Caffeine 30 mg | 1–2 caps q 3–4 hr | Pediatric strength not available | b, e, f |
| Syrup (Schedule III) [U.S.] | Pheniramine maleate 2.5 mg, Pyrilamine maleate 3.33 mg | | Hydrocodone bitartrate 5 mg | | Potassium citrate† 150 mg | | Alcohol 2%, Ascorbic acid 30 mg | 5–10 mL q 3–4 hr | 6–12 yrs: 2.5–5 mL q 3–4 hr | b, c, d, e, f |
| *CoActifed* Syrup (N) [Canada] | Triprolidine HCl 2 mg | Pseudoephedrine HCl 30 mg | Codeine PO$_4$ 10 mg | | | | Alcohol free | 10 mL q 4–6 hr | <6 yrs: 2.5 mL, 6–12 yrs: 5 mL, q 4–6 hr | b, c, d, e, f |

*Specific formulations may vary among the different manufacturers, check product labeling.

†Efficacy as expectorant has not been established.

‡Geriatric patients may be more sensitive to effects of usual adult dose.

§For appropriate *Packaging and storage* and *Auxiliary labeling* information refer to designated letters as follows:

  a—Store below 40 °C (104 °F), preferably between 15 and 30 °C (59 and 86 °F), in a tight container, unless otherwise specified by manufacturer.

  a¹—Store below 30 °C (86 °F), unless otherwise specified by manufacturer. Avoid exposure to excessive heat.

  a²—Store below 25 °C (77 °F), unless otherwise specified by manufacturer.

  b—Store below 40 °C (104 °F), preferably between 15 and 30 °C (59 and 86 °F), in a well-closed container, unless otherwise specified by manufacturer.

  c—Protect from freezing.      f—Auxiliary labeling: • May be habit forming.      h—Dispense in dropper bottle.

  d—Protect from light.      g—Auxiliary labeling: • Shake well.      i—Chew well before swallowing.

  e—Auxiliary labeling: • May cause drowsiness. • Avoid alcoholic beverages.

**Included in subtherapeutic amount to discourage deliberate overdosage.

## Table 3. Oral Dosage Forms (continued)

Note: Content per capsule, tablet, or 5 mL, unless otherwise stated.

| Brand or generic name [availability] | Antihistamines | Decongestants | Antitussives Opioid | Antitussives Non-opioid | Expectorants | Analgesics | Other content information as per product label | Usual Adult and Adolescent Dose prn‡ | Usual Pediatric Dose prn | Packaging, Storage, and Auxiliary labeling§ |
|---|---|---|---|---|---|---|---|---|---|---|
| CoActifed (continued) Tablets (N) [Canada] | Triprolidine HCl 4 mg | Pseudoephedrine HCl 60 mg | Codeine PO$_4$ 20 mg | | | | | 1 tab q 4–6 hr | <6 yrs: See CoActifed Syrup; 6–12 yrs: ½ tab q 4–6 hr | b, d, e, f |
| CoActifed Expectorant Oral Solution (N) [Canada] | Triprolidine HCl 2 mg | Pseudoephedrine HCl 30 mg | Codeine PO$_4$ 10 mg | | Guaifenesin 100 mg | | Alcohol free | 10 mL q 4–6 hr | <6 yrs: 2.5 mL, 6–12 yrs: 5 mL, q 4–6 hr | b, c, d, e, f |
| Co-Apap Tablets (OTC) [U.S.] | Chlorpheniramine maleate 2 mg | Pseudoephedrine HCl 30 mg | | Dextromethorphan HBr 15 mg | | Acetaminophen 325 mg | | 2 tabs q 6 hr | 6–12 yrs: 1 tab q 6 hr | b, e |
| Codamine Syrup (Schedule III) [U.S.] | | Phenylpropanolamine HCl 25 mg | Hydrocodone bitartrate 5 mg | | | | | 5 mL q 4–6 hr | 6–12 yrs: 2.5 mL q 4–6 hr | b, c, d, e, f |
| Codamine Pediatric Syrup (Schedule III) [U.S.] | | Phenylpropanolamine HCl 12.5 mg | Hydrocodone bitartrate 2.5 mg | | | | | Intended for pediatric use. See Codamine Syrup | 2–6 yrs: 2.5 mL, 6–12 yrs: 5 mL, q 4–6 hr | b, c, d, e, f |
| Codan Syrup (Schedule III) [U.S.] | | | Hydrocodone bitartrate 5 mg | | | | Homatropine MBr 1.5 mg** | 5 mL q 4–6 hr | <2 yrs: 1.25 mL, 2–12 yrs: 2.5 mL, q 4–6 hr | b, c, d, e, f |
| Codegest Expectorant Oral Solution (Schedule V) [U.S.] | | Phenylpropanolamine HCl 12.5 mg | Codeine PO$_4$ 10 mg | | Guaifenesin 100 mg | | Alcohol free Sugar free Dye free | 10 mL q 4–6 hr | | b, c, f |
| Codehist DH Elixir (Schedule V) [U.S.] | Chlorpheniramine maleate 2 mg | Pseudoephedrine HCl 30 mg | Codeine PO$_4$ 10 mg | | | | Alcohol 5.7% | 10 mL q 4 hr | 2–6 yrs: 1.25–2.5 mL, 6–12 yrs: 2.5–5 mL, q 4 hr | a, c, d, e, f |

## Table 3. Oral Dosage Forms (*continued*)

Note: Content per capsule, tablet, or 5 mL, unless otherwise stated.

| Brand or generic name [availability] | Antihistamines | Decongestants | Antitussives — Opioid | Antitussives — Non-opioid | Expectorants | Analgesics | Other content information as per product label | Usual Adult and Adolescent Dose prn‡ | Usual Pediatric Dose prn | Packaging, Storage, and Auxiliary labeling§ |
|---|---|---|---|---|---|---|---|---|---|---|
| *Codiclear DH* Syrup (Schedule III) [U.S.] | | | Hydrocodone bitartrate 5 mg | | Guaifenesin 100 mg | | Alcohol free Sugar free Dye free | 5–7.5 mL q 4–6 hr | 3–6 yrs: 1.25–2.5 mL, 6–12 yrs: 2.5–5 mL, q 4–6 hr | b, c, d, e, f |
| *Codimal DH* Syrup (Schedule III) [U.S.] | Pyrilamine maleate 8.33 mg | Phenylephrine HCl 5 mg | Hydrocodone bitartrate 1.66 mg | | | | Alcohol free | 5–10 mL q 4 hr | 6 mos–2 yrs: 1.25 mL q 6 hr 2–6 yrs: 2.5 mL, 6–12 yrs: 5 mL, q 4 hr | b, c, d, e, f |
| *Codimal DM* Syrup (OTC) [U.S.] | Pyrilamine maleate 8.33 mg | Phenylephrine HCl 5 mg | | Dextromethorphan HBr 10 mg | | | Alcohol free Sugar free Dye free | 5–10 mL q 4 hr | 6–12 yrs: 5 mL q 4 hr | b, c, e |
| *Codimal PH* Syrup (Schedule V) [U.S.] | Pyrilamine maleate 8.33 mg | Phenylephrine HCl 5 mg | Codeine PO$_4$ 10 mg | | | | | 5–10 mL q 4 hr | 6–12 yrs: 5 mL q 4 hr | b, c, e, f |
| *Codistan No. 1* Syrup (OTC) [U.S.] | | | | Dextromethorphan HBr 15 mg | Guaifenesin 100 mg | | Alcohol 1.4% | 10 mL q 6–8 hr | 2–6 yrs: 2.5 mL, 6–12 yrs: 5 mL, q 6–8 hr | b, c |
| *Comtrex Cough Formula* Oral Solution (OTC) [U.S.] | | Pseudoephedrine HCl 15 mg | | Dextromethorphan HBr 7.5 mg | Guaifenesin 50 mg | Acetaminophen 125 mg | Alcohol 20% | 20 mL q 4 hr | | b, c |

*Specific formulations may vary among the different manufacturers, check product labeling.

†Efficacy as expectorant has not been established.

‡Geriatric patients may be more sensitive to effects of usual adult dose.

§For appropriate *Packaging and storage* and *Auxiliary labeling* information refer to designated letters as follows:

a—Store below 40 °C (104 °F), preferably between 15 and 30 °C (59 and 86 °F), in a tight container, unless otherwise specified by manufacturer.

a¹—Store below 30 °C (86 °F), unless otherwise specified by manufacturer. Avoid exposure to excessive heat.

a²—Store below 25 °C (77 °F), unless otherwise specified by manufacturer.

b—Store below 40 °C (104 °F), preferably between 15 and 30 °C (59 and 86 °F), in a well-closed container, unless otherwise specified by manufacturer.

c—Protect from freezing.

d—Protect from light.

e—Auxiliary labeling: • May cause drowsiness. • Avoid alcoholic beverages.

f—Auxiliary labeling: • May be habit forming.

g—Auxiliary labeling: • Shake well.

h—Dispense in dropper bottle.

i—Chew well before swallowing.

**Included in subtherapeutic amount to discourage deliberate overdosage.

## Table 3. Oral Dosage Forms (continued)

Note: Content per capsule, tablet, or 5 mL, unless otherwise stated.

| Brand or generic name [availability] | Antihistamines | Decongestants | Antitussives — Opioid | Antitussives — Non-opioid | Expectorants | Analgesics | Other content information as per product label | Usual Adult and Adolescent Dose prn‡ | Usual Pediatric Dose prn | Packaging, Storage, and Auxiliary labeling§ |
|---|---|---|---|---|---|---|---|---|---|---|
| *Comtrex Daytime Caplets* Tablets (OTC) [U.S.] | | Pseudoephedrine HCl 30 mg | | Dextromethorphan HBr 10 mg | | Acetaminophen 325 mg | | 2 tabs q 4 hr | Intended for adult use | b |
| *Comtrex Daytime Maximum Strength Cold, Cough and Flu Relief* Tablets (OTC) [U.S.] | | Pseudoephedrine HCl 30 mg | | Dextromethorphan HBr 15 mg | | Acetaminophen 500 mg | Available in a dual package that also contains *Comtrex Nighttime Maximum Strength Cold, Cough and Flu Relief* | 2 tabs q 6 hr (max 4 tabs daily) | | b |
| *Comtrex Daytime Maximum Strength Cold and Flu Relief* Tablets (OTC) [U.S.] | | Pseudoephedrine HCl 30 mg | | Dextromethorphan HBr 15 mg | | Acetaminophen 500 mg | Available in a dual package that also contains *Comtrex Nighttime Maximum Strength Cold and Flu Relief* | 2 tabs q 6 hr (max 4 tabs daily) | | b |
| *Comtrex Hot Flu Relief for Oral Solution* (OTC) [U.S.] | Chlorpheniramine maleate 4 mg/ packet | Pseudoephedrine HCl 60 mg/ packet | | Dextromethorphan HBr 20 mg/packet | | Acetaminophen 500 mg/ packet | | 1 packet dissolved in 6-oz cup of hot water q 4 hr | | b, e |
| *Comtrex Maximum Strength Liqui-Gels* Capsules (OTC) [U.S.] | Chlorpheniramine maleate 2 mg | Phenylpropanolamine HCl 12.5 mg | | Dextromethorphan HBr 15 mg | | Acetaminophen 500 mg | | 2 caps q 6 hr | | b, c, e |
| *Comtrex Multi-Symptom Cold Reliever* Capsules (OTC) [U.S.] | Chlorpheniramine maleate 1 mg | Phenylpropanolamine HCl 12.5 mg | | Dextromethorphan HBr 10 mg | | Acetaminophen 325 mg | | 2 caps q 4 hr | 6-12 yrs: 1 cap q 4 hr | b, e |
| Oral Solution (OTC) [U.S.] | Chlorpheniramine maleate 0.33 mg | Phenylpropanolamine HCl 4.2 mg | | Dextromethorphan HBr 3.3 mg | | Acetaminophen 108.3 mg | Alcohol 20% | 30 mL q 4 hr | 6-12 yrs: 15 mL q 4 hr | b, c, e |

## Table 3. Oral Dosage Forms (continued)

Note: Content per capsule, tablet, or 5 mL, unless otherwise stated.

| Brand or generic name [availability] | Antihistamines | Decongestants | Antitussives Opioid | Antitussives Non-opioid | Expectorants | Analgesics | Other content information as per product label | Usual Adult and Adolescent Dose prn‡ | Usual Pediatric Dose prn | Packaging, Storage, and Auxiliary labeling§ |
|---|---|---|---|---|---|---|---|---|---|---|
| *Comtrex Multi-Symptom Cold Reliever* (continued) Tablets (OTC) [U.S.] | Chlorpheniramine maleate 1 mg | Phenylpropanolamine HCl 12.5 mg | | Dextromethorphan HBr 10 mg | | Acetaminophen 325 mg | | 2 tabs q 4 hr | 6–12 yrs: 1 tab q 4 hr | b, e |
| *Comtrex Multi-Symptom Non-Drowsy Caplets* (OTC) [U.S.] | | Pseudoephedrine HCl 30 mg | | Dextromethorphan HBr 10 mg | | Acetaminophen 325 mg | | 2 tabs q 4 hr | Intended for adult use | b |
| *Comtrex Nighttime Tablets* (OTC) [U.S.] | Chlorpheniramine maleate 2 mg | Pseudoephedrine HCl 30 mg | | Dextromethorphan HBr 10 mg | | Acetaminophen 325 mg | | 2 tabs hs | Intended for adult use | b, e |
| *Comtrex Nighttime Maximum Strength Cold, Cough and Flu Relief Oral Solution* (OTC) [U.S.] | Chlorpheniramine maleate 4 mg/ 30 mL | Pseudoephedrine HCl 60 mg/ 30 mL | | Dextromethorphan HBr 30 mg/ 30 mL | | Acetaminophen 1000 mg/ 30 mL | Alcohol 10% Available in a dual package that also contains *Comtrex Daytime Maximum Strength Cold, Cough and Flu Relief* | 30 mL hs | | b, c, e |

*Specific formulations may vary among the different manufacturers; check product labeling.

†Efficacy as expectorant has not been established.

‡Geriatric patients may be more sensitive to effects of usual adult dose.

§For appropriate *Packaging and storage* and *Auxiliary labeling* information refer to designated letters as follows:

a—Store below 40 °C (104 °F), preferably between 15 and 30 °C (59 and 86 °F), in a tight container, unless otherwise specified by manufacturer.
a¹—Store below 30 °C (86 °F), unless otherwise specified by manufacturer. Avoid exposure to excessive heat.
a²—Store below 25 °C (77 °F), unless otherwise specified by manufacturer.
b—Store below 40 °C (104 °F), preferably between 15 and 30 °C (59 and 86 °F), in a well-closed container, unless otherwise specified by manufacturer.
c—Protect from freezing.
d—Protect from light.
e—Auxiliary labeling: • May cause drowsiness. • Avoid alcoholic beverages.

f—Auxiliary labeling: • May be habit forming.
g—Auxiliary labeling: • Shake well.
h—Dispense in dropper bottle.
i—Chew well before swallowing.

**Included in subtherapeutic amount to discourage deliberate overdosage.

## Table 3. Oral Dosage Forms (continued)

Note: Content per capsule, tablet, or 5 mL, unless otherwise stated.

| Brand or generic name [availability] | Antihistamines | Decongestants | Antitussives Opioid | Antitussives Non-opioid | Expectorants | Analgesics | Other content information as per product label | Usual Adult and Adolescent Dose prn‡ | Usual Pediatric Dose prn | Packaging, Storage, and Auxiliary labeling§ |
|---|---|---|---|---|---|---|---|---|---|---|
| *Comtrex Nighttime Maximum Strength Cold and Flu Relief* Tablets (OTC) [U.S.] | Chlorpheniramine maleate 2 mg | Pseudoephedrine HCl 30 mg | | Dextromethorphan HBr 15 mg | | Acetaminophen 500 mg | Available in a dual package that also contains *Comtrex Daytime Maximum Strength Cold and Flu Relief* | 2 tabs hs | | b, e |
| *Concentrin* Capsules (OTC) [U.S.] | | Pseudoephedrine HCl 30 mg | | Dextromethorphan HBr 15 mg | Guaifenesin 100 mg | | | 2 caps q 6 hr | 6–12 yrs: 1 cap q 6 hr | b |
| *Conex* Syrup (OTC) [U.S.] | | Phenylpropanolamine HCl 12.5 mg | | | Guaifenesin 100 mg | | | 10 mL q 4–6 hr | 2–6 yrs: 2.5 mL, 6–12 yrs: 5 mL, q 4–6 hr | b, c |
| *Conex with Codeine* Liquid Syrup (Schedule V) [U.S.] | | Phenylpropanolamine HCl 12.5 mg | Codeine PO₄ 10 mg | | Guaifenesin 100 mg | | | 10 mL q 4–6 hr | 2–6 yrs: 1.25–2.5 mL, 6–12 yrs: 2.5–5 mL, q 4–6 hr | b, c, e, f |
| *Congess JR* Extended-release Capsules (Rx) [U.S.] | | Pseudoephedrine HCl 60 mg as extended-release | | | Guaifenesin 125 mg as immediate release | | | Intended for pediatric use. See *Congess SR* Extended-release Capsules | 6–12 yrs: 1 cap q 12 hr | a¹, d |
| *Congess SR* Extended-release Capsules (Rx) [U.S.] | | Pseudoephedrine HCl 120 mg as extended-release | | | Guaifenesin 250 mg as immediate release | | | 1 cap q 12 hr | Intended for adult use. See *Congess JR* Extended-release Capsules | a¹, d |
| *Congestac Caplets* (OTC) [U.S.] | | Pseudoephedrine HCl 60 mg | | | Guaifenesin 400 mg | | | 1 tab q 4 hr (max 4 tabs daily) | | b |

Table 3. Oral Dosage Forms (*continued*)

Note: Content per capsule, tablet, or 5 mL, unless otherwise stated.

| Brand or generic name [availability] | Antihistamines | Decongestants | Antitussives Opioid | Antitussives Non-opioid | Expectorants | Analgesics | Other content information as per product label | Usual Adult and Adolescent Dose prn‡ | Usual Pediatric Dose prn | Packaging, Storage, and Auxiliary labeling§ |
|---|---|---|---|---|---|---|---|---|---|---|
| *Contac Cough & Chest Cold* Oral Solution (OTC) [U.S.] | | Pseudoephedrine HCl 15 mg | | Dextromethorphan HBr 5 mg | Guaifenesin 50 mg | Acetaminophen 125 mg | Alcohol 10% Sugar free | 20 mL q 4–6 hr | | b, c |
| *Contac Cough and Sore Throat* Oral Solution (OTC) [U.S.] | | | | Dextromethorphan HBr 5 mg | | Acetaminophen 125 mg | Alcohol 10% Sugar free | 20 mL q 4–6 hr | | b, c |
| *Contac Day Cold & Flu Caplets* Tablets (OTC) [U.S.] | | Pseudoephedrine HCl 60 mg | | Dextromethorphan HBr 30 mg | | Acetaminophen 650 mg | Available in a dual package that also contains *Contac Night Cold & Flu Caplets* | 1 tab q 6 hr (max 4 tabs daily) | | b |
| *Contac Jr. Children's Cold Medicine* Oral Solution (OTC) [U.S.] | | Phenylpropanolamine HCl 9.4 mg | | Dextromethorphan HBr 5 mg | | Acetaminophen 162.5 mg | Alcohol 10% | Intended for pediatric use | 14.1–21.4 kg: 2.5 mL, 21.4–29.5 kg: 5 mL, 29.5–38.6 kg: 7.5 mL, >38.6 kg: 10 mL, q 4 hr | b, c, e |

*Specific formulations may vary among the different manufacturers; check product labeling.

†Efficacy as expectorant has not been established.

‡Geriatric patients may be more sensitive to effects of usual adult dose.

§For appropriate *Packaging and storage* and *Auxiliary labeling* information refer to designated letters as follows:

  a—Store below 40 °C (104 °F), preferably between 15 and 30 °C (59 and 86 °F), in a tight container, unless otherwise specified by manufacturer.

  a¹—Store below 30 °C (86 °F), unless otherwise specified by manufacturer. Avoid exposure to excessive heat.

  a²—Store below 25 °C (77 °F), unless otherwise specified by manufacturer.

  b—Store below 40 °C (104 °F), preferably between 15 and 30 °C (59 and 86 °F), in a well-closed container, unless otherwise specified by manufacturer.

  c—Protect from freezing.

  d—Protect from light.

  e—Auxiliary labeling: • May cause drowsiness. • Avoid alcoholic beverages.

  f—Auxiliary labeling: • May be habit forming.

  g—Auxiliary labeling: • Shake well.

  h—Dispense in dropper bottle.

  i—Chew well before swallowing.

**Included in subtherapeutic amount to discourage deliberate overdosage.

Table 3. Oral Dosage Forms (*continued*)

Note: Content per capsule, tablet, or 5 mL, unless otherwise stated.

| Brand or generic name [availability] | Antihistamines | Decongestants | Antitussives Opioid | Antitussives Non-opioid | Expectorants | Analgesics | Other content information as per product label | Usual Adult and Adolescent Dose prn‡ | Usual Pediatric Dose prn | Packaging, Storage, and Auxiliary labeling§ |
|---|---|---|---|---|---|---|---|---|---|---|
| *Contac Night Cold & Flu Caplets* Tablets (OTC) [U.S.] | Diphenhydramine HCl 50 mg | Pseudoephedrine HCl 60 mg | | Dextromethorphan HBr 30 mg | | Acetaminophen 650 mg | Available in a dual package that also contains *Contac Cold & Flu Day Caplets* | 1 tab q 6 hr (max 4 tabs daily) | | b, e |
| *Contac Severe Cold and Flu Formula Caplets* Tablets (OTC) [U.S.] | Chlorpheniramine maleate 2 mg | Phenylpropanolamine HCl 12.5 mg | | Dextromethorphan HBr 15 mg | | Acetaminophen 500 mg | | 2 tabs q 6 hr | | b, c, e |
| *Contac Severe Cold & Flu Hot Medicine* Oral Solution (OTC) [U.S.] | Chlorpheniramine maleate 4 mg/ packet | Pseudoephedrine HCl 60 mg/ packet | | Dextromethorphan HBr 20 mg/ packet | | Acetaminophen 650 mg/ packet | | 1 packet dissolved in 6-oz cup of hot water q 4–6 hr (max 4 doses daily) | | b, e |
| *Contac Severe Cold and Flu Non-Drowsy Caplets* Tablets (OTC) [U.S.] | | Pseudoephedrine HCl 30 mg | | Dextromethorphan HBr 15 mg | | Acetaminophen 325 mg | | 2 tabs q 6 hr | | b |
| *Contac Severe Cold Formula* Capsules (OTC) [U.S.] | Chlorpheniramine maleate 2 mg | Pseudoephedrine HCl 30 mg | | Dextromethorphan HBr 15 mg | | Acetaminophen 500 mg | | 2 caps q 6 hr | | b, e |
| *Contac Severe Cold Formula Night Strength* Oral Solution (OTC) [U.S.] | Doxylamine succinate 1.3 mg (7.5 mg/30 mL) | Pseudoephedrine HCl 10 mg (60 mg/30 mL) | | Dextromethorphan HBr 5 mg (30 mg/30 mL) | | Acetaminophen 166.6 mg (1000 mg/ 30 mL) | Alcohol 25% | 30 mL hs or q 6 hr | Not recommended | b, c, e |
| *Contass* Oral Solution (Rx) | | Phenylephrine HCl 5 mg, Phenylpropanolamine HCl 20 mg | | | Guaifenesin 100 mg | | Alcohol 5% | 10 mL qid | | b, c |
| *Cophene-S* Syrup (Schedule V) [U.S.] | Chlorpheniramine maleate 5 mg | Phenylephrine HCl 20 mg, Phenylpropanolamine HCl 20 mg | Dihydrocodeine bitartrate 3 mg | | | | | 5 mL q 4–6 hr | 2–6 yrs: 0.625–1.25 mL, 6–12 yrs: 1.25–2.5 mL, q 4–6 hr | b, c, e, f |

Table 3. Oral Dosage Forms (continued)

Note: Content per capsule, tablet, or 5 mL, unless otherwise stated.

| Brand or generic name [availability] | Antihistamines | Decongestants | Antitussives Opioid | Antitussives Non-opioid | Expectorants | Analgesics | Other content information as per product label | Usual Adult and Adolescent Dose prn‡ | Usual Pediatric Dose prn | Packaging, Storage, and Auxiliary labeling§ |
|---|---|---|---|---|---|---|---|---|---|---|
| *Cophene-X* Capsules (Rx) [U.S.] | | Phenylephrine HCl 10 mg, Phenylpropanolamine HCl 10 mg | | Carbetapentane citrate 20 mg | Potassium guaiacolsulfonate† 45 mg | | | 1–2 caps q 4–6 hr | Pediatric strength not available. See *Cophene-XP* Syrup | b |
| *Cophene XP* Oral Solution (Schedule III) [U.S.] | | Pseudoephedrine HCl 60 mg | Hydrocodone bitartrate 5 mg | | Guaifenesin 200 mg | | Alcohol 12.5% | 5 mL qid | | b, c, e, f |
| *Cophene-XP* Syrup (Rx) [U.S.] | Chlorpheniramine maleate 2.5 mg | Phenylephrine HCl 10 mg, Phenylpropanolamine HCl 10 mg | | Carbetapentane citrate 20 mg | Potassium guaiacolsulfonate† 45 mg | | | 10 mL q 4–6 hr | 2–6 yrs: 1.25–2.5 mL, 6–12 yrs: 2.5–5 mL, q 6 hr | b, c, e |
| *Coristex-DH* Syrup (N) [Canada] | | Phenylephrine HCl 20 mg | Hydrocodone bitartrate 5 mg | | | | Alcohol 4.25% Sucrose 33% | 5 mL q 4 hr | 6–12 yrs: 2.5 mL q 4 hr | a, c, d, e, f |
| *Coristine-DH* Syrup (N) [Canada] | | Phenylephrine HCl 10 mg | Hydrocodone bitartrate 1.7 mg | | | | Alcohol 4.3% Sucrose 33% | 10 mL q 4 hr | 6 mos–1 yr: 1.25–2.5 mL, 1–12 yrs: 2.5–5 mL, q 4 hr | a, c, d, e, f |

*Specific formulations may vary among the different manufacturers, check product labeling.
†Efficacy as expectorant has not been established.
‡Geriatric patients may be more sensitive to effects of usual adult dose.
§For appropriate *Packaging and storage* and *Auxiliary labeling* information refer to designated letters as follows:

a—Store below 40 °C (104 °F), preferably between 15 and 30 °C (59 and 86 °F), in a tight container, unless otherwise specified by manufacturer.
a¹—Store below 30 °C (86 °F), unless otherwise specified by manufacturer. Avoid exposure to excessive heat.
a²—Store below 25 °C (77 °F), unless otherwise specified by manufacturer.
b—Store below 40 °C (104 °F), preferably between 15 and 30 °C (59 and 86 °F), in a well-closed container, unless otherwise specified by manufacturer.
c—Protect from freezing.
d—Protect from light.
e—Auxiliary labeling: • May cause drowsiness. • Avoid alcoholic beverages.

f—Auxiliary labeling: • May be habit forming.
g—Auxiliary labeling: • Shake well.
h—Dispense in dropper bottle.
i—Chew well before swallowing.

**Included in subtherapeutic amount to discourage deliberate overdosage.

Table 3. Oral Dosage Forms (continued)

Note: Content per capsule, tablet, or 5 mL, unless otherwise stated.

| Brand or generic name [availability] | Antihistamines | Decongestants | Antitussives Opioid | Antitussives Non-opioid | Expectorants | Analgesics | Other content information as per product label | Usual Adult and Adolescent Dose prn‡ | Usual Pediatric Dose prn | Packaging, Storage, and Auxiliary labeling§ |
|---|---|---|---|---|---|---|---|---|---|---|
| *CoSudafed Cough Syrup with Decongestant* Syrup (N) [Canada] | | Pseudoephedrine HCl 30 mg | Codeine $PO_4$ 10 mg | | | | | 10 mL q 4–6 hr (max 40 mL daily) | 2–5 yrs: 2.5 mL (max 10 mL daily), 6–11 yrs: 5 mL (max 20 mL daily), q 4–6 hr | a, d, e, f |
| *CoSudafed Cough Tablets with Decongestant* Tablets (N) [Canada] | | Pseudoephedrine HCl 60 mg | Codeine $PO_4$ 20 mg | | | | | ½–1 tab q 4–6 hr (max 4 tabs daily) | | b, d, e, f |
| *CoSudafed Expectorant* Syrup (N) [Canada] | | Pseudoephedrine HCl 30 mg | Codeine $PO_4$ 10 mg | | Guaifenesin 100 mg | | | 10 mL q 4–6 hr (max 40 mL daily) | 2–5 yrs: 2.5 mL (max 10 mL daily), 6–11 yrs: 5 mL (max 20 mL daily), q 4–6 hr | a, d, e, f |
| *Cotridin* Syrup (N) [Canada] | Triprolidine HCl 2 mg | Pseudoephedrine HCl 30 mg | Codeine $PO_4$ 10 mg | | | | Alcohol free | 10 mL q 4–6 hr (max 40 mL daily) | 2–6 yrs: 2.5 mL, 6–12 yrs: 5 mL q 4–6 hr (max 4 doses daily) | a, d, e, f |
| *Cotridin Expectorant* Oral Solution (N) [Canada] | Triprolidine HCl 2 mg | Pseudoephedrine HCl 30 mg | Codeine $PO_4$ 10 mg | | Guaifenesin 100 mg | | | 10 mL q 6 hr | 2–5 yrs: 2.5 mL, 6–11 yrs: 5 mL, q 6 hr | a, d, e, f |
| *Co-Tuss V* Oral Solution (Schedule III) [U.S.] | | | Hydrocodone bitartrate 5 mg | | Guaifenesin 100 mg | | | 5 mL q 4 hr | | b, c, e, f |

## Table 3. Oral Dosage Forms (continued)

Note: Content per capsule, tablet, or 5 mL, unless otherwise stated.

| Brand or generic name [availability] | Antihistamines | Decongestants | Antitussives Opioid | Antitussives Non-opioid | Expectorants | Analgesics | Other content information as per product label | Usual Adult and Adolescent Dose prn‡ | Usual Pediatric Dose prn | Packaging, Storage, and Auxiliary labeling§ |
|---|---|---|---|---|---|---|---|---|---|---|
| *CoTylenol Cold Medication* Capsules (OTC) [U.S.] | Chlorpheniramine maleate 2 mg | Pseudoephedrine HCl 30 mg | | Dextromethorphan HBr 15 mg | | Acetaminophen 325 mg | | 2 caps q 6 hr | 6–12 yrs: 1 cap q 6 hr | b, e |
| Oral Solution (OTC) [U.S.] | Chlorpheniramine maleate 0.66 mg (4 mg/30 mL) | Pseudoephedrine HCl 10 mg (60 mg/30 mL) | | Dextromethorphan HBr 5 mg (30 mg/30 mL) | | Acetaminophen 108 mg (650 mg/30 mL) | Alcohol 7.5% | 30 mL q 4–6 hr | 6–12 yrs: 15 mL q 4–6 hr | b, c, e |
| Tablets (OTC) [U.S.] | Chlorpheniramine maleate 2 mg | Pseudoephedrine HCl 30 mg | | Dextromethorphan HBr 15 mg | | Acetaminophen 325 mg | | 2 tabs q 6 hr | 6–12 yrs: 1 tab q 6 hr | b, e |
| *C-Tussin Expectorant* Oral Solution (Schedule V) [U.S.] | | Pseudoephedrine HCl 30 mg | Codeine PO₄ 10 mg | | Guaifenesin 100 mg | | Alcohol 7.5% | 10 mL q 4 hr | 2–6 yrs: 2.5 mL, 6–12 yrs: 5 mL, q 4 hr | a, c, d, e, f |
| *Decohistine DH* Oral Solution (Schedule V) [U.S.] | Chlorpheniramine maleate 2 mg | Pseudoephedrine HCl 30 mg | Codeine PO₄ 10 mg | | | | Alcohol 5.8% | 5–10 mL q 4–6 hr | | b, c, e, f |
| *Deconsal II* Extended-release Tablets (Rx) [U.S.] | | Pseudoephedrine HCl 60 mg | | | Guaifenesin 600 mg | | Scored | 1–2 tabs q 12 hr | | b |

*Specific formulations may vary among the different manufacturers; check product labeling.

†Efficacy as expectorant has not been established.

‡Geriatric patients may be more sensitive to effects of usual adult dose.

§For appropriate *Packaging and storage* and *Auxiliary labeling* information refer to designated letters as follows:

  a—Store below 40 °C (104 °F), preferably between 15 and 30 °C (59 and 86 °F), in a tight container, unless otherwise specified by manufacturer.

  a¹—Store below 30 °C (86 °F), unless otherwise specified by manufacturer. Avoid exposure to excessive heat.

  a²—Store below 25 °C (77 °F), unless otherwise specified by manufacturer.

  b—Store below 40 °C (104 °F), preferably between 15 and 30 °C (59 and 86 °F), in a well-closed container, unless otherwise specified by manufacturer.

  c—Protect from freezing.

  d—Protect from light.

  e—Auxiliary labeling: • May cause drowsiness. • Avoid alcoholic beverages. • Avoid deliberate overdosage.

  f—Auxiliary labeling: • May be habit forming.

  g—Auxiliary labeling: • Shake well.

  h—Dispense in dropper bottle.

  i—Chew well before swallowing.

**Included in subtherapeutic amount to discourage deliberate overdosage.

Table 3. Oral Dosage Forms (continued)

Note: Content per capsule, tablet, or 5 mL, unless otherwise stated.

| Brand or generic name [availability] | Antihistamines | Decongestants | Antitussives Opioid | Antitussives Non-opioid | Expectorants | Analgesics | Other content information as per product label | Usual Adult and Adolescent Dose prn‡ | Usual Pediatric Dose prn | Packaging, Storage, and Auxiliary labeling§ |
|---|---|---|---|---|---|---|---|---|---|---|
| *Deconsal Pediatric* Syrup (Schedule V) [U.S.] | | Pseudoephedrine HCl 30 mg | Codeine PO$_4$ 10 mg | | Guaifenesin 100 mg | | Alcohol 6% | | | b, c, e, f |
| *Deconsal Sprinkle* Extended-release Capsules (Rx) [U.S.] | | Phenylephrine HCl 10 mg | | | Guaifenesin 300 mg | | | 3 caps q 12 hr | | b |
| *Deproist Expectorant with Codeine* Oral Solution (Schedule V) [U.S.] | | Pseudoephedrine HCl 30 mg | Codeine PO$_4$ 10 mg | | Guaifenesin 100 mg | | Alcohol 8.2% | 10 mL q 4 hr | 2–6 yrs: 2.5 mL, 6–12 yrs: 5 mL, q 4 hr | a, c, d, e, f |
| *Despec* Oral Solution (Rx) [U.S.] | | Phenylephrine HCl 5 mg, Phenylpropanolamine HCl 20 mg | | | Guaifenesin 100 mg | | | 10 mL q 6 hr | | b, c |
| *Despec-SR Caplets* Tablets (Rx) [U.S.] | | Phenylpropanolamine HCl 75 mg | | | Guaifenesin 600 mg | | Scored | 1 tab q 12 hr | 6–12 yrs: ½ tab q 12 hr | a, d |
| *De-Tuss* Syrup (Schedule III) [U.S.] | | Pseudoephedrine HCl 60 mg | Hydrocodone bitartrate 5 mg | | | | Alcohol 5% | 5 mL q 4–6 hr | 2–6 yrs: 1.25 mL, 6–12 yrs: 2.5 mL, q 4–6 hr | b, c, d, e, f |
| *Detussin Expectorant* Oral Solution (Schedule III) [U.S.] | | Pseudoephedrine HCl 60 mg | Hydrocodone bitartrate 5 mg | | Guaifenesin 200 mg | | Alcohol 12.5% | 5 mL q 4–6 hr | Not recommended | b, c, e, f |
| *Detussin Liquid* Oral Solution (Schedule III) [U.S.] | | Pseudoephedrine HCl 60 mg | Hydrocodone bitartrate 5 mg | | | | Alcohol 5% | 5 mL q 4–6 hr | 2–6 yrs: 1.25 mL, 6–12 yrs: 2.5 mL, q 4–6 hr | b, c, d, e, f |
| *Dexafed Cough* Syrup (OTC) [U.S.] | | Phenylephrine HCl 5 mg | | Dextromethorphan HBr 10 mg | Guaifenesin 100 mg | | Alcohol free, Sugar free | 10 mL q 4 hr | | b, c |
| *Diabetic Tussin DM* Oral Solution (OTC) [U.S.] | | | | Dextromethorphan HBr 10 mg | Guaifenesin 100 mg | | Alcohol free, Sugar free, Dye free | 10 mL q 4 hr | | b, c |

## Table 3. Oral Dosage Forms (continued)

Note: Content per capsule, tablet, or 5 mL, unless otherwise stated.

| Brand or generic name [availability] | Antihistamines | Decongestants | Antitussives — Opioid | Antitussives — Non-opioid | Expectorants | Analgesics | Other content information as per product label | Usual Adult and Adolescent Dose prn‡ | Usual Pediatric Dose prn | Packaging, Storage, and Auxiliary labeling§ |
|---|---|---|---|---|---|---|---|---|---|---|
| *Dihistine DH* Elixir (Schedule V) [U.S.] | Chlorpheniramine maleate 2 mg | Pseudoephedrine HCl 30 mg | Codeine PO$_4$ 10 mg | | | | Alcohol 5% | 10 mL q 4 hr | 2–6 yrs: 1.25–2.5 mL, 6–12 yrs: 2.5–5 mL, q 6 hr | a, c, e, f |
| *Dihistine Expectorant* Oral Solution (Schedule V) [U.S.] | | Pseudoephedrine HCl 30 mg | Codeine PO$_4$ 10 mg | | Guaifenesin 100 mg | | | 10 mL q 4 hr | | b, c, e, f |
| *Dilaudid Cough* Syrup (Schedule II) [U.S.] | | | Hydromorphone HCl 1 mg | | Guaifenesin 100 mg | | Alcohol 5% | 5 mL q 3–4 hr | Not recommended | b, c, e, f |
| *Dimacol Caplets* Tablets (OTC) [U.S.] | | Pseudoephedrine HCl 30 mg | | Dextromethorphan HBr 10 mg | Guaifenesin 100 mg | | | 2 tabs q 4 hr (max 4 doses daily) | 6–12 yrs: 1 tab q 4 hr | b |
| *Dimetane-DC Cough* Oral Solution (Schedule V) [U.S.] | Brompheniramine maleate 2 mg | Phenylpropanolamine HCl 12.5 mg | Codeine PO$_4$ 10 mg | | | | Alcohol 0.95% Sugar free | 10 mL q 4 hr | 2–6 yrs: 2.5 mL, 6–12 yrs: 5 mL, q 4 hr | a, c, d, e, f |
| *Dimetane-DX Cough* Syrup (Rx) [U.S.] | Brompheniramine maleate 2 mg | Pseudoephedrine HCl 30 mg | | Dextromethorphan HBr 10 mg | | | Alcohol 0.95% | 10 mL q 4 hr | 2–6 yrs: 2.5 mL, 6–12 yrs: 5 mL, q 4 hr | a, c, d, e |

*Specific formulations may vary among the different manufacturers; check product labeling.

†Efficacy as expectorant has not been established.

‡Geriatric patients may be more sensitive to effects of usual adult dose.

§For appropriate *Packaging and storage* and *Auxiliary labeling* information refer to designated letters as follows:

　a—Store below 40 °C (104 °F), preferably between 15 and 30 °C (59 and 86 °F), in a tight container, unless otherwise specified by manufacturer.
　a¹—Store below 30 °C (86 °F), unless otherwise specified by manufacturer. Avoid exposure to excessive heat.
　a²—Store below 25 °C (77 °F), unless otherwise specified by manufacturer.
　b—Store below 40 °C (104 °F), preferably between 15 and 30 °C (59 and 86 °F), in a well-closed container, unless otherwise specified by manufacturer.
　c—Protect from freezing.
　d—Protect from light.
　e—Auxiliary labeling: • May cause drowsiness. • Avoid alcoholic beverages.
　f—Auxiliary labeling: • May be habit forming.
　g—Auxiliary labeling: • Shake well.
　h—Dispense in dropper bottle.
　i—Chew well before swallowing.

**Included in subtherapeutic amount to discourage deliberate overdosage.

Table 3. Oral Dosage Forms (*continued*)
Note: Content per capsule, tablet, or 5 mL, unless otherwise stated.

| Brand or generic name [availability] | Antihistamines | Decongestants | Antitussives Opioid | Antitussives Non-opioid | Expectorants | Analgesics | Other content information as per product label | Usual Adult and Adolescent Dose prn‡ | Usual Pediatric Dose prn | Packaging, Storage, and Auxiliary labeling§ |
|---|---|---|---|---|---|---|---|---|---|---|
| *Dimetane Expectorant Syrup* (OTC) [Canada] | Brompheniramine maleate 2 mg | Phenylephrine HCl 5 mg, Phenylpropanolamine HCl 5 mg | | | Guaifenesin 100 mg | | Alcohol 3.5% | 5–10 mL q 6 hr | 2–6 yrs: 1.25–2.5 mL, 6–12 yrs: 2.5–5 mL, q 6–8 hr | a, c, e |
| *Dimetane Expectorant-C Syrup* (N) [Canada] | Brompheniramine maleate 2 mg | Phenylephrine HCl 5 mg, Phenylpropanolamine HCl 5 mg | Codeine PO$_4$ 10 mg | | Guaifenesin 100 mg | | Alcohol 3.5% | 5–10 mL q 6 hr | 2–6 yrs: 1.25–2.5 mL, 6–12 yrs: 2.5–5 mL, q 6–8 hr | a, c, d, e, f |
| *Dimetane Expectorant-DC Oral Solution* (N) [Canada] | Brompheniramine maleate 2 mg | Phenylephrine HCl 5 mg, Phenylpropanolamine HCl 5 mg | Hydrocodone bitartrate 1.8 mg | | Guaifenesin 100 mg | | Alcohol 3.5% | 5–10 mL q 6 hr | 2–6 yrs: 1.25–2.5 mL, 6–12 yrs: 2.5–5 mL, q 6–8 hr | b, c, e, f |
| *Dimetapp-C Syrup* (N) [Canada] | Brompheniramine maleate 2 mg | Phenylephrine HCl 5 mg, Phenylpropanolamine HCl 5 mg | Codeine PO$_4$ 10 mg | | | | Alcohol Sodium 3.1 mg, Sugar free | 10 mL q 4 hr | 2–6 yrs: 2.5 mL, 6–12 yrs: 5 mL, q 4 hr | a |
| *Dimetapp DM Oral Solution* (OTC) [U.S.] | Brompheniramine maleate 2 mg | Phenylpropanolamine HCl 12.5 mg | | Dextromethorphan HBr 10 mg | | | Alcohol free | 10 mL q 4 hr | | b, c, e |
| *Dimetapp-DM Elixir* (OTC) [Canada] | Brompheniramine maleate 4 mg | Phenylephrine HCl 5 mg, Phenylpropanolamine HCl 5 mg | | Dextromethorphan HBr 15 mg | | | Alcohol 3% | 5–10 mL q 6–8 hr | 1–6 yrs: 2.5 mL, 6–12 yrs: 5 mL, q 6–8 hr | b, c, e |
| *Tablets* (OTC) [Canada] | Brompheniramine maleate 4 mg | Phenylephrine HCl 5 mg, Phenylpropanolamine HCl 5 mg | | Dextromethorphan HBr 15 mg | | | | 1 tab q 6–8 hr | 4–12 yrs: 1/2–1 tab q 6–8 hr | b |
| *Dimetapp DM Cough and Cold Syrup* (OTC) [U.S.] | Brompheniramine maleate 2 mg | Phenylpropanolamine HCl 12.5 mg | | Dextromethorphan HBr 10 mg | | | Alcohol free | 10 mL q 4 hr | 2–6 yrs: 2.5 mL, 6–12 yrs: 5 mL, q 4 hr | b, c, e |

## Table 3. Oral Dosage Forms (*continued*)

Note: Content per capsule, tablet, or 5 mL, unless otherwise stated.

| Brand or generic name [availability] | Antihistamines | Decongestants | Antitussives — Opioid | Antitussives — Non-opioid | Expectorants | Analgesics | Other content information as per product label | Usual Adult and Adolescent Dose prn‡ | Usual Pediatric Dose prn | Packaging, Storage, and Auxiliary labeling§ |
|---|---|---|---|---|---|---|---|---|---|---|
| *Donatussin* Syrup (Rx) [U.S.] | Chlorpheniramine maleate 2 mg | Phenylephrine HCl 10 mg | | Dextromethorphan HBr 7.5 mg | Guaifenesin 100 mg | | Alcohol free | 5 mL q 4–6 hr (max 6 doses daily) | 2–6 yrs: 1.25 mL, 6–12 yrs: 2.5 mL, q 4–6 hr | b, c, e |
| *Donatussin DC* Syrup (Schedule III) [U.S.] | | Phenylephrine HCl 7.5 mg | Hydrocodone bitartrate 2.5 mg | | Guaifenesin 50 mg | | Alcohol free | 10 mL q 4–6 hr | 3–6 yrs: 2.5 mL, 6–12 yrs: 5 mL, q 4–6 hr | b, c, d, e, f |
| *Donatussin Drops* Oral Solution (Rx) [U.S.] | Chlorpheniramine maleate 5 mg (1 mg/mL) | Phenylephrine HCl 10 mg (2 mg/mL) | | | Guaifenesin 100 mg (20 mg/mL) | | Alcohol free | Intended for pediatric use | <3 mos: 2–3 drops/mo, 3–6 mos: 0.3–0.6 mL, 6 mos–1 yr: 0.6–1 mL, 1–2 yrs: 1–2 mL, q 4–6 hr | b, c, e, h |
| *Dondril* Tablets (OTC) [U.S.] | Chlorpheniramine maleate 1 mg | Phenylephrine HCl 5 mg | | Dextromethorphan HBr 10 mg | | | | 2 tabs q 4 hr | 6–12 yrs: 1 tab q 4 hr | b, e |
| *Dorcol Children's Cough* Syrup (OTC) [U.S.] | | Pseudoephedrine HCl 15 mg | | Dextromethorphan HBr 5 mg | Guaifenesin 50 mg | | Alcohol free | Intended for pediatric use | 2–6 yrs: 5 mL, 6–12 yrs: 10 mL, q 4 hr | b, c |

*Specific formulations may vary among the different manufacturers; check product labeling.

†Efficacy as expectorant has not been established.

‡Geriatric patients may be more sensitive to effects of usual adult dose.

§For appropriate *Packaging and storage* and *Auxiliary labeling* information refer to designated letters as follows:

a—Store below 40 °C (104 °F), preferably between 15 and 30 °C (59 and 86 °F), in a tight container, unless otherwise specified by manufacturer.

a¹—Store below 30 °C (86 °F), unless otherwise specified by manufacturer. Avoid exposure to excessive heat.

a²—Store below 25 °C (77 °F), unless otherwise specified by manufacturer.

b—Store below 40 °C (104 °F), preferably between 15 and 30 °C (59 and 86 °F), in a well-closed container, unless otherwise specified by manufacturer.

c—Protect from freezing.

d—Protect from light.

e—Auxiliary labeling: • May cause drowsiness. • Avoid alcoholic beverages.

f—Auxiliary labeling: • May be habit forming.

g—Auxiliary labeling: • Shake well.

h—Dispense in dropper bottle.

i—Chew well before swallowing.

**Included in subtherapeutic amount to discourage deliberate overdosage.

Table 3. Oral Dosage Forms (continued)

Note: Content per capsule, tablet, or 5 mL, unless otherwise stated.

| Brand or generic name [availability] | Antihistamines | Decongestants | Antitussives Opioid | Antitussives Non-opioid | Expectorants | Analgesics | Other content information as per product label | Usual Adult and Adolescent Dose prn‡ | Usual Pediatric Dose prn | Packaging, Storage, and Auxiliary labeling§ |
|---|---|---|---|---|---|---|---|---|---|---|
| *Dorcol DM* Syrup (OTC) [Canada] | | Phenylpropanolamine HCl 8.75 mg | | Dextromethorphan HBr 7.5 mg | Guaifenesin 37.5 mg | | | Intended for pediatric use | <1 yr: 1.25 mL, 1–6 yrs: 5 mL, 6–12 yrs: 10 mL, q 4–6 hr | b, c |
| *Dristan Cold and Flu* for Oral Solution (OTC) [U.S.] | Chlorpheniramine maleate 4 mg/ packet | Pseudoephedrine HCl 60 mg/ packet | | Dextromethorphan HBr 20 mg/packet | | Acetaminophen 500 mg/ packet | | 1 packet dissolved in 6-oz cup of hot water q 4 hr | | b, e |
| *Dristan Juice Mix-in* Cold, Flu, and Cough for Oral Solution (OTC) [U.S.] | | Pseudoephedrine HCl 60 mg/packet | | Dextromethorphan HBr 20 mg/ packet | | Acetaminophen 500 mg/ packet | | 1 packet dissolved in 6-oz glass of juice q 4 hr | | b |
| *Drixoral Cough & Congestion Liquid Caps* Capsules (OTC) [U.S.] | | Pseudoephedrine HCl 60 mg | | Dextromethorphan HBr 30 mg | | | | 1 cap q 6 hr | Not recommended | a[1], c |
| *Dura-Gest* Capsules (Rx) [U.S.] | | Phenylephrine HCl 5 mg, Phenylpropanolamine HCl 45 mg | | | Guaifenesin 200 mg | | | 1 cap q 6 hr | Not recommended | a |
| *Duratuss* Extended-release Tablets (Rx) [U.S.] | | Pseudoephedrine HCl 120 mg | | | Guaifenesin 600 mg | | Scored Dye free | 1 tab q 12 hr | | b |
| *Duratuss HD* Elixir (Schedule III) [U.S.] | | Pseudoephedrine HCl 30 mg | Hydrocodone bitartrate 2.5 mg | | Guaifenesin 100 mg | | Alcohol 5% | 10 mL q 4–6 hr | | b, c, e, f |
| *Dura-Vent* Extended-release Tablets (Rx) [U.S.] | | Phenylpropanolamine HCl 75 mg | | | Guaifenesin 600 mg | | Dye free Scored | 1 tab q 12 hr | <6 yrs: Not recommended 6–12 yrs: tab q 12 hr | a |
| *ED-TLC* Oral Solution (Schedule III) [U.S.] | Chlorpheniramine maleate 2 mg (12 mg/30 mL) | Phenylephrine HCl 5 mg (30 mg/30 mL) | Hydrocodone bitartrate 1.67 mg (10 mg/30 mL) | | | | | 10 mL q 6–8 hr | 6–12 yrs: 5 mL q 6–8 hr | b, c, e, f |

## Table 3. Oral Dosage Forms (continued)

Note: Content per capsule, tablet, or 5 mL, unless otherwise stated.

| Brand or generic name [availability] | Antihistamines | Decongestants | Antitussives Opioid | Antitussives Non-opioid | Expectorants | Analgesics | Other content information as per product label | Usual Adult and Adolescent Dose prn‡ | Usual Pediatric Dose prn | Packaging, Storage, and Auxiliary labeling§ |
|---|---|---|---|---|---|---|---|---|---|---|
| *ED Tuss HC* Oral Solution (Schedule III) [U.S.] | Chlorpheniramine maleate 4 mg | Phenylephrine HCl 10 mg | Hydrocodone bitartrate 2.5 mg | | | | Alcohol 5% | 5 mL q 6 hr | 2–6 yrs: 1.25 mL; 6–12 yrs: 2.5 mL, q 4–6 hr | b, c, e, f |
| *Effective Strength Cough Formula* Oral Solution (OTC) [U.S.] | Chlorpheniramine maleate 2 mg | | | Dextromethorphan HBr 15 mg | | | Alcohol 10% | 10 mL q 6 hr | | b, c, e |
| *Effective Strength Cough Formula with Decongestant* Oral Solution (OTC) [U.S.] | | Pseudoephedrine HCl 20 mg | | Dextromethorphan HBr 10 mg | | | Alcohol 10% | 15 mL q 6 hr | | b, c, e |
| *Efficol Cough Whip (Cough Suppressant/ Decongestant)* Oral Gel (OTC) [U.S.] | | Phenylpropanolamine HCl 6.25 mg | | Dextromethorphan HBr 2.5 mg | | | Alcohol free | 20 mL q 4 hr | 2–6 yrs: 5 mL, 6–12 yrs: 10 mL, q 4 hr | b, c |
| *Efficol Cough Whip (Cough Suppressant/ Decongestant/Anti-histamine)* Oral Gel (OTC) [U.S.] | Chlorpheniramine maleate 1 mg | Phenylpropanolamine HCl 6.25 mg | | Dextromethorphan HBr 2.5 mg | | | Alcohol free | 20 mL q 4 hr | 6–12 yrs: 10 mL q 4 hr | b, c, e |

*Specific formulations may vary among the different manufacturers; check product labeling.

†Efficacy as expectorant has not been established.

‡Geriatric patients may be more sensitive to effects of usual adult dose.

§For appropriate *Packaging and storage* and *Auxiliary labeling* information refer to designated letters as follows:

a—Store below 40 °C (104 °F), preferably between 15 and 30 °C (59 and 86 °F), in a tight container, unless otherwise specified by manufacturer.

a¹—Store below 30 °C (86 °F), unless otherwise specified by manufacturer. Avoid exposure to excessive heat.

a²—Store below 25 °C (77 °F), unless otherwise specified by manufacturer.

b—Store below 40 °C (104 °F), preferably between 15 and 30 °C (59 and 86 °F), in a well-closed container, unless otherwise specified by manufacturer.

c—Protect from freezing.

d—Protect from light.

e—Auxiliary labeling: • May cause drowsiness. • Avoid alcoholic beverages.

f—Auxiliary labeling: • May be habit forming.

g—Auxiliary labeling: • Shake well.

h—Dispense in dropper bottle.

i—Chew well before swallowing.

**Included in subtherapeutic amount to discourage deliberate overdosage.

## Table 3. Oral Dosage Forms (continued)

Note: Content per capsule, tablet, or 5 mL, unless otherwise stated.

| Brand or generic name [availability] | Antihistamines | Decongestants | Antitussives Opioid | Antitussives Non-opioid | Expectorants | Analgesics | Other content information as per product label | Usual Adult and Adolescent Dose prn‡ | Usual Pediatric Dose prn | Packaging, Storage, and Auxiliary labeling§ |
|---|---|---|---|---|---|---|---|---|---|---|
| Efficol Cough Whip (Cough Suppressant/ Expectorant) Oral Gel (OTC) [U.S.] | | | | Dextromethorphan HBr 2.5 mg | Guaifenesin 50 mg | | Alcohol free | 20 mL q 4 hr | 2–6 yrs: 5 mL, 6–12 yrs: 10 mL, q 4 hr | b, c |
| Endagen-HD Syrup (Schedule III) [U.S.] | Chlorpheniramine maleate 2 mg | Phenylephrine HCl 5 mg | Hydrocodone bitartrate 1.7 mg | | | | | 10 mL q 6–8 hr | 6 12 yrs: 5 mL q 6 8 hr | b, c, e, f |
| Endal Extended-release Tablets (Rx) [U.S.] | | Phenylephrine HCl 20 mg | | | Guaifenesin 300 mg | | | 1 or 2 tabs q 12 hr | | b |
| Endal Expectorant Syrup (Schedule V) [U.S.] | | Phenylpropanolamine HCl 12.5 mg | Codeine PO$_4$ 10 mg | | Guaifenesin 100 mg | | Alcohol 5% Sugar free Dye free | 5–10 mL q 6–8 hr | | b, c, e, f |
| Endal-HD Oral Solution (Schedule III) [U.S.] | Chlorpheniramine maleate 2 mg | Phenylephrine HCl 5 mg | Hydrocodone bitartrate 1.67 mg | | | | | 10 mL q 6–8 hr | 6–12 yrs: 5 mL q 6–8 hr | b, c, e, f |
| Endal-HD Plus Oral Solution (Schedule III) [U.S.] | Chlorpheniramine maleate 2 mg | Phenylephrine HCl 5 mg | Hydrocodone bitartrate 2.5 mg | | | | Alcohol free Dye free | 10 mL q 4 hr | | b, c, e, f |
| Enomine Capsules (Rx) [U.S.] | | Phenylephrine HCl 5 mg, Phenylpropa- nolamine HCl 45 mg | | | Guaifenesin 200 mg | | | 1 cap q 6 hr | | b |
| Entex Capsules (Rx) [U.S.] | | Phenylephrine HCl 5 mg, Phenylpropa- nolamine HCl 45 mg | | | Guaifenesin 200 mg | | | 1 cap q 6 hr | Pediatric strength not available. See *Entex Liquid* Oral Solution | b |
| Entex LA Extended-release Tablets (Rx) [U.S.] | | Phenylpropanolamine HCl 75 mg | | | Guaifenesin 400 mg | | Scored | 1 tab q 12 hr | 6–12 yrs: 1/2 tab q 12 hr | b |

Table 3. Oral Dosage Forms (*continued*)

Note: Content per capsule, tablet, or 5 mL, unless otherwise stated.

| Brand or generic name [availability] | Antihistamines | Decongestants | Antitussives Opioid | Antitussives Non-opioid | Expectorants | Analgesics | Other content information as per product label | Usual Adult and Adolescent Dose prn‡ | Usual Pediatric Dose prn | Packaging, Storage, and Auxiliary labeling§ |
|---|---|---|---|---|---|---|---|---|---|---|
| *Entex LA (continued)* Extended-release Tablets (Rx) [Canada] | | Phenylpropanolamine HCl 75 mg | | | Guaifenesin 600 mg | | Scored | 1 tab q 12 hr | 6–12 yrs: ½ tab q 12 hr | b |
| *Entex Liquid* Oral Solution (Rx) [U.S.] | | Phenylephrine HCl 5 mg, Phenylpropanolamine HCl 20 mg | | | Guaifenesin 100 mg | | Alcohol 5% | 10 mL q 6 hr | 2–4 yrs: 2.5 mL, 4–6 yrs: 5 mL, 6–12 yrs: 7.5 mL, q 6 hr | b, c |
| *Entex PSE* Extended-release Tablets (Rx) [U.S.] | | Pseudoephedrine HCl 120 mg | | | Guaifenesin 600 mg | | Scored | 1 tab q 12 hr | 6–12 yrs: ½ tab q 12 hr | b |
| *Entuss-D* Oral Solution (Schedule III) [U.S.] | | Pseudoephedrine HCl 30 mg | Hydrocodone bitartrate 5 mg | | Guaiacol-sulfonate 300 mg | | Alcohol free Sugar free Dye free | 5–7.5 mL q 4–6 hr | 3–6 yrs: 1.25–2.5 mL, 6–12 yrs: 2.5–5 mL, q 4–6 hr | b, c, d, e, f |
| Tablets (Schedule III) [U.S.] | | Pseudoephedrine HCl 30 mg | Hydrocodone bitartrate 5 mg | | Guaifenesin 300 mg | | Scored | 1–1 tabs q 4–6 hr | 6–12 yrs: ½–1 tab q 4–6 hr | b, d, e, f |
| *Entuss Expectorant* Oral Solution (Schedule III) [U.S.] | | | Hydrocodone bitartrate 5 mg | | Potassium guaiacol-sulfonate† 300 mg | | Alcohol free Sugar free | 5–7.5 mL q 4–6 hr | 3–6 yrs: 1.25–2.5 mL, 6–12 yrs: 2.5–5 mL, q 4–6 hr | b, c, d, e, f |

*Specific formulations may vary among the different manufacturers; check product labeling.

†Efficacy as expectorant has not been established.

‡Geriatric patients may be more sensitive to effects of usual adult dose.

§For appropriate *Packaging and storage* and *Auxiliary labeling* information refer to designated letters as follows:

  a—Store below 40 °C (104 °F), preferably between 15 and 30 °C (59 and 86 °F), in a tight container, unless otherwise specified by manufacturer.

  a¹—Store below 30 °C (86 °F), unless otherwise specified by manufacturer. Avoid exposure to excessive heat.

  a²—Store below 25 °C (77 °F), unless otherwise specified by manufacturer.

  b—Store below 40 °C (104 °F), preferably between 15 and 30 °C (59 and 86 °F), in a well-closed container, unless otherwise specified by manufacturer.

  c—Protect from freezing.

  d—Protect from light.

  e—Auxiliary labeling: • May cause drowsiness. • Avoid alcoholic beverages.

  f—Auxiliary labeling: • May be habit forming.

  g—Auxiliary labeling: • Shake well.

  h—Dispense in dropper bottle.

  i—Chew well before swallowing.

**Included in subtherapeutic amount to discourage deliberate overdosage.

Table 3. Oral Dosage Forms *(continued)*

Note: Content per capsule, tablet, or 5 mL, unless otherwise stated.

| Brand or generic name [availability] | Antihistamines | Decongestants | Antitussives Opioid | Antitussives Non-opioid | Expectorants | Analgesics | Other content information as per product label | Usual Adult and Adolescent Dose prn‡ | Usual Pediatric Dose prn | Packaging, Storage, and Auxiliary labeling§ |
|---|---|---|---|---|---|---|---|---|---|---|
| *Entuss Expectorant (continued)* Tablets (Schedule III) [U.S.] | | | Hydrocodone bitartrate 5 mg | | Guaifenesin 300 mg | | Scored | 1–1 tabs q 4–6 hr | Pediatric strength not available | b, e, f |
| *Entuss Pediatric Expectorant* Oral Solution (Schedule III) [U.S.] | | Pseudoephedrine HCl 30 mg | Hydrocodone bitartrate 2.5 mg | | Guaifenesin 100 mg | | Alcohol 5% | 10 mL q 4–6 hr | 6–12 yrs: 5 mL q 4–6 hr | b, c, d, e, f |
| *Eudal-SR* Extended-release Tablets [Rx] [U.S.] | | Pseudoephedrine HCl 120 mg | | | Guaifenesin 400 mg | | | 1 tab q 12 hr | | b |
| *Exgest LA* Extended-release Tablets [Rx] [U.S.] | | Phenylpropanolamine HCl 75 mg | | | Guaifenesin 400 mg | | Scored | 1 tab q 12 hr | | b |
| *Extra Action Cough* Syrup (OTC) [U.S.] | | | | Dextromethorphan HBr 15 mg | Guaifenesin 100 mg | | Alcohol 1.4% | 10 mL q 6–8 hr | 2–6 yrs: 2.5 mL, 6–12 yrs: 5 mL, q 6–8 hr | b, c |
| *Father John's Medicine Plus* Oral Solution (OTC) [U.S.] | Chlorpheniramine maleate 1 mg | Phenylephrine HCl 2.5 mg | | Dextromethorphan HBr 7.5 mg | Guaifenesin 30 mg, Ammonium Cl† 83.3 mg | | Alcohol free | 5–10 mL q 3–4 hr | 2–6 yrs: 5 mL, 6–12 yrs: 5–10 mL, q 6–8 hr | b, c, e |
| *Fendol* Tablets (OTC) [U.S.] | | Phenylephrine HCl 5 mg | | | Guaifenesin 100 mg | Acetaminophen 355 mg, Salicylamide 65 mg | Caffeine 32 mg | 2 tabs q 4 hr | Pediatric strength not available | a |
| *Fenesin DM* Extended-release Tablets [Rx] [U.S.] | | | | Detromethorphan HBr 30 mg | Guaifenesin 600 mg | | Scored | 1–2 tabs q 12 hr | 2–6 yrs: ½ tab, 6–12 yrs: 1 tab, q 12 hr | a, d |

# Table 3. Oral Dosage Forms (continued)

Note: Content per capsule, tablet, or 5 mL, unless otherwise stated.

| Brand or generic name [availability] | Antihistamines | Decongestants | Antitussives — Opioid | Antitussives — Non-opioid | Expectorants | Analgesics | Other content information as per product label | Usual Adult and Adolescent Dose prn‡ | Usual Pediatric Dose prn | Packaging, Storage, and Auxiliary labeling§ |
|---|---|---|---|---|---|---|---|---|---|---|
| 2/G-DM Cough Syrup (OTC) [U.S.] | | | | Dextromethorphan HBr 15 mg | Guaifenesin 100 mg | | Alcohol 5% | 10 mL q 6–8 hr | 2–6 yrs: 2.5 mL, 6–12 yrs: 5 mL, q 6–8 hr | b, c |
| Genatuss DM Syrup (OTC) [U.S.] | | | | Dextromethorphan HBr 10 mg | Guaifenesin 100 mg | | Alcohol free | 10 mL q 4 hr | | b, c |
| Genite Oral Solution (OTC) [U.S.] | Doxylamine succinate 1.25 mg | Pseudoephedrine HCl 10 mg | | Dextromethorphan HBr 5 mg | | Acetaminophen 167 mg | Alcohol 25% Tartrazine | 30 mL hs or q 6 hr | | b, c |
| Glycofed Tablets (OTC) [U.S.] | | Pseudoephedrine HCl 30 mg | | | Guaifenesin 100 mg | | Scored | 1–2 tabs q 6 hr | | b |
| Glycotuss-dM Tablets (OTC) [U.S.] | | | | Dextromethorphan HBr 10 mg | Guaifenesin 100 mg | | | 1–2 tabs q 4 hr | 6–12 yrs: 1 tab q 4 hr | b |
| Glydeine Cough Syrup USP (Schedule V) [U.S.] | | | Codeine PO₄ 10 mg | | Guaifenesin 100 mg | | Alcohol 3.5% | 5–10 mL q 4 hr | 2–6 yrs: 2.5 mL, 6–12 yrs: 5 mL, q 4 hr | a, d, e, f |
| GP-500 Tablets (Rx) [U.S.] | | Pseudoephedrine HCl 120 mg | | | Guaifenesin 500 mg | | | 1 tab bid | | b |

*Specific formulations may vary among the different manufacturers; check product labeling.
†Efficacy as expectorant has not been established.
‡Geriatric patients may be more sensitive to effects of usual adult dose.
§For appropriate *Packaging and storage* and *Auxiliary labeling* information refer to designated letters as follows:

a—Store below 40 °C (104 °F), preferably between 15 and 30 °C (59 and 86 °F), in a tight container, unless otherwise specified by manufacturer.
a¹—Store below 30 °C (86 °F), unless otherwise specified by manufacturer. Avoid exposure to excessive heat.
a²—Store below 25 °C (77 °F), unless otherwise specified by manufacturer.
b—Store below 40 °C (104 °F), preferably between 15 and 30 °C (59 and 86 °F), in a well-closed container, unless otherwise specified by manufacturer.
c—Protect from freezing.
d—Protect from light.
e—Auxiliary labeling: • May cause drowsiness. • Avoid alcoholic beverages.
f—Auxiliary labeling: • May be habit forming.
g—Auxiliary labeling: • Shake well.
h—Dispense in dropper bottle.
i—Chew well before swallowing.

**Included in subtherapeutic amount to discourage deliberate overdosage.

Table 3. Oral Dosage Forms (*continued*)

Note: Content per capsule, tablet, or 5 mL, unless otherwise stated.

| Brand or generic name [availability] | Antihistamines | Decongestants | Antitussives — Opioid | Antitussives — Non-opioid | Expectorants | Analgesics | Other content information as per product label | Usual Adult and Adolescent Dose prn‡ | Usual Pediatric Dose prn | Packaging, Storage, and Auxiliary labeling§ |
|---|---|---|---|---|---|---|---|---|---|---|
| *Guaifed* Extended-release Capsules (Rx) [U.S.] | | Pseudoephedrine HCl 120 mg (extended-release) | | | Guaifenesin 250 mg (immediate release) | | | 1 cap q 12 hr | Pediatric strength not available | a |
| Syrup (OTC) [U.S.] | | Pseudoephedrine HCl 30 mg | | | Guaifenesin 200 mg | | Sugar free | 10 mL q 4–6 hr | | b |
| *Guaifed-PD* Extended-release Capsules (Rx) [U.S.] | | Pseudoephedrine HCl 60 mg (extended-release) | | | Guaifenesin 300 mg (immediate release) | | | 1–2 caps q 12 hr | 6–12 yrs: 1 cap q 12 hr | a |
| *GuaiMAX-D* Extended-release Tablets (Rx) [U.S.] | | Pseudoephedrine HCl 120 mg | | | Guaifensin 600 mg | | Scored | 1 tab q 12 hr | | b |
| *Guaipax* Extended-release Tablets (Rx) [U.S.] | | Phenylpropanolamine HCl 75 mg | | | Guaifenesin 400 mg | | | 1 tab q 12 hr | 6–12 yrs: ½ tab q 12 hr | b |
| *Guaitab* Tablets (OTC) [U.S.] | | Pseudoephedrine HCl 60 mg | | | Guaifenesin 400 mg | | Scored | 1 tab q 4–6 hr | Pediatric strength not available | b |
| *Guai-Vent/PSE* Extended-release Tablets (Rx) [U.S.] | | Pseudoephedrine HCl 120 mg | | | Guaifenesin 600 mg | | Scored | 1 tab q 12 hr | 6–12 yrs: ½ tab q 12 hr | a, d |
| *GuiaCough CF* Oral Solution (OTC) [U.S.] | | Phenylpropanolamine HCl 12.5 mg | | Dextromethorphan HBr 10 mg | Guaifenesin 100 mg | | Alcohol 4.75% | 10 mL q 4 hr | | b, c |
| *GuiaCough PE* Oral Solution (OTC) [U.S.] | | Pseudoephedrine HCl 30 mg | | | Guaifenesin 100 mg | | Alcohol 1.4% | 10 mL q 4 hr | | b, c |
| *Guiamid D.M. Liquid* Oral Solution (OTC) [U.S.] | | | | Dextromethorphan HBr 15 mg | Guaifenesin 100 mg | | Alcohol 1.4% | 10 mL q 6–8 hr | 2–6 yrs: 2.5 mL, 6–12 yrs: 5 mL q 6–8 hr | b, c |

Table 3. Oral Dosage Forms (*continued*)

Note: Content per capsule, tablet, or 5 mL, unless otherwise stated.

| Brand or generic name [availability] | Antihistamines | Decongestants | Antitussives Opioid | Antitussives Non-opioid | Expectorants | Analgesics | Other content information as per product label | Usual Adult and Adolescent Dose prn‡ | Usual Pediatric Dose prn | Packaging, Storage, and Auxiliary labeling§ |
|---|---|---|---|---|---|---|---|---|---|---|
| *Guiatuss A.C.* Syrup USP (Schedule V) [U.S.] | | | Codeine PO$_4$ 10 mg | | Guaifenesin 100 mg | | Alcohol 3.5% | 5–10 mL q 4–6 hr | 2–6 yrs: 1.25–2.5 mL, 6–12 yrs: 2.5–5 mL, q 4–6 hr | a, d, e, f |
| *Guiatuss CF* Oral Solution (OTC) [U.S.] | | Phenylpropanolamine HCl 12.5 mg | | Dextromethorphan HBr 10 mg | Guaifenesin 100 mg | | Alcohol 4.75% | 10 mL q 4 hr | | b, c |
| *Guiatuss DAC* Oral Solution (Schedule V) [U.S.] | | Pseudoephedrine HCl 30 mg | Codeine PO$_4$ 10 mg | | Guaifenesin 100 mg | | Alcohol | 10 mL q 4 hr | | b, c, e, f |
| *Guiatussin-DM* Syrup (OTC) [U.S.] | | | | Dextromethorphan HBr 10 mg | Guaifenesin 100 mg | | Alcohol 1.4% | 10 mL q 6–8 hr | 2–6 yrs: 2.5 mL, 6–12 yrs: 5 mL, q 6–8 hr | b, c |
| *Guiatussin with Codeine Liquid* Oral Solution (Schedule V) [U.S.] | | | Codeine PO$_4$ 10 mg | | Guaifenesin 100 mg | | Alcohol 3.5% | 5–10 mL q 4–6 hr | 2–6 yrs: 1.25–2.5 mL, 6–12 yrs: 2.5–5 mL, q 4–6 hr | b, c, e, f |
| *Guiatussin DAC* Syrup (Schedule V) [U.S.] | | Pseudoephedrine HCl 30 mg | Codeine PO$_4$ 10 mg | | Guaifenesin 100 mg | | Alcohol 1.6% Sugar free | 10 mL q 4 hr | | b, c, e, f |

*Specific formulations may vary among the different manufacturers; check product labeling.

†Efficacy as expectorant has not been established.

‡Geriatric patients may be more sensitive to effects of usual adult dose.

§For appropriate *Packaging and storage* and *Auxiliary labeling* information refer to designated letters as follows:

  a—Store below 40 °C (104 °F), preferably between 15 and 30 °C (59 and 86 °F), in a tight container, unless otherwise specified by manufacturer.
  a¹—Store below 30 °C (86 °F), unless otherwise specified by manufacturer. Avoid exposure to excessive heat.
  a²—Store below 25 °C (77 °F), unless otherwise specified by manufacturer.
  b—Store below 40 °C (104 °F), preferably between 15 and 30 °C (59 and 86 °F), in a well-closed container, unless otherwise specified by manufacturer.
  c—Protect from freezing.
  d—Protect from light.
  e—Auxiliary labeling: • May cause drowsiness. • Avoid alcoholic beverages.

  f—Auxiliary labeling: • May be habit forming.
  g—Auxiliary labeling: • Shake well.
  h—Dispense in dropper bottle.
  i—Chew well before swallowing.

**Included in subtherapeutic amount to discourage deliberate overdosage.

## Table 3. Oral Dosage Forms (*continued*)

Note: Content per capsule, tablet, or 5 mL, unless otherwise stated.

| Brand or generic name [availability] | Antihistamines | Decongestants | Antitussives Opioid | Antitussives Non-opioid | Expectorants | Analgesics | Other content information as per product label | Usual Adult and Adolescent Dose prn‡ | Usual Pediatric Dose prn | Packaging, Storage, and Auxiliary labeling§ |
|---|---|---|---|---|---|---|---|---|---|---|
| *Guiatussin w/Dextromethorphan* Oral Solution (OTC) [U.S.] | | | | Dextromethorphan HBr 15 mg | Guaifenesin 100 mg | | Alcohol 1.4% | 10 mL q 6–8 hr | | b, c |
| *Guiatuss PE* Syrup (OTC) [U.S.] | | Pseudoephedrine HCl 30 mg | | | Guaifenesin 100 mg | | Alcohol 1.4% | 10 mL q 4 hr | | b, c |
| *Halotussin-DM Expectorant* Syrup (OTC) [U.S.] | | | | Dextromethorphan HBr 10 mg | Guaifenesin 100 mg | | Alcohol free | 10 mL q 6–8 hr | 2–6 yrs: 2.5 mL, 6–12 yrs: 5 mL q 6–8 hr | b, c |
| *Histafed C* Syrup (Schedule V) [U.S.] | Triprolidine HCl 1.25 mg | Pseudoephedrine HCl 30 mg | Codeine PO$_4$ 10 mg | | | | | 10 mL q 4–6 hr | 2–6 yrs: 2.5 mL, 6–12 yrs: 5 mL, q 4–6 hr | b, c, d, e, f |
| *Histatuss Pediatric* Oral Suspension (Rx) [U.S.] | Chlorpheniramine tannate 4 mg | Ephedrine tannate 5 mg, Phenylephrine tannate 5 mg | | Carbetapentane tannate 30 mg | | | | Intended for pediatric use | 2–6 yrs: 2.5–5 mL, 6–12 yrs: 5–10 mL, q 12 hr | b, c, e, g |
| *Histine DM* Syrup (Rx) [U.S.] | Brompheniramine maleate 2 mg | Phenylpropanolamine HCl 12.5 mg | | Dextromethorphan HBr 10 mg | | | | 10 mL q 4 hr | | b, c, e |
| *Histinex HC* Syrup (Schedule III) [U.S.] | Chlorpheniramine maleate 2 mg | Phenylephrine HCl 5 mg | Hydrocodone bitartrate 2.5 mg | | | | Alcohol free Sugar free | 10 mL q 4 hr (max 40 mL daily) | 6–12 yrs: 5 mL q 4 hr (max 20 mL daily) | a, d, e, f |
| *Histussin HC* Syrup (Schedule III) [U.S.] | Chlorpheniramine maleate 2 mg | Phenylephrine HCl 5 mg | Hydrocodone bitartrate 2.5 mg | | | | | 10 mL q 4 hr | 6–12 yrs: 5 mL q 4 hr | b, c, e, f |
| *Humibid DM* Extended-release Tablets (Rx) [U.S.] | | | | Dextromethorphan HBr 30 mg | Guaifenesin 600 mg | | Scored | 1–2 tabs q 12 hr | | b |

Table 3. Oral Dosage Forms (*continued*)
Note: Content per capsule, tablet, or 5 mL, unless otherwise stated.

| Brand or generic name [availability] | Antihistamines | Decongestants | Antitussives — Opioid | Antitussives — Non-opioid | Expectorants | Analgesics | Other content information as per product label | Usual Adult and Adolescent Dose prn‡ | Usual Pediatric Dose prn | Packaging, Storage, and Auxiliary labeling§ |
|---|---|---|---|---|---|---|---|---|---|---|
| *Humibid DM Sprinkle* Extended-release Capsules (Rx) [U.S.] | | | | Dextromethorphan HBr 15 mg | Guaifenesin 300 mg | | | 2–4 caps q 12 hr | | b |
| *HycoClear Tuss* Syrup (Schedule III) [U.S.] | | | Hydrocodone bitartrate 5 mg | | Guaifenesin 100 mg | | Alcohol free Sugar free Dye free | 5 mL q 4 hr (max 30 mL daily) | 2–12 yrs: 2.5 mL q 4 hr | a, e, f |
| *Hycodan* Syrup (Schedule III) [U.S.] | | | Hydrocodone bitartrate 5 mg | | | | Homatropine MBr 1.5 mg** (not in Canadian product) | 5 mL q 4–6 hr | <2 yrs: 1.25 mL, 2–12 yrs: 2.5 mL, q 4–6 hr | b, c, d, e, f |
| Tablets (Schedule III) [U.S.] | | | Hydrocodone bitartrate 5 mg | | | | Homatropine MBr 1.5 mg** Scored | 1 tab q 4–6 hr | <2 yrs: ¼ tab, 2–12 yrs: ½ tab, q 4–6 hr. See also *Hycodan* Syrup | b, d, e, f |
| *Hycomine* Syrup (Schedule III) [U.S.] | | Phenylpropanolamine HCl 25 mg | Hydrocodone bitartrate 5 mg | | | | Sugar free Alcohol free | 5 mL q 4–6 hr | 6–12 yrs: 2.5 mL q 4–6 hr. See also *Hycomine Pediatric Syrup* | b, c, d, e, f |

*Specific formulations may vary among the different manufacturers, check product labeling.
†Efficacy as expectorant has not been established.
‡Geriatric patients may be more sensitive to effects of usual adult dose.
§For appropriate *Packaging and storage* and *Auxiliary labeling* information refer to designated letters as follows:
  a—Store below 40 °C (104 °F), preferably between 15 and 30 °C (59 and 86 °F), in a tight container, unless otherwise specified by manufacturer.
  a¹—Store below 30 °C (86 °F), unless otherwise specified by manufacturer. Avoid exposure to excessive heat.
  a²—Store below 25 °C (77 °F), unless otherwise specified by manufacturer.
  b—Store below 40 °C (104 °F), preferably between 15 and 30 °C (59 and 86 °F), in a well-closed container, unless otherwise specified by manufacturer.
  c—Protect from freezing.
  d—Protect from light.
  e—Auxiliary labeling: • May cause drowsiness. • Avoid alcoholic beverages.
  f—Auxiliary labeling: • May be habit forming.
  g—Auxiliary labeling: • Shake well.
  h—Dispense in dropper bottle.
  i—Chew well before swallowing.
**Included in subtherapeutic amount to discourage deliberate overdosage.

## Table 3. Oral Dosage Forms (continued)

Note: Content per capsule, tablet, or 5 mL, unless otherwise stated.

| Brand or generic name [availability] | Antihistamines | Decongestants | Antitussives — Opioid | Antitussives — Non-opioid | Expectorants | Analgesics | Other content information as per product label | Usual Adult and Adolescent Dose prn‡ | Usual Pediatric Dose prn | Packaging, Storage, and Auxiliary labeling§ |
|---|---|---|---|---|---|---|---|---|---|---|
| Hycomine (continued) Syrup (N) [Canada] | Pyrilamine maleate 12.5 mg | Phenylephrine HCl 10 mg | Hydrocodone bitartrate 5 mg | | Ammonium Cl† 60 mg | | Alcohol free | 5 mL q 4–6 hr | 2–6 yrs: 1.25 mL, 6–12 yrs: 2.5 mL, q 4–6 hr. See also Hycomine-S Pediatric Syrup | b, c, d, e, f |
| Hycomine Compound Tablets (Schedule III) [U.S.] | Chlorpheniramine maleate 2 mg | Phenylephrine HCl 10 mg | Hydrocodone bitartrate 5 mg | | | Acetaminophen 250 mg | Caffeine 30 mg Scored | 1 tab q 4–6 hr | 2–6 yrs: ½ tab q 12 hr 6–12 yrs: ½ tab q 6 hr | b, d, e, f |
| Hycomine Pediatric Syrup (Schedule III) [U.S.] | | Phenylpropanolamine HCl 12.5 mg | Hydrocodone bitartrate 2.5 mg | | | | Sugar free Alcohol free | Intended for pediatric use. See Hycomine Syrup | 2–6 yrs: 2.5 mL, 6–12 yrs: 5 mL, q 4–6 hr | b, c, d, e, f |
| Hycomine-S Pediatric Syrup (N) [Canada] | Pyrilamine maleate 6.25 mg | Phenylephrine HCl 5 mg | Hydrocodone bitartrate 2.5 mg | | Ammonium Cl† 30 mg | | Alcohol free | 10 mL q 4–6 hr | 6 mos–1 yr: 10 drops, 1–3 yrs: 20 drops, 3–6 yrs: 2.5 mL, 6–12 yrs: 5 mL, q 4–6 hr | b, c, d, e, f, h |
| Hycotuss Expectorant Syrup (Schedule III) [U.S.] | | | Hydrocodone bitartrate 5 mg | | Guaifenesin 100 mg | | Alcohol 10% | 5 mL q 4–6 hr | <2 yrs: 0.3 mg of hydrocodone kg/day, 2–12 yrs: 2.5 mL q 4–6 hr | b, c, d, e, f |
| Hydrocodone and Homatropine* Syrup (Schedule III) [U.S.] | | | Hydrocodone bitartrate 5 mg | | | | Homatropine MBr 1.5 mg** | 5 mL q 4–6 hr | <2 yrs: 1.25 mL, 2–12 yrs: 2.5 mL, q 4–6 hr | b, c, d, e, f |

Table 3. Oral Dosage Forms (*continued*)

Note: Content per capsule, tablet, or 5 mL, unless otherwise stated.

| Brand or generic name [availability] | Antihistamines | Decongestants | Antitussives Opioid | Antitussives Non-opioid | Expectorants | Analgesics | Other content information as per product label | Usual Adult and Adolescent Dose prn‡ | Usual Pediatric Dose prn | Packaging, Storage, and Auxiliary labeling§ |
|---|---|---|---|---|---|---|---|---|---|---|
| *Hydromet* Syrup (Schedule III) [U.S.] | | | Hydrocodone bitartrate 5 mg | | | | Homatropine MBr 1.5 mg** | 5 mL q 4–6 hr | | b, c, e, f |
| *Hydromine* Syrup (Schedule III) [U.S.] | | Phenylpropanolamine HCl 25 mg | Hydrocodone bitartrate 5 mg | | | | | 5 mL q 4 hr | Not intended for pediatric use. See *Hycomine Pediatric* | a, c, d, e, f |
| *Hydromine Pediatric* Syrup (Schedule III) [U.S.] | | Phenylpropanolamine HCl 12.5 mg | Hydrocodone bitartrate 2.5 mg | | | | | Intended for pediatric use | 6–12 yrs: 5 mL q 4 hr | a, c, d, e, f |
| *Hydropane* Syrup (Schedule III) [U.S.] | | | Hydrocodone bitartrate 5 mg | | | | Homatropine MBr 1.5 mg** | 5 mL q 4–6 hr | <2 yrs: 1.25 mL, 2–12 yrs: 2.5 mL, q 4–6 hr | b, c, d, e, f |
| *Hydrophen* Oral Solution (Schedule III) [U.S.] | | Phenylpropanolamine HCl 25 mg | Hydrocodone bitartrate 5 mg | | | | | 5 mL q 4–6 hr | 6–12 yrs: 2.5 mL q 4–6 hr | b, c, d, e, f |
| *Improved Sino-Tuss* Tablets (OTC) [U.S.] | Chlorpheniramine maleate 2 mg | Phenylephrine HCl 5 mg | | Dextromethorphan HBr 10 mg | | Acetaminophen 100 mg, Salicylamide 227 mg | | 1 tab q 4 hr | Pediatric strength not available | b, e |

*Specific formulations may vary among the different manufacturers, check product labeling.
†Efficacy as expectorant has not been established.
‡Geriatric patients may be more sensitive to effects of usual adult dose.
§For appropriate *Packaging and storage* and *Auxiliary labeling* information refer to designated letters as follows:

a—Store below 40 °C (104 °F), preferably between 15 and 30 °C (59 and 86 °F), in a tight container, unless otherwise specified by manufacturer.
a¹—Store below 30 °C (86 °F), unless otherwise specified by manufacturer. Avoid exposure to excessive heat.
a²—Store below 25 °C (77 °F), unless otherwise specified by manufacturer.
b—Store below 40 °C (104 °F), preferably between 15 and 30 °C (59 and 86 °F), in a well-closed container, unless otherwise specified by manufacturer.
c—Protect from freezing.
d—Protect from light.
e—Auxiliary labeling: • May cause drowsiness. • Avoid alcoholic beverages.

f—Auxiliary labeling: • May be habit forming.
g—Auxiliary labeling: • Shake well.
h—Dispense in dropper bottle.
i—Chew well before swallowing.

**Included in subtherapeutic amount to discourage deliberate overdosage.

## Table 3. Oral Dosage Forms (*continued*)

Note: Content per capsule, tablet, or 5 mL, unless otherwise stated.

| Brand or generic name [availability] | Antihistamines | Decongestants | Antitussives Opioid | Antitussives Non-opioid | Expectorants | Analgesics | Other content information as per product label | Usual Adult and Adolescent Dose prn‡ | Usual Pediatric Dose prn | Packaging, Storage, and Auxiliary labeling§ |
|---|---|---|---|---|---|---|---|---|---|---|
| *Iophen-C Liquid* Oral Solution (Schedule V) [U.S.] | | | Codeine PO₄ 10 mg | | Iodinated glycerol† 30 mg | | | 5–10 mL q 4 hr | 2–6 yrs: 1.25–2.5 mL, 6–12 yrs: 2.5–5 mL, q 4–6 hr | b, c, e, f |
| *Iophen DM* Oral Solution (Rx) [U.S.] | | | | Dextromethorphan HBr 10 mg | Iodinated glycerol† 30 mg | | | 5–10 mL q 4 hr | | b, c |
| *Ipsatol Cough Formula for Children* Syrup (OTC) [U.S.] | | Phenylpropanolamine HCl 9 mg | | Dextromethorphan HBr 10 mg | Guaifenesin 100 mg | | Alcohol free | Intended for pediatric use | 2–6 yrs: 2.5–5 mL, >6 yrs: 5–10 mL, q 4–6 hr | b, c |
| *Kiddy Koff* Syrup (OTC) [U.S.] | | Phenylpropanolamine HCl 6.25 mg | | Dextromethorphan HBr 5 mg | Guaifenesin 50 mg | | Alcohol 5% | Intended for pediatric use | 2–6 yrs: 5 mL, 6–12 yrs: 10 mL, q 4 hr | b, c |
| *KIE* Syrup (Rx) [U.S.] | | Ephedrine HCl 8 mg | | | Potassium iodide† 150 mg | | Alcohol free | 10 mL q 4 hr | 6–12 yrs: 5 mL, q 4 hr | b, c |
| *Kolephrin/DM Caplets* Tablets (OTC) [U.S.] | Chlorpheniramine maleate 2 mg | Pseudoephedrine HCl 30 mg | | Dextromethorphan HBr 10 mg | | Acetaminophen 325 mg | Caffeine 65 mg | 1 cap q 4–6 hr | Pediatric strength not available | b, e |
| *Kolephrin GG/DM* Oral Solution (OTC) [U.S.] | | | | Dextromethorphan HBr 10 mg | Guaifenesin 150 mg | | Alcohol free | 10 mL q 4 hr | 2–6 yrs: 2.5 mL, 6–12 yrs: 5 mL, q 4 hr | b, c |
| *Kolephrin NN Liquid* Oral Solution (OTC) [U.S.] | Pyrilamine maleate 10 mg | Phenylpropanolamine HCl 12.5 mg | | Dextromethorphan HBr 7.5 mg | | Sodium salicylate 325 mg | Alcohol free | 10 mL q 4 hr | 2–6 yrs: 2.5–5 mL, 6–12 yrs: 5–10 mL, q 6–8 hr | b, c, e |
| *Kophane* Syrup (OTC) [U.S.] | Chlorpheniramine maleate 0.5 mg | Phenylpropanolamine HCl 5 mg | | Dextromethorphan HBr 10 mg | Ammonium Cl† 90 mg | | Sucrose 1.7 gm | 10 mL q 4 hr | 2–6 yrs: 1.25–2.5 mL, 6–12 yrs: 2.5–5 mL, q 4 hr | b, c, e |

## Table 3. Oral Dosage Forms (continued)

Note: Content per capsule, tablet, or 5 mL, unless otherwise stated.

| Brand or generic name [availability] | Antihistamines | Decongestants | Antitussives — Opioid | Antitussives — Non-opioid | Expectorants | Analgesics | Other content information as per product label | Usual Adult and Adolescent Dose prn‡ | Usual Pediatric Dose prn | Packaging, Storage, and Auxiliary labeling§ |
|---|---|---|---|---|---|---|---|---|---|---|
| *Kophane Cough and Cold Formula* Oral Solution (OTC) [U.S.] | Chlorpheniramine maleate 2 mg | Phenylpropanolamine HCl 12.5 mg | | Dextromethorphan HBr 10 mg | | | Alcohol free | 10 mL q 4 hr | 3–12 mos: 1 drop/kg of body weight; 1–2 yrs: 3 drops/kg of body weight; 2–6 yrs: 2.5 mL, 6–12 yrs: 5 mL, q 4 hr | b, c, e |
| *Kwelcof Liquid* Oral Solution (Schedule III) [U.S.] | | | Hydrocodone bitartrate 5 mg | | Guaifenesin 100 mg | | Alcohol free Sugar free Dye free | 5 mL q 4–6 hr | 2–12 yrs: 2.5–5 mL q 4–6 hr | b, c, e, f |
| *Lanatuss Expectorant* Oral Solution (OTC) [U.S.] | Chlorpheniramine maleate 2 mg | Phenylpropanolamine HCl 5 mg | | | Guaifenesin 100 mg, Sodium citrate† 197 mg, Citric acid† 60 mg | | Sugar free | 5 mL q 6–8 hr | 2–6 yrs: 1.25–2.5 mL, 6–12 yrs: 2.5–5 mL, q 6–8 hr | b, c, e |
| *Mapap Cold Formula* Tablets (OTC) [U.S.] | Chlorpheniramine maleate 2 mg | Pseudoephedrine HCl 30 mg | | Dextromethorphan HBr 15 mg | | Acetaminophen 325 mg | | 2 tabs q 6 hr | 6–12 yrs: 1 tab q 6 hr | b, e |

*Specific formulations may vary among the different manufacturers, check product labeling.
†Efficacy as expectorant has not been established.
‡Geriatric patients may be more sensitive to effects of usual adult dose.
§For appropriate *Packaging and storage* and *Auxiliary labeling* information refer to designated letters as follows:
a—Store below 40 °C (104 °F), preferably between 15 and 30 °C (59 and 86 °F), in a tight container, unless otherwise specified by manufacturer.
a¹—Store below 30 °C (86 °F), unless otherwise specified by manufacturer. Avoid exposure to excessive heat.
a²—Store below 25 °C (77 °F), unless otherwise specified by manufacturer.
b—Store below 40 °C (104 °F), preferably between 15 and 30 °C (59 and 86 °F), in a well-closed container, unless otherwise specified by manufacturer.
c—Protect from freezing.
d—Protect from light.
e—Auxiliary labeling: • May cause drowsiness. • Avoid alcoholic beverages.
f—Auxiliary labeling: • May be habit forming.
g—Auxiliary labeling: • Shake well.
h—Dispense in dropper bottle.
i—Chew well before swallowing.
**Included in subtherapeutic amount to discourage deliberate overdosage.

## Table 3. Oral Dosage Forms (continued)

Note: Content per capsule, tablet, or 5 mL, unless otherwise stated.

| Brand or generic name [availability] | Antihistamines | Decongestants | Antitussives Opioid | Antitussives Non-opioid | Expectorants | Analgesics | Other content information as per product label | Usual Adult and Adolescent Dose prn‡ | Usual Pediatric Dose prn | Packaging, Storage, and Auxiliary labeling§ |
|---|---|---|---|---|---|---|---|---|---|---|
| Marcof Expectorant Syrup (Schedule III) [U.S.] | | | Hydrocodone bitartrate 5 mg | | Potassium guaiacol-sulfonate† 300 mg | | | 5–7.5 mL qid | | b, c, e, f |
| Meda Syrup Forte Syrup (OTC) [U.S.] | Chlorpheniramine maleate 1 mg | Phenylephrine HCl 5 mg | | Dextromethorphan HBr 15 mg | Guaifenesin 100 mg | | Alcohol free | 5–10 mL q 4–6 hr | 6–12 yrs: 2.5–5 mL q 4–6 hr | b, c, e, |
| Medi-Flu Oral Solution (OTC) [U.S.] | Chlorpheniramine maleate 0.67 mg (4 mg/30 mL) | Pseudoephedrine HCl 10 mg (60 mg/30 mL) | | Dextromethorphan HBr 5 mg (30 mg/30 mL) | | Acetaminophen 167 mg (1002 mg/30 mL) | Alcohol 19% | 30 mL q 6 hr | Intended for adult use | b, c, e |
| Medi-Flu Caplets Tablets (OTC) [U.S.] | Chlorpheniramine maleate 2 mg | Pseudoephedrine HCl 30 mg | | Dextromethorphan HBr 15 mg | | Acetaminophen 500 mg | | 2 tabs q 6 hr | Intended for adult use | b, e |
| Mediquell Decongestant Formula Chewable Tablets (OTC) [U.S.] | | Pseudoephedrine HCl 30 mg | | Dextromethorphan HBr 15 mg | | | | 2 tabs q 6 hr | 2–6 yrs: ½ tab, 6–12 yrs: 1 tab, q 6 hr | b, i |
| Midahist DH Elixir (Schedule V) [U.S.] | Chlorpheniramine maleate 2 mg | Pseudoephedrine HCl 30 mg | Codeine PO4 10 mg | | | | Alcohol 5% | 10 mL q 4 hr | 2–6 yrs: 1.25–2.5 mL, 6–12 yrs: 2.5–5 mL, q 6 hr | a, c, e, f |
| Mycotussin Oral Solution (Schedule III) [U.S.] | | Pseudoephedrine HCl 60 mg | Hydrocodone bitartrate 5 mg | | | | Alcohol 5% | 5 mL q 4–6 hr | 2–6 yrs: 1.25 mL, 6–12 yrs: 2.5 mL, q 4–6 hr | b, c, d, e, f |
| Myhistine DH Elixir (Schedule V) [U.S.] | Chlorpheniramine maleate 2 mg | Pseudoephedrine HCl 30 mg | Codeine PO4 10 mg | | | | Alcohol 5% | 10 mL q 4 hr | 2–6 yrs: 1.25–2.5 mL, 6–12 yrs: 2.5–5 mL, q 6 hr | a, c, e, f |
| Myhistine Expectorant Oral Solution (Schedule V) [U.S.] | | Pseudoephedrine HCl 30 mg | Codeine PO4 10 mg | | Guaifenesin 100 mg | | Alcohol 7.5% | 10 mL q 4 hr | 2–6 yrs: 2.5 mL, 6–12 yrs: 5 mL, q 4 hr | a, c, e, f |

## Table 3. Oral Dosage Forms (continued)

Note: Content per capsule, tablet, or 5 mL, unless otherwise stated.

| Brand or generic name [availability] | Antihistamines | Decongestants | Antitussives Opioid | Antitussives Non-opioid | Expectorants | Analgesics | Other content information as per product label | Usual Adult and Adolescent Dose prn‡ | Usual Pediatric Dose prn | Packaging, Storage, and Auxiliary labeling§ |
|---|---|---|---|---|---|---|---|---|---|---|
| Myhydromine Syrup (Schedule III) [U.S.] | | Phenylpropanolamine HCl 25 mg | Hydrocodone bitartrate 5 mg | | | | | 5 mL q 4 hr | 6–12 yrs: 2.5 mL q 4–6 hr | a, c, d, e, f |
| Myhydromine Pediatric Syrup (Schedule III) [U.S.] | | Phenylpropanolamine HCl 12.5 mg | Hydrocodone bitartrate 2.5 mg | | | | | Intended for pediatric use. See *Myhydromine Syrup* | 6–12 yrs: 5 mL q 4 hr | a, c, d, e, f |
| Myminic Expectorant Oral Solution (OTC) [U.S.] | | Phenylpropanolamine HCl 12.5 mg | | | Guaifenesin 100 mg | | Alcohol 5% | 10 mL q 4 hr | | b, c |
| Myminicol Oral Solution (OTC) [U.S.] | Chlorpheniramine maleate 2 mg | Phenylpropanolamine HCl 12.5 mg | | Dextromethorphan HBr 10 mg | | | Alcohol free | 10 mL q 4 hr | | b, c, e |
| Myphetane DC Cough Syrup (Schedule V) [U.S.] | Brompheniramine maleate 2 mg | Phenylpropanolamine HCl 12.5 mg | Codeine $PO_4$ 10 mg | | | | Alcohol 1.2% | 10 mL q 4 hr | 2–6 yrs: 2.5 mL, 6–12 yrs: 5 mL, q 4 hr | a, c, d, e, f |
| Myphetane DX Cough Syrup (Rx) [U.S.] | Brompheniramine maleate 2 mg | Pseudoephedrine HCl 30 mg | | Dextromethorphan HBr 10 mg | | | Alcohol 1% | 10 mL q 4 hr | | b, c, e |
| Mytussin AC Oral Solution (Schedule V) [U.S.] | | | Codeine $PO_4$ 10 mg | | Guaifenesin 100 mg | | Alcohol 3.5% | 10 mL q 4 hr | 2–6 yrs: 2.5 mL, 6–12 yrs: 5 mL, q 4 hr | b, c, e, f |

*Specific formulations may vary among the different manufacturers, check product labeling.

‡Efficacy as expectorant has not been established.

†Geriatric patients may be more sensitive to effects of usual adult dose.

§For appropriate *Packaging and storage* and *Auxiliary labeling* information refer to designated letters as follows:

a—Store below 40 °C (104 °F), preferably between 15 and 30 °C (59 and 86 °F), in a tight container, unless otherwise specified by manufacturer.
a¹—Store below 30 °C (86 °F), unless otherwise specified by manufacturer. Avoid exposure to excessive heat.
a²—Store below 25 °C (77 °F), unless otherwise specified by manufacturer
b—Store below 40 °C (104 °F), preferably between 15 and 30 °C (59 and 86 °F), in a well-closed container, unless otherwise specified by manufacturer.
c—Protect from freezing.    f—Auxiliary labeling: • May be habit forming.    h—Dispense in dropper bottle.
d—Protect from light.    g—Auxiliary labeling: • Shake well.    i—Chew well before swallowing.
e—Auxiliary labeling: • May cause drowsiness. • Avoid alcoholic beverages.

**Included in subtherapeutic amount to discourage deliberate overdosage.

Table 3. Oral Dosage Forms (continued)

Note: Content per capsule, tablet, or 5 mL, unless otherwise stated.

| Brand or generic name [availability] | Antihistamines | Decongestants | Antitussives Opioid | Antitussives Non-opioid | Expectorants | Analgesics | Other content information as per product label | Usual Adult and Adolescent Dose prn‡ | Usual Pediatric Dose prn | Packaging, Storage, and Auxiliary labeling§ |
|---|---|---|---|---|---|---|---|---|---|---|
| *Mytussin DAC* Oral Solution (Schedule V) [U.S.] | | Pseudoephedrine HCl 30 mg | Codeine PO$_4$ 10 mg | | Guaifenesin 100 mg | | Alcohol 1.7% Sugar free | 10 mL q 4 hr | 2–6 yrs: 2.5 mL, 6–12 yrs: 5 mL, q 4 hr | a, c, e, f |
| *Mytussin DM* Oral Solution (OTC) [U.S.] | | | | Dextromethorphan HBr 10 mg | Guaifenesin 100 mg | | Alcohol 1.6% | 10 mL q 4 hr | 2–6 yrs: 2.5 mL, 6–12 yrs: 5 mL, q 6–8 hr | a, c, d, e |
| *Naldecon-CX Adult Liquid* Oral Suspension (Schedule V) [U.S.] | | Phenylpropanolamine HCl 12.5 mg | Codeine PO$_4$ 10 mg | | Guaifenesin 200 mg | | Alcohol free Sugar free | 10 mL q 4–6 hr | 2–6 yrs: 1.25–2.5 mL, 6–12 yrs: 2.5–5 mL, q 4–6 hr | b, c, e, f, g |
| *Naldecon-DX Adult Liquid* Oral Solution (OTC) [U.S.] | | Phenylpropanolamine HCl 12.5 mg | | Dextromethorphan HBr 10 mg | Guaifenesin 200 mg | | Alcohol free Sugar free | 10 mL q 4–6 hr | Not intended for pediatric use | b, c |
| *Naldecon-DX Children's Syrup* (OTC) [U.S.] | | Phenylpropanolamine HCl 6.25 mg | | Dextromethorphan HBr 5 mg | Guaifenesin 100 mg | | Alcohol 0.6% | Intended for pediatric use | 2–6 yrs: 5 mL, >6 yrs: 10 mL, q 4–6 hr | b, c |
| *Naldecon-DX Pediatric Drops* Oral Solution (OTC) [U.S.] | | Phenylpropanolamine HCl 6.25 mg/mL | | Dextromethorphan HBr 5 mg/mL | Guaifenesin 50 mg/mL | | Alcohol free Sugar free | Intended for pediatric use | >2 yrs: 1 mL q 4 hr | b, c |
| *Naldecon-EX Syrup* (OTC) [U.S.] | | Phenylpropanolamine HCl 9 mg | | | Guaifenesin 100 mg | | Alcohol free | Intended for pediatric use | 2–6 yrs: 5 mL, 6–12 yrs: 10 mL, q 4 hr | b, c |
| *Naldecon-EX Pediatric Drops* Oral Solution (OTC) [U.S.] | | Phenylpropanolamine HCl 6.25 mg/mL | | | Guaifenesin 50 mg/mL | | Alcohol free Sugar free | Intended for pediatric use | 1–3 mos: 0.25 mL, 4–6 mos: 0.5 mL, 7–9 mos: 0.75 mL, >10 mos: 1 mL q 4–6 hr | b, c, h |

Table 3. Oral Dosage Forms (*continued*)

Note: Content per capsule, tablet, or 5 mL, unless otherwise stated.

| Brand or generic name [availability] | Antihistamines | Decongestants | Antitussives — Opioid | Antitussives — Non-opioid | Expectorants | Analgesics | Other content information as per product label | Usual Adult and Adolescent Dose prn‡ | Usual Pediatric Dose prn | Packaging, Storage, and Auxiliary labeling§ |
|---|---|---|---|---|---|---|---|---|---|---|
| *Naldecon Senior DX* Oral Solution (OTC) [U.S.] | | | | Dextromethorphan HBr 15 mg | Guaifenesin 200 mg | | Alcohol free | 10 mL q 4 hr | 2–6 yrs: 1.25–2.5 mL, 6–12 yrs: 2.5–5 mL, q 6–8 hr | b, c |
| *Naldelate DX Adult* Oral Solution (OTC) [U.S.] | | Phenylpropanolamine HCl 12.5 mg | | Dextromethorphan HBr 10 mg | Guaifenesin 200 mg | | | 10 mL q 4 hr | | b, c |
| *Nasabid* Extended-release Capsules (Rx) [U.S.] | | Pseudoephedrine HCl 90 mg | | | Guaifenesin 250 mg | | | 1 cap q 12 hr | Not recommended | a, d |
| *Nasatab LA* Extended-release Tablets (Rx) [U.S.] | | Pseudoephedrine HCl 120 mg | | | Guaifenesin 500 mg | | Scored Dye free | 1 tab q 12 hr | | b, c |
| *Nasatuss* Syrup (Schedule III) [U.S.] | Chlorpheniramine maleate 2 mg | Phenylephrine HCl 5 mg | Hydrocodone bitartrate 2.5 mg | | | | | 10 mL q 4 hr | 6–12 yrs: 5 mL q 4 hr | b, c, e, f |
| *NeoCitran DM Coughs and Colds* for Oral Solution (OTC) [Canada] | Pheniramine maleate 20 mg/ pouch | Phenylephrine HCl 10 mg/pouch | | Dextromethorphan HBr 30 mg/ pouch | | | Vitamin C 50 mg, Tartrazine | 1 pouch dissolved in 8 oz boiling water q 6–8 hr (max 3 pouches daily) | | e |

*Specific formulations may vary among the different manufacturers; check product labeling.

†Efficacy as expectorant has not been established.

‡Geriatric patients may be more sensitive to effects of usual adult dose.

§For appropriate *Packaging and storage* and *Auxiliary labeling* information refer to designated letters as follows:

  a—Store below 40 °C (104 °F), preferably between 15 and 30 °C (59 and 86 °F), in a tight container, unless otherwise specified by manufacturer.

  a¹—Store below 30 °C (86 °F), unless otherwise specified by manufacturer. Avoid exposure to excessive heat.

  a²—Store below 25 °C (77 °F), unless otherwise specified by manufacturer.

  b—Store below 40 °C (104 °F), preferably between 15 and 30 °C (59 and 86 °F), in a well-closed container, unless otherwise specified by manufacturer.

  c—Protect from freezing.

  d—Protect from light.

  e—Auxiliary labeling: • May cause drowsiness. • Avoid alcoholic beverages.

  f—Auxiliary labeling: • May be habit forming.

  g—Auxiliary labeling: • Shake well.

  h—Dispense in dropper bottle.

  i—Chew well before swallowing.

**Included in subtherapeutic amount to discourage deliberate overdosage.

Table 3. Oral Dosage Forms (*continued*)
Note: Content per capsule, tablet, or 5 mL, unless otherwise stated.

| Brand or generic name [availability] | Antihistamines | Decongestants | Antitussives — Opioid | Antitussives — Non-opioid | Expectorants | Analgesics | Other content information as per product label | Usual Adult and Adolescent Dose prn‡ | Usual Pediatric Dose prn | Packaging, Storage, and Auxiliary labeling§ |
|---|---|---|---|---|---|---|---|---|---|---|
| *Nolex LA* Extended-release Tablets (Rx) [U.S.] | | Phenylpropanolamine HCl 75 mg | | | Guaifenesin 400 mg | | Scored | 1 tab q 12 hr | 6–12 yrs: ½ tab q 12 hr | b |
| *Norastus II Liquid* Oral Solution (OTC) [U.S.] | | Pseudoephedrine HCl 15 mg | | Dextromethorphan HBr 3.75 mg | Guaifenesin 50 mg | | Alcohol free Sodium free Sugar free | Intended for pediatric use | 2–6 yrs: 5 mL, 6–12 yrs: 10 mL, q 4 hr | b, c |
| *Normatane DC* Syrup (Schedule V) [U.S.] | Brompheniramine maleate 2 mg | Phenylpropanolamine HCl 12.5 mg | Codeine PO$_4$ 10 mg | | | | Alcohol 0.95% | 10 mL q 4 hr | 2–6 yrs: 2.5 mL, 6–12 yrs: 5 mL, q 4 hr | a, c, d, e, f |
| *Nortussin with Codeine* Oral Solution (Schedule V) [U.S.] | | | Codeine PO$_4$ 10 mg | | Guaifenesin 100 mg | | Alcohol 3.5% | 5 mL q 3–4 hr | 2–6 yrs: 1.25–2.5 mL, 6–12 yrs: 2.5–5 mL, q 4–6 hr | b, c, e, f |
| *Novagest Expectorant w/Codeine* Oral Solution (Schedule V) [U.S.] | | Pseudoephedrine HCl 30 mg | Codeine PO$_4$ 10 mg | | Guaifenesin 100 mg | | Alcohol 1.4% | 10 mL q 4 hr | | b, c, f |
| *Novahistex C* Oral Solution (N) [Canada] | | Phenylephrine HCl 20 mg | Codeine PO$_4$ 15 mg | | | | Alcohol free | 5 mL q 4–6 hr | 6–12 yrs: 2.5 mL q 4–6 hr | b, c, e, f |
| *Novahistex DH* Oral Solution (N) [Canada] | | Phenylephrine HCl 20 mg | Hydrocodone bitartrate 5 mg | | | | Alcohol free | 5 mL q 4 hr | 1–12 yrs: 1.25–2.5 mL q 4 hr | b, c, e, f |
| *Novahistex DH Expectorant* Oral Solution (N) [Canada] | | Phenylephrine HCl 20 mg | Hydrocodone bitartrate 5 mg | | Guaifenesin 200 mg | | Alcohol free Fructose 10%, Glucose 14.3% | 5 mL q 4 hr | 2–6 yrs: 1.25 mL, 6–12 yrs: 2.5 mL, q 6 hr. See also *Novahistine Expectorant* Oral Solution | b, c, e, f |

Table 3. Oral Dosage Forms *(continued)*
Note: Content per capsule, tablet, or 5 mL, unless otherwise stated.

| Brand or generic name [availability] | Antihistamines | Decongestants | Antitussives Opioid | Antitussives Non-opioid | Expectorants | Analgesics | Other content information as per product label | Usual Adult and Adolescent Dose prn‡ | Usual Pediatric Dose prn | Packaging, Storage, and Auxiliary labeling§ |
|---|---|---|---|---|---|---|---|---|---|---|
| *Novahistex DM* Syrup (OTC) [Canada] | | Pseudoephedrine HCl 30 mg | | Dextromethorphan HBr 15 mg | | | | 10 mL q 4 hr | 6–12 yrs: 5 mL q 6 hr | b, c, e |
| *Novahistex DM Expectorant w/ Decongestant* Oral Solution (OTC) [Canada] | | Pseudoephedrine HCl 30 mg | | Dextromethorphan HBr 15 mg | Guaifenesin 100 mg | | Alcohol free | 10 mL q 4–6 hr (max 40 mL daily) | | b |
| *Novahistex Expectorant w/ Decongestant* Oral Solution (OTC) [Canada] | | Pseudoephedrine HCl 30 mg | | | Guaifenesin 100 mg | | Alcohol free | 10 mL q 4–6 hr (max 40 mL daily) | | b |
| *Novahistine DH* Oral Solution (N) [Canada] | | Phenylephrine HCl 10 mg | Hydrocodone bitartrate 1.7 mg | | | | Alcohol free | 10 mL q 4 hr | 6 mos–1 yr: 1.25–2.5 mL, 1–12 yrs: 2.5–5 mL, q 4 hr | b, c, e, f |
| *Novahistine DH Liquid* Oral Solution (Schedule V) [U.S.] | Chlorpheniramine maleate 2 mg | Pseudoephedrine HCl 30 mg | Codeine PO₄ 10 mg | | | | Alcohol 5% | 10 mL q 4–6 hr | 2–6 yrs: 1.25–2.5 mL, 6–12 yrs: 2.5–5 mL, q 4–6 hr | a, c, d, e, f |

*Specific formulations may vary among the different manufacturers; check product labeling.
†Efficacy as expectorant has not been established.
‡Geriatric patients may be more sensitive to effects of usual adult dose.
§For appropriate *Packaging and storage* and *Auxiliary labeling* information refer to designated letters as follows:
 a—Store below 40 °C (104 °F), preferably between 15 and 30 °C (59 and 86 °F), in a tight container, unless otherwise specified by manufacturer.
 a¹—Store below 30 °C (86 °F), unless otherwise specified by manufacturer. Avoid exposure to excessive heat.
 a²—Store below 25 °C (77 °F), unless otherwise specified by manufacturer.
 b—Store below 40 °C (104 °F), preferably between 15 and 30 °C (59 and 86 °F), in a well-closed container, unless otherwise specified by manufacturer.
 c—Protect from freezing.
 d—Protect from light.
 e—Auxiliary labeling: • May cause drowsiness. • Avoid alcoholic beverages.
 f—Auxiliary labeling: • May be habit forming.
 g—Auxiliary labeling: • Shake well.
 h—Dispense in dropper bottle.
 i—Chew well before swallowing.
**Included in subtherapeutic amount to discourage deliberate overdosage.

Table 3. Oral Dosage Forms (*continued*)
Note: Content per capsule, tablet, or 5 mL, unless otherwise stated.

| Brand or generic name [availability] | Antihistamines | Decongestants | Antitussives — Opioid | Antitussives — Non-opioid | Expectorants | Analgesics | Other content information as per product label | Usual Adult and Adolescent Dose prn‡ | Usual Pediatric Dose prn | Packaging, Storage, and Auxiliary labeling§ |
|---|---|---|---|---|---|---|---|---|---|---|
| *Novahistine DM w/ Decongestant* Oral Solution (OTC) [Canada] | | Pseudoephedrine HCl 15 mg | | Dextromethorphan HBr 7.5 mg | | | Alcohol free | | 2–5 yrs: 5 mL (max 20 mL daily), 6–12 yrs: 10 mL (max 40 mL daily), q 4–6 hr | a |
| *Novahistine DM Expectorant w/ Decongestant* Oral Solution (OTC) [Canada] | | Pseudoephedrine HCl 15 mg | | Dextromethorphan HBr 7.5 mg | Guaifenesin 50 mg | | Alcohol free | | 2–5 yrs: 5 mL (max 20 mL daily), 6–12 yrs: 10 mL (max 40 mL daily), q 4–6 hr | a |
| *Novahistine DMX Liquid* Oral Solution (OTC) [U.S.] | | Pseudoephedrine HCl 30 mg | | Dextromethorphan HBr 10 mg | Guaifenesin 100 mg | | Alcohol 10% | 10 mL q 4–6 hr | 2–6 yrs: 2.5 mL, 6–12 yrs: 5 mL, q 4–6 hr | b, c |
| *Novahistine Expectorant* Oral Solution (Schedule V) [U.S.] | | Pseudoephedrine HCl 30 mg | Codeine PO$_4$ 10 mg | | Guaifenesin 100 mg | | Alcohol 7.5% | 10 mL q 4–6 hr | 2–6 yrs: 2.5 mL, 6–12 yrs: 5 mL, q 4–6 hr | a, c, e, f |
| *Nucochem* Capsules (Schedule III) [U.S.] | | Pseudoephedrine HCl 60 mg | Codeine PO$_4$ 20 mg | | | | | 1 cap q 6 hr | Pediatric strength not available. See *Nucochem* Syrup | b, e, f |
| Syrup (Schedule III) [U.S.] | | Pseudoephedrine HCl 60 mg | Codeine PO$_4$ 20 mg | | | | | 5 mL q 6 hr | 2–6 yrs: 1.25 mL, 6–12 yrs: 2.5 mL, q 6 hr | b, c, e, f |

## Table 3. Oral Dosage Forms (continued)

Note: Content per capsule, tablet, or 5 mL, unless otherwise stated.

| Brand or generic name [availability] | Antihistamines | Decongestants | Antitussives Opioid | Antitussives Non-opioid | Expectorants | Analgesics | Other content information as per product label | Usual Adult and Adolescent Dose prn‡ | Usual Pediatric Dose prn | Packaging, Storage, and Auxiliary labeling§ |
|---|---|---|---|---|---|---|---|---|---|---|
| *Nucochem Expectorant Syrup* (Schedule III) [U.S.] | | Pseudoephedrine HCl 60 mg | Codeine PO$_4$ 20 mg | | Guaifenesin 200 mg | | Alcohol 12.5% | 5 mL q 6 hr | 2–6 yrs: 1.25 mL, 6–12 yrs: 2.5 mL, q 6 hr | b, c, e, f |
| *Nucochem Pediatric Expectorant Syrup* (Schedule V) [U.S.] | | Pseudoephedrine HCl 30 mg | Codeine PO$_4$ 10 mg | | Guaifenesin 100 mg | | Alcohol 6% | 10 mL q 6 hr | 2–6 yrs: 2.5 mL, 6–12 yrs: 5 mL, q 6 hr | b, c, e, f |
| *Nucofed* Capsules (Schedule III) [U.S.] | | Pseudoephedrine HCl 60 mg | Codeine PO$_4$ 20 mg | | | | | 1 cap q 6 hr | Pediatric strength not available. See *Nucofed* Syrup. | b, e, f |
| Syrup (Schedule III) [U.S.] | | Pseudoephedrine HCl 60 mg | Codeine PO$_4$ 20 mg | | | | Alcohol free, Sucrose 2.25 gm/5 mL | 5 mL q 6 hr | 2–6 yrs: 0.62–1.25 mL, 6–12 yrs: 1.25–2.5 mL, q 6 hr | b, c, e, f |
| *Nucofed Expectorant Syrup* (Schedule III) [U.S.] | | Pseudoephedrine HCl 60 mg | Codeine PO$_4$ 20 mg | | Guaifenesin 200 mg | | Alcohol 12.5% | 5 mL q 6 hr | 2–6 yrs: 1.25 mL, 6–12 yrs: 2.5 mL, q 6 hr | b, c, e, f |

*Specific formulations may vary among the different manufacturers; check product labeling.

†Efficacy as expectorant has not been established.

‡Geriatric patients may be more sensitive to effects of usual adult dose.

§For appropriate *Packaging and storage* and *Auxiliary labeling* information refer to designated letters as follows:

a—Store below 40 °C (104 °F), preferably between 15 and 30 °C (59 and 86 °F), in a tight container, unless otherwise specified by manufacturer.

a¹—Store below 30 °C (86 °F), unless otherwise specified by manufacturer. Avoid exposure to excessive heat.

a²—Store below 25 °C (77 °F), unless otherwise specified by manufacturer.

b—Store below 40 °C (104 °F), preferably between 15 and 30 °C (59 and 86 °F), in a well-closed container, unless otherwise specified by manufacturer.

c—Protect from freezing.

d—Protect from light.

e—Auxiliary labeling: • May cause drowsiness. • Avoid alcoholic beverages.

f—Auxiliary labeling: • May be habit forming.

g—Auxiliary labeling: • Shake well.

h—Dispense in dropper bottle.

i—Chew well before swallowing.

**Included in subtherapeutic amount to discourage deliberate overdosage.

## Table 3. Oral Dosage Forms (continued)

Note: Content per capsule, tablet, or 5 mL, unless otherwise stated.

| Brand or generic name [availability] | Antihistamines | Decongestants | Antitussives — Opioid | Antitussives — Non-opioid | Expectorants | Analgesics | Other content information as per product label | Usual Adult and Adolescent Dose prn‡ | Usual Pediatric Dose prn | Packaging, Storage, and Auxiliary labeling§ |
|---|---|---|---|---|---|---|---|---|---|---|
| Nucofed Pediatric Expectorant Syrup (Schedule V) [U.S.] | | Pseudoephedrine HCl 30 mg | Codeine PO₄ 10 mg | | Guaifenesin 100 mg | | Alcohol 6% | 10 mL q 4–6 hr | 2–6 yrs: 1.25–2.5 mL; 6–12 yrs: 2.5–5 mL, q 4–6 hr | a, c, e, f |
| Nucotuss Expectorant Syrup (Schedule III) [U.S.] | | Pseudoephedrine HCl 60 mg | Codeine PO₄ 20 mg | | Guaifenesin 200 mg | | Alcohol 12.5% | 5 mL q 6 hr | | b, c, e, f |
| Nucotuss Pediatric Expectorant Syrup (Schedule V) [U.S.] | | Pseudoephedrine HCl 30 mg | Codeine PO₄ 10 mg | | Guaifenesin 100 mg | | Alcohol 6% | | 2–<12 yrs: 2.5–5 mL q 6 hr | b, c, e, f |
| Nytcold Medicine Oral Solution (OTC) [U.S.] | Doxylamine succinate 1.25 mg | Pseudoephedrine HCl 10 mg | | Dextromethorphan HBr 5 mg | | Acetaminophen 167 mg | Alcohol 25% | 30 mL or 30 mL q 6 hr | | b, c, e |
| Nytime Cold Medicine Liquid Oral Solution (OTC) [U.S.] | Doxylamine succinate 1.2 mg (7.5 mg/30 mL) | Pseudoephedrine HCl 10 mg (60 mg/30 mL) | | Dextromethorphan HBr 5 mg (30 mg/30 mL) | | Acetaminophen 166.6 mg (1000 mg/30 mL) | Alcohol 25% | 30 mL hs or q 6 hr | Not recommended | b, c, e |
| Omnicol Tablets (Rx) [U.S.] | Chlorpheniramine maleate 4 mg, Phenindamine tartrate 4 mg | Phenylephrine HCl 5 mg | | Dextromethorphan HBr 15 mg | | Acetaminophen 100 mg, Salicylamide 227 mg | Caffeine 10 mg, Ascorbic acid 25 mg Sugar coated | 1 tab q 4 hr | Pediatric strength not available | b, e |
| Omni-Tuss Oral Suspension (N) [Canada] | Chlorpheniramine 3 mg, Phenyltoloxamine 5 mg (as cation exchange resin complexes) | Ephedrine 25 mg (as cation exchange resin complex) | Codeine 10 mg (as cation exchange resin complex) | | Guaiacol carbonate† 20 mg | | Sodium 20 mg | 5 mL q 12 hr | 6–12 yrs: 2.5 mL, q 12 hr | b, c, e, f, g |
| Ordrine AT Extended-release Capsules (Rx) [U.S.] | | Phenylpropanolamine HCl 75 mg | | Caramiphen edisylate 40 mg | | | | 1 cap q 12 hr | | b |

Table 3. Oral Dosage Forms (*continued*)
Note: Content per capsule, tablet, or 5 mL, unless otherwise stated.

| Brand or generic name [availability] | Antihistamines | Decongestants | Antitussives — Opioid | Antitussives — Non-opioid | Expectorants | Analgesics | Other content information as per product label | Usual Adult and Adolescent Dose prn‡ | Usual Pediatric Dose prn | Packaging, Storage, and Auxiliary labeling§ |
|---|---|---|---|---|---|---|---|---|---|---|
| *Ornade-DM 10* Oral Solution (OTC) [Canada] | Chlorpheniramine maleate 2 mg | Phenylpropanolamine HCl 15 mg | | Dextromethorphan HBr 10 mg | | | Alcohol 4.7% Sugar free | Intended for pediatric use. See *Ornade-DM 15* and *Ornade DM 30* Oral Solution | 1–5 yrs: 2.5 mL; 6–12 yrs: 5 mL, q 6 hr | b, c, e |
| *Ornade-DM 15* Oral Solution (OTC) [Canada] | Chlorpheniramine maleate 2 mg | Phenylpropanolamine HCl 15 mg | | Dextromethorphan HBr 15 mg | | | Alcohol 3.8% Sugar free | 5–10 mL q 6–8 hr | 2–4 yrs: 1.25 mL, 4–9 yrs: 2.5 mL, 9–12 yrs: 2.5–5 mL, q 6–8 hr | b, c, e |
| *Ornade-DM 30* Oral Solution (OTC) [Canada] | Chlorpheniramine maleate 2 mg | Phenylpropanolamine HCl 15 mg | | Dextromethorphan HBr 30 mg | | | Alcohol free Sugar free | 5 mL q 6–8 hr | Not intended for pediatric use. See *Ornade-DM 10* and *Ornade-DM 15* Oral Solution | b, c, e |
| *Ornade Expectorant* Oral Solution (OTC) [Canada] | Chlorpheniramine maleate 2 mg | Phenylpropanolamine HCl 15 mg | | | Guaifenesin 100 mg | | Alcohol 7% Sugar free | 5–10 mL q 6–8 hr | 1–6 yrs: 2.5 mL, 6–12 yrs: 5 mL, q 6–8 hr | b, c, e |

*Specific formulations may vary among the different manufacturers; check product labeling.
†Efficacy as expectorant has not been established.
‡Geriatric patients may be more sensitive to effects of usual adult dose.
§For appropriate *Packaging and storage* and *Auxiliary labeling* information refer to designated letters as follows:
  a—Store below 40 °C (104 °F), preferably between 15 and 30 °C (59 and 86 °F), in a tight container, unless otherwise specified by manufacturer.
  a¹—Store below 30 °C (86 °F), unless otherwise specified by manufacturer. Avoid exposure to excessive heat.
  a²—Store below 25 °C (77 °F), unless otherwise specified by manufacturer.
  b—Store below 40 °C (104 °F), preferably between 15 and 30 °C (59 and 86 °F), in a well-closed container, unless otherwise specified by manufacturer.
  c—Protect from freezing.
  d—Protect from light.
  e—Auxiliary labeling: • May cause drowsiness. • Avoid alcoholic beverages.
  f—Auxiliary labeling: • May be habit forming.
  g—Auxiliary labeling: • Shake well.
  h—Dispense in dropper bottle.
  i—Chew well before swallowing.
**Included in subtherapeutic amount to discourage deliberate overdosage.

**Table 3. Oral Dosage Forms** *(continued)*
Note: Content per capsule, tablet, or 5 mL, unless otherwise stated.

| Brand or generic name [availability] | Antihistamines | Decongestants | Antitussives — Opioid | Antitussives — Non-opioid | Expectorants | Analgesics | Other content information as per product label | Usual Adult and Adolescent Dose prn‡ | Usual Pediatric Dose prn | Packaging, Storage, and Auxiliary labeling§ |
|---|---|---|---|---|---|---|---|---|---|---|
| *Ornex Severe Cold No Drowsiness Caplets* (OTC) [U.S.] | | Pseudoephedrine HCl 30 mg | | Dextromethorphan HBr 15 mg | | Acetaminophen 500 mg | | 2 tabs q 6 hr | | b |
| *Orthoxicol Cough Syrup* (OTC) [U.S.] | Chlorpheniramine maleate 1.3 mg (4 mg/15 mL) | Phenylpropanolamine HCl 8.3 mg (25 mg/15 mL) | | Dextromethorphan HBr 6.6 mg (20 mg/15 mL) | | | Alcohol 8% | 15 mL q 4 hr | Pediatric strength not available | b, c, e |
| *Para-Hist HD* Oral Solution (Schedule III) [U.S.] | Chlorpheniramine maleate 2 mg | Phenylephrine HCl 5 mg | Hydrocodone bitartrate 1.67 mg | | | | | 10 mL q 6-8 hr | | b, c, e, f |
| *Partuss LA* Extended-release Tablets (Rx) [U.S.] | | Phenylpropanolamine HCl 75 mg | | | Guaifenesin 400 mg | | | 1 tab q 12 hr | | b |
| *PediaCare Children's Cough-Cold* Chewable Tablets (OTC) [U.S.] | Chlorpheniramine maleate 1 mg | Pseudoephedrine HCl 15 mg | | Dextromethorphan HBr 5 mg | | | Phenylalanine 6 mg | Intended for pediatric use | 6-11 yrs: 4 tabs q 4-6 hr | b, e, i |
| *PediaCare Cough-Cold* Oral Solution (OTC) [U.S.] | Chlorpheniramine maleate 1 mg | Pseudoephedrine HCl 15 mg | | Dextromethorphan HBr 5 mg | | | Alcohol free | | 6-11 yrs: 10 mL q 4-6 hr | b, c, e |
| *PediaCare Night Rest Cough-Cold Liquid* Oral Solution (OTC) [U.S.] | Chlorpheniramine maleate 1 mg | Pseudoephedrine HCl 15 mg | | Dextromethorphan HBr 7.5 mg | | | Alcohol free | Intended for pediatric use | 6-11 yrs: 10 mL q 6-8 hr | b, c, e |
| *Pediacof Cough Syrup* (Schedule V) [U.S.] | Chlorpheniramine maleate 0.75 mg | Phenylephrine HCl 2.5 mg | Codeine PO$_4$ 5 mg | | Potassium iodide† 75 mg | | Alcohol 5% | Intended for pediatric use | 6 mos-1 yr: 1.25 mL, 1-3 yrs: 2.5-5 mL, 3-6 yrs: 5-10 mL, 6-12 yrs: 10 mL, q 4-6 hr | b, c, e, f |

## Table 3. Oral Dosage Forms (continued)

Note: Content per capsule, tablet, or 5 mL, unless otherwise stated.

| Brand or generic name [availability] | Antihistamines | Decongestants | Antitussives | | Expectorants | Analgesics | Other content information as per product label | Usual Adult and Adolescent Dose prn‡ | Usual Pediatric Dose prn | Packaging, Storage, and Auxiliary labeling§ |
|---|---|---|---|---|---|---|---|---|---|---|
| | | | Opioid | Non-opioid | | | | | | |
| *Pedituss Cough* Syrup (Schedule V) [U.S.] | Chlorpheniramine maleate .75 mg | Phenylephrine HCl 2.5 mg | Codeine PO₄ 5 mg | | Potassium iodide† 75 mg | | | 6 mos–12 yrs: 1.25–10 mL q 4–6 hr | | b, c, e, f |
| *Pentazine VC w/Codeine* Oral Solution (Schedule V) [U.S.] | Promethazine HCl 6.25 mg | | Codeine PO₄ 10 mg | | | | | 5 mL q 4–6 hr | | b, c, e, f |
| *Pertussin All Night CS* Oral Solution (OTC) [U.S.] | | | | Dextromethorphan HBr 3.5 mg | Guaifenesin 25 mg | | Alcohol 8.5% | 20 mL q 3 hr | 2–5 yrs: 5 mL, 6–12 yrs: 10 mL, q 3 hr | b, c |
| *Pertussin All Night PM* Oral Solution (OTC) [U.S.] | Doxylamine succinate 1.25 mg | Pseudoephedrine HCl 10 mg | | Dextromethorphan HBr 5 mg | | Acetaminophen 167 mg | Alcohol 25% | 30 mL hs | Not recommended | b, c |
| *Phanadex* Syrup (OTC) [U.S.] | Pyrilamine maleate 40 mg | Phenylpropanolamine HCl 25 mg | | Dextromethorphan HBr 15 mg | Guaifenesin 100 mg, Potassium citrate† 75 mg, Citric acid† 35 mg | | Alcohol free Sodium free | 10 mL q 4–6 hr | 2–6 yrs: 2.5 mL, 6–12 yrs: 5 mL, q 4–6 hr | b, c |
| *Phanatuss* Syrup (OTC) [U.S.] | | | | Dextromethorphan HBr 10 mg | Guaifenesin 85 mg, | | Alcohol free Sugar free | 10 mL q 6–8 hr | 6–12 yrs: 5 mL q 6–8 hr | b, c |

*Specific formulations may vary among the different manufacturers, check product labeling.
†Efficacy as expectorant has not been established.
‡Geriatric patients may be more sensitive to effects of usual adult dose.
§For appropriate *Packaging and storage* and *Auxiliary labeling* information refer to designated letters as follows:

a—Store below 40 °C (104 °F), preferably between 15 and 30 °C (59 and 86 °F), in a tight container, unless otherwise specified by manufacturer.
a¹—Store below 30 °C (86 °F), unless otherwise specified by manufacturer. Avoid exposure to excessive heat.
a²—Store below 25 °C (77 °F), unless otherwise specified by manufacturer.
b—Store below 40 °C (104 °F), preferably between 15 and 30 °C (59 and 86 °F), in a well-closed container, unless otherwise specified by manufacturer.
c—Protect from freezing.
d—Protect from light.
e—Auxiliary labeling: • May cause drowsiness. • Avoid alcoholic beverages.
f—Auxiliary labeling: • May be habit forming.
g—Auxiliary labeling: • Shake well.
h—Dispense in dropper bottle.
i—Chew well before swallowing.

**Included in subtherapeutic amount to discourage deliberate overdosage.

## Table 3. Oral Dosage Forms (continued)

Note: Content per capsule, tablet, or 5 mL, unless otherwise stated.

| Brand or generic name [availability] | Antihistamines | Decongestants | Antitussives Opioid | Antitussives Non-opioid | Expectorants | Analgesics | Other content information as per product label | Usual Adult and Adolescent Dose prn‡ | Usual Pediatric Dose prn | Packaging, Storage, and Auxiliary labeling§ |
|---|---|---|---|---|---|---|---|---|---|---|
| *Phenameth DM* Syrup (Rx) [U.S.] | Promethazine HCl 6.25 mg | | | Dextromethorphan HBr 15 mg | | | Alcohol | 5 mL q 4–6 hr | | b, c, e |
| *Phenameth VC with Codeine* Syrup (Schedule V) [U.S.] | Promethazine HCl 6.25 mg | Phenylephrine HCl 5 mg | Codeine PO4 10 mg | | | | Alcohol 7% | 5 mL q 4–6 hr | 2–6 yrs: 1.25–5 mL, 6–12 yrs: 2.5–5 mL q 4–6 hr | a, c, d, e, f |
| *Phenergan with Codeine* Syrup (Schedule V) [U.S.] | Promethazine HCl 6.25 mg | | Codeine PO4 10 mg | | | | Alcohol 7% | 5 mL q 4–6 hr | 2–6 yrs: 1.25–2.5 mL, 6–12 yrs: 2.5 mL, q 4–6 hr | a, c, d, e, f |
| *Phenergan with Dextromethorphan* Syrup (Rx) [U.S.] | Promethazine HCl 6.25 mg | | | Dextromethorphan HBr 15 mg | | | Alcohol 7% | 5 mL q 4–6 hr | 2–6 yrs: 1.25 mL, 6–12 yrs: 2.5 mL, q 4–6 hr | a, c, d, e |
| *Phenergan Expectorant w/Codeine* Syrup (N) [Canada] | Promethazine HCl 5.65 mg | | Codeine PO4 10 mg | | Potassium guaiacolsulfonate† 40 mg | | | 5–10 mL q 4–6 hr | >2 yrs: 2.5–5 mL q 4–6 hr | a, d, e, f, g |
| *Phenergan VC with Codeine* Syrup (Schedule V) [U.S.] | Promethazine HCl 6.25 mg | Phenylephrine HCl 5 mg | Codeine PO4 10 mg | | | | Alcohol 7% | 5 mL q 4–6 hr | 2–6 yrs: 1.25–2.5 mL, 6–12 yrs: 2.5 mL, q 4–6 hr | a, c, d, e, f |
| *Phenergan VC Expectorant* Syrup (OTC) [Canada] | Promethazine HCl 5 mg | Phenylephrine HCl 5 mg | | | Potassium guaiacolsulfonate† 44 mg | | Alcohol | 5–10 mL q 6–8 hr | >2 yrs: 2.5–5 mL q 6–8 hr | a, d, e |
| *Phenergan VC Expectorant w/Codeine* Syrup (N) [Canada] | Promethazine HCl 5 mg | Phenylephrine HCl 5 mg | Codeine PO4 10 mg | | Potassium guaiacolsulfonate† 44 mg | | | 5–10 mL q 4–6 hr | >2 yrs: 2.5–5 mL q 4–6 hr | a, d, e, f |
| *Phenhist DH w/Codeine* Oral Solution (Schedule V) [U.S.] | Chlorpheniramine maleate 2 mg | Pseudoephedrine HCl 30 mg | Codeine PO4 10 mg | | | | Alcohol 5% | 10 mL q 4 hr | | b, c, e, f |

## Table 3. Oral Dosage Forms (continued)

Note: Content per capsule, tablet, or 5 mL, unless otherwise stated.

| Brand or generic name [availability] | Antihistamines | Decongestants | Antitussives | | Expectorants | Analgesics | Other content information as per product label | Usual Adult and Adolescent Dose prn‡ | Usual Pediatric Dose prn | Packaging, Storage, and Auxiliary labeling§ |
|---|---|---|---|---|---|---|---|---|---|---|
| | | | Opioid | Non-opioid | | | | | | |
| *Phenhist Expectorant* Oral Solution (Schedule V) [U.S.] | | Pseudoephedrine HCl 30 mg | Codeine PO$_4$ 10 mg | | Guaifenesin 100 mg | | Alcohol 7.5% | 10 mL q 4-6 hr | 2-6 yrs: 1.25-2.5 mL, 6-12 yrs: 2.5-5 mL, q 4-6 hr | a, c, e, f |
| *Phenylfenesin L.A.* Extended-release Tablets (Rx) [U.S.] | | Phenylpropanolamine HCl 75 mg | | | Guaifenesin 400 mg | | Scored | 1 tab q 12 hr | 6-12 yrs: ½ tab q 12 hr | b |
| *Pherazine w/Codeine* Syrup (Schedule V) [U.S.] | Promethazine HCl 6.25 mg | | Codeine PO$_4$ 10 mg | | | | Alcohol 7% | 5 mL q 4-6 hr | | b, c, e, f |
| *Pherazine DM* Syrup (Rx) [U.S.] | Promethazine HCl 6.25 mg | | | Dextromethorphan HBr 15 mg | | | Alcohol 7% | 5 mL q 4-6 hr | | b, c, e |
| *Pherazine VC with Codeine* Syrup (Schedule V) [U.S.] | Promethazine HCl 6.25 mg | Phenylephrine HCl 5 mg | Codeine PO$_4$ 10 mg | | | | Alcohol 7% | 5 mL q 4-6 hr | 2-6 yrs: 1.25-2.5 mL, 6-12 yrs: 2.5-5 mL, q 4-6 hr | a, c, d, e, f |
| *Pneumotussin HC* Syrup (Schedule III) [U.S.] | | | Hydrocodone bitartrate 5 mg | | Guaifenesin 100 mg | | Alcohol free Sugar free | 5 mL q 4 hr | | b, c, e, f |

*Specific formulations may vary among the different manufacturers, check product labeling.
†Efficacy as expectorant has not been established.
‡Geriatric patients may be more sensitive to effects of usual adult dose.
§For appropriate *Packaging and storage* and *Auxiliary labeling* information refer to designated letters as follows:
a—Store below 40 °C (104 °F), preferably between 15 and 30 °C (59 and 86 °F), in a tight container, unless otherwise specified by manufacturer.
a¹—Store below 30 °C (86 °F), unless otherwise specified by manufacturer. Avoid exposure to excessive heat.
a²—Store below 25 °C (77 °F), unless otherwise specified by manufacturer.
b—Store below 40 °C (104 °F), preferably between 15 and 30 °C (59 and 86 °F), in a well-closed container, unless otherwise specified by manufacturer.
c—Protect from freezing.
d—Protect from light.
e—Auxiliary labeling: • May cause drowsiness. • Avoid alcoholic beverages.
f—Auxiliary labeling: • May be habit forming.
g—Auxiliary labeling: • Shake well.
h—Dispense in dropper bottle.
i—Chew well before swallowing.
**Included in subtherapeutic amount to discourage deliberate overdosage.

## Table 3. Oral Dosage Forms (*continued*)

Note: Content per capsule, tablet, or 5 mL, unless otherwise stated.

| Brand or generic name [availability] | Antihistamines | Decongestants | Antitussives — Opioid | Antitussives — Non-opioid | Expectorants | Analgesics | Other content information as per product label | Usual Adult and Adolescent Dose prn‡ | Usual Pediatric Dose prn | Packaging, Storage, and Auxiliary labeling§ |
|---|---|---|---|---|---|---|---|---|---|---|
| *Polaramine Expectorant* Oral Solution (Rx) [U.S.] | Dexchlorpheniramine maleate 2 mg | Pseudoephedrine sulfate 20 mg | | | Guaifenesin 100 mg | | Alcohol 7.2% | 5–10 mL q 6–8 hr | 2–6 yrs: 1.25–2.5 mL, 6–12 yrs: 2.5–5 mL, q 6–8 hr | a, c, d, e |
| *Poly-Histine-CS* Syrup (Schedule V) [U.S.] | Brompheniramine maleate 2 mg | Phenylpropanolamine HCl 12.5 mg | Codeine PO$_4$ 10 mg | | | | Alcohol free | 5–10 mL q 4 hr | 2–6 yrs: 1.25–2.5 mL, 6–12 yrs: 2.5–5 mL, q 4–6 hr | b, c, e, f |
| *Poly-Histine-DM* Syrup (Rx) [U.S.] | Brompheniramine maleate 2 mg | Phenylpropanolamine HCl 12.5 mg | | Dextromethorphan HBr 10 mg | | | | 5–10 mL q 4 hr | 2–6 yrs: 1.25–2.5 mL, 6–12 yrs: 2.5–5 mL, q 4–6 hr | b, c, e, f |
| *Primatuss Cough Mixture 4* Oral Solution (OTC) [U.S.] | Chlorpheniramine maleate 2 mg | | | Dextromethorphan HBr 15 mg | | | Alcohol 10% | 10 mL q 8 hr | | b, c, e |
| *Primatuss Cough Mixture 4D* Oral Solution (OTC) [U.S.] | | Pseudoephedrine HCl 20 mg | | Dextromethorphan HBr 10 mg | Guaifenesin 67 mg | | Alcohol 10% | 15 mL q 6 hr | | b, c |
| *Promethazine and Codeine** Syrup (Schedule V) [U.S.] | Promethazine HCl 6.25 mg | | Codeine PO$_4$ 10 mg | | | | | 5 mL q 4–6 hr | 2–6 yrs: 1.25–2.5 mL, 6–12 yrs: 2.5–5 mL, q 4–6 hr | a, c, d, e, f |
| *Promethazine DM* Oral Solution (Rx) [U.S.] | Promethazine HCl 6.25 mg | | | Dextromethorphan HBr 15 mg | | | Alcohol | 5 mL q 4–6 hr | | b, c, e |
| *Promethazine VC w/ Codeine* Oral Solution (Schedule V) [U.S.] | Promethazine HCl 6.25 mg | Phenylephrine HCl 5 mg | Codeine PO$_4$ 10 mg | | | | Alcohol | 5 mL q 4–6 hr | | b, c, e, f |
| *Prometh w/Dextromethorphan* Syrup (Rx) [U.S.] | Promethazine HCl 6.25 mg | | | Dextromethorphan HBr 15 mg | | | Alcohol 7% | 5 mL q 4–6 hr | | b, c, e |

Table 3. Oral Dosage Forms (continued)

Note: Content per capsule, tablet, or 5 mL, unless otherwise stated.

| Brand or generic name [availability] | Antihistamines | Decongestants | Antitussives | | Expectorants | Analgesics | Other content information as per product label | Usual Adult and Adolescent Dose prn‡ | Usual Pediatric Dose prn | Packaging, Storage, and Auxiliary labeling§ |
|---|---|---|---|---|---|---|---|---|---|---|
| | | | Opioid | Non-opioid | | | | | | |
| Promethist w/Codeine Syrup (Schedule V) [U.S.] | Promethazine HCl 6.25 mg | Phenylephrine HCl 5 mg | Codeine PO$_4$ 10 mg | | | | Alcohol | 5 mL q 4–6 hr | | b, c, e, f |
| Prometh VC with Codeine Syrup (Schedule V) [U.S.] | Promethazine HCl 6.25 mg | Phenylephrine HCl 5 mg | Codeine PO$_4$ 10 mg | | | | Alcohol 7% | 5 mL q 4–6 hr | 2–6 yrs: 1.25–2.5 mL, 6–12 yrs: 2.5–5 mL, q 4–6 hr | a, c, d, e, f |
| Prominic Expectorant Oral Solution (OTC) [U.S.] | | Phenylpropanolamine HCl 12.5 mg | | | Guaifenesin 100 mg | | Alcohol 5% | 10 mL q 4 hr | 2–6 yrs: 2.5 mL, 6–12 yrs: 5 mL, q 4 hr | b, c |
| Prominicol Cough Syrup (OTC) [U.S.] | Pheniramine maleate 6.25 mg, Pyrilamine maleate 6.25 mg | Phenylpropanolamine HCl 12.5 mg | | Dextromethorphan HBr 15 mg | Ammonium Cl† 90 mg | | | 10 mL q 4 hr | 2–6 yrs: 2.5 mL, 6–12 yrs: 5 mL, q 6–8 hr | b, c, e |
| Promist HD Liquid Oral Solution (Schedule III) [U.S.] | Chlorpheniramine maleate 2 mg | Pseudoephedrine HCl 30 mg | Hydrocodone bitartrate 2.5 mg | | | | Alcohol 5% | 10 mL q 6–8 hr | 2–6 yrs: 2.5 mL, 6–12 yrs: 5 mL, q 6–8 hr | b, c, d, e, f |

*Specific formulations may vary among the different manufacturers, check product labeling.

†Efficacy as expectorant has not been established.

‡Geriatric patients may be more sensitive to effects of usual adult dose.

§For appropriate *Packaging and storage* and *Auxiliary labeling* information refer to designated letters as follows:

a—Store below 40 °C (104 °F), preferably between 15 and 30 °C (59 and 86 °F), in a tight container, unless otherwise specified by manufacturer.

a¹—Store below 30 °C (86 °F), unless otherwise specified by manufacturer. Avoid exposure to excessive heat.

a²—Store below 25 °C (77 °F), unless otherwise specified by manufacturer.

b—Store below 40 °C (104 °F), preferably between 15 and 30 °C (59 and 86 °F), in a well-closed container, unless otherwise specified by manufacturer.

c—Protect from freezing.

d—Protect from light.

e—Auxiliary labeling: • May cause drowsiness. • Avoid alcoholic beverages.

f—Auxiliary labeling: • May be habit forming.

g—Auxiliary labeling: • Shake well.

h—Dispense in dropper bottle.

i—Chew well before swallowing.

**Included in subtherapeutic amount to discourage deliberate overdosage.

Table 3. Oral Dosage Forms (continued)

Note: Content per capsule, tablet, or 5 mL, unless otherwise stated.

| Brand or generic name [availability] | Antihistamines | Decongestants | Antitussives Opioid | Antitussives Non-opioid | Expectorants | Analgesics | Other content information as per product label | Usual Adult and Adolescent Dose prn‡ | Usual Pediatric Dose prn | Packaging, Storage, and Auxiliary labeling§ |
|---|---|---|---|---|---|---|---|---|---|---|
| Pseudo-Car DM Syrup (Rx) [U.S.] | Carbinoxamine maleate 4 mg | Pseudoephedrine HCl 60 mg | | Dextromethorphan HBr 15 mg | | | Alcohol <0.6% | 5 mL q 4–6 hr | 18 mos–6 yrs: 2.5 mL, >6 yrs: 5 mL, q 4–6 hr | a, c, d, e |
| Pseudodine C Cough Syrup (Schedule V) [U.S.] | Triprolidine HCl 1.25 mg | Pseudoephedrine HCl 30 mg | Codeine PO₄ 10 mg | | | | Alcohol 4.3% | 10 mL q 4–6 hr | 2–6 yrs: 2.5 mL, 6–12 yrs: 5 mL, q 4–6 hr | a, c, d, e, f |
| P-V-Tussin Syrup (Schedule III) [U.S.] | Chlorpheniramine maleate 2 mg | Pseudoephedrine HCl 30 mg | Hydrocodone bitartrate 2.5 mg | | | | Alcohol 5% | 10 mL q 4–6 hr | 1–3 yrs: 2.5 mL, 3–6 yrs: 2.5–5 mL, 6–12 yrs: 5 mL, q 4–6 hr | b, c, e, f |
| Tablets (Schedule III) [U.S.] | | Pseudoephedrine 60 mg | Hydrocodone bitartrate 5 mg | | | | Scored | 1 tab q 6 hr | | a, d, e, f |
| Quelidrine Cough Syrup (OTC) [U.S.] | Chlorpheniramine maleate 2 mg | Ephedrine HCl 5 mg, Phenylephrine HCl 5 mg | | Dextromethorphan HBr 10 mg | Ammonium Cl† 40 mg, Ipecac fluidextract† 0.005 mL | | Alcohol 2% | 5 mL q 4–6 hr | 2–6 yrs: 1.25 mL, 6–12 yrs: 2.5 mL, q 4–6 hr | a², c, e |
| Remcol-C Capsules (OTC) [U.S.] | Chlorpheniramine maleate 2 mg | | | Dextromethorphan HBr 15 mg | | Acetaminophen 300 mg | | 1 cap q 4 hr | 6–12 yrs: 1 cap q 6–8 hr | b, e |
| Rentamine Pediatric Oral Suspension (Rx) [U.S.] | Chlorpheniramine tannate 4 mg | Ephedrine tannate 5 mg; Phenylephrine tannate 5 mg | | Carbetapentane tannate 30 mg | | | | Intended for pediatric use | 2–6 yrs: 2.5–5 mL, 6–12 yrs: 5–10 mL, q 12 hr | b, c, e, g |
| Rescaps-D S.R. Extended-release Capsules (Rx) [U.S.] | | Phenylpropanolamine HCl 75 mg | | Caramiphen edisylate 40 mg | | | | 1 cap q 12 hr | Pediatric strength not available | a, d |

## Table 3. Oral Dosage Forms (continued)

Note: Content per capsule, tablet, or 5 mL, unless otherwise stated.

| Brand or generic name [availability] | Antihistamines | Decongestants | Antitussives Opioid | Antitussives Non-opioid | Expectorants | Analgesics | Other content information as per product label | Usual Adult and Adolescent Dose prn‡ | Usual Pediatric Dose prn | Packaging, Storage, and Auxiliary labeling§ |
|---|---|---|---|---|---|---|---|---|---|---|
| Rescon-DM Oral Solution (OTC) [U.S.] | Chlorpheniramine maleate 2 mg | Pseudoephedrine HCl 30 mg | | Dextromethorphan HBr 10 mg | | | Alcohol free Sugar free Dye free | 10 mL q 4-6 hr | | b, c, e |
| Rescon-GG Oral Solution (OTC) [U.S.] | | Phenylephrine HCl 5 mg | | | Guaifenesin 100 mg | | | 10 mL q 4-6 hr | | b, c |
| Respa-1st Extended-release Tablets (Rx) [U.S.] | | Pseudoephedrine HCl 60 mg | | | Guaifenesin 600 mg | | Scored | 1-2 tabs q 12 hr | 6-12 yrs: 1 tab q 12 hr | b |
| Respa-DM Extended-release Tablets (Rx) [U.S.] | | | | Dextromethorphan HBr 30 mg | Guaifenesin 600 mg | | Scored | 1-2 tabs q 12 hr | 6-12 yrs: 1 tab q 12 hr | b |
| Respaire-60 SR Extended-release Capsules (Rx) [U.S.] | | Pseudoephedrine HCl 60 mg | | | Guaifenesin 200 mg | | | 2 caps q 12 hr | 6-12 yrs: 1 cap q 12 hr | b |
| Respaire-120 SR Extended-release Capsules (Rx) [U.S.] | | Pseudoephedrine HCl 120 mg | | | Guaifenesin 250 mg | | | 1 cap q 12 hr | Intended for adult use. See Respaire-60 SR | b |
| Rhinosyn-DM Syrup (OTC) [U.S.] | Chlorpheniramine maleate 2 mg | Pseudoephedrine HCl 30 mg | | Dextromethorphan HBr 15 mg | | | Alcohol 1.4% Dye free | 10 mL q 6 hr | 2-6 yrs: 2.5 mL, 6-12 yrs: 5 mL, q 6 hr | b, c, e |

*Specific formulations may vary among the different manufacturers; check product labeling.

†Efficacy as expectorant has not been established.

‡Geriatric patients may be more sensitive to effects of usual adult dose.

§For appropriate *Packaging and storage* and *Auxiliary labeling* information refer to designated letters as follows:

  a—Store below 40 °C (104 °F), preferably between 15 and 30 °C (59 and 86 °F), in a tight container, unless otherwise specified by manufacturer.

  a¹—Store below 30 °C (86 °F), preferably between 15 and 30 °C (59 and 86 °F), unless otherwise specified by manufacturer. Avoid exposure to excessive heat.

  a²—Store below 25 °C (77 °F), unless otherwise specified by manufacturer.

  b—Store below 40 °C (104 °F), preferably between 15 and 30 °C (59 and 86 °F), in a well-closed container, unless otherwise specified by manufacturer.

  c—Protect from freezing.

  d—Protect from light.

  e—Auxiliary labeling: • May cause drowsiness. • Avoid alcoholic beverages.

  f—Auxiliary labeling: • May be habit forming.

  g—Auxiliary labeling: • Shake well.

  h—Dispense in dropper bottle.

  i—Chew well before swallowing.

**Included in subtherapeutic amount to discourage deliberate overdosage.

## Table 3. Oral Dosage Forms (*continued*)

Note: Content per capsule, tablet, or 5 mL, unless otherwise stated.

| Brand or generic name [availability] | Antihistamines | Decongestants | Antitussives Opioid | Antitussives Non-opioid | Expectorants | Analgesics | Other content information as per product label | Usual Adult and Adolescent Dose prn‡ | Usual Pediatric Dose prn | Packaging, Storage, and Auxiliary labeling§ |
|---|---|---|---|---|---|---|---|---|---|---|
| *Rhinosyn-DMX Expectorant* Syrup (OTC) [U.S.] | | | | Dextromethorphan HBr 15 mg | Guaifenesin 100 mg | | Alcohol 6% Dye free | 10 mL q 6 hr | 2–6 yrs: 2.5 mL, 6–12 yrs: 5 mL, q 6 hr | a, c, d |
| *Rhinosyn-X* Syrup (OTC) [U.S.] | | Pseudoephedrine HCl 30 mg | | Dextromethorphan HBr 10 mg | Guaifenesin 100 mg | | Alcohol 7.5% Dye free | 10 mL q 4 hr | 2–6 yrs: 2.5 mL, 6–12 yrs: 5 mL, q 4 hr | b, c, d |
| *Robafen AC Cough* Syrup USP (Schedule V) [U.S.] | | | Codeine PO₄ 10 mg | | Guaifenesin 100 mg | | Alcohol 3.5% | 5–10 mL q 4–6 hr | | a, c, d, e, f |
| *Robafen CF* Oral Solution (OTC) [U.S.] | | Phenylpropanolamine HCl 12.5 mg | | Dextromethorphan HBr 10 mg | Guaifenesin 100 mg | | | 10 mL q 4 hr | | b, c |
| *Robafen DAC* Syrup (Schedule V) [U.S.] | | Pseudoephedrine HCl 30 mg | Codeine PO₄ 10 mg | | Guaifenesin 100 mg | | Alcohol 1.4% | 10 mL q 4 hr | | b, c, e, f |
| *Robafen DM* Syrup (OTC) [U.S.] | | | | Dextromethorphan HBr 10 mg | Guaifenesin 100 mg | | Alcohol 1.4% | 5–10 mL q 4 hr | | b, c |
| *Robitussin A-C* Syrup USP (Schedule V) [U.S.] | | | Codeine PO₄ 10 mg | | Guaifenesin 100 mg | | Alcohol 3.5% Sugar free | 10 mL q 4 hr | 6–12 yrs: 5 mL, q 4 hr | a, c, d, e, f |
| Syrup (N) [Canada] | Pheniramine maleate 7.5 mg | | Codeine PO₄ 10 mg | | Guaifenesin 100 mg | | Alcohol 3.5% | 5–10 mL q 4–6 mL | 2–6 yrs: 2.5 mL, 6–12 yrs: 5 mL, q 4–6 hr | b, c, e, f |
| *Robitussin-CF* Syrup (OTC) [U.S.] | | Phenylpropanolamine HCl 12.5 mg | | Dextromethorphan HBr 10 mg | Guaifenesin 100 mg | | Alcohol free | 10 mL q 4 hr | 2–6 yrs: 2.5 mL, 6–12 yrs: 5 mL, q 4 hr | b, c |

## Table 3. Oral Dosage Forms (continued)

Note: Content per capsule, tablet, or 5 mL, unless otherwise stated.

| Brand or generic name [availability] | Antihistamines | Decongestants | Antitussives | | Expectorants | Analgesics | Other content information as per product label | Usual Adult and Adolescent Dose prn‡ | Usual Pediatric Dose prn | Packaging, Storage, and Auxiliary labeling§ |
| --- | --- | --- | --- | --- | --- | --- | --- | --- | --- | --- |
| | | | Opioid | Non-opioid | | | | | | |
| Robitussin-CF (continued) Syrup (OTC) [Canada] | | Phenylpropanolamine HCl 12.5 mg | | Dextromethorphan HBr 10 mg | Guaifenesin 100 mg | | Alcohol | 15 mL q 6–8 hr | 2–6 yrs: 3.75 mL, 6–12 yrs: 7.5 mL, q 6–8 hr | b, c |
| Robitussin with Codeine Syrup (N) [Canada] | Pheniramine maleate 7.5 mg | | Codeine PO₄ 3.3 mg | | Guaifenesin 100 mg | | Alcohol 3.5% | 15 mL q 4–6 hr | 2–4 yrs: 2.5 mL, 4–12 yrs: 5 mL, q 4–6 hr | b, c, e, f |
| Robitussin Cold and Cough Liqui-Gels Capsules (OTC) [U.S.] | | Pseudoephedrine HCl 30 mg | | Dextromethorphan HBr 10 mg | Guaifenesin 200 mg | | | 2 caps q 4 hr | 6–12 yrs: 1 cap q 4 hr | b |
| Robitussin-DAC Syrup (Schedule V) [U.S.] | | Pseudoephedrine HCl 30 mg | Codeine PO₄ 10 mg | | Guaifenesin 100 mg | | Alcohol 1.9% Sugar free | 10 mL q 4 hr | 6–12 yrs: 5 mL q 4 hr | a, c, e, f |
| Robitussin-DM Syrup (OTC) [U.S] | | | | Dextromethorphan HBr 10 mg | Guaifenesin 100 mg | | Alcohol free | 10 mL q 4 hr | 2–6 yrs: 2.5 mL, 6–12 yrs: 5 mL, q 4 hr | b, c |

*Specific formulations may vary among the different manufacturers, check product labeling.
†Efficacy as expectorant has not been established.
‡Geriatric patients may be more sensitive to effects of usual adult dose.
§For appropriate *Packaging and storage* and *Auxiliary labeling* information refer to designated letters as follows:
　a—Store below 40 °C (104 °F), preferably between 15 and 30 °C (59 and 86 °F), in a tight container, unless otherwise specified by manufacturer.
　a¹—Store below 30 °C (86 °F), unless otherwise specified by manufacturer. Avoid exposure to excessive heat.
　a²—Store below 25 °C (77 °F), unless otherwise specified by manufacturer.
　b—Store below 40 °C (104 °F), preferably between 15 and 30 °C (59 and 86 °F), in a well-closed container, unless otherwise specified by manufacturer.
　c—Protect from freezing.
　d—Protect from light.
　e—Auxiliary labeling: • May cause drowsiness. • Avoid alcoholic beverages.
　f—Auxiliary labeling: • May be habit forming.
　g—Auxiliary labeling: • Shake well.
　h—Dispense in dropper bottle.
　i—Chew well before swallowing.
**Included in subtherapeutic amount to discourage deliberate overdosage.

Table 3. Oral Dosage Forms *(continued)*
Note: Content per capsule, tablet, or 5 mL, unless otherwise stated.

| Brand or generic name [availability] | Antihistamines | Decongestants | Antitussives — Opioid | Antitussives — Non-opioid | Expectorants | Analgesics | Other content information as per product label | Usual Adult and Adolescent Dose prn‡ | Usual Pediatric Dose prn | Packaging, Storage, and Auxiliary labeling§ |
|---|---|---|---|---|---|---|---|---|---|---|
| *Robitussin-DM (continued)* Syrup (N) [Canada] | | | | Dextromethorphan HBr 15 mg | Guaifenesin 100 mg | | Alcohol 1.4% | 10 mL q 4 hr | 2–6 yrs: 2.5 mL, 6–12 yrs: 5 mL, q 4 hr | b, c |
| *Robitussin Maximum Strength Cough and Cold* Oral Solution (OTC) [U.S.] | | Pseudoephedrine HCl 30 mg | | Dextromethorphan HBr 15 mg | | | Alcohol 1.4% | 10 mL q 6 hr | | b, c |
| *Robitussin Night Relief* Oral Solution (OTC) [U.S.] | Pyrilamine maleate 50 mg/30 mL | Pseudoephedrine HCl 60 mg/ 30 mL | | Dextromethorphan HBr 30 mg/ 30 mL | | Acetaminophen 650 mg/ 30 mL | Alcohol free | 30 mL hs or q 6 hr | | b, e |
| *Robitussin-PE* Syrup (OTC) [U.S.] | | Pseudoephedrine HCl 30 mg | | | Guaifenesin 100 mg | | Alcohol free | 10 mL q 4–6 hr | 2–6 yrs: 2.5 mL, 6–12 yrs: 5 mL, q 4–6 hr | b, c |
| Syrup (OTC) [Canada] | | Pseudoephedrine HCl 30 mg | | | Guaifenesin 100 mg | | Alcohol | 10 mL q 6 hr | 2–6 yrs: 2.5 mL, 6–12 yrs: 5 mL, q 6 hr | b, c |
| *Robitussin Pediatric Cough & Cold* Oral Solution (OTC) [U.S./Canada] | | Pseudoephedrine HCl 15 mg | | Dextromethorphan HBr 7.5 mg | | | Alcohol free | | 2–<6 yrs: 5 mL q 6 hr, 6–12 yrs: 10 mL q 6 hr | b, c |
| *Robitussin Severe Congestion Liqui-Gels* Capsules (OTC) [U.S.] | | Pseudoephedrine HCl 30 mg | | | Guaifenesin 200 mg | | | 2 caps q 4 hr (max 8 caps daily) | 6–12 yrs: 1 cap q 4 hr (max 4 caps daily) | b |
| *Rolatuss Expectorant* Oral Solution (Schedule V) [U.S.] | Chlorpheniramine maleate 2 mg | Phenylephrine HCl 5 mg | Codeine PO₄ 9.85 mg | | Ammonium Cl† 33.3 mg | | Alcohol 5% | 5–10 mL q 6–8 hr | | b, c, e, f |

## Table 3. Oral Dosage Forms (continued)

Note: Content per capsule, tablet, or 5 mL, unless otherwise stated.

| Brand or generic name [availability] | Antihistamines | Decongestants | Antitussives Opioid | Antitussives Non-opioid | Expectorants | Analgesics | Other content information as per product label | Usual Adult and Adolescent Dose prn‡ | Usual Pediatric Dose prn | Packaging, Storage, and Auxiliary labeling§ |
|---|---|---|---|---|---|---|---|---|---|---|
| *Rolatuss w/ Hydrocodone* Oral Solution (Schedule III) [U.S.] | Pheniramine maleate 3.3 mg, Pyrilamine maleate 3.3 mg | Phenylephrine HCL 5 mg, Phenylpropanolamine HCl 3.3 mg | Hydrocodone bitartrate 1.7 mg | | | | | 10 mL q 6 hr | | b, c, e, f |
| *Rondamine-DM Drops* Oral Solution (Rx) [U.S.] | Carbinoxamine maleate 2 mg/mL | Pseudoephedrine HCl 25 mg/mL | | Dextromethorphan HBr 4 mg/mL | | | | | 1–18 mos: 0.25–1 mL q 6 hr | b, c, e |
| *Rondec-DM* Syrup (Rx) [U.S.] | Carbinoxamine maleate 4 mg | Pseudoephedrine HCl 60 mg | | Dextromethorphan HBr 15 mg | | | Alcohol free Sugar free | 5 mL q 4-6 hr | 18 mos-6 yrs: 2.5 mL, >6 yrs: 5 mL, q 6 hr | a¹, c, d, e |
| *Rondec-DM Drops* Oral Solution (Rx) [U.S.] | Carbinoxamine maleate 10 mg (2 mg/mL) | Pseudoephedrine HCl 125 mg (25 mg/mL) | | Dextromethorphan HBr 20 mg (4 mg/mL) | | | Alcohol free Sugar free | Intended for pediatric use. See *Rondec-DM Syrup* | 1–3 mos: 0.25 mL, 3–6 mos: 0.50 mL, 6–9 mos: 0.75 mL, 9–18 mos: 1 mL, q 6 hr, >18 mos: See *Rondec-DM Syrup* | a¹, c, e, h |
| *Ru-Tuss DE* Extended-release Tablets (Rx) [U.S.] | | Pseudoephedrine HCl 120 mg | | | Guaifenesin 600 mg | | | 1 tab q 12 hr | 6 12 yrs: ½ tab q 12 hr | b |

*Specific formulations may vary among the different manufacturers, check product labeling.

†Efficacy as expectorant has not been established.

‡Geriatric patients may be more sensitive to effects of usual adult dose.

§For appropriate *Packaging and storage* and *Auxiliary labeling* information refer to designated letters as follows:

  a—Store below 40 °C (104 °F), preferably between 15 and 30 °C (59 and 86 °F), in a tight container, unless otherwise specified by manufacturer.

  a¹—Store below 30 °C (86 °F), unless otherwise specified by manufacturer. Avoid exposure to excessive heat.

  a²—Store below 25 °C (77 °F), unless otherwise specified by manufacturer.

  b—Store below 40 °C (104 °F), preferably between 15 and 30 °C (59 and 86 °F), in a well-closed container, unless otherwise specified by manufacturer.

  c—Protect from freezing.

  d—Protect from light.

  e—Auxiliary labeling: • May cause drowsiness. • Avoid alcoholic beverages.

  f—Auxiliary labeling: • May be habit forming.

  g—Auxiliary labeling: • Shake well.

  h—Dispense in dropper bottle.

  i—Chew well before swallowing.

**Included in subtherapeutic amount to discourage deliberate overdosage.

## Table 3. Oral Dosage Forms (continued)

Note: Content per capsule, tablet, or 5 mL, unless otherwise stated.

| Brand or generic name [availability] | Antihistamines | Decongestants | Antitussives — Opioid | Antitussives — Non-opioid | Expectorants | Analgesics | Other content information as per product label | Usual Adult and Adolescent Dose prn‡ | Usual Pediatric Dose prn | Packaging, Storage, and Auxiliary labeling§ |
|---|---|---|---|---|---|---|---|---|---|---|
| *Ru-Tuss Expectorant* Oral Solution (OTC) [U.S.] | | Pseudoephedrine HCl 30 mg | | Dextromethorphan HBr 10 mg | Guaifenesin 100 mg | | Alcohol 10% | 10 mL q 4–6 hr (max 40 mL daily) | 2–6 yrs: 2.5 mL, 6–12 yrs: 5 mL, q 4–6 hr (max 4 doses daily) | b, c, e, f |
| *Ru-Tuss with Hydrocodone Liquid* Oral Solution (Schedule III) [U.S.] | Pheniramine maleate 3.3 mg Pyrilamine maleate 3.3 mg | Phenylephrine HCl 5 mg Phenylpropanolamine HCl 3.3 mg | Hydrocodone bitartrate 1.7 mg | | | | Alcohol 5% | 10 mL q 4–6 hr (max 40 mL daily) | 2–6 yrs: 2.5–5 mL, 6–12 yrs: 5 mL, q 4–6 hr (max 4 doses daily) | b, c, d, e, f |
| *Rymed* Capsules (Rx) [U.S.] | | Pseudoephedrine HCl 30 mg | | | Guaifenesin 250 mg | | | 1 cap q 4–6 hr | Pediatric strength not available. See *Rymed Liquid Oral Solution* | b |
| *Rymed Liquid* Oral Solution (OTC) [U.S.] | | Pseudoephedrine HCl 30 mg | | | Guaifenesin 100 mg | | Alcohol 1.4% Sugar free | 10 mL q 4 hr | 2–6 yrs: 2.5 mL, 6–12 yrs: 5 mL, q 4 hr | b, c |
| *Rymed-TR Caplets* Extended-release Tablets (Rx) [U.S.] | | Phenylpropanolamine HCl 75 mg | | | Guaifenesin 400 mg | | | 1 tab q 12 hr | Pediatric strength not available | b |
| *Ryna-C Liquid* Oral Solution (Schedule V) [U.S.] | Chlorpheniramine maleate 2 mg | Pseudoephedrine HCl 30 mg | Codeine $PO_4$ 10 mg | | | | Alcohol free Dye free Sugar free | 10 mL q 4–6 hr | 2–6 yrs: 2.5 mL, 6–12 yrs: 5 mL, q 6 hr | b, c, e, f |
| *Ryna-CX Liquid* Oral Solution (Schedule V) [U.S.] | | Pseudoephedrine HCl 30 mg | Codeine $PO_4$ 10 mg | | Guaifenesin 100 mg | | Alcohol free Dye free Sugar free | 10 mL q 4–6 hr | 2–6 yrs: 1.25–2.5 mL, 6–12 yrs: 2.5–5 mL, q 6 hr | b, c, e, f |

Table 3. Oral Dosage Forms (continued)

Note: Content per capsule, tablet, or 5 mL, unless otherwise stated.

| Brand or generic name [availability] | Antihistamines | Decongestants | Antitussives Opioid | Antitussives Non-opioid | Expectorants | Analgesics | Other content information as per product label | Usual Adult and Adolescent Dose prn‡ | Usual Pediatric Dose prn | Packaging, Storage, and Auxiliary labeling§ |
|---|---|---|---|---|---|---|---|---|---|---|
| *Rynatuss* Tablets (Rx) [U.S.] | Chlorpheniramine tannate 5 mg | Ephedrine tannate 10 mg, Phenylephrine tannate 10 mg | | Carbetapentane tannate 60 mg | | | | 1–2 tabs q 12 hr | 6–12 yrs: ½–1 tab q 12 hr | b, e |
| *Rynatuss Pediatric* Oral Suspension (Rx) [U.S.] | Chlorpheniramine tannate 4 mg | Ephedrine tannate 5 mg, Phenylephrine tannate 5 mg | | Carbetapentane tannate 30 mg | | | | Intended for pediatric use. See *Rynatuss* Tablets | 2–6 yrs: 2.5–5 mL, 6–12 yrs: 5–10 mL, q 12 hr | b, c, e, g |
| *Safe Tussin 30* Oral Solution (OTC) [U.S.] | | | | Dextromethorphan HBr 15 mg | Guaifenesin 100 mg | | Alcohol free Sodium free Sugar free Dye free | 10 mL q 6 hr | 2–6 yrs: 2.5 mL, 6–12 yrs: 5 mL, q 6 hr | b, c |
| *Saleto-CF* Tablets (OTC) [U.S.] | | Phenylpropanolamine HCl 12.5 mg | | Dextromethorphan HBr 10 mg | | Acetaminophen 325 mg | Sodium metabisulfite | 2 tabs q 4 hr | 6–12 yrs: 1 tab q 4 hr | b |
| *Scot-Tussin DM* Oral Solution (OTC) [U.S.] | Chlorpheniramine maleate 2 mg | | | Dextromethorphan HBr 15 mg | | | Alcohol free Sugar free | 5 mL q 4 hr or 10 mL q 6–8 hr | | b, c, e |
| *Silexin Cough* Syrup (OTC) [U.S.] | | | | Dextromethorphan HBr 30 mg | Guaifenesin 200 mg | | Alcohol free Sugar free | 20 mL q 6–8 hr | 6–12 yrs: 10 mL, q 6 8 hr | b, c |
| *Sinufed Timecelles* Extended-release Capsules (Rx) [U.S.] | | Pseudoephedrine HCl 60 mg | | | Guaifenesin 300 mg | | | 1–2 caps q 12 hr | 6–12 yrs: 1 cap q 12 hr | b |

*Specific formulations may vary among the different manufacturers; check product labeling.

†Efficacy as expectorant has not been established.

‡Geriatric patients may be more sensitive to effects of usual adult dose.

§For appropriate *Packaging and storage* and *Auxiliary labeling* information refer to designated letters as follows:

a—Store below 40 °C (104 °F), preferably between 15 and 30 °C (59 and 86 °F), in a tight container, unless otherwise specified by manufacturer.

a¹—Store below 30 °C (86 °F), unless otherwise specified by manufacturer. Avoid exposure to excessive heat.

a²—Store below 25 °C (77 °F), unless otherwise specified by manufacturer.

b—Store below 40 °C (104 °F), preferably between 15 and 30 °C (59 and 86 °F), in a well-closed container, unless otherwise specified by manufacturer.

c—Protect from freezing.

d—Protect from light.

e—Auxiliary labeling: • May cause drowsiness. • Avoid alcoholic beverages.

f—Auxiliary labeling: • May be habit forming.

g—Auxiliary labeling: • Shake well.

h—Dispense in dropper bottle.

i—Chew well before swallowing.

**Included in subtherapeutic amount to discourage deliberate overdosage.

## Table 3. Oral Dosage Forms (continued)

Note: Content per capsule, tablet, or 5 mL, unless otherwise stated.

| Brand or generic name [availability] | Antihistamines | Decongestants | Antitussives Opioid | Antitussives Non-opioid | Expectorants | Analgesics | Other content information as per product label | Usual Adult and Adolescent Dose prn‡ | Usual Pediatric Dose prn | Packaging, Storage, and Auxiliary labeling§ |
|---|---|---|---|---|---|---|---|---|---|---|
| *Sinupan* Extended-release Capsules (Rx) [U.S.] | | Phenylephrine HCl 40 mg | | | Guaifenesin 200 mg | | | 1 cap q 12 hr | | b |
| *Sinutab Non-Drying No Drowsiness Liquid Caps* Capsules (OTC) [U.S.] | | Pseudoephedrine HCl 30 mg | | | Guaifenesin 200 mg | | | 2 caps q 4 hr (max 8 caps daily) | | a² |
| *SINUvent* Extended-release Tablets (Rx) [U.S.] | | Phenylpropanolamine HCl 75 mg | | | Guaifenesin 600 mg | | Scored | 1 tab q 12 hr | | b |
| *Snaplets-DM* Granules (OTC) [U.S.] | | Phenylpropanolamine HCl 6.25 mg/pack | | Dextromethorphan HBr 5 mg/pack | | | | Intended for pediatric use | 2–6 yrs: 1 pack, 6–12 yrs: 2 packs, sprinkled on soft food q 4 hr | b |
| *Snaplets-EX* Granules (OTC) [U.S.] | | Phenylpropanolamine HCl 6.25 mg/pack | | | Guaifenesin 50 mg/pack | | | Intended for pediatric use | | b |
| *Snaplets-Multi* Granules (OTC) [U.S.] | Chlorpheniramine maleate 1 mg/pack | Phenylpropanolamine HCl 6.25 mg/pack | | Dextromethorphan HBr 5 mg/pack | | | | Intended for pediatric use | 2–6 yrs: 1 pack, 6–12 yrs: 2 packs, sprinkled on soft food q 4 hr | b, e |
| *SRC Expectorant* Oral Solution (Schedule III) [U.S.] | | Pseudoephedrine HCl 60 mg | Hydrocodone bitartrate 5 mg | | Guaifenesin 200 mg | | Alcohol 12.5% | 5 mL q 4–6 hr | Not recommended | b, c, e, f |
| *Stamoist E* Extended-release Tablets (Rx) [U.S.] | | Pseudoephedrine HCl 120 mg | | | Guaifenesin 500 mg | | Dye free Scored | 1 tab q 12 hr | | b |

## Table 3. Oral Dosage Forms (continued)

Note: Content per capsule, tablet, or 5 mL, unless otherwise stated.

| Brand or generic name [availability] | Antihistamines | Decongestants | Antitussives — Opioid | Antitussives — Non-opioid | Expectorants | Analgesics | Other content information as per product label | Usual Adult and Adolescent Dose prn‡ | Usual Pediatric Dose prn | Packaging, Storage, and Auxiliary labeling§ |
|---|---|---|---|---|---|---|---|---|---|---|
| *Stamoist LA* Extended-release Tablets (Rx) [U.S.] | | Phenylpropanolamine HCl 75 mg | | | Guaifenesin 400 mg | | Scored | 1 tab q 12 hr | | b |
| *Statuss Expectorant* Syrup (Schedule V) [U.S.] | | Phenylpropanolamine HCl 12.5 mg | Codeine $PO_4$ 10 mg | | Guaifenesin 100 mg | | Alcohol 5% | 5–10 mL q 6–8 hr | 2–6 yrs: 2.5 mL, 6–12 yrs: 5 mL, q 6–8 hr | a, e, f |
| *Statuss Green* Oral Solution (Schedule III) [U.S.] | Pheniramine maleate 3.3 mg, Pyrilamine maleate 3.3 mg | Phenylephrine HCl 5 mg, Phenylpropanolamine HCl 3.3 mg | Hydrocodone bitartrate 1.67 mg | | | | Alcohol 5% | 10 mL q 4–6 hr | | b, c, e, f |
| *S-T Forte* Oral Solution (Schedule III) [U.S.] | Pheniramine maleate 13.33 mg | Phenylephrine HCl 5 mg, Phenylpropanolamine HCl 5 mg | Hydrocodone bitartrate 2.5 mg | | Guaifenesin 80 mg | | Alcohol 5% Sugar free | 5 mL q 6–8 hr | | b, c, e, f |
| *S-T Forte 2* Oral Solution (Schedule III) [U.S.] | Chlorpheniramine maleate 2 mg | | Hydrocodone bitartrate 2.5 mg | | | | Glycerin 99.7% Alcohol free Sugar free Dye free | 5 mL q 6–8 hr | | b, c, e, f |
| *Sudafed Cold & Cough Liquid Caps* (OTC) [U.S.] | | Pseudoephedrine HCl 30 mg | | Dextromethorphan HBr 10 mg | Guaifenesin 100 mg | Acetaminophen 250 mg | | 2 caps q 4 hr (max 8 caps daily) | | b, c |

*Specific formulations may vary among the different manufacturers; check product labeling.

†Efficacy as expectorant has not been established.

‡Geriatric patients may be more sensitive to effects of usual adult dose.

§For appropriate *Packaging and storage* and *Auxiliary labeling* information refer to designated letters as follows:

a—Store below 40 °C (104 °F), preferably between 15 and 30 °C (59 and 86 °F), in a tight container, unless otherwise specified by manufacturer.

a¹—Store below 30 °C (86 °F), unless otherwise specified by manufacturer. Avoid exposure to excessive heat.

a²—Store below 25 °C (77 °F), unless otherwise specified by manufacturer.

b—Store below 40 °C (104 °F), preferably between 15 and 30 °C (59 and 86 °F), in a well-closed container, unless otherwise specified by manufacturer.

c—Protect from freezing.

d—Protect from light.

e—Auxiliary labeling: • May cause drowsiness. • Avoid alcoholic beverages.

f—Auxiliary labeling: • May be habit forming.

g—Auxiliary labeling: • Shake well.

h—Dispense in dropper bottle.

i—Chew well before swallowing.

**Included in subtherapeutic amount to discourage deliberate overdosage.

Table 3. Oral Dosage Forms *(continued)*
Note: Content per capsule, tablet, or 5 mL, unless otherwise stated.

| Brand or generic name [availability] | Antihistamines | Decongestants | Antitussives Opioid | Antitussives Non-opioid | Expectorants | Analgesics | Other content information as per product label | Usual Adult and Adolescent Dose prn‡ | Usual Pediatric Dose prn | Packaging, Storage, and Auxiliary labeling§ |
|---|---|---|---|---|---|---|---|---|---|---|
| *Sudafed Cold & Cough Extra Strength Non-Drowsy* Tablets (OTC) [Canada] | | Pseudoephedrine HCl 60 mg | | Dextromethorphan HBr 30 mg | | Acetaminophen 500 mg | | 1 tab q 4–6 hr (max 4 tabs daily) | | b |
| *Sudafed Cough* Syrup (OTC) [U.S.] | | Pseudoephedrine HCl 15 mg | | Dextromethorphan HBr 5 mg | Guaifenesin 100 mg | | Alcohol 2.4% | 20 mL q 4–6 hr | 2–6 yrs: 5 mL, 6–12 yrs: 10 mL, q 4–6 hr | b, c, d |
| *Sudafed DM* Oral Solution (OTC) [Canada] | | Pseudoephedrine HCl 30 mg | | Dextromethorphan HBr 15 mg | | | Alcohol | 10 mL q 4–6 hr (max 40 mL daily) | 4 mos–2 yr: 1.25 mL, 2–5 yrs: 2.5 mL, 6–11 yrs: 5 mL, q 4–6 hr (max 4 doses daily) | b, c |
| *Sudafed Severe Cold Formula* Caplets (OTC) [U.S.] | | Pseudoephedrine HCl 30 mg | | Dextromethorphan HBr 15 mg | | Acetaminophen 500 mg | | 2 tabs q 6 hr | Intended for adult use | a² |
| *Sudal 60/500* Extended-release Tablets (Rx) [U.S.] | | Pseudoephedrine HCl 60 mg | | | Guaifenesin 500 mg | | Scored | 1–2 tabs q 12 hr | 6–12 yrs: ½–1 tab q 12 hr | a, d |
| *Sudal 120/600* Extended-release Tablets (Rx) [U.S.] | | Pseudoephedrine HCl 120 mg | | | Guaifenesin 600 mg | | Scored | 1 tab q 12 hr | 6–12 yrs: ½ tab q 12 hr | a, d |
| *SYN-Rx AM Treatment* Extended-release Tablets (Rx) [U.S.] | | Pseudoephedrine HCl 60 mg | | | Guaifenesin 600 mg | | Scored Available in a dual package that also contains *SYN-Rx PM Treatment* | 1–2 tabs am | | b |

## Table 3. Oral Dosage Forms (continued)

Note: Content per capsule, tablet, or 5 mL, unless otherwise stated.

| Brand or generic name [availability] | Antihistamines | Decongestants | Antitussives – Opioid | Antitussives – Non-opioid | Expectorants | Analgesics | Other content information as per product label | Usual Adult and Adolescent Dose prn‡ | Usual Pediatric Dose prn | Packaging, Storage, and Auxiliary labeling§ |
|---|---|---|---|---|---|---|---|---|---|---|
| *Syracol CF* Tablets (OTC) [U.S.] | | | | Dextromethorphan HBr 15 mg | Guaifenesin 200 mg | | | 2 tabs q 6–8 hr (max 8 tabs daily) | 2–6 yrs: ½ tab; 6–12 yrs: 1 tab, q 6–8 hr | b |
| *TheraFlu/Flu, Cold and Cough Medicine* for Oral Solution (OTC) [U.S.] | Chlorpheniramine maleate 4 mg/packet | Pseudoephedrine HCl 60 mg/packet | | Dextromethorphan HBr 20 mg/packet | | Acetaminophen 650 mg packet | | 1 packet dissolved in 6-oz cup of hot water q 4 hr | | b, e |
| *TheraFlu Maximum Strength Non-Drowsy Formula Flu, Cold and Cough Medicine* for Oral Solution (OTC) [U.S.] | | Pseudoephedrine HCl 60 mg/packet | | Dextromethorphan HBr 30 mg/packet | | Acetaminophen 1000 mg packet | | 1 packet dissolved in 6-oz cup of hot water q 6 hr (max 4 packets daily) | Not recommended | b |
| Tablets (OTC) [U.S.] | | Pseudoephedrine HCl 30 mg | | Dextromethorphan HBr 15 mg | | Acetaminophen 500 mg | | 2 tabs q 6 hr | | b |

*Specific formulations may vary among the different manufacturers, check product labeling.
†Efficacy as expectorant has not been established.
‡Geriatric patients may be more sensitive to effects of usual adult dose.
§For appropriate *Packaging and storage* and *Auxiliary labeling* information refer to designated letters as follows:
a—Store below 40 °C (104 °F), preferably between 15 and 30 °C (59 and 86 °F), in a tight container, unless otherwise specified by manufacturer.
a¹—Store below 30 °C (86 °F), unless otherwise specified by manufacturer. Avoid exposure to excessive heat.
a²—Store below 25 °C (77 °F), unless otherwise specified by manufacturer.
b—Store below 40 °C (104 °F), preferably between 15 and 30 °C (59 and 86 °F), in a well-closed container, unless otherwise specified by manufacturer.
c—Protect from freezing.
d—Protect from light.
e—Auxiliary labeling: • May cause drowsiness. • Avoid alcoholic beverages.
f—Auxiliary labeling: • May be habit forming.
g—Auxiliary labeling: • Shake well.
h—Dispense in dropper bottle.
i—Chew well before swallowing.
**Included in subtherapeutic amount to discourage deliberate overdosage.

## Table 3. Oral Dosage Forms (continued)

Note: Content per capsule, tablet, or 5 mL, unless otherwise stated.

| Brand or generic name [availability] | Antihistamines | Decongestants | Antitussives Opioid | Antitussives Non-opioid | Expectorants | Analgesics | Other content information as per product label | Usual Adult and Adolescent Dose prn‡ | Usual Pediatric Dose prn | Packaging, Storage, and Auxiliary labeling§ |
|---|---|---|---|---|---|---|---|---|---|---|
| TheraFlu Nighttime Maximum Strength for Oral Solution (OTC) [U.S.] | Chlorpheniramine maleate 4 mg/ packet | Pseudoephedrine HCl 60 mg/packet | | Dextromethorphan HBr 30 mg/packet | | Acetaminophen 1000 mg/ packet | | 1 packet dissolved in 6-oz cup of hot water q 6 hr | | b, e |
| Threamine DM Syrup (OTC) [U.S.] | Chlorpheniramine maleate 2 mg | Phenylpropanolamine HCl 12.5 mg | | Dextromethorphan HBr 10 mg | | | | 10 mL q 4–6 hr | | b, c, e |
| Threamine Expectorant Oral Solution (OTC) [U.S.] | Chlorpheniramine maleate 2 mg | Phenylpropanolamine HCl 12.5 mg | | | Guaifenesin 100 mg | | Alcohol 5% | 10 mL q 4 hr | | b, c |
| T-Koff Syrup (Schedule V) [U.S.] | Chlorpheniramine maleate 5 mg | Phenylephrine HCl 20 mg, Phenylpropanolamine HCl 20 mg | Codeine PO$_4$ 10 mg | | | | | 5 mL, q 4–6 hr | 2–6 yrs: 1.25–2.5 mL, 6–12 yrs: 2.5–5 mL, q 4–6 hr | b, c, e, f |
| Tolu-Sed Cough Syrup USP (Schedule V) [U.S.] | | | Codeine PO$_4$ 10 mg | | Guaifenesin 100 mg | | Alcohol 10% Sugar free | 10 mL q 4 hr | 1–6 yrs: 1.25–2.5 mL, 6–12 yrs: 2.5–5 mL, q 4 hr | a, c, d, e, f |
| Tolu-Sed DM Syrup (OTC) [U.S.] | | | | Dextromethorphan HBr 10 mg | Guaifenesin 100 mg | | Alcohol 10% Sugar free | 10 mL q 4 hr | 1–6 yrs: 1.25–2.5 mL, 6–12 yrs: 2.5–5 mL, q 4 hr | b, c |
| Tauro LA Caplets Extended-release Tablets (Rx) [U.S.] | | Pseudoephedrine HCl 120 mg | | | Guaifenesin 400 mg | | | 1 tab q 12 hr | | b |
| Triacin C Cough Syrup (Schedule V) [U.S.] | Triprolidine HCl 1.25 mg | Pseudoephedrine HCl 30 mg | Codeine PO$_4$ 10 mg | | | | Alcohol 4.3% | 10 mL q 4–6 hr | 2–6 yrs: 2.5 mL, 6–12 yrs: 5 mL, q 4–6 hr | b, c, d, e, f |
| Trifed w/Codeine Syrup (Schedule V) [U.S.] | Triprolidine HCl 1.25 mg | Pseudoephedrine HCl 30 mg | Codeine PO$_4$ 10 mg | | | | | 10 mL q 4–6 hr | | b, c, e, f |

Table 3. Oral Dosage Forms (continued)

Note: Content per capsule, tablet, or 5 mL, unless otherwise stated.

| Brand or generic name [availability] | Antihistamines | Decongestants | Antitussives Opioid | Antitussives Non-opioid | Expectorants | Analgesics | Other content information as per product label | Usual Adult and Adolescent Dose prn‡ | Usual Pediatric Dose prn | Packaging, Storage, and Auxiliary labeling§§ |
|---|---|---|---|---|---|---|---|---|---|---|
| Triaminic AM Oral Solution (OTC) [U.S.] | | Pseudoephedrine HCl 15 mg | | Dextromethorphan HBr 7.5 mg | | | Alcohol free Dye free | 20 mL q 6 hr | 2–6 yrs: 5 mL, 6–12 yrs: 10 mL, q 6 hr | b |
| Triaminic-DM Cough Formula Oral Solution (OTC) [U.S.] | | Phenylpropanolamine HCl 6.25 mg | | Dextromethorphan HBr 5 mg | | | Alcohol free | 20 mL q 4 hr | 3 mos–1 yr: 1.25 mL, 1–2 yrs: 2.5 mL, 2–6 yrs: 5 mL, 6–12 yrs: 10 mL, q 4 hr | b, c |
| Triaminic DM Day Time for Children Syrup (OTC) [Canada] | | Phenylpropanolamine HCl 8.75 mg | | Dextromethorphan HBr 7.5 mg | Guaifenesin 37.5 mg | | | | 2–6 yrs: 5 mL, 6–12 yrs: 10 mL, q 6–8 hr | a, e |
| Triaminic-DM Expectorant Oral Solution (OTC) [Canada] | Pheniramine maleate 6.25 mg, Pyrilamine maleate 6.25 mg | Phenylpropanolamine HCl 12.5 mg | | Dextromethorphan HBr 15 mg | Guaifenesin 100 mg | | Alcohol 7.1% | 5–10 mL q 4 hr | 1–6 yrs: 2.5 mL, 6–12 yrs: 5 mL, q 4 hr | b, c, e |

*Specific formulations may vary among the different manufacturers; check product labeling.

†Efficacy as expectorant has not been established.

‡Geriatric patients may be more sensitive to effects of usual adult dose.

§For appropriate *Packaging and storage* and *Auxiliary labeling* information refer to designated letters as follows:

a—Store below 40 °C (104 °F), preferably between 15 and 30 °C (59 and 86 °F), in a tight container, unless otherwise specified by manufacturer.
a¹—Store below 30 °C (86 °F), unless otherwise specified by manufacturer. Avoid exposure to excessive heat.
a²—Store below 25 °C (77 °F), unless otherwise specified by manufacturer.
b—Store below 40 °C (104 °F), preferably between 15 and 30 °C (59 and 86 °F), in a well-closed container, unless otherwise specified by manufacturer.
c—Protect from freezing.
d—Protect from light.
e—Auxiliary labeling: • May cause drowsiness. • Avoid alcoholic beverages.
f—Auxiliary labeling: • May be habit forming.
g—Auxiliary labeling: • Shake well.
h—Dispense in dropper bottle.
i—Chew well before swallowing.

**Included in subtherapeutic amount to discourage deliberate overdosage.

## Table 3. Oral Dosage Forms (*continued*)

Note: Content per capsule, tablet, or 5 mL, unless otherwise stated.

| Brand or generic name [availability] | Antihistamines | Decongestants | Antitussives — Opioid | Antitussives — Non-opioid | Expectorants | Analgesics | Other content information as per product label | Usual Adult and Adolescent Dose prn‡ | Usual Pediatric Dose prn | Packaging, Storage, and Auxiliary labeling§ |
|---|---|---|---|---|---|---|---|---|---|---|
| *Triaminic DM Night Time for Children* Syrup (OTC) [Canada] | Chlorpheniramine maleate 1.0 mg | Pseudoephedrine HCl 15.0 mg | | Dextromethorphan HBr 7.5 mg | | | | 20 mL q 6–8 hr | 2–6 yrs: 5 mL, 6–12 yrs: 10 mL, q 6–8 hr | a, d, e |
| *Triaminic Expectorant* Oral Solution (OTC) [U.S.] | | Phenylpropanolamine HCl 6.25 mg | | | Guaifenesin 50 mg | | Alcohol free | 20 mL q 4 hr | 3 mos–1 yr: 2 drops/kg body weight, 1–2 yrs: 3 drops/kg body weight, 2–6 yrs: 2.5 mL, 6–12 yrs: 5 mL, q 4 hr | b, c |
| Oral Solution (OTC) [Canada] | Pheniramine maleate 6.25 mg, Pyrilamine maleate 6.25 mg | Phenylpropanolamine HCl 12.5 mg | | | Guaifenesin 100 mg | | Alcohol 7.8% | 10 mL q 4 hr | 1–6 yrs: 2.5 mL, 6–12 yrs: 5 mL, q 4 hr | b, c, e |
| *Triaminic Expectorant w/Codeine* Oral Solution (Schedule V) [U.S.] | | Phenylpropanolamine HCl 12.5 mg | Codeine PO₄ 10 mg | | Guaifenesin 100 mg | | Alcohol 5% | 10 mL q 4 hr | 3 mos–2 yrs: 2 drops/kg body weight, 2–6 yrs: 2.5 mL, 6–12 yrs: 5 mL, q 4 hr | b, c, e, f |
| *Triaminic Expectorant DH* Oral Solution (Schedule III/N) [U.S./Canada] | Pheniramine maleate 6.25 mg, Pyrilamine maleate 6.25 mg | Phenylpropanolamine HCl 12.5 mg | Hydrocodone bitartrate 1.67 mg | | Guaifenesin 100 mg | | Alcohol 5% | 10 mL q 4 hr | 2–6 yrs: 2.5 mL, 6–12 yrs: 5 mL, q 4 hr | b, c, e, f |
| *Triaminicin w/Codeine* Tablets (N) [Canada] | Pheniramine maleate 12.5 mg, Pyrilamine maleate 12.5 mg | Phenylpropanolamine HCl 25 mg | Codeine PO₄ 8 mg | | | Acetaminophen 325 mg | Caffeine 30 mg | 1 tab q 4–6 hr | Pediatric strength not available | b, e, f |

## Table 3. Oral Dosage Forms (*continued*)

Note: Content per capsule, tablet, or 5 mL, unless otherwise stated.

| Brand or generic name [availability] | Antihistamines | Decongestants | Antitussives Opioid | Antitussives Non-opioid | Expectorants | Analgesics | Other content information as per product label | Usual Adult and Adolescent Dose prn‡ | Usual Pediatric Dose prn | Packaging, Storage, and Auxiliary labeling§ |
|---|---|---|---|---|---|---|---|---|---|---|
| *Triaminic Nite Light Oral Solution* (OTC) [U.S.] | Chlorpheniramine maleate 1 mg | Pseudoephedrine HCl 15 mg | | Dextromethorphan HBr 7.5 mg | | | | Intended for pediatric use | 2–6 yrs: 5 mL, 6–12 yrs: 10 mL, 12 yrs or older: 20 mL, q 6 hr | b, c, e |
| *Triaminicol DM Syrup* (OTC) [Canada] | Pheniramine maleate 6.25 mg, Pyrilamine maleate 6.25 mg | Phenylpropanolamine HCl 12.5 mg | | Dextromethorphan HBr 15 mg | | | Alcohol free | 10 mL q 4–6 hr | <1 yr: 1.25 mL, 1–6 yrs: 2.5 mL, 6–12 yrs: 5 mL, q 6–8 hr | b, c, e |
| *Triaminicol Multi-Symptom Relief Syrup* (OTC) [U.S.] | Chlorpheniramine maleate 1 mg | Phenylpropanolamine HCl 6.25 mg | | Dextromethorphan HBr 5 mg | | | Alcohol free | 20 mL q 4 hr | 3 mos–1 yr: 1.25 mL, 1–2 yrs: 2.5 mL, 2–6 yrs: 5 mL, 6–12 yrs: 10 mL, q 4 hr | b, c, e |
| Tablets (OTC) [U.S.] | Chlorpheniramine maleate 2 mg | Phenylpropanolamine HCl 12.5 mg | | Dextromethorphan HBr 10 mg | | | | 2 tabs q 4 hr | 6–12 yrs: 1 tab q 4 hr | b |

*Specific formulations may vary among the different manufacturers, check product labeling.

†Efficacy as expectorant has not been established.

‡Geriatric patients may be more sensitive to effects of usual adult dose.

§For appropriate *Packaging and storage* and *Auxiliary labeling* information refer to designated letters as follows:

a—Store below 40 °C (104 °F), preferably between 15 and 30 °C (59 and 86 °F), in a tight container, unless otherwise specified by manufacturer.

a¹—Store below 30 °C (86 °F), unless otherwise specified by manufacturer. Avoid exposure to excessive heat.

a²—Store below 25 °C (77 °F), unless otherwise specified by manufacturer.

b—Store below 40 °C (104 °F), preferably between 15 and 30 °C (59 and 86 °F), in a well-closed container, unless otherwise specified by manufacturer.

c—Protect from freezing.

d—Protect from light.

e—Auxiliary labeling: • May cause drowsiness. • Avoid alcoholic beverages.

f—Auxiliary labeling: • May be habit forming.

g—Auxiliary labeling: • Shake well.

h—Dispense in dropper bottle.

i—Chew well before swallowing.

**Included in subtherapeutic amount to discourage deliberate overdosage.

## Table 3. Oral Dosage Forms *(continued)*

Note: Content per capsule, tablet, or 5 mL, unless otherwise stated.

| Brand or generic name [availability] | Antihistamines | Decongestants | Antitussives — Opioid | Antitussives — Non-opioid | Expectorants | Analgesics | Other content information as per product label | Usual Adult and Adolescent Dose prn‡ | Usual Pediatric Dose prn | Packaging, Storage, and Auxiliary labeling§ |
|---|---|---|---|---|---|---|---|---|---|---|
| *Triaminicol Multi-Symptom Relief Colds with Coughs* Oral Solution (OTC) [U.S.] | Chlorpheniramine maleate 1 mg | Phenylpropanolamine HCl 6.25 mg | | Dextromethorphan HBr 5 mg | | | Alcohol free | | 6–<12 yrs: 10 mL q 4 hr | b, c, e |
| *Triaminic Sore Throat Formula* Oral Solution (OTC) [U.S.] | | Pseudoephedrine HCl 15 mg | | Dextromethorphan HBr 7.5 mg | | Acetaminophen 160 mg | Alcohol free | | 2–<6 yrs: 5 mL q 6 hr, 6–<12 yrs: 10 mL q 6 hr | b, c |
| *Tricodene Cough & Cold* Oral Solution (Schedule V) [U.S.] | Pyrilamine maleate 12.5 mg | | Codeine PO₄ 8.2 mg | | | | | 10 mL q 6–8 hr | | b, c, e, f |
| *Tricodene Forte* Syrup (OTC) [U.S.] | Chlorpheniramine maleate 2 mg | Phenylpropanolamine HCl 12.5 mg | | Dextromethorphan HBr 10 mg | | | Alcohol free | 10 mL q 4 hr | 2–6 yrs: 1.25–2.5 mL, 6–12 yrs: 2.5–5 mL, q 4 hr | b, c, e |
| *Tricodene NN* Syrup (OTC) [U.S.] | Chlorpheniramine maleate 2 mg | Phenylpropanolamine HCl 12.5 mg | | Dextromethorphan HBr 10 mg | | | | 10 mL q 4 hr | 2–6 yrs: 1.25–2.5 mL, 6–12 yrs: 2.5–5 mL q 4 hr | b, c, e |
| *Tricodene Pediatric* Syrup (OTC) [U.S.] | | Phenylpropanolamine HCl 12.5 mg | | Dextromethorphan HBr 10 mg | | | | 5–10 mL q 4 hr | 2–6 yrs: 1.25–2.5 mL, 6–12 yrs: 2.5–5 mL, q 4 hr | b, c |
| *Tricodene Sugar Free* Oral Solution (OTC) [U.S.] | Chlorpheniramine maleate 2 mg | | | Dextromethorphan HBr 10 mg | | | | 10 mL q 4–6 hr | | b, c, e |
| *Trifed-C Cough* Syrup (Schedule V) [U.S.] | Triprolidine HCl 1.25 mg | Pseudoephedrine HCl 30 mg | Codeine PO₄ 10 mg | | | | Alcohol 4.4.% | 10 mL q 4–6 hr | 2–6 yrs: 2.5 mL, 6–12 yrs: 5 mL, q 4–6 hr | b, c, d, e, f |
| *Triminol Cough* Syrup (OTC) [U.S.] | Chlorpheniramine maleate 2 mg | Phenylpropanolamine HCl 12.5 mg | | Dextromethorphan HBr 10 mg | | | | 10 mL q 4 hr | | b, c, e |

Table 3. Oral Dosage Forms (continued)
Note: Content per capsule, tablet, or 5 mL, unless otherwise stated.

| Brand or generic name [availability] | Antihistamines | Decongestants | Antitussives Opioid | Antitussives Non-opioid | Expectorants | Analgesics | Other content information as per product label | Usual Adult and Adolescent Dose prn‡ | Usual Pediatric Dose prn | Packaging, Storage, and Auxiliary labeling§ |
|---|---|---|---|---|---|---|---|---|---|---|
| *Trinex* Extended-release Tablets (Rx) [U.S.] | Chlorpheniramine maleate 8 mg | Pseudoephedrine HCl 120 mg | | | Guaifenesin 200 mg | | | 1 tab q 8–12 hr | Pediatric strength not available | b, e |
| *Triphenyl Expectorant* Oral Solution (OTC) [U.S.] | | Phenylpropanolamine HCl 12.5 mg | | | Guaifenesin 100 mg | | Alcohol 5% | 10 mL q 4 hr | 2–6 yrs: 2.5 mL, 6–12 yrs: 5 mL, q 4 hr | b, c |
| *Tri-Tannate Plus Pediatric* Oral Suspension (Rx) [U.S.] | Chlorpheniramine tannate 4 mg | Ephedrine tannate 5 mg, Phenylephrine tannate 5 mg | | Carbetapentane tannate 30 mg | | | | | 2–<6 yrs: 2.5–10 mL q 12 hr | b, c, e |
| *Tusquelin* Syrup (Rx) [U.S.] | Chlorpheniramine maleate 2 mg | Phenylephrine HCl 5 mg, Phenylpropanolamine HCl 5 mg | | Dextromethorphan HBr 15 mg | | | Alcohol 5% | 5–10 mL q 4–6 hr | 2–6 yrs: 1.25–2.5 mL, 6–12 yrs: 2.5–5 mL, q 6 hr | b, c, e |
| *Tuss-Ade* Extended-release Capsules (Rx) [U.S.] | | Phenylpropanolamine HCl 75 mg | | Caramiphen edisylate 40 mg | | | | 1 cap q 12 hr | Pediatric strength not available | b |
| *Tussafed* Syrup (Rx) [U.S.] | Carbinoxamine maleate 4 mg | Pseudoephedrine HCl 60 mg | | Dextromethorphan HBr 15 mg | | | Alcohol free Sugar free | 5 mL q 4–6 hr | 18 mos–6 yrs: 2.5 mL, >6 yrs: 5 mL, q 4–6 hr | a, c, d, e |

*Specific formulations may vary among the different manufacturers; check product labeling.

†Efficacy as expectorant has not been established.

‡Geriatric patients may be more sensitive to effects of usual adult dose.

§For appropriate *Packaging and storage* and *Auxiliary labeling* information refer to designated letters as follows:

  a—Store below 40 °C (104 °F), preferably between 15 and 30 °C (59 and 86 °F), in a tight container, unless otherwise specified by manufacturer.

  a¹—Store below 30 °C (86 °F), unless otherwise specified by manufacturer. Avoid exposure to excessive heat.

  a²—Store below 25 °C (77 °F), unless otherwise specified by manufacturer.

  b—Store below 40 °C (104 °F), preferably between 15 and 30 °C (59 and 86 °F), in a well-closed container, unless otherwise specified by manufacturer.

  c—Protect from freezing.

  d—Protect from light.

  e—Auxiliary labeling: • May cause drowsiness. • Avoid alcoholic beverages.

  f—Auxiliary labeling: • May be habit forming.

  g—Auxiliary labeling: • Shake well.

  h—Dispense in dropper bottle.

  i—Chew well before swallowing.

**Included in subtherapeutic amount to discourage deliberate overdosage.

Table 3. Oral Dosage Forms *(continued)*
Note: Content per capsule, tablet, or 5 mL, unless otherwise stated.

| Brand or generic name [availability] | Antihistamines | Decongestants | Antitussives Opioid | Antitussives Non-opioid | Expectorants | Analgesics | Other content information as per product label | Usual Adult and Adolescent Dose prn‡ | Usual Pediatric Dose prn | Packaging, Storage, and Auxiliary labeling§ |
|---|---|---|---|---|---|---|---|---|---|---|
| *Tussafed Drops* Oral Solution (Rx) [U.S.] | Carbinoxamine maleate 2 mg/mL | Pseudoephedrine HCl 25 mg/mL | | Dextromethorphan HBr 4 mg/mL | | | Alcohol free Sugar free | | 1–18 mos: 0.25–1 mL q 6 hr | b, c, e |
| *Tussafin Expectorant* Oral Solution (Schedule III) [U.S.] | | Pseudoephedrine HCl 60 mg | Hydrocodone bitartrate 5 mg | | Guaifenesin 200 mg | | Alcohol 12.5% | 5 mL q 4–6 hr | | b, c, f |
| *Tuss Allergine Modified T.D.* Extended-release Capsules (Rx) [U.S.] | | Phenylpropanolamine HCl 75 mg | | Caramiphen edisylate 40 mg | | | | 1 cap q 12 hr | Pediatric strength not available | b |
| *Tussaminic C* Syrup (N) [Canada] | Pheniramine maleate 12.5 mg, Pyrilamine maleate 12.5 mg | Phenylpropanolamine HCl 25 mg | Codeine PO₄ 15 mg | | | | | 5 mL q 4 hr | Intended for adult use | b, c, e, f |
| *Tussaminic C Pediatric* Syrup (N) [Canada] | Pheniramine maleate 6.25 mg, Pyrilamine maleate 6.25 mg | Phenylpropanolamine HCl 12.5 mg | Codeine PO₄ 5 mg | | | | | Intended for pediatric use | 2–6 yrs: 2.5 mL, 6–12 yrs: 5 mL, q 4 hr | b, c, e, f |
| *Tussaminic DH* Syrup (N) [Canada] | Pheniramine maleate 12.5 mg, Pyrilamine maleate 12.5 mg | Phenylpropanolamine HCl 25 mg | Hydrocodone bitartrate 5 mg | | | | | 5 mL q 4 hr | 2–6 yrs: 1.25 mL, 6–12 yrs: 2.5 mL, q 4–6 hr. See also *Tussaminic DH Pediatric* Oral Solution | b, c, e, f |
| *Tussaminic DH Pediatric* Oral Solution (N) [Canada] | Pheniramine maleate 6.25 mg, Pyrilamine maleate 6.25 mg | Phenylpropanolamine HCl 12.5 mg | Hydrocodone bitartrate 1.66 mg | | | | | Intended for pediatric use. See *Tussaminic DH Forte* Oral Solution | 1–6 yrs: 2.5 mL, 6–12 yrs: 5 mL, q 4 hr | b, c, e, f |

## Table 3. Oral Dosage Forms (*continued*)
Note: Content per capsule, tablet, or 5 mL, unless otherwise stated.

| Brand or generic name [availability] | Antihistamines | Decongestants | Antitussives Opioid | Antitussives Non-opioid | Expectorants | Analgesics | Other content information as per product label | Usual Adult and Adolescent Dose prn‡ | Usual Pediatric Dose prn | Packaging, Storage, and Auxiliary labeling§ |
|---|---|---|---|---|---|---|---|---|---|---|
| *Tussanil DH* Syrup (Schedule III) [U.S.] | Chlorpheniramine maleate 4 mg | Phenylephrine HCl 10 mg | Hydrocodone bitartrate 2.5 mg | | | | Alcohol 5% | 5 mL q 4–6 hr | 2–6 yrs: 1.25 mL, 6–12 yrs: 2.5 mL, q 4–6 hr | b, c, e, f |
| Tablets (Schedule III) [U.S.] | | Phenylpropanolamine HCl 25 mg | Hydrocodone bitartrate 1.66 mg | | Guaifenesin 100 mg | Salicylamide 300 mg | | 1–2 tabs q 4–6 hr | Pediatric strength not available | b, e, f |
| *Tussar-2* Syrup (Schedule V) [U.S.] | | Pseudoephedrine HCl 30 mg | Codeine PO$_4$ 10 mg | | Guaifenesin 100 mg | | Alcohol 2.5% | 10 mL q 4 hr (max 40 mL daily) | 1.25–2.5 mL, 6–12 yrs: 2.5–5 mL, q 4–6 hr | b, c, e, f |
| *Tussar DM* Syrup (OTC) [U.S.] | Chlorpheniramine maleate 2 mg | Pseudoephedrine HCl 30 mg | | Dextromethorphan HBr 15 mg | | | Alcohol free | 10 mL q 6 hr | 6–12 yrs: 5 mL q 6 hrs | b, c, e |
| *Tussar SF* Syrup (Schedule V) [U.S.] | | Pseudoephedrine HCl 30 mg | Codeine PO$_4$ 10 mg | | Guaifenesin 100 mg | | Alcohol 2.5% Sugar free | 10 mL q 4 hr (max 40 mL daily) | Not recommended | b, c, e, f |
| *Tuss-DM* Tablets (OTC) [U.S.] | | | | Dextromethorphan HBr 10 mg | Guaifenesin 200 mg | | | 1–2 tabs q 4 hr | 6–12 yrs: ½–1 tab q 4 hr | b |
| *Tussex Cough* Syrup (OTC) [U.S.] | | Phenylephrine HCl 5 mg | | Dextromethorphan HBr 10 mg | Guaifenesin 100 mg | | | 10 mL q 4 hr | | b |

*Specific formulations may vary among the different manufacturers, check product labeling.

†Efficacy as expectorant has not been established.

‡Geriatric patients may be more sensitive to effects of usual adult dose.

§For appropriate *Packaging and storage* and *Auxiliary labeling* information refer to designated letters as follows:

a—Store below 40 °C (104 °F), preferably between 15 and 30 °C (59 and 86 °F), in a tight container, unless otherwise specified by manufacturer.

a¹—Store below 30 °C (86 °F), unless otherwise specified by manufacturer. Avoid exposure to excessive heat.

a²—Store below 25 °C (77 °F), unless otherwise specified by manufacturer.

b—Store below 40 °C (104 °F), preferably between 15 and 30 °C (59 and 86 °F), in a well-closed container, unless otherwise specified by manufacturer.

c—Protect from freezing.

d—Protect from light.

e—Auxiliary labeling: • May cause drowsiness. • Avoid alcoholic beverages.

f—Auxiliary labeling: • May be habit forming.

g—Auxiliary labeling: • Shake well.

h—Dispense in dropper bottle.

i—Chew well before swallowing.

**Included in subtherapeutic amount to discourage deliberate overdosage.

Table 3. Oral Dosage Forms (*continued*)
Note: Content per capsule, tablet, or 5 mL, unless otherwise stated.

| Brand or generic name [availability] | Antihistamines | Decongestants | Antitussives Opioid | Antitussives Non-opioid | Expectorants | Analgesics | Other content information as per product label | Usual Adult and Adolescent Dose prn‡ | Usual Pediatric Dose prn | Packaging, Storage, and Auxiliary labeling§ |
|---|---|---|---|---|---|---|---|---|---|---|
| *Tussgen* Oral Solution (Schedule III) [U.S.] | | Pseudoephedrine HCl 60 mg | Hydrocodone bitartrate 5 mg | | | | Alcohol 5% | 5 mL q 6 hr | | b, c, e, f |
| *Tuss-Genade Modified* Extended-release Capsules (Rx) [U.S.] | | Phenylpropanolamine HCl 75 mg | | Caramiphen edisylate 40 mg | | | | 1 cap q 12 hr | | b |
| *Tussigon* Tablets (Schedule III) [U.S.] | | | Hydrocodone bitartrate 5 mg | | | | Homatropine MBr** 1.5 mg Scored | 1 tab q 4–6 hr | 2–12 yrs: ½ tab q 4–6 hr | b, d, e, f |
| *Tussilyn DM* Syrup (OTC) [Canada] | Chlorpheniramine maleate 2.5 mg | Pseudoephedrine HCl 30 mg | | Dextromethorphan HBr 15 mg | | | | 10 mL q 8 hr | 2–6 yrs: 2.5 mL; 6–12 yrs: 5 mL, q 8 hr | a |
| *Tussionex* Tablets (N) [Canada] | Phenyltoloxamine as resin complex 10 mg | | Hydrocodone as resin complex 5 mg | | | | | 1 tab q 8–12 hr | >5 yrs: 1 cap q 12 hr | b, e, f |
| Oral Suspension (N) [Canada] | Phenyltoloxamine as resin complex 10 mg | | Hydrocodone as resin complex 5 mg | | | | Sugar free | 5 mL q 8–12 hr | 1–5 yrs: 2.5 mL, >5 yrs: 5 mL, q 12 hr | b, c, e, f, g |
| Oral Suspension (Schedule III) [U.S.] | Chlorpheniramine 8 mg (as polistirex) | | Hydrocodone 10 mg (as polistirex) | | | | Alcohol free | 5 mL q 12 hr | > 6 yrs: 2.5 mL q 12 hr | b, c, e, f |
| *Tussi-Organidin DM NR Liquid* Oral Solution (Rx) [U.S.] | | | | Dextromethorphan HBr 10 mg | Guaifenesin 100 mg | | Alcohol free Sugar free | 10 mL q 4 hr | 6 mos–2 yrs: 0.6–1.25 mL, 2–6 yrs: 2.5 mL, 6–12 yrs: 5 mL, q 4 hr | a, c, d |

Table 3. Oral Dosage Forms (*continued*)

Note: Content per capsule, tablet, or 5 mL, unless otherwise stated.

| Brand or generic name [availability] | Antihistamines | Decongestants | Antitussives Opioid | Antitussives Non-opioid | Expectorants | Analgesics | Other content information as per product label | Usual Adult and Adolescent Dose prn‡ | Usual Pediatric Dose prn | Packaging, Storage, and Auxiliary labeling§ |
|---|---|---|---|---|---|---|---|---|---|---|
| *Tussi-Organidin NR Liquid* Oral Solution (Schedule V) [U.S.] | | | Codeine PO$_4$ 10 mg | | Guaifenesin 100 mg | | Alcohol free Sugar free | 10 mL q 4 hr | 2–6 yrs: 1 mg/kg/day of codeine given in 4 divided doses 6–12 yrs: 5 mL q 4 hr | a, c, d, e, f |
| *Tussirex with Codeine Liquid* Syrup (Schedule V) [U.S.] | Pheniramine maleate 13.3 mg | Phenylephrine HCl 4.2 mg | Codeine PO$_4$ 10 mg | | Sodium citrate† 83.3 mg | Sodium salicylate 83.3 mg | Caffeine citrate 25 mg Alcohol free With or without sugar | 5 mL q 6–8 hr | 2–6 yrs: 1.25–2.5 mL, 6–12 yrs: 2.5–5 mL, q 6–8 hr | b, c, e, f |
| *Tuss-LA* Extended-release Tablets (Rx) [U.S.] | | Pseudoephedrine HCl 120 mg | | | Guaifenesin 500 mg | | | 1 tab q 12 hr | 2–6 yrs: Not recommended 6–12 yrs: tab q 12 hr | b |
| *Tusso-DM* Oral Solution (Rx) [U.S.] | | | | Dextromethorphan HBr 10 mg | Iodinated glycerol† 30 mg | | Alcohol free Sugar free | 5–10 mL q 4 hr | 2–6 yrs: 1.25–2.5 mL, 6–12 yrs: 5 mL, q 4 hr | a, c |
| *Tussogest* Extended-release Capsules (Rx) [U.S.] | | Phenylpropanolamine HCl 75 mg | | Caramiphen edisylate 40 mg | | | | 1 cap q 12 hr | Pediatric strength not available | b |

*Specific formulations may vary among the different manufacturers, check product labeling.

†Efficacy as expectorant has not been established.

‡Geriatric patients may be more sensitive to effects of usual adult dose.

§For appropriate *Packaging and storage* and *Auxiliary labeling* information refer to designated letters as follows:

   a—Store below 40 °C (104 °F), preferably between 15 and 30 °C (59 and 86 °F), in a tight container, unless otherwise specified by manufacturer.

   a¹—Store below 30 °C (86 °F), unless otherwise specified by manufacturer. Avoid exposure to excessive heat.

   a²—Store below 25 °C (77 °F), unless otherwise specified by manufacturer.

   b—Store below 40 °C (104 °F), preferably between 15 and 30 °C (59 and 86 °F), in a well-closed container, unless otherwise specified by manufacturer.

   c—Protect from freezing.

   d—Protect from light.

   e—Auxiliary labeling: • May cause drowsiness. • Avoid alcoholic beverages.

   f—Auxiliary labeling: • May be habit forming.

   g—Auxiliary labeling: • Shake well.

   h—Dispense in dropper bottle.

   i—Chew well before swallowing.

**Included in subtherapeutic amount to discourage deliberate overdosage.

## Table 3. Oral Dosage Forms (continued)

Note: Content per capsule, tablet, or 5 mL, unless otherwise stated.

| Brand or generic name [availability] | Antihistamines | Decongestants | Antitussives Opioid | Antitussives Non-opioid | Expectorants | Analgesics | Other content information as per product label | Usual Adult and Adolescent Dose prn‡ | Usual Pediatric Dose prn | Packaging, Storage, and Auxiliary labeling§ |
|---|---|---|---|---|---|---|---|---|---|---|
| *Tuss-Ornade Spansules* Extended-release Capsules (Rx) [Canada] | Chlorpheniramine maleate 8 mg | Phenylpropanolamine HCl 50 mg | | Caramiphen edisylate 20 mg | | | | 1 cap q 12 hr | Pediatric strength not available | b |
| *Ty-Cold Cold Formula* Tablets (OTC) [U.S.] | Chlorpheniramine maleate 2 mg | Pseudoephedrine HCl 30 mg | | Dextromethorphan HBr 15 mg | | Acetaminophen 325 mg | | 2 tabs q 6 hr | 6–12 yrs: 1 tab q 6 hr | b, e |
| *Tylenol Children's Cold DM* Oral Solution (OTC) [Canada] | Chlorpheniramine maleate 1 mg | Pseudoephedrine HCl 15 mg | | Dextromethorphan HBr 7.5 mg | | Acetaminophen 160 mg | Alcohol free | | 2–5 yrs: 5 mL, 6–12 yrs: 10 mL, q 4–6 hr (max 4 doses daily) | a |
| Chewable Tablets (OTC) [Canada] | Chlorpheniramine maleate 0.5 mg | Pseudoephedrine HCl 7.5 mg | | Dextromethorphan HBr 3.75 mg | | Acetaminophen 80 mg | Phenylalanine | | 2–5 yrs: 2 tabs (max 8 tabs daily), 6–12 yrs: 4 tabs (max 16 tabs daily), q 4–6 hr | b, i |
| *Tylenol Cold and Flu* for Oral Solution (OTC) [U.S.] | Chlorpheniramine maleate 4 mg/packet | Pseudoephedrine HCl 60 mg/packet | | Dextromethorphan HBr 30 mg/packet | | Acetaminophen 650 mg/packet | Phenylalanine 11 mg/packet | 1 packet dissolved in 180 mL of hot water q 6 hr | Intended for adult use | b, e |
| for Oral Solution (OTC) [Canada] | Chlorpheniramine maleate 4 mg/pouch | Pseudoephedrine HCl 60 mg/pouch | | Dextromethorphan HBr 30 mg/pouch | | Acetaminophen 650 mg/pouch | Sugar 19 grams/pouch | 1 pouch dissolved in 225 mL of hot water q 4–6 hr (max 3 pouches daily) | | b, e |
| *Tylenol Cold and Flu No Drowsiness Powder* for Oral Solution (OTC) [U.S.] | | Pseudoephedrine HCl 60 mg/packet | | Dextromethorphan HBr 30 mg/packet | | Acetaminophen 650 mg/packet | Phenylalanine 11 mg/packet | 1 packet dissolved in 180 mL of hot water q 6 hr | | b, c |

Table 3. Oral Dosage Forms (*continued*)

Note: Content per capsule, tablet, or 5 mL, unless otherwise stated.

| Brand or generic name [availability] | Antihistamines | Decongestants | Antitussives Opioid | Antitussives Non-opioid | Expectorants | Analgesics | Other content information as per product label | Usual Adult and Adolescent Dose prn‡ | Usual Pediatric Dose prn | Packaging, Storage, and Auxiliary labeling§ |
|---|---|---|---|---|---|---|---|---|---|---|
| *Tylenol Cold Medication Oral Solution* (OTC) [U.S.] | Chlorpheniramine maleate 0.66 mg (2 mg/15 mL) | Pseudoephedrine HCl 10 mg (30 mg/15 mL) | | Dextromethorphan HBr 5 mg (15 mg/15 mL) | | Acetaminophen 108.3 mg (325 mg/15 mL) | Alcohol 7% | 15–30 mL q 6 hr | Intended for adult use. | b, c, e |
| Tablets (OTC) [U.S./Canada] | Chlorpheniramine maleate 2 mg | Pseudoephedrine HCl 30 mg | | Dextromethorphan HBr 15 mg | | Acetaminophen 325 mg | | 1–2 tabs q 6 hr | 6–12 yrs: 1 tab q 6 hr | b, e |
| | Chlorpheniramine maleate 2 mg | Pseudoephedrine HCl 30 mg | | Dextromethorphan HBr 15 mg | | Acetaminophen 500 mg | | 1–2 tabs q 6 hr | Intended for adult use | b, e |
| *Tylenol Cold Medication, Non-Drowsy* Tablets (OTC) [U.S./Canada] | | Pseudoephedrine HCl 30 mg | | Dextromethorphan HBr 15 mg | | Acetaminophen 325 mg | | 1–2 tabs q 6 hr | 6–12 yrs: 1 tab q 6 hr | b, e |
| | | Pseudoephedrine HCl 30 mg | | Dextromethorphan HBr 15 mg | | Acetaminophen 500 mg | | 1–2 tabs q 6 hr | Intended for adult use | b, e |
| *Tylenol Cough with Decongestant Maximum Strength Oral Solution* (OTC) [U.S.] | | Pseudoephedrine HCl 15 mg | | Dextromethorphan HBr 7.5 mg | | Acetaminophen 250 mg | Alcohol 10% | 20 mL q 6–8 hr | Pediatric strength not available | b, c |

*Specific formulations may vary among the different manufacturers, check product labeling.

†Efficacy as expectorant has not been established.

‡Geriatric patients may be more sensitive to effects of usual adult dose.

§For appropriate *Packaging and storage* and *Auxiliary labeling* information refer to designated letters as follows:

a—Store below 40 °C (104 °F), preferably between 15 and 30 °C (59 and 86 °F), in a tight container, unless otherwise specified by manufacturer.

a¹—Store below 30 °C (86 °F), unless otherwise specified by manufacturer. Avoid exposure to excessive heat.

a²—Store below 25 °C (77 °F), unless otherwise specified by manufacturer.

b—Store below 40 °C (104 °F), preferably between 15 and 30 °C (59 and 86 °F), in a well-closed container, unless otherwise specified by manufacturer.

c—Protect from freezing.

d—Protect from light.

e—Auxiliary labeling: • May cause drowsiness. • Avoid alcoholic beverages.

f—Auxiliary labeling: • May be habit forming.

g—Auxiliary labeling: • Shake well.

h—Dispense in dropper bottle.

i—Chew well before swallowing.

**Included in subtherapeutic amount to discourage deliberate overdosage.

Table 3. Oral Dosage Forms (*continued*)

Note: Content per capsule, tablet, or 5 mL, unless otherwise stated.

| Brand or generic name [availability] | Antihistamines | Decongestants | Antitussives Opioid | Antitussives Non-opioid | Expectorants | Analgesics | Other content information as per product label | Usual Adult and Adolescent Dose prn‡ | Usual Pediatric Dose prn | Packaging, Storage, and Auxiliary labeling§ |
|---|---|---|---|---|---|---|---|---|---|---|
| *Tylenol Extra Strength Cold and Flu* for Oral Solution (OTC) [Canada] | Chlorpheniramine maleate 4 mg/pouch | Pseudoephedrine HCl 60 mg/ pouch | | Dextromethorphan HBr 30 mg/pouch | | Acetaminophen 1000 mg/ pouch | Sugar 17.5 grams/ pouch | 1 pouch dissolved in 225 mL of hot water q 4–6 hr (max 3 pouches daily) | | b, e |
| *Tylenol Junior Strength Cold DM* Chewable Tablets (OTC) [Canada] | Chlorpheniramine maleate 1 mg | Pseudoephedrine HCl 15 mg | | Dextromethorphan HBr 7.5 mg | | Acetaminophen 160 mg | Phenylalanine | | 2–5 yrs: 1 tabs (max 4 tabs daily), 6–11 yrs: 2 tabs (max 8 tabs daily), q 4–6 hr | b, i |
| *Tylenol Maximum Strength Cough* Oral Solution (OTC) [U.S.] | | | | Dextromethorphan HBr 7.5 mg | | Acetaminophen 250 mg | Alcohol 10% | 20 mL q 6–8 hr | | b, c |
| *Tylenol Maximum Strength Flu Gelcaps* Tablets (OTC) [U.S.] | | Pseudoephedrine HCl 30 mg | | Dextromethorphan HBr 15 mg | | Acetaminophen 500 mg | | 2 tabs q 6 hr (max 8 tabs daily) | | b |
| *Tyrodone* Oral Solution (Schedule III) [U.S.] | | Pseudoephedrine HCl 60 mg | Hydrocodone bitartrate 5 mg | | | | Alcohol 5% | 5 mL q 4–6 hr | | a, c, e, f |
| *ULR-LA* Extended-release Tablets (Rx) [U.S.] | | Phenylpropanolamine HCl 75 mg | | | Guaifenesin 400 mg | | | 1 tab q 12 hr | | b |
| *Uni-tussin DM* Syrup (OTC) [U.S.] | | | | Dextromethorphan HBr 10 mg | Guaifenesin 100 mg | | Alcohol free | 10 mL q 4 hr | | b, c |
| *Unproco* Capsules (Rx) [U.S.] | | | | Dextromethorphan HBr 30 mg | Guaifenesin 200 mg | | | 1 cap q 4 hr | Pediatric strength not available | a, d |

## Table 3. Oral Dosage Forms *(continued)*

Note: Content per capsule, tablet, or 5 mL, unless otherwise stated.

| Brand or generic name [availability] | Antihistamines | Decongestants | Antitussives — Opioid | Antitussives — Non-opioid | Expectorants | Analgesics | Other content information as per product label | Usual Adult and Adolescent Dose prn‡ | Usual Pediatric Dose prn | Packaging, Storage, and Auxiliary labeling§ |
|---|---|---|---|---|---|---|---|---|---|---|
| *Utex-S.R.* Extended-release Tablets (Rx) [U.S.] | | Phenylpropanolamine HCl 75 mg | | | Guaifenesin 400 mg | | | 1 tab q 12 hr | Pediatric strength not available | b |
| *Vanex Expectorant* Syrup (Schedule III) [U.S.] | | Pseudoephedrine HCl 30 mg | Hydrocodone bitartrate 2.5 mg | | Guaifenesin 100 mg | | Alcohol 5% | 10 mL q 4 6 hr | 6–12 yrs: 5 mL, q 4 6 hr | b, c, d, e, f |
| *Vanex Grape* Oral Solution (Schedule V) [U.S.] | Chlorpheniramine maleate 5 mg | Phenylpropanolamine HCl 20 mg / Phenylephrine HCl 20 mg | Dihydrocodeine bitartrate 3 mg | | | | | 5 mL q 4 5 hr | 6–12 yrs: 2.5 mL q 4–5 hr | a, e, f |
| *Vanex-HD* Syrup (Schedule III) [U.S.] | Chlorpheniramine maleate 2 mg | Phenylephrine HCl 5 mg | Hydrocodone bitartrate 1.7 mg | | | | | 10 mL q 6–8 hr | 6–12 yrs: 5 mL q 6–8 hr | b, c, e, f |
| *V-Dec-M* Extended-release Tablets (Rx) [U.S.] | | Pseudoephedrine HCl 120 mg | | | Guaifenesin 500 mg | | Scored | 1 tab q 12 hr | | b |
| *Versacaps* Extended-release Capsules (Rx) [U.S.] | | Pseudoephedrine HCl 60 mg | | | Guaifenesin 300 mg | | | 1–2 caps q 12 hr | | b |
| *Vicks 44 Cough and Cold Relief* LiquiCaps Capsules (OTC) [U.S.] | | Pseudoephedrine HCl 60 mg | | Dextromethorphan HBr 30 mg | | | Alcohol free | 1 cap q 6 hr | | b |

\*Specific formulations may vary among the different manufacturers; check product labeling.

†Efficacy as expectorant has not been established.

‡Geriatric patients may be more sensitive to effects of usual adult dose.

§For appropriate *Packaging and storage* and *Auxiliary labeling* information refer to designated letters as follows:

  a—Store below 40 °C (104 °F), preferably between 15 and 30 °C (59 and 86 °F), in a tight container, unless otherwise specified by manufacturer.

  a¹—Store below 30 °C (86 °F), unless otherwise specified by manufacturer. Avoid exposure to excessive heat.

  a²—Store below 25 °C (77 °F), unless otherwise specified by manufacturer.

  b—Store below 40 °C (104 °F), preferably between 15 and 30 °C (59 and 86 °F), in a well-closed container, unless otherwise specified by manufacturer.

  c—Protect from freezing.

  d—Protect from light.

  e—Auxiliary labeling: • May cause drowsiness. • Avoid alcoholic beverages.

  f—Auxiliary labeling: • May be habit forming.

  g—Auxiliary labeling: • Shake well.

  h—Dispense in dropper bottle.

  i—Chew well before swallowing.

\*\*Included in subtherapeutic amount to discourage deliberate overdosage.

Table 3. Oral Dosage Forms *(continued)*

Note: Content per capsule, tablet, or 5 mL, unless otherwise stated.

| Brand or generic name [availability] | Antihistamines | Decongestants | Antitussives Opioid | Antitussives Non-opioid | Expectorants | Analgesics | Other content information as per product label | Usual Adult and Adolescent Dose prn‡ | Usual Pediatric Dose prn | Packaging, Storage, and Auxiliary labeling§ |
|---|---|---|---|---|---|---|---|---|---|---|
| *Vicks 44D Dry Hacking Cough and Head Congestion* Oral Solution (OTC) [U.S.] | | Pseudoephedrine HCl 20 mg (60 mg/15 mL) | | Dextromethorphan HBr 10 mg (30 mg/15 mL) | | | Alcohol 10% | 15 mL q 6 hr | | b, c |
| *Vicks DayQuil Multi-Symptom Cold/Flu LiquiCaps* Capsules (OTC) [U.S.] | | Pseudoephedrine HCl 30 mg | | Dextromethorphan HBr 10 mg | Guaifenesin 100 mg | Acetaminophen 250 mg | | 2 caps q 4 hr (max 8 caps daily) | 6–11 yrs: 1 cap q 4 hr | b, c |
| *Vicks DayQuil Non-Drowsy Cold/Flu* Oral Solution (OTC) [U.S.] | | Pseudoephedrine HCl 30 mg/15 mL | | Dextromethorphan HBr 10 mg/ 15 mL | Guaifenesin 100 mg/ 15 mL | Acetaminophen 325 mg/ 15 mL | Alcohol free | 30 mL q 4 hr | 6–11 yrs: 15 mL q 4 hr (max 4 doses daily) | b, c |
| *Vicks DayQuil Sinus Pressure and Congestion Relief Caplets* Tablets (OTC) [U.S.] | | Phenylpropanolamine HCl 25 mg | | | Guaifenesin 200 mg | | | 1 tab q 4 hr (max 6 tabs daily) | | b |
| *Vicks 44M Cough, Cold and Flu Relief* Oral Solution (OTC) [U.S.] | Chlorpheniramine maleate 1 mg (4 mg/20mL) | Pseudoephedrine HCl 15 mg (60 mg/20 mL) | | Dextromethorphan HBr 7.5 mg (30 mg/20 mL) | | Acetaminophen 130 mg (650 mg/ 20 mL) | Alcohol 10% | 20 mL q 6 hr | | b, c |
| *Vicks 44M Cough, Cold and Flu Relief LiquiCaps* Capsules (OTC) [U.S.] | Chlorpheniramine maleate 2 mg | Pseudoephedrine HCl 30 mg | | Dextromethorphan HBr 10 mg | | Acetaminophen 250 mg | Alcohol free Sugar free | 2 caps q 4 hr | 6–11 yrs: 1 cap q 4 hr | b, e |
| *Vicks NyQuil Hot Therapy for* Oral Solution (OTC) [U.S.] | Doxylamine succinate 12.5 mg/ packet | Pseudoephedrine HCl 60 mg/ packet | | Dextromethorphan HBr 30 mg/ packet | | Acetaminophen 1000 mg/ packet | | 1 packet dissolved in 6-oz cup of hot water q 6 hr | Intended for adult use | b, e |
| *Vicks NyQuil Multi-Symptom Cold/Flu Relief* Oral Solution (OTC) [U.S.] | Doxylamine succinate 2 mg (12.5 mg/30 mL) | Pseudoephedrine HCl 10 mg (60 mg/30 mL) | | Dextromethorphan HBr 5 mg (30 mg/ 30 mL) | | Acetaminophen 166.6 mg (1000 mg/ 30 mL) | Alcohol 10% | 30 mL hs or q 6 hr | Not recommended | b, c, e |

Table 3. Oral Dosage Forms (continued)

Note: Content per capsule, tablet, or 5 mL, unless otherwise stated.

| Brand or generic name [availability] | Antihistamines | Decongestants | Antitussives Opioid | Antitussives Non-opioid | Expectorants | Analgesics | Other content information as per product label | Usual Adult and Adolescent Dose prn‡ | Usual Pediatric Dose prn | Packaging, Storage, and Auxiliary labeling§ |
|---|---|---|---|---|---|---|---|---|---|---|
| Vicks NyQuil Multi-Symptom LiquiCaps Capsules (OTC) [U.S.] | Doxylamine succinate 6.25 mg | Pseudoephedrine HCl 30 mg | | Dextromethorphan HBr 10 mg | | Acetaminophen 250 mg | | 2 caps q 4 hr | Intended for adult use | b, e |
| Vicks Pediatric Formula 44D Cough & Decongestant Oral Solution (OTC) [U.S.] | | Pseudoephedrine HCl 10 mg | | Dextromethorphan HBr 5 mg | | | Alcohol free | | 2–5 yrs: 7.5 mL q 6 hr, 6–11 yrs: 15 mL q 6 hr | b, c |
| Vicks Pediatric Formula 44E Oral Solution (OTC) [U.S.] | | | | Dextromethorphan HBr 3.3 mg | Guaifenesin 33.3 mg | | Alcohol free | | 2–11 yrs: 7.5–15 mL q 4 hr | b, c |
| Vicks Pediatric Formula 44M Multi-Symptom Cough & Cold Oral Solution (OTC) [U.S.] | Chlorpheniramine maleate 0.67 mg | Pseudoephedrine HCl 10 mg | | Dextromethorphan HBr 5 mg | | | Alcohol free | | 6–11 yrs: 15 mL q 6 hr | b, c, e |
| Vicodin Tuss Syrup (Schedule III) [U.S.] | | | Hydrocodone bitartrate 5 mg | | Guaifenesin 100 mg | | Alcohol free Sugar free Dye free | 5 mL q 4 hr | 6–12 yrs: 2.5–5 mL q 4 hr | b, c, e, f |
| Zephrex Tablets (Rx) [U.S.] | | Pseudoephedrine HCl 60 mg | | | Guaifenesin 400 mg | | | 1 tab q 4–6 hr | Pediatric strength not available | b |
| Zephrex-LA Extended-release Tablets (Rx) [U.S.] | | Pseudoephedrine HCl 120 mg | | | Guaifenesin 600 mg | | | 1 tab q 12 hr | Pediatric strength not available | b |

*Specific formulations may vary among the different manufacturers; check product labeling.

†Efficacy as expectorant has not been established.

‡Geriatric patients may be more sensitive to effects of usual adult dose.

§For appropriate *Packaging and storage* and *Auxiliary labeling* information refer to designated letters as follows:

a—Store below 40 °C (104 °F), preferably between 15 and 30 °C (59 and 86 °F), in a tight container, unless otherwise specified by manufacturer.

a¹—Store below 30 °C (86 °F), unless otherwise specified by manufacturer. Avoid exposure to excessive heat.

a²—Store below 25 °C (77 °F), unless otherwise specified by manufacturer.

b—Store below 40 °C (104 °F), preferably between 15 and 30 °C (59 and 86 °F), in a well-closed container, unless otherwise specified by manufacturer.

c—Protect from freezing.

d—Protect from light.

e—Auxiliary labeling: • May cause drowsiness. • Avoid alcoholic beverages.

f—Auxiliary labeling: • May be habit forming.

g—Auxiliary labeling: • Shake well.

h—Dispense in dropper bottle.

i—Chew well before swallowing.

**Included in subtherapeutic amount to discourage deliberate overdosage.

# CROMOLYN   Inhalation-Local

INN: Cromoglicic acid
BAN: Cromoglycic acid
JAN: Sodium cromoglicate
VA CLASSIFICATION (Primary/Secondary): RE101/RE109

Other commonly used names are cromoglicic acid, cromoglycic acid, sodium cromoglicate, and sodium cromoglycate.

Note: For a listing of dosage forms and brand names by country availability, see *Dosage Forms* section(s). For a listing of brand names for the articles in this monograph, refer to the General Index.

## Category

Anti-inflammatory, nonsteroidal (inhalation); mast cell stabilizer; asthma prophylactic; antiallergic (inhalation).

## Indications

### Accepted

Asthma (prophylaxis)—Cromolyn inhalation is indicated as first-line anti-inflammatory medication, either alone or as an adjunct to bronchodilator therapy, for the prevention of airway inflammation and bronchoconstriction in patients with mild to moderate asthma who require daily therapy.

Bronchospasm (prophylaxis)—Cromolyn inhalation is indicated to prevent acute bronchospasm induced by exercise, or by exposure to allergens, cold dry air, environmental pollutants, or other known precipitating factors, whether exposure is episodic or continuous.

### Unaccepted

Cromolyn inhalation is not indicated for the reversal or relief of acute asthma attacks, especially in status asthmaticus; cromolyn has no immediate bronchodilating activity.

## Pharmacology/Pharmacokinetics

### Physicochemical characteristics

Molecular weight—512.34.

### Mechanism of action/Effect

The exact mechanism by which cromolyn prevents immediate-onset and delayed-onset asthmatic reactions following inhaled allergens or non-immunological stimuli is not completely known. Cromolyn inhibits the release of mediators, such as histamine and leukotrienes, from mast cells. Prevention of mediator release is thought to result from indirect blockade of the entry of calcium ions into the cells. Cromolyn has also been shown to inhibit the movement of other inflammatory cells such as neutrophils, eosinophils, and monocytes. Additionally, cromolyn has also been shown in animal studies to inhibit neuronal reflexes within the lung, prevent down-regulation of beta-2-adrenergic receptors on lymphocytes, and to inhibit bronchospasm caused by tachykinins.

Cromolyn has no intrinsic bronchodilator, glucocorticoid, or antihistaminic action.

### Absorption

Following administration of cromolyn by inhalation, approximately 8 to 10% of the radioactively labeled dose of cromolyn penetrates the lungs from which it is readily absorbed into systemic circulation. The remainder is either exhaled or swallowed and excreted via the alimentary tract, with very little medication absorbed.

### Onset of action

Cromolyn inhibits a decrease in forced expiratory volume in one second ($FEV_1$) when inhaled 1 minute before antigen challenge. When cromolyn is used as maintenance therapy, clinical improvement in symptoms and lung function usually occurs within 4 weeks of beginning treatment. However, in some patients, improvement may occur almost immediately.

### Duration of action

Protection against antigen or exercise challenge—Up to 2 hours.

### Elimination

Unchanged, approximately equally divided between urine and bile.

## Precautions to Consider

### Carcinogenicity

Long-term studies in mice (12 months intraperitoneal treatment followed by 6 months observation), hamsters (12 months intraperitoneal treatment followed by 12 months observation), and rats (18 months subcutaneous treatment) showed that cromolyn has no neoplastic effect.

### Mutagenicity

In various mutagenicity studies, there was no evidence of chromosomal damage or cytotoxicity.

### Pregnancy/Reproduction

Fertility—In animal reproduction studies with cromolyn, there was no evidence of impaired fertility.

Pregnancy—Although extensive studies in humans have not been done, some limited data suggest that cromolyn is not associated with an increased incidence of fetal anomalies. Poorly controlled asthma and loss of pulmonary function present a greater risk to the mother and may result in placental hypoxemia and increased perinatal mortality, increased prematurity, and low birth weight.

Reproduction studies in mice, rats, and rabbits with cromolyn administered parenterally in doses of up to 338 times the human clinical dose showed no evidence of fetal malformations. Adverse fetal effects (increased resorptions and decreased fetal weight) were noted only with very high parenteral doses that produced maternal toxicity.

Studies in pregnant mice have shown that the addition of cromolyn (338 times the human dose) to isoproterenol (90 times the human dose) appears to increase the incidence of both resorptions and malformations.

FDA Pregnancy Category B.

### Breast-feeding

It is not known whether cromolyn is distributed into human breast milk; however, problems have not been documented. Since cromolyn reaches very low concentrations in maternal serum, it would be expected to reach even lower and probably undetectable concentrations in breast milk.

In monkeys given intravenous cromolyn, concentrations in breast milk measured less than 0.001% of the administered dose.

### Pediatrics

Appropriate studies performed to date have not demonstrated pediatrics-specific problems that would limit the usefulness of cromolyn in children.

### Geriatrics

Although appropriate studies on the relationship of age to the effects of cromolyn inhalation have not been performed in the geriatric population, no geriatrics-specific problems have been documented to date.

### Laboratory value alterations

The following have been selected on the basis of their potential clinical significance (possible effect in parentheses where appropriate)—not necessarily inclusive (» = major clinical significance):

With diagnostic test results
Bronchial airway hyperreactivity assessment
(cromolyn alters bronchial airway hyperreactivity over time by its proposed anti-inflammatory effect; this may lead to a lessened response to methacholine challenge in some patients)

### Medical considerations/Contraindications

The medical considerations/contraindications included here have been selected on the basis of their potential clinical significance (reasons given in parentheses where appropriate)—not necessarily inclusive (» = major clinical significance):

*Risk-benefit should be considered when the following medical problem exists:*

Sensitivity to cromolyn

## Side/Adverse Effects

Note: Adverse reactions to cromolyn sodium are uncommon. Angioedema, bronchospasm, cough, dizziness, dysuria and urinary frequency, headache, joint swelling and pain, laryngeal edema, lacrimation, nausea, nasal congestion, rash, swollen parotid glands, and urticaria attributed to cromolyn have been reported to occur in less than 1 in 10,000 patients. Anemia, exfoliative dermatitis, hemoptysis, hoarseness, myalgia, nephrosis, periarteritic vasculitis, pericarditis, peripheral neuritis, photodermatitis, polymyositis, pulmonary infiltrates with eosinophilia, and vertigo have been reported in less than 1 in 100,000 patients. In all cases the causal relationship is unclear.

The following side/adverse effects have been selected on the basis of their potential clinical significance (possible signs and symptoms in parentheses where appropriate)—not necessarily inclusive:

**Those indicating need for medical attention**
Incidence rare
   *Anaphylactic reaction* (difficulty in swallowing; hives; itching of skin; swelling of face, lips, or eyelids; increased wheezing or difficulty in breathing; low blood pressure)—reported in less than 1 in 100,000 patients

**Those indicating need for medical attention only if they continue or are bothersome**
Incidence more frequent
   *Bad taste in mouth*—for metered dose inhaler; *throat irritation or dryness*

## Patient Consultation

As an aid to patient consultation, refer to *Advice for the Patient, Cromolyn (Inhalation).*

In providing consultation, consider emphasizing the following selected information (» = major clinical significance):

**Before using this medication**
» Conditions affecting use, especially:
   Sensitivity to cromolyn

**Proper use of this medication**
» Helps prevent, but does not relieve, acute attacks of asthma or bronchospasm
» Importance of not using more medication than the amount prescribed
   Reading patient instructions carefully before using
   Checking periodically with health care professional for proper use of inhaler to prevent incorrect dosage
» Proper dosing
   Missed dose: If used regularly, using as soon as possible; using any remaining doses for that day at regularly spaced intervals
» Proper storage
*For inhalation aerosol dosage form*
   Keeping record of number of sprays used, if possible; not floating canister in water to test fullness
   Testing or priming inhaler before using first time or if not used for a while
   Proper administration technique
   Proper administration technique with spacer device
   Proper cleaning procedure for inhaler
*For inhalation capsule dosage form*
» Not swallowing capsules; medication not effective if swallowed
   Using with Spinhaler or Halermatic inhaler
   Proper loading technique for inhaler
   Proper administration technique
   Proper cleaning procedure for inhaler
*For inhalation solution dosage form*
   Not using if solution cloudy or contains particles
   Proper breaking of ampul
   Using in a power-operated nebulizer with an adequate flow rate and equipped with face mask or mouthpiece; not using hand-squeezed bulb nebulizers
*For patients on scheduled dosing regimen*
» Compliance with therapy; may require up to 4 weeks for full benefit

**Precautions while using this medication**
» Checking with physician if symptoms do not improve within first 4 weeks; checking with physician immediately if condition becomes worse
» Importance of not discontinuing concurrent systemic corticosteroid or bronchodilator therapy without physician's advice
   Possible throat irritation or dryness; gargling and rinsing mouth or taking drink of water after each dose to help prevent these effects

**Side/adverse effects**
   Signs of potential side effects, especially anaphylactic reaction
   Cromolyn inhalation aerosol may cause an unpleasant taste

## General Dosing Information

When cromolyn is introduced into the patient's therapeutic regimen after an acute episode, the episode must be under control, the airway clear, and the patient able to inhale adequately.

A decrease in severity of clinical symptoms or in the need for concomitant therapy is a sign of improvement that will be evident in the first 4 weeks of therapy if patient responds to cromolyn therapy.

In asthmatic patients receiving systemic corticosteroids and/or bronchodilators prior to institution of cromolyn, the corticosteroid and/or bron-

chodilator should be continued following initiation of cromolyn therapy. However, an attempt should be made to reduce the dosage of the systemic corticosteroid and/or institute an alternate-day regimen. The dosage of the corticosteroid should be reduced gradually to avoid an exacerbation of asthma.

*For inhalation solution dosage form only*—Cromolyn solution should be administered from a power-operated nebulizer having an adequate flow rate (6 to 8 liters per minute) and equipped with a suitable face mask or mouthpiece. Hand-squeezed bulb nebulizers are not suitable for administration of cromolyn solution.

## Inhalation Dosage Forms
### CROMOLYN SODIUM INHALATION AEROSOL

**Usual adult and adolescent dose**
Asthma (prophylaxis)—
   Oral inhalation, 2 inhalations (1.6 or 2 mg) four times a day at regular intervals of four to six hours.
   Note: When the patient is stabilized on a maintenance regimen of four times a day, the dosing frequency may be gradually reduced to three times a day, then to two times a day in some patients.
Bronchospasm (prophylaxis)—
   Oral inhalation, 2 inhalations (1.6 or 2 mg) as a single dose administered at least ten to fifteen (but not more than sixty) minutes before exercise or exposure to any precipitating factor.

**Usual adult prescribing limits**
Up to 16 puffs (12.8 or 16 mg) daily.

**Usual pediatric dose**
Children up to 5 years of age—Dosage has not been established.
Children 5 years of age and over—See *Usual adult and adolescent dose.*

**Usual geriatric dose**
See *Usual adult and adolescent dose.*

**Strength(s) usually available**
U.S.—
   800 mcg (0.8 mg) per metered spray (Rx) [*Intal*].
Canada—
   1 mg per metered spray (Rx) [*Intal*].
Note: In Canada, metered dose inhalers are labeled according to the amount of cromolyn delivered at the valve; in the U.S., metered dose inhalers are labeled according to the amount of cromolyn delivered at the mouthpiece or actuator. Therefore, 1 mg of cromolyn delivered at the valve is equivalent to 800 mcg delivered at the mouthpiece.

**Packaging and storage**
Store between 15 and 30 °C (59 and 86 °F), unless otherwise specified by manufacturer. Protect from freezing.

**Auxiliary labeling**
• For oral inhalation only.
• Shake well before using.
• Store away from heat and direct sunlight.

**Note**
Include patient instructions when dispensing.

Demonstrate inhalation technique to patient when dispensing.

**Additional information**
U.S.—Each 8.1-gram canister delivers at least 112 metered sprays; each 14.2-gram canister delivers at least 200 metered sprays.

Canada—Each canister delivers either 112 or 200 metered sprays.

### CROMOLYN SODIUM FOR INHALATION (CAPSULES) USP

**Usual adult and adolescent dose**
Asthma (prophylaxis)—
   Oral inhalation, 20 mg (1 capsule) four times a day at regular intervals of four to six hours.
   Note: When the patient is stabilized on a maintenance regimen of four times a day, the dosing frequency may be gradually reduced to three times a day, then to two times a day in some patients.
Bronchospasm (prophylaxis)—
   Oral inhalation, 20 mg (1 capsule) as a single dose administered at least ten to fifteen (but not more than sixty) minutes before exercise or exposure to the precipitating factor.

**Usual adult prescribing limits**
Up to 160 mg (8 capsules) daily.

**Usual pediatric dose**
Children up to 2 years of age—Dosage has not been established.
Children 2 years of age and over—See *Usual adult and adolescent dose.*

**Usual geriatric dose**
See *Usual adult and adolescent dose.*

**Strength(s) usually available**
U.S.—
Not commercially available.
Canada—
20 mg per inhalation capsule (Rx) [*Intal*].

**Packaging and storage**
Store below 40 °C (104 °F), preferably between 15 and 30 °C (59 and 86 °F), unless otherwise specified by manufacturer. Store in a tight, light-resistant container.

**Auxiliary labeling**
• For inhalation only—Do not swallow capsules.

**Note**
Include patient instructions when dispensing.
Demonstrate administration technique to patient when dispensing.
Demonstration kits may be available.

## CROMOLYN SODIUM INHALATION SOLUTION USP

**Usual adult and adolescent dose**
Asthma (prophylaxis)—
Oral inhalation, 20 mg four times a day at regular intervals of four to six hours.
Note: When the patient is stabilized on a maintenance regimen of four times a day, the dosing frequency may be gradually reduced to three times a day, then to two times a day in some patients.
Bronchospasm (prophylaxis)—
Oral inhalation, 20 mg as a single dose administered at least ten to fifteen (but not more than sixty) minutes before exercise or exposure to the precipitating factor.

**Usual adult prescribing limits**
Up to 160 mg daily.

**Usual pediatric dose**
Children up to 2 years of age—Dosage has not been established.
Children 2 years of age and over—See *Usual adult and adolescent dose.*

**Usual geriatric dose**
See *Usual adult and adolescent dose.*

**Strength(s) usually available**
U.S.—
20 mg per 2-ml ampul (Rx) [*Intal;* GENERIC].
Canada—
20 mg per 2-ml ampul (Rx) [*Intal; Novo-cromolyn; PMS-Sodium Cromoglycate*].

**Packaging and storage**
Store below 40 °C (104 °F), preferably between 15 and 30 °C (59 and 86 °F), unless otherwise specified by manufacturer. Protect from freezing. Protect from light.

**Stability**
Solution should not be used if it is cloudy or contains a precipitate.
Any solution remaining in the nebulizer should be discarded.
Cromolyn sodium inhalation solution has been shown to be physically and chemically compatible with acetylcysteine, albuterol, epinephrine, isoetharine, isoproterenol, metaproterenol, and terbutaline solutions for up to 60 minutes.
When combining cromolyn and ipratropium inhalation solutions, it is recommended that only *preservative-free* ipratropium solution be used. Mixing cromolyn inhalation solution with ipratropium inhalation solution containing the preservative benzalkonium chloride is not recommended because mixing results in cloudiness of the solution, which is due to complexation between cromolyn sodium and benzalkonium chloride, although no precipitation or significant decrease in the concentration of cromolyn or ipratropium occurs.
Cromolyn should not be mixed with bitolterol inhalation solution, since mixing results in cloudiness of the solution.

**Auxiliary labeling**
• For inhalation only.

**Note**
Include patient information when dispensing.
Demonstrate opening and emptying of ampul when dispensing.

## Selected Bibliography

Murphy S. Cromolyn sodium: basic mechanisms and clinical usage. Pediatr Asthma Allergy Immunol 1988; 2: 237-54.
Murphy S, Kelly HW. Cromolyn sodium: a review of mechanisms and clinical use in asthma. DICP 1987; 21: 22-35.

Revised: 04/23/96

---

# CROMOLYN   Nasal

VA CLASSIFICATION (Primary): NT900
Another commonly used name is sodium cromoglycate.
Note: For a listing of dosage forms and brand names by country availability, see *Dosage Forms* section(s). For a listing of brand names for the articles in this monograph, refer to the General Index.

## Category
Mast cell stabilizer (nasal); antiallergic (nasal).

## Indications

**Accepted**
Rhinitis, allergic (prophylaxis and treatment)—Cromolyn sodium nasal solution is indicated for the prophylaxis and treatment of the symptoms of perennial and seasonal allergic rhinitis.
Cromolyn sodium for nasal insufflation is indicated for the prophylaxis of seasonal allergic rhinitis.

## Pharmacology/Pharmacokinetics

**Physicochemical characteristics**
Molecular weight—512.34.
pH—4.5 to 6.5.

**Mechanism of action/Effect**
Cromolyn is a mast cell stabilizer that inhibits the Type I immediate hypersensitivity reaction by preventing the antigen-stimulated release of histamine. Cromolyn also prevents the release of leukotrienes and inhibits eosinophil chemotaxis.
*In vitro* and *in vivo* animal studies have shown that cromolyn inhibits the degranulation of sensitized mast cells that occurs after exposure to specific antigens. Some *in vitro* studies have shown that cromolyn inhibits the degranulation of nonsensitized rat mast cells by phospholipase A and the subsequent release of chemical mediators.

**Other actions/effects**
Cromolyn has no intrinsic bronchodilator, antihistaminic, or anti-inflammatory action.

**Absorption**
Poorly absorbed from the gastrointestinal tract. After instillation of cromolyn nasal solution, less than 7% of the total dose administered is absorbed.

**Onset of therapeutic effect**
Seasonal allergic rhinitis—Results are usually noticeable in less than 1 week.

**Time to peak effect**
Perennial allergic rhinitis—Results are usually noticeable in approximately 1 week; however, in some cases up to 4 weeks may be required.

**Elimination**
Nasal solution—The portion of the dose that is absorbed (7%) is rapidly excreted unchanged in the bile and urine; the remainder of the dose is expelled from the nose, or swallowed and excreted via the alimentary tract.

## Precautions to Consider

**Carcinogenicity**
Long-term studies with cromolyn in mice (12 months intraperitoneal treatment followed by 6 months observation), hamsters (12 months intraperitoneal treatment followed by 12 months observation), and rats (18 months subcutaneous treatment) did not show any neoplastic effect.

**Mutagenicity**
In various mutagenicity studies, there was no evidence of chromosomal damage or cytotoxicity.

## Pregnancy/Reproduction

Fertility—Animal reproduction studies with cromolyn showed no evidence of impaired fertility.

Pregnancy—Adequate and well-controlled studies in humans have not been done.

A ten year study of 296 pregnant asthmatic women in Sri Lanka administered cromolyn by oral inhalation during part or all of their pregnancies resulted in 4 infants (1.35%) with malformations. However, epidemiological studies suggest that the usual incidence of fetal abnormalities in the Sri Lanka population is 2 to 3%.

Reproduction studies in mice, rats, and rabbits with cromolyn administered parenterally in doses up to 338 times the human clinical doses showed no evidence of fetal malformations. (Adverse fetal effects [increased resorptions and decreased fetal weight] were noted only at very high parenteral doses that produced maternal toxicity.)

FDA Pregnancy Category B.

## Breast-feeding

It is not known whether cromolyn is distributed into breast milk; however, cromolyn reaches very low concentrations in maternal serum. Problems in humans have not been documented.

## Pediatrics

Appropriate studies on the relationship of age to the effects of nasal cromolyn have not been performed in the U.S. in children up to 6 years of age (in Canada, up to 5 years of age). In older children, no pediatrics-specific problems have been documented to date.

## Geriatrics

Appropriate studies on the relationship of age to the effects of nasal cromolyn have not been performed in the geriatric population. However, no geriatrics-specific problems have been documented to date.

## Drug interactions and/or related problems

The following drug interactions and/or related problems have been selected on the basis of their potential clinical significance (possible mechanism in parentheses where appropriate)—not necessarily inclusive (» = major clinical significance):

Methacholine, for inhalation
(cromolyn may decrease slightly, but inconsistently, the response to methacholine challenge in the diagnosis of bronchial airway hyperreactivity; however, cromolyn generally does not cause false-negative tests)

## Medical considerations/Contraindications

The medical considerations/contraindications included here have been selected on the basis of their potential clinical significance (reasons given in parentheses where appropriate)—not necessarily inclusive (» = major clinical significance).

*Risk-benefit should be considered when the following medical problems exist:*

Polyps, nasal
(medication may not be effective if nasal passage obstruction exists)
Sensitivity to cromolyn

## Side/Adverse Effects

Note: Eosinophilic pneumonia has been reported rarely with cromolyn nasal products.

Although not reported for cromolyn nasal solution, some side/adverse effects that have occurred with cromolyn formulations for inhalation include joint pain and swelling, and, reported rarely, serum sickness, periarteritic vasculitis, polymyositis, pericarditis, photodermatitis, exfoliative dermatitis, peripheral neuritis, pneumonitis, heart failure, and nephrosis.

The following side/adverse effects have been selected on the basis of their potential clinical significance (possible signs and symptoms in parentheses where appropriate)—not necessarily inclusive:

**Those indicating need for medical attention**
Incidence rare
*Anaphylactic reaction* (coughing; difficulty in swallowing; hives; itching of skin; swelling of face, lips, or eyelids; wheezing or difficulty in breathing); *epistaxis* (nosebleeds); *skin rash*

**Those indicating need for medical attention only if they continue or are bothersome**
Incidence more frequent
*Burning, stinging, or irritation inside of nose; increase in sneezing*
Incidence less frequent
*Cough; headache; postnasal drip; unpleasant taste*

## Patient Consultation

As an aid to patient consultation, refer to *Advice for the Patient, Cromolyn (Nasal).*

In providing consultation, consider emphasizing the following selected information (» = major clinical significance):

**Before using this medication**
» Conditions affecting use, especially:
Sensitivity to cromolyn
Use in children—Safety and efficacy have not been established in the U.S. in children up to 6 years of age (in Canada, up to 5 years of age)

**Proper use of this medication**
Reading patient directions carefully
Clearing nasal passages before use
For *cromolyn nasal solution:* Using with a special spray device; wiping nosepiece with a clean tissue and replacing dust cap after use to keep unit clean
For *cromolyn for nasal insufflation:* Using with a special inhaler; understanding exactly how to use inhaler; wiping nosepiece with a clean tissue and replacing dust cap after use; washing only nosepiece in warm water, drying thoroughly; not washing bulb or dampening bulb interior
» Importance of not using more medication than the amount prescribed
» Using every day in regularly spaced doses in order for medication to work properly; results are usually noticeable in approximately 1 week; however in perennial allergic rhinitis, up to 4 weeks may be required for full benefit
» Proper dosing
Missed dose: Using as soon as possible; using any remaining doses for that day at regularly spaced intervals; not doubling doses
» Proper storage

**Precautions while using this medication**
» Checking with physician if symptoms do not improve or if condition becomes worse

**Side/adverse effects**
Signs of potential side effects, especially anaphylactic reaction, epistaxis, and skin rash

## General Dosing Information

Prior to administration of cromolyn nasal solution or cromolyn for nasal insufflation, the nasal passages should be cleared. During administration, patient should inhale through the nose.

In the management of seasonal allergic rhinitis (pollinosis) and for the prevention of rhinitis caused by other types of specific airborne allergens, treatment with nasal cromolyn is more effective if started prior to exposure to the offending allergen. Therapy should be continued throughout the period of exposure (i.e., until the pollen season is over or until the patient is no longer exposed to the offending allergen).

In the management of perennial allergic rhinitis, improvement of condition may not become apparent for up to 2 to 4 weeks. Concurrent use of an antihistamine and/or a nasal decongestant may be necessary during this time; however, the need for these medications should decrease and these medications may be discontinued when the full effect of nasal cromolyn is achieved.

## Nasal Dosage Forms

### CROMOLYN SODIUM FOR NASAL INSUFFLATION

**Usual adult and adolescent dose**
Allergic rhinitis, seasonal (prophylaxis)—
Initial: Nasal insufflation, 10 mg in each nostril four times a day at four- to six-hour intervals.
Maintenance: Nasal insufflation, 10 mg in each nostril every eight to twelve hours.

**Usual pediatric dose**
Allergic rhinitis, seasonal (prophylaxis)—
Children up to 5 years of age: Dosage has not been established.
Children 5 years of age and over: See *Usual adult and adolescent dose.*

**Usual geriatric dose**
See *Usual adult and adolescent dose.*

**Strength(s) usually available**
U.S.—
Not commercially available.
Canada—
10 mg per cartridge (Rx) [Rynacrom (lactose 10 mg)].

**Packaging and storage**
Store below 30 °C (86 °F), in the original container, in a dry place, unless otherwise specified by manufacturer.

**Stability**
Storage in a damp atmosphere may cause the contents to absorb moisture and render the powder unusable.

**Auxiliary labeling**
• For the nose.

**Note**
Dispense with nasal insufflator.

Include patient instructions when dispensing.

Explain administration technique.

## CROMOLYN SODIUM NASAL SOLUTION USP

**Usual adult and adolescent dose**
Allergic rhinitis, perennial or seasonal (prophylaxis and treatment)—
    Intranasal, 5.2 mg in each nostril three or four times a day at regular intervals. Alternatively, 2.6 mg in each nostril six times a day; when an adequate response has been obtained, the dosage may be reduced to 2.6 mg in each nostril two or three times a day.

**Usual adult prescribing limits**
Up to 5.2 mg in each nostril six times a day.

**Usual pediatric dose**
Allergic rhinitis, perennial or seasonal (prophylaxis and treatment)—
    Children up to 6 years of age (in Canada, up to 5 years of age): Safety and efficacy have not been established.

Children 6 years of age (in Canada, 5 years of age) and over: See *Usual adult and adolescent dose.*

**Usual geriatric dose**
See *Usual adult and adolescent dose.*

**Strength(s) usually available**
U.S.—
    40 mg per mL (5.2 mg per metered spray) (Rx) [*Nasalcrom* (benzalkonium chloride 0.01%; edetate disodium 0.01%)].
Canada—
    20 mg per mL (2.6 mg per metered spray) (Rx) [*Rynacrom* (benzalkonium chloride 0.01%)].

**Packaging and storage**
Store below 40 °C (104 °F), preferably between 15 and 30 °C (59 and 86 °F), unless otherwise specified by manufacturer. Store in a tight, light-resistant container. Protect from freezing.

**Auxiliary labeling**
• For the nose.

**Note**
Include patient instructions when dispensing.

Explain administration technique.

**Additional information**
The nasal spray bottle containing 520 mg/13 mL delivers at least 100 sprays.

Revised: 04/20/94

# CROMOLYN    Ophthalmic

INN: Cromoglicic acid.

BAN: Cromoglycic acid.

VA CLASSIFICATION (Primary): OP900

Another commonly used name is sodium cromoglycate.

Note: For a listing of dosage forms and brand names by country availability, see *Dosage Forms* section(s). For a listing of brand names for the articles in this monograph, refer to the General Index.

## Category
Mast cell stabilizer (ophthalmic); antiallergic (ophthalmic).

## Indications
Note: Bracketed information in the *Indications* section refers to uses that are not included in U.S. product labeling.

**Accepted**
[Conjunctivitis, seasonal allergic (treatment)]
Conjunctivitis, vernal (treatment)[1]
Keratitis, vernal (treatment)[1] or
Keratoconjunctivitis, vernal (treatment)—Cromolyn ophthalmic solution is indicated in the treatment of certain allergic ocular disorders, specifically, seasonal allergic conjunctivitis, vernal conjunctivitis, vernal keratitis, and vernal keratoconjunctivitis.

[1]Not included in Canadian product labeling.

## Pharmacology/Pharmacokinetics

**Physicochemical characteristics**
Molecular weight—512.34.
pH—4.0 to 7.0.

**Mechanism of action/Effect**
Cromolyn is a mast cell stabilizer that inhibits the Type I immediate hypersensitivity reaction by preventing the antigen-stimulated release of histamine. Cromolyn also prevents the release of leukotrienes and inhibits eosinophil chemotaxis.

*In vitro* and *in vivo* animal studies have shown that cromolyn inhibits the degranulation of sensitized mast cells that occurs after exposure to specific antigens. Some *in vitro* studies have shown that cromolyn inhibits the degranulation of nonsensitized rat mast cells by phospholipase A and the subsequent release of chemical mediators. One study has shown that cromolyn does not inhibit the enzymatic action of released phospholipase A on its specific substrate.

**Absorption**
Poorly absorbed.
In normal individuals, approximately 0.03% of cromolyn is absorbed systemically following ophthalmic administration.
Studies in rabbits have shown that less than 0.07% of the administered dose is absorbed systemically following multiple doses. Also, trace amounts (less than 0.01%) of the administered dose penetrate into the aqueous humor, and clearance from this chamber is almost complete within 24 hours following discontinuation of treatment.

**Onset of therapeutic effect**
Usually within a few days.

## Precautions to Consider

**Carcinogenicity**
Long-term studies in mice (12 months of intraperitoneal treatment followed by 6 months of observation), hamsters (12 months of intraperitoneal treatment followed by 12 months of observation), and rats (18 months of subcutaneous treatment) did not show any neoplastic effect associated with administration of cromolyn.

**Mutagenicity**
In various mutagenicity studies, there was no evidence of chromosomal damage or cytotoxicity.

**Pregnancy/Reproduction**
Fertility—In animal reproduction studies with cromolyn, there was no evidence of impaired fertility.
Pregnancy—Adequate and well-controlled studies in humans have not been done.
Reproduction studies in mice, rats, and rabbits with cromolyn administered parenterally in doses up to 338 times the human clinical doses showed no evidence of fetal malformations. Adverse fetal effects (increased resorptions and decreased fetal weight) were noted only at very high parenteral doses that produced maternal toxicity.
FDA Pregnancy Category B.

**Breast-feeding**
It is not known whether cromolyn is distributed into breast milk. However, problems in humans have not been documented. Since cromolyn reaches very low concentrations in maternal serum, it would be expected to reach even lower and probably undetectable concentrations in breast milk.

**Pediatrics**
Appropriate studies on the relationship of age to the effects of ophthalmic cromolyn have not been performed in children up to 4 years of age. Safety and efficacy have not been established. In older children, no pediatrics-specific problems have been documented to date.

### Geriatrics

Appropriate studies on the relationship of age to the effects of cromolyn have not been performed in the geriatric population. However, geriatrics-specific problems that would limit the usefulness of this medication in the elderly are not expected.

### Medical considerations/Contraindications

The medical considerations/contraindications included here have been selected on the basis of their potential clinical significance (reasons given in parentheses where appropriate)—not necessarily inclusive (» = major clinical significance).

*Risk-benefit should be considered when the following medical problem exists:*
   Sensitivity to cromolyn

## Side/Adverse Effects

The following side/adverse effects have been selected on the basis of their potential clinical significance (possible signs and symptoms in parentheses where appropriate)—not necessarily inclusive:

**Those indicating need for medical attention**
Incidence rare
   *Chemosis* (swelling of the membrane covering the white part of the eye); *conjunctival injection* (redness of the white part of the eye); *styes, or other signs of eye irritation not present before therapy; contact dermatitis* (rash or redness around the eyes)

**Those indicating need for medical attention only if they continue or are bothersome**
Incidence more frequent
   *Burning or stinging of eye, mild, temporary*
Incidence less frequent or rare
   *Dryness or puffiness around the eye; watering or itching of eye, increased*

## Patient Consultation

As an aid to patient consultation, refer to *Advice for the Patient, Cromolyn (Ophthalmic)*.

In providing consultation, consider emphasizing the following selected information (» = major clinical significance):

**Before using this medication**
» Conditions affecting use, especially:
      Sensitivity to cromolyn
      Use in children—Safety and efficacy have not been established in children up to 4 years of age

**Proper use of this medication**
   Proper administration technique; not touching applicator tip to any surface; keeping container tightly closed
» Importance of not using more medication than the amount prescribed
» Compliance with therapy; symptomatic response usually occurs within a few days
» Proper dosing
   Missed dose: Using as soon as possible
» Proper storage

**Precautions while using this medication**
» Checking with physician if symptoms do not improve or if condition becomes worse

**Side/adverse effects**
   Signs of potential side effects, especially chemosis, conjunctival injection, styes, or other signs of eye irritation not present before therapy; or contact dermatitis

## General Dosing Information

Symptomatic response to therapy (decreased itching, redness, watering, and discharge) usually occurs within a few days; however, treatment may be required for up to 6 weeks.

Corticosteroids may be used concurrently with cromolyn, if required.

Although the manufacturer recommends that patients not wear soft contact lenses during treatment with cromolyn ophthalmic solution, medical experts do not believe this precaution is necessary unless the patient has corneal epithelial problems and the medication is to be used more often than once every 1 to 2 hours. No significant problems have been documented with ophthalmic solutions containing 0.03% or less of benzalkonium chloride as a preservative, and used as eyedrops in patients with no significant corneal surface problems.

## Ophthalmic Dosage Forms

Note: Bracketed uses in the *Dosage Forms* section refer to categories of use and/or indications that are not included in U.S. product labeling.

### CROMOLYN SODIUM OPHTHALMIC SOLUTION USP

**Usual adult and adolescent dose**
[Conjunctivitis, seasonal allergic]
Conjunctivitis, vernal[1]
Keratitis, vernal or[1]
Keratoconjunctivitis, vernal—
   Topical, to the conjunctiva, 1 drop four to six times a day at regular intervals.

**Usual adult prescribing limits**
Up to 12.8 mg.

**Usual pediatric dose**
[Conjunctivitis, seasonal allergic]
Conjunctivitis, vernal[1]
Keratitis, vernal[1] or
Keratoconjunctivitis, vernal—
   Children up to 4 years of age: Safety and efficacy have not been established.
   Children 4 years of age and older: See *Usual adult and adolescent dose*.

**Usual geriatric dose**
See *Usual adult and adolescent dose*.

**Strength(s) usually available**
U.S.—
   4% (Rx) [*Crolom* (benzalkonium chloride; edetate disodium; hydrochloric acid; sodium hydroxide)].
Canada—
   2% (Rx) [*Opticrom* (benzalkonium chloride); *Vistacrom* (benzalkonium chloride 0.01%; edetate disodium)].
Note: One drop of cromolyn sodium ophthalmic solution 2% contains approximately 0.8 mg of cromolyn sodium; and one drop of cromolyn sodium ophthalmic solution 4% contains approximately 1.6 mg of cromolyn sodium.

**Packaging and storage**
Store below 40 °C (104 °F), preferably between 15 and 30 °C (59 and 86 °F), unless otherwise specified by manufacturer. Store in a tight, light-resistant container. Protect from freezing.

**Auxiliary labeling**
• For the eye.

[1]Not included in Canadian product labeling.

Revised: 04/19/94
Interim revision: 07/10/95

---

# CROMOLYN   Systemic/Oral-Local

VA CLASSIFICATION (Primary): IM900
Another commonly used name is sodium cromoglycate.
Note: For a listing of dosage forms and brand names by country availability, see *Dosage Forms* section(s). For a listing of brand names for the articles in this monograph, refer to the General Index.

## Category
Mast cell stabilizer; antiallergic (systemic).

## Indications

**Accepted**

Mastocytosis (treatment)[1]—Cromolyn administered orally is indicated in the treatment of mastocytosis. It has been shown to improve the symptoms of mastocytosis, such as diarrhea, flushing, headache, vomiting, urticaria, abdominal pain, nausea, and itching.

Note: Although oral cromolyn is approved in Canada for gastrointestinal allergy, the USP DI Advisory Panels believe there is insufficient evidence to support the effectiveness of cromolyn in the prophylaxis of food allergy and the prophylaxis and treatment of chronic inflammatory bowel disease. Further studies are needed to determine the efficacy of oral cromolyn in these conditions. The preferred therapy for gastrointestinal allergy to food is avoidance of those foods to which the patient is allergic. In the prophylaxis and treatment of chronic inflammatory bowel disease, agents that have been proven effective in this condition should be used.

---

[1]Not included in Canadian product labeling.

## Pharmacology/Pharmacokinetics

### Physicochemical characteristics
Molecular weight—512.34.

### Mechanism of action/Effect
Cromolyn inhibits mast cell release of histamine, leukotrienes, and other substances that cause hypersensitivity reactions, probably by interfering with calcium transport across the mast cell membrane.

In vitro and in vivo animal studies have shown that cromolyn inhibits degranulation of sensitized mast cells that occurs after exposure to specific antigens. Some in vitro studies have shown that cromolyn inhibits both degranulation of nonsensitized rat mast cells stimulated by phospholipase A and the subsequent release of chemical mediators.

### Absorption
Poorly absorbed from the gastrointestinal tract; only about 1% of an oral dose is absorbed.

### Half-life
Approximately 80 minutes.

### Elimination
Renal/biliary; unchanged.

## Precautions to Consider

### Carcinogenicity
Long-term studies in mice (12 months intraperitoneal treatment followed by 6 months observation), hamsters (12 months intraperitoneal treatment followed by 12 months observation), and rats (18 months subcutaneous treatment) showed that cromolyn has no neoplastic effect.

### Mutagenicity
In various mutagenicity studies, there was no evidence of chromosomal damage or cytotoxicity.

### Pregnancy/Reproduction
Fertility—In animal reproduction studies with cromolyn, there was no evidence of impaired fertility.

Pregnancy—Adequate and well-controlled studies in humans have not been done.

Studies in mice, rats, and rabbits with cromolyn administered parenterally in doses up to 338 times the human clinical doses showed no evidence of fetal malformations. Adverse fetal effects (increased resorptions and decreased fetal weight) were noted only at very high parenteral doses that produced maternal toxicity.

Studies in pregnant mice have shown that cromolyn alone, administered subcutaneously in doses of 60 to 540 mg per kg of body weight (mg/kg) (38 to 338 times the human dose), does not cause significant increases in resorptions or major malformations; however, the addition of cromolyn (338 times the human dose) to isoproterenol (90 times the human dose) appears to increase the incidence of both resorptions and malformations.

FDA Pregnancy Category B.

### Breast-feeding
It is not known whether cromolyn is distributed into breast milk. However, problems in humans have not been documented. Since cromolyn reaches very low concentrations in maternal serum, it would be expected to reach even lower and probably undetectable concentrations in breast milk.

### Pediatrics
Appropriate studies on the relationship of age to the effects of oral cromolyn have not been performed in the pediatric population. However, no pediatrics-specific problems have been documented to date.

Studies in animals have suggested an increased risk of toxicity in premature animals when cromolyn was administered in doses much higher than those clinically recommended for human use.

Use of oral cromolyn is not recommended in premature to term infants.

Use of oral cromolyn in children less than 2 years of age should be reserved for those patients with severe, incapacitating diseases.

### Geriatrics
Appropriate studies performed to date have not demonstrated geriatrics-specific problems that would limit the usefulness of cromolyn in the elderly. However, elderly patients are more likely to have age-related hepatic function impairment and renal function impairment, which may require reduction of dosage in patients receiving cromolyn.

### Medical considerations/Contraindications
The medical considerations/contraindications included here have been selected on the basis of their potential clinical significance (reasons given in parentheses where appropriate)—not necessarily inclusive (» = major clinical significance).

Risk-benefit should be considered when the following medical problems exist:

Hepatic function impairment
    (excretion via biliary route; dosage reduction may be necessary)
Renal function impairment
    (excretion via renal route; dosage reduction may be necessary)
Sensitivity to cromolyn

## Side/Adverse Effects

Note: Although not reported with oral use of cromolyn, some side/adverse effects that have occurred with cromolyn formulations for inhalation include angioedema, swelling of joints, and, reported rarely, serum sickness, periarteritic vasculitis, polymyositis, pericarditis, photodermatitis, exfoliative dermatitis, peripheral neuritis, and nephrosis.

The following side/adverse effects have been selected on the basis of their potential clinical significance (possible signs and symptoms in parentheses where appropriate)—not necessarily inclusive:

### Those indicating need for medical attention
Incidence less frequent
    *Skin rash*
Incidence rare
    *Anaphylactic reaction, severe* (coughing; difficulty in swallowing; hives; itching of skin; swelling of face, lips, or eyelids; wheezing or difficulty in breathing)

### Those indicating need for medical attention only if they continue or are bothersome
Incidence more frequent
    *Diarrhea; headache*
Incidence less frequent or rare
    *Abdominal pain; irritability; myalgia* (joint pain); *nausea; trouble in sleeping*
    Note: The above side/adverse effects occurring in patients with mastocytosis are usually transient and could represent symptoms of the disease.

## Patient Consultation
As an aid to patient consultation, refer to Advice for the Patient, Cromolyn (Oral).

In providing consultation, consider emphasizing the following selected information (» = major clinical significance):

### Before using this medication
» Conditions affecting use, especially:
    Sensitivity to cromolyn
    Use in children—In premature to term infants, use of oral cromolyn is not recommended; in children less than 2 years of age, use of oral cromolyn should be reserved for those patients with severe, incapacitating diseases

### Proper use of this medication
Proper administration:
    For optimal results, dissolving contents of capsule (s) in one-half glass (4 ounces) of hot water and then adding an equal amount of cold water, unless otherwise directed by physician
    Drinking all of liquid to receive full dose
    Not mixing medication with fruit juice, milk, or foods
» Importance of not using more medication than the amount prescribed
» Proper dosing
    Missed dose: Taking as soon as possible; taking any remaining doses for that day at regularly spaced intervals
» Proper storage

### Precautions while using this medication
» Checking with physician if symptoms do not improve or if condition becomes worse

### Side/adverse effects
Signs of potential side effects, especially skin rash and severe anaphylactic reaction

## General Dosing Information

For optimal results, the contents of the capsules should be dissolved in warm water only and taken as a solution. The powder should not be mixed with fruit juice, milk, or food.

## Oral Dosage Forms

### CROMOLYN SODIUM CAPSULES

**Usual adult and adolescent dose**
Mastocytosis[1]—
  Oral, 200 mg four times a day thirty minutes before meals and at bedtime.

**Usual pediatric dose**
Mastocytosis[1]—
  Premature to term infants:
    Use is not recommended.
  Term infants and children up to 2 years of age:
    Oral, 20 mg per kg of body weight per day in four divided doses. If control of symptoms is not achieved within two to three weeks in children six months to two years of age, dosage may be increased, if necessary, up to 30 mg per kg of body weight per day.
    Note: Use of oral cromolyn in children less than 2 years of age should be reserved for those patients with severe, incapacitating diseases.
  Children 2 to 12 years of age:
    Oral, 100 mg four times a day thirty minutes before meals and at bedtime. If control of symptoms is not achieved within two to

three weeks, dosage may be increased, if necessary, up to 40 mg per kg of body weight per day.

**Usual geriatric dose**
See *Usual adult and adolescent dose*.

**Strength(s) usually available**
U.S.—
  100 mg (Rx) [*Gastrocrom*].
Canada—
  100 mg (Rx) [*Nalcrom*].

**Packaging and storage**
Store below 40 °C (104 °F), preferably between 15 and 30 °C (59 and 86 °F), unless otherwise specified by manufacturer. Store in a tight container.

**Preparation of dosage form**
For optimal results, the contents of the capsule should be dissolved in one-half glass (4 ounces) of hot water, and stirred until completely dissolved. Then, one-half glass (4 ounces) of cold water is added to the solution.

**Auxiliary labeling**
• Do not swallow capsule whole.
• Mix with water only. Do not mix with fruit juice, milk, or food.

[1]Not included in Canadian product labeling.

Revised: 09/06/94

---

# CROTAMITON   Topical

VA CLASSIFICATION (Primary): AP900
Note: For a listing of dosage forms and brand names by country availability, see *Dosage Forms* section(s). For a listing of brand names for the articles in this monograph, refer to the General Index.

## Category

Scabicide.

## Indications

**Accepted**
Scabies (treatment)—Crotamiton is indicated for the treatment of scabies caused by *Sarcoptes scabiei*.

**Unaccepted**
Crotamiton has been used for the symptomatic relief of pruritus associated with various types of dermatoses; however, there are no controlled studies to support claims of crotamiton's antipruritic action.

## Pharmacology/Pharmacokinetics

**Physicochemical characteristics**
Molecular weight—203.28.

**Mechanism of action/Effect**
The mechanisms of the scabicidal and antipruritic actions of crotamiton are not known.

## Precautions to Consider

**Carcinogenicity**
Long-term carcinogenicity studies in animals have not been done.

**Pregnancy/Reproduction**
Pregnancy—Studies have not been done in humans.
Studies have not been done in animals.
FDA Pregnancy Category C.

**Breast-feeding**
Problems in humans have not been documented.

**Pediatrics**
Appropriate studies on the relationship of age to the effects of crotamiton have not been performed in the pediatric population. Safety and efficacy have not been established.

**Geriatrics**
Appropriate studies on the relationship of age to the effects of crotamiton have not been performed in the geriatric population. However, no geriatrics-specific problems have been documented to date.

**Medical considerations/Contraindications**
The medical considerations/contraindications included here have been selected on the basis of their potential clinical significance (reasons given in parentheses where appropriate)—not necessarily inclusive (» = major clinical significance).

*Risk-benefit should be considered when the following medical problems exist:*
» Inflamed skin, acute or
» Raw, oozing skin surfaces
  (condition may be exacerbated)
  Sensitivity to crotamiton

## Side/Adverse Effects

Note: Treatment with crotamiton should be discontinued if severe irritation or sensitization develops.

The following side/adverse effects have been selected on the basis of their potential clinical significance (possible signs and symptoms in parentheses where appropriate)—not necessarily inclusive:

**Those indicating need for medical attention**
Incidence rare
  *Allergic reaction* (skin rash); *skin irritation not present before therapy*

## Patient Consultation

As an aid to patient consultation, refer to *Advice for the Patient, Crotamiton (Topical)*.

In providing consultation, consider emphasizing the following selected information (» = major clinical significance):

**Before using this medication**
» Conditions affecting use, especially:
  Allergy to crotamiton
  Other medical problems, especially acute inflamed skin or raw, oozing skin surfaces

**Proper use of this medication**
» Importance of keeping away from mouth; may be harmful if swallowed
» Importance of not using medication more often than prescribed
» Avoiding contact with eyes and mucous membranes

Reading patient directions carefully before using

Before applying—Drying skin well if bath or shower taken before using medication

*Proper administration of medication in the treatment of scabies*

Applying enough to cover entire skin surface from the chin down; rubbing in well, especially in the body folds and creases, hands, feet (including soles), between fingers and toes, and moist areas (such as underarms and groin)

Not washing off the first coat of medication

Applying a second coat of medication 24 hours after the first one

Taking a cleansing bath 48 hours after second application to remove medication

Putting on freshly washed or dry-cleaned clothing and changing bedding to prevent reinfestation

Concurrent treatment of sexual partners, especially, and all household members may be required if medication is being used to treat scabies

» Proper dosing
» Proper storage

### Precautions while using this medication

» Notifying physician if condition does not improve or if it becomes worse

If medication is being used to treat scabies, using hygienic measures to control reinfestation or spread of infestation such as: Machine washing all underwear, pajamas, sheets, pillowcases, towels, and washcloths in very hot water and drying them by using hot cycle of a dryer; dry cleaning non-washable clothing or bedding

### Side/adverse effects

Signs of potential side effects, especially skin rash or skin irritation not present before use of this medication

## General Dosing Information

If a bath is taken before the cream or lotion is used, the skin should be well dried before medication is applied.

In the treatment of scabies:

• The cream or lotion should be applied in an amount sufficient to cover the entire body surface from the chin down, and rubbed in well. This applies especially to folds and creases in the skin and to the hands, feet (including the soles), between fingers and toes, and moist areas (such as underarms and groin). After 24 hours, a second coat of the cream or lotion should be applied. Patient should put on freshly washed or dry-cleaned clothing and change bedding the morning after the second application to prevent reinfestation. Then, 48 hours after the second application of crotamiton, a cleansing bath should be taken to remove the medication.

• Sexual partners, especially, and all household members may require concurrent therapy, since the infestation may spread to persons in close contact.

• To prevent reinfestation or spreading of the infestation, all underwear, pajamas, sheets, pillowcases, towels, and washcloths should be washed in very hot water and dried using the hot cycle of a dryer. Clothing or bedding that is not washable should be dry cleaned.

### For treatment of systemic toxicity

Recommended treatment includes

• If ingested, gastric lavage should be performed.

• There is no specific antidote to ingestion of crotamiton.

## Topical Dosage Forms

### CROTAMITON CREAM USP

#### Usual adult and adolescent dose

For scabies—

Topical, to the skin, as a 10% cream for two applications at twenty-four-hour intervals.

Note: In resistant cases of scabies, the course of treatment may be repeated one week later, or an alternative scabicide used.

One study has suggested that 5 to 7 days of daily therapy may be more effective than the current treatment of 2 applications at 24-hour intervals.

For pruritus—

Topical, to the skin, as a 10% cream. Repeat as needed.

#### Usual pediatric dose

Safety and efficacy have not been established.

#### Strength(s) usually available

U.S.—

10% (Rx) [*Eurax Cream* (cetyl alcohol)].

Canada—

10% (OTC) [*Eurax Cream* (methylparaben; propylparaben)].

#### Packaging and storage

Store below 40 °C (104 °F), preferably between 15 and 30 °C (59 and 86 °F), unless otherwise specified by manufacturer. Store in a tight, light-resistant container. Protect from freezing.

#### Auxiliary labeling

• For external use only.
• May be harmful if swallowed.

#### Note

When dispensing, include patient instructions.

### CROTAMITON LOTION

#### Usual adult and adolescent dose

See *Crotamiton Cream USP*.

#### Usual pediatric dose

See *Crotamiton Cream USP*.

#### Strength(s) usually available

U.S.—

10% (Rx) [*Eurax Lotion* (cetyl alcohol)].

Canada—

Not commercially available.

#### Packaging and storage

Store below 40 °C (104 °F), preferably between 15 and 30 °C (59 and 86 °F), in a tight, light-resistant container. Protect from freezing.

#### Auxiliary labeling

• For external use only.
• Shake well.
• May be harmful if swallowed.

#### Note

When dispensing, include patient instructions.

Revised: 04/22/94

---

## CUPRIC SULFATE—See *Copper Supplements (Systemic)*

---

## CYANOCOBALAMIN—See *Vitamin B₁₂ (Systemic)*

---

# CYANOCOBALAMIN CO 57   Systemic

VA CLASSIFICATION (Primary): DX201

Note: For a listing of dosage forms and brand names by country availability, see *Dosage Forms* section(s). For a listing of brand names for the articles in this monograph, refer to the General Index.

## Category

Diagnostic aid, radioactive (cyanocobalamin malabsorption syndromes).

## Indications

### Accepted

Anemia (diagnosis)—Cyanocobalamin Co 57 is indicated in the diagnosis of pernicious anemia.

Vitamin B₁₂ deficiency (diagnosis adjunct)—Cyanocobalamin Co 57 is indicated as an adjunct in diagnosing intestinal cyanocobalamin malabsorption syndromes due to lack of intrinsic factor (IF) or other defects in intestinal absorption (e.g., blind loop syndrome and diverticulitis, celiac disease, Crohn's disease, lesions in the small intestine, severe pancreatitis, tropical sprue).

Cyanocobalamin Co 57 may be used either in fecal excretion determinations of unabsorbed cyanocobalamin or urinary excretion determinations (Schilling test) of absorbed cyanocobalamin. However, a normal Schilling test does not rule out the possibility of vitamin $B_{12}$ deficiency.

## Physical Properties

### Nuclear data

| Radionuclide (half-life) | Mode of decay | Principal emissions (keV) | Mean number of emissions/ disintegration |
|---|---|---|---|
| Co 57 (270.9 days) | Electron capture | Gamma (122) | 0.86 |
| Co 58 (71.3 days) | Electron capture 85% | Gamma 99% (810.5) | 0.84 |
| | Positron emission 15% | Annihilation 200% (511) | 0.30 |

## Pharmacology/Pharmacokinetics

### Mechanism of action/Effect
The action of cyanocobalamin Co 57 in the body is identical to that of dietary cyanocobalamin. In order to be readily absorbed from the gastrointestinal tract, it must form a complex with intrinsic factor (IF). The absorption or lack of absorption of radiolabeled cyanocobalamin is determined by the measurement of samples of urine or feces with scintillation counting devices. In patients with pernicious anemia, absorption of cyanocobalamin is less than normal, but it may be normalized by the concurrent administration of IF with cyanocobalamin. Thus, if normal absorption is not obtained, repeat studies may be performed administering IF along with the test dose of cyanocobalamin Co 57 to differentiate pernicious anemia from other causes of cyanocobalamin malabsorption.

### Absorption
Oral—30 to 97% of doses up to 2 micrograms of cyanocobalamin (complexed to IF) are absorbed from the gastrointestinal tract in the distal ileum. At doses greater than 2 micrograms, the IF-dependent absorption process becomes saturated, and the percentage absorbed significantly decreases.

### Protein binding
High (>90%, primarily to the specific transcobalamin II vitamin $B_{12}$-binding protein).

### Half-life
For cyanocobalamin—Biological (in liver): Approximately 500 days.

### Time to peak concentration
6 to 14 hours.

### Radiation dosimetry

| Organ | Co 57 Estimated absorbed radiation dose | | | |
|---|---|---|---|---|
| | Without flushing | | With flushing* | |
| | mGy/ MBq | rad/ microcurie | mGy/ MBq | rad/ microcurie |
| Liver | 36 | 0.13 | 24 | 0.089 |
| Adrenals | 3.8 | 0.014 | 2.5 | 0.0093 |
| Pancreas | 3.8 | 0.014 | 2.6 | 0.0096 |
| Kidneys | 3.5 | 0.013 | 2.3 | 0.0085 |
| Large intestine (upper) | 2.6 | 0.0096 | 1.8 | 0.0067 |
| Lungs | 2.4 | 0.0088 | 1.6 | 0.0059 |
| Red marrow | 2.3 | 0.0085 | 1.5 | 0.0055 |
| Small intestine | 2.0 | 0.0074 | 1.4 | 0.0052 |
| Stomach wall | 2.0 | 0.0074 | 1.4 | 0.0052 |
| Bone surfaces | 1.8 | 0.0067 | 1.2 | 0.0044 |
| Breast | 1.5 | 0.0055 | 0.98 | 0.0036 |
| Spleen | 1.4 | 0.0052 | 0.97 | 0.0036 |
| Large intestine (lower) | 1.3 | 0.0048 | 0.97 | 0.0036 |

| Organ | Co 57 Estimated absorbed radiation dose | | | |
|---|---|---|---|---|
| | Without flushing | | With flushing* | |
| | mGy/ MBq | rad/ microcurie | mGy/ MBq | rad/ microcurie |
| Ovaries | 1.2 | 0.0044 | 0.83 | 0.0031 |
| Uterus | 1.2 | 0.0044 | 0.84 | 0.0031 |
| Bladder wall | 0.95 | 0.0035 | 0.64 | 0.0024 |
| Testes | 0.69 | 0.0025 | 0.46 | 0.0017 |
| Thyroid | 0.66 | 0.0024 | 0.44 | 0.0016 |
| Other tissue | 1.4 | 0.0052 | 0.95 | 0.0035 |
| Effective dose | 4.0 mSv/ MBq | 0.015 rem/ microcurie | 2.7 mSv/ MBq | 0.010 rem/ microcurie |

*The administration of a flushing dose of nonradioactive cyanocobalamin decreases the absorbed radiation dose.

| Organ | Co 58 Estimated absorbed radiation dose | | | |
|---|---|---|---|---|
| | Without flushing | | With flushing* | |
| | mGy/ MBq | rad/ microcurie | mGy/ MBq | rad/ microcurie |
| Liver | 54 | 0.20 | 36 | 0.13 |
| Adrenals | 10 | 0.037 | 6.7 | 0.025 |
| Pancreas | 9.1 | 0.034 | 6.1 | 0.023 |
| Kidneys | 7.9 | 0.029 | 5.3 | 0.020 |
| Large intestine (upper) | 6.3 | 0.023 | 4.4 | 0.016 |
| Lungs | 5.5 | 0.020 | 3.6 | 0.013 |
| Stomach wall | 4.9 | 0.018 | 3.3 | 0.012 |
| Small intestine | 4.7 | 0.017 | 3.2 | 0.012 |
| Breast | 3.7 | 0.014 | 2.5 | 0.0093 |
| Spleen | 3.5 | 0.013 | 2.4 | 0.0088 |
| Large intestine (lower) | 3.4 | 0.013 | 2.7 | 0.010 |
| Red marrow | 3.3 | 0.012 | 2.2 | 0.0081 |
| Uterus | 2.8 | 0.010 | 1.9 | 0.0070 |
| Bone surfaces | 2.6 | 0.0096 | 1.8 | 0.0067 |
| Ovaries | 2.5 | 0.0093 | 1.8 | 0.0067 |
| Bladder wall | 2.4 | 0.0088 | 1.6 | 0.0059 |
| Testes | 2.1 | 0.0078 | 1.4 | 0.0052 |
| Thyroid | 1.8 | 0.0067 | 1.2 | 0.0044 |
| Other tissue | 3.3 | 0.012 | 2.2 | 0.0081 |
| Effective dose | 7.5 mSv/ MBq | 0.028 rem/ microcurie | 5.1 mSv/ MBq | 0.019 rem/ microcurie |

*The administration of a flushing dose of nonradioactive cyanocobalamin decreases the absorbed radiation dose.

### Elimination
In normal patients—Renal (7 to 10% or more); fecal (50% or less).
In patients with reduced absorption—Renal (0 to 7%); fecal (70 to 100%).
Note: Diagnosis of pernicious anemia in patients with reduced absorption is confirmed if abnormal results become normal when IF is administered with the test dose of cyanocobalamin Co 57.

Cyanocobalamin Co 57 is also eliminated in breast milk.

## Precautions to Consider

### Carcinogenicity/Mutagenicity
Long-term animal studies to evaluate carcinogenic or mutagenic potential of cyanocobalamin Co 57 have not been performed.

### Pregnancy/Reproduction
Pregnancy—Adequate and well-controlled studies have not been done in humans. Diagnostic testing should be postponed, if possible, until after delivery since cyanocobalamin Co 57 crosses the placenta and is taken up by the fetus.
To avoid the possibility of radiation exposure to the fetus, in those circumstances where the patient's pregnancy status is uncertain, a pregnancy test will help to prevent inadvertent administration of this preparation during pregnancy.
Studies have not been done in animals.
FDA Pregnancy Category C.

**Breast-feeding**
Cyanocobalamin Co 57 is excreted in breast milk in very small concentrations. Although discontinuation of breast-feeding is not essential, because of the potential risk to the infant from radiation exposure, temporary discontinuation of nursing is recommended for a short period of time.

**Pediatrics**
Although cyanocobalamin Co 57 is used in children, there have been no specific studies evaluating safety and efficacy. When used in children, the diagnostic benefit should be judged to outweigh the potential risk of radiation.

**Geriatrics**
Appropriate studies performed to date have not demonstrated geriatrics-specific problems that would limit the usefulness of cyanocobalamin Co 57 in the elderly. However, elderly patients are more likely to have age-related renal function impairment which may falsely depress Schilling test results; a 48-hour urine collection period (instead of the usual 24-hour period) is recommended in patients with impaired renal function.

Also, in geriatric patients with gastric atrophy that is severe enough to cause a lack of gastric acid and enzymes, the splitting of vitamin $B_{12}$ from its peptide linkages in food cannot be accomplished, thus causing vitamin $B_{12}$ deficiency. However, the gastric atrophy may not be severe enough to cause a lack of gastric intrinsic factor and thus the results of the Schilling test may be normal, unless cyanocobalamin Co 57 is given after incubation with serum protein (e.g., chicken serum).

**Drug interactions and/or related problems**
See *Laboratory value alterations.*

**Laboratory value alterations**
The following have been selected on the basis of their potential clinical significance (possible effect in parentheses where appropriate)—not necessarily inclusive (» = major clinical significance):

With result of *this* test
*Due to other medications*
Alcohol, excessive intake for longer than 2 weeks or
Aminosalicylates or
Antibiotics, especially oral neomycin or
Anticonvulsants, especially phenobarbital, phenytoin, and primidone or
Calcium-chelating agents, such as edetate disodium and penicillamine or
Cholestyramine, prolonged use or
Colchicine or
Potassium, extended-release
(may impair absorption of radioactive cyanocobalamin)
Cyanocobalamin, nonradioactive
(prior administration may impair absorption and excretion of cyanocobalamin Co 57; it is recommended that 24 hours elapse before the administration of cyanocobalamin Co 57)

*Due to medical problems or conditions*
Renal function impairment
(Schilling test results may be falsely depressed)

With results of *other* tests
Bone marrow studies and
Cyanocobalamin determinations, serum and
Reticulocyte counts
(values may be altered because of hematopoietic response resulting from administration of large parenteral doses of cyanocobalamin given in conjunction with Schilling test; it is recommended that these tests be done prior to Schilling test)

**Medical considerations/Contraindications**
The medical considerations/contraindications included here have been selected on the basis of their potential clinical significance (reasons given in parentheses where appropriate)—not necessarily inclusive (» = major clinical significance).
See also *Laboratory value alterations.*

*Risk-benefit should be considered when the following medical problem exists:*
Sensitivity to cyanocobalamin

## Side/Adverse Effects

Note: Presently, there are no known side/adverse effects associated with cyanocobalamin Co 57 used orally as a diagnostic aid. However, side/adverse effects, such as anaphylactic shock, have been reported with the parenteral use of nonradioactive cyanocobalamin.

## Patient Consultation

As an aid to patient consultation, refer to *Advice for the Patient, Radiopharmaceuticals (Diagnostic).*
In providing consultation, consider emphasizing the following selected information (» = major clinical significance):

**Description of use**
Action in the body: Identical to dietary cyanocobalamin
Absorption of radioactive cyanocobalamin determined by measurement of radioactivity in urine or fecal samples
Small amounts used in diagnosis; radiation exposure is considered low

**Before having this test**
» Conditions affecting use, especially:
Sensitivity to cyanocobalamin
Pregnancy—Crosses the placenta; risk to fetus from radiation exposure as opposed to benefit derived from use should be considered
Breast-feeding—Excreted in breast milk; temporary discontinuation of nursing recommended because of risk of radiation exposure to infant
Use in children—Risk of radiation exposure

**Preparation for this test**
Special preparatory instructions may be given; patient should inquire in advance:
Avoiding oral or parenteral cyanocobalamin for at least 24 hours prior to administration of cyanocobalamin Co 57
Fasting for at least 8 to 12 hours prior to administration of cyanocobalamin Co 57

**Precautions after having this test**
No special precautions when used for diagnosis

**Side/adverse effects**
No side effects reported with diagnostic doses

## General Dosing Information

Radiopharmaceuticals are to be administered only by or under the supervision of physicians who have had extensive training in the safe use and handling of radionuclides and who are approved by the appropriate State agency or, outside the U.S., the appropriate authority.

Fasting is recommended for at least 8 to 12 hours prior to the administration of the test dose of cyanocobalamin Co 57. Two hours after the ingestion of the test dose, a light breakfast may be given.

Voiding is recommended immediately prior to the administration of the test dose of cyanocobalamin Co 57. Also, radioactivity measurement of a pre-test urine sample should be obtained prior to starting the study to establish the absence of any potentially interfering radioisotope.

To prevent interference with absorption and elimination, at least 24 hours should elapse prior to the administration of cyanocobalamin Co 57 if a flushing dose for the Schilling test or a therapeutic injection of cyanocobalamin has previously been administered.

In the Schilling test, a flushing dose of 1 mg of nonradioactive cyanocobalamin must be intramuscularly injected within 2 hours following the administration of cyanocobalamin Co 57. A second flushing dose may be injected 24 hours later to help reduce the amount of radioactivity retained by the body.

Manufacturer's package insert or other appropriate literature should be consulted for specific test procedure.

**Safety considerations for handling this radiopharmaceutical**
Improper handling of this radiopharmaceutical may cause radioactive contamination. Guidelines for handling radioactive material have been prepared by scientific, professional, state, federal, and international bodies and are available to the specially qualified and authorized users who have access to radiopharmaceuticals.

## Oral Dosage Forms
### CYANOCOBALAMIN Co 57 CAPSULES USP

**Usual adult and adolescent administered activity**
Diagnosis of cyanocobalamin malabsorption syndromes—
Oral, 0.02 to 0.037 megabecquerel (0.5 to 1 microcurie).

Note: If the test kit containing both the cyanocobalamin Co 57 (bound to intrinsic factor [IF]) and the cyanocobalamin Co 58 capsules is used, both capsules are administered simultaneously. The test is performed in a manner similar to the Schilling test, except that both vitamin $B_{12}$ absorption and response to IF are measured simultaneously.

**Usual pediatric administered activity**
See *Usual adult and adolescent administered activity.*

**Usual geriatric administered activity**
See *Usual adult and adolescent administered activity* .

**Strength(s) usually available**
U.S.—
  0.02 megabecquerel (0.5 microcurie), with a specific activity ranging from 0.02 to 0.037 megabecquerel (0.5 to 1 microcurie) per microgram of cyanocobalamin, per capsule, at time of calibration (Rx) [GENERIC].
  0.02 to 0.037 megabecquerel (0.5 to 1 microcurie), nominal activity per capsule, at time of calibration (Rx) [*Rubratrope-57*].
  0.02 megabecquerel (0.5 microcurie), nominal activity per capsule, at time of calibration (Rx) [*Dicopac*].
  Note: The *Dicopac* test kit also contains a capsule of cyanocobalamin Co 58 with 0.03 megabecquerel (0.8 microcurie), nominal activity at time of calibration.
Canada—
  0.02 megabecquerel (0.5 microcurie) per capsule, at time of calibration (Rx) [GENERIC].

**Packaging and storage**
Store below 40 °C (104 °F), preferably between 15 and 30 °C (59 and 86 °F), unless otherwise specified by manufacturer. Store in a well-closed, light-resistant container.

Note: The *Dicopac* test kit should be stored between 2 and 4 °C (36 and 40 °F).

**Stability**
Deteriorates in presence of strong light, traces of reducing agents, or microorganisms. Decomposes when autoclaved at 115 °C (239 °F) for 30 minutes.

**Note**
Caution—Radioactive material.

**Selected Bibliography**
Zuckier LS, Chervu LR. Schilling evaluation of pernicious anemia: current status. J Nucl Med 1984; 25 (9): 1032-9.

Revised: 08/08/92
Interim revision: 08/02/94

---

# CYCLANDELATE   Systemic

VA CLASSIFICATION (Primary): CV500
Note: For a listing of dosage forms and brand names by country availability, see *Dosage Forms* section(s). For a listing of brand names for the articles in this monograph, refer to the General Index.

## Category
Vasodilator.

## Indications

**Unaccepted**
FDA has classified cyclandelate as being ineffective for its labeled indications, which include use as adjunctive therapy in intermittent claudication, arteriosclerosis obliterans, thrombophlebitis (to control associated vasospasm and muscular ischemia), nocturnal leg cramps, Raynaud's phenomenon, and selected cases of ischemic cerebrovascular disease.

## Pharmacology/Pharmacokinetics

**Physicochemical characteristics**
Molecular weight—276.37.

**Mechanism of action/Effect**
Produces peripheral vasodilation by a direct effect on vascular smooth muscle.

**Absorption**
Well absorbed from the gastrointestinal tract.

**Time to peak effect**
Maximum effect after a single dose occurs within approximately 1.5 hours. Clinical improvement may occur gradually over several weeks.

## Precautions to Consider

**Pregnancy/Reproduction**
Pregnancy—Studies have not been done in humans.
Studies have not been done in animals.

**Breast-feeding**
It is not known whether cyclandelate is distributed into breast milk. However, problems in humans have not been documented.

**Pediatrics**
No information is available on the relationship of age to the effects of cyclandelate in pediatric patients. Safety and efficacy have not been established.

**Geriatrics**
Appropriate studies on the relationship of age to the effects of cyclandelate have not been performed in the geriatric population. However, no geriatrics-specific problems are expected.

**Drug interactions and/or related problems**
The following drug interactions and/or related problems have been selected on the basis of their potential clinical significance (possible mechanism in parentheses where appropriate)—not necessarily inclusive (» = major clinical significance):
Smoking, tobacco
  (concurrent heavy use may interfere with the therapeutic effects of cyclandelate because nicotine constricts blood vessels)

**Medical considerations/Contraindications**
The medical considerations/contraindications included here have been selected on the basis of their potential clinical significance (reasons given in parentheses where appropriate)—not necessarily inclusive (» = major clinical significance).

*Risk-benefit should be considered when the following medical problems exist:*
» Bleeding disorders
  (prolonged bleeding time has been reported with administration of large doses of cyclandelate to animals, although it has not been reported in humans)
» Cerebrovascular disease, severe or
» Myocardial infarction, recent or
» Obliterative coronary artery disease, severe
  (a "steal effect" may occur, since cyclandelate has a greater effect on peripheral than on cerebral and coronary vessels, leading to a further decrease in flow to ischemic areas)
Glaucoma
Sensitivity to cyclandelate

## Side/Adverse Effects
The following side/adverse effects have been selected on the basis of their potential clinical significance (possible signs and symptoms in parentheses where appropriate)—not necessarily inclusive:

**Those indicating need for medical attention only if they continue or are bothersome**
Incidence less frequent—dose-related and occurring more frequently during initial therapy
  *Belching, heartburn, nausea, or stomach pain; dizziness; fast heartbeat; flushing of face; headache; sweating; tingling sensation in face, fingers, or toes; weakness*

## Patient Consultation
As an aid to patient consultation, refer to *Advice for the Patient, Cyclandelate (Systemic)*.

In providing consultation, consider emphasizing the following selected information (» = major clinical significance):

**Before using this medication**
» Conditions affecting use, especially:
    Sensitivity to cyclandelate
    Other medical problems, especially bleeding disorders, severe cerebrovascular disease, recent myocardial infarction, or severe obliterative coronary artery disease

**Proper use of this medication**
» Taking with meals, milk, or antacids to reduce gastrointestinal irritation
» Proper dosing
   Missed dose: Taking as soon as possible; not taking if almost time for next dose; not doubling doses
» Proper storage

**Precautions while using this medication**
   Checking with physician before discontinuing medication
   Avoiding smoking (nicotine constricts blood vessels)
» Caution when getting up from a lying or sitting position, or when climbing stairs

## General Dosing Information

Cyclandelate may be administered with meals, milk, or antacids to reduce gastrointestinal irritation.

## Oral Dosage Forms

### CYCLANDELATE CAPSULES

**Usual adult dose**
Initial: Oral, 1.2 to 1.6 grams a day in divided doses before meals and at bedtime. When a clinical response occurs, the dosage is reduced by decrements of 200 mg until a maintenance dose is reached.
Maintenance: Oral, 400 to 800 mg a day in two to four divided doses.

**Usual pediatric dose**
Safety and efficacy have not been established.

**Strength(s) usually available**
U.S.—
   200 mg (Rx) [*Cyclospasmol*; GENERIC].
   400 mg (Rx) [*Cyclospasmol*; GENERIC].
Canada—
   Not commercially available.

**Packaging and storage**
Store below 40 °C (104 °F), preferably between 15 and 30 °C (59 and 86 °F), in a well-closed container, unless otherwise specified by manufacturer.

### CYCLANDELATE TABLETS

**Usual adult dose**
See *Cyclandelate Capsules.*

**Usual pediatric dose**
See *Cyclandelate Capsules.*

**Strength(s) usually available**
U.S.—
   Not commercially available.
Canada—
   200 mg (OTC) [*Cyclospasmol*].
   400 mg (OTC) [*Cyclospasmol* (scored)].

**Packaging and storage**
Store below 40 °C (104 °F), preferably between 15 and 30 °C (59 and 86 °F), in a well-closed container, unless otherwise specified by manufacturer.

Revised: 10/15/92
Interim revision: 04/14/94

---

# CYCLIZINE   Systemic

VA CLASSIFICATION (Primary): GA700
Note: For a listing of dosage forms and brand names by country availability, see *Dosage Forms* section(s). For a listing of brand names for the articles in this monograph, refer to the General Index.

## Category
Antiemetic.

## Indications

**Accepted**
Motion sickness (prophylaxis and treatment)—Oral cyclizine is indicated for the prophylaxis and treatment of nausea, vomiting, and dizziness associated with motion sickness. Parenteral cyclizine is indicated for the treatment of nausea and vomiting of motion sickness when the oral route cannot be used.

Nausea and vomiting, postoperative (prophylaxis and treatment)—Parenteral cyclizine is used to prevent or relieve postoperative nausea and vomiting.

## Pharmacology/Pharmacokinetics

**Physicochemical characteristics**
Molecular weight—Cyclizine hydrochloride: 302.85.
Cyclizine lactate: 356.46.
pH—Cyclizine lactate: 3.2 to 4.7
pKa—7.7.

**Mechanism of action/Effect**
Antiemetic—The mechanism by which cyclizine exerts its antiemetic and antimotion sickness effects is not precisely known but may be related to its central anticholinergic actions. It diminishes vestibular stimulation and depresses labyrinthine function. An action on the medullary chemoreceptive trigger zone may also be involved in the antiemetic effect.

**Other actions/effects**
Cyclizine also has antihistaminic, anticholinergic, antivertigo, central nervous system (CNS) depressant, and local anesthetic effects.

**Duration of action**
4 to 6 hours.

## Precautions to Consider

**Pregnancy/Reproduction**
Pregnancy—Problems in humans have not been documented. Cyclizine has been shown to be teratogenic in rats at doses above the human therapeutic range.

**Breast-feeding**
It is not known whether cyclizine is distributed into breast milk. However, problems in humans have not been documented. Because of its anticholinergic actions, cyclizine may inhibit lactation.

**Pediatrics**
Appropriate studies on the relationship of age to the effects of cyclizine have not been performed in the pediatric population. However, it is known that pediatric patients exhibit increased sensitivity to anticholinergics, which are related pharmacologically to cyclizine.

**Geriatrics**
No information is available on the relationship of age to the effects of cyclizine in geriatric patients. However, it is known that geriatric patients exhibit increased sensitivity to anticholinergics, which are related pharmacologically to cyclizine. Therefore, constipation, dryness of mouth, and urinary retention (especially in males) are more likely to occur in the elderly.

**Drug interactions and/or related problems**
The following drug interactions and/or related problems have been selected on the basis of their potential clinical significance (possible mechanism in parentheses where appropriate)—not necessarily inclusive (» = major clinical significance):

Note: Combinations containing any of the following medications, depending on the amount present, may also interact with this medication.

» Alcohol or
» CNS depression–producing medications, other (See *Appendix II*)
   (concurrent use may potentiate the CNS depressant effects of either these medications or cyclizine)

   Anticholinergics or other medications with anticholinergic activity (See *Appendix II*)
   (concurrent use with cyclizine may potentiate anticholinergic effects)

   Apomorphine
   (prior administration of cyclizine may decrease the emetic response to apomorphine)

### Laboratory value alterations

The following have been selected on the basis of their potential clinical significance (possible effect in parentheses where appropriate)—not necessarily inclusive (» = major clinical significance):

With diagnostic test results
  Skin tests using allergen extracts
    (may inhibit the cutaneous histamine response, thus producing false-negative results; it is recommended that cyclizine be discontinued at least 72 hours before testing begins)

### Medical considerations/Contraindications

The medical considerations/contraindications included here have been selected on the basis of their potential clinical significance (reasons given in parentheses where appropriate)—not necessarily inclusive (» = major clinical significance).

*Risk-benefit should be considered when the following medical problems exist:*

  Bladder neck obstruction or
  Prostatic hyperplasia, symptomatic
    (anticholinergic effects of cyclizine may precipitate urinary retention)
  Cardiac failure, severe
    (cyclizine may decrease cardiac output and increase heart rate, pulmonary wedge pressure, and mean arterial pressure in patients with cardiac failure)
  Gastroduodenal obstruction
    (decrease in motility and tone may occur, aggravating obstruction and gastric retention)
  Glaucoma, angle-closure, or predisposition to
    (increased intraocular pressure may precipitate an attack of angle-closure glaucoma)
  Glaucoma, open-angle
    (mydriatic effect may cause a slight increase in intraocular pressure; glaucoma therapy may need to be adjusted with continued use of cyclizine)
  Pulmonary disease, chronic obstructive
    (reduction in bronchial secretion may cause inspissation and formation of bronchial plugs)
  Sensitivity to cyclizine

## Side/Adverse Effects

The following side/adverse effects have been selected on the basis of their potential clinical significance (possible signs and symptoms in parentheses where appropriate)—not necessarily inclusive:

**Those indicating need for medical attention only if they continue or are bothersome**
Incidence more frequent
  *Drowsiness*
Incidence less frequent or rare
  *Blurred or double vision; constipation; diarrhea; difficult or painful urination; dizziness; dryness of the mouth, nose, and throat; fast heartbeat; loss of appetite; nervousness, restlessness, or trouble in sleeping; skin rash; upset stomach*

## Patient Consultation

As an aid to patient consultation, refer to *Advice for the Patient, Meclizine/Buclizine/Cyclizine (Systemic).*

In providing consultation, consider emphasizing the following selected information (» = major clinical significance):

**Before using this medication**
» Conditions affecting use, especially:
    Sensitivity to cyclizine
    Pregnancy—Animal studies have shown cyclizine to be teratogenic at doses above human therapeutic range
    Breast-feeding—May inhibit lactation due to anticholinergic effects
    Use in children—Possible increased susceptibility to anticholinergic side effects
    Use in the elderly—Possible increased susceptibility to anticholinergic side effects
    Other medications, especially other CNS depressants

**Proper use of this medication**
  Not taking more medication than the amount prescribed
» Proper dosing

  Missed dose (if on a regular dosing schedule): Taking as soon as possible; not taking if almost time for next dose; not doubling doses
» Proper storage

**Precautions while using this medication**
  Possible interference with skin tests using allergens; need to inform physician of use of this medication
» Avoiding use of alcohol or other CNS depressants
» Caution if drowsiness occurs
  Possible dryness of mouth; using sugarless candy or gum, ice, or saliva substitute for relief; checking with physician or dentist if dry mouth continues for more than 2 weeks

## General Dosing Information

For prophylaxis against motion sickness, this medication should be taken at least 30 minutes before exposure to conditions that may precipitate motion sickness.

## Oral Dosage Forms

### CYCLIZINE HYDROCHLORIDE TABLETS USP

**Usual adult and adolescent dose**
Motion sickness (prophylaxis and treatment)—
  Oral, 50 mg thirty minutes before travel. Dose may be repeated every four to six hours as needed.

**Usual adult prescribing limits**
Up to 200 mg daily.

**Usual pediatric dose**
Motion sickness (prophylaxis and treatment)—
  Children up to 6 years of age:
    Use is not recommended unless directed by a physician.
  Children 6 to 12 years of age:
    Oral, 25 mg thirty minutes before travel. Dose may be repeated every six to eight hours as needed; or
    1 mg per kg of body weight or 33 mg per square meter of body surface area three times a day.
  Children 13 years of age or older:
    See *Usual adult and adolescent dose.*
Note: The total daily dose for pediatric patients should not exceed 75 mg.

**Usual geriatric dose**
See *Usual adult and adolescent dose.*
Note: Geriatric patients may be more sensitive to the effects of the usual adult dose.

**Strength(s) usually available**
U.S.—
  50 mg (OTC) [*Marezine* (scored)].
Canada—
  Not commercially available.

**Packaging and storage**
Store below 40 °C (104 °F), preferably between 15 and 30 °C (59 and 86 °F), unless otherwise specified by manufacturer. Store in a tight, light-resistant container.

**Auxiliary labeling**
• May cause drowsiness.
• Avoid alcoholic beverages.

## Parenteral Dosage Forms

### CYCLIZINE LACTATE INJECTION USP

**Usual adult and adolescent dose**
Motion sickness (prophylaxis and treatment)—
  Intramuscular, 50 mg every four to six hours as needed.
Nausea and vomiting, postoperative (prophylaxis and treatment)—
  Intramuscular, 50 mg fifteen to thirty minutes before end of operation. Dose may be repeated three times a day during the first few postoperative days, if needed.

**Usual pediatric dose**
Motion sickness (prophylaxis and treatment)—
  Intramuscular, 1 mg per kg of body weight or 33 mg per square meter of body surface area three times a day as needed.
Nausea and vomiting, postoperative (prophylaxis and treatment)—
  Children up to 6 years of age:
    Intramuscular, 12.5 mg fifteen to thirty minutes before end of operation. Dose may be repeated three times a day during the first few postoperative days, if needed.

Children 6 to 12 years of age:
Intramuscular, 25 mg fifteen to thirty minutes before end of operation. Dose may be repeated three times a day during the first few postoperative days, if needed.

Children 13 years of age or older:
See *Usual adult and adolescent dose.*

### Usual geriatric dose
See *Usual adult and adolescent dose.*

Note: Geriatric patients may be more sensitive to the effects of the usual adult dose.

### Strength(s) usually available
U.S.—
Not commercially available.
Canada—
50 mg per mL (Rx) [*Marzine*].

### Packaging and storage
Store between 5 and 10 °C (41 and 50 °F), unless otherwise specified by manufacturer. Protect from light. Protect from freezing.

### Preparation of dosage form
Cyclizine may be given intravenously if it is diluted to at least 10 mL with sterile water for injection or 0.9% sodium chloride injection and administered slowly.

### Stability
When stored at room temperature for several months, a slight yellowing of the solution may occur. This does not affect potency.

### Incompatibilities
Cyclizine lactate injection is incompatible with solutions having a pH greater than 6.8.

Revised: 01/03/96

## CYCLIZINE-CONTAINING COMBINATIONS—
Ergotamine, Caffeine, and Cyclizine (Systemic)—See *Vascular Headache Suppressants, Ergot Derivative–containing (Systemic)*

---

# CYCLOBENZAPRINE   Systemic

VA CLASSIFICATION (Primary): MS200

Note: For a listing of dosage forms and brand names by country availability, see *Dosage Forms* section(s). For a listing of brand names for the articles in this monograph, refer to the General Index.

## Category
Skeletal muscle relaxant.

## Indications
Note: Bracketed information in the *Indications* section refers to uses that are not included in U.S. product labeling.

### Accepted
Spasm, skeletal muscle (treatment)—Cyclobenzaprine is indicated as an adjunct to other measures, such as rest and physical therapy, for the relief of muscle spasm associated with acute, painful musculoskeletal conditions. It is not effective in relieving muscle spasm or spasticity caused by central nervous system (CNS) disorders.

[Fibromyalgia syndrome][1]—Cyclobenzaprine is indicated in the treatment of fibromyalgia syndrome (fibrositis, fibrositis syndrome). It has been shown to decrease pain, reduce muscle tightness and the number of tender points, and improve sleep in patients with this condition.

[1]Not included in Canadian product labeling.

## Pharmacology/Pharmacokinetics

### Physicochemical characteristics
Molecular weight—311.85.
pKa—8.47 (25 °C).

### Mechanism of action/Effect
The precise mechanism of action has not been fully determined. Cyclobenzaprine acts primarily at the brain stem to reduce tonic somatic motor activity influencing both gamma and alpha motoneurons. Actions at spinal cord sites may also be involved.

### Other actions/effects
Cyclobenzaprine is structurally related to, and may have actions similar to, the tricyclic antidepressants. These possible effects include central and peripheral anticholinergic actions, a sedative effect, and an increase in heart rate.

### Absorption
Well (but slowly) absorbed following oral administration.

### Protein binding
Very high (93%), with plasma concentrations ranging from 0.1 to 1 mcg per mL (0.32 to 3.21 micromoles per L).

### Biotransformation
Gastrointestinal and hepatic.

### Half-life
1 to 3 days.

### Onset of action
Within 1 hour.

### Time to peak concentration
3 to 8 hours.

### Peak serum concentration
15 to 25 nanograms per mL (0.048 to 0.08 micromoles per L) following a single 10-mg oral dose; subject to large interpatient variation.

### Therapeutic plasma concentration
20 to 30 nanograms per mL (0.064 to 0.096 micromoles per L).

### Time to peak effect
1 to 2 weeks.

### Duration of action
Single dose—12 to 24 hours.

### Elimination
Renal, primarily as conjugated metabolites (<1% of a dose is excreted unchanged); 51% of a single 10-mg dose is excreted within 5 days. Cyclobenzaprine undergoes enterohepatic circulation. Some unchanged cyclobenzaprine is also eliminated via the bile and feces.

## Precautions to Consider

### Carcinogenicity
Cyclobenzaprine did not show evidence of carcinogenicity in an 81-week study in mice or a 105-week study in rats.

### Mutagenicity
No evidence of mutagenicity occurred in male mice receiving up to 20 times the human dose of cyclobenzaprine.

### Pregnancy/Reproduction
Fertility—No evidence of impaired fertility occurred in male or female rats receiving up to 10 times the human dose of cyclobenzaprine.

Pregnancy—Adequate and well-controlled studies in humans have not been done.

Studies in rats, mice, and rabbits have not shown that cyclobenzaprine has adverse effects on the fetus when given in doses up to 20 times the human dose.

FDA Pregnancy Category B.

### Breast-feeding
Problems in humans have not been documented. It is not known whether cyclobenzaprine is distributed into breast milk; however, it is known that some of the structurally related tricyclic antidepressants are distributed into breast milk.

### Pediatrics
No information is available on the relationship of age to the effects of cyclobenzaprine in pediatric patients. Safety and efficacy have not been established.

### Adolescents
No information is available on the relationship of age to the effects of cyclobenzaprine in adolescents up to 15 years of age. Safety and efficacy have not been established.

### Geriatrics
No information is available on the relationship of age to the effects of cyclobenzaprine in geriatric patients. However, it is known that geriatric patients exhibit increased sensitivity to other medications with anticholinergic activity and are more likely than younger adults to

experience adverse reactions to the tricyclic antidepressants, which are structurally related to cyclobenzaprine.

### Dental
The peripheral anticholinergic effects of cyclobenzaprine may inhibit salivary flow, thus contributing to the development of caries, periodontal disease, oral candidiasis, and discomfort.

### Drug interactions and/or related problems
The following drug interactions and/or related problems have been selected on the basis of their potential clinical significance (possible mechanism in parentheses where appropriate)—not necessarily inclusive (» = major clinical significance):

Note: Combinations containing any of the following medications, depending on the amount present, may also interact with this medication.

In addition to the documented interactions listed below, the possibility should be considered that other interactions applying to tricyclic antidepressants may also apply to cyclobenzaprine because they are all chemically related.

» Alcohol or
» Antidepressants, tricyclic or
» CNS depression–producing medications, other (See *Appendix II*)
 (concurrent use with cyclobenzaprine may result in additive CNS depressant effects; caution is recommended, and dosage of one or both agents should be reduced)
 (concurrent use of a tricyclic antidepressant with cyclobenzaprine may also increase the risk of other side effects, such as anticholinergic effects and increased heart rate)

Antidyskinetics or
Anticholinergics or other medications with anticholinergic activity (See *Appendix II*)
 (cyclobenzaprine may potentiate the anticholinergic actions of these medications; patients should be advised to report occurrence of gastrointestinal problems promptly, since paralytic ileus may occur)

Guanadrel or
Guanethidine
 (cyclobenzaprine may decrease or block the antihypertensive effects of these medications)

» Monoamine oxidase (MAO) inhibitors, including furazolidone, procarbazine, and selegiline
 (concurrent use with cyclobenzaprine is not recommended on an outpatient basis, as hyperpyretic crises, severe seizures, and death have resulted when MAO inhibitors were used concurrently with tricyclic antidepressants; a minimum of 14 days should elapse between discontinuance of MAO inhibitors and initiation of cyclobenzaprine therapy, unless the patient is hospitalized; a minimum of 5 to 7 days should elapse between discontinuance of cyclobenzaprine and initiation of MAO inhibitor therapy)

### Medical considerations/Contraindications
The medical considerations/contraindications included here have been selected on the basis of their potential clinical significance (reasons given in parentheses where appropriate)—not necessarily inclusive (» = major clinical significance).

*Except under special circumstances, this medication should not be used when the following medical problems exist:*
» Acute recovery phase of myocardial infarction or
» Cardiac arrhythmias or
» Congestive heart failure or
» Heart block or other conduction disturbances
 (possible adverse cardiovascular effects)
» Hyperthyroidism
 (increased risk of cardiac arrhythmias; also, tachycardia associated with hyperthyroidism may be exacerbated)

*Risk-benefit should be considered when the following medical problems exist:*
Glaucoma or predisposition to or
Urinary retention or history of
 (cyclobenzaprine's anticholinergic effects may be detrimental to patients with these conditions)
Sensitivity to cyclobenzaprine

## Side/Adverse Effects
The following side/adverse effects have been selected on the basis of their potential clinical significance (possible signs and symptoms in parentheses where appropriate)—not necessarily inclusive:

### Those indicating need for medical attention
Incidence rare
 *Anaphylaxis* (changes in facial skin color; skin rash, hives, and/or itching; fast or irregular breathing; puffiness or swelling of the eyelids or the area around the eyes; shortness of breath, troubled breathing, tightness in chest, and/or wheezing); *angioedema* (large, hive-like swellings on face, eyelids, mouth, lips, and/or tongue); *anticholinergic effect* (problems in urinating); *CNS toxicity* (abnormal thinking and dreaming; clumsiness or unsteadiness; severe confusion or disorientation; mental depression; ringing or buzzing in ears); *dermatitis, allergic* (skin rash, hives, or itching); *hepatitis/cholestasis* (yellow eyes or skin); *syncope* (fainting)

Note: *Mania* has also been reported in a few patients with pre-existing psychiatric illness.

### Those indicating need for medical attention only if they continue or are bothersome
Incidence more frequent
 *Anticholinergic effects* (dryness of mouth [7 to 27%] blurred vision [<3%]); *dizziness or lightheadedness*—3 to 11%; *drowsiness*—16 to 39%

Note: *Dizziness, lightheadedness,* and *drowsiness* may be caused by cyclobenzaprine's anticholinergic, as well as its CNS, effects.

Incidence less frequent or rare (<3%)
 *CNS effects* (headache; confusion; excitement or nervousness; general feeling of discomfort or illness; numbness, tingling, pain, or weakness in hands or feet; muscle twitching; trembling; trouble in sleeping; unusual tiredness); *constipation; frequent urination; gastrointestinal irritation* (stomach cramps or pain; bloated feeling or gas; diarrhea; indigestion; nausea; vomiting); *pounding heartbeat; problems in speaking; unpleasant taste or other taste changes; unusual muscle weakness*

## Overdose
For specific information on the agents used in the management of cyclobenzaprine overdose, see:
 • *Benzodiazepines (Systemic)* monograph;
 • *Charcoal, Activated (Oral-Local)* monograph;
 • *Neostigmine* in *Antimyasthenics (Systemic)* monograph;
 • *Physostigmine (Systemic)* monograph;
 • *Propranolol* in *Beta-adrenergic Blocking Agents (Systemic)* monograph; and/or
 • *Pyridostigmine* in *Antimyasthenics (Systemic)* monograph.

For more information on the management of overdose or unintentional ingestion, **contact a Poison Control Center** (see *Poison Control Center Listing*).

### Clinical effects of overdose
The following effects have been on the basis of their potential clinical significance (possible signs and symptoms in parentheses where appropriate)—not necessarily inclusive:

Acute and chronic
 *Cardiotoxicity* (fast or irregular heartbeat; low blood pressure; troubled breathing)—may include bundle branch block or other arrhythmias and congestive heart failure; *CNS toxicity* (severe confusion; delirium; convulsions; severe drowsiness; hallucinations; severe nervousness or restlessness); *dry, hot, flushed skin*—a few cases of paradoxical diaphoresis have also been reported; *increase or decrease in body temperature; unexplained muscle stiffness; vomiting*

### Treatment of overdose
To decrease absorption—Emptying the stomach via induction of emesis, gastric lavage, or activated charcoal.

Monitoring—Taking an electrocardiogram (ECG) and monitoring cardiac function if any signs of dysrhythmia are evident.

Careful monitoring of the patient.

Specific treatment—

Use of physostigmine salicylate for severe or life-threatening anticholinergic effects. Repeating dose as required if life-threatening symptoms (e.g., arrhythmias, convulsions, coma) persist or recur. Because of its toxicity, physostigmine is recommended only in severe cases. See the package insert or *Physostigmine (Systemic)* for specific dosing guidelines for use of this product.

Use of neostigmine, pyridostigmine, or propranolol for cardiac arrhythmias. See the package insert or *Neostigmine* or *Pyridostigmine* in *An-*

*timyasthenics (Systemic)* or *Propranolol* in *Beta-adrenergic Blocking Agents (Systemic)* for specific dosing guidelines for use of this product.

Use of a short-acting digitalis preparation for cardiac failure should be considered. Close monitoring of cardiac function for at least 5 days is recommended. See the package insert or *Digitalis Glycosides (Systemic)* for specific dosing guidelines for use of this product.

Use of an appropriate anticonvulsant for convulsions. Benzodiazepines are most often used. However, because intravenously administered benzodiazepines may cause respiratory and circulatory depression, especially when administered rapidly, medications and equipment needed for support of respiration and for resuscitation must be immediately available. See the package insert or *Benzodiazepines (Systemic)* for specific dosing guidelines for use of this product.

Supportive—May include maintaining an open airway, maintaining adequate fluid intake, regulating body temperature, and treating circulatory shock, convulsions, and metabolic acidosis, if necessary. Patients in whom intentional overdose is known or suspected should be referred for psychiatric consultation.

Note: Dialysis is probably of no value in removing cyclobenzaprine from the body.

## Patient Consultation

As an aid to patient consultation, refer to *Advice for the Patient, Cyclobenzaprine (Systemic)*.

In providing consultation, consider emphasizing the following selected information (» = major clinical significance):

**Before using this medication**
» Conditions affecting use, especially:
    Sensitivity to cyclobenzaprine
    Other medications, especially other CNS depression–producing medications, monoamine oxidase inhibitors, and tricyclic antidepressants
    Other medical problems, especially cardiac arrhythmias, congestive heart failure, heart block or other conduction disturbances, hyperthyroidism, and myocardial infarction (acute recovery phase)

**Proper use of this medication**
Not taking more medication than the amount prescribed, to minimize possibility of side effects
» Proper dosing
    Missed dose: Taking if remembered within an hour; not taking if not remembered until later; not doubling doses
» Proper storage

**Precautions while using this medication**
» Avoiding alcohol or other CNS depressants unless prescribed or otherwise approved by physician
» Caution if blurred vision, drowsiness, or dizziness occurs
    Possible dryness of mouth; using sugarless gum or candy, ice, or saliva substitute for relief; checking with dentist if dry mouth continues for more than 2 weeks

**Side/adverse effects**
Signs and symptoms of potential side effects, especially anaphylaxis, angioedema, allergic dermatitis, hepatitis, and syncope

## General Dosing Information

It is recommended that cyclobenzaprine therapy for acute, painful musculoskeletal conditions be discontinued after 2 to 3 weeks, because evidence of its effectiveness for longer periods is not available. However, studies of the usefulness of cyclobenzaprine in fibromyalgia syndrome have indicated that the medication remains effective for at least 12 weeks.

Cyclobenzaprine is closely related to the tricyclic antidepressants and shares many of their adverse reactions and drug interactions.

## Oral Dosage Forms

Note: Bracketed uses in the *Dosage Forms* section refer to categories of use and/or indications that are not included in U.S. product labeling.

### CYCLOBENZAPRINE HYDROCHLORIDE TABLETS USP

**Usual adult dose**
Acute musculoskeletal conditions—Oral, 20 to 40 mg a day in two to four divided doses, usually 10 mg three times a day.
[Fibromyalgia syndrome][1]—Oral, 5 to 40 mg at bedtime.

**Usual adult prescribing limits**
Not to exceed 60 mg daily.

**Usual pediatric and adolescent dose**
Children up to 15 years of age—Dosage has not been established.
Patients 15 years of age and older—See *Usual adult dose*

**Strength(s) usually available**
U.S.—
    10 mg (Rx) [*Cycoflex; Flexeril;* GENERIC].
Canada—
    10 mg (Rx) [*Flexeril*].

**Packaging and storage**
Store below 40 °C (104 °F), preferably between 15 and 30 °C (59 and 86 °F). Store in a well-closed container.

**Auxiliary labeling**
• May cause drowsiness.
• Avoid alcoholic beverages.

---

[1]Not included in Canadian product labeling.

## Selected Bibliography

Katz WA, Dube J. Cyclobenzaprine in the treatment of acute muscle spasm: review of a decade of clinical experience. Clin Ther 1988; 10: 216-28.

---

Revised: 07/28/94

---

# CYCLOPENTOLATE   Ophthalmic

VA CLASSIFICATION (Primary): OP600

Note: For a listing of dosage forms and brand names by country availability, see *Dosage Forms* section(s). For a listing of brand names for the articles in this monograph, refer to the General Index.

---

## Category
Cycloplegic; mydriatic.

## Indications

Note: Bracketed information in the *Indications* section refers to uses that are not included in U.S. product labeling.

**Accepted**
Refraction, cycloplegic—Indicated for measurement of refractive errors; also indicated for cycloplegia in diagnostic procedures, such as ophthalmoscopy.

Mydriasis, in diagnostic procedures—Indicated for mydriasis in diagnostic procedures, such as ophthalmoscopy.

Mydriasis, preoperative or
Mydriasis, postoperative—May be indicated for mydriasis in some preoperative and postoperative conditions.

[Synechiae, posterior (prophylaxis)][1]—Cyclopentolate is used for prophylaxis of posterior synechiae.

[Uveitis (treatment)][1]—Used in inflammatory conditions of the iris and uveal tract when a shorter-acting mydriatic and cycloplegic is required.

---

[1]Not included in Canadian product labeling.

## Pharmacology/Pharmacokinetics

**Physicochemical characteristics**
Molecular weight—327.85.

**Mechanism of action/Effect**
Cyclopentolate is an anticholinergic drug that blocks the responses of the sphincter muscle of the iris and the accommodative muscle of the ciliary body to stimulation by acetylcholine. Dilation of the pupil (mydriasis) and paralysis of accommodation (cycloplegia) result.

**Onset of action**
Rapid.

**Time to peak effect**
Cycloplegia—Within 25 to 75 minutes.
Mydriasis—Within 30 to 60 minutes.

**Duration of action**
Has a shorter duration of action than atropine.
Complete recovery of accommodation usually takes 6 to 24 hours.
Complete recovery from mydriasis in some persons may take several days.

## Precautions to Consider

### Pregnancy/Reproduction
Pregnancy—Cyclopentolate may be systemically absorbed.
Studies have not been done in humans.
Studies have not been done in animals.

FDA Pregnancy Category C.

### Breast-feeding
It is not known whether cyclopentolate is distributed into breast milk; however, cyclopentolate may be systemically absorbed.

### Pediatrics
An increased susceptibility to cyclopentolate and similar drugs (such as atropine) has been reported in infants and young children and in children with blond hair, blue eyes, Down's syndrome, spastic paralysis, or brain damage; therefore, cyclopentolate should be used with great caution in these patients. In addition, premature and small infants are especially prone to CNS and cardiopulmonary side effects from systemic absorption of cyclopentolate. Also, feeding intolerance may follow ophthalmic use of cyclopentolate in neonates. It is recommended that feeding be withheld for 4 hours following administration of this medication.

### Geriatrics
Geriatric patients are more susceptible to the effects of cyclopentolate and similar drugs (such as atropine), thus increasing the potential for systemic side effects.

Also, cyclopentolate should be used with caution in the elderly because of possible undiagnosed predisposition to angle-closure glaucoma.

### Drug interactions and/or related problems
The following drug interactions and/or related problems have been selected on the basis of their potential clinical significance (possible mechanism in parentheses where appropriate)—not necessarily inclusive (» = major clinical significance):

Note: Combinations containing any of the following medications, depending on the amount present, may also interact with this medication.

Antiglaucoma agents, cholinergic, long-acting, ophthalmic
(cyclopentolate may antagonize the antiglaucoma and miotic actions of ophthalmic long-acting cholinergic antiglaucoma agents, such as demecarium, echothiophate, and isoflurophate)

Carbachol or
Pilocarpine
(cyclopentolate may interfere with the antiglaucoma action of carbachol or pilocarpine; also, these medications counteract the mydriatic effect of cyclopentolate, the result of which may be used to therapeutic advantage)

### Medical considerations/Contraindications
The medical considerations/contraindications included here have been selected on the basis of their potential clinical significance (reasons given in parentheses where appropriate)—not necessarily inclusive (» = major clinical significance).

*Risk-benefit should be considered when the following medical problems exist:*
Brain damage, in children or
Down's syndrome (mongolism), in children and adults or
Spastic paralysis, in children
(increased susceptibility to the effects of cyclopentolate)
» Glaucoma, angle-closure or predisposition to angle closure
Sensitivity to cyclopentolate

## Side/Adverse Effects

Note: An increased susceptibility to cyclopentolate and similar drugs (such as atropine) has been reported in infants, young children, children with blond hair or blue eyes, adults and children with Down's syndrome, children with brain damage or spastic paralysis, and the elderly. This susceptibility increases the potential for systemic side effects.

The following side/adverse effects have been selected on the basis of their potential clinical significance (possible signs and symptoms in parentheses where appropriate)—not necessarily inclusive:

### Those indicating need for medical attention
Symptoms of systemic absorption
*Ataxia* (clumsiness or unsteadiness); *behavioral disturbances; psychotic reactions* (unusual behavior, especially in children using 2% cyclopentolate); *confusion; fast or irregular heartbeat; fever; hallucinations; skin rash; slurred speech; swollen stomach in infants; thirst or dryness of mouth; unusual drowsiness; tiredness or weakness; vasodilation* (flushing or redness of face)

### Those indicating need for medical attention only if they continue or are bothersome
*Blepharoconjunctivitis; conjunctivitis; hyperemia; punctate keratitis; synechiae* (eye irritation not present before therapy); *blurred vision; burning of eye; photophobia* (increased sensitivity of eyes to light)

## Overdose

For specific information on the agents used in the management of ophthalmic cyclopentolate overdose, see:
• *Physostigmine (Systemic)* monograph.

For more information on the management of overdose or unintentional ingestion, **contact a Poison Control Center** (see *Poison Control Center Listing*).

### Treatment of overdose
Cessation of ophthalmic cyclopentolate usually results in spontaneous recovery from adverse systemic effects; for severe toxicity, physostigmine is the antidote of choice.

For children—A dose of 0.5 mg of physostigmine should be slowly administered intravenously. If toxic symptoms persist and no cholinergic symptoms are produced, the dose should be repeated at 5-minute intervals up to a maximum of 2 mg.

For adolescents and adults—A dose of 2 mg of physostigmine should be slowly administered intravenously. A second dose of 1 to 2 mg may be given after 20 minutes if no reversal of toxic manifestations has occurred. Physostigmine may also be administered subcutaneously.

## Patient Consultation

As an aid to patient consultation, refer to *Advice for the Patient, Cyclopentolate (Ophthalmic).*

In providing consultation, consider emphasizing the following selected information (» = major clinical significance):

### Before using this medication
» Conditions affecting use, especially:
Sensitivity to cyclopentolate
Use in children—Infants and young children and children with blond hair or blue eyes may be especially sensitive to the effects of cyclopentolate and similar drugs (such as atropine); this may increase the chance of side effects during treatment; premature and small infants are especially prone to CNS and cardiopulmonary side effects from systemic absorption; feeding intolerance may occur following administration in neonates; it is recommended that feeding be withheld for 4 hours following administration
Use in the elderly—Geriatric patients are more susceptible to the effects of cyclopentolate and similar drugs (such as atropine), thus increasing the potential for systemic side effects
Other medical problems, especially angle-closure glaucoma or predisposition to angle closure

### Proper use of this medication
Proper administration technique
» Importance of nasolacrimal pressure, especially in infants.
Washing hands immediately after application to remove any medicine that may be on them; if applying medication to infants or children, washing their hands also, and not letting any medication get into their mouths
Preventing contamination: Not touching applicator tip to any surface; keeping container tightly closed
» Importance of not using more medication than the amount prescribed
» Proper dosing
Missed dose: Applying as soon as possible; if almost time for next dose, skipping missed dose and going back to regular dosing schedule; not doubling doses
» Proper storage

### Precautions while using this medication
» Medication causes blurred vision; checking with physician if effect continues for longer than 36 hours after discontinuation of medication

» Medication causes increased sensitivity of the eyes to light; wearing sunglasses that block ultraviolet light to protect eyes; checking with physician if effect continues for longer than 36 hours after discontinuation of medication

### Side/adverse effects
Signs of potential side effects, especially symptoms of systemic absorption

## General Dosing Information

Although some manufacturers recommend a dose of 2 drops of an ophthalmic solution at appropriate intervals, the conjunctival sac will usually hold only 1 drop.

More frequent instillation or use of a stronger solution may be required to produce adequate cycloplegia in eyes with brown or hazel irides than in eyes with blue irides.

To avoid excessive systemic absorption, patient should apply digital pressure to the lacrimal sac during and for 2 or 3 minutes following instillation of the solution. This is especially important in infants.

## Ophthalmic Dosage Forms

Note: Bracketed uses in the *Dosage Forms* section refer to categories of use and/or indications that are not included in U.S. product labeling.

### CYCLOPENTOLATE HYDROCHLORIDE OPHTHALMIC SOLUTION USP

#### Usual adult and adolescent dose
Cycloplegic refraction—
Topical, to the conjunctiva, 1 drop of a 0.5 to 2% solution, repeated once in five to ten minutes if necessary, with refraction scheduled for forty to fifty minutes afterward.

For ophthalmoscopy—
Topical, to the conjunctiva, 1 drop of a 0.5 to 2% solution, repeated once in five to ten minutes if necessary.

[Uveitis][1]—
Topical, to the conjunctiva, 1 drop of a 0.5 or 1% solution three or four times a day.

#### Usual pediatric dose
Cycloplegic refraction—
Premature and small infants: Topical, to the conjunctiva, 1 drop of a 0.5% solution, as a single dose.

Children: Topical, to the conjunctiva, 1 drop of a 0.5 to 2% solution, followed by 1 drop of a 0.5 or 1% solution after five to ten minutes if necessary, with refraction scheduled for forty to fifty minutes afterward.

For ophthalmoscopy—
Topical, to the conjunctiva, 1 drop of a 0.5 or 1% solution.

[Uveitis][1]—
Topical, to the conjunctiva, 1 drop of a 0.5 or 1% solution three or four times a day.

Note: In small infants, use of concentrations above 0.5% is not recommended.

Infants should be closely observed for signs of adverse reactions for at least 30 minutes following administration.

To minimize systemic absorption, application of nasolacrimal pressure for 2 or 3 minutes is recommended, especially in infants.

#### Strength(s) usually available
U.S.—
0.5% (Rx) [*Cyclogyl* (benzalkonium chloride 0.01%)].
1% (Rx) [*Ak-Pentolate* (benzalkonium chloride 0.01%); *Cyclogyl* (benzalkonium chloride 0.01%); *I-Pentolate; Ocu-Pentolate; Pentolair; Spectro-Pentolate;* GENERIC].
2% (Rx) [*Cyclogyl* (benzalkonium chloride 0.01%)].
Canada—
0.5% (Rx) [*Ak-Pentolate* (benzalkonium chloride); *Minims Cyclopentolate*].
1% (Rx) [*Ak-Pentolate* (benzalkonium chloride); *Cyclogyl* (benzalkonium chloride); *Minims Cyclopentolate*].

#### Packaging and storage
Store between 15 and 30 °C (59 and 86 °F). Store in a tight container.

#### Auxiliary labeling
• For the eye.
• Keep container tightly closed.

---

[1]Not included in Canadian product labeling.

---

Revised: 03/04/92
Interim revision: 08/30/93

---

# CYCLOPHOSPHAMIDE    Systemic

VA CLASSIFICATION (Primary/Secondary): AN100/DE801; IM600; MS105

Note: For a listing of dosage forms and brand names by country availability, see *Dosage Forms* section(s). For a listing of brand names for the articles in this monograph, refer to the General Index.

## Category
Antineoplastic; immunosuppressant.

## Indications

Note: Bracketed information in the *Indications* section refers to uses that are not included in U.S. product labeling.

### Accepted
Leukemia, acute lymphocytic (treatment)
Leukemia, acute myelocytic (treatment) or
Leukemia, acute monocytic (treatment)—Cyclophosphamide is indicated for treatment of acute lymphoblastic (stem-cell) leukemia in children (including during remission to prolong the duration), and for treatment of acute myelogenous and acute monocytic leukemia.

Leukemia, chronic myelocytic (treatment) or
Leukemia, chronic lymphocytic (treatment)—Cyclophosphamide is indicated for treatment of chronic granulocytic leukemia (it is usually ineffective in acute blastic crisis) and chronic lymphocytic leukemia.

Carcinoma, ovarian (treatment)
Carcinoma, breast (treatment)
Neuroblastoma (treatment)
Retinoblastoma (treatment)
[Carcinoma, lung (treatment)]
[Carcinoma, cervical (treatment)][1]
[Carcinoma, endometrial (treatment)][1]

[Carcinoma, bladder (treatment)][1]
[Carcinoma, prostatic (treatment)][1]
[Carcinoma, testicular (treatment)][1] or
[Wilms' tumor (treatment)][1]—Cyclophosphamide is indicated for treatment of adenocarcinoma of the ovary, breast carcinoma, neuroblastoma [in patients with disseminated disease], retinoblastoma, lung carcinoma, cervical carcinoma, and for endometrial carcinoma, bladder carcinoma, prostatic carcinoma, testicular carcinoma, and Wilms' tumor.

Lymphomas, Hodgkin's (treatment) or
Lymphomas, non-Hodgkin's (treatment)—Cyclophosphamide is indicated for treatment of Stage III and IV (Ann Arbor or Peter's Staging System) Hodgkin's disease and non-Hodgkin's lymphomas including nodular or diffuse lymphocytic lymphoma, mixed-cell type lymphoma, histiocytic lymphoma, Burkitt's lymphoma, [follicular lymphoma, lymphocytic lymphosarcoma, reticulum cell sarcoma, and lymphoblastic lymphosarcoma].

Multiple myeloma (treatment)—Cyclophosphamide is indicated for treatment of multiple myeloma.

Mycosis fungoides (treatment)—Cyclophosphamide is indicated for treatment of advanced mycosis fungoides.

Nephrotic syndrome (treatment)[1]—Cyclophosphamide is indicated as an immunosuppressant in the treatment of steroid-resistant or frequently relapsing steroid-sensitive biopsy proven minimal-change nephrotic syndrome in children [and adults].

[Ewing's sarcoma (treatment)][1]
[Osteosarcoma, (treatment)][1] or
[Sarcomas, soft tissue (treatment)][1]—Cyclophosphamide is used for treatment of various sarcomas, including Ewing's sarcoma, osteosarcoma, and soft tissue sarcomas.

[Tumors, germ cell, ovarian (treatment)]¹—Cyclophosphamide is used for treatment of germ cell ovarian tumors.

[Transplant rejection, organ (prophylaxis)]¹—Cyclophosphamide is used for its immunosuppressant activity, for prevention of rejection in homotransplantation.

[Arthritis, rheumatoid (treatment)]¹
[Wegener's granulomatosis (treatment)]¹
[Lupus erythematosus, systemic]¹
[Dermatomyositis, systemic (treatment)]¹ or
[Multiple sclerosis (treatment)]¹—Cyclophosphamide is used as an immunosuppressant in the treatment of rheumatoid arthritis and other autoimmune diseases such as polymyositis (systemic dermatomyositis), multiple sclerosis, Wegener's granulomatosis, systemic lupus erythematosus (SLE), and other types of vasculitis.

**Extreme caution is recommended in use of cyclophosphamide for non-neoplastic conditions because of potential carcinogenicity with long-term use of this agent.**

¹Not included in Canadian product labeling.

## Pharmacology/Pharmacokinetics

### Physicochemical characteristics
Molecular weight—279.10.

### Mechanism of action/Effect
Cyclophosphamide is classed as an alkylating agent of the nitrogen mustard type. An activated form of cyclophosphamide, phosphoramide mustard, alkylates or binds with many intracellular molecular structures, including nucleic acids. Its cytotoxic action is primarily due to cross-linking of strands of DNA and RNA, as well as inhibition of protein synthesis.

### Other actions/effects
Cyclophosphamide is a potent immunosuppressant. It also causes marked and persistent inhibition of cholinesterase activity.

### Absorption
Well absorbed after oral administration (bioavailability greater than 75%).

### Distribution
Crosses blood-brain barrier to limited extent.

### Protein binding
Very low (some active metabolites—greater than 60%).

### Biotransformation
Hepatic (including initial activation and subsequent degradation).

### Half-life
Unchanged drug—3 to 12 hours.

### Time to peak concentration
Plasma—Metabolites: 2 to 3 hours after intravenous administration.

### Elimination
Renal, 5 to 25% unchanged.
In dialysis—Cyclophosphamide is dialyzable.

## Precautions to Consider

### Carcinogenicity/Mutagenicity
Secondary malignancies are potential delayed effects of many antineoplastic agents, although it is not clear whether the effect is related to their mutagenic or immunosuppressive action. The effect of dose and duration of therapy is also unknown, although risk seems to increase with long-term use. Although information is limited, available data seem to indicate that the carcinogenic risk is greatest with the alkylating agents.

Cyclophosphamide is a potent carcinogen in animals. In humans, it has been associated with development of myeloproliferative and lymphoproliferative carcinomas as well as urinary bladder carcinoma (especially in patients who developed hemorrhagic cystitis while receiving cyclophosphamide) up to several years after administration. One case of carcinoma of the renal pelvis occurred in a patient who received long-term treatment with cyclophosphamide for cerebral vasculitis.

### Pregnancy/Reproduction
Fertility—Gonadal suppression, resulting in amenorrhea or azoospermia, may occur in patients taking antineoplastic therapy, especially with the alkylating agents. In general, these effects appear to be related to dose and length of therapy and may be irreversible. Prediction of the degree of testicular or ovarian function impairment is complicated by the common use of combinations of several antineoplastics, which makes it difficult to assess the effects of individual agents.

However, there have been numerous reports of gonadal suppression with use of cyclophosphamide, which seems to depend on dose, duration,

and state of gonadal function at the time of therapy; sterility may be irreversible in some patients.

Paternal use of cyclophosphamide prior to conception has been associated with cardiac and limb abnormalities in an infant.

Pregnancy—Cyclophosphamide crosses the placenta. Use in humans has resulted in both normal and malformed (missing fingers and/or toes, cardiac anomalies, hernias) newborns; risk seems to be less in the second and third trimesters. Low birth weight is also a risk with exposure of the fetus to antineoplastics.

First trimester: It is usually recommended that use of antineoplastics, especially combination chemotherapy, be avoided whenever possible, especially during the first trimester. Although information is limited because of the relatively few instances of antineoplastic administration during pregnancy, the mutagenic, teratogenic, and carcinogenic potential of these medications must be considered.

Other hazards to the fetus include adverse reactions seen in adults.

In general, use of a contraceptive is recommended during cytotoxic drug therapy.

Studies in animals have shown that cyclophosphamide is teratogenic in mice, rats, rabbits, and monkeys given 0.02, 0.08, 0.5, and 0.07 times the human dose, respectively.

FDA Pregnancy Category D.

### Breast-feeding
Cyclophosphamide is distributed into breast milk. Breast-feeding is not recommended during chemotherapy because of the risks to the infant (adverse effects, mutagenicity, carcinogenicity).

### Pediatrics
Appropriate studies performed to date have not demonstrated pediatrics-specific problems that would limit the usefulness of cyclophosphamide in children.

Prepubescent girls treated with cyclophosphamide usually develop secondary sexual characteristics normally, have regular menses, and subsequently conceive; however, ovarian fibrosis and apparent complete loss of germ cells after prolonged treatment in late prepubescence have been reported. Prepubescent boys treated with cyclophosphamide develop secondary sexual characteristics normally, but may have oligospermia or azoospermia, increased gonadotropin secretion, and some degree of testicular atrophy; azoospermia may be reversible, although possibly not for several years after the end of cyclophosphamide therapy.

### Geriatrics
Although appropriate studies on the relationship of age to the effects of cyclophosphamide have not been performed in the geriatric population, geriatrics-specific problems are not expected to limit the usefulness of this medication in the elderly. However, elderly patients are more likely to have age-related renal function impairment, which may require caution in patients receiving cyclophosphamide.

### Dental
The bone marrow depressant effects of cyclophosphamide may result in an increased incidence of microbial infection, delayed healing, and gingival bleeding. Dental work, whenever possible, should be completed prior to initiation of therapy or deferred until blood counts have returned to normal. Patients should be instructed in proper oral hygiene during treatment, including caution in use of regular toothbrushes, dental floss, and toothpicks.

Cyclophosphamide may also rarely cause stomatitis associated with considerable discomfort.

### Drug interactions and/or related problems
The following drug interactions and/or related problems have been selected on the basis of their potential clinical significance (possible mechanism in parentheses where appropriate)—not necessarily inclusive (» = major clinical significance):

Note: Combinations containing any of the following medications, depending on the amount present, may also interact with this medication.

Allopurinol or
Colchicine or
» Probenecid or
» Sulfinpyrazone
   (cyclophosphamide may raise the concentration of blood uric acid; dosage adjustment of antigout agents may be necessary to control hyperuricemia and gout; uricosuric antigout agents may increase risk of uric acid nephropathy)

   (concurrent use with allopurinol may enhance the bone marrow toxicity of cyclophosphamide; if concurrent use is required, close observation for toxic effects should be considered)

Anticoagulants, oral
(cyclophosphamide may increase anticoagulant activity as a result of decreased hepatic synthesis of procoagulant factors and interference with platelet formation, but may also decrease anticoagulant activity by an unknown mechanism)

Blood dyscrasia–causing medications (See *Appendix II*)
(leukopenic and/or thrombocytopenic effects of cyclophosphamide may be increased with concurrent or recent therapy if these medications cause the same effects; dosage adjustment of cyclophosphamide, if necessary, should be based on blood counts)

» Bone marrow depressants, other (See *Appendix II*) or
» Radiation therapy
(additive bone marrow depression may occur; dosage reduction may be required when two or more bone marrow depressants, including radiation, are used concurrently or consecutively)

» Cocaine
(inhibition of cholinesterase activity by cyclophosphamide reduces or slows cocaine metabolism, thereby increasing and/or prolonging its effects and increasing the risk of toxicity)

» Cytarabine
(concurrent use of high-dose cytarabine with cyclophosphamide for bone marrow transplant preparation has been reported to result in an increase in cardiomyopathy with subsequent death)

Daunorubicin or
Doxorubicin
(concurrent use with cyclophosphamide may result in increased cardiotoxicity; it is recommended that the total dose of daunorubicin or doxorubicin not exceed 400 mg per square meter of body surface)

Hepatic enzyme inducers (See *Appendix II*)
(these agents may induce microsomal metabolism to increase formation of alkylating metabolites of cyclophosphamide, thereby reducing the half-life and increasing the activity of cyclophosphamide)

» Immunosuppressants, other, such as:
Azathioprine
Chlorambucil
Corticosteroids, glucocorticoid
Cyclosporine
Mercaptopurine
Muromonab-CD3
(concurrent use with cyclophosphamide may increase the risk of infection and development of neoplasms)

Lovastatin
(concurrent use in cardiac transplant patients may be associated with an increased risk of rhabdomyolysis and acute renal failure)

Succinylcholine
(cyclophosphamide may decrease plasma concentrations or activity of pseudocholinesterase, the enzyme that metabolizes succinylcholine, thereby enhancing the neuromuscular blockade of succinylcholine. Increased or prolonged respiratory depression or paralysis [apnea] may occur but is of minor clinical significance while the patient is being mechanically ventilated; however, caution and careful monitoring of the patient are recommended during and following concurrent or sequential use, especially if there is a possibility of incomplete reversal of neuromuscular blockade postoperatively)

Vaccines, killed virus
(because normal defense mechanisms may be suppressed by cyclophosphamide therapy, the patient's antibody response to the vaccine may be decreased. The interval between discontinuation of medications that cause immunosuppression and restoration of the patient's ability to respond to the vaccine depends on the intensity and type of immunosuppression-causing medication used, the underlying disease, and other factors; estimates vary from 3 months to 1 year)

» Vaccines, live virus
(because normal defense mechanisms may be suppressed by cyclophosphamide therapy, concurrent use with a live virus vaccine may potentiate the replication of the vaccine virus, may increase the side/adverse effects of the vaccine virus, and/or may decrease the patient's antibody response to the vaccine; immunization of these patients should be undertaken only with extreme caution after careful review of the patient's hematologic status and only with the knowledge and consent of the physician managing the cyclophosphamide therapy. The interval between discontinuation of medications that cause immunosuppression and restoration of the patient's ability to respond to the vaccine depends on the intensity and type of immunosuppression-causing medication used, the un-

derlying disease, and other factors; estimates vary from 3 months to 1 year. Patients with leukemia in remission should not receive live virus vaccine until at least 3 months after their last chemotherapy. In addition, immunization with oral poliovirus vaccine should be postponed in persons in close contact with the patient, especially family members)

**Laboratory value alterations**
The following have been selected on the basis of their potential clinical significance (possible effect in parentheses where appropriate)—not necessarily inclusive (» = major clinical significance):

With diagnostic test results
Candida skin test and
Mumps skin test and
Trichophyton skin test and
Tuberculin PPD skin test
(positive reactions may be suppressed)
Papanicolaou (PAP) test
(false-positive results may be produced)

With physiology/laboratory test values
Pseudocholinesterase
(serum concentrations may be decreased)
Uric acid
(blood and urine concentrations may be increased)

**Medical considerations/Contraindications**
The medical considerations/contraindications included here have been selected on the basis of their potential clinical significance (reasons given in parentheses where appropriate)—not necessarily inclusive (» = major clinical significance).

*Risk-benefit should be considered when the following medical problems exist:*
Adrenalectomy
(toxic effects of cyclophosphamide may be increased; dosage adjustment of both replacement steroids and cyclophosphamide may be necessary)
» Bone marrow depression
» Chickenpox, existing or recent (including recent exposure) or
» Herpes zoster
(risk of severe generalized disease)
Gout, history of or
Urate renal stones, history of
(risk of hyperuricemia)
» Hepatic function impairment
(effect of cyclophosphamide may be reduced because of its dependence on hepatic microsomal enzyme activation)
» Infection
» Renal function impairment
(reduced elimination; dosage reduction usually not necessary)
Sensitivity to cyclophosphamide
» Tumor cell infiltration of bone marrow
(a reduction by one-third to one-half in cyclophosphamide dosage for induction is recommended for patients with bone marrow depression due to tumor cell infiltration)
» Caution should be used also in patients who have had previous cytotoxic drug therapy or radiation therapy; a reduction by one-third to one-half in cyclophosphamide dosage for induction is recommended for patients with bone marrow depression due to cytotoxic or radiation therapy.

**Patient monitoring**
The following are especially important in patient monitoring (other tests may be warranted in some patients, depending on condition; (» = major clinical significance):

Alanine aminotransferase (ALT [SGPT]) values, serum and
Aspartate aminotransferase (AST [SGOT]) values, serum and
Bilirubin values, serum and
Lactate dehydrogenase (LDH) values, serum
(recommended prior to initiation of therapy and at periodic intervals during therapy; frequency varies according to clinical state, agent, dose, and other agents being used concurrently)

Blood urea nitrogen (BUN) concentrations and
Creatinine concentrations, serum
(recommended prior to initiation of therapy and at periodic intervals during therapy; frequency varies according to clinical state, agent, dose, and other agents being used concurrently)

» Examination of urine for microscopic hematuria
(recommended at periodic intervals during therapy, as well as for several hours following a large intravenous dose)

» Hematocrit or hemoglobin and
» Leukocyte count, total and, if appropriate, differential and
» Platelet count
  (determinations recommended prior to initiation of therapy and at periodic intervals during therapy; frequency varies according to clinical state, agent, dose, and other agents being used concurrently)

Uric acid concentrations, serum
  (recommended prior to initiation of therapy and at periodic intervals during therapy; frequency varies according to clinical state, agent, dose, and other agents being used concurrently)

Urinary output and
Urinary specific gravity
  (determinations recommended following high-dose intravenous administration to detect possible syndrome of inappropriate secretion of antidiuretic hormone [SIADH])

## Side/Adverse Effects

Note: Many ''side effects'' of antineoplastic therapy are unavoidable and represent the medication's pharmacologic action. Some of these (for example, leukopenia and thrombocytopenia) are actually used as parameters to aid in individual dosage titration.

The following side/adverse effects have been selected on the basis of their potential clinical significance (possible signs and symptoms in parentheses where appropriate)—not necessarily inclusive:

### Those indicating need for medical attention
Incidence more frequent
  *Gonadal suppression* (missing menstrual periods); *leukopenia or infection* (usually asymptomatic; less frequently, fever or chills; cough or hoarseness; lower back or side pain; painful or difficult urination)
  Note: With *gonadal suppression*, regular menses usually resume within a few months after the end of cyclophosphamide therapy. A marked *leukopenia* usually occurs, with the nadir of the leukocyte count occurring 7 to 12 days after administration and recovery after 17 to 21 days.

With high-dose and/or long-term therapy
  *Cardiotoxicity, including acute myopericarditis* (fast heartbeat; fever or chills; shortness of breath); *hemorrhagic cystitis* (blood in urine; painful urination); *hyperuricemia, uric acid nephropathy, nonhemorrhagic cystitis, or nephrotoxicity* (joint pain; lower back or side pain; swelling of feet or lower legs); *pneumonitis or interstitial pulmonary fibrosis* (cough, shortness of breath); *syndrome resembling inappropriate antidiuretic hormone (SIADH) secretion* (dizziness, confusion, or agitation; unusual tiredness or weakness)
  Note: *Cardiotoxicity* is most severe with use of doses of 180 to 270 mg per kg of body weight (mg/kg) within four to six days.
    A few cases of severe and sometimes fatal *congestive heart failure* have occurred within a few days after the first dose of a high-dose course of cyclophosphamide; histopathologic examination primarily revealed *hemorrhagic myocarditis*. Hemopericardium has occurred secondary to hemorrhagic myocarditis and myocardial necrosis. Pericarditis has been reported independent of any hemopericardium.
    *Hemorrhagic cystitis* may occur within a few hours or be delayed several weeks; thought to be caused by metabolites of cyclophosphamide (chloroacetic acid, acrolein) excreted in the urine. Usually resolves a few days after withdrawal of cyclophosphamide, but may persist; may be fatal. Fibrosis of the urinary bladder, with or without cystitis, may also occur and may be extensive. Atypical urinary bladder epithelial cells may be found in urine. Hemorrhagic ureteritis and renal tubular necrosis, which usually resolve after withdrawal of cyclophosphamide, have also been reported.
    *Hyperuricemia* with uric acid nephropathy occurs most commonly during initial treatment of patients with leukemia or lymphoma, as a result of rapid cell breakdown which leads to elevated serum uric acid concentrations.

Incidence less frequent
  *Anemia; thrombocytopenia* (usually asymptomatic; rarely, unusual bleeding or bruising; black, tarry stools; blood in urine or stools; pinpoint red spots on skin)

Incidence rare
  *Anaphylactic reaction* (sudden shortness of breath); *hemorrhagic colitis* (black, tarry stools); *hepatitis* (yellow eyes or skin); *hyperglycemia* (frequent urination; unusual thirst); *redness, swelling, or pain at site of injection; stomatitis* (sores in mouth and on lips)
  Note: *Anaphylaxis* has resulted in death.

### Those indicating need for medical attention only if they continue or are bothersome
Incidence more frequent
  *Darkening of skin and fingernails; loss of appetite; nausea or vomiting, especially with high oral doses*
Incidence less frequent
  *Diarrhea or stomach pain; flushing or redness of face; headache; increased sweating; myxedema* (swollen lips); *skin rash, hives, or itching*

### Those not indicating need for medical attention
Incidence more frequent
  *Loss of hair*
  Note: Normal *hair growth* usually returns after treatment has ended, although it may be slightly different in color or texture.

### Those indicating the need for medical attention if they occur after medication is discontinued
  *Hemorrhagic cystitis* (blood in urine)

## Patient Consultation

As an aid to patient consultation, refer to *Advice for the Patient, Cyclophosphamide (Systemic)*.

In providing consultation, consider emphasizing the following selected information (» = major clinical significance):

### Before using this medication
» Conditions affecting use, especially:
    Sensitivity to cyclophosphamide
    Pregnancy—Use not recommended because of mutagenic, teratogenic, and carcinogenic potential; advisability of using contraception; telling physician immediately if pregnancy is suspected
    Breast-feeding—Not recommended because of risk of serious side effects
    Other medications, especially probenecid, sulfinpyrazone, other bone marrow depressants, other immunosuppressants, or cytotoxic drug or radiation therapy
    Other medical problems, especially chickenpox, herpes zoster, hepatic function impairment, infection, or renal function impairment

### Proper use of this medication
» Importance of not taking more or less medication than the amount prescribed
  Caution in taking combination therapy; taking each medication at the right time
» Importance of ample fluid intake and subsequent increase in urine output, as well as frequent voiding (including at least once during night), to prevent hemorrhagic cystitis and aid in excretion of uric acid; following physician instructions for recommended fluid intake; some patients may require up to 3000 mL (3 quarts) per day
  Usually best if taken in the morning to reduce risk of hemorrhagic cystitis; however, physician may recommend taking in small doses throughout day to lessen stomach upset; following physician's instructions for timing of doses
» Probability of nausea, vomiting, and loss of appetite; importance of continuing medication despite stomach upset; checking with physician before discontinuing medication
  Checking with physician if vomiting occurs shortly after dose is taken
» Proper dosing
  Missed dose: Not taking at all; not doubling doses; checking with physician
» Proper storage

### Precautions while using this medication
» Importance of close monitoring by physician
» Avoiding immunizations unless approved by physician; other persons in patient's household should avoid immunizations with oral poliovirus vaccine; avoiding persons who have taken oral poliovirus vaccine or wearing a protective mask that covers nose and mouth
  Caution if any kind of surgery, including dental surgery, or emergency treatment with general anesthesia is required within 10 days of treatment
*Caution if bone marrow depression occurs:*
» Avoiding exposure to persons with bacterial infections, especially during periods of low blood counts; checking with physician immediately if fever or chills, cough or hoarseness, lower back or side pain, or painful or difficult urination occur
» Checking with physician immediately if unusual bleeding or bruising; black, tarry stools; blood in urine; or pinpoint red spots on skin occur

Caution in use of regular toothbrush, dental floss, or toothpick; physician, dentist, or nurse may suggest alternatives; checking with physician before having dental work done

Not touching eyes or inside of nose unless hands washed immediately before

Using caution to avoid accidental cuts with use of sharp objects such as safety razor or fingernail or toenail cutters

Avoiding contact sports or other situations where bruising or injury could occur

Caution if any laboratory tests required; possible interference with test results

### Side/adverse effects

May cause adverse effects such as blood problems; loss of hair; toxicity to lungs, heart, or bladder; and cancer; importance of discussing possible effects with physician

Signs of potential side effects, especially gonadal suppression, leukopenia, infection, cardiotoxicity, hemorrhagic cystitis, hyperuricemia, uric acid nephropathy, nonhemorrhagic cystitis, nephrotoxicity, pneumonitis, interstitial pulmonary fibrosis, SIADH secretion, anemia, thrombocytopenia, anaphylactic reaction, hemorrhagic colitis, hepatitis, hyperglycemia, redness or swelling or pain at site of injecton, and stomatitis

Physician or nurse can help in dealing with side effects

Possibility of hair loss; normal hair growth should return after treatment has ended; new hair may be slightly different in color or texture

## General Dosing Information

Patients receiving cyclophosphamide should be under supervision of a physician experienced in cancer chemotherapy or immunosuppressive therapy.

A variety of dosage schedules and regimens of cyclophosphamide, alone or in combination with other antitumor agents, are used. The prescriber may consult the medical literature as well as the manufacturer's literature in choosing a specific dosage.

Dosage must be adjusted to meet the individual requirements of each patient, based on clinical response and appearance or severity of toxicity.

Development of uric acid nephropathy in patients with leukemia or lymphoma may be prevented by adequate oral hydration and, in some cases, administration of allopurinol. Alkalinization of urine may be necessary if serum uric acid concentrations are elevated.

To reduce the risk of hemorrhagic cystitis, adequate hydration is recommended prior to cyclophosphamide treatment and for at least 72 hours following treatment to ensure ample urine output. In addition, the patient should be encouraged to take cyclophosphamide in the morning so that the majority of the metabolites have been excreted by bedtime and to void frequently, to prevent prolonged contact of irritating metabolites with bladder mucosa.

Cyclophosphamide should be discontinued at the first sign of hemorrhagic cystitis. In severe cases, blood replacement may be necessary. Electrocautery diversion of urine flow, cryosurgery, and formaldehyde bladder instillations have been used. Resumption of therapy should be undertaken with caution since recurrence is common.

Initiation of planned maintenance antineoplastic therapy is recommended as soon as the leukocyte count returns to adequate levels following induction.

If marked leukopenia (particularly granulocytopenia) or thrombocytopenia occurs, cyclophosphamide therapy should be withdrawn until leukocyte and platelet counts return to satisfactory levels. Then therapy may be reinstituted, possibly at a lower dose.

In acute leukemia, cyclophosphamide may be administered despite the presence of thrombocytopenia and bleeding; cessation of bleeding and increase in platelet count have occurred in some cases during treatment and platelet transfusions are useful in others.

Special precautions are recommended in patients who develop thrombocytopenia as a result of administration of cyclophosphamide. These may include extreme care in performing invasive procedures; regular inspection of intravenous sites, skin (including perirectal area), and mucous membrane surfaces for signs of bleeding or bruising; limiting frequency of venipuncture and avoiding intramuscular injections; testing urine, emesis, stool, and secretions for occult blood; care in use of regular toothbrushes, dental floss, toothpicks, safety razors, and fingernail and toenail cutters; avoiding constipation; and using caution to prevent falls and other injuries. Such patients should avoid alcohol and aspirin intake because of the risk of gastrointestinal bleeding. Platelet transfusions may be required.

Patients who develop leukopenia should be observed carefully for signs of infection. Antibiotic support may be required. In neutropenic patients who develop fever, broad-spectrum antibiotic coverage should be initiated empirically, pending bacterial cultures and appropriate diagnostic tests.

### For parenteral dosage forms only

Cyclophosphamide may be administered by intravenous push or infusion, intramuscularly, intraperitoneally, or intrapleurally.

### Diet/Nutrition

Oral cyclophosphamide should usually be taken on an empty stomach; however, if stomach upset occurs, doses may be divided and given with meals.

### Safety considerations for handling this medication

There is limited but increasing evidence and concern that personnel involved in preparation and administration of parenteral antineoplastics may be at some risk because of the potential mutagenicity, teratogenicity, and/or carcinogenicity of these agents, although the actual risk is unknown. USP advisory panels recommend cautious handling both in preparation and disposal of antineoplastic agents. Precautions that have been suggested include:

• Use of a biological containment cabinet during reconstitution and dilution of parenteral medications and wearing of disposable surgical gloves and masks.

• Use of proper technique to prevent contamination of the medication, work area, and operator during transfer between containers (including proper training of personnel in this technique).

• Cautious and proper disposal of needles, syringes, vials, ampuls, and unused medication.

A number of medical centers have developed detailed guidelines for handling of antineoplastic agents.

### Combination chemotherapy

Cyclophosphamide may be used in combination with other agents in various regimens. As a result, incidence and/or severity of side effects may be altered and different dosages (usually reduced) may be used. For example, cyclophosphamide is part of the following chemotherapeutic combinations (some commonly used acronyms are in parentheses):

—doxorubicin, cyclophosphamide, vincristine, procarbazine, and prednisone (A-COPP).

—carmustine, cyclophosphamide, vinblastine, procarbazine, and prednisone (BCVPP).

—cyclophosphamide, doxorubicin, and fluorouracil (CAF).

—cyclophosphamide, doxorubicin, methotrexate, and procarbazine (CAMP).

—cyclophosphamide, doxorubicin, and cisplatin (CAP).

—cyclophosphamide, doxorubicin, vincristine, and prednisone (CHOP).

—cyclophosphamide, doxorubicin, and vincristine (CHOR).

—cyclophosphamide, doxorubicin, and cisplatin (CISCA).

—cyclophosphamide, methotrexate, and lomustine (CMC-High dose).

—cyclophosphamide, methotrexate, and fluorouracil (CMF).

—cyclophosphamide, methotrexate, fluorouracil, and prednisone (CMFP).

—cyclophosphamide, methotrexate, fluorouracil, vincristine, and prednisone (CMFVP, Cooper's Regimen).

—cyclophosphamide, vincristine, and prednisone (COP or CVP).

—cyclophosphamide, vincristine, procarbazine, and prednisone (COPP or ''C''MOPP).

—cyclophosphamide, vincristine, doxorubicin, and dacarbazine (CY-VA-DIC).

—fluorouracil, doxorubicin, and cyclophosphamide (FAC).

—methotrexate, mercaptopurine, and cyclophosphamide (MTX + MP + CTX).

—vincristine, dactinomycin, and cyclophosphamide (VAC).

For specific dosages and schedules, consult the literature. For information regarding each agent, consult the individual monographs.

## Oral Dosage Forms

Note: Bracketed uses in the *Dosage Forms* section refer to categories of use and/or indications that are not included in U.S. product labeling.

### CYCLOPHOSPHAMIDE ORAL SOLUTION

Note: In the U.S. and Canada, Cyclophosphamide Injection USP [*Cytoxan; Neosar; Procytox*; GENERIC ] is the dosage form being used to prepare the oral solution dosage form.

### Usual adult dose

Leukemia, acute lymphocytic or

Leukemia, acute myelocytic or

Leukemia, acute monocytic or
Leukemia, chronic myelocytic or
Leukemia, chronic lymphocytic or
Carcinoma, ovarian or
Carcinoma, breast or
Neuroblastoma or
Retinoblastoma or
Carcinoma, lung or
Carcinoma, endometrial or
Carcinoma, bladder or
Carcinoma, prostatic or
Lymphomas, Hodgkin's or
Lymphomas, non-Hodgkin's or
Multiple myeloma or
Mycosis fungoides or
Ewing's sarcoma or
Sarcomas, soft-tissue or
Tumors, germ cell, ovarian—
    Oral, 1 to 5 mg per kg of body weight per day.
Polymyositis—
    Oral, 1 to 2 mg per kg of body weight per day, the dose being adjusted
    on the basis of leukocyte counts.
Rheumatoid arthritis—
    Oral, 1.5 to 2 mg per kg of body weight per day, the dosage being
    increased up to a maximum of 3 mg per kg of body weight per
    day.
Wegener's granulomatosis—
    Oral, 1 to 2 mg per kg of body weight per day, administered in com-
    bination with prednisone.

### Usual pediatric dose
Leukemia, acute lymphocytic or
Leukemia, acute myelocytic or
Leukemia, acute monocytic or
Leukemia, chronic myelocytic or
Leukemia, chronic lymphocytic or
Neuroblastoma or
Retinoblastoma or
Lymphomas, Hodgkin's; or
Lymphomas, non-Hodgkin's—
    Induction: Oral, 2 to 8 mg per kg of body weight or 60 to 250 mg
    per square meter of body surface a day in divided doses for six or
    more days.
    Maintenance: Oral, 2 to 5 mg per kg of body weight or 50 to 150 mg
    per square meter of body surface twice a week.
Nephrotic syndrome—
    Oral, 2.5 to 3 mg per kg of body weight per day.

### Strength(s) usually available
U.S.—
    Dosage form not commercially available. Compounding required for
    prescriptions.
Canada—
    Dosage form not commercially available. Compounding required for
    prescriptions.

### Packaging and storage
Store between 2 and 8 °C (36 and 46 °F). Protect from freezing. Store in
a tight container.

### Preparation of dosage form
Cyclophosphamide oral solution may be prepared by dissolving Cyclophosphamide for Injection USP in Aromatic Elixir NF to a concentration of 1 to 5 mg of cyclophosphamide per mL.

### Stability
Stable for up to 14 days when stored in a glass container in the
refrigerator.

### Auxiliary labeling
• For oral use.
• Take on an empty stomach.
• Drink plenty of water with this medicine.

## CYCLOPHOSPHAMIDE TABLETS USP

### Usual adult dose
Leukemia, acute lymphocytic or
Leukemia, acute myelocytic or
Leukemia, acute monocytic or
Leukemia, chronic myelocytic or
Leukemia, chronic lymphocytic or
Carcinoma, ovarian or
Carcinoma, breast or
Neuroblastoma or
Retinoblastoma or

[Carcinoma, lung] or
[Carcinoma, endometrial][1] or
[Carcinoma, bladder][1] or
[Carcinoma, prostatic][1] or
Lymphomas, Hodgkin's or
Lymphomas, non-Hodgkin's or
Multiple myeloma or
Mycosis fungoides or
[Ewing's sarcoma][1] or
[Sarcomas, soft-tissue][1] or
[Tumors, germ cell, ovarian][1]—
    Oral, 1 to 5 mg per kg of body weight per day.
[Polymyositis][1]—
    Oral, 1 to 2 mg per kg of body weight per day, administered in com-
    bination with prednisone.
[Rheumatoid arthritis][1]—
    Oral, 1 to 2 mg per kg of body weight per day, the dose being adjusted
    on the basis of leukocyte counts.
[Wegener's granulomatosis][1]—
    Oral, 1.5 to 2 mg per kg of body weight per day, the dosage being
    increased up to a maximum of 3 mg per kg of body weight per
    day.

### Usual pediatric dose
Leukemia, acute lymphocytic or
Leukemia, acute myelocytic or
Leukemia, acute monocytic or
Leukemia, chronic myelocytic or
Leukemia, chronic lymphocytic or
Neuroblastoma or
Retinoblastoma or
Lymphomas, Hodgkin's or
Lymphomas, non-Hodgkin's—
    Induction: Oral, 2 to 8 mg per kg of body weight or 60 to 250 mg
    per square meter of body surface a day in divided doses for six or
    more days.
    Maintenance: Oral, 2 to 5 mg per kg of body weight or 50 to 150 mg
    per square meter of body surface twice a week.
Nephrotic syndrome[1]—
    Oral, 2.5 to 3 mg per kg of body weight per day.

### Strength(s) usually available
U.S.—
    25 mg (Rx) [*Cytoxan* (lactose)].
    50 mg (Rx) [*Cytoxan* (lactose)].
Canada—
    25 mg (Rx) [*Cytoxan; Procytox*].
    50 mg (Rx) [*Cytoxan; Procytox*].

### Packaging and storage
Store between 2 and 25 °C (36 and 77 °F). Store in a tight container.

### Auxiliary labeling
• Take on an empty stomach.
• Drink plenty of water with this medicine.

## Parenteral Dosage Forms
Note: Bracketed uses in the *Dosage Forms* section refer to categories of
    use and/or indications that are not included in U.S. product labeling.

## CYCLOPHOSPHAMIDE FOR INJECTION USP

### Usual adult dose
Leukemia, acute lymphocytic or
Leukemia, acute myelocytic or
Leukemia, acute monocytic or
Leukemia, chronic myelocytic or
Leukemia, chronic lymphocytic or
Carcinoma, ovarian or
Carcinoma, breast or
Neuroblastoma or
Retinoblastoma or
[Carcinoma, lung] or
[Carcinoma, endometrial][1] or
[Carcinoma, bladder][1] or
[Carcinoma, prostatic][1] or
Lymphomas, Hodgkin's or
Lymphomas, non-Hodgkin's or
Multiple myeloma or
Mycosis fungoides or
[Ewing's sarcoma][1] or
[Sarcomas, soft-tissue][1] or
[Tumors, germ cell, ovarian][1]—
    Initial: Intravenous, 40 to 50 mg per kg of body weight in divided
    doses over a period of two to five days, or 10 to 15 mg per kg of

body weight every seven to ten days, or 3 to 5 mg per kg of body weight two times a week, or 1.5 to 3 mg per kg of body weight a day.

**Usual adult prescribing limits**

Much higher dosages have been used, depending on the condition being treated. Physicians should consult the medical literature in choosing a specific dosage.

**Usual pediatric dose**

Leukemia, acute lymphocytic or
Leukemia, acute myelocytic or
Leukemia, acute monocytic or
Leukemia, chronic myelocytic or
Leukemia, chronic lymphocytic or
Neuroblastoma or
Retinoblastoma or
Lymphomas, Hodgkin's or
Lymphomas, non-Hodgkin's—

Induction: Intravenous, 2 to 8 mg per kg of body weight or 60 to 250 mg per square meter of body surface a day in divided doses for six or more days (or total dose for seven days once a week).

Maintenance: Intravenous, 10 to 15 mg per kg of body weight every seven to ten days, or 30 mg per kg of body weight at three- to four-week intervals or when bone marrow recovery occurs.

**Strength(s) usually available**

U.S.—

Lyophilized
100 mg (Rx) [*Cytoxan* (mannitol 75 mg)].
200 mg (Rx) [*Cytoxan* (mannitol 150 mg)].
500 mg (Rx) [*Cytoxan* (mannitol 375 mg)].
1 gram (Rx) [*Cytoxan* (mannitol 750 mg)].
2 grams (Rx) [*Cytoxan* (mannitol 1.5 grams)].

Nonlyophilized
100 mg (Rx) [*Cytoxan* (sodium chloride 45 mg [1.9 mmol]); *Neosar* (sodium chloride 45 mg [1.9 mmol]); GENERIC].
200 mg (Rx) [*Cytoxan* (sodium chloride 90 mg [3.9 mmol]); *Neosar* (sodium chloride 90 mg [3.9 mmol]); GENERIC].
500 mg (Rx) [*Cytoxan* (sodium chloride 225 mg [9.7 mmol]); *Neosar* (sodium chloride 225 mg [9.7 mmol]); GENERIC].
1 gram (Rx) [*Cytoxan* (sodium chloride 450 mg [19.5 mmol]); *Neosar* (sodium chloride 450 mg [19.5 mmol]); GENERIC].
2 grams (Rx) [*Cytoxan* (sodium chloride 900 mg [39 mmol]); *Neosar* (sodium chloride 900 mg [39 mmol])].

Canada—

Lyophilized
500 mg (Rx) [*Cytoxan* (mannitol 375 mg)].
750 mg (Rx) [*Cytoxan* (mannitol 562.5 mg)].
1 gram (Rx) [*Cytoxan* (mannitol 750 mg)].
2 grams (Rx) [*Cytoxan* (mannitol 1.5 grams)].

Nonlyophilized
200 mg (Rx) [*Procytox* (sodium chloride 90 mg [3.9 mmol])].

500 mg (Rx) [*Procytox* (sodium chloride 225 mg [9.7 mmol])].
1 gram (Rx) [*Procytox* (sodium chloride 450 mg [19.5 mmol])].

**Packaging and storage**

Store at a temperature not exceeding 25 °C (77 °F).

**Preparation of dosage form**

Nonlyophilized cyclophosphamide for injection may be prepared for parenteral use by adding 5 mL (100-mg vial), 10 mL (200-mg vial), 25 mL (500-mg vial), 50 mL (1-gram vial), or 100 mL (2-gram vial) of sterile water for injection or bacteriostatic water for injection (paraben-preserved only) to the vial and shaking to dissolve (may be difficult and take up to 6 minutes) to provide a solution containing 20 mg of cyclophosphamide per mL. The resulting solution may be added to 5% dextrose injection, 5% dextrose and 0.9% sodium chloride injection, 5% dextrose and Ringer's injection, lactated Ringer's injection, 0.45% sodium chloride injection, or sodium lactate injection for administration by intravenous infusion.

Lyophilized cyclophosphamide for injection may be prepared for parenteral use by adding 5 mL (100-mg vial), 10 mL (200-mg vial), 20 to 25 mL (500-mg vial), 50 mL (1-gram vial), or 80 to 100 mL (2-gram vial) of sterile water for injection or bacteriostatic water for injection (paraben-preserved only) to the vial and shaking to dissolve (takes about 45 seconds) to provide a solution containing 20 mg of cyclophosphamide per mL. The resulting solution may be added to 5% dextrose injection, 5% dextrose and 0.9% sodium chloride injection, 5% dextrose and Ringer's injection, lactated Ringer's injection, 0.45% sodium chloride injection, or sodium lactate injection for administration by intravenous infusion.

Caution: Use of diluents containing benzyl alcohol is not recommended for preparation of medications for use in neonates. A fatal toxic syndrome consisting of metabolic acidosis, central nervous system (CNS) depression, respiratory problems, renal failure, hypotension, and possibly seizures and intracranial hemorrhages has been associated with this use.

**Stability**

Reconstituted solutions of cyclophosphamide are stable for 24 hours at room temperature, or for 6 days if refrigerated. If bacteriostatic water for injection is not used for reconstitution, it is recommended that the solution be used promptly (preferably within 6 hours).

**Note**

Because cyclophosphamide for injection contains no preservative, caution in preparing and storing solutions is required to ensure sterility.

[1]Not included in Canadian product labeling.

## Selected Bibliography

Ahmed AR, Hombal SM. Cyclophosphamide (Cytoxan). A review on relevant pharmacology and clinical uses. J Am Acad Dermatol 1984 Dec; 11: 1115-26.

Revised: 07/11/94

---

# CYCLOSERINE  Systemic†

**VA CLASSIFICATION (Primary): AM500**

Note: For a listing of dosage forms and brand names by country availability, see *Dosage Forms* section(s). For a listing of brand names for the articles in this monograph, refer to the General Index.

†Not commercially available in Canada.

## Category

Antibacterial (antimycobacterial).

## Indications

Note: Bracketed information in the *Indications* section refers to uses that are not included in U.S. product labeling.

**Accepted**

Tuberculosis (treatment)—Cycloserine is indicated in combination with other antituberculars in the treatment of tuberculosis after failure of the primary medications (pyrazinamide, streptomycin, isoniazid, rifampin, and ethambutol).

[Mycobacterial infections, atypical (treatment)]—Cycloserine is used in the treatment of atypical mycobacterial infections, such as *Mycobacterium avium* complex.

Not all species or strains of a particular organism may be susceptible to cycloserine.

**Unaccepted**

Although cycloserine has been used for the treatment of urinary tract infections, it has been superseded by newer, safer, and/or more effective agents (e.g., aminoglycosides, beta-lactams, quinolones, trimethoprim).

## Pharmacology/Pharmacokinetics

**Physicochemical characteristics**

Molecular weight—102.09.

**Mechanism of action/Effect**

Cycloserine, a broad-spectrum antibiotic, may be bactericidal or bacteriostatic, depending on its concentration at the site of infection and the susceptibility of the organism.

Cycloserine is an analog of the amino acid D-alanine. It interferes with an early step in bacterial cell wall synthesis in the cytoplasm by competitive inhibition of 2 enzymes, L-alanine racemase, which forms D-alanine from L-alanine, and D-alanine-D-alanine synthetase, which incorporates D-alanine into the pentapeptide necessary for peptidoglycan formation and bacterial cell wall synthesis.

### Absorption
Rapidly and almost completely (70 to 90%) absorbed from the gastrointestinal tract following oral administration.

### Distribution
Wide, to most body fluids and tissues, including cerebrospinal fluid (CSF), breast milk, bile, sputum, lymph tissue, lungs, and ascitic, pleural, and synovial fluids; crosses the placenta.

CSF concentrations of cycloserine approach those found in the serum.

Urine concentrations—
  High, 55 to 340 mcg per mL.

### Protein binding
None.

### Biotransformation
Up to 35%.

### Half-life
Normal renal function—
  10 hours.
Impaired renal function—
  Prolonged.

### Time to peak serum concentration
3 to 4 hours.

### Peak serum concentration
25 to 30 mcg/mL after a dose of 250 mg every 12 hours.

### Elimination
Renal, by glomerular filtration; 50% excreted unchanged within 12 hours; 65 to 70% excreted unchanged within 24 to 72 hours; accumulates in patients with impaired renal function.

Fecal, small amounts.

Dialysis—
  Cycloserine is removed by hemodialysis.

## Precautions to Consider

### Carcinogenicity/Mutagenicity
Studies have not been performed to determine the carcinogenic potential of cycloserine. The Ames test and unscheduled DNA repair test were negative.

### Pregnancy/Reproduction
Fertility—A study in 2 generations of rats showed no impairment of fertility relative to controls for the first mating, but somewhat lower fertility for the second mating.

Pregnancy—Cycloserine crosses the placenta; fetal serum concentrations may approach maternal serum concentrations.

A study in 2 generations of rats given doses up to 100 mg per kg of body weight per day demonstrated no teratogenic effect in the offspring.

FDA Pregnancy Category C.

### Breast-feeding
Cycloserine is distributed into breast milk; concentrations may approach or exceed maternal serum concentrations.

### Pediatrics
Appropriate studies on the relationship of age to the effects of cycloserine have not been performed in the pediatric population. However, no pediatrics-specific problems have been documented to date.

### Geriatrics
No information is available on the relationship of age to the effects of cycloserine in geriatric patients. However, elderly patients are more likely to have an age-related decrease in renal function, which may require an adjustment of dosage in patients receiving cycloserine.

### Drug interactions and/or related problems
The following drug interactions and/or related problems have been selected on the basis of their potential clinical significance (possible mechanism in parentheses where appropriate)—not necessarily inclusive (» = major clinical significance):

Note: Combinations containing any of the following medications, depending on the amount present, may also interact with this medication.

» Alcohol
  (may increase the risk of seizures, especially in chronic alcohol abuse; patients should be advised to avoid concurrent use)

» Ethionamide
  (concurrent use may result in increased incidence of central nervous system [CNS] effects, especially seizures; dosage adjustments may be necessary and patients should be monitored closely for signs of CNS toxicity)

Isoniazid
  (concurrent use may result in increased incidence of CNS effects such as dizziness or drowsiness; dosage adjustments may be necessary, and patients should be monitored closely for signs of CNS toxicity)

Pyridoxine
  (cycloserine may cause anemia or peripheral neuritis by acting as a pyridoxine antagonist or increasing renal excretion of pyridoxine; requirements for pyridoxine may be increased in patients receiving cycloserine)

### Laboratory value alterations
The following have been selected on the basis of their potential clinical significance (possible effect in parentheses where appropriate)—not necessarily inclusive (» = major clinical significance):

With physiology/laboratory test values
Alanine aminotransferase (ALT [SGPT]) and
Aspartate aminotransferase (AST [SGOT])
  (concentrations may be increased—especially in patients with pre-existing liver disease)

### Medical considerations/Contraindications
The medical considerations/contraindications included here have been selected on the basis of their potential clinical significance (reasons given in parentheses where appropriate)—not necessarily inclusive (» = major clinical significance).

***Risk-benefit should be considered when the following medical problems exist:***

» Alcoholism, active or in remission
  (cycloserine may increase the risk of seizures in alcoholics)

Anxiety, severe or
Mental depression or
Psychosis
  (cycloserine may cause anxiety, mental depression, and psychosis, especially at higher doses)

» Hypersensitivity to cycloserine

» Renal function impairment
  (because cycloserine is renally excreted, cycloserine may accumulate in patients with renal function impairment, leading to an increased risk of side effects; the medication should not be given to patients with renal function impairment [creatinine clearance of <50 mL per minute (0.83 mL per second)])

» Seizure disorders, history of
  (cycloserine may increase the risk of seizures in patients with a seizure disorder)

### Patient monitoring
The following may be especially important in patient monitoring (other tests may be warranted in some patients, depending on condition; » = major clinical significance):

Blood urea nitrogen (BUN) concentrations and
Creatinine concentrations, serum
  (may be required periodically since patients with impaired renal function require a reduction in dose or discontinuation of the medication)

Cycloserine concentrations, serum
  (may be required at least weekly in patients with slightly impaired, but stable, renal function, in patients receiving more than 500 mg daily, or in patients showing signs and symptoms of toxicity; concentrations above 30 mcg/mL should be avoided)

Hemoglobin concentration
  (may be required periodically since administration of cycloserine and other antituberculars has been associated in a few instances with vitamin $B_{12}$ and/or folic acid deficiency, megaloblastic anemia, and sideroblastic anemia)

## Side/Adverse Effects

Note: The side effects of cycloserine, particularly CNS toxicity, may be dose-related and more commonly seen with daily doses greater than 500 mg. Acute toxicity may occur if more than 1 gram is ingested by an adult, and chronic toxicity may occur with ingestion of more than 500 mg daily. The ratio of toxic dose to effective dose is small.

Administraton of 200 to 300 mg of pyridoxine daily may help to prevent cycloserine-related neurotoxicity.

The following side/adverse effects have been selected on the basis of their potential clinical significance (possible signs and symptoms in parentheses where appropriate)—not necessarily inclusive:

**Those indicating need for medical attention**
Incidence more frequent
*CNS toxicity* (anxiety; confusion; dizziness; drowsiness; increased irritability; increased restlessness; mental depression; muscle twitching or trembling; nervousness; nightmares; other mood or mental changes; speech problems; thoughts of suicide)

Incidence less frequent
*Hypersensitivity* (skin rash); *peripheral neuropathy* (numbness, tingling, burning pain, or weakness in the hands or feet); *seizures*

**Those indicating need for medical attention only if they continue or are bothersome**
Incidence more frequent
*Headache*

## Patient Consultation

As an aid to patient consultation, refer to *Advice for the Patient, Cycloserine (Systemic)*.

In providing consultation, consider emphasizing the following selected information (» = major clinical significance):

**Before using this medication**
» Conditions affecting use, especially:
Pregnancy—Cycloserine crosses the placenta and fetal serum concentrations may approach maternal serum concentrations
Breast-feeding—Cycloserine is distributed into breast milk. Concentrations may approach or exceed maternal serum concentrations
Other medications, especially alcohol and ethionamide
Other medical problems, especially alcoholism (active or in remission), a history of seizure disorders, or renal function impairment

**Proper use of this medication**
Taking this medication after meals if gastrointestinal irritation occurs
» Compliance with full course of therapy; in tuberculosis, therapy may take months or years
» Importance of not missing doses and taking at evenly spaced times
» Proper dosing
Missed dose: Taking as soon as possible; not taking if almost time for next dose; not doubling doses
» Proper storage

**Precautions while using this medication**
Regular visits to physician to check progress
Checking with physician if no improvement within 2 to 3 weeks
» Checking with physician immediately if thoughts of suicide occur
» Caution if dizziness or drowsiness occurs
» Avoiding alcoholic beverages while taking this medication

**Side/adverse effects**
Signs of potential side effects, especially CNS toxicity, hypersensitivity reactions, peripheral neuropathy, and seizures

## General Dosing Information

Cycloserine may be taken after meals if gastrointestinal irritation occurs.

Since bacterial resistance may develop rapidly when cycloserine is administered alone in the treatment of tuberculosis, it should only be administered concurrently with other antituberculars.

Patients receiving more than 500 mg of cycloserine daily should be closely observed for symptoms of CNS toxicity.

In the treatment of tuberculosis, therapy may have to be continued for 1 to 2 years and may even be required for up to several years or indefinitely, although in some patients shorter treatment regimens may also be effective.

Serum concentrations should be monitored where possible. Concentrations should be maintained at approximately 25 to 30 mcg/mL in the treatment of tuberculosis. Concentrations above 30 mcg/mL should be avoided since toxicity is closely related to excessive serum concentrations. In addition, the ratio of toxic dose to effective dose is small.

Patients with severe renal function impairment (creatinine clearance of <50 mL per minute [0.83 mL per second]) should not receive cycloserine because of the increased risk of neurotoxicity.

**For treatment of adverse effects**
Recommended treatment consists of the following:
• Inducing emesis and/or use of gastric lavage.
• Administering activated charcoal and cathartic every 4 hours until clinically stable.
• Providing supportive therapy.
• Using anticonvulsants to control seizures.
• Administering 200 to 300 mg of pyridoxine daily to treat neurotoxicity.

## Oral Dosage Forms

### CYCLOSERINE CAPSULES USP

**Usual adult and adolescent dose**
Tuberculosis—
In combination with other antituberculars: Oral, 250 mg every twelve hours for the first two weeks, then cautiously increased as necessary and tolerated, up to 250 mg every six to eight hours and monitored by serum determinations.

**Usual adult prescribing limits**
Up to a maximum of 1 gram daily.
Note: Doses up to 1.5 grams daily have been used.

**Usual pediatric dose**
Tuberculosis—
In combination with other antituberculars: Doses of 10 to 20 mg per kg of body weight per day in divided doses have been used.

**Strength(s) usually available**
U.S.—
250 mg (Rx) [*Seromycin*].
Canada—
Not commercially available.

**Packaging and storage**
Store below 40 °C (104 °F), preferably between 15 and 30 °C (59 and 86 °F), unless otherwise specified by manufacturer. Store in a tight container.

**Stability**
Cycloserine maintains its potency in alkaline solutions, but is rapidly destroyed at neutral or acid pH.

**Auxiliary labeling**
• Avoid alcoholic beverages.
• May cause drowsiness, or dizziness.
• Continue medicine for full time of treatment.

Revised: 05/02/94

# CYCLOSPORINE  Systemic

INN: Ciclosporin
VA CLASSIFICATION (Primary): IM600
Another commonly used name is cyclosporin A.
Note: For a listing of dosage forms and brand names by country availability, see *Dosage Forms* section(s). For a listing of brand names for the articles in this monograph, refer to the General Index.

## Category
Immunosuppressant.

## Indications
Note: Bracketed information in the *Indications* section refers to uses that are not included in U.S. product labeling.

**Accepted**
Transplant rejection, organ (prophylaxis)—Cyclosporine is indicated, usually in combination with corticosteroids, for prevention of rejection of

renal, hepatic, and cardiac transplants (allografts). [Cyclosporine is also being used for prevention of rejection of heart-lung and pancreatic transplants, and for prophylaxis of graft rejection following bone marrow transplantation and prophylaxis of graft-versus-host disease.]

Transplant rejection, organ (treatment)—Cyclosporine is indicated for treatment of chronic rejection in patients previously treated with other immunosuppressants, although corticosteroids are preferred. [It is also being used for treatment of graft-versus-host disease after bone marrow transplantation.]

Although cyclosporine has been used for treatment of severe chronic plaque-type psoriasis in patients who are intolerant of, inappropriate candidates for, or unresponsive to conventional therapy, toxicity is significant, and adequate safety in long-term use for this indication has not been established. USP DI Advisory Panels recommend that cyclosporine be used for severe chronic plaque-type psoriasis only by qualified specialists who are fully aware of and equipped to monitor and treat the potential toxicities of this medication. *Data are insufficient* to prove that cyclosporine is effective for treatment of generalized pustular or erythrodermic psoriasis.

# Pharmacology/Pharmacokinetics

### Physicochemical characteristics
Molecular weight—1202.63.

### Mechanism of action/Effect
The exact mechanism of action is unknown but seems to be related to the inhibition of production and release of interleukin-2, which is a proliferative factor necessary for the induction of cytotoxic T-lymphocytes in response to alloantigenic challenge, and which plays a major role in both cellular and humoral immune responses. Cyclosporine does not affect the nonspecific defense system of the host and does not cause significant myelosuppression.

### Absorption
Variable and incomplete from gastrointestinal tract; bioavailability is about 30% but may increase with increasing dosage and duration of treatment. Absorption may be decreased after liver transplantation or in patients with liver disease or gastrointestinal function impairment (e.g., diarrhea, vomiting, ileus).

### Protein binding
Very high (90%), primarily to lipoproteins.

### Biotransformation
Hepatic, extensive.

### Half-life
Biphasic, variable—
    Terminal:
        Children—Approximately 7 hours (range, 7 to 19 hours).
        Adults—Approximately 19 hours (range, 10 to 27 hours).

### Time to peak concentration
Plasma or blood—Oral: 3.5 hours.

### Peak serum concentration
Plasma or blood—Whole blood concentrations may be 2 to 9 times plasma concentrations.

### Elimination
Biliary/fecal; renal, 6% (0.1% unchanged).
In dialysis—Not dialyzable.

# Precautions to Consider

### Cross-sensitivity and/or related problems
Patients sensitive to polyoxyethylated castor oil may be sensitive to the injectable dosage form also, since the injection contains a polyoxyethylated castor oil vehicle.

### Carcinogenicity/Tumorigenicity
A 78-week study in mice at doses of 1, 4, and 16 mg per kg of body weight (mg/kg) per day found a statistically significant trend for lymphocytic lymphomas in females, and the incidence of hepatocellular carcinomas in mid-dose males significantly exceeded the control value. A 24-month study in rats at doses of 0.5, 2, and 8 mg/kg per day found that incidence of pancreatic islet cell adenomas significantly exceeded the control rate in the low dose level. The hepatocellular carcinomas and pancreatic islet cell adenomas were not dose-related.

Lymphomas and skin malignancies have developed in humans treated with cyclosporine, although a definite causal relationship has not been established; benign breast tumors have also been reported.

### Mutagenicity
No evidence of mutagenicity/genotoxicity was found in the Ames test, the V79-HGPRT test, the micronucleus test in mice and Chinese hamsters, the chromosome-aberration tests in Chinese hamster bone marrow, the

mouse dominant lethal assay, and the DNA-repair test in sperm from treated mice. However, one study analyzing sister chromatid exchange (SCE) induction by cyclosporine using human lymphocytes *in vitro* gave indication of a positive effect (i.e., induction of SCE) at high concentrations in this system.

### Pregnancy/Reproduction
Fertility—Studies in male and female rats found no evidence of impairment of fertility.

Pregnancy—Adequate and well-controlled studies in humans have not been done.

Cyclosporine crosses the placenta.

In a retrospective study of 116 pregnancies of women who received cyclosporine during (and usually throughout) pregnancy, the only consistent patterns of abnormality were premature birth (gestational period of 28 to 36 weeks) and low birth weight for gestational age. Preterm delivery occurred in 47%. Seven malformations were reported in 5 viable infants and in 2 cases of fetal loss. Neonatal complications occurred in 27%. The exact relationship of cyclosporine to these effects has not been established.

Studies in rats and rabbits have shown that cyclosporine is embryotoxic and fetotoxic at doses 2 to 5 times the human dose. At toxic doses (30 mg/kg per day in rats and 100 mg/kg per day in rabbits), cyclosporine was embryotoxic and fetotoxic, as indicated by increased pre- and postnatal mortality and reduced fetal weight together with related skeletal retardations. No embryolethal or teratogenic effects occurred at normal doses (up to 17 mg/kg per day in rats and up to 30 mg/kg per day in rabbits).

FDA Pregnancy Category C.

### Breast-feeding
Cyclosporine is distributed into breast milk. Mothers should be advised to contact physician before nursing infants, since use by nursing mothers is not recommended because of the potential risk of serious adverse effects (e.g., hypertension, nephrotoxicity, malignancy) in the infant.

### Pediatrics
Half-life of cyclosporine is lower in children than in adults. However, appropriate studies performed to date have not demonstrated pediatrics-specific problems that would limit the usefulness of cyclosporine in children.

### Geriatrics
Although appropriate studies on the relationship of age to the effects of cyclosporine have not been performed in the geriatric population, geriatrics-specific problems are not expected to limit the usefulness of this medication in the elderly. However, elderly patients are more likely to have age-related renal function impairment, which may require caution in patients receiving cyclosporine.

### Dental
Gingival hyperplasia, a common complication of cyclosporine therapy, usually starts as gingivitis or gum inflammation in the first month of treatment. The incidence is higher in children under 15 years of age than in adults. Gingival tissue changes are similar to those produced by phenytoin, although with less mature collagen. Tissue overgrowth may be greater anteriorly than posteriorly, creating esthetic and psychological problems for the young patient. A strictly enforced program of teeth cleaning by a professional combined with plaque control by the patient, if begun within 10 days of initiation of cyclosporine therapy, will minimize growth rate and severity of gingival enlargement. Periodontal surgery may be indicated, and should be followed by careful plaque control to inhibit recurrence of gum enlargement.

The immunosuppressant effects of cyclosporine may result in an increased incidence of microbial infection and delayed healing. Dental work, whenever possible should be completed prior to initiation of therapy and undertaken only with great caution during therapy. Patients should be instructed in proper oral hygiene during treatment, including caution in use of regular toothbrushes, dental floss, and toothpicks.

### Drug interactions and/or related problems
The following drug interactions and/or related problems have been selected on the basis of their potential clinical significance (possible mechanism in parentheses where appropriate)—not necessarily inclusive (» = major clinical significance):

Note: Combinations containing any of the following medications, depending on the amount present, may also interact with this medication.

» Androgens or
» Cimetidine or
» Danazol or
» Diltiazem or
» Erythromycin or
» Estrogens or

» Ketoconazole or
  Miconazole
      (have been reported to increase plasma concentrations of cyclo-
      sporine and may increase the risk of hepatotoxicity and nephro-
      toxicity; because of similarity to ketoconazole, miconazole may be
      expected to have the same effect; concurrent use is recommended
      only with great caution and frequent monitoring of blood cyclo-
      sporine concentrations and hepatic and renal function)

  Anti-inflammatory drugs, nonsteroidal (NSAIDs)
      (concurrent use of NSAIDs, especially indomethacin, with cyclo-
      sporine may increase the risk of renal failure; concurrent admin-
      istration with cyclosporine may also result in hyperkalemia)

  Hepatic enzyme inducers (See *Appendix II*)
      (may enhance metabolism of cyclosporine by induction of hepatic
      microsomal enzymes, especially cytochrome P-450; dosage ad-
      justment may be required)

  Hyperkalemia-causing medications, such as:
    Angiotensin-converting enzyme (ACE) inhibitors
    Beta-adrenergic blocking agents
    Digitalis glycosides, with acute overdose
» Diuretics, potassium-sparing
    Heparin
    Penicillins, potassium-containing, with high doses
    Phosphates, potassium-containing
    Potassium citrate–containing medications
    Potassium iodide
    Potassium supplements
    Succinylcholine chloride
      (concurrent administration with cyclosporine may result in
      hyperkalemia)

» Immunosuppressants, other, such as:
    Azathioprine
    Chlorambucil
    Corticosteroids, glucocorticoid
    Cyclophosphamide
    Mercaptopurine
    Muromonab-CD3
      (concurrent use with cyclosporine may increase the risk of infec-
      tion and development of lymphoproliferative disorders; caution is
      recommended)

» Lovastatin
      (concurrent use in cardiac transplant patients may be associated
      with an increased risk of rhabdomyolysis and acute renal failure)

  Nephrotoxic medications (See *Appendix II*)
      (concurrent use with cyclosporine may result in enhanced nephro-
      toxicity; dosage reduction or withdrawal of both medications may
      be necessary if renal impairment occurs)

  Vaccines, killed virus
      (because normal defense mechanisms may be suppressed by cy-
      closporine therapy, the patient's antibody response to the vaccine
      may be decreased. The interval between discontinuation of medi-
      cations that cause immunosuppression and restoration of the pa-
      tient's ability to respond to the vaccine depends on the intensity
      and type of immunosuppression-causing medication used, the un-
      derlying disease, and other factors; estimates vary from 3 months
      to 1 year)

» Vaccines, live virus
      (because normal defense mechanisms may be suppressed by cy-
      closporine therapy, concurrent use with a live virus vaccine may
      potentiate the replication of the vaccine virus, may increase the
      side/adverse effects of the vaccine virus, and/or may decrease the
      patient's antibody response to the vaccine; immunization of these
      patients should be undertaken only with extreme caution after care-
      ful review of the patient's hematologic status and only with the
      knowledge and consent of the physician managing the cyclospor-
      ine therapy. The interval between discontinuation of medications
      that cause immunosuppression and restoration of the patient's abil-
      ity to respond to the vaccine depends on the intensity and type of
      immunosuppression-causing medication used, the underlying dis-
      ease, and other factors; estimates vary from 3 months to 1 year.
      Patients with leukemia in remission should not receive live virus
      vaccine until at least 3 months after their last chemotherapy. Im-
      munization with oral poliovirus vaccine should also be postponed
      in persons in close contact with the patient, especially family
      members)

**Laboratory value alterations**
The following have been selected on the basis of their potential clinical
  significance (possible effect in parentheses where appropriate)—not
  necessarily inclusive (» = major clinical significance):

With physiology/laboratory test values
  Alanine aminotransferase (ALT [SGPT]) values, serum and
  Alkaline phosphatase values, serum and
  Amylase values, serum and
  Aspartate aminotransferase (AST [SGOT]) values, serum and
  Bilirubin concentrations, serum
      (may be increased in association with hepatotoxicity)

  Blood urea nitrogen (BUN) and
  Creatinine, serum
      (concentrations are commonly increased during first few days of
      cyclosporine therapy; does not necessarily indicate rejection in re-
      nal transplant patients)

  Magnesium
      (serum concentrations may be decreased; may be related to
      nephrotoxicity)

  Potassium and
  Uric acid
      (serum concentrations may be increased)

**Medical considerations/Contraindications**
The medical considerations/contraindications included here have been selected on the basis of their potential clinical significance (reasons given
  in parentheses where appropriate)—not necessarily inclusive (» =
  major clinical significance).

*Risk-benefit should be considered when the following medical problems
exist:*
» Chickenpox, existing or recent (including recent exposure) or
» Herpes zoster
      (risk of severe generalized disease)

» Hepatic function impairment
      (reduced biotransformation; reduced absorption; dosage reduction
      may be necessary)

  Hyperkalemia

» Infection
  Malabsorption
      (achieving therapeutic plasma concentrations of cyclosporine may
      be difficult)

» Renal function impairment
» Sensitivity to cyclosporine

**Patient monitoring**
The following may be especially important in patient monitoring (other
  tests may be warranted in some patients, depending on condition;
  » = major clinical significance):

  Alanine aminotransferase (ALT [SGPT]) values, serum and
  Alkaline phosphatase values, serum and
  Amylase values, serum and
  Aspartate aminotransferase (AST [SGOT]) values, serum and
  Bilirubin concentrations, serum
      (determinations recommended at periodic intervals to monitor he-
      patic function)

  Blood pressure measurements
      (recommended at periodic intervals to detect hypertension)

» BUN concentrations and
» Creatinine concentrations, serum and
» Uric acid concentrations, serum
      (determinations recommended at regular intervals to monitor renal
      function)

» Cyclosporine concentrations, plasma or blood, trough, by radioim-
      munoassay (RIA) or high pressure liquid chromatography (HPLC)
      (recommended for all patients, especially those receiving oral cy-
      closporine, because of erratic absorption, or for hepatic transplant
      patients to ensure that the patient is receiving an adequate but not
      toxic dose; because of extreme variability in results achieved de-
      pending on whether plasma or whole blood concentrations are
      measured, timing of samples, handling of samples, and choice of
      RIA or HPLC, determinations must be standardized within each
      individual medical center)

» Dental examinations
      (recommended at 3-month intervals for teeth cleaning and rein-
      forcement of patient's careful plaque control for inhibition of gin-
      gival hyperplasia)

  Magnesium concentrations, serum and
  Potassium concentrations, serum
      (determinations recommended at periodic intervals)

## Side/Adverse Effects

Note: Lymphoproliferative disorders, including lymphomas and skin malignancies, have been reported in patients receiving cyclosporine; some have regressed when the medication was discontinued. Benign breast tumors have been reported in 2 patients.

The following side/adverse effects have been selected on the basis of their potential clinical significance (possible signs and symptoms in parentheses where appropriate)—not necessarily inclusive:

### Those indicating need for medical attention
Incidence more frequent
> *Gingival hyperplasia* (bleeding, tender, or enlarged gums); *hypertension* (asymptomatic); *nephrotoxicity* (asymptomatic)

> Note: *Gingival hyperplasia* is usually reversible within 6 months after withdrawal of cyclosporine.

> *Hypertension* occurs commonly and may be acute, severe, and dose-related (usually associated with doses of 25 to 50 mg per kg of body weight [mg/kg] per day) or chronic and mild to moderate (usually associated with reduced renal function).

> Mild *nephrotoxicity* (presenting as an arrest in the fall of pre-operative elevations of BUN and creatinine at a range of 35 to 45 mg per deciliter and 2.0 to 2.5 mg per deciliter, respectively) usually occurs 2 to 3 months after renal, cardiac, or hepatic transplantation and usually responds to dosage reduction. More overt toxicity, with rapidly rising BUN and creatinine, occurs early after transplantation and must be differentiated from rejection episodes; it also usually responds to dosage reduction. Up to 20% of renal transplant patients may have simultaneous nephrotoxicity and rejection.

> A form of chronic progressive *nephrotoxicity*, characterized by serial deterioration in renal function and morphologic changes in the kidneys (interstitial fibrosis with tubular atrophy) may occur; reduction in a rising serum creatinine will fail to occur despite reduction in dose or withdrawal of cyclosporine in 5 to 15% of patients; in addition, toxic tubulopathy, peritubular capillary congestion, arteriolopathy, and a striped form of interstitial fibrosis with tubular atrophy may be present. Development of chronic nephrotoxicity may be related to high cumulative doses or persistently high circulating trough concentrations of cyclosporine. Effects may be irreversible.

Incidence less frequent
> *Convulsions; hepatotoxicity* (asymptomatic; usually seen as elevations of hepatic enzymes and bilirubin); *infection* (fever or chills; frequent urge to urinate)

> Note: *Convulsions* may be related to nephrotoxicity and hypomagnesemia.

> *Hepatotoxicity* usually responds to dosage reduction.

Incidence rare
> *Anaphylaxis* (flushing of face and neck; wheezing or shortness of breath)—with parenteral use; *hemolytic-uremic syndrome; hyperkalemia* (confusion; irregular heartbeat; numbness or tingling in hands, feet, or lips; shortness of breath or difficult breathing; unexplained nervousness; unusual tiredness or weakness; weakness or heaviness of legs); *pancreatitis* (severe stomach pain with nausea and vomiting); *renal toxicity* (blood in urine)

> Note: *Anaphylaxis* occurs only with intravenous use and may be related to the vehicle. The reaction includes facial flushing, acute respiratory distress, blood pressure changes, and tachycardia. A fatality has been reported. Subsequent oral administration of cyclosporine in patients who have experienced an anaphylactic reaction to intravenous cyclosporine has not produced a reaction.

> The *hemolytic-uremic syndrome* can occur in the absence of rejection, but may result in graft failure. It is accompanied by avid platelet consumption within the graft. It usually responds, if detected early, to dosage reduction or withdrawal of cyclosporine plus administration of streptokinase and heparin or plasmapheresis.

> Irregular heartbeat is usually the earliest clinical indication of *hyperkalemia* and is readily detected by electrocardiogram (ECG). Hyperkalemia may sometimes be associated with hyperchloremic metabolic acidosis.

### Those indicating need for medical attention only if they continue or are bothersome
Incidence more frequent
> *Hirsutism* (increase in hair growth); *tremor* (trembling and shaking of hands)—dose-related

Incidence less frequent
> *Acne or oily skin; headache; leg cramps; nausea or vomiting*

## Overdose

For more information on the management of overdose or unintentional ingestion, **contact a Poison Control Center** (see *Poison Control Center Listing*).

**Treatment of overdose**
Treatment consists of the following:
- In general, treatment is symptomatic and supportive.
- Forced emesis may be useful for up to 2 hours after oral ingestion of toxic doses of cyclosporine.
- Transient hepatotoxicity and nephrotoxicity usually respond to withdrawal.
- Cyclosporine is not removable by hemodialysis or charcoal hemoperfusion.

## Patient Consultation

As an aid to patient consultation, refer to *Advice for the Patient, Cyclosporine (Systemic)*.

In providing consultation, consider emphasizing the following selected information (» = major clinical significance):

### Before using this medication
» Conditions affecting use, especially:
> Sensitivity to cyclosporine
> Pregnancy—Causes birth defects or fetal death in animals
> Breast-feeding—Distributed into breast milk; breast-feeding not recommended because of risk of serious side effects
> Other medications, especially androgens, cimetidine, danazol, diltiazem, potassium-sparing diuretics, erythromycin, estrogens, ketoconazole, other immunosuppressants, or lovastatin
> Other medical problems, especially chickenpox, herpes zoster, hepatic function impairment, infection, or renal function impairment

### Proper use of this medication
» Importance of not taking more or less medication than the amount prescribed
> Getting into the habit of taking at the same time each day to help increase compliance and maintain steady blood concentrations
> Taking solution orally; special dropper to be used for accurate measuring; making sure dropper is properly dried after cleaning before using
> Mixing oral solution with milk, chocolate milk, or orange juice (preferably at room temperature) in a glass (not wax-lined or plastic disposable) container to improve palatability; stirring well and drinking immediately, then rinsing glass and drinking to make sure all medication is taken; wiping pipette dry but not rinsing with water (to prevent cloudiness)
> Taking with meals to reduce gastrointestinal irritation
» Checking with physician before discontinuing medication; possible need for lifelong therapy
» Proper dosing
> Missed dose: Taking as soon as possible if remembered within 12 hours; not taking if almost time for next dose; not doubling doses
» Proper storage

### Precautions while using this medication
» Importance of close monitoring by physician
» Avoiding immunizations unless approved by physician; other persons in patient's household should avoid immunizations with oral poliovirus vaccine; avoiding persons who have taken oral poliovirus vaccine or wearing a protective mask that covers nose and mouth
» Maintaining good dental hygiene and seeing dentist frequently for teeth cleaning to prevent tenderness, bleeding, and gum enlargement

### Side/adverse effects
> Importance of discussing possible effects, including cancer, with physician
> Signs of potential side effects, especially gingival hyperplasia, convulsions, infection, anaphylaxis, hyperkalemia, pancreatitis, and renal toxicity
> Asymptomatic side effects, including hypertension, nephrotoxicity, and hepatotoxicity

## General Dosing Information

Patients receiving cyclosporine should be under the supervision of a physician experienced in immunosuppressive therapy.

If an infection develops, it must be treated promptly; reduction of dosage or withdrawal of cyclosporine may be necessary.

**For parenteral dosage form**

Because of the risk of anaphylaxis, it is recommended that the parenteral dosage form be used only in patients unable to take cyclosporine orally.

Cyclosporine usually should be administered by slow intravenous infusion over a period of 2 to 6 hours; however it may be given over a period of up to 24 hours. Rapid intravenous administration may cause acute nephrotoxicity, as well as less serious side effects such as flushing and nausea.

It is recommended that patients receiving intravenous cyclosporine be under continuous observation for at least the first 30 minutes of the infusion and at frequent intervals after that. Equipment and medications (including epinephrine and oxygen) necessary for treatment of a possible anaphylactic reaction should be immediately available during each administration of cyclosporine.

**For use in prophylaxis and treatment of transplant rejection**

A variety of dosage schedules of cyclosporine in combination with prednisone have been used. The prescriber may consult the medical literature as well as the manufacturer's literature in choosing a specific dosage.

Dosage must be adjusted to meet the individual requirements of each patient, on the basis of clinical response, trough plasma concentrations (especially in patients with hepatic function impairment), and appearance or severity of toxicity.

Dosage adjustment may be necessary if cyclosporine-induced renal function impairment occurs. Cadaveric kidneys frequently develop a tubular necrosis with delayed onset of adequate function, necessitating a reduction in cyclosporine dosage. If persistent negative nitrogen balance occurs, dosage should be reduced.

If signs of allograft rejection occur, a larger dose may be necessary; other therapy should be considered if they persist.

# Oral Dosage Forms

## CYCLOSPORINE CAPSULES

**Usual adult and adolescent dose**

Transplant rejection (prophylaxis)—
    Initial: Oral, 12 to 15 mg per kg of body weight per day beginning four to twelve hours before surgery and continued for one to two weeks postoperatively, then reduced, usually by 5% per week, to the maintenance dose.
    Maintenance: Oral, 5 to 10 mg per kg of body weight per day.

**Usual pediatric dose**

See *Usual adult and adolescent dose*. Pediatric patients may require higher or more frequent dosing because of accelerated clearance.

**Strength(s) usually available**

U.S.—
    25 mg (Rx) [*Sandimmune*].
    100 mg (Rx) [*Sandimmune*].
Canada—
    25 mg [*Sandimmune*].
    100 mg [*Sandimmune*].

**Packaging and storage**

Store below 25 °C (77 °F), in a well-closed container, unless otherwise specified by manufacturer.

## CYCLOSPORINE ORAL SOLUTION USP

**Usual adult and adolescent dose**

See *Cyclosporine Capsules.*.

**Usual pediatric dose**

See *Cyclosporine Capsules*.

**Strength(s) usually available**

U.S.—
    100 mg per mL (Rx) [*Sandimmune* (alcohol 12.5 %)].

Canada—
    100 mg per mL (Rx) [*Sandimmune* (ethanol 100 mg per mL)].

**Packaging and storage**

Store below 30 °C (86 °F), unless otherwise specified by manufacturer. Store in a tight container. Do not refrigerate (according to manufacturer's labeling).

**Stability**

Contents of opened container must be used within 2 months.

**Note**

When dispensing, include a calibrated liquid measuring device provided by the manufacturer.

# Parenteral Dosage Forms

## CYCLOSPORINE CONCENTRATE FOR INJECTION USP

**Usual adult and adolescent dose**

Transplant rejection (prophylaxis)—
    Initial: Intravenous infusion, 2 to 6 mg per kg of body weight per day beginning four to twelve hours prior to surgery and continued postoperatively until the patient can tolerate the oral solution.

**Usual pediatric dose**

See *Usual adult and adolescent dose*. Pediatric patients may require higher or more frequent dosing because of accelerated clearance.

**Strength(s) usually available**

U.S.—
    50 mg per mL (Rx) [*Sandimmune* (polyoxyethylated castor oil 650 mg per mL; alcohol 32.9% v/v)].
Canada—
    50 mg per mL (Rx) [*Sandimmune* (polyoxyethylated castor oil 650 mg per mL; ethanol 278 mg per mL)].

**Packaging and storage**

Store below 30 °C (86 °F), unless otherwise specified by manufacturer. Protect from freezing.

**Preparation of dosage form**

Cyclosporine Concentrate for Injection USP is prepared for intravenous administration by diluting each mL in 20 to 100 mL of 0.9% sodium chloride injection or 5% dextrose injection. Use of glass containers is recommended because of possible leaching of diethylhexylphthalate (DEHP) from polyvinyl chloride (PVC) bags into cyclosporine solutions.

**Stability**

Reconstituted solutions are stable for up to 24 hours in 5% dextrose injection and for 6 hours (in PVC containers) to 12 hours (in glass containers) in 0.9% sodium chloride injection. Significant amounts of cyclosporine are lost when it is administered through PVC tubing.

# Selected Bibliography

Ptachcinski RJ, Burckart GJ, Venkataramanan R. Cyclosporine. Drug Intell Clin Pharm 1985 Feb; 19: 90-100.

Fahey JL, et al. UCLA Conference. Immune interventions in disease. Ann Intern Med 1987 Feb; 106: 257-74.

Scott JP, Higenbottam TW. Adverse reactions and interactions of cyclosporine. Med Toxicol 1988; 3: 107-27.

Revised: 06/09/93
Interim revision: 05/12/94

---

**CYCLOTHIAZIDE**—See *Diuretics, Thiazide (Systemic)*

---

**CYPROHEPTADINE**—See *Antihistamines (Systemic)*

# CYSTEAMINE Systemic†

VA CLASSIFICATION (Primary): XX000

†Not commercially available in Canada; however, it is available by emergency drug release from the Health Protection Branch

Note: For a listing of dosage forms and brand names by country availability, see *Dosage Forms* section(s). For a listing of brand names for the articles in this monograph, refer to the General Index.

## Category

Nephropathic cystinosis therapy.

## Indications

**Accepted**

Cystinosis, nephropathic (prophylaxis)—Cysteamine is indicated for the management of nephropathic cystinosis in children and adults.

## Pharmacology/Pharmacokinetics

**Physicochemical characteristics**

Molecular weight—227.

**Mechanism of action/Effect**

Cysteamine is an aminothiol that converts cystine to cysteine and cysteine-cysteamine mixed disulfide, both of which can pass through the lysosomal membrane of patients with cystinosis. In the nephropathic form of cystinosis, the accumulation of cystine and the formation of crystals damage various organs, especially the kidney. Cysteamine improves glomerular function without affecting tubular function.

**Other actions/effects**

There is some evidence that cysteamine therapy prevents accumulation of cystine in skeletal muscle.

**Protein binding**

Poorly bound to plasma proteins.

## Precautions to Consider

**Cross-sensitivity and/or related problems**

Patients sensitive to penicillamine may be sensitive to this medication also.

**Carcinogenicity**

Long-term carcinogenicity studies in animals have not been performed.

**Mutagenicity**

No evidence of mutagenicity was found in the Ames test. Cysteamine produced a negative response in the *in vitro* sister chromatid exchange assay in human lymphocytes, but a positive response in a similar assay in hamster ovarian cells.

**Pregnancy/Reproduction**

Fertility—Studies in male and female rats given oral cysteamine doses of 75 mg per kg of body weight (mg/kg) per day (450 mg per square meter of body surface area [mg/m$^2$] per day [0.4 times the recommended human dose based on body surface area]) found no evidence of impairment of fertility or reproductive performance. However, another study in male and female rats given 375 mg/kg per day (2250 mg/m$^2$ per day [1.7 times the recommended human dose based on body surface area]) revealed reduced fertility.

Pregnancy—Adequate and well-controlled studies in humans have not been done.

A study in male and female rats given 375 mg/kg per day (2250 mg/m$^2$ per day [1.7 times the recommended human dose based on body surface area]) revealed a reduction in survival of the offspring.

FDA Pregnancy Category C.

**Breast-feeding**

It is not known whether cysteamine is distributed into breast milk. Because of the potential of cysteamine for causing developmental toxicity in suckling rat pups when administered to their lactating mothers at an oral dose of 375 mg/kg per day (2250 mg/m$^2$ per day [1.7 times the recommended human dose based on body surface area]), a decision should be made whether to discontinue nursing or discontinue the drug.

**Pediatrics**

Appropriate studies performed to date have not demonstrated pediatrics-specific problems that would limit the usefulness of cysteamine in children. Cysteamine therapy is most effective when begun early in life, before organ damage has developed.

**Geriatrics**

No information is available on the relationship of age to the effects of cysteamine in geriatric patients.

**Medical considerations/Contraindications**

The medical considerations/contraindications included here have been selected on the basis of their potential clinical significance (reasons given in parentheses where appropriate)—not necessarily inclusive (» = major clinical significance).

**Risk-benefit should be considered when the following medical problems exist:**

Blood disorders (or history of) or
Hepatic function impairment or
» Seizures (or history of)
  (cysteamine may exacerbate these conditions)
Sensitivity to cysteamine or penicillamine

**Patient monitoring**

The following may be especially important in patient monitoring (other tests may be warranted in some patients, depending on condition; » = major clinical significance):

Body height and
Body weight and
Creatinine clearance and
Creatinine, serum
  (determinations recommended every 3 to 4 months to measure effectiveness of cysteamine therapy; creatinine clearance and serum creatinine should stabilize with therapy)

Complete blood count and
Hepatic function
  (determinations recommended every 3 to 4 months because cysteamine has been associated with anemia, leukopenia, and abnormal liver function tests)

» Leukocyte cystine concentrations
  (determinations recommended 5 to 6 hours after a dose, 2 weeks after initiation of therapy, and every 3 months to determine effectiveness of therapy; concentrations should be less than 1 nanomole half-cystine per mg protein; however, patients unable to tolerate doses required to achieve this level may benefit from leukocyte cystine concentrations below 2 nanomole half-cystine per mg protein)

## Side/Adverse Effects

Note: The incidence of side/adverse effects increases with increasing doses.

The following side/adverse effects have been selected on the basis of their potential clinical significance (possible signs and symptoms in parentheses where appropriate)—not necessarily inclusive:

**Those indicating need for medical attention**

Incidence more frequent
  *Abdominal pain; anorexia* (loss of appetite); *diarrhea; fever; lethargy* (drowsiness); *nausea or vomiting; skin rash*
  Note: If *skin rash* develops, cysteamine therapy may need to be withheld, restarted at a lower dose, and slowly titrated to the therapeutic dose. If severe skin rash develops (e.g., erythema multiforme bullosa, toxic epidermal necrolysis), cysteamine therapy should not be readministered. If *abdominal pain, anorexia,* or *nausea or vomiting* develops, therapy should be interrupted and the dose adjusted.

Incidence less frequent
  *Confusion; dizziness; headache; mental depression; sore throat; trembling*
  Note: If *confusion, dizziness, headache,* or *mental depression* develops, therapy should be interrupted and the dose adjusted.

Incidence rare
*Anemia* (unusual tiredness or weakness); *dehydration* (increased thirst); *leukopenia* (sore throat and fever); *seizures* (convulsions)
Note: Development of *seizures* may indicate need to discontinue the drug temporarily and resume at a lower dose.

**Those not indicating need for medical attention**
Incidence less frequent
*Breath odor; constipation*

## Patient Consultation

As an aid to patient consultation, refer to *Advice for the Patient, Cysteamine (Systemic).*

In providing consultation, consider emphasizing the following selected information (» = major clinical significance):

**Before using this medication**
» Conditions affecting use, especially:
Sensitivity to cysteamine or penicillamine
Pregnancy—Studies in animals have shown a decrease in fertility and survival of offspring
Breast-feeding—May be necessary to discontinue medication because of problems in nursing animals
Other medical problems, especially seizures

**Proper use of this medication**
Repeating dose once if vomited within 20 minutes; not repeating if vomiting occurs after 20 minutes
Possible need for dietary supplements
Capsule may be opened and contents sprinkled on food or mixed with formula
» Proper dosing
Missed dose: Taking as soon as possible; not taking if almost time for next dose; not doubling dose
» Proper storage

**Precautions while using this medication**
Regular visits to physician to check progress during therapy
May cause dizziness or drowsiness

**Side/adverse effects**
Signs of potential side effects, especially abdominal pain, anorexia, diarrhea, fever, lethargy, nausea or vomiting, skin rash, confusion, dizziness, headache, mental depression, sore throat, trembling, anemia, dehydration, leukopenia, and seizures

## General Dosing Information

If a dose is vomited within 20 minutes after administration, the dose should be repeated once. If vomiting occurs more than 20 minutes after administration, the dose should be considered absorbed.

**Diet/Nutrition**
Because nephropathic cystinosis may cause the loss of electrolytes from the kidney, the health care professional may recommend that dietary supplements be taken.

For children six years of age and under, the capsule may be opened and the contents of the capsule sprinkled on food or mixed in formula.

## Oral Dosage Forms
### CYSTEAMINE BITARTRATE CAPSULES

**Usual adult and adolescent dose**
Nephropathic cystinosis therapy—
Initially, patients should be started on one-quarter to one-sixth of the maintenance dose; the dose should be raised gradually over four to six weeks. The maintenance dose for patients over 12 years of age and weighing more than 110 pounds (50 kg) is 2 grams a day in four divided doses.

**Usual pediatric dose**
Nephropathic cystinosis therapy—
Initially, patients should be started on one-quarter to one-sixth of the maintenance dose; the dose should be raised gradually over four to six weeks. The maintenance dose of 1.3 grams per square meter of body surface area per day in four divided doses can be approximated using the following table:

Cysteamine Maintenance Dose

| Weight (pounds) | Weight (kg) | Cysteamine free base every 6 hours (mg) |
| --- | --- | --- |
| 0–10 | 0–4.5 | 100 |
| 11–20 | 5–9 | 150 |
| 21–30 | 9.5–13.6 | 200 |
| 31–40 | 14–18 | 250 |
| 41–50 | 18.6–22.7 | 300 |
| 51–70 | 23.2–31.8 | 350 |
| 71–90 | 32.3–40.9 | 400 |
| 91–110 | 41.4–50 | 450 |
| >110 | >50 | 500 |

**Strength(s) usually available**
U.S.—
50 mg (Rx) [*Cystagon*].
150 mg (Rx) [*Cystagon*].
Canada—
Not commercially available; however, it is available by emergency drug release from the Health Protection Branch.

**Packaging and storage**
Store below 40 °C (104 °F), preferably between 15 and 30 °C (59 and 86 °F), unless otherwise specified by manufacturer.

**Preparation of dosage form**
For patients who cannot take oral solids—Capsules may be opened and the contents sprinkled on food or mixed in formula.

Developed: 01/31/96

---

# CYTARABINE Systemic

VA CLASSIFICATION (Primary): AN300
Other commonly used names are ara-C and cytosine arabinoside.
Note: For a listing of dosage forms and brand names by country availability, see *Dosage Forms* section(s). For a listing of brand names for the articles in this monograph, refer to the General Index.

## Category
Antineoplastic.

## Indications
Note: Bracketed information in the *Indications* section refers to uses that are not included in U.S. product labeling.

**Accepted**
Leukemia, acute lymphocytic (treatment)
Leukemia, acute myelocytic (treatment)
Leukemia, meningeal (prophylaxis and treatment)
Erythroleukemia (treatment)
Leukemia, chronic myelocytic (treatment)
Lymphomas, non-Hodgkin's (treatment)
[Lymphomas, Hodgkin's (treatment)][1] or

[Myelodysplastic syndrome (treatment)][1]—Cytarabine is indicated for treatment of acute lymphocytic leukemia, acute myelocytic leukemia, meningeal leukemia (by intrathecal injection), erythroleukemia, chronic myelocytic leukemia (blast phase), non-Hodgkin's lymphomas in children, Hodgkin's disease, and myelodysplastic syndrome.

[1]Not included in Canadian product labeling.

## Pharmacology/Pharmacokinetics

**Physicochemical characteristics**
Molecular weight—243.22.
pKa—4.35 in 60% aqueous ethanol.

**Mechanism of action/Effect**
Cytarabine is an antimetabolite. Cytarabine is cell cycle–specific for the S phase of cell division. Activity occurs as the result of activation to cytarabine triphosphate in the tissues and includes inhibition of DNA synthesis with little effect on RNA and protein synthesis.

**Other actions/effects**
Cytarabine is a potent immunosuppressant.

### Distribution

Only moderate amounts cross the blood-brain barrier with rapid intravenous administration, although cerebrospinal concentrations of 40 to 50% of steady state plasma concentrations are attained after continuous intravenous infusion.

### Protein binding

Low (15%).

### Biotransformation

Rapidly deaminated in blood and tissues, especially the liver, but minimally in the cerebrospinal fluid (CSF).

### Half-life

Varies between individuals; may relate to cytotoxicity.

Alpha phase—10 to 15 minutes.

Beta phase—1 to 3 hours (about 2 hours after intrathecal administration).

### Time to peak plasma concentration

Subcutaneous—20 to 60 minutes.

### Elimination

Renal, less than 10% unchanged.

## Precautions to Consider

### Carcinogenicity

Secondary malignancies are potential delayed effects of many antineoplastic agents, although it is not clear whether the effect is related to their mutagenic or immunosuppressive action. The effect of dose and duration of therapy is also unknown, although risk seems to increase with long-term use. Although information is limited, available data seem to indicate that the carcinogenic risk is greatest with the alkylating agents.

Antimetabolites have been shown to be carcinogenic in animals and may be associated with an increased risk of development of secondary carcinomas in humans, although the risk appears to be less than with alkylating agents.

### Mutagenicity

Cytarabine may cause chromosomal damage, including chromatoid breaks, in humans. Malignant transformation of rodent cells in culture has been reported.

### Pregnancy/Reproduction

Fertility—Gonadal suppression, resulting in amenorrhea or azoospermia, may occur in patients taking antineoplastic therapy, especially with the alkylating agents. In general, these effects appear to be related to dose and length of therapy and may be irreversible. Prediction of the degree of testicular or ovarian function impairment is complicated by the common use of combinations of several antineoplastics, which makes it difficult to assess the effects of individual agents.

Cytarabine has been associated with reversible germ cell toxicity in humans.

Pregnancy—Studies in humans have not been done.

In humans, one case of trisomy, one case of extremity and ear deformities, one case of upper and lower distal limb defects, and one case of enlarged spleen have been reported in infants of mothers who received cytarabine. Other problems reported include pancytopenia; transient depression of leukocyte counts, hematocrit, or platelet counts; electrolyte abnormalities; transient eosinophilia; increased IgM concentrations and hyperpyrexia; fatal gastroenteritis; and prematurity and low birth weight. Several normal births have also been reported.

First trimester: It is usually recommended that use of antineoplastics, especially combination chemotherapy, be avoided whenever possible, especially during the first trimester. Although information is limited because of the relatively few instances of antineoplastic administration during pregnancy, the mutagenic, teratogenic, and carcinogenic potential of these medications must be considered.

Other hazards to the fetus include adverse reactions seen in adults.

In general, use of a contraceptive is recommended during cytotoxic drug therapy.

Cytarabine is teratogenic in some animal species.

FDA Pregnancy Category D.

### Breast-feeding

Although very little information is available regarding distribution of antineoplastic agents into breast milk, breast-feeding is not recommended while cytarabine is being administered because of the risks to the infant (adverse effects, mutagenicity, carcinogenicity). It is not known whether cytarabine is distributed into breast milk.

### Pediatrics

Appropriate studies on the relationship of age to the effects of cytarabine have not been performed in the pediatric population. However, pediatrics-specific problems that would limit the usefulness of this medication in children are not expected.

### Geriatrics

Although appropriate studies on the relationship of age to the effects of cytarabine have not been performed in the geriatric population, geriatrics-specific problems that would limit the usefulness of this medication in the elderly are not expected. However, elderly patients are more likely to have age-related renal function impairment, which may require reduction of dosage in patients receiving cytarabine.

### Dental

The bone marrow depressant effects of cytarabine may result in an increased incidence of microbial infection, delayed healing, and gingival bleeding. Dental work, whenever possible should be completed prior to initiation of therapy or deferred until blood counts have returned to normal. Patients should be instructed in proper oral hygiene during treatment, including caution in use of regular toothbrushes, dental floss, and toothpicks.

Cytarabine also commonly causes stomatitis associated with considerable discomfort.

### Drug interactions and/or related problems

The following drug interactions and/or related problems have been selected on the basis of their potential clinical significance (possible mechanism in parentheses where appropriate)—not necessarily inclusive (» = major clinical significance):

Note: Combinations containing any of the following medications, depending on the amount present, may also interact with this medication.

Allopurinol or
Colchicine or
» Probenecid or
» Sulfinpyrazone
(cytarabine may raise the concentration of blood uric acid; dosage adjustment of antigout agents may be necessary to control hyperuricemia and gout; allopurinol may be preferred to prevent or reverse cytarabine-induced hyperuricemia because of risk of uric acid nephropathy with uricosuric antigout agents)

Blood dyscrasia–causing medications (See *Appendix II*)
(leukopenic and/or thrombocytopenic effects of cytarabine may be increased with concurrent or recent therapy if these medications cause the same effects; dosage adjustment of cytarabine, if necessary, should be based on blood counts)

» Bone marrow depressants, other (See *Appendix II*) or
Radiation therapy
(additive bone marrow depression may occur; dosage reduction may be required when two or more bone marrow depressants, including radiation, are used concurrently or consecutively)

» Cyclophosphamide
(concurrent use with high-dose cytarabine therapy for bone marrow transplant preparation has been reported to result in an increase in cardiomyopathy with subsequent death; the cardiac toxicity may be schedule dependent)

» Immunosuppressants, other, such as:
Azathioprine
Chlorambucil
Corticosteroids, glucocorticoid
Cyclophosphamide
Cyclosporine
Mercaptopurine
Muromonab CD-3
Tacrolimus
(concurrent use with cytarabine may increase the risk of infection)

Methotrexate
(administration of cytarabine 48 hours before or 10 minutes after initiation of methotrexate therapy may result in a synergistic cytotoxic effect; however, evidence is inconclusive and dosage adjustment based on routine hematologic monitoring is recommended)

Vaccines, killed virus
(because normal defense mechanisms may be suppressed by cytarabine therapy, the patient's antibody response to the vaccine may be decreased. The interval between discontinuation of medications that cause immunosuppression and restoration of the patient's ability to respond to the vaccine depends on the intensity and type of immunosuppression-causing medication used, the underlying disease, and other factors; estimates vary from 3 months to 1 year)

» Vaccines, live virus
     (because normal defense mechanisms may be suppressed by cytarabine therapy, concurrent use with a live virus vaccine may potentiate the replication of the vaccine virus, may increase the side/adverse effects of the vaccine virus, and/or may decrease the patient's antibody response to the vaccine; immunization of these patients should be undertaken only with extreme caution after careful review of the patient's hematologic status and only with the knowledge and consent of the physician managing the cytarabine therapy. The interval between discontinuation of medications that cause immunosuppression and restoration of the patient's ability to respond to the vaccine depends on the intensity and type of immunosuppression-causing medication used, the underlying disease, and other factors; estimates vary from 3 months to 1 year. Patients with leukemia in remission should not receive live virus vaccine until at least 3 months after their last chemotherapy. In addition, immunization with oral poliovirus vaccine should be postponed in persons in close contact with the patient, especially family members)

### Laboratory value alterations
The following have been selected on the basis of their potential clinical significance (possible effect in parentheses where appropriate)—not necessarily inclusive (» = major clinical significance):

With physiology/laboratory test values
   Alkaline phosphatase values, serum and
   Aspartate aminotransferase (AST [SGOT]) values, serum and
   Bilirubin concentrations, serum
     (may be increased, indicating possible hepatotoxicity)
   Uric acid
     (concentrations in blood and urine may be increased)

### Medical considerations/Contraindications
The medical considerations/contraindications included here have been selected on the basis of their potential clinical significance (reasons given in parentheses where appropriate)—not necessarily inclusive (» = major clinical significance).

*Risk-benefit should be considered when the following medical problems exist:*
» Bone marrow depression
     (lower dosage may be necessary)
» Chickenpox, existing or recent (including recent exposure) or
» Herpes zoster
     (risk of severe generalized disease)
   Gout, history of or
   Urate renal stones, history of
     (risk of hyperuricemia)
» Hepatic function impairment
     (reduced detoxification of cytarabine; lower dosage may be necessary)
» Infection
   Renal function impairment
     (reduced elimination; lower dosage may be necessary)
   Sensitivity to cytarabine
» Tumor cell infiltration of the bone marrow
» Caution should be used also in patients who have had previous cytotoxic drug therapy or radiation therapy.

### Patient monitoring
The following are especially important in patient monitoring (other tests may be warranted in some patients, depending on condition; (» = major clinical significance):

   Alanine aminotransferase (ALT [SGPT]) values, serum and
   Aspartate aminotransferase (AST [SGOT]) values, serum and
   Bilirubin concentrations, serum and
   Lactate dehydrogenase (LDH) values, serum
     (recommended prior to initiation of therapy and at periodic intervals during therapy; frequency varies according to clinical state, agent, dose, and other agents being used concurrently)
» Bone marrow aspiration
     (recommended at 2-week intervals until remission occurs)
» Hematocrit or hemoglobin and
   Leukocyte count, total and, if appropriate, differential and
» Platelet count
     (determinations recommended prior to initiation of therapy and at periodic intervals during therapy; frequency varies according to clinical state, agent, dose, and other agents being used concurrently)

Uric acid concentrations, serum
     (recommended prior to initiation of therapy and at periodic intervals during therapy; frequency varies according to clinical state, agent, dose, and other agents being used concurrently)

## Side/Adverse Effects
Note:  Many "side effects" of antineoplastic therapy are unavoidable and represent the medication's pharmacologic action. Some of these (for example, leukopenia and thrombocytopenia) are actually used as parameters to aid in individual dosage titration.

   Incidence of side effects (except nausea and vomiting) is higher with continuous intravenous administration than with rapid intravenous administration.

   Intrathecal administration may result in systemic effects.

   Acute pancreatitis has been reported in patients previously treated with asparaginase.

   High-dose therapy has been associated with severe and potentially fatal toxicity, including reversible corneal toxicity and hemorrhagic conjunctivitis (which may be prevented or reduced by prophylactic administration of a local corticosteroid eye drop), cerebral dysfunction (confusion, tiredness, memory loss, seizures), cerebellar dysfunction (trouble in speaking, standing, or walking; tremors), gastrointestinal ulceration, peritonitis (including pneumatosis cystoides intestinalis leading to peritonitis), sepsis and liver abscess, pulmonary edema, hepatic damage with hyperbilirubinemia, bowel necrosis, necrotizing colitis, skin rash leading to desquamation, fatal cardiomyopathy, a potentially fatal syndrome of sudden respiratory distress progressing to pulmonary edema and cardiomegaly, and peripheral motor and sensory neuropathies.

The following side/adverse effects have been selected on the basis of their potential clinical significance (possible signs and symptoms in parentheses where appropriate)—not necessarily inclusive:

### Those indicating need for medical attention
Incidence more frequent—occurring in 15 to 100% of patients
   *Leukopenia or infection* (usually asymptomatic; less frequently, fever or chills; cough or hoarseness; lower back or side pain; painful or difficult urination); *stomatitis* (sores in mouth and on lips); *thrombocytopenia* (usually asymptomatic; less frequently, unusual bleeding or bruising; black, tarry stools; blood in urine or stools; pinpoint red spots on skin)
   Note: With *leukopenia*, leukocyte levels decline in two phases starting in the first 24 hours, with a nadir at days 7 to 9, a brief rise until the twelfth day, and a deeper fall with a nadir at days 15 to 24. Levels rise rapidly to baseline in the next 10 days.
        With *thrombocytopenia*, platelet counts fall noticeably by 5 days following a dose, with the nadir at 12 to 15 days and a rise to baseline over the next 10 days.

Incidence less frequent—occurring in 10% or less of patients
   *Central nervous system (CNS) toxicity, cerebellar or cerebral* (numbness or tingling in fingers, toes, or face; unusual tiredness)—more frequent with high-dose therapy; *hyperuricemia or uric acid nephropathy* (joint pain; lower back or side pain; swelling of feet or lower legs)
   Note: *Hyperuricemia or uric acid nephropathy* occurs most commonly during initial treatment of leukemia or lymphoma, as a result of rapid cell breakdown, which leads to elevated serum uric acid concentrations.

Incidence rare—occurring in 2% or less of patients
   *Cellulitis or thrombophlebitis* (pain at injection site); *drug reaction or ara-C syndrome* (bone or muscle pain; chest pain; fever; general feeling of discomfort or illness or weakness; reddened eyes; skin rash); *esophagitis* (difficulty in swallowing; heartburn); *gastrointestinal hemorrhage* (black, tarry stools); *hepatotoxicity* (yellow eyes or skin); *megaloblastic anemia* (fainting spells; irregular heartbeat; unusual tiredness; weakness); *pulmonary edema or diffuse interstitial pneumonitis* (cough; shortness of breath); *urinary retention* (decrease in urination)
   Note: The *drug reaction or ara-C syndrome* usually occurs 6 to 12 hours after administration; it may be prevented by or respond to steroid treatment.

### Those indicating need for medical attention only if they continue or are bothersome
Incidence more frequent—occurring in 15 to 100% of patients
   *Loss of appetite; nausea and vomiting*
   Note: *Nausea and vomiting* occur more frequently when large intravenous doses are administered quickly than when they are infused.

Incidence less frequent or rare—occurring in 10% or less of patients
*Diarrhea; dizziness; headache, especially after intrathecal administration; itching of skin; skin freckling*

**Those not indicating need for medical attention**
Incidence less frequent or rare
*Loss of hair*
Note: Complete *alopecia* is more frequent with high-dose therapy.

**Those indicating the need for medical attention if they occur after medication is discontinued**
*Bone marrow depression* (black, tarry stools; blood in urine or stools; cough or hoarseness; fever or chills; lower back or side pain; painful or difficult urination; pinpoint red spots on skin; unusual bleeding or bruising)

## Patient Consultation

As an aid to patient consultation, refer to *Advice for the Patient, Cytarabine (Systemic)*.

In providing consultation, consider emphasizing the following selected information (» = major clinical significance):

### Before using this medication
» Conditions affecting use, especially:
  Sensitivity to cytarabine
  Pregnancy—Use not recommended because of mutagenic, teratogenic, and carcinogenic potential; advisability of using contraception; telling physician immediately if pregnancy is suspected
  Breast-feeding—Not recommended because of risk of serious side effects
  Other medications, especially probenecid, sulfinpyrazone, other bone marrow depressants, other immunosuppressants, or other cytotoxic drug or radiation therapy
  Other medical problems, especially chickenpox, herpes zoster, hepatic function impairment, or infection

### Proper use of this medication
  Caution in taking combination therapy; taking each medication at the right time
  Importance of ample fluid intake and subsequent increase in urine output to aid in excretion of uric acid
  Frequency of nausea and vomiting; importance of continuing medication despite stomach upset
» Proper dosing

### Precautions while using this medication
» Importance of close monitoring by the physician
» Avoiding immunizations unless approved by physician; other persons in patient's household should avoid immunizations with oral poliovirus vaccine; avoiding persons who have taken oral poliovirus vaccine or wearing a protective mask that covers nose and mouth
*Caution if bone marrow depression occurs:*
» Avoiding exposure to persons with bacterial infections, especially during periods of low blood counts; checking with physician immediately if fever or chills, cough or hoarseness, lower back or side pain, or painful or difficult urination occur
» Checking with physician immediately if unusual bleeding or bruising; black, tarry stools; blood in urine or stools; or pinpoint red spots on skin occur
  Caution in use of regular toothbrush, dental floss, or toothpick; physician, dentist, or nurse may suggest alternatives; checking with physician before having dental work done
  Not touching eyes or inside of nose unless hands washed immediately before
  Using caution to avoid accidental cuts with use of sharp objects such as safety razor or fingernail or toenail cutters
  Avoiding contact sports or other situations where bruising or injury could occur

### Side/adverse effects
  May cause adverse effects such as blood problems; importance of discussing possible effects with physician
  Signs of potential side effects, especially leukopenia, infection, stomatitis, thrombocytopenia, CNS toxicity, hyperuricemia, uric acid nephropathy, cellulitis, thrombophlebitis, drug reaction, ara-C syndrome, esophagitis, gastrointestinal hemorrhage, hepatotoxicity, megaloblastic anemia, pulmonary edema, diffuse interstitial pneumonitis, and urinary retention
  Physician or nurse can help in dealing with side effects
  Possibility of hair loss; normal hair growth should return after treatment has ended

## General Dosing Information

It is recommended that for induction therapy cytarabine be administered in a hospital setting under supervision of a physician experienced in antimetabolite chemotherapy. Intrathecal therapy should be carried out only by a physician familiar with the regimen.

A variety of dosage schedules and regimens of cytarabine, alone or in combination with other antitumor agents, are used. The prescriber may consult the medical literature as well as the manufacturer's literature in choosing a specific dosage.

Dosage must be adjusted to meet the individual requirements of each patient, on the basis of clinical response and degree of bone marrow depression.

Patients generally tolerate higher doses with less hematologic depression when cytarabine is administered by rapid intravenous injection rather than by slow infusion, although nausea and vomiting may be more severe and may persist for several hours after the injection.

Development of uric acid nephropathy in patients with leukemia or lymphoma may be prevented by adequate oral hydration and, in some cases, administration of allopurinol. Alkalinization of urine may be necessary if serum uric acid concentrations are elevated.

It is recommended that an induction program be continued until either response or toxicity occurs, or until it becomes clear that the patient will not respond. Bone marrow improvement may require 7 to 64 days; treatment is stopped when the bone marrow becomes hypocellular and is resumed when it recovers.

If leukocyte counts fall below 1000 per cubic millimeter or platelet counts below 50,000 per cubic millimeter, cytarabine therapy may need to be withdrawn until definite signs of bone marrow recovery occur. The lowest leukocyte and platelet levels are usually reached after 12 to 24 drug-free days. Therapy should be resumed when appropriate leukocyte and platelet levels are reached; these levels may be lower than normal to avoid patient escape from control.

In acute leukemia, cytarabine may be administered despite the presence of thrombocytopenia and bleeding; cessation of bleeding and increase in platelet count have occurred in some cases during treatment and platelet transfusions are useful in others.

Special precautions are recommended in patients who develop thrombocytopenia as a result of administration of cytarabine. These may include extreme care in performing invasive procedures; regular inspection of intravenous sites, skin (including perirectal area), and mucous membrane surfaces for signs of bleeding or bruising; limiting frequency of venipuncture and avoiding intramuscular injections; testing urine, emesis, stool, and secretions for occult blood; care in use of regular toothbrushes, dental floss, toothpicks, safety razors, and fingernail and toenail cutters; avoiding constipation; and using caution to prevent falls and other injuries. Such patients should avoid alcohol and aspirin intake because of the risk of gastrointestinal bleeding. Platelet transfusions may be required.

Patients who develop leukopenia should be observed carefully for signs of infection. Antibiotic support may be required. In neutropenic patients who develop fever, broad-spectrum antibiotic coverage should be initiated empirically, pending bacterial cultures and appropriate diagnostic tests.

### Safety considerations for handling this medication

There is limited but increasing evidence and concern that personnel involved in preparation and administration of parenteral antineoplastics may be at some risk because of the potential mutagenicity, teratogenicity, and/or carcinogenicity of these agents, although the actual risk is unknown. USP advisory panels recommend cautious handling both in preparation and disposal of antineoplastic agents. Precautions that have been suggested include:
  • Use of a biological containment cabinet during reconstitution and dilution of parenteral medications and wearing of disposable surgical gloves and masks.
  • Use of proper technique to prevent contamination of the medication, work area, and operator during transfer between containers (including proper training of personnel in this technique).
  • Cautious and proper disposal of needles, syringes, vials, ampuls, and unused medication.

A number of medical centers have developed detailed guidelines for handling of antineoplastic agents.

### Combination chemotherapy

Cytarabine is usually used in combination with other agents in various regimens. As a result, incidence and/or severity of side effects may be altered and different dosages (usually reduced) may be used. For example, cytarabine is part of the following chemotherapeutic combinations (some commonly used acronyms are in parentheses):

—cytarabine and doxorubicin (Ara-C + ADR).

—cytarabine, daunorubicin, prednisolone, and mercaptopurine (Ara-C + DNR + PRED + MP).

—cytarabine and thioguanine (Ara-C + 6-TG).

—cytarabine, thioguanine, and daunorubicin.

—cytarabine, doxorubicin, vincristine, and prednisolone.

—cytarabine, daunorubicin, thioguanine, prednisone, and vincristine.

—cytarabine and daunorubicin.

—cytarabine and mitoxantrone.

For specific dosages and schedules, consult the literature. For information regarding each agent, consult the individual monographs.

## Parenteral Dosage Forms

### CYTARABINE STERILE USP

#### Usual adult and adolescent dose

Acute myelocytic leukemia or

Erythroleukemia—

Induction: Intravenous, 100 to 200 mg per square meter of body surface or 3 mg per kg of body weight per day (as a continuous infusion over twenty-four hours or in divided doses by rapid injection) for five to ten days, with the course repeated approximately every two weeks.

Maintenance: Subcutaneous, 1 mg per kg of body weight one or two times a week.

Note: High-dose cytarabine therapy has been used in selected patients with refractory acute leukemia or lymphomas. One commonly used regimen is 2 to 3 grams per square meter of body surface intravenously (over 1 to 3 hours) every twelve hours for two to six days. High-dose cytarabine therapy should be used with extreme caution and only by clinicians familiar with the procedure.

Meningeal leukemia—

Intrathecal, 5 to 75 mg per square meter of body surface at intervals ranging from once a day for four days to once every four days. A frequently used dosage is 30 mg per square meter of body surface once every four days until CSF findings are normal, followed by one additional dose.

#### Usual pediatric dose

See *Usual adult and adolescent dose.*

Note: Safety of use in infants has not been established.

#### Size(s) usually available

U.S.—

100 mg (Rx) [*Cytosar-U;* GENERIC].

500 mg (Rx) [*Cytosar-U;* GENERIC].

1 gram (Rx) [*Cytosar-U*].

2 grams (Rx) [*Cytosar-U*].

Canada—

100 mg (Rx) [*Cytosar*].

500 mg (Rx) [*Cytosar*].

1 gram (Rx) [*Cytosar*].

2 grams (Rx) [*Cytosar*].

#### Packaging and storage

Store below 40 °C (104 °F), preferably between 15 and 30 °C (59 and 86 °F), unless otherwise specified by manufacturer.

#### Preparation of dosage form

Caution: Use of diluents containing benzyl alcohol is not recommended for preparation of medications for use in neonates. A fatal toxic syndrome consisting of metabolic acidosis, CNS depression, respiratory problems, renal failure, hypotension, and possibly seizures and intracranial hemorrhage has been associated with this use. Diluents containing benzyl alcohol should also be avoided in preparation of high-dose and intrathecal therapy.

Sterile Cytarabine USP is reconstituted for *intravenous* or *subcutaneous* (but *not intrathecal*) use by adding 5 mL of bacteriostatic water for injection (with benzyl alcohol) provided by the manufacturer to the 100-mg vial, producing a solution containing 20 mg of cytarabine per mL, or by adding 10 mL of bacteriostatic water for injection to the 500-mg vial, producing a solution containing 50 mg of cytarabine per mL.

Cytarabine solutions may be further diluted with water for injection, 5% dextrose injection, or 0.9% sodium chloride injection for administration by intravenous infusion.

Sterile Cytarabine USP is reconstituted for *intrathecal* use by adding 5 or 10 mL of an isotonic buffered diluent (without preservatives) such as Elliott's B solution, lactated Ringer's injection, or the patient's cerebrospinal fluid (CSF) to the 100- or 500-mg vial, respectively. The volume administered should correspond to an equal volume of CSF removed.

#### Stability

Reconstituted solutions are stable at room temperature for 48 hours. Solutions that develop a slight haze should be discarded. Infusion solutions containing up to 500 mcg (0.5 mg) of cytarabine per mL are stable at room temperature for 7 days. Solutions for intrathecal use should be used immediately after preparation.

## Selected Bibliography

Bolwell BJ, Cassileth PA, Gale RP. High dose cytarabine. A review. Leukemia 1988 May; 2: 253-60.

Revised: 07/15/94

# DACARBAZINE   Systemic

VA CLASSIFICATION (Primary): AN900

Note: For a listing of dosage forms and brand names by country availability, see *Dosage Forms* section(s). For a listing of brand names for the articles in this monograph, refer to the General Index.

## Category
Antineoplastic.

## Indications

Note: Bracketed information in the *Indications* section refers to uses that are not included in U.S. product labeling.

**Accepted**

Melanoma, malignant (treatment)—Dacarbazine is indicated for treatment of metastatic malignant melanoma.

Lymphomas, Hodgkin's (treatment)[1]—Dacarbazine is indicated for treatment of Hodgkin's disease as second-line therapy in combination with other effective agents.

[Sarcomas, soft tissue (treatment)][1]—Dacarbazine is used for treatment of some soft tissue metastatic sarcomas.

[1]Not included in Canadian product labeling.

## Pharmacology/Pharmacokinetics

**Physicochemical characteristics**

Molecular weight—182.19.

pKa—4.42.

**Mechanism of action/Effect**

Dacarbazine is thought to be an alkylating agent. Major action is believed to be alkylation; dacarbazine is cell cycle–phase nonspecific. Dacarbazine may inhibit DNA and RNA synthesis via formation of carbonium ions. Some activity and toxicity may occur as the result of activation by hepatic enzymes.

**Distribution**

Crosses the blood-brain barrier to only a limited extent.

**Protein binding**

Very low.

**Biotransformation**

Hepatic, extensive.

**Half-life**

Normal—

    Alpha phase: 19 minutes.
    Beta phase: 5 hours.

Renal or hepatic function impairment—

    Alpha phase: 55 minutes.
    Beta phase: 7.2 hours.

**Elimination**

Renal; 40% of injected dose in 6 hours, one-half of that unchanged.

## Precautions to Consider

**Carcinogenicity/Mutagenicity**

Secondary malignancies are potential delayed effects of many antineoplastic agents, although it is not clear whether the effect is related to their mutagenic or immunosuppressive action. The effect of dose and duration of therapy is also unknown, although risk seems to increase with long-term use. Although information is limited, available data seem to indicate that the carcinogenic risk is greatest with the alkylating agents.

Dacarbazine is a potent carcinogen in animals and, because it is an alkylating agent, is also likely to be carcinogenic in humans. In rats, dacarbazine produced proliferative endocardial lesions, including fibrosarcomas and sarcomas; in mice, angiosarcomas of the spleen were induced.

**Pregnancy/Reproduction**

Fertility—Gonadal suppression, resulting in amenorrhea or azoospermia, may occur in patients taking antineoplastic therapy, especially with the alkylating agents. In general, these effects appear to be related to dose and length of therapy and may be irreversible. Prediction of the degree of testicular or ovarian function impairment is complicated by the common use of combinations of several antineoplastics, which makes it difficult to assess the effects of individual agents.

Pregnancy—Adequate and well-controlled studies in humans have not been done.

First trimester: It is usually recommended that use of antineoplastics, especially combination chemotherapy, be avoided whenever possible, especially during the first trimester. Although information is limited because of the relatively few instances of antineoplastic administration during pregnancy, the mutagenic, teratogenic, and carcinogenic potential of these medications must be considered.

Other hazards to the fetus include adverse reactions seen in adults.

In general, use of a contraceptive is recommended during cytotoxic drug therapy.

Studies in rats have shown that dacarbazine is teratogenic at doses 20 times the human daily dose given on day 12 of gestation. Administration of 10 times the human daily dose to male rats twice weekly for 9 weeks resulted in an increased incidence of fetal resorptions in female rats mated to them. Dacarbazine caused fetal skeletal anomalies in rabbits given 7 times the human daily dose on days 6 to 15 of gestation.

FDA Pregnancy Category C.

**Breast-feeding**

Although very little information is available regarding distribution of antineoplastic agents into breast milk, breast-feeding is not recommended while dacarbazine is being administered because of the risks to the infant (adverse effects, mutagenicity, carcinogenicity). It is not known whether dacarbazine is distributed into breast milk.

**Pediatrics**

Appropriate studies on the relationship of age to the effects of dacarbazine have not been performed in the pediatric population.

**Geriatrics**

No information is available on the relationship of age to the effects of dacarbazine in geriatric patients. However, elderly patients are more likely to have age-related renal function impairment, which may require reduction of dosage in patients receiving dacarbazine.

**Dental**

The bone marrow depressant effects of dacarbazine may result in an increased incidence of microbial infection, delayed healing, and gingival bleeding. Dental work, whenever possible, should be completed prior to initiation of therapy or deferred until blood counts have returned to normal. Patients should be instructed in proper oral hygiene during treatment, including caution in use of regular toothbrushes, dental floss, and toothpicks.

Dacarbazine may also rarely cause stomatitis associated with considerable discomfort.

**Drug interactions and/or related problems**

The following drug interactions and/or related problems have been selected on the basis of their potential clinical significance (possible mechanism in parentheses where appropriate)—not necessarily inclusive (» = major clinical significance):

Note: Combinations containing any of the following medications, depending on the amount present, may also interact with this medication.

Allopurinol
    (dacarbazine-induced inhibition of xanthine oxidase may cause additive hypouricemic effects when used concurrently with allopurinol)

Blood dyscrasia–causing medications (See *Appendix II*)
    (leukopenic and/or thrombocytopenic effects of dacarbazine may be increased with concurrent or recent therapy if these medications cause the same effects; dosage adjustment of dacarbazine, if necessary, should be based on blood counts)

» Bone marrow depressants, other (See *Appendix II*) or
Radiation therapy
    (additive bone marrow depression may occur; dosage reduction may be required when two or more bone marrow depressants, including radiation, are used concurrently or consecutively)

Hepatic enzyme inducers (See *Appendix II*)
    (may enhance metabolism of dacarbazine by induction of hepatic microsomal enzymes; dosage adjustment may be necessary)

Vaccines, killed virus
    (because normal defense mechanisms may be suppressed by dacarbazine therapy, the patient's antibody response to the vaccine may be decreased. The interval between discontinuation of medications that cause immunosuppression and restoration of the patient's ability to respond to the vaccine depends on the intensity

and type of immunosuppression-causing medication used, the underlying disease, and other factors; estimates vary from 3 months to 1 year)

» Vaccines, live virus
(because normal defense mechanisms may be suppressed by dacarbazine therapy, concurrent use with a live virus vaccine may potentiate the replication of the vaccine virus, may increase the side/adverse effects of the vaccine virus, and/or may decrease the patient's antibody response to the vaccine; immunization of these patients should be undertaken only with extreme caution after careful review of the patient's hematologic status and only with the knowledge and consent of the physician managing the dacarbazine therapy. The interval between discontinuation of medications that cause immunosuppression and restoration of the patient's ability to respond to the vaccine depends on the intensity and type of immunosuppression-causing medication used, the underlying disease, and other factors; estimates vary from 3 months to 1 year. Patients with leukemia in remission should not receive live virus vaccine until at least 3 months after their last chemotherapy. In addition, immunization with oral poliovirus vaccine should be postponed in persons in close contact with the patient, especially family members)

**Laboratory value alterations**
The following have been selected on the basis of their potential clinical significance (possible effect in parentheses where appropriate)—not necessarily inclusive (» = major clinical significance):

With physiology/laboratory test values
Alanine aminotransferase (ALT [SGPT]) and
Alkaline phosphatase and
Aspartate aminotransferase (AST [SGOT])
(serum values may be transiently increased; may indicate hepatotoxicity)
Blood urea nitrogen (BUN)
(concentrations may be transiently increased)

**Medical considerations/Contraindications**
The medical considerations/contraindications included here have been selected on the basis of their potential clinical significance (reasons given in parentheses where appropriate)—not necessarily inclusive (» = major clinical significance).

*Risk-benefit should be considered when the following medical problems exist:*
» Bone marrow depression
» Chickenpox, existing or recent (including recent exposure) or
» Herpes zoster
(risk of severe generalized disease)
» Hepatic function impairment
» Infection
» Renal function impairment
(reduced elimination; dosage reduction may be required)
Sensitivity to dacarbazine
» Caution should be used also in patients who have had previous cytotoxic drug therapy or radiation therapy.

**Patient monitoring**
The following are especially important in patient monitoring (other tests may be warranted in some patients, depending on condition; » = major clinical significance):

Blood urea nitrogen (BUN) concentrations and
Creatinine concentrations, serum
(recommended prior to initiation of therapy and at periodic intervals during therapy; frequency varies according to clinical state, agent, dose, and other agents being used concurrently)
» Hematocrit or hemoglobin and
» Leukocyte count, total and, if appropriate, differential and
» Platelet count
(determinations recommended prior to initiation of therapy and at periodic intervals during therapy; frequency varies according to clinical state, agent, dose, and other agents being used concurrently)
Alanine aminotransferase (ALT [SGPT]) values, serum and
Aspartate aminotransferase (AST [SGOT]) values, serum and
Bilirubin values, serum and
Lactate dehydrogenase (LDH) values, serum
(recommended prior to initiation of therapy and at periodic intervals during therapy; frequency varies according to clinical state, agent, dose, and other agents being used concurrently)

Uric acid concentrations, serum
(recommended prior to initiation of therapy and at periodic intervals during therapy; frequency varies according to clinical state, agent, dose, and other agents being used concurrently)

## Side/Adverse Effects

Note: Many "side effects" of antineoplastic therapy are unavoidable and represent the medication's pharmacologic action. Some of these (for example, leukopenia and thrombocytopenia) are actually used as parameters to aid in individual dosage titration.

According to some investigators, photodegradation products of dacarbazine solution may be responsible for some of its adverse effects, including local toxicity (burning and vein pain), nausea and vomiting, and hepatotoxicity.

The following side/adverse effects have been selected on the basis of their potential clinical significance (possible signs and symptoms in parentheses where appropriate)—not necessarily inclusive:

**Those indicating need for medical attention**
Incidence more frequent
*Anemia; extravasation and tissue damage or pain in injected vein* (redness, swelling, or pain at site of injection); *leukopenia* (usually asymptomatic; less frequently, fever or chills; cough or hoarseness; lower back or side pain; painful or difficult urination); *thrombocytopenia* (usually asymptomatic; less frequently, unusual bleeding or bruising; black, tarry stools; blood in urine or stools; pinpoint red spots on skin)

Note: The fall in leukocyte count usually begins within 16 to 20 days after administration, with the nadir at 21 to 25 days and recovery 3 to 5 days later. *Leukopenia* may be severe enough to be fatal.

The nadir usually occurs 16 days after administration, with recovery 3 to 5 days later. *Thrombocytopenia* may be severe enough to be fatal.

Incidence rare
*Anaphylaxis* (shortness of breath; swelling of face); *hepatotoxicity, including hepatic vein thrombosis; and hepatocellular necrosis* (fever; stomach pain; yellow eyes or skin); *stomatitis* (sores in mouth and on lips)

Note: *Hepatotoxicity* is uniformly fatal. It has been reported with use of dacarbazine alone and in combination with other agents.

**Those indicating need for medical attention only if they continue or are bothersome**
Incidence more frequent—greater than 90%
*Loss of appetite; nausea and vomiting*
Note: *Nausea and vomiting* may last for 1 to 12 hours after administration but usually lessen considerably within 1 to 2 days after treatment is started.

Incidence less frequent
*Flushing of face; influenza-like syndrome* (fever; feelings of uneasiness; joint or muscle pain); *numbness of face*
Note: The *influenza-like syndrome* begins after 7 days and may last 1 to 3 weeks; it may occur with repeated treatments.

**Those not indicating need for medical attention**
Incidence less frequent
*Loss of hair*

**Those indicating the need for medical attention if they occur after medication is discontinued**
*Bone marrow depression* (black, tarry stools; blood in urine or stools; cough or hoarseness; fever or chills; lower back or side pain; painful or difficult urination; pinpoint red spots on skin; unusual bleeding or bruising)

## Patient Consultation

As an aid to patient consultation, refer to *Advice for the Patient, Dacarbazine (Systemic)*.

In providing consultation, consider emphasizing the following selected information (» = major clinical significance):

**Before using this medication**
» Conditions affecting use, especially:
Sensitivity to dacarbazine
Pregnancy—Use not recommended because of mutagenic, teratogenic, and carcinogenic potential; advisability of using contraception; telling physician immediately if pregnancy is suspected

Breast-feeding—Not recommended because of risk of serious side effects

Other medications, especially other bone marrow depressants or previous cytotoxic drug or radiation therapy

Other medical problems, especially chickenpox, herpes zoster, hepatic function impairment, infection, or renal function impairment

## Proper use of this medication

Caution in taking combination therapy; taking each medication at the right time

Frequency of nausea, vomiting, and loss of appetite; importance of continuing medication despite stomach upset; should lessen after 1 or 2 days

» Proper dosing

## Precautions while using this medication

» Importance of close monitoring by the physician

» Avoiding immunizations unless approved by physician; other persons in patient's household should avoid immunizations with oral poliovirus vaccine; avoiding persons who have taken oral poliovirus vaccine or wearing a protective mask that covers nose and mouth

*Caution if bone marrow depression occurs:*

» Avoiding exposure to persons with bacterial infections, especially during periods of low blood counts; checking with physician immediately if fever or chills, cough or hoarseness, lower back or side pain, or painful or difficult urination occur

» Checking with physician immediately if unusual bleeding or bruising; black, tarry stools; blood in urine or stools; or pinpoint red spots on skin occur

Caution in use of regular toothbrush, dental floss, or toothpick; physician, dentist, or nurse may suggest alternatives; checking with physician before having dental work done

Not touching eyes or inside of nose unless hands washed immediately before

Using caution to avoid accidental cuts with use of sharp objects such as safety razor or fingernail or toenail cutters

Avoiding contact sports or other situations where bruising or injury could occur

» Possibility of local tissue injury and scarring if infiltration of intravenous solution occurs; telling doctor or nurse right away about redness, pain, or swelling at injection site

## Side/adverse effects

May cause adverse effects such as blood problems, loss of hair, and cancer; importance of discussing possible effects with physician

Signs of potential side effects, especially anemia, extravasation, pain in injected vein, leukopenia, thrombocytopenia, anaphylaxis, hepatotoxicity, and stomatitis

Physician or nurse can help in dealing with side effects

Possibility of hair loss; normal hair growth should return after treatment has ended

# General Dosing Information

Patients receiving dacarbazine should be under supervision of a physician experienced in cancer chemotherapy.

A variety of dosage schedules and regimens of dacarbazine, alone or in combination with other antitumor agents, are used. The prescriber may consult the medical literature as well as the manufacturer's literature in choosing a specific dosage.

Dosage must be adjusted to meet the individual requirements of each patient, on the basis of clinical response and degree of bone marrow depression.

Dacarbazine may be administered into the tubing of a freely running intravenous solution over a 1- to 2-minute period, or by intravenous infusion over a 15- to 30-minute period. Administration by intravenous infusion may prevent pain along the injected vein.

Care should be taken to avoid extravasation of dacarbazine because of the risk of severe pain and necrosis.

If extravasation of dacarbazine occurs during intravenous administration, as indicated by local burning or stinging, the injection and infusion should be stopped immediately and resumed, completing the dose, in another vein.

If marked leukopenia (particularly granulocytopenia) or thrombocytopenia occurs, dacarbazine should be discontinued until leukocyte and platelet counts return to satisfactory levels, usually within a week after the nadir.

Special precautions are recommended in patients who develop thrombocytopenia as a result of administration of dacarbazine. These may include extra care in performing invasive procedures, regular inspection of intravenous sites, skin (including perirectal area), and mucous

membrane surfaces for signs of bleeding or bruising; limiting frequency of venipuncture and avoiding intramuscular injections; testing urine, emesis, stool, and secretions for occult blood; care in use of regular toothbrushes, dental floss, toothpicks, safety razors, and fingernail and toenail cutters; avoiding constipation; and using caution to prevent falls and other injuries. Such patients should avoid alcohol and aspirin intake because of the risk of gastrointestinal bleeding. Platelet transfusion may be required.

Patients who develop leukopenia should be observed carefully for signs of infection. Antibiotic support may be required. In neutropenic patients who develop fever, broad-spectrum antibiotic coverage should be initiated empirically, pending bacterial cultures and appropriate diagnostic tests.

## Safety considerations for handling this medication

There is limited but increasing evidence and concern that personnel involved in preparation and administration of parenteral antineoplastics may be at some risk because of the potential mutagenicity, teratogenicity, and/or carcinogenicity of these agents, although the actual risk is unknown. USP advisory panels recommend cautious handling both in preparation and disposal of antineoplastic agents. Precautions that have been suggested include:

• Use of a biological containment cabinet during reconstitution and dilution of parenteral medications and wearing of disposable surgical gloves and masks.

• Use of proper technique to prevent contamination of the medication, work area, and operator during transfer between containers (including proper training of personnel in this technique).

• Cautious and proper disposal of needles, syringes, vials, ampuls, and unused medication.

A number of medical centers have developed detailed guidelines for handling of antineoplastic agents.

## Combination chemotherapy

Dacarbazine may be used in combination with other agents in various regimens. As a result, incidence and/or severity of side effects may be altered and different dosages (usually reduced) may be used. For example, dacarbazine is part of the following chemotherapeutic combinations (some commonly used acronyms are in parentheses):

—doxorubicin, bleomycin, vinblastine, and dacarbazine (ABVD).

—cyclophosphamide, vincristine, doxorubicin, and dacarbazine (CY-VA-DIC).

For specific dosages and schedules, consult the literature. For information regarding each agent, consult the individual monographs.

# Parenteral Dosage Forms

## DACARBAZINE FOR INJECTION USP

### Usual adult dose

Melanoma, malignant—

Intravenous, 2 to 4.5 mg per kg of body weight a day for ten days; may be repeated every twenty-eight days, or

Intravenous, up to 250 mg per square meter of body surface a day for five days; may be repeated every twenty-one days.

Lymphomas, Hodgkin's[1]—

Intravenous, 150 mg per square meter of body surface a day for five days, in combination with other agents; may be repeated every twenty-eight days, or

Intravenous, 375 mg per square meter of body surface on Day 1, in combination with other agents, repeated every fifteen days.

Note: Dacarbazine may be as effective at the lower dosage as at the higher dosage.

Dacarbazine has also been administered as a single daily dose of 850 mg per square meter of body surface every twenty-one to forty-two days, with no apparent increase in hematologic toxicity, although extreme nausea and vomiting may occur.

### Usual pediatric dose

Dosage has not been established.

### Strength(s) usually available

U.S.—

100 mg (Rx) [*DTIC-Dome* (mannitol 37.5 mg); GENERIC (mannitol)].

200 mg (Rx) [*DTIC-Dome* (mannitol 75 mg); GENERIC (mannitol)].

Canada—

200 mg [*DTIC*].

### Packaging and storage

Store below 40 °C (104 °F), preferably between 15 and 30 °C (59 and 86 °F), unless otherwise specified by manufacturer. Protect from light.

### Preparation of dosage form

Dacarbazine for Injection USP may be prepared for parenteral use by adding 9.9 mL (100-mg vial), 19.7 mL (200-mg vial), or 49.5 mL

(500-mg vial) of sterile water for injection to the vial, producing a colorless or clear yellow solution containing 10 mg of dacarbazine per mL.

Reconstituted solutions may be further diluted with up to 250 mL of 5% dextrose injection or 0.9% sodium chloride injection for administration by intravenous infusion.

**Stability**

Reconstituted solutions of dacarbazine are stable for up to 72 hours at 4 °C (39 °F) or for up to 8 hours at normal room temperature (temperature and light). Solutions further diluted for administration by intravenous infusion are stable for up to 24 hours at 4 °C (39 °F) or for up to 8

hours at normal room conditions (temperature and light). A change in color of the solution to pink indicates decomposition.

[1]Not included in Canadian product labeling.

## Selected Bibliography

Dorr RT, Fritz WL. Cancer chemotherapy handbook. New York: Elsevier, 1980: 362-7.

Revised: 07/11/94

---

# DACTINOMYCIN  Systemic

VA CLASSIFICATION (Primary): AN200

Another commonly used name is actinomycin-D.

Note: For a listing of dosage forms and brand names by country availability, see *Dosage Forms* section(s). For a listing of brand names for the articles in this monograph, refer to the General Index.

## Category

Antineoplastic.

## Indications

Note: Bracketed information in the *Indications* section refers to uses that are not included in U.S. product labeling.

**Accepted**

Dactinomycin is indicated as a single agent for the following indication(s):
Ewing's sarcoma (treatment).
Sarcoma botryoides (treatment).
Tumors, trophoblastic (treatment).

Dactinomycin may be used in combination with other agents in various regimens. As a result, incidence and/or severity of side effects may be altered and different dosage (usually reduced) may be used. Dactinomycin is indicated in combination with other agents for the following indications (some selected examples of specific chemotherapeutic combinations containing dactinomycin, *not necessarily inclusive*, are also provided):
Carcinoma, endometrial (treatment) or
Tumors, trophoblastic (treatment) or
[Carcinoma, ovarian (treatment)][1]—In combination with one or more of the following: methotrexate, leucovorin, cyclophosphamide, hydroxyurea, vincristine, doxorubicin, etoposide.
  Examples of chemotherapeutic combinations:
  —dactinomycin and methotrexate. Used for treatment of metastatic and nonmetastatic choriocarcinoma.
  —methotrexate, dactinomycin, cyclophosphamide (MAC or MAC III). Used for treatment of gestational trophoblastic neoplasm.
  —cyclophosphamide, hydroxyurea, dactinomycin, methotrexate, vincristine, leucovorin, doxorubicin (CHAMOCA [Modified Bagshawe]). Used for treatment of gestational trophoblastic neoplasm.
  —etoposide, methotrexate, dactinomycin, leucovorin (EMA-CO [High Risk]). Used for treatment of gestational trophoblastic neoplasm.
Carcinoma, testicular (treatment)—In combination with cyclophosphamide, vinblastine, bleomycin, and cisplatin.
  Example of chemotherapeutic combination:
  —vinblastine, dactinomycin, bleomycin, cisplatin, cyclophosphamide (VAB-6).
Wilms' tumor (treatment)—In combination with one or more of the following: vincristine, doxorubicin, cyclophosphamide.
  Example of chemotherapeutic combination:
  —vincristine and dactinomycin.
Ewing's sarcoma (treatment)—In combination with one or more of the following: cyclophosphamide, doxorubicin, vincristine
  Examples of chemotherapeutic combinations:
  —doxorubicin, vincristine, dactinomycin, and cyclophosphamide (T-2 Protocol).
  —dactinomycin and cyclophosphamide.
Rhabdomyosarcoma (treatment)—In combination with vincristine and cyclophosphamide.
  Example of chemotherapeutic combination:
  —vincristine, dactinomycin, and cyclophosphamide (VAC).

[Sarcoma, Kaposi's (treatment)][1]—Examples of chemotherapeutic combinations:
  —doxorubicin, vinblastine, bleomycin, dacarbazine, vincristine, and dactinomycin.
  —vincristine, cyclophosphamide, and dactinomycin.
[Osteosarcoma (treatment)][1]—Examples of chemotherapeutic combinations:
  —cyclophosphamide, bleomycin, and dactinomycin.
  —high-dose methotrexate, leucovorin, doxorubicin, bleomycin, cyclophosphamide, cisplatin, and dactinomycin.
[Melanoma, malignant (treatment)][1]—In combination with one or more of the following: vincristine, cyclophosphamide, dacarbazine, carmustine, lomustine, procarbazine, vinblastine.
  Examples of chemotherapeutic combinations:
  —dactinomycin, vinblastine, procarbazine, lomustine, and vincristine.
  —dactinomycin, dacarbazine, carmustine, and lomustine.
  —dactinomycin, dacarbazine, and carmustine.
  —dactinomycin and dacarbazine.
For specific dosages and schedules, consult the literature. For information regarding each agent, consult the individual monograph.

**Unaccepted**

Although dactinomycin has antibacterial activity, its toxic effects preclude its use in the treatment of infectious diseases.

[1]Not included in Canadian product labeling.

## Pharmacology/Pharmacokinetics

**Physicochemical characteristics**

Molecular weight—1255.43.

**Mechanism of action/Effect**

Dactinomycin is classified as an antibiotic but is not used as an antimicrobial agent. Dactinomycin is considered to be cell cycle–phase nonspecific. Its antineoplastic action may involve binding to DNA by intercalation between base pairs and inhibition of DNA-dependent RNA synthesis.

**Other actions/effects**

Has some bacteriostatic activity on gram-positive and on gram-negative bacteria and on some fungi. Also has some immunosuppressant activity.

**Distribution**

Does not cross the blood-brain barrier.

**Protein binding**

Extensive tissue binding.

**Biotransformation**

Minimal.

**Half-life**

36 hours.

**Elimination**

Biliary/fecal—50% unchanged.
Renal—10% unchanged.
About 30% of a dose is recoverable in urine and feces in one week.

## Precautions to Consider

**Carcinogenicity/Mutagenicity**

Secondary malignancies are potential delayed effects of many antineoplastic agents, although it is not clear whether the effect is related to their mutagenic or immunosuppressive action. The effect of dose and duration of therapy is also unknown, although risk seems to increase with long-term use. Although information is limited, available data seem to indicate that the carcinogenic risk is greatest with the alkylating agents.

Dactinomycin is carcinogenic in mice and rats. Repeated subcutaneous or intraperitoneal injections produced local sarcomas in mice and rats. Intraperitoneal injections of 0.05 mg per kg of body weight (mg/kg) 2 to 5 times per week for 18 weeks in male F344 rats resulted in mesenchymal tumors, the first tumor appearing at 23 weeks.

Dactinomycin has been shown to be mutagenic in both *in vitro* and *in vivo* tests (human fibroblasts and leukocytes, HELA cells) and causes DNA damage and cytogenetic effects in mice and rats.

## Pregnancy/Reproduction

Fertility—Gonadal suppression, resulting in amenorrhea or azoospermia, may occur in patients taking antineoplastic therapy, especially with the alkylating agents. In general, these effects appear to be related to dose and length of therapy and may be irreversible. Prediction of the degree of testicular or ovarian function impairment is complicated by the common use of combinations of several antineoplastics, which makes it difficult to assess the effects of individual agents.

Pregnancy—Dactinomycin crosses the placenta. Adequate and well-controlled studies in humans have not been done.

First trimester: It is usually recommended that use of antineoplastics, especially combination chemotherapy, be avoided whenever possible, especially during the first trimester. Although information is limited because of the relatively few instances of antineoplastic administration during pregnancy, the mutagenic, teratogenic, and carcinogenic potential of these medications must be considered.

Other hazards to the fetus include adverse reactions seen in adults.

In general, use of a contraceptive is recommended during cytotoxic drug therapy.

Some studies in rats, rabbits, and hamsters have shown that dactinomycin causes malformations and embryotoxicity when given intravenously in doses of 50 to 100 mcg (0.05 to 0.1 mg) per kg of body weight (corresponding to 3 to 7 times the maximum recommended human dose).

FDA Pregnancy Category C.

## Breast-feeding

It is not known whether dactinomycin is distributed into breast milk. However, breast-feeding is not recommended while dactinomycin is being administered because of the risks to the infant (adverse effects, mutagenicity, carcinogenicity).

## Pediatrics

Because of the increased risk of toxicity in infants, dactinomycin should be used only in infants older than 6 to 12 months of age, unless potential benefit outweighs risk.

## Geriatrics

No information is available on the relationship of age to the effects of dactinomycin in geriatric patients.

## Dental

The bone marrow depressant effects of dactinomycin may result in an increased incidence of microbial infection, delayed healing, and gingival bleeding. Dental work, whenever possible, should be completed prior to initiation of therapy or deferred until blood counts have returned to normal. Patients should be instructed in proper oral hygiene during treatment, including caution in use of regular toothbrushes, dental floss, and toothpicks.

Dactinomycin commonly causes ulcerative stomatitis and pharyngitis associated with considerable discomfort. Sores often occur under the tongue.

## Drug interactions and/or related problems

The following drug interactions and/or related problems have been selected on the basis of their potential clinical significance (possible mechanism in parentheses where appropriate)—not necessarily inclusive (» = major clinical significance):

Note: Combinations containing any of the following medications, depending on the amount present, may also interact with this medication.

Allopurinol or
Colchicine or
» Probenecid or
» Sulfinpyrazone
    (dactinomycin may raise the concentration of blood uric acid; dosage adjustment of antigout agents may be necessary to control hyperuricemia and gout; allopurinol may be preferred because of risk of uric acid nephropathy with uricosuric antigout agents)

Blood dyscrasia–causing medications (See *Appendix II*)
    (leukopenic and/or thrombocytopenic effects of dactinomycin may be increased with concurrent or recent therapy if these medications

cause the same effects; dosage adjustment of dactinomycin, if necessary, should be based on blood counts)

» Bone marrow depressants, other (See *Appendix II*) or
» Radiation therapy
    (concurrent use with dactinomycin may potentiate the effects of these medications and radiation therapy, including gastrointestinal toxicity, bone marrow depression, and erythema and tanning of the skin; lower doses of each are recommended. Dactinomycin alone may reactivate erythema from previous radiation therapy)

Doxorubicin
    (concurrent or sequential use may result in increased cardiotoxicity; it is recommended that the total dose of doxorubicin not exceed 450 mg per square meter of body surface)

Vaccines, killed virus
    (because normal defense mechanisms may be suppressed by dactinomycin therapy, the patient's antibody response to the vaccine may be decreased. The interval between discontinuation of medications that cause immunosuppression and restoration of the patient's ability to respond to the vaccine depends on the intensity and type of immunosuppression-causing medication used, the underlying disease, and other factors; estimates vary from 3 months to 1 year)

» Vaccines, live virus
    (because normal defense mechanisms may be suppressed by dactinomycin therapy, concurrent use with a live virus vaccine may potentiate the replication of the vaccine virus, may increase the side/adverse effects of the vaccine virus, and/or may decrease the patient's antibody response to the vaccine; immunization of these patients should be undertaken only with extreme caution after careful review of the patient's hematologic status and only with the knowledge and consent of the physician managing the dactinomycin therapy. The interval between discontinuation of medications that cause immunosuppression and restoration of the patient's ability to respond to the vaccine depends on the intensity and type of immunosuppression-causing medication used, the underlying disease, and other factors; estimates vary from 3 months to 1 year. Patients with leukemia in remission should not receive live virus vaccine until at least 3 months after their last chemotherapy. In addition, immunization with oral poliovirus vaccine should be postponed in persons in close contact with the patient, especially family members)

Vitamin K
    (concurrent use with dactinomycin may decrease the effects of vitamin K, although evidence is inconclusive; observation of patients is recommended and a higher dose of vitamin K may be required)

## Laboratory value alterations

The following have been selected on the basis of their potential clinical significance (possible effect in parentheses where appropriate)—not necessarily inclusive (» = major clinical significance):

With diagnostic test results
    Bioassay procedures for determinations of antibacterial drug concentrations
    (may be interfered with)

With physiology/laboratory test values
    Hepatic enzymes
    (serum values may rarely be increased)

    Uric acid concentrations in blood and urine
    (may be increased)

## Medical considerations/Contraindications

The medical considerations/contraindications included here have been selected on the basis of their potential clinical significance (reasons given in parentheses where appropriate)—not necessarily inclusive (» = major clinical significance).

### Risk-benefit should be considered when the following medical problems exist:

» Bone marrow depression

» Chickenpox, existing or recent (including recent exposure) or
» Herpes zoster
    (risk of severe generalized disease)

Gout, history of or
Urate renal stones, history of
    (risk of hyperuricemia)

» Hepatic function impairment
    (some clinicians recommend reduction of dosage by one-third or one-half in patients with hyperbilirubinemia)

» Infection
    Sensitivity to dactinomycin

» Caution should be used also in patients who have had previous cytotoxic drug therapy or radiation therapy.

**Patient monitoring**

The following are especially important in patient monitoring (other tests may be warranted in some patients, depending on condition; (» = major clinical significance):

Alanine aminotransferase (ALT [SGPT]) values, serum and
Aspartate aminotransferase (AST [SGOT]) values, serum and
Bilirubin values, serum and
Lactate dehydrogenase (LDH) values, serum

(recommended prior to initiation of therapy and at periodic intervals during therapy; frequency varies according to clinical state, agent, dose, and other agents being used concurrently)

» Checking patient's mouth for ulceration

(recommended before administration of each dose)

» Hematocrit or hemoglobin and
» Leukocyte count, total and, if appropriate, differential and
» Platelet count

(determinations recommended prior to initiation of therapy and at periodic intervals during therapy; frequency varies according to clinical state, agent, dose, and other agents being used concurrently)

Uric acid concentrations, serum

(recommended prior to initiation of therapy and at periodic intervals during therapy; frequency varies according to clinical state, agent, dose, and other agents being used concurrently)

## Side/Adverse Effects

Note: Many "side effects" of antineoplastic therapy are unavoidable and represent the medication's pharmacologic action. Some of these (for example, leukopenia and thrombocytopenia) are actually used as parameters to aid in individual dosage titration.

Most side effects appear 2 to 4 days after a course is completed and may not be maximal for 1 to 2 weeks.

Combination therapy with radiation may be associated with more frequent and severe side effects of the radiation, including gastric distress and inflammation of mucous membranes at the irradiated site. Severe reactions may occur if high dosages are used. Hepatotoxicity (hepatomegaly, increased serum aspartate aminotransferase [AST (SGOT)], ascites) has occurred when dactinomycin was used within the first 2 months after radiation therapy for right-sided Wilms' tumor.

Complications associated with use of isolation-perfusion administration are mainly related to how much medication reaches the systemic circulation and may include myelosuppression, absorption of toxic products from massive neoplastic tissue destruction, increased risk of infection, impaired wound healing, and superficial gastric mucosal ulceration. Other potential side/adverse effects include edema of the extremity involved, soft tissue damage in the exposed area, and venous thrombosis.

The following side/adverse effects have been selected on the basis of their potential clinical significance (possible signs and symptoms in parentheses where appropriate)—not necessarily inclusive:

**Those indicating need for medical attention**

Incidence more frequent

*Anemia, possibly progressing to aplastic anemia; esophagitis* (difficulty in swallowing; heartburn); *gastrointestinal ulceration or proctitis* (black, tarry stools; continuing diarrhea; continuing stomach pain); *leukopenia* (usually asymptomatic; less frequently, fever or chills, cough or hoarseness, lower back or side pain, painful or difficult urination) *or thrombocytopenia* (usually asymptomatic; less frequently, unusual bleeding or bruising; black, tarry stools; blood in urine or stools; pinpoint red spots on skin); *ulcerative stomatitis or pharyngitis* (sores in mouth and on lips)

Note: *Bone marrow depression* occurs approximately 7 to 10 days after a course of therapy, with the nadir at about 3 weeks and recovery within about 3 weeks. It may be severe and progress to pancytopenia and agranulocytosis, which are potentially fatal.

With *ulcerative stomatitis,* sores often occur under the tongue.

Incidence rare

*Anaphylaxis* (wheezing); *cellulitis or phlebitis* (pain at injection site); *hepatotoxicity, including ascites, hepatomegaly, hepatitis, and hepatic function test abnormalities* (yellow eyes or skin); *hyperuricemia or uric acid nephropathy* (joint pain; lower back or side pain; swelling of feet or lower legs)

Note: *Hepatotoxicity* is usually reversible, but fatalities have been reported.

*Hyperuricemia or uric acid nephropathy* occurs most commonly during initial treatment of patients with leukemia or lymphoma, as a result of rapid cell breakdown which leads to elevated serum uric acid concentrations.

**Those indicating need for medical attention only if they continue or are bothersome**

Incidence more frequent

*Darkening of skin*—if patient has received previous radiation therapy; *nausea and vomiting; redness of skin; skin rash or acne; unusual tiredness*

Note: *Nausea and vomiting* occur during the first few hours after administration, and may last 4 to 20 hours.

**Those not indicating need for medical attention**

Incidence more frequent

*Loss of hair*

Note: *Loss of hair* usually begins 7 to 10 days after administration and may involve scalp and eyebrows.

**Those indicating the need for medical attention if they occur after medication is discontinued**

*Bone marrow depression* (black, tarry stools; blood in urine or stools; cough or hoarseness; fever or chills; lower back or side pain; painful or difficult urination; pinpoint red spots on skin; unusual bleeding or bruising); *gastrointestinal ulceration* (black, tarry stools; diarrhea; stomach pain); *hepatotoxicity* (yellow eyes or skin); *stomatitis* (sores in mouth and on lips)

## Patient Consultation

As an aid to patient consultation, refer to *Advice for the Patient, Dactinomycin (Systemic).*

In providing consultation, consider emphasizing the following selected information (» = major clinical significance):

**Before using this medication**

» Conditions affecting use, especially:

Sensitivity to dactinomycin

Pregnancy—Use not recommended because of mutagenic, teratogenic, and carcinogenic potential; advisability of using contraception; telling physician immediately if pregnancy is suspected

Breast-feeding—Not recommended because of risk of serious side effects

Use in children—Not recommended in infants less than 6 to 12 months of age

Other medications, especially probenecid, sulfinpyrazone, other bone marrow depressants, or previous cytotoxic drug or radiation therapy

Other medical problems, especially chickenpox, herpes zoster, hepatic function impairment, or infection

**Proper use of this medication**

Caution in taking combination therapy; taking each medication at the right time

Frequency of nausea and vomiting; importance of continuing medication despite stomach upset

» Proper dosing

**Precautions while using this medication**

» Importance of close monitoring by physician

» Avoiding immunizations unless approved by physician; other persons in patient's household should avoid immunizations with oral poliovirus vaccine; avoiding persons who have taken oral poliovirus vaccine or wearing a protective mask that covers nose and mouth

*Caution if bone marrow depression occurs:*

» Avoiding exposure to persons with bacterial infections, especially during periods of low blood counts; checking with physician immediately if fever or chills, cough or hoarseness, lower back or side pain, or painful or difficult urination occur

» Checking with physician immediately if unusual bleeding or bruising; black, tarry stools; blood in urine or stools; or pinpoint red spots on skin occur

Caution in use of regular toothbrush, dental floss, or toothpick; physician, dentist, or nurse may suggest alternatives; checking with physician before having dental work done

Not touching eyes or inside of nose unless hands washed immediately before

Using caution to avoid accidental cuts with use of sharp objects such as safety razor or fingernail or toenail cutters

Avoiding contact sports or other situations where bruising or injury could occur

» Possibility of local tissue injury and scarring if infiltration of intravenous solution occurs; telling physician or nurse right away about redness, pain, or swelling at injection site

**Side/adverse effects**

May cause adverse effects such as blood problems, loss of hair, and cancer; importance of discussing possible effects with physician

Signs of potential side effects, especially anemia, esophagitis, gastrointestinal ulceration, proctitis, leukopenia, thrombocytopenia, ulcerative stomatitis, pharyngitis, anaphylaxis, cellulitis, phlebitis, hepatotoxicity, hyperuricemia, and uric acid nephropathy

Physician or nurse can help in dealing with side effects

Possibility of hair loss; normal hair growth should return after treatment has ended

## General Dosing Information

It is recommended that dactinomycin be administered only under supervision of a physician experienced in cancer chemotherapy.

A variety of dosage schedules and regimens of dactinomycin, alone or in combination with other antitumor agents, are used. The prescriber may consult the medical literature as well as the manufacturer's literature in choosing a specific dosage.

Dosage must be adjusted to meet the individual requirements of each patient, based on size and location of the neoplasm, clinical response, and appearance or severity of toxicity.

A lower dosage of dactinomycin (based on body surface area) and daily observation for toxicity is recommended for obese patients, especially if they are receiving dactinomycin by regional isolation perfusion; calculation of dosage on the basis of surface area (i.e., to relate dosage to lean body mass) is recommended. A lower dosage is also recommended for those who are receiving or have received within 3 to 6 weeks other antineoplastic chemotherapy or radiation therapy.

Intravenous fluid therapy and administration of allopurinol for 4 to 5 days may be necessary during a period of severe oral toxicity (i.e., if the patient cannot drink) to prevent hyperuricemia and hyperuricuria resulting from tumor regression.

It is recommended that dactinomycin be given no later than the first 5 to 7 days of radiation therapy because of the risk of severe vesiculation.

Dactinomycin must be given in short intermittent courses to avoid serious toxicity, which may not appear until 2 to 4 days after the last dose and may not be maximal for 1 to 2 weeks.

Reconstituted solutions of dactinomycin may be injected slowly into the tubing of a running intravenous infusion or diluted for administration by intravenous infusion over 10 to 15 minutes in 5% dextrose injection or 0.9% sodium chloride injection.

Prescribers should consult the medical literature in choosing a dosage and technique for isolation-perfusion administration.

Care should be taken to avoid contact of dactinomycin, which is very corrosive, with soft tissues. In at least one case, extravasation has led to contracture of the arms. If the medication is given directly into the vein rather than by infusion, one sterile needle should be used for reconstituting and withdrawing the dose from the vial and another for administration.

If extravasation of dactinomycin occurs during intravenous administration, the injection or infusion should be stopped immediately and the remaining dose given via another vein, care being taken to avoid soft tissue contact.

Systemic absorption of toxic products from neoplastic tissue destruction during administration of dactinomycin by isolation-perfusion can be minimized by removing the perfusate after the procedure.

If marked leukopenia (particularly granulocytopenia), thrombocytopenia, diarrhea, or stomatitis occurs, dactinomycin therapy should be withdrawn immediately. When leukocyte and platelet counts return to satisfactory levels and the patient has recovered, therapy may be reinstituted.

Special precautions are recommended in patients who develop thrombocytopenia as a result of administration of dactinomycin. These may include extreme care in performing invasive procedures; regular inspection of intravenous sites, skin (including perirectal area), and mucous membrane surfaces for signs of bleeding or bruising; limiting frequency of venipuncture and avoiding intramuscular injections; testing urine, emesis, stool, and secretions for occult blood; care in use of regular toothbrushes, dental floss, toothpicks, safety razors, and fingernail and toenail cutters; avoiding constipation; and using caution to prevent falls and other injuries. Such patients should avoid alcohol and aspirin intake because of the risk of gastrointestinal bleeding. Platelet transfusions may be required.

Patients who develop leukopenia should be observed carefully for signs of infection. Antibiotic support may be required. In neutropenic patients who develop fever, broad-spectrum antibiotic coverage should be initiated empirically, pending bacterial cultures and appropriate diagnostic tests.

**Safety considerations for handling this medication**

There is limited but increasing evidence and concern that personnel involved in preparation and administration of parenteral antineoplastics may be at some risk because of the potential mutagenicity, teratogenicity, and/or carcinogenicity of these agents, although the actual risk is unknown. USP advisory panels recommend cautious handling both in preparation and disposal of antineoplastic agents. Precautions that have been suggested include:

• Use of a biological containment cabinet during reconstitution and dilution of parenteral medications and wearing of disposable surgical gloves and masks.

• Use of proper technique to prevent contamination of the medication, work area, and operator during transfer between containers (including proper training of personnel in this technique).

• Cautious and proper disposal of needles, syringes, vials, ampuls, and unused medication.

A number of medical centers have developed detailed guidelines for handling of antineoplastic agents.

## Parenteral Dosage Forms

Note: Bracketed uses in the *Dosage Forms* section refer to categories of use and/or indications that are not included in U.S. product labeling.

### DACTINOMYCIN FOR INJECTION USP

**Usual adult dose**

Carcinoma, testicular or
Carcinoma, endometrial or
Tumors, trophoblastic or
Wilms' tumor or
[Carcinoma, ovarian][1] or
Rhabdomyosarcoma or
Ewing's sarcoma or
Sarcoma botryoides—

     Intravenous, 10 to 15 mcg (0.01 to 0.015 mg) per kg of body weight a day for a maximum of five days every four to six weeks or

     Intravenous, 500 mcg (0.5 mg) per square meter of body surface once a week (maximum 2 mg a week) for three weeks.

Ewing's sarcoma or
Sarcoma botryoides—

     Isolation-perfusion, 50 mcg (0.05 mg) per kg of body weight for lower extremity or pelvis, or 35 mcg (0.035 mg) per kg of body weight for upper extremity.

Note: Dosage should be based on body surface area in obese or edematous patients.

**Usual adult prescribing limits**

Up to 15 mcg (0.015 mg) per kg of body weight or 400 to 600 mcg (0.4 to 0.6 mg) per square meter of body surface per day for five days.

**Usual pediatric dose**

Carcinoma, testicular or
Carcinoma, endometrial or
Tumors, trophoblastic or
Wilms' tumor or
[Carcinoma, ovarian][1] or
Rhabdomyosarcoma or
Ewing's sarcoma or
Sarcoma botryoides—

     Intravenous, 10 to 15 mcg (0.01 to 0.015 mg) per kg of body weight a day or 450 mcg (0.45 mg) per square meter of body surface per day (up to 500 mcg [0.5 mg] per day) for a maximum of five days, or a total dose of 2.5 mg per square meter of body surface in divided daily doses over a seven-day period. A second course may be given after four to six weeks, provided all signs of toxicity have disappeared.

Ewing's sarcoma or
Sarcoma botryoides—

     Isolation-perfusion, 50 mcg (0.05 mg) per kg of body weight for lower extremity or pelvis, or 35 mcg (0.035 mg) per kg of body weight for upper extremity.

Note: Because of the increased risk of toxicity in infants, dactinomycin should be used only in infants older than 6 to 12 months.

**Usual pediatric prescribing limits**

Up to 15 mcg (0.015 mg) per kg of body weight or 400 to 600 mcg (0.4 to 0.6 mg) per square meter of body surface per day for five days.

**Strength(s) usually available**

U.S.—

500 mcg (0.5 mg) (Rx) [*Cosmegen* (mannitol 20 mg)].

Canada—

500 mcg (0.5 mg) (Rx) [*Cosmegen* (mannitol 20 mg)].

**Packaging and storage**

Store below 30 °C (85 °F), unless otherwise specified by manufacturer. Transient temperatures (i.e., for a period not exceeding two weeks) of up to 50 °C (122 °F) are permissible. Protect from light.

**Preparation of dosage form**

Dactinomycin for Injection USP is reconstituted for use by adding 1.1 mL of sterile water for injection (without preservative) to the vial, producing a clear, gold-colored solution containing 500 mcg (0.5 mg) of dactinomycin per mL. Use of sodium chloride injection or water for injection containing preservatives (benzyl alcohol, parabens) for reconstitution results in precipitation.

Reconstituted solutions of dactinomycin may be diluted in 5% dextrose injection or 0.9% sodium chloride injection for administration by intravenous infusion.

**Stability**

Discard any unused portion of reconstituted dactinomycin solutions.

**Note**

Great care should be taken to prevent inhalation of particles of Dactinomycin for Injection USP and exposure of skin to it. If accidental eye contact occurs, immediate copious irrigation with water, followed by an ophthalmologic consultation, is recommended; if accidental skin contact occurs, irrigation with water for at least 15 minutes is recommended.

Use of some intravenous in-line filters containing cellulose ester membrane filters has been reported to partially remove dactinomycin from intravenous solution.

---

[1]Not included in Canadian product labeling.

**Selected Bibliography**

Dorr RT. Fritz WL. Cancer chemotherapy handbook. New York: Elsevier, 1980: 368-72.

Revised: 07/11/94

---

# DANAZOL    Systemic

VA CLASSIFICATION (Primary/Secondary): HS100/IM900

Note: For a listing of dosage forms and brand names by country availability, see *Dosage Forms* section(s). For a listing of brand names for the articles in this monograph, refer to the General Index.

## Category

Gonadotropin inhibitor; angioedema (hereditary) prophylactic.

## Indications

Note: Bracketed information in the *Indications* section refers to uses that are not included in U.S. product labeling.

**Accepted**

Endometriosis (treatment)—Danazol is indicated for the treatment of pain and/or infertility due to endometriosis.

Breast disease, fibrocystic (treatment)—Danazol is indicated for the treatment of fibrocystic breast disease in patients whose symptoms are not relieved by analgesics, the use of well-fitted bras, or other simple methods.

Angioedema, hereditary (prophylaxis)[1]—Danazol is indicated for the prophylactic treatment of hereditary angioedema (cutaneous, abdominal, and laryngeal) in males and females, including prior to surgery.

[Gynecomastia (treatment)][1]

[Menorrhagia (treatment)][1] or

[Puberty, precocious (treatment)][1]—Danazol is being used to treat gynecomastia, menorrhagia, and precocious puberty in females.

---

[1]Not included in Canadian product labeling.

## Pharmacology/Pharmacokinetics

**Physicochemical characteristics**

Chemical group—Synthetic androgen.

Molecular weight—337.46.

**Mechanism of action/Effect**

Gonadotropin inhibitor—May suppress the pituitary-ovarian axis by inhibiting the output of pituitary gonadotropins. Danazol depresses the preovulatory surge in output of follicle-stimulating hormone (FSH) and luteinizing hormone (LH) and therefore reduces ovarian estrogen production. Danazol may also directly inhibit ovarian steroidogenesis, bind to androgen, progesterone, and glucocorticoid receptors, bind to sex-hormone–binding globulin and corticosteroid-binding globulin, and increase the metabolic clearance rate of progesterone.

Endometriosis—As a consequence of suppression of ovarian function, both normal and ectopic endometrial tissues become inactive and atrophic. As a result, anovulation and associated amenorrhea occur.

Fibrocystic breast disease—Exact mechanism of action is unknown, but may be related to suppressed estrogenic stimulation as a result of decreased ovarian production of estrogen; a direct effect on steroid receptor sites in breast tissue is also possible. Disappearance of nodularity, relief of pain and tenderness, and possibly changes in the menstrual pattern result.

Hereditary angioedema—Correction of the underlying biochemical deficiency: Increases serum levels of C1 esterase inhibitor, resulting in increased serum levels of the C4 component of the complement system.

**Other actions/effects**

Weak androgenic effects.

**Biotransformation**

Hepatic, to inactive metabolites.

**Half-life**

Approximately 4.5 hours (variable).

**Onset of action**

Fibrocystic breast disease—Relief of breast pain and tenderness usually begins within 1 month.

**Peak serum concentration**

Following 100-mg dose twice a day—200 to 800 nanograms per mL.

Following 200-mg dose twice a day for 14 days—250 nanograms to 2 mcg per mL.

**Time to peak effect**

Anovulation and amenorrhea—Usually occur after 6 to 8 weeks of therapy.

Fibrocystic breast disease—Breast pain and tenderness are usually eliminated in 2 to 3 months of therapy. Elimination of nodularity usually requires 4 to 6 months of uninterrupted therapy.

**Duration of action**

Anovulation and amenorrhea—Ovulation and cyclic bleeding usually return within 60 to 90 days after therapy is withdrawn.

Fibrocystic breast disease—Symptoms return to some degree within 1 year after therapy is withdrawn in 50% of patients.

**Elimination**

Renal.

## Precautions to Consider

**Pregnancy/Reproduction**

Pregnancy—Danazol is contraindicated during pregnancy. Continuing treatment may result in an androgenic effect (clitoral hypertrophy, labial fusion of the external genitalia, urogenital sinus defect, vaginal atresia, ambiguous genitalia) on the female fetus.

**Breast-feeding**

Nursing mothers should be advised to contact physician before nursing infants. Use by nursing mothers is not recommended because of possible androgenic effects in the infant, such as precocious sexual development in males and virilization in females.

**Pediatrics**

Caution is recommended in children and growing adolescents who are being treated for hereditary angioedema because of possible androgenic effects, such as precocious sexual development in males and virilization in females. Premature epiphyseal closure may also occur.

**Geriatrics**

No information is available on the relationship of age to the effects of danazol in geriatric patients.

Treatment of geriatric male patients with androgens may cause increased risk of prostatic hypertrophy or prostatic carcinoma.

**Drug interactions and/or related problems**

The following drug interactions and/or related problems have been selected on the basis of their potential clinical significance (possible mechanism in parentheses where appropriate)—not necessarily inclusive (» = major clinical significance):

» Anticoagulants, coumarin- or indandione-derivative

   (concurrent use with danazol may enhance effects of anticoagulants because of decreased hepatic synthesis of procoagulant factors, and may cause bleeding)

   Antidiabetic agents, oral or
   Insulin

   (danazol may increase blood glucose concentrations and resistance to insulin due to changes in metabolism of carbohydrates)

   Cyclosporine

   (danazol has been reported to increase plasma concentrations of cyclosporine and may increase the risk of nephrotoxicity)

**Laboratory value alterations**

The following have been selected on the basis of their potential clinical significance (possible effect in parentheses where appropriate)—not necessarily inclusive (» = major clinical significance):

With physiology/laboratory test values

   Alanine aminotransferase (ALT [SGPT]) or
   Aspartate aminotransferase (AST [SGOT])

   (serum concentrations may be increased early in therapy and decrease toward baseline later in therapy; generally return to baseline within one month following therapy)

   Aldosase or
   Creatine kinase (CK)

   (concentrations may be increased in presence of muscle toxicity or rhabdomyolysis)

   Blood pressure

   (may be increased as a result of volume expansion)

   Cholic acid concentration, serum or
   Cholic acid-to-chenodeoxycholic acid serum concentrations ratio

   (fasting levels may be increased during therapy; generally return to baseline within one month following therapy)

   Glucose, blood concentrations or
   Lipoproteins, low-density

   (concentrations may be increased)

   Glucose tolerance

   (may be impaired)

   Lipoproteins, high-density

   (concentrations may be decreased)

   Thyroid function tests

   (may decrease total serum thyroxine [$T_4$] and increase triiodothyroxine [$T_3$] uptake; however, free $T_4$ and thyroid-stimulating hormone [TSH] remain normal because of a concomitant decrease in thyroid-binding globulin [TBG])

**Medical considerations/Contraindications**

The medical considerations/contraindications included here have been selected on the basis of their potential clinical significance (reasons given in parentheses where appropriate)—not necessarily inclusive (» = major clinical significance).

*Risk-benefit should be considered when the following medical problems exist:*

   Cardiac function impairment or
   Epilepsy or
   Migraine headaches or
   Renal function impairment

   (may be aggravated by fluid retention induced by danazol)

» Cardiac function impairment, severe

   Diabetes mellitus

   (possible impairment of glucose tolerance)

» Hepatic function impairment, severe

» Renal function impairment, severe

   Sensitivity to anabolic steroids, androgens, or danazol

» Vaginal bleeding, undiagnosed abnormal

**Patient monitoring**

The following may be especially important in patient monitoring (other tests may be warranted in some patients, depending on condition; » = major clinical significance):

   Biopsy of cysts or
   Mammography

   (recommended prior to initiation of treatment for fibrocystic breast disease to rule out carcinoma; recommended during treatment if nodules persist or enlarge)

» Hepatic function determinations

   (recommended at periodic intervals during therapy)

   Pregnancy test

   (recommended if treatment of endometriosis or fibrocystic breast disease not started during menstruation or in patients with irregular cycles)

   Semen volume and viscosity determinations and
   Sperm count and motility determinations

   (recommended every 3 to 4 months, especially in adolescents)

## Side/Adverse Effects

The following side/adverse effects have been selected on the basis of their potential clinical significance (possible signs and symptoms in parentheses where appropriate)—not necessarily inclusive:

**Those indicating need for medical attention**

Incidence more frequent

   *In females*

   *Amenorrhea* (stopping of menstrual periods); *breakthrough bleeding* (heavier, irregular vaginal bleeding between regular menses); *spotting* (lighter, irregular vaginal bleeding between regular menses); *decreased breast size; irregular menstrual periods; weight gain*

   Note: *Amenorrhea* occurs in most patients treated for endometriosis. Also occurs in 50% of patients treated for fibrocystic breast disease with doses of 100 mg or more; anovulation may not occur. Amenorrhea may be prolonged after danazol therapy is discontinued in any patient.

   *Breakthrough bleeding* or *spotting* may occur in first few months of therapy for endometriosis; does not necessarily indicate lack of efficacy.

   *Irregular menstrual periods* occur in 25% of patients treated for fibrocystic breast disease; anovulation may not occur.

Incidence less frequent

   *In both females and males*

   *Edema* (rapid weight gain; swelling of feet or lower legs)—dose-related; *rhabdomyolysis* (muscle cramps or spasms; unusual tiredness or weakness); *virilism* (acne; oily skin; oily hair)—dose-related

Incidence rare

   *In both females and males*

   *Bladder telangiectasia* (blood in urine); *bleeding gums; carpal tunnel syndrome* (pain, numbness, tingling or burning in all fingers except smallest finger); *cataracts* (gradual blurring or loss of vision); *cholestatic jaundice*—has occurred during long-term treatment with other 17-alkylated androgens; *discharge from nipple; eosinophilia* (general feeling of illness; sudden coughing episodes); *hepatic dysfunction* (yellow eyes or skin)—with doses greater than 400 mg of danazol per day; *intracranial hypertension, benign* (severe headache; decrease in vision; double vision; vomiting); *leukocytosis* (sore throat; headache; general feeling of illness; chills; eye pain; cough; unusual tiredness); *pancreatitis, acute* (sudden, severe, continuing pain in upper or middle of abdomen; nausea; vomiting; unusual tiredness; bloating and tenderness of abdomen; fever; fast heartbeat; transient yellow eyes or skin color); *peliosis hepatis* (dark-colored urine; hives; light-colored stools; continuing loss of appetite; purple- or red-colored spots on body or inside the mouth or nose; sore throat; fever; nausea; vomiting)—has occurred during long-term treatment with other 17-alkylated androgens; *polyneuritis, acute idiopathic* (tingling sensation or weakness in both legs, moving upward to both arms, trunk and face; numbness); *skin rashes; Stevens-Johnson syndrome* (lesions on skin and inside the mouth or nose; fever; general feeling of illness; cough; sore throat; chest pain; vomiting; diarrhea; joint pain; muscle aches); *thrombocytopenia* (unusual bruising or bleeding; more frequent nosebleeds; heavier menstrual periods)

   *In females only*

   *Virilism* (enlarged clitoris; hoarseness or deepening of voice; unnatural hair growth)—dose related

*In males only*
   ***Testicular atrophy*** (decrease in testicle size)

**Those indicating need for medical attention only if they continue
or are bothersome**
Incidence less frequent
   *In both females and males*
      ***Hypoestrogenism*** (flushing or redness of skin; mood or mental
      changes; nervousness; sweating)

Incidence rare
   *In both females and males*
      ***Photosensitivity***

   *In females only*
      ***Monilial vaginitis*** (burning, dryness, or itching of vagina; vaginal
      bleeding)—hypoestrogenic effect

## Patient Consultation

As an aid to patient consultation, refer to *Advice for the Patient, Danazol
(Systemic)*.

In providing consultation, consider emphasizing the following selected
information (» = major clinical significance):

**Before using this medication**
» Conditions affecting use, especially:
   Sensitivity to anabolic steroids, androgens, or danazol
   Pregnancy—Use is not recommended during pregnancy because
      of possible androgenic effects on female fetus
   Breast-feeding—Use is usually not recommended because of pos-
      sible androgenic effects in the infant
   Use in children—Caution is recommended because of possible an-
      drogenic effects
   Other medications, especially coumarin- or indandione-derivative
      anticoagulants
   Other medical problems, especially severe cardiac function im-
      pairment, undiagnosed abnormal vaginal bleeding, severe he-
      patic function impairment, or severe renal function impairment

**Proper use of this medication**
» Taking for full time of therapy
» Proper dosing
   Missed dose: Taking as soon as possible; not taking if almost time for
      next dose; not doubling doses
» Proper storage

**Precautions while using this medication**
   Regular visits to physician to check progress during therapy
   Diabetics: May alter blood sugar levels
» Possible photosensitivity reactions: caution during exposure to sun or
      when using sunlamps, tanning booths or beds
   *For treatment of endometriosis or fibrocystic breast disease*
   Possibility of amenorrhea or irregular menstrual periods; checking
      with physician if regular menstruation does not occur within 60 to
      90 days after discontinuation of medication
   Advisability of using nonhormonal forms of contraception during ther-
      apy; not using oral contraceptives
» Stopping medication and checking with physician if pregnancy is
      suspected

**Side/adverse effects**
   Signs of potential side effects, especially edema, virilism in females,
      liver dysfunction, peliosis hepatis, polyneuritis, pancreatitis, carpal
      tunnel syndrome, hematologic disorders, Stevens-Johnson syn-
      drome, cataracts, intracranial hypertension, bladder telangiectasia,
      testicular atrophy, and irregular menstrual periods

## General Dosing Information

In the treatment of endometriosis and fibrocystic breast disease, it is recommended that therapy begin with the first day of the menstrual cycle
after pregnancy has been ruled out.

Development of amenorrhea is usually evidence of a clinical response to
danazol in the treatment of endometriosis, although spotting or bleeding from the atrophic endometrium can still occur.

In the treatment of endometriosis, therapy should be continued uninterrupted for 3 to 6 months, and may be continued for 9 months if
necessary.

Dosage requirements for continuous treatment of hereditary angioedema
should be individualized on the basis of the patient's clinical response.

It is recommended that danazol treatment be discontinued if signs of virilization (which may not be reversible) occur.

## Oral Dosage Forms

### DANAZOL CAPSULES USP

**Usual adult and adolescent dose**
Endometriosis—
   Moderate to severe: Oral, 400 mg two times a day (beginning Day 1
      of menstruation, if possible) for at least three to six months, and
      may be continued for nine months if necessary.
   Mild: Oral, 100 to 200 mg two times a day (beginning Day 1 of
      menstruation, if possible) for at least three to six months, and may
      be continued for nine months if necessary.
   Note: If symptoms recur after discontinuation of therapy, therapy may
      be reinstituted.
Fibrocystic breast disease—
   Oral, 50 to 200 mg two times a day (beginning Day 1 of menstruation,
      if possible).
   Note: If symptoms recur within one year of discontinuation of ther-
      apy, therapy may be reinstituted.
Angioedema (hereditary) prophylactic[1]—
   Oral, initially 200 mg two or three times a day until the desired initial
      response is obtained; then the maintenance dosage is determined
      by decreasing the initial dosage by 50% or less at intervals of one
      to three months or longer, depending on frequency of attacks prior
      to treatment.
   Note: Daily dosage may be increased by up to 200 mg if condition is
      not controlled at lower doses.

**Usual adult prescribing limits**
Oral, 800 mg per day.

**Usual pediatric dose**
Dosage has not been established.

**Strength(s) usually available**
U.S.—
   50 mg (Rx) [*Danocrine* (benzyl alcohol; lactose; parabens)].
   100 mg (Rx) [*Danocrine* (benzyl alcohol; lactose; parabens)].
   200 mg (Rx) [*Danocrine* (benzyl alcohol; lactose; parabens);
      GENERIC].
Canada—
   50 mg (Rx) [*Cyclomen* (lactose)].
   100 mg (Rx) [*Cyclomen* (lactose)].
   200 mg (Rx) [*Cyclomen* (lactose)].

**Packaging and storage**
Store below 40 °C (104 °F), preferably between 15 and 30 °C (59 and 86
°F), unless otherwise specified by manufacturer. Store in a well-closed
container.

[1]Not included in Canadian product labeling.

Revised: 06/15/93

## DANTHRON-CONTAINING COMBINATIONS—

Danthron and Docusate (Oral-Local)—See *Laxatives (Local)*

# DANTROLENE   Systemic

VA CLASSIFICATION (Primary): MS200
Note: For a listing of dosage forms and brand names by country availability, see *Dosage Forms* section(s). For a listing of brand names for the articles in this monograph, refer to the General Index.

## Category

Malignant hyperthermia therapy adjunct; Antispastic; Neuroleptic malignant syndrome therapy adjunct; Muscle phosphorylase deficiency therapy adjunct; Duchenne muscular dystrophy therapy adjunct.

## Indications

Note: Bracketed information in the *Indications* section refers to uses that are not included in U.S. product labeling.

### Accepted

Hyperthermia, malignant (prophylaxis and treatment adjunct)—Intravenous dantrolene is indicated to reverse the symptoms of the malignant hyperthermic crisis syndrome occurring during or following surgery or anesthesia. However, dantrolene is not a substitute for other measures, including discontinuation of possible triggering agents (such as potent inhalation anesthetics, succinylcholine, or stress), management of increased oxygen requirements and metabolic acidosis, institution of cooling, and correction of fluid and electrolyte imbalances. Oral or intravenous dantrolene is indicated as a follow-up to initial intravenous therapy to prevent recurrence of symptoms, but caution in such use is recommended.

Dantrolene is also indicated for administration prior to surgery or anesthesia to prevent or attenuate the symptoms of the malignant hyperthermic crisis syndrome in patients known or suspected to be at risk for this complication. However, preliminary evidence suggests that prophylactic use of dantrolene is not necessary for most patients, provided that careful patient management procedures are followed (including avoiding known triggering agents during surgery, careful monitoring intra- and postoperatively, and administering intravenous dantrolene if symptoms of malignant hyperthermia develop). Perioperative complications (such as atelectasis, retained secretions, diminished swallow and gag reflexes, impaired postoperative ventilation requiring prolonged endotracheal intubation, and delayed or difficult postoperative ambulation), possibly associated with dantrolene-induced muscle weakness, have been reported following prophylactic use of oral dantrolene and should be considered a possibility following intravenous administration also. Patients with pre-existing myopathy, predisposing neuromuscular disease, or compromised respiratory reserve may be especially at risk for these complications. Although many anesthesiologists advocate prophylactic use of dantrolene, provided that the risk of complications is considered and patients carefully selected, others recommend that dantrolene not be used prophylactically. Patients receiving prophylactic dantrolene should be carefully monitored postoperatively to detect possible prolonged or delayed effects of the medication. The controversy concerning prophylactic use of dantrolene for malignant hyperthermia does *not* extend to its therapeutic use for other indications.

Spasticity (treatment)—Oral dantrolene is indicated to relieve spasticity caused by upper motor neuron disorders such as spinal cord injury, cerebrovascular accident, cerebral palsy, and multiple sclerosis. It may be especially beneficial for patients whose functional rehabilitation is retarded by the sequelae of spasticity. However, baclofen is now more commonly used for this indication.

[Neuroleptic malignant syndrome (treatment)][1]—Dantrolene is used to relieve the symptoms of neuroleptic malignant syndrome, which are similar to those caused by malignant hyperthermia.

[Pain, exercise-induced, in muscle phosphorylase deficiency (treatment)][1]; or

[Pain, exercise-induced, in Duchenne muscular dystrophy (treatment)][1]—Oral dantrolene is used to relieve exercise-induced pain in patients with these conditions.

[Spasms, flexor (treatment)][1]—Oral dantrolene is used in the management of flexor spasms in patients who are confined to bed or a wheelchair.

### Unaccepted

Dantrolene should not be used in patients who require spasticity to sustain upright posture or balance in locomotion, or to obtain increased function.

Dantrolene is not indicated for relief of skeletal muscle spasm caused by rheumatic disorders.

[1]Not included in Canadian product labeling.

## Pharmacology/Pharmacokinetics

### Physicochemical characteristics

Molecular weight—399.29.

### Mechanism of action/Effect

Malignant hyperthermia therapy adjunct—
  By interfering with the release of calcium ion from the sarcoplasmic reticulum, dantrolene prevents or reduces the increase in myoplasmic calcium ion concentration that activates the acute catabolic processes associated with the malignant hyperthermic crisis syndrome.

Antispastic—
  Acts directly on skeletal muscle to dissociate excitation-contraction coupling, probably by interfering with the release of calcium ion from the sarcoplasmic reticulum. Dantrolene reduces muscle contractions mediated via both polysynaptic and monosynaptic reflexes. The extent to which any central nervous system (CNS) actions may contribute to the skeletal muscle relaxant effects is unknown.

### Biotransformation

Hepatic; probably by hepatic microsomal enzymes.

### Half-life

Intravenous—4 to 8 hours
Oral—8.7 hours (100-mg dose)

### Onset of action

Spasticity caused by upper motor neuron disorders—1 week or more.

### Time to peak concentration

Oral—5 hours

### Peak whole blood concentration

300 to 1100 nanograms per mL following administration of 25 to 100 mg; subject to interpatient variation.

### Therapeutic serum concentration

100 to 600 nanograms per mL; subject to interpatient variation.

### Elimination

Renal, as metabolites. Small amounts may also be excreted unchanged.

## Precautions to Consider

### Carcinogenicity/Tumorigenicity

An increased incidence of nonmalignant and malignant mammary tumors occurred with chronic (18 months) administration of dantrolene in doses of 15, 30, or 60 mg per kg of body weight (mg/kg) per day to female Sprague-Dawley rats. Also, an increased incidence of hepatic lymphangiomas and angiosarcomas occurred with chronic administration of 60 mg/kg per day. However, dantrolene did not produce these effects in other studies when administered for 2 years to mice or 2½ years to rats. The risk of carcinogenicity in humans is not known; therefore, risk-benefit with chronic therapy must be considered.

### Pregnancy/Reproduction

Pregnancy—Problems in humans have not been documented.

### Breast-feeding

Dantrolene should not be used in nursing mothers.

### Pediatrics

Appropriate studies performed to date have not demonstrated pediatrics-specific problems that would limit the usefulness of dantrolene in children. However, long-term studies have not been done in children <5 years of age.

### Geriatrics

No information is available on the relationship of age to the effects of dantrolene in geriatric patients.

### Drug interactions and/or related problems

The following drug interactions and/or related problems have been selected on the basis of their potential clinical significance (possible mechanism in parentheses where appropriate)—not necessarily inclusive (» = major clinical significance):

Note: Combinations containing any of the following medications, depending on the amount present, may also interact with this medication.

*For short-term (up to 3 days) or chronic use*
» CNS depression–producing medications (See *Appendix II*)
(concurrent use with dantrolene may result in increased CNS depressant effects; caution is recommended and dosage of one or both agents should be reduced)

*For chronic oral use only*
» Hepatotoxic medications, other (See *Appendix II*)
(concurrent use of these medications with dantrolene may increase the risk of hepatotoxicity; females over 35 years of age may be especially at risk with concurrent use of estrogens)

*For intravenous use in treating malignant hyperthermia only*
Calcium channel blockers
(concurrent administration of therapeutic doses of verapamil with intravenous dantrolene to halothane/alpha-chloralose anesthetized swine has caused ventricular fibrillation and cardiovascular collapse associated with severe hypokalemia; although the relevance of these findings to humans has not been determined, it is recommended that calcium channel blockers not be used concurrently with intravenous dantrolene in the management of a malignant hyperthermic crisis)

**Laboratory value alterations**
The following have been selected on the basis of their potential clinical significance (possible effect in parentheses where appropriate)—not necessarily inclusive (» = major clinical significance):

With physiology/laboratory test values
Liver function tests
(abnormalities may occur indicating hepatotoxicity)

**Medical considerations/Contraindications**
The medical considerations/contraindications included here have been selected on the basis of their potential clinical significance (reasons given in parentheses where appropriate)—not necessarily inclusive (» = major clinical significance).

Note: The following precautions do *not* apply to short-term intravenous use of dantrolene for treatment of a malignant hyperthermic crisis, unless otherwise specified.

*Except under special circumstances, this medication should not be used when the following medical problem exists:*
» Hepatic disease, active, such as hepatitis or cirrhosis
(increased risk of hepatotoxicity)

*Risk-benefit should be considered when the following medical problems exist:*
Cardiac function impairment, especially if due to myocardial disease
(dantrolene may cause pleural effusion and pericarditis)
Hepatic function impairment or history of
(possible increased risk of hepatotoxicity)
Myopathy, pre-existing or
Neuromuscular disease predisposing to respiratory insufficiency
(increased risk of perioperative complications when dantrolene is used as prophylaxis against malignant hyperthermia)
Pulmonary function impairment, especially obstructive pulmonary disease
(dantrolene may cause respiratory depression, possibly associated with muscle weakness, or pleural effusion)
Sensitivity to dantrolene
Caution is also recommended in patients older than 35 years of age, especially females, because of the increased risk of hepatotoxicity.

**Patient monitoring**
The following may be especially important in patient monitoring (other tests may be warranted in some patients, depending on condition; » = major clinical significance):

Blood cell counts and
Renal function determinations
(may be required at periodic intervals during chronic therapy)
» Hepatic function determinations, including:
Alanine aminotransferase (ALT [SGPT]), serum
Alkaline phosphatase
Aspartate aminotransferase (AST [SGOT]), serum
Bilirubin, total
Gammaglutamyl transpeptidase (GGTP)
(may be required before initiation of chronic therapy to determine baseline values and to identify pre-existing hepatic dysfunction or disease and at periodic intervals during chronic therapy)

## Side/Adverse Effects

Note: Dantrolene-induced hepatotoxicity may be caused by an idiosyncratic or allergic reaction to the medication. The risk of hepatotoxicity appears greater with females, patients over 35 years of age, and patients concurrently taking other medications. In particular, females over 35 years of age who are receiving estrogen therapy have an increased frequency of hepatotoxicity. Hepatotoxicity may be less likely to occur in patients taking up to 400 mg per day than in those taking 800 mg or more per day. Even short-term administration of the larger doses within a treatment regimen may increase the risk of hepatotoxicity. Overt hepatitis occurs most frequently between the third and twelfth months of chronic therapy.

The following side/adverse effects have been selected on the basis of their potential clinical significance (possible signs and symptoms in parentheses where appropriate)—not necessarily inclusive:

**Those indicating need for medical attention**
Incidence less frequent
*With short-term (up to 3 days) or chronic oral use*
*Diarrhea, severe; respiratory depression* (shortness of breath or slow or troubled breathing)
Note: *Severe diarrhea* may necessitate temporary discontinuation of therapy. If severe diarrhea recurs when therapy is resumed, therapy should probably be discontinued permanently.

*With chronic oral use only*
*Bloody or dark urine; confusion; constipation, severe*—may cause abdominal distention or other symptoms of bowel obstruction; *convulsions; dermatitis, allergic* (skin rash, hives, or itching); *difficult urination; hepatotoxicity* (yellow eyes or skin)—may be preceded by gastrointestinal symptoms such as nausea, vomiting, anorexia, and abdominal discomfort; *mental depression; phlebitis* (pain, tenderness, changes in skin color, or swelling of foot or leg); *pleural effusion with pericarditis* (chest pain)

**Those indicating need for medical attention only if they continue or are bothersome**
Incidence more frequent
*With short-term (up to 3 days) or chronic oral use*
*Diarrhea, mild; dizziness or lightheadedness; drowsiness; general feeling of discomfort or illness; muscle weakness not affecting muscles of respiration; nausea or vomiting; unusual tiredness*
Incidence less frequent
*Abdominal or stomach cramps or discomfort*
*With chronic oral use only*
Incidence less frequent
*Blurred or double vision or any change in vision; chills and fever; constipation, mild; difficulty in swallowing; frequent urge to urinate or uncontrolled urination; headache; loss of appetite; slurring of speech or other speech problems; sudden decrease in amount of urine; trouble in sleeping; unusual nervousness*

## Overdose

For more information on the management of overdose or unintentional ingestion, **contact a Poison Control Center** (see *Poison Control Center Listing*).

**Treatment of overdose**
To decrease absorption—Removing unabsorbed dantrolene (if ingested orally) via induction of emesis or gastric lavage.

Monitoring—May include monitoring the electrocardiogram (ECG), carefully observing the patient, and instituting supportive treatment of observed symptoms.

Supportive care—Administering large quantities of intravenous fluids to prevent crystalluria.

Maintaining an adequate airway, with equipment for artificial resuscitation at hand. Patients in whom intentional overdose is known or suspected should be referred to for psychiatric consultation.

Note: The possible value of dialysis in treating overdosage has not been determined.

## Patient Consultation

As an aid to patient consultation, refer to *Advice for the Patient, Dantrolene (Systemic)*.

In providing consultation, consider emphasizing the following selected information (» = major clinical significance):

## Before using this medication

» Conditions affecting use, especially:

Other medications, especially CNS depression-producing medications and other hepatotoxic medications

Other medical problems, especially hepatic disease.

## Proper use of this medication

Mixing contents of capsule with fruit juice or other liquid if unable to swallow capsule; drinking immediately after mixing

» Not taking more medication than the amount prescribed, to minimize risk of hepatotoxicity or other adverse effects

» Proper dosing

Missed dose: Taking if remembered within an hour or so; not taking if not remembered within an hour; not doubling doses

» Proper storage

## Precautions while using this medication

Regular visits to physician to check progress during long-term therapy; possibility of blood tests to check for side effects

» Avoiding alcohol or other CNS depressants during therapy unless prescribed or otherwise approved by physician

» Caution if drowsiness, dizziness or lightheadedness, vision disturbances, or muscle weakness occurs

## Side/adverse effects

Signs of potential side effects, especially bloody or dark urine; confusion; constipation, severe; convulsions; allergic dermatitis; diarrhea, severe; difficult urination; hepatitis; mental depression; phlebitis; pleural effusion with pericarditis; and respiratory depression

## General Dosing Information

Side effects such as drowsiness, dizziness, weakness, tiredness, or gastrointestinal irritation may be minimized by initiating therapy with a low dose and gradually increasing the dosage until maximal benefit is achieved.

If no benefit is observed after 45 days of therapy, the medication should be discontinued.

Dantrolene should be discontinued if a patient develops symptoms of hepatitis during therapy. If hepatic function test abnormalities without symptoms of overt hepatitis occur, the medication should probably be discontinued; however, in some patients, hepatic function test values have returned to normal despite continuation of therapy. Reinstitution or continuation of therapy should be considered only for patients receiving major benefit from the medication. Reinstitution of therapy following dantrolene-induced hepatitis should be attempted only after the symptoms and hepatic function test abnormalities have cleared. The patient should be hospitalized. Therapy should be resumed with very small and gradually increasing doses. Liver function tests should be performed frequently and the medication withdrawn immediately if any abnormalities occur.

## For parenteral dosage form only

Extravasation of the intravenous solution into surrounding tissues should be avoided because of the high pH of the solution.

## Oral Dosage Forms

### DANTROLENE SODIUM CAPSULES

#### Usual adult and adolescent dose

Malignant hyperthermic crisis prophylaxis—

Oral, 4 to 8 mg per kg of body weight per day in three or four divided doses for one to two days prior to surgery. The last dose should be given three to four hours prior to scheduled surgery with a minimum of water.

Post-malignant hyperthermic crisis treatment (as a follow-up to intravenous therapy)—

Oral, 4 to 8 mg per kg of body weight per day in four divided doses for one to three days.

Antispastic—

Oral, 25 mg once a day, initially; total daily dose may be increased by 25 mg every four to seven days until optimal response is achieved or until a dosage of 100 mg four times a day is reached. Medication should be administered in four divided daily doses whenever possible.

#### Usual pediatric dose

Antispastic—

Oral, 500 mcg (0.5 mg) per kg of body weight two times a day, initially; total daily dose may be increased by 500 mcg (0.5 mg) per kg of body weight every four to seven days until optimal response is achieved or until a dosage of 3 mg per kg of body weight four times a day is reached. Medication should be administered in four divided daily doses whenever possible.

Note: The maximum recommended pediatric dosage is 400 mg a day.

## Strength(s) usually available

U.S.—

25 mg (Rx) [*Dantrium* (lactose)].

50 mg (Rx) [*Dantrium* (lactose)].

100 mg (Rx) [*Dantrium* (lactose)].

Canada—

25 mg (Rx) [*Dantrium* (lactose)].

100 mg (Rx) [*Dantrium* (lactose)].

## Packaging and storage

Store below 40 °C (104 °F), preferably between 15 and 30 °C (59 and 86 °F), in a well-closed container, unless otherwise specified by manufacturer.

## Preparation of dosage form

For patients who cannot take oral solids

Single dose: Immediately prior to use, add the contents of the required number of capsules to fruit juice or other liquid and stir to mix.

Multiple dose: Empty 5 capsules (100 mg each) into 50 mL of Syrup NF; add 150 mg of citric acid dissolved in 10 mL of water; add enough Syrup NF to make 100 mL of suspension. This suspension will contain 25 mg of dantrolene sodium per 5 mL. Although the stability of such an extemporaneous preparation is unknown, it is thought to be stable for several days when refrigerated. However, since it contains no preservative, care must be taken to avoid contamination.

## Auxiliary labeling

• May cause drowsiness.

• Avoid alcoholic beverages.

## Parenteral Dosage Forms

### DANTROLENE SODIUM FOR INJECTION

#### Usual adult and adolescent dose

Malignant hyperthermia therapy adjunct—

Prophylactic[1]: Intravenous infusion, 2.5 mg per kg of body weight, administered over a one-hour period prior to anesthesia.

Therapeutic: Intravenous, by continuous rapid push, at least 1 mg per kg of body weight, initially, with administration being continued until the symptoms subside or until the maximum cumulative dose of 10 mg per kg of body weight has been reached. Administration may be repeated if symptoms recur.

Note: For treatment of a malignant hyperthermic crisis, some anesthesiologists recommend an initial dose of 2.5 to 3 mg per kg of body weight.

#### Usual pediatric dose

See *Usual adult and adolescent dose.*

#### Size(s) usually available

U.S.—

20 mg (Rx) [*Dantrium Intravenous*].

Canada—

20 mg (Rx) [*Dantrium Intravenous*].

## Packaging and storage

Prior to reconstitution, store below 30 °C (86 °F), protected from prolonged exposure to light, unless otherwise specified by manufacturer.

## Preparation of dosage form

60 mL of sterile water for injection without a bacteriostatic agent should be added to the vial containing 20 mg of dantrolene sodium and shaken until the solution is clear. The solution will contain 333 mcg (0.33 mg) per mL.

## Stability

After reconstitution, protect from temperatures below 15 °C (59 °F) or above 30 °C (86 °F). Protect from direct light. Use within 6 hours following reconstitution.

Precipitate formation has occurred after transfer of reconstituted dantrolene solutions to large glass bottles for preparation of an intravenous infusion. It is recommended that intravenous infusions be prepared in sterile plastic bags, immediately prior to the time of anticipated use. Also, the prepared infusion should be inspected for cloudiness and/or precipitation prior to use, and discarded if either is present.

## Incompatibilities

Dantrolene is incompatible with acidic solutions, including 5% dextrose injection and 0.9% sodium chloride injection. Acidic solutions should not be used for reconstituting the medication.

---

[1]Not included in Canadian product labeling.

---

Revised: 05/10/93

# DAPIPRAZOLE    Ophthalmic

VA CLASSIFICATION (Primary): OP900
Note: For a listing of dosage forms and brand names by country availability, see *Dosage Forms* section(s). For a listing of brand names
for the articles in this monograph, refer to the General Index.

## Category

Antimydriatic.

## Indications

### Accepted

Mydriasis, reversal of—Indicated in the treatment of pharmacologically
induced mydriasis produced by sympathomimetic (phenylephrine) or
parasympatholytic (tropicamide) agents.

### Unaccepted

Dapiprazole is not indicated for the reduction of intraocular pressure, in
the treatment of open angle glaucoma, or for any indication other than
reversal of induced mydriasis.

## Pharmacology/Pharmacokinetics

### Physicochemical characteristics

Molecular weight—361.93.
Description—Dapiprazole hydrochloride is a sterile, white, lyophilized
powder soluble in water.
Dapiprazole hydrochloride solution is a clear, colorless, slightly viscous
solution.
Other characteristics—Reconstituted solution has a pH between 4.5 and 6
and an osmolarity of approximately 415 mOsm.

### Mechanism of action/Effect

Dapiprazole is an alpha-adrenergic blocking agent and acts by blocking
the alpha-adrenergic receptors in smooth muscle. Dapiprazole produces miosis through an effect on the dilator muscle of the iris.
Dapiprazole has demonstrated safe and rapid reversal of mydriasis produced by phenylephrine and, to a lesser degree, of that produced by
tropicamide. It has not been tested against other mydriatics.In patients
with decreased accommodative amplitude due to treatment with tropicamide, the miotic effect of dapiprazole may partially increase the
accommodative amplitude.

### Other actions/effects

Dapiprazole does not significantly alter intraocular pressure in normotensive eyes or in eyes with elevated intraocular pressure.
Dapiprazole does not have any significant effect on ciliary muscle contraction, and therefore does not induce a significant change in the
anterior chamber depth or in the thickness of the lens.

### Onset of action

Eye color affects the rate of pupillary constriction. In individuals with
brown irides, the rate of pupillary constriction may be slightly slower
than in individuals with blue or green irides. Eye color does not appear
to affect the final pupil size.

## Precautions to Consider

### Carcinogenicity

Dapiprazole has been shown to significantly increase the incidence of liver
tumors in rats after continuous dietary administration for 104 weeks.
This effect was found only in male rats treated with the highest dose
administered in the study, i.e., 300 mg per kg of body weight (mg/kg)
per day (80,000 times the human dose). The effect was not observed
in male and female rats at doses of 30 and 100 mg/kg per day or in
female rats at doses of 300 mg/kg per day.

### Mutagenicity

Dapiprazole has not been shown to be mutagenic.

### Pregnancy/Reproduction

Fertility—Studies have not shown that dapiprazole impairs fertility.
Pregnancy—Adequate and well-controlled studies have not been done in
pregnant women.
Reproduction studies have been performed in rats and rabbits at doses up
to 128,000 and 27,000 times the human ophthalmic dose, respectively,
and have revealed no evidence of harm to the fetus due to dapiprazole.
FDA Pregnancy Category B.

### Breast-feeding

It is not known whether dapiprazole is distributed into human milk. However, problems in humans have not been documented.

### Pediatrics

Appropriate studies on the relationship of age to the effects of dapiprazole
have not been performed in the pediatric population. Safety and efficacy have not been established.

### Geriatrics

Appropriate studies on the relationship of age to the effects of dapiprazole
have not been performed in the geriatric population. However, geriatrics-specific problems that would limit the usefulness of this medication in the elderly are not expected.

### Medical considerations/Contraindications

The medical considerations/contraindications included here have been selected on the basis of their potential clinical significance (reasons given
in parentheses where appropriate)—not necessarily inclusive (» =
major clinical significance).

*Except under special circumstances, this medication should not be used
when the following medical problems exist:*
»   Iritis, acute, or other conditions where miosis is undesirable

*Risk-benefit should be considered when the following medical problem
exists:*
Sensitivity to dapiprazole

## Side/Adverse Effects

Note: Miosis produced by dapiprazole may cause difficulty in dark adaptation, may reduce the field of vision, or may reduce central visual acuity.

The following side/adverse effects have been selected on the basis of their
potential clinical significance (possible signs and symptoms in parentheses where appropriate)—not necessarily inclusive:

### Those indicating need for medical attention

Incidence less frequent
*Edema of cornea* (swelling of the clear part of the eye)—incidence
10 to 40%; *punctate keratitis* (severe irritation of the clear part of the
eye)—incidence 10 to 40%

### Those indicating need for medical attention only if they continue
or are bothersome

Incidence more frequent
*Burning of eye upon administration of medication*—incidence 50%;
*conjunctival injection, usually lasting 20 minutes* (redness of the
white part of the eye)—incidence 80%

Incidence less frequent
*Blurring of vision*—incidence <10%; *browache*—incidence 10 to
40%; *chemosis* (swelling of the membrane covering the white part of
the eye)—incidence 10 to 40%; *dryness of eye*—incidence <10%;
*edema of eyelid* (swelling of eyelid)—incidence 10 to 40%; *erythema
of eyelid* (redness of eyelid)—incidence 10 to 40%; *headache*—incidence 10 to 40%; *itching of eye*—incidence 10 to 40%; *photophobia*
(increased sensitivity of eye to light)—incidence 10 to 40%; *ptosis*
(drooping of upper eyelid)—incidence 10 to 40%; *tearing of eye*—
incidence <10%

## Patient Consultation

As an aid to patient consultation, refer to *Advice for the Patient,
Dapiprazole (Ophthalmic).*

In providing consultation, consider emphasizing the following selected
information (» = major clinical significance):

### Before using this medication

»   Conditions affecting use, especially:
Other medical problems, especially acute iritis or other conditions
where miosis is undesirable

### Proper use of this medication

»   Proper dosing

### Precautions while using this medication

»   Medication causes blurred vision or other vision problems; not driving,
using machines, or doing anything else that could be dangerous if
unable to see well
Possible eye photosensitivity; wearing sunglasses that block ultra-vi-
olet light

### Side/adverse effects

Signs of potential side effects, especially edema of cornea and punctate
keratitis

# Ophthalmic Dosage Forms

## DAPIPRAZOLE HYDROCHLORIDE FOR OPHTHALMIC SOLUTION

### Usual adult dose
Antimydriatic—
Topical, to the conjunctiva, 1 drop, followed by another 1 drop after five minutes; administration to start immediately following the retinal examination, to reverse the diagnostic mydriasis.

### Usual adult prescribing limits
Dapiprazole should not be used more frequently than once a week.

### Usual pediatric dose
Safety and efficacy have not been established.

### Strength(s) usually available
U.S.—
0.5% (5 mg of dapiprazole HCl per mL when reconstituted) (Rx) [*Rev-Eyes* (hydroxypropyl methylcellulose 0.4%; benzalkonium chloride 0.01%; mannitol 2%; sodium chloride; edetate sodium 0.01%; sodium phosphate dibasic; sodium phosphate monobasic; water for injection)].

Canada—
0.5% (5 mg of dapiprazole HCl per mL when reconstituted) (Rx) [*Rev-Eyes*].

### Packaging and storage
Store below 40 °C (104 °F), preferably between 15 and 30 °C (59 and 86 °F), unless otherwise specified by manufacturer.

### Preparation of dosage form
Dapiprazole is supplied in a kit consisting of one vial of dapiprazole hydrochloride (25 mg), one vial of diluent (5 mL), and one dropper for dispensing.

To prepare the solution, pour diluent into medication vial, attach dropper assembly to vial, and shake vial for several minutes to dissolve powder.

### Stability
Once the eyedrops have been reconstituted they may be stored at room temperature (15 to 30 °C [59 to 86 °F]) for 21 days. The solution should be discarded if it is not clear and colorless.

### Auxiliary labeling
• For the eye.

## Selected Bibliography
Nyman N, Keates EU. Effects of dapiprazole on the reversal of pharmacologically induced mydriasis. Optom Vis Sci 1990 Sep; 67 (9): 705-9.

Allinson RW et al. Reversal of mydriasis by dapiprazole. Ann Ophthalmol 1990 Apr; 22 (4): 131-3, 138.

Revised: 04/13/92
Interim revision: 08/16/93

---

# DAPSONE   Systemic

VA CLASSIFICATION (Primary/Secondary): AM900/AP101; AP109; AM700

Another commonly used name is DDS.

Note: For a listing of dosage forms and brand names by country availability, see *Dosage Forms* section(s). For a listing of brand names for the articles in this monograph, refer to the General Index.

## Category
Antibacterial (antileprosy agent); dermatitis herpetiformis suppressant; antiprotozoal; antifungal.

## Indications
Note: Bracketed information in the *Indications* section refers to uses that are not included in U.S. product labeling.

### Accepted
Leprosy (treatment)—Dapsone is indicated in combination with other antileprosy agents in the treatment of all types of leprosy (Hansen's disease) caused by *Mycobacterium leprae*.

Dermatitis herpetiformis (treatment)—Dapsone is indicated in the treatment of dermatitis herpetiformis.

[Actinomycotic mycetoma (treatment)]—Dapsone is used in the treatment of actinomycotic mycetoma.

[Cicatricial pemphigoid (treatment)][1]—Dapsone is used in the treatment of desquamative gingival lesions caused by cicatricial pemphigoid.

[Dermatosis, subcorneal pustular (treatment)][1]—Dapsone is used in the treatment of subcorneal pustular dermatosis.

[Granuloma annulare (treatment)][1]—Dapsone is used in the treatment of granuloma annulare.

[Lupus erythematosus, systemic (treatment)][1]—Dapsone is used in the treatment of certain skin lesions of systemic lupus erythematosus, including bullous eruptions and urticarial vasculitis.

[Malaria (prophylaxis)][1]—Dapsone is used in combination with pyrimethamine as secondary agents in the prophylaxis of chloroquine-resistant malaria caused by *Plasmodium falciparum*. Dapsone is also used in combination with pyrimethamine and chloroquine in the prophylaxis of malaria caused by *Plasmodium vivax*.

[Pemphigoid (treatment)][1]—Dapsone is used in the treatment of pemphigoid lesions with oral manifestations.

[Pneumonia, *Pneumocystis carinii* (prophylaxis and treatment)][1]—Dapsone is used in combination with trimethoprim in the treatment of mild to moderate pneumonia caused by *Pneumocystis carinii* (PCP). No difference in efficacy was found in a study comparing the dapsone-trimethoprim combination with oral trimethoprim-sulfamethoxazole.

However, studies have shown that dapsone alone appeared to have inferior efficacy for treatment of PCP.

Dapsone has also been used alone in the prophylaxis of PCP.

[Polychondritis, relapsing (treatment)][1]—Dapsone is used in the treatment of relapsing polychondritis.

[Pyoderma gangrenosum (treatment)][1]—Dapsone is used in the treatment of pyoderma gangrenosum.

---

[1]Not included in Canadian product labeling.

## Pharmacology/Pharmacokinetics

### Physicochemical characteristics
Molecular weight—248.30.

### Mechanism of action/Effect
Antibacterial (antileprosy agent)—Dapsone, a sulfone, is bacteriostatic and probably acts by a mechanism similar to that of the sulfonamides, interfering with folate synthesis. Both have a similar range of antibacterial activity and are antagonized by para-aminobenzoic acid.

Dermatitis herpetiformis suppressant—Mechanism is unknown, but not due to dapsone's bacteriostatic effect. Dapsone may act as an enzyme inhibitor or oxidizing agent. In addition, it has numerous immunologic effects (e.g., immunosuppression), which most likely account for its suppression of dermatitis herpetiformis.

### Absorption
Slowly absorbed from the gastrointestinal tract; absorption half-life of 1.1 hours. Overall bioavailability is 70 to 80%; may be less in patients with severe leprosy. An acidic environment is needed for optimal absorption.

### Distribution
Well distributed throughout total body water and is found in all tissues, especially liver, muscle, kidneys, and skin. Saliva concentrations are 18 to 27% of corresponding plasma dapsone concentrations. Dapsone also crosses the placenta.

$Vol_D$—1.5 L per kg (1.9 L per kg when given with pyrimethamine).

### Protein binding
Dapsone—Moderate to high (70–90%).
Monoacetyl dapsone (MADDS)—Very high (99%).

### Biotransformation
Dapsone is acetylated by *N*-acetyltransferase in the liver to its major metabolite, monoacetyl dapsone (MADDS). MADDS is also deacetylated to dapsone; equilibrium is reached within a few hours. Patients may be divided into slow or fast acetylators. However, unlike with other medications, no relationship has been seen between acetylator type and side effects. There was also no significant difference between the 2 groups in plasma concentrations or pharmacokinetics; therapeutic response was the same in both groups.

Dapsone is also *N*-hydroxylated to dapsone hydroxylamine in the liver by the mixed oxidase system in the presence of oxygen and NADPH, and appears to be responsible for the drug's hematologic toxicity.
Both major metabolites have very low activity and do not contribute to the therapeutic effect of dapsone.

### Half-life
10 to 50 hours (average, 30 hours) for both dapsone and MADDS.

### Time to peak serum concentration
2 to 6 hours, but variable.

### Peak serum concentration
50 mg (single dose)—0.6 to 0.7 mcg/mL.
100 mg (single dose)—1.7 to 1.9 mcg/mL.
100 mg (steady state)—3.1 to 3.3 mcg/mL.

### Elimination
Renal—70 to 85% slowly excreted in the urine as dapsone and metabolites; 5 to 15% of dapsone dose excreted in urine by active tubular secretion, and the remainder excreted as metabolites. Metabolites are partly conjugated, primarily as glucuronides and sulfates.
Biliary—Enterohepatic circulation following biliary excretion of free drug also occurs. Because of this, dapsone may persist in the plasma for up to several weeks after therapy is discontinued.

## Precautions to Consider

### Cross-sensitivity and/or related problems
Patients allergic to dapsone may be allergic to sulfonamides, although this has not been clearly established.

### Carcinogenicity/Tumorigenicity
Studies in male rats and female mice have shown that dapsone causes mesenchymal tumors of the spleen and peritoneum. Dapsone has been shown to cause thyroid carcinoma in female rats as well.

### Mutagenicity
Dapsone has not been shown to be mutagenic in *Salmonella typhimurium* tester strains 1535, 1537, 1538, 98, or 100, when tested with or without microsomal activation.

### Pregnancy/Reproduction
Pregnancy—Dapsone crosses the placenta. Adequate and well-controlled studies in humans and animals have not been done. However, other studies in humans have not shown that dapsone causes adverse effects on reproductive capacity or on the fetus. Dapsone has been recommended for maintenance therapy of pregnant leprosy and dermatitis herpetiformis patients.

FDA Pregnancy Category C.

### Breast-feeding
Dapsone is distributed into breast milk. In one case report, the concentration of dapsone in breast milk was approximately 67% of the corresponding serum concentration. The serum dapsone concentration in the nursing infant reached 27% of the mother's serum concentration. In addition, dapsone could potentially cause hemolytic anemia in glucose-6-phosphate dehydrogenase (G6PD)–deficient neonates.

### Pediatrics
Appropriate studies on the relationship of age to the effects of dapsone have not been performed in the pediatric population. However, no pediatrics-specific problems have been documented to date. Dapsone is generally not considered to have an effect on the later growth, development, and functional development of the child.

### Geriatrics
No information is available on the relationship of age to the effects of dapsone in geriatric patients.

### Drug interactions and/or related problems
The following drug interactions and/or related problems have been selected on the basis of their potential clinical significance (possible mechanism in parentheses where appropriate)—not necessarily inclusive (» = major clinical significance):

Note: Combinations containing any of the following medications, depending on the amount present, may also interact with this medication.

Aminobenzoates (PABA)
(concurrent use in the treatment of leprosy is not recommended since aminobenzoates may be absorbed by bacteria preferentially over sulfones, thereby antagonizing the bacteriostatic effect of sulfones; however, aminobenzoates do not antagonize the effect of dapsone in the treatment of dermatitis herpetiformis)

Blood dyscrasia–causing medications (See *Appendix II*)
(dapsone may, on rare occasions, cause an idiosyncratic agranulocytosis, aplastic anemia, or other blood dyscrasias; if concurrent

use is required, close observation for myelotoxic effects should be considered)

» Didanosine (ddI)
(concurrent administration of dapsone with ddI may decrease the absorption of dapsone; ddI must be given with a buffer to neutralize stomach acidity in order to increase its absorption, and dapsone requires an acidic environment for optimal absorption; until studies are completed that confirm this interaction, dapsone should be administered at least 2 hours before or 2 hours after ddI is given)

» Hemolytics, other (See *Appendix II*)
(concurrent use with dapsone may increase the potential for toxic side effects)

Rifampin
(concurrent use may stimulate hepatic microsomal enzyme activity, resulting in as much as a 7- to 10-fold decrease in dapsone concentrations; however, dapsone dosage adjustments are not required during concurrent rifampin therapy for leprosy since dapsone concentrations are still higher than the MIC, although they may be required in the treatment of other diseases, such as PCP)

Trimethoprim
(concurrent use with dapsone may increase the plasma concentrations of both dapsone and trimethoprim, possibly due to an inhibition in dapsone metabolism, and/or competition for renal secretion between the 2 medications; increased serum dapsone concentrations may increase the frequency and severity of side effects, especially methemoglobinemia and hemolytic anemia)

### Medical considerations/Contraindications
The medical considerations/contraindications included here have been selected on the basis of their potential clinical significance (reasons given in parentheses where appropriate)—not necessarily inclusive (» = major clinical significance).

*Risk-benefit should be considered when the following medical problems exist:*

Allergy to dapsone or sulfonamides

» Anemia, severe or
» Glucose-6-phosphate dehydrogenase (G6PD) deficiency or
» Methemoglobin reductase deficiency
(hemolytic anemia may occur)

Hepatic function impairment
(dapsone may cause toxic hepatitis and cholestatic jaundice; alcoholic liver disease may decrease the plasma protein binding of dapsone, increasing the amount of circulating free drug)

### Patient monitoring
The following may be especially important in patient monitoring (other tests may be warranted in some patients, depending on condition; » = major clinical significance):

» Alanine aminotransferase (ALT [SGPT]) and
» Aspartate aminotransferase (AST [SGOT])
(values should be determined prior to and periodically during treatment; dapsone should be discontinued if there is evidence of progressive hepatic damage)

Blood urea nitrogen and
Creatinine, serum
(determinations required periodically during treatment in patients with severely impaired renal function, who may also require a reduction in dose; dapsone should be discontinued in anuric patients)

» Complete blood counts (CBCs) and
» Platelet counts and
» Reticulocyte count
(required prior to treatment, followed by monthly counts for 1 to 3 months, and semi-annually thereafter; in patients with HIV infection, CBCs are recommended every 2 to 3 days for the first 2 to 3 weeks of therapy; if a significant reduction in leukocytes, platelets, or hematocrit occurs, or if there is an increase in the reticulocyte count, dapsone should be discontinued and the patient should be monitored closely)

Glucose-6-phosphate dehydrogenase (G6PD) concentration
(determination recommended in patients at high risk prior to treatment; if a deficiency is found, dapsone should be given with extreme caution since hemolytic effects may be exaggerated; dosage adjustments may be required)

Methemoglobin, serum
(level should be obtained in patients with cyanosis, lightheadedness, fatigue, headache, or shortness of breath; dapsone should be discontinued at a methemoglobin level of > 20%, and treatment

with methylene blue should be considered in symptomatic patients with levels > 30%)

## Side/Adverse Effects

Note: When dapsone is used in high doses, peripheral motor weakness may occur more frequently.

Fatalities have occurred due to agranulocytosis, aplastic anemia, and other blood dyscrasias. In addition, serious cutaneous reactions, such as exfoliative dermatitis, toxic erythema, erythema multiforme, toxic epidermal necrolysis, morbilliform and scarlatiniform reactions, and erythema nodosum may occur. Dapsone therapy should be promptly discontinued if new or toxic dermatologic reactions occur. However, leprosy reactional states do not require discontinuation of therapy.

A dose-related hemolysis is seen in all patients, with a slight decrease in hemoglobin and an increase in reticulocyte count. Patients with G6PD-deficiency or a decrease in activity in glutathione reductase are more susceptible to hemolysis. A low level of methemoglobinemia also occurs in all patients at recommended doses.

The following side/adverse effects have been selected on the basis of their potential clinical significance (possible signs and symptoms in parentheses where appropriate)—not necessarily inclusive:

### Those indicating need for medical attention
Incidence more frequent
*Hemolytic anemia* (back, leg, or stomach pains; loss of appetite; pale skin; unusual tiredness or weakness; fever); *hypersensitivity* (skin rash); *methemoglobinemia* (cyanosis—bluish fingernails, lips, or skin; difficult breathing; unusual tiredness or weakness)

Incidence rare
*Blood dyscrasias* (fever and sore throat; unusual bleeding or bruising; unusual tiredness and weakness); *exfoliative dermatitis* (itching, dryness, redness, scaling, or peeling of the skin or loss of hair); *hepatic damage* (yellow eyes or skin); *mood or other mental changes; peripheral neuritis* (numbness, tingling, pain, burning, or weakness in hands or feet); *"sulfone syndrome"* (fever; malaise; exfoliative dermatitis; jaundice; lymphadenopathy; methemoglobinemia; anemia)—a hypersensitivity reaction that usually occurs after 6 to 8 weeks of therapy

### Those indicating need for medical attention only if they continue or are bothersome
Incidence rare—usually dose-related
*Central nervous system toxicity* (headache; insomnia; nervousness); *gastrointestinal disturbances* (anorexia; nausea or vomiting)

## Overdose

For more information on the management of overdose or unintentional ingestion, **contact a Poison Control Center** (see *Poison Control Center Listing*).

### Treatment of overdose
Recommended treatment consists of the following:

To decrease absorption—

Performance of gastric lavage. Gastric emptying of dapsone may be delayed after an overdose, and tablet fragments have been found in stomach returns after lavage as late as 5 to 12 hours post-ingestion.

Administration of activated charcoal (30 grams), concurrently with a cathartic, every 6 hours for at least 48 to 72 hours. Repeated doses of activated charcoal reduce the half-life of dapsone and MADDS by approximately 50% to 12.7 hours.

Specific treatment—

In emergency situations, slow, intravenous administration of methylene blue, 1 to 2 mg per kg of body weight (mg/kg). Methylene blue should not be given to fully expressed G6PD-deficient patients. May be repeated if methemoglobin reaccumulates. A continuous infusion of methylene blue has also been used to prevent toxicity from accidental "over-bolusing" of methylene blue, and permit titration of the infusion to methemoglobin levels. A 0.05% solution in 0.9% sodium chloride is usually started at a rate of 0.1 mg/kg per hour.

Supportive care—Patients in whom intentional overdose is known or suspected should be referred for psychiatric consultation.

## Patient Consultation

As an aid to patient consultation, refer to *Advice for the Patient, Dapsone (Systemic)*.

In providing consultation, consider emphasizing the following selected information (» = major clinical significance):

### Before using this medication
» Conditions affecting use, especially:
  Allergy to sulfonamides
  Pregnancy—Dapsone crosses the placenta
  Breast-feeding—Dapsone is distributed into breast milk; it may cause hemolytic anemia in G6PD-deficient neonates
  Other medications, especially other hemolytics and didanosine
  Other medical problems, especially severe anemia, G6PD deficiency, or methemoglobin reductase deficiency

### Proper use of this medication
» Proper dosing
  Missed dose: Taking as soon as possible; not taking if almost time for next dose; not doubling doses
» Proper storage
*For leprosy*
» Compliance with full course of therapy, which may take years
» Importance of not missing doses and taking at same time every day
*For dermatitis herpetiformis*
  Possible need for gluten-free diet
*For Pneumocystis carinii pneumonia*
» Compliance with full course of therapy

### Precautions while using this medication
  Regular visits to physician to check progress
  Checking with physician if no improvement within 2 to 3 months (leprosy), within 1 week (PCP), or within a few days (dermatitis herpetiformis)

### Side/adverse effects
  Signs of potential side effects, especially hemolytic anemia, blood dyscrasias, hypersensitivity reactions, methemoglobinemia, exfoliative dermatitis, peripheral neuropathy, hepatic damage, "sulfone syndrome", and mood and other mental changes

## General Dosing Information

Since bacterial resistance may develop when dapsone is administered alone in the treatment of leprosy, for initial treatment, concurrent administration with rifampin is generally recommended. Clofazimine, ethionamide, or prothionamide (investigational) may be used in place of rifampin, but they are considered less effective.

Dapsone therapy should be discontinued promptly if new or toxic dermatologic reactions occur. However, leprosy reactional states do not require discontinuation of therapy. Large doses of corticosteroids should be given if severe "reversal" reactions (type 1) or neuritis occurs during treatment of leprosy.

Depending on the drug regimen used, therapy may have to be continued for 6 months to 3 years or more in indeterminate and tuberculoid leprosy, 2 to 10 years in borderline (dimorphous) leprosy, and 2 years to life in lepromatous leprosy.

In the treatment of dermatitis herpetiformis, a gluten-free diet for 6 months may allow a reduction in dose by approximately 50% or discontinuation of dapsone.

## Oral Dosage Forms

Note: Bracketed uses in the *Dosage Forms* section refer to categories of use and/or indications that are not included in U.S. product labeling.

### DAPSONE TABLETS USP

**Usual adult and adolescent dose**
Leprosy (Hansen's disease)—
  Oral, in combination with one or more other antileprosy agents, 50 to 100 mg of dapsone once a day; or 1.4 mg per kg of body weight once a day.
Dermatitis herpetiformis suppressant—
  Oral, initially 50 mg daily. Doses may be increased up to 300 mg daily if symptoms are not completely controlled. The dose should then be reduced to the lowest effective maintenance dose as soon as possible.
[Actinomycotic mycetoma]—
  Oral, 100 mg twice a day for several months after clinical symptoms have disappeared.
[Dermatosis, subcorneal pustular][1]—
  Oral, initially 100 mg once a day, increasing the dose by 50 mg every one to two weeks until remission occurs. The dose should then be gradually reduced to the lowest effective maintenance dose.
[Granuloma annulare][1]—
  Oral, 100 mg once a day.

[Malaria (prophylaxis)][1]—
  Oral, 100 mg of dapsone in combination with 12.5 mg of pyrimethamine once every seven days.
[Pneumonia, *Pneumocystis carinii*][1]—
  Treatment: Oral, 100 mg of dapsone once a day in combination with 20 mg per kg of body weight per day of trimethoprim, for twenty-one days.
  Prophylaxis: Oral, 50 to 100 mg once a day.
[Polychondritis, relapsing][1]—
  Oral, 100 mg once or twice a day.
[Pyoderma gangrenosum][1]—
  Oral, 50 to 100 mg once a day, in combination with other medications.

**Usual adult prescribing limits**
Leprosy (Hansen's disease)—
  Up to 100 mg daily.
Dermatitis herpetiformis suppressant—
  Up to 300 mg daily.
Polychondritis, relapsing[1]—
  Up to 200 mg daily.

**Usual pediatric dose**
Leprosy (Hansen's disease)—
  Oral, in combination with one or more other antileprosy agents, 1.4 mg of dapsone per kg of body weight once a day.
Dermatitis herpetiformis suppressant—
  Oral, initially 2 mg per kg of body weight daily. Doses may be increased if symptoms are not completely controlled. The dose

should then be reduced to the lowest effective maintenance dose as soon as possible.
[Pneumonia, *Pneumocystis carinii* (prophylaxis)][1]—
  In children older than 1 month of age: Oral, 1 mg per kg of body weight, up to 100 mg daily.

**Strength(s) usually available**
U.S.—
  25 mg (Rx) [GENERIC (may be scored)].
  100 mg (Rx) [GENERIC (may be scored)].
Canada—
  100 mg (Rx) [*Avlosulfon* (scored)].

**Packaging and storage**
Store below 40 °C (104 °F), preferably between 15 and 30 °C (59 and 86 °F), unless otherwise specified by manufacturer. Store in a well-closed, light-resistant container.

**Auxiliary labeling**
• Continue medicine for full time of treatment (for leprosy and PCP).

---

[1]Not included in Canadian product labeling.

---

Revised: 06/26/92
Interim revision: 03/17/94

---

# DAUNORUBICIN     Systemic

VA CLASSIFICATION (Primary): AN200
Note: For a listing of dosage forms and brand names by country availability, see *Dosage Forms* section(s). For a listing of brand names for the articles in this monograph, refer to the General Index.

## Category
Antineoplastic.

## Indications
Note: Bracketed information in the *Indications* section refers to uses that are not included in U.S. product labeling.

### Accepted
Erythroleukemia (treatment)[1]
Leukemia, acute lymphocytic (treatment)
Leukemia, acute myelocytic (treatment) or
Leukemia, acute monocytic (treatment)[1]—Daunorubicin is indicated, in combination with other antineoplastics, for treatment of acute lymphocytic leukemia and acute nonlymphocytic leukemia (acute myelocytic leukemia, acute monocytic leukemia, erythroleukemia).
[Neuroblastoma (treatment)][1]—Daunorubicin is used for treatment of solid tumors of childhood, such as neuroblastoma.
[Lymphomas, non-Hodgkin's (treatment)]—Daunorubicin is used for treatment of non-Hodgkin's lymphomas such as lymphosarcoma and reticulum cell sarcomas.
[Ewing's sarcoma (treatment)]—Daunorubicin is used for treatment of Ewing's sarcoma.
[Wilms' tumor (treatment)]—Daunorubicin is used for treatment of Wilms' tumor.
[Leukemia, chronic myelocytic (treatment)]—Daunorubicin is used for treatment of chronic myelocytic (myelogenous) leukemia.

---

[1]Not included in Canadian product labeling.

## Pharmacology/Pharmacokinetics

### Physicochemical characteristics
Molecular weight—563.99.
pKa—10.3.

### Mechanism of action/Effect
Daunorubicin is an anthracycline glycoside; it is classified as an antibiotic but is not used as an antimicrobial agent. Daunorubicin is most active in the S phase of cell division, but is not cycle phase–specific. Its exact mechanism of antineoplastic action is unknown but may involve binding to DNA by intercalation between base pairs and inhibition of

DNA and RNA synthesis by template disordering and steric obstruction.

### Other actions/effects
Also has antibacterial and immunosuppressant effects.

### Distribution
Rapidly distributed throughout the body, especially to the kidneys, spleen, liver, and heart, as unchanged medication and metabolites. It does not cross the blood-brain barrier.

### Biotransformation
Rapidly (within 1 hour) in the liver to produce an active metabolite, daunorubicinol. Further metabolism—Hepatic.

### Half-life
Distribution—
  45 minutes.
Elimination—
  Daunorubicin: 18.5 hours.
  Metabolites: 55 hours.
  Daunorubicinol: 26.7 hours.
  Therefore, blood concentrations are prolonged.

### Elimination
Prolonged, in the urine, 25% in an active form; an estimated 40% is eliminated by biliary excretion.

## Precautions to Consider

### Carcinogenicity/Mutagenicity
Secondary malignancies are potential delayed effects of many antineoplastic agents, although it is not clear whether the effect is related to their mutagenic or immunosuppressive action. The effect of dose and duration of therapy is also unknown, although risk seems to increase with long-term use. Although information is limited, available data seem to indicate that the carcinogenic risk is greatest with the alkylating agents.
Daunorubicin subcutaneous injection causes fibrosarcomas at the injection site in mice; however, it did not cause a carcinogenic effect within 22 months of observation after oral or intraperitoneal administration in mice. Daunorubicin is potentially carcinogenic in humans.

### Pregnancy/Reproduction
Fertility—Gonadal suppression, resulting in amenorrhea or azoospermia, may occur in patients taking antineoplastic therapy, especially with the alkylating agents. In general, these effects appear to be related to dose and length of therapy and may be irreversible. Prediction of the degree of testicular or ovarian function impairment is complicated by the common use of combinations of several antineoplastics, which makes it difficult to assess the effects of individual agents.
Daunorubicin causes testicular atrophy in male dogs.

Pregnancy—Adequate and well-controlled studies have not been done in humans.

First trimester: It is usually recommended that use of antineoplastics, especially combination chemotherapy, be avoided whenever possible, especially during the first trimester. Although information is limited because of the relatively few instances of antineoplastic administration during pregnancy, the mutagenic, teratogenic, and carcinogenic potential of these medications must be considered.

Other hazards to the fetus include adverse reactions seen in adults.

In general, use of a contraceptive is recommended during cytotoxic drug therapy.

Studies in rabbits found an increased incidence of fetal abnormalities (parieto-occipital cranioschisis, umbilical hernias, rachischisis) and abortions, and studies in mice showed decreases in fetal birth weight and postdelivery growth rate.

FDA Pregnancy Category D.

**Breast-feeding**

Although very little information is available regarding distribution of antineoplastic agents into breast milk, breast-feeding is not recommended while daunorubicin is being administered because of the risks to the infant (adverse effects, mutagenicity, carcinogenicity).

**Pediatrics**

Appropriate studies on the relationship of age to the effects of daunorubicin have not been performed in the pediatric population.

**Geriatrics**

Although appropriate studies on the relationship of age to the effects of daunorubicin have not been performed in the geriatric population, cardiotoxicity may be more frequent in the elderly. Caution should also used be in patients who have inadequate bone marrow reserves due to old age. In addition, elderly patients are more likely to have age-related renal function impairment, which may require reduction of dosage in patients receiving daunorubicin.

**Dental**

The bone marrow depressant effects of daunorubicin may result in an increased incidence of microbial infection, delayed healing, and gingival bleeding. Dental work, whenever possible, should be completed prior to initiation of therapy or deferred until blood counts have returned to normal. Patients should be instructed in proper oral hygiene during treatment, including caution in use of regular toothbrushes, dental floss, and toothpicks.

Daunorubicin also commonly causes stomatitis which may be associated with considerable discomfort.

**Drug interactions and/or related problems**

The following drug interactions and/or related problems have been selected on the basis of their potential clinical significance (possible mechanism in parentheses where appropriate)—not necessarily inclusive (» = major clinical significance):

Note: Combinations containing any of the following medications, depending on the amount present, may also interact with this medication.

Allopurinol or
Colchicine or
» Probenecid or
» Sulfinpyrazone
(daunorubicin may raise the concentration of blood uric acid; dosage adjustment of antigout agents may be necessary to control hyperuricemia and gout; allopurinol may be preferred to prevent or reverse daunorubicin-induced hyperuricemia because of risk of uric acid nephropathy with uricosuric antigout agents)

Blood dyscrasia–causing medications (See *Appendix II*)
(leukopenic and/or thrombocytopenic effects of daunorubicin may be increased with concurrent or recent therapy if these medications cause the same effects; dosage adjustment of daunorubicin, if necessary, should be based on blood counts)

» Bone marrow depressants, other (See *Appendix II*) or
Radiation therapy
(additive bone marrow depression may occur; dosage reduction may be required when two or more bone marrow depressants, including radiation, are used concurrently or consecutively)

Cyclophosphamide or
Radiation therapy to mediastinal area
(concurrent use may result in increased cardiotoxicity; it is recommended that the total dose of daunorubicin not exceed 400 mg per square meter of body surface)

Doxorubicin
(use of daunorubicin in a patient who has previously received doxorubicin increases the risk of cardiotoxicity; dosage adjustment is necessary. Daunorubicin should not be used in patients who have previously received complete cumulative doses of doxorubicin or daunorubicin; in patients who have previously received less than a complete cumulative dose of doxorubicin, the total cumulative dose of doxorubicin plus daunorubicin should not exceed 550 mg per square meter of body surface)

Hepatotoxic medications, other (See *Appendix II*)
(concurrent use may increase the risk of toxicity; for example, high-dose methotrexate may impair liver function and increase toxicity of subsequently administered daunorubicin)

Vaccines, killed virus
(because normal defense mechanisms may be suppressed by daunorubicin therapy, the patient's antibody response to the vaccine may be decreased. The interval between discontinuation of medications that cause immunosuppression and restoration of the patient's ability to respond to the vaccine depends on the intensity and type of immunosuppression-causing medication used, the underlying disease, and other factors; estimates vary from 3 months to 1 year)

» Vaccines, live virus
(because normal defense mechanisms may be suppressed by daunorubicin therapy, concurrent use with a live virus vaccine may potentiate the replication of the vaccine virus, may increase the side/adverse effects of the vaccine virus, and/or may decrease the patient's antibody response to the vaccine; immunization of these patients should be undertaken only with extreme caution after careful review of the patient's hematologic status and only with the knowledge and consent of the physician managing the daunorubicin therapy. The interval between discontinuation of medications that cause immunosuppression and restoration of the patient's ability to respond to the vaccine depends on the intensity and type of immunosuppression-causing medication used, the underlying disease, and other factors; estimates vary from 3 months to 1 year. Patients with leukemia in remission should not receive live virus vaccine until at least 3 months after their last chemotherapy. In addition, immunization with oral poliovirus vaccine should be postponed in persons in close contact with the patient, especially family members)

**Laboratory value alterations**

The following have been selected on the basis of their potential clinical significance (possible effect in parentheses where appropriate)—not necessarily inclusive (» = major clinical significance):

With physiology/laboratory test values
Alkaline phosphatase and
Aspartate aminotransferase (AST [SGOT]) and
Bilirubin
(serum values may be increased transiently)

Uric acid
(concentrations in blood and urine may be increased)

**Medical considerations/Contraindications**

The medical considerations/contraindications included here have been selected on the basis of their potential clinical significance (reasons given in parentheses where appropriate)—not necessarily inclusive (» = major clinical significance).

*Risk-benefit should be considered when the following medical problems exist:*

» Bone marrow depression
» Chickenpox, existing or recent (including recent exposure) or
» Herpes zoster
(risk of severe generalized disease)

Gout, history of or
Urate renal stones, history of
(risk of hyperuricemia)

» Heart disease
» Hepatic function impairment
(reduction in dosage is recommended; three-quarters of the normal dose is recommended in patients with serum bilirubin concentrations of 1.2 to 3 mg per 100 mL; one-half of the normal dose is recommended in patients with serum bilirubin concentrations of greater than 3 mg per 100 mL)

» Infection
Renal function impairment
(reduced elimination; dosage reduction is recommended; one-half of the normal dose is recommended in patients with serum creatinine concentrations of greater than 3 mg per 100 mL)

Sensitivity to daunorubicin
» Tumor cell infiltration of the bone marrow

» Caution should be used also in patients with inadequate bone marrow reserves due to previous cytotoxic drug or radiation therapy.

### Patient monitoring

The following are especially important in patient monitoring (other tests may be warranted in some patients, depending on condition; » = major clinical significance):

Alanine aminotransferase (ALT [SGPT]) values, serum and
Aspartate aminotransferase (AST [SGOT]) values, serum and
Bilirubin values, serum and
Lactate dehydrogenase (LDH) values, serum
   (recommended prior to initiation of therapy and at periodic intervals during therapy; frequency varies according to clinical state, agent, dose, and other agents being used concurrently)

» Chest x-ray and
» Echocardiography and
   Electrocardiogram (ECG) studies and
» Radionuclide angiography determination of ejection fraction
   (recommended prior to initiation of therapy and at periodic intervals during therapy)

» Hematocrit or hemoglobin and
» Leukocyte count, total and, if appropriate, differential and
» Platelet count
   (determinations recommended prior to initiation of therapy and at periodic intervals during therapy; frequency varies according to clinical state, agent, dose, and other agents being used concurrently)

Uric acid concentrations, serum
   (recommended prior to initiation of therapy and at periodic intervals during therapy; frequency varies according to clinical state, agent, dose, and other agents being used concurrently)

## Side/Adverse Effects

Note: Many "side effects" of antineoplastic therapy are unavoidable and represent the medication's pharmacologic action. Some of these (for example, leukopenia and thrombocytopenia) are actually used as parameters to aid in individual dosage titration.

The following side/adverse effects have been selected on the basis of their potential clinical significance (possible signs and symptoms in parentheses where appropriate)—not necessarily inclusive:

### Those indicating need for medical attention

Incidence more frequent
   *Esophagitis or stomatitis* (sores in mouth and on lips); *leukopenia or infection* (usually asymptomatic; less frequently, fever or chills; cough or hoarseness; lower back or side pain; painful or difficult urination)

   Note: With *esophagitis* or *stomatitis*, sores in mouth and on lips occur 3 to 7 days after administration.

   *Leukopenia* occurs in all patients. The nadir of the leukocyte count occurs 10 to 14 days after a dose. Recovery usually occurs within 21 days after a dose.

   In addition to the risk of *infection*, febrile drug reactions may also occur during or immediately after administration.

Incidence less frequent
   *Cardiotoxicity in the form of congestive heart failure* (irregular heartbeat; shortness of breath; swelling of feet and lower legs); *extravasation, cellulitis, or tissue necrosis* (pain at injection site); *gastrointestinal ulceration* (stomach pain); *hyperuricemia or uric acid nephropathy* (joint pain; lower back or side pain); *thrombocytopenia* (usually asymptomatic; rarely, unusual bleeding or bruising; black, tarry stools; blood in urine or stools; pinpoint red spots on skin)

   Note: Incidence of *cardiotoxicity* is more frequent in adults receiving a total cumulative dosage over 550 mg per square meter of body surface (450 mg per square meter of body surface in patients who have received previous chest irradiation), in the elderly, and in patients with a history of cardiac disease or mediastinal radiation.

   *Cardiotoxicity* usually appears within 1 to 6 months after initiation of therapy. It may develop suddenly and may not be detected by routine ECG. It may be irreversible and fatal but responds to treatment if detected early.

   *Hyperuricemia or uric acid nephropathy* occurs most commonly during initial treatment of patients with leukemia or lymphoma, as a result of rapid cell breakdown which leads to elevated serum uric acid concentrations.

Incidence rare
   *Allergic reaction* (skin rash or itching); *cardiotoxicity in the form of pericarditis-myocarditis*

### Those indicating need for medical attention only if they continue or are bothersome

Incidence more frequent
   *Nausea and vomiting*

   Note: *Nausea and vomiting* are usually mild and transient, occurring soon after administration and lasting 24 to 48 hours.

Incidence less frequent or rare
   *Darkening or redness of skin*—if patient has received previous radiation therapy; *diarrhea*

### Those not indicating need for medical attention

Incidence more frequent
   *Loss of hair; reddish urine*

   Note: *Loss of hair* occurs in most patients. Growth usually resumes 5 or more weeks after therapy is completed.

   *Reddish urine* usually clears within 48 hours.

### Those indicating the need for medical attention if they occur after medication is discontinued

*Cardiotoxicity* (irregular heartbeat; shortness of breath; swelling of feet and lower legs)

## Patient Consultation

As an aid to patient consultation, refer to *Advice for the Patient, Daunorubicin (Systemic)*.

In providing consultation, consider emphasizing the following selected information (» = major clinical significance):

### Before using this medication

» Conditions affecting use, especially:
   Sensitivity to daunorubicin
   Pregnancy—Use not recommended because of mutagenic, teratogenic, and carcinogenic potential; advisability of using a contraceptive; telling physician immediately if pregnancy is suspected
   Breast-feeding—Not recommended because of risk of serious side effects
   Use in the elderly—Increased risk of cardiotoxicity, bone marrow depression
   Other medications, especially probenecid, sulfinpyrazone, other bone marrow depressants, or previous cytotoxic drug or radiation therapy
   Other medical problems, especially chickenpox, herpes zoster, heart disease, hepatic function impairment, or infection

### Proper use of this medication

Caution in taking combination therapy; taking each medication at the right time
Importance of ample fluid intake and subsequent increase in urine output to aid in excretion of uric acid
Frequency of nausea and vomiting; importance of continuing medication despite stomach upset
» Proper dosing

### Precautions while using this medication

» Importance of close monitoring by the physician
» Avoiding immunizations unless approved by physician; other persons in patient's household should avoid immunizations with oral poliovirus vaccine; avoiding persons who have taken oral poliovirus vaccine or wearing a protective mask that covers nose and mouth
*Caution if bone marrow depression occurs:*
» Avoiding exposure to persons with bacterial infections, especially during periods of low blood counts; checking with physician immediately if fever or chills, cough or hoarseness, lower back or side pain, or painful or difficult urination occur
» Checking with physician immediately if unusual bleeding or bruising; black, tarry stools; blood in urine or stools; or pinpoint red spots on skin occur
   Caution in use of regular toothbrush, dental floss, or toothpick; physician, dentist, or nurse may suggest alternatives; checking with physician before having dental work done
   Not touching eyes or inside of nose unless hands washed immediately before
   Using caution to avoid accidental cuts with use of sharp objects such as safety razor or fingernail or toenail cutters
   Avoiding contact sports or other situations where bruising or injury could occur

» Possibility of local tissue injury and scarring if infiltration of intravenous solution occurs; telling doctor or nurse right away about redness, pain, or swelling at injection site

**Side/adverse effects**

May cause adverse effects such as blood problems, loss of hair, heart problems, and cancer; importance of discussing possible effects with physician

Signs of potential side effects, especially esophagitis, stomatitis, leukopenia, infection, cardiotoxicity, extravasation, cellulitis, tissue necrosis, gastrointestinal ulceration, hyperuricemia, uric nephropathy, thrombocytopenia, and allergic reaction

Physician or nurse can help in dealing with side effects

Reddish urine may be alarming to patient although medically insignificant

Possibility of hair loss; normal hair growth should return after treatment has ended

# General Dosing Information

Patients receiving daunorubicin should be under supervision of a physician experienced in cancer chemotherapy. It is recommended that the patient be hospitalized at least during initial treatment.

A variety of dosage schedules of daunorubicin, alone or in combination with other antitumor agents, are used. The prescriber may consult the medical literature as well as the manufacturer's literature in choosing a specific dosage.

Dosage must be adjusted to meet the individual requirements of each patient, on the basis of clinical response and appearance or severity of toxicity.

The desired dose of daunorubicin is withdrawn from the vial of reconstituted solution into a syringe containing 10 to 15 mL of 0.9% sodium chloride injection and then injected over 2 to 3 minutes into the tubing or side arm of a rapidly running intravenous infusion of 5% dextrose injection or 0.9% sodium chloride injection.

Care must be taken to avoid extravasation during intravenous administration. Facial flushing or erythematous streaking along the vein indicates overly rapid injection.

Administration by intravenous infusion is not recommended because of irritation to the vein and the risk of thrombophlebitis.

If extravasation of daunorubicin occurs during intravenous administration, as indicated by local burning or stinging, the injection and infusion should be stopped immediately and resumed, completing the dose, in another vein.

Because it will cause local tissue necrosis, daunorubicin must not be administered intramuscularly or subcutaneously.

Development of uric acid nephropathy in patients with leukemia or lymphoma may be prevented by adequate oral hydration and, in some cases, administration of allopurinol. Alkalinization of urine may be necessary if serum uric acid concentrations are elevated.

In general, it is recommended that a course of daunorubicin be administered no more frequently than every 21 days to allow the bone marrow to recover.

In acute leukemia, daunorubicin may be administered despite the presence of thrombocytopenia and bleeding; stoppage of bleeding and increase in platelet count have occurred during treatment in some cases and platelet transfusions are useful in others.

Special precautions are recommended in patients who develop thrombocytopenia as a result of administration of daunorubicin. These may include extreme care in performing invasive procedures; regular inspection of intravenous sites, skin (including perirectal area), and mucous membrane surfaces for signs of bleeding or bruising; limiting frequency of venipuncture and avoiding intramuscular injections; testing urine, emesis, stool, and secretions for occult blood; care in use of regular toothbrushes, dental floss, toothpicks, safety razors, and fingernail and toenail cutters; avoiding constipation; and using caution to prevent falls and other injuries. Such patients should avoid alcohol and aspirin intake because of the risk of gastrointestinal bleeding. Platelet transfusions may be required.

Patients who develop leukopenia should be observed carefully for signs of infection. Antibiotic support may be required. In neutropenic patients who develop fever, broad-spectrum antibiotic coverage should be initiated empirically, pending bacterial cultures and appropriate diagnostic tests.

**Safety considerations of handling this medication**

There is limited but increasing evidence and concern that personnel involved in preparation and administration of parenteral antineoplastics may be at some risk because of the potential mutagenicity, teratogenicity, and/or carcinogenicity of these agents, although the actual risk is unknown. USP advisory panels recommend cautious handling both in preparation and disposal of antineoplastic agents. Precautions that have been suggested include:

• Use of a biological containment cabinet during reconstitution and dilution of parenteral medications and wearing of disposable surgical gloves and masks.

• Use of proper technique to prevent contamination of the medication, work area, and operator during transfer between containers (including proper training of personnel in this technique).

• Cautious and proper disposal of needles, syringes, vials, ampuls, and unused medication.

A number of medical centers have developed detailed guidelines for handling of antineoplastic agents.

**Combination chemotherapy**

Daunorubicin may be used in combination with other agents in various regimens. As a result, incidence and/or severity of side effects may be altered and different dosages (usually reduced) may be used. For example, daunorubicin is part of the following chemotherapeutic combinations (a commonly used acronym is in parentheses):

—daunorubicin, cytarabine, prednisolone, and mercaptopurine (Ara-C + DNR + PRED + MP).

—daunorubicin, vincristine, and prednisone.

For specific dosages and schedules, consult the literature. For information regarding each agent, consult the individual monographs.

# Parenteral Dosage Forms

## DAUNORUBICIN HYDROCHLORIDE FOR INJECTION USP

**Usual adult dose**

Leukemia, acute lymphocytic—

Intravenous, 45 mg (base) per square meter of body surface on Days 1, 2, and 3 of a thirty-two–day course in combination with vincristine, prednisone, and asparaginase.

Leukemia, acute nonlymphocytic—

Intravenous, 45 mg (base) per square meter of body surface on Days 1, 2, and 3 of the first course and Days 1 and 2 of the second course, in combination with cytarabine.

**Usual adult prescribing limits**

Up to a total lifetime dosage of 550 mg (base) per square meter of body surface, 450 mg per square meter of body surface in patients who have received previous chest irradiation (to reduce risk of cardiotoxicity).

**Usual pediatric dose**

Leukemia, acute lymphocytic—

Intravenous, 25 mg (base) per square meter of body surface once a week, in combination with vincristine and prednisone.

Note: In children less than 2 years of age or below 0.5 square meter of body surface, dosage should be calculated on the basis of mg per kg of body weight rather than body surface area.

**Usual geriatric dose**

For patients 60 years of age and older:

Leukemia, acute nonlymphocytic—

Intravenous, 30 mg (base) per square meter of body surface on Days 1, 2, and 3 of the first course and Days 1 and 2 of the second course, in combination with cytarabine.

Note: This dose is based on a single study and may not be appropriate if optimal supportive care is available.

**Size(s) usually available**

U.S.—

20 mg (base) (21.4 mg as HCl) (Rx) [*Cerubidine* (mannitol 100 mg)].

Canada—

20 mg (base) (21.4 mg as HCl) (Rx) [*Cerubidine*].

**Packaging and storage**

Store below 40 °C (104 °F), preferably between 15 and 30 °C (59 and 86 °F), unless otherwise specified by manufacturer. Protect from light.

**Preparation of dosage form**

Daunorubicin for Injection USP is reconstituted for intravenous administration by adding 4 mL of sterile water for injection to the vial and shaking gently to dissolve, producing a solution containing 5 mg of daunorubicin (base) per mL.

**Stability**

Reconstituted solutions of daunorubicin are stable for 24 hours at room temperature or 48 hours between 2 and 8 °C (36 and 46 °F) when protected from light.

**Note**

Any daunorubicin powder or solution that comes in contact with the skin or mucosae should be washed off thoroughly with soap and water.

**Selected Bibliography**

Dorr RT, Fritz WL. Cancer chemotherapy handbook. New York: Elsevier, 1980: 373-8.

Young RC, Ozols RF, Myers CE. The anthracycline antineoplastic drugs. NEJM 1981 Jul 16; 305: 139-53.

Revised: 07/11/94

---

# DECONGESTANTS AND ANALGESICS   Systemic

This monograph includes information on the following: Phenylephrine and Acetaminophen; Phenylpropanolamine and Acetaminophen; Phenylpropanolamine and Aspirin; Phenylpropanolamine, Acetaminophen, and Aspirin; Phenylpropanolamine, Acetaminophen, and Caffeine; Phenylpropanolamine, Acetaminophen, Salicylamide, and Caffeine; Pseudoephedrine and Acetaminophen; Pseudoephedrine and Aspirin; Pseudoephedrine and Ibuprofen.

VA CLASSIFICATION (Primary): RE599

**NOTE:** The *Decongestants and Analgesics (Systemic)* monograph is maintained on the USP DI electronic data base. For a printed copy of the most recent revision of the complete monograph, contact the USP Division of Information Development, 12601 Twinbrook Parkway, Rockville, MD 20852.

For information on the specific components of this combination, see the *USP DI* monographs for *Acetaminophen (Systemic), Anti-inflammatory Drugs, Nonsteroidal (Systemic), Caffeine (Systemic), Phenylpropanolamine (Systemic), Pseudoephedrine (Systemic), Salicylates (Systemic),* and *Sympathomimetic Agents—Cardiovascular Use (Systemic).*

The information that follows is selectively abstracted from the complete monograph and is provided to facilitate drug use review and patient counseling.

Note: For a listing of dosage forms and brand names by country availability, see *Dosage Forms* section(s). For a listing of brand names for the articles in this monograph, refer to the General Index.

## Category
Decongestant-analgesic.

## Indications

### Accepted
Congestion, nasal (treatment)
Congestion, sinus (treatment) and
Headache, sinus (treatment)—Decongestant and analgesic combinations are indicated for the temporary relief of nasal and sinus congestion and headache pain caused by sinusitis, common colds, allergy, and hay fever.

The therapeutic effectiveness of oral phenylephrine as a nasal decongestant has been questioned, especially at the usual oral dose.

## Patient Consultation

As an aid to patient consultation, refer to *Advice for the Patient, Decongestants and Analgesics (Systemic).*

In providing consultation, consider emphasizing the following selected information (» = major clinical significance):

### Before using this medication
» Conditions affecting use, especially:
Sensitivity to other sympathomimetic amines, salicylates or other nonsteroidal anti-inflammatory drugs
Pregnancy—Concern with high doses and long-term therapy because of salicylate effects; use of aspirin-containing combinations not recommended during third trimester; use of ibuprofen-containing combinations during second half of pregnancy not recommended because of potential adverse effect on fetal blood flow
Breast-feeding—High risk for infants from sympathomimetic amines; also, concern with high doses and chronic use because of high salicylate intake by infant
Use in children—Increased sensitivity to vasopressor and psychiatric effects of sympathomimetic amines; also, increased susceptibility to toxic effects of salicylates, especially if fever and dehydration present; possible association between aspirin usage and Reye's syndrome
Use in adolescents—Possible association between aspirin usage and Reye's syndrome

Use in the elderly—Increased susceptibility to effects of sympathomimetic amines and toxic effects of salicylates; increased risk of toxicity with ibuprofen
Other medications, especially for high blood pressure or depression, CNS depressants or stimulants, and others that may interact with acetaminophen, ibuprofen, and/or salicylates depending on specific ingredients of combination
Other medical problems, especially hypertension (for all combinations); alcoholism or hepatitis (for acetaminophen-containing combinations); hemophilia or other bleeding problems (for aspirin-containing combinations); asthma, gastritis, or peptic ulcer (with salicylate-containing combinations); clotting defects, peptic ulcer or other gastrointestinal tract disease, or stomatitis (for ibuprofen-containing combinations)

### Proper use of this medication
» Importance of not taking more medication than the amount recommended
» Proper dosing
Missed dose: If on scheduled dosing regimen—Taking as soon as possible; not taking if almost time for next dose; not doubling doses
» Proper storage
*For salicylate-containing combinations*
Taking with food or a full glass (240 mL) of water to minimize gastrointestinal irritation
» Not taking combinations containing aspirin if a strong vinegar-like odor is present
*For ibuprofen-containing combinations*
Taking with food or antacids (a magnesium- and aluminum-containing antacid may be preferred) to reduce gastrointestinal irritation; not lying down for 15 to 30 minutes after taking

### Precautions while using this medication
Checking with physician if symptoms persist or become worse, or if high fever is present
» Caution if taking phenylpropanolamine-containing appetite suppressants
» Possible insomnia; taking the medication a few hours before bedtime
Need to inform physician or dentist of use of medication if any kind of surgery (including dental surgery or emergency treatment is required)
» Caution if other medications containing acetaminophen, aspirin, or other salicylates (including diflunisal) are used
» Avoiding use of alcoholic beverages while taking these medications; alcohol consumption may increase risk of ibuprofen- or salicylate-induced gastrointestinal toxicity and acetaminophen-induced liver toxicity
» Suspected overdose: Getting emergency help at once
Not taking products containing aspirin for 5 days prior to any kind of surgery, unless otherwise directed by physician
Diabetics: Aspirin present in some combination formulations may cause false urine sugar test results with prolonged use of 8 or more 325-mg (5-grain) doses per day
*For ibuprofen-containing combinations*
» Caution if drowsiness or dizziness occurs

### Side/adverse effects
Signs of potential side effects, especially allergic reactions, anemia, cardiac effects, CNS stimulation, psychotic episodes, severe dizziness, severe nervousness or restlessness (for all combinations); blood dyscrasias, hepatitis, hepatotoxicity (for acetaminophen-containing); signs of gastrointestinal irritation or bleeding (for ibuprofen- or salicylate-containing); and cutaneous adverse effects, hepatitis, renal impairment (for ibuprofen-containing)

## Oral Dosage Forms
See *Table 1*, page 1141.

Revised: 09/07/94
Interim revision: 07/18/95

## Table 1. Oral Dosage Forms

Note: Content per capsule, tablet, or 5 mL, unless otherwise stated.

| Brand or generic name [availability] | Decongestants | Analgesics | Other content information as per product label | Usual adult and adolescent dose* (prn) | Usual pediatric dose (prn) | Packaging, storage, and auxiliary labeling† |
|---|---|---|---|---|---|---|
| *Actifed Sinus Daytime* Tablets USP (OTC) [U.S.] | Pseudoephedrine HCl 30 mg | Acetaminophen 500 mg | Available in a dual package that also contains *Actifed Sinus Nighttime Tablets* | 2 tabs q 6 hr | Not recommended | a |
| *Actifed Sinus Daytime Caplets* Tablets USP (OTC) [U.S.] | Pseudoephedrine HCl 30 mg | Acetaminophen 500 mg | Available in a dual package that also contains *Actifed Sinus Nighttime Caplets* | 2 tabs q 6 hr | Not recommended | a |
| *Advil Cold and Sinus Caplets* Tablets (OTC) [U.S.] | Pseudoephedrine HCl 30 mg | Ibuprofen 200 mg | | 1–2 tabs q 4–6 hr (max 6 tabs daily) | | a |
| *Alka-Seltzer Plus Sinus Medicine* Effervescent Tablets (OTC) [U.S.] | Phenylpropanolamine bitartrate 20 mg | Aspirin 325 mg | Sodium 504 mg Phenylalanine 12.32 mg | 2 tabs q 4 hr dissolved in 120 mL water (max 8 tabs daily) | | a |
| *Allerest No-Drowsiness* Tablets USP (OTC) [U.S.] | Pseudoephedrine HCl 30 mg | Acetaminophen 325 mg | | 2 tabs q 4–6 hr (max 8 tabs daily) | | a |
| *Bayer Select Head Cold Caplets* Tablets USP (OTC) [U.S.] | Pseudoephedrine HCl 30 mg | Acetaminophen 500 mg | | 2 tabs q 6 hr (max 8 tabs daily) | | a |
| *Bayer Select Maximum Strength Sinus Pain Relief Caplets* Tablets USP (OTC) [U.S.] | Pseudoephedrine HCl 30 mg | Acetaminophen 500 mg | | 2 tabs q 4–6 hr (max 8 tabs daily) | | a |
| *BC Cold Powder Non-Drowsy Formula* for Oral Solution (OTC) [U.S.] | Phenylpropanolamine HCl 25 mg/packet | Aspirin 650 mg/packet | | 1 packet dissolved in water q 6 hr | | a |
| *CoAdvil Caplets* Tablets (OTC) [U.S.] | Pseudoephedrine HCl 30 mg | Ibuprofen 200 mg | | 1 tab q 4–6 hr | | a |
| *Coldrine* Tablets USP (OTC) [U.S.] | Pseudoephedrine HCl 30 mg | Acetaminophen 325 mg | | 2 tabs q 6 hr | | a |

*Geriatric patients may be more sensitive to the effects of usual adult dose.

†For appropriate *Packaging and storage* and *Auxiliary labeling* information refer to designated letters as follows:
    a—Store below 40 °C (104 °F), preferably between 15 and 30 °C (59 and 86 °F), in a tight container, unless otherwise specified by manufacturer.
    b—Protect from freezing.
    c—Auxiliary labeling: • May be chewed.

## Table 1. Oral Dosage Forms *(continued)*

Note: Content per capsule, tablet, or 5 mL, unless otherwise stated.

| Brand or generic name [availability] | Decongestants | Analgesics | Other content information as per product label | Usual adult and adolescent dose* (prn) | Usual pediatric dose (prn) | Packaging, storage, and auxiliary labeling† |
|---|---|---|---|---|---|---|
| *Congespirin for Children Cold Tablets* Chewable Tablets (OTC) [U.S.] | Phenylephrine HCl 1.25 mg | Acetaminophen 81 mg | Scored | Intended for pediatric use | 2–3 yrs: 2 tabs, 4–5 yrs: 3 tabs, 6–8 yrs: 4 tabs, 9–10 yrs: 5 tabs, 11–12 yrs: 6 tabs, q 4 hr | a, c |
| *Congespirin for Children Liquid Cold Medicine* Oral Solution (OTC) [U.S.] | Phenylpropanolamine HCl 6.25 mg | Acetaminophen 130 mg | Alcohol 10% | Intended for pediatric use | 3–5 yrs: 5 mL, 6–12 yrs: 10 mL, q 3–4 hr | a, b |
| *Contac Allergy/Sinus Day Caplets* Tablets USP (OTC) [U.S.] | Pseudoephedrine HCl 60 mg | Acetaminophen 650 mg | Available in a dual package that also contains *Contac Allergy/Sinus Night Caplets* | 1 tab q 6 hr (max 4 tabs daily) | | a |
| *Contac Maximum Strength Sinus Caplets* Tablets USP (OTC) [U.S.] | Pseudoephedrine HCl 30 mg | Acetaminophen 500 mg | | 2 tabs q 6 hr | | a |
| *Contac Non-Drowsy Formula Sinus Caplets* Tablets USP (OTC) [U.S.] | Pseudoephedrine HCl 30 mg | Acetaminophen 500 mg | | 2 tab q 6 hr | | a |
| *Coricidin Non-Drowsy Sinus Formula* Tablets (OTC) [Canada] | Phenylpropanolamine HCl 12.5 mg | Aspirin 325 mg | | 2 tabs q 4 hr (max 8 tabs daily) | | a |
| *Dimetapp Sinus Caplets* Tablets (OTC) [U.S.] | Pseudoephedrine HCl 30 mg | Ibuprofen 200 mg | | 1 tab q 4–6 hr (max 6 tabs daily) | | a |
| *Dristan Cold Caplets* Tablets USP (OTC) [U.S.] | Pseudoephedrine HCl 30 mg | Acetaminophen 500 mg | | 2 tabs q 6 hr | | a |
| *Dristan N.D. Caplets* Tablets USP (OTC) [Canada] | Pseudoephedrine HCl 30 mg | Acetaminophen 325 mg | | 2 tabs q 4 hr (max 8 tabs daily) | | a |
| *Dristan N.D. Extra Strength Caplets* Tablets USP (OTC) [Canada] | Pseudoephedrine HCl 30 mg | Acetaminophen 500 mg | | 1–2 tabs q 4–6 hr (max 8 tabs daily) | | a |
| *Dristan Sinus Caplets* Tablets (OTC) [U.S.] | Pseudoephedrine HCl 30 mg | Ibuprofen 200 mg | | 1 tab q 4–6 hr | | a |
| *Dynafed Maximum Strength* Tablets USP (OTC) [U.S.] | Pseudoephedrine HCl 30 mg | Acetaminophen 500 mg | | 2 tabs q 6 hr | | a |
| *Emertabs* Tablets (OTC) [Canada] | Phenylpropanolamine HCl 16.2 mg | Acetaminophen 325 mg | Caffeine alkaloid 16.2 mg | 1 tab q 4 hr | | a |
| *Genex* Capsules (OTC) [U.S.] | Phenylpropanolamine HCl 18 mg | Acetaminophen 325 mg | | 2 caps q 4 hr | | a |

Table 1. Oral Dosage Forms *(continued)*

Note: Content per capsule, tablet, or 5 mL, unless otherwise stated.

| Brand or generic name [availability] | Decongestants | Analgesics | Other content information as per product label | Usual adult and adolescent dose* (prn) | Usual pediatric dose (prn) | Packaging, storage, and auxiliary labeling† |
|---|---|---|---|---|---|---|
| *Motrin IB Sinus* Tablets (OTC) [U.S.] | Pseudoephedrine HCl 30 mg | Ibuprofen 200 mg | | 1–2 tabs q 4–6 hr (max 6 tabs daily) | | a |
| *Motrin IB Sinus Caplets* Tablets (OTC) [U.S.] | Pseudoephedrine HCl 30 mg | Ibuprofen 200 mg | | 1–2 tabs q 4–6 hr (max 6 tabs daily) | | a |
| *Naldegesic* Tablets USP (OTC) [U.S.] | Pseudoephedrine HCl 15 mg | Acetaminophen 325 mg | Scored | 2 tabs q 4 hr | | a |
| *Neo Citran Extra Strength Sinus* for Oral Solution (OTC) [Canada] | Phenylephrine HCl 10 mg/pouch | Acetaminophen 650 mg/pouch | Vitamin C 50 mg/pouch | Contents of 1 pouch dissolved in 240 mL hot water | | a |
| *Ornex Maximum Strength Caplets* Tablets USP (OTC) [U.S.] | Pseudoephedrine HCl 30 mg | Acetaminophen 500 mg | | 2 tabs q 6 hr (max 8 tabs daily) | | a |
| *Ornex No Drowsiness Caplets* Tablets USP (OTC) [U.S.] | Pseudoephedrine HCl 30 mg | Acetaminophen 325 mg | | 2 tabs q 4 hr (max 8 tabs daily) | 6–11 yrs: 1 tab q 4 hr (max 4 tabs daily) | a |
| *PhenAPAP No. 2* Tablets (OTC) [U.S.] | Phenylpropanolamine HCl 25 mg | Acetaminophen 325 mg | | 1 tab q 4 hr | | a |
| *Rhinocaps* Capsules (OTC) [U.S.] | Phenylpropanolamine HCl 20 mg | Acetaminophen 162 mg, Aspirin 162 mg | | 2 caps q 4 hr | | a |
| *Saleto D* Capsules (OTC) [U.S.] | Phenylpropanolamine HCl 18 mg | Acetaminophen 240 mg, Salicylamide 120 mg | Caffeine 16 mg | 2 caps q 4 hr | | a |
| *Sinarest No-Drowsiness* Tablets USP (OTC) [U.S.] | Pseudoephedrine HCl 30 mg | Acetaminophen 500 mg | | 2 tabs q 6 hr (max 8 tabs daily) | | a |
| *Sine-Aid* Tablets USP (OTC) [U.S.] | Pseudoephedrine HCl 30 mg | Acetaminophen 325 mg | | 2 tabs q 4–6 hr | | a |
| *Sine-Aid IB Caplets* Tablets (OTC) [U.S.] | Pseudoephedrine HCl 30 mg | Ibuprofen 200 mg | | 1–2 tabs q 4–6 hr (max 6 tabs daily) | | a |
| *Sine-Aid Maximum Strength* Tablets USP (OTC) [U.S.] | Pseudoephedrine HCl 30 mg | Acetaminophen 500 mg | | 2 tabs q 4–6 hr (max 8 tabs daily) | | a |
| *Sine-Aid Maximum Strength Caplets* Tablets USP (OTC) [U.S.] | Pseudoephedrine HCl 30 mg | Acetaminophen 500 mg | | 2 tabs q 4–6 hr (max 8 tabs daily) | | a |

*Geriatric patients may be more sensitive to the effects of usual adult dose.

†For appropriate *Packaging and storage* and *Auxiliary labeling* information refer to designated letters as follows:

    a—Store below 40 °C (104 °F), preferably between 15 and 30 °C (59 and 86 °F), in a tight container, unless otherwise specified by manufacturer.

    b—Protect from freezing.

    c—Auxiliary labeling: • May be chewed.

## Table 1. Oral Dosage Forms *(continued)*

Note: Content per capsule, tablet, or 5 mL, unless otherwise stated.

| Brand or generic name [availability] | Decongestants | Analgesics | Other content information as per product label | Usual adult and adolescent dose* (prn) | Usual pediatric dose (prn) | Packaging, storage, and auxiliary labeling† |
|---|---|---|---|---|---|---|
| *Sine-Aid Maximum Strength Gelcaps* Tablets USP (OTC) [U.S.] | Pseudoephedrine HCl 30 mg | Acetaminophen 500 mg | | 2 tabs q 4–6 hr (max 8 tabs daily) | | a |
| *Sine-Off Maximum Strength No Drowsiness Formula Caplets* Tablets USP (OTC) [U.S.] | Pseudoephedrine HCl 30 mg | Acetaminophen 500 mg | | 2 tabs q 6 hr (max 8 tabs daily) | | a |
| *Sinus Excedrin Extra Strength* Tablets USP (OTC) [U.S.] | Pseudoephedrine HCl 30 mg | Acetaminophen 500 mg | | 2 tabs q 6 hr (max 8 tabs daily) | | a |
| *Sinus Excedrin Extra Strength Caplets* Tablets USP (OTC) [U.S.] | Pseudoephedrine HCl 30 mg | Acetaminophen 500 mg | | 2 tabs q 6 hr (max 8 tabs daily) | | a |
| *Sinus-Relief* Tablets USP (OTC) [U.S.] | Pseudoephedrine HCl 30 mg | Acetaminophen 325 mg | | 2 tabs q 4 hr (max 8 tabs daily) | | a |
| *Sinutab II Maximum Strength* Capsules (OTC) [U.S.] | Pseudoephedrine HCl 30 mg | Acetaminophen 500 mg | | 2 caps q 6 hr | | a |
| Tablets USP (OTC) [U.S.] | Pseudoephedrine HCl 30 mg | Acetaminophen 500 mg | | 2 tabs q 6 hr | | a |
| *Sinutab Maximum Strength Without Drowsiness* Tablets USP (OTC) [U.S.] | Pseudoephedrine HCl 30 mg | Acetaminophen 500 mg | | 2 tabs q 6 hr | | a |
| *Sinutab Maximum Strength Without Drowsiness Caplets* Tablets USP (OTC) [U.S.] | Pseudoephedrine HCl 30 mg | Acetaminophen 500 mg | | 2 tabs q 6 hr | | a |
| *Sinutab Sinus Without Drowsiness* Tablets USP (OTC) [U.S.] | Pseudoephedrine HCl 30 mg | Acetaminophen 325 mg | | 2 tabs q 4 hr (max 8 tabs daily) | Not recommended | a |
| *Sinutab No Drowsiness* Tablets USP (OTC) [Canada] | Pseudoephedrine HCl 30 mg | Acetaminophen 325 mg | Scored Tartrazine free | 2 tabs q 4–6 hr (max 8 tabs daily) | >6 yrs: 1 tab q 4–6 hr (max 4 tabs daily) | a |
| *Sinutab No Drowsiness Extra Strength* Tablets USP (OTC) [Canada] | Pseudoephedrine HCl 30 mg | Acetaminophen 500 mg | Tartrazine free | 1–2 tabs q 4–6 hr (max 8 tabs daily) | | a |
| *Sudafed Sinus Extra Strength Caplets* Tablets USP (OTC) [Canada] | Pseudoephedrine HCl 60 mg | Acetaminophen 500 mg | | 1 tab q 4–6 hr (max 4 tabs daily) | | a |
| *Sudafed Sinus Maximum Strength* Tablets USP (OTC) [U.S.] | Pseudoephedrine HCl 30 mg | Acetaminophen 500 mg | | 2 tabs q 6 hr | | a |

## Table 1. Oral Dosage Forms (continued)

Note: Content per capsule, tablet, or 5 mL, unless otherwise stated.

| Brand or generic name [availability] | Decongestants | Analgesics | Other content information as per product label | Usual adult and adolescent dose* (prn) | Usual pediatric dose (prn) | Packaging, storage, and auxiliary labeling† |
|---|---|---|---|---|---|---|
| Sudafed Sinus Maximum Strength Caplets Tablets USP (OTC) [U.S.] | Pseudoephedrine HCl 30 mg | Acetaminophen 500 mg | | 2 tabs q 6 hr | | a |
| Tylenol Sinus Maximum Strength Tablets USP (OTC) [U.S.] | Pseudoephedrine HCl 30 mg | Acetaminophen 500 mg | | 2 tabs q 4–6 hr (max 8 tabs daily) | | a |
| Tylenol Sinus Maximum Strength Caplets Tablets USP (OTC) [U.S.] | Pseudoephedrine HCl 30 mg | Acetaminophen 500 mg | | 2 tabs q 4–6 hr (max 8 tabs daily) | | a |
| Tylenol Sinus Maximum Strength Gelcaps Tablets USP (OTC) [U.S.] | Pseudoephedrine HCl 30 mg | Acetaminophen 500 mg | | 2 tabs q 4–6 hr (max 8 tabs daily) | | a |
| Tylenol Sinus Medication Tablets USP (OTC) [Canada] | Pseudoephedrine HCl 30 mg | Acetaminophen 325 mg | Tartrazine free | 1–2 tabs q 4–6 hr (max 8 tabs daily) | | a |
| Tylenol Sinus Medication Extra Strength Tablets USP (OTC) [Canada] | Pseudoephedrine HCl 30 mg | Acetaminophen 500 mg | Tartrazine free | 1–2 tabs q 4–6 hr (max 8 tabs daily) | | a |
| Ursinus Inlay Tablets (OTC) [U.S.] | Pseudoephedrine HCl 30 mg | Aspirin 325 mg | | 2 tabs q 4 hr | | a |
| Vicks DayQuil Sinus Pressure & Pain Relief Caplets Tablets USP (OTC) [U.S.] | Pseudoephedrine HCl 30 mg | Acetaminophen 500 mg | | 2 tabs q 6 hr | | a |

*Geriatric patients may be more sensitive to the effects of usual adult dose.

†For appropriate Packaging and storage and Auxiliary labeling information refer to designated letters as follows:
   a—Store below 40 °C (104 °F), preferably between 15 and 30 °C (59 and 86 °F), in a tight container, unless otherwise specified by manufacturer.
   b—Protect from freezing.
   c—Auxiliary labeling: • May be chewed.

# DEFEROXAMINE   Systemic

BAN: Desferrioxamine mesylate
JAN: Deferoxamine mesilate
VA CLASSIFICATION (Primary): AD300
Another commonly used name is desferrioxamine.
Note: For a listing of dosage forms and brand names by country availability, see Dosage Forms section(s). For a listing of brand names for the articles in this monograph, refer to the General Index.

## Category
Chelating agent.

## Indications
Note: Bracketed information in the Indications section refers to uses that are not included in U.S. product labeling.

### Accepted
Toxicity, iron, acute (treatment adjunct)—Deferoxamine facilitates the removal of iron from the body in severe, acute iron poisoning. It is used as an adjunct to, not a substitute for, standard treatment measures, which may include induction of emesis with ipecac syrup; gastric lavage; whole bowel irrigation; suction and maintenance of clear airway; control of shock with intravenous fluids, blood, oxygen, and vasopressors; and correction of acidosis.

Acute iron poisoning usually follows a biphasic course. During the first phase, vomiting, sometimes bloody and containing partially digested tablets, may occur within the first half hour and recur for up to several hours. However, enteric-coated iron tablets may pass into the small intestine without causing severe gastric symptoms, but may appear on x-ray. Abdominal pain may or may not occur within the first 6 to 12 hours. Tarry stools or bloody diarrhea and lethargy may occur, and in some cases, leukocytosis, hyperglycemia, and fever may be present. A latent period, lasting from a few to 48 hours after ingestion, may occur between the 2 symptomatic phases, during which time the patient may appear to improve clinically. The second phase, not seen in milder cases, is associated with hepatic injury or failure, hypoglycemia, metabolic acidosis, hypotension, shock, seizures, coma, or death. Several weeks to months after the acute episode, late complications of hepatic cirrhosis or duodenal or pyloric stricture may be seen.

Most iron poisoning cases do not require deferoxamine. However, when deferoxamine is indicated in severe poisoning, the shorter the interval between ingestion of the overdose and administration of deferoxamine, the greater the probability of complete recovery.

Clinical signs suggesting severe iron poisoning that should be treated with deferoxamine include the following:
• Patient is severely symptomatic. Presence of symptoms warrants treatment with deferoxamine regardless of patient's serum iron concentrations, unless symptoms are mild (e.g., minor abdominal upset), or they occur after emesis has been induced by ipecac administration.
• Serum iron concentrations exceeding total iron-binding capacity (TIBC), if obtained within 4 to 6 hours after iron ingestion.
• Serum iron concentrations > 500 mcg per deciliter (mcg/dL) (90 micromoles per liter [micromoles/L]). Serum iron concentrations above 500 mcg/dL (90 micromoles/L) warrant treatment with deferoxamine even if patient is asymptomatic. Use of deferoxamine in asymptomatic patients with serum iron concentrations of 350 to 500 mcg/dL (63 to 90 micromoles/L) has been recommended by some clinicians.
• If serum iron concentrations and TIBC are both unavailable, deferoxamine should be used when a combination of the following occur:
—Diarrhea or vomiting occurs spontaneously within 6 hours of ingestion.
—Leukocyte counts > 15,000 per cubic millimeter (15,000 ×10⁹ per liter).
—Serum glucose > 150 mg per deciliter (8 millimoles per liter).
—There is a positive deferoxamine provocation test. However, a negative test does not rule out iron toxicity, since false negative tests have been reported with deferoxamine.
—Abdominal x-ray reveals presence of tablets/capsules.

Toxicity, iron, chronic (treatment)—Deferoxamine is indicated for promotion of iron excretion in patients who have an iron overload secondary to multiple transfusions associated with some chronic anemias, such as thalassemia, and in secondary hemochromatosis. Ascorbic acid may be administered concurrently in small doses to improve the chelating action of deferoxamine and to increase the amount of iron excreted. Since phlebotomy is precluded in patients with transfusional iron overload, chelation with deferoxamine is the only effective therapeutic alternative.

[Toxicity, aluminum (treatment)]—Deferoxamine, administered intravenously or intraperitoneally, is used to treat aluminum-induced encephalopathy, osteomalacia, and aluminum overload in children and adults with chronic renal failure, but only those who are maintained with hemodialysis or continuous ambulatory peritoneal dialysis (CAPD).

[Toxicity, aluminum (diagnosis)]—Deferoxamine is used to diagnose aluminum toxicity in patients with end-stage renal disease.

#### Unaccepted

Deferoxamine is *not* indicated for the treatment of primary hemochromatosis, since phlebotomy is more effective and is the treatment of choice for this indication.

Deferoxamine is *not* used to remove iron deposits from the cornea and subconjunctiva in the treatment of ocular siderosis, nor to remove rust stains after penetration of the eye by a foreign body.

## Pharmacology/Pharmacokinetics

#### Physicochemical characteristics
Molecular weight—656.79.

#### Mechanism of action/Effect
Iron toxicity—Deferoxamine has a strong affinity for trivalent (ferric) iron, binding with it to form ferrioxamine, a stable, water-soluble complex, which is eliminated via the kidneys. Theoretically, 100 mg of deferoxamine is capable of binding approximately 8.5 mg of ferric iron. Deferoxamine can remove iron from ferritin and hemosiderin *in vitro* and to a lesser extent from transferrin; however, the iron in hemoglobin, myoglobin, or cytochromes is not removed by deferoxamine.
Aluminum toxicity—Deferoxamine combines with tissue-bound aluminum to form aluminoxamine, a stable, water-soluble complex. The formation of aluminoxamine causes blood concentrations of aluminum to rise, resulting in an increased concentration gradient between the blood and dialysate, with the net effect of an increased removal of aluminum during dialysis. Theoretically, 100 mg of deferoxamine is capable of binding approximately 4.1 mg of aluminum.

#### Other actions/effects
Deferoxamine has a low affinity for ferrous iron and a very low affinity for calcium. Studies in man and animals have shown no increase in the excretion of electrolytes or trace metals.

#### Absorption
Poorly absorbed from gastrointestinal tract after oral administration; therefore, parenteral administration is required.

#### Biotransformation
Rapidly metabolized by tissues and by plasma enzymes, but exact mechanism is not known.

#### Half-life
Distribution—About 1 hour.
Elimination—About 6 hours.

#### Elimination
Renal—Deferoxamine is rapidly excreted by the kidneys after intramuscular injection, often without binding any iron. The water-soluble complexes, ferrioxamine and aluminoxamine, pass easily through the kidneys, with ferrioxamine possibly imparting a characteristic orange-rose (vin rosé) color to the urine.
Fecal—About one-third the total quantity of iron excreted in response to deferoxamine therapy is excreted through the bile into the feces.
In dialysis—Dialysis is of no value in removing serum iron alone but may be used to increase excretion of ferrioxamine, the deferoxamine-iron complex. Deferoxamine is readily dialyzable.

## Precautions to Consider

#### Pregnancy/Reproduction
Pregnancy—Problems in humans have not been documented; however, deferoxamine is not recommended for women of child-bearing potential or for use during early pregnancy. However, in cases of moderate to severe, acute iron intoxication, deferoxamine should be used, since iron is also toxic to the fetus.
Skeletal abnormalities were observed in the fetuses of 2 animal species when deferoxamine was administered in doses 4.5 times the maximum daily human dose.

FDA Pregnancy Category C.

#### Breast-feeding
It is not known whether deferoxamine is distributed into breast milk. However, problems in humans have not been documented.

#### Pediatrics
Deferoxamine is used after acute overdose, but is not usually used as chronic therapy in children up to 3 years of age. Younger patients are more likely to experience auditory and ocular toxicity with long-term, high-dose therapy.

#### Geriatrics
In patients with iron overload, when ascorbic acid is administered concurrently with deferoxamine to improve chelation and increase ferrioxamine excretion, older patients may be more prone to cardiac decompensation due to increased tissue iron toxicity; therefore, this regimen should be used with caution in older patients.

#### Drug interactions and/or related problems
The following drug interactions and/or related problems have been selected on the basis of their potential clinical significance (possible mechanism in parentheses where appropriate)—not necessarily inclusive (» = major clinical significance):

Note: Combinations containing any of the following medications, depending on the amount present, may also interact with this medication.

» Ascorbic acid
(vitamin C given orally in doses of 150 to 250 mg per day may improve the chelating action of deferoxamine and increase the amount of iron excreted; however, concurrent use may cause exacerbation of tissue iron toxicity, especially in the heart, causing cardiac decompensation; therefore, this regimen should be used with caution in older patients and patients with cardiac problems; the need for ascorbic acid supplementation should be completely documented by measurements of iron excretion before and after supplements, and the oral dose of ascorbic acid should be given an hour or two after the deferoxamine infusion has been initiated when adequate concentrations of deferoxamine have been achieved)

Epoetin
(aluminum toxicity may reduce erythropoiesis; therefore, dialysis patients with aluminum toxicity may require an adjustment in epoetin dosage)

### Laboratory value alterations

The following have been selected on the basis of their potential clinical significance (possible effect in parentheses where appropriate)—not necessarily inclusive (» = major clinical significance):

With diagnostic test results
    Colorimetric iron assay
       (deferoxamine may interfere with test, resulting in falsely low concentrations of serum iron)
»  Total iron-binding capacity (TIBC)
       (deferoxamine may cause a falsely high TIBC)

### Medical considerations/Contraindications

The medical considerations/contraindications included here have been selected on the basis of their potential clinical significance (reasons given in parentheses where appropriate)—not necessarily inclusive (» = major clinical significance).

*Risk-benefit should be considered when the following medical problems exist:*

»  Anuria or oliguria or
»  Renal disease, severe
       (decreases the excretion of deferoxamine and its chelates; dialysis may be used to increase excretion of the iron-deferoxamine and aluminum-deferoxamine complexes)
    Sensitivity to deferoxamine

### Patient monitoring

The following may be especially important in patient monitoring (other tests may be warranted in some patients, depending on condition; » = major clinical significance):

»  Ferritin concentrations, serum or
»  Iron concentrations, serum
       (recommended periodically to adjust dose of deferoxamine in relation to iron burden; in acute toxicity, blood samples should be obtained within 4 hours after iron ingestion, and repeated, because iron undergoes rapid redistribution into tissues; serum drawn early [within 2 hours after ingestion] may have artificially high concentrations of iron; but achievement of peak serum concentrations is delayed if the iron was in extended-release form, if the patient had a significant amount of food in his/her stomach, and if the dose of iron was large; serum iron concentrations obtained beyond 6 hours after ingestion may not be elevated, even in the presence of severe poisoning; in chronic iron overload, chelation treatment should be continued until the serum iron concentration is < 100 mcg per deciliter [18 micromoles per liter]; it may be important to monitor serum ferritin concentrations in patients with chronic iron overload)

    Iron excretion, urinary, 24-hr
       (recommended periodically for dosage adjustment and to determine duration of therapy)

    Total iron-binding capacity (TIBC)
       (may be useful if evaluated prior to administration of deferoxamine; following deferoxamine therapy, TIBC should not be relied upon as an indicator of acute iron overdose because it cannot provide information on the saturation of iron-binding proteins, and it may be falsely elevated)

*In chronic iron overload only*
»  Audiovisual examinations
       (complete eye examinations, including visual-evoked potentials, and audiologic testing recommended every 3 months, since patients on chronic subcutaneous therapy may be asymptomatic with the loss identified only by careful auditory testing or ophthalmologic examination; slit-lamp eye examinations recommended periodically to detect cataracts in patients treated for chronic iron overload; deficits are usually reversible upon immediate dosage reduction or discontinuation of deferoxamine therapy)

*In aluminum toxicity only*
    Aluminum concentrations, serum
       (recommended before and after administration of deferoxamine; a rise in serum aluminum concentration of > 150 mcg per L, measured 18 to 48 hours after the baseline measurement, is diagnostic of aluminum toxicity)

## Side/Adverse Effects

Note: Iron overload increases susceptibility of patients to *Yersinia enterocolitica* this susceptibility may be enhanced by deferoxamine therapy. Mucormycosis has also been reported in patients receiving deferoxamine while undergoing hemodialysis.

The following side/adverse effects have been selected on the basis of their potential clinical significance (possible signs and symptoms in parentheses where appropriate)—not necessarily inclusive:

**Those indicating need for medical attention**
More frequent
   *Allergic reaction* (hives; itching; skin rash; wheezing); *auditory neurotoxicity* (hearing problems)—especially in younger patients; *convulsions; fast heartbeat; flushing; hives, itching, or skin rash; low blood pressure or shock; ocular toxicity* (blurred vision; decreased acuity; impaired peripheral, color, and night vision; retinal pigmental abnormalities)—more frequent in younger patients; *pain or swelling at site of injection; respiratory distress syndrome* (cyanosis; difficult or fast breathing)—with excessively high intravenous doses for more than 1 day

Note: *Auditory neurotoxicity* may occur in patients on chronic, high-dose therapy. Onset may be acute and may accompany ocular problems. High-frequency hearing loss may occur in some patients after the serum ferritin returns to normal. Usually, but not always, reversible upon reduction of dose.

   *Allergic reaction, convulsions, fast heartbeat, flushing,* or *low blood pressure or shock* may be due to too-rapid a rate of intravenous injection in acute iron intoxication; skin problems may also occur in patients on chronic therapy as an allergic-type reaction.

   *Ocular toxicity* may occur in patients with low ferritin levels who are on chronic, high-dose therapy. Onset may be acute within 4 to 17 days of initiation of therapy and may accompany hearing loss. Usually reversible upon reduction of dose or discontinuation of deferoxamine. Cataracts have been observed on rare occasions in patients on long-term therapy.

Less frequent—with chronic therapy
   *Abdominal or stomach discomfort; diarrhea; difficult urination; fever; hypocalcemia* (abdominal and muscle cramps)—only when used for aluminum toxicity; *leg cramps; thrombocytopenia* (unusual bleeding or bruising)

**Those not indicating need for medical attention**
   *Urine color change to orange-rose or "vin rosé" color*

## Patient Consultation

As an aid to patient consultation, refer to *Advice for the Patient, Deferoxamine (Systemic).*

In providing consultation, consider emphasizing the following selected information (» = major clinical significance):

**Before receiving this medication**
»  Conditions affecting use, especially:
    Sensitivity to deferoxamine
    Pregnancy—Not recommended for use by women of child-bearing potential or during early pregnancy, unless iron poisoning becomes life-threatening
    Use in children—Used after acute overdose, but not usually used as chronic therapy in children up to 3 years of age; also, younger patients on chronic, high-dose therapy are more likely to develop hearing and ocular toxicity
    Use in the elderly—Caution when ascorbic acid used concurrently with deferoxamine; older patients more prone to cardiac decompensation with this regimen
    Other medications, especially ascorbic acid
    Other medical problems, especially renal disease

**Proper use of this medication**
»  Importance of clear understanding and careful following of physician's directions when using medication at home
»  Proper dosing
»  Proper storage

**Precautions while using this medication**
»  Regular visits to physician to check progress of therapy and to prevent adverse effects
»  Checking with doctor as soon as possible if any hearing or vision problems are noticed
    Not taking vitamin C unless ordered by physician

**Side/adverse effects**
    Signs of potential side effects, especially allergic reaction; hearing impairment; convulsions; fast heartbeat; flushing; hives, itching, or skin rash; low blood pressure or shock; vision impairment; pain or swelling at site of injection; respiratory distress syndrome; abdominal or stomach discomfort; diarrhea; difficult urination; fever; hypocalcemia; leg cramps; or thrombocytopenia
    Urine color may change to orange-rose.

# General Dosing Information

### For acute iron intoxication

Slow intravenous infusion should be used for patients in a state of cardiovascular collapse. The rate of infusion should not exceed 15 mg per kg of body weight (mg/kg) per hour. If it is difficult to establish an intravenous line, then the medication may be administered intramuscularly.

Although severe symptoms of iron toxicity do not usually occur when iron measures between 300 and 500 mcg per deciliter (54 and 90 micromoles per liter), a trial dose of deferoxamine may be administered intramuscularly (40 mg/kg) or by intravenous infusion (0.5 to 1 gram) over 4 hours, between 2 to 4 hours after ingestion of iron and after the gastrointestinal tract has been cleaned out. The patient should be observed for ferrioxamine in the urine (orange-rose color change of urine) until the results of serum iron and total iron binding capacity (TIBC) determinations are available, since the color change usually denotes a significant ingestion of iron. If the serum iron and TIBC results are not available, monitoring of urine color change should continue. If the color does not appear by 2 hours after the injection and the patient is asymptomatic, usually no further dose is needed. However, in some cases, the urine color may never change, even in the presence of severe, acute iron poisoning.

Dialysis is of no value in removing serum iron but may be useful in removing the iron-deferoxamine complex in patients who develop renal failure during treatment.

After treatment for acute iron intoxication, some physicians recommend that all treated patients be observed for a minimum of 24 hours after they become asymptomatic and that they be seen again in 2 weeks. This is to check for gastrointestinal symptoms and for iron deficiency caused by blood loss and/or excessive therapy. Delayed effects may include shock (24 to 48 hours) and gastrointestinal obstruction (weeks to months). Residual damage may be ruled out with liver and upper gastrointestinal studies.

### For chronic iron overload

The route of administration, either intramuscular or subcutaneous, must be individualized for each patient.

Because of the short serum half-life of deferoxamine, most of the drug may be rapidly excreted after a single intramuscular injection without binding any iron. However, continuous subcutaneous infusion may be almost as effective in mobilizing iron as continuous intravenous infusion. Therefore, a small mechanical infusion pump may be used to administer deferoxamine into the subcutaneous tissue of the abdomen. Deferoxamine is then infused very slowly over 8 to 16 hours on an outpatient basis. The duration of subcutaneous infusion with a portable mini-infusion pump must be individualized, depending on the rate of the patient's iron excretion. This regimen may remove 2 to 3 times more iron than a single daily intramuscular injection.

Patients who do not tolerate deferoxamine therapy because of cutaneous pain and swelling or hives may receive the medication via an infusion pump in an indwelling central venous line at an adult dose of 2 to 4 grams (40 to 80 mg/kg of body weight) administered over 12 to 16 hours.

If a net negative iron balance in response to deferoxamine can be achieved, long-term therapy should be considered in patients with transfusional iron overload.

If blood is transfused during deferoxamine therapy, it must not be mixed in the same container with deferoxamine.

# Parenteral Dosage Forms

Note: Bracketed uses in the *Dosage Forms* section refer to categories of use and/or indications that are not included in U.S. product labeling.

## DEFEROXAMINE MESYLATE STERILE USP

### Usual adult and adolescent dose

Iron toxicity, acute—
    Intramuscular, initially, 90 mg per kg of body weight, followed by 45 mg per kg of body weight, up to a maximum of 1 gram per dose, every four to twelve hours; not to exceed 6 grams per day.
    Intravenous, 15 mg per kg of body weight per hour, up to a total of 90 mg per kg of body weight every eight hours; not to exceed 6 grams per day.
    Note: The intravenous infusion rate should not exceed 15 mg per kg of body weight per hour.
Iron toxicity, chronic—
    Intramuscular, 500 mg to 1 gram a day.
    Intravenous, in addition to intramuscular administration, 2 grams infused at a rate not to exceed 15 mg per kg of body weight per

hour. This is administered at the same time each unit of blood is transfused, but through a separate line.
    Subcutaneous, 1 to 2 grams (20 to 40 mg per kg of body weight) a day administered over a period of eight to twenty-four hours by means of a portable, continuous mini-infusion pump.
[Aluminum toxicity]—
    Dosage must be individualized; theoretically, 100 mg of deferoxamine can bind 4.1 mg of aluminum.
Note: In hemodialysis or hemofiltration patients with moderate aluminum toxicity, and no concomitant iron toxicity, 1 gram of deferoxamine once a week has been given by slow intravenous infusion during the last two hours of every third dialysis session.

    In peritoneal dialysis patients, 1 to 1.5 grams of deferoxamine have been given in the dialysis fluid once or twice a week, by slow intravenous infusion, or by the intramuscular or subcutaneous route.
[Aluminum toxicity, diagnosis of]—
    Intravenous, 1 gram infused at a rate not to exceed 15 mg per kg of body weight per hour; it is preferably administered during the post-dialysis period, although administration during the last two hours of dialysis is acceptable.

### Usual adult prescribing limits

Up to 6 grams in twenty-four hours.

### Usual pediatric dose

Iron toxicity, acute and chronic—
    Children up to 3 years of age:
        Iron toxicity, acute—Intravenous, 15 mg per kg of body weight per hour.
        Iron toxicity, chronic—Subcutaneous, 10 mg per kg of body weight a day.
        [Aluminum toxicity, diagnosis of]—Intravenous, 15 to 20 mg per kg of body weight, infused at a rate not to exceed 15 mg per kg of body weight per hour; it is preferably administered during the post-dialysis period, although administration during the last two hours of dialysis is acceptable.
    Children over 3 years of age:
        See *Usual adult and adolescent dose.*

### Size(s) usually available

U.S.—
    500 mg (Rx) [*Desferal*].
Canada—
    500 mg (Rx) [*Desferal*].
    2 grams (Rx) [*Desferal*].

### Packaging and storage

Store below 30 °C (86 °F).

### Preparation of dosage form

For intramuscular or subcutaneous use—Add 2 mL of sterile water for injection to each 500-mg vial and 8 mL of sterile water for injection to each 2-gram vial. The powder should be completely dissolved before administration.

For intravenous infusion—Add 2 mL of sterile water for injection to each 500-mg vial and 8 mL of sterile water for injection to each 2-gram vial. The resulting solution should be further diluted in either 0.9% sodium chloride injection, dextrose injection, or lactated Ringer's injection before infusion.

### Stability

Reconstituted solutions should be used within the time period specified by the manufacturer.

### Incompatibilities

Precipitation may result if the solution is reconstituted with solvents or under conditions other than those recommended.

Revised: 05/27/94

# DEHYDROCHOLIC ACID—See *Laxatives (Local)*

# DEHYDROCHOLIC ACID–CONTAINING COMBINATIONS—

Dehydrocholic Acid and Docusate (Oral-Local)—See *Laxatives (Local)*
Dehydrocholic Acid, Docusate, and Phenolphthalein (Oral-Local)—See *Laxatives (Local)*

# DEMECARIUM—See *Antiglaucoma Agents, Cholinergic, Long-acting (Ophthalmic)*

**DEMECLOCYCLINE**—See *Tetracyclines (Systemic)*

**DESERPIDINE**—See *Rauwolfia Alkaloids (Systemic)*

**DESERPIDINE-CONTAINING COMBINATIONS**—

Deserpidine and Hydrochlorothiazide (Systemic)—See *Rauwolfia Alkaloids and Thiazide Diuretics (Systemic)*
Deserpidine and Methyclothiazide (Systemic)—See *Rauwolfia Alkaloids and Thiazide Diuretics (Systemic)*

# DESFLURANE   Inhalation-Systemic†

VA CLASSIFICATION (Primary): CN201

Note: For a listing of dosage forms and brand names by country availability, see *Dosage Forms* section(s). For a listing of brand names for the articles in this monograph, refer to the General Index.

†Not commercially available in Canada.

## Category

Anesthetic (general).

## Indications

### Accepted

Anesthesia, general—Desflurane is indicated for the induction and maintenance of general anesthesia in adults and for maintenance of anesthesia in infants and children. However, inhalation anesthetic agents are rarely used alone; other medications are frequently administered to induce or supplement anesthesia.

When desflurane is used for an inhalation induction in adults, it can cause complications such as coughing, increased secretions, laryngospasm, apnea, and oxyhemoglobin desaturation. The occurrence of such complications may not be decreased, and the risk of hypoxemia may be increased, when nitrous oxide (60 to 66%) is administered concurrently with induction doses of desflurane. However, the risk of severe oxygen desaturation and apnea is decreased when desflurane is administered with 100% oxygen. Therefore, administration of an intravenous induction agent and/or other intravenous adjuvant prior to or concurrently with desflurane, or administration of desflurane with 100% oxygen, should be considered.

### Unaccepted

Desflurane is not recommended for induction of anesthesia in infants and children because of an unacceptably high incidence of moderate to severe adverse effects, such as breath-holding, coughing, severe laryngospasm, increased secretions, oxyhemoglobin desaturation, and excitement. Although these complications may also occur when desflurane is used for an inhalation induction in adults, they occur more frequently and are more severe in pediatric patients.

## Pharmacology/Pharmacokinetics

Note: Concentration-response relationships for inhalation anesthetics are described in terms of the minimum alveolar concentration (MAC), which is defined as the alveolar concentration that prevents movement in 50% of patients subjected to a painful stimulus. The MAC decreases with increasing age (being highest in infants and young children), pregnancy, hypothermia, hypotension, and concurrent use of other CNS depressants, including other inhalation anesthetics. Average MAC values for desflurane (vaporized in oxygen or a mixture of oxygen and air) are 10%, 7.3%, and 5.4% in patients 9 months, 25 years, and 70 years of age, respectively.

### Physicochemical characteristics

Chemical group—A halogenated hydrocarbon (methyl ethel ether) anesthetic, structurally related to isoflurane.
Molecular weight—168.04.
Blood-to-gas partition coefficient (37 °C)—0.42
Note: The blood-to-gas partition coefficient is an indicator of the solubility of the anesthetic in blood, which affects the rate at which the partial pressure of the anesthetic in the blood (and therefore in the brain) equilibrates with that in the alveoli. Low solubility results in rapid rates of induction, changes in depth of anesthesia, and recovery. Desflurane's blood-to-gas partition coefficient is lower than those of other halogenated hydrocarbon anesthetics currently in use.
Oil-to-gas partition coefficient (37 °C)—18.7
Note: The oil-to-gas partition coefficient is an indicator of solubility in fatty tissues. High solubility increases anesthetic potency. Desflur-

ane's oil-to-gas partition coefficient is substantially lower than those of other halogenated hydrocarbon anesthetics currently in use.
Boiling point (1 atm pressure)—22.8 °C

### Mechanism of action/Effect

The precise mechanisms by which inhalation anesthetics produce loss of perception of sensations and unconsciousness have not been established. Inhalation anesthetics probably act on nerve cell membranes to disrupt neuronal transmission in the brain. These agents have been shown to bind to and alter membrane proteins, to alter cellular calcium ion processes, and to augment the activity of the inhibitory neurotransmitter gamma-aminobutyric acid (GABA) on synaptic transmission. The Meyer-Overton theory, which is based on the observation that there is a strong correlation between the potency of an inhalation anesthetic and its solubility in oil, suggests that the effects of these agents may be at least partially mediated via an action at the lipid matrix of the neuronal membrane.

### Other actions/effects

Cardiovascular system effects—
Blood pressure:
Like other potent inhalation anesthetics, desflurane usually causes dose-dependent decreases in blood pressure that may reflect the depth of anesthesia. However, in clinical studies, hypertension occasionally developed during or shortly following induction of anesthesia in patients receiving desflurane.
Cardiac function:
Desflurane depresses myocardial function; it may decrease contractility and possibly compliance. However, after prolonged administration (several hours), some of the cardiovascular depressant effects may be attenuated. Indirect stimulation induced by hypercarbia in spontaneously breathing patients may partially oppose the direct cardiopressant effects of the anesthetic. During desflurane administration indicators of cardiac function (e.g., cardiac index, stroke volume, and central venous pressure) are higher in spontaneously breathing patients than in mechanically ventilated patients.
Use of desflurane for induction of anesthesia may be associated with myocardial ischemia in patients with significant cardiovascular disease unless an agent that blunts the sympathetic response, e.g., an opioid, is administered concurrently.
One study has shown that desflurane is not likely to sensitize the myocardium to the ventricular arrhythmogenic effects of catecholamines or other sympathomimetics.
Heart/pulse rate:
May be increased by desflurane, especially when high concentrations are given during induction, when concentrations are increased rapidly, or after prolonged administration. An increase in heart rate therefore cannot be used as an indication of inadequate anesthesia.
Peripheral vasculature:
Desflurane may cause vasodilatation.
Note: Some of desflurane's cardiovascular effects may be at least partially reversed by surgical stimulation or stress (e.g., skin incision). Also, concurrent use of nitrous oxide (60%) reduces the requirement for desflurane and may therefore attenuate the cardiovascular effects observed with desflurane alone, especially in mechanically ventilated patients.
Central nervous system (CNS) effects—
Electroencephalogram (EEG):
Desflurane produces a dose-dependent decrease in EEG activity. It does not produce convulsive activity in the EEG (as has been observed with enflurane).
Effect on intracranial pressure:
Desflurane dilates cerebral arterioles. In clinical trials, concentrations of 1 MAC or higher (but not 0.5 or 0.8 MAC), increased cerebrospinal fluid pressure in patients undergoing craniotomy for removal of tumors despite use of measures that prevent or attenuate the increase in intracranial pressure induced by equiv-

thetics, i.e., establishment of hypocapnia and barbiturate administration. However, in another study, 1 or 1.5 MAC of desflurane did not increase cerebral blood flow in patients undergoing craniotomies under hypocapnic conditions.

Neuromuscular effects—

Desflurane impairs neuromuscular conduction and decreases muscle contractility. Its neuromuscular blocking activity is equivalent to that of enflurane or isoflurane. Like these other agents, desflurane may produce muscle relaxation sufficient to permit many types of surgery to be performed without a neuromuscular blocking agent.

Respiratory system effects—

Respiration:

Desflurane produces dose-dependent respiratory depression. It increases arterial carbon dioxide tension and respiratory rate and decreases tidal volume. In concentrations higher than 1.5 MAC, desflurane may cause apnea. Respiratory depression induced by inhalation anesthetics may be partially reversed with surgical stimulation or stress.

Effects on the airway:

Desflurane is an irritant to the airway and may cause breath-holding, coughing, increased secretions, and laryngospasm as well as increased sympathetic nervous system activity during induction. These effects may not be attenuated by increasing the inspired concentration slowly, premedicating with an opioid (e.g., fentanyl), and/or administering nitrous oxide concurrently.

## Absorption

Rapidly absorbed into the circulation via the lungs, as indicated by the low blood-to-gas partition coefficient.

## Biotransformation

Hepatic; minimal (approximately 0.02% of the quantity absorbed). In studies performed to date, small quantities of trifluoroacetic acid appeared in the serum and urine of desflurane recipients, but concentrations of inorganic fluoride were not increased. The risk of postoperative renal function impairment, which has occurred in patients with high concentrations of fluoride resulting from administration of other halogenated hydrocarbon anesthetics (primarily methoxyflurane and occasionally enflurane), appears minimal with desflurane.

## Time to peak concentration

The alveolar concentration increases very rapidly toward the inspired concentration. The ratios of the end-tidal alveolar concentration to the inspired concentration (washin ratio) after 10 and 30 minutes of administration are $> 0.8$ and $0.9$, respectively.

## Time to peak effect

Onset of anesthesia—End-tidal concentrations of 4 to 11% of desflurane, administered with or without nitrous oxide, produce anesthesia in 2 to 4 minutes. Desflurane's pungent odor and the airway irritability it causes may limit the rate at which the administered concentration can be increased, resulting in a longer induction time than would be expected with an agent having desflurane's low blood-to-gas partition coefficient.

## Duration of action

Time to recovery—Recovery after administration is discontinued is rapid but subject to interpatient variability. Recovery time also depends on the administered concentration and on whether other CNS depressants have been used concurrently. Whether the duration of administration also affects recovery time has not been studied, but, because of desflurane's rapid elimination, a significant lengthening of the recovery time after prolonged administration would not be expected. In clinical studies, mean emergence times have generally ranged from 5 to 16 minutes. Psychometric testing has shown that patients begin to recover more rapidly after desflurane than after isoflurane. However, other determinants of recovery (e.g., time to sit up or walk) and readiness for discharge from outpatient surgical facilities have not been shown to be significantly more rapid with desflurane than with comparison agents (isoflurane or propofol with nitrous oxide).

## Elimination

Primarily as unchanged desflurane, via exhalation. Less than 0.02% of a dose is eliminated in the urine as metabolites. Also, very small quantities may be eliminated through the skin.

A pharmacokinetic study determined that 5 minutes after discontinuation of desflurane the ratio of the end-tidal alveolar concentration to the last concentration during administration (washout ratio) is 0.14. In other studies, the end-tidal desflurane concentration decreased by about 85% within 2 minutes after discontinuation of administration to pediatric patients and by about 50% within 2.5 minutes after discontinuation of administration to adult patients.

# Precautions to Consider

## Cross-sensitivity and/or related problems

Although this problem has not been documented to date, the possibility exists that patients sensitive to other halogenated hydrocarbon anesthetics (enflurane, halothane, isoflurane, or methoxyflurane) may be sensitive to desflurane also.

## Mutagenicity

No mutagenicity or chromosomal damage was found in *in vitro* and *in vivo* studies, including the Ames mutation assay, metaphase analysis of human lymphocytes, and mouse micronucleus assay.

## Pregnancy/Reproduction

Fertility—Fertility was not affected after exposure of test animals to the equivalent of 1 minimum alveolar concentration (MAC) of desflurane for 1 hour (1 MAC-hour) per day. The cumulative exposure was 63 MAC-hours for males and 14 MAC-hours for females. At higher doses, mortalities and other manifestations of parental toxicity that could affect fertility (e.g., decreased weight gain) occurred.

Pregnancy—
*First trimester*—

Adequate and well-controlled studies in patients have not been done. Studies (by retrospective survey) of operating room personnel chronically exposed to low concentrations of inhalation anesthetics in use at the time the studies were done indicate that pregnancies in female personnel and wives of male personnel may be subject to an increased incidence of spontaneous abortions, stillbirths, and possibly birth defects. However, the methods used in obtaining and interpreting the data in these studies have been questioned. Also, several animal studies (in which operating room conditions were simulated) failed to show fetotoxic or teratogenic effects following chronic exposure of male and/or female animals to low concentrations of inhalation anesthetics prior to and/or during gestation.

Studies in rats and rabbits exposed to 1 MAC-hour per day for 10 and 13 days, respectively, during organogenesis failed to detect evidence of teratogenicity. At higher doses, increased incidences of post-implantation loss and maternal toxicity were observed. Also, at 10 MAC-hours cumulative exposure in rats, the weight of male pups was decreased by about 6% at preterm cesarean delivery.

*Third trimester*—

Rats exposed to 1 MAC-hour of desflurane per day from gestation Day 15 did not show signs of dystocia at delivery. The body weights of the exposed pups were comparable to those of controls.

FDA Pregnancy Category B.

Labor and delivery—The safety of desflurane during labor and delivery has not been established.

## Breast-feeding

Because of its rapid elimination from the body, concentrations of desflurane in breast milk are predicted to be lower than those found with other volatile anesthetics. Concentrations in breast milk are not likely to be of clinical importance 24 hours after anesthesia.

## Pediatrics

Induction—Desflurane is not recommended for induction of anesthesia in pediatric patients because of an unacceptably high incidence of moderate to severe adverse effects, such as breath-holding (68%), coughing (72%), laryngospasm (50%), increased secretions (21%), oxyhemoglobin desaturation (26%), and excitement.

Maintenance—The MAC of desflurane is age-dependent; it is higher in infants and children 2 years of age and younger than in older children and adults. MAC values are highest (about 10%) in infants 6 to 12 months of age, although values in neonates and infants younger than 6 months of age also exceed 9%. In contrast, the MAC values of halothane and isoflurane are highest in infants 1 to 6 months of age. Also, the difference between MAC values in neonates and those in older infants is not as great for desflurane (about 7.7%) as for halothane (25%) or isoflurane (17%). MAC values decrease to approximately 8.7 to 9.1% in children 1 to 3 years of age and to 8.1% in children 7 to 12 years of age.

## Geriatrics

Desflurane has been studied in patients up to 91 years of age. The MAC is lower in geriatric patients than in younger adults, about 5.2% for a patient 70 years of age (compared with 6% and 7.3% for patients 45 and 25 years of age, respectively). Also, although emergence in geriatric patients is approximately 20% more rapid after desflurane than after isoflurane, the difference is not as great as in younger adults.

## Drug interactions and/or related problems

The following drug interactions and/or related problems have been selected on the basis of their potential clinical significance (possible mechanism in parentheses where appropriate)—not necessarily inclusive (» = major clinical significance):

Note: Combinations containing any of the following medications, depending on the amount present, may also interact with this medication.

Many of the following interactions have not been documented with desflurane. However, because they have been reported to occur with other halogenated hydrocarbon anesthetics, the possibility of a significant interaction with desflurane must be considered.

Alcohol, chronic abuse
(anesthetic requirement may be increased)

» Aminoglycosides, systemic, possibly including oral neomycin (if significant quantities are absorbed by patients with renal function impairment) or
Anesthetics, parenteral-local (large doses leading to significant plasma concentrations) or
Bacitracin or
» Capreomycin or
» Citrate-anticoagulated blood, massive transfusions of or
» Clindamycin or
Colistimethate sodium or
Colistin or
Lidocaine (systemic use, with intravenous doses > 5 mg per kg of body weight) or
» Lincomycin, systemic or
» Neuromuscular blocking agents or
» Polymyxins, systemic or
Procaine (systemic use) or
Tetracyclines or
Trimethaphan (large doses)
(neuromuscular blocking activity of these medications may be additive to that of desflurane, with the degree of potentiation being increased as the concentration of desflurane is increased; although increased and/or prolonged skeletal muscle weakness and respiratory depression or paralysis [apnea] may occur, clinical significance is minimal if the patient is being mechanically ventilated)

(administration of desflurane for 15 minutes has been shown to decrease the ED$_{95}$ [dose of a neuromuscular blocking agent required to produce 95% suppression of the adductor pollicis muscle twitch response to ulnar nerve stimulation] of subsequently administered succinylcholine by about 30% and the ED$_{95}$ of subsequently administered atracurium or pancuronium by about 50%; desflurane's effects on ED$_{95}$ values of other nondepolarizing neuromuscular blocking agents and on the duration of action of any neuromuscular blocking agent have not been established; a reduction of dosage, as determined by response to peripheral nerve stimulation, may be needed when a neuromuscular blocking agent is administered after steady-state anesthesia with desflurane has been established)

(concurrent use of succinylcholine with halogenated hydrocarbon anesthetics may increase the risk of malignant hyperthermia; also, repeated concurrent use may increase the risk of bradycardia)

Amiodarone
(concurrent use with inhalation anesthetics may potentiate hypotension and increase the risk of atropine-resistant bradycardia)

Antihypertensive agents, especially diazoxide or ganglionic blockers such as guanadrel, guanethidine, mecamylamine, or trimethaphan or
Chlorpromazine or
Diuretics or
Hypotension-producing medications, other (See Appendix II)
(hypotensive effects may be potentiated when these medications are used concurrently with an inhalation anesthetic; patients should be monitored for excessive fall in blood pressure during and following concurrent use)

Antimyasthenics
(antimyasthenics, especially neostigmine and pyridostigmine, may decrease the neuromuscular blocking activity of halogenated hydrocarbon anesthetics; also, the neuromuscular blocking activity of the anesthetic may interfere with the efficacy of antimyasthenics, and temporary dosage adjustment may be required to control symptoms of myasthenia gravis postoperatively)

Beta-adrenergic blocking agents, including ophthalmic dosage forms
(concurrent use with hydrocarbon inhalation anesthetics may result in prolonged, severe hypotension because beta-blockade reduces the ability of the heart to respond to beta-adrenergically mediated sympathetic reflex stimuli; if necessary to reverse the effects of beta-adrenergic blocking agents during surgery, agonists such as dobutamine, dopamine, isoproterenol, or norepinephrine may be administered)

(it is recommended that high concentrations of halogenated hydrocarbon anesthetics not be administered when labetalol is used to produce controlled hypotension during surgery; possible additive effects may lead to excessive hypotension, large reduction in cardiac output, and increased central venous pressure)

» Catecholamines such as dopamine, epinephrine, or norepinephrine or
» Cocaine or
» Ephedrine or
» Levodopa or
» Metaraminol or
» Methoxamine or
Other sympathomimetic agents
(the increase in heart rate and/or blood pressure induced by these agents may be intensified if desflurane causes the same effects; caution in concurrent use is recommended, especially in patients who are at risk of cardiac ischemia; however, desflurane does not significantly sensitize the myocardium to the ventricular arrhythmogenic effects of catecholamines or other sympathomimetics)

CNS depression–producing medications, other, including those commonly used for pre-anesthetic medication or induction or supplementation of anesthesia (See Appendix II), especially
Benzodiazepines
Nitrous oxide
Opioid analgesics
(concurrent administration with an inhalation anesthetic may cause increased CNS depression, respiratory depression, and/or hypotension, decrease the anesthetic requirement, and prolong recovery from anesthesia; careful attention to the dosage of each agent is required)

(concurrent administration of benzodiazepines and/or opioid analgesics decreases the MAC of desflurane; specifically, midazolam [25 to 50 mcg per kg of body weight (mcg/kg)] decreases the MAC of desflurane by about 16 to 22% and fentanyl [3 to 6 mcg/kg] decreases the MAC of desflurane by 50% or more)

(concurrent administration of nitrous oxide [60%] decreases the MAC of desflurane by about 50% in adult patients [in 1 study, MAC was decreased from 6% to 3%] and by about 25% in pediatric patients; also, concurrent use of 60% nitrous oxide may attenuate many of the cardiovascular effects observed with desflurane alone, especially in mechanically ventilated patients, reduce struggling by patients during induction, and decrease postoperative patient recall of induction)

(2 or more CNS depressants may decrease the MAC of desflurane to a greater extent than a single CNS depressant when used concurrently; in 1 study, MAC values for desflurane were 3.7% when 60% nitrous oxide was given concurrently and 3%, 1.2%, and 0.1% when 3, 6, or 9 mcg/kg, respectively, of fentanyl was added to the desflurane–nitrous oxide regimen)

## Laboratory value alterations

The following have been selected on the basis of their potential clinical significance (possible effect in parentheses where appropriate)—not necessarily inclusive (» = major clinical significance):

With physiology/laboratory test values
Glucose concentrations, blood and
White blood cell count
(may be transiently increased)

## Medical considerations/Contraindications

The medical considerations/contraindications included here have been selected on the basis of their potential clinical significance (reasons given in parentheses where appropriate)—not necessarily inclusive (» = major clinical significance).

### Except under special circumstances, this medication should not be used when the following medical problem exists:

» Malignant hyperthermia, history of or suspected genetic predisposition to
(risk of malignant hyperthermic crisis during or following anesthesia; although this complication has not yet been documented in humans receiving desflurane, the anesthetic has induced malignant hyperthermia in genetically susceptible swine; although prophylactic administration of dantrolene prior to administration of a potent inhalation anesthetic may prevent the occurrence of a malignant hyperthermic crisis during or shortly following surgery in susceptible patients, this use of dantrolene is controversial and should be undertaken with caution [see Dantrolene (Systemic)])

*Risk-benefit should be considered when the following medical problems exist:*

» Coronary artery disease or other conditions in which increases in heart rate and/or blood pressure would be undesirable

(desflurane increased heart rate, arterial blood pressure, and pulmonary blood pressure; decreased stroke volume; and caused ischemia when used as the sole induction agent in patients undergoing cardiovascular surgery; however, ischemia did not occur in studies in patients undergoing cardiovascular surgery when supplemental opioid analgesic was administered concurrently; use of desflurane as the sole induction agent, without premedication with or supplemental administration of an opioid analgesic and/or an appropriate intravenous hypnotic, is not recommended)

Familial periodic paralysis, hypokalemic or hyperkalemic or
» Muscular dystrophy or
» Myasthenia gravis or
Myasthenic syndrome (Eaton-Lambert syndrome) or
Other neuromuscular disease leading to muscle weakness

(the neuromuscular blocking activity of desflurane may cause increased risk of severe muscle weakness or paralysis in patients with these conditions, which may lead to respiratory and other complications; although use of an inhalation anesthetic with substantial neuromuscular blocking activity may be safer than [and may eliminate the need for] a neuromuscular blocking agent in these patients, caution is recommended)

» Head injury or
» Increased intracranial pressure, pre-existing or
» Intracranial lesions, space occupying, or tumors

(desflurane may increase intracranial and/or cerebrospinal fluid [CSF] pressure; in patients undergoing neurosurgery, it is recommended that desflurane be administered in a dose of 0.8 MAC or lower, in conjunction with a barbiturate and hyperventilation [hypocapnia] prior to cranial decompression, and in conjunction with measures to maintain cerebral perfusion; administration of mannitol, in addition to barbiturate administration and reduction of desflurane dosage, may also attenuate the effect of desflurane on CSF pressure)

Sensitivity to desflurane or other halogenated hydrocarbon anesthetics, history of

**Patient monitoring**

The following may be especially important in patient monitoring (other tests may be warranted in some patients, depending on condition; » = major clinical significance):

Note: Various organizations, including medical specialty societies, and institutions have established standards for the pre-, intra-, and postprocedure care, evaluation, and monitoring of patients receiving various forms of anesthesia and/or sedation. The following recommendations represent the minimum standards established by the American Society of Anesthesiologists for monitoring the status of patients receiving general anesthesia. Individual patients may require additional monitoring.

» Blood pressure and
» Body temperature and
» Cardiac/pulse rate and
» Electrocardiographic evaluation and
» Oxygenation and
» Respiratory and ventilatory status

(it is recommended that the patient's blood and tissue oxygenation, ventilation, circulation, and body temperature be monitored continuously during anesthetic administration and as required during the recovery period)

## Side/Adverse Effects

Note: The possibility that malignant hyperthermia may develop during or following anesthesia must be considered. Although this problem has not been documented to date in humans receiving desflurane, the anesthetic has induced malignant hyperthermia in genetically susceptible swine.

Sixty-four percent of adults in clinical studies who received induction of anesthesia with desflurane in oxygen, but a significantly smaller percentage of adults who received nitrous oxide concurrently during induction, reported postoperative recall of induction and of a strong or disagreeable odor.

In addition to the adverse effects reported below, fever, hemorrhage, myalgia, myocardial infarction, and pruritus occurred rarely (incidence of each < 1%) in clinical trials. A causal relationship to use of desflurane has not been established.

Some of the adverse effects that developed during clinical trials, as reported below, may reflect the surgical procedures performed, patient characteristics (including disease), and/or other medications administered concurrently.

The following side/adverse effects have been selected on the basis of their potential clinical significance (possible signs and symptoms in parentheses where appropriate)—not necessarily inclusive:

**Those indicating need for medical attention**

Incidence more frequent (3 to 10%, or as specified)

*During induction by mask (adults only)*
*Apnea*—[15%]; *breath-holding*—[30%]; *coughing*—[34%]; *excitement/struggling; increased secretions; laryngospasm; oxyhemoglobin desaturation; pharyngitis*

*During maintenance or recovery (adult and pediatric patients)*
*Apnea; laryngospasm*

Incidence less frequent (1 to 3%)

*During maintenance or recovery (adult and pediatric patients)*
*Breath-holding; cardiovascular effects, such as bradycardia, hypertension, nodal arrhythmia, and tachycardia*

Incidence rare (less than 1%)

*During maintenance or recovery (adult and pediatric patients)*
*Cardiovascular effects, such as arrhythmias, including bigeminy and other cardiographic abnormalities; myocardial ischemia; respiratory effects, such as asthma, dyspnea, and hypoxia*

**Those indicating need for medical attention only if they continue or are bothersome**

Incidence more frequent (3 to 10%, or as specified)

*During maintenance or recovery (adult and pediatric patients)*
*Coughing; nausea*—[27%]; *vomiting*—[16%]

Incidence less frequent (1 to 3%) or rare (less than 1%)

*During maintenance or recovery (adult and pediatric patients)*
*Agitation* (nervousness or restlessness); *conjunctivitis or conjunctival hyperemia* (red or irritated eyes); *dizziness; excessive salivation; headache; sore throat*

## Overdose

For specific information on the agents used in the management of a desflurane overdose, see:

• *Atropine* in *Anticholinergics/Antispasmodics (Systemic)* monograph; and/or
• *Sympathomimetic Agents—Cardiovascular Use (Parenteral-Systemic)* monograph.

For more information on the management of overdose, **contact a Poison Control Center** (see *Poison Control Center Listing*).

The following effects have been selected on the basis of their potential clinical significance (possible signs and symptoms in parentheses where appropriate)—not necessarily inclusive:

Acute

*Bradycardia; circulatory depression or hypotension, severe; respiratory depression*

**Specific treatment**

For bradycardia—Administering atropine.

For circulatory depression or severe hypotension—Discontinuing or lightening anesthesia (if still being administered) and administering plasma and/or intravenous fluids. If surgical or postsurgical conditions permit, positioning the patient to improve venous return to the heart (i.e., in the Trendelenburg position) is recommended. If necessary, a vasopressor may be administered.

For respiratory depression—Decreasing anesthetic dosage (if still being administered), establishing a clear airway, and instituting assisted or controlled respiration with 100% oxygen.

## Patient Consultation

As an aid to patient consultation, refer to *Advice for the Patient, Desflurane (Systemic)*.

In providing consultation, consider emphasizing the following selected information (» = major clinical significance):

**Before using this medication**
» Conditions affecting use, especially:
Sensitivity to desflurane or other halogenated hydrocarbon anesthetics
Use in children—Not recommended for induction because of the high incidence of severe adverse effects
Other medications, including use of "street" drugs
Other medical problems, especially history of or genetic susceptibility to malignant hyperthermia and neuromuscular diseases leading to muscle weakness (e.g., familial periodic paralysis,

muscular dystrophy, myasthenia gravis, myasthenic syndrome [Eaton-Lambert syndrome])

### Precautions after receiving this medication
*For patients receiving anesthesia in an outpatient facility*
» Possibility of psychomotor impairment following anesthesia; using caution in driving or performing other tasks requiring alertness and coordination for about 24 hours postanesthesia
» Avoiding use of alcohol or central nervous system (CNS) depressants within 24 hours following anesthesia, unless specifically prescribed or otherwise authorized by physician or dentist

### Side/adverse effects
Notifying physician if nausea or vomiting, conjunctivitis, coughing, headache, or pharyngitis occurs or persists after discharge from outpatient surgical unit

## General Dosing Information

Inhalation anesthetics are to be administered only by individuals experienced in airway management and respiratory support. Equipment, medications, and personnel for support of ventilation and circulatory resuscitation must be immediately available.

Desflurane is to be administered only via a vaporizer specifically designed and designated for use with this agent. The anesthetic may be vaporized in oxygen, a mixture of oxygen and air, or a mixture of nitrous oxide and oxygen.

The stated dosages are given as a guideline. **The dosage of inhaled anesthetics must be individualized** according to surgical requirements; concurrent use of adjuvant medications and/or nitrous oxide; patient variables, especially age, body temperature, and physical condition; and patient response.

Anesthetic requirements are increased in very young children and decreased in geriatric patients.

Preanesthetic medications should be selected according to the needs of the individual patient and surgical requirements.

An intravenous induction agent often is administered prior to an inhalation anesthetic to facilitate induction of anesthesia and prevent the transient initial CNS excitation that may occur during induction with the inhalation anesthetic.

During maintenance of anesthesia, the concentration of inhaled anesthetic may be decreased progressively as necessary to prevent further increases in depth of anesthesia and/or hypotension.

Assisted or controlled respiration may be necessary, especially during deep levels of anesthesia, to control respiratory depression and/or respiratory acidosis.

### Safety considerations for handling this medication
Predicted effects in operating room personnel of acute overexposure to anesthetic gases include headache, dizziness, and, in extreme cases, unconsciousness.

The results of some epidemiological studies suggest a link between chronic exposure of operating room personnel to low concentrations of inhalation anesthetics (waste anesthetic gases [WAGs]) and increased health problems, including reproductive problems (increases in spontaneous abortions, stillbirths, and possibly birth defects). Although a causal relationship has not been established, measures to minimize exposure are recommended. Such measures include maintaining adequate general ventilation in the operating room, using a well-designed and well-maintained scavenging system, and minimizing leaks and spills while the anesthetic agent is in use via careful work practices and routine equipment maintenance.

Although no specific work exposure limit has been established for desflurane, the National Institute for Occupational Safety and Health Administration has recommended an 8-hour, time-weighted average limit of 2 parts per million (ppm) for halogenated anesthetic agents in general. The limit for halogenated anesthetics coupled with nitrous oxide is 0.5 ppm.

### For treatment of adverse effects
Recommended treatment includes
• For cardiac arrhythmias—Determining whether the level of anesthesia is adequate for the given surgical stimulus and adjusting (deepening or lightening) the level of anesthesia accordingly or discontinuing anesthesia. Also, determining whether the arrhythmia is caused by electrolyte disturbances (e.g., hypokalemia, hypercarbia, hypocarbia, or hypoxia and correcting as required.
• For malignant hyperthermic crisis—Discontinuing possible triggering agents (e.g., potent inhalation anesthetics, succinylcholine, or stress), managing increased oxygen requirement, cooling the patient, and correcting fluid and electrolyte imbalances and metabolic acidosis. If necessary, administering dantrolene by continu-

ous rapid intravenous push (at least 1 mg per kg of body weight (mg/kg) initially, continued until the symptoms subside or the maximum total dose of 10 mg/kg has been administered). Intravenous dantrolene administration may be repeated if symptoms recur. Dantrolene (4 to 8 mg/kg per day in four divided doses) may be administered orally or intravenously, with caution, for 1 to 3 days postoperatively to prevent recurrence of symptoms.
• For inadequate postoperative ventilation—Decreasing anesthetic dosage (if still being administered), establishing a clear airway, and instituting assisted or controlled respiration with oxygen.
• For emergence delirium—Administering small doses of an opioid (narcotic) analgesic, provided that hypoxemia or hypercarbia is not present.

## Inhalation Dosage Forms
### DESFLURANE

#### Usual adult and adolescent dose
Anesthetic (general)—
Inhalation, vaporized in a flow of oxygen or oxygen and air, or in a flow of nitrous oxide and oxygen:
Induction:
For administration as sole induction agent: 0.5 to 3% initially, to be increased by 0.5 to 1% every two to three breaths, or as tolerated, until onset of anesthesia.
For administration after induction with an intravenous induction agent: 0.5 to 1 minimum alveolar concentration (MAC) initially, then adjusted as necessary.
Maintenance:
To be adjusted according to patient response and surgical requirements, usually 2.5 to 8.5%.

Note: Anesthetic requirements, in terms of administered concentration or of MAC, decrease with increasing age. When the anesthetic is vaporized in 100% oxygen or a mixture of oxygen and air, 1 MAC of desflurane is 7.3% for a 25-year-old adult, 6% for a 45-year-old adult, and 5.2% for a 70-year-old adult. Geriatric patients should require lower total doses of desflurane for induction and maintenance than younger adults.

Concentrations higher than 12% have been administered safely, usually during induction of anesthesia. However, administration of high concentrations of desflurane will reduce proportionally the quantity of oxygen administered. A decrease in the concentration of nitrous oxide and/or air given concurrently may be necessary to ensure adequate oxygenation.

#### Usual pediatric dose
Anesthetic (general)—
Inhalation, vaporized in a flow of oxygen or oxygen and air, or in a flow of nitrous oxide and oxygen:
Induction:
**Use is not recommended.**
Maintenance:
To be adjusted according to patient response and surgical requirements, usually 5.2 to 10%.

Note: Anesthetic requirements, in terms of administered concentration or of minimum alveolar concentration (MAC), are highest in infants 6 to 12 months of age. When desflurane is vaporized in a flow of 100% oxygen, the value of 1 MAC in infants and children of various ages is approximately:

2-week-old neonates—9.2%.
10-week-old infants—9.4%.
9-month-old infants—10%.
2-year-old children—9.1%.
4-year-old children—8.6%.
7-year-old children—8.1%.

#### Usual geriatric dose
See *Usual adult and adolescent dose.*

#### Product(s) usually available
U.S.—
(Rx) [*Suprane*].
Canada—
Not commercially available.

#### Packaging and storage
Store between 15 and 30 °C (59 and 86 °F), unless otherwise specified by manufacturer.

#### Stability
Stable at room temperature. The only known degradation reaction occurs through prolonged direct contact with soda lime. Small quantities of

fluoroform (CHF$_3$) are formed by this reaction. Strong acids do not produce discernible degradation.

## Selected Bibliography

Taylor RH, Lerman J. Minimum alveolar concentration of desflurane and hemodynamic responses in neonates, infants, and children. Anesthesiology 1991; 75 (4S): 975-9.

Zwass MS, Fisher DM, Welborn LG, Coté CJ, Davis PJ, Dinner M, et al. Induction and maintenance characteristics of anesthesia with desflur-

ane and nitrous oxide in infants and children. Anesthesiology 1992; 76: 373-8.

Tinker JH, editor. Clinical pharmacology of desflurane. Anesth Analg 1992; 75 (4S): 1-54.

Developed: 12/21/93

---

**DESIPRAMINE**—See *Antidepressants, Tricyclic (Systemic)*

---

# DESMOPRESSIN   Systemic

VA CLASSIFICATION (Primary/Secondary): HS702/CV900; BL300

Note: For a listing of dosage forms and brand names by country availability, see *Dosage Forms* section(s). For a listing of brand names for the articles in this monograph, refer to the General Index.

## Category

Antidiuretic (central diabetes insipidus)—Desmopressin Acetate Nasal Solution; Desmopressin Acetate Injection.

Antidiuretic (primary nocturnal enuresis)—Desmopressin Acetate Nasal Solution.

Antihemorrhagic—Desmopressin Acetate Injection.

## Indications

**Accepted**

Diabetes insipidus, central (treatment)—Desmopressin is indicated for the prevention or control of polydipsia, polyuria, and dehydration associated with central diabetes insipidus caused by insufficient antidiuretic hormone. Its efficacy, ease of administration, long duration of action, and relative lack of side effects make desmopressin the drug of choice for central diabetes insipidus.

Desmopressin is preferred to vasopressin injection and oral antidiuretics for use in children. Children have been found to respond well to desmopressin therapy.

Desmopressin is also indicated to manage temporary polydipsia and polyuria associated with trauma to, or surgery in, the pituitary region.

Desmopressin is ineffective in the treatment of nephrogenic diabetes insipidus or polyuria associated with psychogenic diabetes insipidus, renal disease, hypokalemia, hypercalcemia, or the administration of demeclocycline or lithium.

Enuresis, primary nocturnal (treatment)—Desmopressin nasal solution is indicated in the treatment of primary nocturnal enuresis.

Hemophilia A (treatment) or

von Willebrand's disease (treatment)—The injectable form of desmopressin is indicated for patients with mild hemophilia A or mild to moderate classic von Willebrand's disease (Type I), with factor VIII concentrations greater than 5%. It is useful when administered 15 to 30 minutes before surgery to maintain hemostasis. Desmopressin will usually stop the bleeding in these patients with episodes of spontaneous or trauma-induced hemarthroses, intramuscular hematomas, or mucosal bleeding.

Desmopressin is not indicated for patients with factor VIII concentrations of 5% or less (except in certain clinical situations with careful monitoring), or in patients who have factor VIII antibodies. Desmopressin is not indicated for treatment of severe classic von Willebrand's disease (Type III) and when there is evidence of an abnormal molecular form of von Willebrand antigen. In patients with Type IIB von Willebrand's disease, desmopressin may induce platelet aggregation, and use is not recommended.

## Pharmacology/Pharmacokinetics

**Physicochemical characteristics**

Source—Synthetic polypeptide structurally related to the posterior pituitary hormone arginine vasopressin (antidiuretic hormone).

Molecular weight—1183.32.

**Mechanism of action/Effect**

Antidiuretic—Increases water reabsorption in the kidney by increasing the cellular permeability of the collecting ducts, resulting in an increase in urine osmolality with a concurrent decrease in urine output.

Antihemorrhagic—Increases plasma levels of clotting factor VIII (antihemophilic factor) and von Willebrand's factor activity as well as a possible direct effect on the blood vessel wall.

**Other actions/effects**

Much less pressor activity than vasopressin and less action on visceral smooth muscle.

**Absorption**

10 to 20% from nasal mucosa. An intravenous dose of desmopressin possesses antidiuretic activity approximately 10 times that of the same nasal desmopressin dose.

**Biotransformation**

Renal.

**Half-life**

Fast phase—7.8 minutes.

Slow phase—75.5 minutes.

**Onset of action**

Antidiuretic—Intranasal: Within 1 hour.

Antihemorrhagic—Increased factor VIII activity and von Willebrand factor levels: Intravenous—15 to 30 minutes.

**Time to peak serum concentration**

Intranasal—1 to 5 hours.

**Time to peak effect**

Antidiuretic—Intranasal: 1 to 5 hours.

Antihemorrhagic—Increased factor VIII activity and von Willebrand factor levels: Intravenous—90 minutes to 2 hours.

**Duration of action**

Antidiuretic—

Intranasal:

Variable, 8 to 20 hours; long duration of action is due to the medication's rate of absorption from nasal mucosa, persistence in plasma, and effect on renal tubules. Effect ends abruptly, over a period of 60 to 90 minutes.

Antihemorrhagic—

Mild hemophilia A: Intravenous—4 to 24 hours.

von Willebrand's disease: Intravenous—Approximately 3 hours.

## Precautions to Consider

**Carcinogenicity/Mutagenicity**

Studies have not been done in either animals or humans.

**Pregnancy/Reproduction**

Pregnancy—Controlled studies in humans have not been done.

Clinical use of desmopressin in pregnant women has been reported, with no adverse effects in the fetus. Desmopressin does not appear to have uterotonic activity.

Studies in rats and rabbits have not shown that desmopressin causes adverse effects on the fetus.

FDA Pregnancy Category B.

**Breast-feeding**

In a study conducted in one woman, desmopressin was distributed into breast milk in minimal amounts, following a 10 mcg intranasal dose. However, problems in humans have not been documented.

**Pediatrics**

Use of desmopressin as an antihemorrhagic in infants less than 3 months of age is not recommended, because of an increased tendency to fluid balance problems in neonates. However, desmopressin may be the drug of choice for use as an antidiuretic in older children because of its low incidence of side effects.

Caution and careful restriction of fluid intake are recommended with use in infants because of the increased risk of hyponatremia and water intoxication.

### Geriatrics

Although appropriate studies have not been performed in the geriatric population, caution and careful restriction of fluid intake are recommended with use in the elderly because of the increased risk of hyponatremia and water intoxication.

### Drug interactions and/or related problems

The following drug interactions and/or related problems have been selected on the basis of their potential clinical significance (possible mechanism in parentheses where appropriate)—not necessarily inclusive (» = major clinical significance):

Note: Combinations containing any of the following medications, depending on the amount present, may also interact with this medication.

Carbamazepine or
Chlorpropamide or
Clofibrate
   (may potentiate the antidiuretic effect of desmopressin when used concurrently)

Demeclocycline or
Lithium or
Norepinephrine
   (may decrease the antidiuretic effect of desmopressin when used concurrently)

### Medical considerations/Contraindications

The medical considerations/contraindications included here have been selected on the basis of their potential clinical significance (reasons given in parentheses where appropriate)—not necessarily inclusive (» = major clinical significance).

*Risk-benefit should be considered when the following medical problems exist:*

Allergic rhinitis or
Nasal congestion or edema or
Upper respiratory infection
   (nasal absorption of desmopressin may be erratic)

Allergy to desmopressin

Coronary artery disease or
Hypertensive cardiovascular disease
   (large doses of desmopressin may rarely produce a slight increase in blood pressure)

Cystic fibrosis or
Dehydration
   (risk of hyponatremia may be increased)

Thrombosis, predisposition to
   (rarely, myocardial infarction and strokes have been reported to occur following the use of desmopressin in patients predisposed to thrombus formation; although it is not known whether these events were related to the use of desmopressin, caution is recommended in the use of desmopressin in this patient population)

### Patient monitoring

The following may be especially important in patient monitoring (other tests may be warranted in some patients, depending on condition; » = major clinical significance):

*For use as an antidiuretic*
Electrolytes
   (measurement of serum concentrations is recommended if therapy is continued beyond 7 days or as determined by physician)

Urine osmolality and/or
Urine volume
   (determinations recommended at appropriate intervals to monitor response and aid in dosage adjustment; in some cases, plasma osmolality determinations may be necessary)

*For use in hemophilia A*
Factor VIII coagulant concentration
   (determinations recommended at appropriate intervals to monitor response)

*For use in von Willebrand's disease*
Bleeding times and
Factor VIII coagulant and
Ristocetin cofactor (von Willebrand factor) and
von Willebrand factor (factor VIII–related antigen)
   (determinations recommended at appropriate intervals to monitor response)

## Side/Adverse Effects

Note: Rarely, thrombotic events (myocardial infarction and strokes) have been reported to occur following the use of desmopressin in patients predisposed to thrombus formation. Although it is not known whether these events were related to the use of desmopressin, caution is recommended in the use of desmopressin in this patient population.

The following side/adverse effects have been selected on the basis of their potential clinical significance (possible signs and symptoms in parentheses where appropriate)—not necessarily inclusive:

### Those indicating need for medical attention
Incidence rare—dose-related
   *Slight hypertension*—with intravenous use; *hyponatremia or water intoxication* (coma; confusion; continuing headache; decreased urination; drowsiness; rapid weight gain; seizures)
   Note: *Hypotension* may be caused by rapid intravenous administration.

### Those indicating need for medical attention only if they continue or are bothersome
Incidence less frequent or rare—dose-related
   *Abdominal or stomach cramps; flushing or redness of skin; pain in vulva*
With high doses
   *Headache; nausea*
With intranasal use
   *Runny or stuffy nose*
With intravenous use
   *Pain, redness, or swelling at site of injection*

## Overdose

For more information on the management of overdose or unintentional ingestion, **contact a Poison Control Center** (see *Poison Control Center Listing*).

### Treatment of overdose

Treatment of overdose consists of reduction of dosage and, if fluid overload is severe, administration of furosemide.

## Patient Consultation

As an aid to patient consultation, refer to *Advice for the Patient, Desmopressin (Systemic)*.

In providing consultation, consider emphasizing the following selected information (» = major clinical significance):

### Before using this medication
» Conditions affecting use, especially:
   Allergy to desmopressin
   Breast-feeding—Distributed into breast milk in minimal amounts
   Use in children—Infants may be more sensitive to effects
   Use in the elderly—Increased risk of hyponatremia and water intoxication

### Proper use of this medication
» Proper dosing
» Proper storage
*For intranasal use only*
» Importance of not using more medication than the amount prescribed
   Proper administration technique; following patient instructions
*Missed dose*
   If dosing schedule is once a day—Using as soon as possible if remembered same day; if not remembered until next day, not using at all and not doubling dose, but going back to regular schedule
   If dosing schedule is more than once a day—Using as soon as possible; not using at all if almost time for next dose; not doubling doses

### Side/adverse effects
   Signs of potential side effects, especially water intoxication and hyponatremia

## General Dosing Information

Fluid intake should be adjusted to decrease the potential for water intoxication and hyponatremia, especially in very young and geriatric patients.

Tolerance may develop with long-term intranasal use or tachyphylaxis may occur when intravenous doses are administered more frequently than every 24 to 48 hours.

**For use in central diabetes insipidus**

Initially, therapy should be directed to control nocturia.

The dosage of desmopressin should be adjusted according to the diurnal pattern of response, with the morning and evening doses being separately adjusted.

Response to therapy can be measured by the volume and frequency of urination and an adequate duration of sleep.

**For intranasal dosage forms**

Desmopressin is administered intranasally as a spray or through a flexible, calibrated catheter known as a rhinyle.

The nasal spray delivery unit should not be used beyond the labeled number of sprays; if it is, the accuracy of the dose delivered cannot be assured.

## Nasal Dosage Forms

### DESMOPRESSIN ACETATE NASAL SOLUTION

**Usual adult and adolescent dose**

Central diabetes insipidus—

Initial: Intranasal, 10 mcg at bedtime; this dose may be increased nightly in increments of 2.5 mcg until a satisfactory sleep response is obtained. If urine volume is still large, a 10-mcg morning dose may be added and adjusted to obtain the desired response.

Maintenance: Intranasal, 10 to 40 mcg per day, as a single dose or in two or three divided doses per day.

Note: In one-quarter to one-third of patients, adequate control is maintained with a single daily dose; however, in some patients, three doses per day are necessary.

Nocturnal enuresis—

Initial: Intranasal, 10 mcg into each nostril at bedtime (total dose per day of 20 mcg).

Maintenance: Dosage is adjusted according to patient response; total dose per day may range from 10 to 40 mcg.

**Usual pediatric dose**

Central diabetes insipidus—

Children up to 3 months of age:

Dosage has not been established.

Children 3 months to 12 years of age:

Initial—Intranasal, 5 mcg at bedtime; this dose may be increased nightly in increments of 2.5 mcg until a satisfactory sleep response is obtained. If urine volume is still large, a 5-mcg morning dose may be added and adjusted to obtain the desired response.

Maintenance—Intranasal, 2 to 4 mcg per kg of body weight per day or 5 to 30 mcg per day, as a single dose or in two divided doses per day.

Nocturnal enuresis—

Children up to 6 years of age:

Dosage has not been established.

Children 6 years of age and older:

Initial—Intranasal, 10 mcg into each nostril at bedtime (total dose per day of 20 mcg).

Maintenance—Dosage is adjusted according to patient response; total dose per day may range from 10 to 40 mcg.

**Strength(s) usually available**

U.S.—

10 mcg per 0.1 mL metered spray (0.01%) (Rx) [*DDAVP Nasal Spray*].

100 mcg per mL (0.01%) (Rx) [*DDAVP Rhinal Tube;* GENERIC].

150 mcg per 0.1 mL metered spray (0.15%) (Rx) [*Stimate Nasal Spray*].

Canada—

10 mcg per 0.1 mL metered spray (0.01%) (Rx) [*DDAVP Spray*].

100 mcg per mL (0.01%) (Rx) [*DDAVP Rhinyle Nasal Solution*].

**Packaging and storage**

Store at about 4 °C (39 °F), unless otherwise specified by manufacturer. Protect from freezing.

**Auxiliary labeling**

• Refrigerate.

**Note**

Include patient instructions when dispensing.

## Parenteral Dosage Forms

### DESMOPRESSIN ACETATE INJECTION

**Usual adult and adolescent dose**

Antidiuretic—

Intravenous (direct) or subcutaneous, 2 to 4 mcg per day, usually in two divided doses in the morning and evening.

Antihemorrhagic—

Intravenous, 0.3 mcg per kg of body weight diluted in 50 mL of 0.9% sodium chloride injection and infused slowly over fifteen to thirty minutes; repeated as needed.

**Usual pediatric dose**

Antihemorrhagic—

Infants less than 3 months of age:

Use is not recommended.

Children 3 months of age and over:

For children weighing 10 kg or less—Intravenous, 0.3 mcg per kg of body weight diluted in 10 mL of 0.9% sodium chloride injection and infused slowly over fifteen to thirty minutes; repeated as needed.

For children weighing more than 10 kg—Intravenous, 0.3 mcg per kg of body weight diluted in 50 mL of 0.9% sodium chloride injection and infused slowly over fifteen to thirty minutes; repeated as needed.

**Strength(s) usually available**

U.S.—

4 mcg per mL (Rx) [*DDAVP; Stimate;* GENERIC].

15 mcg per mL (Rx) [*DDAVP*].

Canada—

4 mcg per mL (Rx) [*DDAVP*].

15 mcg per mL (Rx) [*Octostim*].

**Packaging and storage**

Store at about 4 °C (39 °F), unless otherwise specified by manufacturer. Protect from freezing.

### Selected Bibliography

Miller K, Klauber GT. Desmopressin acetate in children with primary nocturnal enuresis. Clin Ther 1990; 12 (4): 357-66.

Aledort LM. Treatment of von Willebrand's disease [review]. Mayo Clin Proceed 1991; 66: 841-6.

Blevins LS, Jr. Wand GS. Diabetes insipidus [review]. Crit Care Med 1992; 20 (1): 69-79.

Salva KM, Kim HC, Nahum K, et al. DDAVP in the treatment of bleeding disorders. Pharmacother 1988; 8 (2): 94-9.

Revised: 10/26/92

Interim revision: 06/02/94; 07/19/96

---

**DESONIDE**—See *Corticosteroids (Topical)*

---

**DESONIDE-CONTAINING COMBINATIONS—**

Desonide and Acetic Acid (Otic)—See *Corticosteroids and Acetic Acid (Otic)*

---

**DESOXIMETASONE**—See *Corticosteroids (Topical)*

---

**DEXAMETHASONE**—See *Corticosteroids (Inhalation-Local); Corticosteroids (Nasal); Corticosteroids (Ophthalmic); Corticosteroids (Otic); Corticosteroids (Topical); Corticosteroids—Glucocorticoid Effects (Systemic)*

---

**DEXBROMPHENIRAMINE-CONTAINING COMBINATIONS—**

Dexbrompheniramine and Pseudoephedrine (Systemic)—See *Antihistamines and Decongestants (Systemic)*

Dexbrompheniramine, Pseudoephedrine, and Acetaminophen (Systemic)—See *Antihistamines, Decongestants, and Analgesics (Systemic)*

---

**DEXCHLORPHENIRAMINE**—See *Antihistamines (Systemic)*

## DEXCHLORPHENIRAMINE-CONTAINING COMBINATIONS—

Dexchlorpheniramine, Pseudoephedrine, and Guaifenesin (Systemic)—
See *Cough/Cold Combinations (Systemic)*

## DEXTROAMPHETAMINE—See *Amphetamines (Systemic)*

# DEXTROMETHORPHAN    Systemic

VA CLASSIFICATION (Primary): RE302

Note: For a listing of dosage forms and brand names by country availability, see *Dosage Forms* section(s). For a listing of brand names for the articles in this monograph, refer to the General Index.

## Category

Antitussive.

## Indications

**Accepted**

Cough (treatment)—Dextromethorphan is indicated for the symptomatic relief of nonproductive cough due to minor throat and bronchial irritation occurring with colds or inhaled irritants.

## Pharmacology/Pharmacokinetics

**Mechanism of action/Effect**

Suppresses the cough reflex by a direct action on the cough center in the medulla of the brain.

**Biotransformation**

Hepatic. Rapidly and extensively metabolized to dextrorphan (active metabolite).

**Onset of action**

Usually within one-half hour.

**Duration of action**

Up to 6 hours.

Note: The extended-release oral suspension delivers dextromethorphan from an ion-exchange complex over a period of 9 to 12 hours.

**Elimination**

Primarily renal (excreted as unchanged dextromethorphan and demethylated metabolites, including dextrorphan).

## Precautions to Consider

**Pregnancy/Reproduction**

Pregnancy—Problems in humans have not been documented.

**Breast-feeding**

It is not known whether dextromethorphan is distributed into breast milk. However, problems in humans have not been documented.

**Pediatrics**

Appropriate studies on the relationship of age to the effects of dextromethorphan have not been performed in the pediatric population. However, no pediatrics-specific problems have been documented to date.

**Geriatrics**

No information is available on the relationship of age to the effects of dextromethorphan in geriatric patients.

**Drug interactions and/or related problems**

The following drug interactions and/or related problems have been selected on the basis of their potential clinical significance (possible mechanism in parentheses where appropriate)—not necessarily inclusive (» = major clinical significance):

Note: Combinations containing any of the following medications, depending on the amount present, may also interact with this medication.

» Central nervous system (CNS) depression–producing medications, other (see *Appendix II*)
(concurrent use may potentiate the CNS depressant effects of these medications or dextromethorphan)

» Monoamine oxidase (MAO) inhibitors, including furazolidone and procarbazine
(concurrent use with dextromethorphan may cause adrenergic crisis, collapse, coma, dizziness, excitation, hypertension, hyperpyrexia, intracerebral bleeding, lethargy, nausea, psychotic behavior, spasms, and tremors)

Quinidine
(inhibition of the cytochrome P4502D6 enzyme system by quinidine may cause a decrease in the hepatic metabolism of dextromethorphan, which may result in increased dextromethorphan serum concentrations; higher concentrations of dextromethorphan have been associated with an increased incidence of side effects)

**Medical considerations/Contraindications**

The medical considerations/contraindications included here have been selected on the basis of their potential clinical significance (reasons given in parentheses where appropriate)—not necessarily inclusive (» = major clinical significance).

*Risk-benefit should be considered when the following medical problems exist:*

» Asthma
(dextromethorphan may impair expectoration and thus increase airway resistance)

» Cough, productive
(inhibition of cough reflex may lead to retention of secretions)

Hepatic function impairment
(metabolism of dextromethorphan may be impaired)

Sensitivity to dextromethorphan

## Side/Adverse Effects

Note: Toxic psychosis (hyperactivity, visual and auditory hallucinations) has been reported after ingestion of 300 mg or more of dextromethorphan.

Respiratory depression has been reported to occur with very high doses.

Dextromethorphan abuse and dependence may occur rarely, especially following prolonged use of high doses.

The following side/adverse effects have been selected on the basis of their potential clinical significance (possible signs and symptoms in parentheses where appropriate)—not necessarily inclusive:

**Those indicating need for medical attention only if they continue or are bothersome**

Incidence less frequent or rare
*Mild dizziness; mild drowsiness; nausea or vomiting; stomach pain*

## Overdose

For more information on the management of overdose or unintentional ingestion, **contact a Poison Control Center** (see *Poison Control Center Listing*).

Clinical effects of overdose
The following effects have been selected on the basis of their potential clinical significance (possible signs and symptoms in parentheses where appropriate—not necessarily inclusive:

Symptoms of overdose
*Confusion; drowsiness or dizziness; severe nausea or vomiting; severe unusual excitement, nervousness, restlessness, or irritability*

## Patient Consultation

As an aid to patient consultation, refer to *Advice for the Patient, Dextromethorphan (Systemic)*.

In providing consultation, consider emphasizing the following selected information (» = major clinical significance):

**Before using this medication**

» Conditions affecting use, especially:
Sensitivity to dextromethorphan
Other medications, especially other CNS depressants and MAO inhibitors
Other medical problems, especially asthma and productive cough

**Proper use of this medication**

» Importance of not using more medication than the amount prescribed because of habit-forming potential

» Proper dosing
    Missed dose: If on a scheduled dosing regimen—Taking as soon as possible; not taking if almost time for next dose; not doubling doses
» Proper storage

**Precautions while using this medication**
    Checking with physician if cough persists after medication has been used for 7 days or if high fever, skin rash, or continuing headache is present with cough

# Oral Dosage Forms

## DEXTROMETHORPHAN HYDROBROMIDE CAPSULES

**Usual adult and adolescent dose**
Antitussive—
    Oral, 10 to 20 mg every four hours or 30 mg every six to eight hours, as needed.

**Usual adult prescribing limits**
Up to 120 mg per day.

**Usual pediatric dose**
Antitussive—
    Children up to 2 years of age: Use is not recommended.
    Children 2 to 6 years of age: Oral, 2.5 to 5 mg every four hours or 7.5 mg every six to eight hours, as needed, not to exceed 30 mg per day.
    Children 6 to 12 years of age: Oral, 5 to 10 mg every four hours or 15 mg every six to eight hours, as needed, not to exceed 60 mg per day.
Note: Administration of a specific product to a pediatric patient depends upon the ability to achieve suitable dosage for the age of the child.

**Usual geriatric dose**
See *Usual adult and adolescent dose*

**Strength(s) usually available**
U.S.—
    30 mg (OTC) [*Drixoral Cough Liquid Caps*].
Canada—
    30 mg (OTC) [*Ornex•DM 30*].

**Packaging and storage**
Store below 40 °C (104 °F), preferably between 15 and 30 °C (59 and 86 °F), in a well-closed container, unless otherwise specified by manufacturer.

## DEXTROMETHORPHAN HYDROBROMIDE LOZENGES

**Usual adult and adolescent dose**
See *Dextromethorphan Hydrobromide Capsules.*

**Usual adult prescribing limits**
Up to 120 mg per day.

**Usual pediatric dose**
See *Dextromethorphan Hydrobromide Capsules.*
Note: Administration of a specific product to a pediatric patient depends upon the ability to achieve suitable dosage for the age of the child.

**Usual geriatric dose**
See *Dextromethorphan Hydrobromide Capsules.*

**Strength(s) usually available**
U.S.—
    5 mg (OTC) [*Children's Hold; Cough-X* (benzocaine 2 mg); *Hold; Pertussin Cough Suppressant; Robitussin Cough Calmers; Sucrets Cough Control Formula*].
    7.5 mg (OTC) [*Trocal*].
Canada—
    Not commercially available.

**Packaging and storage**
Store below 40 °C (104 °F), preferably between 15 and 30 °C (59 and 86 °F), in a well-closed container, unless otherwise specified by manufacturer.

## DEXTROMETHORPHAN HYDROBROMIDE SYRUP USP

**Usual adult and adolescent dose**
See *Dextromethorphan Hydrobromide Capsules.*

**Usual adult prescribing limits**
Up to 120 mg per day.

**Usual pediatric dose**
Children up to 2 years of age: Dosage must be individualized by physician.
Children 2 to 12 years of age: See *Dextromethorphan Hydrobromide Capsules.*

**Usual geriatric dose**
See *Dextromethorphan Hydrobromide Capsules.*

**Strength(s) usually available**
U.S.—
    3.5 mg per 5 mL (OTC) [*Pertussin CS* (alcohol free)].
    7.5 mg per 5 mL (OTC) [*Benylin Pediatric* (alcohol free; sugar free); *Robitussin Pediatric* (alcohol free); *St. Joseph Cough Suppressant for Children* (alcohol free)].
    10 mg per 15 mL (OTC) [*Creo-Terpin* (alcohol 25%)].
    15 mg per 5 mL (OTC) [*Benylin Adult* (alcohol free; sugar free); *Pertussin ES* (alcohol 9.5%); *Robitussin Maximum Strength Cough Suppressant* (alcohol 1.4%); *Vicks Formula 44 Pediatric Formula*].
Canada—
    7.5 mg per 5 mL (OTC) [*Robitussin Pediatric* (alcohol free)].
    10 mg per 5 mL (OTC) [*Sedatuss*].
    15 mg per 5 mL (OTC) [*Balminil D.M.; Broncho-Grippol-DM; Calmylin #1* (alcohol free; sugar free); *DM Syrup; Koffex; Neo-DM; Ornex•DM 15; Robidex* (alcohol 3.5%)].

**Packaging and storage**
Store between 15 and 30 °C (59 and 86 °F), unless otherwise specified by manufacturer. Store in a tight, light-resistant container. Protect from freezing.

## DEXTROMETHORPHAN HYDROBROMIDE CHEWABLE TABLETS

**Usual adult and adolescent dose**
See *Dextromethorphan Hydrobromide Capsules.*

**Usual adult prescribing limits**
Up to 120 mg per day.

**Usual pediatric dose**
See *Dextromethorphan Hydrobromide Capsules.*
Note: Administration of a specific product to a pediatric patient depends upon the ability to achieve suitable dosage for the age of the child.

**Usual geriatric dose**
See *Dextromethorphan Hydrobromide Capsules.*

**Strength(s) usually available**
U.S.—
    15 mg (OTC) [*Mediquell*].
Canada—
    Not commercially available.

**Packaging and storage**
Store below 40 °C (104 °F), preferably between 15 and 30 °C (59 and 86 °F), in a well-closed container, unless otherwise specified by manufacturer.

**Auxiliary labeling**
• Chew well before swallowing.

## DEXTROMETHORPHAN POLISTIREX EXTENDED-RELEASE ORAL SUSPENSION

**Usual adult and adolescent dose**
Antitussive—
    Oral, 60 mg every twelve hours, as needed.

**Usual adult prescribing limits**
Up to 120 mg per day.

**Usual pediatric dose**
Antitussive—
    Children up to 2 years of age: Dosage must be individualized by physician.
    Children 2 to 6 years of age: Oral, 15 mg every twelve hours, as needed, not to exceed 30 mg per day.
    Children 6 to 12 years of age: Oral, 30 mg every twelve hours, as needed, not to exceed 60 mg per day.

**Usual geriatric dose**
See *Usual adult and adolescent dose*

**Strength(s) usually available**
U.S.—
    30 mg (equivalent of dextromethorphan hydrobromide) per 5 mL (OTC) [*Delsym* (alcohol free)].
Canada—
    30 mg (equivalent of dextromethorphan hydrobromide) per 5 mL (OTC) [*Delsym* (alcohol free)].

**Packaging and storage**
Store below 40 °C (104 °F), preferably between 15 and 30 °C (59 and 86 °F), in a well-closed container, unless otherwise specified by manufacturer. Protect from freezing.

**Auxiliary labeling**
- Shake well.

## Selected Bibliography

Irwin RS, Curley FJ, Bennett FM. Appropriate use of antitussives and protussives. Drugs 1993; 46 (1): 80-91.

Segal S, et al. Use of codeine- and dextromethorphan-containing cough syrups in pediatrics. Pediatrics 1978; 62 (1): 118-22.

Revised: 06/23/94
Interim revision: 06/13/95

## DEXTROMETHORPHAN-CONTAINING COMBINATIONS—

Brompheniramine, Phenylephrine, Phenylpropanolamine, and Dextromethorphan (Systemic)—See *Cough/Cold Combinations (Systemic)*

Brompheniramine, Phenylpropanolamine, and Dextromethorphan (Systemic)—See *Cough/Cold Combinations (Systemic)*

Brompheniramine, Pseudoephedrine, and Dextromethorphan (Systemic)—See *Cough/Cold Combinations (Systemic)*

Carbinoxamine, Pseudoephedrine, and Dextromethorphan (Systemic)—See *Cough/Cold Combinations (Systemic)*

Chlorpheniramine and Dextromethorphan (Systemic)—See *Cough/Cold Combinations (Systemic)*

Chlorpheniramine, Dextromethorphan, and Acetaminophen (Systemic)—See *Cough/Cold Combinations (Systemic)*

Chlorpheniramine, Ephedrine, Phenylephrine, Dextromethorphan, Ammonium Chloride, and Ipecac (Systemic)—See *Cough/Cold Combinations (Systemic)*

Chlorpheniramine, Phenindamine, Phenylephrine, Dextromethorphan, Acetaminophen, Salicylamide, Caffeine, and Ascorbic Acid (Systemic)—See *Cough/Cold Combinations (Systemic)*

Chlorpheniramine, Phenylephrine, and Dextromethorphan (Systemic)—See *Cough/Cold Combinations (Systemic)*

Chlorpheniramine, Phenylephrine, Dextromethorphan, Acetaminophen, and Salicylamide (Systemic)—See *Cough/Cold Combinations (Systemic)*

Chlorpheniramine, Phenylephrine, Dextromethorphan, and Guaifenesin (Systemic)—See *Cough/Cold Combinations (Systemic)*

Chlorpheniramine, Phenylephrine, Dextromethorphan, Guaifenesin, and Ammonium Chloride (Systemic)—See *Cough/Cold Combinations (Systemic)*

Chlorpheniramine, Phenylephrine, Phenylpropanolamine, and Dextromethorphan (Systemic)—See *Cough/Cold Combinations (Systemic)*

Chlorpheniramine, Phenylephrine, Phenylpropanolamine, Dextromethorphan, Guaifenesin, and Acetaminophen (Systemic)—See *Cough/Cold Combinations (Systemic)*

Chlorpheniramine, Phenylpropanolamine, and Dextromethorphan (Systemic)—See *Cough/Cold Combinations (Systemic)*

Chlorpheniramine, Phenylpropanolamine, Dextromethorphan, and Acetaminophen (Systemic)—See *Cough/Cold Combinations (Systemic)*

Chlorpheniramine, Phenylpropanolamine, Dextromethorphan, and Ammonium Chloride (Systemic)—See *Cough/Cold Combinations (Systemic)*

Chlorpheniramine, Phenylpropanolamine, Dextromethorphan, and Aspirin (Systemic)—See *Cough/Cold Combinations (Systemic)*

Chlorpheniramine, Pseudoephedrine, and Dextromethorphan (Systemic)—See *Cough/Cold Combinations (Systemic)*

Chlorpheniramine, Pseudoephedrine, Dextromethorphan, and Acetaminophen (Systemic)—See *Cough/Cold Combinations (Systemic)*

Chlorpheniramine, Pseudoephedrine, Dextromethorphan, Acetaminophen, and Caffeine (Systemic)—See *Cough/Cold Combinations (Systemic)*

Dextromethorphan and Acetaminophen (Systemic)—See *Cough/Cold Combinations (Systemic)*

Dextromethorphan and Guaifenesin (Systemic)—See *Cough/Cold Combinations (Systemic)*

Dextromethorphan and Iodinated Glycerol (Systemic)—See *Cough/Cold Combinations (Systemic)*

Diphenhydramine, Dextromethorphan, and Ammonium Chloride (Systemic)—See *Cough/Cold Combinations (Systemic)*

Diphenhydramine, Pseudoephedrine, Dextromethorphan, and Acetaminophen (Systemic)—See *Cough/Cold Combinations (Systemic)*

Doxylamine, Phenylpropanolamine, Dextromethorphan, and Aspirin (Systemic)—See *Cough/Cold Combinations (Systemic)*

Doxylamine, Pseudoephedrine, Dextromethorphan, and Acetaminophen (Systemic)—See *Cough/Cold Combinations (Systemic)*

Pheniramine, Phenylephrine, and Dextromethorphan (Systemic)—See *Cough/Cold Combinations (Systemic)*

Pheniramine, Pyrilamine, Phenylpropanolamine, and Dextromethorphan (Systemic)—See *Cough/Cold Combinations (Systemic)*

Pheniramine, Pyrilamine, Phenylpropanolamine, Dextromethorphan, and Ammonium Chloride (Systemic)—See *Cough/Cold Combinations (Systemic)*

Pheniramine, Pyrilamine, Phenylpropanolamine, Dextromethorphan, and Guaifenesin (Systemic)—See *Cough/Cold Combinations (Systemic)*

Phenylephrine, Dextromethorphan, and Guaifenesin (Systemic)—See *Cough/Cold Combinations (Systemic)*

Phenylpropanolamine and Dextromethorphan (Systemic)—See *Cough/Cold Combinations (Systemic)*

Phenylpropanolamine, Dextromethorphan, and Acetaminophen (Systemic)—See *Cough/Cold Combinations (Systemic)*

Phenylpropanolamine, Dextromethorphan, and Guaifenesin (Systemic)—See *Cough/Cold Combinations (Systemic)*

Promethazine and Dextromethorphan (Systemic)—See *Cough/Cold Combinations (Systemic)*

Pseudoephedrine and Dextromethorphan (Systemic)—See *Cough/Cold Combinations (Systemic)*

Pseudoephedrine, Dextromethorphan, and Acetaminophen (Systemic)—See *Cough/Cold Combinations (Systemic)*

Pseudoephedrine, Dextromethorphan, and Guaifenesin (Systemic)—See *Cough/Cold Combinations (Systemic)*

Pseudoephedrine, Dextromethorphan, Guaifenesin, and Acetaminophen (Systemic)—See *Cough/Cold Combinations (Systemic)*

Pyrilamine, Phenylephrine, and Dextromethorphan (Systemic)—See *Cough/Cold Combinations (Systemic)*

Pyrilamine, Phenylephrine, Dextromethorphan, and Acetaminophen (Systemic)—See *Cough/Cold Combinations (Systemic)*

Pyrilamine, Phenylpropanolamine, Dextromethorphan, Guaifenesin, Potassium Citrate, and Citric Acid (Systemic)—See *Cough/Cold Combinations (Systemic)*

Pyrilamine, Phenylpropanolamine, Dextromethorphan, and Sodium Salicylate (Systemic)—See *Cough/Cold Combinations (Systemic)*

Triprolidine, Pseudoephedrine, and Dextromethorphan (Systemic)—See *Cough/Cold Combinations (Systemic)*

## DEXTROSE AND ELECTROLYTES—See *Carbohydrates and Electrolytes (Systemic)*

# DEXTROTHYROXINE   Systemic

VA CLASSIFICATION (Primary): CV350

Note: For a listing of dosage forms and brand names by country availability, see *Dosage Forms* section(s). For a listing of brand names for the articles in this monograph, refer to the General Index.

## Category

Antihyperlipidemic.

Note: Dextrothyroxine is a thyroid hormone with only weak thyroid hormone effects, which may be the result of levothyroxine (T₄) contamination.

## Indications

**Unaccepted**

Dextrothyroxine has been used for the treatment of hypercholesterolemia. However, because its use in patients with underlying cardiac disease has been associated with increased mortality and because its use has been replaced by other antihyperlipidemic medications with a more favorable benefit/risk ratio, dextrothyroxine is no longer recommended for the treatment of hypercholesterolemia.

Dextrothyroxine has also been used for treatment of hypothyroidism in patients with cardiac disease who cannot tolerate other thyroid preparations. However, it is seldom used because of the availability of more effective preparations.

Use of dextrothyroxine to treat obesity without laboratory confirmation of contributing hypothyroidism is inappropriate and may cause hyperthyroidism in euthyroid individuals.

## Pharmacology/Pharmacokinetics

### Physicochemical characteristics
Molecular weight—798.86 (anhydrous).

### Mechanism of action/Effect
Antihyperlipidemic—Not completely understood, but dextrothyroxine apparently acts in the liver to stimulate formation of low-density lipoprotein (LDL) and, to a much greater extent, to increase catabolism of LDL; this leads to increased excretion of cholesterol and bile acids via the biliary route into the feces, with a resulting reduction in serum cholesterol and LDL. Dextrothyroxine has no significant effect on high-density lipoproteins (HDL).

### Other actions/effects
Thyroid hormone—The action of thyroid hormones is not completely understood, but they have both catabolic (calorigenic) and anabolic effects and are therefore involved in normal metabolism, growth, and development, especially the development of the central nervous system (CNS) of infants. A feedback system involving the hypothalamus, anterior pituitary, and thyroid normally regulates circulating thyroid hormone concentrations. Most, if not all, of dextrothyroxine's thyroid hormone effects may be the result of levothyroxine ($T_4$) contamination. A dose of 4 mg of dextrothyroxine produces about the same metabolic effects as 0.15 mg of levothyroxine.

### Absorption
About 25% absorbed from gastrointestinal tract.

### Protein binding
Almost completely bound to plasma proteins.

### Biotransformation
As for endogenous thyroid hormone; deiodinated in peripheral tissues; small amounts are metabolized in the liver and excreted in bile.

### Half-life
About 18 hours.

### Time to peak effect
Antihyperlipidemic—1 to 2 months.

### Duration of action
Serum lipid concentrations return to pretreatment concentrations within 6 weeks to 3 months after withdrawal.

### Elimination
Renal; fecal.

## Precautions to Consider

### Pregnancy/Reproduction
Fertility—Reproduction studies in rabbits and rats at doses up to 100 times the maximum daily human dose by weight have revealed no evidence of fertility impairment.

Pregnancy—Thyroid hormones cross the placenta, but only to a limited extent. Adequate and well-controlled studies in humans have not been done.

Studies in 2 animal species have not shown that dextrothyroxine causes adverse effects on the fetus.

FDA Pregnancy Category B.

### Breast-feeding
It is not known whether dextrothyroxine is distributed into breast milk. However, problems in humans have not been documented.

### Pediatrics
Appropriate studies on the relationship of age to the effects of dextrothyroxine have not been performed in the pediatric or adolescent populations. However, use in children under 2 years of age is not recommended since cholesterol is required for normal development.

### Geriatrics
Appropriate studies on the relationship of age to the effects of dextrothyroxine have not been performed in the geriatric population. However, the elderly may be more sensitive to the effects of thyroid hormones. In addition, elderly patients are more likely to have age-related renal function impairment, which may require caution in patients receiving dextrothyroxine.

### Drug interactions and/or related problems
The following drug interactions and/or related problems have been selected on the basis of their potential clinical significance (possible

mechanism in parentheses where appropriate)—not necessarily inclusive (» = major clinical significance):

Note: Combinations containing any of the following medications, depending on the amount present, may also interact with this medication.

» Anticoagulants, coumarin- or indandione-derivative
   (the effects of the oral anticoagulant may be altered, depending on the thyroid status of the patient; effect may consist of alteration of procoagulant synthesis or catabolism or increased receptor affinity for the anticoagulant; administration of dextrothyroxine may necessitate a decrease in anticoagulant dosage; adjustment of anticoagulant dosage on the basis of prothrombin time is recommended)

Antidiabetic agents, oral or
Insulin
   (thyroid hormones may affect insulin or antidiabetic agent requirements; careful monitoring of diabetic control is recommended, especially when dextrothyroxine therapy is started, changed, or discontinued)

Chenodiol or
Ursodiol
   (because dextrothyroxine tends to increase cholesterol saturation of bile, it may decrease the effects of either of these medications if used concurrently)

» Cholestyramine or
» Colestipol
   (concurrent use may decrease the effects of dextrothyroxine by binding and delaying or preventing absorption; an interval of 4 to 5 hours between administration of the two medications is recommended)

Digitalis glycosides
   (administration of a thyroid hormone to a hypothyroid patient receiving a digitalis glycoside may increase the dosage requirements of the digitalis glycoside)

Sodium iodide I 123 or
Sodium iodide I 131
   (thyroid hormones may decrease thyroidal uptake of I 123 or I 131)

Thyroid hormones, other
   (concurrent use may result in additive metabolic effects)

### Laboratory value alterations
The following have been selected on the basis of their potential clinical significance (possible effect in parentheses where appropriate)—not necessarily inclusive (» = major clinical significance):

With physiology/laboratory test values
   Alkaline phosphatase, serum and
   Aspartate aminotransferase (AST [SGOT]), serum and
   Bilirubin, total and direct, serum and
   Glucose, urinary and plasma
      (concentrations may be increased)

   Radioactive iodine uptake (RAIU)
      (may be decreased by the 4th week of treatment, indicating absorption of dextrothyroxine; returns to normal within 10 days after treatment is withdrawn, regardless of the duration of therapy)

   Thyroxine ($T_4$)
      (serum concentrations may be increased by the 4th week of treatment, but increase indicates absorption of dextrothyroxine rather than hyperthyroidism)

### Medical considerations/Contraindications
The medical considerations/contraindications included here have been selected on the basis of their potential clinical significance (reasons given in parentheses where appropriate)—not necessarily inclusive (» = major clinical significance).

*Except under special circumstances, this medication should not be used when the following medical problems exist:*

» Cardiovascular disease, including angina pectoris, arteriosclerosis, coronary artery disease, hypertension, myocardial infarction, cardiac arrhythmia or tachycardia (or history of), rheumatic heart disease, congestive heart failure
   (because of the risks associated with increased metabolic demands caused by thyroid hormone administration, dextrothyroxine should not be used in patients with cardiovascular disease)

*Risk-benefit should be considered when the following medical problems exist:*

» Diabetes mellitus
   (possible reduced glucose tolerance and increased insulin or oral antidiabetic agent requirements)

» Hepatic function impairment or
» Hyperthyroidism or iodism, history of
    (conditions may be exacerbated)
    Hypothyroidism
        (these patients are more sensitive to dextrothyroxine's thyroid hormone effects than euthyroid individuals)
» Renal function impairment
    (may result in reduced clearance of dextrothyroxine)
    Sensitivity to dextrothyroxine

### Patient monitoring
The following may be especially important in patient monitoring (other tests may be warranted in some patients, depending on condition; » = major clinical significance):

Bone age and
» Growth and
» Psychomotor development
    (measurements recommended at periodic intervals in children receiving dextrothyroxine for prolonged periods)

Cholesterol concentrations and
Triglyceride concentrations
    (serum determinations recommended prior to initiation of therapy and every 2 months after stabilization to confirm efficacy and determine that a positive response is maintained)

## Side/Adverse Effects

Note: Incidence of adverse effects is greatest in patients with hypothyroidism and/or organic heart disease, and with doses greater than 8 mg per day.

   Administration of dextrothyroxine has been associated with an increased incidence of both fatal and nonfatal myocardial infarctions and ischemic heart disease. Mortality risk appears to increase with increased duration of treatment.

   Side effects may not occur until 1 to 6 weeks after treatment is begun.

The following side/adverse effects have been selected on the basis of their potential clinical significance (possible signs and symptoms in parentheses where appropriate)—not necessarily inclusive:

### Those indicating need for medical attention
Incidence rare
    *Angina* (chest pain; fast or irregular heartbeat)—especially with high doses; *gallstones* (severe stomach pain with nausea and vomiting)
Signs and symptoms of hyperthyroidism or overdosage
    *Changes in appetite; changes in menstrual periods; diarrhea; fast or irregular heartbeat; fever; hand tremors; headache; increase in urination; irritability, nervousness, or trouble in sleeping; leg cramps; shortness of breath; skin rash or itching; sweating, flushing, or increased sensitivity to heat; vomiting; weight loss, unusual*

## Overdose

For more information on the management of overdose or unintentional ingestion, **contact a Poison Control Center** (see *Poison Control Center Listing*).

### Treatment of overdose
If symptoms of hyperthyroidism occur, it is recommended that dextrothyroxine therapy be withdrawn for 2 to 6 days, then resumed at a lower dose.
    Specific treatment—
        For acute massive overdose: Reducing gastrointestinal absorption, if possible, by means of vomiting, followed by symptomatic and supportive treatment, including administration of oxygen, measures to control fever, hypoglycemia, or fluid loss, and antiadrenergic agents such as propranolol for treatment of increased sympathetic activity.

## Patient Consultation

As an aid to patient consultation, refer to *Advice for the Patient, Dextrothyroxine (Systemic)*.

In providing consultation, consider emphasizing the following selected information (» = major clinical significance):

### Before using this medication
Diet as preferred therapy; importance of following prescribed diet
» Conditions affecting use, especially:
        Sensitivity to dextrothyroxine
        Pregnancy—Crosses placenta to limited extent
        Use in children—Not recommended in children under 2 years of age since cholesterol is required for normal development

Use in the elderly—Elderly patients may be more sensitive to thyroid hormone effects
Other medications, especially anticoagulants, cholestyramine, or colestipol
Other medical problems, especially cardiovascular disease, diabetes mellitus, hepatic function impairment, history of hyperthyroidism or iodism, or renal function impairment

### Proper use of this medication
» Importance of not taking more medication than the amount prescribed; not missing any doses
    Does not cure the condition but rather helps control it; continue taking as directed in order to lower cholesterol level
» Compliance with prescribed diet
» Proper dosing
    Missed dose: Taking as soon as possible; not taking if almost time for next dose; not doubling doses
» Proper storage

### Precautions while using this medication
» Importance of close monitoring by physician
» Checking with physician before discontinuing medication; blood lipid concentrations may increase significantly
» Caution if any kind of surgery (including dental surgery) or emergency treatment is required

### Side/adverse effects
    Signs of potential side effects, especially angina, gallstones, and hyperthyroidism

## General Dosing Information

If signs or symptoms of cardiac disease (angina, tachycardia, extrasystoles) develop, dextrothyroxine should be withdrawn.

It is recommended that dextrothyroxine therapy be discontinued 10 to 14 days prior to scheduled surgery, especially in patients with coronary artery disease or if use of anticoagulants is anticipated. In addition, patients treated with thyroid hormones are at increased risk of precipitation of cardiac arrhythmias.

If response is inadequate after 3 months of treatment, dextrothyroxine therapy should be withdrawn, except in the case of xanthoma tuberosum, which may require up to 1 year of treatment as long as reduction in size and/or number of xanthomata occurs.

Dextrothyroxine therapy may be continued as long as cholesterol concentrations are reduced.

## Oral Dosage Forms

### DEXTROTHYROXINE SODIUM TABLETS USP

#### Usual adult dose
Antihyperlipidemic—
    Oral, initially 1 to 2 mg per day, the dosage being increased in increments of no more than 1 to 2 mg at intervals of no less than one month up to the minimum effective dose.

#### Usual adult prescribing limits
Up to 8 mg per day.

#### Usual pediatric dose
Antihyperlipidemic—
    Children up to 2 years of age:
        Use is not recommended.
    Children 2 years of age and older:
        Initial—Oral, 50 mcg (0.05 mg) per kg of body weight or 1.5 mg per square meter of body surface per day, the dosage being increased in increments of 50 mcg (0.05 mg) per kg of body weight or 1.5 mg per square meter of body surface at intervals of no less than one month up to the minimum effective dose.
        Maintenance—Oral, 100 mcg (0.1 mg) per kg of body weight or 3 mg per square meter of body surface per day.

#### Usual pediatric prescribing limits
Up to 4 mg per day.

#### Strength(s) usually available
U.S.—
    1 mg (Rx) [*Choloxin* (lactose; polysorbate 80)].
    2 mg (Rx) [*Choloxin* (lactose; polysorbate 80; tartrazine)].
    4 mg (Rx) [*Choloxin* (lactose)].
Canada—
    2 mg (Rx) [*Choloxin*].
    4 mg (Rx) [*Choloxin*].

**Packaging and storage**
Store below 40 °C (104 °F), preferably between 15 and 30 °C (59 and 86 °F), unless otherwise specified by manufacturer. Store in a well-closed container.

## Selected Bibliography

The Expert Panel. Report of the National Cholesterol Education Program Expert Panel on Detection, Evaluation and Treatment of High Blood Cholesterol in Adults. Arch Intern Med 1988 Jan; 148: 36-69.

NIH Consensus Conference. Lowering blood cholesterol to prevent heart disease. JAMA 1985 Apr 12; 253: 2080-6.

Knodel LC, Talbert RL. Adverse effects of hypolipidaemic drugs. Med Toxicol 1987; 2: 10-32.

Revised: 04/22/93

---

# DEZOCINE   Systemic†

VA CLASSIFICATION (Primary): CN101

Note: For a listing of dosage forms and brand names by country availability, see *Dosage Forms* section(s). For a listing of brand names for the articles in this monograph, refer to the General Index.

†Not commercially available in Canada.

## Category

Analgesic.

## Indications

### Accepted

Pain (treatment)—Dezocine is indicated for the short-term relief of pain. Dezocine's antagonist activity must be considered prior to administration because it may precipitate withdrawal symptoms if the patient is physically dependent on a mu-receptor opioid analgesic. A patient who has developed a significant degree of tolerance to other opioids during long-term treatment is probably not a suitable candidate for dezocine treatment.

### Unaccepted

Dezocine has not been adequately studied, and is not currently recommended, for treatment of chronic pain.

## Pharmacology/Pharmacokinetics

### Physicochemical characteristics

Chemical group—An opioid agonist/antagonist analgesic of the aminotetralin series.
Molecular weight—245.36.
   *n*-Octanol: Water partition coefficient—1.7

### Mechanism of action/Effect

Analgesic—
   Opioid analgesics bind with stereospecific receptors at many sites within the central nervous system (CNS) to alter processes affecting both the perception of pain and the emotional response to pain. Although precise sites and mechanisms of action have not been fully determined, opioids have been shown to cause alterations in release of various neurotransmitters from afferent nerves sensitive to painful stimuli.
   It has been proposed that there are multiple subtypes of opioid receptors, each mediating various therapeutic and/or side effects of opioid drugs. The actions of an opioid analgesic may therefore depend upon its binding affinity for each type of receptor and whether it acts as a full agonist or a partial agonist or is inactive at each type of receptor. At least 2 of these types of receptors (mu and kappa) mediate analgesia. Mu receptors are widely distributed throughout the CNS, especially in the limbic system (frontal cortex, temporal cortex, amygdala, and hippocampus), thalamus, striatum, hypothalamus, and midbrain as well as laminae I, II, IV, and V of the dorsal horn in the spinal cord. Kappa receptors are localized primarily in the spinal cord and in the cerebral cortex. A third type of receptor (sigma) does not mediate analgesia; actions at this receptor may produce the subjective and psychotomimetic effects characteristic of most opioids having mixed agonist/antagonist activity. Dezocine may act primarily as a partial agonist at the mu receptor. Dezocine has relatively low activity (compared with pentazocine) at the sigma receptor, but psychotomimetic-like effects have been reported after administration of high doses.

Antagonist—
   Dezocine may displace other mu-receptor opioid agonists from their receptor binding sites and competitively inhibit their actions. It may therefore precipitate withdrawal symptoms in physically dependent patients who are chronically receiving these agonists. If administered first, dezocine may also reduce or block the effects of subsequently administered mu-receptor agonists. The antagonist actions of dezocine may impose a ceiling on its analgesic effects.

### Other actions/effects

Dezocine shares the CNS depressant and respiratory depressant effects of opioid analgesics. The respiratory depressant effect of dezocine is subject to a ceiling effect, with maximal respiratory depression occurring at a total cumulative dose of about 30 mg per kg of body weight (mg/kg). Respiratory depression induced by dezocine occurs more rapidly, is more pronounced for about the first 1 to 2 hours, and persists for approximately the same time as that induced by equianalgesic doses of morphine.

Dezocine has not been shown to produce clinically significant cardiovascular adverse effects. However, although cardiac or respiratory performance and systolic and diastolic blood pressures were not significantly altered, increases in cardiac index, stroke volume index, left ventricular stroke work index, and pulmonary vascular resistance occurred in one study when a single dose of 125 mcg per kg of body weight was administered intravenously to patients with stable coronary artery disease. Dezocine has not been studied in patients with severe and/or unstable cardiovascular disease.

Because of its antagonist activity, dezocine may have less potential for causing dependence or abuse than strong opioid analgesics having only agonist activity. However, when dezocine was administered to subjects with a history of opioid abuse, they reported typical subjective opioid effects (e.g., liking, euphoria) and identified the medication as "dope". Also, the medication substituted for morphine in abuse-liability testing in animals. Therefore, dezocine has the potential to be abused, especially by individuals with a history of opioid abuse or dependence.

Although studies in humans have not been done, dezocine did not cause histamine release or bronchoconstriction in an animal study.

Although specific studies with dezocine have not been done, the probability exists that the medication, like other opioid analgesics, may decrease gastrointestinal motility. Also, studies have not been done to determine whether dezocine, like most other opioids, has antitussive or antidiuretic activity or increases biliary tract pressure.

### Absorption

Intramuscular—Rapid and complete.

### Biotransformation

Hepatic, via conjugation (glucuronidation).

### Half-life

Elimination——
   Intramuscular: Average 2.2 hours
   Intravenous:
     5-mg dose—Average 1.7 to 2.6 hours (range 0.6 to 4.4 hours)
     10-mg dose (infused over 5 minutes)—Average 2.4 to 2.6 hours (range 1.2 to 7.4 hours). In patients with hepatic cirrhosis, the half-life is increased by 30 to 50%, probably due to the 30 to 50% expansion of dezocine's volume of distribution in these patients.
     20-mg dose—Average 2.4 to 2.8 hours (range 1.4 to 6.5 hours)

### Onset of action

Intramuscular—Within 30 minutes.
Intravenous—Within 15 minutes.

### Time to peak concentration

Intramuscular—10 to 90 minutes; average about 35 minutes.

### Therapeutic plasma concentration

Steady-state—5 to 9 nanograms per mL.

### Peak serum concentration

Intramuscular (10-mg single dose)—10 to 38 (average 19) nanograms per mL (0.03 to 0.11 [average 0.55] micromoles per L).

### Time to peak effect

Intramuscular—0.6 to 2.5 hours (average 1 to 2 hours).

## Elimination

Renal (66% of a dose), about 1% as unchanged dezocine and the remainder as the glucuronide conjugate. The effect of renal function impairment on clearance has not been studied. Also, in healthy subjects, the total body clearance is greater than the sum of hepatic and renal blood flow, suggesting additional mechanisms of excretion (e.g., biliary).

Total body clearance——

5-mg intravenous dose: 3.52 (range 2.1–6.2) L per hour per kg of body weight (L/hr/kg).

10-mg intravenous dose: 3.33 (range 1.7–7.2) L/hr/kg.

20-mg intravenous dose: 2.76 (range 1.7–4.1) L/hr/kg.

# Precautions to Consider

## Pregnancy/Reproduction

Pregnancy—Adequate and well-controlled studies have not been done in pregnant women. Although there is no experience with long-term administration of dezocine to pregnant women, the possibility must be considered that regular use during pregnancy may cause physical dependence in the fetus, leading to withdrawal symptoms (convulsions, irritability, excessive crying, tremors, hyperactive reflexes, fever, vomiting, diarrhea, sneezing, and yawning) in the neonate.

Studies in mice, rats, and rabbits did not show evidence of teratogenicity. However, intramuscular or intravenous administration of dezocine to rats produced a dose-related decrease in food consumption and body weight in the parental generation and a resultant decrease in pup body weight.

FDA Pregnancy Category C.

Labor and delivery—The safety of dezocine administration during labor has not been established.

## Breast-feeding

It is not known whether dezocine is distributed into breast milk. However, problems in humans have not been documented.

## Pediatrics

No information is available on the relationship of age to the effects of dezocine in pediatric patients. Safety and efficacy in patients up to 18 years of age have not been established.

## Geriatrics

No information is available on the relationship of age to the effects of dezocine in geriatric patients. However, geriatric patients are more susceptible to the effects, especially the respiratory depressant effects, of other opioid analgesics. Also, geriatric patients have been shown to metabolize or eliminate some opioid analgesics more slowly, and/or to be more sensitive to the analgesic effects of opioid analgesics, than younger adults. Therefore, lower doses and/or a longer interval between doses may be sufficient to provide effective analgesia. It is recommended that dezocine therapy in geriatric patients be initiated with lower doses than would be used for younger adults, and that subsequent doses be individualized according to patient tolerance and response.

## Drug interactions and/or related problems

The following drug interactions and/or related problems have been selected on the basis of their potential clinical significance (possible mechanism in parentheses where appropriate)—not necessarily inclusive (» = major clinical significance):

Note: Combinations containing any of the following medications, depending on the amount present, may also interact with this medication.

Other interactions applying to opioid analgesics may apply to dezocine also, although documentation is currently not available.

Antidiarrheals, antiperistaltic, such as:
Difenoxin and atropine
Diphenoxylate and atropine
Kaolin, pectin, belladonna alkaloids and opium
Loperamide
Opium tincture
Paregoric
(repeated administration of both dezocine and any of these antidiarrheals may increase the risk of severe constipation as well as CNS depression)

» CNS depression–producing medications, other (See *Appendix II*) or Monoamine oxidase (MAO) inhibitors, including furazolidone, procarbazine, and selegiline
(concurrent use may increase the CNS depressant, respiratory depressant, and hypotensive effects of these medications and/or dezocine; caution and a reduction in dosage of either or both medications are recommended)

Hydroxyzine
(concurrent use with dezocine may result in increased analgesia as well as increased CNS depressant and hypotensive effects)

Naloxone
(antagonizes the analgesic, CNS, and respiratory depressant effects of dezocine; however, because naloxone may precipitate withdrawal symptoms in physically dependent patients, dosage of naloxone should be carefully titrated when used to treat opioid overdosage in dependent patients)

» Naltrexone
(although not documented, the possibility must be considered that usual doses of dezocine will be ineffective if administered to a patient receiving naltrexone therapy [because naltrexone blocks the therapeutic effects of other potent opioids] and that administration of increased doses of dezocine to override naltrexone-induced blockade of opioid receptors may increase the risk of adverse effects)

» Opioid analgesics, other
(if administered prior to another mu-receptor agonist, dezocine may reduce the therapeutic effects of the other opioid)

(dezocine may precipitate withdrawal symptoms in physically dependent patients who are chronically receiving potent mu-receptor agonists such as morphine)

## Laboratory value alterations

The following have been selected on the basis of their potential clinical significance (possible effect in parentheses where appropriate)—not necessarily inclusive (» = major clinical significance):

With diagnostic test results
Amylase activity, in plasma and
Lipase activity, in plasma
(increases associated with opioid-induced contractions of the sphincter of Oddi and increased biliary tract pressure have been reported with most other opioid analgesics; although these effects have not been reported with dezocine, the possibility should be considered that the diagnostic utility of determinations of these enzymes may be compromised after dezocine administration)

Gastric emptying studies
(opioid analgesics such as dezocine may delay gastric emptying, thereby invalidating test results)

Hepatobiliary imaging, radionuclide
(like most other opioid analgesics, dezocine may prevent or delay delivery of the radionuclide to the small bowel, resulting in delayed visualization and in results resembling obstruction of the common bile duct)

With physiology/laboratory test values
Alkaline phosphatase activity and
Aspartate aminotransferase (AST [SGOT]) activity
(may be increased [incidences <1%])

Cerebrospinal fluid (CSF) pressure
(may be increased; effect is secondary to respiratory depression–induced carbon dioxide retention)

Hemoglobin
(concentrations may be decreased [incidence <1%])

## Medical considerations/Contraindications

The medical considerations/contraindications included here have been selected on the basis of their potential clinical significance (reasons given in parentheses where appropriate)—not necessarily inclusive (» = major clinical significance).

*Except under special circumstances, this medication should not be used when the following medical problem exists:*

» Respiratory depression, acute
(may be exacerbated)

*Risk-benefit should be considered when the following medical problems exist:*

Abdominal conditions, acute
(diagnosis or clinical course may be obscured)

» Asthma, acute attack or

» Respiratory impairment or disease, chronic
(opioid analgesics may decrease respiratory drive and increase airway resistance; a reduction in dosage is recommended)

Cardiovascular disease, severe and/or unstable
(although clinically significant cardiovascular adverse effects have not been reported to date with dezocine, the opioid has not been studied in patients with severe and/or unstable cardiovascular disease; caution is recommended if dezocine is to be administered to

patients with angina pectoris or compromised cardiac function, following cardiac or cardiovascular surgery, or to relieve pain due to acute myocardial infarction)

» Dependence on opioid analgesics, current, confirmed or
Dependence on opioid analgesics, current, suspected
(because of the risk of precipitating withdrawal symptoms, dezocine should be administered only after a suitable period of withdrawal from other opioids)

Diarrhea associated with pseudomembranous colitis caused by cephalosporins, lincomycins (possibly including topical clindamycin) or penicillins or

Diarrhea caused by poisoning, until toxic material has been eliminated from the gastrointestinal tract
(possibility should be considered that dezocine, like other opioid analgesics, may slow elimination of toxic material, thereby worsening and/or prolonging the diarrhea, when administered repeatedly)

Drug abuse or dependence, history of, including acute alcoholism or
Emotional instability or
Suicidal ideation or attempts
(risk of abuse, especially relapse by patients recovering from a drug dependency; it is recommended that dezocine be administered to patients with such problems only in a medically controlled environment)

Gallbladder disease or gallstones
(possibility should be considered that dezocine, like other opioid analgesics, may cause biliary contraction)

Gastrointestinal surgery, recent or
Inflammatory bowel disease, severe
(possibility should be considered that dezocine, like other opioid analgesics, may alter gastrointestinal motility; in patients with severe inflammatory bowel disease, an increased risk of toxic megacolon may result)

Head injury or
Increased intracranial pressure, pre-existing or
Intracranial lesions
(risk of respiratory depression and further elevation of cerebrospinal fluid pressure may be increased; also, opioid analgesics may cause sedation and pupillary changes that may obscure clinical course of head injury)

Hepatic function impairment
(the elimination half-life of dezocine may be prolonged by up to 50% in patients with hepatic cirrhosis, probably because of an increase in the medication's volume of distribution; although any effect of other forms of hepatic function impairment on the pharmacokinetics of dezocine has not been determined, caution and a reduction in dosage are recommended)

Hypothyroidism
(risk of respiratory depression and prolonged CNS depression is greatly increased)

Prostatic hypertrophy or obstruction or
Urethral stricture or
Urinary tract surgery, recent
(possibility must be considered that dezocine, like other opioid analgesics, may cause urinary retention, which may be detrimental to the patient)

Renal function impairment
(although the effect of renal function impairment on the elimination of dezocine has not been determined, caution and a reduction in dose are recommended)

Sensitivity to dezocine, history of

Caution is also advised in administration to geriatric or very ill or debilitated patients, who may be more sensitive to the effects, especially the respiratory depressant effects, of opioid analgesics.

## Side/Adverse Effects

Note: Side effects are more frequent when the dezocine plasma concentration is 45 nanograms per mL (0.13 micromoles per L) or higher. The highest dose administered to nontolerant healthy adults without toxicity is 30 mg per 70 kg of body weight.

Dezocine appears less likely than pentazocine to cause the subjective and psychotomimetic effects characteristic of sigma-receptor agonists. These effects may include several or all of the following, occurring as a group: confusion, delusions, feelings of depersonalization or unreality, hallucinations (usually visual), dysphoria, nightmares, and nervousness or anxiety. However, psychotomimetic-like effects have been reported with high doses of dezocine.

Dezocine may have less dependence or abuse liability than other potent opioid analgesics (i.e., potent mu-receptor agonists). However, the medication has the potential for abuse, especially by individuals with a history of opioid abuse.

The following side/adverse effects have been selected on the basis of their potential clinical significance (possible signs and symptoms in parentheses where appropriate)—not necessarily inclusive:

**Those indicating need for medical attention, unless otherwise referenced**
Incidence rare (<1%)
*Atelectasis* (coughing; difficult breathing); *chest pain; CNS toxicity* (delirium; delusions; mental depression); *dermatitis* (skin rash; itching); *difficult, decreased, or frequent urination; edema* (swelling of face, fingers, lower legs, or feet; weight gain); *hypertension; hypotension* (if severe—dizziness, tiredness); *irregular heartbeat; respiratory depression* (slow, shallow, or difficult breathing); *thrombophlebitis*

**Those indicating need for medical attention only if they continue or are bothersome**
Incidence more frequent (3–9%)
*Drowsiness; gastric upset* (nausea; vomiting)

Incidence less frequent (1–3%) or rare (<1%)
*CNS effects* (anxiety; blurred or double vision; confusion; crying; dizziness or lightheadedness; slurred speech); *flushing or redness of skin; gastrointestinal effects* (abdominal pain or distress; constipation; diarrhea)

**Those indicating possible withdrawal and the need for medical attention if they occur after medication is discontinued**
*Body aches; diarrhea; fast heartbeat; fever, runny nose, or sneezing; gooseflesh; increased sweating; loss of appetite; nausea or vomiting; nervousness, restlessness, or irritability; shivering or trembling; stomach cramps; trouble in sleeping; unusually large pupils of eyes; weakness; yawning*

## Overdose

For specific information on the agents used in the management of dezocine overdose, see *Naloxone (Systemic)* monograph.

For more information on the management of overdose or unintentional ingestion, **contact a Poison Control Center** (see *Poison Control Center Listing*).

**Clinical effects of overdose**
The following effects have been selected on the basis of their potential clinical significance (possible signs and symptoms in parentheses where appropriate)—not necessarily inclusive:

Acute and chronic
*Cold, clammy skin; confusion, nervousness, or restlessness, severe; convulsions; dizziness, severe; drowsiness, severe; low blood pressure; pinpoint pupils of eyes; slow heartbeat; slow or troubled breathing; unconsciousness; weakness, severe*

**Treatment of overdose**
Although there is no experience with dezocine overdose, recommended treatment of overdose of opioid analgesics consists of the following:

Specific treatment—Use of the opioid antagonist naloxone. See the package insert or *Naloxone (Systemic)* monograph for specific dosing guidelines for use of this product. The fact that naloxone may also antagonize the analgesic actions of opioid analgesics and may precipitate withdrawal symptoms in physically dependent patients must be kept in mind.

Monitoring—Continue to monitor the patient (mandatory because the duration of action of the opioid analgesic may exceed that of the antagonist) and administer additional naloxone as needed. Alternatively, initial treatment may be followed by continuous intravenous infusion of naloxone, with the rate of infusion being adjusted according to patient response.

Supportive care—May include establishing adequate respiratory exchange through provision of a patent airway and institution of assisted or controlled respiration.

May also include administering intravenous fluids and/or vasopressors and using other supportive measures as needed. Patients in whom intentional overdose is confirmed or suspected should be referred for psychiatric consultation.

## Patient Consultation

As an aid to patient consultation, refer to *Advice for the Patient, Dezocine (Systemic)*.

In providing consultation, consider emphasizing the following selected information (» = major clinical significance):

### Before using this medication

» Conditions affecting use, especially:

Sensitivity to dezocine, history of

Use in the elderly—Increased risk of respiratory depression or other adverse effects

Other medications, especially other CNS depression–producing medications, other opioids, and naltrexone

Other medical problems, especially asthma or other acute or chronic respiratory problems

### Proper use of this medication

Proper administration technique (if dispensed for home use)

» Importance of not taking more medication than the amount prescribed because of danger of overdose and habit-forming potential

» Proper dosing

» Missed dose (if on scheduled dosing): Using as soon as possible; not using if almost time for next dose; not doubling doses

» Proper storage

### Precautions while using this medication

» Avoiding alcohol or other CNS depressants during therapy

» Caution if dizziness, drowsiness, or lightheadedness occurs

Caution when getting up suddenly from a lying or sitting position

Lying down if nausea, vomiting, dizziness, or lightheadedness occurs

Caution if any kind of surgery (including dental surgery) or emergency treatment is required

» Suspected overdose: Getting emergency help at once

### Side/adverse effects

Signs and symptoms of potential side effects, especially atelectasis; chest pain; CNS toxicity; dermatitis; difficult, decreased, or frequent urination; edema; hypertension; hypotension; irregular heartbeat; respiratory depression; and thrombophlebitis

## General Dosing Information

In recommended doses, dezocine is equipotent with morphine on a mg-per-mg basis.

Dosage and dosing intervals should be adjusted according to the patient's age, weight, and physical status, as well as the severity of pain, other medications given concurrently, and patient response to initial doses.

Dezocine is administered intravenously or intramuscularly. Subcutaneous administration is not recommended. In animal studies, repeated injection at a single site has caused subcutaneous inflammation, vascular irritation, and venous thrombosis.

Opioid analgesics may depress respiration, especially in geriatric, very ill, or debilitated patients and patients with respiratory problems. It is recommended that dosage of dezocine for these patients be reduced initially, then adjusted as required and tolerated. However, geriatric patients may also be more sensitive to the analgesic effects of opioid analgesics so that lower doses and/or a longer interval between doses may be sufficient to provide effective analgesia.

Concurrent administration of a non-opioid analgesic (such as aspirin or other salicylates, other nonsteroidal anti-inflammatory drugs, or acetaminophen) with an opioid analgesic provides additive analgesia and may permit lower doses of the opioid analgesic to be utilized.

Rapid intravenous injection of other strong opioid analgesics has caused anaphylactoid reactions, severe respiratory depression, hypotension, peripheral circulatory collapse, and cardiac arrest. Although these effects have not been documented with dezocine, precautions applying to other opioid analgesics may apply, i.e., administering the medication slowly, with an opioid antagonist and equipment for artificial ventilation available.

When an opioid analgesic is administered parenterally, the patient usually should be lying down and should remain recumbent for a period of time to minimize side effects such as hypotension, dizziness, light-headedness, nausea, and vomiting. If these side effects occur in an ambulatory patient, they may be relieved if the patient lies down.

In patients with shock, impaired perfusion may prevent complete absorption following intramuscular injection. Repeated administration may result in overdose due to an excessive amount suddenly being absorbed when circulation is restored.

## Parenteral Dosage Forms

### DEZOCINE INJECTION

#### Usual adult dose

Analgesic—

Intramuscular, 5 to 20 mg (usually 10 mg, initially). May be repeated every three to six hours as needed.

Intravenous, 2.5 to 10 mg (usually 5 mg, initially). May be repeated every two to four hours as needed.

Note: Lower doses may be required for geriatric, very ill, or debilitated patients and patients with respiratory problems.

#### Usual adult prescribing limits

Single intramuscular dose—20 mg, although there is some evidence that, because of dezocine's antagonist activity, 15 mg may be the maximally effective dose.

Total daily dose—120 mg.

#### Usual pediatric and adolescent dose

Patients up to 18 years of age—Safety and efficacy have not been established.

#### Strength(s) usually available

U.S.—

5 mg per mL (Rx) [*Dalgan* (sodium metabisulfite)].

10 mg per mL (Rx) [*Dalgan* (sodium metabisulfite)].

15 mg per mL (Rx) [*Dalgan* (sodium metabisulfite)].

Canada—

Not commercially available.

#### Packaging and storage

Store below 40 °C (104 °F), preferably between 15 and 30 °C (59 and 86 °F), protected from light, unless otherwise specified by manufacturer.

#### Auxiliary labeling

• May cause drowsiness.

• Avoid alcoholic beverages.

• May be habit-forming.

#### Note

Although a potent opioid (narcotic) analgesic, dezocine is not a controlled substance in the U.S.

## Selected Bibliography

O'Brien JJ, Benfield P. Dezocine. A preliminary review of its pharmacodynamic and pharmacokinetic properties, and therapeutic efficacy. Drugs 1989; 38: 226-48.

Stanbaugh JE, McAdams J. Comparison of intramuscular dezocine with butorphanol and placebo in chronic cancer pain: A method to evaluate analgesia after both single and repeated doses. Clin Pharmacol Ther 1987; 42: 210-9.

Galloway FM, Varma S. Double-blind comparison of intravenous doses of dezocine, butorphanol, and placebo for relief of postoperative pain. Anesth Analg 1986; 65: 283-7.

Revised: 08/29/94

## DIATRIZOATE-CONTAINING COMBINATIONS—

Diatrizoate and Iodipamide (Local)

# DIATRIZOATE AND IODIPAMIDE Local

VA CLASSIFICATION (Primary): DX102

Note: For a listing of dosage forms and brand names by country availability, see *Dosage Forms* section(s). For a listing of brand names for the articles in this monograph, refer to the General Index.

## Category

Diagnostic aid, radiopaque (uterus and fallopian tube disorders; sexual anomalies).

## Indications

Note: Bracketed information in the *Indications* section refers to uses that are not included in U.S. product labeling.

### Accepted

Hysterosalpingography—Diatrizoate and iodipamide combination is indicated for intrauterine instillation to determine the patency of the fallopian tubes and to visualize the uterine and tubal cavities for evaluation of abnormal conditions, such as tumors, of the uterus and fallopian tubes. Hysterosalpingography is used as a diagnostic tool in cases of infertility and other abnormal gynecological conditions; it serves as an adjunct to laparoscopy and ultrasound imaging in discovering subtle abnormalities, such as endometrial polyps and salpingitis isthmica nodosa.

Hysterosalpingography is *not* recommended during the menstrual period or when menstrual flow is imminent, during pregnancy, for at least 6 months after termination of pregnancy, or for 30 days after conization or curettage.

[Sexual anomalies, congenital (diagnosis)][1]—Diatrizoate and iodipamide combination may be indicated in children in the diagnosis of congenital sexual anomalies; however, it is rarely used.

---

[1]Not included in Canadian product labeling.

## Pharmacology/Pharmacokinetics

### Physicochemical characteristics
Molecular weight—Diatrizoate meglumine: 809.13.
Iodipamide meglumine: 1530.20.

### Mechanism of action/Effect
Organic iodine compounds block x-rays as they pass through the body, thereby allowing body structures containing iodine to be delineated in contrast to those structures that do not contain iodine. The degree of opacity produced by these compounds is directly proportional to the total amount (concentration and volume) of the iodinated contrast agent in the path of the x-rays. Installation of diatrizoate and iodipamide solution into the uterus and fallopian tubes allows visualization of these areas.

### Absorption
Intrauterine installation—Most of the medium within the uterine cavity is discharged into the vagina immediately upon termination of procedure. However, any medium retained in the uterine or peritoneal cavity is absorbed systemically within 60 minutes. May not be absorbed for up to 24 hours if tubes are obstructed and dilated.

### Protein binding
Diatrizoate meglumine—Very low.
Iodipamide meglumine—Very high.

### Time to peak opacification:
Immediate.

### Elimination
Absorbed medium—
    Diatrizoate meglumine: Primarily renal.
    Iodipamide meglumine: Primarily fecal.
Unabsorbed medium—Expelled vaginally following the procedure.

## Precautions to Consider

### Cross-sensitivity and/or related problems
Patients sensitive to iodine or other iodinated contrast media may be sensitive to diatrizoate and iodipamide also.

### Pregnancy/Reproduction
Pregnancy—Diatrizoate meglumine and iodipamide meglumine injection for intrauterine installation is not recommended for use during pregnancy since both diatrizoate and iodipamide may cross the placenta, or for at least 6 months after the termination of pregnancy since the procedure may increase the risk of complications such as intrauterine infection.

Also, other organically bound iodine–containing preparations administered near term by intra-amniotic injection have caused hypothyroidism in some newborns.

In addition, elective contrast radiography of the abdomen is usually not recommended during pregnancy because of the risks to the fetus from radiation exposure.

### Breast-feeding
Problems in humans have not been documented. However, since small amounts of this medium may be absorbed and both diatrizoate and iodipamide are known to be distributed unchanged into breast milk when administered intravascularly, breast-feeding is not recommended for at least 24 hours following administration of diatrizoate and iodipamide.

### Pediatrics
No information is available on the relationship of age to the effects of diatrizoate and iodipamide in pediatric patients. Safety and efficacy have not been established.

### Geriatrics
Appropriate studies on the relationship of age to the effects of diatrizoate and iodipamide for intrauterine installation have not been performed in geriatric patients. However, no geriatrics-specific problems have been documented to date.

### Diagnostic Interference
The following have been selected on the basis of their potential clinical significance (possible effect in parentheses where appropriate)—not necessarily inclusive (» = major clinical significance);

With *other* diagnostic test results
    Thyroid function determinations and
    Thyroid imaging
        (absorbed diatrizoate and iodipamide may cause an increase of serum protein–bound iodine [PBI] and a decrease in radioactive iodine or pertechnetate ion uptake for a period varying from 1 week to several months; thyroid test should be performed prior to administration of contrast medium. Other thyroid function tests not based on measurement of iodine, such as resin triiodothyronine uptake, are not affected)

### Medical considerations/Contraindications
The medical considerations/contraindications included here have been selected on the basis of their potential clinical significance (reasons given in parentheses where appropriate)—not necessarily inclusive (» = major clinical significance).

*Except under special circumstances, this medication should not be used when the following medical problem exists:*
» Genital tract infection
    (procedure may increase risk of complications)

*Risk-benefit should be considered when the following medical problems exist:*
    Allergic reaction (anaphylaxis) to penicillins or to skin allergens, previous
        (increased risk of anaphylactoid reaction)
    Allergies or asthma, history of
        (increased risk of idiosyncratic response or anaphylactoid reaction)
» Pelvic inflammatory disease, acute
    (condition may be aggravated)
» Sensitivity to iodinated contrast media
    (increased risk of anaphylactoid reaction in patients with a history of anaphylactoid reaction to iodinated contrast media)
    Caution is also recommended just after cervical or uterine surgery to avoid the risk of complications.

## Side/Adverse Effects

Note: Circulatory collapse may occur.
    Systemic adverse effects, although rare, are possible with intrauterine installation if medium is absorbed systemically after being retained in the uterine cavity or spilled into the peritoneal cavity.

The following side/adverse effects have been selected on the basis of their potential clinical significance (possible signs and symptoms in parentheses where appropriate)—not necessarily inclusive:

### Those indicating need for medical attention
Incidence rare
    *Pseudo-allergic reaction* (increased sweating, skin rash or hives, sneezing, swelling of face or skin, swelling of the larynx, wheezing, tightness in chest, or troubled breathing)—may be due to entry of medium into venous or lymphatic system
    Note: Transient; *pseudo-allergic reactions* may be initial manifestations of more severe anaphylactic reactions.

### Those indicating need for medical attention only if they continue or are bothersome
Incidence more frequent
    *Abdominal or stomach pain and discomfort*
    Note: *Abdominal pain and discomfort* may be associated with the insertion and positioning of the installation device. If occurring later during the procedure, may indicate spillage of contrast medium into the peritoneal cavity.

Incidence less frequent
    *Chills; fever; nausea and vomiting*

## Patient Consultation
As an aid to patient consultation, refer to *Advice for the Patient, Radiopaque Agents (Diagnostic, Local).*

In providing consultation, consider emphasizing the following selected information (» = major clinical significance):

**Description of use**

Instillation into uterus and fallopian tubes; visualization of radiopacity possible with x-rays

**Before having this test**

» Conditions affecting use, especially:

Sensitivity to iodine or other iodinated contrast media

Pregnancy—Diatrizoate and iodipamide cross the placenta; risk to fetus from radiation exposure; intrauterine instillation contraindicated during pregnancy and for at least 6 months after

Breast-feeding—Small amount absorbed and distributed into breast milk; temporary discontinuation of breast-feeding for at least 24 hours after test is recommended

Other medical problems, especially genital tract infection and acute pelvic inflammatory disease

**Preparation for this test**

Enema, vaginal douche, and/or other special preparatory instructions may be given; patient should inquire in advance

Voiding before procedure

**Precautions after having this test**

Possible interference with future thyroid tests

**Side/adverse effects**

Signs of possible side effects, especially pseudo-allergic reaction

## General Dosing Information

Manufacturer's package insert or other appropriate literature should be consulted for specific techniques and procedures for the administration of contrast media.

Sensitivity test doses are not usually recommended since severe or fatal reactions to contrast media are not predictable from a patient's history or a sensitivity test. On some occasions severe or fatal reactions have occurred with a test dose or with a full dose in patients who did not react to the test dose.

Pretreatment with corticosteroids and/or antihistamines is recommended to minimize the incidence and severity of reactions in patients with a history of severe reactions to contrast media or with other high-risk conditions (e.g., asthma or history of allergies, or positive allergy history to skin allergens or penicillin). In some studies, the additional use of ephedrine has been shown to be beneficial in preventing anaphylactoid reactions (except in patients with a history of hypertension or cardiovascular disease). When considering using a contrast agent, the following protocols are recommended:

For high-risk patients

• Use of a high-osmolality contrast agent plus pretreatment with a corticosteroid (oral prednisone, 50 mg administered 13 hours, 7 hours, and 1 hour before the procedure) and an antihistamine (intramuscular, intravenous, or oral diphenhydramine, 50 mg administered 1 hour before procedure); or

• Use of a low-osmolality contrast agent if pretreatment is not feasible; or

• Use of a low-osmolality contrast agent plus corticosteroid pretreatment

For low-risk patients

• Use of a high-osmolality contrast agent; or

• Use of a high-osmolality contrast agent and corticosteroid pretreatment

An enema and vaginal douche before the examination are optional. Patient should empty her bladder before the procedure.

Diatrizoate meglumine and iodipamide meglumine sterile solution is *not* for intravascular injection. It is to be instilled directly into the uterus via a sterile syringe attached to a uterine cannula, or via a tubal insufflator with a salpingogram attachment. It is recommended that in-

stillation into the uterine cavity be performed under controlled pressure with fluoroscopic monitoring. Excessive pressure and overfilling should be avoided.

During and for at least 30 to 60 minutes after administration of contrast media, the patient should be observed for possible severe reactions; competent personnel and emergency facilities should be available during this period.

Any unabsorbed contrast medium is expelled spontaneously upon removal of the cannula.

## Local Dosage Forms

### DIATRIZOATE MEGLUMINE AND IODIPAMIDE MEGLUMINE INJECTION

**Usual adult and adolescent dose**

Hysterosalpingograph—

Intrauterine instillation, up to 3 to 4 mL of a solution containing the equivalent of 380 mg of iodine per mL to fill the uterine cavity and up to an additional 3 to 4 mL to fill the fallopian tubes, administered slowly in fractional doses of 1 mL.

**Usual pediatric dose**

Dosage must be individualized by physician.

**Usual geriatric dose**

See *Usual adult and adolescent dose.*

**Strength(s) usually available**

U.S.—

52.7% (527 mg per mL) of diatrizoate meglumine and 26.8% (268 mg per mL) of iodipamide meglumine with 38% (380 mg per mL) of iodine (Rx) [*Sinografin*].

Canada—

52.7% (527 mg per mL) of diatrizoate meglumine and 26.9% (269 mg per mL) of iodipamide meglumine with 38% (380 mg per mL) of iodine (Rx) [*Sinografin*].

**Packaging and storage**

Store below 40 °C (104 °F), preferably between 15 and 30 °C (59 and 86 °F), in a light-resistant container, unless otherwise specified by manufacturer. Protect from freezing.

**Stability**

Solution may vary from colorless to light amber in color. Solutions that are significantly discolored should not be used.

Any unused portion remaining in the container should be discarded.

## Selected Bibliography

Winfield AC, Henderso-Slayden R, Wentz AC, et al. Hysterosalpingography: comparison of Conray 60 and Sinografin. AJR 1982; 138 (3): 559-60.

Sauer MV. Investigation of the female pelvis. J Reprod Med 1993 Apr; 38 (4): 269-76.

Gutmann JN. Imaging in the evaluation of female infertility. J Reprod Med 1992 Jan; 37 (1): 54-61.

Revised: 06/01/95

---

## DIATRIZOATE MEGLUMINE—See *Diatrizoates (Local)*; *Diatrizoates (Systemic)*

---

## DIATRIZOATE MEGLUMINE AND DIATRIZOATE SODIUM (SYSTEMIC)—See *Diatrizoates (Systemic)*

---

# DIATRIZOATES  Local

VA CLASSIFICATION (Primary): DX102

Note: For a listing of dosage forms and brand names by country availability, see *Dosage Forms* section(s). For a listing of brand names for the articles in this monograph, refer to the General Index.

## Category

Note: Diatrizoate is an ionic radiopaque contrast agent.

Diagnostic aid, radiopaque (urinary tract disorders)—Diatrizoate Meglumine Injection; Diatrizoate Sodium Injection.

Diagnostic aid, radiopaque (uterus and fallopian tube disorders)—Diatrizoate Meglumine Injection; Diatrizoate Sodium Injection.

## Indications

**Accepted**

Cystourethrography, retrograde—Diatrizoate meglumine is indicated in retrograde cystourethrography to evaluate abnormalities of the urethra, bladder, and ureters; and to demonstrate the presence and extent of cystoureteric reflux.

Pyelography, retrograde—Diatrizoate meglumine and diatrizoate sodium solutions are indicated in retrograde pyelography to evaluate abnormalities of the kidneys and ureter.

Hysterosalpingography—Diatrizoate meglumine and diatrizoate sodium are indicated for intrauterine installation to determine the patency of the fallopian tubes and to visualize the uterine and tubal cavities for evaluation of abnormal conditions, such as tumors, of the uterus and fallopian tubes. Hysterosalpingography is used as a diagnostic tool in cases of infertility and other abnormal gynecological conditions; it serves as an adjunct to laparoscopy and ultrasound imaging in discovering subtle abnormalities, such as endometrial polyps and salpingitis isthmica nodosa.

Hysterosalpingography is *not* recommended during the menstrual period or when menstrual flow is imminent, during pregnancy, for at least 6 months after termination of pregnancy, or for 30 days after conization or curettage.

## Pharmacology/Pharmacokinetics

### Physicochemical characteristics
Molecular weight—Diatrizoate meglumine: 809.13.
Diatrizoate sodium: 635.90.

### Mechanism of action/Effect
Organic iodine compounds block x-rays as they pass through the body, thereby allowing body structures containing iodine to be delineated in contrast to those structures that do not contain iodine. The degree of opacity produced by these compounds is directly proportional to the total amount (concentration and volume) of the iodinated contrast agent in the path of the x-rays. The installation of diatrizoate into the urinary bladder, kidneys, ureters, uterus, and fallopian tubes allows visualization of these areas.

### Absorption
Intravesical instillation—Small amounts (less than 2%) absorbed through the bladder.

Intrauterine instillation—Most of the medium within the uterine cavity is discharged into the vagina immediately upon termination of procedure. However, any medium retained in the uterine or peritoneal cavity is absorbed systemically within 60 minutes. May not be absorbed for up to 24 hours if tubes are obstructed and dilated.

### Protein binding
Very low.

### Elimination
Absorbed diatrizoate—Eliminated unchanged through the kidneys by glomerular filtration.

Unabsorbed diatrizoate—Expelled by spontaneous voiding or vaginally, depending on procedure.

## Precautions to Consider

### Cross-sensitivity and/or related problems
Patients sensitive to iodine or other iodinated contrast media may be sensitive to diatrizoates also.

### Carcinogenicity/Mutagenicity
Long-term animal studies to evaluate carcinogenic or mutagenic potential of diatrizoates have not been performed.

### Pregnancy/Reproduction
Pregnancy—Diatrizoates cross the placenta and are evenly distributed in fetal tissue. Other organically bound iodine-containing preparations administered near term by intra-amniotic injection have caused hypothyroidism in some newborns.

Also, elective contrast radiography of the abdomen is usually not recommended during pregnancy because of the risks to the fetus from radiation exposure.

*For intravesical instillation—*
Studies with diatrizoates administered by intravesical instillation have not been done in humans.
Studies have not been done in animals.

FDA Pregnancy Category C.

*For intrauterine instillation—*
Intrauterine instillation is not recommended during pregnancy since diatrizoates may cross the placenta, or for at least 6 months after the termination of pregnancy since the procedure may increase the risk of complications such as intrauterine infection.

### Breast-feeding
Problems in humans have not been documented. However, breast-feeding is not recommended for at least 24 hours following administration of diatrizoates, since small amounts of this medium may be absorbed and diatrizoates are known to be distributed unchanged into breast milk when administered intravascularly.

### Pediatrics
For intravesical instillation—Appropriate studies on the relationship of age to the effects of diatrizoates have not been performed in pediatric patients. However, no pediatrics-specific problems have been documented to date.

For intrauterine instillation—No information is available on the relationship of age to the effects of diatrizoates for intrauterine instillation in pediatric patients.

### Geriatrics
Appropriate studies on the relationship of age to the effects of diatrizoates for intrauterine or intravesical instillation have not been performed in geriatric patients. However, no geriatrics-specific problems have been documented to date.

### Drug interactions and/or related problems
See *Diagnostic interference.*

### Diagnostic interference
The following have been selected on the basis of their potential clinical significance (possible effect in parentheses where appropriate)—not necessarily inclusive (» = major clinical significance):

With results of retrograde pyelography
*Due to other medications*
Dyclonine
(may interfere with visualization when used as a local anesthetic in cystoscopic procedures following pyelography because of possible reaction with the iodine in diatrizoate, which may result in precipitation of iodine)

Sodium alginate
(may interfere with visualization when used as a lubricant in retrograde pyelography because of possible reaction with diatrizoate, which may result in the formation of a white precipitate)

With *other* diagnostic test results
Thyroid function determinations and
Thyroid imaging
(absorbed diatrizoates may cause an increase of serum protein-bound iodine [PBI] and a decrease in radioactive iodine or pertechnetate ion uptake for up to 16 days; thyroid test should be performed prior to administration of contrast medium; other thyroid function tests not based on measurement of iodine, such as resin triiodothyronine uptake, are not affected)

### Medical considerations/Contraindications
The medical considerations/contraindications included here have been selected on the basis of their potential clinical significance (reasons given in parentheses where appropriate)—not necessarily inclusive (» = major clinical significance).

*Except under special circumstances, this medication should not be used when the following medical problems exist:*

*For retrograde pyelography*
» Obstruction to endoscopy or ureteral catheterization, such as in extensive urinary tuberculosis, bladder tumors, ureteral obstructions, and prostate enlargement

» Urinary tract infection, upper, acute
(procedure may increase risk of complications)

*For hysterosalpingography*
» Genital tract infection
(procedure may increase risk of complications)

*Risk-benefit should be considered when the following medical problems exist:*

Allergic reaction (anaphylaxis) to penicillins or to skin allergens, previous
(increased risk of anaphylactoid reaction)

Allergies or asthma, history of
(increased risk of idiosyncratic response or anaphylactoid reaction)

» Sensitivity to iodinated contrast media
(increased risk of anaphylactoid reaction in patients with a history of anaphylactoid reaction to iodinated contrast media)

*For retrograde pyelography*
Renal function impairment, severe
(increased risk of oliguria or anuria)

*For hysterosalpingography*
» Pelvic inflammatory disease, acute
    (condition may be aggravated)
    Caution is also recommended just after cervical or uterine surgery to avoid the risk of complications.

## Side/Adverse Effects

Note: Adverse effects associated with the mechanics of retrograde genitourinary procedures include injury to the urethra, bladder, and ureter, and introduction of infection.

    Systemic adverse effects, similar to those that occur with direct intravascular injection of the diatrizoate salts, may also occur with intravesical or intraureteral instillation as a result of inadvertent intravascular entry of the contrast solution due to either bladder absorption or pyelorenal backflow.

    Systemic adverse effects, although rare, are possible with intrauterine instillation if medium is absorbed systemically after being retained in the uterine cavity or spilled into the peritoneal cavity.

The following side/adverse effects have been selected on the basis of their potential clinical significance (possible signs and symptoms in parentheses where appropriate)—not necessarily inclusive:

### Those indicating need for medical attention
Incidence less frequent
    *Pyelorenal distention* (severe abdominal or stomach pain and discomfort, backache)—resulting from the instillation of an excess volume of contrast solution; renal colic and shock may follow
Incidence rare
    *Pseudo-allergic reaction* (continuing chills, continuing fever, increased sweating, skin rash or hives, sneezing, swelling of face or skin, swelling of larynx, wheezing, tightness in chest, or troubled breathing)—may be due to entry of medium into venous or lymphatic system

### Those indicating need for medical attention only if they continue or are bothersome
Incidence more frequent
    *Abdominal or stomach pain and discomfort*
    Note: *Abdominal pain and discomfort* may be associated with the insertion and positioning of the instillation device. If occurring later during the procedure, may indicate spillage of contrast medium into the peritoneal cavity.
Incidence less frequent
    *Chills; fever; nausea and vomiting*

## Patient Consultation

As an aid to patient consultation, refer to *Advice for the Patient, Radiopaque Agents (Diagnostic, Local)*.

In providing consultation, consider emphasizing the following selected information (» = major clinical significance):

### Description of use
Instillation into bladder or ureters; visualization of radiopacity possible with x-rays

Instillation into uterus and fallopian tubes; visualization of radiopacity possible with x-rays

### Before having this test
» Conditions affecting use, especially:
    Sensitivity to iodine or other iodinated contrast media
    Pregnancy—Diatrizoates cross the placenta; risk to the fetus from radiation exposure; intrauterine instillation contraindicated during pregnancy and for at least 6 months after
    Breast-feeding—Small amount absorbed and distributed into breast milk; temporary discontinuation of breast-feeding for at least 24 hours is recommended
    Other medical problems, especially obstruction or acute upper urinary tract infection (for retrograde pyelography); genital tract infection and acute pelvic inflammatory disease (for hysterosalpingography)

### Preparation for this test
Voiding before procedure
*For retrograde cystourethrography and pyelography*
    Special diet, use of laxative, and/or other preparatory instructions may apply; patient should inquire in advance
*For hysterosalpingography*
    Enema, vaginal douche, and/or other preparatory instructions may apply; patient should inquire in advance

### Precautions after having this test
Possible interference with future thyroid tests
### Side/adverse effects
    Signs of potental side effects, especially pyelorenal distention or pseudo-allergic reaction

## General Dosing Information

Manufacturer's package insert or other appropriate literature should be consulted for specific techniques and procedures for the administration of contrast media.

Sensitivity test doses are not usually recommended since severe or fatal reactions to contrast media are not predictable from a patient's history or a sensitivity test. On some occasions severe or fatal reactions have occurred with a test dose or with a full dose in patients who did not react to the test dose.

Pretreatment with corticosteroids and/or antihistamines is recommended to minimize the incidence and severity of reactions in patients with a history of severe reactions to contrast media or with other high-risk conditions (e.g., asthma or history of allergies, positive allergy history to skin allergens or penicillin). In some studies, the additional use of ephedrine has been shown to be beneficial in preventing anaphylactoid reactions (except in patients with a history of hypertension or cardiovascular disease). When considering the use of a contrast agent, the following protocols are recommended:
For high-risk patients—
    • Use of a high-osmolality contrast agent plus pretreatment with a corticosteroid (oral prednisone, 50 mg administered 13 hours, 7 hours, and 1 hour before procedure) and an antihistamine (intramuscular, intravenous, or oral diphenhydramine, 50 mg administered 1 hour before procedure); or
    • Use of a low-osmolality contrast agent if pretreatment is not feasible; or
    • Use of a low-osmolality contrast agent plus corticosteroid pretreatment.
For low-risk patients—
    • Use of a high-osmolality contrast agent; or
    • Use of a high-osmolality contrast agent and corticosteroid pretreatment.

During and for at least 30 to 60 minutes after administration of contrast media, the patient should be observed for possible severe reactions; competent personnel and emergency facilities should be available during this period.

### For retrograde cystourethrography and pyelography
A low-residue diet the day before and a laxative the night before the procedure are generally recommended.

Diatrizoate meglumine or diatrizoate sodium labeled for retrograde cystourethrography or retrograde pyelography is *not* for intravascular injection. It is to be instilled, after the bladder is emptied, directly into the bladder or ureter and renal pelvis by gravity flow, using an appropriate venoclysis set or syringe. Excessive pressure should be avoided with either method of administration.

Dosage and concentration of diatrizoates for intravesical instillation should be individualized and are usually in proportion to the age of the patient and the technique and equipment used.

### For hysterosalpingography
An enema and vaginal douche before the examination are optional. Patient should empty her bladder before the procedure.

Diatrizoate solutions when used for hysterosalpingography are to be instilled directly into the uterus via a sterile syringe attached to a uterine cannula, or via a tubal insufflator with a salpingogram attachment. It is recommended that instillation into the uterine cavity be performed under controlled pressure with fluoroscopic monitoring. Excessive pressure and overfilling should be avoided.

Any unabsorbed contrast medium is expelled spontaneously upon removal of the cannula.

## Local Dosage Forms

### DIATRIZOATE MEGLUMINE INJECTION USP

**Usual adult and adolescent dose**
Cystourethrography, retrograde—
    Intravesical instillation, 25 to 300 mL or more, depending on age and bladder capacity, of a solution containing the equivalent of 85 mg or 141 mg of iodine per mL.
Pyelography, retrograde—
    Intraureteral instillation, 6 to 10 mL, up to 15 mL, of a solution containing the equivalent of 85 mg or 141 mg of iodine per mL for

unilateral pyelograms. Dose may be doubled for bilateral pyelograms.

Note: The 60% solution (containing the equivalent of 283 mg of iodine per mL) must be diluted to a 20 to 30% solution (containing the equivalent of 94 mg to 141 mg of iodine per mL, respectively) with sterile distilled water prior to use.

In patients with reduced renal function, repeat retrograde pyelography is not recommended for at least 48 hours, because of the possibility of temporary oliguria or anuria.

Hysterosalpingography—

Intrauterine instillation, up to 3 to 4 mL of a solution containing the equivalent of 283 mg of iodine per mL to fill the uterine cavity and up to an additional 3 to 4 mL to fill the Fallopian tubes, administered slowly in fractional doses of 1 mL.

## Usual pediatric dose

Cystourethrography, retrograde—
See *Usual adult and adolescent dose.*
Pyelography, retrograde—
Intraureteral instillation, 1 to 10 mL of a solution containing the equivalent of 85 or 141 mg of iodine per mL. Dosage must be individualized by physician according to size of child.
Hysterosalpingography—
Dosage has not been established.

## Usual geriatric dose
See *Usual adult and adolescent dose.*

## Strength(s) usually available
U.S.—

18% (180 mg per mL) of diatrizoate meglumine with 8.5% (85 mg per mL) of iodine (Rx) [*Cystografin Dilute*].

30% (300 mg per mL) of diatrizoate meglumine with 14.1% (141 mg per mL) of iodine (Rx) [*Cystografin; Hypaque-Cysto; Reno-M-30* (0.3 mg propylparaben and 1 mg methylparaben, per mL); *Urovist Cysto; Urovist Cysto Pediatric*].

Canada—

18% (180 mg per mL) of diatrizoate meglumine with 8.5% (85 mg per mL) of iodine (Rx) [*Hypaque-M 18%*].

30% (300 mg per mL) of diatrizoate meglumine with 14.1% (141 mg per mL) of iodine (Rx) [*Hypaque-M 30%*].

60% (600 mg per mL) of diatrizoate meglumine with 28.3% (283 mg per mL) of iodine (Rx) [*Hypaque-M 60%*].

Note: May also contain edetate disodium or edetate calcium disodium as a sequestering stabilizing agent.

## Packaging and storage
Store below 40 °C (104 °F), preferably between 15 and 30 °C (59 and 86 °F), unless otherwise specified by manufacturer. Protect from light. Protect from freezing.

## Preparation of dosage form
The 30% solution (containing the equivalent of 141 mg of iodine per mL) may be diluted to a 10 to 25% solution (containing the equivalent of 47 mg to 118 mg of iodine per mL, respectively) with sterile water for injection, 5% dextrose injection, or 0.9% sodium chloride injection, according to the manufacturer's instructions.

## Stability
The sterile solution of diatrizoate meglumine is clear and colorless to pale yellow; do not use if discolored.
Crystals may form in the solution at very cold temperatures but are readily redissolved by bringing the container of solution to room temperature and gently shaking it.
Diluted solutions should be used immediately.
Any unused portion remaining in the container should be discarded.

## DIATRIZOATE SODIUM INJECTION USP

### Usual adult and adolescent dose
Pyelography, retrograde—
Intraureteral instillation, 6 to 10 mL of a solution containing the equivalent of 120 mg of iodine per mL for unilateral pyelograms. Dose may be doubled for bilateral pyelograms.

Note: For patients with hydronephrosis, the dose may be increased to 20 mL or more.

The 50% solution (containing the equivalent of 300 mg of iodine per mL) must be diluted to a 20% solution (containing the equivalent of 120 mg of iodine per mL) with sterile distilled water prior to use.

In patients with reduced renal function, repeat retrograde pyelography is not recommended for at least 48 hours, because of the possibility of temporary oliguria or anuria.

Hysterosalpingography—

Intrauterine instillation, up to 3 or 4 mL of a solution containing the equivalent of 300 mg of iodine per mL to fill the uterine cavity and up to an additional 3 or 4 mL to fill the fallopian tubes, administered slowly in fractional doses of 1 mL.

### Usual pediatric dose
Pyelography, retrograde (unilateral)—
Intraureteral instillation of a solution containing the equivalent of 120 mg of iodine per mL for:
Children up to 1 year of age—Less than 1.5 mL.
Children 1 to 5 years of age—1.5 to 3 mL.
Children 5 years of age and over—4 to 5 mL.
Hysterosalpingography—
Dosage has not been established.

### Usual geriatric dose
See *Usual adult and adolescent dose.*

### Strength(s) usually available
U.S.—

20% (200 mg per mL) of diatrizoate sodium with 12% (120 mg per mL) of iodine (Rx) [*Hypaque Sodium 20%*].

50% (500 mg per mL) of diatrizoate sodium with 30% (300 mg per mL) of iodine (Rx) [*Hypaque Sodium 50%; Urovist Sodium 300*].

Canada—

50% (500 mg per mL) of diatrizoate sodium with 30% (300 mg per mL) of iodine (Rx) [*Hypaque Sodium 50%*].

Note: May also contain edetate disodium or edetate calcium disodium as a sequestering stabilizing agent.

### Packaging and storage
Store below 40 °C (104 °F), preferably between 15 and 30 °C (59 and 86 °F), unless otherwise specified by manufacturer. Store in a tight, light-resistant container. Protect from freezing.

### Stability
The diatrizoate sodium injection is clear and pale yellow to light brown; do not use if discolored.
Crystals may form in the solution at very cold temperatures but are readily redissolved by bringing the container of solution to room temperature and gently shaking it.
Any unused portion remaining in the container should be discarded.

### Selected Bibliography
Sauer MV. Investigation of the female pelvis. J Reprod Med 1993 Apr; 38 (4): 269-76.
Gutmann JN. Imaging in the evaluation of female infertility. J Reprod Med 1992 Jan; 37 (1): 54-61.

Revised: 05/11/95

---

# DIATRIZOATES   Systemic

VA CLASSIFICATION (Primary): DX102
Note: For a listing of dosage forms and brand names by country availability, see *Dosage Forms* section(s). For a listing of brand names for the articles in this monograph, refer to the General Index.

## Category
Note: Diatrizoate is an ionic radiopaque contrast agent.

Diagnostic aid, radiopaque (cardiac disease)—Diatrizoate Meglumine Injection; Diatrizoate Meglumine and Diatrizoate Sodium Injection.
Diagnostic aid, radiopaque (vascular disease)—Diatrizoate Meglumine Injection; Diatrizoate Meglumine and Diatrizoate Sodium Injection; Diatrizoate Sodium Injection.
Diagnostic aid, radiopaque (joint disease)—Diatrizoate Meglumine Injection.
Diagnostic aid, radiopaque (biliary tract disorders)—Diatrizoate Meglumine Injection; Diatrizoate Meglumine and Diatrizoate Sodium Injection; Diatrizoate Sodium Injection.

Diagnostic aid, radiopaque (brain disorders)—Diatrizoate Meglumine Injection; Diatrizoate Meglumine and Diatrizoate Sodium Injection; Diatrizoate Sodium Injection.

Diagnostic aid, radiopaque (disk disease)—Diatrizoate Meglumine Injection.

Diagnostic aid, radiopaque (gastrointestinal disorders)—Diatrizoate Meglumine and Diatrizoate Sodium Solution; Diatrizoate Sodium Solution; Diatrizoate Sodium for Solution.

Diagnostic aid, radiopaque (splenic and portal vein disorders)—Diatrizoate Meglumine Injection; Diatrizoate Meglumine and Diatrizoate Sodium Injection; Diatrizoate Sodium Injection.

Diagnostic aid, radiopaque (urinary tract disorders)—Diatrizoate Meglumine Injection; Diatrizoate Meglumine and Diatrizoate Sodium Injection; Diatrizoate Sodium Injection.

Diagnostic aid, radiopaque contrast enhancer in computed tomography—Diatrizoate Meglumine Injection; Diatrizoate Meglumine and Diatrizoate Sodium Injection; Diatrizoate Sodium Injection.

Diagnostic aid, radiopaque contrast enhancer adjunct in computed tomography—Diatrizoate Meglumine and Diatrizoate Sodium Solution.

Diagnostic aid, radiopaque (pregnancy disorders)—Diatrizoate Meglumine Injection.

Osmotic agent (meconium ileus)—Diatrizoate Meglumine and Diatrizoate Sodium Solution; Diatrizoate Sodium Solution.

# Indications

Note: Bracketed information in the *Indications* section refers to uses that are not included in U.S. product labeling.

## Accepted
Oral/Rectal:

Radiography, gastrointestinal—Oral or rectal diatrizoate sodium, and diatrizoate meglumine and diatrizoate sodium combination solutions are indicated for radiographic examination of the gastrointestinal tract when the administration of barium sulfate is not recommended (e.g., for patients with known or suspected gastrointestinal tract perforation in whom barium suspensions could be harmful).

Body imaging, computed tomographic, adjunct—Oral diatrizoate meglumine and diatrizoate sodium combination solution is indicated in low concentration to delineate the stomach and intestinal loops in computed tomography (CT) of the body.

[Meconium ileus (treatment)][1]—Rectal diatrizoate sodium, and diatrizoate meglumine and diatrizoate sodium combination solutions have been used to treat meconium ileus in infants.

Intravascular:

Angiocardiography—Parenteral diatrizoate meglumine and diatrizoate sodium combination is indicated to visualize lesions or malformations of the heart and obstructions or anomalies of the major thoracic blood vessels. Parenteral diatrizoate meglumine is also indicated in angiocardiography; however, the combination containing diatrizoate meglumine and diatrizoate sodium is usually preferred because it causes less severe adverse hemodynamic, neurotoxic, and cardiotoxic effects.

Angiography

Aortography

Arteriography or

Venography—Parenteral diatrizoates are indicated to visualize specific regions of the vascular system and the blood flow in such areas to help in the diagnosis and evaluation of neoplasms (known or suspected) or vascular diseases (congenital or acquired) that may cause changes in normal vascular anatomy or physiology. Parenteral diatrizoate meglumine is indicated in cerebral angiography, aortography, arteriography (peripheral or selective renal[1]), and peripheral venography. Parenteral diatrizoate meglumine and diatrizoate sodium combination is indicated in intravenous digital subtraction arteriography, cerebral angiography, aortography, arteriography (coronary, selective coronary, peripheral, selective renal, and selective visceral), and venography (central, peripheral, or renal)[1]. Parenteral diatrizoate sodium is indicated in cerebral angiography[1], aortography[1], arteriography (peripheral or selective renal)[1], and intraosseous venography.

Diatrizoate meglumine is preferred for cerebral or peripheral angiography because, when administered intra-arterially, it generally causes less severe neurotoxic and local and generalized hemodynamic side effects than diatrizoate sodium or diatrizoate combinations. The sodium ion is probably responsible for the increased neurotoxicity of diatrizoate sodium since it may increase the extravascular diffusion of the medium into the brain tissue. Diatrizoate meglumine is considered at least as safe as, and possibly preferable to, diatrizoate meglumine and diatrizoate sodium combination injection for aortography not involving the ascending aorta. Only in the latter situation may the contrast medium enter the coronary circulation where it is important to have at least some small amount of sodium to prevent cardiotoxic effects.

Cholangiography, direct, operative—Parenteral diatrizoate meglumine, diatrizoate meglumine and diatrizoate sodium combination[1], and diatrizoate sodium are indicated for use during surgery to visualize the biliary ducts and evaluate the cause and location of biliary obstructions such as calculi or strictures, and after surgery to rule out the presence of retained calculi.

Cholangiography, direct, postoperative T-tube—Parenteral diatrizoate meglumine, diatrizoate meglumine and diatrizoate sodium combination[1], and diatrizoate sodium are indicated to visualize, and thus ensure the patency of, the biliary ducts before removal of a surgically placed T-tube.

Cholangiography, percutaneous transhepatic[1]—Parenteral diatrizoate meglumine, diatrizoate meglumine and diatrizoate sodium combination, and diatrizoate sodium are indicated for this procedure. Percutaneous transhepatic cholangiography is used in *some* patients to determine the cause and site of biliary obstruction when other examinations of the biliary system have not provided the needed information.

Brain imaging, computed tomographic—Parenteral diatrizoate meglumine, diatrizoate meglumine and diatrizoate sodium combination, and diatrizoate sodium are indicated for computed tomographic brain imaging (CT of the brain) to determine the presence and extent of neoplasms or other lesions such as cerebral infarction or infection.

Body imaging, computed tomographic—Parenteral diatrizoate meglumine and the diatrizoate meglumine and diatrizoate sodium combination are indicated for computed tomographic body imaging (CT of the body).

Splenoportography—Parenteral diatrizoate meglumine, diatrizoate meglumine and diatrizoate sodium combination, and diatrizoate sodium[1] are indicated for splenoportography, to determine the site of the portal obstruction, or visualize collateral pathways of blood flow or esophageal varices in patients with portal hypertension or portal venous obstruction. It should be noted that splenoportography is being replaced by other procedures in which the portal system may be evaluated by late films of the celiac and superior mesenteric arterial systems (their venous phases). In other cases, it is being replaced by direct portography via the transhepatic (direct percutaneous or transjugular) route.

Urography, excretory—Parenteral diatrizoate meglumine, diatrizoate meglumine and diatrizoate sodium combination, and diatrizoate sodium are indicated by intravenous injection or infusion in excretion urography to evaluate abnormalities of the urinary tract such as urinary tract obstructions.

Urography, retrograde[1]—Parenteral diatrizoate meglumine and parenteral diatrizoate sodium are indicated to determine the site of the urinary tract obstruction when excretion urography has not provided sufficient information or is contraindicated.

Nephrotomography—Parenteral diatrizoate meglumine and diatrizoate sodium combination is indicated at high dosage to prolong and intensify the nephrographic effect, especially with tomography, for the examination of the renal parenchyma when excretion urography has not provided sufficient information. Nephrotomography may be useful in the preoperative differentiation of renal masses and damage to the renal parenchyma such as that caused by infarcts or infections.

[Amniography][1]—Parenteral diatrizoate meglumine has been used for amniography.

Intrasynovial:

Arthrography—Parenteral diatrizoate meglumine is indicated for arthrography in diagnosis of post-traumatic or degenerative joint diseases or synovial rupture, for visualization of communicating bursae or cysts, and in meniscography.

Intradiskal:

Diskography—Parenteral diatrizoate meglumine is indicated for diskography, to determine the presence of disk pathology, degeneration, retropulsion, or rupture.

---

[1]Not included in Canadian product labeling.

# Pharmacology/Pharmacokinetics

## Physicochemical characteristics

Molecular weight—Diatrizoate meglumine: 809.13.
Diatrizoate sodium: 635.90.

Osmolality—High. The osmolality of the injection with iodine concentration of 370 mg per mL ranges from 1940 to 2140 mOsmol per kg of water, depending on product.

## Mechanism of action/Effect

Diagnostic aid, radiopaque—Organic iodine compounds block x-rays as they pass through the body, thereby allowing body structures containing iodine to be delineated in contrast to those structures that do not contain iodine. The degree of opacity produced by these iodinated organic compounds is directly proportional to the total amount (concentration and volume) of the iodinated contrast agent in the path of the x-rays.

Osmotic agent (meconium ileus)—The osmotic effect of diatrizoate sodium, and diatrizoate meglumine and diatrizoate sodium combination solutions draws fluid into the intestine, thus helping to dislodge the meconium impaction.

## Other actions/effects

Anticoagulant (inhibitory effect on platelet aggregation and blood clotting); vasodilating effects.

## Absorption

Oral—Minimally absorbed from gastrointestinal tract.

Intravertebral disk or spleen injection (for diatrizoate meglumine only): Rapidly absorbed.

Intravesical instillation: Small amounts absorbed through the bladder.

## Distribution

Intravascular—Rapidly distributed throughout extracellular fluid following intravascular administration.

## Protein binding

Very low.

## Half-life

Normal renal function—30 to 60 minutes.

Severe renal function impairment—20 to 140 hours.

## Time to peak concentration

Immediate, after rapid intravenous administration, but concentration falls rapidly within 5 to 10 minutes.

## Time to peak opacification

Angiography—
   Immediate, after intravascular administration.

Urography—
   Renal parenchyma including the renal cortex: 1 minute following rapid injection of contrast media. Peak opacification is directly dependent on peak plasma iodine concentration and glomerular filtration rate of the kidney.
   Calyces, pelves, and ureters: 10 to 15 minutes after bolus injection of contrast media. Peak opacification is dependent on both the final urinary iodine concentration and the volume of urine within the respective regions of the urinary tract.

## Elimination

Renal—
   Normal renal function: 95 to 100% of intravascular dose excreted unchanged (via glomerular filtration) within 24 hours.

Fecal—
   Normal renal function: 1 to 2% of intravascular dose excreted via biliary elimination and possibly via the intestinal mucosa.
   Severe renal function impairment: 10 to 50% of intravascular dose; up to 20% of the administered dose has been recovered in feces within 48 hours.

In dialysis—
   Removed by peritoneal dialysis or hemodialysis.

# Precautions to Consider

## Cross-sensitivity and/or related problems

Patients sensitive to iodine or other iodinated contrast media may be sensitive to these agents also.

## Pregnancy/Reproduction

Pregnancy—Diatrizoates, when administered intravenously, cross the placenta and are evenly distributed in fetal tissues. Intra-amniotic injection of diatrizoates has been reported to suppress the fetal thyroid gland.

*For parenteral solutions—*
   Studies with diatrizoates have not been done in humans.
   Studies with diatrizoates have not been done in animals.
   FDA Pregnancy Category C.

*For oral/rectal solutions—*
   Elective contrast radiography of the abdomen is usually not recommended during pregnancy because of the risks to the fetus from radiation exposure. Studies with diatrizoates have not been done in humans.
   For diatrizoate sodium—Studies in animals have not shown that diatrizoate sodium causes adverse effects in the fetus.
   FDA Pregnancy Category B.

## Breast-feeding

Although problems in humans have not been documented, since diatrizoates are distributed unchanged into breast milk, temporary discontinuation of breast-feeding is recommended for at least 24 hours following their administration.

## Pediatrics

Convulsions are more likely to occur in infants than in other age groups with the administration of diatrizoate meglumine, and diatrizoate meglumine and diatrizoate sodium combination injections, especially after repeated injections.

Difficulty in breathing, slow or irregular heartbeat, and unusual feeling of tiredness and depression are more likely to occur in cyanotic infants administered diatrizoate meglumine and diatrizoate meglumine and diatrizoate sodium combination injections.

Dehydration and/or the risk of renal failure may be exacerbated in infants and young children, especially those with polyuria, oliguria, diabetes, or pre-existing dehydration, by the contrast media; adequate hydration is recommended before and subsequent to administration of diatrizoates.

For oral/rectal solutions—In infants and young children (weighing under 10 kg), the hypertonic solutions of contrast media may draw excessive amounts of fluid into the intestine, possibly resulting in hypovolemia, which may cause a shock-like state. Further dilution of contrast solution is recommended for use in pediatric patients.

## Geriatrics

Although overall prevalence of adverse effects has been reported to be less in patients 50 years of age and older, the severity of the reactions may be greater in this age group than in younger patients.

Dehydration and/or the risk of renal failure may be exacerbated in geriatric patients, especially those with polyuria, oliguria, diabetes, or pre-existing dehydration, by the contrast media; adequate hydration is recommended before administration of diatrizoates.

The elderly may be more sensitive to the effects of diatrizoates on thyroid function. Iodine-induced thyrotoxicosis may occur 4 to 12 weeks following contrast radiography. Thyroid function monitoring may be needed in geriatric patients.

For oral/rectal solutions—In elderly patients, the hypertonic solutions of contrast media may draw excessive amounts of fluid into the intestine, possibly resulting in hypovolemia, which may cause a shock-like state. Further dilution of contrast solution is recommended for use in geriatric patients.

## Drug interactions and/or related problems

The following drug interactions and/or related problems have been selected on the basis of their potential clinical significance (possible mechanism in parentheses where appropriate)—not necessarily inclusive ($\gg$ = major clinical significance):

Note: Combinations containing any of the following medications, depending on the amount present, may also interact with this medication.

Beta-adrenergic blocking agents
   (concurrent intravascular administration of diatrizoates with beta-adrenergic blocking agents may increase the risk of moderate to severe anaphylactoid reaction; also, hypotensive effects may be exacerbated; discontinuation of the beta-adrenergic blocking agent may be advisable before administration of contrast media in patients with other risk factors)

Cholecystographic agents, oral
   (may increase the risk of renal toxicity when closely followed by intravenous diatrizoates, especially in patients with hepatic function impairment)

$\gg$ Chymopapain
   (concurrent use with diatrizoates may increase the risk of toxicity, especially if either agent enters the subarachnoid space; it is strongly recommended that diskography not be performed as part of the chemonucleolysis procedure)

Hypotension-producing medications, other (See *Appendix II*)
   (concurrent intravascular administration of diatrizoates with other hypotension-producing medication may result in excessive hypotension)

Interleukin-2
   (incidence of delayed [more than 1 hour after administration] reactions [e.g., hypersensitivity, fever, skin rash, flu-like symptoms, joint pain, flushing, pruritus, emesis, hypotension, dizziness] to intravenous contrast media may be increased in patients who have received interleukin-2; some symptoms may resemble a "recall" reaction to interleukin-2; supportive medical treatment may be necessary if symptoms are significant; there is some evidence that incidence is reduced if contrast media administration is delayed until 6 weeks after interleukin-2 administration)

Nephrotoxic medications, other (See *Appendix II*)
(concurrent intravascular administration of diatrizoates with other nephrotoxic medications may increase the potential for nephrotoxicity)

Vasopressors (See *Appendix II*)
(neurologic effects, including paraplegia, of diatrizoates may increase during aortography when diatrizoates are administered after hypertensive agents used to increase contrast; this increase is due to contraction of vessels in the splanchnic circulation, which forces more of the contrast material into the vessels leading to the spine and spinal cord)

**Diagnostic interference**

The following have been selected on the basis of their potential clinical significance (possible effect in parentheses where appropriate)—not necessarily inclusive (» = major clinical significance):

With *other* diagnostic test results

Blood pool imaging
(imaging of blood pool may be impaired because of decreased technetium Tc 99m-labeling of red blood cells caused by the intravascular administration of diatrizoates)

Leukocyte counts and
Red cell counts
(may be decreased)

Phenolsulfonphthalein (PSP) excretion test
(test results may be affected, especially in patients with severely impaired renal function, who are also given intravascular diatrizoates; diatrizoates are also in part secreted by the renal tubules, thus resulting in decreased tubular excretion of PSP; therefore, concurrent use of intravascular diatrizoates is not recommended in patients receiving PSP excretion test)

Prothrombin time (PT) and
Thromboplastin time
(may be increased since diatrizoates significantly inhibit all stages of coagulation)

Skeletal imaging
(possible renal and hepatic uptake of technetium Tc 99m medronate, technetium Tc 99m oxidronate, technetium Tc 99m pyrophosphate, and technetium Tc 99m [pyro- and trimeta-] phosphates if diatrizoates are administered intravenously immediately after one of these technetium Tc 99m-labeled agents)

Thyroid function determinations and
Thyroid imaging
(diatrizoates may cause an increase of serum protein–bound iodine [PBI] and a decrease in radioactive iodine or pertechnetate ion uptake for a period varying from 1 week to several months; thyroid test should be performed prior to administration of diatrizoates. Other thyroid function tests not based on measurement of iodine, such as resin triiodothyronine uptake, are not affected)

With physiology/laboratory test values

Amylase, serum
(concentrations may be increased temporarily 6 to 18 hours after injection of diatrizoates during direct cholangiography since drug may enter pancreatic duct)

Creatinine, serum
(may be increased temporarily; peak rise in serum creatinine is usually delayed, occurring 3 to 5 days following contrast media administration and generally returning to baseline values in 7 to 10 days)

Platelet aggregation
(may be decreased by high levels of plasma diatrizoates)

Protein, urine
(may be increased; false positive results may occur with Lowry's and sulphosalicylic assays or with protein reagent strips)

**Medical considerations/Contraindications**

The medical considerations/contraindications included here have been selected on the basis of their potential clinical significance (reasons given in parentheses where appropriate)—not necessarily inclusive (» = major clinical significance).

*Risk-benefit should be considered when the following medical problems exist:*

*For all procedures requiring intravascular administration of diatrizoates*
» Allergic reaction (anaphylaxis) to penicillins or to skin allergens, previous
(increased risk of anaphylactoid reaction)
» Allergies or asthma, history of
(increased risk of idiosyncratic response or anaphylactoid reaction)

» Cardiovascular disease, severe
(intravenous administration may produce a transitory increase in circulatory osmotic load and may aggravate condition; increased risk of anaphylactoid reaction)
» Dehydration, especially associated with diabetes mellitus, azotemia, or multiple myeloma
(osmotic diuretic action of diatrizoates may exacerbate dehydration and increase the risk of acute renal failure)

Hyperthyroidism
(intravascular administration may precipitate thyroid storm)
» Pheochromocytoma
(intravascular administration may precipitate severe hypertension; amount of medium injected should be kept to a minimum and blood pressure should be monitored during the procedure; also, pretreatment with the alpha-adrenergic blocking agent phentolamine is recommended)
» Renal function impairment
(intravenous administration may increase risk of acute renal failure in the presence of renal insufficiency [serum creatinine ⩾ 132.6 micromoles/L]; preventive measures recommended to prevent contrast-associated nephropathy include reducing the dose or volume of contrast medium administered, lengthening the time between radiologic procedures, volume expansion with 0.9% sodium chloride, using drug therapy such as furosemide or mannitol or calcium antagonists, and administering low-osmolality contrast media; however, validity of some of these recommendations remains controversial)
» Seizures, recent
(increased risk for reoccurence)
» Sensitivity to iodinated contrast media
(increased risk of anaphylactoid reaction in patients with a history of previous anaphylactoid reaction to iodinated contrast media)

Sickle cell disease
(intravenous or intra-arterial administration may promote sickling in patients who are homozygous for sickle cell disease)

*For gastrointestinal radiography*
Dehydration
(hypertonic solutions of medium may lead to intraluminal movement of fluid with resulting hypovolemia; this loss of plasma fluid may result in a shock-like state)

Gastrointestinal obstruction
(increase in acid concentration due to delayed gastric emptying may precipitate diatrizoates; resultant diatrizoate precipitate may cause gastrointestinal mucosal irritation, erosion, and bleeding; aspiration of gastric contents or alkalinization is recommended before administration of diatrizoates)

*For angiocardiography*
Angina, unstable
(increased risk of severe cardiac reaction)

Aortic stenosis
(intravascular administration may cause decreased coronary artery perfusion due to the systemic hypotension produced)

Cardiac failure, incipient
(fluid overload, pressure changes, and expansion of blood volume may aggravate condition)

Cyanosis, in infants
(increased risk of apnea, bradycardia and other arrhythmias, lethargy and depression, and a tendency to acidosis in cyanotic infants)

Mitral stenosis
(increased blood flow may produce an increase in the mitral diastolic pressure gradient)

Myocardial ischemia
(systemic hypotension and resultant diminished cardiac perfusion may cause increased risk for patient)
» Pulmonary hypertension, severe
(hypervolemic effect of diatrizoates may further increase pulmonary artery and venous pressures due to an increase in cardiac output and a rise in left ventricular end-diastolic and left atrial pressures)

*For cerebral angiography*
Arteriosclerosis, advanced or
Cardiac decompensation or
Cerebral embolism, recent or
Hemorrhage, subarachnoid or
Hypertension, severe or
Migraine or

Senility or
Thrombosis, recent
  (increased risk of vessel occlusion; clinical deterioration, convulsions, and serious temporary or permanent neurological complications may occur)
» Homocystinuria
  (procedure may increase risk of thrombosis and embolism)

*For peripheral arteriography*
» Buerger's disease
  (procedure may induce severe arterial or venous spasm)
» Ischemia, severe, associated with ascending infection

*For percutaneous transhepatic cholangiography*
» Coagulation defects, such as prolonged prothrombin times
  (procedure may increase risk of internal bleeding)

*For CT of the brain*
» Cerebral lesions, primary or metastatic
  (intravascular administration may precipitate convulsions)
» Hemorrhage, cranial subarachnoid
  (intravascular administration may cause death)

*For splenoportography*
» Coagulation defects, such as prolonged prothrombin times and significant thrombocytopenia, or
  Inflammation of spleen
  (procedure may increase risk of rupture of the spleen)

*For excretory urography*
» Anuria or
» Diabetes mellitus
  (may increase risk of acute renal failure)

*For retrograde urography*
» Obstruction to endoscopy or ureteral catheterization, such as in extensive urinary tuberculosis, bladder tumors, ureteral obstructions, and
  prostate enlargement
» Urinary tract infection, upper, acute
  (procedure may increase risk of complications)

*For peripheral venography*
Infection, local, or
Ischemia, severe, or
Phlebitis or
Thrombosis or
Venous stasis or
Venous system obstruction
  (procedure may cause venous inflammatory changes, thrombosis,
  and ischemic changes; irrigation with normal saline is recom-
  mended following the procedure to decrease risk of thrombosis)

*For arthrography*
» Infection, in or near joint to be examined
  (procedure may increase risk of complications)

*For diskography*
» Infection or open injury near region to be examined
  (procedure may increase risk of complications)
» Respiratory infection, upper
  (cervical diskography procedure may increase risk of
  complications)

**Patient monitoring**
The following may be especially important in patient monitoring (other
tests may be warranted in some patients, depending on condition;
» = major clinical significance):

Blood pressure determinations
  (may be required during examination with intravascular administration of diatrizoates, especially in patients with known or suspected pheochromocytoma or hemodynamic compromise or
  instability)
Electrocardiogram (ECG)
  (recommended for early detection of arrhythmias during coronary
  arteriography and angiocardiography)
Thyroid function determinations
  (iodine-induced thyrotoxicosis may occur 4 to 12 weeks following
  contrast radiography in geriatric patients; thyroid function monitoring may be needed)

## Side/Adverse Effects

Note: Adverse effects may vary directly with the concentration of the
  agent, the amount and technique used, and the underlying pathology. Increases in osmolality, volume, concentration, viscosity, and

rate of administration of the solution may tend to increase the incidence and severity of adverse effects.

Systemic adverse effects, similar to those that occur with direct
intravascular injection of diatrizoates, may also occur with oral or
rectal administration in cases of perforation.

Thromboembolic events causing myocardial infarction and stroke
have been reported rarely during angiographic procedures with
ionic contrast media.

Convulsions and death may occur with inadvertent subarachnoid
injection, especially during aortography by the translumbar technique. Use of diatrizoates is contraindicated in myelography or for
examination of dorsal cysts or sinuses that might communicate with
the subarachnoid space.

Skin necrosis of the foot has been reported following extravasation
of diatrizoates injection during administration into a dorsal vein of
the foot.

Acute renal failure has been reported following intravascular administration of diatrizoates during excretory urography, especially
in patients with diabetic nephropathy and susceptible nondiabetic
patients. Also, a higher incidence of contrast-induced renal failure
has been associated with severe congestive heart failure, in patients
who have had multiple contrast studies within 72 hours, those receiving large volumes of contrast agent, and those with elevated
uric acid levels. Renal function may also be slightly and temporarily
impaired following intravascular administration of diatrizoates during selective renal arteriography.

Dehydration and/or the risk of renal failure may be exacerbated,
and in some cases may cause a shock-like state, in infants and
young children, and in geriatric, azotemic, and dehydrated or debilitated patients, by the hypertonic contrast solutions of
diatrizoates.

Cortical blindness has been reported rarely after cardiac angiography; vision has returned within 24 to 48 hours.

In addition to those side/adverse effects listed below as needing
medical attention, other severe reactions such as loss of consciousness, shock, and cardiac arrest may occur rarely during or a few
minutes after intravascular administration of diatrizoates.

The following side/adverse effects have been selected on the basis of their
  potential clinical significance (possible signs and symptoms in parentheses where appropriate)—not necessarily inclusive:

**Those indicating need for medical attention**
Incidence less frequent or rare
  *For all procedures*
    *Pseudo-allergic reaction* (skin rash or hives, stuffy nose, swelling
    of face or skin, thickening of tongue, wheezing, tightness in chest,
    or troubled breathing)
    Note: *Pseudo-allergic reactions* are usually transient. However,
      they may be an initial manifestation of a more severe ana-
      phylactoid reaction. The anaphylactoid reaction may pro-
      gress to respiratory arrest and vasomotor collapse if appro-
      priate treatment is not administered.

  *With intravascular administration*
    *Bronchospasm or pulmonary edema* (severe wheezing or troubled
    breathing); *cardiotoxic effects, with decreased contractile force
    and ventricular fibrillation* (irregular heartbeat); *convulsions, es-
    pecially in patients with convulsive disorders; swelling of the lar-
    ynx; vasovagal effects, with bradycardia and hypotension* (slow
    heartbeat; severe tiredness or weakness)

**Those indicating need for medical attention only if they continue
or are bothersome**
Incidence more frequent
  *With intravascular administration*
    *Cough*—during right ventricular and pulmonary angiography; *ar-
    teriolar vasodilation* (pain or burning at injection site, unusual
    warmth and flushing of skin)
    Note: Vasodilatory activity is directly related to the osmolality of
      the contrast agent's formulation and the volume injected.

  *With intrasynovial administration*
    *Joint pain or exacerbation of existing pain*
  *With intradiskal administration*
    *Pain at injection site*
Incidence less frequent
  *For all procedures*
    *Psychosomatic reaction* (chills, dizziness or lightheadedness,
    headache, nausea or vomiting, sweating, unusual thirst)
    Note: *Psychosomatic reactions* are associated with patient anxiety,
      fatigue, inadequate hydration, and poor nutrition; usually

self-limited and of short duration; may also be initial manifestations of more severe reaction.

*With oral or rectal administration*
   *Hyperosmotic effect* (diarrhea or laxative effect, nausea or vomiting)

## Patient Consultation

As an aid to patient consultation, refer to *Advice for the Patient, Radiopaque Agents (Diagnostic).*

In providing consultation, consider emphasizing the following selected information (» = major clinical significance):

**Description of use**
   Action in the body:
      Oral/rectal administration; visualization of radiopacity in gastrointestinal tract possible with x-rays
      Injection into vein or artery; visualization of radiopacity in blood vessels, heart, brain, and other organs possible with x-rays
      Direct injection into region to be studied; visualization of joint spaces

**Before having this test**
» Conditions affecting use, especially:
      Sensitivity to iodine or other iodinated contrast media
      Pregnancy—Cross the placenta; risk to the fetus from radiation exposure; may cause hypothyroidism in neonate
      Breast-feeding—Distributed into breast milk; temporary discontinuation of breast-feeding for at least 24 hours is recommended
      Use in children—Increased risk of severe adverse reactions, especially in children with other medical problems; possible exacerbation of dehydration
      Use in the elderly—Increased risk of severe adverse effects; possible exacerbation of dehydration; increased risk of thyrotoxicosis
      Other medications, especially chymopapain (for diskography)
      Other medical problems, especially allergies or asthma (history of), anuria, cardiovascular disease, dehydration, diabetes mellitus, pheochromocytoma, previous allergic reaction to penicillins or skin allergens, renal function impairment, and seizures

**Preparation for this test**
   Adequate intake of fluids to prevent dehydration
   Special diet or use of laxative may be prescribed; patient should inquire in advance
   Not eating for several hours before examination to prevent possible aspiration of gastric contents; moderate amounts of clear liquids may be permitted

**Precautions after having this test**
Possible interference with future thyroid tests

**Side/adverse effects**
   Signs of potential side effects, especially pseudo-allergic reaction and cardiac or pulmonary problems that may occur immediately or within minutes of administration

## General Dosing Information

The manufacturer's literature should be consulted for specific techniques and procedures for administering contrast media.

Sensitivity test doses are not usually recommended, since severe or fatal reactions to contrast media are not predictable from a patient's history or a sensitivity test. On some occasions severe or fatal reactions have occurred with a test dose or with a full dose in patients who did not react to the test dose.

Pretreatment with corticosteroids and/or with antihistamines has been used to minimize the incidence and severity of reactions in patients with a history of severe reactions to contrast media and other high-risk conditions (e.g., asthma or history of allergies, positive allergy history to skin allergens or penicillin, dehydration, history of seizures, pheochromocytoma). In some studies, the additional use of ephedrine has been shown to be beneficial in preventing anaphylactoid reactions (except in patients with a history of hypertension or cardiovascular disease). When considering the use of a contrast agent, the following protocols are recommended:
For high-risk patients
   • Use of a high-osmolality contrast agent plus pretreatment with a corticosteroid (oral prednisone, 50 mg administered 13 hours, 7 hours, and 1 hour before procedure) and an antihistamine (intramuscular, intravenous, or oral diphenhydramine, 50 mg administered one hour prior to procedure) or
   • Use of a low-osmolality agent if pretreatment is not feasible or
   • Use of a low-osmolality agent plus corticosteroid pretreatment.

For low-risk patients
   • Use of a high-osmolality contrast agent or
   • Use of a high-osmolality agent and corticosteroid pretreatment.

No food should be ingested for several hours before an examination to prevent aspiration of gastric contents if vomiting occurs. However, moderate amounts of clear liquids are permissible and even recommended by some clinicians to prevent dehydration.

During and for at least 30 to 60 minutes after administration of contrast media, the patient should be observed for possible severe reactions, and competent personnel and emergency facilities should be available during this period.

**For oral dosage forms only**
In very young or debilitated children, and elderly cachectic patients, dilution of the oral solution with water may be necessary to avoid the risk of shock caused by a decrease in circulating plasma volume due to osmosis when the contrast medium passes through the stomach and small intestine.
   For gastrointestinal radiography—
      Adequate hydration of the patient is recommended before and after the examination.

**For parenteral dosage forms only**
Injections of diatrizoate sodium should *not* be prepared from diatrizoate powder or oral or rectal solutions.

Dosage and concentration of diatrizoates for intravascular administration should be individualized and are usually in proportion to the size of the specific region of the vascular system to be visualized and the anticipated degree of hemodilution in the region.

Intravascular or intramuscular administration of diatrizoates may produce osmotic diuresis.

Subcutaneous extravasation of hyperosmolar diatrizoates injections may cause transient stinging, and skin necrosis has also been reported; cold compresses, elevation of the area, or movement of the digits is recommended to promote venous return.

Adequate hydration is especially important in infants, young children, or geriatric or azotemic patients receiving intravascular diatrizoates since dehydration may be further increased by the osmotic diuretic effect of the contrast medium.

Preparatory partial dehydration has been used to increase the urinary concentration of, and contrast produced by, diatrizoates. However, in general, dehydration is not recommended because, with modern contrast media and recommended doses, it is no longer necessary and may do harm. Dehydration is particularly contraindicated in patients with multiple myeloma since it may predispose to irreversible precipitation of myeloma protein in the renal tubules. In these patients fluids should be administered and urine should be made alkaline.

Thromboembolic events causing myocardial infarction and stroke, reported rarely during angiographic procedures, may have resulted from atherosclerotic lesions rather than from coagulation of blood that has come in contact with the contrast agent outside the body. Nonetheless, it is recommended that risk factors for blood cell aggregation be minimized by performing the procedure in the shortest time possible, using plastic rather than glass syringes, and flushing catheters with heparinized saline solutions.
For CT of the brain—
      Administration of parenteral diazepam is recommended immediately prior to injection of contrast medium, when very high doses are used, to prevent seizures in patients with brain metastases.
For splenoportography—
      Fasting is recommended for several hours before examination, in case the patient may require surgery on an emergency basis. Also, a local anesthetic and a sedative may be given before the procedure.
For excretory urography—
      Administration of a laxative at bedtime the evening before the examination is recommended to eliminate gas from the intestine.

**For treatment of adverse effects**
Recommended treatment consists of the following
   • For major or life-threatening reactions, careful monitoring of vital signs and emergency therapy, including artificial respiration with oxygen, if needed for respiratory depression, and cardiac massage in the event of cardiac arrest.
   • To restore blood pressure, administration of intravenous fluids and/or vasopressors. If hypotension requires the use of vasopressors, slow infusion of 0.008 to 0.012 mg per minute of norepinephrine or 0.1 to 0.18 mg per minute of phenylephrine, appropriately diluted. If hypotension is due to increased vagal activity (vasovagal reaction), intravenous administration of 1 mg of atropine, repeated in one to two hours if needed.

• Other specific treatment may include—
*Diphenhydramine:* For minor allergic-like reactions (i.e., urticaria)—
An antihistamine such as diphenhydramine hydrochloride (except in
epileptic patients) may be administered intravenously.
*Epinephrine:* For acute allergic-like or anaphylactoid reactions—Slow
intravenous infusion of 0.1 mg of epinephrine (1:10,000) may be used.
For mild to moderate bronchospasm—0.1 to 0.2 mg of epinephrine (1:
1000) may be administered subcutaneously, except in hypotension. In
extreme emergency, 0.1 mg of epinephrine (1:10,000) may be given
slowly by intravenous route, followed by a continuous intravenous
infusion at an initial rate of 0.001 mg per minute; the rate may be
increased to 0.004 mg per minute if necessary.
Patients on beta-adrenergic blocking agents should not receive epinephrine since they are at risk of unopposed alpha-adrenergic stimulation, which may result in hypertension, reflex bradycardia, and heart
block. In these patients, isoproterenol and norepinephrine are used instead of epinephrine to overcome bronchospasm and hypotension,
respectively.
For cardiac arrest—0.1 to 1 mg of epinepherine may be administered
by the intravenous route.
*Diazepam or phenobarbital:* To control convulsions—5 to 10 mg of
diazepam by slow, intravenous administration or phenobarbital sodium
intravenously or intramuscularly at a rate not to exceed 30 to 60 mg
per minute may be given.

## Oral or Rectal Dosage Forms

### DIATRIZOATE MEGLUMINE AND DIATRIZOATE SODIUM SOLUTION USP

**Usual adult and adolescent dose**
Gastrointestinal tract radiographic examination—
    Oral, 30 to 90 mL.
    Rectal, 240 mL in 1000 mL of tap water.
CT of the body, adjunct—
    Oral, 240 mL of a dilute solution administered fifteen to thirty minutes
        before imaging.
    Note: Solution may be prepared by diluting 25 mL of diatrizoate meg-
        lumine and diatrizoate sodium solution with tap water up to 1
        liter.

**Usual pediatric dose**
Gastrointestinal tract radiographic examination—
Oral:
    Children up to 5 years of age—30 mL.
    Children 5 to 10 years of age—60 mL.
    Note: In debilitated children and in those weighing less than 10
        kg, the dose should be diluted using 1 part of contrast so-
        lution and 3 parts of water. For other children the dose may
        be diluted with an equal volume of water, carbonated bev-
        erage, or milk.
Rectal:
    Children up to 5 years of age—1 part of the contrast solution may
        be diluted with 5 parts of water.
    Children 5 years of age and over—90 mL diluted with 500 mL of
        water.

**Usual geriatric dose**
See *Usual adult and adolescent dose.*
Note: Geriatric patients may be more sensitive to the effects of the usual
    adult dose.
    In elderly cachectic patients, the oral dose may be diluted with an
    equal volume of water, carbonated beverage, or milk.

**Strength(s) usually available**
U.S.—
    66% (660 mg per mL) of diatrizoate meglumine and 10% (100 mg
        per mL) of diatrizoate sodium with 36.7% (367 mg per mL) of
        iodine (Rx) [*Gastrografin; MD-Gastroview*].
Canada—
    66% (660 mg per mL) of diatrizoate meglumine and 10% (100 mg
        per mL) of diatrizoate sodium with 37% (370 mg per mL) of iodine
        (Rx) [*Gastrografin*].

**Packaging and storage**
Store below 40 °C (104 °F), preferably between 15 and 30 °C (59 and 86
°F), unless otherwise specified by manufacturer. Store in a tight, light-
resistant container. Protect from freezing.

**Note**
For oral or rectal use only.

**Additional information**
Oral solution may be ingested directly or given by tube.

### DIATRIZOATE SODIUM SOLUTION USP

**Usual adult and adolescent dose**
Gastrointestinal tract radiographic examination—
    Oral, 90 to 180 mL of a solution containing the equivalent of 155 mg
        to 250 mg of iodine per mL.
    Rectal, 500 to 1000 mL of a solution containing the equivalent of 93
        mg to 155 mg of iodine per mL.

**Usual pediatric dose**
Gastrointestinal tract radiographic examination—
    Oral, 30 to 75 mL of a solution containing the equivalent of 125 mg
        to 250 mg of iodine per mL.
    Rectal, 100 to 500 mL of a solution containing the equivalent of 62
        mg to 93 mg of iodine per mL.

**Usual geriatric dose**
See *Usual adult and adolescent dose*
Note: Geriatric patients may be more sensitive to the effects of the usual
    adult dose.

**Strength(s) usually available**
U.S.—
    41.66% (416.7 mg per mL) of diatrizoate sodium with 24.9% (249 mg
        per mL) of iodine (Rx) [*Hypaque Sodium Oral Solution* (polysor-
        bate 80)].
Canada—
    41.66% (416.7 mg per mL) of diatrizoate sodium with 24.9% (249 mg
        per mL) of iodine (Rx) [*Hypaque Oral* (polysorbate 80)].

**Packaging and storage**
Store below 40 °C (104 °F), preferably between 15 and 30 °C (59 and 86
°F), unless otherwise specified by manufacturer. Store in a tight, light-
resistant container. Protect from freezing.

**Preparation of dosage form**

| Diatrizoate Sodium solution (%)* | Dilution required† | Iodine content of diluted solution (mgI/mL) |
|---|---|---|
| 10 | Dilute each 25 mL to 100 mL | 62 |
| 15 | Dilute each 40 mL to 100 mL | 93 |
| 20 | Dilute each 50 mL to 100 mL | 125 |
| 25 | Dilute each 60 mL to 100 mL | 155 |
| 40 | Use undiluted | 250 |

*Approximate values.
†Oral solutions of different strengths may be prepared by using water,
milk, or a carbonated beverage as diluents.

**Stability**
Solution should be used upon preparation; do not store for future use.

**Note**
For oral or rectal use only.

### DIATRIZOATE SODIUM (FOR SOLUTION) USP

**Usual adult and adolescent dose**
Gastrointestinal tract radiographic examination—
    Oral, 90 to 180 mL of a solution containing the equivalent of 155 mg
        to 250 mg of iodine per mL.
    Rectal, 500 to 1000 mL of a solution containing the equivalent of 93
        mg to 155 mg of iodine per mL.

**Usual pediatric dose**
Gastrointestinal tract radiographic examination—
    Oral, 30 to 75 mL of a solution containing the equivalent of 125 mg
        to 250 mg of iodine per mL.
    Rectal, 100 to 500 mL of a solution containing the equivalent of 62
        mg to 93 mg of iodine per mL.

**Usual geriatric dose**
See *Usual adult and adolescent dose*
Note: Geriatric patients may be more sensitive to the effects of the usual
    adult dose.

**Size(s) usually available**
U.S.—
    250-gram size can containing 59.87% of iodine (approximately 600
        mg of iodine per gram) (Rx) [*Hypaque Sodium Oral Powder* (pol-
        ysorbate 80)].
Canada—
    250-gram size can containing 59.87% of iodine (approximately 600
        mg of iodine per gram) (Rx) [*Hypaque Oral* (polysorbate 80)].

**Packaging and storage**
Store below 40 °C (104 °F), preferably between 15 and 30 °C (59 and 86 °F), in a well-closed container, unless otherwise specified by manufacturer.

**Preparation of dosage form**

| Diatrizoate Sodium solution (%) | Measuring spoons* of powder per 100 mL of diluent† | Iodine content of prepared solution (mgI/mL) |
|---|---|---|
| 10 | 1 | 62 |
| 15 | 1½ | 93 |
| 20 | 2 | 125 |
| 25 | 2½ | 155 |
| 40 | 4 | 250 |

*One level measuring spoon equals approximately 10 grams of powder.
†Oral solutions may be sweetened or flavored (e.g., with vanilla, lemon, chocolate). The diluent may be water, milk, or a carbonated drink.

**Stability**
Solution should be used upon preparation; do not store for future use.

**Note**
Solution for oral or rectal use only.

# Parenteral Dosage Forms
## DIATRIZOATE MEGLUMINE INJECTION USP

**Usual adult and adolescent dose**
Intravascular—
Angiography, cerebral:
For visualization of cerebral vessels—Percutaneous or catheter, 8 to 12 mL of a solution containing the equivalent of 282 mg of iodine per mL, injected into the common carotid artery; repeated as needed.
For visualization of vessels in the posterior fossa or the occipital lobes—Percutaneous or operative method, 6 to 10 mL of a solution containing the equivalent of 282 mg of iodine per mL, injected into the vertebral artery; repeated as needed.
For visualization of vessels in the posterior fossa and/or right cerebral hemisphere (retrograde brachial)—Retrograde catheter, 35 to 50 mL of a solution containing the equivalent of 282 mg of iodine per mL by rapid administration.
Aortography:
Translumbar or retrograde catheter method, 15 to 40 mL of a solution containing the equivalent of 282 mg or 358 mg of iodine per mL administered rapidly into the aorta, as a single dose; may be repeated as needed.
Arteriography:
Peripheral arteriography—Percutaneous or operative methods, 20 to 40 mL of either a solution containing the equivalent of 282 mg or 358 mg of iodine per mL administered into the larger peripheral arteries.
Renal arteriography (selective)—Via catheter, 5 to 8 mL of a diatrizoate meglumine solution containing the equivalent of 282 mg of iodine per mL, administered into the renal artery; may be repeated as needed.
Venography, peripheral:
Upper extremity—Percutaneous, 10 to 20 mL of a solution containing the equivalent of 282 mg of iodine per mL per extremity administered rapidly into a superficial vein of the forearm or hand.
Lower extremity—Intravenous (rapid) or intravenous infusion, 50 to 100 mL of a solution containing the equivalent of 282 mg of iodine per mL, or percutaneous, 20 to 40 mL of a solution (containing the equivalent of 282 mg of iodine per mL) per extremity administered rapidly into a superficial vein on the lateral side of the foot.
Note: To minimize the incidence of pain and phlebitis in the lower extremity, it is recommended that the 60% solution (containing the equivalent of 282 mg of iodine per mL) be diluted to a 45% solution (containing the equivalent of 211.5 mg of iodine per mL) with 5% dextrose injection.
Cholangiography:
Direct cholangiography—Intraductal injection or instillation, 10 to 15 mL of either a solution containing the equivalent of 141 mg or 282 mg of iodine per mL into the cystic duct or common bile duct.
Patients with obstructive jaundice—Intraductal, 40 to 50 mL of a solution containing the equivalent of 282 mg of iodine per mL injected directly after the contents of the gallbladder are aspirated during surgery.

Patients with acute pancreatitis—Intraductal, 5 to 10 mL of a solution containing the equivalent of 282 mg of iodine per mL injected directly.
Percutaneous transhepatic cholangiography[1]—20 to 40 mL (range, 10 to 60 mL, depending on degree of biliary duct dilatation) of either a solution containing the equivalent of 141 mg or 282 mg of iodine per mL administered slowly into the biliary duct.
Note: A 30% solution (containing the equivalent of 141 mg of iodine per mL) may be prepared from a 60% solution (containing the equivalent of 282 mg of iodine per mL) by dilution with 0.9% sodium chloride injection.
CT of the brain:
Intravenous infusion, 1 to 4.4 mL per kg of body weight of a solution containing the equivalent of 141 mg of iodine per mL administered over a period of ten to twenty minutes or longer; or 50 to 150 mL of a solution containing the equivalent of 282 mg of iodine per mL.
CT of the body:
Intravenous infusion, 300 mL of a solution containing the equivalent of 141 mg of iodine per mL administered over a period of approximately twenty minutes.
Splenoportography:
Percutaneous, 20 to 25 mL of a solution containing the equivalent of 282 mg of iodine per mL administered rapidly after a preliminary small dose has been injected to confirm splenic entry.
Urography:
Excretory urography—
Intravenous infusion, 4.4 mL of a solution containing the equivalent of 141 mg of iodine per mL per kg of body weight administered at a rate not to exceed 40 mL per minute. A minimum of 250 mL may be needed for optimum visualization.
Note: Patients with cardiac disease may require a slower infusion rate.
Intravenous, 20 to 60 mL of a solution containing the equivalent of 282 mg of iodine per mL or 20 mL of a solution containing the equivalent of 358 mg of iodine per mL administered over a one- to three-minute period.
Intramuscular, 25 mL of a solution containing the equivalent of 282 mg of iodine per mL.
Note: Intramuscular administration may be very irritating to the tissues.
Retrograde urography (unilateral)[1]—
Via catheter, 15 mL of a solution containing the equivalent of 141 mg of iodine per mL instilled slowly into the ureter and renal pelvis.
Note: The 30% solution (containing the equivalent of 141 mg of iodine per mL) may be diluted with sterile distilled water if less contrast is desired.
Note: In patients with reduced renal function, repeat urography is not recommended for at least forty-eight hours because of the possibility of temporary oliguria or anuria.
Intrasynovial—Arthrography: Intrasynovial, as a solution containing the equivalent of 282 mg of iodine per mL—
Knee, shoulder, or hip joint: 5 to 15 mL.
Temporomandibular joint: 0.5 mL.
Other joints: 1 to 4 mL.
Intradiskal—Diskography: As a solution containing the equivalent of 282 mg of iodine per mL injected slowly—
Cervical disk: Up to 0.5 mL.
Lumbar disk: 1 to 2 mL, not to exceed 2 mL.
Ruptured or abnormal disk: 1 to 2 mL, not to exceed 2 mL.

**Usual pediatric dose**
Intravascular—
Angiocardiography:
Children up to 5 years of age—
Intravenous, 10 to 20 mL of a solution containing the equivalent of 358 mg of iodine per mL administered as a single dose.
Children 5 to 10 years of age—
Intravenous, 20 to 30 mL of a solution containing the equivalent of 358 mg of iodine per mL.
Note: In infants weighing less than 7 kg, especially in those with right-heart strain or failure and with decreased or nonfunctional pulmonary vascular beds, a dose of 10 to 20 mL may be dangerous.
Angiography, cerebral:
Dosage must be individualized by physician in proportion to body weight.

Aortography:
Translumbar or retrograde catheter method, 1 mL per kg of body weight, or 15 to 40 mL as a single injection, of a solution containing the equivalent of 358 mg of iodine per mL.

Arteriography:
Peripheral arteriography—Use is not recommended.
Renal arteriography (selective): Dosage must be individualized by physician in proportion to body weight.

Venography, peripheral:
Dosage must be individualized by physician in proportion to body weight.

Cholangiography, direct:
Dosage must be individualized by physician in proportion to body weight.

Cholangiography, percutaneous transhepatic[1]:
Dosage must be individualized by physician in proportion to body weight.

CT of the brain:
Dosage must be individualized by physician in proportion to body weight.

Splenoportography:
Dosage must be individualized by physician in proportion to body weight.

Urography:
Excretory urography—
Intravenous infusion: Dosage must be individualized by physician in proportion to body weight.
Intravenous, as a solution containing the equivalent of 282 mg of iodine per mL:
Children weighing up to 4.5 kg—5 to 10 mL (or 8 mL of a solution containing the equivalent of 358 mg of iodine per mL).
Children weighing 4.5 to 13.6 kg—10 to 15 mL.
Children weighing 13.6 to 27.3 kg—15 to 30 mL.
Children weighing 27.3 kg and over—30 mL.
Retrograde urography[1]—
Dosage must be individualized by physician in proportion to body weight.

Intrasynovial—
Arthrography: Dosage must be individualized by physician in proportion to body weight.

Intradiskal—
Diskography: Dosage must be individualized by physician in proportion to body weight.

**Usual geriatric dose**
See *Usual adult and adolescent dose*
Note: Geriatric patients may be more sensitive to the effects of the usual adult dose.

**Strength(s) usually available**
U.S.—
30% (300 mg per mL) of diatrizoate meglumine with 14.1% (141 mg per mL) of iodine (Rx) [*Hypaque Meglumine 30%; Reno-Dip; Urovist Meglumine DIU/CT*].
60% (600 mg per mL) of diatrizoate meglumine with 28.2% (282 mg per mL) of iodine (Rx) [*Angiovist 282; Hypaque Meglumine 60%; Reno-M-60*].
76% (760 mg per mL) of diatrizoate meglumine with 35.8% (358 mg per mL) of iodine (Rx) [GENERIC].

Canada—
18% (180 mg per mL) of diatrizoate meglumine with 8.5% (85 mg per mL) of iodine (Rx) [*Hypaque-M 18%*].
30% (300 mg per mL) of diatrizoate meglumine with 14.1% (141 mg per mL) of iodine (Rx) [*Hypaque-M 30%*].
60% (600 mg per mL) of diatrizoate meglumine with 28.3% (283 mg per mL) of iodine (Rx) [*Hypaque-M 60%*].

**Packaging and storage**
Store below 40 °C (104 °F), preferably between 15 and 30 °C (59 and 86 °F), unless otherwise specified by manufacturer. Protect from light. Protect from freezing.

**Stability**
If for intravascular use, any unused portion remaining in the container should be discarded after 6 hours.
Crystals may form in the solution but are readily redissolved by immersing the container in hot water and gently shaking it.

**Incompatibilities**
Diatrizoate meglumine injection is physically incompatible with diphenhydramine hydrochloride injection or promethazine hydrochloride injection.

## DIATRIZOATE MEGLUMINE AND DIATRIZOATE SODIUM INJECTION USP

**Usual adult and adolescent dose**
Intravascular—
Angiocardiography:
Via catheter, administered rapidly within one to two seconds into a large peripheral vein or into the chambers of the heart or associated blood vessels—

| Iodine content of contrast solution (mg I/mL) | mL |
|---|---|
| 310 | 50 |
| 370 | 40–50 |
| 385 | 35–50 |
| 462 | 35–50 |

Intravenous digital subtraction, 30 to 60 mL, with a range of 0.5 to 1 mL per kg of body weight, of a solution containing the equivalent of 370 mg of iodine per mL, administered at a bolus rate of 7.5 to 30 mL per second using a pressure injector.
Left ventriculography—Via catheter, 40 to 50 mL of a solution containing the equivalent of 370 mg of iodine per mL injected rapidly within one to two seconds into the left ventricle of the heart.
Pulmonary angiography—Via catheter, 10 to 56 mL of a solution containing the equivalent of 370 mg of iodine per mL administered rapidly within one to two seconds into the pulmonary artery.
Note: When angiocardiography is combined with other angiographic procedures, the dosage should not exceed 225 mL of a solution containing the equivalent of 370 mg of iodine per mL.

Angiography, cerebral—
For visualization of cerebral vessels—Percutaneous or catheter, 10 mL of a solution containing the equivalent of 290 mg of iodine per mL administered into the common carotid artery.
For visualization of vessels in the posterior fossa or the occipital lobes—Percutaneous or operative method, 6 to 10 mL of a solution containing the equivalent of 290 mg of iodine per mL administered into the vertebral artery.

Aortography—
Translumbar or retrograde catheter method, 20 to 30 mL (some clinicians recommend doses up to 80 mL) of a solution containing the equivalent of 310 mg of iodine per mL; or 15 to 50 mL of a solution containing the equivalent of 370 mg of iodine per mL solution, as a single dose; may be repeated if necessary.
Abdominal aortography:
As a solution containing either the equivalent of 385 mg or 462 mg of iodine per mL:
Translumbar—10 to 15 mL.
Retrograde catheter—15 to 25 mL.
Cannula—35 to 40 mL.

Arteriography—
Coronary arteriography:
Via catheter, 50 mL, administered into the root of the aorta for simultaneous bilateral angiograms, or 15 to 25 mL administered at the sinus of Valsalva on either side, of either a solution containing the equivalent of 385 mg or 462 mg of iodine per mL.
Selective coronary arteriography:
Via catheter, 3 to 5 mL of either a solution containing the equivalent of 385 mg or 462 mg of iodine per mL; or 4 to 10 mL of a solution containing the equivalent of 370 mg of iodine per mL, administered into either coronary artery; may be repeated as needed.
Selective coronary arteriography combined with left ventriculography:
Via catheter, 35 to 50 mL of a solution containing the equivalent of 370 mg of iodine per mL.
Note: Some clinicians recommend that the 60% diatrizoate meglumine and 30% diatrizoate sodium solution (containing the equivalent of 462 mg of iodine per mL) not be used since the risk of ventricular fibrillation may be increased.

Peripheral arteriography:
Entire extremity: Percutaneous or operative method, 20 to 40 mL of a solution containing the equivalent of 290 mg or 370 mg of iodine per mL; or 10 to 25 mL of either a

solution containing the equivalent of 385 mg or 462 mg of iodine per mL; or 30 to 50 mL of a solution containing the equivalent of 310 mg of iodine per mL; as a single dose administered into the femoral or subclavian artery.

Upper or lower extremity: Percutaneous or operative method, 10 to 20 mL of a solution containing the equivalent of 290 mg or 370 mg of iodine per mL; as a single dose.

Renal arteriography (selective):

Via catheter, 5 to 8 mL of a solution containing the equivalent of 385 mg of iodine per mL; or 5 to 10 mL of a solution containing the equivalent of 370 mg of iodine per mL, administered into either or both renal arteries; may be repeated as needed.

Visceral arteriography (selective):

Via catheter, of a solution containing the equivalent of 370 mg of iodine per mL, administered into the appropriate visceral artery

Superior mesenteric artery—20 to 40 mL.

Inferior mesenteric artery—20 to 40 mL.

Celiac artery—30 to 50 mL.

Hepatic artery—15 to 30 mL.

Splenic artery—20 to 50 mL.

Venography[1]—

Central venography[1]:

Inferior or superior venacavography: Percutaneous, 30 to 60 mL of a solution containing the equivalent of 310 mg; or 40 to 50 mL of a solution containing the equivalent of 370 mg of iodine per mL, administered directly or via catheter into the saphenous, femoral, or iliac vein; dose may be repeated if necessary for an additional radiograph.

Renal venography[1]:

Percutaneous, 20 to 40 mL of a solution containing the equivalent of 370 mg of iodine per mL administered via catheter into the vena cava or the renal vein.

Peripheral venography[1]:

Upper extremity: Percutaneous, 20 to 50 mL of either a solution containing the equivalent of 310 mg or 370 mg of iodine per mL; or 10 mL of a solution containing the equivalent of 290 mg of iodine per mL, per extremity, administered rapidly into a superficial vein of the forearm or hand.

Lower extremity: Percutaneous, 20 to 50 mL of a solution containing the equivalent of 290 mg, 310 mg, or 370 mg of iodine per mL, per extremity, administered rapidly into a superficial vein on the lateral side of the foot.

Note: Larger doses than those stated above have been safely used for visualization of veins in the lower extremities.

To minimize the incidence of pain and phlebitis in the lower extremity, it is recommended that 3 parts of a 52% diatrizoate meglumine and 8% diatrizoate sodium injection (containing the equivalent of 290 mg per mL of iodine) be diluted with 1 part of 5% dextrose injection.

Cholangiography[1]—

Direct cholangiography:

Intraductal, 10 mL of a solution containing the equivalent of 290 mg of iodine per mL, diluted or undiluted, injected or instilled into the cystic duct or common bile duct.

In patients with acute pancreatitis: 5 to 10 mL of a solution containing the equivalent of 290 mg of iodine per mL, undiluted.

Transhepatic cholangiography[1]:

Percutaneous, 20 to 40 mL, depending on the degree of biliary duct dilation, of a solution containing the equivalent of 290 mg of iodine per mL, diluted or undiluted, administered slowly into the biliary duct.

CT of the brain—

Intravenous, 2 to 4 mL per kg of body weight of a solution containing the equivalent of 150 mg of iodine per mL; or 50 to 150 mL of a solution containing the equivalent of 290 mg of iodine per mL; or 50 to 125 mL of a solution containing the equivalent of 370 mg of iodine per mL, by rapid administration.

CT of the body—

Intravenous, 50 to 125 mL of a solution containing the equivalent of 370 mg of iodine per mL; or 100 mL of a solution containing the equivalent of 290 mg of iodine per mL.

Note: For vascular opacification, 25 to 50 mL of a solution containing the equivalent of 370 mg of iodine per mL administered as a bolus and repeated if needed.

For prolonged arterial or venous phase enhancement or enhancement of specific lesion, 100 mL of a solution containing the equivalent of 370 mg of iodine per mL by rapid infusion.

Splenoportography—

Percutaneous, 20 to 25 mL of a solution containing the equivalent of 290 mg of iodine per mL administered rapidly after a preliminary small dose has been injected to confirm splenic entry.

Urography, excretory—

Intravenous, 30 mL of a solution containing the equivalent of 310 mg of iodine per mL; or 20 to 50 mL of a solution containing the equivalent of 370 mg of iodine per mL; or 25 mL of a solution containing the equivalent of 290 mg of iodine per mL; or 50 mL of a solution containing the equivalent of 385 mg or 462 mg of iodine per mL, by rapid administration.

Note: In patients with reduced renal function, repeat urography is not recommended for at least 48 hours because of the possibility of temporary oliguria or anuria.

Nephrotomography—

Intravenous, 100 mL of a solution containing the equivalent of 370 mg of iodine per mL, administered rapidly.

**Usual pediatric dose**

Intravascular:

Angiocardiography—

Via catheter, 0.5 to 1 mL per kg of body weight of a solution containing the equivalent of 385 mg of iodine per mL or 0.2 to 0.3 mL per kg of body weight of a solution containing the equivalent of 370 mg of iodine per mL, administered rapidly within one to two seconds into a large peripheral vein or into the chambers of the heart or associated blood vessels.

Or, as a solution containing the equivalent of 310 mg of iodine per mL—

Children up to 2 years of age and weighing 7 kg or more: 10 to 20 mL.

Children 2 to 4 years of age: 20 to 30 mL.

Children 4 to 10 years of age: 30 to 40 mL.

Or, as a solution containing the equivalent of 370 mg of iodine per mL—

Children up to 2 years of age and weighing 7 kg or more: 10 to 15 mL.

Children 2 to 4 years of age: 15 to 20 mL.

Children 4 to 10 years of age: 20 to 30 mL.

Note: In patients with stenotic lesions of the aorta, 0.5 mL per kg of body weight of a solution containing the equivalent of 385 mg of iodine per mL is recommended.

Pulmonary angiography:

Via catheter, 0.3 to 0.9 mL per kg of body weight, not to exceed 1 mL per kg of body weight, of a solution containing the equivalent of 370 mg of iodine per mL administered rapidly within one to two seconds into the pulmonary artery.

Left ventriculography:

Via catheter, 0.2 to 0.3 mL (some clinicians recommend 0.5 to 1.5 mL) per kg of body weight of a solution containing the equivalent of 370 mg of iodine per mL administered rapidly within one to two seconds into the left ventricle of the heart; not to exceed 50 mL.

Note: When angiocardiography is combined with other angiographic procedures, the dosage should not exceed 4 mL per kg of body weight of a solution containing the equivalent of 370 mg of iodine per mL. In young infants the dosage of this solution should not exceed 3 mL per kg of body weight.

Angiography, cerebral—

Dosage must be individualized by physician in proportion to body weight.

Aortography—

Translumbar or retrograde catheter method, 0.3 to 0.9 mL per kg of body weight, not to exceed 1 mL per kg of body weight, of a solution containing the equivalent of 370 mg of iodine per mL.

Arteriography—

Peripheral arteriography—Use is not recommended.

Renal arteriography (selective): Dosage must be individualized by physician in proportion to body weight.

Cholangiography[1]—

Dosage must be individualized by physician in proportion to body weight.

CT of the brain—

Dosage must be individualized by physician in proportion to body weight.

CT of the body—
  Dosage must be individualized by physician in proportion to body weight.
Splenoportography—
  Dosage must be individualized by physician in proportion to body weight.
Urography, excretory—
  Intravenous, 0.5 to 1 mL per kg of body weight, not to exceed 50 mL, of a solution containing the equivalent of 385 mg of iodine per mL; or of a solution containing the equivalent of—

| Children | 290 mgI/mL (mL) | 310 mgI/mL (mL) | 370 mgI/mL (mL) |
|---|---|---|---|
| Up to 6 months | 5 | 6 | 4–5 |
| 6 to 12 months | 8 | 10 | 6–8 |
| 1 to 2 years | 10 | 12 | 8–10 |
| 2 to 5 years | 12 | 15 | 10–12 |
| 5 to 7 years | 15 | 18 | 12–15 |
| 7 to 10 years | 18 | 22 | 14–18 |
| 10 to 15 years | 20 | 24 | 16–20 |

Nephrotomography—
  Dosage must be individualized by physician in proportion to body weight.
Venography, peripheral[1]—
  Dosage must be individualized by physician in proportion to body weight.

### Usual geriatric dose
See *Usual adult and adolescent dose*
Note: Geriatric patients may be more sensitive to the effects of the usual adult dose.

### Strength(s) usually available
U.S.—
  28.5% (285 mg per mL) of diatrizoate meglumine and 29.1% (291 mg per mL) of diatrizoate sodium with 31% (310 mg per mL) of iodine (Rx) [*Renovist II*].
  34.3% (343 mg per mL) of diatrizoate meglumine and 35% (350 mg per mL) of diatrizoate sodium with 37% (370 mg per mL) of iodine (Rx) [*Renovist*].
  52% (520 mg per mL) of diatrizoate meglumine and 8% (80 mg per mL) of diatrizoate sodium with 29% (290 mg per mL) of iodine (Rx) [*Angiovist 292; Renografin-60*].
  66% (660 mg per mL) of diatrizoate meglumine and 10% (100 mg per mL) of diatrizoate sodium with 37% (370 mg per mL) of iodine (Rx) [*Angiovist 370; Hypaque-76; MD-76; Renografin-76*].
Canada—
  50% (500 mg per mL) of diatrizoate meglumine and 25% (250 mg per mL) of diatrizoate sodium with 38.5% (385 mg per mL) of iodine (Rx) [*Hypaque-M 75%*].
  66% (660 mg per mL) of diatrizoate meglumine and 10% (100 mg per mL) of diatrizoate sodium with 37% (370 mg per mL) of iodine (Rx) [*Hypaque-M 76%; MD-76*].

### Packaging and storage
Store below 40 °C (104 °F), preferably between 15 and 30 °C (59 and 86 °F), unless otherwise specified by manufacturer. Protect from light. Protect from freezing.

### Stability
If for intravascular use, any unused portion remaining in the container should be discarded after 6 hours.
Crystals may form in the solution but are readily redissolved by immersing the container in hot water and gently shaking it.

### Incompatibilities
Diatrizoate meglumine and diatrizoate sodium injection is physically incompatible with protamine sulfate solutions or promethazine hydrochloride injection.

## DIATRIZOATE SODIUM INJECTION USP

### Usual adult and adolescent dose
Intravascular—
  Angiography[1]:
    Cerebral angiography—
      For visualization of cerebral vessels: Direct injection, 8 to 12 mL of a solution containing the equivalent of 300 mg of iodine per mL administered into the common carotid artery.
      For visualization of posterior fossa or occipital lobe vessels: Direct injection, 6 to 10 mL of a solution containing the equivalent of 300 mg of iodine per mL administered into the vertebral artery.

For visualization of vessels in the posterior fossa and/or right cerebral hemisphere (retrograde brachial): Retrograde catheter, 35 to 50 mL of a solution containing the equivalent of 300 mg of iodine per mL by rapid administration.
Note: Many clinicians feel the use of pure diatrizoate sodium preparations for cerebral or peripheral angiography is no longer warranted; they recommend diatrizoate meglumine as the salt of choice for these uses.
Aortography[1]:
  As a solution containing the equivalent of 300 mg of iodine per mL—
  Intravenous, 1 mL per kg of body weight.
  Retrograde (catheter), 0.5 to 1 mL per kg of body weight.
  Translumbar, 10 to 30 mL.
Arteriography[1]:
  Peripheral arteriography—
    Percutaneous or operative method, 25 to 35 mL of a solution containing the equivalent of 300 mg of iodine per mL administered into the brachial or femoral artery.
    Note: Many clinicians feel the use of pure diatrizoate sodium preparations for peripheral arteriography is no longer warranted, since their use would result in extreme pain.
  Renal arteriography (selective)—
    Via catheter, 5 to 8 mL of a solution containing the equivalent of 300 mg of iodine per mL administered into the renal artery, repeated as needed.
Cholangiography:
  Operative—
    10 to 15 mL of either a solution containing the equivalent of 150 mg or 300 mg of iodine per mL injected or instilled into the cystic duct or common bile duct.
    In patients with obstructive jaundice: Intravesical instillation, 40 to 50 mL of a solution containing the equivalent of 300 mg of iodine per mL administered directly into the gallbladder after aspiration of its contents.
    In patients with acute pancreatitis: Intravesical instillation, 5 to 10 mL of a solution containing the equivalent of 300 mg of iodine per mL.
  Postoperative T-tube—
    See *Operative cholangiography*.
  Transhepatic cholangiography[1]—
    Percutaneous, 20 to 40 mL (range, 10 to 60 mL, depending on degree of biliary duct dilation) of a solution containing the equivalent of 150 mg or 300 mg of iodine per mL administered slowly into the biliary duct.
    Note: A 25% injection (containing the equivalent of 150 mg of iodine per mL) may be prepared from a 50% injection (containing the equivalent of 300 mg of iodine per mL) by dilution with 0.9% sodium chloride injection.
CT of the brain:
  Intravenous infusion, 300 mL of a solution containing the equivalent of 150 mg of iodine per mL administered over a ten- to twenty-minute period; or 50 to 150 mL of a solution containing the equivalent of 300 mg of iodine per mL.
Splenoportography[1]:
  Percutaneous, 20 to 25 mL of a solution containing the equivalent of 300 mg of iodine per mL administered rapidly after a small preliminary dose has been injected to confirm splenic entry.
Urography:
  Excretory urography—
    Intravenous infusion, 4.4 mL of a solution containing the equivalent of 150 mg of iodine per mL per kg of body weight, not to exceed 400 mL, administered over a three- to ten-minute period. A minimum of 250 mL may be needed for optimum visualization.
    Intravenous, 50 to 60 mL of a solution containing the equivalent of 300 mg of iodine per mL.
  Retrograde urography (unilateral)[1]—
    Via catheter, 6 to 10 mL of a solution containing the equivalent of 120 mg of iodine per mL instilled slowly into the ureter and renal pelvis.
    Note: The above dose is doubled for bilateral examination.
  Note: In patients with reduced renal function, repeat urography is not recommended for at least forty-eight hours because of the possibility of temporary oliguria or anuria.
Venography:
  Peripheral venography[1]—
    Percutaneous, 15 to 40 mL of a solution containing the equivalent of 300 mg of iodine per mL.

Intraosseous venography—
Intraosseous, 10 to 20 mL of a solution containing the equivalent of 300 mg of iodine per mL, administered after aspiration of 4 mL of bone marrow.
Pterygoid venous plexus: Intraosseous, 5 to 8 mL of a solution containing the equivalent of 300 mg of iodine per mL administered into the medullary cavity of the mandible.

Note: Many clinicians feel the use of pure diatrizoate sodium preparations for venography is no longer warranted; they recommend diatrizoate meglumine as the salt of choice for this use.

**Usual pediatric dose**
Intravascular—
Angiography[1]—
Dosage must be individualized by physician in proportion to body weight.
Aortography[1]—
Intravenous—See *Usual adult and adolescent dose.*
Retrograde (catheter)—See *Usual adult and adolescent dose.*
Translumbar—Dosage must be individualized by physician in proportion to body weight.
Arteriography:
Abdominal arteriography—
Translumbar or retrograde catheter method, 1 mL per kg of body weight of a solution containing the equivalent of 300 mg of iodine per mL.
Peripheral arteriography[1]—
Dosage must be individualized by physician in proportion to body weight.
Renal arteriography (selective)[1]—
Dosage must be individualized by physician in proportion to body weight.
Cholangiography:
Dosage must be individualized by physician in proportion to body weight.
CT of the brain:
Dosage must be individualized by physician in proportion to body weight.
Splenoportography[1]:
Dosage must be individualized by physician in proportion to body weight.
Urography:
Excretory urography—
Intravenous, as a solution containing the equivalent of 300 mg of iodine per mL administered rapidly:
Children up to 6 months of age—5 mL.
Children 6 to 12 months of age—6 to 8 mL.
Children 1 to 2 years of age—8 to 10 mL.
Children 2 to 5 years of age—10 to 12 mL.
Children 5 to 7 years of age—12 to 15 mL.
Children 7 to 11 years of age—15 to 18 mL.
Children 11 to 15 years of age—18 to 20 mL.

Note: Some clinicians recommend intravenous administration of 1 to 2 mL per kg of body weight of the solution containing the equivalent of 300 mg of iodine per mL.

Retrograde urography (unilateral)[1]—
Via catheter, as a solution containing the equivalent of 120 mg of iodine per mL:
Children up to 1 year of age—Up to 1.5 mL.
Children 1 to 5 years of age—1.5 to 3 mL.
Children 5 years of age and over—4 to 5 mL.

Note: The above doses are doubled for bilateral examination.
Venography[1]:
Dosage must be individualized by physician in proportion to body weight.

**Usual geriatric dose**
See *Usual adult and adolescent dose*

Note: Geriatric patients may be more sensitive to the effects of the usual adult dose.

**Strength(s) usually available**
U.S.—
25% (250 mg per mL) of diatrizoate sodium with 15% (150 mg per mL) of iodine (Rx) [*Hypaque Sodium 25%*].
50% (500 mg per mL) of diatrizoate sodium with 30% (300 mg per mL) of iodine (Rx) [*Hypaque Sodium 50%; Urovist Sodium 300*].
Canada—
50% (500 mg per mL) of diatrizoate sodium with 30% (300 mg per mL) of iodine (Rx) [*Hypaque Sodium 50%*].

**Packaging and storage**
Store below 40 °C (104 °F), preferably between 15 and 30 °C (59 and 86 °F), unless otherwise specified by manufacturer. Protect from light. Protect from freezing.

**Stability**
If for intravascular use, any unused portion remaining in the container should be discarded.
Crystals may form in the solution but are readily redissolved by immersing the container in hot water and gently shaking it.

**Incompatibilities**
Diatrizoate sodium injection is physically incompatible with diphenhydramine hydrochloride injection.

---

[1] Not included in Canadian product labeling.

## Selected Bibliography
Brinker JA. Selection of a contrast agent in the cardiac catheterization laboratory. Am J Cardiol 1990; 66: 26F-33F.
Wittbrodt ET, Spiner SA. Prevention of anaphylactoid reactions in high-risk patients receiving radiographic contrast media. Ann Pharmacother 1994; 28: 236-41.

---

Revised: 05/11/95

---

**DIATRIZOATE SODIUM**—See *Diatrizoates (Local); Diatrizoates (Systemic)*

---

**DIAZEPAM**—See *Benzodiazepines (Systemic)*

---

# DIAZOXIDE   Oral-Systemic

---

VA CLASSIFICATION (Primary/Secondary): HS503/GA900

Note: For a listing of dosage forms and brand names by country availability, see *Dosage Forms* section(s). For a listing of brand names for the articles in this monograph, refer to the General Index.

## Category
Antihypoglycemic.

## Indications
**Accepted**
Hypoglycemia (treatment)—Diazoxide is indicated orally for the management of hypoglycemia due to hyperinsulinism associated with inoperable islet cell adenoma or carcinoma, or extrapancreatic malignancy; leucine sensitivity; islet cell hyperplasia; nesidioblastosis; or adenomatosis. Diazoxide should only be used in hypoglycemia that is confirmed to be caused by hyperinsulinism unresponsive to other treatment.

**Unaccepted**
Although oral diazoxide reduces blood pressure gradually, it is not used in the chronic treatment of hypertension because of its side effects.

Diazoxide is not recommended for use in the treatment of functional hypoglycemia.

## Pharmacology/Pharmacokinetics
**Physicochemical characteristics**
Chemical group—Diazoxide is a nondiuretic thiazide derivative.
Molecular weight—230.67.
pKa—8.5.

**Mechanism of action/Effect**
Hyperglycemic effect is due primarily to inhibition of insulin release from the pancreas, as well as an extrapancreatic (catecholamine-induced) effect.

**Absorption**
Readily absorbed following oral administration; the suspension may produce higher blood concentrations than the capsule form in some patients.

**Protein binding**
Very high (more than 90%) to serum proteins; reduced in uremia.

**Biotransformation**
Hepatic.

**Half-life**
Normal renal function—28 ± 8.3 hours.
Anuria—20 to 53 hours; may also be prolonged with overdosage.

**Onset of action**
1 hour.

**Duration of action**
Normal renal function— 8 hours or less.

**Elimination**
Renal; approximately 50% unchanged.
In dialysis—Diazoxide is dialyzable; a higher dose or additional doses may be required when patients are being dialyzed.

# Precautions to Consider

**Cross-sensitivity and/or related problems**
Patients sensitive to thiazide diuretics or other sulfonamide-type medications may be sensitive to this medication also.

**Carcinogenicity/Mutagenicity**
Studies have not been done in either animals or humans.

**Pregnancy/Reproduction**
Pregnancy—Diazoxide crosses the placenta. Adequate studies in humans have not been done. Possible adverse effects in infants of mothers who received diazoxide include transient hyperglycemia, hyperbilirubinemia, alopecia, hypertrichosis, and thrombocytopenia.
In rats, increased fetal resorptions, fetal skeletal abnormalities, and delayed parturition were seen. In rabbits, some teratogenic (skeletal, pancreatic, and cardiac) effects have been observed.
FDA Pregnancy Category C.
Labor—Diazoxide may inhibit labor, although oxytocin will reverse this effect.

**Breast-feeding**
It is not known whether diazoxide is distributed into breast milk. However, problems in humans have not been documented.

**Pediatrics**
Diazoxide-induced edema occurs most frequently in infants. In susceptible patients, this may lead to congestive heart failure.
The development of abnormal facial features has been reported in 4 children who were treated chronically (more than 4 years) with diazoxide for hypoglycemia due to hyperinsulinism.

**Geriatrics**
No information is available on the relationship of age to the effects of diazoxide in geriatric patients. However, elderly patients are more likely to have age-related renal function impairment, which may require a reduction in dosage and/or a longer dosing interval.

**Drug interactions and/or related problems**
The following drug interactions and/or related problems have been selected on the basis of their potential clinical significance (possible mechanism in parentheses where appropriate)—not necessarily inclusive (» = major clinical significance):

Note: Combinations containing any of the following medications, depending on the amount present, may also interact with this medication.

Alpha-adrenergic blocking agents, such as:
Labetalol
Phenoxybenzamine
Phentolamine
Prazosin
Tolazoline or
Other medications with alpha-adrenergic blocking action, such as:
Dihydroergotamine
Ergoloid mesylates
Ergotamine
Haloperidol

Loxapine
Phenothiazines
Thioxanthenes
(concurrent use antagonizes the inhibition of insulin release by diazoxide)

Anticoagulants, coumarin- or indandione-derivative
(increased anticoagulant effects may occur because of displacement of the anticoagulant from protein-binding sites; adjustment of anticoagulant dosage may be necessary)

» Anticonvulsants, hydantoin
(concurrent use is generally not recommended since it may result in decreased efficacy of either medication)

Antigout medications
(diazoxide may raise the concentration of blood uric acid; dosage adjustment of antigout medications may be necessary)

Beta-adrenergic blocking agents, ophthalmic, if significant systemic absorption occurs or
Beta-adrenergic blocking agents, systemic
(concurrent use prevents diazoxide-induced tachycardia; however, risk of hypotension may be increased)

Diuretics, loop or
Diuretics, thiazide or
Indapamide
(may potentiate the antihypertensive, hyperglycemic, and hyperuricemic actions of diazoxide; when used concurrently, adjustment of diazoxide dosage may be necessary)

» Hypotension-producing medications, other, (See *Appendix II*) or
» Vasodilators, peripheral, for example, cyclandelate, hydralazine, isoxsuprine, nicotinyl alcohol, nylidrin, papaverine
(concurrent use with diazoxide may result in an additive hypotensive effect, which may be severe; dosage adjustments may be necessary, and patients should be continuously observed for excessive fall in blood pressure for several hours after concurrent administration)

**Laboratory value alterations**
The following have been selected on the basis of their potential clinical significance (possible effect in parentheses where appropriate)—not necessarily inclusive (» = major clinical significance):

With diagnostic test results
Insulin response to glucagon
(false-negative results)

With physiology/laboratory test values
Alkaline phosphatase and
Aspartate aminotransferase (AST [SGOT]) and
Free fatty acid and
Sodium and
Uric acid
(serum concentrations may be increased)

Blood pressure
(may be increased)

Creatinine clearance and
Electrolytes, urine, such as chloride, bicarbonate, potassium, and sodium and
Hematocrit and
Hemoglobin and
Immunoglobulin G (IgG), plasma
(may be decreased)

Glucose and
Urea nitrogen (BUN)
(blood concentrations may be increased)

Heart rate
(may be transiently increased)

**Medical considerations/Contraindications**
The medical considerations/contraindications included here have been selected on the basis of their potential clinical significance (reasons given in parentheses where appropriate)—not necessarily inclusive (» = major clinical significance).

*Risk-benefit should be considered when the following medical problems exist:*

» Acute aortic dissection
» Compensatory hypertension, such as that associated with aortic coarctation or arteriovenous shunt
» Coronary or cerebral insufficiency
Gout, history of or
Hyperuricemia
(may be exacerbated)
Hepatic function impairment

Hypokalemia
(hyperglycemic effects are potentiated)

» Inadequate cardiac reserve, such as uncompensated congestive heart
failure

Renal function impairment
(half-life of diazoxide may be prolonged; reduced dosage may be
necessary with frequent use)

Sensitivity to diazoxide, sulfonamides, or thiazides

### Patient monitoring

The following may be especially important in patient monitoring (other
tests may be warranted in some patients, depending on condition;
» = major clinical significance):

Aspartate aminotransferase (AST [SGOT]), serum and
Creatinine clearance and
Hematocrit and
Leukocyte count, differential and total and
Platelet count and
Urea nitrogen, blood, (BUN) and
Uric acid, serum
(determinations recommended at periodic intervals during pro-
longed therapy)

» Glucose
(measurement of blood or urine concentrations is recommended at
periodic intervals in patients taking diazoxide until hypoglycemia
is corrected and stabilized)

» Ketones
(results of monitoring for ketones in urine reported by the patient
to the physician provides frequent and relatively inexpensive monitoring of the condition)

## Side/Adverse Effects

The following side/adverse effects have been selected on the basis of their
potential clinical significance (possible signs and symptoms in parentheses where appropriate)—not necessarily inclusive:

### Those indicating need for medical attention

Incidence more frequent
*Edema* (decreased urination; rapid weight gain; swelling of feet or
lower legs)
Note: *Edema* occurs most commonly in young infants and adults and
may lead to congestive heart failure in susceptible patients.

Incidence less frequent
*Tachycardia* (fast heartbeat)

Incidence rare
*Allergic reaction* (fever; skin rash); *angina pectoris, myocardial infarction, or myocardial ischemia* (chest pain; unexplained shortness
of breath)—most commonly occurring during physical exertion;
*thrombocytopenia* (unusual bleeding or bruising); *transient focal cerebral ischemic attacks* (confusion; numbness of the hands)

With long-term use
*Extrapyramidal effects* (stiffness of limbs; trembling and shaking of
hands and fingers)

### Those indicating need for medical attention only if they continue or are bothersome

Incidence less frequent
*Changes in ability to taste; ileus* (constipation); *loss of appetite; nausea; stomach pain; vomiting*

With long-term use
*Hypertrichosis* (increased hair growth on forehead, back, arms, and
legs)

## Overdose

For specific information on the agents used in the management of diazoxide overdose, see *Insulin (Systemic)* monograph.

For more information on the management of overdose or unintentional
ingestion, **contact a Poison Control Center** (see *Poison Control Center Listing*).

### Clinical effects of overdose

The following effects have been selected on the basis of their potential
clinical significance (possible signs and symptoms in parentheses
where appropriate)—not necessarily inclusive:
*Hyperglycemia or ketoacidosis* (continuing loss of appetite; drowsiness; flushed, dry skin; fruit-like breath odor; increased urination; unusual thirst)—more likely when administered during intercurrent
illness

### Treatment of overdose

Specific treatment—Administration of insulin to treat hyperglycemia and
prevent ketoacidosis.

Monitoring—Monitoring the patient for up to 7 days, especially if severe
hyperglycemia occurs.

Supportive care—Restoration of fluid and electrolyte balance. Patients in
whom intentional overdose is known or suspected should be referred
for psychiatric consultation.

## Patient Consultation

As an aid to patient consultation, refer to *Advice for the Patient, Diazoxide
(Oral)*.

In providing consultation, consider emphasizing the following selected
information (» = major clinical significance):

### Before using this medication

» Conditions affecting use, especially:
Sensitivity to diazoxide, thiazide diuretics, or other sulfonamide-
type medications
Pregnancy—Studies in animals have demonstrated teratogenicity;
effects on infants born to mothers who received diazoxide may
include hyperglycemia, hyperbilirubinemia, alopecia, hypertrichosis, and thrombocytopenia
Labor—May inhibit labor
Other medications, especially hydantoin anticonvulsants, other hypotension-producing medications, or peripheral vasodilators
Other medical problems, especially acute aortic dissection, compensatory hypertension, coronary or cerebral insufficiency, or
inadequate cardiac reserve

### Proper use of this medication

» Not taking more or less medication than the amount prescribed; taking
at same time each day
» Importance of diet in helping control condition
» Testing for sugar in urine or blood, and ketones in urine
» Proper dosing
Missed dose: Taking as soon as possible; not taking if almost time for
next dose; not doubling doses
» Proper storage

### Precautions while using this medication

» Regular visits to physician to check progress, especially during the
first few weeks of treatment
» Caution if any kind of surgery (including dental surgery) or emergency
treatment is required
» Not taking other medications, especially OTC sympathomimetics, un-
less discussed with physician
» Symptoms of hyperglycemia or ketoacidosis
Symptoms of hypoglycemia

### Side/adverse effects

Possibility of excessive hair growth, which is reversible in several
weeks or months when medication is withdrawn
Signs of potential side effects, especially edema, tachycardia, allergic
reaction, angina pectoris, myocardial infarction or ischemia, thrombocytopenia, transient focal cerebral ischemic attacks, and extrapyramidal effects

## General Dosing Information

Diazoxide is often administered concurrently with a diuretic to prevent
congestive heart failure due to fluid retention.

In some patients, the oral suspension dosage form of diazoxide produces
higher blood concentrations than the capsule form; caution is recommended when a patient is switched from one dosage form to another.

Hyperglycemia is usually transient after intravenous administration of diazoxide (persisting 24 to 48 hours), but may be more persistent after
prolonged oral administration and may rarely progress to ketoacidosis
or hyperosmolar coma.

If diazoxide is not effective within 2 to 3 weeks in the treatment of hypoglycemia, it is recommended that therapy with the medication be
re-evaluated.

## Oral Dosage Forms

### DIAZOXIDE CAPSULES USP

#### Usual adult and adolescent dose

Antihypoglycemic—
Initial: Oral, 1 mg per kg of body weight every eight hours, adjusted
according to clinical response.
Maintenance: Oral, 3 to 8 mg per kg of body weight a day, divided
into two or three equal doses every twelve or eight hours,
respectively.

**Usual adult prescribing limits**
Oral, up to 15 mg per kg of body weight a day.

**Usual pediatric dose**
Antihypoglycemic—
　Neonates and infants:
　　Initial—Oral, 3.3 mg per kg of body weight every eight hours,
　　adjusted according to clinical response.
　　Maintenance—Oral, 8 to 15 mg per kg of body weight a day,
　　divided into two or three equal doses every twelve or eight
　　hours, respectively.
　Children:
　　See *Usual adult and adolescent dose.*

**Strength(s) usually available**
U.S.—
　50 mg (Rx) [*Proglycem*].
Canada—
　50 mg (Rx) [*Proglycem* (lactose)].
　100 mg (Rx) [*Proglycem* (lactose)].

**Packaging and storage**
Store below 40 °C (104 °F), preferably between 15 and 30 °C (59 and 86
°F), unless otherwise specified by manufacturer. Store in a well-closed
container.

## DIAZOXIDE ORAL SUSPENSION USP

**Usual adult and adolescent dose**
See *Diazoxide Capsules USP.*

**Usual pediatric dose**
See *Diazoxide Capsules USP.*

**Strength(s) usually available**
U.S.—
　50 mg per mL (Rx) [*Proglycem* (alcohol 7.25%)].
Canada—
　50 mg per mL (Rx) [*Proglycem* (alcohol 7.25%; parabens)].

**Packaging and storage**
Store below 40 °C (104 °F), preferably between 15 and 30 °C (59 and 86
°F), unless otherwise specified by manufacturer. Store in a tight con-
tainer. Protect from light. Protect from freezing.

**Auxiliary labeling**
• Shake well before using.

Revised: 12/15/92
Interim revision: 05/24/94

---

# DIAZOXIDE   Parenteral-Systemic

VA CLASSIFICATION (Primary): CV490

Note: For a listing of dosage forms and brand names by country availa-
　　bility, see *Dosage Forms* section(s). For a listing of brand names
　　for the articles in this monograph, refer to the General Index.

## Category
Antihypertensive.

## Indications

**Accepted**
Hypertension (treatment)—Diazoxide is indicated intravenously for the
emergency reduction of blood pressure in malignant hypertension or
hypertensive crisis. Diazoxide is ineffective against hypertension associated with monoamine oxidase (MAO) inhibitor therapy or pheochromocytoma, but has been used investigationally by intravenous infusion to treat chronic hypertension in nonemergency situations.

**Unaccepted**
Parenteral diazoxide has only a transient hyperglycemic effect; oral diazoxide is more appropriate for treatment of hypoglycemia.

## Pharmacology/Pharmacokinetics

**Physicochemical characteristics**
Molecular weight—230.67.
pKa—8.5.

**Mechanism of action/Effect**
Exact mechanism of antihypertensive action is unknown. Diazoxide produces arteriolar vasodilation and decreased peripheral resistance.

**Other actions/effects**
Diazoxide has a hyperglycemic effect that is due primarily to inhibition
of insulin release from the pancreas, as well as an extrapancreatic
(catecholamine-induced) effect.

**Protein binding**
High to very high (more than 90%) to albumin; reduced in uremia.

**Biotransformation**
Hepatic.

**Half-life**
Normal—21 to 36 hours (average, 28 hours).
Anuric—20 to 53 hours.
Note: The plasma half-life is much longer than the hypotensive effect;
　　accumulation occurs with repeated doses.

**Onset of action**
1 minute (after intravenous push).

**Time to peak effect**
2 to 5 minutes (after intravenous push).

**Duration of action**
2 to 12 hours.

**Elimination**
Renal; approximately 50% unchanged.
In dialysis—Diazoxide is dialyzable; a higher dose or additional doses
　　may be required when patients are being dialyzed.

## Precautions to Consider

**Cross-sensitivity and/or related problems**
Patients sensitive to thiazide diuretics or other sulfonamide-type medications, including bumetanide, furosemide, and carbonic anhydrase inhibitors, may be sensitive to this medication also.

**Pregnancy/Reproduction**
Pregnancy—Diazoxide crosses the placenta. Studies in humans have not
been done. However, possible adverse effects in infants of mothers
who receive diazoxide include hyperglycemia, hyperbilirubinemia, alopecia or increased hair growth, and thrombocytopenia.
Increased fetal resorptions, delayed parturition, and some teratogenic
(skeletal, pancreatic, and cardiac) effects have been observed in
animals.
Labor—Diazoxide may also inhibit labor, although oxytocin will reverse
this effect.

**Breast-feeding**
It is not known if diazoxide is distributed into breast milk. However,
problems in humans have not been documented.

**Pediatrics**
Studies performed to date have not demonstrated pediatrics-specific problems that would limit the usefulness of parenteral diazoxide in
children.

**Geriatrics**
No information is available on the relationship of age to the effects of
parenteral diazoxide in geriatric patients. However, elderly patients are
more likely to have age-related renal function impairment, which may
require reduction of dose in patients receiving parenteral diazoxide.

**Drug interactions and/or related problems**
The following drug interactions and/or related problems have been selected on the basis of their potential clinical significance (possible
mechanism in parentheses where appropriate)—not necessarily inclusive (» = major clinical significance):
Note: Combinations containing any of the following medications, de-
　　pending on the amount present, may also interact with this
　　medication.

　Allopurinol or
　Colchicine or

Probenecid or
Sulfinpyrazone
  (diazoxide may raise the concentration of blood uric acid; dosage adjustment of antigout medications may be necessary to control hyperuricemia and gout)

Anticoagulants, coumarin- or indandione-derivative
  (concurrent use with diazoxide may result in increased anticoagulant effects because of displacement of the anticoagulant from protein-binding sites; anticoagulant dosage adjustments may be necessary)

Antidiabetic agents, oral or
Insulin
  (concurrent or consecutive use reverses the hyperglycemic effects of diazoxide; in addition, dosage adjustments of hypoglycemic medications may be necessary if diazoxide is administered to diabetics)

Anti-inflammatory drugs, nonsteroidal (NSAIDs), especially indomethacin or
Estrogens or
Sympathomimetics
  (concurrent use antagonizes the hypotensive effects of diazoxide; indomethacin and possibly other NSAIDs may antagonize the hypotensive effect by inhibiting renal prostaglandin synthesis and/or by causing sodium and fluid retention; estrogen-induced fluid retention tends to increase blood pressure)

Beta-adrenergic blocking agents, ophthalmic
  (if significant systemic absorption of ophthalmic beta-blockers occurs, concurrent use may increase the hypotensive effect of diazoxide)

Beta-adrenergic blocking agents, systemic
  (concurrent use prevents the tachycardia produced by diazoxide but may also increase the hypotensive effect)

Diuretics, loop or
Diuretics, thiazide or
Indapamide
  (may potentiate the antihypertensive, hyperglycemic, and hyperuricemic actions of diazoxide; when used concurrently, dosage adjustments may be necessary)

» Hypotension-producing medications, other (see *Appendix II*) or
Ritodrine, intravenous or
» Vasodilators, peripheral, such as cyclandelate, isoxsuprine, nicotinyl alcohol, nylidrin, papaverine
  (concurrent use with diazoxide may result in an additive hypotensive effect, which may be severe; dosage adjustments may be necessary, and patients should be continuously observed for excessive fall in blood pressure for several hours after concurrent administration)

## Laboratory value alterations
The following have been selected on the basis of their potential clinical significance (possible effect in parentheses where appropriate)—not necessarily inclusive (» = major clinical significance):

With diagnostic test results
  Insulin response to glucagon
    (false-negative results)

With physiology/laboratory test values
  Alkaline phosphatase values and
  Aspartate aminotransferase (AST [SGOT]) values and
  Blood urea nitrogen (BUN) concentrations and
  Free fatty acid concentrations, serum and
  Glucose concentrations, blood and
  Sodium concentrations, serum (excretion decreased) and
  Uric acid concentrations, serum
    (may be increased)

  Creatinine clearance and
  Hematocrit and
  Hemoglobin concentrations and
  Immunoglobulin G (IgG) concentrations in plasma and
  Urinary excretion of potassium, chloride, and bicarbonate
    (may be decreased)

## Medical considerations/Contraindications
The medical considerations/contraindications included here have been selected on the basis of their potential clinical significance (reasons given in parentheses where appropriate)—not necessarily inclusive (» = major clinical significance).

*Risk-benefit should be considered when the following medical problems exist:*

» Acute aortic dissection

» Compensatory hypertension, such as that associated with aortic coarctation or arteriovenous shunt
  (decrease in blood pressure may exacerbate this condition)

» Coronary or cerebral insufficiency or
Gout, history of
  (conditions may be exacerbated)

» Diabetes mellitus
  (hyperglycemic effects of diazoxide may require management measures in these patients)

Hepatic function impairment

Hypokalemia
  (hyperglycemic effects potentiated)

» Poor cardiac reserve, such as uncompensated congestive heart failure
  (diazoxide-induced sodium retention may precipitate edema in these patients)

Renal function impairment
  (reduced dosage of diazoxide may be necessary if it is administered repeatedly to patients with renal function impairment, since protein ding is reduced in uremia and the half-life of the medication may be prolonged)

Sensitivity to diazoxide

## Patient monitoring
The following may be especially important in patient monitoring (other tests may be warranted in some patients, depending on condition; » = major clinical significance):

Blood glucose determinations
  (recommended at periodic intervals after parenteral administration to monitor hyperglycemia, especially in diabetics or patients with renal or hepatic function impairment)

» Blood pressure determinations
  (recommended at frequent intervals after parenteral administration until blood pressure has stabilized, then at hourly intervals until the medication is withdrawn)

# Side/Adverse Effects
The following side/adverse effects have been selected on the basis of their potential clinical significance (possible signs and symptoms in parentheses where appropriate)—not necessarily inclusive:

### Those indicating need for medical attention
Incidence more frequent
  *Sodium and water retention and edema* (decrease in urination; swelling of hands, feet, or lower legs)
  Note: *Sodium and water retention* occurs most commonly in young infants and adults after repeated injections and may lead to congestive heart failure in susceptible patients.

Incidence less frequent
  *Hyperglycemia* (drowsiness; fruit-like breath odor; increased urination; unusual thirst); *hypotension; tachycardia* (fast heartbeat)
  Note: *Hyperglycemia* is usually transient after intravenous administration of diazoxide (persisting 24 to 48 hours), but may be more persistent after more than three parenteral doses within a short period (up to 24 hours) and may rarely progress to ketoacidosis and hyperosmolar coma.

Incidence rare
  *Allergic reaction or thrombocytopenia* (fever; skin rash; unusual bleeding or bruising); *cerebral ischemia or thrombosis* (confusion; numbness of hands); *hyperosmolar coma* (confusion); *myocardial ischemia, angina pectoris, or myocardial infarction* (chest pain)

### Those indicating need for medical attention only if they continue or are bothersome
Incidence less frequent
  *Changes in ability to taste; constipation; loss of appetite; nausea and vomiting; stomach pain*

Occurring with intravenous use
  *Back pain; ringing in ears; vasodilation* (flushing or redness of face; headache; weakness); *warmth or pain along injected vein*

Incidence rare
  *Orthostatic hypotension* (dizziness or lightheadedness, especially when getting up from a lying or sitting position)

# Overdose
For more information on the management of overdose or unintentional ingestion, **contact a Poison Control Center** (see *Poison Control Center Listing*).

**Treatment of overdose**
Severe hypotension usually responds to treatment with a vasopressor such as norepinephrine or metaraminol.

## General Dosing Information

It is recommended that diazoxide be administered only into a peripheral vein via an established intravenous line, to prevent cardiac arrhythmia.

Intramuscular, intracavitary, or subcutaneous administration is not recommended since pain may occur at the site of injections.

Diazoxide has been thought to be most effective in reducing blood pressure when intravenous administration is completed within 10 to 30 seconds. Slower administration supposedly reduces or shortens the response because of extensive protein binding. However, recent studies have suggested that administration of diazoxide by intravenous infusion may produce a similar (although usually smaller) but more gradual fall in blood pressure in both chronic hypertension and hypertensive crisis, reducing the risk of impaired perfusion of vital organs that may occur with a sudden fall in blood pressure. One study used a dose of 5 mg per kg of body weight (mg/kg) (15 mg per mL of intravenous infusion) administered at a rate of 15 mg per minute over 20 to 30 minutes. Other studies have found no effect when diazoxide is administered by intravenous infusion; further study is necessary to resolve this controversy.

Care must be taken to avoid extravasation during intravenous administration since cellulitis and pain (but not necrosis) may result. If extravasation occurs, conservative treatment with cold packs is recommended.

It is recommended that diazoxide injection be administered with the patient recumbent during and for 15 to 30 minutes after administration.

Tolerance to the antihypertensive effects of diazoxide may develop unless expansion of plasma and extracellular fluid volume is prevented by use of a diuretic.

Diazoxide is often administered with a diuretic to obtain maximum antihypertensive effect and prevent congestive heart failure due to sodium and water retention. Loop diuretics such as furosemide or ethacrynic acid may be the most useful. Administration of 40 to 80 mg of furosemide intravenously 30 to 60 minutes prior to intravenous diazoxide has been recommended.

Because of the long half-life of diazoxide, patients who develop marked hyperglycemia as a result of overdosage require prolonged monitoring (up to 7 days) while blood sugar concentrations stabilize.

## Parenteral Dosage Forms

### DIAZOXIDE INJECTION USP

**Usual adult and adolescent dose**
Antihypertensive—
Intravenous, up to 150 mg, or 1 to 3 mg per kg of body weight, repeated every five to fifteen minutes if necessary to obtain the desired response. Further doses may be administered every four to twenty-four hours as needed to maintain the desired blood pressure until oral antihypertensive medication is effective, usually within four to five days.

**Usual adult prescribing limits**
Up to 1.2 grams per day.

**Usual pediatric dose**
Antihypertensive—
Intravenous, 1 to 3 mg per kg of body weight or 30 to 90 mg per square meter of body surface, repeated in five to fifteen minutes if necessary to obtain the desired response. Further doses may be administered every four to twenty-four hours as needed to maintain the desired blood pressure until oral antihypertensive medication is effective.

**Strength(s) usually available**
U.S.—
15 mg per mL (Rx) [*Hyperstat* (sodium bisulfite 0.24 mg per mL); GENERIC].
Canada—
15 mg per mL (Rx) [*Hyperstat*].

**Packaging and storage**
Store below 40 °C (104 °F), preferably between 15 and 30 °C (59 and 86 °F), unless otherwise specified by manufacturer. Protect from light. Protect from freezing.

Revised: 05/14/93

---

**DIBUCAINE**—See *Anesthetics (Mucosal-Local)*; *Anesthetics (Topical)*

---

## DICHLORALPHENAZONE-CONTAINING COMBINATIONS—
Isometheptene, Dichloralphenazone, and Acetaminophen (Systemic)

---

**DICHLORPHENAMIDE**—See *Carbonic Anhydrase Inhibitors (Systemic)*

---

**DICLOFENAC**—See *Anti-inflammatory Drugs, Nonsteroidal (Ophthalmic)*; *Anti-inflammatory Drugs, Nonsteroidal (Systemic)*

---

**DICLOXACILLIN**—See *Penicillins (Systemic)*

---

**DICUMAROL**—See *Anticoagulants (Systemic)*

---

**DICYCLOMINE**—See *Anticholinergics/Antispasmodics (Systemic)*

---

# DIDANOSINE Systemic

VA CLASSIFICATION (Primary): AM800

Other commonly used names are ddI and 2,3-dideoxyinosine.

Note: For a listing of dosage forms and brand names by country availability, see *Dosage Forms* section(s). For a listing of brand names for the articles in this monograph, refer to the General Index.

## Category

Antiviral (systemic).

## Indications

Note: Bracketed information in the *Indications* section refers to uses that are not included in U.S. product labeling.

**Accepted**
Human immunodeficiency virus (HIV) infection, advanced (treatment) or Immunodeficiency syndrome, acquired (AIDS) (treatment)—Didanosine is indicated in the treatment of adults and children over 6 months of age with advanced HIV infection who are intolerant of zidovudine therapy or who have demonstrated significant clinical or immunologic deterioration during zidovudine therapy; didanosine is also indicated in the treatment of adults with advanced HIV infection who have received prior zidovudine therapy. [Didanosine is also used in combination with zidovudine.][1]

[1]Not included in Canadian product labeling.

## Pharmacology/Pharmacokinetics

**Physicochemical characteristics**
Molecular weight—236.2.

**Mechanism of action/Effect**
Didanosine (ddI) is metabolized intracellularly by a series of cellular enzymes to its active moiety, 2,3-dideoxyadenosine-5-triphosphate (ddA-TP), which inhibits HIV DNA polymerase (reverse transcriptase). HIV replication is suppressed by chain termination, competitive inhibition of reverse transcriptase, or both. The intracellular half-life of ddA-TP is greater than 12 hours.

## Absorption

Didanosine is acid labile; all oral formulations contain or are compounded with buffering agents to increase the gastric pH; this results in a decreased breakdown of didanosine and a subsequent increase in absorption. All formulations should be taken on an empty stomach. Administration within 5 minutes of a meal decreases the peak plasma concentration ($C_{max}$) and mean area under the plasma concentration versus time curve (AUC) by approximately 50%. If didanosine is not buffered in the stomach, it forms 2,3–dideoxyribose and hypoxanthine, a precursor of uric acid.

Bioavailability was extremely variable in both adults and children after ingestion of a lyophilized formulation similar to the pediatric product for oral solution.—

Adults—Approximately 33% after a single dose and approximately 37% after 4 weeks of therapy in adults receiving 7 mg per kg of body weight (mg/kg) or less.

Children (7 months to 19 years of age)—Average 19 to 42% (range, 2 to 89%).

The chewable/dispersible buffered tablets were found to be 20 to 25% more bioavailable than the buffered powder for oral solution when studied in 18 asymptomatic HIV-seropositive adults.

## Distribution

Crosses blood-brain barrier and distributes into the cerebrospinal fluid (CSF)—

Adults: Approximately 19 to 21% of the simultaneous plasma concentration 1 hour after an intravenous dose.

Children (8 months to 18 years of age): In one study, didanosine distribution into the CSF of 7 children was approximately 46% (range, 12 to 85%) of the simultaneous plasma concentration 1.5 to 3.5 hours after a single dose; however, studies done in rhesus monkeys showed poor CSF penetration, and another study done in children found that didanosine was not detectable in 17 of 20 CSF samples, and penetration into the CSF was limited.

Vol$_D$—

Adults: Average 0.7 to 1 L per kg.

Children (8 months to 18 years of age): Approximately 35.6 L per square meter of body surface (L/m²) [range, 18.4 to 60.7 L/m² ].

## Protein binding

Low (<5%).

## Biotransformation

Rapidly metabolized intracellularly to its active moiety, 2,3–dideoxyadenosine-5-triphosphate (ddA-TP). However, the metabolism of didanosine has not been fully evaluated in humans. Extensive metabolism occurred in dogs administered oral, radiolabeled didanosine; identified urinary metabolites include allantoin, which accounted for approximately 61% of the dose, hypoxanthine, xanthine, and uric acid.

## Half-life

Adults—Approximately 1.5 hours (range, 0.8 to 2.7 hours).

Children (8 months to 18 years of age)—Approximately 0.8 hour (range, 0.5 to 1.2 hours).

Severe renal failure—Approximately 4.5 hours.

Intracellular half-life of ddA-TP is 8 to 24 hours *in vitro*.

## Time to peak concentration

0.5 to 1 hour.

## Peak serum concentration

Adults—

Approximately 1.6 mcg per mL (range, 0.6 to 2.9 mcg per mL) after a single 375-mg dose of buffered powder for oral solution.

Approximately 1.6 mcg per mL (range, 0.5 to 2.6 mcg per mL) after a single 300-mg dose of the buffered chewable/dispersible tablet.

Children (8 months to 18 years of age)—

Steady state values after oral administration of 80, 120, and 180 mg per square meter of body surface were 0.8, 1.4, and 1.7 mcg per mL, respectively.

## Elimination

Renal clearance by glomerular filtration and active tubular secretion makes up approximately 50% of the total body clearance; urinary recovery was approximately 20% (range, 3 to 31%) after a single oral dose in adults and approximately 17% (range, 5 to 30%) at steady state in children. No accumulation was evident in either adults or children.

Dialysis—A 4-hour hemodialysis session reduces the serum didanosine concentration by approximately 20%.

# Precautions to Consider

## Carcinogenicity

Long-term carcinogenicity studies in animals have not been completed.

## Mutagenicity

No evidence of mutagenicity was observed in either the Ames *Salmonella* mutagenicity assays (with or without metabolic activation) or a mutagenicity assay conducted with *Escherichia coli* tester strain WP2 uvrA, where only a slight increase in revertants was observed. In a mammalian cell gene mutation assay conducted in L5178Y/YK+/- mouse lymphoma cells, didanosine was weakly positive in both the presence and absence of metabolic activation at concentrations of approximately 2000 mcg per mL and above. High concentrations of didanosine (≥ 5000 mcg per mL) elevated the frequency of cells bearing chromosome aberrations in an *in vitro* cytogenic study performed in cultured human peripheral lymphocytes. Another *in vitro* mammalian cell chromosome aberrations study using Chinese Hamster Lung cells produced chromosomal aberrations at ≥ 500 mcg per mL after 48 hours of exposure; however, no significant elevations in the frequency of cells with chromosomal aberrations were seen at concentrations up to 250 mcg per mL. In a BALB/c 3T3 *in vitro* transformation assay, didanosine was considered positive only at concentrations of 3000 mcg per mL and above. No evidence of genotoxicity was observed in rat and mouse micronucleus assays.

## Pregnancy/Reproduction

Fertility—No evidence of impaired fertility has been found in rats and rabbits receiving 12 and 14.2 times the estimated human dose of didanosine, based on plasma levels.

Pregnancy—Didanosine crosses the placenta. However, studies in humans have not been done. Unlike zidovudine, it is not known whether didanosine reduces perinatal transmission of HIV infection.

No evidence of harm to the fetus has been found in rats and rabbits receiving 12 and 14.2 times the estimated human dose of didanosine, based on plasma levels. At approximately 12 times the estimated human dose, didanosine was slightly toxic to female rats and their pups during mid and late lactation. The rats showed reduced body weight gains and food intake, but the physical and functional development of the offspring was not impaired and there were no major changes in the F2 generation.

FDA Pregnancy Category B.

## Breast-feeding

It is not known whether didanosine is distributed into breast milk.

There have been case reports of HIV being transmitted from an infected mother to her nursing infant through breast milk. Therefore, breast-feeding is not recommended in HIV-infected mothers where safe infant formula is available and affordable.

## Pediatrics

Data in children over 3 months of age with symptomatic HIV infection suggest that didanosine is well tolerated and may produce an improvement in neuropsychological function, immunological function, p24 antigen levels, and weight gain. However, these data are preliminary. As with adults, the major serious side effect to date in children has been pancreatitis, which usually occurred at doses above 300 mg per square meter of body surface (mg/m²) per day. Retinal depigmentation has been reported in approximately 7% of children treated with didanosine, especially at doses above 300 mg/m² per day.

## Geriatrics

No information is available on the relationship of age to the effects of didanosine in geriatric patients. However, elderly patients are more likely to have an age-related decrease in renal function, which may require a reduction in dose.

## Drug interactions and/or related problems

The following drug interactions and/or related problems have been selected on the basis of their potential clinical significance (possible mechanism in parentheses where appropriate)—not necessarily inclusive (» = major clinical significance):

Note: Combinations containing any of the following medications, depending on the amount present, may also interact with this medication.

» Alcohol or
» Asparaginase or
» Azathioprine or
» Estrogens or
» Furosemide or
» Methyldopa or
» Nitrofurantoin or
» Pentamidine, intravenous or
» Sulfonamides or
» Sulindac or
» Tetracyclines or
» Thiazide diuretics or
» Valproic acid or

Other drugs associated with pancreatitis
(medications associated with the development of pancreatitis should be avoided during didanosine therapy or, if concurrent use is necessary, used with caution since didanosine may cause pancreatitis, which, on rare occasion, has been fatal)

» Chloramphenicol or
» Cisplatin or
» Dapsone or
» Ethambutol or
» Ethionamide or
» Hydralazine or
» Isoniazid or
» Lithium or
» Metronidazole or
» Nitrofurantoin or
» Nitrous oxide or
» Phenytoin or
» Stavudine or
» Vincristine or
» Zalcitabine or
Other drugs associated with peripheral neuropathy
(since didanosine has been shown to cause peripheral neuropathy, medications associated with the development of neuropathy should be avoided during didanosine therapy or, if concurrent use is necessary, used with caution)

» Dapsone or
» Itraconazole or
» Ketoconazole
(concurrent administration of dapsone with didanosine may decrease the absorption of dapsone; didanosine is combined with a buffer to neutralize stomach acidity in order to increase its absorption, while dapsone requires an acidic environment for optimal absorption; dapsone and any other medications that also depend on the gastric acidity for optimal absorption, such as itraconazole and ketoconazole, should be administered at least 2 hours before or 2 hours after didanosine is given)

» Fluoroquinolone antibiotics, such as ciprofloxacin, enoxacin, lomefloxacin, norfloxacin, and ofloxacin or
» Tetracyclines
(concurrent administration of the didanosine chewable/dispersible tablets or pediatric powder for oral solution with fluoroquinolone antibiotics or tetracyclines may cause a decrease in the plasma concentrations of these antibiotics; these 2 didanosine products contain magnesium- and aluminum-containing antacids, which will reduce the absorption of these antibiotics by chelation; fluoroquinolone antibiotics and tetracyclines should be administered at least 2 hours before or 2 hours after didanosine chewable/dispersible tablets or pediatric powder for oral solution is given; buffered didanosine powder for oral solution contains a citrate-phosphate buffer, which will not interact with the fluoroquinolone antibiotics or tetracyclines)

**Laboratory value alterations**
The following have been selected on the basis of their potential clinical significance (possible effect in parentheses where appropriate)—not necessarily inclusive (» = major clinical significance):

With physiology/laboratory test values
Alanine aminotransferase (ALT [SGPT]) and
Alkaline phosphatase and
Aspartate aminotransferase (AST [SGOT]) and
Bilirubin, serum
(values may be increased to greater than 5 times the upper normal limit; the incidence of laboratory abnormalities occurs more frequently in patients with abnormal baseline values)

» Amylase, serum and
Lipase, serum and
Triglycerides, serum
(values may be increased)
Potassium, serum
(concentrations may be decreased; decrease may be secondary to diarrhea from the buffer rather than to didanosine itself)

» Uric acid, serum
(didanosine may cause an asymptomatic increase in uric acid concentrations; may be dose-related; uric acid levels fall with hydration and/or a decrease in dose)

**Medical considerations/Contraindications**
The medical considerations/contraindications included here have been selected on the basis of their potential clinical significance (reasons given in parentheses where appropriate)—not necessarily inclusive (» = major clinical significance).

*Risk-benefit should be considered when the following medical problems exist:*

» Alcoholism, active or
» Hypertriglyceridemia, or history of or
» Pancreatitis, or history of
(didanosine has caused pancreatitis, which, on rare occasion, has been fatal; patients who have pancreatitis or a history of pancreatitis, or are at risk for pancreatitis should either not take didanosine or should take it with extreme caution)

» Conditions requiring sodium-restriction, such as cardiac failure, cirrhosis of the liver or severe hepatic disease, peripheral or pulmonary edema, hypernatremia, hypertension, renal function impairment, or toxemia of pregnancy
(each 2-tablet dose of didanosine chewable/dispersible tablets contains 529 mg of sodium, and each single-dose packet of buffered didanosine powder for oral solution contains 1380 mg of sodium)

Gouty arthritis
(didanosine may cause an increase in uric acid levels, especially in patients who already have an abnormally high baseline before the didanosine therapy is initiated)

Hepatic function impairment
(patients with hepatic function impairment may be at increased risk of toxicity due to altered metabolism; this may require a reduction in dose)

Phenylketonuria
(didanosine chewable/dispersible tablets contain 45 mg or 67.4 mg of phenylalanine per 2-tablet dose, depending on the strength used)

» Peripheral neuropathy
(didanosine may cause peripheral neuropathy, which may require a reduction in dose)

Renal function impairment
(patients with renal function impairment may be at increased risk of toxicity due to decreased clearance through the kidneys, especially patients with a serum creatinine concentration of > 1.5 mg/dL or a creatinine clearance of < 60 mL/min; this may require a reduction in dose; also, each didanosine chewable/dispersible tablet contains 15.7 mEq of magnesium hydroxide, which may lead to a magnesium overload in patients with severe renal disease, especially after prolonged dosing)

**Patient monitoring**
The following may be especially important in patient monitoring (other tests may be warranted in some patients, depending on condition; » = major clinical significance):

» Amylase, serum and
» Lipase, serum and
Triglycerides, serum
(didanosine administration has been associated with pancreatitis; patients should be monitored for laboratory changes consistent with pancreatitis, such as elevated amylase, lipase, and triglyceride concentrations; didanosine should be discontinued if amylase concentration is elevated by 1.5 to 2 times normal limits and/or the patient has symptoms consistent with pancreatitis)

» Ophthalmologic examinations
(dilated ophthalmoscopy should be performed in children every 3 to 6 months, or if there is a change in vision, to monitor for the development and progression of retinal depigmentation; the lesions appear initially in the midperiphery of the fundus; therefore, central vision is not immediately threatened. If retinal lesions are observed, the patient should be re-examined monthly to assess progression; treatment with didanosine may need to be discontinued)

Potassium, serum
(serum potassium should be monitored regularly since hypokalemia has been associated with didanosine administration; however, this may be secondary to diarrhea from the buffer)

Uric acid, serum
(serum uric acid concentrations should be monitored regularly since didanosine may cause an asymptomatic hyperuricemia due to the catabolism of the drug; hyperuricemia occurs more frequently in patients who begin therapy with an abnormal baseline uric acid concentration)

# Side/Adverse Effects

Note: Some side effects, such as pancreatitis, peripheral neuropathy, hepatotoxicity, myalgias, hematologic abnormalities, and elevations in uric acid, may be seen with severe HIV disease; therefore, differentiation between the side effects of didanosine therapy and the complications of HIV disease may be difficult.

The incidence of pancreatitis associated with didanosine administration was 5 to 13% in adults in phase I studies, a controlled trial, and the expanded access program, and approximately 6% in children; the fatality rate of pancreatitis in adults was approximately 0.35%. An increased risk has been found to be associated with higher doses in both adults and children ($\geq$ 12.5 mg/kg per day in adults, $\geq$ 300 mg/m$^2$ per day in children); other risk factors include a history of pancreatitis, renal function impairment (without a dose adjustment), alcoholism, a very low CD4 count, and elevated triglycerides. Pancreatitis usually resolves when didanosine is discontinued.

Peripheral neuropathy also appears to be related to higher daily doses. It has occurred more frequently in adults (34% of patients receiving $\leq$ 12.5 mg/kg per day in phase I trials and 13 to 14% in a controlled trial) than in children (3%), and usually resolves over time, but may persist.

Hematologic abnormalities, such as anemia (hemoglobin < 8.0 grams/dL), granulocytopenia (< 1000/microliter), leukopenia (< 2000/microliter), and thrombocytopenia (< 50,000/microliter) have occurred in 5% or less of patients who started therapy with normal baseline values; however, if the patient began didanosine therapy with abnormal baseline values, the incidence of anemia, granulocytopenia, leukopenia, and thrombocytopenia was 0%, 56%, 37%, and 25%, respectively, in adults, and 27%, 62%, 36%, and 67%, respectively, in children.

Peripheral atrophy of the retinal pigment epithelium has occurred in 3 children receiving high doses of didanosine (> 300 mg/m$^2$ per day) and one child receiving a lower dose. The lesions are described as mottling and atrophy of retinal-pigment epithelium, and later become well circumscribed with hyperpigmented borders in the midperiphery of the fundus. Central visual acuity is not affected. The lesions appear to progress with continued didanosine therapy. When the drug is discontinued, the lesions remain with no progression.

The following side/adverse effects have been selected on the basis of their potential clinical significance (possible signs and symptoms in parentheses where appropriate)—not necessarily inclusive:

**Those indicating need for medical attention**
Incidence more frequent
   *Peripheral neuropathy* (tingling, burning, numbness, and pain in hands or feet)
Incidence less frequent
   *Pancreatitis* (abdominal pain; nausea and vomiting)
Incidence rare
   *Cardiomyopathy* (shortness of breath; swelling of feet or lower legs); *hematologic toxicity, specifically anemia, granulocytopenia or leukopenia, or thrombocytopenia* (unusual tiredness and weakness; fever, chills, or sore throat; unusual bleeding or bruising); *hepatitis* (yellow skin and eyes); *hypersensitivity* (fever and chills; skin rash and itching); *retinal depigmentation; seizures* (convulsions)

**Those indicating need for medical attention only if they continue or are bothersome**
Incidence more frequent
   *CNS toxicity* (anxiety; headache; irritability; insomnia; restlessness); *dryness of mouth; gastrointestinal disturbances* (abdominal pain; nausea; diarrhea)
   Note: Diarrhea occurs frequently and may be related to the buffering agent; if the diarrhea becomes severe, the patient may require medical attention.

## Patient Consultation

As an aid to patient consultation, refer to *Advice for the Patient, Didanosine (Systemic)*.

In providing consultation, consider emphasizing the following selected information (» = major clinical significance):

**Before using this medication**
» Conditions affecting use, especially:
   Use in children—May cause retinal depigmentation, which is more likely to occur in children receiving doses above 300 mg/m$^2$ per day
   Other medications, especially other drugs associated with pancreatitis and peripheral neuropathy, dapsone or medications that require an acidic environment for absorption, tetracyclines, or fluoroquinolone antibiotics
   Other medical problems, especially alcoholism, hypertriglyceridemia, pancreatitis or a history of pancreatitis, conditions requiring sodium-restriction, or peripheral neuropathy

**Proper use of this medication**
» Importance of not taking more medication than prescribed; importance of not discontinuing medication without checking with physician; discontinuing medication and calling physician at first signs and symptoms of pancreatitis
» Importance of not missing doses and of taking at evenly spaced times
» Proper administration:
*For buffered didanosine for oral solution*
   Preparing by opening the packet and dissolving its contents in 1/2 glass (4 ounces) of water. The powder should not be mixed with fruit juice or other acid-containing liquid
   Stirring the mixture for approximately 2 to 3 minutes until the powder is completely dissolved
   Swallowing the entire solution immediately
*For tablets*
   Patients older than 1 year of age must take 2 tablets at each dose to provide adequate buffering and to prevent gastric acid degradation of didanosine
   Children under 1 year of age should receive a 1-tablet dose. The recommended dose for children is based on body surface area and, for adults, on body weight
   Thoroughly chewing, manually crushing, or dispersing in at least 1 ounce of water prior to consumption. Because the tablets are hard, they may be difficult to chew for some patients; manually crushing or dispersing the tablets may be preferable. To disperse tablets, 2 tablets should be added to at least 1 ounce of drinking water. The mixture should be stirred until a uniform dispersion forms and consumed immediately
» Proper dosing
   Missed dose: Taking as soon as possible; not taking if almost time for next dose; not doubling doses
» Proper storage

**Precautions while using this medication**
» Regular visits to physician for blood tests
» Importance of not taking other medications concurrently without checking with physician
» Using a condom to help prevent transmission of the AIDS virus to others; not sharing needles or injectable equipment with anyone

**Side/adverse effects**
   Signs of potential side effects, especially peripheral neuropathy, pancreatitis, cardiomyopathy, hematologic toxicities, hepatitis, hypersensitivity, retinal depigmentation, and seizures

## General Dosing Information

Two tablets must be taken at each dose by patients older than 1 year of age to provide adequate buffering and to prevent gastric acid degradation of didanosine. Children under 1 year of age should receive a 1-tablet dose. The recommended dose for children is based on body surface area and, for adults, on body weight.

It is recommended that patients on hemodialysis receive their dose of didanosine after dialysis.

**Diet/Nutrition**
All didanosine formulations should be taken on an empty stomach. Administration with food decreases absorption by approximately 50%.

Patients on sodium-restricted diets should be made aware that each 2-tablet dose of didanosine tablets contains 529 mg (23 mEq) of sodium, and each single-dose packet of buffered didanosine for oral solution contains 1380 mg (60 mEq) of sodium.

Patients with phenylketonuria should be made aware that each 2-tablet dose of didanosine tablets contains 45 mg or 67.4 mg of phenylalanine, depending on the strength of tablets used.

**Bioequivalence information**
Didanosine tablets are 20 to 25% more bioavailable than the buffered powder for oral solution. Because of this, the dose of the tablets is correspondingly lower and the dosing of the 2 products cannot be interchanged.

## Oral Dosage Forms

### BUFFERED DIDANOSINE FOR ORAL SOLUTION

**Usual adult and adolescent dose**
Antiviral—
   Oral:
      Patients weighing less than 60 kg—167 mg every twelve hours.
      Patients weighing $\geq$60 kg—250 mg every twelve hours.

**Usual pediatric dose**
This product is usually not prescribed for small children. See *Didanosine for Buffered Oral Suspension* or *Didanosine Tablets*.

**Strength(s) usually available**

U.S.—

   100 mg per packet (Rx) [*Videx* (citrate-phosphate buffer; sodium 1380 mg; sucrose)].

   167 mg per packet (Rx) [*Videx* (citrate-phosphate buffer; sodium 1380 mg; sucrose)].

   250 mg per packet (Rx) [*Videx* (citrate-phosphate buffer; sodium 1380 mg; sucrose)].

   375 mg per packet (Rx) [*Videx* (citrate-phosphate buffer; sodium 1380 mg; sucrose)].

Canada—

   Not commercially available.

**Packaging and storage**

Store below 40 °C (104 °F), preferably between 15 and 30 °C (59 and 86 °F), unless otherwise specified by manufacturer.

**Stability**

After preparation, the solution may be stored at room temperature for up to 4 hours.

**Incompatibilities**

Didanosine is unstable in acidic solutions and should not be mixed with fruit juice or other acid-containing liquid.

**Auxiliary labeling**

• Dissolve contents of packet in one-half glass (4 ounces) of water.

• Continue medicine for full time of treatment.

• Take on empty stomach.

## DIDANOSINE FOR BUFFERED ORAL SUSPENSION

**Usual adult and adolescent dose**

This product is usually not used by adults and adolescents. See *Buffered Didanosine for Oral Solution* and *Didanosine Tablets.*

**Usual pediatric dose**

Antiviral—

  Oral:

    Body surface area up to 0.4 square meters—31 mg (3 mL) every eight to twelve hours.

    Body surface area 0.5 to 0.7 square meters—62 mg (6 mL) every eight to twelve hours.

    Body surface area 0.8 to 1.0 square meters—94 mg (9.5 mL) every eight to twelve hours.

    Body surface area 1.1 to 1.4 square meters—125 mg (12.5 mL) every eight to twelve hours.

**Strength(s) usually available**

U.S.—

   2000 mg per 200 mL (when reconstituted according to manufacturer's instructions) (Rx) [*Videx* (aluminum hydroxide; magnesium hydroxide)].

   4000 mg per 400 mL (when reconstituted according to manufacturer's instructions) (Rx) [*Videx* (aluminum hydroxide; magnesium hydroxide)].

Canada—

   2000 mg per 200 mL (when reconstituted according to manufacturer's instructions) (Rx) [*Videx* (aluminum hydroxide; magnesium hydroxide)].

   4000 mg per 400 mL (when reconstituted according to manufacturer's instructions) (Rx) [*Videx* (aluminum hydroxide; magnesium hydroxide)].

**Packaging and storage**

Prior to reconstitution, store below 40 °C (104 °F), preferably between 15 and 30 °C (59 and 86 °F), unless otherwise specified by manufacturer.

**Preparation of dosage form**

Didanosine pediatric powder must initially be diluted by adding 100 mL or 200 mL of purified water to the 2000 mg or 4000 mg bottle of powder, respectively. This produces an initial concentration of 20 mg per mL. This solution must be further diluted as follows:

  One part of the 20 mg per mL solution should be mixed immediately with one part of an aluminum- and magnesium-containing antacid (e.g., Mylanta Double Strength Liquid [formerly Mylanta II] or Maalox TC Suspension). This provides a final dispensing concentration of 10 mg per mL.

For home use, the solution should be dispensed in an appropriately sized, flint-glass bottle with a child-resistant closure.

**Stability**

After reconstitution, the solution may be stored up to 30 days in the refrigerator (2 to 8 °C [36 to 46 °F]). Unused portion should be discarded after 30 days.

**Auxiliary labeling**

• Refrigerate.

• Shake well.

• Continue medicine for full time of treatment.

• Beyond-use date.

• Take on empty stomach.

**Note**

When dispensing, include a calibrated liquid-measuring device.

## DIDANOSINE TABLETS

**Usual adult and adolescent dose**

Antiviral—

  Oral:

    Patients weighing less than 60 kg—125 mg every twelve hours.

    Patients weighing ≥60 kg—200 mg every twelve hours

**Usual pediatric dose**

Antiviral—

  Oral:

    Body surface area up to 0.4 square meters—25 mg every eight to twelve hours.

    Body surface area 0.5 to 0.7 square meters—50 mg every eight to twelve hours.

    Body surface area 0.8 to 1.0 square meters—75 mg every eight to twelve hours.

    Body surface area 1.1 to 1.4 square meters—100 mg every eight to twelve hours.

**Strength(s) usually available**

U.S.—

   25 mg (Rx) [*Videx* (dihydroxyaluminum sodium carbonate; magnesium hydroxide 15.7 mEq; phenylalanine 22.5 mg; sodium 264.5 mg)].

   50 mg (Rx) [*Videx* (dihydroxyaluminum sodium carbonate; magnesium hydroxide 15.7 mEq; phenylalanine 22.5 mg; sodium 264.5 mg)].

   100 mg (Rx) [*Videx* (dihydroxyaluminum sodium carbonate; magnesium hydroxide 15.7 mEq; phenylalanine 22.5 mg; sodium 264.5 mg)].

   150 mg (Rx) [*Videx* (dihydroxyaluminum sodium carbonate; magnesium hydroxide 15.7 mEq; phenylalanine 33.7 mg; sodium 264.5 mg)].

Canada—

   25 mg (Rx) [*Videx* (dihydroxyaluminum sodium carbonate; magnesium hydroxide 15.7 mEq; phenylalanine 22.5 mg; sodium 264.5 mg)].

   50 mg (Rx) [*Videx* (dihydroxyaluminum sodium carbonate; magnesium hydroxide 15.7 mEq; phenylalanine 22.5 mg; sodium 264.5 mg)].

   100 mg (Rx) [*Videx* (dihydroxyaluminum sodium carbonate; magnesium hydroxide 15.7 mEq; phenylalanine 22.5 mg; sodium 264.5 mg)].

   150 mg (Rx) [*Videx* (dihydroxyaluminum sodium carbonate; magnesium hydroxide 15.7 mEq; phenylalanine 33.7 mg; sodium 264.5 mg)].

**Packaging and storage**

Store below 40 °C (104 °F), preferably between 15 and 30 °C (59 and 86 °F), unless otherwise specified by manufacturer.

**Stability**

If dispersed in water, the solution may be stored for up to 1 hour at room temperature.

**Auxiliary labeling**

• Continue medicine for full time of treatment.

• Do not swallow tablets whole.

• Take on empty stomach.

Revised: 06/22/94

Interim revision: 01/11/95

---

**DIENESTROL**—See *Estrogens (Vaginal)*

# DIETHYLCARBAMAZINE   Systemic

VA CLASSIFICATION (Primary): AP200

Note: For a listing of dosage forms and brand names by country availability, see *Dosage Forms* section(s). For a listing of brand names for the articles in this monograph, refer to the General Index.

## Category

Anthelmintic (systemic).

## Indications

### Accepted

Filariasis, Bancroft's (treatment)—Diethylcarbamazine is indicated as a primary agent in the treatment of Bancroft's filariasis caused by *Wuchereria bancrofti.*

Loiasis (treatment)—Diethylcarbamazine is indicated as a primary agent in the treatment of loiasis caused by *Loa loa.*

Onchocerciasis (treatment)—Diethylcarbamazine is indicated as a secondary agent in the curative treatment, given before and after suramin therapy, of onchocerciasis (river blindness) caused by *Onchocerca volvulus.* Ivermectin is considered to be the primary agent in the treatment of onchocerciasis.

Tropical eosinophilia (treatment)—Diethylcarbamazine is indicated as a primary agent in the treatment of tropical eosinophilia (eosinophilic lung; tropical pulmonary eosinophilia).

### Unaccepted

Diethylcarbamazine has been used for the treatment of ascariasis. However, in the opinion of most USP medical experts, it has been superseded by newer, safer, and more effective anthelmintics.

## Pharmacology/Pharmacokinetics

### Mechanism of action/Effect

Filariasis; loiasis—Microfilaricidal and macrofilaricidal.
Onchocerciasis—Microfilaricidal; diethylcarbamazine reduces the number of intrauterine *Onchocerca volvulus* microfilariae by inhibiting the rate of embryogenesis; this agent also increases the rate of loss of *O. volvulus* microfilariae from nematodes and nodules; diethylcarbamazine has no sterilizing effect on adult worms.

### Absorption

Readily absorbed following oral administration.

### Distribution

Widely distributed throughout all body compartments, except adipose tissue.

### Biotransformation

Partially metabolized to diethylcarbamazine *N*-oxide.

### Half-life

Approximately 8 hours.

### Time to peak serum concentration

1 to 2 hours.

### Peak serum concentration

80 to 200 nanograms per mL after a single 50-mg dose.

### Elimination

Renal—Excreted in urine, largely unchanged and as *N*-oxide metabolite, within 48 hours.
Fecal—Approximately 4 to 5% eliminated in feces.

## Precautions to Consider

### Pregnancy/Reproduction

Treatment of pregnant patients with diethylcarbamazine should be deferred until after delivery. However, problems in humans have not been documented.

### Breast-feeding

It is not known whether diethylcarbamazine is distributed into breast milk. However, problems in humans have not been documented.

### Pediatrics

Appropriate studies on the relationship of age to the effects of diethylcarbamazine have not been performed in the pediatric population. However, no pediatrics-specific problems have been documented to date.

### Geriatrics

No information is available on the relationship of age to the effects of diethylcarbamazine in geriatric patients.

### Medical considerations/Contraindications

The medical considerations/contraindications included here have been selected on the basis of their potential clinical significance (reasons given in parentheses where appropriate)—not necessarily inclusive (» = major clinical significance).

***Risk-benefit should be considered when the following medical problem exists:***

Hypersensitivity to diethylcarbamazine

Note: In ocular onchocerciasis, prolonged administration of diethylcarbamazine may result in inflammation and subsequent degenerative changes in the optic disc and retina.

### Patient monitoring

The following may be especially important in patient monitoring (other tests may be warranted in some patients, depending on condition; » = major clinical significance):

*For Bancroft's filariasis and loiasis*
Microfilarial blood concentrations
(may be required prior to and periodically during therapy with diethylcarbamazine; in loiasis, retinal hemorrhage and encephalopathy may occur with very high microfilarial blood concentrations)

*For onchocerciasis*
» Ophthalmologic examinations, including examinations for visual acuity, visual fields, and ophthalmoscopy
(ophthalmologic examinations for visual acuity and visual fields may be required routinely prior to and periodically during therapy with diethylcarbamazine; slit-lamp examinations may be required prior to, periodically during, and following treatment with diethylcarbamazine to assess the number of intraocular microfilariae and adverse reactions such as iridocyclitis)

» Skin snips
(may be required prior to and every 6 to 12 months following treatment with diethylcarbamazine to assess the number of intradermal microfilariae)

## Side/Adverse Effects

Note: In heavily infected patients with onchocerciasis, severe reactions may occur following a single dose of diethylcarbamazine. The Mazzotti reaction, a complex, acute inflammatory response characterized by fever, tachycardia, hypotension, adenitis, and an ocular inflammatory response, usually results from the death of microfilariae. The intensity of the reaction depends on the dose and the microfilarial load. However, it is sometimes difficult to determine whether these reactions are caused by the death of microfilariae or by diethylcarbamazine itself.

In very heavily infected patients with loiasis, encephalopathy and retinal hemorrhage may occur following treatment with diethylcarbamazine.

The following side/adverse effects have been selected on the basis of their potential clinical significance (possible signs and symptoms in parentheses where appropriate)—not necessarily inclusive:

### Those indicating need for medical attention

Incidence more frequent
*Itching and swelling of face, especially eyes*

Incidence less frequent
*Fever; lymphadenopathy* (painful and tender glands in neck, armpits, or groin); *skin rash*

*With prolonged use in onchocerciasis*
*Visual disturbances* (loss of vision; night blindness; tunnel vision)

### Those indicating need for medical attention only if they continue or are bothersome

Incidence more frequent
*Arthralgia* (joint pain); *headache; malaise* (unusual tiredness or weakness)

Incidence less frequent
*Dizziness; nausea or vomiting*

## Patient Consultation

As an aid to patient consultation, refer to *Advice for the Patient, Diethylcarbamazine (Systemic).*

In providing consultation, consider emphasizing the following selected information (» = major clinical significance):

**Before using this medication**
» Conditions affecting use, especially:
    Pregnancy—Treatment of pregnant patients should be deferred until after delivery; however, problems in humans have not been documented

**Proper use of this medication**
    Taking immediately after meals
» Compliance with full course of therapy; second course may be required in some patients
» Proper dosing
    Missed dose: Taking as soon as possible; not taking if almost time for next dose; not doubling doses
» Proper storage

**Precautions while using this medication**
    Checking with physician if no improvement within a few days
    *For river blindness*
    Regular visits to physician to check progress, as well as ophthalmologic examinations
» Caution if dizziness, loss of vision, night blindness, or tunnel vision occurs
    Concurrent administration with systemic corticosteroids to reduce inflammatory response to death of microfilariae

**Side/adverse effects**
    Signs of potential side effects, especially itching and swelling of face, particularly eyes; fever; lymphadenopathy; skin rash; and visual disturbances

## General Dosing Information

Diethylcarbamazine should be taken immediately after meals.

Diethylcarbamazine should be administered with caution (e.g., gradually increasing doses) to prevent or minimize allergic reactions. Most side effects of diethylcarbamazine are not serious and do not generally require discontinuation of therapy. However, it may be necessary to discontinue therapy if severe allergic reactions, in conjunction with skin rash, occur.

Patients who are more heavily infected may require more prolonged treatment.

**For Bancroft's filariasis, loiasis, or onchocerciasis**
In the acute and chronic stages of these infections, treatment should be continued for 2 to 4 weeks. Recurrences require retreatment.

In Bancroft's filariasis, treatment should preferably be given before irreparable damage is done to the lymphatic system and its valves.

In the curative treatment of onchocerciasis, diethylcarbamazine is administered before and after suramin therapy. Diethylcarbamazine is recommended in low initial doses concurrently with systemic corticosteroids to suppress the inflammatory response to the death of microfilariae caused by diethylcarbamazine, especially in moderate to heavy infections with ocular involvement.

In severe onchocerciasis, severe allergic reactions may develop following the administration of a single dose of diethylcarbamazine. Gradually increasing doses are recommended as follows: 25 mg daily, gradually increased to the usual maintenance dose over a period of 7 to 14 days. If very severe allergic reactions occur, diethylcarbamazine should be discontinued and corticosteroids should be given. If severe allergic reactions occur again, diethylcarbamazine should not be used in these patients.

In the suppressive treatment of onchocerciasis, diethylcarbamazine is recommended in low, intermittent doses to preserve eyesight and to relieve pruritus by reducing the microfilarial load.

**For treatment of adverse effects**
Recommended treatment consists of the following:
• Systemic corticosteroids for very severe allergic reactions.

## Oral Dosage Forms

### DIETHYLCARBAMAZINE CITRATE TABLETS USP

**Usual adult dose**
Bancroft's filariasis; or
Loiasis; or
Onchocerciasis—
    Oral, 2 to 3 mg per kg of body weight three times a day.
Tropical eosinophilia—
    Oral, 6 mg per kg of body weight once a day for four to seven days.

**Usual adult prescribing limits**
Onchocerciasis—Up to 9 mg per kg of body weight a day.
Tropical eosinophilia—Up to 13 mg per kg of body weight a day.

**Usual pediatric dose**
Dosage has not been established in the treatment of Bancroft's filariasis, loiasis, onchocerciasis, or tropical eosinophilia. However, doses of 50 mg to 250 mg daily, based on the patient's age, have been used in children between the ages of 1 and 15 years of age.

**Strength(s) usually available**
U.S.—
    50 mg (Rx) [*Hetrazan*].
    200 mg (Rx) [GENERIC].
    400 mg (Rx) [GENERIC].
    Note: The 50-mg tablet is available only through the manufacturer upon request (tel. no.: 914-735-2815).
Canada—
    50 mg (Rx) [*Hetrazan* (scored)].

**Packaging and storage**
Store below 40 °C (104 °F), preferably between 15 and 30 °C (59 and 86 °F), unless otherwise specified by manufacturer. Store in a tight container.

**Auxiliary labeling**
• Take immediately after meals.
• May cause dizziness or vision problems.
• Continue medication for full time of treatment.

Revised: 08/11/95

---

**DIETHYLPROPION**—See *Appetite Suppressants (Systemic)*

---

**DIETHYLSTILBESTROL**—See *Estrogens (Systemic)*

---

**DIETHYLSTILBESTROL-CONTAINING COMBINATIONS**—

Diethylstilbestrol and Methyltestosterone (Systemic)—See *Androgens and Estrogens (Systemic)*

---

# DIETHYLTOLUAMIDE    Topical

VA CLASSIFICATION (Primary): DE900
Other commonly used names are DEET and m-DET
Note: For a listing of dosage forms and brand names by country availability, see *Dosage Forms* section(s). For a listing of brand names for the articles in this monograph, refer to the General Index.

## Category

Insect repellent (topical).

## Indications

**Accepted**
Infections transmitted by bites of insects (prophylaxis) or

Infestations by insects or other arthropods (prophylaxis)—Diethyltoluamide is an insect repellent indicated for the topical prevention of infections transmitted by bites of insects or infestations by insects or other arthropods. Diethyltoluamide is effective against mosquitoes, biting flies (gnats, sandflies, deer flies, stable flies, black flies), ticks, harvest mites, and fleas.

## Pharmacology/Pharmacokinetics

**Physicochemical characteristics**
Molecular weight—191.27.

**Mechanism of action/Effect**
Unknown.

### Absorption

Diethyltoluamide is absorbed through the skin. In one study, approximately 17% of diethyltoluamide was absorbed into the systemic circulation following topical application of 4 mcg per square centimeter of body surface (mcg/cm²) on intact skin (ventral surface of the forearm) of 4 human volunteers. In another study using a 50% solution of diethyltoluamide, approximately 50% was absorbed within 6 hours following topical application of 1 mL of the solution. Factors that may affect the degree of systemic absorption and the risk of toxicity of diethyltoluamide are: the quantity of insect repellent applied, the concentration of diethyltoluamide in the repellent, applying the repellent to broken or abraded skin or onto skin folds, frequency of application, and the use of occlusive covering over the area where the repellent was applied.

Variable penetration of diethyltoluamide into the skin, ranging from 9 to 56% of a topically applied dose, has been reported. It has been postulated that a reservoir depot effect and subsequent slow release of diethyltoluamide into the systemic circulation occur, which may help explain the central nervous system (CNS) and dermatologic effects seen after continuous and repetitive use.

### Biotransformation

Hepatic—Undergoes oxidation of benzylic moiety to produce *m*-carboxyl-*N,N* diethylbenzoylamide and hydroxylation of the sidechain to produce the glucuronide of *N* hydroxyethyl-*N*-ethyl-*m*-toluamide.

### Time to peak concentration

If absorption occurs, peak plasma concentrations are achieved in 1 hour.

### Elimination

Renal—Approximately 50% of the absorbed dose of diethyltoluamide is eliminated in the urine over 5 days following topical application.

## Precautions to Consider

### Carcinogenicity/Tumorigenicity/Mutagenicity

Animal studies with diethyltoluamide have shown no carcinogenic, tumorigenic, or mutagenic effects.

### Pregnancy/Reproduction

Pregnancy—Studies have not been done in humans.

Studies in rats have shown that diethyltoluamide crosses the placenta. Residual diethyltoluamide was observed for 3 months after birth in the body tissues of offspring of female rats that had been administered repeatedly 1000 mg per kg of body weight of the repellent. One animal study reported embryotoxic effects. However, this has not been confirmed by other studies.

### Breast-feeding

It is not known whether diethyltoluamide is distributed into breast milk. However, problems in humans have not been documented.

### Pediatrics

Diethyltoluamide should be used with caution in children. Because of their increased surface-area-to-body-mass ratio, children may be at increased risk for toxicity due to greater skin absorption. Low-concentration products should be used and applied sparingly.

### Geriatrics

No information is available on the relationship of age to the effects of diethyltoluamide in geriatric patients.

### Medical considerations/Contraindications

The medical considerations/contraindications included here have been selected on the basis of their potential clinical significance (reasons given in parentheses where appropriate)—not necessarily inclusive (» = major clinical significance).

*Risk-benefit should be considered when the following medical problem exists:*

Sensitivity to diethyltoluamide

## Side/Adverse Effects

Note: The amount and the concentration of diethyltoluamide are major factors that affect the degree of risks for the development of toxicity. Toxicity may result from administration of large doses or from chronic exposure leading to accumulation of this product. (See also *Absorption* section.) The time to onset of symptoms of toxicity usually ranges from 30 to 60 minutes after exposure. Symptoms of toxicity due to chronic exposure may occur days, weeks, or months after use of diethyltoluamide is begun.

The following side/adverse effects have been selected on the basis of their potential clinical significance (possible signs and symptoms in parentheses where appropriate)—not necessarily inclusive:

**Those indicating need for medical attention**
Incidence rare

> *Cardiovascular toxicity specifically bradycardia* (slow heartbeat) and *hypotension* (low blood pressure; unusual tiredness or weakness); *CNS toxicity, including ataxia* (clumsiness or unsteadiness); *clonic jerking movement* (uncontrolled jerking movement); *coma* (loss of consciousness); *confusion* (mood or mental changes); *insomnia* (trouble in sleeping); *muscle cramping; psychosis* (mood or mental changes); *seizures; slurred speech and tremors; dermatologic/allergic reactions such as anaphylaxis* (changes in facial skin color; skin rash; hives; itching; fast or irregular breathing; puffiness or swelling of the eyelids or around the eyes; shortness of breath; troubled breathing; tightness in chest; wheezing); *bullous skin eruptions* (skin blisters); *contact urticaria* (skin rash; hives; itching); *erythema* (reddening of skin)

> Note: *Cardiovascular, CNS,* and *dermatologic toxicities* are more likely to occur with prolonged or excessive use.

> *Anaphylaxis* may include anaphylactic shock with sudden, severe decrease in blood pressure and collapse

## Patient Consultation

As an aid to patient consultation, refer to *Advice for the Patient, Diethyltoluamide (Topical)*.

In providing consultation, consider emphasizing the following selected information (» = major clinical significance):

**Before using this product**
» Conditions affecting use, especially:
    Sensitivity to diethyltoluamide
    Use in children—Increased risk of toxicity because of greater skin absorption; using low-concentration products of diethyltoluamide and applying sparingly to exposed skin

**Proper use of this product**
» Diethyltoluamide is for external use only.
    Reading directions on the label prior to use
» Using low-concentration products (containing less than 30% of diethyltoluamide) and applying sparingly to exposed area(s) of skin; one application of a low-concentration product lasts about 4 to 8 hours
» If applying product on face, keeping diethyltoluamide away from eyes, lips, or inside of nose; if it accidentally gets into eyes or onto lips or inside of nose, immediately flushing with water and checking with physician if irritation, especially of the eyes, persists; if using aerosol or spray dosage forms, applying carefully to face with hands
» Not applying to wounds or irritated or broken skin because of increased absorption; applying sparingly onto skin folds because of increased risk of irritation
    Wearing long sleeves and long pants when possible and applying diethyltoluamide to clothing; not applying under clothing; washing treated clothing after use or when protection is no longer needed
» Not using products containing alcohol, which is flammable, near fire or open flame or while smoking; not smoking or exposing treated skin to fire until repellent has completely dried; keeping treated clothing away from fire, open flame, or smoking
    Not keeping diethyltoluamide on skin any longer than necessary; washing skin with soap and water after use
    Not using on or near furniture, plastics, watch crystals, leather, or painted or varnished surfaces, including automobiles, to avoid damage to these materials

*Proper administration*
*For liquid or lotion dosage forms*
    Applying enough diethyltoluamide to cover exposed skin, rubbing in gently, and allowing to dry

*For topical aerosol or topical spray dosage forms*
    Holding container 6 to 8 inches from skin or clothing; spraying in a slow, sweeping motion just enough diethyltoluamide to cover exposed skin; spreading evenly with hands to moisten all exposed skin and allowing to dry

*For towelettes dosage form*
    Wiping the towelette over exposed skin and allowing diethyltoluamide to dry

» Proper dosing
» Proper storage

**Precautions while using this product**
  Not breathing in diethyltoluamide
  Not applying diethyltoluamide to hands of young children; taking precautions to prevent children from transferring diethyltoluamide to their eyes or mouth; not applying under diapers of infants; discouraging infants from licking area of application
  » Washing treated skin and checking with physician if side effects seem to have occurred after application; taking product container with you to physician

**Side/adverse effects**
  Signs and symptoms of potential side effects, especially cardiovascular toxicity, CNS toxicity, and dermatologic/allergic reactions

# General Dosing Information

Diethyltoluamide is for external use only.

Application of insect repellent containing high concentrations of diethyltoluamide should be avoided because it carries an increased risk of adverse reactions. Use of lower-concentration products (containing less than 30% of diethyltoluamide) is reported to be equally effective.

Diethyltoluamide should be applied sparingly. Prolonged and excessive use should be avoided. One application using a low-concentration product usually lasts about 4 to 8 hours. The concentration of diethyltoluamide in a product is directly proportional to its duration of action. However, saturation does not increase efficacy.

Diethyltoluamide should not be applied to wounds or irritated or broken skin, because of increased absorption. It should be applied sparingly onto skin folds because the natural occlusive mechanism of skin folds may increase the risk of irritation. Contact with the eyes, lips, or inside of the nose also should be avoided.

It is advisable to apply this product to clothing rather than skin, if possible, to minimize skin exposure to diethyltoluamide.

Diethyltoluamide should be applied sparingly to children because they may be at increased risk of toxicity due to greater skin absorption. Use of a lower-concentration product is also recommended for children.

Diethyltoluamide should not be kept on the skin any longer than necessary. When protection is no longer needed, treated skin should be washed with soap and water.

**For treatment of adverse effects**
  Recommended treatment consists of the following
    • Washing treated skin with soap and water.
    • Symptomatic and supportive treatment.

# Topical Dosage Forms

## DIETHYLTOLUAMIDE LIQUID

**Usual adult and adolescent dose**
Insect repellent (topical)—
  Topical, sparingly to exposed area(s) of skin. Reapply when necessary.

**Usual pediatric dose**
See *Usual adult and adolescent dose.*

**Strength(s) usually available**
U.S.—
  100% (OTC) [*OFF! For Maximum Protection*].
Canada—
  100% (OTC) [*OFF! For Maximum Protection*].

**Packaging and storage**
Store below 40 °C (104 °F), preferably between 15 and 30 °C (59 and 86 °F), unless otherwise specified by manufacturer. Protect from freezing.

**Auxiliary labeling**
• For external use only.
• Keep out of reach of children.

## DIETHYLTOLUAMIDE LOTION

**Usual adult and adolescent dose**
See *Diethyltoluamide Liquid.*

**Usual pediatric dose**
See *Diethyltoluamide Liquid.*

**Strength(s) usually available**
U.S.—
  7.5% (OTC) [*OFF! Skintastic*].
  100% (OTC) [*Muskol*].
Canada—
  7.5% (OTC) [*OFF! Skintastic*].
  25% (OTC) [*Muskol*].

**Packaging and storage**
Store below 40 °C (104 °F), preferably between 15 and 30 °C (59 and 86 °F), unless otherwise specified by manufacturer. Protect from freezing.

**Auxiliary labeling**
• For external use only.
• Keep out of reach of children.

## DIETHYLTOLUAMIDE TOPICAL AEROSOL

**Usual adult and adolescent dose**
Insect repellent (topical)—
  Topical, spray on or apply sparingly to exposed area(s) of skin, or spray onto clothing. Reapply when necessary.

**Usual pediatric dose**
See *Usual adult and adolescent dose.*

**Strength(s) usually available**
U.S.—
  15% (OTC) [*OFF!*].
  23% (OTC) [*Backwoods Cutter*].
  25% (OTC) [*Muskol*].
  30% (OTC) [*Deep Woods OFF!*].
  40% (OTC) [*Deep Woods OFF! For Sportsmen; Ultra Muskol*].
Canada—
  15% (OTC) [*Muskol*].
  25% (OTC) [*Muskol*].
  30% (OTC) [*Deep Woods OFF!*].

**Packaging and storage**
Store below 40 °C (104 °F), preferably between 15 and 30 °C (59 and 86 °F), unless otherwise specified by manufacturer. Protect from freezing or excessive heat.

**Auxiliary labeling**
• For external use only.
• Keep out of reach of children.

**Caution**
Flammable.

## DIETHYLTOLUAMIDE TOPICAL SPRAY SOLUTION

**Usual adult and adolescent dose**
See *Diethyltoluamide Topical Aerosol.*

**Usual pediatric dose**
See *Diethyltoluamide Topical Aerosol.*

**Strength(s) usually available**
U.S.—
  5% (OTC) [*OFF! Skintastic For Kids*].
  6.5% (OTC) [*OFF! Skintastic*].
  10% (OTC) [*Cutter Pleasant Protection*].
  15% (OTC) [*OFF!*].
  25% (OTC) [*Deep Woods OFF!*].
  100% (OTC) [*Muskol*].
Canada—
  7.5% (OTC) [*OFF! Skintastic*].
  15% (OTC) [*OFF!*].
  25% (OTC) [*Deep Woods OFF!*].
  100% (OTC) [*Muskol*].

**Packaging and storage**
Store below 40 °C (104 °F), preferably between 15 and 30 °C (59 and 86 °F), unless otherwise specified by manufacturer. Protect from freezing or excessive heat.

**Auxiliary labeling**
• For external use only.
• Keep out of reach of children.

**Caution**
Flammable.

## DIETHYLTOLUAMIDE TOWELETTES

**Usual adult and adolescent dose**
Insect repellent (topical)—
  Topical, as towelette to exposed area(s) of skin. Reapply when necessary.

**Usual pediatric dose**
See *Usual adult and adolescent dose.*

**Strength(s) usually available**
U.S.—
  7.5% (OTC) [*OFF! Skintastic For Children*].
Canada—
  Not commercially available.

**Packaging and storage**
Store below 40 °C (104 °F), preferably between 15 and 30 °C (59 and 86 °F), unless otherwise specified by manufacturer.

**Auxiliary labeling**
- For external use only.
- Keep out of reach of children.

**Selected Bibliography**
Clem JR, Havemann DF, Raebel MA. Insect repellent (N,N-Diethyl-m-toluamide) cardiovascular toxicity in an adult. Ann Pharmacother 1993; 27: 289-93.
Robbins PJ, Cherniack MG. Review of the biodistribution and toxicity of the insect repellent N,N-diethyl-m-toluamide (DEET). J Toxicol Environ Health 1986; 18: 503-25.

Developed: 06/23/95

# DIFENOXIN AND ATROPINE   Systemic†

VA CLASSIFICATION (Primary): GA400
Note: Controlled substance in the U.S.—Schedule IV.
Note: For a listing of dosage forms and brand names by country availability, see *Dosage Forms* section(s). For a listing of brand names for the articles in this monograph, refer to the General Index.

†Not commercially available in Canada.

## Category
Antidiarrheal (antiperistaltic).

## Indications
Note: The efficacy of any antidiarrheal medication for treatment of most cases of nonspecific diarrhea is questionable, especially in children. **Preferred treatment for acute, nonspecific diarrhea consists of fluid and electrolyte replacement, nutritional therapy, and, if possible, elimination of the underlying cause of the diarrhea.**

**Accepted**
Diarrhea (treatment adjunct)—Difenoxin and atropine combination is indicated in adults, as an adjunct to fluid and electrolyte therapy, in the symptomatic treatment of acute nonspecific diarrhea and acute exacerbations of chronic functional diarrhea.

**Unaccepted**
Difenoxin and atropine combination is not recommended for treatment of diarrhea in children.

## Pharmacology/Pharmacokinetics

**Physicochemical characteristics**
Molecular weight—Atropine sulfate: 694.84.
Difenoxin: 424.54.

**Mechanism of action/Effect**
Difenoxin—Probably acts both locally and centrally to reduce intestinal motility. Antidiarrheal activity is about 5 times that of diphenoxylate.
Atropine—Has anticholinergic activity. However, in this preparation atropine is included in doses below the therapeutic level in an attempt to prevent abuse by deliberate overdosage.

**Biotransformation**
Hepatic.

**Half-life**
Atropine—2.5 hours.
Difenoxin—4.5 hours.

**Time to peak concentration**
Difenoxin—40 to 60 minutes.

**Peak serum concentration**
Difenoxin—2-mg dose produces a serum concentration of 160 nanograms per mL.

**Elimination**
Atropine—Renal; 30 to 50% excreted unchanged.
Difenoxin—Renal/fecal.

## Precautions to Consider

**Carcinogenicity**
Long-term studies in rats with difenoxin and atropine have not shown any evidence of carcinogenesis.

**Mutagenicity**
Studies to evaluate mutagenic potential of difenoxin and atropine have not been performed.

**Pregnancy/Reproduction**
Pregnancy—Studies in humans have not been done.
Reproduction studies in rats and rabbits have not shown evidence of teratogenicity with doses of difenoxin and atropine up to 75 times the human therapeutic dose. However, studies in rats have shown that difenoxin and atropine combination causes an increase in delivery time and a significant increase in the percent of stillbirths when given in doses of 20 times the maximum human dose.
FDA Pregnancy Category C.

**Breast-feeding**
Problems in humans have not been documented. However, risk-benefit must considered since both difenoxin and atropine are distributed into breast milk and have the potential to cause serious adverse effects in the nursing infant. There is no information concerning the concentration of these drugs in breast milk.

**Pediatrics**
Difenoxin and atropine combination is not recommended for treatment of diarrhea in children. Recommended treatment consists of oral rehydration therapy to prevent loss of fluids and electrolytes, nutritional therapy, and, if possible, elimination of the underlying cause of the diarrhea.
Infants and young children exhibit increased sensitivity to the toxic effects of atropine. Children may also be more susceptible to the respiratory depressant effects of difenoxin.

**Geriatrics**
No information is available on the relationship of age to the effects of difenoxin and atropine in geriatric patients. However, elderly patients may be more susceptible to the respiratory depressant effects of difenoxin, and to the mild anticholinergic effects and confusion caused by atropine.
In geriatric patients with diarrhea, caution is recommended because of the risk of fluid and electrolyte loss.

**Drug interactions and/or related problems**
The following drug interactions and/or related problems have been selected on the basis of their potential clinical significance (possible mechanism in parentheses where appropriate)—not necessarily inclusive (» = major clinical significance):
Note: Combinations containing any of the following medications, depending on the amount present, may also interact with this medication.

   Addictive medications, other, especially central nervous system (CNS) depressants with habituating potential
   (concurrent use with difenoxin may increase the risk of habituation; caution is recommended)
» Alcohol or
» CNS depression–producing medications, other (See *Appendix II*)
   (concurrent use with difenoxin may increase the CNS depressant effects of either difenoxin or these medications; also, when tricyclic antidepressants are used concurrently with atropine, their anticholinergic effects may be intensified; dosage adjustment may be required)
» Anticholinergics or other medications with anticholinergic activity (See *Appendix II*)
   (these medications may enhance the effects of atropine during concurrent use; significant interaction is unlikely with usual doses of difenoxin and atropine combination, but may occur with its abuse)
» Monoamine oxidase (MAO) inhibitors, including furazolidone and procarbazine
   (concurrent use with difenoxin may precipitate hypertensive crisis; MAO inhibitors may block detoxification of atropine, thus potentiating its action)

» Naltrexone
  (administration of naltrexone to a patient physically dependent on opioid drugs, such as difenoxin, will precipitate withdrawal symptoms; symptoms may appear within 5 minutes of naltrexone administration, persist for up to 48 hours, and be difficult to reverse)
  (naltrexone blocks the therapeutic effects of opioids, including antidiarrheal effects; naltrexone therapy should not be initiated in patients receiving difenoxin; also, patients receiving naltrexone should be advised to use alternative antidiarrheals when necessary)

Opioid (narcotic) analgesics
  (concurrent use with difenoxin may result in increased risk of severe constipation and additive CNS depressant effects)

**Laboratory value alterations**
The following have been selected on the basis of their potential clinical significance (possible effect in parentheses where appropriate)—not necessarily inclusive (» = major clinical significance):

With diagnostic test results
» Phenolsulfonphthalein (PSP) excretion test
  (atropine utilizes the same tubular mechanism of excretion as PSP, resulting in decreased urinary excretion of PSP; concurrent use of atropine is not recommended in patients receiving a PSP excretion test)

With physiology/laboratory test values
Amylase, serum
  (values may be increased as a result of spasm of the sphincter of Oddi)

**Medical considerations/Contraindications**
The medical considerations/contraindications included here have been selected on the basis of their potential clinical significance (reasons given in parentheses where appropriate)—not necessarily inclusive (» = major clinical significance).

*Except under special circumstances, this medication should not be used when the following medical problems exist:*
» Colitis, severe
  (patient may develop toxic megacolon)
» Diarrhea associated with pseudomembranous colitis resulting from treatment with broad-spectrum antibiotics
  (inhibition of peristalsis may delay the removal of toxin from the colon, thereby prolonging and/or worsening the diarrhea)

*Risk-benefit should be considered when the following medical problems exist:*
Alcoholism, active or in remission or
Drug abuse or dependence, history of
  (difenoxin content may increase chances of drug abuse in patient already predisposed to dependence)
Cardiovascular instability
  (possible increase in heart rate may be undesirable)
» Dehydration
  (may predispose to delayed difenoxin intoxication; inhibition of peristalsis may result in fluid retention in colon and may further aggravate dehydration; discontinuation of medication and rehydration therapy is essential if symptoms of dehydration, such as dryness of mouth, excessive thirst, wrinkled skin, decreased urination, and dizziness or lightheadedness, are present; fluid loss may have serious consequences, such as circulatory collapse and renal failure)
Diarrhea caused by infectious organisms
  (bacterial diarrhea may worsen due to the increased contact time between the mucosa and the penetrating microorganism; however, there is no evidence of this occurring in actual practice)
» Diarrhea caused by poisoning, until toxic material has been eliminated from gastrointestinal tract
Down's syndrome
  (atropine may cause abnormal increase in pupillary dilation and acceleration of heart rate)
» Dysentery, acute, characterized by bloody stools and elevated temperature
  (sole treatment with antiperistaltic antidiarrheals may be inadequate; antibiotic therapy may be required)
Gallbladder disease or gallstones
  (difenoxin may cause biliary tract spasm)
» Gastrointestinal tract obstruction
  (use of atropine and difenoxin combination may result in pseudo-obstruction, or dilation of the large or small bowel)
Glaucoma, angle-closure
  (although unlikely with usual doses of this combination, atropine may precipitate an acute attack of angle-closure glaucoma)

» Hepatic function impairment or jaundice
  (difenoxin may precipitate hepatic coma; it is recommended that dosage be reduced in patients with impaired hepatic function)
Hiatal hernia associated with reflux esophagitis or
Hypertension
  (although unlikely with usual doses of this combination, atropine may aggravate these conditions)
Hyperthyroidism
  (characterized by tachycardia, which may be increased by atropine)
Hypothyroidism
  (difenoxin may increase risk of respiratory depression)
Incontinence, overflow
  (secondary to constipation, but often mistaken for diarrhea; use of difenoxin and atropine may worsen constipation and/or result in pseudo-obstruction of the colon)
Intestinal atony in the elderly or debilitated
  (although unlikely with usual doses of this combination, use of atropine may result in obstruction)
Myasthenia gravis
  (although unlikely with usual doses of this combination, atropine may aggravate condition because of inhibition of acetylcholine action)
Prostatic hypertrophy or
Urethral stricture, acute or
Urinary retention
  (reduction in tone of urinary bladder may aggravate or lead to complete urinary retention)
Renal function impairment
  (decreased elimination of atropine may increase the risk of side effects)
Respiratory disease or impairment
  (increased risk of respiratory depression)
Sensitivity to atropine or difenoxin

**Patient monitoring**
The following may be especially important in patient monitoring (other tests may be warranted in some patients, depending on condition; » = major clinical significance):
» Hepatic function determinations
  (recommended at periodic intervals during long-term therapy, especially for patients with hepatic function impairment)

# Side/Adverse Effects

The following side/adverse effects have been selected on the basis of their potential clinical significance (possible signs and symptoms in parentheses where appropriate)—not necessarily inclusive:

**Those indicating need for medical attention**
Incidence less frequent or rare
  *Paralytic ileus or toxic megacolon* (bloating; constipation; loss of appetite; severe stomach pain with nausea and vomiting)

**Those indicating need for medical attention only if they continue, worsen, or are bothersome**
Incidence less frequent or rare
  *Anticholinergic effects, mild* (blurred vision; difficult urination; dryness of skin and mouth; fever); *confusion; dizziness or lightheadedness; drowsiness; headache; trouble in sleeping; unusual tiredness or weakness*

Note: Since atropine is present in a subtherapeutic dose, symptoms of *mild anticholinergic effects* probably indicate overdosage, although in children they may occur at therapeutic doses.

**Those indicating possible withdrawal and the need for medical attention if they occur after discontinuation of prolonged high-dose therapy**
Incidence rare
  *Increased sweating; muscle cramps; nausea or vomiting; shivering or trembling; stomach cramps*

# Overdose

For specific information on the agents used in the management of difenoxin and atropine overdose, see:
• *Naloxone (Systemic)* monograph.
For more information on the management of overdose or unintentional ingestion, **contact a Poison Control Center** (see *Poison Control Center Listing*).

**Clinical effects of overdose**
The following effects have been selected on the basis of their potential clinical significance (possible signs and symptoms in parentheses where appropriate)—not necessarily inclusive:

*Anticholinergic effects, severe* (continuing blurred vision or changes in near vision; fast heartbeat; severe drowsiness; severe dryness of mouth, nose, and throat; unusual warmth, dryness, and flushing of skin); *coma; respiratory depression* (severe shortness of breath or troubled breathing); *unusual excitement, nervousness, restlessness, or irritability*

Note: *Respiratory depression* may occur as late as 12 to 30 hours after ingestion.

**Treatment of overdose**
Treatment of overdose with difenoxin and atropine is the same as treatment for meperidine or morphine overdosage and involves the following:
To decrease absorption—Gastric lavage if vomiting has not occurred.
Specific treatment—Intravenous administration of 0.4 mg of naloxone, which may be repeated at 2- to 3-minute intervals, for respiratory depression.
Monitoring—Prolonged and careful monitoring for 48 to 72 hours.
Supportive care—Support of respiration. Patients in whom intentional overdose is confirmed or suspected should be referred for psychiatric consultation.

## Patient Consultation

As an aid to patient consultation, refer to *Advice for the Patient, Difenoxin and Atropine (Systemic)*.

In providing consultation, consider emphasizing the following selected information (» = major clinical significance):

**Before using this medication**
» Conditions affecting use, especially:
Sensitivity to atropine or difenoxin
Pregnancy—Studies in rats show increased delivery time and stillbirth at doses 20 times maximum human dose
Breast-feeding—Difenoxin and atropine distributed into breast milk; potential for serious adverse effects in nursing infant
Use in children—Not recommended for use in children; increased susceptibility to toxic effects of atropine and respiratory depressant effects of difenoxin; risk of dehydration
Use in the elderly—Increased risk of respiratory depression; risk of dehydration
Other medications, especially other anticholinergics, CNS depressants, MAO inhibitors, or naltrexone
Other medical problems, especially acute dysentery; dehydration; diarrhea caused by antibiotics or poisoning; gastrointestinal tract obstruction; hepatic function impairment or jaundice; or severe colitis

**Proper use of this medication**
Taking with food or meals if gastric irritation occurs
» Importance of not taking more medication than the amount prescribed because of habit-forming potential
» Importance of maintaining adequate hydration and proper diet
» Proper dosing
Missed dose: If on scheduled dosing regimen—Taking as soon as possible; not taking if almost time for next dose; not doubling doses
» Proper storage

**Precautions while using this medication**
Regular visits to physician to check progress during prolonged therapy
» Consulting physician if diarrhea is not controlled within 48 hours and/or fever develops
» Avoiding use of alcohol or other CNS depressants during therapy
» Suspected overdose: Getting emergency help at once
Need to inform physician or dentist of use of medication if any kind of surgery (including dental surgery) or emergency treatment is required
» Caution if dizziness or drowsiness occurs

**Side/adverse effects**
Signs of potential side effects, especially paralytic ileus or toxic megacolon

## General Dosing Information

If clinical improvement is not observed within 48 hours, treatment with difenoxin and atropine should be discontinued.

Inhibition of peristalsis may produce fluid retention in the bowel, which may aggravate dehydration and depletion of electrolytes, and may also increase variability of response to the medication. If dehydration or electrolyte imbalance occurs, difenoxin and atropine therapy should be withheld until appropriate corrective therapy has begun.

To prevent development of toxic megacolon in patients with acute ulcerative colitis, treatment with difenoxin and atropine should be discontinued promptly if abdominal pain or distention or other specific gastrointestinal symptoms such as anorexia, bloating, constipation, nausea, or vomiting occur.

Prolonged use of larger-than-usual therapeutic doses may result in physical dependence.

Tolerance to the antidiarrheal effects of difenoxin and atropine may develop with prolonged use.

This medication may suppress respiration, especially in the elderly, the very ill, and patients with respiratory problems. Lower doses may be required for these patients.

## Oral Dosage Forms

### DIFENOXIN HYDROCHLORIDE AND ATROPINE SULFATE TABLETS

**Usual adult and adolescent dose**
Antidiarrheal (antiperistaltic)—
Oral, the equivalent of difenoxin hydrochloride, 2 mg initially, then 1 mg after each loose stool or every three or four hours as needed.

**Usual adult prescribing limits**
Up to the equivalent of 8 mg of difenoxin hydrochloride daily.

**Usual pediatric dose**
Use is not recommended.

**Usual geriatric dose**
See *Usual adult and adolescent dose*.
Note: Geriatric patients may be more sensitive to the effects of the usual adult dose.

**Strength(s) usually available**
U.S.—
1 mg of difenoxin hydrochloride and 25 mcg (0.025 mg) of atropine sulfate (Rx) [*Motofen* (scored; calcium stearate; cellulose; lactose; corn starch)].
Canada—
Not commercially available.

**Packaging and storage**
Store below 40 °C (104 °F), preferably between 15 and 30 °C (59 and 86 °F), in a well-closed container, unless otherwise specified by manufacturer.

**Auxiliary labeling**
• May cause drowsiness.
• Avoid alcoholic beverages.
• Keep out of reach of children.
• May be habit-forming.

**Note**
Controlled substance in the U.S.

## Selected Bibliography
Binder HJ. Net fluid and electrolyte secretion: the pathophysiologic basis of diarrhea. In: Binder HJ, editor. Mechanism of intestinal secretion. New York: Alan R Liss Inc., 1979: 1-15.
Brownlee HJ, editor. Proceedings of a symposium: Management of acute nonspecific diarrhea. Am J Med 1990; 88 (Suppl 6A).

Revised: 07/15/94

# DIFENOXIN-CONTAINING COMBINATIONS—
Difenoxin and Atropine (Systemic)

# DIFLORASONE—See *Corticosteroids (Topical)*

# DIFLUCORTOLONE—See *Corticosteroids (Topical)*

# DIFLUNISAL—See *Anti-inflammatory Drugs, Nonsteroidal (Systemic)*

# DIGITALIS GLYCOSIDES    Systemic

This monograph includes information on the following: Digitoxin; Digoxin.

VA CLASSIFICATION (Primary/Secondary): CV050/CV300; CV900

Note: For a listing of dosage forms and brand names by country availability, see *Dosage Forms* section(s). For a listing of brand names for the articles in this monograph, refer to the General Index.

## Category
Antiarrhythmic; cardiotonic.

## Indications

### Accepted
Arrhythmias, cardiac (prophylaxis and treatment)—Digitalis glycosides are indicated for the control of ventricular response rates in atrial fibrillation and atrial flutter. Digitalis glycosides are also indicated for the control of paroxysmal atrioventricular (AV) nodal reentrant tachycardia; digitalis glycosides may convert paroxysmal AV nodal reentrant tachycardia to normal sinus rhythm.

Congestive heart failure (treatment)—Digitalis glycosides are indicated for the treatment of all degrees of congestive heart failure. They are generally most effective in "low output" failure associated with depressed left ventricular function and much less effective in "high output" failure (bronchopulmonary insufficiency, arteriovenous fistula, anemia, beriberi, infection, hyperthyroidism). Their positive inotropic action results in improved cardiac output and an improvement in the signs and symptoms of hemodynamic insufficiency such as dyspnea, edema, and/or venous congestion.

### Unaccepted
The use of digitalis glycosides in the treatment of obesity has been determined unwarranted and dangerous, since these drugs may cause potentially fatal arrhythmias or other adverse effects.

## Pharmacology/Pharmacokinetics

See *Table 1*, page 1204.

### Physicochemical characteristics
Molecular weight—
Digitoxin: 764.95.
Digoxin: 780.95.

### Mechanism of action/Effect
Two major actions are produced by therapeutic doses of digitalis glycosides—
(1) Force and velocity of myocardial contraction are increased (positive inotropic effect). This effect is thought to result from inhibition of movement of sodium and potassium ions across myocardial cell membranes by complexing with adenosine triphosphatase. As a result, there is enhancement of calcium influx and an augmented release of free calcium ions within the myocardial cells to subsequently potentiate the activity of the contractile muscle fibers of the heart.
(2) A decrease in the conduction rate and increase in the effective refractory period of the atrioventricular (AV) node is predominantly due to an indirect effect caused by enhancement of parasympathetic tone and decrease in sympathetic tone.

### Absorption
Digitoxin—Highly lipophilic; almost completely absorbed after oral administration.
Digoxin—Bioavailability is 60 to 80% (tablets), 70 to 85% (oral elixir or intramuscular injection), or 90 to 100% (capsules). The rate, but not the extent, of oral absorption is reduced when the tablets or capsules are taken after meals. In some patients, digoxin is converted to inactive products by colonic bacteria in the gut.

## Precautions to Consider

### Cross-sensitivity and/or related problems
Allergic reactions to a digitalis glycoside preparation occur rarely. Such reactions do not necessarily encompass all digitalis glycosides and therefore may not preclude the trial of another digitalis glycoside.

### Carcinogenicity
Studies have not been done.

### Pregnancy/Reproduction
Pregnancy—Studies have not been done in humans. Digitalis glycosides cross the placenta; at delivery the neonatal serum digoxin concentration is similar to the maternal concentration. Maternal dosage requirements of digitalis glycosides often increase in the final weeks of pregnancy.
Studies have not been done in animals.
FDA Pregnancy Category C.
Postpartum—Following delivery, and for up to 6 weeks thereafter, the maternal dosage often must be reduced to maintain acceptable serum concentrations.

### Breast-feeding
Digoxin is excreted in breast milk. The total amount received daily by the infant is estimated to be less than the usual daily maintenance dose. However, problems in humans have not been documented. It is not known whether digitoxin is excreted in breast milk.

### Pediatrics
Digitalis glycosides are a major cause of accidental poisoning in children. The tolerance of newborn infants to digitalis glycosides is variable, since their renal clearance of the medication is reduced. Premature and immature infants are especially sensitive. Dosage should be reduced and individualized according to the infant's degree of maturity, since renal clearance increases as the infant matures. Children older than 1 month of age generally require proportionally larger doses than adults on the basis of body weight or body surface area.

### Geriatrics
Appropriate studies on the relationship of age to the effects of digitalis glycosides have not been performed in the geriatric population. However, elderly patients are more likely to have age-related hepatic or renal function impairment, which may require lower doses of digitalis glycosides. In addition, elderly patients may also have a decreased volume of distribution for digitalis glycosides and electrolyte imbalances (e.g., hypokalemia), which may require lower doses of digitalis glycosides in order to avoid toxicity. (Digoxin clearance is less affected by hepatic function impairment, while digitoxin clearance is less affected by renal function impairment.)
Digoxin-induced loss of appetite is a significant risk in frail elderly patients.

### Dental
An increased gag reflex may increase the difficulty of taking a dental impression.

### Drug interactions and/or related problems
The following drug interactions and/or related problems have been selected on the basis of their potential clinical significance (possible mechanism in parentheses where appropriate)—not necessarily inclusive (» = major clinical significance):

Note: Combinations containing any of the following medications, depending on the amount present, may also interact with this medication.

» Amiodarone
   (amiodarone increases serum concentrations of digoxin and probably other digitalis glycosides, possibly to toxic levels; when amiodarone therapy is initiated, the digitalis glycoside should be withdrawn or the dose reduced by 50%; if digitalis glycoside therapy is continued, serum concentrations should be carefully monitored; amiodarone and digitalis glycosides may also produce additive effects on sinoatrial [SA] and atrioventricular [AV] nodes)

   Antacids
   (aluminum- and magnesium-containing antacids may inhibit absorption of digitalis glycosides, resulting in decreased plasma concentrations)

» Antiarrhythmics, other, including other digitalis preparations or
» Calcium salts, parenteral or
   Cocaine or
   Pancuronium or
   Rauwolfia alkaloids or
» Succinylcholine or
» Sympathomimetics
   (concurrent use with digitalis glycosides may increase the risk of cardiac arrhythmias; caution and close electrocardiographic [ECG] monitoring are very important if concurrent use is necessary)

» Antidiarrheal adsorbents (e.g., kaolin and pectin) or
» Cholestyramine or
» Colestipol or
   Dietary fiber, such as bran (large quantities) or
   Laxatives, bulk or

Neomycin, oral or
Sulfasalazine
>(concurrent use may inhibit digitalis glycosides absorption, resulting in decreased therapeutic effect of the glycoside; patients should be monitored closely for evidence of altered digitalis effect)

» Calcium channel blocking agents
>(serum digitalis glycoside concentrations may be increased during concurrent use, especially with verapamil and, to a lesser extent, diltiazem; nicardipine and nifedipine do not appear to have a significant effect. Concurrent use of digitalis glycosides with diltiazem and verapamil may result in excessive bradycardia because of additive depression of AV nodal conduction; nicardipine and nifedipine do not produce this effect. Digitalis glycoside dosage may need to be reduced and the patient carefully monitored for digitalis toxicity)

» Diuretics, potassium-depleting (such as bumetanide, ethacrynic acid, furosemide, indapamide, mannitol, or thiazides) or
» Hypokalemia-causing medications, other (See *Appendix II*)
>(hypokalemia caused by these medications may enhance the possibility of digitalis toxicity; frequent potassium determinations are recommended)

Edrophonium
>(when digitalis glycosides are used concurrently with edrophonium, the additive vagomimetic effects may cause excessive slowing of the heart rate)

Erythromycin
>(may increase absorption of digoxin by altering gastrointestinal flora that normally inactivate some digoxin prior to absorption)

Hepatic enzyme inducers (See *Appendix II*)
>(concurrent use may increase the metabolism of digitalis glycosides; may require dosage adjustment of digitalis glycosides, with the possible exception of digoxin)

Indomethacin
>(when indomethacin is administered concurrently with digitalis glycosides to the premature neonate, renal clearance of the digitalis glycoside may be decreased, leading to increased plasma concentrations, elimination half-lives, and risk of digitalis toxicity; it is recommended that digitalis dosage be reduced by 50% when indomethacin therapy is initiated and that further digitalis dosage adjustment be based on monitoring of ECG and digitalis concentration)

>(although not documented, the possibility should be considered that indomethacin may also increase digitalis concentration in adults and that digitalis dosage adjustment may be required)

» Magnesium sulfate, parenteral
>(parenteral magnesium sulfate must be administered with extreme caution in digitalized patients, especially if intravenous calcium salts are also employed; cardiac conduction changes and heart block may occur)

» Potassium salts
>(not recommended for concurrent use with digitalis glycosides in digitalized patients with severe or complete heart block; however, potassium supplements are often used to prevent or correct hypokalemia, especially when potassium-depleting diuretics such as the thiazides are administered concurrently with digitalis glycosides. Careful monitoring of serum potassium during use of supplemental potassium is extremely important in order to avoid hyperkalemia, which is very dangerous in digitalized patients)

» Propafenone
>(concurrent use with digoxin results in an increase in serum digoxin concentrations ranging from 35 to 85%, which appears to be unrelated to digoxin renal clearance but may be related to a decrease in volume of distribution and nonrenal clearance; careful monitoring of digoxin concentrations and dosage reduction of digoxin are recommended when propafenone is initiated; subsequent dosage adjustments should be based on serum digoxin concentrations)

» Quinidine or
Quinine
>(concurrent use may result in substantially increased serum concentrations of digoxin; studies with digitoxin indicate a similar change; serum concentrations should be monitored and dosage adjusted as indicated)

» Spironolactone
>(spironolactone may increase the half-life of digoxin; dosage reduction or increased dosing intervals of digoxin may be necessary and careful monitoring is recommended)

Succinylcholine
>(may cause sudden release of potassium from muscle cells, increasing the risk of digitalis-induced arrhythmias)

» Sucralfate
>(concurrent use with digoxin may decrease the absorption of digoxin; patients should be advised not to take sucralfate within 2 hours of digoxin)

Thallous chloride Tl 201
>(in animal studies, concurrent use of digitalis glycosides decreased myocardial uptake of thallous chloride Tl 201; human data are not available)

**Laboratory value alterations**
The following have been selected on the basis of their potential clinical significance (possible effect in parentheses where appropriate)—not necessarily inclusive (» = major clinical significance):

With diagnostic test results
Electrocardiogram
>(digitalis glycosides may produce false-positive ST-T changes during exercise testing)

**Medical considerations/Contraindications**
The medical considerations/contraindications included here have been selected on the basis of their potential clinical significance (reasons given in parentheses where appropriate)—not necessarily inclusive (» = major clinical significance).

*Except under special circumstances, these medications should not be used when the following medical problems exist:*
» Toxic effects present from prior administration of any digitalis preparation
» Ventricular fibrillation

*Risk-benefit should be considered when the following medical problems exist:*
*For all digitalis glycosides*
» Atrioventricular (AV) block, incomplete, especially in patients with Stokes-Adams attacks
>(may progress to complete block)
» Carotid sinus hypersensitivity
>(digitalis glycosides may cause an increase in vagal tone)
» Glomerulonephritis, acute, accompanied by heart failure
>(use of a low total daily dose is recommended, administered in divided doses, with constant ECG monitoring; use of antihypertensives and diuretics is also recommended and the digitalis glycoside should be withdrawn as soon as possible)
Hepatic function impairment, especially with digitoxin
>(reduced metabolism; dosage reduction may be necessary)
» Hypercalcemia or
» Hyperkalemia
>(increased risk of digitalis-induced arrhythmias, primarily heart block)
» Hypocalcemia
>(digitalis glycosides may be ineffective; administration of calcium may be necessary)
» Hypokalemia (including that resulting from drugs, dialysis, mechanical suction of gastrointestinal secretions, malnutrition, diarrhea, prolonged vomiting, old age, and long-standing heart failure) or
» Hypomagnesemia
>(increased risk of digitalis toxicity)
Hypothyroidism or
Hyperthyroidism
>(altered sensitivity to digitalis; hyperthyroid patients may be less sensitive to digitalis and require larger doses, while hypothyroid patients may be more sensitive and require smaller doses; dosage adjustment may be necessary as patients become euthyroid)
» Idiopathic hypertrophic subaortic stenosis
>(aggravated left ventricular outflow restrictions)
» Ischemic heart disease or
» Myocardial infarction, acute or
» Myocarditis, acute, including rheumatic carditis or viral myocarditis or
» Myxedema or
» Pulmonary disease, severe
>(increased sensitivity of the myocardium to the effects of digitalis glycosides and increased risk of digitalis-induced arrhythmias)
Pericarditis, chronic constrictive
>(patients may fail to respond to digitalis glycosides, and slowing of the heart rate may further reduce cardiac output)

» Premature ventricular contractions or
» Ventricular tachycardia
    (risk of exacerbation; digitalis glycosides should not be used unless congestive heart failure supervenes after a protracted episode not due to digitalis)
    Sensitivity to the digitalis glycoside prescribed
» Sick sinus syndrome
    (possible worsening of sinus bradycardia or sinoatrial [SA] block)
» Wolff-Parkinson-White syndrome, especially when associated with atrial fibrillation
    (possibility of fatal ventricular arrhythmias)
» Caution is also recommended in debilitated patients and patients using electronic cardiac pacemakers; these patients require careful dosage titration, as they may exhibit toxic responses at doses and serum concentrations generally tolerated by other patients.

*For digoxin only*
Renal function impairment
    (reduced excretion and potential toxicity; dosage reduction may be required; in addition, time to achieve a new or steady-state concentration is increased; although digitoxin excretion is also reduced, no dosage reduction is necessary because metabolism and half-life are not affected)

**Patient monitoring**
The following may be especially important in patient monitoring (other tests may be warranted in some patients, depending on condition; » = major clinical significance):
Cardioglycoside, steady-state, trough
    (serum concentrations may be required at periodic intervals, especially in patients with renal function impairment or if digitalis intoxication is suspected; toxicity to digitoxin and digoxin usually occurs at serum concentrations of > 35 and > 2 nanograms per mL, respectively. Individual tolerance and requirements vary; toxicity may occur with < 2 nanograms of digoxin per mL in some patients; others may require > 2 nanograms per mL for effective therapy. Digoxin-like immunoreactive substances have been reported to cause falsely increased serum digitalis glycoside concentration results, especially in infants and neonates, pregnant women, and in patients with hepatic or renal function impairment)
» Electrocardiogram (ECG) monitoring
    (recommended at periodic intervals; if paroxysmal atrial tachycardias with atrioventricular (AV) block or ventricular tachycardia occurs, the digitalis glycoside should be withdrawn and the patient's digitalization and electrolyte status should be evaluated)
Electrolyte, especially potassium, calcium, and magnesium concentrations, serum
    (recommended at periodic intervals, especially in patients also receiving diuretics, to detect possible electrolyte imbalance, which may increase the chance of digitalis toxicity, particularly with regard to arrhythmias, and may affect dosage requirements)
Hepatic function determinations and
Renal function determinations
    (recommended at periodic intervals)
Pulse (apical) check
    (recommended at periodic intervals, especially in patients with atrial fibrillation or when dosage change is made; dosage alteration may be necessary if the pulse rate falls below 60 beats per minute)

## Side/Adverse Effects

Note: Some side/adverse affects, including nausea and vomiting and some arrhythmias, may also be symptoms of toxicity. If there is any doubt about the cause of these symptoms, the digitalis glycoside should be withdrawn until the cause is determined.

The first signs of toxicity in infants and small children are usually cardiac arrhythmias, while in adults and older children, the first symptoms of overdose may be stomach upset, abdominal pain, loss of appetite, or unusually slow heart rate.

In adults, the most common arrhythmia is premature ventricular beats (extrasystoles); paroxysmal and nonparoxysmal nodal rhythms, atrioventricular (AV) (interference) dissociation, and paroxysmal atrial tachycardia with block are also common; increasing AV block may occur; death may occur from ventricular fibrillation. In children, premature ventricular systoles are rare, while nodal and atrial systoles are more frequent; atrial arrhythmias, atrial ectopic rhythms, and paroxysmal atrial tachycardia (particularly with AV block) are more common; ventricular arrhythmias are rare. An increase in PR interval may occur in newborns.

The following side/adverse effects have been selected on the basis of their potential clinical significance (possible signs and symptoms in parentheses where appropriate)—not necessarily inclusive:

**Those indicating need for medical attention**
Incidence rare
    *Allergic reaction* (skin rash or hives)
Signs and/or symptoms of toxicity or intolerance (in order of occurrence)
    *Stimulation of medullary centers* (loss of appetite; nausea or vomiting); *lower stomach pain; diarrhea; electrolyte imbalance, possible* (unusual tiredness or weakness, extreme); *slow or irregular heartbeat*—may be fast heartbeat in children; *blurred vision or other visual disturbances such as colored halos seen around objects*—"yellow," "green," or "white vision"; *drowsiness; confusion or mental depression; headache; fainting*

Note: Large doses may also have a local irritating emetic action.

## Overdose

For more information on the management of overdose or unintentional ingestion, **contact a Poison Control Center** (see *Poison Control Center Listing*).

**Treatment of overdose**
Discontinuation of digitalis medication is often all that is required if symptoms are not severe and occur near the expected time for peak medication effect.

Administration of activated charcoal, cholestyramine, or colestipol may be useful to accelerate clearance of the glycoside.

Potassium salts may be administered if hypokalemia is present and renal function is adequate, but should not be used if hyperkalemia or complete heart block exists unless those conditions are related primarily to supraventricular tachycardia.

For correction of hypokalemia, potassium may be administered:
Orally in divided doses—
    Adults: 40 to 80 mEq (mmol).
    Children: 1 to 1.5 mEq (mmol) per kg of body weight.
Intravenously when correction is urgent—
    Adults: 40 to 80 mEq (mmol) (diluted to 40 mEq [mmol] per 500 mL of 5% dextrose injection) at a rate not exceeding 20 mEq (mmol) per hour and adjusted as indicated by monitoring.
    Children: 1 to 1.5 mEq (mmol) per kg of body weight (diluted in appropriate volume of 5% dextrose injection for patient size) at a rate not exceeding 0.5 mEq (mmol) per kg of body weight per hour and adjusted as indicated by monitoring.

Other agents that have been used to correct arrhythmias caused by digitalis toxicity are lidocaine, procainamide, propranolol, and phenytoin. Ventricular pacing may be temporarily beneficial in cases of advanced heart block.

A chelating agent (e.g., EDTA) may be useful to bind calcium for treatment of arrhythmias caused by digitalis toxicity, hypokalemia, or hypercalcemia.

For life-threatening digoxin or digitoxin overdose—Intravenous administration of digoxin immune Fab (ovine) through a membrane filter. A vial containing 40 mg of digoxin immune Fab (ovine) will bind approximately 0.6 mg of digoxin or digitoxin. See the package insert or *Digoxin Immune Fab (Ovine) (Systemic)* for specific dosing guidelines and precautions in use of the product.

## Patient Consultation

As an aid to patient consultation, refer to *Advice for the Patient, Digitalis Medicines (Systemic)*.

In providing consultation, consider emphasizing the following selected information (» = major clinical significance):

**Before using this medication**
» Conditions affecting use, especially:
    Sensitivity to the digitalis glycoside prescribed
    Pregnancy—Cross placenta
    Use in children—Infant responses vary; careful dosage adjustment required
    Use in the elderly—Increased sensitivity to effects
    Other medications, especially potassium-depleting diuretics or other hypokalemia-causing medications, amiodarone, other antiarrhythmics, sympathomimetics, antidiarrheal adsorbents, calcium channel blocking agents, cholestyramine, colestipol, potassium-containing medications or supplements, quinidine, spironolactone, or sucralfate
    Other medical problems, especially severe pulmonary disease, conduction disturbance, ventricular arrhythmias, ischemic heart disease, recent myocardial infarction, or myocarditis

## Proper use of this medication

» Compliance with therapy; taking exactly as directed, not taking more or less

Proper administration of elixir: Taking orally; special dropper to be used for accurate measuring

Taking medication at the same time each day to help increase compliance

Checking apical pulse as directed (checking with physician if less than 60 beats per minute)

» Proper dosing

Missed dose: Taking as soon as remembered if within 12 hours of scheduled dose; not taking if remembered later; not doubling doses; checking with doctor if dose missed for 2 days or more

» Proper storage

## Precautions while using this medication

Regular visits to physician to check progress

» Checking with physician before discontinuing medication
» Keeping medication out of reach of children
» Reporting to physician any nausea, vomiting, diarrhea, loss of appetite, or extremely slow pulse as possible signs of overdose
» Caution if medical or dental surgery or emergency treatment is required

Carrying medical identification card

» Avoiding other medications unless prescribed by physician

Caution in using medications of similar appearance

## Side/adverse effects

Signs of potential side effects, especially allergic reaction, and signs and symptoms of overdose

## General Dosing Information

Recommended doses are averages only; each dose must be adjusted to meet the individual patient's requirements.

Before a loading dose of a digitalis preparation is administered, it is extremely important to determine whether the patient has taken any form of digitalis during the previous 2 or 3 weeks, since some residual effect may require a reduced dosage to avoid toxicity.

Dosage calculations should be based on ideal (lean) body weight, since digitalis glycosides are not taken up by adipose tissue.

Digoxin may be the preferred cardioglycoside in some patients with liver function impairment because it does not undergo extensive hepatic metabolism.

Reduction of digitalis glycoside dosage prior to cardioversion may be desirable to avoid induction of ventricular arrhythmias; however, the benefit must be weighed against the risk of rapid increase in ventricular response to atrial fibrillation if the digitalis glycoside is withheld 1 to 2 days prior to cardioversion. If digitalis glycoside toxicity is suspected, electrical cardioversion of arrhythmias should be delayed, if possible. When it is considered absolutely necessary, use of the lowest possible energy level and/or pretreatment with lidocaine is recommended.

## For parenteral dosage forms only

The intravenous route is preferred when parenteral administration is indicated. Intramuscular use involves greater local discomfort, slower effect, and erratic bioavailability. Intravenous injections should be administered over a period of at least 5 minutes.

Intramuscular injections are used only when the oral or intravenous routes cannot be used. The injection should be administered deeply into the muscle and preferably should not exceed 2 mL at any one injection site. Following the injection, each site should be massaged well to reduce painful local reactions.

When a patient is transferred from a parenteral digitalis glycoside to an oral digitalis dosage form, dosage adjustments may be necessary to compensate for the pharmacokinetic differences among the medications. One exception is the transfer from digoxin injection to the liquid-filled, soft capsules of digoxin, because both dosage forms have the same bioavailability.

---

### *DIGITOXIN*

## Summary of Differences

Pharmacology/pharmacokinetics:

Hepatically metabolized; renal excretion of inactive metabolites has little effect on digitoxin action.

Protein binding—Very high.

Half-life—120 to 216 hours.

Onset of action—1 to 4 hours.

Time to peak effect—8 to 14 hours.

Duration of action—Approximately 14 days.

Precautions:

Medical considerations/Contraindications—Dosage reduction not necessary in renal function impairment.

## Oral Dosage Forms

### DIGITOXIN TABLETS USP

**Usual adult dose**

Antiarrhythmic or

Cardiotonic—

Digitalization:

Rapid—Oral, 600 mcg (0.6 mg) initially, then 400 mcg (0.4 mg) after four to six hours and 200 mcg (0.2 mg) after another four-to six-hour period, followed by a daily maintenance dose as needed and tolerated, or

Slow—Oral, 200 mcg (0.2 mg) two times a day for four days, followed by a daily maintenance dose as needed and tolerated.

Maintenance:

Oral, 50 to 300 mcg (0.05 to 0.3 mg) once a day, the dosage being adjusted as needed and tolerated.

Note: Geriatric patients, debilitated patients, and patients using electronic cardiac pacemakers require careful dosage titration, as they may exhibit toxic responses at doses and serum concentrations generally tolerated by other patients.

**Usual adult prescribing limits**

Digitalization—Up to a total of 1.6 mg over one or two days.

**Usual pediatric dose**

Prepared oral digitoxin dosage forms are limited and may not be suitable for small children. Other digitalis glycosides may be considered.

**Strength(s) usually available**

U.S.—

100 mcg (0.1 mg) (Rx) [*Crystodigin* (scored); GENERIC].

200 mcg (0.2 mg) (Rx) [GENERIC].

Canada—

100 mcg (0.1 mg) (Rx) [*Digitaline*].

**Packaging and storage**

Store below 40 °C (104 °F), preferably between 15 and 30 °C (59 and 86 °F), unless otherwise specified by manufacturer. Store in a well-closed container.

**Auxiliary labeling**

• Keep out of reach of children.
• Do not take other medicines without advice from your doctor.

---

### *DIGOXIN*

## Summary of Differences

Pharmacology/pharmacokinetics:

Bioavailability—60 to 80% (tablets), 70 to 85% (oral elixir or intramuscular injection), or 90 to 100% (capsules).

Protein binding—Low.

Biotransformation—Minimal hepatic metabolism; excretion and half-life determined by renal function.

Half-life—36 to 48 hours.

Onset of action—5 to 30 minutes (intravenous) or 30 minutes to 2 hours (oral).

Time to peak effect—1 to 4 hours (intravenous) or 2 to 6 hours (oral).

Duration of action—Approximately 6 days.

Precautions:

Medical considerations/Contraindications—Dosage reduction may be required in renal function impairment.

## Additional Dosing Information

**Bioequivalence information**

Bioavailability differences exist among dosage forms of digoxin. Changing therapy from one dosage form to another may require dosage adjustments. A 100-mcg (0.1-mg) dose of the injection or of the digoxin-solution capsule is bioequivalent to a 125-mcg (0.125-mg) dose of the tablet or elixir.

For digoxin tablets—

Variability in the bioavailability of digoxin tablets was recognized as a clinical problem in the early 1970's. These differences in bioavailability were reported among different brands of digoxin tablets as well as among different lots of digoxin tablets produced by the same manufacturer. In response to the problems of bio-inequivalence, official dissolution standards were established. Problems have not been reported following establishment of these standards. However, because bioavailability from any digoxin tablet is incomplete ($\le$ 80%), clinicians should consider this as a possible source of the problem when unexplained difficulty is encountered in the digitalization or maintenance therapy of patients with digoxin tablets.

# Oral Dosage Forms
## DIGOXIN CAPSULES
### Usual adult dose
Antiarrhythmic or
Cardiotonic—
  Digitalization:
    Rapid—Oral, initially, 400 to 600 mcg (0.4 to 0.6 mg) with additional doses of 100 to 300 mcg (0.1 to 0.3 mg) administered every six to eight hours as needed and tolerated until the desired effect is clinically evident.
    Slow—Oral, a total of 50 to 350 mcg (0.05 to 0.35 mg) per day *divided* and administered in two doses, the dosage being repeated for seven to twenty-two days as needed to reach steady-state serum concentrations.
  Maintenance:
    Oral, 50 to 350 mcg (0.05 to 0.35 mg) administered as one or two doses per day as needed and tolerated.
Note: Patients with impaired renal function, geriatric patients, debilitated patients, and patients using electronic cardiac pacemakers require careful dosage titration, as they may exhibit toxic responses at doses and serum concentrations generally tolerated by other patients.

### Usual pediatric dose
Antiarrhythmic or
Cardiotonic—
  Digitalization:
    The following total amounts *divided* into three or more doses, with the initial portion representing approximately one-half the total, doses then being administered every four to eight hours.
    Premature neonates—
      Oral, 15 to 25 mcg (0.015 to 0.025 mg) per kg of body weight.
    Full-term neonates—
      Oral, 20 to 30 mcg (0.02 to 0.03 mg) per kg of body weight.
    Infants 1 month to 2 years of age—
      Oral, 30 to 50 mcg (0.03 to 0.05 mg) per kg of body weight.
    Children 2 to 5 years of age—
      Oral, 25 to 35 mcg (0.025 to 0.035 mg) per kg of body weight.
    Children 5 to 10 years of age—
      Oral, 15 to 30 mcg (0.015 to 0.03 mg) per kg of body weight.
    Children over 10 years of age—
      Oral, 8 to 12 mcg (0.008 to 0.012 mg) per kg of body weight.
  Maintenance:
    Premature neonates: Oral, 20 to 30% of the total digitalizing dose, divided and administered in two or three equal portions per day.
    Full-term neonates, infants, and children up to 10 years of age: Oral, 25 to 35% of the total digitalizing dose, divided and administered in two or three equal portions per day.
    Children 10 years of age and over: Oral, 25 to 35% of the total digitalizing dose administered once a day.
Note: In small children (especially premature and immature infants), careful titration of dosage is required with close monitoring of patient's serum concentrations and ECG readings.

### Strength(s) usually available
U.S.—
  50 mcg (0.05 mg) (Rx) [*Lanoxicaps* (ethyl alcohol 8%)].
  100 mcg (0.1 mg) (Rx) [*Lanoxicaps* (ethyl alcohol 8%)].
  200 mcg (0.2 mg) (Rx) [*Lanoxicaps* (ethyl alcohol 8%)].
  Note: Digoxin capsules consist of a stable digoxin solution enclosed in a soft gelatin capsule.
Canada—
  Not commercially available.

### Packaging and storage
Store between 15 and 30 °C (59 and 86 °F) unless otherwise specified by manufacturer. Store in a tight container.

### Auxiliary labeling
- Keep out of reach of children.
- Keep container tightly closed.
- Do not take other medicines without advice from your doctor.

### Note
When patients are switched from digoxin tablets to digoxin capsules, or vice versa, the difference in bioavailability must be kept in mind.

## DIGOXIN ELIXIR USP
### Usual adult dose
Digitalization:
  Rapid: Oral, a total of 0.75 to 1.25 mg *divided* into two or more doses, each then being administered every six to eight hours.
  Slow: Oral, 125 to 500 mcg (0.125 to 0.5 mg) once a day for seven days.
Maintenance:
  Oral, 125 to 500 mcg (0.125 to 0.5 mg) once a day.
Note: Patients with impaired renal function, geriatric patients, debilitated patients, and patients using electronic cardiac pacemakers require careful dosage titration, as they may exhibit toxic responses at doses and serum concentrations generally tolerated by other patients.

### Usual pediatric dose
Digitalization:
  The following total amounts *divided* into two or more doses, administered at six- to eight-hour intervals:
  Premature and newborn infants up to 1 month of age—
    Oral, 20 to 35 mcg (0.02 to 0.035 mg) per kg of body weight.
  Infants 1 month to 2 years of age—
    Oral, 35 to 60 mcg (0.035 to 0.06 mg) per kg of body weight.
  Children 2 to 5 years of age—
    Oral, 30 to 40 mcg (0.03 to 0.04 mg) per kg of body weight.
  Children 5 to 10 years of age—
    Oral, 20 to 35 mcg (0.02 to 0.035 mg) per kg of body weight.
  Children over 10 years of age—
    Rapid: Oral, a total of 0.75 to 1.25 mg *divided* into two or more doses, each then being administered every six to eight hours.
    Slow: Oral, 125 to 500 mcg (0.125 to 0.5 mg) once a day for seven days.
Maintenance:
  Oral, one-fifth to one-third of the total digitalizing dose administered once a day.
Note: Alternative pediatric dosage (the "small-dose" method)—Oral, 17 mcg (0.017 mg) per kg of body weight per day. This dosage method has the advantage of easier control and therefore less chance for toxicity.
  In small children (especially premature and immature infants) careful titration of dosage is required with close monitoring of patient's serum concentrations and ECG readings.

### Strength(s) usually available
U.S.—
  50 mcg (0.05 mg) per mL (Rx) [*Lanoxin* (alcohol 10%); GENERIC].
Canada—
  50 mcg (0.05 mg) per mL (Rx) [*Lanoxin* (alcohol 11.5%; tartrazine)].

### Packaging and storage
Store below 40 °C (104 °F), preferably between 15 and 30 °C (59 and 86 °F), unless otherwise specified by manufacturer. Store in a tight container.

### Auxiliary labeling
- Keep out of reach of children.
- Keep container tightly closed.
- Do not take other medicines without advice from your doctor.

## DIGOXIN TABLETS USP
Note: Variability in the bioavailability of digoxin tablets was recognized as a clinical problem in the early 1970's. These differences in bioavailability were reported among different brands of digoxin tablets as well as among different lots of digoxin tablets produced by the same manufacturer. In response to the problems of bio-inequivalence, official dissolution standards were established. Problems have not been reported following establishment of these standards. However, because bioavailability from any digoxin tablet is incomplete ($\le$ 80%), clinicians should consider this as a possible source of the problem when unexplained difficulty is encountered in the digitalization or maintenance therapy of patients with digoxin tablets.

**Usual adult dose**

Digitalization:

Rapid: Oral, a total of 0.75 to 1.25 mg *divided* into two or more doses, each then being administered every six to eight hours.

Slow: Oral, 125 to 500 mcg (0.125 to 0.5 mg) once a day for seven days.

Maintenance:

Oral, 125 to 500 mcg (0.125 to 0.5 mg) once a day.

Note: Patients with impaired renal function, geriatric patients, debilitated patients, and patients using electronic cardiac pacemakers require careful dosage titration, as they may exhibit toxic responses at doses and serum concentrations generally tolerated by other patients.

**Usual pediatric dose**

Digitalization:

The following total amounts *divided* into two or more doses, administered at six- to eight-hour intervals:

Premature and newborn infants up to 1 month of age—

Oral, 20 to 35 mcg (0.02 to 0.035 mg) per kg of body weight.

Infants 1 month to 2 years of age—

Oral, 35 to 60 mcg (0.035 to 0.06 mg) per kg of body weight.

Children 2 to 5 years of age—

Oral, 30 to 40 mcg (0.03 to 0.04 mg) per kg of body weight.

Children 5 to 10 years of age—

Oral, 20 to 35 mcg (0.02 to 0.035 mg) per kg of body weight.

Children over 10 years of age—

Rapid: Oral, a total of 0.75 to 1.25 mg *divided* into two or more doses, each then being administered every six to eight hours.

Slow: Oral, 125 to 500 mcg (0.125 to 0.5 mg) once a day for seven days.

Maintenance:

Oral, one-fifth to one-third of the total digitalizing dose administered once a day.

Note: Alternative pediatric dosage (the "small-dose" method)—Oral, 17 mcg (0.017 mg) per kg of body weight per day. This dosage method has the advantage of easier control and therefore less chance for toxicity.

In small children (especially premature and immature infants) careful titration of dosage is required with close monitoring of patient's serum concentrations and ECG readings.

**Strength(s) usually available**

U.S.—

125 mcg (0.125 mg) (Rx) [*Lanoxin* (scored); GENERIC].

250 mcg (0.25 mg) (Rx) [*Lanoxin* (scored); GENERIC].

500 mcg (0.5 mg) (Rx) [*Lanoxin* (scored)].

Canada—

62.5 mcg (0.0625 mg) (Rx) [*Lanoxin*].

125 mcg (0.125 mg) (Rx) [*Lanoxin* (scored)].

250 mcg (0.25 mg) (Rx) [*Lanoxin* (scored)].

**Packaging and storage**

Store below 40 °C (104 °F), preferably between 15 and 30 °C (59 and 86 °F), unless otherwise specified by manufacturer. Store in a tight container.

**Auxiliary labeling**

- Keep out of reach of children.
- Do not take other medicines without advice from your doctor.

**Note**

Caution—The small, white tablets of digoxin 0.25 mg have been confused by numerous patients with other, similar-looking medications such as furosemide, with resultant serious dosage accidents. To reduce this hazard, the dispenser may:

—check with the prescriber; suggest digoxin capsules be used instead of tablets.

—caution the patient about the potential hazard.

—apply auxiliary "Heart medicine" labels to digoxin tablet container.

—use containers of different size or appearance for similar-looking medications.

—suggest that patient not use tablets from both containers at same time.

—suggest that patient never transfer digoxin from original to other containers.

—suggest that patient use separate storage areas for medications that look alike.

When patients are being switched from digoxin capsules to digoxin tablets, or vice versa, the difference in bioavailability must be kept in mind.

## Parenteral Dosage Forms

### DIGOXIN INJECTION USP

**Usual adult dose**

Digitalization—Intravenous, initially, 400 to 600 mcg (0.4 to 0.6 mg) with additional doses of 100 to 300 mcg (0.1 to 0.3 mg) administered every four to eight hours as needed and tolerated until the desired effect is clinically evident.

Maintenance—Intravenous, 125 to 500 mcg (0.125 to 0.5 mg) per day in divided doses or as a single dose.

Note: Patients with impaired renal function, geriatric patients, debilitated patients, and patients using electronic cardiac pacemakers require careful dosage titration, as they may exhibit toxic responses at doses and serum concentrations generally tolerated by other patients.

**Usual pediatric dose**

Digitalization:

The following total amounts *divided* into three or more doses, with the initial portion representing approximately one-half the total, doses then being administered every four to eight hours:

Premature neonates—

Intravenous, 15 to 25 mcg (0.015 to 0.025 mg) per kg of body weight.

Full-term neonates—

Intravenous, 20 to 30 mcg (0.02 to 0.03 mg) per kg of body weight.

Infants 1 month to 2 years of age—

Intravenous, 30 to 50 mcg (0.03 to 0.05 mg) per kg of body weight.

Children 2 to 5 years of age—

Intravenous, 25 to 35 mcg (0.025 to 0.035 mg) per kg of body weight.

Children 5 to 10 years of age—

Intravenous, 15 to 30 mcg (0.015 to 0.03 mg) per kg of body weight.

Children over 10 years of age—

Intravenous, 8 to 12 mcg (0.008 to 0.012 mg) per kg of body weight.

Maintenance (begun within 24 hours after digitalization):

Premature neonates—Intravenous, 20 to 30% of the total digitalizing dose, divided and administered in two or three equal portions per day.

Full-term neonates, infants, and children up to 10 years of age—Intravenous, 25 to 35% of the total digitalizing dose, divided and administered in two or three equal portions per day.

Children over 10 years of age—Intravenous, 25 to 35% of the total digitalizing dose administered once a day.

Note: In small children (especially premature and immature infants) careful titration of dosage is required with close monitoring of patient's serum concentrations and ECG readings.

If parenteral administration is necessary and the intravenous route is not possible, the intravenous dose may be given by the intramuscular route, although this is quite painful and has inconsistent absorption.

**Strength(s) usually available**

U.S.—

100 mcg (0.1 mg) per mL (Rx) [*Lanoxin* (alcohol 10%)].

250 mcg (0.25 mg) per mL (Rx) [*Lanoxin* (alcohol 10%); GENERIC].

Canada—

50 mcg (0.05 mg) per mL (Rx) [*Lanoxin* (alcohol 10%)].

250 mcg (0.25 mg) per mL (Rx) [*Lanoxin* (alcohol 10%)].

**Packaging and storage**

Store below 40 °C (104 °F), preferably between 15 and 30 °C (59 and 86 °F), unless otherwise specified by manufacturer. Protect from freezing.

**Preparation of dosage form**

Digoxin Injection USP may be administered undiluted or may be diluted with a 4-fold or greater volume (to reduce the risk of precipitation) of sterile water for injection, 0.9% sodium chloride injection, or 5% dextrose injection for intravenous administration.

**Stability**

Do not use if markedly discolored or if a precipitate is present. Immediate use of diluted Digoxin Injection USP is recommended.

## Selected Bibliography

Epstein FH. Digitalis. Mechanisms of action and clinical use. N Engl J Med 1988 Feb 11; 318: 358-65.

Revised: 03/10/93
Interim revision: 04/25/95; 08/15/95

---

**DIGITOXIN**—See *Digitalis Glycosides (Systemic)*

---

**DIGOXIN**—See *Digitalis Glycosides (Systemic)*

---

## Table 1. Pharmacology/Pharmacokinetics

| Drug and Route | Protein Binding | Biotransformation | Half-life (hr) | Onset of Action | Time to Peak Effect (hr) | Therapeutic Serum Concentration (nanograms/mL) | Duration of Action (approx. days) | Elimination* |
|---|---|---|---|---|---|---|---|---|
| Digitoxin Oral | Very high (>90%) | Hepatic | 120–216 | 1–4 hr | 8–14 | 13–25 | 14 | Renal (metabolites) |
| Digoxin IV Oral | Low (20–25%) | Hepatic (slight) | 36–48 (4–6 days in anuria) | 5–30 min ¹/₂–2 hr | 1–4 2–6 | 0.5–2.0 | 6 6 | Renal (50–70% unchanged)† |

*Digitalis glycosides are not effectively removed from the body by dialysis, exchange transfusion, or cardiopulmonary bypass.
†The breast milk to plasma ratio of digoxin administered to breast-feeding women is 0.6 to 0.9.

---

# DIGOXIN IMMUNE FAB (OVINE)    Systemic

VA CLASSIFICATION (Primary): AD900

Note: For a listing of dosage forms and brand names by country availability, see *Dosage Forms* section(s). For a listing of brand names for the articles in this monograph, refer to the General Index.

## Category

Antidote, to digitalis glycoside toxicity.

## Indications

### Accepted

Toxicity, digitalis glycoside (treatment)—Digoxin immune Fab (ovine) is indicated for treatment of potentially life-threatening digoxin or digitoxin overdose (i.e., with severe arrhythmias or hyperkalemia).

## Pharmacology/Pharmacokinetics

### Physicochemical characteristics

Source—Produced by a process involving immunization of sheep with digoxin that has been coupled as a hapten to human serum albumin, to stimulate production of digoxin-specific antibodies. After papain digestion of the antibody, digoxin-specific antigen binding (Fab) fragments (molecular weight 46,200 daltons) are isolated and purified by affinity chromatography.
Molecular weight—46,200.

### Mechanism of action/Effect

Preferentially binds molecules of digoxin or digitoxin, and the complex is then excreted by the kidneys. As free serum digoxin is removed, tissue-bound digoxin is also released into the serum to maintain the equilibrium and is bound and removed by digoxin immune Fab. The net result is a reduction in serum and tissue digoxin.

### Half-life

15 to 20 hours.

### Onset of action

Reduction of free active serum digoxin or digitoxin—Less than 1 minute.
Improvement in signs and symptoms of digitalis toxicity—15 to 30 minutes after administration (reversal of inotropic effect is usually slower than reversal of arrhythmias and hyperkalemia and may take several hours).

### Elimination

Renal.

## Precautions to Consider

### Cross-sensitivity and/or related problems

Patients sensitive to sheep or any product of ovine origin may be sensitive to digoxin immune Fab (ovine) also.

### Carcinogenicity

Studies have not been done in either animals or humans.

### Pregnancy/Reproduction

Pregnancy—Studies have not been done in humans.
Studies have not been done in animals.

FDA Pregnancy Category C.

### Breast-feeding

It is not known whether digoxin immune Fab (ovine) passes into breast milk. Problems in humans have not been documented.

### Pediatrics

Studies performed to date have not demonstrated pediatrics-specific problems that would limit the usefulness of digoxin immune Fab (ovine) in children.

### Geriatrics

No information is available on the relationship of age to the effects of digoxin immune Fab (ovine) in geriatric patients. However, elderly patients are more likely to have age-related renal function impairment, which may require caution in patients receiving this medication.

### Laboratory value alterations

The following have been selected on the basis of their potential clinical significance (possible effect in parentheses where appropriate)—not necessarily inclusive (» = major clinical significance):

With diagnostic test results
  Digitalis concentration determinations by immunoassay
    (may be interfered with)

With physiology/laboratory test values
  Digoxin or digitoxin concentrations, serum
    (free active concentrations rapidly fall to undetectable levels)

    (total serum concentrations rise suddenly after administration of Fab antibody but are almost totally bound to the Fab fragment and are inactive; these concentrations decline to undetectable levels several days later as Fab-digoxin complexes are excreted)

  Potassium concentrations, serum
    (may decrease rapidly from high concentrations associated with digitalis toxicity)

### Medical considerations/Contraindications

The medical considerations/contraindications included here have been selected on the basis of their potential clinical significance (reasons given in parentheses where appropriate)—not necessarily inclusive (» = major clinical significance).

*Risk-benefit should be considered when the following medical problems exist:*

Allergy, history of
    (risk of allergic reaction to Fab antibody may be increased)

Renal function impairment
(elimination of Fab-digoxin complexes may be delayed since the complex is eliminated renally. In patients who are functionally anephric, glomerular filtration and renal excretion would not be expected to occur; instead, the complex may be eliminated by the reticuloendothelial system; because it is not clear whether reintoxication would result, prolonged monitoring for digitalis toxicity is recommended in these patients)
» Sensitivity to digoxin immune Fab (ovine)

**Patient monitoring**
The following may be especially important in patient monitoring (other tests may be warranted in some patients, depending on condition; » = major clinical significance):

Body temperature and
Electrocardiogram (ECG)
(monitoring recommended during treatment)
» Digoxin or digitoxin concentrations, serum
(recommended prior to administration of Fab antibody to aid in dosage calculation, but not useful for at least 5 to 7 days after Fab antibody treatment is begun because of interference by the antibody with the test)
» Potassium concentrations, serum
(recommended at frequent intervals during treatment; hypokalemia should be treated promptly)

## Side/Adverse Effects

Allergic or febrile reactions to digoxin immune Fab (ovine) have been reported rarely. Patients previously treated with the product or allergic to ovine proteins appear to be especially at risk.

Side/adverse effects are related more to withdrawal of digitalis effects than to a direct effect of the antibody fragment. Low cardiac output, including congestive heart failure, may be exacerbated as a result of withdrawal of the inotropic effects of digitalis. Ventricular rate may increase as a result of withdrawal of digitalis being used for atrial fibrillation. Hypokalemia may occur as elevated serum potassium concentrations fall rapidly.

## General Dosing Information

It is recommended that equipment and medications necessary for cardio-pulmonary resuscitation be immediately available during administration of digoxin immune Fab (ovine). If necessary, in patients who respond poorly to withdrawal of digoxin's inotropic effect, other intravenous inotropes such as dopamine or dobutamine or cardiac load–reducing agents may be used. Caution is necessary in use of catecholamines because of the risk of aggravation of digitalis toxicity–associated arrhythmias.

Skin-testing for allergy to digoxin immune Fab (ovine) may be performed prior to administration in high-risk patients (i.e., those previously treated with the Fab antibody or with known allergy, especially to sheep proteins). One of two methods may be used:
• Intradermal test: Dilute 0.1 mL of the reconstituted solution (containing 9.5 mg of the Fab antibody per mL) in 9.9 mL of 0.9% sodium chloride injection to produce 10 mL of a solution containing 95 mcg (0.095 mg) per mL; then inject 0.1 mL (9.5 mcg or 0.0095 mg) intradermally. After 20 minutes, inspect the injection site for presence of an urticarial wheal surrounded by a zone of erythema.
• Scratch test: Dilute 0.1 mL of the reconstituted solution (containing 9.5 mg of the Fab antibody per mL) in 9.9 mL of 0.9% sodium chloride injection to produce 10 mL of a solution containing 95 mcg (0.095 mg) per mL; then place 1 drop of the solution on the skin and make a 1/4-inch scratch through the drop with a sterile needle. After 20 minutes, inspect the site for presence of an urticarial wheal surrounded by a zone of erythema.
If a positive skin test occurs, use of digoxin immune Fab (ovine) should be avoided unless absolutely necessary.
If a systemic reaction occurs, measures to treat anaphylaxis should be used.

After reconstitution, digoxin immune Fab (ovine) is administered by intravenous infusion, through a 0.22-micron membrane filter, over 30 minutes. However, it may be given by rapid direct intravenous injection if cardiac arrest is imminent.

Redigitalization of the patient, if necessary, should be delayed until elimination of Fab fragments from the body is complete, usually after several days but may be up to a week or longer in patients with renal function impairment.

## Parenteral Dosage Forms

### DIGOXIN IMMUNE FAB (OVINE) FOR INJECTION

**Usual adult and adolescent dose**
Antidote, to digitalis glycoside toxicity—
Intravenous, in an amount equimolar to the amount of digoxin or digitoxin in the patient's body (total body load [TBL]). A dose of 38 mg of digoxin immune Fab (ovine) binds approximately 0.5 mg of digoxin or digitoxin.
Dosage may be calculated using one of the following formulas:
1) Based on dose of digoxin or digitoxin ingested:
For digoxin tablets, oral solution, or intramuscular injection—
$$\text{Dose (mg)} = (\text{Dose ingested [mg]} \times 0.8)/0.5 \times 38$$
For digitoxin tablets, digoxin capsules, or intravenous injection of digoxin or digitoxin—
$$\text{Dose (mg)} = [\text{Dose ingested (mg)}/0.5] \times 38$$

Table 1. Approximate dose of digoxin immune Fab (ovine) when amount of digoxin ingested is known.

| Number of digoxin tablets or capsules ingested* | Dose of digoxin immune Fab (ovine) | |
|---|---|---|
| | mg | Number of 38-mg vials |
| 25 | 380 | 10 |
| 50 | 760 | 20 |
| 75 | 1140 | 30 |
| 100 | 1520 | 40 |
| 150 | 2280 | 60 |
| 200 | 3040 | 80 |

*0.25-mg tablets with 80% bioavailability, or 0.2-mg capsules.
2) Based on steady-state serum digoxin or digitoxin concentration (SDC):
For digoxin—
$$\text{Dose (mg)} = (\text{SDC [nanograms/mL]} \times \text{body weight [kg]})/100 \times 38$$
For digitoxin—
$$\text{Dose (mg)} = (\text{SDC [nanograms/mL]} \times \text{body weight [kg]})/1000 \times 38$$

Table 2. Approximate *adult and adolescent* dose (number of 38-mg vials) of digoxin immune Fab (ovine) when serum digoxin concentration (SDC) is known.

| SDC (ng/mL) | Patient weight (kg) | | | | |
|---|---|---|---|---|---|
| | 40 | 60 | 70 | 80 | 100 |
| 1 | 0.5 | 0.5 | 1 | 1 | 1 |
| 2 | 1 | 1 | 2 | 2 | 2 |
| 4 | 2 | 3 | 3 | 3 | 4 |
| 8 | 3 | 5 | 6 | 7 | 8 |
| 12 | 5 | 7 | 9 | 10 | 12 |
| 16 | 7 | 10 | 11 | 13 | 16 |
| 20 | 8 | 12 | 14 | 16 | 20 |

Note: Dosage of digoxin immune Fab (ovine) is approximate, since total body digitalis load can be difficult to estimate. After the initial dose, need for and amount of additional dosing should be determined using clinical judgment.

If neither an estimated ingestion amount of digitalis nor the SDC is available, 760 mg of digoxin immune Fab (ovine) may be administered, which will be adequate to treat most life-threatening ingestions.

**Usual pediatric dose**
See *Usual adult and adolescent dose* (including Note).
Note: In small children, monitoring for volume overload is important.

For infants, who can have much smaller dosage requirements, it is recommended that digoxin immune Fab (ovine) be reconstituted as directed and administered with a tuberculin syringe. For very small doses, a reconstituted 38-mg vial can be diluted with 34 mL of 0.9% sodium chloride injection to produce a solution containing 1 mg per mL.

For approximate dose when amount of digoxin ingested is known, see *Usual adult and adolescent dose—Table 1*.

**Table 3.** Approximate *pediatric* dose *(mg)* of digoxin immune Fab (ovine) when serum digoxin concentration (SDC) is known.

| SDC (ng/mL) | Patient weight (kg) | | | | |
|---|---|---|---|---|---|
| | 1 | 3 | 5 | 10 | 20 |
| 1 | 0.4 | 1 | 2 | 4 | 8 |
| 2 | 1 | 2 | 4 | 8 | 15 |
| 4 | 1.5 | 5 | 8 | 15 | 30 |
| 8 | 3 | 9 | 15 | 30 | 61 |
| 12 | 5 | 14 | 23 | 46 | 91 |
| 16 | 6 | 18 | 30 | 61 | 122 |
| 20 | 8 | 23 | 38 | 76 | 152 |

## Size(s) usually available

U.S.—

38 mg (Rx) [*Digibind* (preservative-free)].

Canada—

38 mg (Rx) [*Digibind* (preservative-free)].

## Packaging and storage

Store between 2 and 8 °C (36 and 46 °F). Unreconstituted vials may be stored at up to 30 °C (86 °F) for up to 30 days.

## Preparation of dosage form

Digoxin immune Fab (ovine) for injection is reconstituted for intravenous administration by dissolving 38 mg in 4 mL of sterile water for injection and mixing gently, to produce a solution containing 9.5 mg per mL. The resulting solution may be further diluted with 0.9% sodium chloride injection to a convenient volume for administration by intravenous infusion.

## Stability

Reconstituted solution should be used immediately, but may be stored for up to 4 hours between 2 and 8 °C (36 and 46 °F).

## Selected Bibliography

Stolshek BS, Osterhout SK, Dunham G. The role of digoxin-specific antibodies in the treatment of digitalis poisoning. Med Toxicol 1988; 3: 167-71.

Antman EM, Wenger TL, Butler VP, Haber E, Smith TW. Treatment of 150 cases of life-threatening digitalis intoxication with digoxin-specific Fab antibody fragments. Circulation 1990; 81: 1744-52.

Hickey AR, Wenger TL, Carpenter V, et al. Digoxin immune Fab therapy in the management of digitalis intoxication: safety and efficacy results of an observational study. J Am Coll Cardiol 1991; 17: 590-8.

Revised: 08/17/95

---

# DIHYDROCODEINE-CONTAINING COMBINATIONS—

Aspirin, Caffeine, and Dihydrocodeine (Systemic)—See *Opioid (Narcotic) Analgesics and Aspirin (Systemic)*

Chlorpheniramine, Phenylephrine, Phenylpropanolamine, and Dihydrocodeine (Systemic)—See *Cough/Cold Combinations (Systemic)*

Dihydrocodeine, Acetaminophen, and Caffeine (Systemic)—See *Opioid (Narcotic) Analgesics and Acetaminophen (Systemic)*

---

# DIHYDROERGOTAMINE—See *Vascular Headache Suppressants, Ergot Derivative–containing (Systemic)*

---

# DIHYDROTACHYSTEROL—See *Vitamin D and Analogs (Systemic)*

---

# DIHYDROXYALUMINUM AMINOACETATE—See *Antacids (Oral-Local)*

---

# DIHYDROXYALUMINUM SODIUM CARBONATE—See *Antacids (Oral-Local)*

---

# DILOXANIDE—Since Diloxanide is not commercially available in the U.S. or Canada, the *Diloxanide (Systemic)* monograph is not included in this published version of the USP DI database. Copies of the monograph are available on request from the USP Division of Information Development, 12601 Twinbrook Parkway, Rockville, MD 20852; telephone (301) 816-8351; telefax (301) 816-8374.

---

# DILTIAZEM—See *Calcium Channel Blocking Agents (Systemic)*

---

# DIMENHYDRINATE—See *Antihistamines (Systemic)*

---

# DIMENHYDRINATE-CONTAINING COMBINATIONS—

Ergotamine, Caffeine, and Dimenhydrinate (Systemic)—See *Vascular Headache Suppressants, Ergot Derivative–containing (Systemic)*

---

# DIMERCAPROL    Systemic

## VA CLASSIFICATION (Primary): AD300

Other commonly used names are British Anti-Lewisite and dimercaptopropanol.

Note: For a listing of dosage forms and brand names by country availability, see *Dosage Forms* section(s). For a listing of brand names for the articles in this monograph, refer to the General Index.

## Category

Chelating agent.

## Indications

### Accepted

Toxicity, arsenic (treatment)

Toxicity, gold (treatment) or

Toxicity, mercury (treatment)—Dimercaprol is indicated as a chelating agent in arsenic, gold, and mercury (soluble inorganic compounds) poisoning following ingestion, inhalation, or absorption through the skin of these metals or their salts, or following overdose of therapeutic agents containing the metals.

In arsenic (except for arsine gas) toxicity, early administration of dimercaprol may help reverse the acute and some of the chronic manifestations of poisoning, although polyneuropathy may be refractory. Chelation therapy is recommended if urine arsenic levels are consistently above 200 mcg per liter.

In gold toxicity resulting from therapeutic uses of gold compounds for arthritis, dimercaprol may be effective in enhancing the excretion of accumulated gold salts. In patients with severe renal, hematologic, pulmonary, or enterocolitic complications who do not improve with high-dose corticosteroid treatment or who develop steroid-related adverse reactions, dimercaprol may be considered and has been used successfully. However, patients must be carefully monitored because of the adverse reactions that accompany its use.

In acute inorganic and aryl organic mercury toxicity, dimercaprol therapy is most effective when begun within 1 or 2 hours after ingestion, and ceases to be effective after about 6 hours. Dimercaprol is of questionable efficacy in elemental mercury poisoning.

Toxicity, lead (treatment adjunct)—Dimercaprol is indicated for treatment of acute and chronic lead poisoning when administered in conjunction with edetate calcium disodium (calcium EDTA). When administered promptly, dimercaprol complements edetate calcium disodium by more rapidly removing lead from red blood cells and the central nervous system (CNS) than does edetate calcium disodium alone, and by assisting in mobilization of lead from skeletal stores. This combination is less toxic than edetate calcium disodium alone because lower doses of each can be used. The rate of lead excretion is doubled when the combination is used, thus decreasing the mortality rate and the likelihood of permanent neurologic deficits from lead poisoning.

Signs and symptoms of severe, symptomatic lead poisoning include anemia, gastrointestinal complaints (abdominal pain and vomiting), nephropathy, and encephalopathy. Signs and symptoms of lead encephalopathy include headache and insomnia; persistent vomiting, sometimes projectile; visual disturbances; irritability, restlessness, delirium, hallucinations; ataxia; convulsions and coma; and characteristically high intracranial pressure. Recovery is slow and often incomplete, with residual neurological deficits.

Clinical signs suggesting lead poisoning in children and adults that should be treated with the dimercaprol, edetate calcium disodium combination include the following:
- Patient is severely symptomatic (with or without encephalopathy).
- Blood lead concentrations are greater than or equal to 70 mcg per deciliter.

### Unaccepted
Dimercaprol should not be used in iron, cadmium, selenium, silver, or uranium poisoning because the dimercaprol-metal complexes are more toxic, especially to the kidneys, than the metal alone.

In methylmercury or other short-chain alkyl organic mercury intoxication, dimercaprol enhances the distribution of mercury into the brain, and is contraindicated.

Dimercaprol is of questionable value in poisoning by the heavy metals antimony and bismuth.

Dimercaprol is contraindicated in poisoning from arsine gas ($AsH_3$).

## Pharmacology/Pharmacokinetics

### Physicochemical characteristics
Molecular weight—124.22.

### Mechanism of action/Effect
Chelating agent—
Certain heavy metals, especially arsenic, gold, lead, and mercury, form ligands in the body with the sulfhydryl (-SH) groups of the pyruvate-oxidase enzyme system, and inhibit the normal functioning of the enzymes that are dependent on free sulfhydryl groups for their activity. Dimercaprol, having a greater affinity for the metal than does the protein, reverses the enzyme inhibition by chelating the metal and preventing or reversing its toxic effects by regeneration of free sulfhydryl groups. The resulting dimercaprol-metal complex is relatively stable and rapidly excreted.

In addition, in lead toxicity, dimercaprol causes a fast but short-lived reduction in lead concentrations in red blood cells and CNS, and effects a greater total lead excretion (urinary and fecal) than edetate calcium disodium because of its high fecal lead output. The addition of equimolar amounts of dimercaprol to edetate calcium disodium doubles the ratio of chelants to lead, thus providing the molar excess of chelating agent that is necessary for significant heavy metal excretion.

### Distribution
All tissues, including the brain, but mainly in the intracellular space. The highest concentrations are in the liver and kidneys.

### Biotransformation
About 50% rapidly metabolized to inactive metabolites.

### Onset of action
30 minutes.

### Time to peak concentration
30 to 60 minutes after intramuscular administration.

### Duration of action
About 4 hours. Frequent doses at 3- to 4-hour intervals over prolonged periods are necessary to maintain therapeutic effect.

### Elimination
50% as the dimercaprol-metal complex, via the renal and biliary tracts; as metabolites, in the urine; metabolism and excretion are usually complete within 6 to 24 hours.

## Precautions to Consider

### Cross-sensitivity and/or related problems
Dimercaprol injection should not be used in patients who are allergic to peanuts or peanut products.

### Pregnancy/Reproduction
Pregnancy—Adequate and well-controlled studies have not been done in humans.
Studies have not been done in animals.
FDA Pregnancy Category C.

### Breast-feeding
It is not known whether dimercaprol is distributed into breast milk.

### Pediatrics
Fever, which appears after the second or third dose of dimercaprol, persists throughout therapy, and disappears upon withdrawal of therapy, is more likely to occur in children than in adults. A transient reduction of polymorphonuclear leukocytes may also be seen.

### Geriatrics
No information is available on the relationship of age to the effects of dimercaprol in geriatric patients.

### Drug interactions and/or related problems
The following drug interactions and/or related problems have been selected on the basis of their potential clinical significance (possible mechanism in parentheses where appropriate)—not necessarily inclusive (» = major clinical significance):

» Iron salts
(concurrent administration of medicinal iron with dimercaprol results in the formation of a toxic complex; if iron deficiency is present, its treatment should be postponed until therapy with dimercaprol has been discontinued for at least twenty-four hours; however, severe iron deficiency anemia occurring during dimercaprol therapy should be managed with blood transfusion)

### Laboratory value alterations
The following have been selected on the basis of their potential clinical significance (possible effect in parentheses where appropriate)—not necessarily inclusive (» = major clinical significance):

With diagnostic test results
Thyroid tests
(when test is done during or immediately after dimercaprol therapy, iodine I 131 thyroidal uptake values may be decreased because of dimercaprol interference with normal accumulation of iodine in the thyroid gland)

With physiology/laboratory test values
Alanine aminotransferase (ALT [SGPT]) and
Aspartate aminotransferase (AST [SGOT])
(values may be temporarily elevated)

Polymorphonuclear leukocyte count
(a transient reduction may be seen in children)

### Medical considerations/Contraindications
The medical considerations/contraindications included here have been selected on the basis of their potential clinical significance (reasons given in parentheses where appropriate)—not necessarily inclusive (» = major clinical significance).

*Except under special circumstances, this medication should not be used when the following medical problems exist:*

» Arsine gas poisoning
(chelation with dimercaprol is not useful in acute poisoning because it does not prevent hemolysis)

» Hepatic function impairment
(except in postarsenical jaundice, which may only require a reduction in dosage, metabolism may be reduced)

» Iron, cadmium, selenium, silver, or uranium poisoning
(dimercaprol-metal complexes of these metals are more toxic than the metal alone, and may cause nephrotoxicity)

» Organic (short-chain alkyl) mercury poisoning
(distribution of mercury to the brain is enhanced by dimercaprol)

*Risk-benefit should be considered when the following medical problems exist:*

Glucose-6-phosphate dehydrogenase (G6PD) deficiency
(dimercaprol may induce hemolysis and should be used only in life-threatening situations in patients with this deficiency)

Hypertension
(may be exacerbated)

Renal function impairment or
» Renal insufficiency, acute
(dimercaprol should be used cautiously if acute renal insufficiency develops during therapy because accumulation of dimercaprol may result in toxic serum concentrations; if oliguria is present, dimercaprol should be used with caution and/or in reduced dosage)

Sensitivity to dimercaprol

**Patient monitoring**

The following may be especially important in patient monitoring (other tests may be warranted in some patients, depending on condition; » = major clinical significance):

Alkaline phosphatase concentrations, serum and
Blood urea nitrogen (BUN) concentrations and
Calcium concentrations, serum and
Creatinine concentrations, serum and
Electrolyte concentrations, serum and
Phosphorus concentrations, serum
    (determinations recommended to detect evidence of renal function impairment; hemodialysis may be necessary)

Blood pressure and
Heart rate
    (recommended periodically during therapy, since both may be increased)

Fluid balance
    (recommended for determination of dehydration or impending renal insufficiency; parenteral fluids should be administered, at least during the first 2 or 3 days of dimercaprol therapy, to replace oral feedings that may not be tolerated or to minimize nausea and vomiting caused by either dimercaprol or the toxic agent or both)

Heavy metal concentration in blood and
24-hour urine excretion
    (recommended to determine dosage and duration of therapy)

Hemoglobin
    (recommended periodically in mercury toxicity)

Urinary pH
    (recommended periodically; maintenance of an alkaline pH decreases the risk of nephrotoxicity, which may occur because of dissociation of the dimercaprol-metal complex in acidic urine)

## Side/Adverse Effects

The following side/adverse effects have been selected on the basis of their potential clinical significance (possible signs and symptoms in parentheses where appropriate)—not necessarily inclusive:

**Those indicating need for medical attention**
Incidence more frequent
    *Fast heartbeat; fever*—especially in children; *increased blood pressure*—both systolic and diastolic, roughly dose related
Incidence less frequent
    *Abscesses, usually sterile, at injection site* (painful, red, and pus-containing sores)

**Those indicating need for medical attention only if they continue or are bothersome**
Incidence more frequent
    *Burning feeling in lips, mouth, throat, and penis; conjunctivitis; eyelid twitching; feeling of constriction or pain in throat, chest, or hands; headache; nausea and sometimes vomiting; pain at injection site; runny nose; sweating of forehead and hands; tingling of hands; unpleasant breath odor; watery eyes and mouth*
    Note: All of the effects listed above, except *pain at injection site* and *unpleasant breath odor*, may occur with doses above the recommended dose, may be mild and temporary, and are often accompanied by feelings of anxiety, weakness, and unrest.

Incidence less frequent
    *Abdominal pain; lower back pain; tremors*

## Overdose

For more information on the management of overdose or unintentional ingestion, **contact a Poison Control Center** (see *Poison Control Center Listing*).

**Clinical effects of overdose**
    *Convulsions; severe drowsiness; severe vomiting*
    Note: These symptoms may be seen at doses above 5 mg per kg of body weight (mg/kg), beginning within 30 minutes and usually subsiding within 6 hours following injection.

## General Dosing Information

In any heavy metal poisoning, supportive therapy is as important to survival as chelation therapy. Removal of patient from exposure is the primary therapy for exposed patients. Depending on the metal, supportive treatment may include removal of the residual metal from the body with emesis or gastric lavage; intravenous fluids to correct dehydration and electrolyte deficiencies; bed rest; preservation of body heat; exchange transfusions; abdominal radiographs; and analgesics.

Since dimercaprol is better able to prevent inhibition of sulfhydryl enzymes than to reactivate them, dimercaprol therapy is most effective when begun immediately after exposure. The toxic metal ion is inactivated and its incorporation into binding sites in blood and tissue is prevented. If reactivation of enzymes is necessary, prolonged therapy may be required.

Dimercaprol is always administered by deep intramuscular injection, never by intravenous or subcutaneous injection. Rotating injection sites may minimize development of abscesses.

The dosage of dimercaprol must be repeated frequently for several days. This maintains a plasma concentration of free dimercaprol in the body fluids that enhances the continuous formation of a rapidly excreted stable complex of 2:1 (dimercaprol:metal) until a significant portion of the metal is eliminated from the body.

Because the dimercaprol-metal chelation is reversible and can rapidly dissociate in an acid medium, alkalinization of the urine is necessary to prevent dissociation into the toxic metal and potentially nephrotoxic dimercaprol. After assuring adequate urine volume, a less acid urine may be achieved by oral administration of sodium bicarbonate, with the dosage and frequency being determined by monitoring urinary pH. If patients are placed on parenteral fluids, adjustment of the composition of the solutions may provide a neutral urine, or alkalization of the urine may be achieved by intravenous infusion of sodium bicarbonate over 4 to 8 hours. Such patients may be advanced cautiously to clear oral liquids or oral rehydration solutions.

**For acute lead encephalopathy**

Dimercaprol is combined with edetate calcium disodium because the maximum safe dose of edetate calcium disodium alone may cause a shift of lead into the central nervous system (CNS). The preferred route of administration for edetate calcium disodium is intravenous, and dimercaprol is given by deep intramuscular injection, in divided doses every 4 hours for 5 days. If both medications are given by intramuscular injection, they must be given at separate sites. Dimercaprol is given alone for the first dose 4 hours before the combination is begun. In asymptomatic or mildly symptomatic patients, dimercaprol may be discontinued after 72 hours, with edetate calcium disodium being continued for an additional 48 to 72 hours at reduced dosage.

Oral penicillamine is used for long-term chelation therapy after initial therapy with edetate calcium disodium or combined dimercaprol and edetate calcium disodium, especially if long-bone radiographs show lead lines. The oral chelating agent succimer is used for treatment of children with blood lead concentrations greater than 45 micrograms per deciliter. Although use to date has been limited, toxicity with succimer appears to be less than with other agents.

**For prevention or treatment of adverse effects**
    • For histaminic effects, mild and temporary—Recommended treatment may include administration of diphenhydramine in doses up to 1.5 mg per kg intramuscularly or orally every 6 hours.
    • For nausea or vomiting—May be prevented by giving patient nothing orally and hydrating initially with parenteral fluids. After clinical improvement occurs, clear liquids may be administered orally as parenteral fluids are phased out.
    • For sterile abscesses—May be prevented by rotating sites of injection and always administering *deep* intramuscular injections. If existing abscess does not subside spontaneously, aspiration and drainage may be necessary.

## Parenteral Dosage Forms

### DIMERCAPROL INJECTION USP

**Usual adult and adolescent dose**
Arsenic or gold toxicity—
    Severe: Intramuscular (deep), 3 mg per kg of body weight every four hours for two days, four times on the third day, then twice a day for ten days; or 3 mg per kg of body weight every four hours on the first day, 2 mg per kg of body weight every four hours on the second day, 3 mg per kg of body weight every six hours on the third day, and 3 mg per kg of body weight every twelve hours on each of the following ten days or until recovery.
    Mild: Intramuscular (deep), 2.5 mg per kg of body weight every six hours for two days, every twelve hours on the third day, and once a day on each of the following ten days or until recovery.
Mercury toxicity—
    Intramuscular (deep), 3 to 5 mg per kg of body weight every four hours for two days, then 2.5 to 3 mg per kg of body weight every six hours for two days, then 2.5 to 3 mg per kg of body weight every twelve hours for seven days.
Lead toxicity—
    Severe (encephalopathy): Intramuscular, 4 mg per kg of body weight for the first dose, repeated at four-hour intervals in conjunction

with edetate calcium disodium (calcium EDTA) injection, which is usually administered intravenously, but may be administered intramuscularly at a separate site. This treatment is maintained for two to seven days. If the blood lead concentration after this first course of therapy exceeds 100 mcg per deciliter, treatment may be resumed for an additional five days, following an interval of at least two days without treatment.

Mild: Intramuscular, 4 mg per kg of body weight for the first dose, the dose then being reduced to 3 mg per kg of body weight and administered at four-hour intervals in conjunction with edetate calcium disodium injection, which is administered at a separate site.

### Usual adult prescribing limits
5 mg per kg of body weight.

### Usual pediatric dose
Lead toxicity—
Symptomatic children:
Acute (with or without encephalopathy)—Intramuscular (deep), 75 mg per square meter of body surface area every four hours (up to 450 mg per square meter per twenty-four hours). After four hours, calcium EDTA injection, 1500 mg per square meter of body surface area per twenty-four hours, should be administered on a four-hour schedule, intravenously or intramuscularly at a separate site. This treatment is maintained for five days. If the blood lead concentration after this first course of therapy exceeds 70 mcg per deciliter, treatment may be resumed for an additional five days, following an interval of at least two days without treatment. The cycle may be repeated, depending on the clinical response.

Asymptomatic children:
Intramuscular (deep), 50 mg per square meter of body surface area every four hours. After four hours, calcium EDTA injection, 1000 mg per square meter of body surface area per twenty-four hours, should be administered on a four-hour schedule simultaneously intravenously or intramuscularly at a separate site. This treatment is maintained for five days. Dimercaprol may be discontinued after three days if blood lead concentrations are less than 50 mcg per deciliter. If the blood lead concentration after this first course of therapy exceeds 70 mcg per deciliter, treatment may be resumed for an additional five days, following an interval of at least two days without treatment. Calcium EDTA injection should be continued for five more days. The cycle may be repeated depending on the clinical response.

### Strength(s) usually available
U.S.—
100 mg per mL (Rx) [*BAL in Oil* (benzyl benzoate 200 mg; peanut oil 700 mg)].
Canada—
100 mg per mL (Rx) [*BAL in Oil* (benzyl benzoate 200 mg; peanut oil 700 mg)].

### Packaging and storage
Store below 40 °C (104 °F), preferably between 15 and 30 °C (59 and 86 °F), unless otherwise specified by manufacturer.

Revised: 11/11/94

# DIMETHYL SULFOXIDE    Mucosal-Local

VA CLASSIFICATION (Primary): GU900
Another commonly used name is DMSO.
Note: For a listing of dosage forms and brand names by country availability, see *Dosage Forms* section(s). For a listing of brand names for the articles in this monograph, refer to the General Index.

## Category
Anti-inflammatory, local (interstitial cystitis).

## Indications
### Accepted
Cystitis, interstitial (treatment)—Dimethyl sulfoxide is indicated for the symptomatic relief of interstitial cystitis.

### Unaccepted
Dimethyl sulfoxide has *not* been shown to be effective in the treatment of bacterial infections of the urinary tract.

Also, topical use of dimethyl sulfoxide as a vehicle for enhancing the percutaneous absorption of other drugs has *not* been shown to be effective.

In addition, dimethyl sulfoxide administered topically, orally, or intravenously has *not* been proven to be effective in the treatment of musculoskeletal disorders; diseases of connective tissue (e.g., osteoarthritis, rheumatoid arthritis, cutaneous manifestations of scleroderma, gout, ankylosing spondylitis); viral, bacterial, fungal, or parasitic infections of the skin; burns; postoperative pain; wounds (to promote healing); or mental conditions.

However, investigational studies are being conducted on the transcutaneous carrier properties of dimethyl sulfoxide and on the efficacy of dimethyl sulfoxide in scleroderma, head injury, stroke, spinal cord trauma, arthritis, trauma of acute injuries, such as sprains and strains, and other disorders.

## Pharmacology/Pharmacokinetics
### Physicochemical characteristics
Molecular weight—78.13.

### Mechanism of action/Effect
The mechanism by which dimethyl sulfoxide produces anti-inflammatory effects in interstitial cystitis is not known.

### Absorption
Dimethyl sulfoxide is absorbed systemically following topical application.

### Biotransformation
Metabolized to dimethyl sulfone and dimethyl sulfide.

### Elimination
Dimethyl sulfoxide and one of its metabolites, dimethyl sulfone, are excreted in the urine and feces. The other metabolite, dimethyl sulfide, is eliminated via breath and through the skin.

## Precautions to Consider
### Pregnancy/Reproduction
Pregnancy—Studies in humans have not been done.
Studies in hamsters, rats, and mice have shown that dimethyl sulfoxide causes teratogenic effects when administered intraperitoneally at high doses of 2.5 to 12 grams per kg of body weight. In addition, studies in rabbits have shown that dimethyl sulfoxide causes teratogenic effects when administered topically at doses of 5 grams per kg of body weight for the first 2 days, then 2.5 grams per kg of body weight for the last 8 days. However, in another study using rabbits, dimethyl sulfoxide was not shown to cause any abnormalities when administered topically at doses of 1.1 grams per kg of body weight on Days 3 through 16 of gestation. Furthermore, dimethyl sulfoxide was not shown to cause reproductive problems in hamsters, rats, and mice when administered in oral or topical doses.

FDA Pregnancy Category C.

### Breast-feeding
It is not known whether dimethyl sulfoxide is excreted in breast milk and problems in humans have not been documented; however, dimethyl sulfoxide is systemically absorbed.

### Pediatrics
Appropriate studies on the relationship of age to the effects of this medicine have not been performed in the pediatric population.

### Geriatrics
Appropriate studies on the relationship of age to the effects of this medicine have not been performed in the geriatric population. However, no geriatrics-specific problems have been documented to date.

### Drug interactions and/or related problems
The following drug interactions and/or related problems have been selected on the basis of their potential clinical significance (possible mechanism in parentheses where appropriate)—not necessarily inclusive (» = major clinical significance):
Note: Combinations containing any of the following medications, depending on the amount present, may also interact with this medication.

Medications, intravesical, other
(effects may be increased when these medications are used concurrently with dimethyl sulfoxide)

**Medical considerations/Contraindications**
The medical considerations/contraindications included here have been selected on the basis of their potential clinical significance (reasons given in parentheses where appropriate)—not necessarily inclusive (» = major clinical significance).

*Risk-benefit should be considered when the following medical problems exist:*
Sensitivity to dimethyl sulfoxide
Urinary tract malignancy
(use of dimethyl sulfoxide may be harmful because of drug-induced vasodilation)

**Patient monitoring**
The following may be especially important in patient monitoring (other tests may be warranted in some patients, depending on condition; » = major clinical significance):
Biochemical screening, particularly liver and renal function tests and
Blood cell counts, complete
(recommended approximately every 6 months during therapy)
Ophthalmologic examinations, complete
(recommended prior to and at periodic intervals during therapy, since changes in the refractive index and lens opacities have been documented in animal studies when dimethyl sulfoxide was given chronically)

## Side/Adverse Effects

The following side/adverse effects have been selected on the basis of their potential clinical significance (possible signs and symptoms in parentheses where appropriate)—not necessarily inclusive:

**Those indicating need for medical attention**
*Anaphylactoid reaction* (nasal congestion; shortness of breath or troubled breathing; skin rash, hives, or itching; swelling of face)

**Those not indicating need for medical attention**
*Discomfort, moderate to severe, during administration; garlic-like odor on breath and skin; garlic-like taste*

## Overdose

For information on the management of overdose or unintentional ingestion, **contact a Poison Control Center** (see *Poison Control Center Listing*).

**Treatment of overdose**
If dimethyl sulfoxide is accidently ingested:
To decrease absorption—
Emesis should be induced. Measures that may be considered include gastric lavage and administration of activated charcoal.
To enhance elimination—
Forced diuresis should be considered.

## Patient Consultation

As an aid to patient consultation, refer to *Advice for the Patient, Dimethyl Sulfoxide (Mucosal)*.

In providing consultation, consider emphasizing the following selected information (» = major clinical significance):

**Before using this medication**
» Conditions affecting use, especially:
Allergy to dimethyl sulfoxide

**Proper use of this medication**
» Proper dosing

**Side/adverse effects**
Moderately severe discomfort may occur during administration, but usually lessens with repeated instillations
A garlic-like taste, which may occur within a few minutes after instillation and last for several hours, and a garlic-like odor on the breath and skin, which may last for 72 hours, may be alarming to patient although medically insignificant
Signs of potential side effects, especially anaphylactoid reaction

## General Dosing Information

Dimethyl sulfoxide irrigation is not for intramuscular or intravenous injection or for cutaneous application. It is to be instilled directly into the bladder using a catheter or an asepto syringe.

Prior to inserting the catheter, application of an analgesic lubricant such as lidocaine jelly to the urethra is recommended to avoid spasm.

The medication is expelled by spontaneous voiding.

When symptomatic relief is not complete, 500 mL of a solution containing 1 part of dimethyl sulfoxide and 1 part of sterile water may be used to distend the bladder prior to instillation of the 50-mL dose.

Dimethyl sulfoxide solution 99% is used as a cryopreservative and should not be used for bladder irrigation.

## Topical Dosage Forms

### DIMETHYL SULFOXIDE IRRIGATION USP

**Usual adult and adolescent dose**
Intravesical instillation, 50 mL of a 50% solution, retained in the bladder for fifteen minutes; treatment repeated every two weeks until maximum symptomatic relief is obtained, then time intervals between treatments increased appropriately.

**Usual pediatric dose**
Dosage has not been established.

**Strength(s) usually available**
U.S.—
50% [*Rimso-50;* GENERIC].
Canada—
50% [*Rimso-50*].

**Packaging and storage**
Store between 15 and 30 °C (59 and 86 °F), unless otherwise specified by manufacturer. Protect from strong light.

Revised: 03/04/92
Interim revision: 03/28/94

---

# DINOPROST     Parenteral-Local*

VA CLASSIFICATION (Primary/Secondary): HS875/DX900; GU600
Note: For a listing of dosage forms and brand names by country availability, see *Dosage Forms* section(s). For a listing of brand names for the articles in this monograph, refer to the General Index.

*Not commercially available in the U.S.

## Category

Abortifacient; uterine stimulant; diagnostic aid (angiography).

## Indications

**Accepted**
Abortion, elective—Dinoprost is used for aborting second-trimester pregnancy (between the twelfth to eighteenth week of gestation). Dinoprost can be used for first-trimester and midtrimester abortion, but the procedure is difficult because of the small amount of amniotic fluid pres-

ent and it is associated with an increased incidence of side effects and failures. Dinoprost is sometimes used in combination with hypertonic saline, urea, or oxytocin.

Abortion, incomplete (treatment)[1] or
Abortion, therapeutic[1]—Dinoprost is used in incomplete abortion or for therapeutic abortion in cases of intrauterine fetal death and congenital abnormalities incompatible with life.

Labor, induction of[1]—Low-dose intravenous dinoprost has been used for medically indicated induction of labor at term.

Angiography adjunct[1]—Dinoprost has been injected intra-arterially for use as a vasodilator to assist in angiography.

**Unaccepted**
Dinoprost is generally not useful in the treatment of benign hydatidiform mole because of the lack of fetal membranes and amniotic fluid.

[1]Not included in Canadian product labeling.

# Pharmacology/Pharmacokinetics

## Physicochemical characteristics
Chemical group—Dinoprost tromethamine is the tromethamine salt of naturally occurring prostaglandin $F_{2alpha}$.
Molecular weight—475.62.

## Mechanism of action/Effect
Dinoprost appears to act directly on the myometrium, but this has not been completely established. Dinoprost stimulates myometrial contractions in the gravid uterus that are similar to the contractions that occur in the term uterus during labor. These contractions are usually sufficient to cause abortion. Uterine response to prostaglandins increases gradually throughout pregnancy. Dinoprost also facilitates cervical dilatation and softening.

## Other actions/effects
Dinoprost stimulates the smooth muscle of the gastrointestinal tract, arterioles, and bronchioles.

## Absorption
Dinoprost is slowly absorbed from the amniotic fluid into systemic circulation. Radiolabeled drug studies indicate that dinoprost and its metabolites freely cross the placenta. Because higher drug concentrations were observed in the fetal liver, dinoprost likely selectively enters the liver via the umbilical vein and ductus venosus.

## Biotransformation
Enzymatic dehydrogenation primarily in the maternal lungs and also in the liver.

## Half-life
The half-life of dinoprost in amniotic fluid is 3 to 6 hours. The plasma half-life of dinoprost after intravenous administration is reported to be less than 1 minute.

## Time to peak concentration
6 to 10 hours after single 40 mg intra-amniotic dose.

## Peak blood concentration
3 to 7 nanograms prostaglandin $F_{2alpha}$ equivalents per mL after single 40 mg intra-amniotic dose.

## Time to peak effect
The mean abortion time with dinoprost is about 20 to 24 hours. Intra-amniotic administration of 5 to 10 mg of dinoprost (base) immediately after instillation of hypertonic urea results in a mean abortion time of 16 to 17 hours.

## Elimination
Primarily renal as metabolites, with about 5% excreted in feces.

# Precautions to Consider

## Pregnancy/Reproduction
Pregnancy—Any pregnancy termination with dinoprost that fails should be completed by another method.
Proliferation of bone has been reported with clinical use of prostaglandin $E_1$ during prolonged therapy. There is no evidence to date that the short-term use of dinoprost causes proliferation of bone in the fetus. In animal studies, prostaglandins of the E and F series have caused proliferation of bone with high doses.
Labor and delivery—Use of high doses may result in excessive uterine tone, causing decreased uterine blood flow and fetal distress.

## Drug interactions and/or related problems
The following drug interactions and/or related problems have been selected on the basis of their potential clinical significance (possible mechanism in parentheses where appropriate)—not necessarily inclusive (» = major clinical significance):

Oxytocin or other oxytocics
   (concurrent use with dinoprost may result in uterine hypertonus, possibly causing uterine rupture or cervical laceration, especially in the absence of adequate cervical dilatation; although combinations are sometimes used for therapeutic advantage, when used concurrently, patient should be closely monitored)

## Laboratory value alterations
The following have been selected on the basis of their potential clinical significance (possible effect in parentheses where appropriate)—not necessarily inclusive (» = major clinical significance):

With physiology/laboratory test values
   Blood pressure, maternal or
   Heart rate, maternal
      (may be decreased or increased, especially with large doses)

   White blood cell count
      (may be elevated)

# Medical considerations/Contraindications
The medical considerations/contraindications included here have been selected on the basis of their potential clinical significance (reasons given in parentheses where appropriate)—not necessarily inclusive (» = major clinical significance).

*Except under special circumstances, this medication should not be used when the following medical problem exists:*

» Allergy or intolerance to dinoprost or other oxytocics

» Asthma, or history of
      (increased risk of bronchoconstriction)

   Cephalopelvic disproportion, significant or
   Fetal malpresentation
      (induction of labor is not generally recommended)

» Pelvic inflammatory disease, active
      (induction of uterine contractions is not recommended)

» Pulmonary disease, active
      (use of dinoprost may decrease pulmonary blood flow and increase pulmonary arterial pressure)

» Ruptured membranes—intra-amniotic or extra-amniotic route
      (increased risk of intravascular absorption of dinoprost)

*Risk-benefit should be considered when the following medical problems exist:*

   Anemia, history of
      (increased incidence of excessive uterine bleeding may occur with the use of prostaglandins in performance of abortion)

» Cardiac disease, active
      (decrease in blood pressure and bradycardia may result in cardiovascular collapse and angina pectoris)

   Cardiovascular disease, history of or
   Hypertension, history of or
   Hypotension, history of or
   Preeclampsia
      (may be aggravated by possible vasoconstriction or decreased blood pressure)

   Cervical stenosis or
   Uterine fibroids or
   Uterine surgery, history of
      (increased risk of uterine rupture)

   Diabetes mellitus, history of

   Epilepsy, or history of
      (rarely, seizures have occurred during the use of prostaglandins in epileptics)

   Glaucoma
      (increases in intraocular pressure and miosis have been reported rarely during the use of prostaglandins)

» Hepatic disease, active or
   Hepatic disease, history of
      (metabolism of dinoprost may be impaired, resulting in prolonged half-life)

   Hypersensitivity to dinoprost or
   Multiparity
      (excessive dosage or use with oxytocin may cause uterine hypertonicity with spasm and tetanic contraction, which can lead to posterior cervical perforations, cervical lacerations, uterine rupture, and hemorrhage)

   Jaundice, history of

» Renal disease, active
   Renal disease, history of

## Patient monitoring
The following may be especially important in patient monitoring (other tests may be warranted in some patients, depending on condition; » = major clinical significance):

   Contractions—frequency, duration, and force of and
   Temperature, pulse, and blood pressure determinations and
   Uterine tone, resting
      (monitoring of these parameters is recommended at frequent intervals during abortion procedure or labor and delivery)

   Vaginal examination
      (recommended prior to each intra-amniotic dose to confirm correct positioning of catheter, and after delivery or abortion to check for signs of cervical trauma)

# Side/Adverse Effects

Note: Inadvertent intravascular administration or absorption may result in nausea, vomiting, bronchoconstriction, peripheral vasoconstriction, faintness, hypertension, and feelings of panic. Because dinoprost is rapidly metabolized, these effects are transient (lasting 15 to 30 minutes) and most are not usually a cause for concern.

The following side/adverse effects have been selected on the basis of their potential clinical significance (possible signs and symptoms in parentheses where appropriate)—not necessarily inclusive:

### Those indicating need for medical attention
Incidence less frequent or rare
*Abdominal or stomach pain, severe or continuing; anaphylaxis, generalized* (redness and itching of skin; hives; swelling of face, inside the nose, and eyelids; shortness of breath; trouble in breathing; wheezing; tightness in chest); *bradycardia* (slow heartbeat); *bronchoconstriction* (wheezing; tightness in chest; shortness of breath; sudden coughing)—especially in asthmatics; *burning eyes; chest pain; double vision; dysuria* (difficult or painful urination); *hematuria* (blood in urine); *ileus, adynamic* (constipation, tender or mildly bloated abdomen); *increased uterine pain accompanying abortion*—correlates with efficacy; *pain in legs, back, or shoulder; paresthesias* (numbness in legs or other body parts); *peripheral vasoconstriction* (pale, cool, or blotchy skin on arms or legs; weak or absent pulse in arms or legs); *second-degree heart block* (decreased or irregular heartbeat); *substernal pressure or pain* (pressing or painful feeling in chest); *tachycardia* (fast heartbeat); *urinary retention* (decreased frequency of urination); *uterine tetany* (continuous and severe cramping of the uterus)

### Those indicating need for medical attention only if they continue or are bothersome
Incidence more frequent
*Diarrhea*—about 16%; *nausea*—about 25%; *stomach cramps or pain*—about 25%; *vomiting*—about 57%

Incidence less frequent—<1%
*Anxiety; breast engorgement* (fullness or tenderness of breasts); *burning feeling in breasts; chills or shivering; cough, continuing; dizziness; drowsiness; fever, transient; flushing or redness of face; headache; hiccups; increased sweating; inflammation and pain at injection site; unusual thirst*

### Those indicating possible postabortion complications and the need for medical attention if they occur after medication is discontinued
*Endometritis* (continuing chills or shivering; continuing fever; foul-smelling vaginal discharge; pain in lower abdomen); *unusual increase in uterine bleeding*

## Overdose
For more information on the management of overdose or unintentional ingestion, **contact a Poison Control Center** (see *Poison Control Center Listing*).

### Clinical effects of overdose
Although *overdose* by intra-amniotic administration of dinoprost has not been reported, exaggeration of the nausea, vomiting, and diarrhea that occur with normal doses would be expected.

### Treatment of overdose
Specific treatment—Surgical rupture of the amniotic sac (drug reservoir), if necessary.

Supportive therapy—Emphasis on intravenous fluid replacement.

## Patient Consultation
As an aid to patient consultation, refer to *Advice for the Patient, Dinoprost (Intra-amniotic)*.

In providing consultation, consider emphasizing the following selected information (» = major clinical significance):

### Before using this medication
» Conditions affecting use, especially:
     Allergies or intolerance to dinoprost or other oxytocics
     Pregnancy—Because some prostaglandins are teratogenic in animals, any pregnancy termination with dinoprost that fails should be completed by another method
     Other medical problems, especially pelvic inflammatory disease, ruptured membranes, cardiac disease, hepatic disease, pulmonary disease, or renal disease

### Proper use of this medication
» Proper dosing

### Side/adverse effects
     Signs of potential side effects, especially anaphylaxis; bronchoconstriction; burning eyes; severe and continuing abdominal or stomach pain; double vision; dysuria; hematuria; paresthesias; leg, back,

chest, or shoulder pain; second-degree heart block; urinary retention; endometritis; bradycardia; adynamic ileus; peripheral vasoconstriction; tachycardia; and increased uterine bleeding or pain

## General Dosing Information
Dinoprost is not feticidal and may result in delivery of a live fetus; administration with hypertonic saline or urea results in fetal death.

If dinoprost is ineffective, it is recommended that alternative methods such as hypertonic saline not be used until the uterus has stopped contracting.

It is recommended that antiemetic and antidiarrheal medications be administered prior to or concurrently with dinoprost to decrease the incidence and severity of gastrointestinal side effects. Narcotic analgesics may be given for uterine pain.

Dinoprost has also been administered extra-amniotically (between the fetal membranes and uterine wall), but this method of administration has some disadvantages. Because more frequent dosing and prolonged administration is necessary, the risk of side effects due to systemic absorption of dinoprost and infection is increased. However, some clinicians prefer this route of administration between the thirteenth and fifteenth weeks of gestation when intra-amniotic administration is not feasible, or in cases of intrauterine fetal death.

Dinoprost has been used to terminate pregnancies of more than 20 weeks' gestation in cases of anencephaly. Because of increased uterine sensitivity, lower doses and careful titration are necessary. One group of investigators began with a 5-mg intra-amniotic dose, which was doubled every hour until the appropriate contraction pattern was established.

Confirmation of intrauterine fetal death should be made prior to use of dinoprost for missed abortion or intrauterine fetal death.

Caution should be taken to prevent exposure of skin to dinoprost tromethamine. If dinoprost injection is spilled on the skin, it should be washed off immediately with soap and water.

## Parenteral Dosage Forms
### DINOPROST TROMETHAMINE INJECTION USP
Note: The dosing and strength of the dosage form available are expressed in terms of dinoprost base.

**Usual adult dose**
Abortifacient—
     Intra-amniotic, 40 mg (base). The first 5 mg should be administered at a rate not exceeding 1 mg per minute to determine sensitivity and to confirm that the medication is not being administered intravascularly, with the remaining 35 mg being administered over the next five minutes if there are no adverse reactions.
     An additional dose of 10 to 40 mg (base) may be administered twenty-four hours after the initial dose if the abortion process is not established or completed, provided the membranes are still intact.
     Note: A transabdominal tap of the amniotic sac must be performed before intra-amniotic injection of dinoprost; dinoprost should not be administered if a bloody amniotic fluid sample is obtained.
Induction of labor[1]—
     Intravenous infusion, 2.5 mcg per minute of a 50 mcg-per-mL solution, with the dose being doubled every hour if necessary to a maximum of 20 mcg per minute (total dose is generally 1 to 4 mg).

**Strength(s) usually available**
U.S.—
     Not commercially available.
Canada—
     5 mg (base) per mL (Rx) [*Prostin F₂ Alpha* (benzyl alcohol 9 mg)].

**Packaging and storage**
Store between 2 and 8 °C (36 and 46 °F), unless otherwise specified by manufacturer. Protect from freezing.

**Preparation of dosage form**
To prepare a 50 mcg-per-mL solution—Using standard aseptic technique, dilute each 20 mg with 5% dextrose injection to a total volume of 400 mL.

---

[1]Not included in Canadian product labeling.

Revised: 10/26/92
Interim revision: 05/16/94

# DINOPROSTONE  Cervical/Vaginal

VA CLASSIFICATION (Primary/Secondary): HS875/GU600; GU900

Some other commonly used names are prostaglandin E₂ or PGE₂

Note: For a listing of dosage forms and brand names by country availability, see *Dosage Forms* section(s). For a listing of brand names for the articles in this monograph, refer to the General Index.

## Category

Prostaglandin; oxytocic; abortifacient; antihemorrhagic (postabortion uterine bleeding; postpartum uterine bleeding).

## Indications

Note: Bracketed information in the *Indications* section refers to uses that are not included in U.S. product labeling.

**Accepted**

Abortion, elective—Dinoprostone suppositories are used for aborting midtrimester pregnancy (from the twelfth through the twentieth week of gestation as calculated from the first day of the last normal menstrual period).

Abortion, missed (treatment) or

Abortion, therapeutic—Dinoprostone suppositories are indicated for evacuation of the uterine contents in management of missed abortion or for therapeutic abortion in cases of intrauterine fetal death up to 28 weeks of gestational age as calculated from the first day of the last normal menstrual period. Dinoprostone vaginal gel or suppository is not approved for use as an abortifacient in cases of intrauterine fetal death at more than 28 weeks' gestation because it is associated with an increased risk of uterine rupture. Confirmation of intrauterine fetal death should be made prior to use of dinoprostone for missed abortion or intrauterine fetal death.

Cervical ripening—Dinoprostone cervical gel is used for medically indicated ripening of the cervix in patients at or near term, prior to induction of labor. [Extemporaneously prepared dinoprostone gels have also been used in cervical ripening prior to induction of labor and prior to abortion procedures, such as vacuum curettage].

[Hemorrhage, postpartum (treatment)] or

[Hemorrhage, postabortion (treatment)]—Dinoprostone suppositories are used to reduce blood loss and correct uterine atony postpartum and postabortion in patients unresponsive to conventional treatment such as oxytocin, ergonovine, or methylergonovine.

Hydatidiform mole, benign (treatment)—Although vacuum curettage is preferred, dinoprostone suppositories are indicated for evacuation of the uterine contents in the treatment of nonmetastatic benign hydatidiform mole.

[Labor, induction of]—Dinoprostone suppositories and vaginal gel are used for induction of labor at or near term.

**Unaccepted**

Dinoprostone vaginal suppository is not indicated for use to terminate a pregnancy of greater than 28 weeks gestation or when a fetus *in utero* has reached a stage of viability. Also, the vaginal suppository or vaginal gel should not be used for cervical ripening.

## Pharmacology/Pharmacokinetics

**Physicochemical characteristics**

Chemical group—Dinoprostone is the naturally occurring prostaglandin E₂.

Molecular weight—352.47.

**Mechanism of action/Effect**

For uterine stimulation—

Dinoprostone appears to act directly on the myometrium, but this has not been completely established. It stimulates myometrial contractions in the gravid uterus that are similar to the contractions that occur in the term uterus during natural labor. These contractions are usually sufficient to cause abortion. Uterine response to prostaglandins increases gradually throughout pregnancy. Dinoprostone does not act directly on the fetoplacental unit and is not considered a fetocidal agent.

For cervical ripening—

Dinoprostone has been shown to have a softening effect on the cervix due to stimulation of collagenase secretion, thereby facilitating cervical dilatation. The changes of cervical ripening are independent of myometrial activity.

**Other actions/effects**

Dinoprostone stimulates the smooth muscle of the gastrointestinal tract. It may also cause bronchodilation or bronchoconstriction and vasodilation. Dinoprostone can elevate body temperature due to its effect on hypothalamic thermoregulation.

**Protein binding**

73%, to albumin.

**Biotransformation**

Rapid enzymatic deactivation primarily in the local tissues and maternal lungs, as well as in the kidneys, spleen, and other tissues.

**Half-life**

Less than 1 minute (elimination).

**Onset of action**

Uterine stimulation—Contractions begin within 10 minutes following insertion of a dinoprostone vaginal suppository.

**Time to peak effect**

The mean abortion time with dinoprostone is about 17 hours (range, 12 to 24 hours).

**Duration of action**

Contractions persist for 2 to 6 hours following insertion of a dinoprostone vaginal suppository.

**Elimination**

Primarily renal as metabolites, with a small amount excreted in the feces.

## Precautions to Consider

**Carcinogenicity**

Studies have not been done in animals or humans on the carcinogenicity of dinoprostone.

**Mutagenicity**

The micronucleus test and Ames assay revealed no evidence of mutagenicity with dinoprostone.

**Pregnancy/Reproduction**

Pregnancy—Any pregnancy termination that fails with dinoprostone should be completed by another method.

Proliferation of bone has also been reported with clinical use of prostaglandin E₁ during prolonged therapy. There is no evidence to date that the short-term use of dinoprostone (prostaglandin E₂) causes proliferation of bone in the fetus..

Although animal studies with dinoprostone did not reveal teratogenic properties, dinoprostone has been shown to be embryotoxic in rats and rabbits. In animal studies, prostaglandins of the E and F series have caused proliferation of bone with high doses.

FDA Pregnancy Category C.

Labor and delivery—Use of high doses may result in excessive uterine tone, causing decreased uterine blood flow and fetal distress.

**Drug interactions and/or related problems**

The following drug interactions and/or related problems have been selected on the basis of their potential clinical significance (possible mechanism in parentheses where appropriate)—not necessarily inclusive (» = major clinical significance):

» Oxytocin or other oxytocics

(concurrent or sequential use with dinoprostone may potentiate the effects of oxytocin, possibly resulting in uterine hypertonus, which may cause uterine rupture or cervical laceration, especially in the absence of adequate cervical dilatation; although combinations are sometimes used to therapeutic advantage, oxytocin administration should be begun 6 to 12 hours after administration of dinoprostone vaginal suppository or cervical gel and 12 to 24 hours after administration of the vaginal gel and the patient should be continuously monitored)

**Laboratory value alterations**

The following have been selected on the basis of their potential clinical significance (possible effect in parentheses where appropriate)—not necessarily inclusive (» = major clinical significance):

With physiology/laboratory test values

Blood pressure, maternal or

Heart rate, maternal or fetal

(may be decreased or increased especially with large doses; a decrease in diastolic blood pressure of greater than 20 mm of Hg has been reported in approximately 10% of patients receiving dinoprostone)

Body temperature
(a temperature increase of greater than 1.1 °C [2 °F] usually occurs within 15 to 45 minutes following insertion of suppository or vaginal gel; this has not been seen with the doses of the endocervical gel used for cervical ripening. The temperature returns to normal within 2 to 6 hours after discontinuation of medication or removal of suppository from vagina)

**Medical considerations/Contraindications**

The medical considerations/contraindications included here have been selected on the basis of their potential clinical significance (reasons given in parentheses where appropriate)—not necessarily inclusive (» = major clinical significance).

*Except under special circumstances, this medication should not be used when the following medical problems exist:*

» Allergy to dinoprostone or other oxytocics

» Asthma, or history of
(increased risk of bronchoconstriction)

» Cephalopelvic disproportion, significant or
» Conditions that contraindicate vaginal delivery, other or
» Fetal malpresentation
(induction of labor and vaginal delivery are not generally recommended)

» Pelvic inflammatory disease, acute
(induction of uterine contractions is not recommended)

» Pulmonary disease, active
(use of dinoprostone may decrease pulmonary blood flow and increase pulmonary arterial pressure)

*Risk-benefit should be considered when the following medical problems exist:*

Anemia, or history of
(increased incidence of excessive uterine bleeding postabortion or postpartum with use of prostaglandins)

» Cardiac disease, active
(decrease in blood pressure and bradycardia may result in cardiovascular collapse and angina pectoris)

Cardiovascular disease, history of or
Hypertension, or history of or
Hypotension, history of or
Preeclampsia
(condition may be aggravated by possible vasoconstriction or decreased blood pressure; 2 cases of myocardial infarction have occurred in patients with a history of cardiovascular disease)

Cervical stenosis or
Uterine fibroids or
Uterine surgery, history of
(increased risk of uterine rupture)

Cervicitis or
Endocervical lesions, infected or
Vaginitis, acute
(in some cases, medically induced cervical ripening may increase risk of cervical injury or chronic cervicitis)

Epilepsy, or history of
(rarely, dinoprostone has been reported to cause seizures in epileptics whose seizures were poorly controlled prior to its use)

Exaggerated response to dinoprostone, history of or
Multiparity
(excessive dosage or use with oxytocin may cause uterine hypertonicity with spasm and tetanic contraction, which can lead to posterior cervical perforations, cervical lacerations, uterine rupture, and hemorrhage)

Glaucoma
(increases in intraocular pressure and miosis have been reported rarely during the use of prostaglandins)

» Hepatic disease, active or
Hepatic disease, history of or
» Renal disease, active or
Renal disease, history of
(metabolism and elimination of dinoprostone may be impaired, resulting in prolonged half-life)

**Patient monitoring**

The following may be especially important in patient monitoring (other tests may be warranted in some patients, depending on condition; » = major clinical significance):

Blood pressure, maternal and
Contractions—frequency, duration, and force of and
Heart rate, fetal and maternal and

Temperature, maternal and
Uterine tone, resting
(monitoring of these parameters is recommended at frequent intervals during abortion procedure or labor and delivery; well-hydrating patient with an electrolyte solution counteracts the decreased peripheral-resistance and induced vasodilatation)

(continuous monitoring of uterine activity and fetal state is especially recommended for patients with known history of hypertonic contractility or tetanic uterine contractions)

(maternal temperature increases of greater than 2° F (1.1° C) occurs in 50% of patients 15 to 45 minutes after vaginal suppository administration and normalizes within 2 to 6 hours after therapy is discontinued; differentiation between endometritis pyrexia and dinoprostone-induced pyrexia should be considered)

Vaginal examination
(recommended prior to each dose and after delivery or abortion to monitor cervical response and to check for signs of cervical trauma)

# Side/Adverse Effects

The following side/adverse effects have been selected on the basis of their potential clinical significance (possible signs and symptoms in parentheses where appropriate)—not necessarily inclusive:

**Those indicating need for medical attention**
Incidence less frequent or rare
*Anaphylaxis, generalized* (swelling of face, inside the nose, and eyelids; hives; shortness of breath; trouble in breathing; tightness in chest; wheezing); *bradycardia* (slow heartbeat); *bronchoconstriction* (wheezing; troubled breathing; tightness in chest)—especially in asthmatics; *increased uterine pain accompanying abortion*—correlates with efficacy; *peripheral vasoconstriction* (pale, cool, or blotchy skin on arms or legs; weak or absent pulse in arms or legs)—possibly severe; *substernal pressure or pain* (pressing or painful feeling in chest); *tachycardia* (fast heartbeat); *uterine hypertonus* (severe cramping of the uterus)

**Those indicating need for medical attention only if they continue or are bothersome**
Incidence more frequent
*Abdominal or stomach cramps; diarrhea*—about 40% with use of 20-mg suppositories; *fever, transient*—about 50% with use of 20-mg suppositories; *nausea*—about 33% with use of 20-mg suppositories; *vomiting*—about 67%

Incidence less frequent—about 10% with use of 20-mg suppositories
*Chills or shivering; headache*

Incidence rare
*Flushing; ileus, adynamic* (constipation, tender or mildly bloated abdomen); *vulvar edema*

**Those indicating possible postabortion complications and the need for medical attention if they occur after medication is discontinued**
*Endometritis* (continuing chills; shivering; continuing fever—usually on third day post-abortion; foul-smelling vaginal discharge; pain in lower abdomen); *unusual increase in uterine bleeding*

# Patient Consultation

As an aid to patient consultation, refer to *Advice for the Patient, Dinoprostone (Cervical/Vaginal).*

In providing consultation, consider emphasizing the following selected information (» = major clinical significance):

**Before using this medication**
» Conditions affecting use, especially:
Allergies to dinoprostone or other oxytocics
Pregnancy—Because some prostaglandins are teratogenic in animals, any pregnancy termination that fails with dinoprostone should be completed by another method
Other medical problems, especially asthma, cardiac disease, hepatic disease, pelvic inflammatory disease, pulmonary disease, or renal disease

**Proper use of this medication**
» Remaining in supine position for 10 minutes following insertion of suppository, 10 to 30 minutes following application of cervical gel, or 30 minutes following application of vaginal gel
» Proper dosing

**Side/adverse effects**
Signs of potential side effects, especially anaphylaxis, bradycardia, bronchoconstriction, increased uterine pain accompanying abortion, peripheral vasoconstriction, substernal pressure or pain, tachycardia, uterine hypertonus

Signs of postabortion complications, such as endometritis or unusual increase in uterine bleeding, after medication has been discontinued

## General Dosing Information

Patients receiving dinoprostone should be hospitalized and under the supervision of a physician experienced in its use.

Dinoprostone is not feticidal and may result in delivery of a live fetus.

It is recommended that antiemetic and antidiarrheal medications be administered prior to or concurrently with dinoprostone to decrease the possibility of gastrointestinal side effects. Narcotic analgesics may be given for uterine pain.

Confirmation of intrauterine fetal death should be made prior to use of dinoprostone for missed abortion or intrauterine fetal death.

In those patients with profuse vaginal bleeding or ruptured membranes, blood or fluid present in the cervix and vagina may cause expulsion of the gel or suppository, thereby interfering with the absorption and efficacy of dinoprostone.

### For treatment of adverse effects

Treatment is primarily symptomatic and supportive and may include the following:
- Sponging or irrigation with sterile saline of upper vagina to remove residual dinoprostone and prevent further absorption.
- Using tocolytic therapy, such as ritodrine, terbutaline, or magnesium sulfate, to treat uterine hyperstimulation.

## Cervical Dosage Forms

### DINOPROSTONE CERVICAL GEL

**Usual adult and adolescent dose**
Cervical ripening—
    Intracervical, 0.5 mg placed into the cervical canal, just below the internal cervical os, using the syringe and catheter provided. Patient should remain in supine position for at least fifteen to thirty minutes following administration. A need for an additional dose is determined by the physician and ensuing clinical events.

**Usual adult prescribing limits**
Cervical ripening—
    Maximum cumulative dose is 1.5 mg (7.5 mL) in 24 hours.

**Strength(s) usually available**
U.S.—
    0.5 mg per 2.5 mL (3 grams) prefilled single-use syringe (Rx) [*Prepidil*].
Canada—
    0.5 mg per 2.5 mL (3 grams) prefilled single-use syringe (Rx) [*Prepidil*].

Note: Packaging contains two catheter tips (10 and 20 mm).

**Packaging and storage**
Store between 2 and 8° C (36 and 46° F).

**Preparation of dosage form**
Bring medication to room temperature just prior to administration. Do not force warming by use of external heat source, such as water bath or microwave oven.
Each application is for single use and unused contents should be discarded, including the small amount of gel remaining in the catheter.

## Vaginal Dosage Forms

### DINOPROSTONE VAGINAL GEL

**Usual adult and adolescent dose**
Induction of labor—
    Intravaginal, 1 mg placed into the posterior fornix of the vaginal canal. The patient should remain in supine position for at least fifteen to thirty minutes after administration. A dose of 1 or 2 mg may be repeated once, six hours later, if needed.

**Strength(s) usually available**
U.S.—
    Not commercially available.
Canada—
    1 mg per 2.5 mL (3 grams) applicatorful (Rx) [*Prostin E2*].
    2 mg per 2.5 mL (3 grams) applicatorful (Rx) [*Prostin E2*].

**Packaging and storage**
Store below 2 and 8 °C (36 and 46 °F).

**Preparation of dosage form**
Bring medication to room temperature just prior to administration. Do not force warming by use of external heat source, such as water bath or microwave oven.

## DINOPROSTONE VAGINAL SUPPOSITORIES

**Usual adult and adolescent dose**
Abortifacient—
    Intravaginal, 20 mg, repeated every three to five hours, adjusted according to patient response until abortion occurs. Patient should remain in supine position for at least ten minutes following insertion.

**Usual adult prescribing limits**
Abortifacient—
    Maximum cumulative dose is 240 mg; continuous administration of dinoprostone for more than 2 days is not recommended.

**Strength(s) usually available**
U.S.—
    20 mg (Rx) [*Prostin E₂*].
Canada—
    Not commercially available.

**Packaging and storage**
Store below –20 °C (–4 °F), unless otherwise specified by manufacturer.

**Preparation of dosage form**
Bring medication to room temperature just prior to administration. Do not force warming by use of external heat source, such as water bath or microwave oven.

## Selected Bibliography
Rayburn WF. Prostaglandin E2 gel for cervical ripening and induction of labor: a critical analysis. Am J Obstet Gynecol 1989; 160 (3): 529-34.
Castadot RG. Pregnancy termination: techniques, risks, and complications and their management. Fertil Steril 1986; 45 (1): 5-17.

Revised: 07/26/95

## DIOXYBENZONE-CONTAINING COMBINATIONS—

Dioxybenzone, Oxybenzone, and Padimate O (Topical)—See *Sunscreen Agents (Topical)*

## DIPHENHYDRAMINE—See *Antihistamines (Systemic)*

## DIPHENHYDRAMINE-CONTAINING COMBINATIONS—

Bromodiphenhydramine, Diphenhydramine, Codeine, Ammonium Chloride, and Potassium Guaiacolsulfonate (Systemic)—See *Cough/Cold Combinations (Systemic)*
Diphenhydramine, Codeine, and Ammonium Chloride (Systemic)—See *Cough/Cold Combinations (Systemic)*
Diphenhydramine, Dextromethorphan, and Ammonium Chloride (Systemic)—See *Cough/Cold Combinations (Systemic)*
Diphenhydramine, Phenylpropanolamine, and Aspirin (Systemic)—See *Antihistamines, Decongestants, and Analgesics (Systemic)*
Diphenhydramine and Pseudoephedrine (Systemic)—See *Antihistamines and Decongestants (Systemic)*
Diphenhydramine, Pseudoephedrine, and Acetaminophen (Systemic)—See *Antihistamines, Decongestants, and Analgesics (Systemic)*
Diphenhydramine, Pseudoephedrine, Dextromethorphan, and Acetaminophen (Systemic)—See *Cough/Cold Combinations (Systemic)*
Ergotamine, Caffeine, and Diphenhydramine (Systemic)—See *Vascular Headache Suppressants, Ergot Derivative–containing (Systemic)*

# DIPHENIDOL   Systemic†

INN: Difenidol

VA CLASSIFICATION (Primary/Secondary): CN550/GA700

Note: For a listing of dosage forms and brand names by country availability, see *Dosage Forms* section(s). For a listing of brand names for the articles in this monograph, refer to the General Index.

†Not commercially available in Canada.

## Category

Antiemetic; antivertigo agent.

## Indications

### Accepted

Vertigo (prophylaxis and treatment)—Diphenidol is indicated in the prevention and symptomatic treatment of peripheral (labyrinthine) vertigo and associated nausea and vomiting that occur in such conditions as Meniere's disease and surgery of the middle and inner ear.

Nausea and vomiting (prophylaxis and treatment) and

Nausea and vomiting, cancer chemotherapy–induced (prophylaxis and treatment)—Diphenidol is indicated also for the control of nausea and vomiting associated with postoperative states, malignant neoplasms, labyrinthine disturbances, antineoplastic agent therapy, radiation sickness, and infectious diseases.

### Unaccepted

Diphenidol has been used in the treatment of ventricular tachyarrhythmias; however, the use of diphenidol as an antiarrhythmic is unwarranted because of the frequency and severity of adverse central nervous system (CNS) effects.

Diphenidol is *not* indicated for use in the nausea and vomiting of pregnancy.

## Pharmacology/Pharmacokinetics

### Physicochemical characteristics

Molecular weight—Diphenidol hydrochloride: 345.91.

### Mechanism of action/Effect

The mechanism by which diphenidol exerts its antiemetic and antivertigo effects is not precisely known. It is thought to diminish vestibular stimulation and depress labyrinthine function. An action on the medullary chemoreceptive trigger zone may also be involved in the antiemetic effect.

### Other actions/effects

Diphenidol has no significant sedative, tranquilizing, or antihistaminic action. It has a weak peripheral anticholinergic effect.

### Absorption

Well absorbed from gastrointestinal tract after oral administration.

### Half-life

4 hours.

### Time to peak concentration

$1\frac{1}{2}$ to 3 hours.

### Elimination

Primarily renal (about 90% of drug). Most of an oral dose is excreted within 3 to 4 days.

## Precautions to Consider

### Pregnancy/Reproduction

Pregnancy—Studies in humans and animals have not shown a significant difference in conception rate, litter size, live birth or viability, or birth abnormalities between diphenidol-treated and untreated control groups.

### Breast-feeding

Problems in humans have not been documented.

### Pediatrics

Appropriate studies on the relationship of age to the effects of diphenidol used in the prophylaxis or treatment of vertigo have not been performed in the pediatric population. Also, appropriate studies with diphenidol used in the prophylaxis or treatment of nausea and vomiting in children weighing less than 22.8 kg have not been performed; use in these children is not recommended.

### Geriatrics

No information is available on the relationship of age to the effects of diphenidol in geriatric patients.

### Drug interactions and/or related problems

The following drug interactions and/or related problems have been selected on the basis of their potential clinical significance (possible mechanism in parentheses where appropriate)—not necessarily inclusive (» = major clinical significance):

Note: Combinations containing any of the following medications, depending on the amount present, may also interact with this medication.

Anticholinergics or other medications with anticholinergic activity (See *Appendix II*)
(anticholinergic effects may be potentiated when these medications are used concurrently with diphenidol)

Apomorphine
(prior ingestion of diphenidol may decrease the emetic response to apomorphine in the treatment of poisoning)

» CNS depression–producing medications (See *Appendix II*)
(concurrent use may potentiate the effects of either these medications or diphenidol)

### Medical considerations/Contraindications

The medical considerations/contraindications included here have been selected on the basis of their potential clinical significance (reasons given in parentheses where appropriate)—not necessarily inclusive (» = major clinical significance).

*Except under special circumstances, this medication should not be used when the following medical problem exists:*

» Anuria
(renal shut-down may increase risk of systemic accumulation of diphenidol)

*Risk-benefit should be considered when the following medical problems exist:*

Gastrointestinal tract obstructive disease, such as stenosing peptic ulcer and pyloric or duodenal obstruction
(decrease in motility and tone may occur, resulting in obstruction and gastric retention)

Genitourinary tract obstructive disease, such as prostatic hypertrophy
(use may precipitate urinary retention)

Glaucoma
(use may increase intraocular pressure)

» Hypotension
(may be exacerbated)

» Renal function impairment
(decreased excretion may increase the risk of side effects)

Sensitivity to diphenidol

Caution is recommended when diphenidol is used, since signs of intestinal obstruction, brain tumor, or overdosage of toxic drugs may be obscured by its antiemetic action.

## Side/Adverse Effects

Note: Hallucinations, disorientation, and confusion have been reported with usual doses of diphenidol within the first 3 days of therapy. Upon cessation of therapy, symptoms disappeared within 3 days.

The following side/adverse effects have been selected on the basis of their potential clinical significance (possible signs and symptoms in parentheses where appropriate)—not necessarily inclusive:

### Those indicating need for medical attention

Incidence rare—less than 0.5%
   *Confusion; hallucinations*

### Those indicating need for medical attention only if they continue or are bothersome

Incidence more frequent
   *Drowsiness*

Incidence less frequent or rare
   *Blurred vision; dizziness; dryness of mouth; headache; heartburn; nervousness, restlessness, or trouble in sleeping; skin rash; stomach upset or pain; unusual tiredness or weakness*

## Overdose

For more information on the management of overdose or unintentional ingestion, **contact a Poison Control Center** (see *Poison Control Center Listing*).

### Clinical effects of overdose

The following effects have been selected on the basis of their potential clinical significance (possible signs and symptoms in parentheses where appropriate)–not necessarily inclusive:

*Drowsiness, severe; hypotension* (severe unusual tiredness or weakness); *respiratory depression* (shortness of breath or troubled breathing)

### Treatment of overdose

Treatment of overdosage is essentially supportive, including the following:

To decrease absorption—Early gastric lavage.

Supportive care—Maintenance of blood pressure and respiration. Patients in whom intentional overdose is confirmed or suspected should be referred for psychiatric consultation.

## Patient Consultation

As an aid to patient consultation, refer to *Advice for the Patient, Diphenidol (Systemic)*.

In providing consultation, consider emphasizing the following selected information (» = major clinical significance):

### Before using this medication

» Conditions affecting use, especially:
Sensitivity to diphenidol
Use in children—Not recommended for prophylaxis or treatment of nausea and vomiting in children weighing less than 22.8 kg
Other medications, especially CNS depressants
Other medical problems, especially anuria, hypotension, renal function impairment

### Proper use of this medication

Taking with food, water, or milk to minimize gastric irritation
» Importance of not taking more medication than the amount prescribed
» Proper dosing
Missed dose: If on a regular dosing schedule—using as soon as possible; if almost time for next dose, not using at all; not doubling doses
» Proper storage

### Precautions while using this medication

» Avoiding use of alcohol or other CNS depressants
» Caution if drowsiness or blurred vision occurs

### Side/adverse effects

Signs of potential side effects, especially confusion and hallucinations

## General Dosing Information

Because of its potential to cause hallucinations, disorientation, or confusion, use of diphenidol should be limited to patients who are hospitalized or under comparable continuous close professional supervision.

### Diet/Nutrition

In the preventive treatment of vertigo and associated nausea and vomiting, diphenidol may be taken with food, water, or milk to minimize gastric irritation. However, if nausea and vomiting are present, the further intake of liquids or food may aggravate the condition.

## Oral Dosage Forms

### DIPHENIDOL HYDROCHLORIDE TABLETS

**Usual adult and adolescent dose**
Antiemetic and
Antivertigo—
Oral, 25 to 50 mg every four hours as needed.

**Usual adult prescribing limits**
300 mg a day.

**Usual pediatric dose**
Antiemetic—
Oral, 880 mcg (0.88 mg) per kg of body weight or 25 mg per square meter of body surface every four hours as needed. If symptoms persist, dose may be repeated in one hour after initial dose; subsequent doses should be spaced four hours apart; or,
For children weighing 22.8 to 45.6 kg: Oral, 25 mg every four hours as needed.

Note: Children weighing up to 22.8 kg—Use is not recommended.

**Usual pediatric prescribing limits**
For children weighing 22.8 kg and over: 5.5 mg per kg of body weight a day.

**Strength(s) usually available**
U.S.—

25 mg (Rx) [*Vontrol* (acacia; calcium sulfate; cellulose; FD&C No. 5 [tartrazine]; FD&C Yellow No. 6; magnesium stearate; starch)].
Canada—
Not commercially available.

**Packaging and storage**
Store below 40 °C (104 °F), preferably between 15 and 30 °C (59 and 86 °F), in a tight, light-resistant container, unless otherwise specified by manufacturer.

**Auxiliary labeling**
• May cause drowsiness.
• Avoid alcoholic beverages.

Revised: 04/16/93

---

# DIPHENOXYLATE AND ATROPINE   Systemic

VA CLASSIFICATION (Primary): GA400
Note: Controlled substance classification—

U.S.: V.
Canada: N.

Note: For a listing of dosage forms and brand names by country availability, see *Dosage Forms* section(s). For a listing of brand names for the articles in this monograph, refer to the General Index.

## Category

Antidiarrheal (antiperistaltic).

## Indications

Note: The efficacy of any antidiarrheal medication for treatment of most cases of nonspecific diarrhea is questionable, especially in children. **Preferred treatment for acute, nonspecific diarrhea consists of fluid and electrolyte replacement, nutritional therapy, and, if possible, elimination of the underlying cause of the diarrhea.**

### Accepted

Diarrhea (treatment adjunct)—Diphenoxylate and atropine combination is indicated in adults, as an adjunct to fluid and electrolyte therapy, in the symptomatic treatment of acute and chronic diarrhea.

### Unaccepted

Diphenoxylate and atropine combination is not recommended for treatment of diarrhea in children.

## Pharmacology/Pharmacokinetics

### Physicochemical characteristics

Molecular weight—Atropine sulfate: 694.84.
Diphenoxylate hydrochloride: 489.06.

### Mechanism of action/Effect

Diphenoxylate—Probably acts both locally and centrally to reduce intestinal motility.
Atropine—Has anticholinergic activity. However, in this preparation atropine is included in doses below the therapeutic level in an attempt to prevent abuse by deliberate overdosage.

### Duration of effect

3 to 4 hours.

### Biotransformation

Diphenoxylate—Hepatic; the major metabolite difenoxin (diphenoxylic acid) has similar activity.

**Half-life**
Atropine—2.5 hours.
Diphenoxylate—2.5 hours.
Diphenoxylic acid—4.5 hours.

**Onset of effect**
45 to 60 minutes.

**Elimination**
Atropine—Renal; 30 to 50% excreted unchanged.
Diphenoxylate—Fecal/renal; less than 1% eliminated unchanged in urine.

# Precautions to Consider

## Pregnancy/Reproduction
Pregnancy—Adequate and well-controlled studies in humans have not been done.
Although studies in animals with diphenoxylate and atropine have not shown any evidence of teratogenicity, risk-benefit must be considered since a study in rats showed that maternal weight gain was reduced when diphenoxylate was given at doses of 20 mg per kg per day. Also, at the same dosage, fertility was decreased, and out of 27 matings only 4 rats conceived and bore 25 normal young. Studies in rabbits showed no embryotoxic, teratogenic, or contraceptive effects.
FDA Pregnancy Category C.

## Breast-feeding
Problems in humans have not been documented. However, both diphenoxylate's metabolite, diphenoxylic acid, and atropine are distributed into breast milk.

## Pediatrics
Diphenoxylate and atropine combination is not recommended for treatment of diarrhea in children. Recommended treatment consists of oral rehydration therapy to prevent loss of fluids and electrolytes, nutritional therapy, and, if possible, elimination of the underlying cause of the diarrhea.
Infants and young children are especially susceptible to the toxic effects of atropine.
Children may also be more susceptible to the respiratory depressant effects of diphenoxylate.

## Geriatrics
No information is available on the relationship of age to the effects of diphenoxylate and atropine in geriatric patients. However, elderly patients may be more susceptible to the respiratory depressant effects of diphenoxylate, and to the mild anticholinergic effects and confusion caused by atropine.
In geriatric patients with diarrhea, caution is recommended because of the risk of fluid and electrolyte loss.

## Drug interactions and/or related problems
The following drug interactions and/or related problems have been selected on the basis of their potential clinical significance (possible mechanism in parentheses where appropriate)—not necessarily inclusive (» = major clinical significance):

Note: Combinations containing any of the following medications, depending on the amount present, may also interact with this medication.

Addictive medications, other, especially central nervous system (CNS) depressants with habituating potential
(concurrent use with diphenoxylate may increase the risk of habituation; caution is recommended)

» Alcohol or
» CNS depression–producing medications, other (See *Appendix II*)
(concurrent use with diphenoxylate may increase the CNS depressant effects of either diphenoxylate or these medications; also, when tricyclic antidepressants are used concurrently with atropine, their anticholinergic effects may be intensified; dosage adjustment may be required)

» Anticholinergics or other medications with anticholinergic action (See *Appendix II*)
(these medications may enhance the effects of atropine during concurrent use; significant interaction is unlikely with usual doses of diphenoxylate and atropine combination, but may occur with its abuse)

» Monoamine oxidase (MAO) inhibitors, including furazolidone, procarbazine, and selegiline
(concurrent use with diphenoxylate may precipitate hypertensive crisis; MAO inhibitors may block detoxification of atropine, thus potentiating its action)

» Naltrexone
(administration of naltrexone to a patient physically dependent on opioid drugs, such as diphenoxylate, will precipitate withdrawal symptoms; symptoms may appear within 5 minutes of naltrexone administration, persist for up to 48 hours, and be difficult to reverse)
(naltrexone blocks the therapeutic effects of opioids, including the antidiarrheal effects; also, patients receiving naltrexone should be advised to use alternative antidiarrheals when necessary)

Opioid (narcotic) analgesics
(concurrent use with diphenoxylate may result in increased risk of severe constipation and additive CNS depressant effects)

## Laboratory value alterations
The following have been selected on the basis of their potential clinical significance (possible effect in parentheses where appropriate)—not necessarily inclusive (» = major clinical significance):

With diagnostic test results
» Phenolsulfonphthalein (PSP) excretion test
(atropine utilizes the same tubular mechanism of excretion as PSP, resulting in decreased urinary excretion of PSP; concurrent use of atropine is not recommended in patients receiving PSP excretion test)

With physiology/laboratory test values
Amylase, serum
(values may be increased as a result of spasm of the sphincter of Oddi)

## Medical considerations/Contraindications
The medical considerations/contraindications included here have been selected on the basis of their potential clinical significance (reasons given in parentheses where appropriate)—not necessarily inclusive (» = major clinical significance).

*Except under special circumstances, this medication should not be used when the following medical problems exist:*

» Colitis, severe
(patient may develop toxic megacolon)

» Diarrhea associated with pseudomembranous colitis resulting from treatment with broad-spectrum antibiotics
(inhibition of peristalsis may delay the removal of toxins from the colon, thereby prolonging and/or worsening the diarrhea)

*Risk-benefit should be considered when the following medical problems exist:*

Alcoholism, active or in remission, or
Drug abuse or dependence, history of
(diphenoxylate content may increase chances of drug abuse in patient already predisposed to dependence)

Cardiovascular instability
(possible increase in heart rate may be undesirable)

» Dehydration
(may predispose to delayed diphenoxylate intoxication; inhibition of peristalsis may result in fluid retention in colon and may further aggravate dehydration; discontinuation of medication and rehydration therapy is essential if signs or symptoms of dehydration, such as dryness of mouth, excessive thirst, wrinkled skin, decreased urination, and dizziness or lightheadedness, are present; fluid loss may have serious consequences, such as circulatory collapse and renal failure)

Diarrhea caused by infectious organisms
(bacterial diarrhea may worsen due to the increased contact time between the mucosa and the penetrating microorganism; however, there is no evidence of this occurring in actual practice)

» Diarrhea caused by poisoning, until toxic material has been eliminated from gastrointestinal tract

Down's syndrome
(atropine may cause abnormal increase in pupillary dilation and acceleration of heart rate)

» Dysentery, acute, characterized by bloody stools and elevated temperature
(sole treatment with antiperistaltic antidiarrheals may be inadequate; antibiotic therapy may be required)

Gallbladder disease or gallstones
(diphenoxylate may cause biliary tract spasm)

» Gastrointestinal tract obstruction
(may result in pseudo-obstruction, or in dilation of the large or small bowel)

Glaucoma, angle-closure
(although unlikely with usual doses of this combination, atropine may precipitate an acute attack of angle-closure glaucoma)

» Hepatic function impairment or jaundice
    (diphenoxylate may precipitate hepatic coma; it is recommended that dosage be reduced in patients with impaired hepatic function)

Hiatal hernia associated with reflux esophagitis
    (although unlikely with usual doses of this combination, atropine may aggravate condition)

Hypertension
    (although unlikely with usual doses of this combination, atropine may aggravate condition)

Hyperthyroidism
    (characterized by tachycardia, which may be increased by atropine)

Hypothyroidism
    (diphenoxylate may increase risk of respiratory depression)

Incontinence, overflow
    (secondary to constipation, but often mistaken for diarrhea; use of diphenoxylate and atropine may worsen constipation and/or cause dilation or pseudo-obstruction of the colon)

Intestinal atony of the elderly or debilitated
    (although unlikely with usual doses of this combination, use of atropine may result in obstruction)

Myasthenia gravis
    (although unlikely with usual doses of this combination, atropine may aggravate condition because of inhibition of acetylcholine action)

Prostatic hypertrophy or
Urethral stricture, acute or
Urinary retention
    (reduction in tone of urinary bladder may aggravate or lead to complete urinary retention)

Renal function impairment
    (decreased elimination of atropine may increase the risk of side effects)

Respiratory disease or impairment
    (increased risk of respiratory depression)

Sensitivity to atropine or diphenoxylate

### Patient monitoring

The following may be especially important in patient monitoring (other tests may be warranted in some patients, depending on condition; » = major clinical significance):

» Hepatic function determinations
    (recommended at periodic intervals during long-term therapy, especially for patients with hepatic function impairment)

## Side/Adverse Effects

The following side/adverse effects have been selected on the basis of their potential clinical significance (possible signs and symptoms in parentheses where appropriate)—not necessarily inclusive:

**Those indicating need for medical attention**
Incidence less frequent or rare
    *Paralytic ileus or toxic megacolon* (bloating; constipation; loss of appetite; severe stomach pain with nausea and vomiting)

**Those indicating need for medical attention only if they continue, worsen, or are bothersome**
Incidence less frequent or rare
    *Anticholinergic effects, mild* (blurred vision; difficult urination; dryness of skin and mouth; fever); *CNS depression* (dizziness or lightheadedness; drowsiness; mental depression); *confusion; headache; numbness of hands or feet; skin rash or itching; swelling of the gums*
    Note: Since atropine is present in a subtherapeutic dose, the appearance of these symptoms probably indicates overdosage.

**Those indicating possible withdrawal and the need for medical attention if they occur after discontinuation of prolonged high-dose therapy**
Incidence rare
    *Increased sweating; muscle cramps; nausea or vomiting; shivering or trembling; stomach cramps*

## Overdose

For specific information on the agents used in the management of diphenoxylate and atropine overdose, see:
 • *Charcoal, Activated (Oral-Local)* monograph; and/or
 • *Naloxone (Systemic)* monograph.

For more information on the management of overdose or unintentional ingestion, **contact a Poison Control Center** (see *Poison Control Center Listing*).

### Clinical effects of overdose

The following effects have been selected on the basis of their potential clinical significance (possible signs and symptoms in parentheses where appropriate)–not necessarily inclusive:
    *Anticholinergic effects, severe* (continuing blurred vision or changes in near vision; fast heartbeat; severe drowsiness; severe dryness of mouth, nose, and throat; unusual warmth, dryness, and flushing of skin); *coma; respiratory depression* (severe shortness of breath or troubled breathing); *unusual excitement, nervousness, restlessness, or irritability*
    Note: *Respiratory depression* may occur as late as 12 to 30 hours after ingestion.

Possible symptoms of overdose
    *Anticholinergic effects, mild* (blurred vision; difficult urination; dryness of skin and mouth; fever); *CNS depression* (dizziness or lightheadedness; drowsiness; mental depression); *confusion; headache; numbness of hands or feet; skin rash or itching; swelling of the gums*
    Note: Since atropine is present in a subtherapeutic dose, the appearance of these symptoms probably indicates overdosage.

### Treatment of overdose

Treatment of overdose with diphenoxylate and atropine is the same as treatment for meperidine or morphine overdosage and involves the following:

To decrease absorption—Induction of vomiting, or gastric lavage, if vomiting has not occurred; administration of a slurry of 100 grams of activated charcoal, after induction of vomiting or gastric lavage, in non-comatose patients.

Specific treatment—Intravenous administration of 0.4 mg (0.01 mg per kg of body weight in children) of narcotic antagonist naloxone, which may be repeated at 2- to 3-minute intervals, for respiratory depression.

Monitoring—Careful monitoring for 48 to 72 hours.

Supportive care—Support of respiration. Patients in whom intentional overdose is confirmed or suspected should be referred for psychiatric consultation.

## Patient Consultation

As an aid to patient consultation, refer to *Advice for the Patient, Diphenoxylate and Atropine (Systemic)*.

In providing consultation, consider emphasizing the following selected information (» = major clinical significance):

### Before using this medication

» Conditions affecting use, especially:
    Sensitivity to atropine or diphenoxylate
    Pregnancy—Studies in rats show decreased fertility and decreased maternal weight gain
    Breast-feeding—Diphenoxylate and atropine distributed into breast milk; potential for serious adverse effects in nursing infant
    Use in children—Not recommended for use in children; increased susceptibility to toxic effects of atropine and respiratory depressant effects of diphenoxylate; risk of dehydration
    Use in the elderly—Increased risk of respiratory depression, anticholinergic effects, and confusion; risk of dehydration
    Other medications, especially other anticholinergics, CNS depressants, MAO inhibitors, or naltrexone
    Other medical problems, especially acute dysentery; dehydration; diarrhea caused by antibiotics or poisoning; gastrointestinal tract obstruction; hepatic function impairment or jaundice; or severe colitis

### Proper use of this medication

Taking with food or meals if gastric irritation occurs
» Importance of not taking more medication than the amount prescribed because of habit-forming potential
» Importance of maintaining adequate hydration and proper diet
» Proper dosing
    Missed dose: If on a scheduled dosing regimen—Taking as soon as possible; not taking if almost time for next dose; not doubling doses
» Proper storage
*For liquid dosage form*
    Proper administration technique: Measuring amount with dropper and taking by mouth

### Precautions while using this medication

Regular visits to physician to check progress during prolonged therapy
» Consulting physician if diarrhea is not controlled within 48 hours and/or fever develops
» Avoiding use of alcohol or other CNS depressants during therapy
» Suspected overdose: Getting emergency help at once

Need to inform physician or dentist of use of medication if any kind of surgery (including dental surgery) or emergency treatment is required

» Caution if dizziness or drowsiness occurs

### Side/adverse effects

Signs of potential side effects, especially paralytic ileus or toxic megacolon

## General Dosing Information

Treatment with diphenoxylate and atropine should be continued for 24 to 48 hours before it is considered ineffective in acute diarrhea. If clinical improvement of chronic diarrhea after treatment with a maximum daily dose of 20 mg of diphenoxylate is not observed within 10 days, treatment should be discontinued.

Inhibition of peristalsis may produce fluid retention in the bowel, which may aggravate dehydration and depletion of electrolytes, and may also increase variability of response to the medication. If dehydration or electrolyte imbalance occurs, diphenoxylate and atropine therapy should be withheld until appropriate corrective therapy has begun.

To prevent development of toxic megacolon in patients with acute ulcerative colitis, treatment with diphenoxylate and atropine should be discontinued promptly if abdominal distention or other specific gastrointestinal symptoms such as anorexia, bloating, constipation, nausea, vomiting, or abdominal pain occur.

Prolonged use of larger than usual therapeutic doses may result in physical dependence.

Tolerance to the antidiarrheal effects of diphenoxylate and atropine may develop with prolonged use.

This medication may suppress respiration, especially in the elderly, the very ill, and patients with respiratory problems. Lower doses may be required for these patients.

## Oral Dosage Forms

### DIPHENOXYLATE HYDROCHLORIDE AND ATROPINE SULFATE ORAL SOLUTION USP

#### Usual adult and adolescent dose

Antidiarrheal (antiperistaltic)—
Initial: Oral, 5 mg of diphenoxylate hydrochloride and 50 mcg (0.05 mg) of atropine sulfate three or four times a day.
Maintenance: Oral, 5 mg of diphenoxylate hydrochloride and 50 mcg (0.05 mg) of atropine sulfate once a day, as needed.

#### Usual adult prescribing limits

20 mg per day.

#### Usual pediatric dose

Antidiarrheal (antiperistaltic)—
Children up to 12 years of age: Use is not recommended.
Children 12 years of age and older: See *Usual adult and adolescent dose.*

#### Usual geriatric dose

See *Usual adult and adolescent dose.*
Note: Geriatric patients may be more sensitive to the effects of the usual adult dose.

#### Strength(s) usually available

U.S.—
2.5 mg of diphenoxylate hydrochloride and 25 mcg (0.025 mg) of atropine sulfate, per 5 mL (Rx) [*Lomotil* (alcohol 15%); GENERIC].
Canada—
Not commercially available.

#### Packaging and storage

Store below 40 °C (104 °F), preferably between 15 and 30 °C (59 and 86 °F), unless otherwise specified by manufacturer. Store in a tight, light-resistant container. Protect from freezing.

### Auxiliary labeling

• May cause drowsiness.
• Avoid alcoholic beverages.
• Keep out of reach of children.

### Note

Controlled substance in the U.S.

### DIPHENOXYLATE HYDROCHLORIDE AND ATROPINE SULFATE TABLETS USP

#### Usual adult and adolescent dose

See *Diphenoxylate Hydrochloride and Atropine Sulfate Oral Solution USP.*

#### Usual pediatric dose

Antidiarrheal (antiperistaltic)—
Children up to 12 years of age: Use is not recommended.
Children 12 years of age and older: See *Usual adult and adolescent dose.*

#### Usual geriatric dose

See *Usual adult and adolescent dose.*
Note: Geriatric patients may be more sensitive to the effects of the usual adult dose.

#### Strength(s) usually available

U.S.—
2.5 mg of diphenoxylate hydrochloride and 25 mcg (0.025 mg) of atropine sulfate (Rx) [*Lofene; Logen; Lomocot; Lomotil; Lonox; Vi-Atro;* GENERIC].
Canada—
2.5 mg of diphenoxylate hydrochloride and 25 mcg (0.025 mg) of atropine sulfate (Rx) [*Lomotil*].

#### Packaging and storage

Store below 40 °C (104 °F), preferably between 15 and 30 °C (59 and 86 °F), in a well-closed container, unless otherwise specified by manufacturer. Store in a light-resistant container.

#### Auxiliary labeling

• May cause drowsiness.
• Avoid alcoholic beverages.
• Keep out of reach of children.
• May be habit-forming.

### Note

Controlled substance in the U.S. and Canada.

## Selected Bibliography

Brownlee HJ, editor. Proceedings of a symposium: Management of acute nonspecific diarrhea. Am J Med 1990; 88 (Suppl 6A).
Gaginella TS. Diarrhea: some new aspects of pharmacotherapy. Drug Intell Clin Pharm 1983; 17: 914-6.

Revised: 08/22/94

---

## DIPHENOXYLATE-CONTAINING COMBINATIONS—

Diphenoxylate and Atropine (Systemic)

---

## DIPHENYLPYRALINE—See *Antihistamines (Systemic)*

---

## DIPHENYLPYRALINE-CONTAINING COMBINATIONS—

Diphenylpyraline, Phenylpropanolamine, Acetaminophen, and Caffeine (Systemic)—See *Antihistamines, Decongestants, and Analgesics (Systemic)*

---

## DIPHTHERIA AND TETANUS TOXOIDS (DT)—See *Diphtheria and Tetanus Toxoids (Systemic)*

# DIPHTHERIA AND TETANUS TOXOIDS    Systemic

This monograph includes information on the following: Diphtheria and Tetanus Toxoids for Pediatric Use (DT); Tetanus and Diphtheria Toxoids for Adult Use (Td).

Note: There are some differences in terminology with respect to the use of the terms "primary" and "reinforcing" in some of the manufacturers' labeling used for this monograph. In this monograph, the term "primary immunizing series" will be used to denote the initial doses that are usually given 4 to 8 weeks apart as well as the "reinforcing" dose that is usually given 6 to 12 months thereafter. The dose usually given at 4 to 6 years of age and the doses given every 10 years will be called booster doses.

VA CLASSIFICATION (Primary): IM200

Other commonly used names are: DT [Diphtheria and Tetanus Toxoids], Td [Tetanus and Diphtheria Toxoids]

Note: For a listing of dosage forms and brand names by country availability, see *Dosage Forms* section(s). For a listing of brand names for the articles in this monograph, refer to the General Index.

## Category

Immunizing agent (active).

## Indications

### Accepted

Diphtheria and tetanus (prophylaxis)—Diphtheria and tetanus toxoid combination is indicated for immunization against diphtheria and tetanus.

Diphtheria and tetanus toxoids for pediatric use (DT) is indicated for immunization of infants and children 6 weeks up to 7 years of age who, because of a contraindication to pertussis vaccine, cannot receive diphtheria and tetanus toxoids and pertussis vaccine (DTP) combination. If there is no contraindication to pertussis vaccine, DTP is the vaccine of choice for this age group.

Tetanus and diphtheria toxoids for adult use (Td) is indicated for immunization of adults and children 7 years of age and older.

## Pharmacology/Pharmacokinetics

### Physicochemical characteristics

Source—

Diphtheria toxoid is prepared by first cultivating a suitable strain of *Corynebacterium diphtheriae*. Tetanus toxoid is prepared by first cultivating a suitable strain of *Clostridium tetani* The resulting toxins are detoxified with formaldehyde. The detoxified toxins (toxoids) are adsorbed onto an aluminum salt. This prolongs and enhances the antigenic properties by retarding the rate of absorption of the injected toxoid in the body

### Mechanism of action/Effect

Following intramuscular injection, diphtheria toxoid and tetanus toxoid induce the formation of diphtheria antitoxin and tetanus antitoxin, respectively.

### Protective effect:

Diphtheria antitoxin—

The protective level in serum is 0.01 unit per mL.

Tetanus antitoxin—

The protective level in serum is 0.01 unit per mL.

### Time to protective effect

For diphtheria and tetanus toxoids for pediatric use (DT)—

In a study of 20 children under 1 year of age, protective levels of diphtheria and tetanus antitoxins were detected in 100% of the children after administration of 3 doses of DT. In addition, protective levels of diphtheria and tetanus antitoxins were detected in 100% of the children after administration of 2 doses of DT, but maternal antibody may have contributed to the total neutralizing antibody in some of these children.

For tetanus and diphtheria toxoids for adult use (Td)—

Response to primary immunization:

Diphtheria—In a study of 10 adults who had less than 0.001 unit per mL of diphtheria antitoxin in pre-immunization serum, protective levels of diphtheria antitoxin were detected in 50% of the adults after administration of 2 doses of Td, each containing 2 Lf units of diphtheria toxoid. In a similar study of 6 adults, protective levels of diphtheria antitoxin were detected in 100% of the adults after administration of 3 doses of Td.

Tetanus—In a study of 20 adults who had less than 0.0025 unit per mL of tetanus antitoxin in pre-immunization serum, pro-

tective levels of tetanus antitoxin were detected in 70% of the adults after administration of 2 doses, and in 100% of the adults after administration of 3 doses, of Td, each containing 2 Lf units of tetanus toxoid.

Response to booster doses:

Booster doses of Td given as long as 25 to 30 years after primary immunization series have produced rapid and significant increases in the levels of both tetanus and diphtheria antitoxins.

Diphtheria—In a study of 140 adolescent males, protective levels of diphtheria antitoxin were detected in 100% of the males after administration of a single booster dose of Td containing 1 Lf unit of diphtheria toxoid.

Tetanus—In a study of 36 adults, protective levels of tetanus antitoxin were detected in 100% of the adults after administration of a single booster dose of Td containing 1 Lf unit of tetanus toxoid.

### Duration of protective effect:

At least 10 years for both diphtheria toxoid and tetanus toxoid following a completed primary immunizing series of injections.

## Precautions to Consider

### Cross-sensitivity and/or related problems

Patients sensitive to diphtheria toxoid or tetanus toxoid may be sensitive to diphtheria and tetanus toxoids for pediatric use (DT) or tetanus and diphtheria toxoids for adult use (Td) also.

### Carcinogenicity/Mutagenicity

Studies have not been done.

### Pregnancy/Reproduction

Fertility—Studies have not been done.

Pregnancy—There is no evidence that diphtheria and tetanus toxoid combination is teratogenic.

For DT: Use of DT is not recommended in females of child-bearing age.

For Td: Unimmunized pregnant women should receive 2 properly spaced doses of Td before delivery, preferably during the last 2 trimesters. Incompletely immunized pregnant women should complete the primary immunizing series of Td. Those fully immunized more than 10 years ago should receive a booster dose of Td.

Studies have not been done in animals.

FDA Pregnancy Category C.

### Breast-feeding

Diphtheria and tetanus toxoids have not been isolated from breast milk.

For DT—Use of DT is not recommended in females of child-bearing age.

For Td—There is no evidence that breast milk from women who have received Td is harmful to infants.

### Pediatrics

*For DT—*

Infants up to 6 weeks of age: Use of DT is not recommended.

Infants and children up to 7 years of age: Pediatrics-specific problems that would limit the usefulness of DT in these children are not expected.

Children 7 years of age and older: Use of DT is not recommended in this age group.

*For Td—*

Infants and children up to 7 years of age: Use of Td is not recommended in this age group.

Children 7 years of age and older: Pediatrics-specific problems that would limit the usefulness of Td in these children are not expected.

### Geriatrics

For DT—Use of DT is not recommended in this age group.

For Td—Although appropriate studies on the relationship of age to the effects of Td have not been performed in the geriatric population, geriatrics-specific problems are not expected to limit the usefulness of Td in the elderly. However, the immune response in the elderly may be slightly diminished.

### Drug interactions and/or related problems

The following drug interactions and/or related problems have been selected on the basis of their potential clinical significance (possible mechanism in parentheses where appropriate)—not necessarily inclusive (» = major clinical significance):

Note: Combinations containing any of the following medications, depending on the amount present, may also interact with this medication.

Immunosuppressants or
Radiation therapy
(because normal defense mechanisms are suppressed, the patient's antibody response to DT or Td may be decreased during therapy and deferral of routine DT or Td administration may be considered. The precaution does not apply to corticosteroids used as replacement therapy, for short-term [less than 2 weeks] systemic therapy, or by other routes of administration that do not cause immunosuppression. Where possible, immunosuppressive therapy should be interrupted when immunization is required because of a tetanus-prone wound)

## Medical considerations/Contraindications

The medical considerations/contraindications included here have been selected on the basis of their potential clinical significance (reasons given in parentheses where appropriate)—not necessarily inclusive (» = major clinical significance):

*Except under special circumstances, this medication should not be used when the following medical problems exist:*

» Febrile illness or
» Infection, acute
(routine primary or booster immunization should not be administered until the acute symptoms of the patient's illness have abated; however, emergency tetanus prophylaxis for wounds should be administered as usual. A minor afebrile illness, such as an upper respiratory infection, usually does not preclude administration of DT or Td)

» Sensitivity to DT or Td
» Tetanus infection
(products containing tetanus toxoid should not be used to treat a tetanus infection; tetanus antitoxin, preferably tetanus immune globulin [TIG], should be used instead; after recovery, the primary immunizing series should be initiated or continued, since a tetanus infection does not confer immunity)

*Risk-benefit should be considered when the following medical problem exists:*

» Sensitivity to thimerosal

## Side/Adverse Effects

Note: Although both the diphtheria toxoid and the tetanus toxoid components may evoke local and systemic allergic responses, it has been suggested that the tetanus toxoid component may be the more common cause.

If an Arthus-type hypersensitivity reaction or a fever over 39.4 °C (103 °F) occurs following a dose of diphtheria and tetanus toxoid combination, the patient usually has a very high serum tetanus antitoxin level and no additional doses of tetanus toxoid should be given for any reason, including wound management, more frequently than every 10 years.

Neurological reactions, such as convulsions, encephalopathy, and various mono- and polyneuropathies, have been reported following administration of preparations containing diphtheria toxoid and/or tetanus toxoid. Pallor, coldness, and hyporesponsiveness were reported in 1 child. In the differential diagnosis of polyradiculoneuropathies, previous administration of tetanus toxoid should be considered as a possible cause. If a neurologic reaction or a severe systemic allergic reaction occurs following a dose of diphtheria and tetanus toxoids for pediatric use (DT) or tetanus and diphtheria toxoids for adult use (Td), the person should not be further immunized with DT or Td.

Booster doses of tetanus toxoid administered more frequently than every 10 years have been reported to result in increased occurrence and severity of adverse reactions.

Generally, a history of hypersensitivity reactions other than anaphylaxis, such as delayed-type, cell-mediated allergic reaction (contact dermatitis), does not preclude immunization.

Sterile abscesses have been reported rarely following administration of DT or Td. These are thought to be caused by inadvertent subcutaneous injection of the aluminum adjuvant in the product.

Use of jet injectors, which deposit some toxoid in the subcutaneous tissue, has been associated with a higher frequency of local reactions than has intramuscular injection by needle.

The following side/adverse effects have been selected on the basis of their potential clinical significance (possible signs and symptoms in parentheses where appropriate)—not necessarily inclusive:

### Those indicating need for medical attention
Incidence rare
*For DT and Td*
*Anaphylactic reaction* (difficulty in breathing or swallowing; hives; itching, especially of soles or palms; reddening of skin, especially around ears; swelling of eyes, face, or inside of nose; unusual tiredness or weakness, sudden and severe); *arthralgias* (joint aches or pain); *neurologic reaction* (confusion; excessive sleepiness; fever over 39.4 °C [103 °F]; headache, severe or continuing; seizures; unusual irritability; vomiting, severe or continuing); *pruritus* (itching); *skin rash; urticaria* (hives)

### Additional side/adverse effects that may occur because of very high serum tetanus antitoxin levels and may indicate a need for medical attention
Incidence rare
*Arthus-type reaction* (swelling, blistering, pain, or other severe local reaction at injection site); *fever over 39.4 °C (103 °F)*

Note: *Arthus-type reaction* and *fever over 39.4 °C* usually occur only in patients old enough to receive Td, i.e., persons old enough to have received multiple booster doses of a tetanus toxoid–containing product. An *Arthus-type reaction* generally starts within 2 to 8 hours after the injection and may be severe and extensive.

### Those indicating need for medical attention only if they continue or are bothersome
Incidence more frequent
*For DT and Td*
*Redness or hard lump at injection site*—may persist for a few days
*For DT only*
*Fever under 39.4 °C (103 °F); swelling, pain, or tenderness at injection site*—may persist for a few days
Incidence less frequent
*For DT and Td*
*Nodule (hard lump) at injection site; subcutaneous atrophy (dent or indentation) at injection site*
Note: *Nodule (hard lump) at injection site* probably is caused by the aluminum content of the toxoids and may persist for a few weeks

*For DT only*
*Anorexia* (loss of appetite); *drowsiness; fretfulness; persistent crying; vomiting*

*For Td only*
*Axillary lymphadenopathy* (swelling of glands in armpit); *chills; fever under 39.4 °C (103 °F); headache; hypotension* (unusual tiredness or weakness); *malaise* (general feeling of discomfort or illness); *muscle aches; tachycardia* (fast heartbeat)

## Patient Consultation

As an aid to patient consultation, refer to *Advice for the Patient, Diphtheria and Tetanus Toxoids (Systemic).*

In providing consultation, consider emphasizing the following selected information (» = major clinical significance):

### Before receiving this vaccine
» Conditions affecting use, especially:
Sensitivity to diphtheria toxoid, tetanus toxoid, or thimerosal
Use in children—Not recommended for infants up to 6 weeks of age; only diphtheria and tetanus toxoids for pediatric use (DT) is recommended for infants and children 6 weeks to 7 years of age; only tetanus and diphtheria toxoids for adult use (Td) is recommended for children 7 years of age and older
Use in the elderly—Only tetanus and diphtheria toxoids for adult use (Td) is recommended; the immune response in the elderly may be slightly diminished
Other medical problems, especially acute infection, febrile illness, or tetanus infection

### Proper use of this vaccine
» Proper dosing

### Side/adverse effects
Notifying physician of any side effect that occurs after a dose of DT or Td, even if the side effect has gone away without treatment
Signs of potential side effects, especially anaphylactic reaction; arthralgias; neurologic reaction; pruritus; skin rash; urticaria; Arthus-type reaction; and fever over 39.4 °C (103 °F)

# General Dosing Information

Diphtheria and tetanus toxoid combination is administered by deep intramuscular injection into the deltoid (for adults and older children) or into the area of the midlateral muscles (vastus lateralis) of the thigh (for infants and younger children). The same muscle site should not be used more than once during the course of the primary immunizing series. The vaccine should not be injected subcutaneously or intravenously.

Before each additional dose of diphtheria and tetanus toxoids for pediatric use (DT) or tetanus and diphtheria toxoids for adult use (Td), the health status of the patient should be assessed. In addition, information should be obtained regarding any symptom and/or sign of an adverse reaction that occurred after the previous dose.

Routine immunization of adults and children over 6 months of age should be deferred during an outbreak of poliomyelitis in the community, unless there is also an outbreak of diphtheria. In either case, emergency tetanus prophylaxis for wounds should be administered as usual.

Persons with impaired immune response may be immunized, but may have reduced antibody response to DT or Td. Persons infected with human immunodeficiency virus (HIV) may receive DT or Td whether they have asymptomatic or symptomatic HIV infection.

Diphtheria infection may not (and tetanus infection does not) confer immunity; therefore, initiation or completion of active immunization with DT or Td is indicated at the time of recovery from either of these infections.

Interruption of the recommended schedule for the primary immunizing series of DT or Td by a delay between doses does not interfere with the final immunity achieved and does not necessitate starting the series over again, regardless of the length of time that elapsed between doses.

## Emergency tetanus prophylaxis of wounds

Patients who were unimmunized or inadequately immunized with a tetanus toxoid–containing product prior to a wound should complete their primary immunizing series as soon as possible.

For routine wound management in children under 7 years of age who have not received the primary immunizing series against tetanus, DT (or DTP, if appropriate) should be used instead of single-antigen tetanus toxoid. In addition, children whose wounds are considered to be prone to tetanus infection and who have had fewer than 3 doses (or an unknown number of doses) of a tetanus toxoid–containing product also should be administered tetanus antitoxin, preferably tetanus immune globulin (TIG). A separate syringe and site of administration should be used for DT and TIG.

The decision to administer Td for wound management with or without concomitant passive immunization using tetanus immune globulin (TIG) depends on the condition of the wound and the patient's immunization history. Examples of wounds that are not clean, minor wounds are: wounds contaminated with dirt, feces, soil, or saliva; puncture wounds; wounds caused by tearing; and wounds resulting from missiles, crushing, burns, or frostbite. Tetanus has rarely occurred in persons who have received a documented primary immunizing series of a tetanus toxoid–containing product. Persons who have received the primary immunizing series and whose wounds are minor and uncontaminated should receive a booster dose of a tetanus toxoid–containing product, such as Td, only if they have not received a tetanus toxoid booster dose within the past 10 years. Persons who have received the primary immunizing series and who have wounds that are not minor and uncontaminated should receive a booster dose of a tetanus toxoid–containing product, such as Td, only if they have not received a tetanus toxoid booster dose within the past 5 years. Persons who have not received the primary immunizing series against tetanus (or whose immunization history is unknown) should be immunized with a tetanus toxoid–containing product, such as Td. If persons who have not received the primary immunizing series against tetanus (or whose immunization history is unknown) have wounds that are considered to be prone to tetanus infection, tetanus antitoxin (preferably TIG) should be administered in addition to Td. A separate syringe and site of administration should be used for Td and TIG.

## Emergency diphtheria prophylaxis

Immunization with diphtheria toxoid reduces the risk of developing diphtheria and lessens the severity of clinical illness. However, it does not eliminate *Corynebacterium diphtheriae* from the pharynx or the skin.

Household and other close contacts of persons with diphtheria infection who have received fewer than 3 doses of a diphtheria toxoid–containing product should receive an immediate dose of a diphtheria toxoid–containing product, such as DT or Td (according to their age requirement), and should complete the primary immunizing series according to schedule. Household and other close contacts who have received 3 or more doses of a diphtheria toxoid–containing product and who have

not received an additional dose within 5 years should receive a booster dose of a diphtheria toxoid–containing product, such as DT or Td (according to their age requirement).

## For treatment of adverse effects

Recommended treatment includes:
- For mild hypersensitivity reaction—Administering antihistamines and, if necessary, corticosteroids.
- For severe hypersensitivity or anaphylactic reaction—Administering epinephrine. Antihistamines or corticosteroids may also be administered as required.

---

# *DIPHTHERIA AND TETANUS TOXOIDS (DT)*

## Summary of Differences

Indications: Diphtheria and tetanus toxoids for pediatric use (DT) is indicated for immunization of infants and children 6 weeks up to 7 years of age.

Strength (s) usually available: DT contains 6.6 to 25 Lf units of diphtheria toxoid and 5 to 10 Lf units of tetanus toxoid, per dose.

## Additional Dosing Information

Diphtheria toxoid of the strength used in DT is not recommended for adults and children 7 years of age and older, because of the increased risk of side/adverse effects associated with the use of higher doses of diphtheria toxoid in this age group.

It is recommended that infants and children up to 7 years of age receive diphtheria and tetanus toxoids as part of Diphtheria and Tetanus Toxoids and Pertussis Vaccine Adsorbed (DTP). In those cases in which the pertussis vaccine is contraindicated, it is recommended that DT be administered instead.

The primary immunizing series of DT consists of 4 doses (3 initial and 1 reinforcing) for children 6 weeks up to 1 year of age (in Canada, 2 months up to 7 years of age) or 3 doses (2 initial and 1 reinforcing) for children 1 to 7 years of age.

Preterm infants should be immunized according to their chronological age from birth.

DT can be administered concurrently with the following, using separate body sites and separate syringes (for parenterals), and the precautions that apply to each immunizing agent:
- Hepatitis B recombinant or plasma-derived vaccine.
- Polysaccharide vaccines, such as haemophilus b polysaccharide vaccine, haemophilus b conjugate vaccine, or pneumococcal polyvalent vaccine.
- Live virus vaccines, such as measles, mumps, and rubella (MMR) or oral polio vaccine (OPV).
- Inactivated poliovirus vaccine (IPV) or enhanced-potency inactivated vaccine (enhanced-potency IPV).

## Parenteral Dosage Forms

### DIPHTHERIA AND TETANUS TOXOIDS ADSORBED (DT) (FOR PEDIATRIC USE) USP

Note: DT is indicated for immunization of infants and children 6 weeks up to 7 years of age who cannot receive diphtheria and tetanus toxoids and pertussis vaccine (DTP) combination, because of a contraindication to pertussis vaccine. If there is no contraindication to pertussis vaccine, DTP is the vaccine of choice for this age group.

**Usual adult and adolescent dose**
Use is not recommended. Tetanus and diphtheria toxoids for adult use (Td) should be administered instead.

**Usual pediatric dose**
Diphtheria and tetanus (prophylaxis)—
Intramuscular, preferably into the deltoid or the midlateral muscles of the thigh
U.S.:
Children 6 weeks to 1 year of age: 0.5 mL at four- to eight-week intervals for a total of three doses. A fourth dose of 0.5 mL is administered six to twelve months after the third dose. A booster (fifth) dose of 0.5 mL is usually administered at four through six years of age (i.e., preferably prior to school entry); however, if the fourth dose of the primary immunizing series was administered after the fourth birthday, a booster (fifth) dose is not necessary.
Children 1 to 7 years of age: 0.5 mL followed by 0.5 mL four to eight weeks later for a total of two doses. A third dose of 0.5 mL is administered six to twelve months after the second dose. A booster (fourth) dose of 0.5 mL is usually administered at four through six years of age (i.e., prefer-

ably prior to school entry); however, if the third dose of the primary immunizing series was administered after the fourth birthday, a booster (fourth) dose is not necessary.

Children 7 years of age and older: Use is not recommended. Td should be administered instead.

Canada:

Children 2 months to 7 years of age: 0.5 mL at eight-week intervals for a total of three doses. A fourth dose of 0.5 mL is administered twelve months after the third dose. A booster (fifth) dose of 0.5 mL is usually administered at four through six years of age (i.e., preferably prior to school entry); however, if the fourth dose of the primary immunizing series was administered after the fourth birthday, a booster (fifth) dose is not necessary.

Children 7 years of age and older: Use is not recommended. Td should be administered instead.

## Strength(s) usually available

U.S.—

6.6 Lf units of diphtheria toxoid and 5 Lf units of tetanus toxoid per 0.5 mL dose (Rx) [GENERIC (may contain thimerosal)].

7.5 Lf units of diphtheria toxoid and 7.5 Lf units of tetanus toxoid per 0.5 mL dose (Rx) [GENERIC (may contain thimerosal)].

10 Lf units of diphtheria toxoid and 5 Lf units of tetanus toxoid per 0.5 mL dose (Rx) [GENERIC (may contain thimerosal)].

12.5 Lf units of diphtheria toxoid and 5 Lf units of tetanus toxoid per 0.5 mL dose (Rx) [GENERIC (may contain thimerosal)].

15 Lf units of diphtheria toxoid and 10 Lf units of tetanus toxoid per 0.5 mL dose (Rx) [GENERIC (may contain thimerosal)].

Canada—

25 Lf units of diphtheria toxoid and 5 Lf units of tetanus toxoid in each 0.5 mL dose (Rx) [GENERIC (may contain thimerosal)].

Note: Lf is the quantity of toxoid as assessed by flocculation.

## Packaging and storage

Store between 2 and 8 °C (36 and 46 °F), unless otherwise specified by manufacturer. Store away from the freezer compartment. Protect from freezing.

## Stability

Freezing destroys activity. The product should not be used if it has been exposed to freezing. In addition, the product should not be left out at room temperature (e.g., between patients).

## Auxiliary labeling

• Shake the vial vigorously immediately before each dose is withdrawn in order to resuspend the contents.

• Protect from freezing.

---

### *TETANUS AND DIPHTHERIA TOXOIDS (Td)*

## Summary of Differences

Indications: Tetanus and diphtheria toxoids for adult use (Td) is indicated for immunization of adults and children 7 years of age and older.

Side/adverse effects: Arthus-type reaction and fever over 39.4 °C usually occur only in patients old enough to receive Td, i.e., persons old enough to have received multiple booster doses of a tetanus toxoid–containing product.

Strength (s) usually available: Td contains 2 Lf units of diphtheria toxoid and 2 to 10 Lf units of tetanus toxoid, per dose.

## Additional Dosing Information

The concentration of diphtheria toxoid in Td, which is intended for use in persons 7 years of age and older, is lower than that of the concentration of diphtheria toxoid in diphtheria and tetanus toxoids for pediatric use (DT).

It is recommended that adults and children 7 years of age and older receive Td rather than the single-entity tetanus toxoid for the primary immunizing series, all booster doses, and active tetanus immunization in wound management. This is to help ensure protection against diphtheria infection, since a large proportion of adults is susceptible to diphtheria infection.

The primary immunizing series of Td consists of 3 doses (2 initial and 1 reinforcing) for adults and children 7 years of age and older.

## Parenteral Dosage Forms

### TETANUS AND DIPHTHERIA TOXOIDS ADSORBED FOR ADULT USE (Td) USP

#### Usual adult and adolescent dose

Diphtheria and tetanus (prophylaxis)—Intramuscular, preferably into the deltoid: 0.5 mL followed by 0.5 mL four to eight weeks later (in Canada, eight weeks later) for a total of two doses. A third dose of 0.5 mL is administered six to twelve months after the second dose. A booster dose of 0.5 mL is administered every ten years thereafter.

Note: If a booster dose of Td is administered less than ten years after the previous booster dose (e.g., as part of wound management or after exposure to diphtheria), the next booster dose should be administered ten years after the interim dose.

#### Usual pediatric dose

Diphtheria and tetanus (prophylaxis)—Intramuscular, preferably into the deltoid or the midlateral muscles of the thigh—

Children up to 7 years of age—Use is not recommended. Diphtheria and tetanus toxoids for pediatric use (DT) should be administered instead.

Children 7 years of age and older—See *Usual adult and adolescent dose.*

#### Strength(s) usually available

U.S.—

2 Lf units of tetanus toxoid and 2 Lf units of diphtheria toxoid per 0.5 mL dose (Rx) [GENERIC (may contain thimerosal)].

5 Lf units of tetanus toxoid and 2 Lf units of diphtheria toxoid per 0.5 mL dose (Rx) [GENERIC (may contain thimerosal)].

10 Lf units of tetanus toxoid and 2 Lf units of diphtheria toxoid per 0.5 mL dose (Rx) [GENERIC (may contain thimerosal)].

Canada—

5 Lf units of tetanus toxoid and 2 Lf units of diphtheria toxoid per 0.5 mL dose (Rx) [GENERIC (may contain thimerosal)].

Note: Lf is the quantity of toxoid as assessed by flocculation.

#### Packaging and storage

Store between 2 and 8 °C (36 and 46 °F), unless otherwise specified by manufacturer. Store away from the freezer compartment. Protect from freezing.

#### Stability

Freezing destroys activity. The product should not be used if it has been exposed to freezing. In addition, the product should not be left out at room temperature (e.g., between patients).

#### Auxiliary labeling

• Shake the vial vigorously immediately before each dose is withdrawn in order to resuspend the contents.

• Protect from freezing.

## Selected Bibliography

Centers for Disease Control and Prevention. Diphtheria, tetanus, and pertussis: recommendations for vaccine use and other preventive measures: recommendations of the Immunization Practices Advisory Committee (ACIP). MMWR 1991 Aug 8; 40 (RR-10): 1-28.

Developed: 04/26/95

---

# DIPHTHERIA AND TETANUS TOXOIDS AND PERTUSSIS VACCINE ADSORBED   Systemic

Note:   This monograph describes diphtheria and tetanus toxoids combined with either whole-cell pertussis vaccine or acellular pertussis vaccine. The acellular pertussis-containing vaccine is indicated by the term DTaP or acellular DTP. The whole-cell pertussis-containing vaccine is indicated by the term DTwP or whole-cell DTP. For general statements, the term DTP will be used.

VA CLASSIFICATION (Primary): IM900

Other commonly used names are acellular DTP, DTaP, DTP, DTwP, and whole-cell DTP.

Note: For a listing of dosage forms and brand names by country availability, see *Dosage Forms* section(s). For a listing of brand names for the articles in this monograph, refer to the General Index.

# Category

Immunizing agent (active).

# Indications

## Accepted

Diphtheria, tetanus, and pertussis (prophylaxis)—Whole-cell DTP (DTwP) is indicated for immunization against diphtheria, tetanus, and pertussis. The Immunization Practices Advisory Committee (ACIP) recommends the use of acellular DTP (DTaP) instead of whole-cell DTP for the fourth or fifth dose of the immunization series because of a decreased incidence of side/adverse effects associated with DTaP. The main objective of DTP immunization is to prevent the severe complications, including death, that may arise from the toxins or infections associated with diphtheria, tetanus, and pertussis.

Unless otherwise contraindicated, all children from 2 months up to 7 years of age should be immunized against diphtheria, tetanus, and pertussis, including:
• Those recovering from diphtheria or tetanus. Since a diphtheria or tetanus infection may not confer immunity, active immunization should be initiated or continued at the time of recovery from the illness and the remaining doses of the primary series administered as early as possible according to the schedule of doses.
• Those recovering from a pertussis-like syndrome. Unless a pertussis diagnosis is confirmed by a culture, DTP immunization should be initiated or continued because a pertussis-like syndrome may be caused by another *Bordetella* species, a chlamydia, or a virus. Children who have recovered from a culture-confirmed pertussis infection no longer require pertussis vaccine and should be immunized with diphtheria and tetanus toxoids for pediatric use (DT) according to current labeling.
• Those who have not yet received the recommended number of doses of pertussis vaccine. DTP may be used to immunize these children as long as the total number of doses that the child receives of either the diphtheria or tetanus toxoid does not exceed 6 doses before 7 years of age. Alternatively, a single-antigen pertussis vaccine may be used to complete immunization against pertussis. In the U.S., single-antigen whole-cell pertussis vaccine is currently available only from the Biologics Products Program of the Michigan State Health Department for use within Michigan; however, the vaccine may be available for use outside Michigan under special circumstances as determined by the program.
• Close contacts, household or other, of persons with pertussis. Children who have not completed the 4-dose primary series of DTP should receive an immediate dose of DTP and should subsequently complete the primary series with the minimum recommended intervals between doses. Children who have completed the 4-dose primary series but have not received a dose of DTP within the last 3 years should receive an immediate dose of DTP.

Although some health-care providers inappropriately consider certain conditions as contraindications, the following conditions are *not* contraindications to immunization with DTP:
• Stable neurologic conditions, including well-controlled seizures.
• Resolved or corrected neurologic disorders. DTP is recommended for infants with certain neurologic problems, such as neonatal hypocalcemic tetany or hydrocephalus (following placement of shunt and without seizures), that have been corrected or have subsided without residua.
• A family history of convulsions or other CNS disorders.
• A family history of sudden-infant-death syndrome (SIDS).
• A family history of an adverse reaction to DTP.
• Premature birth. The chronological age from birth should be used for initiating immunization.

Because the incidence and severity of pertussis infection decrease with age, while the chance of side/adverse effects from the pertussis vaccine in DTP still exists, and because the chance of side/adverse effects associated with the strength of diphtheria toxoid used in DTP increases with age, immunization with DTP is not recommended for children 7 years of age and older and adults. Instead, these persons should receive periodic immunizations with tetanus and diphtheria toxoids for adult use (Td) according to current labeling.

# Pharmacology/Pharmacokinetics

## Physicochemical characteristics

Source—Whole-cell DTP vaccine consists of a mixture of the detoxified toxins (toxoids) of diphtheria and tetanus and inactivated *B. pertussis* bacteria that have been adsorbed onto an aluminum salt. The DTaP vaccine consists of a mixture of the detoxified toxins (toxoids) of diphtheria and tetanus and a detoxified acellular pertussis vaccine component, prepared from *B. pertussis* bacteria, that have been adsorbed onto an aluminum salt.

## Mechanism of action/Effect

Diphtheria—Following intramuscular injection, diphtheria toxoid induces the formation of antitoxin.
Tetanus—Following intramuscular injection, tetanus toxoid induces the formation of antitoxin.
Pertussis—Following intramuscular injection, acellular or whole-cell pertussis vaccine induces the formation of several antibodies thought to be clinically protective. The exact mechanism of protection is not known.

## Protective efficacy

Diphtheria—A serum level of antibody greater than approximately 0.01 to 0.1 diphtheria toxin neutralization unit per mL is generally considered protective.
Tetanus—Tetanus toxoid is highly effective, with a failure rate in fully immunized persons of less than 4 per 100 million. Protective levels of serum antitoxin greater than or equal to 0.01 tetanus toxin neutralization unit per mL are achieved after primary immunization with DTP.
Pertussis—Immunization with 3 or more doses of DTP induces immunity against clinical pertussis disease in 80 to 90% of susceptible persons.

## Duration of protective effect

Diphtheria—Primary immunization with DTP protects more than 95% of persons for at least 10 years.
Tetanus—Primary immunization with DTP protects 95% of persons for at least 10 years.
Pertussis—Following primary immunization with DTP vaccine, immunity to pertussis usually persists through childhood, but is thought to decrease over time. Lifelong immunity is probably attained through subsequent mild pertussis infection.

# Precautions to Consider

## Cross-sensitivity and/or related problems

Patients sensitive to diphtheria toxoid, tetanus toxoid, or acellular or whole-cell pertussis vaccine will be sensitive to DTP also.

## Pediatrics

Whole-cell DTP is recommended for children from 2 months up to 7 years of age. The Immunization Practices Advisory Committee (ACIP) recommends the use of DTaP instead of whole-cell DTP for the fourth or fifth dose of the immunization series because of a decreased incidence of side/adverse effects associated with DTaP.

The highest fatality rates from diphtheria and pertussis occur in the very young.

A history of prematurity is not a reason to defer vaccination with DTP.

If a previous dose of DTP caused an immediate anaphylactic reaction, further doses of DTP should not be administered. Because of uncertainty as to which component of the vaccine may be responsible, it is recommended that no further immunization be carried out with any of the three antigens in DTP. Alternatively, because of the importance of tetanus immunization, individuals who had this reaction should be referred for evaluation by an allergist and desensitized to tetanus toxoid if specific allergy can be demonstrated.

If a previous dose of DTP caused any of the following effects (which are most frequently assumed to be attributable to the pertussis vaccine component), subsequent immunization of children up to 7 years of age should consist of only diphtheria and tetanus toxoids for pediatric use (DT) instead of DTP:
• Collapse or shock-like state (hypotonic-hyporesponsive episode), occurring within 48 hours.
• Convulsions, with or without fever, occurring within 3 days.
• Crying, persistent and inconsolable, lasting 3 or more hours and occurring within 48 hours.
• Encephalopathy, not due to another identifiable cause. A causal relationship between DTP and permanent brain damage has not been demonstrated according to ACIP. Encephalopathy is defined as an acute, severe CNS disorder occurring within 7 days following immunization, consisting of major alterations in consciousness, unresponsiveness, generalized or focal seizures that persist more than a few hours, and failure to recover within 24 hours. Even though causation by DTP cannot be established, subsequent doses of pertussis vaccine should not be given. In addition, it may be desirable to delay administering the balance of the doses of DT necessary to complete the primary schedule so that the child's neurological status can clarify.
• Fever of 40.5 °C (105 °F) or more, occurring within 48 hours and not due to other causes.

Because the incidence and severity of pertussis infection decrease with age while the chance of side/adverse effects from the pertussis vaccine in DTP still exists, and because the chance of side/adverse effects associated with the strength of diphtheria toxoid used in DTP increases with age, immunization with DTP is not recommended for children 7 years of age and older and adults. Instead, these persons should receive periodic immunizations with tetanus and diphtheria toxoids for adult use (Td) according to current labeling.

**Drug interactions and/or related problems**

The following drug interactions and/or related problems have been selected on the basis of their potential clinical significance (possible mechanism in parentheses where appropriate)—not necessarily inclusive (» = major clinical significance):

Note: Combinations containing any of the following medications, depending on the amount present, may also interact with this medication.

Immunosuppressive agents or
Radiation therapy
(because normal defense mechanisms are suppressed, concurrent use of immunosuppressive agents or radiation therapy with DTP may decrease the patient's antibody response to DTP or may result in aberrant responses to active immunization procedures. The precaution does not apply to corticosteroids used as replacement therapy, for short-term [less than 2 weeks] systemic therapy, or by other routes of administration that do not cause immunosuppression. If immunosuppressive therapy will be discontinued shortly, immunization with DTP should be deferred until the patient has discontinued therapy for 1 month; otherwise, the patient should be immunized with DTP while still undergoing therapy)

Influenza vaccine, whole or split virus
(influenza vaccine and DTP should not be administered within 3 days of one another, so that the cause of any adverse effect is clear)

**Medical considerations/Contraindications**

The medical considerations/contraindications included here have been selected on the basis of their potential clinical significance (reasons given in parentheses where appropriate)—not necessarily inclusive (» = major clinical significance).

*Except under special circumstances, this medication should not be used when the following medical problems exist:*

» Central nervous system (CNS) disorders, evolving or changing, whether or not the disorder is associated with seizure activity or
» Encephalopathy, progressive or
» Epilepsy, uncontrolled
(increased risk of side/adverse effects)
» Febrile illness, severe
(to avoid confusing manifestations of illness with possible side/adverse effects of vaccine; minor illnesses, such as upper respiratory infection, do not preclude administration of vaccine)

*Risk-benefit should be considered when the following medical problems exist:*

Neurological disease, suspected
(initiation of DTP should be delayed until there is clarification of the child's neurological status; however, the decision whether or not to commence immunization with DTP should be made by the child's first birthday. When making the decision, it should be recognized that children with severe neurological disorders may be at increased risk of pertussis because of their attendance at special schools or clinics where many of the other children attending may not be immunized. In addition, children with neurological disorders may be at increased risk from complications of pertussis)

Seizures, or family history of
(children who have had seizures previously, either febrile or nonfebrile, or who have a family history of seizures, are more likely to have seizures following DTP administration than children without such histories; however, data do not indicate that seizures that occur in the absence of other neurological reactions and that are temporally associated with DTP administration induce permanent brain damage in these children. All children with seizures should be fully evaluated to clarify their medical and neurological status before a decision is made to initiate vaccination with DTP. In addition, acetaminophen, 15 mg/kg, should be administered at the time of immunization and every 4 hours thereafter for 24 hours)

Sensitivity to diphtheria or tetanus toxoids or to pertussis vaccine

## Side/Adverse Effects

Note: DTaP causes fever less often than whole-cell DTP, and it is anticipated that adverse reactions precipitated by fever, such as febrile convulsions, will occur less often in children receiving DTaP.

Although the occurrence of sudden-infant-death syndrome (SIDS) has been related temporally to administration of DTP, studies have not found a causal relationship between DTP immunization and the syndrome.

Claims that DTP may be responsible for transverse myelitis, hyperactivity, learning disorders, infantile autism, and progressive degenerative CNS conditions have no scientific basis. In addition there is no evidence for a causal relationship between DTP immunization and hemolytic anemia or thrombocytopenic purpura.

Children who have had seizures previously, either febrile or nonfebrile, or who have a family history of seizures, are more likely to have seizures following DTP administration than children without such histories. In addition, data do not indicate that seizures that occur in the absence of other neurological reactions and that are temporally associated with DTP administration induce permanent brain damage in these children.

The frequency of fever or local reactions following DTP vaccination is significantly higher with increasing numbers of doses of DTP, whereas other mild to moderate systemic reactions (e.g., vomiting or fretfulness) are significantly less frequent with increasing numbers of doses.

The following side/adverse effects have been selected on the basis of their potential clinical significance (possible signs and symptoms in parentheses where appropriate)—not necessarily inclusive:

**Those indicating need for medical attention**
Incidence rare
*Anaphylactic reaction* (difficulty in breathing or swallowing; hives; itching, especially of soles or palms; reddening of skin, especially around ears; swelling of eyes, face, or inside of nose; unusual tiredness or weakness, sudden and severe); *convulsions, with or without fever, occurring within 3 days; crying, persistent and inconsolable, occurring within 48 hours and lasting 3 or more hours; encephalopathy, occurring within 7 days* (severe alterations in consciousness, with generalized or focal neurological signs; confusion; severe or continuing headache; unusual irritability; excessive sleepiness; severe or continuing vomiting); *fever of 40.5 °C (105 °F) or more, occurring within 48 hours; or hypotonic-hyporesponsive episode, occurring within 48 hours* (collapse or shock-like state)

**Those indicating need for medical attention only if they continue or are bothersome**
Incidence more frequent
*Abscess or local reaction* (redness, swelling, tenderness, or pain at injection site); *fever between 38 and 39 °C (100.4 and 102.2 °F)*—usually lasting up to, but no longer than, 48 hours; may be accompanied by fretfulness, drowsiness, vomiting, and anorexia; *lump at injection site*—may be present for a few weeks after injection

Incidence less frequent
*Fever between 39 and 40 °C (102.2 and 104 °F)*—usually lasting up to, but no longer than, 48 hours; may be accompanied by fretfulness, drowsiness, vomiting, and anorexia

Incidence rare
*Cervical lymphadenopathy* (swollen glands on side of neck following DTP injections into arm); *fever between 40 and 40.5 °C (104 and 105 °F)*—usually lasting up to, but no longer than, 48 hours; may be accompanied by fretfulness, drowsiness, vomiting, and anorexia; *Skin rash*

## Patient Consultation

As an aid to patient consultation, refer to *Advice for the Patient, Diphtheria and Tetanus Toxoids and Pertussis Vaccine Adsorbed (Systemic).*

In providing consultation, consider emphasizing the following selected information (» = major clinical significance):

**Before receiving this vaccine**
» Conditions affecting use, especially:
Sensitivity to diphtheria or tetanus toxoids, pertussis vaccine, or DTP
Other medical problems, especially evolving or changing central nervous system (CNS) disorders, whether or not the disorder is associated with seizure activity; progressive encephalopathy; uncontrolled epilepsy; or severe febrile illness

**Proper use of this vaccine**
» Proper dosing

**After receiving this vaccine**
Possibly receiving acetaminophen at time of injection; possibly continuing acetaminophen every four hours for twenty-four hours following injection; checking with physician if there are questions

### Side/adverse effects

Notifying physician of any side effect that occurs after a dose of DTP, even though the side effect may have gone away without treatment

Signs of potential side effects, especially anaphylactic reaction; convulsions, with or without fever, occurring within 3 days; crying, persistent and inconsolable, occurring within 48 hours and lasting 3 or more hours; encephalopathy occurring within 7 days; fever of 40.5 °C (105 °F) or more, occurring within 48 hours; or hypotonic-hyporesponsive episode occurring within 48 hours

## General Dosing Information

The usual primary immunization against diphtheria, tetanus, and pertussis consists of four 0.5-mL doses of DTP. In addition, a booster dose of DTP is usually administered at 4 through 6 years of age. Either whole-cell DTP or DTaP may be used for the fourth and fifth doses. However, the Immunization Practices Advisory Committee (ACIP) recommends the use of DTaP, because it causes fewer local reactions, less fever, and fewer other common systemic adverse reactions than does the whole-cell DTP.

It is recommended that only full doses (0.5 mL) of DTP be administered. Concern about adverse reactions have led some health care professionals to administer reduced doses of DTP. However, no evidence indicates that decreased doses will decrease the frequency of severe adverse effects. In addition, protection may be compromised.

It is usually recommended that immunization against diphtheria, tetanus, and pertussis be initiated at 2 months of age. However, some sources recommend initiating the DTP series at the infant's 6-week checkup. In addition, pertussis outbreaks may warrant administering the first 3 doses at 6, 10, and 14 weeks of age to provide protection as early as possible.

DTP should be administered by deep intramuscular injection, preferably into the midlateral muscles of the thigh in infants or into the deltoid in children. Each of the 4 primary immunizing doses of DTP should be injected at a different site.

Before each additional dose of DTP, the health status of the child should be reassessed. In addition, information should be obtained regarding any symptom and/or sign of an adverse reaction after the previous dose.

Delay, of any length, in the recommended interval of doses does not interfere with the final immunity achieved and does not require starting the series over again. If a delay occurs, series should be resumed as soon as possible and the doses continued at the recommended intervals, until the total number of doses required is administered.

Although the fourth dose of DTP and the third dose of oral polio vaccine (OPV) have traditionally been administered to children 18 months of age and measles, mumps, and rubella vaccine (MMR) has traditionally been administered to children 15 months of age, it is now recommended that DTP, OPV, and MMR be administered concurrently to children 15 months of age. MMR should not be postponed in order to administer these vaccines concurrently at 18 months of age. In addition, the traditional method is still an acceptable alternative.

Persons infected with human immunodeficiency virus (HIV) may receive DTP whether they have asymptomatic or symptomatic HIV infection.

Diphtheria toxoid, tetanus toxoid, and pertussis vaccine (whole-cell DTP or DTaP), can be administered concurrently with the following, using separate body sites and separate syringes (for parenterals), and the precautions that apply to each immunizing agent:
• Polysaccharide vaccines, such as haemophilus b polysaccharide vaccine, haemophilus b conjugate vaccine, meningococcal polysaccharide vaccine, or pneumococcal polyvalent vaccine.
• Live virus vaccines, such as measles, mumps, rubella, and/or oral polio vaccine (OPV).
• Inactivated poliovirus vaccine (IPV) or enhanced-potency inactivated vaccine (enhanced-potency IPV).
• Hepatitis B recombinant or plasma-derived vaccine.
• Inactivated vaccines, other, except cholera, typhoid (parenteral), and plague. It is recommended that cholera, typhoid (parenteral), and plague vaccines be administered on separate occasions because of these vaccines' propensity to cause side/adverse effects.

Continued use of this medication is contraindicated, according to ACIP, when the following medical problems occur:
• Anaphylactic reaction, immediate (because of uncertainty as to which component of the vaccine may be responsible, it is recommended that no further immunization be carried out with any of the three antigens in DTP. Alternatively, because of the importance of tetanus immunization, such individuals should be referred for evaluation by an allergist and desensitized to tetanus toxoid if specific allergy can be demonstrated).

• Encephalopathy, not due to another identifiable cause (a causal relation between DTP and permanent brain damage has not been demonstrated according to ACIP.Encephalopathy is defined as an acute, severe CNS disorder occurring within 7 days following immunization, consisting of major alterations in consciousness, unresponsiveness, generalized or focal seizures that persist more than a few hours, and failure to recover within 24 hours. Even though causation by DTP cannot be established, subsequent doses of pertussis vaccine should not be given. In addition, it may be desirable to delay administering the balance of the doses of DT necessary to complete the primary schedule so that the child's neurological status can clarify).

Continued use of the pertussis component of this medication, either whole-cell or acellular, should be carefully considered when the following medical problems occur in temporal relation to administration of DTP:
• Convulsions, with or without fever, occurring within 3 days.
• Crying, persistent and inconsolable, lasting 3 or more hours and occurring within 48 hours.
• Fever ≥ 40.5 °C (105 °F) occurring within 48 hours and not due to other causes.
• Hypotonic-hyporesponsive episode (collapse or shock-like state) occurring within 48 hours.

Continued use of this medication should be carefully considered when the following medical problem occurs:
• Neurological event occurring between doses of DTP but not temporally associated (if the child is under 1 year of age and has not received all 3 doses of the primary series, further doses of DTP should be deferred until there is clarification of the child's neurological status; however, the decision whether or not to continue immunization with DTP should be made no later than the child's first birthday and should be based on the nature of the neurological event and the risk/benefit associated with the vaccine. If the child is over 1 year of age, the child's neurological status should be evaluated to ensure that the disorder is stable before immunization with DTP is continued).

### For treatment of adverse effects

Recommended treatment includes:
• For mild hypersensitivity reaction—Administering antihistamines, and, if necessary, glucocorticoids.
• For severe hypersensitivity or anaphylactic reaction—Administering epinephrine. Antihistamines or glucocorticoids may also be administered as required.

## Parenteral Dosage Forms

### DIPHTHERIA AND TETANUS TOXOIDS AND ACELLULAR PERTUSSIS VACCINE ADSORBED

**Usual adult and adolescent dose**
Use is not recommended.

Note: Diphtheria toxoid of the strength used in DTP is not recommended for adults, because of the increased risk of side/adverse effects associated with the use of higher doses of diphtheria toxoid in adults. In addition, at the present time, acellular pertussis vaccine is not recommended for adults. Instead, tetanus and diphtheria toxoids for adult use (Td) should be administered according to its current labeling.

**Usual pediatric dose**
Children 2 to 15 months of age—
Use is not recommended. Whole-cell DTP should be administered instead.

Children 15 months up to 7 years of age who have previously been immunized with three or four doses of whole-cell DTP vaccine—
Intramuscular, 0.5 mL, preferably into the midlateral muscles of the thigh or deltoid, according to one of the following schedules:
If three previous doses of whole-cell DTP have been administered:
One dose at fifteen to eighteen months of age, but not less than six months after the previous dose, followed by another dose at four to six years of age.
If four previous doses of whole-cell DTP have been administered and the fourth dose was administered before the fourth birthday:
One dose at four to six years of age.
Note: If the fourth dose of whole-cell DTP was administered after the fourth birthday, no additional dose is necessary.

If pertussis vaccine is contraindicated in a child under seven years of age, DTP should not be administered. Instead, diphtheria and tetanus toxoids for pediatric use (DT) should be administered according to its current labeling.

Children 7 years of age and older—
Use is not recommended.

Note: Diphtheria toxoid of the strength used in DTP is not recommended for children seven years of age and older, because of the increased risk of side/adverse effects associated with the use of higher doses of diphtheria toxoid in older children. In addition, at the present time, acellular pertussis vaccine is not recommended for children seven years of age and older. Instead, tetanus and diphtheria toxoids for adult use (Td) should be administered according to its current labeling.

**Strength(s) usually available**
U.S.—

6.7 Lf of diphtheria toxoid, 5 Lf of tetanus toxoid, 23.4 mcg protein of filamentous hemagglutinin (FHA), and 23.4 mcg protein of inactivated pertussis toxin (PT) (toxoid), in each 0.5-mL dose. Each 0.5-mL dose contains aluminum present as aluminum potassium sulfate (Rx) [*Tripedia* (thimerosal 1:10,000)].

7.5 Lf of diphtheria toxoid, 5 Lf of tetanus toxoid, and 300 hemagglutinating (HA) units of acellular pertussis vaccine, in each 0.5-mL dose. The acellular pertussis vaccine component contains approximately 40 mcg of pertussis antigens (approximately 86% filamentous hemagglutinin [FHA], approximately 8% lymphocytosis-promoting factor [LPF], approximately 4% 69-kilodalton [69kd] outer membrane protein, and approximately 2% type 2 fimbriae [pertussis-specific agglutinogen]), in each 0.5-mL dose. Each 0.5-mL dose contains not more than 850 mcg (0.85 mg) of aluminum present as aluminum hydroxide and aluminum phosphate (Rx) [*Acel-Imune* (thimerosal 1:10,000)].

Canada—
Not commercially available.

Note: Lf is the quantity of toxoid as assessed by flocculation.

A hemagglutinating (HA) unit is that amount of material that completely agglutinates chicken red blood cells as measured by the HA assay.

**Packaging and storage**
Store between 2 and 8 °C (36 and 46 °F), unless otherwise specified by manufacturer. Protect from freezing.

**Preparation of dosage form**
The product should be shaken well immediately before withdrawing each dose, to obtain a uniform suspension. The product should be discarded if it has remaining clumps after vigorous agitation.

**Stability**
The vaccine should be kept refrigerated, but should not be frozen, exposed to freezing temperatures, or stored near freezing surfaces.

**Auxiliary labeling**
• Shake well.
• Do not freeze.

# DIPHTHERIA AND TETANUS TOXOIDS AND PERTUSSIS VACCINE ADSORBED USP

**Usual adult and adolescent dose**
Use is not recommended.

Note: Diphtheria toxoid of the strength used in DTP is not recommended for adults, because of the increased risk of side/adverse effects associated with the use of higher doses of diphtheria toxoid in adults. In addition, whole-cell pertussis vaccine is not recommended for adults, because the incidence and severity of pertussis infection decrease with age, while the chance of side/adverse effects from the pertussis vaccine still exists. Instead, tetanus and diphtheria toxoids for adult use (Td) should be administered according to its current labeling.

**Usual pediatric dose**
Children 2 months up to 7 years of age—

Intramuscular, preferably into the midlateral muscles of the thigh or deltoid, 0.5 mL at four- to eight-week intervals for three doses, followed by a fourth dose of 0.5 mL six to twelve months after the third dose. A booster (fifth) dose of 0.5 mL is usually administered at four through six years of age; however, if the fourth dose of the basic immunizing series was administered after the fourth birthday, a booster (fifth) dose is not necessary.

Note: Pertussis outbreaks may warrant administering the first three doses at six, ten, and fourteen weeks of age to provide protection as early as possible.

If the child is over one year of age at the time the third dose is due, the third dose should be administered six to twelve

months (instead of the usual four to eight weeks) after the second dose, and the fourth dose should be omitted. The booster dose should be administered as usual.

DTaP is recommended for use instead of whole-cell DTP for the fourth or fifth dose of the immunization series.

If pertussis vaccine is contraindicated in a child under seven years of age, DTP should not be used. Instead, diphtheria and tetanus toxoids for pediatric use (DT) should be administered according to its current labeling.

Children 7 years of age and older—
Use is not recommended.

Note: Diphtheria toxoid of the strength used in DTP is not recommended for children seven years of age and older, because of the increased risk of side/adverse effects associated with the use of higher doses of diphtheria toxoid in older children. In addition, whole-cell pertussis vaccine is not recommended for children seven years of age and older, because the incidence and severity of pertussis infection decrease with age, while the chance of side/adverse effects from the pertussis vaccine still exists. Instead, tetanus and diphtheria toxoids for adult use (Td) should be administered according to its current labeling.

**Strength(s) usually available**
U.S.—

12.5 Lf of diphtheria toxoid aluminum phosphate adsorbed, 5 Lf of tetanus toxoid aluminum phosphate adsorbed, and 4 Protective Units of pertussis vaccine, in each 0.5-mL dose. Each 0.5-mL dose contains not more than 800 mcg (0.8 mg) of aluminum (Rx) [*Tri-Immunol* (thimerosal 1:10,000)].

6.7 Lf of diphtheria toxoid aluminum potassium sulfate adsorbed, 5 Lf of tetanus toxoid aluminum potassium sulfate adsorbed, and 4 Protective Units of pertussis vaccine, in each 0.5-mL dose. Each 0.5-mL dose may contain not more than 250 mcg (0.25 mg) of aluminum in the form of aluminum potassium sulfate (Rx) [GENERIC (may contain thimerosal)].

Canada—

12.5 Lf of diphtheria toxoid aluminum phosphate adsorbed, 5 Lf of tetanus toxoid aluminum phosphate adsorbed, and 4 Protective Units of pertussis vaccine, in each 0.5-mL dose. Each 0.5-mL dose contains not more than 800 mcg (0.8 mg) of aluminum (Rx) [*Tri-Immunol* (thimerosal 1:10,000)].

25 Lf of diphtheria toxoid aluminum phosphate adsorbed, 5 Lf of tetanus toxoid aluminum phosphate adsorbed, and 4 to 12 Protective Units of pertussis vaccine, in each 0.5-mL dose. Each 0.5-mL dose may contain 1.5 mg of aluminum phosphate (Rx) [GENERIC (may contain thimerosal)].

Note: Lf is the quantity of toxoid as assessed by flocculation.

**Packaging and storage**
Store between 2 and 8 °C (36 and 46 °F), unless otherwise specified by manufacturer. Protect from freezing.

**Preparation of dosage form**
The product should be shaken well immediately before withdrawing each dose, since product contains a bacterial suspension and vigorous agitation may be necessary to resuspend the contents of the vial. The product should be discarded if it has remaining clumps after vigorous agitation.

**Stability**
The vaccine should be refrigerated, but should not be frozen, exposed to freezing temperatures, or stored near freezing surfaces. If the vaccine is stored at temperatures below 2 °C (36 °F) or above 25 °C (77 °F) for as little as 24 hours, or if the vaccine is exposed to freezing temperatures or stored near freezing surfaces, subsequent resuspension of the vaccine may be difficult or impossible. Vaccine should not be used if resuspension without any visible clumps cannot be achieved by vigorous shaking.

**Auxiliary labeling**
• Shake well.
• Do not freeze.

Revised: 06/09/93
Interim revision: 03/29/94

# DIPIVEFRIN    Ophthalmic

INN: Dipivefrine

VA CLASSIFICATION (Primary): OP103

Note: For a listing of dosage forms and brand names by country availability, see *Dosage Forms* section(s). For a listing of brand names for the articles in this monograph, refer to the General Index.

## Category

Antiglaucoma agent (ophthalmic).

Note: Dipivefrin belongs to a group of drugs known as prodrugs. Prodrugs are usually not active in themselves, but require biotransformation to the parent compound before being therapeutically active. Dipivefrin is a prodrug of epinephrine.

## Indications

Note: Bracketed information in the *Indications* section refers to uses that are not included in U.S. product labeling.

### Accepted

Glaucoma, open-angle (treatment)—Indicated as initial therapy for the control of intraocular pressure in chronic open-angle glaucoma. Also, for open-angle glaucoma that is difficult to control, the addition of dipivefrin to other antiglaucoma agents, such as pilocarpine, carbachol, echothiophate, timolol, or acetazolamide, has been shown to be effective.

[Glaucoma, secondary (treatment)][1]—Dipivefrin is used in the treatment of secondary glaucoma.

---

[1]Not included in Canadian product labeling.

## Pharmacology/Pharmacokinetics

### Physicochemical characteristics

Source—Dipivefrin is a prodrug formed by the diesterification of epinephrine and pivalic acid.

Molecular weight—387.90.

### Mechanism of action/Effect

Dipivefrin is converted to epinephrine inside the eye by enzyme hydrolysis. The liberated epinephrine, an adrenergic agonist, appears to exert its action by decreasing aqueous production and enhancing aqueous outflow facility.

### Onset of action

About 30 minutes.

### Time to peak effect

About 1 hour.

## Precautions to Consider

### Cross-sensitivity and/or related problems

Patients sensitive to epinephrine may be sensitive to dipivefrin also, since ophthalmic dipivefrin is converted to epinephrine inside the eye by enzyme hydrolysis.

### Tumorigenicity

Studies in rabbits have indicated a dose-related incidence of meibomian gland retention cysts following topical administration of both dipivefrin and epinephrine.

### Pregnancy/Reproduction

Pregnancy—Adequate and well-controlled studies in humans have not been done.

Studies in rats and rabbits at daily oral doses of up to 10 mg per kg of body weight (mg/kg) (5 mg/kg in teratogenicity studies) have not shown that dipivefrin causes impaired fertility or harm to the fetus.

FDA Pregnancy Category B.

### Breast-feeding

It is not known whether dipivefrin is distributed into breast milk; however, dipivefrin may be systemically absorbed.

### Pediatrics

Appropriate studies on the relationship of age to the effects of this medicine have not been performed in the pediatric population. However, no pediatrics-specific problems have been documented to date.

### Geriatrics

Appropriate studies on the relationship of age to the effects of this medicine have not been performed in the geriatric population. However, no geriatrics-specific problems have been documented to date.

### Drug interactions and/or related problems

The following drug interactions and/or related problems have been selected on the basis of their potential clinical significance (possible mechanism in parentheses where appropriate)—not necessarily inclusive (» = major clinical significance):

Note: Combinations containing any of the following medications, depending on the amount present, may also interact with this medication.

Dipivefrin is converted to epinephrine inside the eye by enzyme hydrolysis.

Anesthetics, hydrocarbon inhalation, such as:
   Chloroform
   Cyclopropane
   Enflurane
   Halothane
   Isoflurane
   Methoxyflurane
   Trichloroethylene
     (if significant systemic absorption of ophthalmic epinephrine occurs, concurrent use of cyclopropane, halothane, or possibly chloroform may increase the risk of severe ventricular arrhythmias because these anesthetics greatly sensitize the myocardium to the effects of sympathomimetics; therapy with dipivefrin should be interrupted prior to general anesthesia in patients receiving these anesthetics)
     (enflurane, isoflurane, methoxyflurane, or especially trichloroethylene may also cause some sensitization of the myocardium to the effects of sympathomimetics; caution is recommended during concurrent use with dipivefrin)

Antidepressants, tricyclic or
Maprotiline or
Nomifensine
     (if significant systemic absorption of ophthalmic epinephrine occurs, concurrent use of these medications may potentiate the cardiovascular effects of the epinephrine, possibly resulting in arrhythmias, hypertension, or tachycardia)

Beta-adrenergic blocking agents, ophthalmic
     (concurrent use of ophthalmic betaxolol, levobunolol, or timolol with ophthalmic dipivefrin may provide a beneficial additive effect in lowering intraocular pressure)

Digitalis glycosides
     (if significant systemic absorption of ophthalmic epinephrine occurs, concurrent use of digitalis glycosides may increase the risk of cardiac arrhythmias; caution is recommended if concurrent use is necessary)

Sympathomimetics, systemic
     (if significant systemic absorption of ophthalmic epinephrine occurs, concurrent use of systemic sympathomimetics may result in additive toxic effects)

### Medical considerations/Contraindications

The medical considerations/contraindications included here have been selected on the basis of their potential clinical significance (reasons given in parentheses where appropriate)—not necessarily inclusive (» = major clinical significance).

*Except under special circumstances, this medication should not be used when the following medical problem exists:*

» Glaucoma, angle-closure, predisposition to
     (dilation of pupil may predispose patient to an attack of angle-closure glaucoma)

*Risk-benefit should be considered when the following medical problems exists:*

Aphakic eyes
     (macular edema may occur)

Sensitivity to dipivefrin

### Patient monitoring

The following may be especially important in patient monitoring (other tests may be warranted in some patients, depending on condition; » = major clinical significance):

Fundus examinations and
Visual acuity determinations
(recommended at periodic intervals during therapy in aphakic patients)
Intraocular pressure determinations
(recommended at periodic intervals during therapy)

## Side/Adverse Effects

Note: Therapy with epinephrine (or its prodrug dipivefrin) can lead to adrenochrome deposits in the conjunctiva and cornea.

The following side/adverse effects have been selected on the basis of their potential clinical significance (possible signs and symptoms in parentheses where appropriate)—not necessarily inclusive:

**Those indicating need for medical attention**
Incidence rare
*Systemic absorption* (fast or irregular heartbeat or increase in blood pressure)

**Those indicating need for medical attention only if they continue or are bothersome**
Incidence less frequent
*Burning, stinging, or other eye irritation; increased sensitivity of eyes to light*

## Patient Consultation

As an aid to patient consultation, refer to *Advice for the Patient, Dipivefrin (Ophthalmic).*

In providing consultation, consider emphasizing the following selected information (» = major clinical significance):

**Before using this medication**
» Conditions affecting use, especially:
Sensitivity to dipivefrin or epinephrine
Other medical problems, especially predisposition to angle-closure glaucoma

**Proper use of this medication**
» Importance of not using more medication than the amount prescribed
Proper administration technique
Washing hands immediately after applying eye drops
Preventing contamination: Not touching applicator tip to any surface; keeping container tightly closed
» Proper dosing
Missed dose: Applying as soon as possible; if almost time for next dose, skipping missed dose and going back to regular dosing schedule; not doubling doses
» Proper storage

**Precautions while using this medication**
Regular visits to physician to check eye pressure during therapy

**Side/adverse effects**
Signs of potential side effects, especially fast or irregular heartbeat or increase in blood pressure

## General Dosing Information

Although some manufacturers recommend a dose of 2 drops of an ophthalmic solution at appropriate intervals, the conjunctival sac will usually hold only 1 drop.

When used to replace epinephrine, the epinephrine should be discontinued when dipivefrin therapy is started.

When used to replace an antiglaucoma agent other than epinephrine, the other antiglaucoma agent should be continued on the first day that dipivefrin is used but discontinued on the second day.

When used in addition to other antiglaucoma agents, dipivefrin should be administered at the usual adult dose.

## Ophthalmic Dosage Forms

### DIPIVEFRIN HYDROCHLORIDE OPHTHALMIC SOLUTION USP

**Usual adult and adolescent dose**
Antiglaucoma agent (ophthalmic)—
Topical, to the conjunctiva, 1 drop of a 0.1% solution every twelve hours.

**Usual pediatric dose**
See *Usual adult and adolescent dose.*

**Usual geriatric dose**
See *Usual adult and adolescent dose.*

**Strength(s) usually available**
U.S.—
0.1% (1 mg per mL as the hydrochloride) (Rx) [*Propine C Cap B.I.D.* (benzalkonium chloride 0.005%); GENERIC].
Canada—
0.1% (1 mg per mL as the hydrochloride) (Rx) [*Ophtho-Dipivefrin; Propine C Cap B.I.D.* (benzalkonium chloride 0.004%; sodium metabisulfite); GENERIC].

**Packaging and storage**
Store below 40 °C (104 °F), preferably between 15 and 30 °C (59 and 86 °F), unless otherwise specified by manufacturer. Store in a tight, light-resistant container. Protect from freezing.

**Auxiliary labeling**
• For the eye.
• Keep container tightly closed.

Revised: 05/14/92
Interim revision: 08/16/93; 10/19/93; 12/14/93

---

# DIPYRIDAMOLE    Systemic

VA CLASSIFICATION (Primary/Secondary): BL700/DX900
Note: For a listing of dosage forms and brand names by country availability, see *Dosage Forms* section(s). For a listing of brand names for the articles in this monograph, refer to the General Index.

## Category

Platelet aggregation inhibitor; antithrombotic adjunct; diagnostic aid adjunct (ischemic heart disease); myocardial reinfarction prophylactic adjunct.

## Indications

Note: Bracketed information in the *Indications* section refers to uses that are not included in U.S. product labeling.

**Accepted**
Platelet aggregation (prophylaxis)—Dipyridamole is indicated to inhibit platelet aggregation and correct shortened platelet survival time in the following:
Thromboembolism (prophylaxis adjunct)—Indicated, concurrently with a coumarin- or indandione-derivative anticoagulant, to prevent thromboembolic complications associated with mechanical prosthetic heart valves. Use of dipyridamole for this purpose is optional, but is appropriate if an embolism occurs despite adequate anticoagulation. Also, it is recommended that dipyridamole be used whenever the an-

ticoagulant must be administered in lower dosage than is usually recommended for this indication.
[A few studies have shown that platelet aggregation inhibitors, although not as consistently effective as an anticoagulant or an anticoagulant plus dipyridamole, may provide some protection against the development of thromboembolic complications in patients with mechanical prosthetic heart valves. Therefore, administration of dipyridamole together with aspirin may be considered if anticoagulant therapy is contraindicated for these patients.][1]
[The addition of dipyridamole to therapy with a coumarin- or indandione-derivative anticoagulant may also be considered for patients with documented systemic embolism associated with mitral valve disease if an embolism recurs despite adequate anticoagulation.][1]
[Dipyridamole is also indicated, in conjunction with aspirin, to reduce the risk of thrombosis and/or occlusion of saphenous vein aortocoronary bypass grafts.][1]
[Dipyridamole is also indicated, in conjunction with aspirin, to reduce the risk of thromboembolism that may occur in conjunction with percutaneous transluminal coronary angioplasty. Use of these medications does not eliminate the need for administration of heparin during the procedure. Although the value of this regimen in preventing thromboembolism that may occur in conjunction with peripheral angioplasty has not been established via controlled trials, some clinicians recommend that dipyridamole and aspirin also be used, sequentially with heparin, in patients undergoing peripheral angioplasty.][1]

[Dipyridamole is also indicated, in conjunction with aspirin, to reduce the risk of thrombosis or occlusion of prosthetic or saphenous vein femoral popliteal bypass grafts.][1]

[Dipyridamole is also used, in conjunction with aspirin, in the treatment of lower extremity occlusive vascular disease. This combination of agents has been shown to be more effective than aspirin alone in improving claudication symptoms. Preliminary evidence also suggests that the combination of dipyridamole and aspirin may be more effective than aspirin alone in decreasing the formation of new and/or stenosing vascular lesions.][1]

[Myocardial reinfarction (prophylaxis adjunct)]—Used, concurrently with aspirin, to reduce the risk of reinfarction in patients recovering from myocardial infarction.

[Ischemic attacks, transient, in females and males (treatment)][1]—Used, concurrently with aspirin, to reduce the recurrence of transient ischemic attacks (TIAs) and the risk of stroke and death in patients who have had transient brain ischemia due to fibrin platelet emboli.

Note: Recent studies have shown that the combination of dipyridamole and aspirin for prophylaxis against myocardial reinfarction or treatment of TIAs is not more effective than aspirin used alone. It is recommended that such therapy be re-evaluated and that the use of aspirin alone be considered.

Myocardial perfusion imaging, radionuclide, adjunct and
[Stress echocardiography adjunct][1]—Intravenous dipyridamole is indicated as an adjunct to thallous chloride Tl 201 [and other radionuclides] in myocardial perfusion imaging, [and is also used in conjunction with two-dimensional echocardiography][1], for the diagnosis of perfusion deficits associated with coronary artery disease. Dipyridamole is used primarily as a substitute for exercise in patients who are unable to exercise sufficiently to provide the required level of myocardial stress or when exercise is otherwise not feasible. However, it is sometimes used in conjunction with low levels of exercise, such as isometric handgrip or submaximal treadmill exercise. Intravenous dipyridamole, like exercise, assists assessment via these studies of the risk of new or recurrent coronary events, such as myocardial infarction or ischemia. However, dipyridamole cannot provide the additional physiologic data, such as aerobic capacity, that is obtainable via exercise.

[Oral dipyridamole has also been used as an adjunct to myocardial perfusion imaging, but intravenous administration is preferred because the delayed and variable absorption of orally administered dipyridamole significantly prolongs the time required to perform the study. Also, the high doses used orally generally require prophylactic administration of intravenous aminophylline following the study to minimize the risk and/or severity of unwanted effects. In addition, dipyridamole's effects are more readily reversed by a single dose of intravenous aminophylline when dipyridamole has been administered intravenously than they are after high-dose oral administration.][1]

### Unaccepted

The U.S. Food and Drug Administration (FDA) has classified dipyridamole as lacking substantial evidence of effectiveness for the long-term treatment of chronic angina pectoris. Dipyridamole has generally been replaced by more effective agents as an antianginal agent.

---

[1]Not included in Canadian product labeling.

## Pharmacology/Pharmacokinetics

### Physicochemical characteristics
Molecular weight—504.63.
pKa—6.1.
Other characteristics—Lipophilic.

### Mechanism of action/Effect
Dipyridamole's mechanisms of action have not been fully elucidated, but may involve its ability to increase endogenous concentrations of adenosine, which is a coronary vasodilator and a platelet aggregation inhibitor, and of cyclic adenosine monophosphate (cAMP), which decreases platelet activation. Dipyridamole increases concentrations of adenosine by inhibiting the activity of the enzyme adenosine deaminase, thereby decreasing adenosine metabolism, and by inhibiting adenosine uptake by erythrocytes and vascular endothelial cells. Adenosine stimulates adenylate cyclase activity, leading to increased cAMP synthesis and consequently to reduced platelet function. Additionally, dipyridamole raises the intraplatelet cAMP concentration by increasing prostacyclin-induced stimulation of adenylate cyclase activity, which increases cAMP synthesis, and by inhibiting the enzyme phosphodiesterase, which decreases cAMP breakdown.

Thromboembolism prophylaxis adjunct—Dipyridamole may act by inhibiting platelet aggregation, although studies of the medication's ability to reduce platelet function after oral administration of usual doses have

yielded conflicting results. *In vitro*, high concentrations of dipyridamole are required to inhibit platelet function; the necessary concentrations may not be achieved *in vivo* with recommended doses. There is some evidence that the medication may be more effective in preventing platelet deposition on artificial surfaces (e.g., synthetic prosthetic heart valves) than on natural surfaces. Dipyridamole also restores toward normal the shortened platelet survival time that occurs in patients with thrombosis, prosthetic heart valves, vascular grafts, or vascular abnormalities. However, the relevance of this action to any antithrombotic effect of dipyridamole has not been established.

Diagnostic aid adjunct (ischemic heart disease)—Dipyridamole may preferentially dilate, and increase blood flow through, nondiseased coronary blood vessels, leading to a redistribution of blood flow away from significantly stenotic coronary vessels. This "coronary steal" effect increases the differential in perfusion, and consequently in radiopharmaceutical uptake, between regions of the myocardium supplied by normal coronary arteries and those supplied by stenotic vessels. Dipyridamole-induced changes in perfusion are similar to those produced by exercise stress.

### Absorption
Oral—Slow and subject to interindividual variability; bioavailability varies from 27 to 66%.

### Protein binding
Very high (91 to 99%); primarily to alpha₁-acid glycoprotein and, to a lesser extent, to albumin.

### Biotransformation
Hepatic, to the glucuronic acid conjugate.

### Half-life
Distribution—
   Intravenous: 3 to 12 minutes.
   Oral: About 40 to 90 minutes.
Redistribution—
   Intravenous: 33 to 62 minutes.
Elimination—
   Intravenous: 10 to 15 hours.
   Oral: About 10 to 12 hours.

### Time to peak plasma concentration
Oral—1 to 3 hours; usually about 75 minutes.
Intravenous—2 minutes following completion of a 4-minute infusion.

### Peak plasma concentration
Oral—Dependent on dosage and subject to interindividual variability. Concentrations are reduced when the medication is administered with food.
Single 25-mg dose: 0.5 mcg per mL (0.99 micromoles/L).
Single 75-mg dose: 1.6 mcg per mL (3.17 micromoles/L).
Chronic dosing with 75 mg 3 or 4 times a day: 1 to 2 mcg per mL (1.98 to 3.96 micromoles/L).
Intravenous—4.6 ± 1.3 mcg per mL (9.1 ± 2.57 micromoles/L).

### Time to peak effect
Intravenous infusion of 0.56 mg per kg of body weight (mg/kg), infused over 4 minutes—The peak increase in coronary flow velocity occurs 3.8 to 8.7 (average, 6.5) minutes after the start of the infusion.

### Elimination
Primarily biliary (up to 20% enterohepatic recirculation may occur).
Total body clearance (intravenous administration)—2.3 to 3.5 mL per minute per kg of body weight.

## Precautions to Consider

### Carcinogenicity
Studies in mice for 111 weeks and in rats for 128 to 142 weeks at doses of 8, 25, and 75 mg per kg of body weight (mg/kg) (1, 3.1, and 9.4 times the maximum recommended daily human dose [MRHD]) found no evidence of carcinogenicity.

### Mutagenicity
Mutagenicity studies (cytogenic, microorganism, dominant lethal, and micronucleus tests) were negative.

### Pregnancy/Reproduction
Fertility—Studies in male and female rats receiving oral doses of up to 500 mg/kg per day (63 times the MRHD for a 50-kg individual) revealed no evidence of impaired fertility. However, a significant reduction in the number of corpora lutea, with a consequent reduction in implantations and number of live fetuses, occurred with doses of 1250 mg/kg per day (155 times the MRHD).

Pregnancy—Although adequate and well-controlled studies in humans have not been done, successful pregnancies have been reported in patients who received dipyridamole.

Studies in mice and rats receiving oral doses of up to 125 mg/kg per day (15.6 times the MRHD for a 50-kg person) or in rabbits receiving oral doses of up to 20 mg/kg per day (2.5 times the MRHD for a 50-kg individual) revealed no evidence of harm to the fetus.

FDA Pregnancy Category B.

### Breast-feeding

Dipyridamole is distributed into human breast milk. However, problems in humans have not been documented.

### Pediatrics

No information is available on the relationship of age to the effects of dipyridamole in pediatric patients. Safety and efficacy in children have not been established.

### Geriatrics

Studies of the efficacy of single doses of intravenous dipyridamole for myocardial perfusion imaging revealed no differences in the incidence of chest pain, ST segment depression, or severe ischemia in patients 70 years of age or older compared with patients younger than 70 years of age. Studies on the relationship of age to the effects of dipyridamole in geriatric patients receiving the medication as a platelet aggregation inhibitor have not been done. However, no geriatrics-specific problems have been documented to date with chronic oral administration of dipyridamole.

### Drug interactions and/or related problems

The following drug interactions and/or related problems have been selected on the basis of their potential clinical significance (possible mechanism in parentheses where appropriate)—not necessarily inclusive (» = major clinical significance):

See also *Laboratory value alterations*.

Note: Combinations containing any of the following medications, depending on the amount present, may also interact with this medication.

Adenosine
(dipyridamole potentiates the effects of adenosine by inhibiting adenosine metabolism as well as its uptake by erythrocytes and vascular endothelial cells; a reduction of adenosine dosage may be needed)

» Anticoagulants, coumarin- or indandione-derivative or
» Heparin
(concurrent use with a platelet aggregation inhibitor such as dipyridamole may increase the risk of bleeding; although dipyridamole may be administered in daily doses of up to 400 mg while oral anticoagulants are also being used without affecting prothrombin activity or bleeding time, some clinicians recommend careful monitoring and maintenance of prothrombin activity at the lower end of the therapeutic range to reduce the risk of bleeding)

Anti-inflammatory drugs, nonsteroidal, (NSAIDs), especially
Indomethacin or
Pentoxifylline or
» Platelet aggregation inhibitors, other (See *Appendix II*) or
Salicylates, especially:
» Aspirin
(concurrent use of any of these medications with dipyridamole may increase the risk of bleeding because of additive inhibition of platelet aggregation; in addition, hypoprothrombinemia induced by large doses of salicylates, and the potential occurrence of gastrointestinal ulceration or hemorrhage during therapy with NSAIDs, salicylates [especially aspirin], or sulfinpyrazone, may cause increased risk to patients receiving dipyridamole)

(although aspirin and dipyridamole are commonly used concurrently to provide additional therapeutic benefit, the combination has not been shown to be more effective than aspirin alone for prophylaxis against myocardial reinfarction or treatment of transient ischemic attacks)

(concurrent use of dipyridamole and indomethacin may increase both the risk and the severity of renal function impairment; in one short-term study in well-hydrated individuals with normal renal function, administration of a single dose of both agents produced an 80% reduction in diuresis and decreases in sodium excretion and glomerular filtration rate; the decrements were significantly greater than those occurring with either medication alone; although the risk of a significant effect on renal function with long-term therapy has not been determined, caution is recommended, especially for patients who may be at risk for such complications, e.g., dehydrated individuals or patients with pre-existing renal function impairment)

» Cefamandole or
» Cefoperazone or
» Cefotetan or

» Plicamycin or
» Valproic acid
(these medications may cause hypoprothrombinemia; in addition, plicamycin and valproic acid may inhibit platelet aggregation; concurrent use with dipyridamole may increase the risk of bleeding because of additive interferences with blood clotting)

» Thrombolytic agents, such as:
» Alteplase (tissue-type plasminogen activator, recombinant)
» Anistreplase (anisoylated plasminogen-streptokinase activator complex)
» Streptokinase
» Urokinase
(dipyridamole-induced inhibition of platelet aggregation may increase the risk of severe bleeding in patients receiving thrombolytic therapy)

### Laboratory value alterations

The following have been selected on the basis of their potential clinical significance (possible effect in parentheses where appropriate)—not necessarily inclusive (» = major clinical significance):

With results of dipyridamole-assisted myocardial perfusion studies

*Due to other medications*
» Bronchodilators, xanthine-derivative or
» Caffeine
(these agents reverse the effects of dipyridamole on myocardial blood flow, thereby interfering with test results; dipyridamole-assisted myocardial perfusion studies should not be performed if therapy with a xanthine bronchodilator cannot be withheld for 36 hours prior to the test; also, patients should be instructed to avoid ingesting caffeine [from a dietary or medicinal source] for 8 to 12 hours prior to the test)

### Medical considerations/Contraindications

The medical considerations/contraindications included here have been selected on the basis of their potential clinical significance (reasons given in parentheses where appropriate)—not necessarily inclusive (» = major clinical significance).

### Risk-benefit should be considered when the following medical problems exist:

Angina pectoris, unstable or
Collateral blood vessels, presence of
(increased risk of myocardial ischemia due to a "coronary steal" phenomenon, which may lead to complications such as hypotension, ventricular arrhythmias, or cardiac arrest)

Hypotension or propensity toward
(may be induced or aggravated by excessive doses, which may cause peripheral vasodilation)

Sensitivity to dipyridamole

*For diagnostic use by intravenous injection only (in addition to those medical problems listed above):*
» Asthma, current or history of
(increased risk of bronchospasm)

### Patient monitoring

The following may be especially important in patient monitoring (other tests may be warranted in some patients, depending on condition; » = major clinical significance):

» Electrocardiogram and
Vital signs, especially blood pressure
(monitoring recommended when large single doses of dipyridamole are used adjunctively for myocardial perfusion scanning, because of the risk of severe hypotension and myocardial ischemia, which may lead to ventricular arrhythmias and cardiac arrest; when dipyridamole is administered by intravenous infusion for this purpose, it is recommended that these parameters be monitored for at least 10 to 15 minutes following completion of the infusion)

## Side/Adverse Effects

Note: In addition to the side/adverse effects listed below, asthenia, depersonalization, diaphoresis, dysgeusia, injection site reactions, intermittent claudication, leg cramping, pharyngitis, and pain in the back, breast, eyes, kidneys, muscles, or perineal area have also been reported, very rarely, following intravenous administration of dipyridamole for myocardial perfusion imaging.

The following side/adverse effects have been selected on the basis of their potential clinical significance (possible signs and symptoms in parentheses where appropriate)—not necessarily inclusive:

### Those indicating need for medical attention

Incidence more frequent—with intravenous administration for diagnostic use
*Angina pectoris or exacerbation of* (chest pain)—incidence >19%;
*blood pressure lability*—incidence 1.6%; *extrasystoles*—incidence

5.2%; *hypertension*—incidence 1.5%; *hypotension*—incidence 4.6%; *ST-T segment changes*—incidence 7.5%; *tachycardia*—incidence 3.2%; *other electrocardiographic changes and/or arrhythmias*—very rare

Note: *Angina pectoris* may be induced or exacerbated because of a "coronary steal" phenomenon. Its occurrence following administration of intravenous dipyridamole for diagnostic use is especially likely in patients with significant coronary artery disease, but does not always correlate with or predict the extent of disease. Intravenous dipyridamole has also induced chest pain in individuals without coronary artery disease. Although chest pain without other diagnostic evidence of coronary artery disease is a relatively nonspecific finding, myocardial infarction [incidence 0.1%] and cardiac arrest have occurred rarely.

Rarely, *angina pectoris* has also been reported with oral administration of conventional doses, usually at the beginning of therapy.

*Electrocardiographic changes* and/or *arrhythmias* may include ventricular fibrillation, ventricular tachycardia, bradycardia, atrial fibrillation, supraventricular tachycardia, atrioventricular block or other heart block, and syncope.

Incidence less frequent
   *Allergic reaction* (skin rash [incidence 2.3%]; itching); *dyspnea*—incidence 2.6%; with intravenous administration for diagnostic use

Incidence rare—with intravenous administration for diagnostic use
   *Allergic reaction, including bronchospasm, which may be severe* (shortness of breath; troubled breathing; tightness in chest; wheezing); *cardiomyopathy; cerebral ischemia, transient; edema*—pulmonary edema has also been reported in a patient with a history of pulmonary edema; *hypertonia; hyperventilation; hypoesthesia*—incidence 0.5%; *migraine* (headache, severe and throbbing); *pleural pain; rhinitis* (runny nose; sneezing)

**Those indicating need for medical attention only if they continue or are bothersome**
Incidence more frequent
   *Abdominal cramping*—with high doses; *diarrhea; dizziness or lightheadedness*—incidence of dizziness 11.8% with intravenous administration for diagnostic use and 13.6% with chronic oral therapy; *gastrointestinal irritation*—overall incidence 6.1% with chronic oral administration; *headache*—incidences 12.2% with intravenous administration for diagnostic use and 2.3% with chronic oral therapy; *nausea*—incidence 4.6% with intravenous administration for diagnostic use; *vomiting*—with high doses

Incidence less frequent—more frequent with increase of oral dosage
   *Flushing; weakness*

## Patient Consultation

As an aid to patient consultation, refer to *Advice for the Patient, Dipyridamole—Diagnostic (Systemic)* and *Dipyridamole—Therapeutic (Systemic)*.

In providing consultation, consider emphasizing the following selected information (» = major clinical significance):

**Before using this medication**
»  Conditions affecting use, especially:
      Sensitivity to dipyridamole
      Other medications, especially other platelet aggregation inhibitors, those cephalosporins that may cause hypoprothrombinemia, plicamycin, and valproic acid, and, for myocardial perfusion studies, caffeine and xanthine bronchodilators
      Other medical problems, especially asthma (or history of)—for intravenous use in myocardial perfusion studies

**Proper use of this medication**
»  Importance of taking at evenly spaced times
   Taking medication with water at least 1 hour before or 2 hours after meals for faster absorption; may be taken with meals or milk if gastrointestinal irritation occurs
»  Proper dosing
   Missed dose: Taking as soon as possible unless next scheduled dose is within 4 hours; returning to regular dosing schedule; not doubling doses
»  Proper storage

**Precautions while using this medication**
   Possibility that concurrent use with an anticoagulant or with aspirin may increase the risk of bleeding
»  Not taking aspirin concurrently unless specifically prescribed for concurrent use

»  If taking aspirin concurrently, taking only the amount of aspirin prescribed; checking with physician about proper medication to use for relief of pain, fever
   If taking aspirin concurrently, need for regular visits to physician to check progress during therapy
»  Informing all physicians and dentists of use of dipyridamole and whether taking concurrently with an anticoagulant or aspirin
»  Caution when getting up suddenly from lying or sitting position

**Side/adverse effects**
   Signs of potential side effects, especially angina pectoris and, for diagnostic use only, bronchospasm, dyspnea, and migraine

## General Dosing Information

**For oral dosage form only**
Dipyridamole should preferably be taken with a full glass (240 mL) of water on an empty stomach (either 1 hour before or 2 hours after meals) for faster absorption; however, it may be taken with or immediately after meals or with milk to lessen gastrointestinal irritation.

**For oral or intravenous administration as a diagnostic aid**
Intravenous aminophylline and nitroglycerin should be immediately available for reversal of adverse effects. Routine administration of aminophylline following administration of large doses of dipyridamole (70 mg intravenously or 300 mg orally) has been recommended to minimize the frequency of adverse effects. However, aminophylline should not be given until several (> 2) minutes after the radiopharmaceutical has been injected. Also, because cardiac arrest has occurred (rarely), personnel trained in cardiorespiratory resuscitation and all necessary medications and equipment for handling this emergency should be immediately available.

**For parenteral administration only**
Because small veins may be especially sensitive to the acidic pH of the dipyridamole injection, it is recommended that the medication be infused into an antecubital vein. Also, the injection should not be administered undiluted.

**For treatment of adverse effects**
Recommended treatment consists of the following:
• For angina pectoris, ventricular arrhythmias, or bronchospasm—Administering 50 to 250 mg of aminophylline by intravenous infusion at a rate of 50 to 100 mg over 30 to 60 seconds. If symptoms are relieved, continuing to monitor the patient and administering additional aminophylline if they recur. If chest pain persists, administering nitroglycerin. If angina continues, the possibility of myocardial infarction should be considered and appropriate diagnostic and treatment measures instituted as needed.
• Hypotension, severe—Placing the patient in a supine position, with the head tilted down if necessary, followed by administration of 50 to 250 mg of intravenous aminophylline. Intravenous fluids and/or a vasopressor may also be used if needed.

## Oral Dosage Forms

Note: Bracketed uses in the *Dosage Forms* section refer to categories of use and/or indications that are not included in U.S. product labeling.

**DIPYRIDAMOLE TABLETS USP**

**Usual adult dose**
Platelet aggregation inhibitor—
   Prevention of thromboembolism associated with prosthetic heart valves—
      Oral, 75 to 100 mg four times a day in combination with a coumarin- or indandione-derivative anticoagulant.
      Note: A dose of 100 mg per day is sufficient when given in combination with 1 gram of aspirin per day. However, the combination of aspirin and an anticoagulant for this purpose is not recommended because of the increased risk of severe bleeding.
   [Prevention of thromboembolism associated with prosthetic heart valves in patients for whom anticoagulants are contraindicated][1]—
      Oral, 75 mg three or four times a day, in conjunction with 325 mg of aspirin a day.
   [Prevention of recurrent systemic thromboembolism in patients with mitral valve disease][1]—
      Oral, 225 to 400 mg a day, in conjunction with a coumarin- or indandione-derivative anticoagulant.
   [Prevention of thrombosis or occlusion of coronary bypass graft]—
      Oral, 100 mg four times a day for two days prior to surgery; 100 mg one hour postoperatively; then 75 mg in combination with 325 mg of aspirin seven hours postoperatively (given via nasogastric tube); then 75 mg in combination with 325 mg of aspirin three times a

day. Dipyridamole, but not aspirin, may be discontinued one week postoperatively.

[Myocardial reinfarction prophylactic]—

Oral, 75 mg three times a day in combination with 325 mg of aspirin a day.

Note: Optimum dosage of aspirin as a platelet aggregation inhibitor has not been established. Most studies have utilized doses ranging from 300 mg to 1.5 grams a day. However, there is evidence that doses as low as 160 mg every twenty-four hours or 325 mg every forty-eight hours may effectively inhibit platelet aggregation while minimizing the risk of aspirin-induced side effects. Therefore, lower doses of aspirin than those recommended above are sometimes used in antithrombotic regimens.

[Diagnostic aid adjunct][1]—

Oral, 300 to 400 mg as a single dose, administered approximately forty-five minutes prior to injection of the radiopharmaceutical. However, intravenous administration is preferred for this indication.

### Usual pediatric dose

Safety and efficacy in children have not been established.

### Strength(s) usually available

U.S.—

25 mg (Rx) [*Dipridacot; Persantine;* GENERIC].
50 mg (Rx) [*Persantine;* GENERIC].
75 mg (Rx) [*Persantine;* GENERIC].

Canada—

25 mg (Rx) [*Apo-Dipyridamole; Novodipiradol; Persantine*].
50 mg (Rx) [*Apo-Dipyridamole; Novodipiradol; Persantine*].
75 mg (Rx) [*Apo-Dipyridamole; Novodipiradol; Persantine*].
100 mg (Rx) [*Persantine*].

### Packaging and storage

Store below 40 °C (104 °F), preferably between 15 and 30 °C (59 and 86 °F), unless otherwise specified by manufacturer. Store in a tight, light-resistant container.

## Parenteral Dosage Forms

Note: Bracketed uses in the *Dosage Forms* section refer to categories of use and/or indications that are not included in U.S. product labeling.

### DIPYRIDAMOLE INJECTION

#### Usual adult dose

Diagnostic aid adjunct—

Intravenous infusion, 570 mcg (0.57 mg) per kg of body weight, administered at a rate of 142 mcg (0.142 mg) per kg of body weight per minute for four minutes. The radiopharmaceutical is injected

within three to five minutes after completion of the dipyridamole infusion.

[Platelet aggregation inhibitor]—

Intravenous infusion, 250 mg per day at a rate of 10 mg per hour.

### Usual adult prescribing limits

Diagnostic aid adjunct—60 mg.

[Platelet aggregation inhibitor]—Up to 400 mg per day (lower when given in combination with aspirin).

### Usual pediatric dose

Safety and efficacy in children have not been established.

### Strength(s) usually available

U.S.—

5 mg per mL (10 mg per 2-mL ampul) (Rx) [*I.V. Persantine*].

Canada—

5 mg per mL (50 mg per 10-mL ampul) (Rx) [*Persantine*].

### Packaging and storage

Store between 15 and 25 °C (59 and 77 °F), protected from direct light, unless otherwise specified by manufacturer. Protect from freezing.

### Preparation of dosage form

Diagnostic aid adjunct—The required quantity of dipyridamole injection should be diluted in sufficient 0.45% sodium chloride injection, 0.9% sodium chloride injection, or 5% dextrose injection to yield a total volume of 20 to 50 mL.

[Platelet aggregation inhibitor]—250 mg of dipyridamole (50 mL of dipyridamole injection) should be added to 250 mL of 5% dextrose injection. The resultant solution contains 1 mg per mL. If doses higher than 250 mg per day are required, the concentration of dipyridamole in the infusion solution may be increased.

---

[1]Not included in Canadian product labeling.

### Selected Bibliography

Iskandrian AS, Heo J, Askenase A, Segal BL, Auerbach N. Dipyridamole cardiac imaging. Am Heart J 1988; 115: 432-43.

Leppo JA. Dipyridamole-thallium imaging: the lazy man's stress test. J Nucl Med 1989; 30: 281-7.

FitzGerald GA. Medical intelligence. Dipyridamole. N Engl J Med 1987; 316: 1247-56.

Younis LT, Chaitman BR. Update on intravenous dipyridamole cardiac imaging in the assessment of ischemic heart disease. Clin Cardiol 1990; 13: 3-10.

---

Revised: 01/30/92
Interim revision: 08/17/94; 01/18/95

---

# DIRITHROMYCIN Systemic†

VA CLASSIFICATION (Primary): AM200

Note: For a listing of dosage forms and brand names by country availability, see *Dosage Forms* section(s). For a listing of brand names for the articles in this monograph, refer to the General Index.

---

†Not commercially available in Canada.

## Category

Antibacterial (systemic).

## Indications

### General considerations

Dirithromycin is an oral macrolide antibiotic with *in vitro* activity similar to that of erythromycin. Dirithromycin has a longer elimination half-life than erythromycin does and also achieves a higher concentration in some tissues. The *in vitro* activity of dirithromycin against gram-positive bacteria is similar to that of erythromycin and azithromycin, and generally less than that of clarithromycin. Penicillin-sensitive and methicillin-sensitive *Staphylococcus aureus* are susceptible to dirithromycin; however, methicillin-resistant *S. aureus* is resistant. Dirithromycin is also active against *Streptococcus pyogenes, S. pneumoniae,* and *Listeria monocytogenes. Enterococcus faecalis* and *E. faecium* are generally resistant. Gram-positive organisms that are resistant to erythromycin are also resistant to dirithromycin.

Gram-negative bacteria that are sensitive to dirithromycin include *Helicobacter pylori, H. jejuni, Moraxella catarrhalis, Bordetella pertussis,* and some strains of *Neisseria gonorrhoeae.* Dirithromycin is not active

against *Brucella* species, some strains of *Haemophilus influenzae,* or Enterobacteriaceae. Dirithromycin and erythromycin have comparable activity against *Legionella pneumophila.*

*Chlamydia trachomatis* is moderately susceptible to dirithromycin. It has little *in vitro* activity against most anaerobes and is inactive against *Toxoplasma gondii;* however, like erythromycin, dirithromycin has good activity against *Mycoplasma pneumoniae.*

### Accepted

Bronchitis, bacterial exacerbations (treatment)

Legionnaires' disease (treatment)

Pharyngitis, streptococcal (treatment)

Pneumonia, mycoplasmal (treatment)

Pneumonia, *Streptococcus pneumoniae* (treatment) or

Skin and soft tissue infections (treatment)—Dirithromycin is indicated in the treatment of these disease states when they are caused by susceptible organisms.

### Unaccepted

Dirithromycin should not be used for the treatment of known, suspected, or potential *bacteremia* because serum concentrations are not high enough to provide antibacterial coverage of the blood stream.

## Pharmacology/Pharmacokinetics

### Physicochemical characteristics

Molecular weight—Dirithromycin: 835.09.
Erythromycylamine: 743.97.

## Mechanism of action/Effect

Dirithromycin binds to the 50 S subunit of the 70 S ribosome of susceptible organisms, thereby inhibiting bacterial RNA-dependent protein
synthesis. Macrolide antibiotics are more active at an alkaline pH,
which allows the un-ionized form to penetrate the bacterial cell wall
to a greater extent.

## Absorption

Dirithromycin is rapidly absorbed and converted to the active compound,
erythromycylamine, by nonenzymatic hydrolysis. Dirithromycin
should be administered with food or within one hour of having eaten
a meal. When dirithromycin was administered with food, there was a
slight increase in absorption; in addition, there was a significant decrease in peak plasma concentration (33%) when dirithromycin was
administered one hour before food. Dietary fat had little or no effect
on bioavailability. Absolute bioavailability of dirithromycin is 6 to
14%.

## Distribution

Rapidly and extensively distributed into extravascular tissues. Dirithromycin concentrates in alveolar macrophages and phagocytes; higher
concentrations are found in tissues, such as prostate, tonsils, healthy
lung, infected lung, and bronchial mucosa, than are found in serum or
plasma. Tissue concentrations may be 20 to 30 times higher than simultaneously obtained serum concentrations. No information is available on penetration into the cerebrospinal fluid. Mean apparent volume
of distribution is approximately 800 liters (L).

## Protein binding

Erythromycylamine—Low (15 to 30%).

## Biotransformation

Dirithromycin is converted by nonenzymatic hydrolysis during absorption
to the active compound, erythromycylamine. Sixty to 90% of a dose
is hydrolyzed to erythromycylamine within 35 minutes after dosing,
and conversion is nearly complete after 1.5 hours. Erythromycylamine
undergoes little or no hepatic biotransformation. No other metabolites
of dirithromycin have been detected in the serum.

## Half-life

Erythromycylamine—30 to 50 hours.

## Time to peak concentration

Erythromycylamine—Approximately 4 to 5 hours.

## Peak serum concentration

A single 500-mg dose of dirithromycin produces an erythromycylamine
concentration of 0.3 to 0.48 mcg per mL (0.4 to 0.64 micromole per
L).

## Elimination

Fecal; 81 to 97% of an administered dose of erythromycylamine is eliminated in the bile.
Renal; approximately 1.2 to 2.9% of an administered dose is excreted
renally within 36 hours.
In dialysis—Hemodialysis, forced diuresis, peritoneal dialysis, and hemoperfusion have not been established as being beneficial for an overdose of dirithromycin. Hemodialysis is not effective in the removal of
erythromycylamine in patients with chronic renal failure.

# Precautions to Consider

## Cross-sensitivity and/or related problems

Patients hypersensitive to erythromycin or other macrolide antibiotics may
be sensitive to dirithromycin.

## Carcinogenicity

Studies in animals have not been done.

## Mutagenicity

No mutagenic potential was found when dirithromycin was used in standard tests of genotoxocity, which included in vitro and in vivo bacterial
mutation tests. These tests included the bacterial reverse-mutation test
(Ames test), DNA repair (UDS) in rat hepatocytes, Chinese hamster
lung fibroblast (V79) test, micronucleus test in mice, sister-chromatid
exchange in human lymphocytes, sister-chromatid exchange in Chinese hamsters, and the mouse lymphoma assay.

## Pregnancy/Reproduction

Fertility—Studies done in rats given doses of dirithromycin up to 21 times
the maximum recommended human dose (MRHD) on a mg per square
meter of body surface area (mg/m²) basis and in rabbits at doses up
to 4 times the MRHD on a mg/m² basis revealed no evidence of impaired fertility.

Pregnancy—Adequate and well-controlled studies have not been done in
humans.
Studies in rats given doses of dirithromycin up to 21 times the MRHD
on a mg/m² basis and in rabbits at doses up to 4 times the MRHD on

a mg/m² basis revealed no evidence of harm to the fetus. A study in
CD-1 mice showed that fetal weight was significantly depressed at a
dose of 1000 mg per kg of body weight (mg/kg) (8 times the MRHD
on a mg/m² basis). There was also developmental retardation and increased occurrences of incomplete ossification among these fetuses.
The decrease in ossification was also seen in rats given 1000 mg/kg
per day for 2 weeks prior to mating, throughout the mating period,
and throughout gestation.

FDA Pregnancy Category C.
Labor and delivery—Dirithromycin has not been studied for use during
labor and delivery.

## Breast-feeding

It is not known whether dirithromycin and its metabolite, erythromycylamine, are distributed into breast milk. However, dirithromycin is distributed into the milk of rodents, and other macrolide antibiotics are
distributed into human breast milk.

## Pediatrics

No information is available on the relationship of age to the effects of
dirithromycin in children up to 12 years of age. Safety and effectiveness have not been established.

## Geriatrics

Appropriate studies performed to date have not demonstrated geriatrics-
specific problems that would limit the usefulness of dirithromycin in
the elderly.

## Drug interactions and/or related problems

The following drug interactions and/or related problems have been selected on the basis of their potential clinical significance (possible
mechanism in parentheses where appropriate)—not necessarily inclusive (» = major clinical significance):

Note: Combinations containing any of the following medications, depending on the amount present, may also interact with this
medication.
Unlike erythromycin and some other macrolide antibiotics, dirithromycin and erythromycylamine have not been found to interact
with the cytochrome P-450 system and they do not have a significant effect on oxidative drug metabolism.

Antacids, aluminum-, calcium-, and/or magnesium-containing or
Histamine H₂-receptor antagonists
(the absorption of dirithromycin is slightly enhanced when administered concurrently with antacids or H₂-receptor antagonists due
to increased and faster absorption in the presence of lower gastric
acidity)

Astemizole or
Terfenadine
(in a prospective study done in six healthy volunteers, dirithromycin did not affect the metabolism of terfenadine; however, serious cardiac arrhythmias, some resulting in death, have occurred
in patients taking terfenadine and other macrolide antibiotics; until
further studies are completed, astemizole or terfenadine and dirithromycin should be used with caution)

Contraceptives, estrogen-containing, oral
(concurrent administration of dirithromycin with an estrogen-containing oral contraceptive was found to increase the clearance of
the ethinyl estradiol component of an oral contraceptive; however,
ovulation was not found to have occurred)

Theophylline
(concurrent use of theophylline and dirithromycin in 12 healthy
volunteers resulted in a small, nonsignificant change in the steady-
state plasma concentration of theophylline; in patients with chronic
obstructive pulmonary disease [COPD], there was also no significant change in steady-state theophylline pharmacokinetics; other
macrolide antibiotics have been found to increase the plasma concentration of theophylline; therefore, monitoring of theophylline
serum concentrations is recommended)

## Laboratory value alterations

The following have been selected on the basis of their potential clinical
significance (possible effect in parentheses where appropriate)—not
necessarily inclusive (» = major clinical significance):

With physiology/laboratory test values
Creatine kinase (CK) and
Potassium, serum
(values may be increased)
Platelets
(counts may be increased)

## Medical considerations/Contraindications

The medical considerations/contraindications included here have been selected on the basis of their potential clinical significance (reasons given
in parentheses where appropriate)—not necessarily inclusive (» =
major clinical significance).

*Risk-benefit should be considered when the following medical problems exist:*

Hepatic function impairment
(because dirithromycin and erythromycylamine are hepatically eliminated, dirithromycin should be used with caution in patients with moderate to severe hepatic function impairment; no change in dosing is necessary in patients with mildly impaired hepatic function)

Hypersensitivity to dirithromycin, erythromycin, or other macrolide antibiotics

## Side/Adverse Effects

The following side/adverse effects have been selected on the basis of their potential clinical significance (possible signs and symptoms in parentheses where appropriate)—not necessarily inclusive:

**Those indicating need for medical attention**
Incidence rare
*Clostridium difficile colitis* (severe abdominal or stomach cramps and pain; abdominal tenderness; watery and severe diarrhea, which may also be bloody; fever)

**Those indicating need for medical attention only if they continue or are bothersome**
Incidence less frequent
*Dizziness; gastrointestinal disturbances* (abdominal discomfort or pain; diarrhea; nausea; vomiting); *headache; weakness*

## Overdose

There is no specific information on the overdose of dirithromycin. Symptoms of toxicity after an overdose of other macrolide antibiotics include nausea, epigastric pain, and diarrhea. Forced diuresis, peritoneal dialysis, hemodialysis, or hemoperfusion have not been established as being beneficial in the treatment of an overdose of dirithromycin; hemodialysis is ineffective in increasing the elimination of erythromycylamine from the plasma in patients with chronic renal failure.

For more information on the management of overdose or unintentional ingestion, **contact a Poison Control Center** (see *Poison Control Center Listing*).

## Patient Consultation

As an aid to patient consultation, refer to *Advice for the Patient, Dirithromycin (Systemic)*.

In providing consultation, consider emphasizing the following selected information (» = major clinical significance):

**Before using this medication**
» Conditions affecting use, especially:
Hypersensitivity to dirithromycin or other macrolide antibiotics
Pregnancy—Birth defects were found in animal fetuses in some studies in which high dosages of dirithromycin were used

**Proper use of this medication**
Dirithromycin should be taken with food or within 1 hour after eating
» Compliance with full course of therapy
» Do not cut, crush, or chew tablets

» Proper dosing
Missed dose: Taking as soon as possible; not taking if almost time for next dose; not doubling doses
» Proper storage

**Precautions while using this medication**
Checking with physician if no improvement within a few days

**Side/adverse effects**
Signs of potential side effects, especially *Clostridium difficile* colitis

## General Dosing Information

Dirithromycin should be taken with food or within one hour after eating. Tablets should not be cut, chewed, or crushed.

## Oral Dosage Forms

### DIRITHROMYCIN TABLETS

**Usual adult and adolescent dose**
Antibacterial—
Bronchitis, acute bacterial exacerbations and secondary bacterial infections due to *Moraxella catarrhalis* or *Streptococcus pneumoniae* or
Skin and soft tissue infections due to methicillin-susceptible *Staphylococcus aureus*: Oral, 500 mg once a day for seven days.
Pharyngitis, streptococcal: Oral, 500 mg once a day for ten days.
Pneumonia due to *S. pneumoniae, Legionella pneumophila*, or *Mycoplasma pneumoniae*: Oral, 500 mg once a day for fourteen days.

**Usual pediatric dose**
Antibacterial—
Children up to 12 years of age: Safety and effectiveness have not been established.
Children 12 years of age and older: See *Usual adult and adolescent dose*.

**Usual geriatric dose**
See *Usual adult and adolescent dose*.

**Strength(s) usually available**
U.S.—
250 mg (Rx) [*Dynabac*].
Canada—
Not commercially available.

**Packaging and storage**
Store between 15 and 30 °C (59 and 86 °F).

**Auxiliary labeling**
• Continue medicine for full time of treatment.
• Do not cut, crush, or chew tablets.
• Take with food.

Developed: 06/24/96

---

## DISEASE-SPECIFIC ENTERAL NUTRITION FORMULAS—See *Enteral Nutrition Formulas (Systemic)*

---

# DISOPYRAMIDE   Systemic

VA CLASSIFICATION (Primary): CV300
Note: For a listing of dosage forms and brand names by country availability, see *Dosage Forms* section(s). For a listing of brand names for the articles in this monograph, refer to the General Index.

## Category

Antiarrhythmic.

## Indications

Note: Bracketed information in the *Indications* section refers to uses that are not included in U.S. product labeling.

**Accepted**
Arrhythmias, ventricular (treatment)—Disopyramide is indicated for the treatment of documented, life-threatening ventricular arrhythmias, such as ventricular tachycardia.

[Tachycardia, supraventricular (prophylaxis and treatment)][1]—Disopyramide is used for prophylaxis and treatment of some supraventricular tachycardias.

---

[1]Not included in Canadian product labeling.

## Pharmacology/Pharmacokinetics

**Physicochemical characteristics**
Molecular weight—Disopyramide phosphate: 437.47.
pKa—8.4.

**Mechanism of action/Effect**
Disopyramide depresses myocardial responsiveness and the electrophysiological conduction rate with the exception of the atrioventricular (AV) nodal and the His-Purkinje rates, which are essentially unchanged. Diastolic depolarization is slowed in those tissues having augmented automaticity, and the effective refractory period of the atrium and the ventricles is increased. However, conduction in accessory

pathways is prolonged. In the Vaughan Williams classification of antiarrhythmics, disopyramide is considered to be a class I agent.

### Other actions/effects
Disopyramide has a negative inotropic effect. It possesses anticholinergic activity but no noticeable alpha- or beta-adrenergic effects.

### Absorption
Rapid and nearly complete.

### Protein binding
Moderate (approximately 50% at therapeutic concentrations but may range from 35 to 95% depending largely on serum concentration).

### Biotransformation
Hepatic; primary metabolite has antiarrhythmic and anticholinergic activity.

### Half-life
Normal—7 hours (range 4 to 10 hours in healthy adults).

Renal function impairment (creatinine clearance less than 40 mL per minute)—8 to 18 hours.

### Onset of therapeutic effect
A 300-mg oral loading dose with regular capsules will usually produce a therapeutic effect in 30 minutes to 3.5 hours.

### Time to peak concentration
30 minutes to 3 hours.

### Therapeutic serum concentration
2 to 4 mcg per mL; however, because of variable protein binding and potential toxicity of free unbound drug, serum concentrations should not be used for dosage adjustment.

### Duration of action
After 300-mg oral dose with regular capsules—1.5 to 8.5 hours.

### Elimination
Renal—Approximately 80% (about 50% unchanged and 30% metabolites).

Biliary—Approximately 15%.

In dialysis—Disopyramide is rapidly removed from general circulation during hemodialysis; dialysis patients may require additional dosage following dialysis and should remain under observation until condition is stabilized.

## Precautions to Consider

### Carcinogenicity
No evidence of carcinogenic potential was found in rats given oral disopyramide for 18 months at doses up to 30 times the usual human dose by weight.

### Mutagenicity
The Ames test for mutagenic potential was negative.

### Pregnancy/Reproduction
Fertility—No adverse effect on fertility was found in rats given disopyramide at doses up to 250 mg per kg of body weight (mg/kg) per day.

Pregnancy—Adequate and well-controlled studies in humans have not been done. However, disopyramide has been found in human fetal blood and has been reported to stimulate uterine contractions in pregnant women.

Administration of disopyramide to pregnant rats at doses 20 times the usual daily human dose by weight was associated with decreased numbers of implantation sites and decreased growth and survival of pups. Increased resorption rates were observed in rabbits given disopyramide 60 mg/kg per day.

FDA Pregnancy Category C.

### Breast-feeding
Disopyramide is distributed into human breast milk at a concentration less than that in plasma.

### Pediatrics
Studies performed to date have not demonstrated pediatrics-specific problems that would limit the usefulness of disopyramide in children.

### Geriatrics
Although appropriate studies on the relationship of age to the effects of disopyramide have not been performed in the geriatric population, the elderly may exhibit increased sensitivity to the anticholinergic effects such as urinary retention and dry mouth. In addition, elderly patients are more likely to have age-related renal function impairment, which may require caution and reduction of dosage in patients receiving disopyramide.

### Dental
The secondary anticholinergic effects of disopyramide may decrease or inhibit salivary flow, especially in middle-aged or elderly patients, thus contributing to the development of caries, periodontal disease, oral candidiasis, and discomfort.

### Drug interactions and/or related problems
The following drug interactions and/or related problems have been selected on the basis of their potential clinical significance (possible mechanism in parentheses where appropriate)—not necessarily inclusive (» = major clinical significance):

Note: Combinations containing any of the following medications, depending on the amount present, may also interact with this medication.

Alcohol
(concurrent use of moderate to excessive quantities with disopyramide may enhance the development of hypoglycemia and/or hypotension because of additive effects)

» Antiarrhythmics, other, especially:
Diltiazem or
Encainide or
Flecainide or
Lidocaine or
Procainamide or
Propranolol and other beta-adrenergic blocking agents or
Quinidine or
Tocainide or
Verapamil
(caution is advised when used concurrently with disopyramide, as such usage may result in excessively prolonged electrocardial conduction with decreased cardiac output)

(close monitoring is essential, as clinical heart failure may worsen during use of disopyramide with beta-adrenergic blocking agents in patients with decreased ventricular performance)

(disopyramide should not be administered within 48 hours before or 24 hours following verapamil; deaths have been reported)

Anticholinergics or other medications with anticholinergic activity (See *Appendix II*)
(anticholinergic effects may be intensified when these medications are used concurrently with disopyramide because of secondary anticholinergic activity of disopyramide)

Anticoagulants, coumarin- or indandione-derivative
(concurrent use of warfarin and disopyramide has been reported to increase or decrease the anticoagulant effect; although clinical significance has not been determined, caution is recommended)

Antidiabetic agents, oral or
Insulin
(hypoglycemic effects may be intensified in rare cases by the concurrent use of disopyramide because of additive hypoglycemic effects; patients prone to hypoglycemia should be closely monitored)

Hepatic enzyme inducers (See *Appendix II*)
(concurrent use may reduce serum disopyramide to ineffective concentrations; therefore monitoring of its serum concentrations is necessary during concurrent therapy)

Hypotension-producing medications, other (See *Appendix II*)
(concurrent use with disopyramide may increase the hypotensive effects)

» Pimozide
(concurrent use with disopyramide may potentiate cardiac arrhythmias, which are seen on electrocardiogram [ECG] as prolongation of QT interval)

### Laboratory value alterations
The following have been selected on the basis of their potential clinical significance (possible effect in parentheses where appropriate)—not necessarily inclusive (» = major clinical significance):

With physiology/laboratory test values
Blood glucose concentrations
(may be decreased by an undetermined mechanism)

ECG changes, such as:
QRS widening
QT prolongation
(may occur with overdose)

### Medical considerations/Contraindications
The medical considerations/contraindications included here have been selected on the basis of their potential clinical significance (reasons given in parentheses where appropriate)—not necessarily inclusive (» = major clinical significance).

*Except under special circumstances, this medication should not be used when the following medical problems exist:*
» Atrioventricular (AV) block, pre-existing second or third degree without pacemaker

» Cardiogenic shock

*Risk-benefit should be considered when the following medical problems exist:*

Bladder neck obstruction
    (anticholinergic activity of disopyramide may cause urinary retention)

» Cardiac conduction abnormalities, such as sick sinus syndrome, Wolff-Parkinson-White syndrome, or bundle branch block
    (disopyramide may produce additive cardiac depression)

» Cardiomyopathies
    (risk of congestive heart failure and hypotension with disopyramide; patient should not receive loading dose and dose reduction may be indicated)

» Congestive heart failure, uncompensated or poorly compensated
    (possible aggravation and risk of hypotension)
    (caution use of disopyramide in patients with a very low left ventricular ejection fraction, especially < 30%, because of its cardiodepressant effects)

» Diabetes mellitus
    (disopyramide may significantly lower blood glucose levels)

» Glaucoma, closed-angle, history of
    (anticholinergic activity of disopyramide may result in precipitation of acute condition)

» Hepatic function impairment
    (possible accumulation of disopyramide; dosage reduction may be required)

» Hyperkalemia
    (risk of serious arrhythmias)

» Hypokalemia
    (may reduce efficacy of disopyramide)

» Myasthenia gravis
    (anticholinergic effect of disopyramide may result in myasthenic crisis)

» Prostatic enlargement
    (possible urinary retention; may be exacerbated by anticholinergic effect)

» Renal function impairment
    (accumulation of disopyramide because of reduced excretion; dosage reduction may be required; disopyramide extended-release capsules are not recommended for patients with severe renal insufficiency [creatinine clearance of 40 mL per minute (0.67 mL per second) or less])

Sensitivity to disopyramide

## Patient monitoring

The following may be especially important in patient monitoring (other tests may be warranted in some patients, depending on condition; » = major clinical significance):

Blood glucose concentrations
    (recommended at periodic intervals in patients at risk of developing hypoglycemia, e.g., those with congestive heart failure, chronic malnutrition, or hepatic or renal function impairment, or those taking medications such as beta-blockers)

Blood pressure determinations
    (recommended at periodic intervals during therapy; if hypotension occurs and is not caused by an arrhythmia, disopyramide should be withdrawn and reinstituted at a lower dose only after adequate cardiac compensation is established)

» ECG monitoring
    (recommended at periodic intervals during therapy; if significant QRS widening [> 25%] occurs, disopyramide should be withdrawn; if significant QT prolongation [> 25%] occurs, the patient requires dose monitoring and possible discontinuation of disopyramide)

Hepatic function and
Intraocular pressure and
Potassium concentrations, serum, and
Renal function
    (determinations recommended prior to initiation of therapy and, if necessary, at periodic intervals during therapy)

## Side/Adverse Effects

Note: Overdose may lead to apnea, loss of consciousness, cardiac arrhythmias, loss of spontaneous respiration, and death. Toxic plasma concentrations are associated with excessive widening of the QRS complex and QT interval, worsening of congestive heart failure, hypotension, conduction disturbances, bradycardia, and ultimately asystole; obvious anticholinergic effects also occur.

In the National Heart, Lung, and Blood Institute's Cardiac Arrhythmias Suppression Trial (CAST), treatment with encainide or flecainide was found to be associated with excessive mortality or increased nonfatal cardiac arrest rate, as compared with placebo, in patients with asymptomatic, non–life-threatening arrhythmias who had had a recent myocardial infarction. The implications of these results for other patient populations or other antiarrhythmic agents are uncertain.

The following side/adverse effects have been selected on the basis of their potential clinical significance (possible signs and symptoms in parentheses where appropriate)—not necessarily inclusive:

**Those indicating need for medical attention**
Incidence more frequent—10 to 20%
    *Anticholinergic effect* (difficult urination)
Incidence less frequent—1 to 10%
    *Chest pain; confusion; congestive heart failure, possible, or fluid retention* (fast or slow heartbeat; unexplained shortness of breath; swelling of feet or lower legs; rapid weight gain); *hypotension* (dizziness, lightheadedness, or fainting); *muscle weakness*
Incidence rare—<1%
    *Aggravation of glaucoma, possible* (eye pain); *agranulocytosis* (sore throat and fever); *cholestatic jaundice* (yellow eyes or skin); *hypoglycemia* (anxious feeling; chills; cold sweats; confusion; cool, pale skin; drowsiness; fast heartbeat; headache; hunger, excessive; nausea; nervousness; shakiness; unsteady walk; or unusual tiredness or weakness); *mental depression*

**Those indicating need for medical attention only if they continue or are bothersome**
Incidence more frequent—40%
    *Anticholinergic effect* (dryness of mouth and throat)
Incidence less frequent—1 to 10%
    *Anorexia* (loss of appetite); *anticholinergic effect* (blurred vision; constipation; dry eyes and nose); *bloating or stomach pain; decreased sexual ability; urinary frequency or urgency* (frequent urge to urinate)

## Overdose

For more information on the management of overdose or unintentional ingestion, **contact a Poison Control Center** (see *Poison Control Center Listing*).

**Treatment of overdose**
There is no specific antidote for disopyramide; treatment should be symptomatic and supportive, and may include mechanical respirator and endocardial pacer when indicated or use of cardiac glycosides, diuretics, dopamine, isoproterenol, or neostigmine when indicated. ECG monitoring is essential.

Hemodialysis or charcoal hemoperfusion has been used successfully.

## Patient Consultation

As an aid to patient consultation, refer to *Advice for the Patient, Disopyramide (Systemic).*

In providing consultation, consider emphasizing the following selected information (» = major clinical significance):

**Before using this medication**
» Conditions affecting use, especially:
    Sensitivity to disopyramide
    Pregnancy—May initiate uterine contractions
    Breast-feeding—Passes into breast milk
    Use in the elderly—Increased sensitivity to anticholinergic effects
    Other medications, especially other antiarrhythmics or pimozide
    Other medical problems, especially second or third degree atrioventricular (AV) block, cardiogenic shock, cardiac conduction abnormalities, cardiomyopathies, uncompensated or poorly compensated congestive heart failure, diabetes mellitus, history of closed-angle glaucoma, hepatic function impairment, hyperkalemia or hypokalemia, myasthenia gravis, prostatic enlargement, or renal function impairment

**Proper use of this medication**
» Compliance with therapy; not taking more medication than directed
    Proper administration of extended-release capsules: Swallowing capsule whole, without breaking, crushing, or chewing
    Proper administration of extended-release tablets: Not crushing or chewing
» Importance of not missing doses and taking at evenly spaced intervals
» Proper dosing
» Missed dose: Taking as soon as possible, unless within 4 hours of next dose; not doubling doses
» Proper storage

**Precautions while using this medication**

» Regular visits to physician to check progress
» Checking with physician before stopping medication because of adverse cardiac effects with sudden withdrawal
» Caution when driving or doing things requiring alertness because of possible dizziness, lightheadedness, or fainting, especially when getting up suddenly from lying or sitting position
» Avoiding alcoholic beverages
» Notifying physician and taking sugar if symptoms of hypoglycemia occur
» Possible blurred vision; avoiding driving, using machines, or doing other things requiring clear vision if blurred vision occurs
    Possible dryness of eyes, mouth, and nose; using sugarless candy or gum, ice, or saliva substitute for relief of dry mouth; checking with physician or dentist if dry mouth continues for more than 2 weeks
» Caution during exercise or hot weather because of possible reduced sweating and impaired heat tolerance

**Side/adverse effects**

Signs of potential side effects, especially difficult urination, chest pains, confusion, congestive heart failure, fluid retention, hypotension, muscle weakness, aggravation of glaucoma, agranulocytosis, cholestatic jaundice, mental depression, and hypoglycemia

# General Dosing Information

The dosage for all patients should be individualized within limits of response and tolerance, with required dosage adjustments being made gradually.

Patients of small body size (less than 50 kg body weight) may require reduced dosage.

When a loading dose is used, close monitoring is required for possible development of hypotension and/or congestive heart failure.

Patients receiving quinidine sulfate or procainamide may be changed to disopyramide therapy by starting the regular maintenance dose of disopyramide 6 to 12 hours after the last quinidine sulfate dose or 3 to 6 hours after the last dose of procainamide.

Patients with atrial flutter or fibrillation should be digitalized prior to disopyramide treatment to ensure that drug-induced enhancement of atrioventricular (AV) conduction does not increase the ventricular rate beyond acceptable limits.

Because disopyramide is removed by hemodialysis, additional dosage may be required following dialysis.

If first-degree AV block develops, dosage of disopyramide should be reduced. If block persists or worsens, the medication may have to be withdrawn.

# Oral Dosage Forms

Note: The dosing and strengths of the dosage forms available are expressed in terms of disopyramide base.

## DISOPYRAMIDE CAPSULES

**Usual adult dose**
Antiarrhythmic—
    Loading dose (for rapid control of ventricular arrhythmia):
        Oral, 300 mg (base) (200 mg for body weight less than 50 kg).
        Note: A loading dose is not recommended for patients with cardiomyopathy or possible cardiac decompensation.
    Maintenance:
        Oral, 150 mg (base) every six hours (or 100 mg [base] every six to eight hours for body weight less than 50 kg or in patients with cardiomyopathy or possible cardiac decompensation), the dosage being adjusted as needed and tolerated.
        Note: Geriatric patients may be more sensitive to the effects of the usual adult dose.
            Creatinine clearance is used to determine adjustment of dosing interval in cases of renal insufficiency:

| Creatinine Clearance | | Approximate Maintenance |
| (mL/min) | (mL/s) | Dosing Interval |
| --- | --- | --- |
| 30–40 | 0.5–0.67 | Every 8 hr |
| 15–30 | 0.25–0.5 | Every 12 hr |
| <15 | <0.25 | Every 24 hr |

**Usual adult prescribing limits**
Up to 800 mg (base) daily.
Note: Although total daily doses of up to 1.6 grams (base) have been used in patients with severe refractory ventricular tachycardia, such high doses are restricted to the hospitalized patient.

**Usual pediatric dose**
Antiarrhythmic—
    Oral, the following doses equally divided and administered every six hours (or at other individually appropriate intervals):
        Children up to 1 year of age—10 to 30 mg (base) per kg of body weight per day.
        Children 1 to 4 years of age—10 to 20 mg (base) per kg of body weight per day.
        Children 4 to 12 years of age—10 to 15 mg (base) per kg of body weight per day.
        Children 12 to 18 years of age—6 to 15 mg (base) per kg of body weight per day.
Note: Children should be hospitalized during the initial period of therapy to allow close monitoring until a maintenance dose is established.

**Strength(s) usually available**
U.S.—
    Not commercially available.
Canada—
    100 mg (Rx) [*Rythmodan*].
    150 mg (Rx) [*Rythmodan*].

**Packaging and storage**
Store between 15 and 30 °C (59 and 86 °F), in a well-closed container, unless otherwise specified by manufacturer.

**Auxiliary labeling**
• Avoid alcoholic beverages.
• May cause blurred vision.
• Do not take other medicines without advice from your doctor.

## DISOPYRAMIDE PHOSPHATE CAPSULES USP

**Usual adult dose**
See *Disopyramide Capsules.*

**Usual adult prescribing limits**
See *Disopyramide Capsules.*

**Usual pediatric dose**
See *Disopyramide Capsules.*

**Strength(s) usually available**
U.S.—
    100 mg (base) (Rx) [*Norpace* (lactose); GENERIC].
    150 mg (base) (Rx) [*Norpace* (lactose); GENERIC].
Canada—
    100 mg (base) [*Norpace* (lactose)].
    150 mg (base) [*Norpace* (lactose)].

**Packaging and storage**
Store between 15 and 30 °C (59 and 86 °F), unless otherwise specified by manufacturer. Store in a well-closed container.

**Preparation of dosage form**
For patients who cannot take oral solids—Prepare a liquid suspension for oral use by adding the entire contents from the required number of 100-mg (base) regular Disopyramide Phosphate Capsules USP (do not use extended-release capsules) to an appropriate quantity of Cherry Syrup NF to make a suitable concentration of 1 to 10 mg per mL. Add accessory 'Shake' and 'Refrigerate' labels and dispense in amber glass bottles with child-proof caps.

**Stability**
The extemporaneously prepared oral suspension of disopyramide is stable for one month when refrigerated.

**Auxiliary labeling**
• Avoid alcoholic beverages.
• May cause blurred vision.
• Do not take other medicines without advice from your doctor.
For oral suspension—
    • Avoid alcoholic beverages.
    • May cause blurred vision.
    • Shake well.
    • Refrigerate.
    • Do not take other medicines without advice from your doctor.

## DISOPYRAMIDE PHOSPHATE EXTENDED-RELEASE CAPSULES USP

**Usual adult dose**
Antiarrhythmic—
    Oral, 300 mg (base) every twelve hours (200 mg every twelve hours for body weight less than 50 kg).
Note: Extended-release dosage form is not recommended for initial dosage, but for maintenance dosage only.
    When transferring from the regular oral dosage form, it is recommended that the first dose of the extended-release dosage form be

given six hours after the last regular dose.

**Usual adult prescribing limits**

Up to 800 mg (base) daily.

Note: Although total daily doses of up to 1.6 grams (base) have been used in patients with severe refractory ventricular tachycardia, such high doses are restricted to the hospitalized patient.

**Usual pediatric dose**

Use is not recommended.

**Strength(s) usually available**

U.S.—

100 mg (base) (Rx) [*Norpace CR;* GENERIC].

150 mg (base) (Rx) [*Norpace CR;* GENERIC].

Canada—

Not commercially available.

**Packaging and storage**

Store between 15 and 30 °C (59 and 85 °F), unless otherwise specified by manufacturer. Store in a well-closed container.

**Auxiliary labeling**

• Avoid alcoholic beverages.

• May cause blurred vision.

• Do not take other medicines without advice from your doctor.

• Swallow capsule whole.

## DISOPYRAMIDE PHOSPHATE EXTENDED-RELEASE TABLETS

**Usual adult dose**

See *Disopyramide Phosphate Extended-release Capsules USP.*

**Usual pediatric dose**

Use is not recommended.

**Strength(s) usually available**

U.S.—

Not commercially available.

Canada—

150 mg (base) (Rx) [*Norpace CR; Rythmodan-LA* (scored)].

**Packaging and storage**

Store between 15 and 30 °C (59 and 86 °F), in a well-closed container, unless otherwise specified by manufacturer.

**Auxiliary labeling**

• Avoid alcoholic beverages.

• May cause blurred vision.

• Swallow tablet whole.

• Do not take other medicines without advice from your doctor.

## Parenteral Dosage Forms

### DISOPYRAMIDE INJECTION

Note: Use of the parenteral dosage form may be accompanied by a hypotensive response. This route should be limited to emergencies and the medication should be given in a hospital where intensive coronary care unit facilities are available.

**Usual adult dose**

Antiarrhythmic—

  Loading dose:

    Intravenous—2 mg (base) per kg of body weight (1 mg [base] per kg of body weight for patients with compromised left ventricular function) administered in three equally divided doses; each dose should be injected slowly over a period of three minutes with an interval of three minutes between each dose.

    Intravenous infusion—2 mg (base) per kg of body weight (1 mg [base] per kg of body weight for patients with compromised left ventricular function) administered over fifteen minutes.

    Note: An additional 1 to 2 mg (base) per kg of body weight may be administered by slow infusion over the next forty-five minutes if adequate control of the arrhythmia is not achieved. Careful monitoring of the patient is recommended.

  Maintenance:

    Intravenous infusion, 0.4 mg (400 mcg) (base) per kg of body weight per hour given for up to twenty-four hours.

Note: Total intravenous administration during the first hour should not exceed 300 mg (base) and the total administration during the first twenty-four hours should not exceed 800 mg (base).

**Usual pediatric dose**

Safety and efficacy have not been established.

**Strength(s) usually available**

U.S.—

Not commercially available.

Canada—

10 mg (base) per mL (Rx) [*Rythmodan* (benzyl alcohol 10 mg per mL)].

**Packaging and storage**

Store below 40 °C (104 °F), preferably between 15 and 30 °C (59 and 86 °F), unless otherwise specified by manufacturer. Protect from freezing.

**Preparation of dosage form**

Rythmodan injection is physically compatible with dextrose injection BP, sodium chloride injection BP, compound sodium chloride injection BP, and compound sodium lactate injection BP.

Caution—Use of diluents containing benzyl alcohol is not recommended for preparation of medications for use in neonates. A fatal toxic syndrome consisting of metabolic acidosis, CNS depression, respiratory problems, renal failure, hypotension, and possibly seizures and intracranial hemorrhages has been associated with this use.

## Selected Bibliography

Taylor EH, Pappas AA. Disopyramide: clinical indications, pharmacokinetics and laboratory assessment. Ann Clin Lab Sci 1986 Jul-Aug; 16 (4): 289-95.

Siddoway LA, Woosley RL. Clinical pharmacokinetics of disopyramide. Clin Pharmacokinet 1986 May-Jun; 11 (3): 214-22.

Revised: 05/14/93

Interim revision: 04/13/95

# DISULFIRAM   Systemic

**VA CLASSIFICATION (Primary): AD100**

Note: For a listing of dosage forms and brand names by country availability, see *Dosage Forms* section(s). For a listing of brand names for the articles in this monograph, refer to the General Index.

## Category

Alcohol-abuse deterrent.

## Indications

### Accepted

Alcoholism (treatment)—Disulfiram is used to help maintain sobriety in the treatment of chronic alcoholism in conjunction with supportive and psychotherapeutic measures.

## Pharmacology/Pharmacokinetics

### Physicochemical characteristics

Molecular weight—296.52.

### Mechanism of action/Effect

Produces irreversible inhibition of the enzyme responsible for oxidation of the ethanol metabolite acetaldehyde. The resultant accumulation of acetaldehyde may be responsible for most of the signs and symptoms occurring after ethanol ingestion in disulfiram-treated patients. The hypotensive response may be due to inhibition of norepinephrine synthesis by the major disulfiram metabolite diethyldithiocarbamate.

### Absorption

Slow. 80 to 90% of an oral dose is absorbed.

### Biotransformation

Hepatic.

### Onset of action

A single dose of disulfiram will begin to affect ethanol metabolism within 1 to 2 hours.

### Duration of action

Disulfiram-alcohol reactions may occur up to 14 days following last dose of disulfiram.

### Elimination
Primarily renal, as metabolites. Some of the metabolites are also exhaled as carbon disulfide. Up to 20% of a dose may remain in the body for 1 week or longer. About 5 to 20% of a dose is eliminated unchanged in the feces.

## Precautions to Consider

### Cross-sensitivity and/or related problems
Patients sensitive to other thiuram derivatives (used in rubber, pesticides, or fungicides) may be sensitive to disulfiram also.

### Pregnancy/Reproduction
Pregnancy—Adequate and well-controlled studies in humans have not been done. However, there have been a few reports of congenital defects in infants whose mothers received disulfiram during pregnancy. Further study is needed to determine the relationship between disulfiram and congenital malformations.

Disulfiram is reported to be embryotoxic in animals.

### Breast-feeding
Problems in humans have not been documented.

### Pediatrics
No information is available on the relationship of age to the effects of disulfiram in pediatric patients. Safety and efficacy have not been established.

### Geriatrics
No information is available on the relationship of age to the effects of disulfiram in geriatric patients. However, elderly patients are more likely to have age-related renal function impairment, which may require caution in patients receiving this medication. In addition, elderly patients with cardiac or cerebrovascular disease may not tolerate the hypotension that accompanies the disulfiram-alcohol reaction as well as younger patients.

### Drug interactions and/or related problems
The following drug interactions and/or related problems have been selected on the basis of their potential clinical significance (possible mechanism in parentheses where appropriate)—not necessarily inclusive (» = major clinical significance):

Note: Combinations containing any of the following medications, depending on the amount present, may also interact with this medication.

» Alcohol
   (use of alcohol or alcohol-containing products within 14 days of disulfiram therapy will result in a disulfiram-alcohol reaction)

» Alfentanil
   (chronic preoperative administration or perioperative use of hepatic enzyme inhibitors, such as disulfiram, may decrease plasma clearance and prolong the duration of action of alfentanil)

Amoxicillin and clavulanate combination or
Bacampicillin
   (metabolism of bacampicillin produces low plasma concentrations of alcohol and acetaldehyde; although the risk of a disulfiram-alcohol interaction appears minimal, caution is recommended if concurrent use is unavoidable)

   (a similar reaction is thought to occur with amoxicillin and clavulanate combination)

» Anticoagulants, coumarin- or indandione-derivative
   (anticoagulant effect may be increased during concurrent use with disulfiram because of inhibition of the enzymatic metabolism of the anticoagulant; also, disulfiram may act directly in the liver to increase the hypoprothrombinemia-inducing activity of coumarin derivatives; anticoagulant dosage adjustments based on prothrombin time determinations may be necessary during and following concurrent use)

» Anticonvulsants, hydantoin, especially phenytoin
   (concurrent use with disulfiram may increase the serum concentrations of hydantoins, possibly leading to hydantoin toxicity; hydantoin serum concentrations should be obtained prior to and during concurrent therapy with disulfiram and dosage adjustments made accordingly)

Antidepressants, tricyclic, especially amitriptyline
   (concurrent use with disulfiram may cause transient delirium)

Ascorbic acid
   (may interfere with the disulfiram-alcohol reaction, especially with chronic use or high doses of ascorbic acid; although controversial, this effect has been used beneficially by some clinicians in the management of disulfiram-alcohol reactions)

Central nervous system (CNS) depression–producing medications (See *Appendix II*)
   (concurrent use may enhance the CNS depressant effects of either these medications or disulfiram)

Ethylene dibromide
   (exposure to ethylene dibromide or its vapors concurrently with disulfiram treatment may result in a toxic reaction)

Hepatic enzyme inhibitors (See *Appendix II*)
   (concurrent use of disulfiram with other hepatic enzyme inhibitors may potentiate the effect)

Hepatotoxic medication, other (See *Appendix II*)
   (concurrent use of disulfiram with other hepatotoxic medications may increase the potential for hepatotoxicity)

» Isoniazid
   (concurrent use may result in increased incidence of CNS effects, such as dizziness, incoordination, irritability, or insomnia; a reduction of dosage or discontinuation of disulfiram may be necessary)

» Metronidazole
   (concurrent use with disulfiram may result in confusion and psychotic reactions because of combined toxicity; metronidazole is not recommended concurrently with, and for 2 weeks following, disulfiram)

Midazolam
   (concurrent use may decrease first-pass metabolism and elimination of midazolam in the liver, probably by competitive inhibition at the cytochrome P-450 binding sites, thereby increasing steady-state plasma concentrations of midazolam)

Neurotoxic medications (See *Appendix II*)
   (concurrent use of disulfiram with other neurotoxic medications may increase the potential for neurotoxicity)

» Organic solvents
   (exposure to organic solvents, ingested or inhaled, which may contain alcohol, acetaldehyde, paraldehyde, or structural analogs, may result in a disulfiram-alcohol reaction)

» Paraldehyde
   (concurrent use with disulfiram is not recommended, because inhibition of acetaldehyde dehydrogenase may occur, resulting in decreased metabolism of paraldehyde and increased blood concentrations of paraldehyde and acetaldehyde)

### Laboratory value alterations
The following have been selected on the basis of their potential clinical significance (possible effect in parentheses where appropriate)—not necessarily inclusive (» = major clinical significance):

With physiology/laboratory test values
   Cholesterol concentrations, serum
      (may be increased with doses of 500 mg a day)
   Vanillylmandelic acid (VMA) concentrations, urine
      (may be decreased)

### Medical considerations/Contraindications
The medical considerations/contraindications included here have been selected on the basis of their potential clinical significance (reasons given in parentheses where appropriate)—not necessarily inclusive (» = major clinical significance).

***Risk-benefit should be considered when the following medical problems exist:***

Allergic eczematous contact dermatitis
   (may be exacerbated)
Cardiovascular disorders
   (disulfiram-alcohol reaction may exacerbate condition)
Depression
   (behavioral toxicity may be precipitated)
Diabetes mellitus
   (disulfiram-alcohol reaction may exacerbate condition)
Epilepsy or other seizure disorder, or history of
   (disulfiram-alcohol reaction may exacerbate condition)
Hepatic function impairment or cirrhosis
   (increased potential for hepatotoxicity)
Hypothyroidism
   (disulfiram-alcohol reaction may exacerbate condition)
Psychoses
   (behavioral toxicity may be precipitated)
Pulmonary insufficiency, severe
   (disulfiram-alcohol reaction may exacerbate condition)
Renal function impairment
   (disulfiram elimination may be inhibited)

Sensitivity to disulfiram, rubber, pesticides, or fungicides

**Patient monitoring**

The following may be especially important in patient monitoring (other tests may be warranted in some patients, depending on condition; » = major clinical significance):

Blood cell counts and

Blood chemistry profiles

(recommended at 6-month intervals during therapy)

Hepatic function determinations

(baseline studies are recommended, followed by transaminase tests after 10 to 14 days of therapy; additional liver function tests may also be required at periodic intervals during therapy)

## Side/Adverse Effects

The following side/adverse effects have been selected on the basis of their potential clinical significance (possible signs and symptoms in parentheses where appropriate)—not necessarily inclusive:

**Those indicating need for medical attention**

Incidence less frequent

*Neurotoxicity, including optic neuritis* (eye pain or tenderness or any change in vision); *peripheral neuritis or polyneuritis* (numbness, pain, tingling, or weakness in hands or feet); *psychotic reaction* (mood or mental changes)

Note: *Neurotoxicity* is usually reversible if disulfiram is discontinued.

Incidence rare

*Encephalopathy* (mental changes); *hepatitis* (yellow eyes or skin; darkening of urine; light gray–colored stools; severe stomach pain)

Note: Fulminant hepatic necrosis occurs rarely. Although it cannot be predicted which patients will develop this potentially fatal hepatitis, published experience suggests that the chance of survival is markedly improved if disulfiram is stopped as soon as jaundice is detected. Careful clinical monitoring with discontinuation of disulfiram and laboratory (bilirubin and hepatic enzyme) determinations is recommended when hepatitis is suspected.

**Those indicating need for medical attention only if they continue or are bothersome**

Incidence more frequent

*Drowsiness*

Incidence less frequent or rare

*Headache; impotence* (decreased sexual ability in males); *metallic or garlic-like taste in mouth; skin rash; unusual tiredness*

## Patient Consultation

As an aid to patient consultation, refer to *Advice for the Patient, Disulfiram (Systemic).*

In providing consultation, consider emphasizing the following selected information (» = major clinical significance):

**Before using this medication**

» Conditions affecting use, especially:

Sensitivity to disulfiram, rubber, pesticides, or fungicides

Other medications, especially alcohol; alfentanil; coumarin- or indandione-derivative anticoagulants; hydantoin anticonvulsants, especially phenytoin; isoniazid; metronidazole; organic solvents; or paraldehyde

**Proper use of this medication**

» Not taking this medication within 12 hours of using any alcohol-containing preparation or medication, or if the blood alcohol level is not zero

» Compliance with therapy

» Proper dosing

» Proper storage

**Precautions while using this medication**

» Not drinking or using any alcohol-containing products or medications while taking this medication and for 14 days after discontinuing this medication

Symptoms of disulfiram-alcohol reaction

Blurred vision

Chest pain

Confusion

Dizziness or fainting

Fast or pounding heartbeat

Flushing or redness of face

Increased sweating

Nausea and vomiting

Throbbing headache

Troubled breathing

Weakness, severe

Rarely, seizures, heart attack, unconsciousness, or death if reaction is severe

Carrying medical identification card during therapy

Regular visits to physician to check progress during long-term therapy

» Checking all liquid medications for presence of alcohol

» Caution if drowsiness occurs

» Checking with physician before using other CNS depressants

**Side/adverse effects**

Signs of potential side effects, especially optic neuritis, peripheral neuritis, polyneuritis, or psychotic reaction

## General Dosing Information

The patient should be made fully aware of the nature of this medicine and the disulfiram-alcohol reaction and its consequences.

Disulfiram should not be administered until the patient has abstained from alcohol for at least 12 hours and the blood alcohol level is zero.

The duration of the disulfiram-alcohol reaction is dependent upon the dose of disulfiram and on the quantity of alcohol ingested; it may persist from 30 minutes to several hours.

Reactions to alcohol may occur for up to 2 weeks following withdrawal of disulfiram therapy.

**For treatment of disulfiram-alcohol reaction**

In severe reactions, supportive measures to restore blood pressure and treat shock should be instituted. Other recommendations include:

• Administration of supplemental oxygen.

• Monitoring of serum potassium levels.

• Monitoring of ECG tracings.

Although controversial, administration of intravenous ascorbic acid or intravenous antihistamines has been advocated by some clinicians. Phenothiazines should not be used as they may exacerbate hypotension.

## Oral Dosage Forms

### DISULFIRAM TABLETS USP

**Usual adult and adolescent dose**

Alcohol-abuse deterrent—

Initial: Oral, up to 500 mg once a day for one or two weeks.

Maintenance: Oral, 125 to 500 mg (average of 250 mg) once a day.

Note: Some clinicians recommend the dose be administered at bedtime to reduce daytime drowsiness.

**Usual pediatric dose**

Safety and efficacy have not been established.

**Usual geriatric dose**

See *Usual adult and adolescent dose.*

Note: Geriatric patients may be more sensitive to the effects of the usual adult dose.

**Strength(s) usually available**

U.S.—

250 mg (Rx) [*Antabuse* (scored); GENERIC].

500 mg (Rx) [*Antabuse* (scored); GENERIC].

Canada—

250 mg (Rx) [*Antabuse* (scored)].

500 mg (Rx) [*Antabuse* (scored)].

### Packaging and storage

Store below 40 °C (104 °F), preferably between 15 and 30 °C (59 and 86 °F), in a tight, light-resistant container.

### Note

Patient identification cards may be available from the manufacturer.

## Selected Bibliography

Wright C, Moore RD. Disulfiram treatment of alcoholism. Am J Med 1990; 88: 647-55.

Revised: 01/27/92
Interim revision: 07/20/94

# DIURETICS, LOOP  Systemic

This monograph includes information on the following: Bumetanide†; Ethacrynic Acid; Furosemide.

INN:
  Ethacrynic Acid—Etacrynic acid

JAN:
  Ethacrynic Acid—Etacrynic acid

VA CLASSIFICATION (Primary/Secondary): CV702/CV490; TN900

Note: For a listing of dosage forms and brand names by country availability, see *Dosage Forms* section(s). For a listing of brand names for the articles in this monograph, refer to the General Index.

†Not commercially available in Canada.

## Category

Diagnostic aid adjunct (renal disease)—Furosemide.
Diuretic—Bumetanide; Ethacrynic Acid; Furosemide.
Antihypertensive—Bumetanide; Ethacrynic Acid; Furosemide.
Antihypercalcemic—Bumetanide; Ethacrynic Acid; Furosemide.

## Indications

Note: Bracketed information in the *Indications* section refers to uses that are not included in U.S. product labeling.

### Accepted

Edema (treatment)—Bumetanide, ethacrynic acid, and furosemide are indicated in the treatment of edema associated with congestive heart failure, hepatic cirrhosis, and renal disease (including nephrotic syndrome).

Bumetanide, ethacrynic acid, and furosemide are indicated as adjuncts in the treatment of acute pulmonary edema.

Ethacrynic acid is indicated in the short-term management of ascites due to malignancy, idiopathic edema, and lymphedema; and in the short-term management of hospitalized pediatric patients with congenital heart disease or nephrotic syndrome.

Bumetanide, ethacrynic acid, and furosemide are especially useful in patients refractory to other diuretics or with existing acid-base disorders, congestive heart failure, or renal disease.

Hypertension (treatment)—[Bumetanide], [ethacrynic acid][1], and furosemide are indicated in the treatment of mild to moderate hypertension, usually in combination with other antihypertensive agents, and as adjuncts in the treatment of hypertensive crisis.

Bumetanide, ethacrynic acid, and furosemide are not considered to be primary agents in the treatment of essential hypertension. However, they may be indicated in combination with other antihypertensives in the treatment of hypertension associated with impaired renal function. In the stepped-care approach to antihypertensive treatment, bumetanide, ethacrynic acid, or furosemide may be substituted for a thiazide diuretic in patients with renal function impairment.

For additional information on initial therapeutic guidelines related to the treatment of hypertension, see *Appendix III*.

Hypercalcemia (treatment)—[Bumetanide], [ethacrynic acid][1], and [furosemide][1] are used in the treatment of hypercalcemia.

[Renography, adjunct][1] and
[Renal imaging, radionuclide, adjunct][1]—Furosemide augments radionuclide renography and renal scintigraphy by stimulating the flow of urine and thereby aiding in the differentiation of mechanical obstruction from nonobstructive dilatation in patients with hydroureteronephrosis.

[1]Not included in Canadian product labeling.

## Pharmacology/Pharmacokinetics

### Physicochemical characteristics

Molecular weight—
  Bumetanide: 364.42.

Ethacrynic acid: 303.14.
Furosemide: 330.74.

pKa—
  Ethacrynic acid: 3.5.
  Furosemide: 3.9.

### Mechanism of action/Effect

Diuretic—Bumetanide, ethacrynic acid, and furosemide inhibit reabsorption of sodium and water in the ascending limb of the loop of Henle by interfering with the chloride binding site of the $1Na+$, $1K+$, $2Cl-$ cotransport system. Loop diuretics increase the rate of delivery of tubular fluid and electrolytes to the distal sites of hydrogen and potassium ion secretion, while plasma volume contraction increases aldosterone production. The increased delivery and high aldosterone levels promote sodium reabsorption at the distal tubules, thus increasing the loss of potassium and hydrogen ions. Bumetanide may have a small additional action on sodium reabsorption in the proximal tubule since phosphate reabsorption is reduced.

Antihypertensive—Diuretics lower blood pressure initially by reducing plasma and extracellular fluid volume; cardiac output also decreases. Eventually, cardiac output returns to normal with an accompanying decrease in peripheral resistance.

Antihypercalcemic—Loop diuretics increase the urinary excretion of calcium.

### Absorption

Bumetanide—Almost completely absorbed from gastrointestinal tract. Absorption is probably reduced in patients with edematous bowel caused by congestive heart failure or nephrotic syndrome; parenteral administration may be preferable in these patients.

Furosemide—Approximately 60 to 70% of an oral dose of furosemide is absorbed. Food may slow the rate of absorption but does not appear to alter the bioavailability or diuretic effect. Absorption is reduced to 43 to 46% in patients with end-stage renal disease, and is probably reduced also in patients with edematous bowel caused by congestive heart failure or nephrotic syndrome; parenteral administration may be preferable in these patients.

### Protein binding

Bumetanide—Very high (94 to 96%).
Ethacrynic acid—High.
Furosemide—Very high (91 to 97%; almost totally to albumin).

### Biotransformation

Hepatic; metabolism of bumetanide is limited and produces inactive metabolites.

### Half-life

Bumetanide—
  1 to 1½ hours.
Furosemide—
  Wide variation among individuals.
    Normal:
      ½ to 1 hour.
    Anuric:
      75 to 155 minutes.
      In patients with both renal and hepatic insufficiency, half-lives of 11 to 20 hours have been reported.
      In neonates, reported half-lives are prolonged, probably due to low renal and hepatic clearance.

### Onset of action

Diuretic—
  Bumetanide:
    Oral—30 to 60 minutes.
    Intravenous—Within minutes.
  Ethacrynic acid:
    Oral—30 minutes.
    Intravenous—5 minutes.
  Furosemide:
    Oral—20 to 60 minutes.
    Intravenous—5 minutes.

## Time to peak effect
Diuretic—
  Bumetanide:
    Oral—1 to 2 hours.
    Intravenous—15 to 30 minutes.
  Ethacrynic acid:
    Oral—2 hours.
    Intravenous—15 to 30 minutes.
  Furosemide:
    Oral—1 to 2 hours.
    Intravenous—Within 30 minutes.
Note: The maximum antihypertensive effect may not occur until several
    days after initiation of loop diuretic therapy.

## Duration of action
Diuretic—
  Bumetanide:
    Oral—4 hours with usual doses (1 to 2 mg); 4 to 6 hours with
      higher doses.
    Intravenous—3.5 to 4 hours.
  Ethacrynic acid:
    Oral—6 to 8 hours.
    Intravenous—2 hours.
  Furosemide:
    Oral—6 to 8 hours.
    Intravenous—2 hours.

## Elimination
Bumetanide—
  Renal (81%; 45% unchanged); biliary/fecal (2%).
Ethacrynic acid—
  Renal (67%); biliary/fecal (33%); 20% excreted unchanged.
Furosemide—
  Renal (88%); biliary/fecal (12%).
  In patients with severe renal impairment, renal clearance is reduced
    but overall plasma clearance may be unchanged because nonrenal
    clearance is increased. In patients with uremia, both renal and non-
    renal clearance are reduced, and elimination is delayed.
  In dialysis: Not dialyzable.

# Precautions to Consider

## Cross-sensitivity and/or related problems
Patients sensitive to sulfonamides (including thiazide diuretics) may be
sensitive to bumetanide or furosemide also.

## Carcinogenicity/Tumorigenicity
*Bumetanide*— One study in female rats given 60 mg per kg of body weight
  (mg/kg) of bumetanide for 18 months found an increase in mammary
  adenomas; repetition of the same study did not result in the same
  findings.
*Ethacrynic acid*—A 79-week study in rats at doses up to 45 times the
  human dose revealed no evidence of a tumorigenic effect.

## Mutagenicity
*Bumetanide*—Studies with bumetanide in various strains of *Salmonella
  typhimurium* in the presence or absence of an *in vitro* metabolic activation system found no evidence of mutagenicity.
*Furosemide*—Mutagenicity studies have not been conducted.

## Pregnancy/Reproduction
Pregnancy—Pregnant women should be advised to contact physician before taking this medication, since routine use of diuretics during normal pregnancy is inappropriate and exposes mother and fetus to unnecessary hazard. Diuretics do not prevent development of toxemia of
  pregnancy, and there is no satisfactory evidence that they are useful
  in the treatment of toxemia. Diuretics are indicated only in the treatment of edema due to pathologic causes or as a short course of treatment in patients with severe hypervolemia.
  *Bumetanide*—
    Adequate and well-controlled studies in humans have not been
      done.
    Some studies in animals have shown that bumetanide may cause
      adverse effects on the fetus. Bumetanide has not been shown
      to be teratogenic in mice or hamsters; however, one study in
      rats showed moderate growth retardation and increased inci-
      dence of delayed ossification of sternebrae at doses 3400 times
      the maximum human therapeutic dose. These effects in the rat
      were associated with maternal weight reductions during dosing
      and were not observed at doses 1000 times the maximum hu-
      man therapeutic dose. Delayed ossification of sternebrae was
      also noted in rabbits at doses 10 times the maximum human
      therapeutic dose. A slight embryocidal effect in rats and rabbits
      was evident at doses 3400 and 3.4 times the maximum human

therapeutic dose, respectively. In rabbits, a dose-related de-
  crease in litter size and an increase in resorption rate were
  noted at doses of 3.4 and 10 times the maximum human ther-
  apeutic dose.
  FDA Pregnancy Category C.
*Ethacrynic acid*—
  Adequate and well-controlled studies in humans have not been
    done.
  Studies in mice and rabbits using doses up to 50 times the human
    dose have not shown evidence of external abnormalities of the
    fetus. In rats, a decrease in mean body weights of the fetuses
    was noted at doses 50 times the maximum human dose.
  FDA Pregnancy Category B.
*Furosemide*—
  Furosemide crosses the placenta. Studies in humans have not been
    done.
  Studies in rabbits and mice have shown that furosemide causes an
    increased incidence of hydronephrosis in the fetus. In rabbits,
    unexplained maternal deaths and abortions have occurred at
    doses 2 to 8 times the maximum recommended human dose.
  FDA Pregnancy Category C.

## Breast-feeding
Furosemide is distributed into breast milk; it is not known whether bumetanide or ethacrynic acid is distributed into breast milk.

## Pediatrics
Caution is required in neonates because of the prolonged half-life of furosemide. Usual pediatric doses may be used, but the dosing interval
  should be extended.

## Geriatrics
Although appropriate studies on the relationship of age to the effects of
  loop diuretics have not been performed in the geriatric population, the
  elderly may be more sensitive to the hypotensive and electrolyte effects. In addition, elderly patients are at greater risk of developing
  circulatory collapse and thromboembolic episodes. Elderly patients are
  also more likely to have age-related renal function impairment, which
  may require adjustment of dosage or dosing interval in patients receiving loop diuretics.

## Drug interactions and/or related problems
The following drug interactions and/or related problems have been selected on the basis of their potential clinical significance (possible
  mechanism in parentheses where appropriate)—not necessarily inclusive (» = major clinical significance):
Note: Combinations containing any of the following medications, de-
    pending on the amount present, may also interact with this
    medication.

  Alcohol or
  Hypotension-producing medications, other (See *Appendix II*)
    (hypotensive and/or diuretic effects may be potentiated when these
    medications are used concurrently with loop diuretics; although
    some antihypertensive and/or diuretic combinations are frequently
    used for therapeutic advantage, when used concurrently dosage
    adjustments may be necessary)

  Amiodarone
    (concurrent use of loop diuretics with amiodarone may lead to an
    increased risk of arrhythmias associated with hypokalemia)

  » Amphotericin B, parenteral
    (concurrent and/or sequential administration with loop diuretics
    should be avoided since the potential for ototoxicity and nephro-
    toxicity may be increased, especially in the presence of renal func-
    tion impairment; in addition, concurrent use with loop diuretics
    may intensify electrolyte imbalance, particularly hypokalemia; fre-
    quent electrolyte determinations are recommended and potassium
    supplementation may be required)

  Angiotensin-converting enzyme (ACE) inhibitors
    (sudden and severe hypotension may occur within the first 1 to 5
    hours after the initial dose of captopril, enalapril, or lisinopril, par-
    ticularly in patients who are sodium- and volume-depleted as a
    result of diuretic therapy. Withdrawal of the diuretic or increase
    of salt intake approximately 1 week before start of captopril ther-
    apy or 2 to 3 days before start of benazepril, enalapril, fosinopril,
    lisinopril, quinapril, or ramipril therapy, or initiating ACE inhibitor
    therapy in lower doses, will minimize the reaction; this reaction
    does not usually recur with subsequent doses, although caution in
    increasing doses is recommended; diuretics may be reinstituted as
    necessary)

    (risk of renal failure may be increased in patients who are sodium-
    and volume-depleted as a result of diuretic therapy)

(ACE inhibitors may reduce the secondary aldosteronism and hypokalemia caused by diuretics)

» Anticoagulants, coumarin- or indandione-derivative or
Heparin or
Streptokinase or
Urokinase
(anticoagulant effects may be decreased when these medications are used concurrently with loop diuretics, as a result of reduction of plasma volume leading to concentration of procoagulant factors in the blood; in addition diuretic-induced improvement of hepatic congestion may lead to improved hepatic function, resulting in increased procoagulant factor synthesis; dosage adjustments may be necessary)

(anticoagulant effects may be potentiated when these medications are used concurrently with ethacrynic acid as a result of displacement of anticoagulant from protein-binding sites; dosage adjustments of the anticoagulant may be necessary during and after ethacrynic acid therapy or, alternatively, use of furosemide is recommended)

(gastrointestinal ulcerative or hemorrhagic potential of ethacrynic acid may increase the risk of hemorrhage in patients receiving anticoagulant or thrombolytic therapy; use of a different diuretic is recommended)

Antidiabetic agents, oral or
Insulin
(furosemide, and possibly bumetanide or ethacrynic acid, may rarely raise blood glucose concentrations or interfere with the hypoglycemic effects of these agents; for adult-onset diabetics, dosage adjustment of hypoglycemic medications may be necessary during and after therapy)

Anti-inflammatory drugs, nonsteroidal (NSAIDs), especially indomethacin
(may antagonize the natriuresis and increase in plasma renin activity [PRA] caused by loop diuretics; indomethacin, and possibly other NSAIDs with the exception of diflunisal, may also reduce the increase in urine volume caused by loop diuretics, possibly by inhibiting renal prostaglandin synthesis and/or by causing sodium and fluid retention)

(in addition, concurrent use of NSAIDs with a diuretic may increase the risk of renal failure secondary to a decrease in renal blood flow caused by inhibition of renal prostaglandin synthesis)

(in the premature neonate, administration of 1 mg/kg of furosemide immediately following indomethacin has been shown to prevent or reduce indomethacin-induced adverse renal effects without interfering with ductus arteriosus closure)

Digitalis glycosides
(concurrent use with loop diuretics may enhance the possibility of digitalis toxicity associated with hypokalemia and hypomagnesemia)

» Hypokalemia-causing medications, other (See *Appendix II*)
(risk of severe hypokalemia due to other hypokalemia-causing medications may be increased; monitoring of serum potassium concentrations and cardiac function and potassium supplementation may be required)

» Lithium
(concurrent use with loop diuretics may provoke lithium toxicity because of reduced renal clearance and is not recommended unless patient can be closely monitored)

» Nephrotoxic medications, other (See *Appendix II*) or
Ototoxic medications, other (See *Appendix II*)
(concurrent and/or sequential administration with loop diuretics should be avoided since the potential for ototoxicity and nephrotoxicity may be increased, especially in the presence of renal function impairment)

Neuromuscular blocking agents, nondepolarizing
(loop diuretics may induce hypokalemia, which may enhance the blockade of nondepolarizing neuromuscular blocking agents; serum potassium determinations may be necessary prior to administration of nondepolarizing neuromuscular blocking agents; careful postoperative monitoring of the patient may be necessary following concurrent or sequential use, especially if there is a possibility of incomplete reversal of neuromuscular blockade)

Sympathomimetics
(concurrent use may reduce the antihypertensive effects of the loop diuretics; the patient should be carefully monitored to confirm that the desired effect is being obtained)

*For furosemide only (in addition to those listed above)*
Chloral hydrate
(administration of chloral hydrate followed by intravenous furosemide may result in diaphoresis, hot flashes, and variable blood pressure including hypertension due to a hypermetabolic state caused by displacement of thyroxine from its bound state)

Probenecid
(probenecid has been found to increase serum concentrations of furosemide by inhibiting active renal tubular secretion)

## Laboratory value alterations
The following have been selected on the basis of their potential clinical significance (possible effect in parentheses where appropriate)—not necessarily inclusive (» = major clinical significance):

With physiology/laboratory test values

*For bumetanide, ethacrynic acid, and furosemide*
Blood glucose concentrations and
Urine glucose concentrations
(may be increased; ethacrynic acid increases blood glucose only rarely, especially in diabetics, prediabetics, or patients with compensated cirrhosis; in patients with uremia, large doses of ethacrynic acid may cause severe hypoglycemia; the effect of bumetanide is controversial and possibly variable)

Blood urea nitrogen (BUN) and
Uric acid, serum
(concentrations may be increased)

Calcium and
Chloride and
Magnesium and
Potassium and
Sodium
(serum concentrations may be decreased)

*For bumetanide only (in addition to the above)*
Phosphate
(urinary concentrations may be increased)

## Medical considerations/Contraindications
The medical considerations/contraindications included here have been selected on the basis of their potential clinical significance (reasons given in parentheses where appropriate)—not necessarily inclusive (» = major clinical significance).

*Risk-benefit should be considered when the following medical problems exist:*

*For bumetanide, ethacrynic acid, and furosemide*
» Anuria or
» Renal function impairment, severe
(impaired effectiveness and possible delayed excretion with increased risk of toxicity. Although bumetanide, ethacrynic acid, and furosemide are effective diuretics in patients with renal function impairment, reduced clearance may necessitate use of higher doses combined with more prolonged dosing intervals to prevent accumulation and reduce the risk of ototoxicity)

Diabetes mellitus
(loop diuretics cause impaired glucose tolerance)

Gout, history of, or
Hyperuricemia
(loop diuretics may elevate serum uric acid concentrations)

Hearing function impairment

Hepatic function impairment, including cirrhosis and ascites
(risk of dehydration and electrolyte imbalance, which may precipitate hepatic coma and death; hospitalization during initiation of therapy is recommended)

Myocardial infarction, acute
(excessive diuresis should be avoided because of the danger of precipitating shock)

Pancreatitis, or history of
(pancreatitis has been reported with bumetanide, ethacrynic acid, and furosemide)

Sensitivity to loop diuretic prescribed

Caution is recommended also in patients who are at increased risk if hypokalemia occurs, including those taking digitalis and diuretics and those with:
Certain diarrheal states
Congestive heart failure
Hepatic cirrhosis and ascites
History of ventricular arrhythmias
Potassium-losing nephropathy
States of aldosterone excess with normal renal function

*For ethacrynic acid and furosemide only (in addition to the above)*
Lupus erythematosus, history of
(exacerbation or activation by ethacrynic acid and furosemide has
been reported)

**Patient monitoring**
The following may be especially important in patient monitoring (other
tests may be warranted in some patients, depending on condition;
» = major clinical significance):

Blood pressure measurements
(recommended at periodic intervals in patients being treated for
hypertension; selected patients may be taught to monitor their
blood pressure at home and report the results at regular physician
visits)

Blood urea nitrogen (BUN) and
Carbon dioxide ($CO_2$)
(determinations recommended at periodic intervals during therapy)

Electrolyte concentrations
(determinations recommended at periodic intervals, especially if
patients are also taking cardiac glycosides or systemic steroids, or
when severe hepatic cirrhosis is present)

Glucose, serum and
Hepatic function and
Renal function and
Uric acid, serum
(determinations recommended at periodic intervals)

Hearing examinations
(recommended at periodic intervals in patients receiving prolonged
high-dose intravenous therapy)

Weight measurement
(recommended prior to initiation of therapy and at periodic intervals during therapy to monitor water loss)

# Side/Adverse Effects

See *Table 1*, page 1249.

# Patient Consultation

As an aid to patient consultation, refer to *Advice for the Patient, Diuretics,
Loop (Systemic)*.

In providing consultation, consider emphasizing the following selected
information (» = major clinical significance):

**Before using this medication**
» Conditions affecting use, especially:
Sensitivity to the loop diuretic prescribed, or to sulfonamides (for
bumetanide and furosemide)
Pregnancy—Not recommended for routine use; reported to cause
harmful effects, including birth defects, in animals
Breast-feeding—Furosemide distributed into breast milk
Use in the elderly—Elderly patients may be more sensitive to hypotensive and electrolyte effects, and may be at greater risk of
developing circulatory collapse and thromboembolic episodes
Other medications, especially parenteral amphotericin B, oral anticoagulants, other hypokalemia-causing medications, lithium,
or other nephrotoxic medications
Other medical problems, especially anuria or severe renal function
impairment

**Proper use of this medication**
Diuretic effects of the medication and timing of doses to minimize
inconvenience of diuresis
Getting into habit of taking at same time each day to help increase
compliance
Taking with food or milk to reduce gastrointestinal irritation
» Proper dosing
Missed dose: Taking as soon as possible; not taking if almost time for
next dose; not doubling doses
» Proper storage
*For use as an antihypertensive*
Possible need for control of weight and diet, especially sodium intake
» Patient may not experience symptoms of hypertension; importance of
taking medication even if feeling well
» Does not cure, but controls hypertension; possible need for lifelong
therapy; serious consequences of untreated hypertension
*For oral solution dosage form of furosemide (in addition to the above)*
Taking orally, even if in dropper bottle; importance of accurate
measurement

**Precautions while using this medication**
Regular visits to physician to check progress

» Possibility of hypokalemia; possible need for additional potassium in
diet; not changing diet without first checking with physician
To prevent dehydration, notifying physician if severe nausea, vomit-
ing, or diarrhea occurs and continues
Caution if any kind of surgery (including dental surgery) is required
» Caution when getting up suddenly from a lying or sitting position
» Caution in using alcohol, while standing for long periods or exercising,
and during hot weather because of enhanced orthostatic hypoten-
sive effects
Diabetics: May increase blood sugar levels
*For use as an antihypertensive*
» Not taking other medications, especially nonprescription sympatho-
mimetics, unless discussed with physician
*For furosemide (in addition to the above)*
» Possible skin photosensitivity; avoiding unprotected exposure to sun;
using protective clothing; using a sun block product that includes
protection against both UVA-caused photosensitivity reactions and
UVB-caused sunburn reactions; avoiding use of sunlamp, tanning
bed, or tanning booth

**Side/adverse effects**
Signs of potential side effects, especially allergic reaction, blood in
urine, electrolyte imbalance, gastrointestinal bleeding, gout, hepatic dysfunction, leukopenia, agranulocytosis, ototoxicity, pancreatitis, thrombocytopenia, and xanthopsia

# General Dosing Information

Dosage must be adjusted to meet the individual requirements of each
patient, on the basis of clinical response. The lowest effective dosage
should be utilized to minimize potential fluid and electrolyte
imbalance.

When loop diuretics are used to promote diuresis, intermittent dosage
schedules may reduce the possibility of electrolyte imbalance or hyperuricemia resulting from therapy.

Concurrent administration of potassium supplements or potassium-sparing
diuretics may be indicated in patients considered to be at higher risk
for developing hypokalemia.

If a single daily dose is indicated, it is preferably taken on arising in order
to minimize the effect of increased frequency of urination on sleep.

When bumetanide, ethacrynic acid, or furosemide is added to an antihypertensive regimen, the dose of other antihypertensive agents may
have to be reduced in order to prevent an excessive drop in blood
pressure.

It is recommended that bumetanide, ethacrynic acid, and furosemide be
discontinued if oliguria persists for more than 24 hours at maximal
dosage.

---

## BUMETANIDE

# Summary of Differences

Pharmacology/pharmacokinetics:
Mechanism of action/effect—May have additional action on proximal
tubule.
Biotransformation and elimination—Excreted largely unchanged.
Side/adverse effects:
Muscle pain may occur with large doses. Chest pain, premature ejac-
ulation, and difficulty in keeping an erection have also been
reported.

# Additional Dosing Information

See also *General Dosing Information*.

**For parenteral dosage forms only**
Intravenous administration is generally preferred over intramuscular
administration.
Intravenous administration should be at a slow, controlled rate over a 2-
minute period.

# Oral Dosage Forms

Note: Bracketed uses in the *Dosage Forms* section refer to categories of
use and/or indications that are not included in U.S. product labeling.

**BUMETANIDE TABLETS USP**

**Usual adult dose**
[Antihypertensive or]
Diuretic—
Oral, 500 mcg (0.5 mg) to 2 mg a day as a single daily dose. The
dose may be increased, if necessary, by addition of a second or

third daily dose with intervals of four to five hours between doses. An intermittent dosage schedule (administration on alternate days for three or four days, with one or two days in between) may also be used.

Note: Geriatric patients may be more sensitive to the effects of the usual adult dose.

**Usual adult prescribing limits**
Up to 10 mg a day.

**Usual pediatric dose**
Dosage has not been established.

**Strength(s) usually available**
U.S.—
500 mcg (0.5 mg) (Rx) [*Bumex* (lactose); GENERIC].
1 mg (Rx) [*Bumex* (lactose); GENERIC].
2 mg (Rx) [*Bumex* (lactose); GENERIC].
Canada—
Not commercially available.

**Packaging and storage**
Store below 40 °C (104 °F), preferably between 15 and 30 °C (59 and 86 °F), unless otherwise specified by manufacturer. Store in a tight, light-resistant container.

**Auxiliary labeling**
• Do not take other medicines without your doctor's advice.

## Parenteral Dosage Forms

Note: Bracketed uses in the *Dosage Forms* section refer to categories of use and/or indications that are not included in U.S. product labeling.

### BUMETANIDE INJECTION USP

**Usual adult dose**
[Antihypertensive or]
Diuretic—
Intravenous or intramuscular, 500 mcg (0.5 mg) to 1 mg, repeated at intervals of two to three hours, if necessary.

**Usual adult prescribing limits**
Up to 10 mg a day.

**Usual pediatric dose**
Dosage has not been established.

**Strength(s) usually available**
U.S.—
250 mcg (0.25 mg) per mL (Rx) [*Bumex* (benzyl alcohol 1%)].
Canada—
Not commercially available.

**Packaging and storage**
Store below 40 °C (104 °F), preferably between 15 and 30 °C (59 and 86 °F), unless otherwise specified by manufacturer. Protect from freezing. Protect from light.

**Stability**
Infusion solutions should be freshly prepared and used within a 24-hour period.

---

### *ETHACRYNIC ACID*

---

## Summary of Differences

Indications:
Also indicated for short-term management of ascites due to malignancy, idiopathic edema, and lymphedema, and for treatment of hypercalcemia.
Side/adverse effects:
Greatest risk of ototoxicity. Gastrointestinal bleeding and blood in urine may occur with parenteral use. Higher incidence of gastrointestinal upset. Confusion, loss of appetite, and nervousness were reported more often than with other loop diuretics.

## Additional Dosing Information

See also *General Dosing Information*.

Concurrent administration of ammonium chloride or arginine chloride may be indicated in patients considered to be at higher risk of developing metabolic alkalosis as a result of the chloruretic effect.

Because of the profound effect of ethacrynic acid on sodium excretion, rigid dietary salt restriction is not necessary in most patients and may in fact increase the risk of adverse effects due to hyponatremia.

In patients with renal edema, administration of salt-poor albumin may be helpful in preventing reduced response to ethacrynic acid because of hypoproteinemia.

If severe, watery diarrhea occurs, it is recommended that ethacrynic acid be permanently withdrawn.

**For parenteral dosage forms only**
Intramuscular or subcutaneous administration is not recommended because of local pain and irritation.
Intravenous administration should be at a slow, controlled rate over a period of about 30 minutes.
If a second injection is required, use of a different injection site is recommended to prevent thrombophlebitis.

## Oral Dosage Forms

### ETHACRYNIC ACID ORAL SOLUTION

**Usual adult dose**
Diuretic—
Initial: Oral, 50 to 100 mg a day, in single or divided daily doses with increments of 25 to 50 mg a day as needed.
Maintenance: Oral, reduced to meet individual requirements once dry weight is achieved; usually 50 to 200 mg a day.

Note: Geriatric patients may be more sensitive to the effects of the usual adult dose.

**Usual adult prescribing limits**
Up to 400 mg a day.

**Usual pediatric dose**
Diuretic—
Initial: Oral, 25 mg a day, with increments of 25 mg a day as needed.
Maintenance: Oral, adjusted to meet individual requirements.

Note: Use in infants is not recommended.

**Strength(s) usually available**
U.S.—
Dosage form not commercially available in the U.S. Compounding required for prescriptions.
Canada—
Dosage form not commercially available in Canada. Compounding required for prescriptions.

**Packaging and storage**
Store at or below 24 °C (75 °F). Protect from freezing.

**Preparation of dosage form**
An oral liquid dosage form of ethacrynic acid has been prepared by dissolving ethacrynic acid powder in 10% alcohol in water, then bringing it to volume (to produce a solution containing 1 mg of ethacrynic acid per mL) with a 50% aqueous sorbitol solution (with added 0.005% methylparaben and 0.002% propylparaben as preservatives), and adjusting the pH to 7 with sodium hydroxide.

**Stability**
This product was found to be stable for several weeks when stored at 24 °C (75 °F).

**Auxiliary labeling**
• Take with meals or milk.
• Do not take other medicines without your doctor's advice.

**Note**
Check refill frequency to determine compliance in hypertensive patients.

### ETHACRYNIC ACID TABLETS USP

**Usual adult dose**
See *Ethacrynic Acid Oral Solution*.

**Usual adult prescribing limits**
Up to 400 mg a day.

**Usual pediatric dose**
See *Ethacrynic Acid Oral Solution*.

**Strength(s) usually available**
U.S.—
25 mg (Rx) [*Edecrin* (lactose)].
50 mg (Rx) [*Edecrin* (lactose)].
Canada—
50 mg (Rx) [*Edecrin* (scored; lactose)].

**Packaging and storage**
Store below 40 °C (104 °F), preferably between 15 and 30 °C (59 and 86 °F), unless otherwise specified by manufacturer. Store in a well-closed container.

**Auxiliary labeling**
- Take with meals or milk.
- Do not take other medicines without your doctor's advice.

**Note**
Check refill frequency to determine compliance in hypertensive patients.

## Parenteral Dosage Forms
### ETHACRYNATE SODIUM FOR INJECTION USP

**Usual adult dose**
Diuretic—
    Intravenous, 50 mg (base), or 500 mcg (0.5 mg) to 1 mg per kg of body weight; may be repeated in two to four hours if necessary, then every four to six hours if the patient is responsive. In some emergency situations, the injection may be repeated every hour.
Note: Geriatric patients may be more sensitive to the effects of the usual adult dose.

**Usual adult prescribing limits**
Up to 100 mg (base).

**Usual pediatric dose**
Diuretic—
    Intravenous, 1 mg (base) per kg of body weight.

**Size(s) usually available**
U.S.—
    50 mg (base) (Rx) [*Edecrin* (mannitol 62.5 mg)].
Canada—
    50 mg (base) (Rx) [*Edecrin* (mannitol 62.5 mg)].

**Packaging and storage**
Store below 40 °C (104 °F), preferably between 15 and 30 °C (59 and 86 °F), unless otherwise specified by manufacturer.

**Preparation of dosage form**
Infusion solutions can be prepared using 0.9% sodium chloride injection or 5% dextrose injection, after pH has been adjusted when necessary.

**Stability**
A hazy or opalescent solution may result from use of a diluent with a low pH (below 5); use of such a solution is not recommended.
Unused, reconstituted solution should be discarded after 24 hours at room temperature.

**Incompatibilities**
The solution is physically incompatible with whole blood or its derivatives.

---
### *FUROSEMIDE*
---

## Summary of Differences

Category:
    Furosemide is used as a diagnostic aid adjunct in renal disease.
Precautions:
    Breast-feeding—Distributed into breast milk.
    Pediatrics—Prolonged half-life in neonates.
    Drug interactions and/or related problems—Also interacts with chloral hydrate and probenecid.
Side/adverse effects:
    Also causes xanthopsia and increased sensitivity of skin to sunlight.

## Additional Dosing Information

See also *General Dosing Information*.

When furosemide is used as an antihypercalcemic, body fluid and sodium chloride should be replaced in order to maintain extracellular fluid volume and increase calcium excretion effectively.

**For parenteral dosage forms only**
Intravenous administration is generally preferred over intramuscular administration.
Intravenous administration should be at a slow, controlled rate over a 1- to 2-minute period.
If high-dose parenteral therapy is indicated, administration should be by controlled intravenous infusion at a rate not exceeding 4 mg per minute.

## Oral Dosage Forms

Note: Bracketed uses in the *Dosage Forms* section refer to categories of use and/or indications that are not included in U.S. product labeling.

### FUROSEMIDE ORAL SOLUTION

**Usual adult dose**
Diuretic—
    Oral, initially 20 to 80 mg as a single dose, the dosage then being increased by an additional 20 to 40 mg at six- to eight-hour intervals, until the desired response is obtained. The maintenance dose as determined by titration is then given daily as a single dose or divided into two or three doses, given once a day every other day, or given once a day for two to four consecutive days out of each week.
Antihypertensive—
    Oral, initially 40 mg two times a day, the dosage then being adjusted according to patient response.
[Antihypercalcemic][1]—
    Oral, 120 mg a day as a single dose or divided into two or three doses.
Note: Geriatric patients may be more sensitive to the effects of the usual adult dose.

**Usual adult prescribing limits**
Up to 600 mg a day.
Note: In chronic renal failure, doses of up to 4 grams a day have been used.

**Usual pediatric dose**
Diuretic—
    Oral, initially 2 mg per kg of body weight as a single dose, the dosage then being increased by an additional 1 to 2 mg per kg of body weight at six- to eight-hour intervals, until the desired response is obtained.
Note: Doses as large as 5 mg per kg of body weight may be required in some children with nephrotic syndrome.
    Doses greater than 6 mg per kg of body weight are not recommended.
    Dosing interval should be extended in neonates because of prolonged half-life.

**Strength(s) usually available**
U.S.—
    8 mg per mL (Rx) [GENERIC].
    10 mg per mL (Rx) [*Lasix* (alcohol 11.5%); *Myrosemide* (alcohol 11.5%); GENERIC].
Canada—
    10 mg per mL (Rx) [*Lasix* (sugar-free)].

**Packaging and storage**
Store below 40 °C (104 °F), preferably between 15 and 30 °C (59 and 86 °F), in a well-closed container, unless otherwise specified by manufacturer. Protect from light. Protect from freezing.

**Auxiliary labeling**
- Take by mouth only (when dispensed with graduated dropper).
- Do not take other medicines without your doctor's advice.

**Note**
Do not dispense discolored solution.
When dispensing, include the manufacturer-provided graduated dropper or measuring spoon.
Explain administration technique when dispensed with graduated dropper.
Check refill frequency to determine compliance in hypertensive patients.

### FUROSEMIDE TABLETS USP

**Usual adult dose**
See *Furosemide Oral Solution*.

**Usual adult prescribing limits**
Up to 600 mg a day.
Note: In chronic renal failure, doses of up to 4 grams a day have been used.

**Usual pediatric dose**
See *Furosemide Oral Solution*.

**Strength(s) usually available**
U.S.—
    20 mg (Rx) [*Lasix;* GENERIC (may be scored)].
    40 mg (Rx) [*Lasix* (scored); GENERIC (may be scored)].
    80 mg (Rx) [*Lasix;* GENERIC (may be scored)].
Canada—
    20 mg (Rx) [*Apo-Furosemide; Furoside* (scored); *Lasix; Novosemide* (scored); *Uritol* (scored)].
    40 mg (Rx) [*Apo-Furosemide* (scored); *Furoside* (scored); *Lasix* (scored); *Novosemide* (scored); *Uritol* (scored)].
    80 mg (Rx) [*Apo-Furosemide* (scored); *Novosemide* (scored); *Lasix* (scored)].
    500 mg (Rx) [*Lasix Special* (scored)].

**Packaging and storage**
Store below 40 °C (104 °F), preferably between 15 and 30 °C (59 and 86 °F), unless otherwise specified by manufacturer. Store in a well-closed container. Protect from light.

**Stability**
Exposure to light may cause discoloration. Do not dispense discolored tablets.

**Auxiliary labeling**
• Do not take other medicines without your doctor's advice.

**Note**
Since variations in bioavailability have been found among brands, try to avoid switching brands when dispensing refills.

Check refill frequency to determine compliance in hypertensive patients.

## Parenteral Dosage Forms

Note: Bracketed uses in the *Dosage Forms* section refer to categories of use and/or indications that are not included in U.S. product labeling.

### FUROSEMIDE INJECTION USP

**Usual adult dose**
Diuretic—
Intramuscular or intravenous, initially 20 to 40 mg as a single dose, the dosage then being increased by an additional 20 mg at two-hour intervals until the desired response is obtained. The maintenance dose as determined by titration is then given one or two times a day.

Note: In acute pulmonary edema (not accompanied by hypertensive crisis), the usual initial dose is 40 mg intravenously, followed by 80 mg in one hour if a satisfactory response is not obtained.

Antihypertensive—
Hypertensive crisis in patients with normal renal function: Intravenous, 40 to 80 mg.

Hypertensive crisis accompanied by pulmonary edema or acute renal failure: Intravenous, 100 to 200 mg.

[Antihypercalcemic][1]—
Intramuscular or intravenous, 80 to 100 mg in severe cases, the dosage being repeated if necessary every one to two hours until the desired response is obtained. In less severe cases, smaller doses may be given every two to four hours.

[Diagnostic aid adjunct (renal disease)]—
Intravenous, 0.3 to 0.5 mg per kg of body weight to a maximum of 40 mg.

Note: Geriatric patients may be more sensitive to the effects of the usual adult dose.

**Usual adult prescribing limits**
Although controversial, doses of up to 6 grams a day administered by slow intravenous infusion have been used in acute renal failure by some clinicians.

**Usual pediatric dose**
Diuretic—
Intramuscular or intravenous, initially 1 mg per kg of body weight as a single dose, the dosage then being increased by an additional 1 mg per kg of body weight at two-hour intervals until the desired response is obtained.

[Antihypercalcemic][1]—
Intramuscular or intravenous, 25 to 50 mg, the dosage being repeated if necessary every four hours until the desired response is obtained.

Note: Doses greater than 6 mg per kg of body weight are not recommended.
Dosing interval should be extended in neonates because of prolonged half-life.

**Strength(s) usually available**
U.S.—
10 mg per mL (Rx) [*Lasix;* GENERIC].
Canada—
10 mg per mL (Rx) [*Lasix* (benzyl alcohol); *Lasix Special; Uritol;* GENERIC].

**Packaging and storage**
Store below 40 °C (104 °F), preferably between 15 and 30 °C (59 and 86 °F), unless otherwise specified by manufacturer. Protect from light. Protect from freezing.

**Preparation of dosage form**
Infusion solutions can be prepared using 0.9% sodium chloride injection, lactated Ringer's injection, or 5% dextrose injection, after pH has been adjusted when necessary.

**Stability**
Do not use if solution is yellow.
Infusion solutions should be freshly prepared and used within a 24-hour period.

**Incompatibilities**
Furosemide Injection USP is a mildly buffered alkaline solution and should not be mixed with highly acidic solutions.

---

[1]Not included in Canadian product labeling.

## Selected Bibliography

The fifth report of the Joint National Committee on Detection, Evaluation, and Treatment of High Blood Pressure (JNC V). Arch Intern Med 1993; 153 (2): 154-83.

---

Revised: 08/02/94
Interim revision: 04/24/95

---

## Table 1. Side/Adverse Effects*

Note: Nephrocalcinosis or nephrolithiasis may occur with furosemide administration if hypercalciuria is present.
Ethacrynic acid appears to be more likely to cause ototoxicity than bumetanide or furosemide and less likely to cause hyperglycemia than furosemide.

| The following side/adverse effects have been selected on the basis of their potential clinical significance (possible signs and symptoms in parentheses where appropriate)—not necessarily inclusive: | Legend I=Bumetanide II=Ethacrynic acid III=Furosemide | | |
|---|---|---|---|
| | **I** | **II** | **III** |
| **Those indicating need for medical attention** | | | |
| *Allergic reaction* (skin rash) | R | R | R |
| *Blood in urine*—associated with parenteral use | U | R | U |
| *Electrolyte imbalance such as hyponatremia, hypochloremic alkalosis, and hypokalemia*—occurs frequently, up to 10 to 15% of patients receiving ethacrynic acid (usually not symptomatic; symptoms include dry mouth, increased thirst, irregular heartbeat, mood or mental changes, muscle cramps or pain, nausea or vomiting, unusual tiredness or weakness, weak pulse) | L | L | L |
| *Gastrointestinal bleeding* (black, tarry stools)—associated with parenteral use | U | R | U |
| *Gout* (joint pain, lower back or side pain) | R | R | R |
| *Hepatic dysfunction* (yellow eyes or skin) | R | R | R |

*Differences in frequency of occurrence may reflect either lack of clinical-use data or actual pharmacologic distinctions among agents (although their basic pharmacologic similarity suggests that side effects occurring with one may occur with the others). M = more frequent; L = less frequent; R = rare; U = unknown.
†Dose-related.

## Table 1. Side/Adverse Effects* *(continued)*

| | Legend<br>I = Bumetanide<br>II = Ethacrynic acid<br>III = Furosemide | | |
|---|:---:|:---:|:---:|
| | **I** | **II** | **III** |
| *Leukopenia or agranulocytosis* (fever or chills, cough or hoarseness, lower back or side pain, painful or difficult urination) | R | R | R |
| *Ototoxicity*—more frequent with renal function impairment and in rapid parenteral administration of large doses (ringing or buzzing in ears or any loss of hearing; usually transient, but permanent deafness has occurred, especially in patients receiving other ototoxic drugs) | R | L† | R |
| *Pancreatitis* (severe stomach pain with nausea and vomiting) | R | R | R |
| *Thrombocytopenia* (unusual bleeding or bruising; black, tarry stools; blood in urine or stools; pinpoint red spots on skin) | R | R | R |
| *Xanthopsia* (yellow vision) | U | U | R |
| **Those indicating need for medical attention only if they continue or are bothersome** | | | |
|    *Blurred vision* | L | L | L |
| *Chest pain* | L | U | U |
| *Confusion* | U | L | U |
| *Diarrhea* | L | M† | L |
| *Headache* | L | L | L |
| *Increased sensitivity of skin to sunlight* | U | U | L |
| *Local irritation* (redness or pain at site of injection) | R | R | R |
| *Loss of appetite* | L | M† | L |
| *Nervousness* | U | L | U |
| *Orthostatic hypotension as a result of massive diuresis* (dizziness or lightheadedness when getting up from a lying or sitting position) | M | M | M |
| *Premature ejaculation or difficulty in keeping an erection* | L | U | U |
| *Stomach cramps or pain* | L | L | L |

*Differences in frequency of occurrence may reflect either lack of clinical-use data or actual pharmacologic distinctions among agents (although their basic pharmacologic similarity suggests that side effects occurring with one may occur with the others). M = more frequent; L = less frequent; R = rare; U = unknown.

†Dose-related.

# DIURETICS, POTASSIUM-SPARING   Systemic

This monograph includes information on the following: Amiloride; Spironolactone; Triamterene.

VA CLASSIFICATION (Primary/Secondary):
   Amiloride—CV704/CV490; TN900
   Spironolactone—CV704/CV490; TN900; HS900
   Triamterene—CV704/CV490; TN900

Note: For a listing of dosage forms and brand names by country availability, see *Dosage Forms* section(s). For a listing of brand names for the articles in this monograph, refer to the General Index.

## Category

Diuretic—Amiloride; Spironolactone; Triamterene.
Antihypertensive—Amiloride; Spironolactone; Triamterene.
Aldosterone antagonist—Spironolactone.
Diagnostic aid (primary hyperaldosteronism)—Spironolactone.
Antihypokalemic—Amiloride; Spironolactone; Triamterene.

## Indications

Note: Bracketed information in the *Indications* section refers to uses that are not included in U.S. product labeling.

**Accepted**
Edema (treatment)—Amiloride, spironolactone, and triamterene are indicated as adjuncts in the management of edematous states, especially when a potassium-sparing diuretic effect is desired. These may include congestive heart failure, hepatic cirrhosis, and nephrotic syndrome, which often involve secondary hyperaldosteronism, as well as idiopathic edema.

Hypertension (treatment adjunct)—Amiloride, spironolactone, and [triamterene][1] are indicated as adjuncts in the treatment of hypertension (for spironolactone, with or without accompanying hyperaldosteronism), especially when a potassium-sparing diuretic effect is desired.

For additional information on initial therapeutic guidelines related to the treatment of hypertension, see *Appendix III*.

Hyperaldosteronism, primary (diagnosis and treatment)—Spironolactone is indicated for diagnosis and short- or long-term management of primary hyperaldosteronism.

Hypokalemia (prophylaxis and treatment)—[Amiloride][1], spironolactone, and [triamterene][1] are indicated for prevention and treatment of hypokalemia in patients for whom other measures are inappropriate or inadequate.

[Polycystic ovary syndrome (treatment)][1]—Spironolactone is also used with some success in the treatment of polycystic ovary syndrome.

[Hirsutism, female (treatment)][1]—Spironolactone has been used in the treatment of female hirsutism.

---

[1]Not included in Canadian product labeling.

## Pharmacology/Pharmacokinetics

**Physicochemical characteristics**
Molecular weight—
   Amiloride hydrochloride: 302.12.

Spironolactone: 416.57.
Triamterene: 253.27.

pKa—
Amiloride: 8.7.
Triamterene: 6.2.

## Mechanism of action/Effect

Diuretic or Antihypokalemic—Potassium-sparing diuretics interfere with sodium reabsorption in the distal convoluted tubule, thereby promoting excretion of sodium and water and retention of potassium. Amiloride and triamterene have a direct inhibiting effect on the entry of sodium into the cells, while spironolactone competitively inhibits the action of aldosterone.

Antihypertensive—Diuretics lower blood pressure initially by reducing plasma and extracellular fluid volume; cardiac output also decreases. Eventually, the extracellular fluid volume and the cardiac output return to normal with an accompanying decrease in peripheral resistance.

Aldosterone antagonist or Diagnostic aid (primary hyperaldosteronism)—Spironolactone is a competitive inhibitor of aldosterone; neither amiloride nor triamterene has this effect.

Hirsutism or Polycystic ovary syndrome—May be due to an antiandrogenic effect of spironolactone.

## Absorption

Amiloride—Incompletely (15 to 20%) absorbed from gastrointestinal tract; rate, but not necessarily extent, of absorption is increased after 4 hours of fasting.

Spironolactone—Well absorbed following oral administration; bioavailability is greater than 90%. Absorption is enhanced by concomitant intake of food.

Triamterene—Rapidly but incompletely (30 to 70%) absorbed from the gastrointestinal tract.

## Protein binding

Amiloride—Minimal.
Spironolactone and canrenone—Very high (more than 90%).
Triamterene—Moderate (67%).

## Biotransformation

Amiloride—Not metabolized.
Spironolactone—Hepatic; approximately 25 to 30% converted to canrenone.
Triamterene—Hepatic.

## Half-life

Amiloride—
6 to 9 hours.

Spironolactone—
Canrenone: 13 to 24 hours (average 19 hours) when administered once or twice daily; 9 to 16 hours (average 12.5 hours) when administered 4 times daily.

Triamterene—
Normal, 90 to 120 minutes; anuric, 10 hours. Some active metabolites have a normal half-life of up to 12 hours.
Terminal half-life: 5 to 7 hours.

## Onset of action

Diuretic—
Amiloride: Single dose—Within 2 hours.
Triamterene: Single dose—2 to 4 hours.

## Time to peak concentration

Amiloride—3 to 4 hours.
Triamterene—2 to 4 hours.

## Time to peak effect

Diuretic—
Amiloride: Single dose—6 to 10 hours.
Spironolactone: Multiple doses—2 to 3 days.
Triamterene: Multiple doses—1 day to several days.

## Duration of action

Diuretic—
Amiloride: Single dose—24 hours.
Spironolactone: Multiple doses—2 to 3 days.
Triamterene: Single dose—7 to 9 hours.

## Elimination

Amiloride—Renal, 20 to 50% (unchanged); fecal, 40% (unchanged).
Spironolactone—Metabolites: Primary route, renal (less than 10% unchanged); secondary route, biliary/fecal.
Triamterene—Primary route, biliary/fecal; secondary route, renal.

## Precautions to Consider

### Carcinogenicity/Tumorigenicity

*Amiloride*—
One study in mice at doses up to 25 times the maximum daily human dose and another in male and female rats at doses up to 15 and 20 times the maximum daily human dose for 104 weeks showed no evidence of carcinogenicity or tumorigenicity.

*Spironolactone*—
Breast carcinoma has been reported in men and women taking this medication, but a direct causal relationship has not yet been established.

Spironolactone has been found to be tumorigenic in rats, mainly in endocrine organs and the liver. A statistically significant dose-related increase in benign adenomas of the thyroid and testes was found in male rats given spironolactone in doses up to 250 times the usual daily human dose of 2 mg per kg of body weight (mg/kg). In addition, a dose-related increase in proliferative liver changes was revealed in male rats. Hepatocytomegaly, hyperplastic nodules, and hepatocellular carcinoma were evident at the highest dosage level of 500 mg/kg. In female rats, a statistically significant increase in malignant mammary tumors was seen at the mid-dose level.

*Triamterene*—
Studies evaluating the carcinogenic potential of triamterene have not been done.

### Mutagenicity

*Amiloride*— In Ames tests, no evidence of mutagenicity was found.

### Pregnancy/Reproduction

Fertility—*Amiloride:* Studies in rats given amiloride at 20 times the expected maximum human daily dose revealed no evidence of fertility impairment. However, some toxicity in adult rats and rabbits and a decrease in rat pup growth and survival were seen at doses of 5 or more times the expected maximum daily human dose.

Pregnancy—Pregnant women should be advised to contact physician before taking these medications, since routine use of diuretics during normal pregnancy is inappropriate and exposes mother and fetus to unnecessary hazard. Diuretics do not prevent development of toxemia of pregnancy, and there is no satisfactory evidence that they are useful in the treatment of toxemia. Diuretics are indicated only in the treatment of edema due to pathologic causes or as a short course of treatment in patients with severe hypervolemia.

*Amiloride*—
Adequate and well-controlled studies in humans have not been done.

Amiloride crosses the placenta in modest amounts in rabbits and mice. However, teratogenicity studies in rabbits and mice given 20 and 25 times the maximum human dose, respectively, revealed no evidence of fetal harm.

FDA Pregnancy Category B.

*Spironolactone*—
Spironolactone may cross the placenta. However, problems in humans have not been documented.

*Triamterene*—
Adequate and well-controlled studies in humans have not been done.

Triamterene crosses the placenta and appears in the cord blood of ewes. Studies in rats given triamterene in doses up to 30 times the human dose have revealed no evidence of harm to the fetus.

FDA Pregnancy Category B.

### Breast-feeding

*Amiloride*— It is not known whether amiloride is distributed into human breast milk. However, problems in humans have not been documented. Amiloride has been shown to be distributed into rat's milk.

*Spironolactone*— Problems in humans have not been documented. However, canrenone (an active metabolite of spironolactone) is distributed into breast milk.

*Triamterene*— It is not known whether triamterene is distributed into human breast milk. However, problems in humans have not been documented. Triamterene has been shown to be distributed into animal milk.

### Pediatrics

Studies performed to date have not demonstrated pediatrics-specific problems that would limit the usefulness of potassium-sparing diuretics in children.

### Geriatrics

Although appropriate studies on the relationship of age to the effects of potassium-sparing diuretics have not been performed in the geriatric population, the elderly may be at increased risk of developing hyperkalemia. In addition, elderly patients are more likely to have age-related renal function impairment, which may require caution in patients receiving potassium-sparing diuretics.

**Drug interactions and/or related problems**

The following drug interactions and/or related problems have been selected on the basis of their potential clinical significance (possible mechanism in parentheses where appropriate)—not necessarily inclusive (» = major clinical significance):

Note: Combinations containing any of the following medications, depending on the amount present, may also interact with this medication.

*For all potassium-sparing diuretics*
   Allopurinol or
   Colchicine or
   Probenecid or
   Sulfinpyrazone
      (triamterene may raise the concentration of blood uric acid, but to a lesser extent than thiazide diuretics or ethacrynic acid or furosemide; dosage adjustment of antigout medications may be necessary to control hyperuricemia and gout)
» Anticoagulants, coumarin- or indandione-derivative or
» Heparin
      (anticoagulant effects may be decreased when these medications are used concurrently with potassium-sparing diuretics, as a result of reduction of plasma volume leading to concentration of procoagulant factors in the blood; in addition, diuretic-induced improvement of hepatic congestion may lead to improved hepatic function, resulting in increased procoagulant factor synthesis; dosage adjustments may be necessary)
   Anti-inflammatory drugs, nonsteroidal (NSAIDs), especially indomethacin
      (may reduce the antihypertensive effects of the potassium-sparing diuretics; indomethacin may also reduce the natriuretic and diuretic effects of potassium-sparing diuretics, possibly because of renal prostaglandin synthesis inhibition and/or sodium and fluid retention; the patient should be carefully monitored to confirm that the desired effect is being obtained)
      (concurrent use of NSAIDs with a diuretic may increase the risk of renal failure secondary to a decrease in renal blood flow caused by inhibition of renal prostaglandin synthesis)
» Angiotensin-converting enzyme (ACE) inhibitors or
   Anti-inflammatory drugs, nonsteroidal (NSAIDs), especially indomethacin or
» Blood from blood bank (may contain up to 30 mEq [mmol] of potassium per liter of plasma or up to 65 mEq [mmol] per liter of whole blood when stored for more than 10 days) or
» Cyclosporine or
» Diuretics, potassium-sparing, other or
   Heparin or
» Low-salt milk (may contain up to 60 mEq [mmol] of potassium per liter) or
» Potassium-containing medications or
» Potassium supplements or substances containing high levels of potassium or
   Salt substitutes (most contain substantial amounts of potassium)
      (concurrent administration with potassium-sparing diuretics tends to promote serum potassium accumulation; hyperkalemia may result, especially in patients with renal insufficiency)
   Exchange resins, sodium cycle (such as sodium polystyrene sulfonate)
      (whether administered orally or rectally, these medications reduce serum potassium levels by replacing potassium with sodium; fluid retention may occur in some patients because of the increased sodium intake)
   Hypotension-producing medications, other (See *Appendix II*)
      (antihypertensive and/or diuretic effects may be potentiated when these medications are used concurrently with potassium-sparing diuretics; although some antihypertensive and/or diuretic combinations are frequently used for therapeutic advantage, dosage adjustments may be necessary during concurrent use)
» Lithium
      (concurrent use with potassium-sparing diuretics is not recommended, as they may provoke lithium toxicity by reducing renal clearance)
   Sympathomimetics
      (may reduce the antihypertensive effects of potassium-sparing diuretics; the patient should be carefully monitored to confirm that the desired effect is being obtained)

*For spironolactone only (in addition to those listed for all potassium-sparing diuretics)*
» Digoxin
      (spironolactone may increase the half-life of digoxin; dosage reduction or increased dosing intervals of digoxin may be necessary and careful monitoring is recommended)

*For triamterene only (in addition to those listed for all potassium-sparing diuretics)*
   Amantadine
      (triamterene may reduce the renal clearance of amantadine, resulting in increased plasma concentrations and possible amantadine toxicity)
   Folic acid
      (triamterene may act as a folate antagonist by inhibiting dihydrofolate reductase; most significant with high doses and/or prolonged triamterene use; leucovorin calcium must be used instead of folic acid in patients receiving triamterene)

**Laboratory value alterations**

The following have been selected on the basis of their potential clinical significance (possible effect in parentheses where appropriate)—not necessarily inclusive (» = major clinical significance):

With diagnostic test results
*For spironolactone only*
   Digoxin radioimmunoassays
      (results may be falsely elevated)
   Plasma cortisol concentration determination by Mattingly (fluorometric) assay
      (concentration may be falsely increased; withdrawal of spironolactone 4 to 7 days prior to determinations, or substitution of Ertel, Peterson, or Norymberski method, is recommended)

*For triamterene only*
   Fluorescent measurement of quinidine
      (similar fluorescence spectra)

With physiology/laboratory test values
*For amiloride, spironolactone, and triamterene*
   Blood urea nitrogen (BUN) concentrations (especially in patients with pre-existing renal impairment) and
   Calcium excretion, urinary and
   Creatinine concentrations, serum and
   Magnesium concentrations, serum and
   Plasma renin activity (PRA) and
   Potassium concentrations, serum and
   Uric acid concentrations, serum
      (may be increased)
   Sodium
      (serum concentrations may be decreased)

**Medical considerations/Contraindications**

The medical considerations/contraindications included here have been selected on the basis of their potential clinical significance (reasons given in parentheses where appropriate)—not necessarily inclusive (» = major clinical significance).

*Except under special circumstances, this medication should not be used when the following medical problem exists:*
» Hyperkalemia
      (potassium-sparing diuretics may further increase serum potassium concentrations)

*Risk-benefit should be considered when the following medical problems exist:*
*For amiloride, spironolactone, and triamterene*
» Anuria or
» Renal function impairment
      (potassium-sparing diuretics may aggravate electrolyte imbalance; risk of developing hyperkalemia is increased)
   Diabetes mellitus, especially in patients with confirmed or suspected renal insufficiency or
» Diabetic nephropathy
      (increased risk of hyperkalemia; potassium-sparing diuretic should be discontinued at least 3 days prior to a glucose tolerance test because of the risk of severe hyperkalemia)
» Hepatic function impairment
      (increased sensitivity to electrolyte changes)
   Hyponatremia
   Metabolic or respiratory acidosis, predisposition to
      (acidosis potentiates hyperkalemic effects of potassium-sparing diuretics; potassium-sparing diuretics may potentiate acidosis)

Sensitivity to the potassium-sparing diuretic prescribed

» Caution is also required in severely ill patients and those with relatively small urine volumes, who are at greater risk of developing hyperkalemia.

*For spironolactone only (in addition to those listed above for all potassium-sparing diuretics)*
Menstrual abnormalities or breast enlargement

*For triamterene only (in addition to those listed above for all potassium-sparing diuretics)*
Hyperuricemia or gout
Nephrolithiasis, history of
    (increased risk of forming triamterene stones)

### Patient monitoring

The following may be especially important in patient monitoring (other tests may be warranted in some patients, depending on condition; » = major clinical significance):

*For amiloride, spironolactone, and triamterene*
» Blood pressure measurements
    (recommended at periodic intervals in patients being treated for hypertension; selected patients may be trained to perform blood pressure measurements at home and report the results at regular physician visits)
Blood urea nitrogen (BUN) determinations and/or
Creatinine concentrations, serum
    (determinations recommended prior to initiation of therapy and at periodic intervals during therapy)
Electrocardiograms (ECG) and
» Electrolyte concentrations, serum, especially serum potassium determinations
    (may be required at periodic intervals for patients on long-term therapy, especially if they are also taking systemic steroids, or when congestive heart failure or severe cirrhosis is present)

*For triamterene only*
Platelet count and
Total and differential leukocyte count
    (recommended prior to initiation of therapy and at periodic intervals during therapy, especially in patients with impaired hepatic function)

## Side/Adverse Effects

See *Table 1*, page 1255.

## Overdose

For more information on the management of overdose or unintentional ingestion, **contact a Poison Control Center** (see *Poison Control Center Listing*).

### Treatment of overdose
Overdose should be treated by immediate evacuation of the stomach followed by supportive, symptomatic treatment and monitoring of serum electrolyte concentrations and renal function.

## Patient Consultation

As an aid to patient consultation, refer to *Advice for the Patient, Diuretics, Potassium-sparing (Systemic)*.

In providing consultation, consider emphasizing the following selected information (» = major clinical significance):

### Before using this medication
» Conditions affecting use, especially:
    Sensitivity to the potassium-sparing diuretic prescribed
    Pregnancy—Not recommended for routine use; triamterene crosses placenta; spironolactone may cross placenta
    Breast-feeding—All potassium-sparing diuretics may be distributed into breast milk
    Use in the elderly—Increased risk of hyperkalemia
    Other medications, especially angiotensin-converting enzyme (ACE) inhibitors, cyclosporine, digoxin, other potassium-sparing diuretics, potassium-containing medications or supplements, or lithium
    Other medical problems, especially diabetic nephropathy, hyperkalemia, renal function impairment or hepatic function impairment

### Proper use of this medication
Diuretic effects of the medication and timing of doses to minimize inconvenience of diuresis
Getting into habit of taking at same time each day to help increase compliance

Taking with meals or milk to reduce gastrointestinal irritation
» Proper dosing
    Missed dose: Taking as soon as possible; not taking if almost time for next dose; not doubling doses
» Proper storage

*For use as an antihypertensive (amiloride and spironolactone only)*
Possible need for control of weight and diet, especially sodium intake
» Patient may not experience symptoms of hypertension; importance of taking medication even if feeling well
» Does not cure, but helps control hypertension; possible need for life-long therapy; checking with physician before discontinuing medication; serious consequences of untreated hypertension

### Precautions while using this medication
Regular visits to physician to check progress
Avoiding excessive ingestion of foods high in potassium or use of salt substitutes or other potassium supplements
To prevent dehydration, checking with physician if severe nausea, vomiting, or diarrhea occurs and continues
Caution if any kind of surgery or emergency treatment is required
Caution if any laboratory tests required; possible interference with test results

*For use as an antihypertensive (amiloride and spironolactone only)*
» Not taking other medications, especially nonprescription sympathomimetics, unless discussed with physician

*For triamterene only*
Possible photosensitivity; avoiding unprotected exposure to sun; using protective clothing and sun block product; avoiding use of sunlamp, tanning bed, or tanning booth

### Side/adverse effects
Signs of potential side effects, especially agranulocytosis, allergic reaction, anaphylaxis, and hyperkalemia (for all potassium-sparing diuretics); megaloblastosis, nephrolithiasis, and thrombocytopenia (for triamterene)
*For spironolactone only (in addition to the above)*
Possibility of enlargement of breasts in males; usually reversible within several months

## General Dosing Information

Dosage must be adjusted to meet the individual requirements of each patient, on the basis of clinical response. The lowest effective dose should be utilized to minimize potential electrolyte imbalance.

If a single daily dose is indicated, it is preferably taken on arising in order to minimize the effect of increased frequency of urination on sleep, although the diuretic effect of potassium-sparing diuretics alone is mild.

The normal adult concentration of plasma potassium is 3.5 to 5.0 mEq (mmol) per liter, with 4.5 mEq (mmol) often being used as a reference point. Potassium concentrations exceeding 6 mEq (mmol) per liter are dangerous because of possible initiation of cardiac arrhythmias. Normal potassium concentrations tend to be higher in neonates (7.7 mEq [mmol] per liter) than in adults.

Plasma potassium concentrations do not necessarily indicate the true body potassium concentration. A rise in serum pH may cause a decrease in serum potassium concentration and an increase in the intracellular potassium concentration.

It is recommended that potassium-sparing diuretic therapy be withdrawn if hyperkalemia occurs. If hyperkalemia is associated with ECG changes, prompt additional therapy with intravenous sodium bicarbonate, calcium gluconate, or calcium chloride; with oral or rectal sodium polystyrene sulfonate; or parenteral glucose and insulin may be indicated. It is important to remember that severe hyperkalemia may occur suddenly and may not be preceded by any warning signs.

Recent evidence suggests that withdrawal of antihypertensive therapy prior to surgery is not necessary, but that the anesthesiologist must be aware of such therapy.

### Diet/Nutrition
It is recommended that oral potassium-sparing diuretics be taken with or after meals to minimize stomach upset, and possibly also to enhance bioavailability.

---

### *AMILORIDE*

## Summary of Differences

Pharmacology/pharmacokinetics:
    Protein binding—Minimal.
    Biotransformation—None; excreted unchanged.

Duration of action—Diuretic: Single dose—24 hours.
Side/adverse effects:
No reported cases of agranulocytosis. Amiloride has been reported to cause constipation and muscle cramps.

## Oral Dosage Forms

### AMILORIDE HYDROCHLORIDE TABLETS USP

**Usual adult dose**
Diuretic or
Antihypertensive—
Oral, 5 to 10 mg per day as a single dose.

Note: Geriatric patients may be more sensitive to the effects of the usual adult dose.

**Usual adult prescribing limits**
Up to 20 mg per day.

**Usual pediatric dose**
Dosage has not been established.

**Strength(s) usually available**
U.S.—
5 mg (Rx) [*Midamor*; GENERIC].
Canada—
5 mg (Rx) [*Midamor*].

**Packaging and storage**
Store below 40 °C (104 °F), preferably between 15 and 30 °C (59 and 86 °F), unless otherwise specified by manufacturer. Store in a well-closed container.

**Auxiliary labeling**
• Take with meals or milk.
• Do not take other medicines without your doctor's advice.

**Note**
Check refill frequency to determine compliance in hypertensive patients.

---

### *SPIRONOLACTONE*

## Summary of Differences

Indications:
Diagnosis and treatment of primary hyperaldosteronism. Treatment of polycystic ovary syndrome and female hirsutism.
Pharmacology/pharmacokinetics:
Mechanism of action/effect—Aldosterone antagonist.
Protein binding—Very high (more than 90%).
Biotransformation—Hepatic, extensive, to active metabolite (canrenone).
Duration of action—Diuretic: Multiple doses—2 to 3 days.
Precautions:
Carcinogenicity—Tumorigenic in rats and possibly associated with breast carcinoma in humans.
Drug interactions and/or related problems—Use with digoxin may increase digoxin half-life.
Laboratory value alterations—May falsely increase plasma cortisol determinations by Mattingly (fluorometric) assay. May falsely elevate digoxin radioimmunoassays.
Medical considerations/contraindications—Menstrual abnormalities or breast enlargement.
Side/adverse effects:
Endocrine or antiandrogenic effects more common at doses exceeding 100 mg per day. May cause CNS effects and causes more frequent gastrointestinal irritation.

## Additional Dosing Information

See also *General Dosing Information.*

To reduce delay in onset of effect, a loading dose of 2 to 3 times the daily dose may be administered on the first day of therapy.

When spironolactone is added to therapy with another diuretic or antihypertensive agent, it is recommended that the dosage of the other drug (especially ganglionic blocking agents) be reduced by at least 50% and then adjusted as required.

It is recommended that spironolactone be discontinued several days prior to adrenal vein catheterization for measurement of aldosterone concentrations, for the purpose of attempting lateralization in primary hyperaldosteronism, and for measurements of plasma renin activity.

When high doses of spironolactone are required for treatment of edema due to hepatic cirrhosis, drug dosage may be reduced prior to completion of diuresis to avoid dehydration and precipitation of hepatic coma, although dry weight may be achieved.

## Oral Dosage Forms

Note: Bracketed uses in the *Dosage Forms* section refer to categories of use and/or indications that are not included in U.S. product labeling.

### SPIRONOLACTONE TABLETS USP

**Usual adult dose**
Edema due to congestive heart failure, hepatic cirrhosis, or nephrotic syndrome—
Initial: Oral, 25 to 200 mg a day in two to four divided doses for at least five days.
Maintenance: Oral, 75 to 400 mg a day in two to four divided doses.
Antihypertensive—
Initial: Oral, 50 to 100 mg a day as a single daily dose or in two to four divided doses for at least two weeks, followed by gradual dosage adjustment every two weeks as necessary up to 200 mg a day.
Maintenance: Oral, adjusted to meet individual requirements.
Primary hyperaldosteronism—
Maintenance: Oral, 100 to 400 mg per day in two to four divided daily doses prior to surgery; smaller doses may be used for long-term maintenance in patients unsuitable for surgery.
[Polycystic ovary disease]—
Oral, 100 to 200 mg per day in two divided daily doses.
[Hirsutism, female]—
Oral, 100 mg two times a day.
Diagnostic aid (primary hyperaldosteronism)—
Long test: Oral, 400 mg per day in two to four divided daily doses for three to four weeks.
Short test: Oral, 400 mg per day in two to four divided daily doses for four days.
Antihypokalemic—
Diuretic-induced hypokalemia: Oral, 25 to 100 mg per day as a single daily dose or in two to four divided doses.

Note: Geriatric patients may be more sensitive to the effects of the usual adult dose.

**Usual adult prescribing limits**
Dose may be increased up to three times the initial dose or up to a maximum of 400 mg a day.

**Usual pediatric dose**
Edema
Ascites or
Hypertension—
Initial: Oral, 1 to 3 mg per kg of body weight or 30 to 90 mg per square meter of body surface a day as a single daily dose or in two to four divided doses, the dosage being readjusted after five days. Dosage may be increased up to three times the initial dose.

**Strength(s) usually available**
U.S.—
25 mg (Rx) [*Aldactone*; GENERIC (may be scored)].
50 mg (Rx) [*Aldactone* (scored)].
100 mg (Rx) [*Aldactone* (scored)].
Canada—
25 mg (Rx) [*Aldactone* (scored); *Novospiroton* (scored)].
100 mg (Rx) [*Aldactone* (scored); *Novospiroton* (scored)].

**Packaging and storage**
Store below 40 °C (104 °F), preferably between 15 and 30 °C (59 and 86 °F), unless otherwise specified by manufacturer. Store in a tight, light-resistant container.

**Preparation of dosage form**
For patients who cannot take oral solids—For small children or patients unable to swallow the tablets, Spironolactone Tablets USP may be crushed and dispensed as a suspension in Cherry Syrup NF. This suspension is stable in a refrigerator for 1 month.

**Auxiliary labeling**
• Take with meals or milk.
• Do not take other medicines without your doctor's advice.

**Note**
Check refill frequency to determine compliance in hypertensive patients.

---

### *TRIAMTERENE*

## Summary of Differences

Pharmacology/pharmacokinetics:
Biotransformation—Hepatic.
Duration of action—Diuretic: Single dose—7 to 9 hours.

Precautions:

Drug interactions and/or related problems—Triamterene may increase blood uric acid and antagonize allopurinol, colchicine, probenecid, or sulfinpyrazone.

Laboratory value alterations—May interfere with fluorescent measurement of quinidine.

Medical considerations/contraindications—Hyperuricemia or gout; history of nephrolithiasis.

Side/adverse effects:

Nephrolithiasis; megaloblastosis; photosensitivity; thrombocytopenia. No decrease in sexual ability reported.

## Additional Dosing Information

See also *General Dosing Information.*

Since triamterene is a weak folic acid antagonist, it may contribute to development of megaloblastosis in patients who have depleted folic acid stores (e.g., in pregnancy, hepatic cirrhosis).

When triamterene is combined with another diuretic, it is recommended that the initial dosage of each be reduced and then adjusted as required.

## Oral Dosage Forms

### TRIAMTERENE CAPSULES USP

**Usual adult dose**
Diuretic—
Initial: Oral, 25 to 100 mg a day.
Maintenance: Oral, adjusted to meet individual requirements.

Note: Geriatric patients may be more sensitive to the effects of the usual adult dose.

**Usual adult prescribing limits**
Up to 300 mg daily.

**Usual pediatric dose**
Diuretic—
Initial: Oral, 2 to 4 mg per kg of body weight or 120 mg per square meter of body surface a day or on alternate days in divided doses.
Maintenance: Oral, increased to 6 mg per kg of body weight a day according to individual requirements up to a maximum of 300 mg a day in divided doses.

**Strength(s) usually available**
U.S.—
50 mg (Rx) [*Dyrenium* (lactose)].
100 mg (Rx) [*Dyrenium* (lactose)].
Canada—
Not commercially available.

**Packaging and storage**
Store below 40 °C (104 °F), preferably between 15 and 30 °C (59 and 86 °F), unless otherwise specified by manufacturer. Store in a tight, light-resistant container.

**Auxiliary labeling**
• Take with meals or milk.
• Avoid overexposure to sun or use of sunlamp.
• Do not take other medicines without your doctor's advice.

### TRIAMTERENE TABLETS

**Usual adult dose**
Diuretic—
Initial: Oral, 25 to 100 mg a day.
Maintenance: Oral, adjusted to meet individual requirements.

Note: Geriatric patients may be more sensitive to the effects of the usual adult dose.

**Usual adult prescribing limits**
Up to 300 mg daily.

**Usual pediatric dose**
Diuretic—
Initial: Oral, 2 to 4 mg per kg of body weight or 120 mg per square meter of body surface a day or on alternate days in divided doses.
Maintenance: Oral, increased to 6 mg per kg of body weight a day according to individual requirements up to a maximum of 300 mg a day in divided doses.

**Strength(s) usually available**
U.S.—
Not commercially available.
Canada—
50 mg (Rx) [*Dyrenium*].
100 mg (Rx) [*Dyrenium* (scored)].

**Packaging and storage**
Store below 40 °C (104 °F), preferably between 15 and 30 °C (59 and 86 °F), unless otherwise specified by manufacturer. Store in a tight, light-resistant container.

**Auxiliary labeling**
• Take with meals or milk.
• Avoid overexposure to sun or use of sunlamp.
• Do not take other medicines without your doctor's advice.

## Selected Bibliography

The fifth report of the Joint National Committee on Detection, Evaluation, and Treatment of High Blood Pressure (JNC V). Arch Intern Med 1993; 153 (2): 154-83.

Revised: 10/15/92
Interim revision: 05/18/94

## Table 1. Side/Adverse Effects*

The following side/adverse effects have been selected on the basis of their potential clinical significance (possible signs and symptoms in parentheses where appropriate)—not necessarily inclusive:

Legend:
I=Amiloride
II=Spironolactone
III=Triamterene

| | I | II | III |
|---|---|---|---|
| **Those indicating need for medical attention** | | | |
| *Agranulocytosis* (fever or chills, cough or hoarseness, lower back or side pain, painful or difficult urination) | U | R | R |
| *Allergic reaction or anaphylaxis* (shortness of breath, skin rash or itching) | R | R | R |
| *Hyperkalemia* (confusion; irregular heartbeat; nervousness; numbness or tingling in hands, feet, or lips; shortness of breath or difficult breathing; unusual tiredness or weakness; weakness or heaviness of legs) | | | |
| Note: *Irregular heartbeat* is usually the earliest clinical indication of hyperkalemia and is readily detected by electrocardiogram (ECG). | M† | M† | M† |
| *Megaloblastosis or overdose* (burning, inflamed, or bright red tongue or cracked corners of mouth; weakness) | U | U | R |
| *Nephrolithiasis* (severe lower back or side pain) | U | U | R |
| *Thrombocytopenia* (unusual bleeding or bruising; black, tarry stools; blood in urine or stools; pinpoint red spots on skin) | U | U | R |

*Differences in frequency of occurrence may reflect either lack of clinical-use data or actual pharmacologic distinctions among agents. M = more frequent; L = less frequent; R = rare; U = unknown.

†Signs and symptoms of hyperkalemia may occur even when potassium-sparing diuretics are combined with thiazide diuretics. Hyperkalemia occurs in approximately 10% of patients when amiloride is used alone and may occur in up to 26% of patients receiving spironolactone even when combined with thiazide diuretics.

‡Incidence related to dose and/or duration of therapy.

Table 1. Side/Adverse Effects* *(continued)*

| | Legend:<br>**I** = Amiloride<br>**II** = Spironolactone<br>**III** = Triamterene | | |
| --- | --- | --- | --- |
| | **I** | **II** | **III** |
| **Those indicating need for medical attention only if they continue or are bothersome** | | | |
| *Antiandrogenic or endocrine effect* (breast tenderness in females, deepening of voice in females, enlargement of breasts in males, inability to have or keep an erection, increased hair growth in females, irregular menstrual periods, sweating)<br>Note: *Gynecomastia* occurs frequently after several months of treatment at doses of spironolactone greater than 100 mg per day and rarely may persist even after spironolactone is discontinued. | U | L‡ | U |
| *Central nervous system (CNS) effect* (clumsiness) | U | L‡ | U |
| *CNS effect* (headache) | L | L‡ | L |
| *Constipation* | L | U | U |
| *Decreased sexual ability* | L | L | U |
| *Dizziness* | L | L | L |
| *Gastrointestinal irritation* (nausea or vomiting, stomach cramps and diarrhea) | L | M | L |
| *Hyponatremia* (drowsiness, dryness of mouth, increased thirst, lack of energy) | L | L | L |
| *Increased sensitivity of skin to sunlight* | U | U | L |
| *Muscle cramps* | L | U | U |

*Differences in frequency of occurrence may reflect either lack of clinical-use data or actual pharmacologic distinctions among agents. M = more frequent; L = less frequent; R = rare; U = unknown.

†Signs and symptoms of hyperkalemia may occur even when potassium-sparing diuretics are combined with thiazide diuretics. Hyperkalemia occurs in approximately 10% of patients when amiloride is used alone and may occur in up to 26% of patients receiving spironolactone even when combined with thiazide diuretics.

‡Incidence related to dose and/or duration of therapy.

# DIURETICS, POTASSIUM-SPARING, AND HYDROCHLOROTHIAZIDE    Systemic

This monograph includes information on the following: Amiloride and Hydrochlorothiazide; Spironolactone and Hydrochlorothiazide; Triamterene and Hydrochlorothiazide.

VA CLASSIFICATION (Primary/Secondary): CV704/CV490; TN900

**NOTE:** The *Diuretics, Potassium-sparing, and Hydrochlorothiazide (Systemic)* monograph is maintained on the USP DI electronic data base. For a printed copy of the most recent revision of the complete monograph, contact the USP Division of Information Development, 12601 Twinbrook Parkway, Rockville, MD 20852.

For information on the specific components of this combination, see the *USP DI* monographs for *Diuretics, Potassium-sparing (Systemic)* and *Diuretics, Thiazide (Systemic)*.

The information that follows is selectively abstracted from the complete monograph and is provided to facilitate drug use review and patient counseling.

Note: For a listing of dosage forms and brand names by country availability, see *Dosage Forms* section(s). For a listing of brand names for the articles in this monograph, refer to the General Index.

## Category

Antihypertensive; antihypokalemic; diuretic.

## Indications

### Accepted

Edema (treatment)—These combinations are indicated as adjuncts in the management of edematous states such as congestive heart failure, hepatic cirrhosis, and nephrotic syndrome, as well as in corticosteroid- and estrogen-induced edema and idiopathic edema.

Hypertension (treatment)—Spironolactone and hydrochlorothiazide, triamterene and hydrochlorothiazide, and amiloride and hydrochlorothiazide[1] are also indicated in the treatment of hypertension, especially when a potassium-sparing diuretic effect is desired.

Fixed-dosage combinations are generally not recommended in initial therapy and are useful in subsequent therapy only when the proportion of the component agents corresponds to the dose of the individual agents, as determined by titration.

For additional information on initial therapeutic guidelines related to the treatment of hypertension, see *Appendix III*.

Hypokalemia (treatment)[1]—Amiloride and hydrochlorothiazide, triamterene and hydrochlorothiazide, and spironolactone and hydrochlorothiazide combinations are also indicated for treatment of diuretic-induced hypokalemia in hypertensive patients in whom other measures are inappropriate or inadequate.

[1]Not included in Canadian product labeling.

## Patient Consultation

As an aid to patient consultation, refer to *Advice for the Patient, Diuretics, Potassium-sparing, and Hydrochlorothiazide (Systemic)*.

In providing consultation, consider emphasizing the following selected information (» = major clinical significance):

**Before using this medication**
» Conditions affecting use, especially:
    Sensitivity to the potassium-sparing diuretic prescribed, hydrochlorothiazide or other thiazide diuretics, other sulfonamide-type

medications, bumetanide, furosemide, or carbonic anhydrase inhibitors

Pregnancy—Diuretics not recommended for routine use

Breast-feeding—Hydrochlorothiazide distributed into breast milk; spironolactone may be distributed into breast milk

Use in the elderly—Elderly patients may be more sensitive to hypotensive and electrolyte-depleting effects

Other medications, especially angiotensin-converting enzyme inhibitors, cholestyramine, colestipol, coumarin or indandione anticoagulants, cyclosporine, digitalis glycosides, heparin, lithium, low-salt milk, other potassium-sparing diuretics, potassium-containing medications or supplements, or stored blood from a blood bank

Other medical problems, especially, diabetic nephropathy, hepatic function impairment, renal function impairment or anuria

### Proper use of this medication

Diuretic effects of the medication and timing of doses to minimize inconvenience of diuresis

Getting into habit of taking at same time each day to help increase compliance

Taking with meals or milk to reduce stomach upset

» Proper dosing

Missed dose: Taking as soon as possible; not taking if almost time for next dose; not doubling doses

» Proper storage

*For use as an antihypertensive*

Possible need for control of weight and diet, especially sodium intake

» Patient may not experience symptoms of hypertension; importance of taking medication even if feeling well

» Does not cure, but helps control hypertension; possible need for lifelong therapy; checking with physician before discontinuing medication; serious consequences of untreated hypertension

### Precautions while using this medication

Regular visits to physician to check progress

» Possibility of hypokalemia or hyperkalemia; possible need for monitoring potassium in diet; not changing diet without first checking with physician

To prevent dehydration, checking with physician if severe nausea, vomiting, or diarrhea occurs and continues

Diabetics: May increase blood sugar levels

Possible photosensitivity; avoiding too much sun; using protective clothing and sun block product; avoiding use of sunlamp, tanning bed, or tanning booth

Caution if any kind of surgery or emergency treatment is required

Caution if any laboratory tests required; possible interference with test results

*For triamterene and hydrochlorothiazide combination*

Not changing brands of triamterene and hydrochlorothiazide combination without checking with physician

*For use an an antihypertensive*

» Not taking other medications, especially nonprescription sympathomimetics, unless discussed with physician

### Side/adverse effects

Signs of potential side effects, especially electrolyte imbalance, agranulocytosis, allergic reaction, cholecystitis or pancreatitis, gout or hyperuricemia, hepatic function impairment, thrombocytopenia, megaloblastosis (for triamterene)

*For spironolactone*

Possibility of enlargement of breasts in males and irregular menstrual periods in females; usually reversible within several months

---

## AMILORIDE AND HYDROCHLOROTHIAZIDE

## Oral Dosage Forms

### AMILORIDE HYDROCHLORIDE AND HYDROCHLOROTHIAZIDE TABLETS USP

**Usual adult dose**

Diuretic or

Antihypertensive[1]—

Oral, 1 or 2 tablets a day.

Note: Geriatric patients may be more sensitive to the effects of the usual adult dose.

**Usual pediatric dose**

Dosage has not been established.

**Strength(s) usually available**

U.S.—

5 mg of amiloride hydrochloride and 50 mg of hydrochlorothiazide (Rx) [*Moduretic* (scored); GENERIC (may be scored)].

Canada—

5 mg of amiloride hydrochloride and 50 mg of hydrochlorothiazide (Rx) [*Moduret* (scored)].

**Auxiliary labeling**

• Take with meals or milk.

• Avoid overexposure to the sun or use of sunlamp.

• Do not take other medicines without your doctor's advice.

---

[1]Not included in Canadian product labeling.

---

## *SPIRONOLACTONE AND HYDROCHLOROTHIAZIDE*

## Oral Dosage Forms

### SPIRONOLACTONE AND HYDROCHLOROTHIAZIDE TABLETS USP

**Usual adult dose**

Diuretic—Edema due to congestive heart failure, hepatic cirrhosis, or nephrotic syndrome:—

Maintenance—Oral, 1 to 4 tablets a day, taken as a single dose or in divided doses.

Antihypertensive—

Maintenance: Oral, 2 to 4 tablets a day in divided doses.

Note: Geriatric patients may be more sensitive to the effects of the usual adult dose.

**Usual pediatric dose**

Diuretic—

Maintenance: Oral, 1.65 to 3.3 mg of spironolactone and of hydrochlorothiazide per kg of body weight a day in divided doses.

**Strength(s) usually available**

U.S.—

25 mg of spironolactone and 25 mg of hydrochlorothiazide (Rx) [*Aldactazide*; *Spirozide*; GENERIC (may be scored)].

50 mg of spironolactone and 50 mg of hydrochlorothiazide (Rx) [*Aldactazide* (scored)].

Canada—

25 mg of spironolactone and 25 mg of hydrochlorothiazide (Rx) [*Aldactazide* (scored); *Novo-Spirozine* (scored)].

50 mg of spironolactone and 50 mg of hydrochlorothiazide (Rx) [*Aldactazide* (scored); *Novo-Spirozine* (scored)].

**Auxiliary labeling**

• Take with meals or milk.

• Avoid overexposure to the sun or use of sunlamp.

• Do not take other medicines without your doctor's advice.

---

## *TRIAMTERENE AND HYDROCHLOROTHIAZIDE*

## Oral Dosage Forms

### TRIAMTERENE AND HYDROCHLOROTHIAZIDE CAPSULES USP

**Usual adult dose**

Diuretic or

Antihypertensive—

Oral, 1 or 2 capsules once a day, as determined by individual titration with the component agents; some patients may be maintained on 1 capsule a day or every other day.

Note: Geriatric patients may be more sensitive to the effects of the usual adult dose.

**Usual adult prescribing limits**

Up to 4 capsules daily.

**Usual pediatric dose**

Dosage has not been established.

**Strength(s) usually available**

U.S.—

37.5 mg of triamterene and 25 mg of hydrochlorothiazide (Rx) [*Dyazide* (lactose)].

50 mg of triamterene and 25 mg of hydrochlorothiazide (Rx) [GENERIC].

75 mg of triamterene and 50 mg of hydrochlorothiazide (Rx) [GENERIC].

Canada—

Not commercially available.

**Auxiliary labeling**
• Take with meals or milk.
• Avoid overexposure to the sun or use of sunlamp.
• Do not take other medicines without your doctor's advice.

## TRIAMTERENE AND HYDROCHLOROTHIAZIDE TABLETS USP

**Usual adult dose**
Antihypertensive or
Diuretic—
   *Maxzide*:
      Oral, 1 tablet per day, as determined by individual titration.
   *Apo-Triazide; Dyazide* (Canada); *Novotriamzide*:
      Oral, 1 or 2 tablets two times a day, as determined by individual titration with the component agents; some patients may be maintained on 1 tablet a day or every other day.

Note: Geriatric patients may be more sensitive to the effects of the usual adult dose.

**Usual pediatric dose**
Dosage has not been established.

**Strength(s) usually available**
U.S.—
   37.5 mg of triamterene and 25 mg of hydrochlorothiazide (Rx) [*Maxzide* (scored)].
   75 mg of triamterene and 50 mg of hydrochlorothiazide (Rx) [*Maxzide* (scored); GENERIC (may be scored; may contain lactose)].
Canada—
   50 mg of triamterene and 25 mg of hydrochlorothiazide (Rx) [*Apo-Triazide* (scored); *Dyazide* (scored); *Novo-Triamzide* (scored)].

**Auxiliary labeling**
• Take with meals or milk.
• Avoid overexposure to the sun or use of sunlamp.
• Do not take other medicines without your doctor's advice.

Revised: 08/03/94

# DIURETICS, THIAZIDE    Systemic

This monograph includes information on the following: Bendroflumethiazide; Benzthiazide†; Chlorothiazide†; Chlorthalidone; Cyclothiazide†; Hydrochlorothiazide; Hydroflumethiazide†; Methyclothiazide; Metolazone; Polythiazide†; Quinethazone†; Trichlormethiazide†.

INN:
   Chlorthalidone—Chlortalidone

VA CLASSIFICATION (Primary/Secondary): CV701/CV490; CV900; GU900

Note: For a listing of dosage forms and brand names by country availability, see *Dosage Forms* section(s). For a listing of brand names for the articles in this monograph, refer to the General Index.

   †Not commercially available in Canada.

## Category

Diuretic; antihypertensive; antidiuretic (central and nephrogenic diabetes insipidus); antiurolithic (calcium calculi).

## Indications

Note: Bracketed information in the *Indications* section refers to uses that are not included in U.S. product labeling.

### Accepted

Edema (treatment)—Indications include edema associated with congestive heart failure, hepatic cirrhosis with ascites, corticosteroid and estrogen therapy, and some forms of renal function impairment including nephrotic syndrome, acute glomerulonephritis, and chronic renal failure. However, prompt metolazone tablets are not indicated for treatment of edema because a safe and effective diuretic dosage has not been established.

Hypertension (treatment)—Thiazide diuretics are indicated either alone or as adjunctive therapy in the treatment of hypertension.

For additional information on initial therapeutic guidelines related to the treatment of hypertension, see *Appendix III*.

[Diabetes insipidus, central or nephrogenic (treatment)][1]—Thiazide diuretics are used in the treatment of central and nephrogenic diabetes insipidus.

[Renal calculi, calcium (prophylaxis)][1]—Thiazide diuretics are also used for prevention of calcium-containing renal stones.

   [1]Not included in Canadian product labeling.

## Pharmacology/Pharmacokinetics

Note: Although they are not chemically the same, chlorthalidone, metolazone, and quinethazone have the same actions as the thiazide diuretics.

**Physicochemical characteristics**
Molecular weight—
   Bendroflumethiazide: 421.41.
   Benzthiazide: 431.93.
   Chlorothiazide: 295.72.

   Chlorthalidone: 338.76.
   Cyclothiazide: 389.87.
   Hydrochlorothiazide: 297.73.
   Hydroflumethiazide: 331.28.
   Methyclothiazide: 360.23.
   Metolazone: 365.83.
   Polythiazide: 439.87.
   Quinethazone: 289.74.
   Trichlormethiazide: 380.65.
pKa—
   Bendroflumethiazide: 8.5.
   Chlorothiazide: 6.7 and 9.5.
   Chlorthalidone: 9.4.
   Cyclothiazide: 10.7 in water.
   Hydrochlorothiazide: 7.9 and 9.2.
   Hydroflumethiazide: 8.9 and 10.7.
   Methyclothiazide: 9.4.
   Metolazone: 9.7.
   Quinethazone: 9.3 and 10.7.
   Trichlormethiazide: 8.6.

**Mechanism of action/Effect**
Diuretic—Thiazide diuretics increase urinary excretion of sodium and water by inhibiting sodium reabsorption in the early distal tubules. They increase the rate of delivery of tubular fluid and electrolytes to the distal sites of hydrogen and potassium ion secretion, while plasma volume contraction increases aldosterone production. The increased delivery and increase in aldosterone levels promote sodium reabsorption at the distal tubules, thus increasing the loss of potassium and hydrogen ions.

Antihypertensive—Diuretics lower blood pressure initially by reducing plasma and extracellular fluid volume; cardiac output also decreases. Eventually, cardiac output returns to normal. Thiazide diuretics decrease peripheral resistance by a direct peripheral effect on blood vessels.

Antidiuretic—The antidiuretic effect of thiazide diuretics is a result of mild sodium and water depletion leading to increased reabsorption of glomerular filtrate in the proximal renal tubule and reduced delivery of tubular fluid available for excretion.

Antiurolithic (calcium calculi)—Thiazide diuretics decrease urinary calcium excretion by a direct action on the distal tubule, which may prevent recurrence of calcium-containing renal calculi.

**Absorption**
Thiazide diuretics are absorbed relatively rapidly after oral administration.
Metolazone—The time to peak concentration is 8 hours for extended metolazone tablets and 2 to 4 hours for prompt metolazone tablets. In addition, prompt metolazone tablets have higher bioavailability.

**Protein binding**
Bendroflumethiazide—Very high (94%).
Chlorothiazide—Low to high (20 to 80%).
Chlorthalidone—High (75% [58% to albumin]); increased affinity to carbonic anhydrase in red blood cells.
Hydroflumethiazide—High (74%).

Metolazone—Very high (95%; 50 to 70% to red blood cells).
Polythiazide—High (84%).

**Elimination**

Unchanged; almost totally via the kidneys, with minute quantities in the bile; metolazone undergoes some enterohepatic recycling and slightly greater amounts are excreted in the bile.

| Drug | Half-life (hr) | Diuretic Effect (hr) | | |
|------|---------|-------|------|----------|
| | | Onset | Peak | Duration |
| Bendroflumethiazide | 8.5 | 1–2 | 4 | 6–12 |
| Benzthiazide | | 2 | 4–6 | 12–18 |
| Chlorothiazide | 1–2 | 2 | 4 | 6–12 |
| Chlorthalidone | 35 to 50 | 2 | 2 | 48–72 |
| Cyclothiazide | | 2–4 | 7–12 | 18–24 |
| Hydrochlorothiazide | 5.6–14.8 | 2 | 4 | 6–12 |
| Hydroflumethiazide | 17 | 1–2 | 3–4 | 18–24 |
| Methyclothiazide | | 2 | 6 | >24 |
| Metolazone | 14 | 1* | 2* | 12–24* |
| Polythiazide | | 2 | 6 | 24–48 |
| Quinethazone | | 2 | 6 | 18–24 |
| Trichlormethiazide | | 2 | 6 | ≤24 |

*Information on diuretic effect applies to extended metolazone tablets.

Note: In the absence of edema, negative sodium balance induced by thiazide diuretics lasts for 3 days to 4 weeks with chronic administration. Extracellular fluid volumes remain steady thereafter, although at a lower concentration and volume than before initiation of therapy.

The antihypertensive effects of the thiazide diuretics may be noted after 3 to 4 days of therapy, although up to 3 to 4 weeks may be required for optimal effect. Antihypertensive effects persist for up to 1 week after withdrawal of therapy.

# Precautions to Consider

## Cross-sensitivity and/or related problems

Patients sensitive to other sulfonamide-type medications, bumetanide, furosemide, or carbonic anhydrase inhibitors may be sensitive to this medication also.

## Carcinogenicity/Mutagenicity

*Bendroflumethiazide*—Studies have not been done in either animals or humans.

*Benzthiazide*—Studies have not been done in either animals or humans.

*Chlorothiazide*—Carcinogenicity studies have not been done in either animals or humans. Chlorothiazide was not found to be mutagenic in the Ames microbial mutation test, dominant lethal assay, or a test in *Aspergillus nidulans*.

*Cyclothiazide*—Studies have not been done in either animals or humans.

*Hydrochlorothiazide*—Carcinogenicity studies have not been done in either animals or humans. Hydrochlorothiazide was not found to be mutagenic *in vitro* in the Ames microbial mutation test or on examination of urine from patients who received hydrochlorothiazide; however, it did induce nondisjunction in *Aspergillus nidulans*.

*Hydroflumethiazide*—Studies have not been done in either animals or humans.

*Methyclothiazide*—Studies have not been done in either animals or humans.

*Metolazone*—Studies in mice and rats for 1½ to 2 years at doses of 2, 10, and 50 mg per kg of body weight (mg/kg) per day (100, 500, and 2500 times the maximum recommended human dose [MRHD]) found no evidence of carcinogenicity.

*Trichlormethiazide*—Studies have not been done in either animals or humans.

## Pregnancy/Reproduction

Fertility—*Hydrochlorothiazide*: No adverse effects on fertility were found in rats given doses up to 2 times the maximum recommended human dose of hydrochlorothiazide.

*Methyclothiazide*: No adverse effects on fertility were found in rats given methyclothiazide in doses up to 4 mg per kg of body weight (mg/kg) per day (at least 20 times the maximum recommended human dose).

*Metolazone*: A study in which male rats were given metolazone at doses of 2, 10, and 50 mg/kg for 127 days prior to mating with untreated female rats revealed an increase in the number of resorption sites in dams mated with males given the 50 mg/kg dose. Furthermore, decreased fetal weight and reduced pregnancy rate were observed in dams mated with males from the 10 and 50 mg/kg groups. In mice, there was no evidence that metolazone alters reproductive capacity.

Pregnancy—Thiazide diuretics cross the placenta and appear in cord blood. Although studies in humans have not been done, thiazide diuretics can cause fetal harm when given to pregnant women. Fetal or neonatal jaundice has been reported.

Pregnant women should be advised to contact physician before taking this medication, since routine use of diuretics during normal pregnancy is inappropriate and exposes mother and fetus to unnecessary hazard. Thiazide diuretics do not prevent development of toxemia of pregnancy, and there is no satisfactory evidence that they are useful in the treatment of toxemia. Thiazide diuretics are indicated only in the treatment of edema due to pathologic causes or as a short course of treatment in patients with severe hypervolemia. Possible hazards include fetal or neonatal jaundice, thrombocytopenia, or other adverse reactions seen in adults.

Studies in animals have not shown that thiazide diuretics cause adverse effects on the fetus at several times the human dose.

*Bendroflumethiazide*—
Adequate and well-controlled studies in humans and animals have not been done.

FDA Pregnancy Category C.

*Benzthiazide*—
Has embryocidal effect in rats at doses several hundred times the human dose.

FDA Pregnancy Category C.

*Chlorothiazide*—
Adequate and well-controlled studies in humans have not been done.

Studies in rabbits, mice, and rats at doses up to 500 mg/kg per day (25 times the MRHD) have not shown that chlorothiazide causes adverse effects on the fetus.

FDA Pregnancy Category B.

*Chlorthalidone*—
Adequate and well-controlled studies in humans have not been done.

Studies in rats and rabbits at doses up to 420 times the human dose have not shown that chlorthalidone causes adverse effects on the fetus.

FDA Pregnancy Category B.

*Cyclothiazide*—
Studies have not been done in humans.
Studies have not been done in animals.

FDA Pregnancy Category C.

*Hydrochlorothiazide*—
Adequate and well-controlled studies in humans have not been done.

A study in rats at dosages up to 250 mg/kg per day (62.5 times the MRHD) have not shown that hydrochlorothiazide causes adverse effects on the fetus.

Studies in mice and rabbits with doses up to 100 mg/kg per day (50 times the maximum human dose) revealed no evidence of external abnormalities of the fetus.

FDA Pregnancy Category B.

*Hydroflumethiazide*—
Studies have not been done in humans.
Studies have not been done in animals.

FDA Pregnancy Category C.

*Methyclothiazide*—
Studies have not been done in humans.
Studies in rats and rabbits given methyclothiazide at doses up to 4 mg/kg per day have revealed no evidence of harm to the fetus.

FDA Pregnancy Category B.

*Metolazone*—
Adequate and well-controlled studies in humans have not been done.

Studies in mice, rabbits, and rats at doses up to 50 mg/kg per day (333 times the MRHD) have not shown that metolazone causes adverse effects on the fetus.

FDA Pregnancy Category B.

*Trichlormethiazide*—
Adequate and well-controlled studies in humans have not been done.

Studies in rats at doses 250 to 1250 times the recommended human daily dose have not shown that trichlormethiazide causes adverse effects on the fetus.

FDA Pregnancy Category C.

## Breast-feeding

Thiazide diuretics are distributed into breast milk. The American Academy of Pediatrics recommends that nursing mothers avoid thiazide diuretics during the first month of lactation because of reports of suppression of lactation.

**Pediatrics**

Although appropriate studies on the relationship of age to the effects of thiazide diuretics have not been performed in the pediatric population, pediatrics-specific problems that would limit the usefulness of this medication in children are not expected. However, caution is required in jaundiced infants because of the risk of hyperbilirubinemia.

**Geriatrics**

Although appropriate studies on the relationship of age to the effects of thiazide diuretics have not been performed in the geriatric population, the elderly may be more sensitive to the hypotensive and electrolyte effects. In addition, elderly patients are more likely to have age-related renal function impairment, which may require caution in patients receiving thiazide diuretics.

**Drug interactions and/or related problems**

The following drug interactions and/or related problems have been selected on the basis of their potential clinical significance (possible mechanism in parentheses where appropriate)—not necessarily inclusive (» = major clinical significance):

Note: Combinations containing any of the following medications, depending on the amount present, may also interact with this medication.

Amantadine
(hydrochlorothiazide may reduce the renal clearance of amantadine, resulting in increased plasma concentrations and possible amantadine toxicity)

Amiodarone
(concurrent use of thiazide diuretics with amiodarone may lead to an increased risk of arrhythmias associated with hypokalemia)

Anticoagulants, coumarin- or indandione-derivative
(effects may be decreased when used concurrently with thiazide diuretics as a result of reduction of plasma volume leading to concentration of procoagulant factors in the blood; in addition, diuretic-induced improvement of hepatic congestion may lead to improved hepatic function resulting in increased procoagulant factor synthesis; dosage adjustments may be necessary)

Antidiabetic agents, oral or
Insulin
(thiazide diuretics may raise blood glucose concentrations; for adult-onset diabetics, dosage adjustment of hypoglycemic medications may be necessary during and after thiazide diuretic therapy; insulin requirements may be increased, decreased, or unchanged)

Anti-inflammatory drugs, nonsteroidal (NSAIDs), especially indomethacin
(may antagonize the natriuresis and increase in plasma renin activity [PRA] caused by thiazide diuretics; they may also reduce the antihypertensive effect and increase in urine volume caused by thiazide diuretics, possibly by inhibiting renal prostaglandin synthesis and/or by causing sodium and fluid retention; the patient should be carefully monitored to confirm that the desired effect is being obtained)
(in addition, concurrent use of NSAIDs with a diuretic may increase the risk of renal failure secondary to a decrease in renal blood flow caused by inhibition of renal prostaglandin synthesis)

Calcium-containing medications
(concurrent use of thiazide diuretics with large doses of calcium may result in hypercalcemia because of reduced calcium excretion)

» Cholestyramine or
» Colestipol
(may inhibit gastrointestinal absorption of the thiazide diuretics; administration of thiazide diuretics 1 hour before or 4 hours after cholestyramine or colestipol is recommended)

Diazoxide
(concurrent use with thiazide diuretics may enhance hyperglycemic effects; monitoring of blood glucose levels and/or dosage adjustment of one or both agents may be necessary)
(in addition, concurrent use with thiazide diuretics may enhance hyperuricemic and antihypertensive effects)

Diflunisal
(concurrent use of hydrochlorothiazide with diflunisal produces significantly increased plasma concentrations of hydrochlorothiazide; in addition, the hyperuricemic effect of hydrochlorothiazide is decreased)

» Digitalis glycosides
(concurrent use with thiazide diuretics may enhance the possibility of digitalis toxicity associated with hypokalemia or hypomagnesemia)

Dopamine
(concurrent use may increase the diuretic effect of either thiazide diuretics or dopamine, as a result of dopamine's direct effect on dopaminergic receptors to produce vasodilation of renal vasculature and increase renal blood flow; dopamine also has a direct natriuretic effect)

Hypokalemia-causing medications, other (see *Appendix II*)
(risk of severe hypokalemia due to other hypokalemia-causing medications may be increased; monitoring of serum potassium concentrations and cardiac function and potassium supplementation may be necessary)

Hypotension-producing medications, other (see *Appendix II*)
(antihypertensive and/or diuretic effects may be potentiated when these medications are used concurrently with thiazide diuretics; although some antihypertensive and/or diuretic combinations are frequently used for therapeutic advantage, when used concurrently dosage adjustments may be necessary)

» Lithium
(concurrent use with thiazide diuretics is not recommended, as they may provoke lithium toxicity because of reduced renal clearance; in addition, lithium has nephrotoxic effects)

Neuromuscular blocking agents, nondepolarizing
(thiazide diuretics may induce hypokalemia, which may enhance the blockade of nondepolarizing neuromuscular blocking agents; serum potassium determinations may be necessary prior to administration of nondepolarizing neuromuscular blocking agents; careful postoperative monitoring of the patient may be necessary following concurrent or sequential use, especially if there is a possibility of incomplete reversal of neuromuscular blockade)

Sympathomimetics
(may antagonize the antihypertensive effect of the thiazide diuretics; the patient should be carefully monitored to confirm that the desired effect is being obtained)

**Laboratory value alterations**

The following have been selected on the basis of their potential clinical significance (possible effect in parentheses where appropriate)—not necessarily inclusive (» = major clinical significance):

With diagnostic test results
Bentiromide
(administration of thiazide diuretics during a bentiromide test period will invalidate test results since thiazide diuretics are also metabolized to arylamines and will thus increase the percent of para-aminobenzoic acid [PABA] recovered; discontinuation of thiazide diuretics at least 3 days prior to the administration of bentiromide is recommended)

Phenolsulfonphthalein (PSP) excretion test
(bendroflumethiazide and trichlormethiazide may interfere with PSP excretion)

Phentolamine and tyramine tests
(bendroflumethiazide and trichlormethiazide may produce false negative results)

With physiology/laboratory test values
Bilirubin
(serum concentrations may be increased by displacement from albumin binding)

Calcium
(serum concentrations may be increased; thiazide diuretics should be discontinued before parathyroid function tests are carried out)

Cholesterol, low-density lipoprotein, and triglyceride and
Creatinine
(serum concentrations may be increased)

Glucose, blood and urine
(concentrations may be increased, usually only in patients with a predisposition to glucose intolerance)

Magnesium and
Potassium and
Sodium
(serum concentrations may be decreased; serum magnesium concentrations may increase in uremic patients; a fall in sodium can be life-threatening)

Protein-bound iodine (PBI)
(serum concentrations may be decreased)

Uric acid
(serum concentrations may be increased)

Urinary calcium concentrations
(may be decreased)

## Medical considerations/Contraindications

The medical considerations/contraindications included here have been selected on the basis of their potential clinical significance (reasons given in parentheses where appropriate)—not necessarily inclusive (» = major clinical significance).

*Risk-benefit should be considered when the following medical problems exist:*

» Anuria or severe renal function impairment
   (ineffective; may precipitate azotemia; may produce cumulative effects)

Diabetes mellitus
   (hypoglycemic medication requirements may be altered)

Gout, history of or
Hyperuricemia
   (serum uric acid concentrations may be elevated)

Hepatic function impairment
   (risk of dehydration which may precipitate hepatic coma and death; plasma half-life is unaltered)

Hypercalcemia or
Hypercholesterolemia or
Hypertriglyceridemia or
Hyponatremia
   (conditions may be exacerbated; onset of hyponatremia can be sudden and life-threatening)

Lupus erythematosus, history of
   (exacerbation or activation by thiazide diuretics has been reported)

Pancreatitis

Sensitivity to thiazide diuretics or other sulfonamide-derived medications

Sympathectomy
   (antihypertensive effects may be enhanced)

» Caution is required also in jaundiced infants because of the risk of hyperbilirubinemia.

## Patient monitoring

The following may be especially important in patient monitoring (other tests may be warranted in some patients, depending on condition; » = major clinical significance):

Blood glucose and
Blood urea nitrogen (BUN) and
Creatinine, serum and
Uric acid, serum
   (determinations recommended prior to initiation of therapy and if clinical signs of a significant increase occur)

» Blood pressure measurements
   (recommended at periodic intervals in patients being treated for hypertension; selected patients may be trained to perform blood pressure measurements at home and report the results at regular physician visits)

Cholesterol, serum and
Triglycerides serum
   (determinations recommended after 6 months of therapy and annually thereafter)

Electrolyte, serum, concentrations
   (determinations may be required for patients on long-term therapy, especially if they are also taking cardiac glycosides or systemic steroids, or when severe cirrhosis is present)

## Side/Adverse Effects

Note: Most side effects are dose-related.

The following side/adverse effects have been selected on the basis of their potential clinical significance (possible signs and symptoms in parentheses where appropriate)—not necessarily inclusive:

**Those indicating need for medical attention**
Incidence more frequent
   *Electrolyte imbalance such as hyponatremia,* (confusion; convulsions; decreased mentation; fatigue; irritability; muscle cramps); *hypochloremic alkalosis, and hypokalemia* (dryness of mouth; increased thirst; irregular heartbeat; mood or mental changes; muscle cramps or pain; nausea or vomiting; unusual tiredness or weakness; weak pulse)
   Note: *Hyponatremia* as a complication is rare, but constitutes a medical emergency as onset may be rapid.

Incidence rare
   *Agranulocytosis* (fever or chills; cough or hoarseness; lower back or side pain; painful or difficult urination); *allergic reaction* (skin rash or hives); *cholecystitis or pancreatitis* (severe stomach pain with nau-

sea and vomiting); *gout or hyperuricemia* (joint pain, lower back or side pain); *hepatic function impairment* (yellow eyes or skin); *thrombocytopenia* (unusual bleeding or bruising; black, tarry stools; blood in urine or stools; pinpoint red spots on skin)

**Those indicating need for medical attention only if they continue or are bothersome**
Incidence less frequent
   *Anorexia* (loss of appetite); *decreased sexual ability; diarrhea; orthostatic hypotension* (dizziness or lightheadedness when getting up from a lying or sitting position); *photosensitivity* (increased sensitivity of skin to sunlight); *upset stomach*

## Overdose

For more information on the management of overdose or unintentional ingestion, **contact a Poison Control Center** (see *Poison Control Center Listing*).

### Treatment of overdose

Thiazide diuretic overdose should be treated by immediate evacuation of the stomach followed by supportive, symptomatic treatment and monitoring of serum electrolyte concentrations and renal function.

## Patient Consultation

As an aid to patient consultation, refer to *Advice for the Patient, Diuretics, Thiazide (Systemic)*.

In providing consultation, consider emphasizing the following selected information (» = major clinical significance):

**Before using this medication**
» Conditions affecting use, especially:
   Sensitivity to thiazide diuretics, other sulfonamide-type medications, bumetanide, furosemide, or carbonic anhydrase inhibitors
   Pregnancy—Not recommended for routine use; may cause jaundice, thrombocytopenia, hypokalemia in infant
   Breast-feeding—Distributed into breast milk; recommended that nursing mothers avoid thiazides during first month of breast-feeding because of reports of suppression of lactation
   Use in children—Caution if giving to infants with jaundice
   Use in the elderly—Elderly patients may be more sensitive to hypotensive and electrolyte effects
   Other medications, especially cholestyramine, colestipol, digitalis glycosides, or lithium
   Other medical problems, especially anuria or severe renal function impairment or infants with jaundice

**Proper use of this medication**
   Diuretic effects of the medication and timing of doses to minimize inconvenience of diuresis (except in diabetes insipidus)
   Getting into habit of taking at same time each day to help increase compliance
   Proper administration of concentrated oral hydrochlorothiazide solution: Taking orally; special dropper to be used for accurate measuring
» Proper dosing
   Missed dose: Taking as soon as possible; not taking if almost time for next dose; not doubling doses
» Proper storage
*For use as an antihypertensive*
   Importance of diet; possible need for sodium restriction and/or weight reduction
» Patient may not experience symptoms of hypertension; importance of taking medication even if feeling well
» Does not cure, but helps control hypertension; possible need for life-long therapy; checking with physician before discontinuing medication; serious consequences of untreated hypertension

**Precautions while using this medication**
   Regular visits to physician to check progress
» Possibility of hypokalemia; possible need for additional potassium in diet; not changing diet without first checking with physician
   To prevent dehydration, checking with physician if severe nausea, vomiting, or diarrhea occurs and continues
   Diabetics: May increase blood sugar levels
   Possible photosensitivity; avoiding unprotected exposure to sun; using protective clothing and sun block product; avoiding use of sunlamp, tanning bed, or tanning booth
*For use as an antihypertensive*
» Not taking other medications, especially nonprescription sympathomimetics, unless discussed with physician

### Side/adverse effects

Signs of potential side effects, especially electrolyte imbalance, agranulocytosis, allergic reaction, cholecystitis, pancreatitis, hepatic function impairment, hyperuricemia, gout, and thrombocytopenia

## General Dosing Information

The lowest effective dosage should be utilized to minimize potential electrolyte imbalance and the reflex increase in renin and aldosterone levels.

A single daily dose is preferably taken on arising in order to minimize the effect of increased frequency of urination on sleep. When used to promote diuresis, intermittent dosage schedules (drug-free days) may reduce the possibility of electrolyte imbalance or hyperuricemia resulting from therapy.

Concurrent administration of potassium supplements or potassium-sparing diuretics may be indicated in patients considered to be at higher risk for developing hypokalemia. Caution in administering potassium supplements is recommended, however, since loss of potassium is not clinically significant in most patients, and supplementation leads to a risk of development of hyperkalemia.

Recent evidence suggests that withdrawal of antihypertensive therapy prior to surgery is not necessary, but that the anesthesiologist must be aware of such therapy.

### For hypertension

Low dose thiazide therapy has been found to be effective in the treatment of hypertension.

---

## *BENDROFLUMETHIAZIDE*

## Summary of Differences

Pharmacology/pharmacokinetics:
    Protein binding—Very high.
    Half-life—Normal: 8.5 hours.
    Onset of action—Diuretic: 1 to 2 hours.
    Time to peak effect—Diuretic: 4 hours.
    Duration of action—Diuretic: 6 to 12 hours.
Laboratory value alterations:
    May produce false negative results in phentolamine, phenolsulfonphthalein, and tyramine tests.

## Oral Dosage Forms

Note: Bracketed uses in the *Dosage Forms* section refer to categories of use and/or indications that are not included in U.S. product labeling.

### BENDROFLUMETHIAZIDE TABLETS USP

**Usual adult dose**
Diuretic or
[Antidiuretic (central or nephrogenic diabetes insipidus)][1]—
    Initial: Oral, 2.5 to 10 mg one or two times a day, once every other day, or once a day for three to five days a week.
    Maintenance: Oral, 2.5 to 5 mg once a day, once every other day, or once a day for three to five days a week.
Antihypertensive—
    Oral, 2.5 to 20 mg per day, as a single dose or in two divided daily doses, the dosage being adjusted according to response.
Note: Geriatric patients may be more sensitive to the effects of the usual adult dose.

**Usual pediatric dose**
Diuretic or
[Antidiuretic (central or nephrogenic diabetes insipidus)][1]—
    Initial: Oral, up to 400 mcg (0.4 mg) per kg of body weight or 12 mg per square meter of body surface a day, as a single dose or in two divided daily doses.
    Maintenance: Oral, 50 to 100 mcg (0.05 to 0.1 mg) per kg of body weight or 1.5 to 3 mg per square meter of body surface once a day.
Antihypertensive—
    Oral, 50 to 400 mcg (0.05 to 0.4 mg) per kg of body weight or 1.5 to 12 mg per square meter of body surface per day, as a single dose or in two divided daily doses, the dosage being adjusted according to response.

**Strength(s) usually available**
U.S.—
    5 mg (Rx) [*Naturetin* (scored; lactose)].
    10 mg (Rx) [*Naturetin* (scored; lactose)].
Canada—
    5 mg (Rx) [*Naturetin* (scored; tartrazine)].

### Packaging and storage

Store below 40 °C (104 °F), preferably between 15 and 30 °C (59 and 86 °F), unless otherwise specified by manufacturer. Store in a tight container.

### Auxiliary labeling

• Avoid overexposure to the sun or use of sunlamp.
• Do not take other medicines without your doctor's advice.

### Note

Check refill frequency to determine compliance in hypertensive patients.

---

[1]Not included in Canadian product labeling.

---

## *BENZTHIAZIDE*

## Summary of Differences

Pharmacology/pharmacokinetics:
    Onset of action—Diuretic: 2 hours.
    Time to peak effect—Diuretic: 4 to 6 hours.
    Duration of action—Diuretic: 12 to 18 hours.

## Oral Dosage Forms

Note: Bracketed uses in the *Dosage Forms* section refer to categories of use and/or indications that are not included in U.S. product labeling.

### BENZTHIAZIDE TABLETS USP

**Usual adult dose**
Diuretic or
[Antidiuretic (central or nephrogenic diabetes insipidus)]—
    Oral, 25 to 100 mg two times a day, once every other day, or once a day for three to five days a week.
Antihypertensive—
    Oral, 50 to 100 mg per day, as a single dose or in two divided daily doses, the dosage being adjusted according to response.
Note: Geriatric patients may be more sensitive to the effects of the usual adult dose.

**Usual pediatric dose**
Oral, 900 mcg (0.9 mg) to 3.9 mg per kg of body weight or 30 to 120 mg per square meter of body surface per day, as a single dose or in divided daily doses, adjusted according to response.

**Strength(s) usually available**
U.S.—
    50 mg (Rx) [*Exna* (scored; tartrazine); *Hydrex;* GENERIC].
Canada—
    Not commercially available.

### Packaging and storage

Store below 40 °C (104 °F), preferably between 15 and 30 °C (59 and 86 °F), unless otherwise specified by manufacturer. Store in a tight container.

### Auxiliary labeling

• Avoid overexposure to the sun or use of sunlamp.
• Do not take other medicines without your doctor's advice.

### Note

Check refill frequency to determine compliance in hypertensive patients.

---

## *CHLOROTHIAZIDE*

## Summary of Differences

Pharmacology/pharmacokinetics:
    Protein binding—Low to high.
    Half-life—Normal: 13 hours.
    Onset of action—Diuretic: 2 hours.
    Time to peak effect—Diuretic: 4 hours.
    Duration of action—Diuretic: 6 to 12 hours.

## Additional Dosing Information

See also *General Dosing Information.*
For parenteral dosage forms only—
    • Care must be taken to avoid extravasation during intravenous administration.
    • Chlorothiazide should not be administered intramuscularly or subcutaneously.

## Oral Dosage Forms

Note: Bracketed uses in the *Dosage Forms* section refer to categories of use and/or indications that are not included in U.S. product labeling.

## CHLOROTHIAZIDE ORAL SUSPENSION USP

**Usual adult dose**
Diuretic or
[Antidiuretic (central or nephrogenic diabetes insipidus)]—
    Oral, 250 mg every six to twelve hours.
Antihypertensive—
    Oral, 250 mg to 1 gram per day, as a single dose or in divided daily
    doses, the dosage being adjusted according to response.
Note: Geriatric patients may be more sensitive to the effects of the usual
    adult dose.

**Usual pediatric dose**
Children up to 6 months of age—Oral, 10 to 30 mg per kg of body weight
    per day, as a single dose or in two divided daily doses, the dosage
    being adjusted according to response.
Children 6 months of age and over—Oral, 10 to 20 mg per kg of body
    weight per day, as a single dose or in two divided daily doses, the
    dosage being adjusted according to response.

**Strength(s) usually available**
U.S.—
    50 mg per mL (Rx) [*Diuril* (alcohol 0.5%; glycerin; methylparaben
    0.12%; sodium saccharin; sucrose)].
Canada—
    Not commercially available.

**Packaging and storage**
Store below 40 °C (104 °F), preferably between 15 and 30 °C (59 and 86
    °F), unless otherwise specified by manufacturer. Store in a tight con-
    tainer. Protect from freezing.

**Auxiliary labeling**
• Shake well.
• Avoid overexposure to the sun or use of sunlamp.
• Do not take other medicines without your doctor's advice.

**Note**
Check refill frequency to determine compliance in hypertensive patients.

## CHLOROTHIAZIDE TABLETS USP

**Usual adult dose**
Diuretic or
[Antidiuretic (central or nephrogenic diabetes insipidus)]—
    Oral, 250 mg every six to twelve hours.
Antihypertensive—
    Oral, 250 mg to 1 gram per day, as a single dose or in divided daily
    doses, the dosage being adjusted according to response.
Note: Geriatric patients may be more sensitive to the effects of the usual
    adult dose.

**Usual pediatric dose**
Children up to 6 months of age—Oral, 10 to 30 mg per kg of body weight
    per day, as a single dose or in two divided daily doses, the dosage
    being adjusted according to response.
Children 6 months of age and over—Oral, 10 to 20 mg per kg of body
    weight per day, as a single dose or in two divided daily doses, the
    dosage being adjusted according to response.

**Strength(s) usually available**
U.S.—
    250 mg (Rx) [*Diuril* (scored); GENERIC (may be scored)].
    500 mg (Rx) [*Diuril* (scored); GENERIC (may be scored)].
Canada—
    Not commercially available.

**Packaging and storage**
Store below 40 °C (104 °F), preferably between 15 and 30 °C (59 and 86
    °F), in a well-closed container, unless otherwise specified by
    manufacturer.

**Auxiliary labeling**
• Avoid overexposure to the sun or use of sunlamp.
• Do not take other medicines without your doctor's advice.

**Note**
Check refill frequency to determine compliance in hypertensive patients.

## Parenteral Dosage Forms

Note: Bracketed uses in the *Dosage Forms* section refer to categories of
    use and/or indications that are not included in U.S. product labeling.

## CHLOROTHIAZIDE SODIUM FOR INJECTION USP

**Usual adult dose**
Diuretic or
[Antidiuretic (central or nephrogenic diabetes insipidus)]—
    Intravenous, 250 mg (base) every six to twelve hours.

Antihypertensive—
    Intravenous, 500 mg to 1 gram (base) of chlorothiazide a day, as a
    single dose or in two divided daily doses.
Note: Geriatric patients may be more sensitive to the effects of the usual
    adult dose.

**Usual pediatric dose**
Safety and efficacy have not been established.

**Size(s) usually available**
U.S.—
    500 mg (base) (Rx) [*Diuril* (mannitol 250 mg)].
Canada—
    Not commercially available.

**Packaging and storage**
Store below 40 °C (104 °F), preferably between 15 and 30 °C (59 and 86
    °F), unless otherwise specified by manufacturer.

**Stability**
Reconstituted solution may be stored at room temperature for 24 hours,
    after which it must be discarded.

**Incompatibilities**
Solutions of chlorothiazide are not compatible with whole blood or its
    derivatives.

**Additional information**
Chlorothiazide Sodium for Injection USP is reconstituted for intravenous
    administration by adding no less than 18 mL of sterile water for in-
    jection to the vial and shaking to dissolve, producing a solution con-
    taining 25 mg (base) per mL.
Reconstituted solutions may be further diluted with dextrose injection or
    0.9% sodium chloride injection for administration by intravenous
    infusion.

---

### CHLORTHALIDONE

## Summary of Differences

Pharmacology/pharmacokinetics:
    Although not chemically the same, chlorthalidone has the same actions
    as the thiazide diuretics.
    Protein binding—Very high to carbonic anhydrase in red blood cells.
    Half-life—Normal: 35 to 50 hours.
    Onset of action—Diuretic: 2 hours.
    Time to peak effect—Diuretic: 2 hours.
    Duration of action—Diuretic: 48 to 72 hours.

## Oral Dosage Forms
### CHLORTHALIDONE TABLETS USP

**Usual adult dose**
Diuretic—
    Oral, 25 to 100 mg once a day, or 100 to 200 mg once every other
    day, or once a day for three days a week.
Antihypertensive—
    Oral, 25 to 100 mg once a day, the dosage being adjusted according
    to response.
Note: Geriatric patients may be more sensitive to the effects of the usual
    adult dose.

**Usual pediatric dose**
Oral, 2 mg per kg of body weight or 60 mg per square meter of body
    surface once a day for three days a week, the dosage being adjusted
    according to response.

**Strength(s) usually available**
U.S.—
    25 mg (Rx) [*Hygroton; Thalitone;* GENERIC (may be scored)].
    50 mg (Rx) [*Hygroton;* GENERIC (may be scored)].
    100 mg (Rx) [*Hygroton* (scored); GENERIC (may be scored)].
Canada—
    50 mg (Rx) [*Apo-Chlorthalidone* (scored); *Hygroton* (scored); *Novo-
    Thalidone* (scored); *Uridon* (scored)].
    100 mg (Rx) [*Apo-Chlorthalidone* (scored); *Hygroton* (scored); *Novo-
    Thalidone* (scored); *Uridon* (scored)].

**Packaging and storage**
Store below 40 °C (104 °F), preferably between 15 and 30 °C (59 and 86
    °F), unless otherwise specified by manufacturer. Store in a well-closed
    container.

**Auxiliary labeling**
• Avoid overexposure to the sun or use of sunlamp.
• Do not take other medicines without your doctor's advice.

**Note**
Check refill frequency to determine compliance in hypertensive patients.

---

### CYCLOTHIAZIDE

## Summary of Differences

Pharmacology/pharmacokinetics:
Onset of action—Diuretic: Less than 6 hours.
Time to peak effect—Diuretic: 7 to 12 hours.
Duration of action—Diuretic: 18 to 24 hours.

## Oral Dosage Forms

Note: Bracketed uses in the *Dosage Forms* section refer to categories of use and/or indications that are not included in U.S. product labeling.

### CYCLOTHIAZIDE TABLETS USP

**Usual adult dose**
Diuretic or
[Antidiuretic (central or nephrogenic diabetes insipidus)]—
Oral, 1 to 2 mg once a day, once every other day, or once a day for two or three days a week.
Antihypertensive—
Oral, 2 mg once a day, the dosage being adjusted according to response.
Note: Geriatric patients may be more sensitive to the effects of the usual adult dose.

**Usual adult prescribing limits**
Up to 6 mg daily in divided doses.

**Usual pediatric dose**
Oral, 20 to 40 mcg (0.02 to 0.04 mg) per kg of body weight or 600 mcg (0.6 mg) to 1.2 mg per square meter of body surface once a day, the dosage being adjusted according to response.

**Strength(s) usually available**
U.S.—
2 mg (Rx) [*Anhydron* (scored)].
Canada—
Not commercially available.

**Packaging and storage**
Store below 40 °C (104 °F), preferably between 15 and 30 °C (59 and 86 °F), unless otherwise specified by manufacturer. Store in a well-closed container.

**Auxiliary labeling**
• Avoid overexposure to the sun or use of sunlamp.
• Do not take other medicines without your doctor's advice.

**Note**
Check refill frequency to determine compliance in hypertensive patients.

---

### HYDROCHLOROTHIAZIDE

## Summary of Differences

Pharmacology/pharmacokinetics:
Half-life—Normal: 15 hours.
Onset of action—Diuretic: 2 hours.
Time to peak effect—Diuretic: 4 hours.
Duration of action—Diuretic: 6 to 12 hours.

## Oral Dosage Forms

Note: Bracketed uses in the *Dosage Forms* section refer to categories of use and/or indications that are not included in U.S. product labeling.

### HYDROCHLOROTHIAZIDE ORAL SOLUTION

**Usual adult dose**
Diuretic or
[Antidiuretic (central or nephrogenic diabetes insipidus)]—
Oral, 25 to 100 mg one or two times a day, once every other day, or once a day for three to five days a week.
Antihypertensive—
Oral, 25 to 100 mg a day, as a single dose or in two divided daily doses, the dosage being adjusted according to response.
Note: Geriatric patients may be more sensitive to the effects of the usual adult dose.

**Usual pediatric dose**
Oral, 1 to 2 mg per kg of body weight or 30 to 60 mg per square meter of body surface per day, as a single dose or in two divided daily doses, the dosage being adjusted according to response.

Note: Infants under 6 months of age may receive up to 3 mg per kg of body weight per day.

**Strength(s) usually available**
U.S.—
10 mg per mL (Rx) [GENERIC].
100 mg per mL (Rx) [GENERIC].
Canada—
Not commercially available.

**Packaging and storage**
Store below 40 °C (104 °F), preferably between 15 and 30 °C (59 and 86 °F), in a well-closed container, unless otherwise specified by manufacturer. Protect from freezing.

**Auxiliary labeling**
• Avoid overexposure to the sun or use of sunlamp.
• Do not take other medicines without your doctor's advice.

**Note**
Check refill frequency to determine compliance in hypertensive patients.

Be careful not to confuse oral solution with concentrated oral solution.

Make sure patient understands how to measure dose of concentrated oral solution with calibrated dropper.

### HYDROCHLOROTHIAZIDE TABLETS USP

**Usual adult dose**
Diuretic or
[Antidiuretic (central or nephrogenic diabetes insipidus)][1]—
Oral, 25 to 100 mg one or two times a day, once every other day, or once a day for three to five days a week.
Antihypertensive—
Oral, 25 to 100 mg a day, as a single dose or in two divided daily doses, the dosage being adjusted according to response.
Note: Geriatric patients may be more sensitive to the effects of the usual adult dose.

**Usual pediatric dose**
Oral, 1 to 2 mg per kg of body weight or 30 to 60 mg per square meter of body surface per day, as a single dose or in two divided daily doses, the dosage being adjusted according to response.
Note: Infants under 6 months of age may receive up to 3 mg per kg of body weight per day.

**Strength(s) usually available**
U.S.—
25 mg (Rx) [*Esidrix* (scored); *HydroDIURIL* (scored); *Oretic* (scored); GENERIC (scored)].
50 mg (Rx) [*Esidrix* (scored); *Hydro-chlor; Hydro-D; HydroDIURIL* (scored); *Oretic* (scored); GENERIC (scored)].
100 mg (Rx) [*Esidrix* (scored); *HydroDIURIL* (scored); GENERIC (scored)].
Canada—
25 mg (Rx) [*Apo-Hydro* (scored); *HydroDIURIL* (scored); *Neo-Codema* (scored); *Novo-Hydrazide* (scored); *Urozide* (scored)].
50 mg (Rx) [*Apo-Hydro* (scored); *Diuchlor H* (scored); *HydroDIURIL* (scored); *Neo-Codema* (scored); *Novo-Hydrazide* (scored); *Urozide* (scored)].
100 mg (Rx) [*Apo-Hydro* (scored); *HydroDIURIL* (scored); *Urozide* (scored)].

**Packaging and storage**
Store below 40 °C (104 °F), preferably between 15 and 30 °C (59 and 86 °F), unless otherwise specified by manufacturer. Store in a well-closed container.

**Auxiliary labeling**
• Avoid overexposure to the sun or use of sunlamp.
• Do not take other medicines without your doctor's advice.

**Note**
Check refill frequency to determine compliance in hypertensive patients.

[1]Not included in Canadian product labeling.

---

### HYDROFLUMETHIAZIDE

## Summary of Differences

Pharmacology/pharmacokinetics:
Protein binding—High.
Onset of action—Diuretic: 1 to 2 hours.
Time to peak effect—Diuretic: 3 to 4 hours.
Duration of action—Diuretic: 18 to 24 hours.

# Oral Dosage Forms

Note: Bracketed uses in the *Dosage Forms* section refer to categories of use and/or indications that are not included in U.S. product labeling.

## HYDROFLUMETHIAZIDE TABLETS USP

**Usual adult dose**
Diuretic or
[Antidiuretic (central or nephrogenic diabetes insipidus)]—
    Oral, 25 to 100 mg one or two times a day, once every other day, or once a day for three to five days a week.
Antihypertensive—
    Oral, 50 to 100 mg per day, as a single dose or in two divided daily doses, the dosage being adjusted according to response.

Note: Geriatric patients may be more sensitive to the effects of the usual adult dose.

**Usual adult prescribing limits**
Up to 200 mg per day in divided doses.

**Usual pediatric dose**
Oral, 1 mg per kg of body weight or 30 mg per square meter of body surface once a day, the dosage adjusted according to response.

**Strength(s) usually available**
U.S.—
    50 mg (Rx) [*Diucardin* (scored); *Saluron* (scored); GENERIC (may be scored)].
Canada—
    Not commercially available.

**Packaging and storage**
Store below 40 °C (104 °F), preferably between 15 and 30 °C (59 and 86 °F), unless otherwise specified by manufacturer. Store in a tight container.

**Auxiliary labeling**
• Avoid overexposure to the sun or use of sunlamp.
• Do not take other medicines without your doctor's advice.

**Note**
Check refill frequency to determine compliance in hypertensive patients.

---

## METHYCLOTHIAZIDE

## Summary of Differences

Pharmacology/pharmacokinetics:
    Onset of action—Diuretic: 2 hours.
    Time to peak effect—Diuretic: 6 hours.
    Duration of action—Diuretic: More than 24 hours.

## Oral Dosage Forms

Note: Bracketed uses in the *Dosage Forms* section refer to categories of use and/or indications that are not included in U.S. product labeling.

## METHYCLOTHIAZIDE TABLETS USP

**Usual adult dose**
Diuretic or
[Antidiuretic (central or nephrogenic diabetes insipidus)][1]—
    Oral, 2.5 to 10 mg once a day, once every other day, or once a day for three to five days a week.
Antihypertensive—
    Oral, 2.5 to 5 mg once a day, the dosage being adjusted according to response.

Note: Doses beyond 5 mg once a day will usually not result in further lowering of blood pressure.

Note: Geriatric patients may be more sensitive to the effects of the usual adult dose.

**Usual pediatric dose**
Oral, 50 to 200 mcg (0.05 to 0.2 mg) per kg of body weight or 1.5 to 6 mg per square meter of body surface once a day, the dosage being adjusted according to response.

**Strength(s) usually available**
U.S.—
    2.5 mg (Rx) [*Enduron;* GENERIC (may be scored)].
    5 mg (Rx) [*Aquatensen; Enduron;* GENERIC (may be scored)].
Canada—
    5 mg (Rx) [*Duretic*].

**Packaging and storage**
Store below 40 °C (104 °F), preferably between 15 and 30 °C (59 and 86 °F), unless otherwise specified by manufacturer. Store in a well-closed container.

---

**Auxiliary labeling**
• Avoid overexposure to the sun or use of sunlamp.
• Do not take other medicines without your doctor's advice.

**Note**
Check refill frequency to determine compliance in hypertensive patients.

---

[1]Not included in Canadian product labeling.

---

## METOLAZONE

## Summary of Differences

Pharmacology/pharmacokinetics:
    Although not chemically the same, metolazone has actions similar to the thiazide diuretics.
    Absorption—More rapid and more complete with prompt metolazone tablets than with extended metolazone tablets.
    Protein binding—Very high (50 to 70% to red blood cells).
    Half-life—Normal: 8 hours.
    Onset of action—Diuretic: 1 hour.
    Time to peak effect—Diuretic: 2 hours.
    Duration of action—Diuretic: 12 to 24 hours.
    Elimination—Metolazone undergoes some enterohepatic recycling, and slightly greater amounts are excreted in the bile.

## Additional Dosing Information

*Extended metolazone tablets and prompt metolazone tablets should not be substituted for one another* because of significant differences in rate of absorption and bioavailability.

Absorption of metolazone after oral administration is reduced in patients with cardiac disease (65% in normal subjects as compared with 40% in cardiac disease patients).

Plasma clearance of metolazone is 20 mL per minute in patients with renal failure as compared with 110 mL per minute in healthy subjects.

Duration of diuretic effect is dose-related.

Metolazone may be more effective as a diuretic than other thiazides in patients with severe renal failure. Because of this, metolazone has been added to furosemide therapy in resistant patients; however, caution is necessary because of the risk of severe electrolyte imbalance.

## Oral Dosage Forms

## EXTENDED METOLAZONE TABLETS

**Usual adult dose**
Diuretic—
    Oral, 5 to 20 mg once a day.
Antihypertensive—
    Oral, 2.5 to 5 mg once a day, the dosage being adjusted according to response.

Note: Geriatric patients may be more sensitive to the effects of the usual adult dose.

**Usual pediatric dose**
Dosage has not been established.

**Strength(s) usually available**
U.S.—
    2.5 mg (Rx) [*Diulo; Zaroxolyn*].
    5 mg (Rx) [*Diulo; Zaroxolyn*].
    10 mg (Rx) [*Diulo; Zaroxolyn*].
Canada—
    2.5 mg (Rx) [*Zaroxolyn*].
    5 mg (Rx) [*Zaroxolyn*].
    10 mg (Rx) [*Zaroxolyn*].

**Packaging and storage**
Store below 40 °C (104 °F), preferably between 15 and 30 °C (59 and 86 °F), in a well-closed container, unless otherwise specified by manufacturer.

**Auxiliary labeling**
• Avoid overexposure to the sun or use of sunlamp.
• Do not take other medicines without your doctor's advice.

**Note**
Extended and prompt metolazone tablets are not bioequivalent. *One product should not be substituted for the other.* If patients are to be transferred from one to the other, retitration and appropriate changes in dosage may be necessary.

Check refill frequency to determine compliance in hypertensive patients.

## PROMPT METOLAZONE TABLETS

**Usual adult dose**
Antihypertensive—
  Initial: Oral, 500 mcg (0.5 mg) once a day, the dosage being adjusted according to response.
  Maintenance: Oral, 500 mcg (0.5 mg) to 1 mg once a day.

**Usual adult prescribing limits**
Up to 1 mg per day.

**Usual pediatric dose**
Dosage has not been established.

**Strength(s) usually available**
U.S.—
  500 mcg (0.5 mg) (Rx) [*Mykrox*].
Canada—
  Not commercially available.

**Packaging and storage**
Store below 40 °C (104 °F), preferably between 15 and 30 °C (59 and 86 °F), in a well-closed container, unless otherwise specified by manufacturer.

**Auxiliary labeling**
• Avoid overexposure to the sun or use of sunlamp.
• Do not take other medicines without your doctor's advice.

**Note**
Extended and prompt metolazone tablets are not bioequivalent. *One product should not be substituted for the other.* If patients are to be transferred from one to the other, retitration and appropriate changes in dosage may be necessary.

Check refill frequency to determine compliance in hypertensive patients.

---

### POLYTHIAZIDE

## Summary of Differences
Pharmacology/pharmacokinetics:
  Protein binding—High.
  Onset of action—Diuretic: 2 hours.
  Time to peak effect—Diuretic: 6 hours.
  Duration of action—Diuretic: 24 to 48 hours.

## Oral Dosage Forms
Note: Bracketed uses in the *Dosage Forms* section refer to categories of use and/or indications that are not included in U.S. product labeling.

### POLYTHIAZIDE TABLETS USP

**Usual adult dose**
Diuretic or
[Antidiuretic (central or nephrogenic diabetes insipidus)]—
  Oral, 1 to 4 mg once a day, once every other day, or once a day for three to five days a week.
Antihypertensive—
  Oral, 2 to 4 mg once a day, the dosage being adjusted according to response.
Note: Geriatric patients may be more sensitive to the effects of the usual adult dose.

**Usual pediatric dose**
Oral, 20 to 80 mcg (0.02 to 0.08 mg) per kg of body weight or 500 mcg (0.5 mg) to 2.5 mg per square meter of body surface once a day, the dosage being adjusted according to response.

**Strength(s) usually available**
U.S.—
  1 mg (Rx) [*Renese* (scored; lactose)].
  2 mg (Rx) [*Renese* (scored; lactose)].
  4 mg (Rx) [*Renese* (scored; lactose)].
Canada—
  Not commercially available.

**Packaging and storage**
Store below 40 °C (104 °F), preferably between 15 and 30 °C (59 and 86 °F), unless otherwise specified by manufacturer. Store in a tight, light-resistant container.

**Auxiliary labeling**
• Avoid overexposure to the sun or use of sunlamp.
• Do not take other medicines without your doctor's advice.

**Note**
Check refill frequency to determine compliance in hypertensive patients.

---

### QUINETHAZONE

## Summary of Differences
Pharmacology/pharmacokinetics:
  Although not chemically the same, quinethazone has the same actions as the thiazide diuretics.
  Onset of action—Diuretic: 2 hours.
  Time to peak effect—Diuretic: 6 hours.
  Duration of action—Diuretic: 18 to 24 hours.

## Oral Dosage Forms

### QUINETHAZONE TABLETS USP

**Usual adult dose**
Diuretic or
Antihypertensive—
  Oral, 50 to 200 mg per day, as a single dose or in two divided daily doses, adjusted according to response.

Note: Geriatric patients may be more sensitive to the effects of the usual adult dose.

**Usual adult prescribing limits**
Up to 200 mg daily in divided doses.

**Usual pediatric dose**
Dosage has not been established.

**Strength(s) usually available**
U.S.—
  50 mg (Rx) [*Hydromox* (scored)].
Canada—
  Not commercially available.

**Packaging and storage**
Store below 40 °C (104 °F), preferably between 15 and 30 °C (59 and 86 °F), unless otherwise specified by manufacturer. Store in a tight container.

**Auxiliary labeling**
• Avoid overexposure to the sun or use of sunlamp.
• Do not take other medicines without your doctor's advice.

**Note**
Check refill frequency to determine compliance in hypertensive patients.

---

### TRICHLORMETHIAZIDE

## Summary of Differences
Pharmacology/pharmacokinetics:
  Onset of action—Diuretic: 2 hours.
  Time to peak effect—Diuretic: 6 hours.
  Duration of action—Diuretic: Up to 24 hours.
Laboratory value alterations:
  May produce false negative results in phentolamine, phenolsulfonphthalein, and tyramine tests.

## Oral Dosage Forms
Note: Bracketed uses in the *Dosage Forms* section refer to categories of use and/or indications that are not included in U.S. product labeling.

### TRICHLORMETHIAZIDE TABLETS USP

**Usual adult dose**
Diuretic or
[Antidiuretic (central or nephrogenic diabetes insipidus)]—
  Oral, 1 to 4 mg once a day, once every other day, or once a day for three to five days a week.
Antihypertensive—
  Oral, 2 to 4 mg once a day, the dosage being adjusted according to response.
Note: Geriatric patients may be more sensitive to the effects of the usual adult dose.

**Usual pediatric dose**
For children over 6 months of age—Oral, 70 mcg (0.07 mg) per kg of body weight or 2 mg per square meter of body surface per day, as a single dose or in two divided daily doses, the dosage being adjusted according to response.

**Strength(s) usually available**
U.S.—
  2 mg (Rx) [*Metahydrin; Naqua* (scored); GENERIC].
  4 mg (Rx) [*Metahydrin; Naqua* (scored); *Trichlorex*; GENERIC].

Canada—
  Not commercially available.

**Packaging and storage**
Store below 40 °C (104 °F), preferably between 15 and 30 °C (59 and 86 °F), unless otherwise specified by manufacturer. Store in a tight container.

**Auxiliary labeling**
• Avoid overexposure to the sun or use of sunlamp.
• Do not take other medicines without your doctor's advice.

**Note**
Check refill frequency to determine compliance in hypertensive patients.

## Selected Bibliography

The fifth report of the Joint National Committee on Detection, Evaluation, and Treatment of High Blood Pressure (JNC V). Arch Intern Med 1993; 153 (2): 154-83.
Freis ED. The cardiovascular risks of thiazide diuretics. Clin Pharmacol Ther 1986 Mar; 39: 239-44.
Brater DC. Clinical use of thiazide diuretics. Hosp Form 1983; 18: 788-93.

Revised: 06/07/92
Interim revision: 06/30/94

---

**DIVALPROEX**—See *Valproic Acid (Systemic)*

---

**DOBUTAMINE**—See *Sympathomimetic Agents—Cardiovascular Use (Parenteral-Systemic)*

---

**DOCUSATE**—See *Laxatives (Local)*

---

## DOCUSATE-CONTAINING COMBINATIONS—

Bisacodyl and Docusate (Oral-Local)—See *Laxatives (Local)*
Casanthranol and Docusate (Oral-Local)—See *Laxatives (Local)*
Danthron and Docusate (Oral-Local)—See *Laxatives (Local)*
Dehydrocholic Acid and Docusate (Oral-Local)—See *Laxatives (Local)*
Dehydrocholic Acid, Docusate, and Phenolphthalein (Oral-Local)—See *Laxatives (Local)*
Phenolphthalein and Docusate (Oral-Local)—See *Laxatives (Local)*
Sennosides and Docusate (Oral-Local)—See *Laxatives (Local)*

---

**DOPAMINE**—See *Sympathomimetic Agents—Cardiovascular Use (Parenteral-Systemic)*

---

# DORNASE ALFA  Inhalation-Local

VA CLASSIFICATION (Primary): RE900

Other commonly used names are: recombinant human deoxyribonuclease I (rhDNase) and DNase I.

Note: For a listing of dosage forms and brand names by country availability, see *Dosage Forms* section(s). For a listing of brand names for the articles in this monograph, refer to the General Index.

## Category

Cystic fibrosis therapy adjunct.

## Indications

**Accepted**

Cystic fibrosis (treatment adjunct)—Dornase alfa is indicated in the treatment of cystic fibrosis patients to reduce the frequency of respiratory infections requiring parenteral antibiotics and to improve pulmonary function. It is used in conjunction with standard therapies, including antibiotics and bronchodilators.

Safety and efficacy have not been demonstrated in patients with forced vital capacity (FVC) less than 40% of normal. No studies have been performed with dornase alfa for longer than 12 months.

## Pharmacology/Pharmacokinetics

**Physicochemical characteristics**

Source—Produced by genetically engineered Chinese Hamster Ovary (CHO) cells containing deoxyribonucleic acid (DNA) encoding for DNase

Chemical group—A purified glycoprotein containing 260 amino acids in primary sequence identical to that of the native human enzyme, deoxyribonuclease (DNase)

Molecular weight—37,000 daltons.

**Mechanism of action/Effect**

The bronchial secretions of cystic fibrosis patients contain high levels of highly polymerized, polyanionic DNA, which is released by disintegrating inflammatory cells, especially polymorphonuclear neutrophils, present after lung infections. The excess DNA causes an already abnormal sputum to thicken. The viscous, dehydrated mucus is difficult to expectorate, obstructs airways, and contributes to reduced lung volumes and expiratory flow rates. The accumulation of purulent secretions in the airways provides a continuing growth medium for bacteria, causing chronic pulmonary infections, which are the major cause of morbidity and mortality in cystic fibrosis.

*In vitro* studies have shown that DNase, an enzyme normally produced in small quantities in the pancreas and salivary glands and present in saliva, blood, and urine, significantly reduces the viscoelasticity of sputum in patients with cystic fibrosis by breaking the long extracellular DNA molecule into smaller fragments.

When dornase alfa (rhDNase) is administered every day by inhalation via a nebulizer, lung function is improved and sustained, as evidenced by pulmonary function tests, and the frequency of pulmonary infections requiring the use of parenteral antibiotics is reduced.

**Onset of action**

Significant improvement in lung function—Within 3 days to 1 week.
Reduction in respiratory tract infections—Weeks to months.

## Precautions to Consider

**Carcinogenicity**

No carcinogenicity studies have been completed. A two-year inhalation toxicity study of dornase alfa in rats to assess oncogenic potential is in progress.

**Mutagenicity**

Ames tests using six different strains of bacteria at concentrations of up to 5000 mcg per plate, a cytogenic assay using human peripheral blood lymphocytes at concentrations of up to 2000 mcg per plate, and a mouse lymphoma assay at concentrations of up to 1000 mcg per plate, with and without metabolic activation, showed no evidence of mutagenic potential.

A micronucleus assay in bone marrow cells of mice, conducted after administration of a bolus intravenous dose of 10 mg per kg of body weight (mg/kg) of dornase alfa on two consecutive days, showed no evidence of chromosomal damage.

**Pregnancy/Reproduction**

Fertility—Studies in rats and rabbits given intravenous doses of dornase alfa of up to 10 mg/kg per day (more than 600 times the exposure expected following the recommended human dose) showed no evidence of impairment of fertility in males or females.

Pregnancy—Adequate and well-controlled studies in humans have not been done.

Studies in rats and rabbits given intravenous doses of up to 10 mg/kg per day (more than 600 times the exposure expected following the recommended human dose) showed no evidence of harm or effects on development of the fetus.

FDA Pregnancy Category B.

**Breast-feeding**

It is not known whether dornase alfa is distributed into breast milk.

**Pediatrics**

Appropriate studies on the relationship of age to the effects of dornase alfa have not been performed in children under 5 years of age. Safety and efficacy have not been established.

**Geriatrics**

No information is available on the relationship of age to the effects of dornase alfa in geriatric patients.

**Drug interactions and/or related problems**

Possible drug interactions with dornase alfa have not been studied. However, the medication has been used safely and effectively in conjunction with other medications commonly given orally, parenterally, or via inhalation to patients with cystic fibrosis, including antibiotics, bronchodilators, corticosteroids, enzymes, vitamins, and analgesics.

**Medical considerations/Contraindications**

The medical considerations/contraindications included here have been selected on the basis of their potential clinical significance (reasons given in parentheses where appropriate)—not necessarily inclusive (» = major clinical significance).

*Risk-benefit should be considered when the following medical problem exists:*

Sensitivity to dornase alfa, Chinese Hamster Ovary cell products, or any component of the product

## Side/Adverse Effects

The following side/adverse effects have been selected on the basis of their potential clinical significance (possible signs and symptoms in parentheses where appropriate)—not necessarily inclusive:

**Those indicating need for medical attention only if they continue or are bothersome**

Incidence more frequent
   *Chest pain or discomfort; sore throat; voice changes*
Incidence less frequent
   *Conjunctivitis* (redness, itching, pain, swelling, or other irritation of eyes); *hoarseness; skin rash*

## Patient Consultation

As an aid to patient consultation, refer to *Advice for the Patient, Dornase Alfa (Inhalation)*.

In providing consultation, consider emphasizing the following selected information (» = major clinical significance):

**Before using this medication**
» Conditions affecting use, especially:
   Sensitivity to dornase alfa

**Proper use of this medication**
   Reading patient instructions carefully
» Not using ampul that has been previously opened; not using medication if out of date
» Not using if medication is cloudy or discolored
» Using only with power-operated nebulizer and compressor recommended by manufacturer of medication
» Importance of knowing how to use the medication in the nebulizer; using only with the mouthpiece provided with the nebulizer; not using a face mask
» Compliance with therapy; using at same time every day; some improvement may occur within one week; some patients may require weeks to months for full benefits
» Importance of continuing other cystic fibrosis medications as before; not mixing any other medication with dornase alfa in nebulizer; using other medications, such as inhalation bronchodilators, before or after dornase alfa treatment
   Preparation of nebulizer for use
   Preparation of medication for use in nebulizer; method of opening ampul and emptying ampul contents into nebulizer cup; using all medication in ampul
   Proper administration technique
   Proper care of nebulizer and compressor after use
» Proper dosing
   Missed dose: Taking missed dose as soon as possible; if almost time for next dose, skipping missed dose and going back to regular dosing schedule

» Proper storage: Keeping ampuls in refrigerator in foil pouches at all times; not freezing; not leaving out of refrigerator at room temperature for more than a total of 24 hours

**Precautions while using this medication**
» Checking with physician if condition becomes worse

## General Dosing Information

Dornase alfa inhalation solution is administered by nebulization. The only nebulizers and compressors that should be used are the Hudson T Updraft II disposable jet nebulizer and the Marquest Acorn II disposable jet nebulizer with the Pulmo-Aide compressor, and the reusable PARI LC Jet+ nebulizer with the PARI PRONEB compressor. Safety and efficacy have not been studied with other systems. Therefore, battery-operated systems and ultrasonic nebulizers are not recommended for dornase alfa administration.

A mouthpiece is provided with each nebulizer. A face mask is not recommended because it may reduce delivery of the medication to the lungs.

It is advisable to wash hands thoroughly before assembling the nebulizer and adding the medication. The surface used for assembling the nebulizer must also be clean. The nebulizer and its parts must be kept clean at all times, according to the manufacturer's directions.

Dornase alfa solution should not be mixed or diluted with any other medication in the nebulizer cup because of possible physicochemical incompatibilities. However, other concurrently used medications, such as inhaled bronchodilators, may be administered before or after dornase alfa treatment.

Dornase alfa must be administered every day to maintain its therapeutic effect. A decline in pulmonary function is seen within 48 hours following cessation of therapy.

## Inhalation Dosage Forms

### DORNASE ALFA SOLUTION FOR INHALATION

**Usual adult and adolescent dose**
Cystic fibrosis therapy adjunct—
   Oral inhalation, 2.5 mg per day via nebulization, the dosage being increased to 2.5 mg two times a day if necessary.

**Usual pediatric dose**
Cystic fibrosis therapy adjunct—
   Children up to 5 years of age: Safety and efficacy have not been established.
   Children 5 years of age and over: See *Usual adult and adolescent dose*.

**Strength(s) usually available**
U.S.—
   1 mg per mL (2.5-mL single-use ampul) (Rx) [*Pulmozyme*].
Canada—
   1 mg per mL (2.5-mL single-use ampul) (Rx) [*Pulmozyme*].

**Packaging and storage**
Store between 2 and 8 °C (36 and 46 °F), unless otherwise specified by manufacturer. Protect from light.

**Stability**
Ampul should be discarded if contents are cloudy or discolored.
Unopened ampuls should not be exposed to temperatures over 30 °C (86 °F) for longer than twenty-four hours.
Opened ampul must be used at once or discarded.

**Incompatibilities**
Dornase alfa solution should not be mixed or diluted with any other medication in the nebulizer cup because of possible physicochemical incompatibilities.

**Auxiliary labeling**
• For inhalation only.

Developed: 09/02/94

# DORZOLAMIDE   Ophthalmic†

VA CLASSIFICATION (Primary): OP109

Note: For a listing of dosage forms and brand names by country availability, see *Dosage Forms* section(s). For a listing of brand names for the articles in this monograph, refer to the General Index.

†Not commercially available in Canada.

## Category
Antiglaucoma agent (ophthalmic).

## Indications

### Accepted
Glaucoma, open-angle (treatment) or

Hypertension, ocular (treatment)—Dorzolamide is indicated in the treatment of elevated intraocular pressure in patients with ocular hypertension or open-angle glaucoma.

## Pharmacology/Pharmacokinetics

### Physicochemical characteristics
Chemical group—Sulfonamide.

Molecular weight—360.91.

pH—Dorzolamide hydrochloride ophthalmic solution: Approximately 5.6.

### Mechanism of action/Effect
Dorzolamide is a sulfonamide and a carbonic anhydrase inhibitor. Carbonic anhydrase is an enzyme found in many tissues of the body, including the eye. Carbonic anhydrase catalyzes the reversible reaction involving the hydration of carbon dioxide and the dehydration of carbonic acid. In humans, carbonic anhydrase exists as a number of isoenzymes, the most active of which is carbonic anhydrase II. Carbonic anhydrase II is found primarily in red blood cells, but it also appears in other tissues.

Antiglaucoma agent—Dorzolamide inhibits human carbonic anhydrase II. Inhibition of carbonic anhydrase in the ciliary processes of the eye decreases aqueous humor secretion, presumably by slowing the formation of bicarbonate ions, with subsequent reduction in sodium and fluid transport. The result is a reduction in intraocular pressure. In clinical studies of up to 1 year in duration in patients with glaucoma or ocular hypertension who had baseline intraocular pressure (IOP) of ≥ 23 mm of mercury (mm Hg), dorzolamide had an IOP-lowering effect of approximately 3 to 5 mm Hg throughout the day.

### Other actions/effects
When dorzolamide was administered orally in doses of 2 mg twice a day for up to 20 weeks to 8 healthy volunteers, inhibition of both carbonic anhydrase II activity and total carbonic anhydrase activity was less than the degree of inhibition considered to be necessary for a pharmacological effect on renal function and respiration in healthy persons. (The oral dose of 2 mg twice a day closely approximates the amount of medication delivered systemically by ophthalmic administration of 2% dorzolamide 3 times a day.)

### Absorption
Dorzolamide is systemically absorbed when applied to the eye. In a study designed to simulate systemic absorption during long-term ophthalmic administration, 8 healthy subjects were given 2 mg of oral dorzolamide twice a day for up to 20 weeks. (The oral dose of 2 mg twice a day closely approximates the amount of medication delivered systemically by ophthalmic administration of 2% dorzolamide 3 times a day.) Steady state was reached within 8 weeks.

### Distribution
During chronic dosing, dorzolamide accumulates in red blood cells by binding to carbonic anhydrase II. The N-desethyl metabolite also accumulates in red blood cells by binding primarily to carbonic anhydrase I. Plasma concentrations of dorzolamide and the N-desethyl metabolite are generally below the minimum assay limit of 15 nanomoles.

### Protein binding
Moderate (approximately 33%).

### Biotransformation
The only metabolite is the active N-desethyl derivative, which inhibits carbonic anhydrase II to a lesser extent than does dorzolamide. The N-desethyl metabolite also inhibits carbonic anhydrase I.

### Half-life
After therapy is discontinued, dorzolamide washes out of red blood cells in a nonlinear fashion, resulting in a rapid initial decline in blood concentration, followed by a slower elimination phase having a half-life of about 4 months.

### Time to peak effect
Approximately 2 hours.

### Elimination
Primarily renal, as unchanged dorzolamide and the N-desethyl metabolite.

## Precautions to Consider

### Cross-sensitivity and/or related problems
Patients sensitive to other carbonic anhydrase inhibitors or other sulfonamides, including furosemide, thiazide diuretics, and oral antidiabetic agents, may be sensitive to dorzolamide also.

### Tumorigenicity
In a 21-month study in female and male mice, dorzolamide administered orally in doses of up to 75 mg per kg of body weight (mg/kg) a day (greater than 900 times the recommended human ophthalmic dose) did not result in any treatment-related tumors. In addition, no changes in bladder urothelium were seen in dogs given dorzolamide orally for 1 year at a dose of 2 mg/kg a day (25 times the recommended human ophthalmic dose) or monkeys given dorzolamide topically to the eye for 1 year at a dose of 0.4 mg/kg a day (greater than 5 times the recommended human ophthalmic dose). However, in a 2-year study in male and female Sprague-Dawley rats, dorzolamide administered orally at the highest dose of 20 mg/kg a day (250 times the recommended human ophthalmic dose) produced urinary bladder papillomas in the male rats. Papillomas were not seen in the rats that received the lower oral doses, equivalent to approximately 12 times the recommended human ophthalmic dose. The increased incidence of urinary bladder papillomas seen in the male rats given the highest dose of dorzolamide is also seen in rats given other medications of the carbonic anhydrase inhibitor class. Rats are particularly prone to develop papillomas in response to foreign bodies, compounds causing crystalluria, or diverse sodium salts.

### Mutagenicity
The *in vivo* (mouse) cytogenetic assay, *in vitro* chromosomal aberration assay, alkaline elution assay, V-79 assay, and Ames test were negative for mutagenic potential.

### Pregnancy/Reproduction
Fertility—There were no adverse effects on the reproductive capacity of either male or female rats given oral doses of dorzolamide of up to 188 or 94 times, respectively, the recommended human ophthalmic dose.

Pregnancy—Adequate and well-controlled studies in humans have not been done.

Developmental toxicity studies in rabbits given dorzolamide orally in doses ≥ 2.5 mg/kg a day (31 times the recommended human ophthalmic dose) revealed malformations of the vertebral bodies of the fetuses. Administration of dorzolamide at these doses also caused metabolic acidosis with reduction in body weight gain in dams and decreased weight in fetuses. No treatment-related fetal malformations were seen in rabbits given dorzolamide at a dose of 1 mg/kg a day (13 times the recommended human ophthalmic dose). In addition, there were no treatment-related fetal malformations in developmental toxicity studies in rats given dorzolamide orally at doses of up to 10 mg/kg a day (125 times the recommended human ophthalmic dose).

FDA Pregnancy Category C.

### Breast-feeding
It is not known whether ophthalmic dorzolamide is distributed into breast milk. However, since there is the potential for serious adverse reactions with systemically absorbed carbonic anhydrase inhibitors, including ophthalmic dorzolamide, a decision should be made whether to discontinue breast-feeding or discontinue the medication.

In a study in lactating rats, dorzolamide administered orally at a dose of 7.5 mg/kg a day (94 times the recommended human ophthalmic dose) caused a reduction in body weight gain of 5 to 7% in the pups. In addition, a slight delay in postnatal development (incisor eruption, vaginal canalization, and eye opening) secondary to lower fetal body weight was noted.

### Pediatrics
Appropriate studies on the relationship of age to the effects of dorzolamide have not been performed in the pediatric population. Safety and efficacy have not been established.

## Geriatrics

In clinical studies, 44 and 10% of the total number of patients were 65 and 75 years of age and over, respectively, and no overall differences in effectiveness or safety were observed between these patients and younger patients. Geriatrics-specific problems that would limit the usefulness of this medication in the elderly are not expected.

## Drug interactions and/or related problems

The following drug interactions and/or related problems have been selected on the basis of their potential clinical significance (possible mechanism in parentheses where appropriate)—not necessarily inclusive (» = major clinical significance):

Note: Combinations containing any of the following medications, depending on the amount present, may also interact with this medication.

Amphetamines or
Mecamylamine or
Quinidine

(when amphetamines, mecamylamine, or quinidine are used concurrently with systemic carbonic anhydrase inhibitors, especially acetazolamide, therapeutic and/or side effects may be enhanced or prolonged as a result of decreased elimination caused by alkalinization of urine. A study has shown that ophthalmic dorzolamide does not cause alkalinization of urine when administered in normal therapeutic doses (see *Pharmacology, Other actions/effects*); nonetheless, medical experts suggest that dosage adjustments of amphetamines or quinidine may be needed when ophthalmic dorzolamide therapy is initiated or discontinued. In addition, some medical experts suggest that concurrent use with mecamylamine is not recommended, whereas other medical experts suggest that dosage adjustments of mecamylamine may be needed when ophthalmic dorzolamide therapy is initiated or discontinued)

» Silver preparations, ophthalmic, such as silver nitrate
(topical sulfonamides are incompatible with silver salts; since ophthalmic dorzolamide is a sulfonamide, concurrent use with ophthalmic silver preparations is not recommended)

## Medical considerations/Contraindications

The medical considerations/contraindications included here have been selected on the basis of their potential clinical significance (reasons given in parentheses where appropriate)—not necessarily inclusive (» = major clinical significance).

*Except under special circumstances, this medication should not be used when the following medical problem exists:*

» Sensitivity to dorzolamide

*Risk-benefit should be considered when the following medical problems exist:*

Hepatic function impairment
(dorzolamide has not been studied in patients with hepatic impairment; caution should be used if the medication is used in these patients, since dorzolamide is metabolized by the liver)

» Renal calculi or history of
(may be exacerbated or induced during therapy)

Renal function impairment, severe
(dorzolamide and its metabolite are excreted primarily by the kidney; use of dorzolamide is not recommended in patients with a creatinine clearance of less than 30 mL per minute)

## Side/Adverse Effects

Note: Since dorzolamide is a sulfonamide, the same types of adverse reactions that may occur with other sulfonamides may occur with dorzolamide also. With other sulfonamides, fatalities have occurred rarely because of severe reactions, including Stevens-Johnson syndrome, toxic epidermal necrolysis, fulminant hepatic necrosis, agranulocytosis, aplastic anemia, and other blood dyscrasias. If signs of serious reaction or hypersensitivity occur, *use of dorzolamide should be discontinued.*

In clinical studies, local ocular adverse effects, primarily conjunctivitis and eyelid reactions, were reported with chronic administration of dorzolamide. Many of these reactions had the clinical appearance and course of an allergic-type reaction that resolved upon discontinuation of the medication. If local ocular adverse effects such as conjunctivitis and eyelid reactions occur, *use of dorzolamide should be discontinued and the patient evaluated* before a decision is made whether to restart the medication.

Although acid-base and electrolyte disturbances were not reported in the clinical trials of dorzolamide, they have been reported with use of oral carbonic anhydrase inhibitors and have, in some in-

stances, resulted in drug interactions (e.g., toxicity associated with high-dose salicylate therapy).

Carbonic anhydrase activity has been observed in the cytoplasm and around the plasma membranes of the corneal endothelium. However, the effect of continued administration of dorzolamide on the corneal endothelium has not been evaluated fully.

The following side/adverse effects have been selected on the basis of their potential clinical significance (possible signs and symptoms in parentheses where appropriate)—not necessarily inclusive:

### Those indicating need for medical attention

Incidence more frequent
*Allergic reaction, ocular* (itching, redness, swelling, or other sign of eye or eyelid irritation)—incidence 10%

Incidence rare
*Iridocyclitis* (eye pain, tearing, and blurred vision); *skin rash; urolithiasis* (blood in urine; nausea or vomiting; pain in side, back, or abdomen)

### Those indicating need for medical attention only if they continue or are bothersome

Incidence more frequent
*Bitter taste*—incidence approximately 25%; *burning, stinging, or discomfort when medicine is applied*—incidence 33%; *superficial punctate keratitis* (feeling of something in eye; sensitivity of eyes to light)—incidence 10 to 15%

Incidence less frequent
*Asthenia* (unusual tiredness or weakness)—infrequently; *blurred vision*—incidence 1 to 5%; *dryness of eyes*—incidence 1 to 5%; *fatigue* (unusual tiredness or weakness)—infrequently; *headache*—infrequently; *nausea*—infrequently; *photophobia* (sensitivity of eye to light)—incidence 1 to 5%; *tearing*—incidence 1 to 5%

## Patient Consultation

As an aid to patient consultation, refer to *Advice for the Patient, Dorzolamide (Ophthalmic)*.

In providing consultation, consider emphasizing the following selected information (» = major clinical significance):

### Before using this medication

» Conditions affecting use, especially:
Sensitivity to dorzolamide, other carbonic anhydrase inhibitors, or other sulfonamides
Pregnancy—One study in animals has shown maternal toxicity and fetal birth defects at very high doses
Breast-feeding—Carbonic anhydrase inhibitors (including ophthalmic dorzolamide) have the potential for serious adverse reactions; a decision should be made whether to discontinue breast-feeding or discontinue the medication
Use in children—Safety and efficacy have not been established
Other medications, especially ophthalmic silver preparations such as silver nitrate
Other medical problems, especially renal calculi or history of

### Proper use of this medication

Proper administration technique for ophthalmic solution
» Importance of using medication only as directed
Waiting 10 minutes between the use of 2 different ophthalmic preparations to prevent "washing out" of the first one
» Proper dosing
Missed dose: Using as soon as possible; not using if almost time for next dose; not doubling doses
» Proper storage

### Precautions while using this medication

Regular visits to physician to check progress during therapy
Checking with physician if signs of ocular allergic reaction, such as itching, redness, swelling, or other sign of eye or eyelid irritation, occur
» Caution if blurred vision occurs temporarily; checking with physician if blurred vision continues, since it may be sign of adverse effect
Possible sensitivity of eyes to sunlight or bright light; wearing sunglasses and avoiding exposure to bright light; checking with physician if discomfort continues

### Side/adverse effects

Signs of potential side effects, especially ocular allergic reaction, iridocyclitis, skin rash, and urolithiasis

## General Dosing Information

The efficacy of dorzolamide administered less frequently than 3 times a day (whether alone or in combination with other products) has not been established.

Because of the preservative, benzalkonium chloride, the manufacturer recommends that patients not wear soft contact lenses during treatment with dorzolamide ophthalmic solution. However, medical experts do not believe this precaution is necessary unless the patient has corneal epithelial problems and the medication is to be used more often than once every 1 to 2 hours. No significant problems have been documented with the use of ophthalmic solutions containing 0.03% or less of benzalkonium chloride as a preservative in patients with no significant corneal surface problems.

Dorzolamide may be used concurrently with other medications instilled in the eye to lower intraocular pressure. However, the medications should be administered at least 10 minutes apart.

## Ophthalmic Dosage Forms

### DORZOLAMIDE HYDROCHLORIDE OPHTHALMIC SOLUTION

**Usual adult and adolescent dose**
Antiglaucoma agent (ophthalmic)—
Topical to the conjunctiva, 1 drop three times a day.

**Usual pediatric dose**
Safety and efficacy have not been established.

**Strength(s) usually available**
U.S.—
2% (20 mg base) (22.3 mg as the hydrochloride) (Rx) [*Trusopt* (benzalkonium chloride 0.0075%; hydroxyethyl cellulose; mannitol; sodium citrate dihydrate; sodium hydroxide; water for injection)].
Canada—
Not commercially available.

**Packaging and storage**
Store between 15 and 30 °C (59 and 86 °F), unless otherwise specified by manufacturer. Protect from light and freezing.

**Auxiliary labeling**
• For the eye.

## Selected Bibliography

Serle JB. Pharmacological advances in the treatment of glaucoma. Drugs Aging 1994 Sep; 5 (3): 156-70.
Wilkerson M, Cyrlin M, Lippa EA, et al. Four-week safety and efficacy study of dorzolamide, a novel, active topical carbonic anhydrase inhibitor. Arch Ophthalmol 1993 Oct; 111 (10): 1343-50.

Developed: 01/31/96

# DOXACURIUM Systemic†

VA CLASSIFICATION (Primary): MS300
Note: For a listing of dosage forms and brand names by country availability, see *Dosage Forms* section(s). For a listing of brand names for the articles in this monograph, refer to the General Index.

†Not commercially available in Canada.

## Category
Neuromuscular blocking agent.

## Indications

**Accepted**
Muscle (skeletal) relaxation, for surgery—Doxacurium is indicated as an adjunct to anesthesia to facilitate endotracheal intubation and to induce skeletal muscle relaxation in the surgical field. Doxacurium has a long duration of action in adults; use of doses sufficient to facilitate endotracheal intubation should be considered only for procedures expected to last 90 minutes or longer.

**Unaccepted**
Doxacurium has not been adequately studied for facilitating prolonged mechanical ventilation in intensive-care patients.

## Pharmacology/Pharmacokinetics

**Physicochemical characteristics**
Molecular weight—1106.15.

**Mechanism of action/Effect**
Doxacurium is a nondepolarizing (competitive) neuromuscular blocking agent. Nondepolarizing neuromuscular blocking agents inhibit neuromuscular transmission by competing with acetylcholine for the cholinergic receptors of the motor end plate, thereby reducing the response of the end plate to acetylcholine. This type of neuromuscular block is usually antagonized by anticholinesterase agents. The paralysis is selective initially and usually appears in the following muscles consecutively: levator muscles of eyelids, muscles of mastication, limb muscles, abdominal muscles, muscles of the glottis, and finally, the intercostal muscles and the diaphragm. Neuromuscular blocking agents have no clinically significant effect on consciousness or the pain threshold.

**Distribution**
Volume of distribution (steady-state)—
Normal renal function: About 0.22 L per kg of body weight (L/kg) (range, 0.11–0.43 L/kg), in nongeriatric patients. Values within this range have also been reported for geriatric patients (about 0.22 [range, 0.14 to 0.40] L/kg) and for patients with hepatic failure undergoing hepatic transplantation (about 0.29 [range, 0.17 to 0.35] L/kg).
Renal function impairment: About 0.27 (range, 0.17 to 0.55) L/kg, determined in patients with end-stage renal failure undergoing renal transplantation.

**Protein binding**
Low (about 30%).

**Biotransformation**
Metabolites have not been detected in studies performed to date.

**Half-life**
Elimination—
Normal renal function: About 86 to 123 (range, 25 to 193) minutes, with doses ranging between 15 and 80 mcg per kg of body weight (mcg/kg). Values within this range have also been reported for geriatric patients (about 96 [range, 50 to 114] minutes) and patients undergoing hepatic transplantation (about 115 [range, 69 to 148] minutes).
Renal function impairment: About 221 (range, 84 to 592) minutes, determined following administration to patients with end-stage renal failure undergoing kidney transplantation.

**Onset of action**
Time to achieve intubating conditions—
Note: The onset of action of each dose of doxacurium is dependent on dosage and on the age of the patient. The ED$_{95}$ (dose of a neuromuscular blocking agent required to produce 95% suppression of the adductor pollicis muscle twitch response to ulnar nerve stimulation) is lower after establishment of steady-state anesthesia with a potent volatile inhalation agent (e.g., enflurane, halothane, isoflurane) than during other types of anesthesia. The following values were not obtained during steady-state anesthesia with a volatile agent.
50 mcg/kg: About 5 minutes.
80 mcg/kg: About 4 minutes.
Note: Information on the time to achieve intubating conditions with lower doses of doxacurium has not been published; however, when a dose of 25 mcg/kg is administered after succinylcholine-assisted intubation, 90% suppression of the response to peripheral nerve stimulation occurs in about 6 minutes.

**Time to peak concentration**
About 2 minutes following administration of an initial dose of 30 mcg/kg or a supplemental dose of 5 mcg/kg administered after 25% recovery from the initial dose.

**Peak serum concentration**
30 mcg/kg—About 340 nanograms per mL (0.31 micromoles/L).
5 mcg/kg (supplemental dose)—90 to 100 nanograms per mL (0.08 to 0.09 micromoles/L); values are consistent for all supplemental doses given at 25% recovery from the previous initial (30 mcg/kg) or supplemental (5 mcg/kg) dose, when the doxacurium concentration has decreased to about 44.75 nanograms per mL (0.04 micromoles/L).

**Time to peak effect**
Note: The time to peak effect is dependent on dosage and the age of the patient. Also, it is shorter during anesthesia with a volatile inhalation agent (specified below when applicable) than during other types of anesthesia. However, the time to peak effect is not altered

by prior administration of an intubating dose (1 mg per kg of body weight [mg/kg]) of succinylcholine, provided that doxacurium is administered after recovery of the twitch response to 10% or more of the control value.

In most patients, recommended doses of doxacurium produce maximal responses of 90 to 95% (or even higher) inhibition of the twitch response to peripheral nerve stimulation. However, patients with hepatic failure may be somewhat resistant to the effects of doxacurium; a maximal response of only 70% inhibition of the twitch response was achieved in these patients by a dose that produced higher maximal responses in patients with normal hepatic function.

Time to maximal suppression of the twitch response to peripheral nerve stimulation—
  Children 2 to 12 years of age (halothane anesthesia):
    30 mcg/kg—About 7 minutes.
    50 mcg/kg—About 4 minutes.
  Adults up to 50 years of age with normal hepatic and renal function:
    25 mcg/kg—About 8 to 10 (range, 5.4 to 16) minutes.
    50 mcg/kg—About 4 to 5 (range, 2.5 to 13) minutes.
    80 mcg/kg—About 3.5 (range, 2.4 to 5) minutes.
  Adults up to 55 years of age with end-stage renal failure undergoing renal transplantation:
    Tends to be longer than in nongeriatric adults with normal renal function.
  Adults up to 55 years of age with hepatic failure undergoing hepatic transplantation:
    Tends to be longer than in nongeriatric adults with normal hepatic function.
  Adults older than 65 years of age with normal hepatic and renal function:
    25 mcg/kg (isoflurane anesthesia)—About 11 minutes; slightly more prolonged than in nongeriatric patients with normal hepatic and renal function.

### Duration of action

Note: Doxacurium's duration of action (for both initial and supplemental doses) is dependent on dosage, the age of the patient, and the clearance rate from plasma (which is at least partially dependent on the patient's renal function), as well as being subject to substantial interpatient variability. The duration of action is more prolonged during anesthesia with a volatile anesthetic (specified below when applicable) than during other types of anesthesia. However, cumulative effects on the duration or depth of neuromuscular blockade do not occur when supplemental doses of doxacurium are given after 25% recovery from an initial dose. Also, the duration of action is not significantly altered by prior administration of an intubating dose (1 mg/kg) of succinylcholine, provided that doxacurium is administered after the twitch response has returned to 10% or more of the control value.

Duration of clinical effect (time for spontaneous recovery of the twitch response to peripheral nerve stimulation to 25% of the control value)—
  Children 2 to 12 years of age (halothane anesthesia):
    30 mcg/kg—About 25 to 30 minutes.
    50 mcg/kg—About 45 to 50 minutes.
  Adults up to 50 years of age with normal renal and hepatic function:
    Initial dose—
      25 mcg/kg: About 55 (range, 9 to 145) minutes.
      40 mcg/kg: About 70 to 85 minutes.
      50 mcg/kg: About 100 (range, 39 to 232) minutes.
      60 mcg/kg: About 123 minutes.
      80 mcg/kg: About 160 (range, 110 to 338) minutes.
    Supplemental dose, administered after 25% recovery from an initial 25 mcg/kg dose—
      5 mcg/kg: About 30 (range, 9 to 57) minutes.
      10 mcg/kg: About 45 (range, 14 to 108) minutes.
  Adults older than 65 years of age with normal renal and hepatic function:
    25 mcg/kg (isoflurane anesthesia)—About 97 (range, 36 to 179) minutes; more variable and more prolonged than in younger adults.
  Adults up to 55 years of age with end-stage renal failure undergoing renal transplantation:
    Values tend to be more variable, as well as more prolonged, than in patients with normal renal function.
    Halothane anesthesia—
      25 mcg/kg initial dose: About 120 minutes.
      5 mcg/kg supplemental dose, administered after 25% recovery from the initial dose: About 27.5 minutes.
    Isoflurane anesthesia—
      15 mcg/kg—About 80 (range, 29 to 133) minutes.

Adults up to 55 years of age with hepatic failure undergoing hepatic transplantation:
  15 mcg/kg (isoflurane anesthesia)—About 52 (range, 20 to 91) minutes; longer than in patients with normal hepatic function.
Recovery index (time for the twitch response to peripheral stimulation to increase, spontaneously, from 25% to 75% of the control value)—
  Children 2 to 12 years of age (halothane anesthesia):
    About 27 to 34 minutes (range, 11.2 to 57.5) minutes, with doxacurium doses ranging from 27.5 to 50 mcg/kg.
  Adults up to 50 years of age with normal renal and hepatic function:
    25 mcg/kg—About 51 minutes.
    50 mcg/kg—About 84 (range, 40 to 128) minutes.
Time to spontaneous 95% recovery of the twitch response to peripheral stimulation—Determined in adults up to 50 years of age with normal renal and hepatic function—
    25 mcg/kg—Average 74 minutes, but up to 4 hours in some patients.
    40 mcg/kg—Average 126 minutes.
    50 mcg/kg—Average 204 minutes.

### Elimination

Renal and biliary, as unchanged doxacurium; 24 to 38% of a dose is eliminated in the urine within 6 to 12 hours. The overall extent of biliary excretion is unknown.
  Plasma clearance rate—
    Adults:
      Normal renal function—About 2.2 to 2.6 (range, 1 to 6.6) mL/minute/kg. Values determined over a dose range of 15 to 80 mcg/kg in nongeriatric adults, with 25 mcg/kg in geriatric patients, and with 15 mcg/kg in patients undergoing hepatic transplantation are all within this range.
      Renal failure (patients undergoing transplantation)—About 1.23 (range, 0.48 to 2.4) mL/minute/kg.

## Precautions to Consider

### Carcinogenicity

Carcogenicity studies have not been done.

### Mutagenicity

No mutagenicity was detected in the Ames *Salmonella* assay, mouse lymphoma assay, and human lymphocyte assay. However, statistically significant increases in the incidence of structural abnormalities, relative to vehicle controls, occurred in the *in vivo* rat bone marrow cytogenic assay in male rats receiving 0.1 mg per kg of body weight (mg/kg) (0.625 mg per square meter of body surface area [mg/m$^2$]) when the animals were sacrificed 6 hours, but not 24 or 48 hours, after administration. Structural abnormalities also occurred in female rats administered 0.2 mg/kg (1.25 mg/m$^2$) when the animals were sacrificed 24 hours, but not 6 or 48 hours, after administration. Abnormalities did not occur in male or female rats receiving 0.3 mg/kg (1.875 mg/m$^2$) at any time after administration. Because of the lack of a dose-dependent effect, the likelihood that the abnormalities found in this study were treatment-related or are clinically significant is low.

### Pregnancy/Reproduction

Fertility—Studies have not been done.

Pregnancy—Adequate and well-controlled studies have not been done in pregnant women.

No maternal or fetal toxicity or teratogenicity was found in animal studies performed in nonventilated mice and rats receiving subcutaneous injections of subparalyzing doses.

FDA Pregnancy Category C.

Labor and delivery—Doxacurium has not been studied in obstetrics (labor, vaginal delivery, or Cesarean section). Doxacurium is not recommended for Cesarean section because its duration of action exceeds the expected duration of the surgical procedure.

### Breast-feeding

It is not known whether doxacurium is distributed into breast milk.

### Pediatrics

Neonates—Doxacurium injection contains benzyl alcohol, which is not recommended for administration to neonates. A fatal toxic syndrome consisting of metabolic acidosis, CNS depression, respiratory problems, renal failure, hypotension, and possibly seizures and intracranial hemorrhages has been associated with use of this preservative in neonates.

Children 2 to 12 years of age—These patients are less sensitive to the effects of doxacurium than are adults. Higher doses (on a mcg/kg basis) are required to achieve comparable levels of neuromuscular blockade. Even with higher doses, the onset of action, the duration of clinical effect (time for the twitch response to peripheral stimulation to return to 25% of the control value), and the recovery index (time for the spontaneous recovery from 25% to 75% of the twitch response to peripheral stimulation) are all significantly shorter in children than in adults.

## Geriatrics

Appropriate studies performed to date have shown that elderly patients may be more sensitive than younger adults to the neuromuscular blocking effect of doxacurium. However, the time to maximum block is longer in elderly patients. The duration of clinical effect tends to be longer and more variable in elderly patients. Also, elderly patients are more likely to have age-related renal function impairment, which may also increase sensitivity to, and the duration of action of, doxacurium. The risk of an undesirably prolonged duration of effect in geriatric patients may be reduced by reducing initial dosage and titrating additional doses to achieve the desired response.

## Drug interactions and/or related problems

The following drug interactions and/or related problems have been selected on the basis of their potential clinical significance (possible mechanism in parentheses where appropriate)—not necessarily inclusive (» = major clinical significance):

Note: Combinations containing any of the following medications, depending on the amount present, may also interact with this medication.

Some of the following interactions have not been documented with doxacurium. However, because they have been reported to occur with other nondepolarizing neuromuscular blocking agents, the possibility of a significant interaction with doxacurium must be considered.

» Aminoglycosides, possibly including oral neomycin (if significant quantities are absorbed in patients with renal function impairment) or
Anesthetics, parenteral-local (large doses leading to significant plasma concentrations) or
Bacitracin or
» Capreomycin or
» Citrate-anticoagulated blood (massive transfusions) or
» Clindamycin or
Colistin or
Colistimethate sodium or
Lidocaine (intravenous doses > 5 mg/kg) or
» Lincomycin or
» Polymyxins or
Procaine (intravenous) or
Tetracyclines or
Trimethaphan (large doses)
(neuromuscular blocking activity of these medications may be additive to that of neuromuscular blocking agents; increased or prolonged respiratory depression or paralysis [apnea] may occur, but is of minor clinical significance while the patient is being mechanically ventilated; however, reversal agents have sometimes been ineffective in reversing neuromuscular blockade potentiated by aminoglycosides, clindamycin, lincomycin, or polymyxins; caution and careful monitoring of the patient are recommended during and following concurrent or sequential use, especially if there is a possibility of incomplete reversal of neuromuscular blockade postoperatively)

Analgesics, opioid (narcotic), especially those commonly used as adjuncts to anesthesia
(central respiratory depressant effects of opioid analgesics may be additive to the respiratory depressant effects of neuromuscular blocking agents; increased or prolonged respiratory depression or paralysis [apnea] may occur, but is of minor clinical significance while the patient is being mechanically ventilated; however, caution and careful monitoring of the patient are recommended during and following concurrent or sequential use, especially if there is a possibility of incomplete reversal of neuromuscular blockade postoperatively)

(concurrent use of a neuromuscular blocking agent prevents or reverses muscle rigidity induced by sufficiently high doses of most opioid analgesics, especially alfentanil, fentanyl, or sufentanil)

Anesthetics, hydrocarbon inhalation, such as:
Chloroform
Cyclopropane
Enflurane
Ether
Halothane
Isoflurane
Methoxyflurane
Trichloroethylene
(neuromuscular blocking activity of inhalation hydrocarbon anesthetics, especially enflurane or isoflurane, may be additive to that

of nondepolarizing neuromuscular blocking agents; a reduction of doxacurium dosage may be necessary when it is given after steady-state anesthesia with one of these anesthetics has been established)

Antihypertensives or other hypotension-inducing medications or
Bradycardia-inducing medications
(doxacurium does not counteract hypotension or bradycardia induced by other medications or vagal stimulation; the incidence and/or severity of these effects may be increased, especially in patients with compromised cardiac function and in patients receiving 2 or more medications that may decrease heart rate and/or blood pressure [e.g., benzodiazepines, beta-adrenergic blocking agents, calcium channel blocking agents, opioid analgesics] prior to and/or during surgery)

Antimyasthenics or
Edrophonium
(these agents antagonize the effects of nondepolarizing neuromuscular blocking agents; parenteral neostigmine or pyridostigmine are indicated to reverse neuromuscular blockade following surgery; edrophonium in a dose of 1 mg/kg is not recommended for reversal of moderate to deep levels of doxacurium-induced blockade because it has been reported to be less effective than neostigmine [dose of 60 or 80 mcg/kg (0.06 or 0.08 mg/kg)]; use of pyridostigmine for reversal of doxacurium-induced blockade has not been studied)

(neuromuscular blocking agents may antagonize the effects of antimyasthenics on skeletal muscle; temporary dosage adjustment may be required to control symptoms of myasthenia gravis following surgery)

Calcium channel blocking agents
(although an interaction with doxacurium has not been documented, verapamil and nifedipine have been shown to potentiate the effects of several other neuromuscular blocking agents; also, difficulty in reversing verapamil-potentiated neuromuscular blockade with a single dose of neostigmine has been reported)

Calcium salts
(calcium salts may reverse the effects of nondepolarizing neuromuscular blocking agents)

Carbamazepine and/or
Phenytoin
(resistance to the effects of doxacurium, leading to a lengthening of the time needed to achieve adequate skeletal muscle relaxation and to significantly accelerated recovery from an initial or supplemental dose, may occur in patients receiving chronic carbamazepine and/or phenytoin therapy)

Lithium or
Magnesium salts, parenteral or
» Procainamide or
» Quinidine
(these medications may enhance the blockade of the neuromuscular blocking agents; increased or prolonged respiratory depression or paralysis [apnea] may occur but is of minor clinical significance while the patient is being mechanically ventilated; however, caution and careful monitoring of the patient are recommended during and following concurrent or sequential use, especially if there is a possibility of incomplete reversal of neuromuscular blockade postoperatively)

Neuromuscular blocking agents, other
(prior administration of succinylcholine [for endotracheal intubation] does not potentiate the effects of doxacurium, provided that doxacurium is administered after recovery from the effects of succinylcholine has begun)

(administration of doxacurium in conjunction with other nondepolarizing neuromuscular blocking agents has not been studied)

## Medical considerations/Contraindications

The medical considerations/contraindications included here have been selected on the basis of their potential clinical significance (reasons given in parentheses where appropriate)—not necessarily inclusive (» = major clinical significance).

### Risk-benefit should be considered when the following medical problems exist:

Burns
(doxacurium has not been studied in burn patients; the possibility of resistance, depending on the age and size of the burn, should be considered)

Carcinoma, bronchogenic
(duration of action of neuromuscular blocking agents may be prolonged)

Dehydration or
Electrolyte or acid-base imbalance, especially
Hypokalemia
(action of neuromuscular blocking agents may be altered; neuromuscular blockade is usually counteracted by alkalosis and enhanced by acidosis, but mixed imbalances may be present, leading to unpredictable responses)

(serum potassium determinations may be advisable prior to administration of a nondepolarizing neuromuscular blocking agent, because hypokalemia tends to enhance the blockade produced by these medications; adjustment of dosage of the neuromuscular blocking agent, or correction of potassium concentration prior to administration, may be needed; increased or prolonged respiratory depression or paralysis [apnea] may occur but is of minor clinical significance while the patient is being mechanically ventilated; however, caution and careful monitoring of the patient are recommended during and following concurrent or sequential use, especially if there is a possibility of incomplete reversal of neuromuscular blockade postoperatively)

Hepatic function impairment
(patients with hepatic failure undergoing hepatic transplantation appear less sensitive to the effects of doxacurium than patients with normal hepatic function; a comparative study [in which the same dose was administered under the same type of anesthesia] indicated a tendency toward a slower onset of action and achievement of less intense neuromuscular blockade [maximum block of only 70% and an unusually high incidence of failure to produce more than 50% block] in the hepatic failure patients; however, there was also a tendency toward a prolonged duration of clinical effect in those patients with hepatic failure in whom more than 50% block was achieved)

(doxacurium has not been studied in patients with lesser degrees of hepatic function impairment; caution is recommended)

Hypothermia
(intensity and duration of action of nondepolarizing neuromuscular blocking agents may be increased)

Myasthenia gravis or
Myasthenic syndrome (Eaton-Lambert syndrome)
(increased risk of severe and prolonged muscle paralysis or weakness; a neuromuscular blocking agent with a shorter duration of action may be preferable [although caution is required even with shorter-acting agents])

Pulmonary function impairment or
Respiratory depression
(risk of additive respiratory depression or impairment)

» Renal function impairment
(clearance of doxacurium is decreased, leading to a prolonged elimination half-life and duration of action, in patients with end-stage renal disease undergoing renal transplantation; clearance continues to be decreased after the transplanted kidney begins functioning; these patients may also be more sensitive to the effects of doxacurium than patients with normal renal function; use of a neuromuscular blocking agent with a more predictable duration of action in patients with renal function impairment, i.e., atracurium or vecuronium, may be preferred)

Sensitivity to doxacurium

Caution is also advised if a long-acting neuromuscular blocking agent such as doxacurium is used to assist endotracheal intubation in a patient with a potentially difficult airway; some anesthesiologists recommend that an endotracheal tube be inserted (with the assistance of a short-acting agent) before a long-acting agent is given to such a patient.

## Side/Adverse Effects

Note: Unlike gallamine and pancuronium, doxacurium has no vagolytic activity. Also, histamine release following administration of doxacurium appears minimal, although isolated cases of increased serum histamine or symptoms possibly associated with histamine release (hypotension, cutaneous flushing, urticaria, bronchospasm, or wheezing) have been reported. Therefore, doxacurium causes minimal hemodynamic disturbance, although bradycardia and/or hypotension may occur because doxacurium does not counteract the bradycardia and/or hypotension induced by other medications (e.g., anesthetics, opioid analgesics) or vagal stimulation.

Doxacurium failed to trigger malignant hyperthermia in one study in malignant hyperthermia–susceptible swine (in doses up to 4 times the ED$_{95}$).

The following side/adverse effects have been selected on the basis of their potential clinical significance (possible signs and symptoms in parentheses where appropriate)—not necessarily inclusive:

**Those indicating need for medical attention**
Incidence rare (< 0.1%–0.3%)
*Cardiovascular effects* (flushing; hypotension); *double vision; fever; injection site reaction; respiratory effects* (bronchospasm; wheezing); *urticaria*

## Overdose

For specific information on the agents used in the management of doxacurium overdose see:
- *Atropine* in *Anticholinergics/Antispasmodics (Systemic)* monograph;
- *Glycopyrrolate* in *Anticholinergics/Antispasmodics (Systemic)* monograph; and/or
- *Neostigmine* in *Antimyasthenics (Systemic)* monograph.

For more information on the management of overdose or unintentional ingestion, **contact a Poison Control Center** (see *Poison Control Center Listing*).

**For treatment of overdose**
Specific treatment—
Administering an anticholinesterase agent, e.g., neostigmine (40 to 80 mcg/kg, depending on the dose of doxacurium) to antagonize the action of doxacurium. It is recommended that reversal of doxacurium-induced neuromuscular blockade be attempted only after some spontaneous recovery, as demonstrated using a peripheral nerve stimulator, has taken place. Recovery will not occur as rapidly if the antagonist is administered earlier. Also, higher doses of the anticholinesterase may be needed when more profound levels of block are present (3 or fewer responses to train-of-four stimulation) at the time of reversal. Recovery of the single twitch response to 80% of the control value with recommended doses of neostigmine, when administered after 25% spontaneous recovery has occurred, usually occurs in about 5 minutes; 90 to 95% recovery usually occurs within 20 (range, 7 to 55) minutes. However, recovery of the response to train-of-four stimulation (T$_4$:T$_1$ ratio) is slower than recovery of the response to single twitch stimulation. A T$_4$:T$_1$ ratio of 0.7 generally indicates 90 to 95% recovery. Edrophonium (1 mg per kg of body weight) does not antagonize the effects of doxacurium as rapidly as neostigmine, even when given after > 25% spontaneous recovery has occurred, and is not recommended for reversing moderate to deep levels of block (< 60% recovery). Use of pyridostigmine for antagonism of doxacurium has not been studied. It is recommended that a suitable antimuscarinic agent (e.g., atropine, glycopyrrolate) be administered prior to or concurrently with the antagonist to counteract its muscarinic side effects. However, use of an antagonist is merely an adjunct to, and not to be substituted for, the institution of measures to ensure adequate ventilation.

Monitoring—
Determining the degree of the neuromuscular blockade, using a peripheral nerve stimulator. Monitoring of vital organ function for the period of paralysis and for an extended period post-recovery. Monitoring the patient following successful antagonism, because the duration of action of doxacurium may exceed that of the antagonist.

Supportive care for apnea or prolonged paralysis—
Maintaining an adequate airway and assisting or controlling ventilation. Ventilatory assistance should be continued until adequate spontaneous ventilation can be maintained. Ventilatory assistance must be continued until the patient can maintain an adequate ventilatory exchange unassisted. Administration of a sedative or an anxiolytic may be needed if paralysis continues or recurs and/or mechanical ventilation is maintained after the patient is awake.

## General Dosing Information

Neuromuscular blocking agents have no clinically significant effect on consciousness or the pain threshold; therefore, when used as an adjunct to surgery, the neuromuscular blocking agent should always be used with adequate anesthesia or sedation.

Since neuromuscular blocking agents may cause respiratory depression, they should be used only by those individuals experienced in the techniques of tracheal intubation, artificial respiration, and the administration of oxygen under positive pressure; facilities for these procedures should be immediately available.

Doxacurium is intended for intravenous administration only.

The stated doses are intended as a guideline. Actual dosage must be individualized. It is recommended that a peripheral nerve stimulator be used to monitor response, need for additional doses, and reversal.

The $ED_{95}$ (dose required to produce maximum [95%] suppression of the adductor pollicis muscle twitch response to ulnar nerve stimulation) is about 25 (range, 20 to 33) mcg per kg of body weight (mcg/kg). The $ED_{95}$ may be higher in patients with hepatic failure than in patients with normal hepatic function.

When nondepolarizing neuromuscular blocking agents are administered after anesthesia with a volatile inhalation anesthetic has been established, a reduction in dosage, as determined using a peripheral nerve stimulator, may be required. Halothane may cause less potentiation of doxacurium than either enflurane or isoflurane. However, in one study, administration of 15 mcg/kg of doxacurium with isoflurane (the dose having been selected as approximating the $ED_{95}$ for that anesthetic) produced maximum neuromuscular blockade of only 70% in patients undergoing hepatic transplantation and only 86% in patients with normal hepatic function.

The $ED_{95}$ in children 2 to 12 years of age (halothane anesthesia) is about 30 (range, 12 to 52) mcg/kg.

A reduction of initial dosage may be advisable in geriatric, very ill, or debilitated patients; patients with impaired renal function, neuromuscular disease, severe electrolyte abnormalities, or carcinomatosis; and other patients in whom there is a risk of potentiation of neuromuscular blockade or difficulty with reversal. Supplemental doses should be titrated according to patient response.

Higher initial doses may be needed in burn patients and in patients with hepatic failure. However, clinically effective block, once attained in patients with hepatic failure, may persist somewhat longer than in patients with normal hepatic function.

For obese patients (> 30% above ideal body weight for height), dosage of doxacurium should be calculated on the basis of ideal body weight.

## Parenteral Dosage Forms

Note: The dosing and the strength of the dosage form available are expressed in terms of doxacurium base.

### DOXACURIUM CHLORIDE INJECTION

**Usual adult dose**
Neuromuscular blocking agent—
   Initial:
     For endotracheal intubation and surgical relaxation—
       Intravenous, 50 mcg (0.05 mg) (base) per kg of body weight, to provide adequate intubating conditions in about five minutes and about one hundred minutes of relaxation, or
       Intravenous, 80 mcg (0.08 mg) per kg of body weight, to provide adequate intubating conditions in about four minutes and an average of one hundred sixty minutes of relaxation.
       Note: Satisfactory intubating conditions are attained more slowly when initial doses lower than 50 mcg (0.05 mg) are administered.
     For surgical relaxation only, following succinylcholine-assisted endotracheal intubation—
       Intravenous, 25 mcg (0.025 mg) per kg of body weight, to provide an average of sixty minutes of relaxation. Higher doses may be used if a longer duration of relaxation is required.
   Maintenance:
     Intravenous, to be administered after the twitch response to an initial dose has returned to about 25% of the control value or after reappearance of the second twitch response to train-of-four stimulation—
       5 mcg (0.005 mg) per kg of body weight, to provide about thirty minutes of relaxation, or

10 mcg (0.01 mg) per kg of body weight, to provide about forty-five minutes of relaxation.
       Note: Higher or lower maintenance doses may be given, depending on the desired duration of action.
          The interval between maintenance doses is subject to considerable interindividual variability.

**Usual pediatric dose**
Neuromuscular blocking agent—
   Children up to 2 years of age: Dosage has not been established.
   Children 2 to 12 years of age (inhalation [halothane] anesthesia): Intravenous, 30 mcg (0.03 mg) (base) per kg of body weight, to provide maximum block in about seven minutes and about thirty minutes of relaxation, or
   Intravenous, 50 mcg (0.05 mg) per kg of body weight, to provide maximum block in about four minutes and about forty-five minutes of relaxation.
Note: Maintenance doses are generally required more frequently than in adults.

**Strength(s) usually available**
U.S.—
   1 mg per mL (Rx) [*Nuromax* (0.9% benzyl alcohol)].
Canada—
   Not commercially available.

**Packaging and storage**
Store between 15 and 25 °C (59 and 77 °F), unless otherwise specified by manufacturer. Protect from freezing.

**Preparation of dosage form**
If necessary, doxacurium chloride injection may be diluted up to 1 in 10 with 5% dextrose injection or 0.9% sodium chloride injection.

**Stability**
Doxacurium chloride injection is stable when diluted up to 1 in 10 with 5% dextrose injection or 0.9% sodium chloride injection, when the diluted product is stored in polypropylene syringes and kept at a temperature of 5 to 25 °C (41 to 77 °F) for up to 24 hours.

Diluting the injection diminishes the effectiveness of the preservative in the formulation. Careful attention to aseptic technique is required. It is recommended that the injection be administered immediately after dilution, and that any unused portion of the diluted injection be discarded after 8 hours.

Doxacurium chloride injection is compatible (for Y-site administration) with 5% dextrose injection, 0.9% sodium chloride injection, 5% dextrose and 0.9% sodium chloride injection, and lactated Ringer's injection, and, when the following are diluted as recommended by the manufacturer, with alfentanil hydrochloride injection, fentanyl citrate injection, and sufentanil citrate injection.

**Incompatibilities**
Doxacurium chloride injection is acidic and may not be compatible with alkaline solutions having a pH > 8.5 (e.g., barbiturate injections).

## Selected Bibliography

Estafanous GF, ed. Clinical experience with a new long-acting neuromuscular blocking agent. Proceedings of a symposium. J Cardiothoracic Anesthesia 1990; 4 (Suppl 4): 1-42.

Sarner JB, Brandom BW, Cook DR, et al. Clinical pharmacology of doxacurium chloride (BW A938U) in children. Anesth Analg 1988; 67: 303-6.

Revised: 05/21/92

---

# DOXAPRAM   Systemic

VA CLASSIFICATION (Primary): RE900
Note: For a listing of dosage forms and brand names by country availability, see *Dosage Forms* section(s). For a listing of brand names for the articles in this monograph, refer to the General Index.

---

## Category
Respiratory stimulant.

## Indications

**Accepted**
Respiratory depression (treatment):

Doxapram is indicated as a respiratory stimulant in the following conditions—Drug-induced post-anesthesia respiratory depression or apnea not associated with muscle relaxant medications.

Postoperative patients to stimulate deep breathing.

Acute respiratory insufficiency occurring in patients with chronic obstructive pulmonary disease (COPD). Used (only for about 2 hours) as an aid in the prevention of arterial $CO_2$ tension elevation during the administration of oxygen. Doxapram should not be used in conjunction with mechanical ventilation.

## Unaccepted

Since doxapram hydrochloride injection available in the U.S. contains benzyl alcohol (or chlorobutanol in Canada), its use is contraindicated in newborns and immature infants. The use of benzyl alcohol in the newborn has been associated with a fatal toxic syndrome consisting of metabolic acidosis and central nervous system (CNS), respiratory, circulatory, and renal function impairment.

Although doxapram has been used to treat respiratory and CNS depression (mild to moderate) resulting from drug overdosage, its use for this indication is no longer recommended.

# Pharmacology/Pharmacokinetics

## Physicochemical characteristics
Molecular weight—432.99.

## Mechanism of action/Effect
Doxapram stimulates respiration by an action on peripheral carotid chemoreceptors. As the dosage is increased, the central respiratory centers in the medulla are stimulated with progressive stimulation of other parts of the brain and spinal cord. The respiratory stimulant action is manifested by an increase in tidal volume associated with a slight increase in respiratory rate.

## Other actions/effects
A pressor response may result from doxapram administration due to the improved cardiac output, rather than from peripheral vasoconstriction. An increased release of catecholamines has been noted.

## Onset of action
20 to 40 seconds.

## Time to peak effect
1 to 2 minutes.

## Duration of action
5 to 12 minutes.

## Elimination
Primarily fecal (55%); some renal.

# Precautions to Consider

## Carcinogenicity/Mutagenicity
Studies have not been done.

## Pregnancy/Reproduction
Pregnancy—Adequate and well-controlled studies in humans have not been done.

Studies in animals have not shown that doxapram causes adverse effects on the fetus or impairs fertility.

FDA Pregnancy Category B.

## Breast-feeding
It is not known whether doxapram is distributed into breast milk. However, problems in humans have not been documented.

## Pediatrics
In addition to the adverse effects of benzyl alcohol in the neonate, potential side effects of doxapram when used in neonatal apnea include central neural stimulation, seizures, and possibly hypertension. If use is absolutely necessary, dosages should be kept at a minimum.

## Geriatrics
No geriatrics-specific problems have been documented in studies done to date that have included geriatric patients. However, risk-benefit must be considered in elderly patients with significant cardiac impairment, liver function impairment, or renal insufficiency.

## Drug interactions and/or related problems
The following drug interactions and/or related problems have been selected on the basis of their potential clinical significance (possible mechanism in parentheses where appropriate)—not necessarily inclusive (» = major clinical significance):

Note: Combinations containing any of the following medications, depending on the amount present, may also interact with this medication.

Anesthetics, hydrocarbon inhalation such as:
Chloroform
Cyclopropane
Enflurane
Halothane
Isoflurane
Methoxyflurane
Trichloroethylene
(following discontinuation of anesthetics known to sensitize the myocardium to catecholamines, it is recommended that initiation of doxapram therapy be delayed for at least 10 minutes, since an increase in catecholamine release may occur with doxapram)

CNS stimulation–producing medications, other (See *Appendix II*)
(concurrent use with doxapram may result in additive CNS stimulation to excessive levels, causing nervousness, irritability, insomnia, or possibly convulsions or cardiac arrhythmias; close observation is recommended)

» Monoamine oxidase (MAO) inhibitors, including furazolidone, procarbazine, and selegiline or
» Sympathomimetic agents
(concurrent use may increase the pressor effects of either these medications or doxapram)

## Medical considerations/Contraindications
The medical considerations/contraindications included here have been selected on the basis of their potential clinical significance (reasons given in parentheses where appropriate)—not necessarily inclusive (» = major clinical significance).

*Except under special circumstances, this medicine should not be used when the following medical problems exist:*

» Cerebrovascular accidents or
» Coronary artery disease or
» Epilepsy or other seizure disorders or
» Head injury, evidence of or
» Heart failure, frank, uncompensated or
» Hypertension, severe
(doxapram-induced release of catecholamines may exacerbate condition)

» Incompetence of ventilatory mechanism due to:
Airway obstruction
Dyspnea, extreme
Flail chest
Muscle paresis
Pneumothorax
(may be exacerbated)

» Pulmonary diseases such as:
Asthma, bronchial, acute
Pulmonary embolism
Respiratory failure due to neuromuscular disorders
Restrictive respiratory diseases such as pulmonary fibrosis
(may be exacerbated)

*Risk-benefit should be considered when the following medical problems exist:*

» Asthma, bronchial, history of
(may be exacerbated)

» Cardiac arrhythmia (including severe tachycardia) or
» Cardiac disease or
» Edema, cerebral or
» Hyperthyroidism or
» Pheochromocytoma
(doxapram-induced release of catecholamines may exacerbate condition)

» Liver function impairment
(metabolism may be altered)

» Renal function impairment
(benzyl alcohol, which is excreted in the kidneys, contained in doxapram injection, may be toxic in patients with renal insufficiency)

## Patient monitoring
The following may be especially important in patient monitoring (other tests may be warranted in some patients, depending on condition; » = major clinical significance):

Blood pressure determinations and
Deep tendon reflexes and
Pulse rate determinations
(recommended at periodic intervals to prevent overdosage)

Determinations of arterial blood gases
(recommended prior to administration of doxapram and at least every half hour during the two-hour period of infusion to prevent development of $CO_2$ retention and acidosis when doxapram is used in chronic obstructive pulmonary disease associated with acute hypercapnia; doxapram should be discontinued if the arterial blood gases deteriorate or whenever mechanical ventilation is initiated)

## Side/Adverse Effects

The following side/adverse effects have been selected on the basis of their potential clinical significance (possible signs and symptoms in parentheses where appropriate)—not necessarily inclusive:

**Those indicating need for medical attention**
Incidence less frequent or rare
*Cardiovascular effects* (chest pain; fast or irregular heartbeat; tightness in chest); *hemolysis*—excessive rate of infusion; *thrombophlebitis* (redness, swelling, or pain at injection site); *wheezing, or troubled or unusually fast breathing*

**Those indicating need for medical attention only if they continue or are bothersome**
Incidence less frequent
*Confusion; coughing; diarrhea; dizziness or lightheadedness; feeling of unusual warmth; headache; increased sweating; nausea or vomiting; urination problems*

## Overdose

**Clinical effects of overdose**
The following effects have been selected on the basis of their potential clinical significance (possible signs and symptoms in parentheses where appropriate)—not necessarily inclusive:
*Convulsions; fast heartbeat; increased blood pressure; increase in deep tendon reflexes; trembling or uncontrolled movements of the body*

## General Dosing Information

Rapid infusion of doxapram at a rate faster than that recommended may result in hemolysis.

Vascular extravasation or use of a single injection site over an extended period of time should be avoided since either of these may result in thrombophlebitis or local skin irritation.

## Parenteral Dosage Forms

### DOXAPRAM HYDROCHLORIDE INJECTION USP

**Usual adult and adolescent dose**
Post-anesthesia respiratory depression—
Intravenous, 500 mcg (0.5 mg) to 1 mg per kg of body weight, not to exceed 1.5 mg per kg of body weight, as a single dose; dose may be repeated, if necessary, at five-minute intervals up to a maximum total dose of 2 mg per kg of body weight.

Intravenous infusion, administered initially at a rate of 5 mg per minute until the desired response is obtained, then reduced to a rate of 1 to 3 mg per minute; the recommended maximum total dose is 4 mg per kg of body weight, or approximately 300 mg.
Acute respiratory insufficiency in chronic obstructive pulmonary disease (COPD)—
Intravenous infusion, administered initially at a rate of 1 to 2 mg per minute, the rate of administration being increased up to a maximum of 3 mg per minute if necessary; the maximum time period of infusion should not exceed two hours and additional infusions are not recommended.
Note: The rate of infusion should not be increased in severely ill patients because of the associated increased work in breathing.

**Usual pediatric dose**
Post-anesthesia respiratory depression—
Children up to 12 years of age: Use is not recommended.

**Strength(s) usually available**
U.S.—
20 mg per mL (Rx) [*Dopram* (benzyl alcohol 0.9%); GENERIC].
Canada—
20 mg per mL (Rx) [*Dopram* (chlorobutanol 0.5%)].

**Packaging and storage**
Store below 40 °C (104 °F), preferably between 15 and 30 °C (59 and 86 °F), unless otherwise specified by manufacturer. Protect from freezing.

**Preparation of dosage form**
Post-anesthetic CNS depression—Add 250 mg of doxapram hydrochloride to 250 mL of 5 or 10% dextrose injection or 0.9% sodium chloride injection.
Acute respiratory insufficiency—Add 400 mg of doxapram hydrochloride to 180 mL of 5 or 10% dextrose injection or 0.9% sodium chloride injection.

**Incompatibilities**
Doxapram is incompatible with alkaline solutions such as 2.5% thiopental sodium, aminophylline, or sodium bicarbonate. Precipitation or gas formation will result from these admixtures.

**Additional information**
Doxapram hydrochloride injection that contains benzyl alcohol (in Canada, chlorobutanol) as a preservative must not be used in newborns and immature infants. The use of benzyl alcohol in neonates has been associated with a fatal toxic syndrome consisting of metabolic acidosis and CNS, respiratory, circulatory, and renal function impairment.

Revised: 04/16/93

---

# DOXAZOSIN  Systemic

VA CLASSIFICATION (Primary/Secondary): CV150/CV490; GU900
Note: For a listing of dosage forms and brand names by country availability, see *Dosage Forms* section(s). For a listing of brand names for the articles in this monograph, refer to the General Index.

## Category

Antihypertensive; benign prostatic hyperplasia therapy agent.

## Indications

**Accepted**
Hypertension (treatment)—Doxazosin is indicated in the treatment of hypertension.

For additional information on initial therapeutic guidelines related to the treatment of hypertension, see *Appendix III*.

Benign prostatic hyperplasia (treatment)[1]—Doxazosin is indicated for the treatment of both the urinary outflow obstruction and the obstructive and irritative symptoms associated with benign prostatic hyperplasia (BPH). Doxazosin may be used in normotensive or hypertensive patients. In normotensive patients with BPH, doxazosin does not appear to significantly lower blood pressure. In hypertensive patients with BPH, both conditions are effectively treated with doxazosin. The long-term effects of doxazosin on the incidence of acute urinary obstruction or other complications of BPH or on the need for surgery have not yet been determined.

[1]Not included in Canadian product labeling.

## Pharmacology/Pharmacokinetics

**Physicochemical characteristics**
Molecular weight—547.58.

**Mechanism of action/Effect**
Doxazosin has a selective alpha$_1$-adrenergic blocking action, which is thought to account primarily for its effects.
Hypertension—
Blockade of alpha$_1$-adrenergic receptors by doxazosin results in peripheral vasodilation, which produces a fall in blood pressure because of decreased peripheral vascular resistance.
Benign prostatic hyperplasia—
Relaxation of smooth muscle in the bladder neck, prostate, and prostate capsule produced by alpha$_1$-adrenergic blockade results in a reduction in urethral resistance and pressure, bladder outlet resistance, and urinary symptoms.

**Other actions/effects**
Doxazosin slightly lowers the levels of total cholesterol, low density lipoprotein (LDL) cholesterol, and triglycerides. In addition, doxazosin slightly increases high density lipoprotein (HDL) cholesterol and the HDL/total cholesterol ratio. These lipid effects appear to be the result of doxazosin's effect on lipid metabolism (i.e., increasing LDL receptor activity, decreasing intracellular LDL cholesterol synthesis, decreasing synthesis and secretion of very low density lipoprotein [VLDL] cholesterol, stimulation of lipoprotein lipase activity, and decreasing the rate of cholesterol absorption). However, the implications of these changes are unclear.

**Absorption**
Well-absorbed from gastrointestinal tract; bioavailability is about 65%.

**Protein binding**
Very high (98 to 99%).

**Biotransformation**
Metabolized extensively in the liver. Although several active and inactive metabolites have been identified (2-piperazinyl, 6' and 7'-hydroxy, 6' and 7'-O-desmethyl, and 2-amino), there is no evidence that they are present in substantial amounts.

**Half-life**
Elimination—19 to 22 hours; does not appear to be significantly influenced by age or mild to moderate renal impairment.

**Onset of action**
Hypertension—1 to 2 hours; there is a slight initial fall in blood pressure within the first hour, but the main hypotensive effect is apparent from 2 hours onwards.
Benign prostatic hyperplasia (BPH)—Within 1 to 2 weeks.

**Time to peak concentration**
1.5 to 3.6 hours.

**Peak serum concentration**
At steady state, there is a positive linear relationship between peak serum concentration and dose of doxazosin. Following a 1 mg oral dose of doxazosin, the standardized peak serum concentration was 9.6 mcg per L.

**Time to peak effect**
Antihypertensive—Single dose: 5 to 6 hours.

**Duration of action**
Antihypertensive—Single dose: 24 hours.

**Elimination**
Fecal—Unchanged drug, about 5%; metabolites, 63 to 65%.
Renal—9%.
In dialysis—Doxazosin is not removed by hemodialysis.

# Precautions to Consider

**Cross-sensitivity and/or related problems**
Patients sensitive to other quinazolines (prazosin, terazosin) may also be sensitive to doxazosin.

**Carcinogenicity**
In one 24-month chronic dietary administration study in rats, doxazosin (given at 150 times the maximum recommended human dose) produced no evidence of carcinogenicity. In another similarly conducted study done in mice, up to 18 months of dietary administration produced no evidence of carcinogenicity. The latter study, however, did not use a maximally tolerated dose of doxazosin.

**Mutagenicity**
There is no evidence of drug- or metabolic-related effects at either chromosomal or subchromosomal levels.

**Pregnancy/Reproduction**
Fertility—Studies in rats given oral doses of 20 mg per kg of body weight (mg/kg) per day (about 75 times the maximum recommended human dose) have shown that doxazosin reduces fertility in male rats.
Pregnancy—Adequate and well-controlled studies in humans have not been done.
Studies in rabbits and rats given daily oral doses of 40 and 20 mg/kg, respectively, have shown no evidence of harm to the fetus. The rabbit study, however, did not use a maximally tolerated dose of doxazosin. Reduced fetal survival was associated with a dosage regimen of 82 mg/kg in rabbits. Following oral administration of labeled doxazosin to pregnant rats, radioactivity was found to cross the placenta.
Studies in peri- and postnatal rats, given 40 or 50 mg/kg per day of doxazosin, revealed evidence of delayed postnatal development manifested by slower body weight gain and slightly later appearance of anatomical features and reflexes.
FDA Pregnancy Category C.

**Breast-feeding**
It is not known whether doxazosin is distributed into breast milk. Problems in humans have not been documented. However, in rats given a single oral dose of 1 mg/kg, doxazosin accumulates in rat breast milk with a maximum concentration about 20 times greater than the maternal plasma concentration.

**Pediatrics**
No information is available on the relationship of age to the effects of doxazosin in pediatric patients. Safety and efficacy have not been established.

**Geriatrics**
A study performed in approximately 2000 hypertensive patients older than 65 years of age did not demonstrate geriatrics-specific problems that would limit the usefulness of doxazosin in the elderly. However, the hypotensive effect of doxazosin may be more pronounced in elderly hypertensive individuals, and lower daily maintenance doses may be required.
Experience with use of doxazosin in elderly patients with benign prostatic hyperplasia (BPH) has shown that the safety profile of doxazosin is similar to that in younger patients.

**Drug interactions and/or related problems**
The following drug interactions and/or related problems have been selected on the basis of their potential clinical significance (possible mechanism in parentheses where appropriate)—not necessarily inclusive (» = major clinical significance):

Note: Combinations containing any of the following medications, depending on the amount present, may also interact with this medication.

Anti-inflammatory drugs, nonsteroidal (NSAIDs), especially indomethacin
(antihypertensive effects of doxazosin may be reduced when the medication is used concurrently with these agents; indomethacin, and possibly other NSAIDs, may antagonize the antihypertensive effect by inhibiting renal prostaglandin synthesis and/or by causing sodium and fluid retention; the patient should be carefully monitored to confirm that the desired effect is being obtained)

Cimetidine
(concurrent use may slightly increase the serum concentration of doxazosin; however, the clinical significance of this increase is not known)

Estrogens
(estrogen-induced fluid retention tends to increase blood pressure)

Hypotension-producing medications, other (See *Appendix II*)
(antihypertensive effects may be potentiated when these medications are used concurrently with doxazosin; although some antihypertensive and/or diuretic combinations are frequently used to therapeutic advantage, dosage adjustments are necessary during concurrent use)

Sympathomimetics
(antihypertensive effects of doxazosin may be reduced when it is used concurrently with these agents; the patient should be carefully monitored to confirm that the desired effect is being obtained)
(concurrent use of doxazosin antagonizes the peripheral vasoconstriction produced by high doses of dopamine)
(concurrent use of doxazosin may decrease the pressor response to ephedrine)
(concurrent use of doxazosin may block the alpha-adrenergic effects of epinephrine, possibly resulting in severe hypotension and tachycardia)
(concurrent use of doxazosin usually decreases, but does not reverse or completely block, the pressor effect of metaraminol)
(prior administration of doxazosin may decrease the pressor effect and shorten the duration of action of methoxamine and phenylephrine)

**Medical considerations/Contraindications**
The medical considerations/contraindications included here have been selected on the basis of their potential clinical significance (reasons given in parentheses where appropriate)—not necessarily inclusive (» = major clinical significance).

*Risk-benefit should be considered when the following medical problems exist:*
Hepatic function impairment
(although studies in patients with impaired hepatic function have not been done, doxazosin is primarily metabolized in the liver, and, therefore, increased sensitivity or prolonged doxazosin effect may occur)
Renal function impairment
(small incidence of increased risk of first-dose orthostatic hypotensive reaction and prolonged hypotensive effect)
Sensitivity to doxazosin

**Patient monitoring**
The following may be especially important in patient monitoring (other tests may be warranted in some patients, depending on condition; » = major clinical significance):

» Blood pressure measurements
(recommended at 2 to 6 hours postdose following first dose and with each dosage increase, since postural effects are most likely to occur during this time; dosage to be increased as necessary and tolerated based on individual standing blood pressures taken at 2 to 6 hours and 24 hours postdose)

## Side/Adverse Effects

Note: A "first-dose orthostatic hypotensive reaction" sometimes occurs with the initial dose of doxazosin, especially when the patient is in the upright position. Syncope or other postural symptoms such as dizziness may occur. Subsequent occurrence with dosage increases is also possible. Incidence appears to be dose-related, thus, it is important that therapy be initiated with the 1-mg dose. Patients who are volume-depleted or sodium-restricted may be more sensitive to the orthostatic hypotensive effects of doxazosin, and the effect may be exaggerated after exercise.

Hypotensive side effects are more likely to occur in geriatric patients.

The following side/adverse effects have been selected on the basis of their potential clinical significance (possible signs and symptoms in parentheses where appropriate)—not necessarily inclusive:

**Those indicating need for medical attention**
Incidence more frequent
*Dizziness; vertigo* (dizziness or lightheadedness)
Incidence less frequent
*Arrhythmias* (irregular heartbeat); *dyspnea* (shortness of breath); *orthostatic hypotension* (dizziness or lightheadedness when getting up from a lying or sitting position; sudden fainting); *palpitations* (pounding heartbeat); *peripheral edema* (swelling of feet or lower legs); *tachycardia* (fast heartbeat)

**Those indicating need for medical attention only if they continue or are bothersome**
Incidence more frequent
*Headache; unusual tiredness*
Incidence less frequent
*Nausea; nervousness, restlessness, or unusual irritability; rhinitis* (runny nose); *somnolence* (sleepiness or unusual drowsiness)

## Overdose

For more information on the management of overdose or unintentional ingestion, **contact a Poison Control Center** (see *Poison Control Center Listing*).

**Treatment of overdose**
Treatment of circulatory failure, either by placing the patient in the supine position and elevating the legs or by using additional measures if shock is present, is most important. Volume expanders may be used to treat shock, followed, if necessary, by administration of a vasopressor.
Symptomatic, supportive treatment and monitoring of fluid and electrolyte status.

## Patient Consultation

As an aid to patient consultation, refer to *Advice for the Patient, Doxazosin (Systemic)*.

In providing consultation, consider emphasizing the following selected information (» = major clinical significance):

**Before using this medication**
» Conditions affecting use, especially:
Sensitivity to quinazolines
Use in the elderly—Increased sensitivity to hypotensive effects

**Proper use of this medication**
Getting into the habit of taking at same times each day to help increase compliance
» Proper dosing
Missed dose: Taking as soon as possible; not taking if almost time for next dose; not doubling doses
» Proper storage
*For use as an antihypertensive*
Possible need for control of weight and diet, especially sodium intake
» Patient may not experience symptoms of hypertension; importance of taking medication even if feeling well
» Does not cure, but helps control hypertension; possible need for lifelong therapy; serious consequences of untreated hypertension

*For use in benign prostatic hyperplasia (BPH)*
Relieves symptoms of BPH but does not change the size of the prostate; may not prevent the need for surgery in the future
May require 1 to 2 weeks of therapy before patient experiences improvement of symptoms

**Precautions while using this medication**
Regular visits to physician to check progress
» Not taking other medications, especially nonprescription sympathomimetics, unless discussed with physician
» Caution if dizziness, lightheadedness, or sudden fainting occurs, especially after initial dose; taking first dose at bedtime
» Caution when getting up suddenly from a lying or sitting position
» Caution in using alcohol, while standing for long periods or exercising, and during hot weather, because of enhanced orthostatic hypotensive effects
» Possibility of drowsiness
» Caution when driving or doing anything else requiring alertness because of possible drowsiness, dizziness, or lightheadedness

**Side/adverse effects**
Signs of potential side effects, especially arrhythmias, dizziness, dyspnea, orthostatic hypotension, palpitations, peripheral edema, tachycardia, and vertigo

## General Dosing Information

In order to minimize the "first-dose orthostatic hypotensive reaction," an initial dose of 1 mg is recommended, with gradual increases in dose every 2 weeks as needed. Administration of the initial dose at bedtime is recommended, as well as the initial dose of each increment.

**For use as an antihypertensive**
Dosage of doxazosin should be adjusted to meet the individual requirements of each patient, on the basis of blood pressure response.
Doxazosin may be used alone or in combination with a thiazide diuretic or beta-adrenergic blocking agent, both of which reduce the tendency for sodium and water retention, although they also produce additive hypotension. If combination therapy is indicated, individual titration is required to ensure the lowest possible therapeutic dose of each medication.
Increases in dose beyond 4 mg increase the likelihood of excessive postural effects including syncope, postural dizziness/vertigo, and postural hypotension.
When a diuretic or another antihypertensive agent is added to doxazosin therapy, the dose of doxazosin may be reduced, followed by slow dosage titration of the combination. When doxazosin is added to existing diuretic or antihypertensive therapy, the dose of the other agent may be reduced and doxazosin started at a dose of 1 mg once a day.

**For use in benign prostatic hyperplasia**
Prior to initiation of doxazosin therapy, the presence of prostate carcinoma should be ruled out, since prostate carcinoma can present with symptoms similar to those associated with BPH.

## Oral Dosage Forms

Note: The dosing and strengths of the dosage forms available are expressed in terms of doxazosin base (not the mesylate salt).

### DOXAZOSIN MESYLATE TABLETS

**Usual adult dose**
Antihypertensive—
Initial: Oral, 1 mg (base) once a day, at bedtime.
Maintenance: Oral, the dosage being increased gradually to meet individual requirements; depending on periodic blood pressure measurements, dosage may be increased every two weeks, titrating upwards to 2, 4, 8, and 16 mg (base) once a day as needed and tolerated.
Note: Increases in dose beyond 4 mg (base) increase the likelihood of excessive postural effects including syncope, postural dizziness/vertigo, and postural hypotension.

Geriatric patients may be more sensitive to the effects of the usual adult dose.
Benign prostatic hyperplasia[1]—
Initial: Oral, 1 mg (base) once a day, at bedtime.
Maintenance: Oral, 1 to 8 mg (base) once a day.

**Usual adult prescribing limits**
16 mg once a day.

**Usual pediatric dose**
Safety and efficacy have not been established.

**Strength(s) usually available**
U.S.—
    1 mg (base) (Rx) [*Cardura*].
    2 mg (base) (Rx) [*Cardura*].
    4 mg (base) (Rx) [*Cardura*].
    8 mg (base) (Rx) [*Cardura*].
Canada—
    1 mg (base) (Rx) [*Cardura*].
    2 mg (base) (Rx) [*Cardura*].
    4 mg (base) (Rx) [*Cardura*].

**Packaging and storage**
Store below 30 °C (86 °F), in a well-closed container, unless otherwise
specified by manufacturer.

**Auxiliary labeling**
• Do not take other medicines without your doctor's advice.
• May cause dizziness.

**Note**
Check refill frequency to determine compliance in hypertensive patients.

## Selected Bibliography

Cubeddu LX, Fuenmayor N, Caplan N, Ferry D. Clinical pharmacology
    of doxazosin in patients with essential hypertension. Clin Pharmacol
    Ther 1987; 41: 439-49.
Talseth T, Westlie L, Daae L. Doxazosin and atenolol as monotherapy in
    mild and moderate hypertension: A randomized, parallel study with a
    three year follow-up. Am Heart J 1991; 121: 280-5.
The fifth report of the Joint National Committee on Detection, Evaluation,
    and Treatment of High Blood Pressure. Arch Intern Med 1993; 153:
    154-83.

Revised: 08/02/94
Interim revision: 05/12/95

---

**DOXEPIN**—See *Antidepressants, Tricyclic (Systemic)*

---

# DOXEPIN    Topical

VA CLASSIFICATION (Primary): DE900

Note: For a listing of dosage forms and brand names by country availa-
    bility, see *Dosage Forms* section(s). For a listing of brand names
    for the articles in this monograph, refer to the General Index.

---

## Category
Antipruritic (topical).

## Indications

**Accepted**
Pruritus associated with eczema (treatment)—Doxepin is indicated for the
    short-term (up to 8 days) topical treatment of moderate pruritus in
    adult patients with eczematous dermatitis, e.g., atopic dermatitis and
    lichen simplex chronicus.

## Pharmacology/Pharmacokinetics

**Physicochemical characteristics**
Chemical group—A dibenzoxepin tricyclic antidepressant.
Molecular weight—316.

**Mechanism of action/Effect**
The exact mechanism by which topical doxepin exerts its antipruritic ef-
    fect is unknown. However, doxepin has potent antihistaminic ($H_1$- and
    $H_2$-receptor) activity. As a histamine-blocking agent, doxepin appears
    to bind to histamine receptor sites and competitively inhibits the bio-
    logical activation of histamine receptors. Because topical doxepin pro-
    duces drowsiness in significant numbers of patients, it is believed that
    this sedative property may also have an effect on certain pruritic
    symptoms.

**Other actions/effects**
Topical doxepin may be absorbed into the systemic circulation and, there-
    fore, may have the potential for causing peripheral and central anti-
    cholinergic effects due to its potent and high binding affinity for mus-
    carinic receptors. It may also have the potential to produce prominent
    cardiovascular effects as a result of its anticholinergic activity on the
    heart and a 'quinidine-like' myocardial depressant action, as well as
    inhibition of norepinephrine uptake at adrenergic synapses.

**Absorption**
Doxepin applied topically is absorbed through the skin. As with most
    topical agents, occlusive dressings may increase the absorption of top-
    ical doxepin.

**Distribution**
Once absorbed, doxepin may be distributed in body tissues including
    lungs, heart, brain, and liver.

**Biotransformation**
Once absorbed into the systemic circulation, doxepin undergoes hepatic
    metabolism that results in the conversion to the pharmacologically
    active metabolite, desmethyldoxepin. The parent compound and its
    metabolite also undergo glucuronidation.

**Half-life**
Desmethyldoxepin—Ranges from 28 to 52 hours.

**Peak plasma concentration**
For both doxepin and its active metabolite, desmethyldoxepin, plasma
    concentrations are highly variable and are poorly correlated with dos-
    age. In 19 patients with pruritic eczema treated with topical doxepin,
    plasma doxepin concentrations ranged from nondetectable to 47 nan-
    ograms per mL (168.2 nanomoles per L) with a mean of 10.8 nano-
    grams per mL, (38.6 nanomoles per L) after percutaneous absorption.
    (For oral doxepin, the target therapeutic plasma concentrations for the
    treatment of depression range from 30 to 150 nanograms per mL
    [107.3 to 536.8 nanomoles per L]).

**Elimination**
Renal for both the parent compound and its metabolites.

## Precautions to Consider

**Cross-sensitivity and/or related problems**
Patients sensitive to other dibenzoxepines (tricyclic antidepressants) may
    also be sensitive to doxepin.

**Carcinogenicity**
Studies on carcinogenicity have not been conducted with topical doxepin.

**Mutagenicity**
Studies on mutagenicity have not been conducted with topical doxepin.

**Pregnancy/Reproduction**
Fertility—Studies have not been conducted with topical doxepin in
    humans.
Studies in rats and rabbits given oral doses of doxepin up to 8 times the
    topical human dose (on a milligram per kilogram of body weight [mg/
    kg] basis) have shown no evidence of impaired fertility.
Pregnancy—Adequate and well-controlled studies in humans have not
    been done.
Studies in rats and rabbits given oral doses of doxepin up to 8 times the
    topical human dose (on a milligram per kilogram of body weight [mg/
    kg] basis) have shown no evidence of harm to the fetus.
FDA Pregnancy Category B.

**Breast-feeding**
No studies have been done to determine if doxepin is distributed into
    human milk following topical administration. However, doxepin is dis-
    tributed into human milk after oral administration. Because significant
    systemic concentrations of doxepin are obtained when this agent is
    applied topically, it is possible that this medication could be distributed
    into human milk after topical administration.
Apnea and drowsiness have been reported in 1 nursing infant whose
    mother was taking an oral dosage form of doxepin.

**Pediatrics**
Appropriate studies on the relationship of age to the effects of topical
    doxepin have not been performed in the pediatric population. Safety
    and efficacy have not been established.

**Geriatrics**
Appropriate studies on the relationship of age to the effects of topical
    doxepin have not been performed in the geriatric population. However,
    no geriatrics-specific problems have been documented to date.

## Drug interactions and/or related problems

The following drug interactions and/or related problems have been selected on the basis of their potential clinical significance (possible mechanism in parentheses where appropriate)—not necessarily inclusive (» = major clinical significance):

Note: Combinations containing any of the following medications, depending on the amount present, may also interact with this medication. (See also *Antidepressants, Tricyclic [Systemic]* monograph for oral doxepin drug interactions).

» Alcohol or
» CNS depression-producing medications, other (See *Appendix II*)
   (concurrent use with tricyclic antidepressants may result in serious potentiation of CNS depression, respiratory depression, and hypotensive effects; caution is recommended, and dosage of one or both agents should be reduced)

» Cimetidine
   (cimetidine may inhibit the metabolism and increase the plasma concentration of doxepin, leading to toxicity; serious anticholinergic effects have been associated with concurrent use of cimetidine and tricyclic antidepressants)

» Medications metabolized by cytochrome $P_{450}$isoenzyme $P_{450}IID_6$, such as
   Antiarrhythmic agents, Type 1C, including encainide, flecainide, and propafenone
   Antidepressants, other
   Carbamazepine
   Debrisoquine
   Dextromethorphan
   Phenothiazines
   Quinidine
   (although no studies have been done on the use of topical doxepin with these medications, caution is recommended because experience with oral tricyclic antidepressants has shown that concurrent use with other medications that are metabolized via the cytochrome $P_{450}$isoenzyme $P_{450}11D_6$ may result in mutual inhibition of metabolism and in toxicity of either or both medications, especially in patients known to have genetically determined defects in oxidative metabolism involving this enzyme, if dosage of either or both medications is not reduced; the risk may be particularly high with quinidine and with other tricyclic antidepressants because of additive toxicities)

» Monoamine oxidase (MAO) inhibitors
   (concurrent use with orally administered tricyclic antidepressants has resulted in serious side effects [convulsions, excitation, hyperpyrexia, and mania] and even death [although there have been patients who have received combinations of these medications without ill effects]; MAO inhibitors should be discontinued at least 2 weeks prior to the initiation of treatment with topical doxepin)

## Medical considerations/Contraindications

The medical considerations/contraindications included here have been selected on the basis of their potential clinical significance (reasons given in parentheses where appropriate)—not necessarily inclusive (» = major clinical significance).

*Risk-benefit should be considered when the following medical problems exist:*

» Glaucoma, narrow-angle, untreated or
» Urinary retention
   (doxepin may aggravate these conditions)
   Sensitivity to doxepin or other ingredients of the preparation, or history of

# Side/Adverse Effects

The following side/adverse effects have been selected on the basis of their potential clinical significance (possible signs and symptoms in parentheses where appropriate)—not necessarily inclusive:

**Those indicating need for medical attention**
Incidence more frequent—approximately 1 to 10%
   *Edema at site of application* (swelling at site of application); *exacerbation of pruritus* (worsening of itching); *exacerbation of eczema* (worsening of eczema); *paresthesias* (burning, crawling, or tingling sensation of the skin)

Incidence rare—less than 1%
   *Fever*

**Those indicating need for medical attention only if they continue or are bothersome**
Incidence more frequent—1 to 10%, or as specified
   *Burning and/or stinging at the site of application*—approximately 21%; *changes in taste; dizziness; drowsiness*—22%; *dryness and*

*tightness of skin; dryness of mouth and/or lips; emotional changes; fatigue* (unusual tiredness or weakness); *headache; thirst*

Note: *Drowsiness* is the most common adverse effect reported with the use of topical doxepin, especially in those patients receiving treatment over more than 10% of their body surface area. However, this effect was observed to be mild and temporary, usually lasting 1 or 2 days, as reported by the vast majority of patients who experienced drowsiness during the clinical trials. *Burning and/or stinging at the site of application* is the second most common adverse effect reported. In clinical trials, most patients characterized this reaction as mild and about 25% reported it as severe.

Incidence less frequent or rare—less than 1%
   *Anxiety; irritation, tingling, scaling, or cracking of skin; nausea*

# Overdose

For specific information on the agent used in the management of doxepin overdose, see:
   • *Physostigmine (Systemic)* monograph.

For more information on the management of overdose or unintentional ingestion, **contact a Poison Control Center** (see *Poison Control Center Listing*).

## Clinical effects of overdose

The following effects have been selected on the basis of their potential clinical significance (possible signs and symptoms in parentheses where appropriate)—not necessarily inclusive:

Note: Signs and symptoms of overdose are generally related to the anticholinergic effects of this medication.

Mild effects
   *Blurred vision; drowsiness; dryness of mouth, excessive; stupor* (decreased awareness or responsiveness)

Severe effects
   *Cardiac arrhythmias* (irregular heartbeat); *coma* (unconsciousness); *dilated pupils* (enlarged pupils); *hyperactive reflexes* (increased or excessive unconscious or jerking movements); *hypertension* (increased blood pressure); *hyperthermia* (extremely high fever or body temperature); *hypotension* (dizziness, fainting, or lightheadedness); *hypothermia* (extremely low body temperature; weak or feeble pulse); *paralytic ileus* (abdominal pain and swelling; intractable constipation; vomiting)—may lead to intestinal obstruction; *respiratory depression* (difficulty in breathing); *seizures* (convulsions); *tachycardia* (fast heartbeat); *urinary retention due to bladder atony* (difficulty in passing urine)

## Treatment of overdose

For mild effects, observation and supportive therapy are recommended. It may be necessary to reduce the percent of body surface area treated or the frequency of application. A thinner layer of cream should be applied.

For severe effects, medical management should consist of aggressive supportive therapy.

To decrease absorption—The area of skin covered with topical doxepin should be thoroughly washed with soap and water.

To enhance elimination—Enhancing elimination of absorbed doxepin through dialysis and forced diuresis have not been successful due to the high tissue and protein binding, large volume of distribution, and limited water solubility of this agent.

Specific treatment—Cardiac arrhythmias should be treated with the appropriate antiarrhythmic agents. It has been reported that many of the anticholinergic effects (cardiovascular and central nervous system [CNS] symptoms) of tricyclic antidepressant overdose in adults may be reversed by the slow intravenous administration of physostigmine. The dose should be repeated as required because physostigmine is rapidly metabolized. However, physostigmine should be used with caution because this agent may also increase the risk of cardiac toxicity if used indiscriminately. (See the package insert or *Physostigmine [Systemic]* monograph for specific dosing guidelines for use of this product.) Convulsions may be treated with anticonvulsant agents, such as diazepam or lorazepam; however, barbiturates are not recommended because they may potentiate respiratory depression. If there is any suspicion that the patient may have taken a benzodiazepine in addition to doxepin, flumazenil should not be used to reverse the effects of the benzodiazepine. Administration of flumazenil in such cases has been shown to increase the risk of seizures and/or cardiac arrhythmias.

Monitoring—Vital signs, especially cardiovascular and respiratory functions, should be constantly monitored. Because relapse after apparent recovery has been reported with oral doxepin, electrocardiogram (ECG) monitoring may be required for several days.

Supportive care—For comatose patients, an adequate airway should be established and assisted ventilation should be used if necessary. Patients in whom intentional overdose is known or suspected should be referred for psychiatric consultation.

## Patient Consultation

As an aid to patient consultation, refer to *Advice for the Patient, Doxepin (Topical)*.

In providing consultation, consider emphasizing the following selected information (» = major clinical significance):

### Before using this medication
» Conditions affecting use, especially:
   Sensitivity to doxepin or other ingredients of the preparation
   Breast-feeding—May be distributed into breast milk
   Other medications, especially alcohol and other CNS depression-producing medications, cimetidine, medications metabolized by cytochrome $P_{450}$ isoenzyme $P_{450}11D_6$, and monoamine oxidase (MAO) inhibitors
   Other medical problems, especially untreated narrow-angle glaucoma and urinary retention

### Proper use of this medication
» For external use only; not for ophthalmic, oral, or intravaginal use
» Using this medication exactly as directed; not using more of it, not using it more often, and not using it for more than 8 days; not applying medication to an area of skin larger than recommended by physician
   Applying a thin film of doxepin cream to only affected area(s) of skin and rubbing in gently
   Compliance with full course of therapy
» Not using occlusive dressings, which may increase absorption of medication
» Proper dosing
» Proper storage
   Missed dose

### Precautions while using this medication
   Checking with physician if skin problem does not improve after 8 days or if it becomes worse
» Avoiding alcoholic beverages or other alcohol-containing preparations while using topical doxepin; not taking other medications unless prescribed by physician
» Caution if drowsiness occurs; not driving, using machines, or doing anything else that requires alertness while using topical doxepin; if excessive drowsiness occurs, reducing the number of applications per day, the amount of cream applied, and/or the percentage of body surface area treated, or discontinuing medication after checking with physician
» Possible dryness of mouth; using sugarless gum or candy, ice, or saliva substitute for relief; checking with physician or dentist if dry mouth continues for more than 2 weeks

### Side/adverse effects
   Signs of potential side effects, especially edema at site of application, exacerbation of pruritus, exacerbation of eczema, paresthesias, and fever

## General Dosing Information

Topical doxepin is for external use only. It is not for ophthalmic, oral, or intravaginal use.

A thin film of doxepin cream should be applied to the affected area(s) of skin.

Drowsiness may occur, especially in patients receiving treatment over more than 10% of their body surface area. Patients should be warned of this possibility and cautioned against driving a motor vehicle or operating hazardous machinery while being treated with topical doxepin. If excessive drowsiness occurs, it may be necessary to reduce the body surface area treated, reduce the number of applications per day, reduce the amount of cream applied, or discontinue the medication.

Topical doxepin should not be used for more than 8 days. Chronic use beyond 8 days may result in higher systemic concentrations of the medication because of increased absorption.

## Topical Dosage Forms

### DOXEPIN HYDROCHLORIDE CREAM

#### Usual adult dose
Antipruritic (topical)—
   Topical, a thin film applied to the affected area(s) of skin four times a day, with an interval of at least three to four hours between applications. Treatment may be continued for up to eight days.

#### Usual pediatric dose
Safety and efficacy have not been established.

#### Strength(s) usually available
U.S.—
   5% (Rx) [*Zonalon* (benzyl alcohol; cetyl alcohol; glyceryl stearate; isopropyl myristate; petrolatum; PEG-100 stearate; purified water; sorbitol; titanium dioxide)].
Canada—
   5% (Rx) [*Zonalon*].

#### Packaging and storage
Store at or below 27 °C (80 °F).

#### Auxiliary labeling
• For external use only.
• May cause drowsiness.
• Avoid alcoholic beverages.

## Selected Bibliography
Drake LA, Fallon JD, Sober A, et al. Relief of pruritus in patients with atopic dermatitis after treatment with topical doxepin cream. J Am Acad Dermatol 1994; 31 (4): 613-6.

Developed: 05/26/95

---

# DOXORUBICIN   Systemic

VA CLASSIFICATION (Primary): AN200
Note: For a listing of dosage forms and brand names by country availability, see *Dosage Forms* section(s). For a listing of brand names for the articles in this monograph, refer to the General Index.

## Category
Antineoplastic.

## Indications
Note: Bracketed information in the *Indications* section refers to uses that are not included in U.S. product labeling.

### Accepted
Leukemia, acute lymphocytic (treatment) or
Leukemia, acute myelocytic (treatment)—Doxorubicin is indicated for treatment of acute lymphocytic (lymphoblastic) leukemia and acute myelocytic (myeloblastic) leukemia.
Carcinoma, bladder (treatment)
Carcinoma, breast (treatment)

Neuroblastoma (treatment)
Carcinoma, ovarian (treatment)
Carcinoma, thyroid (treatment)
Wilms' tumor (treatment)
Carcinoma, lung (treatment)
Carcinoma, gastric (treatment)
[Carcinoma, head and neck (treatment)]
[Carcinoma, cervical (treatment)]
[Carcinoma, hepatic (treatment)][1]
[Carcinoma, pancreatic (treatment)][1]
[Carcinoma, prostatic (treatment)][1]
[Carcinoma, testicular (treatment)]
[Carcinoma, endometrial (treatment)] or
[Tumors, germ cell, ovarian (treatment)]—Doxorubicin is indicated for treatment of transitional bladder cell carcinoma, breast carcinoma, neuroblastoma, ovarian carcinoma, thyroid carcinoma, Wilms' tumor, bronchogenic carcinoma (non-oat cell), gastric carcinoma, squamous cell carcinoma of the head and neck, cervical carcinoma, hepatic carcinoma, pancreatic carcinoma, prostatic carcinoma, testicular carcinoma, endometrial carcinoma, and germ cell tumors of the ovary.

Lymphomas, Hodgkin's (treatment) or
Lymphomas, non-Hodgkin's (treatment)—Doxorubicin is indicated for treatment of Hodgkin's and non-Hodgkin's lymphomas.
Sarcomas, soft tissue (treatment)
Osteosarcoma (treatment) or
[Ewing's sarcoma (treatment)][1]—Doxorubicin is indicated for treatment of soft tissue sarcomas, bone sarcomas, and Ewing's sarcoma.
[Multiple myeloma (treatment)][1]—Doxorubicin is used for treatment of multiple myeloma.

---

[1]Not included in Canadian product labeling.

# Pharmacology/Pharmacokinetics

## Physicochemical characteristics
Molecular weight—579.99.
Other characteristics—Unstable in solutions with a pH less than 3 or greater than 7.

## Mechanism of action/Effect
Doxorubicin is an anthracycline glycoside; it is classified as an antibiotic but is not used as an antimicrobial agent. Doxorubicin is cell cycle-specific for the S phase of cell division. Its exact mechanism of antineoplastic activity is unknown but may involve binding to DNA by intercalation between base pairs and inhibition of DNA and RNA synthesis by template disordering and steric obstruction.

## Distribution
Does not cross the blood-brain barrier.

## Protein binding
Extensive tissue binding.

## Biotransformation
Rapidly (within 1 hour) in the liver to produce an active metabolite, adriamycinol. Further metabolism is also hepatic.

## Half-life
Doxorubicin—
   Alpha phase: 0.6 hours.
   Beta phase: 16.7 hours.
Metabolites—
   Alpha phase: 3.3 hours.
   Beta phase: 31.7 hours.

## Elimination
Biliary—
   50% unchanged.
   23% as adriamycinol.
Renal—
   Less than 10%, up to one-half as metabolites.

# Precautions to Consider

## Cross-sensitivity and/or related problems
A case of apparent cross-sensitivity with lincomycin has been reported.

## Carcinogenicity/Mutagenicity
Secondary malignancies are potential delayed effects of many antineoplastic agents, although it is not clear whether the effect is related to their mutagenic or immunosuppressive action. The effect of dose and duration of therapy is also unknown, although risk seems to increase with long-term use. Although information is limited, available data seem to indicate that the carcinogenic risk is greatest with the alkylating agents.
Doxorubicin is carcinogenic in animals and is potentially carcinogenic in humans.

## Pregnancy/Reproduction
Fertility—Gonadal suppression, resulting in amenorrhea or azoospermia, may occur in patients taking antineoplastic therapy, especially with the alkylating agents. In general, these effects appear to be related to dose and length of therapy and may be irreversible. Prediction of the degree of testicular or ovarian function impairment is complicated by the common use of combinations of several antineoplastics, which makes it difficult to assess the effects of individual agents.
Doxorubicin affects gonadal function but has a weaker effect on humans than that seen in experiments with mice.
Pregnancy—Some studies indicate that doxorubicin may cross the placenta in humans.
First trimester: It is usually recommended that use of antineoplastics, especially combination chemotherapy, be avoided whenever possible, especially during the first trimester. Although information is limited because of the relatively few instances of antineoplastic administration during pregnancy, the mutagenic, teratogenic, and carcinogenic potential of these medications must be considered.

Other hazards to the fetus include adverse reactions seen in adults.
In general, use of a contraceptive is recommended during cytotoxic drug therapy.
Doxorubicin is embryotoxic and teratogenic in rats and embryotoxic and abortifacient in rabbits.

## Breast-feeding
Although very little information is available regarding distribution of antineoplastic agents into breast milk, breast-feeding is not recommended while doxorubicin is being administered because of the risks to the infant (adverse effects, mutagenicity, carcinogenicity).

## Pediatrics
Although appropriate studies on the relationship of age to the effects of doxorubicin have not been performed in the pediatric population, cardiotoxicity may be more frequent in children up to 2 years of age.

## Geriatrics
Although appropriate studies on the relationship of age to the effects of doxorubicin have not been performed in the geriatric population, cardiotoxicity may be more frequent in patients 70 years of age or older. Caution should also be used in patients who have inadequate bone marrow reserves due to old age.

## Dental
The bone marrow depressant effects of doxorubicin may result in an increased incidence of microbial infection, delayed healing, and gingival bleeding. Dental work, whenever possible, should be completed prior to initiation of therapy or deferred until blood counts have returned to normal. Patients should be instructed in proper oral hygiene during treatment, including caution in use of regular toothbrushes, dental floss, and toothpicks.
Doxorubicin also commonly causes stomatitis which may be associated with considerable discomfort.

## Drug interactions and/or related problems
The following drug interactions and/or related problems have been selected on the basis of their potential clinical significance (possible mechanism in parentheses where appropriate)—not necessarily inclusive (» = major clinical significance):
Note: Combinations containing any of the following medications, depending on the amount present, may also interact with this medication.

Allopurinol or
Colchicine or
» Probenecid or
» Sulfinpyrazone
   (doxorubicin may raise the concentration of blood uric acid; dosage adjustment of antigout agents may be necessary to control hyperuricemia and gout; allopurinol may be preferred to prevent or reverse doxorubicin-induced hyperuricemia because of risk of uric acid nephropathy with uricosuric antigout agents)
Blood dyscrasia–causing medications (See *Appendix II*)
   (leukopenic and/or thrombocytopenic effects of doxorubicin may be increased with concurrent or recent therapy if these medications cause the same effects; dosage adjustment of doxorubicin, if necessary, should be based on blood counts)
» Bone marrow depressants, other (See *Appendix II*) or
Radiation therapy
   (additive bone marrow depression, including severe dermatitis and/or mucositis, may occur; dosage reduction may be required when two or more bone marrow depressants, including radiation, are used concurrently or consecutively)
Cyclophosphamide or
Dactinomycin or
Mitomycin or
Radiation therapy to mediastinal area
   (concurrent use may result in increased cardiotoxicity; it is recommended that the total dose of doxorubicin not exceed 400 mg per square meter of body surface)
   (concurrent use of cyclophosphamide with doxorubicin may potentiate cyclophosphamide-induced hemorrhagic cystitis)
» Daunorubicin
   (use of doxorubicin in a patient who has previously received daunorubicin increases the risk of cardiotoxicity; dosage adjustment is necessary. Doxorubicin should not be used in patients who have previously received complete cumulative doses of daunorubicin or doxorubicin)
Hepatotoxic medications (See *Appendix II*)
   (concurrent use may increase the risk of toxicity; for example, high-dose methotrexate may impair liver function and increase toxicity of subsequently administered doxorubicin)

Streptozocin
(may prolong the half-life of doxorubicin when used concurrently; dosage reduction of doxorubicin is recommended)

Vaccines, killed virus
(because normal defense mechanisms may be suppressed by doxorubicin therapy, the patient's antibody response to the vaccine may be decreased. The interval between discontinuation of medications that cause immunosuppression and restoration of the patient's ability to respond to the vaccine depends on the intensity and type of immunosuppression-causing medication used, the underlying disease, and other factors; estimates vary from 3 months to 1 year)

» Vaccines, live virus
(because normal defense mechanisms may be suppressed by doxorubicin therapy, concurrent use with a live virus vaccine may potentiate the replication of the vaccine virus, may increase the side/adverse effects of the vaccine virus, and/or may decrease the patient's antibody response to the vaccine; immunization of these patients should be undertaken only with extreme caution after careful review of the patient's hematologic status and only with the knowledge and consent of the physician managing the doxorubicin therapy. The interval between discontinuation of medications that cause immunosuppression and restoration of the patient's ability to respond to the vaccine depends on the intensity and type of immunosuppression-causing medication used, the underlying disease, and other factors; estimates vary from 3 months to 1 year. Patients with leukemia in remission should not receive live virus vaccine until at least 3 months after their last chemotherapy. In addition, immunization with oral poliovirus vaccine should be postponed in persons in close contact with the patient, especially family members)

**Laboratory value alterations**
The following have been selected on the basis of their potential clinical significance (possible effect in parentheses where appropriate)—not necessarily inclusive (» = major clinical significance):

With physiology/laboratory test values
Electrocardiogram (ECG) changes, transient, including:
Arrhythmias
S-T depression
T-wave flattening
(may last up to 2 weeks after a dose or course; withdrawal of doxorubicin is usually not necessary)

QRS reduction
(may be a sign of cardiomyopathy; withdrawal of doxorubicin should be considered)

Uric acid
(concentrations in blood and urine may be increased)

**Medical considerations/Contraindications**
The medical considerations/contraindications included here have been selected on the basis of their potential clinical significance (reasons given in parentheses where appropriate)—not necessarily inclusive (» = major clinical significance).

*Risk-benefit should be considered when the following medical problems exist:*

» Bone marrow depression
» Chickenpox, existing or recent (including recent exposure) or
» Herpes zoster
(risk of severe generalized disease)

Gout, history of or
Urate renal stones, history of
(risk of hyperuricemia)

» Heart disease
(cardiotoxicity may occur at lower cumulative doses)

» Hepatic function impairment
(slowed excretion. Reduction in dosage is recommended; one-half the normal dose is recommended in patients with serum bilirubin concentrations of 1.2 to 3 mg per 100 mL; one-quarter the normal dose is recommended in patients with serum bilirubin concentrations of greater than 3 mg per 100 mL)

Sensitivity to doxorubicin
» Tumor cell infiltration of the bone marrow
» Caution should be used also in patients with inadequate bone marrow reserves due to previous cytotoxic drug or radiation therapy.

**Patient monitoring**
The following are especially important in patient monitoring (other tests may be warranted in some patients, depending on condition; » = major clinical significance:

Alanine aminotransferase (ALT [SGPT]) values, serum and
Aspartate aminotransferase (AST [SGOT]) values, serum and
Bilirubin concentrations, serum and
Lactate dehydrogenase (LDH) values, serum
(recommended prior to initiation of therapy and at periodic intervals during therapy; frequency varies according to clinical state, agent, dose, and other agents being used concurrently)

Chest x-ray and
» Echocardiography and
Electrocardiogram (ECG) studies and
» Radionuclide angiography determination of ejection fraction
(recommended prior to initiation of therapy and at periodic intervals during therapy)

» Examination of patient's mouth for ulceration
(recommended before administration of each dose)

» Hematocrit or hemoglobin and
» Leukocyte count, total and, if appropriate, differential and
» Platelet count
(determinations recommended prior to initiation of therapy and at periodic intervals during therapy; frequency varies according to clinical state, agent, dose, and other agents being used concurrently)

Uric acid concentrations, serum
(recommended prior to initiation of therapy and at periodic intervals during therapy; frequency varies according to clinical state, agent, dose, and other agents being used concurrently)

# Side/Adverse Effects

Note: Many "side effects" of antineoplastic therapy are unavoidable and represent the medication's pharmacologic action. Some of these (for example, leukopenia and thrombocytopenia) are actually used as parameters to aid in individual dosage titration.

A necrotizing colitis (cecal inflammation, bloody stools, severe and sometimes fatal infections) has been associated with a combination regimen of doxorubicin and cytarabine.

Excessively rapid intravenous administration may produce facial flushing.

The following side/adverse effects have been selected on the basis of their potential clinical significance (possible signs and symptoms in parentheses where appropriate)—not necessarily inclusive:

**Those indicating need for medical attention**
Incidence more frequent
*Leukopenia or infection* (usually asymptomatic; less frequently, fever or chills; cough or hoarseness; lower back or side pain; painful or difficult urination); *stomatitis or esophagitis* (sores in mouth and on lips)

Note: With *leukopenia*, the nadir of leukocyte count occurs 10 to 14 days after a dose. Recovery usually occurs within 21 days after a dose.

*Stomatitis or esophagitis* occurs 5 to 10 days after administration. It may be severe and lead to ulceration and the potential for severe infections. It is more severe with dosage regimen of 3 successive days.

Incidence less frequent
*Cardiotoxicity, usually in the form of congestive heart failure* (shortness of breath; swelling of feet and lower legs; fast or irregular heartbeat); *extravasation, cellulitis, or tissue necrosis* (pain at injection site); *gastrointestinal ulceration* (stomach pain); *hyperuricemia or uric acid nephropathy* (joint pain; lower back or side pain); *local reaction* (red streaks along injected vein); *phlebosclerosis* (pain at injection site); *postirradiation erythema, recall* (darkening or redness of skin); *thrombocytopenia* (usually asymptomatic; rarely, unusual bleeding or bruising; black, tarry stools; blood in urine or stools; pinpoint red spots on skin)

Note: Incidence *of cardiotoxicity* is more frequent in patients receiving total dosage over 550 mg per square meter of body surface (400 mg per square meter of body surface in patients who have received previous chest irradiation or medications increasing cardiotoxicity) and in patients with a history of cardiac disease or mediastinal radiation, and may be more frequent in children less than 2 years of age and in the elderly.

*Cardiotoxicity* usually appears within 1 to 6 months after initiation of therapy. Cardiomyopathy has been reported to be associated with persistent voltage reduction in the QRS wave, systolic interval prolongation, and reduction of ejection fraction. It may develop suddenly and may not be detected by routine ECG. It may be irreversible and fatal but responds to treatment if detected early.

Acute life-threatening *arrhythmias* have been reported during or within a few hours after administration.

*Extravasation* may also occur without accompanying stinging or burning and even if blood returns well on aspiration of the infusion needle.

*Hyperuricemia or uric acid nephropathy* occurs most commonly during initial treatment of patients with leukemia or lymphoma, as a result of rapid cell breakdown which leads to elevated serum uric acid concentrations.

A *local reaction* may indicate excessively rapid intravenous administration.

*Phlebosclerosis* occurs especially when small veins are used or a single vein is used repeatedly.

*Recall postirradiation erythema* occurs if patient has received previous radiation therapy; severe dermatitis and/or mucositis in the radiated area may occur with concurrent use.

Incidence rare
   *Allergic reaction* (skin rash or itching; fever; chills); *anaphylaxis* (wheezing)

**Those indicating need for medical attention only if they continue or are bothersome**
Incidence more frequent
   *Nausea and vomiting*—may be severe
Incidence less frequent
   *Darkening of soles, palms, or nails*—especially in children and blacks; *diarrhea*

**Those not indicating need for medical attention**
Incidence more frequent
   *Loss of hair; reddish urine*
   Note: *Loss of hair* is complete and reversible. It occurs in most cases.
      *Reddish urine* clears within 48 hours.

**Those indicating the need for medical attention if they occur after medication is discontinued**
   *Cardiotoxicity* (fast or irregular heartbeat; shortness of breath; swelling of feet and lower legs)

## Patient Consultation

As an aid to patient consultation, refer to *Advice for the Patient, Doxorubicin (Systemic)*.

In providing consultation, consider emphasizing the following selected information (» = major clinical significance):

**Before using this medication**
» Conditions affecting use, especially:
   Sensitivity to doxorubicin or lincomycin
   Pregnancy—Use not recommended because of mutagenic, teratogenic, and carcinogenic potential; advisability of using contraception; telling physician immediately if pregnancy is suspected
   Breast-feeding—Not recommended because of risk of serious side effects
   Use in children—Cardiotoxicity more frequent in children less than 2 years of age
   Use in the elderly—Cardiotoxicity may be more frequent in patients 70 years of age and over
   Other medications, especially probenecid, sulfinpyrazone, other bone marrow depressants, or previous cytotoxic drug or radiation therapy
   Other medical problems, especially chickenpox, herpes zoster, heart disease, or hepatic function impairment

**Proper use of this medication**
   Caution in taking combination therapy; taking each medication at the right time
   Importance of ample fluid intake and subsequent increase in urine output to aid in excretion of uric acid
   Frequency of nausea and vomiting; importance of continuing medication despite stomach upset
» Proper dosing

**Precautions while using this medication**
» Importance of close monitoring by the physician
» Avoiding immunizations unless approved by physician; other persons in patient's household should avoid immunizations with oral po-

liovirus vaccine; avoiding persons who have taken oral poliovirus vaccine or wearing a protective mask that covers nose and mouth
*Caution if bone marrow depression occurs:*
» Avoiding exposure to persons with bacterial infections, especially during periods of low blood counts; checking with physician immediately if fever or chills, cough or hoarseness, lower back or side pain, or painful or difficult urination occur
» Checking with physician immediately if unusual bleeding or bruising; black, tarry stools; blood in urine or stools; or pinpoint red spots on skin occur
   Caution in use of regular toothbrush, dental floss, or toothpick; physician, dentist, or nurse may suggest alternatives; checking with physician before having dental work done
   Not touching eyes or inside of nose unless hands washed immediately before
   Using caution to avoid accidental cuts with use of sharp objects such as safety razor or fingernail or toenail cutters
   Avoiding contact sports or other situations where bruising or injury could occur
» Possibility of local tissue injury and scarring if infiltration of intravenous solution occurs; telling doctor or nurse right away about redness, pain, or swelling at injection site

**Side/adverse effects**
   May cause adverse effects such as blood problems, loss of hair, heart problems, and cancer
   Signs of potential side effects, especially leukopenia, infection, stomatitis, esophagitis, cardiotoxicity, extravasation, cellulitis, tissue necrosis, gastrointestinal ulceration, hyperuricemia, uric acid nephropathy, local reaction, recall of postirradiation erythema, thrombocytopenia, allergic reaction, and anaphylaxis
   Physician or nurse can help in dealing with side effects
   Reddish urine for 1 to 2 days after administration may be alarming to patient although medically insignificant
   Possibility of hair loss; should return after treatment has ended

## General Dosing Information

Patients receiving doxorubicin should be under supervision of a physician experienced in cancer chemotherapy. It is recommended that the patient be hospitalized at least during initial treatment.

Doxorubicin should not be used in patients who have previously received complete cumulative doses of doxorubicin and/or daunorubicin.

A variety of dosage schedules of doxorubicin, alone or in combination with other antitumor agents, are used. The prescriber may consult the medical literature as well as the manufacturer's literature in choosing a specific dosage.

Dosage must be adjusted to meet the individual requirements of each patient, on the basis of clinical response and appearance or severity of toxicity.

Use of a weekly dosage of doxorubicin may be associated with a reduced risk of cardiotoxicity and hematologic toxicity.

It is recommended that doxorubicin be administered slowly into the tubing of a freely running intravenous infusion of 0.9% sodium chloride injection or 5% dextrose injection (over not less than 3 to 5 minutes). If possible, veins over joints or in extremities with compromised venous or lymphatic drainage should be avoided.

Care must be taken to avoid extravasation during intravenous administration because of the risk of severe ulceration and necrosis. Facial flushing indicates too-rapid injection.

If extravasation of doxorubicin occurs during intravenous administration, as indicated by local swelling at the tip of the needle and local burning or stinging (may also be painless), the injection and infusion should be stopped immediately and resumed, completing the dose, in another vein. Local infiltration of antidotes is not recommended. Use of ice packs and elevation of the extremity to reduce swelling are recommended. Surgical excision of the involved area may be necessary.

Because it will cause local tissue necrosis, doxorubicin must not be administered intramuscularly or subcutaneously.

Doxorubicin has also been administered intra-arterially and as a topical bladder instillation.

Development of uric acid nephropathy in patients with leukemia or lymphoma may be prevented by adequate oral hydration and, in some cases, administration of allopurinol. Alkalinization of urine may be necessary if serum uric acid concentrations are elevated.

In acute leukemia, doxorubicin may be administered despite the presence of thrombocytopenia and bleeding; stoppage of bleeding and increase in platelet count have occurred during treatment in some cases and platelet transfusions are useful in others.

Special precautions are recommended in patients who develop thrombocytopenia as a result of administration of doxorubicin. These may include extreme care in performing invasive procedures; regular inspection of intravenous sites, skin (including perirectal area), and mucous membrane surfaces for signs of bleeding or bruising; limiting frequency of venipuncture and avoiding intramuscular injections; testing urine, emesis, stool, and secretions for occult blood; care in use of regular toothbrushes, dental floss, toothpicks, safety razors, and fingernail and toenail cutters; avoiding constipation; and using caution to prevent falls and other injuries. Such patients should avoid alcohol and aspirin intake because of the risk of gastrointestinal bleeding. Platelet transfusions may be required.

Patients who develop leukopenia should be observed carefully for signs of infection. Antibiotic support may be required. In neutropenic patients who develop fever, broad-spectrum antibiotic coverage should be initiated empirically, pending bacterial cultures and appropriate diagnostic tests.

**Safety considerations for handling this medication**

There is limited but increasing evidence and concern that personnel involved in preparation and administration of parenteral antineoplastics may be at some risk because of the potential mutagenicity, teratogenicity, and/or carcinogenicity of these agents, although the actual risk is unknown. USP advisory panels recommend cautious handling both in preparation and disposal of antineoplastic agents. Precautions that have been suggested include:
- Use of a biological containment cabinet during reconstitution and dilution of parenteral medications and wearing of disposable surgical gloves and masks.
- Use of proper technique to prevent contamination of the medication, work area, and operator during transfer between containers (including proper training of personnel in this technique).
- Cautious and proper disposal of needles, syringes, vials, ampuls, and unused medication.

A number of medical centers have developed detailed guidelines for handling of antineoplastic agents.

**Combination chemotherapy**

Doxorubicin may be used in combination with other agents in various regimens. As a result, incidence and/or severity of side effects may be altered and different dosages (usually reduced) may be used. For example, doxorubicin is part of the following chemotherapeutic combinations (some commonly used acronyms are in parentheses):
—doxorubicin, bleomycin, vinblastine, and dacarbazine (ABVD).
—cyclophosphamide and doxorubicin (ACe).
—doxorubicin, cyclophosphamide, vincristine, procarbazine, and prednisone (A-COPP).
—doxorubicin and carmustine (Adria + BCNU).
—cyclophosphamide, doxorubicin, and fluorouracil (CAF).
—cyclophosphamide, doxorubicin, methotrexate, and procarbazine (CAMP).
—lomustine, doxorubicin, and vinblastine (CAVe).
—cyclophosphamide, doxorubicin, vincristine, and prednisone (CHOP).
—cyclophosphamide, doxorubicin, and vincristine (CHOR).
—cyclophosphamide, doxorubicin, and cisplatin (CISCA).
—cyclophosphamide, vincristine, doxorubicin, and dacarbazine (CY-VA-DIC).
—fluorouracil, doxorubicin, and cyclophosphamide (FAC).
—fluorouracil, doxorubicin, and mitomycin (FAM).
—methotrexate, doxorubicin, cyclophosphamide, and lomustine (MACC).
—dactinomycin, doxorubicin, vincristine, and cyclophosphamide (T-2 Protocol).
—doxorubicin and cisplatin.
—doxorubicin, vincristine, and prednisone.
—doxorubicin, cytarabine, vincristine, and prednisone.
—doxorubicin and cytarabine.
—doxorubicin, bleomycin, cyclophosphamide, vincristine, and prednisone.
—vincristine, doxorubicin, cyclophosphamide, and methotrexate.

For specific dosages and schedules, consult the literature. For information regarding each agent, consult the individual monographs.

# Parenteral Dosage Forms

Note: Bracketed uses in the *Dosage Forms* section refer to categories of use and/or indications that are not included in U.S. product labeling.

## DOXORUBICIN HYDROCHLORIDE INJECTION USP

**Usual adult dose**

Leukemia, acute lymphocytic or
Leukemia, acute myelocytic or

Carcinoma, bladder or
Carcinoma, breast or
Neuroblastoma or
Carcinoma, ovarian or
Carcinoma, thyroid or
Wilms' tumor or
Carcinoma, lung or
Carcinoma, gastric or
[Carcinoma, head and neck] or
[Carcinoma, cervical]¹ or
[Carcinoma, pancreatic]¹ or
[Carcinoma, prostatic]¹ or
[Carcinoma, testicular] or
[Carcinoma, endometrial]¹ or
[Tumors, germ cell, ovarian]¹ or
Lymphomas, Hodgkin's or
Lymphomas, non-Hodgkin's or
Sarcomas, soft tissue or
Osteosarcoma or
[Ewing's sarcoma]¹ or
[Multiple myeloma]¹—
    Intravenous, 60 to 75 mg per square meter of body surface, repeated every twenty-one days or
    Intravenous, 25 to 30 mg per square meter of body surface a day on two or three successive days, repeated every three to four weeks or
    Intravenous, 20 mg per square meter of body surface once a week.

**Usual adult prescribing limits**

Total cumulative dosage of 550 mg per square meter of body surface, 400 mg per square meter of body surface in patients who have received previous chest irradiation or medications increasing cardiotoxicity (to reduce risk of cardiotoxicity).

**Usual pediatric dose**

Intravenous, 30 mg per square meter of body surface a day on three successive days every four weeks.

**Strength(s) usually available**

U.S.—
    2 mg per mL (5-, 10-, and 25-mL single-dose vials, and 100-mL multidose vial) (Rx) [*Adriamycin PFS* (sodium chloride 0.9%); GENERIC (sodium chloride 0.9%)].

Canada—
    2 mg per mL (15-, 17.5-, 20-, and 25-mL prefilled syringes; 5- and 25-mL single-dose vials, and 200-mL multidose vial) (Rx) [*Adriamycin PFS* (sodium chloride 0.9%)].

**Packaging and storage**

Store between 2 and 8 °C (36 and 46 °F). Protect from light.

**Incompatibilities**

Doxorubicin should not be mixed with heparin, dexamethasone, fluorouracil, hydrocortisone sodium succinate, aminophylline, or cephalothin, since a precipitate may form.

Caution—
    Caution in handling of the 100-mL (200-mg) multidose vial is recommended to prevent confusion with the single-dose vial and possible inadvertent overdose. For example, the manufacturer recommends that the vial be stored in the original carton until the contents are used.

**Note**

Great care should be taken to prevent exposure of the skin to doxorubicin. The use of gloves is recommended. Any doxorubicin solution that comes in contact with the skin or mucosae should be washed off thoroughly with soap and water.

## DOXORUBICIN HYDROCHLORIDE FOR INJECTION USP

**Usual adult dose**

Leukemia, acute lymphocytic or
Leukemia, acute myelocytic or
Carcinoma, bladder or
Carcinoma, breast or
Neuroblastoma or
Carcinoma, ovarian or
Carcinoma, thyroid or
Wilms' tumor or
Carcinoma, lung or
Carcinoma, gastric or
[Carcinoma, head and neck] or
[Carcinoma, cervical] or
[Carcinoma, pancreatic]¹ or
[Carcinoma, prostatic]¹ or

[Carcinoma, testicular] or
[Carcinoma, endometrial] or
[Tumors, germ cell, ovarian] or
Lymphomas, Hodgkin's or
Lymphomas, non-Hodgkin's or
Sarcomas, soft tissue or
Osteosarcoma or
[Ewing's sarcoma][1] or
[Multiple myeloma][1]—
  Intravenous, 60 to 75 mg per square meter of body surface, repeated
    every twenty-one days or
  Intravenous, 25 to 30 mg per square meter of body surface a day on
    two or three successive days, repeated every three to four weeks
    or
  Intravenous, 20 mg per square meter of body surface once a week.

**Usual adult prescribing limits**
Total cumulative dosage of 550 mg per square meter of body surface, 400
mg per square meter of body surface in patients who have received
previous chest irradiation or medications increasing cardiotoxicity (to
reduce risk of cardiotoxicity).

**Usual pediatric dose**
Intravenous, 30 mg per square meter of body surface a day on three successive days every four weeks.

**Size(s) usually available**
U.S.—
  10 mg (single-dose vial) (Rx) [Adriamycin RDF (lactose; methylpar-
    aben); Rubex (lactose); GENERIC (lactose)].
  20 mg (single-dose vial) (Rx) [Adriamycin RDF (lactose; methylpar-
    aben); GENERIC (lactose)].
  50 mg (single-dose vial) (Rx) [Adriamycin RDF (lactose; methylpar-
    aben); Rubex (lactose); GENERIC (lactose)].
  100 mg (single-dose vial) (Rx) [Rubex (lactose)].
  150 mg (multidose vial) (Rx) [Adriamycin RDF (lactose;
    methylparaben)].
Canada—
  10 mg (single-dose vial) (Rx) [Adriamycin RDF (lactose;
    methylparaben)].
  20 mg (single-dose vial) (Rx) [Adriamycin RDF (lactose;
    methylparaben)].
  50 mg (single-dose vial) (Rx) [Adriamycin RDF (lactose;
    methylparaben)].
  150 mg (multidose vial) (Rx) [Adriamycin RDF (lactose;
    methylparaben)].

**Packaging and storage**
Store below 40 °C (104 °F), preferably between 15 and 30 °C (59 and 86
°F), unless otherwise specified by manufacturer. Protect from light.

**Preparation of dosage form**
Doxorubicin Hydrochloride for Injection USP is reconstituted for intravenous administration by adding 5 mL (10-mg vial), 10 mL (20-mg
vial), 25 mL (50-mg vial), 50 mL (100-mg vial), or 75 mL (150-mg
vial) of 0.9% sodium chloride injection to the vial and shaking to
dissolve, producing a solution containing 2 mg of doxorubicin hydrochloride per mL. Use of bacteriostatic diluents is not recommended.
An appropriate volume of air should be withdrawn from the vial during reconstitution to avoid excessive pressure buildup.

**Stability**
Reconstituted solutions of Adriamycin RDF are stable for 7 days at room
temperature and under normal room light (100 foot-candles) or 15 days
between 2 and 8 °C (36 and 46 °F) when protected from sunlight.
Unused solution from single-dose vials or unused solution from the
multiple-dose vial remaining beyond the recommended storage time
should be discarded.
Reconstituted solutions of Rubex or generic doxorubicin are stable for 24
hours at room temperature or 48 hours between 2 and 8 °C (36 and
46 °F). The solution should be protected from light and any unused
solution should be discarded.

**Incompatibilities**
Doxorubicin should not be mixed with heparin, dexamethasone, fluorouracil, hydrocortisone sodium succinate, aminophylline, or cephalothin,
since a precipitate may form.

**Note**
Great care should be taken to prevent inhalation of particles of doxorubicin hydrochloride and exposure of the skin to it. The use of gloves
is recommended. Any doxorubicin powder or solution that comes in
contact with the skin or mucosae should be washed off thoroughly
with soap and water.

[1]Not included in Canadian product labeling.

## Selected Bibliography

Dorr RT, Fritz WL. Cancer chemotherapy handbook. New York: Elsevier,
  1980: 388-401.
Young RC, Ozols RF, Myers CE. The anthracycline antineoplastic drugs.
  NEJM 1981 Jul 16; 305: 139-53.

Revised: 07/11/94
Interim revision: 01/19/95

## DOXYCYCLINE—See Tetracyclines (Systemic)

## DOXYLAMINE—See Antihistamines (Systemic)

## DOXYLAMINE-CONTAINING COMBINATIONS—

Doxylamine, Phenylpropanolamine, Dextromethorphan, and Aspirin (Sys-
temic)—See Cough/Cold Combinations (Systemic)
Doxylamine, Pseudoephedrine, Dextromethorphan, and Acetaminophen
(Systemic)—See Cough/Cold Combinations (Systemic)

# DRONABINOL  Systemic

VA CLASSIFICATION (Primary/Secondary): GA700/GA900
Note: Controlled substance classification—
  U.S.: Schedule II.
  Canada: N.
Another commonly used name is delta-9-tetrahydrocannabinol (THC).
Note: For a listing of dosage forms and brand names by country availa-
  bility, see Dosage Forms section(s). For a listing of brand names
  for the articles in this monograph, refer to the General Index.

## Category
Antiemetic; appetite stimulant.

## Indications

**Accepted**
Nausea and vomiting, cancer chemotherapy-induced (prophylaxis)—
  Dronabinol is indicated in selected patients for the prevention of nausea and vomiting associated with emetogenic cancer chemotherapy
  when other antiemetic medications are not effective.

Anorexia, AIDS-associated (treatment)—Dronabinol is indicated for the
  treatment of anorexia associated with weight loss in patients with acquired immunodeficiency syndrome (AIDS). Tachyphylaxis and tolerance to some effects of dronabinol develop with chronic use; unlike
  cardiovascular and subjective adverse CNS effects, the appetite stimulant effects of dronabinol have been sustained for up to 5 months in
  AIDS patients receiving doses ranging from 2.5 to 20 mg per day.

## Pharmacology/Pharmacokinetics

**Physicochemical characteristics**
Chemical group—A cannabinoid.
Molecular weight—314.47.
pKa—10.6.

**Mechanism of action/Effect**
The exact mechanism of action of dronabinol is not known. Cannabinoid
receptors in neural tissues may mediate the effects of dronabinol and
other cannabinoids. Animal studies with other cannabinoids suggest
that dronabinol's antiemetic effects may be due to inhibition of the
vomiting control mechanism in the medulla oblongata.

## Other actions/effects

Central sympathomimetic activity may result in tachycardia and/or conjunctival injection. Dose-related reversible effects on appetite, mood, cognition, memory, and perception also occur, subject to great interpatient variability.

## Absorption

Although dronabinol is 90 to 95% absorbed after administration of single oral doses, only 10 to 20% reaches the systemic circulation, due to first-pass hepatic metabolism and high lipid solubility.

## Distribution

Apparent volume of distribution is approximately 10 liters per kilogram (L/kg).
Distributed into breast milk.

## Protein binding

Very high (97%).

## Biotransformation

Extensive first-pass hepatic metabolism, primarily by microsomal hydroxylation, yields both active and inactive metabolites. Dronabinol and its principal active metabolite, 11-OH-delta-9-THC, are present in approximately equal concentrations in plasma.

## Half-life

Elimination—
   Alpha phase: 4 hours.
   Terminal (beta) phase: 25 to 36 hours.

## Time to peak concentration

2 to 4 hours.

## Duration of action

Psychoactive effects—4 to 6 hours.
Appetite stimulant effects—24 hours or longer.

## Elimination

Primarily fecal; approximately 50% of an oral dose appears in the feces and 10 to 15% in the urine (either as unchanged drug or as metabolite), within 72 hours.

# Precautions to Consider

## Cross-sensitivity and/or related problems

Patients sensitive to other marijuana products or sesame oil may be sensitive to this preparation also.

## Carcinogenicity

Studies to evaluate the carcinogenic potential of dronabinol have not been performed.

## Mutagenicity

Dronabinol was not shown to be mutagenic in an Ames test.

## Pregnancy/Reproduction

Fertility—In a long-term study in rats at doses 0.3 to 1.5 times the maximum recommended human dose (MRHD) in cancer patients or 2 to 10 times the MRHD in AIDS patients, a decrease in seminal fluid volume, as well as reduced ventral prostate, seminal vesicle, and epididymal weights were reported. Decreases in spermatogenesis, number of developing germ cells, and number of Leydig cells in the testes were also observed. However, sperm count, mating success, and testosterone levels were not affected. The significance of these animal findings for use in humans is not known.

Pregnancy—Adequate and well-controlled studies in humans have not been done.

Reproduction studies in mice (at doses 0.2 to 5 times the MRHD in cancer patients and 1 to 30 times the MRHD in AIDS patients) and in rats (at doses 0.8 to 3 times the MRHD in cancer patients and 5 to 20 times the MRHD in AIDS patients) have revealed no evidence of teratogenicity. However, dose-dependent effects of dronabinol, including decreased maternal weight gain and number of viable pups, and increased fetal mortality and early resorptions were observed.

FDA Pregnancy Category C.

## Breast-feeding

Use is not recommended since dronabinol is distributed into and concentrated in breast milk and is absorbed by the nursing infant.

## Pediatrics

No information is available on whether the risk of dronabinol-induced adverse effects is increased in children. However, because of this medication's psychoactive effects and potential for dependence, it should be used with caution, after less toxic alternatives have been considered and found ineffective. Recommended doses should not be exceeded, and children should be carefully monitored during therapy.

## Geriatrics

Studies performed in a limited number of patients up to 82 years of age have not demonstrated geriatrics-specific problems that would limit the usefulness of dronabinol in the elderly. However, because of this medication's psychoactive effects and potential for creating dependency, therapy could be more troublesome in the elderly and should be used with caution, after less toxic alternatives have been considered and found ineffective. Recommended doses should not be exceeded, and the elderly patient should be carefully monitored during therapy.

## Drug interactions and/or related problems

The following drug interactions and/or related problems have been selected on the basis of their potential clinical significance (possible mechanism in parentheses where appropriate)—not necessarily inclusive (» = major clinical significance):

Note: Combinations containing any of the following medications, depending on the amount present, may also interact with this medication.

Alcohol or
» Central nervous system (CNS) depression–producing medications, other (See *Appendix II*)
   (concurrent use may potentiate the CNS depressant effects of either these medications or dronabinol)

Apomorphine
   (prior administration of dronabinol may decrease the emetic response to apomorphine; also, concurrent use may potentiate the CNS depressant effects of either apomorphine or dronabinol)

## Medical considerations/Contraindications

The medical considerations/contraindications included here have been selected on the basis of their potential clinical significance (reasons given in parentheses where appropriate)—not necessarily inclusive (» = major clinical significance).

*Risk-benefit should be considered when the following medical problems exist:*

Cardiac disorders
   (dronabinol may cause cardiac effects including occasional hypotension, hypertension, syncope, and tachycardia)

Drug abuse or dependence, history of, including acute alcoholism
   (increased risk of dronabinol abuse and dependence)

Hypertension
   (increase in sympathomimetic activity may exacerbate condition)

Manic or depressive states or
Schizophrenia
   (symptoms may be exacerbated)

Sensitivity to dronabinol or sesame oil

## Patient monitoring

The following may be especially important in patient monitoring (other tests may be warranted in some patients, depending on condition; » = major clinical significance):

Blood pressure determinations and
Cardiac function monitoring
   (recommended for early detection of tachycardia and changes in blood pressure, especially in patients with hypertension or cardiac disease)

# Side/Adverse Effects

Note: Following abrupt withdrawal of dronabinol, an abstinence syndrome manifested by irritability, insomnia, and restlessness was observed within 12 hours in volunteers receiving dosages of 210 mg per day for 12 to 16 consecutive days; approximately 24 hours later, the withdrawal syndrome intensified with such symptoms as hot flashes, sweating, rhinorrhea, loose stools, hiccups, and anorexia. Withdrawal symptoms dissipated gradually over the next 48 hours. Electroencephalographic changes consistent with the hyperexcitation effects of drug withdrawal were recorded in patients after abrupt discontinuation.

Sleep disturbances, which continued for several weeks after discontinuation of high-dose dronabinol therapy, have been reported.

Although chronic abuse of cannabis has been associated with decreases in motivation, cognition, judgment, and perception, no such decrements in psychological, social, or neurological status have been associated with the administration of dronabinol for therapeutic purposes. In an open-label study in patients with AIDS who received dronabinol for up to 5 months, no abuse, diversion, or systematic change in personality or social functioning was observed, even in those patients with a history of drug abuse.

The following side/adverse effects have been selected on the basis of their potential clinical significance (possible signs and symptoms in parentheses where appropriate)—not necessarily inclusive:

### Those indicating need for medical attention
Incidence less frequent
*Fast or pounding heartbeat; psychotomimetic effects* (changes in mood; confusion, including delusions and feelings of depersonalization or unreality; hallucinations; mental depression; nervousness or anxiety)

Note: The above side/adverse effects may also be symptoms of overdose.

An initial tachycardia may be followed by normal sinus rhythm and then bradycardia. These effects may disappear when tolerance develops after continued use.

### Those indicating need for medical attention only if they continue or are bothersome
Incidence more frequent
*Clumsiness or unsteadiness; dizziness; drowsiness; nausea; trouble thinking; vomiting*
Incidence less frequent or rare
*Blurred vision or any changes in vision; dryness of mouth; orthostatic hypotension* (feeling faint or lightheaded; unusual tiredness or weakness); *restlessness*

## Overdose

For specific information on the agents used in the management of dronabinol overdose, see:
• *Diazepam* in *Benzodiazepines (Systemic)* monograph.

For more information on the management of overdose or unintentional ingestion, **contact a Poison Control Center** (see *Poison Control Center Listing*).

### Clinical effects of overdose
The following effects have been selected on the basis of their potential clinical significance (possible signs and symptoms in parentheses where appropriate)—not necessarily inclusive:

*Mild intoxication*
*Heightened sensory awareness* (change in your sense of smell, taste, sight, sound, or touch); *altered time perception* (change in how fast you think time is passing); *reddened conjunctiva* (redness of eyes)

*Moderate intoxication*
*Memory impairment* (being forgetful); *urinary retention* (problems in urinating); *reduced bowel motility* (constipation)

*Severe intoxication*
*Slurred speech*

### Treatment of overdose
Overdose may occur either with therapeutic doses or with higher, nontherapeutic doses. Recommended treatment includes:

To decrease absorption—Gut decontamination, if ingestion is recent.

Specific treatment—Treatment of hypertension or hypotension, if necessary. Hypotension usually responds to Trendelenburg position and administration of IV fluids. Pressors are rarely required. Administration of benzodiazepines (5 to 10 mg of diazepam orally) may be used to treat extreme agitation.

Monitoring—Observation of patient in a quiet environment. Continuous blood pressure monitoring. Cardiac monitoring.

Supportive care—Supportive therapy. Patients in whom intentional overdose is confirmed or suspected should be referred for psychiatric consultation.

## Patient Consultation

As an aid to patient consultation, refer to *Advice for the Patient, Dronabinol (Systemic)*.

In providing consultation, consider emphasizing the following selected information (» = major clinical significance):

### Before using this medication
» Conditions affecting use, especially:
Sensitivity to marijuana products or sesame oil
Pregnancy—No studies in humans; increased risk of fetal mortality and resorptions in animal studies with doses many times the usual human dose
Breast-feeding—Not recommended; distributed into breast milk
Use in children—Caution recommended because of psychoactive effects and potential for dependence
Use in the elderly—Caution recommended because of psychoactive effects and potential for dependence
Other medications, especially CNS depressants

### Proper use of this medication
» Importance of not taking more medication than the amount prescribed because of danger of overdose
» Proper dosing
» Missed dose: Taking as soon as possible; not taking if almost time for next dose; not doubling doses
» Proper storage

### Precautions while using this medication
» Avoiding use of alcohol or other CNS depressants during therapy
» Caution if dizziness, drowsiness, lightheadedness, or false sense of well-being occurs
» Caution when getting up suddenly from a lying or sitting position
» Suspected overdose: Getting emergency help at once

### Side/adverse effects
Signs of potential side effects, especially psychotomimetic effects and tachycardia

## General Dosing Information

Because of the potential for abuse and risk of diversion, the amount of dronabinol dispensed should be limited to the amount necessary for the period between clinic visits.

Patients should remain under the supervision of a responsible adult during initial use of dronabinol and following dosage adjustments. Also, patients taking dronabinol should be advised of possible changes in mood and other adverse behavioral effects of the medication, so that occurrence of such effects will not be alarming.

Psychological and physical dependence may occur with high doses or chronic administration of dronabinol; an abstinence syndrome may be precipitated when dronabinol is discontinued. However, this is very unlikely to occur with therapeutic doses and short-term use of dronabinol.

## Oral Dosage Forms

### DRONABINOL CAPSULES USP

#### Usual adult and adolescent dose
Antiemetic—
Oral, 5 mg per square meter of body surface one to three hours prior to the administration of chemotherapy, then every two to four hours after chemotherapy, for a total of four to six doses a day.

Note: The dose may be increased by increments of 2.5 mg per square meter of body surface if initial dose is ineffective and side effects are not significant.

Appetite stimulant—
Oral, initially 2.5 mg two times a day, before lunch and supper. Patients unable to tolerate this dose may be given 2.5 mg a day, administered as a single dose in the evening or at bedtime. The dose may be increased, if clinically indicated and in the absence of significant adverse effects, to a maximum of 20 mg a day; however, the incidence of psychiatric symptoms increases significantly at maximum doses.

#### Usual adult prescribing limits
Antiemetic—
Up to 15 mg per square meter of body surface per dose.
Appetite stimulant—
20 mg a day.

#### Usual pediatric dose
See *Usual adult and adolescent dose.*

#### Usual geriatric dose
See *Usual adult and adolescent dose.*

#### Strength(s) usually available
U.S.—
2.5 mg (Rx) [*Marinol* (sesame oil)].
5 mg (Rx) [*Marinol* (sesame oil)].
10 mg (Rx) [*Marinol* (sesame oil)].
Canada—
2.5 mg (Rx) [*Marinol*].
5 mg (Rx) [*Marinol*].

#### Packaging and storage
Store between 8 and 15 °C (46 and 59 °F), in a well-closed container, unless otherwise specified by manufacturer. Protect from freezing.

#### Auxiliary labeling
• Refrigerate.
• May cause drowsiness.
• Avoid alcoholic beverages.
• May be habit-forming.

**Note**
Controlled substance in the U.S.

Revised: 06/07/93

**DYCLONINE**—See *Anesthetics (Mucosal-Local)*

# DYPHYLLINE   Systemic†

INN: Diprophylline
BAN: Diprophylline
JAN: Diprophylline

VA CLASSIFICATION (Primary): RE104

Another commonly used name is diprophylline.

Note: For a listing of dosage forms and brand names by country availability, see *Dosage Forms* section(s). For a listing of brand names for the articles in this monograph, refer to the General Index.

†Not commercially available in Canada.

## Category

Bronchodilator.

## Indications

### Unaccepted
Dyphylline has been used in the treatment of acute and chronic bronchial asthma, chronic bronchitis, and emphysema; however, aminophylline, oxtriphylline, and theophylline are considered safer and more effective.

Dyphylline is not indicated for management of status asthmaticus or neonatal apnea.

## Pharmacology/Pharmacokinetics

### Physicochemical characteristics
Source—Dyphylline is a chemical derivative of theophylline, but is not a theophylline salt, as are aminophylline and oxtriphylline.
Molecular weight—254.25.

### Mechanism of action/Effect
Dyphylline is a xanthine derivative presumed to have a mechanism of action similar to that of theophylline, although this has not been proven. Dyphylline has only about one-tenth the bronchodilator effect of theophylline.

### Absorption
Oral—Rapid and incomplete.
Intramuscular—Rapid.

### Distribution
Distributed into breast milk.

### Protein binding
Unknown.

### Biotransformation
Not metabolized to theophylline *in vivo*.

### Half-life
Approximately 2 hours, except in patients with impaired renal function. In anuric patients, elimination half-life can be increased to 3 to 4 times that in patients with normal renal function.

### Time to peak concentration
Within 1 hour following oral or intramuscular administration.

### Peak serum concentration
Therapeutic range has not been determined.

### Elimination
Renal; approximately 88% excreted unchanged in the urine.
In dialysis—Hemodialysis accelerates removal of dyphylline.

## Precautions to Consider

### Cross-sensitivity and/or related problems
Patients allergic to another xanthine compound, such as aminophylline, caffeine, oxtriphylline, or theophylline, may be allergic to dyphylline.

### Carcinogenicity/Tumorigenicity/Mutagenicity
Studies have not been done.

### Pregnancy/Reproduction
Fertility—Studies have not been done.
Pregnancy—Studies have not been done in humans.
Studies have not been done in animals.
FDA Pregnancy Category C.

### Breast-feeding
Dyphylline is distributed into breast milk and accumulates to concentrations approximately twice those in plasma. However, dyphylline is considered to be compatible with breast-feeding.

### Pediatrics
As in other patients, aminophylline, oxtriphylline, and theophylline are the preferred xanthine bronchodilators.

### Geriatrics
As in younger patients, aminophylline, oxtriphylline, and theophylline are the preferred xanthine bronchodilators. Since dyphylline is renally eliminated, caution is recommended in older patients who may have age-related renal function impairment.

### Drug interactions and/or related problems
The following drug interactions and/or related problems have been selected on the basis of their potential clinical significance (possible mechanism in parentheses where appropriate)—not necessarily inclusive (» = major clinical significance):

Note: Because dyphylline is not hepatically metabolized, its clearance is not affected by concurrent tobacco or marijuana smoking, or by altered physiologic states, medications, or diets known to affect the hepatic metabolism of theophylline.

Combinations containing any of the following medications, depending on the amount present, may interact with this medication.

» Anesthetics, hydrocarbon inhalation, especially halothane
 (concurrent use with dyphylline may increase the risk of ventricular arrhythmias)

» Beta-adrenergic blocking agents, including ophthalmic agents
 (concurrent use with dyphylline may result in inhibition of dyphylline bronchodilator effect; although agents with beta-1-selectivity may be less antagonistic, extreme caution is recommended if these agents are used in patients with bronchospasm)

Ephedrine
 (concurrent use with dyphylline may result in increased frequency of nausea, nervousness, and insomnia)

» Probenecid
 (caution is recommended if probenecid is used concurrently with dyphylline, since probenecid competes for renal tubular secretion, resulting in decreased elimination of dyphylline)

Sucralfate
 (concurrent use with dyphylline may result in adsorption of the xanthine if these 2 medications are administered less than 2 hours apart)

» Xanthine-derivatives, other
 (concurrent use of aminophylline, oxtriphylline, or theophylline with dyphylline is not recommended)

### Laboratory value alterations
The following have been selected on the basis of their potential clinical significance (possible effect in parentheses where appropriate)—not necessarily inclusive (» = major clinical significance):

With diagnostic test results

Note: Dyphylline does not interfere with serum theophylline concentrations determined by immunoassay or high pressure liquid chromatography.

» Dipyridamole-assisted myocardial perfusion studies
 (dyphylline may reverse the effects of dipyridamole on myocardial blood flow, thereby interfering with test results; dipyridamole-assisted myocardial perfusion studies should not be performed if therapy with dyphylline cannot be withheld for 36 hours prior to the test)

### Medical considerations/Contraindications

The medical considerations/contraindications included here have been selected on the basis of their potential clinical significance (reasons given in parentheses where appropriate)—not necessarily inclusive (» = major clinical significance):

*Risk-benefit should be considered when the following medical problems exist:*

Cardiovascular disease, severe, including acute myocardial injury
(high dyphylline serum concentrations may worsen condition)

Congestive heart failure
(plasma clearance may be decreased, resulting in increased serum concentrations and risk of adverse effects)

» Gastritis, active or
» Peptic ulcer disease, active or history of
(may be exacerbated because the xanthines increase gastric acid secretion)

» Renal function impairment
(elimination half-life of dyphylline is prolonged with decreasing renal function)

» Sensitivity to dyphylline

### Patient monitoring

The following may be especially important in patient monitoring (other tests may be warranted in some patients, depending on condition; » = major clinical significance):

Dyphylline concentration, serum
(assay methods used for measuring serum theophylline concentrations will not measure dyphylline and should not be used; however, dyphylline serum concentration can be determined using high pressure liquid chromatography [HPLC] or gas-liquid chromatography; therapeutic range has not been determined; theophylline does not interfere with serum dyphylline concentrations determined by HPLC)

Pulmonary function tests
(objective measures of lung function are essential for diagnosing and guiding therapeutic decision-making in asthma; measurement of forced expiratory airflow, using a spirometer or peak expiratory flowmeter, is recommended at periodic intervals)

Renal function determinations
(may be required upon initiation of therapy and at periodic intervals during therapy, depending upon the individual patient's condition)

## Side/Adverse Effects

Note: The following side effects have been reported with theophylline. Some may not have been recognized with dyphylline; however, because of pharmacologic similarities among xanthines, they should be considered as potential side effects when dyphylline is administered.

With dyphylline, as with theophylline, the less severe signs or symptoms of toxicity may not always precede the more serious ones such as sinus tachycardia, ventricular arrhythmias, or seizures.

The following side/adverse effects have been selected on the basis of their potential clinical significance (possible signs and symptoms in parentheses where appropriate)—not necessarily inclusive:

### Those indicating need for medical attention
Incidence less frequent
*Gastroesophageal reflux* (heartburn; vomiting)
Note: Theophylline has been shown to relax the gastroesophageal sphincter, possibly resulting in *heartburn* and/or *vomiting*. Although this effect has not been documented with dyphylline, if vomiting occurs, toxicity should be considered.

### Those indicating need for medical attention only if they continue or are bothersome
Incidence less frequent
*Headache; increased urination; insomnia* (trouble in sleeping); *nausea; nervousness; tachycardia* (fast heartbeat); *trembling*

## Overdose

For more information on the management of overdose or unintentional ingestion, **contact a Poison Control Center** (see *Poison Control Center Listing*).

### Clinical effects of overdose
*Abdominal pain, continuing or severe; agitation* (nervousness or restlessness); *confusion or change in behavior; diarrhea; hematemesis* (dark or bloody vomit); *hyperglycemia; hypokalemia; hypotension;*

*metabolic acidosis; seizures; tachyarrhythmias* (fast and irregular heartbeat); *tachycardia* (fast heartbeat); *trembling, continuing; vomiting*

### Treatment of overdose
See *Bronchodilators, Theophylline (Systemic)* monograph.

## Patient Consultation

As an aid to patient consultation, refer to *Advice for the Patient, Dyphylline (Systemic).*

In providing consultation, consider emphasizing the following selected information (» = major clinical significance):

### Before using this medication
» Conditions affecting use, especially:
Allergy to dyphylline or other xanthines
Other medications, especially anesthetics, beta-adrenergic blocking agents, probenecid, or other xanthine-derivatives
Other medical problems, especially gastritis, peptic ulcer disease, or renal function impairment

### Proper use of this medication
Importance of not using more medication than the amount prescribed
Compliance with therapy; not missing any doses
Proper administration: Taking on an empty stomach with a glass of water for faster absorption or, if necessary, taking with meals or immediately after meals to lessen gastrointestinal irritation, unless otherwise directed.

» Proper dosing
Missed dose: Taking as soon as possible; not taking if almost time for next dose; not doubling doses
» Proper storage

### Precautions while using this medication
Regular visits to physician to check progress during therapy
Caution in eating or drinking large amounts of xanthine-containing foods or beverages during therapy with this medication
Caution if any kind of surgery requiring general anesthesia is required.

### Side/adverse effects
Signs of potential side effects, especially gastroesophageal reflux and symptoms of toxicity

## General Dosing Information

Although the molecular weight of dyphylline is 70% of the molecular weight of theophylline, the amount of dyphylline equivalent to a given amount of theophylline is not known. *Use of 70% as a conversion factor in changing a patient from dyphylline to theophylline can result in a serious dosing error.*

### For oral dosage forms only
Alcohol content of the oral liquid dosage forms is significant.

### For parenteral dosage forms only
Dyphylline injection is for intramuscular use only.

Exposure of this dosage form to excessive cold may cause formation of a precipitate. Do not use injection if precipitate is present.

### Diet/Nutrition
Large amounts of caffeine-containing foods or beverages should be avoided during dyphylline therapy, since they may increase the central nervous system stimulant effects of xanthine-derivative bronchodilators.

## Oral Dosage Forms
### DYPHYLLINE ELIXIR USP

**Usual adult dose**
Bronchodilator—Oral, 15 mg per kg of body weight every six hours.

**Usual pediatric dose**
Use is not recommended in children due to high alcohol content and since other medications are more appropriate.

**Strength(s) usually available**
U.S.—
33.3 mg per 5 mL (Rx) [*Lufyllin* (alcohol 20% [by volume])].
53.3 mg per 5 mL (Rx) [*Dilor* (alcohol 18%)].
Canada—
Not commercially available.

**Packaging and storage**
Store below 40 °C (104 °F), preferably between 15 and 30 °C (59 and 86 °F), unless otherwise specified by manufacturer. Store in a tight container. Protect from freezing.

# DYPHYLLINE TABLETS USP

**Usual adult dose**
Bronchodilator—Oral, up to 15 mg per kg of body weight every six hours.

**Usual pediatric dose**
Use is not recommended in children since other medications are more appropriate.

**Strength(s) usually available**
U.S.—
200 mg (Rx) [*Dilor* (scored); *Lufyllin* (scored)].
400 mg (Rx) [*Dilor-400* (scored); *Lufyllin-400* (scored)].
Canada—
Not commercially available.

**Packaging and storage**
Store below 40 °C (104 °F), preferably between 15 and 30 °C (59 and 86 °F), unless otherwise specified by manufacturer. Store in a tight container.

# Parenteral Dosage Forms

## DYPHYLLINE INJECTION USP

**Usual adult dose**
Bronchodilator—Intramuscular, 500 mg initially, followed by 250 to 500 mg every two to six hours as indicated by patient's response.

**Usual adult prescribing limits**
15 mg per kg of body weight.

**Usual pediatric dose**
Use is not recommended in children since other medications are more appropriate.

**Strength(s) usually available**
U.S.—
250 mg per mL (Rx) [*Dilor* (benzyl alcohol; sodium metabisulfite); *Lufyllin*].
Canada—
Not commercially available.

**Packaging and storage**
Store between 15 and 40 °C (59 and 104 °F). Protect from light.

**Stability**
Excessive cold may cause formation of a precipitate. Do not use the injection if precipitate is present.

Developed: 07/10/95

**ECHOTHIOPHATE**—See *Antiglaucoma Agents, Cholinergic, Long-acting (Ophthalmic)*

**ECONAZOLE**—See *Antifungals, Azole (Vaginal)*; *Econazole (Topical)*

# ECONAZOLE Topical

VA CLASSIFICATION (Primary/Secondary): DE102

Note: For a listing of dosage forms and brand names by country availability, see *Dosage Forms* section(s). For a listing of brand names for the articles in this monograph, refer to the General Index.

## Category

Antifungal (topical)

Note: Econazole is a broad-spectrum antifungal, which has an antifungal spectrum similar to that of miconazole.

.

## Indications

Note: Bracketed information in the *Indications* section refers to uses that are not included in U.S. product labeling.

**Accepted**

Candidiasis, cutaneous (treatment)—Econazole is indicated as a primary agent in the topical treatment of cutaneous candidiasis (moniliasis) caused by *Candida (Monilia)* species.

Tinea corporis (treatment)

Tinea cruris (treatment) or

Tinea pedis (treatment)—Econazole is indicated as a primary agent in the topical treatment of tinea corporis (ringworm of the body), tinea cruris (ringworm of the groin; jock itch), or tinea pedis (ringworm of the foot; athlete's foot) caused by *Trichophyton rubrum, T. mentagrophytes, T. tonsurans, Microsporum canis, M. audouini, M. gypseum,* and *Epidermophyton floccosum (Acrothesium floccosum).*

Tinea versicolor (treatment)—Econazole is indicated as a primary agent in the topical treatment of tinea versicolor (pityriasis versicolor; "sun fungus") caused by *Pityrosporon orbiculare (Malassezia furfur).*

[Paronychia (treatment)][1]—Econazole is used in the topical treatment of paronychia caused by fungi.

[Tinea barbae (treatment)][1] or

[Tinea capitis (treatment)][1]—Econazole is used in combination with griseofulvin or systemic ketoconazole (for griseofulvin-resistant cases) in the treatment of tinea barbae and tinea capitis.

Not all species or strains of a particular organism may be susceptible to econazole.

---

[1]Not included in Canadian product labeling.

## Pharmacology/Pharmacokinetics

**Physicochemical characteristics**

Chemical group—Synthetic chlorinated imidazole derivative, structurally related to clotrimazole, ketoconazole, and miconazole.

Molecular weight—444.70.

**Mechanism of action/Effect**

Fungistatic; may be fungicidal, depending on concentration; inhibits biosynthesis of ergosterol or other sterols, damaging the fungal cell wall membrane and altering its permeability; as a result, loss of essential intracellular elements may occur; also inhibits biosynthesis of triglycerides and phospholipids by fungi; in addition, inhibits oxidative and peroxidative enzyme activity, resulting in intracellular buildup of toxic concentrations of hydrogen peroxide, which may contribute to deterioration of subcellular organelles and cellular necrosis. In *Candida albicans,* inhibits transformation of blastospores into invasive mycelial form.

**Other actions/effects**

Also has some activity against gram-positive bacteria.

**Absorption**

Minimal systemic absorption following topical application to normal skin.

**Stratum corneum concentration**

Far exceeded minimum inhibitory concentrations (MICs) for dermatophytes; inhibitory concentrations found in epidermis and as deep as middle region of dermis.

**Elimination**

Renal and fecal; < 1% of applied dose recovered in urine and feces.

## Precautions to Consider

**Carcinogenicity**

Long-term studies in animals have not been done.

**Pregnancy/Reproduction**

Fertility—Studies in rats have shown that econazole given orally causes prolonged gestation. However, studies in humans have not shown that econazole given intravaginally causes prolonged gestation or other adverse reproductive effects.

Pregnancy—Adequate and well-controlled studies in humans have not been done.

Segment I studies in rats have shown that econazole is fetotoxic or embryotoxic when given orally in doses 10 to 40 times the usual human dermal dose. Similar effects were seen in mice, rabbits, and/or rats in Segment II or Segment III studies when econazole was given orally in doses 80 or 40 times the usual human dermal dose, respectively. However, no teratogenic effects were seen in mice, rabbits, or rats when econazole was given orally.

FDA Pregnancy Category C.

**Breast-feeding**

It is not known whether econazole is distributed into human breast milk. However, problems in humans have not been documented. Econazole and/or its metabolites are distributed into the milk of rats following oral administration and were found in the nursing pups. Also, in lactating rats given large oral doses of econazole (40 or 80 times the usual human dermal dose), a decrease in the postpartum viability of pups and survival to weaning was seen.

**Pediatrics**

Appropriate studies on the relationship of age to the effects of econazole have not been performed in the pediatric population. However, pediatrics-specific problems that would limit the usefulness of this medicine in children are not expected.

**Geriatrics**

Appropriate studies on the relationship of age to the effects of econazole have not been performed in the geriatric population. However, geriatrics-specific problems that would limit the usefulness of this medicine in the elderly are not expected.

**Medical considerations/Contraindications**

The medical considerations/contraindications included here have been selected on the basis of their potential clinical significance (reasons given in parentheses where appropriate)—not necessarily inclusive (» = major clinical significance).

*Risk-benefit should be considered when the following medical problem exists:*

Sensitivity to econazole

## Side/Adverse Effects

The following side/adverse effects have been selected on the basis of their potential clinical significance (possible signs and symptoms in parentheses where appropriate)—not necessarily inclusive:

**Those indicating need for medical attention**

Incidence less frequent

*Hypersensitivity* (burning, itching, stinging, redness, or other signs of irritation not present before therapy)

## Patient Consultation

As an aid to patient consultation, refer to *Advice for the Patient, Econazole (Topical).*

In providing consultation, consider emphasizing the following selected information (» = major clinical significance):

**Before using this medication**

» Conditions affecting use, especially:

Pregnancy—Fetotoxic and embryotoxic reactions were seen in rats, mice, and rabbits given large oral doses

Breast-feeding—Econazole was distributed into breast milk of rats given large oral doses

**Proper use of this medication**

Applying sufficient medication to cover affected and surrounding areas, and rubbing in gently

» Avoiding contact with the eyes

» Not applying occlusive dressing over this medication unless directed to do so by physician

» Compliance with full course of therapy; fungal infections may require prolonged therapy

» Proper dosing

Missed dose: Applying as soon as possible; not applying if almost time for next dose

» Proper storage

**Precautions while using this medication**

Checking with physician if no improvement within 2 weeks or more

» Using hygienic measures to help cure infection or to help prevent reinfection

*For tinea cruris*

Avoiding underwear that is tight-fitting or made from synthetic materials; wearing loose-fitting cotton underwear instead

Using a bland, absorbent powder or an antifungal powder on the skin; not using cream and powder concurrently

*For tinea pedis*

Carefully drying feet, especially between toes, after bathing

Avoiding socks made from wool or synthetic materials; wearing clean, cotton socks and changing them daily or more often if feet perspire excessively

Wearing well-ventilated shoes or sandals

Using a bland, absorbent powder or an antifungal powder between toes, on feet, and in socks and shoes liberally once or twice daily; not using cream and powder concurrently

**Side/adverse effects**

Signs of potential side effects, especially hypersensitivity reactions

## General Dosing Information

Use of topical antifungals may lead to skin sensitization, resulting in hypersensitivity reactions with subsequent topical use of the medication.

To reduce the possibility of recurrence, *Candida* infections, tinea cruris, and tinea corporis should be treated for at least 2 weeks and tinea pedis should be treated for at least 1 month.

When this medication is used in the treatment of candidiasis, occlusive dressings should be avoided since they provide conditions that favor growth of yeast and release of its irritating endotoxin.

## Topical Dosage Forms

### ECONAZOLE NITRATE CREAM

**Usual adult and adolescent dose**

Candidiasis, cutaneous—

Topical, to the skin, two times a day, morning and evening.

Tinea corporis; or

Tinea cruris; or

Tinea pedis; or

Tinea versicolor—

Topical, to the skin, once a day.

**Usual pediatric dose**

See *Usual adult and adolescent dose*.

**Strength(s) usually available**

U.S.—

1% (Rx) [*Spectazole*].

Canada—

1% (Rx) [*Ecostatin*].

**Packaging and storage**

Store below 30 °C (86 °F), in a well-closed container, unless otherwise specified by manufacturer. Protect from freezing.

**Auxiliary labeling**

• For external use only.

• Continue medicine for full time of treatment.

Revised: 04/14/92
Interim revision: 06/06/94

---

# EDETATE CALCIUM DISODIUM    Systemic

INN: Sodium calcium edetate

VA CLASSIFICATION (Primary/Secondary): AD300/DX900

Other commonly used names are calcium EDTA, edathamil calcium disodium, and sodium calcium edetate.

Note: For a listing of dosage forms and brand names by country availability, see *Dosage Forms* section(s). For a listing of brand names for the articles in this monograph, refer to the General Index.

## Category

Chelating agent; diagnostic aid, lead mobilization.

## Indications

Note: Bracketed information in the *Indications* section refers to uses that are not included in U.S. product labeling.

**Accepted**

Toxicity, lead (treatment)—Edetate calcium disodium is indicated for the treatment of acute and chronic lead poisoning (plumbism) and lead encephalopathy.

Dimercaprol complements edetate calcium disodium by rapidly removing lead from red blood cells and by assisting in mobilizing lead from skeletal stores. When the combination is used, the rate of lead excretion is doubled, thus decreasing the mortality rate and likelihood of permanent neurologic deficits from lead poisoning.

Signs and symptoms of lead poisoning include anemia, gastrointestinal complaints (abdominal pain and vomiting), nephropathy, and encephalopathy. Symptoms of lead encephalopathy include headache and insomnia; persistent vomiting, sometimes projectile; visual disturbances; irritability, restlessness, delirium, hallucinations; ataxia; convulsions and coma; and characteristically high intracranial pressure. Recovery is slow and often incomplete, with residual neurologic deficit.

Edetate calcium disodium may be used as sole therapy when blood lead levels fall between 45 and 69 mcg per deciliter, unless serious symptoms such as encephalopathy are present. Clinical signs and symptoms

suggesting lead poisoning that should be treated with the dimercaprol, edetate calcium disodium combination include the following:

• Patient is symptomatic (with or without encephalopathy).

• Blood lead concentrations are greater than or equal to 70 mcg per deciliter.

[Lead mobilization determination][1]—Edetate calcium disodium may be used as a diagnostic agent to identify patients who qualify for a full course of chelation therapy by determining the magnitude of lead stores in high-risk, asymptomatic children with mild to moderate increases in lead absorption (25 to 44 mcg of lead per deciliter of whole blood). However, use of the lead mobilization test is controversial because of variable results, difficulty in collecting urine from non-toilet-trained children, possible increase in brain lead levels, and risk of iron deficiency causing a negative mobilization result.

**Unaccepted**

To a lesser extent, cadmium, manganese, iron, copper, chromium, and nickel are also chelated, but the value of edetate calcium disodium in poisoning caused by these metals is questionable or unproven.

Edetate calcium disodium is *not* effective in arsenic, gold, or mercury poisoning.

Edetate calcium disodium is *not* effective in preventing or retarding the progression of atherosclerosis.

---

[1]Not included in Canadian product labeling.

## Pharmacology/Pharmacokinetics

**Physicochemical characteristics**

Molecular weight—374.27.

**Mechanism of action/Effect**

Edetate calcium disodium reduces blood concentrations and depot stores of lead. The calcium is replaced by divalent and trivalent metals, especially any available lead, to form stable, soluble complexes that are readily excreted. Edetate calcium disodium is saturated with calcium but can be administered intravenously in large quantities without causing any significant changes in serum or total body calcium concentrations.

## Other actions/effects
Edetate calcium disodium greatly increases chelation and urinary excretion of zinc, but this action is considered clinically insignificant unless therapy is continued for more than 5 days or zinc stores are low prior to treatment. Edetate calcium disodium has been found to chelate iron, copper, calcium, and manganese.

## Absorption
Well absorbed after parenteral administration; poorly absorbed from the gastrointestinal tract. The oral route of administration is no longer used because of poor GI absorption. The absorption of any lead in the intestines may be increased upon oral administration of edetate calcium disodium because the lead chelate formed is more soluble than the lead itself. After absorption, the chelate dissociates and releases free lead ions, producing increased symptoms of lead toxicity.

## Distribution
Extracellular fluid (90%); edetate calcium disodium does not penetrate erythrocytes and only slowly diffuses into the cerebrospinal fluid.

## Biotransformation
No metabolism occurs; after parenteral administration, edetate calcium disodium is excreted in the urine either unchanged or as the metal chelates.

## Half-life
Plasma—
Intravenous administration: 20 to 60 minutes.
Intramuscular administration: 1.5 hours.

## Elimination
Renal, by glomerular filtration; 50% of the chelate that is formed appears in urine within the first hour after parenteral administration; 70% or more during first 4 hours; and 95% in 24 hours. Excretion is unaffected by urinary pH. Theoretically, one gram of edetate calcium disodium chelates 620 mg of lead, but only 3 to 5 mg of lead is excreted in the urine after parenteral administration of one gram to patients with symptoms of acute lead poisoning or with high concentrations of lead in soft tissues.

# Precautions to Consider

## Pregnancy/Reproduction
Pregnancy—Studies in humans have not been done. Risk-benefit must be considered during early pregnancy or in women of child-bearing potential.
One reproduction study in rats at doses up to 13 times the human dose revealed no evidence of impaired fertility or harm to the fetus. Another reproduction study performed in rats at doses up to 25 to 40 times the human dose revealed evidence of fetal malformations, which were prevented by simultaneous administration of zinc supplements.
FDA Pregnancy Category B.

## Breast-feeding
It is not known whether edetate calcium disodium is distributed into breast milk.

## Pediatrics
Because the intramuscular route is painful and there may be poor blood flow to muscle, the intravenous route is recommended for children. In cases of lead encephalopathy, fluid restriction may necessitate giving edetate calcium disodium intramuscularly. Children may require repeated courses of therapy if blood lead levels are greater than 45 mcg per deciliter.
The preferred treatment for children with lead encephalopathy is combined therapy with edetate calcium disodium and dimercaprol.

## Geriatrics
No information is available on the relationship of age to the effects of edetate calcium disodium in geriatric patients.

## Drug interactions and/or related problems
The following drug interactions and/or related problems have been selected on the basis of their potential clinical significance (possible mechanism in parentheses where appropriate)—not necessarily inclusive (» = major clinical significance):
Insulin
   (concurrent use will decrease the duration of action of zinc insulin preparations by chelation of zinc)
Zinc supplements
   (concurrent use may decrease the effectiveness of edetate calcium disodium and zinc supplements due to chelation; zinc supplement therapy should be withheld until edetate calcium disodium therapy is completed)

## Laboratory value alterations
The following have been selected on the basis of their potential clinical significance (possible effect in parentheses where appropriate)—not necessarily inclusive (» = major clinical significance):
With diagnostic test results
   Electrocardiogram (ECG) readings
      (inversion of T-wave may occur)

## Medical considerations/Contraindications
The medical considerations/contraindications included here have been selected on the basis of their potential clinical significance (reasons given in parentheses where appropriate)—not necessarily inclusive (» = major clinical significance).

### Except under special circumstances, this medication should not be used when the following medical problems exist:
» Anuria or
» Oliguria, severe
      (fatal lower nephron necrosis may result; if anuria occurs during therapy or is present before therapy, urine flow should be restored before starting edetate calcium disodium therapy)

### Risk-benefit should be considered when the following medical problems exist:
» Dehydration
      (when acutely ill patients are dehydrated from vomiting and/or diarrhea, urine flow must be established before administering the first dose of edetate calcium disodium; once the flow is established, intravenous fluids must be restricted to basal water and electrolyte requirements)
   Hypercalcemia
      (transitory hypercalcemia during treatment may exacerbate an existing condition)
» Renal function impairment
      (reduced glomerular filtration may delay the excretion of the chelate and increase the risk of nephrotoxicity)

## Patient monitoring
The following may be especially important in patient monitoring (other tests may be warranted in some patients, depending on condition; » = major clinical significance):
   Blood urea nitrogen (BUN) concentrations and
   Calcium concentrations, serum and
   Creatinine concentrations, serum and
   Hepatocellular enzymes and
   Phosphorus concentrations, serum and
   Urine output
      (determinations recommended prior to treatment and on the first, third, and fifth day of each course of therapy for evidence of renal function impairment)
   Cardiac monitoring
      (may be recommended periodically to find irregularities of cardiac rhythm, especially if edetate calcium disodium is given intravenously)
   Fluid intake
      (must be kept to a minimum if cerebral edema is present; volume of urine and flow must be adequate for elimination of lead chelate)
   Urinalysis, routine
      (recommended daily during each course of therapy; since severe, acute lead poisoning and edetate calcium disodium may both produce the same signs of renal damage, urinalyses should be performed to determine if proteinuria or hematuria is improving or if evidence of renal tubular injury is worsening; edetate calcium disodium must be discontinued immediately if large renal epithelial cells or increasing numbers of red blood cells are present in urinary sediment, or if there is evidence of increased proteinuria)

# Side/Adverse Effects
The following side/adverse effects have been selected on the basis of their potential clinical significance (possible signs and symptoms in parentheses where appropriate)—not necessarily inclusive:

## Those indicating need for medical attention
Incidence more frequent
*Systemic febrile reaction* (chills or sudden fever; fatigue; headache; increased thirst; loss of appetite; malaise); *histamine-like reaction* (sneezing; stuffy nose; watery eyes)—possibly occurring 4 to 8 hours after intravenous infusion; *low blood pressure; nausea or vomiting; renal damage or renal tubular necrosis* (cloudy urine); *thrombophlebitis* (pain or swelling at site of injection)

Note: *Febrile reaction* has been observed in some patients 4 to 8 hours after infusion; it may accompany *histamine-like reaction*.

*Renal damage* or *tubular necrosis* may occur when daily dose is excessive. Microscopic hematuria, proteinuria, or large renal epithelial cells may be observed in urine.

*Thrombophlebitis* may be a result of inadequate dilution of injection. Concentration of solution should not exceed 0.5%.

**Incidence less frequent**

*Transient anemia or bone marrow depression* (bleeding and bruising; sore throat and fever; unusual tiredness or weakness); *dermatitis* (cracking and dry, scaly skin, or sores in mouth and on lips); *hypercalcemia* (constipation; drowsiness; dry mouth; continuing headache; loss of appetite; metallic taste)

Note: *Dermatitis* lesions are similar to those caused by vitamin $B_6$ deficiency; results from prolonged administration at high doses and may be due to zinc depletion.

*Hypercalcemia* is usually transitory and accompanied by a significant increase in urinary excretion of calcium from endogenous sources. However, since recurring hypercalcemia may be causally related to renal tubular injury, discontinuation of edetate calcium disodium therapy is recommended when hypercalcemia occurs in susceptible patients.

**Incidence rare**

*Frequent or sudden urge to urinate; secondary gout* (severe pain in feet, knees, hands, elbows)—hyperuricemia may result from renal tubular toxicity

## General Dosing Information

**Warning:** The dosage schedule should be followed and the recommended daily dose must not be exceeded because of the toxic and potentially fatal effects of edetate calcium disodium.

Edetate calcium disodium is equally effective when administered intramuscularly or intravenously. However, the intravenous route is preferred because the intramuscular route is painful and children have poor blood flow to muscle.

In patients with lead encephalopathy or cerebral edema, intravenous infusion is preferred, but rapid infusion may be lethal because of a sudden increase in intracranial pressure. An excess of fluids must be avoided in such patients, and the intramuscular route should be used.

If edetate calcium disodium is given intramuscularly, pain at site of intramuscular injection may be reduced by mixing a 20% solution of edetate calcium disodium with procaine or lidocaine. A final procaine or lidocaine concentration of 5 mg per mL (0.5%) can be obtained by mixing 0.25 mL of a 10% lidocaine solution per 5 mL of edetate calcium disodium or 1 mL of 1% procaine or lidocaine solution per mL of edetate calcium disodium. Crystalline procaine may be used instead to maintain minimum fluid volume.

Urine flow should be established before the first dose of edetate calcium disodium is administered to acutely ill, dehydrated patients. When urine flow has been established, further intravenous fluids should be restricted to basal water and electrolyte requirements.

Each course of therapy should not exceed 5 to 7 days, with a drug-free interval of at least 2 days (preferably 2 weeks) between courses. This allows redistribution of lead from inaccessible storage sites, such as soft tissue or bone, and will result in a greater amount of lead available for elimination.

In cases of lead encephalopathy, children may require repeated courses of therapy if blood lead levels are greater than 45 mcg per deciliter.

Successful chelation therapy requires the administration of a sufficient molar excess of chelating agent over lead. Since the maximum safe dose of edetate calcium disodium alone may cause a shift of lead into the CNS, dimercaprol is combined with edetate calcium disodium. The preferred route of administration for edetate calcium disodium is intravenous and dimercaprol is given by deep intramuscular injection in divided doses every 4 hours for 5 days. If both drugs are given by intramuscular injection, then they must be given at separate sites. Dimercaprol is given alone for the first dose 4 hours before the combination is begun. Injection sites should be rotated. In asymptomatic or mildly symptomatic patients, dimercaprol may be discontinued after 48 hours, with edetate calcium disodium being continued for an additional 48 to 72 hours at reduced dosage.

Oral penicillamine is used after initial therapy with edetate calcium disodium or combined dimercaprol and edetate calcium disodium for long-term chelation therapy, especially if long-bone radiographs show lead lines. The oral chelating agent succimer has recently been approved for treatment of children with blood lead levels greater than 45 mcg per deciliter. Although use to date has been limited, toxicity appears to be less than with other agents.

**For lead mobilization test**

Use of the lead mobilization test is controversial because of variable results, difficulty in collecting urine from non–toilet-trained children, possible increase in brain lead levels, and risk of iron deficiency causing a negative mobilization result.

Since the blood lead (BL) concentrations may not be a sensitive indicator of the body burden of lead in asymptomatic children with BL 25 to 44 mcg per dL, diagnostic tests may be performed as follows:

• Edetate calcium disodium is given intravenously at a dose of 15 mg per kg of body weight (mg/kg) (500 mg per square meter) in 5% dextrose over 1 hour; or edetate calcium disodium given intramuscularly at a dose of 15 mg/kg (500 mg per square meter) mixed with an equivalent amount of procaine so that the final concentration of procaine is 0.5%.

• An 8-hour urine sample, collected in lead-free equipment, is obtained.

• The test is considered positive for increased body burden of lead when the 8-hour urinary excretion of lead is greater than 0.6 mcg per mg of edetate calcium disodium administered.

• If the diagnostic mobilization test is positive, a five-day course of therapy is administered. The test may be repeated if another course of therapy is necessary.

• The upper limit for acceptable blood lead concentrations is 10 mcg per deciliter of whole blood. At 20 mcg per deciliter, medical evaluation should occur.

• In symptomatic patients or those with whole blood lead concentrations greater than or equal to 45 mcg per dL, appropriate chelation therapy should be given immediately without performing the mobilization test.

**For treatment of adverse effects**

Recommended treatment consists of the following:

• Cessation of urine flow during therapy—Administration of edetate calcium disodium must be stopped to avoid excessively high tissue concentrations of the chelating agent.

• Sores in mouth and on lips—Subside when edetate calcium disodium is discontinued; replacement of zinc by supplementation may be advisable during drug-free interval between courses of therapy.

## Parenteral Dosage Forms

Note: Bracketed uses in the *Dosage Forms* section refer to categories of use and/or indications that are not included in U.S. product labeling.

### EDETATE CALCIUM DISODIUM INJECTION USP

**Usual adult and adolescent dose**

Lead toxicity—

Intravenous or intramuscular, in conjunction with dimercaprol, 30 to 50 mg of edetate calcium disodium per kg of body weight (1 to 1.5 grams per square meter of body surface area) per day in two divided doses twelve hours apart for three to five days.

Note: Patients with blood lead levels between 45 and 69 mcg per deciliter may be treated with edetate calcium disodium alone using the same dosage given above for use with dimercaprol.

A second course of treatment may be administered for up to five additional days after at least a two-day drug-free interval (preferably two weeks).

When serum creatinine is 2 mg per deciliter or less, the dosage is 1 gram a day for 5 days. If the serum creatinine is 2 to 3 mg per deciliter, the dosage is 500 mg a day.

For intravenous administration, the dilution must be infused slowly over a period of at least two hours for symptomatic patients and one hour for asymptomatic patients.

[Lead mobilization test][1]—

Intravenous, 1 gram over 1 hour. The same dose can be mixed with procaine, so that the final concentration of procaine is 0.5%; and given intramuscularly.

**Usual adult prescribing limits**

The maximum dose is 2 grams a day.

**Usual pediatric dose**

Lead toxicity—

For blood lead levels greater than 70 mcg per deciliter or serious symptoms: Intravenous or intramuscular, in conjunction with dimercaprol, 1500 mg of edetate calcium disodium per square meter of body surface area a day, administered on a four-hour schedule for 5 days.

Note: Some clinicians prefer that edetate calcium disodium be given by continuous intravenous infusion. If given by intramuscular route, it must be given at a separate site from dimercaprol.

Children with blood lead levels between 45 and 69 mcg per deciliter may be treated with edetate calcium disodium alone, using a dose of 1000 mg of edetate calcium disodium per square meter of body surface area a day for 5 days.

A second course of treatment may be administered after a drug-free interval of at least two days.

Children with lead encephalopathy may require additional courses of therapy. Therapy should continue if blood lead levels are greater than 45 mcg per dL.

[Lead mobilization test][1]—

Intravenous, 15 mg per kg of body weight (500 mg per square meter of body surface area) up to a maximum dose of 1 gram over 1 hour. The same dose can be mixed with procaine, so that the final concentration of procaine is 0.5%, and given intramuscularly.

### Strength(s) usually available
U.S.—

200 mg per mL (Rx) [*Calcium Disodium Versenate*].

Canada—

200 mg per mL (Rx) [*Calcium Disodium Versenate*].

### Packaging and storage
Store below 40 °C (104 °F), preferably between 15 and 30 °C (59 and 86 °F), unless otherwise specified by manufacturer.

### Preparation of dosage form
Intravenous—Dilute 1 gram of edetate calcium disodium with 250 to 500 mL of 0.9% sodium chloride injection or 5% dextrose injection.

### Incompatibilities
Edetate calcium disodium injection is physically incompatible with 10% dextrose injection, 10% invert sugar, 10% invert sugar in sodium chloride injection, lactated Ringer's injection, Ringer's injection, one-sixth molar sodium lactate injection, and injectable preparations of amphotericin B and hydralazine hydrochloride.

### Additional information
Contains 5.3 mEq of sodium per gram of edetate calcium disodium.

[1]Not included in Canadian product labeling.

Revised: 07/06/92

---

# EDETATE DISODIUM   Ophthalmic*†

VA CLASSIFICATION (Primary): OP900.

Some commonly used names are disodium EDTA, edathamil disodium, and sodium edetate.

Note: For a listing of dosage forms and brand names by country availability, see *Dosage Forms* section(s). For a listing of brand names for the articles in this monograph, refer to the General Index.

*Not commercially available in the U.S.
†Not commercially available in Canada.

## Category
Chelating agent (ophthalmic).

## Indications
Note: Bracketed information in the *Indications* section refers to uses that are not included in U.S. product labeling.

### Accepted
[Calcium deposits, corneal (treatment)][1]—Edetate disodium is used topically to remove exogenous or endogenous calcific corneal deposits that may cause pain or impair vision. Removal of superficial calcium deposits may improve vision, unless scarring and vascularization have occurred.

[Calcium hydroxide burns, in eye (treatment)][1] or
[Zinc chloride injury, in eye (treatment)][1]—Edetate disodium has been used as emergency treatment to decontaminate the eye after injury by zinc chloride and for emergency management and follow-up treatment of calcium hydroxide burns in the eye.

[1]Not included in Canadian product labeling.

## Pharmacology/Pharmacokinetics

### Physicochemical characteristics
Molecular weight—372.24.

### Mechanism of action/Effect
Calcium deposits, corneal—Deposits from band keratopathy and other corneal calcium deposits associated with chronic uveitis, advanced interstitial keratitis, or hypercalcemia are dissolved from the conjunctiva, corneal epithelium, and anterior layers of the stroma.

### Distribution
Calcium deposits in the deep stroma are not affected. Edetate disodium does not penetrate the corneal epithelium. The epithelium must be completely removed before application, unless the deposit extends to the surface.

## Precautions to Consider

### Pregnancy/Reproduction
Problems in humans have not been documented.

### Breast-feeding
Problems in humans have not been documented.

### Pediatrics
No information is available on the relationship of age to the effects of edetate disodium in pediatric patients.

### Geriatrics
No information is available on the relationship of age to the effects of edetate disodium in geriatric patients.

## Side/Adverse Effects
The following side/adverse effects have been selected on the basis of their potential clinical significance (possible signs and symptoms in parentheses where appropriate)—not necessarily inclusive:

**Those indicating need for medical attention**
Incidence less frequent
   *Swelling of the stroma*—usually with the higher concentrations

**Those indicating need for medical attention only if they continue or are bothersome**
Incidence less frequent
   *Stinging in the eye; swelling of the eyelids*

## General Dosing Information

To remove calcium deposits from the anterior layers of the stroma, a local anesthetic is administered before the procedure. Since cocaine facilitates the removal of the corneal epithelium, it is often preferred.

After the complete removal of the epithelium, the edetate disodium solution is applied to the cornea as a corneal bath, by continuous irrigation, or by a solution-soaked pledget for 15 to 20 minutes.

The eye is irrigated after the procedure with 0.9% sodium chloride injection or a balanced salt solution.

Since edetate disodium does not solubilize calcium well, treatment usually needs to be combined with mechanical scraping.

For treatment of calcium hydroxide burns or zinc chloride injury, the eye should first be flushed with water as quickly as possible and then irrigated with edetate disodium solution for 15 minutes. Treatment for zinc chloride injury may be ineffective unless started within 2 minutes of injury.

Edetate disodium is toxic to the corneal stroma, causing swelling of the cornea and severe inflammation. To avoid overuse, only as much as necessary should be applied for the shortest possible duration, varying from patient to patient.

## Ophthalmic Dosage Forms
Note: Bracketed uses in the *Dosage Forms* section refer to categories of use and/or indications for drugs that are not commercially available in the U.S.

### EDETATE DISODIUM OPHTHALMIC SOLUTION
Note: In the U.S. and Canada, edetate disodium injection [*Disotate; Endrate*; GENERIC ] is being used to prepare the ophthalmic solution dosage form. Edetate disodium injection is not commercially available in Canada; however, it is available by drug emergency release from the Health Protection Branch.

**Usual adult and adolescent dose**
[Corneal calcium deposits]¹or
[Calcium hydroxide burns]¹—
    Topical, to the cornea, a 0.35 to 1.85% solution as irrigation for fifteen
      to twenty minutes.
[Zinc chloride injury]¹—
    Topical, to the cornea, a 1.7% solution as irrigation for fifteen minutes.

**Usual pediatric dose**
See *Usual adult and adolescent dose.*

**Strength(s) usually available**
U.S.—
    Dosage form not commercially available. Compounding required for
      prescriptions.

Canada—
    Dosage form not commercially available. Compounding required for
      prescriptions.

**Preparation of dosage form**
Dilute edetate disodium injection to the desired concentration with 0.9%
  sodium chloride injection.

¹Not included in Canadian product labeling.

Revised: 02/20/92

---

# EDETATE DISODIUM   Systemic†

VA CLASSIFICATION (Primary): AD300

Other commonly used names are disodium EDTA, edathamil disodium,
  and sodium edetate.

Note: For a listing of dosage forms and brand names by country availa-
      bility, see *Dosage Forms* section(s). For a listing of brand names
      for the articles in this monograph, refer to the General Index.

†Not commercially available in Canada; however, it is available by
emergency drug release from the Health Protection Branch.

## Category
Chelating agent.

## Indications

**Accepted**

Hypercalcemia (treatment)—Edetate disodium is indicated in selected patients for the emergency treatment of acute hypercalcemia, but is recommended only when the severity of the clinical condition (as when
  there has been a judgment of imminent death from hypercalcemic crisis) justifies the aggressive measures associated with this therapy.
  Other therapies should be started simultaneously so that treatment with
  edetate disodium will not exceed 48 hours. Some physicians recommend not using edetate disodium for hypercalcemia, especially when
  it is associated with metastatic bone disease, because of minimal and
  temporary beneficial effects and the great risk of renal damage.

Toxicity, digitalis glycoside (treatment)—Edetate disodium is indicated
  for the control of ventricular arrhythmias associated with digitalis toxicity. Although its onset of action is rapid, the short-term effects require that alternative therapy be undertaken quickly. Edetate disodium
  is rarely used to treat digitalis-induced ventricular arrhythmias since
  other more effective agents are available. Although edetate disodium
  may have been useful when other medications, such as potassium or
  phenytoin, were contraindicated or ineffective, or when controlling
  arrhythmias caused by digitalis poisoning in children who had ingested
  massive doses, it has now been replaced by digoxin immune fab as
  the first-line agent for treatment of life-threatening digitalis glycoside
  toxicity.

**Unaccepted**

Edetate disodium is *not* indicated for the treatment of arteriosclerosis or
  atherosclerotic vascular disease involving coronary or peripheral vessels associated with advancing age, since it has not been proven effective and severe nephrotoxicity may occur.

Edetate disodium is *not* indicated for the treatment of lead poisoning because, unlike edetate calcium disodium, it causes hypocalcemia.

Edetate disodium is *not* indicated for the treatment of renal calculi by
  retrograde irrigation.

## Pharmacology/Pharmacokinetics

**Mechanism of action/Effect**

Hypercalcemia—Edetate disodium forms soluble complexes with calcium
  in the blood, which are filtered by the glomeruli and not reabsorbed
  by the renal tubules. Chelation with calcium produces a lowering of
  serum calcium concentrations and a mobilization of extracirculatory
  calcium stores, especially from bone, during slow intravenous infusion. Theoretically, 1 gram of edetate disodium will chelate 120 mg
  of calcium. Hypocalcemic tetany, seizures, severe cardiac arrhythmias,
  and respiratory arrest may occur with the rapid decrease in serum
  calcium concentrations. However, the mobilization of calcium from

bone may lessen the risk of hypocalcemia. Calcium ion concentrations
  in cerebrospinal fluid are not affected by edetate disodium.

Digitalis toxicity—Edetate disodium exerts a negative inotropic effect on
  the heart. The chronotropic and inotropic effects of digitalis glycosides
  on the ventricles of the heart are transiently antagonized by the hypocalcemia induced by edetate disodium.

**Other actions/effects**

Edetate disodium also forms chelates with and increases urinary excretion
  of other polyvalent metals, such as magnesium, zinc, and other trace
  elements.

Although edetate disodium does not form a chelate with potassium, the
  serum concentration of potassium may be decreased and the urinary
  excretion of potassium increased.

**Biotransformation**
None.

**Elimination**
Rapidly excreted by the kidneys, principally as the calcium chelate; 95%
  of a dose appears in the urine within 24 hours; changes in urine flow
  and pH do not affect the rate of excretion of the chelate.

## Precautions to Consider

**Pregnancy/Reproduction**

Pregnancy—Edetate disodium crosses the placenta. Adequate and well-
  controlled studies in humans have not been done.

Studies in rats have shown that edetate disodium causes impaired reproduction and fetal malformations. Since these effects were prevented
  by simultaneous supplementation of dietary zinc, it is believed that
  zinc deficiency may be the cause.

FDA Pregnancy Category C.

**Breast-feeding**
Problems in humans have not been documented.

**Pediatrics**
No information is available on the relationship of age to the effects of
  edetate disodium in pediatric patients.

**Geriatrics**
No information is available on the relationship of age to the effects of
  edetate disodium in geriatric patients.

**Drug interactions and/or related problems**
The following drug interactions and/or related problems have been selected on the basis of their potential clinical significance (possible
  mechanism in parentheses where appropriate)—not necessarily inclusive (» = major clinical significance):

» Digitalis glycosides
      (sudden drop in serum calcium concentrations induced by edetate
      disodium may reverse effects of digitalis)

  Insulin
      (concurrent use may require adjustments in dosage of insulin due
      to decreased serum glucose and possible chelation of zinc in
      insulin)

**Laboratory value alterations**
The following have been selected on the basis of their potential clinical
  significance (possible effect in parentheses where appropriate)—not
  necessarily inclusive (» = major clinical significance):

With diagnostic test results

Electrocardiograms (ECGs)

(changes such as sagging of the S-T segment, depression of the T wave, and elevation of the U wave may occur as a result of reduced serum potassium concentrations)

Calcium determinations, serum

(the oxalate method of determining serum calcium tends to give low readings in the presence of edetate disodium; sampling just before a subsequent dose will produce the least interference; acidifying the sample or using an alternate method may be necessary)

With physiology/laboratory test values

Alkaline phosphatase, serum

(concentration may be lowered because of hypomagnesemia induced by edetate disodium)

Glucose, serum

(treatment with edetate disodium may cause a lowering of blood sugar concentrations)

Glucose, urine

(concentration may be increased)

Magnesium, serum or

Potassium, serum

(concentration may be decreased)

### Medical considerations/Contraindications

The medical considerations/contraindications included here have been selected on the basis of their potential clinical significance (reasons given in parentheses where appropriate)—not necessarily inclusive (» = major clinical significance).

*Except under special circumstances, this medication should not be used when the following medical problems exist:*

» Anuria or
» Renal function impairment

(excretion of edetate disodium may be delayed by reduced glomerular filtration, increasing the risk of nephrotoxicity)

» Hypocalcemia

(may be exacerbated)

*Risk-benefit should be considered when the following medical problems exist:*

Diabetes mellitus

(treatment with edetate disodium may reduce blood sugar concentrations and require adjustment of insulin dosage in diabetic patients)

» Heart disease

(myocardial contractility may be affected)

Hypokalemia

(edetate disodium may exacerbate hypokalemia and produce ECG changes)

Intracranial lesions or
» Seizure disorders, history of

(edetate disodium may induce seizures because of hypocalcemia)

Sensitivity to edetate disodium

Tuberculosis, active or with healed calcified lesions

(may be provoked)

### Patient monitoring

The following may be especially important in patient monitoring (other tests may be warranted in some patients, depending on condition; » = major clinical significance):

Blood pressure determinations

(recommended prior to and periodically during therapy)

Blood urea nitrogen (BUN) concentrations and
Creatinine concentrations, serum

(determinations recommended prior to and during therapy for evidence of renal function impairment)

Cardiac function studies, including ECG and
Electrolyte determinations, serum and urinary, especially potassium and magnesium

(recommended prior to administration of edetate disodium and periodically, as clinically indicated, during therapy, especially in patients with ventricular arrhythmias, limited cardiac reserve, congestive heart failure, or a history of seizure disorders or intracranial lesions; reduced serum potassium concentrations may produce ECG changes; serum magnesium determinations may be required during prolonged therapy)

Liver function tests

(recommended if there is any clinical evidence of liver function impairment during treatment)

Urinalysis

(recommended daily during treatment)

## Side/Adverse Effects

The following side/adverse effects have been selected on the basis of their potential clinical significance (possible signs and symptoms in parentheses where appropriate)—not necessarily inclusive:

### Those indicating need for medical attention

Incidence more frequent

*Thrombophlebitis* (pain, burning, or swelling at site of injection)

Incidence less frequent

*Anemia* (unusual tiredness or weakness); *exfoliative dermatitis* (skin rash or other skin and mucous membrane lesions); *febrile reaction, systemic* (chills or sudden fever; fatigue; headache; malaise; muscle cramps; excessive thirst; weakness); *gout, secondary* (severe pain or inflammation in feet, knees, hands, or elbows)—hyperuricemia may result from renal tubular toxicity; *hypocalcemia* (convulsions; difficulty in breathing; irregular heartbeats; mood or mental changes; muscle spasms [tetany] in hands, arms, feet, legs, or face; numbness and tingling around the mouth, fingertips, or feet)—due to sudden decrease in serum calcium concentration caused by rapid intravenous infusion or high dose of edetate disodium; *hypokalemia or hypomagnesemia* (drowsiness; loss of appetite; muscle twitching or trembling; nausea or vomiting; unusual tiredness or weakness)—may be accompanied by hypocalcemia; *nephrotoxicity* (cloudy urine; frequent or sudden urge to urinate; large or small volume of urine; painful or difficult urination)

Note: Prolonged use may cause lesions similar to those seen with pyridoxine deficiency, such as cracking and dry scaly skin and sores in mouth and on lips, possibly due to zinc depletion.

*Nephrotoxicity* may be due to damage to the reticuloendothelial system with hemorrhagic tendencies, or may indicate possible renal tubular necrosis. Microscopic hematuria, proteinuria, and/or large renal epithelial cells in urine may be observed. Nephrotoxicity is usually associated with high doses of edetate disodium. Signs are often reversible within a few days after discontinuation of medication.

### Those indicating need for medical attention only if they continue or are bothersome

Incidence more frequent

*Abdominal or stomach pain or cramps; diarrhea; hypotension, postural* (dizziness or lightheadedness)

Incidence less frequent

*Headache, without other symptoms of a febrile reaction*

## General Dosing Information

Because of its irritant effect on the tissues and the danger of hypocalcemia, edetate disodium must be diluted before infusion.

Dilute solution must be infused slowly over three hours or more, preferably four to six hours, and the cardiac reserve of the patient not exceeded. Rapid intravenous infusion or high serum concentrations of edetate disodium may cause a sudden drop in serum calcium concentration, resulting in hypocalcemic tetany, convulsions, severe cardiac arrhythmias, and death from respiratory arrest.

### For treatment of adverse effects

Recommended treatment consists of the following:

• Hypocalcemia—A parenteral calcium salt, such as calcium gluconate, should be immediately available before administration of edetate disodium for calcium ion replacement. However, intravenous calcium should be administered with caution, especially in patients who are digitalized, since a reversal of digitalis effects may occur.

• Nephrotoxicity—Edetate disodium must be discontinued; maximum hydration compatible with patient's cardiovascular reserve may be necessary.

• Postural hypotension—Patient should remain in bed for a short time after infusion.

## Parenteral Dosage Forms

### EDETATE DISODIUM INJECTION USP

**Usual adult dose**

Hypercalcemia or
Digitalis toxicity—

Intravenous, 50 mg per kg of body weight in twenty-four hours. The dosage may be repeated for four more consecutive daily doses followed by a two-day drug-free interval, with repeated courses, as necessary, up to fifteen doses.

**Usual adult prescribing limits**
3 grams in twenty-four hours.

**Usual pediatric dose**
Hypercalcemia or
Digitalis toxicity—
Intravenous, 40 mg per kg of body weight in twenty-four hours.

Note:  The pediatric dose may go as high as 70 mg per kg in twenty-four
hours.

**Strength(s) usually available**
U.S.—
150 mg per mL (Rx) [*Disotate; Endrate;* GENERIC].
Canada—
Edetate disodium injection is not commercially available in Canada;
however, it is available by emergency drug release from the Health
Protection Branch.

**Packaging and storage**
Store below 40 °C (104 °F), preferably between 15 and 30 °C (59 and 86
°F), unless otherwise specified by manufacturer. Protect from freezing.

**Preparation of dosage form**
Adult use—The calculated dose is dissolved in 500 mL of 5% dextrose
injection or sodium chloride injection.
Pediatric use—The calculated dose is dissolved in a sufficient volume of
5% dextrose injection or sodium chloride injection to make a final
concentration of not more than 3% (30 mg per mL).

**Additional information**
Injection contains 5.4 mEq of sodium per gram of edetate disodium.

Revised: 02/20/92

---

# EDROPHONIUM   Systemic

VA CLASSIFICATION (Primary/Secondary): AU300/DX900; AD900

Note:  For a listing of dosage forms and brand names by country availability, see *Dosage Forms* section(s). For a listing of brand names
for the articles in this monograph, refer to the General Index.

## Category

Cholinergic (cholinesterase inhibitor); diagnostic aid (myasthenia gravis);
antidote (to nondepolarizing neuromuscular block).

Note:  Cholinergic (cholinesterase inhibitor) is the basic category; the
other categories are specific categories of use.

## Indications

**Accepted**
Myasthenia gravis (diagnosis)—Edrophonium is indicated in the differential diagnosis of myasthenia gravis and as an adjunct in the evaluation of treatment requirements in the disease. It is also indicated for
evaluating emergency treatment in myasthenic crisis. Edrophonium is
not recommended for maintenance therapy in myasthenia gravis because of its short duration of action.

Neuromuscular blockade, nondepolarizing, (treatment); and
Toxicity, curare (treatment)—Edrophonium is indicated to reverse the
neuromuscular block produced by many nondepolarizing agents including atracurium, gallamine, metocurine, pancuronium, tubocurarine, and vecuronium. Although edrophonium is frequently used to reverse moderate degrees of residual neuromuscular blockade, other
agents (such as neostigmine) may better antagonize profound levels
of neuromuscular blockade.

Edrophonium is not effective against depolarizing agents such as de-
camethonium and succinylcholine.

Also, edrophonium is indicated as an adjunct in the treatment of respiratory depression caused by overdosage of nondepolarizing neuromuscular blocking agents.

**Unaccepted**
Edrophonium has been used to terminate supraventricular tachycardias
(SVT; paroxysmal atrial tachycardia) but has generally been replaced
by other antiarrhythmic agents.

## Pharmacology/Pharmacokinetics

**Physicochemical characteristics**
Molecular weight—201.70.
Other characteristics—Edrophonium injection: pH approximately 5.4.

**Mechanism of action/Effect**
Cholinergic (cholinesterase inhibitor)—
Inhibits destruction of acetylcholine by acetylcholinesterase, thereby
facilitating transmission of impulses across the myoneural junction.
Diagnostic aid (myasthenia gravis): By prolonging the duration of action of acetylcholine at the motor end plate, edrophonium transiently increases muscle strength in patients with myasthenia
gravis, whereas patients with other disorders develop either no increase in strength or even a slight weakness and possibly
fasciculations.
Antidote (to nondepolarizing neuromuscular block): Since nondepolarizing neuromuscular blocking agents combine reversibly with
the receptors, preventing access of acetylcholine, antagonism can

be overcome by increasing the amount of agonist at the receptors;
therefore, muscle paralysis induced by nondepolarizing neuromuscular blocking agents is reversed by edrophonium, which increases
the concentration of acetylcholine at the receptors.

**Distribution**
The volume of distribution (Vol$_D$) of edrophonium is $1.1 \pm 0.2$ L per kg.

**Half-life**
Distribution—7 to 12 minutes.
Elimination—33 to 110 minutes.

**Onset of action**
Intramuscular—2 to 10 minutes.
Intravenous—Within 30 to 60 seconds.

**Duration of action**
In the diagnosis of myasthenia gravis—
Intramuscular: 5 to 30 minutes.
Intravenous: About 10 minutes.

**Elimination**
Renal. The clearance of edrophonium is about 0.5 L per hour per kg.

## Precautions to Consider

**Pregnancy/Reproduction**
Pregnancy—Studies have not been done in humans.
Studies have not been done in animals.

FDA Pregnancy Category C.

**Breast-feeding**
It is not known whether edrophonium is distributed into breast milk. However, problems in humans have not been documented.

**Pediatrics**
Appropriate studies on the relationship of age to the effects of edrophonium have not been performed in the pediatric population. However,
no pediatrics-specific problems have been documented to date.

**Geriatrics**
Extensive studies on the relationship of age to the effects of edrophonium
have not been performed in the geriatric population. However, in 2
studies comparing small numbers of patients 76 to 87 years of age
with younger adults, the onset of action and the duration of antagonism
of neuromuscular blockade by edrophonium in the older group were
no different than they were in younger patients.

**Drug interactions and/or related problems**
The following drug interactions and/or related problems have been selected on the basis of their potential clinical significance (possible
mechanism in parentheses where appropriate)—not necessarily inclusive (» = major clinical significance):
Cholinesterase inhibitors, other, including antimyasthenics, demecarium, echothiophate, and isoflurophate and possibly topical malathion in excessive quantities
(caution is recommended when administering edrophonium to patients with symptoms of myasthenic weakness who are also receiving these medications, since symptoms of cholinergic crisis
[overdosage] may be similar to those occurring with myasthenic
crisis [underdosage], and the patient's condition may be worsened
by use of edrophonium)

Digitalis glycosides
  (when used concurrently with edrophonium, the additive vagomimetic effects may cause excessive slowing of the heart rate)
Neuromuscular blocking agents
  (phase I block of depolarizing neuromuscular blocking agents such as succinylcholine may be prolonged when these medications are used concurrently with edrophonium; however, if these blocking agents have been used over a prolonged period of time and the depolarization block has changed to a nondepolarization block, edrophonium may reverse the nondepolarization block)
  (effects of many nondepolarizing neuromuscular blocking agents are antagonized by edrophonium, especially moderate degrees of residual neuromuscular blockade; profound levels of neuromuscular blockade may be better antagonized by other agents such as neostigmine)

### Medical considerations/Contraindications
The medical considerations/contraindications included here have been selected on the basis of their potential clinical significance (reasons given in parentheses where appropriate)—not necessarily inclusive (» = major clinical significance).

*Except under special circumstances, this medication should not be used when the following medical problems exist:*
» Asthma, bronchial
  (increase in bronchial secretions and other respiratory effects of edrophonium may aggravate condition)
» Intestinal or urinary tract obstruction, mechanical

*Risk-benefit should be considered when the following medical problems exist:*
Cardiac dysrhythmias such as bradycardia and atrioventricular (AV) block
  (increased risk of cardiac arrhythmias)
Sensitivity to edrophonium

## Side/Adverse Effects

Note: Severe side/adverse effects occur rarely with usual doses of edrophonium. Any side effects that may occur with edrophonium are usually short-lived because of its short duration of action and are usually less severe than those that occur with neostigmine, pyridostigmine, or ambenonium.

The following side/adverse effects have been selected on the basis of their potential clinical significance (possible signs and symptoms in parentheses where appropriate)—not necessarily inclusive:

**Those indicating need for medical attention**
Incidence rare
  *Muscarinic effects* (shortness of breath, troubled breathing, wheezing or tightness in chest; slow heartbeat; unusual tiredness or weakness); *nicotinic effects* (muscle weakness, cramps, or twitching)
  Note: Cholinergic reaction includes severe muscarinic side effects in addition to nicotinic effects.

**Those indicating need for medical attention only if they continue or are bothersome**
Incidence less frequent or rare
  *Muscarinic effects* (blurred vision; diarrhea; frequent urge to urinate; increased sweating; increased watering of eyes or mouth; increase in bronchial secretions; nausea or vomiting; stomach cramps or pain)

## Overdose

For specific information on the agents used in the management of edrophonium overdose, see *Atropine* in *Anticholinergic/Antispasmodics (Systemic)* monograph.

For more information on the management of overdose or unintentional ingestion, **contact a Poison Control Center** (see *Poison Control Center listing*).

**Treatment of overdose**
Discontinuation of edrophonium.

Specific treatment—Administration of intravenous atropine sulfate to control muscarinic effects.

May include treatment of seizures or shock as appropriate.

Monitoring—Monitoring of cardiac function.

Supportive care—May include maintaining an open airway (possible suction of bronchial secretions); use of assisted respiration.

## General Dosing Information

When edrophonium is used for testing, atropine injection should always be readily available to counteract severe cholinergic reactions, which may occur in hypersensitive individuals.

Atropine will prevent or relieve the muscarinic side effects, but is usually not required, except in patients older than 50 years of age, who should be given atropine before myasthenic testing to prevent bradycardia and hypotension.

Atropine may be administered to relieve the transient bradycardia that may occur with the use of edrophonium.

When used to reverse the effects of nondepolarizing neuromuscular blockade, edrophonium should not be administered prior to the nondepolarizing neuromuscular blocking agent but at the time the effect is needed.

When used as a test for the evaluation of treatment requirements in myasthenia gravis:
• In patients who require additional anticholinesterase medication, a transient increase in muscle strength without fasciculation or muscarinic side effects will occur (myasthenic response).
• In patients who have been overtreated with anticholinesterase agents, muscle strength is decreased, muscle fasciculations may occur, and severe muscarinic effects usually occur (cholinergic response).
• In patients being adequately treated with anticholinesterase agents, there is no change in muscle strength, muscle fasciculations may occur, and side effects, if any occur, are mild.

When used to differentiate myasthenic crisis from cholinergic crisis, edrophonium may temporarily increase muscle strength if treatment has been inadequate (myasthenic crisis), whereas in overtreatment (cholinergic crisis) the condition may worsen.

## Parenteral Dosage Forms
### EDROPHONIUM CHLORIDE INJECTION USP

**Usual adult and adolescent dose**
For evaluation of treatment requirements in myasthenia gravis—
  Intravenous, 1 to 2 mg one hour after administration of anticholinesterase agent.
To differentiate cholinergic crisis from myasthenic crisis—
  Intravenous, initially 1 mg, followed after one minute by an additional 1 mg if the initial dose does not further impair patient.
Diagnostic aid (myasthenia gravis)—
  Intramuscular, 10 mg.
  Note: If cholinergic reaction occurs, test should be repeated after thirty minutes using a dose of 2 mg, to rule out a false-negative reaction.
  Intravenous, initially 2 mg administered within fifteen to thirty seconds, followed by 8 mg if no response after forty-five seconds.
  Note: If cholinergic reaction occurs after initial dose of 2 mg, test should be discontinued and 400 mcg (0.4 mg) of atropine given intravenously. Test may be repeated after thirty minutes.
Reversal of nondepolarizing neuromuscular block—
  Intravenous, 10 mg administered over a period of thirty to forty-five seconds, repeated as needed, up to a maximum total dose of 40 mg. Alternatively, doses of 0.5 to 1 mg of edrophonium per kg of body weight are used.

**Usual pediatric dose**
Diagnostic aid (myasthenia gravis)—
  Infants:
    Intramuscular or subcutaneous, 500 mcg (0.5 mg) to 1 mg.
    Intravenous, 500 mcg (0.5 mg).
  Children up to 34 kg of body weight:
    Intramuscular, 2 mg.
    Intravenous, 1 mg initially; if no response within forty-five seconds, then 1 mg every thirty to forty-five seconds up to a total dose of 5 mg.
  Children 34 kg of body weight and over:
    Intramuscular, 5 mg.
    Intravenous, 2 mg initially; if no response within forty-five seconds, then 1 mg every thirty to forty-five seconds up to a total dose of 10 mg.

**Usual geriatric dose**
See *Usual adult and adolescent dose.*
Note: Patients older than 50 years of age should be given atropine before myasthenic testing to prevent bradycardia and hypotension.

**Strength(s) usually available**
U.S.—
  10 mg per mL (Rx) [*Enlon* (phenol 0.45%; sodium sulfite 0.2%; sodium citrate; citric acid); *Reversol* (phenol 0.45%; sodium sulfite

0.2%; sodium citrate; citric acid); *Tensilon* (sodium sulfite 0.2%; sodium citrate; citric acid—in 1-mL ampuls; or phenol 0.45%; sodium sulfite 0.2%; sodium citrate; citric acid—in 10-mL vials)].

Canada—
10 mg per mL (Rx) [*Enlon* (sodium sulfite 0.2%; sodium citrate; citric acid—in 5-mL ampuls; or phenol 0.45%; sodium sulfite 0.2%; sodium citrate, citric acid—in 15-mL vials); *Tensilon* (phenol 0.45%,

sodium sulfite 0.2%, sodium citrate, citric acid; sodium <1 mmol per mL)].

**Packaging and storage**
Store below 40 °C (104 °F), preferably between 15 and 30 °C (59 and 86 °F), unless otherwise specified by manufacturer. Protect from freezing.

Revised: 08/10/94

# EFLORNITHINE    Systemic†

VA CLASSIFICATION (Primary): AP109

Other commonly used names are DFMO and alpha-difluoromethylornithine.

Note: For a listing of dosage forms and brand names by country availability, see *Dosage Forms* section(s). For a listing of brand names for the articles in this monograph, refer to the General Index.

†Not commercially available in Canada.

## Category
Antiprotozoal (systemic).

## Indications
### Accepted
Trypanosomiasis, African (treatment)—Eflornithine is indicated in the treatment of the meningoencephalitic stage of *Trypanosoma brucei gambiense* infection (West African sleeping sickness).

Not all species or strains of a particular organism may be susceptible to eflornithine.

## Pharmacology/Pharmacokinetics
### Physicochemical characteristics
Molecular weight—236.65.

### Mechanism of action/Effect
Eflornithine is an enzyme-activated, irreversible inhibitor of ornithine decarboxylase (ODC), the key enzyme in the conversion of ornithine to polyamines. Polyamines (putrescine, spermidine, and spermine) play an essential role in the growth, differentiation, and replication of cells by participating in nucleic acid and protein synthesis in protozoa, as well as in normal tissue and tumors in humans. Eflornithine's inhibition of ODC results in complete intracellular elimination of putrescine and a 60–75% reduction in spermidine, producing morphologic changes of trypanosomes in the bloodstream. Because the clearance of parasites from the bloodstream is slow, it is likely that eflornithine is cytostatic rather than cytolytic; in addition, animal studies have suggested that an intact immune response is probably necessary for complete elimination of the parasites from the bloodstream.

### Absorption
Well absorbed after oral administration; bioavailability approximately 50%.

### Distribution
Crosses the blood-brain barrier, with cerebrospinal fluid (CSF) concentrations reaching 6 to 51% of corresponding blood concentrations. One very small study found higher penetration into the CSF of patients with the most severe form of the disease, suggesting that penetration into the CSF may be related to the degree of CNS involvement. $Vol_D = 0.30$ to 0.43 L per kg.

### Protein binding
No significant plasma protein binding.

### Half-life
Normal renal function—Elimination: 3.2 to 3.6 hours.

### Time to peak serum concentration:
End of infusion.

### Mean peak serum concentration
196.6 to 317.9 mcg per mL after 100 mg per kg of body weight every 6 hours.

### Elimination
Renal; approximately 80% excreted unchanged in the urine within 24 hours. The renal clearance of eflornithine approximates that of creatinine clearance.

## Precautions to Consider
### Carcinogenicity
Long-term studies in animals have not been performed to evaluate the carcinogenic potential of eflornithine.

### Mutagenicity
Eflornithine did not induce mutagenic changes in *in vitro* studies using *Salmonella* and 2 strains of *Saccharomyces*.

### Pregnancy/Reproduction
Fertility—Decreased spermatogenic effects and impaired fertility were found in rats and rabbits at doses equivalent to one-half the recommended human dose and in mice at approximately 2 times the human dose.

Pregnancy—Adequate and well-controlled studies in humans have not been done. Eflornithine should only be used during pregnancy if the potential benefit justifies the potential risk to the fetus. The meningoencephalitic stage of African trypanosomiasis has such a high mortality rate if left untreated that treatment with eflornithine may justify the potential risk to the fetus.

Eflornithine has been shown to be contragestational in rats, rabbits, and mice given doses of 0.5, 0.5, and 2 times the human dose, respectively. In postnatal studies, retarded development was reported in rat pups receiving doses slightly higher than the human dose.

FDA Pregnancy Category C.

### Breast-feeding
It is not known whether eflornithine is distributed into breast milk. However, problems in humans have not been documented.

### Pediatrics
No information is available on the relationship of age to the effects of eflornithine in pediatric patients. Safety and efficacy have not been established.

### Geriatrics
No information is available on the relationship of age to the effects of eflornithine in geriatric patients.

### Dental
The bone marrow–depressant effects of eflornithine may result in an increased incidence of microbial infection, delayed healing, and gingival bleeding.

### Drug interactions and/or related problems
The following drug interactions and/or related problems have been selected on the basis of their potential clinical significance (possible mechanism in parentheses where appropriate)—not necessarily inclusive (» = major clinical significance):

Note: Combinations containing any of the following medications, depending on the amount present, may also interact with this medication.

» Bone marrow depressants, other (See *Appendix II*)
(concurrent use with eflornithine may increase the bone marrow-depressant effects of these medications and radiation therapy)

Ototoxic medications, other (See *Appendix II*)
(concurrent use of these medications with long-term eflornithine therapy may increase the potential for ototoxicity)

### Medical considerations/Contraindications
The medical considerations/contraindications included here have been selected on the basis of their potential clinical significance (reasons given in parentheses where appropriate)—not necessarily inclusive (» = major clinical significance).

*Risk-benefit should be considered when the following medical problems exist:*

Eighth-cranial-nerve impairment, pre-existing
(hearing loss has occurred in patients receiving long-term therapy with eflornithine for treatment of cancer and *Pneumocystis carinii*

pneumonia [conditions in which efficacy of eflornithine has not been clearly demonstrated]; although treatment for African trypanosomiasis is relatively short, the risk of hearing loss may still exist)

» Hematologic abnormalities, pre-existing
(eflornithine may cause anemia, leukopenia, or thrombocytopenia, worsening any pre-existing hematologic abnormalities)

» Renal function impairment
(because eflornithine is excreted primarily through the kidneys and its renal clearance approximates that of the creatinine clearance, the dose of eflornithine may need to be reduced in patients with renal function impairment)

**Patient monitoring**

The following may be especially important in patient monitoring (other tests may be warranted in some patients, depending on condition; » = major clinical significance):

Audiograms, serial
(may be required prior to, periodically during, and following treatment, especially in patients with pre-existing eighth-cranial-nerve impairment or patients receiving long-term therapy)

» Complete blood counts (CBCs) and
» Platelet counts
(because eflornithine may cause anemia, leukopenia, and thrombocytopenia, a complete blood count and platelet count should be performed before treatment, 2 times a week during therapy, and then weekly, thereafter, until blood counts return to baseline)

## Side/Adverse Effects

Note: Most side effects are transient and reversible by discontinuing the drug or decreasing the dose. Hematologic abnormalities occur frequently, ranging from 10–55%. These abnormalities are dose-related and usually reversible. Thrombocytopenia is thought to be due to a production defect rather than to peripheral destruction. Seizures were seen in approximately 8% of patients, but may be related to the disease state rather than the drug.

Reversible sensorineural hearing loss has occurred in 30–70% of patients receiving long-term therapy (more than 4–8 weeks of therapy or a total dose of >300 grams); high-frequency hearing is lost first, followed by middle- and low-frequency hearing. Because treatment for African trypanosomiasis is short-term, patients are unlikely to experience hearing loss.

The following side/adverse effects have been selected on the basis of their potential clinical significance (possible signs and symptoms in parentheses where appropriate)—not necessarily inclusive:

**Those indicating need for medical attention**

Incidence more frequent
*Hematologic abnormalities, specifically anemia* (unusual tiredness or weakness); *leucopenia* (sore throat and fever); *or thrombocytopenia* (unusual bleeding or bruising)

Incidence rare
*Ototoxicity* (sensorineural hearing loss); *seizures*

**Those indicating need for medical attention only if they continue or are bothersome**

Incidence more frequent
*Gastrointestinal disturbances* (diarrhea; nausea; abdominal pain; vomiting)

Incidence rare
*Alopecia* (hair loss); *headache*

## Patient Consultation

As an aid to patient consultation, refer to *Advice for the Patient, Eflornithine (Systemic)*.

In providing consultation, consider emphasizing the following selected information (» = major clinical significance):

**Before receiving this medication**

» Conditions affecting use, especially:
Pregnancy—Because the meningoencephalitic stage of African trypanosomiasis has such a high mortality rate if left untreated, treatment with eflornithine justifies the potential risk to the fetus
Dental—The neutropenic and thrombocytopenic effects of eflornithine may result in an increased incidence of microbial infection, delayed healing, and gingival bleeding
Other medications, especially other bone marrow depressants
Other medical problems, especially hematologic disturbances or renal function impairment

**Proper use of this medication**

» Importance of receiving medication for full course of therapy and on a regular schedule
» Proper dosing

**Precautions after receiving this medication**

Regular visits to physician to check progress
Caution if bone marrow depression occurs:
» Checking with physician immediately if fever or chills occur or if you think you are getting an infection
» Checking with physician immediately if unusual bleeding or bruising; black, tarry stools; blood in urine or stools; or pinpoint red spots on skin occur
Caution in use of regular toothbrushes, dental floss, and toothpicks; physician, dentist, or nurse may suggest alternative methods for cleaning teeth and gums; checking with physician before having dental work done
Using caution to avoid accidental cuts with use of sharp objects such as a safety razor or fingernail or toenail cutters

**Side/adverse effects**

Signs of potential side effects, especially hematologic disturbances, ototoxicity, and seizures

## General Dosing Information

Severe anemia, leukopenia or thrombocytopenia requires an interruption in therapy until there is evidence of bone marrow recovery.

Because eflornithine's excretion through the kidneys is approximately the same as creatinine clearance, patients with renal function impairment may need an adjustment in dosage, based on their creatinine clearance.

## Parenteral Dosage Forms

### EFLORNITHINE HYDROCHLORIDE CONCENTRATE FOR INJECTION

**Usual adult and adolescent dose**

Trypanosomiasis, African (treatment)—
Intravenous infusion, 100 mg per kg of body weight, infused over at least forty-five minutes, every six hours for fourteen days.

**Usual pediatric dose**

Safety and efficacy have not been established.

**Strength(s) usually available**

U.S.—
20,000 mg in 100 mL (Rx) [*Ornidyl*].
Canada—
Not commercially available.

**Packaging and storage**

Store below 30 °C (86 °F), unless otherwise specified by manufacturer. Protect from freezing and light.

**Preparation of dosage form**

Eflornithine hydrochloride concentrate for injection is hypertonic and must be diluted with sterile water for injection before infusion. To prepare initial dilution for intravenous infusion, withdraw the entire 100 mL from the vial and add 25 mL of eflornithine into each of 4 containers with 100 mL of sterile water for injection. This produces a concentration of 40 mg per mL (5000 mg in 125 mL).

**Stability**

After dilution with sterile water for injection, eflornithine must be used within 24 hours. Bags containing diluted eflornithine should be stored at 4 °C (39 °F) to minimize the risk of microbial proliferation.

**Incompatibilities**

Eflornithine hydrochloride for injection should not be administered intravenously with any other drugs.

Revised: 06/26/95

---

**ENALAPRIL**—See *Angiotensin-converting Enzyme (ACE) Inhibitors (Systemic)*

---

## ENALAPRIL-CONTAINING COMBINATIONS—

Enalapril and Hydrochlorothiazide (Systemic)—See *Angiotensin-converting Enzyme (ACE) Inhibitors and Hydrochlorothiazide (Systemic)*

# ENCAINIDE Systemic*†

VA CLASSIFICATION (Primary): CV300

Note: For a listing of dosage forms and brand names by country availability, see *Dosage Forms* section(s). For a listing of brand names for the articles in this monograph, refer to the General Index.

Although this product is no longer commercially available, the manufacturer is making it available to physicians who had patients well managed on encainide prior to market withdrawal.

*Not commercially available in the U.S.
†Not commercially available in Canada.

## Category
Antiarrhythmic.

## Indications

### Accepted
Arrhythmias, ventricular (treatment)—Encainide is indicated for suppression of documented life-threatening ventricular arrhythmias, including sustained ventricular tachycardia.

### Unaccepted
Use of encainide is no longer accepted for treatment of less severe arrhythmias such as nonsustained ventricular tachycardias or frequent premature ventricular contractions, even if patients are symptomatic, because of results of a trial that found increased mortality in patients with non–life-threatening arrhythmias treated with encainide compared to those treated with placebo.

## Pharmacology/Pharmacokinetics

### Physicochemical characteristics
Molecular weight—388.94.

### Mechanism of action/Effect
Decreases excitability, conduction velocity, and automaticity as a result of slowed atrial, atrioventricular (AV) nodal, His-Purkinje, and intraventricular conduction, and causes a slight but significant prolongation of refractory periods in these tissues. The greatest effect is on the His-Purkinje system. Decreases the rate of rise of the action potential without markedly affecting its duration. Electrophysiologic effects are greater in ischemic than in normal myocardial tissue. In the Vaughan Williams classification of antiarrhythmics, encainide is considered to be a class IC agent.

### Other actions/effects
Very little negative inotropic effect.

### Absorption
Nearly complete; slowed by food, but bioavailability is unchanged.

### Protein binding
Encainide and O-demethylencainide (ODE)—High (75 to 85%).
3-Methoxy-O-demethylencainide (MODE)—Very high (92%).

### Biotransformation
Hepatic. In over 90% of patients, rapidly and extensively metabolized to two active metabolites, ODE and MODE. In less than 10% of patients, more slowly metabolized (these patients also have a diminished ability to metabolize debrisoquin); little, if any, MODE and only small amounts of ODE are present in plasma.

### Half-life
In normal metabolizers—
Encainide: 1 to 2 hours.
ODE: 3 to 4 hours.
MODE: 6 to 12 hours.
In slow metabolizers—
Encainide: 6 to 11 hours.

### Onset of action
1 to 3 hours.

### Time to peak plasma concentration
30 to 90 minutes.

### Time to steady-state plasma concentration
Multiple doses—3 to 5 days.

### Elimination
Renal/fecal (in slow metabolizers, more predominantly renal and mainly unchanged).

## Precautions to Consider

### Carcinogenicity
Studies in rats and mice at oral doses of up to 30 mg per kg of body weight (mg/kg) per day and 135 mg/kg per day, respectively, found no evidence of carcinogenicity.

### Mutagenicity
Bacterial and mammalian mutagenicity tests were negative.

### Pregnancy/Reproduction
Fertility—Studies in male and female rats at oral doses of 28 mg/kg per day (approximately 13 times the average human dose) prior to mating found a reduction in fertility; doses up to 14 mg/kg per day did not reduce fertility.

Pregnancy—Adequate and well-controlled studies in humans have not been done.

Studies in rats and rabbits at doses of up to 13 and 9 times the average human dose, respectively, have not shown that encainide causes adverse effects in the fetus.

FDA Pregnancy Category B.

### Breast-feeding
Encainide is distributed into the milk of laboratory animals and has been reported to be present in human milk. However, problems in humans have not been documented.

### Pediatrics
Appropriate studies on the relationship of age to the effects of encainide have not been performed in the pediatric population. Safety and efficacy have not been established.

### Geriatrics
Appropriate studies on the relationship of age to the effects of encainide have not been performed in the geriatric population. However, elderly patients are more likely to have age-related renal function impairment, which may require dosage reduction and increase in dosage intervals in patients receiving encainide.

### Drug interactions and/or related problems
The following drug interactions and/or related problems have been selected on the basis of their potential clinical significance (possible mechanism in parentheses where appropriate)—not necessarily inclusive (» = major clinical significance):

Antiarrhythmics, other
(concurrent use with encainide may result in increased cardiac effects)

Cimetidine
(concurrent use of cimetidine increases plasma concentrations of encainide and its active metabolites; dosage reduction of encainide is recommended if concurrent use with cimetidine is necessary)

### Laboratory value alterations
The following have been selected on the basis of their potential clinical significance (possible effect in parentheses where appropriate)—not necessarily inclusive (» = major clinical significance):

With physiology/laboratory test values
Electrocardiogram (ECG) changes such as:
QRS widening and
PR prolongation
(occur in most patients; dose-related)
QT prolongation
(may occur secondary to QRS widening)
Note: ECG changes produced by encainide do not necessarily indicate efficacy, toxicity, or overdose.

### Medical considerations/Contraindications
The medical considerations/contraindications included here have been selected on the basis of their potential clinical significance (reasons given in parentheses where appropriate)—not necessarily inclusive (» = major clinical significance).

*Except under special circumstances, this medication should not be used when the following medical problems exist:*

» Atrioventricular (AV) block, pre-existing second or third degree without pacemaker or
» Right bundle branch block associated with a left hemiblock (bifascicular block) without pacemaker
(risk of complete heart block)

*Risk-benefit should be considered when the following medical problems exist:*

» Cardiogenic shock

Cardiomyopathy or
Congestive heart failure
(encainide may exacerbate these conditions)

Diabetes mellitus
(encainide may in rare cases increase serum glucose levels, resulting in symptomatic hyperglycemia, especially in patients with pre-existing glucose intolerance; monitoring of serum glucose levels is recommended)

Hepatic function impairment
(reduced conversion to metabolites O-demethylencainide [ODE] and 3-methoxy-O-demethylencainide [MODE], but concentrations of metabolites are not significantly changed; no specific dosage adjustment recommendations can be made, but dosage should be increased cautiously)

Hypokalemia or hyperkalemia
(effects of encainide may be altered; any electrolyte imbalance should be corrected prior to beginning therapy with encainide)

Myocardial infarction, history of, with associated left ventricular function impairment
(increased risk of encainide-induced arrhythmias)

Renal function impairment
(reduced elimination; in patients with renal function impairment, the interval between dosage increments should be greater than 3 to 5 days, usually at least 7 days, and dosage reduction may be necessary)

Sensitivity to encainide

» Sick sinus syndrome
(sinus node recovery time prolonged; sinus bradycardia, sinus pause, or sinus arrest may occur)

Caution is also recommended in patients with permanent pacemakers or temporary pacing electrodes because encainide may increase endocardial pacing thresholds and may suppress ventricular escape rhythms; use is not recommended in patients with existing poor thresholds or nonprogrammable pacemakers unless suitable pacing rescue is available.

### Patient monitoring

The following may be especially important in patient monitoring (other tests may be warranted in some patients, depending on condition; » = major clinical significance):

» ECG
(Holter monitoring or 24-hour ambulatory ECG recommended prior to initiation of therapy and at periodic intervals during therapy to help assess efficacy and detect possible proarrhythmic effects)

Glucose
(serum concentrations recommended, especially in diabetic patients)

## Side/Adverse Effects

Note: In the National Heart Lung and Blood Institute's Cardiac Arrhythmia Suppression Trial (CAST), encainide treatment was found to be associated with excessive mortality or increased nonfatal cardiac arrest rate as compared with placebo in patients with asymptomatic, non–life-threatening arrhythmias who had a recent myocardial infarction.

Adverse cardiac effects reported with encainide administration include new or exacerbated ventricular arrhythmias in about 10% of patients and, in 1% or less of patients, new or exacerbated congestive heart failure, second or third degree atrioventricular (AV) block, sinus bradycardia, sinus pause, or sinus arrest.

Incidence of cardiac and other effects is at least partially dose-related. Proarrhythmic effects are much more frequent at doses exceeding 200 mg per day.

Signs of overdose include excessive QRS widening and QT prolongation, AV dissociation, hypotension, and bradycardia; asystole may develop. Seizures have been reported. Deaths have occurred.

The following side/adverse effects have been selected on the basis of their potential clinical significance (possible signs and symptoms in parentheses where appropriate)—not necessarily inclusive:

**Those indicating need for medical attention**
Incidence more frequent
*Chest pain; ventricular tachyarrhythmias* (fast or irregular heartbeat)
Note: *Ventricular tachyarrhythmias* are dose-related and potentially fatal; incidence increased in patients with sustained ventricular tachycardia, cardiomyopathy, congestive heart failure, or history of myocardial infarction with associated left ventricular function impairment. Proarrhythmic effects usually occur during the first week of therapy.

Incidence rare
*Central nervous system (CNS) effect* (trembling or shaking); *congestive heart failure* (shortness of breath; swelling of feet or lower legs)

**Those indicating need for medical attention only if they continue or are bothersome**
Incidence less frequent
*CNS effects* (blurred or double vision; dizziness; headache; unusual tiredness or weakness); *nausea; pain in arms or legs; skin rash*

## Overdose

For more information on the management of overdose or unintentional ingestion, **contact a Poison Control Center** (see *Poison Control Center Listing*).

**Treatment of overdose**
Treatment is primarily supportive and symptomatic and includes immediate evacuation of the stomach (gastric lavage followed by activated charcoal) and cardiac monitoring

## Patient Consultation

As an aid to patient consultation, refer to *Advice for the Patient, Encainide (Systemic)*.

In providing consultation, consider emphasizing the following selected information (» = major clinical significance):

**Before using this medication**
» Conditions affecting use, especially:
Sensitivity to encainide
Pregnancy—Reduces fertility in rats
Other medical problems, especially second or third degree atrioventricular (AV) block, right bundle branch block associated with a left hemiblock, cardiogenic shock, or sick sinus syndrome

**Proper use of this medication**
» Compliance with therapy; taking as directed even if feeling well
» Importance of not missing doses and taking at evenly spaced intervals
» Proper dosing
Missed dose: Taking as soon as possible if remembered within 4 hours; not taking if remembered later; not doubling doses
» Proper storage

**Precautions while using this medication**
Regular visits to physician to check progress
Carrying medical identification card or bracelet
» Caution if any kind of surgery (including dental surgery) or emergency treatment is required
Caution when driving or doing things requiring alertness because of possible dizziness

**Side/adverse effects**
Signs of potential side effects, especially chest pain, ventricular tachyarrhythmias, congestive heart failure, and trembling or shaking

## General Dosing Information

Because of the long half-life of encainide's metabolites and the long half-life of encainide in slow metabolizers, dosage increments should be made no more frequently than every 3 to 5 days.

In general, it is recommended that previous antiarrhythmic therapy be withdrawn 2 to 4 plasma half-lives before initiation of encainide therapy.

In patients with pacemakers, it is recommended that the pacing threshold be determined prior to initiation of therapy, after one week of administration, and then at regular intervals.

## Oral Dosage Forms

### ENCAINIDE HYDROCHLORIDE CAPSULES

**Usual adult dose**
Antiarrhythmic—
Oral, initially 25 mg every eight hours, the dosage being increased, if necessary, after three to five days to 35 mg every eight hours; may be further increased after an additional three to five days, if necessary, to 50 mg every eight hours.

Note: Patients well controlled by doses of 50 mg every eight hours or less may be changed to every-twelve-hour dosing if necessary to aid in compliance. No more than 75 mg should be taken in each dose.

Occasional patients may require doses of 50 mg every six hours or, for life-threatening arrhythmias, 75 mg every six hours.

In patients with severe renal function impairment (serum creatinine greater than 3.5 mg per deciliter or creatinine clearance less than 20 mL per minute), therapy should be initiated at a dose of 25 mg once a day. If necessary, dosage may be increased to 25 mg every twelve hours after at least seven days, followed by 25 mg every eight hours after an additional seven days (up to a maximum of 150 mg per day).

**Usual pediatric dose**
Safety and efficacy have not been established.

**Strength(s) usually available**
U.S.—
Note: Although this product is no longer commercially available, the manufacturer is making it available to physicians who had patients adequately maintained on encainide prior to market withdrawal.

Canada—
Not commercially available.

**Packaging and storage**
Store below 30 °C (85 °F), in a well-closed container, unless otherwise specified by manufacturer.

## Selected Bibliography

Brogden RN, Todd PA. Encainide. A review of its pharmacological properties and therapeutic efficacy. Drugs 1987; 34: 519-38.

Chase SL, Sloskey GE. Encainide hydrochloride and flecainide acetate: two class 1c antiarrhythmic agents. Clin Pharm 1987 Nov; 6: 839-50.

Woosley RL, Wood AJJ, Roden DM. Encainide. New Engl J Med 1988 Apr 28; 318: 1107-15.

Revised: 06/08/93
Interim revision: 01/26/95

---

## ENFLURANE—See *Anesthetics, Inhalation (Systemic)*

---

## ENOXACIN—See *Fluoroquinolones (Systemic)*

---

# ENOXAPARIN    Systemic

**VA CLASSIFICATION (Primary): BL900**

Another commonly used name is low molecular weight heparin. However, enoxaparin is only one of a group of substances known by this designation.

Note: For a listing of dosage forms and brand names by country availability, see *Dosage Forms* section(s). For a listing of brand names for the articles in this monograph, refer to the General Index.

## Category

Antithrombotic.

## Indications

Note: Bracketed information in the *Indications* section refers to uses that are not included in U.S. product labeling.

**Accepted**
Thromboembolism, pulmonary (prophylaxis); and
Thrombosis, deep venous (prophylaxis)—Enoxaparin is indicated to prevent deep venous thrombosis and to reduce the risk of pulmonary embolism following hip [or knee] replacement surgery.

[Enoxaparin has been shown to be as effective as unfractionated heparin in preventing deep venous thrombosis following general surgical procedures, such as abdominal, thoracic, or other surgical procedures that leave the patient immobilized.][1]

[1]Not included in Canadian product labeling.

## Pharmacology/Pharmacokinetics

**Physicochemical characteristics**
Source—Obtained by alkaline depolymerization of heparin benzyl ester derived from porcine intestinal mucosa.
Molecular weight—3500 to 5500 daltons (average 4500 daltons).
pH—5.5 to 7.5
Specific activity—
Anti-factor Xa: 100 to 160 International Units (IU) per mg.
Anti-factor IIa: 20 to 40 IU per mg.

**Mechanism of action/Effect**
Enoxaparin, like unfractionated heparin, potentiates the actions of an endogenous inhibitor of blood coagulation, antithrombin III (heparin cofactor). Antithrombin III combines in a 1:1 molar ratio with activated serine proteases of the intrinsic and common coagulation pathways (primarily thrombin [factor IIa] and factor Xa, and, to a lesser extent, factors IXa, XIa, and XIIa) to form inactive complexes. Enoxaparin binds to antithrombin III, producing a conformational change in the cofactor molecule that results in significantly more rapid binding with and inactivation of the clotting factors than is achieved by the endogenous inhibitor alone.

Enoxaparin acts primarily by increasing antithrombin III–mediated inhibition of the formation and activity of factor Xa. This activity, in turn, reduces thrombin generation. These actions decrease thrombin-mediated events in coagulation, including the conversion of fibrinogen to fibrin, thereby inhibiting fibrin clot formation. Unlike unfractionated heparin, which has an anti-factor Xa (antithrombotic) to anti-factor IIa (anticoagulant) activity ratio of approximately 1 to 1, enoxaparin has an anti-factor Xa to anti-factor IIa activity ratio of approximately 3 to 1. Enoxaparin's higher ratio of antithrombotic to anticoagulant activity is thought to result in an antithrombotic effect equivalent to that of unfractionated heparin with a lower risk of bleeding. However, it has not been consistently demonstrated that the risk of bleeding is lower with enoxaparin than with unfractionated heparin. Enoxaparin also decreases inhibition of platelet function and disrupts vascular permeability to a lesser extent than does unfractionated heparin.

**Other actions/effects**
Enoxaparin has been shown to increase the plasma concentration of nonesterified fatty acids, without affecting plasma cholesterol, triglycerides, or phospholipids.

**Absorption**
Absorbed rapidly and almost completely following subcutaneous injection, with approximately 90% bioavailability.

**Distribution**
The volume of distribution is between 5.2 and 9.3 L.

**Biotransformation**
Hepatic; weakly metabolized by desulfation and depolymerization.

**Half-life**
Elimination, based on anti-factor Xa activity—3 to 6 hours. May be prolonged in the presence of chronic, severe renal failure.

**Time to peak effect**
3 to 5 hours following subcutaneous injection.

**Duration of action**
Up to 24 hours following subcutaneous injection.

**Elimination**
Primarily renal. Total clearance is decreased in patients with chronic, severe renal failure.

# Precautions to Consider

## Cross-sensitivity and/or related problems
Patients with a history of allergies, especially those who are allergic to heparin, or to pork or pork products, may be allergic to this medication also.

## Carcinogenicity
The carcinogenic potential of enoxaparin has not been investigated.

## Mutagenicity
No mutagenicity was demonstrated *in vitro*, in the Ames test, mouse lymphoma cell forward mutation test, or human lymphocyte chromosomal aberration test; or *in vivo*, in the rat bone marrow chromosomal aberration test.

No disruption of chromosomes was demonstrated *in vitro*, in rat bone marrow cells, or *in vivo*, in human peripheral lymphocytes.

## Pregnancy/Reproduction
Pregnancy—Enoxaparin does not appear to cross the placenta. Adequate and well-controlled studies in humans have not been done.

No evidence of teratogenicity was found in studies in mice receiving 30 mg per kg of body weight per day or 211 mg per square meter of body surface area per day, or in rabbits receiving 410 mg per square meter of body surface area per day.

FDA Pregnancy Category B.

## Breast-feeding
It is not known whether enoxaparin is distributed into breast milk.

## Pediatrics
Appropriate studies on the relationship of age to the effects of enoxaparin have not been performed in the pediatric population. Safety and efficacy have not been established.

## Geriatrics
Elderly patients, especially females, may be more susceptible than other patients to bleeding during enoxaparin therapy. Also, the time to peak concentration and the half-life of enoxaparin may be prolonged in elderly patients. However, it is not necessary to modify the dose or the frequency of dosing.

## Drug interactions and/or related problems
The following drug interactions and/or related problems have been selected on the basis of their potential clinical significance (possible mechanism in parentheses where appropriate)—not necessarily inclusive (» = major clinical significance):

Note: Combinations containing any of the following medications, depending on the amount present, may also interact with this medication.

In addition to the interactions listed below, the possibility should be considered that multiple effects leading to further impairment of blood clotting and/or increased risk of bleeding may occur if enoxaparin is administered to a patient receiving any medication having a significant potential for causing hypoprothrombinemia, thrombocytopenia, or gastrointestinal ulceration or hemorrhage.

Anticoagulants, coumarin- or indandione-derivative
(concurrent use may increase the risk of bleeding)

Anti-inflammatory drugs, nonsteroidal (NSAIDs) or
» Platelet aggregation inhibitors, other, (See *Appendix II*) especially:
» Aspirin
» Sulfinpyrazone
» Ticlopidine
(inhibition of platelet function by these agents may increase the risk of bleeding)

(hypoprothrombinemia induced by large [antirheumatic] doses of aspirin, and the potential occurrence of gastrointestinal ulceration or hemorrhage during therapy with NSAIDs, aspirin, or sulfinpyrazone, also may increase the risk of bleeding in patients receiving enoxaparin)

Cefamandole or
Cefoperazone or
Cefotetan or
» Plicamycin or
» Valproic acid
(these medications may cause hypoprothrombinemia; in addition, plicamycin or valproic acid may inhibit platelet aggregation; concurrent use with enoxaparin may increase the risk of hemorrhage and is not recommended)

» Thrombolytic agents, such as:
» Alteplase (tissue-type plasminogen activator, recombinant)
» Anistreplase (anisoylated plasminogen-streptokinase activator complex; APSAC)
» Streptokinase

» Urokinase
(concurrent or sequential use with enoxaparin may increase the risk of bleeding complications)

## Laboratory value alterations
The following have been selected on the basis of their potential clinical significance (possible effect in parentheses where appropriate)—not necessarily inclusive (» = major clinical significance):

With physiology/laboratory test values
Alanine aminotransferase (ALT [SGPT]) and
Alkaline phosphatase and
Aspartate aminotransferase (AST [SGOT])
(serum values may be increased)

Hemoglobin concentration and
Hematocrit value and
Red blood cell count
(values may be decreased)

## Medical considerations/Contraindications
The medical considerations/contraindications included here have been selected on the basis of their potential clinical significance (reasons given in parentheses where appropriate)—not necessarily inclusive (» = major clinical significance).

***Except under special circumstances, this medication should not be used when the following medical problems exist:***
» Abortion, threatened, or
» Aneurysm, cerebral or dissecting aorta, except in conjunction with corrective surgery, or
» Cerebrovascular hemorrhage, confirmed or suspected
(increased risk of uncontrollable hemorrhage)
» Hemorrhage, active uncontrollable
» Hypertension, severe uncontrolled
(increased risk of cerebral hemorrhage)
» Thrombocytopenia, severe, enoxaparin- or heparin-induced, within past several months
(risk of recurrence, which may cause resistance to enoxaparin and new thromboembolic complications)

***Risk-benefit should be considered when the following medical problems exist:***
Any medical or dental procedure or condition in which the risk of bleeding or hemorrhage is present, such as:
» Anesthesia, regional or lumbar block
» Blood dyscrasias, hemorrhagic, especially thrombocytopenia, hemophilia, or von Willebrand disease; or other hemorrhagic tendency
» Childbirth, recent
Diabetes, severe
» Endocarditis, acute or subacute bacterial
Gastrointestinal ulceration, history of
Intrauterine contraceptive device, use of
» Neurosurgery, recent or contemplated
» Ophthalmic surgery, recent or contemplated
» Pericarditis or pericardial effusion
Radiation therapy, recent
Renal function impairment, mild to moderate
» Renal function impairment, severe
» Retinopathy, diabetic or hemorrhagic
» Spinal puncture, recent
» Trauma, severe, especially to the central nervous system (CNS)
Tuberculosis, active
» Ulceration or other lesions of the gastrointestinal, respiratory, or urinary tract, active
» Vasculitis, severe
» Wounds resulting in large open surfaces
Hepatic function impairment, mild to moderate
» Hepatic function impairment, severe
Hypertension, mild to moderate
(increased risk of cerebral hemorrhage)
Sensitivity to enoxaparin or to heparin

## Patient monitoring
The following may be especially important in patient monitoring (other tests may be warranted in some patients, depending on condition; » = major clinical significance):
» Blood coagulation tests
(although enoxaparin, in therapeutic doses, does not alter activated partial thromboplastin time [APTT], prothrombin time [PT], or thrombin time test values, these tests should be performed prior to therapy to establish a baseline or control value; also recommended to identify pre-existing coagulation defects and aid in determining whether the patient is a suitable candidate for treatment)

Blood pressure measurement
Hemoglobin concentration and
Hematocrit value
(recommended periodically during therapy; an unexplained fall in the blood pressure or hematocrit may signal occult bleeding; bleeding should be considered major if the hemoglobin concentration is decreased by more than 2 grams per deciliter [20 grams per liter], or if a transfusion of 2 or more units of blood is required)

» Platelet aggregation test
(recommended prior to initiation of therapy in patients who have developed thrombocytopenia following administration of unfractionated heparin; if the result is negative, enoxaparin therapy may be instituted, with daily monitoring of the platelet count; however, if the result is positive, enoxaparin should not be given)

» Platelet count
(recommended prior to initiation of therapy, then twice weekly for the duration of therapy to detect thrombocytopenia)

Stool tests for occult blood loss
(recommended periodically during therapy)

## Side/Adverse Effects

The following side/adverse effects have been selected on the basis of their potential clinical significance (possible signs and symptoms in parentheses where appropriate)—not necessarily inclusive:

**Those indicating need for medical attention**
Incidence less frequent
*Bleeding complications which may include; blood in urine; bloody or black, tarry stools; bruising; coughing up blood; ecchymosis* (large, nonelevated blue or purplish patches in the skin); *hematoma* (collection of blood under the skin); *hypochromic anemia* (fatigue; headache; irritability; lightheadedness); *nosebleed; persistent bleeding or oozing from mucous membranes or surgical wound; shortness of breath; vomiting of blood or material that looks like coffee grounds; confusion; fever; peripheral edema* (swelling of ankles, feet, fingers); *thrombocytopenia which may cause; gangrene* (moderate to severe pain or numbness in the arms, legs, hands, feet); *organ infarction; pulmonary embolism* (chest discomfort; convulsions; dizziness or lightheadedness when getting up from a lying or sitting position; shortness of breath or fast breathing); *and stroke*—caused by excessive platelet aggregation

Incidence rare
*Angioedema* (swelling of the face, genitalia, larynx [voice box], mouth, tongue); *cardiovascular toxicity* (chest pain; dizziness or lightheadedness when getting up from a lying or sitting position; fast or irregular heartbeat; shortness of breath; sudden fainting); *skin rash or hives*

**Those indicating need for medical attention only if they continue or are bothersome**
Incidence less frequent or rare
*Increased menstrual bleeding; irritation, pain, or redness at injection site; nausea; vomiting*

## Overdose

For specific information on the agents used in the management of enoxaparin overdose, see the *Protamine (Systemic)* monograph.

For more information on the management of overdose or unintentional ingestion, **contact a Poison Control Center** (see *Poison Control Center Listing*).

**Clinical effects of overdose**
The following effects have been selected on the basis of their potential clinical significance (possible signs and symptoms in parentheses where appropriate)—not necessarily inclusive:

Acute
*Bleeding complications*

**Treatment of overdose**
Specific treatment—Administration of protamine sulfate by slow intravenous injection. The dose of protamine sulfate should be equivalent, on a mg-per-mg basis, to the dose of enoxaparin. An equivalent dose of protamine sulfate will neutralize the anti-factor IIa (anticoagulant) activity of enoxaparin, but will only neutralize approximately 60% of its anti-factor Xa (antithrombotic) activity. However, studies in animals indicate that protamine sulfate stops microvascular bleeding produced by very high concentrations of enoxaparin.

## Patient Consultation

As an aid to patient consultation, refer to *Advice for the Patient, Enoxaparin (Systemic)*.

In providing consultation, consider emphasizing the following selected information (» = major clinical significance):

**Before using this medication**
» Conditions affecting use, especially:
Sensitivity to enoxaparin or to heparin
Other medications, especially platelet aggregation inhibitors, hypoprothrombinemia-inducing medications, and thrombolytic agents
Other medical problems, especially threatened abortion; aneurysm; hemorrhage; hypertension; thrombocytopenia; hemorrhagic blood dyscrasias; recent childbirth; endocarditis; pericarditis or pericardial effusion; severe renal function impairment; diabetic or hemorrhagic retinopathy; spinal puncture, surgery, or other trauma; ulcers or other lesions of the gastrointestinal, respiratory, or urinary tract; severe vasculitis; wounds resulting in large open surfaces; and severe hepatic function impairment

**Proper use of this medication**
» Proper injection technique
» Safe handling and disposal of syringe
» Proper dosing
Missed dose: Using as soon as possible; not using if almost time for next dose; not doubling doses
» Proper storage

**Precautions while using this medication**
» Need to inform all physicians and dentists that this medicine is being used

**Side/adverse effects**
Signs and symptoms of potential side effects, including bleeding complications, confusion, fever, peripheral edema, thrombocytopenia, angioedema, cardiovascular toxicity, and skin rash or hives

## General Dosing Information

Enoxaparin is administered by deep subcutaneous (intrafat) injection into the abdominal fat layer; injection sites should be rotated. Enoxaparin must not be administered intramuscularly or intravenously.

A controlled, comparative study found that in non-dialyzed patients with severe renal impairment (mean creatinine clearance 11.4 mL per minute), the total clearance of enoxaparin was 1.9 times slower and the apparent half-lives of absorption and elimination were 1.7 times longer than in healthy subjects. Dosage modifications are therefore recommended in patients with severe renal impairment who are not receiving hemodialysis. However, dosage modifications are not required in dialysis patients.

## Parenteral Dosage Forms
### ENOXAPARIN INJECTION

**Usual adult dose:**
Thromboembolism, pulmonary (prophylaxis); and
Thrombosis, deep venous (prophylaxis)—
Subcutaneously, 30 mg twice a day for an average of seven to ten days. The initial dose should be given as soon as possible after surgery, but no more than twenty-four hours postoperatively.

**Usual pediatric dose:**
Safety and efficacy have not been established.

**Usual geriatric dose:**
See *Usual adult dose*.

**Strength(s) usually available**
U.S.—
30 mg in 0.3 mL of Water for Injection (Rx) [*Lovenox*].
Canada—
30 mg in 0.3 mL of Water for Injection (Rx) [*Lovenox*].

**Packaging and storage**
Store between 15 and 25 °C (59 and 77 °F), unless otherwise specified by manufacturer. Protect from freezing.

**Stability**
Because the injection contains no preservative, each syringe should be used to administer a single dose only.

**Incompatibilities**
Enoxaparin should not be admixed with intravenous fluids or other medications.

## Selected Bibliography

Buckley MM, Sorkin EM. Enoxaparin. A review of its pharmacology and clinical applications in the prevention and treatment of thromboembolic disorders. Drugs 1992; 44: 465-97.

Hirsh J, Levine MN. Low molecular weight heparin. Blood 1992; 79: 1-17.

Developed: 11/22/93

---

# ENTERAL NUTRITION FORMULAS

This monograph includes information on the following: Blenderized Enteral Nutrition Formulas; Disease-specific Enteral Nutrition Formulas§; Fiber-containing Enteral Nutrition Formulas; Milk-based Enteral Nutrition Formulas; Modular Enteral Nutrition Formulas; Monomeric (Elemental) Enteral Nutrition Formulas; Polymeric Enteral Nutrition Formulas.

VA CLASSIFICATION (Primary): TN200

Note: For a listing of dosage forms and brand names by country availability, see *Dosage Forms* section(s). For a listing of brand names for the articles in this monograph, refer to the General Index.

---

§Use for product as stated in product information.

---

## Category

Nutritional replacement.

## Indications

### Accepted

Nutritional deficiency (prophylaxis and treatment)—Enteral nutritional formulas are indicated to provide nutritional support for individuals with impaired digestion or specialized nutritional support for individuals with special nutritional needs. Enteral nutrition formulas may be the sole source of nutrition or a partial supplement to the diet. Under most circumstances, enteral feeding is preferred over parenteral feeding. Enteral nutrition may be necessary in certain persons or conditions, such as:

Acquired immunodeficiency syndrome (AIDS)
Burns
Cancer
Dysphagia
Gastrointestinal disorders—bowel resection, Crohn's, inflammatory bowel disease, malabsorption, partial gastrointestinal obstruction, stricture, ulcerative colitis
Hepatic dysfunction
Pancreatic insufficiency
Pancreatitis
Pulmonary dysfunction
Renal dysfunction
Sepsis, prolonged
Surgery, major
Trauma, major

*For Blenderized Formulas* Blenderized enteral nutrition formulas are made from selected, blended, foods. These formulas use milk or beef or a combination of the 2 as the main source of protein, and may contain pectins, some saturated fat, and cholesterol. These formulas are made from a limited range of foods.

*For Disease-specific Formulas* Disease-specific enteral nutrition formulas are formulated to meet nutrient requirements for patients with specific medical diseases and can be divided into products containing branched-chain amino acids, high-fat formulas, essential amino acid-as-protein-source formulas, and formulas high in omega fatty acids. Branched-chain amino acids may have beneficial effects on nitrogen balance. High-fat formulas provide calories through fat rather than through carbohydrates, and thus may be beneficial in patients with respiratory problems. Essential amino acid formulas minimize nitrogen waste because they contain only essential amino acids; these formulas may be beneficial to patients with renal dysfunction. Omega-3 fatty acid formulas are believed by some clinicians to modify the immune response and diminish inflammation. While polymeric and blenderized formulas are used for a variety of disease states, disease-specific formulas should only be administered for their claimed use. In general, scientific evidence for efficacy of these products for a specific disease state is weak and requires further study.

*For Fiber-containing Formulas* Fiber-containing enteral nutrition formulas may be beneficial in modulating stool consistency. However, fiber-containing formulas may cause gastrointestinal symptoms.

## Systemic

*For Milk-based Formulas* Milk-based enteral nutrition formulas contain the same nutrients as polymeric formulas but in a milk-based formula. They should not be used in patients who are lactose intolerant.

*For Modular Formulas* Modular enteral nutrition formulas provide carbohydrates, proteins, fats, vitamins, and minerals separately and in varying combinations for addition to foods or other formulas. These are not nutritionally complete.

*For Monomeric (Elemental) Formulas* Monomeric (elemental) enteral nutrition formulas contain fats, carbohydrates, and proteins in a more easily absorbed state. The term "elemental" is being replaced by "monomeric" because these formulas are not truly elemental in nature. These products contain protein in the form of peptides and/or amino acids; fat as medium-chain triglycerides and/or polyunsaturated oils such as safflower, corn, soy, or sunflower; and carbohydrates in the form of intermediate starches such as maltodextrins and glucose oligosaccharides. Monomeric (elemental) enteral formulas may be useful in patients with compromised digestive or absorptive capabilities, but, because of cost, they should be used only in patients who cannot tolerate polymeric enteral formulas.

*For Polymeric Formulas* Polymeric enteral nutrition formulas are the most common and are all lactose-free. Some polymeric formulas have a high caloric density and provide more calories per volume for patients on fluid restriction. However, patients receiving high-caloric-density formulas are more prone to dehydration and nitrogen or electrolyte retention problems due to an increased renal solute load.

### Unaccepted

There is no documented benefit for use of enteral products in healthy populations.

## Precautions to Consider

### Pregnancy/Reproduction

Pregnancy—Studies have not been done in humans or animals; however, problems would not be expected.

### Breast-feeding

Problems in humans would not be expected.

### Pediatrics

Appropriate studies performed to date have not demonstrated pediatrics-specific problems that would limit the usefulness of enteral feedings in children. However, children up to one year of age are known to have immature gastrointestinal, hepatic, and renal systems, which may determine the type of enteral formula the infant should receive. Pediatric patients may also have milk sensitivity and metabolic disorders.

### Geriatrics

Studies performed to date indicate that the elderly may be more at risk of developing nasogastric tube problems such as aspiration pneumonia, especially with prolonged use of enteral feeding. The elderly are also more likely to remove the nasogastric tube.

### Drug interactions and/or related problems

The following drug interactions and/or related problems have been selected on the basis of their potential clinical significance (possible mechanism in parentheses where appropriate)—not necessarily inclusive (» = major clinical significance):

Note: Combinations containing any of the following medications, depending on the amount present, may also interact with enteral nutrition formulas.

Only specific interactions between enteral formulas and other oral medications have been identified in this monograph. However, enteral formulas that are administered continuously may reduce the rate and/or extent of absorption of medications that must be given on an empty stomach.

Ciprofloxacin
(concurrent administration of ciprofloxacin and enteral formulas has been found to decrease the absorption of ciprofloxacin; ciprofloxacin administration should be separated from enteral feedings if possible)

Phenytoin, oral

(enteral formulas have been found to decrease the absorption of phenytoin; the enteral feeding should be held and the nasogastric tube should be flushed 2 hours before and 2 hours after administration of phenytoin; monitoring of phenytoin blood levels is recommended)

Sucralfate

(concurrent use of sucralfate and enteral nutrition formulas in a nasogastric feeding tube has resulted in bezoar formation due to the protein-binding properties of sucralfate)

Warfarin, oral

(warfarin resistance has been reported with concurrent administration of enteral feedings, possibly due to the vitamin K found in some products; more frequent monitoring of prothrombin times may be recommended)

## Laboratory value alterations

The following have been selected on the basis of their potential clinical significance (possible effect in parentheses where appropriate)—not necessarily inclusive (» = major clinical significance):

With physiology/laboratory test values

Alkaline phosphatase, serum and
Cholesterol, serum and
Glucose, serum and
Phospholipids, serum and
Transaminase, serum and
Triglycerides, serum

(concentrations may be increased)

Electrolytes, serum

(concentrations may be increased or decreased)

## Medical considerations/Contraindications

The medical considerations/contraindications included here have been selected on the basis of their potential clinical significance (reasons given in parentheses where appropriate)—not necessarily inclusive (» = major clinical significance).

*Except under special circumstances, this enteral nutrition formula should not be used when the following medical problems exist:*

» Bowel obstruction, total or
» Ileus preventing nutrient absorption or
» Ischemic bowel or
» Pancreatitis, severe or
» Perforated bowel

(some patients may require post-pyloric feeding to achieve enteral nutrition; patients with pancreatitis must be fed beyond the Ligament of Treitz)

*Risk-benefit should be considered when the following medical problems exist:*

Note: Administration of enteral formulas in patients with the following medical problems may be accomplished by careful selection of an enteral formula or by changing the manner of administration.

Aspiration pneumonitis, especially in the presence of severe pulmonary disease

(condition may be exacerbated by introduction of nasogastric tube, especially in the elderly)

Cardiac insufficiency

(condition may be exacerbated, especially during initiation of feeding in severely malnourished patients; adjustment of infusion rate may be required)

Dehydration

(condition may be exacerbated, especially if supplementary fluids are not given; patients should be monitored for signs of dehydration)

Diabetes mellitus or
Hyperglycemia

(the carbohydrate content of many enteral formulas may require adjustment of antidiabetic therapy or addition of insulin or other antidiabetic medications to the treatment regimen in patients with diabetes mellitus or hyperglycemia)

Diarrhea, severe

(condition may be exacerbated by enteral feedings; use of formulas with a low osmolality may decrease the risk of diarrhea)

Electrolyte abnormalities

(electrolyte disturbances may occur with enteral feedings; patient monitoring may be necessary)

» Gastric function abnormalities

(gastric emptying may be delayed with certain disease processes, which may lead to retention, nausea, and/or vomiting; passing the tube into the duodenum or switching to a formula with a low osmolality may be necessary)

Hepatic function impairment

(enteral formulas have been reported to alter hepatic function)

Hyperlipidemia

(the fat content of some enteral formulas may exacerbate the condition)

Lactose intolerance

(some enteral formulas contain lactose)

» Malnutrition, severe

(severe cardiopulmonary and neurologic complications have been reported when refeeding severely malnourished patients; adjustment of infusion rate may be required)

Pancreatic insufficiency with fat malabsorption

(condition may be exacerbated; use of an enteral supplement with a low fat content may be necessary)

Phenylketonuria

(some enteral formulas contain phenylalanine, which may exacerbate the condition)

Renal function impairment

(certain components such as fluid, proteins, electrolytes, vitamins, and minerals may need to be used with caution in patients with compromised renal function)

Respiratory difficulty

(condition may be exacerbated, especially with high carbohydrate formulas in patients who retain carbon dioxide, or during initiation of feeding in severely malnourished patients; adjustment of infusion rate may be required)

» Vomiting, severe

## Patient monitoring

The following may be especially important in patient monitoring (other tests may be warranted in some patients, depending on condition; » = major clinical significance):

The following (listed in order of progression) may be especially important in patient monitoring (other tests may be warranted in some patients, depending on condition; (» = major clinical significance):

Anthropometric measurements and
Body weight

(recommended periodically as a measure of lean body or adipose tissue mass or fluid status; body weight should be determined daily for patients on short-term enteral nutrition therapy and weekly for patients on long-term therapy)

Albumin, serum and
Prealbumin, serum and
Transferrin, serum and
Urea nitrogen, 24-hour, urinary

(recommended periodically to assess protein status; transferrin should be monitored in patients receiving short-term enteral nutrition therapy and albumin in those receiving long-term enteral nutrition therapy; some clinicians recommend monitoring prealbumin, but this test is expensive and may not be available in some institutions)

Energy expenditure

(may be necessary, to determine success of short-term enteral nutrition therapy)

Complete blood count and
Electrolytes, serum and
Glucose, serum and
Hepatic function determinations and
Renal function determinations and
Vitamin and mineral status

(recommended periodically depending on patient condition; abnormal serum glucose may require an adjustment of insulin dosage in diabetic patients; mineral status determinations may be necessary in patients receiving long-term enteral nutrition therapy; if a patient has an abnormal renal function, there may be a need to restrict fluids, electrolytes, vitamins, and/or trace minerals)

## Side/Adverse Effects

Note: Aspiration pneumonitis may occur with enteral tube feedings, and is more common in the elderly.

The following side/adverse effects have been selected on the basis of their potential clinical significance (possible signs and symptoms in parentheses where appropriate)—not necessarily inclusive:

**Those indicating need for medical attention**
Incidence more frequent
> *Dehydration* (decrease in urine volume; unusual tiredness or weakness); *hyperglycemia* (frequent urination or unusual thirst); *hyperkalemia* (confusion; irregular heartbeat; numbness or tingling in hands, feet, or lips; shortness of breath or difficulty breathing; unexplained nervousness; unusual tiredness or weakness; weakness or heaviness of legs); *hypokalemia* (dryness of mouth; increased thirst; irregular heartbeat; mood or mental changes; muscle cramps or pain; weak pulse); *hypophosphatemia* (convulsions; respiratory distress; unusual tiredness or weakness)

Incidence less frequent
> *Hyperphosphatemia* (muscle cramps; numbness, tingling, pain, or weakness in hands or feet; shortness of breath or troubled breathing)

**Those indicating need for medical attention only if they continue or are bothersome**
Incidence more frequent
> *Gastrointestinal disturbances, specifically constipation; or diarrhea; nausea and vomiting*

> Note: *Gastrointestinal disturbances* may also be a complication of feeding tube use, with or without pneumonitis.

## Patient Consultation

As an aid to patient consultation, refer to *Advice for the Patient, Enteral Nutrition Formulas (Systemic)*.

In providing consultation, consider emphasizing the following selected information (» = major clinical significance):

**Before using this enteral nutrition formula**
» Conditions affecting use, especially:
> Sensitivity to any ingredient in the enteral nutrition formula
> Use in children—Use with caution in children up to one year of age because of their decreased ability to metabolize certain components of enteral feeding
> Use in the elderly—Elderly more at risk of developing aspiration pneumonitis or of self-extubation
> Other medical problems, especially bowel obstruction, gastric function abnormalities, ileus preventing nutrient absorption, ischemic or perforated bowel, severe pancreatitis, severe malnutrition, or severe vomiting

**Precautions while using this enteral nutrition formula**
> Caution about bacterial contamination, particularly with home use

**Side/adverse effects**
> Dehydration, hyperglycemia, hyperkalemia, hypokalemia, hyperphosphatemia, and hypophosphatemia

## General Dosing Information

Bacterial contamination of enteral feedings may occur due to improper handling. Enteral formulas for tube-feeding use should not be hung or left for longer than 12 hours at room temperature.

Some products may be given either orally or by feeding tube; other products are designed to be given only by feeding tube.

The complication of aspiration can be reduced by confirming the anatomic position of the feeding tube, elevating the patient's head to 30° while feeding, and limiting the administration rate to 150 mL per hour or less.

Formulas that are dense in consistency are more likely to clog the feeding tube.

## Oral Dosage Forms

**Usual adult and adolescent dose**
The administration of enteral formula by continuous or intermittent feeding and the dosage are very individualized and are a decision of the prescribing physician.

**Usual pediatric dose**
The administration of enteral formula by continuous or intermittent feeding and the dosage are very individualized and are a decision of the prescribing physician.

**Strength(s) usually available**
U.S.—
> See *Tables 1–7*, pages 1312—1322.
Canada—
> See *Tables 1–7*, pages 1312—1322.

**Packaging and storage**
The unopened product should be stored below 40 °C (104 °F), preferably between 15 and 30 °C (59 and 86 °F), unless otherwise specified by the manufacturer.

**Preparation of dosage form**
For formulas in the powder form—This product must be reconstituted before administration. Follow carefully the directions for mixing on the product container.

**Stability**
For formulas in the ready-to-use form—Formulas should be refrigerated after opening. Any unused portions should be discarded within 24 to 48 hours after opening.

For formulas in the powder form—Any unused solution should be refrigerated and used within 24 to 48 hours after preparation, depending on the manufacturer's instructions.

**Auxiliary labeling**
Shake container well before opening.

## Selected Bibliography

Mobarhan S, Trumbore L. Enteral tube feeding: a clinical perspective on recent advances. Nutr Rev 1991; 49 (5): 129-40.

Smith J, Heymsfield S. Enteral nutrition support: formula preparation from modular ingredients. JPEN 1983; 7 (3): 280-8.

Revised: 8/31/93
Interim revision: 08/03/95

## Table 1. Blenderized Formulas

Note: Some products may be given either orally or by feeding tube; others are designed to be given by feeding tube only.

| Brand name [availability] | KCal (kJoules) per mL | mOsm per kg water | Protein Grams per 1000 mL | Protein Source; % KCal | Nonprotein KCal per gm of Nitrogen | Carbohydrates Grams per 1000 mL | Carbohydrates Source; % KCal | Fat Grams per 1000 mL | Fat Source; % KCal | Na+ mg (mEq) per L | K+ mg (mEq) per L | Ca++ mg (mEq) per L | Mg++ mg (mEq) per L | Phos mg per L | mL to supply 100% RDI for vitamins | Comments |
|---|---|---|---|---|---|---|---|---|---|---|---|---|---|---|---|---|
| *Compleat Modified* Oral Solution [U.S.] | 1.07 (4.5) | 300 | 43 | Beef, calcium caseinate; 16 | 131:1 | 140 | Maltodextrin, vegetables, fruits; 53 | 37 | Beef, canola oil; 31 | 1000 (43) | 1400 (36) | 670 (33.5) | 270 (22) | 870 | 1500 | Lactose-free, contains 4.2 grams fiber per 1000 mL |
| Oral solution [Canada] | 1.07 (4.5) | 300 | 43 | Beef, calcium caseinate; 16 | 131:1 | 140 | Maltodextrin, vegetables, fruits; 53 | 37 | Beef, corn oil; 31 | 850 (37) | 1400 (36) | 730 (36) | 270 (22) | 930 | N/A | Lactose-free, contains 4.2 grams fiber per 1000 mL |
| *Compleat Regular* Oral Solution [U.S.] | 1.07 (4.5) | 450 | 43 | Beef, nonfat milk; 16 | 131:1 | 130 | Maltodextrin, vegetables, fruits, nonfat milk; 48 | 43 | Beef, corn oil; 36 | 1300 (57) | 1400 (36) | 670 (33) | 270 (22) | 1200 | 1500 | Contains lactose, contains 4.2 grams fiber per 1000 mL |
| *Vitaneed* Oral Solution [U.S.] | 1 (4.2) | 300 | 40 | Beef, calcium and sodium caseinates; 16 | 134:1 | 128 | Maltodextrin, vegetables, fruits, soy fiber; 48 | 40 | Corn oil; 36 | 680 (30) | 1250 (32) | 667 (33.4) | 267 (21.4) | 667 | 1500 | Lactose-free, contains 8 grams fiber per 1000 mL |

## Table 2. Disease-specific Formulas

Note: Some products may be given either orally or by feeding tube; others are designed to be given by feeding tube only.

| Brand name [availability] | KCal (kJoules) per mL | mOsm per kg water | Protein Grams per 1000 mL | Protein Source; % KCal | Nonprotein KCal per gm of Nitrogen | Carbohydrates Grams per 1000 mL | Carbohydrates Source; % KCal | Fat Grams per 1000 mL | Fat Source; % KCal | Na+ mg (mEq) per L | K+ mg (mEq) per L | Ca++ mg (mEq) per L | Mg+ mg (mEq) per L | Phos mg per L | mL to supply 100% RDI for vitamins | Comments |
|---|---|---|---|---|---|---|---|---|---|---|---|---|---|---|---|---|
| **For Patients with Hepatic Disease\*** | | | | | | | | | | | | | | | | |
| *Hepatic-Aid II* for Oral Solution [U.S.] | 1.2 (5) | 560 | 44.1 | Crystalline amino acids; 15 | 148:1 | 168.5 | Maltodextrins, sucrose; 57.3 | 36.2 | Soybean oil, lecithin monodiglycerides; 27.7 | Less than 339 (14.7) | Less than 230.3 (5.9) | N/A | N/A | N/A | N/A | Contains phenylalanine, contains tartrazine |

Table 2. Disease-specific Formulas *(continued)*
Note: Some products may be given either orally or by feeding tube; others are designed to be given by feeding tube only.

| Brand name [availability] | KCal (kJoules) per mL | mOsm per kg water | Protein Grams per 1000 mL | Protein Source; % KCal | Nonprotein KCal per gm of Nitrogen | Carbohydrates Grams per 1000 mL | Carbohydrates Source; % KCal | Fat Grams per 1000 mL | Fat Source; % KCal | Na⁺ mg (mEq) per L | K⁺ mg (mEq) per L | Ca⁺⁺ mg (mEq) per L | Mg⁺ mg (mEq) per L | Phos mg per L | mL to supply 100% RDI for vitamins | Comments |
|---|---|---|---|---|---|---|---|---|---|---|---|---|---|---|---|---|
| *NutriHep* Oral Solution [U.S.] | 1.5 (6.3) | 690 | 40 | Crystalline L-amino acids, whey protein concentrate; 11 | 209:1 | 290 | Maltodextrin, modified cornstarch; 77 | 21.2 | MCT† oil, canola oil, lecithin, corn oil; 12 | 320 (14) | 1320 (34) | 1000 (50) | 400 (32) | 1000 | 1000 | Lactose-free |
| **For Immunocompromised Patients or Patients with Metabolic Stress/Trauma*** | | | | | | | | | | | | | | | | |
| *Advera* Oral Solution [U.S.] | 1.28 | 680 | 60 | Soy protein hydrolysate, sodium caseinate; 18.7 | 108:1 | 215.8 | Maltodextrin, sucrose, soy fiber; 65.5 | 22.8 | Canola oil, MCT† oil, refined deodorized sardine oil; 15.8 | 1056 (45.9) | 2827 (72.5) | 1083 (54.2) | 338 (27.5) | 1083 | 1184 | |
| *Crucial* Oral Solution [U.S.] | 1.5 (6.3) | 490 | 94 | Enzymatically hydrolyzed casein; L-arginine; 25 | 75:1 | 135 | Maltodextrin, cornstarch; 36 | 68 | MCT†, fish oil, soy oil; 39 | 1168 (51) | 1872 (48) | 1000 (50) | 400 (32) | 1000 | 1000 | Lactose-free |
| *Immun-Aid* for Oral Solution [U.S.] | 1 (4.2) | 580 | 37 | Amino acids; 15 | 167:1 | 120 | Maltodextrin; 48 | 22 | MCT† oil, canola oil; 20 | 800 (35) | 1756 (45) | 600 (30) | 200 (16) | 600 | 2000 | |
| *Impact* Oral Solution [U.S./Canada] | 1 (4.2) | 375 | 56 | Sodium and calcium caseinates; L-arginine; 22 | 71:1 | 130 | Hydrolyzed cornstarch; 53 | 28 | Structured lipid, menhaden oil; 25 | 1100 (48) | 1400 (36) | 800 (40) | 270 (22) | 800 (26) | 1500 | Lactose-free |
| *Impact with Fiber* Oral Solution [U.S.] | 1 (4.2) | 375 | 56 | Sodium and calcium caseinates, L-arginine; 22 | 71:1 | 140 | Hydrolyzed cornstarch, soy fiber, enzymatically modified guar; 53 | 28 | Structured lipid, menhaden oil; 25 | 1100 (48) | 1400 (36) | 800 (40) | 270 (22) | 800 (26) | 1500 | Lactose-free, contains 10 grams fiber per 1000 mL |

*Manufacturer suggested use as stated in the product information
†Medium-chain triglyceride

Table 2. Disease-specific Formulas (continued)

Note: Some products may be given either orally or by feeding tube; others are designed to be given by feeding tube only.

| Brand name [availability] | KCal (kJoules) per mL | mOsm per kg water | Protein Grams per 1000 mL | Protein Source; % KCal | Nonprotein KCal per gm of Nitrogen | Carbohydrates Grams per 1000 mL | Carbohydrates Source; % KCal | Fat Grams per 1000 mL | Fat Source; % KCal | Na$^+$ mg (mEq) per L | K$^+$ mg (mEq) per L | Ca$^{++}$ mg (mEq) per L | Mg$^+$ mg (mEq) per L | Phos mg per L | mL to supply 100% RDI for vitamins | Comments |
|---|---|---|---|---|---|---|---|---|---|---|---|---|---|---|---|---|
| *Perative* Oral Solution [U.S.] | 1.3 (5.4) | 385 | 66.6 | Partially hydrolyzed sodium caseinate, lactalbumin hydrolysate, L-arginine; 20.5 | 97:1 | 177.2 | Maltodextrin; 54.5 | 37.4 | Canola oil, MCT† oil, corn oil; 25 | 1040 (45.2) | 1730 (44.2) | 867 (43.3) | 347 (28.9) | 867 | 1155 | |
| *Protain XL* Oral Solution [U.S.] | 1 (4.2) | 340 | 55 | Sodium and calcium caseinates; 14 | 92:1 | 138 | Maltodextrin, soy fiber; 51 | 30 | MCT†, corn oil; 27 | 860 (37.4) | 1500 (38.4) | 800 (40) | 320 (25.6) | 800 | 1250 | Lactose-free |
| *TraumaCal* Oral Solution [U.S.] | 1.5 (6.3) | 560 | 82 | Sodium and calcium caseinates; 22 | 91:1 | 142 | Corn syrup, sugar; 38 | 68 | MCT† oil, soy oil; 40 | 1180 (51) | 1390 (36) | 750 (37) | 200 (16.5) | 750 | 2000 | Lactose-free |
| *Traum-Aid HBC* for Oral Solution [U.S.] | 1 (4.2) | 640 | 56 | Crystalline amino acids; 22.4 | 132:1 | 166 | Maltodextrin; 66.4 | 12.4 | Soybean oil, MCT† oil, lecithin; 11.2 | 530 (23) | 1173 (30) | 400 | 133 | 400 | 3000 | |
| **For Patients with Fat Malabsorption*** | | | | | | | | | | | | | | | | |
| *Citrotein* for Oral Solution [Canada] orange punch | 0.67 (2.8) | 490 480 | 41 | Egg white solids: 25 | 76:1 | 120 | Maltodextrin sugar; 73 | 1.6 | Partially hydrogenated soybean oil; 2 | 670 (29) | 550 (14) | 1100 (56) | 420 (35) | 1100 | N/A | Lactose-free, cholesterol-free |
| *Lipisorb* for Oral Solution [U.S.] | Dilution #1 1 (4.2) | 320 | 35 | Sodium caseinate; 14 | 157:1 | 116 | Corn syrup, sucrose; 46 | 48 | MCT† oil, corn oil; 40 | 740 (32) | 1260 (32) | 710 (36) | 200 (16.5) | 710 | 2000 | Lactose-free |
| | Dilution #2 1.35 (5.6) | 470 | 47 | Sodium caseinate; 14 | 157:1 | 155 | Corn syrup, sucrose; 46 | 65 | MCT† oil, corn oil; 40 | 990 (43) | 1690 (43) | 950 (48) | 270 (22) | 950 | 1480 | Lactose-free |

Table 2. Disease-specific Formulas *(continued)*

Note: Some products may be given either orally or by feeding tube; others are designed to be given by feeding tube only.

| Brand name [availability] | KCal (kJoules) per mL | mOsm per kg water | Protein Grams per 1000 mL | Protein Source; % KCal | Nonprotein KCal per gm of Nitrogen | Carbohydrates Grams per 1000 mL | Carbohydrates Source; % KCal | Fat Grams per 1000 mL | Fat Source; % KCal | Na+ mg (mEq) per L | K+ mg (mEq) per L | Ca++ mg (mEq) per L | Mg+ mg (mEq) per L | Phos mg per L | mL to supply 100% RDI for vitamins | Comments |
|---|---|---|---|---|---|---|---|---|---|---|---|---|---|---|---|---|
| *Lipisorb (continued)* Oral Solution [U.S.] | 1.35 (5.6) | 630 | 57 | Sodium and calcium caseinates; 17 | 125:1 | 161 | Maltodextrin, sucrose; 48 | 57 | MCT† oil, soy oil; 35 | 1350 (59) | 1690 (43) | 850 (43) | 340 (28) | 850 | 1180 | Lactose-free |
| *Nutren 2.0* Oral Solution [U.S.] | 2 (8.4) | 720 | 80 | Calcium and potassium caseinates; 16 | 131:1 | 196 | Corn syrup solids, maltodextrin, sucrose; 39 | 106 | MCT† oil, canola oil, corn oil; 45 | 1300 (56.5) | 1920 (49.2) | 1340 (67) | 536 (42.9) | 1340 | 750 | Lactose-free, vanilla |
| *Peptamen* Oral Solution [U.S.] | 1 (4.2) | 270 | 40 | Hydrolyzed whey; 16 | 131:1 | 127 | Maltodextrin, starch; 51 | 39 | MCT† oil, sunflower oil; 33 | 500 (22) | 1250 (32) | 800 (40) | 400 (32) | 700 | 1500 | Lactose-free |
| *Peptamen Junior* Oral Solution [U.S.] | 1 (4.2) | 260 | 30 | Enzymatically hydrolyzed whey protein; 12 | 183:1 | 137.5 | Maltodextrin, cornstarch; 55 | 38.5 | MCT†, soybean oil, canola oil; 33 | 460 (20) | 1320 (34) | 1000 (50) | 200 (16) | 800 | 1000 | Lactose-free |
| *Peptamen VHP* Oral Solution [U.S.] | 1 (4.2) | 300 | 62.5 | Enzymatically hydrolyzed whey protein; 25 | 75:1 | 104.5 | Maltodextrin, cornstarch; 42 | 39 | MCT†, soybean oil; 33 | 560 (24) | 1500 (38.5) | 800 (40) | 300 (24) | 700 | 1500 | Lactose-free |
| **For Patients with Glucose Intolerance*** | | | | | | | | | | | | | | | | |
| *DiabetiSource* Oral Solution [U.S.] | 1 (4.2) | 360 | 50 | Beef and calcium caseinates; 20 | 100:1 | 90 | Maltodextrin, fructose; 36 | 49 | High-oleic sunflower oil, canola oil; beef fat; 44 | 1000 (43) | 1400 (36) | 670 (33) | 270 (22) | 670 | 1500 | Lactose-free, contains 6.4 grams fiber per 1500 mL |
| *Glucerna* Oral Solution [U.S./Canada] | 1 (4.2) | 375 | 41.8 | Sodium and calcium caseinates; 16.7 | 125:1 | 93.7 | Hydrolyzed cornstarch, soy fiber, fructose; 33.3 | 55.7 | High-oleic safflower oil, soy oil; 50 | 930 (40.5) | 1560 (40) | 704 (35.2) | 282 (23.5) | 704 | 1422 | Lactose-free, contains 14.4 grams fiber per 1000 mL |

*Manufacturer suggested use as stated in the product information

†Medium-chain triglyceride

## Table 2. Disease-specific Formulas (continued)

Note: Some products may be given either orally or by feeding tube; others are designed to be given by feeding tube only.

| Brand name [availability] | KCal (kJoules) per mL | mOsm per kg water | Protein Grams per 1000 mL | Protein Source; % KCal | Nonprotein KCal per gm of Nitrogen | Carbohydrates Grams per 1000 mL | Carbohydrates Source; % KCal | Fat Grams per 1000 mL | Fat Source; % KCal | Na+ mg (mEq) per L | K+ mg (mEq) per L | Ca++ mg (mEq) per L | Mg+ mg (mEq) per L | Phos mg per L | mL to supply 100% RDI for vitamins | Comments |
|---|---|---|---|---|---|---|---|---|---|---|---|---|---|---|---|---|
| *Glytrol* Oral Solution [U.S.] | 1 (4.2) | 380 | 45 | Calcium and potassium caseinates; 18 | 114:1 | 100 | Maltodextrin, modified cornstarch, fructose; 40 | 47.5 | Canola oil, high-oleic safflower oil, MCT†; 42 | 740 (32) | 1400 (36) | 720 (36) | 286 (23) | 720 | 1400 | Lactose-free, contains 15 grams fiber per 1000 mL |
| **For Patients with Pulmonary Disease\*** | | | | | | | | | | | | | | | | |
| *NutriVent* Oral Solution [U.S.] | 1.5 (6.3) | 330 | 67.5 | Calcium and potassium caseinates; 18 | 113:1 | 100 | Maltodextrin, sugar; 27 | 94 | MCT† oil, canola oil, corn oil, lecithin; 55 | 1170 (51) | 1872 (48) | 1200 (60) | 480 (38) | 1200 | 1000 | Lactose-free |
| *Pulmocare* Oral Solution [U.S./Canada] | 1.5 (6.3) | 475 | 62.6 | Sodium and calcium caseinates; 16.7 | 125:1 | 105.7 | Sucrose, maltodextrin; 28.2 | 93.3 | Canola oil, MCT† oil, corn oil, high-oleic safflower oil; 55.1 | 1310 (57) | 1730 (44.2) | 1056 (52.8) | 423 (35.3) | 1056 | 947 | Lactose-free |
| *Respalor* Oral Solution [U.S.] | 1.52 (6.4) | 580 | 76 | Sodium and calcium caseinates; 20 | 102:1 | 148 | Corn syrup, sucrose; 39 | 71 | MCT† oil, canola oil; 41 | 1270 (55) | 1480 (38) | 710 (36) | 280 (23) | 710 | 1420 | |
| **For Patients with Renal Disease\*** | | | | | | | | | | | | | | | | |
| *Amin-Aid* for Oral Solution [U.S.] | 2 (8.4) | 510 | 19.4 | Crystalline, amino acids; 4 | 640:1 | 365.6 | Malto-dextrins, sucrose; 74.8 | 46.2 | Partially hydrogenated soybean oil, lecithin, mono- and diglycerides | Less than 339 (14.7) | Less than 230.3 (5.9) | N/A | N/A | N/A | N/A | Contains tartrazine |
| *Magnacal* Oral Solution [U.S.] | 2 | 590 | 70 | Sodium and calcium caseinates; 14 | 154:1 | 250 | Maltodextrin, sucrose; 50 | 80 | Soy oil; 36 | 1000 (43.5) | 1250 (32) | 1000 (50) | 400 (32) | 1000 | 1000 | |
| *Nepro* Oral Solution [U.S/Canada] | 2 (8.4) | 635 | 69.9 | Calcium, magnesium, and sodium caseinates; 14 | 154:1 | 215.2 | Corn syrup, sucrose; 43 | 95.6 | High-oleic safflower oil, soy oil; 43 | 829 (36.1) | 1057 (27) | 1373 (68.6) | 211 (17.6) | 686 | 947 | |

Table 2. Disease-specific Formulas *(continued)*
Note: Some products may be given either orally or by feeding tube; others are designed to be given by feeding tube only.

| Brand name [availability] | KCal (kJoules) per mL | mOsm per kg water | Protein Grams per 1000 mL | Protein Source; % KCal | Nonprotein KCal per gm of Nitrogen | Carbohydrates Grams per 1000 mL | Carbohydrates Source; % KCal | Fat Grams per 1000 mL | Fat Source; %KCal | Na⁺ mg (mEq) per L | K⁺ mg (mEq) per L | Ca⁺⁺ mg (mEq) per L | Mg⁺ mg (mEq) per L | Phos mg per L | mL to supply 100% RDI for vitamins | Comments |
|---|---|---|---|---|---|---|---|---|---|---|---|---|---|---|---|---|
| *Suplena* Oral Solution [U.S./Canada] | 2 (8.4) | 600 | 30 | Sodium and calcium caseinates; 6 | 393:1 | 255.2 | Maltodextrin, sucrose; 51 | 95.6 | High-oleic safflower oil, soy oil; 43 | 783 (34) | 1116 (28.5) | 1385 (69.2) | 211 (17.6) | 728 | 947 | |
| *Travasorb Renal Diet* for Oral Solution [U.S.] | 1.35 (5.6) | 590 | 22.9 | Amino acids; 6.9 | 339:1 | 270.5 | Glucose oligo-saccharides, sucrose; 81.1 | 17.7 | MCT† oil, sunflower oil; 12 | N/A | N/A | N/A | N/A | N/A | N/A | |

*Manufacturer suggested use as stated in the product information
†Medium-chain triglyceride

Table 3. Fiber-containing Formulas
Note: Some products may be given either orally or by feeding tube; others are designed to be given by feeding tube only.

| Brand name [availability] | KCal (kJoules) per mL | mOsm per kg water | Protein Grams per 1000 mL | Protein Source; % KCal | Nonprotein KCal per gm of Nitrogen | Carbohydrates Grams per 1000 mL | Carbohydrates Source; % KCal | Fat Grams per 1000 mL | Fat Source; %KCal | Na⁺ mg (mEq) per L | K⁺ mg (mEq) per L | Ca mg (mEq) per L | Mg⁺⁺ mg (mEq) per L | Phos mg per L | mL to supply 100% RDI for vitamins | Comments |
|---|---|---|---|---|---|---|---|---|---|---|---|---|---|---|---|---|
| *Ensure with Fiber* Oral Solution [U.S./Canada] | 1.1 (4.6) | 480 | 39.7 | Sodium and calcium caseinates, soy protein isolate; 14.5 | 148:1 | 162 | Maltodextrin, sucrose, soy fiber; 55 | 37.2 | Corn oil; 30.5 | 846 (36.8) | 1693 (43.3) | 719 (35.9) | 288 (24) | 719 | 1391 | Lactose-free, contains 14.4 grams fiber per 1000 mL |
| *Fiberlan* Oral Solution [U.S.] | 1.2 (5) | 310 | 50 | Caseinates; 16.7 | 122:1 | 160 | Maltodextrin; 53.3 | 40 | MCT† oil, corn oil; 27.8 | 1012 (44) | 1716 (44) | 800 (40) | 320 (25.6) | 800 | 1250 | Lactose-free, contains 14 grams fiber per 1000 mL |
| *Fibersource* Oral Solution [U.S.] | 1.2 (5) | 390 | 43 | Sodium and calcium caseinates; 14 | 151:1 | 170 | Hydrolyzed cornstarch, soy fiber; 56 | 41 | MCT† oil, canola oil; 30 | 1100 (48) | 1800 (46) | 670 (33) | 270 (22) | 670 | 1500 | Lactose-free, contains 10 grams fiber per 1000 mL |

†Medium-chain triglyceride

## Table 3. Fiber-containing Formulas *(continued)*

Note: Some products may be given either orally or by feeding tube; others are designed to be given by feeding tube only.

| Brand name [availability] | KCal (kJoules) per mL | mOsm per kg water | Protein Grams per 1000 mL | Protein Source; % KCal | Nonprotein KCal per gm of Nitrogen | Carbohydrates Grams per 1000 mL | Carbohydrates Source; % KCal | Fat Grams per 1000 mL | Fat Source; % KCal | Na+ mg (mEq) per L | K+ mg (mEq) per L | Ca mg (mEq) per L | Mg++ mg (mEq) per L | Phos mg per L | mL to supply 100% RDI for vitamins | Comments |
|---|---|---|---|---|---|---|---|---|---|---|---|---|---|---|---|---|
| *Fibersource HN* Oral Solution [U.S.] | 1.2 (5) | 390 | 53 | Sodium and calcium caseinates; 18 | 118:1 | 160 | Hydrolyzed cornstarch, soy fiber; 52 | 41 | MCT† oil, canola oil; 30 | 1100 (48) | 1800 (46) | 670 (33) | 270 (22) | 670 | 1500 | Lactose-free, contains 6.7 grams fiber per 1000 mL |
| *Glytrol* Oral Solution [U.S.] | 1.0 (4.2) | 380 | 45 | Calcium and potassium caseinate; 18 | 114:1 | 100 | Maltodextrin, modified cornstarch, fructose; 40 | 47.5 | Canola oil, high-oleic safflower oil, MCT†; 42 | 740 (32) | 1400 (36) | 720 (36) | 286 (23) | 720 | 1400 | Lactose-free, 15 grams fiber/1000 mL |
| *Impact with Fiber* Oral Solution [U.S.] | 1 (4.2) | 375 | 56 | Sodium and calcium caseinates, L-arginine; 22 | 71:1 | 140 | Hydrolyzed cornstarch, soy fiber, enzymatically modified guar; 53 | 28 | Structural lipid menhaden oil; 25 | 1100 (48) | 1400 (36) | 800 (40) | 270 (22) | 800 (26) | 1500 | Lactose-free, contains 10 grams fiber per 1000 mL |
| *IsoSource VHN* Oral Solution [U.S.] | 1 (4.2) | 300 | 62 | Sodium and calcium caseinates; 25 | 77:1 | 130 | Hydrolyzed cornstarch, soy fiber and hydrolyzed guar fiber; 50 | 29 | MCT† oil, canola oil; 25 | 1300 (57) | 1600 (41) | 800 (40) | 320 (25.6) | 800 | 1250 | Lactose-free, contains 12.5 grams fiber per 1250 mL |
| *Jevity* Oral Solution [U.S.] | 1.06 (4.4) | 310 | 44.3 | Sodium and calcium caseinates; 16.7 | 125:1 | 154.4 | Maltodextrin, soy fiber; 54.3 | 34.7 | High-oleic safflower oil, canola oil, MCT† oil; 29 | 930 (40.5) | 1570 (40.2) | 909 (45.4) | 304 (25.3) | 758 | 1321 | Lactose-free, contains 14.4 grams fiber per 1000 mL |
| Oral Solution [Canada] | 1.06 (4.4) | 310 | 44 | Sodium and calcium caseinates; 16.7 | 125:1 | 152 | Hydrolyzed cornstarch, soy fiber; 53.3 | 37 | MCT† oil, corn oil; 30 | 740 (32) | 1240 (32) | 908 (45.4) | 302 (24.2) | 748.8 | 1321 | Lactose-free, contains 14.4 grams fiber per 1000 mL |
| *Kindercal* Oral Solution [U.S.] | 1.06 (4.4) | 310 | 34 | Sodium and calcium caseinates, milk protein concentrate; 13 | 171:1 | 135 | Maltodextrin, sucrose; 50 | 44 | MCT† oil, canola oil, corn oil, high-oleic safflower oil; 37 | 370 (16.1) | 1310 (34) | 850 (43) | 210 (17.4) | 850 | 950 | Lactose-free, contains 6.3 grams fiber per 1000 mL |

Table 3. Fiber-containing Formulas (continued)

Note: Some products may be given either orally or by feeding tube; others are designed to be given by feeding tube only.

| Brand name [availability] | KCal (kJoules) per mL | mOsm per kg water | Protein | | | Nonprotein KCal per gm of Nitrogen | Carbohydrates | | | Fat | | | Na+ mg (mEq) per L | K+ mg (mEq) per L | Ca mg (mEq) per L | Mg++ mg (mEq) per L | Phos mg per L | mL to supply 100% RDI for vitamins | Comments |
|---|---|---|---|---|---|---|---|---|---|---|---|---|---|---|---|---|---|---|---|
| | | | Grams per 1000 mL | Source; % KCal | | | Grams per 1000 mL | Source; % KCal | | Grams per 1000 mL | Source; % KCal | | | | | | | | |
| NuBasics with Fiber Oral Solution [U.S.] | 1 (4.2) | 520 | 35 | Calcium and potassium caseinates; 14 | | 153:1 | 132.4 | Corn syrup solids, sucrose; 53 | | 36.8 | Canola oil, corn oil; 33 | | 876 (38) | 1248 (32) | 500 (25) | 200 (16) | 500 | 2000 | Lactose-free, contains 14 grams fiber per 1000 mL |
| Nutren 1.0 with Fiber Oral Solution [U.S.] | 1 (4.2) | 310 | 40 | Calcium and potassium caseinates; 16 | | 131:1 | 127 | Maltodextrin, corn syrup solids; 51 | | 38 | MCT† oil, canola oil, corn oil; 33 | | 876 (38) | 1250 (32) | 668 (33) | 268 (21.4) | 668 | 1500 | Contains 14 grams fiber per 1000 mL |
| NutriSource Oral Solution [Canada] | 1.2 (5) | 390 | 43 | Sodium and calcium caseinates; 14 | | 151:1 | 170 | Maltodextrin, corn syrup solids, soy fiber; 56 | | 41 | MCT† oil, canola oil; 30 | | 1100 (48) | 1800 (46) | 670 (33) | 270 (22) | 670 | N/A | Lactose-free, contains 10 grams fiber per 1000 mL |
| NutriSource HN Oral Solution [Canada] | 1.2 (5) | 390 | 53 | Sodium and calcium caseinates; 18 | | 118:1 | 160 | Maltodextrin, corn syrup solids, soy fiber; 52 | | 41 | MCT† oil, canola oi; 30 | | 1100 (48) | 1800 (46) | 670 (33) | 270 (22) | 670 | N/A | Lactose-free, contains 6.7 grams fiber per 1000 mL |
| Pediasure with Fiber Oral Solution [U.S.] | 1 (4.2) | <345 | 30 | Sodium caseinate, whey protein concentrate; 12 | | 185:1 | 113.5 | Hydrolyzed cornstarch, sucrose, soy fiber; 43.9 | | 49.7 | High-oleic safflower oil, soy oil, MCT† oil; 44.1 | | 380 (16.5) | 1310 (33.5) | 970 (48.5) | 200 (16.7) | 800 | 1000 | Trace lactose, contains 5 grams fiber per 1000 mL |
| ProBalance Oral Solution [U.S.] | 1.2 (5) | 350 | 54 | Calcium and potassium caseinates; 18 | | 114:1 | 156 | Maltodextrin; 52 | | 40.6 | Canola oil, MCT†, corn oil; 30 | | 763 (33) | 1560 (40) | 1250 (62.5) | 400 (32) | 1000 | 1000 | Lactose-free, contains 10 grams fiber per 1000 mL |
| Profiber Oral Solution [U.S.] | 1 (4.2) | 300 | 40 | Sodium and calcium caseinates; 16 | | 134:1 | 147 | Maltodextrin, soy fiber; 54 | | 35 | Corn oil, MCT† oil; 30 | | 800 (34.8) | 1500 (38.4) | 800 (40) | 320 (25.6) | 800 | 1250 | Lactose-free, contains 12 grams fiber per 1000 mL |
| Promote with Fiber Oral Solution [U.S.] | 1 | 370 | 62.5 | Sodium and calcium caseinates; 25 | | 75:1 | 139.4 | Hydrolyzed cornstarch, sucrose, oat fiber, soy fiber; 50 | | 28.2 | High-oleic safflower oil, canola oil, MCT† oil; 25 | | 1300 (56.6) | 1980 (50.6) | 1200 (60) | 400 (32.6) | 1200 | 1000 | Lactose-free, contains 14.4 grams fiber per 1000 mL |
| Replete with Fiber Oral Solution [U.S.] | 1 (4.2) | 300 | 62.5 | Calcium and potassium caseinates; 25 | | 75:1 | 113 | Maltodextrin, corn syrup solids; 45 | | 34 | Canola oil; MCT† oil; 30 | | 876 (38) | 1500 (38) | 1000 (50) | 400 (32) | 1000 | 1000 | Lactose-free, contains 14 grams fiber per 1000 mL |

†Medium-chain triglyceride

## Table 3. Fiber-containing Formulas

Note: Some products may be given either orally or by feeding tube; others are designed to be given by feeding tube only.

| Brand name [availability] | KCal (kJoules) per mL | mOsm per kg water | Protein Grams per 1000 mL | Protein Source; % KCal | Nonprotein KCal per gm of Nitrogen | Carbohydrates Grams per 1000 mL | Carbohydrates Source; % KCal | Fat Grams per 1000 mL | Fat Source; % KCal | Na+ mg (mEq) per L | K+ mg (mEq) per L | Ca mg (mEq) per L | Mg++ mg (mEq) per L | Phos mg per L | mL to supply 100% RDI for vitamins | Comments |
|---|---|---|---|---|---|---|---|---|---|---|---|---|---|---|---|---|
| *Sustacal with Fiber* Oral Solution [U.S.] | 1.06 (4.4) | 490 | 46 | Sodium and calcium caseinates, soy protein isolates; 17 | 120:1 | 139 | Maltodextrin, sugar; 53 | 35 | Corn oil; 30 | 720 (31) | 1390 (36) | 850 (43) | 280 (23) | 710 | 1420 | Lactose-free, contains 10.6 grams fiber per 1000 mL |
| *Ultracal* Oral Solution [U.S.] | 1.06 (4.4) | 310 | 44 | Sodium and calcium caseinates; 17 | 128:1 | 123 | Maltodextrin; 46 | 45 | MCT† oil, canola oil; 37 | 930 (40) | 1610 (41) | 850 (43) | 340 (28) | 850 | 1180 | Lactose-free, contains 14.4 grams fiber per 1000 mL |

†Medium-chain triglyceride

## Table 4. Milk-based Formulas

Note: Some products may be given either orally or by feeding tube; others are designed to be given by feeding tube only.

| Brand name [availability] | KCal (kJoules) per mL | mOsm per kg water | Protein Grams per 1000 mL | Protein Source; % KCal | Nonprotein KCal per gm of Nitrogen | Carbohydrates Grams per 1000 mL | Carbohydrates Source; % KCal | Fat Grams per 1000 mL | Fat Source; % KCal | Na+ mg (mEq) per L | K+ mg (mEq) per L | Ca++ mg (mEq) per L | Mg++ mg (mEq) per L | Phos mg per L | mL to supply 100% RDI for vitamins | Comments |
|---|---|---|---|---|---|---|---|---|---|---|---|---|---|---|---|---|
| *Carnation Instant Breakfast* for Oral Solution [U.S.] | 1 (4.2) | — | 63.3 | Nonfat dry milk, fluid milk§ | — | 149.6 | Lactose, sucrose§ | 34.6 | Milk fat§ | 1062.5 (45.8) | 3083.3 (78.8) | 2045.8 (102.3) | 470.8 (37.7) | 1700 | N/A | Contains lactose |
| *Carnation Instant Breakfast No Sugar Added* for Oral Solution [U.S.] | 0.7 (2.9) | — | 62.5 | Casein, nonfat dry milk, fluid milk§ | — | 86.3 | Lactose,§ maltodextrin | 20.8 | Milk fat§ | 1041.7 (45.4) | 2822.9 (72.5) | 1716.7 (85.8) | 470.8 (37.7) | 1362.5 | N/A | Contains lactose, sugar-free, contains aspartame |
| *Great Shake* Oral Solution [U.S.] | 1.67 (7.04) | 910 | 50 | Nonfat milk, skim milk; 12 | 183:1 | 261 | Corn syrup, high fructose corn syrup, lactose; 62.7 | 50 | Partially hydrogenated soybean oil, milk-fat; 27 | 1100 (48.1) | 1940 (49.5) | 1670 (83.5) | 670 (54.7) | 1110 | 900 | Contains lactose |

## Table 4. Milk-based Formulas (continued)

Note: Some products may be given either orally or by feeding tube; others are designed to be given by feeding tube only.

| Brand name [availability] | KCal (kJoules) per mL | mOsm per kg water | Protein Grams per 1000 mL | Protein Source; % KCal | Nonprotein KCal per gm of Nitrogen | Carbohydrates Grams per 1000 mL | Carbohydrates Source; % KCal | Fat Grams per 1000 mL | Fat Source; % KCal | Na+ mg (mEq) per L | K+ mg (mEq) per L | Ca++ mg (mEq) per L | Mg++ mg (mEq) per L | Phos mg per L | mL to supply 100% RDI for vitamins | Comments |
|---|---|---|---|---|---|---|---|---|---|---|---|---|---|---|---|---|
| *Great Shake Jr.* Oral Solution [U.S./Canada] | 1.92 (7.95) | 890 | 66.7 | Nonfat milk, skim milk; 13.9 | 155:1 | 165 | Corn syrup, high fructose corn syrup, lactose; 57.4 | 35 | Partially hydrogenated soybean oil, milk-fat; 27.4 | 800 (35) | 1500 (38.3) | 1000 (50) | 400 (32) | 1000 | 800 | Contains lactose |
| *Menu Magic Instant Breakfast* for Oral Solution [U.S.] | 1.12 (5) | — | 64 | Nonfat milk, whole milk, isolated soy protein; 22.1 | 113:1 | 144 | Sucrose, lactose; 49.9 | 36 | Milk fat; 28 | 900 (39) | 2960 (75) | 3600 (180) | 320 (25.6) | 1800 | 715 | Contains lactose |
| *Menu Magic Milk Shake* Oral Solution [U.S.] | 1 (4.2) | — | 32 | Nonfat milk, whole milk; 13.5 | 187.5:1 | 136 | Lactose, dextrose, maltodextrin; 56.5 | 32 | Milk fat; 30 | 600 (26.3) | 1600 (41.1) | 1400 (67) | 560 (45.7) | 1200 | 1000 | Contains lactose |
| *Meriene* for Oral Solution [U.S.] | 1.06 (4.4) | 690 | 69 | Nonfat milk, whole milk; 26 | 71:1 | 120 | Lactose, sugar, hydrolyzed corn starch; 45 | 34 | Milk fat; 29 | 1100 (48) | 2800 (72) | 2200 (110) | 380 (31) | 1900 | 1040 | Contains lactose |
| for Oral Solution [Canada] | 1.06 (4.4) | 690 | 72 | Nonfat milk, whole milk; 26 | 96:1 | 120 | Corn syrup solids; 45 | 35 | Partially hydrogenated soybean oil; 29 | 960 (42) | 3000 (77) | 2300 (110) | 380 (31) | 1900 | N/A | Contains lactose |
| *206 Shake* Oral Solution [U.S.] | 1.67 (7.04) | 910 | 50 | Nonfat milk, skim milk; 12 | 183:1 | 261 | Corn syrup, high fructose corn syrup, lactose; 62.7 | 50 | Partially hydrogenated soybean oil, milkfat; 27 | 1100 (48.1) | 1940 (49.5) | 1670 (83.5) | 670 (54.7) | 1110 | 900 | Contains lactose |
| *Sustagen* for Oral Solution [U.S./Canada] | 1.86 (7.8) | 1130 | 115 | Nonfat milk, whole milk, calcium caseinate; 25 | 78:1 | 320 | Lactose, dextrose, corn syrup solids; 67 | 16.8 | Milk fat; 8 | 1060 (46) | 3400 (87) | 3400 (170) | 420 (35) | 2500 | 950 | Contains lactose |

§The percent KCal for protein, carbohydrates, and fat depends on the fat content of the beverage used to prepare the product.

## Table 4. Milk-based Formulas

Note: Some products may be given either orally or by feeding tube; others are designed to be given by feeding tube only.

| Brand name [availability] | KCal (kJoules) per mL | mOsm per kg water | Protein Grams per 1000 mL | Protein Source; % KCal | Nonprotein KCal per gm of Nitrogen | Carbohydrates Grams per 1000 mL | Carbohydrates Source; % KCal | Fat Grams per 1000 mL | Fat Source; % KCal | Na+ mg (mEq) per L | K+ mg (mEq) per L | Ca++ mg (mEq) per L | Mg++ mg (mEq) per L | Phos mg per L | mL to supply 100% RDI for vitamins | Comments |
|---|---|---|---|---|---|---|---|---|---|---|---|---|---|---|---|---|
| *Tasty Shake* Oral Solution [U.S.] | 1.2 (5) | — | 64 | Whole milk, nonfat milk, isolated soy protein; 22.1 | 113.3:1 | 144 | Sucrose, lactose; 49.9 | 36 | Milk fat; 28 | 900 (39.5) | 2960 (75) | 3600 (180) | 320 (26.7) | 1800 | 715 | Contains lactose |

§The percent KCal for protein, carbohydrates, and fat depends on the fat content of the beverage used to prepare the product.

## Table 5. Modular Formulas

Note: Some products may be given either orally or by feeding tube; others are designed to be given by feeding tube only.

| Brand name [availability] | KCal (kJoules) per gram | Protein Grams per 100 grams | Protein Source | Carbohydrates Grams per 100 grams | Carbohydrates Source | Fat Grams per 100 grams | Fat Source | Na+ mg (mEq) per 100 grams | K+ mg (mEq) per 100 grams | Ca++ mg (mEq) per 100 grams | Mg++ mg (mEq) per 100 grams | Phos mg per 100 grams | Comments |
|---|---|---|---|---|---|---|---|---|---|---|---|---|---|
| *Casec* Oral Powder [U.S.] | 3.8 (15.9) | 90 | Calcium caseinate | | | 2 | Milk fat | 100 (4.3) | 10 (0.26) | 1400 (70) | N/A | 800 | |
| *Elementra* Oral Powder [U.S.] | 3.8 (16) | 79 | Hydrolyzed whey protein | | | | | 39 (1.7) | 1515 (39) | 909 (45) | 35 (2.8) | 454 | |
| *MCT Oil* Oral Solution [U.S./Canada] | 7.7 (32) per mL | | | | | | Fractionated coconut oil | N/A | N/A | N/A | N/A | N/A | |
| *Microlipid* Oral Solution [U.S.] | 4.5 (18.8) per mL | | | | | 0.5 gm per mL | Safflower oil | N/A | N/A | N/A | N/A | N/A | |
| *Moducal* Oral Powder [U.S.] | 3.8 (15.9) | | | 95 | Maltodextrin | | | 70 (3) | Less than 10 mg (0.26) | N/A | N/A | N/A | |

# Table 5. Modular Formulas (continued)

Note: Some products may be given either orally or by feeding tube; others are designed to be given by feeding tube only.

| Brand name [availability] | KCal (kJoules) per gram | Protein Grams per 100 grams | Protein Source | Carbohydrates Grams per 100 grams | Carbohydrates Source | Fat Grams per 100 grams | Fat Source | Na+ mg (mEq) per 100 grams | K+ mg (mEq) per 100 grams | Ca++ mg (mEq) per 100 grams | Mg++ mg (mEq) per 100 grams | Phos mg per 100 grams | Comments |
|---|---|---|---|---|---|---|---|---|---|---|---|---|---|
| *Polycose* Oral Solution [U.S./Canada] | 2 (8.4) per mL | | | 50 gm per 100 mL | Glucose polymers | | | Does not exceed 70 (3) per 100 mL | Does not exceed 6 (.15) per 100 mL | Does not exceed 20 (1) per 100 mL | N/A | Does not exceed 3 mg per 100 mL | Lactose-free |
| Oral Powder [U.S./Canada] | 3.8 (15.9) | | | 94 | Glucose polymers | | | Does not exceed 110 (4.8) | Does not exceed 10 (0.3) | Does not exceed 30 (1.5) | N/A | Does not exceed 5 mg | Lactose-free |
| *ProMod* Oral Powder [U.S./Canada] | 4.2 (23.4) | 75 | Whey protein concentrate | Does not exceed 10.2 | | Does not exceed 9 | Soy lecithin | Does not exceed 227 (9.8) | Does not exceed 985 (25.2) | Does not exceed 667 (33.4) | N/A | Does not exceed 500 mg | |
| *Propac Plus* Oral Powder [U.S.] | 3.7 | 88.5 | Milk protein from skimmed milk | <1 | Lactose | <2 | Milk protein, soy, lecithin | 30 | 50 | 1350 | 20 | 700 | Lactose-free, protein from casein and whey |
| *Sumacal* Oral Powder [U.S.] | 3.8 (15.9) | | | 95 | Maltodextrin | | | 100 (4.3) | N/A | N/A | N/A | N/A | |

## Table 6. Monomeric (Elemental) Formulas

Note: Some products may be given either orally or by feeding tube; others are designed to be given by feeding tube only.

| Brand name [availability] | KCal (kJoules) per mL | mOsm per kg water | Protein Grams per 1000 mL | Protein Source; % KCal | Nonprotein KCal per gm of Nitrogen | Carbohydrates Grams per 1000 mL | Carbohydrates Source; % KCal | Fat Grams per 1000 mL | Fat Source; % KCal | Na$^+$ mg (mEq) per L | K$^+$ mg (mEq) per L | Ca$^{++}$ mg (mEq) per L | Mg$^{++}$ mg (mEq) per L | Phos mg per L | mL to supply 100% RDI for vitamins | Comments |
|---|---|---|---|---|---|---|---|---|---|---|---|---|---|---|---|---|
| Accupep HPF for Oral Solution [U.S.] | 1 (4.2) | 490 | 40 | Hydrolyzed lactalbumin; 16 | 132:1 | 188 | Maltodextrin; 75.5 | 10 | MCT† oil, corn oil; 8.5 | 680 (29.6) | 1150 (29.5) | 625 (31.3) | 250 (20) | 625 | 1600 | |
| Alitraq for Oral Solution [U.S.] | 1 (4.2) | 575 | 52.5 | Soy hydrolysate, L-glutamine, whey protein concentrate, lactalbumin hydrolysate, free amino acids; 21 | 94:1 | 165 | Maltodextrin, sucrose, fructose; 66 | 15.5 | MCT† oil, safflower oil; 13 | 1000 (43.5) | 1200 (30.7) | 733 (36.6) | 267 (22.3) | 733 | 1500 | |
| Criticare HN Oral Solution [U.S.] | 1.06 (4.4) | 650 | 38 | Hydrolyzed casein, amino acids; 14 | 149:1 | 220 | Maltodextrin, cornstarch; 81.5 | 5.3 | Safflower oil; 4.5 | 630 (27) | 1310 (34) | 530 (26) | 210 (17) | 530 | 1890 | Lactose-free |
| Peptamen Oral Solution [U.S.] | 1 (4.2) | 270 | 40 | Hydrolyzed whey; 16 | 131:1 | 127 | Maltodextrin, starch; 51 | 39 | MCT† oil, sunflower oil; 33 | 500 (22) | 1250 (32) | 800 (40) | 400 (32) | 700 | 1500 | Lactose-free |
| Peptamen Junior Oral Solution [U.S.] | 1 (4.2) | 260 | 30 | Enzymatically hydrolyzed whey protein; 12 | 183:1 | 137.5 | Maltodextrin, cornstarch; 55 | 38.5 | MCT†, soybean oil, canola oil; 33 | 460 (20) | 1320 (34) | 1000 (50) | 200 (16) | 800 | 1000 | Lactose-free |
| Peptamen VHP Oral Solution [U.S.] | 1.0 (4.2) | 300 | 62.5 | Enzymatically hydrolyzed whey protein; 25 | 75:1 | 104.5 | Maltodextrin, cornstarch; 42 | 39 | MCT†, soybean oil; 33 | 560 (24) | 1500 (38.5) | 800 (40) | 300 (24) | 700 | 1500 | Lactose-free |
| Reabilan Oral Solution [U.S.] | 1 (4.2) | 350 | 31.5 | Whey peptides, casein peptides; 12.5 | 175:1 | 131.5 | Maltodextrin, tapicoa starch; 52.5 | 40.5 | MCT† oil, soy oil, canola oil; 35 | 700 (30.4) | 1250 (32) | 500 (25) | 250 (20.1) | 500 | 2000 | Lactose-free |
| Reabilan HN Oral Solution [U.S.] | 1.33 (5.6) | 490 | 58.2 | Whey peptides, casein peptides; 17.5 | 125:1 | 158 | Maltodextrin, tapioca starch; 47.5 | 54 | MCT† oil, soy oil, canola oil; 35 | 1000 (43.5) | 1662 (42.4) | 665 (33.3) | 332 (26.5) | 665 | 1500 | Lactose-free |

Table 6. Monomeric (Elemental) Formulas *(continued)*

Note: Some products may be given either orally or by feeding tube; others are designed to be given by feeding tube only.

| Brand name [availability] | KCal (kJoules) per mL | mOsm per kg water | Protein Grams per 1000 mL | Protein Source; % KCal | Nonprotein KCal per gm of Nitrogen | Carbohydrates Grams per 1000 mL | Carbohydrates Source; % KCal | Fat Grams per 1000 mL | Fat Source; % KCal | Na+ mg (mEq) per L | K+ mg (mEq) per L | Ca++ mg (mEq) per L | Mg++ mg (mEq) per L | Phos mg per L | mL to supply 100% RDI for vitamins | Comments |
|---|---|---|---|---|---|---|---|---|---|---|---|---|---|---|---|---|
| SandoSource Peptide Oral Solution [U.S./Canada] | 1 (4.2) | 500 | 50 | Hydrolyzed casein caseinates; 20 | 100:1 | 160 | Hydrolyzed cornstarch; 65 | 17 | MCT†, soybean oil; 15 | 1100 (48) | 1490 (38) | 570 (28.5) | 230 (18.7) | 570 | 1750 | Lactose-free |
| Tolerex Oral Solution [U.S./Canada] | 1 (4.2) | 550 | 21 | Amino acids; 8 | 282:1 | 230 | Glucose, oligosaccharides; 91 | 1.5 | Safflower oil; 1 | 470 (20) | 1200 (31) | 560 (28) | 220 (18) | 560 | 3160 | Lactose-free |
| Travasorb HN for Oral Solution [U.S.] | 1 (4.2) | 560 | 45 | Hydrolyzed lactalbumin; 18 | 126:1 | 175 | Glucose, oligosaccharides; 70 | 13.5 | MCT† oil, sunflower oil; 12 | 920 (40) | 1170 (30) | 500 (25) | 200 (16.5) | 500 | 2000 | Lactose-free |
| Travasorb STD for Oral Solution [U.S.] | 1 (4.2) | 560 | 30 | Hydrolyzed lactalbumin; 12 | 171:1 | 190 | Glucose, oligosaccharides; 76 | 13.5 | MCT† oil, sunflower oil; 12 | 920 (40.1) | 1170 (30) | 500 (25) | 200 (16.5) | 500 | 2000 | Lactose-free |
| Vital High Nitrogen Oral Solution [U.S./Canada] | 1 (4.2) | 500 | 41.7 | Partially hydrolyzed whey, meat and soy protein, free amino acids; 16.7 | 125:1 | 185 | Hydrolyzed cornstarch, sucrose; 73.9 | 10.8 | Safflower oil, MCT† oil; 9.4 | 566 (24.6) | 1400 (35.8) | 667 33.3 | 267 (22.3) | 667 | 1500 | |
| Vivonex Pediatric Oral Solution [U.S./Canada] | 0.8 (3.3) | 360 | 24 | Amino acids; 12 | 200:1 | 130 | Maltodextrin, modified starch; 63 | 24 | MCT†, soybean oil; 25 | 400 (17) | 1200 (31) | 970 (48.5) | 200 (16.4) | 800 | 1000 | Lactose-free |
| Vivonex Plus Oral Solution [U.S./Canada] | 1 (4.2) | 650 | 45 | Amino acids; 18 | 115:1 | 190 | Maltodextrin, modified starch; 76 | 6.7 | Soybean oil; 6 | 610 (27) | 1100 (28) | 560 (28) | 220 (17.6) | 560 | 1800 | Lactose-free |
| Vivonex T.E.N. Oral Solution [U.S./Canada] | 1 (4.2) | 630 | 38 | Amino acids; 15 | 149:1 | 210 | Maltodextrin; 82 | 2.8 | Safflower oil; 3 | 460 (20) | 780 (20) | 500 (25) | 200 (16) | 500 | 2000 | Lactose-free |

†Medium-chain triglyceride

## Table 7. Polymeric Formulas

Note: Some products may be given either orally or by feeding tube; others are designed to be given by feeding tube only.

| Brand name [availability] | KCal (kJoules) per mL | mOsm per kg water | Protein Grams per 1000 mL | Protein Source; % KCal | Nonprotein KCal per gm of Nitrogen | Carbohydrates Grams per 1000 mL | Carbohydrates Source; % KCal | Fat Grams per 1000 mL | Fat Source; % KCal | Na+ mg (mEq) per L | K+ mg (mEq) per L | Ca++ mg (mEq) per L | Mg++ mg (mEq) per L | Phos mg per L | mL to supply 100% RDI for vitamins | Comments |
|---|---|---|---|---|---|---|---|---|---|---|---|---|---|---|---|---|
| Attain Oral Solution [U.S.] | 1 (4.2) | 300 | 40 | Sodium and calcium caseinates; 16 | 134:1 | 135 | Maltodextrin; 54 | 35 | MCT† oil, corn oil; 30 | 805 (35) | 1600 (41) | 960 (48) | 320 (25.6) | 800 | 1250 | Lactose-free |
| CitriSource Oral Solution [U.S.] | 0.76 (3.2) | 700 | 37 | Whey protein concentrate; 20 | 105:1 | 150 | Sugar, hydrolyzed corn starch; 80 | 0 | 0 | 230 (10) | 63 (1.6) | 570 (28) | 210 (17) | 680 | 1890 | Not appropriate for total feeding |
| Oral Solution [Canada] | 0.77 (3.2) | 700 | 37 | Whey protein concentrate; 20 | 107:1 | 150 | Sugar, corn syrup solids; 79 | 2 | soybean oil; 2 | 230 (10) | 63 (1.6) | 570 (28) | 210 (17) | 680 | 1890 | Lactose-free, not appropriate for total feeding |
| Citrotein for Oral Solution [U.S.] grape orange punch | 0.67 (2.8) | 510 490 480 | 41 | Egg white solids; 25 | 76:1 | 120 | Maltodextrin, sugar; 73 | 1.6 | Partially hydrogenated soybean oil; 2 | 670 (29) | 550 (14) | 1100 (55) | 420 (34) | 1100 | 1100 | Lactose-free, cholesterol-free |
| Comply Oral Solution [U.S.] | 1.5 (6.3) | 410 | 60 | Sodium and calcium caseinates; 16 | 131:1 | 180 | Hydrolyzed cornstarch; 48 | 60 | Corn oil; 36 | 1100 (48) | 1850 (47) | 1000 (50) | 400 (32) | 1000 | 1000 | Lactose-free |
| Deliver 2.0 Oral Solution [U.S.] | 2 (8.4) | 640 | 75 | Sodium and calcium caseinates; 15 | 145:1 | 200 | Corn syrup; 40 | 102 | MCT† oil, soy oil; 45 | 800 (35) | 1690 (43) | 1010 (51) | 400 (33) | 1010 | 1000 | Lactose-free |
| Enercal Oral Solution [Canada] | 1 (4.2) | 370 | 38 | Whey protein concentrate, soy protein isolate; 15 | 144:1 | 144 | Maltodextrin, sucrose; 55 | 34 | Soybean oil; oleic oil, 30 | 500 (22) | 1250 (32) | 670 | 270 | 670 | | Lactose-free |

# Table 7. Polymeric Formulas (continued)

Note: Some products may be given either orally or by feeding tube; others are designed to be given by feeding tube only.

| Brand name [availability] | KCal (kJoules) per mL | mOsm per kg water | Protein Grams per 1000 mL | Protein Source; % KCal | Nonprotein KCal per gm of Nitrogen | Carbohydrates Grams per 1000 mL | Carbohydrates Source; % KCal | Fat Grams per 1000 mL | Fat Source; % KCal | Na$^+$ mg (mEq) per L | K$^+$ mg (mEq) per L | Ca$^{++}$ mg (mEq) per L | Mg$^{++}$ mg (mEq) per L | Phos mg per L | mL to supply 100% RDI for vitamins | Comments |
|---|---|---|---|---|---|---|---|---|---|---|---|---|---|---|---|---|
| *Ensure* Oral Solution [U.S.] | 1.06 (4.4) | 470 | 37.2 | Sodium and calcium caseinates, soy protein isolate; 14 | 153:1 | 145 | Corn syrup, sucrose; 54.5 | 37.2 | Corn oil; 31.5 | 846 (36.8) | 1564 (40) | 530 (26.5) | 212 (17.7) | 530 | 1887 | Lactose-free |
| Oral Solution [Canada] | 1.06 (4.4) | 470 | 37.2 | Sodium and calcium caseinates, soy protein isolate; 14 | 153:1 | 145 | Maltodextrin, corn syrup, sucrose; 54.5 | 37.2 | Corn oil; 31.5 | 700 (30.4) | 1200 (30.7) | 500 (25) | 200 (16) | 500 | | Lactose-free |
| *Ensure High Protein* Oral Solution [U.S./Canada] | 0.95 (4) | 610 | 50.7 | Calcium and sodium caseinates, soy protein isolate; 21.3 | 92:1 | 130 | Sucrose, maltodextrin; 54.7 | 25.4 | High-oleic safflower oil, canola oil, soy oil; 24 | 1224 (53.2) | 2110 (53.9) | 1055 (52.7) | 422 (35.2) | 1055 | 948 | Lactose-free |
| *Ensure HN* Oral Solution [U.S.] | 1.06 (4.4) | 470 | 44.4 | Sodium and calcium caseinates, soy protein isolate; 16.7 | 125:1 | 141.2 | Corn syrup, maltodextrin, sucrose; 53.2 | 35.5 | Corn oil; 30.1 | 802 (34.9) | 1564 (40) | 758 (37.9) | 303 (25.3) | 758 | 1321 | Lactose-free |
| *Ensure Plus* Oral Solution [U.S./Canada] | 1.5 (6.3) | 690 | 54.9 | Sodium and calcium caseinates, soy protein isolate; 14.7 | 146.1 | 200 | Corn syrup, maltodextrin sucrose; 53.3 | 53.3 | Corn oil; 32 | 1050 (45.7) | 1940 (49.6) | 705 (35.2) | 282 (23.5) | 705 | 1420 | Lactose-free |
| *Ensure Plus HN* Oral Solution [U.S.] | 1.5 (6.3) | 650 | 62.6 | Sodium and calcium caseinates, soy protein isolate; 16.7 | 125:1 | 199.9 | Maltodextrin, sucrose; 53.3 | 50 | Corn oil; 30 | 1180 (51.3) | 1820 (46.5) | 1056 (52.8) | 423 (35.3) | 1056 | 947 | Lactose-free |
| *Entrition Half-Strength* Oral Solution [U.S.] | 0.5 (2.1) | 120 | 17.5 | Sodium and calcium caseinates; 14 | 153:1 | 68 | Maltodextrin; 54.5 | 17.5 | Corn oil; 31.5 | 350 (15.2) | 600 (15.4) | 250 (12.5) | 100 (8) | 250 | N/A | Lactose-free |

†Medium-chain triglyceride

## Table 7. Polymeric Formulas (continued)

Note: Some products may be given either orally or by feeding tube; others are designed to be given by feeding tube only.

| Brand name [availability] | KCal (kJoules) per mL | mOsm per kg water | Protein Grams per 1000 mL | Protein Source; % KCal | Nonprotein KCal per gm of Nitrogen | Carbohydrates Grams per 1000 mL | Carbohydrates Source; % KCal | Fat Grams per 1000 mL | Fat Source; % KCal | Na⁺ mg (mEq) per L | K⁺ mg (mEq) per L | Ca⁺⁺ mg (mEq) per L | Mg⁺⁺ mg (mEq) per L | Phos mg per L | mL to supply 100% RDI for vitamins | Comments |
|---|---|---|---|---|---|---|---|---|---|---|---|---|---|---|---|---|
| *Entrition HN* Oral Solution [U.S.] | 1 (4.2) | 300 | 44 | Sodium and calcium caseinates, soy; 17.6 | 117:1 | 114 | Maltodextrin; 45.6 | 41 | Corn oil; 36.8 | 845 (36.7) | 1579 (40.5) | 770 (38.5) | 308 (24.6) | 770 | 1300 | Lactose-free |
| *Introlan* Oral Solution [U.S.] | .5 (2.2) | 150 | 22.5 | Sodium and calcium caseinates; 17 | 125:1 | 70 | Maltodextrin; 53 | 18 | MCT† oil, corn oil; 30 | 344.4 (15) | 589.3 (15) | 500 (25) | 200 (16) | 500 | 2000 | Lactose-free |
| *Introlite* Oral Solution [U.S.] | 0.53 (2.2) | 220 | 22.2 | Sodium and calcium caseinates, soy protein isolate; 16.7 | 125:1 | 70.5 | Hydrolyzed cornstarch; 53.3 | 18.4 | MCT† oil, corn oil, soy oil; 30 | 930 (40.5) | 1570 (40.2) | 758 (37.9) | 304 (25.3) | 758 | 1321 | Lactose-free |
| *Isocal* Oral Solution [U.S.] | 1.06 (4.4) | 270 | 34 | Sodium and calcium caseinates, soy protein isolate; 13 | 167:1 | 135 | Maltodextrin; 50 | 44 | MCT† oil, soy oil; 37 | 530 (23) | 1310 (34) | 630 (32) | 210 (17.4) | 530 | 1890 | Lactose-free, fiber-free |
| *Isocal HN* Oral Solution [U.S.] | 1.06 (4.4) | 270 | 44 | Sodium and calcium caseinates, soy protein isolate; 17 | 125:1 | 124 | Maltodextrin; 46 | 45 | MCT† oil, soy oil; 37 | 930 (40) | 1610 (41) | 850 (43) | 340 (28) | 850 | 1180 | Lactose-free |
| *Isolan* Oral Solution [U.S.] | 1.06 (4.4) | 300 | 40 | Caseinates; 16 | 141:1 | 144 | Maltodextrin; 54 | 36 | MCT† oil, corn oil; 28 | 897 (39) | 1200 (52) | 800 (40) | 320 (25.6) | 800 | 1250 | Lactose-free |
| *Isosource* Oral Solution [U.S./Canada] | 1.2 (5) | 360 | 43 | Sodium and calcium caseinates, soy protein isolate; 14 | 148:1 | 170 | Hydrolyzed cornstarch; 56 | 41 | MCT† oil, canola oil; 30 | 1200 (52) | 1700 (43) | 670 (33) | 270 (22) | 670 | 1500 | Lactose-free, fiber-free |
| *Isosource HN* Oral Solution [U.S./Canada] | 1.2 (5) | 330 | 53 | Sodium and calcium caseinates, soy protein isolate; 18 | 116:1 | 160 | Hydrolyzed cornstarch; 52 | 41 | MCT† oil, canola oil; 30 | 1100 (48) | 1700 (43) | 670 (33) | 270 (22) | 670 | 1500 | Lactose-free, fiber-free |

## Table 7. Polymeric Formulas (continued)

Note: Some products may be given either orally or by feeding tube; others are designed to be given by feeding tube only.

| Brand name [availability] | KCal (kJoules) per mL | mOsm per kg water | Protein Grams per 1000 mL | Protein Source; % KCal | Nonprotein KCal per gm of Nitrogen | Carbohydrates Grams per 1000 mL | Carbohydrates Source; % KCal | Fat Grams per 1000 mL | Fat Source; % KCal | Na$^+$ mg (mEq) per L | K$^+$ mg (mEq) per L | Ca$^{++}$ mg (mEq) per L | Mg$^{++}$ mg (mEq) per L | Phos mg per L | mL to supply 100% RDI for vitamins | Comments |
|---|---|---|---|---|---|---|---|---|---|---|---|---|---|---|---|---|
| Isotein HN for Oral Solution [U.S.] | 1.2 (5) | 300 | 68 | Delactosed lactalbumin; 23 | 86:1 | 160 | Hydrolyzed cornstarch, monosaccharides; 52 | 34 | MCT† oil, partially hydrogenated soybean oil; 25 | 620 (27) | 1100 (28) | 560 (28) | 230 (19) | 560 | 1770 | Lactose-free |
| Magnacal Oral Solution [U.S.] | 2 (8.4) | 590 | 70 | Sodium and calcium caseinates; 14 | 154:1 | 250 | Maltodextrin, sucrose; 50 | 80 | Partially hydrogenated soy oil; 36 | 1000 (43.5) | 1250 (32) | 1000 (50) | 400 (32) | 1000 | 1000 | Lactose-free |
| NuBasics Oral Solution [U.S.] | 1 (4.2) | 500 | 35 | Calcium and potassium caseinates; 14 | 153:1 | 132.4 | Corn syrup solids, sucrose; 53 | 36.8 | Canola oil, corn oil; 33 | 876 (38) | 1248 (32) | 500 (25) | 200 (16) | 500 | 2000 | Lactose-free |
| NuBasics Plus Oral Solution [U.S.] | 1.5 (6.3) | 620 | 52.4 | Calcium and potassium caseinates; 14 | 153:1 | 176.4 | Corn syrup solids, sucrose; 47 | 64.8 | Canola oil, corn oil; 39 | 1168 (51) | 1868 (48) | 748 (37.4) | 300 (24) | 748 | 1333 | Lactose-free |
| NuBasics VHP Oral Solution [U.S.] | 1 (4.2) | 460 | 62.4 | Calcium and potassium caseinates; 25 | 75:1 | 112.8 | Corn syrup solids, sucrose; 45 | 33.2 | Canola oil, corn oil; 30 | 876 (38) | 1248 (32) | 580 (25) | 200 (16) | 580 | 2000 | Lactose-free |
| Nutren 1.0 Oral Solution [U.S.] | 1 (4.2) | 300 | 40 | Calcium and potassium caseinates; 16 | 131:1 | 127 | Maltodextrin, corn syrup solids; 51 | 38 | MCT† oil, canola oil, corn oil; 33 | 876 (38) | 1248 (32) | 668 (33.4) | 268 (21.4) | 668 | 1500 | Lactose-free |
| Nutren 1.5 Oral Solution [U.S.] | 1.5 (6.3) | 430 | 60 | Calcium and potassium caseinates; 16 | 131:1 | 169.2 | Maltodextrin, sucrose; 45 | 67.6 | MCT† oil, canola oil, corn oil; 39 | 1170 (50.9) | 1872 (48) | 1000 (50) | 400 (32) | 1000 | 1000 | Lactose-free |
| Nutren 2.0 Oral Solution [U.S.] | 2 (8.4) | 720 | 80 | Calcium and potassium caseinates; 16 | 131:1 | 196 | Corn syrup solids, maltodextrin; sucrose; 39 | 106 | MCT† oil, canola oil, corn oil; 45 | 1300 (56.5) | 1920 (49.2) | 1340 (67) | 536 (42.9) | 1340 | 750 | Lactose-free |
| Nutrilan Oral Solution [U.S.] | 1.06 (4.4) | 520 | 38 | Sodium and calcium caseinates; 14 | 149:1 | 143 | Maltodextrin, sugar; 54 | 37 | MCT† oil, corn oil; 31 | 690 (30) | 1326 (34) | 630 (31.5) | 253 (20.2) | 630 | 1585 | Lactose-free |

†Medium-chain triglyceride

# Table 7. Polymeric Formulas (continued)

Note: Some products may be given either orally or by feeding tube; others are designed to be given by feeding tube only.

| Brand name [availability] | KCal (kJoules) per mL | mOsm per kg water | Protein Grams per 1000 mL | Protein Source; % KCal | Nonprotein KCal per gm of Nitrogen | Carbohydrates Grams per 1000 mL | Carbohydrates Source; % KCal | Fat Grams per 1000 mL | Fat Source; % KCal | Na+ mg (mEq) per L | K+ mg (mEq) per L | Ca++ mg (mEq) per L | Mg++ mg (mEq) per L | Phos mg per L | mL to supply 100% RDI for vitamins | Comments |
|---|---|---|---|---|---|---|---|---|---|---|---|---|---|---|---|---|
| *Osmolite* Oral Solution [U.S.] | 1.06 (4.4) | 300 | 37.1 | Sodium and calcium caseinates, soy protein isolate; 14 | 153:1 | 151.1 | Maltodextrin; 57 | 34.7 | High-oleic safflower oil, canola oil, MCT† oil; 29 | 640 (27.8) | 1020 (26.1) | 530 (26.5) | 212 (17.7) | 530 | 1887 | Lactose-free |
| *Osmolite HN* Oral Solution [U.S./Canada] | 1.06 (4.4) | 300 | 44.3 | Sodium and calcium caseinates, soy protein isolate; 16.7 | 125:1 | 143.9 | Maltodextrin; 54.3 | 34.7 | High-oleic safflower oil, canola oil, MCT† oil; 29 | 930 (40.5) | 1570 (40.2) | 758 (37.9) | 304 (25.3) | 758 | 1321 | Lactose-free |
| *Pediasure* Oral Solution [U.S./Canada] | 1 (4.2) | <310 | 30 | sodium caseinate, whey protein concentrate; 12 | 185:1 | 109.7 | Hydrolyzed cornstarch, sucrose; 43.9 | 49.7 | High-oleic safflower oil, soy oil, MCT† oil; 44.1 | 380 (16.5) | 1310 (33.5) | 970 (48.5) | 200 (16.7) | 800 | 1000 | Trace lactose |
| *Pre-Attain* Oral Solution [U.S.] | .5 (2.1) | 150 | 20 | Sodium caseinate; 16 | 131:1 | 60 | Maltodextrin; 48 | 20 | Corn oil; 36 | 340 (15) | 575 (15) | 312.5 (15.6) | 250 (20) | 312.5 | 2000 | Lactose-free |
| *Promote* Oral Solution [U.S.] | 1 (4.2) | 340 | 62.5 | Sodium and calcium caseinates, soy protein isolate; 25 | 75:1 | 130 | Hydrolyzed cornstarch, sucrose; 52 | 26 | High-oleic safflower oil, canola oil; MCT† oil; 23 | 1000 (43.5) | 1980 (50.6) | 1200 (60) | 400 (33.3) | 1200 | 1000 | Lactose-free |
| *Replete* Oral Solution [U.S.] | 1 (4.2) | 300 | 62.5 | Calcium and potassium caseinates; 25 | 75:1 | 113 | Maltodextrin, sucrose; 45 | 34 | Canola oil, MCT† oil; 30 | 876 (38) | 1500 (38) | 1000 (50) | 400 (32) | 1000 | 1000 | Lactose-free |
| *Resource* Oral Solution [U.S./Canada] | 1.06 (4.4) | 430 | 37 | Sodium and calcium caseinates, soy protein isolate; 14 | 154:1 | 140 | Hydrolyzed cornstarch, sugar; 54 | 37 | Corn oil; 32 | 890 (39) | 1600 (41) | 530 (27) | 210 (17) | 530 | 1890 | Lactose-free |

## Table 7. Polymeric Formulas (continued)

Note: Some products may be given either orally or by feeding tube; others are designed to be given by feeding tube only.

| Brand name [availability] | KCal (kJoules) per mL | mOsm per kg water | Protein Grams per 1000 mL | Protein Source; % KCal | Nonprotein KCal per gm of Nitrogen | Carbohydrates Grams per 1000 mL | Carbohydrates Source; % KCal | Fat Grams per 1000 mL | Fat Source; % KCal | Na⁺ mg (mEq) per L | K⁺ mg (mEq) per L | Ca⁺⁺ mg (mEq) per L | Mg⁺⁺ mg (mEq) per L | Phos mg per L | mL to supply 100% RDI for vitamins | Comments |
|---|---|---|---|---|---|---|---|---|---|---|---|---|---|---|---|---|
| Resource Plus Oral Solution [U.S./Canada] | 1.5 (6.3) | 600 | 55 | Sodium and calcium caseinates, soy protein isolate; 15 | 146:1 | 200 | Hydrolyzed cornstarch, sugar; 53 | 53 | Corn oil; 32 | 1300 (57) | 2100 (54) | 700 (35) | 310 (26) | 700 | 1400 | Lactose-free |
| Sustacal Oral Solution (All flavors but chocolate) [U.S.] | 1 (4.2) | 650 | 61 | Sodium and calcium caseinates, soy protein isolate; 24 | 78:1 | 140 | Corn syrup, sugar; 55 | 23 | Partially hydrogenated soy oil; 21 | 930 (40) | 2100 (54) | 1010 (50) | 380 (31) | 930 | 1060 | Lactose-free, fiber-free |
| Sustacal Oral Solution (Chocolate) [U.S.] | 1 (4.2) | 690 | 61 | Sodium and calcium caseinates, soy protein isolate; 24 | 78:1 | 140 | Corn syrup, sugar; 55 | 23 | Partially hydrogenated soy oil; 21 | 930 (40) | 2100 (54) | 1010 (50) | 380 (31) | 930 | 1060 | Lactose-free, fiber-free |
| Sustacal Basic Oral Solution (Chocolate) [U.S.] | 1.06 (4.4) | 470 | 37 | Casein, soy protein isolate; 14 | 153:1 | 148 | Corn syrup, sucrose; 56 | 35 | Soy oil; 30 | 850 (37) | 1610 (41) | 530 (27) | 210 (17.4) | 530 | 1890 | Lactose-free |
| Oral Solution (Vanilla) [U.S./Canada] | 1.06 (4.4) | 500 | 37 | Casein, soy protein isolate; 14 | 153:1 | 148 | Corn syrup, sucrose; 56 | 35 | Soy oil; 30 | 850 (37)/ U.S. 740 (32)/ Canada | 1610 (41)/ U.S. 1240 (32)/ Canada | 530 (27) | 210 (17.4) | 530 | 1890 | Lactose-free |
| Sustacal Plus Oral Solution (All flavors but chocolate) [U.S.] | 1.52 (6.4) | 670 | 61 | Sodium and calcium caseinates; 16 | 134:1 | 190 | Corn syrup solids, sugar; 50 | 58 | Corn oil; 34 | 850 (37) | 1480 (38) | 850 (43) | 340 (28) | 850 | 1180 | Lactose-free, fiber-free |
| Oral Solution (Chocolate) [U.S.] | 1.52 (6.4) | 630 | 61 | Sodium and calcium caseinates; 16 | 134:1 | 190 | Corn syrup solids, sugar; 50 | 58 | Corn oil; 34 | 850 (37) | 1480 (38) | 850 (43) | 340 (28) | 850 | 1180 | Lactose-free, fiber-free |

†Medium-chain triglyceride

## Table 7. Polymeric Formulas (continued)

Note: Some products may be given either orally or by feeding tube; others are designed to be given by feeding tube only.

| Brand name [availability] | KCal (kJoules) per mL | mOsm per kg water | Protein | | | Nonprotein KCal per gm of Nitrogen | Carbohydrates | | | Fat | | | Na+ mg (mEq) per L | K+ mg (mEq) per L | Ca++ mg (mEq) per L | Mg++ mg (mEq) per L | Phos mg per L | mL to supply 100% RDI for vitamins | Comments |
|---|---|---|---|---|---|---|---|---|---|---|---|---|---|---|---|---|---|---|---|
| | | | Grams per 1000 mL | Source; % KCal | | | Grams per 1000 mL | Source; % KCal | | Grams per 1000 mL | Source; % KCal | | | | | | | | |
| *TwoCal HN* Oral Solution [U.S.] | 2 (8.4) | 690 | 83.7 | Sodium and calcium caseinates; 16.7 | | 125:1 | 217.3 | Maltodextrin, sucrose; 43.2 | | 90.9 | Corn oil, MCT† oil; 40.1 | | 1310 (57) | 2456 (62.8) | 1052 (52.6) | 421 (35.1) | 1052 | 947 | Lactose-free |
| *Ultralan* Oral Solution [U.S.] | 1.5 (6.3) | 540 | 60 | Sodium and calcium caseinates, soy protein isolate; 16 | | 131:1 | 202 | Maltodextrin; 54 | | 50 | MCT† oil, corn oil; 50 | | 1173 (51) | 1911 (49) | 1000 (50) | 400 (32) | 1000 | 1000 | Lactose-free |

†Medium-chain triglyceride

## ENZYME IMMUNOASSAY PREGNANCY TEST
KITS—See *Pregnancy Test Kits for Home Use*

---

## EPHEDRINE—See *Bronchodilators, Adrenergic (Systemic); Sympathomimetic Agents—Cardiovascular Use (Parenteral-Systemic)*

---

## EPHEDRINE-CONTAINING COMBINATIONS—
Chlorpheniramine, Ephedrine, and Guaifenesin (Systemic)—See *Cough/Cold Combinations (Systemic)*
Chlorpheniramine, Ephedrine, Phenylephrine, and Carbetapentane (Systemic)—See *Cough/Cold Combinations (Systemic)*
Chlorpheniramine, Ephedrine, Phenylephrine, Dextromethorphan, Ammonium Chloride, and Ipecac (Systemic)—See *Cough/Cold Combinations (Systemic)*

Chlorpheniramine, Phenyltoloxamine, Ephedrine, Codeine, and Guaiacol Carbonate (Systemic)—See *Cough/Cold Combinations (Systemic)*
Ephedrine and Guaifenesin (Systemic)—See *Cough/Cold Combinations (Systemic)*
Ephedrine and Potassium Iodide (Systemic)—See *Cough/Cold Combinations (Systemic)*
Theophylline, Ephedrine, Guaifenesin, and Phenobarbital (Systemic)
Theophylline, Ephedrine, and Hydroxyzine (Systemic)
Theophylline, Ephedrine, and Phenobarbital (Systemic)

---

## EPINEPHRINE—See *Bronchodilators, Adrenergic (Systemic); Sympathomimetic Agents—Cardiovascular Use (Parenteral-Systemic)*

---

# EPINEPHRINE    Ophthalmic

This monograph includes information on the following: Epinephrine; Epinephryl Borate.

VA CLASSIFICATION (Primary): OP103

Note: For a listing of dosage forms and brand names by country availability, see *Dosage Forms* section(s). For a listing of brand names for the articles in this monograph, refer to the General Index.

## Category

Antiglaucoma agent (ophthalmic); Surgical aid, ophthalmic.

## Indications

Note: Bracketed information in the *Indications* section refers to uses that are not included in U.S. product labeling.

### Accepted

Glaucoma, open-angle (treatment)—Ophthalmic epinephrine is indicated primarily in the treatment of open-angle (chronic simple) glaucoma, either alone or in combination with miotics, beta-blockers, hyperosmotic agents, or carbonic anhydrase inhibitors.

[Congestion, conjunctival, during surgery (treatment)][1]—Ophthalmic epinephrine is used in the treatment of conjunctival congestion during surgery.

[Glaucoma, secondary (treatment)][1]—Ophthalmic epinephrine is used in the treatment of secondary glaucoma.

### Unaccepted

Epinephrine is not an effective mydriatic when used topically in the eye.

[1]Not included in Canadian product labeling.

## Pharmacology/Pharmacokinetics

### Physicochemical characteristics

Molecular weight—
   Epinephrine: 183.21.
   Epinephryl borate: 209.01.

pH—
   Epinephryl borate ophthalmic solution: 7.4.

### Mechanism of action/Effect

Epinephrine is a direct-acting sympathomimetic amine.

Antiglaucoma agent (ophthalmic)—The mechanism by which epinephrine lowers intraocular pressure is not completely known, but appears to involve both a decrease in production of aqueous humor and an increase in aqueous outflow facility.

Surgical aid (antihemorrhagic; mydriatic)—Epinephrine acts on alpha-adrenergic receptors in the conjunctiva to produce vasoconstriction and hemostasis in bleeding from small vessels. It contracts the dilator muscle of the pupil by acting on alpha-adrenergic receptors, resulting in dilation of the pupil (mydriasis).

### Onset of action

Reduction in intraocular pressure—Within 1 hour.
Vasoconstriction—Within 5 minutes.

### Time to peak effect

Reduction in intraocular pressure—4 to 8 hours.

### Duration of action

Reduction in intraocular pressure—Up to 24 hours.
Vasoconstriction—Less than 1 hour.

## Precautions to Consider

### Carcinogenicity/Tumorigenicity

Studies have not been done in either animals or humans.

### Pregnancy/Reproduction

Pregnancy—Ophthalmic epinephrine may be systemically absorbed.
Studies have not been done in humans.
Studies have not been done in animals.

FDA Pregnancy Category C.

### Breast-feeding

It is not known whether epinephrine is distributed into breast milk; however, ophthalmic epinephrine may be systemically absorbed.

### Pediatrics

Appropriate studies on the relationship of age to the effects of this medication have not been performed in the pediatric population. Safety and efficacy have not been established.

### Geriatrics

Appropriate studies on the relationship of age to the effects of this medication have not been performed in the geriatric population. However, no geriatrics-specific problems have been documented to date.

### Dental

Epinephrine is used in gingival retraction cords, and systemic absorption may occur, especially from application of topical cords to abraded surfaces. Concurrent systemic absorption of ophthalmic epinephrine will result in an additive effect.

### Drug interactions and/or related problems

The following drug interactions and/or related problems have been selected on the basis of their potential clinical significance (possible mechanism in parentheses where appropriate)—not necessarily inclusive (» = major clinical significance):

Note: Combinations containing any of the following medications, depending on the amount present, may also interact with this medication.

Anesthetics, hydrocarbon inhalation, such as:
   Chloroform
   Cyclopropane
   Desflurane
   Enflurane
   Halothane
   Isoflurane
   Methoxyflurane
   Trichloroethylene
      (if significant systemic absorption of ophthalmic epinephrine occurs, concurrent use of cyclopropane, halothane, or possibly chloroform may increase the risk of severe ventricular arrhythmias because these anesthetics greatly sensitize the myocardium to the effects of sympathomimetics; therapy with ophthalmic epinephrine should be interrupted prior to general anesthesia in patients receiving these anesthetics)

(enflurane, methoxyflurane, or especially trichloroethylene may cause some sensitization of the myocardium to the effects of sympathomimetics; caution is recommended during concurrent use with ophthalmic epinephrine)

(desflurane and isoflurane do not significantly sensitize the myocardium to the ventricular arrhythmogenic effects of epinephrine)

Antidepressants, tricyclic or
Maprotiline or
Nomifensine
(if significant systemic absorption of ophthalmic epinephrine occurs, concurrent use of these medications may potentiate the cardiovascular effects of epinephrine, possibly resulting in arrhythmias, hypertension, or tachycardia)

Beta-adrenergic blocking agents, ophthalmic
(concurrent use of ophthalmic betaxolol, levobunolol, or timolol with ophthalmic epinephrine may provide a beneficial additive effect in lowering intraocular pressure)

Digitalis glycosides
(if significant systemic absorption of ophthalmic epinephrine occurs, concurrent use of digitalis glycosides may increase the risk of cardiac arrhythmias; caution is recommended if concurrent use is necessary)

Monoamine oxidase (MAO) inhibitors, including furazolidone, procarbazine, and selegiline
(if significant systemic absorption of ophthalmic epinephrine occurs, concurrent use of MAO inhibitors may result in exaggerated adrenergic effects; adjustment of the ophthalmic epinephrine dose is required when it is administered concurrently or within 21 days after administration of MAO inhibitors)

Sympathomimetics, systemic or local
(if significant systemic absorption of ophthalmic epinephrine occurs, concurrent use of systemic sympathomimetics may result in additive toxic effects; in addition, local anesthetics with vasoconstrictors should be avoided or a minimal amount of the vasoconstrictor should be used with the local anesthetic)

## Medical considerations/Contraindications

The medical considerations/contraindications included here have been selected on the basis of their potential clinical significance (reasons given in parentheses where appropriate)—not necessarily inclusive (» = major clinical significance).

*Risk-benefit should be considered when the following medical problems exist:*

Aphakia
(epinephrine therapy may cause reversible macular edema)

Asthma, bronchial
» Cardiovascular disease or
Cerebral arteriosclerosis or
Hypertension or
Hyperthyroidism
(if systemic absorption occurs, the vasoconstrictive action of epinephrine may make condition worse)

Diabetes mellitus

» Glaucoma, angle-closure, or predisposition to
(may precipitate an acute attack of angle-closure glaucoma)

Sensitivity to epinephrine or sulfites

## Patient monitoring

The following may be especially important in patient monitoring (other tests may be warranted in some patients, depending on condition; » = major clinical significance):

Gonioscopy
(recommended prior to initiating therapy)

Intraocular pressure determinations
(recommended at periodic intervals during therapy)

## Side/Adverse Effects

Note: Pigmentary deposits in the conjunctiva may occur after prolonged use of ophthalmic epinephrine; on rare occasions, deposits in the eyelids or cornea may also occur.

The following side/adverse effects have been selected on the basis of their potential clinical significance (possible signs and symptoms in parentheses where appropriate)—not necessarily inclusive:

### Those indicating need for medical attention
Incidence less frequent
*Maculopathy in aphakic eyes* (blurred or decreased vision); *systemic absorption* (fast, irregular, or pounding heartbeat; feeling faint; increased sweating; paleness; trembling; increased blood pressure)

### Those indicating need for medical attention only if they continue or are bothersome
Incidence more frequent
*Headache or browache; stinging, burning, redness, or other eye irritation; watering of eyes*
Incidence less frequent
*Blurred vision or other vision change; eye pain or ache*

## Overdose

For specific information on the agents used in the management of ophthalmic epinephrine overdose, see:
• *Beta-adrenergic Blocking Agents (Systemic)* monograph.

For more information on the management of overdose or unintentional ingestion, **contact a Poison Control Center** (see *Poison Control Center Listing*).

### Treatment of overdose
Systemic effects should be treated symptomatically; however, overdosage is not likely to occur due to the limited rate of absorption and rapid inactivation of epinephrine once it enters the bloodstream. If tachycardia occurs and persists, a beta-adrenergic blocker may be administered.

Overdosage in eyes should be treated by immediately flushing eyes with water or normal saline.

## Patient Consultation

As an aid to patient consultation, refer to *Advice for the Patient, Epinephrine (Ophthalmic)*.

In providing consultation, consider emphasizing the following selected information (» = major clinical significance):

### Before using this medication
» Conditions affecting use, especially:
Sensitivity to epinephrine or sulfites
Other medical problems, especially cardiovascular disease, angle-closure glaucoma, or predisposition to angle-closure glaucoma

### Proper use of this medication
» Importance of not using more medication than the amount prescribed
Proper administration technique
Preventing contamination: Not touching applicator tip to any surface; keeping container tightly closed
Not using if medication becomes discolored or contains a precipitate
» Proper dosing
Missed dose: Applying as soon as possible; if almost time for next dose, skipping missed dose and returning to regular dosing schedule; not doubling doses
» Proper storage

### Precautions while using this medication
Regular visits to physician to check eye pressure during therapy
» Blurred vision may occur for short time after application; not driving, using machines, or doing anything else that could be dangerous if unable to see well

### Side/adverse effects
Signs of potential side effects, especially maculopathy in aphakic eyes or signs of systemic absorption

## General Dosing Information

Although some manufacturers recommend a dose of 2 drops of an ophthalmic solution at appropriate intervals, the conjunctival sac will usually hold only 1 drop.

To avoid excessive systemic absorption, patient should press finger to the lacrimal sac during and for 1 or 2 minutes following instillation of medication.

Caution is recommended when epinephrine is used in aphakic eyes, since maculopathy may occur rarely, resulting in decreased visual acuity. In this event, medication should be promptly discontinued.

Although some manufacturers recommend that patients not wear soft contact lenses during treatment with ophthalmic epinephrine, USP medical experts do not believe this precaution is necessary unless the patient has corneal epithelial problems and the medication is to be used more often than once every 1 to 2 hours. No significant problems have been documented with ophthalmic solutions containing 0.03% or less of benzalkonium chloride as a preservative, and used as eye drops in patients with no significant corneal surface problems.

## EPINEPHRINE

## Ophthalmic Dosage Forms

### EPINEPHRINE OPHTHALMIC SOLUTION USP

**Usual adult and adolescent dose**
Antiglaucoma agent (ophthalmic)—
  Topical, to the conjunctiva, 1 drop one or two times a day.

**Usual pediatric dose**
Safety and efficacy have not been established.

**Usual geriatric dose**
See *Usual adult and adolescent dose.*

**Strength(s) usually available**
U.S.—
  0.1% (Rx) [GENERIC].
  0.5% (Rx) [*Epifrin* (benzalkonium chloride; sodium metabisulfite)].
  1% (Rx) [*Epifrin* (benzalkonium chloride; sodium metabisulfite); *Glaucon* (benzalkonium chloride 0.01%; sodium metabisulfite)].
  2% (Rx) [*Epifrin* (benzalkonium chloride; sodium metabisulfite); *Glaucon* (benzalkonium chloride 0.01%; sodium metabisulfite)].
Canada—
  1% (Rx) [*Epifrin* (benzalkonium chloride 0.004%; sodium metabisulfite)].

**Packaging and storage**
Store below 40 °C (104 °F), preferably between 15 and 30 °C (59 and 86 °F), unless otherwise specified by manufacturer. Store in a tight, light-resistant container. Protect from freezing.

**Stability**
Do not use if solution is pinkish or brownish in color or contains a precipitate.

**Auxiliary labeling**
• For the eye.
• Keep container tightly closed.

## EPINEPHRYL BORATE

## Ophthalmic Dosage Forms

### EPINEPHRYL BORATE OPHTHALMIC SOLUTION USP

**Usual adult and adolescent dose**
Antiglaucoma agent (ophthalmic)—
  Topical, to the conjunctiva, 1 drop one or two times a day.

# EPOETIN   Systemic

VA CLASSIFICATION (Primary): BL400

Other commonly used names are human erythropoietin, recombinant; EPO; and r-HuEPO.

Note: For a listing of dosage forms and brand names by country availability, see *Dosage Forms* section(s). For a listing of brand names for the articles in this monograph, refer to the General Index.

## Category
Antianemic.

## Indications
Note: Bracketed information in the *Indications* section refers to uses that are not included in U.S. product labeling.

**Accepted**
Anemia associated with renal failure (treatment)—Epoetin is indicated for the treatment of anemia associated with chronic renal failure. It is used for patients who do not require dialysis as well as patients receiving dialysis (continuous peritoneal dialysis, high-flux short-time hemodialysis, or conventional hemodialysis). However, in patients not receiving dialysis, use of epoetin should be limited to individuals having hematocrit values below 30%.

**Usual pediatric dose**
Safety and efficacy have not been established.

**Usual geriatric dose**
See *Usual adult and adolescent dose.*

**Strength(s) usually available**
U.S.—
  0.5% (base) (Rx) [*Epinal* (benzalkonium choloride 0.01%)].
  1% (base) (Rx) [*Epinal* (benzalkonium chloride 0.01%); *Eppy/N* (benzalkonium chloride 0.01%)].
  2% (base) (Rx) [*Eppy/N* (benzalkonium chloride 0.01%)].
Canada—
  Not commercially available.

**Packaging and storage**
Store below 40 °C (104 °F), preferably between 15 and 30 °C (59 and 86 °F), unless otherwise specified by manufacturer. Store in a tight, light-resistant container. Protect from freezing.

**Stability**
The color of this solution may vary from colorless to amber yellow. Do not use if solution is dark brown or contains a precipitate.

**Auxiliary labeling**
• For the eye.
• Keep container tightly closed.

Revised: 11/28/94

## EPINEPHRINE-CONTAINING COMBINATIONS—

Bupivacaine and Epinephrine (Parenteral-Local)—See *Anesthetics (Parenteral-Local)*
Etidocaine and Epinephrine (Parenteral-Local)—See *Anesthetics (Parenteral-Local)*
Lidocaine and Epinephrine (Parenteral-Local)—See *Anesthetics (Parenteral-Local)*
Prilocaine and Epinephrine (Parenteral-Local)—See *Anesthetics (Parenteral-Local)*

## EPINEPHRYL BORATE—See *Epinephrine (Ophthalmic)*

Anemia, severe, associated with acquired immunodeficiency syndrome (AIDS) (treatment)[1]—Epoetin is indicated for the treatment of severe anemia associated with AIDS or with zidovudine therapy for AIDS.

[Anemia associated with frequent blood donation (prophylaxis)][1]—Epoetin is indicated to prevent anemia in patients who donate blood (for future autologous transfusion) prior to elective surgery. The medication has been found effective in females, patients with low packed-cell volumes due to anemia or small body size, and patients requiring donation of 4 units or more of blood.

[Anemia associated with malignancy (treatment)][1]—Epoetin is indicated for treatment of chronic anemia associated with neoplastic diseases.

Note: Epoetin is not a substitute for blood transfusions, which may be required for the emergency treatment of severe anemia. However, with chronic use, epoetin reduces the need for repeated maintenance blood transfusions.

[1]Not included in Canadian product labeling.

## Pharmacology/Pharmacokinetics

**Physicochemical characteristics**
Molecular weight—Epoetin alfa: About 30,400 daltons.

## Mechanism of action/Effect

Epoetin alfa is a glycoprotein, produced by recombinant DNA technology, that contains 165 amino acids in a sequence identical to that of endogenous human erythropoietin. Recombinant epoetin has the same biological activity as the endogenous hormone, which induces erythropoiesis by stimulating the division and differentiation of committed erythroid progenitor cells, including burst-forming units–erythroid, colony-forming units–erythroid, erythroblasts, and reticulocytes, in bone marrow. Erythropoietin also induces the release of reticulocytes from the bone marrow into the blood stream, where they mature into erythrocytes.

Endogenous erythropoietin is produced primarily in the kidney. The anemia associated with chronic renal failure is caused primarily by inadequate production of the hormone. Administration of epoetin corrects the erythropoietin deficiency in patients with chronic renal failure. Epoetin also stimulates red blood cell production in patients who do not have a documented erythropoietin deficiency, i.e., patients with normal or slightly elevated concentrations of endogenous erythropoietin. However, it may not be effective in patients who are anemic despite having significantly elevated concentrations of erythropoietin.

## Other actions/effects

The increase in hematocrit induced by epoetin may increase blood viscosity and peripheral vascular resistance, leading to a rise in blood pressure. The medication does not appear to have a direct pressor effect.

Epoetin may correct the bleeding tendency associated with chronic renal failure, which may be caused partially by red blood cell deficiency. However, the medication may also increase the thrombotic tendency in some patients.

Correction of anemia by epoetin may result in an improved feeling of well-being; increased appetite; relief of anemia-induced fatigue, tachycardia, headache, weakness, or angina pectoris; increased exercise tolerance and physical activity; and improved sleep, sexual function, and cognitive function.

Administration of epoetin alfa apparently does not induce antibody formation, because antibodies have not been detected in the blood of patients treated with the recombinant hormone for up to 12 months.

Endogenous erythropoietin production may be suppressed by chronic administration of recombinant epoetin.

## Half-life

Elimination—May average 4 to 13 hours following intravenous or subcutaneous administration. The elimination half-life is generally higher after the first few doses (>7.5 hours) than after 2 or more weeks of treatment (6.2 hours after 7 doses; 4.6 hours after 24 doses).

## Onset of action

Increase in reticulocyte count (initial effect)—Within 7 to 10 days.

Increase in red cell count, hematocrit, hemoglobin—Clinically significant increases generally occur in 2 to 6 weeks The rate and extent of the response are dependent on dosage and availability of iron stores. Over a 2-week period, administration of 50 Units per kg of body weight 3 times weekly increases the hematocrit by an average of 1.5 points, administration of 100 Units per kg of body weight 3 times weekly increases the hematocrit by an average of 2.5 points, and administration of 150 Units per kg of body weight 3 times weekly increases the hematocrit by an average of 3.5 points.

## Time to peak concentration

Single intravenous dose—15 minutes.

Single subcutaneous dose—5 to 24 hours. Peak concentrations may be maintained for 12 to 16 hours, and detectable quantities are present for at least 24 hours, after administration.

Note: With repeated subcutaneous administration, peak concentrations are achieved and maintained over the same time periods as with single subcutaneous doses, but are substantially lower than those achieved by a single dose. However, the lower epoetin concentrations are sufficient for achieving, and even lower concentrations are sufficient for maintaining, the desired response.

## Time to peak effect

Increase in hematocrit to target area—Dose dependent; usually within 2 months with administration of 100 or 150 Units per kg of body weight 3 times weekly.

## Duration of action

The hematocrit may begin to decrease about 2 weeks after treatment has been discontinued.

# Precautions to Consider

## Carcinogenicity

The carcinogenic potential of epoetin alfa has not been investigated.

## Mutagenicity

Epoetin alfa does not induce bacterial gene mutation (Ames test), chromosomal aberrations in mammalian cells, micronuclei in mice, or gene mutation at the HGPRT locus. Also, examination of the bone marrow of patients receiving epoetin for up to 8 weeks has revealed no evidence of karyotypic abnormalities or alteration in the sister chromatid exchange rate.

## Pregnancy/Reproduction

Fertility—Administration of 100 or 500 Units per kg of body weight intravenously to male and female rats showed a trend toward slightly increased fetal wastage, but the trend was not statistically significant.

Pregnancy—Adequate and well-controlled studies in humans have not been done. However, administration of 500 Units per kg of body weight to female rats caused decreases in weight gain, delays in the appearance of abdominal hair, delayed eyelid opening, delayed ossification, and decreases in the number of caudal vertebrae in first generation fetuses. Administration of up to 500 Units per kg of body weight to female rabbits from Day 6 to Day 18 of gestation produced no adverse effects.

FDA Pregnancy Category C.

## Breast-feeding

It is not known whether epoetin alfa is excreted in human breast milk. However, in animal studies, administration of up to 500 Units per kg of body weight to female rats during lactation produced no adverse effects in the pups.

## Pediatrics

No pediatrics-specific information is available for children up to 12 years of age.

## Geriatrics

No published geriatrics-specific information is available.

## Drug interactions and/or related problems

The following drug interactions and/or related problems have been selected on the basis of their potential clinical significance (possible mechanism in parentheses where appropriate)—not necessarily inclusive (» = major clinical significance):

Note: Combinations containing any of the following medications, depending on the amount present, may also interact with this medication.

Antihypertensive agents
(epoetin may increase blood pressure, possibly to hypertensive levels, especially when the hematocrit is rising rapidly; more intensive antihypertensive therapy [increase in dosage, administration of additional and/or more potent medications] may be required to control blood pressure)

Heparin
(an increase in heparin dosage may be required in patients receiving hemodialysis, because epoetin-induced increases in red blood cell volume may lead to blood clotting in the dialyzer and/or vascular access [arteriovenous shunt])

Iron supplements
(iron requirement may be increased as existing iron stores are used for erythropoiesis; some clinicians recommend supplementation for all patients who are not overloaded with iron because of frequent blood transfusions; in some patients, oral iron supplementation may be insufficient and intravenous iron dextran may be required)

## Laboratory value alterations

The following have been selected on the basis of their potential clinical significance (possible effect in parentheses where appropriate)—not necessarily inclusive (» = major clinical significance):

With physiology/laboratory test values
Bleeding time
(may be decreased; also, the prolonged bleeding time associated with chronic renal failure in some patients may be corrected during epoetin treatment)

Blood pressure
(may be increased, possibly to hypertensive levels)

Blood urea nitrogen (BUN) and
Serum creatinine concentrations and
Serum phosphorus concentrations and
Serum potassium concentrations and
Serum sodium concentrations and
Serum uric acid concentrations
(may be increased; however, whether the increases reported in patients with chronic renal failure are caused by a direct effect of epoetin on the renal clearance of these substances or the efficacy of dialysis and/or by noncompliance with required dietary restrictions, which may occur when improvement of anemia increases

the patient's appetite and feeling of well-being, has not been established)

Iron concentration and
Serum ferritin
(usually are decreased, unless the patient is receiving adequate iron supplementation, as iron stores are utilized for hemoglobin synthesis functional iron deficiency may occur and lead to a decrease or loss of epoetin efficacy)

### Medical considerations/Contraindications
The medical considerations/contraindications included here have been selected on the basis of their potential clinical significance (reasons given in parentheses where appropriate)—not necessarily inclusive (» = major clinical significance).

*Except under special circumstances, this medication should not be used when the following medical problems exist:*

» Hypersensitivity to human albumin or to mammalian cell–derived products
(risk of a serious allergic reaction to the albumin present in the commercial formulation or to the recombinant product itself)

» Hypertension, uncontrolled
(may be exacerbated, especially during the early phase of treatment or when the hematocrit is rising too rapidly [>4 points within 2 weeks]; a few cases of hypertensive encephalopathy have occurred in patients with poorly controlled blood pressure during epoetin therapy; initiation of therapy should be delayed until blood pressure is adequately controlled)

*Risk-benefit should be considered when the following medical problems exist:*

Any condition that may decrease or delay the response to epoetin alfa, such as:
Aluminum intoxication
Folic acid deficiency
Hemolysis
Infection
Inflammation
Malignancy
Osteitis fibrosa cystica
Vitamin $B_{12}$ deficiency

Cardiovascular system abnormalities caused by hypertension or
» Hypertension, previous, controlled
(increased risk of hypertension, which may lead to hypertensive encephalopathy)

Hematologic disorders, such as:
Hypercoagulable disorders
Myelodysplastic syndromes
Sickle cell anemia or
Vascular disease
(caution and close monitoring are recommended because of an increased thrombotic tendency or other potential complications associated with increases in blood viscosity and peripheral vascular resistance that may occur as a result of epoetin-induced increases in hematocrit)
(the safety and efficacy of epoetin therapy in patients with hematologic disorders have not been determined; also, the presence of myelodysplastic disorders may slow or decrease the bone marrow response to the medication)

Seizure disorders, history of
(seizures not associated with hypertensive encephalopathy have been reported during epoetin therapy; although a causal association has not been established [in clinical studies, seizures occurred at the same rate in both epoetin-treated and placebo-treated patients with chronic renal failure], caution is recommended)

### Patient monitoring
The following may be especially important in patient monitoring (other tests may be warranted in some patients, depending on condition; » = major clinical significance):

» Blood pressure determinations
(recommended at frequent intervals because epoetin may increase blood pressure, possibly to hypertensive levels; although the risk may be greatest in patients with pre-existing hypertension [even if optimally controlled at the time epoetin therapy is initiated], epoetin may also increase blood pressure in previously normotensive patients; control of blood pressure is essential because a few cases of hypertensive encephalopathy have occurred during epoetin therapy in patients with poorly controlled hypertension and because hypertension may be especially hazardous to patients with chronic renal failure, who are predisposed to cardiovascular complications including myocardial ischemia, myocardial infarction, heart fail-

ure, and/or stroke; initiation of or increase in antihypertensive therapy, reduction in dosage or temporary withdrawal of epoetin alfa, or even phlebotomy may be required to control hypertension)

Complete blood count and
Platelet count
(recommended periodically because increases in white blood cell and platelet counts have been reported, although the counts have generally remained within the normal range)

» Hematocrit
(determinations recommended prior to initiation of therapy, then twice weekly during therapy as a guide to efficacy and dosage; because a too-rapid rise in hematocrit may be associated with an increased risk of adverse effects, it is recommended that epoetin dosage be reduced if the hematocrit increases by more than 4 points in a 2-week period; after the hematocrit has been stabilized in the target range [30 to 33%], the frequency of monitoring may be decreased; however, after each dosage adjustment, determinations should be performed twice a week for at least 2 to 6 weeks, until the hematocrit has stabilized at the new level; also, to prevent adverse effects, therapy should be discontinued if the hematocrit exceeds 36%)

» Iron status, including:
Serum ferritin
Transferrin saturation
(determination recommended prior to initiation of therapy, because epoetin's efficacy is decreased when the available iron is insufficient to support erythropoiesis; serum ferritin should be at least 100 nanograms per mL, and transferrin saturation at least 20%, before therapy is initiated)
(monitoring recommended at regular intervals throughout therapy to determine whether iron supplementation should be initiated or increased, because incorporation of iron into hemoglobin may decrease iron stores to the point of functional iron deficiency, leading to a decrease or loss of epoetin efficacy)

Neurologic evaluation
(recommended periodically, especially during the first 90 days of therapy, to detect premonitory signs indicative of a risk of seizures; although a causal association between a rapid rise in hematocrit and seizures has not been established, it is recommended that epoetin dosage be reduced if the hematocrit increases by more than 4 points within 2 weeks)

» Renal function, including:
Blood urea nitrogen (BUN) and
Serum creatinine and
Serum phosphorous and
Serum potassium and
Serum sodium and
Serum uric acid
(close monitoring recommended in patients with renal function impairment to determine the need for initiating or increasing dialysis; however, whether the increases in concentrations of these substances that have been reported during epoetin therapy are caused by a direct effect of the hormone on renal function or the efficacy of dialysis and/or by noncompliance with dietary restrictions required by patients with chronic renal failure, which may occur when improvement of anemia produces increased appetite and feeling of well-being, has not been established)

## Side/Adverse Effects

Note: Some of the side effects listed below are known sequelae of chronic renal failure; therefore, a causal association with epoetin therapy has not always been established.

Menses have resumed during treatment in some female patients. Therefore, the risk of pregnancy should be evaluated and an appropriate method of contraception instituted if necessary.

The following side/adverse effects have been selected on the basis of their potential clinical significance (possible signs and symptoms in parentheses where appropriate)—not necessarily inclusive:

### Those indicating need for medical attention
Incidence more frequent
*Chest pain*—incidence 7%; *edema* (swelling of face, fingers, ankles, feet, or lower legs; weight gain)—incidence 9%; *fast heartbeat; headache*—incidence 16%; may rarely indicate hypertensive encephalopathy; *increased blood pressure*—incidence 24%; may reach hypertensive levels and, rarely, lead to cerebral ischemia or to hypertensive encephalopathy (blurred vision or other change in vision, grand mal seizures, headache); *polycythemia*—may lead to hyperviscosity resulting in increased peripheral vascular resistance, hypertension, and

thrombotic complications, e.g., clotting of arteriovenous (AV) shunts [incidence 6.8%] and/or dialyzer, and rarely, transient ischemic attacks or cerebrovascular accident [incidence 0.4%] or myocardial infarction [incidence 0.4%]

Incidence less frequent

*Seizures*—incidence 1.1% overall, but 2.5% during the first 90 days of treatment in patients receiving dialysis; *shortness of breath*

Incidence rare

*Skin rash or hives*

**Those indicating need for medical attention only if they continue or are bothersome**

Incidence more frequent

*Arthralgias* (bone pain)—incidence 11%; *asthenia* (muscle weakness, severe)—incidence 7%; *diarrhea*—incidence 8.5%; *nausea*—incidence 10.5%; *skin reaction at administration site*—incidence 7%; *tiredness*—incidence 9%; *vomiting*—incidence 8%

Incidence less frequent or rare

*Influenza-like syndrome, mild* (bone pain; muscle aches; chills; shivering; sweating)—may appear 1 to 2 hours after intravenous administration and persist for up to 12 hours

## Patient Consultation

As an aid to patient consultation, refer to *Advice for the Patient, Epoetin (Systemic)*.

In providing consultation, consider emphasizing the following selected information (» = major clinical significance):

**Before using this medication**

» Conditions affecting use, especially:
   Other medical problems, especially hypertension and a history of hypersensitivity to albumin or to mammalian cell–derived products

**Proper use of this medication**

» Proper injection technique (if dispensed for home use)
» Proper dosing
   Missed dose: Administering as soon as possible; not administering if almost time for next dose; not doubling doses
» Proper storage

**Precautions while receiving this medication**

Risk of seizures, especially during the first 90 days of treatment; avoiding activities that may be hazardous should a seizure occur
» Importance of keeping medical and dialysis appointments
» Importance of compliance with antihypertensive regimen (medications and diet), if prescribed, and dietary restrictions pertinent to patients with chronic renal failure
» Importance of compliance with iron or other vitamin supplementation

**Side/adverse effects**

Signs of potential side effects, especially chest pain, edema, fast heartbeat, headache, hypertension, seizures, shortness of breath, and skin rash or hives

## General Dosing Information

Epoetin alfa is administered intravenously or subcutaneously. In general, it is given intravenously to patients with an available intravenous access, i.e., patients receiving hemodialysis, and either intravenously or subcutaneously to other patients.

An increase in dosage may be required if aluminum intoxication, which is not uncommon in patients with chronic renal failure, is present.

**Diet/Nutrition**

Failure to achieve an adequate response to the medication, or loss of efficacy during therapy, may indicate a lack of sufficient iron to support erythropoiesis. Iron supplementation should be initiated or increased as needed. Also, folic acid and/or vitamin $B_{12}$ deficiency may reduce or delay the response to the medication; supplementation with these nutrients may also be required.

Correction of anemia often results in increased appetite and a feeling of well-being, which, in turn, may lead to noncompliance with dietary restrictions (e.g., regulated protein, sodium, and potassium intake) that are necessary in patients with chronic renal failure. Noncompliance with such restrictions may require institution of, or an increase in, dialysis.

**For treatment of adverse effects**

Recommended treatment consists of the following
   • For clotting of arteriovenous (AV) shunt and/or dialyzer—Clotting complications should be managed according to the dialysis center's policy and procedures. AV shunts may be cleared by use of a syringe with heparinized saline solution. If this is unsuccessful, a thrombolytic agent (streptokinase or urokinase) may be used,

after allowing the effects of prior anticoagulation to diminish. Increasing heparin dosage helps prevent recurrent clotting complications.
   • For hypertension—Instituting or increasing administration of antihypertensive medications. In some patients, a decrease in dosage or temporary withdrawal of epoetin and/or phlebotomy may be needed.
   • For polycythemia—Decreasing the dosage of, or temporarily suspending therapy with, epoetin. In some patients, phlebotomy may be needed.

## Parenteral Dosage Forms

### EPOETIN ALFA, RECOMBINANT, INJECTION

**Usual adult and adolescent dose**

Anemia associated with renal failure—
   Initial: Intravenous or subcutaneous, 50 to 100 Units per kg of body weight three times a week. Dosage may be increased if, after eight weeks of therapy, the hematocrit has not increased by five to six points and is still below the desired range (30 to 33%). Adjustments in dosage are generally made in increments of 25 Units per kg of body weight.
   Note: Some clinicians begin therapy with lower doses, e.g., 40 Units per kg of body weight three times a week.
      An interval of at least four weeks should elapse between dosage adjustments, unless clinical circumstances dictate otherwise, because the response to a change in dosage may require two to six weeks.
      Because of a possible risk of hypertensive and/or thrombotic complications, it is recommended that dosage be decreased if the hematocrit increases by more than four points in a two-week period.
      Administration of epoetin should be discontinued temporarily if the hematocrit reaches or exceeds the maximum recommended level of 36%. When the hematocrit has returned to the desired range, therapy may be resumed using a dose that is 25 Units per kg of body weight lower than the previous dose.
   Maintenance: Dosage should be decreased gradually, by 25 Units per kg of body weight at intervals of four weeks or more, to the lowest dose that will maintain the hematocrit at the desired level (30 to 33%).
   Note: Although maintenance doses of up to 525 Units per kg of body weight three times a week have been administered, the maximum maintenance dose recommended by the manufacturer is 300 Units per kg of body weight three times a week.
      Once-weekly subcutaneous administration of the entire week's dosage requirement may be sufficient to maintain some patients at the desired hematocrit range.

**Usual pediatric dose**

Children up to 12 years of age—Dosage has not been established.

**Strength(s) usually available**

U.S.—
   In 1-mL single-dose vials
      2000 Units per mL (Rx) [*Epogen* (human albumin 2.5 mg); *Procrit* (human albumin 2.5 mg)].
      3000 Units per mL (Rx) [*Epogen* (human albumin 2.5 mg); *Procrit* (human albumin 2.5 mg)].
      4000 Units per mL (Rx) [*Epogen* (human albumin 2.5 mg); *Procrit* (human albumin 2.5 mg)].
      10,000 Units per mL (Rx) [*Epogen* (human albumin 2.5 mg); *Procrit* (human albumin 2.5 mg)].

Canada—
      4000 Units per mL (Rx) [*Eprex* (human albumin 2.5 mg)].
      10,000 Units per mL (Rx) [*Eprex* (human albumin 2.5 mg)].

**Packaging and storage**

Store at 2 to 8 °C (36 to 46 °F), unless otherwise specified by manufacturer. Protect from freezing.

**Stability**

*Do not shake the vial of epoetin alfa, recombinant, injection.* Shaking may denature the glycoprotein and render it biologically inactive.

Because the injection contains no preservative, each vial should be used to administer a single dose only. Any unused portion of the solution must be discarded.

**Incompatibilities**

It is recommended that epoetin alfa, recombinant, not be admixed with other medications.

## Selected Bibliography

Eschbach JW, Egrie JC, Downing MR, et al. Correction of the anemia of end-stage renal disease with recombinant human erythropoietin: results of a combined phase I and II clinical trial. N Engl J Med 1987; 316: 73-8.

Mohini R. Clinical efficacy of recombinant human erythropoietin in hemodialysis patients. Semin Nephrol 1989; 9 Suppl 1: 16-21.

Schwenk MH, Halstenson CE. Recombinant human erythropoietin. DICP 1989; 23: 528-36.

Revised: 07/07/92
Interim revision: 05/02/94

**ERGOCALCIFEROL**—See *Vitamin D and Analogs (Systemic)*

---

# ERGOLOID MESYLATES    Systemic

VA CLASSIFICATION (Primary): CN900

Another commonly used name is dihydrogenated ergot alkaloids.

Note: For a listing of dosage forms and brand names by country availability, see *Dosage Forms* section(s). For a listing of brand names for the articles in this monograph, refer to the General Index.

---

## Category

Dementia symptoms treatment adjunct.

## Indications

### Accepted

Dementia, early (treatment adjunct)—Ergoloid mesylates has been used to treat symptoms of an idiopathic decline in mental capacity (such as cognitive and interpersonal skills, mood, self-care, and apparent motivation) related to aging or to an underlying dementing condition such as primary progressive dementia, Alzheimer's dementia, or senile-onset multi-infarct dementia. Careful diagnosis is recommended prior to use to rule out other causes of the presenting symptoms.

The role of this medication in the therapy of dementia is controversial. A recent controlled study in patients with Alzheimer's disease found no advantage to the use of ergoloid mesylates as compared to placebo, and suggested that ergoloid mesylates may worsen scores on certain cognitive and behavioral rating scales. More study is needed to determine the risk-benefit profile of ergoloid mesylates in the treatment of dementia.

## Pharmacology/Pharmacokinetics

### Physicochemical characteristics

Molecular weight—Dihydroergocornine mesylate: 659.80.
Dihydroergocristine mesylate: 707.84.
Dihydro-alpha-ergocryptine mesylate: 673.82.
Dihydro-beta-ergocryptine mesylate: 673.82.

### Mechanism of action/Effect

Not established with regard to indications. Ergoloid mesylates acts centrally to decrease vascular tone and slow the heart rate, and acts peripherally to block alpha-receptors. Another possible mechanism is the effect of ergoloid mesylates on neuronal cell metabolism, possibly resulting in improved oxygen uptake and improved cerebral metabolism, which in turn may normalize depressed neurotransmitter levels.

### Absorption

Ergoloid mesylates is rapidly but incompletely (approximately 25%) absorbed from the gastrointestinal tract. Approximately 50% of an absorbed dose is removed by first-pass metabolism.

### Biotransformation

Hepatic.

### Half-life

2 to 5 hours.

### Onset of action

Clinical improvement may not be apparent for 3 to 4 weeks or longer.

### Time to peak plasma concentration

1 to 2 hours.

## Precautions to Consider

### Medical considerations/Contraindications

The medical considerations/contraindications included here have been selected on the basis of their potential clinical significance (reasons given in parentheses where appropriate)—not necessarily inclusive (» = major clinical significance).

*Risk-benefit should be considered when the following medical problems exist:*

» Bradycardia or
» Hypotension
   (may be exacerbated)
   Hepatic function impairment
   (impaired elimination and possible toxicity)
» Psychosis, acute or chronic
   (bradycardia reported; dopamine agonist activity may aggravate existing psychosis)
   Sensitivity to ergoloid mesylates or other ergot alkaloids

### Patient monitoring

The following may be especially important in patient monitoring (other tests may be warranted in some patients, depending on condition; » = major clinical significance):

Blood pressure and
Pulse count
   (determinations recommended prior to initiation of therapy and at periodic intervals during therapy)

## Side/Adverse Effects

Note: At recommended dosage, side effects usually are rare. Incidence and severity of side effects tend to be related to dose and duration of treatment and are usually reversible after therapy is discontinued.

    Ergot alkaloids have been reported to precipitate attacks of acute intermittent porphyria in susceptible patients.

The following side/adverse effects have been selected on the basis of their potential clinical significance (possible signs and symptoms in parentheses where appropriate)—not necessarily inclusive:

### Those indicating need for medical attention

Incidence less frequent or rare
   *Bradycardia* (drowsiness; slow heartbeat); *orthostatic hypotension* (dizziness or lightheadedness when getting up from a lying or sitting position); *skin rash*

### Those indicating need for medical attention only if they continue or are bothersome

Incidence less frequent or rare
   *Soreness under tongue*—with sublingual use

Incidence dose-related—possible symptoms of overdose
   *Blurred vision; dizziness; fainting; flushing; headache; loss of appetite; nausea or vomiting; stomach cramps; stuffy nose*

## Patient Consultation

As an aid to patient consultation, refer to *Advice for the Patient, Ergoloid Mesylates (Systemic).*

In providing consultation, consider emphasizing the following selected information (» = major clinical significance):

### Before using this medication

» Conditions affecting use, especially:
   Sensitivity to ergoloid mesylates
   Other medical problems, especially bradycardia, hypotension, or acute or chronic psychosis

### Proper use of this medication

» Importance of not using more or less medication than the amount prescribed
   Proper administration of sublingual tablet: Dissolving tablet under tongue; not eating, drinking or smoking while tablet is dissolving
» Proper dosing
   Missed dose: Not taking missed dose; not doubling doses; checking with physician if two or more doses in a row are missed
» Proper storage

**Precautions while using this medication**
Importance of regular monitoring by physician
» May require several weeks before clinical response is noted; checking with physician before discontinuing medication

**Side/adverse effects**
Signs of potential side effects, especially bradycardia, orthostatic hypotension, and skin rash

## General Dosing Information

Clinical improvement may not be apparent for 3 to 4 weeks or longer. Continued clinical evaluation of the patient during ergoloid mesylates therapy is required to determine whether there is any initial benefit of the medication and if the benefits continue with time.

If marked bradycardia or hypotension occurs, it is recommended that therapy with ergoloid mesylates be permanently withdrawn.

Ergoloid mesylates does not have the vasoconstrictor properties of the natural ergot alkaloids.

## Oral Dosage Forms
### ERGOLOID MESYLATES CAPSULES

**Usual adult dose**
Dementia symptoms treatment adjunct—
Oral, 1 to 2 mg three times a day.

**Strength(s) usually available**
U.S.—
1 mg (Rx) [*Hydergine LC* (methyl paraben; propyl paraben; sorbitol)].
Note: 0.333 mg each of dihydroergocornine mesylate, dihydroergocristine mesylate, and dihydroergocryptine mesylate, per capsule.
Canada—
Not commercially available.

**Packaging and storage**
Store below 30 °C (86 °F), preferably between 15 and 30 °C (59 and 86 °F), unless otherwise specified by manufacturer. Store in a tight container. Protect from light.

### ERGOLOID MESYLATES ORAL SOLUTION USP

**Usual adult dose**
See *Ergoloid Mesylates Capsules.*

**Strength(s) usually available**
U.S.—
1 mg per mL (Rx) [*Hydergine* (alcohol 28.5%; glycerin; propylene glycol; purified water)].
Note: 0.333 mg each of dihydroergocornine mesylate, dihydroergocristine mesylate, and dihydroergocryptine mesylate, per mL.
Canada—
Not commercially available.

**Packaging and storage**
Store below 30 °C (86 °F), preferably between 15 and 30 °C (59 and 86 °F), unless otherwise specified by manufacturer. Store in a tight, light-resistant container. Protect from freezing.

### ERGOLOID MESYLATES TABLETS USP

**Usual adult dose**
See *Ergoloid Mesylates Capsules.*

**Strength(s) usually available**
U.S.—
0.5 mg (Rx) [GENERIC].
1 mg (Rx) [*Gerimal; Hydergine* (lactose); GENERIC].
Canada—
1 mg (Rx) [*Hydergine* (scored)].
Note: An equal quantity of dihydroergocornine mesylate, dihydroergocristine mesylate, and dihydroergocryptine mesylate (that is, 0.167 or 0.333 mg of each) per tablet.

**Packaging and storage**
Store below 40 °C (104 °F), preferably between 15 and 30 °C (59 and 86 °F), unless otherwise specified by manufacturer. Store in a tight, light-resistant container.

## Sublingual Dosage Forms
### ERGOLOID MESYLATES TABLETS (SUBLINGUAL) USP

**Usual adult dose**
Dementia symptoms treatment adjunct—
Sublingual, 1 to 2 mg three times a day.

**Strength(s) usually available**
U.S.—
0.5 mg (Rx) [*Gerimal; Hydergine* (sucrose); GENERIC].
1 mg (Rx) [*Gerimal; Hydergine* (sucrose); GENERIC].
Note: An equal quantity of dihydroergocornine mesylate, dihydroergocristine mesylate, and dihydroergocryptine mesylate (that is, 0.167 or 0.333 mg of each) per tablet.
Canada—
Not commercially available.

**Packaging and storage**
Store below 40 °C (104 °F), preferably between 15 and 30 °C (59 and 86 °F), unless otherwise specified by manufacturer. Store in a tight, light-resistant container.

**Auxiliary labeling**
• Dissolve under the tongue.
• Do not swallow tablets whole.

Revised: 04/16/93

---

# ERGONOVINE   Systemic

INN: Ergometrine
VA CLASSIFICATION (Primary/Secondary): GU600/GU900; DX900
Another commonly used name is ergometrine.
Note: For a listing of dosage forms and brand names by country availability, see *Dosage Forms* section(s). For a listing of brand names for the articles in this monograph, refer to the General Index.

## Category
Uterine stimulant; diagnostic aid (coronary vasospasm).

## Indications
Note: Bracketed information in the *Indications* section refers to uses that are not included in U.S. product labeling.

**Accepted**
Hemorrhage, postpartum and postabortal (prophylaxis and treatment)—
Ergonovine is indicated in the prevention or treatment of postpartum or postabortal uterine bleeding due to uterine atony or subinvolution. Its use is not recommended prior to delivery of the placenta since placental entrapment may occur.

[Abortion, incomplete (treatment)][1]—In cases of incomplete abortion, ergonovine may be used to hasten expulsion of uterine contents.

[Angina pectoris (diagnosis)][1]—Ergonovine is used as an aid in the diagnosis of variant angina pectoris. Use of ergonovine for this indication should only be undertaken by cardiologists experienced in this use. Careful monitoring is required, as myocardial infarction and death have been reported with the use of ergonovine during this procedure.

**Unaccepted**
Ergonovine is not as effective in treatment of migraine as other ergot alkaloids and, therefore, its use for this indication is not recommended.

Ergonovine is not indicated for induction or augmentation of labor, to induce abortion, or in cases of threatened spontaneous abortion because of its propensity to produce nonphysiologic, tetanic contractions and its long duration of action.

Ergonovine has been used in the diagnosis of esophageal spasm. However, its use for this procedure is not generally recommended.

---

[1]Not included in Canadian product labeling.

## Pharmacology/Pharmacokinetics

**Physicochemical characteristics**
Chemical group—Amine ergot alkaloid.
Molecular weight—441.48.

## Mechanism of action/Effect

Uterine stimulant—

Ergonovine directly stimulates the uterine muscle to increase force and frequency of contractions. With usual doses, these contractions precede periods of relaxation; with larger doses, basal uterine tone is elevated and these relaxation periods will be decreased. Contraction of the uterine wall around bleeding vessels at the placental site produces hemostasis. Ergonovine also induces cervical contractions. The sensitivity of the uterus to the oxytocic effect is much greater toward the end of pregnancy. The oxytocic actions of ergonovine are greater than its vascular effects.

Vasoconstriction—

Ergonovine, like other ergot alkaloids, produces arterial vasoconstriction by stimulation of alpha-adrenergic and serotonin receptors and inhibition of endothelial-derived relaxation factor release. It is a less potent vasoconstrictor than ergotamine.

Diagnostic aid (coronary vasospasm)—

Ergonovine causes vasoconstriction of coronary arteries.

## Other actions/effects

Ergonovine has minor actions on the central nervous system (CNS). In the CNS, ergonovine is a partial agonist and partial antagonist at some serotonin and dopamine receptors. Ergonovine also possesses weak dopaminergic antagonist actions in certain blood vessels and partial agonist actions at serotonin receptors in umbilical and placental blood vessels. It does not possess significant alpha-adrenergic blocking activity.

## Absorption

Absorption is rapid and complete after oral or intramuscular administration.

## Biotransformation

Hepatic.

## Onset of action

Contraction of uterus, postpartum—
Oral: 6 to 15 minutes.
Intramuscular: 2 to 3 minutes.
Intravenous: One minute or less.

## Time to peak concentration

60 to 90 minutes (plasma), after oral dosing.

## Duration of action

Contraction of uterus, postpartum—
Oral: Approximately 3 hours.
Intramuscular: Approximately 3 hours.
Intravenous: 45 minutes (although rhythmic contractions may persist for up to 3 hours).

## Elimination

Renal excretion of metabolites.

Note: It is not known if use of forced diuresis, peritoneal dialysis, hemodialysis, or charcoal hemoperfusion will hasten the elimination of ergonovine, especially in overdose.

# Precautions to Consider

## Cross-sensitivity and/or related problems

Patients sensitive to other ergot derivatives may be sensitive to this medication also, although there is some degree of variation among ergot alkaloids in their ability to elicit oxytocic, CNS, or vasoconstrictive effects.

## Pregnancy/Reproduction

Fertility—Ergonovine has been shown to increase fallopian tube motility.

Pregnancy—Use of ergonovine is contraindicated during pregnancy. Tetanic contractions may result in decreased uterine blood flow and fetal distress.

Labor and delivery—High doses of ergonovine administered prior to delivery may cause uterine tetany and problems in the infant (hypoxia, intracranial hemorrhage). Ergonovine should *not* be administered prior to delivery of the placenta. Administration prior to delivery of the placenta may cause captivation of the placenta or missed diagnosis of a second infant, due to excessive uterine contraction.

## Breast-feeding

Problems in humans have not been documented. However, ergot alkaloids are excreted in breast milk. Although inhibition of lactation has not been reported for ergonovine, other ergot alkaloids inhibit lactation. Also, studies have shown that ergonovine interferes with the secretion of prolactin (to a lesser degree than bromocriptine) in the immediate postpartum period. This could result in delayed or diminished lactation with prolonged use.

Ergot alkaloids have the potential to cause chronic ergot poisoning in the infant if used in higher-than-recommended doses or if used for a longer period of time than is generally recommended.

## Pediatrics

Elimination of ergonovine may be prolonged in newborns. Neonates inadvertently administered ergonovine in overdose amounts have developed respiratory depression, cyanosis, seizures, decreased urine output, and severe peripheral vasoconstriction.

## Geriatrics

No information is available on the effects of ergonovine in geriatric patients.

## Drug interactions and/or related problems

The following drug interactions and/or related problems have been selected on the basis of their potential clinical significance (possible mechanism in parentheses where appropriate)—not necessarily inclusive (» = major clinical significance):

Note: Combinations containing any of the following medications, depending on the amount present, may also interact with this medication.

Anesthetics, general, especially halothane
(peripheral vasoconstriction may be potentiated by the concurrent use of general anesthetics)

(concurrent use of halothane in concentrations greater than 1% may interfere with the oxytocic actions of ergonovine, resulting in severe uterine hemorrhage)

Bromocriptine or
Ergot alkaloids, other
(the incidence of rare cases of hypertension, strokes, seizures, and myocardial infarction associated with the postpartum use of bromocriptine may be increased with the use of ergot alkaloids)

Nicotine or
Smoking, tobacco
(nicotine absorption from heavy smoking may result in enhanced vasoconstriction)

Nitroglycerin or
Antianginal agents, other
(ergot alkaloids may induce coronary vasospasm, lowering the efficacy of nitroglycerin or other antianginal agents; increased doses of nitroglycerin or antianginal agents and/or use of intracoronary nitroglycerin may be necessary)

Vasoconstrictors, other, including those present in some local anesthetics or
Vasopressors
(concurrent use may result in enhanced vasoconstriction; dosage adjustments may be necessary)

(the pressor effect of sympathomimetic pressor amines may be potentiated, resulting in potentially severe hypertension, headache, and rupture of cerebral blood vessels; gangrene developed in a patient receiving both dopamine and ergonovine infusions)

## Laboratory value alterations

The following have been selected on the basis of their potential clinical significance (possible effect in parentheses where appropriate)—not necessarily inclusive (» = major clinical significance):

With physiology/laboratory test values
Blood pressure or
Central venous pressure
(may be elevated due to peripheral vasoconstriction, primarily of postcapillary vessels; has sometimes been associated with preeclampsia, history of hypertension, intravenous administration of ergonovine, or concurrent use of local anesthetics containing vasoconstrictors; hypotension has also been reported)

Heart rate
(may be decreased due primarily to an increase in vagal tone, and possibly to decreased central sympathetic activity and direct depression of the myocardium)

Prolactin
(serum concentrations may be decreased during the postpartum period)

## Medical considerations/Contraindications

The medical considerations/contraindications included here have been selected on the basis of their potential clinical significance (reasons given in parentheses where appropriate)—not necessarily inclusive (» = major clinical significance).

*Except under special circumstances, this medication should not be used when the following medical problems exist:*

*For all indications*
» Angina pectoris, unstable or
» Myocardial infarction, recent
    (vasospasm caused by ergonovine may precipitate angina or myocardial infarction)
» Cerebrovascular accident, history of or
» Transient ischemic attack, history of
    (patients may be susceptible to recurrence due to increases in blood pressure)
» Hypertension, severe, or history of
    (may be exacerbated)

*For obstetric uses only*
» Coronary artery disease
    (patients may be more susceptible to angina or myocardial infarction caused by ergonovine-induced vasospasm)
» Eclampsia or
» Preeclampsia
    (may be exacerbated; patients may be more likely to develop ergonovine-induced hypertension; headaches, severe cardiac arrhythmias, seizures, and cerebrovascular accidents have occurred)
» Occlusive peripheral vascular disease or
» Raynaud's phenomenon, severe
    (may be exacerbated; a patient with Raynaud's phenomenon developed impalpable arterial pulses)

*Risk-benefit should be considered when the following medical problems exist:*
Allergy, hypersensitivity, or intolerance to ergonovine or other ergot alkaloids
» Cardiovascular disease or
» Coronary artery disease (in diagnosis of angina) or
» Mitral valve stenosis or
» Venoatrial shunts
    (vasospasm caused by ergonovine may precipitate angina or myocardial infarction)
    (in patients with pre-existing coronary artery disease, careful monitoring is critical during the diagnosis of angina because severe chest pain, myocardial ischemia, myocardial infarction, and death may occur more frequently and/or as a result of overdose)
» Hepatic function impairment
    (impaired metabolism of ergonovine may result in ergot overdose)
Hypocalcemia
    (oxytocic response to ergonovine may be reduced; cautious use of intravenous calcium gluconate may restore oxytocic response to ergonovine)
» Positive response to ergonovine testing, history of or
» Electrocardiograph abnormalities such as ST changes during exercise or episodes of chest pain or prolonged QT interval (atrioventricular block) during chest pain, rest, or activity
    (ergonovine should not be used routinely in the diagnosis of variant angina in these patients because prolonged coronary vasoconstriction may precipitate angina, acute myocardial infarction, or heart failure)
» Renal function impairment
» Sepsis
    (possible increased sensitivity to the effects of ergonovine)

**Patient monitoring**
The following may be especially important in patient monitoring (other tests may be warranted in some patients, depending on condition; » = major clinical significance):

*For obstetric uses*
Blood pressure determinations and
Pulse rate determinations and
Uterine response
    (recommended at frequent intervals after parenteral therapy to monitor for adverse reactions; especially important with intravenous administration)

*For diagnosis of variant angina pectoris*
Blood pressure and
Electrocardiogram (ECG)
    (recommended throughout procedure)

## Side/Adverse Effects

Note: Because the duration of therapy with ergonovine is generally short, many of the side effects seen with other ergot alkaloids do not occur.

The following side/adverse effects have been selected on the basis of their potential clinical significance (possible signs and symptoms in parentheses where appropriate)—not necessarily inclusive:

**Those indicating need for medical attention**
Incidence less frequent
    *Bradycardia* (slow heartbeat); *coronary vasospasm* (chest pain)
Incidence rare
    *Allergic reaction, including shock; cardiac arrest or ventricular arrhythmias, including fibrillation and tachycardia* (irregular heartbeat); *dyspnea* (unexplained shortness of breath); *hypertension, sudden and severe* (sudden, severe headache; blurred vision; seizures); *myocardial infarction* (crushing chest pain; unexplained shortness of breath)—has occurred with the use of ergot preparations in the postpartum period and with the use of ergonovine for the diagnosis of variant angina; *peripheral vasospasm* (itching of skin; pain in arms, legs, or lower back; pale or cold hands or feet; weakness in legs)—dose-related

**Those indicating need for medical attention only if they continue or are bothersome**
Incidence more frequent
    *Nausea*—especially after intravenous use; *uterine cramping; vomiting*—especially after intravenous use
    Note: *Uterine cramping* will occur to some degree in all patients and is indicative of efficacy. However, dosage reduction may be required in occasional patients with severe or intolerable uterine cramps.
Incidence less frequent
    *Abdominal or stomach pain; diarrhea; dizziness; headache, mild and transient; nasal congestion; sweating; tinnitus* (ringing in the ears); *unpleasant taste*

## Overdose

For specific information on the agents used in the management of ergonovine overdose, see:
- *Charcoal, Activated (Oral-Local)* monograph;
- *Chlorpromazine* in *Phenothiazines (Systemic)* monograph;
- *Diazepam* in *Benzodiazepines (Systemic)* monograph;
- *Hydralazine (Systemic)* monograph;
- *Laxatives (Local)* monograph;
- *Nitroglycerin* in *Nitrates (Systemic)* monograph;
- *Nitroprusside (Systemic)* monograph;
- *Phentolamine (Systemic)* monograph;
- *Phenytoin* in *Anticonvulsants, Hydantoin (Systemic)* monograph; and/or
- *Tolazoline (Parenteral-Systemic)* monograph.

For more information on the management of overdose or unintentional ingestion, **contact a Poison Control Center** (see *Poison Control Center Listing*).

**Clinical effects of overdose**
The following effects have been selected on the basis of their potential clinical significance (possible signs and symptoms in parentheses where appropriate)—not necessarily inclusive:

Acute
    *Angina* (chest pain); *bradycardia* (slow heartbeat); *confusion; drowsiness; fast, weak pulse; miosis* (small pupils); *peripheral vasoconstriction, severe* (cool, pale, or numb arms or legs; muscle pain; weak or absent arterial pulse in arms or legs; tingling, itching, and cool skin); *respiratory depression* (decreased breathing rate or trouble in breathing; bluish color of skin or inside of nose or mouth); *seizures; tachycardia* (fast heartbeat); *unconsciousness; unusual thirst; uterine tetany* (severe cramping of the uterus)

Chronic
    *Formication* (false feeling of insects crawling on the skin); *gangrene* (dry, shriveled appearance of skin on hands, lower legs, or feet); *hemiplegia* (paralysis of one side of the body); *thrombophlebitis* (pain and redness in an arm or leg)
    Note: *Chronic overdose symptoms* are unlikely with proper use since treatment is of short duration.

### Treatment of overdose

Immediate discontinuation of ergonovine. Since there is no specific antidote for the management of ergonovine overdose, treatment is primarily supportive and symptomatic and may include the following:

To decrease absorption—Gastrointestinal decontamination for oral overdose, preferably with multiple doses of activated charcoal and an appropriate cathartic. Gastric lavage may also be considered. It is not known if use of forced diuresis, peritoneal dialysis, hemodialysis, or charcoal hemoperfusion will hasten the elimination of ergonovine, especially in overdose.

Specific treatment—

Use of nitroglycerin for treatment of myocardial ischemia. Intracoronary nitroglycerin may be necessary.

Use of diazepam or phenytoin for treatment of seizures.

Use of sodium nitroprusside, tolazoline, or phentolamine for treatment of peripheral ischemia.

Use of sodium nitroprusside, chlorpromazine 15 mg, or hydralazine for treatment of severe hypertension.

Monitoring—Frequent monitoring of vital signs, arterial blood gases, and electrolytes. Monitoring of serum ergonovine levels is not predictive of the outcome of overdose. Electrocardiogram monitoring to assess cardiac function and perfusion.

Supportive care—May include maintaining an open airway and breathing, maintaining proper fluid and electrolyte balance, correcting hypertension, and controlling seizures. Patients in whom intentional overdose is known or suspected should be referred for psychiatric consultation.

## Patient Consultation

As an aid to patient consultation, refer to *Advice for the Patient, Ergonovine/Methylergonovine (Systemic)*.

In providing consultation, consider emphasizing the following selected information (» = major clinical significance):

**Before using this medication**
» Conditions affecting use, especially:
   Allergies, hypersensitivity, or intolerance to ergonovine or other ergot alkaloids
   Pregnancy—Should not be administered prior to delivery or delivery of the placenta
   Breast-feeding—Ergot alkaloids are excreted in breast milk
   Other medical problems, especially cardiac or vascular disease, hepatic function impairment, severe hypertension or history of hypertension, renal function impairment, and sepsis

**Proper use of this medication**
» Importance of not using more medication or for longer than prescribed; risk of ergotism and gangrene with prolonged use
» Proper dosing
   Missed dose: Not taking at all; not doubling doses
» Proper storage

**Precautions while using this medication**
   Notifying physician if infection develops, since infection may cause increased sensitivity to medication

**Side/adverse effects**
   Signs of potential side effects, especially allergic reaction, coronary vasospasm or other cardiovascular complications, dyspnea, severe hypertension, or peripheral vasospasm

## General Dosing Information

Antiemetic medications such as prochlorperazine may be administered prior to use of ergonovine.

### For parenteral dosage forms only

Because the risk of severe adverse effects is increased with intravenous use of ergonovine, its use is recommended only for emergencies such as excessive uterine bleeding.

If intravenous use is warranted, administration must be done slowly, over a period of at least 1 minute. Some clinicians recommend dilution of the solution before administration.

In some patients who do not respond to ergonovine because of hypocalcemia, cautious intravenous administration of calcium gluconate (provided the patient is not receiving digitalis) may restore the oxytocic action.

## Oral Dosage Forms

### ERGONOVINE MALEATE TABLETS USP

**Usual adult and adolescent dose**
Uterine stimulant—
   Oral or sublingual, 200 to 400 mcg (0.2 to 0.4 mg) two to four times a day (every six to twelve hours) until the danger of uterine atony and hemorrhage has passed.
Note: Generally, a treatment course of 48 hours is sufficient. Oral or sublingual administration usually follows an initial parenteral dose.

**Strength(s) usually available**
U.S.—
   200 mcg (0.2 mg) (Rx) [*Ergotrate*].
Canada—
   200 mcg (0.2 mg) (Rx) [*Ergotrate Maleate*].

**Packaging and storage**
Store below 40 °C (104 °F), preferably between 15 and 30 °C (59 and 86 °F), unless otherwise specified by manufacturer. Store in a well-closed container.

## Parenteral Dosage Forms

Note: Bracketed uses in the *Dosage Forms* section refer to categories of use and/or indications that are not included in U.S. product labeling.

### ERGONOVINE MALEATE INJECTION USP

**Usual adult and adolescent dose**
Uterine stimulant—
   Intravenous, administered over at least one minute, or intramuscular, 200 mcg (0.2 mg), repeated in two to four hours if necessary, up to five doses.
[Angina pectoris (diagnosis)][1]—
   Intravenous, 50 mcg (0.05 mg), repeated every five minutes until chest pain occurs or a total dose of 400 mcg (0.4 mg) has been given.

**Strength(s) usually available**
U.S.—
   200 mcg (0.2 mg) per mL (Rx) [*Ergotrate*].
Canada—
   250 mcg (0.25 mg) per mL (Rx) [GENERIC].

**Packaging and storage**
Store below 8 °C (46 °F), preferably between 2 and 8 °C (36 and 46 °F), unless otherwise specified by manufacturer. Protect from light. Protect from freezing.

**Stability**
Ergonovine maleate ampules may be stored at room temperature for up to 60 days. At any time, discolored solutions or solutions containing visible particles should not be used.

---

[1]Not included in Canadian product labeling.

---

Revised: 06/07/93

---

**ERGOTAMINE**—See *Vascular Headache Suppressants, Ergot Derivative-containing (Systemic)*

# ERGOTAMINE, BELLADONNA ALKALOIDS, AND PHENOBARBITAL   Systemic

VA CLASSIFICATION (Primary/Secondary): CN105/AU900

**NOTE:** The *Ergotamine, Belladonna Alkaloids, and Phenobarbital (Systemic)* monograph is maintained on the USP DI electronic data base. For a printed copy of the most recent revision of the complete monograph, contact the USP Division of Information Development, 12601 Twinbrook Parkway, Rockville, MD 20852.

For information on the specific components of this combination, see the *USP DI* monographs for *Anticholinergics/Antispasmodics (Systemic), Barbiturates (Systemic),* and *Vascular Headache Suppressants, Ergot Derivative-containing (Systemic).*

The information that follows is selectively abstracted from the complete monograph and is provided to facilitate drug use review and patient counseling.

Note: For a listing of dosage forms and brand names by country availability, see *Dosage Forms* section(s). For a listing of brand names for the articles in this monograph, refer to the General Index.

## Category

Vascular headache prophylactic; menopausal symptoms suppressant.

## Indications

### Accepted

Headache, vascular (prophylaxis)—Ergotamine, belladonna alkaloids, and phenobarbital combination is used in the prevention of vascular (migraine or cluster) headaches.

Menopausal symptoms (treatment)—Ergotamine, belladonna alkaloids, and phenobarbital combination is indicated to ameliorate symptoms such as hot flushes, sweating, restlessness, and insomnia in menopausal women. It is usually used for women who are unable to take estrogens. However, unlike estrogen replacement therapy, the ergotamine, belladonna, and phenobarbital combination does not protect against postmenopausal osteoporosis.

The ergotamine, belladonna alkaloids, and phenobarbital combination has also been used for its autonomic effects in the treatment of various cardiovascular, gastrointestinal, and genitourinary disorders. However, it generally *has been replaced* by more specific agents for these uses.

## Patient Consultation

As an aid to patient consultation, refer to *Advice for the Patient, Ergotamine, Belladonna Alkaloids, and Phenobarbital (Systemic).*

In providing consultation, consider emphasizing the following selected information (» = major clinical significance):

### Before using this medication
» Conditions affecting use, especially:

Allergies to ergotamine, belladonna alkaloids, or barbiturates

Pregnancy—Use is not recommended because of ergotamine's oxytocic activity; also, belladonna alkaloids and barbiturates cross placenta; phenobarbital may cause fetal abnormalities and neonatal hemorrhage

Breast-feeding—Ergot alkaloids inhibit lactation; also, they are distributed into breast milk and may cause ergotism in the infant; belladonna alkaloids may also inhibit lactation; phenobarbital is distributed into breast milk and may cause CNS depression in the infant

Use in children—Increased susceptibility to toxic effects of belladonna alkaloids; increased response to belladonna alkaloids in children with spastic paralysis or brain damage; also, risk of paradoxical phenobarbital-induced excitement in hypersensitive children

Use in the elderly—Increased risk of hypothermia and other adverse effects associated with peripheral vasoconstriction; also, increased susceptibility to mental and other toxic effects of anticholinergics and barbiturates; danger of precipitating undiagnosed glaucoma; possible memory impairment

Other medications, especially other anticholinergics, antacids, anticoagulants, antidiarrheals, carbamazepine, CNS depressants, corticosteroids or corticotropin, estrogen- and progestin-containing oral contraceptives, other ergot alkaloids, ketoconazole, monoamine oxidase (MAO) inhibitors, potassium chloride, and other vasoconstrictors (including those present in local anesthetic solutions)

Other medical problems, especially angina pectoris, coronary artery disease, gastrointestinal obstructive disease, glaucoma, hepatic function impairment, hypertension, severe infection, peripheral vascular disease, pruritus, renal function impairment, urinary retention, and recent or contemplated angioplasty or vascular surgery

### Proper use of this medication
» Importance of not using more medication than the amount prescribed; risk of ergotism with overdosage; habit-forming potential

Proper administration of extended-release tablets: Swallowing whole without crushing, breaking, or chewing

» Proper dosing

Missed dose: Not taking missed dose at all; not doubling doses

» Proper storage

### Precautions while using this medication
» Checking with physician before discontinuing medication after prolonged use; gradual dosage reduction may be necessary to avoid the possibility of withdrawal symptoms

Avoiding antacids and antidiarrheal medication within 1 hour of taking this medication

» Avoiding use of alcohol or other central nervous system (CNS) depressants; alcohol also aggravates headache

» Caution when driving or doing jobs requiring alertness because of possible dizziness, lightheadedness, or drowsiness

Avoiding smoking, since nicotine constricts blood vessels

Avoiding exposure to excessive cold, which may aggravate peripheral vasoconstriction

» Caution during exercise and hot weather; overheating may result in heat stroke

Possible increased sensitivity of eyes to light

Notifying physician if infection develops, since infection may cause increased sensitivity to medication

Possible dryness of mouth, nose, and throat; using sugarless candy or gum, ice or saliva substitute for relief; checking with physician or dentist if dry mouth continues for more than 2 weeks

### Side/adverse effects

Signs and symptoms of potential side effects, especially agranulocytosis, allergic reactions, edema, fast or slow heartbeat, gangrene, hepatitis, increased intraocular pressure, cerebral or peripheral ischemia, thrombocytopenia, and coronary or ocular vasospasm

## Oral Dosage Forms

### ERGOTAMINE TARTRATE, BELLADONNA ALKALOIDS, AND PHENOBARBITAL SODIUM TABLETS

#### Usual adult dose

Vascular headache prophylactic and

Menopausal symptoms suppressant—

Oral, 1 tablet in the morning and at noon and 2 tablets at bedtime. In more resistant cases, therapy may begin with 6 tablets per day, the dosage being gradually reduced at weekly intervals to the lowest effective dose.

Note: Geriatric and debilitated patients may react to usual doses of barbiturates with excitement, confusion, or mental depression. Lower doses may be required in these patients.

#### Usual adult prescribing limits

Not to exceed 33 tablets per week.

#### Usual pediatric dose

Safety and efficacy have not been established.

#### Strength(s) usually available

U.S.—

Not commercially available.

Canada—

300 mcg (0.3 mg) of ergotamine tartrate, 100 mcg (0.1 mg) of belladonna alkaloids, and 20 mg of phenobarbital (Rx) [*Bellergal* (lactose; tartrazine)].

#### Auxiliary labeling

• May cause drowsiness.

• Avoid alcoholic beverages.

## ERGOTAMINE TARTRATE, BELLADONNA ALKALOIDS, AND PHENOBARBITAL SODIUM EXTENDED-RELEASE TABLETS

### Usual adult dose
Vascular headache prophylactic and
Menopausal symptoms suppressant—
    Oral, 1 tablet in the morning and 1 tablet in the evening.

Note: Geriatric and debilitated patients may react to usual doses of barbiturates with excitement, confusion, or mental depression. Lower doses may be required in these patients.

### Usual pediatric dose
Safety and efficacy have not been established.

### Strength(s) usually available
U.S.—
    600 mcg (0.6 mg) of ergotamine tartrate, 200 mcg (0.2 mg) of belladonna alkaloids, and 40 mg of phenobarbital (Rx) [*Bellergal-S* (scored; lactose)].
Canada—
    600 mcg (0.6 mg) of ergotamine tartrate, 200 mcg (0.2 mg) of belladonna alkaloids, and 40 mg of phenobarbital (Rx) [*Bellergal Spacetabs* (scored; lactose; tartrazine)].

### Auxiliary labeling
- May cause drowsiness.
- Avoid alcoholic beverages.
- Swallow whole.

Revised: 08/30/94

## ERGOTAMINE-CONTAINING COMBINATIONS—

Ergotamine, Belladonna Alkaloids, and Phenobarbital (Systemic)
Ergotamine and Caffeine (Systemic)—See *Vascular Headache Suppressants, Ergot Derivative–containing (Systemic)*
Ergotamine, Caffeine, and Belladonna Alkaloids (Systemic)—See *Vascular Headache Suppressants, Ergot Derivative–containing (Systemic)*
Ergotamine, Caffeine, Belladonna Alkaloids, and Pentobarbital (Systemic)—See *Vascular Headache Suppressants, Ergot Derivative–containing (Systemic)*
Ergotamine, Caffeine, and Cyclizine (Systemic)—See *Vascular Headache Suppressants, Ergot Derivative–containing (Systemic)*
Ergotamine, Caffeine, and Dimenhydrinate (Systemic)—See *Vascular Headache Suppressants, Ergot Derivative–containing (Systemic)*
Ergotamine, Caffeine, and Diphenhydramine (Systemic)—See *Vascular Headache Suppressants, Ergot Derivative–containing (Systemic)*

## ERYTHRITYL TETRANITRATE—See *Nitrates (Systemic)*

# ERYTHROMYCIN    Ophthalmic

VA CLASSIFICATION (Primary): OP201
Note: For a listing of dosage forms and brand names by country availability, see *Dosage Forms* section(s). For a listing of brand names for the articles in this monograph, refer to the General Index.

## Category
Antibacterial (ophthalmic).

## Indications
Note: Bracketed information in the *Indications* section refers to uses that are not included in U.S. product labeling.

### Accepted
Conjunctivitis, neonatal (prophylaxis)—Erythromycin is indicated in the topical prophylaxis of neonatal conjunctivitis caused by *Chlamydia trachomatis*.

Ocular infections (treatment)—Erythromycin is indicated in the topical treatment of superficial ocular infections of the conjunctiva and/or cornea caused by susceptible organisms.

Ophthalmia neonatorum (prophylaxis)—Erythromycin is indicated alone in the prophylaxis of ophthalmia neonatorum caused by *Neisseria gonorrhoeae* or *C. trachomatis*. However, in infants born to mothers who have clinically apparent gonorrhea, ophthalmic erythromycin is indicated concurrently with parenteral aqueous penicillin G.

[Blepharitis, bacterial (treatment)][1]
[Blepharoconjunctivitis (treatment)][1]
[Chlamydial infections (treatment)][1]
[Conjunctivitis, bacterial (treatment)][1]
[Keratitis, bacterial (treatment)][1]
[Keratoconjunctivitis, bacterial (treatment)][1]
[Meibomianitis (treatment)][1] or
[Trachoma (treatment)][1]—Erythromycin is used in the topical treatment of bacterial blepharitis, blepharoconjunctivitis, chlamydial infections, bacterial conjunctivitis, bacterial keratitis, bacterial keratoconjunctivitis, meibomianitis, and trachoma.

Not all species or strains of a particular organism may be susceptible to erythromycin.

[1]Not included in Canadian product labeling.

## Pharmacology/Pharmacokinetics

### Physicochemical characteristics
Molecular weight—733.94.
Family—Macrolide group of antibiotics.

### Mechanism of action/Effect
Erythromycin is a bacteriostatic macrolide antibiotic. However, it may be bactericidal in high concentrations or when used against highly susceptible organisms. It is thought to penetrate the bacterial cell membrane and to reversibly bind to the 50 S subunit of bacterial ribosomes or near the "P" or donor site so that binding of tRNA (transfer RNA) to the donor site is blocked. Translocation of peptides from the "A" or acceptor site to the "P" or donor site is prevented, and subsequent protein synthesis is inhibited.
Erythromycin is effective only against actively dividing organisms.

### Absorption
Topical application of the ophthalmic ointment to the eye may result in absorption into the cornea and aqueous humor.

## Precautions to Consider

### Cross-sensitivity and/or related problems
Patients intolerant of one erythromycin may be intolerant of other erythromycins also.

### Tumorigenicity
Two-year studies of rats administered erythromycin orally showed no evidence of tumorigenicity.

### Mutagenicity
Studies have not been done.

### Pregnancy/Reproduction
Fertility—Studies of rats, mice, and rabbits given high doses of systemic erythromycin showed no evidence of impaired fertility
Pregnancy—Problems in humans have not been documented.
Studies of rats, mice, and rabbits given high doses of systemic erythromycin showed no evidence of harm to the fetus.
FDA Pregnancy Category B.

### Breast-feeding
Problems in humans have not been documented.

### Pediatrics
Appropriate studies on the relationship of age to the effects of this medicine have not been performed in the pediatric population. However, no pediatrics-specific problems have been documented to date.

### Geriatrics
Appropriate studies on the relationship of age to the effects of this medicine have not been performed in the geriatric population. However, no geriatrics-specific problems have been documented to date.

### Medical considerations/Contraindications
The medical considerations/contraindications included here have been selected on the basis of their potential clinical significance (reasons given in parentheses where appropriate)—not necessarily inclusive (» = major clinical significance).

*Risk-benefit should be considered when the following medical problem exists:*

Intolerance to erythromycin or parabens

## Side/Adverse Effects

The following side/adverse effects have been selected on the basis of their potential clinical significance (possible signs and symptoms in parentheses where appropriate)—not necessarily inclusive:

**Those indicating need for medical attention**
Incidence rare
*Eye irritation not present before therapy*

## Patient Consultation

As an aid to patient consultation, refer to *Advice for the Patient, Erythromycin (Ophthalmic).*

In providing consultation, consider emphasizing the following selected information (» = major clinical significance):

**Before using this medication**
» Conditions affecting use, especially:
    Allergy to this or any of the other erythromycins

**Proper use of this medication**
   Proper administration technique for ophthalmic ointment
» Compliance with full course of therapy
» Proper dosing
   Missed dose: Applying as soon as possible; not applying if almost time for next dose
» Proper storage

**Precautions while using this medication**
   Checking with physician if no improvement within a few days
   Blurred vision after application of ophthalmic ointments

**Side/adverse effects**
   Signs of potential side effects, especially eye irritation not present before therapy

## General Dosing Information

Use of topical antibacterials may lead to skin sensitization, resulting in hypersensitivity reactions with subsequent topical or systemic use of the medication.

In the prophylaxis of ophthalmia neonatorum, erythromycin ophthalmic ointment should not be flushed from the eye following administration. In addition, ophthalmic erythromycin is given concurrently with parenteral aqueous penicillin G in infants born to mothers who have clinically apparent gonorrhea.

## Ophthalmic Dosage Forms
### ERYTHROMYCIN OPHTHALMIC OINTMENT USP

**Usual adult and adolescent dose**
Ocular infections—
   Topical, to the conjunctiva, a thin strip (approximately 1 cm) of ointment up to six times a day, depending on the severity of the infection.

**Usual pediatric dose**
Conjunctivitis, neonatal or
Ophthalmia neonatorum—
   Topical, to each conjunctiva, a thin strip (approximately 0.5 to 1 cm) of ointment as a single dose following cesarean or vaginal delivery.
Ocular infections—
   See *Usual adult and adolescent dose.*

**Strength(s) usually available**
U.S.—
   0.5% (Rx) [*Ilotycin* (methylparaben, propylparaben); GENERIC].
Canada—
   0.5% (Rx) [*Ilotycin;* GENERIC].

**Packaging and storage**
Store below 40 °C (104 °F), preferably between 15 and 30 °C (59 and 86 °F), unless otherwise specified by manufacturer. Protect from freezing.

**Auxiliary labeling**
• For the eye.
• Continue medicine for full time of treatment.

Revised: 11/28/94

---

# ERYTHROMYCIN   Topical

VA CLASSIFICATION (Primary/Secondary): DE752/DE101
Note: For a listing of dosage forms and brand names by country availability, see *Dosage Forms* section(s). For a listing of brand names for the articles in this monograph, refer to the General Index.

## Category

Antiacne agent (topical)—Erythromycin Ointment; Erythromycin Pledgets; Erythromycin Topical Gel; Erythromycin Topical Solution.
Antibacterial (topical)—Erythromycin Ointment.

## Indications

Note: Bracketed information in the *Indications* section refers to uses that are not included in U.S. product labeling.

**Accepted**
Acne vulgaris (treatment)—Topical erythromycin is indicated in the topical treatment of acne vulgaris. It may be effective in grades II and III acne, which are characterized by inflammatory lesions such as papules and pustules. Topical antibacterials are not generally considered to be as effective as systemic antibacterials in the treatment of acne, especially more severe inflammatory acne.

[Skin infections, bacterial, minor (prophylaxis)][1] or
[Skin infections, bacterial, minor (treatment)][1]—Erythromycin ointment is used in the topical prophylaxis and treatment of superficial pyogenic infections of the skin.

**Unaccepted**
Topical erythromycin is not effective in deep cystic lesions or in noninflammatory lesions.

---
[1]Not included in Canadian product labeling.

## Pharmacology/Pharmacokinetics

**Physicochemical characteristics**
Molecular weight—733.94.

**Mechanism of action/Effect**
Antiacne agent (topical)—Probably due to its antibacterial activity. Topical erythromycin is thought to suppress the growth of *Propionibacterium acnes (Corynebacterium acnes)*, an anaerobe found in sebaceous glands and follicles. *P. acnes* produces proteases, hyaluronidases, lipases, and chemotactic factors, all of which can produce inflammatory components or inflammation directly.

## Precautions to Consider

**Cross-sensitivity and/or related problems**
Patients sensitive to one erythromycin may be sensitive to other erythromycins also.

**Carcinogenicity**
*For erythromycin pledgets; erythromycin topical gel; erythromycin topical solution—*
   Long-term studies in animals have not been done to evaluate carcinogenicity.

**Mutagenicity**
*For erythromycin pledgets; erythromycin topical gel—*
   Long-term studies in animals have not been done to evaluate mutagenicity.
*For erythromycin topical solution—*
   Erythromycin topical solution has not been shown to be mutagenic in the Ames Salmonella/Microsome Plate Test.

## Pregnancy/Reproduction

Pregnancy—

*For erythromycin pledgets—*

Fertility; pregnancy:

Studies have not been done in humans or animals.

FDA Pregnancy Category C.

*For erythromycin topical gel; erythromycin topical solution—*

Fertility; pregnancy:

Erythromycin crosses the placenta, although fetal serum concentrations are generally low. Adequate and well-controlled studies in humans have not been done.

Studies in rats, fed erythromycin base in amounts up to 0.25% of their diet prior to and during mating, during gestation, and through weaning, have not shown that erythromycin causes adverse effects on the fetus. In addition, studies in rats and rabbits, given 1.5, 4, and 13 times the estimated human dose, have not shown that erythromycin causes impaired fertility or adverse effects on the fetus.

FDA Pregnancy Category B.

## Breast-feeding

*For erythromycin pledgets; erythromycin topical gel—*

It is not known whether erythromycin, applied topically, is distributed into breast milk. Erythromycin, given systemically, is distributed into breast milk. However, problems in humans have not been documented.

## Pediatrics

*For erythromycin topical gel—*

Appropriate studies on the relationship of age to the effects of this medicine have not been performed in the pediatric population.

*For erythromycin topical solution—*

Appropriate studies on the relationship of age to the effects of this medicine have not been performed in children up to 12 years of age.

## Geriatrics

Appropriate studies on the relationship of age to the effects of this medicine have not been performed in the geriatric population. However, geriatrics-specific problems that would limit the usefulness of this medication in the elderly are not expected.

## Drug interactions and/or related problems

The following drug interactions and/or related problems have been selected on the basis of their potential clinical significance (possible mechanism in parentheses where appropriate)—not necessarily inclusive (» = major clinical significance):

Note: Combinations containing any of the following medications, depending on the amount present, may also interact with this medication.

Abrasive or medicated soaps or cleansers or

Acne preparations or preparations containing a peeling agent, such as:

Benzoyl peroxide

Resorcinol

Salicylic acid

Sulfur

Tretinoin or

Alcohol-containing preparations, topical, such as:

After-shave lotions

Astringents

Perfumed toiletries

Shaving creams or lotions or

Cosmetics or soaps with a strong drying effect or

Isotretinoin or

Medicated cosmetics or ''cover-ups''

(concurrent use with erythromycin pledgets, topical gel, or topical solution may cause a cumulative irritant or drying effect, especially with the application of peeling, desquamating, or abrasive agents, resulting in excessive irritation of the skin)

## Medical considerations/Contraindications

The medical considerations/contraindications included here have been selected on the basis of their potential clinical significance (reasons given in parentheses where appropriate)—not necessarily inclusive (» = major clinical significance).

*Risk-benefit should be considered when the following medical problem exists:*

Sensitivity to erythromycin

## Side/Adverse Effects

The following side/adverse effects have been selected on the basis of their potential clinical significance (possible signs and symptoms in parentheses where appropriate)—not necessarily inclusive:

**Those indicating need for medical attention only if they continue or are bothersome**

For ointment

*Incidence less frequent*

**Peeling; redness**

For pledgets, topical gel, and topical solution

*Incidence more frequent*

**Dry or scaly skin; irritation; itching; stinging or burning feeling**

*Incidence less frequent*

**Peeling; redness**

## Patient Consultation

As an aid to patient consultation, refer to *Advice for the Patient, Erythromycin (Topical).*

In providing consultation, consider emphasizing the following selected information (» = major clinical significance):

**Before using this medication**

» Conditions affecting use, especially:

Sensitivity to erythromycins

Pregnancy—Erythromycin crosses the placenta

Breast-feeding—Erythromycin enters breast-milk

**Proper use of this medication**

Proper administration technique

» Compliance with full course of therapy, which may take months or longer

» Proper dosing

Missed dose: Applying as soon as possible; not applying if almost time for next dose

» Proper storage

*For pledgets, topical gel, and topical solution*

» Not using near heat or open flame or while smoking

Not using medication more often than prescribed

Avoiding too frequent washing of affected areas

» Importance of applying medication to entire affected area

» Not using in eyes, nose, mouth, or on other mucous membranes

**Precautions while using this medication**

Checking with physician if no improvement in acne within 3 to 4 weeks; may take up to 8 to 12 weeks before full therapeutic benefit is seen

*For pledgets, topical gel, and topical solution*

Waiting at least 1 hour before applying any other topical medication for acne

Possibility of stinging or burning after application

Checking with physician if treated skin becomes excessively dry

Proper use of cosmetics

## General Dosing Information

**For topical solution dosage form**

If the treated area(s) become uncomfortable because of excessive dryness or irritation, the dosage of erythromycin topical solution may be reduced to once a day or less often until the symptoms have subsided.

In the treatment of acne with erythromycin topical solution, noticeable improvement may be seen in 3 to 4 weeks. However, 8 to 12 weeks of treatment may be required before maximum benefit is seen.

## Topical Dosage Forms

### ERYTHROMYCIN OINTMENT USP

Note: The composition of *Akne-Mycin* available in the U.S. is different from that of *Akne-Mycin* available in Europe.

**Usual adult and adolescent dose**

Acne vulgaris—

Topical, to the skin, two times a day, morning and evening.

**Usual pediatric dose**

See *Usual adult and adolescent dose.*

**Strength(s) usually available**

U.S.—

2% (Rx) [*Akne-Mycin*].

Canada—

Not commercially available.

**Packaging and storage**
Store preferably between 15 and 30 °C (59 and 86 °F). Store in a collapsible tube or in another tight container. Protect from freezing.

**Auxiliary labeling**
• For external use only.
• Continue medication for full time of treatment.

## ERYTHROMYCIN PLEDGETS USP

**Usual adult and adolescent dose**
Acne vulgaris—
   Topical, to the skin, two times a day.

**Usual pediatric dose**
See *Usual adult and adolescent dose.*

**Strength(s) usually available**
U.S.—
   2% (Rx) [*Erycette* (alcohol 66%; propylene glycol); *T-Stat* (alcohol 71.2%; propylene glycol)].
Canada—
   Not commercially available.
Note: Supplied as foil-covered pledgets (swabs) saturated with 2% erythromycin topical solution.

**Packaging and storage**
Store below 40 °C (104 °F), preferably between 15 and 30 °C (59 and 86 °F), unless otherwise specified by manufacturer. Store in a tight container.

**Auxiliary labeling**
• For external use only.
• Continue medication for full time of treatment.
• Flammable—Keep from heat and flame.

## ERYTHROMYCIN TOPICAL GEL

**Usual adult and adolescent dose**
See *Erythromycin Ointment USP.*

**Usual pediatric dose**
Dosage has not been established.

**Strength(s) usually available**
U.S.—
   2% (Rx) [*A/T/S* (alcohol 92%); *Erygel* (alcohol 92%)].
Canada—
   Not commercially available.

**Packaging and storage**
Store below 40 °C (104 °F), preferably between 15 and 30 °C (59 and 86 °F), unless otherwise specified by manufacturer. Protect from freezing.

**Auxiliary labeling**
• For external use only.
• Continue medication for full time of treatment.
• Flammable—Keep from heat and flame.

## ERYTHROMYCIN TOPICAL SOLUTION USP

**Usual adult and adolescent dose**
See *Erythromycin Ointment USP.*

**Usual pediatric dose**
Infants and children up to 12 years of age—Dosage has not been established.
Children 12 years of age and over—See *Usual adult and adolescent dose.*

**Strength(s) usually available**
U.S.—
   1.5% (Rx) [*Staticin* (alcohol 55%; propylene glycol); GENERIC].
   2% (Rx) [*Akne-Mycin* (alcohol 66%; propylene glycol); *A/T/S* (alcohol 66%; propylene glycol); *EryDerm* (alcohol 77%; propylene glycol); *Erymax* (alcohol 66%; propylene glycol); *Ery-Sol*; *ETS* (alcohol 66%; propylene glycol); *T-Stat* (alcohol 71.2%; propylene glycol); GENERIC].
Canada—
   1.5% (Rx) [*Staticin* (alcohol 55%)].
   2% (Rx) [*Sans-Acne* (alcohol 44%)].

**Packaging and storage**
Store below 40 °C (104 °F), preferably between 15 and 30 °C (59 and 86 °F), unless otherwise specified by manufacturer. Store in a tight container.

**Auxiliary labeling**
• For external use only.
• Continue medication for full time of treatment.
• Keep container tightly closed.
• Flammable—Keep from heat and flame.

**Note**
Explain administration technique.

Revised: 06/23/92
Interim revision: 07/06/94

---

**ERYTHROMYCIN BASE**—See *Erythromycin (Ophthalmic);
Erythromycin (Topical); Erythromycins (Systemic)*

---

# ERYTHROMYCIN AND BENZOYL PEROXIDE   Topical

**VA CLASSIFICATION (Primary): DE752**

**NOTE:** The *Erythromycin and Benzoyl Peroxide (Topical)* monograph is maintained on the USP DI electronic data base. For a printed copy of the most recent revision of the complete monograph, contact the USP Division of Information Development, 12601 Twinbrook Parkway, Rockville, MD 20852.

For information on the specific components of this combination, see the *USP DI* monographs for *Benzoyl Peroxide (Topical)* and *Erythromycin (Topical).*

The information that follows is selectively abstracted from the complete monograph and is provided to facilitate drug use review and patient counseling.

Note: For a listing of dosage forms and brand names by country availability, see *Dosage Forms* section(s). For a listing of brand names for the articles in this monograph, refer to the General Index.

## Category
Antiacne agent (topical).

## Indications
Note: Bracketed information in the *Indications* section refers to uses that are not included in U.S. product labeling.

**Accepted**
Acne vulgaris (treatment)—Erythromycin and benzoyl peroxide combination is indicated [as a primary agent] in the topical treatment of acne vulgaris. [It may be effective in grades II and III acne, which are characterized by inflammatory lesions such as papules and pustules.] [Topical antibacterials are not generally considered to be as effective as systemic antibacterials in the treatment of acne, especially more severe inflammatory acne.]

**Unaccepted**
Topical erythromycin-containing preparations are not as effective in deep cystic lesions or in noninflammatory lesions.

## Patient Consultation
As an aid to patient consultation, refer to *Advice for the Patient, Erythromycin and Benzoyl Peroxide (Topical).*

In providing consultation, consider emphasizing the following selected information (» = major clinical significance):

**Before using this medication**
» Conditions affecting use, especially:
   Sensitivity to erythromycins

**Proper use of this medication**
» Not applying medication to raw or irritated skin
   Before applying, thoroughly washing affected area(s), rinsing well, and patting dry; after washing or shaving, waiting 30 minutes before applying medication
   Avoiding too frequent washing of affected area(s)
*To use*
» Importance of not using more medication than the amount prescribed
   After washing affected area(s), applying medication with fingertips; however, washing medication off hands afterward
» Importance of applying medication to entire affected area

» Not using in or around eyes, nose, or mouth, or on other mucous membranes

Not using medication after expiration date

» Compliance with full course of therapy, which may take months or longer

» Proper dosing

Missed dose: Applying as soon as possible; not applying if almost time for next dose

» Proper storage

**Precautions while using this medication**

Checking with physician if no improvement in acne within 3 to 4 weeks; may take up to 8 to 12 weeks before full therapeutic benefit is seen

Waiting at least 1 hour after applying the first medication before applying the second topical medication for acne

Possibility of mild stinging or burning of the skin after application; checking with physician if irritation continues; using medication less frequently

Checking with physician if treated skin becomes excessively dry

» Medication may bleach hair or colored fabrics

Using only "oil-free" cosmetics to avoid worsening acne

**Side/adverse effects**

Signs of potential side effects, especially allergic contact dermatitis, painful irritation of the skin, or skin rash

## Topical Dosage Forms

### ERYTHROMYCIN AND BENZOYL PEROXIDE TOPICAL GEL USP

**Usual adult and adolescent dose**

Acne vulgaris—

Topical, to the affected area(s), two times a day, morning and evening; or as directed by physician.

**Usual pediatric dose**

Acne vulgaris—

Infants and children up to 12 years of age: Dosage has not been established.

Children 12 years of age and over: See *Usual adult and adolescent dose.*

**Strength(s) usually available**

**When reconstituted and mixed according to manufacturer's instructions**

U.S.—

3% of erythromycin and 5% of benzoyl peroxide (Rx) [*Benzamycin* (alcohol 22%; fragrance)].

Note: Erythromycin and benzoyl peroxide topical gel is supplied in a package containing 20 grams of benzoyl peroxide gel and a plastic vial containing 800 mg of active erythromycin powder.

After reconstitution and mixing, the combined weight is 23.3 grams.

Canada—

Not commercially available.

**Preparation of dosage form**

Prior to dispensing—

1) Add 3 mL of ethyl alcohol (to the mark) to the vial containing the erythromycin powder.

2) Shake the vial well to dissolve the erythromycin powder.

3) Add the erythromycin-containing solution to the benzoyl peroxide gel. Stir the mixture until it is homogeneous in appearance (approximately 1 to 1½ minutes).

**Auxiliary labeling**

• Refrigerate.

• For external use only.

• Keep container tightly closed.

• Continue medication for full time of treatment.

• Beyond-use date.

Revised: 06/26/92
Interim revision: 07/06/94

## ERYTHROMYCIN-CONTAINING COMBINATIONS—

Erythromycin and Benzoyl Peroxide (Topical)
Erythromycin and Sulfisoxazole (Systemic)

## ERYTHROMYCIN ESTOLATE—See *Erythromycins (Systemic)*

## ERYTHROMYCIN ETHYLSUCCINATE—See *Erythromycins (Systemic)*

## ERYTHROMYCIN GLUCEPTATE—See *Erythromycins (Systemic)*

## ERYTHROMYCIN LACTOBIONATE—See *Erythromycins (Systemic)*

# ERYTHROMYCINS   Systemic

This monograph includes information on the following: Erythromycin Base; Erythromycin Estolate; Erythromycin Ethylsuccinate; Erythromycin Gluceptate; Erythromycin Lactobionate; Erythromycin Stearate.

BAN:

Erythromycin ethylsuccinate—Erythromycin ethyl succinate

VA CLASSIFICATION (Primary/Secondary):

Erythromycin Base—AM200/DE751
Erythromycin Estolate—AM200/DE751
Erythromycin Ethylsuccinate—AM200/DE751
Erythromycin Gluceptate—AM200
Erythromycin Lactobionate—AM200
Erythromycin Stearate—AM200/DE751

Note: For a listing of dosage forms and brand names by country availability, see *Dosage Forms* section(s). For a listing of brand names for the articles in this monograph, refer to the General Index.

## Category

Antibacterial (systemic)—Erythromycin Base; Erythromycin Estolate; Erythromycin Ethylsuccinate; Erythromycin Gluceptate; Erythromycin Lactobionate; Erythromycin Stearate.

Antiacne agent—Erythromycin Base; Erythromycin Estolate; Erythromycin Ethylsuccinate; Erythromycin Stearate.

Bowel preparation (preoperative) adjunct—Erythromycin Base.

## Indications

Note: Bracketed information in the *Indications* section refers to uses that are not included in U.S. product labeling.

**General considerations**

Erythromycin is a broad-spectrum antibiotic with activity against gram-positive and gram-negative bacteria, and other infectious agents, including *Chlamydia trachomatis*, mycoplasmas (*Mycoplasma pneumoniae* and *Ureaplasma urealyticum*), and spirochetes (*Treponema pallidum* and *Borrelia* species).

Erythromycin has good activity against *Streptococcus pneumoniae*, *S. pyogenes* (group A beta-hemolytic streptococci), and *Staphylococcus aureus*. Resistant strains of both streptococci have been encountered, especially in populations recently exposed to erythromycin. The incidence of resistance to group A streptococci has ranged from 1 to 18% in small studies to up to 60% in a population that had been widely treated with erythromycin for respiratory infections. Most strains of *S. aureus* are currently sensitive to erythromycin. However, the incidence of resistance is increasing. Resistance may develop to erythromycin alone, or may be the result of cross-resistance to other macrolides.

Erythromycin also has good activity against certain gram-negative bacteria, including *Legionella pneumophila*, *Campylobacter jejuni*, and *Bordetella pertussis*, and somewhat lower activity against *Haemophilus influenzae*. There is activity against some gram-negative anaerobes, but most strains of *Bacteroides fragilis* are resistant. Enterobacteriaceae are usually resistant.

### Accepted

Bowel preparation, preoperative—Enteric-coated erythromycin base is indicated concurrently with oral-local neomycin as part of an adjunctive regimen for the suppression of normal bacterial flora in the preoperative preparation of the bowel.

Bronchitis, bacterial exacerbations (treatment)

Otitis media, acute (treatment) or

Sinusitis (treatment)—Erythromycins are indicated in the treatment of bacterial exacerbations of bronchitis and in the treatment of sinusitis caused by susceptible organisms. Erythromycins are indicated concurrently with sulfonamides in the treatment of acute otitis media caused by susceptible organisms.

Chlamydial infections, endocervical and urethral (treatment)—Erythromycins are indicated in the treatment of endocervical and urethral chlamydial infections caused by *Chlamydia trachomatis*. Erythromycins are recommended for the treatment of chlamydia in pregnant women. However, erythromycin estolate is contraindicated in pregnancy because of drug-related hepatotoxicity.

Conjunctivitis, chlamydial (treatment) or

Pneumonia, chlamydial (treatment)—Erythromycins are indicated in the treatment of conjunctivitis in newborns and pneumonia in infants caused by *Chlamydia trachomatis*. The efficacy of erythromycin treatment for these uses is approximately 80%; a second course of therapy may be required.

Diphtheria (prophylaxis and treatment)—Erythromycins are indicated as an adjunct to antitoxin, to prevent establishment of chronic carriers and to eradicate the organsim in carriers of diphtheria caused by *Corynebacterium diphtheriae*.

Endocarditis, bacterial (prophylaxis)—Erythromycins are indicated in the prophylaxis of bacterial endocarditis in penicillin-allergic patients who have congenital heart disease, rheumatic or other acquired valvular heart disease, prosthetic heart valves, previous bacterial endocarditis, hypertrophic cardiomyopathy, mitral valve prolapse with valvular regurgitation, and who undergo certain dental or surgical procedures.

Erythrasma (treatment)—Erythromycins are indicated in the treatment of erythrasma caused by *Corynebacterium minutissimum*.

Gonorrhea, endocervical (treatment) or

Gonorrhea, urethral (treatment)—Erythromycins are indicated in the treatment of gonorrhea caused by *Neisseria gonorrhoeae*; cephalosporins and fluoroquinolones are recommended for first-line treatment.

Legionnaires' disease (treatment)—Erythromycins are indicated in the treatment of Legionnaires' disease caused by *Legionella pneumophila*.

Listeriosis (treatment)—Erythromycins are indicated in the treatment of listeriosis caused by *Listeria monocytogenes*.

Pertussis (treatment)—Erythromycins are indicated in the treatment of pertussis (whooping cough) caused by *Bordetella pertussis*.

Pharyngitis, streptococcal (treatment)—Erythromycins are indicated in the treatment of pharyngitis caused by *Streptococcus pyogenes* (group A beta-hemolytic streptococci) in patients allergic to penicillin.

Pneumonia, mycoplasmal (treatment) or

Pneumonia, pneumococcal (treatment)—Erythromycins are indicated in the treatment of pneumonia caused by *Mycoplasma pneumoniae* and *Streptococcus pneumoniae*.

Rheumatic fever (prophylaxis)—Erythromycins are indicated as an alternative to penicillin in the long-term prophylaxis of rheumatic fever.

Skin and soft tissue infections (treatment)—Erythromycins are indicated in the treatment of skin and soft tissue infections, including burn wound infections, caused by *S. pyogenes* (group A beta-hemolytic streptococci).

Syphilis (treatment)—Erythromycins are indicated in the treatment of syphilis caused by *Treponema pallidum* in penicillin-allergic patients. However, erythromycin is less effective than other recommended regimens, and its use in pregnancy has failed to prevent congenital syphilis.

Urethritis, nongonococcal (treatment)—Erythromycins are indicated in the treatment of nongonococcal urethritis caused by *Chlamydia trachomatis* and *Ureaplasma urealyticum*.

[Acne vulgaris (treatment)]—Oral erythromycins are used in the treatment of acne vulgaris.

[Actinomycosis (treatment)][1];

[Anthrax (treatment)][1];

[Chancroid (treatment)][1];

[Lymphogranuloma venereum (treatment)][1]; or

[Relapsing fever (treatment)][1]—Erythromycins are used in the treatment of actinomycosis, anthrax, chancroid, lymphogranuloma venereum, and relapsing fever caused by *Borrelia* species.

[Enteritis, *Campylobacter* (treatment)][1]—Erythromycins are used in the treatment of enteritis caused by *Campylobacter jejuni*. Erythromycin therapy shortened the excretion of *C. jejuni* in the feces, but had no effect on the clinical course of the disease.

[Gastroparesis (treatment)][1]—Erythromycins are used in the treatment of gastroparesis, including severe diabetic gastroparesis, gastroparesis associated with progressive systemic sclerosis, and postvagotomy gastroparesis. Intravenous erythromycin appears to be more effective than oral erythromycin at increasing gastric emptying.

[Lyme disease (treatment)][1]—Erythromycins are used in the treatment of early stage Lyme disease in patients who are allergic to penicillin and in children under 9 years of age; however, erythromycins may be less effective than amoxicillin or doxycycline, possibly due to erratic absorption.

Not all species or strains of a particular organism may be susceptible to erythromycins.

---

[1]Not included in Canadian product labeling.

## Pharmacology/Pharmacokinetics

### Physicochemical characteristics

Molecular weight—

   Erythromycin base: 733.94.

   Erythromycin estolate: 1056.39.

   Erythromycin ethylsuccinate: 862.06.

   Erythromycin gluceptate: 960.12.

   Erythromycin lactobionate: 1092.23.

   Erythromycin stearate: 1018.42.

### Mechanism of action/Effect

Antibacterial—Erythromycin is a bacteriostatic macrolide antibiotic. However, it may be bactericidal in high concentrations or when used against highly susceptible organisms. It is thought to penetrate the bacterial cell membrane and to reversibly bind to the 50 S subunit of bacterial ribosomes; it does not directly inhibit peptide formation, but rather inhibits the translocation of peptides from the acceptor site on the ribosome to the donor site, inhibiting subsequent protein synthesis. Erythromycin is effective only against actively dividing organisms.

Gastroparesis—Erythromycin is thought to bind to motilin receptors and to act as an agonist. Erythromycin administration accelerates gastric emptying by increasing the amplitude of antral contractions and improving antroduodenal coordination. The effect appears to be dose-related. In patients with diabetic gastroparesis, low intravenous doses (40 mg) induce phase 3 of the migrating motor complex in the antrum of the stomach; and higher doses (200 mg) elicit prolonged periods of strong antral contractions. Faster emptying from the proximal stomach contributes to more rapid gastric emptying.

### Absorption

Bioavailability varies between 30 and 65%, depending on the salt. Erythromycin film-coated tablets (base and stearate) are subject to gastric acid inactivation and are best absorbed on an empty stomach. However, enteric-coated erythromycin base and erythromycin estolate are acid-stable and may be taken without regard to meals, and erythromycin ethylsuccinate is better absorbed when taken with meals.

### Distribution

Widely distributed to most tissues and fluids, including middle ear exudate, prostatic fluid, and semen. Highest concentrations are found in the liver, bile, and spleen. Low concentrations are found in the cerebrospinal fluid (CSF); however, penetration into CSF increases with meningeal inflammation.

Vol $_D$ = 0.9 L per kg.

### Protein binding

High (70 to 90%).

### Biotransformation

Hepatic; > 90% is hepatically metabolized, partially to inactive metabolites; may accumulate in patients with severe hepatic disease.

Erythromycin estolate (lauryl sulfate salt of the propinoate ester)—Propinoate ester is partially hydrolyzed in the gastrointestinal tract, then hydrolyzed in the blood to produce 20 to 40% of the dose as base in the serum.

Erythromycin ethylsuccinate—Absorbed into the blood as the ethylsuccinate salt and hydrolyzed to erythromycin base in the gastrointestinal tract and in the blood to produce 56 to 69% of the dose as base in the serum. Also, despite the high rate of biotransformation of erythromycin ethylsuccinate to active base, the area-under-the-curve (AUC) of active base generated from the ethylsuccinate salt was 1.6 times lower than that generated from a comparable dose of erythromycin estolate.

Erythromycin stearate—Dissociated to erythromycin base in the duodenum.

### Half-life
Normal renal function—1.4 to 2 hours.

Anuric patients—Approximately 5 hours.

### Time to peak concentration
2 to 4 hours, depending on the specific product (see *Peak serum concentration*).

### Peak serum concentration
Erythromycin base—
Delayed-release capsules: Single dose of 250 mg—1.1 to 1.7 mcg per mL (mcg/mL) at 3 hours.
Delayed-release tablets: Single dose of 250 mg—Approximately 0.9 mcg/mL at 4 hours.
Delayed-release tablets: Multiple doses of 250 mg—Approximately 2.8 mcg/mL at 2 hours.
Erythromycin estolate—
Single dose of 250 mg: Approximately 0.8 to 1.2 mcg/mL at 2 to 4 hours.
Erythromycin ethylsuccinate—
Single dose of 400 mg: Approximately 0.8 mcg/mL at 1 hour.
Multiple doses (400 mg twice a day), fasting: Approximately 1.4 mcg/ mL.
Multiple doses (400 mg twice a day), with food: Approximately 3 mcg/mL.
Erythromycin gluceptate—
Single dose of 200 mg: 3 to 4 mcg/mL.
Erythromycin lactobionate—
Single dose of 500 mg: Approximately 10 mcg/mL.
Erythromycin stearate—
Single dose of 250 mg: Approximately 0.8 mcg/mL at 3 hours.

### Elimination
Biliary; primarily excreted into the bile.

Renal, by glomerular filtration; 2 to 5% excreted unchanged following oral administration; 12 to 15% excreted unchanged following intravenous administration.

Erythromycins are not removed by hemodialysis or peritoneal dialysis.

## Precautions to Consider

### Cross-sensitivity and/or related problems
Patients intolerant of one erythromycin or other macrolides may be intolerant of other erythromycins also.

### Tumorigenicity/Mutagenicity
Long-term (20 month) oral studies done in rats did not demonstrate erythromycin base to be tumorigenic. Mutagenicity studies have not been conducted.

### Pregnancy/Reproduction
Fertility—Adequate and well-controlled studies in humans have not been done.

Studies in rats fed erythromycin base at concentrations up to 0.25% of their diet found no apparent effect on male or female fertility.

Pregnancy—Erythromycins cross the placenta, resulting in low fetal plasma concentrations (5 to 20% of maternal plasma concentrations). Erythromycin estolate has been associated with an increased risk of reversible, subclinical hepatotoxicity in approximately 10% of pregnant women; its use during pregnancy is not recommended. However, problems with other erythromycins have not been documented.

There was no evidence of teratogenicity or any other adverse effect on reproduction in female rats fed erythromycin base (up to 0.25% of their diet) prior to and during mating, during gestation, and through weaning of 2 successive litters.

FDA Pregnancy Category B.

### Breast-feeding
Erythromycins are distributed into breast milk. However, problems in humans have not been documented.

### Pediatrics
Studies performed to date have not demonstrated pediatrics-specific problems that would limit the usefulness of erythromycin in children.

### Geriatrics
Studies performed to date have not demonstrated geriatrics-specific problems that would limit the usefulness of erythromycin in the elderly. However, elderly patients may be at increased risk of hearing loss if they also have decreased renal or hepatic function associated with aging and are receiving high doses of erythromycin.

### Dental
Systemic erythromycins may lead to oral candidiasis in patients undergoing long-term therapy.

### Drug interactions and/or related problems
The following drug interactions and/or related problems have been selected on the basis of their potential clinical significance (possible mechanism in parentheses where appropriate)—not necessarily inclusive (» = major clinical significance):

Note: Combinations containing any of the following medications, depending on the amount present, may also interact with this medication.

Alcohol
(concurrent use with intravenous erythromycin was found to increase the peak blood alcohol concentration by 40%; erythromycin is not known to affect alcohol metabolism directly, but is thought to be related to more rapid gastric emptying. Less exposure to alcohol dehydrogenase in the gastric mucosa and slower small intestine transit time may also favor the increase of alcohol absorption. There may be less of an effect with oral erythromycin)

» Alfentanil
(chronic preoperative or perioperative use of erythromycins, which are hepatic enzyme inhibitors, may decrease the plasma clearance and prolong the duration of action of alfentanil)

» Astemizole or
» Terfenadine
(concurrent use of astemizole or terfenadine with erythromycins is contraindicated; concurrent use may increase the risk of cardiotoxicity, such as torsades de pointes and ventricular tachycardia, and death)

» Carbamazepine or
Valproic acid
(erythromycins may inhibit carbamazepine and valproic acid metabolism, resulting in increased anticonvulsant plasma concentrations and toxicity; it is recommended that erythromycins be used with caution if at all in patients receiving carbamazepine or valproic acid)

» Chloramphenicol or
» Lincomycins
(erythromycins may displace these medications from, or prevent them from binding to, 50 S subunits of bacterial ribosomes, thus antagonizing the effects of chloramphenicol and lincomycins; concurrent use is not recommended)

» Cyclosporine
(erythromycin has been reported to increase cyclosporine plasma concentrations and may increase the risk of nephrotoxicity)

Digoxin
(erythromycin may alter gut flora, which prevents inactivation of digoxin, allowing more digoxin to be absorbed; this results in increased digoxin levels)

Ergotamine
(erythromycin inhibits the metabolism of ergotamine and has been reported to increase the vasospasm associated with ergotamines)

» Hepatotoxic medications, other (see *Appendix II*)
(concurrent use of other hepatotoxic medications with erythromycins may increase the potential for hepatotoxicity)

Lovastatin
(concurrent use of lovastatin with erythromycin may increase the risk of rhabdomyolysis, which typically occurs after the completion of erythromycin therapy; this is thought to be due to erythromycin's inhibition of lovastatin metabolism, which increases lovastatin serum concentrations; simultaneous administration of erythromycin and lovastatin should be used with caution)

Midazolam or
Triazolam
(concurrent use with erythromycin may decrease the clearance of these medications, increasing the pharmacological effect of midazolam or triazolam)

Ototoxic medications, other (see *Appendix II*)
(concurrent use of other ototoxic medications with high-dose erythromycin in patients with renal function impairment may increase the potential for ototoxicity)

Penicillins
(since bacteriostatic drugs may interfere with the bactericidal effect of penicillins in the treatment of meningitis or in other situations where a rapid bactericidal effect is necessary, it is best to avoid concurrent therapy)

» Warfarin
    (use of erythromycins in patients receiving chronic warfarin ther-
    apy may result in excessive prolongation of prothrombin time and
    increased risk of hemorrhage, especially in elderly patients, be-
    cause of possible decreased warfarin metabolism and clearance;
    warfarin dosage adjustments may be necessary during and after
    therapy with erythromycins, and prothrombin times should be
    monitored closely)

» Xanthines, such as:
    Aminophylline
    Caffeine
    Oxtriphylline
    Theophylline
    (concurrent use of the xanthines [except dyphylline] with eryth-
    romycins may decrease hepatic clearance of theophylline, resulting
    in increased serum theophylline concentrations and/or toxicity; this
    effect may be more likely to occur after 6 days of concurrent ther-
    apy because the magnitude of theophylline clearance reduction is
    proportional to the peak serum erythromycin concentrations; dos-
    age adjustment of the xanthines may be necessary during and after
    therapy with erythromycins)

**Laboratory value alterations**
The following have been selected on the basis of their potential clinical
significance (possible effect in parentheses where appropriate)—not
necessarily inclusive (» = major clinical significance):

With diagnostic test results
    Aspartate aminotransferase (AST [SGOT])
    (use of erythromycin may interfere with AST [SGOT] determina-
    tions if azonefast violet B or diphenylhydrazine colorimetric tests
    are used)

    Catecholamines, urinary
    (erythromycin may produce false elevations of urinary catechola-
    mines because of interference with the fluorometric determination)

With physiology/laboratory test values
    Alanine aminotransferase (ALT [SGPT]) and
    Alkaline phosphatase and
    Aspartate aminotransferase (AST [SGOT]) and
    Bilirubin, serum
    (values may be increased by all erythromycins, but more com-
    monly by erythromycin estolate)

**Medical considerations/Contraindications**
The medical considerations/contraindications included here have been selected on the basis of their potential clinical significance (reasons given
in parentheses where appropriate)—not necessarily inclusive (» =
major clinical significance).

*Risk-benefit should be considered when the following medical problems
exist:*
» Cardiac arrhythmias, history of, or QT prolongation
    (patients with a history of cardiac arrhythmias or QT prolongation
    may be at risk for arrhythmias or torsades de pointes while re-
    ceiving high doses of erythromycin)

» Hepatic function impairment, especially with erythromycin estolate
    (erythromycins, especially erythromycin estolate, may be hepato-
    toxic on rare occasion)

    Hypersensitivity to erythromycins

    Loss of hearing
    (patients with a history of hearing loss may be at increased risk of
    further hearing loss, especially if the patient has renal or hepatic
    function impairment, is elderly, and is receiving high doses of
    erythromycin)

**Patient monitoring**
The following may be especially important in patient monitoring (other
tests may be warranted in some patients, depending on condition;
» = major clinical significance):

Electrocardiogram
    (monitoring of QT interval recommended, especially in patients
    receiving high doses of parenteral erythromycin)

» Hepatic function determinations
    (may be required periodically if signs of hepatic dysfunction occur
    with any of the erythromycins; erythromycins should be discontin-
    ued promptly if signs of hepatic dysfunction occur)

## Side/Adverse Effects

Note: Hepatotoxicity has been associated, rarely, with all erythromycin
    salts, but more frequently with erythromycin estolate. Reports sug-
    gest that a hypersensitivity mechanism may be involved. Symptoms
    include malaise, nausea, vomiting, abdominal cramps, skin rash,

and fever. Jaundice may or may not be present. Liver function tests
often indicate cholestasis. Symptoms typically appear within a few
days to 1 or 2 weeks after the start of continuous therapy, and are
reversible when erythromycin is discontinued. However, hepatotoxicity reappears promptly on readministration to sensitive patients.

Hearing loss is more likely to occur with administration of high
doses (≥ 4 grams per day) in patients with renal or hepatic disease
and/or in elderly patients. It appears to be related to high peak
plasma concentrations, usually exceeding 12 mcg per mL. Hearing
loss is usually reversible, although irreversible deafness has occurred. It occurs from 36 hours to 8 days after treatment is started,
and begins to recover within 1 to 14 days after erythromycin is
discontinued.

The following side/adverse effects have been selected on the basis of their
potential clinical significance (possible signs and symptoms in parentheses where appropriate)—not necessarily inclusive:

**Those indicating need for medical attention**
Incidence less frequent
    *Hepatotoxicity* (fever; nausea; skin rash; stomach pain, severe; unusual
    tiredness or weakness; yellow eyes or skin; vomiting); *hypersensitivity*
    (skin rash, redness, or itching)
Incidence less frequent—parenteral erythromycins only
    *Inflammation or phlebitis at the injection site*
Incidence rare
    *Cardiac toxicity, especially QT prolongation and torsades de pointes*
    (irregular or slow heart rate; recurrent fainting; sudden death); *loss of
    hearing, usually reversible; pancreatitis* (severe abdominal pain, nau-
    sea, and vomiting)

**Those indicating need for medical attention only if they continue
or are bothersome**
Incidence more frequent
    *Gastrointestinal disturbances* (abdominal or stomach cramping and
    discomfort; diarrhea, nausea or vomiting)
Incidence less frequent
    *Oral candidiasis* (sore mouth or tongue; white patches in mouth and/or
    on tongue); *vaginal candidiasis* (vaginal itching and discharge)

## Overdose

For specific information on the agents used in the management of erythromycin overdose, see:
    • *Epinephrine (Systemic)* monograph;
    • *Corticosteroids (Systemic)* monograph; and/or
    • *Antihistamines (Systemic)* monograph.

For more information on the management of overdose or unintentional
ingestion, **contact a Poison Control Center** (see *Poison Control Center Listing*).

**Treatment of overdose**
Recommended treatment consists of the following:

To decrease absorption—Evacuating the stomach to eliminate unabsorbed
drug.

Specific treatment—Administering epinephrine, corticosteroids, and antihistamines for allergic reactions.

Supportive care—Using supportive measures as needed. Patients in whom
intentional overdose is known or suspected should be referred for psy-
chiatic consultation.

## Patient Consultation

As an aid to patient consultation, refer to *Advice for the Patient,
Erythromycins (Systemic)*.

In providing consultation, consider emphasizing the following selected
information (» = major clinical significance):

**Before using this medication**
» Conditions affecting use, especially:
    Hypersensitivity to erythromycins or other macrolides
    Pregnancy—Erythromycins cross the placenta; erythromycin es-
        tolate has been associated with an increased risk of reversible,
        subclinical hepatotoxicity in pregnant women
    Breast-feeding—Erythromycins are distributed into breast milk
    Dental—Oral candidiasis may occur with long-term therapy
    Other medications, especially alfentanil, astemizole, carbamaze-
        pine, chloramphenicol, cyclosporine, other hepatotoxic medi-
        cations, lincomycins, terfenadine, warfarin, and xanthines
    Other medical problems, especially a history of cardiac arrhyth-
        mias or QT prolongation or hepatic function impairment

**Proper use of this medication**
Taking with a full glass of water, on an empty stomach; may be taken
    with food if stomach upset occurs

Proper administration technique for oral liquids and/or pediatric drops, chewable tablets, delayed-release capsules and tablets

Not using oral liquids and/or pediatric drops after expiration date

» Compliance with full course of therapy, especially in streptococcal infections

» Importance of not missing doses and taking at evenly spaced times

» Proper dosing

Missed dose: Taking as soon as possible; not taking if almost time for next dose; not doubling dose

» Proper storage

**Precautions while using this medication**

Checking with physician if no improvement within a few days

**Side/adverse effects**

Signs of potential side effects, especially, hepatotoxicity, hypersensitivity, inflammation or phlebitis at the injection site, cardiac toxicity, loss of hearing, or pancreatitis

# General Dosing Information

Therapy should be continued for at least 10 days in group A beta-hemolytic streptococcal infections to help prevent the occurrence of acute rheumatic fever.

## For oral dosage forms only

Doses greater than 1 gram per dose are not recommended with twice-a-day dosing.

Erythromycin film-coated tablets (base and stearate) are best absorbed on an empty stomach; however, if gastrointestinal irritation occurs, they may be taken with food. Enteric-coated erythromycin base and erythromycin estolate may be taken without regard to meals; and erythromycin ethylsuccinate is better absorbed when taken with meals.

---

## ERYTHROMYCIN BASE

---

# Oral Dosage Forms

Note: Bracketed uses in the *Dosage Forms* section refer to categories of use and/or indications that are not included in U.S. product labeling.

## ERYTHROMYCIN DELAYED-RELEASE CAPSULES USP

### Usual adult and adolescent dose

Antibacterial—

Oral, 250 mg (base) every six hours; 333 mg every eight hours; or 500 mg every twelve hours if twice-a-day dosage is desired.

Note: Acne vulgaris—Oral, 250 mg (base) every six hours; 333 mg every eight hours; or 500 mg every twelve hours for four weeks. This dose may be reduced to 333 to 500 mg once a day for a maintenance dose.

Bowel preparation (preoperative) adjunct—Oral, 1 gram (base) administered at nineteen hours, eighteen hours, and nine hours (total of 3 grams) before the start of surgery.

Chlamydial infections, endocervical and urethral—Oral, 333 mg (base) every eight hours, or 500 mg every six hours for seven days; or 250 mg every six hours for fourteen days. Erythromycin base may be used in pregnant women.

[Chancroid][1]—Oral, 500 mg (base) every six hours for seven days.

Endocarditis prophylaxis—Oral, 1 gram (base) two hours prior to the procedure, and 500 mg six hours after the initial dose.

[Enteritis, *Campylobacter*][1]—Oral, 250 mg (base) four times a day for five days.

[Gastroparesis][1]—Oral, 250 mg (base) taken thirty minutes before meals, three times a day.

Legionnaires' disease—Oral, 500 mg (base) to 1 gram every six hours.

[Lyme disease][1]—Oral, 250 mg (base) four times a day for ten to twenty-one days.

[Lymphogranuloma venereum][1]—Oral, 500 mg (base) every six hours for twenty-one days.

Pelvic inflammatory disease, caused by *Neisseria gonorrhoeae* — Oral, 250 mg (base) every six hours for seven days, after intravenous administration of erythromycin 500 mg every six hours for three days.

[Relapsing fever][1]—Oral, 10 mg (base) per kg of body weight every six hours for ten days.

Streptococcal prophylaxis—Continuous prophylaxis of streptococcal infections in patients with a history of rheumatic heart disease: Oral, 250 mg (base) every twelve hours.

Syphilis, primary—Oral, 30 to 40 grams (base) over a ten- to fifteen-day period.

Urethritis, nongonococcal, caused by *Ureaplasma urealyticum* — Oral, 500 mg (base) every six hours for seven days; or 250 mg every six hours for fourteen days.

### Usual adult prescribing limits

Antibacterial—

Up to 4 grams (base) a day.

### Usual pediatric dose

Antibacterial—

Oral, 7.5 to 12.5 mg (base) per kg of body weight every six hours; or 15 to 25 mg per kg of body weight every twelve hours.

Severe infections, 15 to 25 mg (base) per kg of body weight every six hours.

Note: Chlamydial infections, endocervical and urethral—

Children up to 45 kg of body weight: Oral, 10 mg (base) per kg of body weight every six hours for ten to fourteen days.

Children 45 kg of body weight and over but less than 8 years of age: See *Usual adult and adolescent dose.*

Conjunctivitis, chlamydial[1]—Oral, 12.5 mg (base) per kg of body weight every six hours for at least ten to fourteen days.

Diphtheria—Oral, 10 to 12.5 mg (base) per kg of body weight every six hours for fourteen days.

Endocarditis prophylaxis—Oral, 20 mg (base) per kg of body weight two hours prior to the procedure, and 10 mg per kg of body weight six hours after the initial dose.

[Enteritis, *Campylobacter*][1]—Oral, 10 mg (base) per kg of body weight every six hours for five days.

[Lyme disease][1]—Oral, 7.5 mg (base) per kg of body weight every six hours for ten to twenty-one days.

Pertussis—Oral, 10 to 12.5 mg (base) per kg of body weight every six hours for fourteen days.

Pneumonia, chlamydial[1]—Oral, 12.5 mg (base) per kg of body weight every six hours for two weeks.

[Relapsing fever][1]—Oral, 10 mg (base) per kg of body weight every six hours for ten days.

Streptococcal pharyngitis—Oral, 5 to 7.5 mg (base) per kg of body weight every six hours; or 10 to 15 mg per kg of body weight every twelve hours for at least ten days.

### Strength(s) usually available

U.S.—

250 mg (base) (Rx) [*ERYC*; GENERIC].

Canada—

250 mg (base) (Rx) [*Apo-Erythro E-C*; *ERYC-250*; *Novo-rythro Encap*].

333 mg (base) (Rx) [*Apo-Erythro E-C*; *ERYC-333*].

### Packaging and storage

Store below 40 °C (104 °F), preferably between 15 and 30 °C (59 and 86 °F), unless otherwise specified by manufacturer. Store in a tight container.

### Auxiliary labeling

• Continue medicine for full time of treatment.

• Swallow capsules whole.

### Note

Erythromycin delayed-release capsules contain enteric-coated pellets. The entire contents of a capsule may be sprinkled on applesauce, jelly, or ice cream immediately prior to ingestion. Subdividing the contents of the capsule is not recommended.

## ERYTHROMYCIN TABLETS USP

### Usual adult and adolescent dose

See *Erythromycin Delayed-release Capsules USP.*

### Usual adult prescribing limits

See *Erythromycin Delayed-release Capsules USP.*

### Usual pediatric dose

See *Erythromycin Delayed-release Capsules USP.*

### Strength(s) usually available

U.S.—

250 mg (base) (Rx) [GENERIC].

500 mg (base) (Rx) [GENERIC].

Canada—

250 mg (base) (Rx) [*Apo-Erythro*; *Erythromid*].

**Packaging and storage**
Store below 40 °C (104 °F), preferably between 15 and 30 °C (59 and 86 °F), unless otherwise specified by manufacturer. Store in a tight container.

**Auxiliary labeling**
• Continue medicine for full time of treatment.

## ERYTHROMYCIN DELAYED-RELEASE TABLETS USP

**Usual adult and adolescent dose**
See *Erythromycin Delayed-release Capsules USP*.

Note: Endocarditis prophylaxis—The manufacturer of E-Mycin recommends taking 1 gram three to four hours prior to the procedure because of the pharmacokinetics of their enteric-coated product.

**Usual adult prescribing limits**
See *Erythromycin Delayed-release Capsules USP*.

**Usual pediatric dose**
See *Erythromycin Delayed-release Capsules USP*.

Note: Endocarditis prophylaxis—The manufacturer of E-Mycin recommends taking 1 gram three to four hours prior to the procedure because of the pharmacokinetics of their enteric-coated product.

**Strength(s) usually available**
U.S.—
   250 mg (base) (Rx) [*E-Mycin; Ery-Tab; Ilotycin;* GENERIC].
   333 mg (base) (Rx) [*E-Base; E-Mycin; Ery-Tab; PCE;* GENERIC].
   500 mg (base) (Rx) [*E-Base; Ery-Tab; PCE*].
Canada—
   250 mg (base) (Rx) [*E-Mycin;* GENERIC].
   333 mg (base) (Rx) [*PCE*].
   500 mg (base) (Rx) [*Erybid*].

**Packaging and storage**
Store below 40 °C (104 °F), preferably between 15 and 30 °C (59 and 86 °F), unless otherwise specified by manufacturer. Store in a tight container.

**Auxiliary labeling**
• Continue medicine for full time of treatment.
• Swallow tablets whole.

---

[1]Not included in Canadian product labeling.

---

### *ERYTHROMYCIN ESTOLATE*

## Summary of Differences

Precautions:
   Pregnancy—Associated with increased risk of reversible, subclinical hepatotoxicity.
   Laboratory value alterations—Serum alkaline phosphatase, bilirubin, AST (SGOT), and ALT (SGPT) concentrations may be increased more frequently than with other erythromycins.
Side/adverse effects:
   May also cause cholestatic jaundice less frequently (rare with other erythromycins).

## Oral Dosage Forms

Note: Bracketed uses in the *Dosage Forms* section refer to categories of use and/or indications that are not included in U.S. product labeling.
   The dosing and strengths of the dosage forms available are expressed in terms of erythromycin base (not the estolate salt).

## ERYTHROMYCIN ESTOLATE CAPSULES USP

**Usual adult and adolescent dose**
Antibacterial—
   Oral, 250 mg (base) every six hours; or 500 mg every twelve hours if twice a day dosage is desired.

Note: Chlamydial infections, endocervical and urethral—Oral, 500 mg (base) every six hours for seven days; or 250 mg every six hours for fourteen days. Erythromycin estolate is not recommended for use in pregnant women.
   Endocarditis prophylaxis—Oral, 1 gram (base) two hours prior to the procedure, and 500 mg six hours after the initial dose.
   [Gastroparesis][1]—Oral, 250 mg (base) taken thirty minutes before meals, three times a day.
   Legionnaires' disease—Oral, 500 mg (base) to 1 gram every six hours.
   Streptococcal prophylaxis—Continuous prophylaxis of streptococcal infections in patients with a history of rheumatic heart disease: Oral, 250 mg (base) every twelve hours.

Syphilis, primary—Oral, 20 to 30 grams (base) over a ten-day period.

**Usual adult prescribing limits**
Antibacterial—
   Up to 4 grams (base) daily.

**Usual pediatric dose**
Antibacterial—
   Oral, 7.5 to 12.5 mg (base) per kg of body weight every six hours; or 15 to 25 mg per kg of body weight every twelve hours.
   Severe infections, 15 to 25 mg (base) per kg of body weight every six hours.

Note: Conjunctivitis, chlamydial[1]—Oral, 12.5 mg (base) per kg of body weight every six hours for at least two weeks.
   Diphtheria—Oral, 10 to 12.5 mg (base) per kg of body weight every six hours for fourteen days.
   Endocarditis prophylaxis—Oral, 20 mg (base) per kg of body weight two hours prior to the procedure, and 10 mg per kg of body weight six hours after the initial dose.
   Pertussis—Oral, 10 to 12.5 mg (base) per kg of body weight every six hours for fourteen days.
   Pneumonia, chlamydial[1]—Oral, 12.5 mg (base) per kg of body weight every six hours for two weeks.
   Streptococcal pharyngitis—Oral, 5 to 7.5 mg (base) per kg of body weight every six hours; or 10 to 15 mg per kg of body weight every twelve hours for at least ten days.

**Strength(s) usually available**
U.S.—
   250 mg (base) (Rx) [*Ilosone;* GENERIC].
Canada—
   250 mg (base) (Rx) [*Ilosone; Novo-rythro*].

**Packaging and storage**
Store below 40 °C (104 °F), preferably between 15 and 30 °C (59 and 86 °F), unless otherwise specified by manufacturer. Store in a tight container.

**Auxiliary labeling**
• Continue medicine for full time of treatment.

## ERYTHROMYCIN ESTOLATE ORAL SUSPENSION USP

**Usual adult and adolescent dose**
See *Erythromycin Estolate Capsules USP*.

**Usual adult prescribing limits**
See *Erythromycin Estolate Capsules USP*.

**Usual pediatric dose**
See *Erythromycin Estolate Capsules USP*.

**Strength(s) usually available**
U.S.—
   125 mg (base) per 5 mL (Rx) [*Ilosone* (methylparaben; propylparaben); GENERIC].
   250 mg (base) per 5 mL (Rx) [*Ilosone* (methylparaben; propylparaben); GENERIC].
Canada—
   125 mg (base) per 5 mL (Rx) [*Ilosone; Novo-rythro*].
   250 mg (base) per 5 mL (Rx) [*Ilosone; Novo-rythro*].

**Packaging and storage**
Store between 2 and 8 °C (36 and 46 °F). Store in a tight container.

**Auxiliary labeling**
• Refrigerate.
• Shake well.
• Continue medicine for full time of treatment.
• Take by mouth only (pediatric drops).

**Note**
Explain administration technique for pediatric drops (100 mg per mL).
When dispensing, include a calibrated liquid-measuring device.

## ERYTHROMYCIN ESTOLATE TABLETS USP

**Usual adult and adolescent dose**
See *Erythromycin Estolate Capsules USP*.

**Usual adult prescribing limits**
See *Erythromycin Estolate Capsules USP*.

**Usual pediatric dose**
See *Erythromycin Estolate Capsules USP*.

**Strength(s) usually available**
U.S.—
   250 mg (base) (Rx) [GENERIC].
   500 mg (base) (Rx) [*Ilosone*].

Canada—
500 mg (base) (Rx) [*Ilosone*].

**Packaging and storage**
Store below 40 °C (104 °F), preferably between 15 and 30 °C (59 and 86 °F), unless otherwise specified by manufacturer. Store in a tight container.

**Auxiliary labeling**
• Continue medicine for full time of treatment.

---

[1]Not included in Canadian product labeling.

---

## *ERYTHROMYCIN ETHYLSUCCINATE*

## Summary of Differences

1.6 grams of erythromycin ethylsuccinate produce approximately the same blood levels as 1 gram erythromycin base.

In pediatric patients, equivalent doses of erythromycin ethylsuccinate and erythromycin base produce comparable blood levels.

## Oral Dosage Forms

Note: Bracketed uses in the *Dosage Forms* section refer to categories of use and/or indications that are not included in U.S. product labeling.

The dosing and dosage forms available are expressed in terms of ethylsuccinate salt. 400 mg of erythromycin ethylsuccinate produces approximately the same blood levels as 250 mg erythromycin base.

## ERYTHROMYCIN ETHYLSUCCINATE ORAL SUSPENSION USP

**Usual adult and adolescent dose**
Antibacterial—
Oral, 400 mg every six hours; or 800 mg every twelve hours if twice-a-day dosing is desired.

Note: Chlamydial infections, endocervical and urethral—Oral, 800 mg (base) every six hours for seven days, or 400 mg every six hours for fourteen days. Erythromycin ethylsuccinate may be used in pregnant women.

Endocarditis prophylaxis—Oral, 1.6 grams two hours prior to the procedure, and 800 mg six hours after the initial dose.

[Gastroparesis][1]—Oral, 400 mg taken thirty minutes before meals, three times a day.

Legionnaires' disease—Oral, 400 mg to 1 gram every six hours.

Streptococcal prophylaxis—Continuous prophylaxis of streptococcal infections in patients with a history of rheumatic heart disease: Oral, 400 mg every twelve hours.

Syphilis, primary—Oral, 48 to 64 grams (base) over a ten- to fifteen-day period.

Urethritis, nongonococcal, caused by *Ureaplasma urealyticum*—Oral, 800 mg every eight hours for seven days; or 400 mg every six hours for fourteen days.

**Usual adult prescribing limits**
Antibacterial—
Up to 4 grams daily.

**Usual pediatric dose**
Antibacterial—
Oral, 7.5 to 12.5 mg per kg of body weight every six hours; or 15 to 25 mg per kg of body weight every twelve hours.
Severe infections, 15 to 25 mg per kg body weight every six hours.

Note: Conjunctivitis, chlamydial[1]—Oral, 12.5 mg (base) per kg of body weight every six hours for ten to fourteen days.

Diphtheria—Oral, 10 to 12.5 mg (base) per kg of body weight every six hours for fourteen days.

Endocarditis prophylaxis—Oral, 20 mg per kg of body weight two hours prior to the procedure, and 10 mg per kg of body weight six hours after the initial dose.

[Enteritis, *Campylobacter*][1]—Oral, 10 mg (base) per kg of body weight every six hours for five days.

Pertussis—Oral, 10 to 12.5 mg per kg of body weight every six hours for fourteen days.

Pneumonia, chlamydial[1]—Oral, 12.5 mg (base) per kg of body weight every six hours for ten to fourteen days.

**Strength(s) usually available**
U.S.—
200 mg per 5 mL (Rx) [*E.E.S.* (methylparaben; propylparaben); *Erythro*; GENERIC].

400 mg per 5 mL (Rx) [*E.E.S.* (methylparaben; propylparaben); *Erythro*; GENERIC].
Canada—
Not commercially available.

**Packaging and storage**
Store between 2 and 8 °C (36 and 46 °F). Store in a tight container.

Note: After dispensing, suspensions do not require refrigeration if used within 14 days. Some manufacturers recommend storage in light-resistant containers to prevent discoloration.

**Auxiliary labeling**
• Shake well.
• Continue medicine for full time of treatment.
• Beyond-use date.

**Note**
When dispensing, include a calibrated liquid-measuring device.

## ERYTHROMYCIN ETHYLSUCCINATE FOR ORAL SUSPENSION USP

**Usual adult and adolescent dose**
See *Erythromycin Ethylsuccinate Oral Suspension USP*.

**Usual adult prescribing limits**
See *Erythromycin Ethylsuccinate Oral Suspension USP*.

**Usual pediatric dose**
See *Erythromycin Ethylsuccinate Oral Suspension USP*.

**Strength(s) usually available**
U.S.—
200 mg per 5 mL (when reconstituted according to manufacturer's instructions) (Rx) [*E.E.S.*; *EryPed*; GENERIC].
400 mg per 5 mL (when reconstituted according to manufacturer's instructions) (Rx) [*EryPed*; GENERIC].
Canada—
100 mg per 5 mL (when reconstituted according to manufacturer's instructions) (Rx) [*Novo-Rythro*].
200 mg per 5 mL (when reconstituted according to manufacturer's instructions) (Rx) [*E.E.S.*; *Novo-Rythro*].
400 mg per 5 mL (when reconstituted according to manufacturer's instructions) (Rx) [*E.E.S.*].

**Packaging and storage**
Prior to reconstitution, store below 40 °C (104 °F), preferably between 15 and 30 °C (59 and 86 °F), unless otherwise specified by manufacturer. Store in a tight container.

Note: After reconstitution, depending on manufacturer or specific product, suspensions do not require refrigeration if used within 14 days.

**Auxiliary labeling**
• Shake well.
• Continue medicine for full time of treatment.
• Beyond-use date.
• Take by mouth only (pediatric drops).

**Note**
Explain administration technique for pediatric drops.
When dispensing, include a calibrated liquid-measuring device.

## ERYTHROMYCIN ETHYLSUCCINATE TABLETS USP

**Usual adult and adolescent dose**
See *Erythromycin Ethylsuccinate Oral Suspension USP*.

**Usual adult prescribing limits**
See *Erythromycin Ethylsuccinate Oral Suspension USP*.

**Usual pediatric dose**
See *Erythromycin Ethylsuccinate Oral Suspension USP*.

**Strength(s) usually available**
U.S.—
400 mg (Rx) [*E.E.S.*; GENERIC].
Canada—
600 mg (Rx) [*Apo-Erythro-ES*; *E.E.S.*].

**Packaging and storage**
Store below 40 °C (104 °F), preferably beween 15 and 30 °C (59 and 86 °F), unless otherwise specified by manufacturer. Store in a tight container.

**Auxiliary labeling**
• Continue medicine for full time of treatment.

## ERYTHROMYCIN ETHYLSUCCINATE TABLETS (CHEWABLE) USP

**Usual adult and adolescent dose**
See *Erythromycin Ethylsuccinate Oral Suspension USP*.

**Usual adult prescribing limits**
See *Erythromycin Ethylsuccinate Oral Suspension USP.*

**Usual pediatric dose**
See *Erythromycin Ethylsuccinate Oral Suspension USP.*

**Strength(s) usually available**
U.S.—
200 mg (Rx) [*EryPed*].
400 mg (Rx) [*Erythro*].
Canada—
200 mg (Rx) [*E.E.S.* (scored); *EryPed*].

**Packaging and storage**
Store below 40 °C (104 °F), preferably between 15 and 30 °C (59 and 86 °F), unless otherwise specified by manufacturer. Store in a tight container.

**Auxiliary labeling**
• Chew or crush tablets before swallowing.
• Continue medicine for full time of treatment.

¹Not included in Canadian product labeling.

---

## *ERYTHROMYCIN GLUCEPTATE*

## Summary of Differences

Category: Indicated only as an antibacterial.

## Parenteral Dosage Forms

Note: Bracketed uses in the *Dosage Forms* section refer to categories of use and/or indications that are not included in U.S. product labeling.
The dosing and strengths of the dosage forms available are expressed in terms of erythromycin base (not the gluceptate salt).

## STERILE ERYTHROMYCIN GLUCEPTATE USP

**Usual adult and adolescent dose**
Antibacterial—
Intravenous infusion, 250 to 500 mg (base) every six hours; or 3.75 to 5 mg per kg of body weight every six hours.
Note: [Gastroparesis]¹—Oral, 200 mg taken thirty minutes before meals, three times a day.
Legionnaires' disease—Intravenous infusion, 1 gram (base) every six hours.
Pelvic inflammatory disease, caused by *Neisseria gonorrhoeae* — Intravenous infusion, 500 mg (base) every six hours for three days, then oral administration of erythromycin 250 mg every six hours for seven days.

**Usual adult prescribing limits**
Up to 4 grams (base) daily.

**Usual pediatric dose**
Antibacterial—
Intravenous infusion, 3.75 to 5 mg (base) per kg of body weight every six hours.
Note: Diphtheria—Oral, 10 to 12.5 mg (base) per kg of body weight every six hours for fourteen days.

**Size(s) usually available**
U.S.—
1 gram (base) (Rx) [*Ilotycin*].
Canada—
500 mg (base) (Rx) [*Ilotycin*].
1 gram (base) (Rx) [*Ilotycin*].

**Packaging and storage**
Prior to reconstitution, store below 40 °C (104 °F), preferably between 15 and 30 °C (59 and 86 °F), unless otherwise specified by manufacturer.

**Preparation of dosage form**
To prepare initial dilution, add at least 10 mL of sterile water for injection (without preservatives) to each 500-mg vial and at least 20 mL of diluent to each 1-gram vial.
After initial dilution, solution may be further diluted to a concentration of 1 gram per liter in 0.9% sodium chloride injection or 5% dextrose injection for slow, continuous infusion.

**Stability**
After reconstitution, initial dilutions (25 to 50 mg per mL) retain their potency for 7 days if refrigerated.

**Additional information**
Infusions with a pH below 5.5 tend to lose potency rapidly and should be administered completely within 4 hours after dilution.

---

If administration time is prolonged, infusions should be buffered to neutrality with a suitable buffer and administered completely within 24 hours after dilution.
If administered by intermittent infusion, dose may be diluted in 100 to 250 mL of 0.9% sodium chloride injection or 5% dextrose injection and administered slowly over a 20- to 60-minute period.

---

¹Not included in Canadian product labeling.

---

## *ERYTHROMYCIN LACTOBIONATE*

## Summary of Differences

Category: Indicated only as an antibacterial.

## Parenteral Dosage Forms

Note: Bracketed uses in the *Dosage Forms* section refer to categories of use and/or indications that are not included in U.S. product labeling.
The dosing and strengths of the dosage forms available are expressed in terms of erythromcyin base (not the lactobionate salt).

## ERYTHROMYCIN LACTOBIONATE FOR INJECTION USP

**Usual adult and adolescent dose**
Antibacterial—
Intravenous infusion, 250 to 500 mg (base) every six hours; or 3.75 to 5 mg per kg of body weight every six hours.
Note: [Gastroparesis]¹—Oral, 200 mg administered thirty minutes before meals, three times a day.
Legionnaires' disease—Intravenous infusion, 1 gram (base) every six hours.
Pelvic inflammatory disease, caused by *Neisseria gonorrhoeae*—Intravenous infusion, 500 mg (base) every six hours for three days, then oral administration of erythromycin 250 mg every six hours for seven days.

**Usual adult prescribing limits**
Up to 4 grams (base) daily.

**Usual pediatric dose**
Antibacterial—
Intravenous infusion, 3.75 to 5 mg (base) per kg of body weight every six hours. This product should be used with caution in neonates since it contains benzyl alcohol.
Note: Diphtheria—Oral, 10 to 12.5 mg (base) per kg of body weight every six hours for fourteen days.

**Size(s) usually available**
U.S.—
500 mg (base) (Rx) [*Erythrocin* (may contain benzyl alcohol 90 mg per 500 mg vial); GENERIC].
1 gram (base) (Rx) [*Erythrocin* (may contain benzyl alcohol 180 mg per 1 gram vial); GENERIC].
Canada—
500 mg (base) (Rx) [*Erythrocin* (may contain benzyl alcohol 0.9% per vial)].
1 gram (base) (Rx) [*Erythrocin* (may contain benzyl alcohol 0.9% per vial)].

**Packaging and storage**
Prior to reconstitution, store below 40 °C (104 °F), preferably between 15 and 30 °C (59 and 86 °F), unless otherwise specified by manufacturer.

**Preparation of dosage form**
To prepare initial dilution, add 10 mL of sterile water for injection (without preservatives) to each 500-mg vial and 20 mL of diluent to each 1-gram vial.
After initial dilution, solution may be further diluted to a concentration of 1 to 5 mg per mL in 0.9% sodium chloride injection, lactated Ringer's injection, or other electrolyte solutions (see manufacturer's package insert) for slow, continuous infusion. Dextrose-containing solutions may also be used if suitably buffered by adding 1 mL of 4% sodium bicarbonate per 100 mL of solution.
For reconstitution of piggyback infusion bottles, see manufacturer's labeling for instructions.
Caution: Use of diluents containing benzyl alcohol is not recommended for preparation of medications for use in neonates. A fatal toxic syndrome consisting of metabolic acidosis, CNS depression, respiratory problems, renal failure, hypotension, and possibly seizures and intracranial hemorrhages has been associated with this use.

## Stability

After reconstitution, initial dilutions (50 mg per mL) retain their potency for 14 days if refrigerated, or for 24 hours at room temperature.

Infusions prepared in piggyback infusion bottles retain their potency for 8 hours at room temperature, for 24 hours if refrigerated, or for 30 days if frozen.

Infusions prepared in the ADD-vantage system should not be stored.

### Additional information

Acidic infusions are unstable and lose potency rapidly. A pH of at least 5.5 is recommended for final dilutions, which should be administered completely within 8 hours after dilution.

If administered by intermittent infusion, dose may be diluted to a maximum concentration of 5 mg per mL with specified diluent and administered slowly over a 20- to 60-minute period.

---

¹Not included in Canadian product labeling.

---

### ERYTHROMYCIN STEARATE

## Oral Dosage Forms

Note: Bracketed uses in the *Dosage Forms* section refer to categories of use and/or indications that are not included in U.S. product labeling.

The dosing and strengths of the dosage forms available are expressed in terms of erythromycin base (not the stearate salt).

### ERYTHROMYCIN STEARATE ORAL SUSPENSION

#### Usual adult and adolescent dose

Antibacterial—

Oral, 250 mg (base) every six hours; or 500 mg every twelve hours if twice a day dosage is desired.

Note: Chlamydial infections, endocervical and urethral—Oral, 500 mg (base) every six hours for seven days; or 250 mg every six hours for fourteen days. Erythromycin stearate may be used in pregnant women.

Endocarditis prophylaxis—Oral, 1 gram (base) two hours prior to the procedure, and 500 mg six hours after the initial dose.

Legionnaires' disease—Oral, 500 mg (base) to 1 gram every six hours.

Pelvic inflammatory disease, caused by *Neisseria gonorrhoeae*—Oral, 250 mg (base) every six hours for seven days, after intravenous administration of erythromycin 500 mg (base) every six hours for three days.

Streptococcal prophylaxis—Continuous prophylaxis of streptococcal infections in patients with a history of rheumatic heart disease: Oral, 250 mg (base) every twelve hours.

Syphilis, primary—Oral, 30 to 40 grams (base) over a ten- to fifteen-day period.

[Gastroparesis]¹—Oral, 150 to 250 mg (base) taken thirty minutes before meals, three times a day.

#### Usual adult prescribing limits

Antibacterial—

Up to 4 grams (base) daily.

#### Usual pediatric dose

Antibacterial—

Oral, 7.5 to 12.5 mg (base) per kg of body weight every six hours; or 15 to 25 mg per kg of body weight every twelve hours.

Severe infections, 15 to 25 mg (base) per kg of body weight every six hours.

Note: Conjunctivitis, chlamydial¹—Oral, 12.5 mg (base) per kg of body weight every six hours for at least two weeks.

Endocarditis prophylaxis—Oral, 20 mg (base) per kg of body weight two hours prior to the procedure, and 10 mg per kg of body weight six hours after the initial dose.

Pertussis—Oral, 10 to 12.5 mg (base) per kg of body weight every six hours for fourteen days.

Pneumonia, chlamydial¹—Oral, 12.5 mg (base) per kg of body weight every six hours for two weeks.

Streptococcal pharyngitis—Oral, 5 to 7.5 mg (base) per kg of body weight every six hours; or 10 to 15 mg per kg of body weight every twelve hours for at least ten days.

### Strength(s) usually available

U.S.—

Not commercially available.

Canada—

125 mg per 5 mL (base) (Rx) [*Erythrocin* (parabens); *Novo-rythro*].

250 mg per 5 mL (base) (Rx) [*Erythrocin* (parabens); *Novo-rythro*].

### Packaging and storage

Prior to reconstitution, store below 40 °C (104 °F), preferably between 15 and 30 °C (59 and 86 °F), unless otherwise specified by manufacturer. Store in a tight container.

### Auxiliary labeling

- Refrigerate.
- Shake well.
- Continue medicine for full time of treatment.
- Beyond-use date.

### Note

When dispensing, include a calibrated liquid-measuring device.

### ERYTHROMYCIN STEARATE TABLETS USP

#### Usual adult and adolescent dose

See *Erythromycin Stearate Oral Suspension*.

#### Usual adult prescribing limits

See *Erythromycin Stearate Oral Suspension*.

#### Usual pediatric dose

See *Erythromycin Stearate Oral Suspension*.

### Strength(s) usually available

U.S.—

250 mg (base) (Rx) [*Erythrocin; Erythrocot; My-E; Wintrocin;* GENERIC].

500 mg (base) (Rx) [*Erythrocin;* GENERIC].

Canada—

250 mg (base) (Rx) [*Apo-Erythro-S; Erythrocin; Novo-rythro*].

500 mg (base) (Rx) [*Apo-Erythro-S; Erythrocin*].

### Packaging and storage

Store below 40 °C (104 °F), preferably between 15 and 30 °C (59 and 86 °F), unless otherwise specified by manufacturer. Store in a tight container.

Note: Some manufacturers recommend storage in light-resistant containers to prevent discoloration.

### Auxiliary labeling

- Continue medicine for full time of treatment.

---

¹Not included in Canadian product labeling.

---

Revised: 07/22/94

---

**ERYTHROMYCIN STEARATE**—See *Erythromycins (Systemic)*

---

# ERYTHROMYCIN AND SULFISOXAZOLE   Systemic

VA CLASSIFICATION (Primary): AM900

**NOTE:** The *Erythromycin and Sulfisoxazole (Systemic)* monograph is maintained on the USP DI electronic data base. For a printed copy of the most recent revision of the complete monograph, contact the USP Division of Information Development, 12601 Twinbrook Parkway, Rockville, MD 20852.

For information on the specific components of this combination, see the *USP DI* monographs for *Erythromycins (Systemic)* and *Sulfonamides (Systemic)*.

The information that follows is selectively abstracted from the complete monograph and is provided to facilitate drug use review and patient counseling.

Note: For a listing of dosage forms and brand names by country availability, see *Dosage Forms* section(s). For a listing of brand names for the articles in this monograph, refer to the General Index.

## Category

Antibacterial (systemic).

## Indications

Note: Bracketed information in the *Indications* section refers to uses that are not included in U.S. product labeling.

### Accepted

Otitis media, acute (treatment)—Erythromycin and sulfisoxazole combination is indicated in the treatment of acute otitis media caused by *Haemophilus influenzae*, [pneumococci, group A streptococci, and *Branhamella catarrhalis*] in children.

[Sinusitis (treatment)][1]—Erythromycin and sulfisoxazole combination is used in the treatment of acute sinusitis caused by *H. influenzae*, pneumococci, group A streptococci, and *B. catarrhalis* in children.

Not all species or strains of a particular organism may be susceptible to erythromycin and sulfisoxazole combination.

---

[1]Not included in Canadian product labeling.

## Patient Consultation

As an aid to patient consultation, refer to *Advice for the Patient, Erythromycin and Sulfisoxazole (Systemic)*.

In providing consultation, consider emphasizing the following selected information (» = major clinical significance):

### Before using this medication

» Conditions affecting use, especially:

   Allergy to erythromycins or sulfonamides; patients allergic to furosemide, thiazide diuretics, sulfonylureas, or carbonic anhydrase inhibitors may also be allergic to this medication

   Pregnancy—Erythromycin crosses the placenta; sulfisoxazole also crosses the placenta and should not be used at term because it may cause kernicterus in the infant; it has also been associated with cleft palates and skeletal defects in the offspring of mice and rats

   Breast-feeding—Erythromycins are distributed into breast milk in concentrations that may exceed maternal serum concentrations; sulfisoxazole is also distributed into breast-milk and is not recommended in nursing women since sulfonamides may cause kernicterus in nursing infants

   Use in children—Sulfonamides should not be used in children up to 2 months of age because they may cause kernicterus

   Dental—Systemic erythromycins may cause oral candidiasis; the leukopenic and thrombocytopenic effects of sulfonamides may result in an increased incidence of certain microbial infections, delayed healing, and gingival bleeding

   Other medications, especially alfentanil; coumarin- or indandione-derivative anticoagulants; hydantoin anticonvulsants; oral antidiabetic agents; carbamazepine; chloramphenicol; cyclosporine; other hemolytics; other hepatotoxic medications; lincomycins; methenamine; methotrexate; or xanthines, especially theophylline

   Other medical problems, especially blood dyscrasias, glucose-6-phosphate dehydrogenase (G6PD) deficiency, hepatic function impairment, porphyria, or renal function impairment

### Proper use of this medication

» Maintaining adequate fluid intake; taking with food
» Not giving to infants under 2 months of age
   Proper administration technique for oral liquids; not using after expiration date
» Compliance with full course of therapy
» Importance of not missing doses and taking at evenly spaced times
» Proper dosing
   Missed dose: Taking as soon as possible; not taking if almost time for next dose; not doubling dose
» Proper storage

### Precautions while using this medication

» Regular visits to physician to check blood counts, especially in long-term therapy

Checking with physician if no improvement within a few days
» Possible photosensitivity reactions
   Using caution in use of regular toothbrushes, dental floss, and toothpicks; delaying dental work until blood counts have returned to normal; checking with physician or dentist concerning proper oral hygiene

### Side/adverse effects

Signs of potential side effects, especially blood dyscrasias, crystalluria, goiter, hematuria, hepatitis, hypersensitivity reactions, interstitial nephritis, Lyell's syndrome, Stevens-Johnson syndrome, thyroid function disturbance, and tubular necrosis

## Oral Dosage Forms

### ERYTHROMYCIN ETHYLSUCCINATE AND SULFISOXAZOLE ACETYL FOR ORAL SUSPENSION USP

#### Usual adult and adolescent dose

Use is not indicated in adults.

#### Usual pediatric dose

Antibacterial—

Infants up to 2 months of age:
   Use is contraindicated since sulfonamides may cause kernicterus in neonates.
Infants and children 2 months of age and over:
   The dose can be calculated, based on either the equivalent of erythromycin or sulfisoxazole base, as follows—
   Oral, 12.5 mg (erythromycin) per kg of body weight every six hours for ten days; or
   Oral, 37.5 mg (sulfisoxazole) per kg of body weight every six hours for ten days.
The following dosage schedule can also be used:

| Body Weight | Dose (Every 6 hours) |
|---|---|
| Less than 8 kg<br>   Less than 18 lb | Adjust dosage by body weight |
| 8 kg (18 lb) | 1/2 teaspoonful (2.5 mL) |
| 16 kg (35 lb) | 1 teaspoonful (5 mL) |
| 24 kg (53 lb) | 1 1/2 teaspoonfuls (7.5 mL) |
| Over 45 kg<br>   (over 100 lb) | 2 teaspoonfuls (10 mL) |

Note: The maximum dose for children should not exceed 6 grams (sulfisoxazole) daily.

#### Strength(s) usually available

U.S.—

   200 mg of erythromycin and 600 mg of sulfisoxazole per 5 mL (when reconstituted according to manufacturer's instructions) (Rx) [*Eryzole; Pediazole; Sulfimycin;* GENERIC].

Canada—

   200 mg of erythromycin and 600 mg of sulfisoxazole per 5 mL (when reconstituted according to manufacturer's instructions) (Rx) [*Pediazole*].

#### Auxiliary labeling

• Refrigerate.
• Shake well.
• Take with water.
• Avoid too much sun or use of sunlamp.
• Continue medicine for full time of treatment.
• Beyond-use date.

---

Revised: 08/27/92
Interim revision: 03/18/94

---

# ESMOLOL   Systemic†

VA CLASSIFICATION (Primary/Secondary): CV100/CV300

Note: For a listing of dosage forms and brand names by country availability, see *Dosage Forms* section(s). For a listing of brand names for the articles in this monograph, refer to the General Index.

---

†Not commercially available in Canada.

## Category

Antiadrenergic; antiarrhythmic.

## Indications

Note: Bracketed information in the *Indications* section refers to uses that are not included in U.S. product labeling.

**Accepted**

Arrhythmias, cardiac (treatment)—Esmolol is indicated for rapid and short-term control of ventricular rate in patients with atrial fibrillation or atrial flutter in perioperative, postoperative, or other emergency situations. It is also indicated in noncompensatory sinus tachycardia judged by the physician to need intervention. [Esmolol is used for control of heart rate in patients with myocardial ischemia.] It is not recommended for use in chronic situations where transfer to another agent is anticipated.

Tachycardia, intraoperative and postoperative (treatment)—Esmolol is indicated for the treatment of refractory tachycardia that occurs during surgery, on emergence from anesthesia, and in the postoperative period. It is recommended for use only when other treatable causes of tachycardia, such as bleeding or hypovolemia, have been ruled out.

Hypertension, intraoperative and postoperative (treatment)—Esmolol is indicated for the treatment of refractory hypertension that occurs during surgery, on emergence from anesthesia, and in the postoperative period. Esmolol is not considered to be a first-line agent and should be reserved for situations in which agents known to be effective in treating the etiology of the hypertension have failed. It is not recommended for use in patients with hypertension secondary to the vasoconstriction associated with hypothermia.

## Pharmacology/Pharmacokinetics

**Physicochemical characteristics**

Molecular weight—331.84.

**Mechanism of action/Effect**

Like other beta-blockers, esmolol blocks the agonistic effect of the sympathetic neurotransmitters by competing for receptor binding sites. Because it predominantly blocks the beta-1 receptors in cardiac tissue, it is said to be cardioselective. In general, so-called cardioselective beta-blockers are relatively cardioselective; at lower doses they block beta-1 receptors only but begin to block beta-2 receptors as the dose increases. At therapeutic dosages, esmolol does not have intrinsic sympathomimetic activity (ISA) or membrane-stabilizing (quinidine-like) activity.

Antiarrhythmic activity is due to blockade of adrenergic stimulation of cardiac pacemaker potentials. In the Vaughan Williams classification of antiarrhythmics, beta-blockers are considered to be class II agents.

**Protein binding**

Moderate (55%).

**Biotransformation**

Rapid hydrolysis by esterases in red blood cells to a free acid metabolite (with 1/1500 the activity of esmolol) and methanol.

**Half-life**

Esmolol—
Distribution: Approximately 2 minutes.
Elimination: Approximately 9 minutes.
Free acid metabolite—
Approximately 3.7 hours (increased up to tenfold in renal failure).

**Time to steady-state blood concentration**

With loading dose—Within 5 minutes.

Without loading dose—Approximately 30 minutes.

Note: Use of a loading dose expedites achievement of constant plasma drug concentrations, but true steady-state occurs at 30 minutes, with or without a loading dose.

**Duration of action**

10 to 20 minutes after infusion is discontinued.

**Elimination**

Renal, almost entirely as metabolite.

## Precautions to Consider

**Carcinogenicity/Mutagenicity**

Studies have not been done in either animals or humans.

**Pregnancy/Reproduction**

Fertility—Studies have not been done in either animals or humans.

Pregnancy—Adequate and well-controlled studies in humans have not been done.

Studies in rats and rabbits at intravenous doses of up to 10 and 3 times the maximum human maintenance dose (MHMD), respectively, for 30 minutes daily showed no evidence of maternal toxicity, embryotoxicity, or teratogenicity. However, doses of approximately 30 and 8 times the MHMD in rats and rabbits, respectively, caused maternal toxicity, death, and increased fetal resorptions.

FDA Pregnancy Category C.

**Breast-feeding**

Although it is not known whether esmolol is distributed into human breast milk, problems have not been documented.

**Pediatrics**

Appropriate studies on the relationship of age to the effects of esmolol have not been performed in the pediatric population. However, limited experience with esmolol in the evaluation and management of pediatric tachyarrhythmias have not demonstrated pediatrics-specific problems that would limit the usefulness of esmolol in children.

**Geriatrics**

Although appropriate studies on the relationship of age to the effects of esmolol have not been performed in the geriatric population, the elderly may be less sensitive to some of the effects of beta-blockers. However, reduced metabolic and excretory capabilities in many elderly patients may lead to increased myocardial depression and require dosage reduction of beta-blockers. The net effect is uncertain; dosage adjustment should be based on clinical response.

**Drug interactions and/or related problems**

The following drug interactions and/or related problems have been selected on the basis of their potential clinical significance (possible mechanism in parentheses where appropriate)—not necessarily inclusive (» = major clinical significance):

Note: Combinations containing any of the following medications, depending on the amount present, may also interact with this medication.

Because of esmolol's short duration of action and the short periods of time over which it is used, many of the drug interactions associated with other beta-blockers do not apply.

» Antidiabetic agents, sulfonylurea or
» Insulin
(esmolol may mask certain symptoms of developing hypoglycemia, such as increases in pulse rate and blood pressure)

Gallamine or
Metocurine or
Pancuronium or
Tubocurarine
(esmolol may potentiate and prolong the action of nondepolarizing neuromuscular blocking agents when used concurrently; careful postoperative monitoring of the patient may be necessary following concurrent or sequential use, especially if there is a possibility of incomplete reversal of neuromuscular blockade)

Hypotension-producing medications, other (See *Appendix II*)
(antihypertensive effects may be potentiated when these medications are used concurrently with esmolol; dosage adjustments should be based on blood pressure measurements)

» Monoamine oxidase (MAO) inhibitors, including furazolidone, procarbazine, and selegiline
(possible significant hypertension may theoretically occur up to 14 days following discontinuation of the MAO inhibitor; although sufficient clinical reports are lacking, concurrent use with esmolol is not recommended)

Phenytoin
(concurrent use of esmolol with intravenous phenytoin may produce additive cardiac depressant effects)

Reserpine
(concurrent use with esmolol may result in additive and possibly excessive beta-adrenergic blockade; close observation is recommended since bradycardia and hypotension may occur)

» Sympathomimetics
(concurrent use of esmolol with sympathomimetic amines having beta-adrenergic stimulant activity may result in mutual but short-lived inhibition of therapeutic effects)

» Xanthines, especially aminophylline or theophylline
(concurrent use with esmolol may result in mutual inhibition of therapeutic effects; in addition, concurrent use of beta-blockers with the xanthines [except dyphylline] may decrease theophylline clearance, especially in patients with increased theophylline clearance induced by smoking; concurrent use requires careful monitoring)

**Medical considerations/Contraindications**

The medical considerations/contraindications included here have been selected on the basis of their potential clinical significance (reasons given in parentheses where appropriate)—not necessarily inclusive (» = major clinical significance).

*Except under special circumstances, this medication should not be used when the following medical problems exist:*

» Cardiac failure, overt or
» Cardiogenic shock or
» Heart block, 2nd- or 3rd-degree atrioventricular (AV) block or
» Sinus bradycardia (heart rate less than 45 beats per minute)
(risk of further myocardial depression; may be used with extreme caution in some patients with cardiac failure [e.g., high output failure associated with thyrotoxicosis])

*Risk-benefit should be considered when the following medical problems exist:*

» Allergy, history of or
» Asthma, bronchial or
» Emphysema or nonallergenic bronchitis
(esmolol may promote bronchospasm and block the bronchodilating effect of epinephrine; however, because esmolol is cardioselective and may be less likely to cause such effects than less cardioselective beta-blockers, it may be used with caution)
» Congestive heart failure
(risk of further depression of myocardial contractility)
» Diabetes mellitus
(all beta-blockers may mask tachycardia associated with hypoglycemia, but not dizziness and sweating)
    Renal function impairment
    Sensitivity to esmolol

### Patient monitoring

The following may be especially important in patient monitoring (other tests may be warranted in some patients, depending on condition; » = major clinical significance):

» Blood pressure and
» Electrocardiogram (ECG) and
» Heart rate
(should be carefully monitored during intravenous administration)

## Side/Adverse Effects

The following side/adverse effects have been selected on the basis of their potential clinical significance (possible signs and symptoms in parentheses where appropriate)—not necessarily inclusive:

**Those indicating need for medical attention**
Incidence less frequent
*Confusion; redness or swelling at place of injection; reduced peripheral circulation* (cold hands and feet)
Incidence rare
*Bradycardia, especially less than 50 beats per minute; breathing difficulty and/or wheezing; chest pain; fainting; fever; mental depression*

**Those indicating need for medical attention only if they continue or are bothersome**
Incidence more frequent
*Hypotension* (dizziness; sweating)—symptomatic in about 12% of patients, asymptomatic in about 25% of patients
Note: *Hypotension* can occur at any dose, but is dose-related.

Incidence less frequent
*Anxiety or nervousness; drowsiness or tiredness; flushing or pale skin; headache; nausea or vomiting*

## Overdose

For specific information on the agents used in the management of esmolol overdose, see:
• *Atropine* in *Anticholinergics/Antispasmodics (Systemic)* monograph;
• *Bronchodilators, Theophylline (Systemic)* monograph;
• *Glucagon (Systemic)* monograph;
• *Isoproterenol* in *Bronchodilators, Adrenergic (Systemic)* monograph;
• *Lidocaine (Systemic)* monograph; and/or
• *Sympathomimetic Agents—Cardiovascular Use (Parenteral-Systemic)* monograph.

For more information on the management of overdose or unintentional ingestion, **contact a Poison Control Center** (see *Poison Control Center Listing*).

### Clinical effects of overdose (in order of occurrence)
The following effects have been selected on the basis of their potential clinical significance (possible signs and symptoms in parentheses where appropriate)—not necessarily inclusive:
*Slow heartbeat; dizziness, severe, or fainting; drowsiness, severe; difficulty in breathing; bluish-colored fingernails or palms of hands; seizures*

### Treatment of overdose
In most cases, symptoms of esmolol overdose disappear quickly after esmolol is withdrawn.
Specific treatment—
Clinical reports are increasing for the successful use of glucagon to counteract the cardiovascular effects (bradycardia, hypotension) resulting from overdose with beta-blockers. An intravenous dose of 2 to 3 mg is administered over a period of 30 seconds and repeated if necessary, followed by an intravenous glucagon infusion at the rate of 5 mg per hour until the patient has been stabilized.
Supportive care—
Bradycardia—Atropine sulfate may be administered intravenously to correct severe bradycardia if the patient is hypotensive. If vagal blockade is unresponsive, atropine may be repeated or intravenous isoproterenol or dobutamine may be given cautiously. Intravenous epinephrine or a transvenous pacemaker may be necessary.
Premature ventricular contractions—Intravenous lidocaine or phenytoin (quinidine, procainamide, and disopyramide should be avoided since they may further depress myocardial function).
Cardiac failure—Provision of oxygen. Digitalization of patient and/or administration of diuretic.
Hypotension—Trendelenburg position and intravenous fluids (unless pulmonary edema is present). Intravenous administration of a vasopressor such as epinephrine, norepinephrine, dopamine, or dobutamine (some reports indicate epinephrine may be the agent of choice). Serial monitoring of blood pressure. Hypotension does not respond to beta-2 agonists. (See *Drug interactions and/or related problems* for precautions in use of sympathomimetic vasopressors.)
Bronchospasm—Administration of a beta-2 agonist such as isoproterenol and/or a theophylline derivative.

## General Dosing Information

The 250-mg-per-mL strength of esmolol hydrochloride injection must be diluted before it is administered by intravenous infusion. Concentrations of greater than 10 mg of esmolol hydrochloride per mL may produce irritation. The 10-mg-per-mL strength may be given by direct infusion.
If a reaction occurs at the infusion site, the infusion should be stopped and resumed at another site. Use of butterfly needles for administration is not recommended.
To convert to other antiarrhythmic therapy after control has been achieved with esmolol
—30 minutes after administration of the first dose of the alternative agent, infusion rate of esmolol should be reduced by one-half, and
—after the second dose of the alternative agent, if a satisfactory response is maintained for 1 hour, esmolol should be discontinued.

### For treatment of adverse effects
Hypotension is usually reversed within 30 minutes after dosage reduction or withdrawal of esmolol.
Dosage reduction or withdrawal of esmolol is recommended at the first sign of congestive heart failure.

## Parenteral Dosage Forms
### ESMOLOL HYDROCHLORIDE INJECTION

**Usual adult dose**
Antiarrhythmic—
Dosage is established by means of a series of loading and maintenance doses
Loading: Intravenous infusion, 500 mcg (0.5 mg) per kg of body weight per minute for one minute, followed by
Maintenance: Intravenous infusion, 50 mcg (0.05 mg) per kg of body weight per minute for four minutes.
If an adequate response is observed at the end of five minutes, the infusion dosage should be maintained with periodic adjustments as needed.
If an adequate response is not observed at the end of the five minutes, the sequence is repeated with an increment of 50 mcg (0.05 mg) per kg of body weight per minute in the maintenance dose
Loading: Intravenous infusion, 500 mcg (0.5 mg) per kg of body weight per minute for one minute, followed by
Maintenance: Intravenous infusion, 100 mcg (0.1 mg) per kg of body weight per minute for four minutes.
The sequence is repeated until an adequate response is obtained, with an increment of 50 mcg (0.05 mg) per kg of body weight per minute in the maintenance dose at each step. As the desired endpoint (defined by desired heart rate or undesirable decrease in blood pressure) is approached, the loading dose may be omitted

and increments in the maintenance dose reduced to 25 mcg (0.025 mg) per kg of body weight per minute or less. If desired, the interval between titration steps may be increased from five to ten minutes. The established maintenance dose usually does not exceed 200 mcg (0.2 mg) per kg of body weight per minute and can be given for up to forty-eight hours.

Note: Because of the time required for titration, the above dosage regimen may not be optimal for intraoperative use.

Tachycardia, intraoperative or postoperative or
Hypertension, intraoperative or postoperative
Initial: Intravenous, 250 to 500 mcg (0.25 to 0.5 mg) per kg of body weight over one minute.
Maintenance: Intravenous infusion, 50 mcg (0.05 mg) per kg of body weight per minute for four minutes.
If an adequate response is not observed, the sequence may be repeated, with an increment of 50 mcg (0.05 mg) per kg of body weight per minute in the maintenance dose
Initial: Intravenous, 250 to 500 mcg (0.25 to 0.5 mg) per kg of body weight over one minute.
Maintenance: Intravenous infusion, 100 mcg (0.1 mg) per kg of body weight per minute for four minutes.

The sequence may be repeated up to four times if needed, with an increment of 50 mcg (0.05 mg) per kg of body weight per minute in the maintenance dose at each step.

**Usual adult prescribing limits**
Maintenance—Up to 200 mcg (0.2 mg) per kg of body weight per minute (because of the risk of hypotension).

**Usual pediatric dose**
Arrhythmias, supraventricular—
Intravenous infusion, 50 mcg (0.05 mg) per kg of body weight per minute; dosage may be titrated upwards every ten minutes up to 300 mcg (0.3 mg) per kg of body weight per minute.

**Strength(s) usually available**
U.S.—
10 mg per mL (100 mg per 10-mL single-dose vial) (Rx) [*Brevibloc*].
Note: The 10-mg-per-mL strength is prediluted and may be used for the loading dose.
250 mg per mL (2500 mg per 10-mL ampul) (Rx) [*Brevibloc* (alcohol 25%)].
Note: The 250-mg-per-mL strength must be diluted before use. It is not intended for direct intravenous injection.
Canada—
Not commercially available.

**Packaging and storage**
Store below 40 °C (104 °F), preferably between 15 and 30 °C (59 and 86 °F), unless otherwise specified by manufacturer. Not adversely affected by freezing.

**Preparation of dosage form**
Esmolol hydrochloride injection (250-mg-per-mL strength) is prepared for administration by intravenous infusion by aseptically removing 20 mL from a 500-mL bottle of intravenous fluid (5% dextrose injection, 5% dextrose in Ringer's injection, 5% dextrose and 0.45% sodium chloride injection, 5% dextrose and 0.9% sodium chloride injection, lactated Ringer's injection, 0.45% sodium chloride injection, or 0.9% sodium chloride injection) and then adding 5 grams of esmolol hydrochloride injection to the bottle, producing a solution containing 10 mg of esmolol hydrochloride per mL.

**Stability**
Diluted solutions of esmolol hydrochloride are stable for at least 24 hours at room temperature.

**Incompatibilities**
Not compatible with 5% sodium bicarbonate injection.

**Auxiliary labeling**
For 250-mg-per-mL vial
• Must be diluted before administration.

**Caution**
Confusion caused by two significantly different concentrations of esmolol has resulted in massive overdoses, including several deaths. The incidents occurred when the 250-mg-per-mL ampul, which requires dilution prior to administration, was given undiluted. The 250-mg-per-mL ampul of esmolol must be diluted before administration. Caution should be utilized when dispensing, using, and storing this medication.

**Selected Bibliography**
Angaran DM, Schultz NJ, Tschida VH. Esmolol hydrochloride: an ultrashort-acting, beta-adrenergic blocking agent. Clin Pharm 1986 Apr; 5: 288-303.
Covinsky JO. Esmolol: a novel cardioselective, titratable, intravenous beta-blocker with ultrashort half-life. DICP, Ann Pharmacother 1987; 21: 316-21.
Murthy VS, Frishman WH. Controlled beta-receptor blockade with esmolol and flestolol. Pharmacother 1988; 8 (3): 168-82.

Revised: 09/13/94
Interim revision: 04/19/96

**ESTAZOLAM**—See *Benzodiazepines (Systemic)*

**ESTERIFIED ESTROGEN–CONTAINING COMBINATIONS**—
Esterified Estrogens and Methyltestosterone (Systemic)—See *Androgens and Estrogens (Systemic)*

**ESTRADIOL**—See *Estrogens (Systemic)*; *Estrogens (Vaginal)*

**ESTRADIOL-CONTAINING COMBINATIONS**—
Testosterone and Estradiol (Systemic)—See *Androgens and Estrogens (Systemic)*

# ESTRAMUSTINE  Systemic

VA CLASSIFICATION (Primary): AN900
Note: For a listing of dosage forms and brand names by country availability, see *Dosage Forms* section(s). For a listing of brand names for the articles in this monograph, refer to the General Index.

## Category
Antineoplastic.

## Indications
**Accepted**
Carcinoma, prostatic (treatment)—Estramustine is indicated for palliative treatment of metastatic and/or progressive carcinoma of the prostate gland.

## Pharmacology/Pharmacokinetics
**Physicochemical characteristics**
Molecular weight—Estramustine phosphate sodium: 564.35.

**Mechanism of action/Effect**
Exact mechanism of antineoplastic action is unknown. Structurally, estramustine is a phosphorylated combination of estradiol and mechlorethamine (nitrogen mustard). However, estramustine has very weak alkylating activity and may be effective in some patients refractory to estrogen therapy. Therefore, its antineoplastic activity may be due to the estrogen component, a direct effect of estramustine or one of its metabolites, other antimitotic activity, or a combination of effects. Prolonged use elevates total plasma estradiol concentrations to within ranges similar to those produced in prostatic carcinoma patients given conventional estradiol therapy. Estrogenic effects (changes in circulating concentrations of steroids and pituitary hormones) are also similar to those produced by estradiol. A suppressive effect on the hypothalamic-hypophyseal-gonadal axis with a resultant reduction in serum testosterone concentrations may also be involved. Estramustine is highly localized in prostatic tissue because of binding to an estramustine-specific protein.

## Absorption

Well absorbed (up to 75%) from the gastrointestinal tract; impaired by milk, milk products, and other substances high in calcium.

## Biotransformation

Rapidly dephosphorylated during absorption into peripheral circulation, then estramustine is oxidized and hydrolyzed to estromustine, with low levels of estradiol and estrone, and to mechlorethamine; metabolism is by conjugation in the liver.

## Half-life

Multiphasic; 20 hours (terminal phase).

## Elimination

Biliary/fecal; renal (minor).

# Precautions to Consider

## Cross-sensitivity and/or related problems

Patients sensitive to estradiol or mechlorethamine may be sensitive to estramustine also.

## Carcinogenicity/Mutagenicity

Secondary malignancies are potential delayed effects of many antineoplastic agents, although it is not clear whether the effect is related to their mutagenic or immunosuppressive action. The effect of dose and duration of therapy is also unknown, although risk seems to increase with long-term use. Although information is limited, available data seem to indicate that the carcinogenic risk is greatest with the alkylating agents.

Studies with estramustine have not been done. Antimitotic agents have been associated with an increased risk of development of secondary carcinomas in humans. Long-term continuous administration of estrogens in some animals has been associated with an increased frequency of carcinomas of the breast and liver. Compounds structurally similar to estramustine are carcinogenic in mice.

Although estramustine was not found to be mutagenic in Ames tests, both estradiol and nitrogen mustard alone are mutagenic.

## Pregnancy/Reproduction

Fertility—Gonadal suppression, resulting in azoospermia, has been reported in patients taking estramustine. These effects appear to be related to dose and length of therapy and may be irreversible. On the other hand, patients impotent from previous therapy may regain potency when taking estramustine.

Antimitotic agents have been reported to cause alterations in sperm cells, which could result in mutagenicity and teratogenicity.

## Geriatrics

Appropriate studies on the relationship of age to the effects of estramustine have not been performed in the geriatric population. However, elderly patients are more likely to have age-related renal function impairment and/or peripheral vascular disease, which may require caution in patients receiving estrogens.

## Drug interactions and/or related problems

The following drug interactions and/or related problems have been selected on the basis of their potential clinical significance (possible mechanism in parentheses where appropriate)—not necessarily inclusive (» = major clinical significance):

Note: Combinations containing any of the following medications, depending on the amount present, may also interact with this medication.

Calcium-containing medications or
Calcium supplements
   (calcium binds with estramustine in the gastrointestinal tract and forms an insoluble calcium phosphate salt, which is not absorbed; simultaneous administration should be avoided)

Corticosteroids, glucocorticoid
   (concurrent use with estrogens may alter the metabolism and protein binding of the glucocorticoids, leading to decreased clearance, increased elimination half-life, and increased therapeutic and toxic effects of the glucocorticoids; glucocorticoid dosage adjustment may be required during and following concurrent use)

Corticotropin (chronic therapeutic use)
   (concurrent use with estrogens may potentiate the anti-inflammatory effects of endogenous cortisol [adrenal secretion of endogenous cortisol is increased by corticotropin])

» Hepatotoxic medications (See *Appendix II*)
   (concurrent use of these medications with estrogens may increase the risk of hepatotoxicity)

» Smoking, tobacco
   (not recommended during estrogen therapy because of the increased risk of serious cardiovascular side effects, including cerebrovascular accident, transient ischemic attacks, thrombophlebitis, and pulmonary embolism; risk increases with increasing tobacco usage and with age)

Vaccines, killed virus
   (because normal defense mechanisms may be suppressed by estramustine therapy, the patient's antibody response to the vaccine may be decreased. The interval between discontinuation of medications that cause immunosuppression and restoration of the patient's ability to respond to the vaccine depends on the intensity and type of immunosuppression-causing medication used, the underlying disease, and other factors; estimates vary from 3 months to 1 year)

Vaccines, live virus
   (because normal defense mechanisms may be suppressed by estramustine therapy, concurrent use with a live virus vaccine may potentiate the replication of the vaccine virus, may increase the side/adverse effects of the vaccine virus, and/or may decrease the patient's antibody response to the vaccine; immunization of these patients should be undertaken only with extreme caution after careful review of the patient's hematologic status and only with the knowledge and consent of the physician managing the estramustine therapy. The interval between discontinuation of medications that cause immunosuppression and restoration of the patient's ability to respond to the vaccine depends on the intensity and type of immunosuppression-causing medication used, the underlying disease, and other factors; estimates vary from 3 months to 1 year. Patients with leukemia in remission should not receive live virus vaccine until at least 3 months after their last chemotherapy. In addition, immunization with oral poliovirus vaccine should be postponed in persons in close contact with the patient, especially family members)

## Laboratory value alterations

The following have been selected on the basis of their potential clinical significance (possible effect in parentheses where appropriate)—not necessarily inclusive (» = major clinical significance):

With diagnostic test results
» Metyrapone test
   (reduced response)
Norepinephrine-induced platelet aggregability
   (may be increased)
Sulfobromophthalein (BSP) test
   (increased BSP retention)
Thyroid function test
   (protein-bound thyroxine [$T_4$] is increased; serum free $T_4$ concentrations may be unchanged or decreased; triiodothyronine [$T_3$] serum resin uptake is decreased, because estrogens increase serum thyroid-binding globulin [TBG]; serum $T_3$ may be increased)

With physiology/laboratory test values
Alanine aminotransferase (AST [SGOT]) values, serum and
Bilirubin concentrations, serum and
Lactate dehydrogenase (LDH) values, serum
   (may be increased)

Antithrombin 3 concentrations and
Folate concentrations, serum and
Pregnanediol excretion and
Pyridoxine concentrations
   (may be decreased)

Ceruloplasmin and
Cortisol and
Glucose and
Phospholipids and
Prolactin and
Prothrombin and clotting factors VII, VIII, IX, and X and
Sodium and
Triglycerides
   (serum concentrations may be increased)
Phosphate
   (serum concentrations may be decreased)

## Medical considerations/Contraindications

The medical considerations/contraindications included here have been selected on the basis of their potential clinical significance (reasons given in parentheses where appropriate)—not necessarily inclusive (» = major clinical significance).

*Except under special circumstances, this medication should not be used when the following medical problems exist:*
- » Thromboembolic disorders, active, including recent myocardial infarction or stroke or
- » Thrombophlebitis, active
  (may be aggravated by estrogen component; an exception may be made when the actual tumor mass is the cause of the thromboembolic phenomenon)

*Risk-benefit should be considered when the following medical problems exist:*

Asthma or
Cardiac insufficiency or
Epilepsy or
Mental depression, or history of or
Migraine headaches or
Renal function impairment
(fluid retention sometimes caused by estrogen component may aggravate these conditions)

Bone disease, metabolic, associated with hypercalcemia or
Renal insufficiency
(estrogens influence metabolism of calcium and phosphorus)

Bone marrow depression, moderate to severe

Cerebrovascular disease or
Coronary artery disease or
- » Thrombophlebitis, thrombosis, or thromboembolic disorders, history of, especially if associated with estrogen therapy
  (risk of thromboembolic disorders caused by estrogens)
- » Chickenpox, existing or recent (including recent exposure) or
- » Herpes zoster
  (risk of severe generalized disease)

Cholestatic jaundice, history of, including previous jaundice that occurred with estrogens or as a reaction to other medication

Diabetes mellitus
(glucose tolerance may be decreased)

Gallbladder disease, or history of, especially gallstones

Hepatic function impairment
(reduced metabolism and possible hepatotoxicity)
- » Hypercalcemia associated with metastatic breast disease
- » Peptic ulcer
- » Sensitivity to estramustine

### Patient monitoring
The following are especially important in patient monitoring (other tests may be warranted in some patients, depending on condition; (» = major clinical significance):

Acid phosphatase values, serum and/or

Alkaline phosphatase values, serum
(to assess response; elevated concentrations should be reduced)

Blood counts, complete and
Platelet counts
(may be appropriate at periodic intervals, although leukopenia and thrombocytopenia are rare with estramustine)

Blood pressure and
Hepatic function
(determinations recommended at periodic intervals)

Calcium concentrations, serum and
Phosphate concentrations, serum
(recommended at periodic intervals, especially in patients with bone metastases)

## Side/Adverse Effects

The following side/adverse effects have been selected on the basis of their potential clinical significance (possible signs and symptoms in parentheses where appropriate)—not necessarily inclusive:

**Those indicating need for medical attention**
Incidence more frequent
*Sodium and fluid retention* (swelling of feet or lower legs)
Incidence rare
*Allergic reaction* (skin rash or fever); *anemia* (unusual tiredness or weakness); *leukopenia* (usually asymptomatic; rarely, fever or chills; cough or hoarseness; lower back or side pain; painful or difficult urination); *thrombocytopenia* (usually asymptomatic; rarely, unusual bleeding or bruising; black, tarry stools; blood in urine or stools; pinpoint red spots on skin); *thrombosis* (severe or sudden headaches; sudden loss of coordination; pains in chest, groin, or leg, especially

calf of leg; sudden and unexplained shortness of breath; sudden slurred speech; sudden vision changes; weakness or numbness in arm or leg)

**Those indicating need for medical attention only if they continue or are bothersome**
Incidence more frequent
*Breast tenderness or enlargement*—incidence 20 to 50%; *decreased interest in sex*—occurs in most patients; *diarrhea*—incidence 20 to 50%; *nausea*—incidence 20 to 50%
Incidence less frequent
*Trouble in sleeping; vomiting*
Note: *Vomiting* is intolerable in approximately 8% of patients.

## Overdose
For more information on the management of overdose or unintentional ingestion, **contact a Poison Control Center** (see *Poison Control Center Listing*).

**Treatment of overdose**
Treatment of overdose is symptomatic and supportive and should include:
Removal of gastric contents by gastric lavage.
Monitoring of hematologic and hepatic parameters for at least 6 weeks.

## Patient Consultation
As an aid to patient consultation, refer to *Advice for the Patient, Estramustine (Systemic)*.

In providing consultation, consider emphasizing the following selected information (» = major clinical significance):

**Before using this medication**
- » Conditions affecting use, especially:
  Sensitivity to estramustine, estradiol, or mechlorethamine
  Pregnancy—Use not recommended because of mutagenic and teratogenic potential
  Other medications, especially hepatotoxic medications
  Other medical problems, especially chickenpox, herpes zoster, active or history of thromboembolic disorders (including recent myocardial infarction or stroke), active or history of thrombophlebitis, or peptic ulcer
  Smoking

**Proper use of this medication**
- » Importance of not taking more or less medication than the amount prescribed
  For best results, taking 1 hour before or 2 hours after meals or milk or milk products
- » Frequently causes nausea and sometimes causes vomiting; checking with physician before discontinuing medication
  Checking with physician if vomiting occurs shortly after dose is taken
- » Proper dosing
  Missed dose: Not taking at all; not doubling doses
- » Proper storage

**Precautions while using this medication**
- » Importance of close monitoring by physician
- » Avoiding immunizations unless approved by physician; other persons in patient's household should avoid immunizations with oral poliovirus vaccine; avoiding persons who have taken oral poliovirus vaccine or wearing a protective mask that covers nose and mouth

**Side/adverse effects**
Signs of potential side effects, especially allergic reaction, anemia, leukopenia, thrombocytopenia, and thrombosis

## General Dosing Information
Patients receiving estramustine should be under supervision of a physician experienced in cancer chemotherapy.

A trial period of 30 to 90 days is usually considered adequate for determining whether or not a response will occur.

Estramustine therapy may be continued for as long as a favorable response is maintained.

Nausea and vomiting sometimes responds to treatment with phenothiazines but may be severe enough to necessitate withdrawal of estramustine in some patients.

### Diet/Nutrition
It is recommended that estramustine be taken 1 hour before or 2 hours after meals. Milk, milk products, calcium-rich foods, or calcium-containing medications should not be taken simultaneously.

## Oral Dosage Forms

### ESTRAMUSTINE PHOSPHATE SODIUM CAPSULES

**Usual adult dose**
Carcinoma, prostatic—
　Oral, 600 mg (base) per square meter of body surface per day in three divided doses (one hour before or two hours after meals) or 14 mg per kg of body weight (range 10 to 16 mg per kg) per day in three or four divided doses (one hour before or two hours after meals).

**Strength(s) usually available**
U.S.—
　140 mg (base) (Rx) [*Emcyt*].
Canada—
　140 mg (base) (Rx) [*Emcyt*].

**Packaging and storage**
Store between 2 and 8 °C (36 and 46 °F), in a tight container, unless otherwise specified by manufacturer. Protect from light.

**Auxiliary labeling**
• Take 1 hour before or 2 hours after meals.
• Avoid milk or milk products.

### Selected Bibliography

Hauser AR, Merryman R. Estramustine phosphate sodium. Drug Intell Clin Pharm 1984 May; 18: 368-74.
Dorr RT, Fritz WL. Cancer chemotherapy handbook. New York: Elsevier, 1980: 406-9.

Revised: 07/11/94

---

# ESTROGENS   Systemic

This monograph includes information on the following: Chlorotrianisene†; Conjugated Estrogens; Diethylstilbestrol; Estradiol; Esterified Estrogens; Estrone†; Estropipate; Ethinyl Estradiol; Quinestrol†.

VA CLASSIFICATION (Primary/Secondary):
Chlorotrianisene—HS300/AN500
Diethylstilbestrol—HS300/AN500; HS200; MS900
Estradiol—HS300/AN500; MS900
Estrogens, Conjugated—HS300/AN500; HS200; MS900
Estrogens, Esterified—HS300/AN500; MS900
Estrone—HS300/AN500
Estropipate—HS300/MS900
Ethinyl Estradiol—HS300/AN500; HS200; MS900
Quinestrol—HS300

Other commonly used names are: DES [Diethylstilbestrol] , Piperazine Estrone Sulfate [Estropipate]

Note: For a listing of dosage forms and brand names by country availability, see *Dosage Forms* section(s). For a listing of brand names for the articles in this monograph, refer to the General Index.

---

†Not commercially available in Canada.

---

## Category

Estrogen (systemic)—Chlorotrianisene; Conjugated Estrogens; Diethylstilbestrol; Esterified Estrogens; Estradiol; Estrone; Estropipate; Ethinyl Estradiol; Quinestrol.
Antineoplastic—Chlorotrianisene; Conjugated Estrogens Tablets USP; Diethylstilbestrol; Esterified Estrogens; Estradiol; Estradiol Valerate; Estrone; Ethinyl Estradiol.
Osteoporosis prophylactic—Conjugated Estrogens Tablets USP; Diethylstilbestrol Tablets USP; Diethylstilbestrol Tablets USP (Enteric-coated); Esterified Estrogens; Estradiol Tablets USP; Estradiol Transdermal System; Estropipate; Ethinyl Estradiol.

## Indications

Note: Bracketed information in the *Indications* section refers to uses that are not included in U.S. product labeling.

**Accepted**
Estrogen deficiency (treatment)
Vaginitis, atrophic (treatment)
Hypogonadism, female (treatment)
Vulvar squamous hyperplasia (treatment)
Ovarian failure, primary (treatment)
Menopause, vasomotor symptoms of (treatment)—Conjugated estrogens tablets, estradiol, estradiol valerate, esterified estrogens, estrone, estropipate, and quinestrol are indicated as estrogen replacement therapy in the treatment of atrophic vaginitis, female hypogonadism or castration, vulvar squamous hyperplasia, primary ovarian failure, and moderate to severe vasomotor symptoms associated with menopause.
　Chlorotrianisene is indicated as estrogen replacement therapy in the treatment of atrophic vaginitis, female hypogonadism, vulvar squamous hyperplasia, and moderate to severe vasomotor symptoms of menopause.
　Estradiol cypionate[1] and ethinyl estradiol[1] are indicated as estrogen replacement therapy in the treatment of female hypogonadism and moderate to severe vasomotor symptoms of menopause.
Bleeding, uterine, hormonal imbalance–induced (treatment)—Conjugated estrogens for injection, [estradiol valerate], estrone, and [ethinyl estra-diol] are indicated in the treatment of inorganic abnormal uterine bleeding caused by hormonal imbalance.
Carcinoma, breast (treatment)—Conjugated estrogens tablets, diethylstilbestrol tablets and enteric-coated tablets, [estradiol valerate], esterified estrogens[1], estradiol tablets, and [ethinyl estradiol] are indicated for treatment of metastatic breast carcinoma in selected men and postmenopausal women.
Carcinoma, prostatic (treatment)—Chlorotrianisene, conjugated estrogens tablets, diethylstilbestrol tablets, esterified estrogens[1], estradiol, estradiol valerate, estrone, and [ethinyl estradiol] are indicated for treatment of advanced prostatic carcinoma.
Osteoporosis, postmenopausal (prophylaxis)—Conjugated estrogens tablets, [diethylstilbestrol tablets][1], [diethylstilbestrol enteric-coated tablets][1], [esterified estrogens][1], estradiol tablets[1] and transdermal system, [ethinyl estradiol][1], and estropipate[1] are indicated in postmenopausal women to retard bone loss and estrogen deficiency–induced osteoporosis. Estrogen replacement therapy can reduce the rate of bone loss and fractures in postmenopausal women. Proper diet, calcium supplementation, and physical activity should also be encouraged along with estrogen replacement therapy.
[Osteoporosis, premenopausal, estrogen deficiency–induced (prophylaxis)][1]—Conjugated estrogens tablets, diethylstilbestrol tablets[1], diethylstilbestrol enteric-coated tablets[1], esterified estrogens[1], estradiol tablets[1] and transdermal estradiol system, ethinyl estradiol[1], and estropipate[1] are also used in premenopausal women who are estrogen-deficient to protect them against bone loss.
[Atherosclerotic disease (prophylaxis)][1]—Estrogens may be effective in the prevention of cardiovascular disease in postmenopausal women.
[Turner's syndrome (treatment)][1]—Ethinyl estradiol is used in the treatment of Turner's syndrome (gonadal dysgenesis).

Chlorotrianisene, estropipate, and quinestrol are infrequently prescribed for estrogen replacement therapy. Also, there is very little use for estrogens administered parenterally.

**Unaccepted**
The use of estrogens to reduce postpartum breast engorgement is not recommended. In many patients, postpartum breast engorgement is a benign, self-limited condition that may respond to breast support and mild analgesics, such as acetaminophen and ibuprofen. Evidence supporting the efficacy of estrogens for this indication is lacking. Therefore, the questionable benefits of administering the large doses of estrogens required for this indication are outweighed by the risk of increasing the incidence of puerperal thromboembolism.
Ethinyl estradiol, conjugated estrogens, and diethylstilbestrol tablets have been used as postcoital contraceptives (the "morning-after pill"), primarily in emergency care situations, such as the management of rape or incest victims. However, the combination oral contraceptive, norgestrel and ethinyl estradiol, is more commonly prescribed for this indication.

---

[1]Not included in Canadian product labeling.

## Pharmacology/Pharmacokinetics

**Physicochemical characteristics**
Source—
　Naturally occurring compounds include estradiol ($E_2$), conjugated estrogens (sodium estrone sulfate, sodium equilin sulfate, and others

as found in equine urine), esterified estrogens (sodium sulfate esters of estrogenic substances, primarily estrone), and estrone ($E_1$).
Semisynthetic compounds include estradiol cypionate, estradiol valerate, estropipate, ethinyl estradiol, and quinestrol.
Synthetic compounds include chlorotrianisene, diethylstilbestrol, and diethylstilbestrol phosphate.

Molecular weight—
Chlorotrianisene: 380.87.
Diethylstilbestrol: 268.35.
Diethylstilbestrol diphosphate: 428.31.
Estradiol: 272.39.
Estradiol cypionate: 396.57.
Estradiol valerate: 356.50.
Estrone: 270.37.
Estropipate: 436.56.
Ethinyl estradiol: 296.41.
Quinestrol: 364.53.

## Mechanism of action/Effect

At the cellular level, estrogens increase the synthesis of DNA, RNA, and various proteins in target tissues. Pituitary mass is also increased. Estrogens reduce the release of gonadotropin-releasing hormone from the hypothalamus, leading to a reduction in release of follicle-stimulating hormone and luteinizing hormone from the pituitary.

For estrogen replacement—
In healthy females, endogenous estrogens maintain genitourinary function and vasomotor stability. Estrogens are used as replacement therapy to alleviate or prevent symptoms caused by the decreased amounts of estrogens produced by the ovaries after natural or surgical menopause or other estrogen-deficiency states.

For prevention of postmenopausal osteoporosis—
During periods of estrogen deficiency, the rate of bone resorption by osteoclasts greatly exceeds the rate of bone formation by osteoblasts. Estrogen replacement therapy prevents this accelerated bone loss by inhibiting bone resorption to a level where the near equilibrium between bone resorption and formation is restored. However, estrogens do not replace previously lost bone or significantly increase total bone mass.

For prostatic carcinoma—
Inhibition of pituitary secretion of luteinizing hormone and a possible minor, direct effect on the testis, resulting in decreased serum concentrations of testosterone.

## Distribution

To most tissues; higher affinity for adipose tissue.

## Protein binding

Moderate to high (50 to 80% to albumin and sex hormone binding globulin).

## Biotransformation

Primarily hepatic; some metabolism also occurs in muscle, kidneys, and gonads. The metabolic sites for all synthetic estrogens have not been completely determined, although some seem to undergo hepatic change.

## Elimination

Primarily renal excretion of metabolites, some fecal; undergo extensive enterohepatic recirculation. Prolonged in obese patients.

# Precautions to Consider

## Carcinogenicity

Independent studies have shown an increased risk of endometrial cancer in postmenopausal women placed on unopposed (without a progestin) estrogen replacement therapy for prolonged periods. The risk of endometrial cancer in estrogen users, which appears to depend on duration of treatment and dose, was 5 to 10 times greater than in nonusers. However, studies have shown that administration of a progestin for 10 to 14 days of an estrogen cycle is associated with a lower incidence of endometrial hyperplasia and endometrial carcinoma than an estrogen-only cycle. There is no risk of endometrial cancer in patients who have undergone hysterectomies and, therefore, no documented need for concurrent progestin therapy.

Whether the use of systemic estrogens increases the incidence of breast cancer in some postmenopausal women is unresolved. Some large studies reported an increase in the relative risk for development of breast cancer. At present, however, the majority of data available does not seem to support this conclusion.

In certain animal species, long-term, continuous administration of estrogens increases the frequency of cancers of the breast, cervix, testis, uterus, vagina, and liver.

Estrogens have been reported to be associated with carcinoma of the male breast. Males treated with estrogens should have regular breast examinations.

## Pregnancy/Reproduction

Pregnancy—Estrogens are not recommended for use during pregnancy. Studies suggest an association of congenital malformations with use of some estrogens.

Diethylstilbestrol: Daughters of women who took diethylstilbestrol (DES) during pregnancy have developed abnormalities of the reproductive tract and, in rare cases, cancer of the vagina and/or uterine cervix upon reaching childbearing age. In addition, sons of women who took DES during pregnancy have developed urogenital tract abnormalities. Patients who become pregnant while taking estrogens should be informed of the potential risks to the fetus.

FDA Pregnancy Category X.

## Breast-feeding

Estrogens are distributed into breast milk. Use by nursing mothers is not recommended. Potential adverse effects in the nursing infant are not predictable.

Ethinyl estradiol—When used in high doses as an antineoplastic, traces of ethinyl estradiol are distributed into breast milk. Also, use of combination oral contraceptives containing ethinyl estradiol during lactation has been associated with a decrease in milk production and in the milk protein and nitrogen content. However, the magnitude of these effects was small and would only likely be of clinical significance in malnourished mothers.

## Pediatrics

Estrogens may accelerate epiphyseal closure. Therefore, estrogens should be used with caution in children and adolescents in whom bone growth is not complete.

## Geriatrics

Studies performed to date have not demonstrated geriatrics-specific problems that would limit the usefulness of estrogens in the elderly.

## Dental

Estrogens may predispose the patient to bleeding of the gingival tissues. In addition, gingival hyperplasia may occur during estrogen therapy, usually starting as gingivitis or gum inflammation. A strictly enforced program of teeth cleaning by a professional, combined with plaque control by the patient, will minimize growth rate and severity of gingival enlargement.

## Drug interactions and/or related problems

The following drug interactions and/or related problems have been selected on the basis of their potential clinical significance (possible mechanism in parentheses where appropriate)—not necessarily inclusive (» = major clinical significance):

Note: Combinations containing any of the following medications, depending on the amount present, may also interact with this medication.

» Bromocriptine
(estrogens may cause amenorrhea, interfering with effects of bromocriptine; concurrent use is not recommended)

Calcium supplements
(concurrent use with estrogens may increase calcium absorption; this can be used to therapeutic advantage)

Corticosteroids, glucocorticoid
(concurrent use with estrogens may alter the metabolism and protein binding of the glucocorticoids, leading to decreased clearance, increased elimination half-life, and increased therapeutic and toxic effects of the glucocorticoids; glucocorticoid dosage adjustment may be required during and following concurrent use)

Corticotropin (chronic therapeutic use)
(concurrent use with estrogens may potentiate the anti-inflammatory effects of endogenous cortisol induced by corticotropin)

» Cyclosporine
(estrogens have been reported to inhibit cyclosporine metabolism and thereby increase plasma concentrations of cyclosporine, possibly increasing the risk of hepatotoxicity and nephrotoxicity; concurrent use is recommended only with great caution and frequent monitoring of blood cyclosporine concentrations and liver and renal function)

» Hepatotoxic medications, especially dantrolene (See *Appendix II*)
(concurrent use of these medications with estrogens may increase the risk of hepatotoxicity; risk may be further increased with use in females over 35 years of age, prolonged use, or use in patients with a history of liver disease)

Smoking, tobacco
(data from studies on tobacco smoking and the use of high-dose
estrogen oral contraceptives indicate that there is an increased risk
of serious cardiovascular side effects, including cerebrovascular
accident, transient ischemic attacks, thrombophlebitis, and pulmonary embolism; risk increases with increasing tobacco usage
and with age, especially in women over 35 years of age; it is not
known whether any elevation of risk occurs with tobacco smoking
during the use of estrogen replacement therapy)
(metabolism of estrogens may also be increased by smoking, resulting in a decreased estrogenic effect)

Somatrem or
Somatropin
(in prepubertal patients, concurrent use of estrogens with somatrem
or somatropin may accelerate epiphyseal maturation)

Tamoxifen
(concurrent use may interfere with therapeutic effect of tamoxifen)

## Laboratory value alterations
The following have been selected on the basis of their potential clinical
significance (possible effect in parentheses where appropriate)—not
necessarily inclusive (» = major clinical significance):

With diagnostic test results
Fasting blood sugar (FBS) and
Glucose tolerance test
(may be altered by large doses of estrogens)

Metyrapone test
(reduced response)

Norepinephrine-induced platelet aggregability
(may be increased)

Thyroid function tests, such as:
Thyroxine ($T_4$) determinations
(protein-bound $T_4$ is increased; serum free $T_4$ concentrations may
be unchanged or decreased)
Triiodothyronine ($T_3$) determinations
(serum concentration may be increased, but $T_3$ resin uptake is decreased because estrogens increase serum thyroid-binding globin
[TBG]; free thyroid hormone levels remain unchanged; TBG is not
affected by transdermal estradiol)

With physiology/laboratory test values
Antithrombin III, serum and
Cholesterol, total, serum and
Folate, serum and
Lipoproteins, low density (LDL), serum and
Pregnanediol, urine and
Pyridoxine, serum
(concentrations may be decreased)

Calcium
(serum concentrations may be markedly elevated in immobilized
patients or in patients with breast cancer and bone metastases who
are treated with estrogens)

Ceruloplasmin and
Clotting factors VII, VIII, IX, and X and
Cortisol and
Glucose—especially in diabetic or prediabetic patients taking larger
doses of estrogens, and
Lipoproteins, high density (HDL) and
Phospholipids and
Prolactin and
Prothrombin and
Sodium and
Triglycerides
(serum concentrations may be increased)

Renin substrate
(may be increased by conjugated estrogens and ethinyl estradiol;
this effect may also occur with other estrogens; however, transdermal estradiol does not affect renin substrate)

## Medical considerations/Contraindications
The medical considerations/contraindications included here have been selected on the basis of their potential clinical significance (reasons given
in parentheses where appropriate)—not necessarily inclusive (» =
major clinical significance).

*Except under special circumstances, this medication should not be used
when the following medical problems exist:*

» Breast cancer, known or suspected, except in selected patients treated
for metastatic diseases
(possible promotion of tumor growth in breast cancer)

» Vaginal bleeding, abnormal and undiagnosed
(may indicate the presence of endometrial hyperplasia or carcinoma, which may be exacerbated or promoted by the use of
estrogens)

*Risk-benefit should be considered when the following medical
problems exist:*

Endometriosis
(endometrial implants may be aggravated by use of estrogens)

Gallbladder disease, or history of, especiallylstones
(conflicting evidence exists as to whether an increased risk of recurrence or exacerbation occurs secondary to estrogen use)

Hepatic dysfunction
(metabolism of estrogens may be impaired)

» Hypercalcemia associated with metastatic breast disease
(severe hypercalcemia may occur in patients with breast cancer
and bone metastases who are treated with estrogens; estrogens may
aggravate breast cancer–induced hypercalcemia, through alterations in the metabolism of calcium and phosphorus; appropriate
monitoring is recommended)

Jaundice, or history of during pregnancy
(estrogens may increase risk of recurrence)

Porphyria, hepatic—acute intermittent or variegate
(may be exacerbated)

Sensitivity to estrogens

» Thrombophlebitis or thromboembolic disorders, active
(may be exacerbated)

Uterine fibroids
(may increase in size during estrogen therapy)

*For all indications, except for the treatment of breast cancer or prostatic
cancer*

» Thrombophlebitis, thrombosis, or thromboembolic disorders, estrogen-
induced, history of
(resumption of estrogen therapy may result in recurrence)

*For treatment of male breast cancer or prostatic cancer only, in addition
to those conditions listed above*

Cerebrovascular disease or
Coronary artery disease
Thrombophlebitis, active or
Thromboembolic disorders
(the large doses of estrogens used in males to treat breast and
prostate cancer have been associated with an increased risk of myocardial infarction, pulmonary embolism, and thrombophlebitis)

## Patient monitoring
The following may be especially important in patient monitoring (other
tests may be warranted in some patients, depending on condition;
» = major clinical significance):

Blood pressure determinations
(blood pressure elevations that generally occur within a short time
after initiation of therapy are due to a reversible effect on the renin-
angiotensin system and have only been documented during the use
of high-dose combination oral contraceptives; hypertension occurring during the treatment of gonadal dysgenesis may also be a
result of worsening of the disease state itself, and may not necessarily be attributable to estrogen therapy)

Bone age determinations
(x-ray of hand and wrist recommended every 6 months for children
and adolescents to determine rate of bone maturation and effects
on epiphyseal centers)

Breast examinations
(should be performed routinely by patient and physician for early
detection of possible breast cancer)

Endometrial biopsy
(should be considered periodically in patients with an intact uterus
who are not also receiving progestins, or if continuous, rather than
cyclical, estrogen therapy is prescribed; patients with a uterus
should be monitored for signs of endometrial cancer and malignancy should be ruled out in cases of persistent or abnormal vaginal bleeding; there is no risk of endometrial cancer in patients
who have undergone a hysterectomy)

Hepatic function determinations
(recommended at regular intervals, especially during therapy in
patients who have or are suspected of having hepatic disease)

Lipid profile determinations, serum
(recommended annually in women who are receiving estrogen replacement therapy, especially if taking a progestin)

Mammogram
(every 12 months, or as determined by physician)

Papanicolaou (Pap) test and
Physical examinations
(every year or more frequently when so determined by physician,
with special attention being given to abdomen, breast, and pelvic
organs)

## Side/Adverse Effects

The following side/adverse effects have been selected on the basis of their
potential clinical significance (possible signs and symptoms in parentheses where appropriate)—not necessarily inclusive:

**Those indicating need for medical attention**
Incidence more frequent
*Breast pain or tenderness*—in females as well as in males treated for
prostatic cancer; *enlargement of breasts*—in females; *gynecomastia*
(increased breast size)—in males treated for prostatic cancer; *peripheral edema* (swelling of feet and lower legs; rapid weight gain)

Incidence less frequent or rare
*Amenorrhea* (stopping of menstrual bleeding); *breakthrough bleeding*
(heavier vaginal bleeding between regular menses); *menorrhagia or*
(prolonged or heavier menses); *spotting* (lighter vaginal bleeding between regular menses); *breast tumors* (breast lumps; discharge from
breast); *chorea* (involuntary jerky muscular movements); *gallbladder
obstruction or hepatitis* (yellow eyes or skin; pains in stomach, side,
or abdomen)

Note: If persistent or recurring *abnormal vaginal bleeding* occurs, malignancy should be ruled out. However, *withdrawal bleeding*
will frequently occur in patients placed on cyclic estrogen therapy with a progestin who have not undergone hysterectomy.

For treatment of male breast cancer or prostatic cancer only, in addition
to those listed above
*Thromboembolism or thrombus formation* (severe or sudden headache; sudden loss of coordination; pains in chest, groin, or leg, especially calf; sudden and unexplained shortness of breath; sudden slurred
speech; sudden vision changes; weakness or numbness in arm or leg)

Note: The use of large doses of estrogens in males to treat breast and
prostate cancer has been associated with an increased risk of
*myocardial infarction*, *pulmonary embolism*, and
*thrombophlebitis*.

**Those indicating need for medical attention only if they continue
or are bothersome**
Incidence more frequent
*Abdominal cramping or bloating; anorexia* (loss of appetite); *nausea;
skin irritation and redness*—with transdermal system

Incidence less frequent
*Diarrhea, mild; dizziness, mild; headaches, mild; intolerance to con-
tact lenses; libido, decrease*—in males; *libido, increase*—in females;
*migraine headaches; vomiting*—primarily of central origin; usually
with high doses

## Patient Consultation

As an aid to patient consultation, refer to *Advice for the Patient, Estrogens
(Systemic)*.

In providing consultation, consider emphasizing the following selected
information (» = major clinical significance):

**Before using this medication**
» Reading patient package insert carefully
» Conditions affecting use, especially:
Sensitivity to estrogens
Increased risk of endometrial cancer for patients with intact uteri
placed on unopposed estrogen replacement therapy; decreased
risk occurs when used with a progestin; male breast cancer has
occurred in association with estrogen use; continuous, long-
term estrogen use in animal studies increased frequency of cancers of the breast, cervix, and liver
Pregnancy—Use of some estrogens suggested to be associated with
congenital abnormalities
Breast-feeding—Use is not recommended because estrogens are
distributed into breast milk and may have unpredictable effects
Use in children—Use in children or growing adolescents may slow
or stop growth
Other medications, especially bromocriptine, cyclosporine, or hepatotoxic medications; smoking tobacco may increase risk of
cardiovascular side effects and increase metabolism of estrogen
Other medical problems, especially some types of breast cancer;
abnormal and undiagnosed vaginal bleeding; history of estrogen-induced thrombophlebitis, thrombosis, or thromboembolic

disorders; or active thrombophlebitis or thromboembolic
disorders

**Proper use of this medication**
» Proper storage
*For oral or parenteral dosage forms*
» Compliance with therapy
Taking with or immediately after food to reduce nausea
Missed dose: Taking as soon as possible; not taking if almost time for
next dose; not doubling doses
*For transdermal estradiol*
Reading patient directions
Washing and drying hands thoroughly before and after application
Applying to clean, dry, non-oily, hairless, intact area of skin on the
abdomen or buttocks; not applying over cuts or irritation
» Not applying to breasts; not applying to waistline or other areas where
tight clothes may rub disk loose
Pressing the disk firmly in place with palm for about 10 seconds;
making sure there is good contact, especially around edges
Reapplying disk if it comes loose, or discarding and applying a new
one
Applying each patch to different area of skin on abdomen or buttocks
so at least 1 week elapses before the area is used again to help
prevent skin irritation
» Proper dosing
Missed dose: Using as soon as possible; not using if almost time for
next dose; not doubling doses

**Precautions while using this medication**
» Regular visits to physician every year, or more often, as determined
by physician
Possibility of dental problems, such as tenderness, swelling, or bleeding of gums; brushing and flossing teeth, massaging gums, and
having dentist clean teeth regularly; checking with dentist if there
are questions about care of teeth or gums or if tenderness, swelling,
or bleeding of gums is noticed
» Stopping medication immediately and checking with physician if pregnancy is suspected
Importance of not giving medication to anyone else

**Side/adverse effects**
Withdrawal bleeding will occur in many postmenopausal patients with
an intact uterus who are placed on cyclic estrogen therapy with a
progestin
Signs of potential side effects, especially menstrual irregularities, chorea, breast pain or tenderness, breast tumors, enlargement of
breasts in females, gynecomastia in males treated for prostatic cancer, peripheral edema, gallbladder obstruction, hepatitis; for treatment of prostatic cancer and male breast cancer only—thromboembolism or thrombus formation

## General Dosing Information

As a general rule, unopposed (without a progestin) estrogen therapy
should be administered at the lowest effective dosage. When prolonged
therapy is necessary, the patient should be re-evaluated at least every
year to determine the need for continued therapy.

An estrogen may be administered for the entire period of estrogen deficiency. With chronic administration of estrogens in patients with the
uterus *in situ*, the concurrent use of a progestin during the last 10 to
14 days of the cycle should be considered. Administration of a progestin decreases the risk of occurrence of endometrial hyperplasia and
endometrial carcinoma. There is no risk of endometrial hyperplasia or
endometrial carcinoma in patients who do not have an intact uterus.
In the prevention of conditions such as osteoporosis or atherosclerotic
disease, estrogen and progestin therapy may continue for several years
or for the remainder of the life of the patient. With prolonged therapy,
the patient should be evaluated at least every year.

Estrogens may be administered on a cyclic or continuous regimen when
used to treat estrogen deficiency states, for prevention of osteoporosis,
and for prevention of atherosclerotic disease. Some patients are placed
on a cyclic regimen consisting of three weeks of estrogen therapy,
with a progestin being concurrently administered (if indicated) for 10
to 14 days of the three-week period. The fourth and final week of the
cycle, no medication is administered. An alternative cyclical schedule
consists of the administration of an estrogen for the first 25 days of
each calendar month, with no drug being administered for the remainder of the month (3 to 6 days). A progestin may be administered
concurrently during the final 10 to 14 days of each estrogen cycle
(monthly dates 12 or 16 through 25). Other physicians advocate the
use of continuous estrogen dosing with a progestin administered (if
indicated) for 10 to 14 days of each month.

Estrogen therapy may cause nausea, especially in the morning, when either oral or parenteral dosage is used. Although this nausea is primarily of central origin, eating solid food often provides some relief.

**For parenteral dosage forms only**
Intramuscular injections should be administered slowly and deeply into a large muscle area such as the upper outer quadrant of the buttock.

Rapid intravenous injections may cause perineal or vaginal burning.

A dry syringe and needle of at least 21 gauge should be used for the oil-vehicle preparations.

**For transdermal dosage forms of estradiol only**
Patients who are currently taking oral estrogens should wait 1 week after withdrawal of oral estrogens before the transdermal dosage system is initiated.

Transdermal estradiol is generally administered on a continuous regimen, with a progestin administered (if indicated) for 10 to 14 days of each month.

The adhesive side of the transdermal system should be placed on a clean, dry area of the skin on the trunk of the body. The abdomen is the preferred site, though the patch may also be applied to the buttocks. It should not be applied to the breasts or waistline. The area selected should not be oily or irritated and the skin should not be broken. The application site should be rotated, and no site should be reused until 1 week has passed.

The system should be applied immediately after removal from the pouch and removal of the protective liner. It should not be stored unpouched. The system should be pressed firmly in place with the palm of the hand for about 10 seconds, making sure there is good contact, especially around the edges.

If a transdermal system loosens or falls off, it may be reapplied or a new system may be applied instead. In either case, the patient should continue with the original treatment schedule.

---

### CHLOROTRIANISENE

## Oral Dosage Forms
### CHLOROTRIANISENE CAPSULES USP

**Usual adult dose**
Atrophic vaginitis or
Menopausal symptoms (vasomotor) or
Vulvar squamous hyperplasia—
    Oral, 12 to 25 mg a day, cyclically or continuously.
Female hypogonadism—
    Oral, 12 to 25 mg a day, cyclically or continuously.
Prostatic carcinoma—
    Oral, 12 to 25 mg a day.
Note: Chlorotrianisene provides a long-acting effect, which sometimes makes cyclical therapy difficult.

**Strength(s) usually available**
U.S.—
    12 mg (Rx) [*TACE* (methylparaben; propylparaben; tartrazine)].
    25 mg (Rx) [*TACE* (tartrazine)].
Canada—
    Not commercially available.

**Packaging and storage**
Store below 40 °C (104 °F), preferably between 15 and 30 °C (59 and 86 °F), unless otherwise specified by manufacturer. Store in a well-closed container. Store in a dry place.

**Note**
Include mandatory patient package insert (PPI) when dispensing.

---

### DIETHYLSTILBESTROL

## Oral Dosage Forms
### DIETHYLSTILBESTROL TABLETS USP

**Usual adult dose**
Breast carcinoma (inoperable and progressing in selected men and post-menopausal women)—
    Oral, 15 mg a day.
Prostatic carcinoma (inoperable and progressing)—
    Oral, 1 to 3 mg initially and increased as needed in advanced cases, with the dosage later being reduced to 1 mg a day.
Note: The doses in prostatic carcinoma have been found to have a maximal effect in maintenance doses of up to 1 mg a day. Higher doses

do not appreciably increase the therapeutic results, but may increase the risk of cardiovascular embolism.

**Strength(s) usually available**
U.S.—
    1 mg (Rx) [GENERIC (Lilly—lactose)].
    5 mg (Rx) [GENERIC (Lilly—lactose)].
Canada—
    Not commercially available.

**Packaging and storage**
Store below 40 °C (104 °F), preferably between 15 and 30 °C (59 and 86 °F), unless otherwise specified by manufacturer. Store in a well-closed container.

**Note**
Include mandatory patient package insert (PPI) when dispensing.

### DIETHYLSTILBESTROL TABLETS (ENTERIC-COATED) USP

**Usual adult dose**
Breast carcinoma (inoperable and progressing in selected men and post-menopausal women)—
    Oral, 15 mg a day.
Prostatic carcinoma (inoperable and progressing)—
    Oral, 1 to 3 mg initially and increased as needed in advanced cases, with the dosage later being reduced to 1 mg a day.
Note: The doses in prostatic carcinoma have been found to have a maximal effect in maintenance doses of up to 1 mg a day. Higher doses do not appreciably increase the therapeutic results, but may increase the risk of thromboembolism or myocardial toxicity.

**Strength(s) usually available**
U.S.—
    1 mg (Rx) [GENERIC (Lilly—lactose, sucrose)].
    5 mg (Rx) [GENERIC (Lilly—lactose, sucrose)].
Canada—
    Not commercially available.

**Packaging and storage**
Store below 40 °C (104 °F), preferably between 15 and 30 °C (59 and 86 °F), in a well-closed container, unless otherwise specified by manufacturer.

**Auxiliary labeling**
• Do not break, crush, or chew tablets.

**Note**
Include mandatory patient package insert (PPI) when dispensing.

### DIETHYLSTILBESTROL DIPHOSPHATE TABLETS

**Usual adult dose**
Prostatic carcinoma (inoperable and progressing)—
    Oral, 50 to 166 mg three times a day, the dosage being increased gradually to 200 mg or more, three times a day as needed and tolerated.

**Usual adult prescribing limits**
Oral, 1 gram a day.

**Strength(s) usually available**
U.S.—
    50 mg (Rx) [*Stilphostrol* (scored; lactose)].
Canada—
    83 mg (diethylstilbestrol diphosphate sodium 100 mg) (Rx) [*Honvol* (scored; lactose)].

**Packaging and storage**
Store below 40 °C (104 °F), preferably between 15 and 30 °C (59 and 86 °F), in a well-closed container, unless otherwise specified by manufacturer.

**Note**
Include mandatory patient package insert (PPI) when dispensing.

## Parenteral Dosage Forms
### DIETHYLSTILBESTROL DIPHOSPHATE INJECTION USP

**Usual adult dose**
Prostatic carcinoma (inoperable and progressing)—
    Induction: Intravenous infusion, initially 500 mg in 250 mL of Sodium Chloride Injection USP or 5% Dextrose Injection USP administered at a rate of 1 mL per minute during the first ten to fifteen minutes, the flow then being adjusted to permit dose completion within one hour. The dosage is increased to 1 gram a day for the subsequent five or more days as needed for relief.

Maintenance: Intravenous infusion, 250 to 500 mg in 250 mL of Sodium Chloride Injection USP or 5% Dextrose Injection USP administered once or twice a week at same rate as during induction.

**Strength(s) usually available**

U.S.—

50 mg per mL (Rx) [*Stilphostrol*].

Canada—

50 mg per mL (diethylstilbestrol diphosphate sodium 60 mg) (Rx) [*Honvol*].

**Packaging and storage**

Store below 21 °C (70 °F), unless otherwise specified by manufacturer. Protect from freezing.

**Note**

Include mandatory patient package insert (PPI) if dispensed to patient.

---

## *ESTRADIOL*

# Oral Dosage Forms
## ESTRADIOL TABLETS USP

**Usual adult dose**

Atrophic vaginitis or
Female hypogonadism or
Menopausal (vasomotor) symptoms or
Ovariectomy or
Primary ovarian failure or
Vulvar squamous hyperplasia—
    Oral, 500 mcg (0.5 mg) to 2 mg a day, cyclically or continuously.
Breast carcinoma (inoperable and progressing in selected men and postmenopausal women)—
    Oral, 10 mg three times a day for at least three months.
Prostatic carcinoma (inoperable and progressing)—
    Oral, 1 to 2 mg three times a day.
Osteoporosis prophylactic—
    Oral, 0.5 mg (500 mcg) a day, cyclically or continuously.

**Strength(s) usually available**

U.S.—

500 mcg (0.5 mg) (Rx) [*Estrace* (scored; lactose)].

1 mg (Rx) [*Estrace* (scored; lactose)].

2 mg (Rx) [*Estrace* (scored; lactose; tartrazine)].

Canada—

1 mg (Rx) [*Estrace* (scored)].

2 mg (Rx) [*Estrace* (scored)].

**Packaging and storage**

Store below 40 °C (104 °F), preferably between 15 and 30 °C (59 and 86 °F), unless otherwise specified by manufacturer. Store in a tight, light-resistant container.

**Note**

Include mandatory patient package insert (PPI) when dispensing.

# Parenteral Dosage Forms

Note: Bracketed uses in the *Dosage Forms* section refer to categories of use and/or indications that are not included in U.S. product labeling.

## ESTRADIOL CYPIONATE INJECTION USP

**Usual adult dose**

Female hypogonadism—
    Intramuscular, 1.5 to 2 mg administered at monthly intervals.
Menopausal (vasomotor) symptoms—
    Intramuscular, 1 to 5 mg administered at three- to four-week intervals.

**Strength(s) usually available**

U.S.—

5 mg per mL (Rx) [*depGynogen* (chlorobutanol; cottonseed oil); *Depo-Estradiol* (chlorobutanol 5.4 mg; cottonseed oil); *Depogen* (chlorobutanol; cottonseed oil); *Dura-Estrin* (chlorobutanol; cottonseed oil); *E-Cypionate; Estragyn LA 5; Estro-Cyp* (chlorobutanol; cottonseed oil); *Estrofem* (chlorobutanol; cottonseed oil); *Estroject-LA* (chlorobutanol; cottonseed oil); *Estro-L.A.;* GENERIC].

Canada—

Not commercially available.

**Packaging and storage**

Store below 40 °C (104 °F), preferably between 15 and 30 °C (59 and 86 °F), in a light-resistant container, unless otherwise specified by manufacturer. Protect from freezing.

**Note**

Include mandatory patient package insert (PPI) if dispensed to patient.

## ESTRADIOL VALERATE INJECTION USP

**Usual adult dose**

Atrophic vaginitis or
Female hypogonadism or
Menopausal (vasomotor) symptoms or
Ovariectomy or
Primary ovarian failure or
Vulvar squamous hyperplasia—
    Intramuscular, 10 to 20 mg repeated every four weeks as needed.
Prostatic carcinoma (inoperable and progressing)—
    Intramuscular, 30 mg every one or two weeks, the dose being adjusted as needed.

**Strength(s) usually available**

U.S.—

10 mg per mL (Rx) [*Delestrogen* (chlorobutanol 5 mg; sesame oil); *Valergen-10* (chlorobutanol; sesame oil); GENERIC].

20 mg per mL (Rx) [*Delestrogen* (benzyl alcohol; benzyl benzoate; castor oil); *Dioval XX* (benzyl alcohol; benzyl benzoate; castor oil); *Duragen-20* (benzyl alcohol; benzyl benzoate; castor oil); *Gynogen L.A. 20* (benzyl alcohol; benzyl benzoate; castor oil); *Menaval-20; Valergen-20* (benzyl alcohol; benzyl benzoate; castor oil); GENERIC].

40 mg per mL (Rx) [*Clinagen LA 40; Deladiol-40* (benzyl alcohol; benzyl benzoate; castor oil); *Delestrogen* (benzyl alcohol; benzyl benzoate; castor oil); *Dioval 40* (benzyl alcohol; benzyl benzoate; castor oil); *Duragen-40* (benzyl alcohol; benzyl benzoate; castor oil); *Estra-L 40* (benzyl alcohol; benzyl benzoate; castor oil); *Estro-Span; Gynogen L.A. 40* (benzyl alcohol; benzyl benzoate; castor oil); *Valergen-40* (benzyl alcohol; benzyl benzoate; castor oil); GENERIC].

Canada—

10 mg per mL (Rx) [*Delestrogen* (chlorobutanol 0.5%; sesame oil)].

20 mg per mL (Rx) [*Femogex* (chlorobutanol 0.5%)].

**Packaging and storage**

Store below 40 °C (104 °F), preferably between 15 and 30 °C (59 and 86 °F), unless otherwise specified by manufacturer. Store in a light-resistant container. Protect from freezing.

**Note**

Include mandatory patient package insert (PPI) if dispensed to patient.

# Topical Dosage Forms
## ESTRADIOL TRANSDERMAL SYSTEM

**Usual adult dose**

Atrophic vaginitis or
Female hypogonadism or
Menopausal (vasomotor) symptoms or
Osteoporosis, postmenopausal (prophylaxis) or
Ovariectomy or
Primary ovarian failure or
Vulvar squamous hyperplasia—
    Topical, to the skin, one transdermal dosage system delivering per day 50 mcg (0.05 mg) or 100 mcg (0.10 mg), worn continuously and replaced twice a week. Treatment is usually initiated with 50 mcg (0.05 mg), the dosage being adjusted as necessary to control symptoms.

**Strength(s) usually available**

U.S.—

50 mcg (0.05 mg) delivered per day (Rx) [*Estraderm*].

100 mcg (0.1 mg) delivered per day (Rx) [*Estraderm*].

Canada—

25 mcg (0.025 mg) delivered per day (Rx) [*Estraderm*].

50 mcg (0.05 mg) delivered per day (Rx) [*Estraderm*].

100 mcg (0.1 mg) delivered per day (Rx) [*Estraderm*].

**Packaging and storage**

Store below 30 °C (86 °F).

**Note**

Include mandatory patient package insert (PPI) when dispensing.

---

## *ESTROGENS, CONJUGATED*

# Oral Dosage Forms
## CONJUGATED ESTROGENS TABLETS USP

**Usual adult dose**

Atrophic vaginitis or
Vulvar squamous hyperplasia—
    Oral, 300 mcg (0.3 mg) to 1.25 mg or more a day, cyclically or continuously.

Note: May be used in conjunction with vaginal dosage forms.

Female hypogonadism—
Oral, 2.5 to 7.5 mg a day, in divided doses, cyclically.

Menopausal (vasomotor) symptoms—
Oral, 625 mcg (0.625 mg) to 1.25 mg a day, cyclically or continuously.

Ovariectomy or

Primary ovarian failure—
Oral, 1.25 mg a day, cyclically or continuously. For maintenance, adjust estrogen dose to lowest level that provides control.

Breast carcinoma (inoperable and progressing in selected men and post-menopausal women)—
Oral, 10 mg three times a day for at least three months.

Prostatic carcinoma (inoperable and progressing)—
Oral, 1.25 to 2.5 mg three times a day.

Osteoporosis prophylactic—
Oral, 300 mcg (0.3 mg) to 1.25 mg a day, cyclically or continuously.

### Strength(s) usually available

U.S.—
300 mcg (0.3 mg) (Rx) [*Premarin*].

625 mcg (0.625 mg) (Rx) [*Premarin; Premphase; Prempro*].

Note: *Premphase* (cyclical hormone replacement therapy) contains a 28-day supply of 0.625 mg conjugated estrogens tablets (*Premarin* brand name) packaged with a 14-day supply of 5 mg medroxyprogesterone tablets (*Cycrin* brand name).

*Prempro* (continuous hormone replacement therapy) contains a 28-day supply of 0.625 mg conjugated estrogens tablets (*Premarin* brand name) packaged with a 28-day supply of 2.5 mg medroxyprogesterone tablets (*Cycrin* brand name).

900 mcg (0.9 mg) (Rx) [*Premarin*].

1.25 mg (Rx) [*Premarin*].

2.5 mg (Rx) [*Premarin*].

Canada—
300 mcg (0.3 mg) (Rx) [*C.E.S; Congest; Premarin*].

625 mcg (0.625 mg) (Rx) [*C.E.S; Congest; Premarin;* GENERIC].

900 mcg (0.9 mg) (Rx) [*C.E.S; Congest; Premarin*].

1.25 mg (Rx) [*C.E.S; Congest; Premarin;* GENERIC].

2.5 mg (Rx) [*C.E.S; Congest; Premarin*].

### Packaging and storage

Store below 40 °C (104 °F), preferably between 15 and 30 °C (59 and 86 °F), unless otherwise specified by manufacturer. Store in a well-closed container.

### Note

Include mandatory patient package insert (PPI) when dispensing.

## Parenteral Dosage Forms

### CONJUGATED ESTROGENS FOR INJECTION

#### Usual adult dose

Abnormal uterine bleeding (hormonal imbalance)—
Intramuscular or intravenous, 25 mg, repeated in six to twelve hours if needed.

Note: Intravenous administration is preferred because of the more rapid response obtained. To reduce the possibility of a flushing reaction, the medication should be administered slowly.

#### Strength(s) usually available

U.S.—
25 mg (Rx) [*Premarin Intravenous* (benzyl alcohol 2%—diluent; lactose 200 mg; simethicone 200 mcg [0.2 mg]; sodium citrate 12.2 mg; sodium hydroxide or hydrochloric acid)].

Canada—
25 mg (Rx) [*Premarin Intravenous* (lactose 200 mg; simethicone 200 mcg [0.2 mg]; sodium citrate 12.5 mg; sodium hydroxide or hydrochloric acid)].

#### Packaging and storage

Prior to reconstitution, store between 2 and 8 °C (36 and 46 °F), unless otherwise specified by manufacturer.

#### Preparation of dosage form

Using aseptic technique, withdraw at least 5 mL of air from the dry container. Slowly add 5 mL of the sterile diluent provided against the container side. Gently agitate vial to dissolve contents—*do not shake container vigorously.*

#### Stability

When stored between 2 and 8 °C (36 and 46 °F), the reconstituted solution retains potency for about 60 days. Do not use if solution has darkened or if a precipitate is present.

### Incompatibilities

The prepared injection is compatible with normal saline, dextrose, and invert sugar solutions. It is *not* compatible with solutions having an acid pH, such as protein hydrolysate or ascorbic acid.

### Note

Include mandatory patient package insert (PPI) if dispensed to patient.

---

## ESTROGENS, ESTERIFIED

## Oral Dosage Forms

Note: Bracketed uses in the *Dosage Forms* section refer to categories of use and/or indications that are not included in U.S. product labeling.

### ESTERIFIED ESTROGENS TABLETS USP

#### Usual adult dose

Atrophic vaginitis or

Vulvar squamous hyperplasia—
Oral, 300 mcg (0.3 mg) to 1.25 mg or more a day, depending on response of patient, cyclically or continuously.

Note: May be used in conjunction with vaginal dosage forms.

Female hypogonadism—
Oral, 2.5 to 7.5 mg a day, in divided doses, cyclically or continuously.

Menopausal (vasomotor) symptoms—
Oral, 625 mcg (0.625 mg) to 1.25 mg a day, cyclically or continuously.

Ovariectomy or

Primary ovarian failure—
Oral, 1.25 mg a day, cyclically or continuously. For maintenance, adjust estrogen dose to lowest level that provides control.

Breast carcinoma (inoperable and progressing in selected men and post-menopausal women)—
Oral, 10 mg three times a day for at least three months.

Prostatic carcinoma (inoperable and progressing)—
Oral, 1.25 to 2.5 mg three times a day.

[Osteoporosis (prophylaxis)][1]—
Oral, 300 mcg (0.3 mg) to 1.25 mg a day, cyclically or continuously.

#### Strength(s) usually available

U.S.—
300 mcg (0.3 mg) (Rx) [*Estratab; Menest*].

625 mcg (0.625 mg) (Rx) [*Estratab; Menest*].

1.25 mg (Rx) [*Estratab; Menest*].

2.5 mg (Rx) [*Estratab; Menest*].

Canada—
300 mcg (0.3 mg) (Rx) [*Neo-Estrone*].

625 mcg (0.625 mg) (Rx) [*Neo-Estrone*].

1.25 mg (Rx) [*Neo-Estrone*].

#### Packaging and storage

Store below 40 °C (104 °F), preferably between 15 and 30 °C (59 and 86 °F), unless otherwise specified by manufacturer. Store in a well-closed container.

### Note

Include mandatory patient package insert (PPI) when dispensing.

---

[1]Not included in Canadian product labeling.

---

## ESTRONE

## Parenteral Dosage Forms

### STERILE ESTRONE SUSPENSION USP

#### Usual adult dose

Abnormal uterine bleeding (hormonal imbalance)—
Intramuscular, 2 to 5 mg a day for several days.

Female hypogonadism or

Ovariectomy or

Primary ovarian failure—
Intramuscular, 100 mcg (0.1 mg) to 2 mg a week, administered as a single dose or in divided doses, cyclically or continuously.

Atrophic vaginitis or

Menopausal (vasomotor) symptoms or

Vulvar squamous hyperplasia—
Intramuscular, 100 to 500 mcg (0.1 to 0.5 mg) two or three times a week, cyclically or continuously.

Prostatic carcinoma (inoperable and progressing)—
Intramuscular, 2 to 4 mg two or three times a week.

**Strength(s) usually available**
U.S.—
2 mg estrone per mL (Rx) [*Aquest; Wehgen* (benzyl alcohol; methylparaben; propylparaben); GENERIC].
5 mg estrone per mL (Rx) [*Estragyn 5; Estro-A; Estrone '5'* (benzyl alcohol; methylparaben; propylparaben); *Kestrone-5* (benzyl alcohol; methylparaben; propylparaben); GENERIC].
Canada—
Not commercially available.

**Packaging and storage**
Store below 40 °C (104 °F), preferably between 15 and 30 °C (59 and 86 °F), unless otherwise specified by manufacturer. Protect from freezing.

**Note**
Include mandatory patient package insert (PPI) if dispensed to patient.

---

### ESTROPIPATE

## Oral Dosage Forms
### ESTROPIPATE TABLETS USP

**Usual adult dose**
Atrophic vaginitis or
Vulvar squamous hyperplasia—
Oral, 750 mcg (0.75 mg) to 6 mg of estropipate a day, cyclically or continuously.
Female hypogonadism—
Oral, 1.5 to 9 mg of estropipate a day, cyclically or continuously.
Menopausal (vasomotor) symptoms—
Oral, 750 mcg (0.75 mg) to 6 mg of estropipate a day, cyclically or continuously.
Ovariectomy or
Primary ovarian failure—
Oral, 1.5 to 9 mg of estropipate a day, cyclically or continuously. For maintenance, adjust dose to lowest level that provides control.

**Strength(s) usually available**
U.S.—
750 mcg (0.75 mg) estropipate—equivalent to 625 mcg (0.625 mg) estrone sodium sulfate (Rx) [*Ogen.625* (scored); *Ortho-Est;* GENERIC].
1.5 mg estropipate—equivalent to 1.25 mg estrone sodium sulfate (Rx) [*Ogen 1.25* (scored); *Ortho-Est;* GENERIC].
3 mg estropipate—equivalent to 2.5 mg estrone sodium sulfate (Rx) [*Ogen 2.5* (scored); GENERIC].
Canada—
750 mcg (0.75 mg) estropipate—equivalent to 625 mcg (0.625 mg) estrone sodium sulfate (Rx) [*Ogen* (scored)].
1.5 mg estropipate—equivalent to 1.25 mg estrone sodium sulfate (Rx) [*Ogen* (scored; lactose; parabens)].
3 mg estropipate—equivalent to 2.5 mg estrone sodium sulfate (Rx) [*Ogen* (scored; lactose; parabens)].

**Packaging and storage**
Store below 40 °C (104 °F), preferably between 15 and 30 °C (59 and 86 °F), unless otherwise specified by manufacturer. Store in a well-closed container.

**Note**
Include mandatory patient package insert (PPI) when dispensing.

---

### ETHINYL ESTRADIOL

## Oral Dosage Forms
### ETHINYL ESTRADIOL TABLETS USP

**Usual adult dose**
Female hypogonadism—
Oral, 50 mcg (0.05 mg) one to three times a day, cyclically or continuously, the dosage being repeated for three to six months to establish a normal menses.

Menopausal (vasomotor) symptoms—
Oral, 20 to 50 mcg (0.02 to 0.05 mg) a day, cyclically or continuously.
Breast carcinoma (inoperable and progressing in selected postmenopausal women)—
Oral, 1 mg three times a day.
Prostatic carcinoma (inoperable and progressing)—
Oral, 150 mcg (0.15 mg) to 3 mg a day.

**Strength(s) usually available**
U.S.—
20 mcg (0.02 mg) (Rx) [*Estinyl* (butylparaben; lactose; sucrose; tartrazine)].
50 mcg (0.05 mg) (Rx) [*Estinyl* (butylparaben; lactose; sucrose)].
500 mcg (0.5 mg) (Rx) [*Estinyl* (scored; lactose)].
Canada—
20 mcg (0.02 mg) (Rx) [*Estinyl* (lactose; sucrose 57 mg)].
50 mcg (0.05 mg) (Rx) [*Estinyl* (lactose; sucrose 81 mg)].
500 mcg (0.5 mg) (Rx) [*Estinyl* (scored; lactose 162 mg)].

**Packaging and storage**
Store below 40 °C (104 °F), preferably between 15 and 30 °C (59 and 86 °F), unless otherwise specified by manufacturer. Store in a well-closed container.

**Note**
Include mandatory patient package insert (PPI) when dispensing.

---

### QUINESTROL

## Oral Dosage Forms
### QUINESTROL TABLETS

**Usual adult dose**
Atrophic vaginitis or
Female hypogonadism or
Menopausal (vasomotor) symptoms or
Ovariectomy or
Primary ovarian failure or
Vulvar squamous hyperplasia—
Oral, 100 mcg (0.1 mg) *a day* for seven days, followed by one *week* of no medication, after which a maintenance dose of 100 mcg (0.1 mg) once *a week* is taken.
Note: CAUTION patient regarding the unusual dosage: 1 tablet *a day* for induction and then usually 1 tablet *a week* for maintenance.
The weekly maintenance dose may be increased to 200 mcg (0.2 mg) if needed and tolerated.

**Strength(s) usually available**
U.S.—
100 mcg (0.1 mg) (Rx) [*Estrovis* (lactose)].
Canada—
Not commercially available.

**Packaging and storage**
Store below 40 °C (104 °F), preferably between 15 and 30 °C (59 and 86 °F), in a well-closed container, unless otherwise specified by manufacturer.

**Note**
Affirm that patient understands physician instructions.
Include mandatory patient package insert (PPI) when dispensing.

Revised: 06/18/93
Interim revision: 06/30/94; 02/17/95; 08/02/95; 09/22/95

---

# ESTROGENS   Vaginal

This monograph includes information on the following: Dienestrol; Estradiol; Estrogens, Conjugated; Estrone*; Estropipate†.
VA CLASSIFICATION (Primary/Secondary): GU500/HS300
Another commonly used name for estropipate is piperazine estrone sulfate.

Note: For a listing of dosage forms and brand names by country availability, see *Dosage Forms* section(s). For a listing of brand names for the articles in this monograph, refer to the General Index.

*Not commercially available in the U.S.
†Not commercially available in Canada.

# Category

Estrogen (vaginal).

# Indications

## Accepted

Vaginitis, atrophic (treatment) or

Vulvar squamous hyperplasia (treatment)—Vaginal application of estrogens is indicated in the treatment of atrophic vaginitis or vulvar squamous hyperplasia associated with estrogen deficiency, such as that resulting from menopause or ovariectomy.

# Pharmacology/Pharmacokinetics

## Physicochemical characteristics

Source—

Naturally occurring compounds include estradiol, conjugated estrogens (sodium estrone sulfate, sodium equilin sulfate, and others as found in equine urine), and estrone.

Semi-synthetic compounds include estropipate.

Synthetic compounds include dienestrol.

Molecular weight—

Dienestrol: 266.34.

Estradiol: 272.39.

Estrone: 270.37.

Estropipate: 436.56.

## Mechanism of action/Effect

At the cellular level, estrogens increase the cellular synthesis of DNA, RNA, and various proteins in responsive tissues. Estrogens reduce the release of gonadotropin-releasing hormone (GnRH) from the hypothalamus, leading to a reduction in release of follicle-stimulating hormone (FSH) and luteinizing hormone (LH) from the pituitary.

For estrogen replacement—

In healthy females, endogenous estrogens maintain genitourinary function and vasomotor stability. Estrogens are used as replacement therapy to alleviate or prevent symptoms caused by the decreased amounts of estrogens produced by the ovaries after natural or surgical menopause or other estrogen-deficiency states.

## Absorption

Clinical studies have shown that vaginally administered estrogens are extensively absorbed (approximately 50%) into the systemic circulation. Vaginal estrogen products are better absorbed than non-vaginal estrogen products. Consistent use of vaginal preparations generally results in higher blood concentrations than with the use of non-vaginal products. However, the amount of estrogen absorbed from vaginal preparations may vary dramatically, unless they are used consistently and correctly.

## Distribution

To most tissues; higher affinity for adipose tissue.

## Protein binding

Moderate to high (50 to 80% to albumin and sex hormone binding globulin). Tissue-specific receptor proteins form complexes with estrogens in estrogen-responsive tissues.

## Biotransformation

Primarily hepatic; some metabolism also occurs in muscle, kidneys, and gonads.

## Elimination

Primarily renal (excretion of metabolites), some fecal; undergo extensive enterohepatic recirculation. Prolonged in obese patients.

# Precautions to Consider

Note: Recent studies have shown that vaginal estrogen preparations are extensively absorbed. Therefore, some of the same estrogenic effects may be anticipated whether administration is systemic or vaginal.

## Carcinogenicity

Independent studies have shown an increased risk of endometrial cancer in postmenopausal women placed on unopposed (without a progestin) systemic estrogen replacement therapy for prolonged periods. Since estrogens applied vaginally are extensively absorbed, the risk may apply to them also. The risk of endometrial cancer in systemic estrogen users, which appears to depend on duration of treatment and dose, was 5 to 10 times greater than in nonusers. However, studies have shown that administration of a progestin for 10 to 14 days of an estrogen cycle is associated with a lower incidence of endometrial hyperplasia

and endometrial carcinoma than an estrogen-only cycle. There is no risk of endometrial cancer in patients who have undergone hysterectomies and, therefore, no documented need for concurrent progestin therapy exists in these patients.

Whether the use of systemic estrogens increases the incidence of breast cancer in some postmenopausal women is unresolved. Some large studies reported an increase in the relative risk for development of breast cancer. At present, however, the majority of data available does not seem to support this conclusion.

In certain animal species, long-term, continuous systemic administration of estrogens increases the frequency of cancers of the breast, cervix, vagina, and liver.

## Pregnancy/Reproduction

Pregnancy—Estrogens are not recommended during pregnancy, since studies suggest an association of systemic usage of some estrogens with congenital malformations. Precautions should also be taken for vaginal usage.

Daughters of women who took systemic diethylstilbestrol (DES) during pregnancy have developed abnormalities of the reproductive tract and, in rare cases, cancer of the vagina and/or uterine cervix upon reaching childbearing age. In addition, sons of women who took systemic DES during pregnancy have developed urogenital tract abnormalities. Patients who become pregnant while taking estrogens should be informed of the potential risks to the fetus.

FDA Pregnancy Category X.

## Breast-feeding

Estrogens are distributed into breast milk. Use of estrogens by nursing mothers is not recommended. Potential adverse effects in the nursing infant are not predictable.

When used in high doses as an antineoplastic, traces of ethinyl estradiol are distributed into breast milk. Also, use of combination oral contraceptives containing ethinyl estradiol during lactation has been associated with a decrease in milk production and in the milk protein and nitrogen content. However, the magnitude of these effects was small and would only likely be of clinical significance in malnourished mothers.

## Geriatrics

Studies performed to date have not demonstrated geriatrics-specific problems that would limit the usefulness of vaginal estrogens in the elderly.

## Dental

Estrogens may predispose the patient to bleeding of the gingival tissues. In addition, gingival hyperplasia may occur during estrogen therapy, usually starting as gingivitis or gum inflammation. A strictly enforced program of teeth cleaning by a professional, combined with plaque control by the patient, will minimize growth rate and severity of gingival enlargement.

## Drug interactions and/or related problems

The following drug interactions and/or related problems have been selected on the basis of their potential clinical significance (possible mechanism in parentheses where appropriate)—not necessarily inclusive (» = major clinical significance):

Note: Combinations containing any of the following medications, depending on the amount present, may also interact with this medication.

» Bromocriptine

(estrogens may cause amenorrhea, interfering with effects of bromocriptine; concurrent use is not recommended)

Calcium supplements

(concurrent use with estrogens may increase calcium absorption; this can be used to therapeutic advantage)

Corticosteroids, glucocorticoid

(concurrent use with estrogens may alter the metabolism and protein binding of glucocorticoids, leading to decreased clearance, increased elimination half-life, and increased therapeutic and toxic effects of the glucocorticoids; glucocorticoid dosage adjustment may be required during and following concurrent use)

Corticotropin (chronic therapeutic use)

(concurrent use with estrogens may potentiate the anti-inflammatory effects of endogenous cortisol induced by corticotropin)

» Cyclosporine

(systemic estrogens have been reported to inhibit cyclosporine metabolism and thereby increase plasma concentrations of cyclosporine, possibly increasing the risk of hepatotoxicity and nephrotoxicity; concurrent use is recommended only with great caution and frequent monitoring of blood cyclosporine concentrations and liver and renal function)

» Hepatotoxic medications, especially dantrolene (See *Appendix II*)
   (concurrent use of these medications with estrogens may increase
   the risk of hepatotoxicity; with concurrent use of dantrolene, use
   in females over 35 years of age, prolonged use, or use in patients
   with a history of liver disease, risk may be further increased)

   Smoking, tobacco
   (data from studies on tobacco smoking and the use of high-dose
   estrogen oral contraceptives indicate that there is an increased risk
   of serious cardiovascular side effects, including cerebrovascular
   accident, transient ischemic attacks, thrombophlebitis, and pulmonary embolism; risk increases with increasing tobacco usage
   and with age, especially in women over 35 years of age; it is not
   known whether any elevation of risk occurs with tobacco smoking
   during the use of vaginal estrogens for estrogen deficiency)

   (metabolism of estrogens may also be increased by smoking, resulting in a decreased estrogenic effect)

   Tamoxifen
   (concurrent use may interfere with therapeutic effect of tamoxifen)

## Laboratory value alterations

The following have been selected on the basis of their potential clinical
significance (possible effect in parentheses where appropriate)—not
necessarily inclusive (» = major clinical significance):

With diagnostic test results
Fasting blood sugar (FBS) and
Glucose tolerance test
   (may be altered by large doses of estrogens)

Metyrapone test
   (reduced response)

Norepinephrine-induced platelet aggregability
   (may be increased)

*Thyroid function tests, such as*
Thyroxine [$T_4$] determinations:
   (protein-bound $T_4$ is increased; serum free $T_4$ concentrations may
   be unchanged or decreased)

Triiodothyronine [$T_3$] determinations:
   (serum concentration may be increased, but $T_3$ resin uptake is decreased because estrogens increase serum thyroid-binding globulin
   [TBG]; free thyroid hormone levels remain unchanged)

With physiology/laboratory test values
Antithrombin III, serum and
Cholesterol, total, serum and
Folate, serum and
Lipoproteins, low density (LDL), serum and
Pregnanediol, urine and
Pyridoxine, serum
   (concentrations may be decreased)

Calcium
   (serum concentrations may be markedly elevated in immobilized
   patients)

Ceruloplasmin and
Clotting factors VII, VIII, IX, and X and
Cortisol and
Glucose—especially in diabetic or prediabetic patients using larger
   doses of estrogens and
Lipoproteins, high density (HDL) and
Phospholipids and
Prolactin and
Prothrombin and
Sodium and
Triglycerides
   (serum concentrations may be increased)

Renin substrate
   (may be increased by conjugated estrogens)

## Medical considerations/Contraindications

The medical considerations/contraindications included here have been selected on the basis of their potential clinical significance (reasons given
in parentheses where appropriate)—not necessarily inclusive (» =
major clinical significance).

*Except under special circumstances, this medication should not be used
when the following medical problems exist:*

» Breast cancer, known or suspected
   (possible promotion of tumor growth in breast cancer)

» Vaginal bleeding, abnormal and undiagnosed
   (may indicate the presence of endometrial hyperplasia or carcinoma, which may be exacerbated or promoted by the use of
   estrogens)

*Risk-benefit should be considered when the following medical problems
exist:*
Endometriosis
   (endometrial implants may be aggravated by use of estrogens)

Gallbladder disease, or history of, especially gallstones
   (conflicting evidence exists as to whether an increased risk of recurrence or exacerbation occurs secondary to estrogen use)

Hepatic dysfunction
   (metabolism of estrogens may be impaired)

Jaundice, or history of during pregnancy
   (estrogens may increase risk of recurrence)

Porphyria, hepatic—acute, intermittent, or variegate
   (may be exacerbated)

Sensitivity to estrogens
» Thrombophlebitis or thromboembolic disorders, active
   (may be exacerbated)

» Thrombophlebitis, thrombosis, or thromboembolic disorders, estrogen-
   induced, history of
   (resumption of estrogen therapy may result in recurrence)

Uterine fibroids
   (may increase in size during estrogen therapy)

## Patient monitoring

The following may be especially important in patient monitoring (other
tests may be warranted in some patients, depending on condition;
» = major clinical significance):

Blood pressure determinations
   (blood pressure elevations that generally occur within a short time
   after initiation of therapy are due to a reversible effect on the renin-
   angiotensin system and have been documented only during the use
   of high-dose combination oral contraceptives; hypertension occurring during the treatment of gonadal dysgenesis may also be a
   result of worsening of the disease state itself, and may not necessarily be attributable to estrogen therapy)

Breast examinations
   (should be performed routinely by patient and physician, for early
   detection of possible breast cancer)

Endometrial biopsy
   (should be considered periodically in patients with an intact uterus
   who are not also receiving progestins, or if continuous, rather than
   cyclical, estrogen therapy is prescribed; patients with a uterus
   should be monitored for signs of endometrial cancer and malignancy should be ruled out in cases of persistent or abnormal vaginal bleeding; there is no risk of endometrial cancer in patients
   who have undergone a hysterectomy)

Hepatic function determinations
   (recommended at regular intervals, especially during therapy in
   patients who have or are suspected of having hepatic disease)

Lipid profile determinations, serum
   (recommended annually in women who are receiving estrogen replacement therapy, especially if taking a progestin)

Mammogram
   (every 12 months, or as determined by physician)

Papanicolaou (Pap) test and
Physical examinations
   (every 6 to 12 months or more frequently when so determined by
   physician, with special attention being given to abdomen, breasts,
   and pelvic organs)

# Side/Adverse Effects

Note: Recent studies have shown that vaginal estrogen preparations are
   extensively absorbed. Therefore, some of the same estrogenic effects may be anticipated whether administration is systemic or
   vaginal.

The following side/adverse effects have been selected on the basis of their
   potential clinical significance (possible signs and symptoms in parentheses where appropriate)—not necessarily inclusive:

## Those indicating need for medical attention
Incidence more frequent
   *Breast pain or tenderness; enlargement of breasts; peripheral edema*
   (swelling of feet and lower legs; rapid weight gain)

Incidence less frequent or rare
   *Amenorrhea* (stopping of menstrual bleeding); *breakthrough bleeding*
   (heavier vaginal bleeding between regular menses); *menorrhagia* (prolonged or heavier menses); *or spotting* (lighter vaginal bleeding between regular menses); *breast tumors* (breast lumps; discharge from
   breast); *chorea* (involuntary jerky muscular movements); *gallbladder*

*obstruction or hepatitis* (yellow eyes or skin; pains in stomach, side, or abdomen); *local irritation, such as swelling, redness, or itching*

Note: If *persistent or recurring abnormal vaginal bleeding* occurs, malignancy should be ruled out. However, withdrawal bleeding will frequently occur in patients placed on cyclic estrogen therapy with a progestin who have not undergone hysterectomy.

**Those indicating need for medical attention only if they continue or are bothersome**
Incidence more frequent
*Abdominal cramping or bloating; anorexia* (loss of appetite)

Incidence less frequent
*Diarrhea, mild; dizziness, mild; headaches, mild; intolerance to contact lenses; increased libido; migraine headaches*

## Patient Consultation

As an aid to patient consultation, refer to *Advice for the Patient, Estrogens (Vaginal)*.

In providing consultation, consider emphasizing the following selected information (» = major clinical significance):

**Before using this medication**
» Conditions affecting use, especially:
   Sensitivity to estrogens
   Carcinogenicity—Increased risk of endometrial cancer for patients with an intact uterus placed on unopposed estrogen replacement therapy; decreased risk occurs when used with a progestin; continuous, long-term estrogen use in animal studies increased frequency of cancers of the breast, cervix, and liver
   Pregnancy—Use of some estrogens suggested to be associated with congenital abnormalities
   Breast-feeding—Use is not recommended because estrogens are distributed into breast milk and may have unpredictable effects
   Other medications, especially bromocriptine, cyclosporine, hepatotoxic medications; smoking tobacco may increase risk of cardiovascular side effects and increase metabolism of estrogen
   Other medical problems, especially some types of breast cancer; abnormal and undiagnosed vaginal bleeding; history of estrogen-induced thrombophlebitis, thrombosis, or thromboembolic disorders; or active thrombophlebitis or thromboembolic disorders

**Proper use of this medication**
» Reading patient package insert carefully
» Compliance with therapy
   Using medication at bedtime to increase effectiveness; wearing sanitary napkin to protect clothing
   Proper administration technique
» Proper dosing
   Missed dose: Not using missed dose at all but returning to regular dosing schedule
» Proper storage

**Precautions while using this medication**
» Regular visits to physician at least every year, or more often, as determined by physician
   Possibility of dental problems, such as tenderness, swelling, or bleeding of gums; brushing and flossing teeth, massaging gums, and having dentist clean teeth regularly; checking with dentist if there are questions about care of teeth or gums or if tenderness, swelling, or bleeding of gums is noticed
» Stopping medication immediately and checking with physician if pregnancy is suspected
   Importance of not giving medication to anyone else

**Side/adverse effects**
   Withdrawal bleeding will occur in many postmenopausal patients with an intact uterus who are placed on cyclic estrogen therapy with a progestin
   Signs of potential side effects, especially menstrual irregularities, chorea, breast tumors, peripheral edema, gallbladder obstruction, or hepatitis

## General Dosing Information

Detailed instructions for inserting or applying estrogens vaginally should be furnished to the patient. The manufacturer provides such information on the medication carton or in a patient package insert (PPI).

As a general rule, unopposed estrogen therapy should be administered at the lowest effective dosage. When prolonged therapy is necessary, the patient should be re-evaluated at least every year to determine the need for continued therapy.

In order to avoid overstimulation of estrogen-sensitive tissues, estrogens are applied vaginally each day for 10 days to 3 weeks. During the third and/or fourth weeks of the cycle, the dose is either reduced or the medication discontinued. This schedule is repeated cyclically until improvement of the condition allows a reduced regimen. With chronic use of vaginal estrogens in patients with the uterus *in situ*, the concurrent use of a progestin during the last 10 to 14 days of the cycle should be considered. Administration of a progestin decreases the risk of occurrence of endometrial hyperplasia and endometrial carcinoma. There is no risk of endometrial hyperplasia or endometrial carcinoma in patients who do not have an intact uterus.

The vehicles for some vaginal estrogen products contain lipid-based components. It is not known whether these products adversely affect the performance of latex contraceptive devices, such as cervical caps, condoms, or diaphragms.

---

### *DIENESTROL*

## Vaginal Dosage Forms
### DIENESTROL CREAM USP

**Usual adult dose**
Atrophy, vaginal and vulval—
   Initial: Intravaginal, one applicatorful one or two times a day for one or two weeks, the dose then being reduced to either one-half to one applicatorful a day or one applicatorful every other day, for an additional one or two weeks.
   Maintenance: Intravaginal, one applicatorful one to three times a week for three weeks with no medication used the fourth week may be used after restoration of vaginal mucosa is achieved.

**Strength(s) usually available**
U.S.—
   0.01% (Rx) [*Ortho Dienestrol*].
Canada—
   0.01% (Rx) [*Ortho Dienestrol*].

**Packaging and storage**
Store below 40 °C (104 °F), preferably between 15 and 30 °C (59 and 86 °F), unless otherwise specified by manufacturer. Store in a collapsible tube or tight container. Protect from freezing.

**Auxiliary labeling**
• For vaginal use only.

**Note**
Include mandatory patient package insert (PPI) when dispensing.

---

### *ESTRADIOL*

## Vaginal Dosage Forms
### ESTRADIOL VAGINAL CREAM

**Usual adult dose**
Atrophy, vaginal and vulval—
   Initial: Intravaginal, 200 to 400 mcg of estradiol daily for one or two weeks, the dosage then being gradually reduced to one half the initial dosage for one or two weeks.
   Maintenance: Intravaginal, 100 mcg one to three times a week for three weeks with no medication used the fourth week may be used after restoration of vaginal mucosa is achieved.

**Strength(s) usually available**
U.S.—
   100 mcg per gram (Rx) [*Estrace*].

**Packaging and storage**
Store below 40 °C (104 °F), preferably between 15 and 30 °C (59 and 86 °F). Store in a collapsible tube or tight container. Protect from freezing.

**Auxiliary labeling**
• For vaginal use only.

**Note**
Include mandatory patient package insert (PPI) when dispensing.

## ESTROGENS, CONJUGATED

# Vaginal Dosage Forms
## CONJUGATED ESTROGENS VAGINAL CREAM

**Usual adult dose**
Atrophy, vaginal and vulval—
Intravaginal or topical, 1.25 to 2.5 mg of conjugated estrogens daily for three weeks with no medication used the fourth week, the schedule being repeated cyclically as indicated.

**Strength(s) usually available**
U.S.—
625 mcg (0.625 mg) per gram (Rx) [*Premarin*].
Canada—
625 mcg (0.625 mg) per gram (Rx) [*Premarin*].

**Packaging and storage**
Store below 40 °C (104 °F), preferably between 15 and 30 °C (59 and 86 °F), unless otherwise specified by manufacturer. Protect from freezing.

**Auxiliary labeling**
• For vaginal use only.

**Note**
Include mandatory patient package insert (PPI) when dispensing.

## ESTRONE

# Vaginal Dosage Forms
## ESTRONE VAGINAL CREAM

**Usual adult dose**
Atrophy, vaginal and vulval—
Intravaginal, 2 to 4 mg of estrone daily.

**Strength(s) usually available**
U.S.—
Not commercially available.
Canada—
1 mg per gram (Rx) [*Oestrilin* (methylparaben; propylparaben)].

**Packaging and storage**
Store below 40 °C (104 °F), preferably between 15 and 30 °C (59 and 86 °F), in a well-closed container, unless otherwise specified by manufacturer. Protect from freezing.

**Auxiliary labeling**
• For vaginal use only.

**Note**
Include mandatory patient package insert (PPI) when dispensing.

## ESTRONE VAGINAL SUPPOSITORIES

**Usual adult dose**
Atrophy, vaginal and vulval—
Intravaginal, 250 to 500 mcg daily.

**Strength(s) usually available**
U.S.—
Not commercially available.
Canada—
250 mcg (Rx) [*Oestrilin*].

**Packaging and storage**
Store below 40 °C (104 °F), preferably between 15 and 30 °C (59 and 86 °F), in a well-closed container, unless otherwise specified by manufacturer. Protect from freezing.

**Auxiliary labeling**
• For vaginal use only.

**Note**
Include mandatory patient package insert (PPI) when dispensing.

## ESTROPIPATE

# Vaginal Dosage Forms
## ESTROPIPATE VAGINAL CREAM USP

**Usual adult dose**
Atrophy, vaginal and vulval—
Intravaginal, 3 to 6 mg of estropipate daily for three weeks with no medication used the fourth week, the schedule being repeated cyclically as indicated.

**Strength(s) usually available**
U.S.—
1.5 mg per gram (Rx) [*Ogen* (parabens)].
Canada—
Not commercially available.

**Packaging and storage**
Store below 40 °C (104 °F), preferably between 15 and 30 °C (59 and 86 °F), unless otherwise specified by manufacturer. Protect from freezing.

**Auxiliary labeling**
• For vaginal use only.

**Note**
Include mandatory patient package insert (PPI) when dispensing.

Revised: 06/16/93

---

**ESTROGENS, CONJUGATED**—See *Estrogens (Systemic)*; *Estrogens (Vaginal)*

---

**ESTROGENS, ESTERIFIED**—See *Estrogens (Systemic)*

---

# ESTROGENS AND PROGESTINS Oral Contraceptives    Systemic

This monograph includes information on the following: Desogestrel and Ethinyl Estradiol; Ethynodiol Diacetate and Ethinyl Estradiol; Levonorgestrel and Ethinyl Estradiol; Norethindrone Acetate and Ethinyl Estradiol; Norethindrone and Ethinyl Estradiol; Norethindrone and Mestranol; Norgestimate and Ethinyl Estradiol; Norgestrel and Ethinyl Estradiol.

INN:
Ethinyl estradiol—Ethinylestradiol
Ethynodiol diacetate—Etynodiol
Norethindrone—Norethisterone

BAN:
Ethinyl estradiol—Ethinyloestradiol
Ethynodiol diacetate—Ethynodiol
Norethindrone—Norethisterone

JAN:
Ethinyl estradiol—Ethinylestradiol
Ethynodiol diacetate—Etynodiol acetate
Norethindrone—Norethisterone

VA CLASSIFICATION (Primary/Secondary): HS200/HS900

Other commonly used names are
Ethinylestradiol [Ethinyl estradiol]
Ethinyloestradiol [Ethinyl estradiol]
Ethynodiol [Ethynodiol diacetate]
Etynodiol [Ethynodiol diacetate]
Etynodiol acetate [Ethynodiol diacetate]
Norethindrone [Norethisterone]

Note: For a listing of dosage forms and brand names by country availability, see *Dosage Forms* section(s). For a listing of brand names for the articles in this monograph, refer to the General Index.

## Category

Contraceptive, systemic; Antiendometriotic; Estrogen-progestin; Gonadotropin inhibitor, female, noncontraceptive use—Desogestrel and Ethinyl Estradiol; Ethynodiol Diacetate and Ethinyl Estradiol; Levonorgestrel and Ethinyl Estradiol; Norethindrone Acetate and Ethinyl Estradiol; Norethindrone and Ethinyl Estradiol; Norethindrone and

Mestranol; Norgestimate and Ethinyl Estradiol; Norgestrel and Ethinyl Estradiol.

Contraceptive, postcoital (systemic)—Levonorgestrel and Ethinyl Estradiol; Norgestrel and Ethinyl Estradiol.

## Indications

Note: Bracketed information in the *Indications* section refers to uses that are not included in U.S. product labeling.

### Accepted

Pregnancy, prevention of (prophylaxis)—Combination estrogen-progestin oral contraceptives are indicated for the prevention of pregnancy. The lowest expected failure rate for women who use oral contraceptives consistently and correctly under clinical conditions is 0.1% in the first year of use; however, under nonclinical conditions the typical use is less perfect and typical failures may range from 0 to 6%. All regimens are considered equally effective for preventing pregnancy.

The following table presents the results of studies examining contraceptive failure rates calculated using the life-table method. The first column lists the contraceptive method used. The second column indicates the percentage of women experiencing an accidental pregnancy in the first year of use of a contraceptive method while using the method perfectly under clinical conditions. The range of failure rates in the clinical trials may be explained by interstudy variations in study design or patient population characteristics, such as motivation, fecundity, or socioeconomic factors (including education). The third column indicates contraceptive failure rates in the first year of contraceptive use under clinical conditions for typical couples who start using a method (not necessarily for the first time). Failure rates among adolescents may be higher due to poorer compliance than in other age groups.

| Method used | Failure rate range (over 12 months) in clinical studies (%) | Typical first year failure rate (%) |
|---|---|---|
| None | 78–94 | 85 |
| Spermicides[1] | 0.3–37 | 21 |
| Periodic abstinence[2] | 13–35 | 20 |
| Withdrawal | 7–22 | 19 |
| Cervical cap with spermicide | 6–27 | 18 |
| Diaphragm with spermicide | 2–23 | 18 |
| Condom without spermicide | 2–14 | 12 |
| IUD | | |
| Progesterone-releasing | 1.9–2.0 | 2 |
| Copper-T 200 | 3.0–3.6 | |
| Copper-T 200Ag[3] | 0–1.2 | |
| Copper-T 220C[4] | 0.9–1.8 | |
| Copper-T 380A | 0.5–0.8 | 0.8 |
| Copper-T 380S | 0.9 | |
| Oral contraceptive | | 3 |
| Estrogen and progestin | 0–6 | |
| Progestin only | 1–10 | |
| Medroxyprogesterone injection (90-day) | 0–0.3 | 0.3 |
| Levonorgestrel (subdermal) | | |
| Six capsules | 0–0.09 | 0.09 |
| Two rods | 0–0.2 | 0.3 |
| Sterilization | | |
| Female[5] | 0–8 | 0.4 |
| Male | 0–0.5 | 0.15 |

[1]Spermicides studied include creams, foams, gels, jellies, and suppositories.

[2]Methods studied include calendar, ovulation method, and symptothermal (cervical mucus method supplemented by basal body temperature post-ovulation).

[3]Life-table method rate is unavailable for Copper-T 200Ag and the Pearl method rate at 12 months was reported; these methods at 12 months are considered comparable.

[4]Copper-T 220C is manufactured with copper sleeves instead of copper wire; often used as a control in clinical studies.

[5]Methods studied include culdotomy laparoscopy, minilaparotomy, electrocoagulation, laparotomy, tubal diathermy and/or use of rings or clips.

[Contraception, emergency postcoital (prophylaxis)][1]—A combination of levonorgestrel or norgestrel with ethinyl estradiol is used as *emergency contraception* (also called intraception, morning-after treatment, or postcoital contraception) for postcoital birth control after pregnancy has been ruled out. The dosing method using high doses of estrogen-progestin hormones is commonly called the Yuzpe method. Using oral contraceptives for emergency postcoital contraception is preferable to

using ethinyl estradiol alone because, although the failure rate is higher (2% versus 1%) with oral contraceptives, they cause fewer and less severe side effects to occur. Treatment is initiated within the first 72 hours, preferably within the first 12 hours, after unprotected intercourse.

[Amenorrhea (treatment)] or
[Dysfunctional uterine bleeding (DUB) (treatment)] or
[Dysmenorrhea (treatment)] or
[Hypermenorrhea (treatment)]—[Norethindrone and mestranol tablets (dose of 1/50)] are indicated [and other estrogen-progestin combinations and doses are used][1] as a hormonal treatment for hypoestrogenic or hyperandrogenic conditions, which may present as menstrual cycle abnormalities or unusual uterine bleeding, such as amenorrhea, dysfunctional uterine bleeding, or hypermenorrhea. When treating amenorrhea and hypermenorrhea, the abnormality should be diagnosed first and then treated appropriately; oral contraceptives have limited use for treating conditions not caused by a hypoestrogenic or hyperandrogenic state. Patients who require contraception as well as relief from primary dysmenorrhea may benefit from treatment with oral contraceptives. If contraception is not needed, prostaglandin-inhibiting medications, such as nonsteroidal anti-inflammatory drugs (NSAIDs), are used. If dysmenorrhea is not relieved by oral contraceptives or NSAIDs, endometriosis or another organic cause should be considered.

[Endometriosis (prophylaxis and treatment)]—[Norethindrone and mestranol tablets (dose of 1/50)] are indicated [and other estrogen-progestin combinations and doses are used][1] to reduce the size and growth of endometrial tissue.

[Hirsutism, female (treatment and treatment adjunct)][1] or
[Hyperandrogenism, ovarian (treatment and treatment adjunct)][1] or
[Polycystic ovary syndrome (treatment)][1]—When treating these conditions, the basic cause should be ascertained first, if possible, and treated accordingly. When contraception is needed as well, oral contraceptives are used to help suppress hypothalamic-pituitary function in LH-dependent hyperandrogenism in conditions such as polycystic ovary syndrome. Oral contraceptive treatment results in regularity of the menstrual cycle and lessening of hirsutism in these conditions.

### Acceptance not established

Only limited data are available evaluating the use of oral contraceptives as adjunct agents to replace the estrogen component as *add-back* therapy when gonadotropin-releasing hormone agonists are used to suppress the hypothalamic-pituitary axis. Using oral contraceptives as the estrogen replacement may be especially useful in women needing contraception as well. By replacing estrogen, hypoestrogenic side effects caused by the gonadotropin-releasing hormone agonist, such as bone loss and the associated vasomotor symptoms, are reduced. Further studies are needed to evaluate the safety and efficacy of this use.

Oral contraceptives, which are effective in dysmenorrhea, have been used to reduce premenstrual pain associated with the premenstrual syndrome in some patients, but generally oral contraceptives are not considered useful for this indication.

### Unaccepted

Administration of oral contraceptives to induce withdrawal bleeding should not be used as a test for pregnancy.

Oral contraceptives should not be used during pregnancy for the treatment of threatened or habitual abortion.

[1]Not included in Canadian product labeling.

## Pharmacology/Pharmacokinetics

### Physicochemical characteristics

Chemical group—
    Estrogens—
        Ethinyl estradiol.
        Mestranol.
    Progestins, 19-nortestosterone derivatives—
        Desogestrel.
        Ethynodiol diacetate.
        Levonorgestrel (levorotatory isomer).
        Norethindrone.
        Norethindrone acetate.
        Norgestimate.
        Norgestrel (racemic mixture).
Molecular weight—
    Desogestrel: 310.48.
    Ethinyl estradiol: 296.41.
    Ethynodiol diacetate: 384.52.
    Levonorgestrel: 312.45.
    Mestranol: 310.44.
    Norethindrone: 298.43.

Norethindrone acetate: 340.47.
Norgestimate: 369.51.
Norgestrel: 312.45.

## Mechanism of action/Effect

Estrogen-progestin—Estrogens increase the cellular synthesis of chromatin (DNA), RNA, and various proteins in responsive tissues, and progestins increase the synthesis of RNA by means of interaction with DNA.

Contraceptive, systemic—The synergistic anti-ovulatory effect from the combined use of estrogen and progestin directly decreases the secretion of the gonadotropin-releasing hormone (GnRH) from the hypothalamus and is considered the main action. This negative feedback mechanism disrupts ovulation by interfering with the hypothalamus-pituitary-ovary axis and gonadotropin secretion from the pituitary. Specifically, the progestin component blunts or suppresses luteinizing hormone (LH) release and the LH surge, which is necessary for ovulation, and the estrogen component blunts or suppresses the follicle-stimulating hormone (FSH), which prevents the selection and maturation of the dominant follicle. Neither the estrogen nor the progestin hormone dose used in combination hormonal oral contraceptives alone would be able to suppress ovulation but together the estrogen and progestin hormones work synergistically to suppress ovulation successfully. Other contributing effects include delayed maturation of the endometrium, which prevents implantation of ova; and the development of viscous cervical mucus, which slows spermatic ingress. The effects on the endometrium and cervical mucus are considered the mechanisms of action for the estrogen-progestin oral contraceptives used for emergency contraception (intraception).

Antiendometriotic—Oral contraceptives can produce a pseudopregnant state (especially when used continuously) in which the uterine endometrium and ectopic endometriotic implants undergo decidual reaction, necrosis, and eventual atrophy. Sometimes endometriotic symptoms may increase before improvement is noted.

Gonadotropin inhibitor, female, noncontraceptive use—Suppressed ovarian steroidogenesis secondary to LH concentration reduction prevents ovarian cyst formation in functional ovarian cysts, corpus luteum cysts, or polycystic ovary syndrome. Although a decrease in occurrence of repetitively forming functional ovarian cysts is possible, treatment to either speed the resolution of existing ovarian cysts or to treat functional ovarian cysts secondary to ovulation induction has not been established. The likelihood of suppressing ovarian cyst formation is greatest with 50-mcg ethinyl estradiol–containing monophasic formulations but 35-mcg ethinyl estradiol–containing monophasic formulations are used effectively, also. Suppression is least likely with triphasic formulations. In addition to suppression of ovarian steroidogenesis, there is an increase in sex–hormone-binding globulin, which binds testosterone and decreases the quantity of free hormone. This effectively reduces the androgenic symptoms of hirsutism, polycystic ovary syndrome, and hyperandrogenism. Desogestrel and norgestimate additionally improve acne or hirsutism conditions because of their high level of progestational effects and absence of androgenic effects. Other progestins having androgenic properties, such as levonorgestrel, norgestrel, or norethindrone, may or may not worsen acne or hirsutism, depending on the progestin-estrogen dose relationship.

## Other actions/effects

The following noncontraceptive effects have been observed with the use of oral contraceptives: menstrual cycle regularity, fewer occurrences of iron-deficient anemia associated with heavy menses flow or pelvic inflammatory disease; and fewer ectopic pregnancies. Although low-dose oral contraceptives may have less effect, high-dose formulations (containing ≥ 50 mcg [0.05 mg] estrogen) used long-term have decreased the occurrence of benign breast disease, including fibroadenomas and fibrocystic breast disease. Also, oral contraceptives may protect against or delay development of benign or malignant endometrial and ovarian cancers, atherosclerosis, or rheumatoid arthritis (although some of these are still controversial).

Norgestrel and levonorgestrel have the most androgenic activity of all the progestins. Norethindrone and ethynodiol diacetate possess slight estrogenic activity, and norethindrone has some androgenic activity. Norgestimate and desogestrel have high progestational activity and are low in androgenicity.

## Absorption

Both estrogen and progestin components are rapidly and well absorbed.

Ethinyl estradiol or

Mestranol—Relative bioavailability is 83% because these estrogens have both a first-pass effect and enterohepatic recirculation with similar blood concentrations achieved for both 50 mcg of mestranol-containing and 35 mcg of ethinyl estradiol–containing oral contraceptives.

Desogestrel—Desogestrel is primarily absorbed in the intestine as its active metabolite, 3-keto-desogestrel, but because of a significant first-pass effect, the relative bioavailability of 3-keto-desogestrel is 84%.

Ethynodiol diacetate or

Norethindrone or

Norethindrone acetate—Ethynodiol diacetate and norethindrone acetate are completely hydrolyzed by intestinal tissue to norethindrone, which is then absorbed. All of these progestins are rapidly and well absorbed but because of a first-pass effect, 53% bioavailability results.

Levonorgestrel or

Norgestimate or

Norgestrel—Intestinal absorption within 2 hours; completely bioavailable because these progestins do not exhibit a first-pass effect.

## Distribution

Oral contraceptives are widely distributed.

Ethinyl estradiol—Distributed into the uterus (0.9%), blood (8.8%), adipose tissue (28.2%), and other tissues. Fifty mcg of ethinyl estradiol taken orally would yield a concentration of 10 nanograms/100 mL a day in breast milk, which is not considered clinically significant.

Desogestrel (with ethinyl estradiol administration)—Volume of distribution ($Vol_D$) is 143 ± 61 liters (L).

Norethindrone (with ethinyl estradiol)—$Vol_D$ is approximately 236 ± 60 L.

## Protein binding

Oral contraceptives differ in their ability to increase the concentration of sex hormone–binding globulin (SHBG) that is induced by estrogen because contraceptive progestins differ in their ability to suppress this estrogen effect. Also, contraceptive progestins have different affinities for albumin and SHBG. Therefore, progestins binding to serum proteins again differ relative to how the estrogen and the progestin together affect serum proteins, i.e., a progestin with greater affinity for albumin than SHBG but faced with greater serum concentration of SHBG induced by estrogen would result in greater binding of progestin to SHBG.

Ethinyl estradiol—High; specifically, ethinyl estradiol is 95% bound to albumin, but not to SHBG; ethinyl estradiol induces production of SHBG. Tissue-specific receptor proteins form complexes with estrogens in estrogen-responsive tissues.

Desogestrel (with ethinyl estradiol administration)—High; albumin (66 ± 12%), SHBG (31 ± 12%), unbound (2.5 ± 0.2%). Because desogestrel does not counteract the increase of SHBG caused by daily estrogen administration, nonlinear kinetics result; desogestrel binds to a threefold increase of SHBG, which is highest between the third and sixth months of treatment.

Levonorgestrel (with ethinyl estradiol administration)—High; proportion bound to albumin or SHBG varies by strength and phasic relationship of both levonorgestrel and estrogen. Specifically, 250 mcg levonorgestrel and 50 mcg ethinyl estradiol have decreased SHBG by 24%, 150 mcg levonorgestrel and 30 mcg ethinyl estradiol decreased SHBG by 10%, and triphasic formulations increased SHBG. Levonorgestrel's affinity for SHBG is greater than its affinity for albumin.

Norethindrone—Without use of estrogen, norethindrone binds 61% to albumin and 35.5% to SHBG while 3.5% is unbound. With use of ethinyl estradiol, an 80 to 100% increase in SHBG may be expected, which will increase the SHBG-bound proportion of norethindrone.

## Biotransformation

Desogestrel—In Phase I hydroxylation, desogestrel, a prodrug, is metabolized in the intestinal tract and by hepatic first-pass metabolism to the biologically active metabolite 3-keto-desogestrel and several inactive metabolites. The metabolism is completed in Phase II, resulting in polar conjugated glucuronide and sulfate metabolites.

Ethinyl estradiol or

Mestranol—Exhibits Phase I and Phase II metabolism. Seventy percent of the prodrug, mestranol, converts to ethinyl estradiol by demethylation. Estrogen metabolites, mainly conjugates, are hydroxylated by enzymes of intestinal bacteria, which are then reabsorbed via enterohepatic recirculation.

Ethynodiol diacetate or

Norethindrone or

Norethindrone acetate—Hydrolysis of ethynodiol diacetate and norethindrone acetate to norethindrone occurs mainly in the intestines, but also in the liver. Norethindrone is metabolized to sulfate (predominately in plasma) and glucuronide conjugates, which may prolong activity if active metabolites are discovered. Also, it is postulated that the aromatization of norethindrone to ethinyl estradiol by tissues such as the liver, ovaries, and placenta may be of clinical significance.

Levonorgestrel or

Norgestrel—Metabolism of the inactive isomer L-(d)-norgestrel differs considerably from metabolism of the active isomer L-(l)-norgestrel; the latter is sulfated more rapidly than is the inactive isomer.

Norgestimate—Considered an incomplete prodrug for levonorgestrel; has biological activity, but 85% of activity is thought to be due to norgestrel acetate and, to a much lesser extent, norgestrel. Metabolized to active metabolites, levonorgestrel and 17-deactyl norgestimate (has activity similar to norgestimate), as well as other hydroxy-compounds.

**Half-life**

Desogestrel (with ethinyl estradiol administration) or

Levonorgestrel (with ethinyl estradiol administration)—Elimination, plasma: 8 to 13 hours.

Ethinyl estradiol (with desogestrel administration)—Elimination, plasma: 26 hours.

Ethinyl estradiol (with norgestimate administration)—Elimination: 6 to 14 hours.

Ethynodiol diacetate (with ethinyl estradiol administration) or

Norethindrone (with ethinyl estradiol administration) or

Norethindrone acetate (with ethinyl estradiol administration)—Elimination, plasma: 8 hours.

Norgestimate (with ethinyl estradiol administration)—Elimination, plasma: 30 to 71 hours for norgestimate; 17 to 30 hours for 17-deactyl norgestimate, a metabolite.

**Elimination**

Desogestrel—Renal: 45%, of which 14 to 28% is unchanged, and 38 to 61% is excreted as glucuronide and 23 to 39% as sulfate conjugates. Fecal: Up to 30%.

Ethinyl estradiol or

Mestranol—Renal: 22 to 58%.
Fecal: 30 to 53%.
Biliary: 26 to 43%

Ethynodiol diacetate or

Norethindrone acetate or

Norethindrone—Renal: 37 to 87%, of which 3% is unchanged, and 40% is excreted as glucuronide and 15% as sulfate conjugates.
Fecal: Up to 40%.

Levonorgestrel or

Norgestrel—Renal, as inactive metabolites.

Norgestimate—Renal: 45 to 49%
Fecal: 16 to 49%

# Precautions to Consider

## Carcinogenicity

Recent and current users of high-dose oral contraceptives (containing 50 mcg or more of estrogen) for at least 2 years have shown a progressive reduction of up to 40% in incidence of benign fibrocystic breast disease; it is unknown if low-dose oral contraceptives (containing less than 50 mcg of estrogen) have similar effects.

Use of oral contraceptives in women between 25 and 39 years of age does not increase the risk of developing breast cancer at 45 years of age or older. Whether oral contraceptives increase the risk of breast cancer in certain subgroups of women, such as women under 20 years of age using oral contraceptives for more than 4 years or women 46 to 54 years of age using oral contraceptives for more than 3 years, is unresolved. Some case-control studies have shown no association between oral contraceptive use and breast cancer in women under 20 years of age and a protective effect or no enhancement of risk in women 46 to 54 years of age. Because risk factors vary for women of different age groups, parity, environment, and age at first use, controlling for these and other confounding factors and establishing whether additional risk occurs is difficult. The magnitude of increased risk, if it exists at all, is considered very small, and does not warrant withholding the use of oral contraceptives in any subgroup of women (including those women having a family history of either breast cancer or benign breast disease, or women having a history of benign breast disease) or restricting use for young nulliparous women. Further analyses of risks associated with using low-dose oral contraceptives as compared to high-dose contraceptives and to characterize effects of duration of use are being evaluated.

If an oral contraceptive containing 50 mcg of estrogen is taken for at least 12 months, a 15-year protective effect against the development of endometrial cancer persists after stopping the oral contraceptive treatment; similar effects for low-dose oral contraceptives are expected but need to be evaluated.

High and low doses of monophasic oral contraceptives used continuously for at least 3 years have shown a protective effect against ovarian cancer that is fully developed in 6 years and may persist for at least 10 years; shorter-term use has not shown a protective effect. Similar effects for short- and long-term, low-dose bi- and triphasic oral contraceptives are expected since they suppress ovulation, but this theory needs to be evaluated.

Epidemiologic studies suggest that women taking oral contraceptives for 8 or more years have an increased risk of developing hepatocellular

carcinoma as compared to women not taking oral contraceptives. However, these cancers are extremely rare and cases caused by long-term oral contraceptive use are less than one per million users of oral contraceptives.

Risk for dysplasia and carcinoma of the cervix is increased with oral contraceptive use for more than 1 year. The risk of invasive cervical cancer could increase twofold after 5 years of use; the greatest risk is in women using oral contraceptives for longer than 10 years. A great portion of the risk is thought to be due to the number of sexual partners a woman has and the age at first coitus, a factor that may be different between users and never-users.

## Tumorigenicity

Although benign and rare, liver cell adenomas, many of which regressed with the cessation of oral contraceptive use, have occurred in women using oral contraceptives for longer than 5 years. Liver cell adenomas should be suspected in patients having abdominal pain and tenderness, abdominal mass, or hypovolemic shock. These adenomas may rupture and may cause death through intra-abdominal hemorrhage.

## Mutagenicity

It is generally believed that there is no increased risk of mutagenicity or teratogenicity, including any development of fetal sexual malformation, when oral contraceptives are inadvertently taken in early pregnancy. This information is based on a small number of case reports, and well-designed studies still are needed.

## Pregnancy/Reproduction

Fertility—Delayed fertility has been shown to occur rarely in users of oral contraceptives, especially in nulliparous women. In one study, the rate of impaired fertility normalized by 48 and 72 months for two groups of nulliparous women (25 to 29 years of age and 30 to 34 years of age, respectively). Infertility rates have not been shown to increase.

Pregnancy—Studies have shown that combination oral contraceptives do not appear to increase the risk of birth defects when they are used before pregnancy. Studies have also shown that oral contraceptives, when taken inadvertently during early pregnancy, do not seem to have a teratogenic effect. However, oral contraceptives are not recommended for use during pregnancy and should be discontinued immediately if pregnancy is suspected.

Any patient who has missed two consecutive menstrual periods while taking oral contraceptives should discontinue their use; a nonhormonal contraceptive method should be used until pregnancy is ruled out. If the patient has not followed the dosing schedule, pregnancy should be ruled out after the first missed menstrual period.

When considering pregnancy, it is recommended that conception be delayed for one or two months after cessation of oral contraceptives or until after the first regular menses to accurately date the gestation period.

FDA Pregnancy Category X.

Postpartum or postabortion—Oral contraceptive use and the immediate postpartum period are both associated with an increased risk of thromboembolism occurrence. Therefore, to lessen any potential risk that may exist, oral contraceptives should be started no sooner than two weeks after delivery in women choosing to not breast-feed. Also, ovulation usually does not occur before this time and contraception is not needed. However, the chance of early ovulation is high following abortion but the risk of thromboembolic phenomena is not great. Therefore, some clinicians recommend that use of a low-dose oral contraceptive may begin immediately after a first-trimester or second-trimester abortion. Also, immediate use of an oral contraceptive is recommended following a second-trimester premature delivery or after a pregnancy of less than 12 weeks; however, for a pregnancy of 12 or more weeks, use of a low-dose oral contraceptive is recommended after 2 weeks.

## Breast-feeding

Oral contraceptives are distributed into breast milk, and may diminish its quantity or quality or shorten the time of lactation, especially for those women who are only partially breast-feeding and have less physical stimulus for lactation. Use of oral contraceptives by nursing mothers in the early postpartum period is generally not recommended. When used by mothers who are exclusively breast-feeding, oral contraceptive therapy is recommended to begin after the third postpartum month or, if only partially or not breast-feeding, to begin in the third postpartum week. If contraception is needed prior to this, some clinicians begin low-dose oral contraceptives after lactation has been well-established.

## Adolescents

One of the most accepted, frequently prescribed and, when used regularly, effective contraceptive methods for adolescents is oral contraceptives. However, the pregnancy rate for adolescents using oral contraceptives is estimated at 6 to 12 per 100 woman years, which is higher than the pregnancy rate, 0.3 to 0.7 per 100 woman years, for all age groups of women.

Studies generally have shown that adolescents tend to be less compliant users of any type of contraceptive. Any psychosocial factors involved and discussion of preconceived thoughts on side effects, including weight gain, fluid retention, or breakthrough uterine bleeding, are important areas for patient counseling to help aid in this age group's compliance problem with using oral contraceptives.

## Dental

Increased concentrations of progestins increase the normal oral flora growth rate, leading to an increase in inflammation of the gingival tissues and increased bleeding. A strictly enforced program of teeth cleaning by a professional, combined with plaque control by the patient, will minimize severity.

An increased incidence of local alveolar osteitis (dry socket) after dental extractions has been seen with the use of estrogen and progestin combination oral contraceptives. A direct correlation exists between the incidence of dry socket occurrence and increasing estrogen dose. Therefore, it is recommended that patients inform their dentist or oral surgeon that they are taking an estrogen and progestin contraceptive.

## Drug interactions and/or related problems

The following drug interactions and/or related problems have been selected on the basis of their potential clinical significance (possible mechanism in parentheses where appropriate)—not necessarily inclusive (» = major clinical significance):

Note: Combinations containing any of the following medications, depending on the amount present, may also interact with this medication.

Amoxicillin or
Ampicillin or
Doxycycline or
Penicillin V or
Tetracycline
(there have been rare case reports of reduced oral contraceptive effectiveness in women taking amoxicillin, ampicillin, doxycycline, penicillin V, or tetracycline, resulting in unplanned pregnancy. This is thought to be due to a reduction in enterohepatic circulation of estrogens, which may cause a lower estrogen plasma concentration than expected. Although the association is very weak, patients, especially long-term users of antibiotic therapy, should be advised of this information and given the option of using an alternate or additional method of contraception while taking any of these antibiotics, especially if the duration of antibiotic therapy is greater than 2 weeks)

Anticoagulants, coumarin- or indandione-derivative
(concurrent use with oral contraceptives has modestly increased, and in some cases decreased, the effectiveness of anticoagulants; however, the mechanism is unknown and appropriate studies have not been done. Because estrogens increase hepatic synthesis of procoagulant factors and decrease antithrombin III, it is possible that adjustment of the anticoagulant dosage based on prothrombin time determinations may be needed)

Antidiabetic agents, sulfonylurea or
Insulin
(estrogen-containing oral contraceptives may cause glucose or insulin resistance in diabetic patients, resulting in a loss, probably slight, of metabolic control of plasma glucose concentration; unless the changes can be controlled with diet, this may necessitate an increased sulfonylurea or insulin dose and regular monitoring)

Benzodiazepines
(metabolism of those benzodiazepines, such as diazepam and alprazolam, that undergo oxidation may be inhibited, resulting in delayed diazepam elimination and increased concentration of plasma diazepam, which may increase the side effects of diazepam. Although the pharmacokinetics of alprazolam were not affected with long-term use, a study has shown a greater sensitivity to alprazolam and psychomotor impairment with single doses of alprazolam in long-term contraceptive users; pharmacokinetic factors were not believed to contribute to this effect. Metabolism of those benzodiazepines that undergo conjugation, such as oxazepam, lorazepam, and temazepam, is not impaired)

(reduction of oral contraceptive effectiveness has not been shown with concurrent use of benzodiazepines)

Caffeine
(oral contraceptives reduce or inhibit the hepatic metabolism of caffeine, thereby increasing the plasma concentration of caffeine up to 30 to 40%; patient may need to be counseled about the increased effects of caffeine if warranted)

Clofibrate
(concurrent use with oral contraceptives may lower the effectiveness of clofibrate)

» Corticosteroids, glucocorticoid
(concurrent use with estrogens may lower the metabolism of glucocorticoids, decrease the elimination of potent metabolites, decrease the protein binding of glucocorticoids, and increase the production of the protein-binding globulin, transcortin (also called cortisol-binding globulin), leading to decreased clearance [approximately 30 to 50% for prednisolone] of the glucocorticoid free fraction, prolonged elimination half-life, and increased effects of the glucocorticoids; lower doses of the glucocorticoid are needed with concurrent use of estrogen-containing oral contraceptives)

» Cyclosporine
(a case report has shown that concurrent use with oral contraceptives increased the plasma concentration of cyclosporine, which may increase its effects; monitoring of plasma cyclosporine concentration and hepatic factors for toxicity, reducing cyclosporine dose, or changing to nonhormonal contraception may be required to minimize the risk of cyclosporine toxicity)

» Hepatic enzyme inducers (See *Appendix II*), especially:
Barbiturates
Carbamazepine
Griseofulvin
Phenytoin
Primidone
Rifampicin
Rifampin
(concurrent use of these medications with oral contraceptives may induce hepatic enzyme oral contraceptive metabolism, especially of the estrogen component, which could result in reduced contraceptive reliability and increased incidence of breakthrough bleeding; high interindividual variability in hepatic enzyme induction exists but patients should be advised to use a high-dose estrogen-containing contraceptive if oral contraceptives are used, or an alternative or additional method of contraception during use of any these medications, especially if breakthrough bleeding occurs)

(additionally, phenobarbital and phenytoin have been shown to increase sex hormone–binding globulin [SHBG], which may lower the amount of free progestin available for biological action and contribute to the lowered effectiveness of the oral contraceptive)

» Hepatotoxic medications, especially troleandomycin (See *Appendix II*)
(the estrogen component of oral contraceptives increases hepatic blood flow and size of the liver with increased vesiculation of the smooth and rough endoplasmic reticulum, which results in altered hepatic metabolism; it is possible that concurrent use of these medications with estrogens may increase the risk of hepatotoxicity; more frequent monitoring of hepatic function is needed)

» Ritonavir
(area under the plasma concentration–time curve [AUC] of estrogen is decreased by 40% during use of ritonavir; the estrogen dose of the oral contraceptive should be increased or an alternative form of birth control used with concurrent use of ritonavir)

» Smoking, tobacco
(polycyclic hydrocarbons in cigarette smoke are potent inducers of certain hepatic cytochrome P450 isoenzymes; the consequences of this effect on metabolism have not been fully explored but may influence the associated risks of using oral contraceptives and smoking concurrently. Although some studies showed inhibition of metabolism of a metabolite of ethinyl estradiol, smoking did not affect the metabolism of ethinyl estradiol)

(oral contraceptives are not recommended with heavy tobacco use because of an increased risk of serious cardiovascular side effects, including cerebrovascular accident, transient ischemic attacks, thrombophlebitis, and pulmonary embolism; risk increases with increased tobacco usage and with age, especially in women over 35 years of age; the mechanisms for these outcomes are still being explored. Some clinicians have used low-dose estrogen oral contraceptives in women who are light smokers or who use a nicotine patch)

Tamoxifen
(concurrent use with estrogens may interfere with the antiestrogenic therapeutic effect of tamoxifen)

» Theophylline
(although theophylline reduced the apparent clearance of ethinyl estradiol 30 to 35% in oral contraceptive users, clinical significance was not noted because of the wide interindividual variability in metabolism of the estrogen; however, reduction of the total plasma clearance of theophylline by 25 to 35% by oral contraceptives was considered clinically significant. These effects result in an increase of both the theophylline and ethinyl estradiol plasma concentration; a lower dose of the theophylline may be needed)

Tricyclic antidepressants
(inhibition of imipramine oxidation by oral contraceptives results in higher plasma concentrations of imipramine; imipramine dose may need to be adjusted)

(estrogen has facilitated the development of neuroleptic antipsychotic or tricyclic antidepressant medication–associated movement disorders, such as akathisia, but not tardive dyskinesia. It is not known if the low doses of estrogen used in oral contraceptives are also implicated in akathisia)

(rare cases of chorea have developed in women with chorea gravidarum using oral contraceptives, but oral contraceptives do not appear to create any additional risk in women not predisposed to develop chorea)

## Laboratory value alterations
The following have been selected on the basis of their potential clinical significance (possible effect in parentheses where appropriate)—not necessarily inclusive (» = major clinical significance):

With diagnostic test results
Aldosterone, serum or
Aldosterone, urine or
Renin, plasma
(the estrogen component decreases the plasma concentration of plasma renin but increases plasma renin activity; oral contraceptives should be discontinued at least 2 weeks, and preferably 4 weeks, before testing plasma renin activity)

Antipyrine test
(lower values result because oral contraceptives significantly reduce antipyrine metabolism, particularly the oxidative mechanism)

Corticotropin-releasing hormone stimulation test or
Metyrapone test
(corticotropin plasma levels were reduced approximately 25% overall in a study of women using triphasic oral contraceptives who had been given a morning corticotropin-releasing hormone [CRH] stimulation test; normal basal levels were unchanged; reduced response also has been noted for the metyrapone test with other oral contraceptives)

Dexamethasone suppression test
(oral contraceptive users had a significantly higher plasma cortisol level pre- and post-dexamethasone testing; this effect caused by estrogen may persist for up to 1 month after oral contraceptive treatment ends)

Glucose tolerance test, oral
(significantly higher 2-hour oral glucose tolerance test results)

Norepinephrine-induced platelet aggregability
(may be increased)

*Thyroid function tests*
Thyroxine ($T_4$) determinations
(estrogen-induced thyroid-binding globulin elevates the amount of $T_4$ that is protein bound; this effect reverses in about 2 months after discontinuation of oral contraceptives; serum free $T_4$ concentrations are unchanged. Specifically, triphasic oral contraceptives containing 30 micrograms of ethinyl estradiol have increased thyroid-binding globulin by about 20% and elevated total $T_4$ by 40%)

Triiodothyronine ($T_3$) determinations
(free $T_3$ and reverse $T_3$ are unchanged, but $T_3$ resin uptake is decreased because estrogens increase serum thyroid-binding globulin [TBG]; total $T_3$ radioimmunoassay [RIA] values are increased but proportionately less than serum $T_4$ values)

With physiology/laboratory test values
Albumin
(monophasic norethindrone-ethinyl estradiol 1/35 decreased albumin levels throughout the treatment period; this was not seen with monophasic levonorgestrel-ethinyl estradiol 0.15/30)

Alkaline phosphatase
(monophasic norethindrone-ethinyl estradiol 1/35 decreased alkaline phosphatase levels throughout a 1-year treatment period; this was not seen with monophasic levonorgestrel-ethinyl estradiol 0.15/30)

Androstenedione or
Ceruloplasmin, serum or
Dehydroepiandrosterone sulfate (DHEA-S) or
Pregnenolone or
Sex hormone–binding globulin (SHBG), serum or
Testosterone or
Thyroid-binding globulin or
Transferrin or cortisol-binding globulin, serum
(oral contraceptives increase protein synthesis of SHBG, thyroid-binding globulin, transferrin, and ceruloplasmin; the serum con-

centrations of total sex steroids, copper, and cortisol may also increase while the free thyroid concentration remains unchanged and thyroid function remains unaltered; response of free non–protein-bound component may be variable)

(oral contraceptives' net effect on SHBG is the result of the opposing actions of the estrogen and progestin. A dose-related response to progestins of greater androgenicity, such as norgestrel, has a greater suppressive effect on the estrogen-induced increases of SHBG than do those with low androgenic effect, such as desogestrel or norgestimate, which have little suppressive effect on estrogen-induced SHBG levels and result in a three- to fourfold increase of SHBG. However, further elevations of SHBG above some level that remains undetermined do not appear to result in any further decrease in free testosterone. For instance, one study showed that an elevation of SHBG by 92% and 175% decreased free testosterone similarly [by 35%]. Monophasic ethinyl estradiol and norethindrone 1/35 and 1/50 increased SHBG levels 183 to 390%; ethinyl estradiol and norgestrel increased SHBG 12%. Testosterone levels are further changed by those progestins that have greater affinity for SHBG, such as levonorgestrel-containing oral contraceptives, that can displace testosterone from its SHBG binding site)

(also, norgestrel-, ethynodiol diacetate–, and norethindrone-containing oral contraceptives reduce circulating DHEA-S 28%, androstenedione 47%, and testosterone 40%, including the precursor, pregnenolone, by causing a decrease in corticotropin stimulation or by direct effect on hepatic enzyme inhibition; the complexity of these factors causes a variable clinical effect among individuals taking oral contraceptives)

Antithrombin III
(may be decreased by most oral contraceptives, which contributes to decreased anticoagulant or increased fibrinolytic activity of oral contraceptives. A study showed that desogestrel increased fibrinolytic activity less than did triphasic levonorgestrel but still significantly more than did controls; however, the increase was generally within normal laboratory ranges; extreme values among individuals may need to be taken into consideration. Specifically, triphasic levonorgestrel and ethinyl estradiol showed a slight increase of antithrombin III at 12 weeks, then a decrease until the end of the 48-week study, while the amount of antithrombin III was decreased at 24 weeks for desogestrel and ethinyl estradiol but returned to normal at 48 weeks)

Apolipoprotein $A_1$, $A_2$, or B or
Cholesterol, total or
Triglycerides
(in general, the net effect on lipoproteins is the result of the opposing actions of the estrogen and progestin and depends on the ratio between the two hormones; the estrogen component increases triglyceride, very low density lipoproteins (VLDL), and total cholesterol concentrations and decreases low density lipoproteins (LDL), while the progestin component, if androgenic, decreases high density lipoproteins (HDL) and increases LDL. The low concentrations of the androgenic progestins in oral contraceptives have slight effect, which is only of clinical significance for some predisposed individuals. Sometimes, older women with higher serum concentrations of cholesterol may experience a reduction caused by a lowering of the serum LDL concentrations. Triglycerides are increased by all oral contraceptives because of the predominant estrogen effects. The increase of total cholesterol caused by desogestrel- and norgestimate-containing oral contraceptives is considered favorable because it is the net result of the increase of $HDL_3$-C (an estrogen effect) without an increase of $HDL_2$-C concentrations. The increase of $HDL_2$-C caused by other low-dose oral contraceptives is considered an androgenic effect of some of the 19–nortestosterone-derived progestins)

*For monophasics*
(monophasic ethynodiol diacetate-ethinyl estradiol 1/35 showed the greatest increase in apolipoprotein $A_1$ and monophasic levonorgestrel-ethinyl estradiol 0.15/30 showed the smallest increase; monophasic ethinyl estradiol-norgestrel has shown significant decrease in apolipoproteins $A_1$ and $A_2$)

(in one study, monophasic norethindrone-ethinyl estradiol 1/35 increased triglycerides to levels that continued throughout a 1-year treatment period while monophasic levonorgestrel-ethinyl estradiol 0.15/30 caused no change in triglyceride levels over a 1-year treatment period; total cholesterol levels were slightly decreased for norethindrone-ethinyl estradiol 1/35 but returned toward baseline within the 1-year treatment period, while monophasic levonorgestrel-ethinyl estradiol 0.15/30 slightly reduced total cholesterol levels at 3-month and 1-year treatment periods)

*For triphasics*

(in a study with triphasics, levonorgestrel-ethinyl estradiol [7/7/7- and 9/5/7-day regimens] and norethindrone-ethinyl estradiol, significant increases in plasma triglyceride [28 to 52%] and plasma apolipoprotein B levels [20 to 23%] were shown in each treatment group at 6 months with less of an increase in total plasma cholesterol [3 to 11%] than occurs in nonhormonal contraceptive users; similarly, plasma apolipoprotein $A_1$ values increased 5 to 12% in the contraceptive users. A 12-month study showed increased values also but considered them within acceptable clinical limits; another study showed a significant decrease of total cholesterol, thought to be due to a decrease in LDL, during the first week of oral triphasic contraceptive use; the total serum cholesterol returned to baseline over the next 3 weeks)

Aspartate aminotransferase (SGOT), serum or
Bilirubin, total, serum or
Urobilinogen, urine

(these values are decreased with oral contraceptives containing 50 mcg of ethinyl estradiol; the incidence of abnormal liver test values is lower for oral contraceptives containing 35 mcg of ethinyl estradiol or 50 mcg of mestranol; total bilirubin, urinary urobilinogen, and serum SGOT were significantly decreased at 3 months for monophasic norethindrone-ethinyl estradiol 1/35, but returned to baseline at 12 months, while users of monophasic levonorgestrel-ethinyl estradiol 0.15/30 showed only slightly decreased concentrations that were not considered clinically significant)

Clotting factors VII, VIII, IX, and X or
Prothrombin time or
Thromboplastin time, partial

(oral contraceptives shorten partial thromboplastin and prothrombin time, but these results are neither consistent nor do they occur in all individuals. Activation of the segments of the intrinsic and extrinsic system of coagulation by oral contraceptives enhances, depending on the factor, either the fibrinolysis or procoagulation or affects both. If baseline values were increased, the increase was within normal laboratory ranges in most cases and did not consistently alter bleeding or clotting times)

Cortisol, serum or urine

(the net effect of oral contraceptives on serum cortisol is the result of the opposing actions of the estrogen and progestin and depends on the ratio between the two hormones. Progestins, such as norethindrone, having glucocorticoid effects decrease corticotropin release and adrenal cortisol production. Estrogens augment corticotropin release by downregulating pituitary glucocorticoid receptors and increase adrenal cortisol responsiveness to corticotropin stimulation. This results in an increase in serum cortisol concentrations and a decrease in urinary cortisol clearance)

Glucose, plasma or serum or
Insulin

(reduced glucose tolerance and elevated fasting insulin and C-peptide values can occur with use of low-dose oral contraceptives during the first 12 months of use, returning to normal between 12 and 24 months of continued use. These changes from baseline were clinically nonsignificant in most prospective studies of low-dose oral contraceptives as many values were still within the normal range. Levonorgestrel- or norgestrel-containing combinations caused the greatest insulin resistance followed by combinations of desogestrel and low-dose norethindrone oral contraceptives. Levonorgestrel significantly increased second-phase pancreatic insulin production while desogestrel and norgestimate did not)

Growth hormone

(physiologic levels may increase during the first year)

High density lipoproteins (HDL), serum

(low-dose oral contraceptives show a trend of no change or a decrease in value of HDL; the estrogen component increases HDL and the progestin component, if androgenic, lowers HDL. If the progestin is nonandrogenic, HDL is not influenced. In studies clinically comparing oral contraceptives, formulations containing levonorgestrel and norgestrel had a greater adverse effect on lipids than did less androgenic formulations such as those containing ethynodiol diacetate, norethindrone, or norethindrone acetate. However, if levonorgestrel or norgestrel is given in low doses or if the total dose given is limited, such as in biphasic or triphasic formulations, these potent androgenic progestins exhibit only mild lipid changes similar to those of less potent androgenic progestins given in monophasic formulations. Nonandrogenic formulations, such as desogestrel and norgestimate, had little effect on lipid profile)

Low density lipoproteins (LDL), serum or
Very low density lipoproteins (VLDL), serum

(low-dose oral contraceptives show a trend of no change or an increase in value of LDL; the estrogen component decreases LDL and the progestin component, if androgenic, raises LDL. If the progestin is nonandrogenic, LDL is not influenced. In clinical studies comparing oral contraceptives, formulations containing levonorgestrel and norgestrel had a greater adverse effect on lipids than did less androgenic formulations, such as those containing ethynodiol diacetate, norethindrone, or norethindrone acetate. However, if levonorgestrel or norgestrel is given in low doses or if the total dose given is limited, such as in biphasic or triphasic formulations, these potent androgenic progestins exhibit only mild lipid changes similar to those of less potent androgenic progestins given in monophasic formulations. Nonandrogenic formulations, such as desogestrel and norgestimate, had little effect)

(low-dose oral contraceptives increase serum concentrations of large triglyceride-rich VLDL threefold and production rates fivefold compared with serum concentrations in nonusers, and serum concentrations of small VLDL increase 2.2-fold and production rates 3.4-fold over those of nonusers, all without slowing VLDL catabolism)

Oxytocin, serum

(mean basal oxytocin levels were higher in women on oral contraceptives)

Plasminogen activity

(activity is increased above normal laboratory reference values)

## Medical considerations/Contraindications

The medical considerations/contraindications included here have been selected on the basis of their potential clinical significance (reasons given in parentheses where appropriate)—not necessarily inclusive ($\gg$ = major clinical significance).

*Except under special circumstances, this medication should not be used when the following medical problems exist:*

$\gg$ Carcinoma, breast, known or suspected or
$\gg$ Carcinoma, endometrium or
$\gg$ Neoplasia, estrogen-dependent, known or suspected

(may worsen conditions; estrogen-containing oral contraceptives should be discontinued and nonhormonal contraceptives initiated, although sometimes progestin-only contraceptives are used for selected patients)

$\gg$ Cardiac insufficiency

(oral contraceptives should not be used in patients with marginal cardiac reserve; fluid retention sometimes caused by estrogens may aggravate this condition)

$\gg$ Cerebrovascular disease, active, or history of or
$\gg$ Coronary artery disease, active or history of

(the estrogen component of oral contraceptives has a protective effect against atherosclerosis. Any association with risk in these conditions has been related to thrombosis or interference with cholesterol-lipoprotein profile, such as with levonorgestrel, a progestin, in doses greater than 150 to 250 micrograms for those individuals predisposed to thrombosis. No correlation has been seen between coronary artery disease and use of low-dose oral contraceptives, including those formulated with levonorgestrel, in these women or in women who are not predisposed to these conditions. Oral contraceptives should be discontinued or strictly avoided if any cardiovascular or cerebrovascular accidents occur; users should switch to nonhormonal contraception. If oral contraceptives are used in women at risk, special monitoring may be required)

(the progestins norgestimate and desogestrel have minimal negative impact and may improve the cholesterol-lipoprotein profile, which is thought to additionally protect against cardiovascular disease along with the estrogen component of oral contraceptives)

$\gg$ Hepatic disease, cholestatic, active or
$\gg$ Hepatic tumors, benign or malignant, or history of

(metabolism of estrogens may be impaired; also, estrogens may worsen the condition. Oral contraceptives should be discontinued and nonhormonal contraception initiated; for those women with active hepatic disease, oral contraceptive use may be resumed after liver function tests return to normal)

$\gg$ Thrombophlebitis, thrombosis, or thromboembolic disorders, active or history of

(oral contraceptives are not recommended for women with predisposing factors, especially those who smoke tobacco or who have an underlying abnormality of the coagulation system, that place them at special risk for thrombosis. Although hormones can increase thrombin formation, the coagulation effect is offset by an increase in fibrolytic activity. Some women with coagulation disorders may successfully use oral contraceptives as evaluated by the physician if only a slight risk for a thrombogenic condition exists. Problems generally have not been associated with the low doses of hormones used for contraception for women not at risk for these conditions)

» Uterine bleeding, abnormal or undiagnosed
(malignancy should be ruled out in cases of persistent or recurring abnormal uterine bleeding; use of a progestin-containing oral contraceptive may delay diagnosis by masking underlying conditions, including cancer)

*Risk-benefit should be considered when the following medical problems exist:*

Breast cancer, strong family history of or
Breast disease, benign
(although studies have failed to conclusively prove that use of oral contraceptives causes any excess risk for developing breast disease in these women, caution and more frequent monitoring for potential problems may be warranted)

Chorea gravidarum
(oral contraceptives do not cause chorea gravidarum but rarely they have aggravated pre-existing conditions)

Diabetes mellitus
(use of oral contraceptives may slightly decrease glucose tolerance, slightly increase insulin release in patients with non–insulin-dependent diabetes mellitus, or mildly change the cholesterol-lipoprotein profile adversely; change in the dose of the antidiabetic agent or more frequent monitoring for plasma glucose or lipid profile may be needed, depending on the oral contraceptive used; if adverse metabolic effects cannot be controlled, the oral contraceptive should be discontinued)

(norethindrone-, ethynodiol diacetate-, norgestimate-, and desogestrel-containing oral contraceptives affect carbohydrate metabolism less than do levonorgestrel- or norgestrel-containing oral contraceptives; many clinicians recommend low-dose oral contraceptives, such as the triphasic oral contraceptives, for patients with diabetes mellitus)

(use of oral contraceptives in patients with insulin-dependent diabetes mellitus who are 35 years of age or older or in any patient having diabetes mellitus complications is generally not recommended because of the potential increased risk of thrombosis; otherwise healthy patients under 35 years of age have minimal risk, but more frequent monitoring for cholesterol-lipoprotein profile and plasma glucose may still be needed, although insulin dose is usually unaffected)

Epilepsy
(oral contraceptives can be used effectively with this condition but their use may affect the pharmacokinetics of certain antiepileptic medications; dose changes for both medications and special monitoring may be needed)

Gallbladder disease, or history of, especially gallstones
(estrogens may alter the composition of gallbladder bile and cause a rise in cholesterol saturation, which may result in modestly accelerated development of gallstones during the first 2 years of use in predisposed individuals; overall risk is low and thought to be of minimal clinical importance; however, cautious use of oral contraceptives is recommended with known gallbladder disease)

» Hepatic dysfunction
(metabolism of estrogens may be impaired; also, estrogens may worsen the condition; therefore, oral contraceptives should be discontinued and nonhormonal contraception initiated with active disease and resumed after liver function tests return to normal. Oral contraceptives are not thought to aggravate cirrhosis or exacerbate previous hepatitis)

Hypertension
(low-dose monophasic oral contraceptives have been shown to raise blood pressure in some normotensive women considered to be at high risk [although these women cannot be easily identified] or further raise blood pressure in hypertensive women; using low-dose multiphasic contraceptives can lower risk)

Immobilization, extended or
Surgery, major
(although controversial, many guidelines suggest that concurrent oral contraceptive usage increases the risk of postoperative thromboembolism in predisposed women, especially for smokers of tobacco or for those women having a history of thromboembolism; when possible or if appropriate, oral contraceptives should be discontinued at least 4 weeks before and for 2 weeks after an extended period of immobilization or scheduled major elective surgery. If

not possible, prophylactic low-dose heparin therapy should be considered prior to surgery)

Jaundice, obstructive or history of during pregnancy
(estrogens may increase risk of recurrence but low-dose contraceptives have not done so consistently; risk is higher shortly after hormone exposure; increased monitoring may be needed)

Mental depression, or history of
(may be aggravated; however, low-dose contraceptives are considered to have minimal effect on mental depression; the oral contraceptive should be discontinued if significant depression occurs, especially in women with a history of depression)

Migraine headaches
(since migraine headaches have been associated with an increased risk of stroke, discontinuation of oral contraceptives may be warranted if migraine headaches are recurring, persistent, or more severe with use of oral contraceptives, especially for those individuals predisposed to thrombosis)

**Patient monitoring**
The following may be especially important in patient monitoring (other tests may be warranted in some patients, depending on condition; » = major clinical significance):

Blood pressure determinations and
Hepatic function determinations and
Papanicolaou (Pap) test and
Physical examinations
(recommended as determined by physician—generally every 12 months for healthy women with no risk factors but every 6 months if needed when such risk factors exist, although breast and pelvic examinations are needed only annually; also, new oral contraceptive users should be reassessed at 3 months; special attention should be given to breast, liver, and pelvic area in physical exam and patient should be encouraged to self-examine breasts monthly)

(special attention to rule out malignancy should be given to patients complaining of persistent or recurring uterine bleeding)

Glucose, serum and
Lipid profile, serum and
Lipoprotein profile, serum
(routine assessment is needed only for women at special risk, including the following: 35 years of age or older; having personal or strong family history of heart disease, diabetes mellitus, or hypertension; having history of gestational diabetes; having xanthomatosis; being obese; or having diabetes mellitus)

*For perimenopausal women using oral contraceptives*
Gonadotropin determination
(FSH levels should be measured annually to determine when menopause occurs.)

# Side/Adverse Effects

Note: The risk of any serious adverse effect is minimal for healthy women using low-dose oral contraceptives. Some women who are at special risk have successfully used low-dose oral contraceptives, although in others the use of oral contraceptives rarely will increase the incidence of life-threatening effects, such as benign hepatic adenomas, hepatocellular carcinoma, or thromboembolism or thromboembolic events such as deep vein thrombosis, cerebral or coronary ischemia and/or infarction, pulmonary embolism, or stroke. Most of these events may be exacerbated when pre-existing factors, such as genetic predisposition (i.e., antiestrogen antibodies, activated protein C or antithrombin deficiencies or resistance, or genetic thrombotic disorder), hypertension, hyperlipidemia, obesity, diabetes, or smoking of cigarettes, exist. Low-dose oral contraceptives are recommended for most women throughout their reproductive years without need for discontinuance. Mortality rates in oral contraceptive users are lower than those that are associated with childbirth. This is true even for smokers 35 years and older and nonsmokers 40 years and older.

There is no evidence of an etiological relationship between oral contraceptive use and pituitary prolactinoma; however, the appearance of galactorrhea while on oral contraceptives merits investigation.

The following side/adverse effects have been selected on the basis of their potential clinical significance (possible signs and symptoms in parentheses where appropriate)—not necessarily inclusive:

**Those indicating need for immediate medical attention**
Incidence rare
*Thromboembolism or thrombosis* (abdominal pain, sudden, severe, or continuing; coughing up blood; headache, severe or sudden; loss of coordination, sudden; pains in chest, groin, or leg, especially calf of

leg; shortness of breath, sudden, unexplained; slurring of speech, sudden; vision changes, sudden; weakness, numbness, or pain in arm or leg, unexplained)—mainly exhibited in women having predisposing or pre-existing conditions, especially for those who smoke tobacco, but may be idiopathic

### Those indicating need for medical attention
Incidence more frequent, especially during the first three months of oral contraceptive use
*Changes in the uterine bleeding pattern of menses or intermenstrual bleeding, such as; amenorrhea* (complete stoppage of menstrual bleeding over several months); *absence of withdrawal bleeding* (occasional stoppage of menses over nonconsecutive months); *breakthrough bleeding* (vaginal bleeding between regular menstrual periods, which may require the use of a pad or a tampon); *metrorrhagia* (prolonged bleeding); *scanty menses* (very light menstrual bleeding); *or spotting* (light vaginal bleeding between regular menstrual periods); *dysmenorrhea* (increased pain or cramping during menstrual period)

Note: Malignancy should be ruled out as the cause if persistent or recurring abnormal *uterine bleeding* occurs.

Up to 46% of women using oral contraceptives experience *changes in the intermenstrual uterine bleeding pattern*. These problems become less frequent with duration of use; women who use high-dose oral contraceptives or who are changing formulations have fewer uterine bleeding problems than do women who are new users. *Breakthrough bleeding* occurs in 6 to 12% of women; some may require a change to a higher formulation with progestin or a change to a monophasic oral contraceptive after 3 months. Intervention with therapeutic doses of estrogen and/or progestin may be necessary if breakthrough bleeding is heavy or further prolonged. Six to 12%, 6 to 10%, and less than 1% of women will experience *spotting, scanty menses,* or *metrorrhagia*, respectively. Up to 12% of women using norethindrone-containing oral contraceptives and less than 2% of women using desogestrel-, norgestimate-, or levonorgestrel-containing oral contraceptives will experience an *absence of withdrawal bleeding*. Early or mid-cycle spotting or absence of withdrawal bleeding may be seen with use of low doses of monophasic contraceptives and may not be an unexpected side effect but is a major reason for discontinuance. A change to a different formulation with a greater estrogen:progestin ratio or less progestin, such as multiphasic formulations, or temporary supplementation with an estrogen, may improve these adverse effects. Failure of oral contraceptives to induce *withdrawal uterine bleeding* may be caused by insufficient estrogen activity to induce endometrial development; a change to a different formulation with increased estrogen:progestin ratio may improve this effect.

Incidence less frequent
*Glucose tolerance, mildly reduced* (faintness; nausea; skin paleness; sweating)—usually for women with predisposing conditions; *headaches or migraines, worsening or increased frequency of*—21%; *hypertension, worsening or exacerbation; vaginal candidiasis or vaginitis, sporadic or recurrent* (vaginal discharge, thick, white, or curd-like, or vaginal itching or other irritation)—10 to 16%

Note: Several studies have confirmed that 15 to 18% of oral contraceptive users will experience an increase, but not a clinically significant elevation, in blood pressure. Another study has observed that 4% of contraceptive users will develop *hypertension*, especially when either a history of hypertension in pregnancy or a family history of hypertension exists; severe or *malignant hypertension* has been rarely seen.

Although one large cross-sectional study has shown a 43 to 61% increase in the area under the plasma concentration–time curve for glucose, past or current use of oral contraceptives does not increase risk for developing non–insulin-dependent diabetes mellitus; the effect of the increase is considered transitory and reversible with discontinuation. Oral contraceptive formulations vary in the degree to which they cause *reduced glucose tolerance,* which is usually mild, and may be of clinical importance only for a subset of women at particular risk. In separate studies, norgestimate-containing oral contraceptives showed minimal decreases in glucose tolerance of 6.6% after 24 months and monophasic desogestrel-containing oral contraceptives showed an increase in the area under the plasma concentration–time curve of only 26%.

Frequency and severity of *headaches or migraines* have been reduced in some patients using oral contraceptives and have slightly worsened in others because of fluid retention; however, if headaches or migraines worsen considerably, discontinuation of oral contraceptives should be considered since this may be a prodomal symptom of stroke.

Withdrawal of oral contraceptives does not seem to affect the frequency of *recurrent vaginal candidiasis or vaginitis;* the increased risk may depend on other factors, such as lifestyle.

Incidence rare
*Breast tumors* (lumps in breast)—primarily in women having a predisposing or pre-existing condition; *hepatic focal nodular hyperplasia, hepatitis, or hepatocellular carcinoma* (pains in stomach, side, or abdomen, or yellow eyes or skin)—primarily in women having a predisposing or pre-existing condition, especially those who smoke tobacco; *hepatic cell adenomas, benign* (swelling, pain, or tenderness in upper abdominal area); *mental depression, slight worsening*—in pre-existing conditions

Note: Association of increased incidence of *breast tumors* is controversial. One study of women 20 to 34 years of age who were long-term oral contraceptive users (10 or more years of use) or recent users (within 5 years of breast cancer diagnosis) found only 1 more case of invasive breast cancer per year among oral contraceptive users than in nonusers for every 100,000 women. It still has not been determined whether the risk of breast cancer increases for early users under 20 years of age or for long-term users.

Although very rare, *hepatic cell adenomas* should be considered in patients having abdominal pain and tenderness, abdominal mass, or hypovolemic shock, although one-third of patients are asymptomatic at diagnosis. Studies of developing countries that have a high incidence of primary liver cancer have not associated oral contraceptives with an increased risk; however, Western countries, with a low incidence of hepatic carcinoma, have shown a fivefold increase in long-term (5 to 10 years) users of oral contraceptives that persisted for 10 years or more after stopping treatment; studies in the U.S., also a country with low incidence of hepatic carcinoma, have not confirmed this finding. Whether hepatic cell adenomas are premalignant is disputed. On occurrence, discontinuing the oral contraceptives is necessary and may result in spontaneous regression of the adenoma.

*Mental depression* has improved for many women with pre-existing conditions; otherwise, no effect with oral contraceptive use usually is noted but severe depression should be reported to and treatment continuance evaluated by physician.

### Those indicating need for medical attention only if they continue or are bothersome
Incidence more frequent
*Abdominal cramping or bloating; acne*—usually less frequent after the first 3 months of use; *breast pain, tenderness, or swelling*—8.5 to 25%; *dizziness*—10 to 14%; *nausea or vomiting*—6 to 12%; *sodium and fluid retention* (swelling of ankles and feet); *unusual tiredness or weakness*

Note: Increased *acne* was absent, less severe, or acne was improved with desogestrel and norgestimate compared with levonorgestrel, norgestrel, or norethindrone.*Nausea, vomiting, breast tenderness,* and *sodium and fluid retention* diminish after the first 2 or 3 months.

Incidence less frequent
*Gain or loss of body or facial hair; increased skin sensitivity to sun; libido changes* (increase or decrease of interest in sexual intercourse); *melasma* (brown, blotchy spots on exposed skin); *weight gain or loss*—1%

Note: *Melasma* usually is temporary but can be permanent; women having dark complexions, having a history of melasma during pregnancy, or having prolonged exposure to sunlight are most susceptible to developing melasma.

## Overdose
Serious adverse effects generally do not occur with an acute overdosage. When children have accidently ingested a large amount of an oral contraceptive, more serious adverse effects also did not result. Withdrawal bleeding has occasionally occurred in young girls and does not require treatment.

For more information on the management of overdose or unintentional ingestion, **contact a Poison Control Center** (see *Poison Control Center Listing*).

### Clinical effects of overdose
The following effects have been selected on the basis of their potential clinical significance (possible signs and symptoms in parentheses where appropriate)—not necessarily inclusive:
*Irregular bleeding cycle; nausea or vomiting*—occuring in less than 10% of patients; *withdrawal bleeding*

**Treatment of overdose**

Specific treatment—Nausea or vomiting is treated for symptomatic relief.

Supportive care—Patients in whom intentional overdose is known or suspected should be referred for psychiatric consultation.

# Patient Consultation

As an aid to patient consultation, refer to *Advice for the Patient, Estrogens and Progestins (Oral Contraceptives) (Systemic)*.

Consider advising the patient on the following (» = major clinical significance):

**Before using this medication**
» Conditions affecting use, especially:
  Sensitivity to estrogens or progestins
  Pregnancy—Not recommended for use during pregnancy
  Breast-feeding—Oral contraceptives are distributed into breast milk
  Use in adolescents—Careful counseling may be required to increase compliance
  Dental—May increase possibility of bleeding of gingival tissues, gingival hyperplasia, or local alveolar osteitis (dry socket)
  Other medications, especially corticosteroids, cyclosporine, hepatic enzyme inducers, hepatotoxic medications (especially troleandomycin), ritonavir, theophylline, or tobacco smoking
  Other medical problems, especially carcinoma of the breast (known or suspected); carcinoma of the endometrium; cardiac insufficiency; cerebrovascular disease—especially if patient smokes cigarettes (active or history of); coronary artery disease; hepatic disease, cholestatic (active); estrogen-dependent neoplasia (known or suspected); hepatic tumors, benign or malignant (active or history of); thrombophlebitis, thrombosis, or thromboembolic disorders (active or history of); uterine bleeding (abnormal or undiagnosed); hepatic dysfunction

**Proper use of this medication**
» Reading patient package insert carefully
  Taking with or immediately after food to reduce nausea
  Using an additional method of birth control for the first 7 days; some clinicians may recommend that an additional method of birth control be used during the first cycle of oral contraceptive use
» Compliance with therapy; taking medication at the same time each day, at 24-hour intervals
  Keeping an extra 1-month supply available when possible
  Taking tablets in proper (color-coded) sequence
» Proper dosing
  Missed doses for the monophasic, biphasic, or triphasic cycle—
    Missing the first tablet of a new cycle—Taking as soon as possible; if not remembered until next day, taking two tablets; continuing on regular dosing schedule and using another birth control method for seven days after the last missed dose
    Missing one day—Taking as soon as possible; if not remembered until next day, taking 2 tablets; continuing on regular dosing schedule
    Missing two days in a row in the first or second week—Taking 2 tablets a day for next two days, then continuing on regular dosing schedule; using additional method of birth control for remainder of cycle
    Missing two days in a row in the third week or
    Missing three days in a row—
      Using Day-1 start: Discarding remaining doses for current cycle; beginning a new cycle following the recommended dosing schedule and using a second method of birth control, additionally, for seven days after the last missed dose; contacting health care professional if two menstrual periods are missed
      Using Sunday start: Continuing on regular dosing schedule for current cycle until Sunday; on Sunday, throwing out remaining doses for current cycle and beginning a new cycle; using an additional method of birth control for seven days after the last missed dose; contacting health care professional if two menstrual periods are missed
    Missing any of the last seven tablets of a twenty-eight–day cycle is not important, but beginning new cycle on time is essential
» Proper storage

**Precautions while using this medication**
» Regular visits to physician at least every 6 to 12 months to check progress
» Caution if medical or dental surgery or emergency treatment is required—increased risk of thrombotic complications

» Using an additional method of birth control during each cycle in which the following medications are used: ampicillin, hepatic enzyme inducers, penicillin V, or tetracyclines
  What to expect and do if vaginal bleeding occurs
  What to expect and do if a menstrual period is missed; contacting health professional if two menstrual periods are missed
  Possibility of dental problems, such as tenderness, swelling, or bleeding of gums; brushing and flossing teeth, massaging gums, and having dentist clean teeth regularly; checking with dentist if there are questions about care of teeth or gums or if tenderness, swelling, or bleeding of gums is noticed
  Possibility of photosensitivity
» Stopping medication immediately and checking with physician if pregnancy is suspected
  If scheduled for laboratory tests, telling physician if taking birth control pills; certain blood tests may be affected by oral contraceptives
  Not refilling an old prescription for oral contraceptives without having a physical examination by physician, especially after a pregnancy

**Side/adverse effects**
  Signs of potential side effects, especially thromboembolism or thrombosis; changes in the uterine bleeding pattern of the menses or intermenstrual bleeding; dysmenorrhea; headaches or migraines; hypertension, worsening; mildly reduced glucose tolerance (usually for predisposed individuals); vaginal candidiasis or vaginitis; breast tumors (usually for predisposed individuals); hepatic focal nodular hyperplasia, hepatitis, or hepatocellular carcinoma; hepatic cell adenomas, benign; slight worsening of mental depression
  Cigarette smoking combined with oral contraceptive use causes increased risk of serious thromboembolic or hepatic side effects, especially for heavy smokers or women over age 35

# General Dosing Information

The doses of estrogens and progestins used for contraception are much greater than those doses of estrogens and progestins used for hormone replacement therapy. Perimenopausal women should be tested for serum FSH levels annually for accurate dating of menopause; oral contraceptives should be discontinued and hormone replacement therapy started if or when appropriate.

Low doses of estrogen (doses containing 35 mcg or less of ethinyl estradiol or 50 mcg mestranol) are preferred to higher doses (equal to 50 mcg of ethinyl estradiol). Many side effects are related to the dominance of either the estrogen or progestin present in the preparation. By changing to preparations of differing component ratios, side effects can often be lessened or eliminated. In some instances low-dose estrogen formulations are not acceptable and the high-dose estrogen formulations should be used, such as when the effectiveness of oral contraceptives is compromised because of increased hepatic metabolism; this may occur when some anticonvulsant medications are used concurrently. All effects of long-term use of the lower-dose oral contraceptives have not been determined; most long-term studies performed have been in patients using higher doses of estrogens and progestins than are used commonly at present.

Thirty-five mcg of ethinyl estradiol and 50 mcg of mestranol are considered to have equal therapeutic potency as the estrogen component for contraception. Norgestrel (d,l-norgestrel) is a racemic mixture of dextro- and levonorgestrel and has one-half the potency of levonorgestrel on a weight basis. Dextronorgestrel can be considered an inactive isomer.

The multiphasic formulations were developed to supply the lowest possible total hormone dose over a treatment cycle. Monophasic, biphasic, and triphasic regimens are considered equally effective for preventing pregnancy and choice may be unique to an individual's lifestyle, health risks, or other factors. The success of an oral contraceptive is also highly dependent on proper selection of the formulation for an individual, according to her menstrual cycle regularity, her ability to be compliant, and her tolerance for side effects. When possible, the lowest dose of hormones should be used to achieve these goals.
• The *monophasic regimen* provides constant doses of estrogen and progestin.
• The *biphasic regimen* provides 2 different dose ratios of the estrogen:progestin and includes a constant estrogen dose throughout the cycle with a progestin dose increase either at the 7th or the 10th day, depending on the product.
• The *triphasic regimen* provides 3 different dose ratios of estrogen:progestin and includes either variable doses of estrogen and progestin changing at the 6th and 11th days, a constant estrogen dose throughout the cycle plus an increase of the progestin dose for only 9 days (8th through the 16th day), or a constant estrogen dose throughout with an increase of the progestin dose every 7 days.

### For routine contraception

To begin taking oral contraceptives, the first tablet is taken either on Day 1 (first day of menstrual bleeding) of the menstrual cycle or the first Sunday following the start of menses. Dosage schedules are arranged on a 21- or 28-day cycle to correspond with the 28 days of the menstrual cycle. The 21-day regimens provide 21 active tablets containing estrogen and progestin hormone therapy. The 28-day cycle adds 7 inactive (nonhormonal) tablets to the 21-day regimen for either 7 days of placebo tablets for ease of daily counting or 7 days of iron (ferrous fumarate) companion tablets to supplement the diet. To help the patient to comply with this schedule, most manufacturers integrate the schedule into a non-childproof dispensing container, which should be utilized whenever possible. Tablets containing different strengths of hormones are colored differently to help the patient differentiate between the tablet strengths; this is especially helpful for biphasic and triphasic formulations. Also, the active and inactive tablets are different colors. Patients should be informed of the necessity of taking different colored tablets in the proper sequence and not mixing tablets of different colors indiscriminately. Also, even if the hormone formulation is the same for 2 products of different manufacturers, tablet colors do not always correspond.

Maximum contraceptive effect is obtained by taking doses at 24-hour intervals and beginning the new regimen on time; this enhances patient compliance, also. When initiating oral contraceptive treatment, many clinicians instruct patients to use a nonhormonal backup method for 7 days if contraceptive therapy is started within the first 5 days of the menstrual cycle. Other clinicians counsel patients to use a nonhormonal backup method of contraception for the first month. Contraceptive effectiveness is continued when transferring patients between oral contraceptive formulations when initiated at the beginning of the menstrual cycle, with minimal side effects. Breakthrough bleeding or spotting may recur for several months when an oral contraceptive is started, but is usually less for those patients transferred between formulations than for initial users.

A periodic pill-free *rest period* is not recommended, since it appears to provide no therapeutic advantage and does not enhance the resumption of ovulatory cycles after cessation of oral contraceptive therapy. Such intervals may result in noncompliance with the substituted contraceptive and unwanted pregnancies.

### For emergency postcoital contraception

Therapy is initiated as soon as possible or up to 72 hours after intercourse; repeated courses in a single cycle are not recommended as efficacy may be compromised.

The use of norgestrel or levonorgestrel and ethinyl estradiol tablets as a postcoital contraceptive (the *morning-after pill*) has been employed primarily in emergency situations, such as when possible contraceptive method failure is realized early or when any unprotected sexual intercourse is of concern to patient. Effectiveness depends on the time interval between coitus and administration of the medication. A pregnancy test should be performed prior to administering medication. A patient requesting treatment should be fully informed of the risks involved, such as potential increased risk of blood clot formation because of the higher dosage of hormone required, although treatment is of short duration. Also, nausea and vomiting may result, increasing the possibility of contraceptive failure because of the difficulty of maintaining compliance.

### For patients with hirsutisim

Treatment with oral contraceptives for 6 months to 1 year may be required before effects are apparent. Although hormones suppress new hair growth, normal androgen levels maintain hair that is already present.

### For patients with endometriosis

Oral contraceptives can be given continuously or cyclically for 6 to 9 months to aid in ectopic implant atrophy. Low-dose estrogen preparations containing a high progestational progestin, such as desogestrel, are probably best for this. Endometriotic symptoms may increase before improvement is noted by patient.

### Diet

Should be taken with food or milk to lessen gastrointestinal irritation if it occurs or tablets may be taken at bedtime.

---

*DESOGESTREL AND ETHINYL ESTRADIOL*

## Summary of Differences

Pharmacology/pharmacokinetics—Desogestrel is a prodrug that is metabolized to a more active form, 3-keto-desogestrel. Exhibits first-pass effect. Highly progestational and does not counteract the estrogen increase in sex hormone–binding globulin (SHBG) levels; highly bound to SHBG and albumin; low androgenicity.

Laboratory value alterations—Little effect on lipoproteins.

Medical considerations/contraindications—Desogestrel plus ethinyl estradiol increases glucose tolerance but does not affect 2-hour insulin release; had less effect on carbohydrate metabolism than other oral contraceptives did.

Side/adverse effects—Absence of withdrawal menstrual bleeding is low; improves pre-existing acne.

## Oral Dosage Forms

Note: Bracketed uses in the *Dosage Forms* section refer to categories of use and/or indications that are not included in U.S. product labeling.

### DESOGESTREL AND ETHINYL ESTRADIOL TABLETS

**Usual adult and adolescent dose**

Contraceptive, systemic or
Estrogen-progestin or
[Antiendometriotic][1] or
[Gonadotropin inhibitor, female, noncontraceptive use][1]—

Twenty-one–day cycle: Oral, 1 tablet a day for twenty-one days commencing on Day 1 of the menstrual cycle or on the first Sunday after the menstrual cycle begins; the next round of treatment is begun on the eighth day after the last tablet of the previous cycle has been taken.

Twenty-eight–day cycle: Oral, 1 tablet a day for twenty-eight days commencing on Day 1 of the menstrual cycle, or on the first Sunday after the menstrual cycle begins; the next round of treatment is begun on the day after the last tablet of the previous cycle has been taken.

Note: With a Sunday-start schedule, the patient should take her first tablet on the first Sunday after the onset of menstruation. If the patient's period begins on a Sunday, she should take her first tablet that same day.

With a Day 1 start schedule, the patient should take her first tablet on Day 1 of the menstrual cycle.

The last seven tablets of the twenty-eight–day cycle contain no hormones. These seven companion tablets are a different color from those containing hormones.

Oral contraceptives may be given continuously or cyclically for endometriosis.

**Strength(s) usually available**

U.S.—

150 mcg (0.15 mg) of desogestrel and 30 mcg (0.03 mg) of ethinyl estradiol (Rx) [*Desogen; Ortho-Cept*].

Canada—

150 mcg (0.15 mg) of desogestrel and 30 mcg (0.03 mg) of ethinyl estradiol (Rx) [*Marvelon; Ortho-Cept*].

Note: Marvelon and Ortho-Cept are available in twenty-one– or twenty-eight–day cycles. The twenty-eight–day cycle includes an additional seven days of placebo tablets.

**Packaging and storage**

Store below 40 °C (104 °F), preferably between 15 and 30 °C (59 and 86 °F), unless otherwise specified by manufacturer. Store in a well-closed container.

**Auxiliary labeling**
• Take with food.
• Avoid too much sun or use of sunlamp.

**Note**

Include mandatory patient package inserts (PPIs) (the brief summary of patient labeling and the detailed patient labeling) when dispensing.

Caution first-time users to use an additional form of birth control as directed by their physician until maximal contraception protection begins.

---

[1]Not included in Canadian product labeling.

---

*ETHYNODIOL DIACETATE AND ETHINYL ESTRADIOL*

## Summary of Differences

Pharmacology/pharmacokinetics—Ethynodiol diacetate hydrolyzed to norethindrone; aromatization by tissues may be clinically significant. Greater affinity for albumin but significant SHBG binding occurs because of estrogen-induced SHBG levels. Exhibits first-pass effect. Slightly estrogenic.

Laboratory value alterations—Triglycerides increase; shows the greatest increase of apolipoprotein $A_1$ of all contraceptives.

Dosage forms—High estrogen dose formulation available.

## Oral Dosage Forms

Note: Bracketed uses in the *Dosage Forms* section refer to categories of use and/or indications that are not included in U.S. product labeling.

### ETHYNODIOL DIACETATE AND ETHINYL ESTRADIOL TABLETS USP

**Usual adult and adolescent dose**
Contraceptive, systemic or
Estrogen-progestin or
[Antiendometriotic][1] or
[Gonadotropin inhibitor, female, noncontraceptive use][1]—

Twenty-one–day cycle: Oral, 1 tablet a day for twenty-one days commencing on Day 1 of the menstrual cycle or on the first Sunday after the menstrual cycle begins; the next round of treatment is begun on the eighth day after the last tablet of the previous cycle has been taken.

Twenty-eight–day cycle: Oral, 1 tablet a day for twenty-eight days commencing on Day 1 of the menstrual cycle, or on the first Sunday after the menstrual cycle begins; the next round of treatment is begun on the day after the last tablet of the previous cycle has been taken.

Note: With a Sunday-start schedule, the patient should take her first tablet on the first Sunday after the onset of menstruation. If the patient's period begins on a Sunday, she should take her first tablet that same day.

With a Day 1 start schedule, the patient should take her first tablet on Day 1 of the menstrual cycle.

The last seven tablets of the twenty-eight–day cycle contain no hormones. These seven companion tablets are of a different color from those containing hormones.

Oral contraceptives may be given continuously or cyclically for endometriosis.

**Strength(s) usually available**
U.S.—

1 mg of ethynodiol diacetate and 35 mcg (0.035 mg) of ethinyl estradiol (Rx) [*Demulen 1/35; Zovia 1/35E*].

1 mg of ethynodiol diacetate and 50 mcg (0.05 mg) of ethinyl estradiol (Rx) [*Demulen 1/50; Zovia 1/50E*].

Canada—

1 mg of ethynodiol diacetate and 50 mcg (0.05 mg) of ethinyl estradiol (Rx) [*Demulen 50*].

2 mg of ethynodiol diacetate and 30 mcg (0.03 mg) of ethinyl estradiol (Rx) [*Demulen 30*].

Note: Available in twenty-one– or twenty-eight–day cycles. The twenty-eight–day cycle includes an additional seven days of placebo tablets.

**Packaging and storage**
Store below 40 °C (104 °F), preferably between 15 and 30 °C (59 and 86 °F), unless otherwise specified by manufacturer. Store in a well-closed container.

**Auxiliary labeling**
• Take with food.
• Avoid too much sun or use of sunlamp.

**Note**
Include mandatory patient package inserts (PPIs) (the brief summary of patient labeling and the detailed patient labeling) when dispensing.

Caution first-time users to use additional form of birth control as directed by their physician until maximal contraception protection begins.

[1]Not included in Canadian product labeling.

---

### LEVONORGESTREL AND ETHINYL ESTRADIOL

## Summary of Differences

Indications—Also used for emergency postcoital contraception.
Pharmacology/pharmacokinetics—Levonorgestrel is the active enantiomer of norgestrel. Proportion bound to SHBG depends on both estrogen and levonorgestrel dose; suppresses estrogen-induced increase of SHBG levels except when the triphasic formulation is used, which slightly increase SHBG levels. No first-pass effect. One of the most androgenic progestins; androgenic effects depend on both progestin and estrogen dose.
Laboratory value alterations—No change in triglycerides over 1 year; may slightly decrease or increase total cholesterol; negatively affected lipoprotein, increases LDL and lowers HDL; increases apolipoprotein $A_1$

the least of all contraceptives; can increase free testosterone by displacing it from SHBG.
Dosage forms—High estrogen dose formulation available.

## Oral Dosage Forms

Note: Bracketed uses in the *Dosage Forms* section refer to categories of use and/or indications that are not included in U.S. product labeling.

### LEVONORGESTREL AND ETHINYL ESTRADIOL TABLETS USP

**Usual adult and adolescent dose**
Contraceptive, systemic or
Estrogen-progestin or
[Antiendometriotic][1] or
[Gonadotropin inhibitor, female, noncontraceptive use][1]—

Twenty-one–day cycle: Oral, 1 tablet a day for twenty-one days commencing on Day 1 of the menstrual cycle or on the first Sunday after the menstrual cycle begins; the next round of treatment is begun on the eighth day after the last tablet of the previous cycle has been taken.

Twenty-eight–day cycle: Oral, 1 tablet a day for twenty-eight days commencing on Day 1 of the menstrual cycle, or on the first Sunday after the menstrual cycle begins; the next round of treatment is begun on the day after the last tablet of the previous cycle has been taken.

Note: With a Sunday-start schedule, the patient should take her first tablet on the first Sunday after the onset of menstruation. If the patient's period begins on a Sunday, she should take her first tablet that same day.

With a Day 1 start schedule, the patient should take her first tablet on Day 1 of the menstrual cycle.

The last seven tablets of the twenty-eight–day cycle contain no hormones. These seven companion tablets are a different color from those containing hormones.

Oral contraceptives may be given continuously or cyclically for endometriosis.

[Contraceptive, postcoital, systemic][1]—

Four tablets (150 mcg levonorgestrel and 30 mcg of ethinyl estradiol per tablet) taken as soon as possible after unprotected coitus, preferably within twelve hours but not longer than seventy-two hours later. Then, four more tablets are taken twelve hours after the first dose.

Note: Monophasic or only phase-three tablets of the triphasic oral contraceptives contain sufficient hormone doses for postcoital emergency contraception use.

**Strength(s) usually available**
U.S.—

Monophasic twenty-one–day cycle formula
   150 mcg (0.15 mg) of levonorgestrel and 30 mcg (0.03 mg) of ethinyl estradiol (Rx) [*Levlen; Levora 0.15/30; Nordette*].
Triphasic twenty-one–day cycle formula
   **Phase one (six days)**—50 mcg (0.05 mg) of levonorgestrel and 30 mcg (0.03 mg) of ethinyl estradiol.
   **Phase two (five days)**—75 mcg (0.075 mg) of levonorgestrel and 40 mcg (0.04 mg) of ethinyl estradiol.
   **Phase three (ten days)**—125 mcg (0.125 mg) of levonorgestrel and 30 mcg (0.03 mg) of ethinyl estradiol. (Rx) [*Tri-Levlen; Triphasil*].

Canada—

Monophasic twenty-one–day cycle formula
   150 mcg (0.15 mg) of levonorgestrel and 30 mcg (0.03 mg) of ethinyl estradiol (Rx) [*Min-Ovral*].
Triphasic twenty-one–day cycle formula
   **Phase one (six days)**—50 mcg (0.05 mg) of levonorgestrel and 30 mcg (0.03 mg) of ethinyl estradiol.
   **Phase two (five days)**—75 mcg (0.075 mg) of levonorgestrel and 40 mcg (0.04 mg) of ethinyl estradiol.
   **Phase three (ten days)**—125 mcg (0.125 mg) of levonorgestrel and 30 mcg (0.03 mg) of ethinyl estradiol. (Rx) [*Triphasil; Triquilar*].

Note: Available in twenty-one– or twenty-eight–day cycles. The twenty-eight–day cycle includes an additional seven days of placebo tablets.

**Packaging and storage**
Store below 40 °C (104 °F), preferably between 15 and 30 °C (59 and 86 °F), unless otherwise specified by manufacturer. Store in a well-closed container.

**Auxiliary labeling**
- Take with food.
- Avoid too much sun or use of sunlamp.

**Note**

Include mandatory patient package inserts (PPIs) (the brief summary of patient labeling and the detailed patient labeling) when dispensing.

Explain sequence of administration of triphasic cycle formula when dispensing, especially for twenty-eight–day cycle (colored tablet sequence).

Caution first-time users to use an additional form of birth control as directed by their physician until maximal contraception protection begins.

---

[1]Not included in Canadian product labeling.

---

## NORETHINDRONE ACETATE AND ETHINYL ESTRADIOL

## Summary of Differences

Pharmacology/pharmacokinetics—Proportion bound to SHBG depends on both estrogen and norethindrone dose; does not suppress estrogen-induced increase of SHBG levels. Norethindrone acetate metabolized to norethindrone, which exhibits no first-pass effect. Androgenic effect depends on both progestin and estrogen dose; androgenic effects less than those of levonorgestrel or norgestrel; possesses slight estrogenic activity.

Laboratory value alterations—Slightly increases total cholesterol; negatively affects lipoproteins—increases LDL and lowers HDL; increases apolipoprotein $A_1$.

Dosage forms—High estrogen dose formulation available.

## Oral Dosage Forms

Note: Bracketed uses in the *Dosage Forms* section refer to categories of use and/or indications that are not included in U.S. product labeling.

### NORETHINDRONE ACETATE AND ETHINYL ESTRADIOL TABLETS USP

**Usual adult and adolescent dose**

Contraceptive, systemic or

Estrogen-progestin or

[Antiendometriotic][1] or

[Gonadotropin inhibitor, female, noncontraceptive use][1]—

    Twenty-one–day cycle: Oral, 1 tablet a day for twenty-one days commencing on Day 1 of the menstrual cycle or on the first Sunday after the menstrual cycle begins; the next round of treatment is begun on the eighth day after the last tablet of the previous cycle has been taken.

    Twenty-eight–day cycle: Oral, 1 tablet a day for twenty-eight days commencing on Day 1 of the menstrual cycle, or on the first Sunday after the menstrual cycle begins; the next round of treatment is begun on the day after the last tablet of the previous cycle has been taken.

Note: With a Sunday-start schedule, the patient should take her first tablet on the first Sunday after the onset of menstruation. If the patient's period begins on a Sunday, she should take her first tablet that same day.

    With a Day 1 start schedule, the patient should take her first tablet on Day 1 of the menstrual cycle.

    The last seven tablets of the twenty-eight–day cycle contain no hormones. Although in most preparations these tablets are placebos, in a few preparations they contain 75 mg of ferrous fumarate. These seven companion tablets are a different color from those containing hormones.

    Oral contraceptives may be given continuously or cyclically for endometriosis.

**Strength(s) usually available**

U.S.—

    1 mg of norethindrone acetate and 20 mcg (0.02 mg) of ethinyl estradiol (Rx) [*Loestrin 1/20*].

    1.5 mg of norethindrone acetate and 30 mcg (0.03 mg) of ethinyl estradiol (Rx) [*Loestrin 1.5/30*].

Canada—

    1 mg of norethindrone acetate and 20 mcg (0.02 mg) of ethinyl estradiol (Rx) [*Minestrin 1/20*].

    1.5 mg of norethindrone acetate and 30 mcg (0.03 mg) of ethinyl estradiol (Rx) [*Loestrin 1.5/30*].

---

Note: Available in twenty-one– or twenty-eight–day cycles. The twenty-eight–day cycle includes an additional seven days of either placebo tablets (for *Loestrin* or *Minestrin*) or tablets containing 75 mg ferrous fumarate each (for *Loestrin Fe*).

**Packaging and storage**

Store below 40 °C (104 °F), preferably between 15 and 30 °C (59 and 86 °F), unless otherwise specified by manufacturer. Store in a well-closed container.

**Auxiliary labeling**
- Take with food.
- Avoid too much sun or use of sunlamp.

**Note**

Include mandatory patient package inserts (PPIs) (the brief summary of patient labeling and the detailed patient labeling) when dispensing.

Caution first-time users to use an additional form of birth control as directed by their physician until maximal contraception protection begins.

---

[1]Not included in Canadian product labeling.

---

## NORETHINDRONE AND ETHINYL ESTRADIOL

## Summary of Differences

Pharmacology/pharmacokinetics—Proportion bound to SHBG depends on both estrogen and norethindrone dose; does not suppress estrogen-induced increase of SHBG levels. Norethindrone exhibits no first-pass effect; less androgenic than levonorgestrel or norgestrel; its androgenic effect depends on both progestin and estrogen doses; slight estrogenic activity.

Laboratory value alterations—Triglycerides increase as with all oral contraceptives; slightly increases total cholesterol; negatively affects lipoproteins—increases LDL and lowers HDL; increases apolipoprotein $A_1$.

Dosage forms—High estrogen dose formulation available.

## Oral Dosage Forms

Note: Bracketed uses in the *Dosage Forms* section refer to categories of use and/or indications that are not included in U.S. product labeling.

### NORETHINDRONE AND ETHINYL ESTRADIOL TABLETS USP

**Usual adult and adolescent dose**

Contraceptive, systemic or

Estrogen-progestin or

[Antiendometriotic][1] or

[Gonadotropin inhibitor, female, noncontraceptive use][1]—

    Twenty-one–day cycle: Oral, 1 tablet a day for twenty-one days commencing on Day 1 of the menstrual cycle or on the first Sunday after the menstrual cycle begins; the next round of treatment is begun on the eighth day after the last tablet of the previous cycle has been taken.

    Twenty-eight–day cycle: Oral, 1 tablet a day for twenty-eight days commencing on Day 1 of the menstrual cycle, or on the first Sunday after the menstrual cycle begins; the next round of treatment is begun on the day after the last tablet of the previous cycle has been taken.

Note: With a Sunday-start schedule, the patient should take her first tablet on the first Sunday after the onset of menstruation. If the patient's period begins on a Sunday, she should take her first tablet that same day.

    With a Day 1 start schedule, the patient should take her first tablet on Day 1 of the menstrual cycle.

    The last seven tablets of the twenty-eight–day cycle contain no hormones. These seven companion tablets are a different color from those containing hormones.

    Oral contraceptives may be given continuously or cyclically for endometriosis.

**Strength(s) usually available**

U.S.—

    Monophasic twenty-one–day cycle formula

        400 mcg (0.4 mg) of norethindrone and 35 mcg (0.035 mg) of ethinyl estradiol (Rx) [*Ovcon-35*].

        500 mcg (0.5 mg) of norethindrone and 35 mcg (0.035 mg) of ethinyl estradiol (Rx) [*Brevicon; Genora 0.5/35; Intercon 0.5/35; ModiCon; Necon 0.5/35; Nelova 0.5/35E*].

        1 mg of norethindrone and 35 mcg (0.035 mg) of ethinyl estradiol (Rx) [*Genora 1/35; Intercon 1/35; Necon 1/35; N.E.E. 1/35;*

*Nelova 1/35E; Norethin 1/35E; Norinyl 1+35; Ortho-Novum 1/35].*

1 mg of norethindrone and 50 mcg (0.05 mg) of ethinyl estradiol (Rx) [*N.E.E. 1/50; Ovcon-50*].

Biphasic twenty-one–day cycle formula, Option one

**Phase one (ten days):** 500 mcg (0.5 mg) of norethindrone and 35 mcg (0.035 mg) of ethinyl estradiol.

**Phase two (eleven days):** 1 mg of norethindrone and 35 mcg (0.035 mg) of ethinyl estradiol. (Rx) [*Necon 10/11; Nelova 10/11; Ortho-Novum 10/11*].

Biphasic twenty-one–day cycle formula, Option two

**Phase one (seven days):** 500 mcg (0.5 mg) of norethindrone and 35 mcg (0.035 mg) of ethinyl estradiol.

**Phase two (fourteen days):** 1 mg of norethindrone and 35 mcg (0.035 mg) of ethinyl estradiol. (Rx) [*Jenest*].

Triphasic twenty-one–day cycle formula, Option one

**Phase one (seven days):** 500 mcg (0.5 mg) of norethindrone and 35 mcg (0.035 mg) of ethinyl estradiol.

**Phase two (nine days):** 1 mg of norethindrone and 35 mcg (0.035 mg) of ethinyl estradiol.

**Phase three (five days):** 500 mcg (0.5 mg) of norethindrone and 35 mcg (0.035 mg) of ethinyl estradiol. (Rx) [*Tri-Norinyl*].

Triphasic twenty-one–day cycle formula, Option two

**Phase one (seven days):** 500 mcg (0.5 mg) of norethindrone and 35 mcg (0.035 mg) of ethinyl estradiol.

**Phase two (seven days):** 750 mcg (0.75 mg) of norethindrone and 35 mcg (0.035 mg) of ethinyl estradiol.

**Phase three (seven days):** 1 mg of norethindrone and 35 mcg (0.035 mg) of ethinyl estradiol. (Rx) [*Ortho-Novum 7/7/7*].

Canada—

Monophasic twenty-one–day cycle formula

500 mcg (0.5 mg) of norethindrone and 35 mcg (0.035 mg) of ethinyl estradiol (Rx) [*Brevicon 0.5/35; Ortho 0.5/35*].

1 mg of norethindrone and 35 mcg (0.035 mg) of ethinyl estradiol (Rx) [*Brevicon 1/35; Ortho 1/35*].

Biphasic twenty-one–day cycle formula

**Phase one (ten days)**—500 mcg (0.5 mg) of norethindrone and 35 mcg (0.035 mg) of ethinyl estradiol.

**Phase two (eleven days)**—1 mg of norethindrone and 35 mcg (0.035 mg) of ethinyl estradiol. (Rx) [*Ortho 10/11; Synphasic*].

Triphasic twenty-one–day cycle formula

**Phase one (seven days)**—500 mcg (0.5 mg) of norethindrone and 35 mcg (0.035 mg) of ethinyl estradiol.

**Phase two (seven days)**—750 mcg (0.75 mg) of norethindrone and 35 mcg (0.035 mg) of ethinyl estradiol.

**Phase three (seven days)**—1 mg of norethindrone and 35 mcg (0.035 mg) of ethinyl estradiol. (Rx) [*Ortho 7/7/7*].

Note: Most products are available in twenty-one– or twenty-eight–day cycles. The twenty-eight–day cycle includes an additional seven days of placebo tablets.

**Packaging and storage**
Store below 40 °C (104 °F), preferably between 15 and 30 °C (59 and 86 °F), unless otherwise specified by manufacturer. Store in a well-closed container.

**Auxiliary labeling**
• Take with food.
• Avoid too much sun or use of sunlamp.

**Note**
Include mandatory patient package inserts (PPIs) (the brief summary of patient labeling and the detailed patient labeling) when dispensing.

Explain sequence of administration of biphasic or triphasic cycle formula when dispensing, especially for twenty-eight–day cycle (colored tablet sequence).

Caution first-time users to use an additional form of birth control as directed by their physician until maximal contraception protection begins.

[1]Not included in Canadian product labeling.

---

### NORETHINDRONE AND MESTRANOL

## Summary of Differences

Pharmacology/pharmacokinetics—Proportion bound to SHBG depends on both estrogen and norethindrone dose; does not suppress estrogen-induced increase of SHBG levels. Norethindrone exhibits no first-pass effect. Mestranol is a prodrug metabolized to ethinyl estradiol at about 83% conversion rate; high first-pass effect and enterohepatic recirculation. Norethindrone is less androgenic than levonorgestrel or nor-

---

gestrel; its androgenic effect depends on both progestin and estrogen doses; slight estrogenic activity.

Laboratory value alterations—Triglycerides increase as with all oral contraceptives; slightly increases total cholesterol; negatively affects lipoproteins—increases LDL and lowers HDL; increases apolipoprotein A₁.

Dosage forms—High estrogen dose formulation available.

## Oral Dosage Forms

Note: Bracketed uses in the *Dosage Forms* section refer to categories of use and/or indications that are not included in U.S. product labeling.

### NORETHINDRONE AND MESTRANOL TABLETS USP

**Usual adult and adolescent dose**
Contraceptive, systemic or
Estrogen-progestin or
[Antiendometriotic] or
[Gonadotropin inhibitor, female, noncontraceptive use][1]—

Twenty-one–day cycle: Oral, 1 tablet a day for twenty-one days commencing on Day 1 of the menstrual cycle or on the first Sunday after the menstrual cycle begins; the next round of treatment is begun on the eighth day after the last tablet of the previous cycle has been taken.

Twenty-eight–day cycle: Oral, 1 tablet a day for twenty-eight days commencing on Day 1 of the menstrual cycle, or on the first Sunday after the menstrual cycle begins; the next round of treatment is begun on the day after the last tablet of the previous cycle has been taken.

Note: With a Sunday-start schedule, the patient should take her first tablet on the first Sunday after the onset of menstruation. If the patient's period begins on a Sunday, she should take her first tablet that same day.

With a Day 1 start schedule, the patient should take her first tablet on Day 1 of the menstrual cycle.

The last seven tablets of the twenty-eight–day cycle contain no hormones. These seven companion tablets are a different color from those containing hormones.

Oral contraceptives may be given continuously or cyclically for endometriosis.

**Strength(s) usually available**
U.S.—
Monophasic twenty-one–day cycle formula
1 mg of norethindrone and 50 mcg (0.05 mg) of mestranol (Rx) [*Genora 1/50; Intercon 1/50; Necon 1/50; Nelova 1/50M; Norethin 1/50M; Norinyl 1+50; Ortho-Novum 1/50*].

Canada—
Monophasic twenty-one–day cycle formula
1 mg of norethindrone and 50 mcg (0.05 mg) of mestranol (Rx) [*Norinyl 1/50; Ortho-Novum 1/50*].

Note: Most products are available in twenty-one– or twenty-eight–day cycles. The twenty-eight–day cycle includes an additional seven days of placebo tablets.

**Packaging and storage**
Store below 40 °C (104 °F), preferably between 15 and 30 °C (59 and 86 °F), unless otherwise specified by manufacturer. Store in a well-closed container.

**Auxiliary labeling**
• Take with food.
• Avoid too much sun or use of sunlamp.

**Note**
Include mandatory patient package inserts (PPIs) (the brief summary of patient labeling and the detailed patient labeling) when dispensing.

Caution first-time users to use an additional form of birth control as directed by their physician until maximal contraception protection begins.

[1]Not included in Canadian product labeling.

---

### NORGESTIMATE AND ETHINYL ESTRADIOL

## Summary of Differences

Pharmacology/pharmacokinetics—Norgestimate is an incomplete prodrug, which is metabolized to other active forms, such as levonorgestrel, norgestrel acetate, and norgestrel. No first-pass effect. Highly progestational; does not counteract the estrogen increase in SHBG levels—highly bound to SHBG and albumin; low androgenicity.

Laboratory value alterations—Triglycerides increase but little effect on lipoproteins.

Medical considerations/contraindications—Norgestimate plus ethinyl estradiol increase glucose tolerance; do not affect 2-hour insulin release; had one of the smallest effects on both areas of carbohydrate metabolism compared with other oral contraceptives.

Side/adverse effects—Absence of withdrawal menstrual bleed was low with norgestimate and ethinyl estradiol formulation; improves pre-existing acne.

## Oral Dosage Forms

Note: Bracketed uses in the *Dosage Forms* section refer to categories of use and/or indications that are not included in U.S. product labeling.

### NORGESTIMATE AND ETHINYL ESTRADIOL TABLETS

#### Usual adult and adolescent dose
Contraceptive, systemic or
Estrogen-progestin or
[Antiendometriotic][1] or
[Gonadotropin inhibitor, female, noncontraceptive use][1]—
  Twenty-one-day cycle: Oral, 1 tablet a day for twenty-one days commencing on Day 1 of the menstrual cycle or on the first Sunday after the menstrual cycle begins; the next round of treatment is begun on the eighth day after the last tablet of the previous cycle has been taken.
  Twenty-eight-day cycle: Oral, 1 tablet a day for twenty-eight days commencing on Day 1 of the menstrual cycle, or on the first Sunday after the menstrual cycle begins; the next round of treatment is begun on the day after the last tablet of the previous cycle has been taken.

Note: With a Sunday-start schedule, the patient should take her first tablet on the first Sunday after the onset of menstruation. If the patient's period begins on a Sunday, she should take her first tablet that same day.

  With a Day 1 start schedule, the patient should take her first tablet on Day 1 of the menstrual cycle.

  The last seven tablets of the twenty-eight-day cycle contain no hormones. These seven companion tablets are a different color from those containing hormones.

  Oral contraceptives may be given continuously or cyclically for endometriosis.

#### Strength(s) usually available
U.S.—
  Monophasic twenty-one-day cycle formula
    250 mcg (0.25 mg) of norgestimate and 35 mcg (0.035 mg) of ethinyl estradiol (Rx) [Ortho-Cyclen].
  Triphasic twenty-one-day cycle formula
    **Phase one (seven days)**—180 mcg (0.18 mg) of norgestimate and 35 mcg (0.035 mg) of ethinyl estradiol.
    **Phase two (seven days)**—215 mcg (0.215 mg) of norgestimate and 35 mcg (0.035 mg) of ethinyl estradiol.
    **Phase three (seven days)**—250 mcg (0.25 mg) of norgestimate and 35 mcg (0.035 mg) of ethinyl estradiol. (Rx) [Ortho Tri-Cyclen].
Canada—
  Monophasic twenty-one-day cycle formula: 250 mcg (0.25 mg) of norgestimate and 35 mcg (0.035 mg) of ethinyl estradiol (Rx) [Cyclen].
  Triphasic twenty-one-day cycle formula
    **Phase one (seven days)**—180 mcg (0.18 mg) of norgestimate and 35 mcg (0.035 mg) of ethinyl estradiol.
    **Phase two (seven days)**—215 mcg (0.215 mg) of norgestimate and 35 mcg (0.035 mg) of ethinyl estradiol.
    **Phase three (seven days)**—250 mcg (0.25 mg) of norgestimate and 35 mcg (0.035 mg) of ethinyl estradiol. (Rx) [Tri-Cyclen].

Note: Available in twenty-one- or twenty-eight-day cycles. The twenty-eight-day cycle includes an additional seven days of placebo tablets.

#### Packaging and storage
Store below 40 °C (104 °F), preferably between 15 and 30 °C (59 and 86 °F), unless otherwise specified by manufacturer. Store in a well-closed container.

#### Auxiliary labeling
• Take with food.
• Avoid too much sun or use of sunlamp.

#### Note
Include mandatory patient package inserts (PPIs) (the brief summary of patient labeling and the detailed patient labeling) when dispensing.

Explain sequence of administration of biphasic or triphasic cycle formula when dispensing, especially for twenty-eight-day cycle (colored tablet sequence).

Caution first-time users to use an additional form of birth control as directed by their physician until maximal contraception protection begins.

[1]Not included in Canadian product labeling.

---

### *NORGESTREL AND ETHINYL ESTRADIOL*

## Summary of Differences
Indications:
  Also, used for emergency postcoital contraception.
Pharmacology/pharmacokinetics:
  Proportion bound to SHBG depends on both estrogen and norgestrel dose; suppressed estrogen-induced increase of SHBG levels in most contraceptive doses except for triphasic formulation which only slightly increased SHBG levels. No first-pass effect.
  Norgestrel is one of the most androgenic progestins; its androgenic effect depends on both progestin and estrogen doses.
Laboratory value alterations:
  No change of triglycerides over 1 year; may slightly decrease or increase total cholesterol; negatively affects lipoprotein, increases LDL and lowers HDL; increases apolipoprotein A$_1$ the least of all contraceptives; can increase free testosterone by displacing it from SHBG.
Dosage forms:
  High estrogen dose formulation available.

## Oral Dosage Forms
Note: Bracketed uses in the *Dosage Forms* section refer to categories of use and/or indications that are not included in U.S. product labeling.

### NORGESTREL AND ETHINYL ESTRADIOL TABLETS USP

#### Usual adult and adolescent dose
Contraceptive, systemic or
Estrogen-progestin or
[Antiendometriotic][1] or
[Gonadotropin inhibitor, female, noncontraceptive use][1]—
  Twenty-one-day cycle: Oral, 1 tablet a day for twenty-one days commencing on Day 1 of the menstrual cycle or on the first Sunday after the menstrual cycle begins; the next round of treatment is begun on the eighth day after the last tablet of the previous cycle has been taken.
  Twenty-eight-day cycle: Oral, 1 tablet a day for twenty-eight days commencing on Day 1 of the menstrual cycle, or on the first Sunday after the menstrual cycle begins; the next round of treatment is begun on the day after the last tablet of the previous cycle has been taken.

Note: With a Sunday-start schedule, the patient should take her first tablet on the first Sunday after the onset of menstruation. If the patient's period begins on a Sunday, she should take her first tablet that same day.

  With a Day 1 start schedule, the patient should take her first tablet on Day 1 of the menstrual cycle.

  The last seven tablets of the twenty-eight-day cycle contain no hormones. These seven companion tablets are a different color from those containing hormones.

  Oral contraceptives may be given continuously or cyclically for endometriosis.

[Contraceptive, postcoital, systemic][1]—
  Two tablets (500 mcg norgestrel and 50 mcg of ethinyl estradiol per tablet) or four tablets (300 mcg norgestrel and 30 mcg ethinyl estradiol per tablet) taken as soon as possible after unprotected coitus, preferably within twelve hours but not longer than seventy-two hours later. Then, repeat the dose twelve hours after the first dose.

#### Strength(s) usually available
U.S.—
  300 mcg (0.3 mg) of norgestrel and 30 mcg (0.03 mg) of ethinyl estradiol (Rx) [Lo/Ovral].
  500 mcg (0.5 mg) of norgestrel and 50 mcg (0.05 mg) of ethinyl estradiol (Rx) [Ovral].
Canada—
  500 mcg (0.50 mg) of norgestrel and 50 mcg (0.05 mg) of ethinyl estradiol (Rx) [Ovral].

Note: Available in twenty-one– or twenty-eight–day cycles. The twenty-eight–day cycle includes an additional seven days of placebo tablets.

**Packaging and storage**
Store below 40 °C (104 °F), preferably between 15 and 30 °C (59 and 86 °F), unless otherwise specified by manufacturer. Store in a well-closed container.

**Auxiliary labeling**
• Take with food.
• Avoid too much sun or use of sunlamp.

**Note**
Include mandatory patient package inserts (PPIs) (the brief summary of patient labeling and the detailed patient labeling) when dispensing.

Caution first-time users to use an additional form of birth control as directed by their physician until maximal contraception protection begins.

___

[1]Not included in Canadian product labeling.

## Selected Bibliography

**General**
Fraser IS. Contraceptive choice for women with 'risk factors.' Drug Safety 8 (4): 271-9.
Speroff L, DeCherney A, The Advisory Board for the New Progestins. Evaluation of a new generation of oral contraceptives. Obstet Gynecol 1993 Jun; 81 (6): 1034-47.
World Health Organization. Oral contraceptives and neoplasia. WHO Technical Report Series 1992; 817: 1-45.

**For desogestrel and ethinyl estradiol**
Burkman RT, editor. Desogestrel: a progestin for the 1990s. Am J Obstet Gynecol 1993 May; 168 (3 pt 2): 1009-52.

**For ethynodiol diacetate and ethinyl estradiol**
Burkman RT, Robinson CJ, Kruszone-Moran DA, et al. Lipid and lipo-protein changes associated with oral contraceptive use: a randomized clinical trial. Obstet Gynecol 1988 Jan; 71 (1): 33-8.

**For levonorgestrel and ethinyl estradiol**
Godsland IF, Walton C, Felton C, et al. Insulin resistance, secretion, and metabolism in users of oral contraceptives. J Clin Endocrinol Metab 1992; 74 (1): 64-70.

**For norethindrone acetate and ethinyl estradiol**
Goldzieher JW. Pharmacokinetics and metabolism of ethynyl estrogens. In: Goldzieher JW, editor. Pharmacology of the contraceptive steroids. New York: Raven Press, 1994: 127-51.

**For norethindrone and ethinyl estradiol**
Godsland IF, Crook D, Simpson R, et al. The effects of different formulations of oral contraceptive agents on lipid and carbohydrate metabolism. N Engl J Med 1990 Nov 15; 1375-81.

**For norgestrel and ethinyl estradiol**
Ayangade O, Akinyemi A. A comparative study of Norinyl 1/35 versus Lo-Ovral in Ile-Ife, Nigeria. Int J Gynaecol Obstet 1989; 30: 165-70.

**For norethindrone and mestranol**
Policar M. Clinical experience with multiphasic oral contraceptives. J Reprod Med 1986; 31 (9): 939-45.

**For norgestimate and ethinyl estradiol**
McGuire JL, Phillips A, Hahn DW, et al. Pharmacologic and pharmacokinetic characteristics of norgestimate and its metabolites. Am J Obstet Gynecol 1990; 163 (6 pt 2): 2127-31.

Revised: 06/28/96
Interim revision: 09/27/96

___

**ESTRONE**—See *Estrogens (Systemic); Estrogens (Vaginal)*

___

**ESTROPIPATE**—See *Estrogens (Systemic); Estrogens (Vaginal)*

___

**ETHACRYNIC ACID**—See *Diuretics, Loop (Systemic)*

___

# ETHAMBUTOL Systemic

VA CLASSIFICATION (Primary): AM500
Note: For a listing of dosage forms and brand names by country availability, see *Dosage Forms* section(s). For a listing of brand names for the articles in this monograph, refer to the General Index.

## Category
Antibacterial (antimycobacterial).

## Indications
Note: Bracketed information in the *Indications* section refers to uses that are not included in U.S. product labeling.

**Accepted**
Tuberculosis (treatment)—Ethambutol is indicated in combination with other antituberculosis medications in the treatment of all forms of tuberculosis, including tuberculous meningitis, caused by *Mycobacterium tuberculosis*.

[Mycobacterial infections, atypical (treatment)]—Ethambutol is used in the treatment of atypical mycobacterial infections, such as *Mycobacterium avium* complex (MAC).

No cross-resistance with other available antimycobacterial agents has been demonstrated.

Not all species or strains of a particular organism may be susceptible to ethambutol.

## Pharmacology/Pharmacokinetics

**Physicochemical characteristics**
Molecular weight—277.23.

**Mechanism of action/Effect**
Ethambutol is a synthetic, bacteriostatic antitubercular agent. Its mechanism of action is not fully known. It diffuses into mycobacteria and appears to suppress multiplication by interfering with RNA synthesis. It is effective only against mycobacteria that are actively dividing.

**Absorption**
Rapidly absorbed (75 to 80%) from the gastrointestinal tract following oral administration.

**Distribution**
Widely distributed to most tissues and fluids, except cerebrospinal fluid (CSF). CSF concentrations are 10 to 50% of the corresponding serum concentrations.
Erythrocytes—
Equal to or double the plasma concentrations, which provide a depot effect for 24 hours.
Distributed into breast milk.
CSF—
Does not penetrate intact meninges, but 10 to 50% may penetrate the meninges of patients with tuberculous meningitis.
$Vol_D$ = 1.6 liters per kg.

**Protein binding**
Low (20-30%).

**Biotransformation**
Hepatic; up to 15% metabolized to inactive metabolites.

**Half-life**
Normal renal function—
3 to 4 hours.
Impaired renal function—
Up to 8 hours.

**Time to peak serum concentration:**
2 to 4 hours.

**Peak serum concentration:**
2 to 5 mcg per mL after a single oral dose of 25 mg per kg of body weight (mg/kg).

**Elimination**
Renal—
By glomerular filtration and tubular secretion; up to 80% excreted within 24 hours (at least 50% excreted unchanged and up to 15% as inactive metabolites).

Fecal—
20% excreted unchanged.
In dialysis—
Ethambutol is removed from the blood by hemodialysis and peritoneal dialysis.

## Precautions to Consider

### Pregnancy/Reproduction
Pregnancy—It is recommended that pregnant women with tuberculosis be treated for a minimum of 9 months with multi-drug therapy, including ethambutol. Ethambutol crosses the placenta, resulting in fetal plasma concentrations approximately 30% of maternal plasma concentrations. However, problems in humans have not been documented.

Studies in mice given high doses have shown that ethambutol causes a low incidence of cleft palate, exencephaly, and vertebral column abnormalities. In addition, studies in rats given high doses have shown that ethambutol causes minor abnormalities of the cervical vertebrae. Studies in rabbits given high doses have shown that ethambutol may cause monophthalmia, limb reduction defects, hare lip, and cleft palate.

### Breast-feeding
Ethambutol is distributed into breast milk in concentrations approximating maternal serum concentrations. However, problems in humans have not been documented.

### Pediatrics
Appropriate studies on the relationship of age to the effects of ethambutol have not been performed in children up to 13 years of age. Ethambutol is generally not recommended in children whose visual acuity cannot be monitored (younger than 6 years of age). However, ethambutol should be considered for all children with organisms resistant to other medications, and in whom susceptibility to ethambutol has been demonstrated or is likely.

### Geriatrics
No information is available on the relationship of age to the effects of ethambutol in geriatric patients. However, elderly patients are more likely to have an age-related decrease in renal function, which may require an adjustment of dosage in patients receiving ethambutol.

### Drug interactions and/or related problems
The following drug interactions and/or related problems have been selected on the basis of their potential clinical significance (possible mechanism in parentheses where appropriate)—not necessarily inclusive (» = major clinical significance):

Note: Combinations containing any of the following medications, depending on the amount present, may also interact with this medication.

Neurotoxic medications, other (See *Appendix II*)
(concurrent administration of ethambutol with other neurotoxic medications may increase the potential for neurotoxicity, such as optic and peripheral neuritis)

### Laboratory value alterations
The following have been selected on the basis of their potential clinical significance (possible effect in parentheses where appropriate)—not necessarily inclusive (» = major clinical significance):

With physiology/laboratory test values
Uric acid, serum
(concentrations may be increased)

### Medical considerations/Contraindications
The medical considerations/contraindications included here have been selected on the basis of their potential clinical significance (reasons given in parentheses where appropriate)—not necessarily inclusive (» = major clinical significance).

*Risk-benefit should be considered when the following medical problems exist:*
Gouty arthritis
(ethambutol may increase uric acid concentrations)
» Hypersensitivity to ethambutol
» Optic neuritis
(ethambutol may cause retrobulbar optic neuritis)
» Renal function impairment
(because ethambutol is excreted primarily through the kidneys, patients with renal function impairment may require a reduction in dosage)

### Patient monitoring
The following may be especially important in patient monitoring (other tests may be warranted in some patients, depending on condition; » = major clinical significance):
Ophthalmologic examinations
(tests for visual fields and acuity and red-green discrimination may be required prior to and monthly during treatment, especially if treatment is prolonged or if dosage is greater than 15 mg per kg of body weight [mg/kg] daily)
Uric acid concentrations, serum
(may be required during treatment since elevated serum uric acid concentrations frequently occur, possibly resulting in precipitation of acute gout)

## Side/Adverse Effects

Note: Retrobulbar optic neuritis is thought to be dose-related, occurring most frequently with daily doses of 25 mg per kg of body weight (mg/kg) and after 2 months of therapy; however, optic neuritis has occurred after only a few days of treatment. Most cases are reversible after several weeks or months. Visual changes may be unilateral or bilateral; therefore, each eye must be tested separately and both eyes tested together.

The following side/adverse effects have been selected on the basis of their potential clinical significance (possible signs and symptoms in parentheses where appropriate)—not necessarily inclusive:

### Those indicating need for medical attention
Incidence less frequent
*Acute gouty arthritis* (chills; pain and swelling of joints, especially big toe, ankle or knee; tense, hot skin over affected joints)
Incidence rare
*Hypersensitivity* (skin rash; fever; joint pain); *peripheral neuritis* (numbness, tingling, burning pain, or weakness in hands or feet); *retrobulbar optic neuritis* (blurred vision, eye pain, red-green color blindness, or any loss of vision)

### Those indicating need for medical attention only if they continue or are bothersome
Incidence less frequent
*Confusion; disorientation; gastrointestinal disturbances* (abdominal pain; loss of appetite; nausea and vomiting); *headache*

## Patient Consultation
As an aid to patient consultation, refer to *Advice for the Patient, Ethambutol (Systemic)*.

In providing consultation, consider emphasizing the following selected information (» = major clinical significance):

### Before using this medication
» Conditions affecting use, especially:
Pregnancy—Ethambutol crosses the placenta. However, problems in humans have not been documented
Breast-feeding—Ethambutol is distributed into breast milk
Use in children—Appropriate studies have not been done in children up to 13 years of age. Ethambutol is generally not recommended in children whose visual acuity cannot be monitored (younger than 6 years of age)
Other medical problems, especially optic neuritis and renal function impairment

### Proper use of this medication
Taking with food if gastrointestinal irritation occurs
» Compliance with full course of therapy, which may take months or years
» Proper dosing
Missed dose: Taking as soon as possible; not taking if almost time for next dose; not doubling doses
» Proper storage

### Precautions while using this medication
Checking with physician if no improvement within 2 or 3 weeks
» Regular visits to physician to check progress; need to report promptly to physician signs of optic neuritis and prodromal signs of peripheral neuritis; need for ophthalmologic examinations if signs of optic neuritis occur
» Caution if blurred vision or loss of vision occurs

### Side/adverse effects
Signs of potential side effects, especially acute gouty arthritis, hypersensitivity, peripheral neuritis, or retrobulbar optic neuritis

## General Dosing Information

Ethambutol may be taken with food if gastrointestinal irritation occurs.

Since daily administration in divided doses may not result in therapeutic serum concentrations, ethambutol should be administered only in a single daily dose.

Since bacterial resistance may develop rapidly when ethambutol is administered alone, it should only be administered concurrently with other antituberculosis medications.

Tuberculosis therapy must be continued for 6 months to 2 years, depending on the treatment regimen. Uncomplicated pulmonary tuberculosis is often successfully treated within 6 to 12 months. Several different treatment regimens are currently recommended.

• The Infectious Diseases Society of America recommends standard triple-drug therapy for patients born in the United States who have never been treated, do not reside in communities with a known high prevalence of drug-resistant *Mycobacterium* strains, and have no risk factors for drug-resistant tuberculosis.

—Isoniazid, rifampin, and, usually, pyrazinamide are given together daily for the first 2 months, then isoniazid and rifampin are continued daily or twice a week for the remainder of the treatment period. Directly observed therapy is recommended for patients suspected of being noncompliant. If a patient is at risk of being infected with drug-resistant organisms, 4-drug therapy, consisting of isoniazid, rifampin, pyrazinamide, and ethambutol, is recommended.

• The Centers for Disease Control recommend 3 other treatment regimen options available for non–HIV-infected patients:

—In geographic areas where the isoniazid resistance rate is documented to be ≥ 4%, an initial 4-drug regimen of isoniazid, rifampin, pyrazinamide, and streptomycin or ethambutol, taken under direct observation, is recommended. This should be administered for 8 weeks. After that time and provided that the organism is found to be susceptible, isoniazid and rifampin are administered daily, or 2 or 3 times a week, under direct observation, for 16 weeks. When results of susceptibility tests for these medications become available, the regimen should be altered as appropriate.

—Isoniazid, rifampin, pyrazinamide, and streptomycin or ethambutol taken daily under direct observation for 2 weeks, followed by twice-weekly administration of all 4 medications for 6 weeks, under direct observation. This is then followed by twice-weekly administration, directly observed, of isoniazid and rifampin for 16 weeks.

—Isoniazid, rifampin, pyrazinamide, and streptomycin or ethambutol taken 3 times a week under direct observation for 6 months.

HIV-infected patients may use any of the 3 options recommended by the CDC; however, treatment regimens should continue for a total of 9 months and at least 6 months beyond culture conversion.

Healthcare or correctional institutions experiencing outbreaks of tuberculosis that are resistant to isoniazid and rifampin, or that are resuming therapy for a patient with a prior history of antitubercular therapy, may need to begin 5- or 6-drug regimens as initial therapy. These regimens should include the 4-drug regimen and at least 3 medications to which the suspected multi-drug–resistant strain may be susceptible.

The regimen for treating pulmonary tuberculosis should be effective in treating extrapulmonary tuberculosis. Some experts recommend extending the duration of therapy to 9 months in patients with disseminated disease, miliary tuberculosis, disease involving bones or joints, or tuberculosis lymphadenitis. Adjunctive therapies, such as surgery and corticosteroids, may be beneficial.

Serum concentrations may be increased and half-life prolonged in patients with impaired renal function. Therefore, patients with impaired renal function may require a reduction in dose.

## Oral Dosage Forms

Note: Bracketed uses in the *Dosage Forms* section refer to categories of use and/or indications that are not included in U.S. product labeling.

### ETHAMBUTOL HYDROCHLORIDE TABLETS USP

**Usual adult and adolescent dose**
Tuberculosis—
   In combination with other antituberculosis medications: Oral, 15 to 25 mg per kg of body weight once a day; or 50 mg per kg of body weight, up to 2.5 grams, two times a week; or 25 to 30 mg per kg of body weight, up to 2.5 grams, three times a week.
   [Mycobacterial infections, atypical]—Oral, 15 to 25 mg per kg of body weight once a day.

**Usual adult prescribing limits**
Tuberculosis—
   2.5 grams daily.

**Usual pediatric dose**
Children up to 13 years of age—Dosage has not been established. However, ethambutol should be considered for all children with organisms resistant to other medications, and in whom susceptibility to ethambutol has been demonstrated or is likely. Ethambutol is generally not recommended in children whose visual acuity cannot be monitored (younger than 6 years of age).
Children 13 years of age and over—See *Usual adult and adolescent dose*.

**Strength(s) usually available**
U.S.—
   100 mg (Rx) [*Myambutol*].
   400 mg (Rx) [*Myambutol* (scored)].
Canada—
   100 mg (Rx) [*Etibi* (scored); *Myambutol*].
   400 mg (Rx) [*Etibi* (scored); *Myambutol* (scored)].

**Packaging and storage**
Store below 40 °C (104 °F), preferably between 15 and 30 °C (59 and 86 °F), unless otherwise specified by manufacturer. Store in a well-closed container.

**Auxiliary labeling**
   • Continue medicine for full time of treatment.

Revised: 06/22/94

---

# ETHANOLAMINE OLEATE   Parenteral-Local

VA CLASSIFICATION (Primary): CV600
Note: For a listing of dosage forms and brand names by country availability, see *Dosage Forms* section(s). For a listing of brand names for the articles in this monograph, refer to the General Index.

## Category
Sclerosing agent.

## Indications

**Accepted**
Esophageal varices, bleeding (treatment)—Ethanolamine oleate is indicated in the treatment of bleeding esophageal varices, and the prevention of recurrent bleeding in patients whose varices have recently bled.

   Ethanolamine oleate does not correct portal hypertension, the underlying cause of esophageal varices. Recanalization of varices and collateralization may therefore occur, requiring further treatment.

**Acceptance not established**
Ethanolamine oleate sclerotherapy has been used to treat *cystic lesions* including testicular hydroceles, spermatoceles, and renal cysts. In the case of scrotal lesions, improved results were obtained when treatment was limited to a maximum of 3 cysts. In addition, sclerotherapy for the treatment of spermatoceles was not recommended for men in their reproductive years who wish to have children because of the danger of its causing infertility. Even though results have generally been good, data is limited and further study is required to define the role of ethanolamine oleate in these conditions.

**Unaccepted**
Ethanolamine oleate is not indicated for the prophylactic treatment of esophageal varices that have not bled. Trials of prophylactic sclerotherapy have shown mixed results and varied greatly in design; the early favorable results were obtained from poor quality studies.

## Pharmacology/Pharmacokinetics

**Physicochemical characteristics**
Molecular weight—343.55.

## Mechanism of action/Effect

Injection of ethanolamine oleate causes an acute, dose-related inflammatory reaction of the intimal endothelium of the vein. This leads to scarring and possible occlusion of the vein. An acute, dose-related extravascular inflammatory reaction also occurs as ethanolamine oleate rapidly diffuses through the venous wall.

Ethanolamine oleate also causes a transient activation of the coagulation and fibrinolytic systems. The oleic acid component, which is responsible for the inflammatory response, may initiate coagulation by activation of Hageman factor and release of tissue factor. However, the ethanolamine component may inhibit clot formation by chelating calcium, which is necessary for coagulation. Therefore, a procoagulant effect of ethanolamine oleate has not been demonstrated.

## Absorption

After injection into an esophageal varix, ethanolamine oleate is cleared from the injection site within five minutes via the portal vein. Some of the medication also flows into the azygos vein through the periesophageal vein if more than 20 mL is injected.

# Precautions to Consider

## Cross-sensitivity and/or related problems

Patients allergic to ethanolamine, oleic acid, or morrhuate sodium may be allergic to ethanolamine oleate also.

## Carcinogenicity

There have been a few case reports of esophageal carcinoma following endoscopic injection sclerotherapy for esophageal varices. However, an association between sclerotherapy and carcinoma is difficult to determine. In the reported cases, various sclerosants were used and other risk factors such as age and alcohol/tobacco abuse were present. There were also geographic differences in the sites of sclerosis and the development of carcinoma. Present information is insufficient to establish a causal relationship between endoscopic sclerotherapy and development of esophageal carcinoma. Further study and observation are required, and periodic long-term follow-up should be performed following endoscopic sclerotherapy.

## Pregnancy/Reproduction

Pregnancy—Studies have not been done in humans.
Studies have not been done in animals.
FDA Pregnancy Category C.

## Breast-feeding

It is not known whether ethanolamine oleate is distributed into breast milk.

## Pediatrics

Appropriate studies performed to date have not demonstrated pediatrics-specific problems that would limit the usefulness of ethanolamine oleate in children.

## Geriatrics

Appropriate studies performed to date have not demonstrated geriatrics-specific problems that would limit the usefulness of ethanolamine oleate in the elderly.

## Medical considerations/Contraindications

The medical considerations/contraindications included here have been selected on the basis of their potential clinical significance (reasons given in parentheses where appropriate)—not necessarily inclusive (» = major clinical significance).

*Except under special circumstances, this medication should not be used when the following medical problems exist:*

» Allergy to ethanolamine, oleic acid, ethanolamine oleate, or morrhuate sodium

# Side/Adverse Effects

Note: Many of these complications are related to injection sclerotherapy in general and are not necessarily a result of ethanolamine oleate therapy specifically.

Portal gastropathy may develop following endoscopic injection sclerotherapy of esophageal varices, with a peak incidence 6 to 9 months after treatment. Its development may be a result of the transmission of pressure to gastric mucosal and submucosal veins and the formation of gastric capillary ectasia with obstruction of the esophageal varices.

Overdosage of ethanolamine oleate during injection sclerotherapy of esophageal varices can result in severe intramural necrosis of the esophagus. Complications occurring after such an overdose have resulted in death.

The following side/adverse effects have been selected on the basis of their potential clinical significance (possible signs and symptoms in parentheses where appropriate)—not necessarily inclusive:

**Those indicating need for medical attention**
Incidence less frequent
*Esophageal stricture; pneumonia, including aspiration pneumonia; portal vein thrombosis*
Incidence rare
*Allergic reactions, including anaphylaxis; urticaria; and generalized skin reactions; CNS infection, including brain abscess and meningitis; disseminated intravascular coagulation; esophageal perforation; renal failure, acute; spinal cord paralysis*
Note: A case of fatal *anaphylactic shock* occurred in a patient who had a known allergic disposition and received a larger than normal volume of ethanolamine oleate.

**Those indicating need for medical attention only if they continue or are bothersome**
Note: The following adverse effects are generally transient, self-limiting, and inconsequential. In the case of fever and bacteremia, antibiotic therapy is not indicated unless fever is high, has erratic swings, persists beyond 48 hours, or is associated with other signs of infection.
Incidence more frequent
*Chest pain; dysphagia; fever*
Incidence less frequent
*Bacteremia*

**Those not indicating need for medical attention**
Incidence more frequent
*Abnormal chest x-rays, including pulmonary infiltrates and pleural effusions; esophageal ulceration*

# General Dosing Information

Ethanolamine oleate should be administered only by physicians who are experienced with the use of an acceptable injection technique.

**For treatment of esophageal varices**
Careful monitoring and reduction of the total dose per session is recommended in patients with concomitant cardiorespiratory or significant liver disease (Child Class C).

Esophageal ulceration following ethanolamine oleate sclerotherapy is more common in patients in Child Class C.

Esophageal ulceration, necrosis, and delayed perforation appear to occur more often when the medication is injected submucosally. This route of administration is not recommended.

Because fatal aspiration pneumonia has occurred following ethanolamine oleate sclerotherapy, precautions should be taken to prevent its occurrence, particularly in the elderly and critically ill patients.

Antibiotic prophylaxis is recommended for immunosuppressed patients or for patients with valvular heart disease or prosthetic graft material because of the potential for bacteremia associated with endoscopy. *Staphylococcus aureus* and alpha hemolytic streptococci are the most commonly identified organisms associated with bacteremia following upper gastrointestinal endoscopy.

**Safety considerations for handling this medication**
The physician should wear protective eye gear during procedures to prevent eye damage by spattered sclerosant.

**For treatment of adverse effects**
Serious anaphylactic reactions require emergency treatment, which consists of the following
• 0.25 mL of a 1:1,000 intravenous solution of epinephrine (0.25 mg).
• Oxygen.
• Parenteral antihistamines.
• Intravenous corticosteroids.
• Airway management (including intubation).

# Parenteral Dosage Forms
## ETHANOLAMINE OLEATE INJECTION

**Usual adult dose**
Esophageal varices, bleeding—
Intravenous, 1.5 to 5 mL per varix, up to a maximum dose of 20 mL per treatment session.
To obliterate the varix, injections may be given at the time of the acute bleeding episode and then one week, six weeks, three months, and six months later as indicated.

**Usual adult prescribing limits**
20 mL per treatment session.

**Usual pediatric dose**
Esophageal varices, bleeding—
   Intravenous, 2 to 3 mL per varix, up to a maximum dose of 10 to 20 mL per treatment session.

**Usual pediatric prescribing limits**
10 to 20 mL per treatment session.

**Strength(s) usually available**
U.S.—
   5% (50 mg [approximate] per mL) (Rx) [*Ethamolin* (benzyl alcohol, 2% by volume)].
Canada—
   5% (50 mg [approximate] per mL) (Rx) [*Ethamolin* (benzyl alcohol, 2% by volume)].

**Packaging and storage**
Store at controlled room temperature, between 15 and 30 °C (59 and 86 °F). Protect from light.

**Note**
Injection should be inspected visually for particulate matter and discoloration prior to administration.

## Selected Bibliography

Bornman PC, Krige JEJ, Terblanche J. Management of oesophageal varices. Lancet 1994; 343: 1079-84.

Developed: 08/10/95

# ETHCHLORVYNOL  Systemic

VA CLASSIFICATION (Primary): CN309

Note: For a listing of dosage forms and brand names by country availability, see *Dosage Forms* section(s). For a listing of brand names for the articles in this monograph, refer to the General Index.

## Category
Sedative-hypnotic.

## Indications

**Accepted**

Ethchlorvynol has been used for short-term hypnotic therapy in the management of insomnia for periods of up to one week in duration; however, this medication generally *has been replaced* by other sedative-hypnotic agents. If ethchlorvynol is used for the treatment of insomnia and retreatment is necessary after drug-free intervals of one or more weeks, the patient should be further evaluated.

## Pharmacology/Pharmacokinetics

**Physicochemical characteristics**
Molecular weight—144.60.

**Mechanism of action/Effect**
Unknown.

**Absorption**
Rapidly absorbed from gastrointestinal tract.

**Distribution**
Extensive tissue localization of ethchlorvynol, especially in adipose tissue. Ethchlorvynol and/or its metabolites have also been found in the liver, kidneys, spleen, brain, bile, and cerebrospinal fluid.

**Protein binding**
Moderate (35 to 50%).

**Biotransformation**
About 90% of a dose is metabolized in the liver. Some ethchlorvynol may also be metabolized in the kidneys.

**Half-life**
Plasma half-life is approximately 10 to 20 hours.

**Onset of action**
Within 15 minutes to 1 hour.

**Time to peak plasma concentration**
Within 2 hours following a single oral fasting dose.

**Duration of action**
About 5 hours.

**Elimination**
Renal.

## Precautions to Consider

**Carcinogenicity/Tumorigenicity**
A study in mice showed ethchlorvynol, at doses up to 7 times the maximum human daily dose for 22 to 24 months, to cause a statistically significant increase in total lung tumors in female mice. However, a study in rats did not show ethchlorvynol to be potentially carcinogenic when the medication was administered at 5 to 15 times the maximum human daily dose for up to 2 years.

**Pregnancy/Reproduction**
Pregnancy—First and second trimesters: Ethchlorvynol crosses the placenta. Adequate and well-controlled studies have not been done in humans. Use of ethchlorvynol is not recommended during the first and second trimesters of pregnancy since studies in animals have shown a higher percentage of stillbirths and a lower survival rate of offspring when ethchlorvynol was given in doses of 40 mg per kg of body weight (mg/kg) per day.
Third trimester: Use during the third trimester of pregnancy may produce central nervous system (CNS) depression and withdrawal symptoms in the neonate.

FDA Pregnancy Category C.

**Breast-feeding**
It is not known whether ethchlorvynol is excreted in breast milk.

**Pediatrics**
Appropriate studies on the relationship of age to the effects of ethchlorvynol have not been performed in the pediatric population. Safety and efficacy have not been established.

**Geriatrics**
Elderly patients may be more sensitive to the effects of ethchlorvynol; therefore, they should receive the minimum effective dose. Also, elderly patients are more likely to have age-related hepatic function impairment and renal function impairment, which may require reduction of dosage in patients receiving ethchlorvynol.

**Drug interactions and/or related problems**
The following drug interactions and/or related problems have been selected on the basis of their potential clinical significance (possible mechanism in parentheses where appropriate)—not necessarily inclusive (» = major clinical significance):

Note: Combinations containing any of the following medications, depending on the amount present, may also interact with this medication.

Addictive medications, other, especially CNS depressants with habituating potential
   (prolonged concurrent use may increase the risk of habituation; caution is recommended)
» Alcohol or
» CNS depression–producing medications, other (See *Appendix II*)
   (concurrent use may increase the CNS depressant effects of either these medications or ethchlorvynol; caution is recommended and dosage of one or both agents should be reduced)
» Anticoagulants, coumarin- or indandione-derivative
   (hypoprothrombinemic effects may be decreased when these medications are used concurrently with ethchlorvynol because of accelerated metabolism of anticoagulant secondary to stimulation of hepatic microsomal enzyme activity; dosage adjustments of anticoagulants may be necessary during and after ethchlorvynol therapy)
Antidepressants, tricyclic, especially amitriptyline
   (in addition to possibly increasing CNS depressant effects, concurrent use with ethchlorvynol may cause transient delirium)

## Laboratory value alterations

The following have been selected on the basis of their potential clinical significance (possible effect in parentheses where appropriate)—not necessarily inclusive (» = major clinical significance):

With physiology/laboratory test values

Phentolamine test

(ethchlorvynol may cause false-positive phentolamine test; it is recommended that all medications be withdrawn at least 24 hours, preferably 48 to 72 hours, prior to a phentolamine test)

## Medical considerations/Contraindications

The medical considerations/contraindications included here have been selected on the basis of their potential clinical significance (reasons given in parentheses where appropriate)—not necessarily inclusive (» = major clinical significance).

*Risk-benefit should be considered when the following medical problems exist:*

» Alcoholism, active or in remission or
» Drug abuse or dependence, history of
   (predisposition of patient to habituation and dependence)
   Hepatic function impairment
   (ethchlorvynol metabolized in liver)
» Mental depression
   Pain, uncontrolled
» Porphyria
   Renal function impairment
   (ethchlorvynol excreted via kidneys)
   Sensitivity to ethchlorvynol

## Side/Adverse Effects

The following side/adverse effects have been selected on the basis of their potential clinical significance (possible signs and symptoms in parentheses where appropriate)—not necessarily inclusive:

### Those indicating need for medical attention
Incidence less frequent
   *Allergic reaction* (skin rash or hives); *paradoxical reaction* (unusual excitement, nervousness, or restlessness); *thrombocytopenia* (unusual bleeding or bruising)
Incidence rare
   *Cholestatic jaundice* (darkening of urine; itching; pale stools; yellow eyes or skin)

### Those indicating need for medical attention only if they continue or are bothersome
Incidence more frequent
   *Blurred vision; dizziness or lightheadedness; indigestion; nausea or vomiting; numbness of face; stomach pain; unpleasant aftertaste; unusual tiredness or weakness*
Incidence less frequent
   *Clumsiness or unsteadiness; confusion; drowsiness, daytime*

### Those indicating possible withdrawal and the need for medical attention if they occur (usually after 2 weeks) after medication is discontinued
   *Convulsions; hallucinations; muscle twitching; nausea or vomiting; restlessness, nervousness, or irritability; sweating; trembling; trouble in sleeping; weakness*

## Overdose

For more information on the management of overdose or unintentional ingestion, **contact a Poison Control Center** (see *Poison Control Center Listing*).

### Clinical effects of overdose
The following effects have been selected on the basis of their potential clinical significance (possible signs and symptoms in parentheses where appropriate)–not necessarily inclusive:

Acute
   *Low body temperature; shortness of breath or slow or troubled breathing; slow heartbeat; weakness, severe*
Chronic
   *Confusion, continuing; double vision; numbness, tingling, pain, or weakness in hands or feet; slurred speech; staggering; trembling; unusual movements of the eyes*

### Treatment of overdose
Recommended treatment for acute ethchlorvynol toxicity includes the following:
   To decrease absorption—
      Gastric evacuation should be immediately performed. In the unconscious patient, gastric lavage should be preceded by tracheal intubation with a cuffed tube to prevent aspiration of vomitus.
   To enhance elimination—
      Hemoperfusion using the Amberlite column technique has been reported to be effective.
      Hemodialysis and peritoneal dialysis also may be effective. Aqueous and oil dialysates have been used.
   Monitoring—
      Pulmonary function and blood gases should be monitored.
   Supportive care—
      Supportive measures such as assisted ventilation, frequent monitoring of vital signs, and control of blood pressure are essential.
      Patients in whom intentional overdose is known or suspected should be referred for psychiatric consultation.

## Patient Consultation

As an aid to patient consultation, refer to *Advice for the Patient, Ethchlorvynol (Systemic)*.

In providing consultation, consider emphasizing the following selected information (» = major clinical significance):

### Before using this medication
» Conditions affecting use, especially:
   Sensitivity to ethchlorvynol
   Carcinogenicity/tumorigenicity—A study in mice showed ethchlorvynol, at doses up to 7 times the maximum human daily dose for 22 to 24 months, to significantly increase total lung tumors in female mice
   Pregnancy—Ethchlorvynol crosses placenta; use not recommended during first and second trimesters, because studies in animals have shown a higher percentage of stillbirths and a lower survival rate of offspring when ethchlorvynol was given in doses of 40 mg per kg of body weight (mg/kg) per day; also, use during third trimester may produce CNS depression and withdrawal symptoms in neonate
   Use in the elderly—Elderly patients may be more sensitive to effects of ethchlorvynol
   Other medications, especially alcohol or other CNS depression–producing medications or coumarin- or indandione-derivative anticoagulants
   Other medical problems, especially alcohol or drug abuse or dependence, mental depression, or porphyria

### Proper use of this medication
» Taking medication with food or milk to minimize dizziness or ataxia
» Importance of not taking more medication than the amount prescribed because of habit-forming potential
» Proper dosing
» Proper storage

### Precautions while using this medication
   Regular visits to physician to check progress during prolonged therapy
   Checking with physician before discontinuing medication after prolonged use; gradual dosage reduction may be necessary to avoid possibility of withdrawal symptoms
» Avoiding use of alcohol or other CNS depressants
» Suspected overdose: Getting emergency help at once
» Caution if dizziness, lightheadedness, or daytime drowsiness occurs

### Side/adverse effects
   Signs of potential side effects, especially allergic reaction, cholestatic jaundice, paradoxical reaction, and thrombocytopenia
   Side/adverse effects more likely to occur in elderly patients, who may be more sensitive to effects of ethchlorvynol

## General Dosing Information

A single supplemental dose of 200 mg may be taken to reinstitute sleep in patients who awaken after the original bedtime dose of 500 or 750 mg.

For patients with insomnia characterized by untimely awakening during the early morning hours, a single dose of 200 mg may be taken upon awakening.

Since prolonged use of ethchlorvynol may result in tolerance and psychological or physical dependence, the medication should not be used for periods exceeding 1 week.

If prolonged administration is necessary, ethchlorvynol should be withdrawn gradually in order to avoid the possibility of precipitating withdrawal symptoms.

**Diet/Nutrition**
Ethchlorvynol may be administered with food or milk to lessen dizziness or ataxia caused by very rapid absorption.

**For treatment of dependence**
Treatment of physical dependence consists of cautious and gradual withdrawal of ethchlorvynol. Withdrawal may be accomplished by administering a stabilizing dose of ethchlorvynol (or a barbiturate, such as phenobarbital), which is then reduced gradually over a period of days or weeks. In addition to this regimen, a phenothiazine compound may be administered to those patients who exhibit psychotic symptoms during the withdrawal period. The patient should be closely monitored, preferably hospitalized, and general supportive therapy given as needed.

## Oral Dosage Forms
### ETHCHLORVYNOL CAPSULES USP

**Usual adult dose**
For insomnia—
    Oral, 500 mg to 1 gram at bedtime.

Note: Geriatric or debilitated patients may be more sensitive to the effects of the usual adult dose.

**Usual pediatric dose**
Safety and efficacy have not been established.

**Strength(s) usually available**
U.S.—
    200 mg (Rx) [*Placidyl* (methylparaben; propylparaben)].
    500 mg (Rx) [*Placidyl* (methylparaben; propylparaben); GENERIC].
    750 mg (Rx) [*Placidyl* (methylparaben; propylparaben; tartrazine); GENERIC].
Canada—
    200 mg (Rx) [*Placidyl* (tartrazine)].
    500 mg (Rx) [*Placidyl* (tartrazine)].
    750 mg (Rx) [*Placidyl* (tartrazine)].

**Packaging and storage**
Store below 40 °C (104 °F), preferably between 15 and 30 °C (59 and 86 °F), unless otherwise specified by manufacturer. Store in a tight, light-resistant container.

**Auxiliary labeling**
• Avoid alcoholic beverages.
• May cause drowsiness.

**Note**
Controlled substance in the U.S.

Revised: 03/09/93

---

**ETHINAMATE**—Since Ethinamate is not commercially available in the U.S. or Canada, the *Ethinamate (Systemic)* monograph is not included in this published version of the USP DI database. Copies of the monograph are available on request from the USP Division of Information Development, 12601 Twinbrook Parkway, Rockville, MD 20852; telephone (301) 816-8351; telefax (301) 816-8374.

---

**ETHINYL ESTRADIOL**—See *Estrogens (Systemic)*

---

## ETHINYL ESTRADIOL–CONTAINING COMBINATIONS—
Desogestrel and Ethinyl Estradiol (Systemic)—See *Estrogens and Progestins (Systemic)*
Ethynodiol Diacetate and Ethinyl Estradiol (Systemic)—See *Estrogens and Progestins (Systemic)*
Fluoxymesterone and Ethinyl Estradiol (Systemic)—See *Androgens and Estrogens (Systemic)*
Levonorgestrel and Ethinyl Estradiol (Systemic)—See *Estrogens and Progestins (Systemic)*
Norethindrone Acetate and Ethinyl Estradiol (Systemic)—See *Estrogens and Progestins (Systemic)*
Norethindrone and Ethinyl Estradiol (Systemic)—See *Estrogens and Progestins (Systemic)*
Norgestimate and Ethinyl Estradiol (Systemic)—See *Estrogens and Progestins (Systemic)*
Norgestrel and Ethinyl Estradiol (Systemic)—See *Estrogens and Progestins (Systemic)*

---

# ETHIONAMIDE    Systemic†

VA CLASSIFICATION (Primary): AM500
Note: For a listing of dosage forms and brand names by country availability, see *Dosage Forms* section(s). For a listing of brand names for the articles in this monograph, refer to the General Index.

†Not commercially available in Canada.

## Category
Antibacterial (antimycobacterial; antileprosy agent).

## Indications
Note: Bracketed information in the *Indications* section refers to uses that are not included in U.S. product labeling.

**Accepted**
Tuberculosis (treatment)—Ethionamide is indicated in combination with other antituberculosis medications in the treatment of tuberculosis, including tuberculous meningitis, after failure with the primary medications (streptomycin, isoniazid, rifampin, and ethambutol) or when these cannot be used because of toxicity or development of resistant tubercle bacilli. Ethionamide is effective only against mycobacteria.

[Leprosy (treatment)]—Ethionamide is used in combination with other antileprosy agents in the treatment of Hansen's disease.

[Mycobacterial infections, atypical (treatment)]—Ethionamide is used in the treatment of atypical mycobacterial infections, such as *Mycobacterium avium* complex (MAC).

Not all species or strains of a particular organism may be susceptible to ethionamide.

## Pharmacology/Pharmacokinetics

**Physicochemical characteristics**
Molecular weight—166.24.

**Mechanism of action/Effect**
Ethionamide's mechanism of action is not known, but it appears to inhibit peptide synthesis. Ethionamide is bacteriostatic against *Mycobacterium tuberculosis*.

**Absorption**
Rapidly absorbed from the gastrointestinal tract following oral administration. Bioavailability approximately 100%.

**Distribution**
Widely distributed to most tissues and fluids, including liver, kidneys, and spleen. Concentrations in various organs and cerebrospinal fluid (CSF) are approximately equal to plasma concentrations. Readily crosses the placenta, also.
$Vol_D$ =Approximately 2.8 L/kg.

**Protein binding**
Low (10%).

**Biotransformation**
Probably hepatic; metabolized to sulfoxide, which is active, and to inactive metabolites.

**Half-life**
Approximately 2 to 3 hours.

**Time to peak concentration**
Approximately 1.8 hours.

**Peak serum concentration**
Approximately 2.2 mcg/mL after a single oral 500-mg dose.

## Elimination
Renal; 1% excreted unchanged; up to 5% excreted as active metabolite; the remainder excreted as inactive metabolites.

# Precautions to Consider

### Cross-sensitivity and/or related problems
Patients sensitive to isoniazid, pyrazinamide, niacin (nicotinic acid), or other chemically related medications may be sensitive to this medication also.

### Pregnancy/Reproduction
Pregnancy—Ethionamide crosses the placenta.

Ethionamide has been shown to be teratogenic in rabbits and rats given doses greater than the usual human dose.

### Breast-feeding
It is not known whether ethionamide is distributed into breast milk. However, problems in humans have not been documented.

### Pediatrics
Appropriate studies on the relationship of age to the effects of ethionamide have not been performed in the pediatric population. However, no pediatrics-specific problems have been documented to date.

### Geriatrics
No information is available on the relationship of age to the effects of ethionamide in geriatric patients.

### Dental
Ethionamide may cause a metallic taste and stomatitis (sore mouth).

### Drug interactions and/or related problems
The following drug interactions and/or related problems have been selected on the basis of their potential clinical significance (possible mechanism in parentheses where appropriate)—not necessarily inclusive (» = major clinical significance):

Note: Combinations containing any of the following medications, depending on the amount present, may also interact with this medication.

» Cycloserine
(concurrent use may result in increased incidence of central nervous system [CNS] effects, especially seizures; dosage adjustments may be necessary and patients should be monitored closely for signs of CNS toxicity)

Neurotoxic medications, other (See *Appendix II*)
(concurrent administration of ethionamide with other neurotoxic medications may increase the potential for neurotoxicity, such as optic and peripheral neuritis)

### Laboratory value alterations
The following have been selected on the basis of their potential clinical significance (possible effect in parentheses where appropriate)—not necessarily inclusive (» = major clinical significance):

With physiology/laboratory test values
Alanine aminotransferase (ALT [SGPT]) and
Aspartate aminotransferase (AST [SGOT])
(serum values may be increased)

### Medical considerations/Contraindications
The medical considerations/contraindications included here have been selected on the basis of their potential clinical significance (reasons given in parentheses where appropriate)—not necessarily inclusive (» = major clinical significance).

*Risk-benefit should be considered when the following medical problems exist:*

» Diabetes mellitus
(management of diabetes mellitus may be more difficult in patients taking ethionamide)

» Hepatic function impairment, severe
(may increase risk of hepatotoxicity)

» Hypersensitivity to ethionamide

### Patient monitoring
The following may be especially important in patient monitoring (other tests may be warranted in some patients, depending on condition; » = major clinical significance):

Hepatic function determinations
(AST [SGOT] and ALT [SGPT] concentrations may increase during therapy; however, elevated serum enzyme values may not be predictive of clinical hepatitis and may return to normal despite continued treatment; patients with impaired hepatic function may require a reduction in dose)

Ophthalmologic examinations
(if loss of vision and other symptoms of optic neuritis occur during treatment, ophthalmologic examinations should be performed immediately and periodically thereafter)

# Side/Adverse Effects

Note: Peripheral neuritis may be alleviated by administering pyridoxine.

The following side/adverse effects have been selected on the basis of their potential clinical significance (possible signs and symptoms in parentheses where appropriate)—not necessarily inclusive:

### Those indicating need for medical attention
Incidence less frequent
*Hepatitis or jaundice* (yellow eyes or skin); *peripheral neuritis* (clumsiness or unsteadiness; numbness, tingling, burning, or pain in hands and feet); *psychiatric disturbances* (mental depression, confusion, mood or other mental changes)

Incidence rare
*Goiter or hypothyroidism* (changes in menstrual periods; coldness; decreased sexual ability—males; dry, puffy skin; swelling of front part of neck; weight gain); *hypoglycemia* (difficulty in concentrating, faster heartbeat, increased hunger, nervousness, shakiness); *optic neuritis* (blurred vision or loss of vision, with or without eye pain); *skin rash*

### Those indicating need for medical attention only if they continue or are bothersome
Incidence more frequent
*Gastrointestinal disturbances* (loss of appetite, metallic taste, nausea or vomiting, sore mouth); *orthostatic hypotension* (dizziness, especially when getting up from a lying or sitting position)

Incidence less frequent or rare
*gynecomastia* (enlargement of the breasts in males)

# Patient Consultation

As an aid to patient consultation, refer to *Advice for the Patient, Ethionamide (Systemic)*.

In providing consultation, consider emphasizing the following selected information (» = major clinical significance):

### Before using this medication
» Conditions affecting use, especially:
Hypersensitivity to ethionamide
Pregnancy—Ethionamide crosses the placenta
Dental—Ethionamide may cause a metallic taste and stomatitis
Other medications, especially cycloserine
Other medical problems, especially diabetes mellitus or hepatic function impairment

### Proper use of this medication
Taking with or after meals if gastrointestinal irritation occurs
» Compliance with full course of therapy, which may take months or years
» Taking pyridoxine concurrently to prevent or minimize signs of peripheral neuritis
» Proper dosing
Missed dose: Taking as soon as possible; not taking if almost time for next dose; not doubling doses
» Proper storage

### Precautions while using this medication
Checking with physician if no improvement within 2 or 3 weeks
» Regular visits to physician to check progress, as well as ophthalmologic examinations if signs of optic neuritis occur
» Caution if blurred vision or loss of vision occurs
» Need to report promptly to physician signs of optic neuritis and prodromal signs of peripheral neuritis

### Side/adverse effects
Signs of potential side effects, especially hepatitis or jaundice, peripheral neuritis, psychiatric disturbances, goiter or hypothyroidism, hypoglycemia, optic neuritis, and skin rash

# General Dosing Information

Ethionamide may be given with or after meals if gastrointestinal irritation occurs.

Ethionamide has been given as a single daily dose after the evening meal or at bedtime. Serum concentrations are higher and effectiveness may be greater than with divided doses. However, gastrointestinal irritation may also be increased.

Ethionamide has also been given rectally as suppositories, resulting in fewer side effects. However, serum concentrations may be inadequate.

Ethionamide should generally be given in the maximum daily dose that the patient can tolerate. However, approximately one-third of the patients taking ethionamide are unable to tolerate therapeutic doses and the dose must be reduced by $^1/_3$ to $^1/_2$ or the medication must be discontinued.

Since bacterial resistance may develop rapidly when ethionamide is administered alone in the treatment of tuberculosis, it should only be administered concurrently with other antituberculars.

Therapy may have to be continued for 1 to 2 years, and may even be required for up to several years or indefinitely, although in some patients shorter treatment regimens may be effective.

### For treatment of adverse effects

Recommended treatment consists of the following:

• Administration of pyridoxine concurrently with ethionamide to help prevent or minimize the symptoms of peripheral neuritis, especially in patients with prior isoniazid-induced peripheral neuritis.

## Oral Dosage Forms

Note: Bracketed uses in the *Dosage Forms* section refer to categories of use and/or indications that are not included in U.S. product labeling.

### ETHIONAMIDE TABLETS USP

#### Usual adult and adolescent dose

Tuberculosis; or

[Mycobacterial infections, atypical]—In combination with other antituberculosis medications: Oral, 250 mg every eight to twelve hours, as tolerated.

[Leprosy]—In combination with other antileprosy agents: Oral, 250 mg every eight to twelve hours.

#### Usual adult prescribing limits

Up to a maximum of 1 gram daily.

#### Usual pediatric dose

Tuberculosis—In combination with other antituberculosis medications: Oral, 4 to 5 mg per kg of body weight every eight hours, as tolerated.

Note: Some children have received up to 20 mg per kg of body weight per day. However, the maximum daily dose should not exceed 750 mg.

#### Strength(s) usually available

U.S.—

250 mg (Rx) [*Trecator-SC*].

Canada—

Not commercially available.

### Packaging and storage

Store below 40 °C (104 °F), preferably between 15 and 30 °C (59 and 86 °F), unless otherwise specified by manufacturer. Store in a tight container.

### Auxiliary labeling

• Continue medicine for full time of treatment.

Revised: 06/22/94

---

## ETHOPROPAZINE—See *Antidyskinetics (Systemic)*

---

## ETHOSUXIMIDE—See *Anticonvulsants, Succinimide (Systemic)*

---

## ETHOTOIN—See *Anticonvulsants, Hydantoin (Systemic)*

---

## ETHYLNOREPINEPHRINE—See *Bronchodilators, Adrenergic (Systemic)*

---

## ETHYNODIOL DIACETATE–CONTAINING COMBINATIONS—

Ethynodiol Diacetate and Ethinyl Estradiol (Systemic)—See *Estrogens and Progestins (Systemic)*

---

## ETIDOCAINE—See *Anesthetics (Parenteral-Local)*

---

## ETIDOCAINE-CONTAINING COMBINATIONS—

Etidocaine and Epinephrine (Parenteral-Local)—See *Anesthetics (Parenteral-Local)*

---

# ETIDRONATE  Systemic

VA CLASSIFICATION (Primary): HS900

Another commonly used name is EHDP.

Note: For a listing of dosage forms and brand names by country availability, see *Dosage Forms* section(s). For a listing of brand names for the articles in this monograph, refer to the General Index.

## Category

Bone resorption inhibitor; antihypercalcemic.

## Indications

### Accepted

Paget's disease of bone (treatment)—Oral etidronate is indicated for the treatment of symptomatic Paget's disease (osteitis deformans), characterized by abnormal and accelerated bone turnover in one or more bones. Signs and symptoms may include bone pain, deformity, and/or fractures; increased concentrations of serum alkaline phosphatase and/or urinary hydroxyproline; neurologic disorders associated with skull lesions and vertebral deformities; and elevated cardiac output and other vascular disorders associated with increased vascularity of bones.

Although studies have not been done on etidronate's effects in *asymptomatic* Paget's disease, treatment may be considered for such patients if extensive involvement of the skull or vertebral column might lead to neurologic damage; if extensive involvement of weight-bearing bones threatens their integrity; or if juxta-articular involvement threatens the integrity of adjacent joints.

Ossification, heterotopic (prophylaxis and treatment)—Oral etidronate is indicated for the prevention and treatment of heterotopic ossification (myositis ossificans—circumscripta, progressiva, or traumatica; ectopic calcification; periarticular ossification; or paraosteoarthropathy) following total hip replacement or caused by spinal cord injury. Het-

erotopic ossification is characterized by metaplastic osteogenesis, and may be accompanied by localized inflammation and pain, and elevated skin temperature or redness. Also, loss of joint function or reduction in range of motion may occur when tissues near joints are involved.

Hypercalcemia, associated with neoplasms (treatment adjunct)—Parenteral etidronate is indicated as adjunctive therapy for the treatment of hypercalcemia of malignancy that is inadequately managed by dietary changes and/or oral hydration alone. It is used in conjunction with adequate saline hydration and with "high ceiling" or loop diuretics, such as bumetanide, ethacrynic acid, and furosemide. Limited clinical study results show that oral etidronate may be used in some patients after the last dose of etidronate infusion to maintain clinically acceptable serum calcium concentrations and to prolong normocalcemia.

### Unaccepted

Hypercalcemia caused by hyperparathyroidism, where increased tubular reabsorption of calcium may be a factor in the hypercalcemia, is refractory to parenteral etidronate.

Note: Oral etidronate is presently being used experimentally in the U.S. to treat osteoporosis in adults. A small increase in bone mineral density has been noted. Some studies with continuous dosing of etidronate have found abnormal mineralization of osteoid and microfractures that might potentially result in increased susceptibility to fractures, especially nonvertebral fractures. Further studies are needed to determine the safety profile and dosing information.

## Pharmacology/Pharmacokinetics

### Physicochemical characteristics

Molecular weight—249.99.

### Mechanism of action/Effect

Although the exact mechanism is not completely understood, etidronate chemisorbs to calcium phosphate surfaces of calcium hydroxyapatite crystals and their amorphous precursors, and, *in vitro*, blocks the aggregation, growth, and mineralization of the crystals. A similar process is believed to be responsible *in vivo* for retarding the mineralization and growth of heterotopic ossification. This process may also be responsible for retarding bone resorption, and, secondarily, for retarding the accelerated rate of bone turnover in Paget's disease.

Paget's disease—Etidronate induces a reduction of bone resorption, which is accompanied by a reduction in the number of osteoclasts. Secondarily, coupled bone formation is reduced, which is associated with a reduction in the number of osteoblasts. New bone formed following the reduction in bone turnover is histologically more normal. Lamellar bone is formed, and the marrow becomes less vascular and fibrotic. Etidronate reduces serum alkaline phosphatase and urinary hydroxyproline concentrations, reduces radionuclide uptake at pagetic lesions, decreases elevated cardiac output by reducing bone vascularity, and reduces elevated skin temperature over pagetic lesions. The incidence of pagetic fractures may be reduced when etidronate is administered intermittently over a period of years.

Heterotopic ossification—Etidronate slows the progression of immature bone lesions, thus reducing the severity of the disease.

Hypercalcemia of malignancy—Bone resorption is increased in the presence of neoplastic tissue. Etidronate inhibits abnormal bone resorption and reduces the flow of calcium from the resorbing bone into the blood, effectively decreasing total and ionized serum calcium. When kidney function is adequate for the fluid load, hydration with saline increases urine output and the use of diuretics increases the rate of calcium excretion.

### Duration of therapeutic effect

Paget's disease—Possibly up to a year or more after discontinuation of therapy.

Heterotopic ossification—Several months after discontinuation of therapy.

Hypercalcemia—Clinical studies indicate a median duration of normocalcemia of 11 days.

### Absorption

Lower doses (5 mg per kg of body weight (mg/kg) a day)—1% (average).

Higher doses (10 to 20 mg per kg a day)—2.5 to 6% (average).

### Distribution

Approximately half of absorbed dose is chemically adsorbed to bone, presumably upon hydroxyapatite crystals, in areas of elevated osteogenesis.

### Biotransformation

None.

### Half-life

Elimination—Approximately 50% of the absorbed/infused dose is eliminated from the body within 24 hours. The remainder is presumably chemisorbed to bone and slowly eliminated.

Plasma—5 to 7 hours.

### Onset of action

Paget's disease—May be observed after 1 month of treatment; initially observed as a reduction in urinary hydroxyproline.

Hypercalcemia—Reductions in urinary calcium excretion, which accompany reductions in bone resorption, may become apparent after 24 hours.

### Time to peak effect

Hypercalcemia—Decreases in serum calcium are maximal on the day following the third infusion, in most patients.

### Elimination

Absorbed dose—50% excreted intact in the urine via the kidneys.

Unabsorbed dose—Intact in the feces.

## Precautions to Consider

### Carcinogenicity

Long-term studies in rats have shown no evidence of carcinogenicity.

### Pregnancy/Reproduction

Pregnancy—

*For oral etidronate—*

Adequate and well-controlled studies in humans have not been done.

Studies in rats and rabbits administered oral doses up to 5 times the maximum human dose have shown no evidence of impaired fertility or harm to the fetus. However, studies in rats administered doses 22 times the maximum human dose of etidronate have shown a decrease in live fetuses.

FDA Pregnancy Category B.

*For parenteral etidronate—*

Reproductive studies have not been done in either animals or humans. Rats administered large parenteral doses showed skeletal

malformations, which were attributed to the pharmacologic action of the drug

FDA Pregnancy Category C.

### Breast-feeding

It is not known if etidronate is distributed into breast milk. However, problems in humans have not been documented.

### Pediatrics

Appropriate studies have not been performed in the pediatric population. However, in children treated for heterotopic ossification or soft tissue calcifications at doses of 10 mg or more per kg of body weight a day for prolonged periods (approaching or exceeding a year), signs of a rachitic syndrome were infrequently reported. Epiphyseal radiologic changes associated with retarded mineralization of new osteoid and cartilage have been reversible upon discontinuation of etidronate.

### Geriatrics

Appropriate studies have not been performed in the geriatric population. However, elderly patients may be more prone to overhydration when treated with parenteral etidronate in conjunction with hydration therapy. Careful monitoring of fluid and electrolyte status is recommended.

### Drug interactions and/or related problems

The following drug interactions and/or related problems have been selected on the basis of their potential clinical significance (possible mechanism in parentheses where appropriate)—not necessarily inclusive (» = major clinical significance):

Note: Combinations containing any of the following medications, depending on the amount present, may also interact with this medication.

»  Antacids containing calcium, magnesium, or aluminum or
»  Foods containing large amounts of calcium, such as milk or other dairy products or
»  Mineral supplements or other medications containing calcium, iron, magnesium, or aluminum
     (concurrent use may prevent absorption of oral etidronate; patients should be advised to avoid using within 2 hours of etidronate)

### Laboratory value alterations

The following have been selected on the basis of their potential clinical significance (possible effect in parentheses where appropriate)—not necessarily inclusive (» = major clinical significance):

With diagnostic test results
Technetium Tc 99m medronate or
Technetium Tc 99m oxidronate or
Technetium Tc 99m pyrophosphate
     (etidronate may theoretically interfere with bone uptake of these diagnostic agents; clinical significance is unknown)

### Medical considerations/Contraindications

The medical considerations/contraindications included here have been selected on the basis of their potential clinical significance (reasons given in parentheses where appropriate)—not necessarily inclusive (» = major clinical significance).

*Except under special circumstances, this medication should not be used when the following medical problem exists:*

*For hypercalcemia*

»  Renal function impairment when serum creatinine is 5 mg per dL or greater
     (kidney function may be inadequate for the increased fluid load and the excretion of etidronate)

*Risk-benefit should be considered when the following medical problems exist:*

»  Bone fractures, especially of long bones
     (mineralization of osteoid laid down during the bone accretion process may be retarded because of the inhibition of hydroxyapatite crystal growth; delay or interruption of etidronate treatment for Paget's disease may be necessary until callus formation and calcification are evident)

»  Cardiac failure
     (overhydration should be avoided with use of parenteral etidronate in patients with cardiac failure)

»  Enterocolitis
     (risk of diarrhea is increased, particularly at higher doses)

Hyperphosphatemia
     (high doses of oral etidronate may increase the tubular reabsorption of phosphate; occurs less frequently with parenteral therapy)

Hypocalcemia or
Hypovitaminosis D
     (patients with restricted intake of calcium or vitamin D may be more sensitive to medications that affect calcium homeostasis)

» Renal function impairment when serum creatinine is 2.5 to 4.9 mg per dL

(excretion of etidronate may be reduced; reduction of dose may be necessary; in addition, renal function impairment may be exacerbated by etidronate infusion)

Sensitivity to etidronate

### Patient monitoring

The following may be especially important in patient monitoring (other tests may be warranted in some patients, depending on condition; » = major clinical significance):

*For Paget's disease and hypercalcemia*

Renal function determinations, especially glomerular filtration rate (GFR) and/or blood urea nitrogen (BUN)

(recommended at periodic intervals during therapy; reduction in dosage in patients with impairment of renal function [GFR] should be considered and such patients closely monitored; occasional mild to moderate abnormalities in renal function [increases of serum creatinine >0.5 mg per dL and elevated BUN] may occur when etidronate infusion is given to patients with hypercalcemia; these increases are reversible or may remain stable without worsening after completion of the course of infusion)

*For Paget's disease only*

Pain relief, assessment of

(pain may be an indication of Paget's disease activity; however, in elderly patients, biochemical indices, periodically monitored during therapy, are more valuable)

» Serum alkaline phosphatase concentrations and

» Urine hydroxyproline concentrations

(determinations recommended every 3 to 6 months during therapy; decreases in urine hydroxyproline result from decreased collagen resorption following reduced osteoclastic activity and reduced bone resorption; decreases in alkaline phosphatase result from a secondary reduction in osteoblastic activity; reduction in both parameters are an indication of improvement; sustained decreases during drug-free period are evidence of remission; retreatment is started when biochemical indices re-elevate to 75% of pretreatment values or symptoms recur)

Serum phosphate concentrations

(determinations recommended prior to and 4 weeks after initiation of therapy; at higher doses [10 mg or more per kg of body weight per day], a rise of greater than 0.5 mg per deciliter over pretreatment is normal and without clinical consequence and is probably related to an alteration in renal tubular reabsorption of phosphate [normal values return within 2 to 4 weeks after discontinuation of etidronate]; a rise of 0.5 mg per deciliter or greater at lower doses [5 mg or less per kg of body weight per day] is uncommon and may indicate above average bioavailability; if such a rise is seen at the lower dose, the serum alkaline phosphatase and urinary hydroxyproline values should be examined for evidence that the drug is reducing bone turnover as expected; if there are no significant declines in these values, etidronate dosage should be reduced or the medication discontinued to avoid possible reduced mineralization of osteoid with no accompanying clinical benefit)

*For hypercalcemia only*

Serum albumin concentrations and

Serum calcium concentrations

(determinations recommended periodically during therapy; since serum proteins, especially albumin, may influence the ratio of free and bound calcium, corrected serum calcium values should be calculated by using an established algorithm; albumin-corrected serum calcium determinations may be useful when the signs and symptoms of hypercalcemia are inconsistent with unadjusted calcium values)

## Side/Adverse Effects

The following side/adverse effects have been selected on the basis of their potential clinical significance (possible signs and symptoms in parentheses where appropriate)—not necessarily inclusive:

### Those indicating need for medical attention

Incidence more frequent

*Bone pain or tenderness, increased, continuing, or recurrent*—in patients with Paget's disease

Note: Usually occurs over the site of pagetic lesions, but sometimes occurs at previously asymptomatic sites, beginning within 4 to 6 weeks of initiation of therapy; more common with doses of 5 mg per kg of body weight (mg/kg) or greater for more than six months. Pain may persist in some patients, even with con-

tinued therapy; usually subsides days to months after etidronate is discontinued.

Incidence less frequent

*Osteomalacia* (bone fractures, especially of the femur)

Note: Usually occur in patients taking doses higher than 20 mg/kg or continuous administration of etidronate for longer than 6 months. Microfractures may be due to decreased strength of active pagetic bone or may be caused by a mineralization defect accompanying etidronate therapy.

Incidence rare

*Allergic reaction, specifically; angioedema* (swelling of the extremities, face, lips, tongue, glottis, and/or larynx); *skin rash or itching; urticaria* (hives)

### Those indicating need for medical attention only if they continue or are bothersome

Incidence more frequent—at higher doses

*Diarrhea; nausea*

Incidence less frequent—with parenteral dosage form

*Loss of taste or metallic or altered taste*

## Patient Consultation

As an aid to patient consultation, refer to *Advice for the Patient, Etidronate* (Systemic).

In providing consultation, consider emphasizing the following selected information (» = major clinical significance):

### Before using this medication

» Conditions affecting use, especially:

Sensitivity to etidronate

Use in children—Children given adult dosages for nearly a year or more were reported to have signs of a rachitic syndrome that were reversible upon discontinuation of etidronate

Use in the elderly—Elderly patients may be more prone to overhydration when treated with parenteral etidronate in conjunction with hydration therapy

Other medications, especially antacids or mineral supplements

Other medical problems, especially renal function impairment, bone fractures, cardiac failure, or enterocolitis

### Proper use of this medication

» Taking with water on an empty stomach, at least 2 hours before or after food (upon arising, midmorning, or at bedtime)

» Compliance with therapy; not taking more or less medication or for longer period of time than prescribed

Checking with physician before discontinuing medication; may require 1 to 3 months for symptomatic improvement

» Maintaining a well-balanced diet with adequate intake of calcium and vitamin D; not taking within 2 hours of milk or milk products, antacids, mineral supplements, or other medicines high in calcium, magnesium, iron, or aluminum

» Proper dosing

Missed dose: Taking as soon as possible; not taking if almost time for next dose; not doubling doses

» Proper storage

### Precautions while using this medication

» Regular visits to physician to check progress even if between treatments

Checking with physician if nausea or diarrhea occurs and continues; dosage adjustment may be necessary

» Checking with physician if bone pain appears or worsens during treatment

### Side/adverse effects

Signs of potential side effects, especially increased or continuing bone pain, fractures, or allergic reaction

## General Dosing Information

See also *Patient monitoring*.

### For Paget's disease

Symptomatic improvement as evidence of therapeutic response may not be seen for 1 to 3 months; dosage should not be prematurely increased or discontinued during that time.

Although etidronate is usually taken as a single dose, divided doses may be preferred if diarrhea or nausea occurs.

In patients with Paget's disease, retreatment should be initiated only after a medication-free period of at least 3 months and only if there is evidence of active disease or if the biochemical indices have become re-elevated to 75% of pretreatment values or symptoms recur.

Analgesics may be required at any time if patient experiences bone pain.

In many patients with Paget's disease, the disease process may be suppressed for a year or more after discontinuing therapy.

Etidronate therapy in patients with total hip replacement does not promote loosening of the prosthesis or impede trochanteric reattachment.

The dosage of etidronate should be reduced when there is a decrease in the glomerular filtration rate

**For hypercalcemia**

Retreatment with parenteral etidronate for more than 3 days and the safety and effectiveness of more than 2 courses of therapy have not been studied.

The daily dose must be diluted in at least 250 mL of normal saline solution or 5% dextrose injection. More of the diluent may be used, if convenient. The diluted dose should be administered over a period of at least 2 hours.

Limited clinical studies suggest that oral administration of etidronate in some patients may be started on the day following the last dose of parenteral therapy. If serum calcium levels remain normal, treatment may be extended for up to 90 days. Normocalcemia may be defined as serum calcium concentrations usually within 8.5 to 10.5 mg per dL.

**Diet/Nutrition**

Etidronate should be taken with water on an empty stomach, at least 2 hours before or after food (e.g., upon arising, midmorning, or at bedtime) for maximum absorption.

A well-balanced diet with adequate intake of calcium and vitamin D should be maintained.

Foods containing large amounts of calcium, such as milk or other dairy products, mineral supplements, or other medicines high in calcium, magnesium, iron, or aluminum, may prevent absorption of etidronate and should not be taken within 2 hours of etidronate.

## Oral Dosage Forms

### ETIDRONATE DISODIUM TABLETS USP

**Usual adult dose**

Paget's disease of bone—

Oral, initially 5 mg per kg of body weight a day, usually as a single dose, for a period of time not to exceed six months; or 6 to 10 mg per kg of body weight a day, for a period of time not to exceed six months; or 11 to 20 mg per kg of body weight a day, for no longer than three months.

Note: Doses above 5 mg per kg of body weight are recommended only when lower doses are ineffective or there is an overriding requirement for suppression of increased bone turnover or when a more prompt reduction of elevated cardiac output is required.

The retreatment dose after a drug-free period remains the same as the initial dose for most patients.

Heterotopic ossification—

Patients with total hip replacement: Oral, 20 mg per kg of body weight a day for one month prior to and for three months after surgery.

Patients with spinal cord injury: Oral, initially 20 mg per kg of body weight a day for two weeks, beginning as soon as medically feasible after injury and preferably before evidence of heterotopic ossification, the dosage then being decreased to 10 mg per kg of body weight a day for an additional ten weeks.

Hypercalcemia—

Maintenance: Oral, 20 mg per kg of body weight a day for thirty days, up to a maximum of ninety days.

**Usual adult prescribing limits**

20 mg per kg of body weight a day.

**Usual pediatric dose**

Dosage has not been established.

**Strength(s) usually available**

U.S.—

200 mg (Rx) [*Didronel*].

400 mg (Rx) [*Didronel* (scored)].

Canada—

200 mg (Rx) [*Didronel*].

**Packaging and storage**

Store below 40 °C (104 °F), preferably between 15 and 30 °C (59 and 86 °F), unless otherwise specified by manufacturer. Store in a tight container.

**Auxiliary labeling**

• Take on an empty stomach.

• Do not take with milk or antacids.

## Parenteral Dosage Forms

### ETIDRONATE DISODIUM INJECTION

Note: Etidronate disodium injection is not commercially available in Canada.

**Usual adult dose**

Hypercalcemia—

Intravenous infusion, initially 7.5 mg per kg of body weight per day, administered over a period of at least two hours, for three consecutive days.

Note: Some patients may be treated for up to seven days, but the risk of hypocalcemia is increased after three days.

The retreatment dose after a seven-day drug-free interval remains the same as the initial dose for most patients.

**Usual pediatric dose**

Dosage has not been established.

**Strength(s) usually available**

U.S.—

50 mg per mL (Rx) [*Didronel*].

**Packaging and storage**

Store below 40 °C (104 °F), preferably between 15 and 30 °C (59 and 86 °F), unless otherwise specified by manufacturer. Protect from freezing.

**Preparation of dosage form**

Dilute the daily dose in at least 250 mL of 0.9% sodium chloride injection or 5% dextrose injection.

**Stability**

Diluted solution may be stored at controlled room temperature for at least 48 hours without loss of drug.

Revised: 8/19/92
Interim revision: 08/10/94

---

**ETODOLAC**—See *Anti-inflammatory Drugs, Nonsteroidal (Systemic)*

---

# ETOMIDATE   Systemic†

VA CLASSIFICATION (Primary/Secondary): CN203/CN205

Note: For a listing of dosage forms and brand names by country availability, see *Dosage Forms* section(s). For a listing of brand names for the articles in this monograph, refer to the General Index.

†Not commercially available in Canada.

## Category

Anesthetic, general; anesthesia adjunct.

## Indications

Note: Bracketed information in the *Indications* section refers to uses that are not included in U.S. product labeling.

**Accepted**

Anesthesia, general or

Anesthesia, general, adjunct—Etomidate is indicated for the induction of general anesthesia. It is also indicated to supplement low-potency anesthetics, such as nitrous oxide and oxygen, during maintenance of anesthesia for short operative procedures such as dilation and curettage or cervical conization.

Etomidate may be especially useful in patients with compromised cardiopulmonary function because of its minimal cardiovascular and respiratory depressant effects and lack of histamine release at usual doses.

Etomidate is a sedative-hypnotic, which has no analgesic action.

# Pharmacology/Pharmacokinetics

### Physicochemical characteristics
Molecular weight—244.29.

### Mechanism of action/Effect
Etomidate is a short-acting hypnotic, which appears to have gamma-aminobutyric acid (GABA)–like effects. Unlike the barbiturates, etomidate reduces subcortical inhibition at the onset of hypnosis while inducing neocortical sleep. Studies in animals suggest that a part of the action of etomidate consists of a depression of the activity and reactivity of the brain stem reticular formation.

### Other actions/effects
Etomidate does not cause significant cardiovascular or respiratory depression, but may cause a brief period of apnea. Also, it does not appear to elevate plasma histamine or cause histamine release when administered in recommended dosage. The decrease in cerebral blood flow produced by etomidate is approximately the same as that produced by thiopental and methohexital; this reduction appears to be uniform in the absence of intracranial tumors. Etomidate slightly lowers intracranial pressure and preliminary data suggest that it usually causes a moderate decrease in intraocular pressure. Also, etomidate (at induction doses of 0.3 mg per kg of body weight [mg/kg]) has been reported to reduce plasma cortisol concentrations; this effect persists for 6 to 8 hours and appears to be unresponsive to adrenocorticotropic hormone (ACTH).

### Protein binding
High (76%), primarily to serum albumin.

### Biotransformation
Hepatic; rapidly metabolized by ester hydrolysis to inactive metabolites.

### Half-life
About 75 minutes.

### Onset of action
Rapid, usually within 1 minute.

### Plasma concentration
Minimal hypnotic plasma concentrations of unchanged drug are equal to or higher than 0.23 mcg per mL; they decrease rapidly for up to 30 minutes following injection and more slowly thereafter.

### Duration of action
Dose dependent, but usually 3 to 5 minutes with an average dose of 0.3 mg/kg; may be prolonged by a sedative premedication or by repeated injections of etomidate.

### Time to recovery
As rapid as, or slightly faster than, immediate recovery after similar use of thiopental. The immediate recovery period will usually be shortened in adults by intravenous administration of approximately 0.1 mg of fentanyl 1 or 2 minutes before induction of anesthesia, possibly because less etomidate is generally required.

### Elimination
Renal; approximately 75% of a dose excreted in the urine the first day after injection. The major inactive acid metabolite accounts for approximately 80% of the urinary excretion.

## Precautions to Consider

### Carcinogenicity/Mutagenicity
Studies have not been done.

### Pregnancy/Reproduction
Fertility—Reproduction studies showed no impairment of fertility in male and female rats when etomidate was administered prior to pregnancy at 0.31, 1.25, and 5 mg per kg of body weight (mg/kg) (approximately 1, 4, and 16 times the human dose, respectively).

Pregnancy—Studies in humans have not been done. However, studies in animals have shown that etomidate causes an embryocidal effect in rats when given in doses 1 and 4 times the human dose; decreases pup survival in rats at doses of 0.3 and 5 mg per kg (approximately 1 and 16 times the human dose) and in rabbits at doses of 1.5 and 4.5 mg per kg (approximately 5 and 15 times the human dose); slightly increases the incidence of stillborn fetuses in rats at doses of 0.3 and 1.25 mg per kg (approximately 1 and 4 times the human dose); and causes maternal toxicity with deaths in 6 out of 20 rats at a dose of 5 mg per kg (approximately 16 times the human dose) and in 6 out of 20 rabbits at a dose of 4.5 mg per kg (approximately 15 times the human dose). However, studies in animals have not shown that etomidate causes teratogenic effects.

FDA Pregnancy Category C.

Labor and delivery—Use of etomidate is not recommended since data are insufficient to support its use in obstetrics, including cesarean section deliveries.

### Breast-feeding
It is not known whether etomidate is distributed into breast milk. However, problems in humans have not been documented.

### Pediatrics
Appropriate studies with etomidate have not been performed in children up to 10 years of age. Safety and efficacy have not been established.

### Geriatrics
Elderly patients are more sensitive to the effects of etomidate than are younger patients. In addition, geriatric patients are more likely to have age-related hepatic function impairment, which may require reduction of dosage in patients receiving etomidate.

### Drug interactions and/or related problems
The following drug interactions and/or related problems have been selected on the basis of their potential clinical significance (possible mechanism in parentheses where appropriate)—not necessarily inclusive (» = major clinical significance):

Note: Combinations containing any of the following medications, depending on the amount present, may also interact with this medication.

» Alcohol or
» Central nervous system (CNS) depression–producing medications, other (See *Appendix II*)
   (concurrent use may increase the CNS depressant effects of either these medications or etomidate; dosage adjustment of etomidate may be necessary)

Hypotension-producing medications, other (See *Appendix II*)
   (concurrent use may potentiate the hypotensive effect of etomidate; dosage adjustments may be necessary)

   (caution is advised during titration of calcium channel blocker dosage for those patients taking medication, such as etomidate, known to promote hypotension, since the combination may result in excessive hypotension)

   (concurrent use of diazoxide with etomidate may result in an additive hypotensive effect, which may be severe; dosage adjustments may be necessary, and patient should be continuously observed for excessive fall in blood pressure for several hours after concurrent use)

   (concurrent use of mecamylamine or trimethaphan with etomidate may potentiate the hypotensive response, with increased risk of severe hypotension, shock, and cardiovascular collapse during surgery)

Ketamine
   (concurrent use of ketamine, especially in high doses or when rapidly administered, with etomidate may increase the risk of hypotension and/or respiratory depression)

### Medical considerations/Contraindications
The medical considerations/contraindications included here have been selected on the basis of their potential clinical significance (reasons given in parentheses where appropriate)—not necessarily inclusive (» = major clinical significance).

*Risk-benefit should be considered when the following medical problems exist:*

Immunosuppression or
Sepsis or
Transplantation
   (potential effects on adrenal function)

Sensitivity to etomidate

## Side/Adverse Effects

Note: Etomidate can block the adrenal gland's production of cortisol and other steroid hormones, possibly resulting in temporary adrenal gland failure. This may cause abnormal salt and water balance, lowered blood pressure, and, ultimately, shock. Postoperative or critically ill patients may require adrenocorticoid supplementation.
Etomidate may cause brief periods of apnea.

The following side/adverse effects have been selected on the basis of their potential clinical significance (possible signs and symptoms in parentheses where appropriate)—not necessarily inclusive:

**Those indicating need for medical attention**
Incidence more frequent
   *Nausea and/or vomiting*
     Note: Incidence of postoperative *nausea* and *vomiting* more frequent than with thiopental when etomidate is used for both induction and maintenance of anesthesia in short procedures or when analgesia is insufficient.

Incidence less frequent or rare
   *Fast or slow breathing; increase or decrease in blood pressure; irregular or fast or slow heartbeat*

**Those indicating need for medical attention only if they continue or are bothersome**
Incidence more frequent—less frequent when fentanyl is given immediately before induction
   *Involuntary muscle movements, temporary*—observed incidence 32%; reported incidence 22.7 to 63%; *pain, temporary, at injection site*—observed incidence 20%; reported incidence 1.2 to 42%
     Note: May last for less than 1 minute; self-limiting without residual effects; appear to be more frequent with occurrence of venous pain on injection.
     Bilateral movements are possibly a manifestation of disinhibition of cortical activity; unilateral movements sometimes resemble localized response to stimuli such as venous pain on injection.
     *Pain at injection site* occurs immediately and appears to be less frequent when larger, more proximal arm veins are used.

Incidence less frequent or rare
   *Hiccups*

## Overdose

For more information on the management of overdose or unintentional ingestion, **contact a Poison Control Center** (see *Poison Control Center Listing*).

**Treatment of overdose**
Recommended treatment for suspected or apparent overdosage of etomidate includes the following:

Discontinuation of medication.

Supportive care—Supportive measures such as establishing and maintaining a patent airway (intubating, if necessary) and administering oxygen with assisted ventilation, if necessary. Patients in whom intentional overdose is known or suspected should be referred for psychiatric consultation.

## Patient Consultation

As an aid to patient consultation, refer to *Advice for the Patient, Anesthetics, General (Systemic)*.

In providing consultation, consider emphasizing the following selected information (» = major clinical significance):

**Before using this medicine**
» Conditions affecting use, especially:
   Sensitivity to etomidate
   Pregnancy—Studies in animals have shown etomidate to cause embryocidal effects in rats, decrease pup survival in rats, slightly increase incidence of stillborn fetuses in rats, and cause maternal toxicity in rats and rabbits
   Labor and delivery—Use of etomidate is not recommended since data are insufficient to support its use in obstetrics
   Other medications, especially alcohol or other CNS depression–producing medications

**Proper use of this medication**
   Proper dosing

**Precautions after receiving this medication**
» Possibility of psychomotor impairment following use of anesthetics; using caution in driving or performing other tasks requiring alertness and coordination for about 24 hours following anesthesia

» Avoiding use of alcohol or other CNS depressants within 24 hours following anesthesia except as directed by physician or dentist

**Side/adverse effects**
   Signs of potential side effects, especially fast or slow breathing; increase or decrease in blood pressure; irregular, fast, or slow heartbeat; and nausea and/or vomiting

## General Dosing Information

Etomidate injection is for intravenous administration only. It is not intended for administration by prolonged infusion because of potential prolonged suppression of endogenous cortisol and aldosterone production.

Although clinical experience and animal studies have shown that inadvertent intra-arterial injection of etomidate usually will not cause necrosis of tissue, intra-arterial injection of etomidate is not recommended.

**Intravenous etomidate should be administered only by individuals trained in the administration of general anesthetics and in the management of complications encountered during general anesthesia.**

Dosage of etomidate must be individualized for each patient.

Etomidate injection is compatible with commonly administered preanesthetics, which may be used as indicated.

Immediately before anesthesia induction with etomidate, narcotic analgesics (e.g., fentanyl) may be administered to provide analgesia and to minimize pain on injection and involuntary muscle movements. Diazepam also may be used to reduce the incidence and magnitude of involuntary muscle movements.

Concurrent use of etomidate with neuromuscular blocking agents does not significantly alter the usual dosage requirements of these agents when used for endotracheal intubation or other procedures shortly after induction of anesthesia.

## Parenteral Dosage Forms

### ETOMIDATE INJECTION

Note: Etomidate injection is not commercially available in Canada.

**Usual adult and adolescent dose**
Anesthesia, general (induction of anesthesia)—
   Dosage must be individualized by physician; however, as a general guideline: Intravenous, 300 mcg (0.3 mg) (range, 200 to 600 mcg [0.2 to 0.6 mg]) per kg of body weight, administered over a period of thirty to sixty seconds.
   Note: Smaller increments of etomidate may be administered during short operative procedures to supplement low-potency anesthetics, such as nitrous oxide and oxygen. Although the dosage is usually much smaller than the initial induction dose, it must be individualized.

**Usual pediatric dose**
Anesthesia, general (induction of anesthesia)—
   Children up to 10 years of age: Safety and efficacy have not been established.
   Children 10 years of age and over—See *Usual adult and adolescent dose.*

**Usual geriatric dose**
See *Usual adult and adolescent dose.*

**Strength(s) usually available**
U.S.—
   2 mg per mL (Rx) [*Amidate* (propylene glycol 35% v/v)].

**Packaging and storage**
Store below 40 °C (104 °F), preferably between 15 and 30 °C (59 and 86 °F), unless otherwise specified by manufacturer. Protect from freezing.

**Stability**
Any unused portion should be discarded.

---

Revised: 06/26/90
Interim revision: 08/10/94

# ETOPOSIDE    Systemic

**VA CLASSIFICATION (Primary):** AN900

Another commonly used name is VP-16.

Note: For a listing of dosage forms and brand names by country availability, see *Dosage Forms* section(s). For a listing of brand names for the articles in this monograph, refer to the General Index.

## Category

Antineoplastic.

## Indications

Note: Bracketed information in the *Indications* section refers to uses that are not included in U.S. product labeling.

**Accepted**

Carcinoma, testicular (treatment)—Etoposide injection is indicated, in combination with other antineoplastics, for treatment of refractory testicular tumors in patients who have already received appropriate surgical, chemotherapeutic, and radiation therapy.

Carcinoma, lung (treatment)—Etoposide is indicated in combination with other agents for treatment of small cell lung carcinoma.

[Carcinoma bladder (treatment)][1]—Etoposide is used for treatment of bladder carcinoma.

[Lymphomas, Hodgkin's (treatment)]

[Lymphomas, non-Hodgkin's (treatment)] or

[Leukemia, acute myelocytic (treatment)][1]—Etoposide is also used, alone and in combination with other agents, for treatment of Hodgkin's and non-Hodgkin's lymphomas and acute nonlymphocytic (myelocytic) leukemia.

[Ewing's sarcoma (treatment)][1] or

[Kaposi's sarcoma, AIDS-associated (treatment)][1]—Etoposide is used for treatment of Ewing's sarcoma and AIDS-associated Kaposi's sarcoma.

---

[1]Not included in Canadian product labeling.

## Pharmacology/Pharmacokinetics

**Physicochemical characteristics**

Molecular weight—588.56.

Other characteristics—Lipophilic.

**Mechanism of action/Effect**

The exact mechanism of etoposide's antineoplastic effect is unknown. Etoposide is a topoisomerase II inhibitor. It seems to act at the premitotic stage of cell division to inhibit DNA synthesis; it is cell cycle–dependent and phase–specific, with maximum effect on the S and $G_2$ phases of cell division.

**Absorption**

Variable oral bioavailability; mean 50% (range, 25 to 75%).

**Distribution**

Low and variable into cerebrospinal fluid (CSF). Concentrations are higher in normal lung than in lung metastases, and are similar in primary tumors and normal tissues of the myometrium.

**Protein binding**

Very high (97%) *in vitro*. Etoposide binding ratio correlates directly with serum albumin in normal individuals and cancer patients. The unbound fraction has been found to correlate significantly with bilirubin in a group of cancer patients. Phenylbutazone, sodium salicylate, and aspirin displaced protein-bound etoposide *in vitro*.

**Biotransformation**

Hepatic.

**Half-life**

Terminal (biphasic)—7 hours (range, 3 to 12 hours).

**Elimination**

Renal—44 to 60% (67% of that unchanged).

Fecal—Up to 16% (as unchanged drug and metabolites).

Biliary—6% or less.

## Precautions to Consider

**Carcinogenicity**

Secondary malignancies are potential delayed effects of many antineoplastic agents, although it is not clear whether the effect is related to their mutagenic or immunosuppressive action. The effect of dose and duration of therapy is also unknown, although risk seems to increase with long-term use. Although information is limited, available data

seem to indicate that the carcinogenic risk is greatest with the alkylating agents.

Acute leukemia, with or without a preleukemic phase, has been reported rarely in patients treated with etoposide in association with other antineoplastic agents.

**Mutagenicity**

Etoposide is mutagenic and genotoxic in mammalian cells. Etoposide caused aberrations in chromosome number and structure in embryonic murine cells and human hematopoietic cells, gene mutations in Chinese hamster ovary cells, and DNA damage by strand breakage and DNA-protein cross-links in mouse leukemia cells; it also caused a dose-related increase in sister chromatid exchanges in Chinese hamster ovary cells.

**Pregnancy/Reproduction**

Fertility—Gonadal suppression, resulting in amenorrhea or azoospermia, may occur in patients receiving antineoplastic therapy, especially with the alkylating agents. In general, these effects appear to be related to dose and length of therapy and may be irreversible. Prediction of the degree of testicular or ovarian function impairment is complicated by the common use of combinations of several antineoplastics, which makes it difficult to assess the effects of individual agents.

Pregnancy—Adequate and well-controlled studies in humans have not been done.

First trimester: It is usually recommended that use of antineoplastics, especially combination chemotherapy, be avoided whenever possible, especially during the first trimester. Although information is limited because of the relatively few instances of antineoplastic administration during pregnancy, the mutagenic, teratogenic, and carcinogenic potential of these medications must be considered.

Other hazards to the fetus include adverse reactions seen in adults.

In general, use of a contraceptive is recommended during cytotoxic drug therapy.

Etoposide has been shown to be teratogenic and embryotoxic in mice and rats at doses of 1 to 3% of the recommended clinical dose based on body surface. Dose-related maternal toxicity, embryotoxicity (prenatal mortality, fetal resorptions, decreased fetal weights), and teratogenicity (major skeletal abnormalities, exencephaly, encephalocele, and anophthalmia) have been reported with intravenous administration of 0.4, 1.2, and 3.6 mg of etoposide per kg of body weight on Days 6 to 15 of gestation to SPF rats; a dose of 0.13 mg per kg of body weight (mg/kg) caused an increase in retarded ossification. Dose-related embryotoxicity (intrauterine fetal death, decreased fetal weights) and teratogenicity (cranial abnormalities, major skeletal abnormalities) have also been reported with intraperitoneal administration of 1, 1.5, or 2 mg/kg on Day 6, 7, or 8 of gestation to Swiss-Albino mice. Risk-benefit must be carefully considered when this medication is required in life-threatening situations or in serious diseases for which other medications cannot be used or are ineffective.

FDA Pregnancy Category D.

**Breast-feeding**

Etoposide is distributed into breast milk. Breast-feeding is not recommended during chemotherapy because of the risks to the infant (adverse effects, mutagenicity, carcinogenicity).

**Pediatrics**

Appropriate studies on the relationship of age to the effects of etoposide have not been performed in the pediatric population. However, there are numerous reports of etoposide use in children and no pediatrics-specific problems have been documented to date.

**Geriatrics**

No information is available on the relationship of age to the effects of etoposide in geriatric patients.

**Dental**

The bone marrow depressant effects of etoposide may result in an increased incidence of microbial infection, delayed healing, and gingival bleeding. Dental work, whenever possible, should be completed prior to initiation of therapy or deferred until blood counts have returned to normal. Patients should be instructed in proper oral hygiene during treatment, including caution in use of regular toothbrushes, dental floss, and toothpicks.

Etoposide may also cause stomatitis which may be associated with considerable discomfort.

**Drug interactions and/or related problems**

The following drug interactions and/or related problems have been selected on the basis of their potential clinical significance (possible mechanism in parentheses where appropriate)—not necessarily inclusive (» = major clinical significance):

Note: Combinations containing any of the following medications, depending on the amount present, may also interact with this medication.

Blood dyscrasia–causing medications (See *Appendix II*)
(leukopenic and/or thrombocytopenic effects of etoposide may be increased with concurrent or recent therapy if these medications cause the same effects; dosage adjustment of etoposide, if necessary, should be based on blood counts)

» Bone marrow depressants, other (See *Appendix II*) or
Radiation therapy
(additive bone marrow depression may occur; dosage reduction may be required when two or more bone marrow depressants, including radiation, are used concurrently or consecutively)

Vaccines, killed virus
(because normal defense mechanisms may be suppressed by etoposide therapy, the patient's antibody response to the vaccine may be decreased. The interval between discontinuation of medications that cause immunosuppression and restoration of the patient's ability to respond to the vaccine depends on the intensity and type of immunosuppression-causing medication used, the underlying disease, and other factors; estimates vary from 3 months to 1 year)

» Vaccines, live virus
(because normal defense mechanisms may be suppressed by etoposide therapy, concurrent use with a live virus vaccine may potentiate the replication of the vaccine virus, may increase the side/adverse effects of the vaccine virus, and/or may decrease the patient's antibody response to the vaccine; immunization of these patients should be undertaken only with extreme caution after careful review of the patient's hematologic status and only with the knowledge and consent of the physician managing the etoposide therapy. The interval between discontinuation of medications that cause immunosuppression and restoration of the patient's ability to respond to the vaccine depends on the intensity and type of immunosuppression-causing medication used, the underlying disease, and other factors; estimates vary from 3 months to 1 year. Patients with leukemia in remission should not receive live virus vaccine until at least 3 months after their last chemotherapy. In addition, immunization with oral poliovirus vaccine should be postponed in persons in close contact with the patient, especially family members)

**Medical considerations/Contraindications**
The medical considerations/contraindications included here have been selected on the basis of their potential clinical significance (reasons given in parentheses where appropriate)—not necessarily inclusive (» = major clinical significance).

*Risk-benefit should be considered when the following medical problems exist:*

» Bone marrow depression
» Chickenpox, existing or recent (including recent exposure) or
» Herpes zoster
(risk of severe generalized disease)
Hepatic function impairment
(reduced clearance)
» Infection
Renal function impairment
(reduced elimination; lower dosage may be necessary)
Sensitivity to etoposide
Caution should be used also in patients who have had previous cytotoxic drug therapy or radiation therapy.

**Patient monitoring**
The following are especially important in patient monitoring (other tests may be warranted in some patients, depending on condition; (» = major clinical significance):

» Examination of patient's mouth for ulceration
(recommended prior to each dose)
» Hematocrit or hemoglobin and
» Leukocyte count, total and, if appropriate, differential and
» Platelet count
(determinations recommended prior to initiation of therapy and at periodic intervals during therapy; frequency varies according to clinical state, agent, dose, and other agents being used concurrently)

## Side/Adverse Effects

Note: Many "side effects" of antineoplastic therapy are unavoidable and represent the medication's pharmacologic action. Some of these (for example, leukopenia and thrombocytopenia) are actually used as parameters to aid in individual dosage titration.

Hypotension may occur temporarily with intravenous infusion periods of less than 30 minutes.

Use of higher than recommended doses has been associated with hepatic toxicity and metabolic acidosis.

The following side/adverse effects have been selected on the basis of their potential clinical significance (possible signs and symptoms in parentheses where appropriate)—not necessarily inclusive:

**Those indicating need for medical attention**
Incidence more frequent
*Anemia; leukopenia* (usually asymptomatic; less frequently, fever or chills; cough or hoarseness; lower back or side pain; painful or difficult urination); *thrombocytopenia* (usually asymptomatic; less frequently, unusual bleeding or bruising; black, tarry stools; blood in urine or stools; pinpoint red spots on skin)
Note: With *leukopenia*, the nadir of the granulocyte count occurs 7 to 14 days after administration, and recovery is usually complete by the 20th day; cumulative myelosuppression has not been reported.
With *thrombocytopenia*, the nadir of the platelet count occurs 9 to 16 days after administration, and recovery is usually complete by the 20th day; cumulative myelosuppression has not been reported.

Incidence less frequent
*Anaphylaxis* (fast heartbeat; fever or chills; shortness of breath or wheezing; rarely, back pain; cough; loss of consciousness; sweating; swelling of face or tongue; tightness in throat); *stomatitis* (sores in mouth or on lips)
Note: *Anaphylaxis* is also associated with hypotension; hypertension and flushing have also been reported; blood pressure usually returns to normal within a few hours after the intravenous infusion is discontinued. An apparent hypersensitivity-associated apnea has been reported rarely. Anaphylaxis may rarely be fatal.

Incidence rare
*Chemical phlebitis* (pain at site of injection); *neurotoxicity* (difficulty in walking; numbness or tingling in fingers and toes; weakness); *skin rash or itching*
Note: At investigational doses, a generalized pruritic erythematous maculopapular *rash*, consistent with perivasculitis, has been reported.

**Those indicating need for medical attention only if they continue or are bothersome**
Incidence more frequent
*Loss of appetite; nausea and vomiting*
Incidence less frequent
*Central nervous system (CNS) toxicity* (unusual tiredness); *diarrhea*

**Those not indicating need for medical attention**
Incidence more frequent
*Loss of hair*
Note: *Loss of hair* sometimes progresses to total baldness; it is reversible.

## Patient Consultation

As an aid to patient consultation, refer to *Advice for the Patient, Etoposide (Systemic).*

In providing consultation, consider emphasizing the following selected information (» = major clinical significance):

**Before using this medication**
» Conditions affecting use, especially:
Sensitivity to etoposide
Pregnancy—Use not recommended because of mutagenic, teratogenic, and carcinogenic potential; advisability of using contraception; telling physician immediately if pregnancy is suspected
Breast-feeding—Not recommended because of risk of serious side effects
Other medications, especially other bone marrow depressants or previous cytotoxic drug or radiation therapy
Other medical problems, especially chickenpox, herpes zoster, or infection

## Proper use of this medication
» Importance of not taking more or less medication than the amount
   prescribed
   Caution in taking combination therapy; taking each medication at the
   right time
   Frequency of nausea, vomiting, and loss of appetite; importance of
   continuing medication despite stomach upset
   Checking with physician if vomiting occurs shortly after dose is taken
» Proper dosing
   Missed dose: Not taking at all; not doubling doses
» Proper storage

## Precautions while using this medication
» Importance of close monitoring by physician
» Avoiding immunizations unless approved by physician; other persons
   in patient's household should avoid immunizations with oral poliovirus vaccine; avoiding persons who have taken oral poliovirus
   vaccine or wearing a protective mask that covers nose and mouth
*Caution if bone marrow depression occurs:*
» Avoiding exposure to persons with bacterial infections, especially during periods of low blood counts; checking with physician immediately if fever or chills, cough or hoarseness, lower back or side
   pain, or painful or difficult urination occur
» Checking with physician immediately if unusual bleeding or bruising;
   black, tarry stools; blood in urine or stools; or pinpoint red spots
   on skin occur
   Caution in use of regular toothbrush, dental floss, or toothpick; physician, dentist, or nurse may suggest alternatives; checking with
   physician before having dental work done
   Not touching eyes or inside of nose unless hands washed immediately
   before
   Using caution to avoid accidental cuts with use of sharp objects such
   as safety razor or fingernail or toenail cutters
   Avoiding contact sports or other situations where bruising or injury
   could occur

## Side/adverse effects
   Importance of discussing possible effects, including cancer, with
   physician
   Signs of potential side effects, especially leukopenia, thrombocytope-
   nia, anaphylaxis, stomatitis, chemical phlebitis, neurotoxicity, and
   skin rash or itching
   Physician or nurse can help in dealing with side effects
   Possibility of hair loss; should return after treatment has ended

# General Dosing Information

Patients receiving etoposide should be under supervision of a physician
   experienced in cancer chemotherapy.

A variety of dosage schedules of etoposide, alone or in combination with
   other antitumor agents, are used. The prescriber may consult the medical literature as well as the manufacturer's literature in choosing a
   specific dosage.

Dosage must be adjusted to meet the individual requirements of each
   patient, based on clinical response and appearance or severity of
   toxicity.

Frequency and duration of nausea and vomiting may be reduced in some
   patients by administration of antiemetics prior to dosing.

Special precautions are recommended in patients who develop thrombocytopenia as a result of administration of etoposide. These may include
   extreme care in performing invasive procedures; regular inspection of
   intravenous sites, skin (including perirectal area), and mucous
   membrane surfaces for signs of bleeding or bruising; limiting frequency of venipuncture and avoiding intramuscular injections; testing
   urine, emesis, stool, and secretions for occult blood; care in use of
   regular toothbrushes, dental floss, toothpicks, safety razors, and fingernail and toenail cutters; avoiding constipation; and using caution to
   prevent falls and other injuries. Such patients should avoid alcohol and
   aspirin intake because of the risk of gastrointestinal bleeding. Platelet
   transfusions may be required.

Patients who develop leukopenia should be observed carefully for signs
   of infection. Antibiotic support may be required. In neutropenic patients who develop fever, broad-spectrum antibiotic coverage should
   be initiated empirically, pending bacterial cultures and appropriate diagnostic tests.

## For parenteral dosage form only
It is recommended that etoposide injection be diluted prior to use, and
   that it be administered by slow intravenous infusion over a period of
   30 to 60 minutes to prevent hypotension. Etoposide should not be
   administered by rapid intravenous injection or any other route.

## Safety considerations for handling this medication
There is limited but increasing evidence and concern that personnel involved in preparation and administration of parenteral antineoplastics
   may be at some risk because of the potential mutagenicity, teratogenicity, and/or carcinogenicity of these agents, although the actual risk
   is unknown. USP advisory panels recommend cautious handling both
   in preparation and disposal of antineoplastic agents. Precautions that
   have been suggested include:
• Use of a biological containment cabinet during reconstitution and
   dilution of parenteral medications and wearing of disposable surgical gloves and masks.
• Use of proper technique to prevent contamination of the medication,
   work area, and operator during transfer between containers (including proper training of personnel in this technique).
• Cautious and proper disposal of needles, syringes, vials, ampuls, and
   unused medication.
A number of medical centers have developed detailed guidelines for
   handling of antineoplastic agents.

## Combination chemotherapy
Etoposide may be used in combination with other agents in various regimens. As a result, incidence and/or severity of side effects may be
   altered and different dosages (usually reduced) may be used. For example, etoposide is part of the following chemotherapeutic combinations (some commonly used acronyms are in parentheses):
—doxorubicin, procarbazine, and etoposide (APE).
—etoposide, cyclophosphamide, doxorubicin, and vincristine (CAVE,
   ECHO, CAPO, EVAC, or VOCA).
—cyclophosphamide, doxorubicin, and etoposide (CAE or ACE).
—cisplatin, bleomycin, doxorubicin, and etoposide.
—cisplatin, bleomycin, and etoposide (BEP).
—cisplatin and etoposide (PE).
For specific dosages and schedules, consult the literature. For information
   regarding each agent, consult the individual monographs.

## For treatment of adverse effects
Hypotension may be treated by stopping the infusion, administering fluids
   and other supportive treatment, then resuming the infusion at a slower
   rate.

Anaphylaxis should be treated by stopping the infusion and administering
   pressor agents, adrenocorticoids, antihistamines, or volume expanders
   as necessary.

# Oral Dosage Forms
## ETOPOSIDE CAPSULES

### Usual adult dose
Small cell lung carcinoma—
   Oral, 70 mg per square meter of body surface (rounded to the nearest
   50 mg) per day for four days to 100 mg per square meter of body
   surface (rounded to the nearest 50 mg) per day for five days, repeated every three to four weeks.

### Usual pediatric dose
Dosage has not been established.

### Strength(s) usually available
U.S.—
   50 mg (Rx) [*VePesid*].
Canada—
   50 mg (Rx) [*VePesid*].
   100 mg (Rx) [*VePesid*].

### Packaging and storage
Store between 2 and 8 °C (36 and 46 °F), in a well-closed container, unless
   otherwise specified by manufacturer.

# Parenteral Dosage Forms
## ETOPOSIDE INJECTION

### Usual adult dose
Testicular carcinoma—
   Intravenous infusion, 50 to 100 mg per square meter of body surface
   per day on Days 1 to 5 to 100 mg per square meter of body surface
   on Days 1, 3, and 5 of a regimen which is repeated every three to
   four weeks.
Small cell lung carcinoma—
   Intravenous infusion, 35 mg per square meter of body surface per day
   for four days to 50 mg per square meter of body surface per day
   for five days, repeated every three to four weeks.

### Usual pediatric dose
Dosage has not been established.

**Strength(s) usually available**
U.S.—
    20 mg per mL (Rx) [*VePesid* (benzyl alcohol 30 mg per mL; poly-
        sorbate 80; alcohol 30.5% v/v)].
Canada—
    20 mg per mL (Rx) [*VePesid* (benzyl alcohol 30 mg per mL; poly-
        sorbate 80; ethanol); GENERIC].

**Packaging and storage**
Store below 40 °C (104 °F), preferably between 15 and 30 °C (59 and 86
°F), unless otherwise specified by manufacturer. Protect from freezing.

**Preparation of dosage form**
Etoposide injection may be diluted for administration by intravenous in-
    fusion in either 5% dextrose injection or 0.9% sodium chloride injec-
    tion to produce a solution containing 200 to 400 mcg (0.2 to 0.4 mg)
    of etoposide per mL (precipitation may occur with concentrations
    greater than 400 mcg per mL).
Cracking and leaking of plastic containers made of ABS (a polymer com-
    posed of acrylonitrile, butadiene, and styrene) has been reported when
    used with undiluted (but not diluted) etoposide injection.
    Caution—
        Use of products containing benzyl alcohol is generally not rec-
        ommended for preparation of medications for use in neonates.
        A fatal toxic syndrome consisting of metabolic acidosis, CNS
        depression, respiratory problems, renal failure, hypotension,
and possibly seizures and intracranial hemorrhages has been
associated with this use.
Use of products containing polysorbate 80 is generally not rec-
    ommended for preparation of medications for use in premature
    infants. A life-threatening syndrome consisting of hepatic and
    renal failure, pulmonary deterioration, thrombocytopenia, and
    ascites has been associated with this use.

**Stability**
When diluted as recommended, 0.2 and 0.4 mg per mL solutions are stable
    for 96 and 24 hours, respectively, at 25 °C (77 °F) under normal room
    fluorescent light in glass or plastic containers.

## Selected Bibliography

Phillips NC. Oral etoposide. Drug Intell Clin Pharm 1988 Nov; 22: 860-
3.
Sinkule JA. Etoposide: a semisynthetic epipodophyllotoxin. Chemistry,
    pharmacology/pharmacokinetics, adverse effects and use as an anti-
    neoplastic agent. Pharmacother 1984 Mar/Apr; 4: 61-73.
Fleming RA, Miller AA, Stewart CF. Etoposide: an update. Clin Pharm
    1989 Apr; 8: 274-93.

Revised: 08/09/92
Interim revision: 08/08/94

# ETRETINATE   Systemic

VA CLASSIFICATION (Primary/Secondary): DE801/DE890
Note: For a listing of dosage forms and brand names by country availa-
    bility, see *Dosage Forms* section(s). For a listing of brand names
    for the articles in this monograph, refer to the General Index.

## Category
Antipsoriatic (systemic).

## Indications
Note: Bracketed information in the *Indications* section refers to uses that
    are not included in U.S. product labeling.

**FOR WOMEN OF CHILD-BEARING POTENTIAL, SEE THE
*PREGNANCY/REPRODUCTION* SECTION OF *PRECAUTIONS
TO CONSIDER* FOR RESTRICTIONS ON THE USE OF
ETRETINATE.**

**Accepted**
Psoriasis (treatment)—Etretinate is indicated for the treatment of severe
    recalcitrant psoriasis, including the erythrodermic and generalized pus-
    tular types, in patients who are unresponsive to or intolerant of the
    standard therapies.
    [Etretinate is also used in combination with psoralens plus ultraviolet
    light A (PUVA), ultraviolet light B (UVB), selective ultraviolet light,
    topical adrenocorticoids, anthralin, or coal tar in the treatment of
    psoriasis.]

[Lichen planus, oral (treatment)][1]—Etretinate is used for the treatment of
    severe, intractable oral lichen planus.

Etretinate is also used in correcting severe intractable forms of keratini-
    zation disorders, such as
[Dermatoses, ichthyosiform]
[Erythroderma, congenital ichthyosiform]
[Ichthyosis, lamellar, and other ichthyoses]
[Keratosis follicularis (Darier's disease)]
[Keratosis palmaris et plantaris]
[Pityriasis rubra pilaris (PRP)]
[Pustulosis, palmoplantar]

[1]Not included in Canadian product labeling.

## Pharmacology/Pharmacokinetics

**Physicochemical characteristics**
Molecular weight—354.49.

**Mechanism of action/Effect**
The mechanism of action of etretinate is not known. However, improve-
    ment in psoriatic patients occurs in association with a decrease in
    scaling, erythema, and thickness of lesions, and there is histological
    evidence of normalization of epidermal differentiation, decreased stra-
tum corneum thickness, and decreased inflammation in the epidermis
and dermis.

**Absorption**
Etretinate is absorbed in the small intestine.
Studies in normal volunteers indicate that the absorption of etretinate is
    greater in patients consuming whole milk or a high-fat diet than in
    patients in a fasting state.

**Distribution**
Etretinate accumulates in high concentrations in adipose tissue, especially
    in the liver and in subcutaneous fat.
Liver concentrations of etretinate in patients who had received therapy for
    six months were generally higher than accompanying plasma concen-
    trations and tended to be higher still in livers with a higher degree of
    fatty infiltration.
Concentrations of etretinate and its active metabolite in epidermal speci-
    mens obtained after 1 to 36 months of therapy were a function of
    location: subcutis much greater than serum greater than epidermis
    greater than dermis.
Because of the large number of binding sites available for etretinate, dis-
    placement from binding sites by other medications is not important.

**Protein binding**
Etretinate is more than 99% bound to plasma proteins, predominantly
    lipoproteins, whereas its active metabolite, acetretin (etretin), is pre-
    dominantly bound to albumin.

**Biotransformation**
Following oral administration, etretinate is extensively metabolized, with
    significant first-pass metabolism to the pharmacologically active acid
    form. Subsequent metabolism results in the inactive 13-*cis* acid form,
    chain-shortened breakdown products, and conjugates that are ulti-
    mately excreted.

**Half-life**
In one study, the apparent terminal half-life of etretinate after 6 months
    of therapy was approximately 120 days.
In another study of 47 patients who had undergone chronic therapy with
    etretinate, 5 patients had detectable serum drug concentrations (0.5 to
    12 nanograms per mL) 2.1 to 2.9 years after therapy was completed.
The long half-life of etretinate appears to be due to its storage in adipose
    tissue.

**Time to peak concentration**
2 to 6 hours during chronic therapy with doses ranging from 25 mg once
    daily to 25 mg four times daily.

**Peak serum concentration**
102 to 389 nanograms per mL during chronic therapy with doses ranging
    from 25 mg once daily to 25 mg four times daily.

**Elimination**
Primarily biliary; also renal.

## Precautions to Consider

Note: **Patients receiving etretinate should not donate blood during therapy or for an undetermined length of time (several years or longer) after therapy, because of the possible risk to the developing fetus of a pregnant patient who may receive such blood.**

### Cross-sensitivity and/or related problems

Patients sensitive to isotretinoin, tretinoin, or vitamin A derivatives may be sensitive to this medication also, since etretinate is related to both retinoic acid and retinol (vitamin A).

### Carcinogenicity/Tumorigenicity

In a 2-year study, Sprague-Dawley rats given etretinate at doses up to 3 mg per kg of body weight (mg/kg) per day (2 times the maximum recommended human therapeutic dose) had no increase in tumor incidence.

In an 80-week study, the high-dose male group, but not the high-dose female group, of Crl:CD-1 (ICR) BR mice given doses of 4 to 5 mg/kg per day of etretinate had an increased incidence of blood vessel tumors.

### Mutagenicity

Except for a weakly positive response in the Ames test when the tester strain TA 100 was used, there was no evidence of genotoxicity when etretinate was evaluated by the Ames test in a host-mediated assay, in the micronucleus test, and in a 'treat and plate' test using the diploid yeast strain *S. cerevisiae* D7. In addition, no differences were noted in the rate of sister chromatid exchange (SCE) in the lymphocytes of patients examined before and after 4 weeks of treatment with etretinate.

### Pregnancy/Reproduction

Fertility—In human males, no adverse effects on sperm production were observed in 12 psoriatic patients who were treated with 75 mg per day of etretinate for 1 month and 50 mg per day for an additional 2 months.

However, in male animal studies, testicular atrophy was observed in subchronic and chronic rat studies and in a chronic dog study, in some cases at doses approaching those recommended for use in humans. In addition, decreased sperm counts were reported in a 13-week dog study at doses as low as 3 mg/kg per day (approximately 2 times the maximum recommended human dose [MRHD]). Also in dogs, spermatogenic arrest was observed with chronic administration of the all-*trans* metabolite.

In female animal studies, at doses up to 2.5 mg/kg per day, a study of fertility and general reproductive performance in rats showed no etretinate-related effects. In addition, no adverse effects on various parameters of late gestation were noted in rats given doses of etretinate up to 4 mg/kg per day (approximately 3 times the MRHD). However, at 5 mg/kg per day, the readiness of the treated rats to copulate was reduced, although the pregnancy rate was unaffected. In addition, at this higher dose, the number of live young at birth was reduced, their postnatal weight gain and survival were adversely affected, and the pregnancy rate of the untreated first generation rats and postnatal weight gain of the untreated second generation rats were reduced. Furthermore, at doses of 8 mg/kg per day (approximately 5 times the MRHD), the rate of stillbirths was increased and neonatal weight gain and survival rate were markedly reduced. The relevance of these findings to human females is not known.

Pregnancy—**Etretinate is contraindicated during pregnancy,** since it has caused major human fetal abnormalities, including meningomyelocoele; meningoencephalocoele; multiple synostoses; facial dysmorphia; syndactyly; absence of terminal phalanges; malformations of hip, ankle, and forearm; abnormalities of the heart and thymus; low set ears; high palate; decreased cranial volume; and alterations of the skull and cervical vertebrae.

**In addition, it has not been determined how long pregnancy should be avoided after discontinuation of treatment;** patients have been followed for as long as 2 years after treatment was discontinued, and fetal abnormalities associated with etretinate have occurred during this 2-year period. **Therefore, etretinate should not be used in women who plan to have children in the future.**

**In women of childbearing potential, etretinate should not be used until the possibility of pregnancy is ruled out. In addition, etretinate should not be used in women who, while undergoing treatment and for an indefinite period of time thereafter, are deemed unreliable in their use of contraception or who may not use reliable contraception.**

It is strongly recommended that a pregnancy test be performed within 2 weeks prior to etretinate therapy. Etretinate therapy should then be initiated on the second or third day of the next normal menstrual period. It is also recommended that an effective form of contraception

be used for at least 1 month before therapy, during therapy, and for an indefinite period of time following completion of therapy.

**Etretinate imposes serious risks to the fetus for an indefinite period of time following completion of therapy.** Etretinate blood concentrations of 0.5 to 12 nanograms per mL have been reported in 5 of 47 patients 2.1 to 2.9 years after treatment was concluded. It has not been determined how long it is necessary to wait after discontinuation of treatment to assure that no drug will be detectable in the blood. In addition, the significance of undetectable blood concentrations relative to the risk of teratogenicity is unknown.

**Women of child-bearing potential should be fully counseled on the serious risks to the fetus should they become pregnant during therapy and for an indefinite period of time following completion of therapy.** If pregnancy does occur, patients should be counseled about the risks of continuing the pregnancy.

FDA Pregnancy Category X.

### Breast-feeding

Problems in humans have not been documented. Although it is not known whether etretinate is distributed into breast milk, use is not recommended during breast-feeding or if breast-feeding is anticipated in the future, because of the potential for adverse effects in nursing babies. In addition, studies have shown that etretinate is distributed into the milk of lactating rats, although no adverse effects on various parameters of lactation were noted at doses of etretinate up to 4 mg/kg per day (approximately 3 times the MRHD).

### Pediatrics

Because of the shortage of data on etretinate treatment in children and the possibility that children may be more sensitive to the effects of the medication, etretinate should not be used in children unless all alternative therapies have been exhausted.

Ossification of interosseous ligaments and tendons of the limbs has been reported in children. In addition, in at least 2 children there were x-ray changes suggestive of premature epiphyseal closure during treatment with etretinate. It is not known whether these adverse effects occur more commonly in children, but they may be more significant because of the growth process.

Before therapy with etretinate is initiated in children, x-rays for bone age, including x-rays of the knees, should be done, and yearly monitoring thereafter is advised. In addition, during treatment children experiencing pain or limitation of motion should be thoroughly evaluated.

### Geriatrics

No information is available on the relationship of age to the effects of etretinate in geriatric patients.

### Dental

Gingival bleeding and inflammation and dry mouth have occurred in up to 10% of patients treated with etretinate.

Since use of etretinate decreases or inhibits salivary flow, it contributes to the development of caries, periodontal disease, oral candidiasis, and discomfort.

### Drug interactions and/or related problems

The following drug interactions and/or related problems have been selected on the basis of their potential clinical significance (possible mechanism in parentheses where appropriate)—not necessarily inclusive (» = major clinical significance):

Note: Combinations containing any of the following medications, depending on the amount present, may also interact with this medication.

Abrasive or medicated soaps or cleansers or
Acne preparations or preparations containing a peeling agent, such as:
  Benzoyl peroxide
  Resorcinol
  Salicylic acid
  Sulfur
  Tretinoin or
Alcohol-containing preparations, topical, such as:
  After-shave lotions
  Astringents
  Perfumed toiletries
  Shaving creams or lotions or
Cosmetics or soaps with a strong drying effect or
Medicated cosmetics or "cover-ups"
  (may cause a cumulative irritant or drying effect, especially with the application of peeling, desquamating, or abrasive agents, resulting in excessive irritation of the skin)

» Alcohol
  (consumption during etretinate therapy may result in hypertriglyceridemia, since both alcohol and etretinate may increase plasma triglyceride concentration)

High-fat diet or
Milk
    (concomitant consumption of milk or a high-fat meal increases the
    absorption of etretinate; intermittent consumption may make it dif-
    ficult to accurately titrate the dosage; patients should consistently
    take each dose of etretinate with milk or high-fat foods)
» Isotretinoin or
» Tretinoin or
» Vitamin A
    (may result in additive toxic effects)
» Methotrexate or
» Hepatotoxic medications, other (See *Appendix II*)
    (concurrent use with other hepatotoxic medications, especially
    methotrexate, may increase the potential for hepatotoxicity)
    Photosensitizing medications, other
    (concurrent use may cause additive photosensitizing effects)
» Tetracyclines
    (may increase the potential for pseudotumor cerebri)

**Laboratory value alterations**
The following have been selected on the basis of their potential clinical
significance (possible effect in parentheses where appropriate)—not
necessarily inclusive (» = major clinical significance):
With physiology/laboratory test values
    Acetonuria and
    Casts in urine and
    Glycosuria and
    Hemoglobinuria and
    Microscopic hematuria and
    Proteinuria and
    White blood cells (WBC) in urine
        (have occurred; in clinical trials, 1 to 10% [for WBC's in urine,
        10 to 25%] of patients treated with etretinate have experienced
        these effects)
» Alanine aminotransferase (ALT [SGPT]) and
» Aspartate aminotransferase (AST [SGOT]) and
» Lactate dehydrogenase (LDH)
        (serum values may be increased; in clinical trials, elevations of
        ALT, AST, and LDH have occurred in 23%, 18%, and 15%, re-
        spectively, of patients treated with etretinate; in most cases the
        elevations were slight to moderate, and concentrations became nor-
        mal again either during or after cessation of therapy)
    Albumin concentration and
    Calcium concentration and
    Chloride concentration and
    Fasting blood sugar (FBS) concentration and
    Phosphorus concentration and
    Potassium concentration and
    Prothrombin time and
    Sodium concentration and
    Total protein concentration and
    Venous $CO_2$ concentration and
    WBC counts
        (may be increased or decreased. In clinical trials, changes in cal-
        cium, phosphorus, and potassium have occurred in 25 to 50%;
        changes in chloride, FBS, prothrombin time, sodium, venous $CO_2$,
        and WBC's have occurred in 10 to 25%; and changes in albumin
        and total protein have occurred in 1 to 10% of patients treated with
        etretinate)
    Alkaline phosphatase value and
    Bilirubin concentration and
    Blood urea nitrogen (BUN) concentration and
    Creatinine concentration and
    Creatine kinase (CK) concentration and
    Erythrocyte sedimentation rate (ESR) and
    Gamma glutamyl transpeptidase (GGTP) and
    Globulin concentration and
    Reticulocyte counts
        (may be increased. In clinical trials, elevations of ESR and retic-
        ulocytes have occurred in 25 to 50%; elevations of GGTP, glob-
        ulin, and alkaline phosphatase have occurred in 10 to 25%; and
        elevations of bilirubin, BUN, creatinine, and CK have occurred in
        1 to 10% of patients treated with etretinate)
    Hemoglobin and hematocrit and
    Red blood cell counts
        (may be decreased or increased, mainly decreased; in clinical trials,
        decreases have occurred in 10 to 25% and elevations have occurred
        in 1 to 10% of patients treated with etretinate)

» High-density lipoprotein (HDL)
        (serum concentrations may be decreased; in clinical trials, de-
        creases in HDL have occurred in about 37% of patients [54% of
        these had decreases below 36 mg%]; the effect is reversible upon
        discontinuation of medication)
    Mean corpuscular hemoglobin (MCH) and
    Mean corpuscular hemoglobin concentration (MCHC) and
    Partial thromboplastin time (PTT) and
    Platelet counts
        (may be increased or decreased, mainly increased; in clinical trials,
        elevations of MCH and MCHC and increases in PTT have oc-
        curred in 25 to 50% [elevations of platelets have occurred in 10
        to 25%] and decreases have occurred in 1 to 10% of patients
        treated with etretinate)
    Mean corpuscular volume (MCV)
        (may be decreased; in clinical trials, decreases have occurred in
        10 to 25% of patients treated with etretinate)
» Triglyceride concentrations, plasma and
» Cholesterol concentrations, serum
        (may be increased; in clinical trials, elevated plasma triglyceride
        concentration has occurred in about 45% of patients [46% of these
        had elevations above 250 mg per dL and 1 case had a concentra-
        tion greater than 1000 mg%] and increased cholesterol concentra-
        tion has occurred in about 16% of patients [19% of these had
        elevations above 300 mg%]; elevation of serum triglycerides in
        excess of 800 mg per dL has been associated with acute pancre-
        atitis; these effects are reversible upon discontinuation of
        medication)

**Medical considerations/Contraindications**
The medical considerations/contraindications included here have been selected on the basis of their potential clinical significance (reasons given
in parentheses where appropriate)—not necessarily inclusive (» =
major clinical significance).

***Risk-benefit should be considered when the following medical problems
    exist:***
» Cardiovascular disease, or family history of or
» Cardiovascular risk, history of or family history of
        (etretinate may increase plasma triglyceride concentration, possibly
        increasing patient's cardiovascular risk status)
    Diabetes mellitus, or family history of
        (possibility of alteration in blood sugar concentration; etretinate
        may increase plasma triglyceride concentration in patients with di-
        abetes mellitus, possibly increasing their cardiovascular risk status)
    Hepatic disease, history of or family history of
» Hypertriglyceridemia or
» Conditions predisposing to hypertriglyceridemia, such as:
    High alcohol intake, or history of
    Hypertriglyceridemia, family history of
    Obesity
        (etretinate may increase plasma triglyceride concentration, possibly
        increasing patient's cardiovascular risk status)
    Sensitivity to etretinate

**Patient monitoring**
The following may be especially important in patient monitoring (other
tests may be warranted in some patients, depending on condition;
» = major clinical significance):
» Alanine aminotransferase (ALT [SGPT]) values, serum and
» Aspartate aminotransferase (AST [SGOT]) values, serum and
» Lactate dehydrogenase (LDH) values
        (determinations recommended prior to therapy, at 1- to 2-week
        intervals for the first 1 to 2 months of therapy, and thereafter at 1-
        to 3-month intervals, depending on the patient's response to etre-
        tinate administration; if hepatotoxicity is suspected, etretinate
        should be discontinued until the etiology of the hepatotoxicity is
        determined)
    Bone x-rays, especially of the ankles, pelvis, and knees
        (recommended because of the possibility of hyperostosis occurring
        in patients undergoing long-term or recurrent courses of etretinate
        therapy)
    Bone-age determinations, including x-rays of knees
        (recommended in children prior to therapy and yearly during ther-
        apy to determine effects on epiphyseal centers)
» Lipid concentrations, blood
        (determinations recommended in patients under fasting conditions
        prior to therapy and at 1- to 2-week intervals during therapy until
        the lipid response to etretinate is determined [usually within 4 to
        8 weeks]. Following consumption of alcohol, 36 hours should
        elapse before blood lipid determination)

Ophthalmologic examinations
(patient should be examined for papilledema if early symptoms of pseudotumor cerebri, such as severe or continuing headache, nausea and vomiting, and blurred vision or other changes in vision, occur)

Sugar concentrations, blood
(determinations recommended during therapy in known or suspected diabetics because minor elevations in fasting blood sugar concentrations have been reported)

## Side/Adverse Effects

Note: Nearly all of the side/adverse effects reported with etretinate to date resemble those of hypervitaminosis A syndrome, which primarily produces signs and symptoms related to the mucocutaneous, musculoskeletal, hepatic, and central nervous systems.

An elevation of plasma triglycerides has occurred in approximately 45% of patients; a decrease in high density lipoproteins (HDL) has occurred in approximately 37% of patients; and an increase in cholesterol concentrations has occurred in approximately 16% of patients receiving etretinate. These effects on triglycerides, HDL, and cholesterol were reversible after therapy was discontinued. Hypertriglyceridemia, hypercholesterolemia, and lowered HDL may increase cardiovascular risk, and elevation of serum triglycerides in excess of 800 mg per dL has been associated with acute pancreatitis. Every attempt should be made to control significant elevations of triglycerides or cholesterol or significant decreases in HDL during therapy with etretinate, possibly through weight reduction or restriction of dietary fat and alcohol.

In clinical trials, 84% of patients receiving etretinate for an average of 60 months had radiographic evidence of extraspinal tendon and ligament calcification. The most common sites of this hyperostosis were the ankles (76%), pelvis (53%), and knees (42%). Spinal changes were uncommon. In 47% of the affected patients, there were no bone or joint symptoms.

Studies in rodents have shown an increased incidence of bone fractures with etretinate use, although no evidence of fractures was observed in a 1-year study in dogs. Other dose-related changes in some animals treated with etretinate at subchronic- or chronic-toxicity doses include alopecia, erythema, reductions in body weight and food consumption, stiffness, altered gait, hematologic changes, elevations in serum alkaline phosphatase, and testicular atrophy with microscopic evidence of reduced spermatogenesis. In general, etretinate toxicity in studies in rats, mice, and dogs was dose-related with respect to incidence, onset, and severity.

The following side/adverse effects have been selected on the basis of their potential clinical significance (possible signs and symptoms in parentheses where appropriate)—not necessarily inclusive:

**Those indicating need for medical attention**
Incidence more frequent
*Bone or joint pain, tenderness, or stiffness; cramps or pain in upper abdomen or stomach area; eyelid abnormalities* (burning, redness, itching, feeling of dryness, pain, tenderness, excessive tearing, or other sign of inflammation or irritation of eyes); *muscle cramps; unusual bruising*
Incidence less frequent
*Abnormalities of conjunctiva, cornea, lens, retina, extraocular musculature, ocular tension, pupil, or vitreous humor* (blurred or double vision or other changes in vision); *conjunctivitis or mucous membrane abnormalities* (burning, redness, itching, feeling of dryness, pain, tenderness, excessive tearing, or other sign of inflammation or irritation of eyes); *hepatitis* (dark-colored urine, flu-like symptoms, or yellow eyes or skin); *otitis externa* (change in hearing; earache or pain in ear; ear drainage)
Note: If *visual difficulties* occur, etretinate should be discontinued and patient should have an ophthalmologic examination.

*Hepatitis* occurred in approximately 1.5% of patients treated with etretinate in clinical trials. In addition, pathology findings consisting of hepatic fibrosis, necrosis, and cirrhosis have been reported that may be related to etretinate therapy. If signs and symptoms of hepatitis occur, etretinate should be discontinued and the etiology investigated.

Incidence rare
*Amnesia, anxiety, confusion, or depression* (mood or mental changes); *bleeding or inflammation of gums; blot retinal hemorrhage, iritis, posterior subcapsular cataract, pseudotumor cerebri, or scotoma* (blurred or double vision or other changes in vision); pseudotumor cerebri may also cause severe or continuing headache or nausea and vomiting); *ear infection* (change in hearing; earache or pain

in ear; ear drainage); *photophobia* (burning, redness, itching, feeling of dryness, pain, tenderness, excessive tearing, or other sign of inflammation or irritation of eyes)
Note: If *visual difficulties* occur, etretinate should be discontinued and patient should have an ophthalmologic examination.
If signs and symptoms of *pseudotumor cerebri* occur, etretinate should be discontinued immediately and the patient should be referred for neurologic diagnosis and care.

**Those indicating need for medical attention only if they continue or are bothersome**
Incidence more frequent
*Changes in appetite; chapped lips; dryness of nose; dryness, redness, scaling, itching, rash, or other sign of inflammation or irritation of the skin; headache, mild; increased sensitivity to contact lenses—*may occur during and after therapy; *increased sensitivity of skin to sunlight; nosebleeds; peeling of skin on fingertips, palms of hands, or soles of feet; thinning of hair; unusual thirst; unusual tiredness*
Incidence less frequent
*Dizziness; dryness of mouth; fever; nausea, mild; onycholysis or paronychia* (redness or soreness around fingernails or loosening of the fingernails); *soreness, cracking, swelling, or inflammation of lips; soreness of tongue*

## Patient Consultation

As an aid to patient consultation, refer to *Advice for the Patient, Etretinate (Systemic)*.

In providing consultation, consider emphasizing the following selected information (» = major clinical significance):

**Before using this medication**
» Conditions affecting use, especially:
Sensitivity to etretinate, isotretinoin, tretinoin, or vitamin A–like preparations
Pregnancy—Not taking etretinate during pregnancy, because it causes birth defects in humans. In addition, since it is not known how long pregnancy should be avoided after treatment stops, planning on never having children after treatment with etretinate. Not taking etretinate unless an effective form of contraception is used for at least 1 month before beginning treatment. Continuing contraception during treatment and for as long as pregnancy is possible after etretinate is stopped. Discussing this information with doctor
Breast-feeding—Although it is not known whether etretinate passes into the breast milk, etretinate is not recommended during breast-feeding, or if breast-feeding is planned in the future, because it may cause unwanted effects in nursing babies
Use in children—Because of the shortage of data on etretinate treatment in children and the possibility that children may be more sensitive to the effects of the medication, etretinate should not be used in children unless all alternative therapies have been exhausted
Other medications, especially alcohol, methotrexate or other hepatotoxic medications, isotretinoin, tretinoin, vitamin A, and tetracyclines
Other medical problems, especially personal or family history of cardiovascular risk or disease or hypertriglyceridemia or conditions predisposing to hypertriglyceridemia, such as high alcohol intake or history of high alcohol intake, family history of hypertriglyceridemia, or obesity

**Proper use of this medication**
» Taking each dose with milk or fatty food because fats help medication to be absorbed better; rest of time following low-fat diet because of possible hypertriglyceridemia and consequent cardiovascular risks
» Importance of not taking more medication than the amount prescribed
» Proper dosing
Missed dose: Taking as soon as possible with milk or fatty food; not taking if almost time for next dose; not doubling doses
» Proper storage

**Precautions while using this medication**
» Regular visits to physician to check progress during therapy
» Using a reliable form of contraception and not changing contraception method during therapy and for as long as able to become pregnant after therapy ends, since etretinate causes birth defects in humans during its use and for at least several years afterwards (it is not known how long after therapy is discontinued that birth defects may occur); stopping medication immediately and checking with physician if pregnancy is suspected during therapy; checking with physician as soon as possible if pregnancy occurs anytime in the

future after therapy is discontinued; talking to physician in either case about the risks of continuing the pregnancy

» To prevent the possibility of a pregnant patient receiving blood containing etretinate, never donating blood to a blood bank during or after treatment with etretinate, since it is not known how long etretinate stays in the body

» Avoiding concurrent use of vitamin A and vitamin supplements containing vitamin A

» Not drinking, or at least reducing consumption of, alcoholic beverages, because of possible hypertriglyceridemia and consequent cardiovascular risks

Diabetics: May alter blood sugar concentrations

» Caution if decrease in night vision, which may be sudden, occurs; not driving, using machines, or doing other things that could be dangerous if unable to see well; checking with physician if this occurs

Possibility of dryness of eyes; may decrease tolerance to contact lenses during therapy and for several weeks or longer after discontinuation of therapy; checking with physician if inflammation occurs and about using ocular lubricant to relieve dryness of eyes

Possibility of photosensitivity; avoiding unprotected exposure to sunlight and not using sunlamp; checking with physician if severe reaction occurs

Possible dryness of mouth and nose; for relief of mouth dryness, using sugarless gum or candy, ice, or saliva substitute for relief; checking with dentist if dry mouth continues for more than 2 weeks

Possibility that psoriasis may appear to worsen, with increased redness or itching, during initial therapy; checking with physician if irritation or other symptoms of condition become severe; possibly having to take medication for 2 or 3 months before full effects are seen

### Side/adverse effects

Signs of potential side effects, especially abnormalities of conjunctiva, cornea, lens, retina, extraocular musculature, ocular tension, pupil, or vitreous humor; amnesia; anxiety; bleeding or inflammation of gums; blot retinal hemorrhage; bone or joint pain, tenderness, or stiffness; conjunctivitis; cramps or pain in upper abdomen or stomach area; depression; ear infection; eyelid abnormalities; hepatitis; iritis; mucous membrane abnormalities; muscle cramps; otitis externa; photophobia; posterior subcapsular cataract; pseudotumor cerebri; scotoma; or unusual bruising

## General Dosing Information

It is recommended that etretinate be prescribed only by physicians knowledgeable in the systemic use of retinoids.

Each dose of etretinate should be taken with milk or fatty food. This increases the absorption of the medication and allows smaller doses to be given. However, the rest of the day a low-fat diet should be followed.

During the initial period of etretinate therapy, transient exacerbation of psoriasis commonly occurs.

Clinical improvement has been observed in the majority of patients treated with etretinate. In approximately 10% of all patients treated for severe psoriasis, complete clearing of the disease was observed after 4 to 9 months of therapy; this included complete clearing in 16% of patients with erythrodermic psoriasis and 37% of patients with generalized pustular psoriasis.

Generally, therapy should be terminated in patients whose lesions have adequately resolved.

After therapy with etretinate is discontinued, the majority of patients experience some degree of relapse by the end of 2 months. However, subsequent 4- to 9-month courses of etretinate have resulted in approximately the same clinical response as was experienced during the initial course of therapy.

When treating relapses, the same dosage should be used as was used for the initial therapy.

Various treatment protocols are being used for combination therapy using etretinate and other antipsoriatics:

• Either etretinate or another antipsoriatic is used as initial treatment. If satisfactory results do not occur after a reasonable length of time, another antipsoriatic or etretinate, respectively, is added to the therapy regimen.

• When etretinate is used in combination with psoralens plus ultraviolet light A (PUVA), ultraviolet light B (UVB), or selective ultraviolet light (SUP), standard phototherapy protocols can be used, a reduced dosage of etretinate can be administered, and the total number of ultraviolet treatments can be reduced.

• Etretinate is also being administered starting 1 to 2 weeks prior to phototherapy. Some clinicians believe that the reduction in scaling and skin thickness derived from the etretinate therapy improves the efficacy of the subsequent phototherapy.

• Etretinate is being administered in doses as low as 10 to 20 mg per day initially. Each week thereafter, the daily dose is increased by 10 mg until cheilitis is observed. If satisfactory healing does not occur from this therapy, PUVA, a topical corticosteroid, or anthralin is added to the regimen while maintaining the same dosage of etretinate. After the patient's condition has satisfactorily improved, the additional antipsoriatic is discontinued and the patient is maintained at the same dosage of etretinate.

• Patients who are successfully treated for psoriasis with a combination of etretinate and up to 18 PUVA treatments are being subsequently treated for an additional year with a maintenance dose of etretinate equal to half of the highest tolerated dose of etretinate used during the combination therapy, which in most patients is reported to be 0.5 mg per kg of body weight (mg/kg) per day. It is reported that 80% of these patients remain clear after one year. However, among patients requiring more than 18 PUVA treatments during the combination therapy, little or no benefit was seen from this maintenance therapy.

• When etretinate is used in combination with topical adrenocorticoids or anthralin, better therapeutic results are reported to occur and it may be possible to reduce etretinate doses more rapidly than during etretinate therapy alone. In addition, average maintenance doses of etretinate have been reported to be as low as 0.3 mg/kg per day during combination therapy with topical adrenocorticoids or anthralin. Also, when etretinate is used in combination therapy with topical adrenocorticoids, the cutaneous side effects associated with etretinate therapy may be reduced.

## Oral Dosage Forms
### ETRETINATE CAPSULES

#### Usual adult and adolescent dose

Initial—Oral, 750 mcg (0.75 mg) to 1 mg per kg of body weight per day in divided doses.

Note: Erythrodermic psoriasis may respond to initial doses of 250 mcg (0.25 mg) per kg of body weight a day, increased by 250 mcg (0.25 mg) per kg of body weight per day each week until optimal initial response is attained.

Maintenance—Oral, 500 to 750 mcg (0.5 to 0.75 mg) per kg of body weight per day may be initiated after initial response, generally after 8 to 16 weeks of therapy.

Note: Because of interpatient variation in absorption and metabolism of etretinate, the fact that psoriasis is an unpredictable disease, and the possible concurrent use of other antipsoriatics, the dosage of etretinate and any other antipsoriatic that may be used concurrently should be individualized to achieve the maximal therapeutic response with a tolerable level of side effects.

Patients may respond to doses of etretinate as low as 200 mcg (0.2 mg) per kg of body weight per day when etretinate is administered concurrently with psoralens plus ultraviolet light A (PUVA), ultraviolet light B (UVB), selective ultraviolet light (SUP), topical adrenocorticoids, or anthralin. In addition, it may be possible to reduce the other medication's dosage.

#### Usual adult prescribing limits
Oral, 1.5 mg per kg of body weight per day.

#### Usual pediatric dose
Use is not recommended unless all alternative therapies have proven ineffective.

#### Strength(s) usually available
U.S.—

  10 mg (Rx) [*Tegison* (lactose; methylparaben; propylparaben)].

  25 mg (Rx) [*Tegison* (lactose; methylparaben; propylparaben)].

Canada—

  10 mg (Rx) [*Tegison*].

  25 mg (Rx) [*Tegison*].

#### Packaging and storage
Store below 40 °C (104 °F), preferably between 15 and 30 °C (59 and 86 °F), unless otherwise specified by manufacturer. Protect from light.

#### Auxiliary labeling
• Do not take this medication if you are pregnant.
• Take with milk or fatty food.
• Avoid too much sun or use of sunlamp.
• May cause dizziness or blurred vision.

#### Note
Include patient instructions when dispensing.

Revised: June 1990
Interim revision: 06/17/94

# FACTOR IX    Systemic

BAN: Factor IX Fraction

VA CLASSIFICATION (Primary): BL300

Other commonly used names are Christmas factor, plasma thromboplastin component (PTC), and prothrombin complex concentrate (PCC).

Note: For a listing of dosage forms and brand names by country availability, see *Dosage Forms* section(s). For a listing of brand names for the articles in this monograph, refer to the General Index.

## Category

Antihemorrhagic.

## Indications

Note: Some of the indications for factor IX formulations vary among different brand name products because of differences in composition. Some brand name products contain clinically useful quantities of clotting factors other than factor IX; other brand name products contain only factor IX, or factor IX with clinically insignificant quantities of other clotting factors.

### Accepted

Hemophilia B, hemorrhagic complications of (prophylaxis) or

Hemophilia B, hemorrhagic complications of (treatment)—Factor IX is indicated for the control and prevention of bleeding in patients with hemophilia B (Christmas disease).

Hemophilia A, hemorrhagic complications of (prophylaxis) or

Hemophilia A, hemorrhagic complications of (treatment)—Factor IX complex concentrates may be indicated for the control and prevention of bleeding in patients with hemophilia A (classical hemophilia) who have developed inhibitor antibodies to, and therefore will not respond to treatment with, factor VIII.

Hemorrhagic complications of factor VII deficiency (prophylaxis) or

Hemorrhagic complications of factor VII deficiency (treatment)—*Proplex T* is indicated for the replacement of factor VII in patients lacking this clotting factor.

Hemorrhage, anticoagulant-induced (treatment)—Factor IX complex concentrates may be indicated to reverse life-threatening hemorrhage induced by coumarin- and indandione-derivative anticoagulants.

## Pharmacology/Pharmacokinetics

### Physicochemical characteristics

Source—Factor IX products are sterile, dried concentrates derived from pooled human plasma. One type of factor IX product, which is also called prothrombin complex concentrate (PCC), may contain clinically useful quantities of vitamin K–dependent clotting factors II, VII, and X in addition to factor IX. PCCs also may contain other proteins, including proteins C and S; high molecular weight kininogen; and small quantities of activated clotting factors II, VII, IX, or X.

A second type of factor IX product, which is called coagulation factor IX, is purified of extraneous plasma proteins, including clotting factors II, VII, and X, by affinity chromatography (*AlphaNine* and *AlphaNine SD*) or by immunoaffinity chromatography utilizing murine monoclonal antibodies to factor IX (*Mononine*). Products of this type contain clinically useful quantities of factor IX only.

Molecular weight—Factor IX: 55,000 to 71,000.

### Mechanism of action/Effect

Hemorrhagic complications of Hemophilia B—Factor IX is a vitamin K–dependent clotting factor synthesized in the liver. It is part of the intrinsic pathway of blood coagulation. Factor IX is converted to its activated form, factor IXa, by factor XIa in the presence of calcium ions. Factor IXa, in combination with activated factor VIII, calcium ions, and phospholipids, converts factor X to its activated form, factor Xa, resulting ultimately in the conversion of prothrombin to thrombin, and the formation of a fibrin clot. Hemophilia B is an inherited, X chromosome–linked disorder in which there is a deficiency of factor IX. Hemophilia B is classified as mild, moderate, or severe when plasma factor IX concentrations are more than 5%, 1 to 5%, or less than 1% of normal, respectively. The average normal plasma activity of factor IX is designated as 60 to 100%, and a plasma factor IX concentration of 25 to 40% of normal is required for hemostasis. The administration of factor IX products temporarily replaces the deficient clotting factor to correct or prevent bleeding episodes.

Hemorrhagic complications of hemophilia A—The exact mechanism of action is unclear. However, the clotting factors present in the pro-

thrombin complex concentrates are believed to bypass the factor VIII inhibitors and directly activate factor X.

Hemorrhagic complications of factor VII deficiency—Factor VII is part of the extrinsic pathway of blood coagulation. It is activated to factor VIIa by factor Xa. Factor VIIa, in combination with tissue factor, activates factors IX and X. The administration of the factor VII present in factor IX complex replaces the deficient clotting factor to correct or prevent bleeding episodes.

Anticoagulant-induced hemorrhage—Coumarin- and indandione-derivative anticoagulants act indirectly in the liver by inhibiting the vitamin K–mediated gamma-carboxylation of precursor proteins, thus preventing the activation of clotting factors II, VII, IX, and X. The administration of factor IX complex concentrates containing additional vitamin K–dependent clotting factors increases the plasma concentration of these clotting factors to overcome the effect of the anticoagulant.

### Half-life

Factor IX—

Distribution: 3 to 6 hours.

Elimination: 18 to 32 hours.

### Time to peak effect

10 to 30 minutes after intravenous administration.

## Precautions to Consider

### Pregnancy/Reproduction

Pregnancy—Studies have not been done in humans.

Studies have not been done in animals.

FDA Pregnancy Category C.

### Breast-feeding

It is not known whether the proteins present in factor IX products are distributed into breast milk. However, distribution into breast milk would be highly unlikely because of the large size of the protein molecules.

### Pediatrics

Premature infants and neonates may be at increased risk of developing thrombotic complications following the administration of factor IX products.

### Geriatrics

Appropriate studies performed to date have not demonstrated geriatrics-specific problems that would limit the usefulness of factor IX products in the elderly.

### Drug interactions and/or related problems

The following drug interactions and/or related problems have been selected on the basis of their potential clinical significance (possible mechanism in parentheses where appropriate)—not necessarily inclusive (» = major clinical significance):

Note: Combinations containing any of the following medications, depending on the amount present, may also interact with this medication.

Aminocaproic acid or

Tranexamic acid

(although these antifibrinolytic agents are used commonly in conjunction with clotting factor replacement to control and prevent excessive bleeding in hemophiliacs undergoing tooth extraction or other surgical procedures, concurrent use with factor IX products may increase the risk of thrombotic complications; some hematologists recommend that the administration of aminocaproic acid or tranexamic acid be delayed 8 hours following injection of factor IX products)

### Medical considerations/Contraindications

The medical considerations/contraindications included here have been selected on the basis of their potential clinical significance (reasons given in parentheses where appropriate)—not necessarily inclusive (» = major clinical significance):

### *Risk-benefit should be considered when the following medical problems exist:*

Hepatic function impairment or

Surgery, recent

(increased risk of disseminated intravascular coagulation, fibrinolysis, or thrombosis)

Sensitivity to factor IX

Sensitivity to mouse protein
(risk of allergic reaction to protein, which is present in monoclonal antibody–derived product, *Mononine*)

**Patient monitoring**

The following may be especially important in patient monitoring (other tests may be warranted in some patients, depending on condition; » = major clinical significance):

Activated partial thromboplastin time (APTT) tests
Plasma fibrinogen determinations
Platelet count and
Prothrombin time (PT) tests
(recommended daily during therapy to detect disseminated intravascular coagulation [DIC]; prolonged APTT and PT test results in combination with a reduced fibrinogen concentration and thrombocytopenia are highly suggestive of DIC; additional laboratory findings that further corroborate the diagnosis of DIC include prolonged thrombin time, an increase in plasma D-dimer and fibrinogen degradation products, and a decrease in plasma clotting factors)

Factor IX plasma, determinations
(recommended daily during therapy to assure that adequate factor IX concentrations have been achieved and are maintained)

## Side/Adverse Effects

Note: To reduce the risk of transmission of viruses by blood and blood components, potential blood donors are screened, and donor blood is tested and must be found negative for antibodies to human immunodeficiency virus (HIV), hepatitis B core antigen, hepatitis C (non-A, non-B) virus, and for hepatitis B surface antigen. The concentration of alanine aminotransferase (ALT) also must be within normal limits. However, these precautions are not totally effective in eliminating viral infectivity. To further reduce the risk, factor IX products are treated utilizing one or more methods of viral inactivation. Some of the methods employed include dry heating, vapor heating, heating in solvent suspension, use of solvent detergent, immunoaffinity chromatography, and ultrafiltration. These processes substantially decrease the risk of transmission of HIV, hepatitis B, and hepatitis C (non-A, non-B) viruses.

Approximately 1 to 3% of patients treated with factor IX products develop inhibitors, or antibodies, which neutralize the procoagulant activity of factor IX. Patients with inhibitor antibodies to factor IX may be treated with increased quantities of factor IX, which complex with and thereby inactivate the antibodies, or with an anti-inhibitor coagulant complex, which directly activates factor X. However, the success of either of these treatment options is variable. Recombinant activated factors VII and X are currently undergoing clinical trials to assess safety and efficacy in the treatment of patients with factor IX inhibitor antibodies.

The following side/adverse effects have been selected on the basis of their potential clinical significance (possible signs and symptoms in parentheses where appropriate)—not necessarily inclusive:

**Those indicating need for medical attention**

Incidence more frequent
*Disseminated intravascular coagulation* (cyanosis [bluish coloring], especially of the hands and feet; ecchymoses at injection sites [large, nonelevated blue or purplish patches in the skin]; excessive sweating; persistent bleeding or oozing from puncture sites or mucous membranes [bowel, mouth, nose, or urinary bladder]); *myocardial infarction* (anxiety; cold sweating; increased heart rate; nausea or vomiting; severe pain or pressure in the chest and/or the neck, back, or left arm; shortness of breath); *pulmonary embolism* (chest discomfort; convulsions; dizziness or lightheadedness when getting up from a lying or sitting position; shortness of breath or fast breathing); *thrombosis or thromboembolism* (pains in chest, groin, or legs [especially calves]; severe, sudden headache; sudden and unexplained shortness of breath; slurred speech; vision changes; and/or weakness or numbness in arm or legs; sudden loss of coordination)—depending on site of thrombus formation or embolization

Note: The nonactivated clotting factors II, VII, and X; activated clotting factors II, VII, IX, and X; and coagulant-active phospholipids present in prothrombin complex concentrates are thought to be largely responsible for the *thrombotic complications* described. These complications are less likely to occur after the administration of purified coagulation factor IX products *AlphaNine, AlphaNine SD,* and *Mononine*.

Incidence less frequent
*Anaphylaxis or other allergic reaction* (changes in facial skin color; fast or irregular breathing; puffiness or swelling of the eyelids or

around the eyes; shortness of breath, troubled breathing, tightness in chest, and/or wheezing; skin rash, hives, and/or itching)—may include anaphylactic shock with sudden, severe decrease in blood pressure and collapse; *injection reaction* (burning or stinging at injection site; changes in blood pressure or pulse rate; chills; drowsiness; fever; flushing [redness of face]; headache; nausea or vomiting; shortness of breath)—occurs with too rapid an injection rate

Note: An *allergic reaction* to mouse protein (incidence rare) may occur after the administration of the monoclonal antibody–derived product, *Mononine*.

## Patient Consultation

As an aid to patient consultation, refer to *Advice for the Patient, Factor IX (Systemic)*.

In providing consultation, consider emphasizing the following selected information (» = major clinical significance):

**Before using this medication**

» Conditions affecting use, especially:
Sensitivity to factor IX or to mouse protein
Use in children—Thrombotic complications are more likely to occur in premature infants and neonates, who are usually more sensitive than adults to the effects of factor IX

**Proper use of this medication**

» Proper preparation of medication: bringing dry concentrate and diluent to room temperature before reconstitution; when reconstituting, directing stream of diluent against side of vial of concentrate to prevent foaming; gently swirling vial to dissolve contents; not shaking vigorously
» Administering within 3 hours of reconstitution
» Use of plastic disposable syringe and filter needle; safe handling and disposal of syringe and needle
» Proper dosing
Missed dose: Contacting physician immediately for instructions
» Proper storage

**Precautions while using this medication**

Need for patients newly diagnosed with hemophilia to receive hepatitis B vaccine
» Notifying physician if medication seems less effective than usual; this may indicate the development of antibodies to factor IX
» Need to carry identification stating condition

**Side/adverse effects**

Signs and symptoms of potential adverse effects, including disseminated intravascular coagulation, myocardial infarction, pulmonary embolism, thrombosis or thromboembolism, and allergic reaction to factor IX or mouse protein

## General Dosing Information

Factor IX products are recommended for intravenous use only.

Factor IX products should be administered via plastic disposable syringes because the proteins present tend to adhere to the ground-glass surface of all-glass syringes.

Factor IX products should be filtered before administration.

Each vial of factor IX concentrate is labeled with the factor IX activity expressed in International Units (IU) per vial. This potency assignment is referenced to the World Health Organization International Standard. One IU of factor IX activity per kg of body weight is approximately equal to the factor IX activity in 1 mL of fresh plasma, and increases the plasma concentration of factor IX by 1%. The specific factor IX activity of the prothrombin complex concentrates ranges from 0.7 to 3 IU per mg of total protein. The specific factor IX activities of coagulation factor IX products *AlphaNine* and *AlphaNine SD* are ≥ 50 IU per mg of total protein, whereas the specific factor IX activity of *Mononine* is 180 to 200 IU per mg of total protein. Although the dose of factor IX should be individualized for each patient based on body weight, type of hemorrhage, and desired plasma factor IX concentration, the following formula may be used as a guide in determining dosage:

Dose factor IX (IU) = Body weight (kg) × Desired factor IX increase (% of normal) × 1 IU/kg

## Parenteral Dosage Forms

### FACTOR IX COMPLEX USP

Note: *Bebulin VH* may be administered at a rate ≤2 mL per minute, *Konÿne 80* at a rate of 100 IU per minute, *Profilnine Heat-Treated* at a rate ≤10 mL per minute, and *Proplex T* at a rate between 2 and 3 mL per minute. However, the rate at which factor IX complex is administered should be guided by the comfort of the patient.

**Usual adult and adolescent dose**
Hemophilia B—
 Prophylaxis of spontaneous hemorrhage:
  Intravenous, 20 to 40 IU per kg of body weight, administered twice
   a week.
 Treatment of hemorrhage:
  Mild to moderate hemorrhage: Intravenous, 25 to 55 IU per kg of
   body weight, or a quantity sufficient to raise the plasma factor
   IX concentration to 20 to 40% of normal, administered once a
   day for one to two days.
  Severe hemorrhage: Intravenous, 60 to 70 IU per kg of body
   weight, or a quantity sufficient to raise the plasma factor IX
   concentration to 20 to 60% of normal, administered every ten
   to twelve hours for two to three days.
 Control of perisurgical hemostasis:
  Tooth extraction: Intravenous, 50 to 60 IU per kg of body weight,
   or a quantity sufficient to raise the plasma factor IX concentration to 40 to 60% of normal, administered one hour prior to
   the procedure. The dose may be repeated if bleeding occurs.
  Other surgery: Intravenous, 50 to 95 IU per kg of body weight, or
   a quantity sufficient to raise the plasma factor IX concentration
   to 25 to 60% of normal, administered one hour prior to surgery
   and repeated every twelve to twenty-four hours after surgery
   for at least seven days.
Hemophilia A—
 Prevention and control of bleeding in patients with inhibitors to factor
  VIII:
  Intravenous, 75 IU per kg of body weight. The dose may be repeated after twelve hours, if necessary.
Factor VII deficiency—
 Control of perisurgical hemostasis:
  *Proplex T:* Intravenous, a quantity sufficient to raise the plasma
   factor VII concentration to 25% of normal, administered prior
   to the procedure with repeat doses every four to six hours after
   the procedure, as needed, for at least seven days. To estimate
   the dose of factor IX complex required to treat factor VII deficiency, the following formula may be used:
   Dose factor IX complex (IU) = Body weight (kg) × Desired factor
    VII increase (% of normal) × 0.5 IU/kg
Anticoagulant-induced hemorrhage—
 Intravenous, 1500 IU, administered with vitamin K₁, if needed in severe cases.

**Usual pediatric dose**
See *Usual adult and adolescent dose.*

**Size(s) usually available**
U.S.—
 500 IU of factor IX with sterile water for injection provided as diluent
  (Rx) [*Konȳne 80* (diluent 20 mL)].
 1000 IU or less of factor IX, as specified on the label, with sterile
  water for injection provided as diluent (Rx) [*Proplex T* (heparin
  ≤1.5 USP units per mL; diluent 10 mL)].
 1000 IU of factor IX, with sterile water for injection provided as diluent (Rx) [*Konȳne 80* (diluent 40 mL); *Profilnine Heat-Treated*
  (diluent 10 mL)].
 1200 IU or less of factor IX, as specified on the label, with sterile
  water for injection provided as diluent (Rx) [*Bebulin VH* (heparin
  ≤0.15 IU per IU of factor IX; diluent 20 mL)].
 1500 IU of factor IX, with sterile water for injection provided as diluent (Rx) [*Profilnine Heat-Treated* (diluent 10 mL)].
Canada—
 1200 IU or less of factor IX, as specified on the label, with sterile
  water for injection provided as diluent (Rx) [*Bebulin VH* (heparin
  ≤0.15 IU per IU of factor IX; diluent 20 mL)].
Note: The products listed also contain factors II, VII, and X. The quantities may be specified on the individual product labels.

**Packaging and storage**
The dry concentrates are stored preferably between 2 and 8 °C (36 and
 46 °F). However, *Konȳne 80* and *Profilnine Heat-Treated* may be
 stored at room temperatures not exceeding 25 °C (77 °F) for up to 1
 month. The solution should not be refrigerated after reconstitution. The
 diluent should be protected from freezing.

**Preparation of dosage form**
The diluent and dry concentrate should be brought to room temperature
 prior to reconstitution. The solution should be gently swirled, not
 shaken, until all of the concentrate is dissolved. Reconstitution generally requires 5 to 10 minutes. The reconstituted solution should be
 approximately at room temperature at the time of administration.

Note: Heparin may be added to prothrombin complex concentrates at a
 concentration of 5 to 10 USP units per mL of reconstituted product.

The addition of heparin has been shown, in some cases, to reduce
 the likelihood of development of thrombotic complications.

**Stability**
Administration should begin within 3 hours after reconstitution. Partially
 used vials should be discarded.

**Incompatibilities**
It is recommended that factor IX complex, after reconstitution with the
 provided diluent, be administered through a separate line, by itself,
 and without mixing with other intravenous fluids or medications.

## COAGULATION FACTOR IX ( (HUMAN))

Note: *AlphaNine* and *AlphaNine SD* may be administered at a rate not
 exceeding 10 mL per minute, and *Mononine* at a rate of 2 mL per
 minute. However, the rate at which coagulation factor IX is administered should be guided by the comfort of the patient.

**Usual adult and adolescent dose**
Hemophilia B—
 Prophylaxis of spontaneous hemorrhage:
  Intravenous, 20 to 30 IU per kg of body weight, or a quantity
   sufficient to raise the plasma factor IX concentration to 15 to
   25% of normal. The dose may be repeated after twenty-four
   hours, if necessary.
 Treatment of hemorrhage:
  Mild to moderate hemorrhage: Intravenous, a quantity sufficient to
   raise the plasma factor IX concentration to 20 to 30% of normal, administered as a single dose.
  Severe hemorrhage: Intravenous, up to 75 IU per kg of body
   weight, or a quantity sufficient to raise the plasma factor IX
   concentration to 25 to 50% of normal, administered every
   eighteen to thirty hours, as needed.
 Control of perisurgical hemostasis:
  Tooth extraction: Intravenous, a quantity sufficient to raise the
   plasma factor IX concentration to 50% of normal, administered
   immediately prior to the procedure. The dose may be repeated
   if bleeding occurs.
  Other surgery: Intravenous, up to 75 IU per kg of body weight, or
   a quantity sufficient to raise the plasma factor IX concentration
   to 25 to 50% of normal, administered prior to surgery and
   repeated every eighteen to thirty hours after surgery for seven
   to ten days.

**Usual pediatric dose**
See *Usual adult and adolescent dose.*

**Size(s) usually available**
U.S.—
 250 IU, with sterile water for injection provided as diluent (Rx) [*Mononine* (factors II, VII, and X ≤0.0025 units per unit of factor IX;
  sodium chloride 66 mmol; mouse protein ≤50 nanograms per 100
  units of factor IX; diluent 2.5 mL)].
 500 IU, with sterile water for injection provided as diluent (Rx)
  [*AlphaNine* (factors II and VII <5 units per 100 IU of factor IX;
  factor X <20 units per IU of factor IX; heparin ≤0.04 USP units
  per IU of factor IX; dextrose ≤1 mg per IU of factor IX; diluent
  10 mL); *AlphaNine SD* (factors II and VII <5 units per 100 IU of
  factor IX; factor X <20 units per IU of factor IX; heparin ≤0.04
  USP units per IU of factor IX; dextrose ≤1 mg per IU of factor
  IX; diluent 10 mL); *Mononine* (factors II, VII, and X ≤0.0025
  units per unit of factor IX; sodium chloride 66 mmol; mouse protein ≤50 nanograms per 100 units of factor IX; diluent 5 mL)].
 1000 IU, with sterile water for injection provided as diluent (Rx)
  [*AlphaNine* (factors II and VII <5 units per 100 IU of factor IX;
  factor X <20 units per IU of factor IX; heparin ≤0.04 USP units
  per IU of factor IX; dextrose ≤1 mg per IU of factor IX; diluent
  10 mL); *AlphaNine SD* (factors II and VII <5 units per 100 IU of
  factor IX; factor X <20 units per IU of factor IX; heparin ≤0.04
  USP units per IU of factor IX; dextrose ≤1 mg per IU of factor
  IX; diluent 10 mL); *Mononine* (factors II, VII, and X ≤0.0025
  units per unit of factor IX; sodium chloride 66 mmol; mouse protein ≤50 nanograms per 100 units of factor IX; diluent 10 mL)].
 1500 IU, with sterile water for injection provided as diluent (Rx)
  [*AlphaNine* (factors II and VII <5 units per 100 IU of factor IX;
  factor X <20 units per IU of factor IX; dextrose ≤1 mg per IU
  of factor IX; diluent 10 mL); *AlphaNine SD* (factors II and VII
  <5 units per 100 IU of factor IX; factor X <20 units per IU of
  factor IX; dextrose ≤1 mg per IU of factor IX; diluent 10 mL)].
Canada—
 500 IU, with sterile water for injection provided as diluent (Rx)
  [*AlphaNine* (factors II and VII <5 units per 100 IU of factor IX;
  factor X <20 units per IU of factor IX; dextrose ≤1 mg per IU
  of factor IX; diluent 10 mL)].

1000 IU, with sterile water for injection provided as diluent (Rx) [*AlphaNine* (factors II and VII <5 units per 100 IU of factor IX; factor X <20 units per IU of factor IX; dextrose ≤1 mg per IU of factor IX; diluent 10 mL)].

1500 IU, with sterile water for injection provided as diluent (Rx) [*AlphaNine* (factors II and VII <5 units per 100 IU of factor IX; factor X <20 units per IU of factor IX; dextrose ≤1 mg per IU of factor IX; diluent 10 mL)].

## Packaging and storage

The dry concentrates preferably are stored between 2 and 8 °C (36 and 46 °F). However, *Mononine* may be stored at room temperatures not exceeding 30 °C (86 °F) for up to 1 month. The diluent should be protected from freezing.

## Preparation of dosage form

The diluent and dry concentrate should be brought to room temperature prior to reconstitution. The reconstituted solution should be gently swirled, not shaken, until all of the concentrate is dissolved. Recon-

stitution generally requires 1 to 5 minutes. The reconstituted solution should be approximately at room temperature at the time of administration.

## Stability

Administration should begin within 3 hours after reconstitution. Partially used vials should be discarded.

## Incompatibilities

It is recommended that coagulation factor IX, after reconstitution with the provided diluent, be administered through a separate line, by itself, and without mixing with other intravenous fluids or medications.

## Selected Bibliography

Thompson AR. Factor IX concentrates for clinical use. Semin Thromb Hemost 1993; 19: 25-36.

Revised: 08/27/93

---

# FAMCICLOVIR Systemic†

VA CLASSIFICATION (Primary): AM800

Note: For a listing of dosage forms and brand names by country availability, see *Dosage Forms* section(s). For a listing of brand names for the articles in this monograph, refer to the General Index.

†Not commercially available in Canada.

## Category

Antiviral (systemic).

## Indications

### Accepted

Herpes zoster (treatment)—Famciclovir is indicated in the treatment of herpes zoster infections (shingles) caused by varicella-zoster virus (VZV). Famciclovir has been found to decrease the duration of post-herpetic neuralgia (defined as pain at or following healing) when compared to placebo (55 to 62 days versus 128 days, respectively). Famciclovir has also been found to be equivalent to acyclovir in decreasing the duration of acute pain. Therapy is most effective when started within 48 hours of the onset of rash. Famciclovir has been studied only in healthy adults. There are no data on its safety and efficacy in children or in immunocompromised persons, or on its efficacy in the treatment of ophthalmic zoster or disseminated zoster.

## Pharmacology/Pharmacokinetics

### Physicochemical characteristics

Molecular weight—321.3.

### Mechanism of action/Effect

Famciclovir is a pro-drug; it is the diacetyl 6-deoxy analog of the active antiviral compound, penciclovir. Penciclovir is phosphorylated by viral thymidine kinase to penciclovir monophosphate, which is then converted to penciclovir triphosphate by cellular kinases. Penciclovir inhibits herpes viral DNA synthesis, and, therefore, replication. Penciclovir does not inhibit DNA synthesis in uninfected cells because it is phosphorylated only in herpes-infected cells.

Penciclovir has antiviral activity against herpes simplex virus type 1 (HSV-1), HSV-2, varicella-zoster virus (VZV), and Epstein-Barr virus. *In vitro* studies have shown that penciclovir triphosphate has greater intracellular stability in HSV-2–infected cells than does acyclovir triphosphate. Also, unlike acyclovir, the antiviral activity of penciclovir persists in the absence of extracellular drug.

### Absorption

Famciclovir is absorbed in the upper intestine and rapidly converted in the intestinal wall to the active compound, penciclovir. The bioavailability of penciclovir after oral administration of famciclovir is approximately 77%.

Famciclovir may be taken without regard to meals; although a decrease in the time to peak serum concentration and peak serum concentration of penciclovir was seen when famciclovir was taken with food or after a meal, there was no decrease in the extent of systemic availability.

### Distribution

The steady-state volume of distribution of penciclovir is approximately 1 liter per kilogram (L/kg).

### Protein binding

Low (20 to 25%).

### Biotransformation

Famciclovir is deacetylated, and then oxidized to form the active agent, penciclovir. Little or no famciclovir is detected in the plasma or urine. Inactive metabolites include 6-deoxy penciclovir, monoacetylated penciclovir, and monoacetylated 6-deoxypenciclovir, all of which account for < 1.5% of the dose.

### Half-life

Normal renal function—
2.1 to 3 hours.
Severe renal failure (creatinine clearance < 30 mL/min [0.33 mL/sec]—
10 to 13 hours.
Intracellular half-life of penciclovir triphosphate—
In HSV-1–infected cells—Approximately 10 hours.
In HSV-2–infected cells—Approximately 20 hours.
In VZV-infected cells—Approximately 7 hours.

### Time to peak plasma concentration

0.7 to 0.9 hours.

### Peak plasma concentration

3.3 to 4.2 mcg/mL [10.3 to 13.1 micromoles/L] after a single oral dose (fasting) of 500 mg.

### Elimination

Renal (glomerular filtration and tubular secretion); 60 to 65% of an oral dose is recovered as penciclovir in the urine; 27% in the feces over 72 hours.

In dialysis—It is not known if hemodialysis removes penciclovir from the blood.

## Precautions to Consider

### Carcinogenicity

Dietary carcinogenicity studies of famciclovir were conducted in rats and mice at the doses listed below for approximately 1.5 years. A significant increase in the incidence of mammary adenocarcinoma was seen in female rats receiving 600 mg per kg (mg/kg) per day (1.5 times the human systemic exposure at 500 mg three times a day, based on the area under the plasma-concentration-time curve [AUC] for penciclovir). Marginal increases in the incidence of subcutaneous tissue fibrosarcomas or squamous cell carcinomas of the skin were seen in female rats and male mice dosed at 600 mg/kg per day (0.4 times the human exposure, based on AUC for penciclovir). There was no increase in tumor incidence reported in male rats treated with doses of up to 240 mg/kg per day (0.9 times the human AUC), or in female mice treated with doses of up to 600 mg/kg per day (0.4 times the human AUC).

### Mutagenicity

Famciclovir and penciclovir were negative in *in vitro* tests for gene mutations in bacteria (*S. typhimurium* and *E. coli*) and unscheduled DNA synthesis in mammalian HeLa 83 cells. Famciclovir was also negative in the L5178Y mouse lymphoma assay, the *in vivo* mouse micronucleus test, and rat dominant lethal study. Famciclovir induced increases in polyploidy in human lymphocytes *in vitro* in the absence of chromosomal damage.

Penciclovir was positive in the L5178Y mouse lymphoma assay for gene mutation/chromosomal aberrations, with and without metabolic activation. In human lymphocytes, penciclovir caused chromosomal aberrations in the absence of metabolic activation. Penciclovir caused an increased incidence of micronuclei in mouse bone marrow *in vivo* when administered intravenously at doses highly toxic to bone marrow, but not when administered orally.

## Pregnancy/Reproduction

Fertility—Testicular toxicity was observed in rats, mice, and dogs following repeated administration of famciclovir or penciclovir. Testicular changes included atrophy of the seminiferous tubules, reduction in sperm count, and/or increased incidence of sperm with abnormal morphology or reduced motility. The degree of toxicity was related to dose and duration of exposure. In male rats, decreased fertility was observed after 10 weeks of dosing at 500 mg/kg per day (1.9 times the human AUC). Testicular toxicity was observed following chronic administration to mice (104 weeks) and dogs (26 weeks) at doses of 600 mg/kg per day (0.4 times the human AUC) and 150 mg/kg per day (107 times the human AUC), respectively.

Famciclovir had no effect on general reproductive performance or fertility in female rats at doses up to 1000 mg/kg per day (3.6 times the human AUC).

Pregnancy—No adequate and well-controlled studies have been done in pregnant women.

No adverse effects were observed on embryo-fetal development in rats and rabbits given oral famciclovir at doses up to 1000 mg/kg per day (approximately 3.6 and 1.8 times the human exposure based on AUC, respectively), and intravenous doses of 360 mg/kg per day in rats (2 times the human exposure based on body surface area [BSA]) and 120 mg/kg per day in rabbits (1.5 times the human exposure based on BSA). Also, no adverse effects were observed after intravenous administration of penciclovir to rats given 80 mg/kg per day (0.4 times the human exposure based on BSA), and rabbits given 60 mg/kg per day (0.7 times the human exposure based on BSA).

FDA Pregnancy Category B.

## Breast-feeding

Following oral administration of famciclovir, it is not known whether penciclovir is distributed into human breast milk. However, it has been found to pass into the milk of lactating rats at concentrations higher than those seen in the plasma. Also, because of the tumorigenicity seen in rats, it is recommended that either breast-feeding or administration of famciclovir to the mother be discontinued.

## Pediatrics

Safety and efficacy have not been established in children up to 18 years of age.

## Geriatrics

Studies performed to date have not demonstrated geriatric-specific problems that would limit the usefulness of famciclovir in the elderly. However, elderly patients are more likely to have an age-related decrease in renal function, which may require an adjustment of famciclovir dosage or dosing interval.

## Drug interactions and/or related problems

The following drug interactions and/or related problems have been selected on the basis of their potential clinical significance (possible mechanism in parentheses where appropriate)—not necessarily inclusive (» = major clinical significance):

Note: Combinations containing any of the following medications, depending on the amount present, may also interact with this medication.

Probenecid
(probenecid may compete with penciclovir for active tubular secretion, resulting in increased plasma concentrations of penciclovir)

## Medical considerations/Contraindications

The medical considerations/contraindications included here have been selected on the basis of their potential clinical significance (reasons given in parentheses where appropriate)—not necessarily inclusive (» = major clinical significance).

*Risk-benefit should be considered when the following medical problem exists:*

» Renal function impairment
(because penciclovir is renally excreted, patients with renal function impairment may be at increased risk of toxicity; patients with a creatinine clearance of < 60 mL/min [1 mL/sec] require a reduction in dose)

## Side/Adverse Effects

Note: No serious side effects have been noted to date with the administration of famciclovir.

**Those indicating need for medical attention only if they continue or are bothersome**
Incidence more frequent
   *Headache*
Incidence less frequent
   *Dizziness; fatigue* (unusual tiredness or weakness); *gastrointestinal disturbances* (diarrhea; nausea; vomiting)

## Patient Consultation

As an aid to patient consultation, refer to *Advice for the Patient, Famciclovir (Systemic).*

In providing consultation, consider emphasizing the following selected information (» = major clinical significance):

**Before using this medication**
» Conditions affecting use, especially:
   Breast-feeding—Because of the potential for tumorigenicity seen in rats, it is recommended that either breast-feeding or famciclovir be discontinued
   Use in children—Safety and efficacy have not been established in children up to 18 years of age
   Other medical problems, especially renal function impairment

**Proper use of this medication**
   Initiating use of famciclovir at the earliest sign or symptom; it is most effective when started within 48 hours of the onset of rash
   Famciclovir may be taken with meals
» Compliance with full course of therapy; not using more often or for longer than prescribed
» Proper dosing
   Missed dose: Taking as soon as possible; not taking if almost time for next dose; not doubling doses
» Proper storage

**Precautions while using this medication**
   Checking with physician if no improvement within a few days
   Keeping affected areas as clean and dry as possible; wearing loose-fitting clothing to avoid irritation of lesions

## General Dosing Information

Therapy should be initiated as soon as possible following the onset of signs and symptoms of varicella-zoster infection. Treatment was started within 72 hours of the onset of rash in clinical studies; however, famciclovir was found to be more useful if started within 48 hours.

In clinical trials, the effect of famciclovir on the resolution of rash was most pronounced in patients over 50 years of age.

Famciclovir tablets may be taken with meals since absorption has not been shown to be significantly affected by food.

Adults with impaired renal function may require a change in dosing, as follows:

| Creatinine Clearance (mL/min)/ (mL/sec) | Recommended dose |
| --- | --- |
| ≥60/1.0 | 500 mg every 8 hours |
| 40–59/0.67–0.98 | 500 mg every 12 hours |
| 20–39/0.33–0.65 | 500 mg every 24 hours |

There are not enough data to recommend a dosage for patients with a creatinine clearance of less than 20 mL/min (0.33 mL/sec).

## Oral Dosage Forms

### FAMCICLOVIR TABLETS

**Usual adult dose**
Antiviral—
   Oral, 500 mg every eight hours for seven days.

**Usual pediatric dose**
Safety and efficacy have not been established for patients less than 18 years of age.

**Strength(s) usually available**
U.S.—
   500 mg (Rx) [*Famvir*].
Canada—
   Not commercially available.

**Packaging and storage**
Store between 15 and 25 °C (59 and 77 °F), in a tight container, unless otherwise specified by manufacturer.

**Auxiliary labeling**
• Continue medicine for full time of treatment.

Developed: 11/28/94

---

**FAMOTIDINE**—See *Histamine H₂-receptor Antagonists (Systemic)*

# FAT EMULSIONS   Systemic

VA CLASSIFICATION (Primary): TN300

Note: For a listing of dosage forms and brand names by country availability, see *Dosage Forms* section(s). For a listing of brand names for the articles in this monograph, refer to the General Index.

## Category

Nutritional supplement (fatty acid).

## Indications

### Accepted

Fatty acid deficiency (prophylaxis and treatment)—Intravenous fat emulsions are used to prevent or reverse fatty acid deficiency and provide a source of calories for patients requiring parenteral nutrition.

Deficiency of essential fatty acids may lead to anemia, desquamative dermatitis, growth retardation in infants, hepatic dysfunction, impaired wound healing, loss of hair, and thrombocytopenia.

## Pharmacology/Pharmacokinetics

### Mechanism of action/Effect

Infused fat particles cause a transient increase in plasma triglyceride concentrations. The triglycerides are then hydrolyzed to free fatty acids and glycerol by the enzyme lipoprotein lipase. The free fatty acids either enter the tissues (to be oxidized or resynthesized to triglycerides for storage) or circulate bound to albumin in the plasma, and subsequently may undergo hepatic oxidation or conversion to very low–density lipoproteins (VLDL) that re-enter the bloodstream.

### Other actions/effects

Fat emulsions also contain phosphatides (a component of which is choline) as an emulsifier, and glycerin to adjust tonicity. Phosphatides are involved in the formation of membrane structures; choline prevents deposition of fat in the liver; and glycerin is metabolized to carbon dioxide and glycogen or is used in the synthesis of fats.

### Protein binding

Bound to albumin.

### Biotransformation

Hepatic.

## Precautions to Consider

### Cross-sensitivity and/or related problems

Patients sensitive to eggs, soybeans, or legumes may be sensitive to fat emulsions.

### Pregnancy/Reproduction

Pregnancy—Adequate and well-controlled studies in humans have not been done. It is not known if fat emulsions can cause fetal harm when administered to a pregnant woman or can affect reproduction capacity.

Adequate and well-controlled studies have not been done in animals.

FDA Pregnancy Category C.

### Breast-feeding

It is not known whether fat emulsions are distributed into human breast milk. However, problems in humans have not been documented.

### Pediatrics

Fat emulsions must be administered to preterm infants with extreme caution. These infants have poor clearance of intravenous fat emulsions. The resultant increase of free fatty acid plasma concentrations may lead to fat accumulation in the lungs and possibly death.

### Geriatrics

Appropriate studies on the relationship of age to the effects of fat emulsions have not been performed in the geriatric population. However, no geriatrics-specific problems have been documented to date.

### Laboratory value alterations

The following have been selected on the basis of their potential clinical significance (possible effect in parentheses where appropriate)—not necessarily inclusive (» = major clinical significance):

With diagnostic test results

Colorimetric laboratory analysis

     (serum lipids may interfere with colorimetric laboratory analysis; blood samples should be drawn in the morning prior to infusion of fat emulsions)

With physiology/laboratory test values

Alkaline phosphatase, serum and

Bilirubin, serum and

Cholesterol, serum and

Phospholipid, serum and

Transaminase, serum and

Triglyceride, plasma

     (concentrations may be increased)

### Medical considerations/Contraindications

The medical considerations/contraindications included here have been selected on the basis of their potential clinical significance (reasons given in parentheses where appropriate)—not necessarily inclusive (» = major clinical significance).

*Risk-benefit should be considered when the following medical problems exist:*

Anemia

     (condition may be exacerbated)

Blood coagulation disorders or

» Conditions in which there is a disturbance in normal fat metabolism, such as:

Diabetes, uncompensated or

Hyperlipidemia, pathologic or

Lipid nephrosis or

Pancreatitis, acute, if accompanied by hyperlipemia or

Renal insufficiency

     (fat emulsions may increase serum lipids and exacerbate these conditions)

Hepatic damage, severe

     (fat emulsions undergo biotransformation in the liver)

Immunocompromised patient

     (fat emulsions have been reported to alter the immune response)

Jaundice

     (fat emulsions increase free fatty acids, which may displace bilirubin bound to albumin)

Platelet dysfunction disorders

     (fat emulsions have been reported to cause hypercoagulability)

Pulmonary disease

     (fat emulsions may exacerbate condition; slowing infusion rate has been found to reduce pulmonary problems)

Sensitivity to fat emulsions

Sepsis

     (fat emulsions have been found to alter the immune response and decrease reticuloendothelial system function, which could exacerbate the condition)

### Patient monitoring

The following may be especially important in patient monitoring (other tests may be warranted in some patients, depending on condition; » = major clinical significance):

Blood coagulation tests and

Hemogram and

Platelet counts

     (determinations may be required at weekly intervals, especially during continuous therapy)

Bilirubin concentrations, serum and

Cholesterol concentrations, serum and

Hepatic function determinations and

Phospholipid concentrations, serum and

Triglyceride concentrations, plasma

     (determinations may be required at weekly intervals, especially in premature infants, to prevent hyperlipemia)

## Side/Adverse Effects

The following side/adverse effects have been selected on the basis of their potential clinical significance (possible signs and symptoms in parentheses where appropriate)—not necessarily inclusive:

### Those indicating need for medical attention

Incidence more frequent

     *Sepsis* (chills, fever, or sore throat)

Incidence rare
   *Allergic reactions, specifically chills; dyspnea,* (difficulty in breathing); *fever; or urticaria* (hives); *hematologic abnormalities, specifically anemia* (unusual tiredness or weakness); *hypercoagulability; or thrombocytopenia* (unusual bleeding or bruising)—more frequent with prolonged use; *hyperlipemia* (fever; headache; unusual irritability)—more frequent with prolonged use; *jaundice* (yellow eyes or skin)—more frequent with prolonged use; *pulmonary effects, specifically chest or back pain, or cyanosis* (bluish color of skin)

**Those indicating need for medical attention only if they continue or are bothersome**
Incidence more frequent
   *Thrombophlebitis* (redness, swelling, or pain at injection site)
Incidence less frequent
   *Diarrhea; dizziness; flushing; nausea and vomiting*

## Overdose

For more information on the management of overdose or unintentional ingestion **contact a Poison Control Center** (see *Poison Control Center Listing*).

**Treatment of overdose**
Discontinue therapy.
Plasma lipid clearance should be determined before restarting therapy.

## Patient Consultation

As an aid to patient consultation, refer to *Advice for the Patient, Fat Emulsions (Systemic).*

In providing consultation, consider emphasizing the following selected information (» = major clinical significance):

**Before using this medication**
» Conditions affecting use, especially:
      Sensitivity to eggs, legumes, soybeans, or fat emulsions
      Use in children—May cause or worsen lung problems or jaundice in premature infants
      Other medical problems, especially problems with lipid metabolism

**Proper use of this medication**
» Proper dosing
» Proper storage

**Precautions while using this medication**
   Importance of close monitoring by physician
   Importance of reporting any infections to physician

**Side/adverse effects**
   Signs of potential side effects, especially allergic reactions, hematologic abnormalities, hyperlipemia, jaundice, pulmonary effects, and sepsis

## General Dosing Information

Although the manufacturer does not recommend the use of a filter during administration of fat emulsions, 1.2 micron filters are used in practice by some clinicians. Filters smaller than 1.2 microns may filter out lipids, or disrupt the stability of the emulsion.

Fat emulsions extract small amounts of plasticizer from PVC containers.

Fat emulsions can be infused into the same central or peripheral vein as amino acids by use of a Y-type infusion set, which allows mixing of the 2 just before they enter the vein.

The combination of parenteral amino acids, dextrose, and fat emulsions in one container (known as 3-in-1, or total nutrient admixture [TNA]) is stable for short periods of time, usually 24 hours, depending on the formulation. The compatibility of electrolytes, vitamins, trace metals, and a few drugs has been evaluated in some combinations, but the stability depends on the formulation used. The order of mixing, final pH, and cation content are important; product information should be consulted.

The addition of 1 or 2 units of heparin per mL to fat emulsions may result in a more rapid clearance of lipemia, may minimize the risks associated with hypercoagulability, and may prevent catheter thrombosis; however, its use is generally not recommended by most clinicians.

## Parenteral Dosage Forms

### FAT EMULSIONS INJECTION

**Usual adult and adolescent dose**
Nutritional supplement—
   Intravenous, 0.5 mL of 20% fat emulsions per minute or 1 mL of 10% fat emulsions per minute for the first fifteen to thirty minutes with the rate then increased to allow no more than 500 mL of the 10% fat emulsions or 250 mL of the 20% fat emulsions to be infused over a period of four to six hours.

Note: Fat emulsions should be administered via peripheral vein or central venous catheter.

**Usual adult prescribing limits**
The daily dose of fat emulsions should not exceed 3 grams per kilogram of body weight.

**Usual pediatric dose**
Nutritional supplement—
   Intravenous, 0.1 mL of 10% or 20% fat emulsions per minute for the first fifteen minutes with the rate then increased to allow no more than 100 mL of 10% fat emulsions per hour or 50 mL of the 20% fat emulsions per hour.

Note: Fat emulsions should be administered via peripheral vein or central venous catheter. A syringe pump unit is used to control administration rates for infants who require small volumes of fat emulsions.

**Usual pediatric prescribing limits**
The daily dose of fat emulsions should not exceed 4 grams per kilogram of body weight.

**Strength(s) usually available**
   See *Table 1*, page 1419.

**Packaging and storage**
Store below 40 °C (104 °F), preferably between 15 and 30 °C (59 and 86 °F), unless otherwise specified by manufacturer. Protect from freezing.

**Stability**
Fat emulsions have been shown to support bacterial and fungal growth; visual changes in the emulsion were not noted. The addition of fat emulsions to total parenteral nutrition (TPN) solutions has been found to enhance the ability of these solutions to support bacterial growth.

**Incompatibilities**
Depending on the product used, the concentration, the temperature, and the length of mixing time, albumin, amikacin, aminophylline, ampicillin, calcium salts, cephalothin, gentamicin, iron dextran, magnesium chloride, methicillin, penicillin, phenytoin, potassium chloride, tetracycline, tobramycin, and vitamin B complex have been found to be physically incompatible with fat emulsions when mixed directly with the emulsion. Amikacin, methyldopate, and tetracycline have been found to be physically incompatible with Y-site injection. Consult the medical literature for additional information.

## Selected Bibliography

Wan J. Invited comment: lipids and the development of immune dysfunction and infection. JPEN 1988; 12[6]: 43S-52S.

Revised: 05/12/93

## Table 1. Strengths Usually Available

| | Safflower Oil | Soybean Oil | Fatty Acid Component (%) Linoleic Acid | Oleic Acid | Palmitic Acid | Linolenic Acid | Stearic Acid | Egg Phospholipid (%) | Glycerin (%) | Calories per mL | Osmolarity (mOsm) per Liter | pH |
|---|---|---|---|---|---|---|---|---|---|---|---|---|
| ***Intralipid*** | | | | | | | | | | | | |
| 10% [U.S.] (Rx) | | 10 | 50 | 26 | 10 | 9 | 3.5 | 1.2 | 2.25 | 1.1 | 260 | 6–8.9 |
| 10% [Canada] (Rx) | | 10 | 50 | 26.5 | 10.5 | 8.5 | 3.5 | 1.2 | 2.25 | 1.1 | 300 | 8 |
| 20% [U.S.] (Rx) | | 20 | 50 | 26 | 10 | 9 | 3.5 | 1.2 | 2.25 | 2 | 260 | 6–8.9 |
| 20% [Canada] (Rx) | | 20 | 50 | 26.5 | 10.5 | 8.5 | 3.5 | 1.2 | 2.25 | 2 | 350 | 8 |
| ***Liposyn II*** | | | | | | | | Up to: | | | | |
| 10% [U.S.] (Rx) | 5 | 5 | 65.8 | 17.7 | 8.8 | 4.2 | 3.4 | 1.2 | 2.5 | 1.1 | 276 | 8 |
| 10% [Canada] (Rx) | 5 | 5 | 65.8 | 17.7 | 8.8 | 4.2 | 3.4 | 0.7 | 2.5 | 1.1 | 276 | 8.3 |
| 20% [U.S.] (Rx) | 10 | 10 | 65.8 | 17.7 | 8.8 | 4.2 | 3.4 | 1.2 | 2.5 | 1.1 | 258 | 8.3 |
| 20% [Canada] (Rx) | 10 | 10 | 65.8 | 17.7 | 8.8 | 4.2 | 3.4 | 1.2 | 2.5 | 2 | 258 | 8.3 |
| ***Liposyn III*** | | | | | | | | | | | | |
| 10% [U.S.] (Rx) | | 10 | 54.5 | 22.4 | 10.5 | 8.3 | 4.2 | 1.2 | 2.5 | 1.1 | 284 | 8.3 |
| 20% [U.S.] (Rx) | | 20 | 54.5 | 22.4 | 10.5 | 8.3 | 4.2 | 1.2 | 2.5 | 2 | 292 | 8.3 |

# FECAL OCCULT BLOOD TEST KITS

This monograph includes information on the following: Fecal Occult Blood Test Kits for Clinic Use†; Fecal Occult Blood Test Kits for Home Use.

VA CLASSIFICATION (Primary): DX900

Note: For a listing of dosage forms and brand names by country availability, see *Dosage Forms* section(s). For a listing of brand names for the articles in this monograph, refer to the General Index.

†Not commercially available in Canada.

## Category

Diagnostic aid (occult bleeding).

## Indications

### Accepted

Carcinoma, colorectal (diagnosis adjunct) and

Bleeding, gastrointestinal (diagnosis)—When used as a screening device, a fecal occult blood test detects a small amount of blood in the feces, which may be from intermittently bleeding colon or rectal lesions. This bleeding may be an early sign of neoplasias, which are frequently fatal when allowed to reach the stage at which they produce symptoms such as abdominal complaints, anemia, or change in bowel habits.

Current American Cancer Society recommendations for colorectal cancer detection in asymptomatic persons not at increased risk include digital rectal examination yearly for persons age 40 and over and a stool guaiac test annually and sigmoidoscopy every 3 to 5 years for persons over 50.

Persons at increased risk for colorectal cancer include those with a family history of colon polyps or cancer, prior cured colon or rectal cancers, prior breast, uterine, or ovarian cancer, inflammatory bowel disease, familial polyposis syndromes, or a history of adenomatous polyps. These patients should begin screening with fecal occult blood tests earlier than others, along with digital, radiologic, and endoscopic examinations according to their physicians' recommendations.

Fecal occult blood test is also used for the detection of other gastrointestinal bleeding.

### Unaccepted

Not intended for use in detecting blood in gastric contents.

## Pharmacology/Pharmacokinetics

### Physicochemical characteristics

Test consists of chromogen-impregnated slide or tape (*Colo-Rectal Test, ColoScreen, Hemoccult, HemaChek*), paper pad floated in toilet (*ColoCare, ColoScreen Self-Test, EZ Detect*), or pad wiped on anal area (*HemaWipe*). Most tests require the addition of a developer, an alcohol-hydrogen peroxide solution. The developer is usually sold only to the health professional. The test is easily developed by the addition of drops of the solution and observation for a color reaction. The appearance of color indicates the presence of small amounts of blood in the feces.

Gum guaiac, a heterogeneous natural compound, is used in most test kits. The active component, alpha-guaiaconic acid, is a colorless phenolic structure that is oxidized by hydrogen peroxide in the presence of peroxidases or catalases such as hemoglobin to a colored quinone, usually blue.

*ColoScreen Self-Test* uses a guaiacol derivative which turns red-orange. Tetramethylbenzidine is the chromogen for *EZ Detect* and *ColoCare*, producing a blue-green color. All available products include control areas to verify reactivity of the test kit.

*HemeSelect* is an immunochemical hemagglutination method specific for human hemoglobin, and is developed in professional laboratories.

## Precautions to Consider

### Laboratory value alterations

The following have been selected on the basis of their potential clinical significance (possible effect in parentheses where appropriate)—not necessarily inclusive (» = major clinical significance):

With results of *this* test
  *Due to other medications*
    Anti-inflammatories, nonsteroidal or
    Aspirin and other salicylates or
    Corticosteroids or

Reserpine or
Other gastrointestinal irritants
    (drugs which alter the integrity of the gastrointestinal tract may cause sufficient bleeding to produce positive fecal occult blood tests)
Ascorbic acid
    (ascorbic acid in excess of 250 mg per day may inhibit the guaiac test reaction, causing a false-negative result)
Rectal medications
    (medications given rectally may interfere with test results)
  *Due to diet (for guaiac tests only)*
Ascorbic acid
    (ascorbic acid in excess of 250 mg per day may inhibit the guaiac test reaction, causing a false-negative result)
Meat, red, rare
    (hemoglobin which is not completely denatured, such as in rare red meats, may cause false-positive tests)
Peroxidase-containing vegetables and fruits
    (when fecal samples are tested immediately after collection, some vegetables and fruits contain peroxidases which may cause false-positive reactions if eaten in very large quantities; these include turnips, horseradish, radishes, mushrooms, carrots, broccoli, cucumbers, cauliflower, cantaloupes, and grapefruit)
  *Due to medical problems or conditions*
Anal fissure or
Constipation or
Diarrhea or
Diverticulitis or
Esophageal irritation or varices or
Hematuria or
Hemorrhoids or
Menses or
Nosebleeds or
Polyps, benign or
Ulcerative colitis or
Ulcer, peptic or
Uterine bleeding
    (other sources of blood in the feces may give a positive reaction)
Non-bleeding tumors
    (tumors bleed intermittently and may not bleed during the test period, therefore producing a false-negative test; some experts suggest the use of additional dietary fiber, such as bran, peanuts, and popcorn, to abrade possible bleeding sites)
  *Due to test procedures*
Storage, prolonged
    (prolonged storage of the sample before developing may produce false-negative results)
    (deteriorated, heat-exposed, or outdated test materials may produce false-negative results)
Toilet bowl cleansers
    (bowl tests may be affected by toilet bowl cleansers)

## Patient Consultation

As an aid to patient consultation, refer to *Advice to the Patient, Fecal Occult Blood Test Kits.*

In providing consultation, consider emphasizing the following selected information (» = major clinical significance):

### Before using this test

Following kit directions about diet; kits vary in their instructions on rare meats and peroxidase-containing foods

Checking with physician about other medical conditions that may interfere with test results

Modifying medication therapy only as advised by physician

### Proper use of this test

Checking expiration date on kits and not using outdated materials

Reading kit instructions before starting the test; consulting a physician, nurse, or pharmacist, or calling the toll-free number in the kit for any questions

Following instructions carefully in taking 2 samples from different parts of the stool and sampling 3 consecutive bowel movements, unless diarrhea, constipation, or menses ensue

Avoiding prolonged storage of samples; card tests should be returned as soon as collected, if possible, and definitely not stored more than 5 days (14 days for *HemaWipe, HemeSelect, Hemoccult, Hemoccult SENSA*)

For tests being developed at home (bowl tests):

    Flushing toilet several times to clear bowl of cleansers or detergent, and flushing away urine, before using the bowl tests

    Timing test results carefully, as the color reactions may fade quickly

    Observing carefully for the color changes, and getting assistance if vision-impaired

    Observing control areas of the test materials to ensure proper reactivity of test materials

    Recording results for discussion with health care professional

For test being mailed to clinic or physician's office: Instructing patient about postal regulations (special pouch required)

» Proper storage

**Follow-up**

All positive tests need careful follow-up, with reassurance that not all positive tests indicate cancer. There are many other sources of bleeding and other causes of positive results. Only 5 to 10 percent of patients with positive tests are found to have cancer.

Negative tests do not necessarily prove the patient free of cancer, since tumors bleed intermittently. Therefore, patients should be counseled to comply with test instructions which state that a number of consecutive samples be taken, or tests run. Patients should be taught to report any persistent changes in bowel habits and to have an annual cancer check-up starting at age 40.

---

## FECAL OCCULT BLOOD TEST KITS FOR CLINIC USE

## Diagnostic Product Forms

### FECAL OCCULT BLOOD TEST KITS FOR CLINIC USE

**Administration**

Patient should comply with diet and drug modifications for 2 days before and through the test period.

    Card tests:

        Guaiac test: With an applicator, take a small amount of stool from 2 separate areas of the stool. Apply each sample in a thin smear to each window. Wait 3 to 5 minutes before adding developer. Open flap in back of card and apply 2 drops of developer to the guaiac paper directly over each smear. In 60 seconds observe for any trace of blue color (positive) on or at the edge of the smear.

        Immunochemical test: With an applicator, take a small amount of stool from 2 separate areas of the stool. Place both samples on the collection paper. Spread thinly and evenly over the paper. Wait 10 minutes before proceeding with test. Follow manufacturer's directions for test procedure and interpretation of results.

    Tape:

        Apply a thin smear to a strip of tape. Wait 3 to 5 minutes before adding developer. Apply 2 drops of developer to the reverse side of the tape, directly behind the smear. In 60 seconds observe for any trace of blue color (positive) on or at the edge of the smear.

**Product(s) usually available**

U.S.—

    Cards [*DigiWipe; Hemoccult; Hemoccult SENSA*].

    Tape [*ColoScreen; Hemoccult*].

Canada—

    Not commercially available.

Note: See *Table 1*, page 1421.

**Packaging and storage**

Store at room temperature, 15 to 30 °C (59 to 86 °F). Avoid freezing, direct sunlight, and excess humidity.

---

## FECAL OCCULT BLOOD TEST KITS FOR HOME USE

## Diagnostic Product Forms

### FECAL OCCULT BLOOD TEST KITS FOR HOME USE

**Administration**

Patient should comply with diet and drug modifications for 2 days before beginning collection and during collection of 3 consecutive bowel movements.

    *Bowl tests*: Flush toilet several times (at least 3 times) to clear of detergent or cleanser residues. Flush any urine that is voided, then have bowel movement. Carefully float test pad on toilet bowl water, observing for color development for the designated time (blue-green, 30 seconds for *ColoCare*, 2 minutes for *EZ Detect*; red-orange, 30 seconds for *ColoScreen Self-Test*).

    *Card tests*: With an applicator, take a small amount of stool from 2 separate areas of the stool. Apply each sample in a thin smear to each window of the card. Return promptly to clinic for development.

    *Tablet tests*: For *Hematest*, smear a small amount of stool on the filter paper. Place 1 reagent tablet in the center of the specimen area. Add 2 drops of water onto the tablet so that they run down the sides onto the filter paper. Observe for appearance of blue color in 2 minutes. Blue color in the paper around the tablet indicates a positive test.

    *Wipe tests*: For *HemaWipe*, pat anal area gently after bowel movement to obtain light smear of stool, fold over sample tissue and seal. Return sample to clinic for development.

**Product(s) usually available**

U.S.—

    Bowl Tests [*ColoCare; ColoScreen Self-Test; EZ Detect*].

    Tablets [*Hematest*].

    Cards/Slides [*ColoScreen; ColoScreen III; HemaChek; HemeSelect; Hemoccult; Hemoccult II; Hemoccult SENSA; Hemoccult II SENSA*].

    Wipe Tests [*HemaWipe*].

Canada—

    Tablets [*Hematest*].

    Cards/Slides [*Colo-Rectal Test*].

Note: Except for the *bowl tests*, which are completed at home, test kits are usually sent home with patient and returned to the health clinic or physician's office for development. *HemeSelect* requires laboratory development.

    See *Table 1*, page 1421.

**Packaging and storage**

Store at room temperature, 15 to 30 °C (59 to 86 °F). Avoid freezing, direct sunlight, and excess humidity.

## Selected Bibliography

Anon. Tests for Occult Blood. Medical Letter 28 (705): 5, 1986.

Simon JB. Occult blood screening for colorectal carcinoma: a critical review. Gastroenterology 88: 820, 1985.

Simon JB. The pros and cons of fecal occult blood testing for colorectal neoplasms. Cancer and Metastasis Reviews 6: 397, 1987.

Revised: 06/18/92

---

## Table 1. Diagnostic Product Forms

| Form | Indicator | Development Office/Clinic* | Development Home | Number of Tests/Unit |
|------|-----------|--------------------------|------------------|----------------------|
| **Bowl** | | | | |
| *ColoCare* | Tetramethylbenzidine (blue-green) | | X | 3 pads, instructions, and reply card in kit |
| *ColoScreen Self-Test* | Guaiacol derivative (red-orange) | | X | 3 pads, instructions, and reply card in kit |
| *EZ Detect* | Tetramethylbenzidine (blue-green) | | X | 5 pads (1 for negative control), 1 positive control test pad, instructions, and result card in kit |

*Usually sent home with patient and returned to health clinic or physician's office for development.

## Table 1. Diagnostic Product Forms (continued)

| Form | Indicator | Development Office/Clinic* | Development Home | Number of Tests/Unit |
|------|-----------|---------------------------|------------------|----------------------|
| **Cards/Slides** | | | | |
| Colo-Rectal Test | Guaiac | X | | 2 areas/card, triple card pack |
| ColoScreen | Guaiac | X | | 2 areas/card, single card |
| ColoScreen III | Guaiac | X | | 2 areas/card, triple card pack |
| DigiWipe | Guaiac | X | | Single card, in 150-unit examination room dispenser |
| HemaChek | Guaiac | X | | 2 areas/card, single and triple cards |
| HemeSelect | Immunochemical (hemagglutination) | X (Laboratory required) | | 1 sample collection card |
| Hemoccult | Guaiac | X | X | 2 areas/card, single card |
| Hemoccult II | Guaiac | X | X | 2 areas/card, triple card pack |
| Hemoccult SENSA | Guaiac | X | | 2 areas/card, single card |
| Hemoccult II SENSA | Guaiac | X | | 2 areas/card, triple card pack |
| **Tablets** | | | | |
| Hematest | Orthotolidine, strontium peroxide | X | | 50 reagent tablets and filter papers |
| **Tape** | | | | |
| ColoScreen | Guaiac | X | | 100 tests/tape roll, examination room dispenser |
| Hemoccult | Guaiac | X | | 100 tests/tape roll |
| **Wipe** | | | | |
| HemaWipe | Guaiac | X | | Single pads in 150-unit dispenser (reports 14-day stability after collection) |

*Usually sent home with patient and returned to health clinic or physician's office for development.

# FELBAMATE   Systemic†

VA CLASSIFICATION (Primary): CN400

Another commonly used name is FBM.

Note: For a listing of dosage forms and brand names by country availability, see *Dosage Forms* section(s). For a listing of brand names for the articles in this monograph, refer to the General Index.

†Not commercially available in Canada.

## Category

Anticonvulsant.

## Indications

**Accepted**

Epilepsy (treatment)—Felbamate is indicated as monotherapy or as an adjunct to other anticonvulsants for the treatment of partial seizures with or without generalization in adults with severe epilepsy that has not responded to other treatment.

Epilepsy, Lennox-Gastaut syndrome (treatment adjunct)—Felbamate is indicated as adjunctive therapy in the treatment of partial and generalized seizures associated with Lennox-Gastaut syndrome in children who have not responded to other treatment.

## Pharmacology/Pharmacokinetics

**Physicochemical characteristics**

Chemical group—Dicarbamate. Structurally similar to meprobamate.
Molecular weight—238.24.

**Mechanism of action/Effect**

*In vitro* receptor binding studies suggest that felbamate may be an antagonist at the strychnine-insensitive glycine-recognition site of the N-methyl-D-aspartate (NMDA) receptor-ionophore complex. Antagonism of the NMDA receptor glycine binding site may block the effects of the excitatory amino acids and suppress seizure activity. Animal studies indicate that felbamate may increase the seizure threshold and may decrease seizure spread.

**Other actions/effects**

Animal studies have shown felbamate to induce the cytochrome P-450 enzyme system to some extent. In clinical studies, however, felbamate has acted as an enzyme inhibitor, possibly through competitive inhibition. In rat studies, felbamate has been shown to possess some neuroprotective activity against hypoxic-ischemic damage, probably through interaction with the strychnine-insensitive glycine receptor, at plasma concentrations achieved during clinical use; the relevance to humans is unknown.

**Absorption**

Complete (>90%). Absorption is unaffected by food, and both tablet and suspension dosage forms exhibit similar kinetics.

**Distribution**

Felbamate enters the central nervous system (CNS), with a brain/plasma coefficient of approximately 0.9. The apparent volume of distribution ($Vol_D$) ranged from 0.73 to 0.85 L per kg of body weight (L/kg) in single and multiple dose studies. Felbamate is distributed into breast milk.

**Protein binding**

Low (20-36%).

**Biotransformation**

Hepatic, probably by the cytochrome P-450 system; primarily by hydroxylation and conjugation to metabolites that are neither pharmacologically active nor neurotoxic.

**Half-life**

Elimination—13 to 23 hours.

**Time to peak concentration**

1 to 6 hours.

**Therapeutic serum concentration**

The therapeutic concentration range for felbamate has yet to be established. Plasma concentrations in 21 patients receiving monotherapy with 3600 mg of felbamate per day ranged from 23.7 to 136.6 mcg per mL (mcg/mL) (99.5 to 573.7 micromoles per L [micromoles/L]), with a mean of 78.4 mcg/mL (329.3 micromoles/L).

## Elimination

Renal—About 90% of an orally administered radioactive dose of felbamate was recovered in the urine, 40 to 50% of which was recovered unchanged.

Fecal—Less than 5% of an orally administered radioactive dose of felbamate was recovered in the feces.

# Precautions to Consider

## Cross-sensitivity and/or related problems

Patients sensitive to other carbamate derivatives (for example, carbromal, carisoprodol, meprobamate, mebutamate, or tybamate) may also be sensitive to felbamate. Felbamate should be used cautiously in patients who have demonstrated hypersensitivity reactions to other carbamate derivatives.

## Carcinogenicity/Tumorigenicity

In lifetime carcinogenicity studies, rats and mice received dosages of felbamate that resulted in steady state plasma concentrations less than or equal to those of humans receiving 3600 mg per day. The mice and the female rats showed a significant increase in hepatic cell adenomas, the mice showed a significant increase in hepatic hypertrophy, and the male rats showed a significant increase in benign interstitial cell tumors of the testes. The significance to humans is unknown.

As a result of the manufacturing process of felbamate, small amounts of two known animal carcinogens, ethyl carbamate (urethane) and methyl carbamate, may be present in the final dosage forms. The amounts present in felbamate used in lifetime carcinogenic studies were inadequate to cause tumors in rats and mice. A patient receiving 3600 mg per day of felbamate could be exposed to up to 0.72 mcg of urethane and 1800 mcg of methyl carbamate per day. These amounts are 1/10,000 and 1/1,600, respectively, of the dose levels shown to be carcinogenic in rodents, on a mg per square meter of body surface area (mg/m²) basis.

## Mutagenicity

No evidence of mutagenesis was revealed in microbial and mammalian cell assays.

## Pregnancy/Reproduction

Fertility—No effect on male or female fertility was seen in rats at oral doses up to 3 times the human maximum daily dose on a mg/m² basis.

Pregnancy—Studies in humans have not been done.

Felbamate crosses the placenta in rats. Incidence of malformation in offspring was not increased in rats at doses up to 3 times, or in rabbits at doses less than 2 times, the human maximum daily dose on a mg/m² basis. However, rat pup weight was decreased, and pup mortality during lactation was increased. The cause of these deaths is unknown. No effect was seen in rats given 1.5 times the human maximum daily dose of felbamate on a mg/m² basis.

FDA Pregnancy Category C.

Labor and delivery—The effect of felbamate on labor and delivery is not known.

## Breast-feeding

Felbamate is distributed into breast milk. However, the effect on the nursing infant is unknown.

## Pediatrics

Felbamate has been associated with several deaths due to aplastic anemia and acute liver failure. It is not known whether children are at increased risk for developing these adverse effects. However, children may be less able than adults to articulate symptoms should these effects occur. Felbamate should be used in children only if other medications have failed to control seizures.

## Geriatrics

Although appropriate studies on the relationship of age to the effects of felbamate have not been performed in the geriatric population, no geriatrics-specific problems have been documented to date. However, elderly patients are more likely to have age-related renal function impairment and other concomitant diseases, and to use other medications, which may require more cautious dosing of felbamate.

## Drug interactions and/or related problems

The following drug interactions and/or related problems have been selected on the basis of their potential clinical significance (possible mechanism in parentheses where appropriate)—not necessarily inclusive (» = major clinical significance):

Note: Possible interactions with hepatic enzyme inducers, hepatic enzyme inhibitors, and medications that are metabolized by the hepatic P-450 enzyme system, other than those listed below, have not been studied, but the possibility of a significant interaction should be considered and the patient should be carefully monitored during and following concurrent use.

» Carbamazepine

(enzyme induction by carbamazepine may lead to decreased felbamate plasma concentrations; increased felbamate plasma concentrations may occur when carbamazepine dosage is reduced or carbamazepine is discontinued; concurrent use may also decrease carbamazepine plasma concentrations by about 20 to 30% and may increase the plasma concentrations of carbamazepine-10,11-epoxide, an active metabolite of carbamazepine, by about 60%, leading to an increase in adverse effects; carbamazepine dosage should be reduced by 20 to 33% when felbamate therapy is initiated, and plasma concentrations of carbamazepine should be monitored, with further dosage adjustments made as clinically necessary)

Methsuximide

(felbamate may increase plasma concentrations of N-desmethyl-methsuximide, an active metabolite of methsuximide, leading to increased adverse effects; methsuximide dosage should be reduced by 20 to 33% when felbamate therapy is initiated, with further dosage adjustments made as clinically necessary)

Phenobarbital

(felbamate may increase phenobarbital plasma concentrations, leading to increased adverse effects; phenobarbital dosage should be reduced by 20 to 33% when felbamate therapy is initiated, and plasma phenobarbital concentrations should be monitored, with further dosage adjustments made as clinically necessary

» Phenytoin

(enzyme induction by phenytoin may lead to decreased felbamate plasma concentrations during concurrent use; increased felbamate plasma concentrations may occur when phenytoin dosage is reduced or phenytoin is discontinued; since both felbamate and phenytoin are hydroxylated by the cytochrome P-450 system, possible competitive inhibition of phenytoin metabolism may result in phenytoin plasma concentrations being increased by 20 to 40%, leading to increased adverse effects; phenytoin dosage should be reduced by 20 to 33% when felbamate therapy is initiated, and plasma concentrations of phenytoin should be monitored, with further dosage adjustments made as necessary to maintain therapeutic plasma concentrations and limit adverse effects)

» Valproic acid

(felbamate may increase valproic acid plasma concentrations by approximately 20 to 40%, leading to increased adverse effects; valproic acid dosage should be reduced by 20 to 33% when felbamate therapy is initiated, and plasma concentrations of valproic acid should be monitored, with further dosage adjustments made as clinically necessary)

## Medical considerations/Contraindications

The medical considerations/contraindications included here have been selected on the basis of their potential clinical significance (reasons given in parentheses where appropriate)—not necessarily inclusive (» = major clinical significance).

*Except under special circumstances, this medication should not be used when the following medical problems exist:*

» Blood disorders characterized by serious abnormalities in blood count, platelets, or serum iron or

» Bone marrow depression, or history of or

» Hepatic function impairment or history of
   (condition may be exacerbated)

*Risk-benefit should be considered when the following medical problems exist:*

» Hematologic reactions to other medications, history of
   (patients may be especially at risk for felbamate-induced bone marrow depression)

» Sensitivity to felbamate or other carbamate derivatives

## Patient monitoring

The following may be especially important in patient monitoring (other tests may be warranted in some patients, depending on condition; » = major clinical significance):

Note: Monitoring may not detect aplastic anemia or liver failure before serious illness has developed; however, early detection of these life-threatening adverse effects may facilitate optimal treatment.

» Hepatic function determinations

(ALT [SGPT], AST [SGOT], and serum bilirubin determinations are recommended prior to initiation of felbamate treatment, and regularly thereafter. Felbamate should be discontinued immediately if any indication of liver injury develops)

» Blood counts, complete (CBCs), including platelet and possibly reticulocyte counts and

» Iron concentrations, serum

(determinations recommended prior to initiation of therapy as a baseline. Patients who develop low or decreased white blood cell or platelet counts during the course of treatment should be monitored closely and felbamate discontinued if there is any evidence of significant bone marrow depression)

## Side/Adverse Effects

Note: There have been reports of deaths due to both aplastic anemia and acute liver failure associated with felbamate use. However, causal relationships have not been definitively established. Appropriate monitoring, including complete blood cell counts, determinations of serum iron concentrations, and liver function tests, should be conducted.

In clinical trials, the frequency of adverse effects was much lower during felbamate monotherapy than during polytherapy with other anticonvulsant medications. The adverse effects seen most frequently during felbamate monotherapy were anorexia, headache, insomnia, and weight loss.

The following side/adverse effects have been selected on the basis of their potential clinical significance (possible signs and symptoms in parentheses where appropriate)—not necessarily inclusive:

### Those indicating need for medical attention
Incidence more frequent
*Fever; gait abnormality* (walking in unusual manner); *purpura* (purple or red spots on skin)

Incidence less frequent
*CNS toxicity, specifically agitation, aggression or other mood or mental changes, ataxia* (clumsiness or unsteadiness); *or tremor* (trembling or shaking); *skin rash*

Incidence rare
*Anaphylactoid reaction* (nasal congestion; shortness of breath or troubled breathing; skin rash, hives or itching; swelling of face); *blood dyscrasias, including agranulocytosis* (chills; fever; sore throat; general feeling of tiredness or weakness); *aplastic anemia* (shortness of breath, troubled breathing, wheezing, or tightness in chest; sores, ulcers, or white spots on lips or in mouth; swollen or painful glands; unusual bleeding or bruising); *leukopenia* (chills; fever; sore throat); *pancytopenia* (nosebleeds or other unusual bleeding or bruising); *thrombocytopenia* (unusual bleeding or bruising; black, tarry stools; blood in urine or stools; pinpoint red spots on skin); *or qualitative platelet disorder* (unusual bruising or bleeding; black or tarry stools); *bone marrow depression* (chills; fever; sore throat; unusual bleeding or bruising); *liver failure, acute* (continuing headache; continuing stomach pain; continuing vomiting; dark-colored urine; general feeling of tiredness or weakness; light-colored stools; yellow eyes or skin); *lymphadenopathy* (swollen lymph nodes); *photosensitivity* (sensitivity of skin to sunlight); *psychosis* (severe mood or mental changes); *Stevens-Johnson syndrome* (skin rash or itching; sores or white spots on lips or in mouth; sore throat; fever; chills; muscle cramps; pain; weakness; chest pain)

Note: *Thrombocytopenia* is usually asymptomatic; rarely, symptoms are present.

### Those indicating need for medical attention only if they continue or are bothersome
Incidence more frequent
*Dizziness; gastrointestinal effects, specifically abdominal pain* (stomach pain); *anorexia* (loss of appetite); *constipation; dyspepsia* (indigestion); *nausea or vomiting; headache; insomnia* (trouble in sleeping); *taste perversion* (change in sense of taste)

Incidence less frequent
*Anxiety; diarrhea; drowsiness; nervousness; rhinitis* (runny nose); *upper respiratory tract infection* (coughing; ear congestion or pain; fever; head congestion; nasal congestion; runny nose; sneezing; sore throat); *vision abnormalities, including blurred vision and diplopia* (double vision); *weight loss*

## Overdose

For information on the management of overdose or unintentional ingestion, **contact a Poison Control Center** (see *Poison Control Center Listing*).

### Clinical effects of overdose
Experience with felbamate overdose is limited. One patient who ingested 12 grams of felbamate over 12 hours experienced mild gastric distress and a resting heart rate of 100 beats per minute.

### Treatment of overdose
There is no specific antidote for felbamate overdose. Recommended treatment includes:

To decrease absorption—Emesis or gastric lavage.

Supportive care—Patients in whom intentional overdose is confirmed or suspected should be referred for psychiatric consultation.

## Patient Consultation

As an aid to patient consultation, refer to *Advice for the Patient, Felbamate (Systemic)*.

In providing consultation, consider emphasizing the following selected information (» = major clinical significance):

### Before using this medication
» Conditions affecting use, especially:
Sensitivity to felbamate or to other carbamate derivatives
Pregnancy—Crosses the placenta in rats. Animal studies using up to 3 times the maximum human dose in mg/m$^2$ have shown decreased rat pup weight and decreased survival; clinical significance is unknown
Breast-feeding—Distributed into breast milk
Use in children—Children may be unable to articulate symptoms of aplastic anemia or acute liver failure; use only if other medications have failed to control seizures
Other medications, especially carbamazepine, phenytoin, and valproic acid
Other medical problems, especially blood disorders, bone marrow depression, or hepatic function impairment

### Proper use of this medication
» Compliance with therapy; not taking more or less medicine than prescribed
Proper administration for liquid dosage form: Shaking well; using an accurate measuring device, such as a specially marked measuring spoon, a plastic syringe, or a small graduated cup
» Proper dosing
Missed dose: Taking as soon as possible; if almost time for next dose, skipping missed dose and going back to regular dosing schedule; not doubling doses
» Proper storage

### Precautions while using this medication
» Regular visits to physician to check progress of therapy and to monitor for severe adverse effects
» Not discontinuing felbamate abruptly; consulting physician about gradually reducing dosage
» Possible dizziness, drowsiness, impairment of judgment, thinking, or motor skills; caution when driving or doing jobs requiring alertness

### Side/adverse effects
Fever; gait abnormality; purpura; CNS toxicity, specifically agitation, aggression, or other mood or mental changes, ataxia, tremor; skin rash; anaphylactoid reaction; blood dyscrasias, including agranulocytosis, aplastic anemia, leukopenia, pancytopenia, thrombocytopenia, qualitative platelet disorder; bone marrow depression; liver failure, acute; lymphadenopathy; photosensitivity; psychosis; Stevens-Johnson syndrome

## General Dosing Information

Most adverse effects that emerge when adding felbamate to an anticonvulsant regimen resolve as dosages of concomitant anticonvulsant medications are reduced.

Adverse gastrointestinal effects may be reduced by taking felbamate after meals. If nausea persists, felbamate dosage may be decreased until tolerance to the gastrointestinal effects develops.

Neither felbamate nor other anticonvulsant medications should be suddenly discontinued because of the possibility of increased seizure frequency. The dosage should be reduced gradually when an anticonvulsant medication is being withdrawn.

### For treatment of adverse effects
Treatment of bone marrow depression includes the following:
• Discontinuing felbamate therapy.
• Daily CBC, platelet and reticulocyte counts.
• Performing a bone marrow aspiration and trephine biopsy immediately and repeating with sufficient frequency to monitor recovery.
• Considering other studies that may be helpful, including white cell and platelet antibodies; $^{59}$Fe—ferrokinetic studies; peripheral blood cell typing; cytogenic studies on marrow and peripheral blood; bone marrow culture studies for colony-forming units; hemoglobin electrophoresis for A$^2$ and F hemoglobin; and serum folic acid and B$_{12}$ concentrations. If aplastic anemia develops, spe-

cialized consultation should be sought for appropriate monitoring and treatment.

## Oral Dosage Forms

### FELBAMATE ORAL SUSPENSION

**Usual adult and adolescent dose**
Anticonvulsant—
Oral, initially 1200 mg per day, usually divided into three or four doses, the dosage being gradually increased over several weeks based on clinical response.

**Usual adult and adolescent prescribing limits**
3600 mg per day.

**Usual pediatric dose**
Anticonvulsant—
Children 2 to 14 years of age: Oral, initially 15 mg per kg of body weight per day, usually divided into three or four doses, the dosage being gradually increased over a few weeks based on clinical response.

**Usual pediatric prescribing limits**
Children 2 to 14 years of age—45 mg per kg per day or 3600 mg per day, whichever is less.

**Strength(s) usually available**
U.S.—
600 mg per 5 mL (Rx) [*Felbatol* (sorbitol; glycerin; microcrystalline cellulose; carboxymethylcellulose sodium; simethicone; polysorbate 80; methylparaben; saccharin sodium; propylparaben; FD&C Yellow No. 6; FD&C Red No. 40; flavorings; purified water)].
Canada—
Not commercially available.

**Packaging and storage**
Store below 40 °C (104 °F), preferably between 15 and 30 °C (59 and 86 °F), in a tight container, unless otherwise specified by manufacturer.

**Auxiliary labeling**
• Shake well before using.
• May cause dizziness or drowsiness.

**Additional information**
Use a specially marked measuring spoon, a plastic syringe, or a small marked measuring cup to measure each dose accurately.

### FELBAMATE TABLETS

**Usual adult and adolescent dose**
See *Felbamate Oral Suspension.*

**Usual adult and adolescent prescribing limits**
See *Felbamate Oral Suspension.*

**Usual pediatric dose**
See *Felbamate Oral Suspension.*

**Usual pediatric prescribing limits**
See *Felbamate Oral Suspension.*

**Strength(s) usually available**
U.S.—
400 mg (Rx) [*Felbatol* (scored; starch; microcrystalline cellulose; croscarmellose sodium; lactose; magnesium stearate; FD&C Yellow No. 6)].
600 mg (Rx) [*Felbatol* (scored; starch; microcrystalline cellulose; croscarmellose sodium; lactose; magnesium stearate; FD&C Yellow No. 6; D&C Yellow No. 10; FD&C Red No. 40)].
Canada—
Not commercially available.

**Packaging and storage**
Store below 40 °C (104 °F), preferably between 15 and 30 °C (59 and 86 °F), in a tight container, away from moisture, unless otherwise specified by manufacturer.

**Auxiliary labeling**
• May cause dizziness or drowsiness.

## Selected Bibliography

Palmer KJ, McTavish D. Felbamate: A review of its pharmacodynamic and pharmacokinetic properties, and therapeutic efficacy in epilepsy. Drugs 1993; 45(6): 1041-65.

Graves NM. Felbamate. Ann Pharmacother 1993 Sep; 27: 1073-81.

Developed: 08/30/94
Interim revision: 10/06/94; 03/28/95

---

**FELODIPINE**—See *Calcium Channel Blocking Agents (Systemic)*

---

**FENFLURAMINE**—See *Appetite Suppressants (Systemic)*

---

**FENOPROFEN**—See *Anti-inflammatory Drugs, Nonsteroidal (Systemic)*

---

**FENOTEROL**—See *Bronchodilators, Adrenergic (Systemic)*

---

**FENTANYL**—See *Fentanyl (Transdermal-Systemic); Fentanyl and Derivatives (Systemic)*

---

# FENTANYL    Transdermal-Systemic

VA CLASSIFICATION (Primary): CN101

Note: Controlled substance classification—
U.S.: II.
Canada: N.

Note: For a listing of dosage forms and brand names by country availability, see *Dosage Forms* section(s). For a listing of brand names for the articles in this monograph, refer to the General Index.

## Category
Analgesic.

## Indications
Note: **Transdermal fentanyl should be prescribed, and its use monitored, only by persons knowledgeable in the continuous administration of potent opioid analgesics, in the care of patients requiring such treatment, and in the detection and management of hypoventilation.**

Use of this formulation requires that the advantages of providing a continuous, prolonged analgesic effect via a noninvasive, nonoral route of administration outweigh the disadvantage of being unable to adjust dosage rapidly should analgesic requirements change or adverse effects occur.

**Accepted**
Pain, chronic (treatment)—Transdermal fentanyl is indicated to relieve chronic pain that requires continuous treatment with a potent opioid analgesic. Most patients will need supplemental administration of an analgesic with a rapid onset and a short duration of action for pain relief during the interval between application of the first transdermal system and the onset of effective analgesia (24 hours or longer) and for relief of breakthrough pain.

**Unaccepted**
**Transdermal fentanyl is not recommended for treatment of acute pain (including postoperative pain).** Use of this formulation for postoperative pain may cause severe hypoventilation; a few fatalities have been reported. Also, clinical trials have shown that application of transdermal fentanyl 2 hours prior to anesthesia does not eliminate the need for postoperative administration of a rapidly acting analgesic, especially in the first 12 to 24 hours after surgery. However, transdermal fentanyl need not be discontinued perioperatively if a patient being treated for chronic pain requires surgery.

This formulation is **not** recommended for treatment of mild or intermittent pain that can be managed with less potent analgesics or with as-needed administration of short- or intermediate-acting opioid analgesics.

# Pharmacology/Pharmacokinetics

## Physicochemical characteristics
Source—Synthetic.
Chemical group—Phenylpiperidine derivative; chemically related to meperidine.
Molecular weight—336.5.
pKa—8.4.
*n*-Octanol:water partition coefficient—860:1.
Note: Physicochemical characteristics that facilitate percutaneous absorption of a medication include high lipid solubility (as indicated by a high *n*-octanol:water partition coefficient) and relatively low molecular weight ($< 1000$ daltons). Lipophilic opioid analgesics such as fentanyl are well absorbed through intact skin; hydrophilic opioid analgesics (e.g., morphine, codeine, and hydromorphone) are not.

## Mechanism of action/Effect
Opioid analgesics such as fentanyl bind with stereospecific receptors at many sites within the central nervous system (CNS) to alter processes affecting both the perception of and emotional response to pain. Although the precise sites and mechanisms of action have not been fully determined, alterations in the release of various neurotransmitters from afferent nerves sensitive to painful stimuli may be partially responsible for the analgesic effects.

Multiple subtypes of opioid receptors, each mediating various therapeutic and/or side effects of opioid analgesics, have been identified. The actions of an opioid analgesic may therefore depend on whether it acts as a full agonist or a partial agonist or is inactive at each type of receptor. Fentanyl probably produces its effects predominantly via agonist actions at the mu receptor.

On a weight basis, fentanyl is considerably more potent than morphine. Transdermal administration of fentanyl at a delivery rate of 100 mcg per hour (mcg/hr) is therapeutically equivalent to intramuscular administration of 60 mg of morphine, chronic oral administration of 180 mg of morphine, or intermittent oral administration of 360 mg of morphine per day in 6 divided doses administered at 4-hour intervals. This high potency permits a therapeutic dose to be applied to a relatively small skin area.

## Other actions/effects
Fentanyl, like other opioid analgesics, may cause respiratory depression (characterized by decreases in respiratory rate, tidal volume, minute ventilation, and ventilatory response to carbon dioxide), increased biliary tone, increased smooth muscle tone in the urinary tract, decreased gastrointestinal motility, euphoria, miosis, hypotension, and bradycardia. However, unlike many other opioid analgesics, fentanyl does not cause clinically significant histamine release with therapeutic doses (as determined by intravenous administration of single doses of up to 50 mcg per kg of body weight [mcg/kg]).

## Absorption
Following application of a transdermal system, some fentanyl is released relatively rapidly from the adhesive layer of the system. Most of the fentanyl is located in a reservoir layer within the system, from which it is released gradually at a rate controlled by a restrictive copolymer membrane located between the reservoir and adhesive layers. A very small quantity of alcohol present in the formulation enhances passage of the medication through both the rate-limiting restrictive membrane and the skin. Less than 0.2 mL of alcohol is released from a transdermal system. The rate at which fentanyl is delivered to the skin may vary across the 72-hour application time. The labeled strength of a transdermal system represents the average quantity of fentanyl delivered to the systemic circulation per hour across intact skin.

Absorption of fentanyl after application of a transdermal system is initially slow because a depot of fentanyl, from which the medication is subsequently absorbed into the systemic circulation, must first form in the upper skin layers. Absorption is subject to intra- as well as interindividual variability. The rate and/or extent of absorption may be altered by the temperature, state of hydration, and integrity of the skin at the application site. Also, absorption may depend on blood flow in the area of application, which may increase or decrease with the patient's level of activity. Despite these variables, the average quantity of fentanyl absorbed per hour into the systemic circulation of an individual patient is sufficiently consistent to permit dosage titration over extended periods of time.

Approximately 92% of the fentanyl contained in a transdermal system is absorbed into the systemic circulation over 72 hours (calculated value). In a multiple-dose study, absorption from the fifth consecutive transdermal system to be applied and kept in place for 72 hours was 47% complete after 24 hours, 88% complete after 48 hours, and 94% complete after 72 hours.

Absorption of fentanyl from the depot in the skin continues after removal of the transdermal system. When application sites are rotated, continued absorption prevents plasma concentrations from decreasing to subtherapeutic values while another depot is forming below the new application site. Failure to rotate application sites may lead to more rapid absorption and higher fentanyl concentrations, which may increase the risk of toxicity.

## Distribution
Fentanyl is distributed to and accumulates in adipose tissue and skeletal muscle. The medication is slowly released from these tissues to the systemic circulation. Fentanyl readily crosses the blood/brain barrier. Alterations in pH may affect the medication's distribution between CNS tissues and plasma.
Volume of distribution (determined with intravenous administration to surgical patients)—6 (range, approximately 3 to 8) L per kg of body weight.

## Protein binding
High (79 to 87%), primarily to albumin and lipoproteins; dependent on plasma pH.

## Biotransformation
Primarily hepatic, mostly via N-dealkylation to norfentanyl and other inactive metabolites. Fentanyl is not metabolized in the skin.

## Half-life
Elimination—Transdermal—
    Single application—17 (range, 13 to 22) hours
    Multiple applications—$21.9 \pm 8.9$ hours, determined after 5 consecutive 72-hour applications.
Note: The prolonged elimination half-life with transdermal administration (relative to that with intravenous administration—about 3.6 hours) is due to prolonged continued absorption from the skin depot below the transdermal system.

    Values may be greatly prolonged in geriatric patients. In a single-dose study the mean value for patients 78 to 88 years of age was $43.1 \pm 23.4$ hours.

    The half-life of transdermal fentanyl has not been assessed in patients with renal or hepatic function impairment.

## Onset of action
Very slow (12 to 24 hours in most studies) because of delayed absorption following application of an initial transdermal dose.

## Time to peak concentration
Single 72-hour application—Generally between 24 and 72 hours.
Multiple applications—Concentrations continue to increase during the first few 72-hour applications.

## Peak serum concentration
Serum concentrations achieved with transdermal fentanyl have been studied primarily in clinical trials that investigated whether the formulation might be useful for postoperative pain control. In general, the studies found fentanyl concentrations to be proportional to the transdermal delivery rate in mcg per hour, subject to substantial interpatient variability, and significantly higher in geriatric patients than in younger adults. The concentrations produced were similar to those measured during continuous intravenous infusion of fentanyl at the same rate of administration, but took considerably longer to achieve. In many studies, measurable quantities of fentanyl were not present in serum within the first 2 hours after application of an initial transdermal system. Specific values determined during short-term use in postoperative patients are not likely to be relevant to prolonged use of this medication in chronic pain patients.

## Steady-state concentrations
A multiple-dose study in which pharmacokinetics of fentanyl were assessed during 5 consecutive 72-hour applications of a system designed to deliver 100 mcg per hour reported mean trough concentrations of $0.91 \pm 0.55$ nanograms/mL ($0.0027 \pm 0.0016$ micromoles/L) prior to, and mean maximum concentrations of $2.6 \pm 1.3$ nanograms/mL ($0.0077 \pm 0.0039$ micromoles/L) during, application of the fifth dose. Steady-state concentrations are subject to substantial interpatient variability because of individual differences in skin permeability and clearance of fentanyl. Although several sequential 72-hour applications may be required to achieve steady-state, measurement of trough concentrations prior to application of each dose in the multiple-dose study suggested that steady-state concentrations are approached by the second dose.

## Therapeutic concentrations
Generally 0.2 to 1.2 nanograms/mL (0.0006 to 0.0036 micromoles/L) in patients who are not tolerant to opioid analgesics. Required concentrations increase with the degree of tolerance to opioid analgesics.

Fentanyl requirements are highly subject to intrapatient variability and dependent on the intensity of pain.

Effective concentrations were reached between 1.2 and 37.3 hours after application of a transdermal system in various postoperative pain studies. In 1 of these studies, concentrations decreased to subtherapeutic values between 2.3 and > 24.9 hours (mean, $16.1 \pm 7.1$ hours) after the system was removed.

### Duration of action
Individual transdermal systems are designed to release fentanyl over 72 hours. Analgesic effects may persist for several hours after a system is removed because of continued absorption. This provides relatively constant analgesia during the time required for an effective quantity of fentanyl to be absorbed from the next dose.

### Elimination
Studies with intravenously administered fentanyl have shown that approximately 75% of a dose is eliminated in the urine (10% as unchanged fentanyl and the remainder as metabolites) and another 9% in the feces, mostly as metabolites. These studies also indicated that clearance rates are more variable and prolonged in patients with hepatic or renal function impairment than in patients with normal hepatic and renal function. Clearance rates for transdermally administered fentanyl have not been published.

## Precautions to Consider

### Cross-sensitivity and/or related problems
Patients hypersensitive to alfentanil or sufentanil may be hypersensitive to fentanyl also.

### Carcinogenicity
Long-term studies with fentanyl have not been done.

### Mutagenicity
No evidence of mutagenicity was demonstrated in the Ames test, primary rat hepatocyte unscheduled DNA synthesis assay, BALB/c-3T3 transformation test, and the human lymphocyte and CHO chromosomal aberration *in vitro* assays. In the mouse lymphoma assay, fentanyl concentrations more than 2000 times greater than those occurring with chronic systemic use were mutagenic only in the presence of metabolic activation.

### Pregnancy/Reproduction
Fertility—Intravenous administration of 0.3 times the human dose of fentanyl for 12 days impaired fertility in rats.

Pregnancy—Adequate and well-controlled studies with transdermal fentanyl have not been done in pregnant women. Chronic use of other opioids by pregnant women has caused physical dependence in the fetus, leading to withdrawal symptoms (convulsions, irritability, excessive crying, tremors, hyperactive reflexes, fever, vomiting, diarrhea, sneezing, and yawning) in the neonate. Also, use of opioid analgesics shortly before or during labor may cause respiratory depression in the neonate.

Studies in rats have not shown that fentanyl is teratogenic.

FDA Pregnancy Category C.

Labor and delivery—Use of transdermal fentanyl to provide analgesia during labor and delivery is not recommended.

### Breast-feeding
Fentanyl is distributed into human breast milk. Nursing infants may ingest quantities of fentanyl sufficient to produce adverse effects typical of potent opioid analgesics, including sedation, respiratory depression, and physical dependence when the mother is receiving chronic, high-dose treatment. Use of transdermal fentanyl by nursing women is therefore not recommended.

### Pediatrics
No information is available on the relationship of age to the effects of transdermal fentanyl in pediatric patients. Safety and efficacy have not been established. Administration to children younger than 12 years of age is not recommended except in an authorized investigational research setting.

### Adolescents
No information is available on the relationship of age to the effects of transdermal fentanyl in adolescents up to 18 years of age. Safety and efficacy have not been established. Administration to patients younger than 18 years of age who weigh less than 50 kg is not recommended except in an authorized investigational research setting.

### Geriatrics
No information is available on the relationship of age to the effects of transdermal fentanyl in geriatric patients with chronic pain. However, it is known that geriatric patients are generally more susceptible to the effects, especially the respiratory depressant effects, of opioid analgesics. Short-term pharmacokinetic studies with transdermal fentanyl

have shown that the elimination half-life and serum concentrations are significantly higher in elderly individuals than in younger people. Also, in a study that utilized an investigational 24-hour transdermal system with a delivery rate of 50 mcg per hour, the systems were removed earlier than anticipated from all of the elderly subjects (planned application time 24 hours; mean time of removal $11.7 \pm 4.9$ hours), but none of the younger individuals, because of adverse effects. Caution and careful attention to dosage are recommended, especially if the patient is not tolerant to opioid analgesics.

### Drug interactions and/or related problems
The following drug interactions and/or related problems have been selected on the basis of their potential clinical significance (possible mechanism in parentheses where appropriate)—not necessarily inclusive ($\gg$ = major clinical significance):

Note: Combination containing any of the following medications, depending on the amount present, may also interact with this medication.

$\gg$ Alcohol or

$\gg$ CNS depression–producing medications, other (See *Appendix II*)
(concurrent or sequential use with fentanyl may result in increased CNS depressant, respiratory depressant, and hypotensive effects; caution and careful titration of the dose of each agent are recommended)

(concurrent use of fentanyl with other CNS depressants that may cause habituation may increase the risk of habituation)

Anticholinergics or other medications with anticholinergic activity (See *Appendix II*)
(concurrent use with fentanyl may result in increased risk of severe constipation, which may lead to paralytic ileus, and/or urinary retention)

Antidiarrheals, antiperistaltic, such as:
Difenoxin and atropine
Diphenoxylate and atropine
Loperamide
Opium tincture
Paregoric
(repeated administration of any of these antidiarrheals with fentanyl, especially during chronic, high-dose fentanyl therapy, may increase the risk of severe constipation and CNS depression)

Antihypertensives, especially ganglionic blockers such as guanadrel, guanethidine, and mecamylamine or
Diuretics or
Hypotension-producing medications, other (see *Appendix II*)
(hypotensive effects of these medications may be potentiated when they are used concurrently with fentanyl; patients should be monitored for excessive fall in blood pressure)

(concurrent use of a beta-adrenergic blocking agent with fentanyl may also increase the risk of bradycardia)

Hydroxyzine
(concurrent use with fentanyl may result in increased analgesia as well as increased CNS depressant and hypotensive effects)

Metoclopramide
(fentanyl may antagonize the effects of metoclopramide on gastrointestinal motility)

Monoamine oxidase (MAO) inhibitors, including furazolidone, procarbazine, and selegiline
(caution is recommended when any opioid analgesic is given to patients who have received an MAO inhibitor within 14 days because administration of meperidine to patients receiving MAO inhibitors has caused unpredictable, severe, and sometimes fatal reactions, including immediate excitation, sweating, rigidity, and severe hypertension, or, in some patients, hypotension, severe respiratory depression, coma, seizures, hyperpyrexia, and vascular collapse; although a few reports indicated that intravenous injections of fentanyl did not cause adverse reactions when administered perioperatively to patients receiving MAO inhibitor therapy, administration of an intravenous test dose of fentanyl [to detect any possible interaction] may be advisable prior to initiation of transdermal therapy because the effects of transdermal fentanyl cannot be terminated rapidly)

Naloxone
(antagonizes the analgesic, CNS, and respiratory depressant effects of opioid analgesics; however, because naloxone may precipitate withdrawal symptoms in physically dependent patients, dosage of naloxone should be carefully titrated when it is used to treat opioid overdosage in dependent patients; also, because absorption of fentanyl from the depot that forms in the skin layers below the transdermal system continues after the system has been removed, prolonged infusion or repeated administration of naloxone may be required)

» Naltrexone
  (fentanyl will be ineffective if administered to a patient receiving naltrexone, which blocks the therapeutic effects of opioid analgesics; administration of increased doses of an opioid analgesic to override naltrexone blockade of opioid receptors may result in increased and prolonged respiratory depression and/or circulatory collapse and is not recommended)

  (administration of naltrexone to a patient who is physically dependent on fentanyl will precipitate withdrawal symptoms; symptoms may appear within 5 minutes of naltrexone administration, persist for up to 48 hours, and be very difficult to reverse)

Neuromuscular blocking agents and possibly other medications having some neuromuscular blocking activity
  (respiratory suppressant effects of neuromuscular blockade may be additive to the central respiratory depressant effects of opioid analgesics; increased or prolonged respiratory depression [apnea] may occur but is of minor clinical significance if the patient is being ventilated mechanically; however, caution and careful monitoring of the patient are recommended during and following concurrent or sequential use, especially if there is a possibility of incomplete reversal of neuromuscular blockade)

» Opioid analgesics, other
  (although most patients require supplemental administration of an analgesic with a rapid onset of action for pain relief during the interval between application of the first transdermal system and the onset of effective analgesia [24 hours or longer] and for relief of breakthrough pain, the risk of additive CNS and/or respiratory depression or other adverse effects must be considered, especially in patients who are not tolerant to opioid analgesics; use of long-acting opioid analgesics [or extended-release dosage forms of short-acting opioids] in conjunction with transdermal fentanyl may be especially hazardous and is not recommended)

  (in addition to their potential for causing additive effects when used concurrently with fentanyl, opioids having partial mu-receptor activity [e.g., buprenorphine and dezocine] and some opioids having mixed agonist/antagonist activity [i.e., nalbuphine and pentazocine] have the potential to antagonize fentanyl's therapeutic and adverse effects; whether additive or antagonistic effects occur may depend on the dose of each medication as well as on the order in which the medications are given and the extent to which physical dependence has developed; administration of a partial mu-receptor agonist prior to an initial dose of fentanyl may reduce the therapeutic response to fentanyl, whereas administration of a partial mu-receptor agonist, nalbuphine, or pentazocine to a patient who is receiving fentanyl may antagonize fentanyl's effects to the extent of precipitating withdrawal symptoms in physically dependent patients)

**Laboratory value alterations**
The following have been selected on the basis of their potential clinical significance (possible effect in parentheses where appropriate)—not necessarily inclusive (» = major clinical significance):

With diagnostic test results
  Gastric emptying studies
    (opioid analgesics may delay gastric emptying, thereby invalidating test results)
  Hepatobiliary imaging using a technetium Tc 99m–labeled iminodiacetic acid derivative
    (delivery of the radiopharmaceutical to the small bowel may be slowed because of fentanyl-induced constriction of the sphincter of Oddi and increased biliary tract pressure; these actions result in delayed visualization, which may be falsely interpreted as indicating obstruction of the common bile duct)

With physiology/laboratory test values
  Amylase, plasma and
  Lipase, plasma
    (enzyme values may be increased because fentanyl can cause contractions of the sphincter of Oddi and increased biliary tract pressure; the diagnostic utility of determinations of these enzymes may be compromised during, and for a time following discontinuation of, transdermal fentanyl therapy)
  Cerebrospinal fluid pressure
    (fentanyl may increase cerebrospinal fluid pressure; effect is secondary to respiratory depression–induced carbon dioxide retention)

**Medical considerations/Contraindications**
The medical considerations/contraindications included here have been selected on the basis of their potential clinical significance (reasons given in parentheses where appropriate)—not necessarily inclusive (» = major clinical significance).

*Except under special circumstances, this medication should not be used when the following medical problems exist:*
» Diarrhea associated with pseudomembranous colitis caused by cephalosporins, lincomycins (possibly including topical clindamycin), or penicillins or
» Diarrhea caused by poisoning, until toxic material has been eliminated from the gastrointestinal tract
  (opioid analgesics may slow elimination of toxic material, thereby worsening and/or prolonging the diarrhea)
» Respiratory depression, acute
  (may be exacerbated)

*Risk-benefit should be considered when the following medical problems exist:*
  Abdominal conditions, acute
    (diagnosis or clinical course may be obscured)
  Allergic reaction to fentanyl, alfentanil, or sufentanil, or to the adhesives in the transdermal system
    (risk of hypersensitivity reaction)
» Asthma, acute attack or
» Respiratory impairment or disease, chronic
    (opioids may decrease respiratory drive and increase airway resistance in patients with these conditions)
  Bradyarrhythmias
    (may be exacerbated)
  Drug abuse or dependence, current or history of, including alcoholism or
  Emotional instability or
  Suicidal ideation or attempts
    (patient predisposition to drug abuse; possibility of adverse effects if patient uses nonprescribed CNS depressants concurrently with fentanyl)
    (although this medication should not be withheld from known opioid addicts who require treatment for chronic pain, caution is recommended; addicts treated with fentanyl transdermal systems have been reported to increase the rate of fentanyl release by disrupting the restrictive membrane and to remove fentanyl from the reservoir for rapid administration by other routes)
  Fever
    (temperature-dependent changes in fentanyl release from the transdermal system and increased skin permeability may result in a 33% increase in fentanyl plasma concentrations in patients with a fever of 40 °C [102 °F]; patients who develop a fever while a system is in place should be monitored for adverse effects and fentanyl dosage adjusted and/or treatment instituted as needed)
  Gallbladder disease or gallstones
    (fentanyl may cause biliary contraction and increased biliary tract pressure; biliary colic may be exacerbated rather than relieved)
  Gastrointestinal tract surgery, current or recent
    (alteration of gastrointestinal motility by fentanyl may be undesirable)
  Head injury or
  Increased intracranial pressure, pre-existing or
  Intracranial lesions
    (risk of respiratory depression and further elevation of cerebrospinal fluid pressure, which may lead to complications such as impaired consciousness, is increased; also, opioid analgesics may cause sedation and pupillary changes that may obscure the clinical course of patients with head injury)
  Hepatic function impairment or
  Renal function impairment
    (potential for reduced clearance of fentanyl, leading to higher plasma concentrations; pharmacokinetic studies on which recommendations regarding use of transdermal fentanyl could be based have not been done in patients with these conditions)
    (fluid retention associated with renal function impairment may be exacerbated because fentanyl may also cause urinary retention)
  Hypothyroidism
    (risk of respiratory depression and prolonged CNS depression is greatly increased)
» Inflammatory bowel disease, severe
    (risk of toxic megacolon, especially with prolonged use of fentanyl)
  Prostatic hypertrophy or obstruction or
  Urethral stricture or
  Urinary tract surgery, current or recent
    (patient predisposition to urinary retention)

Caution is also recommended in administration to elderly or very ill or debilitated patients, who may be more sensitive to the effects, especially the respiratory depressant effects, of opioid analgesics.

### Patient monitoring

The following may be especially important in patient monitoring (other tests may be warranted in some patients, depending on condition; » = major clinical significance):

Blood pressure and
Heart rate and
» Respiratory rate and
» Sedation, degree of

(should be monitored at periodic intervals, especially at the beginning of therapy and after increases in dosage; if the system is removed because of adverse effects, monitoring should continue for at least 12 hours because absorption of fentanyl continues, and serum concentrations decrease slowly, after the system is removed)

## Side/Adverse Effects

Note: The frequencies of the adverse effects reported below were obtained in clinical studies in 510 patients (153 cancer patients, 56% of whom received treatment lasting from 30 days to more than a year, and 357 surgical patients who received the medication for 1 to 3 days), almost all of whom received supplemental doses of other opioid analgesics. The relative contribution of fentanyl, other opioid analgesic (s), the patient's underlying condition, and/or various surgical procedures to the occurrence of specific symptoms has not been established.

The risk of hypoventilation and of CNS adverse effects in opioid-naive individuals is increased when serum concentrations of fentanyl reach 2 nanograms per mL (nanograms/mL) (0.006 micromoles/liter [micromoles/L]) and more than 3 nanograms/mL (0.009 micromoles/L), respectively. The concentration at which toxicity occurs increases with increasing tolerance to the opioid analgesic.

In addition to the side/adverse effects listed below, a case of toxic delirium has been reported in an elderly patient receiving 125 mcg per hour of transdermal fentanyl together with other CNS depressants.

Physical dependence, with or without psychological dependence, may occur with chronic administration of fentanyl; an abstinence syndrome may occur when the medication is discontinued abruptly.

The following side/adverse effects have been selected on the basis of their potential clinical significance (possible signs and symptoms in parentheses where appropriate)—not necessarily inclusive:

### Those indicating need for medical attention
Incidence more frequent (3 to 10%)
*Apnea; CNS depression; difficult breathing; hypoventilation*—respiratory rate < 8 breaths per minute, pCO$_2$ > 55 mm Hg; *hallucinations* (seeing, hearing, or feeling things that are not there); *urinary retention* (decreased frequency of urination; decrease in urine volume)

Note: The risk of *hypoventilation* is higher in nontolerant women than in men, in patients weighing less than 63 kg, in patients with pre-existing respiratory function impairment, and in patients receiving doses of 75 mcg per hour or higher.

Incidence less frequent (1 to 3%)
*Chest pain; CNS effects* (abnormal thinking; difficulty in speaking; fainting; problems with coordination or gait); *paranoia* (delusions of persecution, mistrust, suspiciousness, and/or combativeness)—frequency of CNS effects and paranoia symptoms is 1 to 3% in clinical studies; *irregular heartbeat; localized skin reaction* (redness, swelling, and/or bumps on the skin, with or without itching, at place of application); *spitting blood*

Note: *Fainting* occurs more frequently in ambulatory than in recumbent patients and may be associated with postural hypotension. Localized reactions to the transdermal system are probably caused by the adhesive rather than by fentanyl. These reactions have been characterized as mild, transient (generally disappearing within 6 to 24 hours after removal of the transdermal system), and more typical of local irritation and occlusion than of allergic contact dermatitis. Generalized skin reactions also may occur; at least 1 case of diffuse, nonpruritic macular papules has been attributed to transdermal fentanyl therapy.

Incidence rare (less than 1%)
*Abdominal distention* (swelling of abdominal area); *amblyopia* (any change in vision); *bladder pain; bradycardia* (slow heartbeat); *cessation of urination; CNS toxicity* (inability to speak; depersonalization; stupor); *dermatitis, exfoliative* (fever with or without chills; red, thickened, or scaly skin; swollen and/or painful glands; unexplained

bruising); *fluid-filled blisters; frequent urge to urinate; respiratory problems, including asthma* (noisy breathing; shortness of breath; troubled breathing; tightness in chest; wheezing)

### Those indicating need for medical attention only if they continue or are bothersome
Incidence more frequent (each symptom 3% or higher)
*CNS effects* (anxiety; confusion; dizziness; drowsiness; false sense of well-being; nervousness; weakness); *gastrointestinal effects* (abdominal pain; constipation; diarrhea; indigestion; loss of appetite); *headache; itching of skin; nausea; sweating; vomiting*

Note: *Nausea* and *vomiting* are more likely to occur in ambulatory than in recumbent patients. These effects may be induced by a direct effect on the chemoreceptor trigger zone in the CNS.

Incidence less frequent (1 to 3%)
*Agitation* (feeling anxious and restless); *bloated feeling or gas; feeling of crawling, tingling, or burning of the skin; memory loss; unusual dreams*

### Those indicating possible withdrawal and the need for medical attention if they occur after medication is discontinued
*Body aches; diarrhea; fast heartbeat; fever, runny nose, or sneezing; gooseflesh; increased sweating; increased yawning; loss of appetite; nausea or vomiting; nervousness, restlessness, or irritability; shivering or trembling; stomach cramps; trouble in sleeping; unusually large pupils; weakness*

## Overdose

For specific information on the agents used in the management of fentanyl overdose, see:
• *Atropine* in *Anticholinergics/Antispasmodics (Systemic)* monograph; and/or
• *Naloxone (Systemic)* monograph.

For more information on the management of overdose or unintentional ingestion, **contact a Poison Control Center** (see *Poison Control Listing*).

### Clinical effects of overdose
Clinical effects of overdose
The following effects have been selected on the basis of their potential clinical significance (possible signs and symptoms in parentheses where appropriate)—not necessarily inclusive:

Acute and chronic
*Cold, clammy skin; confusion; convulsions; severe dizziness, drowsiness, nervousness, restlessness, or weakness; low blood pressure; pinpoint pupils of eyes; slow heartbeat; slow or troubled breathing; unconsciousness*

### Treatment of overdose
General measures—Removing the transdermal system (if symptoms are judged sufficiently severe to warrant removal) and monitoring the patient, keeping in mind that fentanyl absorption continues and plasma concentrations decline slowly after the system has been removed. Prolonged monitoring may be needed.

Specific treatment—

For hypoventilation:

Verbal stimulation or waking the patient (if bradypnea occurs during sleep) may be sufficient to increase the respiratory rate and provide adequate ventilation.

Use of the opioid antagonist naloxone if necessary. However, usual doses of naloxone may reverse analgesia and precipitate withdrawal in opioid-dependent patients. Since naloxone's duration of action is considerably shorter than that of transdermal fentanyl, administration via continuous intravenous infusion at a rate titrated to the needs of the individual patient may be necessary.

For bradycardia: Use of atropine.

For hypotension: Use of intravenous fluids and/or vasopressors and using other supportive measures as needed.

Supportive care—May include establishing adequate respiratory exchange through provision of a patent airway and institution of assisted or controlled respiration.

## Patient Consultation

As an aid to patient consultation, refer to *Advice for the Patient, Fentanyl (Transdermal-Systemic)*.

In providing consultation, consider emphasizing the following selected information (» = major clinical significance):

### Before using this medication
» Conditions affecting use, especially:
Sensitivity to fentanyl, alfentanil, or sufentanil

Pregnancy—Opioids cross the placenta; use by pregnant women may cause physical dependence in the fetus and withdrawal symptoms and/or respiratory depression in the neonate

Breast-feeding—Fentanyl is distributed into breast milk; opioid effects including sedation, respiratory depression, and physical dependence may occur in the infant if the mother is receiving chronic, high-dose therapy

Use in the elderly—Geriatric patients are more susceptible to the effects of opioids, especially respiratory depression

Other medications, especially alcohol or other CNS depressants (including other opioid analgesics) and naltrexone

Other medical problems, especially asthma or other acute or chronic respiratory problems, diarrhea caused by poisoning or antibiotic therapy, and severe inflammatory bowel disease

**Proper use of this medication**

» Reading patient instructions carefully before using
» Proper application technique

Keeping medication in sealed pouch until ready to apply

Using caution in handling; not touching adhesive surface with the hand; washing area with clear water if medication does touch the skin in an unintended location

Using care not to damage (puncture or tear) the surface of the transdermal system

Applying to clean, dry skin area of upper arm or torso that is free of oil, hair, scars, cuts, burns, or irritation; avoiding areas that have been irradiated

Clipping, not shaving, hair at application site, if necessary

If cleansing site prior to application, using only clear water (not soaps, lotions, or cleansers that contain oils, alcohol, or other agents) and allowing area to dry completely prior to application

Removing liner from adhesive layer, then pressing system in place with palm of hand for about 30 seconds; making sure that good contact is achieved, especially around the edges

If dose requires applying 2 or more systems, keeping them far enough apart so that the edges do not touch or overlap

Washing hands with clear water after applying or handling transdermal system

Removing system after 3 days; applying next system, if treatment is being continued, at new site, preferably on opposite side of the body; not reusing a site for at least 3 days

Disposing of used or unneeded systems by folding in half with adhesive layer inside the fold, then flushing down the toilet

» Not using more transdermal fentanyl than directed, even if medication appears ineffective; onset of action may require 24 hours or longer and several dosage adjustments may be required to achieve maximum effectiveness

» Taking "rescue" doses of short-acting opioid for first few days after initiation of therapy and for breakthrough pain, but not using more than prescribed because of danger of overdose

» Proper dosing

Missed dose: Applying as soon as possible

» Proper storage

**Precautions while using this medication**

Regular consultations with health care professional during long-term therapy

» Checking with health care professional before increasing dose of transdermal fentanyl and/or "rescue" medication if treatment becomes less effective

» Avoiding use of alcoholic beverages or other CNS depressants during therapy, unless prescribed or otherwise approved by physician

» Caution if dizziness, drowsiness, lightheadedness, or false sense of well-being occurs; checking with health care professional if severe drowsiness persists for more than a few days

» Getting up slowly from a lying or sitting position; lying down for a while may provide relief if patient becomes dizzy, lightheaded, or faint

Caution that nausea or vomiting may occur, especially during first several days of treatment, and may be relieved by lying down; checking with health care professional if severe, since an antiemetic may be needed

» Compliance with regimen for preventing severe constipation, if prescribed

» Avoiding external sources of heat (e.g., heating pad, sunlamps, heated water beds, electric blankets, sunbathing, prolonged baths or showers in hot water) and checking with health care professional if fever occurs; absorption of fentanyl may be accelerated

» Informing physician or dentist of use of medication if any kind of surgery (including dental surgery) or emergency treatment is required

System may be worn while bathing, showering, or swimming, but should not be rubbed vigorously because it may become loose or

detached; discarding system and applying a new one in an alternate, dry location if this occurs

» Not discontinuing medication abruptly after prolonged use; checking with physician instead, since gradual withdrawal may be needed to minimize risk of precipitating abstinence syndrome

» Suspected overdose: Getting emergency help at once

**Side/adverse effects**

Getting emergency help if symptoms of overdose occur, i.e., very slow (fewer than 8 breaths per minute) or troubled breathing, extreme drowsiness, convulsions, low blood pressure, or slow heartbeat

Other potential side effects, especially hallucinations or other CNS effects, urinary retention, chest pain, irregular heartbeat, localized skin reactions, skin rash or blisters, spitting blood, abdominal distention, amblyopia, bladder pain, bradycardia, exfoliative dermatitis, and urinary frequency

# General Dosing Information

Transdermal fentanyl may cause respiratory depression, especially in elderly, very ill, or debilitated patients and patients with pre-existing respiratory problems. Lower doses may be required for these patients, at least initially. However, elderly patients may also be more sensitive to the analgesic effects of opioid analgesics, and lower doses may be sufficient to provide effective analgesia.

Dosage must be individualized. Pre-existing tolerance to opioid analgesics is the primary factor to be considered in determining the appropriate initial dose of transdermal fentanyl. The rate at which tolerance develops varies widely among individuals. For patients who have been receiving chronic therapy with another opioid analgesic, initial dosage of transdermal fentanyl should be based on the patient's daily opioid requirement.

The transdermal system should be kept in the protective packaging until it is used. It should be applied to a dry, flat, nonirritated, non-irradiated skin surface of the upper arm or torso. If necessary, hair at the application site may be clipped (but not shaved) prior to application. Also, if the site is cleansed prior to application, clear water should be used; soaps, oils, lotions, alcohol, or other agents that may irritate the skin or change its characteristics should be avoided. The system should be pressed firmly in place with the palm of the hand for about 30 seconds, making sure that contact is complete, especially around the edges.

Because of the delayed onset of action after initial application of a fentanyl transdermal system, the adequacy of analgesia cannot be evaluated for 24 hours. A short-acting opioid analgesic must be administered as needed to relieve pain. If necessary, a higher dose may be applied for the second 72 hours, based on the quantity of supplemental opioid required during the second or third day of the first 72-hour application. Subsequent increases in dosage, if needed, should be made at 6-day intervals, with "rescue" doses continuing to be administered as needed until maximum analgesia has been attained. Some patients may require "rescue" dosing with a short-acting opioid analgesic for breakthrough pain throughout transdermal fentanyl therapy.

The fentanyl transdermal system should be removed after 72 hours. If treatment is being continued, a new system should be applied at a new site after the prior one has been removed.

Concurrent administration of a nonopioid analgesic (such as aspirin or other salicylates, other nonsteroidal anti-inflammatory drugs, or acetaminophen) with opioid analgesics provides additive analgesia and may permit lower doses of the opioid analgesic to be utilized.

The overall treatment regimen for chronic pain patients who are receiving long-term opioid analgesic therapy includes management of common side effects such as sedation, nausea and vomiting, and constipation. An antiemetic may be needed, especially during the first few weeks of therapy. Also, measures to prevent constipation and decrease the risk of intestinal obstruction may be needed, such as administration of a laxative (a bowel stimulant and/or a stool softener), a high fluid intake, and an increase in dietary fiber. Appropriate medications and dosages must be determined according to the physical condition and the needs of the individual patient.

Increases in the dosage of transdermal fentanyl and/or "rescue" medications may be required as tolerance to the medication develops or increases and/or the intensity of pain increases. Tolerance to the respiratory depressant effects of an opioid analgesic develops concurrently with tolerance to its analgesic effects. Careful adjustment of dosage as required to provide adequate analgesia is not likely to increase the risk of respiratory depression. However, a reduction in dose may be needed to prevent respiratory depression, which may occur even at a previously well-tolerated opioid dose, if the intensity of pain decreases because of changes in the patient's condition or institution of other pain-relieving treatments.

Psychological and physical dependence may occur with chronic administration of an opioid analgesic; an abstinence syndrome may occur when the medication is discontinued. However, physical dependence in patients receiving prolonged therapy for severe chronic pain rarely leads to true addiction, i.e., a desire to continue taking the medication (for its euphoric effect) after it is no longer required for pain relief. **Fear of causing addiction should not result in failure to provide adequate pain relief,** although caution is advised if patient predisposition toward drug abuse is known or strongly suspected. Reducing the dose gradually prior to discontinuation may minimize the development of withdrawal symptoms following prolonged use.

If a patient is being changed from transdermal fentanyl to another opioid analgesic, the transdermal system should be removed and the new analgesic administered in a low dose that may be gradually increased according to the patient's report of pain until adequate analgesia is achieved. The fact that fentanyl concentrations decrease very slowly after removal of the system must be considered when selecting a starting dose of the new agent. Also, the oral morphine–to–transdermal fentanyl conversion ratios recommended by the manufacturer for determining initial doses of transdermal fentanyl for opioid-tolerant patients are very conservative. Using the reverse of these ratios to calculate an appropriate dose of a subsequently administered opioid could result in an overdose and is not recommended.

### Safety considerations for handling this medication

The transdermal system is supplied in sealed systems that pose little risk of exposure to health care personnel. If any of the gel in the reservoir should contact the skin, the area should be flushed with copious quantities of water. Soap, alcohol, or other solvents may enhance penetration of fentanyl through the skin and should not be used.

## Transdermal Dosage Forms

### FENTANYL TRANSDERMAL SYSTEM

Note: The doses and strengths of the fentanyl transdermal system are expressed in terms of the delivery rate in mcg per hour.

### Usual adult dose

Analgesic—

For chronic pain: Transdermal, the appropriate number of transdermal systems to be applied and kept in place for seventy-two hours.

For patients who are not opioid-tolerant—Not more than one transdermal system rated to deliver 25 mcg (0.025 mg) per hour, initially. Dosage may be increased gradually as needed and tolerated until an adequate response has been attained.

For opioid-tolerant patients—Initially, a quantity of fentanyl (in mcg per hour) equivalent to the patient's current twenty-four-hour oral morphine requirement, as follows:

| Fentanyl (mcg/hr) | Morphine* (mg/24 hr) |
|---|---|
| | Oral |
| 25 | 45–134 |
| 50 | 135–224 |
| 75 | 225–314 |
| 100 | 315–404 |
| 125 | 405–494 |
| 150 | 495–584 |
| 175 | 585–674 |
| 200 | 675–764 |
| 225 | 765–854 |
| 250 | 855–944 |
| 275 | 945–1034 |
| 300 | 1035–1124 |

*A 10-mg intramuscular (IM) dose of morphine is therapeutically equivalent to 30 mg of chronically administered oral morphine or 60 mg of intermittently administered oral morphine. For patients who are receiving opioid analgesics other than morphine, the patient's twenty-four-hour opioid requirement should be determined, then converted to the equianalgesic oral morphine dose. The following quantities are equivalent to 30 mg of chronically administered oral morphine or 60 mg of intermittently administered oral morphine:

For buprenorphine—300 mcg (0.3 mg) IM.
For butorphanol—2 mg IM.

For codeine—200 mg orally; 130 mg IM.
For dezocine—10 mg IM.
For heroin—60 mg orally; 5 mg IM.
For hydromorphone—7.5 mg orally; 1.5 mg IM.
For levorphanol—4 mg orally; 2 mg IM.
For meperidine—300 mg orally; 75 mg IM.
For methadone—20 mg orally; 10 mg IM.
For nalbuphine—10 mg IM.
For oxycodone—30 mg orally.
For oxymorphone—1 mg IM; 10 mg rectally.
For pentazocine—180 mg orally; 60 mg IM.

Note: The oral morphine-to-transdermal fentanyl conversion ratios listed above are conservative; the need for an increase in dose should be anticipated. The second dose of transdermal fentanyl may be increased by 25 mcg per hour for each 90 mg per day of supplemental oral morphine (or equivalent dosage of other opioid analgesics) required during the second or third day of the first application. Six days may be required to reach equilibrium after each increase in dose; therefore, the higher dose should be worn for seventy-two-hour applications before further increases are made. If necessary, more than one transdermal system may be applied at a time.

A few patients may need replacement of the transdermal system (s) every forty-eight hours. Before the interval between applications is decreased, an attempt should be made to maintain the seventy-two-hour interval.

### Usual pediatric dose

Children up to 18 years of age—Safety and efficacy have not been established.

### Usual geriatric dose

See *Usual adult dose*

Note: It is recommended that initial dosage not exceed 25 mcg (0.025 mg) per hour unless the patient has been receiving chronic therapy with more than 135 mg per day of oral morphine or an equivalent dose of another opioid analgesic.

### Strength(s) usually available

U.S.—

25 mcg (0.025 mg) per hour (a total of 2.5 mg of fentanyl per 10 square centimeters [cm$^2$]) (Rx) [*Duragesic* (alcohol 0.1 mL)].

50 mcg (0.05 mg) per hour (a total of 5 mg of fentanyl per 20 cm$^2$) (Rx) [*Duragesic* (alcohol 0.2 mL)].

75 mcg (0.075 mg) per hour (a total of 7.5 mg of fentanyl per 30 cm$^2$) (Rx) [*Duragesic* (alcohol 0.3 mL)].

100 mcg (0.1 mg) per hour (a total of 10 mg of fentanyl per 40 cm$^2$) (Rx) [*Duragesic* (alcohol 0.4 mL)].

Canada—

25 mcg (0.025 mg) per hour (a total of 2.5 mg of fentanyl per 10 cm$^2$) (Rx) [*Duragesic* (alcohol 0.1 mL)].

50 mcg (0.05 mg) per hour (a total of 5 mg of fentanyl per 20 cm$^2$) (Rx) [*Duragesic* (alcohol 0.2 mL)].

75 mcg (0.075 mg) per hour (a total of 7.5 mg of fentanyl per 30 cm$^2$) (Rx) [*Duragesic* (alcohol 0.3 mL)].

100 mcg (0.1 mg) per hour (a total of 10 mg of fentanyl per 40 cm$^2$) (Rx) [*Duragesic* (alcohol 0.4 mL)].

### Packaging and storage

Store below 30 °C (59 °F), unless otherwise specified by manufacturer.

### Auxiliary labeling

• May cause drowsiness.
• Avoid alcoholic beverages.
• May be habit-forming.

## Selected Bibliography

Calis KA, Kohler DR, Corso DM. Transdermally administered fentanyl for pain management. Clin Pharm 1992; 11: 22-36.

Yee LY, Lopez JR. Transdermal fentanyl. Ann Pharmacother 1992; 26: 1393-9.

Payne R. Transdermal fentanyl: Suggested recommendations for clinical use. J Pain Symptom Manage 1992; 7 No 3 (suppl): S40-S44.

Developed: 07/27/94

# FENTANYL DERIVATIVES    Systemic

This monograph includes information on the following: Alfentanil; Fentanyl; Sufentanil.

VA CLASSIFICATION (Primary/Secondary): CN101/CN205

Note: Controlled substance classification—

U.S.: II.
Canada: N.

Note: For a listing of dosage forms and brand names by country availability, see *Dosage Forms* section(s). For a listing of brand names for the articles in this monograph, refer to the General Index.

## Category

Anesthesia adjunct (opioid analgesic)—Alfentanil, Fentanyl, Sufentanil.
Analgesic—Fentanyl.

## Indications

Note: Bracketed information in the *Indications* section refers to uses that are not included in U.S. product labeling.

### Accepted

Anesthesia, general [or local][1] adjunct—Fentanyl and its derivatives are indicated as opioid analgesic supplements to general anesthesia. During surgery, they are often used in conjunction with other agents, such as a combination of an ultrashort-acting barbiturate, a neuromuscular blocking agent, and an inhalation anesthetic (usually nitrous oxide), for the maintenance of "balanced" anesthesia.

Fentanyl and its derivatives are also indicated as primary agents for the induction of anesthesia in patients undergoing general surgery.

Fentanyl and sufentanil are also indicated as primary agents for the maintenance of anesthesia in selected patients undergoing major surgery. In these cases, they are administered in high doses with 100% oxygen or nitrous oxide plus oxygen and a neuromuscular blocking agent.

Fentanyl [and sufentanil][1] are indicated to provide neuroleptanalgesia (in conjunction with a neuroleptic agent such as droperidol) or neuroleptanesthesia (in conjunction with a neuroleptic agent and nitrous oxide).

Fentanyl [and sufentanil][1] are indicated to supplement regional or local anesthesia.

Fentanyl is approved by U.S. and Canadian regulatory agencies for use as presurgical medication. However, because of its short duration of action (following administration of single analgesic doses), fentanyl may be less desirable than longer acting opioid analgesics for this purpose.

Pain, postoperative (treatment)—Fentanyl is also approved by U.S. and Canadian regulatory agencies for prevention or relief of pain in the immediate postoperative period; however, longer acting opioid analgesics are more commonly used in this situation.

### Unaccepted

Alfentanil has also been investigated for use as the primary agent, administered in conjunction with 100% oxygen and a neuromuscular blocking agent, for the maintenance of anesthesia in selected patients undergoing cardiovascular surgery. Preliminary information indicates that the patient must be heavily premedicated and that continuous intravenous infusion of extremely high doses is required. Further study is needed to determine efficacy and appropriate dosage for such use.

[1]Not included in Canadian product labeling.

## Pharmacology/Pharmacokinetics

### Physicochemical characteristics

Molecular weight—
Alfentanil hydrochloride: 452.98.
Fentanyl citrate: 528.60.
Sufentanil citrate: 578.68.
pKa—
Alfentanil: 6.5.
Fentanyl: 8.43.
Sufentanil: 8.01.
Partition coefficient (octanol:water; pH 7.4)—
Alfentanil hydrochloride: 130
Fentanyl citrate: 816
Sufentanil citrate: 1727

### Mechanism of action/Effect

Low to moderate doses of fentanyl and its derivatives produce analgesia. During surgery, analgesic actions provide dose-related protection against hemodynamic responses to surgical stress; however, patient responsiveness to the pharmacodynamic actions of these medications is highly variable. Although high doses of these medications produce loss of consciousness, the ability of opioid analgesics (when used alone) to induce a true anesthetic state has been questioned.

Opioid analgesics bind with stereospecific receptors at many sites within the central nervous system (CNS) to alter processes affecting both the perception of and emotional response to pain. Although the precise sites and mechanisms of action have not been fully determined, alterations in the release of various neurotransmitters from afferent nerves sensitive to painful stimuli may be partially responsible for the analgesic effects.

It has been proposed that there are multiple subtypes of opioid receptors, each mediating various therapeutic and/or side effects of opioid drugs. The actions of an opioid analgesic may therefore depend upon whether it acts as a full agonist or a partial agonist or is inactive at each type of receptor. Fentanyl and its derivatives probably produce their effects via agonist actions at the mu receptor.

### Other actions/effects

Fentanyl and its derivatives may produce signs and symptoms common to opioid analgesics including respiratory depression (characterized by decreases in respiratory rate, tidal volume, minute ventilation, and ventilatory response to carbon dioxide), ureteral spasm, biliary spasm, decreased gastrointestinal motility, euphoria, miosis, hypotension, and bradycardia. However, unlike many other opioid analgesics, fentanyl and its derivatives have not been shown to cause histamine release (in doses used clinically).

Fentanyl and its derivatives, especially in moderate or high doses, may induce skeletal muscle rigidity.

Fentanyl and its derivatives may produce a dose-related decrease in certain hormonal responses during surgery, such as increased blood concentrations of circulating growth hormone, catecholamines, cortisol, antidiuretic hormone, and prolactin. However, alfentanil's effects on endocrine responses to surgical stimulation have not been fully evaluated. Also, in patients undergoing coronary bypass surgery, these agents may not suppress such endocrine responses, especially increased catecholamine concentrations, during the period of cardiopulmonary bypass.

### Volume of distribution

Alfentanil—Usually 0.6 to 1.0 liter per kg of body weight but subject to interpatient variability; values ranging from 0.23 to 2.47 liters per kg of body weight have been reported. The volume of distribution may be increased during aortocoronary bypass or decreased in children, but is not altered by obesity or hepatic function impairment. However, the distribution volume of total alfentanil (but not of the unbound [free] fraction) may be increased in patients with renal failure.

Fentanyl—Usually 4 liters per kg of body weight, although values ranging from 3.1 to 7.8 liters per kg of body weight have been reported.

Sufentanil—1.08 to 2.78 liters per kg of body weight.

Note: Fentanyl and its derivatives readily cross the blood/brain barrier; however, because of alfentanil's lower degree of lipophilicity (and therefore lower degree of tissue binding) and its lower pKa, alfentanil reaches receptors in the brain significantly more rapidly than fentanyl.

Fentanyl and sufentanil are rapidly distributed to body tissues. The relatively poor blood flow to fatty tissues limits the rate of the medications' accumulation in these tissues. However, accumulation in body fat, as well as in other tissues, may occur with large or multiple doses or prolonged administration. Clearance of either of these agents from tissues may result in therapeutic blood concentrations being maintained following discontinuation of administration, leading to a prolonged duration of action.

Alfentanil is also rapidly distributed to body tissues. Although accumulation of alfentanil may occur with prolonged continuous infusion or with repeated administration of single doses and may lead to a prolonged duration of action, alfentanil's accumulation in body tissues is significantly less than that of fentanyl or sufentanil. Therefore, alfentanil's duration of action is less likely than that of fentanyl or sufentanil to be substantially prolonged by clearance from body tissues.

### Protein binding

Alfentanil—About 92%; primarily to glycoproteins (especially alpha-1-acidglycoprotein [AAG]). Although independent of alfentanil plasma concentration or plasma pH, alfentanil protein binding is subject to interpatient variability and may be decreased in patients with alcoholic hepatic cirrhosis or renal failure and during cardiopulmonary bypass.

Fentanyl—80 to 89%, primarily to albumin and lipoproteins; dependent on plasma pH.

Sufentanil—92.5%, primarily to AAG; independent of sufentanil plasma concentration but highly dependent on plasma pH.

### Biotransformation

Hepatic; sufentanil may also undergo some metabolism in the small intestine. The rate of metabolism is dependent on total dosage, hepatic function, and factors affecting hepatic blood flow (possibly including certain surgical manipulations or, to a much lesser extent, concurrent use of a potent inhalation anesthetic). The rate of fentanyl or sufentanil metabolism is also dependent on the rate of their release from various body tissues. The rate of alfentanil metabolism is decreased in geriatric patients, obese patients, and patients with hepatic function impairment. In addition, genetic polymorphism has been suspected as a cause of unusually slow alfentanil metabolism in a few patients.

### Half-life

Alfentanil—
  Triphasic (with a dose of 50 or 125 mcg per kg of body weight):
    Distribution—0.4 to 3.1 minutes.
    Redistribution—4.6 to 21.6 minutes.
    Elimination—Generally 1 to 2.1 hours, although values well outside this range have been reported. The elimination half-life is not altered in patients with renal failure but may be decreased in children. Also, the elimination half-life is highly dependent on factors affecting the rate of metabolism. Increased values have been reported in patients with reduced hepatic function (up to 4.9 hours in asymptomatic patients with abnormal liver function test values and up to 5.8 hours in patients with active hepatic [alcoholic] cirrhosis), geriatric patients (about 2.3 hours), and obese patients (about 3 hours).

Fentanyl—
  Triphasic (with a dose of 6.4 mcg per kg of body weight):
    Distribution—1.7 minutes.
    Redistribution—13 minutes.
    Elimination—3.6 hours; may be greatly prolonged during and following cardiopulmonary bypass and in geriatric patients. One study showed an average elimination half-life of 15.75 hours following administration of 10 mcg per kg of body weight to patients 60 years of age or older.

Sufentanil—
  Triphasic (with a dose of 5 mcg per kg of body weight):
    Distribution—1.4 minutes.
    Redistribution—18 minutes.
    Elimination—2.7 hours; may be greatly prolonged during and following cardiopulmonary bypass.

### Onset of action

Alfentanil—
  Analgesic effects (anesthesia adjunct doses):
    Within 1 minute.
  Time to loss of consciousness (induction doses):
    Dependent on rate of administration; generally within 1 to 2 minutes.

Fentanyl—
  Analgesic effects (anesthesia adjunct doses):
    Intramuscular—7 to 15 minutes.
    Intravenous—1 to 2 minutes.
  Time to loss of consciousness (induction doses):
    Dependent on rate of administration; 4 to 5 minutes when administered intravenously at a rate of 400 mcg per minute.

Sufentanil—
  Analgesic effects (anesthesia adjunct doses):
    Within 1 minute.
  Time to loss of consciousness (induction doses):
    Dependent on rate of administration; 1 to 1.6 minutes when administered intravenously at a rate of 300 mcg per minute.

Note: The time to loss of consciousness with induction doses of these medications may be substantially decreased by premedication with a benzodiazepine.

### Therapeutic plasma concentration

Requirements are highly subject to interpatient variability and dependent on the intensity of the surgical stimulus. With alfentanil, it has been shown that the highest plasma concentrations are required near the beginning of surgery (with intubation requiring higher concentrations than incision) and the lowest toward the end of surgery (i.e., during skin closure). Studies of therapeutic plasma concentrations of fentanyl or sufentanil required for different types of surgery, or at different times during a surgical procedure, have not been done.

For use of alfentanil as a supplement to inhalation (nitrous oxide/oxygen) anesthesia—
  For superficial surgery: 100 to >300 nanograms per mL.
  For intra-abdominal surgery: 310 to >400 nanograms per mL.

### Time to peak effect

Alfentanil—
  Single analgesic dose of up to 500 mcg:
    Within 1.5 to 2 minutes (for both analgesia and respiratory depression).

Fentanyl—
  Analgesic effects:
    Intramuscular—20 to 30 minutes.
    Intravenous—3 to 5 minutes.
  Respiratory depressant effects:
    5 to 15 minutes following administration of a single intravenous dose.

### Duration of action

Alfentanil—
  Analgesic effects (single dose of up to 500 mcg):
    5 to 10 minutes.
  Time to awakening (when used as a supplement to nitrous oxide/oxygen anesthesia):
    Usually within 10 minutes following the end of surgery when administered either as single injections or as a variable-rate infusion that is discontinued approximately 15 minutes before the end of surgery.

  Note: Alfentanil's duration of action may be decreased in children.

Fentanyl—
  Analgesic effects (anesthesia adjunct doses):
    Intramuscular—1 to 2 hours.
    Intravenous—0.5 to 1 hour (single dose of up to 100 mcg).
  Time to awakening (high doses):
    0.7 to 3.5 hours following an average total dose of 122 mcg per kg of body weight.

Sufentanil—
  Analgesic effects (anesthesia adjunct doses):
    5 minutes.
  Time to awakening (high doses):
    0.7 to 2.9 hours following an average total dose of 12.9 mcg per kg of body weight.

Note: The duration of action of fentanyl and its derivatives is dose-dependent. The effects of a low to moderate single dose of any of these medications are terminated rapidly because of redistribution.

With high or multiple doses or prolonged administration of fentanyl or sufentanil, the duration of action is prolonged because substantial plasma concentrations of these agents may be maintained during their clearance from tissue storage sites (although accumulation of sufentanil is less than that of fentanyl). Accumulation of alfentanil resulting in a prolonged duration of action may occur with prolonged continuous infusion or, to a lesser extent, with repeated administration of single injections during lengthy surgical procedures. However, because accumulation of alfentanil in body tissues is significantly less extensive than that of fentanyl or sufentanil, alfentanil's duration of action after multiple doses or prolonged continuous infusion is more highly dependent on total body clearance than on redistribution and subsequent removal from tissue storage sites. Therefore, alfentanil's duration of action may be affected to a greater extent than that of fentanyl or sufentanil by factors that tend to decrease the rate of metabolism (See *Biotransformation*).

When fentanyl or sufentanil is administered in high doses as the primary agent for maintenance of anesthesia, respiratory depression requiring continued mechanical ventilation may persist for many hours after the patient awakens.

### Elimination

Alfentanil—Hepatic; only 0.2% of a dose is excreted in the urine as unchanged alfentanil. Inactive metabolites are also excreted in the urine. Approximately 81% of a dose is excreted within 24 hours.

Fentanyl—Primarily hepatic; 10 to 25% of a dose may be excreted in the urine as unchanged fentanyl. About 70% of a dose is excreted within 4 days.

Sufentanil—Via metabolism; about 2% of a dose is excreted in the urine as unchanged sufentanil. About 80% of a dose is excreted within 24 hours.

## Precautions to Consider

### Cross-sensitivity and/or related problems

Patients hypersensitive to fentanyl may be hypersensitive to the chemically related alfentanil or sufentanil also, and vice versa.

**Carcinogenicity**

Long-term animal studies of the carcinogenic potential of alfentanil have not been done.

**Mutagenicity**

For alfentanil—No evidence of mutagenicity was demonstrated in the Ames *Salmonella* metabolic activating test. Also, no mutagenicity was demonstrated in the micronucleus test in female rats or the dominant lethal assay in female and male mice with single intravenous doses up to 20 mg per kg of body weight (mg/kg) (approximately 40 times the upper recommended human dose).

For sufentanil—Sufentanil has not been shown to have mutagenic potential in the micronucleus test in female rats (with single intravenous doses up to 80 mcg per kg) or in the Ames test.

**Pregnancy/Reproduction**

Pregnancy—

*First trimester—*

For alfentanil:

Although adequate and well-controlled studies in humans have not been done, one study demonstrated that alfentanil readily crosses the placenta. Studies in rats and rabbits have not shown that alfentanil is teratogenic. However, embryocidal effects (possibly related to maternal toxicity) occurred following administration of 2.5 times the upper recommended human dose for 10 to more than 30 days.

FDA Pregnancy Category C.

For fentanyl:

Although studies on the teratogenic potential of fentanyl have not been done in either animals or humans, one study showed that fentanyl crosses the placenta when it is administered to the mother prior to cesarean section.

FDA Pregnancy Category C.

For sufentanil:

Although adequate and well-controlled studies in humans have not been done, studies in rats and rabbits have not shown that sufentanil is teratogenic. However, embryocidal effects (possibly related to maternal toxicity, decreased food consumption, and anoxia) occurred in rats and rabbits following administration of up to 2.5 times the upper human dose for 10 to more than 30 days.

FDA Pregnancy Category C.

Labor and delivery—The safety of fentanyl derivatives in obstetrics has not been established. However, in one study, drowsiness (but no other adverse effect) was observed in 4-hour-old neonates after administration of fentanyl to the mother prior to cesarean section. This effect was associated with a concentration of 0.8 nanograms (or more) of fentanyl per mL of cord blood. Drowsiness was not present 24 hours after birth.

**Breast-feeding**

Problems in humans have not been documented.

*For alfentanil—*

In one study, 0.88 nanograms of alfentanil per mL was measured in colostrum 4 hours following maternal administration of 60 mcg per kg of body weight. Measurable concentrations were not present 28 hours following administration.

*For sufentanil—*

It is not known whether sufentanil is excreted in breast milk.

**Pediatrics**

Neonates may be more susceptible to the effects, especially the respiratory depressant effects, of opioid analgesics. Caution is recommended if fentanyl is used as presurgical or postsurgical medication in these patients.

Neonates have been found to have low concentrations of alpha-1-acidglycoprotein, leading to a reduced protein-binding capacity for alfentanil and an increase in the quantity of the medication available to receptor sites. However, one study has demonstrated an increased alfentanil dosage requirement in neonates.

The elimination half-life and duration of action of alfentanil may be decreased in pediatric patients. More frequent administration of supplemental doses than is usually needed by adults may be required.

**Geriatrics**

Geriatric patients may be more susceptible to the effects, especially the respiratory depressant effects, of opioid analgesics. Also, elderly patients are more likely to have age-related renal function impairment, which may require caution in patients receiving alfentanil (because of decreased protein-binding, which increases the effects of alfentanil by increasing its concentration at receptor sites) or fentanyl (because excretion of fentanyl may be slowed). Lower initial and supplemental doses, a slower infusion rate, and/or a longer interval between doses than are usually recommended for younger adults may be required for

these patients. However, geriatric patients may also be more sensitive to the therapeutic effects of opioid analgesics so that lower doses may be sufficient. In one study, possible increased brain sensitivity to alfentanil was demonstrated in geriatric patients (compared with healthy young adults) as shown by a 40% reduction in the dose required to produce delta waves in the electroencephalogram (EEG).

Many studies have indicated that clearance of opioid analgesics is significantly reduced in geriatric patients. Specifically, studies have shown that alfentanil clearance is reduced by approximately 30% (leading to a prolonged elimination half-life) in patients older than 65 years of age, and that the elimination half-life of fentanyl may be greatly prolonged (in one study, to 15.75 hours) because of reduced clearance in patients 60 years of age and older. Reduced clearance may lead to a risk of delayed postoperative recovery.

**Drug interactions and/or related problems**

The following drug interactions and/or related problems have been selected on the basis of their potential clinical significance (possible mechanism in parentheses where appropriate)—not necessarily inclusive (» = major clinical significance):

Note: Combinations containing any of the following medications, depending on the amount present, may also interact with this medication.

Anesthetics, peridural conduction or
Anesthetics, spinal

(alterations in respiration caused by high levels of spinal or peridural blockade may be additive to fentanyl derivative–induced alterations in respiratory rate and alveolar ventilation; also, the vagal effects of fentanyl derivatives may be more pronounced in patients with high levels of spinal or epidural anesthesia, possibly leading to bradycardia and/or hypotension)

Antihypertensives or
Diuretics or
Hypotension-producing medications, other (See *Appendix II*)

(hypotensive effects of these medications may be potentiated when they are used concurrently with a fentanyl derivative; patients should be monitored for excessive fall in blood pressure during and following concurrent use)

» Benzodiazepines

(premedication with a benzodiazepine such as diazepam, lorazepam, or midazolam may decrease the dose of a fentanyl derivative required for induction of anesthesia and decrease the time to loss of consciousness with induction doses; also, administration of a benzodiazepine prior to or during surgery may decrease the risk of patient recall of surgical events postoperatively; however, these potential benefits must be weighed against the potential risks of concurrent use, such as an increased risk of severe hypotension associated with decreases in systemic vascular resistance, increased risk of respiratory depression, and delayed recovery time, especially when the benzodiazepine is administered intravenously)

Beta-adrenergic blocking agents

(preoperative chronic use of systemic beta-adrenergic blocking agents may decrease the frequency and/or severity of hypertensive responses to surgery, especially during sternotomy and sternal spread in cardiac or coronary artery surgery; however, chronic preoperative use of systemic beta-adrenergic blocking agents or ophthalmic beta-adrenergic blocking agents [especially levobunolol or timolol] may also increase the risk of initial bradycardia following induction doses of a fentanyl derivative)

» Buprenorphine and other partial mu-receptor agonists

(use of buprenorphine as presurgical medication prior to opioid analgesic–assisted anesthesia should be undertaken with caution because this partial mu-receptor agonist has high affinity for, and dissociates slowly from, the mu receptor and may therefore decrease the therapeutic effects of subsequently administered mu-receptor agonist)

(buprenorphine and other partial mu-receptor agonists have the potential to reverse respiratory depressant effects induced by high doses of other opioid analgesics [while providing adequate postoperative analgesia] or to cause additive respiratory depression, hypotension, and/or CNS depression if administered in conjunction with low doses of other opioids; although the effects of buprenorphine administered following alfentanil- or sufentanil-assisted anesthesia have not been determined, in one study, administration of 0.3 or 0.45 mg of buprenorphine intramuscularly every 6 hours following opioid-assisted anesthesia with total doses of 0.2 or 0.3 mg of fentanyl caused a higher incidence of hypotension, respiratory depression, and CNS depression than equianalgesic doses [10 or 15 mg] of morphine intramuscularly every 6 hours)

» CNS depression–producing medications, other, including those commonly used as preanesthetic medication or for induction, supplementation, or maintenance of anesthesia (See *Appendix II*)

(concurrent use with a fentanyl derivative may result in increased CNS depressant, respiratory depressant, and hypotensive effects; caution is recommended and the dosage of each agent should be carefully titrated)

(it is recommended that initial dosage of other opioid agonist analgesics used during recovery from fentanyl- or sufentanil-assisted anesthesia be decreased to as low as one-fourth to one-third of the usual recommended dose)

(dosage requirements of volatile inhalation anesthetics may be decreased by 30 to 50% for the first hour of maintenance following administration of anesthetic induction doses of alfentanil)

» Hepatic enzyme inhibitors (See *Appendix II*)

(chronic preoperative administration or perioperative use of hepatic enzyme inhibitors may decrease plasma clearance and prolong the duration of action of alfentanil)

Monoamine oxidase (MAO) inhibitors, including furazolidone, pargyline, and procarbazine

(caution is recommended when using a fentanyl derivative in patients who have received an MAO inhibitor within 14 days because concurrent use of MAO inhibitors with meperidine has resulted in unpredictable, severe, and sometimes fatal reactions, including immediate excitation, sweating, rigidity, and severe hypertension, or, in some patients, hypotension, severe respiratory depression, coma, seizures, hyperpyrexia, and vascular collapse; the risk of a significant reaction with fentanyl-derivative opioid analgesics has been questioned because a few reports indicate that fentanyl caused no adverse reactions when administered to patients receiving MAO inhibitor therapy; however, administration of a small test dose of a fentanyl derivative [to detect any possible interaction] may be advisable until the relative risk of concurrent use has been better defined)

Nalbuphine or
Pentazocine

(these opioid agonist/antagonist analgesics may partially antagonize the analgesic, respiratory depressant, and CNS depressant effects of fentanyl derivatives; however, because of their agonist activity, concurrent use of these agents also has the potential to produce additive CNS, respiratory, and hypotensive effects; the extent to which antagonistic or additive effects will predominate may depend upon dosage of the fentanyl derivative, with antagonism being more likely with low to moderate doses)

Naloxone

(naloxone antagonizes the analgesic, hypotensive, CNS, and respiratory depressant effects of fentanyl derivatives; dosage of the antagonist should be carefully titrated when used to reverse the effects of opioid analgesics used during surgery in order to achieve the desired effect without interfering with control of postoperative pain or inducing other adverse effects)

(naloxone also reverses skeletal muscle rigidity induced by fentanyl derivatives)

» Naltrexone

(usual doses of opioid analgesics will be ineffective if administered to a patient receiving naltrexone, which blocks the therapeutic effects of opioid analgesics; if possible, alternative [nonopioid] medications should be used prior to, during, and following surgery, because administration of increased doses of opioids to override naltrexone blockade of opioid receptors may result in increased and more prolonged respiratory depression and/or circulatory collapse; naltrexone should be discontinued several days prior to elective surgery if administration of an opioid is unavoidable)

Neuromuscular blocking agents

(concurrent use with high doses of sufentanil may reduce the initial dosage requirements for a nondepolarizing neuromuscular blocking agent; it is recommended that a peripheral nerve stimulator be used to determine dosage)

(concurrent use of a neuromuscular blocking agent prevents or reverses muscle rigidity induced by fentanyl derivatives)

(a neuromuscular blocking agent having vagolytic activity such as pancuronium or gallamine may decrease the risk of fentanyl derivative–induced bradycardia or hypotension, especially in patients receiving chronic therapy with beta-adrenergic blocking agents and/or vasodilators for treatment of coronary artery disease; however, concurrent use may also increase the risk of tachycardia or hypertension in some patients)

(a nonvagolytic neuromuscular blocking agent such as succinylcholine will not decrease the risk of bradycardia or hypotension

induced by a fentanyl derivative; however, in some patients, especially those with compromised cardiac function and/or those receiving a beta-adrenergic blocking agent preoperatively, concurrent use may increase the incidence and/or severity of these effects)

(respiratory depressant effects of neuromuscular blocking agents may be additive to respiratory depressant effects of fentanyl derivatives; although increased or prolonged respiratory depression or paralysis [apnea] may occur, clinical significance is minimal while the patient is being mechanically ventilated; however, patients should be carefully monitored during and following concurrent use, especially if there is a possibility of incomplete reversal of neuromuscular blockade postoperatively)

Nitrous oxide

(in addition to the increased CNS depressant, respiratory depressant, and hypotensive effects that may occur when a fentanyl derivative is used concurrently with any CNS depressant, concurrent use of nitrous oxide with high doses of these agents may decrease mean arterial pressure, heart rate, and cardiac output; these effects may be more pronounced in patients with poor left ventricular function)

Phenothiazines

(in addition to the increased CNS depressant, respiratory depressant, and hypotensive effects that may occur when a phenothiazine is used concurrently with an opioid analgesic, some phenothiazines increase, while others decrease, the effects of opioid analgesic supplements to anesthesia; however, the effect of various phenothiazines on fentanyl derivative–assisted anesthesia has not been determined)

## Laboratory value alterations

The following have been selected on the basis of their potential clinical significance (possible effect in parentheses where appropriate)—not necessarily inclusive (» = major clinical significance):

With diagnostic test results

Gastric emptying studies

(opioid analgesics may delay gastric emptying, thereby invalidating test results)

Hepatobiliary imaging using technetium Tc 99m disofenin

(delivery of technetium Tc 99m disofenin to the small bowel may be prevented because of opioid analgesic–induced constriction of the sphincter of Oddi and increased biliary tract pressure; these actions result in delayed visualization and thus resemble obstruction of the common bile duct; contraction of the sphincter of Oddi has been demonstrated with alfentanil and fentanyl and, although not yet documented, should be considered a possibility with sufentanil also)

Plasma amylase determinations and
Plasma lipase determinations

(activity of these enzymes may be increased because alfentanil and fentanyl can cause contractions of the sphincter of Oddi and increased biliary tract pressure; the possibility should be considered that the diagnostic utility of determinations of these enzymes may be compromised for up to 24 hours after fentanyl administration or for several hours after alfentanil administration; although documentation is not yet available, the possibility exists that similar effects may occur with sufentanil)

With physiology/laboratory test values

Cerebrospinal fluid pressure

(opioid analgesics may increase cerebrospinal fluid pressure; effect is secondary to respiratory depression–induced carbon dioxide retention)

## Medical considerations/Contraindications

The medical considerations/contraindications included here have been selected on the basis of their potential clinical significance (reasons given in parentheses where appropriate)—not necessarily inclusive (» = major clinical significance).

*Risk-benefit should be considered when the following medical problems exist:*

*For all indications*

Allergic reaction to fentanyl or its derivatives, history of

Cardiac bradyarrhythmias

(may be induced or exacerbated)

Cardiac conditions leading to compromised cardiac reserve

(increased risk of severe bradycardia and/or undesirably large decreases in mean blood pressure, especially following rapid administration of induction doses of a fentanyl derivative)

Head injury or
Increased intracranial pressure, pre-existing or
Intracranial lesions
>    (risk of respiratory depression and further elevation of cerebrospinal fluid pressure is increased; also, opioid analgesic–induced sedation and pupillary changes may obscure clinical course of head injury)

» Hepatic function impairment or cirrhosis
>    (studies have demonstrated that alfentanil clearance rate is reduced, leading to increased elimination half-life and prolonged duration of action; although clearance of fentanyl or sufentanil may not be altered as greatly as that of alfentanil, caution is advised)
>    (alfentanil's effects may also be increased because of decreased protein-binding leading to increased concentration of medication at receptor sites; a reduction of alfentanil dosage may be required)

Hypothyroidism
>    (risk of respiratory depression and prolonged CNS depression is greatly increased; a reduction in dosage of the fentanyl derivative may be required)

Renal function impairment
>    (elimination of fentanyl [up to 25% of a dose is excreted unchanged in the urine] may be slowed)
>    (alfentanil's effects may be increased because of decreased protein-binding leading to increased concentration of medication at receptor sites; however, alfentanil's clearance rate and duration of action are not affected)

Respiratory impairment or pulmonary disease, pre-existing
>    (opioid analgesics may further decrease respiratory drive and increase airway resistance; although clinical significance is minimal if the patient is being mechanically ventilated during surgery, respiratory support may be required with doses that usually permit spontaneous breathing)

Caution is also advised in elderly, very ill, or debilitated patients, who may be more sensitive to the effects, especially the respiratory depressant effects, of opioid analgesics.

*For use of a fentanyl derivative for indications other than as a component of anesthesia*
Abdominal conditions, acute
>    (diagnosis or clinical course may be obscured)

Gallbladder disease or gallstones
>    (opioid analgesics may cause biliary tract spasm)

Gastrointestinal tract surgery
>    (opioid analgesics may decrease gastrointestinal motility)

Prostatic hypertrophy or obstruction or
Urethral stricture or
Urinary tract surgery
>    (opioid analgesics may cause urinary retention)

» Respiratory impairment or pulmonary disease, pre-existing
>    (opioid analgesics may further decrease respiratory drive and increase airway resistance)

» Caution is also advised in elderly, very ill, or very young patients, who may be more sensitive to the effects, especially the respiratory depressant effects, of opioid analgesics.

**Patient monitoring**
The following may be especially important in patient monitoring (other tests may be warranted in some patients, depending on condition; » = major clinical significance):

Monitoring of vital signs, especially blood pressure and respiratory status
>    (required during and following administration; prolonged postoperative surveillance may be necessary following high or multiple doses or prolonged administration because of the risk of prolonged respiratory depression, especially after use of fentanyl or sufentanil; also, following high or multiple doses or prolonged administration of alfentanil or fentanyl, respiratory depression, respiratory arrest, bradycardia, asystole, arrhythmias, and hypotension have occurred or recurred following initial recovery)

## Side/Adverse Effects

Note: *Fentanyl derivatives may cause rigidity in muscles of respiration in the chest and pharynx, which may lead to difficulty in establishing pulmonary ventilation. Rigidity may occur more rapidly with alfentanil than with fentanyl or sufentanil. In addition, alfentanil may cause rigidity of abdominal muscles; flexion of the fingers, wrists, and elbows; extension of the toes, ankles, knees, and hips; contraction of neck muscles; immobility of the head; and/or clenching of the jaw. These effects are dose-dependent and must be an-*

ticipated with anesthetic induction doses. Abnormal eye movements (i.e., disconjugate gaze) have also been reported during induction with alfentanil. Chest wall rigidity has also been reported during emergence from fentanyl- or sufentanil-assisted anesthesia.

Delayed respiratory depression, respiratory arrest, bradycardia, asystole, arrhythmias, and hypotension have been reported to occur or recur following initial recovery from alfentanil- or fentanyl-assisted anesthesia and should be considered a possibility following sufentanil-assisted anesthesia also.

Like other opioid analgesics, fentanyl derivatives may cause physical dependence following prolonged use. It has been proposed that adverse effects (such as tachycardia, hypertension, hyperpnea, hyperalgesia, nausea, and vomiting) occurring (rarely) after naloxone is administered for reversal of opioid effects following lengthy surgical procedures may be manifestations of an induced abstinence syndrome in acutely dependent individuals. However, other symptoms more commonly associated with an opioid withdrawal syndrome have not been reported following perisurgical use.

In addition to the side effects listed below, hypertension, tachycardia, and skeletal muscle movements (not related to onset of rigidity) may occur during surgery. These effects may be indicative of a failure to suppress autonomic responses to surgical stimulation rather than a direct effect of the medication. The incidence and severity of these effects are lower with sufentanil than with alfentanil or fentanyl.

Although not all of the side/adverse effects listed below have been reported with all of the fentanyl derivatives, they have been reported with at least one of these medications and/or encountered during administration of other opioid analgesics. Therefore, they should be considered potential side effects of any of the fentanyl derivatives.

The following side/adverse effects have been selected on the basis of their potential clinical significance (possible signs and symptoms in parentheses where appropriate)—not necessarily inclusive:

**Those indicating need for medical attention**
*Bradycardia; hypotension*—most likely to occur shortly after administration; blood pressure may return to preadministration values with surgical stimulation; *respiratory depression, intra- or postoperative*—may progress to apnea
Incidence less frequent
*Cardiac arrhythmia*—incidence 2% with alfentanil or fentanyl; <1% with sufentanil; *confusion, postoperative*—rare with alfentanil
Incidence rare
*Bronchospasm, allergic*—not caused by histamine release; *circulatory depression*—may lead to cardiac arrest; *convulsions*—reported with fentanyl and sufentanil only; *dermatitis, allergic* (skin rash [fentanyl], hives [alfentanil, fentanyl], and/or itching [alfentanil, fentanyl, sufentanil]); *dysesthesia, opioid analgesic–induced* (itching, especially of the face); *laryngospasm*—may be a form of rigidity; *mental depression, postoperative; paradoxical CNS excitation or delirium*

**Those common to opioid analgesics (but not necessarily reported specifically with fentanyl derivatives) and indicating need for medical attention only if they continue or are bothersome**
Incidence more frequent
*Drowsiness, postoperative*—less frequent with alfentanil; *nausea or vomiting*—lower incidence reported with sufentanil than with alfentanil or fentanyl but highly variable; may depend on the specific surgical procedure performed, e.g., especially likely following gynecologic surgery
Incidence less frequent or rare
*Biliary spasm; blurred or double vision or other changes in vision; chills; CNS depression or hypotension, orthostatic* (dizziness, lightheadedness, feeling faint, unusual tiredness or weakness); *constipation; ureteral spasm* (decreased or difficult urination)

## Overdose

For specific information on the agents used in the management of an overdose, see:
• *Atropine* in *Anticholinergics/Antispasmodics (Systemic)* monograph;
• *Naloxone (Systemic)* monograph; and/or
• *Neuromuscular Blocking Agents (Systemic)* monograph; and/or
• *Sympathomimetic Agents—Cardiovascular Use (Parenteral-Systemic)* monograph.

For more information on the management of overdose or unintentional ingestion, **contact a Poison Control Center** (see *Poison Control Center Listing*).

## Clinical effects of overdose

The following effects have been selected on the basis of their potential clinical significance (possible signs and symptoms in parentheses where appropriate)—not necessarily inclusive:

Acute

> *Bradycardia; circulatory depression; cold, clammy skin; dizziness, severe; drowsiness, severe; hypotension; nervousness or restlessness, severe; pinpoint pupils of eyes; respiratory depression; weakness, severe*

## Treatment of overdose

Specific treatment—

>    For bradycardia—Administering atropine. Alternatively, if a neuromuscular blocking agent is being used, administration of a neuromuscular blocking agent with vagolytic activity, such as pancuronium or gallamine, may antagonize fentanyl derivative–induced bradycardia.

>    For respiratory depression—During surgery, respiratory depression may be managed via endotracheal intubation and assisted or controlled respiration. If respiratory depression persists following surgery, prolonged mechanical ventilation may be required. Also, intravenous administration of the opioid antagonist naloxone may be required. Dosage of naloxone should be carefully titrated to achieve the desired effect without interfering with control of postoperative pain or causing other adverse effects; hypertension and tachycardia, sometimes resulting in left ventricular failure and pulmonary edema, have occurred following naloxone administration in these circumstances (especially in cardiac patients). Initial doses as small as 0.5 mcg (0.0005 mg) of naloxone per kg of body weight have been recommended. Because the duration of respiratory depression may exceed the duration of action of a single intravenous dose of the antagonist, continued monitoring of the patient is mandatory so that additional antagonist may be administered as necessary. Continuous intravenous infusion of naloxone may provide continuing control of undesirable opioid effects.

>    For hypotension—Administration of appropriate parenteral fluid therapy is recommended. Repositioning of the patient to improve venous return to the heart should be considered when surgical conditions permit. If necessary, a vasopressor (during or following surgery) and/or naloxone (postoperatively only) may be administered.

>    For muscle rigidity—Administering a neuromuscular blocking agent and assisting respiration via controlled ventilation with oxygen. Alternatively, if muscle rigidity should occur upon emergence, naloxone may be administered.

Supportive care—

>    Other supportive measures should also be employed as needed. Patients in whom intentional overdose is confirmed or suspected should be referred for psychiatric consultation.

## Patient Consultation

As an aid to patient consultation, refer to *Advice for the Patient, Narcotic Analgesics—For Surgery and Obstetrics (Systemic)*.

In providing consultation, consider emphasizing the following selected information (» = major clinical significance):

### Before receiving this medication

» Conditions affecting use, especially:

Allergic reaction to fentanyl or its derivatives

Pregnancy—Alfentanil and fentanyl cross the placenta

Breast-feeding—Fentanyl is excreted in breast milk

Use in children—Increased sensitivity to the effects of opioid analgesics in neonates

Use in the elderly—Increased sensitivity to the effects of opioid analgesics

Any other medications, including ''street'' drugs

Other medical problems, especially hepatic function impairment or cirrhosis and pulmonary disease

### Precautions after receiving this medication

*To be followed for about 24 hours after receiving this medication as part of an outpatient regimen*

» Caution if dizziness, drowsiness, lightheadedness, or blurred vision occurs

» Avoiding use of alcohol or other CNS depressants unless specifically prescribed or otherwise approved by physician or dentist

### Side/adverse effects

Signs and symptoms of potential side effects, especially postoperative CNS depression and allergic dermatitis

## General Dosing Information

Fentanyl derivatives should be administered only by personnel experienced in the use of intravenous anesthetics and in the management of the respiratory effects of opioid analgesics.

*An opioid antagonist, resuscitative medications, intubation equipment, and oxygen should be readily available during and following administration of a fentanyl derivative. Careful monitoring of the patient's respiratory status is necessary during and following surgery.* These medications suppress respiration, especially in elderly, very ill, or debilitated patients and those with respiratory problems. Postoperative respiratory depression may be prolonged or may recur following initial recovery, especially following use of moderate or high doses. Following administration of fentanyl or sufentanil, respiratory depression requiring mechanical ventilation may be greatly prolonged. Alfentanil-induced respiratory depression is of shorter duration than that induced by fentanyl or sufentanil. The peak respiratory depressant effect of fentanyl occurs 5 to 15 minutes following administration of a single intravenous dose and may persist longer than the analgesic effect.

Sufentanil is approximately 5 to 7 times more potent than fentanyl on a mcg-to-mcg (and mL-to-mL) basis. 100 mcg of fentanyl or 13 to 20 mcg of sufentanil produce analgesic effects equivalent to 10 mg of morphine. Alfentanil has been reported to be 3 to 10 times less potent than fentanyl on a mcg-to-mcg basis (as determined by dosage requirements). However, because of alfentanil's considerably smaller volume of distribution, much higher plasma concentrations are achieved with alfentanil than with equal doses of fentanyl; studies comparing plasma concentrations of fentanyl or alfentanil required to produce similar effects have indicated that fentanyl may be up to 75 times more potent than alfentanil. Also, interpatient variability in responsiveness to these medications and/or differences in analytic methodology may have contributed to the difficulty in determining relative potency.

The usual adult and pediatric doses stated below are intended as a guideline only. Dosage must be individualized on the basis of the age, weight, body size, and physical status of the patient; underlying pathology; other medications used concurrently, especially the type of anesthesia to be used; type and anticipated duration of the surgical procedure involved; and patient response. Also, for obese patients (more than 20% above ideal body weight), the dosage of alfentanil or sufentanil should be determined on the basis of lean body weight.

It is recommended that initial dosage be reduced in elderly or debilitated patients. The effects of the initial dose should be considered in determining supplemental doses. Lower doses may also be required in patients with chronic hepatic disease (especially for alfentanil) or hypothyroidism.

Fentanyl derivatives may cause rigidity of chest and abdominal muscles, which may interfere with pulmonary ventilation. Alfentanil may also cause rigidity in other muscles. The risk of muscle rigidity may be reduced if intravenous injections are administered slowly. A neuromuscular blocking agent compatible with the patient's condition may be administered prophylactically to prevent muscle rigidity or to induce muscle relaxation after rigidity occurs. Rigidity has also been reported upon emergence from fentanyl- or sufentanil-assisted anesthesia and should be considered a possibility upon emergence from alfentanil-assisted anesthesia.

It is recommended that intravenous injections of fentanyl or sufentanil be given slowly over a period of at least 1 to 2 minutes, especially if high doses are being administered. It is recommended that induction doses of alfentanil also be given slowly. Although the manufacturer's prescribing information recommends that induction doses of alfentanil be administered over a period of approximately 3 minutes, many investigators have administered induction doses within 90 seconds. Slow intravenous administration of these medications may reduce the incidence and/or severity of rigidity, bradycardia, and hypotension. Also, rapid intravenous administration of other opioid analgesics has caused anaphylactoid reactions, severe respiratory depression, hypotension, peripheral circulatory collapse, and cardiac arrest.

Premedication with a benzodiazepine may reduce induction dose requirements and decrease the time to loss of consciousness. In addition, administration of a benzodiazepine or other amnestic agent may help to prevent patient recall of intrasurgical events postoperatively. Patient recall of intrasurgical events despite the absence of autonomic or hormonal responses indicative of light or inadequate anesthesia has been reported following use of high-dose fentanyl with 100% oxygen and, although not reported to date, should be considered a possibility following use of high-dose sufentanil with 100% oxygen or following administration of alfentanil also. However, the fact that concurrent use of a benzodiazepine with a fentanyl derivative may increase the risk of hypotension, respiratory depression, or delayed recovery must be kept in mind. Alternatively, detection of signs of inadequate anesthesia may be facilitated if the neuromuscular blocking agent being used is administered in doses titrated to avoid complete paralysis.

Fentanyl derivatives, even in very high doses, may fail to suppress autonomic responses to surgical stimulation. Tachycardia and hypertension may occur and are more likely to respond rapidly to additional doses of alfentanil or sufentanil than to additional fentanyl. However, administration of a suitable antihypertensive agent may be required in some patients. In patients undergoing cardiac surgery, administration of a beta-adrenergic blocking agent with the presurgical medication (or continuation of previously instituted therapy with a beta-adrenergic blocking agent up to the time of surgery) may reduce or prevent these responses.

Tolerance to the effects of fentanyl or sufentanil may occur with repeated dosing; in addition, patients who have become tolerant to other opioid analgesics may be at least partially cross-tolerant to the effects of a fentanyl derivative also.

Like other opioid analgesics, fentanyl derivatives may cause physical dependence following prolonged use. Rarely, symptoms possibly indicating a type of withdrawal syndrome (e.g., tachycardia, hypertension, hyperpnea, hyperalgesia, nausea, and vomiting) may occur following administration of naloxone (especially in high doses) for reversal of opioid effects postoperatively. However, other symptoms commonly associated with an opioid withdrawal syndrome do not occur.

**For treatment of adverse effects**
Recommended treatment may include:
• For hypotension—Administration of appropriate parenteral fluid therapy is recommended. Repositioning of the patient to improve venous return to the heart should be considered when surgical conditions permit. If necessary, a vasopressor (during or following surgery) and/or naloxone (postoperatively only) may be administered.
• For muscle rigidity—Administering a neuromuscular blocking agent and assisting respiration via controlled ventilation with oxygen. Alternatively, if muscle rigidity should occur upon emergence, naloxone may be administered.

Other supportive measures should also be employed as needed.

---

*ALFENTANIL*

## Summary of Differences

Indications: See *Indications*.
Pharmacology/pharmacokinetics: See *Pharmacology/Pharmacokinetics*.
Pediatrics: Duration of action may be reduced in children.
Drug interactions and/or related problems: Hepatic enzyme inhibitors may prolong duration of action.
Side/adverse effects: See *Side/Adverse Effects*.

## Additional Dosing Information

See also *General Dosing Information*.

The anesthetic $ED_{90}$ in unpremedicated patients (induction dose required to attenuate or abolish the response to placement of a nasopharyngeal airway in 90% of the patients) is approximately 169 to 182 mcg per kg of body weight (using a rapid induction); however, values ranging from 137 to 383 mcg per kg of body weight have been reported.

An initial loading dose of alfentanil is required to achieve therapeutic plasma concentrations rapidly. Administration of the induction or loading dose may be followed by continuous intravenous infusion of the medication and/or administration of supplemental single injections as required. Continuous intravenous infusion, with the rate of infusion adjusted according to the observed clinical effect, may reduce the total maintenance dosage requirement, decrease the risk of postoperative respiratory depression, and speed recovery time, and may be the preferred method of administration. If necessary, small single doses may be administered in addition to or instead of increasing the infusion rate as required to prevent or abolish responses to surgical stimuli or other signs of light or inadequate anesthesia.

Because alfentanil requirements are lowest near the end of surgery, it is recommended that the maintenance infusion be discontinued 10 to 20 minutes before the end of surgery. If further administration of alfentanil is required after the infusion is discontinued, single injections of 7 to 15 mcg per kg of body weight may be given.

Because of alfentanil's short duration of action, postoperative pain requiring treatment may occur relatively early in the recovery period.

## Parenteral Dosage Forms
### ALFENTANIL HYDROCHLORIDE INJECTION
**Usual adult dose**
Anesthesia adjunct (opioid analgesic)—
    Induction of anesthesia (for procedures lasting 45 minutes or longer): Intravenous, 130 to 245 mcg (0.13 to 0.245 mg) (base) per kg of body weight. Induction with alfentanil may be followed by administration of an inhalation anesthetic (with the required concentration of inhalation anesthetic generally being reduced by 30 to 50% during the first hour of maintenance) or by further administration of alfentanil in maintenance doses.
    Maintenance of anesthesia (in conjunction with nitrous oxide and oxygen):
        Procedures lasting up to 30 minutes—Intravenous, 8 to 20 mcg (0.008 to 0.02 mg) (base) per kg of body weight as an initial loading dose, followed by administration of single doses of 3 to 5 mcg (0.003 to 0.005 mg) per kg of body weight as required or by continuous infusion at a rate of 0.5 to 1 mcg (0.0005 to 0.001 mg) per kg of body weight per minute.
        Procedures lasting longer than 30 minutes—Intravenous, 20 to 75 mcg (0.02 to 0.075 mg) (base) per kg of body weight as an initial loading dose (if an agent other than alfentanil has been used for induction), followed by continuous infusion at a rate of 0.5 to 4 mcg (0.0005 to 0.004 mg) per kg of body weight per minute and/or by single injections of 5 to 15 mcg (0.005 to 0.015 mg) per kg of body weight as required. Following induction with alfentanil, infusion rate requirements may be reduced by 30 to 50% during the first hour of maintenance.
        Note: For maintenance of anesthesia, continuous infusions of alfentanil are generally administered at an average rate of 0.5 to 1.5 mcg (0.0005 to 0.0015 mg) (base) per kg of body weight per minute. However, a variable rate of infusion is recommended, with the rate being increased in response to signs of light or inadequate anesthesia or decreased when signs of light or inadequate anesthesia have been absent for a suitable period of time.

**Usual pediatric dose**
Anesthesia adjunct (opioid analgesic) for maintenance of anesthesia—Intravenous, 30 to 50 mcg (0.03 to 0.05 mg) (base) per kg of body weight as an initial loading dose, followed by supplemental single doses of 10 to 15 mcg (0.01 to 0.015 mg) per kg of body weight as required, or by continuous infusion at a rate of 0.5 to 1.5 mcg (0.0005 to 0.0015 mg) per kg of body weight per minute.

Note: Alfentanil half-life and duration of action are decreased in children as compared with adults; therefore, more frequent supplemental dosing may be required.

**Strength(s) usually available**
U.S.—
    Without preservative: 500 mcg (0.5 mg) (base) per mL (Rx) [*Alfenta*].
Canada—
    Without preservative: 500 mcg (0.5 mg) (base) per mL (Rx) [*Alfenta*].

**Packaging and storage**
Store between 15 and 30 °C (59 and 86 °F), protected from light, unless otherwise specified by manufacturer. Protect from freezing.

**Preparation of dosage form**
Alfentanil hydrochloride injection may be diluted with 0.9% sodium chloride injection, 5% dextrose and sodium chloride injection (0.9% sodium chloride), 5% dextrose injection, or lactated Ringer's injection to a convenient concentration. As an example, 20 mL of alfentanil hydrochloride injection may be added to 230 mL of diluent to provide a solution containing 40 mcg (0.04 mg) of alfentanil per mL.

**Stability**
Alfentanil hydrochloride injection is stable when diluted to a concentration of 25 to 80 mcg of alfentanil base per mL using any of the solutions listed in *Preparation of dosage form* above.

**Note**
Controlled substance in the U.S., Canada, and the U.K.

---

*FENTANYL*

## Summary of Differences

Indications: See *Indications*.
Pharmacology/pharmacokinetics: See *Pharmacology/Pharmacokinetics*.
Pediatrics: Neonates may be more susceptible to respiratory depressant effects, especially if used as presurgical or postsurgical medication.
Side/adverse effects: See *Side/Adverse Effects*.

# Additional Dosing Information

See also *General Dosing Information.*

A reduction in dosage may be required in very young patients receiving fentanyl as presurgical or postsurgical medication.

## Parenteral Dosage Forms

### FENTANYL CITRATE INJECTION USP

**Usual adult dose**
Anesthesia, general, adjunct—
  For minor surgery:
    Intravenous, 2 mcg (0.002 mg) (base) per kg of body weight.
  For major surgery:
    Moderate dose—Intravenous, 2 to 20 mcg (0.002 to 0.02 mg) (base) per kg of body weight.
    High dose (for open-heart surgery or complicated neurological or orthopedic procedures requiring prolonged anesthesia and abolition of stress response)—Intravenous, 20 to 50 mcg (0.02 to 0.05 mg) (base) per kg of body weight.
    Note: The total moderate or high dosage recommended during major surgery may be given as a single dose or in divided doses. The quantity of fentanyl given as an initial loading dose and as subsequent maintenance doses must be individualized, depending upon the anesthetic regimen being used, the type and anticipated duration of the surgical procedure involved, and the occurrence of signs of surgical stress or lightening of anesthesia during surgery. Although fentanyl may be administered intramuscularly during surgery, it is usually administered intravenously.
Anesthesia, local, adjunct—
  Intravenous, 0.7 to 1.4 mcg (0.0007 to 0.0014 mg) (base) per kg of body weight.
Anesthesia, as primary agent in major surgery—
  Intravenous, 50 to 100 mcg (0.05 to 0.1 mg) (base) per kg of body weight, to be administered with 100% oxygen or oxygen plus nitrous oxide and a neuromuscular blocking agent.
  Note: Up to 150 mcg (0.15 mg) (base) per kg of body weight may be required in some patients.
    In order to provide both immediate and sustained effects throughout a prolonged surgical procedure, administration of an initial loading dose of fentanyl simultaneously with or followed by continuous intravenous infusion is recommended.
Presurgical medication—
  Intramuscular, 0.7 to 1.4 mcg (0.0007 to 0.0014 mg) (base) per kg of body weight thirty to sixty minutes prior to surgery.
Postoperative (in recovery room period)—
  Intramuscular, 0.7 to 1.4 mcg (0.0007 to 0.0014 mg) (base) per kg of body weight; may be repeated in one or two hours as needed.

**Usual pediatric dose**
Anesthesia, as primary agent in major surgery—
  Children up to 2 years of age: Dosage has not been established.
  Children 2 to 12 years of age: Intravenous, 2 to 3 mcg (0.002 to 0.003 mg) (base) per kg of body weight.

**Strength(s) usually available**
U.S.—
  Without preservative: 50 mcg (0.05 mg) (base) per mL (Rx) [*Sublimaze;* GENERIC].
Canada—
  Without preservative: 50 mcg (0.05 mg) (base) per mL (Rx) [*Sublimaze*].

**Packaging and storage**
Store below 40 °C (104 °F), preferably between 15 and 30 °C (59 and 86 °F), unless otherwise specified by manufacturer. Protect from light. Protect from freezing.

**Note**
Controlled substance in the U.S., Canada, and the U.K.

## SUFENTANIL

## Summary of Differences

Indications: See *Indications.*
Pharmacology/pharmacokinetics: See *Pharmacology/Pharmacokinetics.*
Drug interactions and/or related problems: See *interaction with neuromuscular blocking agents* for information that may not apply to alfentanil or fentanyl.
Side/adverse effects: See *Side/Adverse Effects.*

## Parenteral Dosage Forms

### SUFENTANIL CITRATE INJECTION USP

**Usual adult dose**
Anesthesia, general, adjunct—
  Low dose: Intravenous, 0.5 to 1 mcg (0.0005 to 0.001 mg) (base) per kg of body weight initially. Supplemental doses of 10 to 25 mcg (0.01 to 0.025 mg) may be administered as needed.
  Moderate dose (for major surgical procedures requiring some attenuation of sympathetic response to surgical stimuli): Intravenous, 2 to 8 mcg (0.002 to 0.008 mg) (base) per kg of body weight initially. Supplemental doses of 10 to 50 mcg (0.01 to 0.05 mg) may be administered as needed.
  Note: When administered with nitrous oxide and oxygen for procedures lasting up to 8 hours, total doses of 1 mcg (0.001 mg) per kg of body weight per hour, or less, are recommended.
Anesthesia, as primary agent in major surgery—
  Intravenous, 8 to 30 mcg (0.008 to 0.03 mg) (base) per kg of body weight initially, administered with 100% oxygen. Supplemental doses of 25 to 50 mcg (0.025 to 0.05 mg) may be administered as needed.
  Note: In order to provide both immediate and sustained effects throughout a prolonged surgical procedure, administration of an initial loading dose of sufentanil simultaneously with or followed by continuous intravenous infusion is recommended.

**Usual pediatric dose**
Anesthesia, as primary agent in cardiovascular surgery—
  Initial: Intravenous, 10 to 25 mcg (0.01 to 0.025 mg) (base) per kg of body weight, administered with 100% oxygen.
  Maintenance: Intravenous, up to 25 to 50 mcg (0.025 to 0.05 mg) (base).

**Strength(s) usually available**
U.S.—
  Without preservative: 50 mcg (0.05 mg) (base) per mL (Rx) [*Sufenta;* GENERIC].
Canada—
  Without preservative: 50 mcg (0.05 mg) (base) per mL (Rx) [*Sufenta*].

**Packaging and storage**
Store below 40 °C (104 °F), preferably between 15 and 30 °C (59 and 86 °F), protected from light, unless otherwise specified by manufacturer. Protect from freezing.

**Note**
Controlled substance in both the U.S. and Canada.

Revised: 06/19/90
Interim revision: 07/26/96

---

# FERROUS CITRATE FE 59   Systemic*

VA CLASSIFICATION (Primary): DX201
Note: For a listing of dosage forms and brand names by country availability, see *Dosage Forms* section(s). For a listing of brand names for the articles in this monograph, refer to the General Index.

*Not commercially available in the U.S.

## Category

Diagnostic aid (iron metabolism; iron absorption).

## Indications

**Accepted**
Anemia (diagnosis) and
Iron metabolism studies—Ferrous citrate Fe 59 is indicated, by intravenous administration, to determine various parameters of the kinetics

of iron metabolism, including plasma iron clearance, plasma iron turn-over rate, and the utilization of iron in new red blood cells. The values of serum iron obtained from these studies provide diagnostic information in patients with anemias. Ferrous citrate Fe 59 is also useful to assess the role of the spleen in red blood cell production and destruction, and thus to help determine the advisability of splenectomy. Also, organ uptake measurements are used to measure the sites of red cell production (or lack thereof) in extramedullary erythropoiesis in myeloproliferative disorders.

Iron absorption studies—Ferrous citrate Fe 59 is indicated, by oral administration, to measure the absorption of iron from the intestine.

## Physical Properties

### Nuclear data

| Radionu-clide (half-life) | Decay constant | Mode of decay | Principal emissions (meV) | Mean number of emissions/ disintegration |
|---|---|---|---|---|
| Fe 59 (44.6 days) | 0.000649 hr⁻¹ | Beta emission | Beta-2 (mean 0.081) | 0.45 |
| | | | Beta-3 (mean 0.149) | 0.53 |
| | | | Gamma-2 (0.192) | 0.03 |
| | | | Gamma-5 (1.099) | 0.56 |
| | | | Gamma-6 (1.292) | 0.43 |

## Pharmacology/Pharmacokinetics

### Mechanism of action/Effect

Iron from ferrous citrate is bound to plasma protein (transferrin) and carried to the blood-forming organs where it is utilized to form hemoglobin or is deposited in the reticuloendothelial cells of the liver and spleen. The amount of radioactive iron absorbed, transported, stored, utilized, and excreted can then be measured by the periodic collection of blood specimens and external counting.

### Protein binding
Very high.

### Half-life
Plasma iron clearance (biological)—
   Normal: 1 to 2 hours.
   Polycythemia, iron deficiency anemia, chronic blood loss, and hemolytic anemia: < 1 hour.
   Hypoplastic anemia, myelofibrosis, and hemachromatosis: > 2 hours.

Note: Transferrin-bound radioactive iron concentration in plasma decreases as radioactive iron accumulates in the bone marrow. Rate of disappearance reflects erythropoiesis.

### Radiation dosimetry

| Mode of administration | Estimated absorbed radiation dose* | | |
|---|---|---|---|
| | Target organ | mGy/MBq | rad/mCi |
| Intravenous | Spleen | 55 | 200 |
| | Heart wall | 24 | 90 |
| | Liver | 12 | 44 |
| | Red marrow | 12 | 43 |
| | Kidneys | 8.6 | 32 |
| | Ovaries | 6.4 | 24 |
| | Testes | 5.3 | 20 |
| | Total body | 6.4 | 24 |

*In normal subjects.

### Elimination
No significant physiological system of excretion exists for iron. Very slowly excreted, mostly in feces; remainder excreted within cells shed by skin and gastrointestinal mucosa.

## Precautions to Consider

### Pregnancy/Reproduction
Pregnancy—The possibility of pregnancy should be assessed in women of child-bearing potential. Clinical situations exist where the benefit to the patient and fetus derived from radiopharmaceutical use outweighs the risks from radiation exposure to the fetus. In these situa-

tions, the physician should use discretion and reduce the radiopharmaceutical dose to the lowest possible amount.

### Breast-feeding
Ferrous citrate Fe 59 is excreted in breast milk. Because of the potential risk of radiation exposure to the infant, temporary discontinuation of nursing is recommended for a length of time that may be assessed by measuring the activity of breast milk and estimating the radiation exposure to the infant.

### Pediatrics
There have been no specific studies evaluating safety and efficacy of ferrous citrate Fe 59 in children. When this radiopharmaceutical is used in children, the diagnostic benefit should be judged to outweigh the potential risk of radiation.

### Geriatrics
Appropriate studies on the relationship of age to the effects of ferrous citrate Fe 159 have not been performed in the geriatric population. However, no geriatrics-specific problems have been documented to date.

### Diagnostic interference
With results of *this* test
   Foods
      (absorption of oral ferrous citrate Fe 59 may be decreased by presence of food in the stomach; overnight fasting is recommended prior to its administration for iron absorption studies)

## Side/Adverse Effects

At present, there are no known side/adverse effects associated with the use of ferrous citrate Fe 59.

## Patient Consultation

As an aid to patient consultation, refer to *Advice for the Patient, Radiopharmaceuticals (Diagnostic)*.

In providing consultation, consider emphasizing the following selected information (» = major clinical significance):

### Description of use
   Action in the body: Utilization by body of radioactive iron same as dietary iron
   Collection of blood specimen allows measurement of iron
   Small amounts of radioactivity used in diagnosis; radiation received is low and considered safe

### Before having this test
» Conditions affecting use, especially:
      Pregnancy—Risk of radiation exposure to fetus
      Breast-feeding—Excreted in breast milk; temporary discontinuation of nursing recommended because of risk of radiation exposure to infant
      Use in children—Risk of radiation exposure

### Preparation for this test
   Special preparatory instructions may be given; patient should inquire in advance

### Precautions after having this test
   No special precautions

## General Dosing Information

Radiopharmaceuticals are to be administered only by or under the supervision of physicians who have had extensive training in the safe use and handling of radionuclides and who are licensed by the Nuclear Regulatory Commission (NRC) or the appropriate Agreement State agency or, outside the U.S., the appropriate authority.

Overnight fasting is recommended prior to the oral administration of ferrous citrate Fe 59 for iron absorption studies.

### Safety considerations for handling this radiopharmaceutical

Improper handling of this radiopharmaceutical may cause radioactive contamination. Guidelines for handling radioactive material have been prepared by scientific, professional, state, federal, and international bodies and are available to the specially qualified and authorized users who have access to radiopharmaceuticals.

## Parenteral Dosage Forms

### FERROUS CITRATE Fe 59 INJECTION USP

### Usual adult and adolescent administered activity
Diagnostic aid—
   Intravenous or oral, 0.185 to 0.555 megabecquerel (5 to 15 microcuries).

**Usual pediatric administered activity**
Diagnostic aid—
   Dosage must be individualized by physician.

**Usual geriatric administered activity**
See *Usual adult and adolescent administered activity*.

**Strength(s) usually available**
U.S.—
   Not commercially available.
Canada—
   0.185 to 3.7 megabecquerels (5 to 100 microcuries) per mL, having a
   specific activity ranging from 0.185 to 1.11 megabecquerels (5 to
   30 microcuries) per microgram of iron, at time of calibration (Rx)
   [GENERIC].

**Packaging and storage**
Store below 40 °C (104 °F), preferably between 15 and 30 °C (59 and 86
°F), unless otherwise specified by manufacturer.

**Note**
Caution—Radioactive material.

Revised: 06/23/92
Interim revision: 08/02/94

---

**FERROUS FUMARATE**—See *Iron Supplements (Systemic)*

---

**FERROUS GLUCONATE**—See *Iron Supplements (Systemic)*

---

**FERROUS SULFATE**—See *Iron Supplements (Systemic)*

---

**FIBER-CONTAINING ENTERAL NUTRITION
FORMULAS**—See *Enteral Nutrition Formulas (Systemic)*

---

**FILGRASTIM**—See *Colony Stimulating Factors (Systemic)*

---

# FINASTERIDE   Systemic

VA CLASSIFICATION (Primary): GU900
Note: For a listing of dosage forms and brand names by country availa-
      bility, see *Dosage Forms* section(s). For a listing of brand names
      for the articles in this monograph, refer to the General Index.

## Category
Benign prostatic hyperplasia therapy agent.

## Indications

**Accepted**
Benign prostatic hyperplasia (treatment)—Finasteride is indicated for the
treatment of symptomatic benign prostatic hyperplasia (BPH).

   Although regression of the enlarged prostate gland occurs in most
   treated patients, significant increases in urinary flow and improvement
   in symptoms of BPH are slight and occur in only about one-third of
   treated patients. The long-term effect on the incidence of surgery,
   acute urinary obstruction, or other complications of BPH has not been
   determined.

   Because finasteride causes only slight improvement in symptoms, it is
   probably less useful in patients with severe symptoms than in patients
   with mild to moderate symptoms.

   Prior to initiation of finasteride therapy, infection, prostate cancer,
   stricture disease, hypotonic bladder, or other neurogenic disorders that
   might mimic BPH should be ruled out.

**Unaccepted**
Finasteride is not useful in patients with obstructive uropathy accompanied
by urinary retention.

## Pharmacology/Pharmacokinetics

**Physicochemical characteristics**
Source—Synthetic.
Chemical group—A 4-azasteroid compound.
Molecular weight—372.55.

**Mechanism of action/Effect**
Finasteride competitively and specifically inhibits 5-alpha-reductase, an
enzyme that metabolizes testosterone to dihydrotestosterone (DHT) in
the prostate gland, liver, and skin. Development of the prostate gland
is dependent on DHT, which is a potent androgen. After administration
of finasteride, 5-alpha–reduced steroid metabolites in blood and urine
are decreased; serum DHT is reduced by approximately 70% by daily
dosing. Concentrations of both DHT and prostate specific antigen
(PSA) are decreased in prostatic tissue. Finasteride has no affinity for
the androgen receptor and the hypothalamic-pituitary-testicular axis
does not appear to be affected.

**Absorption**
Mean bioavailability of a 5-mg tablet was 63% (range 34 to 108%) in a
study in healthy male subjects. Bioavailability is not affected by food.

**Distribution**
Finasteride crosses the blood-brain barrier. It also appears in semen; however, the amount in patients receiving 5 mg per day has been estimated
to be less than 1/50 of the dose of finasteride (5 mcg) that had no
effect on circulating DHT concentrations in adults.

**Protein binding**
Plasma—Very high (90%).

**Biotransformation**
Hepatic. The major metabolite isolated from urine is the monocarboxylic
acid metabolite; the t-butyl side chain monohydroxylated metabolite
has been isolated from plasma. These metabolites have no more than
20% of the 5-alpha-reductase inhibiting activity of finasteride.

**Half-life**
Mean 6 hours (range 3 to 16 hours) following a single 5-mg dose in
healthy male subjects 45 to 60 years of age; approximately 8 hours in
subjects 70 years of age or older.

**Time to peak concentration**
Plasma—1 to 2 hours.

**Peak serum concentration**
Plasma—Slow accumulation occurs with multiple dosing; in one study,
mean plasma concentrations were approximately 50% higher after 17
days of treatment than after the first dose, and mean trough concentrations in another study after 1 year were even higher. In one study,
mean AUC (0-24 hours) after 17 days' dosing was 15% higher in
subjects 70 years of age or older.

**Time to peak effect**
Reduction in serum DHT concentration—8 hours after the first dose.

**Duration of action**
Single dose—Reduction in serum DHT concentration: 24 hours.
Multiple doses—DHT concentrations return to pretreatment levels within
approximately 2 weeks after withdrawal of daily therapy. The prostate
returns to pretreatment size in about 4 months.

**Elimination**
Fecal, 57% (range 51 to 64%), as metabolites; renal, 39% (range 32 to
46%), as metabolites. In renal function impairment, urinary excretion
of metabolites is decreased, but fecal excretion of metabolites is increased; therefore, no dosage adjustment is necessary.
In dialysis—Unknown.

## Precautions to Consider

**Carcinogenicity**
A 19-month study in CD-1 mice at a dose of 250 mg per kg of body
weight (mg/kg) per day (228 times the human exposure) found a statistically significant increase in incidence of testicular Leydig cell adenomas. An increase in the incidence of Leydig cell hyperplasia was
observed in mice at a dose of 25 mg/kg per day (23 times the human
exposure, estimated) and in rats at a dose greater than or equal to 40
mg/kg per day (39 times the human exposure). A positive correlation

between the proliferative changes in the Leydig cells and an increase in serum luteinizing hormone (LH) concentrations (2- to 3-fold above control) has been demonstrated in both rodent species treated with high doses. No drug-related Leydig cell changes were seen in either rats or dogs treated for 1 year at doses of 20 mg/kg per day and 45 mg/kg per day (30 and 350 times, respectively, the human exposure) or in mice treated for 19 months at a dose of 2.5 mg/kg per day (2.3 times the human exposure, estimated).

### Tumorigenicity

A 24-month study in Sprague-Dawley rats at doses up to 160 mg/kg per day in males and 320 mg/kg per day in females (producing 111 and 274 times, respectively, the systemic exposure observed in man receiving the recommended human dose) found no evidence of tumorigenicity.

### Mutagenicity

No evidence of mutagenicity was found in an *in vitro* bacterial mutagenesis assay, a mammalian cell mutagenesis assay, or an *in vitro* alkaline elution assay. In an *in vitro* chromosome aberration assay, when Chinese hamster ovary cells were treated with high concentrations (450 to 550 micromoles, corresponding to 4000 to 5000 times the peak plasma concentrations in humans given a total dose of 5 mg) of finasteride, there was a slight increase in chromosome aberrations. In addition, the concentrations (450 to 550 micromoles) used in *in vitro* studies are not achievable in a biological system. In an *in vivo* chromosome aberration assay in mice, no treatment-related increase in chromosome aberration was observed at the maximum tolerated dose of 250 mg/kg per day (228 times the human exposure) as determined in the carcinogenicity studies.

### Pregnancy/Reproduction

Fertility—Volume of ejaculate may be decreased in some patients during therapy, but the decrease does not appear to interfere with normal sexual function.

No effect on fertility, sperm count, or ejaculate volume was found in sexually mature male rabbits and no effect on fertility was found in sexually mature male rats treated with 80 mg/kg per day for up to 12 weeks. However, with continued treatment for up to 24 or 30 weeks, there was an apparent decrease in fertility, fecundity, and an associated significant decrease in the weights of the seminal vesicles and prostate, which were reversible within 6 weeks of withdrawal of finasteride. No drug-related effect on testes or on mating performance has been seen in rats or rabbits. The decrease in fertility in rats is secondary to an effect on accessory sex organs (prostate and seminal vesicles) that results in failure to form a seminal plug, which is essential for normal fertility in rats but is not relevant in man.

Pregnancy—Finasteride is not indicated for use in women.

Because of the ability of 5-alpha-reductase inhibitors to inhibit conversion of testosterone to dihydrotestosterone (DHT), finasteride administration to a pregnant woman may cause abnormalities of the external genitalia of a male fetus.

Because of the potential risk to a male fetus, a woman who is pregnant or who may become pregnant should not handle crushed finasteride tablets.

When a patient's sexual partner is or may become pregnant, the patient should either avoid exposure of his sexual partner to semen or should discontinue finasteride.

Administration to pregnant rats at doses ranging from 100 mcg per kg of body weight per day (mcg/kg) to 100 mg/kg per day (1 to 1000 times the recommended human dose) produced dose-dependent development of hypospadias in 3.6 to 100% of male offspring. Pregnant rats given doses greater than or equal to 30 mcg/kg (3/10 of the recommended human dose) produced male offspring with decreased prostatic and seminal vesicular weights, delayed preputial separation, and transient nipple development; doses of greater than or equal to 3 mcg/kg per day (3/100 of the recommended dose) produced decreased anogenital distance. All changes are expected pharmacologic effects of 5-alpha-reductase inhibitors and are similar to those reported in male infants with a genetic deficiency of 5-alpha-reductase. The critical period during which these effects can be induced in male rats has been defined to be days 16 to 17 of gestation. No abnormalities were observed in female offspring exposed *in utero* to any dose of finasteride.

In studies of male rats treated with 80 mg/kg per day (61 times the human exposure), no developmental abnormalities were observed in first filial generation ($F_1$) male or female offspring resulting from mating with untreated females. Administration of 3 mg/kg per day (30 times the recommended human dose) during the late gestation and lactation period resulted in slightly decreased fertility in $F_1$ male offspring; no effects were seen in female offspring. In rabbit fetuses exposed to finasteride *in utero* from days 6 to 18 of gestation at doses up to 100 mg/kg per day (1000 times the recommended human dose), no evidence of malformations was observed; however, effects on male gen-

italia would not be expected since the rabbits were not exposed during the critical period of genital system development.

FDA Pregnancy Category X.

### Breast-feeding

Finasteride is not indicated for use in women. It is not known whether finasteride is distributed into breast milk.

### Pediatrics

Finasteride is not indicated for use in children. No information is available on the relationship of age to the effects of finasteride in pediatric patients.

### Geriatrics

The elimination rate of finasteride is decreased in the elderly (70 years of age or older); however, no dosage adjustment is necessary.

### Drug interactions and/or related problems

The following drug interactions and/or related problems have been selected on the basis of their potential clinical significance (possible mechanism in parentheses where appropriate)—not necessarily inclusive (» = major clinical significance):

Note: Combinations containing any of the following medications, depending on the amount present, may also interact with this medication.

» Anticholinergics or other medications with anticholinergic activity (See *Appendix II*) or
» Bronchodilators, adrenergic or
» Bronchodilators, xanthine-derivative or
   Sympathomimetic decongestants, especially ephedrine, phenylpropanolamine, and pseudoephedrine
   (may precipitate or aggravate urinary retention, reducing the effectiveness of finasteride in BPH, and should be avoided)

### Laboratory value alterations

The following have been selected on the basis of their potential clinical significance (possible effect in parentheses where appropriate)—not necessarily inclusive (» = major clinical significance):

With diagnostic test results
   Prostate specific antigen (PSA)
      (serum concentrations are decreased by finasteride, even in the presence of prostatic cancer; the effect on usefulness of PSA determinations for prostatic cancer detection is unknown)

With physiology/laboratory test values
   Dihydrotestosterone (DHT)
      (serum and prostatic concentrations are rapidly reduced)

   Follicle-stimulating hormone (FSH) and
   Luteinizing hormone (LH) and
   Testosterone
      (median circulating serum concentrations are increased by 10% but remain within the physiologic range; testosterone concentrations in prostatic tissue increase up to ten-fold)

### Medical considerations/Contraindications

The medical considerations/contraindications included here have been selected on the basis of their potential clinical significance (reasons given in parentheses where appropriate)—not necessarily inclusive (» = major clinical significance).

*Risk-benefit should be considered when the following medical problems exist:*

Hepatic function impairment
   (reduced metabolism)

Large residual urinary volume or
Reduced urinary flow
   (because of possible presence of obstructive uropathy, patients with these conditions may not be candidates for finasteride therapy)

» Sensitivity to finasteride

### Patient monitoring

The following may be especially important in patient monitoring (other tests may be warranted in some patients, depending on condition; » = major clinical significance):

» Digital rectal examination
   (recommended prior to initiation of therapy and at periodic intervals during therapy, to detect possible prostate cancer)

## Side/Adverse Effects

Note: Most side/adverse effects are mild and transient.

The following side/adverse effects have been selected on the basis of their potential clinical significance (possible signs and symptoms in parentheses where appropriate)—not necessarily inclusive:

**Those indicating need for medical attention only if they continue or are bothersome**
Incidence less frequent or rare
*Decreased libido; decreased volume of ejaculate; impotence*

## Patient Consultation

As an aid to patient consultation, refer to *Advice for the Patient, Finasteride (Systemic)*.

In providing consultation, consider emphasizing the following selected information (» = major clinical significance):

**Before using this medication**
» Conditions affecting use, especially:
  Sensitivity to finasteride
  Carcinogenicity—Increased incidence of testicular tumors in mice and rats receiving very high doses
  Pregnancy—When sexual partner is or may become pregnant, patient should either avoid exposure of sexual partner to semen or discontinue finasteride
  Other medications, especially anticholinergics or medications with anticholinergic effects, adrenergic bronchodilators, xanthine bronchodilators, or sympathomimetic decongestants

**Proper use of this medication**
  Getting into the habit of taking at same time each day to help increase compliance
» Does not cure, but helps control BPH; possible need for lifelong therapy; checking with physician before discontinuing medication
  Tablets may be crushed
  All patients with BPH should avoid drinking fluids, especially coffee or alcohol, in the evening, to reduce nocturia
» Proper dosing
  Missed dose: Taking as soon as possible; not taking if almost time for next dose; not doubling doses
» Proper storage

**Precautions while using this medication**
» Not taking other medications, especially nonprescription sympathomimetics, unless discussed with physician
  Women who are or who may become pregnant should not handle crushed tablets

**Side/adverse effects**
  Signs of potential side effects, especially decreased libido, decreased volume of ejaculate, or impotence (these side effects occur less frequently or rarely, and usually do not need medical attention)

## General Dosing Information

**Diet/Nutrition**
Finasteride may be taken with or without food.

## Oral Dosage Forms

### FINASTERIDE TABLETS

**Usual adult dose**
Benign prostatic hyperplasia—
  Oral, 5 mg once a day.

Note: At least six to twelve months of therapy may be required to assess clinical response.

**Strength(s) usually available**
U.S.—
  5 mg (Rx) [*Proscar* (lactose)].
Canada—
  5 mg (Rx) [*Proscar*].

**Packaging and storage**
Store below 30 °C (86 °F), unless otherwise specified by manufacturer. Store in a tight container. Protect from light.

## Selected Bibliography

Gormley GJ, Stoner E, Bruskewitz RC, et al. The effect of finasteride in men with benign prostatic hyperplasia. New Engl J Med 1992 Oct 22; 327: 1185-91.

Stoner E, The Finasteride Study Group. The clinical effects of a 5-alpha-reductase inhibitor, finasteride, on benign prostatic hyperplasia. J Urol 1992 May; 147: 1298-1302.

Proceedings of meeting of the Endocrinology and Metabolic Drugs Advisory Committee, Center for Drug Evaluation and Research, Food and Drug Administration, Bethesda, MD. February 3, 1992: Drugs for the treatment of benign prostatic hypertrophy: efficacy and safety criteria. February 4, 1992: Proscar (finasteride) for the treatment of BPH.

Revised: 03/03/93
Interim revision: 11/12/93

---

# FLAVOXATE   Systemic

VA CLASSIFICATION (Primary): GU201
Note: For a listing of dosage forms and brand names by country availability, see *Dosage Forms* section(s). For a listing of brand names for the articles in this monograph, refer to the General Index.

## Category

Antispasmodic (urinary tract).

## Indications

**Accepted**
Urologic disorders, symptoms of (treatment); and
Irritative voiding, symptoms of (treatment)—Flavoxate is indicated for the symptomatic relief, but not the definitive treatment, of dysuria, urgency, nocturia, suprapubic pain, and frequency and incontinence associated with cystitis, prostatitis, urethritis, urethrocystitis, or urethrotrigonitis.

## Pharmacology/Pharmacokinetics

**Physicochemical characteristics**
Molecular weight—427.93.

**Mechanism of action/Effect**
Exerts direct antispasmodic (relaxant) effect on smooth muscle, mainly of the urinary tract.

**Other actions/effects**
Also has weak antihistaminic, local anesthetic, and analgesic action. With high doses, flavoxate has weak anticholinergic properties.

**Absorption**
Well absorbed from gastrointestinal tract.

**Elimination**
Renal (10 to 30% eliminated within 6 hours).

## Precautions to Consider

**Pregnancy/Reproduction**
Pregnancy—Adequate and well-controlled studies in humans have not been done.
Reproduction studies in rats and rabbits at doses up to 34 times the recommended human dose have not shown that flavoxate causes impaired fertility or adverse effects on the fetus.
FDA Pregnancy Category B.

**Breast-feeding**
Problems in humans have not been documented.

**Pediatrics**
Appropriate studies on the relationship of age to the effects of flavoxate have not been performed in the pediatric population.

**Geriatrics**
Confusion is more likely to occur in geriatric patients taking flavoxate.

**Dental**
Prolonged use or use of large doses of flavoxate may decrease or inhibit salivary flow, thus contributing to the development of caries, periodontal disease, oral candidiasis, and discomfort.

**Medical considerations/Contraindications**
The medical considerations/contraindications included here have been selected on the basis of their potential clinical significance (reasons given in parentheses where appropriate)—not necessarily inclusive (» = major clinical significance).

***Risk-benefit should be considered when the following medical problems exist:***

» Gastrointestinal tract obstructive disease as in achalasia and pylorod-uodenal stenosis
(decrease in motility and tone may occur, resulting in obstruction and gastric retention)

Glaucoma, angle-closure
(mydriatic effect of flavoxate resulting in increased intraocular pressure may precipitate an acute attack of angle-closure glaucoma)

» Hemorrhage, gastrointestinal
(may exacerbate condition)

» Paralytic ileus
(may result in obstruction)

Sensitivity to flavoxate

» Uropathy, obstructive, such as bladder neck obstruction due to pro-static hypertrophy
(urinary retention may be precipitated)

## Side/Adverse Effects

Note: Although weak, flavoxate's anticholinergic action should be taken into consideration when it is given to patients where the environmental temperature is high, since there is risk of a rapid increase in body temperature because of suppression of sweat gland activity.

The following side/adverse effects have been selected on the basis of their potential clinical significance (possible signs and symptoms in parentheses where appropriate)—not necessarily inclusive:

**Those indicating need for medical attention**
Incidence rare
*Confusion*—especially in the elderly; *hypersensitivity* (skin rash or hives); *increased intraocular pressure* (eye pain); *leukopenia* (sore throat and fever)

**Those indicating need for medical attention only if they continue or are bothersome**
Incidence more frequent
*Drowsiness; dryness of mouth and throat*

Incidence less frequent or rare
*Constipation*—more frequent with doses of 800 mg or above; *difficult urination; difficulty concentrating; difficulty in eye accommodation* (blurred vision); *dizziness; fast heartbeat; headache; increased sweating; mydriatic effect* (increased sensitivity of eyes to light); *nausea or vomiting; nervousness; stomach pain*

## Overdose

For specific information on the agents used in the management of flavox-ate overdose, see:
*Thiopental in Anesthetics, Barbiturate (Systemic)* monograph;
*Benzodiazepines (Systemic)* monograph;
*Charcoal, Activated (Oral-Local)* monograph;
*Chloral Hydrate (Systemic)* monograph

For more information on the management of overdose or unintentional ingestion, **contact a Poison Control Center** (see *Poison Control Center Listing*).

**Clinical effects of overdose**
The following effects have been selected on the basis of their potential clinical significance (possible signs and symptoms in parenthesis where appropriate)—not necessarily inclusive:

*Anticholinergic effects* (clumsiness or unsteadiness; severe dizziness; severe drowsiness; fever; flushing or redness of face; hallucinations; shortness of breath or troubled breathing; unusual excitement; nervousness; restlessness; or irritability)

**Treatment of overdose**
Recommended treatment for overdose with flavoxate includes:
• To decrease absorption—Emesis or gastric lavage with 4% tannic acid solution or administration of an aqueous slurry of activated charcoal.
• Specific treatment—Administration of small doses of short-acting barbiturate (100 mg thiopental sodium) or benzodiazepines, or rectal infusion of 100 to 200 mL of a 2% solution of chloral hydrate, to

control excitement. Artificial respiration with oxygen if needed for respiratory depression. Adequate hydration. Symptomatic treatment as necessary.
• Supportive care—Patients in whom intentional overdose is known or suspected should be referred for psychiatric consultation.

## Patient Consultation

As an aid to patient consultation, refer to *Advice for the Patient, Flavoxate (Systemic)*.

In providing consultation, consider emphasizing the following selected information (» = major clinical significance):

**Before using this medication**
» Conditions affecting use, especially:
Sensitivity to flavoxate
Use in the elderly—Confusion more likely
Dental—Possible development of dental problems because of decreased salivary flow
Other medical problems, especially gastrointestinal hemorrhage, paralytic ileus, or obstruction in gastrointestinal or urinary tract

**Proper use of this medication**
Taking medication on an empty stomach with water, or with food or milk to reduce gastric irritation
» Importance of not taking more medication than the amount prescribed
» Proper dosing
Missed dose: Taking as soon as possible; if almost time for next dose, not taking at all; not doubling doses
» Proper storage

**Precautions while using this medication**
Possible increased sensitivity of eyes to light
» Caution if drowsiness or blurred vision occurs
» Caution during exercise or hot weather; overheating may result in heat stroke
Possible dryness of mouth and throat; using sugarless gum or candy, ice, or saliva substitute for relief; checking with physician or dentist if dry mouth continues for more than 2 weeks

**Side/adverse effects**
Signs of potential side effects, especially hypersensitivity, confusion, increased intraocular pressure, and leukopenia

## General Dosing Information

Flavoxate may be taken on an empty stomach with water; however, if gastric irritation occurs it may be taken with food or milk.

If urinary tract infection is present, appropriate antibacterial therapy should be administered.

## Oral Dosage Forms

### FLAVOXATE HYDROCHLORIDE TABLETS

**Usual adult and adolescent dose**
Urologic disorders or
Irritative voiding—
Oral, 100 to 200 mg three or four times a day, the dosage being adjusted as needed and tolerated.

**Usual pediatric dose**
Dosage has not been established.

**Usual geriatric dose**
See *Usual adult and adolescent dose.*

**Strength(s) usually available**
U.S.—
100 mg (Rx) [*Urispas*].
Canada—
200 mg (Rx) [*Urispas*].

**Packaging and storage**
Store below 40 °C (104 °F), preferably between 15 and 30 °C (59 and 86 °F), unless otherwise specified by manufacturer.

**Auxiliary labeling**
• May cause drowsiness or blurred vision.

Revised: 01/18/93

# FLECAINIDE    Systemic

VA CLASSIFICATION (Primary): CV300

Note: For a listing of dosage forms and brand names by country availability, see *Dosage Forms* section(s). For a listing of brand names for the articles in this monograph, refer to the General Index.

## Category

Antiarrhythmic.

## Indications

### Accepted

Arrhythmias, supraventricular (prophylaxis)[1]—In patients without structural heart disease, flecainide is indicated for the prevention of paroxysmal supraventricular tachycardias, including atrioventricular nodal reentrant tachycardia, atrioventricular reentrant tachycardia, and other supraventricular tachycardias of unspecified mechanism associated with disabling symptoms. It is also indicated for the prevention of paroxysmal atrial fibrillation/flutter associated with disabling symptoms in patients without structural heart disease.

Arrhythmias, ventricular (prophylaxis and treatment)—Flecainide is indicated for the prevention and suppression of documented life-threatening ventricular arrhythmias, such as sustained ventricular tachycardia.

### Unaccepted

Use of flecainide is no longer accepted for treatment of less severe arrhythmias such as nonsustained ventricular tachycardias or frequent premature ventricular contractions, even if patients are symptomatic, because of results of a trial that found increased mortality in patients with non–life-threatening arrhythmias treated with flecainide.

Flecainide is not accepted for use in the treatment of chronic atrial fibrillation because of the increased risk for development of ventricular arrhythmias such as ventricular tachycardia and ventricular fibrillation.

[1]Not included in Canadian product labeling.

## Pharmacology/Pharmacokinetics

### Physicochemical characteristics
Molecular weight—474.40.
pKa—9.3.

### Mechanism of action/Effect
Decreases excitability, conduction velocity, and automaticity as a result of slowed atrial, atrioventricular (AV) nodal, His-Purkinje, and intraventricular conduction, and causes a slight but significant prolongation of refractory periods in these tissues. The greatest effect is on the His-Purkinje system. Decreases the rate of rise of the action potential without affecting its duration. In the Vaughan Williams classification of antiarrhythmics, flecainide is considered to be a class IC agent.

### Other actions/effects
Mild to moderate negative inotropic effect; local anesthetic activity.

### Absorption
Nearly complete; not affected by food or antacids.

### Protein binding
Moderate (40%).

### Biotransformation
Hepatic.

### Half-life
Elimination—Approximately 20 hours (range, 12 to 27 hours); increased with renal or hepatic function impairment or congestive heart failure. In addition, elimination is slowed significantly in those rare conditions where urinary pH is 8 or higher (e.g., renal tubular acidosis, strict vegetarian diet).

### Time to peak plasma concentration
Single dose—Approximately 3 hours (range, 1 to 6 hours).

### Time to steady-state plasma concentration
Multiple doses—3 to 5 days.

### Therapeutic trough plasma concentration
0.2 to 1.0 mcg per mL.

### Elimination
Renal—Approximately 30% (range, 10 to 50%) unchanged.
Fecal—5%.
In dialysis—Hemodialysis removes only about 1% of a dose as unchanged drug.

## Precautions to Consider

### Cross-sensitivity and/or related problems
Patients sensitive to other amide-type anesthetics may rarely be sensitive to flecainide also. Cross-sensitivity with procainamide or quinidine has not been reported.

### Carcinogenicity
Studies with flecainide in rats and mice at doses up to 8 times the usual human dose found no evidence of carcinogenicity.

### Mutagenicity
Mutagenicity studies (Ames test, mouse lymphoma, *in vivo* cytogenetics) found no evidence of mutagenicity.

### Pregnancy/Reproduction
Fertility—A reproduction study in male and female rats given flecainide in doses up to 50 mg per kg of body weight (mg/kg) per day (7 times the usual human dose) did not reveal fertility impairment.

Pregnancy—Adequate and well-controlled studies in humans have not been done.

Studies in New Zealand White rabbits given doses of 30 and 35 mg/kg per day revealed teratogenic and embryotoxic effects. Teratogenic effects did not occur in Dutch Belted rabbits at the same dose or in rats and mice given doses up to 50 and 80 mg/kg per day, respectively. However, delayed sternebral and vertebral ossification was seen at the high dose in rats.

FDA Pregnancy Category C.

### Breast-feeding
Flecainide is distributed into human breast milk in concentrations as high as 4 times the corresponding plasma concentrations. The potential dose to a nursing infant, assuming a maternal plasma concentration of 1 mcg per mL (mcg/mL) and infant ingestion of 700 mL of breast milk over 24 hours, would be less than 3 mg.

### Pediatrics
Appropriate studies on the relationship of age to the effects of flecainide have not been performed in the pediatric population. Safety and efficacy have not been established.

### Geriatrics
The half-life of flecainide may be somewhat prolonged in the elderly, although dosage adjustment is usually not necessary. In addition, incidence of proarrhythmic effects may be increased in the elderly, who are more likely to have underlying cardiac function impairment. Elderly patients are also more likely to have age-related renal function impairment, which may require caution in patients receiving flecainide.

### Drug interactions and/or related problems
The following drug interactions and/or related problems have been selected on the basis of their potential clinical significance (possible mechanism in parentheses where appropriate)—not necessarily inclusive (» = major clinical significance):

Note: Combinations containing any of the following medications, depending on the amount present, may also interact with this medication.

Acidifiers, urinary
(by decreasing urine pH, may increase elimination of flecainide; dosage adjustment of flecainide may be necessary)

Alkalizers, urinary
(by increasing urine pH, may decrease elimination of flecainide; dosage adjustment of flecainide may be necessary)

» Antiarrhythmics, other
(concurrent use with flecainide may produce additive cardiac effects; irreversible ventricular tachycardia/fibrillation has been reported in patients with hypotensive ventricular tachycardia)

(concurrent use of amiodarone with flecainide has resulted in a twofold or greater increase in plasma flecainide concentrations; it is recommended that the usual dose of flecainide be reduced by 50% and plasma flecainide concentrations monitored carefully during concurrent use)

Beta-adrenergic blocking agents
(concurrent use with flecainide may result in additive negative inotropic effects; in addition, concurrent use of propranolol with flecainide has resulted in increased plasma concentrations of both, but less depression of heart rate than occurs with propranolol alone)

Bone marrow depressants (See *Appendix II*)
   (although problems have not been reported, concurrent use with flecainide may increase the risk of leukopenia and thrombocytopenia)

Digoxin
   (concurrent use with flecainide has resulted in transiently increased plasma digoxin concentrations; no adverse effects have been reported)

## Laboratory value alterations

The following have been selected on the basis of their potential clinical significance (possible effect in parentheses where appropriate)—not necessarily inclusive (» = major clinical significance):

With physiology/laboratory test values
   Electrocardiogram (ECG) changes such as:
      QRS widening and
      PR prolongation and
      QT prolongation secondary to QRS widening
      (occur in most patients)

      Note: ECG changes produced by flecainide do not necessarily indicate efficacy, toxicity, or overdose.

## Medical considerations/Contraindications

The medical considerations/contraindications included here have been selected on the basis of their potential clinical significance (reasons given in parentheses where appropriate)—not necessarily inclusive (» = major clinical significance).

*Except under special circumstances, this medication should not be used when the following medical problems exist:*

» Atrioventricular (AV) block, pre-existing second or third degree without pacemaker or
» Right bundle branch block associated with a left hemiblock (bifascicular block) without pacemaker
   (risk of complete heart block)

*Risk-benefit should be considered when the following medical problems exist:*

» Cardiogenic shock
   (negative inotropic effect of flecainide; increased risk of flecainide-induced arrhythmias)

Congestive heart failure
   (may be aggravated as a result of small negative inotropic effect; elimination may be delayed; increased risk of flecainide-induced arrhythmias; dosage reduction may be necessary)

» Hepatic function impairment
   (elimination may be significantly slowed; the interval between dosage increments should be greater than 4 days, and dosage reduction may be necessary; dosage adjustments should be made on the basis of plasma flecainide determinations)

Hypokalemia or hyperkalemia
   (effects of flecainide may be altered; pre-existing hypokalemia or hyperkalemia should be corrected before administration of flecainide)

Myocardial infarction, history of, with associated left ventricular function impairment
   (increased risk of flecainide-induced arrhythmias)

Renal function impairment
   (reduced elimination; the interval between dosage increments should be greater than 4 days, and dosage reduction may be necessary; dosage adjustments should be made on the basis of plasma flecainide determinations)

Sensitivity to flecainide

» Sick sinus syndrome
   (flecainide prolongs sinus node recovery time; may cause sinus bradycardia, sinus pause, or sinus arrest)

Caution is also recommended in patients with permanent pacemakers or temporary pacing electrodes because flecainide increases endocardial pacing thresholds and may suppress ventricular escape rhythms; use is not recommended in patients with existing high thresholds or nonprogrammable pacemakers unless suitable pacing rescue is available. In patients with pacemakers, it is recommended that the pacing threshold be determined prior to initiation of therapy, after one week of administration, and then at regular intervals.

## Patient monitoring

The following may be especially important in patient monitoring (other tests may be warranted in some patients, depending on condition; » = major clinical significance):

Blood counts
   (recommended at periodic intervals to detect bone marrow depression)

» ECG
   (Holter monitoring or 24-hour ambulatory ECG recommended prior to initiation of therapy and at periodic intervals during therapy to assess efficacy and detect possible proarrhythmic effects)

Plasma flecainide determinations, trough
   (recommended at frequent intervals to aid in dosage adjustment in patients with severe renal or hepatic disease; may also be useful in patients with congestive heart failure or moderate renal disease)

# Side/Adverse Effects

Note: In the National Heart Lung and Blood Institute's Cardiac Arrhythmias Suppression Trial (CAST), flecainide treatment was found to be associated with excessive mortality or increased nonfatal cardiac arrest rate as compared with placebo in patients with asymptomatic, non–life-threatening arrhythmias who had a recent myocardial infarction.

Adverse cardiac effects reported with flecainide administration include new or exacerbated ventricular or supraventricular arrhythmias, new or exacerbated congestive heart failure, second or third degree atrioventricular (AV) block, and rarely, sinus bradycardia, sinus pause, or sinus arrest.

Incidence of cardiac and other effects is at least partially dose-related and is increased at plasma flecainide concentrations greater than 0.7 to 1.0 mcg per mL.

The following side/adverse effects have been selected on the basis of their potential clinical significance (possible signs and symptoms in parentheses where appropriate)—not necessarily inclusive:

### Those indicating need for medical attention

Incidence less frequent
   *Arrhythmias, including new or worsened ventricular tachyarrhythmias, increased frequency of premature ventricular contractions, or new supraventricular arrhythmias* (irregular heartbeat); *chest pain; congestive heart failure* (shortness of breath; swelling of feet or lower legs); *trembling or shaking*
   Note: *Arrhythmias* are dose-related and potentially fatal; incidence increased in patients with congestive heart failure or history of myocardial infarction with associated left ventricular function impairment.

Incidence rare
   *Hepatic function impairment* (yellow eyes or skin)

### Those indicating need for medical attention only if they continue or are bothersome

Incidence more frequent
   *Blurred vision or seeing spots; dizziness or lightheadedness*

Incidence less frequent
   *Anxiety or mental depression; constipation; headache; nausea or vomiting; skin rash; stomach pain or loss of appetite; unusual tiredness or weakness*

# Overdose

For specific information on the agents used in the management of flecainide overdose, see:
• *Dobutamine, Dopamine,* or *Isoproterenol* in *Sympathomimetic Agents–Cardiovascular Use (Parenteral-Systemic)* monograph.

For more information on the management of overdose or unintentional ingestion, **contact a Poison Control Center** (see *Poison Control Center Listing*).

### Treatment of overdose

To decrease absorption—Treatment should begin with immediate evacuation of the stomach.

Specific treatment—Treatment is primarily supportive and symptomatic and may include oxygen, mechanical respiratory assistance, circulatory assistance (e.g., intra-aortic balloon pumping), transvenous conduction pacing, administration of inotropic agents (dopamine, dobutamine, or isoproterenol), cardioversion defibrillation if sustained ventricular tachycardia attributable to flecainide's effects occurs, and if the sustained ventricular tachycardia has caused or may lead to hemodynamic decomposition and/or ventricular fibrillation.

Supportive care—Patients in whom intentional overdose is confirmed or suspected should be referred for psychiatric consultation.

# Patient Consultation

As an aid to patient consultation, refer to *Advice for the Patient, Flecainide (Systemic).*

In providing consultation, consider emphasizing the following selected information (»= major clinical significance):

**Before using this medication**
» Conditions affecting use, especially:
   Sensitivity to flecainide or amide-type anesthetics
   Pregnancy—Teratogenic in rabbits
   Use in the elderly—Increased duration of action; increased risk of proarrhythmic effects
   Other medications, especially other antiarrhythmics
   Other medical problems, especially hepatic function impairment

**Proper use of this medication**
» Compliance with therapy; taking as directed even if feeling well
» Importance of not missing doses and taking at evenly spaced intervals
» Proper dosing
   Missed dose: Taking as soon as possible if remembered within 6 hours; not taking if remembered later; not doubling doses
» Proper storage

**Precautions while using this medication**
   Regular visits to physician to check progress
   Carrying medical identification card or bracelet
» Caution if any kind of surgery (including dental surgery) or emergency treatment is required
» Caution when driving or doing things requiring alertness because of possible dizziness
   Checking with physician before discontinuing medication; gradual dosage reduction may be necessary

**Side/adverse effects**
   Signs of potential side effects, especially arrhythmias, chest pain, congestive heart failure, trembling or shaking, and hepatic function impairment

## General Dosing Information

Previous antiarrhythmic therapy should be withdrawn 2 to 4 half-lives before initiation of flecainide therapy (except lidocaine, which can be used for interim control).

Occasionally, patients intolerant to or not adequately controlled by every-twelve-hour dosing may be dosed at eight-hour intervals.

Because of flecainide's long half-life, dosage increments should be made no more frequently than every 4 days.

It is recommended that treatment be initiated in the hospital because of the increased risk of proarrhythmic effects associated with flecainide administration.

It is recommended that flecainide therapy be withdrawn if bone marrow depression occurs.

**For treatment of adverse effects**
Digitalis or diuretic therapy may be useful in patients with flecainide-induced or -aggravated congestive heart failure. Dosage reduction or withdrawal of flecainide may be necessary.

## Oral Dosage Forms

### FLECAINIDE ACETATE TABLETS

**Usual adult dose**
Paroxysmal supraventricular tachycardias or paroxysmal atrial fibrillation/flutter—
   Oral, 50 mg every twelve hours, the dosage being increased in increments of 50 mg two times a day every four days as needed and tolerated.
Sustained ventricular tachycardia—
   Initial: Oral, 100 mg every twelve hours, the dosage being increased in increments of 50 mg two times a day every four days as needed and tolerated.

   Note: In patients with severe renal function impairment (creatinine clearance of 35 mL per minute per 1.73 square meters of body surface or less), an initial dose of 100 mg once a day or 50 mg every twelve hours is recommended, and dosage should be adjusted on the basis of frequent plasma concentration determinations. In patients with less severe renal function impairment, an initial dose of 100 mg every twelve hours may be used; plasma concentration determinations may be useful in dosage adjustment.
   Maintenance: Oral, up to 150 mg every twelve hours.

**Usual adult prescribing limits**
Paroxysmal supraventricular arrhythmias—Up to 300 mg per day.
Sustained ventricular tachycardia—Up to 400 mg per day.

**Usual pediatric dose**
Safety and efficacy have not been established.

**Strength(s) usually available**
U.S.—
   50 mg (Rx) [*Tambocor*].
   100 mg (Rx) [*Tambocor* (scored)].
   150 mg (Rx) [*Tambocor* (scored)].
Canada—
   100 mg (Rx) [*Tambocor* (scored)].

**Packaging and storage**
Store below 40 °C (104 °F), preferably between 15 and 30 °C (59 and 86 °F), unless otherwise specified by manufacturer. Store in a tight container. Protect from light.

## Selected Bibliography

Nappi JM, Anderson JL. Flecainide: a new prototype antiarrhythmic agent. Pharmacother 1985; 5: 209-21.
A symposium. Flecainide. Am J Cardiol 1988 Aug 25; 62: 1D-66D.
Roden DM, Woosley AL. Flecainide. N Engl J Med 1986 Jul 3; 315: 36-41.

Revised: 09/24/92
Interim revision: 04/29/94

---

**FLOCTAFENINE**—See *Anti-inflammatory Drugs, Nonsteroidal (Systemic)*

---

# FLOXURIDINE   Systemic†

**VA CLASSIFICATION (Primary): AN300**
Note: For a listing of dosage forms and brand names by country availability, see *Dosage Forms* section(s). For a listing of brand names for the articles in this monograph, refer to the General Index.

---

†Not commercially available in Canada.

---

## Category
Antineoplastic.

## Indications
Note: Bracketed information in the *Indications* section refers to uses that are not included in U.S. product labeling.

**Accepted**
Carcinoma, gastrointestinal (treatment)
Carcinoma, hepatic (treatment)
[Carcinoma, breast (treatment)]

[Carcinoma, ovarian (treatment)]
[Carcinoma, cervical (treatment)]
[Carcinoma, bladder (treatment)]
[Carcinoma, renal (treatment)] or
[Carcinoma, prostatic (treatment)]—Floxuridine, given by continuous regional intra-arterial infusion, is indicated for palliative management of gastrointestinal adenocarcinoma (including [colorectal carcinoma]) metastatic to the liver that has not responded to other treatment. Floxuridine is most useful when the disease has not extended beyond an area capable of infusion via a single artery.

Floxuridine has also been used for carcinoma of the breast, ovary, cervix, urinary bladder, kidney, and prostate not responsive to other antimetabolites.

## Pharmacology/Pharmacokinetics

**Physicochemical characteristics**
Molecular weight—246.19.

### Mechanism of action/Effect

Floxuridine is an antimetabolite of the pyrimidine analog type. Floxuridine is considered to be cell cycle–specific for the S-phase of cell division. Activity occurs as the result of activation in the tissues, and includes inhibition of DNA and, as a result of action of the fluorouracil metabolite, RNA synthesis.

### Distribution

Some crosses the blood-brain barrier; active metabolites are localized intracellularly.

### Biotransformation

Hepatic and in tissues, extensive, to the monophosphate derivative and fluorouracil; after continuous intra-arterial infusion, conversion to the monophosphate derivative is enhanced; largely converted to fluorouracil after rapid intravenous or intra-arterial injection.

### Elimination

Respiratory (as carbon dioxide), about 60%.
Renal, 10 to 13% (as unchanged drug and metabolites).

## Precautions to Consider

### Carcinogenicity

Secondary malignancies are potential delayed effects of many antineoplastic agents, although it is not clear whether the effect is related to their mutagenic or immunosuppressive action. The effect of dose and duration of therapy is also unknown, although risk seems to increase with long-term use. Although information is limited, available data seem to indicate that the carcinogenic risk is greatest with the alkylating agents.
Studies with floxuridine have not been done.
Antimetabolites have been shown to be carcinogenic in animals and may be associated with an increased risk of development of secondary carcinomas in humans, although the risk appears to be less than with alkylating agents.

### Mutagenicity

Floxuridine produces oncogenic transformation of fibroblasts in cultured C3H/10T1/2 mouse embryo cells.
Floxuridine is mutagenic in human leukocytes *in vitro* and in the *Drosophila* test system.

### Pregnancy/Reproduction

Fertility—Gonadal suppression, resulting in amenorrhea or azoospermia, may occur in patients taking antineoplastic therapy, especially with the alkylating agents. In general, these effects appear to be related to dose and length of therapy and may be irreversible. Prediction of the degree of testicular or ovarian function impairment is complicated by the common use of combinations of several antineoplastics, which makes it difficult to assess the effects of individual agents.
Studies with floxuridine have not been done. However, fluorouracil, which is a metabolite of floxuridine, has significant effects on fertility in animals.
Pregnancy—Adequate and well-controlled studies in humans have not been done.
First trimester: It is usually recommended that use of antineoplastics, especially combination chemotherapy, be avoided whenever possible, especially during the first trimester. Although information is limited because of the relatively few instances of antineoplastic administration during pregnancy, the mutagenic, teratogenic, and carcinogenic potential of these medications must be considered.
Other hazards to the fetus include adverse reactions seen in adults.
In general, use of a contraceptive is recommended during cytotoxic drug therapy.
Floxuridine is teratogenic in chick embryos, mice (at doses of 100 mg per kg of body weight [mg/kg]), and rats (at doses of 75 to 150 mg/kg); doses were 4.2 to 125 times the recommended human therapeutic dose. Malformations included cleft palates, skeletal defects, and deformed appendages, paws, and tails.
FDA Pregnancy Category D.

### Breast-feeding

It is not known whether floxuridine is distributed into breast milk. Although very little information is available regarding distribution of antineoplastic agents into breast milk, breast-feeding is not recommended during chemotherapy, because of the risks to the infant (adverse effects, mutagenicity, carcinogenicity).

### Pediatrics

No information is available on the relationship of age to the effects of floxuridine in pediatric patients.

### Geriatrics

Although appropriate studies on the relationship of age to the effects of floxuridine have not been performed in the geriatric population, geri-atrics-specific problems are not expected to limit the usefulness of this medication in the elderly. However, elderly patients are more likely to have age-related renal function impairment, which may require reduction of dosage in patients receiving floxuridine.

### Dental

The bone marrow depressant effects of floxuridine may result in an increased incidence of microbial infection, delayed healing, and gingival bleeding. Dental work, whenever possible, should be completed prior to initiation of therapy or deferred until blood counts have returned to normal. Patients should be instructed in proper oral hygiene during treatment, including caution in use of regular toothbrushes, dental floss, and toothpicks.
Floxuridine also commonly causes stomatitis, which may be associated with considerable discomfort.

### Drug interactions and/or related problems

The following drug interactions and/or related problems have been selected on the basis of their potential clinical significance (possible mechanism in parentheses where appropriate)—not necessarily inclusive (» = major clinical significance):

Blood dyscrasia–causing medications
   (leukopenic and/or thrombocytopenic effects of floxuridine may be increased with concurrent or recent therapy if these medications cause the same effects; dosage adjustment of floxuridine, if necessary, should be based on blood counts)

» Bone marrow depressants, other or
Radiation therapy
   (additive bone marrow depression may occur; dosage reduction may be required when two or more bone marrow depressants, including radiation, are used concurrently or consecutively)

Vaccines, killed virus
   (because normal defense mechanisms may be suppressed by floxuridine therapy, the patient's antibody response to the vaccine may be decreased. The interval between discontinuation of medications that cause immunosuppression and restoration of the patient's ability to respond to the vaccine depends on the intensity and type of immunosuppression-causing medication used, the underlying disease, and other factors; estimates vary from 3 months to 1 year)

» Vaccines, live virus
   (because normal defense mechanisms may be suppressed by floxuridine therapy, concurrent use with a live virus vaccine may potentiate the replication of the vaccine virus, may increase the side/adverse effects of the vaccine virus, and/or may decrease the patient's antibody response to the vaccine; immunization of these patients should be undertaken only with extreme caution after careful review of the patient's hematologic status and only with the knowledge and consent of the physician managing the floxuridine therapy. The interval between discontinuation of medications that cause immunosuppression and restoration of the patient's ability to respond to the vaccine depends on the intensity and type of immunosuppression-causing medication used, the underlying disease, and other factors; estimates vary from 3 months to 1 year. Patients with leukemia in remission should not receive live virus vaccine until at least 3 months after their last chemotherapy. Immunization with oral poliovirus vaccine should also be postponed in persons in close contact with the patient, especially family members)

### Laboratory value alterations

The following have been selected on the basis of their potential clinical significance (possible effect in parentheses where appropriate)—not necessarily inclusive (» = major clinical significance):

With physiology/laboratory test values
   Alanine aminotransferase (ALT [SGPT]) values, serum and
   Alkaline phosphatase values, serum and
   Aspartate aminotransferase (AST [SGOT]) values, serum and
   Bilirubin concentrations, serum and
   Lactate dehydrogenase (LDH) values, serum
      (may be increased; possible chemical hepatitis or biliary sclerosis)

### Medical considerations/Contraindications

The medical considerations/contraindications included here have been selected on the basis of their potential clinical significance (reasons given in parentheses where appropriate)—not necessarily inclusive (» = major clinical significance).

### *Risk-benefit should be considered when the following medical problems exist:*

» Bone marrow depression
» Chickenpox, existing or recent (including recent exposure) or
» Herpes zoster
      (risk of severe generalized disease)

» Hepatic function impairment
  (reduced biotransformation; lower dosage is recommended)
» Hepatitis, history of
  (increased risk of chemical hepatitis)
» Infection
» Renal function impairment
  (reduced elimination; lower dosage is recommended)
  Sensitivity to floxuridine
» Extreme caution should be used also in patients who have had previous cytotoxic drug therapy with alkylating agents or high-dose pelvic radiation therapy; a lower dosage is recommended.

**Patient monitoring**
The following are especially important to patient monitoring (other tests may be warranted in some patients, depending on condition; » = major clinical significance):

  Alanine aminotransferase (ALT [SGPT]) values, serum and
  Aspartate aminotransferase (AST [SGOT]) values, serum and
  Bilirubin concentrations, serum and
  Lactate dehydrogenase (LDH) values, serum
    (recommended prior to initiation of therapy and at periodic intervals during therapy; frequency varies according to clinical state, agent, dose, and other agents being used concurrently)
» Examination of patient's mouth for ulceration
    (recommended before administration of each dose)
» Hematocrit or hemoglobin and
» Leukocyte count, total and, if appropriate, differential and
» Platelet count
    (determinations recommended prior to initiation of therapy and at periodic intervals during therapy; frequency varies according to clinical state, agent, dose, and other agents being used concurrently)

# Side/Adverse Effects

Note:  Many "side effects" of antineoplastic therapy are unavoidable and represent the medication's pharmacologic action. Some of these (for example, leukopenia and thrombocytopenia) are actually used as parameters to aid in individual dosage titration.

  Floxuridine is a highly toxic medication and serious toxic effects frequently occur. When floxuridine is administered intra-arterially, local reactions are more prominent than systemic reactions.

  Because floxuridine is converted to fluorouracil, there is a possibility that some side/adverse effects associated with fluorouracil may also occur.

  Adverse effects associated with prolonged use of an arterial catheter include arterial ischemia, thrombosis, bleeding at the catheter site, blocked catheters, leakage at the site, embolism, fibromyositis, infection at the catheter site, abscesses, thrombophlebitis, and perforation of the duodenum or stomach.

  Floxuridine administered via hepatic artery infusion may cause a chemical hepatitis, characterized by elevated hepatic enzymes and nausea and vomiting. However, elevated hepatic enzymes may also be a sign of biliary sclerosis.

The following side/adverse effects have been selected on the basis of their potential clinical significance (possible signs and symptoms in parentheses where appropriate)—not necessarily inclusive:

**Those indicating need for medical attention**
Incidence more frequent
  *Aphthous stomatitis* (sores in mouth and on lips); *enteritis* (diarrhea; stomach pain or cramps)
Incidence less frequent
  *Displaced hepatic artery catheter* (heartburn; black tarry stools); *esophagopharyngitis* (heartburn); *gastrointestinal ulceration or gastritis* (black tarry stools); *glossitis* (swelling or soreness of tongue); *nausea and vomiting; scaling or redness of hands or feet*—with prolonged infusion therapy
Incidence rare
  *Hepatotoxicity or intra- and extrahepatic biliary sclerosis or acalculus cholecystitis* (yellow eyes or skin); *leukopenia or infection* (usually asymptomatic; rarely, fever or chills; cough or hoarseness; lower back or side pain; painful or difficult urination); *thrombocytopenia or anemia* (usually asymptomatic; rarely, unusual bleeding or bruising;

black, tarry stools; blood in urine or stools; pinpoint red spots on skin); *trouble in walking*

**Those indicating need for medical attention only if they continue or are bothersome**
Incidence less frequent or rare
  *Loss of appetite; skin rash or itching*

**Those not indicating need for medical attention**
Incidence less frequent or rare
  *Thinning of hair*

# Patient Consultation

As an aid to patient consultation, refer to *Advice for the Patient, Floxuridine (Systemic)*.

In providing consultation, consider emphasizing the following selected information (» = major clinical significance):

**Before using this medication**
» Conditions affecting use, especially:
    Sensitivity to floxuridine
    Pregnancy—Use not recommended because of mutagenic, teratogenic, and carcinogenic potential; advisability of using contraception; telling physician immediately if pregnancy is suspected
    Breast-feeding—Not recommended because of risk of serious side effects
    Other medications, especially other bone marrow depressants or previous cytotoxic drug or radiation therapy
    Other medical problems, especially chickenpox, herpes zoster, hepatic function impairment, history of hepatitis, infection, or renal function impairment

**Proper use of this medication**
» Telling physician about nausea and vomiting, especially with stomach pain
» Proper dosing

**Precautions while using this medication**
» Importance of close monitoring by physician
» Avoiding immunizations unless approved by physician; other persons in patient's household should avoid immunizations with oral poliovirus vaccine; avoiding persons who have taken oral poliovirus vaccine or wearing a protective mask that covers nose and mouth

**Side/adverse effects**
  May cause adverse effects such as blood problems, inflammation of gastrointestinal tract, chemical hepatitis, and cancer; importance of discussing possible effects with physician
  Signs of potential side effects, especially aphthous stomatitis, enteritis, esophagopharyngitis, displaced hepatic artery catheter, gastrointestinal ulceration, gastritis, glossitis, nausea and vomiting, scaling or redness of hands or feet, hepatotoxicity, leukopenia, infection, thrombocytopenia, anemia, and trouble in walking
  Physician or nurse can help in dealing with side effects
  Possibility of thinning of hair; should return after treatment has ended

# General Dosing Information

Patients receiving floxuridine should be under supervision of a physician experienced in antimetabolite chemotherapy and the technique of intra-arterial infusion.

Floxuridine is recommended mainly for intra-arterial use. Use of an appropriate infusion pump is recommended to ensure a uniform rate of infusion. In selected patients, a portable or implantable pump may be used.

Therapy with floxuridine is continued as long as a response occurs, which may vary from 1 week to several months (with appropriate rest periods). However, floxuridine is an extremely toxic medication; therapy should be discontinued promptly at the first sign of:
  Diarrhea (five or more loose stools daily)
  Esophagopharyngitis
  Gastrointestinal ulceration and bleeding
  Hemorrhage from any site
  Leukopenia (particularly granulocytopenia), marked
  Myocardial ischemia
  Stomatitis
  Thrombocytopenia, marked
  Vomiting, intractable
Therapy may be reinitiated at a lower dosage when side effects have subsided.

Floxuridine should be withdrawn if signs of obstructive jaundice occur and reinstituted only after careful evaluation of the patient.

Special precautions are recommended in patients who develop thrombocytopenia as a result of administration of floxuridine. These may include extreme care in performing invasive procedures; regular inspection of intravenous sites, skin (including perirectal area), and mucous membrane surfaces for signs of bleeding or bruising; limiting frequency of venipuncture and avoiding intramuscular injections; testing urine, emesis, stool, and secretions for occult blood; care in use of regular toothbrushes, dental floss, toothpicks, safety razors, and fingernail and toenail cutters; avoiding constipation; and using caution to prevent falls and other injuries. Such patients should avoid alcohol and aspirin intake because of the risk of gastrointestinal bleeding. Platelet transfusions may be required.

Patients who develop leukopenia should be observed carefully for signs of infection. Antibiotic support may be required. In neutropenic patients who develop fever, broad-spectrum antibiotic coverage should be initiated empirically, pending bacterial cultures and appropriate diagnostic tests.

### Safety considerations for handling this medication

There is limited but increasing evidence and concern that personnel involved in preparation and administration of parenteral antineoplastics may be at some risk because of the potential mutagenicity, teratogenicity, and/or carcinogenicity of these agents, although the actual risk is unknown. USP advisory panels recommend cautious handling both in preparation and disposal of antineoplastic agents. Precautions that have been suggested include:
• Use of a biological containment cabinet during reconstitution and dilution of parenteral medications and wearing of disposable surgical gloves and masks.
• Use of proper technique to prevent contamination of the medication, work area, and operator during transfer between containers (including proper training of personnel in this technique).
• Cautious and proper disposal of needles, syringes, vials, ampuls, and unused medication.
A number of medical centers have developed detailed guidelines for handling of antineoplastic agents.

## Parenteral Dosage Forms

### FLOXURIDINE STERILE USP

#### Usual adult dose
Carcinoma, gastrointestinal or
Carcinoma, hepatic—
    Intra-arterial, 100 to 600 mcg (0.1 to 0.6 mg) per kg of body weight per day continuously over twenty-four hours, continued until tox-
icity or a response occurs, usually for fourteen to twenty-one days, with a rest period of two weeks between courses.

#### Usual pediatric dose
Safety and efficacy have not been established.

#### Size(s) usually available
U.S.—
    500 mg (Rx) [FUDR; GENERIC].
Canada—
    Not commercially available.

#### Packaging and storage
Store below 40 °C (104 °F), preferably between 15 and 30 °C (59 and 86 °F), unless otherwise specified by manufacturer. Protect from light.

#### Preparation of dosage form
Sterile Floxuridine USP is reconstituted for use by adding 5 mL of sterile water for injection to the vial; may be further diluted in 5% dextrose injection or 0.9% sodium chloride injection for administration by infusion.

#### Stability
Reconstituted solutions of floxuridine are stable at 2 to 8 °C (36 to 46 °F) for not more than 2 weeks.

### Selected Bibliography
Dorr RT, Fritz WL. Cancer chemotherapy handbook. New York: Elsevier, 1980: 429-34.

Revised: 07/26/94

---

## FLUCLOXACILLIN—See Penicillins (Systemic)

---

## FLUCONAZOLE—See Antifungals, Azole (Systemic)

---

# FLUCYTOSINE   Systemic

VA CLASSIFICATION (Primary): AM700
Other commonly used names are 5-fluorocytosine and 5-FC.
Note: For a listing of dosage forms and brand names by country availability, see Dosage Forms section(s). For a listing of brand names for the articles in this monograph, refer to the General Index.

## Category
Antifungal (systemic).

## Indications
Note: Bracketed information in the Indications section refers to uses that are not included in U.S. product labeling.

### Accepted
Endocarditis, fungal (treatment)—Flucytosine is indicated in the treatment of endocarditis caused by Candida species.

Meningitis, fungal (treatment)—Flucytosine is indicated in the treatment of meningitis caused by Cryptococcus species.

Pneumonia, fungal (treatment)
Septicemia, fungal (treatment) or
Urinary tract infections, fungal (treatment)—Flucytosine is indicated in the treatment of pneumonia, septicemia, and urinary tract infections caused by Candida and Cryptococcus species.

[Candidiasis, disseminated (treatment)][1]
[Chromomycosis (treatment)][1] or
[Cryptococcosis (treatment)][1]—Flucytosine is used in the treatment of disseminated candidiasis, chromomycosis, and cryptococcosis.

In the treatment of disseminated fungal disease, flucytosine is usually administered concurrently with parenteral amphotericin B because of

rapid development of resistance when flucytosine is administered alone.

Not all species or strains of a particular organism may be susceptible to flucytosine.

[1]Not included in Canadian product labeling.

## Pharmacology/Pharmacokinetics

### Physicochemical characteristics
Chemical group—Fluorinated pyrimidine derivative; chemically related to fluorouracil and floxuridine
Molecular weight—129.09.

### Mechanism of action/Effect
Flucytosine penetrates into fungal cells and is converted to fluorouracil, an antimetabolite. By interfering with pyrimidine metabolism, flucytosine interrupts nucleic acid and protein synthesis. The cells of the host do not convert large quantities of flucytosine to fluorouracil, accounting for the selective toxicity of the compound against fungi.

### Absorption
Rapidly and well absorbed from the gastrointestinal tract. Bioavailability—78 to 90%.

### Distribution
Flucytosine is distributed widely throughout the body. The exact distribution in body fluids and organs is not known. However, cerebrospinal fluid (CSF) concentrations may range from about 60 to 90% of those achieved in the serum. Concentrations in the liver, kidneys, spleen, heart, and lungs appear to equal those in the serum.

### Protein binding
Very low (2–4%).

**Biotransformation**

Flucytosine is not significantly metabolized.

**Half-life**

Normal renal function—2.5 to 6 hours.

Impaired renal function—12 to 250 hours.

**Time to peak serum concentration**

1 to 2 hours.

**Peak serum concentration**

30 to 40 mcg/mL 2 to 4 hours after a 2-gram dose in adults.

**Elimination**

Renal; more than 90% excreted by glomerular filtration as unchanged drug.

## Precautions to Consider

### Carcinogenicity/Mutagenicity

Adequate studies in animals have not been performed to evaluate the carcinogenic potential of flucytosine. No mutagenicity was detected in Ames-type studies in the presence or absence of activating enzymes.

### Pregnancy/Reproduction

Pregnancy—Flucytosine crosses the placenta. Problems in humans have not been documented.

However, studies in rats have shown that flucytosine, which is metabolized in rats to fluorouracil, is teratogenic.

FDA Pregnancy Category C.

### Breast-feeding

It is not known whether flucytosine is excreted in breast milk. However, problems in humans have not been documented.

### Pediatrics

Appropriate studies on the relationship of age to the effects of flucytosine have not been performed in the pediatric population. However, no pediatrics-specific problems have been documented to date.

### Geriatrics

No information is available on the relationship of age to the effects of flucytosine in geriatric patients. However, elderly patients are more likely to have an age-related decrease in renal function, which may require an adjustment of dosage in patients receiving flucytosine.

### Dental

The bone marrow–depressant effects of flucytosine may result in an increased incidence of microbial infection, delayed healing, and gingival bleeding. Dental work, whenever possible, should be completed prior to initiation of therapy or deferred until blood counts have returned to normal. Patients should be instructed in proper oral hygiene during treatment, including caution in use of regular toothbrushes, dental floss, and toothpicks.

### Drug interactions and/or related problems

The following drug interactions and/or related problems have been selected on the basis of their potential clinical significance (possible mechanism in parentheses where appropriate)—not necessarily inclusive (» = major clinical significance):

Note: Combinations containing any of the following medications, depending on the amount present, may also interact with this medication.

Amphotericin B, parenteral

(concurrent use of amphotericin B and flucytosine may have additive or slightly synergistic effects; amphotericin B-induced renal dysfunction may increase the bone marrow toxicity of flucytosine. However, 2-drug therapy may allow the total daily dose of amphotericin B to be lowered, decreasing its risk of nephrotoxicity)

Blood dyscrasia–causing medications (See *Appendix II*) or

» Bone marrow depressants, other, (See *Appendix II*) or

» Radiation therapy

(concurrent use with flucytosine may increase the bone marrow–depressant effects of these medications and radiation therapy; dosage reduction may be required)

Cytarabine

(cytarabine has been reported to antagonize the antifungal activity of flucytosine by competitive inhibition)

### Medical considerations/Contraindications

The medical considerations/contraindications included here have been selected on the basis of their potential clinical significance (reasons given in parentheses where appropriate)—not necessarily inclusive (» = major clinical significance).

*Except under special circumstances, this medication should not be used when the following medical problem exists:*

» Allergy to flucytosine

*Risk-benefit should be considered when the following medical problems exist:*

» Bone marrow depression or
Hematologic disease
(flucytosine may cause bone marrow depression, resulting in anemia, leukopenia, and thrombocytopenia)
Hepatic function impairment
(flucytosine may cause jaundice or hepatic dysfunction, worsening any pre-existing hepatic function impairment)

» Renal function impairment
(because flucytosine is excreted renally, it is recommended that this medication be administered in a reduced dosage to patients with impaired renal function)

» Risk-benefit should be considered in patients who have had previous cytotoxic drug therapy or radiation therapy also.

### Patient monitoring

The following may be especially important in patient monitoring (other tests may be warranted in some patients, depending on condition; » = major clinical significance):

Alanine aminotransferase (ALT [SGPT]), serum and
Alkaline phosphatase, serum and
Aspartate aminotransferase (AST [SGOT]), serum and
Bilirubin, serum
(concentrations are recommended prior to initiation of therapy and at frequent intervals during therapy)

Blood urea nitrogen (BUN) and
Creatinine, serum
(recommended prior to initation of therapy and at periodic intervals during therapy since flucytosine may cause azotemia or an increase in these values; dosage must be reduced in renal function impairment)
(flucytosine may interfere with serum creatinine determinations that are measured by the Kodak Ektachem-700 analyzer, falsely elevating creatinine values; an analyzer that uses the Jaffe procedure should be used to measure serum creatinine)

Flucytosine concentrations, serum
(serum flucytosine concentrations are recommended in patients with renal function impairment [e.g., creatinine clearance <40 mL per min or 0.67 mL per sec], to assess the adequacy of renal excretion and to prevent flucytosine accumulation in the serum; side effects are more common with serum concentrations >100 mcg/mL)

## Side/Adverse Effects

The following side/adverse effects have been selected on the basis of their potential clinical significance (possible signs and symptoms in parentheses where appropriate)—not necessarily inclusive:

**Those indicating need for medical attention**

Incidence more frequent
*Anemia* (unusual tiredness or weakness); *hepatitis or jaundice* (yellow eyes or skin); *hypersensitivity* (skin rash, redness, or itching); *leukopenia* (sore throat and fever); *thrombocytopenia* (unusual bleeding or bruising)

Incidence less frequent
*Confusion; hallucinations; photosensitivity* (increased sensitivity of skin to sunlight)

**Those indicating need for medical attention only if they continue or are bothersome**

Incidence more frequent
*Gastrointestinal disturbances* (abdominal pain; diarrhea; loss of appetite; nausea; vomiting)

Incidence less frequent
*CNS effects* (dizziness or lightheadedness; drowsiness; headache)

## Overdose

For more information on the management of overdose or unintentional ingestion, **contact a Poison Control Center** (see*Poison Control Center Listing*).

### Treatment of overdose

Recommended treatment is symptomatic and supportive and consists of the following:

· Gastric lavage.

· Diuresis.

• Frequent monitoring of hematologic parameters.
• Using hemodialysis to reduce serum concentrations rapidly, especially in anuric patients.

## Patient Consultation

As an aid to patient consultation, refer to *Advice for the Patient, Flucytosine (Systemic)*.

In providing consultation, consider emphasizing the following selected information (» = major clinical significance):

**Before using this medication**
» Conditions affecting use, especially:
    Allergy to flucytosine
    Pregnancy—Flucytosine crosses the placenta; studies in rats have shown this medication to be teratogenic
    Dental—Bone marrow depression effects of flucytosine may result in an increased incidence of microbial infection, delayed healing, and gingival bleeding
    Other medication, especially bone marrow depressants or radiation therapy
    Other medical problems, especially bone marrow depression or renal function impairment
    Previous cytotoxic drug therapy or radiation therapy

**Proper use of this medication**
    Taking multiple dosage units, prescribed as a single dose, over a period of 15 minutes to minimize nausea or vomiting
» Compliance with full course of therapy
» Proper dosing
    Missed dose: Taking as soon as possible; not taking if almost time for next dose; not doubling doses
» Proper storage

**Precautions while using this medication**
    Regular visits to physician to check progress during therapy
    Using caution in use of regular toothbrushes, dental floss, and toothpicks; completing dental work prior to initiation of therapy or delaying it until blood counts have returned to normal; checking with physician or dentist concerning proper oral hygiene
» Possible photosensitivity reactions
» Caution if dizziness, lightheadedness, or drowsiness occurs

**Side/adverse effects**
    Signs of potential side effects, especially anemia, confusion, hallucinations, hepatitis, hypersensitivity, jaundice, leukopenia, photosensitivity and thrombocytopenia

## General Dosing Information

If multiple dosage units are prescribed as a single dose, administration may be spaced over a period of 15 minutes to prevent or reduce nausea or vomiting.

Since fungal resistance may develop rapidly when flucytosine is administered alone, it is usually administered concurrently with parenteral amphotericin B.

Dosing intervals may be adjusted according to creatinine clearance as follows:

| Creatinine Clearance (mL/min)/ (mL/sec) | Dosing Interval (hr) |
|---|---|
| >40/0.67 | 6 |
| 20–40/0.33–0.67 | 12 |
| 10–20/0.17–0.33 | 24 |
| <10/0.17 | >24 |

## Oral Dosage Forms

### FLUCYTOSINE CAPSULES USP

**Usual adult and adolescent dose**
Antifungal—
    Oral, 12.5 to 37.5 mg per kg of body weight every six hours.

**Usual pediatric dose**
Antifungal—
    Oral, 12.5 to 37.5 mg per kg of body weight or 375 to 562.5 mg per square meter of body surface every six hours.

**Strength(s) usually available**
U.S.—
    250 mg (Rx) [*Ancobon*].
    500 mg (Rx) [*Ancobon*].
Canada—
    500 mg (Rx) [*Ancotil*].

**Packaging and storage**
Store below 40 °C (104 °F), preferably between 15 and 30 °C (59 and 86 °F), unless otherwise specified by manufacturer. Store in a tight, light-resistant container.

**Auxiliary labeling**
• Continue medicine for full time of treatment.

Revised: 07/24/92
Interim revision: 03/17/94

---

# FLUDARABINE Systemic

VA CLASSIFICATION (Primary): AN300
Note: For a listing of dosage forms and brand names by country availability, see *Dosage Forms* section(s). For a listing of brand names for the articles in this monograph, refer to the General Index.

## Category

Antineoplastic.

## Indications

**Accepted**
Leukemia, chronic lymphocytic (treatment)—Fludarabine is indicated for treatment of patients with B-cell chronic lymphocytic leukemia (CLL) who have not responded to or whose disease has progressed during treatment with at least one standard alkylating agent–containing regimen.

## Pharmacology/Pharmacokinetics

**Physicochemical characteristics**
Chemical group—Fludarabine is a fluorinated adenine analog (a fluorinated nucleotide analog of vidarabine [Ara-A], which differs from vidarabine in that it is resistant to deactivation by adenosine deaminase).
Molecular weight—365.21.

**Mechanism of action/Effect**
Fludarabine is a purine antimetabolite. Activity occurs as the result of activation to 2-fluoro-ara-ATP and includes inhibition of DNA synthesis (primarily in the S-phase of cell division) by inhibition of ribonucleotide reductase and the DNA polymerases. It is also postulated that fludarabine interferes with RNA by decreased incorporation of uridine and leucine into RNA and protein, respectively. Fludarabine is also active against non-proliferating cells.

**Other actions/effects**
Fludarabine appears to have immunosuppressant activity by inhibiting lymphocytes.

**Biotransformation**
Rapidly dephosphorylated in serum to 2-fluoro-ara-A (9-beta-D-arabinofuranosyl-2-fluoroadenine) within minutes after intravenous infusion, then phosphorylated intracellularly by deoxycytidine kinase to the active triphosphate, 2-fluoro-ara-ATP, the principal active metabolite.

**Half-life**
2-Fluoro-ara-A—Triphasic: Terminal—Approximately 10 hours.

**Onset of action**
In two studies, the median time to response was 7 weeks (range, 1 to 68 weeks) and 21 weeks (range, 1 to 53 weeks).

**Elimination**
2-Fluoro-ara-A—Renal, approximately 23% unchanged.

## Precautions to Consider

**Carcinogenicity**
Secondary malignancies are potential delayed effects of many antineoplastic agents, although it is not clear whether the effect is related to their mutagenic or immunosuppressive action. The effect of dose and duration of therapy is also unknown, although risk seems to increase with long-term use. Although information is limited, available data

seem to indicate that the carcinogenic risk is greatest with the alkylating agents.

Antimetabolites have been shown to be carcinogenic in animals and may be associated with an increased risk of development of secondary carcinomas in humans, although the risk appears to be less than with alkylating agents.

Studies with fludarabine in animals have not been done.

### Mutagenicity

Fludarabine was not found to be mutagenic in several strains of *Salmonella typhimurium*, including TA-98, TA-100, TA-1535, and TA-1537. It was also nonmutagenic to Chinese hamster ovary (CHO) cells at the hypoxanthine-guanine-phosphororibosyltransferase (HGPRT) locus under both activated and nonactivated metabolic conditions. However, chromosomal aberrations were observed in an *in vitro* assay using CHO cells under metabolically activated conditions. It was also determined to cause increased sister chromatid exchanges in an *in vitro* sister chromatid exchange (SCE) assay under both metabolically activated and non-activated conditions.

### Pregnancy/Reproduction

Fertility—Gonadal suppression, resulting in amenorrhea or azoospermia, may occur in patients taking antineoplastic therapy, especially with the alkylating agents. In general, these effects appear to be related to dose and length of therapy and may be irreversible. Prediction of the degree of testicular or ovarian function impairment is complicated by the common use of combinations of several antineoplastics, which makes it difficult to assess the effects of individual agents.

Dose-related adverse effects on the male reproductive system have been demonstrated in mice, rats, and dogs; effects consisted of a decrease in mean testicular weights in mice and rats with a trend toward decreased testicular weights in dogs, and degeneration and necrosis of spermatogenic epithelium of the testes in mice, rats, and dogs.

Pregnancy—Adequate and well-controlled studies in women have not been done.

First trimester: It is usually recommended that use of antineoplastics, especially combination chemotherapy, be avoided whenever possible, especially during the first trimester. Although information is limited because of the relatively few instances of antineoplastic administration during pregnancy, the mutagenic, teratogenic, and carcinogenic potential of these medications must be considered.

Other hazards to the fetus include adverse reactions seen in adults.

In general, use of a contraceptive is recommended during cytotoxic drug therapy.

Studies in rats at intravenous doses of 0, 1, 10, or 30 mg per kg of body weight (mg/kg) per day on days 6 to 15 of gestation found an increased incidence of skeletal malformations. Studies in rabbits at doses of 5 and 8 mg/kg per day found dose-related teratogenic effects (external deformities and skeletal malformations).

FDA Pregnancy Category D.

### Breast-feeding

Although very little information is available regarding distribution of antineoplastic agents into breast milk, breast-feeding is not recommended during chemotherapy because of the potential risks to the infant (adverse effects, mutagenicity, carcinogenicity). It is not known whether fludarabine is distributed into breast milk.

### Pediatrics

No information is available on the relationship of age to the effects of fludarabine in pediatric patients. Safety and efficacy have not been established.

### Geriatrics

Although appropriate studies on the relationship of age to the effects of fludarabine have not been performed in the geriatric population, clinical trials have included elderly patients and geriatrics-specific problems that would limit the usefulness of this medication in the elderly are not expected. However, elderly patients are more likely to have age-related renal function impairment, which may require reduction of dosage in patients receiving fludarabine.

### Dental

The bone marrow depressant effects of fludarabine may result in an increased incidence of microbial infection, delayed healing, and gingival bleeding. Dental work, whenever possible, should be completed prior to initiation of therapy or deferred until blood counts have returned to normal. Patients should be instructed in proper oral hygiene during treatment, including caution in use of regular toothbrushes, dental floss, and toothpicks.

Fludarabine also sometimes causes stomatitis associated with considerable discomfort.

### Drug interactions and/or related problems

The following drug interactions and/or related problems have been selected on the basis of their potential clinical significance (possible mechanism in parentheses where appropriate)—not necessarily inclusive (» = major clinical significance):

Note: Combinations containing any of the following medications, depending on the amount present, may also interact with this medication.

Allopurinol or
Colchicine or
» Probenecid or
» Sulfinpyrazone
(fludarabine may raise the concentration of blood uric acid as part of a tumor lysis syndrome; dosage adjustment of antigout agents may be necessary to control hyperuricemia and gout; allopurinol may be preferred to prevent or reverse fludarabine-induced hyperuricemia because of risk of uric acid nephropathy with uricosuric antigout agents)

Blood dyscrasia–causing medications (See *Appendix II*)
(leukopenic and/or thrombocytopenic effects of fludarabine may be increased with concurrent or recent therapy if these medications cause the same effects; dosage adjustment of fludarabine, if necessary, should be based on blood counts)

» Bone marrow depressants, other (See *Appendix II*) or
Radiation therapy
(additive bone marrow depression may occur; dosage reduction may be required when two or more bone marrow depressants, including radiation, are used concurrently or consecutively)

» Pentostatin
(concurrent use with fludarabine is not recommended because of a possible increased risk of fatal pulmonary toxicity)

Vaccines, killed virus
(because normal defense mechanisms may be suppressed by fludarabine therapy, the patient's antibody response to the vaccine may be decreased. The interval between discontinuation of medications that cause immunosuppression and restoration of the patient's ability to respond to the vaccine depends on the intensity and type of immunosuppression-causing medication used, the underlying disease, and other factors; estimates vary from 3 months to 1 year)

» Vaccines, live virus
(because normal defense mechanisms may be suppressed by fludarabine therapy, concurrent use with a live virus vaccine may potentiate the replication of the vaccine virus, may increase the side/adverse effects of the vaccine virus, and/or may decrease the patient's antibody response to the vaccine; immunization of these patients should be undertaken only with extreme caution after careful review of the patient's hematologic status and only with the knowledge and consent of the physician managing the fludarabine therapy. The interval between discontinuation of medications that cause immunosuppression and restoration of the patient's ability to respond to the vaccine depends on the intensity and type of immunosuppression-causing medication used, the underlying disease, and other factors; estimates vary from 3 months to 1 year. Patients with leukemia in remission should not receive live virus vaccine until at least 3 months after their last chemotherapy. In addition, immunization with oral poliovirus vaccine should be postponed in persons in close contact with the patient, especially family members)

### Laboratory value alterations

The following have been selected on the basis of their potential clinical significance (possible effect in parentheses where appropriate)—not necessarily inclusive (» = major clinical significance):

With physiology/laboratory test values
Alkaline phosphatase and
Aspartate aminotransferase (AST [SGOT])
(serum values may rarely be increased)

Uric acid concentrations in blood and urine
(may be increased as part of a tumor lysis syndrome in patients with large tumor burdens)

### Medical considerations/Contraindications

The medical considerations/contraindications included here have been selected on the basis of their potential clinical significance (reasons given in parentheses where appropriate)—not necessarily inclusive (» = major clinical significance).

*Risk-benefit should be considered when the following medical problems exist:*

» Bone marrow depression
    (lower dosage may be necessary)
» Chickenpox, existing or recent (including recent exposure) or
» Herpes zoster
    (risk of severe generalized disease)
  Gout, history of or
  Urate renal stones, history of
    (risk of hyperuricemia as part of tumor lysis syndrome in patients with large tumor burdens)
» Infection
» Renal function impairment
    (reduced elimination; dosage adjustment may be necessary)
» Sensitivity to fludarabine
» Caution should be used also in patients who have had previous cytotoxic drug therapy or radiation therapy.

## Patient monitoring

The following are especially important in patient monitoring (other tests may be warranted in some patients, depending on condition; » = major clinical significance):

» Hematocrit or hemoglobin and
» Leukocyte count, total and, if appropriate, differential and
» Platelet count
    (determinations recommended prior to initiation of therapy and at periodic intervals during therapy; frequency varies according to clinical state, agent, dose, and other agents being used concurrently)
  Uric acid concentrations, serum
    (recommended prior to initiation of therapy and at periodic intervals during therapy in patients with large tumor burdens, because of the risk of tumor lysis syndrome; frequency varies according to clinical state, agent, dose, and other agents being used concurrently)

## Side/Adverse Effects

Note: Many "side effects" of antineoplastic therapy are unavoidable and represent the medication's pharmacologic action. Some of these (for example, leukopenia and thrombocytopenia) are actually used as parameters to aid in individual dosage titration.

Dose-related bone marrow depression occurs in the majority of patients treated with fludarabine and may be severe and cumulative. Bone marrow fibrosis occurred in one patient.

High single doses (above 75 mg per square meter of body surface) have been associated with severe, delayed, irreversible, and potentially fatal toxicity, including central nervous system (CNS) toxicity (cortical blindness, incontinence, seizure, continued deterioration of mental status, coma). Most patients experiencing neurotoxicity were found to have progressive CNS demyelination; leukoencephalopathy involving the subcortical white matter, optic nerves, and optic tract was found. High doses are also associated with severe thrombocytopenia and neutropenia.

The following side/adverse effects have been selected on the basis of their potential clinical significance (possible signs and symptoms in parentheses where appropriate)—not necessarily inclusive:

### Those indicating need for medical attention

Incidence more frequent
  *Anemia* (usually asymptomatic); *leukopenia or infection* (usually asymptomatic; fever or chills; cough or hoarseness; lower back or side pain; painful or difficult urination); *pain; pneumonia* (cough; fever; shortness of breath); *thrombocytopenia* (usually asymptomatic; rarely, unusual bleeding or bruising; black, tarry stools; blood in urine or stools; pinpoint red spots on skin)
  Note: In *leukopenia,* the median time to nadir of granulocyte counts in a phase I study in solid tumor patients was 13 days (range, 3 to 25 days). Cumulative and severe myelosuppression may occur.

  *Infections* may be caused by opportunistic organisms including herpes zoster, cytomegalovirus, Pneumocystis carinii, and candida, among others. In a study in patients with chronic lymphocytic leukemia (CLL), immunodeficiency in the form of a marked and prolonged decrease in CD4+ and CD8+ T cells, associated with delayed severe infection, was reported after two courses of fludarabine in all 17 patients.

  In *thrombocytopenia,* the median time to nadir of platelet counts in a phase I study in solid tumor patients was 16 days (range,

2 to 32 days). Cumulative and severe myelosuppression may occur.

Incidence less frequent
  *Edema* (swelling of feet or lower legs); *neurologic effects, including agitation or confusion; blurred vision; loss of hearing; peripheral neuropathy* (numbness or tingling in fingers, toes, or face); *or weakness; stomatitis or mucositis* (sores in mouth and on lips)

Incidence rare
  *Delayed severe neurologic effects* (blindness; coma); *hemolytic anemia* (unusual tiredness or weakness); *hemorrhagic cystitis* (blood in urine; painful urination); *pulmonary edema or diffuse interstitial hypersensitivity pneumonitis* (cough; fever; shortness of breath); *tumor lysis syndrome, including hyperuricemia; hyperphosphatemia; hypocalcemia; metabolic acidosis; hyperkalemia; hematuria; urate crystalluria; renal failure* (blood in urine, lower back or side pain)

  Note: Death may also occur as a result of *delayed neurologic effects.* This syndrome is rare in patients receiving fludarabine for chronic lymphocytic leukemia. However, it occurred commonly in patients treated for acute leukemia with high doses of fludarabine (approximately 4 times greater than the recommended dose); symptoms occurred 21 to 60 days following the last dose.

  *Hemolytic anemia* has been reported after one or more cycles of fludarabine in patients with or without a history of autoimmune hemolytic anemia or a positive Coombs' test. Hospitalization and transfusion have been necessary in severe cases and a fatality has occurred.

  *Tumor lysis syndrome* has been reported in chronic lymphocytic leukemia patients with large tumor burdens.

### Those indicating need for medical attention only if they continue or are bothersome

Incidence more frequent
  *Diarrhea; nausea or vomiting; skin rash; unusual tiredness*

Incidence less frequent
  *Aching muscles; headache; loss of appetite; malaise* (general feeling of discomfort or illness)

### Those not indicating need for medical attention

Incidence less frequent or rare
  *Loss of hair*

## Overdose

For more information on the management of overdose or unintentional ingestion, **contact a Poison Control Center** (see *Poison Control Center Listing*).

**Treatment of overdose**
Treatment consists of withdrawal of fludarabine and supportive therapy.

## Patient Consultation

As an aid to patient consultation, refer to *Advice for the Patient, Fludarabine (Systemic).*

In providing consultation, consider emphasizing the following selected information (» = major clinical significance):

### Before using this medication
» Conditions affecting use, especially:
    Sensitivity to fludarabine
    Pregnancy—Use not recommended because of mutagenic, teratogenic, and carcinogenic potential; advisability of using contraception; telling physician immediately if pregnancy is suspected
    Breast-feeding—Not recommended because of risk of serious side effects
    Other medications, especially probenecid, sulfinpyrazone, other bone marrow depressants, or other cytotoxic drug or radiation therapy
    Other medical problems, especially chickenpox, herpes zoster, renal function impairment, or infection

### Proper use of this medication
    Possibility of nausea and vomiting; importance of continuing medication despite stomach upset
» Proper dosing

### Precautions while using this medication
» Importance of close monitoring by the physician
» Avoiding immunizations unless approved by physician; other persons in patient's household should avoid immunizations with oral poliovirus vaccine; avoiding persons who have taken oral poliovirus vaccine or wearing a protective mask that covers nose and mouth

*Caution if bone marrow depression occurs:*
- » Avoiding exposure to persons with bacterial infections, especially during periods of low blood counts; checking with physician immediately if fever or chills, cough or hoarseness, lower back or side pain, or painful or difficult urination occur
- » Checking with physician immediately if unusual bleeding or bruising; black, tarry stools; blood in urine or stools; or pinpoint red spots on skin occur

Caution in use of regular toothbrush, dental floss, or toothpick; physician, dentist, or nurse may suggest alternatives; checking with physician before having dental work done

Not touching eyes or inside of nose unless hands washed immediately before

Using caution to avoid accidental cuts with use of sharp objects such as safety razor or fingernail or toenail cutters

Avoiding contact sports or other situations where bruising or injury could occur

### Side/adverse effects

May cause adverse effects such as blood problems; importance of discussing possible effects with physician

Signs of potential side effects, especially leukopenia, infection, pneumonia, pain, thrombocytopenia, edema, neurologic effects, stomatitis, pulmonary edema, pneumonitis, and tumor lysis syndrome

Physician or nurse can help in dealing with side effects

Possibility of hair loss; normal hair growth should return after treatment has ended

## General Dosing Information

Patients receiving fludarabine should be under supervision of a physician experienced in cancer chemotherapy.

A variety of dosage schedules and regimens of fludarabine, alone or in combination with other antitumor agents, are used. The prescriber may consult the medical literature as well as the manufacturer's literature in choosing a specific dosage.

Dosage must be adjusted to meet the individual requirements of each patient, on the basis of clinical response and degree of bone marrow depression.

If neurotoxicity occurs, consideration should be given to delaying or discontinuing fludarabine.

Development of uric acid nephropathy in patients with leukemia or lymphoma may be prevented by adequate oral hydration and, in some cases, administration of allopurinol. Alkalinization of urine may be necessary if serum uric acid concentrations are elevated.

Special precautions are recommended in patients who develop thrombocytopenia as a result of administration of fludarabine. These may include extreme care in performing invasive procedures; regular inspection of intravenous sites, skin (including perirectal area), and mucous membrane surfaces for signs of bleeding or bruising; limiting frequency of venipuncture and avoiding intramuscular injections; testing urine, emesis, stool, and secretions for occult blood; care in use of regular toothbrushes, dental floss, toothpicks, safety razors, and fingernail and toenail cutters; avoiding constipation; and using caution to prevent falls and other injuries. Such patients should avoid alcohol and aspirin intake because of the risk of gastrointestinal bleeding. Platelet transfusions may be required.

Patients who develop leukopenia should be observed carefully for signs of infection. Antibiotic support may be required. In neutropenic patients who develop fever, broad-spectrum antibiotic coverage should be initiated empirically, pending bacterial cultures and appropriate diagnostic tests.

### Safety considerations for handling of medication

There is limited but increasing evidence and concern that personnel involved in preparation and administration of parenteral antineoplastics may be at some risk because of the potential mutagenicity, teratogenicity, and/or carcinogenicity of these agents, although the actual risk is unknown. USP advisory panels recommend cautious handling both in preparation and disposal of antineoplastic agents. Precautions that have been suggested include:
- Use of a biological containment cabinet during reconstitution and dilution of parenteral medications and wearing of disposable surgical gloves and masks.
- Use of proper technique to prevent contamination of the medication, work area, and operator during transfer between containers (including proper training of personnel in this technique).
- Cautious and proper disposal of needles, syringes, vials, ampuls, and unused medication.

A number of medical centers have developed detailed guidelines for handling of antineoplastic agents.

The manufacturer recommends use of latex gloves and safety glasses during handling and preparation of fludarabine to avoid exposure in case of breakage of the vial or other accidental spillage. If the solution contacts the skin or mucous membranes, they should be washed thoroughly with soap and water; eyes should be rinsed thoroughly with plain water. Exposure by inhalation or by direct contact of the skin or mucous membranes should be avoided.

## Parenteral Dosage Forms

### FLUDARABINE PHOSPHATE FOR INJECTION

#### Usual adult dose
Chronic lymphocytic leukemia—
     Intravenous (over approximately thirty minutes), 25 mg per square meter of body surface per day for five consecutive days. Each five-day course of treatment should begin every twenty-eight days.

Note: Dosage may be decreased or delayed based on evidence of hematologic or nonhematologic toxicity.

#### Usual pediatric dose
Safety and efficacy have not been established.

#### Size(s) usually available
U.S.—
     50 mg (Rx) [*Fludara* (mannitol 50 mg; sodium hydroxide)].
Canada—
     50 mg (Rx) [*Fludara* (mannitol 50 mg; sodium hydroxide)].

#### Packaging and storage
Store between 2 and 8 °C (36 and 46 °F), unless otherwise specified by manufacturer.

#### Preparation of dosage form
Fludarabine phosphate for injection is prepared for intravenous use by aseptically adding 2 mL of sterile water for injection to the 50-mg vial, producing a solution containing 25 mg of fludarabine phosphate per mL (the solid cake should fully dissolve within 15 seconds).

Fludarabine phosphate solutions may be further diluted in 100 or 125 mL of 5% dextrose injection or 0.9% sodium chloride injection for administration by intravenous infusion.

#### Stability
Reconstituted solutions contain no preservative and should be used within 8 hours of reconstitution.

## Selected Bibliography

Hood MA, Finley RS. Fludarabine: a review. DICP Ann Pharmacother 1991 May; 25: 518-24.

Chun HG, Leyland-Jones B, Cheson BD. Fludarabine phosphate: a synthetic purine antimetabolite with significant activity against lymphoid malignancies. J Clin Oncol 1991 Jan; 9: 175-88.

Multiple authors. Fludarabine phosphate: an effective therapy for lymphoid malignancies. Semin Oncol 1990 Oct; 17 (5 Suppl 8): 1-78.

Revised: 08/02/94

---

# FLUDEOXYGLUCOSE F 18    Systemic*†

VA CLASSIFICATION (Primary): DX201

Note: For a listing of dosage forms and brand names by country availability, see *Dosage Forms* section(s). For a listing of brand names for the articles in this monograph, refer to the General Index.

*Not commercially available in the U.S.
†Not commercially available in Canada.

## Category

Diagnostic aid, radioactive (brain disorders; cardiac disease; neoplastic disease).

## Indications

Note: Because fludeoxyglucose F 18 (FDG) is not commercially available in the U.S. or Canada, the bracketed information and the use of the superscript 1 in this monograph reflect the lack of labeled (approved) indications for this product.

## Accepted

[Brain imaging, positron emission tomographic][1]—Positron emission tomography (PET) using FDG is used in studies of cerebral glucose metabolism in various physiological and pathological states. FDG-PET is currently used for the following diagnostic studies:

[Tumors, brain (diagnosis)][1]—FDG-PET is used to locate and differentiate primary brain tumors. It is helpful in staging the extent of malignant growth. It also provides indications of prognosis, as well as an ongoing means of assessing therapeutic response. Also, in patients with cerebral tumors who have undergone radiation therapy, FDG-PET is the primary means, other than biopsy, available to differentiate tumor recurrence from radiation necrosis and edema.

[Seizures (diagnosis)][1]—FDG-PET is used in patients with partial complex seizures who do not respond adequately to medication, in order to establish the site of the epileptogenic focus, when temporal lobectomy or focal resection are being considered. In interictal FDG-PET scans of patients with partial seizures, regions of focal or lateralized hypometabolism have been shown to correlate with the site of epileptogenic lesions. PET can complement electroencephalographic (EEG) studies in the preoperative evaluation of patients with partial seizures, making invasive depth electrode studies unnecessary in about 50% of the cases. In intractable childhood seizures, FDG-PET is used to identify site(s) for surgical resection, from focal resections to hemispherectomies. In large area resections, FDG-PET is also used to assess functional status of uninvolved areas of the brain before and after surgery. It provides a direct means of predicting postsurgical developmental response.

[Depression, mental (diagnosis)][1]—FDG-PET can be used to differentiate unipolar from bipolar depression, as well as to differentiate chronic depression (pseudodementia) from Alzheimer's.

[Behavior-metabolism relationship studies][1]—FDG-PET is used in behavior-metabolism relationship studies, since differences in regional rates of glucose metabolism are associated with different behavioral tasks. It can be used to test for normal function or deficits in motor, visual, sensory, memory, and cognitive functions in the brain.

[Dementia, Alzheimer-type (diagnosis)][1]—FDG-PET is used to examine glucose metabolism in dementia. Regional alterations, particularly in the temporal-parietal cortex, provide means of detecting early to late stage Alzheimer's, and provide differential diagnosis from confounding conditions, such as multi-infarct dementia, pseudodementia, thyroid disease, normal-pressure hydrocephalus, as well as normal aging.

[Stroke (diagnosis)][1]—FDG-PET can be used to determine the degree and extent of injury in acute and chronic stages. Also, the technique provides criteria for reversible injury and provides a means of establishing proper selection and evaluation of therapy.

[Cardiac imaging, positron emission tomographic][1]—FDG-PET is currently used for the following diagnostic studies:

[Ischemia, myocardial (diagnosis)][1]—FDG-PET is used to evaluate the extent and degree of regional alterations in myocardial metabolism associated with acute and chronic ischemia. These data are used to distinguish viable, but functionally impaired, ischemic myocardium from nonviable (infarcted) myocardium and are critical in deciding between angioplasty or surgical bypass versus a more conservative medical treatment. The technique is also useful for follow-up studies to determine therapeutic outcome.

[Cardiac wall-motion abnormalities assessment][1]—PET using ammonia N 13 ($^{13}NH_3$) or rubidium Rb 82 ($^{82}Rb$) to assess the distribution of blood flow in conjunction with FDG-PET to estimate myocardial metabolic viability in dysfunctional myocardial segments serves to predict, preoperatively, the presence of reversible regional wall-motion abnormalities, which is helpful in the selection of patients in whom revascularization may lead to improved ventricular function.

[Cardiac bypass surgery assessment][1]—FDG-PET is used in conjunction with $^{13}NH_3$-PET or $^{82}Rb$-PET before and after aortocoronary bypass surgery to help evaluate the effect of surgery on myocardial glucose metabolism. Also, graft patency can be established with postoperative images.

[Percutaneous transluminal coronary angioplasty assessment][1]—FDG-PET is used in conjunction with $^{13}NH_3$-PET or $^{82}Rb$-PET, before and after percutaneous transluminal coronary angioplasty, to evaluate the infarcted areas and assess the recovery of myocardial blood flow and metabolism in the ischemic myocardium.

[Carcinoma, thyroid (diagnosis)][1]—FDG-PET is used in imaging of metastases of advanced thyroid carcinoma. FDG-PET may reveal metastases that do not accumulate I 131. Also, FDG-PET may be useful for confirmation of complete remission after treatment with radioiodine.

[Carcinoma, hepatic (diagnosis)][1]—FDG-PET is used to detect and characterize liver tumors and to monitor liver tumor therapy.

[Lymphomas, non-Hodgkin's (diagnosis)][1]; or

[Sarcomas, soft tissue (diagnosis)][1]—FDG-PET can be used for the detection of non-Hodgkin's lymphoma (especially high-grade malignancy) and soft tissue sarcomas.

[Tumors, musculoskeletal (diagnosis)][1]—FDG-PET is helpful in determining the degree of malignancy of neoplasms of the musculoskeletal system.

[Carcinoma, breast (diagnosis)][1];

[Carcinoma, lung (diagnosis)][1];

[Carcinoma, colorectal (diagnosis)][1]; or

[Tumors, head and neck (diagnosis)][1]—FDG-PET is used to characterize various tumors, monitor effects of treatment regimens, and differentiate recurrent or residual tumor from therapy-induced changes.

---

[1]Not included in Canadian product labeling.

## Physical Properties

### Nuclear data

| Radionuclide (half-life) | Decay constant | Mode of decay | Principal photon emissions (keV) | Mean number of photons emissions/ disintegration |
|---|---|---|---|---|
| F 18 (110 min) | 0.0063 min$^{-1}$ | Positron decay | Gamma* (511) | 1.94 |

*The 2 gamma rays emitted in opposite directions at the moment of positron annihilation are used for imaging purposes. Detection devices usually used are positron emission tomography (PET) units; however, conventional planar scintillation cameras have also been used for some studies.

## Pharmacology/Pharmacokinetics

### Physicochemical characteristics
Molecular weight—182.

### Mechanism of action/Effect
FDG is transported from blood to tissues in a manner similar to glucose and competes with glucose for hexokinase phosphorylation to FDG-6-phosphate. However, since FDG-6-phosphate is not a substrate for subsequent glycolytic pathways and has a very low membrane permeability, the FDG becomes trapped in tissue in proportion to the rate of glycolysis or glucose utilization of that tissue.

Brain imaging; and

Neoplastic disease (diagnosis)—The rate of anaerobic glycolysis in tumors increases with higher degree of malignancy. It is believed that increased FDG uptake is caused by a shift in energy metabolism within malignant tumors from high yield oxidative pathways to inefficient anaerobic glycolysis, resulting in an increase in glucose utilization for a given energy demand. Accumulation of FDG in malignant tissue not only helps to locate and differentiate tumors, but can also be used to help distinguish recurrent malignant cerebral tumors from foci of radiation necrosis and edema, since glucose uptake takes place in tumors and in normal brain tissue, while active uptake is absent in an area of necrosis and reduced in edema.

Ischemia, myocardial (diagnosis)—The amount of FDG-6-phosphate accumulated in myocardial tissue is proportional to the tissue's rate of glucose consumption. Significant glucose consumption and uptake of FDG occurs in ischemic tissue because in severe oxygen deprived states the primary source of energy for the myocardium shifts from fatty acids to anaerobic glucose metabolism.

### Distribution
FDG accumulates mainly in the heart and brain because of the high glycolytic rate of these tissues; also, accumulates throughout the body in proportion to glucose metabolism. FDG also has been shown to accumulate in bone tumors and in primary and metastatic carcinomas of the liver. Accumulation of FDG in tumors may be related to the degree of tumor differentiation.

### Protein binding
Minimal.

### Biotransformation
FDG is phosphorylated to FDG-6-phosphate by hexokinase, with no further metabolism taking place throughout the remainder of the study.

### Half-life
75% of administered dose of FDG is retained with an effective half-life of 1.83 hours; 19% has an effective half-life of 0.26 hour; and the remaining 6% has an effective half-life of 1.53 hours.

**Time to peak concentration**

Approximately 30 minutes to peak tissue concentration.

**Time to peak diagnostic effect**

High tumor-to-background ratio has been obtained one hour after injection of FDG. Brain and heart are the only major organs showing high uptake of FDG. Low background activity is expected in the abdominal region with the exception of the urinary tract.

**Radiation dosimetry**

| Estimated absorbed radiation dose*† | | |
|---|---|---|
| Organ | mGy/MBq | mrad/mCi |
| Bladder wall | 0.17 | 629 |
| Heart | 0.065 | 240 |
| Brain | 0.026 | 96 |
| Kidneys | 0.021 | 77 |
| Uterus | 0.020 | 74 |
| Ovaries | 0.015 | 55 |
| Testes | 0.015 | 55 |
| Adrenals | 0.014 | 51 |
| Small intestine | 0.013 | 48 |
| Liver | 0.012 | 44 |
| Pancreas | 0.012 | 44 |
| Spleen | 0.012 | 44 |
| Red marrow | 0.011 | 41 |
| Lungs | 0.011 | 41 |
| Thyroid | 0.0097 | 36 |
| Other tissue | 0.011 | 41 |

Effective dose: 0.027mSv/MBq (0.1 rem/mCi)

*For adults; intravenous injection.

†Data based on the International Commission on Radiological Protection (ICRP) Publication 53—Radiation Dose to Patients from Radiopharmaceuticals.

**Elimination**

Renal (approximately 20% of administered dose excreted within the first 2 hours).

## Precautions to Consider

**Pregnancy/Reproduction**

Pregnancy—The possibility of pregnancy should be assessed in women of child-bearing potential. Clinical situations exist where the benefit to the patient and fetus, based on information derived from radiopharmaceutical use, outweighs the risks from fetal exposure to radiation. In this situation, the physician should use discretion and reduce the radiopharmaceutical dose to the lowest possible amount.

**Breast-feeding**

It is not known whether FDG is excreted in breast milk; however, it is expected that some will be present. Temporary discontinuation of nursing for a period of 12 to 24 hours is considered adequate.

**Pediatrics**

Although FDG is used in children, there have been no specific studies evaluating safety and efficacy. When used in children, the diagnostic benefit should be judged to outweigh the potential risk of radiation.

**Geriatrics**

Diagnostic studies performed to date have not demonstrated geriatrics-specific problems that would limit the usefulness of FDG in the elderly.

**Drug interactions and/or related problems**

See *Diagnostic interference*.

**Diagnostic interference**

The following have been selected on the basis of their potential clinical significance (possible effect in parentheses where appropriate)—not necessarily inclusive (» = major clinical significance):

With results of *cardiac imaging*
*Due to other medications*
 Dopamine and
 Insulin
  (concurrent intravenous administration of these medications with FDG may alter myocardial extraction of FDG)

*Due to medical problems or conditions*
 Diabetes mellitus
  (patients with diabetes mellitus may require normalization of plasma glucose levels and insulin therapy for optimal myocardial image quality)

**Medical considerations/Contraindications**

See *Diagnostic interference*.

## Side/Adverse Effects

There are no known side/adverse effects associated with the use of FDG.

## Patient Consultation

As an aid to patient consultation, refer to *Advice for the Patient, Radiopharmaceuticals (Diagnostic)*.

In providing consultation, consider emphasizing the following selected information (» = major clinical significance):

**Description of use**

Action in the body: Concentration of radioactivity in brain, heart, and other sites of high glucose utilization (e.g., certain tumors) allows images to be obtained

Small amounts of radioactivity used in diagnosis; radiation received is low and considered safe

**Before having this test**

» Conditions affecting use, especially:
  Pregnancy—Risk to fetus from radiation exposure as opposed to benefit derived from use should be considered
  Breast-feeding—Not known if excreted in breast milk; temporary discontinuation of nursing recommended because of risk of radiation exposure to infant
  Use in children—Risk to child from radiation exposure as opposed to benefit derived from use should be considered

**Preparation for this test**

Special preparatory instructions may be given; patient should inquire in advance

**Precautions after having this test**

No special precautions

## General Dosing Information

Radiopharmaceuticals are to be administered only by or under the supervision of physicians who have had extensive training in the safe use and handling of radioactive materials and who are authorized by the appropriate Federal or State regulatory agency, if required, or, outside the U.S., the appropriate authority.

**For brain imaging**

Fasting for about 4 to 6 hours prior to the examination is sometimes recommended to increase the amount of FDG delivered to the brain.

To minimize the influence of external stimulation on the brain uptake of FDG, prior to, and during the initial 30 minutes following, the injection of FDG, the patient should be kept lying or sitting still in a quiet room.

Imaging is usually performed 30 minutes after administration of FDG.

**For cardiac imaging**

Optimal cardiac FDG-PET (e.g., better image quality) may be obtained if patients are in a glucose-loaded state rather than in the fasting state. Under fasting conditions with normal plasma levels of nonesterified fatty acids, only the ischemic areas of the myocardium use glucose preferentially, and thus, only these areas will accumulate FDG. This renders an image in which the myocardial outline is not well seen, making it difficult to locate the ischemic area.

**For tumor imaging**

Fasting overnight or for at least 6 hours prior to the examination is recommended to increase the relative uptake of FDG by the tumor.

**Safety considerations for handling this radiopharmaceutical**

Improper handling of this radiopharmaceutical may cause radioactive contamination. Guidelines for handling radioactive material have been prepared by scientific, professional, state, federal, and international bodies and are available to the specially qualified and authorized users who have access to radiopharmaceuticals.

## Parenteral Dosage Forms

### FLUDEOXYGLUCOSE F 18 INJECTION USP

**Usual adult and adolescent administered activity**

Brain imaging
Cardiac imaging or
Tumor imaging—Intravenous, 370 megabecquerels (10 millicuries).

**Usual pediatric administered activity**

Brain imaging
Cardiac imaging or
Tumor imaging—Intravenous, up to 5.3 megabecquerels (0.14 millicuries) per kg of body weight.

**Usual geriatric administered activity**
See *Usual adult and adolescent administered activity*

**Strength(s) usually available**
U.S.—
Prepared on-site at various clinical facilities.
Canada—
Prepared on-site at various clinical facilities.

**Packaging and storage**
Store below 40 °C (104 °F), preferably between 15 and 30 °C (59 and 86 °F). Protect from freezing.

**Note**
Caution—Radioactive material.

## Selected Bibliography

Chan SY, Brunken RC, Buxton DB. Cardiac positron emission tomography: the foundations and clinical applications. J Thorac Imaging 1990; 5 (3): 9-19.

Jamieson D, Alavi A, Jolles P, et al. Positron emission tomography in the investigation of central nervous system disorders. Radiol Clin North Am 1988; 26 (5): 1075-88.

Hawkins RA, Phelps ME. PET in clinical oncology. Cancer Metastasis Rev 1988; 7 (2): 119-42.

Revised: 11/13/92
Interim revision: 08/02/94

---

# FLUDROCORTISONE   Systemic

VA CLASSIFICATION (Primary/Secondary): HS052/CV900; DX900
Note: For a listing of dosage forms and brand names by country availability, see *Dosage Forms* section(s). For a listing of brand names for the articles in this monograph, refer to the General Index.

## Category

Corticosteroid (mineralocorticoid); antihypotensive (idiopathic orthostatic); diagnostic aid (renal tubular acidosis).

## Indications

Note: Bracketed information in the *Indications* section refers to uses that are not included in U.S. product labeling.

**Accepted**
Adrenocortical insufficiency, chronic primary (treatment) or
Adrenocortical insufficiency, chronic secondary (treatment)—Fludrocortisone is indicated as partial replacement therapy in the treatment of adrenocortical insufficiency.
Adrenogenital syndrome, congenital (treatment)—Fludrocortisone is indicated in salt-losing forms of adrenogenital syndrome.
[Hypotension, idiopathic orthostatic (treatment)][1]—Fludrocortisone is used in conjunction with increased sodium intake in the treatment of idiopathic orthostatic hypotension.
[Acidosis, in renal tubular disorders (diagnosis and treatment)][1]—Fludrocortisone is used in the treatment of Type IV renal tubular acidosis associated with hyporeninemic hypoaldosteronism. Fludrocortisone is also used as an aid in diagnosing the cause of the condition. Effectiveness of fludrocortisone therapy indicates that the condition is caused by hyporeninemic hypoaldosteronism rather than by renal tubular transport dysfunction.

[1]Not included in Canadian product labeling.

## Pharmacology/Pharmacokinetics

**Physicochemical characteristics**
Molecular weight—422.49.

**Mechanism of action/Effect**
Fludrocortisone acetate is an adrenal cortical steroid that has very high levels of mineralocorticoid activity and moderate levels of glucocorticoid activity. However, it is used only for its mineralocorticoid effects.
Mineralocorticoids act on the distal tubules to increase potassium excretion, hydrogen ion excretion, and sodium reabsorption and subsequent water retention. Cation transport in other secretory cells is similarly affected; excretion of water and electrolytes by the large intestine and by salivary and sweat glands is also altered, but to a lesser extent.
At the cellular level, corticosteroids diffuse across cell membranes and complex with specific cytoplasmic receptors. These complexes then enter the cell nucleus, bind to DNA (chromatin), and stimulate transcription of mRNA (messenger RNA) and subsequent protein synthesis of various enzymes thought to be ultimately responsible for the physiological effects of these hormones.

**Protein binding**
High.

**Biotransformation**
Hepatic, renal.

**Half-life**
≥3.5 hours (plasma); 18–36 hours (biological).

**Duration of action**
1–2 days.

**Elimination**
Renal, mostly as inactive metabolites.

## Precautions to Consider

**Carcinogenicity/Mutagenicity**
Adequate animal studies have not been conducted on the carcinogenicity or mutagenicity of fludrocortisone.

**Pregnancy/Reproduction**
Pregnancy—Studies on use of fludrocortisone during pregnancy have not been done in humans.
Infants born to mothers who have received substantial doses of corticosteroids during pregnancy should be closely observed for signs of hypoadrenalism.
Studies on use of fludrocortisone during pregnancy have not been done in animals.
FDA Pregnancy Category C.

**Breast-feeding**
Problems in humans have not been documented. However, corticosteroids are distributed into breast milk and may cause unwanted effects in the infant such as growth suppression and inhibition of endogenous steroid production.

**Pediatrics**
Although adequate and well-controlled studies have not been done in the pediatric population, corticosteroids may cause unwanted effects in children and growing adolescents, such as growth suppression and inhibition of endogenous steroid production.

**Geriatrics**
Appropriate studies have not been performed in the geriatric population. One published report described the use of fludrocortisone in the treatment of severe hyponatremia that occurred following head injury in 3 geriatric patients in whom syndrome of inappropriate antidiuretic hormone (SIADH) had been ruled out as the cause of the hyponatremia. Doses ranged from 0.1 to 0.4 mg of fludrocortisone per day.

**Drug interactions and/or related problems**
The following drug interactions and/or related problems have been selected on the basis of their potential clinical significance (possible mechanism in parentheses where appropriate)—not necessarily inclusive (» = major clinical significance):

Note: Combinations containing any of the following medications, depending on the amount present, may also interact with this medication.

» Digitalis glycosides
(risk of cardiac arrhythmias or digitalis toxicity associated with hypokalemia may be increased; serum potassium concentrations and cardiac function should be monitored; potassium supplements may be required)

» Hepatic enzyme inducers (See *Appendix II*)
(phenytoin and rifampin have been reported to increase 6-beta-hydroxylation of fludrocortisone, via induction of P-450 liver enzymes; fludrocortisone dosage increase may be required)

» Hypokalemia-causing medications (See *Appendix II*)
(risk of severe hypokalemia due to other hypokalemia-causing medications may be increased; monitoring of serum potassium concentrations and cardiac function and potassium supplementation may be required)

Lithium
(in one published case report, lithium antagonized the mineralocorticoid effects of fludrocortisone; increased fludrocortisone dose and dietary sodium supplementation were required during concurrent use)

» Sodium-containing medications or foods
(concurrent use with fludrocortisone in the treatment of Type IV renal tubular acidosis may result in hypernatremia, edema, and potentially severe increases in blood pressure; adjustment of sodium intake may be required)

**Laboratory value alterations**

The following have been selected on the basis of their potential clinical significance (possible effect in parentheses where appropriate)—not necessarily inclusive (» = major clinical significance):

With physiology/laboratory test values

Blood pressure
(may be increased)

Hematocrit percentage
(may be decreased due to increased blood volume)

Potassium
(serum concentration may be decreased due to increased potassium excretion)

Sodium
(serum concentration may be increased due to sodium retention)

**Medical considerations/Contraindications**

The medical considerations/contraindications included here have been selected on the basis of their potential clinical significance (reasons given in parentheses where appropriate)—not necessarily inclusive (» = major clinical significance).

*Risk-benefit should be considered when the following medical problems exist:*

» Cardiac disease or
» Congestive heart failure or
» Hypertension or
Peripheral edema or
» Renal function impairment, except when fludrocortisone is used to treat Type IV renal tubular acidosis
(sodium- and fluid-retaining effects detrimental to these patients)

Glomerulonephritis, acute

Hepatic function impairment or
Hypothyroidism
(clearance of fludrocortisone may be decreased)

Hyperthyroidism
(clearance of fludrocortisone may be increased)

Nephritis, chronic

Osteoporosis
(may be exacerbated by increased calcium excretion)

Sensitivity to fludrocortisone

**Patient monitoring**

The following may be especially important in patient monitoring (other tests may be warranted in some patients, depending on condition; » = major clinical significance):

Blood pressure determinations and
Serum electrolyte concentrations
(recommended at onset of therapy and at periodic intervals during prolonged therapy)

## Side/Adverse Effects

The following side/adverse effects have been selected on the basis of their potential clinical significance (possible signs and symptoms in parentheses where appropriate)—not necessarily inclusive:

**Those indicating need for medical attention**

Incidence less frequent or rare

*Anaphylaxis, generalized* (cough; difficulty swallowing; hives; redness and itching of skin; redness of conjunctivae; shortness of breath; swelling of nasal membranes, face, and eyelids); *congestive heart failure* (cough; dilated neck veins; extreme fatigue; irregular breathing; irregular heartbeat); *dizziness; headache, severe or continuing; hypokalemic syndrome* (irregular heartbeat; loss of appetite; muscle cramps or pain; nausea; severe weakness of extremities and trunk; vomiting); *peripheral edema* (rapid weight gain; swelling of feet or lower legs)

## Patient Consultation

As an aid to patient consultation, refer to *Advice for the Patient, Fludrocortisone (Systemic)*.

In providing consultation, consider emphasizing the following selected information (» = major clinical significance):

**Before using this medication**

» Conditions affecting use, especially:
Sensitivity to fludrocortisone
Pregnancy—Infants born to mothers who received substantial doses of corticosteroids during pregnancy require close observation for signs of hypoadrenalism
Use in children and growing adolescents—May cause growth suppression and inhibition of endogenous steroid production
Other medications, especially hypokalemia-causing medications, digitalis glycosides, hepatic enzyme inducers, or sodium-containing medications or food
Other medical problems, especially cardiac disease, congestive heart failure, hypertension, or renal function impairment

**Proper use of this medication**

» Importance of not taking more medication than the amount prescribed
Missed dose: Taking as soon as possible; not taking if almost time for next dose; not doubling doses
» Proper dosing
» Proper storage

**Precautions while using this medication**

» Regular visits to physician to check progress during therapy
Carrying medical identification card during long-term therapy

**Side/adverse effects**

Signs of potential side effects, especially generalized anaphylaxis, congestive heart failure, dizziness, severe headache, hypokalemic syndrome, or peripheral edema

## General Dosing Information

When used in the treatment of adrenocortical insufficiency or salt-losing forms of adrenogenital syndrome, fludrocortisone should be administered with appropriate glucocorticoid therapy such as 10 to 30 mg of hydrocortisone per day or 10 to 37.5 mg of cortisone per day. Sodium supplementation may also be necessary.

In the treatment of Type IV renal tubular acidosis, concurrent use of a diuretic may be necessary to decrease the risk of sodium and fluid retention, especially in patients with hypertension, congestive heart failure, or renal function impairment.

## Oral Dosage Forms

Note: Bracketed uses in the *Dosage Forms* section refer to categories of use and/or indications that are not included in U.S. product labeling.

### FLUDROCORTISONE ACETATE TABLETS USP

**Usual adult and adolescent dose**

Adrenocortical insufficiency, chronic—
Oral, 100 mcg (0.1 mg) per day.

Note: Dose should be reduced to 50 mcg (0.05 mg) per day if transient hypertension occurs. Dosages of 100 mcg (0.1 mg) three times a week to 200 mcg (0.2 mg) once a day have been employed.

Adrenogenital syndrome, congenital—
Oral, 100 to 200 mcg (0.1 to 0.2 mg) per day.

[Antihypotensive, idiopathic orthostatic][1]—
Oral, 50 to 200 mcg (0.05 to 0.2 mg) per day.

**Usual pediatric dose**

Oral, 50 to 100 mcg (0.05 to 0.1 mg) per day.

**Strength(s) usually available**

U.S.—
100 mcg (0.1 mg) (Rx) [*Florinef* (scored; lactose)].

Canada—
100 mcg (0.1 mg) (Rx) [*Florinef* (scored; lactose)].

**Packaging and storage**

Store below 40 °C (104 °F), preferably between 15 and 30 °C (59 and 86 °F), unless otherwise specified by manufacturer. Store in a well-closed container.

---

[1]Not included in Canadian product labeling.

---

Revised: 06/15/93

# FLUMAZENIL    Systemic

VA CLASSIFICATION (Primary): AD900

Note: For a listing of dosage forms and brand names by country availability, see *Dosage Forms* section(s). For a listing of brand names for the articles in this monograph, refer to the General Index.

## Category

Benzodiazepine antagonist.

## Indications

### General considerations

**Administering flumazenil to reverse the effects of benzodiazepines does not eliminate the need for monitoring and evaluating the patient and instituting needed interventions,** e.g., establishing an airway, assisting ventilation, and supporting circulation. Although flumazenil partially reverses benzodiazepine-induced hypoventilation, **it should not be relied upon to provide complete or sustained reversal of hypoventilation,** especially if the patient has also received an opioid analgesic. Also, resedation may occur after initial recovery, although most patients remain more alert than they were before flumazenil administration.

Before flumazenil is administered, the advantages of reversing benzodiazepine-induced sedation should be weighed against the possible disadvantages, especially in high-risk patients. The risks of antagonizing the anticonvulsant effects of benzodiazepines and/or of precipitating a withdrawal syndrome in physically dependent patients must be considered because seizures may result.

### Accepted

Sedation, benzodiazepine-induced, reversal—Flumazenil is indicated for partial or complete reversal of post-procedure residual sedation resulting from use of benzodiazepines for induction and/or maintenance of anesthesia, conscious sedation, or deep sedation. The benefits of reversing post-procedure residual sedation are more apparent in patients who are heavily sedated at the time of administration than in patients who are only mildly or moderately sedated. Flumazenil facilitates patient management most significantly during the first hour following administration. After 1 hour, significant spontaneous recovery is also apparent in patients who have not received the medication. Flumazenil has been shown to speed recovery of patients who have received benzodiazepines concurrently with opioid analgesics, inhalation anesthetics, or local, regional, spinal, or topical anesthetics. However, its efficacy may be decreased when multiple anesthetic agents have been used or sedating medications are required post-procedure.

Flumazenil is indicated to reverse the effects of benzodiazepines used to sedate critical care patients.

Toxicity, benzodiazepine (treatment)—Flumazenil is indicated for the management of benzodiazepine overdose. However, if the patient has been intubated flumazenil may be unnecessary and may complicate patient management by causing agitation. In addition to reversing central nervous system (CNS) depression, flumazenil has been reported to reverse benzodiazepine-induced hypotension and bradycardia unresponsive to administration of intravenous fluids, atropine, and dopamine. Flumazenil is most effective in intoxications caused by a benzodiazepine alone, although resedation occurs frequently. Flumazenil may also be at least partially effective in treating mixed overdoses, but its efficacy depends on the extent to which a benzodiazepine contributes to the intoxication, especially if significant quantities of other sedating medications have been used concurrently. Flumazenil is not a substitute for other measures that may be necessary, but in some clinical trials its use decreased the need for interventions such as gastric lavage, urinary catheterization, and diagnostic tests.

**Extreme caution is recommended if flumazenil is considered for treating mixed overdoses in which medications with potential seizurogenic and/or arrhythmogenic activity or unidentified medications may have been taken.** Reversal of the protective effect of the benzodiazepine in such cases has resulted in seizures and/or arrhythmias, usually in mixed overdoses with tricyclic antidepressants. Some emergency care physicians recommend that flumazenil not be used until after a diagnostic electrocardiogram and/or quantitative analytical testing has ruled out severe cyclic (tricyclic or tetracyclic) antidepressant overdosage.

Note: Flumazenil does not reverse benzodiazepine-induced amnesia for events occurring prior to administration of the antagonist (retrograde amnesia). Although flumazenil may partially reverse amnesia for events occurring after it is given (anterograde amnesia), its ef-

fects on memory are less complete, less consistent, and of shorter duration than its effects on sedation. Also, although flumazenil may reverse post-procedure psychomotor deficits associated with benzodiazepine administration, normal levels of performance may not be achieved.

### Acceptance not established

Flumazenil has been used to reverse benzodiazepine-maintained anesthesia intraoperatively during spinal surgery, to arouse the patient temporarily for assessment of sensory and motor function. Assessments could be performed within 1 or 2 minutes after administration of flumazenil. Postoperatively, the patients did not recall having been aroused. However, flumazenil has been used for this purpose in relatively few patients; more experience is needed before the risks and benefits of this procedure can be determined.

### Unaccepted

Flumazenil should not be administered in mixed overdoses if signs of severe cyclic (tricyclic or tetracyclic) antidepressant toxicity are present. Instead, respiration and circulation should be supported until signs of cyclic antidepressant toxicity have abated.

Use of flumazenil for the treatment of benzodiazepine dependence is not recommended. Efficacy has not been established.

Because of the unacceptably high risk of adverse effects, flumazenil should not be used to determine whether dependence on sedating benzodiazepines has occurred in critical care patients.

Flumazenil is not recommended for treatment of hepatic encephalopathy. Although intravenously administered flumazenil has produced partial improvement of neurologic status in some patients, the beneficial effect was not sustained, and several patients became worse after treatment was discontinued. One patient who received twice-daily administration of oral flumazenil in an attempt to prevent return of symptoms experienced a psychotic reaction that began 48 hours after treatment was started and resolved within 12 hours after the medication was discontinued.

## Pharmacology/Pharmacokinetics

### Physicochemical characteristics

Chemical group—Flumazenil is a 1,4-imidazobenzodiazepine derivative. It is structurally related to benzodiazepine agonists.

Molecular weight—303.29.

pKa—1.78.

Octanol:buffer partition coefficient—14.1.

### Mechanism of action/Effect

Flumazenil selectively antagonizes or attenuates the effects of benzodiazepines in the CNS by competitively inhibiting their actions at the benzodiazepine binding site of the gamma aminobutyric acid (GABA)–benzodiazepine receptor complex. Flumazenil does not antagonize the effects of CNS-active substances that act via other receptors. Also, flumazenil does not alter the pharmacokinetics of benzodiazepines.

The extent to which flumazenil reverses the effects of a benzodiazepine depends on the dose and plasma concentration of both medications and on the effect being assessed. Flumazenil reverses some components of benzodiazepine-induced hypoventilation, leading to at least partial improvement in respiratory function. One study showed that midazolam's effect on respiration results primarily (but not exclusively) from a reduction in tidal volume, and that flumazenil completely reverses this effect. However, several studies have shown that flumazenil may not affect other measures of respiratory function, especially measures that are independent of patient effort or wakefulness. Also, amnesia is antagonized less consistently and less completely than psychomotor deficits, which may be reversed less completely than sedation.

### Other actions/effects

Animal studies have shown that flumazenil may have some weak agonist or inverse agonist activity when given in high doses. However, therapeutic doses of flumazenil have not produced clinically significant effects other than antagonism of administered benzodiazepines in humans.

### Distribution

Flumazenil is rapidly distributed into the brain. Concentrations are highest in the cerebral cortex (which contains the largest number of benzodiazepine receptors), intermediate in the inferior temporal lobe and cerebellum, and lowest in white matter.

Volume of distribution (Vol$_D$)—
  Initially, 0.5 L per kg of body weight (L/kg). After redistribution, the apparent Vol$_D$ is approximately 1 L/kg (range, 0.77 to 1.6 L/kg). One study in children 5 to 9 years of age also reported a mean Vol$_D$ at steady-state of 1 ± 0.2 L/kg. These values are not altered in patients with moderately impaired hepatic function, but are increased by approximately 37% in patients with severe hepatic function impairment.

**Protein binding**
Moderate (approximately 50%, of which 66% is bound to albumin). Protein binding is reduced in patients with hepatic cirrhosis; in one study, the free fraction was increased from 55% in controls to 64 and 79% in patients with moderate and severe hepatic function impairment, respectively.

**Biotransformation**
Hepatic; rapid and extensive. Clearance is dependent on hepatic blood flow.

**Half-life**
In plasma—
  Distribution: 7 to 15 minutes.
  Elimination: Approximately 54 minutes (range, 41 to 79 minutes) in adults. One study in children 5 to 9 years of age reported a mean elimination half-life of 35.3 ± 13.8 minutes. Prolonged to about 1.3 hours and 2.5 hours in patients with moderate and severe hepatic function impairment, respectively, but not affected by renal function impairment or by hemodialysis beginning 1 hour after flumazenil administration.
In brain—
  Elimination: 20 to 30 minutes.

**Onset of action**
Approximately 1 to 2 minutes.

**Time to peak concentration**
In the CNS—Approximately 1 to 3 minutes.

**Peak serum concentration**
1-mg dose, infused over 5 minutes—24 (range, 11 to 43) nanograms per mL (nanograms/mL) (0.08 [range, 0.036 to 0.14] micromoles/L); substantially higher in patients with moderate, stable, alcoholic cirrhosis. The concentration in the brain may be higher than the simultaneous plasma concentration.

**Therapeutic serum concentration**
Dependent on the benzodiazepine being reversed and its concentration. In patients receiving usual sedating doses of benzodiazepines, partial reversal generally occurs at flumazenil concentrations of 3 to 6 nanograms/mL (0.01 to 0.02 micromoles/L) and complete reversal usually occurs at concentrations of 12 to 28 nanograms/mL (0.036 to 0.09 micromoles/L). These concentrations are generally produced by doses of 100 to 200 mcg (0.1 to 0.2 mg) and 400 mcg (0.4 mg) to 1 mg, respectively.

**Time to peak effect**
6 to 10 minutes after completion of the injection.

**Duration of action**
Dependent on the doses and concentrations of the benzodiazepine being antagonized and of flumazenil. In various clinical trials that assessed flumazenil's ability to reverse post-procedure residual sedation, the level of alertness achieved was maintained during the 3-hour observation period in 60 to 95% of the responders. Although up to 40% of the patients experienced partial resedation, most retained an adequate level of alertness. Up to 3% of the patients experienced clinically significant resedation, generally 1 to 2 hours after flumazenil administration. In a study that assessed flumazenil's ability to reverse much larger quantities (i.e., overdoses) of various benzodiazepines, resedation occurred in > 60% of the patients, generally 60 to 90 minutes after flumazenil administration.

**Elimination**
Renal—90 to 95% of a dose, primarily as metabolites (following hepatic metabolism). In adults, < 1% of a dose is eliminated in the urine as unchanged flumazenil. However, in a study in children 5 to 9 years of age, 5.8 to 13.8% of a dose was eliminated in the urine as unchanged flumazenil.
Biliary/fecal—In adults: 5 to 10% of a dose.
Note: About 70% of a dose is excreted within 2 hours, and 86% of a dose is excreted within 4 hours, after administration. Elimination is complete within 72 hours.
  Plasma clearance in healthy adult subjects ranges from 0.7 to 1.3 (mean, 1) L per hour per kg of body weight (L/hr/kg). Values in pediatric patients undergoing minor surgery are similar; a study in

a small number of children 5 to 9 years of age reported a mean clearance rate of 1.2 L/hr/kg.
  Ingestion of food during an infusion has been shown to increase flumazenil clearance by 50%, probably by increasing hepatic blood flow. The clinical significance of this effect is not known. Clearance rates may be increased by approximately 25% in patients with chronic stable renal failure (with or without dialysis), but are not affected by hemodialysis beginning 1 hour after administration of flumazenil or by advanced age. However, clearance rates are decreased to approximately 40 to 60% of normal values in patients with moderate hepatic function impairment and to 25% of normal values in patients with severely impaired hepatic function.

## Precautions to Consider

**Carcinogenicity**
Studies have not been done.

**Mutagenicity**
Flumazenil was not mutagenic in the Ames test (performed with 5 different test strains), assays in *S. cerevisiae* D7 and Chinese hamster cells, blastogenesis assays in peripheral human lymphocytes *in vitro*, and in a mouse micronucleus assay *in vivo*. Cytotoxic concentrations of flumazenil caused a slight increase in unscheduled DNA synthesis in rat hepatocyte culture, but no increase in DNA repair occurred in male mouse germ cells in an *in vivo* assay.

**Pregnancy/Reproduction**
Fertility—Flumazenil did not impair fertility in male or female rats given oral doses of 125 mg per kg of body weight (mg/kg) per day. This dose is considered, on the basis of area under the concentration-time curve (AUC) comparisons, to represent 120 times the human exposure provided by the maximum recommended intravenous dose of 5 mg.

Pregnancy—Adequate and well-controlled studies in humans have not been done. However, after administration to a pregnant woman who took an overdose of diazepam, flumazenil (300 mcg [0.3 mg] intravenously) reversed tachycardia and occasional decelerations in the fetus as well as antagonizing sedation in the woman. Fetal cardiac abnormalities and maternal drowsiness recurred about 15 hours later and responded to a second dose of flumazenil.

Studies in rats given up to 150 mg/kg per day orally from Day 6 to Day 15 of gestation and in rabbits given up to 150 mg/kg per day orally from Day 6 to Day 18 of gestation (120 to 600 times the human exposure from an intravenous dose of 5 mg, based on AUC comparisons) found no evidence of teratogenicity. Embryocidal effects (higher rates of pre-implantation and post-implantation losses) occurred in rabbits given 50 mg/kg (200 times the human exposure to a 5-mg intravenous dose) but did not occur in rabbits given 15 mg/kg (60 times the human exposure to a 5-mg intravenous dose). Also, decreased survival during lactation, increased liver weight at weaning, delayed incisor eruption, and delayed ear opening (and, consequently, delayed appearance of the auditory startle response) were observed in offspring of rats given 125 mg/kg per day (120 times the human exposure to a 5-mg intravenous dose), but not in offspring of rats given 5 or 25 mg/kg per day (up to 24 times the human exposure to a 5-mg intravenous dose).

FDA Pregnancy Category C.

Labor and delivery—The safety of administering flumazenil to reverse the effects of benzodiazepines used during labor and delivery has not been established.

**Breast-feeding**
It is not known whether flumazenil is distributed into breast milk.

**Pediatrics**
Flumazenil has been administered to a limited number of pediatric patients up to 14 years of age, including a neonate with apnea (born at 38 weeks' gestation) who had been exposed to diazepam *in utero* during the last 3 weeks of pregnancy as well as children receiving the medication for reversal of benzodiazepine sedation or for treatment of benzodiazepine overdose. Although appropriate dosage has not been established, preliminary data indicate that the pharmacokinetics and pharmacodynamics of flumazenil in children (in doses ranging between 10 and 100 mcg/kg) are similar to those in adults, and that pediatrics-specific problems that would limit use of flumazenil in children are not expected.

**Geriatrics**
Flumazenil was found to be safe and effective in geriatric patients in clinical trials, which included patients up to 91 years of age. Other studies have shown that the pharmacokinetics of flumazenil are not altered, and no adjustment of dosage is needed, in geriatric patients. However, particularly careful monitoring of the patient may be needed

because benzodiazepine-induced sedation tends to be deeper and more prolonged in geriatric patients than in younger adults.

## Drug interactions and/or related problems

The following drug interactions and/or related problems have been selected on the basis of their potential clinical significance (possible mechanism in parentheses where appropriate)—not necessarily inclusive (» = major clinical significance):

Note: Combinations containing any of the following medications, depending on the amount present, may also interact with this medication.

Benzodiazepines, chronic use of
(the risk of precipitating withdrawal symptoms and of other adverse effects, including those associated with reversal of the therapeutic effects of a benzodiazepine, is increased when flumazenil is administered to patients taking a benzodiazepine chronically)

Seizurogenic medications, especially:
» Cyclic (tricyclic or tetracyclic) antidepressants
(high risk of seizures, especially in a mixed overdose with a seizurogenic medication and a benzodiazepine, because flumazenil reverses the anticonvulsant, as well as the sedative, effects of benzodiazepines)

## Medical considerations/Contraindications

The medical considerations/contraindications included here have been selected on the basis of their potential clinical significance (reasons given in parentheses where appropriate)—not necessarily inclusive (» = major clinical significance).

*Risk-benefit should be considered when the following medical problems exist:*

Anxiety, chronic or episodic, history of or
Anxiety, existing or
Panic disorder
(reversal of benzodiazepines may cause anxiety and has precipitated panic attacks in susceptible patients; caution and careful titration of dosage to clinical response are recommended, especially in patients with cardiac disease)

Cardiac disease, especially with increased left ventricular end-diastolic pressure
(although studies in patients with cardiac disease undergoing cardiac catheterization or surgery have not shown that administration of flumazenil produces significant alterations in cardiac function or evidence of ischemia, caution is recommended if the patient has displayed significant pre-procedure nervousness because stress and/or anxiety associated with abrupt reversal of benzodiazepines has led to increased blood pressure in some patients, especially after cardiac surgery; also, flumazenil has increased left ventricular end-diastolic pressure in some patients with coronary artery disease who received the medication to reverse benzodiazepine-induced sedation after cardiac catheterization; although the increases generally represented a return to presedation values, caution is recommended in patients with pre-existing increases in left ventricular end-diastolic pressure)

Drug abuse or history of, especially:
» Benzodiazepine abuse or chronic use
(risk of precipitating withdrawal symptoms, including seizures, since the patient may be dependent on benzodiazepines; also, flumazenil administration may complicate treatment for withdrawal from alcohol, barbiturates, and sedatives to which cross-tolerance may exist)

» Head injury, severe
(flumazenil may induce seizures and/or alter cerebral blood flow in patients with head injury; flumazenil has increased intracranial pressure significantly in patients with severe head injuries when intracranial pressure was not well controlled [but not when intracranial pressure was adequately controlled]; it should therefore be used with caution, if at all, in cases of severe head injury with known or suspected increases in intracranial pressure or poor intracranial compliance)

Hepatic function impairment
(clearance of flumazenil is decreased to 40 to 60% of normal in patients with mild to moderate hepatic function impairment, and to 25% of normal in patients with severely impaired hepatic function; although no alteration of initial dosage is necessary, a reduction in the size or frequency of subsequent doses may be needed)

» Hypersensitivity to benzodiazepines or to flumazenil

» Seizure disorders, especially if treated with benzodiazepines
(high risk of precipitating seizures)

## Patient monitoring

The following may be especially important in patient monitoring (other tests may be warranted in some patients, depending on condition; » = major clinical significance):

» Electrocardiographic determinations
(may be advisable to detect QRS prolongation, a possible sign of cyclic [tricyclic or tetracyclic] antidepressant toxicity, prior to flumazenil administration in overdose situations, especially when mixed overdosage with a cyclic antidepressant is suspected)

» Oxygenation, determined via pulse oximetry
(monitoring for an adequate period of time, depending on the dose and duration of action of the benzodiazepine being antagonized, is essential following flumazenil administration because benzodiazepine-induced hypoventilation may not be completely antagonized or may recur; it cannot be assumed that residual respiratory depression is not present in an alert patient; ventilatory assistance and/or supplemental oxygen may be required)

» Patient alertness
(monitoring for at least 1 to 2 hours following flumazenil administration is essential, although more prolonged monitoring may be needed, depending on the dose and the duration of action of the benzodiazepine being antagonized and whether other CNS depressants have been or are being given; resedation requiring additional treatment may occur, especially after initial reversal of the effects of large quantities of a benzodiazepine or of a benzodiazepine with a long elimination half-life or active metabolites; patients who do not show signs of resedation within 2 hours after post-procedure administration of 1 mg of flumazenil are not likely to experience severe resedation at a later time; however, resedation may occur 3 to 5 hours or longer [15 hours, in 1 reported case] after reversal of an overdose)

» Vital signs
(monitoring of blood pressure, heart rate, and respiratory rate is recommended so that supplemental treatment can be instituted as required)

# Side/Adverse Effects

Note: Flumazenil caused no serious adverse effects when administered in large intravenous doses to volunteers who had not received a benzodiazepine agonist. Many side/adverse effects are caused by abrupt reversal of the effects of benzodiazepines.

Reversal of the effects of benzodiazepines in physically dependent patients may precipitate a withdrawal syndrome with symptoms ranging from anxiety, headache, and/or emotional lability to seizures, depending on the degree of dependence. Other possible signs and symptoms of benzodiazepine withdrawal include hypertension, dizziness, involuntary movements, irritability, muscle tension, palpitations, panic, paresthesias, perceptual disturbances, sweating, tachycardia, and tinnitus. The risk of precipitating a withdrawal syndrome is increased with flumazenil doses higher than 1 mg and/or rapid administration. Severe symptoms, especially seizures, may be more likely to occur in patients who have been receiving long-term benzodiazepine therapy, especially for seizure disorders. However, benzodiazepine dependence resulting in an increased risk of seizures or other withdrawal symptoms may develop after relatively short exposure (3 to 5 days) when a benzodiazepine is used to provide continuous sedation in critical care patients.

In addition to the side/adverse effects reported below, arrhythmias including atrial, nodal, and ventricular extrasystoles, bradycardia, and tachycardia; hypertension; and chest pain have been reported (frequencies of occurrence less than 1%). Arrhythmias have been reported mostly in mixed overdoses with potentially arrhythmogenic medications, including chloral hydrate and tricyclic antidepressants. Also, complete heart block occurred in a patient who overdosed on temazepam, atenolol, and nifedipine. It has been proposed that arrhythmias may occur in association with hypoxic seizures after other medications taken together with a benzodiazepine in an overdose have sensitized the myocardium to such complications.

The following side/adverse effects have been selected on the basis of their potential clinical significance (possible signs and symptoms in parentheses where appropriate)—not necessarily inclusive:

## Those indicating need for medical attention
Incidence more frequent (3 to 9%)
*Agitation* (anxiety; dry mouth; dyspnea; hyperventilation; insomnia; nervousness; palpitations; tremor); *headache*

Incidence less frequent (1 to 3%)
*Emotional lability* (crying; depersonalization; dysphoria; euphoria; mental depression; paranoia); *hypertension; resedation, severe; skin rash*

Note: *Anxiety* and *emotional lability,* in addition to being symptoms of benzodiazepine withdrawal, may reflect reversal of the anxiolytic effects for which a benzodiazepine may have been prescribed.

Overall *resedation* rates of 3 to 9% and 10 to 15% were reported in clinical studies in which flumazenil was used to reverse conscious sedation and deep sedation or anesthesia, respectively, although substantially higher rates of partial resedation have been reported in individual studies. Resedation severe enough to be considered clinically significant occurred less frequently. Resedation may occur in 40 to > 60% of patients being treated for an overdose. The risk of resedation in critical care patients receiving flumazenil for reversal of prolonged sedation is also high. Clinically significant resedation is more likely to occur when large or repeated doses of a benzodiazepine have been administered, especially during a long procedure during which multiple anesthetics have been used, after initial reversal of a long-acting benzodiazepine, and in overdose situations.

Incidence rare (less than 1%)
*Convulsions without other signs or symptoms of withdrawal; hallucinations; hives or itching of skin*

Note: The risk of *convulsions* is increased in benzodiazepine-dependent patients, in patients with seizure disorders (especially if a benzodiazepine is being used for long-term treatment or for control of a convulsive episode), in patients treated for a mixed overdose with a cyclic (tricyclic or tetracyclic) antidepressant or other potentially seizurogenic medication, and in patients who are undergoing withdrawal from nonbenzodiazepine sedative-hypnotic agents.

**Those indicating need for medical attention only if they continue or are bothersome**
Incidence more frequent (3 to 11%, unless otherwise specified)
*Blurred vision or other vision disturbance; dizziness, possibly with ataxia and/or vertigo; drowsiness, residual or re-emergent*—incidence up to 40 to 60%; *nausea; pain at injection site; vomiting*

Incidence less frequent (1 to 3%) or rare (less than 1%)
*Fatigue, possibly with asthenia and malaise; flushing or hot flashes; hearing disturbances; thrombophlebitis at injection site*

## General Dosing Information

**Flumazenil administration is not a substitute for interventions such as establishing an airway, assisting ventilation, and supporting circulation.** Equipment and medications needed to institute such measures should be available for immediate use.

Equipment required for patient management, such as endotracheal tubes and intravenous access lines, should be securely in place before flumazenil is given. Some patients become confused and agitated when aroused, and may attempt to remove them.

**Preparation for managing seizures should be made prior to flumazenil administration,** especially when flumazenil is used to reverse long-term or high-dose use of a benzodiazepine for sedation in critical care patients or to treat a mixed overdose in which a potentially seizurogenic medication may have been ingested.

Flumazenil is to be administered intravenously. To minimize injection pain, it should be injected into a large vein through a freely flowing intravenous infusion. Extravasation may result in local irritation and should be avoided.

To allow control over the rate and degree of reversal while avoiding complications associated with too-rapid awakening or other adverse effects, it is recommended that flumazenil be administered as a series of small injections rather than as a single dose.

Dosage must be individualized according to the needs of the patient and clinical circumstances. Doses higher than the minimally effective dose are tolerated well by most patients, but administration of more flumazenil than is necessary increases the risk of adverse effects resulting from reversal of a benzodiazepine's therapeutic effects and may complicate the management of physically dependent patients.

The effects of a neuromuscular blocking agent, if used during surgery or for facilitating assisted ventilation in an intensive care patient, should be reversed completely before flumazenil is administered. Neuromuscular blocking agents should not be used without adequate sedation because the respiratory paralysis they induce is highly distressing to aware patients.

Post-procedure analgesic requirements are not increased in patients who have received flumazenil, but awake patients may report pain, and require earlier treatment, than patients who have not received the reversal agent.

Because psychomotor and memory deficits may persist after sedation has been completely reversed, patients receiving flumazenil following an outpatient procedure should be advised not to resume normal activities for at least 18 to 24 hours after discharge. Also, post-procedure instructions should be given to the patient in writing or given to a responsible caretaker.

### For treatment of adverse effects
Recommended treatment consists of the following:
• For convulsions—Benzodiazepines are usually recommended for treatment of convulsions, but higher than usual doses may be needed after flumazenil has been administered. Therefore, the risk of substantial resedation after the effects of flumazenil have subsided must be considered. Administration of a barbiturate or phenytoin instead of a benzodiazepine should be considered.
• For CNS effects possibly associated with benzodiazepine withdrawal, e.g., anxiety and emotional lability—Signs and symptoms are usually mild and short-lived and may not require treatment. If severe, continuing symptoms occur, administration of a barbiturate, benzodiazepine, or other sedative may be required.

## Parenteral Dosage Forms
### FLUMAZENIL INJECTION

**Usual adult dose**
Benzodiazepine antagonist—
Reversal of benzodiazepine-induced sedation:
Intravenous, 200 mcg (0.2 mg), administered over fifteen seconds, initially. If the desired response has not been attained after forty-five seconds to one minute, additional 200-mcg (0.2-mg) doses may be administered over fifteen seconds at one-minute intervals, up to a maximum cumulative dose of 1 mg. Most patients require 600 mcg (0.6 mg) to 1 mg.
If resedation occurs, additional flumazenil may be administered at a rate of 200 mcg (0.2 mg) per minute, up to a total cumulative dose of 1 mg. This dose may be repeated at twenty-minute intervals, up to a maximum of 3 mg in a one-hour period.
Treatment of benzodiazepine overdose:
Intravenous, 200 mcg (0.2 mg), administered over thirty seconds, initially. If the desired response has not been obtained after thirty seconds to one minute, 300 mcg (0.3 mg) may be administered over thirty seconds. If necessary, additional doses of 500 mcg (0.5 mg) may be administered over thirty seconds at one-minute intervals, up to a maximum cumulative dose of 3 mg. Most patients respond to a cumulative dose of 1 to 3 mg. Higher doses do not reliably produce additional benefit, but patients who have responded partially to 3 mg may obtain additional benefit from a total dose of 4 or 5 mg; occasional patients have required as much as 8 mg to achieve full reversal. If no response is attained after a cumulative dose of 5 mg, it can be assumed that a benzodiazepine was not responsible for the overdose and that further administration of flumazenil is not likely to be helpful. If resedation occurs, additional doses of up to a total of 1 mg of flumazenil may be administered at a rate of 500 mcg (0.5 mg) per minute. This dose may be repeated at twenty-minute intervals, up to a maximum of 3 mg in a one-hour period. Alternatively, flumazenil may be administered as an intravenous infusion at a rate adjusted to provide the desired level of arousal, generally 100 to 400 mcg (0.1 to 0.4 mg) per hour.

Note: Dosage should be titrated to produce the desired degree of arousal. Complete reversal may not be needed or desirable in certain circumstances.

For patients who may be tolerant to or dependent on benzodiazepines, a slower rate of administration (100 mcg [0.1 mg] per minute) and lower total doses may be required to minimize the risk of adverse effects.

The recommended one-minute interval between doses may not be sufficiently long for high-risk patients.

No adjustment of initial dosage is required for patients with significant hepatic function impairment, but a reduction in the size and/or frequency of subsequent doses is recommended.

To prevent resedation after initial reversal, up to 1 mg of flumazenil may be administered intravenously at a rate of 200 mcg (0.2 mg) per minute thirty minutes and possibly sixty minutes later.

### Usual adult prescribing limits

For reversal of benzodiazepine-induced sedation—
Not more than 1 mg at any one time or 3 mg per hour.

### Usual pediatric dose

Dosage has not been established. However, the medication is being administered intravenously to pediatric patients in doses ranging from 10 mcg (0.01 mg) per kg of body weight (for reversing sedation) to 100 mcg (0.1 mg) per kg of body weight (for life-threatening overdose), up to a maximum cumulative dose of 1 mg. Some investigators have also administered flumazenil by intravenous infusion at a rate of 5 to 10 mcg (0.005 to 0.01 mg) per kg of body weight per hour.

### Usual geriatric dose

See *Usual adult dose.*

### Strength(s) usually available

U.S.—

100 mcg (0.1 mg) per mL (Rx) [*Romazicon* (methylparaben 1.8 mg per mL; propylparaben 0.2 mg per mL; sodium chloride 0.9%; edetate disodium 0.01%; acetic acid 0.01%)].

Canada—

100 mcg (0.1 mg) per mL (Rx) [*Anexate* (edetate disodium 0.1 mg per mL; sodium chloride; glacial acetic acid; sodium hydroxide)].

### Packaging and storage

Store between 15 and 30 °C (59 and 86 °F), unless otherwise specified by manufacturer.

### Preparation of dosage form

Flumazenil injection may be diluted with 5% dextrose injection, 0.9% sodium chloride injection, 0.45% sodium chloride and 2.5% dextrose injecton, or lactated Ringer's injection.

### Stability

Infusion solutions prepared with 5% dextrose injection, 0.9% sodium chloride injection, or 0.45% sodium chloride and 2.5% dextrose injection are stable for up to 24 hours at room temperature. Flumazenil injections that have been drawn into a syringe or mixed with intravenous infusion solutions should be discarded after 24 hours.

One study has shown that stability of 20 mcg per mL (mcg/mL) of flumazenil in 5% dextrose injection is maintained for 12 hours at 23 °C (73 to 74 °F) when admixed with 3.2 mcg/mL of dopamine hydrochloride and for 24 hours when admixed with 2 mg per mL (mg/mL) of aminophylline, 2 mg/mL of dobutamine, 2.4 mg/mL of cimetidine, 0.08 mg/mL of famotidine, 50 USP Units per mL of heparin sodium, 4 mg/mL of lidocaine hydrochloride, 4 mg/mL of procainamide hydrochloride, or 0.3 mg/mL of ranitidine. Whether flumazenil affected the stability of the other medications was not determined.

## Selected Bibliography

Brogden RN, Goa KL. Flumazenil. A reappraisal of its pharmacological properties and therapeutic efficacy as a benzodiazepine antagonist. Drugs 1991; 42: 1061-89.

Ghouri AF, Ruiz MAR, White PF. Effect of flumazenil on recovery after midazolam and propofol sedation. Anesthesiology 1994; 81: 333-9.

Miller RD, supplemental section editor. U.S. clinical trials of flumazenil, a benzodiazepine antagonist. Clin Ther 1992; 14: 860-995.

Developed: 02/28/95

---

**FLUMETHASONE**—See *Corticosteroids (Topical)*

---

**FLUNARIZINE**—See *Calcium Channel Blocking Agents (Systemic)*

---

**FLUNISOLIDE**—See *Corticosteroids (Inhalation-Local)*; *Corticosteroids (Nasal)*

---

**FLUOCINOLONE**—See *Corticosteroids (Topical)*

---

**FLUOCINONIDE**—See *Corticosteroids (Topical)*

---

**FLUOROMETHOLONE**—See *Corticosteroids (Ophthalmic)*

---

# FLUOROQUINOLONES    Systemic

This monograph includes information on the following: Ciprofloxacin; Enoxacin; Lomefloxacin; Norfloxacin; Ofloxacin.

VA CLASSIFICATION (Primary): AM900

Note: For a listing of dosage forms and brand names by country availability, see *Dosage Forms* section(s). For a listing of brand names for the articles in this monograph, refer to the General Index.

## Category

Antibacterial (systemic).

## Indications

Note: Bracketed information in the *Indications* section refers to uses that are not included in U.S. product labeling.

### General considerations

Fluoroquinolones are broad-spectrum anti-infectives, active against a wide range of aerobic gram-positive and gram-negative organisms. They are active *in vitro* against most Enterobacteriaceae, including *Citrobacter* species (including *C. diversus* and *C. freundii*), *Enterobacter* species (including *E. cloacae* and *E. aerogenes*), *Escherichia coli*, *Klebsiella* species, *Morganella morganii*, *Proteus* species (including *P. mirabilis* and *P. vulgaris*), *Salmonella*, *Shigella*, and *Vibrio* species, and *Yersinia enterocolitica*. All of the fluoroquinolones also have good *in vitro* activity against multiply resistant gram-negative bacilli, penicillin-resistant strains of *Neisseria gonorrhoeae* and beta-lactamase-producing strains of *Haemophilus influenzae* and *Moraxella catarrhalis*. Ciprofloxacin appears to have the greatest *in vitro* activity of the fluoroquinolones against most organisms. Ciprofloxacin is the most active against *Pseudomonas aeruginosa*. It is not generally effective against most strains of *Ps. cepacia* and some strains of *Ps. maltophilia*. Ofloxacin's potency against *Ps. aeruginosa* is similar to that of norfloxacin, and greater than that of enoxacin and lomefloxacin.

Fluoroquinolones also have good *in vitro* activity against *Staphylococcus aureus*, including methicillin-resistant (MRSA) strains, *S. saprophyti-* cus, *S. epidermidis*, and other staphylococci. However, resistance to fluoroquinolones develops rapidly and MRSA strains cannot be assumed to be fluoroquinolone-susceptible; any bacteria that is resistant to one fluoroquinolone also may be resistant to another. Streptococci, including *S. pneumoniae*, *S. pyogenes*, and *Enterococcus faecalis*, are all moderately susceptible to ofloxacin and ciprofloxacin *in vitro*. Therapeutic failures have been reported in patients taking ciprofloxacin for the treatment of pneumococcal pneumonia.

Ciprofloxacin and ofloxacin have been found to have good *in vitro* activity against *Chlamydia trachomatis*, *Mycoplasma*, and *Legionella* species. These two medications are also active *in vitro* against *Mycobacterium tuberculosis* and atypical mycobacteria. The susceptibility of *M. avium-intracellulare*, however, is only fair to poor, and inhibition requires significantly higher drug concentrations.

### Accepted

Bone and joint infections (treatment)—Ciprofloxacin is indicated in the treatment of bone and joint infections caused by susceptible organisms.

Bronchitis, bacterial exacerbations (treatment)—Ciprofloxacin, lomefloxacin, and ofloxacin are indicated in the treatment of bacterial exacerbations of bronchitis caused by susceptible organisms.

Chlamydial infections, endocervical and urethral (treatment)—Ofloxacin is indicated in the treatment of endocervical and urethral infections caused by *Chlamydia trachomatis*.

Gastroenteritis, bacterial (treatment)—Ciprofloxacin and [norfloxacin][1] are indicated in the treatment of bacterial gastroenteritis caused by *Aeromonas hydrophilia*, enterotoxigenic *E. coli*, *Salmonella* species, *Shigella flexneri*, *S. sonnei*, and *Vibrio parahaemolyticus*.

Gonorrhea, endocervical and urethral (treatment)—Ciprofloxacin, enoxacin, norfloxacin, and ofloxacin are indicated in the treatment of endocervical and urethral infections caused by *Neisseria gonorrhoeae*.

Pneumonia, bacterial, gram-negative and streptococcal (treatment)—Ciprofloxacin and ofloxacin are indicated in the treatment of gram-negative bacterial and streptococcal pneumonia.

Caution should be used in treating streptococcal and pneumococcal pneumonia with fluoroquinolones. Although they have been effective in limited trials, treatment failures have been reported; fluoroquinolones should not be considered the drug of first choice in the treatment of presumed or confirmed pneumococcal pneumonia.

Prostatitis, bacterial (treatment)—[Ciprofloxacin][1], norfloxacin[1], and ofloxacin are indicated in the treatment of bacterial prostatitis caused by susceptible organisms.

Skin and soft tissue infections (treatment)—Ciprofloxacin and ofloxacin are indicated in the treatment of skin and soft tissue infections caused by susceptible organisms.

Typhoid fever (treatment)—Ciprofloxacin is indicated in the treatment of typhoid fever caused by susceptible strains of *Salmonella typhi*.

Urinary tract infections, bacterial (prophylaxis)—Lomefloxacin is indicated pre-operatively for the prophylaxis of urinary tract infections in patients undergoing transurethral surgical procedures.

Urinary tract infections, bacterial (treatment)—Ciprofloxacin, enoxacin, lomefloxacin, norfloxacin, and ofloxacin are indicated in the treatment of complicated and uncomplicated urinary tract infections caused by susceptible organisms.

[Chancroid (treatment)][1]—Ciprofloxacin and enoxacin are used in the treatment of chancroid caused by *Haemophilus ducreyi*.

Not all species or strains of a particular organism may be susceptible to a particular fluoroquinolone.

### Unaccepted
Fluoroquinolones have not been shown to be effective in the treatment of syphilis and have poor activity against most anaerobic bacteria (including *Bacteroides fragilis* and *Clostridium difficile*).

[1]Not included in Canadian product labeling.

## Pharmacology/Pharmacokinetics

See *Table 1*, page 1471, and *Table 2*, page 1472.

### Physicochemical characteristics
Molecular weight—
  Ciprofloxacin: 385.82.
  Enoxacin: 320.32.
  Lomefloxacin: 387.8.
  Norfloxacin: 319.34.
  Ofloxacin: 361.4.

### Mechanism of action/Effect
Bactericidal; fluoroquinolones act intracellularly by inhibiting DNA gyrase. DNA gyrase is an essential bacterial enzyme that is a critical catalyst in the duplication, transcription, and repair of bacterial DNA.

### Distribution
Fluoroquinolones are widely distributed to most body fluids and tissues; high concentrations are attained in the kidneys, gallbladder, liver, lungs, gynecological tissue, prostatic tissue, phagocytic cells, urine, sputum, and bile. Ciprofloxacin is also distributed to skin, fat, muscle, bone, and cartilage. The skin, fascia, and subcutaneous fat concentrations of ofloxacin are less than 50% of that found in the serum.

Ciprofloxacin and ofloxacin have been found to penetrate into the cerebrospinal fluid (CSF). CSF concentrations of ciprofloxacin reach 10% of peak serum concentration with non-inflamed meninges, and 14 to 37% with inflamed meninges. Ofloxacin penetrates into the CSF in the presence and absence of meningeal inflammation (range, 14 to 60%). This has resulted in bactericidal CSF titers that have ranged from inadequate to high, depending on the organism and its sensitivity.

## Precautions to Consider

### Cross-sensitivity and/or related problems
Patients allergic to one fluoroquinolone or other chemically related quinolone derivatives (e.g., cinoxacin, nalidixic acid) may be allergic to other fluoroquinolones also.

### Carcinogenicity/Tumorigenicity
*Ciprofloxacin*—Long-term carcinogenicity studies (up to 2 years) in rats and mice with oral ciprofloxacin have shown no evidence that ciprofloxacin had any carcinogenic or tumorigenic effects.
*Enoxacin*—Long-term studies to determine the carcinogenic potential of enoxacin in animals have not been conducted.
*Lomefloxacin*—Long-term studies to determine the carcinogenic potential of lomefloxacin in animals have not been conducted.
*Norfloxacin*—Studies lasting up to 96 weeks in rats given doses of 8 to 9 times the usual human dose have shown that norfloxacin causes no increase in neoplastic changes, compared with controls.
*Ofloxacin*—Long-term studies to determine the carcinogenic potential of ofloxacin have not been conducted.

### Mutagenicity
*Ciprofloxacin*—In vitro mutagenicity studies have shown both positive and negative results. Negative results were obtained in the Salmonella/Microsome Test, *Escherichia coli* DNA Repair Assay, Chinese Hamster $V_{79}$ Cell HGPRT Test, Syrian Hamster Embryo Cell Transformation Assay, *Saccharomyces cerevisiae* Point Mutation Assay, and the *S. cerevisiae* Mitotic Crossover and Gene Conversion Assay. Positive results were obtained in the Mouse Lymphoma Cell Forward Mutation Assay and the Rat Hepatocyte DNA Repair Assay. Although positive results were obtained in 2 of 8 *in vitro* studies, negative results were obtained in the *in vivo* Rat Hepatocyte DNA Repair Assay, Micronucleus Test in mice, and the Dominant Lethal Test in mice.
*Enoxacin*—Enoxacin did not induce point mutations in bacterial cells or mitotic gene conversion in yeast cells, with or without metabolic activation. Enoxacin did not induce sister chromatid exchanges or structural chromosomal aberrations in mammalian cells *in vitro*, with or without metabolic activation. Also, it did not induce chromosomal aberrations in mice. There was a minimal, dose-related, statistically significant increase in micronuclei at high doses in mice; however, the significance of these findings, in the absence of effects in other test systems, is not established.
*Lomefloxacin*—One *in vitro* mutagenicity test (CHO/HGPRT assay) was weakly positive at concentrations of 226 mcg per mL (mcg/mL) and higher, and negative at concentrations of less than 226 mcg/mL. Mutagenicity tests were negative in two other *in vitro* tests (chromosomal aberrations in Chinese hamster ovary cells and chromosomal aberrations in human lymphocytes). Two *in vivo* mouse micronucleus mutagenicity tests were also negative.
*Norfloxacin*—Studies in mice have shown that norfloxacin causes no mutagenic effects in the dominant lethal test. Studies in hamsters and rats given doses of 30 to 60 times the usual human dose have shown that norfloxacin causes no chromosomal aberrations. The Ames microbial mutagen test, studies in Chinese hamster fibroblasts, and the V-79 mammalian cell assay have shown that norfloxacin causes no mutagenic activity *in vitro*.
*Ofloxacin*—Ofloxacin was not found to be mutagenic in the Ames bacterial test, *in vitro* and *in vivo* cytogenic assay, sister chromatid exchange (Chinese Hamster and Human Cell Lines), unscheduled DNA Repair, or dominant lethal assays.

### Pregnancy/Reproduction
Fertility—
  *Ciprofloxacin*—
    Adequate and well-controlled studies in humans have not been done. Studies in rats and mice given doses of up to 6 times the usual daily human dose have not shown that ciprofloxacin causes adverse effects on fertility.
  *Enoxacin*—
    No consistent effects on fertility and reproductive parameters were noted in female rats given oral doses up to 1000 mg per kg of body weight (mg/kg) of enoxacin. Decreased spermatogenesis and subsequent impaired fertility were noted in male rats given oral doses of 1000 mg/kg.
  *Lomefloxacin*—
    The fertility of male and female rats was not affected when lomefloxacin was given at oral doses of up to 8 times the recommended human dose based on mg per square meter of body surface area ($mg/m^2$), or 34 times the recommended human dose based on mg/kg.
  *Norfloxacin*—
    Studies in male and female mice given oral doses of up to 30 times the usual human dose have not shown that norfloxacin causes adverse effects on fertility.

Pregnancy—
  *Ciprofloxacin*—
    Ciprofloxacin crosses the placenta. Adequate and well-controlled studies in humans have not been done. However, since ciprofloxacin has been shown to cause arthropathy in immature animals, use is not recommended in pregnancy.
    Studies in rats and mice given doses of up to 6 times the usual daily human dose have not shown that ciprofloxacin causes adverse effects on the fetus. Studies in rabbits given oral doses of 30 and 100 mg/kg have shown that ciprofloxacin causes gastrointestinal disturbances, resulting in maternal weight loss and an increased incidence of abortion. However, these studies have not shown that ciprofloxacin is teratogenic at either dose. Studies using intravenous doses of up to 20 mg/kg have not shown that ciprofloxacin causes maternal toxicity, embryotoxicity, or teratogenic effects.

  FDA Pregnancy Category C.

*Enoxacin—*

Adequate and well-controlled studies in humans have not been done. Since enoxacin has been shown to cause arthropathy in immature animals, use is not recommended in pregnancy.

Rats and mice given oral enoxacin have shown no evidence of teratogenic potential. Intravenous infusion of enoxacin into pregnant rabbits at doses of 10 to 50 mg/kg caused dose-related maternal toxicity (venous irritation, weight loss, and reduced food intake). At 50 mg/kg, there were increased post-implantation losses and stunted fetuses. The incidence of fetal malformations was also significantly increased at this dose in the presence of overt maternal and fetal toxicity.

FDA Pregnancy Category C.

*Lomefloxacin—*

Adequate and well-controlled studies in humans have not been done. Since lomefloxacin has been shown to cause arthropathy in immature animals, use is not recommended in pregnancy.

Reproduction studies done on rats given oral doses of lomefloxacin at up to 34 times the recommended human dose based on mg/kg reported no harm to the fetus. An increased incidence of fetal loss in monkeys has been observed at approximately 6 to 12 times the recommended human dose based on mg/kg. No teratogenicity has been observed in rats and monkeys at up to 16 times the recommended human dose exposure. In the rabbit, maternal toxicity and associated fetotoxicity, decreased placental weight, and variations of the coccygeal vertebrae occurred at doses 2 times the recommended human exposure based on mg/m$^2$.

FDA Pregnancy Category C.

*Norfloxacin—*

Adequate and well-controlled studies in humans have not been done. The umbilical cord serum concentration ranged from undetectable to 0.5 mg per mL (mg/mL) and the amniotic fluid concentration ranged from undetectable to 0.92 mg/mL following the administration of a single 200-mg dose of norfloxacin. Since norfloxacin has been shown to cause arthropathy in immature animals, use is not recommended in pregnancy.

Studies in monkeys given doses of 10 times the maximum human dose (800 mg daily) have shown that norfloxacin causes embryonic loss. Peak plasma concentrations were 2 to 3 times those seen in humans. Studies in cynomolgus monkeys given doses of 150 mg/kg per day or more have shown that norfloxacin is embryocidal and causes slight maternal toxicity (vomiting and anorexia) as well. However, studies in rats, rabbits, mice, and monkeys given doses of 6 to 50 times the usual human dose have not shown that norfloxacin is teratogenic.

FDA Pregnancy Category C.

*Ofloxacin—*

Ofloxacin crosses the placenta. In one small study, umbilical cord serum concentrations reached 80 to 90% of maternal serum concentrations after mothers received 200-mg doses. Ofloxacin was also detected in the amniotic fluid from over half the mothers. Another small study found that ofloxacin concentrated in the amniotic fluid, reaching 35 to 257% of the simultaneous maternal serum concentration. Adequate and well-controlled studies in humans have not been done. However, since ofloxacin and other quinolones have been shown to cause arthropathy in immature animals, use is not recommended in pregnancy.

Studies in rats and rabbits given doses of up to 810 mg/kg per day and 160 mg/kg per day have not shown ofloxacin to be teratogenic. Studies in rats given doses of up to 360 mg/kg per day showed no adverse effect on late fetal development, labor, delivery, lactation, neonatal viability, or growth of the newborn. Doses equivalent to 50 to 100 times the maximum human recommended dose (MHRD) were fetotoxic in rats (decreased fetal body weight) and rabbits (increased fetal mortality). Rats given 810 mg/kg per day, more than 50 times the MHRD, were reported to have minor skeletal variations.

FDA Pregnancy Category C.

**Breast-feeding**

Ciprofloxacin and ofloxacin are known to be distributed into human breast milk. The concentration of ofloxacin in breast milk was similar to that found in plasma. One small study found that ofloxacin was highly concentrated in breast milk, reaching 98% of the simultaneous maternal serum level within 2 hours of administration. It is not known whether enoxacin, lomefloxacin, or norfloxacin is distributed into breast milk. Norfloxacin has not been detected in breast milk when it was given in low (200-mg) doses to nursing mothers. However, other quinolone derivatives are distributed into human breast milk. Fluoro-

quinolones have been shown to cause permanent lesions of the cartilage of weight-bearing joints, as well as other signs of arthropathy in immature animals. Therefore, if an alternative antibiotic cannot be given and a fluoroquinolone must be administered, breast-feeding is not recommended.

**Pediatrics**

*For all fluoroquinolones—*

Fluoroquinolones are not recommended for use in infants and children. Patients up to age 18 have not been included in clinical trials because fluoroquinolones caused lameness in immature dogs due to permanent lesions of the cartilage of weight-bearing joints. These medications and other related quinolones have been reported to cause arthropathy in immature animals of various species.

Fluoroquinolones have been used in children with serious infections that have not responded to other therapeutic regimens, or infections caused by multiple organisms resistant to other antibiotics, without reported damage to cartilage tissue. However, there have been case reports of arthropathy that was thought to be due to ciprofloxacin developing in children with pseudomonal pneumonias associated with cystic fibrosis. The arthropathy completely resolved soon after the drug was discontinued.

**Adolescents**

*For all fluoroquinolones—*

Fluoroquinolones are not recommended for use in adolescents. Patients up to age 18 have not been included in clinical trials because fluoroquinolones caused lameness in immature dogs due to permanent lesions of the cartilage of weight-bearing joints. These medications and other related quinolones have been reported to cause arthropathy in immature animals of various species.

Fluoroquinolones have been used in children and adolescents with serious infections that have not responded to other therapeutic regimens, or infections caused by multiple organisms resistant to other antibiotics, without reported damage to cartilage tissue. However, there have been case reports of arthropathy that was thought to be due to ciprofloxacin developing in children with pseudomonal pneumonias associated with cystic fibrosis. The arthropathy completely resolved soon after the drug was discontinued.

**Geriatrics**

*For all fluoroquinolones—*

Studies performed to date have not demonstrated geriatrics-specific problems that would limit the usefulness of fluoroquinolones in the elderly. However, elderly patients are more likely to have an age-related decrease in renal function, which may require an adjustment of dosage in patients receiving any of these medications.

**Drug interactions and/or related problems**

The following drug interactions and/or related problems have been selected on the basis of their potential clinical significance (possible mechanism in parentheses where appropriate)—not necessarily inclusive (» = major clinical significance):

Note: Combinations containing any of the following medications, depending on the amount present, may also interact with this medication.

Alkalizers, urinary, such as:
 Carbonic anhydrase inhibitors
 Citrates
 Sodium bicarbonate
 (urinary alkalizers may reduce the solubility of ciprofloxacin and norfloxacin in the urine; patients should be observed for signs of crystalluria and nephrotoxicity, although the incidence is rare)

» Aminophylline or
» Oxtriphylline or
» Theophylline
 (concurrent use of aminophylline, oxtriphylline, or theophylline with ciprofloxacin and enoxacin significantly reduces the hepatic metabolism and clearance of theophylline, probably by competitive inhibition at the cytochrome P-450 binding sites; this may result in a prolonged theophylline elimination half-life, increased serum concentration, and increased risk of theophylline-related toxicity; enoxacin has the greatest effect on theophylline clearance and it is recommended that the dose of theophylline be decreased by 50%; ciprofloxacin may also increase the risk of toxicity, especially in patients with theophylline concentrations at the upper end of the therapeutic range; serum theophylline concentrations should be monitored and dosage adjustments may be required; norfloxacin and ofloxacin have a minor effect on theophylline clearance; one study with ofloxacin found an increase of approximately 10% in the theophylline serum concentration; however, other studies have found that ofloxacin has a negligible effect on theophylline metabolism; theophylline dosage adjustment is usually not necessary in

patients receiving norfloxacin or ofloxacin; theophylline clearance has not been found to be significantly altered by lomefloxacin)

» Antacids, aluminum-, calcium-, and/or magnesium-containing or
» Ferrous sulfate or
    Laxatives, magnesium-containing or
» Sucralfate or
    Zinc

(antacids, ferrous sulfate, zinc, and sucralfate may reduce absorption of fluoroquinolones by chelation, resulting in lower serum and urine concentrations; therefore, concurrent use is not recommended; because the bioavailability of enoxacin is decreased the most by concurrent administration of these medicines, it is recommended that enoxacin be taken at least 2 hours before or 8 hours after any of these medications; ciprofloxacin and lomefloxacin should be taken at least 2 hours before or 6 hours after any of these medications; and norfloxacin and ofloxacin should be taken at least 2 hours before or after any of these medications)

Bismuth

(concomitant administration of bismuth subsalicylate, or administration 60 minutes following enoxacin administration, decreased enoxacin bioavailability by approximately 25%)

» Caffeine

(concurrent use of caffeine with enoxacin has been found to decrease the hepatic metabolism of caffeine, resulting in a dose-related increase in the half-life of caffeine of up to 5 times normal; ciprofloxacin and, to a lesser extent, norfloxacin also reduce the hepatic metabolism and clearance of caffeine, increasing its half-life and the risk of caffeine-related CNS stimulation; lomefloxacin and ofloxacin have not produced any significant change in caffeine metabolism)

Cyclosporine

(concurrent use with ciprofloxacin or norfloxacin has been reported to elevate serum creatinine and serum cyclosporine concentrations; other studies have not found ciprofloxacin or enoxacin to alter the pharmacokinetics of cyclosporine; cyclosporine concentrations should be monitored, and dosage adjustments may be required)

» Didanosine

(concurrent use of didanosine with ciprofloxacin has been shown to reduce the absorption of ciprofloxacin due to chelation of ciprofloxacin by the aluminum and magnesium buffers in didanosine; didanosine should not be administered concurrently with any fluoroquinolone)

Digoxin

(enoxacin may raise serum digoxin concentrations in some patients; digoxin serum concentrations should be monitored)

Probenecid

(concurrent use of probenecid decreases the renal tubular secretion of fluoroquinolones, resulting in decreased urinary excretion of the fluoroquinolone, prolonged elimination half-life, and increased risk of toxicity; this interaction is more significant with ofloxacin, which is excreted largely unchanged in the urine, and of less clinical significance with fluoroquinolones that have larger nonrenal elimination, such as ciprofloxacin and enoxacin)

» Warfarin

(concurrent use of warfarin with ciprofloxacin or norfloxacin has been reported to increase the anticoagulant effect of warfarin, increasing the chance of bleeding; other studies have not found fluoroquinolones to alter the prothrombin time [PT] significantly; enoxacin decreased the clearance of R-warfarin, the less active isomer of racemic warfarin, but not the active S-isomer; changes in clotting time have not been observed when enoxacin and warfarin were coadministered; the PT of patients receiving warfarin should be carefully monitored in all patients receiving fluoroquinolones)

**Laboratory value alterations**

The following have been selected on the basis of their potential clinical significance (possible effect in parentheses where appropriate)—not necessarily inclusive (» = major clinical significance):

With physiology/laboratory test values

    Alanine aminotransferase (ALT [SGPT]), serum, and
    Alkaline phosphatase, serum, and
    Aspartate aminotransferase (AST [SGOT]), serum, and
    Lactate dehydrogenase (LDH), serum
      (values may be increased)

**Medical considerations/Contraindications**

The medical considerations/contraindications included here have been selected on the basis of their potential clinical significance (reasons given in parentheses where appropriate)—not necessarily inclusive (» = major clinical significance).

*Except under special circumstances, this medication should not be used when the following medical problem exists:*

» Previous allergic reaction to fluoroquinolones or other chemically related quinolone derivatives

*Risk-benefit should be considered when the following medical problems exist:*

    CNS disorders, including cerebral arteriosclerosis or epilepsy
      (fluoroquinolones may cause CNS stimulation or toxicity)

    Hepatic function impairment
      (patients with severe hepatic function impairment, such as cirrhosis with ascites, may have decreased clearance of ofloxacin, resulting in an increase in peak serum concentration and elimination half-life; patients with *both* hepatic and renal function impairment may require a reduction in the dosage of ciprofloxacin; cirrhosis has not been found to decrease the nonrenal clearance of lomefloxacin)

» Renal function impairment
      (fluoroquinolones are primarily excreted renally; it is recommended that a reduced dose be administered to patients with impaired renal function)

## Side/Adverse Effects

Note: The relative insolubility of ciprofloxacin and norfloxacin at an alkaline pH has resulted in crystalluria, usually when the urinary pH exceeds 7.0. Because normal urinary pH is acidic, approximately 5–6, crystalluria is very unlikely to occur unless the patient's urine has become alkalinized.

Seizures have been reported very rarely with ciprofloxacin therapy; however, the patients who did have seizures either had a previous seizure history, were alcoholic, or were taking ciprofloxacin concurrently with theophylline.

Achilles tendinitis and tendon rupture have been reported in patients receiving fluoroquinolones. The ruptures occurred 2 to 42 days after the start of therapy. These injuries may require surgical repair or result in prolonged disability. It is recommended that fluoroquinolone treatment be discontinued at the first sign of tendon pain or inflammation and that patients refrain from exercising until the diagnosis of tendinitis has been excluded.

The following side/adverse effects have been selected on the basis of their potential clinical significance (possible signs and symptoms in parentheses where appropriate)—not necessarily inclusive:

**Those indicating need for medical attention**
Incidence rare
    *Central nervous system (CNS) stimulation* (acute psychosis; agitation; confusion; hallucinations; tremors); *hypersensitivity reactions* (skin rash, itching, or redness; Stevens-Johnson syndrome; shortness of breath; swelling of face or neck; vasculitis); *interstitial nephritis* (bloody or cloudy urine; fever; rash; swelling of feet or lower legs); *phlebitis* (pain at site of injection)—for intravenous ciprofloxacin and ofloxacin; *tendinitis or tendon rupture* (pain in calves, radiating to heels; swelling of calves or lower legs)

**Those indicating need for medical attention only if they continue or are bothersome**
Incidence more frequent
    *CNS toxicity* (dizziness or lightheadedness; headache; nervousness; drowsiness; insomnia); *gastrointestinal reactions* (abdominal or stomach pain or discomfort; diarrhea; nausea or vomiting)

Incidence less frequent or rare
    *Photosensitivity* (increased sensitivity of skin to sunlight)—more common with lomefloxacin

## Overdose

**Treatment of overdose**

Since there is no specific antidote for ciprofloxacin overdose, treatment should be symptomatic and supportive and may include the following:

To decrease absorption—Induction of emesis or use of gastric lavage to empty the stomach.

Specific treatment—Maintenance of adequate hydration.

Supportive care—Supportive therapy. Patients in whom intentional overdose is known or suspected should be referred for psychiatric consultation.

## Patient Consultation

As an aid to patient consultation, refer to *Advice for the Patient, Fluoroquinolones (Systemic)*.

In providing consultation, consider emphasizing the following selected information (» = major clinical significance):

## Before using this medication
» Conditions affecting use, especially:
   Allergies to fluoroquinolones or other quinolone derivatives
   Pregnancy—Fluoroquinolones are not recommended for use during pregnancy because they have been shown to cause arthropathy in immature animals
   Breast-feeding—Not recommended since fluoroquinolones have been shown to cause arthropathy in immature animals
   Use in children—Use of fluoroquinolones is not recommended in infants and children since these medications have been shown to cause arthropathy in immature animals
   Use in adolescents—Use of fluoroquinolones is not recommended in adolescents since these medications have been shown to cause arthropathy in immature animals
   Other medications, especially aluminum-, calcium-, and/or magnesium-containing antacids, caffeine-containing products, didanosine, ferrous sulfate, sucralfate, aminophylline, oxtriphylline, theophylline, or warfarin
   Other medical problems, especially allergy to quinolones and renal function impairment

## Proper use of this medication
» Not giving to infants, children, adolescents, or pregnant women; fluoroquinolones have been shown to cause arthropathy in immature animals
» Taking with full glass (240 mL) of water; maintaining adequate fluid intake
» For enoxacin, norfloxacin, and ofloxacin—taking on an empty stomach
» For ciprofloxacin and lomefloxacin—taking with meals or on an empty stomach
» Compliance with full course of therapy
» Importance of not missing doses and taking at evenly spaced times
» Proper dosing
   Missed dose: Taking as soon as possible; not taking if almost time for next dose; not doubling doses
» Proper storage

## Precautions while using this medication
   Checking with physician if no improvement within a few days
» Avoiding concurrent use of antacids or sucralfate and fluoroquinolones; taking antacids or sucralfate at least 6 hours before or 2 hours after administration of ciprofloxacin or lomefloxacin, 2 hours before or after administration of norfloxacin or ofloxacin, and 8 hours before or 2 hours after administration of enoxacin
» Possible photosensitivity reactions
» Caution if blurred vision or other vision problems, dizziness, lightheadedness, or drowsiness occurs

## Side/adverse effects
   Signs of potential side effects, especially central nervous system stimulation, hypersensitivity reactions, interstitial nephritis, phlebitis, tendinitis, and tendon rupture

## General Dosing Information

Patients with impaired renal function may require a reduction in dosage based on creatinine clearance. Creatinine clearance (in mL per minute) may be calculated as follows:

Adult males: Creatinine clearance

$$= [(140 - age) \times (ideal\ body\ weight\ in\ kg)]/[72 \times serum\ creatinine\ (in\ milligrams\ per\ dL)]$$

Adult females: Creatinine clearance

$$= [(140 - age) \times (ideal\ body\ weight\ in\ kg)]/[72 \times serum\ creatinine\ (in\ milligrams\ per\ dL)] \times 0.85$$

Creatinine clearance may also be calculated in SI units (as mL per second) as follows:

Adult males: Creatinine clearance

$$= [(140 - age) \times (ideal\ body\ weight\ in\ kg)]/[50 \times serum\ creatinine\ (in\ micromoles\ per\ L)]$$

Adult females: Creatinine clearance

$$= [(140 - age) \times (ideal\ body\ weight\ in\ kg)]/[50 \times serum\ creatinine\ (in\ micromoles\ per\ L)] \times 0.85$$

## CIPROFLOXACIN

## Additional Dosing Information

### Diet/Nutrition
The presence of food in the stomach may delay the rate of absorption of oral ciprofloxacin; however, the overall absorption is not affected. Therefore, ciprofloxacin may be taken with meals or on an empty stomach. Ciprofloxacin should be taken with a full glass (240 mL) of water.

Intravenous ciprofloxacin should be administered over at least 60 minutes to minimize patient discomfort and reduce the risk of venous irritation.

Crystalluria has been reported, especially in patients with alkaline urine (pH 7 or above). Therefore, alkalinization of the urine should be avoided. Although crystalluria has been reported only rarely in humans, fluid intake should be sufficient to maintain urine output of at least 1200 to 1500 mL per day in adults.

## Oral Dosage Forms
Note: The dosing and strengths of the dosage forms available are expressed in terms of ciprofloxacin base.

### CIPROFLOXACIN HYDROCHLORIDE TABLETS USP

**Usual adult dose**
Bone and joint infections
Pneumonia, gram-negative, bacterial or
Skin and soft tissue infections—Oral, 500 to 750 mg (base) every twelve hours for seven to fourteen days. Severe or complicated infections may require prolonged therapy. Bone infections may require treatment for four to six weeks or longer.
Diarrhea, bacterial—Oral, 500 mg (base) every twelve hours for five to seven days.
Gonorrhea, endocervical and urethral—Oral, 250 mg (base) as a single dose.
Typhoid fever—Oral, 500 mg (base) every twelve hours for ten days.
Urinary tract infections, bacterial—Oral, 250 to 500 mg (base) every twelve hours for seven to fourteen days. Severe or complicated infections may require prolonged therapy.
Note: Adults with impaired renal function may require a reduction in dose as follows:

| Creatinine Clearance (mL/min)/(mL/sec) | Dose (base) |
|---|---|
| >50/0.83 | See *Usual adult dose* |
| 30–50/0.50–0.83 | 250–500 mg every 12 hours |
| 5–29/0.08–0.48 | 250–500 mg every 18 hours |
| Hemodialysis or Peritoneal dialysis patients | 250–500 mg every 24 hours after dialysis |

**Usual adult prescribing limits**
Up to 1.5 grams (base) daily.

**Usual pediatric dose**
Children up to 18 years of age—Use is not recommended in infants, children, or adolescents since ciprofloxacin causes arthropathy in immature animals. However, ciprofloxacin has been given to children at doses of 10 to 20 mg (base) per kg of body weight every twelve hours when alternative therapy could not be used.

**Strength(s) usually available**
U.S.—
   250 mg (base) (Rx) [*Cipro*].
   500 mg (base) (Rx) [*Cipro*].
   750 mg (base) (Rx) [*Cipro*].
Canada—
   250 mg (base) (Rx) [*Cipro*].
   500 mg (base) (Rx) [*Cipro*].
   750 mg (base) (Rx) [*Cipro*].

**Packaging and storage**
Store below 30 °C (86 °F), unless otherwise specified by manufacturer. Store in a well-closed container.

**Auxiliary labeling**
• Take with a full glass of water.
• May cause dizziness or lightheadedness.
• Continue medicine for full time of treatment.
• Avoid too much sun or use of sunlamp.
• Do not take antacids or iron preparations within 4 hours of this medicine.

## Parenteral Dosage Forms
### CIPROFLOXACIN FOR INJECTION
**Usual adult dose**
Bone and joint infections
Pneumonia, gram-negative, bacterial or
Skin and soft tissue infections—Intravenous injection, 400 mg every twelve hours. Administer over at least sixty minutes. Severe or complicated infections may require prolonged therapy. Bone infections may require treatment for four to six weeks or longer.
Urinary tract infections, bacterial—Intravenous injection, 200 to 400 mg every twelve hours for seven to fourteen days. Severe or complicated infections may require prolonged therapy.

Note: Adults with impaired renal function may require a reduction in dose as follows:

| Creatinine Clearance (mL/min)/(mL/sec) | Dose (base) |
|---|---|
| ≥30/0.50 | See *Usual adult dose* |
| 5–29/0.08–0.48 | 200–400 mg every 18 to 24 hours |

**Usual pediatric dose**
Children up to 18 years of age—Use is not recommended in infants, children, or adolescents since ciprofloxacin causes arthropathy in animals. However, ciprofloxacin has been given to children at doses of 10 to 20 mg (base) per kg of body weight every twelve hours when alternative therapy could not be used.

**Strength(s) usually available**
U.S.—
  200 mg in 100 mL (Rx) [*Cipro IV*].
  400 mg in 200 mL (Rx) [*Cipro IV*].
Canada—
  Not commercially available.

**Packaging and storage**
Store between 5 and 25 °C (41 and 77 °F). Protect from light and freezing.

### CIPROFLOXACIN IN DEXTROSE INJECTION
**Usual adult dose**
See *Ciprofloxacin for Injection.*

**Usual pediatric dose**
See *Ciprofloxacin for Injection.*

**Strength(s) usually available**
U.S.—
  200 mg per 20 mL (Rx) [*Cipro IV*].
  400 mg per 40 mL (Rx) [*Cipro IV*].
  1200 mg per 120 mL (Rx) [*Cipro IV*].
Canada—
  200 mg per 20 mL (Rx) [*Cipro IV*].
  400 mg per 40 mL (Rx) [*Cipro IV*].

**Packaging and storage**
Store between 5 and 25 °C (41 and 77 °F). Protect from light and freezing.

**Preparation of dosage form**
To prepare initial dilution for direct intravenous use, withdraw the appropriate volume of concentrate from the vial. Dilute with 5% dextrose injection or 0.9% sodium chloride injection to a final concentration of 1 to 2 mg per mL. The resulting solution should be infused over a period of 60 minutes.

**Stability**
Diluted solutions (0.5 to 2 mg per mL) are stable for up to 14 days at room temperature or if refrigerated.

---

### *ENOXACIN*

## Summary of Differences
Precautions: Drug interactions—Enoxacin has the greatest effect in decreasing the clearance of caffeine and theophylline, increasing the risk of toxicity for these medications.

## Additional Dosing Information

**Diet/Nutrition**
The effect of food on the absorption of enoxacin tablets has not been studied; it is recommended that enoxacin be taken at least one hour before or two hours after a meal; however, decreased gastric acidity has been shown to decrease the bioavailability of enoxacin.

## Oral Dosage Forms
### ENOXACIN TABLETS
**Usual adult dose**
Gonorrhea or
Urethritis, gonococcal—Oral, 400 mg as a single dose.
Urinary tract infections (uncomplicated)—Oral, 200 mg every twelve hours for seven days.
Urinary tract infections (complicated)—Oral, 400 mg every twelve hours for fourteen days.

Note: Adults with impaired renal function may require a reduction in dose as follows:

| Creatinine Clearance (mL/min)/(mL/sec) | Dose |
|---|---|
| ≥30/0.50 | See *Usual adult dose* |
| <30/0.50 | 50% of dose every 12 hours |

**Usual pediatric dose**
Children up to 18 years of age—Use is not recommended in infants, children, or adolescents since enoxacin causes arthropathy in immature animals.

**Strength(s) usually available**
U.S.—
  200 mg (Rx) [*Penetrex*].
  400 mg (Rx) [*Penetrex*].
Canada—
  200 mg (Rx) [*Penetrex*].
  400 mg (Rx) [*Penetrex*].

**Packaging and storage**
Store below 40 °C (104 °F), preferably between 15 and 30 °C (59 and 86 °F), in a tight container, unless otherwise specified by manufacturer.

**Auxiliary labeling**
• Take with a full glass of water.
• May cause dizziness, lightheadedness, or drowsiness.
• Continue medicine for full time of treatment.

---

### *LOMEFLOXACIN*

## Summary of Differences
Pharmacology/pharmacokinetics: Longer half-life; may be dosed once a day.
Precautions: Drug interactions—Does not significantly interfere with the clearance of caffeine and theophylline.
Side/adverse effects: More likely to cause phototoxicity.

## Additional Dosing Information

**Diet/Nutrition**
When lomefloxacin was administered with food, the extent of absorption was only slightly decreased. Lomefloxacin may be taken with or without food.

## Oral Dosage Forms
### LOMEFLOXACIN TABLETS
**Usual adult dose**
Treatment:
  Bronchitis, bacterial exacerbations: Oral, 400 mg once a day for ten days.
  Urinary tract infections (uncomplicated): Oral, 400 mg once a day for ten days.
  Urinary tract infections (complicated): Oral, 400 mg once a day for fourteen days.

Note: Adults with impaired renal function may require a reduction in dose as follows:

| Creatinine Clearance (mL/min)/(mL/sec) | Dose (base) |
|---|---|
| >40/0.67 | See *Usual adult dose* |
| ≤40/0.67 or Hemodialysis | 400 mg for first dose, then 200 mg once a day |

Prophylaxis, transuretheral surgery:
  Oral, 400 mg as a single dose two to six hours before the start of surgery.

**Usual pediatric dose**

Children up to 18 years of age—Use is not recommended in infants, children, and adolescents since lomefloxacin causes arthropathy in immature animals.

**Strength(s) usually available**

U.S.—

400 mg (Rx) [*Maxaquin* (scored)].

Canada—

400 mg (Rx) [*Maxaquin* (scored)].

**Packaging and storage**

Store below 40 °C (104 °F), preferably between 15 and 30 °C (59 and 86 °F), in a tight container, unless otherwise specified by manufacturer.

**Auxiliary labeling**

• Take with a full glass of water.
• May cause dizziness, lightheadedness, or drowsiness.
• Continue medicine for full time of treatment.

---

## NORFLOXACIN

## Additional Dosing Information

**Diet/Nutrition**

The presence of food in the stomach may slightly decrease or delay absorption of norfloxacin. Therefore, norfloxacin should preferably be taken with a full glass (240 mL) of water on an empty stomach (either 1 hour before or 2 hours after meals).

In studies with volunteers, crystalluria has been reported, especially with high doses (1200 or 1600 mg) and alkaline urine (pH 7 or above). Although crystalluria has not been reported with usual adult doses (400 mg twice a day), fluid intake should be sufficient to maintain urine output of at least 1200 to 1500 mL per day in adults.

## Oral Dosage Forms

Note: Bracketed uses in the *Dosage Forms* section refer to categories of use and/or indications that are not included in U.S. product labeling.

### NORFLOXACIN TABLETS USP

**Usual adult dose**

Gonorrhea or
Urethritis, gonococcal—Oral, 800 mg as a single dose.
Prostatitis[1]—Oral, 400 mg every twelve hours for twenty-eight days.
Urinary tract infections (uncomplicated)—Oral, 400 mg every twelve hours for three days.
Urinary tract infections (complicated)—Oral, 400 mg every twelve hours for ten to twenty-one days.
[Gastroenteritis, bacterial][1]—Oral, 400 mg every eight to twelve hours for five days.

Note: Adults with impaired renal function may require a reduction in dose as follows:

| Creatinine Clearance (mL/min)/(mL/sec) | Dose |
| --- | --- |
| >30/0.50 | See *Usual adult dose* |
| ≤30/0.50 | 400 mg once a day |

**Usual adult prescribing limits**

Urinary tract infections—Up to a maximum of 800 mg daily.
[Gastroenteritis][1]—Up to 1.2 grams daily.

**Usual pediatric dose**

Use is not recommended in infants and children since norfloxacin causes arthropathy in immature animals.

**Strength(s) usually available**

U.S.—

400 mg (Rx) [*Noroxin*].

Canada—

400 mg (Rx) [*Noroxin*].

**Packaging and storage**

Store below 40 °C (104 °F), preferably between 15 and 30 °C (59 and 86 °F), in a tight container, unless otherwise specified by manufacturer.

**Auxiliary labeling**

• Take with a full glass of water.
• Take on empty stomach.
• May cause dizziness, lightheadedness, or drowsiness.
• Continue medicine for full time of treatment.

[1]Not included in Canadian product labeling.

---

## OFLOXACIN

## Summary of Differences

Precautions: Drug interactions—Has a minor effect on the metabolism of theophylline.
General dosing information: Unlike intravenous ciprofloxacin, the dose of intravenous ofloxacin does not need to be changed from the oral dose.

## Additional Dosing Information

**Diet/Nutrition**

Food has minor influence on the absorption of ofloxacin, causing only a slight decrease in the peak serum concentration and the area under the serum concentration-time curve (AUC).

Ofloxacin injection should only be administered by slow intravenous infusion over 60 minutes. Rapid or bolus injection may result in hypotension.

## Oral Dosage Forms

### OFLOXACIN TABLETS

**Usual adult dose**

Bronchitis, bacterial exacerbations, or Pneumonia:
   Oral, 400 mg every twelve hours for ten days.
Chlamydial infections, endocervical and urethral, with or without concurrent gonorrhea:
   Oral, 300 mg every twelve hours for seven days.
Gonorrhea, uncomplicated:
   Oral, 400 mg as a single dose.
Prostatitis:
   Oral, 300 mg every twelve hours for six weeks.
Skin and soft tissue infections:
   Oral, 400 mg every twelve hours for ten days.
Urinary tract infections:
   Cystitis due to *E. coli* or *K. pneumoniae*: Oral, 200 mg every twelve hours for three days.
   Cystitis due to other organisms: Oral, 200 mg every twelve hours for seven days.
   Complicated urinary tract infections: Oral, 200 mg every twelve hours for ten days.

Note: Adults with impaired renal function may require a reduction in dose as follows:

| Creatinine Clearance (mL/min)/(mL/sec) | Dose % | Dosing Interval (hr) |
| --- | --- | --- |
| >50/0.83 | 100 | 12 |
| 10–50/0.17–0.83 | 100 | 24 |
| <10/0.17 | 50 | 24 |

**Usual pediatric dose**

Children up to 18 years of age—Use is not recommended in infants, children, or adolescents since ofloxacin and other quinolones have been shown to cause arthropathy in immature animals.

**Strength(s) usually available**

U.S.—

200 mg (Rx) [*Floxin*].
300 mg (Rx) [*Floxin*].
400 mg (Rx) [*Floxin*].

Canada—

200 mg (Rx) [*Floxin*].
300 mg (Rx) [*Floxin*].
400 mg (Rx) [*Floxin*].

**Packaging and storage**

Store below 30 °C (86 °F), unless otherwise specified by manufacturer. Store in a well-closed container.

**Auxiliary labeling**

• Take with a full glass of water.
• Continue medicine for full time of treatment.
• Do not take antacids, or zinc or iron preparations within 2 hours of this medicine.

## Parenteral Dosage Forms

### OFLOXACIN IN DEXTROSE INJECTION

**Usual adult dose**

Bronchitis, bacterial exacerbations, or Pneumonia:
   Intravenous infusion, 400 mg, administered over sixty minutes, every twelve hours for ten days.

Chlamydial infections, endocervical and urethral, with or without concurrent gonorrhea:
Intravenous infusion, 300 mg, administered over sixty minutes, every twelve hours for seven days.

Gonorrhea, uncomplicated:
Intravenous infusion, 400 mg, administered over sixty minutes, as a single dose.

Prostatitis:
Intravenous infusion, 300 mg, administered over sixty minutes, every twelve hours for six weeks.

Skin and soft tissue infections:
Intravenous infusion, 400 mg, administered over sixty minutes, every twelve hours for ten days.

Urinary tract infections:
Cystitis due to *E. coli* or *K. pneumoniae*: Intravenous infusion, 200 mg, administered over sixty minutes, every twelve hours for three days.
Cystitis due to other organisms: Intravenous infusion, 200 mg, administered over sixty minutes, every twelve hours for seven days.
Complicated urinary tract infections: Intravenous infusion, 200 mg, administered over sixty minutes, every twelve hours for ten days.

Note: Adults with impaired renal function may require a reduction in dose as follows:

| Creatinine Clearance (mL/min)/(mL/sec) | Dose % | Dosing Interval (hr) |
|---|---|---|
| >50/0.83 | 100 | 12 |
| 10–50/0.17–0.83 | 100 | 24 |
| <10/0.17 | 50 | 24 |

**Usual pediatric dose**
Children up to 18 years of age—Use is not recommended in infants, children, or adolescents since ofloxacin and other quinolones have been shown to cause arthropathy in immature animals.

**Strength(s) usually available**
U.S.—
200 mg in 50 mL (Rx) [*Floxin IV*].
400 mg in 100 mL (Rx) [*Floxin IV*].
Canada—
Not commercially available.

**Packaging and storage**
Store below 30 °C (86 °F), unless otherwise specified by manufacturer. Protect from freezing and light.

**Preparation of dosage form**
Premixed ofloxacin in dextrose injection in bottles and flexible containers requires no further dilution prior to administration (see manufacturer's labeling for instructions). Since these injections contain no preservatives or bacteriostatic agent, they should be used promptly after opening; unused portions should be discarded.

**Stability**
When diluted to a concentration between 0.4 mg/mL and 4 mg/mL, ofloxacin in dextrose injection is stable for 72 hours when stored at or below 24 °C (75 °F) and for 14 days when refrigerated at 5 °C (41 °F) in glass bottles or plastic intravenous containers. Solutions that are diluted and frozen are stable for 6 months when stored at −20 °C (−4

°F). Once thawed, the solution is stable for up to 14 days, if it is refrigerated.
Thaw frozen solutions at room temperature or in a refrigerator. Do not force thawing by microwave irradiation or immersion in water baths. Do not refreeze after initial thawing.
Ofloxacin in dextrose injection contains no preservatives or bacteriostatic agent. Do not use if injection is discolored or contains a precipitate.

**Incompatibilities**
Because only limited data are available on the compatibility of ofloxacin in dextrose injection with other intravenous substances, additives or other medications should not be added to the preparation or infused simultaneously through the same intravenous line.

## OFLOXACIN INJECTION

**Usual adult dose**
See *Ofloxacin in Dextrose Injection*.

**Usual pediatric dose**
See *Ofloxacin in Dextrose Injection*.

**Strength(s) usually available**
U.S.—
20 mg per mL (Rx) [*Floxin IV*].
40 mg per mL (Rx) [*Floxin IV*].
Canada—
Not commercially available.

**Packaging and storage**
Store below 30 °C (86 °F), unless otherwise specified by manufacturer. Protect from freezing and light.

**Preparation of dosage form**
To prepare for intravenous use, withdraw the appropriate dose of ofloxacin from the vial. Add each dose to 50 to 100 mL of 0.9% sodium chloride injection, 5% dextrose injection, or other compatible intravenous fluid to provide a concentration of 4 mg per mL.

**Stability**
When diluted to a concentration between 0.4 mg/mL and 4 mg/mL, ofloxacin injection is stable for 72 hours when stored at or below 24 °C (75 °F) and for 14 days when refrigerated at 5 °C (41 °F) in glass bottles or plastic intravenous containers. Solutions that are diluted and frozen are stable for 6 months when stored at −20 °C (−4 °F). Once thawed, the solution is stable for up to 14 days, if it is refrigerated.
Thaw frozen solutions at room temperature or in a refrigerator. Do not force thawing by microwave irradiation or immersion in water baths. Do not refreeze after initial thawing.
Ofloxacin injection contains no preservatives or bacteriostatic agent. Do not use if injection is discolored or contains a precipitate.

**Incompatibilities**
Because only limited data are available on the compatibility of ofloxacin injection with other substances, additives or other medications should not be added to the preparation or infused simultaneously through the same intravenous line.

Revised: 05/20/93
Interim revision: 04/24/95; 07/29/95

## Table 1. Pharmacology/Pharmacokinetics

| Drug | Bioavailability (%) | Half-life (hr) Normal Renal Function | Half-life (hr) Impaired Renal Function | Time to Peak Serum Concentration (hr) | Peak Serum Concentration After Dose mcg/mL | Peak Serum Concentration After Dose Dose (mg) | Peak Urine Concentration After Dose mcg/mL | Peak Urine Concentration After Dose Dose (mg) |
|---|---|---|---|---|---|---|---|---|
| **Ciprofloxacin** | | | | | | | | |
| Oral | 70–80* | 4† | 6–8 | 1–2 | 1.2–1.4 | 250 | >200 | 250 |
| | | | | | 2.4–2.6 | 500 | | |
| | | | | | 3.4–4.3 | 750 | | |
| IV | | 5–6 | | End of Infusion | 2.1 | 200 | >200 | 200 |
| | | | | | 4.6 | 400 | | |

*Absorption delayed in presence of food, although overall absorption not substantially affected.
†Half-life of ciprofloxacin slightly prolonged in elderly patients (approximately 6 hours).
‡Half-life of ofloxacin slightly prolonged in elderly patients (approximately 6 to 8.5 hours).
§Half-life of ofloxacin also prolonged in patients who have cirrhosis with ascites (approximately 7.3 to 19.5 hours).

## Table 1. Pharmacology/Pharmacokinetics *(continued)*

| Drug | Bioavailability (%) | Half-life (hr) Normal Renal Function | Half-life (hr) Impaired Renal Function | Time to Peak Serum Concentration (hr) | Peak Serum Concentration After Dose mcg/mL | Peak Serum Concentration After Dose Dose (mg) | Peak Urine Concentration After Dose mcg/mL | Peak Urine Concentration After Dose Dose (mg) |
|---|---|---|---|---|---|---|---|---|
| Enoxacin Oral | 90 | 3–6 | 9–10 | 1–3 | 0.9 2.0 | 200 400 | | |
| Lomefloxacin Oral | 95–98 | 7–8 | 21–45 | 1.5 | 3–5.2 | 400 | >300 | 400 |
| Norfloxacin Oral | 30–70* | 3–4 | 6–9 | 1–2 | 1.4–1.6 2.5 | 400 800 | 98–200 | 400 |
| Ofloxacin Oral | 95–100 | 4.7–7.0‡ | 15–60§ | 1–2 | 1.5–2.6 4.6–5.0 | 200 400 | | |
| IV | | | | End of Infusion | 2.3–2.7 5.5–7.2 | 200 400 | | |

*Absorption delayed in presence of food, although overall absorption not substantially affected.
†Half-life of ciprofloxacin slightly prolonged in elderly patients (approximately 6 hours).
‡Half-life of ofloxacin slightly prolonged in elderly patients (approximately 6 to 8.5 hours).
§Half-life of ofloxacin also prolonged in patients who have cirrhosis with ascites (approximately 7.3 to 19.5 hours).

## Table 2. Pharmacology/Pharmacokinetics*

| Drug | Protein Binding (%) | Renal Excretion (% unchanged/hrs) | Metabolism (%) | Biliary Excretion (%) | Vol_D (liter/kg) | Removal by Dialysis HD (%) | Removal by Dialysis PD (%) |
|---|---|---|---|---|---|---|---|
| Ciprofloxacin Oral IV | 20–40 | 40–50/24 50–70/24 | 20 | 20–35 15 | 2.0 | <10 | <10 |
| Enoxacin | 40† | 40–60/48 | 20 | 18 | 1.6 | <5 | |
| Lomefloxacin | 10 | 60–80/48 | 5 | 10 | 1.8–2.5 | <3 | <3 |
| Norfloxacin | 10–15 | 26–40/24–48 | 20 | 28–30 | 3.2 | <10 | |
| Ofloxacin | 20–25 | 70–90/36 | 3 | 4–8 | 0.9–1.8 | 10–30 | 2–10 |

*Abbreviations: Vol_D = volume of distribution; HD = hemodialysis; PD = peritoneal dialysis; NS = not significant.
†Approximately 14% of enoxacin is bound to plasma proteins in patients with impaired renal function.

# FLUOROURACIL Systemic

VA CLASSIFICATION (Primary): AN300
Another commonly used name is 5-FU.

Note: For a listing of dosage forms and brand names by country availability, see *Dosage Forms* section(s). For a listing of brand names for the articles in this monograph, refer to the General Index.

## Category

Antineoplastic.

## Indications

Note: Bracketed information in the *Indications* section refers to uses that are not included in U.S. product labeling.

**Accepted**
Carcinoma, colorectal (treatment)
Carcinoma, breast (treatment)
Carcinoma, gastric (treatment)
Carcinoma, pancreatic (treatment)
[Carcinoma, bladder (treatment)]
[Carcinoma, prostatic (treatment)]
[Carcinoma, ovarian (treatment)]
[Carcinoma, cervical (treatment)][1]
[Carcinoma, endometrial (treatment)][1]
[Carcinoma, lung (treatment)][1]

[Carcinoma, hepatic (treatment)][1] or
[Carcinoma, head and neck (treatment)]—Fluorouracil is indicated for palliative treatment of carcinoma of the colon, rectum, breast, stomach, and pancreas in patients considered to be incurable by surgery or other means.

Fluorouracil is also used for treatment of bladder carcinoma, prostatic carcinoma, ovarian carcinoma, cervical carcinoma, endometrial carcinoma, lung carcinoma, and by intra-arterial injection for treatment of liver tumors and head and neck tumors.

[Malignant effusions, pericardial (treatment)][1]
[Malignant effusions, peritoneal (treatment)][1] or
[Malignant effusions, pleural (treatment)][1]—Fluorouracil is used by intracavitary administration for treatment of malignant pleural, peritoneal, and pericardial effusions.

[1]Not included in Canadian product labeling.

## Pharmacology/Pharmacokinetics

### Physicochemical characteristics
Molecular weight—130.08.
pKa—8.0 and 13.0.

### Mechanism of action/Effect
Fluorouracil is an antimetabolite of the pyrimidine analog type. Fluorouracil is considered to be cell cycle–specific for the S phase of cell

division. Activity occurs as the result of conversion to an active metabolite in the tissues and includes inhibition of DNA and RNA synthesis.

**Distribution**
Crosses the blood-brain barrier; active metabolites are localized intracellularly.

**Biotransformation**
Rapidly (within 1 hour), via a complicated pathway in the tissues to produce an active metabolite, floxuridine monophosphate. Catabolic degradation occurs in the liver.

**Half-life**
Intravenous—
 Alpha phase: 10 to 20 minutes (fluorouracil).
 Beta phase: Prolonged because of storage in the tissues (metabolites); postulated to be approximately 20 hours.

**Elimination**
Primary route—Respiratory (60 to 80% as carbon dioxide).
Secondary route—Renal (approximately 7 to 20% unchanged, 90% in the first hour).

## Precautions to Consider

### Carcinogenicity
Secondary malignancies are potential delayed effects of many antineoplastic agents, although it is not clear whether the effect is related to their mutagenic or immunosuppressive action. The effect of dose and duration of therapy is also unknown, although risk seems to increase with long-term use. Although information is limited, available data seem to indicate that the carcinogenic risk is greatest with the alkylating agents.

Antimetabolites have been shown to be carcinogenic in animals and may be associated with an increased risk of development of secondary carcinomas in humans, although the risk appears to be less than with alkylating agents.

Long-term carcinogenicity studies in animals have not been done. However, studies in rats at oral doses of 0.01 0.3, 1, or 3 mg per rat 5 days a week for 52 weeks, followed by a 6-month observation period, found no evidence of carcinogenicity. In addition, studies in male rats at intravenous doses of 33 mg per kg of body weight (mg/kg) once a week for 52 weeks, followed by observation for the rest of their lifetimes, found no evidence of carcinogenicity. Incidence of lung adenomas was unchanged in female mice given 1 mg intravenously once a week for 16 weeks.

### Mutagenicity
Very high levels of fluorouracil produce oncogenic changes in cultured C3H/10T1/2 mouse embryo cells. In addition, fluorouracil has been found to be mutagenic in several strains of *Salmonella typhimurium*, including TA 1535, TA 1537, and TA 1538, and in *Saccharomyces cerevisiae*, but not in *Salmonella typhimurium* strains TA 92, TA 98, and TA 100. A positive effect was also observed in the micronucleus test on bone marrow cells of the mouse, and very high concentrations of fluorouracil produced chromosomal breaks in hamster fibroblasts *in vitro*.

### Pregnancy/Reproduction
Fertility—Gonadal suppression, resulting in amenorrhea or azoospermia, may occur in patients taking antineoplastic therapy, especially with the alkylating agents. In general, these effects appear to be related to dose and length of therapy and may be irreversible. Prediction of the degree of testicular or ovarian function impairment is complicated by the common use of combinations of several antineoplastics, which makes it difficult to assess the effects of individual agents.

Fluorouracil causes reversible germ cell toxicity.

In male rats given intraperitoneal doses of 125 or 250 mg/kg, fluorouracil induced chromosomal aberrations and changes in chromosomal organization of spermatogonia. In addition, inhibition of spermatogonial differentiation by fluorouracil resulted in transient infertility. However, fluorouracil did not produce any abnormalities at doses of up to 80 mg/kg per day in a strain of mouse that is sensitive to the induction of sperm head abnormalities after exposure to a range of chemical mutagens and carcinogens.

In female rats given intraperitoneal doses of 25 or 50 mg/kg per week for three weeks during the pre-ovulatory phase of oogenesis, fluorouracil significantly reduced the incidence of fertile matings, delayed the development of pre- and post-implantation embryos, increased the incidence of pre-implantation lethality, and induced chromosomal anomalies in these embryos. A limited study in rabbits with single doses of 25 mg/kg or five daily doses of 5 mg/kg found no effect on ovulation, no apparent effect on implantation, and only a limited effect in producing zygote destruction.

Pregnancy—Adequate and well-controlled studies in humans have not been done.
 *First trimester—*
  It is usually recommended that use of antineoplastics, especially combination chemotherapy, be avoided whenever possible, especially during the first trimester. Although information is limited because of the relatively few instances of antineoplastic administration during pregnancy, the mutagenic, teratogenic, and carcinogenic potential of these medications must be considered.
  One case of multiple congenital anomalies has been reported with fluorouracil administration in the first trimester.
  Other hazards to the fetus include adverse reactions seen in adults.
  In general, use of a contraceptive is recommended during cytotoxic drug therapy.
 *Teratogenic effects—*
  Fluorouracil has been reported to be teratogenic in mice given single intraperitoneal doses of 10 to 40 mg/kg, in rats given 12 to 37 mg/kg intraperitoneally between days 9 and 12 of gestation, and in hamsters given 3 to 9 mg intramuscularly between days 8 and 11 of gestation; these dosages, which are 1 to 3 times the maximum recommended human dose (MRHD) produced malformations including cleft palates, skeletal defects, and deformed appendages, paws, and tails. Teratogenicity did not occur in monkeys given divided doses of 40 mg/kg between days 20 and 24 of gestation.
 *Nonteratogenic effects—*
  Studies of effects of fluorouracil on peri- and postnatal development in animals have not been done. However, in rats fluorouracil crosses the placenta and enters into fetal circulation, and use has resulted in increased resorptions and embryolethality. In monkeys, abortion of all embryos exposed to fluorouracil at maternal doses higher than 40 mg/kg occurred.

FDA Pregnancy Category D.

### Breast-feeding
It is not known whether fluorouracil is distributed into breast milk. Although very little information is available regarding distribution of antineoplastic agents into breast milk, breast-feeding is not recommended during chemotherapy because of the risks to the infant (adverse effects, mutagenicity, carcinogenicity).

### Pediatrics
Appropriate studies on the relationship of age to the effects of fluorouracil have not been performed in the pediatric population. However, pediatrics-specific problems that would limit the usefulness of this medication in children are not expected.

### Geriatrics
Although appropriate studies on the relationship of age to the effects of fluorouracil have not been performed in the geriatric population, geriatrics-specific problems are not expected to limit the usefulness of this medication in the elderly. However, elderly patients are more likely to have age-related renal function impairment, which may require reduction of dosage in patients receiving fluorouracil.

### Dental
The bone marrow depressant effects of fluorouracil may result in an increased incidence of microbial infection, delayed healing, and gingival bleeding. Dental work, whenever possible, should be completed prior to initiation of therapy or deferred until blood counts have returned to normal. Patients should be instructed in proper oral hygiene during treatment, including caution in use of regular toothbrushes, dental floss, and toothpicks.

Fluorouracil also commonly causes ulcerative stomatitis, which may be associated with considerable discomfort.

### Drug interactions and/or related problems
The following drug interactions and/or related problems have been selected on the basis of their potential clinical significance (possible mechanism in parentheses where appropriate)—not necessarily inclusive (» = major clinical significance):

Blood dyscrasia–causing medications (See *Appendix II*)
 (leukopenic and/or thrombocytopenic effects of fluorouracil may be increased with concurrent or recent therapy if these medications cause the same effects; dosage adjustment of fluorouracil, if necessary, should be based on blood counts)

» Bone marrow depressants, other (See *Appendix II*) or
 Radiation therapy
 (additive bone marrow depression may occur; dosage reduction may be required when two or more bone marrow depressants, including radiation, are used concurrently or consecutively)

Leucovorin
(concurrent use may increase the therapeutic and toxic effects of fluorouracil; although the two medications may be used together for therapeutic advantage, dosage adjustment may be necessary)

Vaccines, killed virus
(because normal defense mechanisms may be suppressed by fluorouracil therapy, the patient's antibody response to the vaccine may be decreased. The interval between discontinuation of medications that cause immunosuppression and restoration of the patient's ability to respond to the vaccine depends on the intensity and type of immunosuppression-causing medication used, the underlying disease, and other factors; estimates vary from 3 months to 1 year)

» Vaccines, live virus
(because normal defense mechanisms may be suppressed by fluorouracil therapy, concurrent use with a live virus vaccine may potentiate the replication of the vaccine virus, may increase the side/adverse effects of the vaccine virus, and/or may decrease the patient's antibody response to the vaccine; immunization of these patients should be undertaken only with extreme caution after careful review of the patient's hematologic status and only with the knowledge and consent of the physician managing the fluorouracil therapy. The interval between discontinuation of medications that cause immunosuppression and restoration of the patient's ability to respond to the vaccine depends on the intensity and type of immunosuppression-causing medication used, the underlying disease, and other factors; estimates vary from 3 months to 1 year. Patients with leukemia in remission should not receive live virus vaccine until at least 3 months after their last chemotherapy. Immunization with oral poliovirus vaccine should also be postponed in persons in close contact with the patient, especially family members)

**Laboratory value alterations**
The following have been selected on the basis of their potential clinical significance (possible effect in parentheses where appropriate)—not necessarily inclusive (» = major clinical significance):

With physiology/laboratory test values
Albumin, plasma
(may be decreased because of drug-induced protein malabsorption)

Excretion of 5-hydroxyindoleacetic acid (5-HIAA) in urine
(may be increased)

**Medical considerations/Contraindications**
The medical considerations/contraindications included here have been selected on the basis of their potential clinical significance (reasons given in parentheses where appropriate)—not necessarily inclusive (» = major clinical significance).

*This medication should be used with extreme caution when the following medical problems exist:*
» Bone marrow depression
» Chickenpox, existing or recent (including recent exposure) or
» Herpes zoster
(risk of severe generalized disease)
» Hepatic function impairment
(reduced biotransformation; lower dosage is recommended)
» Infection
» Renal function impairment
(reduced elimination; lower dosage is recommended)
» Sensitivity to fluorouracil
» Tumor cell infiltration of bone marrow
» Extreme caution should be used also in patients who have had previous cytotoxic drug therapy with alkylating agents or high-dose pelvic radiation therapy; a lower dosage is recommended.

**Patient monitoring**
The following are especially important in patient monitoring (other tests may be warranted in some patients, depending on condition; (» = major clinical significance):

Alanine aminotransferase (ALT [SGPT]) values, serum and
Aspartate aminotransferase (AST [SGOT]) values serum and
Bilirubin concentrations, serum and
Lactate dehydrogenase (LDH) values, serum
(recommended prior to initiation of therapy and at periodic intervals during therapy; frequency varies according to clinical state, agent, dose, and other agents being used concurrently)
» Examination of patient's mouth for ulceration
(recommended before administration of each dose)
» Hematocrit or hemoglobin and
» Leukocyte count, total and, if appropriate, differential and

» Platelet count
(determinations recommended prior to initiation of therapy and at periodic intervals during therapy; frequency varies according to clinical state, agent, dose, and other agents being used concurrently)

## Side/Adverse Effects

Note: Many "side effects" of antineoplastic therapy are unavoidable and represent the medication's pharmacologic action. Some of these (for example, leukopenia and thrombocytopenia) are actually used as parameters to aid in individual dosage titration.

Adverse effects associated with prolonged use of an arterial catheter include arterial ischemia, thrombosis, bleeding at the catheter site, blocked catheters, leakage at the site, embolism, fibromyositis, infection at the catheter site, abscesses, and thrombophlebitis.

The following side/adverse effects have been selected on the basis of their potential clinical significance (possible signs and symptoms in parentheses where appropriate)—not necessarily inclusive:

**Those indicating need for medical attention**
Incidence more frequent
*Diarrhea; esophagopharyngitis* (heartburn); *leukopenia or infection* (usually asymptomatic; less frequently, fever or chills; cough or hoarseness; lower back or side pain; painful or difficult urination); *ulcerative stomatitis* (sores in mouth and on lips)

Note: *Esophagopharyngitis* may lead to sloughing and ulceration.

*Leukopenia* usually occurs by 9 to 14 days after each course of treatment; the nadir of leukocyte count occurs about 9 to 14 days after the first day of a course of therapy (uncommonly, as long as 20 days) and usually recovers by about 30 days. Severity of bone marrow depression varies and determines subsequent dosage of fluorouracil.

Incidence less frequent
*Gastrointestinal ulceration* (black, tarry stools; severe nausea and vomiting; stomach cramps); *thrombocytopenia* (usually asymptomatic; rarely, unusual bleeding or bruising; black, tarry stools; blood in urine or stools; pinpoint red spots on skin)

Incidence rare
*Acute cerebellar syndrome* (trouble with balance); *myocardial ischemia* (chest pain; shortness of breath); *palmar-plantar erythrodysesthesia syndrome* (tingling of hands and feet, followed by pain, redness, and swelling); *pneumopathy* (cough; shortness of breath)

Note: *Myocardial ischemia* may occur several hours after a dose; it usually develops after the second or later doses.

The *palmar-plantar erythrodysesthesia syndrome* is also known as hand-foot syndrome. It begins with tingling of hands and feet and may progress over the next few days to pain when holding objects or walking. Symmetrical swelling and erythema of palms and soles, with tenderness of the distal phalanges, occurs, possibly accompanied by desquamation. Symptoms gradually resolve over 5 to 7 days following withdrawal of fluorouracil. The syndrome may also be treatable with oral pyridoxine.

**Those indicating need for medical attention only if they continue or are bothersome**
Incidence more frequent
*Dermatitis* (skin rash and itching, usually on extremities and less frequently on trunk); *loss of appetite; nausea and vomiting; weakness*

Note: *Gastrointestinal distress* usually occurs on about the fourth day of therapy and subsides 2 or 3 days after the medication is stopped. Weakness usually occurs immediately and persists 12 to 36 hours after administration.

Incidence less frequent
*Dry skin and fissuring*

**Those not indicating need for medical attention**
Incidence more frequent
*Loss of hair*

**Those indicating the need for medical attention if they occur after medication is discontinued**
*Bone marrow depression* (black, tarry stools; blood in urine or stools; cough or hoarseness; fever or chills; lower back or side pain; painful or difficult urination; pinpoint red spots on skin; unusual bleeding or bruising)

## Patient Consultation

As an aid to patient consultation, refer to *Advice for the Patient, Fluorouracil (Systemic).*

In providing consultation, consider emphasizing the following selected information (» = major clinical significance):

**Before using this medication**
» Conditions affecting use, especially:
   Sensitivity to fluorouracil
   Pregnancy—Use not recommended because of mutagenic, terato-genic, and carcinogenic potential; advisability of using contra-ception; telling physician immediately if pregnancy is suspected
   Breast-feeding—Not recommended because of risk of serious side effects
   Other medications, especially other bone marrow depressants or previous cytotoxic drug or radiation therapy
   Other medical problems, especially chickenpox, herpes zoster, he-patic function impairment, infection, or renal function impairment

**Proper use of this medication**
   Caution with combination therapy; taking each medication at the right time
   Frequency of nausea and vomiting; importance of continuing medi-cation despite stomach upset
» Proper dosing

**Precautions while using this medication**
» Importance of close monitoring by the physician
» Avoiding immunizations unless approved by physician; other persons in patient's household should avoid immunizations with oral po-liovirus vaccine; avoiding persons who have taken oral poliovirus vaccine or wearing a protective mask that covers nose and mouth
*Caution if bone marrow depression occurs:*
» Avoiding exposure to persons with bacterial infections, especially dur-ing periods of low blood counts; checking with physician imme-diately if fever or chills, cough or hoarseness, lower back or side pain, or painful or difficult urination occur
» Checking with physician immediately if unusual bleeding or bruising; black, tarry stools; blood in urine or stools; or pinpoint red spots on skin occur
   Caution in use of regular toothbrush, dental floss, or toothpick; phy-sician, dentist, or nurse may suggest alternatives; checking with physician before having dental work done
   Not touching eyes or inside of nose unless hands washed immediately before
   Using caution to avoid accidental cuts with use of sharp objects such as safety razor or fingernail or toenail cutters
   Avoiding contact sports or other situations where bruising or injury could occur

**Side/adverse effects**
   May cause adverse effects such as blood problems, loss of hair, and cancer; importance of discussing possible effects with physician
   Signs of potential side effects, especially diarrhea, esophagopharyn-gitis, leukopenia, infection, ulcerative stomatitis, gastrointestinal ulceration, thrombocytopenia, acute cerebellar syndrome, myocar-dial ischemia, palmar-plantar erythrodysesthesia, and pneumopathy
   Physician or nurse can help in dealing with side effects
   Possibility of hair loss; should return after treatment has ended

# General Dosing Information

Patients receiving fluorouracil should be under supervision of a physician experienced in antimetabolite chemotherapy and should be hospital-ized at least during the first course of treatment.

Dosage subsequent to the initial dose should be adjusted to meet the in-dividual requirements of each patient, based on hematological re-sponse of the patient to the previous dose. An additional course of fluorouracil should be given only after toxic effects from the first course have subsided.

Fluorouracil is recommended for parenteral use only. Fluorouracil should not be administered intrathecally because of neurotoxicity.

Administration of fluorouracil by slow intravenous infusion over 2 to 24 hours appears to reduce the toxicity, although rapid injections (over 1 to 2 minutes) may be more effective.

When fluorouracil is given intra-arterially, use of an appropriate infusion pump is recommended to ensure a uniform rate of infusion. In selected patients, a portable pump may be used.

Fluorouracil is an extremely toxic medication; therapy should be discon-tinued promptly at the first sign of:
   Diarrhea
   Esophagopharyngitis
   Gastrointestinal ulceration and bleeding
   Hemorrhage from any site

   Leukopenia, marked, or rapidly falling leukocyte (particularly granu-locyte) count
   Stomatitis
   Thrombocytopenia
   Vomiting, intractable
Therapy may be reinitiated at a lower dose when side effects have subsided.

Special precautions are recommended in patients who develop thrombo-cytopenia as a result of administration of fluorouracil. These may in-clude extreme care in performing invasive procedures; regular inspec-tion of intravenous sites, skin (including perirectal area), and mucous membrane surfaces for signs of bleeding or bruising; limiting fre-quency of venipuncture and avoiding intramuscular injections; testing urine, emesis, stool, secretions for occult blood; care in use of regular toothbrushes, dental floss, toothpicks, safety razors, and fingernail and toenail cutters; avoiding constipation; and using caution to prevent falls and other injuries. Such patients should avoid alcohol and aspirin intake because of the risk of gastrointestinal bleeding. Platelet trans-fusions may be required.

Patients who develop leukopenia should be observed carefully for signs of infection. Antibiotic support may be required. In neutropenic pa-tients who develop fever, broad-spectrum antibiotic coverage should be initiated empirically, pending bacterial cultures and appropriate di-agnostic tests.

**Safety considerations for handling this medication**

There is limited but increasing evidence and concern that personnel in-volved in preparation and administration of parenteral antineoplastics may be at some risk because of the potential mutagenicity, teratoge-nicity, and/or carcinogenicity of these agents, although the actual risk is unknown. USP advisory panels recommend cautious handling both in preparation and disposal of antineoplastic agents. Precautions that have been suggested include:
• Use of a biological containment cabinet during reconstitution and dilution of parenteral medications and wearing of disposable surgical gloves and masks.
• Use of proper technique to prevent contamination of the medication, work area, and operator during transfer between containers (including proper training of personnel in this technique).
• Cautious and proper disposal of needles, syringes, vials, ampuls, and unused medication.
A number of medical centers have developed detailed guidelines for handling of antineoplastic agents.

**Combination chemotherapy**

Fluorouracil may be used in combination with other agents in various regimens. As a result, incidence and/or severity of side effects may be altered and different dosages (usually reduced) may be used. For example, fluorouracil is part of the following chemotherapeutic com-binations (some commonly used acronyms are in parentheses):
—cyclophosphamide, doxorubicin, and fluorouracil (CAF).
—cyclophosphamide, methotrexate, and fluorouracil (CMF).
—cyclophosphamide, methotrexate, fluorouracil, and prednisone (CMFP).
—cyclophosphamide, methotrexate, fluorouracil, vincristine, and pred-nisone (CMFVP, Cooper's Regimen).
—fluorouracil, doxorubicin, and cyclophosphamide (FAC).
—fluorouracil, doxorubicin, and mitomycin (FAM).
—fluorouracil and leucovorin.
For specific dosages and schedules, consult the literature. For information regarding each agent, consult the individual monographs.

**For treatment of side/adverse effects**
The palmar-plantar erythrodysesthesia syndrome may be treated with oral pyridoxine in a dose of 100 to 150 mg per day.

# Parenteral Dosage Forms

Note: Bracketed uses in the *Dosage Forms* section refer to categories of use and/or indications that are not included in U.S. product labeling.

### FLUOROURACIL INJECTION USP

**Usual adult and adolescent dose**
Carcinoma, colorectal or
Carcinoma, breast or
Carcinoma, gastric or
Carcinoma, pancreatic or
[Carcinoma, bladder] or
[Carcinoma, prostatic] or
[Carcinoma, ovarian] or—
   Initial:
      Intravenous, 7 to 12 mg per kg of body weight per day for four days, then after three days if no toxicity has occurred, 7 to 10

mg per kg of body weight every three or four days for a total course of two weeks or

Intravenous, 12 mg per kg of body weight per day for four days, then after one day if no toxicity has occurred, 6 mg per kg of body weight every other day for four or five doses, for a total course of twelve days.

Note: Poor-risk patients should receive a dose of 3 to 6 mg per kg of body weight per day for three days, then after one day if no toxicity has occurred, 3 mg per kg of body weight every other day for three doses.

Maintenance:

Intravenous, 7 to 12 mg per kg of body weight every seven to ten days or

Intravenous, 300 to 500 mg per square meter of body surface per day for four or five days, repeated monthly.

Note: Although dosages are based on the patient's actual weight, use of estimated lean body mass (dry weight) is recommended in obese patients or those with weight gain due to edema, ascites, or other abnormal fluid retention.

Fluorouracil has also been administered on a regimen containing no loading dose, at an intravenous dose of 15 mg per kg of body weight or 500 to 600 mg per square meter of body surface a week.

**Usual adult prescribing limits**
Up to 800 mg daily (400 mg daily in poor-risk patients).

**Usual pediatric dose**
See *Usual adult and adolescent dose.*

**Strength(s) usually available**
U.S.—
　50 mg per mL (10-, 50-, and 100-mL vials) (Rx) [*Adrucil;* GENERIC].

Canada—
　50 mg per mL (10-mL vials) (Rx) [*Adrucil;* GENERIC].

**Packaging and storage**
Store below 40 °C (104 °F), preferably between 15 and 30 °C (59 and 86 °F), unless otherwise specified by manufacturer. Protect from light. Protect from freezing.

**Preparation of dosage form**
Fluorouracil Injection USP may be mixed with 5% dextrose injection or 0.9% sodium chloride injection for administration by intravenous infusion.

Note: The 50- and 100-mL vials are intended for intravenous admixture service use only. Entry into the vial should be made with a sterile dispensing device or transfer set that will accept a syringe hub; use of a syringe and needle is not recommended because of the risk of leakage and microbial and particulate contamination. Proper aseptic technique, under a laminar flow hood, should be used. Any unused portion should be discarded within 1 hour.

**Stability**
Although Fluorouracil Injection USP may discolor slightly during storage, potency and safety are not adversely affected. If a precipitate forms because of exposure to low temperatures, redissolve the medication by heating to 60 °C (140 °F) and shaking vigorously, then allow to cool to body temperature before using.

**Selected Bibliography**
Pinedo HM, Peters GFJ. Fluorouracil: biochemistry and pharmacology. J Clin Oncol 1988 Oct; 6: 1653-64.

Revised: 07/26/94

---

# FLUOROURACIL　Topical

VA CLASSIFICATION (Primary): DE600

Another commonly used name is 5-FU.

Note: For a listing of dosage forms and brand names by country availability, see *Dosage Forms* section(s). For a listing of brand names for the articles in this monograph, refer to the General Index.

## Category
Antineoplastic, topical.

## Indications
Note: Bracketed information in the *Indications* section refers to uses that are not included in U.S. product labeling.

**Accepted**
Actinic keratoses, multiple (treatment)
[Actinic cheilitis (treatment)][1]
[Leukoplakia, mucosal (treatment)][1]
[Radiodermatitis (treatment)][1]
[Bowen's disease (treatment)][1] or
[Erythroplasia of Queyrat (treatment)][1]—Topical fluorouracil is indicated for treatment of precancerous skin conditions including multiple actinic (solar) keratoses, actinic cheilitis, mucosal leukoplakia, radiodermatitis, Bowen's disease, and erythroplasia of Queyrat.

Carcinoma, skin (treatment)—Topical fluorouracil is indicated for treatment of superficial basal cell carcinomas (multiple lesions or difficult access sites), although conventional treatment is preferred whenever possible.

[1]Not included in Canadian product labeling.

## Pharmacology/Pharmacokinetics

**Physicochemical characteristics**
Molecular weight—130.08.
pKa—8.0 and 13.0.

**Mechanism of action/Effect**
Fluorouracil is an antimetabolite of the pyrimidine analog type. Fluorouracil is considered to be cell cycle–specific for the S phase of cell division. Activity occurs as a result of activation in the tissues and includes inhibition of DNA and RNA synthesis. Topical fluorouracil selectively destroys rapidly proliferating cells.

**Absorption**
Approximately 6% (not enough to produce systemic side effects).

**Onset of action**
2 to 3 days. A treatment period of 2 to 6 weeks is usually required to reach the erosion and necrosis stage, or up to 12 weeks in some patients with superficial basal cell carcinomas. Complete healing may not occur for 1 to 2 months after therapy is stopped.

## Precautions to Consider

**Carcinogenicity**
Studies have not been done. However, morphological transformation of cells was produced by fluorouracil in three *in vitro* cell transformation assays. In one of these assays, a metabolite of fluorouracil produced morphological transformation, and injection of the transformed cells into immunosuppressed syngeneic mice produced malignant tumors.

**Mutagenicity**
Parenteral administration of fluorouracil in humans at cumulative doses of 240 mg to 1 gram has produced an increase in numerical and structural chromosome aberrations in peripheral blood lymphocytes. Fluorouracil is mutagenic in yeast cells, *Bacillus subtilis*, and *Drosophila* assays. It produced chromosome damage in an *in vitro* hamster fibroblast assay at concentrations of 1.0 and 2.0 mcg per liter and increased micronuclei formation in the bone marrow of mice at intraperitoneal doses within the human therapeutic dose range of 12 to 15 mg per kg of body weight (mg/kg) per day. Results of the dominant lethal mutation assay performed in mice were negative.

**Pregnancy/Reproduction**
Fertility—Parenteral fluorouracil impairs fertility in rats. In mice, single-dose intravenous and intraperitoneal injections of fluorouracil killed differentiated spermatogonia and spermatocytes at a dose of 500 mg/kg and produced abnormalities in spermatids at a dose of 50 mg/kg.

Pregnancy—Because some systemic absorption occurs, topical fluorouracil is not recommended during pregnancy.

First trimester: Problems in humans have not been documented; however, risk-benefit must be considered, especially during the first trimester, since some systemic absorption occurs, and all antineoplastics affect cell kinetics and can theoretically cause mutagenicity or teratogenicity.

Systemic fluorouracil has been reported to be teratogenic in mice, rats, and hamsters, and embryolethal in monkeys.

FDA Pregnancy Category X.

### Breast-feeding

Problems in humans have not been documented. However, because some systemic absorption occurs, breast-feeding is not recommended while topical fluorouracil is being administered.

### Pediatrics

Appropriate studies on the relationship of age to the effects of topical fluorouracil have not been performed in the pediatric population.

### Geriatrics

Appropriate studies on the relationship of age to the effects of topical fluorouracil have not been performed in the geriatric population. However, geriatrics-specific problems that would limit the usefulness of this medication in elderly patients are not expected.

### Laboratory value alterations

The following have been selected on the basis of their potential clinical significance (possible effect in parentheses where appropriate)—not necessarily inclusive (» = major clinical significance):

With physiology/laboratory test values
    Eosinophilia and
    Leukocytosis and
    Thrombocytopenia and
    Toxic granulation
        (may occur)

### Medical considerations/Contraindications

The medical considerations/contraindications included here have been selected on the basis of their potential clinical significance (reasons given in parentheses where appropriate)—not necessarily inclusive (» = major clinical significance).

*Risk-benefit should be considered when the following medical problems exist:*

    Hemorrhagic ulcerated tissues
        (significant systemic absorption and toxicity may occur)
    Pre-existing dermatoses, especially chloasma and rosacea
        (may be accentuated by the inflammatory response to fluorouracil)
»  Sensitivity to fluorouracil

### Patient monitoring

The following may be especially important in patient monitoring (other tests may be warranted in some patients, depending on condition; » = major clinical significance):

    Biopsy
        (recommended to confirm diagnosis if solar keratoses do not respond or if they recur after treatment, and to confirm cure of superficial basal cell carcinomas)

## Side/Adverse Effects

The following side/adverse effects have been selected on the basis of their potential clinical significance (possible signs and symptoms in parentheses where appropriate)—not necessarily inclusive:

### Those indicating need for medical attention

Incidence more frequent
    *Inflammatory response or allergic reaction* (redness and swelling of normal skin)
    Note: A delayed *hypersensitivity* reaction may occur. Patch testing for hypersensitivity may be inconclusive.

### Those indicating need for medical attention only if they continue or are bothersome

Incidence more frequent
    *Burning feeling at site of application; contact dermatitis* (skin rash); *increased sensitivity of skin to sunlight; itching; oozing; soreness or tenderness of skin*
Incidence less frequent or rare
    *Darkening of skin; scaling; watery eyes*

## Patient Consultation

As an aid to patient consultation, refer to *Advice for the Patient, Fluorouracil (Topical).*

In providing consultation, consider emphasizing the following selected information (» = major clinical significance):

### Before using this medication

»  Conditions affecting use, especially:
    Sensitivity to fluorouracil
    Pregnancy—Use not recommended because of teratogenic potential; some systemic absorption occurs
    Breast-feeding—Not recommended because of risk of serious side effects; some systemic systemic absorption occurs

### Proper use of this medication

»  Compliance with therapy; applying enough medication to cover affected areas
    Washing area to be treated with soap and water and drying thoroughly; using cotton-tipped applicator or fingertips to apply
»  Washing hands immediately after application if fingertips are used
    Possible unsightly and uncomfortable reaction during therapy and for several weeks after therapy is completed; possible temporary pink, smooth spot left during healing; checking with physician before discontinuing medication
»  Proper dosing
    Missed dose: Applying as soon as remembered; not applying if not remembered within a few hours; checking with physician if more than one dose is missed
»  Proper storage

### Precautions while using this medication

»  Importance of close monitoring by physician
»  Caution in applying medication; avoiding eyes, nose, and mouth
»  Possible photosensitivity reactions during therapy and for 1 or 2 months after therapy is completed; avoiding sun; using protective clothing and sun block product; avoiding use of sunlamp, tanning bed, or tanning booth

### Side/adverse effects

    Signs of potential side effects, especially inflammatory response or allergic reaction

## General Dosing Information

Patients using topical fluorouracil should be under supervision of a physician experienced in use of the medication.

Increased frequency of application may be required on areas other than the head and neck.

Application of fluorouracil to easily irritated areas such as around the eyes, nasolabial folds, and wrinkles is not recommended.

Inflammatory and clinical response to fluorouracil in diseased skin areas after topical application is indicated by the following sequence: erythema, usually followed by vesiculation, tenderness, erosion, necrosis, and epithelialization. Use of the medication is terminated when the reaction reaches the stage of erosion, necrosis, and ulceration.

Application of a topical adrenocorticoid after completion of treatment with fluorouracil may hasten healing.

Responses in areas that appear clinically normal may indicate subclinical solar keratoses or an adverse reaction.

Use of occlusive dressings may result in increased incidence of inflammatory reactions on adjacent normal skin and is not recommended.

It is recommended that treatment with fluorouracil be discontinued if an excessive inflammatory response occurs on normal skin.

## Topical Dosage Forms

### FLUOROURACIL CREAM USP

#### Usual adult dose

Actinic or solar keratoses—
    Topical, to the skin, as a 1% cream once or twice a day in a sufficient amount to cover the lesions. Usually the 1% strength is effective on the head, neck, and chest; 2 to 5% may be needed on the hands.
Superficial basal cell carcinomas—
    Topical, to the skin, as a 5% cream twice a day in a sufficient amount to cover the lesions, for at least three to six weeks, and possibly up to twelve weeks.

#### Usual pediatric dose

Safety and efficacy have not been established.

#### Strength(s) usually available

U.S.—
    1% (Rx) [*Fluoroplex* (benzyl alcohol)].
    5% (Rx) [*Efudex* (methylparaben; propylparaben)].
Canada—
    1% (Rx) [*Fluoroplex* (benzyl alcohol)].
    5% (Rx) [*Efudex*].

#### Packaging and storage

Store below 40 °C (104 °F), preferably between 15 and 30 °C (59 and 86 °F), unless otherwise specified by manufacturer. Store in a tight container.

#### Auxiliary labeling

- For the skin.
- Continue medicine for full course of treatment.
- Avoid overexposure to sun.

## FLUOROURACIL TOPICAL SOLUTION USP

### Usual adult dose
Actinic or solar keratoses—
Topical, to the skin, as a 1 or 2% solution once or twice a day in a sufficient amount to cover the lesions. Usually the 1% strength is effective on the head, neck, and chest; 2 to 5% may be needed on the hands.

Superficial basal cell carcinomas—
Topical, to the skin, as a 5% solution twice a day in a sufficient amount to cover the lesions, for at least three to six weeks, and possibly up to twelve weeks.

### Usual pediatric dose
Safety and efficacy have not been established.

### Strength(s) usually available
U.S.—
1% (Rx) [Fluoroplex].

2% (Rx) [Efudex (methylparaben; propylparaben)].
5% (Rx) [Efudex (methylparaben; propylparaben)].
Canada—
1% (Rx) [Fluoroplex].

### Packaging and storage
Store between 15 and 30 °C (59 and 86 °F), unless otherwise specified by manufacturer. Store in a tight container. Protect from freezing.

### Auxiliary labeling
• For the skin.
• Continue medicine for full course of treatment.
• Avoid overexposure to sun.

Revised: 06/09/93
Interim revision: 05/02/94

---

# FLUOXETINE   Systemic

VA CLASSIFICATION (Primary): CN609

Note: For a listing of dosage forms and brand names by country availability, see Dosage Forms section(s). For a listing of brand names for the articles in this monograph, refer to the General Index.

## Category
Antidepressant; antiobsessional agent.

## Indications
Note: Bracketed information in the Indications section refers to uses that are not included in U.S. product labeling.

### Accepted
Depression, mental (treatment)—Fluoxetine is indicated for the treatment of major depressive disorder.

Obsessive-compulsive disorder (treatment)—Fluoxetine is used to relieve symptoms of obsessive-compulsive disorder.

## Pharmacology/Pharmacokinetics

### Physicochemical characteristics
Chemical group—Cyclic, propylamine-derivative antidepressant. Chemically unrelated to tricyclic, tetracyclic, or other available antidepressants.
Molecular weight—345.79.

### Mechanism of action/Effect
Fluoxetine is a potent and selective inhibitor of serotonin (5-HT) uptake, but not of norepinephrine uptake, in the central nervous system (CNS). Because uptake inactivates serotonin by removing it from the synaptic cleft, uptake inhibition by fluoxetine enhances serotonergic function. As a consequence, the 5-HT$_1$ receptors are desensitized or downregulated after chronic fluoxetine administration. Fluoxetine does not interact directly with serotonergic receptors, muscarinic-cholinergic receptors, histaminergic H$_1$ receptors, or alpha-adrenergic receptors. Fluoxetine, unlike most other antidepressant medications, does not appear to cause downregulation of postsynaptic beta-adrenergic receptors.

### Other actions/effects
Fluoxetine has an anorectic effect and potentially causes weight loss proportional to the degree of initial obesity as measured by the body mass index (BMI).

### Absorption
Well absorbed with a small first-pass effect. Food does not affect the extent of absorption, although the rate may be slightly decreased.

### Distribution
Readily crosses the blood-brain barrier.

### Protein binding
High (94.5%).

### Biotransformation
Metabolized by demethylation in the liver to the active metabolite, norfluoxetine, and other unidentified metabolites.

### Half-life
Elimination—
Fluoxetine: 2 to 3 days.
Norfluoxetine: 7 to 9 days.

### Onset of action
Between 1 and 4 weeks.

### Time to peak concentration
6 to 8 hours after a single oral dose of 40 mg.

### Peak serum concentration
Single dose (40 mg)—
Fluoxetine: 15 to 55 nanograms per mL.
Multiple dose (40 mg a day for 30 days)—
Fluoxetine: 91 to 302 nanograms per mL.
Norfluoxetine: 72 to 258 nanograms per mL.

### Elimination
Renal—
80% excreted in the urine (11.6% fluoxetine, 7.4% fluoxetine glucuronide, 6.8% norfluoxetine, 8.2% norfluoxetine glucuronide, >20% hippuric acid, 46% other).
Biliary—
Approximately 15% in the feces.
In dialysis—
Not dialyzable because of high protein binding.

## Precautions to Consider

### Carcinogenicity
Studies in rats and mice given dietary fluoxetine in doses equivalent to 7.5 to 9 times the maximum human dose showed no evidence of carcinogenicity.

### Mutagenicity
Fluoxetine and norfluoxetine have shown no genotoxic effects in the bacterial mutation assay; DNA repair assay in cultured rat hepatocytes; mouse lymphoma assay; or in vivo sister chromatid exchange assay in Chinese hamster bone marrow cells.

### Pregnancy/Reproduction
Fertility—No evidence of adverse effects on fertility was shown in rats given fluoxetine doses of 5 to 9 times the maximum human dose.

Pregnancy—Studies in humans have not been done.

However, studies in animals have not shown that fluoxetine causes adverse effects on the fetus. Studies in rats given fluoxetine doses of 5 to 9 times the maximum human dose showed a slight decrease in neonatal survival, which was possibly associated with decreased maternal food consumption and lack of weight gain.

FDA Pregnancy Category B.

Labor and delivery—The effect of fluoxetine on labor and delivery is not known.

### Breast-feeding
Fluoxetine is distributed into breast milk. In one case report, vomiting, watery stools, crying, and sleep disorders were reported in the infant of a nursing mother taking 20 mg of fluoxetine a day; these symptoms recurred when the infant was rechallenged with breast milk. Use of fluoxetine in nursing mothers is not recommended.

**Pediatrics**
Appropriate studies on the relationship of age to the effects of fluoxetine have not been performed in the pediatric population. Safety and efficacy have not been established.

**Geriatrics**
No geriatrics-related problems have been documented in studies done to date that included elderly patients.

**Drug interactions and/or related problems**
The following drug interactions and/or related problems have been selected on the basis of their potential clinical significance (possible mechanism in parentheses where appropriate)—not necessarily inclusive (» = major clinical significance):

Note: Combinations containing any of the following medications, depending on the amount present, may also interact with this medication.

» Alcohol or
» CNS depression–producing medications, other (See *Appendix II*)
    (concurrent use with fluoxetine may result in potentiation of CNS depressant effects)

Antidepressants, tricyclic or
Maprotiline or
Trazodone
    (plasma concentrations of these medications may be doubled when fluoxetine is used concurrently; some clinicians recommend dosage reductions of about 50% in tricyclic antidepressants if these agents are given concurrently with fluoxetine)

Diazepam
    (concurrent use may prolong the half-life of diazepam in some patients but the psychomotor and physiological responses may be unaffected)

Electroconvulsive therapy
    (prolonged seizures have been reported in patients on concomitant fluoxetine therapy)

Haloperidol or
Loxapine or
Molindone or
Phenothiazines or
Pimozide or
Thioxanthenes
    (caution in concurrent use of other CNS-active medications with fluoxetine is recommended because of a potentially increased risk of side effects)

» Highly protein-bound medications, especially:
Anticoagulants
Digitalis or digitoxin
    (caution in concurrent use with fluoxetine is recommended because of possible displacement of either medication from protein-binding sites, leading to increased plasma concentrations of the free [unbound] medications and increased risk of adverse effects)

Lithium
    (lithium concentrations may be altered, leading to toxicity; close monitoring of lithium concentrations is recommended)

» Monoamine oxidase (MAO) inhibitors, including furazolidone, procarbazine, and selegiline
    (a potentially lethal hyperserotonergic state known as the serotonin syndrome may occur as the result of combining a serotonergic agent such as fluoxetine with MAO inhibitors. The syndrome may be manifest by mental status changes [confusion, hypomania], restlessness, myoclonus, hyperreflexia, diaphoresis, shivering, tremor, diarrhea, incoordination, and/or fever. If recognized early, the syndrome usually resolves quickly upon withdrawal of the offending agents)
    (concurrent use of fluoxetine with MAO inhibitors may result in confusion, agitation, restlessness, and gastrointestinal symptoms, or possibly hyperpyretic episodes, severe convulsions, and hypertensive crises. Based on experience with tricyclic antidepressants, at least 14 days should elapse between discontinuation of an MAO inhibitor and initiation of fluoxetine. However, because of the long half-lives of fluoxetine and its active metabolite, at least 5 weeks [approximately 5 half-lives of norfluoxetine] should elapse between discontinuation of fluoxetine and initiation of therapy with an MAO inhibitor. Administration of an MAO inhibitor within 5 weeks of discontinuation of fluoxetine may increase the risk of serious events. While a causal relationship to fluoxetine has not been established, death has been reported following the initiation of an MAO inhibitor shortly after fluoxetine administration was stopped)

» Phenytoin
    (elevated plasma phenytoin concentrations resulting in symptoms of toxicity have been reported when fluoxetine was used concurrently with phenytoin; caution and close monitoring are suggested)
» Tryptophan
    (concurrent use may potentiate agitation, restlessness, and gastrointestinal problems)

**Medical considerations/Contraindications**
The medical considerations/contraindications included here have been selected on the basis of their potential clinical significance (reasons given in parentheses where appropriate)—not necessarily inclusive (» = major clinical significance).

*Risk-benefit should be considered when the following medical problems exist:*

Diabetes mellitus
    (glycemic control may be altered)
» Hepatic function impairment
    (metabolism of fluoxetine is delayed; lower doses or less frequent dosing is recommended in patients with liver disease)
» Renal function impairment
    (excretion of fluoxetine may be delayed; lower doses or less frequent dosing is recommended in patients with renal disease)
Seizure disorders, history of
    (seizures may be induced by fluoxetine in patients with a history of seizure disorders)
Sensitivity to fluoxetine

Caution should also be used in debilitated patients or in patients taking multiple CNS-active medications, who may be more susceptible to fluoxetine-induced seizures.

**Patient monitoring**
The following may be especially important in patient monitoring (other tests may be warranted in some patients, depending on condition; » = major clinical significance):

Careful supervision of depressed patients with suicidal tendencies
    (recommended especially during early treatment phase prior to peak effectiveness of fluoxetine; prescribing the smallest number of capsules necessary for good patient management is recommended to prevent overdosing)
    (there have been recent anecdotal reports of a few cases of suicidal ideation occurring in patients on fluoxetine therapy; patients who have previously been treated with other antidepressants, or who develop intense fatigue, hypersomnia, or restlessness on fluoxetine therapy may be at greatest risk)

# Side/Adverse Effects

Note: There have been recent anecdotal reports of suicidal ideation occurring in a few patients receiving fluoxetine. However, controversy exists regarding the role of fluoxetine in these episodes, and a causal relationship has not been established.

The following side/adverse effects have been selected on the basis of their potential clinical significance (possible signs and symptoms in parentheses where appropriate)—not necessarily inclusive:

**Those indicating need for medical attention**
Incidence less frequent
    *Chills or fever; joint or muscle pain; skin rash, hives, or itching; trouble in breathing*
Incidence rare
    *Allergic reaction or serum sickness–like syndrome* (skin rash or hives associated with burning or tingling in fingers, hands, or arms [carpal tunnel syndrome]; chills or fever; swollen glands; joint or muscle pain; swelling of feet or lower legs; trouble in breathing); *hypoglycemia* (anxiety; chills; cold sweats; confusion; cool pale skin; difficulty in concentration; drowsiness; excessive hunger; fast heartbeat; headache; nervousness; shakiness; unsteady walk; unusual tiredness or weakness); *hyponatremia* (lack of energy)—especially in geriatric or volume-depleted patients; *mania or hypomania* (unusual excitement); *seizures; swollen glands*

Note: *Allergic reaction* or *serum sickness–like syndrome* may be associated with proteinuria, leukocytosis, and mild transaminase elevation.

**Those indicating need for medical attention only if they continue or are bothersome**
Incidence more frequent
    *Anxiety and nervousness; diarrhea; drowsiness; headache; increased sweating; insomnia* (trouble in sleeping); *nausea*

Incidence less frequent
*Abnormal dreams; change in taste; changes in vision; chest pain; constipation; cough; decreased appetite or weight loss; decrease in concentration; decreased sexual drive or ability; dizziness or lightheadedness; dryness of mouth; fast or irregular heartbeat; feeling of warmth or heat; flushing or redness of skin, especially on face and neck; frequent urination; increased appetite; menstrual pain; stomach cramps, gas, or pain; stuffy nose; tiredness or weakness; tremor; vomiting*

## Overdose

For specific information on the agents used in the management of fluoxetine overdose, see:
*Charcoal, Activated (Oral-Local)* monograph; and/or
*Diazepam* in *Benzodiazepines (Systemic)* monograph.

For more information on the management of overdose or unintentional ingestion, **contact a Poison Control Center** (see *Poison Control Center Listing*).

### Clinical effects of overdose
The following effects have been selected on the basis of their potential clinical significance (possible signs and symptoms in parentheses where appropriate)—not necessarily inclusive:

*Agitation and restlessness; hypomania* (unusual excitement); *nausea and vomiting, severe; seizures*

### Treatment of overdose
Treatment is essentially symptomatic and supportive, possibly including:
To decrease absorption—
Administering activated charcoal with sorbitol.
Specific treatment—
Administering an anticonvulsant such as diazepam, if necessary, for seizure control.
Monitoring—
Monitoring cardiovascular function (ECG).
Supportive care—
Maintaining respiratory and cardiac function.
Maintaining body temperature.
Patients in whom intentional overdose is known or suspected should be referred for psychiatric consultation.
Note: Dialysis, forced diuresis, hemoperfusion or exchange transfusions are unlikely to be of benefit due to the large volume of distribution and high degree of protein binding of fluoxetine.

## Patient Consultation

As an aid to patient consultation, refer to *Advice for the Patient, Fluoxetine (Systemic)*.

In providing consultation, consider emphasizing the following selected information (» = major clinical significance):

### Before using this medication
» Conditions affecting use, especially:
Sensitivity to fluoxetine
Breast-feeding—Not recommended
Other medications, especially CNS depression–causing medications; highly protein-bound medications such as anticoagulants, digitalis, or digitoxin; monoamine oxidase (MAO) inhibitors; phenytoin; or tryptophan
Other medical problems, especially hepatic or renal function impairment
Recent anecdotal reports of fluoxetine use possibly related to suicidal ideation in a few patients

### Proper use of this medication
» Compliance with therapy; not taking more or less medicine than prescribed
May be taken with food to lessen possible stomach upset
» May require up to 4 weeks or longer of therapy to obtain antidepressant effects
» Proper dosing
Missed dose: Skipping the missed dose and continuing on regular schedule with next dose; not doubling doses
» Proper storage

### Precautions while using this medication
Regular visits to physician to check progress of therapy
» Avoiding use of alcoholic beverages; not taking other CNS depressants unless prescribed by physician
» Stopping fluoxetine and checking with physician as soon as possible if skin rash or hives occurs
» Possible drowsiness, impairment of judgment, thinking, or motor skills; caution when driving or doing jobs requiring alertness

» Possible dizziness or lightheadedness; caution when getting up suddenly from a lying or sitting position
» Possible dryness of mouth; using sugarless gum or candy, ice, or saliva substitute for relief; checking with physician or dentist if dry mouth continues for more than 2 weeks

### Side/adverse effects
Signs of potential side effects, especially chills or fever, swollen glands, joint or muscle pain, skin rash, hives, or itching, trouble in breathing, allergic reaction, serum sickness–like syndrome, convulsions, mania, or hypomania

## General Dosing Information

Because of the long elimination half-lives of fluoxetine and norfluoxetine, dosing changes are not reflected in plasma for several weeks. This must be taken into consideration when titrating to a final dose. In addition, it is unlikely that any withdrawal effect would develop upon cessation of therapy, since fluoxetine is essentially self-tapering. However, a gradual return of symptoms of depression may occur after discontinuation.

Potentially suicidal patients should not have access to large quantities of this medication since depressed patients, particularly those who may use alcohol excessively, may continue to exhibit suicidal tendencies until significant improvement occurs. Some clinicians recommend that the patient be supplied with the least amount of medication necessary for satisfactory patient management.

### Diet/Nutrition
Fluoxetine may be taken with food to lessen possible stomach upset.

### For treatment of adverse effects
Skin rash or hives—Fluoxetine should be discontinued on appearance of skin rash or hives. Treatment with antihistamines and/or steroids may be necessary.

## Oral Dosage Forms
### FLUOXETINE HYDROCHLORIDE CAPSULES

#### Usual adult dose
For depression or obsessive-compulsive disorder—
Oral, initially 20 mg (base) a day as a single morning dose. After several weeks, the dose may be increased by 20 mg a day at weekly intervals, as needed and tolerated.
Note: The manufacturer recommends that doses over 20 mg a day be taken in two divided doses, in the morning and at noon.

#### Usual adult prescribing limits
80 mg (base) a day.

#### Usual pediatric dose
Safety and efficacy have not been established.

#### Usual geriatric dose
See *Usual adult dose*.
Note: Dosage for elderly patients is often initiated at 10 mg (base) a day and should not exceed 60 mg (base) a day.

#### Strength(s) usually available
U.S.—
10 mg (base) (Rx) [*Prozac* (FD&C Blue No.1; gelatin; iron oxide; silicon; starch; titanium dioxide)].
20 mg (base) (Rx) [*Prozac* (FD&C Blue No.1; gelatin; iron oxide; silicon; starch; titanium dioxide)].
Canada—
10 mg (base) (Rx) [*Prozac*].
20 mg (base) (Rx) [*Prozac*].

#### Packaging and storage
Store below 40 °C (104 °F), preferably between 15 and 30 °C (59 and 86 °F), in a well-closed container, unless otherwise specified by manufacturer.

#### Auxiliary labeling
• May cause drowsiness.
• Avoid alcoholic beverages.

### FLUOXETINE HYDROCHLORIDE ORAL SOLUTION

#### Usual adult dose
See *Fluoxetine Hydrochloride Capsules*.

#### Usual adult prescribing limits
See *Fluoxetine Hydrochloride Capsules*.

#### Usual pediatric dose
See *Fluoxetine Hydrochloride Capsules*.

#### Usual geriatric dose
See *Fluoxetine Hydrochloride Capsules*.

**Strength(s) usually available**
U.S.—
   20 mg (base) per 5 mL (Rx) [*Prozac* (alcohol 0.23%; benzoic acid; flavoring agent; glycerin; purified water; sucrose)].
Canada—
   20 mg (base) per 5 mL (Rx) [*Prozac*].

**Packaging and storage**
Store below 40 °C (104 °F), preferably between 15 and 30 °C (59 and 86 °F), in a tight light-resistant container, unless otherwise specified by manufacturer.

**Auxiliary labeling**
• May cause drowsiness.
• Avoid alcoholic beverages.

**Additional information**
The oral solution is mint-flavored.

Developed: 08/04/92
Interim revision: 04/29/94

---

**FLUOXYMESTERONE**—See *Androgens (Systemic)*

---

## FLUOXYMESTERONE-CONTAINING COMBINATIONS—

Fluoxymesterone and Ethinyl Estradiol (Systemic)—See *Androgens and Estrogens (Systemic)*

---

**FLUPENTHIXOL**—See *Thioxanthenes (Systemic)*

---

**FLUPHENAZINE**—See *Phenothiazines (Systemic)*

---

**FLURANDRENOLIDE**—See *Corticosteroids (Topical)*

---

**FLURAZEPAM**—See *Benzodiazepines (Systemic)*

---

**FLURBIPROFEN**—See *Anti-inflammatory Drugs, Nonsteroidal (Ophthalmic); Anti-inflammatory Drugs, Nonsteroidal (Systemic)*

---

# FLUTAMIDE Systemic

VA CLASSIFICATION (Primary): AN900
Note: For a listing of dosage forms and brand names by country availability, see *Dosage Forms* section(s). For a listing of brand names for the articles in this monograph, refer to the General Index.

## Category
Antineoplastic.

## Indications
**Accepted**
Carcinoma, prostatic (treatment)—Flutamide is indicated, in combination with luteinizing hormone–releasing hormone (LHRH) analogs such as leuprolide, for treatment of metastatic prostatic carcinoma (stage $D_2$).

**Unaccepted**
Use of flutamide for hirsutism, benign prostatic hyperplasia (BPH), or other benign disorders is not recommended because of the risk of acute, severe, potentially fatal hepatotoxicity.

## Pharmacology/Pharmacokinetics
**Physicochemical characteristics**
Molecular weight—276.21.

**Mechanism of action/Effect**
Flutamide has antiandrogenic effects, including inhibition of androgen uptake and/or inhibition of nuclear binding of androgen in target tissues. Its interference with testosterone at the cellular level complements the medical castration produced by LHRH analogs.

**Absorption**
Rapidly and completely absorbed.

**Protein binding**
Very high (94 to 96% for flutamide; 92 to 94% for the alpha-hydroxylated metabolite).

**Biotransformation**
Hepatic (rapid and extensive). At least 6 metabolites have been identified; the major one found in plasma is a biologically active alpha-hydroxylated derivative (2-hydroxyflutamide).

**Half-life**
Alpha-hydroxylated metabolite—6 hours.
Note: In geriatric patients, half-life is 8 hours after a single dose and 9.6 hours at steady-state.

**Time to peak concentration**
Alpha-hydroxylated metabolite—2 hours.

**Elimination**
Renal/fecal (4.2%).
In dialysis—Because of extensive protein binding, unlikely to be significantly removed by hemodialysis or peritoneal dialysis.

## Precautions to Consider
**Carcinogenicity**
Studies have not been done. However, testicular interstitial cell adenomas occurred at all doses in rats given 3, 8, or 17 times the human dose daily for 52 weeks.

**Mutagenicity**
No evidence of mutagenicity was found in the Ames *Salmonella* /microsome Mutagenesis Assay. Dominant lethal tests in rats were also negative.

**Pregnancy/Reproduction**
Fertility—Flutamide therapy results in reduced sperm counts in humans. In male rats, flutamide interfered with mating behavior and caused suppression of spermatogenesis and decreased conception rates.
Leuprolide, which is used in combination with flutamide, suppresses testosterone secretion and impairs fertility; it is not known whether fertility is restored after leuprolide is withdrawn.
Pregnancy—Studies in rats at doses of 3, 9, and 19 times the human dose found a decrease in 24-hour survival of offspring. In addition, at the two higher doses, a slight increase in minor variations in the development of the sternebra and vertebra occurred in the fetuses and feminization of males occurred. Studies in rabbits at doses of 1.4 times the human dose found a decreased survival rate in offspring.
FDA Pregnancy Category D.

**Geriatrics**
Half-life is increased in the elderly.

**Laboratory value alterations**
The following have been selected on the basis of their potential clinical significance (possible effect in parentheses where appropriate)—not necessarily inclusive (» = major clinical significance):
With physiology/laboratory test values
  Alanine aminotransferase (ALT [SGPT]) values, serum and
  Aspartate aminotransferase (AST [SGOT]) values, serum
    (may be increased transiently during long-term treatment or in acute hepatotoxicity)
  Bilirubin concentrations, serum and
  Creatinine concentrations, serum
    (may be increased transiently during long-term treatment)
  Estradiol and
  Testosterone
    (plasma concentrations may be increased)

**Medical considerations/Contraindications**

The medical considerations/contraindications included here have been selected on the basis of their potential clinical significance (reasons given
in parentheses where appropriate)—not necessarily inclusive (» =
major clinical significance).

*Risk-benefit should be considered when the following medical problem
exists:*

» Sensitivity to flutamide

**Patient monitoring**

The following may be especially important in patient monitoring (other
tests may be warranted in some patients, depending on condition;
» = major clinical significance):

» Hepatic function tests
   (recommended at periodic intervals)

## Side/Adverse Effects

Note: Side/adverse effects listed (except for hepatotoxicity) are for combined flutamide and LHRH analog therapy. Hepatotoxicity has occurred with use of flutamide as a single agent.

During LHRH analog therapy, some signs and symptoms of prostatic carcinoma, including difficult urination, may worsen transiently. In addition, worsening of neurologic signs and symptoms
in patients with vertebral metastases may result in temporary weakness and paresthesias of the lower extremities. There is some evidence that flutamide attenuates these effects of LHRH analogs.

The following side/adverse effects have been selected on the basis of their
potential clinical significance (possible signs and symptoms in parentheses where appropriate)—not necessarily inclusive:

**Those indicating need for medical attention**
Incidence rare
   *Hepatotoxicity, acute, including abnormal liver function tests; hep-
   atitis; cholestatic jaundice; hepatic necrosis; and hepatic encephalopathy* (usually asymptomatic; may progress to dark urine; itching;
   loss of appetite; nausea or vomiting; pain in right side; yellow eyes or
   skin); *hypertension* (usually not symptomatic); *methemoglobinemia*
   (usually asymptomatic; symptoms include bluish-colored lips, fingernails, or palms of hands; dizziness, extreme, or fainting; feeling of
   extreme pressure in head; shortness of breath; weak and fast heartbeat)
   Note: *Hepatotoxicity* usually resolves when flutamide is withdrawn,
   but may be progressive and fatal. Symptoms require immediate
   medical attention.

**Those indicating need for medical attention only if they continue
or are bothersome**
Incidence more frequent
   *Diarrhea; hot flashes* (sudden sweating and feelings of warmth); *im-
   potence or decrease in sexual desire*
   Note: Flutamide alone causes little *impairment of sexual function.*

Incidence less frequent
   *Gynecomastia* (swelling and increased tenderness of breasts); *loss of
   appetite; numbness or tingling of hands or feet; swelling of feet or
   lower legs*

## Overdose

For more information on the management of overdose or unintentional
ingestion, **contact a Poison Control Center** (see *Poison Control Center Listing*).

**Treatment of overdose**
Recommended treatment consists of the following:
   • Induction of vomiting, if patient is alert and vomiting has not already
     occurred.
   • Supportive treatment.

## Patient Consultation

As an aid to patient consultation, refer to *Advice for the Patient, Flutamide
(Systemic).*

In providing consultation, consider emphasizing the following selected
information (» = major clinical significance):

**Before using this medication**
» Conditions affecting use, especially:
   Sensitivity to flutamide
   Pregnancy/Fertility—Flutamide reduces sperm count and leuprol-
      ide causes potentially irreversible impairment of fertility
   Use in the elderly—Half-life increased, but no precautions
      necessary

**Proper use of this medication**
» Importance of not using more or less medication than the amount
   prescribed
» Importance of following physician's instructions for simultaneous use
   with LHRH analog
» Importance of continuing medication despite side effects
   Checking with physician if vomiting occurs shortly after dose is taken
» Proper dosing
   Missed dose: Taking as soon as possible; not taking if almost time for
      next dose; not doubling doses
» Proper storage

**Precautions while using this medication**
» Importance of close monitoring by the physician

**Side/adverse effects**
   Signs of potential side effects, especially hepatotoxicity, hypertension,
      and methemoglobinemia

## General Dosing Information

Patients taking flutamide should be under supervision of a physician experienced in cancer chemotherapy.

Flutamide therapy should begin simultaneously with LHRH analog
therapy.

## Oral Dosage Forms

### FLUTAMIDE CAPSULES

**Usual adult dose**
Prostatic carcinoma—
   Oral, 250 mg every eight hours.

Note: Flutamide should be given simultaneously with LHRH analog (e.g.,
   leuprolide) therapy. The usual dose of leuprolide is 1 mg subcutaneously per day or 7.5 mg intramuscularly once a month.

**Strength(s) usually available**
U.S.—
   125 mg (Rx) [*Eulexin* (lactose)].
Canada—
   Not commercially available.

**Packaging and storage**
Store below 40 °C (104 °F), preferably between 15 and 30 °C (59 and 86
°F), in a well-closed container, unless otherwise specified by
manufacturer.

### FLUTAMIDE TABLETS

**Usual adult dose**
See *Flutamide Capsules.*

**Strength(s) usually available**
U.S.—
   Not commercially available.
Canada—
   250 mg (Rx) [*Euflex* (scored; lactose)].

**Packaging and storage**
Store below 40 °C (104 °F), preferably between 15 and 30 °C (59 and 86
°F), in a well-closed container, unless otherwise specified by
manufacturer.

## Selected Bibliography

Sogani PC, Fair WR. Treatment of advanced prostatic cancer. Urol Clin
   N Am 1987 May; 14 (2): 353-71.
Namer M. Clinical applications of antiandrogens. J Steroid Biochem 1988
   Oct; 31 (4B): 719-29.
Labrie F, et al. Combination therapy with flutamide and CD-Trpb, des-
   Gly-NH₂ (10) LHRH ethylamide in Stage C and D prostate cancer:
   today's therapy of choice—rationale and 5-year clinical experience.
   Prog Clin Biol Res 1988; 262: 11-63.

Revised: 08/03/94

---

**FLUTICASONE**—See *Corticosteroids (Topical)*

---

**FLUVASTATIN**—See *HMG-CoA Reductase Inhibitors (Systemic)*

# FOLIC ACID    Systemic

VA CLASSIFICATION (Primary): VT102

Another commonly used name is Vitamin B₉.

Note: For a listing of dosage forms and brand names by country availability, see *Dosage Forms* section(s). For a listing of brand names for the articles in this monograph, refer to the General Index.

## Category

Nutritional supplement (vitamin); diagnostic aid (folate deficiency).

Note: Folic acid (vitamin B₉) is a water-soluble vitamin.

## Indications

Note: Bracketed information in the *Indications* section refers to uses that are not included in U.S. product labeling.

### Accepted

Folic acid deficiency (prophylaxis and treatment)—Folic acid is indicated for prevention and treatment of folic acid deficiency states. Folic acid deficiency may occur as a result of inadequate nutrition or intestinal malabsorption but does not occur in healthy individuals receiving an adequate balanced diet. Simple nutritional deficiency of individual B vitamins is rare since dietary inadequacy usually results in multiple deficiencies. For prophylaxis of folic acid deficiency, dietary improvement, rather than supplementation, is advisable. For treatment of folic acid deficiency, supplementation is preferred.

Folic acid should not be given until the diagnosis of pernicious anemia has been ruled out, since it corrects the hematologic manifestations and masks pernicious anemia while allowing neurologic damage to progress.

Deficiency of folic acid may lead to megaloblastic and macrocytic anemias and glossitis.

Recommended intakes may be increased and/or supplementation may be necessary in the following persons or conditions (based on documented folic acid deficiency):
Alcoholism
Anemia, hemolytic
Fever, chronic
Gastrectomy
Hemodialysis, chronic
Infants—low-birthweight, breast-fed, or those receiving unfortified formulas such as evaporated milk or goat's milk
Intestinal diseases—celiac disease, tropical sprue, persistent diarrhea
Malabsorption syndromes associated with hepatic-biliary disease—hepatic function impairment, alcoholism with cirrhosis
Stress, prolonged

Some unusual diets (e.g., reducing diets that drastically restrict food selection) may not supply minimum daily requirements of folic acid. Supplementation is necessary in patients receiving total parenteral nutrition (TPN) or undergoing rapid weight loss or in those with malnutrition, because of inadequate dietary intake.

Recommended intakes for all vitamins and most minerals are increased during pregnancy. Many physicians recommend that pregnant women receive multivitamin and mineral supplements, especially those pregnant women who do not consume an adequate diet and those in high-risk categories (i.e., women carrying more than one fetus, heavy cigarette smokers, and alcohol and drug abusers). Taking excessive amounts of a multivitamin and mineral supplement may be harmful to the mother and/or fetus and should be avoided.

Some studies have found that folic acid supplementation alone or in combination with other vitamins given before conception and during early pregnancy may reduce the incidence of neural tube defects in infants.

Recommended intakes for all vitamins and most minerals are increased during breast-feeding.

Recommended intakes may be increased by the following medications: Analgesics (long-term use), anticonvulsants, epoetin, estrogens, sulfasalazine.

[Folate deficiency (diagnosis)]¹—Folic acid is being used in the diagnosis of folate deficiency.

### Unaccepted

Folic acid has not been proven effective for prevention of mental disorders or in the treatment of normocytic, refractory, or aplastic anemias.

¹Not included in Canadian product labeling.

## Pharmacology/Pharmacokinetics

### Physicochemical characteristics

Molecular weight—441.41.

### Mechanism of action/Effect

Folic acid, after conversion to tetrahydrofolic acid, is necessary for normal erythropoiesis, synthesis of purine and thymidylates, metabolism of amino acids such as glycine and methionine, and the metabolism of histidine.

### Absorption

Commercially available folic acid is almost completely absorbed from the gastrointestinal tract (mostly in the upper duodenum), even in the presence of malabsorption due to tropical sprue. However, absorption of food folates is impaired in malabsorption syndromes.

### Protein binding

Extensive (to plasma proteins).

### Storage

Hepatic (large proportion).

### Biotransformation

Hepatic. Folic acid is converted (in the presence of ascorbic acid) in the liver and plasma to its metabolically active form (tetrahydrofolic acid) by dihydrofolate reductase.

### Peak serum concentration

30 to 60 minutes.

### Elimination

Renal (almost entirely as metabolites). Excess beyond daily needs is excreted, largely unchanged, in urine.

In dialysis—Folic acid is removed by hemodialysis; therefore, dialysis patients should receive increased amounts (100 to 300% of USRDA [United States Recommended Daily Allowances]).

## Precautions to Consider

### Pregnancy/Reproduction

Pregnancy—Problems in humans have not been documented with intake of normal daily recommended amounts. Folic acid crosses the placenta. However, adequate and well-controlled studies in humans have not shown that folic acid causes adverse effects on the fetus.

Some studies have found that folic acid supplementation alone or in combination with other vitamins given before conception and during early pregnancy may reduce the incidence of neural tube defects in infants.

FDA Pregnancy Category A.

### Breast-feeding

Folic acid is distributed into breast milk. However, problems in humans have not been documented with intake of normal daily recommended amounts.

### Pediatrics

Problems in pediatrics have not been documented with intake of normal daily recommended amounts.

Folic acid injection that contains benzyl alcohol as a preservative should not be used in newborn and immature infants. The use of benzyl alcohol in neonates has been associated with a fatal toxic syndrome consisting of metabolic acidosis and CNS, respiratory, circulatory, and renal function impairment.

### Geriatrics

Problems in geriatrics have not been documented with intake of normal daily recommended amounts.

### Drug interactions and/or related problems

The following drug interactions and/or related problems have been selected on the basis of their potential clinical significance (possible mechanism in parentheses where appropriate)—not necessarily inclusive (» = major clinical significance):

Note: Combinations containing any of the following medications, depending on the amount present, may also interact with this medication.

Analgesics, long-term use or
Anticonvulsants, hydantoin or
Carbamazepine or
Estrogens or
Oral contraceptives
    (requirements for folic acid may be increased in patients receiving these medications)

(concurrent use with folic acid may decrease the effects of hydantoin anticonvulsants by antagonism of their central nervous system [CNS] effects; an increase in hydantoin dosage may be necessary for patients who receive folic acid supplementation)

Antacids, aluminum- or magnesium-containing

(prolonged use of aluminum- and/or magnesium-containing antacids may decrease folic acid absorption by lowering the pH of the small intestine; patients should be advised to take antacids at least 2 hours after folic acid)

Antibiotics

(may interfere with the microbiologic method of assay for serum and erythrocyte folic acid concentrations and cause falsely low results)

Cholestyramine

(concurrent use with folic acid may interfere with absorption of folic acid; folic acid supplementation taken at least 1 hour before or 4 to 6 hours after cholestyramine is recommended in patients receiving cholestyramine for prolonged periods)

Methotrexate or
Pyrimethamine or
Triamterene or
Trimethoprim

(act as folate antagonists by inhibiting dihydrofolate reductase; most significant with high doses and/or prolonged use; leucovorin calcium must be used instead of folic acid in patients receiving these medications)

Sulfonamides, including sulfasalazine

(inhibit absorption of folate; folic acid requirements may be increased in patients receiving sulfasalazine)

Zinc supplements

(some studies have found that folate may decrease the absorption of zinc, but not in the presence of excessive zinc; other studies have found no inhibition)

### Laboratory value alterations

The following have been selected on the basis of their potential clinical significance (possible effect in parentheses where appropriate)—not necessarily inclusive (» = major clinical significance):

With physiology/laboratory test values

Vitamin $B_{12}$ concentrations in blood

(may be reduced by large and continuous doses of folic acid)

### Medical considerations/Contraindications

The medical considerations/contraindications included here have been selected on the basis of their potential clinical significance (reasons given in parentheses where appropriate)—not necessarily inclusive (» = major clinical significance).

*Risk-benefit should be considered when the following medical problems exist:*

» Pernicious anemia

(folic acid will correct hematologic abnormalities but neurologic problems will progress irreversibly; doses of folic acid greater than 0.4 mg per day are not recommended until pernicious anemia has been ruled out, except during pregnancy and lactation)

Sensitivity to folic acid

## Side/Adverse Effects

Note: No side effects other than an allergic reaction have been reported with folic acid administration, even at doses of up to 10 times the recommended dietary allowances (RDA) for 1 month.

The following side/adverse effects have been selected on the basis of their potential clinical significance (possible signs and symptoms in parentheses where appropriate)—not necessarily inclusive:

**Those indicating need for medical attention**
Incidence rare
*Allergic reaction, specifically; bronchospasm* (shortness of breath; troubled breathing; tightness of chest; wheezing); *erythema* (reddened skin); *fever; skin rash or itching*

## Patient Consultation

As an aid to patient consultation, refer to *Advice for the Patient, Folic Acid (Vitamin B₉) (Systemic).*

In providing consultation, consider emphasizing the following selected information (» = major clinical significance):

**Description of use**
Description should include function in the body, signs of deficiency, and unproven uses

**Importance of diet**
Importance of proper nutrition; supplement may be needed because of inadequate dietary intake
Food sources of folic acid; effects of processing
Not using vitamins as substitute for balanced diet
Recommended daily intake for folic acid

**Before using this dietary supplement**
» Conditions affecting use, especially:
Other medical problems, especially pernicious anemia

**Proper use of this dietary supplement**
» Proper dosing
Missed dose: No cause for concern because of length of time necessary for depletion; remembering to take as directed
» Proper storage

**Side/adverse effects**
Signs of potential side effects, especially allergic reaction

## General Dosing Information

Because of the infrequency of single B vitamin deficiencies, combinations are commonly administered. Many commercial combinations of B vitamins are available.

**For parenteral dosage forms only**
In most cases, parenteral administration is indicated only when oral administration is not acceptable (for example, in nausea, vomiting, preoperative and postoperative conditions) or possible (for example, in malabsorption syndromes or following gastric resection).

**Diet/Nutrition**
Recommended dietary intakes for folic acid are defined differently worldwide.
For U.S.—

The Recommended Dietary Allowances (RDAs) for vitamins and minerals are determined by the Food and Nutrition Board of the National Research Council and are intended to provide adequate nutrition in most healthy persons under usual environmental stresses. In addition, a different designation may be used by the FDA for food and dietary supplement labeling purposes, as with Daily Value (DV). DVs replace the previous labeling terminology United States Recommended Daily Allowances (USRDAs).

For Canada—

Recommended Nutrient Intakes (RNIs) for vitamins, minerals, and protein are determined by Health and Welfare Canada and provide recommended amounts of a specific nutrient while minimizing the risk of chronic diseases.

Daily recommended intakes for folic acid are generally defined as follows:

| Persons | U.S. (mcg) | Canada (mcg) |
|---|---|---|
| Infants and children | | |
| Birth to 3 years of age | 25–50 | 50–80 |
| 4 to 6 years of age | 75 | 90 |
| 7 to 10 years of age | 100 | 125–180 |
| Adolescent and adult males | 150–200 | 150–220 |
| Adolescent and adult females | 150–180 | 145–190 |
| Pregnant females | 400 | 445–475 |
| Breast-feeding females | 260–280 | 245–275 |

These are usually provided by adequate diets.

Best dietary sources of folic acid include vegetables, especially green vegetables; potatoes; cereal and cereal products; fruits; and organ meats (liver, kidney). Heat destroys folic acid (50 to 90%) in foods.

## Oral Dosage Forms

Note: Bracketed uses in the *Dosage Forms* section refer to categories of use and/or indications that are not included in U.S. product labeling.

### FOLIC ACID TABLETS USP

**Usual adult and adolescent dose**
Deficiency (prophylaxis)—
Oral, amount based on normal daily recommended intakes:

| Persons | U.S. (mcg) | Canada (mcg) |
|---|---|---|
| Adolescent and adult males | 150–200 | 150–220 |
| Adolescent and adult females | 150–180 | 145–190 |
| Pregnant females | 400 | 445–475 |
| Breast-feeding females | 260–280 | 245–275 |

Deficiency (treatment)—
    Treatment dose is individualized by prescriber based on severity of deficiency.

[Diagnostic aid (folate deficiency)][1]—
    Oral, 100 to 200 mcg (0.1 to 0.2 mg) a day for ten days plus low dietary folic acid and vitamin $B_{12}$.

### Usual pediatric dose

Deficiency (prophylaxis)—
    Oral, amount based on normal daily recommended intakes:

| Persons | U.S. (mcg) | Canada (mcg) |
|---|---|---|
| Infants and children | | |
| Birth to 3 years of age | 25–50 | 50–80 |
| 4 to 6 years of age | 75 | 90 |
| 7 to 10 years of age | 100 | 125–180 |

Deficiency (treatment)—
    Treatment dose is individualized by prescriber based on severity of deficiency.

### Strength(s) usually available

U.S.—
    100 mcg (Rx) [GENERIC].
    400 mcg (Rx) [GENERIC].
    800 mcg (Rx) [GENERIC].
    1 mg (Rx) [*Folvite;* GENERIC].

Canada—
    5 mg (Rx) [*Apo-Folic* (scored); *Folvite* (scored); *Novo-Folacid;* GENERIC].

Note: Some strengths of these folic acid preparations may exceed the dosage range recommended by USP DI Advisory Panels based on the amount necessary to meet normal nutritional needs.

### Packaging and storage

Store below 40 °C (104 °F), preferably between 15 and 30 °C (59 and 86 °F), unless otherwise specified by manufacturer. Store in a well-closed container.

## Parenteral Dosage Forms

Note: Bracketed uses in the *Dosage Forms* section refer to categories of use and/or indications that are not included in U.S. product labeling.

### FOLIC ACID INJECTION USP

#### Usual adult and adolescent dose

Deficiency (prophylaxis)—
    Intravenous infusion, as part of total parenteral nutrition solutions, the specific amount determined by individual patient need.

Deficiency (treatment)—
    Intramuscular, intravenous, or deep subcutaneous: 250 mcg (0.25 mg) to 1 mg a day until a hematologic response occurs.

[Diagnostic aid (folate deficiency)][1]—
    Intramuscular, 100 to 200 mcg (0.1 to 0.2 mg) a day for ten days plus low dietary folic acid and vitamin $B_{12}$.

#### Usual pediatric dose

See *Usual adult and adolescent dose.*

Note: Folic acid injection that contains benzyl alcohol as a preservative should not be used in newborn and immature infants. The use of benzyl alcohol in neonates has been associated with a fatal toxic syndrome consisting of metabolic acidosis and CNS, respiratory, circulatory, and renal function impairment.

#### Strength(s) usually available

U.S.—
    5 mg (base) per mL (Rx) [*Folvite* (benzyl alcohol 1.5%); GENERIC].
    10 mg per mL (Rx) [GENERIC].

Canada—
    5 mg (base) per mL (Rx) [*Folvite*].

#### Packaging and storage

Store below 40 °C (104 °F), preferably between 15 and 30 °C (59 and 86 °F), unless otherwise specified by manufacturer. Protect from light. Protect from freezing.

---

[1]Not included in Canadian product labeling.

---

Revised: 05/20/92
Interim revision: 08/17/94; 05/01/95

---

# FOSCARNET    Systemic†

VA CLASSIFICATION (Primary): AM800
Other commonly used names are PFA, phosphonoformic acid, and trisodium phosphonoformate.

Note: For a listing of dosage forms and brand names by country availability, see *Dosage Forms* section(s). For a listing of brand names for the articles in this monograph, refer to the General Index.

†Not commercially available in Canada.

---

## Category

Antiviral (systemic).

## Indications

Note: Bracketed information in the *Indications* section refers to uses that are not included in U.S. product labeling.

### Accepted

Cytomegalovirus retinitis (treatment)—Foscarnet is indicated in the treatment of cytomegalovirus (CMV) retinitis in patients with acquired immunodeficiency syndrome (AIDS).

[Cytomegalovirus disease (treatment)]—Foscarnet is used in the treatment of severe, life-threatening CMV disease, including CMV pneumonia, CMV gastrointestinal disease, and disseminated CMV infections, in immunocompromised patients.

[Herpes simplex (treatment)]—Foscarnet is used in the treatment of acyclovir-resistant mucocutaneous herpes simplex virus (HSV-1 and HSV-2) infections in human immunodeficiency virus (HIV)-infected patients.

[Varicella-zoster (treatment)]—Foscarnet is used in the treatment of acyclovir-resistant varicella-zoster virus infection in HIV-infected patients.

### Unaccepted

Foscarnet is not active against bacteria or mycoplasma.

## Pharmacology/Pharmacokinetics

### Physicochemical characteristics

Molecular weight—Foscarnet sodium hexahydrate: 300.1.

### Mechanism of action/Effect

Virostatic. Foscarnet inhibits viral replication by noncompetitively blocking the pyrophosphate binding site of viral DNA polymerase, preventing cleavage of pyrophosphate from deoxynucleoside triphosphate and elongation of the viral DNA chain. Unlike acyclovir and ganciclovir, foscarnet does not require viral thymidine kinase for activation. Viral replication resumes after foscarnet is discontinued.

### Other actions/effects

*In vitro* studies show that foscarnet inhibits the viral replication of all known herpes viruses—herpes simplex virus (HSV-1 and HSV-2), varicella-zoster, Epstein-Barr virus, human herpesvirus 6 (HHV-6), and cytomegalovirus. It has also been found to noncompetitively inhibit human immunodeficiency virus (HIV) reverse transcriptase and hepatitis B virus DNA polymerase. However, the use of foscarnet in clinical practice for many of these viral infections has not been fully evaluated.

Foscarnet is also a specific competitive inhibitor of the sodium-phosphate cotransport by renal cortical brush border membrane vesicles. The inhibition is dose-dependent and specific for phosphate, which may decrease the tubular reabsorption and thus increase renal excretion of phosphate.

### Absorption

Foscarnet is poorly absorbed after oral administration; bioavailability ranges from 12 to 22%.

### Distribution

Foscarnet is sequestered into bone and cartilage; however, the extent to which this occurs is not known. Cerebrospinal fluid (CSF) concentration was approximately 43% (13 to 68%) of plasma concentration in HIV-infected patients receiving a continuous intravenous infusion;

other CSF-to-plasma ratios have been 35 to 103%; variable penetration may be due to disease-related defects in the blood-brain barrier.
Vol$_D$ =0.3 to 0.7 L per kg.

**Protein binding**
14 to 17%.

**Biotransformation**
Not metabolized.

**Half-life**
Normal renal function—
    Distribution: 0.4 to 1.4 hours.
    Elimination: 3.3 to 6.8 hours.
    Terminal: 18 to 88 hours.
Renal function impairment—
    Prolonged.

**Time to peak concentration**
End of infusion.

**Peak serum concentration**
Approximately 575 micromoles per L on both days 1 and 14 or 15 after administration of 57 (on day 1) and 47 mg (on days 14 or 15) per kg of body weight (mg/kg), infused over 1 hour, every 8 hours.

**Elimination**
Renal; approximately 80 to 87% excreted unchanged in the urine; in one study, glomerular filtration accounted for 44% of total renal excretion, and net tubular secretion accounted for 56%. Tubular reabsorption may also occur. Apparent extrarenal clearance reflects the uptake of foscarnet into bone matrix.
Dialysis—Foscarnet is cleared through hemodialysis; clearance is approximately 80 mL per minute.

## Precautions to Consider

### Carcinogenicity
No evidence of carcinogenicity was found in rats and mice given oral doses of 500 mg per kg of body weight (mg/kg) per day and 250 mg/kg per day, respectively, resulting in plasma concentrations equal to one-third and one-fifth of those in humans as measured by area under the plasma concentration time curve (AUC).

### Mutagenicity
Foscarnet was found to be genotoxic in the BALB/3T3 *in vitro* transformation assay at concentrations greater than 0.5 mcg per mL; there was also an increased frequency of chromosome aberrations in the sister chromatid exchange assay at 1000 mcg per mL. Foscarnet caused an increase in micronucleated polychromatic erythrocytes *in vivo* in mice at doses (350 mg/kg) that produced exposures (AUC) comparable to those anticipated clinically.

### Pregnancy/Reproduction
Fertility—Foscarnet did not adversely affect the fertility and general reproductive performance of rats; however, because of the doses used, these studies do not adequately define the potential for fertility impairment at human doses.

Pregnancy—It is not known whether foscarnet crosses the placenta. Studies in humans have not been done.
A slight increase (< 5%) in the number of skeletal anomalies compared with controls was seen in female rats given daily subcutaneous doses of up to 75 mg/kg administered prior to and during mating, during gestation, and 21 days postpartum. An increase in the frequency of skeletal anomalies/variations was found in rats and rabbits given daily subcutaneous doses of up to 75 mg/kg and 150 mg/kg, respectively. On the basis of estimated drug exposure (AUC), these doses were approximately one-eighth (rat) and one-third (rabbit) the estimated maximal daily human exposure. These studies are inadequate to define the potential teratogenicity at levels to which women will be exposed.

FDA Pregnancy Category C.

### Breast-feeding
It is not known whether foscarnet is distributed into human breast milk. However, in lactating rats administered 75 mg/kg, foscarnet was distributed into milk at concentrations 3 times higher than peak maternal blood concentrations.

### Pediatrics
No information is available on the relationship of age to the effects of foscarnet in pediatric patients. Safety and efficacy have not been established. Post mortem data show that foscarnet is deposited in the bones of human adults; 40% of an intravenous dose is also deposited in the teeth and bones of young and growing animals; therefore, it is likely that foscarnet also will deposit in developing bone in children.

### Geriatrics
No information is available on the relationship of age to the effects of foscarnet in geriatric patients. However, elderly patients are more likely to have age-related renal function impairment, which may require adjustment of dosage or dosing interval in patients receiving foscarnet.

### Drug interactions and/or related problems
The following drug interactions and/or related problems have been selected on the basis of their potential clinical significance (possible mechanism in parentheses where appropriate)—not necessarily inclusive (» = major clinical significance):

Note: Combinations containing any of the following medications, depending on the amount present, may also interact with this medication.

» Nephrotoxic medications, other (See *Appendix II*)
    (concurrent use of foscarnet with other nephrotoxic drugs, such as aminoglycosides or amphotericin B, may increase the risk of renal toxicity)

» Pentamidine
    (concurrent use of foscarnet with intravenous pentamidine may result in severe but reversible hypocalcemia, hypomagnesemia, and nephrotoxicity)

Zidovudine
    (concurrent use of foscarnet with zidovudine may produce an additive effect, increasing the risk of anemia; however, there is no evidence of increased myelosuppression when these 2 drugs are used concurrently)

### Laboratory value alterations
The following have been selected on the basis of their potential clinical significance (possible effect in parentheses where appropriate)—not necessarily inclusive (» = major clinical significance):

With physiology/laboratory test values
    Alanine aminotransferase (ALT [SGPT]) and
    Alkaline phosphatase and
    Aspartate aminotransferase (AST [SGOT]) and
    Bilirubin, serum
        (values may be increased)

» Calcium, ionized, serum and
» Calcium, total, serum and
» Phosphate, serum
    (concentrations of phosphate may be increased or decreased; concentrations of total calcium may be decreased; although the total calcium concentration may also appear normal, the level of ionized calcium may be decreased and result in symptomatic hypocalcemia)

» Creatinine, serum
    (concentration may be increased)

» Magnesium, serum
    (concentration may be decreased)

Potassium, serum
    (concentration may be decreased)

### Medical considerations/Contraindications
The medical considerations/contraindications included here have been selected on the basis of their potential clinical significance (reasons given in parentheses where appropriate)—not necessarily inclusive (» = major clinical significance).

#### Risk-benefit should be considered when the following medical problems exist:
Anemia
    (foscarnet may cause a decrease in hemoglobin concentration, worsening pre-existing anemia)

» Dehydration
    (to help avoid renal toxicity, patients must be well hydrated both before and during treatment with foscarnet)

Hypersensitivity to foscarnet

» Renal function impairment
    (because foscarnet is nephrotoxic and is excreted through the kidneys, patients with renal function impairment must receive a reduction in dosage or dosing interval)

### Patient monitoring
The following may be especially important in patient monitoring (other tests may be warranted in some patients, depending on condition; » = major clinical significance):

» Calcium, ionized and total, serum and
» Magnesium, serum and

» Phosphate, serum and
  Potassium, serum
    (should be monitored 2 to 3 times a week during induction, and
    once a week during maintenance therapy; total serum calcium lev-
    els may appear normal in some patients; however, ionized calcium
    levels may be decreased, resulting in symptoms of hypocalcemia,
    such as perioral tingling, numbness in the extremities and pares-
    thesias; there is an inverse linear relationship between the plasma
    foscarnet concentration and ionized calcium, not seen with total
    calcium concentrations; this is thought to be due to foscarnet com-
    plexing with ionized calcium; if abnormal neurologic or cardiac
    events occur, ionized calcium levels ideally should be measured at
    the end of the foscarnet infusion)

    (decreases in magnesium and potassium, and an increase and de-
    crease in calcium and phosphate have been observed; this may be
    a result of foscarnet replacing phosphate in the bone or of foscarnet
    inhibiting the tubular reabsorption of phosphate)

  Complete blood counts (CBCs)
    (foscarnet may cause a decrease in serum hemoglobin concentra-
    tions, resulting in anemia; there have also been rare reports of
    thrombocytopenia and leukopenia)

» Ophthalmologic examinations
    (ophthalmologic examinations should be performed at the start of
    treatment, at the conclusion of induction, and every 4 weeks during
    maintenance; since foscarnet is virostatic and not a cure for cyto-
    megalovirus [CMV] retinitis, progression of retinitis is expected to
    eventually occur during or following foscarnet treatment; exami-
    nations during maintenance therapy should be more frequent if
    there is residual disease activity [whitening of lesion borders] or
    if lesions are close to the macula or optic nerve head; in selected
    cases, examinations could be less frequent if lesions are completely
    inactive and located only in the peripheral retina)

» Renal function tests
    (blood urea nitrogen and serum creatinine concentrations should
    be monitored at least 2 to 3 times a week during induction, and at
    least once a week during maintenance therapy since foscarnet is
    nephrotoxic and patients with renal function impairment will re-
    quire an adjustment in dosage or discontinuation of the drug)

## Side/Adverse Effects

Note: Renal function impairment is the major dose-limiting side effect of
      foscarnet therapy. Acute tubular necrosis is the most common type
      of nephrotoxicity; however, nephrogenic diabetes insipidus and fos-
      carnet crystal formation in the glomerular capillary lumen have also
      been described. Hydration with 0.5 to 1 liter of 0.9% sodium chlo-
      ride per dose, throughout the course of foscarnet treatment, has
      been found to lessen the nephrotoxic effects.

The following side/adverse effects have been selected on the basis of their
potential clinical significance (possible signs and symptoms in parentheses where appropriate)—not necessarily inclusive:

**Those indicating need for medical attention**
Incidence more frequent
  *Nephrotoxicity* (decreased urination, or increased thirst and urination)
Incidence less frequent
  *Anemia* (unusual tiredness and weakness); *granulocytopenia or leu-
  kopenia* (fever, chills, or sore throat); *neurotoxicity* (muscle twitching;
  tremor; seizures; tingling sensation around mouth; pain or numbness
  in hands or feet); *phlebitis* (pain at site of injection)
  Note: *Anemia* was reported in 33% of 189 patients in the 5 controlled
        U.S. clinical trials. Only 1 patient required discontinuation of
        drug.

        *Granulocytopenia or leukopenia* was reported in 17% of 189
        patients in the 5 controlled U.S. clinical trials. Only 2 patients
        required discontinuation of drug.

        *Neurotoxicity* may be related to drug-induced alterations in se-
        rum minerals and electrolytes, especially a decrease in ionized
        calcium concentrations.

Incidence rare
  *Sores or ulcers of the mouth or throat, penis, or vulva*
**Those indicating need for medical attention only if they continue
or are bothersome**
Incidence more frequent
  *Gastrointestinal disturbances* (abdominal pain; anorexia; nausea and
  vomiting); *neurotoxicity* (anxiety; confusion; dizziness; fatigue;
  headache)

## Patient Consultation

As an aid to patient consultation, refer to *Advice for the Patient, Foscarnet
(Systemic)*.

In providing consultation, consider emphasizing the following selected
information (» = major clinical significance):

**Before using this medication**
» Conditions affecting use, especially:
    Hypersensitivity to foscarnet
    Other medications, especially other nephrotoxic medications or
      pentamidine
    Other medical problems, especially dehydration or renal function
      impairment

**Proper use of this medication**
» Importance of receiving medication for full course of therapy and on
    a regular schedule
» Maintaining adequate fluid intake
    Washing genitals after urination to decrease risk of genital ulceration
» Proper dosing

**Precautions while using this medication**
» Regular visits to ophthalmologist to examine eyes since progression
    of retinitis and visual loss may occur during foscarnet therapy
**Side/adverse effects**
  Signs of potential side effects, especially nephrotoxicity, anemia, gran-
  ulocytopenia, leukopenia, neurotoxicity, phlebitis, and sores or ul-
  cers of the mouth or throat, penis, or vulva

## General Dosing Information

Foscarnet must be administered at a constant rate by an infusion pump
and must not be administered by rapid intravenous injection. Rapid
administration may result in excessive plasma levels of foscarnet and
increased risk of acute hypocalcemia or other toxicity. Doses of 60
mg per kg of body weight (mg/kg) or less may be infused over 1 hour;
higher doses should be infused over at least a 2-hour period. The
recommended dosage, frequency, or infusion rate should not be
exceeded.

Patients must be adequately hydrated during treatment to avoid
nephrotoxicity.

Foscarnet may be administered undiluted (24 mg/mL) but only through a
central venous line. When a peripheral vein is used, the solution must
be diluted to 12 mg/mL (1:1) with 5% dextrose in water or 0.9%
sodium chloride for injection prior to administration to avoid local
irritation of peripheral veins.

Intravitreal administration of foscarnet has been used in patients with a
history of intolerance to acyclovir and advanced renal function impairment. Intravitreal doses of 1200 to 2400 mcg of undiluted foscarnet (0.05 mL) were injected into the eye 6 times at 72-hour intervals,
followed by a single, weekly maintenance injection. Intravitreal administration has resulted in improvement of patients' visual acuity and
appeared to be well tolerated. The elimination half-life of foscarnet
from the vitreous fluid was estimated to be approximately 32 hours,
and the intravitreal concentration was calculated to remain above the
mean 50% inhibition level for cytomegalovirus for approximately 41
hours after a single injection.

## Parenteral Dosage Forms

Note: Bracketed uses in the *Dosage Forms* section refer to categories of
      use and/or indications that are not included in U.S. product labeling.

### FOSCARNET SODIUM INJECTION

**Usual adult and adolescent dose**
Cytomegalovirus (CMV) retinitis—
  Induction:
    Intravenous infusion, 60 mg per kg of body weight, administered
    over at least 1 hour with an infusion pump, every eight hours
    for fourteen to twenty-one days, depending on the clinical
    response.
  Note: Induction doses of 90 and 100 mg per kg of body weight
        every twelve hours also have been used; dosing twice a day
        was found to be as effective as the three-times-a-day dosing,
        and was more convenient.

Adults with impaired renal function require a reduction in dose as follows:

| Creatinine clearance (mL/min/kg)/ (mL/sec/kg) | Equivalent to 60 mg/kg dose every 8 hours |
|---|---|
| ≥1.6/0.027 | 60 |
| 1.5/0.025 | 57 |
| 1.4/0.023 | 53 |
| 1.3/0.022 | 49 |
| 1.2/0.020 | 46 |
| 1.1/0.018 | 42 |
| 1.0/0.017 | 39 |
| 0.9/0.015 | 35 |
| 0.8/0.013 | 32 |
| 0.7/0.012 | 28 |
| 0.6/0.010 | 25 |
| 0.5/0.008 | 21 |
| 0.4/0.007 | 18 |

Maintenance:

Intravenous infusion, 90 to 120 mg per kg of body weight, administered over 2 hours with an infusion pump, once a day.

Note: It is recommended that most patients be started on maintenance treatment with a dose of 90 mg per kg of body weight per day since the superiority of 120 mg per kg of body weight per day has not been established in controlled trials, and higher plasma levels may lead to increased toxicity. Treatment with 120 mg per kg of body weight per day may be considered if early reinduction is required because of retinitis progression. Patients who show excellent tolerance to foscarnet may benefit from a maintenance dose of 120 mg per kg of body weight per day early in their treatment.

If CMV retinitis progresses during maintenance therapy, patients should be retreated with the induction regimen.

Adults with impaired renal function receiving a 90 mg per kg of body weight maintenance dose require a reduction in dose as follows:

| Creatinine clearance (mL/min/kg)/ (mL/sec/kg) | Equivalent to 90 mg/kg dose every 24 hours |
|---|---|
| ≥1.4/0.023 | 90 |
| 1.2–1.4/0.020–0.023 | 78 |
| 1.0–1.2/0.017–0.020 | 75 |
| 0.8–1.0/0.013–0.017 | 71 |
| 0.6–0.8/0.010–0.013 | 63 |
| 0.4–0.6/0.007–0.010 | 57 |

Adults with impaired renal function receiving a 120 mg per kg of body weight maintenance dose require a reduction in dose as follows:

| Creatinine clearance (mL/min/kg)/ (mL/sec/kg) | Equivalent to 120 mg/kg dose every 24 hours |
|---|---|
| ≥1.4/0.023 | 120 |
| 1.2–1.4/0.020–0.023 | 104 |
| 1.0–1.2/0.017–0.020 | 100 |
| 0.8–1.0/0.013–0.017 | 94 |
| 0.6–0.8/0.010–0.013 | 84 |
| 0.4–0.6/0.007–0.010 | 76 |

[Herpes simplex (treatment)] and [Varicella-zoster (treatment)]—

Intravenous infusion, 40 mg per kg of body weight, administered over at least 1 hour with an infusion pump, every eight hours for four-teen to twenty-one days, depending on the clinical response. The dose should be adjusted if the calculated creatinine clearance is less than 1.6 mL per kg of body weight.

**Usual pediatric dose**
See *Usual adult and adolescent dose.*

**Strength(s) usually available**
U.S.—
6000 mg in 250 mL (Rx) [*Foscavir*].
12,000 mg in 500 mL (Rx) [*Foscavir*].
Canada—
Not commercially available.

**Packaging and storage**
Store below 40 °C (104 °F), preferably between 15 and 30 °C (59 and 86 °F), unless otherwise specified by manufacturer. Do not freeze. Refrigeration of stock or diluted solutions may result in crystallization of drug.

**Preparation of dosage form**
Undiluted foscarnet (24 mg per mL) can only be administered through a central line due to its potential for causing venous irritation.

For peripheral administration, dilute stock solution of foscarnet with an equal amount (1:1) of 5% dextrose injection or 0.9% sodium chloride injection, for a final concentration of 12 mg per mL. After calculation of the dose, based on body weight, it is advisable to remove and discard any excess foscarnet from the bottle before starting the infusion, to avoid accidental overdosage.

**Stability**
Undiluted foscarnet is stable for 24 months at 25 °C.

Because foscarnet contains no preservatives, diluted foscarnet should be discarded after 24 hours.

Foscarnet must not be frozen because precipitation is likely to occur. Any drug that has been frozen must be discarded.

**Incompatibilities**
Foscarnet must not be mixed with anything other than 5% dextrose injection or 0.9% sodium chloride injection. It is incompatible with 30% dextrose injection, lactated Ringer's solution, or any solution containing calcium.

Foscarnet has been found to precipitate immediately with acyclovir, amphotericin B, ganciclovir, pentamidine isethionate, trimethoprim-sulfamethoxazole, trimetrexate, and vancomycin. Delayed precipitation was observed when foscarnet was combined with dobutamine hydrochloride, droperidol, and haloperidol. Gas production was observed when foscarnet was combined with diazepam, digoxin, lorazepam, midazolam, and promethazine hydrochloride. Cloudiness and/or color change was observed when foscarnet was combined with diphenhydramine hydrochloride, leucovorin calcium, and prochlorperazine.

## Selected Bibliography
Minor JR, Baltz JK. Foscarnet sodium. DICP, Ann Pharmacother 1991; 25: 41-7.
Chrisp P, Clissold SP. Foscarnet. Drugs 1991; 41 (1): 104-29.

Revised: 07/22/94

**FOSINOPRIL**—See *Angiotensin-converting Enzyme (ACE) Inhibitors (Systemic)*

# FRUCTOSE, DEXTROSE, AND PHOSPHORIC ACID    Oral-Local

VA CLASSIFICATION (Primary): GA700

Note: For a listing of dosage forms and brand names by country availability, see *Dosage Forms* section(s). For a listing of brand names for the articles in this monograph, refer to the General Index.

## Category
Antiemetic.

## Indications

### Accepted
Fructose, dextrose, and phosphoric acid oral solution is used for the symptomatic relief of nausea and vomiting. However, to date, there is insufficient evidence to establish effectiveness (FDA Category III).

## Pharmacology/Pharmacokinetics

### Physicochemical characteristics
Molecular weight—
    Fructose: 180.16.
    Dextrose: 198.17.
    Phosphoric acid: 98.0.

### Mechanism of action/Effect
Exact mechanism has not been determined. Appears to have a direct local action on the wall of the gastrointestinal tract that reduces smooth muscle contraction and delays gastric emptying time through the high osmotic pressure exerted by the solution of simple sugars. Phosphoric acid is added to adjust pH to between 1.5 and 1.6.

### Absorption
Fructose—Slowly absorbed from gastrointestinal tract.
Dextrose—Rapidly absorbed from gastrointestinal tract.

### Biotransformation
Fructose—Hepatic, by phosphorylation; partly converted to liver glycogen and glucose.
Dextrose—Hepatic; metabolized to carbon dioxide and water.

## Precautions to Consider

### Pregnancy/Reproduction
Pregnancy—Studies have not been done in humans.
Studies have not been done in animals.

### Breast-feeding
Problems in humans have not been documented.

### Pediatrics
In infants and children up to 3 years of age with vomiting, caution is recommended because of the risk of fluid and electrolyte loss; these patients should be referred to a physician.

### Geriatrics
In geriatric patients with vomiting, caution is recommended because of the risk of fluid and electrolyte loss; these patients should be referred to a physician.

### Laboratory value alterations
The following have been selected on the basis of their potential clinical significance (possible effect in parentheses where appropriate)—not necessarily inclusive (» = major clinical significance):
With physiology/laboratory test values
    Glucose
      (blood concentrations may be elevated)

### Medical considerations/Contraindications
The medical considerations/contraindications included here have been selected on the basis of their potential clinical significance (reasons given in parentheses where appropriate)—not necessarily inclusive (» = major clinical significance).

*Except under special circumstances, this medication should not be used when the following medical problems exist:*
»  Appendicitis, symptoms of or
»  Inflamed bowel, symptoms of
    (proper diagnosis required or severe condition may develop)
»  Fructose intolerance, hereditary
    (severe side effects may occur)

*Risk-benefit should be considered when the following medical problems exist:*
»  Diabetes mellitus
    (condition may be aggravated because of solution's high carbohydrate content)
Intolerance to dextrose or phosphoric acid

## Side/Adverse Effects
The following side/adverse effects have been selected on the basis of their potential clinical significance (possible signs and symptoms in parentheses where appropriate)—not necessarily inclusive:

### Those indicating need for medical attention
Incidence rare
    *Fructose intolerance* (fainting; swelling of face, arms, and legs; unusual bleeding; vomiting; weight loss; yellow eyes or skin)

### Those indicating need for medical attention only if they continue or are bothersome
Incidence less frequent—more frequent with large doses
    *Diarrhea; stomach or abdominal pain*

## Patient Consultation
As an aid to patient consultation, refer to *Advice for the Patient, Fructose, Dextrose, and Phosphoric Acid (Oral).*

In providing consultation, consider emphasizing the following selected information (» = major clinical significance):

### Before using this medication
»  Conditions affecting use, especially:
    Intolerance to fructose, dextrose, or phosphoric acid
    Use in children—Risk of fluid and electrolyte loss due to vomiting
    Use in the elderly—Risk of fluid and electrolyte loss due to vomiting
    Other medical problems, especially diabetes mellitus, symptoms of appendicitis, or inflamed bowel

### Proper use of this medication
    Following physician's or manufacturer's instructions
    Not diluting or taking fluids before or after dose
»  Proper dosing
»  Proper storage

### Precautions while using this medication
»  Checking with physician if symptoms do not improve or become worse
»  Not taking if symptoms of appendicitis or inflamed bowel are present; checking with physician for proper diagnosis

### Side/adverse effects
Signs of potential side effects, especially fructose intolerance

## General Dosing Information
The fructose, dextrose, and phosphoric acid oral solution should not be diluted. Also, oral fluids should not be taken immediately before or for at least 15 minutes after the dose.

## Oral Dosage Forms

### FRUCTOSE, DEXTROSE, AND PHOSPHORIC ACID ORAL SOLUTION

#### Usual adult and adolescent dose
Antiemetic—Oral, 15 to 30 mL. Dose may be repeated every fifteen minutes until distress subsides, but should not be taken for more than one hour (five doses) without consulting a physician.

Note: For morning sickness, dose should be taken on arising and repeated every three hours as needed.

#### Usual pediatric dose
Antiemetic—
    Children up to 3 years of age: Use is not recommended.
    Children over 3 years of age: Oral, 5 to 10 mL. Dose may be repeated every fifteen minutes until distress subsides, but should not be taken for more than one hour (five doses) without consulting a physician.

#### Usual geriatric dose
See *Usual adult and adolescent dose.*

## Strength(s) usually available

U.S.—

1.87 grams of fructose, 1.87 grams of dextrose, and 21.5 mg of phosphoric acid, per 5 mL (OTC) [*Emetrol*].

Canada—

1.87 grams of fructose, 1.87 grams of dextrose, and 21.5 mg of phosphoric acid, per 5 mL (OTC) [*Emetrol*].

## Packaging and storage

Store below 40 °C (104 °F), preferably between 15 and 30 °C (59 and 86 °F), in a well-closed container, unless otherwise specified by manufacturer. Protect from freezing.

Revised: 05/12/93

# FURAZOLIDONE   Oral-Local†

VA CLASSIFICATION (Primary/Secondary): AM600/AP109

Note: For a listing of dosage forms and brand names by country availability, see *Dosage Forms* section(s). For a listing of brand names for the articles in this monograph, refer to the General Index.

†Not commercially available in Canada.

## Category

Antibacterial (oral-local); antiprotozoal.

Note: Furazolidone is a broad-spectrum anti-infective that is effective against most gastrointestinal tract pathogens.

## Indications

### Accepted

Cholera (treatment)—Furazolidone is indicated as a secondary agent in the treatment of cholera caused by *Vibrio cholerae (V. comma)*.

Diarrhea, bacterial (treatment)—Furazolidone is indicated as a secondary agent in the treatment of bacterial diarrhea caused by susceptible organisms. Furazolidone is active *in vitro* against *Campylobacter jejuni, Enterobacter aerogenes, Escherichia coli, Proteus* species, *Salmonella* species, *Shigella* species, and staphylococci. However, clinical studies on the effectiveness of furazolidone in some types of bacterial diarrhea have been inconclusive or conflicting.

Giardiasis (treatment)—Furazolidone is indicated as a secondary agent in the treatment of giardiasis caused by *Giardia lamblia*.

Not all species or strains of a particular organism may be susceptible to furazolidone.

## Pharmacology/Pharmacokinetics

### Physicochemical characteristics

Molecular weight—225.16.

### Mechanism of action/Effect

Microbicidal. Furazolidone interferes with several bacterial enzyme systems. It neither significantly alters normal bowel flora nor results in fungal overgrowth.

### Other actions/effects

Furazolidone also acts as a monoamine oxidase inhibitor (MAOI). MAOIs prevent the inactivation of tyramine by hepatic and gastrointestinal monoamine oxidase. Tyramine in the bloodstream releases norepinephrine from the sympathetic nerve terminals and produces a sudden increase in blood pressure.

### Absorption

Radiolabeled drug studies indicate that furazolidone is well absorbed following oral administration.

### Distribution

Limited pharmacokinetic information is available in humans; however, recent data have reported that variable plasma concentrations were measured in subjects given therapeutic doses. One study of 8 meningitis patients showed that cerebral spinal fluid (CSF) concentrations reached levels comparable to serum concentrations. Also, significant concentrations have been measured in the bile of rats.

### Biotransformation

Furazolidone is rapidly and extensively metabolized; the primary metabolic pathway identified begins with nitro-reduction to the aminofuran derivative.

### Elimination

Radiolabeled drug studies showed that more than 65% of an oral dose was recovered in the urine of humans and animals. Also found in feces.

## Precautions to Consider

### Cross-sensitivity and/or related problems

Patients hypersensitive to other nitrofurans may be hypersensitive to this medication also.

### Carcinogenicity/Tumorigenicity

Several studies in rodents, given chronic, high-dose furazolidone orally, have shown that this medication is tumorigenic. Furazolidone has been shown to cause mammary neoplasia in two strains of rats. In addition, furazolidone has been shown to cause pulmonary tumors in mice.

### Pregnancy/Reproduction

Pregnancy—Studies in humans have not been done. However, teratogenic effects on the human fetus or newborn infants have not been reported. Studies in animals have not shown that furazolidone, given in doses far exceeding recommended human doses for long periods of time, causes adverse effects on the fetus.

### Breast-feeding

It is not known whether furazolidone is distributed into breast milk. However, breast-feeding is not recommended in nursing infants up to 1 month of age because of the possibility of hemolytic anemia due to glutathione instability in the early neonatal period.

### Pediatrics

Use of furazolidone is not recommended in infants up to 1 month of age because of the possibility of hemolytic anemia due to immature enzyme systems (glutathione instability) in the early neonatal period.

### Geriatrics

No information is available on the relationship of age to the effects of furazolidone in geriatric patients.

### Drug interactions and/or related problems

The following drug interactions and/or related problems have been selected on the basis of their potential clinical significance (possible mechanism in parentheses where appropriate)—not necessarily inclusive (» = major clinical significance):

Note: Combinations containing any of the following medications, depending on the amount present, may also interact with this medication.

» Alcohol

(concurrent use of alcohol with furazolidone may rarely result in a disulfiram-like reaction, characterized by facial flushing, difficult breathing, slight fever, and tightness of the chest; these effects usually subside spontaneously within 24 hours with no lasting ill effects; patients should be advised not to drink alcoholic beverages while taking furazolidone and for 4 days after discontinuing it)

» Antidepressants, tricyclic or
» Monoamine oxidase (MAO) inhibitors, other or
» Sympathomimetics, direct- or indirect-acting, such as amphetamines, ephedrine, or phenylephrine or
» Tyramine- or other high pressor amine–containing foods and beverages, such as aged cheese; beer; reduced-alcohol and alcohol-free beer and wine; red and white wine; sherry; liqueurs; yeast or protein extracts; fava or broad bean pods; smoked or pickled meat, poultry, or fish; fermented sausage (bologna, pepperoni, salami, summer sausage) or other fermented meat; and any overripe fruit
(concurrent use of these medications, foods, and beverages with furazolidone may theoretically precipitate sudden and severe hypertensive reactions due to furazolidone's MAO inhibitory properties; a dose of 400 mg daily for 5 days was required to experimentally enhance tyramine and amphetamine sensitivity by 2- to 3-fold; this dose does not usually cause an undue risk of hypertensive crises in adults due to MAO inhibition, and no clinical reports of this interaction have been reported; however, if furazolidone is given in larger-than-recommended doses or for more than 5 days, there may be an increased risk of hypertensive crises due to accumulation of monoamine oxidase)

(because of furazolidone's MAO inhibitory properties, dietary restrictions must be continued for at least 2 weeks after the medication is discontinued; other tyramine- or high pressor amine–containing foods, such as yogurt, sour cream, cream cheese, cottage cheese, chocolate, and soy sauce, if eaten when fresh and in moderation, are considered unlikely to cause serious problems)

### Medical considerations/Contraindications
The medical considerations/contraindications included here have been selected on the basis of their potential clinical significance (reasons given in parentheses where appropriate)—not necessarily inclusive (» = major clinical significance).

#### Risk-benefit should be considered when the following medical problems exist:
Glucose-6-phosphate dehydrogenase (G6PD) deficiency
   (mild, reversible, hemolytic anemia may occur in G6PD-deficient patients; it is recommended that furazolidone be discontinued if hemolytic anemia occurs in patients with G6PD deficiency)
Hypersensitivity to furazolidone or other nitrofurans

### Patient monitoring
The following may be especially important in patient monitoring (other tests may be warranted in some patients, depending on condition; » = major clinical significance):

Glucose-6-phosphate dehydrogenase (G6PD) determinations
   (recommended prior to treatment in Caucasians of Mediterranean and Near Eastern origin, Orientals, and blacks; if a deficiency is found, furazolidone should be given with caution since hemolytic effects may be exacerbated in these patients; dosage adjustments and/or discontinuation of the medication may be required)

*For giardiasis*
» Stool examinations
   (3 stool examinations, taken several days apart, beginning 3 to 4 weeks following treatment are recommended if symptoms persist; however, in some successfully treated patients, the lactose intolerance brought on by infection may persist for a period of some weeks or months, mimicking the symptoms of giardiasis; in cases of treatment failure, alternate medications may be used)

## Side/Adverse Effects

Note: Furazolidone may cause mild, reversible hemolytic anemia in G6PD-deficient patients. Furazolidone should be discontinued if hemolytic anemia occurs in these patients.

The following side/adverse effects have been selected on the basis of their potential clinical significance (possible signs and symptoms in parentheses where appropriate)—not necessarily inclusive:

### Those indicating need for medical attention
Incidence rare
   *Hypersensitivity reactions* (fever; itching; joint pain; skin rash or redness)—incidence approximately 0.6%; *leukopenia* (sore throat and fever)—incidence approximately 0.2%

### Those indicating need for medical attention only if they continue or are bothersome
Incidence less frequent
   *Gastrointestinal disturbances* (abdominal pain, diarrhea, nausea, or vomiting); *headache*

### Those not indicating need for medical attention
Incidence more frequent
   *Dark yellow to brown discoloration of urine*

## Patient Consultation

As an aid to patient consultation, refer to *Advice for the Patient, Furazolidone (Oral).*

In providing consultation, consider emphasizing the following selected information (» = major clinical significance):

### Before using this medication
» Conditions affecting use, especially:
   Sensitivity to furazolidone or other nitrofurans
   Breast-feeding—Not recommended in infants up to 1 month of age because of possibility of hemolytic anemia
   Use in children—Not recommended in infants up to 1 month of age because of possibility of hemolytic anemia
   Other medications, especially direct-acting and indirect-acting sympathomimetics, other MAO inhibitors, or tricyclic antidepressants

### Proper use of this medication
» Not giving to infants up to 1 month of age; may cause hemolytic anemia
   May be taken with food to reduce gastrointestinal irritation
   Proper administration technique for oral suspension: Using a specially marked measuring spoon or other device
» Compliance with full course of therapy
» Proper dosing
   Missed dose: Taking as soon as possible; not taking if almost time for next dose; not doubling doses
» Proper storage

### Precautions while using this medication
Regular visits to physician to check progress
Checking with physician if no improvement within a week
» Avoiding alcoholic beverages or other alcohol-containing preparations while taking, and for 4 days after discontinuing, furazolidone
» Avoiding tyramine- and other high pressor amine–containing foods and beverages, OTC appetite suppressants, cough and cold medications, and other medications unless prescribed by physician; also avoiding these products for at least 2 weeks after discontinuing furazolidone; asking health care professional to provide list of products that may or may not cause serious problems with furazolidone

### Side/adverse effects
Signs of potential side effects, especially hypersensitivity reactions and leukopenia
Dark yellow to brown discoloration of urine may be alarming to patient, although medically insignificant

## General Dosing Information

Furazolidone has been used as adjunctive therapy with other antibacterial agents or bismuth salts with no problems reported.

### Diet/Nutrition
Gastrointestinal intolerance may be decreased if furazolidone is taken with food or if the dose is reduced.

After discontinuation of furazolidone, the MAO inhibiting effects may persist for at least 2 weeks. During this time, food, beverage, and medication precautions must be observed by patients receiving larger-than-recommended doses or prolonged therapy (See *Drug interactions and/or related problems*).

### For treatment of adverse effects:
Recommended treatment consists of the following:
   • Administering direct-acting vasopressor agents (e.g., norepinephrine) to counteract hypotensive episodes. Avoiding indirect-acting vasopressor agents.
   • Administering phentolamine or parenteral chlorpromazine to counteract hypertensive crises.

## Oral Dosage Forms

### FURAZOLIDONE ORAL SUSPENSION USP

#### Usual adult and adolescent dose
Cholera or
Diarrhea, bacterial—
   Oral, 100 mg four times a day for five to seven days.
   Note: Some medical experts recommend shorter courses of treatment (e.g., two to five days) for the above-listed infections.
Giardiasis—
Oral, 100 mg four times a day for seven to ten days.

#### Usual pediatric dose
Cholera or
Diarrhea, bacterial—
   Infants up to 1 month of age: Use is not recommended because of the possibility of hemolytic anemia due to immature enzyme systems (glutathione instability) in these infants.
   Infants and children 1 month of age and over: Oral, 1.25 mg per kg of body weight four times a day for five to seven days.
Giardiasis—
   Infants up to 1 month of age: Use is not recommended because of the possibility of hemolytic anemia due to immature enzyme systems (glutathione instability) in these infants.
   Infants and children 1 month of age and over: Oral, 1.25 to 2 mg per kg of body weight four times a day for seven to ten days.
Note: The maximum dose for children should not exceed 8.8 mg per kg of body weight daily because of the possibility of nausea or vomiting.

**Strength(s) usually available**

U.S.—

50 mg per 15 mL (Rx) [*Furoxone Liquid* (methylparaben; propylparaben)].

Canada—

Not commercially available.

**Packaging and storage**

Store below 40 °C (104 °F) in a tight, light-resistant container. Protect from freezing.

**Auxiliary labeling**

- Shake well.
- Avoid alcoholic beverages.
- Continue medication for full time of treatment.
- May discolor urine.

## FURAZOLIDONE TABLETS USP

**Usual adult and adolescent dose**

See *Furazolidone Oral Suspension USP.*

**Usual pediatric dose**

See *Furazolidone Oral Suspension USP.*

**Strength(s) usually available**

U.S.—

100 mg (Rx) [*Furoxone* (scored; sucrose)].

Canada—

Not commercially available.

**Packaging and storage**

Store below 40 °C (104 °F) in a tight, light-resistant container.

**Preparation of dosage form**

*For patients who cannot take oral solids*—Furazolidone tablets may be crushed and given in a teaspoonful of corn syrup.

**Auxiliary labeling**

- Avoid alcoholic beverages.
- Continue medication for full time of treatment.
- May discolor urine.

## Selected Bibliography

Strickland GT, editor. Hunter's tropical medicine. 6th ed. Philadelphia: W. B. Saunders Company, 1984: 279-82, 305-12.

Rabbani GH, Butler T, Shahrier M, et al. Efficacy of a single dose of furazolidone for treatment of cholera in children. Antimicrob Agents Chemother 1991; 35 (9): 1864-7.

Revised: 08/11/95

## FUROSEMIDE—See *Diuretics, Loop (Systemic)*

# GABAPENTIN Systemic

VA CLASSIFICATION (Primary): CN400

Another commonly used name is GBP

Note: For a listing of dosage forms and brand names by country availability, see *Dosage Forms* section(s). For a listing of brand names for the articles in this monograph, refer to the General Index.

## Category

Anticonvulsant.

## Indications

### Accepted

Epilepsy (treatment adjunct)—Gabapentin is indicated as an adjunct to other anticonvulsant medications in the treatment of partial seizures with or without secondary generalization in adults and adolescents over 12 years of age with epilepsy.

## Pharmacology/Pharmacokinetics

### Physicochemical characteristics

Chemical group—Cyclohexane-acetic acid derivative. Structural analog to gamma-aminobutyric acid (GABA).

Molecular weight—171.24.

pKa—3.68 and 10.70.

### Mechanism of action/Effect

The mechanism of action is unknown. Gabapentin does not interact with GABA receptors, is not metabolized to a GABA agonist or to GABA, and does not inhibit GABA uptake or degradation. In rats, gabapentin interacts with a novel binding site on cortical neurons that may be associated with the L-system amino acid transporter of brain cell membranes.

### Absorption

Rapid. Gabapentin is absorbed in part by the L-amino acid transport system, which is a saturable transport system, and as the dose increases, bioavailability decreases. Bioavailability ranges from approximately 60% for a 300 mg dose, to approximately 35% for a 1600 mg dose. Therefore, as the total daily dosage is increased, it may be necessary to divide the total dosage into smaller doses given more frequently. Absorption is unaffected by food.

### Distribution

Volume of distribution ($Vol_D$) is approximately 50 to 60 L Gabapentin penetrates the blood-brain barrier, yielding cerebrospinal fluid (CSF) concentrations approximately equal to 20% of corresponding steady state plasma trough concentrations in patients with epilepsy. Brain tissue concentrations in one patient undergoing temporal lobectomy were approximately 80% of corresponding plasma concentrations.

### Protein binding

Very low (<5%).

### Biotransformation

Gabapentin is not metabolized.

### Half-life

Elimination—

Normal renal function: 5 to 7 hours.

In hemodialysis: In 11 anuric patients, a single 400 mg oral dose of gabapentin had an elimination half-life of 132 hours on days when patients did not receive dialysis, and 3.8 hours during dialysis.

### Time to peak concentration

2 to 4 hours.

### Therapeutic serum concentration

The therapeutic concentration range for gabapentin is not well defined. However, in one study it was noted that seizure frequency decreased significantly only in patients with gabapentin serum concentrations > 2 mg/L (11.7 micromoles/L). After receiving gabapentin 400 mg three times per day for one week, patients maintained on phenytoin had minimum gabapentin plasma concentrations of 2 to 4.8 mg/L (11.7 to 28 micromoles/L) and maximum gabapentin plasma concentrations of 3.6 to 8.6 mg/L (21 to 50.2 micromoles/L). Titration of dosage is based on clinical response.

### Elimination

Renal—Entire absorbed dose, as unchanged drug. Gabapentin clearance is directly proportional to creatinine clearance.

In dialysis—Gabapentin can be removed from plasma by hemodialysis.

## Precautions to Consider

### Carcinogenicity/Tumorigenicity

In 2 year carcinogenicity studies, a statistically significant increase in the incidence of pancreatic acinar cell adenomas and carcinomas was found in male rats receiving doses of gabapentin that produced plasma concentrations 10 times higher than those seen in humans receiving 3600 mg per day. Tumors were noninvasive, did not metastasize, did not affect survival, and did not occur in female rats or in mice. The significance to humans is unknown.

### Mutagenicity

No evidence of mutagenicity was found in appropriate *in vitro* and *in vivo* testing.

### Pregnancy/Reproduction

Fertility—No adverse effect on fertility was seen in rats given up to 5 times an equivalent human dose of 3600 mg on a mg per square meter of body surface area (mg/m²) basis.

Pregnancy—Gabapentin should be used during pregnancy only if the benefit justifies the potential risk to the fetus.

Studies have not been done in humans.

Mice given 1 to 4 times an equivalent human dose of 3600 mg on a mg/m² basis produced offspring with delayed ossification of several bones in the skull, vertebrae, and limbs. Rats given approximately 1 to 5 times an equivalent human dose of 3600 mg on a mg/m² basis produced offspring with an increased incidence of hydroureter and hydronephrosis. In rabbits given < ¼ to 8 times an equivalent human dose of 3600 mg on a mg/m² basis an increased incidence of postimplantation fetal loss occurred.

FDA Pregnancy Category C.

### Breast-feeding

It is not known whether gabapentin is distributed into breast milk.

### Pediatrics

No information is available on the relationship of age to the effects of gabapentin in children up to 12 years of age. Safety and efficacy have not been established.

### Adolescents

Appropriate studies on the relationship of age to the effects of gabapentin have not been performed in the adolescent population. However, clinical trials that included a limited number of patients aged 12 to 18 years revealed no adolescence-specific problems.

### Geriatrics

Plasma clearance of gabapentin is reduced in the elderly, probably due to age-related renal function decline. Dosage reduction based on creatinine clearance is recommended. Further dosage adjustments should be based on clinical response.

### Drug interactions and/or related problems

The following drug interactions and/or related problems have been selected on the basis of their potential clinical significance (possible mechanism in parentheses where appropriate)—not necessarily inclusive (» = major clinical significance):

Note: Combinations containing any of the following medications, depending on the amount present, may also interact with this medication.

Alcohol or

Central nervous system (CNS) depression–producing medications, other (See *Appendix II*)
(increased CNS depression may occur)

Antacids, especially aluminum- and magnesium-containing
(antacid taken with or within 2 hours after gabapentin reduces gabapentin's bioavailability by 20%; gabapentin should be taken at least 2 hours after antacid)

### Laboratory value alterations

The following have been selected on the basis of their potential clinical significance (possible effect in parentheses where appropriate)—not necessarily inclusive (» = major clinical significance):

With diagnostic test results

Dipstick tests for urinary protein (e.g., Ames N-Multistix SG, Chemstrip 3)
(gabapentin causes a false positive result; the sulfosalicylic acid precipitation procedure should be used to detect urinary protein in patients taking gabapentin)

With physiology/laboratory test values
    White blood cell counts
        (may be decreased)

## Medical considerations/Contraindications

The medical considerations/contraindications included here have been selected on the basis of their potential clinical significance (reasons given in parentheses where appropriate)—not necessarily inclusive (» = major clinical significance).

*Risk-benefit should be considered when the following medical problems exist:*

» Renal function impairment
        (elimination may be prolonged in patients not receiving hemodialysis, and shortened in patients during hemodialysis; dosage adjustment based on creatinine clearance is recommended)
    Sensitivity to gabapentin

## Side/Adverse Effects

The following side/adverse effects have been selected on the basis of their potential clinical significance (possible signs and symptoms in parentheses where appropriate)—not necessarily inclusive:

### Those indicating need for medical attention
Incidence more frequent
    *Ataxia* (clumsiness or unsteadiness); *nystagmus* (continuous, uncontrolled back and forth and/or rolling eye movements)

Incidence less frequent
    *Amnesia* (loss of memory); *depression, irritability, or other mood or mental changes*

Incidence rare
    *Leukopenia* (usually asymptomatic; rarely, fever or chills; cough or hoarseness; lower back or side pain; painful or difficult urination)

### Those indicating need for medical attention only if they continue or are bothersome
Incidence more frequent
    *Dizziness; drowsiness; fatigue* (unusual tiredness or weakness); *myalgia* (muscle ache or pain); *peripheral edema* (swelling of hands, feet, or lower legs); *tremor* (trembling or shaking); *vision abnormalities, including blurred vision and diplopia* (double vision)

Incidence less frequent or rare
    *Asthenia* (weakness or loss of strength); *dryness of mouth or throat; dysarthria* (slurred speech); *frequent urination; gastrointestinal effects, including diarrhea dyspepsia* (indigestion); *nausea and vomiting; headache; hypotension* (low blood pressure); *insomnia* (trouble in sleeping); *rhinitis* (runny nose); *tinnitus* (noise in ears); *trouble in thinking; weight gain*

## Overdose

For more information on the management of overdose or unintentional ingestion, **contact a Poison Control Center** (see *Poison Control Center Listing*).

### Clinical effects of overdose
The following effects have been selected on the basis of their potential clinical significance (possible signs and symptoms in parentheses where appropriate)—not necessarily inclusive:

    *Diarrhea, severe; diplopia* (double vision); *dizziness, severe; drowsiness, severe; dysarthria, severe* (slurred speech); *lethargy* (sluggishness)

### Treatment of overdose
Note: There is no specific antidote for gabapentin overdose.

Specific treatment—Hemodialysis (may be indicated by clinical state or in patients with significant renal impairment)

Supportive care—Patients in whom intentional overdose is confirmed or suspected should be referred for psychiatric consultation.

## Patient Consultation

As an aid to patient consultation, refer to *Advice for the Patient, Gabapentin (Systemic)*

In providing consultation, consider emphasizing the following selected information (» = major clinical significance):

### Before using this medication
» Conditions affecting use, especially:
        Sensitivity to gabapentin
        Use in the elderly—Elderly patients may excrete gabapentin more slowly; dosage reduction based on creatinine clearance, and dosage adjustment based on clinical response are recommended

Other medications, especially antacids
Other medical problems, especially renal function impairment

### Proper use of this medication
» Compliance with therapy; not taking more or less medicine than prescribed; not missing any doses
» Importance of not exceeding 12 hour interval between any 2 doses while on 3 times a day dosing schedule
» Importance of dissolving each dose as needed when a liquid dosage form is required; not dissolving any doses to save for later use
    Missed dose: Taking as soon as possible; if less than 2 hours until next dose, taking missed dose immediately and taking next dose 1 to 2 hours later, then resuming regular dosing schedule; not doubling doses
» Proper storage

### Precautions while using this medication
» Importance of regular visits to physician to check progress of therapy
    Discussing alcohol use or use of other CNS depressants with physician
» Possible blurred or double vision, dizziness, drowsiness, impairment of thinking or motor skills; caution when driving or doing jobs requiring alertness
    Possible false positive results with dipstick tests for urinary protein; using the sulfosalicylic acid precipitation procedure to determine presence of urinary protein
» Not discontinuing gabapentin abruptly; consulting physician about gradually reducing dosage

### Side/adverse effects
Ataxia; nystagmus; amnesia; depression, irritability, or other mood or mental changes; leukopenia

## General Dosing Information

Gabapentin dosage is titrated to clinical effect, not to plasma concentration.

Adverse effects are generally mild to moderate in severity, and tend to diminish with continued use of gabapentin.

Anticonvulsant medications should not be discontinued abruptly because of the possibility of increased seizure frequency. If gabapentin is to be discontinued, or if another anticonvulsant medication is to be added to the patient's therapy, the change should be made gradually, over a minimum period of one week, to avoid loss of seizure control.

## Oral Dosage Forms

### GABAPENTIN CAPSULES

#### Usual adult and adolescent dose
Anticonvulsant—
    Oral, 300 mg on the first day, 600 mg divided into two doses on the second day, 900 mg divided into three doses on the third day. The dosage may be gradually increased based on clinical response. Dosages of 900 to 1800 mg per day are effective for most patients. However, dosages as high as 2400 to 3600 mg per day have been well tolerated.

Note: Taking the initial dose at bedtime will minimize adverse effects.

    Dosage may be increased more slowly to avoid CNS adverse effects.

    When taking gabapentin three times a day, the maximum time between doses should not exceed twelve hours.

    For patients with renal function impairment: See *Usual geriatric dose*

    For patients undergoing hemodialysis: Oral, 300 to 400 mg initially for patients who have never received gabapentin, then 200 to 300 mg following each four hours of hemodialysis.

#### Usual adult and adolescent prescribing limits
Up to 3600 mg per day.

#### Usual pediatric dose
Anticonvulsant—
    Children up to 12 years of age: Safety and efficacy have not been established.
    Children 12 years of age and over: See *Usual adult and adolescent dose.*

#### Usual geriatric dose
Anticonvulsant—
    Oral, initial dosage recommendations, based on creatinine clearance, are as follows. Dosage adjustments may be made based on clinical response.

| Creatinine Clearance (mL per minute) | Total Daily Dose (mg per day) | Dosage Regimen (mg) |
|---|---|---|
| >60 | 1200 | 400 three times a day |
| 30 to 60 | 600 | 300 two times a day |
| 15 to 30 | 300 | 300 once a day |
| <15 | 150 | 300 once every other day |

## Strength(s) usually available
U.S.—

100 mg (Rx) [*Neurontin* (lactose; corn starch; talc; gelatin; titanium dioxide; FD&C Blue No.2)].

300 mg (Rx) [*Neurontin* (lactose; corn starch; talc; gelatin; titanium dioxide; yellow iron oxide; FD&C Blue No.2)].

400 mg (Rx) [*Neurontin* (lactose; corn starch; talc; gelatin; red iron oxide; titanium dioxide; yellow iron oxide; FD&C Blue No.2)].

Canada—

100 mg (Rx) [*Neurontin* (lactose; corn starch; talc)].

300 mg (Rx) [*Neurontin* (lactose; corn starch; talc)].

400 mg (Rx) [*Neurontin* (lactose; corn starch; talc)].

Note: Capsule shells may contain gelatin, titanium dioxide, silicon dioxide, sodium lauryl sulfate, yellow iron oxide, red iron oxide, and FD&C Blue No. 2.

## Packaging and storage
Store below 40 °C (104 °F), preferably between 15 and 30 °C (59 and 86 °F), in a well closed container, unless otherwise specified by manufacturer.

## Preparation of dosage form
For patients who cannot take oral solids—Individual doses may be dissolved in juice or sprinkled over soft foods, such as applesauce, immediately before use. However, gabapentin solutions degrade over time and should be taken immediately after preparation.

## Auxiliary labeling
• May cause blurred vision.
• May cause dizziness.
• May cause drowsiness. Alcohol may intensify this effect.

## Selected Bibliography
Goa KL, Sorkin EM. Gabapentin: A review of its pharmacological properties and clinical potential in epilepsy. Drugs 1993; 46 (3): 409-27.

Developed: 02/28/95

# GADODIAMIDE   Systemic

VA CLASSIFICATION (Primary): DX900

Note: For a listing of dosage forms and brand names by country availability, see *Dosage Forms* section(s). For a listing of brand names for the articles in this monograph, refer to the General Index.

## Category
Diagnostic aid, paramagnetic (brain disorders; spine disorders).
Note: Gadodiamide is a nonionic paramagnetic contrast agent.

## Indications
### Accepted
Brain imaging, magnetic resonance—Gadodiamide is indicated to provide contrast enhancement during magnetic resonance imaging (MRI) and thus facilitate visualization of intracranial lesions with abnormal vascularity or those suspected of causing an abnormality in the blood-brain barrier.

Spinal lesions imaging, magnetic resonance—Gadodiamide is indicated to provide contrast enhancement during MRI and thus facilitate visualization of lesions in the spine and associated tissues.

## Pharmacology/Pharmacokinetics
### Physicochemical characteristics
Molecular weight—591.68.
Osmolality—789 mOsmol per kg of water.
pH—5.5 to 7.0.

### Mechanism of action/Effect
Based on the behavior of protons when placed in a strong magnetic field, which is interpreted and transformed into images by magnetic resonance (MR) instruments. Paramagnetic agents have unpaired electrons that generate a magnetic field about 700 times larger than the proton's field, thus disturbing the proton's local magnetic field. When the local magnetic field around a proton is disturbed, its relaxation process is altered. MR images are based on proton density and proton relaxation dynamics. MR instruments can record 2 different relaxation processes, the T1 (spin-lattice or longitudinal relaxation time) and the T2 (spin-spin or transverse relaxation time). In magnetic resonance imaging (MRI), visualization of normal and pathological brain tissue depends in part on variations in the radiofrequency signal intensity that occur with changes in proton density, alteration of the T1, and variation in the T2. When placed in a magnetic field, gadodiamide shortens both the T1 and the T2 relaxation times in tissues where it accumulates. At clinical doses, gadodiamide primarily affects the T1 relaxation time, thus producing an increase in signal intensity. Gadodiamide does not cross the intact blood-brain barrier; therefore, it does not accumulate in normal brain tissue or in central nervous system (CNS) lesions that have not caused an abnormal blood-brain barrier (e.g., cysts, mature post-operative scars). Abnormal vascularity or disruption of the blood-

brain barrier allows accumulation of gadodiamide in lesions such as neoplasms, abscesses, and subacute infarcts.

### Half-life
Distribution—$3.7 \pm 2.7$ minutes (mean).
Elimination—$77.8 \pm 16$ minutes (mean).

### Elimination
Renal (approximately 96% of dose excreted within 24 hours).

## Precautions to Consider
### Carcinogenicity
Animal studies to evaluate the carcinogenic potential of gadodiamide have not been performed.

### Pregnancy/Reproduction
Pregnancy—Adequate and well-controlled studies with gadodiamide have not been done in humans. Also, although there is no evidence that the magnetic and electric fields associated with MRI have an effect on human development, *in vitro* studies and theoretical predictions raise concern regarding the risk of exposure of the developing embryo and fetus to MR. More studies are needed to establish the safety of MRI in pregnant patients.

Studies in rabbits showed that gadodiamide at doses 5 times the maximum recommended human dose increased the incidence of skeletal and visceral abnormalities in the offspring.

FDA Pregnancy Category C.

### Breast-feeding
It is not known whether gadodiamide is distributed into breast milk.

### Pediatrics
Appropriate studies on the relationship of age to the effects of gadodiamide have not been performed in the pediatric population. However, pediatrics-specific problems that would limit the usefulness of this agent in children are not expected.

### Geriatrics
Appropriate studies on the relationship of age to the effects of gadodiamide have not been performed in the geriatric population. However, clinical trials conducted to date, which included older patients, have not demonstrated geriatrics-specific problems that would limit the usefulness of this agent in the elderly.

### Medical considerations/Contraindications
The medical considerations/contraindications included here have been selected on the basis of their potential clinical significance (reasons given in parentheses where appropriate)—not necessarily inclusive (» = major clinical significance).

*Risk-benefit should be considered when the following medical problems exist:*

» Allergies or asthma, history of
(increased risk of idiosyncratic response)

Anemia, hemolytic
  (although this effect has not been specifically reported for gadodiamide, the use of gadopentetate dimeglumine, another paramagnetic contrast agent, has been associated with an increased risk of
  hemolysis; until more conclusive evidence is available, caution is
  recommended)
» Renal function impairment, severe
  (excretion of gadodiamide may be impaired)
» Sensitivity to gadodiamide
  Sickle cell disease
    (in *in vitro* studies, deoxygenated sickle erythrocytes have been
    shown to align perpendicular to a magnetic field, which may result
    in vascular occlusion *in vivo*; however, more studies are needed to
    establish extent of risk)

## Side/Adverse Effects

The following side/adverse effects have been selected on the basis of their
potential clinical significance (possible signs and symptoms in parentheses where appropriate)—not necessarily inclusive:

**Those indicating need for medical attention**
Incidence less frequent or rare
  *Pseudo-allergic reaction* (itching, watery eyes; skin rash or hives;
  swelling of face; thickening of tongue; wheezing, tightness in chest,
  or troubled breathing)

**Those indicating need for medical attention only if they continue
or are bothersome**
Incidence more frequent
  *Dizziness; headache; nausea*
Incidence less frequent or rare
  *Changes in taste; chest pains; CNS effects* (anxiety; confusion; con-
  vulsions); *diarrhea; dryness of mouth; pain at injection site; vaso-
  dilation* (unusual warmth and flushing of skin)

## Patient Consultation

As an aid to patient consultation, refer to *Advice for the Patient, MRI
Contrast Agents (Diagnostic)*.

In providing consultation, consider emphasizing the following selected
information (» = major clinical significance):

**Description of use**
  Action in the body: Accumulates in brain and spinal lesions creating
  a local magnetic field; visualization of lesions possible with MR
  instruments

**Before having this test**
» Conditions affecting use, especially:
    Sensitivity to gadodiamide
    Other medical problems, especially allergies or asthma (history of)
    or severe renal function impairment

**Preparation for this test**
  Special preparatory instructions may apply; patient should inquire in
  advance

**Side/adverse effects**
  Signs of possible side effects, especially pseudo-allergic reaction

## General Dosing Information

The manufacturer's package insert or other appropriate literature should
be consulted for specific techniques and procedures for the administration of gadodiamide.

During and for at least 30 to 60 minutes after injection of gadodiamide,
the patient should be observed for possible severe reactions. Competent personnel and emergency facilities should be available during this
period.

Imaging procedures should be completed within 1 hour of injection of
gadodiamide.

## Parenteral Dosage Forms
### GADODIAMIDE INJECTION

**Usual adult and adolescent dose**
Brain and spinal lesions imaging, magnetic resonance—
  Intravenous, by direct injection (at a rate >60 mL per minute), 0.2
  mL (0.1 mmol) per kg of body weight.
Note: To insure complete injection of gadodiamide, a 5-mL flush using
  0.9% sodium chloride injection should be administered following
  injection of gadodiamide.
  If repeat examinations are required, an interval of time should
  elapse between injections to allow for normal clearance of
  gadodiamide.

**Usual adult prescribing limits**
Up to a total dose of 5.74 grams (20 mL).

**Usual pediatric dose**
Brain and spinal lesions imaging, magnetic resonance—
  Dosage must be individualized by physician.
Note: Doses based on 0.2 mL (0.1 mmol) of gadodiamide per kg of body
  weight have been used in pediatric patients.

**Usual geriatric dose**
See *Usual adult and adolescent dose*.

**Strength(s) usually available**
U.S.—
  287 mg (0.5 mmol) per mL of gadodiamide (Rx) [*Omniscan* (12 mg
  of caldiamide sodium per mL)].
Canada—
  287 mg (0.5 mmol) per mL of gadodiamide (Rx) [*Omniscan*].

**Packaging and storage**
Store between 15 and 30 °C (59 and 86 °F), in a light-resistant container,
unless otherwise specified by manufacturer. Protect from freezing.

## Selected Bibliography

Sze G, Brant-Zawadzki M, Haughton VM, et al. Multicenter study of
  gadodiamide as a contrast agent in MR imaging of the brain and spine.
  Radiology 1991; 181 (3): 693-9.

Revised: 08/17/93
Interim revision: 08/30/94

---

# GADOPENTETATE   Systemic†

INN: Gadopentetic Acid
VA CLASSIFICATION (Primary): DX900
Note: For a listing of dosage forms and brand names by country availability, see *Dosage Forms* section(s). For a listing of brand names
  for the articles in this monograph, refer to the General Index.

  †Not commercially available in Canada.

## Category

Diagnostic aid, paramagnetic (brain disorders; spine disorders; breast disease; cardiac disease; liver disorders; musculoskeletal disease; uterus
  disorders).
Note: Gadopentetate meglumine is an ionic paramagnetic agent.

## Indications

Note: Bracketed information in the *Indications* section refers to uses that
  are not included in U.S. product labeling.

**Accepted**
Brain imaging, magnetic resonance—Gadopentetate dimeglumine is indicated in adults and children 2 years of age and older to provide
  contrast enhancement during magnetic resonance imaging (MRI) of
  intracranial lesions with abnormal vascularity or those suspected of
  causing an abnormality in the blood-brain barrier. Gadopentetate-enhanced MRI helps in the diagnosis and characterization of neoplastic
  disease, acoustic neuroma, subacute infarction, inflammatory disease,
  certain vascular abnormalities, and certain demyelinating abnormalities
  (e.g., multiple sclerosis).

Gadopentetate dimeglumine is used in magnetic resonance (MR) studies to help differentiate changes that occur secondary to brain tumor resection (e.g., encephalomalacia, gliosis) or to postoperative irradiation or chemotherapy (e.g., edema, ischemia, demyelination, necrosis) from changes that represent residual or recurrent tumors, to accurately assess treatment results.

MRI with gadopentetate dimeglumine is particularly useful in patients with normal unenhanced studies who have central nervous system (CNS) symptoms, in patients with CNS tumors that are difficult to separate from surrounding edema, and in patients who have undergone surgery, to differentiate recurrence of the lesions from postoperative changes.

In patients with suspected meningitis, gadopentetate-enhanced MRI may be particularly useful in defining the active inflammatory process of the meninges and focal lesions.

Spinal lesions imaging, magnetic resonance—Gadopentetate dimeglumine is indicated in adults and children 2 years of age and older to provide contrast enhancement and facilitate visualization of lesions in the spine and associated tissues.

Gadopentetate dimeglumine provides enhanced contrast of epidural abscesses, which makes it possible to differentiate them from adjacent compressed thecal sac; it facilitates the diagnosis of disk space infection and osteomyelitis; it helps localize portions of paraspinal masses most likely to yield a positive percutaneous biopsy; and it helps distinguish active spinal infections from those that have responded adequately to antibiotic therapy.

MRI with gadopentetate dimeglumine may be useful in differentiating postoperative epidural fibrosis (scar tissue) from recurrent disk herniation in patients with symptoms of failed back surgery syndrome, to avoid unnecessary, and possibly damaging, reoperation if scar tissue is the cause.

Body imaging, magnetic resonance—Gadopentetate dimeglumine is indicated in adults to improve lesion contrast during MR body imaging (excluding the heart) in the evaluation of suspected hepatic lesions, endometrial or cervical carcinomas or pelvic masses, breast lesions (suspected or known), and musculoskeletal lesions.

MRI of the breast is also used in patients with postoperative scarring and silicon implants to exclude or demonstrate malignancy, especially in patients with uncertain mammographic and/or clinical findings.

[Cardiac imaging, magnetic resonance]—Gadopentetate-enhanced MRI is used in the evaluation of patients with great vessel disease (e.g., aortic aneurysm, aortic dissection, congenital abnormalities, vena cava obstruction); in patients with ischemic cardiac disease to examine the heart for regions of wall thinning and intracardiac thrombus, to assess chamber size, myocardial mass, wall motion, and wall thickening, and to detect regions of acute infarction; and in patients with congenital heart disease to evaluate malrotations of the heart and for post-surgery assessment. Also, gadopentetate-enhanced MRI helps in the assessment of coronary artery reperfusion after thrombolysis.

## Pharmacology/Pharmacokinetics

### Physicochemical characteristics
Molecular weight—938.01.

### Mechanism of action/Effect
Based on the behavior of protons when placed in a strong magnetic field, which is interpreted and transformed into images by magnetic resonance (MR) instruments. MR images are based primarily on proton density and proton relaxation dynamics. MR instruments are sensitive to two different relaxation processes, the T1 (spin-lattice or longitudinal relaxation time) and T2 (spin-spin or transverse relaxation time). Paramagnetic agents contain one or more unpaired electrons that enhance the T1 and T2 relaxation rates of protons in their molecular environment. The proton relaxation effect (PRE) of an unpaired electron is 700 times stronger than that of a proton itself. In MRI, visualization of normal and pathological brain tissue depends in part on variations in the radio frequency signal intensity that occur with changes in proton density, alteration of the T1, and variation in T2. When placed in a magnetic field, gadopentetate dimeglumine shortens the T1 and T2 relaxation times in tissues where it accumulates. In the central nervous system (CNS), gadopentetate dimeglumine enhances visualization of normal tissues that lack a blood-brain barrier, such as the pituitary gland and the meninges. Gadopentetate dimeglumine does not cross the intact blood-brain barrier; therefore, it does not accumulate in normal brain tissue or in CNS lesions that have not caused an abnormal blood-brain barrier (e.g., cysts, mature post-operative scars). Abnormal vascularity or disruption of the blood-brain barrier

allows accumulation of gadopentetate dimeglumine in lesions such as neoplasms, abscesses, and subacute infarcts. Outside the CNS, gadopentetate dimeglumine rapidly reaches equilibrium in the interstitial compartment and enhances signal in all tissues as a function of delivery and size of the interstitial compartment.

### Distribution
Rapidly cleared from blood after intravenous administration and distributed in extracellular space.

### Half-life
Elimination—$1.6 \pm 0.13$ hours (mean).

### Elimination
Renal, by passive filtration (approximately 83% of dose excreted within 6 hours).

## Precautions to Consider

### Carcinogenicity/Mutagenicity
Long-term animal studies to evaluate carcinogenic or mutagenic potential of gadopentetate dimeglumine have not been performed.

### Pregnancy/Reproduction
Pregnancy—Adequate and well-controlled studies in humans have not been done. Also, although there is no evidence that the magnetic and electric fields associated with MRI have an effect on human development, *in vitro* studies and theoretical predictions raise concern regarding the risk of exposure to MR to the developing embryo and fetus. More studies are needed to establish the safety of MRI in pregnant patients.

Studies in rats with gadopentetate dimeglumine at doses 2.5 times, and in rabbits at doses 7.5 and 12.5 times, the human dose have shown that this agent causes slight retardation in development.

FDA Pregnancy Category C.

### Breast-feeding
Problems in humans have not been documented. Since gadopentetate is distributed in small amounts into breast milk, temporary discontinuation of breast-feeding should be considered for at least 24 hours following its administration.

### Pediatrics
Appropriate studies have not been performed in children up to 2 years of age. In older children, pediatrics-specific problems that would limit the usefulness of this agent are not expected.

### Geriatrics
Appropriate studies on the relationship of age to the effects of gadopentetate dimeglumine have not been performed in the geriatric population. However, clinical trials, which included older patients, were conducted and geriatrics-specific problems that would limit the usefulness of this medication in the elderly are not expected.

### Laboratory value alterations
The following have been selected on the basis of their potential clinical significance (possible effect in parentheses where appropriate)—not necessarily inclusive (» = major clinical significance):

With physiology/laboratory test values
  Bilirubin and
  Iron
     (serum concentrations may be transiently increased)

### Medical considerations/Contraindications
The medical considerations/contraindications included here have been selected on the basis of their potential clinical significance (reasons given in parentheses where appropriate)—not necessarily inclusive (» = major clinical significance).

*Risk-benefit should be considered when the following medical problems exist:*
» Anemia, hemolytic
     (possible risk of increased hemolysis)
  Epilepsy
     (gadopentetate dimeglumine may precipitate seizure)
  Hypotension
     (may be exacerbated)
» Renal function impairment, severe
     (excretion of gadopentetate dimeglumine may be impaired)
» Sensitivity to gadopentetate dimeglumine

## Side/Adverse Effects

The following side/adverse effects have been selected on the basis of their potential clinical significance (possible signs and symptoms in parentheses where appropriate)—not necessarily inclusive:

**Those indicating need for medical attention**
Incidence less frequent
*Convulsions; pseudo-allergic reaction* (skin rash or hives; wheezing, tightness in chest, or troubled breathing); *severe hypotension* (unusual tiredness or weakness)

**Those indicating need for medical attention only if they continue or are bothersome**
Incidence more frequent
*Coldness at injection site*—2.8%; *dizziness*—less than 2%; *headache*—5.5%; *nausea*—2.5%

Incidence less frequent or rare
*Agitation; dryness of mouth; fever; increased salivation; pain and/ or burning sensation at injection site; ringing or buzzing in ears; stomach pain; vasodilation* (unusual warmth and flushing of skin); *vomiting; weakness or tiredness*

## Patient Consultation

As an aid to patient consultation, refer to *Advice for the Patient, MRI Contrast Agents (Diagnostic)*.

In providing consultation, consider emphasizing the following selected information (» = major clinical significance):

**Description of use**
Action in the body: Accumulates in brain and spinal lesions creating a local magnetic field; visualization of lesions possible with MR instruments

**Before having this test**
» Conditions affecting use, especially:
Sensitivity to gadopentetate dimeglumine
Breast-feeding—Distributed in small amounts into breast milk; temporary discontinuation of breast-feeding should be considered
Other medical problems, especially hemolytic anemia or severe renal function impairment

**Preparation for this test**
Special preparatory instructions may apply; patient should inquire in advance

**Side/adverse effects**
Signs of possible side effects, especially convulsions, pseudo-allergic reaction, or severe hypotension

## General Dosing Information

The manufacturer's package insert or other appropriate literature should be consulted for specific techniques and procedures for the administration of gadopentetate.

Imaging procedures of the CNS should be completed within 1 hour of injection of gadopentetate. Maximal lesion-liver contrast occurs within the first few minutes after administration of gadopentetate dimeglumine; thus liver scans should be obtained immediately after contrast administration and, preferably, with rapid image acquisition sequences.

Gadopentetate dimeglumine injection, although hypertonic as compared to plasma (6.8 times the osmolality of plasma), is subject to rapid hemodilution.

## Parenteral Dosage Forms

Note: Bracketed uses in the *Dosage Forms* section refer to categories of use and/or indications that are not included in U.S. product labeling.

### GADOPENTETATE DIMEGLUMINE INJECTION

**Usual adult and adolescent dose**
Brain and spinal lesions imaging, magnetic resonance; Body imaging, magnetic resonance; and [Cardiac imaging, magnetic resonance]— Intravenous, 93.8 mg (0.1 mmol [0.2 mL]) per kg of body weight, administered at a rate not to exceed 10 mL per minute.

Note: Injection rates that exceed 10 mL per minute have been associated with nausea.

To insure complete injection of gadopentetate, a 5-mL normal saline flush should be administered following injection of gadopentetate.

If repeat examinations are required, an interval of time should elapse between injections to allow for normal clearance of gadopentetate.

**Usual adult prescribing limits**
Up to a total dose of 9.38 grams (20 mL).

**Usual pediatric dose**
Brain and spinal lesions imaging, magnetic resonance—
Children up to 2 years of age: Safety and efficacy have not been established.
Children 2 years of age and older: See *Usual adult and adolescent dose*.
Body imaging, magnetic resonance—
Dosage has not been established.

**Usual geriatric dose**
See *Usual adult and adolescent dose*.

**Strength(s) usually available**
U.S.—
469.01 mg (0.5 mmol) per mL (Rx) [*Magnevist* (meglumine 0.39 mg; diethylenetriamine pentaacetic acid 0.15 mg)].
Canada—
Not commercially available.

**Packaging and storage**
Store between 15 and 30 °C (59 and 86 °F), in a light-resistant container, unless otherwise specified by manufacturer. Protect from freezing.

## Selected Bibliography

Runge VM, Carollo BR, Wolf CR, et al. GdDTPA: a review of clinical indications in central nervous system magnetic resonance imaging. Radiographics 1989; 9 (5): 929-58.
Goldstein HA, et al. Safety assessment of gadopentetate dimeglumine in U.S. clinical trials. Radiology Jan 1990; 174 (1): 17-23.

Revised: 08/19/94

# GADOTERIDOL  Systemic†

VA CLASSIFICATION (Primary): DX900
Note: For a listing of dosage forms and brand names by country availability, see *Dosage Forms* section(s). For a listing of brand names for the articles in this monograph, refer to the General Index.

†Not commercially available in Canada.

## Category

Diagnostic aid, paramagnetic (brain disorders; spine disorders).
Note: Gadoteridol is a nonionic paramagnetic agent.

## Indications

**Accepted**
Brain imaging, magnetic resonance—Gadoteridol is indicated to provide contrast enhancement during magnetic resonance imaging (MRI) and facilitate visualization of intracranial lesions with abnormal vascularity

or those suspected of causing an abnormality in the blood-brain barrier.
Spinal lesions imaging, magnetic resonance—Gadoteridol is indicated to provide contrast enhancement during MRI and facilitate visualization of lesions in the spine and associated tissues.

## Pharmacology/Pharmacokinetics

**Physicochemical characteristics**
Molecular weight—558.7.
Osmolality—630 mOsmol per kg of water
pH—6.5 to 8.0

**Mechanism of action/Effect**
Based on the behavior of protons when placed in a strong magnetic field, which is interpreted and transformed into images by magnetic resonance (MR) instruments. Paramagnetic agents have unpaired electrons

that generate a magnetic field about 700 times larger than the proton's field, thus disturbing the proton's local magnetic field. When the local magnetic field around a proton is disturbed its relaxation process is altered. MR images are based on proton density and proton relaxation dynamics. MR instruments can record two different relaxation processes, the T1 (spin-lattice or longitudinal relaxation time) and T2 (spin-spin or transverse relaxation time). In MRI, visualization of normal and pathological brain tissue depends in part on variations in the radiofrequency signal intensity that occur with changes in proton density, alteration of the T1, and variation in T2. When placed in a magnetic field, gadoteridol shortens the T1 relaxation time in tissues where it accumulates. Gadoteridol does not cross the intact blood-brain barrier; therefore, it does not accumulate in normal brain tissue or in central nervous system (CNS) lesions that have not caused an abnormal blood-brain barrier (e.g., cysts, mature post-operative scars). Abnormal vascularity or disruption of the blood-brain barrier allows accumulation of gadoteridol in lesions such as neoplasms, abscesses, and subacute infarcts.

### Half-life
Distribution—$0.20 \pm 0.04$ hours (mean).
Elimination—$1.57 \pm 0.08$ hours (mean).

### Elimination
Renal (approximately 94% of dose excreted within 24 hours).

## Precautions to Consider

### Carcinogenicity
Animal studies to evaluate the carcinogenic potential of gadoteridol have not been performed.

### Pregnancy/Reproduction
Pregnancy—Adequate and well-controlled studies in humans have not been done. Also, although there is no evidence that the magnetic and electric fields associated with MRI have an effect on human development, *in vitro* studies and theoretical predictions raise concern regarding the risk of exposure of the developing embryo and fetus to MR. More studies are needed to establish the safety of MRI in pregnant patients.
Studies in rats showed that gadoteridol at doses 33 times the maximum recommended human dose for 12 days during gestation doubled the incidence of postimplantation loss. Also, when rats were administered gadoteridol at doses 20 to 33 times the maximum human dose for 12 days, an increase in spontaneous locomotor activity was observed in the offspring.

FDA Pregnancy Category C.

### Breast-feeding
It is not known whether gadoteridol is distributed into breast milk.

### Pediatrics
Appropriate studies on the relationship of age to the effects of gadoteridol have not been performed in the pediatric population. However, clinical trials conducted to date in a limited number of pediatric patients have not demonstrated pediatrics-specific problems that would limit the usefulness of gadoteridol in children.

### Geriatrics
Appropriate studies on the relationship of age to the effects of gadoteridol have not been performed in the geriatric population. However, clinical trials conducted to date, which included older patients, have not demonstrated geriatrics-specific problems that would limit the usefulness of this agent in the elderly.

### Medical considerations/Contraindications
The medical considerations/contraindications included here have been selected on the basis of their potential clinical significance (reasons given in parentheses where appropriate)—not necessarily inclusive (» = major clinical significance).

*Risk-benefit should be considered when the following medical problems exist:*
» Allergies or asthma, history of
    (increased risk of idiosyncratic response)
  Anemia, hemolytic
    (although this effect has not been specifically reported for gadoteridol, the use of gadopentetate dimeglumine, another paramagnetic contrast agent, has been associated with an increased risk of hemolysis; until more conclusive evidence is available, caution is recommended)
» Renal function impairment, severe
    (excretion of gadoteridol may be impaired)
» Sensitivity to gadoteridol

Sickle cell disease
    (in *in vitro* studies deoxygenated sickle erythrocytes have been shown to align perpendicular to a magnetic field, which may result in vascular occlusion *in vivo*; however, more studies are needed to establish extent of risk)

## Side/Adverse Effects
The following side/adverse effects have been selected on the basis of their potential clinical significance (possible signs and symptoms in parentheses where appropriate)—not necessarily inclusive:

**Those indicating need for medical attention**
Incidence less frequent or rare
    *Cardiovascular effects* (low blood pressure; fast or irregular heartbeat); *pseudo-allergic reaction* (itching, watery eyes; skin rash or hives; swelling of face; thickening of tongue; wheezing, tightness in chest, or troubled breathing)

**Those indicating need for medical attention only if they continue or are bothersome**
Incidence more frequent
    *Changes in taste; nausea or vomiting*
Incidence less frequent or rare
    *CNS effects* (anxiety; confusion; dizziness); *diarrhea; headache; pain at injection site; vasodilation* (unusual warmth and flushing of skin)

## Patient Consultation
As an aid to patient consultation, refer to *Advice for the Patient, MRI Contrast Agents (Diagnostic)*.

In providing consultation, consider emphasizing the following selected information (» = major clinical significance):

**Description of use**
    Action in the body: Accumulates in brain and spinal lesions creating a local magnetic field; visualization of lesions possible with MR instruments

**Before having this test**
» Conditions affecting use, especially:
    Sensitivity to gadoteridol
    Other medical problems, especially allergies or asthma (history of) or severe renal function impairment

**Preparation for this test**
    Special preparatory instructions may apply; patient should inquire in advance

**Side/adverse effects**
    Signs of possible side effects, especially cardiovascular effects and pseudo-allergic reaction

## General Dosing Information
The manufacturer's package insert or other appropriate literature should be consulted for specific techniques and procedures for the administration of gadoteridol.

During and for at least 30 to 60 minutes after injection of gadoteridol, the patient should be observed for possible severe reactions; competent personnel and emergency facilities should be available during this period.

Imaging procedures should be completed within 1 hour of injection of gadoteridol.

## Parenteral Dosage Forms

### GADOTERIDOL INJECTION

**Usual adult and adolescent dose**
Brain and spinal lesions imaging, magnetic resonance—
    Intravenous, as rapid infusion or direct injection (bolus, >60 mL per minute), 0.2 mL (0.1 mmol) per kg of body weight.
Note: To insure complete injection of gadoteridol, a 5-mL flush using 0.9% sodium chloride injection should be administered following injection of gadoteridol.
    A second dose of 0.4 mL (0.2 mmol) per kg of body weight may be administered up to 30 minutes after the first dose in patients suspected of having cerebral metastases or other poorly enhancing lesions, or in the presence of negative or equivocal scans.

**Usual pediatric dose**
Brain and spinal lesions imaging, magnetic resonance—
    Dosage must be individualized by physician.
Note: In clinical trials, 0.2 mL (0.1 mmol) of gadoteridol per kg of body weight was used in pediatric patients.

**Usual geriatric dose**
See *Usual adult and adolescent dose*.

**Strength(s) usually available**
U.S.—
   279.3 mg (0.5 mmol) per mL of gadoteridol (Rx) [*ProHance* (0.23 mg of calteridol calcium; 1.21 mg tromethamine, per mL)].
Canada—
   Not commercially available.

**Packaging and storage**
Store between 15 and 30 °C (59 and 86 °F), in a light-resistant container, unless otherwise specified by manufacturer. Protect from freezing.

## Selected Bibliography

Carvlin MJ, De Simone DN, Meeks MJ. Phase II clinical trial of gadoteridol injection, a low-osmolal magnetic resonance imaging contrast agent. Invest Radiol (suppl) 1992; 1: 16S-21S.

McLachlan SJ, Eaton S, De Simone DN. Pharmacokinetic behavior of gadoteridol injection. Invest Radiol (suppl) 1992; 1: 12S-15S.
Runge VM, Bronen RA, Davis KR. Efficacy of gadoteridol for magnetic resonance imaging of the brain and spine. Invest Radiol (suppl) 1992; 1: 22S-32S.

Revised: 08/17/93
Interim revision: 08/30/94

**GALLAMINE**—See *Neuromuscular Blocking Agents (Systemic)*

# GALLIUM CITRATE Ga 67   Systemic

VA CLASSIFICATION (Primary): DX201

Note: For a listing of dosage forms and brand names by country availability, see *Dosage Forms* section(s). For a listing of brand names for the articles in this monograph, refer to the General Index.

## Category

Diagnostic aid, radioactive (neoplastic disease; focal inflammatory lesions).

## Indications

Note: Bracketed information in the *Indications* section refers to uses that are not included in U.S. product labeling.

**Accepted**
Neoplastic disease (diagnosis)—Gallium citrate Ga 67 is indicated to demonstrate the presence and extent of lymphoma, bronchogenic carcinoma, [acute myelocytic leukemia], [chronic myelocytic leukemia], [hepatoma], and [bone sarcoma]. May also be useful in the detection of [epithelial, head, and neck carcinoma]; [malignant melanoma]; [malignant fibrous histiocytoma]; and [testicular tumors].

Inflammatory lesions, focal (diagnosis)—Gallium citrate Ga 67 is indicated for the localization of focal inflammatory lesions, such as abscess, osteomyelitis, pneumonia, pyelonephritis, and granulomatous diseases (sarcoidosis). May also be useful in the detection of active tuberculosis; and for assessing the activity of the inflammatory process in certain interstitial pulmonary diseases, including sarcoidosis and fibrosing alveolitis.

In combination with thallous chloride Tl 201 imaging, gallium citrate Ga 67 imaging may be useful in the diagnosis of myocardial sarcoidosis and in predicting the response to corticosteroid therapy.

[Immunodeficiency syndrome, acquired, related disorders of (diagnosis)][1]— Gallium citrate Ga 67 is useful in the diagnosis and monitoring of *Pneumocystis carinii* pneumonia, tuberculosis, and other infections in acquired immunodeficiency syndrome (AIDS) patients.

[Fever, unknown origin, source of (diagnosis)][1]—Gallium citrate Ga 67 is useful as a diagnostic screening test in cases of prolonged fever, when physical examination, laboratory tests, and other imaging studies have failed to disclose the source of the fever.

In the absence of pre-existing symptoms, a positive uptake of gallium citrate Ga 67 justifies additional testing for potential disease.

[1]Not included in Canadian product labeling.

## Physical Properties

**Nuclear data**

| Radionu-clide (half-life) | Decay constant | Mode of decay | Principal photon emissions (keV) | Mean number of emissions/ disintegration (≥0.01) |
|---|---|---|---|---|
| Ga 67 (78.26 hr) | 0.00886 hr-1 | Electron capture | Gamma-3 (93.3) | 0.37 |
| | | | Gamma-4 (184.6) | 0.20 |
| | | | Gamma-5 (300.2) | 0.17 |

## Pharmacology/Pharmacokinetics

**Mechanism of action/Effect**
Diagnosis of neoplastic disease and

Diagnosis of inflammatory lesions—The exact mechanism of action is unknown, but gallium citrate Ga 67 has been found to concentrate in certain viable primary and metastatic tumors as well as focal sites of inflammation. Studies of Ga 67 accumulation in acute inflammatory lesions suggest that a number of factors are involved in the accumulation and retention of Ga 67 at the site of inflammation. Adequate blood supply is essential for delivery of Ga 67 to the lesion. Ga 67, mainly in the form of transferrin-Ga-67 complex, is delivered to the lesion through capillaries with increased permeability. Some Ga 67 is taken up by the leukocytes and bacteria, if present at the site of inflammation.

**Distribution**
Rapidly distributed throughout body; concentrating first in tumors and sites of infection, and renal cortex. Maximum concentration shifts to bone (including marrow) and lymph nodes after the first day, and to liver and spleen after the first week.

**Protein binding**
High (mainly to plasma transferrin; to a lesser extent to albumins and globulins).

**Half-life**
Biological—Approximately 2 to 3 weeks.

| Estimated absorbed radiation dose* | | |
|---|---|---|
| Organ | mGy/MBq | rad/mCi |
| Bone surfaces | 0.59 | 2.18 |
| Intestine wall (lower) | 0.20 | 0.74 |
| Red marrow | 0.19 | 0.70 |
| Spleen | 0.15 | 0.55 |
| Adrenals | 0.14 | 0.52 |
| Liver | 0.12 | 0.44 |
| Intestine wall (upper) | 0.12 | 0.44 |
| Kidneys | 0.11 | 0.41 |
| Pancreas | 0.083 | 0.31 |
| Ovaries | 0.082 | 0.30 |
| Bladder wall | 0.081 | 0.30 |
| Uterus | 0.079 | 0.29 |
| Stomach wall | 0.072 | 0.27 |
| Lungs | 0.065 | 0.24 |
| Breast | 0.062 | 0.23 |
| Small intestine | 0.059 | 0.22 |
| Testes | 0.057 | 0.21 |
| Thyroid | 0.056 | 0.21 |
| Other tissue | 0.063 | 0.23 |

Effective dose: 0.12 mSv/MBq (0.44 rem/mCi)

*For adults; intravenous injection.

**Elimination**
Slow—
   Primary:
      Renal (26% of the administered dose of which 10 to 15% is eliminated within 24 hours).

Secondary:

    Fecal (10% within the first week). Fecal excretion becomes primary route of excretion after the first 24 hours.

Note: Bowel radioactivity may interfere with the interpretation of abdominal scans. To cleanse the bowel prior to imaging, laxatives and/or enemas are recommended on the day of gallium citrate Ga 67 administration and/or subsequent days prior to imaging. Imaging is usually done 48 to 72 hours after administration of the radiotracer.

## Precautions to Consider

### Carcinogenicity/Mutagenicity

Long-term animal studies to evaluate carcinogenic or mutagenic potential of gallium citrate Ga 67 have not been performed.

### Pregnancy/Reproduction

Pregnancy—Gallium citrate Ga 67 crosses the placenta. Adequate and well-controlled studies have not been done in humans.

The possibility of pregnancy should be assessed in women of child-bearing potential. Clinical situations exist where the benefit to the patient and fetus, based on information derived from radiopharmaceutical use, outweighs the risks from fetal exposure to radiation. In these situations, the physician should use discretion and reduce the radiopharmaceutical dose to the lowest possible amount.

Studies have not been done in animals.

FDA Pregnancy Category C.

### Breast-feeding

Gallium citrate Ga 67 is excreted in breast milk. It has been recommended that nursing be resumed, after administration of a radiopharmaceutical, when the infant's ingested effective dose equivalent (EDE) is below 1 mSv (100 mrem). A method to calculate the EDE has been proposed based on the effective half-life of the radionuclide, the activity administered to the mother, the fraction of administered activity ingested by the infant, and the total body effective dose equivalent to the newborn infant per unit of activity ingested. According to this method, it has been estimated that, for gallium citrate Ga 67, the time to reduce the EDE to the infant to below 1 mSv (100 mrem) is approximately 3 weeks after administration to the mother. Because of the difficulty of maintaining the maternal milk supply for such an extended period of time, complete cessation of nursing is usually recommended.

### Pediatrics

There have been no specific studies evaluating safety and efficacy of gallium citrate Ga 67 in children. When this radiopharmaceutical is used in children, the diagnostic benefit should be judged to outweigh the potential risk of radiation.

Caution is recommended when using preparations that contain benzyl alcohol as preservative in neonates, particularly infants born prematurely.

### Geriatrics

Appropriate studies on the relationship of age to the effects of gallium citrate Ga 67 have not been performed in the geriatric population. However, no geriatrics-specific problems have been documented to date.

### Drug interactions and/or related problems

See *Diagnostic interference.*

### Diagnostic interference

The following have been selected on the basis of their potential clinical significance (possible effect in parentheses where appropriate)—not necessarily inclusive (» = major clinical significance):

With results of *this* test

  *Due to other medications*

    Antineoplastics, which cause an elevation of serum iron, such as:
      Cytarabine
      Fluorouracil
      Methotrexate or
      Iron
      (concurrent use may result in more unbound Ga 67, thus increasing renal excretion and bone uptake of Ga 67, possibly by elevating serum iron, which in turn may displace Ga 67 from plasma protein-binding sites; tumor or abscess localization of gallium citrate Ga 67 is decreased)

    Calcium gluconate, parenteral
    (soft tissue accumulation of gallium citrate Ga 67 may occur as a result of extravasated calcium gluconate)

    COPP chemotherapy
    (thymic uptake of gallium citrate Ga 67 may occur during or after cyclophosphamide-vincristine-procarbazine-prednisone [COPP] chemotherapy)

    Corticosteroids, glucocorticoid
    (concurrent use may decrease gallium citrate Ga 67 uptake by brain tumor or abscess because of reduced peritumor edema caused by the steroid)
    (thymic uptake of gallium citrate Ga 67 may occur with concurrent use of prednisone)

    Gallium nitrate
    (gallium nitrate competes with gallium citrate Ga 67 for plasma protein binding sites, resulting in reduced tumor or abscess uptake and increased skeletal uptake, increased renal excretion, and reduced liver uptake of gallium citrate Ga 67)

    Iron dextran
    (abscess-to-muscle ratio may be increased when iron dextran is given 24 hours after the injection of gallium citrate Ga 67, but may be decreased if given before or concurrently with it; this effect is probably due to a displacement of Ga 67 from plasma protein-binding sites by the iron, which results in increased elimination of the radiopharmaceutical)

    Mechlorethamine or
    Vincristine
    (concurrent use may decrease whole body retention and increase bone deposition and urinary excretion of gallium citrate Ga 67)

*Due to medical problems or conditions*

    Cardiotoxicity, doxorubicin-induced
    (doxorubicin-induced cardiotoxicity may enhance myocardial uptake of gallium citrate Ga 67)

    Gynecomastia or hyperprolactinemia, diethylstilbestrol-, imipramine-, metoclopramide-, oral contraceptive-, phenothiazine-, or reserpine-induced
    (possible localization of gallium citrate Ga 67 in breast [females and males])

    Lymphadenopathy, phenytoin-induced
    (false positive images that resemble true lymphoma may occur since phenytoin has been associated with the development of local or generalized lymphadenopathy; condition should be differentiated from other types of lymph node pathology and the patient observed for an extended period of time)

    Nephritis, drug-induced
    (interstitial nephritis induced by drugs [e.g., allopurinol, cephalosporins, erythromycin, furosemide, gold compounds, nonsteroidal anti-inflammatory drugs, pentamidine, phenobarbital, rifampin, sulfonamides, thiazide diuretics] may result in kidney uptake of gallium citrate Ga 67 that resembles that observed with other inflammatory kidney disease and possibly may be mistaken for glomerulonephritis, pyelonephritis, or the nephrotoxic syndrome)

    Pseudomembranous colitis, antibiotic-induced
    (inflammation of the colon induced by antibiotics or other drugs may result in colonic uptake of gallium citrate Ga 67 that resembles that observed with other inflammatory bowel diseases)

    Pulmonary disease, amiodarone-, bleomycin-, busulfan-, combination chemotherapeutic agent-, or nitrofurantoin-induced
    (pulmonary interstitial pneumonitis and/or fibrosis induced by therapy with these medications may result in diffuse pulmonary localization of gallium citrate Ga 67 that resembles that observed with other diffuse pulmonary diseases not related to drug therapy)

### Medical considerations/Contraindications

The medical considerations/contraindications included here have been selected on the basis of their potential clinical significance (reasons given in parentheses where appropriate)—not necessarily inclusive (» = major clinical significance).

See also *Diagnostic interference.*

***Risk-benefit must be considered when the following medical problem exists:***

Sensitivity to the radiopharmaceutical preparation

## Side/Adverse Effects

The following side/adverse effects have been selected on the basis of their potential clinical significance (possible signs and symptoms in parentheses where appropriate)—not necessarily inclusive:

**Those indicating need for medical attention**

Incidence rare

    *Fast heartbeat; nausea or vomiting; skin rash, hives, or itching*

## Patient Consultation

As an aid to patient consultation, refer to *Advice for the Patient, Radiopharmaceuticals (Diagnostic).*

In providing consultation, consider emphasizing the following selected information (» = major clinical significance):

### Description of use

Action in the body: Concentration of radioactivity in certain tumors and sites of inflammation allows images to be obtained

Small amounts of radioactivity used in diagnosis; radiation received is low and considered safe

### Before having this test

» Conditions affecting use, especially:

Sensitivity to the radiopharmaceutical preparation

Pregnancy—Crosses the placenta; risk to fetus from radiation exposure as opposed to benefit derived from use should be considered

Breast-feeding—Excreted in breast milk; cessation of nursing recommended because of risk to infant from radiation exposure

Use in children—Risk from radiation exposure as opposed to benefit derived from use should be considered

### Preparation for this test

Special preparatory instructions may apply; laxatives or enemas may be prescribed

### Precautions after having this test

No special precautions

### Side/adverse effects

Signs of potential side effects, especially fast heartbeat; nausea or vomiting; or skin rash, hives, or itching

## General Dosing Information

Radiopharmaceuticals are to be administered only by or under the supervision of physicians who have had extensive training in the safe use and handling of radioactive materials and who are authorized by the appropriate Federal or State agency, if required or, outside the U.S., the appropriate authority.

Gallium citrate Ga 67 is to be administered intravenously only.

Imaging is usually done 48 to 72 hours after administration of the radiotracer.

Abnormal gallium citrate Ga 67 concentration usually implies the existence of underlying pathology, but further diagnostic studies may be required to distinguish benign from malignant lesions.

To cleanse the bowel of radioactive material and minimize the possibility of false-positive test results, laxatives and/or enemas may be given daily until final images are obtained.

### Safety considerations for handling this radiopharmaceutical

Improper handling of this radiopharmaceutical may cause radioactive contamination. Guidelines for handling radioactive material have been prepared by scientific, professional, state, federal, and international bodies and are available to the specially qualified and authorized users who have access to radiopharmaceuticals.

## Parenteral Dosage Forms

### GALLIUM CITRATE Ga 67 INJECTION USP

#### Usual adult and adolescent administered activity

Diagnostic aid, radioactive (neoplastic); and

Diagnostic aid, radioactive (focal inflammatory lesions)—

Intravenous, 74 to 185 megabecquerels (2 to 5 millicuries).

Note: In patients with known tumors, doses of 370 megabecquerels (10 millicuries) are used, to facilitate tomography (SPECT) and delayed imaging (>96 hours).

#### Usual pediatric administered activity

Dosage must be individualized by physician.

#### Usual geriatric administered activity

See *Usual adult and adolescent administered activity.*

#### Strength(s) usually available

U.S.—

74 megabecquerels (2 millicuries) ± 10% of gallium Ga 67 per mL at time of calibration (Rx) [Neoscan; GENERIC].

Canada—

As per labeling of supplier [GENERIC].

#### Packaging and storage

Store below 40 °C (104 °F), preferably between 15 and 30 °C (59 and 86 °F), unless otherwise specified by manufacturer. Protect from freezing.

#### Note

Caution—Radioactive material.

### Selected Bibliography

Tsan M. Mechanism of gallium 67 accumulation in inflammatory lesions. J Nucl Med 1985; 26: 88-92.

McNeil BJ, Sanders R, Alderson PO, et al. A prospective study of computed tomography, ultrasound, and gallium imaging in patients with fever. Radiology 1981; 139: 647-53.

Ganz WI, Serafini AN. The diagnostic role of nuclear medicine in the acquired immunodeficiency syndrome. J Nucl Med 1989; 30: 1935-45.

Revised: 10/21/92
Interim revision: 08/02/94

---

# GALLIUM NITRATE   Systemic†

VA CLASSIFICATION (Primary): HS900

Note: For a listing of dosage forms and brand names by country availability, see *Dosage Forms* section(s). For a listing of brand names for the articles in this monograph, refer to the General Index.

†Not commercially available in Canada.

## Category

Antihypercalcemic.

## Indications

### Accepted

Hypercalcemia, associated with neoplasms (treatment)—Gallium nitrate is indicated in the treatment of hypercalcemia of malignancy that is inadequately managed by oral hydration alone. It is used with saline hydration and may be used with diuretics.

### Acceptance not established

Gallium nitrate has been used to treat moderate to severe symptoms of Paget's disease of bone (osteitis deformans), characterized by abnormal and accelerated bone metabolism in one or more bones. However, data are limited and further study is required to define the role of gallium nitrate in this condition.

## Pharmacology/Pharmacokinetics

### Physicochemical characteristics

Source—Gallium nitrate is a hydrated nitrate salt of the group IIIa element gallium.

Molecular weight—417.87.

### Mechanism of action/Effect

*In vivo* studies indicate that gallium nitrate preferentially accumulates in metabolically active areas of high bone turnover, where it reversibly inhibits osteoclast-mediated bone resorption.

Hypercalcemia of malignancy—Bone resorption is increased in the presence of neoplastic tissue. Gallium nitrate inhibits abnormal bone resorption and reduces the flow of calcium from the resorbing bone into the blood, effectively decreasing total and ionized serum calcium. When kidney function is adequate for the fluid load, hydration with saline increases urine output and the use of diuretics increases the rate of calcium excretion.

### Distribution

$Vol_D$—1.27 liters per kg of body weight (L/kg).

### Biotransformation

None.

### Half-life

Alpha—1 hour.

Beta—24 hours, but lengthens to 72 to 115 hours with prolonged intravenous infusion.

**Duration of action**
Studies have reported a median duration of 6 to 8 days (range, 0 to 15+ days).

**Elimination**
Renal.

## Precautions to Consider

### Carcinogenicity
Long-term carcinogenicity studies have not been performed in animals.

### Mutagenicity
Gallium nitrate has not been found to be mutagenic in standard tests such as Ames and chromosomal aberration studies on human lymphocytes.

### Pregnancy/Reproduction
Pregnancy—Studies have not been done in humans.
Studies have not been done in animals.
FDA Pregnancy Category C.

### Breast-feeding
It is not known whether gallium nitrate is distributed into breast milk. It is recommended that mothers taking gallium nitrate not breast-feed because of potentially serious adverse effects in nursing infants.

### Pediatrics
No information is available on the relationship of age to the effects of gallium nitrate in pediatric patients. Safety and efficacy have not been established.

### Geriatrics
Although appropriate studies on the relationship of age to the effects of gallium nitrate have not been performed in the geriatric population, no geriatrics-specific problems have been documented to date. However, elderly patients are more likely to have age-related renal function impairment, which may require caution in patients receiving gallium nitrate.

### Drug interactions and/or related problems
The following drug interactions and/or related problems have been selected on the basis of their potential clinical significance (possible mechanism in parentheses where appropriate)—not necessarily inclusive (» = major clinical significance):

» Nephrotoxic medications, other (See *Appendix II*)
(the possibility of additive toxicity should be considered if these medications are used concurrently with gallium nitrate)

### Laboratory value alterations
The following have been selected on the basis of their potential clinical significance (possible effect in parentheses where appropriate)—not necessarily inclusive (» = major clinical significance):

With diagnostic test results
Gallium citrate Ga 67 scintigraphy for tumor or abscess localization
(gallium nitrate competes with gallium citrate Ga 67 for plasma protein binding sites, resulting in reduced tumor or abscess uptake and increased skeletal uptake, increased renal excretion, and reduced liver uptake of gallium citrate Ga 67)

### Medical considerations/Contraindications
The medical considerations/contraindications included here have been selected on the basis of their potential clinical significance (reasons given in parentheses where appropriate)—not necessarily inclusive (» = major clinical significance):

*Except under special circumstances, this medication should not be used when the following medical problem exists:*

» Renal function impairment when serum creatinine is greater than 2.5 mg per deciliter (mg/dL)
(condition may be exacerbated)

*Risk-benefit should be considered when the following medical problem exists:*

» Renal function impairment when serum creatinine is 2 to 2.5 mg/dL
(frequent monitoring of patient's renal status is recommended; gallium nitrate treatment should be discontinued if serum creatinine exceeds 2.5 mg/dL)

### Patient monitoring
The following may be especially important in patient monitoring (other tests may be warranted in some patients, depending on condition; » = major clinical significance):

Albumin concentrations, serum and
Calcium concentrations, serum and
Phosphorus concentrations, serum
(serum calcium should be monitored daily, serum phosphorus two times a week, and serum albumin before and after each course of therapy; serum proteins, especially albumin, may influence the ra-

tio of free and bound calcium; corrected serum calcium values should be calculated by using an established algorithm; albumin-corrected serum calcium determinations may be useful when the signs and symptoms of hypercalcemia are inconsistent with unadjusted calcium values)

» Renal function determinations, especially serum creatinine and blood urea nitrogen (BUN)
(recommended daily to every 2 to 3 days during therapy; treatment should be discontinued if serum creatinine is greater than 2.5 mg per dL)

## Side/Adverse Effects
The following side/adverse effects have been selected on the basis of their potential clinical significance (possible signs and symptoms in parentheses where appropriate)—not necessarily inclusive:

Note: Decreased serum bicarbonate, possibly secondary to mild respiratory alkalosis, has been reported. It has been asymptomatic and has not required specific treatment.

**Those indicating need for medical attention**
Incidence more frequent
*Hypophosphatemia* (bone pain; loss of appetite; muscle weakness); *nephrotoxicity* (blood in urine; greatly increased or decreased frequency of urination or amount of urine; increased thirst; loss of appetite; nausea; vomiting)

Incidence less frequent
*Hypocalcemia* (abdominal cramps; confusion; muscle spasms)

Incidence rare
*Anemia* (unusual tiredness or weakness)—with doses of up to 1400 mg per square meter of body surface area

**Those indicating need for medical attention only if they continue or are bothersome**
Incidence more frequent
*Diarrhea; metallic taste; nausea; vomiting*

## Patient Consultation
As an aid to patient consultation, refer to *Advice for the Patient, Gallium Nitrate (Systemic)*.

In providing consultation, consider emphasizing the following selected information (» = major clinical significance):

**Before using this medication**
» Conditions affecting use, especially:
Breast-feeding—Not known if distributed into breast milk; may cause potentially serious adverse effects in nursing infants
Other medications, especially nephrotoxic medications
Other medical problems, especially renal function impairment

**Proper use of this medication**
» Proper dosing
» Proper storage

**Precautions while using this medication**
Importance of close monitoring by physician

**Side/adverse effects**
Signs of potential adverse effects, especially hypophosphatemia, nephrotoxicity, hypocalcemia, and anemia

## General Dosing Information
The daily dose is usually diluted in 1000 mL of 0.9% sodium chloride injection or 5% dextrose injection. The diluted dose should be administered over a period of twenty-four hours. The solution can also be delivered undiluted via a metered ambulatory infusion pump.

During acute therapy for hypercalcemia, patients should maintain a urinary output of at least 2000 mL per day to decrease the chance of nephrotoxicity.

## Parenteral Dosage Forms

### GALLIUM NITRATE INJECTION

**Usual adult and adolescent dose**
Hypercalcemia (treatment)—
Intravenous infusion, 100 to 200 mg per square meter of body surface area per day, administered over a period of twenty-four hours, for five days.

Note: If serum calcium concentrations decrease to normal in less than five days, treatment should be discontinued.

Some clinicians recommend that therapy be repeated, if needed, after a waiting period of two to four weeks.

**Usual pediatric dose**
Safety and efficacy have not been established.

**Usual geriatric dose**
Safety and efficacy have not been established.

**Strength(s) usually available**
U.S.—
    25 mg per mL (Rx) [*Ganite*].
Canada—
    Gallium nitrate is not commercially available in Canada; however, it is available by emergency drug release from the Health Protection Branch.

**Packaging and storage**
Store below 40 °C (104 °F), preferably between 15 and 30 °C (59 and 86 °F), unless otherwise specified by manufacturer.

**Preparation of dosage form**
The daily dose is usually diluted in 1000 mL of 0.9% sodium chloride injection or 5% dextrose injection.

**Stability**
Diluted solution may be stored at controlled room temperature for 48 hours and under refrigeration for 7 days without loss of potency.

Revised: 06/28/96

---

# GANCICLOVIR   Systemic

VA CLASSIFICATION (Primary): AM800
Another commonly used name is DHPG.
Note: For a listing of dosage forms and brand names by country availability, see *Dosage Forms* section(s). For a listing of brand names for the articles in this monograph, refer to the General Index.

## Category
Antiviral (systemic).

## Indications
Note: Bracketed information in the *Indications* section refers to uses that are not included in U.S. product labeling.

**Accepted**
Cytomegalovirus retinitis (treatment)—Parenteral ganciclovir is indicated for induction and maintenance in the treatment of cytomegalovirus (CMV) retinitis in immunocompromised patients, including patients with acquired immunodeficiency syndrome (AIDS). Oral ganciclovir is indicated only for the maintenance of CMV retinitis in patients who have had a complete resolution of active retinitis after an induction course of parenteral ganciclovir; however, oral ganciclovir has been associated with a shorter time to CMV retinitis progression. [Intravitreal administration of ganciclovir has also been used in patients who have been unresponsive to intravenous ganciclovir, or in whom serious myelosuppression has precluded the continuation of intravenous therapy.]

Cytomegalovirus disease (prophylaxis)[1]—Parenteral ganciclovir is indicated for the prophylaxis of CMV disease in transplant patients who are at risk for the disease.

[Cytomegalovirus disease (treatment)][1]—Parenteral ganciclovir is used in the treatment of severe CMV disease, including CMV pneumonia, CMV gastrointestinal disease, and disseminated CMV infections, in immunocompromised patients.

[Polyradiculopathy (treatment)][1]—Parenteral ganciclovir is used in the treatment of polyradiculopathy caused by CMV in patients with AIDS.

Resistance to ganciclovir has been reported. One paper described CMV disease refractory to ganciclovir therapy due to infections with a resistant virus, a susceptible virus that became resistant, and an infection first by a susceptible strain, and later by a genetically distinct, resistant one. The primary mechanism of resistance to ganciclovir is the decreased ability to form the active triphosphate moiety. Recurrence may be more frequent in patients treated with ganciclovir for prolonged periods, (> 3 to 6 months).

[1]Not included in Canadian product labeling.

## Pharmacology/Pharmacokinetics

**Physicochemical characteristics**
High pH (11).
Molecular weight—Ganciclovir: 255.23.
    Ganciclovir sodium: 277.22.

**Mechanism of action/Effect**
Ganciclovir is a prodrug that is structurally similar to acyclovir. Its antiviral activity results from its intracellular conversion to the triphosphate form. In cytomegalovirus (CMV)-infected cells, ganciclovir is thought to be rapidly phosphorylated to the monophosphate form by a CMV-encoded enzyme, then subsequently converted to the diphosphate and triphosphate forms by cellular kinases. Ganciclovir is phosphorylated much more rapidly in infected cells; however, uninfected cells can also produce low levels of ganciclovir-triphosphate. Ganci-clovir-triphosphate competitively inhibits DNA polymerase by acting as a substrate and becoming incorporated into the DNA. This inhibits DNA synthesis by suppressing DNA chain elongation. The drug inhibits viral DNA polymerases more effectively than it does cellular polymerase. Chain elongation resumes when ganciclovir is removed.

**Absorption**
Ganciclovir is poorly absorbed after oral administration; bioavailability under fasting conditions is approximately 5%, and when administered with food, 6 to 9%.

**Distribution**
Ganciclovir is widely distributed to all tissues and crosses the placenta; however, there is no marked accumulation in any one type of tissue. Penetration into the cerebral spinal fluid averaged 38% in one study, and ranged from 7 to 67% in others. Ganciclovir also appears to have good intraocular penetration. In one patient, the subretinal fluid ganciclovir concentration was 7.2 micromoles per L with a corresponding plasma concentration of 8.2 micromoles per L 5.5 hours after a dose of 5 mg per kg of body weight (mg/kg), and 2.58 micromoles per L with a corresponding plasma concentration of 1.3 micromoles per L 8 hours after a subsequent dose of 5 mg/kg.
Vol$_D$ (steady state) —Adults and neonates: Approximately 0.74 L per kg.

**Protein binding**
Low (1 to 2%).

**Biotransformation**
Little to no metabolism.

**Half-life**
Serum—
    Intravenous:
        Adults—Normal renal function: 2.5 to 3.6 hours (average, 2.9 hours).
        Adults—Renal function impairment: 9 to 30 hours (creatinine clearance of 20 to 50 mL per minute [0.33 to 0.83 mL per second]).
        Neonates—Approximately 2.4 hours.
    Oral:
        Normal renal function—3.1 to 5.5 hours.
        Renal function impairment—15.7 to 18.2 hours (creatinine clearance of 10 to 50 mL per minute [0.17 to 0.83 mL per second]).
Vitreous fluid—
    Approximately 13 hours.

**Time to peak concentration**
Intravenous—
    End of infusion (approximately 1 hour).
Oral—
    Fasting: Approximately 1.8 hours.
    With food: Approximately 3 hours.

**Peak concentrations**
Intravenous—
    Adults: 5 mg/kg over 1 hour—8.3 to 9 mcg/mL.
    Neonates: 4 and 6 mg/kg over 1 hour—Approximately 5.5 and 7 mcg/mL, respectively.
Oral—
    3 grams per day: 1 to 1.2 mcg/mL.
Intravitreal injection—
    1000 mcg administered in 5 divided doses over 15 days: 16.2 mcg/mL; ganciclovir was not detected in plasma.

**Elimination**
Renal; almost 100% excreted unchanged in the urine by glomerular filtration and tubular secretion.

In dialysis—Plasma ganciclovir concentrations are reduced by approximately 50% after a single, 4-hour hemodialysis.

# Precautions to Consider

## Cross-sensitivity and/or related problems

Patients hypersensitive to acyclovir may also be hypersensitive to ganciclovir because of the chemical similarity of the 2 medications.

## Carcinogenicity/Tumorigenicity

Ganciclovir is carcinogenic in animals and should be considered a potential carcinogen in humans. Ganciclovir was carcinogenic in the mouse at oral doses of 20 and 1000 mg/kg per day (approximately 0.1 and 1.4 times, respectively, the mean drug exposure in humans following the recommended intravenous dose of 5 mg/kg, based on the area under the concentration-time curve [AUC]) comparisons. Mice given oral doses of 20 mg per kg of body weight (mg/kg) per day showed a slightly increased incidence of tumors in the preputial and harderian glands in males, forestomach in males and females, and liver in females. Studies in mice given oral doses of 1000 mg/kg per day showed an increased incidence of tumors of the forestomach in males and females, preputial gland in males, and reproductive tissues and liver in females. All ganciclovir-induced tumors were of epithelial or vascular origin, except for histiocytic sarcoma of the liver. No carcinogenic effect occurred at a dose of 1 mg/kg per day.

## Mutagenicity

Ganciclovir was mutagenic in mouse lymphoma cells at concentrations between 50 and 500 mcg/mL, and caused chromosomal damage *in vitro* in human lymphocytes at concentrations between 250 and 2000 mcg/mL. Parenteral ganciclovir was also clastogenic in the mouse micronucleus assay at doses of 150 and 500 mg/kg (2.8 to 10 times the human exposure based on area under the concentration-time curve [AUC] of a single intravenous dose of 5 mg/kg), but not at a dose of 50 mg/kg (exposure approximately comparable to the human dose based on AUC). Ganciclovir was not mutagenic in the Ames Salmonella assay at concentrations of 500 to 5000 mcg/mL.

## Pregnancy/Reproduction

Fertility—Although data in humans have not been obtained, temporary or permanent suppression of fertility in women and spermatogenesis in men may occur.

In female mice, ganciclovir caused decreased mating behavior, decreased fertility, and increased death *in utero* at doses approximately 1.7 times the recommended human dose (based on the AUC of a single intravenous dose of 5 mg/kg). Ganciclovir was also found to cause decreased fertility in male mice, and hypospermatogenesis in mice and dogs following daily oral or intravenous administration of doses ranging from 0.2 to 10 mg/kg. Inhibition of spermatogenesis and subsequent infertility was reversible at lower doses and irreversible at higher doses in animals. Systemic drug exposure (as measured by AUC) at the lowest dose showing toxicity in each species ranged from 0.03 to 0.1 times the AUC of the recommended human intravenous dose.

Pregnancy—Adequate and well-controlled studies in humans have not been done. However, ganciclovir has been found to cross the placenta. Due to the high toxicity and mutagenic and teratogenic potential of ganciclovir, use during pregnancy should be avoided whenever possible. Women of childbearing age should use effective contraception. Men should use barrier contraception during, and for at least 90 days following, treatment with ganciclovir.

Ganciclovir was found to be carcinogenic in animals and teratogenic in rabbits, causing cleft palate, anophthalmia/microphthalmia, aplastic organs (kidneys and pancreas), hydrocephaly, bradygnathia, and fetal growth retardation. It also was found to be embryotoxic in mice, and to cause death in utero and maternal toxicity in both rabbits and mice. Fetal resorptions occurred in at least 85% of rabbits and mice administered 60 mg/kg per day and 108 mg/kg per day (2 times the human exposure based on AUC comparisons), respectively. Daily intravenous doses of 90 mg/kg administered to female mice prior to mating, during gestation, and during lactation caused hypoplasia of the testes and seminal vesicles in the month-old male offspring, as well as pathologic changes in the nonglandular region of the stomach. The drug exposure in mice as estimated by the AUC was approximately 1.7 times the human AUC.

FDA Pregnancy Category C.

## Breast-feeding

It is not known whether ganciclovir is distributed into breast milk; however, it is likely that some drug will accumulate because of its pharmacokinetic properties. Because of the potential for serious adverse effects in nursing infants, breast-feeding should be stopped during ganciclovir therapy. Ganciclovir has caused irreversible toxicity in nursing animal pups.

## Pediatrics

There is little information currently available on the use of ganciclovir in children, especially those up to the age of 12. At this time, the side effects seen in children appear to be similar to those seen in adults, especially granulocytopenia (17%) and thrombocytopenia (10%). However, the probability of long-term carcinogenicity and reproductive toxicity seen in animal studies should also be considered.

## Geriatrics

No information is available on the relationship of age to the effects of ganciclovir in geriatric patients. However, elderly patients are more likely to have an age-related decrease in renal function, which may require an adjustment of dosage or dosing interval in patients receiving ganciclovir.

## Dental

The neutropenic and thrombocytopenic effects of ganciclovir may result in an increased incidence of microbial infection, delayed healing, and gingival bleeding. Patients should be instructed in proper oral hygiene, including caution in use of regular toothbrushes, dental floss, and toothpicks.

## Drug interactions and/or related problems

The following drug interactions and/or related problems have been selected on the basis of their potential clinical significance (possible mechanism in parentheses where appropriate)—not necessarily inclusive (» = major clinical significance):

Note: Combinations containing any of the following medications, depending on the amount present, may also interact with this medication.

Blood dyscrasia–causing medications (See *Appendix II*) or
» Bone marrow depressants, other (See *Appendix II*) or
Radiation therapy
    (concurrent use with ganciclovir may increase the bone marrow–depressant effects of these medications and radiation therapy)

Didanosine
    (concurrent and sequential [2 hours apart] administration of didanosine with ganciclovir results in a significant increase in the steady-state area under the concentration-time curve [AUC] of didanosine [range, 72 to 111%]; when didanosine was administered 2 hours before oral ganciclovir, the steady-state AUC of ganciclovir was decreased by approximately 21%; there was no significant change in renal clearance of either medication)

Imipenem and cilastatin combination
    (generalized seizures have been reported in patients receiving ganciclovir and imipenem and cilastatin combination concurrently)

» Nephrotoxic medications (See *Appendix II*)
    (concurrent use with ganciclovir may increase serum creatinine; concurrent use with nephrotoxic medications, such as cyclosporine or amphotericin B, may increase the chance of renal function impairment; this may also decrease elimination of ganciclovir and increase the risk of toxicity)

Probenecid
    (concurrent use with probenecid increases the AUC of ganciclovir by approximately 53% and decreases its renal clearance by approximately 22%; concurrent use of ganciclovir with probenecid, or other medications that inhibit renal tubular secretion, may reduce the renal clearance of ganciclovir and lead to toxicity)

» Zidovudine
    (concurrent use of ganciclovir with zidovudine has been associated with severe hematologic toxicity in some patients, even when the zidovudine dose was reduced to 300 mg per day; concurrent use increases the AUC of zidovudine by approximately 14 to 19%; *in vitro* studies found concurrent use of these 2 drugs to be synergistically cytotoxic; concurrent administration should be used with caution)

## Laboratory value alterations

The following have been selected on the basis of their potential clinical significance (possible effect in parentheses where appropriate)—not necessarily inclusive (» = major clinical significance):

With physiology/laboratory test values
Alanine aminotransferase (ALT [SGPT]), serum and
Alkaline phosphatase, serum and
Aspartate aminotransferase (AST [SGOT]), serum and
Bilirubin, serum
    (values may be increased)

Blood urea nitrogen (BUN) or
Creatinine, serum
    (values may be increased)

## Medical considerations/Contraindications

The medical considerations/contraindications included here have been selected on the basis of their potential clinical significance (reasons given in parentheses where appropriate)—not necessarily inclusive (» = major clinical significance).

*Risk-benefit should be considered when the following medical problems exist:*

» Absolute neutrophil count (ANC) <500 cells/mm³ or platelet count <25,000 cells/mm³

» Hypersensitivity to acyclovir or ganciclovir

» Renal function impairment
    (because ganciclovir is excreted through the kidneys, the dose of ganciclovir should be reduced or the dosing interval increased in patients with renal function impairment)

## Patient monitoring

The following may be especially important in patient monitoring (other tests may be warranted in some patients, depending on condition; » = major clinical significance):

» Complete blood counts (CBCs) and
» Platelet counts
    (because ganciclovir may cause granulocytopenia and thrombocytopenia, neutrophil and platelet counts should be monitored prior to treatment, every 2 days during induction therapy, then at least weekly thereafter. Neutrophil and platelet counts should be performed daily in patients undergoing hemodialysis, patients with neutrophil counts less than 1000 cells/mm³ at the beginning of treatment, and those in whom use of ganciclovir or other nucleoside analogs previously resulted in leukopenia. When severe neutropenia [absolute neutrophil count < 500 cells/mm³ ] or severe thromboctyopenia [platelet count < 25,000 cells/mm³ ] occurs, discontinuation of ganciclovir may be necessary; however, a small number of patients have been successfully treated with concurrent use of sargramostim [GM-CSF; granulocyte-macrophage colony stimulating factor] or filgrastin [G-CSF; granulocyte colony stimulating factor])

    Liver function tests
    (liver function tests, including serum ALT [SGPT] and AST [SGOT] values, and serum bilirubin concentration, should be monitored periodically since elevations, usually reversible, have occurred during ganciclovir therapy)

» Renal function determinations
    (blood urea nitrogen and serum creatinine determinations should be monitored at least every 2 weeks since patients with renal function impairment will require an adjustment in dosage or dosage interval)

*For treatment of cytomegalovirus [CMV] retinitis, in addition to the above*
» Ophthalmologic examinations
    (ophthalmologic examinations should be performed weekly during induction and every 4 weeks during maintenance since ganciclovir is not a cure for cytomegalovirus [CMV] retinitis, and progression of retinitis may occur during or following ganciclovir treatment; however, the frequency of examinations may vary, depending on the extent of disease, activity, and proximity to the macula and optic disc)

# Side/Adverse Effects

The following side/adverse effects have been selected on the basis of their potential clinical significance (possible signs and symptoms in parentheses where appropriate)—not necessarily inclusive:

**Those indicating need for medical attention**
Incidence more frequent
    *For intravenous and oral administration*
    **Granulocytopenia** (sore throat and fever); **thrombocytopenia** (unusual bleeding or bruising)
        Note: *Granulocytopenia* is usually reversible, with an overall incidence of approximately 40%; the incidence of dose-limiting toxicity is <20%.
        *Thrombocytopenia* is also usually reversible, with an overall incidence of approximately 20%; the incidence of dose-limiting toxicity is 5 to 10%.

Incidence less frequent
    *For intravenous and oral administration*
    **Anemia** (unusual tiredness and weakness); *central nervous system (CNS) effects* (mood or other mental changes; nervousness; tremor); *hypersensitivity* (fever; skin rash); *phlebitis* (pain at site of injection)

*For intravitreal administration*
    **Bacterial endophthalmitis; conjunctival scarring, mild; foreign body sensation; retinal detachment; scleral induration; or subconjunctival hemorrhage** (decreased vision or any change in vision)

**Those indicating need for medical attention only if they continue or are bothersome**
Incidence less frequent
    *Gastrointestinal disturbances* (abdominal pain; loss of appetite; nausea and vomiting)

# Patient Consultation

As an aid to patient consultation, refer to *Advice for the Patient, Ganciclovir (Systemic).*

In providing consultation, consider emphasizing the following selected information (» = major clinical significance):

**Before using this medication**
» Conditions affecting use, especially:
    Hypersensitivity to acyclovir or ganciclovir
    Pregnancy—Use of ganciclovir during pregnancy should be avoided whenever possible. Ganciclovir crosses the placenta and has been found to be carcinogenic and teratogenic in animals. Use of effective contraception by men and women who are undergoing treatment and in men for 90 days following treatment is recommended
    Breast-feeding—Because of ganciclovir's potential for severe toxicity, breast-feeding should be stopped during therapy
    Use in children—There is little information currently available on the use of ganciclovir in children, especially those up to the age of 12; long-term carcinogenicity and reproductive toxicity due to ganciclovir use in children is unknown
    Dental—The neutropenic and thrombocytopenic effects of ganciclovir may result in an increased incidence of microbial infection, delayed healing, and gingival bleeding
    Other medications, especially other bone marrow depressants, nephrotoxic medications, or zidovudine
    Other medical problems, especially renal function impairment, an absolute neutrophil count (ANC) <500 cells/mm³, or platelet count <25,000 cells/mm³

**Proper use of this medication**
» Taking ganciclovir capsules with food
» Importance of receiving medication for full course of therapy and on a regular schedule
» Proper dosing

**Precautions while using this medication**
*To reduce the risk of bleeding during periods of low blood counts:*
» Checking with physician immediately if getting an infection or fever or chills
» Checking with physician immediately if unusual bleeding or bruising; black, tarry stools; blood in urine or stools; or pinpoint red spots on skin occur
    Using caution in use of regular toothbrushes, dental floss, and toothpicks; physician, dentist, or nurse may suggest alternative methods for cleaning teeth and gums; checking with physician before having dental work done
    Using caution to avoid accidental cuts with use of sharp objects such as a safety razor or fingernail or toenail cutters

» Using contraception since ganciclovir has mutagenic and teratogenic potential; women should use effective contraception during treatment, and men should use barrier contraception during and for at least 90 days following treatment
» Regular visits to physician to check blood counts
» *For CMV retinitis*— Regular visits to ophthalmologist to examine eyes since progression of retinitis and visual loss may occur during ganciclovir therapy

**Side/adverse effects**
    Signs of potential side effects, especially granulocytopenia, thrombocytopenia, anemia, CNS effects, hypersensitivity, and phlebitis when ganciclovir is administered intravenously or orally; and bacterial endophthalmitis, mild conjunctival scarring, foreign body sensation, retinal detachment, scleral induration, and subconjunctival hemorrhage when it is administered intravitreally

# General Dosing Information

Ganciclovir is not a cure for cytomegalovirus infections. Maintenance therapy is almost always necessary in AIDS patients to prevent relapse, which is very common once the medication has been withdrawn.

Monitoring of serum ganciclovir concentrations has not been shown to be useful for ensuring efficacy or avoiding toxicity.

Ganciclovir sodium should be administered by intravenous infusion only. Intramuscular or subcutaneous injection will result in severe tissue irritation due to ganciclovir's high pH (11).

Intravenous infusions of ganciclovir should be administered at a constant rate *over at least a 1-hour period*, and patients must be adequately hydrated, to avoid increased toxicity. The recommended dosage, frequency, and infusion rate should not be exceeded.

Severe neutropenia or thrombocytopenia (absolute neutrophil count [ANC] <500 cells/mm³ or platelet count <25,000 cells/mm³) requires an interruption in therapy until there is evidence of bone marrow recovery (ANC ≥750 cells/mm³); however, a small number of patients have been successfully treated with concurrent use of sargramostim (GM-CSF; granulocyte-macrophage colony stimulating factor).

Ganciclovir capsules should be taken with food for maximum absorption.

The dose of ganciclovir must be decreased in patients with renal function impairment.

Patients undergoing hemodialysis should not receive a dose in excess of 1.25 mg per kg of body weight (mg/kg) every 24 hours. On dialysis days, the dose of ganciclovir should be administered after hemodialysis has been performed since dialysis will reduce plasma ganciclovir concentrations by approximately 50%.

Ganciclovir capsules are indicated as an alternative to intravenous ganciclovir for maintenance therapy of CMV retinitis in immunocompromised patients, including those with AIDS. Oral ganciclovir should be used in patients in whom retinitis is stable and quiescent following appropriate induction therapy and for whom the risk of more rapid progression is balanced by the benefit associated with avoiding long-term daily intravenous infusions, usually requiring indwelling intravenous catheters.

Intravitreal administration of ganciclovir has been used in patients who have been unresponsive to intravenous ganciclovir, or in whom serious myelosuppression has precluded the continuation of intravenous therapy. Intravitreal doses of 200 micrograms have resulted in improvement or stabilization of retinitis, and have been well tolerated. In one report describing a patient who received 28 intravitreal injections, plasma concentrations after intravitreal injections showed no significant systemic absorption. The elimination half-life of ganciclovir from the vitreous fluid was estimated to be 13.3 hours, and the intravitreal concentration remained above the $ID_{50}$ of cytomegalovirus for approximately 62 hours after a single injection.

### Safety considerations for handling this medication

Caution should be exercised in the handling and preparation of ganciclovir. Because ganciclovir shares some properties of anti-tumor agents (i.e., carcinogenicity and mutagenicity), it should be handled and disposed of according to guidelines issued for cytotoxic drugs. Ganciclovir solution is alkaline (pH 11). Avoid inhalation, ingestion, or direct contact of ganciclovir with the skin or mucous membranes. If contact does occur, wash area thoroughly with soap and water; rinse eyes thoroughly with plain water. Ganciclovir capsules should not be opened or crushed.

## Oral Dosage Forms

### GANCICLOVIR CAPSULES

**Usual adult and adolescent dose**
Cytomegalovirus retinitis—
    Induction: Ganciclovir capsules should not be used for induction therapy. See *Sterile Ganciclovir Sodium*
    Maintenance: Oral, 1000 mg three times a day with food, or 500 mg six times a day every three hours with food, during waking hours.
    Note: For maintenance, patients with impaired renal function may require a reduction in dose as follows:

| Creatinine Clearance (mL/min)/ (mL/sec) | Dose |
| --- | --- |
| ≥70/1.17 | See *Usual adult and adolescent dose* |
| 50–69/0.83–1.15 | 1500 mg once a day, or 500 mg three times a day |
| 25–49/0.42–0.82 | 1000 mg once a day, or 500 mg twice a day |
| 10–24/0.17–0.40 | 500 mg once a day |
| <10/0.17 | 500 mg three times a week, following hemodialysis |

**Usual pediatric dose**
Dosage has not been established.

**Strength(s) usually available**
U.S.—
    250 mg (Rx) [*Cytovene*].
Canada—
    Not commercially available.

**Packaging and storage**
Store below 40 °C (104 °F), preferably between 15 and 30 °C (59 and 86 °F), unless otherwise specified by manufacturer.

**Auxiliary labeling**
• Continue medicine for full time of treatment.

**Note**
Ganciclovir capsules should not be opened or crushed.

## Parenteral Dosage Forms

### GANCICLOVIR SODIUM STERILE

**Usual adult and adolescent dose**
Cytomegalovirus retinitis (treatment)—
    Induction:
        Intravenous infusion, 5 mg per kg of body weight, administered over at least one hour, every twelve hours for fourteen to twenty-one days.
        Note: Doses of 7.5 to 15 mg per kg of body weight per day divided into two or three doses have been used, and treatment has been continued for longer than twenty-one days; if retinitis does not show significant improvement, the possibility of viral resistance should be considered.
    Intravitreal injection, 200 mcg two times a week for three weeks.
    Note: For induction, patients with impaired renal function may require a reduction in dose as follows:

| Creatinine Clearance (mL/min)/(mL/sec) | Dose |
| --- | --- |
| ≥70/1.17 | See *Usual adult and adolescent dose* |
| 50–69/0.83–1.15 | 2.5 mg per kg every twelve hours |
| 25–49/0.42–0.82 | 2.5 mg per kg every twenty-four hours |
| 10–24/0.17–0.40 | 1.25 mg per kg every twenty-four hours |
| <10 | 1.25 mg per kg three times a week, following hemodialysis |

    Maintenance:
        Intravenous infusion, 5 mg per kg of body weight a day, administered over at least one hour, once a day for seven days per week; or 6 mg per kg of body weight, administered over at least one hour, once a day for five days of the week.
        Note: If CMV retinitis progresses during maintenance therapy, patients should be retreated with the twice-a-day induction regimen.
    Intravitreal injection, 200 mcg once a week.
    Note: For maintenance, patients with impaired renal function may require a reduction in dose as follows:

| Creatinine Clearance (mL/min)/ (mL/sec) | Dose |
| --- | --- |
| ≥70/1.17 | See *Usual adult and adolescent dose* |
| 50–69/0.83–1.15 | 2.5 mg per kg every twelve hours |
| 25–49/0.42–0.82 | 1.25 mg per kg every twenty-four hours |
| 10–24/0.17–0.40 | 0.625 mg per kg every twenty-four hours |
| <10 | 0.625 mg per kg three times a week, following hemodialysis |

Cytomegalovirus disease (prophylaxis)—
    Intravenous infusion, 5 mg per kg of body weight, administered over at least one hour, every twelve hours for seven to fourteen days; then 5 mg per kg of body weight, administered over at least one hour, once a day for seven days of the week, or 6 mg per kg of body weight, administered over at least one hour, once a day for five days of the week.

**Usual pediatric dose**
Dosage has not been established. However, induction doses of 7.5 to 10 mg per kg of body weight divided into two or three doses, and maintenance doses of 2.5 to 5 mg per kg of body weight a day have been used in children.

**Strength(s) usually available**

U.S.—

500 mg (Rx) [*Cytovene-IV* (sodium 46 mg)].

Canada—

500 mg (Rx) [*Cytovene*].

**Packaging and storage**

Store below 40 °C (104 °F), preferably between 15 and 30 °C (59 and 86 °F), unless otherwise specified by manufacturer.

**Preparation of dosage form**

To prepare initial dilution for intravenous infusion, 10 mL of sterile water for injection (without parabens) should be added to each 500-mg vial to provide 50 mg per mL. To ensure complete dissolution, the vial should be shaken until solution is clear. The resulting solution should be further diluted, usually with 100 mL of 0.9% sodium chloride injection, 5% dextrose injection, Ringer's injection, or lactated Ringer's injection. Final concentrations of 10 mg per mL or less are recommended.

Note: Caution should be exercised in the handling and preparation of ganciclovir. Because ganciclovir shares some properties of antitumor agents (i.e., carcinogenicity and mutagenicity), it should be handled and disposed of according to guidelines issued for cytotoxic drugs. Ganciclovir solution is alkaline (pH 11). Avoid inhalation, ingestion, or direct contact of ganciclovir with the skin or mucous membranes. If contact does occur, wash area thoroughly with soap and water; rinse eyes thoroughly with plain water.

**Stability**

The manufacturer states that after reconstitution, solutions at concentrations of 50 mg per mL retain their potency for 12 hours at room temperature. Refrigeration is not recommended. After further dilution for intravenous infusion, it is recommended that solutions be used within 24 hours since nonbacteriostatic infusion solutions must be used; refrigerate the diluted solution; do not freeze.

However, studies have found that ganciclovir, when diluted to concentrations of 1, 5, and 10 mg per mL in 5% dextrose injection and 0.9% sodium chloride injection, was stable when assayed at 28 and 35 days. These solutions were refrigerated in polyvinyl chloride (PVC) bags and syringes. Ganciclovir was also stable when 5 and 10 mg per mL solutions were frozen in PVC bags for 28 days.

**Incompatibilities**

Parabens are incompatible with ganciclovir sodium and may cause precipitation.

## Selected Bibliography

Markham A, Faulds D. Ganciclovir. An update of its therapeutic use in cytomegalovirus infections. Drugs 1994; 48 (3): 455-84.

Revised: 08/08/95

---

# GEMFIBROZIL    Systemic

VA CLASSIFICATION (Primary): CV350

Note: For a listing of dosage forms and brand names by country availability, see *Dosage Forms* section(s). For a listing of brand names for the articles in this monograph, refer to the General Index.

## Category

Antihyperlipidemic.

## Indications

**Accepted**

Hyperlipidemia (treatment)—Gemfibrozil is indicated in the treatment of hyperlipidemia and to reduce the risk of coronary heart disease *only* in those patients with type IIb hyperlipidemia without history of or symptoms of existing coronary heart disease, who have not responded to diet, exercise, weight loss, or other pharmacologic therapy (bile acid sequestrants and niacin) alone *and* who have the triad of low high density lipoprotein (HDL) cholesterol levels, elevated low density lipoprotein (LDL) cholesterol levels, and elevated triglycerides.

Gemfibrozil is also recommended for use in patients with severe primary hyperlipidemia (types IV and V hyperlipidemia) and a significant risk of coronary artery disease, abdominal pain typical of pancreatitis, or pancreatitis, who have not responded to diet or other measures alone. Its use is limited in type III hyperlipidemia because of its limited effect on cholesterol concentrations. It is not useful in the treatment of type I hyperlipidemia.

Gemfibrozil is not indicated for treatment of patients with type IIa hyperlipidemia or patients with low HDL cholesterol as their only lipid abnormality because the potential benefits do not outweigh the risks.

Caution and close observation are recommended in patients with high triglyceride concentrations, since in some of these patients treatment with gemfibrozil is associated with significant increases in low density lipoprotein (LDL)-cholesterol concentrations.

For additional information on initial therapeutic guidelines related to the treatment of hyperlipidemia, see *Appendix III.*

Gemfibrozil is not recommended for community-wide prevention of ischemic heart disease.

Studies have suggested that control of elevated cholesterol and triglycerides may not lessen the danger of cardiovascular disease and mortality, although incidence of nonfatal myocardial infarctions may be decreased.

## Pharmacology/Pharmacokinetics

**Physicochemical characteristics**

Molecular weight—250.34.

**Mechanism of action/Effect**

Gemfibrozil reduces plasma triglyceride (very low–density lipoprotein [VLDL]) concentrations and increases high-density lipoprotein (HDL) concentrations. Although gemfibrozil may slightly reduce total and low-density lipoprotein (LDL) cholesterol concentrations, use of gemfibrozil in patients with elevated triglycerides associated with type IV hyperlipidemia often results in significant increases in LDL; LDL concentrations are not significantly affected by gemfibrozil in patients with Type IIb hyperlipidemia (although HDL is significantly increased). The mechanism of this action is not completely understood but may involve inhibition of peripheral lipolysis; reduced hepatic extraction of free fatty acids, which reduces hepatic triglyceride production; inhibition of synthesis and increased clearance of VLDL carrier, apolipoprotein B, which also reduces VLDL production; and, according to animal studies, reduced incorporation of long-chain fatty acids into newly formed triglycerides, accelerated turnover and removal of cholesterol from the liver (stimulates incorporation of cholesterol precursors into liver sterols), and increased excretion of cholesterol in the feces.

**Absorption**

Well absorbed from gastrointestinal tract.

**Biotransformation**

Hepatic.

**Half-life**

Single dose—1.5 hours.

Multiple doses—1.3 hours.

**Onset of action**

Reduction of plasma VLDL concentrations—2 to 5 days.

**Time to peak concentration**

1 to 2 hours.

**Time to peak effect**

Reduction of plasma VLDL concentrations—4 weeks (major effect; further decreases occur over several months).

**Elimination**

Renal (70%; largely unchanged)/fecal (6%).

## Precautions to Consider

**Carcinogenicity/Tumorigenicity**

During long term follow-up of patients in the Helsinki Heart Study, there was a trend toward an increased incidence of basal cell carcinomas and deaths attributed to cancer in the group of patients originally randomized to gemfibrozil. However, these data did not reach statistical significance.

Long term studies in male rats have shown gemfibrozil to have a tumorigenic effect. Studies in rats given gemfibrozil for prolonged periods found an increased incidence of benign and malignant hepatic tumors in male and female rats, as well as benign testicular (Leydig cell) tumors in male rats, at doses of 1 and 10 times the human dose.

### Pregnancy/Reproduction

Fertility—Studies in male rats given gemfibrozil at doses 0.6 to 2 times the human dose (based on surface area) for 10 weeks revealed a dose-related decrease in fertility.

Pregnancy—Studies in humans have not been done.

Studies in female rats given gemfibrozil at 0.6 to 2 times the human dose (based on surface area) before and throughout gestation resulted in a dose-related decrease in conception rate and an increase in skeletal variations, including anophthalmia. At the high dose level an increase in stillbirths and reduction in pup weight during lactation were observed. In addition, similar doses given to female rats from gestation day 15 through weaning resulted in decreased birth weights and pup growth suppression during lactation.

Gemfibrozil, given at doses 1 to 3 times the human dose (based on surface area) to female rabbits during organogenesis, caused decreased litter sizes and, at the high dose, an increased incidence of parietal bone variations.

FDA Pregnancy Category C.

### Breast-feeding

It is not known whether gemfibrozil is excreted in breast milk. Problems in humans have not been documented; however, any decision regarding breast-feeding during therapy should take into account that gemfibrozil has a tumorigenic effect in rats.

### Pediatrics

Appropriate studies on the relationship of age to the effects of gemfibrozil have not been performed in the pediatric population. However, use in children under 2 years of age is not recommended since cholesterol is required for normal development.

### Geriatrics

No information is available on the relationship of age to the effects of gemfibrozil in geriatric patients. However, elderly patients are more likely to have age-related renal function impairment, which may require reduction of dosage in patients receiving gemfibrozil.

### Drug interactions and/or related problems

The following drug interactions and/or related problems have been selected on the basis of their potential clinical significance (possible mechanism in parentheses where appropriate)—not necessarily inclusive (» = major clinical significance):

» Anticoagulants, coumarin- or indandione-derivative
   (concurrent use with gemfibrozil may significantly increase the anticoagulant effect of these medications; adjustment of anticoagulant dosage based on frequent prothrombin-time determinations is recommended)

Chenodiol or
Ursodiol
   (effect may be decreased when chenodiol or ursodiol is used concurrently with gemfibrozil, which tends to increase cholesterol saturation of bile)

» Lovastatin
   (concurrent use with gemfibrozil may be associated with an increased risk of rhabdomyolysis, significant increases in creatine kinase [CK] concentrations, and myoglobinuria that leads to acute renal failure; may be seen as early as 3 weeks or as late as several months after initiation of combined therapy; monitoring of CK has not been shown to prevent severe myopathy or renal damage)

### Laboratory value alterations

The following have been selected on the basis of their potential clinical significance (possible effect in parentheses where appropriate)—not necessarily inclusive (» = major clinical significance):

With physiology/laboratory test values
Alanine aminotransferase (ALT [SGPT]), serum and
Alkaline phosphatase, serum and
Aspartate aminotransferase (AST [SGOT]), serum and
Bilirubin, serum and
Creatine kinase (CK), plasma and
Lactate dehydrogenase (LDH), serum
   (concentrations may be increased, indicating liver function abnormalities)

Hematocrit and
Hemoglobin concentrations and
Leukocyte counts
   (may be mildly decreased, but usually stabilize with continued administration)

Potassium
   (serum concentrations may be decreased)

### Medical considerations/Contraindications

The medical considerations/contraindications included here have been selected on the basis of their potential clinical significance (reasons given in parentheses where appropriate)—not necessarily inclusive (» = major clinical significance).

*Except under special circumstances, this medication should not be used when the following medical problem exists:*

» Primary biliary cirrhosis
   (use of gemfibrozil may further raise the cholesterol)

*Risk-benefit should be considered when the following medical problems exist:*

Gallbladder disease or
Gallstones
   (increased risk of biliary complications, including possible formation of gallstones)

» Hepatic function impairment
   (reduced biotransformation; reduced dosage is recommended)

» Renal function impairment, severe
   (reduced clearance leads to increased incidence of side effects; reduced dosage is recommended)
   (gemfibrozil may worsen pre-existing renal insufficiency)

Sensitivity to gemfibrozil

### Patient monitoring

The following may be especially important in patient monitoring (other tests may be warranted in some patients, depending on condition; » = major clinical significance):

Blood counts, complete and
Cholesterol, serum and
Liver function tests and
Triglycerides, serum
   (determinations recommended prior to initiation of therapy and at periodic intervals during therapy)

## Side/Adverse Effects

Note: Because of the chemical, pharmacologic, and clinical similarity of gemfibrozil to clofibrate, the possibility of similar long-term effects should be kept in mind. Studies with clofibrate have associated long-term use of the medication with an increased incidence of deaths from noncardiovascular causes and have also found a greatly increased incidence of cholelithiasis and cholecystitis requiring surgery in clofibrate users (see *Clofibrate [Systemic]*). In addition, studies have suggested that control of elevated cholesterol and triglycerides may not lessen the danger of cardiovascular disease and mortality, although incidence of nonfatal myocardial infarctions may be decreased.

Subcapsular bilateral cataracts and unilateral cataracts have been reported in 10% and 6.3%, respectively, of male rats given 10 times the human dose.

The following side/adverse effects have been selected on the basis of their potential clinical significance (possible signs and symptoms in parentheses where appropriate)—not necessarily inclusive:

### Those indicating need for immediate medical attention

Incidence rare
   *Anemia or leukopenia* (cough or hoarseness; fever or chills; lower back or side pain; painful or difficult urination); *gallstones* (severe stomach pain with nausea and vomiting); *myositis* (muscle pain, unusual tiredness or weakness)

   Note: Gemfibrozil may increase cholesterol secretion into the bile.

### Those indicating need for medical attention only if they continue or are bothersome

Incidence more frequent
   *Stomach pain, gas, or heartburn*

Incidence less frequent
   *Diarrhea; nausea or vomiting; skin rash; unusual tiredness*

## Patient Consultation

As an aid to patient consultation, refer to *Advice for the Patient, Gemfibrozil (Systemic)*.

In providing consultation, consider emphasizing the following selected information (» = major clinical significance):

### Before using this medication

Potential serious toxicity because of similarity to clofibrate
» Diet as preferred therapy
» Conditions affecting use, especially:
   Sensitivity to gemfibrozil

Pregnancy—High doses in animals cause birth defects and an increase in fetal deaths

Breast-feeding—High doses associated with increased incidence of tumors in rats; consider when deciding whether to breast-feed

Use in children—Not recommended in children under 2 years of age since cholesterol is required for normal development

Other medications, especially lovastatin or oral anticoagulants

Other medical problems, especially primary biliary cirrhosis, hepatic function impairment, or severe renal function impairment

## Proper use of this medication

» Importance of not taking more or less medication than the amount prescribed

Taking 30 minutes before morning and evening meal

» Compliance with prescribed diet

» Proper dosing

Missed dose: Taking as soon as possible; not taking if almost time for next dose; not doubling doses

» Proper storage

## Precautions while using this medication

» Importance of close monitoring by physician

» Checking with physician before discontinuing medication; blood lipid concentrations may increase significantly

## Side/adverse effects

Signs of potential side effects, especially gallstones, leukopenia, anemia, and myositis

## General Dosing Information

If response is inadequate after 3 months of treatment, gemfibrozil therapy should be withdrawn.

When gemfibrozil is discontinued, an appropriate hypolipidemic diet and monitoring of serum lipids are recommended until the patient stabilizes, since a rise in serum triglyceride and cholesterol concentrations to the original base may occur.

If results of hepatic function tests rise significantly or show significant abnormalities, it is recommended that gemfibrozil therapy be withdrawn and not resumed; laboratory abnormalities are usually reversible.

If gallstones are found, gemfibrozil therapy should be withdrawn.

If patients receiving gemfibrozil experience muscle pain or weakness, evaluation for myositis (including serum CK determinations) is recommended. It is recommended that gemfibrozil be withdrawn if myositis is suspected or diagnosed.

## Diet/Nutrition

Gemfibrozil should be taken 30 minutes before the morning and evening meals.

## Oral Dosage Forms

### GEMFIBROZIL CAPSULES USP

**Usual adult dose**
Antihyperlipidemic—
Oral, 1.2 grams a day in two divided doses thirty minutes before the morning and evening meals.

**Usual pediatric dose**
Dosage has not been established.

**Strength(s) usually available**
U.S.—
Not commercially available.
Canada—
300 mg (Rx) [*Lopid*].

**Packaging and storage**
Store below 30 °C (86 °F), unless otherwise specified by manufacturer. Store in a tight container.

### GEMFIBROZIL TABLETS

**Usual adult dose**
Antihyperlipidemic—
Oral, 1.2 grams a day in two divided doses thirty minutes before the morning and evening meals.

**Usual pediatric dose**
Dosage has not been established.

**Strength(s) usually available**
U.S.—
600 mg (Rx) [*Lopid* (scored; methylparaben; propylparaben)].
Canada—
600 mg (Rx) [*Lopid*].

**Packaging and storage**
Store below 30 °C (86 °F), unless otherwise specified by manufacturer. Store in a tight container.

## Selected Bibliography

National Cholesterol Education Program. Second Report of the Expert Panel on Detection, Evaluation, and Treatment of High Blood Cholesterol in Adults (Adult Treatment Panel II). Circulation 1994; 89 (3): 1329-445.

Knodel LC, Talbert RL. Adverse effects of hypolipidaemic drugs. Med Toxicol 1987; 2: 10-32.

Frick MH, Elo O, Haapa K, et al. Helsinki Heart Study: Primary-prevention trial with gemfibrozil in middle-aged men with dyslipidemia. N Engl J Med 1987; 317: 1237-45.

Revised: 05/24/93
Interim revision: 06/28/95

---

**GENTAMICIN**—See *Aminoglycosides (Systemic)*; *Gentamicin (Ophthalmic)*; *Gentamicin (Otic)*; *Gentamicin (Topical)*

---

# GENTAMICIN   Ophthalmic

VA CLASSIFICATION (Primary): OP201

Another commonly used name is gentamycin.

Note: For a listing of dosage forms and brand names by country availability, see *Dosage Forms* section(s). For a listing of brand names for the articles in this monograph, refer to the General Index.

## Category

Antibacterial (ophthalmic).

## Indications

### Accepted

Blepharitis, bacterial (treatment)
Blepharoconjunctivitis (treatment)
Conjunctivitis, bacterial (treatment)
Dacryocystitis (treatment)
Keratitis, bacterial (treatment)
Keratoconjunctivitis, bacterial (treatment) or
Meibomianitis (treatment)—Ophthalmic gentamicin is indicated in the treatment of blepharitis, blepharoconjunctivitis, conjunctivitis, dacryocystitis, keratitis, keratoconjunctivitis, and acute meibomianitis caused by coagulase-negative and coagulase-positive staphylococci, *Pseudomonas aeruginosa*, indole-positive and indole-negative *Proteus* species, *Escherichia coli*, *Klebsiella pneumoniae*, *Hemophilus influenzae*, *H. aegyptius*, *Enterobacter aerogenes (Aerobacter aerogenes)*, *Moraxella lacunata* (Morax-Axenfeld bacillus), and *Neisseria* species, including *N. gonorrhoeae*.

Note: Not all species or strains of a particular organism may be susceptible to gentamicin.

## Pharmacology/Pharmacokinetics

### Physicochemical characteristics

Chemical group—Aminoglycosides.
pH—Gentamicin sulfate ophthalmic solution is buffered to pH of approximately 7.

### Mechanism of action/Effect

Aminoglycoside; actively transported across the bacterial cell membrane, binds to a specific receptor protein on the 30 S subunit of bacterial ribosomes, and interferes with an initiation complex between mRNA (messenger RNA) and the 30 S subunit, inhibiting protein synthesis. DNA may be misread, thus producing nonfunctional proteins; polyribosomes are split apart and are unable to synthesize protein.

Note: Aminoglycosides are bactericidal, while most other antibiotics that interfere with protein synthesis are bacteriostatic.

### Absorption
May be absorbed in minute quantities following topical application to the eye.

## Precautions to Consider

### Cross-sensitivity and/or related problems
Patients sensitive to one aminoglycoside may be sensitive to other aminoglycosides also.

### Pregnancy/Reproduction
Problems in humans have not been documented.

### Breast-feeding
Problems in humans have not been documented.

### Pediatrics
Appropriate studies on the relationship of age to the effects of this medicine have not been performed in the pediatric population. However, no pediatrics-specific problems have been documented to date.

### Geriatrics
Appropriate studies on the relationship of age to the effects of this medicine have not been performed in the geriatric population. However, no geriatrics-specific problems have been documented to date.

### Medical considerations/Contraindications
The medical considerations/contraindications included here have been selected on the basis of their potential clinical significance (reasons given in parentheses where appropriate)—not necessarily inclusive (» = major clinical significance).

*Risk-benefit should be considered when the following medical problem exists:*
Sensitivity to gentamicin

## Side/Adverse Effects
The following side/adverse effects have been selected on the basis of their potential clinical significance (possible signs and symptoms in parentheses where appropriate)—not necessarily inclusive:

### Those indicating need for medical attention
Incidence less frequent
*Hypersensitivity* (itching, redness, swelling, or other sign of irritation not present before therapy)

### Those indicating need for medical attention only if they continue or are bothersome
Incidence less frequent
*Burning or stinging*

### Those not indicating need for medical attention
For ophthalmic ointment dosage form only
*Blurred vision*

## Patient Consultation
As an aid to patient consultation, refer to *Advice for the Patient, Gentamicin (Ophthalmic).*

In providing consultation, consider emphasizing the following selected information (» = major clinical significance):

### Before using this medication
» Conditions affecting use, especially:
Sensitivity to gentamicin or to any related antibiotic, such as amikacin, kanamycin, neomycin, netilmicin, streptomycin, or tobramycin

### Proper use of this medication
Proper administration technique
» Compliance with full course of therapy
» Proper dosing
Missed dose: Applying as soon as possible; not applying if almost time for next dose
» Proper storage

### Precautions while using this medication
Checking with physician if no improvement within a few days

### Side/adverse effects
Blurred vision may occur for a few minutes after application of ophthalmic ointments
Signs of potential side effects, especially hypersensitivity

## General Dosing Information
Gentamicin sulfate ophthalmic solution is not for subconjunctival injection or for direct injection into the anterior chamber of the eye.

Although some manufacturers recommend a dose of 2 drops of an ophthalmic solution at appropriate intervals, the conjunctival sac will usually hold only 1 drop.

At night the ophthalmic ointment may be used as an adjunct to the ophthalmic solution to provide prolonged contact with the medication.

In infections of the tear sacs (dacryocystitis), often occurring in children with nonpatent tear passages, hot compresses and gentle massage of the area over the tear duct may be useful adjuncts to treatment with the ophthalmic solution.

## Ophthalmic Dosage Forms
### GENTAMICIN SULFATE OPHTHALMIC OINTMENT USP

#### Usual adult and adolescent dose
Antibacterial (ophthalmic)—
Topical, to the conjunctiva, a thin strip (approximately 1 cm) of ointment every eight to twelve hours.

#### Usual pediatric dose
See *Usual adult and adolescent dose.*

#### Strength(s) usually available
U.S.—
5 mg of gentamicin sulfate, equivalent to 3 mg of gentamicin base, per gram (Rx) [*Garamycin* (methylparaben; propylparaben); *Genoptic S.O.P.* (methylparaben; propylparaben); *Gentacidin; Gentafair* (may contain methylparaben; may contain propylparaben); *Gentak* (methylparaben; propylparaben); *Gentrasul* (methylparaben 0.05%; propylparaben 0.01%); *Ocu-Mycin;* GENERIC (may contain methylparaben; may contain propylparaben)].

Canada—
5 mg of gentamicin sulfate, equivalent to 3 mg of gentamicin base, per gram (Rx) [*Garamycin* (methylparaben; propylparaben); *Gentrasul*].

#### Packaging and storage
Store below 40 °C (104 °F). Store in a collapsible ophthalmic ointment tube. Protect from freezing.

#### Auxiliary labeling
• For the eye.
• Continue medicine for full time of treatment.

### GENTAMICIN SULFATE OPHTHALMIC SOLUTION USP

#### Usual adult and adolescent dose
Antibacterial (ophthalmic)—
Mild to moderate infections: Topical, to the conjunctiva, 1 drop every four hours.
Severe infections: Topical, to the conjunctiva, 1 drop every hour.

#### Usual pediatric dose
See *Usual adult and adolescent dose.*

#### Strength(s) usually available
U.S.—
5 mg of gentamicin sulfate, equivalent to 3 mg of gentamicin base, per mL (Rx) [*Garamycin* (benzalkonium chloride); *Genoptic Liquifilm* (polyvinyl alcohol 1.4%; benzalkonium chloride); *Gentacidin* (benzalkonium chloride); *Gentafair* (may contain benzalkonium chloride); *Gentak* (benzalkonium chloride 0.01%); *Gentrasul* (benzalkonium chloride 0.01%); *Ocu-Mycin; Spectro-Genta;* GENERIC (may contain benzalkonium chloride)].

Canada—
5 mg of gentamicin sulfate, equivalent to 3 mg of gentamicin base, per mL (Rx) [*Alcomicin* (benzalkonium chloride 0.01%); *Garamycin* (benzalkonium chloride); *Gentrasul*].

#### Packaging and storage
Store below 40 °C (104 °F). Store in a tight container. Protect from freezing.

#### Auxiliary labeling
• For the eye.
• Continue medicine for full time of treatment.

#### Note
Dispense in original unopened container.

Revised: 6/23/92
Interim revision: 8/30/93

# GENTAMICIN Otic*

VA CLASSIFICATION (Primary): OT101

Note: For a listing of dosage forms and brand names by country availability, see *Dosage Forms* section(s). For a listing of brand names for the articles in this monograph, refer to the General Index.

*Not commercially available in the U.S.

## Category
Antibacterial (otic).

## Indications
### Accepted
Mastoidectomy cavity infections (treatment) or
Otitis media, chronic suppurative (treatment) or
Otitis media, subacute purulent (treatment) or
Otitis, external (treatment)—Gentamicin otic preparations are used in the treatment of mastoidectomy cavity infections, chronic suppurative otitis media, subacute purulent otitis media with tympanic membrane perforation, or external otitis.

Note: Not all species or strains of a particular organism may be susceptible to gentamicin.

## Pharmacology/Pharmacokinetics
### Physicochemical characteristics
Chemical group—Aminoglycosides.

### Mechanism of action/Effect
Aminoglycoside; actively transported across the bacterial cell membrane, binds to a specific receptor protein on the 30 S subunit of bacterial ribosomes, and interferes with an initiation complex between mRNA (messenger RNA) and the 30 S subunit, inhibiting protein synthesis. DNA may be misread, thus producing nonfunctional proteins; polyribosomes are split apart and are unable to synthesize protein.

Note: Aminoglycosides are bactericidal, while most other antibiotics that interfere with protein synthesis are bacteriostatic.

### Absorption
May be absorbed in minute quantities following topical application to the ear, especially if the eardrum is perforated or if tissue damage is present.

## Precautions to Consider
### Cross-sensitivity and/or related problems
Patients sensitive to one aminoglycoside may be sensitive to other aminoglycosides also.

### Pregnancy/Reproduction
Problems in humans have not been documented.

### Breast-feeding
It is not known whether otic gentamicin is excreted in breast milk. However, problems in humans have not been documented.

### Pediatrics
Appropriate studies on the relationship of age to the effects of this medicine have not been performed in the pediatric population. However, no pediatrics-specific problems have been documented to date.

### Geriatrics
Appropriate studies on the relationship of age to the effects of this medicine have not been performed in the geriatric population. However, no geriatrics-specific problems have been documented to date.

### Medical considerations/Contraindications
The medical considerations/contraindications included here have been selected on the basis of their potential clinical significance (reasons given in parentheses where appropriate)—not necessarily inclusive (» = major clinical significance).

*Risk-benefit should be considered when the following medical problems exist:*

Perforated eardrum

Sensitivity to aminoglycosides

## Side/Adverse Effects
The following side/adverse effects have been selected on the basis of their potential clinical significance (possible signs and symptoms in parentheses where appropriate)—not necessarily inclusive:

### Those indicating need for medical attention
Incidence less frequent
*Hypersensitivity* (itching, redness, swelling, or other sign of irritation not present before therapy)

### Those indicating need for medical attention only if they continue or are bothersome
Incidence less frequent
*Burning or stinging*

## Patient Consultation
As an aid to patient consultation, refer to *Advice for the Patient, Gentamicin (Otic).*

In providing consultation, consider emphasizing the following selected information (» = major clinical significance):

### Before using this medication
» Conditions affecting use, especially:
    Sensitivity to aminoglycosides

### Proper use of this medication
Proper administration technique
» Compliance with full course of therapy
» Proper dosing
    Missed dose: Applying as soon as possible; not applying if almost time for next dose
» Proper storage

### Precautions while using this medication
Checking with physician if no improvement within a few days

### Side/adverse effects
Signs of potential side effects, especially hypersensitivity

## Otic Dosage Forms
### GENTAMICIN SULFATE OTIC SOLUTION

**Usual adult and adolescent dose**
Topical, to the ear canal, 3 or 4 drops three times a day.

**Usual pediatric dose**
See *Usual adult and adolescent dose.*

**Strength(s) usually available**
U.S.—
    Not commercially available. Gentamicin sulfate ophthalmic solution is being used for otic application.
Canada—
    0.3% (base) (Rx) [*Garamycin Otic Solution*].

Note: Each mL of solution contains 5 mg of gentamicin sulfate, equivalent to 3 mg of gentamicin base.

**Packaging and storage**
Store below 40 °C (104 °F), preferably between 15 and 30 °C (59 and 86 °F), unless otherwise specified by manufacturer. Store in a tight container. Protect from freezing.

**Auxiliary labeling**
• For the ear.
• Continue medicine for full time of treatment.

**Note**
Dispense in original unopened container.

Revised: 08/12/92
Interim revision: 04/11/94

# GENTAMICIN   Topical

VA CLASSIFICATION (Primary): DE101
Note: For a listing of dosage forms and brand names by country availability, see *Dosage Forms* section(s). For a listing of brand names for the articles in this monograph, refer to the General Index.

## Category
Antibacterial (topical).

## Indications
Note: Bracketed information in the *Indications* section refers to uses that are not included in U.S. product labeling.

### Accepted
Folliculitis (treatment)
Furunculosis (treatment)
Paronychia (treatment) or
Skin infections, bacterial, other minor (treatment)—Topical gentamicin is indicated in the topical treatment of folliculitis, furunculosis, paronychia, and other minor bacterial skin infections (including infected insect bites, infected minor burns, infected contact dermatitis, infectious eczematoid dermatitis, infected seborrheic dermatitis, infected excoriation, infected lacerations, infected skin abscesses and cysts, infected skin ulcers, infected stasis ulcers, infected stings, bacterial superinfections of minor fungal and viral infections, sycosis barbae, and minor surgical wounds) caused by staphylococci, streptococci, *Proteus vulgaris*, *Escherichia coli*, *Pseudomonas aeruginosa*, and *Enterobacter aerogenes (Aerobacter aerogenes)*.

[Skin infections, bacterial, minor (prophylaxis)][1] or
[Ulcer, dermal (treatment)]—Topical gentamicin is used in the prophylaxis of minor bacterial skin infections and in the treatment of dermal ulcer.

Not all species or strains of a particular organism may be susceptible to gentamicin.

### Unaccepted
Indiscriminate use of topical gentamicin may lead to the emergence of aminoglycoside-resistant organisms. Therefore, use in immunocompromised or other high-risk patients is not recommended.

Gentamicin is not effective against anaerobes, fungi, or viruses.

[1]Not included in Canadian product labeling.

## Pharmacology/Pharmacokinetics

### Physicochemical characteristics
Chemical group—Aminoglycosides.

### Mechanism of action/Effect
Aminoglycoside; actively transported across the bacterial cell membrane, binds to a specific receptor protein on the 30 S subunit of bacterial ribosomes, and interferes with an initiation complex between mRNA (messenger RNA) and the 30 S subunit, inhibiting protein synthesis. DNA may be misread, thus producing nonfunctional proteins; polyribosomes are split apart and are unable to synthesize protein.

Note: Aminoglycosides are bactericidal, while most other antibiotics that interfere with protein synthesis are bacteriostatic.

### Absorption
Although not absorbed through intact skin, topical gentamicin is readily absorbed from large denuded, burned, or granulating areas. Greater and more rapid absorption occurs with gentamicin cream than with the ointment.

## Precautions to Consider

### Cross-sensitivity and/or related problems
Patients sensitive to one aminoglycoside may be sensitive to other aminoglycosides also. However, patients who are sensitive to neomycin have been treated with gentamicin without apparent adverse effects.

### Pregnancy/Reproduction
Problems in humans have not been documented.

### Breast-feeding
It is not known whether topical gentamicin is distributed into breast milk. However, problems in humans have not been documented.

### Pediatrics
Appropriate studies on the relationship of age to the effects of this medicine have not been performed in infants and children up to 1 year of age. In children over 1 year of age, appropriate studies performed to

date have not demonstrated pediatrics-specific problems that would limit the usefulness of this medicine.

### Geriatrics
Appropriate studies on the relationship of age to the effects of this medicine have not been performed in the geriatric population. However, no geriatrics-specific problems have been documented to date.

### Medical considerations/Contraindications
The medical considerations/contraindications included here have been selected on the basis of their potential clinical significance (reasons given in parentheses where appropriate)—not necessarily inclusive (» = major clinical significance).

*Risk-benefit should be considered when the following medical problem exists:*
Sensitivity to topical gentamicin

## Side/Adverse Effects
The following side/adverse effects have been selected on the basis of their potential clinical significance (possible signs and symptoms in parentheses where appropriate)—not necessarily inclusive:

### Those indicating need for medical attention
Incidence less frequent
*Hypersensitivity* (itching, redness, swelling, or other sign of irritation not present before therapy)

## Patient Consultation
As an aid to patient consultation, refer to *Advice for the Patient, Gentamicin (Topical)*.

In providing consultation, consider emphasizing the following selected information (» = major clinical significance):

### Before using this medication
» Conditions affecting use, especially:
    Sensitivity to aminoglycosides

### Proper use of this medication
    Before applying, washing affected area with soap and water and drying thoroughly; applying small amount and rubbing in gently
    After applying, covering with gauze dressing if desired
» Compliance with full course of therapy
» Proper dosing
    Missed dose: Applying as soon as possible; not applying if almost time for next dose
» Proper storage

### Precautions while using this medication
Checking with physician if no improvement within 1 week

### Side/adverse effects
Signs of potential side effects, especially hypersensitivity

## General Dosing Information
The treated area(s) may be covered with a gauze dressing if desired.

Serum concentrations up to 4 mcg per mL or more have been reported following topical administration. Nephrotoxicity and moderate to severe ototoxicity may occur, especially if renal function is impaired and systemic nephrotoxic and/or ototoxic drugs are given concurrently.

Use of topical antibacterials may lead to skin sensitization, resulting in hypersensitivity reactions with subsequent topical or systemic use of the medication.

## Topical Dosage Forms

### GENTAMICIN SULFATE CREAM USP

#### Usual adult and adolescent dose
Antibacterial—
Topical, to the skin, three or four times a day.

#### Usual pediatric dose
Antibacterial—
Infants and children over 1 year of age: See *Usual adult and adolescent dose*.

#### Strength(s) usually available
U.S.—
    0.1% (base) (Rx) [*Garamycin* (butylparaben 0.4%; methylparaben 0.1%); *Gentamar*; *G-Myticin*; GENERIC].
Canada—
    0.1% (base) (Rx) [*Garamycin* (chlororesol 0.1%)].

Note: Each gram of cream contains 1.7 mg of gentamicin sulfate, equivalent to 1 mg of gentamicin base.

**Packaging and storage**
Store below 40 °C (104 °F). Store in a collapsible tube or other tight container. Protect from freezing.

**Auxiliary labeling**
• For external use only.
• Continue medication for full time of treatment.

**Note**
Gentamicin sulfate cream is water-washable and may be useful in treating wet, oozing primary infections and greasy, secondary infections of the skin, such as pustular acne or infected seborrheic dermatitis.

## GENTAMICIN SULFATE OINTMENT USP

**Usual adult and adolescent dose**
See *Gentamicin Sulfate Cream USP.*

**Usual pediatric dose**
See *Gentamicin Sulfate Cream USP.*

**Strength(s) usually available**
U.S.—
    0.1% (base) (Rx) [*Garamycin* (methylparaben 0.05%; propylparaben 0.01%); *Gentamar; G-Myticin;* GENERIC].
Canada—
    0.1% (base) (Rx) [*Garamycin* (methylparaben 0.05%; propylparaben 0.01%)].
Note: Each gram of ointment contains 1.7 mg of gentamicin sulfate, equivalent to 1 mg of gentamicin base.

**Packaging and storage**
Store below 40 °C (104 °F). Store in a collapsible tube or other tight container. Protect from freezing.

**Auxiliary labeling**
• For external use only.
• Continue medication for full time of treatment.

**Note**
Gentamicin sulfate ointment helps retain moisture and may be useful in treating infections of dry, eczematous, or psoriatic skin.

Revised: 06/23/92
Interim revision: 06/08/94

---

# GENTIAN VIOLET   Topical†

VA CLASSIFICATION (Primary): DE102
Note: For a listing of dosage forms and brand names by country availability, see *Dosage Forms* section(s). For a listing of brand names for the articles in this monograph, refer to the General Index.

---

†Not commercially available in Canada.

## Category
Antifungal (topical).

## Indications
**Unaccepted**
Although gentian violet has been superseded by more effective and nonstaining antifungal agents, it has been used in the topical treatment of cutaneous and mucocutaneous infections caused by *Candida (Monilia) albicans*, such as oral (thrush), intertriginous and paronychial candidiasis. It is usually not recommended for use in dermatophytic infections because of its local irritant and staining properties.

## Pharmacology/Pharmacokinetics

**Physicochemical characteristics**
Molecular weight—407.99.

## Precautions to Consider

**Carcinogenicity/Mutagenicity**
Studies conducted in rodents suggest that gentian violet is carcinogenic and mutagenic with chronic exposure. However, there have been no studies on or reports of carcinogenicity or mutagenicity in humans exposed to gentian violet.

**Pregnancy/Reproduction**
Problems in humans have not been documented.

**Breast-feeding**
It is not known whether topical gentian violet is distributed into breast milk. However, problems in humans have not been documented.

**Pediatrics**
When gentian violet is used in infants for oral candidiasis, the infant should be turned face downward following application to minimize the possibility of swallowing the medication.

**Geriatrics**
Appropriate studies on the relationship of age to the effects of this medicine have not been performed in the geriatric population. However, no geriatrics-specific problems have been documented to date.

**Medical considerations/Contraindications**
The medical considerations/contraindications included here have been selected on the basis of their potential clinical significance (reasons given in parentheses where appropriate)—not necessarily inclusive (» = major clinical significance).

*Risk-benefit should be considered when the following medical problems exist:*
Sensitivity to gentian violet
Ulcerative lesions of face
    (gentian violet may cause tattooing of the skin)

## Side/Adverse Effects
The following side/adverse effects have been selected on the basis of their potential clinical significance (possible signs and symptoms in parentheses where appropriate)—not necessarily inclusive:

**Those indicating need for medical attention**
*Skin irritation not present before therapy*

## Patient Consultation
As an aid to patient consultation, refer to *Advice for the Patient, Gentian Violet (Topical).*

In providing consultation, consider emphasizing the following selected information (» = major clinical significance):

**Before using this medication**
» Conditions affecting use, especially:
    Use in children—The infant should be turned face downward after application to minimize the possibility of swallowing the medication

**Proper use of this medication**
Applying enough medication to cover only affected area
Avoiding swallowing medication if used in the mouth
» Not applying an occlusive dressing over this medication
» Compliance with full course of therapy
» Proper dosing
    Missed dose: Applying as soon as possible; not applying if almost time for next dose
» Proper storage

**Precautions while using this medication**
» Medication will stain skin and clothing

**Side/adverse effects**
Signs of potential side effects, especially skin irritation not present before therapy

## General Dosing Information
When gentian violet is used in infants for oral candidiasis, the infant should be turned face downward following application to minimize the possibility of swallowing the medication.

Use of topical antifungals may lead to skin sensitization, resulting in hypersensitivity reactions with subsequent topical use of the medication.

This medication is not recommended for use on ulcerative lesions of the face since application of gentian violet to granulation tissue may result in tattooing of the skin.

When used in the treatment of oral candidiasis (thrush), gentian violet should be painted only on the individual lesions since esophagitis, laryngitis, or tracheitis may result from swallowing the solution.

Frequent and prolonged use of this medication in the treatment of oral candidiasis may result in laryngeal obstruction.

Occlusive dressings should be avoided in the treatment of candidiasis since they provide conditions that favor growth of yeast and release of its irritating endotoxin.

## Topical Dosage Forms

### GENTIAN VIOLET TOPICAL SOLUTION USP

**Usual adult and adolescent dose**
Candidiasis—
     Topical, to the oral mucous membranes or skin, two or three times a day for three days.

**Usual pediatric dose**
See *Usual adult and adolescent dose.*

---

# GENTIAN VIOLET    Vaginal

VA CLASSIFICATION (Primary): GU300
Note: For a listing of dosage forms and brand names by country availability, see *Dosage Forms* section(s). For a listing of brand names for the articles in this monograph, refer to the General Index.

## Category
Antifungal (vaginal).

## Indications

**Accepted**
Candidiasis, vulvovaginal (treatment)—Vaginal gentian violet is used occasionally for a short duration as second-line therapy in the treatment of vulvovaginal candidiasis caused by *Candida* species. It is used specifically in those patients in whom conventional therapies (such as vaginal imidazoles) have failed.

Not all species or strains of a particular organism may be susceptible to gentian violet.

## Pharmacology/Pharmacokinetics

**Physicochemical characteristics**
Chemical group—Gentian violet is a dye consisting of a mixture of crystal and methyl violets, which are aniline derivatives.
Molecular weight—407.99.

**Mechanism of action/Effect**
Gentian violet possesses antifungal and anthelmintic activity, as well as bactericidal and bacteriostatic activities against gram-positive bacteria.

## Precautions to Consider

**Carcinogenicity/Mutagenicity**
Studies in rodents have been conducted that suggest that gentian violet is carcinogenic and mutagenic with chronic exposure. However, there have been no studies on or reports of carcinogenicity or mutagenicity in humans exposed to gentian violet. Also, the use of gentian violet in humans is generally for short durations.

**Pregnancy/Reproduction**
Fertility—Studies have not been done in either animals or humans.

Pregnancy—Studies have not been done in either animals or humans.

FDA Pregnancy Category C.

**Breast-feeding**
It is not known whether gentian violet, applied vaginally, is absorbed systemically and distributed into breast milk. However, problems in humans have not been documented.

**Pediatrics**
No information is available on the relationship of age to the effects of vaginal gentian violet in pediatric patients.

**Geriatrics**
Appropriate studies on the relationship of age to the effects of vaginal gentian violet have not been performed in the geriatric population. However, no geriatrics-specific problems have been documented to date.

**Strength(s) usually available**
U.S.—
     1% (OTC) [GENERIC].
     2% (OTC) [GENERIC].
Canada—
     Not commercially available.

**Packaging and storage**
Store below 40 °C (104 °F), preferably between 15 and 30 °C (59 and 86 °F), unless otherwise specified by manufacturer. Store in a tight container. Protect from freezing.

**Auxiliary labeling**
• For external use only.
• Continue medication for full time of treatment.
• Will stain skin and clothing.

---

Revised: 06/23/92
Interim revision: 06/29/94

---

## Side/Adverse Effects

Note: The use of tampons has been associated with toxic shock syndrome (TSS), a rare but serious side effect that may result in death.

The following side/adverse effects have been selected on the basis of their potential clinical significance (possible signs and symptoms in parentheses where appropriate)—not necessarily inclusive:

**Those indicating need for medical attention**
*Vaginal burning, itching, pain, or other sign of irritation not present before therapy*

## Patient Consultation

As an aid to patient consultation, refer to *Advice for the Patient, Gentian Violet (Vaginal)*.

In providing consultation, consider emphasizing the following selected information (» = major clinical significance):

**Proper use of this medication**
     Reading patient directions before using medication
     After inserting, removing tampon after 3 to 4 hours
» Compliance with full course of therapy
     Not using regular tampons if menstrual period occurs during therapy; use of sanitary napkins instead
» Proper dosing
     Missed dose: Inserting as soon as possible; not inserting if almost time for next dose
» Proper storage

**Precautions while using this medication**
» Checking with physician if no improvement in a few days
     Using hygienic measures to control sources of infection or reinfection
     Use of condom for partner if patient has intercourse during therapy
     Checking with physician about douching
» Medication will stain the skin and clothing
     Protection of clothing because of possible vaginal drainage

**Side/adverse effects**
     Vaginal burning, itching, pain, or other sign of irritation not present before therapy

## General Dosing Information

Pregnant patients may require a slightly longer period of treatment.

Treatment with gentian violet tampons may be repeated if infection persists.

## Vaginal Dosage Forms

### GENTIAN VIOLET VAGINAL TAMPONS

**Usual adult and adolescent dose**
Antifungal—
     Intravaginal, 5 mg, retained for three to four hours, one or two times a day for twelve consecutive days.

Note: In resistant cases, an additional tampon may be used overnight.

**Usual pediatric dose**
Dosage has not been established.

**Strength(s) usually available**

U.S.—

5 mg (Rx) [*Genapax*].

**Packaging and storage**

Store between 15 and 30 °C (59 and 86 °F), in a well-closed container, unless otherwise specified by manufacturer.

**Auxiliary labeling**

- For vaginal use only.
- Continue medicine for full time of treatment.
- Will stain skin and clothing.

---

**Note**

Include patient instructions when dispensing.

---

Revised: 10/26/92

Interim revision: 06/04/94

---

**GLICLAZIDE**—See *Antidiabetic Agents, Sulfonylurea (Systemic)*

---

**GLIPIZIDE**—See *Antidiabetic Agents, Sulfonylurea (Systemic)*

---

# GLUCAGON    Systemic

VA CLASSIFICATION (Primary/Secondary): HS503/AD900; DX900; GA801

Note: For a listing of dosage forms and brand names by country availability, see *Dosage Forms* section(s). For a listing of brand names for the articles in this monograph, refer to the General Index.

## Category

Antihypoglycemic; diagnostic aid adjunct (antispasmodic); antispasmodic; antidote (to beta-adrenergic blocking agents; to calcium channel blocking agents).

## Indications

Note: Bracketed information in the *Indications* section refers to uses that are not included in U.S. product labeling.

**Accepted**

Hypoglycemia (treatment)—Glucagon is indicated in the correction of severe hypoglycemic conditions. Glucagon is helpful in hypoglycemia only if liver glycogen is available. Glucagon and glucose may be used together without decreasing the effects of either. When glucagon is used for patients in a very deep state of coma (such as Stage IV or Stage V of Himwich), intravenous glucose is given in addition to glucagon for a more immediate response.

Radiography, gastrointestinal, adjunct—Glucagon is indicated in barium radiographic examinations to produce hypotonicity and relaxation of the esophagus, stomach, duodenum, small bowel, and colon. Glucagon is administered to provide relaxation of smooth musculature, and to decrease peristalsis thereby reducing patient discomfort, slowing emptying, and improving the examination quality.

[Abdominal imaging, digital angiographic, adjunct][1] or

[Abdominal imaging, computed tomographic, adjunct][1] or

[Abdominal imaging, magnetic resonance, adjunct][1] or

[Pelvic imaging, magnetic resonance, adjunct][1]—Glucagon is being used to inhibit bowel peristalsis in abdominal digital vascular imaging, abdominal and pelvic magnetic resonance imaging, and in abdominal CT scanning to prevent motion-related artifact.

[Bleeding, gastrointestinal (diagnosis adjunct)][1]—Glucagon may be beneficial as an adjuvant to Tc 99m–labeled red blood cells in the scintigraphic diagnosis of small bowel hemorrhage.

[Hysterosalpingography, adjunct][1]—Glucagon is used rarely by some clinicians to eliminate possible spasm of the fallopian tubes during hysterosalpingography in those patients whose fallopian tubes are not visualized during examination.

[Toxicity, beta-adrenergic blocking agent (treatment)][1]—Glucagon administered in large intravenous doses is used to treat the cardiotoxic effects, specifically bradycardia and hypotension, in overdoses of beta-adrenergic blocking agents. Glucagon may be used with isoproterenol or dobutamine. Supplemental potassium may be necessary for treated patients since glucagon tends to reduce serum potassium.

[Toxicity, calcium channel blocking agent (treatment)][1]—Glucagon may be of use in treating myocardial depression due to calcium channel blocking agents in those patients in whom conventional therapies have been ineffective.

[Esophageal obstruction, foreign body (treatment)][1]—Glucagon is used in the treatment of lower esophageal obstruction due to foreign bodies, including food boluses.

**Unaccepted**

Glucagon is of little or no help in the treatment of hypoglycemia in conditions where hepatic glycogen stores are depleted, such as starvation, adrenal insufficiency, or chronic hypoglycemia.

Glucagon should not be used to treat birth asphyxia or hypoglycemia in premature infants or in infants who have had intrauterine growth retardation.

Glucagon has been used as an aid in the diagnosis of insulinoma and pheochromocytoma; however, USP advisory panels do not generally recommend this use because of questions about safety.

[1]Not included in Canadian product labeling.

## Pharmacology/Pharmacokinetics

**Physicochemical characteristics**

Source—Beef or porcine pancreas.

Chemical group—Glucagon is a single-chain polypeptide containing 29 amino acid residues. Chemically unrelated to insulin. One USP Unit of glucagon is equivalent to 1 International Unit of glucagon and also to about 1 mg of glucagon.

Molecular weight—3482.78.

**Mechanism of action/Effect**

Promotes hepatic glycogenolysis and gluconeogenesis. Stimulates adenylate cyclase to produce increased cyclic-AMP, which is involved in a series of enzymatic activities. The resultant effects are increased concentrations of plasma glucose, a relaxant effect on smooth musculature, and an inotropic myocardial effect. Hepatic stores of glycogen are necessary for glucagon to elicit an antihypoglycemic effect.

**Biotransformation**

Primarily hepatic and renal through enzymatic proteolysis.

**Half-life**

10 minutes (plasma).

**Onset of action**

Hyperglycemic action—

Intravenous: 5 to 20 minutes.

Intramuscular: 15 minutes.

Subcutaneous: 30 to 45 minutes.

Smooth muscle relaxation—

Intravenous:

0.25 to 2 USP Units—45 seconds.

Intramuscular:

1 USP Unit—8 to 10 minutes.

2 USP Units—4 to 7 minutes.

**Duration of action**

Hyperglycemic action—

90 minutes.

Smooth muscle relaxation—

Intravenous:

0.25 to 0.5 USP Units—9 to 17 minutes.

2 USP Units—22 to 25 minutes.

Intramuscular:

1 USP Unit—12 to 27 minutes.

2 USP Units—21 to 32 minutes.

## Precautions to Consider

**Cross-sensitivity and/or related problems**

Patients who are allergic to beef or porcine proteins may be allergic to glucagon, since glucagon is either of beef or porcine origin.

### Carcinogenicity/Mutagenicity

No studies have been done on carcinogenicity or mutagenicity.

### Pregnancy/Reproduction

*Fertility*—Studies in rats have not shown that glucagon causes impaired fertility.

*Pregnancy*—Adequate and well-controlled studies in humans have not been done.

Studies in rats have not shown that glucagon causes adverse effects on the fetus.

FDA Pregnancy Category B.

### Breast-feeding

Problems in humans have not been documented. It is not known whether glucagon is distributed into breast milk. However, because glucagon is inactivated by gastric acid, problems are unlikely. Also, glucagon has a short half-life and is usually used for a short duration.

### Pediatrics

Appropriate studies performed to date have not demonstrated pediatrics-specific problems that would limit the usefulness of glucagon in children.

### Geriatrics

Appropriate studies on the relationship of age to the effects of glucagon have not been performed in the geriatric population. However, geriatrics-specific problems that would limit the usefulness of this medication in the elderly are not expected.

### Drug interactions and/or related problems

The following drug interactions and/or related problems have been selected on the basis of their potential clinical significance (possible mechanism in parentheses where appropriate)—not necessarily inclusive (» = major clinical significance):

Anticoagulants, coumarin- or indandione-derivative

(concurrent use with glucagon may potentiate the anticoagulant effects; enhanced anticoagulant activity has been reported with unusually high doses such as 25 mg or more per day for 2 or more days)

### Laboratory value alterations

The following have been selected on the basis of their potential clinical significance (possible effect in parentheses where appropriate)—not necessarily inclusive (» = major clinical significance):

With physiology/laboratory test values

Potassium

(serum concentrations may be decreased with use of large doses)

### Medical considerations/Contraindications

The medical considerations/contraindications included here have been selected on the basis of their potential clinical significance (reasons given in parentheses where appropriate)—not necessarily inclusive (» = major clinical significance).

*Risk-benefit should be considered when the following medical problems exist:*

Allergy to beef or porcine proteins, history of

» Diabetes mellitus

(risk of hyperglycemia when glucagon is used as a diagnostic adjunct; however, glucagon is commonly used by diabetic patients to treat hypoglycemia resulting from overdose of oral antidiabetic agents or insulin)

» Insulinoma, or history of

(may paradoxically decrease blood glucose concentrations)

» Pheochromocytoma

(may cause hypertension due to stimulation of the release of catecholamines)

Sensitivity to glucagon

## Side/Adverse Effects

The following side/adverse effects have been selected on the basis of their potential clinical significance (possible signs and symptoms in parentheses where appropriate)—not necessarily inclusive:

### Those indicating need for medical attention

Incidence less frequent

*Allergic reaction* (dizziness; lightheadedness; skin rash; trouble in breathing)

### Those indicating need for medical attention only if they continue or are bothersome

*Nausea or vomiting*—incidence is generally dependent upon dose and (with intravenous use) the rate of injection; these effects may be diminished by slower intravenous administration

## Overdose

For specific information on the agents used in the management of glucagon overdose, see *Potassium Supplements (Systemic)* monograph.

For more information on the management of overdose or unintentional ingestion, **contact a Poison Control Center** (see *Poison Control Center Listing*).

### Clinical effects of overdose (in order of usual occurrence)

The following effects have been selected on the basis of their potential clinical significance (possible signs and symptoms in parentheses where appropriate)—not necessarily inclusive:

*Continuing nausea; continuing vomiting; hypokalemic syndrome* (severe weakness of extremities and trunk; loss of appetite; nausea; vomiting; irregular heartbeat; muscle cramps or pain)

### Treatment of overdose

Due to the short half-life of glucagon, treatment of glucagon overdose is primarily symptomatic and supportive.

*Specific treatment*—Treating hypokalemia with potassium supplementation as required.

*Monitoring*—Monitoring of serum electrolytes, especially potassium; monitoring blood glucose concentrations and blood pressure.

*Supportive care*—Replacing fluids as necessary, due to excessive nausea and vomiting. Patients in whom intentional overdose is confirmed or suspected should be referred for psychiatric consultation.

## Patient Consultation

As an aid to patient consultation, refer to *Advice for the Patient, Glucagon (Systemic)*.

In providing consultation, consider emphasizing the following selected information (» = major clinical significance):

### Before using this medication

» Conditions affecting use, especially:

Sensitivity to glucagon

Other medical problems, especially diabetes mellitus (for diagnostic procedures only), insulinoma or history of, or pheochromocytoma

### Proper use of this medication

» Using medication only as directed by physician; need to explain use to family or friend; reviewing use on a regular basis

» Reading directions in glucagon kit before medication is actually needed; knowing how to reconstitute and inject properly

» Knowing which type of syringe to use; keeping sterile syringe and needles always readily available; knowing how to use syringe supplied with some kits

May be reconstituted when emergency occurs or ahead of time, but must be used within 48 hours of reconstitution

» Not keeping after expiration date on vial; checking date regularly; replacing medication before it expires

» Proper dosing

*Proper storage*

» Storing unmixed medication at room temperature

Storing mixed solution in refrigerator for no longer than 48 hours and protecting from freezing

### Precautions while using this medication

» Importance of knowing symptoms of hypoglycemia: mild abdominal or stomach pain; anxious feeling; continuing chills; cold sweats; confusion; convulsions; cool, pale skin; difficulty in concentrating; drowsiness; fast heartbeat; continuing headache; excessive hunger; continuing nausea or vomiting; nervousness; shakiness; unconsciousness; unsteady walk; vision changes; unusual tiredness or weakness

» Importance of eating some form of sugar (glucose tablets or gel; fruit juice; corn syrup; honey; nondiet soft drinks; sugar cubes or table sugar dissolved in water) if symptoms of hypoglycemia occur

*Steps to be taken after glucagon is injected for hypoglycemia in unconscious patient:*

» After injection, turning patient on one side to avoid choking if emesis occurs

Contacting an emergency medical service and physician

Monitoring blood glucose concentrations throughout episode, treatment, and for 3 to 4 hours after patient becomes conscious

If patient not conscious in 5 minutes (intravenous use) or 15 minutes (intramuscular use), giving second dose; simultaneously, getting emergency help

When patient conscious enough to swallow, initially giving some form of sugar to take orally then having patient eat crackers and cheese or half a sandwich or drink a glass of milk to prevent hypoglycemia from recurring before the next scheduled meal or snack

If nausea and vomiting prevent a patient from swallowing some form of sugar for an hour after injection, getting medical assistance

» Importance of keeping physician informed of hypoglycemic episodes and use of glucagon

» Replacing supply of glucagon as soon as possible

**Side/adverse effects**

Signs of potential side effects, especially allergic reaction

## General Dosing Information

### For use as an antihypoglycemic

For ambulatory-care use of glucagon kits that do not supply the user with a syringe, USP medical advisory panelists generally recommend that a standard 1-mL insulin syringe be used for injection. Using an insulin syringe will ensure availability when needed and reduce the potential for confusion or improper injection. However, the injection should be made at a 90-degree angle rather than the standard subcutaneous approach. Although the standard insulin syringe will not generally allow for a true intramuscular injection, the deeper injection may provide for a more rapid response time than would the subcutaneous route. A different syringe may be considered if the user is able to make such an injection in an appropriate manner and/or if the insulin syringe being used will not hold the appropriate amount of glucagon solution required.

A rapid blood glucose test should be performed to confirm that the patient has low blood sugar. Emergency medical assistance should also be obtained as soon as possible. Blood glucose should also be monitored throughout the hypoglycemic episode, treatment period, and for 3 to 4 hours after the patient regains consciousness.

Patient response usually occurs 5 minutes following intravenous administration or 15 minutes following intramuscular administration. Dose may be repeated if no response is evident within this time. Medical care will be needed if response is not obtained following a second glucagon dose; intravenous glucose will be required if the patient fails to respond to glucagon.

After the patient is sufficiently alert and oriented, oral supplemental sugar (glucose or sucrose) must be given to prevent secondary hypoglycemia. Patients with insulin-dependent diabetes (type I) do not have as great a response in blood glucose levels as do the non-insulin-dependent (type II), stable diabetic patients. Therefore, it is especially important that supplemental carbohydrates be given as soon as possible to patients with type I diabetes. Emergency room evaluation and/or hospital admission should be considered for all patients experiencing a hypoglycemic episode from oral antidiabetic agents (especially chlorpropamide), since hypoglycemia may recur after blood glucose concentrations are normalized.

If nausea and vomiting result from glucagon administration and the patient is unable to ingest some form of sugar for 1 hour, medical assistance should be obtained immediately. Severe hypoglycemia may rapidly recur under these circumstances.

## Parenteral Dosage Forms

Note: Bracketed uses in the *Dosage Forms* section refer to categories of use and/or indications that are not included in U.S. product labeling.

### GLUCAGON FOR INJECTION USP

**Usual adult and adolescent dose**

Antihypoglycemic—

Intramuscular, intravenous, or subcutaneous, 0.5 to 1 mg (0.5 to 1 USP Unit), repeated in twenty minutes if necessary.

Diagnostic aid—Radiography, gastrointestinal or

[Abdominal imaging, computed tomographic or magnetic resonance][1] or

[Pelvic imaging, computed tomographic or magnetic resonance][1] or

[Hysterosalpingography]—

Intravenous, 0.25 to 1 mg (0.25 to 1 USP Unit).

Note: Doses in the upper range and/or intramuscular dosing may be preferred by some clinicians to achieve hypotonicity during the prolonged scan times associated with magnetic resonance imaging. The duration of action of glucagon is longer with intramuscular dosing.

[Antidote (to beta-adrenergic blocking agents)][1]—

Intravenous, initially, 50 to 150 mcg (0.05 to 0.15 USP Unit) per kg of body weight over one minute, to be followed by a 1 to 5 mg-per-hour infusion.

[Antidote (to calcium channel blocking agents)][1]—

Intravenous, initially 2 mg (2 USP Units). Maintenance dosing is then titrated according to patient response.

[Antispasmodic (esophageal obstruction due to foreign body)][1]—

Intravenous, 0.5 to 2 mg (0.5 to 2 USP Units), repeated in ten to twenty minutes if necessary.

**Usual pediatric dose**

Antihypoglycemic—

Intramuscular, intravenous, or subcutaneous, 25 mcg (0.025 USP Unit) per kg of body weight, up to a maximum dose of 1 mg (1 USP Unit), repeated in twenty minutes if necessary.

**Size(s) usually available**

U.S.—

1 mg (1 USP Unit) (Rx) [*Glucagon Emergency Kit* (phenol 0.2%, in diluent); GENERIC (Lilly—phenol 0.2%, in diluent)].

10 mg (10 USP Units) (Rx) [GENERIC (Lilly—phenol 0.2%, in diluent)].

Canada—

1 mg (1 USP Unit) (Rx) [*Glucagon Emergency Kit* (phenol 0.2%, in diluent); GENERIC (Lilly—phenol 0.2%, in diluent)].

**Packaging and storage**

Prior to reconstitution, store between 15 and 30 °C (59 and 86 °F), unless otherwise specified by manufacturer.

**Preparation of dosage form**

Check expiration dating.

See patient instruction sheet in glucagon package.

Use the diluent provided in the package for doses of 2 USP Units (2 mg) or less. When more than 2 USP Units (2 mg) are needed, sterile water for injection should be used, rather than the diluent provided, to minimize the possibility of thrombophlebitis, central nervous system toxicity, or myocardial depression, which may be caused by the phenol preservative in the manufacturer-supplied diluent.

**Stability**

When stored between 2 and 8 °C (36 and 46 °F) and reconstituted with diluent provided, the reconstituted solution retains potency for 48 hours.

Solutions prepared with sterile water for injection should be used immediately.

**Incompatibilities**

Glucagon may precipitate from saline solution and solutions having a pH of 3 to 9.5.

**Auxiliary labeling**

• Refrigerate after reconstituting.

• After reconstituting, discard after 48 hours.

**Note**

Make sure patient has syringe and needles or understands use of syringe supplied with kit.

Check patient's understanding of preparing and administering medication.

Make sure patient routinely checks expiration date of medication.

---

[1]Not included in Canadian product labeling.

Revised: 01/13/93

---

## GLUCOSE OXIDASE URINE GLUCOSE TEST—See *Urine Glucose and Ketone Test Kits for Home Use*

---

# GLUTETHIMIDE   Systemic†

VA CLASSIFICATION (Primary): CN309

Note: Controlled substance in the U.S.—Schedule II.

Note: For a listing of dosage forms and brand names by country availability, see *Dosage Forms* section(s). For a listing of brand names for the articles in this monograph, refer to the General Index.

---

†Not commercially available in Canada.

## Category

Sedative-hypnotic.

## Indications

**Unaccepted**

Glutethimide has been used for the short-term treatment of insomnia; however, it has been replaced by safer and more effective sedative-hypnotic agents.

# Pharmacology/Pharmacokinetics

**Physicochemical characteristics**
Molecular weight—217.27.

**Mechanism of action/Effect**
Unknown.

**Other actions/effects**
Glutethimide exhibits pronounced anticholinergic activity, which is manifested by decreased intestinal motility, inhibition of salivary secretions, and mydriasis.

**Absorption**
Absorbed erratically from the gastrointestinal tract.

**Protein binding**
Moderate (about 50%).

**Biotransformation**
Hepatic. Glutethimide is almost completely metabolized.

**Half-life**
About 10 to 12 hours.

**Onset of action**
Within 30 minutes.

**Time to peak plasma concentration**
1 to 6 hours following a single oral dose of 500 mg.

**Duration of action**
4 to 8 hours.

**Elimination**
Renal—
    Less than 2% of a dose is excreted unchanged.
Fecal—
    Up to 2% of a dose may be excreted in the feces.

# Precautions to Consider

**Carcinogenicity**
No carcinogenicity studies in animals have been done.

**Pregnancy/Reproduction**
Pregnancy—Studies have not been done in either humans or animals. Chronic usage during pregnancy may lead to withdrawal symptoms in the neonate.
FDA Pregnancy Category C.

**Breast-feeding**
Glutethimide is excreted in breast milk; use by nursing mothers may cause sedation in the infant.

**Pediatrics**
Appropriate studies on the relationship of age to the effects of glutethimide have not been performed in the pediatric population. Safety and efficacy have not been established.

**Geriatrics**
Elderly patients may be more sensitive to the effects of glutethimide. Also, elderly patients are more likely to have age-related prostatic hypertrophy and renal function impairment, which may require adjustment of dosage in patients receiving glutethimide.

**Drug interactions and/or related problems**
The following drug interactions and/or related problems have been selected on the basis of their potential clinical significance (possible mechanism in parentheses where appropriate)—not necessarily inclusive (» = major clinical significance):

Note: Combinations containing any of the following medications, depending on the amount present, may also interact with this medication.

Addictive medications, other, especially central nervous system (CNS) depressants with habituating potential
    (prolonged concurrent use may increase the risk of habituation; caution is recommended)

» Alcohol or
» CNS depression–producing medications, other (See *Appendix II*)
    (concurrent use may increase the CNS depressant effects of either these medications or glutethimide; caution is recommended and dosage of one or both agents should be reduced)

» Anticoagulants, coumarin- or indandione-derivative
    (effects may be decreased when these medications are used concurrently with glutethimide because of accelerated metabolism of anticoagulant secondary to stimulation of hepatic microsomal enzymes; dosage adjustments of anticoagulants may be necessary during and after glutethimide therapy)

**Laboratory value alterations**
The following have been selected on the basis of their potential clinical significance (possible effect in parentheses where appropriate)—not necessarily inclusive (» = major clinical significance):

With diagnostic test results
    Phentolamine
        (glutethimide may cause false-positive phentolamine test; it is recommended that all medications be withdrawn at least 24 hours, preferably 48 to 72 hours, prior to a phentolamine test)
    Urinary steroid determinations
        (glutethimide may interfere with the assay for urine 17-ketosteroids or 17-ketogenic steroids, and with the absorbance of urinary 17-hydroxycorticosteroids using the modified Glenn-Nelson technique)

**Medical considerations/Contraindications**
The medical considerations/contraindications included here have been selected on the basis of their potential clinical significance (reasons given in parentheses where appropriate)—not necessarily inclusive (» = major clinical significance).

*Risk-benefit should be considered when the following medical problems exist:*
    Conditions that might be aggravated by anticholinergic activity, such as:
        Bladder neck obstruction
        Cardiac arrhythmias
        Glaucoma, narrow-angle, predisposition to
        Peptic ulcer, stenosing
        Prostatic hypertrophy
        Pyloroduodenal obstruction
    Drug abuse or dependence, history of
    Pain, uncontrolled
» Porphyria
    Renal function impairment, severe
    Sensitivity to glutethimide

# Side/Adverse Effects

The following side/adverse effects have been selected on the basis of their potential clinical significance (possible signs and symptoms in parentheses where appropriate)—not necessarily inclusive:

**Those indicating need for medical attention**
Incidence less frequent
    *Skin rash*
Incidence rare
    *Blood dyscrasias* (sore throat and fever; unusual bleeding or bruising; unusual tiredness or weakness); *paradoxical reaction* (unusual excitement)

**Those indicating need for medical attention only if they continue or are bothersome**
Incidence more frequent
    *Drowsiness, daytime*
Incidence less frequent
    *Blurred vision; clumsiness or unsteadiness; confusion; dizziness; "hangover" effect; headache; nausea; vomiting*

**Those indicating possible withdrawal and the need for medical attention if they occur after medication is discontinued**
    *Convulsions; fast heartbeat; hallucinations; increased dreaming; muscle cramps or spasms; nausea or vomiting; nightmares; stomach cramps or pain; trembling; trouble in sleeping*

# Overdose

For specific information on the agents used in the management of glutethimide overdose, see:
    • *Castor oil* in *Laxatives (Local)* monograph; and/or
    • *Charcoal, Activated (Oral-Local)* monograph.

For more information on the management of overdose or unintentional ingestion, **contact a Poison Control Center** (see *Poison Control Center Listing*).

**Clinical effects of overdose**
The following effects have been selected on the basis of their potential clinical significance (possible signs and symptoms in parentheses where appropriate)—not necessarily inclusive:

Acute
    *Bluish coloration of skin; convulsions; fever; low body temperature; muscle spasms or twitching; shortness of breath or slow or troubled*

*breathing; slow heartbeat; slowness or loss of reflexes; weakness, severe*

Chronic

*Confusion, continuing; memory problems; slurred speech; staggering; trembling; trouble in concentrating*

## Treatment of overdose

Recommended treatment for glutethimide overdose consists of the following:

To decrease absorption—

If the patient is fully conscious, vomiting should be induced.

If emesis or gastric lavage cannot be effected in the fully conscious patient, absorption of glutethimide may be delayed by giving 1 pint of water, milk, or fruit juice; flour or cornstarch suspension; or activated charcoal in water. Then emesis should be induced or gastric lavage performed as soon as possible. Intestinal lavage (100 to 250 mL of 25 to 40% sorbitol or mannitol) should be used to remove unabsorbed glutethimide from the intestines.

In the unconscious patient, gastric lavage should be done, regardless of time elapsed since ingestion of glutethimide, using caution to prevent aspiration of gastric contents or respiratory arrest during manipulation (including prior insertion of a cuffed endotracheal tube or employment of tracheostomy). A 1:1 mixture of castor oil and water should be used as a lavage since larger amounts of glutethimide are removed from the stomach than with aqueous lavage. Fifty mL of castor oil should be left in the stomach as a cathartic.

To enhance elimination—

In severe glutethimide overdosage, in addition to supportive measures and symptomatic treatment, hemodialysis or hemoperfusion should be considered in Grade III or Grade IV coma, when renal shutdown or impaired renal function is manifest, and in life-threatening conditions complicated by pulmonary edema, heart failure, circulatory collapse, significant liver disease, major metabolic disturbance, or uremia.

Although aqueous hemodialysis is less effective for glutethimide than for readily water-soluble compounds, glutethimide blood concentrations may be decreased more rapidly with hemodialysis and the duration of coma may be shortened; however, the efficacy of this procedure is controversial.

Peritoneal dialysis removes some glutethimide; however, it is minimally effective.

Charcoal hemoperfusion has been reported to be more effective than hemodialysis. Also, resin hemoperfusion has been reported to be more effective than hemodialysis, especially in patients with life-threatening coma and lethal blood concentrations of intoxicant drugs.

Drug extraction techniques should be continued for at least 2 hours after the patient regains consciousness since glutethimide is highly lipid soluble and, therefore, rapidly accumulates in lipoid tissue. As glutethimide is removed from the bloodstream by any technique, it is gradually released from fat storage back into the bloodstream. After substantial amounts of glutethimide have been extracted, this blood-concentration rebound may cause coma to persist or recur.

Specific treatment—

If coma is prolonged, appropriate antibiotic therapy is indicated if pulmonary or other infection occurs.

Monitoring—

Continuous electrocardiogram monitoring should be done to detect arrhythmias.

Urinary output should be monitored and maintained, if coma is prolonged.

Supportive care—

Cardiopulmonary supportive measures should be used and include: maintenance of a patent airway with assisted ventilation, if necessary; monitoring of vital signs and level of consciousness; continuous electrocardiogram to detect arrhythmias; and maintenance of blood pressure with plasma volume expanders and, if necessary, pressor agents.

Adequate respiratory gas exchange should be maintained and may require tracheostomy and mechanical assistance.

If coma is prolonged, urinary output should be monitored and maintained while preventing overhydration, which might contribute to pulmonary or cerebral edema.

Patients in whom intentional overdose is known or suspected should be referred for psychiatric consultation.

## Patient Consultation

As an aid to patient consultation, refer to *Advice for the Patient, Glutethimide (Systemic).*

In providing consultation, consider emphasizing the following selected information (» = major clinical significance):

### Before using this medication

» Conditions affecting use, especially:

Sensitivity to glutethimide

Pregnancy—Chronic usage of glutethimide during pregnancy may cause withdrawal symptoms in the neonate

Breast-feeding—Glutethimide excreted in breast milk; use by nursing mothers may cause sedation in the infant

Use in the elderly—Elderly patients may be more sensitive to effects of glutethimide

Other medications, especially alcohol or other CNS depression–producing medications or coumarin- or indandione-derivative anticoagulants

Other medical problems, especially porphyria

### Proper use of this medication

» Importance of not using more medication than the amount prescribed because of habit-forming potential

» Proper dosing

» Proper storage

### Precautions while using this medication

Regular visits to physician to check progress during prolonged therapy

Checking with physician before discontinuing medication after prolonged use; gradual dosage reduction may be necessary to avoid possibility of withdrawal symptoms

» Avoiding use of alcohol or other CNS depressants

Caution if any laboratory tests required; possible interference with results of metyrapone test.

» Suspected overdose: Getting emergency help at once

» Caution if dizziness or daytime drowsiness occurs

### Side/adverse effects

Signs of potential side effects, especially blood dyscrasias, paradoxical reaction, and skin rash

Side/adverse effects more likely to occur in elderly patients, who may be more sensitive to effects of glutethimide

## General Dosing Information

Prolonged use of larger-than-usual therapeutic doses may result in psychic or physical dependence.

Following prolonged administration, glutethimide should be withdrawn gradually to avoid the possibility of precipitating withdrawal symptoms.

### For treatment of dependence

Glutethimide dependence may be treated by gradual, stepwise reduction of dosage over a period of days or weeks. If withdrawal symptoms occur, they may be controlled by readministration of glutethimide, or substitution of pentobarbital, and subsequent gradual withdrawal.

## Oral Dosage Forms

### GLUTETHIMIDE CAPSULES USP

#### Usual adult dose

Sedative-hypnotic—

Oral, 500 mg at bedtime; dose may be repeated if necessary, but not less than four hours before patient arises.

Note: Geriatric or debilitated patients may be more sensitive to the effects of the usual adult dose. The initial daily dose should not exceed 500 mg at bedtime.

#### Usual pediatric dose

Sedative-hypnotic—

Safety and efficacy have not been established.

#### Strength(s) usually available

U.S.—

500 mg (Rx) [GENERIC].

Canada—

Not commercially available.

#### Packaging and storage

Store below 40 °C (104 °F), preferably between 15 and 30 °C (59 and 86 °F), unless otherwise specified by manufacturer. Store in a well-closed container.

#### Auxiliary labeling

• Avoid alcoholic beverages.

• May cause drowsiness.

#### Note

Controlled substance in the U.S.

## GLUTETHIMIDE TABLETS USP

**Usual adult dose**

Sedative-hypnotic—

Oral, 250 to 500 mg at bedtime; dose may be repeated if necessary, but not less than four hours before patient arises.

Note: Debilitated patients may be more sensitive to the effects of the usual adult dose. The initial daily dose should not exceed 500 mg at bedtime.

**Usual pediatric dose**

Sedative-hypnotic—

Safety and efficacy have not been established.

**Usual geriatric dose**

Sedative-hypnotic—

Oral, initially 250 mg, not to exceed 500 mg, at bedtime, the dosage being adjusted as needed and tolerated.

**Strength(s) usually available**

U.S.—

500 mg (Rx) [GENERIC].

Canada—

Not commercially available.

**Packaging and storage**

Store below 40 °C (104 °F), preferably between 15 and 30 °C (59 and 86 °F), unless otherwise specified by manufacturer. Store in a well-closed container.

**Auxiliary labeling**

• Avoid alcoholic beverages.

• May cause drowsiness.

**Note**

Controlled substance in the U.S.

Revised: 05/12/93

---

**GLYBURIDE**—See *Antidiabetic Agents, Sulfonylurea (Systemic)*

---

**GLYCERIN**—See *Glycerin (Systemic); Laxatives (Local)*

---

# GLYCERIN Systemic

VA CLASSIFICATION (Primary/Secondary): CV709/OP106

Note: For a listing of dosage forms and brand names by country availability, see *Dosage Forms* section(s). For a listing of brand names for the articles in this monograph, refer to the General Index.

## Category

Diuretic; antiglaucoma agent (systemic).

## Indications

Note: Bracketed information in the *Indications* section refers to uses that are not included in U.S. product labeling.

**Accepted**

Glaucoma (treatment)—Glycerin is indicated for short-term reduction of intraocular pressure in treatment of an acute attack of glaucoma or during or after ophthalmic surgery.

[Edema, cerebral (treatment)]—Glycerin is used to reduce elevated intracranial pressure due to a variety of causes.

## Pharmacology/Pharmacokinetics

**Physicochemical characteristics**

Molecular weight—92.09.

**Mechanism of action/Effect**

Cerebral edema—Glycerin elevates blood plasma osmolality, resulting in enhanced flow of water from extravascular spaces into plasma. Reduction of intracranial pressure is attributed to the establishment of an osmotic gradient between blood, cerebrospinal fluid (CSF), and brain, resulting in withdrawal of fluid from the brain and CSF.

Glaucoma—Glycerin elevates blood plasma osmolality, resulting in enhanced flow of water from the eye into plasma and a consequent reduction in intraocular pressure.

**Biotransformation**

Hepatic.

**Onset of action**

Reduction in intraocular pressure—Within 10 minutes.

**Time to peak effect**

Reduction in intraocular pressure and vitreous volume—60 to 90 minutes.

Reduction in intracranial pressure—60 to 90 minutes.

**Duration of action**

Reduction in intraocular pressure—Approximately 5 hours.

**Elimination**

Renal; about 7 to 14% of a dose may be excreted unchanged within 2.5 hours.

## Precautions to Consider

**Pregnancy/Reproduction**

Pregnancy—Studies have not been done in humans.

Studies have not been done in animals.

FDA Pregnancy Category C.

**Breast-feeding**

It is not known whether glycerin is distributed into breast milk. However, problems in humans have not been documented.

**Pediatrics**

Appropriate studies on the relationship of age to the effects of oral glycerin have not been performed in the pediatric population. However, pediatrics-specific problems that would limit the usefulness of this medication in children are not expected.

**Geriatrics**

Although appropriate studies on the relationship of age to the effects of oral glycerin have not been performed in the geriatric population, the possibility of dehydration may be increased in elderly patients. In addition, elderly patients are more likely to have age-related renal function impairment, which may require caution in patients receiving glycerin.

**Drug interactions and/or related problems**

The following drug interactions and/or related problems have been selected on the basis of their potential clinical significance (possible mechanism in parentheses where appropriate)—not necessarily inclusive (» = major clinical significance):

Note: Combinations containing any of the following medications, depending on the amount present, may also interact with this medication.

Diuretics, including carbonic anhydrase inhibitors

(diuretic and intraocular pressure–reducing effects may be potentiated when used concurrently with glycerin; dosage adjustments may be necessary)

**Medical considerations/Contraindications**

The medical considerations/contraindications included here have been selected on the basis of their potential clinical significance (reasons given in parentheses where appropriate)—not necessarily inclusive (» = major clinical significance).

*Risk-benefit should be considered when the following medical problems exist:*

Cardiac disease

(sudden expansion of extracellular fluid may lead to congestive heart failure)

Confused mental states or

Dehydration, severe or

Hypovolemia

(conditions may be exacerbated)

Diabetes mellitus

(patients may already be dehydrated)

Hypervolemia
(expansion of extracellular fluid may lead to circulatory overload, which may produce congestive symptoms in patients with reduced cardiac function)

Renal disease
(accumulation may lead to overexpansion of extracellular fluid and circulatory overload)

Sensitivity to glycerin

### Patient monitoring
The following may be especially important in patient monitoring (other tests may be warranted in some patients, depending on condition; » = major clinical significance):

Intraocular pressure determinations
(may be required at periodic intervals when glycerin is used in the treatment of glaucoma)

## Side/Adverse Effects

Note: Severe dehydration, cardiac arrhythmias, and hyperosmolar non-ketotic coma have been reported and may be fatal.

The following side/adverse effects have been selected on the basis of their potential clinical significance (possible signs and symptoms in parentheses where appropriate)—not necessarily inclusive:

### Those indicating need for medical attention
Incidence less frequent
*Confusion*

Incidence rare
*Arrhythmias* (irregular heartbeat)

### Those indicating need for medical attention only if they continue or are bothersome
Incidence more frequent
*Headache; nausea or vomiting*

Incidence less frequent
*Diarrhea; dizziness; dryness of mouth or increased thirst*

## Patient Consultation

As an aid to patient consultation, refer to *Advice for the Patient, Glycerin (Systemic)*.

In providing consultation, consider emphasizing the following selected information (» = major clinical significance):

### Before using this medication
» Conditions affecting use, especially:
Sensitivity to glycerin
Use in the elderly—Possibility of dehydration may be increased

### Proper use of this medication
» Importance of not taking more medication than the amount prescribed
May be mixed with unsweetened fruit juice, poured over cracked ice, and sipped through a straw to improve taste
» Proper dosing
Missed dose: Taking as soon as possible; not taking if almost time for next dose; not doubling doses
» Proper storage

### Precautions while using this medication
Regular visits to physician to check progress during therapy

Possibility of headache; lying down while and for a short time after taking to minimize this effect

### Side/adverse effects
Signs of potential side effects, especially confusion and arrhythmias

## General Dosing Information

To improve the taste, the solution may be mixed with a small amount of unsweetened lemon, lime, or orange juice, poured over cracked ice, and sipped through a straw.

When used preoperatively, the dose should be administered 1 to 1½ hours prior to surgery. Precautions should be taken to avoid acute urinary retention.

To help prevent or relieve headache resulting from cerebral dehydration, the patient should lie down during and after administration of glycerin.

## Oral Dosage Forms

### GLYCERIN ORAL SOLUTION USP

#### Usual adult dose
Oral, 1 to 1.5 grams per kg of body weight as a single dose. Initial doses up to 2 grams per kg of body weight have been used. Additional doses of 500 mg per kg of body weight may be administered at approximately six-hour intervals, if necessary.

#### Usual pediatric dose
Oral, 1 to 1.5 grams per kg of body weight or 40 grams per square meter of body surface as a single dose. Dose may be repeated in four to eight hours, if necessary.

#### Strength(s) usually available
U.S.—
50% (v/v) (equivalent to 3.1 grams per 5 mL) (Rx) [*Osmoglyn*].
75% (v/v) (equivalent to 4.7 grams per 5 mL) (Rx) [*Glyrol*].

#### Packaging and storage
Store below 40 °C (104 °F), preferably between 15 and 30 °C (59 and 86 °F), unless otherwise specified by manufacturer. Store in a tight container. Protect from freezing.

## Selected Bibliography
Tourtellotte WW, Reinglass JL, Newkirk TA. Cerebral dehydration action of glycerol. I. Historical aspects with emphasis on toxicity and intravenous administration. Clin Pharmacol Ther 1971; 13: 159-71.

Revised: 08/03/94

## GLYCERIN-CONTAINING COMBINATIONS—
Mineral Oil and Glycerin (Oral-Local)—See *Laxatives (Local)*
Mineral Oil, Glycerin, and Phenolphthalein (Oral-Local)—See *Laxatives (Local)*

## GLYCOPYRROLATE—See    *Anticholinergics/Antispasmodics (Systemic)*

# GOLD COMPOUNDS    Systemic

This monograph includes information on the following: Auranofin; Aurothioglucose; Gold Sodium Thiomalate.
INN:
Gold Sodium Thiomalate—Sodium Aurothiomalate
VA CLASSIFICATION (Primary): MS106
A commonly used name for gold sodium thiomalate is sodium aurothiomalate.
Note: For a listing of dosage forms and brand names by country availability, see *Dosage Forms* section(s). For a listing of brand names for the articles in this monograph, refer to the General Index.

## Category
Antirheumatic (disease-modifying).

## Indications
Note: Bracketed information in the *Indications* section refers to uses that are not included in U.S. product labeling.

### Accepted
Arthritis, rheumatoid (treatment) or
Arthritis, juvenile (treatment)—Auranofin is indicated in the treatment of adult rheumatoid arthritis and is used in the treatment of [juvenile arthritis][1] Aurothioglucose and gold sodium thiomalate are indicated in the treatment of adult or juvenile rheumatoid arthritis. These agents are usually used for treating patients who show evidence of continued or additional disease activity despite conservative therapy, e.g., with salicylates (especially aspirin) or other nonsteroidal anti-inflammatory agents, glucocorticoids, etc. Gold compounds may induce remission or suppression of rheumatoid arthritis. In chronic advanced rheumatoid arthritis, they may prevent further damage to affected joints; however,

they do not reverse existing damage.

[Arthritis, psoriatic (treatment)][1] or

[Felty's syndrome (treatment)][1]—Gold compounds are used in the treatment of these rheumatic conditions.

---

[1]Not included in Canadian product labeling.

## Pharmacology/Pharmacokinetics

### Physicochemical characteristics
Molecular weight—
Auranofin: 678.48.
Aurothioglucose: 392.18.
Gold sodium thiomalate: 758.16.

### Mechanism of action/Effect
The predominant clinical effect of the gold compounds appears to be suppression of the synovitis of the active stage of rheumatoid disease. The precise mechanism of anti-inflammatory effect is unknown, but it has been suggested that these agents alter cellular mechanisms by inhibiting sulfhydryl systems. Other proposed mechanisms for gold compounds' effects in patients with rheumatoid arthritis include alteration or inhibition of various enzyme systems, suppression of the phagocytic activity of macrophages and polymorphonuclear leukocytes, alteration of immune response, and alteration of collagen biosynthesis. *In vitro*, the gold compounds have been shown to inhibit prostaglandin synthesis.

### Absorption
Approximately 25% of the gold in a dose of auranofin is absorbed from the gastrointestinal tract.

### Protein binding
Auranofin—Moderate. In blood, approximately 60% of the gold is bound to plasma proteins; the remainder is present in red blood cells.
Aurothioglucose and
Gold sodium thiomalate—Very high; to plasma proteins only.

### Biotransformation
Auranofin—Metabolized so rapidly that the intact molecule has not been detected in blood.
Aurothioglucose and
Gold sodium thiomalate—The metabolic fate is unknown, but it is believed that these compounds are not broken down to elemental gold.

### Half-life
Elimination—
Oral (determined [as gold] after reaching steady-state blood concentrations):
Blood—21 to 31 days; average 26 days.
Tissue (body)—42 to 128 days; average 80 days.
Parenteral:
Dependent on dose and duration of therapy.

### Onset of action
Oral—Usually 3 to 4 months but up to 6 months in some patients.
Parenteral—At least 6 to 8 weeks.

### Time to steady-state blood concentration
Auranofin (measured as blood gold concentration)—3 months.

### Steady-state blood concentration
Auranofin—Blood gold concentrations of about 68 mcg per mL are achieved with administration of 6 mg per day.

### Elimination
Oral—60% of the absorbed gold (15% of the administered dose) is excreted in the urine; the remainder of the dose is excreted in the feces.
Parenteral—60 to 90% renal, very slowly; 10 to 40% fecal, mostly via biliary secretion.

## Precautions to Consider

### Cross-sensitivity and/or related problems
Patients sensitive to gold or other heavy metals may be sensitive to this medication also.
Patients sensitive to sesame products may also be sensitive to the sesame oil vehicle of parenteral aurothioglucose.
Patients intolerant of parabens may be intolerant of parenteral aurothioglucose, which may contain propylparaben, also.

### Carcinogenicity/Tumorigenicity
For auranofin—Renal tubular cell karyomegaly and cytomegaly, renal adenoma, and malignant renal epithelial tumors have been reported in rats receiving 1 and 2.5 mg per kg of body weight (mg/kg) per day (8 and 21 times the usual human dose, respectively) for 24 months. In another study, renal tubular epithelial tumors occurred in rats receiving 23 mg/kg per day (192 times the human dose) for 12 months.

In a third study, no tumorigenicity was demonstrated in mice receiving 1, 3, or 9 mg/kg per day (8, 24, and 72 times the human dose, respectively) for 18 months.

For aurothioglucose and gold sodium thiomalate—Renal adenoma and adenocarcinoma have been reported in rats with prolonged administration of frequent, high doses of parenteral gold compounds (2 mg per kg weekly for 45 weeks followed by 6 mg per kg daily for 47 weeks in one study; 3 mg per kg or 6 mg per kg daily for up to 2 years in a second study). The adenomas were similar to those produced in rats by chronic administration of other heavy metals such as lead or nickel. Renal adenoma has not been reported in humans receiving these medications therapeutically.

### Mutagenicity
High concentrations (313 to 700 nanograms per mL) of auranofin increased the frequency of mutations in the mouse lymphoma forward mutation assay in the presence of a rat liver microsomal preparation. No mutagenic activity was observed in the Ames (salmonella) test, the forward and reverse mutation inducement assay with *Saccharomyces*, the *in vitro* transformation of BALB/T3 cell mouse assay, or the dominant lethal assay.

### Pregnancy/Reproduction
Fertility—Studies in rats have shown that auranofin decreases litter size, probably because of maternal toxicity, when given in doses of 5 mg/kg per day (42 times the human dose) but not when given in doses of 2.5 mg/kg per day (21 times the human dose).

Pregnancy—For auranofin: Well-controlled and adequate studies in humans have not been done. However, studies in rabbits have shown that auranofin increases the incidence of resorptions and abortions, decreases fetal weight, and causes congenital abnormalities, mainly abdominal defects such as gastrochisis and umbilical hernia, when administered in doses of 0.5, 3, or 6 mg/kg per day (up to 50 times the usual human dose). Other studies in animals have shown that auranofin increases the incidence of resorptions and decreases fetal weight in rats receiving 5 mg/kg per day (42 times the human dose), probably because of maternal toxicity, but not in those receiving 2.5 mg/kg per day (21 times the human dose). Studies in mice receiving 5 mg/kg per day (42 times the human dose) showed no teratogenic effects

FDA Pregnancy Category C.

For aurothioglucose and gold sodium thiomalate: Studies in humans have not been done. However, studies in animals have shown parenteral gold compounds to cause hydrocephalus and microphthalmia in rats (at a dose of 25 mg per kg per day from Day 6 through Day 15 of gestation); and gastrochisis; umbilical hernia; anomalies of the brain, heart, lung, and skeleton; microphthalmia; and limb defects in rabbits (at a dose of 20 to 45 mg per kg per day from Day 6 through Day 18 of gestation)

FDA Pregnancy Category C.

### Breast-feeding
Problems in humans have not been documented. However, use by nursing mothers is not recommended because of the potential for serious adverse effects in the infant. Parenterally administered gold is excreted in human breast milk and has been detected in the blood of a nursing infant. It is not known whether auranofin is excreted in human breast milk, but gold has been detected in the milk of lactating rats and mice following auranofin administration.

### Pediatrics
For auranofin—Although appropriate studies have not been done in the pediatric population, auranofin is being used in the treatment of juvenile arthritis.
For aurothioglucose and gold sodium thiomalate—Studies performed to date have not demonstrated pediatrics-specific problems that would limit the usefulness of these medications in children.

### Geriatrics
Studies performed to date have not demonstrated geriatrics-specific problems that would limit the usefulness of these medications in the elderly. However, elderly patients are more likely to have age-related renal function impairment, which may require caution in patients receiving gold compounds.

### Dental
The leukopenic and/or thrombocytopenic effects of gold compounds may result in an increased incidence of microbial infection, delayed healing, and gingival bleeding. If leukopenia or thrombocytopenia occurs, dental work should be deferred until blood counts have returned to normal and patients should be instructed in proper oral hygiene, including caution in use of regular toothbrushes, dental floss, and toothpicks.
Gold compounds may cause glossitis, gingivitis, or stomatitis.

**Drug interactions and/or related problems**

The following drug interactions and/or related problems have been selected on the basis of their potential clinical significance (possible mechanism in parentheses where appropriate)—not necessarily inclusive (» = major clinical significance):

Bone marrow depressants (See *Appendix II*) or

Dermatitis-causing medications, other or

Hepatotoxic medications, other (See *Appendix II*) or

Nephrotoxic medications, other (See *Appendix II*)

(the possibility of additive toxicity should be considered if these medications are used concurrently with gold compounds)

» Penicillamine

(concurrent use of penicillamine with gold compounds may be especially likely to increase the risk of serious hematologic and/or renal adverse effects; concurrent use is not recommended)

**Laboratory value alterations**

The following have been selected on the basis of their potential clinical significance (possible effect in parentheses where appropriate)—not necessarily inclusive (» = major clinical significance):

With physiology/laboratory test values

Hematocrit and

Hemoglobin concentration and

Platelet count and

White blood cell count

(may be decreased)

Liver function tests

(abnormalities may occur)

Urine protein concentrations

(may be increased)

**Medical considerations/Contraindications**

The medical considerations/contraindications included here have been selected on the basis of their potential clinical significance (reasons given in parentheses where appropriate)—not necessarily inclusive (» = major clinical significance).

*Except under special circumstances, this medication should not be used when the following medical problems exist:*

» Serious adverse effects associated with previous gold therapy, such as bone marrow aplasia or other severe hematologic disorders, exfoliative dermatitis, necrotizing enterocolitis, or pulmonary fibrosis, history of

(high risk of recurrence)

*Risk-benefit should be considered when the following medical problems exist:*

» Blood dyscrasias or a history of agranulocytosis or hemorrhagic diathesis

Blood dyscrasias, such as granulocytopenia or anemia caused by drug sensitivity, history of

Colitis—especially for auranofin

» Debilitation, severe

Inadequate or compromised cerebral or cardiovascular circulation

Renal disease, or history of

» Sensitivity to any of the gold compounds, history of

» Sjögren's syndrome in rheumatoid arthritis

Skin rash

» Systemic lupus erythematosus

» Urticaria or eczema

**Patient monitoring**

The following may be especially important in patient monitoring (other tests may be warranted in some patients, depending on condition; » = major clinical significance):

Hepatic function tests and

Renal function tests

(recommended prior to initiation of auranofin therapy and at appropriate intervals during therapy)

Platelet counts and

Total white blood cell counts and

Urinalyses, especially urinary protein determination

(recommended prior to therapy; urinalysis or urinary protein determination recommended prior to each injection and blood and platelet counts [or platelet estimations] recommended before every second injection; also, blood and platelet counts and urinalysis recommended at least monthly during auranofin administration)

## Side/Adverse Effects

See *Table 1*, page 1526.

## Patient Consultation

As an aid to patient consultation, refer to *Advice for the Patient, Gold Compounds (Systemic)*.

In providing consultation, consider emphasizing the following selected information (» = major clinical significance):

**Before using this medication**

» Conditions affecting use, especially:

Sensitivity to gold, other heavy metals, or sesame products

Pregnancy—Studies in humans have not been done, but gold compounds have caused teratogenic and fetotoxic effects in animal studies

Breast-feeding—Use is not recommended because of potential adverse effects in the nursing infant; aurothioglucose and gold sodium thiomalate are excreted in human breast milk; it is not known whether auranofin is excreted in human breast milk

Dental—Risk of adverse effects such as infection, delayed healing, and gingival bleeding associated with blood dyscrasias, as well as gold compound–induced gingivitis, glossitis, and/or stomatitis

Other medications, especially penicillamine

Other medical problems, especially serious adverse effects to prior gold therapy, blood dyscrasias (especially hemorrhagic or caused by sensitivity to a medication), severe debilitation, Sjögren's syndrome, systemic lupus erythematosus, eczema, or urticaria

**Proper use of this medication**

Compliance with therapy; symptomatic relief may not occur until after three to six months of continuous use

» Proper dosing

*For auranofin (oral dosage form) only*

» Not taking more medication than amount prescribed

Missed dose: If dosing schedule is

Once a day: Taking as soon as possible; not taking if not remembered until next day; not doubling doses

More than once a day: Taking as soon as possible; not taking if almost time for next dose; not doubling doses

» Proper storage

**Precautions while using this medication**

Possibility of phototoxicity

*For oral dosage form only*

Regular visits to physician to check progress during therapy; blood and urine tests may be required to detect possible adverse effects

*For parenteral dosage forms only*

Possibility of nitritoid reactions immediately following injection

Possibility of joint pain occurring for 1 or 2 days after injection

**Side/adverse effects**

Signs and symptoms of potential side effects, especially allergic reactions, blood dyscrasias, central nervous system or neurologic effects, cutaneous or dermatologic effects, difficulty in swallowing, fever, ulcerative enterocolitis, gastrointestinal bleeding, hepatotoxicity, mucous membrane reactions, ocular effects, pulmonary effects, and renal effects

Possibility of side effects occurring up to many months after discontinuation of medication

## General Dosing Information

Concurrent therapy with salicylates or other nonsteroidal anti-inflammatory drugs or glucocorticoids is necessary, especially during the first few months of gold therapy, to provide symptomatic relief.

Following mild adverse reactions, therapy should be discontinued temporarily. After the reactions have cleared, therapy may be resumed using a reduced dosage schedule.

Therapy should not be reinstituted after severe or idiosyncratic reactions.

**For treatment of adverse effects**

Recommended treatment may include

• Discontinuing the medication promptly.

• Administering appropriate therapy, such as topical adrenocorticoids, soothing lotions, or local anesthetics, for relief of mild to moderately severe skin or mucous membrane reactions.

• Administering systemic glucocorticoids (i.e., 10 to 40 mg of prednisone daily in divided doses) for severe or generalized dermatitis or stomatitis.

• Administering high doses of glucocorticoids (i.e., 40 to 100 mg of prednisone daily in divided doses) if required for severe pulmonary or other complications. If symptoms do not improve with high-dose glucocorticoid treatment, or if significant glucocorticoid-

induced adverse effects develop, use of a chelating agent such as dimercaprol (BAL) to enhance gold excretion may be considered. However, the efficacy of BAL has not been established. Also, caution in use of BAL is recommended because of its toxicity.
• Administering other supportive treatment as required for specific complications.

---

## AURANOFIN

## Summary of Differences

Pharmacology/pharmacokinetics:
    Protein-binding—Less extensive than with parenteral gold formulations.
    Onset of action—Usually 3 to 4 months, but up to 6 months in some patients.
Precautions:
    Patient monitoring—
      Hepatic and renal function tests also recommended.
Side/adverse effects:
    Nitritoid reactions and temporary joint pain that sometimes occur following injections have not been reported.
    Lower incidence of mucous membrane reactions (other than stomatitis) than with injectible gold formulations.
    Higher incidence of gastrointestinal irritation (e.g., cramping, indigestion, constipation, diarrhea, nausea) than with injectible gold products.

## Additional Dosing Information

See also *General Dosing Information.*

Diarrhea occurring during auranofin therapy may respond to a reduction in dosage.

## Oral Dosage Forms
### AURANOFIN CAPSULES

**Usual adult dose**
Oral, 6 mg once a day or 3 mg twice a day.

Note: Initiation of therapy with doses higher than 6 mg per day is associated with an increased incidence of diarrhea and is not recommended.

If an adequate response has not been achieved after six months, the daily dose may be increased to 9 mg, administered in three divided doses. If an adequate response has not been achieved after three months of treatment at the higher dose, therapy should be discontinued.

**Usual adult prescribing limits**
9 mg per day.

**Usual pediatric dose**
Dosage has not been established.

**Strength(s) usually available**
U.S.—
    3 mg (Rx) [*Ridaura* (lactose)].
Canada—
    3 mg (Rx) [*Ridaura* (lactose)].

**Packaging and storage**
Store below 40 °C (104 °F), preferably between 15 and 30 °C (59 and 86 °F), unless otherwise specified by manufacturer.

---

## AUROTHIOGLUCOSE

## Summary of Differences

Pharmacology/pharmacokinetics:
    Protein-binding—More extensive than with auranofin.
    Onset of action—Usually 6 to 8 weeks.
Side/adverse effects:
    May cause nitritoid reactions and temporary joint pain after an injection.
    Higher incidence of mucous membrane reactions (other than stomatitis) than with auranofin.
    Lower incidence of gastrointestinal irritation (e.g., cramping, indigestion, constipation, diarrhea, nausea) than with auranofin.

## Additional Dosing Information

See also *General Dosing Information.*

Aurothioglucose is for intramuscular injection only. Injections should be administered deeply into the upper outer quadrant of the gluteal region, using an 18-gauge, 1¹/₂-inch (2-inch for obese patients) needle.

Before withdrawing the dose, the vial should be thoroughly shaken to obtain a uniform suspension.

The needle and syringe used to withdraw the dose from the vial must be dry.

To facilitate withdrawing the suspension from the vial, the vial may be heated by immersing in warm water.

## Parenteral Dosage Forms
### STERILE AUROTHIOGLUCOSE SUSPENSION USP

**Usual adult and adolescent dose**
Initial—
    Intramuscular, 10 mg the first week, 25 mg the second and third weeks, then 25 to 50 mg once a week until a total dose of 800 mg to 1 gram has been given.
Maintenance—
    Intramuscular, 25 to 50 mg every two weeks for two to twenty weeks, then 25 to 50 mg every three to four weeks.

**Usual adult prescribing limits**
Up to 50 mg per week.

**Usual pediatric dose**
Children up to 6 years of age—Dosage has not been established.
Children 6 to 12 years of age—Intramuscular, 2.5 mg the first week, 6.25 mg the second and third weeks, then 12.5 mg every week until a total dose of 200 to 250 mg has been given; thereafter, 6.25 to 12.5 mg every three to four weeks.

**Strength(s) usually available**
U.S.—
    50 mg per mL (Rx) [*Solganal* (propylparaben)].

**Packaging and storage**
Store below 40 °C (104 °F), preferably between 15 and 30 °C (59 and 86 °F), unless otherwise specified by manufacturer. Protect from light. Protect from freezing.

**Auxiliary labeling**
• Shake well.

---

## GOLD SODIUM THIOMALATE

## Summary of Differences

Pharmacology/pharmacokinetics:
    Protein-binding—More extensive than with auranofin.
    Onset of action—Usually 6 to 8 weeks.
Side/adverse effects:
    May cause nitritoid reactions and temporary joint pain after an injection.
    Higher incidence of mucous membrane reactions (other than stomatitis) than with auranofin.
    Lower incidence of gastrointestinal irritation (e.g., cramping, indigestion, constipation, diarrhea, nausea) than with auranofin.

## Additional Dosing Information

See also *General Dosing Information.*

Gold sodium thiomalate should be administered only by intramuscular injection, preferably intragluteally.

To reinstitute therapy following mild adverse reactions, an initial dose of 5 mg is given. If the medication is well tolerated, the dose may be increased in 5- to 10-mg increments at weekly to monthly intervals until a dose of 25 to 50 mg is reached.

Maintenance treatment at intervals of 1 to 3 weeks may be required for some patients.

## Parenteral Dosage Forms
### GOLD SODIUM THIOMALATE INJECTION USP

**Usual adult and adolescent dose**
Initial—
    Intramuscular, 10 mg the first week, 25 mg the second week, then 25 to 50 mg once a week until the desired therapeutic response is obtained or until toxicity occurs, up to a total dose of 1 gram.

**Maintenance—**
Intramuscular, 25 to 50 mg every two weeks for two to twenty weeks, then 25 to 50 mg every three or four weeks.

**Usual pediatric dose**
Intramuscular, 10 mg the first week, then 1 mg per kg of body weight, not to exceed 50 mg per dose. See *Usual adult and adolescent dose* for recommended spacing of doses.

**Strength(s) usually available**
U.S.—
10 mg per mL (Rx) [GENERIC].
25 mg per mL (Rx) [Myochrysine (benzyl alcohol); GENERIC].
50 mg per mL (Rx) [Myochrysine (benzyl alcohol); GENERIC].
Canada—
10 mg per mL (Rx) [Myochrysine].
25 mg per mL (Rx) [Myochrysine].
50 mg per mL (Rx) [Myochrysine].

**Packaging and storage**
Store below 40 °C (104 °F), preferably between 15 and 30 °C (59 and 86 °F), unless otherwise specified by manufacturer. Protect from light. Protect from freezing.

**Stability**
Do not use if solution has darkened to more than a pale yellow.

Revised: June 1990
Interim revision: 08/22/94

# GOLD SODIUM THIOMALATE—See *Gold Compounds (Systemic)*

## Table 1. Side/Adverse Effects*

The following side/adverse effects have been selected on the basis of their potential clinical significance (possible signs and symptoms in parentheses where appropriate)—not necessarily inclusive:

Legend:
I = Auranofin
II = Aurothioglucose
III = Gold Sodium Thiomalate

| | I | II | III |
|---|---|---|---|
| **Medical attention needed** | | | |
| **Allergic reactions** | | | |
| *Anaphylactic shock* (changes in facial skin color; skin rash, hives, and/or itching; fast or irregular breathing; puffiness or swelling of the eyelids or around the eyes; shortness of breath, troubled breathing, tightness in chest, and/or wheezing; sudden, severe decrease in blood pressure and collapse) | U | R | R |
| *Angioedema* without other signs and symptoms of nitritoid or allergic reaction (large hive-like swellings on face, eyelids, mouth, lips, and/or tongue) | R | U | U |
| *Nitritoid or allergic reaction, severe* (difficulty in breathing or swallowing; fainting; slow heartbeat; large hive-like swellings on face, eyelids, mouth, lips, and/or tongue; thickening of tongue)—may occur up to 10 minutes after injection | † | R | R |
| **Central nervous system (CNS)/Neurologic effects** | | | |
| *Confusion* | U | U | R |
| *Convulsions* | U | U | R |
| *Encephalitis* | U | R | U |
| *Electroencephalographic (EEG) abnormalities* | U | R | U |
| *Guillain-Barre syndrome* (tingling, numbness, and weakness in arms, trunk, or face; problems with muscle coordination) | U | U | R |
| *Hallucinations* | U | U | R |
| *Neuropathy, peripheral* (numbness, tingling, pain, or weakness in hands or feet)‡ | R | R | R |
| **Cutaneous/dermatologic effects** | | | |
| **Dermatitis, allergic**‡ | | | |
| (hives) | L | U | U |
| (itching)—may occur first and indicate an impending cutaneous reaction | M (17%) | M | M |
| (skin rash)—both papular and vesicular dermatitis have been reported with aurothioglucose; in some patients, skin rash may indicate toxicity rather than an allergic reaction; also, skin rash may be caused or aggravated by exposure to sunlight | M (24%) | M | M |
| *Dermatitis, exfoliative* (fever with or without chills; red, thickened, or scaly skin; swollen and/or painful glands; unusual bruising)—may lead to alopecia and shedding of nails | U | R | R |
| *Hair loss without symptoms of exfoliative dermatitis* | L | U | U |
| *Reddened skin* | U | M | U |
| *Difficulty in swallowing* without other symptoms of nitritoid or allergic reaction | R | U | U |
| *Fever* | U | R | R |
| **Gastrointestinal effects** | | | |
| *Enterocolitis, ulcerative* (abdominal pain, cramping, or burning, severe; bloody or black tarry stools; vomiting of blood or material that looks like coffee grounds; nausea, heartburn, and/or indigestion, severe and continuing) | R | R | R |

## Table 1. Side/Adverse Effects* (continued)

| | Legend: I=Auranofin II=Aurothioglucose III=Gold Sodium Thiomalate | | |
|---|:---:|:---:|:---:|
| | **I** | **II** | **III** |
| *Gastrointestinal bleeding* without other signs and symptoms of ulcerative enterocolitis (bloody or black tarry stools)—occult blood in the stool has also been reported with auranofin | R | U | U |
| *Hematologic effects*—may occur individually or in combination | | | |
| *Agranulocytosis* (sore throat and fever with or without chills; sores, ulcers, or white spots on lips or in mouth) | R | R | R |
| *Anemia* (unusual tiredness or weakness)‡ | R | U | U |
| *Anemia, aplastic [anemia, hypoplastic; pancytopenia; red cell aplasia]* (shortness of breath, troubled breathing, tightness in chest, and/or wheezing; sores, ulcers, or white spots on lips or in mouth; swollen and/or painful glands; unusual bleeding or bruising; unusual tiredness or weakness)‡ | R | R | R |
| *Eosinophilia* | L | R | R |
| *Leukopenia [neutropenia]* (usually asymptomatic; rarely, fever or chills, cough or hoarseness, lower back or side pain, painful or difficult urination)‡ | L | M | U |
| *Thrombocytopenia with or without purpura* (usually asymptomatic; rarely, unusual bleeding or bruising; black, tarry stools; blood in urine or stools; pinpoint red spots on skin)‡ | L | R | R |
| *Hepatotoxicity* (dark urine, pale stools, and/or yellow eyes or skin)—cholestatic hepatitis and toxic hepatitis have both been reported‡ | R | R | R |
| *Mucous membrane reactions* | | | |
| *Gingivitis* (redness, soreness, swelling, or bleeding of gums)‡ | R | M | M |
| *Glossitis* (irritation or soreness of tongue)‡ | L | M | M |
| *Metallic taste*—may indicate impending gingivitis, glossitis, or stomatitis‡ | R | M | M |
| *Pharyngitis, tracheitis, or upper respiratory tract inflammation* (irritation of nose, throat, and/or upper chest area, possibly with hoarseness and/or coughing) | U | R | U |
| *Stomatitis*‡ (ulcers, sores, or white spots in mouth or throat)—indicative of toxicity | M (13%) | M | M |
| *Vaginitis* (irritation of vagina) | U | R | U |
| *Ocular effects* | | | |
| *Conjunctivitis* (redness, itching, or tearing of eyes; feeling of something in the eye)‡ | M | R | R |
| *Corneal ulcers* | U | R | R |
| *Iritis* (eye pain, tearing, decreased vision) | U | R | R |
| *Pulmonary effects* (coughing, shortness of breath) *Bronchitis [gold bronchitis], or* *Fibrosis, pulmonary*‡, or *Pneumonitis*‡, *interstitial* | U U R | R R R | R R R |
| *Renal effects*‡ *Glomerulitis* (pain in lower back or abdomen; bloody urine; difficulty in breathing; decreased urination; swelling of face and/or legs) | U | R | R |
| *Hematuria* without other signs or symptoms of renal toxicity (bloody urine)—may be detected microscopically before bleeding is visually apparent | L | R | R |
| *Nephrotic syndrome* (swelling of face, fingers, ankles, lower legs, and/or feet; cloudy urine) | U | R | R |
| *Proteinuria* without other signs or symptoms of renal toxicity (cloudy urine) | M | L | L |
| **Medical attention needed only if continuing or bothersome** **Allergic reaction** *Nitritoid or allergic reaction, mild* (dizziness, feeling faint, flushing or redness of face, increased sweating, nausea with or without vomiting, weakness)—may occur immediately after injection | † | R | R |

*Differences in frequency of occurrence may reflect either lack of clinical-use data or actual pharmacologic distinctions among agents (although their pharmacologic similarity suggests that side effects occurring with one may occur with the others).

For auranofin: M=3–9%; L=1–3%; R=<1%; U=unknown; unless otherwise specified.

For aurothioglucose and gold sodium thiomalate (actual percentages not available): M=more frequent; F=less frequent; R=rare; U=unknown.

†Has not been reported with auranofin.

‡May occur during therapy or up to several months after cessation of therapy.

§If severe, may indicate overdose (parenteral dosage forms only).

Table 1. Side/Adverse Effects* *(continued)*

| | Legend:<br>**I**=Auranofin<br>**II**=Aurothioglucose<br>**III**=Gold Sodium Thiomalate | | |
|---|---|---|---|
| | **I** | **II** | **III** |
| *Gastrointestinal effects* | | | |
| *Abdominal or stomach cramps or pain, mild to moderate‡* | M (14%) | R | R |
| *Bloated feeling, gas, or indigestion, mild to moderate* | M | U | U |
| *Constipation* | L | U | U |
| *Decrease or loss of appetite* | M | R | R |
| *Diarrhea or loose stools‡* | M (47%) | R§ | R§ |
| *Loss of or other change in taste sense* | L | U | U |
| *Nausea with or without vomiting, mild to moderate* | M (10%) | R§ | R§ |
| *Joint pain*—may occur for 1 or 2 days after injection | — | L | L |

*Differences in frequency of occurrence may reflect either lack of clinical-use data or actual pharmacologic distinctions among agents (although their pharmacologic similarity suggests that side effects occurring with one may occur with the others).

For auranofin: M=3–9%; L=1–3%; R=<1%; U=unknown; unless otherwise specified.

For aurothioglucose and gold sodium thiomalate (actual percentages not available): M=more frequent; F=less frequent; R=rare; U=unknown.

†Has not been reported with auranofin.

‡May occur during therapy or up to several months after cessation of therapy.

§If severe, may indicate overdose (parenteral dosage forms only).

# GONADORELIN    Systemic

VA CLASSIFICATION (Primary/Secondary): HS900/DX900

Other commonly used names are gonadotropin-releasing hormone (GnRH), luteinizing hormone–releasing hormone (LHRH), and luteinizing hormone-/follicle-stimulating hormone–releasing hormone (LH/FSH–RH).

Note: For a listing of dosage forms and brand names by country availability, see *Dosage Forms* section(s). For a listing of brand names for the articles in this monograph, refer to the General Index.

## Category

Gonad-stimulating principle; diagnostic aid (hypothalamic-pituitary-gonadal axis function).

## Indications

Note: Bracketed information in the *Indications* section refers to uses that are not included in U.S. product labeling.

**Accepted**

Hypogonadism (diagnosis)—Gonadorelin is indicated as an adjunct to other laboratory tests and physical examination for diagnosis of hypogonadism in males or females, whether due to hypothalamic function impairment alone or in combination with anterior pituitary failure, and for evaluating residual gonadotropic function of the pituitary following removal of a pituitary tumor by surgery and/or irradiation.

The single-injection gonadorelin test is not useful for distinguishing between hypothalamic and pituitary function impairment, but a multiple dose (priming) test may be valuable for this purpose. In addition, the single-injection gonadorelin test indicates the presence of functional pituitary gonadotropes but does not measure pituitary gonadotropic reserve.

[Puberty, delayed (treatment)]¹ or
Amenorrhea (treatment)¹ or
[Infertility (treatment)]¹—Intermittent gonadorelin administration is also being investigated, alone and with other agents, for treatment of delayed puberty, amenorrhea, and infertility due to hypogonadotropic hypogonadism in males and females with adequate pituitary reserve. The most promising results have been obtained using a pulse-dosing schedule of intravenous gonadorelin administration, which is postulated to simulate normal release of gonadotropin-releasing hormone from the hypothalamus.

¹Not included in Canadian product labeling.

## Pharmacology/Pharmacokinetics

**Physicochemical characteristics**

Source—Gonadorelin is synthetic gonadotropin-releasing hormone (GnRH).

Molecular weight—Base: 1182.33.

**Mechanism of action/Effect**

Like naturally occurring gonadotropin-releasing hormone (GnRH), gonadorelin primarily stimulates the synthesis and release of luteinizing hormone (LH) from the anterior pituitary gland. Follicle-stimulating hormone (FSH) production and release is also increased by gonadorelin, but to a lesser degree. In prepubertal females and some gonadal function disorders, the FSH response may be greater than the LH response.

For the treatment of amenorrhea, delayed puberty, and infertility—

Administration of gonadorelin is used to simulate the physiologic release of GnRH from the hypothalamus in treatment of delayed puberty, treatment of infertility caused by hypogonadotropic hypogonadism, and induction of ovulation in those women with hypothalamic amenorrhea. This results in increased levels of pituitary gonadotropins LH and FSH, which subsequently stimulate the gonads to produce reproductive steroids.

For diagnosis of hypogonadism—

Quantitation of LH response (See *Table 1*, page 1530) allows for detection of hypothalamic or pituitary dysfunction, possibly resulting from a variety of causes.

**Biotransformation**

Rapid metabolism to various biologically inactive peptide fragments.

**Half-life**

Initial, 2 to 10 minutes; terminal, 10 to 40 minutes.

**Duration of action**

3 to 5 hours.

**Elimination**

Renal excretion of inactive metabolites.

## Precautions to Consider

**Pregnancy/Reproduction**

Fertility—Repeated high doses in humans may lead to luteolysis and inhibition of spermatogenesis.

**Pregnancy**—Adequate and well-controlled studies in humans have not been done. However, studies in mice, rats, and rabbits have not shown that gonadorelin causes adverse effects on the fetus.

FDA Pregnancy Category B.

**Breast-feeding**
Problems in humans have not been documented.

**Pediatrics**
Studies performed to date have not demonstrated pediatrics-specific problems that would limit the usefulness of gonadorelin in pediatric patients.

Newborn infants are very sensitive to the effects of GnRH (peak responsiveness is at 1 to 3 months of age). Responsiveness declines dramatically until puberty (except for FSH in prepubertal females). However, there are no medically accepted indications for the use of gonadorelin in newborn infants.

**Drug interactions and/or related problems**
See *Laboratory value alterations*.

**Laboratory value alterations**
The following have been selected on the basis of their potential clinical significance (possible effect in parentheses where appropriate)—not necessarily inclusive (» = major clinical significance):

With results of *this* test
  *Due to other medications*
    Adrenocorticoids, glucocorticoid or
    Androgens or
    Estrogens or
    Progestins
      (may alter results of the gonadorelin test by affecting pituitary secretion of gonadotropins through feedback mechanism)

    Contraceptives, oral or
    Digoxin
      (may suppress serum gonadotropin concentrations)

    Levodopa or
    Spironolactone
      (may elevate serum gonadotropin concentrations)

    Metoclopramide or
    Phenothiazines
      (may blunt the response to gonadorelin by increasing serum prolactin concentrations)

With physiology/laboratory test values
  Estradiol in females
    (serum concentrations may initially decrease within the first 90 minutes after gonadorelin administration, then increase, reaching a peak at 6 hours and returning to normal by 18 hours)

  Testosterone in males
    (serum concentrations may increase transiently)

**Medical considerations/Contraindications**
The medical considerations/contraindications included here have been selected on the basis of their potential clinical significance (reasons given in parentheses where appropriate)—not necessarily inclusive (» = major clinical significance).

*Risk-benefit should be considered when the following medical problem exists:*
  Allergy to gonadorelin

**Patient monitoring**
The following may be especially important in patient monitoring (other tests may be warranted in some patients, depending on condition; » = major clinical significance):

  Luteinizing hormone (LH)
    (measurement of serum concentrations recommended at timed intervals before and after gonadorelin administration for diagnostic procedures)

## Side/Adverse Effects

The following side/adverse effects have been selected on the basis of their potential clinical significance (possible signs and symptoms in parentheses where appropriate)—not necessarily inclusive:

**Those indicating need for medical attention**
  *Anaphylaxis, generalized* (difficulty in breathing; persistent flushing; hives; hardening of tissue at injection site)—following multiple doses; *skin rash, generalized or local*—after chronic subcutaneous use

**Those indicating need for medical attention only if they continue or are bothersome**
Incidence less frequent
  *Itching, pain, or swelling at subcutaneous injection site*

Incidence rare
  *Abdominal or stomach discomfort; flushing, transient; headaches; lightheadedness; nausea*

## Patient Consultation

As an aid to patient consultation, refer to *Advice for the Patient, Gonadorelin (Systemic)*.

In providing consultation, consider emphasizing the following selected information (» = major clinical significance):

**Before using this medication**
» Conditions affecting use, especially:
    Allergy to gonadorelin

**Proper use of this medication**
  Test procedure: Blood samples taken; injection given; several blood samples taken again; measurement of medication in blood
» Proper dosing

**Side/adverse effects**
  Signs of potential side effects, especially anaphylaxis

## General Dosing Information

**For use in diagnosis of hypogonadism**
Results of the gonadorelin test should be interpreted by someone familiar with hypothalamic-pituitary-gonadal physiology and the clinical status of the patient.

To determine the baseline luteinizing hormone (LH) concentration, the LH concentrations of 2 samples of venous blood drawn 15 minutes and immediately prior to gonadorelin administration are averaged.

Following gonadorelin administration, venous blood samples are drawn at regular intervals (for example, at 15, 30, 45, 60, and 120 minutes after administration) and analyzed for serum LH concentration.

If results are blunted or borderline, the gonadorelin test should be repeated.

Lack of specificity of the assays used by various laboratories may result in variability in LH concentration results reported. Therefore, controls for the laboratory being used should be established and the physician made aware of these values, to aid in accurate interpretation of the test.

The peak change in LH concentration is the most useful single clinical parameter since it is easily calculated and correlates well with the other parameters.

A subnormal response or lack of response may occur in individuals with pituitary and/or hypothalamic function impairment.

Normal baseline serum LH concentrations are usually 5 to 25 mIU per mL (depending on the laboratory and assay method used) in postpubertal males and females and in premenopausal females.

In menopausal and postmenopausal females, baseline LH concentrations are elevated and the maximum LH increases are exaggerated compared to premenopausal concentrations.

Basal LH and follicle-stimulating hormone (FSH) concentrations increase with age (over 50 years) in males; however, time to peak LH response after gonadorelin administration in older males is significantly delayed and may be diminished.

LH response in females varies, depending on the time during the menstrual cycle that gonadorelin is given. Females given gonadorelin during the follicular phase respond the same as males; LH response is greatest when gonadorelin is given during the luteal phase.

## Parenteral Dosage Forms

### GONADORELIN HYDROCHLORIDE FOR INJECTION

**Usual adult dose**
Hypogonadism (diagnosis)—
  Subcutaneous or intravenous, 100 mcg (0.1 mg) (base).

  Note: In females, gonadorelin should be administered within the early follicular phase of the menstrual cycle, if that can be determined.

**Usual pediatric dose**
Hypogonadism (diagnosis)—
  Children 12 years of age and over: Intravenous or subcutaneous, 100 mcg (0.1 mg) (base).

**Size(s) usually available**
U.S.—
  100 mcg (0.1 mg) (base) (Rx) [*Factrel* (diluent—benzyl alcohol 2%)].
  500 mcg (0.5 mg) (base) (Rx) [*Factrel* (diluent—benzyl alcohol 2%)].

Canada—
100 mcg (0.1 mg) (base) (Rx) [*Factrel* (diluent—benzyl alcohol 2%)].
500 mcg (0.5 mg) (base) (Rx) [*Factrel* (diluent—benzyl alcohol 2%)].

**Packaging and storage**
Store below 40 °C (104 °F), preferably between 15 and 30 °C (59 and 86 °F), unless otherwise specified by manufacturer.

**Preparation of dosage form**
Using standard aseptic technique, add 1 or 2 mL of diluent provided to the 100- or 500-mcg vial, respectively. The solution should be made immediately before use. Unused reconstituted solution and diluent should be discarded.

**Stability**
Reconstituted gonadorelin injection should be stored at room temperature and used within 24 hours.

Revised: August 1990
Interim revision: 05/16/94

## Table 1. Pharmacology/Pharmacokinetics*

| | Males | | Females (in early follicular phase of cycle) | |
|---|---|---|---|---|
| | SC | IV | SC | IV |
| Time to peak serum LH concentration (minutes) | 34 ± 13 | 27 ± 14 | 71.5 ± 49.6 | 36 ± 24 |
| Peak serum LH concentration (mIU/mL) | 60.3 ± 26.2 | 63.8 ± 40.3 | 67.9 ± 27.5 | 57.6 ± 36.7 |
| Maximum LH increase (mIU/mL) | 46.7 ± 20.8 | 51.3 ± 35.2 | 52.8 ± 26.4 | 44.5 ± 31.8 |
| LH percent response | 437 ± 243 | 481 ± 184 | 374 ± 221 | 356 ± 282 |

*Normal responses to single 100-mcg doses of gonadorelin (mean values).

Note: SC=subcutaneous; IV=intravenous; LH=luteinizing hormone.

It is necessary to use mean values because of the pulsating secretory pattern of endogenous LH.

LH percent increase is calculated using the following formula:

$$\frac{\text{peak LH} - \text{baseline LH}}{\text{baseline LH}} \times 100$$

Constant infusion of gonadorelin may result in pituitary desensitization and a reduced LH response.

There is wide variation in individual LH response to gonadorelin. Peak serum LH concentration and 50% decay time for the LH response are dose-related.

# GOSERELIN   Systemic

VA CLASSIFICATION (Primary): AN500

Note: For a listing of dosage forms and brand names by country availability, see *Dosage Forms* section(s). For a listing of brand names for the articles in this monograph, refer to the General Index.

## Category
Antineoplastic.

## Indications

**Accepted**
Carcinoma, prostatic (treatment)—Goserelin is indicated for the palliative treatment of advanced prostatic carcinoma, especially as an alternative to orchiectomy or estrogen administration.

## Pharmacology/Pharmacokinetics

**Physicochemical characteristics**
Molecular weight—Goserelin: 1269.43.
Goserelin acetate: 1328.
pKa—Goserelin: 6.2.

**Mechanism of action/Effect**
Goserelin is a synthetic luteinizing hormone–releasing hormone (LHRH) analog. Like naturally occurring LHRH that is produced by the hypothalamus, initial or intermittent administration of goserelin stimulates release of luteinizing hormone (LH) and follicle-stimulating hormone (FSH) from the anterior pituitary, which in turn transiently increases testosterone concentrations in males. However, continuous daily administration of goserelin in the treatment of prostatic carcinoma suppresses secretion of LH and FSH, with a resultant fall in testosterone concentrations and a "medical castration".

**Absorption**
Slower during the first 8 days after injection than during the remainder of the 28-day dosing period.

**Half-life**
4.2 hours; increased slightly in renal failure, but no dosage adjustment required.

**Onset of action**
Testosterone concentrations—Transient increase occurs within first week of therapy; a decline to castrate levels occurs within 2 to 4 weeks.

**Time to peak serum concentration**
12 to 15 days. Released continuously over a 28-day period.

**Peak serum concentration**
3.6-mg dose—2.5 nanograms per mL.

**Duration of action**
Suppression of testosterone concentrations to castrate levels persists for the duration of therapy.

## Precautions to Consider

**Carcinogenicity**
Studies in male and female rats at subcutaneous doses of 31.5 or 62.4 and 21.5 or 42.4 times the recommended monthly dose for a 70-kg human, respectively, every 4 weeks for 1 year found an increased incidence of benign pituitary macroadenomas. No increased incidence of pituitary adenomas was found in mice given doses of 1200 and 2400 micrograms per kg of body weight per day (600 and 1200 times the recommended human dose, respectively) every 3 weeks for 2 years; however, an increased incidence of histiocytic sarcomas of the bone marrow in vertebral column and femur was observed at both doses. Studies in dogs at doses up to 100 times the human dose for 1 year and in monkeys at doses up to 200 times the human dose for 6 months found no increased incidence of pituitary adenomas.

**Mutagenicity**
Mutagenicity tests using bacterial and mammalian systems for point mutations and cytogenetic effects were negative.

**Pregnancy/Reproduction**
Fertility—Suppression of testosterone secretion results in impairment of fertility. Although it is not known whether fertility is restored after

goserelin is withdrawn, reversal of fertility suppression does occur after withdrawal of similar analogs.

Studies in male rats found that goserelin produced changes consistent with gonadal suppression as a result of its endocrine action, including decreased weight and atrophic histological changes in the testes, epididymis, seminal vesicle, and prostate gland with complete suppression of spermatogenesis. Except for the testes, almost complete histologic reversal of these changes occurred several weeks after the end of dosing. In male dogs, suppression of fertility was fully reversible after continuous administration of goserelin at 100 times the recommended monthly dose for 1 year.

### Geriatrics

Appropriate studies on the relationship of age to the effects of goserelin have not been performed in the geriatric population. However, clinical trials were conducted mainly in older patients and geriatrics-specific problems that would limit the usefulness of this medication in the elderly are not expected.

### Laboratory value alterations

The following have been selected on the basis of their potential clinical significance (possible effect in parentheses where appropriate)—not necessarily inclusive (» = major clinical significance):

With physiology/laboratory test values
Serum acid phosphatase concentrations
(transient increases may occur early in treatment, but concentrations usually decrease to or near baseline by the fourth week; may decrease to below baseline levels if elevated concentrations were present before treatment)
Serum testosterone concentrations
(usually increased during the first week of therapy but then decrease; castrate levels are reached within 2 to 4 weeks)

### Medical considerations/Contraindications

The medical considerations/contraindications included here have been selected on the basis of their potential clinical significance (reasons given in parentheses where appropriate)—not necessarily inclusive (» = major clinical significance).

*Risk-benefit should be considered when the following medical problems exist:*

Obstructive uropathy, history of
(increased incidence of disease flare during initial goserelin treatment because of the initial increase in serum testosterone concentrations)
Sensitivity to goserelin
Vertebral metastases
(risk of spinal cord compression as a result of disease flare during initial goserelin treatment)

### Patient monitoring

The following may be especially important in patient monitoring (other tests may be warranted in some patients, depending on condition; » = major clinical significance):

Acid phosphatase concentrations, plasma prostatic or serum or
Serum prostatic specific antigen concentrations and
Serum testosterone concentrations
(recommended at periodic intervals to monitor response)

## Side/Adverse Effects

The following side/adverse effects have been selected on the basis of their potential clinical significance (possible signs and symptoms in parentheses where appropriate)—not necessarily inclusive:

**Those indicating need for medical attention**
Incidence more frequent—approximately 10%
*Possible disease flare* (bone pain; numbness or tingling of hands or feet; trouble in urinating; weakness in legs)
Note: A transient, sometimes severe, increase in bone or tumor pain may occur shortly after initiation of therapy, usually associated with the increase in serum testosterone, but usually subsides with continued goserelin treatment. Analgesics may be required during this time. Other signs and symptoms of prostatic carcinoma, including difficult urination, may also worsen transiently. In addition, worsening of neurologic signs and symptoms in patients with vertebral metastases may result in temporary weakness and paresthesias of the lower extremities.

Incidence less frequent
*Anemia; cardiovascular effects, including arrhythmias* (irregular heartbeat); *cerebrovascular accident* (sudden weakness); *hypertension; myocardial infarction* (chest pain; shortness of breath); *or pe-*

*ripheral vascular disorder* (painful or cold hands or feet); *gout* (joint pain); *skin rash*

**Those indicating need for medical attention only if they continue or are bothersome**
Incidence more frequent
*Hot flashes* (sudden sweating and feelings of warmth)—incidence about 60%; *impotence or decrease in sexual desire*—incidence about 20%
Incidence less frequent
*Anxiety or mental depression; chronic obstructive pulmonary disease (COPD) or upper respiratory infection* (shortness of breath); *congestive heart failure or edema* (swelling of feet or lower legs); *constipation; diarrhea; dizziness; headache; loss of appetite; nausea or vomiting; swelling and increased tenderness of breasts; trouble in sleeping; unusual tiredness or weakness; weight gain*

## Patient Consultation

As an aid to patient consultation, refer to *Advice for the Patient, Goserelin (Systemic)*.

In providing consultation, consider emphasizing the following selected information (» = major clinical significance):

**Before using this medication**
» Conditions affecting use, especially:
Sensitivity to goserelin
Pregnancy—Pregnancy/Reproduction—May cause sterility

**Proper use of this medication**
» Importance of continuing medication despite side effects
» Proper dosing
Missed dose: Getting as soon as possible

**Precautions while using this medication**
» Importance of close monitoring by the physician

**Side/adverse effects**
Signs of potential side effects, especially transient disease flare, anemia, cardiovascular effects, gout, and skin rash

## General Dosing Information

Patients receiving goserelin should be under supervision of a physician experienced in cancer therapy. Administration of goserelin should be carried out, using sterile technique, under supervision of a physician.

Goserelin has a longer duration of action than naturally occurring luteinizing hormone–releasing hormone.

**For treatment of side/adverse effects**
Bone pain associated with transient disease flare can be treated symptomatically.

Spinal cord compression or renal impairment due to ureteral obstruction should receive standard treatment; in extreme cases, an immediate orchiectomy may be necessary.

## Parenteral Dosage Forms

### GOSERELIN ACETATE IMPLANTS

**Usual adult dose**
Prostatic carcinoma—
Subcutaneous (into upper abdominal wall), 3.6 mg (base) every twenty-eight days.
Note: If the implant needs to be removed for any reason, it can be located by ultrasound.

**Size(s) usually available**
U.S.—
3.6 mg (base) (preloaded in a special single use syringe) (Rx) [*Zoladex*].
Canada—
3.6 mg (base) (preloaded in a special single use syringe) (Rx) [*Zoladex*].
Note: Goserelin acetate is available in a biodegradable and biocompatible, sterile, white to cream colored cylinder, dispersed in a matrix of D,L-lactic and glycolic acids copolymer (13.3–14.3 mg per dose) containing less than 2.5% acetic acid and up to 15% goserelin-related substances.

**Packaging and storage**
Store below 25 °C (77 °F), unless otherwise specified by manufacturer.

## Selected Bibliography

The management of clinically localized prostate cancer. National Institutes of Health Consensus Development Conference Statement 1987 June 15-17; 6 (10).

Korman LB. Treatment of prostate cancer. Clin Pharm 1989 Jun; 8: 412-24.

Furr BJA, Woodburn JR. Luteinizing hormone–releasing hormone and its analogues: a review of biological properties and clinical uses. J Endocrinol Invest 1988 Jul-Aug; 11: 535-57.

Schroder FH (ed.). New treatment modalities in prostatic cancer: LHRH superagonists. Symposium held during World Congress of Oncology, Budapest, Hungary, August 26, 1986. Am J Clin Oncol 1988; 11 (Suppl 1): S1-46.

Revised: 07/90
Interim revision: 07/08/94

## GRAMICIDIN-CONTAINING COMBINATIONS—
Neomycin, Polymyxin B, and Gramicidin (Ophthalmic)

# GRANISETRON Systemic†

VA CLASSIFICATION (Primary): GA700

Note: For a listing of dosage forms and brand names by country availability, see *Dosage Forms* section(s). For a listing of brand names for the articles in this monograph, refer to the General Index.

†Not commercially available in Canada.

## Category
Antiemetic.

## Indications
Note: Bracketed information in the *Indications* section refers to uses that are not included in U.S. product labeling.

### Accepted
Nausea and vomiting, cancer chemotherapy–induced (prophylaxis)—Granisetron is indicated for the prevention of nausea and vomiting associated with initial and repeat courses of moderately or severely emetogenic cancer chemotherapy, including high-dose cisplatin.

Studies have found intravenous granisetron to be as effective as high-dose metoclopramide plus dexamethasone, and superior to dexamethasone plus chlorpromazine or prochlorperazine in preventing nausea and vomiting induced by high-dose cisplatin, and by moderately emetogenic chemotherapy, respectively, during the acute phase lasting 24 hours after the start of chemotherapy. However, the dose of granisetron used in many of these studies was higher than the dose that is currently recommended. Unlike metoclopramide, granisetron has no dopamine receptor antagonist activity and thus does not induce extrapyramidal side effects.

[Nausea and vomiting, cancer radiotherapy–induced (prophylaxis)]—Granisetron injection may be used to prevent the nausea and vomiting associated with total body or upper hemibody irradiation in patients undergoing bone marrow transplantation.

## Pharmacology/Pharmacokinetics

### Physicochemical characteristics
Molecular weight—348.9.
pH—4.7 to 7.3

### Mechanism of action/Effect
Antiemetic—Granisetron is a potent, selective antagonist of 5-hydroxytryptamine (serotonin) subtype 3 (5-HT$_3$) receptors. 5-HT$_3$ receptors are present peripherally on vagal nerve terminals and centrally in the area postrema of the brain. Cytotoxic drugs and radiation damage gastrointestinal mucosa causing the release of serotonin from the enterochromaffin cells of the gastrointestinal tract. Stimulation of 5-HT$_3$ receptors causes transmission of sensory signals to the vomiting center via vagal afferent fibers to induce vomiting. By binding to 5-HT$_3$ receptors, granisetron blocks vomiting mediated by serotonin release.

### Other actions/effects
Granisetron may slow colonic transit time, perhaps by antagonizing the effects of serotonin on the cholinergic neurons of the colon.

### Distribution
The volume of distribution in cancer patients following a 5-minute infusion of 40 mcg of granisetron per kg of body weight was 2 to 3 L/kg. Granisetron distributes freely between plasma and erythrocytes.

### Protein binding
Moderate (65%).

### Biotransformation
Hepatic; undergoes *N*-demethylation and aromatic ring oxidation followed by conjugation. Animal studies suggest that some of the metabolites may have 5-HT$_3$ receptor antagonist activity.

### Half-life
Intravenous—The elimination half-life in healthy volunteers following a single intravenous dose of 40 mcg per kg of body weight has been reported as 4 to 5 hours. The elimination half-life in cancer patients following a single intravenous dose of 40 mcg per kg of body weight has been reported as 9 to 12 hours. However, there is wide intra- and interpatient variability.

Oral—The elimination half-life in healthy volunteers following a single 1-mg dose has been reported as 6.23 hours.

### Peak serum concentration
Intravenous—Following a 5-minute infusion of 40 mcg of granisetron per kg of body weight, a mean peak plasma concentration of 63.8 nanograms per mL (ng/mL) was reported in adult cancer patients, and a mean value of 42.8 ng/mL was reported in healthy volunteers. Following a 3-minute infusion of 40 mcg of granisetron per kg of body weight to healthy volunteers, a mean peak plasma concentration of 64.3 ng/mL was reported in subjects 21 to 42 years of age, and a mean value of 57 ng/mL was reported in subjects 65 to 81 years of age.

Oral—Following an oral dose of 1 mg twice a day for 7 days, a mean peak plasma concentration of 5.99 ng/mL was reported in adult cancer patients. Following a single oral dose of 1 mg, a mean value of 3.63 ng/mL was reported in healthy volunteers.

### Elimination
Predominantly hepatic. In healthy volunteers, approximately 8 to 15% of an intravenous dose, and 11% of an oral dose, of granisetron is recovered unchanged in the urine. The remainder of the dose is excreted as metabolites, 48 to 49% in the urine and 34 to 38% in the feces.

## Precautions to Consider

### Cross-sensitivity and/or related problems
Patients sensitive to ondansetron may also be sensitive to granisetron.

### Carcinogenicity/Tumorigenicity
In a 2-year study in rats, granisetron—given orally in doses corresponding to 20 and 101 times the recommended human oral dose (81 and 405 times the recommended human intravenous dose, respectively) —produced a statistically significant increase in the incidence of hepatocellular carcinomas and adenomas in males and females. In a 1-year study in rats, granisetron given orally in a dose corresponding to 405 times the recommended human oral dose (1622 times the recommended human intravenous dose) produced hepatocellular adenomas in males and females.

### Mutagenicity
Granisetron was not mutagenic in the *in vitro* Ames test and mouse lymphoma cell forward mutation assay, the *in vivo* mouse micronucleus test, and *in vitro* and *ex vivo* rat hepatocyte unscheduled DNA synthesis (UDS) assays. However, granisetron produced a significant increase in UDS in HeLa cells *in vitro* and a significantly increased incidence of cells with polyploidy in an *in vitro* human lymphocyte chromosomal aberration test.

### Pregnancy/Reproduction
Fertility—Granisetron was found to have no effect on the fertility and reproductive performance of male or female rats when given subcutaneously a dose corresponding to 97 times the recommended human intravenous dose (405 times the recommended human oral dose).

Pregnancy—Adequate and well-controlled studies have not been done in humans.

Studies in pregnant rats and rabbits given intravenous doses corresponding to 146 and 96 times the recommended human intravenous dose (507 and 255 times the recommended human oral dose), respectively, have not shown that granisetron causes adverse effects in the fetus.

FDA Pregnancy Category B.

**Breast-feeding**

It is not known whether granisetron is distributed into breast milk.

**Pediatrics**

Appropriate studies performed to date have not demonstrated pediatrics-specific problems that would limit the use of intravenous granisetron in children 2 years of age and older.

Appropriate studies on the relationship of age to the effects of oral granisetron have not been performed in the pediatric population. Safety and efficacy have not been established.

**Geriatrics**

Studies performed in approximately 700 patients 65 years of age or older have not demonstrated geriatrics-specific problems that would limit the usefulness of granisetron in the elderly.

**Drug interactions and/or related problems**

The following drug interactions and/or related problems have been selected on the basis of their potential clinical significance (possible mechanism in parentheses where appropriate)—not necessarily inclusive (» = major clinical significance):

Note: Combinations containing any of the following medications, depending on the amount present, may also interact with this medication.

Hepatic enzyme inducers (See *Appendix II*) or
Hepatic enzyme inhibitors (See *Appendix II*)
 (because granisetron is metabolized by hepatic cytochrome P-450 3A enzymes, inducers or inhibitors of this enzyme may alter granisetron's clearance and half-life)

**Laboratory value alterations**

The following have been selected on the basis of their potential clinical significance (possible effect in parentheses where appropriate)—not necessarily inclusive (» = major clinical significance):

With physiology/laboratory test values
Alanine aminotransferase (ALT [SGPT]) and
Aspartate aminotransferase (AST [SGOT])
 (values may be increased)

**Medical considerations/Contraindications**

The medical considerations/contraindications included here have been selected on the basis of their potential clinical significance (reasons given in parentheses where appropriate)—not necessarily inclusive (» = major clinical significance).

*Risk-benefit should be considered when the following medical problem exists:*

» Sensitivity to granisetron

## Side/Adverse Effects

The following side/adverse effects have been selected on the basis of their potential clinical significance (possible signs and symptoms in parentheses where appropriate)—not necessarily inclusive:

**Those indicating need for medical attention**

Incidence less frequent
 *Fever*
Incidence rare
 *Arrhythmias* (irregular heartbeat); *chest pain; fainting; hypersensitivity reaction* (shortness of breath; skin rash, hives, and itching)

 Note: *Alopecia, anemia, anorexia, leukopenia,* and *thrombocytopenia* have also been reported. However, it is not clear whether these effects were caused by granisetron or by the chemotherapy.

**Those indicating need for medical attention only if they continue or are bothersome**

Incidence more frequent
 *Abdominal pain; constipation; diarrhea; headache; unusual tiredness or weakness*
Incidence less frequent
 *Agitation; dizziness; drowsiness; insomnia* (trouble in sleeping); *unusual taste in mouth*

## Patient Consultation

As an aid to patient consultation, refer to *Advice for the Patient, Granisetron (Systemic).*

In providing consultation, consider emphasizing the following selected information (» = major clinical significance):

**Before receiving this medication**

» Conditions affecting use, especially:
 Sensitivity to granisetron

**Proper use of this medication**

» Proper dosing

**Precautions while receiving this medication**

 Consulting physician if severe nausea and vomiting occur after administration of chemotherapy

**Side/adverse effects**

 Signs of potential side effects, especially fever, arrhythmias, chest pain, fainting, and hypersensitivity reaction

## Oral Dosage Forms

Note: The dosing and strength of the dosage form available are expressed in terms of granisetron base (not the hydrochloride salt).

### GRANISETRON HYDROCHLORIDE TABLETS

**Usual adult and adolescent dose**

Nausea and vomiting, cancer chemotherapy–induced, prophylaxis—
 Oral, 1 mg (base) administered up to one hour prior to chemotherapy, then 1 mg administered twelve hours after the initial dose.

Note: Dosage adjustment is not required in the elderly, or in patients with hepatic or renal function impairment.

**Usual pediatric dose**

Dosage has not been established.

**Usual geriatric dose**

See *Usual adult and adolescent dose.*

**Strength(s) usually available**

U.S.—
 1 mg (base) (Rx) [*Kytril* (hydroxypropyl methylcellulose; lactose; magnesium stearate; microcrystalline cellulose; polyethylene glycol; polysorbate 80; sodium starch glycolate; titanium dioxide)].
Canada—
 Not commercially available.

**Packaging and storage**

Store between 15 and 30 °C (59 and 86 °F), unless otherwise specified by manufacturer. Protect from light.

## Parenteral Dosage Forms

Note: Bracketed uses in the *Dosage Forms* section refer to categories of use and/or indications that are not included in U.S. product labeling.

 The dosing and strength of the dosage form available are expressed in terms of granisetron base (not the hydrochloride salt).

### GRANISETRON HYDROCHLORIDE INJECTION

**Usual adult and adolescent dose**

Nausea and vomiting, cancer chemotherapy–induced, prophylaxis; or
[Nausea and vomiting, cancer radiotherapy–induced, prophylaxis]—
 Intravenous, 10 mcg (base) per kg of body weight, administered over five minutes beginning within thirty minutes before initiation of emetogenic chemotherapy or radiotherapy.

Note: Dosage adjustment is not required in the elderly, or in patients with hepatic or renal function impairment.

**Usual pediatric dose**

Children up to 2 years of age—Dosage has not been established.
Children 2 years of age and older—See *Usual adult and adolescent dose.*

**Usual geriatric dose**

See *Usual adult and adolescent dose.*

**Strength(s) usually available**

U.S.—
 1 mg (base) per mL (Rx) [*Kytril* (sodium chloride 9 mg)].
Canada—
 Not commercially available.

**Packaging and storage**

Store between 2 and 30 °C (36 and 86 °F), unless otherwise specified by manufacturer. Protect from light.

**Preparation of dosage form**

Granisetron should be diluted in 20 to 50 mL of 5% dextrose injection or 0.9% sodium chloride injection.

**Stability**

Intravenous infusions of granisetron retain their potency for 48 hours at room temperature under normal lighting after dilution with 5% dextrose injection or 0.9% sodium chloride injection.

## Incompatibilities

The chemical stability of granisetron with the following medications injected into Y-sites of administration sets has been verified:

| Medication | Concentration |
|---|---|
| Cyclophosphamide | 2 mg/mL |
| Cytarabine | 2 mg/mL |
| Dacarbazine | 1.7 mg/mL |
| Dexamethasone | 0.24 mg/mL |
| Doxorubicin | 0.2 mg/mL |
| Fluorouracil | 2 mg/mL |
| Furosemide | 0.4 mg/mL |
| Ifosfamide | 4 mg/mL |
| Magnesium sulfate | 4 grams/250 mL |
| Methotrexate | 12.5 mg/mL |
| Potassium chloride | 40 mEq/L |

Additionally, granisetron admixed with dexamethasone and mannitol is stable for 24 hours. However, no data are available on the compatibility of granisetron injection with other substances; therefore, other medications should not be added to the preparation or infused simultaneously through the same intravenous line.

## Caution

Granisetron dosage is expressed in terms of mcg; however, the vial concentration is identified in terms of mg per mL.

## Selected Bibliography

Plosker GL, Goa KL. Granisetron. A review of its pharmacological properties and therapeutic use as an antiemetic. Drugs 1991; 42: 805-24.

Joss RA, Dott CS, on behalf of the Granisetron Study Group. Clinical studies with granisetron, a new 5-HT$_3$ receptor antagonist for the treatment of cancer chemotherapy–induced emesis. Eur J Cancer 1993; 29A (1 Suppl): S22-S29.

Developed: 12/16/94
Interim revision: 08/02/95

---

# GRISEOFULVIN Systemic

VA CLASSIFICATION (Primary): AM700

Note: For a listing of dosage forms and brand names by country availability, see *Dosage Forms* section(s). For a listing of brand names for the articles in this monograph, refer to the General Index.

## Category

Antifungal (systemic).

## Indications

### Accepted

Tinea barbae (treatment)
Tinea capitis (treatment)
Tinea corporis (treatment)
Tinea cruris (treatment)
Tinea pedis (treatment) or
Tinea unguium—Griseofulvin is indicated in the treatment of tinea barbae, tinea capitis, tinea corporis, tinea cruris, tinea pedis, and tinea unguium (onychomycosis) caused by *Trichophyton rubrum, T. tonsurans, T. mentagrophytes, T. interdigitale, T. verrucosum, T. megninii, T. gallinae, T. schoenleinii, Microsporum audouinii, M. canis, M. gypseum,* and *Epidermophyton floccosum.*

Not all species or strains of a particular organism may be susceptible to griseofulvin. In addition, griseofulvin may not be effective because of poor absorption or inadequate tissue concentrations of griseofulvin.

### Unaccepted

Griseofulvin is not indicated in the treatment of minor or trivial infections that will respond to topical antifungals alone.

Griseofulvin is not effective in the treatment of bacterial infections, candidiasis, histoplasmosis, actinomycosis, sporotrichosis, chromoblastomycosis, coccidioidomycosis, North American blastomycosis, cryptococcosis, tinea versicolor, or nocardiosis.

## Pharmacology/Pharmacokinetics

### Physicochemical characteristics

Molecular weight—352.77.

### Mechanism of action/Effect

Fungistatic; griseofulvin inhibits fungal cell mitosis by causing disruption of the mitotic spindle structure, thereby arresting the metaphase of cell division. It is deposited in varying concentrations in the keratin precursor cells of skin, hair, and nails, rendering the keratin resistant to fungal invasion. As the infected keratin is shed, it is replaced with healthy tissue.

### Absorption

Microsize—Variable, ranging from 25 to 70% of an oral dose.
Ultramicrosize—Almost completely absorbed.
Absorption is significantly enhanced by administration with or after a fatty meal.

### Distribution

Griseofulvin is deposited in varying concentrations in the keratin layer of the skin, hair, and nails. It can be detected in the stratum corneum of the skin within a few hours following administration. Only a very small fraction of an oral dose is distributed in the body fluids and tissues.

### Biotransformation

Hepatic; major metabolites are 6-methyl-griseofulvin and its glucuronide conjugate.

### Half-life

Approximately 24 hours.

### Time to peak serum concentration

Approximately 4 hours following administration of a single dose of 250 mg of ultramicrosize griseofulvin or 500 mg of microsize griseofulvin.

### Elimination

Renal. Less than 1% of a dose is excreted as unchanged drug in the urine. Approximately 36% of griseofulvin is excreted unchanged in the feces.

## Precautions to Consider

### Cross-sensitivity and/or related problems

Since griseofulvin is derived from a species of *Penicillium,* it is theoretically possible that patients intolerant of penicillins or penicillamine may be intolerant of griseofulvin also. However, cross-sensitivity between griseofulvin and penicillins or penicillamine has not been clinically substantiated. In addition, penicillin-sensitive patients have received griseofulvin without difficulty.

### Carcinogenicity/Tumorigenicity/Mutagenicity

Griseofulvin has been shown to cause hepatomas in several strains of mice, particularly males, that were chronically fed griseofulvin at levels ranging from 0.5% to 2.5% of their diet. Smaller particle-size griseofulvin resulted in an enhanced tumorigenic effect. Griseofulvin, given subcutaneously in relatively small doses once a week during the first 3 weeks of life, has also been shown to cause hepatomas in mice.

Griseofulvin has been shown to cause thyroid tumors, mostly adenomas but also some carcinomas, in male rats that were fed griseofulvin at levels of 0.2%, 1%, and 2% of their diet. Thyroid tumors were also reported in female rats that were fed the two higher dosage levels of griseofulvin.

Studies in other animal species have not shown that griseofulvin is tumorigenic, however.

Griseofulvin has been shown to have a colchicine-like effect on mitosis and to be cocarcinogenic with methylcholanthrene in cutaneous tumor induction studies in laboratory animals.

### Pregnancy/Reproduction

Fertility—Griseofulvin has been shown to suppress spermatogenesis in rats, although this has not been confirmed in humans.

Pregnancy—Griseofulvin crosses the placenta. Conjoined twins have been reported rarely in patients taking griseofulvin during the first trimester of pregnancy. Therefore, this medication is not recommended for use during pregnancy.

Studies in rats have shown that griseofulvin is embryotoxic and teratogenic. In addition, studies in dogs have shown that griseofulvin may cause adverse effects in pups.

### Breast-feeding

It is not known whether griseofulvin is excreted in breast milk. However, problems in humans have not been documented.

**Pediatrics**

Appropriate studies on the relationship of age to the effects of griseofulvin have not been performed in children up to 2 years of age.

**Geriatrics**

Appropriate studies on the relationship of age to the effects of griseofulvin have not been performed in the geriatric population. However, no geriatrics-specific problems have been documented to date.

**Dental**

Griseofulvin may cause oral thrush (soreness or irritation of mouth or tongue).

**Drug interactions and/or related problems**

The following drug interactions and/or related problems have been selected on the basis of their potential clinical significance (possible mechanism in parentheses where appropriate)—not necessarily inclusive (» = major clinical significance):

Note: Combinations containing any of the following medications, depending on the amount present, may also interact with this medication.

Alcohol

(effects may be potentiated when alcohol is used concurrently with griseofulvin; also, concurrent use with griseofulvin may result in tachycardia, diaphoresis, and flushing)

» Anticoagulants, coumarin- or indandione-derivative

(anticoagulant effects may be decreased when these agents are used concurrently with griseofulvin; decrease is thought to be due to accelerated metabolism of anticoagulants secondary to stimulation of hepatic microsomal enzyme activity; prothrombin time should be monitored until a stable level is maintained; dosage adjustments may be necessary during and after griseofulvin therapy)

Barbiturates or
Primidone

(antifungal effects of griseofulvin may be decreased when it is used concurrently with primidone or barbiturates, especially phenobarbital, because of impaired absorption, resulting in decreased serum concentrations; although the effect of decreased serum concentrations on therapeutic response has not been established, concurrent use is preferably avoided)

» Contraceptives, estrogen-containing, oral

(concurrent long-term use of griseofulvin may decrease the effectiveness of oral contraceptives, possibly because of stimulation of hepatic microsomal enzyme activity, resulting in decreased serum estrogen concentrations; this may lead to intermenstrual bleeding, amenorrhea, or unplanned pregnancies; patients should be advised to use an alternate or additional method of contraception while taking griseofulvin concurrently with estrogen-containing oral contraceptives and for 1 month after stopping griseofulvin)

**Medical considerations/Contraindications**

The medical considerations/contraindications included here have been selected on the basis of their potential clinical significance (reasons given in parentheses where appropriate)—not necessarily inclusive (» = major clinical significance).

*Risk-benefit should be considered when the following medical problems exist:*

» Hepatic dysfunction
(griseofulvin may on rare occasion be hepatotoxic)

Hypersensitivity to griseofulvin

Lupus erythematosus or lupus-like syndromes
(griseofulvin may precipitate or exacerbate lupus)

» Porphyria
(griseofulvin may precipitate porphyria attacks)

**Patient monitoring**

The following may be especially important in patient monitoring (other tests may be warranted in some patients, depending on condition; » = major clinical significance):

Complete blood count (CBC) and
Creatinine concentration, serum and
Hepatic function determinations
(recommended at periodic intervals during therapy)

Urinalysis
(recommended at periodic intervals during therapy since proteinuria has been rarely reported)

**Side/Adverse Effects**

The following side/adverse effects have been selected on the basis of their potential clinical significance (possible signs and symptoms in parentheses where appropriate)—not necessarily inclusive:

**Those indicating need for medical attention**

Incidence less frequent
*Confusion; hypersensitivity* (skin rash, hives, or itching); *oral thrush* (soreness or irritation of mouth or tongue); *photosensitivity* (increased sensitivity of skin to sunlight)

Incidence rare—more frequent with prolonged use and/or high doses
*Granulocytopenia or leukopenia* (sore throat and fever); *hepatitis* (yellow eyes or skin); *peripheral neuritis* (numbness, tingling, pain, or weakness in hands or feet)

**Those indicating need for medical attention only if they continue or are bothersome**

Incidence more frequent
*Headache*

Incidence less frequent
*Dizziness; gastrointestinal reactions* (diarrhea; nausea or vomiting; stomach pain); *insomnia* (trouble in sleeping); *unusual tiredness*

## Patient Consultation

As an aid to patient consultation, refer to *Advice for the Patient, Griseofulvin (Systemic)*.

In providing consultation, consider emphasizing the following selected information (» = major clinical significance):

**Before using this medication**

» Conditions affecting use, especially:
Hypersensitivity to griseofulvin; theoretic cross-sensitivity with penicillin, however, penicillin-sensitive patients have received griseofulvin without difficulty
Pregnancy—Griseofulvin crosses the placenta; use is not recommended during pregnancy since griseofulvin has been shown to be embryotoxic and teratogenic in rats
Dental—Griseofulvin may cause oral thrush
Other medications, especially coumarin- or indandione-derivative anticoagulants or estrogen-containing oral contraceptives
Other medical problems, especially hepatic dysfunction or porphyria

**Proper use of this medication**

» Taking with or after meals, especially fatty ones, to minimize gastrointestinal irritation and to increase absorption; checking with physician if on low-fat diet
Proper administration technique for oral suspension
» Compliance with full course of therapy
» Proper dosing
Missed dose: Taking as soon as possible; not taking if almost time for next dose; not doubling doses
» Proper storage

**Precautions while using this medication**

Regular visits to physician to check progress during therapy
» Use of an alternate or additional means of contraception if taking estrogen-containing oral contraceptives concurrently and for 1 month after stopping griseofulvin
Caution in drinking alcoholic beverages during griseofulvin therapy
» Caution if dizziness occurs
» Possible photosensitivity reactions

**Side/adverse effects**

Signs of potential side effects, especially confusion, hypersensitivity, photosensitivity, oral thrush, granulocytopenia, leukopenia, and peripheral neuritis

## General Dosing Information

An oral dose of 250 to 330 mg of ultramicrosize griseofulvin produces serum concentrations equal to 500 mg of microsize griseofulvin.

Griseofulvin should be administered with or after meals (preferably meals high in fat content) to minimize possible gastrointestinal irritation and to increase absorption.

To help prevent relapse, therapy should be continued until the infecting organism is completely eradicated as determined by clinical or laboratory examination. Representative treatment periods are: tinea capitis, 8 to 10 weeks; tinea corporis, 2 to 4 weeks; tinea pedis, 4 to 8 weeks; onychomycosis, at least 4 months for fingernails and at least 6 months for toenails. However, recurrence rates in the treatment of onychomycosis of the toenails are very high.

Concurrent use of an appropriate topical agent is usually required, particularly in the treatment of tinea pedis, since both yeasts and bacteria as well as fungi may be involved in some forms of athlete's foot. Also, griseofulvin is not effective against bacterial or monilial infections. In addition, concurrent use with a topical antifungal agent may reduce the likelihood of relapse.

# Oral Dosage Forms

## GRISEOFULVIN CAPSULES (MICROSIZE) USP

### Usual adult and adolescent dose

Antifungal—
Onychomycosis; or
Tinea pedis: Oral, 500 mg every twelve hours.
Tinea capitis
Tinea corporis or
Tinea cruris: Oral, 250 mg every twelve hours; or 500 mg once a day.

### Usual pediatric dose

Antifungal—
Oral, 5 mg per kg of body weight or 150 mg per square meter of body surface every twelve hours; or 10 mg per kg of body weight or 300 mg per square meter of body surface once a day; or for
Children 14 to 23 kg: Oral, 62.5 to 125 mg every twelve hours; or 125 to 250 mg once a day.
Children 23 kg and over: Oral, 125 to 250 mg every twelve hours; or 250 to 500 mg once a day.

### Strength(s) usually available

U.S.—
250 mg (Rx) [*Grisactin*].
Canada—
Not commercially available.

### Packaging and storage

Store below 40 °C (104 °F), preferably between 15 and 30 °C (59 and 86 °F), unless otherwise specified by manufacturer. Store in a tight container.

### Auxiliary labeling

• May cause dizziness.
• Avoid alcoholic beverages.
• Avoid too much sun or use of sunlamp.
• Continue medicine for full time of treatment.
• Take with or after meals or milk.

## GRISEOFULVIN ORAL SUSPENSION (MICROSIZE) USP

### Usual adult and adolescent dose

See *Griseofulvin Capsules USP (Microsize)*.

### Usual pediatric dose

See *Griseofulvin Capsules USP (Microsize)*.

### Strength(s) usually available

U.S.—
125 mg per 5 mL (Rx) [*Grifulvin V* (alcohol 0.008%; methylparaben; propylparaben)].
Canada—
Not commercially available.

### Packaging and storage

Store below 40 °C (104 °F), preferably between 15 and 30 °C (59 and 86 °F), unless otherwise specified by manufacturer. Store in a tight container. Protect from freezing.

### Auxiliary labeling

• Shake well.
• May cause dizziness.
• Avoid alcoholic beverages.
• Avoid too much sun or use of sunlamp.
• Continue medicine for full time of treatment.
• Take with or after meals or milk.

### Note

When dispensing, include a calibrated liquid-measuring device.

## GRISEOFULVIN TABLETS (MICROSIZE) USP

### Usual adult and adolescent dose

See *Griseofulvin Capsules USP (Microsize)*.

### Usual pediatric dose

See *Griseofulvin Capsules USP (Microsize)*.

### Strength(s) usually available

U.S.—
250 mg (Rx) [*Fulvicin-U/F* (scored); *Grifulvin V* (scored)].
500 mg (Rx) [*Fulvicin-U/F* (scored); *Grifulvin V* (scored); *Grisactin*].
Canada—
125 mg (Rx) [*Fulvicin U/F* (scored); *Grisovin-FP*].
250 mg (Rx) [*Fulvicin U/F* (scored); *Grisovin-FP*].
500 mg (Rx) [*Fulvicin U/F* (scored); *Grisovin-FP*].

### Packaging and storage

Store below 40 °C (104 °F), preferably between 15 and 30 °C (59 and 86 °F), unless otherwise specified by manufacturer. Store in a tight container.

### Auxiliary labeling

• May cause dizziness.
• Avoid alcoholic beverages.
• Avoid too much sun or use of sunlamp.
• Continue medicine for full time of treatment.
• Take with or after meals or milk.

## ULTRAMICROSIZE GRISEOFULVIN TABLETS USP

### Usual adult and adolescent dose

Antifungal—
Onychomycosis or
Tinea pedis: Oral, 250 to 375 mg every twelve hours.
Tinea capitis
Tinea corporis or
Tinea cruris: Oral, 125 to 187.5 mg every twelve hours; or 250 to 375 mg once a day.

### Usual pediatric dose

Antifungal—
Oral, 2.75 to 3.65 mg per kg of body weight every twelve hours; or 5.5 to 7.3 mg per kg of body weight once a day; or for
Children 14 to 23 kg: Oral, 31.25 to 82.5 mg every twelve hours; or 62.5 to 165 mg once a day.
Children 23 kg and over: Oral, 62.5 to 165 mg every twelve hours; or 125 to 330 mg once a day.

Note: Infants and children up to 2 years of age—Dosage has not been established.

### Strength(s) usually available

U.S.—
100 mg (Rx) [GENERIC].
125 mg (Rx) [*Fulvicin P/G* (scored); *Gris-PEG* (scored; methylparaben)].
165 mg (Rx) [*Fulvicin P/G* (scored); GENERIC].
250 mg (Rx) [*Fulvicin P/G* (scored); *Grisactin Ultra* (scored); *Gris-PEG* (scored; methylparaben)].
330 mg (Rx) [*Fulvicin P/G* (scored); *Grisactin Ultra* (scored); GENERIC].
Canada—
165 mg (Rx) [*Fulvicin P/G*].
330 mg (Rx) [*Fulvicin P/G*].

### Packaging and storage

Store below 40 °C (104 °F), preferably between 15 and 30 °C (59 and 86 °F), unless otherwise specified by manufacturer. Store in a well-closed container.

### Auxiliary labeling

• May cause dizziness.
• Avoid alcoholic beverages.
• Avoid too much sun or use of sunlamp.
• Continue medicine for full time of treatment.
• Take with or after meals or milk.

Revised: 09/06/92
Interim revision: 03/17/94; 04/24/95

# GROWTH HORMONE   Systemic

This monograph includes information on the following: Somatrem; Somatropin, Recombinant.

VA CLASSIFICATION (Primary): HS701

Other commonly used names are GH and human growth hormone (hGH)

Note: For a listing of dosage forms and brand names by country availability, see *Dosage Forms* section(s). For a listing of brand names for the articles in this monograph, refer to the General Index.

## Category
Growth hormone.

## Indications
Note: Bracketed information in the *Indications* section refers to uses that are not included in U.S. product labeling.

### Accepted
Growth failure (treatment)—Somatrem and recombinant somatropin are indicated for long-term treatment of growth failure in children caused by pituitary growth hormone (GH) deficiency (pituitary dwarfism), including GH deficiency caused by cranial irradiation. Failure to grow must be documented by a subnormal growth rate, and GH deficiency is usually identified by a lack of response to 2 standard pharmacologic stimuli that would normally provoke the release of somatropin or evidence of impaired spontaneous secretion or bioactivity of endogenous GH.

Human growth hormone is ineffective in patients with closed epiphyses; use in patients with epiphyseal maturation of greater than 15 to 16 years in males or 14 to 15 years in females is not generally recommended, although therapy may be useful in some older patients if epiphyses have not closed.

[Human growth hormone is also being used to treat growth failure associated with Turner's syndrome.]

There are currently insufficient data to establish the efficacy and the long-term safety of the use of human growth hormone in treating idiopathic short stature.

### Unaccepted
The use of human growth hormone in older males to change body composition (e.g., to decrease adiposity and to prevent decline in muscle mass) is not recommended.

## Pharmacology/Pharmacokinetics

### Physicochemical characteristics
Source—
Somatrem: Biosynthetic. A single polypeptide chain of 192 amino acids, one more (methionine) than naturally occurring human growth hormone, produced by a recombinant DNA process in *Escherichia coli.*
Somatropin, recombinant: Biosynthetic, produced by a recombinant DNA process in *Escherichia coli*; same amino acid sequence as naturally occurring human growth hormone. A single polypeptide chain of 191 amino acids.
Chemical name—
Somatrem: Somatotropin (human), *N*-L-methionyl-.
Somatropin, recombinant: Somatotropin (human).

### Mechanism of action/Effect
Human growth hormone is an anterior pituitary hormone. Most anabolic actions are thought to be mediated by insulin-like growth factor-I (IGF-I, which has also been known as somatomedin-C), synthesized in the liver and other tissues in response to growth hormone stimulation.
Stimulates linear growth by affecting cartilaginous growth areas of long bones. Also stimulates growth by increasing the number and size of skeletal muscle cells, influencing the size of organs, and increasing red cell mass through erythropoietin stimulation.
Influences metabolism of carbohydrates by decreasing insulin sensitivity and possibly by affecting glucose transport; of fats by causing mobilization of fatty acids; of minerals by causing the retention of phosphorus, sodium, and potassium through promotion of cellular growth; and of proteins by increasing protein synthesis, which results in nitrogen retention.

### Biotransformation
Hepatic, approximately 90%.

### Half-life
Intravenous injection—Approximately 20 to 30 minutes (elimination).
Intramuscular or subcutaneous injection—Serum concentrations decline with a half-life of approximately 3 to 5 hours, reflecting continued release of the hormone from the injection site.

### Duration of action
Approximately 12 to 48 hours.

### Elimination
Biliary (approximately 0.1% of a dose as unchanged drug).

## Precautions to Consider

### Carcinogenicity/Mutagenicity
Carcinogenicity and mutagenicity testing has not been performed in animals or humans. Mutagenicity testing *in vitro* with recombinant somatropin did not reveal any mutagenic effects.
Anecdotal cases of acute and chronic leukemia have been reported in patients treated with human growth hormone, at an incidence slightly higher than that expected in the overall population. However, the exact relationship to human growth hormone therapy is unknown. Leukemia has also been reported in hypopituitary patients who have not been treated with growth hormone.

### Drug interactions and/or related problems
The following drug interactions and/or related problems have been selected on the basis of their potential clinical significance (possible mechanism in parentheses where appropriate)—not necessarily inclusive (» = major clinical significance):

Note: Combinations containing any of the following medications, depending on the amount present, may also interact with this medication.

Anabolic steroids or
Androgens or
Estrogens or
Thyroid hormones
(concurrent use of excessive doses of these hormones may accelerate epiphyseal closure, although supplemental use of these hormones may be necessary in patients with those deficiencies, to maintain the growth response to human growth hormone)

» Corticosteroids, glucocorticoid or
» Corticotropin (ACTH), especially with chronic therapeutic use
(inhibition of the growth response to human growth hormone may occur with chronic therapeutic use of corticotropin or with daily oral doses [per square meter of body surface] in excess of:

Betamethasone: 300 to 450 mcg
Cortisone: 12.5 to 18.8 mg
Dexamethasone: 250 to 500 mcg
Hydrocortisone: 10 to 15 mg
Methylprednisolone: 2 to 3 mg
Paramethasone: 1 to 1.5 mg
Prednisolone: 2.5 to 3.75 mg
Prednisone: 2.5 to 3.75 mg
Triamcinolone: 2 to 3 mg

Maximum parenteral corticosteroid doses are approximately one-half maximum oral doses. In general, it is recommended that these doses not be exceeded during human growth hormone therapy and if larger doses are required, administration of human growth hormone should be postponed, except for brief administration of stress dosages during acute febrile illness or other acute stress; however, there is great interindividual variation. Also, concurrent use with corticotropin is not recommended; of the others, hydrocortisone or cortisone is usually preferred, except in extenuating circumstances)

### Laboratory value alterations
The following have been selected on the basis of their potential clinical significance (possible effect in parentheses where appropriate)—not necessarily inclusive (» = major clinical significance):
With physiology/laboratory test values
Glucose tolerance
(may be reduced by high doses)

Inorganic phosphate
(serum concentrations may be increased to normal during treatment with growth hormone as a result of metabolic activity associated with bone growth as well as increased tubular reabsorption of phosphate by the kidney)

Nonesterified fatty acids
(plasma concentrations may be increased as a result of lipid mobilization from body fat stores)

Thyroid function
(serum thyroxine [$T_4$] concentration, radioactive iodine uptake [RAIU], and thyroxine-binding capacity may be slightly decreased; asymptomatic hypothyroidism usually occurs in less than 5%, but possibly up to 10 to 20%, of patients with hypopituitarism)

**Medical considerations/Contraindications**

The medical considerations/contraindications included here have been selected on the basis of their potential clinical significance (reasons given in parentheses where appropriate)—not necessarily inclusive (» = major clinical significance).

*Risk-benefit should be considered when the following medical problems exist:*

Hypothyroidism, untreated
(interferes with growth response to human growth hormone; prior and/or concurrent thyroid hormone replacement therapy is recommended)

Malignancy, especially intracranial tumor, actively growing within the previous 12 months
(human growth hormone should not be used if there is evidence of progression or recurrent growth of an underlying tumor; antitumor therapy and a reasonable period of observation should be complete before growth hormone therapy is initiated)

Sensitivity to the growth hormone product prescribed

**Patient monitoring**

The following may be especially important in patient monitoring (other tests may be warranted in some patients, depending on condition; » = major clinical significance):

Antibodies to growth hormone, serologic evaluation for
(in some cases, where growth rate falls during therapy and all other sources of growth inhibition have been ruled out, serologic evaluation for the presence of antibodies to growth hormone may be performed, with emphasis on binding capacity; antibodies to somatrem may be formed in the first 3 to 6 months of treatment, but only rarely cause failure to respond to therapy; antibodies to recombinant somatropin have been detected in patients treated for 6 months or more; relative incidence of antibody formation is difficult to compare because different assays have been used; however, growth inhibition appears to be correlated more with high binding capacity than with titer, and differences in antibody formation have demonstrated minimal clinical significance to date)

Bone age determinations
(recommended annually during therapy, especially in pubertal patients on concurrent androgen, estrogen, or thyroid replacement therapy since concurrent use may accelerate epiphyseal maturation)

Examinations to monitor intracranial lesion
(recommended at frequent intervals in patients with growth hormone deficiency secondary to an intracranial lesion)

Growth rate determinations from stadiometer measurements
(recommended every 3 to 6 months during therapy; if the growth rate does not exceed the pretreatment growth rate by at least 2 cm per year, the patient should be checked for noncompliance or the presence of antibodies or other medical problems such as hypothyroidism or malnutrition)

Thyroid function determinations
(recommended at regular intervals during therapy to detect hypothyroidism that develops during treatment; untreated hypothyroidism interferes with response to human growth hormone)

## Side/Adverse Effects

Note: Prolonged use of excessive doses of human growth hormone in patients who are not growth hormone deficient may theoretically cause acromegalic features (face, hands, feet), and other problems associated with acromegaly, including organ enlargement, diabetes mellitus, atherosclerosis, hypertension, and nerve entrapment syndrome (carpal tunnel syndrome).

The following side/adverse effects have been selected on the basis of their potential clinical significance (possible signs and symptoms in parentheses where appropriate)—not necessarily inclusive:

**Those indicating need for medical attention**

Incidence rare
*Allergic reaction* (skin rash or itching); *pain and swelling at site of injection; slipped capital femoral epiphysis* (limp; pain in hip or knee)

Note: *Slipped femoral epiphyses* may also occur in growth hormone–deficient children not treated with growth hormone.

## Patient Consultation

As an aid to patient consultation, refer to *Advice for the Patient, Growth Hormone (Systemic).*

In providing consultation, consider emphasizing the following selected information (» = major clinical significance):

**Before using this medication**
» Conditions affecting use, especially:
Sensitivity to growth hormone
Other medications, especially corticosteroids or corticotropin (ACTH)

**Proper use of this medication**
» Proper dosing

**Precautions while using this medication**
» Importance of regular visits to physician

**Side/adverse effects**
Signs of potential side effects, especially allergic reaction, and pain and swelling at site of injection

## General Dosing Information

Patients receiving human growth hormone should be under the supervision of a physician trained in the use of and familiar with growth hormone therapy.

The dosage and schedule of administration must be individualized for each patient.

The dosage of human growth hormone may be increased above the recommended dosage in older children with hypopituitarism, especially those who have open epiphyses.

Generally, after 2 or more years of treatment, growth rate will decrease, if therapy is continued. Attenuation of growth may be spontaneous. However, if this occurs, the patient should be checked for poor compliance with therapy, other medical problems (such as malnutrition or hypothyroidism), or the presence of antibodies. An increased dose of human growth hormone may be effective. In some patients, low doses of androgens or estrogens may be given concomitantly to restore the response, as long as epiphyseal maturation of 11 years or greater is present.

Human growth hormone therapy should be continued as long as the patient is responsive, until the patient reaches a mature adult height or until epiphyses close.

---

*SOMATREM*

## Parenteral Dosage Forms
### SOMATREM FOR INJECTION

Note: The specific activity of growth hormone is defined as International Units (IU) per mg of protein. In October 1994, a new standard was developed that changed the conversion amount from 2.6 IU per mg of growth hormone to 3 IU per mg of growth hormone. This change did not affect the milligram-per-kg dosing or the quantity (mg) of growth hormone per vial. The only change was the increase of IUs per mg.

**Usual pediatric dose**
Growth hormone—
Intramuscular or subcutaneous, up to 0.3 mg (0.9 International Unit [IU]) per kg of body weight a week with dosing and dosing regimen individualized according to the patient's needs. It is recommended by the manufacturer that this dose be divided into the appropriate dose for daily injection (six or seven times per week). The subcutaneous route of administration is preferred to the intramuscular route.

Note: If the growth rate does not exceed the pretreatment growth rate by at least 2 cm per year, the patient should be checked for noncompliance or the presence of antibodies or other medical problems such as hypothyroidism or malnutrition. If increasing the dose is not effective, treatment should be discontinued and the patient reevaluated.

**Size(s) usually available**
U.S.—
5 mg (approximately 15 IU) per vial (Rx) [*Protropin* (diluent—benzyl alcohol)].
10 mg (approximately 30 IU) per vial (Rx) [*Protropin* (diluent—benzyl alcohol)].

Canada—
    5 mg (approximately 15 IU) per vial (Rx) [*Protropin* (diluent—benzyl alcohol)].
    10 mg (approximately 30 IU) per vial (Rx) [*Protropin* (diluent—benzyl alcohol)].

**Packaging and storage**
Prior to and following reconstitution, store between 2 and 8 °C (36 and 46 °F). Protect the reconstituted solution and diluent from freezing.

**Preparation of dosage form**
Using standard aseptic technique, add 1 to 5 mL of Bacteriostatic Water for Injection USP (benzyl alcohol preserved only) to a 5-mg vial or 1 to 10 mL to a 10-mg vial. Swirl gently to dissolve. The vial should not be shaken. Cloudy solution should not be used.
If somatrem is to be administered to a neonate, Water for Injection should be used for reconstitution; benzyl alcohol used as a preservative has been associated with toxicity in neonates. Each vial should then be used only for one dose and any unused portion discarded.

**Stability**
When prepared with the diluent provided by the manufacturer, reconstituted solutions should be stored in the refrigerator and used within 14 days. If water for injection is used for reconstitution, each vial should be used only for one dose and any unused portion discarded. If these procedures are not followed, sterility of the solution cannot be assured.

---

### SOMATROPIN, RECOMBINANT

## Parenteral Dosage Forms

### SOMATROPIN, RECOMBINANT, FOR INJECTION

Note: The specific activity of growth hormone is defined as International Units (IU) per mg of protein. In October 1994, a new standard was developed that changed the conversion amount from 2.6 IU per mg of growth hormone to 3 IU per mg of growth hormone. This change did not affect the milligram-per-kg dosing or the quantity (mg) of growth hormone per vial. The only change was the increase of IUs per mg.

**Usual pediatric dose**
Growth hormone—
    Intramuscular or subcutaneous, 0.18 to 0.3 mg (0.54 to 0.9 International Unit [IU]) per kg of body weight a week with dosing and dosing regimen individualized according to the patient's needs. This can be divided into the appropriate dose for daily injection (six or seven times per week) or, as an alternative, divided and injected three times a week (every other day). The subcutaneous route of administration is preferred to the intramuscular route.

Note: If the growth rate does not exceed the pretreatment growth rate by at least 2 cm per year, the patient should be checked for noncompliance or the presence of antibodies or other medical problems such as hypothyroidism or malnutrition. If increasing the dose is not effective, treatment should be discontinued and the patient reevaluated.

**Size(s) usually available**
U.S.—
    5 mg (approximately 15 IU) per vial (Rx) [*Humatrope* (diluent—m-cresol; glycerin); *Nutropin* (diluent—benzyl alcohol)].
    10 mg (approximately 30 IU) per vial (Rx) [*Nutropin* (diluent—benzyl alcohol)].
Canada—
    2 mg (approximately 6 IU) per vial (Rx) [*Humatrope* (diluent—m-cresol; glycerin)].
    5 mg (approximately 15 IU) per vial (Rx) [*Humatrope* (diluent—m-cresol; glycerin)].

**Packaging and storage**
Prior to and following reconstitution, store between 2 and 8 °C (36 and 46 °F). Protect the reconstituted solution and diluent from freezing.

**Preparation of dosage form**
Some brands of *Humatrope* are packaged in a system with the diluent and somatropin in the same vial, with a rubber stopper separating each component. The product can be reconstituted by depressing the stopper, which allows the two components to mix.
For products that package the diluent and somatropin in separate vials, using standard aseptic technique the following amount of diluent should be added:
    For *Humatrope*—1.5 to 5 mL of the diluent provided by the manufacturer is added to a 2-mg or 5-mg vial.
    For *Nutropin*—1 to 10 mL of the diluent provided by the manufacturer or Bacteriostatic Water for Injection USP (benzyl alcohol preserved only) is added to a 5-mg or 10-mg vial.
To mix the diluent with the somatropin, the diluent must be injected while aimed against the glass wall of the vial, then swirled gently to dissolve the contents of the vial. The vial should not be shaken. Cloudy solutions or those containing particulate matter should not be used.
If somatropin is to be administered to a neonate, Water for Injection should be used for reconstitution; benzyl alcohol used as a preservative has been associated with toxicity in neonates. Each vial should then be used only for one dose and any unused portion discarded.

**Stability**
Somatropin is stable for up to 14 days if stored in the refrigerator following reconstitution with the diluent provided by the manufacturer. If sterile water for injection is used for reconstitution, each vial should be refrigerated and used within 24 hours.

## Selected Bibliography

Frasier SD, Lippe BM. The rational use of growth hormone during childhood [review]. J Clin Endocrinol Metab 1990; 71 (2): 269-73.
Laron Z, Butenandt O. Optimum use of growth hormone in children [review]. Drugs 1991; 42 (1): 1-8.

---

Revised: 11/18/92
Interim revision: 06/30/94; 08/15/95

---

# GUAIFENESIN  Systemic

VA CLASSIFICATION (Primary): RE302
Another commonly used name is glyceryl guaiacolate.
Note: For a listing of dosage forms and brand names by country availability, see *Dosage Forms* section(s). For a listing of brand names for the articles in this monograph, refer to the General Index.

---

## Category
Expectorant.

## Indications

**Accepted**
Cough (treatment)—Guaifenesin is indicated as an expectorant in the temporary symptomatic management of cough due to minor upper respiratory infections and related conditions, such as sinusitis, pharyngitis, and bronchitis, when these conditions are complicated by viscous mucus and congestion. However, because supporting data are very limited, there is some controversy about its effectiveness.

## Pharmacology/Pharmacokinetics

**Physicochemical characteristics**
Molecular weight—198.22.

**Mechanism of action/Effect**
Guaifenesin is thought to act as an expectorant by increasing the volume and reducing the viscosity of secretions in the trachea and bronchi. Thus, it may increase the efficiency of the cough reflex and facilitate removal of the secretions; however, objective evidence for this is limited and conflicting.

**Absorption**
Readily absorbed from gastrointestinal tract.

**Elimination**
Renal, as inactive metabolites.

## Precautions to Consider

**Carcinogenicity/Tumorigenicity/Mutagenicity**
Studies to determine the carcinogenicity, tumorigenicity, or mutagenicity of guaifenesin in animals have not been conducted.

**Pregnancy/Reproduction**

Pregnancy—Although adequate and well-controlled studies in pregnant women have not been done, the Collaborative Perinatal Project monitored 197 mother-child pairs exposed to guaifenesin during the first trimester. An increased occurrence of inguinal hernias was found in the neonates. However, congenital defects were not strongly associated with guaifenesin use during pregnancy in 2 large groups of mother-child pairs.

Studies have not been done in animals.

FDA Pregnancy Category C.

**Breast-feeding**

It is not known whether guaifenesin is distributed into breast milk. However, problems in humans have not been documented.

**Pediatrics**

Appropriate studies on the relationship of age to the effects of guaifenesin have not been performed in the pediatric population. However, no pediatrics-specific problems have been documented to date.

Caution is recommended in children up to 12 years of age with persistent or chronic cough, such as occurs with asthma, or if the cough is accompanied by excessive phlegm (mucus). The condition of these children may need a physician's evaluation before guaifenesin is administered.

Guaifenesin should not be given to children younger than 2 years of age unless recommended by a physician.

**Geriatrics**

Appropriate studies on the relationship of age to the effects of guaifenesin have not been performed in the geriatric population. However, no geriatrics-specific problems have been documented to date.

**Laboratory value alterations**

The following have been selected on the basis of their potential clinical significance (possible effect in parentheses where appropriate)—not necessarily inclusive (» = major clinical significance):

With diagnostic test results

5-hydroxyindoleacetic acid (5-HIAA), urine

(urinary determinations may be falsely increased when nitrosonaphthol reagent is used because of color interference by guaifenesin metabolites; guaifenesin should be discontinued 48 hours before collection of urine for this test)

Vanillylmandelic acid (VMA), urine

(guaifenesin or its metabolites may cause color interference with urinary determinations and may falsely elevate VMA test for catechols; guaifenesin should be discontinued 48 hours before collection of urine for this test)

**Medical considerations/Contraindications**

The medical considerations/contraindications included here have been selected on the basis of their potential clinical significance (reasons given in parentheses where appropriate)—not necessarily inclusive (» = major clinical significance):

*Risk-benefit should be considered when the following medical problem exists:*

Sensitivity to guaifenesin

# Side/Adverse Effects

The following side/adverse effects have been selected on the basis of their potential clinical significance (possible signs and symptoms in parentheses where appropriate)—not necessarily inclusive:

**Those indicating need for medical attention only if they continue or are bothersome**

Less frequent or rare

*Diarrhea; dizziness; headache; nausea or vomiting; skin rash; stomach pain; urticaria* (hives)

# Patient Consultation

As an aid to patient consultation, refer to *Advice for the Patient, Guaifenesin (Systemic).*

In providing consultation, consider emphasizing the following selected information (» = major clinical significance):

**Before using this medication**

» Conditions affecting use, especially:

Sensitivity to guaifenesin

Pregnancy—Increased incidence of inguinal hernias in the babies of one group of women taking guaifenesin during pregnancy; however, this did not occur in other groups

Use in children—For self-medication, caution if cough is persistent or occurs with excessive phlegm; not administering to children younger than 2 years of age unless directed by a physician

**Proper use of this medication**

*Proper administration*

Importance of maintaining adequate fluid intake

» For extended-release dosage forms

Swallowing capsules whole or opening capsules and sprinkling contents on soft food, then swallowing without crushing or chewing

Not breaking (unless scored for breakage), crushing, or chewing tablets; swallowing tablet whole

» Proper dosing

Missed dose (if on a scheduled dosing regimen): Taking as soon as possible; not taking if almost time for next dose; not doubling doses

» Proper storage

**Precautions while using this medication**

Checking with physician if cough persists after medication has been used for 7 days or if fever, skin rash, continuing headache, or sore throat is present with cough

# General Dosing Information

Before prescribing or recommending medication to suppress or modify cough, it is important that the underlying cause of the cough be assessed.

For self-medication, guaifenesin should not be taken for chronic cough unless directed by a physician.

Patient should be advised to maintain adequate hydration.

# Oral Dosage Forms

## GUAIFENESIN CAPSULES USP

**Usual adult and adolescent dose**

Expectorant—

Oral, 200 to 400 mg every four hours, not to exceed 2400 mg a day.

**Usual pediatric dose**

Expectorant—

Children 2 to 6 years of age: The liquid or extended-release capsule dosage forms may be preferable for children in this age group.

Children 6 to 12 years of age: Oral, 100 to 200 mg every four hours, not to exceed 1200 mg a day.

**Usual geriatric dose**

See *Usual adult and adolescent dose.*

**Strength(s) usually available**

U.S.—

200 mg (OTC) [*Breonesin; GG-CEN; Hytuss-2X*].

Canada—

Not commercially available.

**Packaging and storage**

Store below 40 °C (104 °F), preferably between 15 and 30 °C (59 and 86 °F), unless otherwise specified by manufacturer. Store in a tight container.

## GUAIFENESIN EXTENDED-RELEASE CAPSULES

**Usual adult and adolescent dose**

Expectorant—

Oral, 600 to 1200 mg every twelve hours, not to exceed 2400 mg a day.

**Usual pediatric dose**

Expectorant—

Children 2 to 6 years of age: Oral, 300 mg every twelve hours, not to exceed 600 mg a day.

Note: The liquid dosage forms may be preferable for children 2 to 6 years of age, who cannot always be relied upon to swallow the contents of the capsule without chewing.

Children 6 to 12 years of age: Oral, 600 mg every twelve hours, not to exceed 1200 mg a day.

**Usual geriatric dose**

See *Usual adult and adolescent dose.*

**Strength(s) usually available**

U.S.—

300 mg (Rx) [*Humibid Sprinkle*].

Canada—

Not commercially available.

**Packaging and storage**

Store between 15 and 30 °C (59 and 86 °F), unless otherwise specified by manufacturer. Store in a tight container.

**Additional information**

Extended-release capsules may be swallowed whole or opened and the contents sprinkled on soft food immediately prior to ingestion, then swallowed without crushing or chewing. Capsule contents should not be subdivided.

## GUAIFENESIN ORAL SOLUTION

**Usual adult and adolescent dose**

See *Guaifenesin Capsules USP*.

**Usual pediatric dose**

Expectorant—

Children 6 months to 2 years of age—Dosage must be individualized by physician. A commonly used regimen is 25 to 50 mg every four hours, not to exceed 300 mg a day.

Children 2 to 6 years of age—Oral, 50 to 100 mg every four hours, not to exceed 600 mg a day.

Children 6 to 12 years to age—See *Guaifenesin Capsules USP*.

**Usual geriatric dose**

See *Usual adult and adolescent dose*.

**Strength(s) usually available**

U.S.—

100 mg per 5 mL (OTC) [*Diabetic Tussin EX* (alcohol free; sugar free); *Scot-tussin Expectorant* (alcohol 3.5%; sugar free)].

100 mg per 5 mL (Rx) [*Organidin NR* (sorbitol; alcohol free)].

200 mg per 5 mL (OTC) [*Naldecon Senior EX* (alcohol free; sugar free)].

Canada—

Not commercially available.

**Packaging and storage**

Store below 40 °C (104 °F), preferably between 15 and 30 °C (59 and 86 °F), unless otherwise specified by manufacturer. Store in a tight container. Protect from freezing.

## GUAIFENESIN SYRUP USP

**Usual adult and adolescent dose**

See *Guaifenesin Capsules USP*.

**Usual pediatric dose**

See *Guaifenesin Oral Solution*.

**Usual geriatric dose**

See *Usual adult and adolescent dose*.

**Strength(s) usually available**

U.S.—

100 mg per 5 mL (OTC) [*Anti-Tuss* (alcohol 3.5%); *Genatuss* (alcohol 3.5%); *Guiatuss; Halotussin* (alcohol 3.5%); *Robitussin* (alcohol 3.5%); *Uni-tussin* (alcohol 3.5%); GENERIC].

Canada—

100 mg per 5 mL (OTC) [*Balminil Expectorant; Benylin-E* (alcohol 5%); *Calmylin Expectorant* (sorbitol; alcohol free); *Robitussin* (alcohol 3.5%)].

**Packaging and storage**

Store below 40 °C (104 °F), preferably between 15 and 30 °C (59 and 86 °F), unless otherwise specified by manufacturer. Store in a tight container. Protect from freezing.

## GUAIFENESIN TABLETS USP

**Usual adult and adolescent dose**

See *Guaifenesin Capsules USP*.

**Usual pediatric dose**

See *Guaifenesin Capsules USP*.

**Usual geriatric dose**

See *Usual adult and adolescent dose*.

**Strength(s) usually available**

U.S.—

100 mg (OTC) [*Glycotuss; Hytuss* (scored; sugar free)].

200 mg (OTC) [*Gee-Gee; Glytuss*].

200 mg (Rx) [*Organidin NR* (scored)].

Canada—

100 mg (OTC) [*Resyl*].

**Packaging and storage**

Store below 40 °C (104 °F), preferably between 15 and 30 °C (59 and 86 °F), unless otherwise specified by manufacturer. Store in a tight container.

## GUAIFENESIN EXTENDED-RELEASE TABLETS

**Usual adult and adolescent dose**

See *Guaifenesin Extended-release Capsules*.

**Usual pediatric dose**

See *Guaifenesin Extended-release Capsules*.

**Strength(s) usually available**

U.S.—

600 mg (Rx) [*Fenesin* (scored); *Humibid L.A* (scored); *Pneumomist* (scored); *Sinumist-SR* (scored); *Touro EX* (scored); GENERIC].

Canada—

Not commercially available.

**Packaging and storage**

Store between 15 and 30 °C (59 and 86 °F), unless otherwise specified by manufacturer. Store in a tight container.

## Selected Bibliography

Irwin RS, Curley FJ, Bennett FM. Appropriate use of antitussives and protussives. Drugs 1993; 46 (1): 80-91.

Revised: 08/04/95

# GUAIFENESIN-CONTAINING COMBINATIONS—

Brompheniramine, Phenylephrine, Phenylpropanolamine, Codeine, and Guaifenesin (Systemic)—See *Cough/Cold Combinations (Systemic)*

Brompheniramine, Phenylephrine, Phenylpropanolamine, and Guaifenesin (Systemic)—See *Cough/Cold Combinations (Systemic)*

Brompheniramine, Phenylephrine, Phenylpropanolamine, Hydrocodone, and Guaifenesin (Systemic)—See *Cough/Cold Combinations (Systemic)*

Chlorpheniramine, Ephedrine, and Guaifenesin (Systemic)—See *Cough/Cold Combinations (Systemic)*

Chlorpheniramine, Phenylephrine, Dextromethorphan, and Guaifenesin (Systemic)—See *Cough/Cold Combinations (Systemic)*

Chlorpheniramine, Phenylephrine, Dextromethorphan, Guaifenesin, and Ammonium Chloride (Systemic)—See *Cough/Cold Combinations (Systemic)*

Chlorpheniramine, Phenylephrine, and Guaifenesin (Systemic)—See *Cough/Cold Combinations (Systemic)*

Chlorpheniramine, Phenylephrine, Phenylpropanolamine, Dextromethorphan, Guaifenesin, and Acetaminophen (Systemic)—See *Cough/Cold Combinations (Systemic)*

Chlorpheniramine, Phenylpropanolamine, Codeine, Guaifenesin, and Acetaminophen (Systemic)—See *Cough/Cold Combinations (Systemic)*

Chlorpheniramine, Phenylpropanolamine, and Guaifenesin (Systemic)—See *Cough/Cold Combinations (Systemic)*

Chlorpheniramine, Phenylpropanolamine, Guaifenesin, Sodium Citrate, and Citric Acid (Systemic)—See *Cough/Cold Combinations (Systemic)*

Chlorpheniramine, Pseudoephedrine, and Guaifenesin (Systemic)—See *Cough/Cold Combinations (Systemic)*

Codeine, Ammonium Chloride, and Guaifenesin (Systemic)—See *Cough/Cold Combinations (Systemic)*

Codeine and Guaifenesin (Systemic)—See *Cough/Cold Combinations (Systemic)*

Dexchlorpheniramine, Pseudoephedrine, and Guaifenesin (Systemic)—See *Cough/Cold Combinations (Systemic)*

Dextromethorphan and Guaifenesin (Systemic)—See *Cough/Cold Combinations (Systemic)*

Ephedrine and Guaifenesin (Systemic)—See *Cough/Cold Combinations (Systemic)*

Hydrocodone and Guaifenesin (Systemic)—See *Cough/Cold Combinations (Systemic)*

Hydromorphone and Guaifenesin (Systemic)—See *Cough/Cold Combinations (Systemic)*

Oxtriphylline and Guaifenesin (Systemic)

Pheniramine, Codeine, and Guaifenesin (Systemic)—See *Cough/Cold Combinations (Systemic)*

Pheniramine, Phenylephrine, Phenylpropanolamine, Hydrocodone, and Guaifenesin (Systemic)—See *Cough/Cold Combinations (Systemic)*

Pheniramine, Pyrilamine, Phenylpropanolamine, Dextromethorphan, and Guaifenesin (Systemic)—See *Cough/Cold Combinations (Systemic)*

Pheniramine, Pyrilamine, Phenylpropanolamine, and Guaifenesin (Systemic)—See *Cough/Cold Combinations (Systemic)*

Pheniramine, Pyrilamine, Phenylpropanolamine, Hydrocodone, and Guaifenesin (Systemic)—See *Cough/Cold Combinations (Systemic)*

Phenylephrine, Dextromethorphan, and Guaifenesin (Systemic)—See *Cough/Cold Combinations (Systemic)*

Phenylephrine and Guaifenesin (Systemic)—See *Cough/Cold Combinations (Systemic)*

Phenylephrine, Guaifenesin, Acetaminophen, Salicylamide, and Caffeine (Systemic)—See *Cough/Cold Combinations (Systemic)*

Phenylephrine, Hydrocodone, and Guaifenesin (Systemic)—See *Cough/ Cold Combinations (Systemic)*

Phenylephrine, Phenylpropanolamine, and Guaifenesin (Systemic)—See *Cough/Cold Combinations (Systemic)*

Phenylpropanolamine, Codeine, and Guaifenesin (Systemic)—See *Cough/ Cold Combinations (Systemic)*

Phenylpropanolamine, Dextromethorphan, and Guaifenesin (Systemic)— See *Cough/Cold Combinations (Systemic)*

Phenylpropanolamine and Guaifenesin (Systemic)—See *Cough/Cold Combinations (Systemic)*

Phenylpropanolamine, Hydrocodone, Guaifenesin, and Salicylamide (Systemic)—See *Cough/Cold Combinations (Systemic)*

Pseudoephedrine, Codeine, and Guaifenesin (Systemic)—See *Cough/Cold Combinations (Systemic)*

Pseudoephedrine, Dextromethorphan, and Guaifenesin (Systemic)—See *Cough/Cold Combinations (Systemic)*

Pseudoephedrine, Dextromethorphan, Guaifenesin, and Acetaminophen (Systemic)—See *Cough/Cold Combinations (Systemic)*

Pseudoephedrine and Guaifenesin (Systemic)—See *Cough/Cold Combinations (Systemic)*

Pseudoephedrine, Hydrocodone and Guaifenesin (Systemic)—See *Cough/ Cold Combinations (Systemic)*

Pyrilamine, Phenylpropanolamine, Dextromethorphan, Guaifenesin, Potassium Citrate, and Citric Acid (Systemic)—See *Cough/Cold Combinations (Systemic)*

Theophylline, Ephedrine, Guaifenesin, and Phenobarbital (Systemic)

Theophylline and Guaifenesin (Systemic)

Triprolidine, Pseudoephedrine, Codeine, and Guaifenesin (Systemic)—See *Cough/Cold Combinations (Systemic)*

---

# GUANABENZ    Systemic†

VA CLASSIFICATION (Primary): CV490

Note: For a listing of dosage forms and brand names by country availability, see *Dosage Forms* section(s). For a listing of brand names for the articles in this monograph, refer to the General Index.

---

†Not commercially available in Canada.

## Category

Antihypertensive.

## Indications

### Accepted

Hypertension (treatment)—Guanabenz is indicated for treatment of hypertension. Because it usually does not cause postural hypotension, guanabenz may be useful as a substitute for other central adrenergic blockers in patients who cannot tolerate these agents because of severe orthostatic hypotension.

For additional information on initial therapeutic guidelines related to the treatment of hypertension, see *Appendix III*.

## Pharmacology/Pharmacokinetics

### Physicochemical characteristics

Molecular weight—Guanabenz acetate: 291.14.

### Mechanism of action/Effect

Guanabenz is a centrally acting alpha-2 adrenergic agonist. The antihypertensive effect is thought to be due to central alpha-adrenergic stimulation, which results in a decreased sympathetic outflow to the heart, kidneys, and peripheral vasculature; decreased systolic and diastolic blood pressure; and slight slowing of pulse rate. Chronic administration of guanabenz also causes a decrease in peripheral vascular resistance.

### Absorption

Approximately 75% absorbed from gastrointestinal tract; however, bioavailability is very low because of extensive first-pass metabolism.

### Protein binding

Very high (90%).

### Biotransformation

Hepatic.

### Half-life

Average, 6 hours.

### Onset of action

Within 60 minutes (after a single dose).

### Time to peak plasma concentration

2 to 5 hours.

### Time to peak effect

2 to 4 hours.

### Duration of action

12 hours (after a single dose).

### Elimination

Renal (less than 1% unchanged); fecal, about 16%.

## Precautions to Consider

### Carcinogenicity

Studies in rats at doses up to 10 times the maximum recommended human dose have not shown that guanabenz causes carcinogenic effects.

### Mutagenicity

Dose-related increases in the number of mutants occurred in one (TA 1537) of five *Salmonella typhimurium* strains in the Ames test at doses of 200 to 500 mcg per plate or 30 to 50 mcg per mL in suspension. No mutagenic activity was seen in other assays.

### Pregnancy/Reproduction

Fertility—Guanabenz has been found to impair fertility in both male and female rats given high doses (9.6 mg per kg of body weight [mg/kg]).

Pregnancy—Studies have not been done in humans.

Animal studies suggest that guanabenz crosses the placenta. Studies in mice have shown that guanabenz at doses of 3 to 6 times the maximum recommended human dose of 1 mg/kg causes an increase in skeletal abnormalities; these did not occur in rabbits or rats. Other studies have found increased fetal loss in rats and rabbits given 14 to 20 mg/kg. Slightly decreased live-birth indexes, decreased fetal survival rate, and decreased pup body weight occurred in rats given 6.4 to 9.6 mg/kg.

FDA Pregnancy Category C.

### Breast-feeding

It is not known whether guanabenz is distributed into breast milk. However, problems in humans have not been documented.

### Pediatrics

Appropriate studies on the relationship of age to the effects of guanabenz have not been performed in the pediatric population. Safety and efficacy have not been established.

### Geriatrics

Although appropriate studies on the relationship of age to the effects of guanabenz have not been performed in the geriatric population, no geriatrics-specific problems have been documented to date. However, elderly patients are more likely to have age-related renal function impairment, which may require caution in patients receiving guanabenz. In addition, elderly patients may be more sensitive to the hypotensive and sedative effects of guanabenz.

### Dental

Use of guanabenz may decrease or inhibit salivary flow, thus contributing to the development of caries, periodontal disease, oral candidiasis, and discomfort.

### Drug interactions and/or related problems

The following drug interactions and/or related problems have been selected on the basis of their potential clinical significance (possible mechanism in parentheses where appropriate)—not necessarily inclusive (» = major clinical significance):

Note: Combinations containing any of the following medications, depending on the amount present, may also interact with this medication.

Alcohol or
Central nervous system (CNS) depression–producing medications (See *Appendix II*)
(concurrent use may enhance the CNS depressant effects of either these medications or guanabenz)

Anti-inflammatory drugs, nonsteroidal (NSAIDs), especially indomethacin
(concurrent use may reduce antihypertensive effects of guanabenz; indomethacin, and possibly other NSAIDs, may antagonize the antihypertensive effect by inhibiting renal prostaglandin synthesis and/or by causing sodium and fluid retention; the patient should be carefully monitored to confirm that the desired effect is being obtained)

Beta-adrenergic blocking agents, ophthalmic
(if significant systemic absorption of ophthalmic beta-blockers occurs, concurrent use may increase the hypotensive effect of guanabenz)

» Beta-adrenergic blocking agents, systemic or
Hypotension-producing medications, other (See *Appendix II*)
(antihypertensive effects may be potentiated when these medications are used concurrently with guanabenz; although some antihypertensive and/or diuretic combinations are frequently used for therapeutic advantage, dosage adjustments may be necessary during concurrent use)
(when therapy is discontinued in patients receiving a beta-blocker and guanabenz concurrently, the beta-blocker should be gradually discontinued in order to avoid beta-adrenergic blocking agent–withdrawal hypertensive crisis; blood pressure control may also be impaired when the two are combined)

Estrogens
(estrogen-induced fluid retention may increase blood pressure)

Sympathomimetics
(concurrent use may reduce the antihypertensive effects of guanabenz; the patient should be carefully monitored to confirm that the desired effect is being obtained)

### Laboratory value alterations
The following have been selected on the basis of their potential clinical significance (possible effect in parentheses where appropriate)—not necessarily inclusive (» = major clinical significance):

With physiology/laboratory test values
Cholesterol and total triglyceride
(serum values may be reduced with chronic administration)

### Medical considerations/Contraindications
The medical considerations/contraindications included here have been selected on the basis of their potential clinical significance (reasons given in parentheses where appropriate)—not necessarily inclusive (» = major clinical significance).

*Risk-benefit should be considered when the following medical problems exist:*
Cerebrovascular disease or
Coronary insufficiency or
Myocardial infarction, recent
(may be aggravated by reduced blood pressure)
Hepatic function impairment
(plasma concentrations of guanabenz may increase; careful monitoring of blood pressure during dosage titration is recommended)
Renal function impairment
(half-life of guanabenz is increased and clearance is decreased; careful monitoring of blood pressure during dosage titration is recommended)
Sensitivity to guanabenz

### Patient monitoring
The following may be especially important in patient monitoring (other tests may be warranted in some patients, depending on condition; » = major clinical significance):

» Blood pressure measurements
(recommended at periodic intervals in patients being treated for hypertension; selected patients may be trained to perform blood pressure measurements at home and report the results at regular physician visits)

## Side/Adverse Effects
The following side/adverse effects have been selected on the basis of their potential clinical significance (possible signs and symptoms in parentheses where appropriate)—not necessarily inclusive:

**Those indicating need for medical attention only if they continue or are bothersome**
Incidence more frequent
*Dizziness; drowsiness; dryness of mouth; weakness*
Note: Incidence of *drowsiness* is dose-related and usually declines with continued administration.

Incidence less frequent or rare
*Decreased sexual ability; headache; nausea*

**Those indicating possible withdrawal and the need for medical attention if they occur after medication is abruptly discontinued**
*Anxiety or tenseness; chest pain; fast or irregular heartbeat; headache; increased salivation; increase in sweating; nausea or vomiting; nervousness or restlessness; shaking or trembling of hands or fingers; stomach cramps; trouble in sleeping*

Note: The above are symptoms of sympathetic overactivity; elevation of blood pressure above baseline levels occurs rarely. The risk appears to be increased in patients receiving doses of greater than 32 mg of guanabenz per day.

## Overdose
For specific information on the agents used in the management of guanabenz overdose, see:
• *Atropine* in *Anticholinergics/Antispasmodics (Systemic)* monograph;
• *Charcoal (Oral-Local)* monograph; and/or
• *Dopamine* in *Sympathomimetic Agents—Cardiovascular Use (Systemic)* monograph.

For more information on the management of overdose or unintentional ingestion, **contact a Poison Control Center** (see *Poison Control Center Listing*).

### Clinical effects of overdose
The following effects have been selected on the basis of their potential clinical significance (possible signs and symptoms in parentheses where appropriate)—not necessarily inclusive:

*Bradycardia* (slow heartbeat); *hypotension* (dizziness, severe); *irritability; lethargy* (unusual tiredness or weakness); *miosis* (pinpoint pupils); *somnolence*

### Treatment of overdose
To decrease absorption—
Gastric lavage and administration of activated charcoal.
Specific treatment—
Treatment is mainly supportive. Maintaining adequate airway and fluid balance is recommended.
For bradycardia: Atropine has been used successfully.
For hypotension: Vasopressor agents, such as dopamine, have been used successfully.
Monitoring—
Carefully monitor vital signs and fluid balance.
Supportive care—
Patients in whom intentional overdose is known or suspected should be referred for psychiatric evaluation.

## Patient Consultation
As an aid to patient consultation, refer to *Advice for the Patient, Guanabenz (Systemic)*.

In providing consultation, consider emphasizing the following selected information (» = major clinical significance):

**Before using this medication**
» Conditions affecting use, especially:
Sensitivity to guanabenz
Pregnancy—High doses in animals cause decreased fertility, birth defects, and fetal death
Use in the elderly—Increased sensitivity to hypotensive and sedative effects
Dental—May decrease or inhibit salivary flow
Other medications, especially systemic beta-adrenergic blocking agents

**Proper use of this medication**
Possible need for control of weight and diet, especially sodium intake
» Patient may not experience symptoms of hypertension; importance of taking medication even if feeling well
» Does not cure but helps control hypertension; possible need for lifelong therapy; serious consequences of untreated hypertension
Getting into the habit of taking at same time each day to help increase compliance
» Proper dosing
Missed dose: Taking as soon as possible; not taking if almost time for next dose; checking with physician if two or more doses in a row are missed; possible unpleasant effects if stopped abruptly
» Proper storage

**Precautions while using this medication**
Regular visits to physician to check progress
Checking with physician before discontinuing medication; possible need for gradual dosage reduction

Caution if any kind of surgery (including dental surgery) or emergency treatment is required
» Not taking other medications, especially nonprescription sympathomimetics, unless discussed with physician
» Caution in taking alcohol or other CNS depressants
» Caution when driving or doing things requiring alertness because of possible dizziness or drowsiness
Possible dryness of mouth; using sugarless candy or gum, ice, or saliva substitute for relief; checking with physician or dentist if dry mouth continues for more than 2 weeks

### Side/adverse effects
Signs of potential side effects, especially signs and symptoms of overdose or withdrawal reaction

## General Dosing Information

It is recommended that the last daily dose be taken at bedtime to ensure overnight control of blood pressure and reduce daytime drowsiness.

Recent evidence suggests that withdrawal of antihypertensive therapy prior to surgery is not necessary, but that the anesthesiologist must be aware of such therapy.

The possibility of withdrawal syndrome should be kept in mind if guanabenz is discontinued abruptly, since rebound hypertension occurs rarely.

## Oral Dosage Forms

### GUANABENZ ACETATE TABLETS USP

**Usual adult dose**
Antihypertensive—
Oral, 4 mg two times a day initially, the dosage being increased if necessary in increments of 4 to 8 mg per day every one to two weeks up to the minimum effective dose.

Note: Geriatric patients may be more sensitive to the effects of the usual adult dose.

**Usual adult prescribing limits**
Up to 32 mg per day.

**Usual pediatric dose**
Safety and efficacy have not been established.

**Strength(s) usually available**
U.S.—
4 mg (Rx) [*Wytensin* (lactose)].
8 mg (Rx) [*Wytensin* (lactose)].
Canada—
Not commercially available.

**Packaging and storage**
Store below 40 °C (104 °F), preferably between 15 and 30 °C (59 and 86 °F), unless otherwise specified by manufacturer. Store in a tight, light-resistant container.

**Auxiliary labeling**
• Do not take other medicines without your doctor's advice.
• May cause dizziness.
• May cause drowsiness.

## Selected Bibliography

The fifth report of the Joint National Committee on Detection, Evaluation, and Treatment of High Blood Pressure (JNC V). Arch Intern Med 1993; 153 (2): 154-83.

Revised: 07/22/96

# GUANADREL   Systemic†

VA CLASSIFICATION (Primary): CV490
Note: For a listing of dosage forms and brand names by country availability, see *Dosage Forms* section(s). For a listing of brand names for the articles in this monograph, refer to the General Index.

†Not commercially available in Canada.

## Category

Antihypertensive.

## Indications

### Accepted
Hypertension (treatment)—Guanadrel is indicated in the treatment of hypertension.

For additional information on initial therapeutic guidelines related to the treatment of hypertension, see *Appendix III*.

## Pharmacology/Pharmacokinetics

### Physicochemical characteristics
Molecular weight—524.63.

### Mechanism of action/Effect
Guanadrel is a postganglionic adrenergic blocking agent. Uptake of guanadrel and storage in sympathetic neurons occurs via the norepinephrine pump; guanadrel slowly displaces norepinephrine from its storage in nerve endings and thereby blocks the release of norepinephrine normally produced by nerve stimulation. The reduction in neurotransmitter release in response to sympathetic nerve stimulation, as a result of catecholamine depletion, leads to reduced arteriolar vasoconstriction, especially the reflex increase in sympathetic tone that occurs with a change in position.

### Absorption
Rapidly and well absorbed from gastrointestinal tract.

### Protein binding
Low (approximately 20%).

### Biotransformation
Hepatic.

### Half-life
Approximately 10 hours, with wide interindividual variability; may be prolonged up to 19.2 hours in the presence of renal function impairment.

### Onset of action
2 hours (after a single dose).

### Time to peak concentration
1.5 to 2 hours.

### Time to peak effect
4 to 6 hours (after a single dose).

### Duration of action
Average—9 hours (range 4 to 14 hours) after a single dose.

### Elimination
Renal, 85% (about 40% unchanged).

## Precautions to Consider

### Carcinogenicity
Two-year studies in mice found no carcinogenic effect of guanadrel. In a 2-year study in rats, an increased incidence of benign testicular interstitial cell tumors was observed at doses of 100 mg per kg of body weight (mg/kg) per day and 400 mg/kg per day. However, the significance of these findings is not known since these spontaneous tumors are common in aged rats.

### Mutagenicity
*Salmonella* testing (Ames test) showed no evidence of mutagenicity.

### Pregnancy/Reproduction
Fertility—Suppressed libido and reduced fertility were observed in male and female rats at a dose of 100 mg/kg per day (12 times the maximum human dose in a 50-kg person). Suppressed libido was evident to a lesser extent at a dose of 30 mg/kg per day.

Pregnancy—Studies in humans have not been done.
Studies in rats and rabbits at doses up to 12 times the maximum recommended human dose have not shown that guanadrel causes adverse effects in the fetus.

FDA Pregnancy Category B.

**Breast-feeding**
It is not known whether guanadrel is distributed into breast milk. However, problems in humans have not been documented.

**Pediatrics**
Appropriate studies on the relationship of age to the effects of guanadrel have not been performed in the pediatric population. Safety and efficacy have not been established.

**Geriatrics**
Appropriate studies on the relationship of age to the effects of guanadrel have not been performed in the geriatric population. However, the elderly may be more sensitive to the hypotensive effects of guanadrel.

**Drug interactions and/or related problems**
The following drug interactions and/or related problems have been selected on the basis of their potential clinical significance (possible mechanism in parentheses where appropriate)—not necessarily inclusive (» = major clinical significance):

Note:  Because of the similarity of guanadrel's actions to those of guanethidine, some of the following potential interactions are stated for cautionary reference.

   Combinations containing any of the following medications, depending on the amount present, may also interact with this medication.

Alcohol or
Barbiturates or
Opioid (narcotic) analgesics
   (concurrent use with guanadrel will produce additive orthostatic hypotensive effects)

Alpha-adrenergic blocking agents or
Other medications with alpha-adrenergic blocking action, such as:
   Dihydroergotamine
   Ergoloid mesylates
   Ergotamine
   Haloperidol
   Loxapine
   Phenothiazines
   Thioxanthenes or
Beta-adrenergic blocking agents or
Rauwolfia alkaloids
   (concurrent use with guanadrel may cause an increased incidence of orthostatic hypotension or bradycardia)

Amphetamines or
» Antidepressants, tricyclic or
Appetite suppressants, with the exception of fenfluramine or
Cyclobenzaprine or
Haloperidol or
» Loxapine or
Maprotiline or
Methylphenidate or
Phenothiazines, especially chlorpromazine or
» Thioxanthenes or
» Trimeprazine
   (concurrent use may decrease the hypotensive effects of guanadrel because of its displacement from and inhibition of uptake by adrenergic neurons; caution is recommended when these medications are discontinued, especially if discontinued abruptly, because effects of guanadrel might be suddenly increased)

Anticholinergics, especially atropine and related compounds
   (concurrent use with guanadrel may antagonize the inhibitory action of these medications on gastric acid secretion)

Anti-inflammatory drugs, nonsteroidal (NSAIDs), especially indomethacin
   (antihypertensive effects of guanadrel may be reduced when it is used concurrently with these agents; indomethacin, and possibly other NSAIDs, may antagonize the antihypertensive effect by inhibiting renal prostaglandin synthesis and/or by causing sodium and fluid retention; the patient should be carefully monitored to confirm that the desired effect is being obtained)

Estrogens
   (concurrent use may decrease the antihypertensive effect of guanadrel because estrogen-induced fluid retention may lead to increased blood pressure)

Fenfluramine
   (concurrent use with guanadrel may produce additive hypotensive effects, and may result in postural hypotension; dosage adjustments of the antihypertensive may be necessary)

Hypotension-producing medications, other (See *Appendix II*)
   (antihypertensive effects may be potentiated when these medications are used concurrently with guanadrel; although some antih-

ypertensive and/or diuretic combinations are frequently used for therapeutic advantage, dosage adjustments may be necessary during concurrent use)

» Monoamine oxidase (MAO) inhibitors, including furazolidone, procarbazine, and selegiline
   (concurrent use with guanadrel may result in moderate to severe hypertension due to release of catecholamines; withdrawal of MAO inhibitors at least 1 week prior to initiation of guanadrel therapy is recommended)

Sympathomimetic agents, such as:
   Cocaine or
   Dobutamine or
   Dopamine or
   Ephedrine or
   Epinephrine or
» Metaraminol or
   Methoxamine or
   Norepinephrine or
   Phenylephrine or
   Phenylpropanolamine
   (concurrent use of any sympathomimetics with guanadrel may reduce the antihypertensive effects of guanadrel; the patient should be carefully monitored to confirm that the desired effect is being obtained)

   (in addition to possibly decreasing the hypotensive effects of guanadrel, concurrent use of cocaine, dobutamine, dopamine, ephedrine, epinephrine, metaraminol, methoxamine, norepinephrine, phenylephrine, or phenylpropanolamine with guanadrel may potentiate the pressor effect of these medications, as a result of inhibition of sympathomimetic uptake by adrenergic neurons, possibly resulting in hypertension and cardiac arrhythmias)

   (concurrent use of ephedrine or phenylpropanolamine with guanadrel may decrease the hypotensive effects of guanadrel because of its displacement from and inhibition of uptake by adrenergic neurons)

   (concurrent use of metaraminol with guanadrel may cause a hypertensive crisis. When metaraminol is used within 5 days after discontinuation of guanadrel, a hypertensive potential may remain)

   (concurrent use of phenylephrine ophthalmic solution with guanadrel may increase the pupillary response)

**Medical considerations/Contraindications**
The medical considerations/contraindications included here have been selected on the basis of their potential clinical significance (reasons given in parentheses where appropriate)—not necessarily inclusive (» = major clinical significance).

*Risk-benefit should be considered when the following medical problems exist:*

Asthma, history of
   (may be aggravated because of hypersensitivity to catecholamine depletion)

Cerebrovascular insufficiency or
Coronary insufficiency or
Myocardial infarction, recent
   (ischemia may be aggravated as a result of reduced blood pressure)

» Congestive heart failure, frank, not due to hypertension
   (may be aggravated by fluid retention; in addition, guanadrel may directly depress the myocardium)

Diarrhea
   (may be aggravated)

Fever
   (dosage requirements may be reduced)

Peptic ulcer, history of
   (may be aggravated by relative increase in parasympathetic tone)

» Pheochromocytoma
   (release of catecholamines and increased sensitivity to circulating norepinephrine may exacerbate symptoms)

Sensitivity to guanadrel

Sinus bradycardia
   (may be aggravated)

**Patient monitoring**
The following may be especially important in patient monitoring (other tests may be warranted in some patients, depending on condition; » = major clinical significance):

» Blood pressure measurements
   (recommended at periodic intervals in patients being treated for hypertension; selected patients may be trained to perform blood

pressure measurements at home and report the results at regular physician visits)

## Side/Adverse Effects

Note: Side/adverse effects are largely due to selective sympathetic blockade and unopposed parasympathetic activity.

Side/adverse effects are usually reduced after the first 8 weeks of therapy.

The following side/adverse effects have been selected on the basis of their potential clinical significance (possible signs and symptoms in parentheses where appropriate)—not necessarily inclusive:

**Those indicating need for medical attention**
Incidence more frequent
   *Edema, peripheral* (swelling of feet or lower legs)
Incidence less frequent or rare
   *Angina* (chest pain); *dyspnea* (shortness of breath)

**Those indicating need for medical attention only if they continue or are bothersome**
Incidence more frequent
   *Difficulty in ejaculating; drowsiness; fatigue* (unusual tiredness or weakness); *orthostatic hypotension* (dizziness, lightheadedness, or fainting, especially when getting up from a lying or sitting position); *weight gain or loss, excessive*
   Note: Morning *orthostatic hypotension* is less frequent with guanadrel than with guanethidine.
Incidence less frequent or rare
   *Diarrhea or increase in bowel movements; dryness of mouth; headache; muscle pain or tremors; nocturia* (nighttime urination)
   Note: *Diarrhea* is more commonly reported with guanethidine than with guanadrel.

## Overdose

For specific information on the agents used in the management of guanadrel overdose, see *Phenylephrine* in *Sympathomimetic Agents—Cardiovascular Use (Parenteral-Systemic)* monograph.

For more information on the management of overdose or unintentional ingestion, **contact a Poison Control Center** (see *Poison Control Center Listing*).

**Clinical effects of overdose**
The following effects have been selected on the basis of their potential clinical significance (possible signs and symptoms in parentheses where appropriate)—not necessarily inclusive:
   *Orthostatic hypotension, marked* (marked dizziness, blurred vision, or syncope when getting up from a lying or sitting position)

**Treatment of overdose**
For excessive hypotension—A vasoconstrictor, such as phenylephrine, may be necessary, keeping in mind that patients may be extra sensitive to these agents; symptomatic and supportive.

## Patient Consultation

As an aid to patient consultation, refer to *Advice for the Patient, Guanadrel (Systemic).*

In providing consultation, consider emphasizing the following selected information (» = major clinical significance):

**Before using this medication**
» Conditions affecting use, especially:
      Sensitivity to guanadrel
      Use in the elderly—Increased sensitivity to hypotensive effects
      Other medications, especially loxapine, MAO inhibitors, thioxanthenes, tricyclic antidepressants, or trimeprazine
      Other medical problems, especially congestive heart failure or pheochromocytoma

**Proper use of this medication**
   Importance of diet; possible need for sodium restriction and/or weight reduction
» Patients may not experience symptoms of hypertension; importance of taking medication even if feeling well
» Does not cure, but helps control hypertension; possible need for lifelong therapy; checking with physician before discontinuing medication; serious consequences of untreated hypertension
   Getting into the habit of taking at same time each day to help increase compliance
» Proper dosing

Missed dose: Taking as soon as possible; not taking if almost time for next dose; not doubling doses
» Proper storage

**Precautions while using this medication**
   Regular visits to physician to check progress
» Caution when getting up suddenly from a lying or sitting position, especially in the morning
» Caution in using alcohol, while standing for long periods or exercising, and during hot weather because of enhanced orthostatic hypotensive effects
» Not taking other medications, especially nonprescription sympathomimetics, unless discussed with physician
   Caution if any kind of surgery (including dental surgery) or emergency treatment is required
   Reporting fever to physician; dosage adjustment may be required

**Side/adverse effects**
   Signs of potential side effects, especially peripheral edema, angina, and dyspnea

## General Dosing Information

Because of wide variation in response to guanadrel, dosage must be adjusted to meet the requirements of each patient on the basis of clinical response.

The hypotensive effect of guanadrel is especially pronounced when the patient is standing. If feasible, blood pressure readings should be taken in the supine position, after standing for 10 minutes, and immediately after exercise. Dosage increases should be made only if there has been no decrease in the standing blood pressure from previous levels.

Hospitalized patients should not be discharged until the effect of guanadrel on their standing blood pressure has been determined.

With continuing use, apparent tolerance to the antihypertensive effects of guanadrel may develop as a result of fluid retention and expanded plasma volume. Concurrent administration of a diuretic is recommended.

Recent evidence suggests that withdrawal of antihypertensive therapy prior to surgery is not necessary, but that the anesthesiologist must be aware of such therapy.
   Dosage reduction is indicated if the patient has:
   • Excessive orthostatic fall in pressure
   • Normal supine pressure
   • Severe diarrhea

## Oral Dosage Forms

### GUANADREL SULFATE TABLETS USP

**Usual adult dose**
Antihypertensive—
   Initial: Oral, 5 mg two times a day, the dosage being increased at weekly or monthly intervals as necessary to control blood pressure.
   Maintenance: Oral, 20 to 75 mg per day in two to four divided doses.

Note: Geriatric patients may be more sensitive to the effects of the usual adult dose.

**Usual pediatric dose**
Safety and efficacy not been established.

**Strength(s) usually available**
U.S.—
   10 mg (Rx) [*Hylorel* (scored; lactose)].
   25 mg (Rx) [*Hylorel* (scored; lactose)].
Canada—
   Not commercially available.

**Packaging and storage**
Store below 40 °C (104 °F), preferably between 15 and 30 °C (59 and 86 °F), unless otherwise specified by manufacturer. Store in a tight, light-resistant container.

**Auxiliary labeling**
• Avoid alcoholic beverages.
• Do not take other medicines without your doctor's advice.

**Note**
Check refill frequency to determine compliance in hypertensive patients.

## Selected Bibliography

Finnerty FA, Brogden RN. Guanadrel. A review of its pharmacodynamic and pharmacokinetic properties and therapeutic use in hypertension. Drugs 1985 Jul; 30: 22-31.

Palmer JD, Nugent CA. Guanadrel sulfate: a postganglionic sympathetic inhibitor for the treatment of mild to moderate hypertension. Pharmacotherapy 1983; 3 (4): 220-9.

The fifth report of the Joint National Committee on Detection, Evaluation, and Treatment of High Blood Pressure (JNC V). Arch Intern Med 1993; 153 (2): 154-83.

Revised: 01/03/96

# GUANETHIDINE   Systemic

VA CLASSIFICATION (Primary): CV490

Note: For a listing of dosage forms and brand names by country availability, see *Dosage Forms* section(s). For a listing of brand names for the articles in this monograph, refer to the General Index.

## Category

Antihypertensive.

## Indications

### Accepted

Hypertension (treatment)—Guanethidine is indicated in the treatment of moderate to severe hypertension.

For additional information on initial therapeutic guidelines related to the treatment of hypertension, see *Appendix III*.

Guanethidine is also indicated in the treatment of renal hypertension, including that secondary to pyelonephritis, renal amyloidosis, and renal artery stenosis.

## Pharmacology/Pharmacokinetics

### Physicochemical characteristics

Molecular weight—296.38.

pKa—9 and 12.

### Mechanism of action/Effect

Guanethidine is a postganglionic adrenergic blocking agent. Uptake of guanethidine and storage in sympathetic neurons occur via the norepinephrine pump. Guanethidine slowly displaces norepinephrine from its storage in nerve endings and thereby blocks the release of norepinephrine normally produced by nerve stimulation. Catecholamine depletion leads to reduced arteriolar vasoconstriction, especially the reflex increase in sympathetic tone that occurs with a change in position.

### Absorption

With chronic oral administration, absorption of guanethidine is highly variable among patients; between 3 and 30% of an oral dose is absorbed.

### Biotransformation

Hepatic, to 3 metabolites that are pharmacologically less active than guanethidine.

### Half-life

Following chronic oral administration, the initial phase of elimination with a half-life of 1.5 days is followed by a second phase of elimination with a half-life of 4 to 8 days.

### Time to peak effect

Single dose—The peak effect occurs within 8 hours after a single dose.

Multiple doses—The full therapeutic effects may not be noticed until 1 to 3 weeks after initiation of therapy.

### Duration of action

Multiple doses—Blood pressure returns gradually to pretreatment levels within 1 to 3 weeks after withdrawal.

### Elimination

Renal, 25 to 50% unchanged.

## Precautions to Consider

### Carcinogenicity/Mutagenicity

Studies have not been done.

### Pregnancy/Reproduction

Fertility—Reversible inhibition of ejaculation has been reported in men taking guanethidine.

Guanethidine given to rats and rabbits, subcutaneously or intraperitoneally, for several weeks at doses of 5 or 10 mg per kg of body weight (mg/kg) per day has been shown to inhibit sperm passage and result in accumulation of sperm debris. However, recovery of ejaculatory function and fertility has been shown in rats given guanethidine intramuscularly for 8 weeks at a dose of 25 mg/kg per day.

Pregnancy—Studies have not been done in humans.

Studies have not been done in animals.

FDA Pregnancy Category C.

### Breast-feeding

Small quantities of guanethidine are distributed into breast milk. However, problems in humans have not been documented.

### Pediatrics

Appropriate studies on the relationship of age to the effects of guanethidine have not been performed in the pediatric population. However, pediatrics-specific problems that would limit the usefulness of this medication in children are not expected.

### Geriatrics

Although appropriate studies on the relationship of age to the effects of guanethidine have not been performed in the geriatric population, the elderly may be more sensitive to the hypotensive effects. In addition, elderly patients are more likely to have age-related renal function impairment, which may require caution in patients receiving guanethidine.

### Drug interactions and/or related problems

The following drug interactions and/or related problems have been selected on the basis of their potential clinical significance (possible mechanism in parentheses where appropriate)—not necessarily inclusive (» = major clinical significance):

Note: Combinations containing any of the following medications, depending on the amount present, may also interact with this medication.

Alcohol or

Barbiturates or

Methotrimeprazine or

Opioid (narcotic) analgesics

(concurrent use with guanethidine will contribute to additive orthostatic hypotensive effects)

Alpha-adrenergic blocking agents or

Other medications with alpha-adrenergic blocking action, such as:

Dihydroergotamine

Ergoloid mesylates

Ergotamine

Haloperidol

Loxapine

Phenothiazines

Thioxanthenes or

Beta-adrenergic blocking agents or

Rauwolfia alkaloids

(concurrent use with guanethidine may cause an increased incidence of orthostatic hypotension or bradycardia)

Amphetamines or

» Antidepressants, tricyclic or

Appetite suppressants, with the exception of fenfluramine or

Cyclobenzaprine or

Haloperidol or

» Loxapine or

Maprotiline or

Methylphenidate or

Phenothiazines, especially chlorpromazine or

» Thioxanthenes or

» Trimeprazine

(concurrent use may decrease the hypotensive effects of guanethidine because of its displacement from and inhibition of uptake by adrenergic neurons)

(however, up to 150 mg of doxepin a day can be given without antagonizing the antihypertensive effect of guanethidine)

Anticholinergics, especially atropine and related compounds
(concurrent use with guanethidine may antagonize the inhibitory action of these medications on gastric acid secretion)

» Antidiabetic agents, sulfonylurea or
Insulin
(concurrent use with guanethidine may enhance the hypoglycemic effect, in part through displacement of sulfonylurea antidiabetic agents from serum proteins; dosage adjustments may be necessary)

Anti-inflammatory drugs, nonsteroidal (NSAIDs), especially indomethacin
(antihypertensive effects of guanethidine may be reduced when it is used concurrently with these agents; indomethacin, and possibly other NSAIDs, may antagonize the antihypertensive effect by inhibiting renal prostaglandin synthesis and/or by causing sodium and fluid retention; the patient should be carefully monitored to confirm that the desired effect is being obtained)

Estrogens
(concurrent use may decrease the antihypertensive effect of guanethidine because estrogen-induced fluid retention may lead to increased blood pressure)

Fenfluramine
(concurrent use with guanethidine may produce additive hypotensive effects, and may result in postural hypotension; dosage adjustments of the antihypertensive may be necessary)

Hypotension-producing medications, other (See *Appendix II*) or
» Minoxidil
(antihypertensive effects may be potentiated when these medications are used concurrently with guanethidine; although some antihypertensive and/or diuretic combinations are frequently used for therapeutic advantage, when used concurrently dosage adjustments may be necessary; concurrent use with minoxidil is not recommended)

» Monoamine oxidase (MAO) inhibitors, including furazolidone, procarbazine, and selegiline
(concurrent use with guanethidine may result in moderate to severe hypertension due to release of catecholamines; withdrawal of MAO inhibitors at least 1 week prior to initiation of guanethidine therapy is recommended)

Sympathomimetic agents, such as:
Cocaine
Dobutamine
Dopamine
Ephedrine
Epinephrine
» Metaraminol
Methoxamine
Norepinephrine
Phenylephrine
Phenylpropanolamine
(antihypertensive effects of guanethidine may be reduced when it is used concurrently with any sympathomimetics; the patient should be carefully monitored to confirm that the desired effect is being obtained)

(in addition to possibly decreasing the hypotensive effects of guanethidine, concurrent use of cocaine, dobutamine, dopamine, epinephrine, metaraminol, methoxamine, norepinephrine, or phenylephrine may potentiate the pressor effect of these medications as a result of inhibition of sympathomimetic uptake by adrenergic neurons, possibly resulting in hypertension and cardiac arrhythmias)

(concurrent use of ephedrine or phenylpropanolamine with guanethidine may decrease the hypotensive effects of guanethidine because of its displacement from and inhibition of uptake by adrenergic neurons)

(concurrent use of metaraminol with guanethidine may cause a hypertensive crisis. When metaraminol is used within 5 days of discontinuation of guanethidine, a hypertensive potential may remain)

(concurrent use of phenylephrine ophthalmic solution with guanethidine may increase the pupillary response)

**Medical considerations/Contraindications**
The medical considerations/contraindications included here have been selected on the basis of their potential clinical significance (reasons given in parentheses where appropriate)—not necessarily inclusive (» = major clinical significance).

*Risk-benefit should be considered when the following medical problems exist:*
Asthma, history of
(may be aggravated because of hypersensitivity to catecholamine depletion)
Cerebrovascular insufficiency or
Coronary insufficiency or
Myocardial infarction, recent
(ischemia may be aggravated as a result of reduced blood pressure)
» Congestive heart failure, frank, not due to hypertension or
» Congestive heart failure, severe
(may be aggravated by fluid retention; in addition, guanethidine may interfere with the compensatory response of the adrenergic system in these patients)
Diabetes mellitus
(guanethidine may enhance effects of hypoglycemic medications)
Diarrhea or
Sinus bradycardia
(may be aggravated)
Fever
(dosage requirements may be reduced)
Hepatic function impairment
(reduced metabolism and excessive accumulation of guanethidine may occur; lower doses may be required)
Peptic ulcer, history of
(may be aggravated by relative increase in parasympathetic tone)
» Pheochromocytoma
(release of catecholamines may exacerbate symptoms)
Renal function impairment
(guanethidine further reduces glomerular filtration rate and renal plasma flow; may produce transient urinary retention; severe orthostatic hypotension may occur because of excessive accumulation)
Sensitivity to guanethidine

**Patient monitoring**
The following may be especially important in patient monitoring (other tests may be warranted in some patients, depending on condition; » = major clinical significance):

» Blood pressure measurements
(recommended at periodic intervals in patients being treated for hypertension; selected patients may be trained to perform blood pressure measurements at home and report the results at regular physician visits)

# Side/Adverse Effects

Note: Side effects are largely due to selective sympathetic blockade and unopposed parasympathetic activity.

The following side/adverse effects have been selected on the basis of their potential clinical significance (possible signs and symptoms in parentheses where appropriate)—not necessarily inclusive:

**Those indicating need for medical attention**
Incidence more frequent
*Edema, peripheral* (swelling of feet or lower legs)

Incidence less frequent or rare
*Angina* (chest pain); *edema, pulmonary* (shortness of breath)

**Those indicating need for medical attention only if they continue or are bothersome**
Incidence more frequent
*Bradycardia* (slow heartbeat); *diarrhea or increase in bowel movements; difficulty in ejaculating; nasal congestion* (stuffy nose); *orthostatic hypotension* (dizziness, lightheadedness, or fainting, especially when getting up from a lying or sitting position); *unusual tiredness or weakness*

Note: *Orthostatic hypotension* may be most marked in the morning possibly due to an early morning reduction in vascular volume or by an inhibitory effect of guanethidine on the diurnal rhythm of catecholamine excretion. Hot weather, alcohol, or exercise may accentuate this effect.

Incidence less frequent or rare
*Blurred vision; drooping eyelids; dryness of mouth; headache; loss of hair on scalp; muscle pain or tremors; nausea or vomiting; nocturia* (nighttime urination); *skin rash*

## Overdose

For specific information on the agents used in the management of guanethidine overdose, see:
- *Atropine (Systemic)* monograph;
- *Charcoal, Activated (Oral-Local)* monograph; and/or
- *Laxatives (Local)* monograph.

For more information on the management of overdose or unintentional ingestion, **contact a Poison Control Center** (see *Poison Control Center Listing*).

### Clinical effects of overdose

The following effects have been selected on the basis of their potential clinical significance (possible signs and symptoms in parentheses where appropriate)—not necessarily inclusive:

*Bradycardia; diarrhea; nausea; orthostatic hypotension; shock*

### Treatment of overdose

To decrease absorption—
Gastric lavage. If conditions permit, activated charcoal and laxatives may be administered.

Specific treatment—
For sinus bradycardia: Atropine should be administered.
For diarrhea: If severe and persistent, anticholinergic agents may be administered to reduce intestinal hypermotility. Hydration and electrolyte balance should be maintained.

Monitoring—
Cardiovascular and renal function should be monitored for several days.

Supportive care—
For previously normotensive patients: Restoring blood pressure and heart rate to normal by keeping patient in supine position. Normal homeostatic control usually returns over a 72-hour period.
For previously hypertensive patients: Supporting vital functions and controlling cardiac irregularities that might present. Keeping patient in supine position. Use of vasopressors, if necessary, with extreme caution since guanethidine may increase the responsiveness to these agents, potentially resulting in a rise in blood pressure and cardiac arrhythmias.

## Patient Consultation

As an aid to patient consultation, refer to *Advice for the Patient, Guanethidine (Systemic)*.

In providing consultation, consider emphasizing the following selected information (» = major clinical significance):

### Before using this medication

» Conditions affecting use, especially:
   Sensitivity to guanethidine
   Breast-feeding—Small quantities distributed into breast milk
   Use in the elderly—Increased sensitivity to hypotensive effects
   Other medications, especially loxapine, MAO inhibitors, minoxidil, sulfonylurea antidiabetic agents, thioxanthenes, tricyclic antidepressants, or trimeprazine
   Other medical problems, especially congestive heart failure or pheochromocytoma
   Fertility—Reversible inhibition of ejaculation

### Proper use of this medication

Possible need for control of weight and diet, especially sodium intake
» Patient may not experience symptoms of hypertension; importance of taking medication even if feeling well
» Does not cure, but helps control hypertension; possible need for lifelong therapy; checking with physician before discontinuing medication; serious consequences of untreated hypertension
Getting into the habit of taking at same time each day to help increase compliance
» Proper dosing
Missed dose: Taking as soon as possible; not taking if almost time for next dose; not doubling doses
» Proper storage

### Precautions while using this medication

Regular visits to physician to check progress
» Caution when getting up suddenly from a lying or sitting position, especially in the morning
» Caution in using alcohol, while standing for long periods or exercising, and during hot weather because of enhanced orthostatic hypotensive effects
» Not taking other medications, especially nonprescription sympathomimetics, unless discussed with physician
Caution if any kind of surgery (including dental surgery) or emergency treatment is required

Reporting fever to physician; dosage adjustment may be required
Male patients: Guanethidine may interfere with ejaculation

### Side/adverse effects

Signs of potential side effects, especially peripheral and pulmonary edema and angina

## General Dosing Information

Because of wide individual variation in response to guanethidine, dosage must be adjusted to meet the requirements of each patient on the basis of clinical response.

Because of its long half-life, the effects of guanethidine are cumulative over long periods. Initial doses should be small with gradual increases being made if necessary. Unless the patient is hospitalized, dosage increases should not be made more often than every 5 to 7 days.

The hypotensive effect of guanethidine is especially pronounced when the patient is standing. If feasible, blood pressure readings should be taken in the supine position, after standing for 10 minutes, and immediately after exercise. Dosage increases should be made only if there has been no decrease in the standing blood pressure from previous levels.

Hospitalized patients should not be discharged until the effect of guanethidine on their standing blood pressure has been determined.

With continuing use, apparent tolerance to the antihypertensive effects of guanethidine may develop as a result of fluid retention and expanded plasma volume. Concurrent administration of a diuretic is recommended.

Recent evidence suggests that withdrawal of antihypertensive therapy prior to surgery is not necessary, but that the anesthesiologist must be aware of such therapy.
Dosage reduction is indicated if the patient has:
- Excessive orthostatic fall in pressure
- Normal supine pressure
- Severe diarrhea

## Oral Dosage Forms

### GUANETHIDINE MONOSULFATE TABLETS USP

**Usual adult dose**
Antihypertensive—
Ambulatory patients:
   Initial—Oral, 10 or 12.5 mg once a day, the daily dosage being increased by 10 or 12.5 mg at five- to seven-day intervals if necessary for control of blood pressure.
   Maintenance—Oral, 25 to 50 mg once a day.
Hospitalized patients:
   Initial—Oral, 25 to 50 mg once a day, the daily dosage being increased by 25 to 50 mg at daily or every-other-day intervals if necessary for control of blood pressure.

Note: Geriatric patients may be more sensitive to the effects of the usual adult dose.

**Usual pediatric dose**
Antihypertensive—
Oral, 200 mcg (0.2 mg) per kg of body weight or 6 mg per square meter of body surface area once a day, the daily dosage being increased by 200 mcg (0.2 mg) per kg of body weight or 6 mg per square meter of body surface area at seven- to ten-day intervals if necessary for control of blood pressure.

**Strength(s) usually available**
U.S.—
   10 mg (Rx) [*Ismelin* (scored; lactose); GENERIC (may be scored; may contain lactose)].
   25 mg (Rx) [*Ismelin* (scored; lactose); GENERIC (may be scored; may contain lactose)].
Canada—
   10 mg (Rx) [*Apo-Guanethidine* (scored); *Ismelin* (scored)].
   25 mg (Rx) [*Apo-Guanethidine* (scored); *Ismelin* (scored)].

**Packaging and storage**
Store below 40 °C (104 °F), preferably between 15 and 30 °C (59 and 86 °F), unless otherwise specified by manufacturer. Store in a well-closed container.

**Auxiliary labeling**
- Avoid alcoholic beverages.
- Do not take other medicines without your doctor's advice.

**Note**
Check refill frequency to determine compliance in hypertensive patients.

## Selected Bibliography

The fifth report of the Joint National Committee on Detection, Evaluation, and Treatment of High Blood Pressure (JNC V). Arch Intern Med 1993; 153 (2): 154-83.

Revised: 01/03/96

## GUANETHIDINE-CONTAINING COMBINATIONS—

Guanethidine and Hydrochlorothiazide (Systemic)

---

# GUANETHIDINE AND HYDROCHLOROTHIAZIDE    Systemic

**VA CLASSIFICATION (Primary): CV400**

**NOTE:** The *Guanethidine and Hydrochlorothiazide (Systemic)* monograph is maintained on the USP DI electronic data base. For a printed copy of the most recent revision of the complete monograph, contact the USP Division of Information Development, 12601 Twinbrook Parkway, Rockville, MD 20852.

> For information on the specific components of this combination, see the *USP DI* monographs for *Diuretics, Thiazide (Systemic)* and *Guanethidine (Systemic)*.

> The information that follows is selectively abstracted from the complete monograph and is provided to facilitate drug use review and patient counseling.

Note: For a listing of dosage forms and brand names by country availability, see *Dosage Forms* section(s). For a listing of brand names for the articles in this monograph, refer to the General Index.

## Category

Antihypertensive.

## Indications

**Accepted**

Hypertension (treatment)—This medication is indicated for treatment of hypertension.

> Fixed-dosage combinations are generally not recommended for initial therapy and are useful for subsequent therapy only when the proportion of the component agents corresponds to the dose of the individual agents, as determined by titration.

> For additional information on initial therapeutic guidelines related to the treatment of hypertension, see *Appendix III*.

## Patient Consultation

As an aid to patient consultation, refer to *Advice for the Patient, Guanethidine and Hydrochlorothiazide (Systemic)*.

In providing consultation, consider emphasizing the following selected information (» = major clinical significance):

**Before using this medication**

» Conditions affecting use, especially:
   Sensitivity to guanethidine, hydrochlorothiazide, other sulfonamide-type medications, bumetanide, furosemide, or carbonic anhydrase inhibitors
   Pregnancy—Hydrochlorothiazide may cause jaundice, thrombocytopenia, hypokalemia in infant
   Breast-feeding—Hydrochlorothiazide is distributed into breast milk; small quantities of guanethidine are distributed into breast milk
   Use in children—Caution if giving to infants with jaundice
   Use in the elderly—Increased sensitivity to hypotensive and electrolyte effects
   Other medications, especially tricyclic antidepressants, loxapine, thioxanthenes, trimeprazine, minoxidil, MAO inhibitors, cholestyramine or colestipol, digitalis glycosides, lithium, or oral antidiabetic agents
   Other medical problems, especially congestive heart failure, pheochromocytoma, or anuria or severe renal function impairment

**Proper use of this medication**

   Diuretic effects of the medication and timing of doses to minimize inconvenience of diuresis
   Possible need for control of weight and diet, especially sodium intake

» Patient may not experience symptoms of hypertension; importance of taking medication even if feeling well

» Does not cure, but helps control hypertension; possible need for lifelong therapy; checking with physician before discontinuing medication; serious consequences of untreated hypertension
   Getting into the habit of taking at same time each day to help increase compliance

» Proper dosing
   Missed dose: Taking as soon as possible; not taking if almost time for next dose; not doubling doses

» Proper storage

**Precautions while using this medication**

» Regular visits to physician to check progress
» Not taking other medications, especially nonprescription sympathomimetics, unless discussed with physician
» Possibility of hypokalemia; possible need for additional potassium in diet; not changing diet without first checking with physician
   To prevent dehydration, checking with physician if severe nausea, vomiting, or diarrhea occurs and continues
» Caution when getting up suddenly from a lying or sitting position, especially in the morning
» Caution in using alcohol, while standing for long periods or exercising, and during hot weather because of enhanced orthostatic hypotensive effects
   Diabetics: May increase blood sugar levels
   Possible photosensitivity; avoiding unprotected exposure to sun; using protective clothing and sun block product; avoiding use of sunlamp, tanning bed, or tanning booth
   Reporting fever to physician; dosage adjustment may be required
   Caution if any kind of surgery (including dental surgery) or emergency treatment is required

**Side/adverse effects**

   Signs of potential side effects, especially electrolyte imbalance, angina, agranulocytosis, allergic reaction, cholecystitis, pancreatitis, hepatic function impairment, hyperuricemia, gout, thrombocytopenia, peripheral and pulmonary edema

## Oral Dosage Forms

### GUANETHIDINE MONOSULFATE AND HYDROCHLOROTHIAZIDE TABLETS

**Usual adult dose**

Antihypertensive—
   Oral, 2 tablets a day as determined by individual titration with the component agents.

Note: Geriatric patients may be more sensitive to the effects of the usual adult dose.

**Usual adult prescribing limits**

Up to 4 tablets daily.

**Usual pediatric dose**

Oral, as determined by individual titration with the component agents.

**Strength(s) usually available**

U.S.—
   10 mg of guanethidine monosulfate and 25 mg of hydrochlorothiazide (Rx) [*Esimil* (scored; lactose; sucrose)].

Canada—
   10 mg of guanethidine monosulfate and 25 mg of hydrochlorothiazide (Rx) [*Ismelin-Esidrix*].

**Auxiliary labeling**

• Avoid alcoholic beverages.
• Do not take other medicines without your doctor's advice.

Revised: 07/14/92
Interim revision: 04/29/94

# GUANFACINE   Systemic†

VA CLASSIFICATION (Primary): CV490

Note: For a listing of dosage forms and brand names by country availability, see *Dosage Forms* section(s). For a listing of brand names for the articles in this monograph, refer to the General Index.

---

†Not commercially available in Canada.

---

## Category

Antihypertensive.

## Indications

### Accepted

Hypertension (treatment)—Guanfacine is indicated, usually in combination with a thiazide diuretic, in the treatment of hypertension.

> For additional information on initial therapeutic guidelines related to the treatment of hypertension, see *Appendix III*.

## Pharmacology/Pharmacokinetics

### Physicochemical characteristics

Molecular weight—282.56.

### Mechanism of action/Effect

Thought to be due to central alpha$_2$-adrenergic stimulation, which results in a decreased sympathetic outflow to the heart, kidneys, and peripheral vasculature; decreased systolic and diastolic blood pressure; and slightly decreased heart rate.

### Other actions/effects

Growth hormone secretion stimulated by single doses (no effect with long-term use).

### Absorption

Rapid and complete; bioavailability approximately 80%.

### Protein binding

Moderate (70%; 50% to erythrocytes).

### Biotransformation

Hepatic.

### Half-life

Approximately 17 hours (range, 10–30 hours); 13 to 14 hours in younger patients.

### Onset of action

Multiple doses—Within 1 week.

### Time to peak plasma concentration

1 to 4 hours (average, 2.6 hours).

### Time to peak effect

Single dose—8 to 12 hours.
Multiple doses—1 to 3 months.

### Duration of action

Single dose—24 hours.

### Elimination

Renal, approximately 40% unchanged.
In dialysis—Not significantly removed by dialysis (2.4%).

## Precautions to Consider

### Carcinogenicity

Studies in mice for 78 weeks at doses greater than 150 times the maximum recommended human dose and in rats for 102 weeks at doses greater than 100 times the maximum recommended human dose found no evidence of carcinogenicity.

### Mutagenicity

Mutagenicity studies were negative.

### Pregnancy/Reproduction

Fertility—Studies in male and female rats found no adverse effects on fertility.

Pregnancy—Adequate and well-controlled studies in humans have not been done.

Studies in rats and rabbits at doses 70 and 20 times the maximum recommended human dose, respectively, have not shown that guanfacine causes adverse effects in the fetus. Studies with doses of 100 and 200 times the maximum recommended human dose in rabbits and rats re-

spectively, showed maternal toxicity and reduced fetal survival. Guanfacine crosses the placenta in rats.

FDA Pregnancy Category B.

### Breast-feeding

It is not known whether guanfacine is distributed into human breast milk. However, problems have not been documented. Guanfacine is distributed into the milk of lactating rats.

### Pediatrics

Appropriate studies on the relationship of age to the effects of guanfacine have not been performed in the pediatric population. Safety and efficacy have not been established.

### Geriatrics

Appropriate studies on the relationship of age to the effects of guanfacine have not been performed in the geriatric population. However, the elderly may be more sensitive to the hypotensive and sedative effects.

### Dental

Use of guanfacine may decrease or inhibit salivary flow, thus contributing to the development of caries, periodontal disease, oral candidiasis, and discomfort.

### Drug interactions and/or related problems

The following drug interactions and/or related problems have been selected on the basis of their potential clinical significance (possible mechanism in parentheses where appropriate)—not necessarily inclusive (» = major clinical significance):

Note: Combinations containing any of the following medications, depending on the amount present, may also interact with this medication.

Alcohol or
Central nervous system (CNS) depression–producing medications (See *Appendix II*)
   (concurrent use may enhance the CNS depressant effects of either these medications or guanfacine)

Anti-inflammatory drugs, nonsteroidal (NSAIDs), especially indomethacin
   (may reduce antihypertensive effects of guanfacine; indomethacin, and possibly other NSAIDs, may antagonize the antihypertensive effect by inhibiting renal prostaglandin synthesis and/or by causing sodium and fluid retention; the patient should be carefully monitored to confirm that the desired effect is being obtained)

Estrogens
   (estrogen-induced fluid retention may increase blood pressure)

Hypotension-producing medications, other (See *Appendix II*)
   (concurrent use may potentiate antihypertensive effects; although some antihypertensive and/or diuretic combinations are frequently used for therapeutic advantage, dosage adjustments may be necessary during concurrent use)

Sympathomimetics
   (may reduce antihypertensive effects of guanfacine; the patient should be carefully monitored to confirm that the desired effect is being obtained)

### Laboratory value alterations

The following have been selected on the basis of their potential clinical significance (possible effect in parentheses where appropriate)—not necessarily inclusive (» = major clinical significance):

With physiology/laboratory test values
   Catecholamine concentrations, urinary, and
   Vanillylmandelic acid (VMA), urinary, excretion
      (values may be decreased but may increase on abrupt withdrawal)

   Growth hormone, plasma
      (concentrations may be increased transiently because of stimulation of growth hormone release, but are not elevated chronically with long-term use of guanfacine)

### Medical considerations/Contraindications

The medical considerations/contraindications included here have been selected on the basis of their potential clinical significance (reasons given in parentheses where appropriate)—not necessarily inclusive (» = major clinical significance).

*Risk-benefit should be considered when the following medical problems exist:*

Cerebrovascular disease or
Coronary insufficiency or
Myocardial infarction, recent
   (may be aggravated by reduced blood pressure)

Hepatic function impairment, chronic
   (increased sensitivity or prolonged guanfacine effect may occur, since guanfacine undergoes hepatic biotransformation)

Mental depression, history of
   (may be aggravated by CNS effects of guanfacine)

Sensitivity to guanfacine

## Patient monitoring

The following may be especially important in patient monitoring (other tests may be warranted in some patients, depending on condition; » = major clinical significance):

» Blood pressure measurements
   (recommended at periodic intervals in patients being treated for hypertension; selected patients may be trained to perform blood pressure measurements at home and report the results at regular physician visits)

## Side/Adverse Effects

Note: Side/adverse effects are dose-related and incidence usually declines with continued administration.

The following side/adverse effects have been selected on the basis of their potential clinical significance (possible signs and symptoms in parentheses where appropriate)—not necessarily inclusive:

**Those indicating need for medical attention**
Incidence less frequent
   *Confusion; mental depression*
Signs and symptoms of overdose
   *Difficulty in breathing; dizziness, extreme, or faintness; slow heartbeat; unusual tiredness or weakness, severe*

**Those indicating need for medical attention only if they continue or are bothersome**
Incidence more frequent
   *Constipation; dizziness; drowsiness; dryness of mouth*
Incidence less frequent
   *Conjunctivitis* (dry, itching, or burning eyes); *decreased sexual ability; headache; nausea or vomiting; trouble in sleeping; unusual tiredness or weakness*

**Those indicating possible withdrawal and the need for medical attention if they occur after medication is discontinued**
   *Sympathetic overactivity* (anxiety or tenseness; chest pain; fast or irregular heartbeat; headache; increased salivation; nausea; nervousness; restlessness; shaking or trembling of hands and fingers; stomach cramps; sweating; trouble in sleeping; vomiting)
   Note: *Sympathetic overactivity* is usually infrequent and mild and does not occur until 2 to 7 days after abrupt withdrawal of guanfacine. The risk appears to be increased in patients receiving divided doses totaling more than 4 mg per day. Rebound hypertension occurs less frequently.

## Overdose

For more information on the management of overdose or unintentional ingestion, **contact a Poison Control Center** (see *Poison Control Center Listing*).

**Treatment of overdose**
Guanfacine overdose should be treated symptomatically, with careful cardiovascular monitoring. Treatment may include gastric lavage; isoproterenol infusion, as appropriate.

## Patient Consultation

As an aid to patient consultation, refer to *Advice for the Patient, Guanfacine (Systemic)*.

In providing consultation, consider emphasizing the following selected information (» = major clinical significance):

**Before using this medication**
» Conditions affecting use, especially:
   Sensitivity to guanfacine
   Pregnancy—Use of extremely high doses in animals caused increased fetal deaths
   Use in the elderly—Increased sensitivity to hypotensive effects

**Proper use of this medication**
   Possible need for control of weight and diet, especially sodium intake
» Patient may not experience symptoms of hypertension; importance of taking medication even if feeling well
» Does not cure, but helps control hypertension; possible need for lifelong therapy; serious consequences of untreated hypertension
   Taking at bedtime to reduce daytime drowsiness
» Proper dosing
» Missed dose: Taking as soon as possible; checking with physician if two or more doses in a row are missed; possible reaction if stopped abruptly
» Proper storage

**Precautions while using this medication**
   Regular visits to physician to check progress
   Checking with physician before discontinuing medication; gradual dosage reduction may be necessary to avoid rebound hypertension
   Having enough medication on hand to get through weekends, holidays, and vacations; possibly carrying second prescription for emergency use
   Caution if any kind of surgery (including dental surgery) or emergency treatment is required
» Not taking other medications, especially nonprescription sympathomimetics, unless discussed with physician
» Avoiding use of alcohol or other CNS depressants
» Caution when driving or doing things requiring alertness because of possible drowsiness
   Possible dryness of mouth; using sugarless gum or candy, ice, or saliva substitute for relief; checking with dentist if dry mouth continues for more than 2 weeks

**Side/adverse effects**
   Signs of potential side effects, especially confusion, mental depression, and withdrawal reaction

## General Dosing Information

It is recommended that the daily dose be taken at bedtime to reduce daytime drowsiness.

Recent evidence suggests that withdrawal of antihypertensive therapy prior to surgery is not necessary, but that the anesthesiologist must be aware of such therapy. In addition, the possibility of withdrawal syndrome should be kept in mind if guanfacine is discontinued abruptly, although the syndrome does not generally occur until the patient has been without the drug for more than 2 days.

Guanfacine therapy should be discontinued if drug-related mental depression occurs.

## Oral Dosage Forms

### GUANFACINE HYDROCHLORIDE TABLETS

Note: The dosing and strengths of the dosage form available are expressed in terms of guanfacine base.

**Usual adult dose**
Antihypertensive—
   Oral, 1 mg (base) once a day at bedtime, the dosage being increased after three to four weeks, if necessary, to 2 mg per day. If necessary, dosage may be further increased after an additional three to four weeks to 3 mg per day.

Note: If reduction in blood pressure is not maintained over 24 hours, divided daily dosing may be more effective, although the incidence of side/adverse effects may be increased.

**Usual pediatric dose**
Dosage has not been established.

**Strength(s) usually available**
U.S.—
   1 mg (base) (Rx) [*Tenex* (lactose)].
   2 mg (base) (Rx) [*Tenex* (lactose)].
   3 mg (base) (Rx) [*Tenex* (lactose)].
Canada—
   Not commercially available.

**Packaging and storage**
Store below 40 °C (104 °F), preferably between 15 and 30 °C (59 and 86 °F), in a tight container, unless otherwise specified by manufacturer. Protect from light.

**Auxiliary labeling**
• Avoid alcoholic beverages.
• Keep container tightly closed.

**Note**
Check refill frequency to determine compliance in hypertensive patients.

## Selected Bibliography

Sorkin EM, Heel RC. Guanfacine: A review of its pharmacodynamic and pharmacokinetic properties, and therapeutic efficacy in the treatment of hypertension. Drugs 1986; 31: 301-36.

Cornish LA. Guanfacine hydrochloride: a centrally acting antihypertensive agent. Clin Pharm 1988 Mar; 7: 187-97.

The fifth report of the Joint National Committee on Detection, Evaluation, and Treatment of High Blood Pressure (JNC V). Arch Intern Med 1993; 153 (2): 154-83.

Revised: 10/21/92

Interim revision: 07/05/94

# HAEMOPHILUS B CONJUGATE VACCINE   Systemic

This monograph includes information on the following: Haemophilus b conjugate vaccine (HbOC—diptheria CRM$_{197}$ protein conjugate); Haemophilus b conjugate vaccine (PRP-D—diphtheria toxoid conjugate); Haemophilus b conjugate vaccine (PRP-OMP—meningococcal protein conjugate); Haemophilus b conjugate vaccine (PRP-T—tetanus protein conjugate).

Note: It is recommended that, whenever possible, persons with indications for haemophilus b (Hib) vaccine be immunized with this newer, more immunogenic conjugate vaccine instead of with the polysaccharide vaccine. This is especially important for children 2 months to 24 months of age. See *Haemophilus b Polysaccharide Vaccine (Systemic)* for information on the polysaccharide vaccine.

This vaccine is not an immunizing agent against diphtheria, meningococcal disease, or tetanus.

VA CLASSIFICATION (Primary): IM100

Other commonly used names for HbOC are oligo-CRM and PRP-HbOC.

Note: For a listing of dosage forms and brand names by country availability, see *Dosage Forms* section(s). For a listing of brand names for the articles in this monograph, refer to the General Index.

## Category
Immunizing agent (active).

## Indications

### Accepted
*Haemophilus influenzae* type b disease (prophylaxis)—Haemophilus b conjugate vaccine is indicated for routine immunization of all children 2 to 59 months of age against diseases caused by *Haemophilus influenzae* type b (Hib).

Note: *Act-Hib* (PRP-T), *Hibtiter* (HbOC), and *Pedvaxhib* (PRP-OMP) are licensed for use in infants and children 2 months of age and older.

*Prohibit* (PRP-D) is licensed for use in children 15 months of age and older (U.S.) and in children 18 months of age and older (Canada).

There are no efficacy data available on the use of Hib vaccine for children 5 years of age and older and adults. Moreover, healthy adults and children 5 and older are not at risk for invasive Hib disease. However, studies suggest that patients in this age group who have chronic conditions associated with an increased risk of Hib disease, such as sickle cell disease, leukemia, splenectomy, or HIV infection, demonstrate good immune responses when immunized with Hib vaccine and may benefit from such immunization. Persons infected with human immunodeficiency virus (HIV) may receive this vaccine whether they are asymptomatic or symptomatic.

The following children should be included:
• Children attending day-care facilities.
• Children in residential institutions, such as orphanages.
• Children with chronic illnesses associated with increased risk of Hib disease. These illnesses include asplenia, sickle cell disease, antibody deficiency syndromes, immunosuppression, and Hodgkin's disease. Children scheduled to undergo immunosuppressive therapy, including that for Hodgkin's disease, should receive the conjugate vaccine at least 10 to 14 days prior to the therapy's initiation. The interval between discontinuation of therapy that causes immunosuppression and the restoration of the patient's ability to respond to an active immunizing agent depends on the intensity and type of immunosuppressive therapy used, the underlying disease, and other factors; estimates vary from 3 months to 1 year. Children with immunodeficiency syndromes secondary to deficient synthesis of immunoglobulins (e.g., agammaglobulinemia) probably will not benefit from immunization with the conjugate vaccine. Instead, passive immunity should be considered in these children.
• Infants and children under 24 months of age who have already had invasive Hib disease. Many infants and children under 24 months of age do not develop an adequate immune response to Hib disease and may contract the disease again if they are not immunized. The vaccine series can be initiated, or continued, at the time of discharge from the hospital. Children 24 months of age or older who contract Hib disease do not need to be immunized, since most children in this age group will develop protective levels of antibody from their illnesses.
• Children with asymptomatic or symptomatic human immunodeficiency virus (HIV) infection. Immunization is recommended even

though immunization may be less effective than it would be for immunocompetent children.
• Children of certain racial groups, such as American Indian and Alaskan Eskimo. These racial groups appear to be at increased risk of Hib disease.
• Children of low socioeconomic status. Low socioeconomic status is often associated with crowded living conditions, which increase a child's risk of contact with Hib-infected persons.
• Children who have been previously immunized with the polysaccharide vaccine. Children previously immunized before 24 months of age should be reimmunized with the conjugate vaccine. Reimmunization should take place at least 2 months after the polysaccharide immunization. Children previously immunized at 24 months of age or older do not need to be reimmunized.

Even though they may be protected from invasive disease themselves, household, nursery, and day-care contacts, both adults and children, exposed to children with Hib disease may become asymptomatic carriers of Hib organisms and may infect unimmunized contacts. Therefore, the Immunization Practices Advisory Committee (ACIP) recommends that all contacts (whether immunized or unimmunized) of children with Hib disease receive rifampin chemoprophylaxis with the precautions that apply to the medication. Immunization of unimmunized contacts should not be used to prevent Hib disease in these contacts, because of the time required to generate an immunologic response. In addition, routinely immunizing health-care and day-care workers who may come into close contact with children with invasive Hib disease is not necessary, because healthy adults are not at risk for invasive Hib disease.

### Unaccepted
This vaccine should not be used as an immunizing agent against diphtheria, tetanus, or meningococcal disease, even though there will be some increase in serum diphtheria or tetanus antitoxin levels or antibody levels to the outer membrane protein complex (OMPC) of *Neisseria meningitidis*, respectively, following immunization. No changes in the schedule for administration of diphtheria or tetanus toxoid or meningococcal vaccine are necessitated by the administration of this vaccine.

The conjugate vaccine protects against only *Haemophilus influenzae* type b (Hib). Protection against other strains of *H. influenzae*, such as nonencapsulated strains associated with recurrent upper respiratory disease (including otitis media and sinusitis) should not be anticipated following administration of this vaccine.

## Pharmacology/Pharmacokinetics

### Physicochemical characteristics
Source—
Purified capsular polysaccharide, a polymer of ribose, ribitol, and phosphate (PRP), from the bacterium *Haemophilus influenzae* type b (Hib). It has been conjugated in one of the following ways:
• For the diphtheria toxoid conjugate—The polysaccharide has been conjugated to the diphtheria toxoid via a 6-carbon linker molecule
• For the diphtheria CRM$_{197}$ protein conjugate—The oligosaccharide has been derived from the polysaccharide and has been bound directly to CRM$_{197}$ (a nontoxic variant of diphtheria toxin) by reductive amination
• For the meningococcal protein conjugate—The polysaccharide has been covalently bound to an outer membrane protein complex (OMPC) of the B11 strain of *Neisseria meningitidis* serogroup B
• For the tetanus protein conjugate—The polysaccharide has been covalently bound to tetanus toxoid protein

### Mechanism of action/Effect
*Haemophilus influenzae* type b (Hib) bacteria are surrounded by polysaccharide capsules, which make these bacteria resistant to attack by white blood cells. However, human blood serum contains antibodies that render the bacteria vulnerable to attack. The vaccine, which is derived from the purified polysaccharide from Hib cells, stimulates production of anticapsular antibodies and provides active immunity to the *Haemophilus influenzae* type b bacteria.

Whereas the nonconjugated polysaccharide vaccine predominantly stimulates B-cells to produce antibodies (known as being T-cell independent), haemophilus b conjugate vaccine stimulates T-cells also. The additional stimulation of T-cells (known as being T-cell dependent) is particularly important in young children to ensure an adequate and persistent antibody response. Stimulation of T-cells also results in an anamnestic response to future doses of the conjugate or nonconjugate vaccine and to future natural exposure to *Haemophilus influenzae* type b, resulting in elevated antibody levels.

**Protective effect**

The exact protective level of anti-Haemophilus b polysaccharide antibody has not been established; however, 0.15 mcg per mL is considered by many experts to be protective, and 1 mcg per mL in post-immunization sera is considered indicative of long-term protection.

Antibody response to the vaccine is age related in children, with the immune response improving with increasing age.

Some differences in immunogenicity may exist among the different conjugates of haemophilus b conjugate vaccine; however, further studies are needed to confirm these differences and to evaluate their clinical relevance.

Haemophilus b conjugate vaccine is significantly more immunogenic than the nonconjugated polysaccharide vaccine.

**Time to protective effect**

Approximately 1 to 2 weeks for onset of a detectable antibody response to the vaccine.

**Duration of protective effect**

The duration of immunity of the conjugate vaccine is unknown.

## Precautions to Consider

**Cross-sensitivity and/or related problems**

Patients sensitive to haemophilus b polysaccharide vaccine may be sensitive to the conjugate vaccine also.

Patients sensitive to diphtheria toxoid, meningococcal vaccine, or tetanus toxoid protein may be sensitive to the conjugate vaccines available in the U.S. and Canada. These vaccines contain either diphtheria toxoid, a nontoxic variant of diphtheria toxin, an outer membrane protein complex (OMPC) of *Neisseria meningitidis*, or tetanus toxoid protein.

**Carcinogenicity/Mutagenicity**

The conjugate vaccine has not been evaluated for its carcinogenic or mutagenic potential.

**Pregnancy/Reproduction**

Pregnancy—Studies have not been done in humans or animals.

FDA Pregnancy Category C.

**Breast-feeding**

Problems in humans have not been documented.

**Pediatrics**

Immunization is not recommended for children less than 2 months of age, since the safety and efficacy of the conjugate vaccine have not been established in this age group.

**Geriatrics**

Appropriate studies on the relationship of age to the effects of Hib vaccine have not been performed in the geriatric population. However, no geriatrics-specific problems have been documented to date.

**Drug interactions and/or related problems**

The following drug interactions and/or related problems have been selected on the basis of their potential clinical significance (possible mechanism in parentheses where appropriate)—not necessarily inclusive (» = major clinical significance):

Note: Combinations containing any of the following medications, depending on the amount present, may also interact with this medication.

Immunosuppressive agents or
Radiation therapy
(because normal defense mechanisms are suppressed by immunosuppressive agents or radiation treatment, the patient's antibody response to the conjugate vaccine may be decreased. If possible, children who are to undergo therapy with agents that cause immunosuppression, including treatment for Hodgkin's disease, should receive the vaccine at least 10 days, and preferably more than 14 days, before receiving the immunosuppressive agent; otherwise, it may be preferable to postpone the immunization until after the immunosuppressive therapy is completed. The interval between discontinuation of therapy that causes immunosuppression and the restoration of the patient's ability to respond to an active immunizing agent depends on the intensity and type of immunosuppressive therapy used, the underlying disease, and other factors; estimates vary from 3 months to 1 year. The precaution does not apply to corticosteroids used as replacement therapy, for short-term [less than 2 weeks] systemic therapy, or by other routes of administration that do not cause immunosuppression)

**Laboratory value alterations**

The following have been selected on the basis of their potential clinical significance (possible effect in parentheses where appropriate)—not necessarily inclusive (» = major clinical significance):

With diagnostic test results
Antigen detection tests
(there is a possibility that the conjugate vaccine may interfere with interpretation of antigen detection tests, such as latex agglutination and countercurrent immunoelectrophoresis, that are used for diagnosis of systemic Hib disease. PRP [a polymer of ribose, ribitol, and phosphate] derived from haemophilus b meningococcal protein conjugate vaccine may be detected in the urine of some persons for up to 7 days following immunization)

**Medical considerations/Contraindications**

The medical considerations/contraindications included here have been selected on the basis of their potential clinical significance (reasons given in parentheses where appropriate)—not necessarily inclusive (» = major clinical significance).

*Except under special circumstances, this medication should not be used when the following medical problems exist:*

» Illness, acute or febrile
(administration of the conjugate vaccine should be postponed to avoid confusing the symptoms of the illness with the side effects of the vaccine; minor illnesses, such as mild upper respiratory infections, do not preclude administration of the vaccine)

*Risk-benefit should be considered when the following medical problem exists:*

Sensitivity to haemophilus b conjugate vaccine

## Side/Adverse Effects

Note: Side effects generally are minor and last 48 hours or less; in addition, no serious systemic reactions have been observed.

In one person, thrombocytopenia was temporally noted; however, no causative relationship was established.

There are no significant differences in the frequency or types of side effects between haemophilus b polysaccharide vaccine and haemophilus b conjugate vaccine.

The following side/adverse effects have been selected on the basis of their potential clinical significance (possible signs and symptoms in parentheses where appropriate)—not necessarily inclusive:

**Those indicating need for medical attention**
Incidence rare
*Anaphylactic reaction* (difficulty in breathing or swallowing; hives; itching, especially of soles or palms; reddening of skin, especially around ears; swelling of eyes, face, or inside of nose; unusual tiredness or weakness, sudden and severe); *convulsions*

**Those indicating need for medical attention only if they continue or are bothersome**
Incidence more frequent
*Anorexia* (loss of appetite); *erythema at injection site* (redness); *fever up to 39 °C (102.2 °F)* (usually resolves within 48 hours); *irritability; lethargy* (lack of interest; reduced physical activity); *tenderness at injection site*
Incidence less frequent
*Diarrhea; fever over 39 °C (over 102.2 °F)* (usually resolves within 48 hours); *induration* (hard lump); *swelling, or warm feeling at injection site; skin rash; urticaria* (hives); *vomiting*

## Patient Consultation

As an aid to patient consultation, refer to *Advice for the Patient, Haemophilus b Conjugate Vaccine (Systemic).*

In providing consultation, consider emphasizing the following selected information (» = major clinical significance):

**Before receiving this vaccine**
» Conditions affecting use, especially:
Sensitivity to haemophilus b conjugate vaccine, haemophilus b polysaccharide vaccine, diphtheria toxoid, meningococcal vaccine, or tetanus toxoid
Use in children—Not recommended for use in children up to 2 months of age
Other medical problems, especially fever or serious illness

**Proper use of this vaccine**
» Proper dosing

## Side/adverse effects

Signs of potential side effects, especially anaphylactic reaction or convulsions

# General Dosing Information

When sterilizing syringes before vaccination, care should be taken to avoid use of preservatives, antiseptics, detergents, and disinfectants, since the conjugate vaccine may be inactivated by these substances. Disposable syringes and needles are recommended.

The conjugate vaccine is for intramuscular administration only. It should not be administered intravenously.

This vaccine should not be used as an immunizing agent against diphtheria, meningococcal meningitis, or tetanus, even though there may be some slight increase in serum antitoxin or antibody levels following immunization. No changes in the schedule for administration of diphtheria or tetanus toxoid or meningococcal vaccine are necessitated by the administration of this vaccine.

Polysaccharide vaccines, including haemophilus b conjugate vaccine, may be administered concurrently with the vaccines listed below, using separate syringes for the parenterals, and the precautions that apply to each immunizing agent. If DTP, MMR, and IPV are administered concurrently with Hib conjugate vaccine, any 2 of the vaccines may be administered in the same deltoid, and any of these vaccines may be administered in the thigh. If any of the other vaccines listed below is to be administered concurrently with Hib conjugate vaccine, each parenteral vaccine should be administered at a separate body site.

- Polysaccharide vaccines, other, such as meningococcal polysaccharide vaccine or pneumococcal polyvalent vaccine.
- Influenza vaccine, whole or split virus.
- Diphtheria toxoid, tetanus toxoid, and/or pertussis vaccine.
- Live virus vaccines, such as measles, mumps, and/or rubella vaccines.
- Poliovirus vaccines (oral [OPV], inactivated [IPV], or enhanced-potency inactivated [enhanced-potency IPV]).
- Hepatitis B recombinant or plasma-derived vaccine.
- Immune globulin and disease-specific immune globulins.
- Inactivated vaccines, except cholera, typhoid (parenteral), and plague. It is recommended that cholera, typhoid (parenteral), and plague vaccines be administered on separate occasions because there are no data available on the concurrent administration of haemophilus b conjugate vaccine and these vaccines and because of these vaccines' propensity for causing side/adverse effects.

The first conjugate vaccine was licensed for use in the U.S. in December 1987. Persons immunized against Hib disease before that date can be presumed to have received the polysaccharide vaccine.

## For treatment of adverse effects

Recommended treatment includes:
- For mild hypersensitivity reaction—Administering antihistamines, and, if necessary, glucocorticoids.
- For severe hypersensitivity or anaphylactic reaction—Administering epinephrine. Antihistamines or glucocorticoids may also be administered as required.

---

## *HAEMOPHILUS B CONJUGATE VACCINE (HbOC— DIPTHERIA CRM<sub>197</sub> PROTEIN CONJUGATE)*

*HAEMOPHILUS B CONJUGATE VACCINE (HbOC—DIPTHERIA CRM$_{197}$ PROTEIN CONJUGATE)*

---

# Parenteral Dosage Forms

## HAEMOPHILUS B CONJUGATE VACCINE INJECTION (HbOC—diphtheria CRM$_{197}$ protein conjugate)

### Usual adult and adolescent dose

Active immunizing agent—

Use is not recommended in these age groups, except for patients with certain chronic conditions associated with an increased risk of Hib disease.

### Usual pediatric dose

Active immunizing agent—

Intramuscular, 0.5 mL, into the outer aspect of the upper arm (deltoid) or into the lateral mid thigh (vastus lateralis), according to the following dosage schedules:

In the U.S.—

Infants:

First dose—At 2 months of age.

Note: The vaccine series may be initiated as early as 6 weeks of age.

Second dose—At 4 months of age.
Third dose—At 6 months of age.
Booster—At 15 months of age.

Children up to 59 months of age who did not follow the above schedule:

Age 2 to 6 months of age at first dose—Three doses, two months apart, then a booster dose at 15 months of age or as soon as possible thereafter, but not less than two months after previous dose.

Age 7 to 11 months of age at first dose—Two doses, two months apart, then a booster dose at 15 months of age or as soon as possible thereafter, but not less than two months after previous dose.

Age 12 to 14 months of age at first dose—One dose, then a booster dose at 15 months of age or as soon as possible thereafter, but not less than two months after previous dose.

Age 15 to 59 months of age at first dose—One dose.

Note: An interval as short as 1 month between doses is acceptable, but is not optimal.

Any of the other conjugate vaccines may be used for the booster dose; however, there are no data demonstrating that a booster response will occur if one of these other vaccines is used. Ideally, the same conjugate vaccine should be used throughout the vaccination series, including the booster.

Children 5 years of age and older:

Use is not recommended, except for patients with certain chronic conditions associated with an increased risk of Hib disease.

In Canada—

Infants:

First dose—At 2 months of age.

Note: The vaccine series may be initiated as early as 6 weeks of age.

Second dose—At 4 months of age.
Third dose—At 6 months of age.
Booster—At 15 to 18 months of age.

Children up to 59 months of age who did not follow the above schedule:

Age 2 to 6 months of age at first dose—Three doses, two months apart, then a booster dose at 15 to 18 months of age or as soon as possible thereafter, but not less than two months after previous dose.

Age 7 to 11 months of age at first dose—Two doses, two months apart, then a booster dose at 15 to 18 months of age or as soon as possible thereafter, but not less than two months after previous dose.

Age 12 to 17 months of age at first dose—One dose, then a booster dose at 15 to 18 months of age or as soon as possible thereafter, but not less than two months after previous dose.

Age 18 to 59 months of age at first dose—One dose.

Note: An interval as short as 1 month between doses is acceptable, but is not optimal.

Any of the other conjugate vaccines may be used for the booster dose; however, there are no data demonstrating that a booster response will occur if one of these other vaccines is used. Ideally, the same conjugate vaccine should be used throughout the vaccination series, including the booster.

Children 5 years of age and older:

Use is not recommended.

Note: Children 5 years of age and older with certain chronic conditions associated with an increased risk of Hib disease may profit from Hib immunization.

### Strength(s) usually available

U.S.—

10 mcg (0.01 mg) of purified haemophilus b saccharide and approximately 25 mcg (0.025 mg) of CRM$_{197}$ protein, a nontoxic variant of diphtheria toxin, per 0.5 mL dose (Rx) [*Hibtiter* (in multidose vials—thimerosal 1:10,000)].

Canada—

10 mcg (0.01 mg) of purified haemophilus b saccharide and approximately 25 mcg (0.025 mg) of CRM$_{197}$ protein, a nontoxic variant of diphtheria toxin, per 0.5 mL dose (Rx) [*Hibtiter*].

### Packaging and storage

Store between 2 and 8 °C (35 and 46 °F), unless otherwise specified by manufacturer. Do not freeze.

## HAEMOPHILUS B CONJUGATE VACCINE (PRP-D—DIPHTHERIA TOXOID CONJUGATE)

## Parenteral Dosage Forms

### HAEMOPHILUS B CONJUGATE VACCINE INJECTION (PRP-D—diphtheria toxoid conjugate)

**Usual adult and adolescent dose**
Active immunizing agent—
    Use is not recommended in these age groups, except for patients with certain chronic conditions associated with an increased risk of Hib disease.

**Usual pediatric dose**
Active immunizing agent—
    Intramuscular, 0.5 mL, into the outer aspect of the upper arm (deltoid) or into the lateral mid thigh (vastus lateralis), according to the following dosage schedules:
    In the U.S.—
        Infants and children up to 15 months of age: Use is not recommended.
        Children 15 to 59 months of age who were not previously immunized: One dose.
        Children 5 years of age and older: Use is not recommended, except for patients with certain chronic conditions associated with an increased risk of Hib disease.
    In Canada—
        Infants and children up to 18 months of age: Use is not recommended.
        Children 18 to 60 months of age who were not previously immunized: One dose.
        Children 5 years of age and older: Use is not recommended, except for patients with certain chronic conditions associated with an increased risk of Hib disease.

**Strength(s) usually available**
U.S.—
    25 mcg (0.025 mg) of purified haemophilus b capsular polysaccharide and 18 mcg (0.018 mg) of diphtheria toxoid protein, per 0.5 mL dose (Rx) [*Prohibit* (thimerosal 1:10,000)].
Canada—
    25 mcg (0.025 mg) of purified haemophilus b capsular polysaccharide and 18 mcg (0.018 mg) of diphtheria toxoid protein, per 0.5 mL dose (Rx) [*Prohibit* (thimerosal 1:10,000)].

**Packaging and storage**
Store between 2 and 8 °C (35 and 46 °F), unless otherwise specified by manufacturer. Do not freeze.

## HAEMOPHILUS B CONJUGATE VACCINE (PRP-OMP—MENINGOCOCCAL PROTEIN CONJUGATE)

## Parenteral Dosage Forms

### HAEMOPHILUS B CONJUGATE VACCINE INJECTION (PRP-OMP—meningococcal protein conjugate)

**Usual adult and adolescent dose**
Active immunizing agent—
    Use is not recommended in these age groups, except for patients with certain chronic conditions associated with an increased risk of Hib disease.

**Usual pediatric dose**
Active immunizing agent—
    Intramuscular, 0.5 mL, into the outer aspect of the upper arm (deltoid) or into the lateral mid thigh (vastus lateralis), according to the following dosage schedules:
    In the U.S.—
        Infants:
            First dose—At 2 months of age.
            Note: the vaccine series may be initiated as early as 6 weeks of age.
            Second dose—At 4 months of age.
            Booster—At 12 months of age.
        Children up to 59 months of age who did not follow the above schedule:
            Age 2 to 6 months of age at first dose—Two doses, two months apart, then a booster dose at 12 months of age or as soon as possible thereafter, but not less than two months after previous dose.

Age 7 to 11 months of age at first dose—Two doses, two months apart, then a booster dose at 15 months of age or as soon as possible thereafter, but not less than two months after previous dose.
Age 12 to 14 months of age at first dose—One dose, then a booster dose at 15 months of age or as soon as possible thereafter, but not less than two months after previous dose.
Age 15 to 59 months of age at first dose—One dose.
Note: The U.S. manufacturer's labeling gives the age ranges and dosages as: 2 to 10 months of age at first dose—2 doses, 2 months apart, with a booster at 12 to 15 months; 11 to 14 months of age at first dose—2 doses, 2 months apart; 15 to 71 months of age at first dose—1 dose. These recommendations differ somewhat from those of the Immunization Practices Advisory Committee (ACIP) that are used above.
    An interval as short as 1 month between doses is acceptable, but is not optimal.
    Any of the other conjugate vaccines may be used for the 15-month booster dose; however, there are no data demonstrating that a booster response will occur if one of these other vaccines is used. Ideally, the same conjugate vaccine should be used throughout the vaccination series, including the booster.
Children 5 years of age and older:
    Use is not recommended, except for patients with certain chronic conditions associated with an increased risk of Hib disease.
In Canada—
    Infants:
        First dose—At 2 months of age.
        Note: The vaccine series may be initiated as early as 6 weeks of age.
        Second dose—At 4 months of age.
        Booster—At 12 months of age.
    Children up to 59 months of age who did not follow the above schedule:
        Age 2 to 6 months of age at first dose—Two doses, two months apart, then a booster dose at 12 months of age or as soon as possible thereafter, but not less than two months after previous dose.
        Age 7 to 11 months of age at first dose—Two doses, two months apart, then a booster dose at 15 months of age or as soon as possible thereafter, but not less than two months after previous dose.
        Age to 12 to 17 months of age at first dose—One dose, then a booster dose at 18 months of age or as soon as possible thereafter, but not less than two months after previous dose.
        Age 18 to 59 months of age at first dose—One dose.
        Note: An interval as short as 1 month between doses is acceptable, but is not optimal.
            Any of the other conjugate vaccines may be used for the 15- or 18-month booster dose; however, there are no data demonstrating that a booster response will occur if one of these other vaccines is used. Ideally, the same conjugate vaccine should be throughout the vaccination series, including the booster.
Children 5 years of age and older:
    Use is not recommended.
    Note: Children 5 years of age and older with certain chronic conditions associated with an increased risk of Hib disease may profit from Hib immunization.

**Strength(s) usually available**
U.S.—
    15 mcg (0.015 mg) of purified haemophilus b capsular polysaccharide and 250 mcg (0.25 mg) of an outer membrane protein complex (OMPC) of the B11 strain of *Neisseria meningitidis* serogroup B, per 0.5 mL dose (Rx) [*Pedvaxhib* (in lyophilized product—lactose 2 mg; in diluent—aluminum 225 mcg as aluminum hydroxide; thimerosal 1:20,000)].
Canada—
    15 mcg (0.015 mg) of purified haemophilus b capsular polysaccharide and 250 mcg (0.25 mg) of an outer membrane protein complex (OMPC) of the B11 strain of *Neisseria meningitidis* serogroup B, per 0.5 mL dose (Rx) [*Pedvaxhib* (in lyophilized product—lactose 2 mg; in diluent—aluminum 225 mcg as aluminum hydroxide; thimerosal 1:20,000)].

## Packaging and storage

Store between 2 and 8 °C (35 and 45 °F), unless otherwise specified by manufacturer. Do not freeze reconstituted vaccine or aluminum hydroxide diluent.

## Preparation of dosage form

*Pedvaxhib* should be reconstituted only with the aluminum hydroxide diluent that is supplied. The diluent should be agitated prior to its withdrawal. The vaccine should be agitated at the time of reconstitution, prior to withdrawal of the vaccine dose into the syringe, and prior to injection.

## Stability

*Pedvaxhib* should be used as soon as possible after reconstitution. Reconstituted vaccine should be stored between 2 and 8 °C (35 and 46 °F) and discarded if not used within 24 hours.

## Auxiliary labeling

• Shake gently before use.

---

## HAEMOPHILUS B CONJUGATE VACCINE (PRP-T— TETANUS PROTEIN CONJUGATE)

---

# Parenteral Dosage Forms

## HAEMOPHILUS B CONJUGATE VACCINE INJECTION (PRP-T—tetanus protein conjugate)

### Usual adult and adolescent dose

Active immunizing agent—

Use is not recommended in these age groups, except for patients with certain chronic conditions associated with an increased risk of Hib disease.

### Usual pediatric dose

Active immunizing agent—

Intramuscular, 0.5 mL, into the outer aspect of the upper arm (deltoid) or into the lateral mid thigh (vastus lateralis), according to the following dosage schedules:

In the U.S.—

Infants:

First dose—At 2 months of age.

Note: The vaccine series may be initiated as early as 6 weeks of age.

Second dose—At 4 months of age.

Third dose—At 6 months of age.

Booster—At 15 months of age.

Children up to 59 months of age who did not follow the above schedule:

Age 2 to 6 months of age at first dose—Three doses, two months apart, then a booster dose at 15 months of age or as soon as possible thereafter, but not less than two months after previous dose.

Age 7 to 11 months of age at first dose—Two doses, two months apart, then a booster dose at 15 months of age or as soon as possible thereafter, but not less than two months after previous dose.

Age 12 to 14 months of age at first dose—One dose, then a booster dose at 15 months of age or as soon as possible thereafter, but not less than two months after previous dose.

Age 15 to 59 months of age at first dose—One dose.

Note: An interval as short as 1 month between doses is acceptable, but is not optimal.

Any of the other conjugate vaccines may be used for the booster dose; however, there are no data demonstrating that a booster response will occur if one of these other vaccines is used. Ideally, the same conjugate vaccine should be used throughout the vaccination series, including the booster.

Children 5 years of age and older:

Use is not recommended, except for patients with certain chronic conditions associated with an increased risk of Hib disease.

In Canada—

Infants:

First dose—At 2 months of age.

Note: The vaccine series may be initiated as early as 6 weeks of age.

Second dose—At 4 months of age.

Third dose—At 6 months of age.

Booster—At 18 months of age.

Children up to 59 months of age who did not follow the above schedule:

Age 3 to 6 months of age at first dose—Three doses, two months apart, then a booster dose at 18 months of age or as soon as possible thereafter, but not less than two months after previous dose.

Age 7 to 11 months of age at first dose—Two doses, two months apart, then a booster dose at 18 months of age or as soon as possible thereafter, but not less than two months after previous dose.

Age 12 to 14 months of age at first dose—One dose, then a booster dose at 18 months of age or as soon as possible thereafter, but not less than two months after previous dose.

Age 15 to 59 months of age at first dose—One dose.

Note: An interval as short as 1 month between doses is acceptable, but is not optimal.

The booster dose may be given as early as 15 months of age or as soon as possible thereafter, but not less than two months after previous dose.

Any of the other conjugate vaccines may be used for the booster dose; however, there are no data demonstrating that a booster response will occur if one of these other vaccines is used. Ideally, the same conjugate vaccine should be used throughout the vaccination series, including the booster.

Children 5 years of age and older:

Use is not recommended, except for patients with certain chronic conditions associated with an increased risk of Hib disease.

### Strength(s) usually available

U.S.—

10 mcg (0.01 mg) of purified haemophilus b capsular polysaccharide and 20 mcg (0.02 mg) of tetanus protein, per 0.5 mL dose (Rx) [*Act-Hib*].

Canada—

10 mcg (0.01 mg) of purified haemophilus b capsular polysaccharide and 20 mcg (0.02 mg) of tetanus protein, per 0.5 mL dose (Rx) [*Act-Hib*].

### Packaging and storage

Store between 2 and 8 °C (35 and 46 °F), unless otherwise specified by manufacturer. Do not freeze the reconstituted vaccine.

### Preparation of dosage form

*Act-Hib* should be reconstituted only with the 0.4% saline diluent that is supplied. The vaccine should be shaken gently until a clear, colorless solution results. (In Canada, *Act-Hib* may be reconstituted also with the Connaught-Canada brand of DTP vaccine.)

### Stability

*Act-Hib* should be discarded if it is not used immediately after reconstitution.

## Selected Bibliography

Centers for Disease Control. ACIP update: prevention of Haemophilus influenzae type b disease. MMWR 1988 Jan 22; 37: 13-6.

Berkowitz CD, et al. Safety and immunogenicity of Haemophilus influenzae type b polysaccharide and polysaccharide diphtheria toxoid conjugate vaccines in children 15 to 24 months of age. J Pediatr 1987 Apr: 509-14.

Weinberg GA, Granoff DM. Polysaccharide-protein conjugate vaccines for the prevention of Haemophilus influenzae type b disease. J Pediatr 1988 Oct; 113 (4): 621-31.

Centers for Disease Control. Haemophilus b conjugate vaccines for prevention of Haemophilus influenzae type b disease among infants and children two months of age and older: recommendation of the Immunization Practices Advisory Committee (ACIP). MMWR 1991 Jan 11: 40 (RR-1).

Centers for Disease Control. Update on adult immunization: recommendations of the Immunization Practices Advisory Committee (ACIP). MMWR 1991 Nov 15: 40 (RR-12).

Revised: 06/21/93

Interim revision: 03/29/94

## HAEMOPHILUS B CONJUGATE VACCINE (HBOC— DIPHTHERIA CRM₁₉₇ PROTEIN CONJUGATE)—See
*Haemophilus b Conjugate Vaccine (Systemic)*

## HAEMOPHILUS B CONJUGATE VACCINE (PRP-D— DIPHTHERIA TOXOID CONJUGATE)—See *Haemophilus b Conjugate Vaccine (Systemic)*

## HAEMOPHILUS B CONJUGATE VACCINE (PRP- OMP—MENINGOCOCCAL PROTEIN CONJUGATE)—See *Haemophilus b Conjugate Vaccine (Systemic)*

## HAEMOPHILUS B CONJUGATE VACCINE (PRP-T— TETANUS PROTEIN CONJUGATE)—See *Haemophilus b Conjugate Vaccine (Systemic)*

---

# HAEMOPHILUS B POLYSACCHARIDE VACCINE    Systemic*†

VA CLASSIFICATION (Primary): IM100

Note: This monograph applies only to the polysaccharide vaccine.

It is recommended that, whenever possible, children with indications for haemophilus b vaccine be immunized with the more immunogenic conjugate vaccine instead of with this polysaccharide vaccine. This is especially important for children under 24 months of age. See *Haemophilus b Conjugate Vaccine (Systemic)* for information on the conjugate vaccine.

Commonly used names are: Haemophilus influenzae type b polysaccharide vaccine; HbPV; Hib CPS; Hib polysaccharide vaccine; and PRP.

Note: For a listing of dosage forms and brand names by country availability, see *Dosage Forms* section(s). For a listing of brand names for the articles in this monograph, refer to the General Index.

---

*Not commercially available in the U.S.
†Not commercially available in Canada.

---

## Category
Immunizing agent (active).

## Indications

### Accepted
*Haemophilus influenzae* type b disease (prophylaxis)—Haemophilus b polysaccharide vaccine is indicated for routine immunization of children 24 months to 5 years of age (i.e., up to the 5th birthday) against diseases caused by *Haemophilus influenzae* type b (Hib). Although the polysaccharide vaccine was licensed for use up to the 6th birthday, pediatric experts recommend that the vaccine be used only up to the 5th birthday.

In addition, immunization with haemophilus b polysaccharide vaccine should be considered for children 18 to 24 months of age, especially those in known high-risk groups, only if the more immunogenic conjugate vaccine is not available. These groups include:
• Children attending day-care facilities.
• Children in residential institutions, such as orphanages.
• Children with chronic illnesses associated with increased risk of Hib disease. These illnesses include asplenia, sickle cell disease, antibody deficiency syndromes, immunosuppression, and Hodgkin's disease. Children scheduled to undergo immunosuppressive therapy, including that for Hodgkin's disease, should receive the polysaccharide vaccine at least 10 to 14 days prior to the initiation of therapy. The interval between discontinuation of immunosuppressive therapy and the restoration of the patient's ability to respond to an active immunizing agent depends on the intensity and type of immunosuppression-causing therapy, the underlying disease, and other factors; estimates vary from 3 months to 1 year. Children with immunodeficiency syndromes secondary to deficient synthesis of immunoglobulins (e.g., agammaglobulinemia) probably will not benefit from immunization with the polysaccharide vaccine. Instead, passive immunity should be maintained in these children.
• Children under 24 months of age who have already had invasive Hib disease. Most children under 24 months of age do not develop an immune response to Hib disease and may contract the disease again if they are not immunized. The vaccine should be administered to these children no sooner than 2 months following Hib disease and not until they have reached 24 months of age. Children 24 months of age or older who contract Hib disease do not need to be immunized, since most children in this age group will develop protective levels of antibody from their illnesses.
• Children with asymptomatic or symptomatic human immunodeficiency virus (HIV) infection. Immunization is recommended even though immunization of symptomatic children may be less effective than it would be for immunocompetent children.
• Children of certain racial groups, such as American Indian and Alaskan Eskimo. These racial groups appear to be at increased risk of Hib disease.
• Children of low socioeconomic status. Low socioeconomic status is often associated with crowded living conditions, which increase a child's risk of contact with Hib-infected persons.

Even though they may be protected from invasive disease themselves, household, nursery, and day-care contacts, both adults and children, exposed to children with Hib disease may become asymptomatic carriers of Hib organisms and may infect unimmunized contacts. There is an increased risk of invasive Hib disease among unimmunized household contacts less than 4 years of age; in addition, unimmunized nursery and day-care contacts may also be at increased risk, especially if they are younger than 2 years of age. In households where there is at least one contact younger than 48 months of age, it is recommended that all household contacts, both adults and children, receive rifampin chemoprophylaxis, regardless of the immunization status of any of the contacts. For nursery and day-care contacts where the facility provides for children less than 2 years of age for at least 25 hours per week, rifampin chemoprophylaxis is recommended for all contacts, both adults and children, regardless of the immunization status of any of the contacts. For nursery and day-care facilities where all contacts are more than 2 years of age, rifampin chemoprophylaxis is not necessary.

Since satisfactory response to the polysaccharide vaccine is not consistent among children 18 to 24 months of age, most authorities believe that these children should be reimmunized. The optimal timing of this second dose is not known; however, it appears that reimmunization of these children should occur at or after 24 months of age, with 2 to 18 months having elapsed between the first immunization and the second one. Previous immunization does not affect the immune response or adverse reaction to a subsequent dose of the vaccine.

### Unaccepted
Because the polysaccharide vaccine protects against only *Haemophilus influenzae* type b (Hib), protection against other strains of *H. influenzae*, such as nonencapsulated strains associated with recurrent upper respiratory disease (including otitis media and sinusitis), should not be anticipated following administration of this vaccine.

## Pharmacology/Pharmacokinetics

### Physicochemical characteristics
Source—Purified capsular polysaccharide, a polymer of ribose, ribitol, and phosphate (PRP), from the bacterium *Haemophilus influenzae* type b (Hib).

### Mechanism of action/Effect
*Haemophilus influenzae* type b (Hib) bacteria are surrounded by polysaccharide capsules, which make the bacteria resistant to attack by white blood cells. However, human blood serum contains antibodies, which render the bacteria vulnerable to attack. The vaccine, which is composed of the purified polysaccharide from Hib bacterial cells, stimulates production of anticapsular antibodies and provides active immunity to the *Haemophilus influenzae* type b bacteria represented by the polysaccharide in the vaccine.

Haemophilus b polysaccharide vaccine, unlike the conjugate vaccine, predominantly stimulates B-cells to produce antibodies. This is known as being T-cell independent and is characteristic of polysaccharide vaccines. The initial stimulation of T-cells followed by stimulation of B cells (known as a T-cell response) is particularly important in young children to ensure adequate and persisting antibody production. Stimulation of T-cells also results in an anamnestic response to future doses of the vaccine and future natural exposure to *Haemophilus influenzae* type b. The poor T-cell response stimulated by the polysaccharide vaccine is thought to be one reason why the polysaccharide vaccine is not adequately immunogenic in children up to 18 months of age and may not be fully immunogenic in children 18 to 24 months of age. In addition, lack of initial T-cell stimulation probably is the reason that repeat doses of the polysaccharide vaccine do not boost the antibody response consistently.

### Protective efficacy
The exact protective level of anti-Haemophilus b polysaccharide antibody has not been established; however, 0.15 mcg/mL is considered by many experts to be protective, and 1 mcg/mL in post-immunization sera is considered indicative of long-term protection.

Antibody response to the vaccine is age related in children. Children up to 18 months of age develop very little immunologic response to the vaccine. Children 18 to 24 months of age have inconsistent and less than optimal response to the vaccine. Children over 24 months of age have a high rate of seroconversion. Antibody response continues to improve until it reaches adult levels in children approximately 6 years of age.

### Time to protective efficacy
Approximately 1 week for onset of an antibody response to the vaccine; approximately 3 weeks for attainment of the protective level of 1 mcg per mL, which is considered indicative of long-term protection.

### Duration of protective effect
The duration of immunity after a single dose of the polysaccharide vaccine has not been completely described. However, it may be less than the duration of immunity following administration of the conjugate vaccine, which is expected to be at least 1.5 to 3 years.

Duration of antibody response is age related in children. In one study of children 15 to 24 months of age, an antibody concentration of 1 mcg per mL, which is considered indicative of long-term protection, was reached in less than 30% of children.

## Precautions to Consider

### Cross-sensitivity and/or related problems
Patients sensitive to haemophilus b conjugate vaccine may be sensitive to the polysaccharide vaccine also.

### Pediatrics
For children up to 18 months of age—Immunization is not recommended, since children in this age group will not have an adequate antibody response to the polysaccharide vaccine.

For children 18 to 24 months of age—Immunization is recommended for children in this age group, especially those in known high risk groups. However, the efficacy of the polysaccharide vaccine in these children appears to be less than in children 24 months of age or older, and some of these children will not have an adequate antibody response to the polysaccharide vaccine. It is recommended that, whenever possible, the more immunogenic conjugate vaccine be used instead of the polysaccharide vaccine.

### Drug interactions and/or related problems
The following drug interactions and/or related problems have been selected on the basis of their potential clinical significance (possible mechanism in parentheses where appropriate)—not necessarily inclusive (» = major clinical significance):

Note: Combinations containing any of the following medications, depending on the amount present, may also interact with this medication.

Immunosuppressive agents or
Radiation therapy
   (because immunosuppressive agents and radiation therapy suppress normal defense mechanisms, the patient's antibody response to the polysaccharide vaccine may be decreased. If possible, children who are to undergo therapy with agents that cause immunosuppression, including that for Hodgkin's disease, should receive the vaccine at least 10 days, and preferably more than 14 days, prior to receiving the immunosuppression-causing agent; otherwise, it may be preferable to postpone the immunization until after the immunosuppression-causing therapy is completed. The interval between discontinuation of therapy that causes immunosuppression and the restoration of the patient's ability to respond to an active immunizing agent depends on the intensity and type of immunosuppression-causing therapy, the underlying disease, and other factors; estimates vary from 3 months to 1 year. The precaution does not apply to corticosteroids used as replacement therapy, for short-term [less than 2 weeks] systemic therapy, or by other routes of administration that do not cause immunosuppression)

### Laboratory value alterations
The following have been selected on the basis of their potential clinical significance (possible effect in parentheses where appropriate)—not necessarily inclusive (» = major clinical significance):

With diagnostic test results
   Antigen detection tests
      (the polysaccharide vaccine may interfere with interpretation of antigen detection tests, such as latex agglutination and countercurrent immunoelectrophoresis, that are used for diagnosis of systemic Hib disease. Antigenuria from administration of the haemophilus b polysaccharide vaccine can produce positive urinary latex agglutination tests for up to 11 days after immunization)

### Medical considerations/Contraindications
The medical considerations/contraindications included here have been selected on the basis of their potential clinical significance (reasons given in parentheses where appropriate)—not necessarily inclusive (» = major clinical significance).

*Except under special circumstances, this medication should not be used when the following medical problem exists:*
»   Illness, acute or febrile
      (administration of the polysaccharide vaccine should be postponed to avoid confusing the symptoms of the illness with the side effects of the vaccine; minor illnesses, such as mild upper respiratory infections, do not preclude administration of the vaccine)

*Risk-benefit should be considered when the following medical problem exists:*
   Sensitivity to haemophilus b polysaccharide vaccine

## Side/Adverse Effects

Note: Side effects generally are minor, occur within 24 hours, and last 24 hours or less.

   There are no significant differences in the frequency or types of side effects between haemophilus b polysaccharide vaccine and haemophilus b conjugate vaccine.

The following side/adverse effects have been selected on the basis of their potential clinical significance (possible signs and symptoms in parentheses where appropriate)—not necessarily inclusive:

### Those indicating need for medical attention
Incidence rare
   *Anaphylactic reaction* (difficulty in breathing or swallowing; hives; itching, especially of soles or palms; reddening of skin, especially around ears; swelling of eyes, face, or inside of nose; unusual tiredness or weakness, sudden and severe); *convulsions*

### Those indicating need for medical attention only if they continue or are bothersome
Incidence more frequent
   *Anorexia* (lack of appetite); *diarrhea; erythema at injection site* (redness at place of injection); *fever up to 39 °C (102.2 °F)*—usually resolves within 48 hours; *irritability; lethargy* (lack of interest; reduced physical activity); *tenderness at injection site*

Incidence less frequent or rare
   *Fever over 39 °C (over 102.2 °F)*—usually resolves within 48 hours; *induration at injection site* (hard lump at place of injection); *serum sickness–like reaction* (itching; skin rash; swelling of face; arthralgia; joint pain); *sleep disturbance* (trouble in sleeping); *swelling at injection site; vomiting*

## Patient Consultation

As an aid to patient consultation, refer to *Advice for the Patient, Haemophilus b Polysaccharide Vaccine (Systemic)*.

In providing consultation, consider emphasizing the following selected information (» = major clinical significance):

### Before receiving this vaccine
»   Conditions affecting use, especially:
      Sensitivity to haemophilus b polysaccharide vaccine or haemophilus b conjugate vaccine
      Use in children—Not recommended for use in children up to 18 months of age
      Other medical problems, especially fever or serious illness

### Proper use of this vaccine
»   Proper dosing

### Side/adverse effects
      Signs of potential side effects, especially anaphylactic reaction or convulsions

# General Dosing Information

When sterilizing syringes and skin before vaccination, care should be taken to avoid use of preservatives, antiseptics, detergents, and disinfectants, since the polysaccharide vaccine may be inactivated by these substances.

The polysaccharide vaccine is for intramuscular or subcutaneous administration. It should not be administered intradermally or intravenously.

To prevent inactivation of the vaccine, it is recommended that only the diluent provided by the manufacturer be used for vaccine reconstitution.

Persons infected with human immunodeficiency virus (HIV) may receive this vaccine whether they have asymptomatic or symptomatic HIV infection.

Polysaccharide vaccines, including haemophilus b polysaccharide vaccine, may be administered concurrently with the following, using separate body sites, separate syringes, and the precautions that apply to each immunizing agent:
• Polysaccharide vaccines, other, such as meningococcal polysaccharide vaccine or pneumococcal polyvalent vaccine.
• Influenza vaccine, whole or split virus.
• Diphtheria toxoid, tetanus toxoid, and/or pertussis vaccine.
• Live virus vaccines, such as measles, mumps, and/or rubella vaccines.
• Poliovirus vaccines (oral [OPV], inactivated [IPV], or enhanced-potency inactivated [enhanced-potency IPV]).
• Hepatitis B recombinant or plasma-derived vaccine.
• Immune globulin and disease-specific immune globulins.
• Inactivated vaccines, except cholera, typhoid, and plague. It is recommended that cholera, typhoid, and plague vaccines be administered on separate occasions because there are no data available on the concurrent administration of haemophilus b polysaccharide vaccine and these vaccines and because of these vaccines' propensity to cause side/adverse effects.

Parents should be informed that the polysaccharide vaccine is not as effective in children 18 to 24 months of age as it is in older children and that reimmunization may be necessary.

Most authorities believe that children immunized between 18 and 24 months of age should be reimmunized. The optimal timing of this second dose is not known; however, it appears that reimmunization of these children should occur at or after 24 months of age, with 2 to 18 months having elapsed between the first immunization and the second one. Previous immunization does not affect the immune response or adverse reaction to a subsequent dose of the vaccine.

## For treatment of adverse effects

Recommended treatment consists of the following—
For children
• If anaphylaxis occurs, 0.01 mg of epinephrine per kg of body weight or 0.3 mg of epinephrine per square meter of body surface, up to a maximum of 0.5 mg per dose, may be administered subcutaneously, the dose being repeated every fifteen minutes for two doses, then administered every four hours as needed.
• If anaphylactic shock occurs, 0.01 mg of epinephrine per kg of body weight, up to a maximum of 0.3 mg, may be administered intramuscularly or subcutaneously, the dose being repeated every five minutes if necessary. If there is an inadequate response to the intramuscular or subcutaneous dosage, 0.01 mg of epinephrine per kg of body weight may be administered intravenously every five to fifteen minutes as needed.

# Parenteral Dosage Forms

## HAEMOPHILUS B POLYSACCHARIDE VACCINE (FOR INJECTION)

### Usual adult and adolescent dose
Use is not recommended.

### Usual pediatric dose
Children up to 18 months of age—Use is not recommended.
Children 18 to 24 months of age (especially if they are in known high risk groups) and
Children 24 months to 5 years of age (i.e., up to the 5th birthday)—Intramuscular or subcutaneous, 0.5 mL, into the outer aspect of the upper arm (deltoid) or into the lateral mid thigh (vastus lateralis).
Note: Since satisfactory response to the polysaccharide vaccine is not consistent among children 18 to 24 months of age, most authorities believe that these children should be reimmunized. The optimal timing of this second dose is not known; however, it appears that reimmunization of these children should occur at or after 24 months of age with 2 to 18 months having elapsed between the first immunization and the second one. Previous immunization does not affect the immune response or adverse reaction to a subsequent dose of the vaccine.

### Strength(s) usually available
U.S.—
Not commercially available.
Canada—
Not commercially available.

### Packaging and storage
Store lyophilized and reconstituted polysaccharide vaccine and diluent between 2 to 8 °C (35 to 46 °F), unless otherwise specified by manufacturer. Do not freeze.

### Preparation of dosage form
The appropriate measured amount of the sterile diluent supplied by the manufacturer should be injected into the vial of lyophilized polysaccharide vaccine and then the vial should be gently shaken to dissolve the contents; the lyophilized vaccine dissolves rapidly. The reconstituted solution is clear and colorless.

### Stability
The reconstituted polysaccharide vaccine should be administered as soon as possible; discard unused reconstituted vaccine after 8 hours.
The date and time of reconstitution should be recorded on the label of the vaccine vial.

# Selected Bibliography

Centers for Disease Control and Prevention. ACIP: Polysaccharide vaccine for prevention of haemophilus influenzae type b disease. MMWR 1985 Apr 19: 201-5.
Preblud, et al. Progress in haemophilus type b polysaccharide vaccine use in the United States. Pediatrics 1988 Jan; 81 (1): 166-8.
Centers for Disease Control and Prevention. ACIP Update: Prevention of haemophilus influenzae type b disease. MMWR 1986 Mar 21: 170-80.

Revised: 06/21/93
Interim revision: 03/29/94

---

**HALAZEPAM**—See *Benzodiazepines (Systemic)*

---

**HALCINONIDE**—See *Corticosteroids (Topical)*

---

**HALOBETASOL**—See *Corticosteroids (Topical)*

# HALOFANTRINE   Systemic*†

VA CLASSIFICATION (Primary): AP101

Note: For a listing of dosage forms and brand names by country availability, see *Dosage Forms* section(s). For a listing of brand names for the articles in this monograph, refer to the General Index.

---

\*Not commercially available in the U.S.

†Not commercially available in Canada.

---

## Category

Antimalarial.

## Indications

Note: Because halofantrine is not commercially available in the U.S or Canada, the bracketed information and the use of the superscript 1 in this monograph reflect the lack of labeled (approved) indications for this medication.

### Accepted

[Malaria (treatment)][1]—Halofantrine is indicated as alternative treatment for acute malaria (single or mixed infections) caused by chloroquine-resistant or multi-drug resistant strains of *Plasmodium falciparum* or *P. vivax*. Limited data indicate favorable results with the use of halofantrine in the treatment of malaria caused by *Plasmodium ovale* and *Plasmodium malariae*. Halofantrine does not exert any effect on the exoerythrocytic (intrahepatic) stage of *Plasmodium ovale* or *Plasmodium vivax* infection; therefore, subsequent treatment with an 8-aminoquinoline derivative such as primaquine is recommended to eliminate the hepatic forms and thus effect a cure.

### Unaccepted

Halofantrine is not recommended for use as a causal or suppressive prophylactic medication against malaria. Indiscriminate use of halofantrine should be avoided to prevent or minimize the emergence of resistance to the drug by some strains of *Plasmodium falciparum*. A recent study on the large scale use of halofantrine in the Congo confirmed the existence of a high frequency and degree of resistance of *Plasmodium falciparum* to halofantrine. Use of halofantrine should be restricted to those individuals with suspected chloroquine, or multi-drug resistant malaria.

---

[1]Not included in Canadian product labeling.

---

## Pharmacology/Pharmacokinetics

### Physicochemical characteristics

Molecular weight—536.89.

### Mechanism of action/Effect

Blood schizontocidal; halofantrine acts on the erythrocytic stage of the life cycle (trophozoites and schizonts) of the parasite.

Although the mechanism of action is still uncertain, it is believed that halofantrine forms complexes with ferriprotoporphyrin IX, which is formed during digestion of hemoglobin by plasmodia. The resulting toxic complex damages cell membranes, thereby causing lysis and death of the schizont.

Halofantrine also may act by inhibiting the proton pump, which is believed to be present at the host-parasite interface in the intraerythrocytic stage of the parasite's life cycle. Halofantrine is not effective against exoerythrocytic or hepatic schizonts and hypnozoites, or against the sporozoites, merozoites, or gametocytic stages of the life cycle of the *Plasmodium* species studied.

### Absorption

Following oral administration—Slow with wide intra- and intersubject variability, which may be attributed to poor drug solubility in water (<0.01%), notably at high pH; food enhances the rate and extent of absorption, especially food with high fat content, which increases absorption approximately 6-fold.

### Distribution

Large volume of distribution both in healthy volunteers and in patients with malaria; animal studies have shown that halofantrine is widely distributed in the tissues, with drug-related material persisting for at least 72 hours.

### Biotransformation

Metabolized primarily to N-desbutyl halofantrine, the desbutyl derivative of halofantrine; animal studies have shown that at peak concentrations, N-desbutyl halofantrine may represent 20 to 30% of all halofantrine-related material.

### Half-life

Highly variable for both halofantrine and its principal metabolite, N-desbutyl halofantrine.

Mean half-life in healthy volunteers—
  Halofantrine: Approximately 1 to 2 days.
  N-desbutyl halofantrine: Approximately 3 to 5 days.

Mean half-life in patients with malaria—
  Halofantrine: Approximately 4 to 5 days.
  N-desbutyl halofantrine: Approximately 4 to 5 days.

### Time to peak concentration

Oral doses of 250 to 2000 mg—
  Halofantrine: Approximately 6 hours.
  N-desbutyl halofantrine: Approximately 10 to 18 hours (range 6 to 32 hours).

### Peak serum concentration

Variable.

Following three 500-mg oral doses—
  Halofantrine: Averages 1134 nanograms per mL.
  N-desbutyl halofantrine: Averages about one-half the concentration of halofantrine.

### Elimination

Eliminated mainly in the feces as unchanged drug.

## Precautions to Consider

### Mutagenicity

Halofantrine has not been shown to be mutagenic either in animals or in *in vitro* tests utilizing the following assay techniques: Ames test, HGPRT gene mutation assay, CHO chromosome aberration test, mouse micronucleus test, and dominant lethal assays in rats. There were no adverse effects observed at the proposed clinical doses in the animal tests.

### Pregnancy/Reproduction

Fertility—Studies in male rats given halofantrine hydrochloride at doses of 15 to 30 mg per kg of body weight (mg/kg) per day for 16 weeks have not shown that halofantrine causes adverse effects on fertility.

Pregnancy—Adequate and well-controlled studies in humans have not been done. Halofantrine is not recommended for use in pregnancy since it has been found to be embryotoxic in animals.

Studies in animals have shown that halofantrine is not teratogenic at doses below 45 mg/kg of body weight per day (halofantrine base) in rats and 120 mg/kg per day (halofantrine base) in rabbits. However, halofantrine base was found to be embryotoxic at doses of 30 mg/kg per day in rats and 60 mg/kg per day in rabbits. In addition to the increased frequency of post-implantation embryonic death, reduced fetal body weight was observed at doses in excess of 15 mg/kg given for 5 days.

### Breast-feeding

Halofantrine may be distributed into breast milk. Animal studies have shown that halofantrine is distributed into milk in quantities sufficient to cause a reduced rate of weight gain, growth, and survival of the nursing offspring. In rats, these dose-related decreases were observed in pups exposed to the milk of dams receiving halofantrine at a dose of 50 mg/kg per day. However, no adverse effect was seen at a dose of 25 mg/kg per day.

### Pediatrics

Appropriate studies on the relationship of age to the effects of halofantrine have not been performed in the pediatric population. However, no pediatrics-specific problems have been documented to date.

### Geriatrics

Appropriate studies on the relationship of age to the effects of halofantrine have not been performed in the geriatric population. However, no geriatrics-specific problems have been documented to date.

### Drug interactions and/or related problems

The following drug interactions and/or related problems have been selected on the basis of their potential clinical significance (possible mechanism in parentheses where appropriate)—not necessarily inclusive (» = major clinical significance):

Note: Combinations containing any of the following medications, depending on the amount present, may also interact with this medication.

» Mefloquine
  (recent or concomitant treatment with mefloquine further prolongs the QT interval and may potentiate the risk of adverse cardiac effects)

#### Laboratory value alterations

The following have been selected on the basis of their potential clinical significance (possible effect in parentheses where appropriate)—not necessarily inclusive (» = major clinical significance):

With physiology/laboratory test values

Alanine aminotransferase (ALT [SGPT]), serum, and

Aspartate aminotransferase (AST [SGOT]), serum

(values may be transiently increased; however, their relation to medication is not clear since such enzymic changes are also commonly seen in acute malaria; values return to normal usually within 1 week after treatment)

Electrocardiogram (ECG) changes, such as prolongation of QT interval (occur at both the recommended therapeutic and higher doses)

#### Medical considerations/Contraindications

The medical considerations/contraindications included here have been selected on the basis of their potential clinical significance (reasons given in parentheses where appropriate)—not necessarily inclusive (» = major clinical significance).

*Except under special circumstances, this medication should not be used when the following medical problem exists:*

» Known congenital QT prolongation, or family history of (risk of arrhythmia)

*Risk-benefit should be considered when the following medical problems exist:*

» Atrioventricular (AV) conduction disorders or
» Syncope, unexplained, or
» Thiamine deficiency or
» Ventricular dysrhythmias

(these conditions prolong the QT interval which may cause an increased risk of arrhythmia)

Cerebral malaria and other complicated malarial conditions
(caution is required since there is no experience with the use of halofantrine in these conditions)

Hypersensitivity to halofantrine

#### Patient monitoring

The following may be especially important in patient monitoring (other tests may be warranted in some patients, depending on condition; » = major clinical significance):

Electrocardiogram (ECG)
(may be advisable to check arrhythmia)

## Side/Adverse Effects

Note: Side/adverse effects of halofantrine may be difficult to distinguish from the symptoms of acute malarial infection, since most of these side effects also occur in clinical malaria.

The following side/adverse effects have been selected on the basis of their potential clinical significance (possible signs and symptoms in parentheses where appropriate)—not necessarily inclusive:

#### Those indicating need for medical attention

Incidence rare

*Acute intravascular hemolysis* (anxiety; chest or lower back pain; fast heartbeat; flushing; nausea; rapid breathing; restlessness; scanty and black urine); *cardiovascular toxicity, specifically prolonged QT interval* (fast and irregular heartbeat)

#### Those indicating need for medical attention only if they continue or are bothersome

Incidence less frequent

*Gastrointestinal disturbances* (abdominal pain, diarrhea, nausea, and vomiting); *hypersensitivity* (skin itching or rash)

## Overdose

For more information on the management of overdose or unintentional ingestion, **contact a Poison Control Center** (See *Poison Control Center Listing*).

#### Treatment of overdose

Recommended treatment consists of the following:

To decrease absorption—
Immediate induction of emesis and/or gastric lavage may be performed.

Specific treatment—
Symptomatic treatment may be given.

Monitoring—
ECG monitoring should be done.

Supportive care—
Supportive measures such as maintaining an open airway, respiration, and circulation may be administered. Patients in whom intentional

overdose is known or suspected should be referred for psychiatric consultation.

## Patient Consultation

As an aid to patient consultation, refer to *Advice for the Patient, Halofantrine (Systemic)*.

In providing consultation, consider emphasizing the following selected information (» = major clinical significance):

#### Before using this medication

» Conditions affecting use, especially:

Hypersensitivity to halofantrine

Pregnancy—Not recommended for use in pregnancy because of its embryotoxic effects in animals

Breast-feeding—May be distributed into breast milk, resulting in reduced rate of weight gain, growth, and survival of nursing offspring as shown in animals; breast-feeding is not recommended while the patient is taking halofantrine

Other medications, especially mefloquine

Other medical problems, especially, atrioventricular conduction disorders, prolonged QT interval, thiamine deficiency, unexplained syncope, or ventricular dysrhythmias

#### Proper use of this medication

» Taking on an empty stomach due to cardiotoxicity
» Compliance with full course of therapy
» Repeating treatment after 1 week
» Proper dosing

Missed dose: Taking as soon as possible; not taking if almost time for next dose; not doubling doses

» Proper storage

#### Precautions while using this medication

Regular visits to physician to check progress

Checking with physician if symptoms persist or if no improvement occurs after the full course of treatment

*Self-protection measures against mosquitoes to help prevent infection or reinfection:*

Avoiding exposure to mosquitoes, especially at peak feeding times (between dusk and dawn)

Wearing suitable clothing (long-sleeved shirt and long trousers) to protect arms and legs when mosquitoes are out

Applying insect repellant (containing diethylmetatoluamide [DEET]) sparingly to exposed skin

Sleeping in screened or air-conditioned room

Using bed netting impregnated with repellant or permethrin

Using mosquito coils or sprays

#### Side/adverse effects

Signs of potential side effects, especially acute intravascular hemolysis and cardiovascular toxicity

## General Dosing Information

Halofantrine has been shown to prolong QT interval at the recommended therapeutic dose. Higher than recommended doses or recent or concomitant treatment with mefloquine further prolongs the QT interval.

Because of the variability of absorption of halofantrine within individuals, oral halofantrine should be given in three doses over a 12-hour period every six hours to ensure adequate blood concentration. Due to its cardiotoxic effects, it is recommended that halofantrine be taken on an empty stomach, because food enhances its absorption.

Since halofantrine does not exert any effect on the exoerythrocytic or intrahepatic stage of *Plasmodium ovale* or *P. vivax*, subsequent treatment with an 8-aminoquinoline derivative such as primaquine is recommended to eliminate the hepatic forms of these parasites.

A second course of treatment with halofantrine is recommended one week after the first course to prevent recrudescence.

## Oral Dosage Forms

Note: Bracketed uses in the *Dosage Forms* section refer to categories of use and/or indications that are not included in U.S. product labeling.

#### HALOFANTRINE HYDROCHLORIDE ORAL SUSPENSION

#### Usual adult and adolescent dose

[Malaria][1]—

Oral, 500 mg taken on an empty stomach every six hours three times a day for one day. Treatment should be repeated after one week.

**Usual pediatric dose**

[Malaria)][1]——

Children weighing less than 40 kg: Oral, 8 mg per kg of body weight taken on an empty stomach every six hours three times a day for one day. Treatment should be repeated after one week. The following doses also have been given—

Children 1 to 2 years of age (10 to 12 kg of body weight): Oral, 100 mg taken on an empty stomach every six hours three times a day for one day. Treatment should be repeated after one week.

Children 2 to 5 years of age (13 to 18 kg of body weight): Oral, 150 mg taken on an empty stomach every six hours three times a day for one day. Treatment should be repeated after one week.

Children 5 to 8 years of age (19 to 25 kg of body weight): Oral, 200 mg taken on an empty stomach every six hours three times a day for one day. Treatment should be repeated after one week.

Children 8 to 10 years of age (26 to 31 kg of body weight): Oral, 250 mg taken on an empty stomach every six hours three times a day for one day. Treatment should be repeated after one week.

Children 10 to 12 years of age (32 to 40 kg of body weight): Oral, 300 mg taken on an empty stomach every six hours three times a day for one day. Treatment should be repeated after one week.

Children 12 years of age and over (over 40 kg of body weight): See *Usual adult and adolescent dose.*

**Strength(s) usually available**

U.S.—

Not commercially available.

Canada—

Not commercially available.

Other (United Kingdom)—

100 mg (93 mg base) per 5 mL (Rx) [*Halfan*].

**Packaging and storage**

Store below 40 °C (104 °F), preferably between 15 and 30 °C (59 and 86 °F), in a well-closed light-resistant container, unless otherwise specified by manufacturer. Protect from freezing.

**Auxiliary labeling**

• Shake well.

## HALOFANTRINE HYDROCHLORIDE TABLETS

**Usual adult and adolescent dose**

See *Halofantrine Hydrochoride Oral Suspension.*

**Usual pediatric dose**

[Malaria)][1]——

Children weighing less than 40 kg: Oral, 8 mg per kg of body weight taken on an empty stomach every six hours three times a day for one day. Treatment should be repeated after one week. The following doses also have been given

Children up to 23 kg of body weight: Dosage has not been established.

Children 23 to 31 kg of body weight: Oral, 250 mg taken on an empty stomach every six hours three times a day for one day. Treatment should be repeated after one week.

Children 32 to 37 kg of body weight: Oral, 375 mg taken on an empty stomach every six hours three times a day for one day. Treatment should be repeated after one week.

Children 37 kg of body weight and over: See *Usual adult and adolescent dose.*

**Strength(s) usually available**

U.S.—

Not commercially available.

Canada—

Not commercially available.

Other (United Kingdom)—

250 mg (233 mg base) (Rx) [*Halfan*].

**Packaging and storage**

Store below 40 °C (104 °F), preferably between 15 and 30 °C (59 and 86 °F), in a well-closed container. Protect from light.

[1]Not included in Canadian product labeling.

### Selected Bibliography

Bryson HM, Goa KL. Halofantrine: a review of its antimalarial activity, pharmacokinetic properties and therapeutic potential. Drugs 1992; 43 (2): 236-58.

Weinke T, Loscher T, Fleischer K, Kretschmer H, Pohle HD, Kohler B, et al. The efficacy of halofantrine in the treatment of acute malaria in nonimmune travelers. Am J Trop Med Hyg 1992; 47 (1): 1-5.

Shanks GD, Watt G, Edstein MD, Webster HK, Suriyamongkol V, Watanasook C, et al. Halofantrine for the treatment of mefloquine chemoprophylaxis failures in Plasmodium falciparum infections. Am J Trop Med Hyg 1991; 45 (4): 488-91.

Revised: 8/27/93

---

# HALOPERIDOL    Systemic

VA CLASSIFICATION (Primary/Secondary): CN709/CN900; GA700

Note: For a listing of dosage forms and brand names by country availability, see *Dosage Forms* section(s). For a listing of brand names for the articles in this monograph, refer to the General Index.

## Category

Antipsychotic; antidyskinetic (Gilles de la Tourette's syndrome; Huntington's chorea); antiemetic.

## Indications

Note: Bracketed information in the *Indications* section refers to uses that are not included in U.S. product labeling.

**Accepted**

Psychotic disorders (treatment)—Haloperidol is indicated for the management of the manifestations of acute and chronic psychotic disorders including schizophrenia, manic states, and drug-induced psychoses, such as steroid psychosis. It may also be useful in the management of aggressive and agitated patients, including patients with organic mental syndrome or mental retardation. Haloperidol decanoate, a long-acting parenteral form, is intended for maintenance use in the management of patients requiring prolonged parenteral therapy, as in chronic schizophrenia.

Behavior problems, severe (treatment)—Haloperidol is effective in the treatment of children with severe behavior problems of apparently unprovoked, combative, explosive hyperexcitability. It is also effective in the *short-term* treatment of hyperactivity in children who show excessive motor activity with accompanying conduct disorders such as aggressiveness, impulsiveness, easy frustration, short attention span, and/or rapid mood fluctuations. In these 2 groups of children, haloperidol should be tried only in patients who fail to respond to psychotherapy or other non-neuroleptic medication.

Gilles de la Tourette's syndrome (treatment)—Haloperidol is used to control tics and vocalizations of Tourette's syndrome in children and adults.

[Autism, infantile (treatment)][1]—Haloperidol has been used to reduce abnormal behaviors, such as withdrawal, stereotypy, abnormal object relationships, fidgetiness, hyperactivity, negativism, angry affect, and labile affect, and may improve learning, in some patients with autism.

[Chorea, Huntington's (treatment)][1]—Because of its strong extrapyramidal effects, haloperidol is used to reduce disabling choreiform movements in Huntington's disease.

[Nausea and vomiting, cancer chemotherapy–induced (prophylaxis and treatment)][1]—Haloperidol is used as a second-line agent to control nausea and vomiting associated with antineoplastic therapy and surgery.

[1]Not included in Canadian product labeling.

## Pharmacology/Pharmacokinetics

Note: Pharmacological effects of haloperidol are similar to the effects of piperazine-derivative phenothiazines, which include aceto-phenazine, fluphenazine, perphenazine, prochlorperazine, and trifluoperazine.

**Physicochemical characteristics**

Chemical group—A butyrophenone derivative

Molecular weight—Haloperidol: 375.87.

Haloperidol decanoate: 530.12.

Other characteristics—Haloperidol oral solution: pH 2.75–3.75

Haloperidol injection: pH 3.0–3.8

**Mechanism of action/Effect**

Although the complex mechanism of the therapeutic effect is not clearly established, haloperidol is known to produce a selective effect on the central nervous system (CNS) by competitive blockade of postsynaptic dopamine ($D_2$) receptors in the mesolimbic dopaminergic system and an increased turnover of brain dopamine to produce its tranquilizing effects. With subchronic therapy, depolarization blockade, or diminished firing rate of the dopamine neuron (decreased release) along with $D_2$ postsynaptic blockade results in the antipsychotic action.

The long-acting decanoate form acts as a pro-drug, slowly and steadily releasing haloperidol from the vehicle.

### Other actions/effects

Blockade of dopamine receptors in the nigrostriatal dopamine pathway produces extrapyramidal motor reactions; blockade of dopamine receptors in the tuberoinfundibular system decreases growth hormone release and increases prolactin release by the pituitary. There is also some blockade of alpha-adrenergic receptors of the autonomic system.

### Absorption

Oral—60%.

### Distribution

The volume of distribution of haloperidol at steady state ($Vd_{ss}$) is 18 L per kg.

### Protein binding

Very high (92%).

### Biotransformation

Hepatic; extensive.

### Half-life

Haloperidol—Elimination—
    Oral—24 hours (range, 12 to 37 hours).
    Intramuscular—21 hours (range, 17 to 25 hours).
    Intravenous—14 hours (range, 10 to 19 hours).
Haloperidol decanoate—Elimination—
    Approximately 3 weeks (single or multiple doses).

### Time to peak plasma concentration

Oral—3 to 6 hours
Intramuscular—10 to 20 minutes.
Long-acting intramuscular—3 to 9 days, although variable. May occur on first day in some patients, notably the elderly.

### Therapeutic plasma concentration

4 to 20 nanograms per mL (10.6 to 53.2 micromoles per L).

### Elimination

Renal—
    About 40% of a single oral dose is excreted in the urine within 5 days, 1% of which is unchanged drug. A mean clearance value of 12 mL per kg per minute has been reported.
Biliary—
    15% of an oral dose is excreted in the feces by biliary elimination.

## Precautions to Consider

### Carcinogenicity/Tumorigenicity

Neuroleptic drugs (including haloperidol) elevate prolactin concentrations; the elevation persists during chronic administration. Tissue culture experiments indicate that approximately one-third of human breast cancers are prolactin dependent *in vitro*, a factor of potential importance if the prescription of these drugs is contemplated in a patient with a previously detected breast cancer. Although disturbances such as galactorrhea, amenorrhea, gynecomastia, and impotence have been reported, the clinical significance of elevated serum prolactin concentrations is unknown for most patients. An increase in mammary neoplasms has been found in rodents after chronic administration of neuroleptic drugs. However, neither clinical studies nor epidemiologic studies conducted to date have shown an association between chronic administration of these drugs and mammary tumorigenesis; the available evidence is considered too limited to be conclusive at this time.

### Mutagenicity

Haloperidol decanoate—No mutagenic potential was found in the Ames Salmonella microsomal activation assay.

### Pregnancy/Reproduction

Fertility—Animal reproduction studies have shown decreased fertility with doses 2 to 20 times the usual maximum human dose of haloperidol.

Pregnancy—
  *For haloperidol—*
    Adequate studies in humans have not been done. However, there have been some reports of limb malformations with maternal use of haloperidol along with other drugs of suspected teratogenicity during the first trimester.
    Some rodent studies have shown an increase in incidence of fetal resorption, delayed delivery, and neonatal death with doses 2 to 20 times the usual maximum human dose of haloperidol.

    Cleft palate has been observed in a study with mice given 15 times the human dose of haloperidol.
  *For haloperidol decanoate—*
    Adequate studies in humans have not been done.
    Studies in rats given up to 3 times the usual maximum human dose showed an increase in incidence of fetal resorption, fetal mortality, and neonatal mortality.
    FDA Pregnancy Category C.

### Breast-feeding

Haloperidol is excreted in breast milk. Animal studies have shown that haloperidol is excreted in milk in quantities sufficient to cause sedation and motor function impairment in the nursing offspring. Breast-feeding during haloperidol therapy is not recommended.

### Pediatrics

Haloperidol is not recommended for use in children up to 3 years of age. Children are highly susceptible to the extrapyramidal side effects, especially dystonias, of haloperidol.

### Geriatrics

Geriatric patients tend to develop higher plasma concentrations of haloperidol because of changes in distribution due to decreases in lean body mass, total body water, and albumin, and often an increase in total body fat composition. These patients usually require lower initial dosage and a more gradual titration of dose.

Elderly patients appear to be more prone to orthostatic hypotension and exhibit an increased sensitivity to the anticholinergic and sedative effects of haloperidol. In addition, they are more prone to develop extrapyramidal side effects, such as tardive dyskinesia and parkinsonism. The symptoms of tardive dyskinesia are persistent, difficult to control, and, in some patients, appear to be irreversible. The symptoms may be masked during long-term treatment, but may appear if haloperidol is discontinued. There is no known effective treatment. Careful observation during haloperidol therapy for early signs of tardive dyskinesia and reduction of dosage or discontinuation of medication may prevent a more severe manifestation of the syndrome.

It has been suggested that elderly patients receive half the usual adult dose. Patients with organic mental syndrome or acute confusional states, should initially receive one-third to one-half the usual adult dose, with the dose being increased no more frequently than every 2 or 3 days, and preferably at intervals of 7 to 10 days. A periodic attempt should be made to discontinue medication as soon as the patient improves.

### Dental

The peripheral anticholinergic effects of haloperidol may decrease or inhibit salivary flow, especially in middle-aged or elderly patients, thus contributing to the development of caries, periodontal disease, oral candidiasis, and discomfort.

Extrapyramidal reactions induced by haloperidol will result in increased motor activity of the head, face, and neck. Occlusal adjustments, bite registrations, and treatment for bruxism may be made less reliable.

The leukopenic and thrombocytopenic effects of haloperidol may result in an increased incidence of microbial infection, delayed healing, and gingival bleeding. If leukopenia or thrombocytopenia occurs, dental work should be deferred until blood counts have returned to normal. Patients should be instructed in proper oral hygiene, including caution in use of regular toothbrushes, dental floss, and toothpicks.

### Drug interactions and/or related problems

The following drug interactions and/or related problems have been selected on the basis of their potential clinical significance (possible mechanism in parentheses where appropriate)—not necessarily inclusive (» = major clinical significance):

Note: Combinations containing any of the following medications, depending on the amount present, may also interact with this medication.

» Alcohol or
» CNS depression–producing medications, other (See *Appendix II*)
    (concurrent use with haloperidol may result in increased CNS and respiratory depression and increased hypotensive effects)
    (concurrent use with haloperidol may potentiate alcohol intoxication)

  Amphetamines
    (concurrent use may decrease stimulant effects of amphetamines due to alpha-adrenergic blockade by haloperidol; also, the antipsychotic effects of haloperidol may be reduced when amphetamines and haloperidol are used concurrently)

Anticholinergics or other medications with anticholinergic activity
(See *Appendix II*) or
Antidyskinetic agents or
Antihistamines
(concurrent use with haloperidol may intensify anticholinergic side
effects, especially those of confusion, hallucinations, nightmares,
and increased intraocular pressure, because of secondary anticholinergic effects of haloperidol; also, patients should be advised to
report occurrence of gastrointestinal problems since paralytic ileus
may occur with concurrent therapy; in addition, antipsychotic effectiveness of haloperidol may be decreased because of reduced
gastrointestinal absorption; dosage adjustments may be necessary)

Anticoagulants, coumarin- or indandione-derivative
(concurrent use with haloperidol may either increase or decrease
anticoagulant activity; although the clinical significance has not
been determined, caution is recommended)

Anticonvulsants, including barbiturates
(concurrent use with haloperidol may cause a change in the pattern
and/or frequency of epileptiform seizures; dosage adjustments of
anticonvulsants may be necessary; serum concentrations of haloperidol may be significantly reduced)

Antidepressants, tricyclic or
Maprotiline or
Monoamine oxidase (MAO) inhibitors, including furazolidone, procarbazine, or selegiline or
Trazodone
(concurrent use with haloperidol may prolong and intensify the
sedative and anticholinergic effects of either these medications or
haloperidol)

Bromocriptine
(concurrent use with haloperidol may increase serum prolactin concentrations and interfere with effects of bromocriptine; dosage adjustment of bromocriptine may be necessary)

Bupropion
(concurrent use of bupropion with haloperidol may lower the seizure threshold and increase the risk of major motor seizures)

Diazoxide
(concurrent use antagonizes the inhibition of insulin release by
diazoxide)

Dopamine
(concurrent use may antagonize peripheral vasoconstriction produced by high doses of dopamine because of the alpha-adrenergic
blocking action of haloperidol)

Ephedrine
(concurrent use may decrease the pressor response to ephedrine)

» Epinephrine
(concurrent use may block the alpha-adrenergic effects of epinephrine, possibly resulting in severe hypotension and tachycardia)

» Extrapyramidal reaction–causing medications, other (See *Appendix II*)
(concurrent use with haloperidol may increase the severity and
frequency of extrapyramidal effects)

Fluoxetine
(caution in concurrent use of fluoxetine with haloperidol is recommended because of a potentially increased risk of CNS side
effects, particularly extrapyramidal reactions)

Guanadrel or
Guanethidine
(concurrent use with haloperidol may decrease the hypotensive effects of these agents because of displacement from and inhibition
of uptake into alpha-adrenergic neurons)

» Levodopa or
Pergolide
(concurrent use may decrease the therapeutic effects of these
agents because of blockade of dopamine receptors by haloperidol)

» Lithium
(lithium is frequently used concurrently with haloperidol during
the first week or two of treatment for acute manic episodes; lithium
alone may be adequate thereafter, although some patients may continue to need both; however, concurrent use with haloperidol has
been associated with irreversible neurological toxicity and brain
damage, especially in patients with organic mental syndrome or
other CNS impairment, although this interaction has been reported
only with high doses; extrapyramidal symptoms may be increased
by haloperidol's enhancement of dopamine blockade; patients
should be monitored closely during concurrent use; dosage adjustments or discontinuation of treatment may be necessary)

(admixture of the liquid forms of lithium and haloperidol may result in precipitation of free haloperidol)

Metaraminol
(concurrent use with haloperidol usually decreases, but does not
reverse or completely block, the pressor response to metaraminol,
because of the alpha-adrenergic blocking action of haloperidol)

Methoxamine
(prior administration of haloperidol may decrease the pressor effect
and duration of action of methoxamine because of the alpha-adrenergic blocking action of haloperidol)

Methyldopa
(concurrent use with haloperidol may cause unwanted mental effects such as disorientation and slowed or difficult thought
processes)

Phenylephrine
(prior administration of haloperidol may decrease the pressor response to phenylephrine because of the alpha-adrenergic blocking
action of haloperidol)

**Laboratory value alterations**
The following have been selected on the basis of their potential clinical
significance (possible effect in parentheses where appropriate)—not
necessarily inclusive (» = major clinical significance):

With diagnostic test results
ECG
(prolongation of the Q-T interval and changes compatible with
configuration of torsades de pointes may occur)

**Medical considerations/Contraindications**
The medical considerations/contraindications included here have been selected on the basis of their potential clinical significance (reasons given
in parentheses where appropriate)—not necessarily inclusive (» =
major clinical significance).

*Except under special circumstances, this medication should not be used
when the following medical problem exists:*
» CNS depression, toxic, drug-induced, severe
(may be potentiated)

*Risk-benefit should be considered when the following medical problems
exist:*
Alcoholism, active
(CNS depression may be potentiated; risk of heat stroke may be
increased)
» Cardiovascular disease, severe, especially angina
(transient hypotension and anginal pain may be provoked)
» Epilepsy
(seizure threshold may be lowered)
Glaucoma or predisposition to
(may be potentiated because of secondary anticholinergic effects
of haloperidol)
Hepatic function impairment
(metabolism may be altered)
Hyperthyroidism or thyrotoxicosis
(severe neurotoxicity such as rigidity and inability to walk or talk
may result)
» Parkinson's disease
(may be potentiated)
Pulmonary insufficiency, such as asthma, emphysema, or acute pulmonary infections
(potentiation of breathing impairment may possibly lead to "silent
pneumonias")
Renal function impairment
(excretion may be altered; more applicable to higher dosage since
renal clearance of unchanged drug is relatively low)
» Sensitivity to haloperidol
(patients with known allergies or with a history of allergic reactions to other medications may also be sensitive to haloperidol)
» Urinary retention
(may be potentiated)

**Patient monitoring**
The following may be especially important in patient monitoring (other
tests may be warranted in some patients, depending on condition;
» = major clinical significance):

Blood cell counts and differential in patients with sore throat and fever
or infections
(may be required during high-dose or prolonged therapy when
symptoms of infection develop; if significant cellular depression
occurs, medication should be discontinued and appropriate therapy
initiated; rechallenge in recovered patients will usually cause a
recurrence of agranulocytosis)

Careful observation for early signs of dehydration, such as lethargy and decreased sensation of thirst
(recommended at periodic intervals, especially in elderly or debilitated persons, for prevention of bronchopneumonia)

Careful observation for early symptoms of tardive dyskinesia
(recommended at periodic intervals, especially in the elderly and patients on high or extended maintenance dosage; since there is no known effective treatment if syndrome should develop, haloperidol should be discontinued, if clinically feasible, at earliest signs, usually fine, worm-like movements of the tongue, to stop further development)

Careful observation for early symptoms of tardive dystonia
(recommended at periodic intervals; since there is no known effective treatment if syndrome should develop, haloperidol should be discontinued, if clinically feasible, at the earliest signs)

Careful observation for signs of overdose or insufficient dosing with haloperidol decanoate
(recommended during initial dosing adjustments; since haloperidol decanoate slowly increases to steady state plasma concentration over 2 to 4 months, accumulation to excessive levels may occur; if psychotic symptoms reappear before next dose, therapy can be supplemented with short-acting forms of haloperidol)

Hepatic function determinations
(may be required at periodic intervals during high-dose or prolonged therapy or if jaundice or grippe-like symptoms occur, to detect liver function impairment)

## Side/Adverse Effects

Note: A few cases of sudden and unexpected death have been reported in patients who were receiving haloperidol therapy. However, there is no definite evidence that haloperidol is a causative factor.

Children are highly susceptible to extrapyramidal effects.

Geriatric and debilitated patients are more prone to develop extrapyramidal side effects and orthostatic hypotension and usually require a lower initial dosage and a more gradual titration of dose.

The following side/adverse effects have been selected on the basis of their potential clinical significance (possible signs and symptoms in parentheses where appropriate)—not necessarily inclusive:

**Those indicating need for medical attention**
Incidence more frequent
*Akathisia* (restlessness or need to keep moving); *dystonic extrapyramidal effects* (muscle spasms of face, neck, and back; tic-like or twitching movements; twisting movements of body; inability to move eyes; weakness of arms and legs); *parkinsonian extrapyramidal effects* (difficulty in speaking or swallowing; loss of balance control; mask-like face; shuffling walk; stiffness of arms or legs; trembling and shaking of hands and fingers)

Note: *Akathisia* may appear within first 6 hours after dose; often indistinguishable from psychotic agitation; differentiation with benztropine may improve haloperidol-induced akathisia but not psychotic agitation.

*Dystonic extrapyramidal effects* appear most often in children and young adults and early in treatment; may subside within 24 to 48 hours after drug has been discontinued.

*Parkinsonian extrapyramidal effects* are more frequent in the elderly; symptoms may be seen in the first few days of treatment or after prolonged treatment, and can recur after even a single dose.

Incidence less frequent
*Allergic reaction* (red and raised, or acne-like skin rash); *anticholinergic effects* (difficult urination; hallucinations); *CNS effect* (hallucinations); *decreased thirst, or unusual tiredness or weakness; orthostatic hypotension* (dizziness, lightheadedness, or fainting); *persistent tardive dyskinesia* (lip smacking or puckering; puffing of cheeks; rapid or worm-like movements of tongue; uncontrolled chewing movements; uncontrolled movements of the arms and legs)

Note: *Decreased thirst* or *unusual tiredness or weakness* may precede dehydration, hemoconcentration, reduced pulmonary ventilation, and bronchopneumonia; occur most often in elderly or debilitated patients.

*Tardive dyskinesia* is more frequent in elderly patients, women, and patients with brain damage; initially dose related, but may increase with long-term treatment and total cumulative dose; may persist after discontinuation of haloperidol.

Incidence rare
*Agranulocytosis* (sore throat and fever; unusual bleeding or bruising); *heat stroke* (hot, dry skin; inability to sweat; muscle weakness; confusion); *obstructive jaundice* (yellow eyes or skin); *neuroleptic malignant syndrome (NMS)* (difficult or unusually fast breathing; fast heartbeat or irregular pulse; high fever; high or low [irregular] blood pressure; increased sweating; loss of bladder control; severe muscle stiffness; seizures; unusual tiredness or weakness; unusually pale skin); *tardive dystonia* (increased blinking or spasms of eyelid; unusual facial expressions or body positions; uncontrolled twisting movements of neck, trunk, arms, or legs)

Note: *Heat stroke,* caused by haloperidol-induced suppression of central and peripheral temperature regulation in the hypothalamus, may occur during environmental conditions of high heat and high humidity. The effectiveness of sweating as a cooling mechanism may be reduced by humid conditions and by the anticholinergic effects of haloperidol, used alone or in combination with other anticholinergic medications such as nonprescription cold medications or antihistamines. Adequate interior temperature control (air conditioning) must be maintained for institutionalized patients during hot weather because of the increased risk of heat stroke and NMS. Patients should be advised to avoid exertion, stay in cool areas, and avoid dehydration and other anticholinergic medications.

*NMS* may occur at any time during neuroleptic therapy, but is more commonly seen soon after start of therapy, or after patient has switched from one neuroleptic to another, during combined therapy with another psychotropic medication, or after a dosage increase. Along with the overt signs of skeletal muscle rigidity, hyperthermia, autonomic dysfunction, and altered consciousness, differential diagnosis may reveal leukocytosis (9500 to 26,000 cells per cubic millimeter), elevated liver function test values, and elevated creatine phosphokinase (CPK).

**Those indicating need for medical attention only if they continue or are bothersome**
Incidence more frequent
*Blurred vision; changes in menstrual period; constipation; dryness of mouth; swelling or soreness in breasts in females; unusual secretion of milk; weight gain*
Incidence less frequent
*Decreased sexual ability; drowsiness; increased sensitivity of skin to sun; nausea or vomiting*

**Those indicating the need for medical attention if they occur after the medication is discontinued**
*Withdrawal emergent dyskinesia* (trembling of fingers and hands; uncontrolled, repetitive movements of mouth, tongue, and jaw)—more frequent in elderly patients, women, and patients with brain damage

## Overdose

For specific information on the agents used in the management of haloperidol overdose, see:
• *Albumin Human (Systemic)* monograph;
• *Benztropine* in *Antidyskinetics (Systemic)* monograph;
• *Charcoal, Activated (Oral-Local)* monograph;
• *Diphenhydramine* in *Antihistamines (Systemic)* monograph; and/or
• *Norepinephrine* in *Sympathomimetic Agents—Cardiovascular Use (Parenteral-Systemic)* monograph.

For more information on the management of overdose or unintentional ingestion, **contact a Poison Control Center** (see *Poison Control Center Listing*).

**Clinical effects of overdose**
In general, symptoms of overdose may be an exaggeration of adverse effects. Patient would appear comatose with respiratory depression and hypotension severe enough to produce a shock-like state.
The following effects have been selected on the basis of their potential clinical significance (possible signs and symptoms in parentheses where appropriate)—not necessarily inclusive:
*Severe breathing difficulty; dizziness; severe drowsiness or comatose state; severe muscle trembling, jerking, stiffness, or uncontrolled movements; severe tiredness or weakness*

**Treatment of overdose**
Treatment is essentially symptomatic and supportive with possible utilization of the following:
To decrease absorption—
Inducing emesis or initiating gastric lavage, immediately followed by administration of activated charcoal.
Specific treatment—
Counteracting hypotension and circulatory collapse by use of intravenous fluids, plasma, or concentrated albumin, and vasopressor agents such as norepinephrine. Epinephrine should *not* be used since it may cause paradoxical hypotension.

Administering benztropine or diphenhydramine to manage severe extrapyramidal reactions.

Monitoring—
Monitoring ECG for signs of Q-T prolongation or torsades de pointes.
Severe arrhythmias should be treated with appropriate antiar-
rhythmic measures.

Supportive care—
Establishing a patent airway.
Mechanically assisting respiration, if necessary.
Patients in whom intentional overdose is known or suspected should
be referred for psychiatric consultation.

Note: Dialysis is not effective in removing excessive systemic
haloperidol.

## Patient Consultation

As an aid to patient consultation, refer to *Advice for the Patient,
Haloperidol (Systemic)*.

In providing consultation, consider emphasizing the following selected
information (» = major clinical significance):

**Before using this medication**
» Conditions affecting use, especially:
   Sensitivity to haloperidol
   Pregnancy—Reports of limb malformations after maternal use of
   haloperidol with other drugs of suspected teratogenicity during
   first trimester; animal reproduction studies have shown a decrease in fertility, increased incidence of fetal resorption, delayed delivery, and neonatal death with very high doses
   Breast-feeding—Excreted in breast milk; animal studies have
   shown sedation, impaired motor function in nursing offspring;
   not recommended for use during breast-feeding
   Use in children—Children are more prone to extrapyramidal symptoms, especially dystonias
   Use in the elderly—Elderly patients are more likely to develop
   extrapyramidal, anticholinergic, hypotensive, and sedative effects; reduced dosage recommended
   Dental—Haloperidol-induced blood dyscrasias may result in infections, delayed healing, and bleeding; dry mouth may cause caries, candidiasis, periodontal disease, and discomfort; increased
   motor activity of face, head, and neck may interfere with some
   dental procedures
   Other medications, especially alcohol, other CNS depression–producing medications, epinephrine, other extrapyramidal reaction–producing medications, levodopa, or lithium
   Other medical problems, especially severe cardiovascular disease,
   severe CNS depression, Parkinson's disease, allergies, epilepsy, or urinary retention

**Proper use of this medication**
   Taking with food or milk to reduce gastrointestinal irritation
   Proper administration of oral liquid form:
      Using special dropper
      Mixing with water or a beverage such as orange juice, apple juice,
      tomato juice, or cola; not mixing with tea or coffee
» Importance of not taking more or less medication than the amount
   prescribed
» Compliance with therapy; may require several weeks of therapy to
   obtain desired effects
» Proper dosing
   Missed dose: Taking as soon as possible; taking any remaining doses
   for that day at regularly spaced intervals; not doubling doses
» Proper storage

**Precautions while using this medication**
   Regular visits to physician to check progress of therapy
» Checking with physician before discontinuing medication; gradual
   dosage reduction may be needed
» Avoiding use of alcoholic beverages or other CNS depressants during
   therapy
» Possible drowsiness or dizziness; caution when driving, using machin-
   ery, or doing things requiring alertness
   Possible dizziness or lightheadedness: caution when getting up suddenly from a lying or sitting position
» Possible heat stroke: caution during exercise, hot baths, or hot weather
   Avoiding the use of over-the-counter medications for colds or allergies, to prevent increased anticholinergic effects and risk of heat
   stroke
» Caution if any kind of surgery, dental treatment, or emergency treatment is required; telling physician or dentist in charge about taking
   haloperidol because of possible drug interactions or blood
   dyscrasias

Possible skin photosensitivity; avoiding unprotected exposure to sun;
using protective clothing; using a sun block product that includes
protection against both UVA-caused photosensitivity reactions and
UVB-caused sunburn reactions; avoiding use of sunlamp, tanning
bed, or tanning booth

Possible dryness of mouth; using sugarless gum or candy, ice, or saliva
substitute for relief; checking with physician or dentist if dry
mouth continues for more than 2 weeks

If taking liquid form, avoiding contact with skin (to prevent contact
dermatitis)

Observing precautions for up to 6 weeks with long-acting parenteral
form

**Side/adverse effects**
» Stopping medication and notifying physician immediately if symptoms
   of neuroleptic malignant syndrome (NMS) appear
   Extrapyramidal effects are more likely to occur in children, the elderly,
   and debilitated patients
   Notifying physician as soon as possible if early symptoms of tardive
   dyskinesia appear
   Possibility of withdrawal symptoms
   Signs of potential side effects, especially akathisia, dystonias, parkinsonism, allergic reaction, anticholinergic effects, CNS effect, decreased thirst, unusual tiredness or weakness, orthostatic hypotension, tardive dyskinesia or dystonia, blood dyscrasias, heat stroke,
   obstructive jaundice, and neuroleptic malignant syndrome (NMS)

## General Dosing Information

See also *Patient monitoring*.

Dosage must be individualized by titration from the lower dose range.
After a favorable response is noted (usually within 3 weeks), the
proper maintenance dosage should be determined by gradually decreasing to the lowest level of therapeutic dosage that will maintain
an adequate clinical response.

The antiemetic effect of haloperidol may mask signs of drug toxicity or
may obscure diagnosis of conditions in which the primary symptom
is nausea.

When extended therapy is discontinued, a gradual reduction in haloperidol
dosage over several weeks is recommended, since abrupt withdrawal
may cause some patients on high or long-term dosage to experience
withdrawal-emergent neurological symptoms.

Avoid skin contact with haloperidol oral solution; contact dermatitis has
been reported.

**For oral dosage forms only**
Because undiluted haloperidol concentrated oral solution may irritate mucous membranes, the dose should be diluted with water or beverages
having a pH less than 4 (such as orange juice, apple juice, tomato
juice, or cola). The dilution should be prepared immediately prior to
administration to prevent precipitation. If mixed with coffee, tea, or
lithium citrate syrup, free haloperidol will precipitate.

**For long-acting dosage form only**
Patients being considered for haloperidol decanoate therapy should be first
converted to oral haloperidol from any other neuroleptic they may
have been taking to prevent unexpected adverse sensitivity to
haloperidol.

Variations in patient response may require adjustments of dose and dosing
intervals. Each patient must be carefully supervised to determine the
optimal dosing interval and lowest effective dose, depending on patient's response, age, physical condition, symptoms, severity of illness,
and drug history.

Effects of the extended-action injectable form may last up to 6 weeks in
some patients. The side effects information and precautions apply during this period of time.

**Diet/Nutrition**
Haloperidol tablets may be taken with food or a full glass (240 mL) of
water or milk if necessary to lessen gastrointestinal irritation.

To prevent mucosal irritation, haloperidol oral solution should be diluted
in water or beverages such as orange juice, apple juice, tomato juice,
or cola immediately prior to administration.

**For treatment of adverse effects**
Neuroleptic malignant syndrome (NMS)—
   Treatment is essentially symptomatic and supportive and includes
   the following
      • *Discontinuing haloperidol immediately*. Neuroleptic malig-
      nant syndrome after injection of long-acting haloperidol de-
      canoate may be difficult to treat because of this dosage form's
      long half-life.
      • Hyperthermia—Administering antipyretics (aspirin or aceta-
      minophen); using cooling blanket.

• Dehydration—Restoring fluids and electrolytes.
• Cardiovascular instability—Monitoring blood pressure and cardiac rhythm closely.
• Hypoxia—Administering oxygen; considering airway insertion and assisted ventilation.
• Muscle rigidity—Dantrolene sodium may be administered (100 to 300 mg per day in divided doses; 1.25 to 1.5 mg per kg of body weight, intravenously). Bromocriptine (5 to 7.5 mg every eight hours) has been used to reverse hyperpyrexia and muscle rigidity.

Parkinsonism, severe—
Many authorities advise that the only appropriate treatment of extrapyramidal symptoms is reduction of the antipsychotic dosage, if possible. Oral antidyskinetic agents such as trihexyphenidyl, 2 mg three times per day, or benztropine, may be effective in treating more severe parkinsonism and acute motor restlessness but are used sparingly, and then usually for no longer than 3 months. Extrapyramidal symptoms may reappear if both haloperidol and the antidyskinetic agent are discontinued simultaneously. The antidyskinetic agent may have to be continued after haloperidol is discontinued because of different excretion rates. Milder effects may be treated by adjusting dosage.

Akathisia—
May be treated with antiparkinsonian medications, or with propranolol (30 to 120 mg per day), nadolol (40 mg per day), pindolol (5 to 60 mg per day), lorazepam (1 or 2 mg two or three times a day), or diazepam (2 mg two or three times a day).

Dystonia—
Acute dystonic postures or oculogyric crisis may be relieved by parenteral administration of benztropine (2 mg intramuscularly); or diphenhydramine (50 mg intramuscularly); or diazepam (5 to 7.5 mg intravenously), to be followed by oral antidyskinetic medication for one or two days to prevent recurrent dystonic episodes. Dosage adjustments of haloperidol may control these effects, and discontinuation of haloperidol may reverse severe symptoms in weeks to months.

Tardive dyskinesia or tardive dystonia—
No known effective treatment. Dosage of haloperidol should be lowered or medication discontinued, if clinically feasible, at earliest signs of tardive dyskinesia or tardive dystonia, to prevent possible irreversible effects.

# Oral Dosage Forms

Note: Bracketed uses in the *Dosage Forms* section refer to categories of use and/or indications that are not included in U.S. product labeling.

## HALOPERIDOL ORAL SOLUTION USP

**Usual adult and adolescent dose**
Antipsychotic; antidyskinetic—
Oral, 500 mcg (0.5 mg) to 5 mg two or three times a day initially, the dosage being gradually adjusted as needed and tolerated.

**Usual adult prescribing limits**
100 mg a day.

**Usual pediatric dose**
Children up to 3 years of age: Safety and efficacy have not been established.
Children 3 to 12 years of age or 15 to 40 kg of body weight:
Psychotic disorders—
Oral, initially 50 mcg (0.05 mg) per kg of body weight a day (in two or three divided doses), the daily dose being increased as needed and tolerated by 500-mcg (0.5 mg) increments at five- to seven-day intervals up to a total of 150 mcg (0.150 mg) per kg of body weight a day.
Nonpsychotic behavior disorders and Tourette's syndrome—
Oral, initially 50 mcg (0.05 mg) per kg of body weight a day (in two or three divided doses), the daily dose being increased as needed and tolerated by 500-mcg (0.5 mg) increments at five- to seven-day intervals up to a total of 75 mcg (0.075 mg) per kg of body weight a day. Alternatively, some clinicians recommend that, in the treatment of Tourette's syndrome, the initial daily dose be administered at bedtime to avoid daytime sedation.
[Infantile autism][1]—
Oral, 25 mcg (0.025 mg) per kg of body weight a day, up to 50 mcg (0.05 mg) per kg of body weight a day.
Note: There is little evidence that pediatric dosages exceeding 6 mg a day produce additional improvement in behavior or in tics.

**Usual geriatric dose**
Oral, 500 mcg (0.5 mg) to 2 mg two or three times a day, the dosage being increased gradually as needed and tolerated.
Note: The dose for debilitated patients is the same as the geriatric dose.

**Strength(s) usually available**
U.S.—
2 mg per mL (Rx) [*Haldol* (methylparaben); GENERIC].
Canada—
2 mg per mL (Rx) [*Apo-Haloperidol; Novo-Peridol; Peridol; PMS Haloperidol;* GENERIC].

**Packaging and storage**
Store below 40 °C (104 °F), preferably between 15 and 30 °C (59 and 86 °F), unless otherwise specified by manufacturer. Store in a tight, light-resistant container. Protect from freezing.

**Incompatibilities**
Insoluble precipitate of haloperidol is formed when mixed with coffee, tea or lithium citrate syrup.

**Auxiliary labeling**
• May cause drowsiness.
• Avoid alcoholic beverages.

**Note**
Avoid skin contact with liquid forms of this medication; contact dermatitis has been reported.

Each dose must be diluted in water or a beverage such as orange juice, apple juice, tomato juice, or cola, immediately prior to administration.

Provide patient with specially marked dosage dropper and explain use if necessary.

## HALOPERIDOL TABLETS USP

**Usual adult and adolescent dose**
See *Haloperidol Oral Solution USP.*

**Usual adult prescribing limits**
See *Haloperidol Oral Solution USP.*

**Usual pediatric dose**
See *Haloperidol Oral Solution USP.*

**Usual geriatric dose**
See *Haloperidol Oral Solution USP.*

**Strength(s) usually available**
U.S.—
500 mcg (0.5 mg) (Rx) [*Haldol;* GENERIC].
1 mg (Rx) [*Haldol* (tartrazine); GENERIC].
2 mg (Rx) [*Haldol;* GENERIC].
5 mg (Rx) [*Haldol* (tartrazine); GENERIC].
10 mg (Rx) [*Haldol* (tartrazine); GENERIC].
20 mg (Rx) [*Haldol;* GENERIC].
Canada—
500 mcg (0.5 mg) (Rx) [*Apo-Haloperidol; Haldol; Novo-Peridol; Peridol* (scored); GENERIC].
1 mg (Rx) [*Apo-Haloperidol; Haldol* (tartrazine); *Novo-Peridol; Peridol* (scored); GENERIC].
2 mg (Rx) [*Apo-Haloperidol; Haldol* (metabisulfite); *Novo-Peridol; Peridol* (scored); GENERIC].
5 mg (Rx) [*Apo-Haloperidol; Haldol* (tartrazine); *Novo-Peridol; Peridol* (scored); GENERIC].
10 mg (Rx) [*Apo-Haloperidol; Haldol* (tartrazine); *Novo-Peridol; Peridol* (scored); GENERIC].
20 mg (Rx) [*Haldol* (metabisulfite); *Novo-Peridol;* GENERIC].

**Packaging and storage**
Store below 40 °C (104 °F), preferably between 15 and 30 °C (59 and 86 °F), unless otherwise specified by manufacturer. Store in a tight, light-resistant container.

**Auxiliary labeling**
• May cause drowsiness.
• Avoid alcoholic beverages.

# Parenteral Dosage Forms

## HALOPERIDOL INJECTION USP

**Usual adult and adolescent dose**
Acute psychosis—
Intramuscular, 2 to 5 mg initially, the dosage being repeated at one-hour intervals if necessary, or at four- to eight-hour intervals if symptoms are satisfactorily controlled.
Note: For the rapid control of acute psychosis or delirium, haloperidol has also been administered intravenously, in doses of 0.5 to 50 mg at a rate of 5 mg per minute, the dose being repeated as needed at 30-minute intervals. Alternatively, the dose of haloperidol can be diluted in 30 to 50 mL of compatible intravenous fluid and administered over 30 minutes.

**Usual adult prescribing limits**
Intramuscular: 100 mg daily.

**Usual pediatric dose**
Safety and efficacy have not been established.

**Strength(s) usually available**
U.S.—
5 mg per mL (Rx) [*Haldol* (methylparaben 1.8 mg; propylparaben 0.2 mg; lactic acid); GENERIC].
Canada—
5 mg per mL (Rx) [*Haldol* (methylparaben 1.8 mg; propylparaben 0.2 mg; lactic acid); GENERIC].

**Packaging and storage**
Store below 40 °C (104 °F), preferably between 15 and 30 °C (59 and 86 °F), unless otherwise specified by manufacturer. Protect from light. Protect from freezing.

**Incompatibilities**
Haloperidol injection may be precipitated by phenytoin or heparin.

## HALOPERIDOL DECANOATE INJECTION

Note: The dosing of haloperidol decanoate injection is expressed in terms of haloperidol base (not the decanoate).

**Usual adult and adolescent dose**
Chronic psychosis—
Intramuscular, initially 10 to 15 times the previous daily oral dose of haloperidol, up to a maximum initial dose of 100 mg (base), at monthly intervals, the dosing interval and dose being adjusted as needed and tolerated.
Note: Administration is by deep intramuscular injection into gluteal region using Z-track technique. A 2-inch long, 21-gauge needle is recommended.

The maximum volume per injection site should not exceed 3 mL.

**Usual adult prescribing limits**
300 mg (base) per month.
Note: Monthly doses as high as 900 mg (base) have been reported.

**Usual pediatric dose**
Safety and efficacy have not been established.

**Strength(s) usually available**
U.S.—
50 mg (base) (70.52 mg of haloperidol decanoate) per mL (Rx) [*Haldol Decanoate* (benzyl alcohol 1.2%; sesame oil)].
100 mg (base) (141.04 mg of haloperidol decanoate) per mL (Rx) [*Haldol Decanoate* (benzyl alcohol 1.2%; sesame oil)].
Canada—
50 mg (base) (70.52 mg of haloperidol decanoate) per mL (Rx) [*Haldol LA* (benzyl alcohol 15 mg/mL)].
100 mg (base) (141.04 mg of haloperidol decanoate) per mL (Rx) [*Haldol LA* (benzyl alcohol 15 mg/mL)].

**Packaging and storage**
Store below 40 °C (104 °F), preferably between 15 and 30 °C (59 and 86 °F), unless otherwise specified by manufacturer. Protect from light. Protect from freezing. Do not refrigerate.

**Note**
Not to be administered intravenously.

---

[1]Not included in Canadian product labeling.

Revised: 03/19/93
Interim revision: 08/04/95

---

# HALOPROGIN    Topical

VA CLASSIFICATION (Primary): DE102
Note: For a listing of dosage forms and brand names by country availability, see *Dosage Forms* section(s). For a listing of brand names for the articles in this monograph, refer to the General Index.

---

## Category

Antifungal (topical).

## Indications

Note: Bracketed information in the *Indications* section refers to uses that are not included in U.S. product labeling.

**Accepted**
Tinea corporis (treatment)
Tinea cruris (treatment)
Tinea manuum (treatment) or
Tinea pedis (treatment)—Haloprogin is indicated in the topical treatment of tinea corporis, tinea cruris, tinea manuum, and tinea pedis caused by *Trichophyton rubrum*, *T. tonsurans*, *T. mentagrophytes*, *Microsporum canis*, and *Epidermophyton floccosum*.

Pityriasis versicolor (treatment)—Haloprogin is indicated in the topical treatment of pityriasis versicolor (tinea versicolor;''sun fungus'') caused by *Pityrosporon orbiculare (Malassezia furfur)*.

[Tinea barbae (treatment)][1] or
[Tinea capitis (treatment)][1]—Haloprogin is used in the topical treatment of tinea barbae and tinea capitis.

Not all species or strains of a particular organism may be susceptible to haloprogin.

[1]Not included in Canadian product labeling.

## Pharmacology/Pharmacokinetics

**Physicochemical characteristics**
Molecular weight—361.39.

## Precautions to Consider

**Carcinogenicity**
Carcinogenicity studies have not been done in animals.

**Mutagenicity**
Haloprogin has not been shown to be mutagenic in the Ames-Salmonella/Microsome Plate Assay.

**Pregnancy/Reproduction**
Fertility—Adequate and well-controlled studies in humans have not been done.
Studies in rats and rabbits, given 10 daily topical applications equivalent to up to 3 times the estimated total human dose for a 30-day course of therapy, have not shown that haloprogin causes impaired fertility.
Pregnancy—Adequate and well-controlled studies in humans have not been done.
Studies in rats and rabbits, given 10 daily topical applications equivalent to up to 3 times the estimated total human dose for a 30-day course of therapy, have not shown that haloprogin causes adverse effects on the fetus.
FDA Pregnancy Category B.

**Breast-feeding**
It is not known whether haloprogin, applied topically, is absorbed systemically and distributed into breast milk. However, problems in humans have not been documented.

**Pediatrics**
Appropriate studies on the relationship of age to the effects of haloprogin have not been performed in the pediatric population. Safety and efficacy have not been established.

**Geriatrics**
Appropriate studies on the relationship of age to the effects of haloprogin have not been performed in the geriatric population. However, no geriatrics-specific problems have been documented to date.

**Medical considerations/Contraindications**
The medical considerations/contraindications included here have been selected on the basis of their potential clinical significance (reasons given in parentheses where appropriate)—not necessarily inclusive (» = major clinical significance).

*Risk-benefit should be considered when the following medical problem exists:*
Sensitivity to haloprogin

## Side/Adverse Effects

The following side/adverse effects have been selected on the basis of their potential clinical significance (possible signs and symptoms in parentheses where appropriate)—not necessarily inclusive:

**Those indicating need for medical attention**
   *Blistering, burning, itching, or other sign of skin irritation not present before therapy*

## Patient Consultation

As an aid to patient consultation, refer to *Advice for the Patient, Haloprogin (Topical)*.

In providing consultation, consider emphasizing the following selected information (» = major clinical significance):

**Before using this medication**
» Conditions affecting use, especially:
      Sensitivity to haloprogin

**Proper use of this medication**
   Applying enough medication to cover affected area and rubbing in gently
» Avoiding contact with the eyes
» Compliance with full course of therapy
» Proper dosing
   Missed dose: Applying as soon as possible; not applying if almost time for next dose
» Proper storage

**Precautions while using this medication**
   Checking with physician if no improvement within 4 weeks

**Side/adverse effects**
   Possible stinging when solution form of medication is applied
   Signs of potential side effects, especially blistering, burning, itching, or other signs of skin irritation not present before therapy

## General Dosing Information

Use of topical antifungals may lead to skin sensitization, resulting in hypersensitivity reactions with subsequent topical use of the medication.

## Topical Dosage Forms

### HALOPROGIN CREAM USP

**Usual adult and adolescent dose**
Topical antifungal—
   Topical, to the skin, two times a day for two to four weeks.

---

**Usual pediatric dose**
Safety and efficacy have not been established.

**Strength(s) usually available**
U.S.—
   1% (Rx) [*Halotex*].
Canada—
   1% (Rx) [*Halotex*].

**Packaging and storage**
Store between 15 and 30 °C (59 and 86 °F). Store in a tight, light-resistant container. Protect from freezing.

**Auxiliary labeling**
• For external use only.
• Continue medicine for full time of treatment.

### HALOPROGIN TOPICAL SOLUTION USP

**Usual adult and adolescent dose**
Topical antifungal—
   Topical, to the skin, two times a day for two to four weeks.

**Usual pediatric dose**
Safety and efficacy have not been established.

**Strength(s) usually available**
U.S.—
   1% (Rx) [*Halotex* (alcohol 75%)].
Canada—
   1% (Rx) [*Halotex* (alcohol)].

**Packaging and storage**
Store between 15 and 30 °C (59 and 86 °F). Store in a tight, light-resistant container. Protect from freezing.

**Auxiliary labeling**
• For external use only.
• Keep container tightly closed.
• Continue medicine for full time of treatment.

Revised: 06/21/93

---

**HALOTHANE**—See *Anesthetics, Inhalation (Systemic)*

---

## HEMAGGLUTINATION INHIBITION PREGNANCY TEST KITS—See *Pregnancy Test Kits for Home Use*

---

# HEPARIN   Systemic

**VA CLASSIFICATION (Primary): BL100**
Note: For a listing of dosage forms and brand names by country availability, see *Dosage Forms* section(s). For a listing of brand names for the articles in this monograph, refer to the General Index.

## Category

Anticoagulant.

## Indications

Note: Bracketed information in the *Indications* section refers to uses that are not included in U.S. product labeling.

Note: Some of the indications for heparin therapy are identical to those for thrombolytic (alteplase [tissue-type plasminogen activator, recombinant], anistreplase [anisoylated plasminogen-streptokinase activator complex, APSAC], streptokinase, or urokinase) or coumarin- or indandione-derivative anticoagulant therapy. However, thrombolytic agents are used primarily to lyse obstructive thrombi and restore blood flow in a recently occluded blood vessel, whereas anticoagulants are used primarily to prevent thrombus formation and extension of existing thrombi. For treatment of acute deep venous thrombosis and acute pulmonary embolism, a thrombolytic agent may be the treatment of choice in selected patients. However, the selection of thrombolytic therapy or anticoagulant therapy as opposed to other forms of treatment, including vascular surgery, must be based on determination of the severity of thrombotic disease and assessment of patient condition and history.

Heparin is the anticoagulant of choice when an immediate effect is required. When long-term anticoagulant therapy is required, a cou-

marin or indandione derivative is usually administered as a follow-up to heparin therapy. However, in some patients (especially pregnant women) long-term anticoagulation with heparin may be desirable.

**Accepted**
Thrombosis, deep venous (prophylaxis and treatment) and
Thromboembolism, pulmonary (prophylaxis and treatment)—Heparin is indicated using a full-dose regimen in the treatment of patients with recent thrombosis or thrombophlebitis of the deep veins to prevent extension and embolization of the thrombus and to reduce the risk of pulmonary embolism or recurrent thrombus formation. In acute pulmonary embolism, full-dose heparin is indicated to decrease the risk of extension, recurrence, or death.

Heparin is also indicated using a low-dose regimen to prevent the development of venous thrombosis and pulmonary embolism following major abdominal or thoracic surgery in high-risk patients, such as patients with a history of thromboembolism and patients requiring prolonged immobilization following surgery, especially if they are 40 years of age or older. Low-dose heparin may be ineffective for this purpose in some patients, especially following hip surgery. Many clinicians question the validity of data showing the efficacy and safety of low-dose heparin prophylaxis.

[Low-dose heparin prophylaxis is also used to prevent thrombus formation in selected immobilized medical patients who are not at risk of hemorrhage.]

Heparin is also administered using an adjusted-dose regimen for prophylaxis against thromboembolic complications when low-dose heparin may not be effective, e.g., for general abdominal or thoracic surgery in very high-risk patients, high-risk orthopedic procedures such as elective hip surgery or knee reconstruction, and [the second half of the third trimester in pregnant women with a history of venous thrombosis or pulmonary embolism][1].

Adjusted-dose subcutaneous heparin is also recommended when long-term anticoagulation is required and use of a coumarin- or indandione-derivative anticoagulant is contraindicated or inadvisable (e.g., during pregnancy). In addition, after the dosage of heparin has been stabilized (i.e., the desired level of anticoagulation has been achieved and maintained for a 2-week period without additional dosage adjustment), further anticoagulant monitoring and dosage adjustment are not needed (except during pregnancy, when heparin requirements increase with the patient's blood volume as pregnancy progresses). Therefore, this regimen can be utilized for the long-term treatment of nonpregnant patients when anticoagulant therapy cannot be monitored on a regular basis.

Thromboembolism (prophylaxis)—Heparin is indicated prior to and during attempted cardioversion or surgery to prevent systemic thromboembolism that may occur in patients with chronic atrial fibrillation, especially those with rheumatic mitral stenosis, congestive heart failure, left atrial enlargement, or cardiomyopathy.

Heparin is indicated as adjunctive therapy in acute myocardial infarction to reduce the risk of thromboembolic complications, especially in high-risk patients such as those with shock, congestive heart failure, prolonged arrhythmias (especially atrial fibrillation), previous myocardial infarction, or history of venous thrombosis or pulmonary embolism. Also, heparin may be administered to help prevent reocclusion following thrombolytic therapy in patients with acute myocardial infarction.

[Heparin is also used to prevent catheter-induced thromboembolism during coronary angiography and percutaneous transluminal angioplasty.][1]

Blood clotting (prophylaxis)—Heparin is indicated to prevent blood clotting during extracorporeal circulation in cardiac surgery and dialysis procedures.

Heparin is indicated to prevent blood clotting during and following arterial surgery. It is administered systemically or by local intra-arterial injection.

Heparin is indicated to prevent blood clotting during blood transfusions and in blood sampling for laboratory purposes. However, heparinized blood should not be used for isoagglutinin, complement, or erythrocyte fragility tests, or for platelet counts. In addition, leukocyte counts should be performed within 2 hours after heparin is added to the blood sample.

Heparin is also available as a lock flush solution, which is not intended for anticoagulant therapy. This solution is used to maintain the patency of an indwelling intravascular device.

Coagulation, disseminated intravascular (treatment)—Although heparin is indicated as a temporary measure in the treatment of disseminated intravascular coagulation, especially if there is clinical evidence of intravascular thrombosis, its use in this condition is controversial. The underlying cause of the condition must be determined and treated.

Thromboembolism, arterial (treatment)—Heparin is indicated as adjunctive therapy for peripheral arterial embolism. It may prevent further thrombus formation when surgery must be delayed.

Thrombosis, cerebral (prophylaxis)—Heparin is indicated to decrease the risk of cerebral thrombosis and death in patients with progressive stroke (stroke-in-evolution).

[Thromboembolism, cerebral, recurrence (prophylaxis)][1]—Heparin is also used in the treatment of patients with recent cerebral embolism to decrease the risk of recurrence and death; however, this use is controversial. Although administration of an anticoagulant too soon after a cerebral embolism may increase the risk of cerebral hemorrhage, recent studies have indicated that the risk of early recurrence may be greater than the risk of anticoagulant therapy. It is recommended that heparin therapy be initiated only if the patient is not hypertensive and a computerized tomographic (CT) scan performed 24 hours or longer following the onset of the stroke shows no evidence of hemorrhagic transformation. If severe hypertension is present, or the embolic stroke is large, there is a risk of late hemorrhagic transformation and anticoagulant therapy should be delayed for several days. If hemorrhagic transformation is documented, anticoagulant therapy should be postponed for at least 8 to 10 days. Long-term anticoagulation is recommended.

**Unaccepted**

Prophylactic use of heparin (low-dose or full-dose) is not recommended for patients with bleeding disorders; patients having neurosurgery, ophthalmic surgery, or spinal anesthesia; or patients who are receiving

a coumarin- or indandione-derivative anticoagulant or a platelet active agent.

[Heparin has also been used to reduce the risk of thrombosis and/or occlusion of the aortocoronary bypass following coronary bypass surgery; however, its efficacy has not been established and this use is controversial. Also, platelet aggregation inhibitors, especially aspirin, are more commonly used for this indication.]

---

[1]Not included in Canadian product labeling.

## Pharmacology/Pharmacokinetics

### Mechanism of action/Effect

Heparin acts indirectly at multiple sites in both the intrinsic and extrinsic blood clotting systems to potentiate the inhibitory action of antithrombin III (heparin cofactor) on several activated coagulation factors, including thrombin (factor IIa) and factors IXa, Xa, XIa, and XIIa, by forming a complex with and inducing a conformational change in the antithrombin III molecule. Inhibition of activated factor Xa interferes with thrombin generation and thereby inhibits the various actions of thrombin in coagulation. Heparin also accelerates the formation of an antithrombin III–thrombin complex, thereby inactivating thrombin and preventing the conversion of fibrinogen to fibrin; these actions prevent extension of existing thrombi. Larger doses of heparin are required to inactivate thrombin than are required to inhibit thrombin formation. Heparin also prevents formation of a stable fibrin clot by inhibiting the activation of the fibrin stabilizing factor by thrombin. Heparin has no fibrinolytic activity.

Full-dose heparin prolongs partial thromboplastin time, thrombin time, whole blood clotting time, and activated clotting time (ACT).

### Other actions/effects

Heparin reduces the concentration of triglycerides in plasma by releasing the enzyme lipoprotein lipase from tissues and stabilizing the enzyme. The resultant hydrolysis of triglycerides leads to increased blood concentrations of free fatty acids.

### Protein binding

Very high; primarily to low-density lipoproteins; also bound to globulins and to fibrinogen.

### Biotransformation

Hepatic; however, the primary route of removal from the circulation is uptake by the reticuloendothelial system.

### Half-life

1 to 6 hours (average 1.5 hours); dose and route dependent and subject to inter- and intrapatient variation. May be increased above the average in patients with renal failure, hepatic function impairment, or obesity. May be decreased in patients with pulmonary embolism, infections, or malignancy.

### Onset of action

Direct intravenous injection—Immediate.

Intravenous infusion—Immediate when infusion is preceded by the recommended intravenous loading dose. If no loading dose is given, the onset of action may depend upon the rate of infusion.

Subcutaneous—Generally within 20 to 60 minutes but subject to interpatient variability.

### Elimination

Renal, usually as metabolites. However, after intravenous administration of high doses, up to 50% of a dose may be excreted unchanged.

In dialysis—Not removed via hemodialysis.

## Precautions to Consider

### Cross-sensitivity and/or related problems

Patients with a history of allergies, especially those who are allergic to swine, beef, or other animal proteins, may be allergic to this medication also (depending on heparin source).

### Pregnancy/Reproduction

Pregnancy—Heparin does not cross the placenta and is the anticoagulant of choice for use during pregnancy because it does not affect blood clotting mechanisms in the fetus. Although heparin has not been reported to cause birth defects, use during pregnancy has been reported to increase the risk of stillbirth or prematurity. However, the underlying condition, rather than heparin itself, may have been responsible. Also, the reported incidence (13 to 22%) of these complications is lower than that reported with coumarin-derivative anticoagulants (31%). In addition, caution is recommended when heparin is used during the last trimester of pregnancy or during the postpartum period because of the increased risk of maternal bleeding.

Especially careful monitoring of the patient and attention to dosage are recommended during pregnancy. Heparin requirements increase, because of expansion of the patient's blood volume, as pregnancy progresses. Readjustment of heparin dosage may be needed following delivery.

FDA Pregnancy Category C.

### Breast-feeding

Heparin is not distributed into breast milk. However, administration to lactating women has rarely been reported to cause rapid (within 2 to 4 weeks) development of severe osteoporosis and vertebral collapse.

### Pediatrics

Appropriate studies performed to date have not demonstrated pediatrics-specific problems that would limit the usefulness of heparin in children. However, heparin injections that contain benzyl alcohol should not be administered to premature neonates because the preservative has been associated with a fatal "gasping syndrome" in these patients.

### Geriatrics

Patients 60 years of age or older, especially females, may be more susceptible to hemorrhaging during heparin therapy. Also, elderly patients are more likely to have age-related renal function impairment, which may increase the risk of bleeding in patients receiving anticoagulants.

### Dental

Bleeding from gingival tissue may be a symptom of heparin overdose.

Heparin therapy increases the risk of localized hemorrhage during and following oral surgical procedures. Consultation with the prescribing physician may be advisable prior to oral surgery, to determine whether a temporary dosage reduction or withdrawal of heparin therapy is feasible. Also, local measures to minimize bleeding should be used at the time of surgery.

### Drug interactions and/or related problems

The following drug interactions and/or related problems have been selected on the basis of their potential clinical significance (possible mechanism in parentheses where appropriate)—not necessarily inclusive (» = major clinical significance):

Note: Combinations containing any of the following medications, depending on the amount present, may also interact with this medication.

Interactions listed below may not apply to short-term use of heparin followed by protamine reversal, as in cardiovascular surgery.

In addition to the documented interactions listed below, the possibility should be considered that multiple effects leading to further impairment of blood clotting and/or increased risk of bleeding may occur if heparin is administered to a patient receiving any medication having a significant potential for causing hypoprothrombinemia, thrombocytopenia, or gastrointestinal ulceration or hemorrhage.

Acid citrate dextrose (ACD)–converted blood—blood collected in heparin and later converted to ACD blood
 (heparin anticoagulant activity lasts for up to 22 days after conversion to ACD blood when refrigerated; use of ACD blood in heparin-treated patients may increase the risk of hemorrhage)

Adrenocorticoids, glucocorticoid or
Corticotropin, especially chronic therapeutic use or
Ethacrynic acid or
Salicylates, nonacetylated
 (the potential occurrence of gastrointestinal ulceration or hemorrhage during therapy with these medications may cause increased risk of bleeding in patients receiving anticoagulant therapy)

 (large [antirheumatic] doses of salicylates may cause hypoprothrombinemia, which may increase the risk of bleeding in patients receiving anticoagulant therapy)

Anticoagulants, coumarin- or indandione-derivative
 (although these medications are commonly used concurrently with heparin, the fact that concurrent use may lead to a severe deficiency of vitamin K–dependent procoagulant factors, leading to increased risk of bleeding, must be considered)

 (heparin may prolong the prothrombin time used for dosage adjustments of these agents)

Antihistamines or
Digitalis glycosides or
Nicotine or
Tetracyclines
 (these medications may partially counteract the anticoagulant effect of heparin; heparin dosage adjustment may be required during and following concurrent use)

Anti-inflammatory drugs, nonsteroidal (NSAIDs) or
» Platelet aggregation inhibitors, other, (See *Appendix II*) especially:
» Aspirin
» Sulfinpyrazone
 (inhibition of platelet function by these agents may lead to hem-

orrhage because it impairs a hemostatic mechanism on which heparin-treated patients depend to prevent bleeding)

 (hypoprothrombinemia induced by large [antirheumatic] doses of aspirin, and the potential occurrence of gastrointestinal ulceration or hemorrhage during therapy with NSAIDs, aspirin, or sulfinpyrazone, may also cause increased risk of bleeding in patients receiving heparin therapy)

» Cefamandole or
» Cefoperazone or
» Cefotetan or
» Plicamycin or
» Valproic acid
 (these medications may cause hypoprothrombinemia; in addition, plicamycin or valproic acid may inhibit platelet aggregation; concurrent use with heparin may increase the risk of hemorrhage and is not recommended)

Chloroquine or
Hydroxychloroquine
 (these agents may cause thrombocytopenia, which may increase the risk of hemorrhage because heparin-treated patients depend on platelet aggregation to prevent bleeding)

» Methimazole or
» Propylthiouracil
 (these medications may cause hypoprothrombinemia, which may enhance the anticoagulant effect of heparin and increase the risk of bleeding)

Nitroglycerin, intravenous
 (the anticoagulant effect of heparin may be decreased in patients receiving nitroglycerin via intravenous infusion; adjustment of heparin dosage may be required to maintain the desired degree of anticoagulation during and following administration of a nitroglycerin infusion)

» Probenecid
 (probenecid may increase and prolong the anticoagulant effect of heparin)

» Thrombolytic agents, such as:
» Alteplase (tissue-type plasminogen activator, recombinant)
» Anistreplase (anisoylated plasminogen-streptokinase activator complex; APSAC)
» Streptokinase
» Urokinase
 (concurrent or sequential use with heparin increases the risk of bleeding complications; although heparin is sometimes given before, and is usually given to decrease the risk of reocclusion following, thrombolytic therapy, caution and especially careful monitoring of the patient are recommended)

### Diagnostic interference

With diagnostic test results
 Blood pool imaging studies
  (heparin may impair blood pool images by decreasing the radiolabeling of red blood cells with sodium pertechnetate Tc 99m)

 $^{125}$I-fibrinogen uptake test
  (some reports have indicated that heparin may cause false-negative test results in patients with actively forming or established venous thrombosis)

 Platelet scintigraphy using indium In 111 oxyquinoline
  (although studies of the effect of heparin on In 111–labeled platelet accumulation on venous thrombi have yielded contradictory results, the possibility should be considered that false negative test results may occur in heparin-treated patients)

 Prothrombin-time test, one-stage
  (may be prolonged; single intravenous injections or subcutaneous injection of full therapeutic doses of heparin may prolong the prothrombin time considerably because of the high concentrations of heparin in the blood, whereas usual prophylactic [low] doses of heparin given subcutaneously or full therapeutic doses given by continuous intravenous infusion usually do not increase the prothrombin time by more than a few seconds; to minimize problems, draw blood for the prothrombin time test just prior to, or at least 5 hours after, a single intravenous dose or 12 to 24 hours following subcutaneous injection of a full therapeutic dose)

 Radionuclide imaging using technetium Tc 99m sulfur colloid
  (heparin may reduce the quantity of technetium Tc 99m sulfur colloid reaching the site being studied by causing the radiotracer to accumulate in the lung, probably by increasing the number of free intravascular macrophages, which may migrate to, and phagocytize colloidal particles in, the pulmonary capillary bed)

Skeletal imaging, radionuclide
(subcutaneously administered heparin calcium may cause extraosseous accumulation of technetium Tc 99m medronate, technetium Tc 99m oxidronate, or technetium Tc 99m pyrophosphate, thereby interfering with the bone scan, if injected near the site to be studied; the interference involves precipitation of calcium, which may occur if the tissue concentration of calcium exceeds its solubility limits, and therefore does not occur with subcutaneously administered heparin sodium)

Thyroid function tests
(increases in serum thyroxine concentrations may occur, depending on the test method used; also, resin $T_3$ uptake may be increased)

With physiology/laboratory test values
Plasma free fatty acid concentration
(may be increased)

Plasma triglyceride concentration
(may be decreased)

Serum alanine aminotransferase (ALT [SGPT]) activity and
Serum aspartate aminotransferase (AST [SGOT]) activity
(may be increased during, and for a time following, heparin therapy; the usefulness of determinations of these enzymes in the differential diagnosis of myocardial infarction, pulmonary embolism, or liver disease may therefore be decreased)

Serum cholesterol concentration
(may be decreased with doses of 15,000 to 20,000 USP Units of heparin)

## Medical considerations/Contraindications

The medical considerations/contraindications included here have been selected on the basis of their potential clinical significance (reasons given in parentheses where appropriate)—not necessarily inclusive (» = major clinical significance).

*Except under special circumstances, this medication should not be used when the following medical problems exist:*

» Abortion, threatened or
» Aneurysm, cerebral or dissecting aorta, except in conjunction with corrective surgery or
» Cerebrovascular hemorrhage, confirmed or suspected
(increased risk of uncontrollable hemorrhage)
» Hemorrhage, active uncontrollable, except in disseminated intravascular coagulation
» Hypertension, severe uncontrolled
(increased risk of cerebral hemorrhage)
» Thrombocytopenia, severe, heparin-induced, within past several months
(risk of recurrence, which may cause resistance to heparin and new thromboembolic complications)

*Risk-benefit should be considered when the following medical problems exist:*

Allergic reaction to heparin, history of
Allergy or asthma, history of
(increased risk of allergic reactions because heparin is derived from animal tissue)
Any medical or dental procedure or condition in which the risk of bleeding or hemorrhage is present, such as:
» Anesthesia, regional or lumbar block
» Blood dyscrasias, hemorrhagic, especially thrombocytopenia or hemophilia; or other hemorrhagic tendency
» Childbirth, recent
Diabetes, severe
» Endocarditis, subacute bacterial
Gastrointestinal ulceration, history of
Intrauterine contraceptive device, use of
» Neurosurgery, recent or contemplated
» Ophthalmic surgery, recent or contemplated
» Pericarditis or pericardial effusion
Radiation therapy, recent
Renal function impairment, mild to moderate
» Renal function impairment, severe
» Spinal puncture, recent
» Surgery, major, or wounds resulting in large open surfaces
» Trauma, severe, especially to the central nervous system (CNS)
Tuberculosis, active
» Ulceration or other lesions of the gastrointestinal, respiratory, or urinary tract, active
» Vasculitis, severe
Hepatic function impairment, mild to moderate
» Hepatic function impairment, severe

Hypertension, mild to moderate
(increased risk of cerebral hemorrhage)

» Caution in use is also recommended for lactating women, who may develop severe osteoporosis after only 2 to 4 weeks of heparin therapy, and geriatric patients, who may be at increased risk of heparin-induced hemorrhage.

**Patient monitoring**

The following may be especially important in patient monitoring (other tests may be warranted in some patients, depending on condition; » = major clinical significance):

» Blood coagulation tests
(except in rare acute or emergency situations, should be performed prior to full-dose therapy to establish a baseline or control value; also, recommended prior to initiation of low-dose prophylaxis to identify pre-existing coagulation defects and aid in determining whether the patient is a suitable candidate for such treatment)

» Blood coagulation tests, heparin-specific, such as:
Activated clotting time (ACT) test or
Partial thromboplastin time (PTT) tests
(must be performed at periodic intervals during full-dose therapy as a guide to dosage, efficacy, and safety)

(PTT tests are used to establish dosage requirements during the initial phase of adjusted-dose therapy; they are also required at periodic intervals throughout adjusted-dose therapy, as a guide to dosage and efficacy, if the patient is pregnant)

Hematocrit determinations and
Stool tests for occult blood loss
(should be performed at regular intervals during full-dose therapy)

» Platelet counts
(recommended prior to initiation of therapy and at intervals of every 2 to 3 days during full-dose, adjusted-dose, or low-dose therapy to detect thrombocytopenia)

# Side/Adverse Effects

Note: The occurrence of hemorrhage (especially in the gastrointestinal tract) during heparin therapy, especially if blood coagulation tests are within the therapeutic range, may indicate the presence of an underlying occult lesion such as a tumor or ulcer.

Two forms of reversible thrombocytopenia related to heparin therapy have been identified, either of which may occur in up to 30% of patients receiving the medication. A mild form may occur on the second to fourth day of heparin therapy and may improve despite continuing heparin usage. This condition is characterized by a moderate decrease in platelet count and by the absence of thrombotic or hemorrhagic complications; it may occur more frequently with bovine lung heparin than with porcine mucosal heparin. A severe form of thrombocytopenia, associated with the development of heparin-dependent antiplatelet antibodies resulting in greatly increased platelet aggregation, has also been reported. This condition usually occurs after the eighth day of therapy, although it has occurred within as little as 2 days in some patients, and is characterized by reduction of platelet count to as low as 5000 per cu. mm. and by increased resistance to heparin therapy. Continued use of heparin may lead to the "white clot syndrome", i.e., the formation of new thrombi composed primarily of fibrin platelet aggregates, which may cause thrombotic complications including organ infarction, skin necrosis, gangrene of the extremities, pulmonary embolism, and stroke. Rarely, hemorrhage may occur. This severe form of thrombocytopenia is independent of the source of heparin, dosage, or route of administration; however, patients who have recently received a prior course of heparin therapy may be at greater risk of developing this complication. Heparin should be discontinued immediately if severe thrombocytopenia occurs or is suspected. Severe thrombocytopenia may recur if heparin is administered to the patient within several months following the development of this complication.

Adrenal hemorrhage resulting in acute adrenal insufficiency has been reported to occur rarely during anticoagulant therapy. Diagnosis may be difficult because the initial symptoms (abdominal pain, apprehension, diarrhea, dizziness or fainting, headache, loss of appetite, nausea or vomiting, and weakness) are nonspecific and variable. If acute adrenal insufficiency is suspected, anticoagulant therapy must be discontinued and high-dose adrenocorticoid therapy (preferably with hydrocortisone, since other glucocorticoids do not provide sufficient sodium retention) instituted immediately. Delay of treatment while laboratory confirmation of the diagnosis is awaited may prove fatal to the patient. It has been proposed that abdominal computerized axial tomographic (CAT) scanning may be of use in diagnosing this condition more rapidly.

Heparin may suppress aldosterone synthesis. Rarely, with prolonged use, inhibition of renal function, hyperkalemia, and metabolic acidosis may result.

The following side/adverse effects have been selected on the basis of their potential clinical significance (possible signs and symptoms in parentheses where appropriate)—not necessarily inclusive:

### Those indicating need for medical attention
Incidence less frequent or rare

*Allergic reaction* (fever with or without chills; runny nose; headache; nausea with or without vomiting; shortness of breath, troubled breathing, wheezing, or tightness in chest; skin rash, itching, or hives; tearing of eyes); *anaphylactoid reaction, possibly including anaphylactic shock* (changes in facial skin color; skin rash, hives, and/or itching; fast or irregular breathing; puffiness or swelling of the eyelids or around the eyes; shortness of breath, troubled breathing, tightness in chest, and/or wheezing; sudden, severe decrease in blood pressure and collapse); *chest pain; frequent or persistent erection; itching and burning feeling, especially on the plantar site of the feet; pain, coldness, and blue color of skin of arms or legs; peripheral neuropathy* (numbness or tingling in hands or feet)

Note: Signs and symptoms suggestive of *ischemia* may occur in one or more limbs approximately 6 to 10 days following initiation of therapy. If heparin therapy is continued, progression of the reaction may lead to cyanosis, tachypnea, and headache. Protamine sulfate will not reverse these effects, which in the past have been attributed to an allergic vasospastic reaction. Whether these effects are actually identical to complications associated with heparin-induced thrombocytopenia has not been determined.

### Signs and symptoms of hemorrhage indicating need for medical attention
Early signs of hemorrhage

*Bleeding from gums when brushing teeth; heavy bleeding or oozing from cuts or wounds; unexplained bruising or purplish areas on skin; unexplained nosebleeds; unusually heavy or unexpected menstrual bleeding*

Note: *Unexplained bleeding or bruising* may also indicate thrombocytopenia.

Signs and symptoms of internal bleeding—incidence 5 to 15%

*Abdominal pain or swelling; back pain or backaches; blood in urine; bloody or black, tarry stools; constipation caused by hemorrhage-induced paralytic ileus or intestinal obstruction; coughing up blood; dizziness; headaches, severe or continuing; joint pain, stiffness, or swelling; vomiting of blood or material that looks like coffee grounds*

### Those occurring during long-term (6 months or longer) therapy and indicating need for medical attention
*Osteoporosis* (back or rib pain; decrease in height); *unusual hair loss*

### Those occurring at site of administration and indicating need for medical attention
Incidence less frequent or rare with deep subcutaneous injections

*Hematoma* (collection of blood under skin [blood blister]); *histamine-like reaction; hives, localized; irritation, pain, redness, or ulceration; necrosis, cutaneous* (peeling or sloughing of skin)—several cases of tissue necrosis, possibly associated with cutaneous hemorrhage, have also been reported following intravenous administration

## Overdose
For specific information on the agents used in the management of heparin overdose, see the *Protamine (Systemic)* monograph.

For more information on the management of overdose, **contact a Poison Control Center** (see *Poison Control Center Listing*).

### Clinical effects of overdose
The following effects have been selected on the basis of their potential clinical significance (possible signs and symptoms in parentheses where appropriate)—not necessarily inclusive:

Early signs of excessive anticoagulation

*Bleeding from gums when brushing teeth; heavy bleeding or oozing from cuts or wounds; unexplained bruising or purplish areas on skin; unexplained nosebleeds; unusually heavy or unexpected menstrual bleeding*

Note: *Unexplained bleeding or bruising* may also indicate thrombocytopenia.

Signs and symptoms of internal bleeding

*Abdominal pain or swelling; back pain or backaches; blood in urine; bloody or black, tarry stools; constipation caused by hemorrhage-induced paralytic ileus or intestinal obstruction; coughing up blood;*

*dizziness; headaches, severe or continuing; joint pain, stiffness, or swelling; vomiting of blood or material that looks like coffee grounds*

### Treatment of overdose
For mild effects of heparin overdose, withdrawal of heparin therapy may be sufficient.

Specific treatment—

For more severe overdose, administration of the heparin antagonist protamine is required. One milligram of protamine sulfate will neutralize approximately 100 USP Units of heparin. However, heparin blood concentrations decrease rapidly following intravenous administration; 30 minutes after intravenous administration of heparin, half as much protamine sulfate may be sufficient to neutralize the remaining heparin. In most cases, it is recommended that protamine sulfate be administered intravenously, slowly (over a one- to three-minute period), and in doses not exceeding 50 mg in any ten-minute period. It is strongly recommended that blood coagulation tests be used to determine optimum protamine dosage, especially when neutralizing large doses of heparin given during cardiac or arterial surgery.

Because absorption of heparin may be prolonged following subcutaneous administration, it has been recommended that protamine (when used to neutralize heparin administered via that route) be administered as an initial loading dose of 25 to 50 mg that is followed by continuous intravenous infusion (over a period of 8 to 16 hours) of the remainder of the calculated dose. It is recommended that blood coagulation tests and/or direct titration of a sample of the patient's blood with protamine be used as a guide to protamine dosage.

When protamine is used to neutralize large doses of heparin, such as those used during cardiopulmonary bypass surgery, a rebound of heparin activity resulting in hemorrhage may occur despite initial complete neutralization of heparin. Prolonged monitoring of the patient is necessary; additional protamine should be administered as determined by coagulation test results. Also, it is recommended that no more than 100 mg of protamine sulfate be administered over a short period of time (2 hours) unless accurate titrations or other tests indicate that larger doses are required.

For severe hemorrhaging, transfusion of whole blood or plasma may also be required. This may dilute, but will not neutralize the effects of, heparin.

## Patient Consultation
As an aid to patient consultation, refer to *Advice for the Patient, Heparin (Systemic)*.

In providing consultation, consider emphasizing the following selected information (» = major clinical significance):

### Before using this medication
» Conditions affecting use, especially:

Allergies, especially to heparin or to swine, beef, or other animal proteins

Pregnancy—Although heparin does not cross the placenta and is not likely to adversely affect the fetus or neonate, there is a risk of maternal bleeding

Breast-feeding—Although heparin is not distributed into breast milk and poses no danger to the infant, severe osteoporosis and vertebral collapse may develop rapidly in lactating women

Use in the elderly—Increased risk of hemorrhage, especially in elderly females

Other medications, especially platelet aggregation inhibitors, hypoprothrombinemia-inducing medications, and probenecid

Other medical problems, especially hypertension; hemorrhagic blood dyscrasias; recent childbirth, spinal puncture, surgery, or other trauma; endocarditis; hepatic function impairment; renal function impairment; ulcers or other lesions of the gastrointestinal, respiratory, or urinary tract; and history of heparin-induced thrombocytopenia

### Proper use of this medication
» Proper administration of injections at home (if applicable)
» Importance of strict compliance with dosage measurement and dosage schedule to achieve maximum effectiveness and to lessen chance of bleeding
» Regular visits to physician and regular blood coagulation tests to check progress during therapy
» Proper dosing
» Missed dose: Using as soon as possible; not using if almost time for next dose; not doubling doses; keeping record of doses taken to avoid mistakes; keeping record of missed doses to give physician
» Proper storage—if dispensed to patient

**Precautions while using this medication**

» Not taking aspirin while using this medication; checking all medications for aspirin content; not taking ibuprofen or other platelet-active medications (unless prescribed by physician) while using heparin

» Need to inform all physicians and dentists that this medication is being used

Need to carry identification stating that medication is being used

Avoiding activities that may lead to injuries

Using care in brushing teeth and shaving

**Side/adverse effects**

Signs of potential side effects, especially allergic reactions, including anaphylaxis and anaphylactic shock; bleeding, including internal bleeding; chest pain; pain, coldness, or blue color of skin of arms or legs; peripheral neuropathy; skin necrosis; and local reactions at the injection site

Notifying physician immediately if signs and symptoms of bleeding are evident

## General Dosing Information

Full-dose heparin is administered by deep subcutaneous (intrafat) injection, direct intravenous injection, or intravenous infusion. Heparin should not be administered by intramuscular injection because of the increased incidence of hematomas, irritation, and pain at the injection site. Low-dose heparin is generally administered by deep subcutaneous injection.

The deep subcutaneous (intrafat) injections should be made deep into fatty tissue such as above the iliac crest or into the abdominal fat layer, and the sites should be rotated to prevent formation of hematomas. Aspiration of blood should not be attempted, and the needle should not be moved while the solution is being injected. Other measures recommended to reduce the risk of tissue trauma during subcutaneous injections include use of a small needle, use of a concentrated heparin solution to minimize the injection volume, and injection of the solution into a 2 to 2.5 cm (l to 2 inch) area of fat which is grasped and held away from deeper tissues. The injection sites should not be massaged before or after the injections; however, application of pressure over the injection sites for up to two minutes following each injection has been recommended.

For intravenous administration, many clinicians prefer continuous intravenous infusion because several studies have indicated that a more constant degree of anticoagulation may be achieved with lower total daily dosages and that the incidence of bleeding complications may be decreased. However, other clinicians prefer intermittent intravenous administration. Use of an indwelling, rubber-capped needle (heparin-lock) has been recommended for intermittent intravenous therapy. Use of a constant infusion pump or mechanical syringe pump has been recommended for administration of the continuous intravenous infusion, to control the flow rate and infusion volume. **It is recommended that other medications not be added to infusion solutions containing heparin**, even if compatibility has been established, because changes in the infusion rate that may be needed to adjust heparin dosage will also affect the delivery rate of other medications present in the solution.

When heparin is administered using a full-dose regimen, the dosage must be individualized and adjusted according to the results of periodic coagulation tests. *Full-dose heparin therapy is contraindicated whenever suitable blood coagulation tests cannot be performed at the required intervals.* However, the effect of low-dose heparin usually does not require monitoring if the patient has normal pretreatment coagulation parameters. During the first day of treatment, a coagulation test is usually performed prior to each injection (if given via an intermittent dosage schedule). When the medication is given by continuous intravenous infusion, the test is usually performed $1^{1}/_{2}$ to 2 hours after the infusion is started, then every 4 hours during the early stages of treatment. However, the frequency of testing must be adjusted to the needs of the individual patient. Coagulation tests should be performed at least once daily for the duration of therapy; however, increased monitoring may be necessary in patients who may be more sensitive to the effects of heparin, such as elderly patients or those with hypertension, renal function impairment, or hepatic function impairment.

When heparin is administered using an adjusted-dose regimen, dosage must be established according to the results of daily coagulation tests. When no dosage adjustments have been needed for two weeks, further monitoring at regular frequent intervals may be unnecessary for most patients. However, pregnant women should be monitored throughout therapy because their dosage requirements increase as pregnancy progresses.

The standard tests used for measuring heparin's general effect on clotting include the Lee-White whole blood clotting time, the whole blood

activated partial thromboplastin time (WBAPTT), the activated partial thromboplastin time (APTT), and the activated clotting time (ACT). Other tests may be used in some cases. The Lee-White whole blood clotting time has been reported to be less reproducible than other tests and has largely been replaced by partial thromboplastin time tests. If the Lee-White whole blood clotting time is used to monitor therapy, the clotting time should be elevated to $2^{1}/_{2}$ to 3 times the control value in minutes. The generally accepted value for the APTT is $1^{1}/_{2}$ to $2^{1}/_{2}$ times the control value in seconds. However, the specific reagent used must be considered when evaluating APTT test results because the various reagents used in the APTT test vary widely in their sensitivity to heparin. The generally accepted value for the ACT test is 2 to 3 times the control value in seconds. The ACT has been recommended as being particularly useful during extracorporeal circulation because it can be performed at the bedside; however, one study has indicated that the ACT may be ineffective for monitoring heparin dosage and protamine neutralization during cardiopulmonary bypass procedures in which hypothermia has been induced. Hypothermia may also interfere with the results of other coagulation tests. It is recommended that a single laboratory be employed for each patient, and that the laboratory understand the test will be used to monitor heparin therapy.

Because heparin is derived from animal tissue, it is recommended that patients with a history of allergies or asthma be given a test dose of 1000 USP Units before therapy is initiated.

Postsurgical patients and those with active thromboembolic disease (especially pulmonary embolism or myocardial infarction), infections with thrombosing tendency, malignancy, or a fever may be resistant to the effects of heparin and may require larger doses than other patients. Resistance to the effects of heparin also occurs in patients with familial antithrombin III deficiency. However, this type of resistance cannot always be overcome by increasing the dosage of heparin; a coumarin- or indandione-derivative anticoagulant is indicated for such patients. Also, local antithrombin III depletion resulting in loss of heparin effect may occur when heparin is administered intraperitoneally during peritoneal dialysis procedures.

If clinical evidence of thromboembolism occurs in a patient receiving low-dose heparin prophylaxis, full therapeutic doses of an anticoagulant should be administered. However, before full therapeutic doses of heparin are given, the possibility that the thrombosis may be due to the severe form of heparin-induced thrombocytopenia must be ruled out.

Heparin may be administered prior to or following thrombolytic therapy with alteplase (tissue-type plasminogen activator, recombinant), streptokinase, or urokinase. However, heparin should be discontinued and the patient's TT or APTT should be less than twice the control value prior to initiation of intravenous thrombolytic therapy. Also, following thrombolytic therapy, the patient's TT or APTT should return to less than twice the control value prior to administration of heparin.

When anticoagulant therapy is initiated with heparin and continued with a coumarin or indandione derivative, it is recommended that both agents be given concurrently until prothrombin time determinations indicate an adequate response to the coumarin or indandione derivative. The fact that early changes in prothrombin time may reflect initial depletion of factor VII rather than peak antithrombogenic activity must be kept in mind. Some clinicians recommend continuation of heparin therapy for several days after prothrombin time determinations have shown a reduction of activity to ensure that peak antithrombogenic activity has been reached.

Intramuscular injection of other medications is not recommended in patients receiving heparin because hematomas and bleeding into adjacent areas may occur.

A concentration of 400 to 600 USP Units of heparin per 100 mL of whole blood is usually used to prevent clotting during blood transfusion; a concentration of 70 to 150 USP Units of heparin per 10 to 20 mL of whole blood is usually used to prevent clotting in blood used for laboratory sampling. Consult manufacturers' prescribing information for specific directions. For use of heparin lock-flush solution in maintaining the patency of an indwelling venipuncture device, consult manufacturers' prescribing information. For use of heparin to prevent clotting during extracorporeal dialysis procedures, consult the equipment manufacturers' operating directions.

## Parenteral Dosage Forms

Note: The following doses are given in USP Heparin Units. The strengths of heparin preparations available in the U.S. are labeled in USP Heparin Units per mL. The strengths of heparin preparations available in Canada may be labeled in USP Units or in International Units (IU) per mL. The strengths of heparin preparations available in many other countries, including the U.K., are labeled only in IU per mL. *USP Heparin Units are not identical to IU.* The relative potency between USP Units and IU may vary, depending upon the test method and specific reagents used to measure heparin activity. Also, a new International Standard for Heparin (used to calibrate potency in IU) was adopted in 1983. Therefore, equivalence in USP Units of dosages in clinical studies using heparin preparations labeled in IU may be difficult to determine.

Consult current labeling for specific dosage recommendations for heparin preparations labeled in IU.

At one time, 1 mg of heparin sodium was equivalent to 100 USP Units. However, this is no longer the case because of increased purification.

# HEPARIN CALCIUM INJECTION USP

## Usual adult dose

Full-dose (therapeutic) regimen—

Subcutaneous, deep (intrafat), 10,000 to 20,000 USP Units initially, then 8000 to 10,000 USP Units every eight hours or 15,000 to 20,000 USP Units every twelve hours, or as determined by coagulation test results. This dosage schedule is usually preceded by a loading dose of 5000 USP Units administered by intravenous injection.

Intravenous, 10,000 USP Units initially, then 5000 to 10,000 USP Units every four to six hours or 100 USP Units per kg of body weight every four hours, or as determined by coagulation test results. The dose may be administered undiluted or diluted with 50 to 100 mL of 0.9% sodium chloride injection.

Intravenous infusion, 20,000 to 40,000 USP Units in 1000 mL of 0.9% sodium chloride injection, administered over a twenty-four-hour period. This dosage schedule is usually preceded by a loading dose of 35 to 70 USP Units per kg of body weight or 5000 USP Units, administered by intravenous injection. The infusion is often administered at a rate of 1000 USP Units per hour; however, dosage must be adjusted as determined by coagulation test results.

Note: Recommendations for specific indications include:

Heart and blood vessel surgery—Intravenous, initially not less than 150 USP Units per kg of body weight. Doses of 300 USP Units per kg of body weight are often used for procedures expected to last less than 60 minutes and doses of 400 USP units per kg of body weight are often used for procedures expected to last longer than 60 minutes. It is recommended that subsequent doses be based on coagulation test results.

Disseminated intravascular coagulation—Intravenous, 50 to 100 USP Units per kg of body weight every four hours, administered by continuous infusion or as a single injection. The medication should be discontinued if no improvement occurs within 4 to 8 hours.

Adjusted-dose regimen—

Subcutaneous, deep (intrafat), an established dose to be injected every twelve hours. The required dose is determined by adjusting heparin dosage until the midinterval (six hours after an injection) activated partial thromboplastin time (APTT) is maintained at one and one-half times the control value.

Low-dose (prophylactic) regimen—

Subcutaneous, deep (intrafat), 5000 USP Units two hours before surgery and every eight to twelve hours thereafter for seven days or until the patient is fully ambulatory, whichever is longer.

## Usual pediatric dose

Intravenous, 50 USP Units per kg of body weight initially, then 50 to 100 USP Units per kg of body weight every four hours, or as determined by coagulation test results.

Intravenous infusion, 50 USP Units per kg of body weight as a loading dose initially, then 100 USP Units per kg of body weight added and absorbed every four hours or 20,000 USP Units per square meter of body surface every twenty-four hours, or as determined by coagulation test results.

Note: Recommendations for specific indications include:

Disseminated intravascular coagulation—Intravenous, 25 to 50 USP Units per kg of body weight every four hours, administered by continuous infusion or as a single injection. The medication should be discontinued if no improvement occurs within 4 to 8 hours.

Heart and blood vessel surgery—Intravenous, initially not less than 150 USP Units per kg of body weight. Doses of 300 USP Units per kg of body weight are often used for procedures expected to last less than 60 minutes. It is recommended that subsequent doses be based on coagulation test results.

## Strength(s) usually available

U.S.—

Derived from porcine intestinal mucosa

25,000 USP Units per mL (Rx) [*Calciparine* (in single unit-dose

containers providing 5000 USP Units per 0.2 mL; 12,500 USP Units per 0.5 mL; and 20,000 USP Units per 0.8 mL)].

Canada—

Derived from porcine intestinal mucosa

25,000 International Units (IU) per mL (Rx) [*Calcilean* (in single unit-dose containers providing 20,000 IU per 0.8 mL); *Calciparine* (in single unit-dose containers providing 5000 IU per 0.2 mL; 12,500 IU per 0.5 mL; and 20,000 IU per 0.8 mL)].

## Packaging and storage

Store below 40 °C (104 °F), preferably between 15 and 30 °C (59 and 86 °F), unless otherwise specified by manufacturer. Protect from freezing.

## Stability

Do not use if the solution is discolored or contains a precipitate. Some studies have indicated that loss of heparin activity may occur if heparin is diluted with 5% dextrose injection and the diluted solution is not used within 24 hours, or if diluted solutions of heparin in any diluent are stored in glass containers.

## Incompatibilities

Heparin is strongly acidic and is incompatible with many solutions containing medications, although no loss of activity occurs when the agents are given via separate administration sites. Also, heparin may be incompatible with solutions containing a phosphate buffer, sodium carbonate, or sodium oxalate. It is recommended that heparin not be mixed, or administered through the same intravenous line, with other medications unless compatibility has first been established. In addition, heparin may be inactivated when used in conjunction with an artificial kidney because of an influx of calcium, magnesium, and acetate ions from the dialysate.

## Note

When preparing the label, indicate that heparin calcium is of porcine mucosal origin.

# HEPARIN SODIUM INJECTION USP

## Usual adult dose

Full-dose (therapeutic) regimen—

Subcutaneous, deep (intrafat), 10,000 to 20,000 USP Units initially, then 8000 to 10,000 USP Units every eight hours or 15,000 to 20,000 USP Units every twelve hours, or as determined by coagulation test results. This dosage schedule is usually preceded by a loading dose of 5000 USP Units administered by intravenous injection.

Intravenous, 10,000 USP Units initially, then 5000 to 10,000 USP Units every four to six hours or 100 USP Units per kg of body weight every four hours, or as determined by coagulation test results. The dose may be administered undiluted or diluted with 50 to 100 mL of 0.9% sodium chloride injection.

Intravenous infusion, 20,000 to 40,000 USP Units in 1000 mL of 0.9% sodium chloride injection, administered over a twenty-four-hour period. This dosage schedule is usually preceded by a loading dose of 35 to 70 USP Units per kg of body weight or 5000 USP Units, administered by intravenous injection. The infusion is often administered at a rate of 1000 USP Units per hour; however, dosage must be adjusted as determined by coagulation test results.

Note: Recommendations for specific indications include:

Heart and blood vessel surgery—Intravenous, initially not less than 150 USP Units per kg of body weight. Doses of 300 USP Units per kg of body weight are often used for procedures expected to last less than 60 minutes and doses of 400 USP units per kg of body weight are often used for procedures expected to last longer than 60 minutes. It is recommended that subsequent doses be based on coagulation test results.

Disseminated intravascular coagulation—Intravenous, 50 to 100 USP Units per kg of body weight every four hours, administered by continuous infusion or as a single injection. The medication should be discontinued if no improvement occurs within 4 to 8 hours.

Adjusted-dose regimen—

Subcutaneous, deep (intrafat), an established dose to be injected every twelve hours. The required dose is determined by adjusting heparin dosage until the midinterval (six hours after an injection) activated partial thromboplastin time (APTT) is maintained at one and one-half times the control value.

Low-dose (prophylactic) regimen—

Subcutaneous, deep (intrafat), 5000 USP Units two hours before surgery and every eight to twelve hours thereafter for seven days or until the patient is fully ambulatory, whichever is longer.

**Usual pediatric dose**

Intravenous, 50 USP Units per kg of body weight initially, then 50 to 100 USP Units per kg of body weight every four hours, or as determined by coagulation test results.

Intravenous infusion, 50 USP Units per kg of body weight as a loading dose initially, then 100 USP Units per kg of body weight added and absorbed every four hours or 20,000 USP Units per square meter of body surface every twenty-four hours, or as determined by coagulation test results.

Note: Recommendations for specific indications include:

Disseminated intravascular coagulation—Intravenous, 25 to 50 USP Units per kg of body weight every four hours, administered by continuous infusion or as a single injection. The medication should be discontinued if no improvement occurs within 4 to 8 hours.

Heart and blood vessel surgery—Intravenous, initially not less than 150 USP Units per kg of body weight. Doses of 300 USP Units per kg of body weight are often used for procedures expected to last less than 60 minutes. It is recommended that subsequent doses be based on coagulation test results. .

**Strength(s) usually available**

U.S.—

Derived from beef lung: With preservative

1000 USP Units per mL (Rx) [GENERIC].

5000 USP Units per mL (Rx) [GENERIC].

10,000 USP Units per mL (Rx) [GENERIC].

20,000 USP Units per mL (Rx) [GENERIC].

Derived from beef lung: Without preservative

1000 USP Units per mL (Rx) [GENERIC].

5000 USP Units per mL (Rx) [GENERIC].

Derived from porcine intestinal mucosa: With preservative

1000 USP Units per mL (Rx) [*Liquaemin* (benzyl alcohol); GENERIC].

2500 USP Units per mL (Rx) [GENERIC].

5000 USP Units per mL (Rx) [*Liquaemin* (benzyl alcohol); GENERIC].

7500 USP Units per mL (Rx) [GENERIC].

10,000 USP Units per mL (Rx) [*Liquaemin* (benzyl alcohol); GENERIC].

15,000 USP Units per mL (Rx) [GENERIC].

20,000 USP Units per mL (Rx) [*Liquaemin* (benzyl alcohol); GENERIC].

25,000 USP Units per mL (Rx) [GENERIC].

40,000 USP Units per mL (Rx) [*Liquaemin* (benzyl alcohol); GENERIC].

Derived from porcine intestinal mucosa: Without preservative

1000 USP Units per mL (Rx) [*Liquaemin;* GENERIC].

5000 USP Units per mL (Rx) [*Liquaemin;* GENERIC].

Note: Single unit-dose containers may also provide the quantities of heparin sodium listed above in volumes other than 1 mL.

Canada—

Derived from porcine intestinal mucosa: With preservative

1000 International Units (IU) per mL (Rx) [*Heparin Leo* (chlorobutanol)].

1000 USP Units per mL (Rx) [*Hepalean* (benzyl alcohol); GENERIC].

10,000 IU per mL (Rx) [*Heparin Leo* (chlorobutanol)].

10,000 USP Units per mL (Rx) [*Hepalean* (benzyl alcohol); GENERIC].

25,000 IU per mL (Rx) [*Heparin Leo* (in 2-mL containers; chlorobutanol)].

25,000 USP Units per mL (Rx) [*Hepalean* (in single-dose containers providing 5000 USP Units in 0.2 mL and in 2-mL containers; benzyl alcohol)].

Derived from porcine intestinal mucosa: Without preservative

1000 IU per mL (Rx) [*Heparin Leo*].

1000 USP Units per mL (Rx) [*Hepalean*].

10,000 IU per mL (Rx) [*Heparin Leo*].

25,000 IU per mL (Rx) [*Heparin Leo* (in single-dose containers providing 5000 IU in 0.2 mL)].

**Packaging and storage**

Store below 40 °C (104 °F), preferably between 15 and 30 °C (59 and 86 °F), unless otherwise specified by manufacturer. Protect from freezing.

**Stability**

Do not use if the solution is discolored or contains a precipitate. Some studies have indicated that loss of heparin activity may occur if heparin is diluted with 5% dextrose injection and the diluted solution is not used within 24 hours, or if diluted solutions of heparin in any diluent are stored in glass containers.

**Incompatibilities**

Heparin is strongly acidic and is incompatible with many solutions containing medications, although no loss of activity occurs when the agents are given via separate administration sites. Also, heparin may be incompatible with solutions containing a phosphate buffer, sodium carbonate, or sodium oxalate. It is recommended that heparin not be mixed, or administered through the same intravenous line, with other medications unless compatibility has first been established. In addition, heparin may be inactivated when used in conjunction with an artificial kidney because of an influx of calcium, magnesium, and acetate ions from the dialysate.

**Note**

When preparing the label, indicate the organ and species from which the heparin is derived.

**Additional information**

Heparin sodium injections that contain benzyl alcohol should not be administered to premature neonates because the preservative has been associated with a fatal "gasping syndrome" in these patients.

## HEPARIN SODIUM IN DEXTROSE INJECTION

**Usual adult dose**

Intravenous infusion, 20,000 to 40,000 USP Units, administered over a twenty-four-hour period. This dosage schedule is usually preceded by a loading dose of 35 to 70 USP Units per kg of body weight or 5000 USP Units, administered by intravenous injection. The infusion is often administered at a rate of 1000 USP Units per hour; however, dosage must be adjusted as determined by coagulation test results.

**Usual pediatric dose**

Intravenous infusion, 50 USP Units per kg of body weight as a loading dose initially, then 100 USP Units per kg of body weight added and absorbed every four hours or 20,000 USP Units per square meter of body surface every twenty-four hours, or as determined by coagulation test results..

**Strength(s) usually available**

U.S.—

Derived from porcine intestinal mucosa

20 USP Units per mL (10,000 USP Units per 500 mL), with 5% of dextrose (Rx) [GENERIC].

40 USP Units per mL (20,000 USP Units per 500 mL), with 5% of dextrose (Rx) [GENERIC].

50 USP Units per mL (12,500 USP Units per 250 mL and 25,000 USP Units per 500 mL), with 5% of dextrose (Rx) [GENERIC].

100 USP Units per mL (10,000 USP Units per 100 mL and 25,000 USP Units per 250 mL), with 5% of dextrose (Rx) [GENERIC].

Canada—

Derived from porcine intestinal mucosa

40 USP Units per mL (20,000 USP Units per 500 mL), with 5% of dextrose (Rx) [GENERIC].

**Packaging and storage**

Store below 40 °C (104 °F), preferably between 15 and 30 °C (59 and 86 °F), unless otherwise specified by manufacturer. Protect from freezing.

**Incompatibilities**

Heparin is strongly acidic and is incompatible with many solutions containing medications, although no loss of activity occurs when the agents are given via separate administration sites. Also, heparin may be incompatible with solutions containing a phosphate buffer, sodium carbonate, or sodium oxalate. It is recommended that heparin not be mixed, or administered through the same intravenous line, with other medications unless compatibility has first been established.

## HEPARIN SODIUM IN SODIUM CHLORIDE INJECTION

**Usual adult dose**

Intravenous infusion, 20,000 to 40,000 USP Units, administered over a twenty-four-hour period. This dosage schedule is usually preceded by a loading dose of 35 to 70 USP Units per kg of body weight or 5000 USP Units, administered by intravenous injection. The infusion is often administered at a rate of 1000 USP Units per hour; however, dosage must be adjusted as determined by coagulation test results.

**Usual pediatric dose**

Intravenous infusion, 50 USP Units per kg of body weight as a loading dose initially, then 100 USP Units per kg of body weight added and absorbed every four hours or 20,000 USP Units per square meter of body surface every twenty-four hours, or as determined by coagulation test results.

**Strength(s) usually available**

U.S.—

Derived from porcine intestinal mucosa

2 USP Units per mL (1000 USP Units per 500 mL and 2000 USP Units per mL (1000 mL), with 0.9% of sodium chloride (Rx) [GENERIC].

50 USP Units per mL (12,500 USP Units per 250 mL and 25,000 USP Units per 500 mL), with 0.45% of sodium chloride (Rx) [GENERIC].

100 USP Units per mL (25,000 USP Units per 250 mL), with 0.45% of sodium chloride (Rx) [GENERIC].

Canada—

Derived from porcine intestinal mucosa

2 USP Units per mL (1000 USP Units per 500 mL and 2000 USP Units per mL (1000 mL), with 0.9% of sodium chloride (Rx) [GENERIC].

5 USP Units per mL (5000 USP Units per 1000 mL), with 0.9% of sodium chloride (Rx) [GENERIC].

**Packaging and storage**

Store below 40 °C (104 °F), preferably between 15 and 30 °C (59 and 86 °F), unless otherwise specified by manufacturer. Protect from freezing.

**Incompatibilities**

Heparin is strongly acidic and is incompatible with many solutions containing medications, although no loss of activity occurs when the agents are given via separate administration sites. Also, heparin may be incompatible with solutions containing a phosphate buffer, sodium carbonate, or sodium oxalate. It is recommended that heparin not be mixed, or administered through the same intravenous line, with other medications unless compatibility has first been established.

Revised: August 1990
Interim revision: 08/23/94

---

# HEPATITIS B VACCINE RECOMBINANT    Systemic

**VA CLASSIFICATION (Primary): IM100**

Note: This monograph applies to the recombinant hepatitis B vaccine. The plasma-derived hepatitis B vaccine is no longer being produced in the U.S., and its availability is limited by the manufacturer to hemodialysis patients, other immunocompromised patients, and persons with a known allergy to yeast.

Recombinant hepatitis B vaccine has been shown to induce antibody to hepatitis B surface antigen (anti-HBs) that is biochemically and immunologically comparable to antibody induced by the plasma-derived hepatitis B vaccine. In addition, recommended doses of recombinant hepatitis B vaccine (*Recombivax HB*) and plasma-derived hepatitis B vaccine (*Heptavax-B*, MSD) have resulted in similar seroconversion rates in healthy adults.

In one study of 31 healthy adults immunized 5 to 7 years previously with plasma-derived hepatitis B vaccine (*Heptavax-B*, MSD), a single injection of the recommended dose of recombinant hepatitis B vaccine (*Recombivax HB*) induced significant anamnestic antibody responses in 97% of the subjects.

Based on the comparability of the plasma-derived and the recombinant hepatitis B vaccines, these 2 types of vaccine may be used interchangeably, with the precautions and dosages that pertain to each.

Another commonly used name is HB vaccine.

Note: For a listing of dosage forms and brand names by country availability, see *Dosage Forms* section(s). For a listing of brand names for the articles in this monograph, refer to the General Index.

---

## Category

Immunizing agent (active).

## Indications

**Accepted**

Hepatitis B virus (prophylaxis)—Hepatitis B recombinant vaccine is indicated for immunization of persons of all ages against infection caused by all subtypes of hepatitis B virus. The dialysis formulation of hepatitis B recombinant vaccine is indicated for immunization of adult predialysis and dialysis patients.

Hepatitis B recombinant vaccine is also recommended in conjunction with hepatitis B immune globulin (HBIG) for postexposure prophylaxis.

Unless otherwise contraindicated, hepatitis B recombinant vaccine is recommended for all infants (whether at high or low risk), adolescents, and persons of all ages who live in areas of high prevalence of hepatitis B infection or who are or will be at increased risk of infection from hepatitis B virus. Regarding the immunization of adolescents, the Immunization Practices Advisory Committee (ACIP) recommends immunization of adolescents who live in areas of high prevalence of hepatitis B infection; the American Academy of Pediatrics (AAP) recommends immunization of all adolescents with emphasis on adolescents who live in areas of high prevalence of hepatitis B infection. In areas with high prevalence of infection, most of the population is at risk of acquiring hepatitis B infection at a young age.

Examples of groups identified as being at increased risk of infection include:

• Infants born to hepatitis B surface antigen (HBsAg) positive mothers. Transmission of hepatitis B virus (HBV) from mother to infant during the perinatal period represents one of the most efficient modes of HBV infection and often leads to severe long-term consequences in these children. It is, therefore, recommended that all pregnant women be routinely tested for HBsAg.

• Health care personnel. HBV infection is a major infectious occupational hazard for health-care and public-safety workers. The risk of acquiring HBV infection from occupational exposures is dependent on the frequency of percutaneous and permucosal exposures to blood or blood products. Risk is often highest during the professional training period of medical personnel. Therefore, immunization should be completed during training in the schools of medicine, dentistry, nursing, laboratory technology, and other allied health professions before workers have their first contact with human blood.

• Employees in medical facilities, such as paramedical personnel and custodial staff, who may be exposed to the virus via blood, blood products, or other patient specimens.

• Patients and staff of institutions or residential settings for the developmentally disabled. Staff who work closely with patients, and the patients themselves, should be immunized. The risk in institutional environments is associated not only with blood exposure, but also with bites and contact with skin lesions and other infective secretions.

• Staff of nonresidential day-care programs for the developmentally disabled, such as schools and sheltered workshops. Staff who have clients who are HBV carriers are at a risk of HBV infection comparable to that among health-care workers. Although the risk of HBV infection to clients appears to be lower than the risk to staff, immunization of clients is recommended if a client who is an HBV carrier is aggressive or has special medical problems that increase the risk of exposure to his or her blood or serous secretions.

• Sexually active homosexual and bisexual males, including those with human immunodeficiency virus (HIV) infection. Sexually active homosexual males and bisexual males should be immunized regardless of their age or the duration of their homosexual practices. Males should be immunized as soon as possible after their homosexual activity begins or if they anticipate initiating homosexual activity in the future.

• Sexually active heterosexual persons with multiple sexual partners. Heterosexual persons with multiple sexual partners are at increased risk of HBV infection, the risk increasing with the number of sexual partners. Immunization is recommended for prostitutes, persons with a history of multiple sexual partners in the last 6 months, and persons who have recently or repeatedly acquired other sexually transmitted diseases.

• Hemodialysis patients. Although seroconversion rates and antibody to hepatitis B surface antigen (anti-HBs) titers are lower in hemodialysis patients than in healthy persons, for the patients who do respond, hepatitis B recombinant vaccine will protect them from HBV infection and reduce the need for frequent serologic screening.

• Patients with renal disease. Some studies have shown higher seroconversion rates and antibody titers for patients with uremia who were immunized before they required dialysis. Therefore, it is recommended that patients be immunized early in the course of their renal disease.

• Users of illicit injectable drugs. Injectable drug abusers should be immunized as soon as possible after their drug abuse begins.

• Patients with clotting disorders who receive clotting-factor concentrates. These patients are at increased risk of HBV infection and should be immunized at the time that their specific clotting disorder is identified. Preimmunization testing for HBsAg may be cost effective in patients who have already received multiple infusions of these blood products.

• Household and sexual contacts of HBV carriers. Household contacts of HBV carriers are at high risk, and sexual contacts appear to be at the greatest risk of HBV infection.

• Persons accepting orphans or adoptees from countries of high or intermediate HBV endemicity. The children should be tested for HBsAg. If the children are found to be positive, the adopting family members should be immunized.

• Populations with high endemicity of HBV infection, such as Alaskan Eskimos, Pacific Islanders, and refugees from HBV-endemic areas.

• Inmates of long-term correctional facilities.

• International travelers. Immunization should be considered for travelers who plan to reside abroad for more than 6 months and have close contact with the local population in areas with high levels of endemic HBV. Immunization should also be considered for short-term travelers who are likely to have sexual contact with, or contact with blood from, members of the local population of endemic areas.

• Military personnel identified as being at increased risk.

• Morticians and embalmers.

• Police and fire department personnel. Paramedical or other personnel who render first aid or medical assistance may be exposed to the hepatitis B virus.

Hepatitis D virus (prophylaxis)—Since hepatitis D infection (caused by the delta virus) can only occur in the presence of hepatitis B infection, it can be expected that hepatitis D infection will be prevented by immunization with hepatitis B recombinant vaccine.

### Unaccepted
Because this vaccine protects only against subtypes of hepatitis B virus (and indirectly against hepatitis D virus), immunization with hepatitis B recombinant vaccine is not an indication for, and will not provide protection against, hepatitis caused by other hepatitis viruses or by other viruses known to infect the liver.

## Pharmacology/Pharmacokinetics

### Physicochemical characteristics
Hepatitis B recombinant vaccines are produced from *Saccharomyces cerevisiae* (baker's yeast), into which a plasmid containing the gene for the hepatitis B surface antigen (HBsAg) has been inserted. Purified HBsAg is obtained by lysing the yeast cells and separating the HBsAg from the yeast components. These vaccines contain more than 95% HBsAg protein. Yeast-derived protein constitutes no more than 5% of the final product. Hepatitis B recombinant vaccines are adsorbed with aluminum hydroxide (0.5 mg per mL). No substances of human origin are used in their manufacture.

### Protective effect
An adequate antibody response to HBsAg is defined as greater than or equal to 10 milliInternational Units (mIU); 10 sample ratio units (SRU) by radioimmunoassay (RIA); or a positive result as determined by enzyme immunoassay (EIA).

The recommended series of 3 intramuscular doses of the vaccine (given at 0, 1, and 6 months) induces an adequate antibody response in more than 90% of healthy adults and in more than 95% of children from birth through 19 years of age.

### Duration of protective effect
The duration of protection and the need for booster doses are not yet fully defined. However, data show that vaccine-induced antibody levels decline steadily with time and that up to 50% of adults who develop adequate antibody initially will have low or undetectable antibody levels within 7 years; however, protection against viremic infection and clinical disease appears to persist.

Immunogenicity and efficacy of the vaccines among hemodialysis patients are much lower than among normal adults. Protection in this group may last only as long as detectable antibody levels persist.

## Precautions to Consider

### Cross-sensitivity and/or related problems
Patients sensitive to the plasma-derived hepatitis B vaccine may be sensitive to the recombinant vaccine also.

### Pregnancy/Reproduction
Pregnancy—Adequate and well-controlled studies have not been done in humans. Although data are not available on the safety of hepatitis B recombinant vaccine for the developing fetus, there should be no risk to the fetus, because the vaccine contains only noninfectious HBsAg particles. In contrast, hepatitis B infection in a pregnant female may result in severe disease in the mother and chronic infection in the newborn. Therefore, pregnancy should not be considered a contraindication to the use of hepatitis B recombinant vaccine in females for whom the vaccine is otherwise indicated.

Studies have not been done in animals.

FDA Pregnancy Category C.

### Breast-feeding
It is not known whether the vaccine is distributed into breast milk. However, problems in humans have not beeen documented.

Although data are not available, there should be no risk to breast-fed infants, because the vaccine contains only noninfectious HBsAg particles.

### Pediatrics
Hepatitis B recombinant vaccine has been shown to be well tolerated and highly immunogenic in infants and children of all ages. Newborns also respond well, and maternally transferred antibodies do not interfere with the active immune response to the vaccine. No published pediatrics-specific information is available for the dialysis formulation of hepatitis B recombinant vaccine. Safety and efficacy have not been established.

### Geriatrics
Studies have shown that the adult response to hepatitis B vaccine is inversely related to age: more than 90% in young adults, 70% in persons 50 to 59 years of age, and 50 to 70% in persons 60 years of age and over. Other geriatrics-specific problems that would limit the usefulness of this medication in the elderly are not expected.

### Drug interactions and/or related problems
The following drug interactions and/or related problems have been selected on the basis of their potential clinical significance (possible mechanism in parentheses where appropriate)—not necessarily inclusive (» = major clinical significance):

Note: Combinations containing any of the following medications, depending on the amount present, may also interact with this medication.

Immunosuppressive agents or
Radiation therapy
(because normal defense mechanisms are suppressed, the patient's antibody response to hepatitis B recombinant vaccine may be decreased. Larger vaccine doses [2 to 4 times normal adult dose] or an increased number of doses [4 doses] may be required to induce protective antibody in immunocompromised persons)

### Laboratory value alterations
The following have been selected on the basis of their potential clinical significance (possible effect in parentheses where appropriate)—not necessarily inclusive (» = major clinical significance):

With physiology/laboratory test values
Erythrocyte sedimentation (SED) rate
(may be increased)

### Medical considerations/Contraindications
The medical considerations/contraindications included here have been selected on the basis of their potential clinical significance (reasons given in parentheses where appropriate)—not necessarily inclusive (» = major clinical significance).

*Risk-benefit should be considered when the following medical problems exist:*

Allergy to yeast
(hepatitis B recombinant vaccine is produced by using baker's yeast; up to a maximum of 1 or 5%, depending on the manufacturer, of yeast-derived protein may be present in the final vaccine; although there have not been any proven allergic reactions to the yeast, the possibility that they may occur exists)

Cardiopulmonary status, severely compromised
(a febrile or systemic reaction to the vaccine could pose a significant risk to persons with this condition)

Illness, moderate or severe, with or without a fever
(administration of the vaccine should be delayed except when withholding the vaccine entails a greater risk to the patient than a possible superimposed reaction to the vaccine)

Immune deficiency condition
(antibody response to hepatitis B recombinant vaccine may be decreased; larger vaccine doses [2 to 4 times normal adult dose] or an increased number of doses [4 doses] may be required to induce protective antibody in immunocompromised persons)

Sensitivity to hepatitis B recombinant vaccine

## Side/Adverse Effects

Note: Cases of Guillain-Barre syndrome following administration of the recombinant hepatitis B vaccine have been reported, but their relationship to the vaccine is unclear. However, for the plasma-derived hepatitis B vaccine, postvaccination surveillance has shown an association of borderline significance between the Guillain-Barre syndrome and receipt of the first dose. The rate of this occurrence was very low (0.5 per 100,000 vaccine recipients).

Agitation, conjunctivitis, constipation, erythrocyte sedimentation rate increase, hepatic enzymes elevation, herpes zoster, hypesthesia, irritability, keratitis, migraine, myelitis, petechiae, radiculopathy, somnolence, Stevens-Johnson Syndrome, syncope, tachycardia, thrombocytopenia, tinnitus, and visual disturbances also have been reported in temporal association with administration of recombinant hepatitis B vaccine, but their relationship to the vaccine is unclear.

The following side/adverse effects have been selected on the basis of their potential clinical significance (possible signs and symptoms in parentheses where appropriate)—not necessarily inclusive:

**Those indicating need for medical attention**
Incidence rare
  *Anaphylactic reaction* (difficulty in breathing or swallowing; hives; itching, especially of soles or palms; reddening of skin, especially around ears; swelling of eyes, face, or inside of nose; unusual tiredness or weakness, sudden and severe); *neuropathy* (muscle weakness or numbness or tingling of limbs); *optic neuritis* (blurred vision or other vision changes); *serum sickness–like reaction* (aches or pain in joints, fever, or skin rash or welts)—may occur days to weeks following administration of the vaccine

**Those indicating need for medical attention only if they continue or are bothersome**
Incidence more frequent
  *Soreness at injection site*—20 to 30%
Incidence less frequent (1 to 10% frequency)
  *Fatigue* (unusual tiredness or weakness); *fever 37.7 °C (100 °F) or over; headache; induration* (hard lump); *erythema* (redness); *swelling; pain; pruritus* (itching); *ecchymosis* (purple spot); *tenderness; or warmth at injection site; vertigo* (dizziness)
Incidence rare (less than 1% frequency)
  *Anorexia* (lack of appetite); *or decreased appetite; arthralgia, arthritis, or myalgia* (aches or pain in joints or muscles); *back pain; chills; diarrhea or abdominal cramps or pain* (stomach pain); *flushing* (sudden redness of skin); *hypotension* (unusual tiredness or weakness); *increased sweating; influenza-like symptoms or upper respiratory tract illness* (headache, sore throat, runny nose, or fever); *insomnia or sleep disturbance* (trouble in sleeping); *lymphadenopathy* (swelling of glands in armpit or neck); *malaise* (feeling of bodily discomfort); *nausea or vomiting; nodule at injection site* (lump)—probably from the aluminum content of the vaccine; may persist for a few weeks; *pruritus* (itching); *urticaria* (welts); *or skin rash; stiffness or pain in neck or shoulder*

## Patient Consultation

As an aid to patient consultation, refer to *Advice for the Patient, Hepatitis B Vaccine Recombinant (Systemic)*.

In providing consultation, consider emphasizing the following selected information (» = major clinical significance):

**Before using this medication**
» Conditions affecting use, especially:
    Sensitivity to plasma-derived hepatitis B vaccine or recombinant hepatitis B vaccine or allergy to baker's yeast
    Use in the elderly—Compared with younger adults, persons over 50 years of age may be less likely to develop a protective antibody level following immunization with hepatitis B recombinant vaccine

**Proper use of this medication**
» Proper dosing

**Side/adverse effects**
    Signs of potential side effects, especially anaphylactic reaction, neuropathy, optic neuritis, or serum sickness–like reaction

## General Dosing Information

Only persons who have not been infected with hepatitis B virus (HBV) previously need to be immunized with hepatitis B recombinant vaccine. Therefore, as a cost-effective measure, testing for prior HBV infection should be considered for adults in groups having a high prevalence of HBV infection (e.g., injecting drug users, homosexual men, and household contacts of HBV carriers). If the group to be tested is also expected to have a high prevalence of carriers, it may be preferable to test for antibody to hepatitis B core antigen (anti-HBc), since this test identifies previously infected persons, both carriers and noncarriers. If the group to be tested is not expected to have a high rate of carriers, the test for antibody to hepatitis B surface antigen (anti-

HBs) will be adequate, since this test identifies previously infected persons, except for carriers.

For persons who already possess antibodies against HBV from a previous infection, immunization is neither necessary nor harmful. Such persons will have a postimmunization increase in their anti-HBs levels.

For HBV carriers, hepatitis B recombinant vaccine is neither necessary nor harmful.

Although the dosages are different for the products of different manufacturers, the resulting immunogenicity of each is comparable. An immunization schedule started with one manufacturer's vaccine and dose may be completed with the other manufacturer's vaccine and dose.

Because of the long incubation period of hepatitis B virus (HBV), unrecognized infection may be present at the time of immunization; the vaccine may not prevent hepatitis B in already infected patients.

Passively acquired antibody, whether from administration of immune globulins or from the transplacental route, will not interfere with active immunization with hepatitis B recombinant vaccine. In addition, there is no interference with the induction of protective antibodies elicited by hepatitis B recombinant vaccine when hepatitis B immune globulin (HBIG) is administered at the same time at different body sites.

Neonates born to hepatitis B surface antigen (HBsAg) positive mothers should receive HBIG within 12 hours after birth. In addition, immunization with the appropriate dosage of hepatitis B recombinant vaccine should be initiated. If hepatitis B recombinant vaccine and HBIG are administered at the same time, they should be administered in opposite anterolateral thighs.

If within 7 days of delivery a mother of unknown HBsAg status is determined to be HBsAg positive, the infant should receive HBIG immediately. In addition, immunization with the appropriate dosage of hepatitis B recombinant vaccine should be initiated or continued. If hepatitis B recombinant vaccine and HBIG are administered at the same time, they should be administered in opposite anterolateral thighs. If a mother of unknown HBsAg status is determined not to be HBsAg positive, the infant should complete the immunization series with the appropriate dosage of hepatitis B recombinant vaccine.

For known or presumed exposure to the hepatitis B virus, HBIG should be administered according to its directions as soon as possible after exposure and within 24 hours if possible. (HBIG's value if given later than 7 days after exposure is unclear; in addition, the period after sexual exposure to HBV during which HBIG is effective is unknown, but extrapolation from other data suggests that this period would not exceed 14 days.) In addition, hepatitis B recombinant vaccine should be administered at a separate body site, using one of the following dosage schedules and the dosage that applies to it:
• If using *Recombivax HB*—At the same time as HBIG or within 7 days after exposure, then 1 month and 6 months after the first dose, for a total of 3 doses.
• If using *Engerix-B*—
  —At the same time as HBIG or within 7 days after exposure, then 1 month and 6 months after the first dose, for a total of 3 doses.
  —Alternatively, at the same time as HBIG or within 7 days after exposure, then 1 month, 2 months, and 12 months after the first dose, for a total of 4 doses.

  If the exposed person has begun, but not completed, immunization with hepatitis B recombinant vaccine, HBIG should be given as usual, and immunization with the vaccine should be completed as scheduled.

For travelers: Ideally, immunization with hepatitis B recombinant vaccine should begin at least 6 months before travel to allow completion of the full 3-dose vaccine series (given at 0, 1, and 6 months). However, if 6 months of time before travel is not available, the first 3 doses of an alternative 4-dose schedule (given at 0, 1, 2, and 12 months) may provide earlier protection during travel if they can be delivered before travel begins.

Although the alternative 4-dose schedule (given at 0, 1, 2, and 12 months) (*Engerix-B*) provides a more rapid induction of immunity, there is no clear evidence that this schedule provides greater long-term protection than the standard 3-dose schedule (given at 0, 1, and 6 months).

Vaccine doses administered at longer-than-recommended intervals (recommended intervals being 0, 1, and 6 months) provide equally satisfactory protection. However, optimal protection is not conferred until after the third dose. If the vaccine series is interrupted after the first dose, the second dose should be given as soon as possible, followed by the third dose 3 to 5 months later. Persons who are late for the third dose should be given this dose as soon as practical. In healthy persons, it is not considered necessary to do postvaccination testing to ensure an adequate antibody response in either of the above situations.

When sterilizing syringes and skin before vaccination, care should be taken to avoid contact of the vaccine with preservatives, antiseptics, detergents, and disinfectants, since the vaccine virus particles may be easily denatured by these substances.

The hepatitis B recombinant vaccine should be administered by intramuscular (IM) injection. The needle should be of sufficient length and bore to reach the muscle mass itself and to prevent vaccine from seeping into subcutaneous tissue. For adults, the suggested needle length is 1½ inches. For children, a 20- or 22-gauge needle 1 to 1¼ inches long is recommended. For small infants, a 25-gauge needle 5/8 inch long may be adequate. However, for persons at risk of hemorrhage following IM injections, the vaccine may be administered subcutaneously, although the subsequent antibody titer may be lower and there may be an increased risk of local reactions. The vaccine should not be administered intravenously or intradermally.

The deltoid muscle (outer aspect of the upper arm) is the recommended site for the immunization of adults and older children. For infants and young children, the anterolateral thigh muscle is the recommended site. The vaccine should not be administered in the gluteal region (buttock), because the immunogenicity of the vaccine is substantially lower.

The 40 mcg/mL strength (*Recombivax HB Dialysis Formulation*) is intended only for adult predialysis and dialysis patients; the 20 mcg/mL strength (*Engerix-B*) may be used for either adult predialysis and dialysis patients or for regular immunizations; the lower strengths are not intended for adult predialysis and dialysis patients.

Larger vaccine doses (2 to 4 times normal adult dose) or an increased number of doses (4 doses) may be necessary for immunocompromised persons (such as those on immunosuppressive drugs or with human immunodeficiency virus [HIV] infection). However, although persons with HIV infection have an impaired response to hepatitis B recombinant vaccine, the immunogenicity of higher doses of the vaccine is unknown in these persons and specific recommendations on dosage are not available.

Although postimmunization testing for serologic response and immunity is not routinely recommended, it is recommended for the following:
• Persons whose subsequent management depends on knowledge of their immune status, such as dialysis patients, medical staff, and infants born to HBsAg positive mothers.
• Persons in whom a less than optimal response may be anticipated, such as those who were administered the vaccine in the buttock or subcutaneously, persons over 50 years of age, and persons with HIV infection or other immune deficiencies.
• Persons at occupational risk who may have hepatitis B virus exposures necessitating postexposure prophylaxis.
Postimmunization testing should be done 1 to 6 months after completion of the immunization series to provide definitive information on the response to the vaccine.
Reimmunization of persons who did not originally respond to the primary series produces adequate antibody in 15 to 25% after 1 additional dose and in 30 to 50% after 3 additional doses, when the original immunization was administered in the deltoid. For persons who did not adequately respond to a primary vaccine series given in the buttock, data suggest that reimmunization in the arm induces adequate antibody in greater than 75%.

In adult predialysis and dialysis patients, hepatitis B recombinant vaccine-induced protection is less complete and may persist only as long as antibody levels remain at or above 10 milliInternational Units (mIU) per mL. The need for additional doses of the vaccine should be assessed by annual antibody testing. It is recommended that additional doses of 40 mcg of hepatitis B recombinant vaccine be given when antibody levels decline below 10 mIU per mL.

Hepatitis B recombinant vaccine, an inactivated product, can be administered concurrently with the following, using separate body sites (in infants, selecting separate sites in the same anterolateral thigh muscle is preferable to administering hepatitis B recombinant vaccine in the buttock or deltoid muscle), separate syringes (for parenterals), and the precautions that apply to each immunizing agent:
• Polysaccharide vaccines, such as haemophilus b polysaccharide vaccine, haemophilus b conjugate vaccine, meningococcal polysaccharide vaccine, or pneumococcal polyvalent vaccine.
• Influenza vaccine, whole or split virus.
• Diphtheria toxoid, tetanus toxoid, and/or pertussis (whole cell or acellular) vaccine.
• Live virus vaccines, such as measles, mumps, and/or rubella vaccines.
• Poliovirus vaccines (oral [OPV], inactivated [IPV], or enhanced-potency inactivated [enhanced-potency IPV]).
• Immune globulin and disease-specific immune globulins.
• Inactivated vaccines, other, except cholera, typhoid (parenteral), and plague. It is recommended that cholera, typhoid (parenteral), and

plague vaccines be administered on separate occasions because of these vaccines' propensity to cause side/adverse effects.

**For treatment of adverse effects**

Recommended treatment includes:
• For mild hypersensitivity reaction—Administering antihistamines, and, if necessary, corticosteroids.
• For severe hypersensitivity or anaphylactic reaction—Administering epinephrine. Antihistamines or corticosteroids may also be administered as required.

# Parenteral Dosage Forms

## STERILE HEPATITIS B VACCINE RECOMBINANT SUSPENSION

### Usual adult and adolescent dose

Immunizing agent (active)—
Adolescents 11 to 20 years of age: Intramuscular, into the deltoid, 5 mcg (*Recombivax HB*—U.S. and Canada) or 20 mcg (*Engerix-B*—U.S. and Canada), at initial visit, then one month and six months after the first dose, for a total of three doses.
Adults 20 years of age and older: Intramuscular, into the deltoid, 10 mcg (*Recombivax HB*—U.S. and Canada) or 20 mcg (*Engerix-B*—U.S. and Canada), at initial visit, then one month and six months after the first dose, for a total of three doses.
Adult predialysis and dialysis patients—Intramuscular, into the deltoid
40 mcg (*Recombivax HB Dialysis Formulation*—U.S. and Canada), at initial visit, then one month and six months after the first dose, for a total of three doses.
Or;
40 mcg (*Engerix-B*—U.S. and Canada), at initial visit, then one month, two months, and six months after the first dose, for a total of four doses. The dose may be given as two injections of 20 mcg/mL each and administered at separate body sites or as one injection of 40 mcg/2 mL.

### Usual pediatric dose

Immunizing agent (active)—
Neonates born to hepatitis B surface antigen (HBsAg) positive mothers—Intramuscular, into the anterolateral thigh:
5 mcg (*Recombivax HB*—U.S. and Canada), 10 mcg (*Engerix-B*—U.S.), or 20 mcg (*Engerix-B*—Canada), within twelve hours after birth (preferably) or within seven days after birth, then one month and six months after the first dose, for a total of three doses.
Or;
10 mcg (*Engerix-B*—U.S.) or 20 mcg (*Engerix-B*—Canada), within twelve hours after birth (preferably) or within seven days after birth, then one month, two months, and twelve months after the first dose, for a total of four doses.
Neonates born to mothers of unknown HBsAg status—Intramuscular, into the anterolateral thigh:
5 mcg (*Recombivax HB*—U.S.), 10 mcg (*Engerix-B*—U.S.), or 20 mcg (*Engerix-B*—Canada), within twelve hours after birth (preferably) or within seven days after birth, then:
Infants of mothers subsequently determined to be HBsAg positive:
5 mcg (*Recombivax HB*—U.S.), 10 mcg (*Engerix-B*—U.S.), or 20 mcg (*Engerix-B*—Canada), one month and six months after the first dose, for a total of three doses.
Or;
10 mcg (*Engerix-B*—U.S.) or 20 mcg (*Engerix-B*—Canada), one month, two months, and twelve months after the first dose, for a total of four doses.
Infants of mothers subsequently determined to be HBsAg negative:
2.5 mcg (*Recombivax HB*—U.S.), 10 mcg (*Engerix-B*—U.S.), or 20 mcg (*Engerix-B*—Canada), one month and six months after the first dose, for a total of three doses.
Neonates born to HBsAg negative mothers; or
Infants and children up to 11 years of age: Intramuscular, into the anterolateral thigh for neonates, infants, and young children and into the deltoid for older children, 2.5 mcg (*Recombivax HB*—U.S. and Canada), 10 mcg (*Engerix-B*—U.S.), or 20 mcg (*Engerix-B*—Canada), at initial visit, then one month and six months after the first dose, for a total of three doses.

### Strength(s) usually available

U.S.—
2.5 mcg (0.0025 mg) of hepatitis B surface antigen (HBsAg) protein per 0.5 mL (Rx) [*Recombivax HB* (0.25 mg aluminum as aluminum hydroxide; thimerosal 1:20,000)].

5 mcg (0.005 mg) of HBsAg protein per 0.5 mL (Rx) [*Recombivax HB* (0.25 mg aluminum as aluminum hydroxide; thimerosal 1: 20,000)].

10 mcg (0.01 mg) of HBsAg protein per mL (Rx) [*Recombivax HB* (0.5 mg aluminum as aluminum hydroxide; thimerosal 1:20,000)].

10 mcg (0.01 mg) of HBsAg protein per 0.5 mL (Rx) [*Engerix-B* (0.25 mg aluminum as aluminum hydroxide; thimerosal 1:20,000)].

20 mcg (0.02 mg) of HBsAg protein per mL (Rx) [*Engerix-B* (0.5 mg aluminum as aluminum hydroxide; thimerosal 1:20,000)].

40 mcg (0.04 mg) of HBsAg protein per mL (Rx) [*Recombivax HB Dialysis Formulation* (0.5 mg aluminum as aluminum hydroxide; thimerosal 1:20,000)].

Canada—

5 mcg (0.005 mg) of HBsAg protein per 0.5 mL (Rx) [*Recombivax HB* (alum adjuvant; thimerosal 1:20,000)].

10 mcg (0.01 mg) of HBsAg protein per mL (Rx) [*Recombivax HB* (alum adjuvant; thimerosal 1:20,000)].

20 mcg (0.02 mg) of HBsAg protein per mL (Rx) [*Engerix-B* (0.5 mg aluminum as aluminum hydroxide; thimerosal 1:20,000)].

40 mcg (0.04 mg) of HBsAg protein per mL (Rx) [*Recombivax HB Dialysis Formulation* (thimerosal 1:20,000)].

### Packaging and storage

Store between 2 and 8 °C (36 and 46 °F), unless otherwise specified by manufacturer. Protect from freezing.

### Preparation of dosage form

The vaccine should be used as supplied, and should not be diluted. The vial should be shaken well immediately before withdrawal of the dose.

In addition, thorough agitation at the time of administration is necessary to maintain suspension of the vaccine. After agitation, the vaccine is a slightly opaque, white suspension.

### Stability

Storage above or below the recommended temperature may reduce potency. Freezing destroys potency, and the vaccine should be discarded if freezing occurs.

### Auxiliary labeling

• Do not freeze; discard if freezing occurs.
• Shake well.

### Selected Bibliography

Centers for Disease Control. Hepatitis B virus: a comprehensive strategy for eliminating transmission in the United States through universal childhood vaccination: recommendations of the Immunization Practices Advisory Committee (ACIP). MMWR 1991 Nov 22; 40 (RR-13): 1-25.

Centers for Disease Control. Update on adult immunization: recommendations of the Immunization Practices Advisory Committee (ACIP). MMWR 1991 Nov 15; 40 (RR-12).

Committee on Infectious Diseases. Universal hepatitis B immunization. Pediatrics 1992 Apr; 89 (4): 795.

Revised: 02/23/94

---

# HISTAMINE   Systemic*

VA CLASSIFICATION (Primary): DX900

Note: For a listing of dosage forms and brand names by country availability, see *Dosage Forms* section(s). For a listing of brand names for the articles in this monograph, refer to the General Index.

*Not commercially available in the U.S.

## Category

Diagnostic aid (gastric function).

## Indications

### Accepted

Anacidity (diagnosis) or

Gastric histamine test or

Hypersecretory conditions, gastric (diagnosis)—Histamine phosphate is indicated as a diagnostic aid for evaluation of gastric acid secretory function. Anacidity (achlorhydria) in response to histamine may indicate pernicious anemia, atrophic gastritis, adenomatous polyps of stomach, or gastric carcinoma. Gastric hypersecretion in response to histamine may indicate duodenal ulcer or the Zollinger-Ellison syndrome. Use of this diagnostic aid for evaluation of gastric acid secretory function has generally been replaced by the pentagastrin test.

### Unaccepted

Histamine phosphate has been used for the presumptive diagnosis of pheochromocytoma; however, the use of histamine in patients suspected of having pheochromocytoma is hazardous and unwarranted due to the risk of precipitating a hypertensive crisis. Other tests, such as fluorometric measurements of unconjugated catecholamines, spectrophotometric measurement of total metanephrines, vanillylmandelic acid (VMA) in urine collections, or plasma catecholamine measurements, provide a safer alternative in the diagnosis of pheochromocytoma.

Histamine phosphate has been used to produce short-term improvement in patients with vertigo, tinnitus, and deafness. However, it has not been proven effective in the symptomatic treatment of Menière's disease.

Also, histamine phosphate has not been proven effective as a desensitizing agent in allergic diseases.

## Pharmacology/Pharmacokinetics

### Physicochemical characteristics

Molecular weight—307.14.

### Mechanism of action/Effect

Diagnostic aid (gastric function)—Histamine stimulates gastric gland secretion, causing an increased secretion of gastric juice of high acidity.

This action is probably due mainly to a direct action on parietal and chief gland cells.

### Other actions/effects

Histamine acts directly on the blood vessels to dilate arteries and capillaries; this action is apparently mediated by both $H_1$- and $H_2$-receptors. Capillary dilatation may produce flushing of the face, a decrease in systemic blood pressure, and an increase in skin temperature. Increased capillary permeability accompanies capillary dilatation, producing an outward passage of plasma protein and fluid into the extracellular spaces, an increase in lymph flow and protein content, and the formation of edema. Histamine increases rate and force of myocardial contraction as well as increasing cardiac output; it also tends to slow A-V conduction and (in large concentrations) may cause arrhythmias. Histamine also has a stimulant effect on chromaffin cells in the adrenal medulla or other extra-adrenal tissue, which causes the release of epinephrine and norepinephrine. In addition, histamine has a direct stimulant action on smooth muscle, producing contraction if $H_1$-receptors are activated, or mostly relaxation if $H_2$-receptors are activated. Smooth muscle response varies considerably among the different species. In humans, bronchoconstriction is more pronounced in patients with bronchial asthma, emphysema, or bronchitis. Also in humans, the stimulant effect of histamine may cause contraction of the intestinal muscle. However, little effect is noticed on the uterus, bladder, or gallbladder. Histamine has some stimulant effect on duodenal, salivary, pancreatic, bronchial, and lacrimal glands, but the effect of histamine on these glands is not clinically important.

### Absorption

Readily absorbed after parenteral administration.

### Distribution

Rapid diffusion into body tissues. The mast cell is the primary storage site for histamine in most tissues.

### Biotransformation

Primarily hepatic. Histamine is rapidly metabolized by methylation and oxidation. Methylation involves ring methylation and catalyzation by the enzyme histamine-N-methyltransferase, producing N-methylhistamine, which is mostly converted to N-methyl imidazole acetic acid. Oxidative deamination produces imidazole acetic acid and its riboside. Metabolites produced have no significant pharmacologic activity.

### Onset of action

Rapid after subcutaneous or intramuscular administration.

### Duration of action

Transient.

# Precautions to Consider

## Pregnancy/Reproduction
Pregnancy—Studies have not been done in humans.
Studies have not been done in animals.

## Breast-feeding
It is not known whether histamine is distributed into breast milk. However, problems in humans have not been documented.

## Pediatrics
Appropriate studies on the relationship of age to the effects of histamine have not been performed in the pediatric population. Safety and efficacy have not been established.

## Geriatrics
Appropriate studies on the relationship of age to the effects of histamine have not been performed in the geriatric population. No geriatrics-specific problems have been documented to date with the use of the gastric histamine test. However, elderly patients are more likely to have age-related renal function impairment, which may require careful monitoring in patients receiving histamine.

## Drug interactions and/or related problems
See *Diagnostic interference.*

## Diagnostic interference
The following have been selected on the basis of their potential clinical significance (possible effect in parentheses where appropriate)—not necessarily inclusive (» = major clinical significance):

With results of *this* test
*Due to other medications*
»  Antacids
     (administration on the morning of the test may decrease the total effect of histamine on gastric acidity and output)
»  Anticholinergics or other medications with anticholinergic activity
     (See *Appendix II*) or
»  Histamine H$_2$-receptor antagonists, such as cimetidine, famotidine, nizatidine, ranitidine
     (concurrent use may antagonize the effect of histamine on gastric secretion; administration of these medications is not recommended during the 24 hours preceding the test)
»  Omeprazole
     (concurrent use may antagonize the effect of histamine on gastric acid secretion; administration of omeprazole is not recommended during the 96 hours preceding the test)

## Medical considerations/Contraindications
The medical considerations/contraindications included here have been selected on the basis of their potential clinical significance (reasons given in parentheses where appropriate)—not necessarily inclusive (» = major clinical significance):

*Except under special circumstances, this medication should not be used when the following medical problems exist:*
»  Cardiac disease, severe
     (may be aggravated due to histamine-induced cardiovascular effects)
»  Hypertension, severe or
»  Hypotension or
»  Vasomotor instability
     (may be exacerbated)
»  Pheochromocytoma
     (irreversible vascular and cerebral damage may be produced by prolonged paroxysms of hypertension)
»  Respiratory disease, especially bronchial disease, or history of
     (bronchial constriction induced by histamine may precipitate severe asthma attack)

*Risk-benefit should be considered when the following medical problems exist:*
     Cardiac disease or abnormality
         (condition may be exacerbated)
»    Renal function impairment, severe
         (may decrease excretion of histamine)

## Patient monitoring
The following may be especially important in patient monitoring (other tests may be warranted in some patients, depending on condition; » = major clinical significance):

     Blood pressure determination and
     Pulse rate determination
         (recommended frequently during and/or immediately following administration of histamine)

# Side/Adverse Effects
The following side/adverse effects have been selected on the basis of their potential clinical significance (possible signs and symptoms in parentheses where appropriate)—not necessarily inclusive:

## Those indicating need for medical attention
Incidence more frequent
     *Dilatation of cerebral vessels* (continuing or severe headache); *hypertension* (dizziness, continuing or severe headache); *hypotension* (dizziness, lightheadedness, or fainting); *nervousness; tachycardia* (fast or pounding heartbeat)

     Note: The above side effects may occur with average or large doses.

Incidence less frequent or rare
     *Difficulty in breathing; flushing or redness of face; seizures*
*With large doses*
     *Bluish coloration of face; blurred vision; chest discomfort or pain; decrease in blood pressure, sudden; diarrhea, severe; difficulty in breathing, severe; flushing or redness of face; nausea and vomiting, severe*

## Those indicating need for medical attention only if they continue or are bothersome
Incidence more frequent
     *Abdominal or stomach spasms or cramps; diarrhea; gastrointestinal effects resembling symptoms of peptic ulcer due to increased acid secretion* (nausea or vomiting, stomach pain); *metallic taste; swelling or redness at injection site*—with subcutaneous administration

     Note: With subcutaneous administration, *swelling or redness at injection site* is a characteristic intracutaneous effect of histamine known as the triple response. Involves erythema from capillary dilatation, wheal due to local edema from increased capillary permeability, and a flare from a neuronal reflex mechanism producing a surrounding area of arteriolar vasodilatation.

# Overdose
For specific information on the agents used in the management of histamine overdose, see:
     • *Antihistamines (Systemic)* monograph;
     *Epinephrine* in *Sympathomimetic Agents—Cardiovascular Use (Parenteral Systemic)* monograph; and/or
     • *Histamine H$_2$-receptor Antagonists (Systemic)* monograph.

For more information on the management of overdose or unintentional ingestion, **contact a Poison Control Center** (see *Poison Control Center Listing*).

## Treatment of overdose
Recommended treatment consists of the following:
     Specific treatment—
         Applying a temporary tourniquet near the injection site to slow down the absorption of histamine.
         Administering 0.3 to 0.5 mL of epinephrine hydrochloride injection (1:1000) subcutaneously to treat hypotension, repeating every 20 minutes for two doses as needed. Legs of patient should be raised.
         Administering antihistamines (H$_1$- and H$_2$-receptor blockers).
     Supportive care—
         Maintaining an adequate airway, with assisted respiration and administration of oxygen as needed. Patients in whom intentional overdose is confirmed or suspected should be referred for psychiatric consultation.

# Patient Consultation
As an aid to patient consultation, refer to *Advice for the Patient, Histamine (Diagnostic).*

In providing consultation, consider emphasizing the following selected information (» = major clinical significance):

## Description of use
Test procedure for gastric histamine test: Possible administration of an antihistamine prior to test. Stomach contents emptied through stomach tube before administration of histamine; dose of histamine, based on body weight, is then injected subcutaneously; 5 minutes after injection, stomach contents emptied and tested for volume and acidity; stomach emptying and testing repeated every 15 minutes up to total of 4 times

## Before having this test
»  Conditions affecting use, especially:
     Other medications, especially antacids, anticholinergics, histamine H$_2$-receptor antagonists, or omeprazole

mine, based on body weight, is then injected subcutaneously; 5 minutes after injection, stomach contents emptied and tested for volume and acidity; stomach emptying and testing repeated every 15 minutes up to total of 4 times

### Before having this test
» Conditions affecting use, especially:
Other medications, especially antacids, anticholinergics, histamine H₂-receptor antagonists, or omeprazole
Other medical problems, especially severe cardiac disease, severe hypertension, hypotension, pheochromocytoma, severe renal function impairment, respiratory disease, urticaria, or vasomotor instability

### Preparation for this test
» Importance of following physician's instructions about not taking certain medications before the histamine test
» Fasting for 12 hours before histamine test is administered

### Precautions during administration of this test
» Not swallowing saliva during administration of test

### Side/adverse effects
Signs of potential side effects, especially, dilatation of cerebral vessels, difficulty in breathing, flushing or redness of face, hypertension, hypotension, nervousness, seizures, and tachycardia ＼

## General Dosing Information

No food should be ingested for 12 hours before the administration of the gastric histamine test.

Care should be taken to prevent the patient from swallowing salivary secretions. The alkalinity of the saliva may interfere with the test results.

During and after the administration of histamine, epinephrine hydrochloride should be available in case of a severe hypotensive reaction.

The test is performed after the patient has rested in bed under standard basal conditions. Fasting gastric contents are then aspirated through a stomach tube. Histamine is administered subcutaneously, and 5 minutes afterwards gastric contents are collected and tested for volume, acidity, pH, and acid output. Stomach emptying and testing are repeated every 15 minutes until 4 collections have been made. If no

acidity is detected, a maximum histamine stimulation test can be performed.

For the augmented histamine test, an appropriate dose of antihistamine (e.g., 10 mg of chlorpheniramine maleate, 50 mg of diphenhydramine hydrochloride, or 50 mg of pyrilamine maleate) is administered intramuscularly prior to the basal secretion study. After the basal study is completed, histamine is administered subcutaneously.

Pulse rate and blood pressure should be determined immediately after histamine injection.

## Parenteral Dosage Forms

### HISTAMINE PHOSPHATE INJECTION USP

**Usual adult and adolescent dose**
Diagnostic aid (gastric function)—
Subcutaneous, 500 to 750 mcg, administered after collection of basal gastric secretion.

Note: If no acidity is detected, a maximum histamine stimulation test can be performed using 40 mcg per kg of body weight subcutaneously, administered after basal secretion study.

For augmented histamine test: Subcutaneous, 40 mcg of histamine phosphate per kg of body weight, administered after basal secretion study.

**Usual pediatric dose**
Safety and efficacy have not been established.

**Usual geriatric dose**
See *Usual adult and adolescent dose*.

**Strength(s) usually available**
U.S.—
Not commercially available.
Canada—
1 mg (0.36 mg base) (Rx) [GENERIC].

**Packaging and storage**
Store below 40 °C (104 °F), preferably between 15 and 30 °C (59 and 86 °F), unless otherwise specified by manufacturer. Protect from freezing.

Revised: 06/02/93
Interim revision: 06/23/94

# HISTAMINE H₂-RECEPTOR ANTAGONISTS  Systemic

This monograph includes information on the following: Cimetidine; Famotidine; Nizatidine; Ranitidine.

VA CLASSIFICATION (Primary/Secondary):
Cimetidine—GA301/DE890
Famotidine—GA301
Nizatidine—GA301
Ranitidine—GA301

Note: For a listing of dosage forms and brand names by country availability, see *Dosage Forms* section(s). For a listing of brand names for the articles in this monograph, refer to the General Index.

## Category

Histamine H₂-receptor antagonist—All drugs in this monograph are used as histamine H₂-receptor antagonists.
Antiulcer agent—All drugs in this monograph are used as antiulcer agents.
Gastric acid secretion inhibitor—All drugs in this monograph are used as gastric acid secretion inhibitors.
Urticaria therapy adjunct—Cimetidine.

## Indications

Note: Bracketed information in the *Indications* section refers to uses that are not included in U.S. product labeling.

### Accepted
Ulcer, duodenal (prophylaxis and treatment)—Histamine H₂-receptor antagonists are indicated in the short-term treatment of active duodenal ulcer. They are also indicated (at reduced dosage) in the prevention of duodenal ulcer recurrence in selected patients.

Ulcer, gastric (treatment)—Cimetidine, famotidine, nizatidine, and ranitidine are indicated in the short-term treatment of active benign gastric ulcer.

Ulcer, gastric (prophylaxis)—Ranitidine is indicated (at reduced dosage) in the prevention of gastric ulcer recurrence after the healing of acute ulcers.

Heartburn, acid indigestion, and sour stomach associated with hyperacidity (prophylaxis and treatment)—Nonprescription strengths of the histamine H₂-receptor antagonists cimetidine, famotidine, and ranitidine are indicated for relief of symptoms associated with hyperacidity, including heartburn, acid indigestion, and sour stomach. Nonprescription strengths of cimetidine, famotidine, and nizatidine are also indicated in prevention of hyperacidity symptoms brought on by the consumption of food or beverages.

Hypersecretory conditions, gastric (treatment)
Zollinger-Ellison syndrome (treatment)
Mastocytosis, systemic (treatment) or
Adenoma, multiple endocrine (treatment)—Cimetidine, famotidine, [nizatidine][1], and ranitidine are indicated in the treatment of pathological gastric hypersecretion associated with Zollinger-Ellison syndrome (alone or as part of multiple endocrine neoplasia Type-1), systemic mastocytosis, and multiple endocrine adenoma.

Reflux, gastroesophageal (treatment)—Cimetidine, famotidine nizatidine[1], and ranitidine are indicated in the treatment of acute gastroesophageal reflux disease, which may or may not cause erosive or ulcerative esophagitis.

[Pancreatic insufficiency (treatment adjunct)][1]—Cimetidine is used to enhance pancreatic replacement by reducing peptic acid deactivation and to enhance the efficacy of orally administered pancreatic enzymes in patients with pancreatic insufficiency by reducing the secretion of hydrochloric acid. However, the efficacy of cimetidine in acute pancreatitis has not been established, and some studies have demonstrated that cimetidine may increase and prolong hyperamylasemia.

Bleeding, upper gastrointestinal (treatment)—Cimetidine, [famotidine][1], and [ranitidine] are used to treat upper gastrointestinal bleeding secondary to gastric ulcer, duodenal ulcer, or hemorrhagic gastritis.

Stress-related mucosal damage (prophylaxis and treatment)—[Parenteral ranitidine] is used to prevent and treat and parenteral cimetidine is use of nonsteroidal anti-inflammatory drugs in the treatment of rheumatoid arthritis.

[Urticaria, acute (treatment adjunct)][1]—Cimetidine is used in combination with an antihistamine to treat acute urticaria.

[1]Not included in Canadian product labeling.

## Pharmacology/Pharmacokinetics

See *Table 1*, page 1594 and *Table 2*, page 1594.

### Physicochemical characteristics

Molecular weight—
Cimetidine: 252.34.
Famotidine: 337.43.
Nizatidine: 331.45.
Ranitidine: 350.87.

pKa—
Cimetidine: 7.09.
Cimetidine hydrochloride: 7.11.
Ranitidine: 8.2 and 2.7.

### Mechanism of action/Effect

H$_2$-receptor antagonists inhibit basal and nocturnal gastric acid secretion by competitive inhibition of the action of histamine at the histamine H$_2$-receptors of the parietal cells. They also inhibit gastric acid secretion stimulated by food, betazole, pentagastrin, caffeine, insulin, and physiological vagal reflex.

Urticaria therapy adjunct—Cimetidine blocks H$_2$-receptors, which in part are responsible for the inflammatory response, in the cutaneous blood vessels of humans.

### Other actions/effects

Cimetidine—Inhibits hepatic cytochrome P-450 and P-448 mixed function oxidase (microsomal enzyme) systems; antagonizes dihydrotestosterone (antiandrogenic action); produces transient and clinically insignificant increases in prolactin concentrations (with intravenous bolus administration only). May enhance gastromucosal defense and healing in acid-related disorders, particularly stress-induced ulceration and bleeding, by increasing production of gastric mucus, content of mucus glycoprotein, mucosal secretion of bicarbonate, gastric mucosal blood flow, endogenous mucosal prostaglandin synthesis, and rate of epithelial cell renewal.

Famotidine—Weak inhibitor of hepatic cytochrome P-450 mixed function oxidase system.

Nizatidine—Weak inhibitor of hepatic cytochrome P-450 mixed function oxidase system.

Ranitidine—Weak inhibitor of hepatic cytochrome P-450 mixed function oxidase system; produces small, transient, and clinically insignificant increases in serum prolactin concentrations (reported with intravenous bolus administration of 100 mg or more).

### Distribution

All H$_2$-receptor antagonists are distributed in breast milk and cerebral spinal fluid.

### Onset of action

Famotidine—Oral: 1 hour.

## Precautions to Consider

### Cross-sensitivity and/or related problems

Patients sensitive to one of the histamine H$_2$-receptor antagonists may be sensitive to the other histamine H$_2$-receptor antagonists also.

### Carcinogenicity/Mutagenicity/Tumorigenicity

It is not known whether the histamine H$_2$-receptor antagonists are carcinogenic or mutagenic in humans.

For cimetidine—Long-term toxicity studies in rats have shown a significantly higher incidence of benign Leydig cell tumors in cimetidine-treated groups than in controls at doses approximately 8 to 48 times the recommended human dose.

For famotidine—Studies in rats and mice with oral doses approximately 2500 times the recommended human dose showed no evidence of carcinogenicity. Studies in mice with a micronucleus test and a chromosomal aberration test showed no evidence of mutagenicity.

For nizatidine—Studies in rats and mice with oral doses many times the recommended human dose showed no evidence of carcinogenicity.

For ranitidine—Long-term studies in mice and rats with doses up to 2 grams per kg of body weight have not shown ranitidine to be carcinogenic.

### Pregnancy/Reproduction

Fertility—For cimetidine: There has been no evidence of impaired mating performance or fertility at doses 40 times the human dose in rats, rabbits, and mice.

For famotidine: Studies in rats and rabbits with oral doses of up to 2000 and 500 mg per kg of body weight (mg/kg) per day, respectively, have not shown that famotidine impairs fertility.

For nizatidine: Studies in rats and rabbits with oral doses up to 300 and 55 times the human dose, respectively, have not shown that nizatidine impairs fertility.

For ranitidine: Studies in rats and rabbits at doses up to 160 times the human dose have not shown that ranitidine impairs fertility.

Pregnancy—
*For cimetidine*—
Adequate and well-controlled studies in humans have not been done.

Animal studies have shown that cimetidine crosses the placenta. Also, a study in rats exposed to cimetidine during intrauterine life and the immediate neonatal period showed a hypoandrogenization in adult life with decreased weights of androgen-dependent tissues and decreased concentrations of testosterone.

FDA Pregnancy Category B.

*For famotidine*—
Famotidine crosses the placenta. Adequate and well-controlled studies in humans have not been done.

Studies in rats and rabbits with oral doses of up to 2000 and 500 mg/kg per day, respectively, have not shown that famotidine has adverse effects on the fetus.

FDA Pregnancy Category B.

*For nizatidine*—
Nizatidine crosses the placenta. Adequate and well-controlled studies in humans have not been done.

Rabbits treated with a dose equivalent to 300 times the human dose had abortions, a decreased number of live fetuses, and depressed fetal weights.

FDA Pregnancy Category C.

*For ranitidine*—
Ranitidine crosses the placenta. Adequate and well-controlled studies in humans have not been done.

Studies in rats and rabbits at doses up to 160 times the human dose have not shown that ranitidine causes adverse effects on the fetus.

FDA Pregnancy Category B.

### Breast-feeding

Problems in humans have not been documented; however, cimetidine, famotidine, nizatidine, and ranitidine are distributed into breast milk and could possibly suppress gastric acidity, inhibit drug metabolism, and cause central nervous system (CNS) stimulation in the nursing infant. It has been found that very high acute and chronic milk/plasma ratios occur with the use of cimetidine; therefore, the Committee on Drugs of the American Academy of Pediatrics has recommended that cimetidine not be taken by mothers while they are breast-feeding. Although, at present, data for ranitidine are insufficient, it appears that high milk/plasma ratios may also occur with ingestion of ranitidine.

### Pediatrics

For cimetidine, famotidine, and ranitidine—Studies performed to date have not demonstrated pediatrics-specific problems that would limit the usefulness of cimetidine, famotidine, and ranitidine in children for short-term (6 to 8 weeks) use. Cimetidine, famotidine, and ranitidine have been used for long-term treatment of chronic gastroesophageal reflux disease in children; however, cimetidine-induced cerebral toxicity and reported cimetidine effects on the hormonal system in adults may be of concern with long-term use in children.

For nizatidine—Appropriate studies have not been performed in children up to 16 years of age.

### Geriatrics

For cimetidine, famotidine, and ranitidine—Although appropriate studies on the relationship of age to the effects of these medicines have not been performed in the geriatric population, no geriatrics-specific problems have been documented to date. However, confusion is more likely to occur in elderly patients with impaired hepatic or renal function.

For nizatidine—Studies performed to date have not demonstrated geriatrics-specific problems that would limit the usefulness of nizatidine in the elderly.

### Drug interactions and/or related problems

The following drug interactions and/or related problems have been selected on the basis of their potential clinical significance (possible

mechanism in parentheses where appropriate)—not necessarily inclusive (» = major clinical significance):

Note: Only specific interactions between histamine H₂-receptor antagonists and other medications have been identified in this monograph. However, histamine H₂-receptor antagonists, by increasing gastric pH, have the potential to affect the bioavailability of those medications and dosage forms (e.g., enteric-coated) whose absorption is pH-dependent. Also, histamine H₂-receptor antagonists may prevent the degradation of acid-labile drugs.

In addition, because of cimetidine's documented ability to inhibit hepatic microsomal drug metabolism, elimination of other medications that require hepatic metabolism via the cytochrome (P-450) system or that are highly extracted by the liver, may be decreased during concurrent use with cimetidine. This same possibility should be kept in mind for ranitidine, although ranitidine's ability to inhibit hepatic microsomal drug metabolism is significantly less than that for cimetidine. To date, there is no evidence that famotidine or nizatidine binds to cytochrome P-450 to a significant extent, and interactions with medications metabolized by this system have not been reported; however, clinical experience with famotidine and nizatidine is very limited.

Combinations containing any of the following medications, depending on the amount present, may also interact with this medication.

*For all histamine H₂-receptor antagonists*
Antacids
(concurrent use with histamine H₂-receptor antagonists in the treatment of peptic ulcer may be indicated for the relief of pain; however, simultaneous administration of antacids of medium to high potency [80 mmol to 150 mmol HCl] is not recommended since absorption of histamine H₂-receptor antagonists may be decreased; patients should be advised not to take any antacids within one-half to one hour of histamine H₂-receptor antagonists)

Bone marrow depressants (See *Appendix II*)
(concurrent use with H₂-receptor antagonists may increase the risk of neutropenia or other blood dyscrasias)

» Itraconazole or
» Ketoconazole
(histamine H₂-receptor antagonists may increase gastrointestinal pH; concurrent administration with histamine H₂-receptor antagonists may result in a marked reduction in absorption of itraconazole or ketoconazole; patients should be advised to take histamine H₂-receptor antagonists at least 2 hours after itraconazole or ketoconazole)

Sucralfate
(although a decrease in absorption is only reported in the literature for cimetidine and ranitidine, concurrent use with sucralfate may decrease the absorption of any H₂-receptor antagonist; patients should be advised to take an H₂-receptor antagonist 2 hours before sucralfate)

*For cimetidine*
Alcohol
(some studies in humans have found increased blood alcohol levels when oral cimetidine was given in conjunction with alcohol; the clinical significance of this effect has not been documented)

» Anticoagulants, coumarin- or indandione-derivative or
» Antidepressants, tricyclic or
Benzodiazepines, especially chlordiazepoxide, diazepam, and midazolam or
Glipizide or
Glyburide or
» Metoprolol or
Metronidazole or
» Phenytoin or
» Propranolol or
» Xanthines, such as:
  Aminophylline
  Caffeine
  Oxtriphylline
  Theophylline
(inhibition of the cytochrome P-450 enzyme system by cimetidine may cause a decrease in the hepatic metabolism of these medications, which may result in delayed elimination and increased blood concentrations, when these medications are used concurrently with cimetidine)

(monitoring of blood concentrations, or prothrombin time for anticoagulants, as a guide to dosage is recommended since dosage adjustment of these medications may be necessary during and after

cimetidine therapy to prevent bleeding due to anticoagulant potentiation)

(concurrent use of phenytoin with cimetidine may increase the risk of ataxia due to increased blood concentrations of phenytoin)

(concurrent use of metoprolol or propranolol with cimetidine may require monitoring of blood pressure)

Calcium channel blocking agents
(concurrent use with cimetidine may result in accumulation of the calcium channel blocking agent as a result of inhibition of first-pass metabolism; caution and careful titration of the calcium channel blocking agent dose is recommended on initiation of therapy in patients receiving cimetidine)

Cyclosporine
(although this effect is rare, cimetidine has been reported to increase plasma concentrations of cyclosporine and may increase the risk of nephrotoxicity)

Lidocaine
(concurrent administration of lidocaine with cimetidine may result in reduced hepatic clearance of lidocaine, possibly resulting in delayed elimination and increased blood concentrations; lower doses of lidocaine may be required)

Procainamide
(renal elimination of procainamide may be decreased due to competition between cimetidine and procainamide for active tubular secretion, resulting in increased blood concentration of procainamide)

Quinine
(concurrent use of quinine with cimetidine may reduce the clearance of quinine)

*For ranitidine*
Alcohol
(some studies in humans have found increased blood alcohol levels when oral ranitidine was given in conjunction with alcohol; the clinical significance of this effect has not been documented)

Glipizide or
Glyburide or
Metoprolol or
Midazolam or
Nifedipine or
Phenytoin or
Theophylline or
Warfarin
(ranitidine is a weak inhibitor of hepatic drug metabolism; isolated cases of drug interactions have been reported between ranitidine and glipizide, glyburide, metoprolol, midazolam, nifedipine, phenytoin, theophylline, and warfarin)

(monitoring of blood concentrations or prothrombin time for anticoagulants as a guide to dosage is recommended since dosage adjustment of these medications may be necessary during and after ranitidine therapy to prevent bleeding due to anticoagulant potentiation)

(concurrent use of phenytoin with ranitidine may increase the risk of ataxia due to increased blood concentrations of phenytoin)

Procainamide
(renal elimination of procainamide may be decreased due to competition between ranitidine and procainamide for active tubular secretion, resulting in increased blood concentration of procainamide)

**Laboratory value alterations**
The following have been selected on the basis of their potential clinical significance (possible effect in parentheses where appropriate)—not necessarily inclusive (» = major clinical significance):

With diagnostic test results

*For all histamine H₂-receptor antagonists*
» Gastric acid secretion test
(histamine H₂-receptor antagonists may antagonize the effect of pentagastrin and histamine in the evaluation of gastric acid secretory function; administration of histamine H₂-receptor antagonists is not recommended during the 24 hours preceding the test)

Skin tests using allergen extracts
(histamine H₂-receptor antagonists may inhibit the cutaneous histamine response, thus producing false-negative results; it is recommended that histamine H₂-receptor antagonists be discontinued before the diagnostic use of immediate skin tests)

*For nizatidine only (in addition to those listed above for all histamine H₂-receptor antagonists)*

Urine urobilinogen test

(a false-positive reaction may be produced during nizatidine therapy)

*For ranitidine only (in addition to those listed above for all histamine H$_2$-receptor antagonists)*

Urine protein test
(a false-positive reaction may be produced during ranitidine therapy; testing with sulphosalicylic acid is recommended)

With physiology/laboratory test values

*For cimetidine*

Creatinine and
Transaminase
(serum values may be increased)

Parathyroid hormone
(concentrations may be decreased, especially when abnormally elevated as in primary hyperparathyroidism)

Prolactin
(serum concentrations may be increased after intravenous bolus administration)

*For famotidine*

Transaminase
(serum values may be increased)

*For nizatidine*

Alanine aminotransferase (ALT [SGPT]) and
Alkaline phosphatase and
Aspartate aminotransferase (AST [SGOT])
(serum values may be increased)

*For ranitidine*

Creatinine and
Gamma-glutamyl transpeptidase and
Transaminase
(serum values may be increased)

**Medical considerations/Contraindications**

The medical considerations/contraindications included here have been selected on the basis of their potential clinical significance (reasons given in parentheses where appropriate)—not necessarily inclusive (» = major clinical significance).

*Risk-benefit should be considered when the following medical problems exist:*

Cirrhosis, with history of portal systemic encephalopathy or
Hepatic function impairment or
» Renal function impairment
(decreased hepatic or renal clearance of histamine H$_2$-receptor antagonists may result in increased plasma concentrations thus increasing the risk of side effects, especially CNS effects; dosage reduction of histamine H$_2$-receptor antagonists or longer intervals between doses are recommended with renal function impairment and may be necessary with hepatic function impairment)

Immunocompromised patients
(decreased gastric acidity may increase the possibility of a hyperinfection of stongyloidiasis)

Sensitivity to any of the histamine H$_2$-receptor antagonists

**Patient monitoring**

The following may be especially important in patient monitoring (other tests may be warranted in some patients, depending on condition; » = major clinical significance):

Cyanocobalamin (vitamin B$_{12}$) concentration determinations
(monitoring may be needed in long-term treatment of patients likely to have impaired secretion of intrinsic factor, such as those with severe fundic gastritis, to prevent malabsorption of cyanocobalamin)

## Side/Adverse Effects

See *Table 3*, page 1595.

Note: Rapid intravenous bolus administration (an infusion time of less than 5 minutes) of histamine H$_2$-receptor antagonists may cause significant, transient hypotension. Also, rare instances of cardiac arrhythmias have been reported with intravenous boluses of cimetidine and ranitidine.

Rare cases of hepatitis, with or without jaundice, have been reported in patients using histamine H$_2$-receptor antagonists; however, a direct association with the use of histamine H$_2$-receptor antagonists has not been established.

## Overdose

For specific information on the agents used in the management of overdose with histamine H$_2$-receptor antagonists, see:
  • *Atropine* in *Anticholinergics/Antispasmodics (Systemic)* monograph;
  • *Diazepam* in *Benzodiazepines (Systemic)* monograph; and/or
  • *Lidocaine Hydrochloride (Systemic)* monograph.

For more information on the management of overdose or unintentional ingestion, **contact a Poison Control Center** (see *Poison Control Center Listing*).

**Clinical effects of overdose**

Experience with overdose in humans is limited. In animals, toxic doses of cimetidine have caused respiratory failure and tachycardia. Toxic doses of famotidine given intravenously to dogs caused emesis, restlessness, pallor of mucous membranes or redness of mouth and ears, hypotension, tachycardia, and collapse. Muscular tremors, vomiting, and rapid respiration have been reported with daily doses in excess of 225 mg of ranitidine per kg of body weight in animals.

**Treatment of overdose**

Since there is no specific antidote for overdose with histamine H$_2$-receptor antagonists, treatment is symptomatic and supportive with possible utilization of the following:

To decrease absorption—
Induction of emesis and/or use of gastric lavage.

Specific treatment—
For seizures—Treatment with intravenous diazepam.
For bradycardia—Treatment with atropine.
For ventricular arrhythmias—Treatment with lidocaine.

Monitoring—
Possible laboratory monitoring for adverse reactions.

Supportive care—
Patients in whom intentional overdose is confirmed or suspected should be referred for psychiatric consultation.

## Patient Consultation

As an aid to patient consultation, refer to *Advice for the Patient, Histamine H$_2$-receptor Antagonists (Systemic)*.

In providing consultation, consider emphasizing the following selected information (» = major clinical significance):

**Before using this medication**
» Conditions affecting use, especially:
Sensitivity to any of the H$_2$-receptor antagonists
Pregnancy—All cross placenta
Breast-feeding—Cimetidine, famotidine, nizatidine, and ranitidine distributed into breast milk; nursing not recommended during cimetidine therapy, because of high concentration in breast milk
Use in the elderly—Confusion more likely with cimetidine, famotidine, and ranitidine in elderly patients with impaired hepatic or renal function
Other medications, especially itraconazole, ketoconazole (with all histamine H$_2$-receptor antagonists); anticoagulants, metoprolol, phenytoin, xanthines (with cimetidine and possibly ranitidine only); propranolol or tricyclic antidepressants (with cimetidine only)
Other medical problems, especially renal function impairment

**Proper use of this medication**
For patients taking nonprescription strengths: not taking maximum daily dose continuously for more than 2 weeks unless directed by physician; seeing physician promptly if having trouble swallowing or persistent abdominal pain
Dosing schedule for patients taking prescription strengths:
1 dose a day—Taking at bedtime
2 doses a day—Taking in the morning and at bedtime
Several doses a day—Taking with meals and at bedtime
For patients taking ranitidine effervescent granules or tablets, removing foil wrapping and dissolving dose in 6 to 8 ounces of water before drinking
Taking antacids for relief of ulcer pain; not taking within one-half to one hour of histamine H$_2$-receptor antagonists
» Compliance with full course of therapy
» Proper dosing
Missed dose: Taking as soon as possible; not taking if almost time for next dose; not doubling doses
» Proper storage

**Precautions while using this medication**
Possible interference with gastric acid secretion tests or skin tests using allergens; need to inform physician of use of medication

Avoiding use of foods, drinks, or other medication that may cause
gastrointestinal irritation

Discontinuing smoking or at least avoiding smoking after last dose of
day

Avoiding alcoholic beverages

Checking with physician if condition does not improve or worsens

**Side/adverse effects**

Signs of possible side effects, especially allergic reaction, bradycardia
or tachycardia, bronchospasm, confusion, fever, and neutropenia
or other blood dyscrasias

# General Dosing Information

Use of histamine H₂-receptor antagonists in the treatment of duodenal
ulcer rarely continues beyond 8 weeks, since no long-term, carefully
monitored studies have been done with these medications. Also, most
patients taking histamine H₂-receptor antagonists heal within 6 to 8
weeks.

Although the symptoms of duodenal ulcers may subside within 1 or 2
weeks after initiation of therapy, therapy should be continued for at
least 4 to 6 weeks, unless healing has been documented by endoscopic
examination or x-rays.

Histamine H₂-receptor antagonists may be used, in reduced doses, to prevent ulcer recurrence. However, until consequences of very long term
use are fully determined, such use should be limited to patients likely
to need surgical treatment, patients with concomitant illnesses in
whom surgery would constitute a greater-than-usual risk, and patients
with recurrent ulcers.

Initial titration of doses and subsequent dosage adjustment of histamine
H₂-receptor antagonists is recommended in the long-term treatment of
pathological hypersecretory conditions (e.g., Zollinger-Ellison syndrome, systemic mastocytosis, multiple endocrine adenomas). Doses
of cimetidine should generally not exceed 2.4 grams per day; however,
doses up to 12 grams per day have been used. Up to 160 mg of
famotidine every 6 hours and up to 6 grams of ranitidine per day have
been administered to some patients with severe Zollinger-Ellison
syndrome.

The efficacy of histamine H₂-receptor antagonists in inhibiting nocturnal
gastric acid secretion may be decreased by cigarette smoking. Patients
with peptic ulcer disease should discontinue smoking, or at least avoid
smoking after their last dose of the day.

Dosage of histamine H₂-receptor antagonists may need to be increased in
burn patients to achieve adequate control of gastric pH, because of
enhanced clearance of histamine H₂-receptor antagonists in these patients. Individualization of dosage should be based on monitoring of
gastric pH and/or plasma concentrations of histamine H₂-receptor antagonists since their clearance varies in proportion to burn size.

No dosage adjustment of histamine H₂-receptor antagonists is necessary
for hemodialysis and peritoneal dialysis patients, since only small
amounts of the medications are removed.

**For oral dosage forms only**

In the treatment of peptic ulcer and other hypersecretory conditions, optimal therapeutic effect is obtained when histamine H₂-receptor antagonists are taken with meals and at bedtime. By administering histamine
H₂-receptor antagonists with meals, maximum serum concentrations
and antisecretory effects are achieved when the stomach is no longer
protected by the buffering capacity of the food. However, more recent
information indicates that ulcer healing rates may be greatest with a
bedtime-only dosage regimen.

If required, antacids of standard neutralizing capacity (e.g., 13 mEq per
15 mL) may be administered concurrently with histamine H₂-receptor
antagonists for the relief of pain. However, spacing of doses one-half
to one hour apart is recommended, especially with antacids of greater
neutralizing capacity, since absorption of histamine H₂-receptor antagonists may be decreased.

**For parenteral dosage forms only**

Parenteral administration may be indicated in hospitalized patients with
pathological hypersecretory disorders or intractable ulcers, or in patients who are unable to take oral medication.

Rapid intravenous bolus administration of cimetidine, famotidine, or ranitidine is not recommended because it may increase the risk of cardiac
arrhythmias and hypotension.

---

## CIMETIDINE

# Summary of Differences

Indications:

Also used in treatment of pancreatic insufficiency and as a treatment
adjunct in acute urticaria.

Pharmacology/pharmacokinetics:

Other actions/effects—Inhibits hepatic cytochrome P-450 and P-448
mixed function oxidase (microsomal enzyme) systems; possesses
antiandrogenic activity; increases prolactin concentration (with IV
bolus injection); enhances gastromucosal defense and healing in
stress-induced ulceration and bleeding.

Precautions:

Drug interactions and/or related problems—May interact with alcohol,
anticoagulants, tricyclic antidepressants, benzodiazepines, glipizide, glyburide, metoprolol, metronidazole, phenytoin, propranolol,
xanthines, calcium channel blocking agents, cyclosporine, lidocaine, procainamide, sucralfate, quinine.

Laboratory value alterations—May increase serum prolactin concentrations; may decrease parathyroid hormone concentrations.

Side/adverse effects:

Constipation has not been reported. Bronchospasms have not been
reported as a side/adverse effect with cimetidine.

# Oral Dosage Forms

Note: Bracketed uses in the *Dosage Forms* section refer to categories of
use and/or indications that are not included in U.S. product labeling.

## CIMETIDINE TABLETS USP

**Usual adult and adolescent dose**

Duodenal ulcer—

Treatment: Oral, 300 mg four times a day, with meals and at bedtime;
400 or 600 mg two times a day, in the morning and at bedtime;
or 800 mg at bedtime.

Note: A 1600-mg dose of cimetidine at bedtime has been found to
produce a more rapid healing in some ulcer patients who have
an endoscopically demonstrated ulcer larger than 1 cm and are
also heavy smokers.

Prophylaxis of recurrent duodenal ulcer: Oral, 300 mg two times a
day, in the morning and at bedtime; or 400 mg at bedtime. Patients
have been maintained on continued treatment with 400 mg at bedtime for periods of up to five years.

Gastric ulcer, benign, active—

Oral, 300 mg four times a day, with meals and at bedtime; or 600 mg
two times a day, in the morning and at bedtime; or 800 mg at
bedtime.

Heartburn, acid indigestion, and sour stomach—

Treatment: Oral, 200 mg with water as symptoms occur; dose may be
repeated once in twenty-four hours

Prophylaxis: Oral, 200 mg with water one hour before consuming food
or beverages expected to cause symptoms

Gastric hypersecretory conditions (e.g., Zollinger-Ellison syndrome, systemic mastocytosis, multiple endocrine adenomas)—

Oral, 300 mg four times a day, with meals and at bedtime, the dosage
being adjusted as needed, and therapy continued for as long as
clinically indicated.

Gastroesophageal reflux—

Oral, 800 to 1600 mg per day in divided doses for 12 weeks.

Upper gastrointestinal bleeding—

Oral, 300 mg every six hours; or 600 mg two times a day, in the
morning and at bedtime.

Note: For patients with impaired renal function—Oral, 300 mg every
twelve hours, the dosage being increased to 300 mg every eight
hours or more frequently, if necessary. Further reduction in dosage
may be required if hepatic function impairment is also present.

**Usual adult prescribing limits**

Up to 2.4 grams daily; however, doses up to 12 grams per day have been
used in the treatment of pathological hypersecretory conditions.

**Usual pediatric dose**

Duodenal ulcer; or

Gastric ulcer—

Oral, 20 to 40 mg per kg of body weight a day in divided doses
four times a day, with meals and at bedtime.

Gastroesophageal reflux—

Oral, 40 to 80 mg per kg of body weight a day in divided doses four
times a day.

Note: In certain circumstances, doses may be titrated based on gastric pH.

Clinical experience with the use of cimetidine in children up to 16
years of age is limited; risk-benefit must be considered.

In children with impaired renal function, dosage should be reduced to 10 to 15 mg per kg of body weight a day, and the dosing interval increased to eight hours.

**Usual geriatric dose**
See *Usual adult and adolescent dose.*

**Strength(s) usually available**
U.S.—
100 mg (OTC) [*Tagamet HB*].
200 mg (Rx) [*Tagamet;* GENERIC].
300 mg (Rx) [*Tagamet;* GENERIC].
400 mg (Rx) [*Tagamet;* GENERIC].
800 mg (Rx) [*Tagamet;* GENERIC].
Canada—
200 mg (Rx) [*Apo-Cimetidine; Novocimetine; Peptol; Tagamet*].
300 mg (Rx) [*Apo-Cimetidine; Novocimetine; Peptol; Tagamet*].
400 mg (Rx) [*Apo-Cimetidine; Novocimetine; Peptol; Tagamet*].
600 mg (Rx) [*Apo-Cimetidine; Novocimetine; Peptol; Tagamet*].
800 mg (Rx) [*Apo-Cimetidine; Novocimetine; Peptol; Tagamet*].

**Packaging and storage**
Store between 15 and 30 °C (59 and 86 °F), in a tight, light-resistant container.

**Auxiliary labeling**
• Continue medicine for full time of treatment.

**Note**
Tablets have a characteristic odor, which does not represent any risk to the patient.

## CIMETIDINE HYDROCHLORIDE ORAL SOLUTION

**Usual adult and adolescent dose**
See *Cimetidine Tablets USP.*

**Usual adult prescribing limits**
See *Cimetidine Tablets USP.*

**Usual pediatric dose**
See *Cimetidine Tablets USP.*

**Usual geriatric dose**
See *Usual adult and adolescent dose.*

**Strength(s) usually available**
U.S.—
300 mg (base) per 5 mL (Rx) [*Tagamet* (alcohol 2.8%); GENERIC].
Canada—
300 mg (base) per 5 mL (Rx) [*Tagamet* (alcohol 2.8%)].

**Packaging and storage**
Store between 15 and 30 °C (59 and 86 °F), in a tight, light-resistant container, unless otherwise specified by manufacturer. Protect from freezing.

**Auxiliary labeling**
• Continue medicine for full time of treatment.

## Parenteral Dosage Forms

Note: Bracketed uses in the *Dosage Forms* section refer to categories of use and/or indications that are not included in U.S. product labeling.

## CIMETIDINE HYDROCHLORIDE INJECTION

Note: The dosing and strengths of the dosage forms available are expressed in terms of cimetidine base (not the hydrochloride salt).

**Usual adult and adolescent dose**
Duodenal ulcer or
Gastric ulcer or
Gastric hypersecretory conditions (e.g., Zollinger-Ellison syndrome, systemic mastocytosis, multiple endocrine adenomas) or
Upper gastrointestinal bleeding—
Intramuscular, 300 mg (base) every six to eight hours.
Intravenous, 300 mg (base) every six to eight hours, diluted with a compatible intravenous solution and administered over a period of not less than five minutes.
Intravenous infusion, 300 mg (base) every six to eight hours, diluted in a compatible intravenous solution and administered over a fifteen- to twenty-minute period.
Note: If necessary, increases in dosage should be made by more frequent administration of a 300 mg dose.
Continuous intravenous infusion, 37.5 (base) mg per hour (900 mg per day), diluted in a compatible intravenous solution. The infusion rate should be adjusted to individual patient requirements.
Note: For patients requiring a rapid elevation of gastric pH, a loading dose of 150 mg may be administered by intravenous infusion before continuous infusion is begun.

Prophylaxis of stress-related mucosal bleeding—
Continuous intravenous infusion, 50 mg (base) per hour, diluted in a compatible intravenous solution for up to 7 days.
Note: Patients with a creatinine clearance less than 30 mL per minute should receive 25 mg per hour.
[Prophylaxis of aspiration pneumonitis]—
Intramuscular, 300 mg (base) one hour before induction of anesthesia, and 300 mg (base) given intramuscularly or intravenously every four hours until patient responds to verbal commands.
[Urticaria therapy adjunct]—
Intravenous, 300 mg over 15 to 20 minutes.

Note: For patients with impaired renal function—Intravenous, 300 mg (base) every twelve hours, the dosage being increased to 300 mg every eight hours or more frequently, if necessary. Further reduction in dosage may be required if hepatic function impairment is also present.

**Usual adult prescribing limits**
Up to 2.4 grams (base) daily.

**Usual pediatric dose**
Duodenal ulcer or;
Gastric ulcer—
Intramuscular, 5 to 10 mg (base) per kg of body weight every six to eight hours.
Intravenous, 5 to 10 mg (base) per kg of body weight every six to eight hours, diluted to a suitable volume with a compatible intravenous solution and administered over a period of not less than two minutes.
Intravenous infusion, 5 to 10 mg (base) per kg of body weight every six to eight hours, diluted to a suitable volume with a compatible intravenous solution and administered over a fifteen- to twenty-minute period.

Note: In certain circumstances, doses may be titrated based on gastric pH.
Clinical experience with the use of cimetidine in children up to 16 years of age is limited; risk-benefit must be considered.
In children with impaired renal function, doses should be reduced and dosing interval increased.

**Usual geriatric dose**
See *Usual adult and adolescent dose.*

**Strength(s) usually available**
U.S.—
300 mg (base) per 2 mL (Rx) [*Tagamet;* GENERIC].
300 mg (base) per 50 mL (premixed) (Rx) [*Tagamet*].
Canada—
300 mg (base) per 2 mL (Rx) [*Tagamet*].
300 mg (base) per 50 mL (premixed) (Rx) [*Tagamet*].

**Packaging and storage**
Store between 15 and 30 °C (59 and 86 °F), unless otherwise specified by manufacturer. Protect from light. Protect from freezing.

**Preparation of dosage form**
Not for premixed dosage form
• For intravenous use, cimetidine hydrochloride injection must be diluted prior to use with a compatible intravenous solution, such as sodium chloride injection (0.9%).
• For intermittent intravenous infusion, cimetidine hydrochloride injection must be diluted prior to use in 50 mL of a compatible intravenous solution, such as dextrose injection (5%).

**Stability**
Diluted solutions of cimetidine hydrochloride injection are stable for 48 hours at room temperature.
Exposure to cold may lead to development of cloudiness. However, this is of no clinical significance, and solution clears on returning to room temperature.
Injection should not be used if discolored or if a precipitate is present.

---

### *FAMOTIDINE*

## Summary of Differences

Side/adverse effects: Loss of appetite, dryness of mouth or skin, ringing or buzzing in ears have been reported. A decrease in sexual ability has not been reported with famotidine.

# Oral Dosage Forms

## FAMOTIDINE FOR ORAL SUSPENSION

### Usual adult and adolescent dose
Duodenal ulcer—
    Treatment: Oral, 40 mg once a day at bedtime or 20 mg two times a day.
    Prophylaxis of recurrent duodenal ulcer: Oral, 20 mg at bedtime.
Gastric ulcer, benign, active—
    Treatment: Oral, 40 mg once a day at bedtime.
Gastric hypersecretory conditions (e.g., Zollinger-Ellison syndrome, systemic mastocytosis, multiple endocrine adenomas)—
    Oral, 20 mg every six hours, the dosage being adjusted as needed and therapy continued for as long as clinically indicated. Doses up to 160 mg every six hours have been administered to some patients with severe Zollinger-Ellison syndrome.
Gastroesophageal reflux—
    Oral, 20 mg two times a day for up to six weeks.
    Note: The recommended oral dose for esophagitis due to gastroesophageal reflux disease is 20 to 40 mg two times a day for up to twelve weeks.
[Prophylaxis of aspiration pneumonitis]—
    Oral, 40 mg given either the night before or the morning of surgery.
Note: For patients with severely impaired renal function (creatinine clearance less than 10 mL per minute)—Oral, 20 mg at bedtime. Depending on patient's response, the dosing interval may have to be increased to thirty-six to forty-eight hours.

### Usual pediatric dose
Gastroesophageal reflux disease—
    For children weighing more than 10 kg: Oral, 1 to 2 mg per kg of body weight a day, in two divided doses.
    For children weighing less than 10 kg: Oral, 1 to 2 mg per kg per day, in three divided doses.
Note: In certain circumstances, doses may be titrated based on gastric pH.

### Usual geriatric dose
See *Usual adult and adolescent dose.*

### Strength(s) usually available
U.S.—
    40 mg per 5 mL (Rx) [*Pepcid*].
Canada—
    Not commercially available.

### Packaging and storage
Prior to constitution, store below 40 °C (104 °F), preferably between 15 and 30 °C (59 and 86 °F), unless otherwise specified by manufacturer.
After constitution, store below 30 °C (86 °F), unless otherwise specified by manufacturer. Protect from freezing.

### Preparation of dosage form
At time of dispensing, slowly add 46 mL of purified water. Shake vigorously for 5 to 10 seconds immediately after adding the water and immediately before use.

### Stability
Unused oral suspension of famotidine should be discarded after 30 days.

### Auxiliary labeling
• Shake well.
• Continue medicine for full time of treatment.

## FAMOTIDINE TABLETS USP

### Usual adult and adolescent dose
Duodenal ulcer—
    Treatment: Oral, 40 mg once a day at bedtime or 20 mg two times a day.
    Prophylaxis of recurrent duodenal ulcer: Oral, 20 mg at bedtime.
Gastric ulcer, benign, active—
    Treatment: Oral, 40 mg once a day at bedtime.
Heartburn, acid indigestion, and sour stomach—
    Treatment: Oral, 10 mg at onset of symptoms; dose may be repeated once in twenty-four hours.
    Prophylaxis: Oral, 10 mg one hour before consuming food or beverages expected to cause symptoms.
Gastric hypersecretory conditions (e.g., Zollinger-Ellison syndrome, systemic mastocytosis, multiple endocrine adenomas)—
    Oral, 20 mg every six hours, the dosage being adjusted as needed and therapy continued for as long as clinically indicated. Doses up to 160 mg every six hours have been administered to some patients with severe Zollinger-Ellison syndrome.
Gastroesophageal reflux—
    Oral, 20 mg two times a day for up to six weeks.

Note: The recommended oral dose for esophagitis due to gastroesophageal reflux disease is 20 to 40 mg two times a day for up to twelve weeks.
[Prophylaxis of aspiration pneumonitis]—
    Oral, 40 mg given either the night before or the morning of surgery.
Note: For patients with severely impaired renal function (creatinine clearance less than 10 mL per minute)—Oral, 20 mg at bedtime. Depending on patient's response, the dosing interval may have to be increased to thirty-six to forty-eight hours

### Usual pediatric dose
See *Famotidine for Oral Suspension.*

### Usual geriatric dose
See *Usual adult and adolescent dose.*

### Strength(s) usually available
U.S.—
    10 mg (OTC) [*Pepcid AC*].
    20 mg (Rx) [*Pepcid*].
    40 mg (Rx) [*Pepcid*].
Canada—
    20 mg (Rx) [*Pepcid*].
    40 mg (Rx) [*Pepcid*].

### Packaging and storage
Store below 40 °C (104 °F), preferably between 15 and 30 °C (59 and 86 °F), in a well-closed container, unless otherwise specified by manufacturer. Protect from light.

### Auxiliary labeling
• Continue medicine for full time of treatment.

# Parenteral Dosage Forms

## FAMOTIDINE INJECTION

### Usual adult and adolescent dose
Duodenal ulcer
Gastric ulcer, benign, active and
Gastric hypersecretory conditions (e.g., Zollinger-Ellison syndrome, systemic mastocytosis, multiple endocrine adenomas)—
    Intravenous, 20 mg every twelve hours, diluted with a compatible intravenous solution and administered over a period of not less than two minutes.
    Intravenous infusion, 20 mg every twelve hours, diluted with a compatible intravenous solution and administered over a fifteen- to thirty-minute period.
[Prophylaxis of aspiration pneumonitis]—
    Intramuscular, 20 mg given either the night before or the morning of surgery.

### Usual pediatric dose
Dosage has not been established.

### Usual geriatric dose
See *Usual adult and adolescent dose.*

### Strength(s) usually available
U.S.—
    10 mg per mL (Rx) [*Pepcid I.V.*].
    20 mg per 50 mL (premixed) [*Pepcid*].
Canada—
    10 mg per mL (Rx) [*Pepcid I.V.*].

### Packaging and storage
Store between 2 and 8 °C (36 and 46 °F), unless otherwise specified by manufacturer. Protect from freezing.

### Preparation of dosage form
For intravenous use, famotidine must be diluted prior to use with a compatible intravenous solution, such as sodium chloride injection (0.9%) to a total volume of either 5 or 10 mL.
For intravenous infusion, famotidine must be diluted prior to use in 100 mL of a compatible intravenous solution, such as dextrose injection (5%).

### Stability
Diluted solutions of famotidine injection are stable for 48 hours at room temperature.
Injection should not be used if discolored or if a precipitate is present.

---

### *NIZATIDINE*

# Summary of Differences

Pharmacology/pharmacokinetics: Nizatidine is moderately protein bound, approximately 35%.

Precautions: Laboratory value alterations—Increases serum aspartate aminotransferase concentrations. May cause false-positive reaction with urine urobilinogen test.

Side/adverse effects: Agranulocytosis, diarrhea, joint or muscle pain, and loss of hair have not been reported with nizatidine. Increase in sweating has been reported.

## Oral Dosage Forms

### NIZATIDINE CAPSULES USP

**Usual adult and adolescent dose**
Duodenal ulcer—
    Treatment: Oral, 300 mg once a day at bedtime or 150 mg two times a day.
    Note: For patients with impaired renal function:
        With creatinine clearance less than 20 mL per minute: Oral, 150 mg every other day.
        With creatinine clearance from 20 to 50 mL per minute: Oral, 150 mg every day.
Duodenal ulcer, recurrent—
    Prophylaxis: Oral, 150 mg once a day at bedtime.
    Note: For patients with impaired renal function:
        With creatinine clearance less than 20 mL per minute: Oral, 150 mg every three days.
        With creatinine clearance from 20 to 50 mL per minute: Oral, 150 mg every other day.
Gastric ulcer, benign, active—
    Treatment: Oral, 300 mg once a day at bedtime or 150 mg two times a day.
Gastroesophageal reflux[1]—
    Oral, 150 mg two times a day.

**Usual pediatric dose**
Dosage has not been established.

**Usual geriatric dose**
See *Usual adult and adolescent dose.*

**Strength(s) usually available**
U.S.—
    150 mg (Rx) [*Axid*].
    300 mg (Rx) [*Axid*].
Canada—
    150 mg (Rx) [*Axid*].
    300 mg (Rx) [*Axid*].

**Packaging and storage**
Store between 15 and 30 °C (59 and 86 °F), in a well-closed container, unless otherwise specified by manufacturer.

**Auxiliary labeling**
• Continue medicine for full time of treatment.

### NIZATIDINE TABLETS

**Usual adult and adolescent dose**
Heartburn, acid indigestion, and sour stomach—
    Prophylaxis: Oral, 75 mg thirty to sixty minutes before consuming food or beverages expected to cause symptoms.

**Usual pediatric dose**
Dosage has not been established.

**Usual geriatric dose**
See *Usual adult and adolescent dose.*

**Strength(s) usually available**
U.S.—
    75 mg (OTC) [*Axid AR*].
Canada—
    Not commercially available.

**Packaging and storage**
Store between 20 and 25 °C (68 and 77 °F), in a well-closed container, unless otherwise specified by manufacturer. Protect from light.

[1]Not included in Canadian product labeling.

---

## *RANITIDINE*

## Summary of Differences

Pharmacology/pharmacokinetics:
    Other actions/effects—
        Weak inhibitor of P-450 mixed function oxidase (microsomal enzyme) system; produces small, transient increase in prolactin concentration (with IV bolus injection).

Precautions:
    Laboratory value alterations—May increase glutamyl transpeptidase. May cause false-positive reaction with urine protein test.
    Drug interactions and/or related problems—May interact with alcohol, antacids, glipizide, glyburide, metoprolol, midazolam, nifedipine, phenytoin, theophylline, warfarin, procainamide, sucralfate.

Side/adverse effects:
    Blurred vision has been reported.

## Oral Dosage Forms

### RANITIDINE CAPSULES

**Usual adult and adolescent dose**
Duodenal ulcer—
    Treatment: Oral, 150 mg two times a day or 300 mg at bedtime.
    Prophylaxis of recurrent duodenal ulcer: Oral, 150 mg at bedtime.
Gastric ulcer, benign, active—
    Treatment: Oral, 150 mg two times a day.
    Prophylaxis of recurrent gastric ulcer: Oral, 150 mg at bedtime.
Gastric hypersecretory conditions (e.g., Zollinger-Ellison syndrome, systemic mastocytosis, multiple endocrine adenomas)—
    Oral, 150 mg two times a day, the dosage being adjusted as needed and therapy continued as long as clinically indicated. Doses up to 6 grams per day have been used in severe cases.
Gastroesophageal reflux—
    Oral, 150 mg two times a day.
    Note: The recommended oral dose for erosive esophagitis is 150 mg four times a day.
Note: For patients with impaired renal frunction (creatinine clearance of less than 50 mL per minute)—Oral, 150 mg every twenty-four hours, the frequency of the dosage being increased to every twelve hours or more frequently, if necessary. Reductions in dosage may also be required if hepatic function impairment is present.

**Usual pediatric dose**
Duodenal ulcer or
Gastric ulcer—
    Oral, 2 to 4 mg per kg of body weight, two times a day up to a maximum dose of 300 mg per day.
Gastroesophageal reflux—
    Oral, 2 to 8 mg per kg of body weight per dose three times a day.
Note: In certain circumstances, doses may be titrated based on gastric pH.

**Usual geriatric dose**
See *Usual adult and adolescent dose.*

**Strength(s) usually available**
U.S.—
    150 mg (Rx) [*Zantac 150 GELdose*].
    300 mg (Rx) [*Zantac 300 GELdose*].
Canada—
    150 mg (Rx) [*Zantac-C*].
    300 mg (Rx) [*Zantac-C*].

**Packaging and storage**
Store between 2 and 25 °C (36 and °F), unless otherwise specified by manufacturer. Store in a tight, light-resistant container.

**Auxiliary labeling**
• Continue medicine for full time of treatment.

### RANITIDINE EFFERVESCENT GRANULES

**Usual adult and adolescent dose**
See *Ranitidine Capsules.*

**Usual pediatric dose**
See *Ranitidine Capsules.*

**Usual geriatric dose**
See *Ranitidine Capsules.*

**Strength(s) usually available**
U.S.—
    150 mg (Rx) [*Zantac EFFERdose Granules*].
Canada—
    Not commercially available.

**Packaging and storage**
Store between 2 and 30 °C (36 and 86 °F), unless otherwise specified by manufacturer.

**Preparation of dosage form**
Dissolve each dose in 6 to 8 ounces (180 to 240 mL) of water before drinking.

**Auxiliary labeling**
• Continue medicine for full time of treatment.

## RANITIDINE HYDROCHLORIDE SYRUP

**Usual adult and adolescent dose**
See *Ranitidine Capsules.*

**Usual pediatric dose**
See *Ranitidine Capsules.*

**Usual geriatric dose**
See *Ranitidine Capsules.*

**Strength(s) usually available**
U.S.—
    150 mg (base) per 10 mL (Rx) [*Zantac* (alcohol 7.5%)].
Canada—
    75 mg (base) per 5 mL (Rx) [*Zantac* (alcohol 7.5%)].

**Packaging and storage**
Store between 4 and 25 °C (39 and 77 °F), in a tight, light-resistant container, unless otherwise specified by manufacturer. Protect from freezing.

**Auxiliary labeling**
• Continue medicine for full time of treatment.

## RANITIDINE TABLETS USP

**Usual adult and adolescent dose**
Duodenal ulcer—
    Treatment: Oral, 150 mg two times a day or 300 mg at bedtime.
    Prophylaxis of recurrent duodenal ulcer: Oral, 150 mg at bedtime.
Gastric ulcer, benign, active—
    Treatment: Oral, 150 mg two times a day.
Heartburn, acid indigestion, and sour stomach—
    Oral, 75 mg at onset of symptoms; dose may be repeated once in twenty-four hours.
Gastric hypersecretory conditions (e.g., Zollinger-Ellison syndrome, systemic mastocytosis, multiple endocrine adenomas)—
    Oral, 150 mg two times a day, the dosage being adjusted as needed and therapy continued as long as clinically indicated. Doses up to 6 grams per day have been used in severe cases.
Gastroesophageal reflux—
    Oral, 150 mg two times a day.
    Note: The recommended oral dose for erosive esophagitis is 150 mg four times a day.
Note: For patients with impaired renal function (creatinine clearance of less than 50 mL per minute)—Oral, 150 mg every twenty-four hours, the frequency of the dosage being increased to every twelve hours or more frequently, if necessary. Reductions in dosage may also be required if hepatic function impairment is present.

**Usual pediatric dose**
Duodenal ulcer or
Gastric ulcer—
    Oral, 2 to 4 mg per kg of body weight, two times a day up to a maximum dose of 300 mg per day.
Gastroesophageal reflux—
    Oral, 2 to 8 mg per kg of body weight per dose three times a day.
Note: In certain circumstances, doses may be titrated based on gastric pH.

**Usual geriatric dose**
See *Usual adult and adolescent dose.*

**Strength(s) usually available**
U.S.—
    75 mg (OTC) [*Zantac 75*].
    150 mg (Rx) [*Zantac*].
    300 mg (Rx) [*Zantac*].
Canada—
    150 mg (Rx) [*Apo-Ranitidine; Zantac*].
    300 mg (Rx) [*Apo-Ranitidine; Zantac*].

**Packaging and storage**
Store between 15 and 30 °C (59 and 86 °F), unless otherwise specified by manufacturer. Store in a tight, light-resistant container.

**Auxiliary labeling**
• Continue medicine for full time of treatment.

## RANITIDINE EFFERVESCENT TABLETS

**Usual adult and adolescent dose**
See *Ranitidine Capsules.*

**Usual pediatric dose**
See *Ranitidine Capsules.*

**Usual geriatric dose**
See *Ranitidine Capsules.*

**Strength(s) usually available**
U.S.—
    150 mg (Rx) [*Zantac EFFERdose Tablets*].
Canada—
    Not commercially available.

**Packaging and storage**
Store between 2 and 30 °C (36 and 86 °F), unless otherwise specified by manufacturer.

**Preparation of dosage form**
Dissolve each dose in 6 to 8 ounces (180 to 240 mL) of water before drinking.

**Auxiliary labeling**
• Continue medicine for full time of treatment.

# Parenteral Dosage Forms

Note: Bracketed uses in the *Dosage Forms* section refer to categories of use and/or indications that are not included in U.S. product labeling.

## RANITIDINE INJECTION USP

**Usual adult and adolescent dose**
Duodenal ulcer
Gastric ulcer
Gastric hypersecretory conditions (e.g., Zollinger-Ellison syndrome, systemic mastocytosis, multiple endocrine adenomas) and
[Prophylaxis of stress-related mucosal bleeding]—
    Intramuscular, 50 mg every six to eight hours.
    Intravenous, 50 mg every six to eight hours, diluted to a total volume of 20 mL with a compatible intravenous solution and administered over a period of not less than five minutes.
    Intravenous infusion, 50 mg every six to eight hours, diluted in 100 mL of a compatible intravenous solution and administered over a fifteen- to twenty-minute period.
    Continuous intravenous infusion, 6.25 mg per hour, diluted in a compatible intravenous solution.
Note: For gastric hypersecretory conditions, the infusion should be started at 1 mg per kg of body weight per hour and increased by 0.5 mg per kg of body weight per hour increments (if gastric acid output is greater than 10 mEq per hour or patient is symptomatic), up to 2.5 mg per kg of body weight per hour.
[Prophylaxis of aspiration pneumonitis]—
    Intramuscular or slow intravenous injection, 50 mg administered forty-five to sixty minutes before induction of general anesthesia.
Note: For patients with impaired renal function (creatinine clearance of less than 50 mL per minute)—Intravenous, 50 mg every eighteen to twenty-four hours, the frequency of the dosage being increased to every twelve hours or more frequently, if necessary. Further reduction in dosage may be required if hepatic function impairment is also present.

**Usual adult prescribing limits**
Up to 400 mg a day.

**Usual pediatric dose**
Duodenal ulcer or
Gastric ulcer—
    Intravenous infusion, 2 to 4 mg per kilogram of body weight a day, diluted to a suitable volume with a compatible intravenous solution and administered over a fifteen- to twenty-minute period
Gastroesophageal reflux—
    Intravenous infusion, 2 to 8 mg per kg of body weight, diluted in a suitable volume with a compatible intravenous solution and administered over a fifteen- to twenty-minute period, three times a day.
Note: In certain circumstances, doses may be titrated based on gastric pH.

**Usual geriatric dose**
See *Usual adult and adolescent dose.*

**Strength(s) usually available**
U.S.—
    50 mg per 2 mL (Rx) [*Zantac*].
Canada—
    50 mg per 2 mL (Rx) [*Zantac*].

**Packaging and storage**
Store below 30 °C (86 °F), unless otherwise specified by manufacturer. Protect from light. Protect from freezing.

**Preparation of dosage form**
For 50 mg per 2 mL strength—
    For intravenous use, ranitidine injection must be diluted prior to use to a total volume of 20 mL with a compatible intravenous solution, such as sodium chloride injection (0.9%).

For intermittent intravenous infusion, ranitidine injection must be diluted prior to use in 100 mL of a compatible intravenous solution, such as dextrose injection (5%).

**Stability**

Diluted solutions of ranitidine injection are stable for 48 hours at room temperature.

Injection should not be used if discolored or if a precipitate is present.

The bulk package of ranitidine should be discarded within twenty-four hours after it is opened.

## RANITIDINE IN SODIUM CHLORIDE INJECTION

**Usual adult and adolescent dose**

See *Ranitidine Injection USP*

**Usual adult prescribing limits**

See *Ranitidine Injection USP*

**Usual pediatric dose**

See *Ranitidine Injection USP*

**Usual geriatric dose**

See *Ranitidine Injection USP*

**Strength(s) usually available**

U.S.—

50 mg per 50 mL (premixed), in 0.45% sodium chloride (Rx) [*Zantac*].

Canada—

50 mg per 50 mL (premixed), in 0.45% sodium chloride (Rx) [*Zantac*].

**Packaging and storage**

Store between 2 °C and 25 °C (36 °F and 77 °F). Protect from light. Protect from freezing.

Note: Brief exposure to temperatures up to 40 °C (104 °F) has not adversely affected the premixed product.

## Selected Bibliography

Feldman M, Burton M. Histamine$_2$-receptor antagonists standard therapy for acid-peptic diseases (first of two parts). N Engl J Med 1990; 323 (24): 1672-80.

Feldman M, Burton M. Histamine$_2$-receptor antagonists standard therapy for acid-peptic diseases (second of two parts). N Engl J Med 1990; 323 (25): 1749-55.

Revised: 08/08/96

## Table 1. Pharmacology/Pharmacokinetics

| Drug | Absorption* (% oral bioavailability) | Protein binding | Biotransformation | Half-life (elimination) | |
|---|---|---|---|---|---|
| | | | | With normal renal function (hr) | With reduced creatinine clearance (mL/min: hr) |
| Cimetidine | Rapid (60–70) | Low (15–20%) | Hepatic (30–40% of oral dose) | Oral: 2.0 Parenteral: 1.6–2.1† | 20–50: 2.9 <20: 3.7 Anephric: 5 |
| Famotidine | Rapid; incomplete (40–45) | Low (15–20%) | Hepatic (minimal first pass metabolism) | Oral/Parenteral: 2.5–3.5 | <10: 20 or more |
| Nizatidine | Rapid (>90) | Moderate (35%) | Hepatic (minimal first pass metabolism) | Oral: 1–2 | Anephric: 3.5–11 |
| Ranitidine | Rapid (39–87) | Low (15%) | Hepatic | Oral: 2.5 Parenteral: 2–2.5 | Oral—20–30: 8–9 Parenteral—25–35: 4.8 |

*Rate of absorption, but not extent, is delayed by food. Younger patients usually have better absorption of cimetidine than elderly patients. Absorption of famotidine and nizatidine is slightly increased by food, while the absorption of ranitidine is not significantly affected by the presence of food.

†In burn patients with thermal injury ranging from 6 to 80% of the body surface, and with normal renal function, elimination half-life of cimetidine has been found to be significantly reduced.

## Table 2. Pharmacology/Pharmacokinetics

| Drug | Mean serum concentration resulting in 50% inhibition* (ng/mL) | Time to peak concentration after oral dose (hr) | Time to peak effect (hr) | Duration of action (hr) | Elimination† (% excreted unchanged) |
|---|---|---|---|---|---|
| Cimetidine | 500 | ³/₄–1 | Oral: 1–2 | Nocturnal: 6–8 Basal: 4–5 | Primarily renal (48% of oral dose; 75% of parenteral dose)‡ |
| Famotidine | 13 | 1–3 | Oral: 1–3 Parenteral: ¹/₂ | Nocturnal and basal: 10–12 (oral and IV) | Primarily renal (30–35% of oral dose; 65–70% of parenteral dose) |
| Nizatidine | 295 | ¹/₂–3 | Oral: ¹/₂–3 | Nocturnal: Up to 12 Basal: Up to 8 | Primarily renal (60% of oral dose) |
| Ranitidine | 100 | 2–3 | Oral: 1–3 | Nocturnal: 13 Basal: 4 | Primarily renal (30% of oral dose; 70% of parenteral dose) |

*Refers to inhibition of pentagastrin-stimulated acid secretion.

†Trace amounts of H$_2$-receptor antagonists are removable by hemodialysis and peritoneal dialysis.

‡In burn patients with thermal injury ranging from 6 to 80% of the body surface, and with normal renal function, total clearance of cimetidine has been found to be significantly increased.

# Table 3. Side/Adverse Effects*

The following side/adverse effects have been selected on the basis of their potential clinical significance (possible signs and symptoms in parentheses where appropriate)—not necessarily inclusive:

Legend:
**I** = Cimetidine
**II** = Famotidine
**III** = Nizatidine
**IV** = Ranitidine

| | I | II | III | IV |
|---|---|---|---|---|
| **Medical attention needed** | | | | |
| *Agranulocytosis* (fever, sore throat, or unusual tiredness or weakness) | R§ | R§ | – | R§ |
| *Allergic reaction* (burning, redness, skin rash, or swelling) | ✔ | R | R | ✔ |
| *Bradycardia* (slow heartbeat) | R‡ | R | R | R |
| *Bronchospasm* (tightness in chest) | – | R | R | R |
| *Confusion* | R† | ✔ | R | R† |
| *Fever* | R | R | R | R |
| *Neutropenia* (sore throat and fever) | R§ | R§ | R§ | R§ |
| *Tachycardia* (fast, pounding, or irregular heartbeat) | R | R | R | R |
| *Thrombocytopenia* (unusual bleeding or bruising) | R§ | R§ | R§ | R§ |
| **Medical attention needed only if continuing or bothersome** | | | | |
| *Antiandrogenic effect* | | | | |
|   (decreased sexual ability) | R** | – | ✔ | ✔ |
|   (swelling of the breasts or breast soreness in females and males) | R†† | ✔ | ✔ | ✔ |
| *Blurred vision* | | | | ✔ |
| *Constipation* | – | <2% | ✔ | <2% |
| *Decrease in sexual desire* | ✔ | ✔ | ✔ | ✔ |
| *Diarrhea* | <2% | <2% | – | <2% |
| *Dizziness* | <2% | <2% | ✔ | <2% |
| *Drowsiness* | <2% | ✔ | 2.4% | <2% |
| *Dryness of mouth or skin* | – | ✔ | | |
| *Headache* | <3.5% | <5% | ✔ | 2% |
| *Increased sweating* | – | – | 1% | – |
| *Joint or muscle pain* | ✔ | ✔ | | ✔ |
| *Loss of appetite* | ✔ | ✔ | – | – |
| *Loss of hair* | ✔ | ✔ | – | ✔ |
| *Nausea or vomiting* | <2% | ✔ | ✔ | <2% |
| *Ringing or buzzing in ears* | – | ✔ | – | – |
| *Skin rash* | <2% | ✔ | ✔ | <2% |

*Differences in frequency of occurrence may reflect either lack of clinical-use data or actual pharmacologic distinctions among agents (although their pharmacologic similarity suggests that side effects occurring with one may occur with the others). M = more frequent; L = less frequent; R = rare; – = not reported; ✔ = reported, but percentage of occurrence and/or direct relationship to therapy has not been established.

†More likely to occur in severely ill patients or in patients with impaired hepatic or renal function, particularly elderly patients. Reversible within 3 to 4 days following discontinuation of medication. This side effect may mimic alcohol withdrawal syndrome (delirium tremens) in patients treated for gastrointestinal complications of alcoholism.

‡Cardiac effects after intravenous bolus injection.

§Neutropenia or other blood dyscrasias are more likely to occur in patients with serious concomitant illnesses or in those who also received antimetabolites, alkylating agents, or other medications and/or treatment known to produce neutropenia. Appear to be reversible and tend to occur within the first 30 days of administration.

**Rare; more likely to occur in patients with Zollinger-Ellison syndrome receiving high doses (3 to 10 grams of cimetidine a day) for at least 1 year.

††Rare; more frequent (about 4%) with long-term therapy.

# HMG-COA REDUCTASE INHIBITORS    Systemic

This monograph includes information on the following: Fluvastatin†; Lovastatin; Pravastatin; Simvastatin.

VA CLASSIFICATION (Primary): CV350

Other commonly used names are: Epistatin [Simvastatin], Eptastatin [Pravastatin], Mevinolin [Lovastatin] , Synvinolin [Simvastatin]

Note: For a listing of dosage forms and brand names by country availability, see *Dosage Forms* section(s). For a listing of brand names for the articles in this monograph, refer to the General Index.

---

†Not commercially available in Canada.

---

## Category

HMG-CoA reductase inhibitor; antihyperlipidemic.

## Indications

### Accepted

Hyperlipidemia (treatment)—3-Hydroxy-3-methylglutaryl coenzyme A (HMG-CoA) reductase inhibitors are indicated as adjuncts to diet in the treatment of primary hypercholesterolemia (type IIa and IIb hyperlipoproteinemia) caused by elevated low-density lipoprotein (LDL) cholesterol concentrations in patients with a significant risk of coronary artery disease, who have not responded to diet or other measures alone. The HMG-CoA reductase inhibitors may also be useful for the reduction of elevated LDL cholesterol concentrations in patients with combined hypercholesterolemia and hypertriglyceridemia.

For additional information on initial therapeutic guidelines related to the treatment of hyperlipidemia, see *Appendix III*.

## Pharmacology/Pharmacokinetics

### Physicochemical characteristics

Source—
    Fluvastatin: Synthetic.
    Lovastatin, pravastatin, simvastatin: Fungus-derived.
Molecular weight—
    Fluvastatin sodium: 433.45.
    Lovastatin: 404.55.
    Pravastatin sodium: 446.52.
    Simvastatin: 418.57.

### Mechanism of action/Effect

The active beta-hydroxy acid form of the 3-hydroxy-3-methylglutaryl coenzyme A (HMG-CoA) reductase inhibitors competitively inhibits the enzyme HMG-CoA reductase. Fluvastatin and pravastatin are administered in the active (open acid) form, while lovastatin and simvastatin must be hydrolyzed to the beta-hydroxyacid in tissues.

Inhibition of HMG-CoA reductase prevents conversion of HMG-CoA to mevalonate, the rate-limiting step in cholesterol biosynthesis. The primary site of action of HMG-CoA reductase inhibitors is the liver. Inhibition of cholesterol synthesis in the liver leads to upregulation of LDL receptors and an increase in catabolism of LDL cholesterol. There may also be some reduction in LDL production as a result of inhibition of hepatic synthesis of very low-density lipoprotein (VLDL), the precursor of LDL. HMG-CoA reductase inhibitors reduce LDL cholesterol, VLDL cholesterol, and to a lesser extent, plasma triglyceride concentrations, and slightly increase high-density lipoprotein (HDL) concentrations.

### Absorption

Fluvastatin—Rapidly and almost completely absorbed from the gastrointestinal tract (greater than 90%); bioavailability 19 to 29%.
Lovastatin—Reduced by approximately 30% when administered on an empty stomach rather than with food.
Pravastatin—Approximately 34%; bioavailability approximately 18%.

### Protein binding

Fluvastatin—Very high (greater than 98%).
Lovastatin—Very high (greater than 95%).
Pravastatin—Moderate (50%).
Simvastatin—Very high (approximately 95%).

### Biotransformation

Fluvastatin—Administered in active (open acid) form. Biotransformation by hydroxylation, N-dealkylation, and beta-oxidation; the major metabolic products present in plasma are pharmacologically inactive.
Lovastatin and simvastatin—By hydrolysis in tissues, to several metabolites, including a major active beta-hydroxy metabolite.

Pravastatin—Administered in active (open acid) form and converted to inactive metabolites and active metabolites with minimal activity.

### Half-life

Fluvastatin—Approximately 1.2 hours (range, 0.5 to 3.1 hours).
Lovastatin—3 hours.
Pravastatin—1.3 to 2.7 hours.

### Time to peak concentration

Fluvastatin—0.5 to 0.7 hour.
Lovastatin—2 to 4 hours.
Pravastatin—Approximately 1 hour.
Simvastatin—1.3 to 2.4 hours.

### Duration of action

Lovastatin—After withdrawal of continuous therapy: 4 to 6 weeks.

### Elimination

Fluvastatin—
    Fecal (biliary): 90%.
    Renal: 5%.
Lovastatin—
    Fecal (biliary and unabsorbed): 83%.
    Renal: 10%.
Pravastatin—
    Fecal (biliary and unabsorbed): 70%.
    Renal: 20%.
Simvastatin—
    Fecal (biliary and unabsorbed): 60%.
    Renal: 13%.

## Precautions to Consider

### Carcinogenicity

*Fluvastatin*—A study in rats given fluvastatin in doses of 6, 9, and 18 to 24 mg per kg of body weight (mg/kg) per day (plasma drug concentrations of approximately 9, 13, and 26 to 35 times the mean human plasma drug concentration after a 40-mg dose) found a low incidence of forestomach squamous papillomas and one carcinoma of the forestomach at the 24 mg/kg dose. However, these results were thought to reflect prolonged hyperplasia induced by direct contact with fluvastatin sodium rather than a systemic drug effect. Similar results were found in mice studies. In addition, an increased incidence of thyroid follicular cell adenomas and carcinomas was found in male rats treated with the 18 to 24 mg/kg doses.

*Lovastatin*—Studies in male and female mice given lovastatin in doses of 500 mg/kg per day (a total plasma drug exposure [total HMG-CoA reductase inhibitory activity in extracted plasma] 3 to 4 times that of humans given the highest recommended dose) for 21 months found an increased incidence of hepatocellular carcinomas and adenomas. In female mice, an increase in pulmonary adenomas was observed at approximately 4 times the human drug exposure. The incidence of papillomas in nonglandular mucosa of the stomach was also increased beginning at exposures 1 to 2 times that of humans; however, the human stomach contains only glandular mucosa. In rats given lovastatin for 24 months at drug exposures between 2 and 7 times human exposure at 80 mg per day, a positive dose–response relationship for hepatocellular carcinogenicity was observed in males.

*Pravastatin*—A study in rats given pravastatin doses producing serum drug concentrations 6 to 10 times higher than those in humans receiving 40 mg showed an increased incidence of hepatocellular carcinomas in male rats at the highest dose. Administration of pravastatin (producing plasma drug concentrations 0.5 to 5 times the human drug concentrations at 40 mg) in mice for 22 months resulted in an increased incidence of malignant lymphomas in females.

*Simvastatin*—A 72-week study in mice given simvastatin at doses producing serum concentrations 3, 15, and 33 times higher than the mean human plasma drug concentration after a 40-mg dose revealed increased incidences of liver adenomas, liver carcinomas, and lung adenomas in the middle- and high-dose groups. In addition, a higher incidence of Harderian gland (a gland of the eye in rodents) adenomas was observed in the high-dose group.

A 2-year study in rats exposed to simvastatin concentrations 45 times higher than those in humans given 40 mg revealed an increased incidence of thyroid follicular adenomas.

### Mutagenicity

*Fluvastatin*—No evidence of mutagenicity was observed in *in vitro* studies with or without rat-liver activation, including microbial mutagen tests, unscheduled DNA synthesis in rat primary hepatocytes, and chromosomal aberration tests. Additionally, there was no evidence of mutagenicity in *in vivo* rat or mouse micronucleus tests.

*Lovastatin* and *simvastatin*—A microbial mutagen test using mutant strains of *Salmonella typhimurium* with or without rat or mouse liver metabolic activation found no evidence of mutagenicity. There was also no evidence of damage to genetic material in *in vitro* alkaline elution assays using rat or mouse hepatocytes, a V-79 mammalian cell forward mutation study, an *in vitro* chromosome aberration study in CHO cells, or an *in vivo* chromosomal aberration assay in mouse bone marrow.

*Pravastatin*—No evidence of mutagenicity was observed in *in vitro* tests with or without liver metabolic activation, including microbial mutagen tests, a chromosomal aberration test, a gene conversion assay, a dominant lethal test in mice, and a micronucleus test in mice.

## Pregnancy/Reproduction

Fertility—*Fluvastatin:* No adverse effects on fertility or reproductive performance were observed in rats given fluvastatin sodium at doses of up to 6 mg/kg per day in females and 20 mg/kg per day in males.

*Lovastatin:* Testicular atrophy, decreased spermatogenesis, spermatocytic degeneration, and giant cell formation were seen in dogs given lovastatin starting at doses of 20 mg/kg per day. However, no adverse effects on fertility were observed in rats.

*Pravastatin:* No adverse effects on fertility or general reproductive performance were observed in rats given pravastatin at doses of up to 500 mg/kg per day.

*Simvastatin:* Decreased fertility was noted in rats given simvastatin for 34 weeks at 15 times the maximum human exposure level. However, this effect was not observed in another study in rats given simvastatin for 11 weeks at the same dosage level. Seminiferous tubule degeneration was observed in rats given simvastatin at a dose of 180 mg/kg per day (44 times the exposure level of humans given 40 mg per day). Testicular atrophy, decreased spermatogenesis, spermatocytic degeneration, and giant cell formation were observed in dogs given simvastatin at a dose of 10 mg/kg per day (7 times the human exposure level at a dose of 40 mg per day).

Pregnancy—HMG-CoA reductase inhibitors are not recommended for use during pregnancy or in women who plan to become pregnant in the near future.

Adequate and well-controlled studies in humans have not been done. However, because HMG-CoA reductase inhibitors interfere with biosynthesis of mevalonic acid, a cholesterol precursor that may have an essential function in DNA replication and, therefore, may be closely tied to fetal development (including synthesis of steroids and cell membranes), there is a possibility that fetal harm may be caused by administration of these medications during pregnancy. Vertebral anomalies, anal atresia, tracheo-esophageal fistula with esophageal atresia, and renal and radial dysplasias occurred in a neonate born to a mother who took lovastatin during the first trimester of pregnancy. However, a direct causal relationship has not been proven.

Use of birth control is recommended during use of these medications. If pregnancy occurs during HMG-CoA reductase inhibitor therapy, it is recommended that the HMG-CoA reductase inhibitor be discontinued for the duration of the pregnancy. Because of the long-term nature of antihyperlipidemic treatment, temporary suspension of therapy is not expected to be deleterious.

*Fluvastatin—*
No evidence of teratogenicity was found in rats or rabbits given doses of up to 36 mg/kg and 10 mg/kg per day, respectively. Administration of fluvastatin at 12 and 24 mg/kg per day to female rats during the third trimester resulted in maternal mortality at or near term and postpartum. Fetal and neonatal deaths were also observed. These results were confirmed by a second study.

FDA Pregnancy Category X.

*Lovastatin—*
Studies in mice and rats at doses producing plasma concentrations 40 (mouse fetus) and 80 (rat fetus) times the human exposure found an increased incidence of skeletal malformations. No changes occurred in rats or mice at multiples of 8 and 4 times, respectively, or in rabbits at exposures up to 3 times the highest tolerated human exposure.

FDA Pregnancy Category X.

*Pravastatin—*
Studies in rats and rabbits given pravastatin at doses of 1000 mg/kg per day (240 times the human exposure based on surface area) and 50 mg/kg per day (20 times the human exposure based on surface area), respectively, did not reveal teratogenic effects.

FDA Pregnancy Category X.

*Simvastatin—*
No teratogenic effects were observed in rats or rabbits given simvastatin at doses of 25 mg/kg per day (6 times the human exposure based on surface area) and 10 mg/kg per day (4 times the human exposure based on surface area), respectively.

FDA Pregnancy Category X.

## Breast-feeding

Use of HMG-CoA reductase inhibitors while breast-feeding is not recommended, because of the potential for serious adverse effects in nursing infants.

*Fluvastatin—*
Fluvastatin is distributed into breast milk and is present in breast milk in a 2 to 1 ratio (milk to plasma).

*Lovastatin—*
It is not known whether lovastatin is distributed into human breast milk, but it is distributed into the milk of rats.

*Pravastatin—*
Trace amounts of pravastatin are distributed into human breast milk.

*Simvastatin—*
It is not known whether simvastatin is distributed into human breast milk.

## Pediatrics

Appropriate studies on the relationship of age to the effects of HMG-CoA reductase inhibitors have not been performed in the pediatric population. Safety and efficacy have not been established.

Limited experience with use of lovastatin and simvastatin in children younger than 18 years of age seems to indicate that these medications are well tolerated and may be useful in severely hypercholesterolemic children who need medication therapy. However, the long-term safety of HMG-CoA reductase inhibitor use in children has not been studied. Use of these agents should be reserved for severe cases under the care of a lipid specialist. Caution is recommended in use of cholesterol-lowering agents in children younger than 10 years of age.

## Geriatrics

Studies performed to date in a limited number of patients 65 years of age or older have not demonstrated geriatrics-specific problems that would limit the usefulness of HMG-CoA reductase inhibitors in the elderly.

## Drug interactions and/or related problems

The following drug interactions and/or related problems have been selected on the basis of their potential clinical significance (possible mechanism in parentheses where appropriate)—not necessarily inclusive (» = major clinical significance):

Note: Combinations containing any of the following medications, depending on the amount present, may also interact with this medication.

Anticoagulants, coumarin- or indandione-derivative
(concurrent use with HMG-CoA reductase inhibitors may increase bleeding or prothrombin time; prothrombin time should be monitored in patients taking HMG-CoA reductase inhibitors with anticoagulants)

Cholestyramine or
Colestipol
(concurrent use may decrease the bioavailability of HMG-CoA reductase inhibitors; therefore, when these agents are used with HMG-CoA reductase inhibitors for therapeutic advantage, it is recommended that the HMG-CoA reductase inhibitor be given 4 hours after cholestyramine or colestipol)

» Cyclosporine or
Erythromycin or
» Gemfibrozil or
Immunosuppressants or
» Niacin
(concurrent use with HMG-CoA reductase inhibitors may be associated with an increased risk of rhabdomyolysis and acute renal failure; although cases have been reported only with lovastatin, the potential also exists with other HMG-CoA reductase inhibitors; combined therapy of HMG-CoA reductase inhibitors with gemfibrozil, niacin, or immunosuppressants should include careful monitoring for symptoms of myopathy or rhabdomyolysis)

*For simvastatin (in addition to those listed above)*
Digoxin
(concurrent use with simvastatin may cause a slight elevation in serum digoxin concentrations)

## Laboratory value alterations

The following have been selected on the basis of their potential clinical significance (possible effect in parentheses where appropriate)—not necessarily inclusive (» = major clinical significance):

With physiology/laboratory test values
   Creatine kinase (CK) concentrations
      (mild transient increases are common and may not be drug-related; drug-related marked increases, with myositis and possible renal failure, occur in about 0.5 to 1% of patients, although the incidence may be higher in organ transplant patients treated concurrently with immunosuppressants or gemfibrozil)
   Transaminase, serum
      (values may be increased, usually to less than 3 times the upper limit of normal; in slightly less than 1 to 2% of patients receiving HMG-CoA reductase inhibitors for at least 1 year, marked increases to more than 3 times the upper limit of normal have occurred)

**Medical considerations/Contraindications**
The medical considerations/contraindications included here have been selected on the basis of their potential clinical significance (reasons given in parentheses where appropriate)—not necessarily inclusive (» = major clinical significance).

*Except under special circumstances, this medication should not be used when the following medical problem exists:*
» Hepatic disease, active
      (condition may be exacerbated)

*Risk-benefit should be considered when the following medical problems exist:*
   Alcoholism, active or in remission or
   Hepatic disease, history of
      (further increases in liver enzymes may occur)
» Organ transplant, with immunosuppressant therapy
      (increased risk of rhabdomyolysis and renal failure)
   Sensitivity to any HMG-CoA reductase inhibitor
» Serious conditions predisposing to the development of renal failure secondary to rhabdomyolysis, such as hypotension, severe acute infection, severe metabolic, endocrine, or electrolyte disorders, uncontrolled seizures, major surgery, or trauma
      (increased risk of secondary renal failure if rhabdomyolysis occurs)

**Patient monitoring**
The following may be especially important in patient monitoring (other tests may be warranted in some patients, depending on condition; » = major clinical significance):
» Cholesterol, serum
      (determinations recommended 4 weeks after initiation of therapy and at periodic intervals during therapy)
» Creatine kinase (CK), serum
      (determinations recommended if patient develops muscle tenderness during therapy or during concurrent therapy with niacin or immunosuppressive medications)
» Liver function tests, including serum transaminase
      (determinations recommended prior to initiation of therapy, every 6 weeks during the first 3 months of therapy, every 8 weeks during the remainder of the first year of therapy, and then at periodic intervals [approximately every 6 months])

# Side/Adverse Effects

Note: Recent data on patients receiving lovastatin do not reveal clinically significant differences between lovastatin and placebo in the incidence, type, or progression of lens opacities. To date, no increased incidence of lens opacities has been found with fluvastatin, pravastatin, or simvastatin.

Acute *pancreatitis* has been reported during clinical use with simvastatin and lovastatin. A causal relationship with the HMG-CoA reductase inhibitors has not been clearly established. However, onset of symptoms appears to occur within 3 months of initiation of therapy. Rapid regression of symptoms and laboratory anomalies has been observed upon discontinuation of the HMG-CoA reductase inhibitor. Patients should be advised to report immediately to physician acute onset of severe abdominal pain. Although reports of fluvastatin- or pravastatin-associated pancreatitis are lacking, patients taking these medications should also be properly advised, since the mechanism of the effect is poorly understood.

The following side/adverse effects have been selected on the basis of their potential clinical significance (possible signs and symptoms in parentheses where appropriate)—not necessarily inclusive:

**Those indicating need for medical attention**
Incidence less frequent or rare
   *Myalgia, myositis, or rhabdomyolysis* (fever; muscle aches or cramps; unusual tiredness or weakness)
   Note: *Rhabdomyolysis* may lead to renal failure. Incidence may be increased in patients treated with immunosuppressants, gemfibrozil, erythromycin, or niacin. Onset may occur weeks to months after initiation of treatment. Patients should be advised to report immediately to physician any unexplained muscle pain, tenderness, or weakness, especially if it is accompanied by malaise or fever.

**Those indicating need for medical attention only if they continue or are bothersome**
Incidence more frequent
   *Constipation, diarrhea, gas, heartburn, or stomach pain; dizziness; headache; nausea; skin rash*
Incidence rare
   *Impotence* (decreased sexual ability); *insomnia* (trouble in sleeping)

# Patient Consultation

As an aid to patient consultation, refer to *Advice for the Patient, HMG-CoA Reductase Inhibitors (Systemic).*

In providing consultation, consider emphasizing the following selected information (» = major clinical significance):

**Before using this medication**
   Diet as preferred therapy; importance of following prescribed diet
» Conditions affecting use, especially:
      Sensitivity to any HMG-CoA reductase inhibitor
      Pregnancy—Use not recommended in pregnancy or in women who plan to become pregnant in near future, because inhibited formation of cholesterol may impair fetal development; birth defects reported with lovastatin
      Breast-feeding—Use not recommended, because of potentially serious adverse effects in nursing infants
      Other medications, especially cyclosporine, gemfibrozil, or niacin
      Other medical problems, especially active hepatic disease; hypotension; major surgery; organ transplant with immunosuppressant therapy; severe infection; severe metabolic, endocrine, or electrolyte disorders; trauma; or uncontrolled seizures

**Proper use of this medication**
*For all HMG-CoA reductase inhibitors*
» Importance of not taking more or less medication than the amount prescribed
   This medication does not cure the condition but instead helps control it
» Compliance with prescribed diet
» Proper dosing
   Missed dose: Taking as soon as possible; not taking if almost time for next dose; not doubling doses
» Proper storage
*For lovastatin*
   Taking with meals, since medication is more effective with food

**Precautions while using this medication**
» Importance of close monitoring by physician
» Notifying physician immediately if pregnancy is suspected
» Checking with physician before discontinuing medications; blood lipid levels may increase significantly
» Caution if any kind of surgery (including dental surgery) or emergency treatment is required

**Side/adverse effects**
   Signs of potential side effects, especially myalgia, myositis, or rhabdomyolysis

# General Dosing Information

If serum transaminase concentrations increase to 3 times the upper limit of normal, HMG-CoA reductase inhibitor therapy should be withdrawn.

If creatine kinase (CK) concentrations are markedly increased or myositis occurs, HMG-CoA reductase inhibitor therapy should be withdrawn.

**Diet/Nutrition**
Nonpharmacologic management (dietary and weight control) of hypercholesterolemia is recommended as an adjunct to all pharmacologic therapy.

## FLUVASTATIN

## Summary of Differences

Pharmacology/pharmacokinetics:
> Biotransformation—By hydroxylation, N-dealkylation, and beta-oxidation to inactive metabolites.
> Time to peak concentration—0.5 to 0.7 hour.

## Additional Dosing Information

Can be taken with meals or on an empty stomach.

## Oral Dosage Forms

Note: The dosing and strengths of the dosage forms available are expressed in terms of fluvastatin base (not the sodium salt).

### FLUVASTATIN SODIUM CAPSULES

**Usual adult and adolescent dose**
Antihyperlipidemic—
> Initial: Oral, 20 mg (base) once a day at bedtime, the dosage being adjusted at four-week intervals as needed and tolerated.
> Maintenance: Oral, 20 to 40 mg (base) once a day in the evening.
> Note: A 40-mg (base) daily dose may be split and taken two times a day.

**Usual pediatric dose**
Safety and efficacy have not been established.

**Strength(s) usually available**
U.S.—
> 20 mg (base) (Rx) [*Lescol* (lactose)].
> 40 mg (base) (Rx) [*Lescol* (lactose)].

Canada—
> Not commercially available.

**Packaging and storage**
Store below 30 °C (86 °F) in a tight container. Protect from light.

## LOVASTATIN

## Summary of Differences

Pharmacology/pharmacokinetics:
> Absorption—Reduced by one-third on empty stomach.
> Biotransformation—By hydrolysis to active metabolites.
> Time to peak concentration—2 to 4 hours.
> Duration of action—After withdrawal of continuous therapy: 4 to 6 weeks.

## Additional Dosing Information

Should be taken with meals to maximize absorption.

## Oral Dosage Forms

### LOVASTATIN TABLETS USP

**Usual adult and adolescent dose**
Antihyperlipidemic—
> Initial: Oral, 20 mg once a day with the evening meal, the dosage being adjusted at four-week intervals as needed and tolerated.
> Maintenance: Oral, 20 to 80 mg per day, as a single dose or in divided doses, with meals.

Note: For patients on concomitant immunosuppressive therapy, it is recommended that lovastatin therapy begin with 10 mg per day and not exceed 20 mg per day.

> For patients with severe renal function impairment (creatinine clearance less than 30 mL per min), doses above 20 mg per day should be carefully considered and dosage titration should proceed cautiously.

**Usual adult prescribing limits**
Up to 80 mg per day.

**Usual pediatric dose**
Safety and efficacy have not been established.

**Strength(s) usually available**
U.S.—
> 10 mg (Rx) [*Mevacor* (lactose)].
> 20 mg (Rx) [*Mevacor* (lactose)].
> 40 mg (Rx) [*Mevacor* (lactose)].

Canada—
> 20 mg (Rx) [*Mevacor* (lactose)].
> 40 mg (Rx) [*Mevacor* (lactose)].

**Packaging and storage**
Store below 40 °C (104 °F), preferably between 15 and 30 °C (59 and 86 °F), in a tight, light-resistant container, unless otherwise specified by manufacturer.

**Auxiliary labeling**
• Take with meals.

## PRAVASTATIN

## Summary of Differences

Pharmacology/pharmacokinetics:
> Biotransformation—Administered in active form.
> Time to peak concentration—1 hour.

## Additional Dosing Information

Can be taken with meals or on an empty stomach.

## Oral Dosage Forms

### PRAVASTATIN SODIUM TABLETS

**Usual adult and adolescent dose**
Antihyperlipidemic—
> Initial:
>> Oral, 10 to 20 mg once a day at bedtime, the dosage being adjusted at four-week intervals as needed and tolerated.
>> Note: An initial dose of 10 mg once a day at bedtime is recommended in patients with significant renal function impairment or hepatic function impairment, and for the elderly.
> Maintenance:
>> 10 to 40 mg once a day at bedtime.
>> Note: In the elderly, maintenance doses of 20 mg a day or less are usually effective.

**Usual pediatric dose**
Safety and efficacy have not been established.

**Strength(s) usually available**
U.S.—
> 10 mg (Rx) [*Pravachol*].
> 20 mg (Rx) [*Pravachol*].
> 40 mg (Rx) [*Pravachol*].

Canada—
> 10 mg (Rx) [*Pravachol*].
> 20 mg (Rx) [*Pravachol*].

**Packaging and storage**
Store below 40 °C (104 °F), preferably between 15 and 30 °C (59 and 86 °F), in a well-closed container, unless otherwise specified by manufacturer.

## SIMVASTATIN

## Summary of Differences

Pharmacology/pharmacokinetics:
> Biotransformation—By hydrolysis to active metabolites.
> Time to peak concentration—1.3 to 2.4 hours.
Precautions:
> Drug interactions and/or related problems—Elevation of serum digoxin.

## Additional Dosing Information

Can be taken with meals or on an empty stomach.

## Oral Dosage Forms

### SIMVASTATIN TABLETS

**Usual adult and adolescent dose**
Antihyperlipidemic—
> Initial: Oral, 5 to 10 mg once a day in the evening, the dosage being adjusted at four-week intervals.
> Maintenance: 5 to 40 mg once a day in the evening.

Note: For patients taking concurrent immunosuppressive medications, it is recommended that simvastatin therapy begin with 5 mg per day and not exceed 10 mg per day.

**Usual adult prescribing limits**
40 mg per day.

**Usual pediatric dose**
Safety and efficacy have not been established.

**Strength(s) usually available**
U.S.—

5 mg (Rx) [*Zocor*].
10 mg (Rx) [*Zocor*].
20 mg (Rx) [*Zocor*].
40 mg (Rx) [*Zocor*].

Canada—

5 mg (Rx) [*Zocor*].
10 mg (Rx) [*Zocor*].
20 mg (Rx) [*Zocor*].

**Packaging and storage**
Store below 40 °C (104 °F), preferably between 15 and 30 °C (59 and 86 °F), in a well-closed container, unless otherwise specified by manufacturer.

## Selected Bibliography

**General**
Grundy SM. HMG-CoA reductase inhibitors for treatment of hypercholesterolemia. N Engl J Med 1988 Jul 7; 319: 24-33.

**For Fluvastatin**
Levy RI, Troendle AJ, Fattu JM. A quarter century of drug treatment of dyslipoproteinemia, with a focus on the new HMG-CoA reductase inhibitor fluvastatin. Circulation 1993; 87 (Suppl III): III45-III53.

**For Lovastatin**
Zeller FP, Uvodich KC. Lovastatin for hypercholesterolemia. Drug Intell Clin Pharm 1988 Jul/Aug; 2: 542-5.

**For Pravastatin**
Jungnickel PW, Cantral KA, Maloley PA. Pravastatin: a new drug for the treatment of hypercholesterolemia. Clin Pharm 1992; 11: 677-89.

**For Simvastatin**
Todd P, Goa K. Simvastatin: a review of its pharmacological properties and therapeutic potential in hypercholesterolaemia. Drugs 1990; 40 (4): 583-607.

Revised: 03/06/95

**HOMATROPINE**—See *Anticholinergics/Antispasmodics (Systemic)*; *Homatropine (Ophthalmic)*

# HOMATROPINE   Ophthalmic

VA CLASSIFICATION (Primary): OP600

Note: For a listing of dosage forms and brand names by country availability, see *Dosage Forms* section(s). For a listing of brand names for the articles in this monograph, refer to the General Index.

## Category
Cycloplegic; mydriatic.

## Indications

**Accepted**
Refraction, cycloplegic—Homatropine is indicated for measurement of refractive errors.

Uveitis (treatment)—Homatropine is indicated for pupil dilation and ciliary muscle relaxation, which are desirable in acute inflammatory conditions of the uveal tract.

Mydriasis, postoperative or
Mydriasis, preoperative—Homatropine may be indicated to produce mydriasis in some preoperative and postoperative conditions.

Lens opacities, axial—Homatropine is indicated as an optical aid in some cases of axial lens opacities.

## Pharmacology/Pharmacokinetics

**Mechanism of action/Effect**
Homatropine (a belladonna alkaloid) is an anticholinergic agent that blocks the responses of the sphincter muscle of the iris and the accommodative muscle of the ciliary body to stimulation by acetylcholine. Dilation of the pupil (mydriasis) and paralysis of accommodation (cycloplegia) result.

**Duration of action**
Moderately long-acting cycloplegic and mydriatic.
Has a shorter duration of action than atropine.
Residual cycloplegia and mydriasis may persist for 24 to 72 hours following instillation of medication.

## Precautions to Consider

**Cross-sensitivity and/or related problems**
Patients sensitive to any of the other belladonna alkaloids may be sensitive to homatropine also.

**Carcinogenicity**
No long-term studies in animals have been done.

**Pregnancy/Reproduction**
Pregnancy—Studies have not been done in humans; however, ophthalmic homatropine may be systemically absorbed.
Studies have not been done in animals.
FDA Pregnancy Category C.

**Breast-feeding**
It is not known whether homatropine is distributed into breast milk. Problems in humans have not been documented; however, ophthalmic homatropine may be systemically absorbed.

**Pediatrics**
An increased susceptibility to homatropine and similar drugs (such as atropine) has been reported in infants and young children and in children with blond hair, blue eyes, Down's syndrome, spastic paralysis, or brain damage; therefore, homatropine should be used with great caution in these patients.

**Geriatrics**
Geriatric patients are more susceptible to the effects of homatropine and similar drugs (such as atropine), thus increasing the potential for systemic side effects.

**Drug interactions and/or related problems**
The following drug interactions and/or related problems have been selected on the basis of their potential clinical significance (possible mechanism in parentheses where appropriate)—not necessarily inclusive (» = major clinical significance):

Note: Combinations containing any of the following medications, depending on the amount present, may also interact with this medication.

Anticholinergics or medications with anticholinergic activity, other (See *Appendix II*)
(if significant systemic absorption of ophthalmic homatropine occurs, concurrent use of other anticholinergics or medications with anticholinergic activity may result in potentiated anticholinergic effects)

Antiglaucoma agents, cholinergic, long-acting, ophthalmic
(concurrent use with homatropine may antagonize the antiglaucoma and miotic actions of ophthalmic long-acting cholinergic antiglaucoma agents, such as demecarium, echothiophate, and isoflurophate; concurrent use with homatropine may also antagonize the antiaccommodative convergence effects of these medications when they are used for the treatment of strabismus)

Antimyasthenics or
Potassium citrate or
Potassium supplements
(if significant systemic absorption of ophthalmic homatropine occurs, concurrent use may increase the chance of toxicity and/or side effects of these systemic medications because of the anticholinergic-induced slowing of gastrointestinal motility)

Carbachol or
Physostigmine or
Pilocarpine
(concurrent use with homatropine may interfere with the antiglaucoma action of carbachol, physostigmine, or pilocarpine. Also, concurrent use counteracts the mydriatic effect of homatropine; this counteraction may be used to therapeutic advantage)

CNS depression–producing medications (See *Appendix II*)
(if significant systemic absorption of ophthalmic homatropine occurs, concurrent use of medications having CNS effects, such as antiemetic agents, phenothiazines, or barbiturates, may result in opisthotonos, convulsions, coma, and extrapyramidal symptoms)

### Medical considerations/Contraindications

The medical considerations/contraindications included here have been selected on the basis of their potential clinical significance (reasons given in parentheses where appropriate)—not necessarily inclusive (» = major clinical significance).

*Risk-benefit should be considered when the following medical problems exist:*

Brain damage, in children

Down's syndrome (mongolism), in children and adults

» Glaucoma, primary, or predisposition to angle closure

Keratoconus
(homatropine may produce fixed dilated pupil)

Sensitivity to homatropine

Spastic paralysis, in children

Synechiae between the iris and lens

## Side/Adverse Effects

Note: An increased susceptibility to homatropine and similar drugs (such as atropine) has been reported in infants, young children, children with blond hair or blue eyes, adults and children with Down's syndrome, children with brain damage or spastic paralysis, and the elderly. This susceptibility increases the potential for systemic side effects.

Prolonged use of homatropine may produce local irritation, resulting in follicular conjunctivitis, vascular congestion, edema, exudate, contact dermatitis, or an eczematoid dermatitis.

The following side/adverse effects have been selected on the basis of their potential clinical significance (possible signs and symptoms in parentheses where appropriate)—not necessarily inclusive:

### Those indicating need for medical attention

Symptoms of systemic absorption

*Clumsiness or unsteadiness; confusion or unusual behavior; dryness of skin; fever; flushing or redness of face; hallucinations; skin rash; slurred speech; swollen stomach in infants; tachycardia* (fast or irregular heartbeat); *unusual drowsiness; tiredness or weakness; xerostomia* (thirst or dryness of mouth)

### Those indicating need for medical attention only if they continue or are bothersome

*Blurred vision; eye irritation not present before therapy; increased sensitivity of eyes to light; swelling of the eyelids*

## Overdose

For specific information on the agents used in the management of ophthalmic homatropine overdose, see:
- *Atropine* in *Anticholinergics/Antispasmodics (Systemic)* monograph;
- *Diazepam* in *Benzodiazepines (Systemic)* monograph; and/or
- *Physostigmine (Systemic)* monograph.

For more information on the management of overdose or unintentional ingestion, **contact a Poison Control Center** (see *Poison Control Center Listing*).

### Treatment of overdose

For accidental ingestion, emesis or gastric lavage with 4% tannic acid solution is recommended.

For systemic effects, 0.2 to 1 mg (0.2 mg in children) physostigmine should be administered intravenously, as a dilution containing 1 mg in 5 mL of normal saline. The solution should be injected over a period of not less than 2 minutes. Dosage may be repeated every 5 minutes up to a total dose of 2 mg in children and 6 mg in adults in each 30-minute period.

Physostigmine is contraindicated in hypotensive reactions.

ECG monitoring is recommended during physostigmine administration.

Excitement may be controlled by diazepam or a short-acting barbiturate.

It is recommended that 1 mg of atropine be available for immediate injection if the physostigmine causes bradycardia, convulsion, or bronchoconstriction.

Supportive therapy may require oxygen and assisted respiration; cool water baths for fever, especially in children; and catheterization for urinary retention. In infants and small children, the body surface should be kept moist.

## Patient Consultation

As an aid to patient consultation, refer to *Advice for the Patient, Atropine/Homatropine/Scopolamine (Ophthalmic)*.

In providing consultation, consider emphasizing the following selected information (» = major clinical significance):

### Before using this medication

» Conditions affecting use, especially:

Sensitivity to atropine, homatropine, or scopolamine

Use in children—Infants and young children and children with blond hair or blue eyes may be especially sensitive to the effects of homatropine; this may increase the chance of side effects during treatment

Use in the elderly—Geriatric patients are more susceptible to the effects of homatropine and similar drugs (such as atropine), thus increasing the potential for systemic side effects

Other medical problems, especially primary glaucoma or predisposition to angle closure

### Proper use of this medication

Proper administration technique

Washing hands immediately after application to remove any medication that may be on them; if applying medication to infants or children, washing their hands immediately afterwards also, and not letting any medication get into their mouths; wiping off any medication that may have accidentally gotten on the infant or child, including his or her face and eyelids

Preventing contamination: Not touching applicator tip to any surface; keeping container tightly closed

» Importance of not using more medication than the amount prescribed

» Proper dosing

Missed dose: If dosing schedule is—

Once a day: Applying as soon as possible if remembered same day; if remembered later, skipping missed dose and going back to regular dosing schedule; not doubling doses

More than once a day: Applying as soon as possible; if almost time for next dose, skipping missed dose and going back to regular dosing schedule; not doubling doses

» Proper storage

### Precautions while using this medication

» Medication causes blurred vision and increased sensitivity of the eyes to light; checking with physician if these effects continue longer than 3 days after discontinuation of homatropine

### Side/adverse effects

Signs of potential side effects, especially symptoms of systemic absorption

## General Dosing Information

Although some manufacturers recommend a dose of 2 drops of an ophthalmic solution at appropriate intervals, the conjunctival sac will usually hold only 1 drop.

More frequent instillation or use of a stronger solution may be required to produce adequate cycloplegia in eyes with brown or hazel irides than in eyes with blue irides.

To avoid excessive systemic absorption, patient should press finger to the lacrimal sac during, and for 2 or 3 minutes following, instillation of the solution.

## Ophthalmic Dosage Forms

### HOMATROPINE HYDROBROMIDE OPHTHALMIC SOLUTION USP

**Usual adult and adolescent dose**

Cycloplegic refraction—

Topical, to the conjunctiva, 1 drop of a 2 or 5% solution. May be repeated every five to ten minutes if needed for two or three doses immediately prior to refraction.

Uveitis—

Topical, to the conjunctiva, 1 drop of a 2 or 5% solution two or three times a day. In some cases, a frequency of up to every 3 or 4 hours may be required.

**Usual pediatric dose**

Cycloplegic refraction—

Topical, to the conjunctiva, 1 drop of a 2 to 5% solution every ten minutes for two or threedoses immediately prior to refraction.

Uveitis—

Topical, to the conjunctiva, 1 drop of a 2 to 5% solution two or three times a day.

## Strength(s) usually available

U.S.—

2% (Rx) [*Isopto Homatropine* (benzalkonium chloride 0.01%); *Spectro-Homatropine* (benzalkonium chloride 0.01%); GENERIC].

5% (Rx) [*AK-Homatropine* (benzalkonium chloride 0.01%); *I-Homatrine; Isopto Homatropine* (benzethonium chloride 0.005%); *Spectro-Homatropine;* GENERIC].

Canada—

2% (Rx) [*Isopto Homatropine* (benzalkonium chloride); *Minims Homatropine;* GENERIC].

5% (Rx) [*Isopto Homatropine* (benzethonium chloride); GENERIC].

## Packaging and storage

Store below 40 °C (104 °F), preferably between 15 and 30 °C (59 and 86 °F), unless otherwise specified by manufacturer. Store in a tight container. Protect from freezing.

## Auxiliary labeling

• For the eye.

• Keep container tightly closed.

Revised: 06/21/94

## HOMATROPINE-CONTAINING COMBINATIONS—

Hydrocodone and Homatropine (Systemic)—See *Cough/Cold Combinations (Systemic)*

## HOMOSALATE—See *Sunscreen Agents (Topical)*

## HOMOSALATE-CONTAINING COMBINATIONS—

Homosalate, Menthyl Anthranilate, and Octyl Methoxycinnamate (Topical)—See *Sunscreen Agents (Topical)*

Homosalate, Menthyl Anthranilate, Octyl Methoxycinnamate, Octyl Salicylate, and Oxybenzone (Topical)—See *Sunscreen Agents (Topical)*

Homosalate, Octocrylene, Octyl Methoxycinnamate, and Oxybenzone (Topical)—See *Sunscreen Agents (Topical)*

Homosalate, Octyl Methoxycinnamate, Octyl Salicylate, and Oxybenzone (Topical)—See *Sunscreen Agents (Topical)*

Homosalate, Octyl Methoxycinnamate, and Oxybenzone (Topical)—See *Sunscreen Agents (Topical)*

Homosalate and Oxybenzone (Topical)—See *Sunscreen Agents (Topical)*

# HYDRALAZINE   Systemic

VA CLASSIFICATION (Primary/Secondary): CV490/CV900

Note: For a listing of dosage forms and brand names by country availability, see *Dosage Forms* section(s). For a listing of brand names for the articles in this monograph, refer to the General Index.

## Category

Antihypertensive; vasodilator, congestive heart failure.

## Indications

Note: Bracketed information in the *Indications* section refers to uses that are not included in U.S. product labeling.

### Accepted

Hypertension (treatment)—Hydralazine is indicated orally for the treatment of hypertension.

For additional information on initial therapeutic guidelines related to the treatment of hypertension, see *Appendix III*.

Hydralazine is indicated intravenously when oral therapy cannot be given or when there is an urgent need to lower blood pressure, such as in hypertensive crisis or pre-eclampsia or eclampsia.

[Congestive heart failure (treatment)][1]—Hydralazine may be used in combination with isosorbide dinitrate plus diuretics and digitalis in the treatment of congestive heart failure. Hydralazine and isosorbide dinitrate combination has been shown to improve 3-year mortality when compared to placebo. A more favorable effect on 2-year mortality was shown with an angiotensin-converting enzyme (ACE) inhibitor than with hydralazine and isosorbide dinitrate combination in a subsequent study. However, hydralazine plus isosorbide dinitrate still improved survival and exerted a more favorable effect on exercise performance and left ventricular ejection fraction than the ACE inhibitor. This combination may be considered in patients with left ventricular systolic dysfunction who cannot tolerate ACE inhibitors.

[1]Not included in Canadian product labeling.

## Pharmacology/Pharmacokinetics

### Physicochemical characteristics

Molecular weight—Hydralazine hydrochloride: 196.64.

pKa—7.3.

### Mechanism of action/Effect

Antihypertensive—The exact mechanism of antihypertensive action is not fully understood. The predominant effect of hydralazine is direct vasodilation of arterioles with little effect on veins, resulting in a decrease in peripheral resistance and an increase in heart rate, stroke volume, and cardiac output.

Vasodilator, congestive heart failure—Beneficial effects are due to increased cardiac output, decreased systemic resistance, and afterload

reduction when hydralazine is used in combination with isosorbide dinitrate.

### Absorption

Hydralazine is well absorbed (up to 90%) after oral administration, although plasma concentrations are considerably lower than after intramuscular or intravenous administration of the same dose because of first-pass metabolism. Oral bioavailability is approximately 50% (slow acetylators) or 30% (fast acetylators).

### Protein binding

High (87%).

### Biotransformation

Hydralazine undergoes extensive hepatic metabolism. Hydralazine is subject to polymorphic acetylation, although this does not appear to be the major metabolic pathway. Formation of hydrazone metabolites constitutes the other important metabolic pathway. The active metabolites, hydralazine acetonide hydrazone and hydralazine pyruvate hydrazone, are equipotent with the parent, hydralazine.

### Half-life

3 to 7 hours; prolonged in renal failure.

Some references state a difference in half-life between slow and fast acetylators, but there is generally thought to be little difference.

The half-life of antihypertensive action is much longer than the plasma half-life, possibly because hydralazine persists within muscular arterial walls.

### Onset of action

Oral—45 minutes.

Intravenous—10 to 20 minutes.

### Time to peak concentration

Oral—1 to 2 hours.

### Time to peak effect

Intravenous—15 to 30 minutes.

### Duration of action

Oral or intravenous—3 to 8 hours.

### Elimination

Renal, 2 to 4% unchanged after oral administration and 11 to 14% unchanged after intravenous administration.

## Precautions to Consider

### Cross-sensitivity and/or related problems

Patients sensitive to tartrazine may be sensitive to the tablet dosage form also, since some tablets contain tartrazine.

### Carcinogenicity

In a 2-year carcinogenicity study of rats, hydralazine given at dose levels of 15, 30, and 60 mg per kg of body weight (mg/kg) per day (about 5 to 20 times the recommended human daily dose) produced a small, but statistically significant, increase in benign neoplastic nodules in male and female rats from the high-dose group and in female rats from the intermediate-dose group. Furthermore, benign interstitial cell tumors of the testes were significantly increased in male rats from the high-dose group.

### Tumorigenicity

A lifetime study in Swiss male and female albino mice given hydralazine continuously in their drinking water at a dose of about 250 mg/kg per day (approximately 80 times the maximum recommended human dose) revealed an increase in the incidence of lung tumors (adenomas and adenocarcinomas).

### Mutagenicity

Hydralazine was shown to be mutagenic in bacterial systems (gene mutation and DNA repair). Mutagenicity was also found in 1 of 2 rat and 1 rabbit hepatocyte *in vitro* DNA repair studies. However, *in vivo* and *in vitro* studies using mice lymphoma cells, germinal cells, and fibroblasts, Chinese hamster bone marrow cells, and human cell fibroblasts did not reveal any mutagenic potential for hydralazine.

### Pregnancy/Reproduction

Pregnancy—Hydralazine crosses the placenta. Studies in humans have not been done. However, thrombocytopenia, leukopenia, petechial bleeding, and hematomas have been reported in newborns whose mothers took hydralazine; symptoms resolved spontaneously in 1 to 3 weeks. Furthermore, there have been some reports of fetal distress following intravenous use of hydralazine to control maternal hypertension. The risk of fetal distress appears to be greater when vasodilation with hydralazine is undertaken without prior volume expansion. Preterm infants and growth-retarded infants appear to be particularly at risk.

Studies in mice given hydralazine at 20 to 30 times the maximum daily human dose of 200 to 300 mg revealed teratogenic effects. Furthermore, studies in rabbits indicate teratogenic effects at doses 10 to 15 times the maximum daily human dose. Teratogenic effects observed were cleft palate and malformations of facial and cranial bones. However, hydralazine was not shown to be teratogenic in rats.

FDA Pregnancy Category C.

### Breast-feeding

It is not known whether hydralazine is distributed into human milk.

### Pediatrics

Appropriate studies on the relationship of age to the effects of hydralazine have not been performed in the pediatric population. However, pediatrics-specific problems that would limit the usefulness of this medication in children are not expected.

### Geriatrics

Although appropriate studies on the relationship of age to the effects of hydralazine have not been performed in the geriatric population, geriatrics-specific problems are not expected to limit the usefulness of hydralazine in the elderly. However, elderly patients may be more sensitive to the hypotensive effects of hydralazine and are more likely to have age-related renal function impairment, both of which may require dosage reduction.

### Pharmacogenetics

All patients may be divided into two groups, slow and fast acetylators of hydralazine. Patients who are slow acetylators may be more prone to develop adverse effects (especially the systemic lupus erythematosus [SLE]–like syndrome) and may require lower-than-usual doses. Eskimo, Oriental, and American Indian populations have the lowest prevalence of slow acetylators, while Egyptian, Israeli, Scandanavian, other Caucasian, and black populations have the highest prevalence of slow acetylators.

### Drug interactions and/or related problems

The following drug interactions and/or related problems have been selected on the basis of their potential clinical significance (possible mechanism in parentheses where appropriate)—not necessarily inclusive (» = major clinical significance):

Note: Combinations containing any of the following medications, depending on the amount present, may also interact with this medication.

Anti-inflammatory drugs, nonsteroidal (NSAIDs), especially indomethacin
(may reduce antihypertensive effects of hydralazine; indomethacin, and possibly other NSAIDs, may antagonize the antihypertensive effect by inhibiting renal prostaglandin synthesis and/or by causing sodium and fluid retention; the patient should be carefully monitored to confirm that the desired effect is being obtained)

» Diazoxide or
Hypotension-producing medications, other (See *Appendix II*)
(antihypertensive effects may be potentiated when these medications are used concurrently with hydralazine; concurrent use of diazoxide or other potent parenteral antihypertensives with hydralazine may result in a severe, additive hypotensive effect; although some antihypertensive and/or diuretic combinations are frequently used for therapeutic advantage, dosage adjustments may be necessary during concurrent use)
(patients should be continuously observed for excessive fall in blood pressure for several hours after concurrent administration of diazoxide or other potent parenteral antihypertensives)

Estrogens
(estrogen-induced fluid retention may increase blood pressure)

Sympathomimetics
(may reduce antihypertensive effects of hydralazine; the patient should be carefully monitored to confirm that the desired effect is being obtained)

### Laboratory value alterations

The following have been selected on the basis of their potential clinical significance (possible effect in parentheses where appropriate)—not necessarily inclusive (» = major clinical significance):

With physiology/laboratory test values
Direct antiglobulin (Coombs') tests
(may produce positive results)

### Medical considerations/Contraindications

The medical considerations/contraindications included here have been selected on the basis of their potential clinical significance (reasons given in parentheses where appropriate)—not necessarily inclusive (» = major clinical significance).

### *Risk-benefit should be considered when the following medical problems exist:*

Aortic aneurysm or
» Aortic dissection, acute
(reflexive increase in heart rate, cardiac output, and shear stress associated with hydralazine may exacerbate condition)

Cerebrovascular disease or accident
(decreased blood pressure may increase cerebral ischemia)

Congestive heart failure
(use of hydralazine alone is not recommended, although it may improve cardiac performance in some patients with intractable left ventricular failure)

» Coronary artery disease
(myocardial stimulation and increased myocardial oxygen demands may cause or aggravate ischemia and angina and reportedly may precipitate myocardial infarction)

Renal function impairment, advanced
(accumulation of hydralazine may occur because of slower acetylation and reduced elimination, although incidence of toxic side effects is not increased; lower dosage may be required)

» Rheumatic heart disease, mitral valvular
(hydralazine may increase pulmonary artery pressure)

Sensitivity to hydralazine

Note: There is no substantial evidence that use of hydralazine in the treatment of hypertension in patients with systemic vasculitis or systemic lupus erythematosus exacerbates the underlying disease process.

### Patient monitoring

The following may be especially important in patient monitoring (other tests may be warranted in some patients, depending on condition; » = major clinical significance):

Antinuclear antibody (ANA) titer determinations and
Complete blood counts and
Lupus erythematosus cell preparations
(may be indicated if patient develops arthralgia, fever, chest pain, continued malaise, or other unexplained symptoms)

» Blood pressure measurements
(recommended at periodic intervals in patients being treated for hypertension; selected patients may be trained to perform blood pressure measurements at home and report the results at regular physician visits)

## Side/Adverse Effects

Note: Side/adverse effects are rare at lower dosages and are generally reversible.

Hepatotoxicity has been reported in a few patients.

The following side/adverse effects have been selected on the basis of their potential clinical significance (possible signs and symptoms in parentheses where appropriate)—not necessarily inclusive:

**Those indicating need for medical attention**
Incidence less frequent
*Allergic reaction* (skin rash or itching); *angina pectoris* (chest pain); *cutaneous vasculitis* (blisters on skin); *lymphadenopathy* (swelling of lymph glands); *peripheral neuritis* (numbness, tingling, pain, or weakness in hands or feet); *sodium and water retention and edema* (swelling of feet or lower legs); *systemic lupus erythematosus (SLE)–like syndrome, including glomerulonephritis* (blisters on skin; chest pain; general feeling of discomfort, illness, or weakness; muscle pain; joint pain; skin rash or itching; sore throat and fever)

Note: The *SLE-like syndrome* is a pharmacologic rather than an allergic effect. Risk factors include high daily doses of hydralazine (greater than 200 mg per day), slow acetylator or HLA-DRw4 phenotype, and family history of autoimmune disease. It is rarely seen with doses lower than 200 mg per day. The most common symptoms associated with hydralazine-induced SLE-like syndrome involve the musculoskeletal system, including arthralgias, arthritis, and myalgias. Other symptoms may include malaise, fever, or skin changes. Renal or central nervous system involvement is rare. A positive antinuclear antibody (ANA) is evident in virtually all cases of hydralazine-induced SLE-like syndrome. However, approximately 30% of all patients receiving hydralazine develop a positive ANA within one year of continuous therapy. Therefore, an isolated positive ANA does not necessarily mean that hydralazine-induced SLE-like syndrome is present. The clinical manifestations of hydralazine-induced SLE-like syndrome resolve within days to weeks of medication withdrawal. Resolution of positive ANA usually takes several months.

Incidence rare
*Blood dyscrasias, including agranulocytosis, leukopenia, and purpura* (fever; general feeling of discomfort or illness; sore throat; weakness)

**Those indicating need for medical attention only if they continue or are bothersome**
Incidence more frequent
*Anorexia* (loss of appetite); *diarrhea; headache; nausea or vomiting; palpitations* (pounding heartbeat); *tachycardia* (fast heartbeat)

Note: In patients with severe heart failure, sympathetic tone is already high and there will be little or no change in heart rate.

Incidence less frequent
*Constipation; dyspnea* (shortness of breath); *hypotension* (dizziness or lightheadedness); *lacrimation* (watering eyes); *nasal congestion* (stuffy nose); *redness or flushing of face*

## Overdose

For specific information on the agents used in the management of hydralazine overdose, see:
• *Beta-adrenergic Blocking Agents (Systemic) monograph;*
• *Charcoal, Activated (Oral-Local) monograph; and/or*
• *Sympathomimetic Agents—Cardiovascular Use (Parenteral-Systemic) monograph.*

For more information on the management of overdose or unintentional ingestion, **contact a Poison Control Center** (see *Poison Control Center Listing*).

**Clinical effects of overdose**
The following effects have been selected on the basis of their potential clinical significance (possible signs and symptoms in parentheses where appropriate)—not necessarily inclusive:

*Headache; hypotension; myocardial infarction; myocardial ischemia* (chest pain); *skin flushing; shock; tachycardia* (fast heartbeat)

Note: *Myocardial ischemia* with marked ST segment depression has been reported.

**Treatment of overdose**
To decrease absorption—
Evacuation of gastric contents. If conditions permit, activated charcoal may be administered.

Specific treatment—
For shock: Plasma expanders. If a vasopressor is required, care should be taken not to precipitate or aggravate cardiac arrhythmia.
For tachycardia: Beta-adrenergic blocking agents.
Monitoring—
Fluid and electrolyte status and renal function should be monitored.
Supportive care—
Support of cardiovascular system is most important. Patients in whom intentional overdose is known or suspected should be referred for psychiatric consultation.

## Patient Consultation

As an aid to patient consultation, refer to *Advice for the Patient, Hydralazine (Systemic).*

In providing consultation, consider emphasizing the following selected information (» = major clinical significance):

**Before using this medication**
» Conditions affecting use, especially:
Sensitivity to hydralazine
Pregnancy—Blood problems and fetal distress reported in infants of mothers who took hydralazine; causes birth defects in animals
Use in the elderly—Increased sensitivity to hypotensive effects
Other medications, especially diazoxide
Other medical problems, especially acute aortic dissection, coronary artery disease, or rheumatic heart disease

**Proper use of this medication**
Getting into the habit of taking at same times each day to help increase compliance
» Proper dosing
Missed dose: Taking as soon as possible; not taking if almost time for next dose; not doubling doses
» Proper storage
*For use as an antihypertensive*
Possible need for control of weight and diet, especially sodium intake
» Patient may not experience symptoms of hypertension; importance of taking medication even if feeling well
» Does not cure, but helps control hypertension; possible need for lifelong therapy; checking with physician before discontinuing medication; serious consequences of untreated hypertension

**Precautions while using this medication**
Regular visits to physician to check progress
» Caution when driving or doing things requiring alertness because of possible headache or dizziness
*For use as an antihypertensive*
» Not taking other medications, especially nonprescription sympathomimetics, unless discussed with physician

**Side/adverse effects**
Signs of potential side effects, especially allergic reaction, angina pectoris, cutaneous vasculitis, lymphadenopathy, peripheral neuritis, sodium and water retention, edema, SLE-like syndrome, and blood dyscrasias

## General Dosing Information

Apparent tolerance to the antihypertensive effects of hydralazine may develop with chronic administration, as a result of fluid retention and expanded plasma volume and reflex activation of the sympathetic nervous system, which increases heart rate and cardiac output. Concurrent administration of a diuretic may decrease this likelihood and will enhance the antihypertensive effects of hydralazine.

If combination therapy is indicated, individual titration is required to ensure the lowest possible therapeutic dose of each drug.

Incidence and severity of some of the side effects of hydralazine can be minimized if the dosage is increased slowly to its therapeutic level. In addition, some side effects (especially tachycardia, headache, and dizziness) may be less pronounced if beta-adrenergic blocking agents are administered concurrently.

Recent evidence suggests that withdrawal of antihypertensive therapy prior to surgery is not necessary, but that the anesthesiologist must be aware of such therapy.

Peripheral neuritis has been observed in some patients on hydralazine therapy. Evidence suggests that this may be due to an antipyridoxine effect. Discontinuation of hydralazine or continuation of hydralazine with supplemental vitamin B₆ (pyridoxine)—100 to 200 mg per day—usually results in remission of the neuritis over a period of 4 to 6 weeks.

It is recommended that hydralazine therapy be discontinued if a systemic lupus erythematosus (SLE)-like syndrome occurs.

To avoid a sudden increase in blood pressure, patients on hydralazine who have shown a significant decrease in blood pressure should have the medication withdrawn gradually at cessation of therapy.

**For oral dosage forms**
Food may enhance the bioavailability of hydralazine by reducing first-pass metabolism in the gastrointestinal wall. Consistent administration in relation to meals is recommended.

**For parenteral dosage forms**
Most patients can be transferred to the oral dosage form of hydralazine within 24 to 48 hours after initiation of parenteral therapy.

## Oral Dosage Forms

Note: Bracketed uses in the *Dosage Forms* section refer to categories of use and/or indications that are not included in U.S. product labeling.

### HYDRALAZINE HYDROCHLORIDE TABLETS USP

**Usual adult dose**
Hypertension—
   Initial: Oral, 10 mg four times a day for the first two to four days, followed by 25 mg four times a day for the balance of the first week.
   Maintenance: Oral, 50 mg four times a day for the second and subsequent weeks; dosage should be adjusted to the lowest effective levels.
[Congestive heart failure][1]—
   Initial: Oral, 25 to 37.5 mg four times a day. This dose may be increased as tolerated.
   Maintenance: Oral, 75 mg four times a day; or 100 mg three times a day.
Note: Geriatric patients may be more sensitive to the effects of the usual adult dose.

**Usual adult prescribing limits**
Up to 300 mg daily (higher doses have been used in treatment of congestive heart failure).

**Usual pediatric dose**
Hypertension—
   Oral, 750 mcg (0.75 mg) per kg of body weight a day divided into four doses, the dosage being increased gradually over three to four weeks as needed, up to a maximum of 7.5 mg per kg of body weight or 200 mg a day.

**Strength(s) usually available**
U.S.—
   10 mg (Rx) [*Apresoline* (lactose); GENERIC].
   25 mg (Rx) [*Apresoline* (lactose); GENERIC].
   50 mg (Rx) [*Apresoline* (lactose); GENERIC].
   100 mg (Rx) [*Apresoline* (tartrazine; lactose); GENERIC].
Canada—
   10 mg (Rx) [*Apresoline* (scored; tartrazine)].
   25 mg (Rx) [*Apresoline* (lactose); *Novo-Hylazin*].
   50 mg (Rx) [*Apresoline* (lactose); *Novo-Hylazin*].

**Packaging and storage**
Store below 40 °C (104 °F), preferably between 15 and 30 °C (59 and 86 °F), unless otherwise specified by manufacturer. Store in a tight, light-resistant container.

**Auxiliary labeling**
• Do not take other medicines without your doctor's advice.

**Note**
Check refill frequency to determine compliance in hypertensive patients.

## Parenteral Dosage Forms

### HYDRALAZINE HYDROCHLORIDE INJECTION USP

**Usual adult dose**
Antihypertensive—
   Intramuscular or intravenous, 5 to 40 mg, repeated as needed.
   Pre-eclampsia or eclampsia: Intravenous, 5 mg every fifteen to twenty minutes. If a therapeutic response is not achieved after a total dose of 20 mg, another agent should be considered.
Note: Geriatric patients may be more sensitive to the effects of the usual adult dose.

**Usual pediatric dose**
Antihypertensive—
   Intramuscular or intravenous, 1.7 to 3.5 mg per kg of body weight a day, divided into four to six daily doses.

**Strength(s) usually available**
U.S.—
   20 mg per mL (Rx) [GENERIC].
Canada—
   Not commercially available.
Note: The brand name product is no longer commercially available in the U.S. or Canada. However, the manufacturer is making it available to physicians on an emergency basis.

**Packaging and storage**
Store below 40 °C (104 °F), preferably between 15 and 30 °C (59 and 86 °F), unless otherwise specified by manufacturer. Protect from freezing.

**Stability**
Hydralazine hydrochloride injection should be used immediately after the ampul is opened.

**Incompatibilities**
Hydralazine hydrochloride injection may undergo color changes when added to infusion fluids. It is recommended that hydralazine hydrochloride injection not be added to infusion solutions.

---

[1] Not included in Canadian product labeling.

## Selected Bibliography

Stratton MA. Drug-induced systemic lupus erythematosus. Clin Pharm 1985; 4; 657-63.
The fifth report of the Joint National Committee on Detection, Evaluation, and Treatment of High Blood Pressure (JNC V), Arch Intern Med 1993; 153 (2); 154-83.

---

Revised: 08/22/96

---

## HYDRALAZINE-CONTAINING COMBINATIONS—
Hydralazine and Hydrochlorothiazide (Systemic)
Reserpine, Hydralazine and Hydrochlorothiazide (Systemic)

---

# HYDRALAZINE AND HYDROCHLOROTHIAZIDE    Systemic

VA CLASSIFICATION (Primary): CV400
**NOTE:** The *Hydralazine and Hydrochlorothiazide (Systemic)* monograph is maintained on the USP DI electronic data base. For a printed copy of the most recent revision of the complete monograph, contact the USP Division of Information Development, 12601 Twinbrook Parkway, Rockville, MD 20852.

   For information on the specific components of this combination, see the *USP DI* monographs for *Diuretics, Thiazide (Systemic)* and *Hydralazine (Systemic)*.

   The information that follows is selectively abstracted from the complete monograph and is provided to facilitate drug use review and patient counseling.

Note: For a listing of dosage forms and brand names by country availability, see *Dosage Forms* section(s). For a listing of brand names for the articles in this monograph, refer to the General Index.

## Category
Antihypertensive.

## Indications

**Accepted**
Hypertension (treatment)—Hydralazine and hydrochlorothiazide combination is indicated in the treatment of hypertension.

   Fixed-dosage combinations are generally not recommended for initial therapy and are useful for subsequent therapy only when the proportion of the component agents corresponds to the dose of the individual agents, as determined by titration.

For additional information on initial therapeutic guidelines related to the treatment of hypertension, see *Appendix III*.

## Patient Consultation

As an aid to patient consultation, refer to *Advice for the Patient, Hydralazine and Hydrochlorothiazide (Systemic)*.

In providing consultation, consider emphasizing the following selected information (» = major clinical significance):

### Before using this medication

» Conditions affecting use, especially:

Sensitivity to hydralazine, hydrochlorothiazide, sulfonamide-type medications, bumetanide, furosemide, or carbonic anhydrase inhibitors

Pregnancy—Blood problems reported in infants of mothers who took hydralazine and birth defects found in animals; hydrochlorothiazide may cause jaundice, thrombocytopenia, hypokalemia in infant

Breast-feeding—Hydrochlorothiazide is distributed into breast milk

Use in the elderly—Increased sensitivity to hypotensive and electrolyte effects; increased risk of hydralazine-induced hypothermia

Other medications, especially diazoxide, digitalis glycosides, lithium

Other medical problems, especially coronary artery disease, rheumatic heart disease, anuria or severe renal function impairment, or infants with jaundice

### Proper use of this medication

Diuretic effects of the medication and timing of doses to minimize inconvenience of diuresis

Possible need for control of weight and diet, especially sodium intake

» Patient may not experience symptoms of hypertension; importance of taking medication even if feeling well

» Does not cure, but helps control hypertension; possible need for lifelong therapy; checking with physician before discontinuing medication; serious consequences of untreated hypertension

Getting into the habit of taking at same times each day to help increase compliance

» Proper dosing

Missed dose: Taking as soon as possible; not taking if almost time for next dose; not doubling doses

» Proper storage

### Precautions while using this medication

Regular visits to physician to check progress

» Not taking other medications, especially nonprescription sympathomimetics, unless discussed with physician

» Caution when driving or doing things requiring alertness because of possible headache or dizziness

» Caution when getting up suddenly from a lying or sitting position

» Caution in using alcohol, while standing for long periods or exercising, and during hot weather because of enhanced orthostatic hypotensive effects

» Possibility of hypokalemia; possible need for additional potassium in diet; not changing diet without first checking with physician

To prevent dehydration, checking with physician if severe nausea, vomiting, or diarrhea occurs and continues

Diabetics: May increase blood sugar levels

Possible photosensitivity; avoiding unprotected exposure to sun; using protective clothing and sun block product; avoiding use of sunlamp, tanning bed, or tanning booth

### Side/adverse effects

Signs of potential side effects, especially electrolyte imbalance, agranulocytosis, allergic reaction, angina pectoris, cutaneous vasculitis, lymphadenopathy, peripheral neuritis, SLE-like syndrome, agranulocytosis, cholecystitis, pancreatitis, hepatic function impairment, hyperuricemia, gout, and thrombocytopenia

## Oral Dosage Forms

### HYDRALAZINE HYDROCHLORIDE AND HYDROCHLOROTHIAZIDE CAPSULES

#### Usual adult dose

Antihypertensive—

Oral, 1 capsule two times a day, as determined by individual titration with the component agents.

Note: Geriatric patients may be more sensitive to the effects of the usual adult dose.

#### Usual pediatric dose

Antihypertensive—

Oral, as determined by individual titration with the component agents.

#### Strength(s) usually available

U.S.—

25 mg of hydralazine hydrochloride and 25 mg of hydrochlorothiazide (Rx) [*Apresazide* (sodium bisulfite); *Aprozide; Hydra-zide;* GENERIC].

50 mg of hydralazine hydrochloride and 50 mg of hydrochlorothiazide (Rx) [*Apresazide* (sodium bisulfite); *Aprozide; Hydra-zide;* GENERIC].

100 mg of hydralazine hydrochloride and 50 mg of hydrochlorothiazide (Rx) [*Apresazide* (sodium bisulfite); *Hydra-zide;* GENERIC].

Canada—

Not commercially available.

#### Auxiliary labeling

• Do not take other medicines without your doctor's advice.

### HYDRALAZINE HYDROCHLORIDE AND HYDROCHLOROTHIAZIDE TABLETS

#### Usual adult dose

Antihypertensive—

Oral, 1 tablet two times a day, as determined by individual titration with the component agents.

Note: Geriatric patients may be more sensitive to the effects of the usual adult dose.

#### Usual pediatric dose

Antihypertensive—

Oral, as determined by individual titration with the component agents.

#### Strength(s) usually available

U.S.—

25 mg of hydralazine hydrochloride and 15 mg of hydrochlorothiazide (Rx) [*Apresoline-Esidrix* (lactose; sucrose); GENERIC].

25 mg of hydralazine hydrochloride and 25 mg of hydrochlorothiazide (Rx) [GENERIC (may contain tartrazine)].

50 mg of hydralazine hydrochloride and 50 mg of hydrochlorothiazide (Rx) [GENERIC (may contain tartrazine)].

100 mg of hydralazine hydrochloride and 50 mg of hydrochlorothiazide (Rx) [GENERIC].

Canada—

Not commercially available.

#### Auxiliary labeling

• Do not take other medicines without your doctor's advice.

Revised: 08/24/92
Interim revision: 04/29/94

## HYDROCHLOROTHIAZIDE—See *Diuretics, Thiazide (Systemic)*

## HYDROCHLOROTHIAZIDE-CONTAINING COMBINATIONS—

Amiloride and Hydrochlorothiazide (Systemic)—See *Diuretics, Potassium-sparing, and Hydrochlorothiazide (Systemic)*

Bisoprolol and Hydrochlorothiazide (Systemic)—See *Beta-adrenergic Blocking Agents and Thiazide Diuretics (Systemic)*

Captopril and Hydrochlorothiazide (Systemic)—See *Angiotensin-converting Enzyme (ACE) Inhibitors and Hydrochlorothiazide (Systemic)*

Deserpidine and Hydrochlorothiazide (Systemic)—See *Rauwolfia Alkaloids and Thiazide Diuretics (Systemic)*

Enalapril and Hydrochlorothiazide (Systemic)—See *Angiotensin-converting Enzyme (ACE) Inhibitors and Hydrochlorothiazide (Systemic)*

Guanethidine and Hydrochlorothiazide (Systemic)

Hydralazine and Hydrochlorothiazide (Systemic)

Lisinopril and Hydrochlorothiazide (Systemic)—See *Angiotensin-converting Enzyme (ACE) Inhibitors and Hydrochlorothiazide (Systemic)*

Methyldopa and Hydrochlorothiazide (Systemic)—See *Methyldopa and Thiazide Diuretics (Systemic)*

Metoprolol and Hydrochlorothiazide (Systemic)—See *Beta-adrenergic Blocking Agents and Thiazide Diuretics (Systemic)*

Pindolol and Hydrochlorothiazide (Systemic)—See *Beta-adrenergic Blocking Agents and Thiazide Diuretics (Systemic)*

Propranolol and Hydrochlorothiazide (Systemic)—See *Beta-adrenergic Blocking Agents and Thiazide Diuretics (Systemic)*

Reserpine, Hydralazine, and Hydrochlorothiazide (Systemic)

Reserpine and Hydrochlorothiazide (Systemic)—See *Rauwolfia Alkaloids and Thiazide Diuretics (Systemic)*

Spironolactone and Hydrochlorothiazide (Systemic)—See *Diuretics, Potassium-sparing, and Hydrochlorothiazide (Systemic)*

Timolol and Hydrochlorothiazide (Systemic)—See *Beta-adrenergic Blocking Agents and Thiazide Diuretics (Systemic)*

Triamterene and Hydrochlorothiazide (Systemic)—See *Diuretics, Potassium-sparing, and Hydrochlorothiazide (Systemic)*

---

# HYDROCODONE—See *Opioid (Narcotic) Analgesics (Systemic)*

---

# HYDROCODONE-CONTAINING COMBINATIONS—

Brompheniramine, Phenylephrine, Phenylpropanolamine, Hydrocodone, and Guaifenesin (Systemic)—See *Cough/Cold Combinations (Systemic)*

Chlorpheniramine and Hydrocodone (Systemic)—See *Cough/Cold Combinations (Systemic)*

Chlorpheniramine, Pheniramine, Pyrilamine, Phenylephrine, Hydrocodone, Salicylamide, Caffeine, and Ascorbic Acid (Systemic)—See *Cough/Cold Combinations (Systemic)*

Chlorpheniramine, Phenylephrine, and Hydrocodone (Systemic)—See *Cough/Cold Combinations (Systemic)*

Chlorpheniramine, Phenylephrine, Hydrocodone, Acetaminophen, and Caffeine (Systemic)—See *Cough/Cold Combinations (Systemic)*

Chlorpheniramine, Pseudoephedrine, and Hydrocodone (Systemic)—See *Cough/Cold Combinations (Systemic)*

Hydrocodone and Acetaminophen (Systemic)—See *Opioid (Narcotic) Analgesics and Acetaminophen (Systemic)*

Hydrocodone and Aspirin (Systemic)—See *Opioid (Narcotic) Analgesics and Aspirin (Systemic)*

Hydrocodone and Guaifenesin (Systemic)—See *Cough/Cold Combinations (Systemic)*

Hydrocodone and Homatropine (Systemic)—See *Cough/Cold Combinations (Systemic)*

Hydrocodone and Potassium Guaiacolsulfonate (Systemic)—See *Cough/Cold Combinations (Systemic)*

Pheniramine, Phenylephrine, Phenylpropanolamine, Hydrocodone, and Guaifenesin (Systemic)—See *Cough/Cold Combinations (Systemic)*

Pheniramine, Pyrilamine, Hydrocodone, Potassium Citrate, and Ascorbic Acid (Systemic)—See *Cough/Cold Combinations (Systemic)*

Pheniramine, Pyrilamine, Phenylephrine, Phenylpropanolamine, and Hydrocodone (Systemic)—See *Cough/Cold Combinations (Systemic)*

Pheniramine, Pyrilamine, Phenylpropanolamine, and Hydrocodone (Systemic)—See *Cough/Cold Combinations (Systemic)*

Pheniramine, Pyrilamine, Phenylpropanolamine, Hydrocodone, and Guaifenesin (Systemic)—See *Cough/Cold Combinations (Systemic)*

Phenylephrine and Hydrocodone (Systemic)—See *Cough/Cold Combinations (Systemic)*

Phenylephrine, Hydrocodone, and Guaifenesin (Systemic)—See *Cough/Cold Combinations (Systemic)*

Phenylpropanolamine and Hydrocodone (Systemic)—See *Cough/Cold Combinations (Systemic)*

Phenylpropanolamine, Hydrocodone, Guaifenesin, and Salicylamide (Systemic)—See *Cough/Cold Combinations (Systemic)*

Phenyltoloxamine and Hydrocodone (Systemic)—See *Cough/Cold Combinations (Systemic)*

Pseudoephedrine and Hydrocodone (Systemic)—See *Cough/Cold Combinations (Systemic)*

Pseudoephedrine, Hydrocodone, and Guaiacolsulfonate (Systemic)—See *Cough/Cold Combinations (Systemic)*

Pseudoephedrine, Hydrocodone, and Guaifenesin (Systemic)—See *Cough/Cold Combinations (Systemic)*

Pyrilamine, Phenylephrine, and Hydrocodone (Systemic)—See *Cough/Cold Combinations (Systemic)*

Pyrilamine, Phenylephrine, Hydrocodone, and Ammonium Chloride (Systemic)—See *Cough/Cold Combinations (Systemic)*

---

# HYDROCORTISONE—See *Corticosteroids (Ophthalmic); Corticosteroids (Otic); Corticosteroids (Topical); Corticosteroids—Glucocorticoid Effects (Systemic)*

---

# HYDROCORTISONE-CONTAINING COMBINATIONS—

Clioquinol and Hydrocortisone (Topical)

Colistin, Neomycin, and Hydrocortisone (Otic)

Hydrocortisone and Acetic Acid (Otic)—See *Corticosteroids and Acetic Acid (Otic)*

Neomycin, Polymyxin B, and Hydrocortisone (Ophthalmic)

Neomycin, Polymyxin B, and Hydrocortisone (Otic)

---

# HYDROFLUMETHIAZIDE—See *Diuretics, Thiazide (Systemic)*

---

# HYDROFLUMETHIAZIDE-CONTAINING COMBINATIONS—

Reserpine and Hydroflumethiazide (Systemic)—See *Rauwolfia Alkaloids and Thiazide Diuretics (Systemic)*

---

# HYDROMORPHONE—See *Opioid (Narcotic) Analgesics (Systemic)*

---

# HYDROMORPHONE-CONTAINING COMBINATIONS—

Hydromorphone and Guaifenesin (Systemic)—See *Cough/Cold Combinations (Systemic)*

---

# HYDROXOCOBALAMIN—See *Vitamin B₁₂ (Systemic)*

---

# HYDROXYCHLOROQUINE   Systemic

VA CLASSIFICATION (Primary/Secondary): AP101/MS103; TN900

Note: For a listing of dosage forms and brand names by country availability, see *Dosage Forms* section(s). For a listing of brand names for the articles in this monograph, refer to the General Index.

## Category

Antiprotozoal; antirheumatic (disease-modifying); lupus erythematosus suppressant; antihypercalcemic; polymorphous light eruption suppressant; porphyria cutanea tarda suppressant.

## Indications

Note: Bracketed information in the *Indications* section refers to uses that are not included in U.S. product labeling.

### Accepted

Malaria (prophylaxis and treatment)—Hydroxychloroquine is indicated in the suppressive treatment and the treatment of acute attacks of malaria caused by *Plasmodium vivax, P. malariae, P. ovale*, and susceptible strains of *P. falciparum*. The radical cure of *P. vivax* and *P. ovale* malaria requires the concurrent or subsequent administration of primaquine.

Arthritis, rheumatoid (treatment)—Hydroxychloroquine is indicated in the treatment of acute and chronic rheumatoid arthritis in patients who do not respond adequately to other less toxic antirheumatics. [It may be used in addition to nonsteroidal anti-inflammatory agents.]

Lupus erythematosus, discoid (treatment) or

Lupus erythematosus, systemic (treatment)—Hydroxychloroquine is indicated as a suppressant for chronic discoid and systemic lupus erythematosus.

[Arthritis, juvenile (treatment)][1]—Hydroxychloroquine is used in the treatment of juvenile arthritis.

[Hypercalcemia, sarcoid-associated (treatment)][1]—Hydroxychloroquine is used to reduce urinary calcium excretion and the levels of 1,25-dihydroxyvitamin D in the serum of sarcoid patients who are unable to take corticosteroids.

[Polymorphous light eruption (treatment)][1]—Hydroxychloroquine is used as a suppressant for polymorphous light eruption.

[Porphyria cutanea tarda (treatment)][1]—Hydroxychloroquine is used in the treatment of porphyria cutanea tarda.

[Urticaria, solar (treatment)][1] or
[Vasculitis, chronic cutaneous (treatment)][1]—Hydroxychloroquine is used in the treatment of solar urticaria and chronic cutaneous vasculitis unresponsive to other therapy.

Chloroquine-resistant strains of *P. falciparum*, originally seen only in Southeast Asia and South America, are now documented in all malarious areas except Central America west of the Canal Zone, the Middle East, and the Caribbean. Chloroquine is still the drug of choice for the treatment of susceptible strains of *P. falciparum* and the other 3 malarial species; however, chloroquine-resistant *P. vivax* has recently been reported.

### Unaccepted
Hydroxychloroquine does not prevent relapses in patients with *P. vivax* or *P. ovale* malaria since it is not effective against exo-erythrocytic forms of the parasite. In these species, "hypnozoites," which remain dormant in the liver, are responsible for relapses.

[1]Not included in Canadian product labeling.

## Pharmacology/Pharmacokinetics

Note: Because hydroxychloroquine concentrates in the cellular fraction of blood, hydroxychloroquine concentrations measured in the blood are higher than those measured in the plasma.

### Physicochemical characteristics
Molecular weight—433.95.

### Mechanism of action/Effect
Antiprotozoal—Malaria: Unknown, but may be based on ability of hydroxychloroquine to bind to and alter the properties of DNA. Also has been found to be taken up into the acidic food vacuoles of the parasite in the erythrocyte. This increases the pH of the acid vesicles, interfering with vesicle functions and possibly inhibiting phospholipid metabolism. In suppressive treatment, hydroxychloroquine inhibits the erythrocytic stage of development of plasmodia. In acute attacks of malaria, it interrupts erythrocytic schizogony of the parasite. Its ability to concentrate in parasitized erythrocytes may account for their selective toxicity against the erythrocytic stages of plasmodial infection.

Antirheumatic—Hydroxychloroquine is thought to act as a mild immunosuppressant, inhibiting the production of rheumatoid factor and acute phase reactants. It also accumulates in white blood cells, stabilizing lysosomal membranes and inhibiting the activity of many enzymes, including collagenase and the proteases that cause cartilage breakdown.

### Absorption
Variable rate of absorption; absorption half-life of 3.6 hours (range, 1.9 to 5.5 hours). Bioavailability is approximately 74%.

### Distribution
Widely distributed in body tissues such as the eyes, kidneys, liver, and lungs where retention is prolonged. Concentrations are 2 to 5 times higher in erythrocytes than in plasma. Very low concentrations in intestinal wall. Crosses the placenta, also.
Apparent $Vol_D$ =5,522 L (measured in blood); 44,257 L (measured in plasma).

### Protein binding
Moderate (approximately 45%).

### Biotransformation
Hepatic (partially), to active de-ethylated metabolites.

### Half-life
Terminal elimination half-life—
    In blood: Approximately 50 days.
    In plasma: Approximately 32 days.

### Time to peak concentration
Approximately 3.2 hours (range, 2 to 4.5 hours).

### Peak concentrations
Steady state concentration in whole blood (achieved at 6 months)—
    155 mg (base) daily: 948 nanograms per mL.
    310 mg (base) daily: 1895 nanograms per mL.

### Elimination
Renal; 23 to 25% of hydroxychloroquine excreted unchanged in the urine. Hydroxychloroquine is excreted very slowly; may persist in urine for months or years after medication is discontinued. Also excreted in bile.
Hemodialysis does not remove appreciable amounts of hydroxychloroquine from blood.

## Precautions to Consider

### Cross-sensitivity and/or related problems
Patients hypersensitive to chloroquine, a 4-aminoquinoline compound structurally similar to hydroxychloroquine, may also be hypersensitive to hydroxychloroquine.

### Pregnancy/Reproduction
Pregnancy—Hydroxychloroquine crosses the placenta. Use is not recommended during pregnancy except in the suppression or treatment of malaria or hepatic amebiasis since malaria poses greater potential danger to the mother and fetus (i.e., abortion and death) than prophylactic administration of hydroxychloroquine. Hydroxychloroquine, given in weekly chemoprophylactic doses, has not been shown to cause adverse effects on the fetus. However, risk-benefit must be considered since 4-aminoquinolines, given in therapeutic doses, have been shown to cause central nervous system (CNS) damage, including ototoxicity (auditory and vestibular); congenital deafness; retinal hemorrhages; and abnormal retinal pigmentation. In addition, hydroxychloroquine has been shown to accumulate selectively in melanin structures of fetal eyes. It may be retained in ocular tissues for up to 5 months after elimination from the blood.

### Breast-feeding
One case report found that a very small amount of hydroxychloroquine is distributed into breast milk; chloroquine is also distributed into breast milk. Although problems in humans have not been documented, risk-benefit must be considered since infants and children are especially sensitive to the effects of 4-aminoquinolines.

### Pediatrics
Infants and children are especially sensitive to the effects of hydroxychloroquine and chloroquine. Fatalities have been reported following the ingestion of as little as 750 mg to 1 gram of chloroquine; hydroxychloroquine is assumed to be equally toxic. Long-term therapy with hydroxychloroquine is not generally recommended in children. However, it has been used in juvenile arthritis for as long as 6 months with little or no toxicity.

### Geriatrics
No information is available on the relationship of age to the effects of hydroxychloroquine in geriatric patients.

### Drug interactions and/or related problems
The following drug interactions and/or related problems have been selected on the basis of their potential clinical significance (possible mechanism in parentheses where appropriate)—not necessarily inclusive (» = major clinical significance):

Note: Combinations containing any of the following medications, depending on the amount present, may also interact with this medication.

Penicillamine
    (concurrent use of penicillamine with hydroxychloroquine may increase penicillamine plasma concentrations, increasing the potential for serious hematologic and/or renal adverse reactions, as well as the possibility of severe skin reactions)

### Medical considerations/Contraindications
The medical considerations/contraindications included here have been selected on the basis of their potential clinical significance (reasons given in parentheses where appropriate)—not necessarily inclusive (» = major clinical significance).

### *Risk-benefit should be considered when the following medical problems exist:*
» Blood disorders, severe
    (hydroxychloroquine may cause blood dyscrasias, including agranulocytosis, aplastic anemia, neutropenia, or thrombocytopenia)

Gastrointestinal disorders, severe
    (hydroxychloroquine may cause gastrointestinal irritation)

Glucose-6-phosphate dehydrogenase (G6PD) deficiency
    (hydroxychloroquine may cause hemolytic anemia in G6PD-deficient patients, although this is unlikely when hydroxychloroquine is given in therapeutic doses)

» Hepatic function impairment
    (because hydroxychloroquine is metabolized in the liver, hepatic function impairment may increase blood concentrations of hydroxychloroquine, increasing the risk of side effects)

Hypersensitivity to hydroxychloroquine or chloroquine
» Neurological disorders, severe
    (hydroxychloroquine may cause neuromyopathy, ototoxicity, polyneuritis, or seizures)
Porphyria
    (hydroxychloroquine may cause exacerbation of porphyria)
Psoriasis
    (hydroxychloroquine may precipitate severe attacks of psoriasis)
» Retinal or visual field changes, presence of
    (hydroxychloroquine may cause corneal opacities, keratopathy, or retinopathy)

**Patient monitoring**
The following may be especially important in patient monitoring (other tests may be warranted in some patients, depending on condition; » = major clinical significance):
» Complete blood counts (CBCs)
    (recommended periodically during prolonged daily therapy with hydroxychloroquine; if severe blood dyscrasias occur that are not attributable to the disease being treated, discontinuation of hydroxychloroquine should be considered)
» Neuromuscular examinations, including knee and ankle reflexes
    (recommended periodically during long-term therapy with hydroxychloroquine to detect muscle weakness; if muscle weakness occurs, hydroxychloroquine should be discontinued)
» Ophthalmologic examinations, including visual acuity, expert slitlamp, funduscopic, and visual field tests
    (recommended before and at least every 3 to 6 months during prolonged daily therapy since irreversible retinal damage has been reported with long-term or high-dosage therapy; serious ocular injury has been thought to be correlated with a total cumulative dose of greater than 100 grams (base) of chloroquine; however, a daily dose of greater than 310 mg (base), or 5 mg (base) per kg daily, of hydroxychloroquine may be a more important determinant; any retinal or visual abnormality that is not fully explainable by difficulties of accommodation or corneal opacities should be monitored following discontinuation of therapy, since retinal changes and visual disturbances may progress even after cessation of therapy)

## Side/Adverse Effects

Note: Side/adverse effects of hydroxychloroquine are usually dose-related. When hydroxychloroquine is used for the short-term treatment of malaria or other parasitic diseases, side/adverse effects are usually mild and reversible. However, following prolonged use and/or high-dose therapy such as in the treatment of rheumatoid arthritis, lupus erythematosus, or polymorphous light eruption, side/adverse effects may be serious and sometimes irreversible.

Irreversible retinal damage may be more likely to occur when the daily dosage equals or exceeds the equivalent of 310 mg (base), or 5 mg (base) per kg daily, of hydroxychloroquine.

The following side/adverse effects have been selected on the basis of their potential clinical significance (possible signs and symptoms in parentheses where appropriate)—not necessarily inclusive:

**Those indicating need for medical attention**
Incidence less frequent
    *Ocular toxicity specifically corneal opacities* (blurred vision or any other change in vision); *keratopathy* (blurred vision or any other change in vision); *or retinopathy* (blurred vision or any other change in vision)
Incidence rare
    *Blood dyscrasias, specifically agranulocytosis* (sore throat and fever); *aplastic anemia* (fatigue; weakness); *neutropenia* (sore throat and fever); *or thrombocytopenia* (unusual bleeding or bruising); *emotional changes or psychosis* (mood or other mental changes); *neuromyopathy* (increased muscle weakness); *ototoxicity* (any loss of hearing; ringing or buzzing in ears)—usually in patients with pre-existing auditory damage; *seizures*

**Those indicating need for medical attention only if they continue or are bothersome**
Incidence more frequent
    *Ciliary muscle dysfunction* (difficulty in reading); *gastrointestinal irritation* (diarrhea; loss of appetite; nausea; stomach cramps or pain; vomiting); *headache; itching* (especially in black patients)—not an indication for discontinuation of therapy in black patients

Incidence less frequent
    *Bleaching of hair or increased hair loss; blue-black discoloration of skin, fingernails, or inside of mouth; dizziness or lightheadedness; nervousness or restlessness; skin rash or itching*

**Those indicating possible retinal changes, visual disturbances and the need for medical attention if they occur or progress after medication is discontinued**
    *Blurred vision or any other change in vision*

## Overdose

For specific information on the agents used in the management of hydroxychloroquine overdose, see:
  • *Charcoal, Activated (Oral-Local)* monograph;
  • *Diazepam* in *Benzodiazepines (Systemic)* monograph; and/or
  • *Sympathomimetic Agents—Cardiovascular Use (Parenteral-Systemic)* monograph.

For more information on the management of overdose or unintentional ingestion, **contact a Poison Control Center** (see *Poison Control Center Listing*).

**Clinical effects of overdose**
After ingestion of an overdose of hydroxychloroquine, toxic symptoms may occur within 30 minutes. These include drowsiness, visual disturbances, cardiovascular collapse, and seizures, followed by sudden respiratory and cardiac arrest.
Doses of chloroquine phosphate as small as 0.75 to 1 gram in children, and 2.25 to 3 grams in adults, may be fatal. It is assumed that hydroxychloroquine is equally toxic.
The following effects have been selected on the basis of their potential clinical significance (possible signs and symptoms in parenthesis where appropriate)—not necessarily inclusive:
Acute
    *Cardiovascular toxicities, specifically conduction disturbances or hypotension; neurotoxicity, specifically drowsiness; headache; hyperexcitability; seizures; or coma; respiratory and cardiac arrest; visual disturbances* (blurred vision)

**Treatment of overdose**
Since there is no specific antidote, treatment of hydroxychloroquine overdose should be symptomatic and supportive with possible utilization of the following:
To decrease absorption—
    Emptying stomach with gastric lavage.
    Administering activated charcoal with a cathartic. The dose of activated charcoal should be 5 to 10 times the estimated dose of the drug ingested.
To enhance elimination—
    Forcing diuresis and acidifying the urine, with ammonium chloride, for example, can help promote urinary excretion of 4-aminoquinolines. Adjusting the dose of the acidifying agent to maintain a urinary pH of 5.5 to 6.5. Monitoring of plasma potassium is recommended. Using with caution in patients with renal function impairment and/or metabolic acidosis.
Specific treatment—
    For seizures—Treating repetitive seizures or status epilepticus with intravenous diazepam (in 2.5 to 5 mg increments).
    For arrhythmias—Managing life-threatening ventricular arrhythmias or cardiac arrest appropriately, as per Advanced Cardiac Life Support guidelines.
    For hypotension and circulatory shock—Administering fluids at a sufficient rate to maintain urine output. Administering intravenous pressors and/or inotropic drugs, such as norepinephrine, dopamine, isoproterenol, or dobutamine, if required. One study found that administration of a high-dose diazepam infusion improved hemodynamic function, and epinephrine decreased the myocardial depressant and vasodilatory effects of chloroquine overdose. This may also apply to a hydroxychloroquine overdose.
Monitoring—
    Monitoring of plasma potassium is recommended.
Supportive care—
    Securing and maintaining a patent airway, administering oxygen, and instituting assisted or controlled respiration as required. In severe overdoses, early mechanical ventilation has been suggested to prevent hypoxemia. Patients in whom intentional overdose is known or suspected should be referred for psychiatric consultation.

## Patient Consultation

As an aid to patient consultation, refer to *Advice for the Patient, Hydroxychloroquine (Systemic)*.

In providing consultation, consider emphasizing the following selected information (» = major clinical significance):

**Before using this medication**
» Conditions affecting use, especially:
Hypersensitivity to hydroxychloroquine or chloroquine
Pregnancy—May cause toxicity to the fetus when given to mother in therapeutic doses; however, hydroxychloroquine has not been shown to cause adverse effects in the fetus when used as a prophylactic agent against malaria
Use in children—Infants and children are especially sensitive to effects of hydroxychloroquine
Other medical problems, especially impaired hepatic function, presence of retinal or visual field changes, severe blood disorders, or severe neurologic disorders

**Proper use of this medication**
» Taking with meals or milk to minimize possible gastrointestinal irritation
» Keeping medication out of reach of children; fatalities reported with as few as 3 or 4 tablets (250-mg strength) of chloroquine phosphate; hydroxychloroquine is assumed to be equally toxic
» Importance of not taking more medication than the amount prescribed
» Compliance with full course of therapy
» Importance of not missing doses and taking medication on regular schedule
» Proper dosing
Missed dose: Taking as soon as possible; not taking if almost time for next dose; not doubling doses
» Proper storage
*For prevention of malaria*
Starting medication 1 to 2 weeks before entering malarious area to ascertain patient response and allow time to substitute another medication if reactions occur
» Continuing medication while staying in area and for 4 to 6 weeks after leaving area; checking with physician immediately if fever develops while traveling or within 2 months after departure from endemic area
*For arthritis and lupus erythematosus*
Importance of taking medication on regular schedule
May require up to 6 months for full benefit
*For patients unable to swallow hydroxychloroquine tablets*
Crushing tablets and putting each dose in capsules; contents of capsules may be mixed with jam, jelly, or jello

**Precautions while using this medication**
» Regular visits to physician to check for blood problems, muscle weakness, and ophthalmologic examinations during or after long-term therapy
Checking with physician if no improvement within a few days (or a few weeks or months for arthritis)
» Caution if blurred vision, difficulty in reading, other change in vision, dizziness, or lightheadedness occurs
Mosquito-control measures to reduce the chance of getting malaria:
Sleeping under mosquito netting
Wearing long-sleeved shirts or blouses and long trousers to protect arms and legs between dusk and dawn
Applying mosquito repellent to uncovered areas of skin between dusk and dawn

**Side/adverse effects**
Signs of potential side effects, especially ocular toxicity, blood dyscrasias, emotional or psychological changes, neuromyopathy, ototoxicity, and seizures

# General Dosing Information

Long-term and/or high-dosage therapy may cause irreversible retinal damage and/or neurosensorial deafness.

Hydroxychloroquine should be discontinued if any of the following problems occur: any abnormality in visual acuity, visual fields, retinal macular changes, or any visual symptoms; muscle weakness; or severe blood disorders.

Malaria-suppressive therapy should be started 1 to 2 weeks before the patient enters a malarious area and should be continued for 4 to 6 weeks after patient leaves the area. Starting the medication in advance will help to determine the patient's tolerance to the medication and allow time to substitute other antimalarials if the patient develops allergies to the medication or develops other adverse effects.

Hydroxychloroquine should be taken with meals or milk to minimize the possibility of gastrointestinal irritation.

Corticosteroids and/or nonsteroidal anti-inflammatory analgesics (including salicylates) may be given concurrently with hydroxychloroquine in the treatment of rheumatoid arthritis. These medications can usually be reduced gradually in dosage or discontinued after hydroxychloroquine has been given for several weeks.

When hydroxychloroquine is used in the treatment of rheumatoid arthritis, several months of therapy may be required for it to reach its maximum effectiveness. If improvement (such as reduced joint swelling and increased mobility) does not occur within 6 months, the medication should be discontinued.

# Oral Dosage Forms

Note: Bracketed uses in the *Dosage Forms* section refer to categories of use and/or indications that are not included in U.S. product labeling.

### HYDROXYCHLOROQUINE SULFATE TABLETS USP

**Usual adult and adolescent dose**
Malaria—
Suppressive: Oral, 400 mg (310 mg base) once every seven days.
Therapeutic: Oral, 800 mg (620 mg base) as a single dose; or 800 mg (620 mg base) initially, followed by 400 mg (310 mg base) in six to eight hours, and 400 mg (310 mg base) once a day on the second and third days.
Antirheumatic (disease-modifying)—
Oral, up to 6.5 mg (5 mg base) per kg of lean body weight daily, with meals or a glass of milk.

Note: In a small number of patients who experience side effects with the usual initial dose in the treatment of rheumatoid arthritis, a temporary reduction in the initial dose of hydroxychloroquine may be required. After five to ten days the dose may be gradually increased until the desired response is obtained.

If relapse occurs after withdrawal of hydroxychloroquine, therapy may be resumed or continued on an intermittent schedule if there are no ocular contraindications.
Lupus erythematosus suppressant—
Oral, up to 6.5 mg (5 mg base) per kg of lean body weight daily.
[Polymorphous light eruption suppressant][1]—
Oral, 200 mg (155 mg base) two or three times a day.

**Usual pediatric dose**
Malaria—
Suppressive: Oral, 6.4 mg (5 mg base) per kg of body weight, not to exceed the adult dose, once every seven days.
Therapeutic: Oral, 32 mg (25 mg base) per kg of body weight administered over a period of three days as follows: 12.9 mg (10 mg base) per kg of body weight, not to exceed a single dose of 800 mg (620 mg base); then 6.4 mg (5 mg base) per kg of body weight, not to exceed a single dose of 400 mg (310 mg base), six, twenty-four, and forty-eight hours after the first dose.

Note: Children are especially sensitive to the effects of the 4-aminoquinolines.

Long-term therapy with hydroxychloroquine is not recommended in children.

**Strength(s) usually available**
U.S.—
200 mg (equivalent to 155 mg base) (Rx) [*Plaquenil*].
Canada—
200 mg (equivalent to 155 mg base) (Rx) [*Plaquenil* (scored)].

**Packaging and storage**
Store below 40 °C (104 °F), preferably between 15 and 30 °C (59 and 86 °F), unless otherwise specified by manufacturer. Store in a well-closed container.

**Preparation of dosage form**
According to the manufacturer, the tablets may be crushed and each dose placed in a capsule. The contents of each compounded capsule may then be mixed with a teaspoonful of jam, jelly, or jello prior to administration. Preparation of hydroxychloroquine sulfate oral suspensions is not recommended.

**Auxiliary labeling**
• Continue medication for full time of treatment.
• Keep out of reach of children.
• Take with food or milk.
• May cause dizziness.

**Note**
Explain potential danger of accidental overdose in children.

Consider dispensing in unit-dose packaging in child-resistant containers ("double-barrier" packaging).

---

[1]Not included in Canadian product labeling.

---

Revised: 12/30/94

---

# HYDROXYPROPYL CELLULOSE  Ophthalmic

**VA CLASSIFICATION (Primary): OP500**

Note: For a listing of dosage forms and brand names by country availability, see *Dosage Forms* section(s). For a listing of brand names for the articles in this monograph, refer to the General Index.

## Category

Protectant (ophthalmic); tears (artificial).

## Indications

Note: Bracketed information in the *Indications* section refers to uses that are not included in U.S. product labeling.

**Accepted**

Keratoconjunctivitis sicca (treatment)—Hydroxypropyl cellulose is indicated in patients with moderate to severe dry eye syndromes associated with deficient tear production, including keratoconjunctivitis sicca. It is indicated especially in patients who remain symptomatic following an adequate trial of therapy with artificial tear solutions.

Corneal erosions, recurrent (treatment)[1]
Corneal sensitivity, decreased (treatment) or
Keratitis, exposure (treatment)—Hydroxypropyl cellulose is indicated in the treatment of recurrent corneal erosions, decreased corneal sensitivity, and exposure keratitis.

[Keratitis, neuroparalytic (treatment)][1]—Hydroxypropyl cellulose is used in the treatment of neuroparalytic keratitis.

[Ocular lubrication][1]—Hydroxypropyl cellulose is used as an ocular lubricant for artificial eyes.

---

[1]Not included in Canadian product labeling.

## Pharmacology/Pharmacokinetics

**Mechanism of action/Effect**

Acts to stabilize and thicken the precorneal tear film and prolong the tear film breakup time, which is usually shortened in dry eye conditions. Also acts to lubricate and protect the eye.

## Precautions to Consider

**Carcinogenicity/Mutagenicity**

No histospathologic changes or other negative effects occurred when hydroxypropyl cellulose was fed to rats at levels of up to 5% of their diet.

**Pregnancy/Reproduction**

Problems in humans have not been documented.

**Breast-feeding**

Problems in humans have not been documented.

**Pediatrics**

Appropriate studies on the relationship of age to the effects of hydroxypropyl cellulose have not been performed in the pediatric population. However, pediatrics-specific problems that would limit the usefulness of this medication in children are not expected.

**Geriatrics**

Appropriate studies on the relationship of age to the effects of hydroxypropyl cellulose have not been performed in the geriatric population. However, geriatrics-specific problems that would limit the usefulness of this medication in the elderly are not expected.

**Medical considerations/Contraindications**

The medical considerations/contraindications included here have been selected on the basis of their potential clinical significance (reasons given in parentheses where appropriate)—not necessarily inclusive (» = major clinical significance).

**HYDROXYPROGESTERONE**—See *Progestins (Systemic)*

*Risk-benefit should be considered when the following medical problem exists:*
    Sensitivity to hydroxypropyl cellulose

## Side/Adverse Effects

Note: Side/adverse effects of hydroxypropyl cellulose are usually mild and transient.

The following side/adverse effects have been selected on the basis of their potential clinical significance (possible signs and symptoms in parentheses where appropriate)—not necessarily inclusive:

**Those indicating need for medical attention only if they continue or are bothersome**
Incidence less frequent
    *Blurred vision; eye redness or discomfort or other irritation not present before therapy; increased sensitivity of eyes to light; matting or stickiness of eyelashes; swelling of eyelids; watering of eyes*

## Patient Consultation

As an aid to patient consultation, refer to *Advice for the Patient, Hydroxypropyl Cellulose (Ophthalmic).*

In providing consultation, consider emphasizing the following selected information (» = major clinical significance):

**Before using this medication**
» Conditions affecting use, especially:
        Sensitivity to hydroxypropyl cellulose

**Proper use of this medication**
    Proper administration technique:
        Reading patient instructions carefully before use
        Importance of inserting ocular system properly
        Checking with physician if administration technique not understood
        Accidentally expelled ocular system:
            Not inserting in eye again, because of possible contamination
            Inserting another ocular system if necessary
» Proper dosing
        Missed dose: Inserting as soon as possible
» Proper storage

**Precautions while using this medication**
» Caution if blurred vision occurs
        Possible increased sensitivity of eyes to light; wearing sunglasses for relief
» Removing eye system and checking with physician if eye symptoms worsen or new symptoms appear

## General Dosing Information

Some patients may have difficulty in understanding the proper administration technique of this ocular system; therefore, it is important that the administration technique be thoroughly explained.

If the hydroxypropyl cellulose ocular system is inadvertently expelled, as sometimes occurs in patients with shallow conjunctival fornices or when the eye is rubbed, another ocular system may be inserted if necessary.

If experience with the ocular system indicates that transient blurred vision occurs, the ocular system may be removed a few hours after insertion to prevent this. Then another ocular system may be inserted, if necessary.

Some persons may require several weeks of therapy before symptoms improve.

## Ophthalmic Dosage Forms

### HYDROXYPROPYL CELLULOSE OCULAR SYSTEM USP

**Usual adult and adolescent dose**
Artificial tears or
Ophthalmic protectant—
    Topical, to the conjunctiva, 1 ocular system delivering 5 mg, once a day.

Note:  Some patients may require 5 mg two times a day for optimal results.

**Usual pediatric dose**
See *Usual adult and adolescent dose.*

**Strength(s) usually available**
U.S.—
    5 mg (Rx) [*Lacrisert*].
Canada—
    5 mg (Rx) [*Lacrisert*].

**Packaging and storage**
Store below 30 °C (86 °F), unless otherwise specified by manufacturer.

**Auxiliary labeling**
• For the eye.

**Note**
Include patient instructions when dispensing.

Revised: 06/21/93

# HYDROXYPROPYL METHYLCELLULOSE    Ophthalmic

INN: Hypromellose

VA CLASSIFICATION (Primary): OP500

Note:  For a listing of dosage forms and brand names by country availability, see *Dosage Forms* section(s). For a listing of brand names for the articles in this monograph, refer to the General Index.

## Category

Protectant (ophthalmic); tears (artificial); lubricant (ophthalmic); diagnostic aid (contact lens procedures; gonioscopy).

## Indications

Note:  Bracketed information in the *Indications* section refers to uses that are not included in U.S. product labeling.

**Accepted**
Keratitis, exposure (treatment)
Keratitis, neuroparalytic (treatment) or
Keratoconjunctivitis sicca (treatment)—Hydroxypropyl methylcellulose is indicated for the relief of dry eyes and eye irritation associated with deficient tear production in order to prevent corneal damage.

[Corneal erosions, recurrent (treatment)][1] or
[Corneal sensitivity, decreased (treatment)][1]—Hydroxypropyl methylcellulose is used in the treatment of recurrent corneal erosions and decreased corneal sensitivity.

Ocular lubrication[1]—Hydroxypropyl methylcellulose is indicated as an ocular lubricant for hard contact lenses and artificial eyes and to protect the cornea during gonioscopy and procedures involving use of a diagnostic contact lens, such as laser photocoagulation of the retina, laser gonioplasty, and laser iridectomy.

[1]Not included in Canadian product labeling.

## Pharmacology/Pharmacokinetics

**Mechanism of action/Effect**
Promotes corneal wetting by stabilizing and thickening the precorneal tear film and prolonging the tear film breakup time, which is usually shortened in dry eye conditions. Also acts to lubricate and protect the eye.

## Precautions to Consider

**Pregnancy/Reproduction**
Problems in humans have not been documented.

**Breast-feeding**
Problems in humans have not been documented.

**Pediatrics**
Appropriate studies on the relationship of age to the effects of hydroxypropyl methylcellulose have not been performed in the pediatric population. However, pediatrics-specific problems that would limit the usefulness of this medication in children are not expected.

**Geriatrics**
Appropriate studies on the relationship of age to the effects of hydroxypropyl methylcellulose have not been performed in the geriatric population. However, geriatrics-specific problems that would limit the usefulness of this medication in the elderly are not expected.

**Medical considerations/Contraindications**
The medical considerations/contraindications included here have been selected on the basis of their potential clinical significance (reasons given in parentheses where appropriate)—not necessarily inclusive (» = major clinical significance).

*Risk-benefit should be considered when the following medical problem exists:*
    Sensitivity to hydroxypropyl methylcellulose

## Side/Adverse Effects

The following side/adverse effects have been selected on the basis of their potential clinical significance (possible signs and symptoms in parentheses where appropriate)—not necessarily inclusive:

**Those indicating need for medical attention**
    *Eye irritation not present before therapy*

**Those indicating need for medical attention only if they continue or are bothersome**
Incidence less frequent—more frequent with 1% solution
    *Blurred vision; matting or stickiness of eyelashes*

## Patient Consultation

As an aid to patient consultation, refer to *Advice for the Patient, Hydroxypropyl Methylcellulose (Ophthalmic).*

In providing consultation, consider emphasizing the following selected information (» = major clinical significance):

**Before using this medication**
»  Conditions affecting use, especially:
        Sensitivity to hydroxypropyl methylcellulose

**Proper use of this medication**
    Proper administration technique
    Preventing contamination: Not touching applicator tip to any surface; keeping container tightly closed
»  Proper dosing
»  Proper storage
*For patients wearing hard contact lenses*
    Taking care not to float lens from eye when applying medication

**Precautions while using this medication**
»  Checking with physician if eye pain, changes in vision, or continued redness or irritation of the eye occurs, or if present symptoms continue for more than 3 days or become worse

**Side/adverse effects**
    Signs of potential side effects, especially eye irritation not present before use of medication

## General Dosing Information

Although some manufacturers recommend that patients not wear soft contact lenses during treatment with ophthalmic hydroxypropyl methylcellulose, USP medical experts do not believe this precaution is necessary unless the patient has corneal epithelial problems and the medication is to be used more often than once every 1 to 2 hours. No significant problems have been documented with the use of ophthalmic solutions containing 0.03% or less of benzalkonium chloride as a preservative in patients with no significant corneal surface problems.

## Ophthalmic Dosage Forms

### HYDROXYPROPYL METHYLCELLULOSE OPHTHALMIC SOLUTION USP

**Usual adult and adolescent dose**
Keratitis, exposure (treatment)
Keratitis, neuroparalytic (treatment) or
Keratoconjunctivitis sicca (treatment)—
   Topical, to the conjunctiva, 1 drop of a 0.3 to 1% solution three or
   four times a day or as needed.

Note: The 2 and 2.5% solutions of hydroxypropyl methylcellulose are
   used in gonioscopic examinations, the gonioscopic prism being
   filled with solution as needed.

**Usual pediatric dose**
See *Usual adult and adolescent dose.*

**Strength(s) usually available**
U.S.—
   0.3% (OTC) [*Bion Tears; Tears Naturale; Tears Naturale II; Tears
   Naturale Free*].
   0.4% (OTC) [*Artificial Tears; Nature's Tears*].

0.5% (OTC) [*Isopto Plain; Isopto Tears; Just Tears; Lacril; Moisture
   Drops; Tearisol; Tears Renewed*].
0.8% (OTC) [*Ocucoat; Ocucoat PF*].
1% (OTC) [*Isopto Alkaline; Ultra Tears*].
2.5% [*Gonak* (OTC); *Goniosoft* (Rx); *Goniosol* (OTC)].
Canada—
   0.3% (OTC) [*Tears Naturale; Tears Naturale II; Tears Naturale
   Free*].
   0.5% (OTC) [*Eyelube; Isopto Tears; Moisture Drops; Ocutears*].
   1% (OTC) [*Eyelube; Isopto Tears*].
   2% (OTC) [*Methocel*].

**Packaging and storage**
Store below 40 °C (104 °F), preferably between 15 and 30 °C (59 and 86
   °F), unless otherwise specified by manufacturer. Store in a tight con-
   tainer. Protect from freezing.

**Auxiliary labeling**
• For the eye.
• Keep container tightly closed.

Revised: 08/14/95

---

# HYDROXYUREA   Systemic

VA CLASSIFICATION (Primary): AN300
Note: For a listing of dosage forms and brand names by country availability, see *Dosage Forms* section(s). For a listing of brand names
   for the articles in this monograph, refer to the General Index.

## Category
Antineoplastic.

## Indications

Note: Bracketed information in the *Indications* section refers to uses that
   are not included in U.S. product labeling.

**Accepted**
Carcinoma, head and neck (treatment)
Carcinoma, ovarian (treatment) or
[Carcinoma, cervical (treatment)][1]—Hydroxyurea is indicated, in combination with radiation therapy, for local control of primary squamous
   cell (epidermoid) carcinomas of the head and neck, excluding the lip.
   Hydroxyurea is also indicated for treatment of recurrent, metastatic,
   or inoperable carcinoma of the ovary, and is used for treatment of
   advanced prostatic carcinoma.

Leukemia, chronic myelocytic (treatment)—Hydroxyurea is indicated for
   treatment of resistant chronic myelocytic leukemia.

Melanoma, malignant (treatment)—Hydroxyurea is indicated for treatment
   of melanoma.

[Polycythemia vera (treatment)][1]—Hydroxyurea is used for treatment of
   polycythemia vera.

[1]Not included in Canadian product labeling.

## Pharmacology/Pharmacokinetics

**Physicochemical characteristics**
Molecular weight—76.05.

**Mechanism of action/Effect**
Hydroxyurea is classified as an antimetabolite. Hydroxyurea is thought to
   be cell cycle–specific for the S phase of cell division. The exact mechanism of antineoplastic activity is unknown but is thought to involve
   interference with synthesis of DNA, with no effect on synthesis of
   RNA or protein.

**Absorption**
Well absorbed from the gastrointestinal tract.

**Distribution**
Crosses the blood-brain barrier.

**Biotransformation**
Hepatic.

**Half-life**
3 to 4 hours.

**Time to peak serum concentration**
2 hours.

**Elimination**
Renal—80% within 12 hours (50% unchanged).
Respiratory—As carbon dioxide.

## Precautions to Consider

**Cross-sensitivity and/or related problems**
Patients sensitive to tartrazine may be sensitive to the capsule dosage form
   available in Canada also, since the capsules may contain tartrazine.

**Carcinogenicity/Mutagenicity**
Secondary malignancies are potential delayed effects of many antineoplastic agents, although it is not clear whether the effect is related to
   their mutagenic or immunosuppressive action. The effect of dose and
   duration of therapy is also unknown, although risk seems to increase
   with long-term use. Although information is limited, available data
   seem to indicate that the carcinogenic risk is greatest with the alkylating agents.
Antimetabolites have been shown to be carcinogenic in animals and may
   be associated with an increased risk of development of secondary carcinomas in humans, although the risk appears to be less than with
   alkylating agents.

**Pregnancy/Reproduction**
Fertility—Gonadal suppression, resulting in amenorrhea or azoospermia,
   may occur in patients taking antineoplastic therapy, especially with the
   alkylating agents. In general, these effects appear to be related to dose
   and length of therapy and may be irreversible. Prediction of the degree
   of testicular or ovarian function impairment is complicated by the
   common use of combinations of several antineoplastics, which makes
   it difficult to assess the effects of individual agents. Hydroxyurea
   causes reversible germ cell toxicity.

Pregnancy—First trimester: It is usually recommended that use of antineoplastics, especially combination chemotherapy, be avoided whenever possible, especially during the first trimester. Although information is limited because of the relatively few instances of antineoplastic
   administration during pregnancy, the mutagenic, teratogenic, and carcinogenic potential of these medications must be considered.
Other hazards to the fetus include adverse reactions seen in adults.
In general, use of a contraceptive is recommended during cytotoxic drug
   therapy.
Hydroxyurea is teratogenic in animals.

**Breast-feeding**
Although very little information is available regarding excretion of antineoplastic agents in breast milk, breast-feeding is not recommended
   during chemotherapy because of the risks to the infant (adverse effects,
   mutagenicity, carcinogenicity).

**Pediatrics**
Although appropriate studies on the relationship of age to the effects of
   hydroxyurea have not been performed in the pediatric population, children may be more sensitive to the effects of hydroxyurea.

**Geriatrics**
Although appropriate studies on the relationship of age to the effects of
   hydroxyurea have not been performed in the geriatric population, the

elderly may be more sensitive to effects of hydroxyurea. In addition, elderly patients are more likely to have age-related renal function impairment, which may require reduction of dosage in patients receiving hydroxyurea.

**Dental**

The bone marrow depressant effects of hydroxyurea may result in an increased incidence of microbial infection, delayed healing, and gingival bleeding. Dental work, whenever possible, should be completed prior to initiation of therapy or deferred until blood counts have returned to normal. Patients should be instructed in proper oral hygiene during treatment, including caution in use of regular toothbrushes, dental floss, and toothpicks.

Hydroxyurea may also cause stomatitis associated with considerable discomfort.

**Drug interactions and/or related problems**

The following drug interactions and/or related problems have been selected on the basis of their potential clinical significance (possible mechanism in parentheses where appropriate)—not necessarily inclusive (» = major clinical significance):

Allopurinol or
Colchicine or
» Probenecid or
» Sulfinpyrazone
(hydroxyurea may raise the concentration of blood uric acid; dosage adjustment of antigout agents may be necessary to control hyperuricemia and gout; allopurinol may be preferred to prevent or reverse hydroxyurea-induced hyperuricemia because of risk of uric acid nephropathy with uricosuric antigout agents)

Blood dyscrasia–causing medications (See *Appendix II*)
(leukopenic and/or thrombocytopenic effects of hydroxyurea may be increased with concurrent or recent therapy if these medications cause the same effects; dosage adjustment of hydroxyurea, if necessary, should be based on blood counts)

» Bone marrow depressants, other (See *Appendix II*) or
Radiation therapy
(additive bone marrow depression may occur; dosage reduction may be required when two or more bone marrow depressants, including radiation, are used concurrently or consecutively)

Vaccines, killed virus
(because normal defense mechanisms may be suppressed by hydroxyurea therapy, the patient's antibody response to the vaccine may be decreased. The interval between discontinuation of medications that cause immunosuppression and restoration of the patient's ability to respond to the vaccine depends on the intensity and type of immunosuppression-causing medications used, the underlying disease, and other factors; estimates vary from 3 months to 1 year)

» Vaccines, live virus
(because normal defense mechanisms may be suppressed by hydroxyurea therapy, concurrent use with a live virus vaccine may potentiate the replication of the vaccine virus, may increase the side/adverse effects of the vaccine virus, and/or may decrease the patient's antibody response to the vaccine; immunization of these patients should be undertaken only with extreme caution after careful review of the patient's hematologic status and only with the knowledge and consent of the physician managing the hydroxyurea therapy. The interval between discontinuation of medications that cause immunosuppression and restoration of the patient's ability to respond to the vaccine depends on the intensity and type of immunosuppression-causing medications used, the underlying disease, and other factors; estimates vary from 3 months to 1 year. Patients with leukemia in remission should not receive live virus vaccine until at least 3 months after their last chemotherapy. Immunization with oral poliovirus vaccine should also be postponed in persons in close contact with the patient, especially family members)

**Laboratory value alterations**

The following have been selected on the basis of their potential clinical significance (possible effect in parentheses where appropriate)—not necessarily inclusive (» = major clinical significance):

With physiology/laboratory test values
Blood urea nitrogen (BUN) and
Creatinine, serum
(concentrations may occasionally be temporarily increased as a result of impairment of renal tubular function)
Uric acid, serum
(concentrations may be increased)

**Medical considerations/Contraindications**

The medical considerations/contraindications included here have been selected on the basis of their potential clinical significance (reasons given in parentheses where appropriate)—not necessarily inclusive (» = major clinical significance).

*Risk-benefit should be considered when the following medical problems exist:*

» Anemia
(if severe, must be corrected with whole blood replacement before initiation of hydroxyurea therapy)
» Bone marrow depression
» Chickenpox, existing or recent (including recent exposure) or
» Herpes zoster
(risk of severe generalized disease)
Gout, history of or
Urate renal stones, history of
(risk of hyperuricemia)
» Infection
» Renal function impairment
(reduced elimination; lower dosage is recommended)
Sensitivity to hydroxyurea
» Caution should be used in patients who have had previous cytotoxic drug therapy and radiation therapy.

**Patient monitoring**

The following are especially important in patient monitoring (other tests may be warranted in some patients, depending on condition; » = major clinical significance):

Blood urea nitrogen (BUN) concentrations and
Creatinine concentrations, serum
(recommended prior to initiation of therapy and at periodic intervals during therapy; frequency varies according to clinical state, agent, dose, and other agents being used concurrently)
» Hematocrit or hemoglobin and
» Leukocyte count, total and, if appropriate, differential and
» Platelet count
(determinations recommended prior to initiation of therapy and at periodic intervals during therapy; frequency varies according to clinical state, agent, dose, and other agents being used concurrently)
Uric acid concentrations, serum
(recommended prior to initiation of therapy and at periodic intervals during therapy; frequency varies according to clinical state, agent, dose, and other agents being used concurrently)

## Side/Adverse Effects

Note: Many "side effects" of antineoplastic therapy are unavoidable and represent the medication's pharmacologic action. Some of these (for example, leukopenia and thrombocytopenia) are actually used as parameters to aid in individual dosage titration.

Administration of hydroxyurea to patients with severe renal function impairment may produce visual and auditory hallucinations and pronounced hematologic toxicity.

Skin changes resembling atrophic lichen planus, including atrophy, brittle nails, darkening or redness of skin, and skin ulcers, have been reported rarely in patients receiving prolonged (over several years) daily treatment with hydroxyurea.

The following side/adverse effects have been selected on the basis of their potential clinical significance (possible signs and symptoms in parentheses where appropriate)—not necessarily inclusive:

**Those indicating need for medical attention**
Incidence more frequent
*Anemia or erythrocytic abnormalities; leukopenia* (usually asymptomatic; less frequently, fever or chills; cough or hoarseness; lower back or side pain; painful or difficult urination)

Note: Self-limiting *megaloblastic erythropoiesis* occurs commonly early in the course of therapy; morphologic changes resemble pernicious anemia, but are not related to vitamin $B_{12}$ or folic acid deficiency. Plasma iron clearance may be delayed and rate of iron utilization by erythrocytes reduced, but hydroxyurea does not appear to alter red blood cell survival time.

Onset of *leukopenia* occurs about 10 days after initiation of therapy.

Incidence less frequent
> *Stomatitis* (sores in mouth and on lips); *thrombocytopenia* (usually asymptomatic; rarely, unusual bleeding or bruising; black, tarry stools; blood in urine or stools; pinpoint red spots on skin)

Incidence rare
> *Hyperuricemia or uric acid nephropathy* (joint pain; lower back or side pain; swelling of feet or lower legs); *neurotoxicity or cerebral metastatic disease* (confusion; convulsions; dizziness; hallucinations; headache); *renal function impairment*

> Note: *Hyperuricemia* or *uric acid nephropathy* occurs most commonly during initial treatment of patients with leukemia or lymphoma, as a result of rapid cell breakdown, which leads to elevated serum uric acid concentrations.

**Those indicating need for medical attention only if they continue or are bothersome**
Incidence more frequent—dose-related
> *Diarrhea; drowsiness*—large doses; *loss of appetite; nausea or vomiting*

Incidence less frequent
> *Constipation; exacerbation of postirradiation erythema* (redness of skin); *skin rash and itching*

**Those indicating the need for medical attention if they occur after medication is discontinued**
> *Bone marrow depression* (black, tarry stools; blood in urine; cough or hoarseness; fever or chills; lower back or side pain; painful or difficult urination; pinpoint red spots on skin; unusual bleeding or bruising)

## Patient Consultation

As an aid to patient consultation, refer to *Advice for the Patient, Hydroxyurea (Systemic)*.

In providing consultation, consider emphasizing the following selected information (» = major clinical significance):

**Before using this medication**
> Conditions affecting use, especially:
>> Sensitivity to hydroxyurea
>> Pregnancy—Use not recommended because of mutagenic, teratogenic, and carcinogenic potential; advisability of using contraception; telling physician immediately if pregnancy is suspected
>> Breast-feeding—Not recommended because of risk of serious side effects
>> Use in children—Children may be more sensitive to effects
>> Use in the elderly—Elderly patients may be more sensitive to effects
>> Other medications, especially probenecid, sulfinpyrazone, other bone marrow depressants, or previous cytotoxic drug or radiation therapy
>> Other medical problems, especially chickenpox, herpes zoster, anemia, infection, or renal function impairment

**Proper use of this medication**
> Importance of not taking more or less medication than the amount prescribed
>> For patients who cannot swallow capsules: Contents of capsules may be emptied into glass of water and taken immediately; some inert material may not dissolve and may float on surface
>> Caution in taking combination chemotherapy; taking each medication at the right time
>> Importance of ample fluid intake and subsequent increase in urine output to aid in excretion of uric acid
> Frequency of nausea, vomiting, and diarrhea; importance of continuing medication despite stomach upset
>> Checking with physician if vomiting occurs shortly after dose is taken
> Proper dosing
>> Missed dose: Not taking at all; not doubling doses
> Proper storage

**Precautions while using this medication**
> Importance of close monitoring by the physician
> Avoiding immunizations unless approved by physician; other persons in patient's household should avoid immunizations with oral poliovirus vaccine; avoiding other persons who have taken oral poliovirus vaccine or wearing a protective mask that covers nose and mouth

*Caution if bone marrow depression occurs:*
> Avoiding exposure to persons with bacterial infections, especially during period of low blood counts; checking with physician immediately if fever or chills, cough or hoarseness, lower back or side pain, or painful or difficult urination occur

> Checking with physician immediately if unusual bleeding or bruising; black, tarry stools; blood in urine; or pinpoint red spots on skin occur
>> Caution in use of regular toothbrush, dental floss, or toothpick; physician, dentist, or nurse may suggest alternatives; checking with physician before having dental work done
>> Not touching eyes or inside of nose unless hands washed immediately before
>> Using caution to avoid accidental cuts with use of sharp objects such as safety razor or fingernail or toenail cutters
>> Avoiding contact sports or other situations where bruising or injury could occur

**Side/adverse effects**
> May cause adverse effects such as blood problems and cancer; importance of discussing possible effects with physician
> Signs of potential side effects, especially leukopenia, stomatitis, thrombocytopenia, neurotoxicity, cerebral metastatic disease, hyperuricemia, and uric acid nephropathy
> Physician or nurse can help in dealing with side effects

## General Dosing Information

Patients receiving hydroxyurea should be under supervision of a physician experienced in antimetabolite chemotherapy.

Dosage must be adjusted to meet the individual requirements of each patient, based on clinical response and appearance or severity of toxicity.

Dosage reduction may be necessary in children and in the elderly, who may be more sensitive to effects of the drug.

If the patient is unable to swallow capsules, the contents of the capsule may be emptied into a glass of water (some inert material may float on the surface) and taken immediately.

Development of uric acid nephropathy in patients with leukemia or lymphoma may be prevented by adequate oral hydration and, in some cases, administration of allopurinol. Alkalinization of urine may be necessary if serum uric acid concentrations are elevated.

If there is no clinical response after 6 weeks of therapy, the medication should be discontinued; if a response occurs, the medication may be continued indefinitely.

Combination therapy with radiation may be associated with more frequent and severe side effects of the radiation, including gastric distress and inflammation of mucous membranes at the irradiated site. Severe reactions may require temporary withdrawal of hydroxyurea therapy.

It is recommended that hydroxyurea therapy be temporarily withdrawn if marked leukopenia (particularly granulocytopenia) or thrombocytopenia occurs. Therapy may be resumed if, after 3 days, the counts rise significantly towards normal values; counts usually return to normal within 10 to 30 days after discontinuation of hydroxyurea. If anemia occurs, it may be corrected with whole blood replacement, without interruption of hydroxyurea therapy.

Special precautions are recommended in patients who develop thrombocytopenia as a result of administration of hydroxyurea. These may include extreme care in performing invasive procedures; regular inspection of intravenous sites, skin (including perirectal area), and mucous membrane surfaces for signs of bleeding or bruising; limiting frequency of venipuncture and avoiding intramuscular injections; testing urine, emesis, stool, and secretions for occult blood; care in use of regular toothbrushes, dental floss, toothpicks, safety razors, and fingernail and toenail cutters; avoiding constipation; and using caution to prevent falls and other injuries. Such patients should avoid alcohol and any aspirin intake because of the risk of gastrointestinal bleeding. Platelet transfusions may be required.

Patients who develop leukopenia should be observed carefully for signs of infection. Antibiotic support may be required. In neutropenic patients who develop fever, broad-spectrum antibiotic coverage should be initiated empirically, pending bacterial cultures and appropriate diagnostic tests.

## Oral Dosage Forms

### HYDROXYUREA CAPSULES USP

**Usual adult dose**
Carcinoma, head and neck or
Carcinoma, ovarian or
Melanoma, malignant—
> Oral, 60 to 80 mg per kg of body weight or 2000 to 3000 mg per square meter of body surface in a single dose every third day, alone or in combination with radiation therapy, or 20 to 30 mg per kg of body weight per day in a single dose.

Note: Administration of hydroxyurea should begin at least seven days prior to initiation of radiation therapy, and should be continued during radiation therapy and indefinitely afterwards.

Leukemia, chronic myelocytic, resistant—
Oral, 20 to 30 mg per kg of body weight a day in a single dose or two divided daily doses.

Note: Although dosages are based on the patient's actual weight, use of estimated lean body mass (dry weight) is recommended in obese patients or those with abnormal fluid retention.

In general, use of intermittent dosage is associated with less risk of serious toxicity than continuous daily dosage.

**Usual pediatric dose**
Dosage has not been established.

**Strength(s) usually available**
U.S.—
500 mg (Rx) [*Hydrea* (lactose)].
Canada—
500 mg (Rx) [*Hydrea* (tartrazine 3 mg)].

**Packaging and storage**
Store below 40 °C (104 °F), preferably between 15 and 30 °C (59 and 86 °F), unless otherwise specified by manufacturer. Store in a tight container.

**Auxiliary labeling**
• Keep container tightly closed.

## Selected Bibliography
Dorr RT, Fritz WL. Cancer chemotherapy handbook. New York: Elsevier, 1980: 468-71.

Revised: 06/16/92
Interim revision: 06/21/94

---

# HYDROXYZINE—See *Antihistamines (Systemic)*

---

# HYDROXYZINE-CONTAINING COMBINATIONS—
Theophylline, Ephedrine, and Hydroxyzine (Systemic)

---

# HYOSCYAMINE—See                 *Anticholinergics/Antispasmodics (Systemic)*

---

# HYOSCYAMINE-CONTAINING COMBINATIONS—
Atropine, Hyoscyamine, Methenamine, Methylene Blue, Phenyl Salicylate, and Benzoic Acid (Systemic)
Atropine, Hyoscyamine, Scopolamine, and Phenobarbital (Systemic)—See *Belladonna Alkaloids and Barbiturates (Systemic)*
Chlorpheniramine, Phenylephrine, Phenylpropanolamine, Atropine, Hyoscyamine, and Scopolamine (Systemic)—See *Antihistamines, Decongestants, and Anticholinergics (Systemic)*
Hyoscyamine and Phenobarbital (Systemic)—See *Belladonna Alkaloids and Barbiturates (Systemic)*
Kaolin, Pectin, Hyoscyamine, Atropine, and Scopolamine (Systemic)—See *Kaolin, Pectin, and Belladonna Alkaloids (Systemic)*

**IBUPROFEN**—See *Anti-inflammatory Drugs, Nonsteroidal* (Systemic)

**IBUPROFEN-CONTAINING COMBINATIONS**—
Pseudoephedrine and Ibuprofen (Systemic)—See *Decongestants and Analgesics (Systemic)*

---

# IDARUBICIN    Systemic

VA CLASSIFICATION (Primary): AN200

Note: For a listing of dosage forms and brand names by country availability, see *Dosage Forms* section(s). For a listing of brand names for the articles in this monograph, refer to the General Index.

## Category
Antineoplastic.

## Indications

### Accepted
Leukemia, acute myelocytic (treatment)—Idarubicin is indicated for treatment of acute myelocytic leukemia (including French-American-British [FAB] classifications M1 through M7).

## Pharmacology/Pharmacokinetics

### Physicochemical characteristics
Source—Synthetic. Analog of daunorubicin.
Molecular weight—Idarubicin hydrochloride: 533.96.
Other characteristics—Lipophilic.

### Mechanism of action/Effect
Idarubicin is an anthracycline glycoside; it is classified as an antibiotic but is not used as an antimicrobial agent. Its exact mechanism of antineoplastic activity is unknown; however, it intercalates DNA and inhibits DNA synthesis, interacts with RNA polymerases, and inhibits topoisomerase II (an enzyme that promotes DNA strand supercoiling).

### Distribution
High volume of distribution (approximately 2225 liters). Concentrations of both idarubicin and idarubicinol (the primary metabolite) are 400- and 200-fold higher, respectively, in nucleated blood and bone marrow cells than in plasma. Data about whether idarubicin crosses the blood-brain barrier are conflicting.

### Protein binding
Extensive tissue binding.
    Plasma—
        Idarubicin: Very high (97%).
        Idarubicinol: Very high (94%).

### Biotransformation
Rapidly and extensively, both hepatically and extrahepatically, to produce the primary metabolite, idarubicinol, which is equipotent with idarubicin.

### Half-life
Idarubicin—
    As a single agent: Average, 22 hours (range, 4 to 46 hours).
    In combination with cytarabine: Average, 20 hours (range, 7 to 38 hours).
Idarubicinol—
    Approximately double the half-life of idarubicin.

### Time to peak concentration
Cellular (nucleated blood and bone marrow cells)—Within a few minutes after injection.

### Elimination
Biliary, as idarubicinol.
Renal, less than 5%.
In dialysis—Studies have not been done. However, because of the multicompartment behavior, along with the extensive extravascular distribution and tissue binding, it is unlikely that significant amounts of idarubicin would be removable by dialysis.

## Precautions to Consider

### Carcinogenicity/Mutagenicity
Secondary malignancies are potential delayed effects of many antineoplastic agents, although it is not clear whether the effect is related to their mutagenic or immunosuppressive action. The effect of dose and duration of therapy is also unknown, although risk seems to increase with long-term use. Although information is limited, available data seem to indicate that the carcinogenic risk is greatest with the alkylating agents.

Long-term carcinogenicity studies have not been done. However, studies in experimental models (including bacterial systems, mammalian cells in culture, and female Sprague-Dawley rats) indicate that idarubicin has mutagenic and carcinogenic properties.

### Pregnancy/Reproduction
Fertility—Gonadal suppression, resulting in amenorrhea or azoospermia, may occur in patients taking antineoplastic therapy, especially with the alkylating agents. In general, these effects appear to be related to dose and length of therapy and may be irreversible. Prediction of the degree of testicular or ovarian function impairment is complicated by the common use of combinations of several antineoplastics, which makes it difficult to assess the effects of individual agents.

Idarubicin caused testicular atrophy (with inhibition of spermiogenesis and sperm maturation, resulting in few or no mature sperm) in male dogs given 1.8 mg per square meter of body surface per day or more 3 times a week for 13 weeks. Effects were not readily reversible after an 8-week recovery period.

Pregnancy—Adequate and well-controlled studies in humans have not been done.

First trimester: It is usually recommended that use of antineoplastics, especially combination chemotherapy, be avoided whenever possible, especially during the first trimester. Although information is limited because of the relatively few instances of antineoplastic administration during pregnancy, the mutagenic, teratogenic, and carcinogenic potential of these medications must be considered.

Other hazards to the fetus include adverse reactions seen in adults.

Studies in rats at a dose of 1.2 mg per square meter of body surface per day (one-tenth the human dose), which was nontoxic to dams, found idarubicin to be embryotoxic and teratogenic. Studies in rabbits at a dose of 2.4 mg per square meter of body surface (two-tenths the human dose), which was toxic to dams, found idarubicin to be embryotoxic but not teratogenic.

FDA Pregnancy Category D.

In general, use of contraception is recommended during cytotoxic drug therapy.

### Breast-feeding
It is not known whether idarubicin is distributed into breast milk. Although very little information is available regarding distribution of antineoplastic agents into breast milk, breast-feeding is not recommended during chemotherapy because of the potential risks to the infant (adverse effects, mutagenicity, carcinogenicity).

### Pediatrics
Appropriate studies on the relationship of age to the effects of idarubicin have not been performed in the pediatric population. In two small studies of the pharmacokinetics, conflicting results were obtained about a possible difference in clearance rate. Safety and efficacy have not been established.

### Geriatrics
Although appropriate studies on the relationship of age to the effects of idarubicin have not been performed in the geriatric population, cardiotoxicity may be more frequent in older persons (over 60 years of age). Caution should also be used in patients who have inadequate bone marrow reserves due to old age. In addition, elderly patients are more likely to have age-related renal function impairment, which when severe may require reduction of dosage in patients receiving idarubicin.

### Dental
The bone marrow depressant effects of idarubicin may result in an increased incidence of microbial infection, delayed healing, and gingival bleeding. Dental work, whenever possible, should be completed prior to initiation of therapy or deferred until blood counts have returned to normal. Patients should be instructed in proper oral hygiene during treatment, including caution in use of regular toothbrushes, dental floss, and toothpicks.

Idarubicin also commonly causes mucositis, which may be associated with considerable discomfort.

**Drug interactions and/or related problems**
The following drug interactions and/or related problems have been selected on the basis of their potential clinical significance (possible mechanism in parentheses where appropriate)—not necessarily inclusive (» = major clinical significance):

Note: Combinations containing any of the following medications, depending on the amount present, may also interact with this medication.

Allopurinol or
Colchicine or
» Probenecid or
» Sulfinpyrazone
  (idarubicin may raise the concentration of blood uric acid; dosage adjustment of antigout agents may be necessary to control hyperuricemia and gout; allopurinol may be preferred to prevent or reverse idarubicin-induced hyperuricemia because of risk of uric acid nephropathy with uricosuric antigout agents)

Blood dyscrasia–causing medications (See *Appendix II*)
  (leukopenic and/or thrombocytopenic effects of idarubicin may be increased with concurrent or recent therapy if these medications cause the same effects; dosage adjustment of idarubicin, if necessary, should be based on blood counts)

» Bone marrow depressants, other (See *Appendix II*) or
Radiation therapy
  (additive bone marrow depression may occur; dosage reduction may be required when two or more bone marrow depressants, including radiation, are used concurrently or consecutively)

Daunorubicin or
Doxorubicin
  (use of idarubicin in a patient who has previously received daunorubicin or doxorubicin increases the risk of cardiotoxicity; in general, idarubicin should not be used in patients who have previously received complete cumulative doses of daunorubicin or doxorubicin)

Radiation therapy to mediastinal area
  (concurrent use with idarubicin may result in increased cardiotoxicity)

Vaccines, killed virus
  (because normal defense mechanisms may be suppressed by idarubicin therapy, the patient's antibody response to the vaccine may be decreased. The interval between discontinuation of medications that cause immunosuppression and restoration of the patient's ability to respond to the vaccine depends on the intensity and type of immunosuppression-causing medication used, the underlying disease, and other factors; estimates vary from 3 months to 1 year)

» Vaccines, live virus
  (because normal defense mechanisms may be suppressed by idarubicin therapy, concurrent use with a live virus vaccine may potentiate the replication of the vaccine virus, may increase the side/adverse effects of the vaccine virus, and/or may decrease the patient's antibody response to the vaccine; immunization of these patients should be undertaken only with extreme caution after careful review of the patient's hematologic status and only with the knowledge and consent of the physician managing the idarubicin therapy. The interval between discontinuation of medications that cause immunosuppression and restoration of the patient's ability to respond to the vaccine depends on the intensity and type of immunosuppression-causing medication used, the underlying disease, and other factors; estimates vary from 3 months to 1 year. Patients with leukemia in remission should not receive live virus vaccine until at least 3 months after their last chemotherapy. In addition, immunization with oral poliovirus vaccine should be postponed in persons in close contact with the patient, especially family members)

**Laboratory value alterations**
The following have been selected on the basis of their potential clinical significance (possible effect in parentheses where appropriate)—not necessarily inclusive (» = major clinical significance):

With physiology/laboratory test values
Alanine aminotransferase (ALT [SGPT]), serum and
Alkaline phosphatase, serum and
Aspartate aminotransferase (AST [SGOT]), serum and
Bilirubin, serum
  (values may be increased transiently)

Electrocardiogram (ECG) changes, transient, including:
Arrhythmias (atrial or ventricular premature beats, tachycardia)
ST-T wave changes
T-wave flattening
T-wave inversion
  (may occur)

Left ventricular ejection fraction (LVEF)
  (decrease from pretreatment baseline values usually occurs with idarubicin-induced cardiomyopathy)

Uric acid concentrations in blood and urine
  (may be increased)

**Medical considerations/Contraindications**
The medical considerations/contraindications included here have been selected on the basis of their potential clinical significance (reasons given in parentheses where appropriate)—not necessarily inclusive (» = major clinical significance).

*Risk-benefit should be considered when the following medical problems exist:*

» Bone marrow depression
» Chickenpox, existing or recent (including recent exposure) or
» Herpes zoster
  (risk of severe generalized disease)

Gout, history of or
Urate renal stones, history of
  (risk of hyperuricemia)

» Heart disease
  (increased risk of cardiotoxicity)

» Hepatic function impairment
  (reduction in dosage is recommended; one-half the normal dose is recommended in patients with serum bilirubin values of 2.6 to 5 mg per 100 mL; administration of idarubicin is not recommended in patients with serum bilirubin values of greater than 5 mg per 100 mL)

» Infection
  (should be controlled before initiation of idarubicin treatment)

Renal function impairment
  (dosage reduction should be considered in patients with a serum creatinine of greater than 2.5 mg per 100 mL)

Sensitivity to idarubicin

» Caution should be used also in patients with inadequate bone marrow reserves due to previous cytotoxic drug or radiation therapy.

**Patient monitoring**
The following are especially important in patient monitoring (other tests may be warranted in some patients, depending on condition; » = major clinical significance):

Alanine aminotransferase (ALT [SGPT]) values, serum and
Alkaline phosphatase values, serum and
Aspartate aminotransferase (AST [SGOT]) values, serum and
Bilirubin values, serum and
Lactate dehydrogenase (LDH) values, serum
  (recommended prior to initiation of therapy and at periodic intervals during therapy to monitor hepatic function; frequency varies according to clinical state, agent, dose, and other agents being used concurrently)

Chest x-ray and
» Echocardiography and
Electrocardiogram (ECG) studies and
» Radionuclide angiography determination of ejection fraction
  (recommended prior to initiation of therapy and at periodic intervals during therapy)

Creatinine concentrations, serum
  (recommended prior to treatment and at periodic intervals during treatment to monitor renal function)

» Examination of patient's mouth for ulceration
  (recommended before administration of each dose)

» Hematocrit or hemoglobin and
» Platelet count and
» Leukocyte count, total and, if appropriate, differential
  (determinations recommended prior to initiation of therapy and at periodic intervals during therapy; frequency varies according to clinical state, agent, dose, and other agents being used concurrently)

Uric acid concentrations, serum
  (recommended prior to initiation of therapy and at periodic intervals during therapy; frequency varies according to clinical state,
  agent, dose, and other agents being used concurrently)

## Side/Adverse Effects

Note: Many ''side effects'' of antineoplastic therapy are unavoidable and
  represent the medication's pharmacologic action. Some of these (for
  example, leukopenia and thrombocytopenia) are actually used as
  parameters to aid in individual dosage titration.

The following side/adverse effects have been selected on the basis of their
  potential clinical significance (possible signs and symptoms in parentheses where appropriate)—not necessarily inclusive:

### Those indicating need for medical attention
Incidence more frequent
  *Leukopenia or infection* (fever or chills; cough or hoarseness; lower
  back or side pain; painful or difficult urination); *mucositis* (sores in
  mouth and on lips); *thrombocytopenia* (unusual bleeding or bruising;
  black, tarry stools; blood in urine or stools; pinpoint red spots on skin)
  Note: Severe *leukopenia* occurs in all patients; deaths due to infection
    have been reported. Nadir of leukocyte counts occurs 10 to 14
    days after a dose; recovery usually occurs within 21 days after
    a dose.
    Severe *thrombocytopenia* occurs in all patients; deaths due to
    bleeding have been reported. Nadir of platelet counts occurs 10
    to 14 days after a dose; recovery usually occurs within 21 days
    after a dose.

Incidence less frequent
  *Cardiotoxicity, in the form of arrhythmias, congestive heart failure,*
  *or other cardiomyopathies* (shortness of breath; swelling of feet and
  lower legs; fast or irregular heartbeat); *extravasation or tissue necrosis*
  (pain at injection site); *hyperuricemia or uric acid nephropathy* (joint
  pain, lower back or side pain)
  Note: Incidence of *cardiotoxicity* is more frequent in patients who
    have received previous chest irradiation or medications increas-
    ing cardiotoxicity and in patients with a history of cardiac dis-
    ease or mediastinal radiation, and may be more frequent in the
    elderly. Cumulative cardiotoxicity has not been studied.
    *Extravasation* may occur with or without accompanying sting-
    ing or burning and even if blood returns well on aspiration of
    the infusion needle.
    *Hyperuricemia or uric acid nephropathy* occurs most com-
    monly during initial treatment of patients with leukemia or lym-
    phoma, as a result of rapid cell breakdown which leads to el-
    evated serum uric acid concentrations.

Incidence rare
  *Enterocolitis, with perforation* (severe stomach pain); *skin rash or*
  *hives*

### Those indicating need for medical attention only if they continue or are bothersome
Incidence more frequent
  *Diarrhea or stomach cramps; headache; nausea and vomiting*
  Note: *Nausea and vomiting* are usually mild.

Incidence less frequent
  *Peripheral neuropathy* (numbness or tingling of fingers, toes, or face);
  *recall postirradiation erythema* (darkening or redness of skin)
  Note: *Recall postirradiation erythema* occurs if patient has received
    previous radiation therapy.

### Those not indicating need for medical attention
Incidence more frequent
  *Loss of hair; reddish urine*
  Note: *Loss of hair* occurs in most patients.

### Those indicating the need for medical attention if they occur after medication is discontinued
  *Cardiotoxicity* (fast or irregular heartbeat; shortness of breath; swelling
  of feet and lower legs)

## Overdose

For more information on the management of overdose or unintentional
  ingestion, **contact a Poison Control Center** (see *Poison Control Cen-*
  *ter Listing*).

### Treatment of overdose
Treatment of overdose involves supportive care, including:
Platelet transfusions and antibiotics for severe and prolonged
  myelosuppression.
Symptomatic treatment of mucositis.
It is unlikely that dialysis would remove significant amounts of idarubicin
  or its metabolites.

## Patient Consultation

As an aid to patient consultation, refer to *Advice for the Patient, Idarubicin*
  *(Systemic)*.

In providing consultation, consider emphasizing the following selected
  information (» = major clinical significance):

### Before using this medication
» Conditions affecting use, especially:
    Sensitivity to idarubicin
    Pregnancy—Use not recommended because of mutagenic, terato-
      genic, and carcinogenic potential; advisability of using contra-
      ception; telling physician immediately if pregnancy is
      suspected
    Breast-feeding—Not recommended because of risk of serious side
      effects
    Use in the elderly—Cardiotoxicity may be more frequent in pa-
      tients over 60 years of age
    Other medications, especially probenecid, sulfinpyrazone, other
      bone marrow depressants, or previous cytotoxic drug or radi-
      ation therapy
    Other medical problems, especially chickenpox, herpes zoster,
      heart disease, hepatic function impairment, or infection

### Proper use of this medication
    Caution in taking combination therapy; taking each medication at the
      right time
    Importance of ample fluid intake and subsequent increase in urine
      output to aid in excretion of uric acid
    Frequency of nausea and vomiting; importance of continuing medi-
      cation despite stomach upset
» Proper dosing

### Precautions while using this medication
» Importance of close monitoring by the physician
» Avoiding immunizations unless approved by physician; other persons
    in patient's household should avoid immunizations with oral po-
    liovirus vaccine; avoiding persons who have taken oral poliovirus
    vaccine or wearing a protective mask that covers nose and mouth
*Caution if bone marrow depression occurs:*
» Avoiding exposure to persons with bacterial infections, especially dur-
    ing periods of low blood counts; checking with physician imme-
    diately if fever or chills, cough or hoarseness, lower back or side
    pain, or painful or difficult urination occur
» Checking with physician immediately if unusual bleeding or bruising;
    black, tarry stools; blood in urine or stools; or pinpoint red spots
    on skin occur
    Caution in use of regular toothbrush, dental floss, or toothpick; phy-
      sician, dentist, or nurse may suggest alternatives; checking with
      physician before having dental work done
    Not touching eyes or inside of nose unless hands washed immediately
      before
    Using caution to avoid accidental cuts with use of sharp objects such
      as safety razor or fingernail or toenail cutters
    Avoiding contact sports or other situations where bruising or injury
      could occur
» Possibility of local tissue injury and scarring if infiltration of intra-
    venous solution occurs; telling doctor or nurse right away about
    redness, pain, or swelling at injection site

### Side/adverse effects
    Importance of discussing possible effects, including cancer, with
      physician
    Signs of potential side effects, especially leukopenia, infection, mu-
      cositis, thrombocytopenia, cardiotoxicity, extravasation, tissue ne-
      crosis, hyperuricemia, uric acid nephropathy, enterocolitis, and
      skin rash or hives
    Physician or nurse can help in dealing with side effects
    Possibility of hair loss; should return after treatment has ended

# General Dosing Information

Patients receiving idarubicin should be under supervision of a physician experienced in cancer chemotherapy.

A variety of dosage schedules of idarubicin, alone or in combination with other antitumor agents, are used. The prescriber may consult the medical literature as well as the manufacturer's literature in choosing a specific dosage.

Dosage must be adjusted to meet the individual requirements of each patient, on the basis of clinical response and appearance or severity of toxicity.

The desired dose of idarubicin is withdrawn from the vial of reconstituted solution and then injected over 10 to 15 minutes into the tubing of a freely running intravenous infusion of 5% dextrose injection or 0.9% sodium chloride injection. The tubing should be attached to a butterfly needle or other suitable device and inserted preferably into a large vein.

Care must be taken to avoid extravasation during intravenous administration because of the risk of severe ulceration and necrosis.

If extravasation of idarubicin occurs during intravenous administration, possibly indicated by local burning or stinging (may also be painless), the injection and infusion should be stopped immediately and resumed, completing the dose, in another vein. Treatment of known or suspected subcutaneous extravasation may include intermittent ice packs (one-half hour immediately, then one-half hour 4 times a day for 3 days) over the area of extravasation and elevation of the affected extremity. Frequent examination of the area, as well as an early plastic surgery consultation are recommended if there is any sign of a local reaction such as pain, erythema, edema, or vesication. Early excision of the involved area should be considered if ulceration begins or there is severe persistent pain at the site.

Because it will cause local tissue necrosis, idarubicin must not be administered intramuscularly or subcutaneously.

Development of uric acid nephropathy in patients with leukemia or lymphoma may be prevented by adequate oral hydration and, in some cases, administration of allopurinol. Alkalinization of urine may be necessary if serum uric acid concentrations are elevated.

In patients who experience severe mucositis, a second course of idarubicin should be delayed until recovery has occurred and a dose reduction of 25% is recommended.

In acute leukemia, idarubicin may be administered despite the presence of thrombocytopenia and bleeding; stoppage of bleeding and increase in platelet count can occur during or after treatment. Platelet transfusions may be necessary.

Special precautions are recommended in patients who develop thrombocytopenia as a result of administration of idarubicin. These may include extreme care in performing invasive procedures; regular inspection of intravenous sites, skin (including perirectal area), and mucous membrane surfaces for signs of bleeding or bruising; limiting frequency of venipuncture and avoiding intramuscular injections; testing urine, emesis, stool, and secretions for occult blood; care in use of regular toothbrushes, dental floss, toothpicks, safety razors, and fingernail and toenail cutters; avoiding constipation; and using caution to prevent falls and other injuries. Such patients should avoid alcohol and aspirin intake because of the risk of gastrointestinal bleeding. Platelet transfusions may be required.

Patients who develop leukopenia should be observed carefully for signs of infection. Antibiotic support may be required. In neutropenic patients who develop fever, broad-spectrum antibiotic coverage should be initiated empirically, pending bacterial cultures and appropriate diagnostic tests.

## Safety considerations for handling this medication

There is concern and limited evidence that personnel involved in preparation and administration of parenteral antineoplastics may be at some risk because of the potential mutagenicity, teratogenicity, and/or carcinogenicity of these agents, although the actual risk is unknown. USP advisory panels recommend cautious handling both in preparation and disposal of antineoplastic agents. Precautions that have been suggested include:

- Use of a biological containment cabinet during reconstitution and dilution of parenteral medications and wearing of disposable surgical gloves and masks.
- Use of proper technique to prevent contamination of the medication, work area, and operator during transfer between containers (including proper training of personnel in this technique).
- Cautious and proper disposal of needles, syringes, vials, ampuls, and unused medication.

A number of medical centers have developed detailed guidelines for handling of antineoplastic agents.

## Combination chemotherapy

Idarubicin may be used in combination with other agents in various regimens. As a result, incidence and/or severity of side effects may be altered and different dosages (usually reduced) may be used. For example, idarubicin is part of the following chemotherapeutic combination:

— Idarubicin, cytarabine.

For specific dosages and schedules, consult the literature. For information regarding each agent, consult the individual monographs.

# Parenteral Dosage Forms

## IDARUBICIN HYDROCHLORIDE FOR INJECTION USP

### Usual adult dose

Leukemia, acute myelocytic—
Intravenous, slow (over ten to fifteen minutes), 12 mg per square meter of body surface per day for three days. This is given in combination with cytarabine in a dose of either 100 mg per square meter of body surface per day by continuous intravenous infusion for seven days or 25 mg per square meter of body surface intravenously followed by 200 mg per square meter of body surface per day by continuous intravenous infusion for five days.

Note: A second course may be given to patients with unequivocal evidence of leukemia after the first course.

### Usual pediatric dose

Safety and efficacy have not been established.

### Size(s) usually available

U.S.—
5 mg (Rx) [*Idamycin* (lactose 50 mg)].
10 mg (Rx) [*Idamycin* (lactose 100 mg)].
Canada—
5 mg (Rx) [*Idamycin* (lactose 50 mg)].
10 mg (Rx) [*Idamycin* (lactose 100 mg)].

### Packaging and storage

Store below 40 °C (104 °F), preferably between 15 and 30 °C (59 and 86 °F), unless otherwise specified by manufacturer. Protect from light.

### Preparation of dosage form

Idarubicin Hydrochloride for Injection USP is reconstituted for intravenous administration by adding 5 or 10 mL, respectively, of 0.9% sodium chloride injection to the 5- or 10-mg vial, producing a solution containing 1 mg of idarubicin hydrochloride per mL. Use of bacteriostatic diluents is not recommended. Care should be taken when the needle is inserted in the vial, whose contents are under negative pressure to minimize aerosol formation during reconstitution.

### Stability

Reconstituted solutions of idarubicin are physically and chemically stable for 72 hours at room temperature or at least 168 hours (7 days) between 2 and 8 °C (36 and 46 °F) when protected from light.

### Incompatibilities

Idarubicin should not be mixed with heparin, since a precipitate may form.

### Note

Great care should be taken to prevent exposure of the skin to idarubicin. Any idarubicin powder or solution that comes in contact with the skin or mucosae should be washed off thoroughly with soap and water.

# Selected Bibliography

Fields SM, Koeller JM. Idarubicin: a second generation anthracycline. DICP, Ann Pharmacother 1991 May; 25: 505-17.

Revised: 06/18/93
Interim revision: 11/22/93; 06/21/94

# IDOXURIDINE    Ophthalmic

VA CLASSIFICATION (Primary): OP203

Note: For a listing of dosage forms and brand names by country availability, see *Dosage Forms* section(s). For a listing of brand names for the articles in this monograph, refer to the General Index.

## Category

Antiviral (ophthalmic).

## Indications

Note: Bracketed information in the *Indications* section refers to uses that are not included in U.S. product labeling.

### Accepted

Keratitis, herpes simplex virus (treatment) or

[Keratitis, vaccinia virus (treatment)][1]—Idoxuridine is indicated in the treatment of keratitis caused by herpes simplex virus (HSV) and [vaccinia virus].

[Keratoconjunctivitis, herpes simplex virus (treatment)][1]—Idoxuridine is used in the treatment of keratoconjunctivitis caused by herpes simplex virus (HSV).

### Unaccepted

Idoxuridine has no effect on accumulated scarring, vascularization, or progressive loss of vision that may result from the infection. It also has no effect on corneal inflammation that may follow HSV keratitis when the virus is absent, nor on adenoviral keratoconjunctivitis.

[1]Not included in Canadian product labeling.

## Pharmacology/Pharmacokinetics

### Physicochemical characteristics

Chemical group—Chemically related to thymidine.
Molecular weight—354.10.

### Mechanism of action/Effect

Idoxuridine, which closely resembles thymidine, inhibits thymidylic phosphorylase and specific DNA polymerases, which are necessary for the incorporation of thymidine into viral DNA. Idoxuridine is incorporated in place of thymidine into viral DNA, resulting in faulty DNA and the inability to infect or destroy tissue or to reproduce. Idoxuridine is incorporated into mammalian DNA as well.

### Distribution

Idoxuridine penetrates the cornea poorly and therefore is ineffective in the treatment of iritis or deep stromal infections.

### Biotransformation

Idoxuridine is rapidly inactivated by deaminases or nucleotidases.

## Precautions to Consider

### Cross-sensitivity and/or related problems

Patients sensitive to iodine or iodine-containing preparations may be sensitive to this medication also.

### Pregnancy/Reproduction

Pregnancy—Idoxuridine crosses the placenta. Studies in humans have not been done.
Fetal malformations in rabbits (including exophthalmos and clubbing of forelegs) and chromosomal aberrations in mice have been reported.

### Breast-feeding

It is not known whether idoxuridine is distributed into breast milk. However, problems in humans have not been documented.

### Pediatrics

Appropriate studies on the relationship of age to the effects of this medicine have not been performed in the pediatric population. However, no pediatrics-specific problems have been documented to date.

### Geriatrics

Appropriate studies on the relationship of age to the effects of this medicine have not been performed in the geriatric population. However, no geriatrics-specific problems have been documented to date.

### Drug interactions and/or related problems

The following drug interactions and/or related problems have been selected on the basis of their potential clinical significance (possible

mechanism in parentheses where appropriate)—not necessarily inclusive (» = major clinical significance):

Note: Combinations containing any of the following medications, depending on the amount present, may also interact with this medication.

» Boric acid

(concurrent use of boric acid with idoxuridine formulations is not recommended; boric acid may interact with inactive ingredients in some idoxuridine formulations, resulting in precipitate formation; in addition, boric acid may interact with preservatives, especially higher concentrations of thimerosal, in other idoxuridine formulations, resulting in increased ocular toxicity)

### Medical considerations/Contraindications

The medical considerations/contraindications included here have been selected on the basis of their potential clinical significance (reasons given in parentheses where appropriate)—not necessarily inclusive (» = major clinical significance).

*Risk-benefit should be considered when the following medical problem exists:*

Sensitivity to idoxuridine

### Patient monitoring

The following may be especially important in patient monitoring (other tests may be warranted in some patients, depending on condition; » = major clinical significance):

Ophthalmologic, including slit-lamp, examinations
(may be required periodically during therapy)

## Side/Adverse Effects

The following side/adverse effects have been selected on the basis of their potential clinical significance (possible signs and symptoms in parentheses where appropriate)—not necessarily inclusive:

### Those indicating need for medical attention

Incidence less frequent
*Hypersensitivity* (itching, redness, swelling, pain, or other sign of irritation not present before therapy); *increased sensitivity of eyes to light*

Incidence rare
*Corneal clouding* (blurring, dimming, or haziness of vision)

### Those indicating need for medical attention only if they continue or are bothersome

Incidence less frequent
*Lacrimal punctal stenosis or occlusion* (excess flow of tears)

### Those not indicating need for medical attention

For ophthalmic ointment dosage form only
*Blurred vision*

## Patient Consultation

As an aid to patient consultation, refer to *Advice for the Patient, Idoxuridine (Ophthalmic).*

In providing consultation, consider emphasizing the following selected information (» = major clinical significance):

### Before using this medication

» Conditions affecting use, especially:
Sensitivity to idoxuridine or to iodine or iodine-containing preparations
Pregnancy—Ophthalmic idoxuridine crosses the placenta and has been shown to cause protruding eyes and deformed forelegs in rabbits. However, the medication has not been shown to cause birth defects or other problems in humans
Other medications, especially boric acid

### Proper use of this medication

Proper administration technique for ophthalmic ointment and solution
» Not administering more frequently or for longer than ordered by physician
» Compliance with full course of therapy
» Proper dosing
Missed dose: Applying as soon as possible; not applying if almost time for next dose
» Proper storage

### Precautions while using this medication

Regular visits to physician to check progress
Checking with physician if no improvement within a week

Possible photophobic reactions; wearing sunglasses and avoiding prolonged exposure to bright light

**Side/adverse effects**

Blurred vision may occur for a few minutes after application of ophthalmic ointments

Signs of potential side effects, especially hypersensitivity, increased sensitivity of eyes to light, or corneal clouding

## General Dosing Information

At night the ophthalmic ointment may be used as an adjunct to the ophthalmic solution to provide prolonged contact with the medication.

Although some manufacturers recommend a dose of 2 drops of an ophthalmic solution at appropriate intervals, the conjunctival sac will usually hold only 1 drop.

Idoxuridine may be administered concurrently with cycloplegics, antibiotics, or corticosteroids. Corticosteroids can accelerate the spread of viral infections and are usually contraindicated in superficial herpes simplex virus keratitis. However, steroids may be used concurrently with idoxuridine in the treatment of herpes simplex infections with stromal lesions, corneal edema, or iritis. Prolonged administration with corticosteroids may be required. Idoxuridine should be continued for a few days after the steroid has been discontinued.

Since idoxuridine inhibits the formation of DNA in the cornea, prolonged administration of idoxuridine alone may damage the corneal epithelium and prevent healing of the ulcers. Treatment should usually not be continued for more than 21 days total or for more than 3 to 5 days after healing is complete. However, chronic or particularly difficult infections may require up to 3 to 6 weeks of treatment. Too frequent administration may result in small punctate defects in the cornea.

Burning after application or failure to respond to treatment may suggest deterioration of the ophthalmic solution; replace with fresh solution.

Herpetic keratitis may recur if idoxuridine is discontinued before microscopic staining with fluorescein has cleared.

## Ophthalmic Dosage Forms

Note: Bracketed uses in the *Dosage Forms* section refer to categories of use and/or indications that are not included in U.S. product labeling.

### IDOXURIDINE OPHTHALMIC OINTMENT USP

**Usual adult and adolescent dose**

Keratitis, herpes simplex virus—

Topical, to the conjunctiva, a thin strip (approximately 1 cm) of ointment every four hours (five times a day) during the day. The last dose may be administered at bedtime. Treatment should be continued until definite improvement occurs, as demonstrated by loss of staining with fluorescein.

[Keratitis, vaccinia virus][1] or
[Keratoconjunctivitis, herpes simplex virus][1]—

Topical, to the conjunctiva, a thin strip (approximately 1 cm) of ointment five times a day.

**Usual adult prescribing limits**

Up to 8 times daily.

**Usual pediatric dose**

See *Usual adult and adolescent dose.*

**Strength(s) usually available**

U.S.—

0.5% (Rx) [*Stoxil*].

Canada—

0.5% (Rx) [*Stoxil*].

**Packaging and storage**

Store between 8 and 15 °C (46 and 59 °F). Store in a collapsible ophthalmic ointment tube.

Note: Some manufacturers indicate that the ointment does not require refrigeration.

**Stability**

Idoxuridine is rapidly inactivated by deaminases or nucleotidases.

**Auxiliary labeling**

• Store in a cool place. May be refrigerated.
• For the eye.
• Continue medicine for full time of treatment.
• Do not use more often or longer than ordered.

### IDOXURIDINE OPHTHALMIC SOLUTION USP

**Usual adult and adolescent dose**

Keratitis, herpes simplex virus—

Topical, to the conjunctiva, 1 drop every hour during the day and every two hours during the night; or 1 drop every minute for five minutes with the dosage schedule repeated every four hours day and night. Treatment should be continued until definite improvement occurs, as demonstrated by loss of staining with fluorescein. Dose may then be reduced to 1 drop every two hours during the day and every four hours during the night.

[Keratitis, vaccinia virus][1] or
[Keratoconjunctivitis, herpes simplex virus][1]—

Topical, to the conjunctiva, 1 drop every hour during the day and every two hours during the night.

**Usual pediatric dose**

See *Usual adult and adolescent dose.*

**Strength(s) usually available**

U.S.—

0.1% (Rx) [*Herplex Liquifilm* (polyvinyl alcohol 1.4%; benzalkonium chloride); *Stoxil* (thimerosal 1:50,000)].

Canada—

0.1% (Rx) [*Herplex Liquifilm* (polyvinyl alcohol 1.4%; benzalkonium chloride 0.004%); *Stoxil* (thimerosal 1:50,000)].

**Packaging and storage**

Store between 2 and 8 °C (36 and 46 °F). Store in a tight, light-resistant container.

**Stability**

Idoxuridine is rapidly inactivated by deaminases or nucleotidases. To ensure stability, the ophthalmic solution should not be mixed with other medications. Burning after application or failure to respond to treatment may suggest deterioration of the ophthalmic solution; replace with fresh solution.

**Auxiliary labeling**

• Refrigerate.
• For the eye.
• Continue medicine for full time of treatment.
• Do not use more often or longer than ordered.

**Note**

Dispense in original unopened container.

---

[1]Not included in Canadian product labeling.

Revised: 06/21/93

---

# IFOSFAMIDE   Systemic

VA CLASSIFICATION (Primary): AN100

Note: For a listing of dosage forms and brand names by country availability, see *Dosage Forms* section(s). For a listing of brand names for the articles in this monograph, refer to the General Index.

---

## Category

Antineoplastic.

## Indications

Note: Bracketed information in the *Indications* section refers to uses that are not included in U.S. product labeling.

**Accepted**

Tumors, germ cell, testicular (treatment)[1]—Ifosfamide is indicated, in combination with other antineoplastics and a prophylactic agent against hemorrhagic cystitis (such as mesna), for third line treatment of germ cell testicular tumors.

[Sarcomas, soft-tissue (treatment)]
[Ewing's sarcoma (treatment)][1] or
[Lymphomas, non-Hodgkin's (treatment)][1]—Ifosfamide is used for treatment of soft-tissue sarcomas, Ewing's sarcoma, and non-Hodgkin's lymphomas.

[Carcinoma, lung (treatment)][1]

[Carcinoma, pancreatic (treatment)]—Ifosfamide is used for treatment of lung carcinoma and pancreatic carcinoma.

---

[1]Not included in Canadian product labeling.

## Pharmacology/Pharmacokinetics

### Physicochemical characteristics
Molecular weight—261.09.

### Mechanism of action/Effect
Ifosfamide is classed as an alkylating agent of the nitrogen mustard type. After metabolic activation, active metabolites of ifosfamide alkylate or bind with many intracellular molecular structures, including nucleic acids. The cytotoxic action is primarily due to cross-linking of strands of DNA and RNA, as well as inhibition of protein synthesis.

### Distribution
Active metabolites cross blood-brain barrier to only a limited extent.

### Biotransformation
Hepatic (including initial activation and subsequent degradation). Metabolic pathways appear to be saturated at high doses.

### Half-life
At single doses of 3.8 to 5.0 grams per square meter of body surface— Biphasic: Terminal—15 hours.

At doses of 1.6 to 2.4 grams per square meter of body surface per day— Monophasic: 7 hours.

### Elimination
Renal, 70 to 86%—
  61% unchanged at single doses of 5 grams per square meter of body surface.
  12 to 18% unchanged at doses of 1.2 to 2.4 grams per square meter of body surface.

## Precautions to Consider

### Carcinogenicity
Secondary malignancies are potential delayed effects of many antineoplastic agents, although it is not clear whether the effect is related to their mutagenic or immunosuppressive action. The effect of dose and duration of therapy is also unknown, although risk seems to increase with long-term use. Although information is limited, available data seem to indicate that the carcinogenic risk is greatest with the alkylating agents.

Studies in rats have found ifosfamide to be carcinogenic, with female rats showing a significant incidence of leiomyosarcomas and mammary fibroadenomas.

### Mutagenicity
Ifosfamide has been shown to be mutagenic in bacterial studies *in vitro* and mammalian cells *in vivo*. *In vivo*, ifosfamide has induced mutagenic effects in mice and *Drosophila melanogaster* germ cells, and has induced a significant increase in dominant lethal mutations in male mice as well as recessive sex-linked lethal mutations in *Drosophila*.

### Pregnancy/Reproduction
Fertility—Gonadal suppression, resulting in amenorrhea or azoospermia, may occur in patients taking antineoplastic therapy, especially with the alkylating agents. In general, these effects appear to be related to dose and length of therapy and may be irreversible. Prediction of the degree of testicular or ovarian function impairment is complicated by the common use of combinations of several antineoplastics, which makes it difficult to assess the effects of individual agents.

Pregnancy—First trimester: It is usually recommended that use of antineoplastics, especially combination chemotherapy, be avoided whenever possible, especially during the first trimester. Although information is limited because of the relatively few instances of antineoplastic administration during pregnancy, the mutagenic, teratogenic, and carcinogenic potential of these medications must be considered.

Other hazards to the fetus include adverse reactions seen in adults.

In general, use of a contraceptive is recommended during cytotoxic drug therapy.

Studies in animals have shown that ifosfamide is teratogenic in mice, rats, and rabbits given 0.05 to 0.075 times the human dose.

FDA Pregnancy Category D.

### Breast-feeding
Ifosfamide is excreted in breast milk. Breast-feeding is not recommended during chemotherapy because of the risks to the infant (adverse effects, mutagenicity, carcinogenicity).

### Pediatrics
Appropriate studies on the relationship of age to the effects of ifosfamide have not been performed in the pediatric population. However, no pediatrics-specific problems have been documented to date.

### Geriatrics
No information is available on the relationship of age to the effects of ifosfamide in geriatric patients. However, elderly patients are more likely to have age-related renal function impairment, which may require caution.

### Dental
The bone marrow depressant effects of ifosfamide may result in an increased incidence of microbial infection, delayed healing, and gingival bleeding. Dental work, whenever possible, should be completed prior to initiation of therapy or deferred until blood counts have returned to normal. Patients should be instructed in proper oral hygiene during treatment, including caution in use of regular toothbrushes, dental floss, and toothpicks.

Ifosfamide may also rarely cause stomatitis associated with considerable discomfort.

### Drug interactions and/or related problems
The following drug interactions and/or related problems have been selected on the basis of their potential clinical significance (possible mechanism in parentheses where appropriate)—not necessarily inclusive (» = major clinical significance):

Note: Combinations containing any of the following medications, depending on the amount present, may also interact with this medication.

Blood dyscrasia–causing medications (See *Appendix II*)
  (leukopenic and/or thrombocytopenic effects of ifosfamide may be increased with concurrent or recent therapy if these medications cause the same effects; dosage adjustment of ifosfamide, if necessary, should be based on blood counts)

» Bone marrow depressants, other (See *Appendix II*) or
» Radiation therapy
  (additive bone marrow depression may occur; dosage reduction may be required when two or more bone marrow depressants, including radiation, are used concurrently or consecutively)

Hepatic enzyme inducers (See *Appendix II*)
  (these agents may induce microsomal metabolism to increase formation of alkylating metabolites of ifosfamide; although it is unknown whether activity of ifosfamide is increased, neurotoxicity may be increased; caution is recommended)

Nephrotoxic medications
  (prior or concurrent use with ifosfamide may increase its nephrotoxic effects)
  (previous use of large cumulative doses of cisplatin may increase the risk of CNS toxicity with ifosfamide)

Vaccines, killed virus
  (because normal defense mechanisms may be suppressed by ifosfamide therapy, the patient's antibody response to the vaccine may be decreased. The interval between discontinuation of medications that cause immunosuppression and restoration of the patient's ability to respond to the vaccine depends on the intensity and type of immunosuppression-causing medication used, the underlying disease, and other factors; estimates vary from 3 months to 1 year)

» Vaccines, live virus
  (because normal defense mechanisms may be suppressed by ifosfamide therapy, concurrent use with a live virus vaccine may potentiate the replication of the vaccine virus, may increase the side/ adverse effects of the vaccine virus, and/or may decrease the patient's antibody response to the vaccine; immunization of these patients should be undertaken only with extreme caution after careful review of the patient's hematologic status and only with the knowledge and consent of the physician managing the ifosfamide therapy. The interval between discontinuation of medications that cause immunosuppression and restoration of the patient's ability to respond to the vaccine depends on the intensity and type of immunosuppression-causing medication used, the underlying disease, and other factors; estimates vary from 3 months to 1 year. Patients with leukemia in remission should not receive live virus vaccine until at least 3 months after their last chemotherapy. In addition, immunization with oral poliovirus vaccine should be postponed in persons in close contact with the patient, especially family members)

## Laboratory value alterations

The following have been selected on the basis of their potential clinical significance (possible effect in parentheses where appropriate)—not necessarily inclusive (» = major clinical significance):

With physiology/laboratory test values

Alanine aminotransferase (ALT [SGPT]) and
Aspartate aminotransferase (AST [SGOT]) and
Bilirubin and
Lactate dehydrogenase (LDH)
    (serum values may be increased as a sign of hepatotoxicity)

Blood urea nitrogen (BUN) concentrations or
Creatinine concentrations, serum
    (may be increased transiently as a sign of renal toxicity)

Creatinine clearance
    (may be decreased transiently as a sign of renal toxicity)

## Medical considerations/Contraindications

The medical considerations/contraindications included here have been selected on the basis of their potential clinical significance (reasons given in parentheses where appropriate)—not necessarily inclusive (» = major clinical significance).

*Risk-benefit should be considered when the following medical problems exist:*

» Bone marrow depression

» Chickenpox, existing or recent (including recent exposure) or

» Herpes zoster
    (risk of severe generalized disease)

» Hepatic function impairment
    (effect of ifosfamide may be reduced or enhanced because of its dependence on hepatic microsomal enzyme activation and degradation)

» Infection

» Renal function impairment
    (reduced elimination; incidence of central nervous system [CNS] toxicity and renal toxicity may be increased; dosage reduction may be necessary)

Sensitivity to ifosfamide

Tumor cell infiltration of bone marrow
    (bone marrow depression)

» Caution should be used also in patients who have had previous cytotoxic drug therapy or radiation therapy.

### Patient monitoring

The following are especially important in patient monitoring (other tests may be warranted in some patients, depending on condition; » = major clinical significance):

Alanine aminotransferase (ALT [SGPT]) values, serum and
Alkaline phosphatase values, serum and
Aspartate aminotransferase (AST [SGOT]) values, serum and
Bilirubin values, serum and
Lactate dehydrogenase (LDH) values, serum
    (recommended prior to initiation of therapy and at periodic intervals during therapy; frequency varies according to clinical state, agent, dose, and other agents being used concurrently)

Blood urea nitrogen (BUN) concentrations and
Creatinine concentrations, serum
    (recommended prior to initiation of therapy and at periodic intervals during therapy; frequency varies according to clinical state, agent, dose, and other agents being used concurrently)

» Examination of urine for microscopic hematuria
    (recommended prior to each dose)

» Hematocrit or hemoglobin and

» Leukocyte count, total and, if appropriate, differential and

» Platelet count
    (determinations recommended prior to initiation of therapy and at periodic intervals during therapy; frequency varies according to clinical state, agent, dose, and other agents being used concurrently)

Phosphate concentrations, serum and
Potassium concentrations, serum
    (recommended at periodic intervals during therapy)

## Side/Adverse Effects

Note: Many "side effects" of antineoplastic therapy are unavoidable and represent the medication's pharmacologic action. Some of these (for example, leukopenia and thrombocytopenia) are actually used as parameters to aid in individual dosage titration.

The following side/adverse effects have been selected on the basis of their potential clinical significance (possible signs and symptoms in parentheses where appropriate)—not necessarily inclusive:

### Those indicating need for medical attention

Incidence more frequent—dose-related

*CNS effects or encephalopathy* (agitation; confusion; hallucinations; unusual tiredness; less frequently, dizziness; rarely, seizures; coma); *leukopenia; thrombocytopenia* (rarely associated with unusual bleeding or bruising; black, tarry stools; blood in urine or stools; pinpoint red spots on skin); *urotoxicity, including hemorrhagic cystitis; dysuria; urinary frequency* (blood in urine; frequent urination; painful urination)

Note: *CNS effects or encephalopathy* do not appear to be dose-related. They may be associated with electroencephalogram (EEG) changes. Signs and symptoms usually return to normal within 3 days after withdrawal of ifosfamide, but may persist for longer. Fatalities have been reported.

*Leukopenia* is usually mild to moderate. Nadir of leukocyte count occurs within 7 to 14 days and counts usually recover by 21 days after a course.

With *thrombocytopenia*, nadir of platelet count occurs within 7 to 14 days and counts usually recover by 21 days after a course.

*Urotoxicity* may occur within a few hours or be delayed several weeks; thought to be caused by metabolite of ifosfamide (acrolein). Usually resolves a few days after withdrawal of ifosfamide, but may persist; may be fatal. Incidence is reduced by fractionation of dosage, adequate hydration, and administration of mesna.

Incidence less frequent

*Hepatotoxicity* (usually asymptomatic; detected on laboratory tests); *infection, resulting from leukopenia* (fever or chills; cough or hoarseness; lower back or side pain; painful or difficult urination); *nephrotoxicity* (usually asymptomatic; signs of tubular damage detected on laboratory tests); *phlebitis* (redness, swelling, or pain at site of injection)

Note: Metabolic acidosis as a manifestation of *nephrotoxicity* has been reported to occur frequently in patients receiving high doses of ifosfamide. Renal tubular acidosis, Fanconi syndrome, and renal rickets have been reported.

Incidence rare

*Cardiotoxicity; polyneuropathy; pulmonary toxicity* (cough or shortness of breath); *stomatitis* (sores in mouth and on lips)

### Those indicating need for medical attention only if they continue or are bothersome

Incidence more frequent

*Nausea and vomiting*

Note: *Nausea and vomiting* are usually controlled by antiemetics.

### Those not indicating need for medical attention

Incidence more frequent

*Loss of hair*

### Those indicating the need for medical attention if they occur after medication is discontinued

*Hemorrhagic cystitis* (blood in urine)

## Patient Consultation

As an aid to patient consultation, refer to *Advice for the Patient, Ifosfamide (Systemic)*.

In providing consultation, consider emphasizing the following selected information (» = major clinical significance):

### Before using this medication

» Conditions affecting use, especially:

Sensitivity to ifosfamide

Pregnancy—Use not recommended because of mutagenic, teratogenic, and carcinogenic potential; advisability of using contraception; telling physician immediately if pregnancy is suspected

Breast-feeding—Not recommended because of risk of serious side effects

Other medications, especially other bone marrow depressants, previous cytotoxic drug therapy or radiation therapy

Other medical problems, especially chickenpox, herpes zoster, hepatic function impairment, infection, renal function impairment

### Proper use of this medication

Caution in taking combination therapy; taking each medication at the right time

Importance of ample fluid intake and subsequent increase in urine output, as well as frequent voiding (including at least once during night), to prevent hemorrhagic cystitis and aid in excretion of uric acid; following physician instructions for recommended fluid intake; some patients may require up to 3000 mL (3 quarts) per day

Probability of nausea and vomiting; importance of continuing medication despite stomach upset

» Proper dosing

### Precautions while using this medication

» Importance of close monitoring by physician

» Avoiding immunizations unless approved by physician; other persons in patient's household should avoid immunizations with oral poliovirus vaccine; avoiding other persons who have taken oral poliovirus vaccine or wearing a protective mask that covers nose and mouth

*Caution if bone marrow depression occurs:*

» Avoiding exposure to persons with bacterial infections, especially during periods of low blood counts; checking with physician immediately if fever or chills, cough or hoarseness, lower back or side pain, or painful or difficult urination occur

» Checking with physician immediately if unusual bleeding or bruising; black, tarry stools; blood in urine or stools; or pinpoint red spots on skin occur

Caution in use of regular toothbrush, dental floss, or toothpick; physician, dentist, or nurse may suggest alternatives; checking with physician before having dental work done

Not touching eyes or inside of nose unless hands washed immediately before

Using caution to avoid accidental cuts with use of sharp objects such as safety razor or fingernail or toenail cutters

Avoiding contact sports or other situations where bruising or injury might occur

### Side/adverse effects

May cause adverse effects such as blood problems; loss of hair; toxicity to lungs, heart, or bladder; and cancer; importance of discussing possible effects with physician

Signs of potential side effects, especially CNS effects, leukopenia or infection, thrombocytopenia, hemorrhagic cystitis, phlebitis, pulmonary toxicity, and stomatitis

Physician or nurse can help in dealing with side effects

Possibility of hair loss; normal hair growth should return after treatment has ended

## General Dosing Information

Patients receiving ifosfamide should be under supervision of a physician experienced in cancer chemotherapy.

A variety of dosage schedules and regimens of ifosfamide, alone or in combination with other antitumor agents, are used. The prescriber may consult the medical literature as well as the manufacturer's literature in choosing a specific dosage.

Dosage must be adjusted to meet the individual requirements of each patient, based on clinical response and appearance or severity of toxicity.

To reduce the risk of hemorrhagic cystitis, adequate hydration is recommended prior to ifosfamide treatment and for at least 72 hours following treatment to ensure ample urine output. Concurrent use of an agent to prevent hemorrhagic cystitis (such as mesna) is recommended. In addition, the patient should be encouraged to void frequently, to prevent prolonged contact of irritating metabolites with bladder mucosa.

Development of mild bladder irritation (microscopic hematuria) may require adjustment of mesna dosage. Although concurrent use of mesna greatly reduces the risk, ifosfamide should be discontinued at the first sign of hemorrhagic cystitis. In severe cases, blood replacement may be necessary. Electrocautery diversion of urine flow, cryosurgery, and formaldehyde bladder instillations have been used. Resumption of therapy should be undertaken with caution since recurrence is common.

Each subsequent dose should be given only after microscopic hematuria, if present (defined as greater than 10 red blood cells per high power field), has resolved.

Ifosfamide therapy should be discontinued if severe CNS symptoms occur.

Special precautions are recommended in patients who develop thrombocytopenia as a result of administration of ifosfamide. These may include extreme care in performing invasive procedures; regular inspection of intravenous sites, skin (including perirectal area), and mucous membrane surfaces for signs of bleeding or bruising; limiting frequency of venipuncture and avoiding intramuscular injections; testing urine, emesis, stool, and secretions for occult blood; care in use of

regular toothbrushes, dental floss, toothpicks, safety razors, and fingernail and toenail cutters; avoiding constipation; and using caution to prevent falls and other injuries. Such patients should avoid alcohol and any aspirin intake because of the risk of gastrointestinal bleeding. Platelet transfusions may be required.

Patients who develop leukopenia should be observed carefully for signs of infection. Antibiotic support may be required. In neutropenic patients who develop fever, broad-spectrum antibiotic coverage should be initiated empirically, pending bacterial cultures and appropriate diagnostic tests.

If marked leukopenia (particularly granulocytopenia) or thrombocytopenia occurs, ifosfamide therapy should be withdrawn until leukocyte and platelet counts return to satisfactory levels. Then therapy may be reinstituted, possibly at a lower dose.

### Safety considerations for handling this medication

There is limited but increasing evidence and concern that personnel involved in preparation and administration of parenteral antineoplastics may be at some risk because of the potential mutagenicity, teratogenicity, and/or carcinogenicity of these agents, although the actual risk is unknown. USP advisory panels recommend cautious handling both in preparation and disposal of antineoplastic agents. Precautions that have been suggested include:

• Use of a biological containment cabinet during reconstitution and dilution of parenteral medications and wearing of disposable surgical gloves and masks.

• Use of proper technique to prevent contamination of the medication, work area, and operator during transfer between containers (including proper training of personnel in this technique).

• Cautious and proper disposal of needles, syringes, vials, ampuls, and unused medication.

A number of medical centers have developed detailed guidelines for handling of antineoplastic agents.

### Combination chemotherapy

Ifosfamide may be used in combination with other agents in various regimens. As a result, incidence and/or severity of side effects may be altered and different dosages (usually reduced) may be used. For example, ifosfamide is part of the following chemotherapeutic combinations (some commonly used acronyms are in parentheses):

—etoposide, ifosfamide, and cisplatin (VIP).

—vinblastine, ifosfamide, and cisplatin (VeIP).

For specific dosages and schedules, consult the literature. For information regarding each agent, consult the individual monographs.

## Parenteral Dosage Forms

### IFOSFAMIDE STERILE USP

#### Usual adult and adolescent dose
Germ cell testicular tumors[1]—

Intravenous infusion (over at least 30 minutes), 1.2 grams per square meter of body surface per day for five consecutive days, the course being repeated every three weeks or after hematologic recovery.

Note: Mesna is also administered during ifosfamide therapy to reduce hemorrhagic cystitis.

#### Usual pediatric dose
Dosage has not been established.

#### Size(s) usually available
U.S.—

1 gram (Rx) [*IFEX* (plus 200-mg ampul of mesna)].

3 grams (Rx) [*IFEX* (plus 400-mg ampul of mesna)].

Canada—

1 gram (Rx) [*IFEX*].

2 grams (Rx) [*IFEX*].

3 grams (Rx) [*IFEX*].

#### Packaging and storage
Store below 40 °C (104 °F), preferably between 15 and 30 °C (59 and 86 °F), unless otherwise specified by manufacturer.

#### Preparation of dosage form
May be prepared for parenteral use by adding 20, 40, or 60 mL of sterile water for injection or bacteriostatic water for injection (benzyl alcohol– or paraben-preserved) to the 1-gram, 2-gram, or 3-gram vial, respectively, and shaking to dissolve, to provide a solution containing 50 mg of ifosfamide per mL. The resulting solution may be added to 5% dextrose injection, 0.9% sodium chloride injection, lactated Ringer's injection, or sterile water for injection for administration by intravenous infusion. Use of intermediate concentrations or mixtures of excipients (e.g., 2.5% dextrose injection, 0.45% sodium chloride injection, 5% dextrose and 0.9% sodium chloride injection) is also acceptable.

Caution: Use of diluents containing benzyl alcohol is not recommended for preparation of medications for use in neonates. A fatal toxic syndrome consisting of metabolic acidosis, CNS depression, respiratory problems, renal failure, hypotension, and possibly seizures and intracranial hemorrhages has been associated with this use.

**Stability**
Reconstituted solutions of ifosfamide are stable for at least 1 week at 30 °C (86 °F) or 6 weeks at 5 °C (41 °F). If bacteriostatic water for injection is not used for reconstitution, it is recommended that the solution be refrigerated and used promptly (preferably within 6 hours).

**Note**
Because ifosfamide for injection contains no preservative, caution in preparing and storing solutions is required to ensure sterility.

Ifosfamide and mesna may be mixed in the same infusion.

¹Not included in Canadian product labeling.

**Selected Bibliography**
Zalupski M, Baker LH. Ifosfamide. J Natl Cancer Inst 1988 Jun 15; 80 (8): 556-66.
Brade WP, Herdrich K, Varini M. Ifosfamide—pharmacology/pharmacokinetics, safety and therapeutic potential. Cancer Treat Rev 1985; 12: 1-47.

Revised: 09/09/92
Interim revision: 06/21/94

# IMIGLUCERASE Systemic†

VA CLASSIFICATION (Primary): BL900
Note: For a listing of dosage forms and brand names by country availability, see *Dosage Forms* section(s). For a listing of brand names for the articles in this monograph, refer to the General Index.

†Not commercially available in Canada.

## Category
Enzyme (glucocerebrosidase) replenisher.

## Indications
**Accepted**
Gaucher's disease, (treatment)—Imiglucerase is indicated as enzyme replacement therapy in Type I Gaucher's disease, in which glucocerebrosidase is deficient, resulting in an accumulation of glycolipids in the spleen, liver, and bone marrow. Clinical manifestations requiring treatment include moderate to severe anemia, thrombocytopenia with bleeding tendency, bone disease, and/or significant hepatomegaly or splenomegaly.

## Pharmacology/Pharmacokinetics
**Mechanism of action/Effect**
Imiglucerase catalyzes the hydrolysis of the glycolipid, glucocerebroside, to glucose and ceramide as part of the normal degradation pathway for membrane lipids.

**Distribution**
Vol$_D$—0.09 to 0.15 L per kg of body weight.

**Half-life**
Elimination—3.6 to 10.4 minutes.

**Time to peak effect:**
During one-hour intravenous infusions of four doses (7.5, 15, 30, 60 Units per kg of body weight) steady-state enzymatic activity was achieved by 30 minutes.

## Precautions to Consider
**Cross-sensitivity and/or related problems**
Patients sensitive to alglucerase may be sensitive to imiglucerase also.

**Carcinogenicity/Mutagenicity**
Carcinogenicity and mutagenicity studies have not been performed in either animals or humans.

**Pregnancy/Reproduction**
Pregnancy—Studies have not been done in humans.
Studies have not been done in animals.
FDA Pregnancy Category C.

**Breast-feeding**
It is not known whether imiglucerase is distributed into breast milk.

**Pediatrics**
Appropriate studies on the relationship of age to the effects of imiglucerase have not been performed in the pediatric population. However, pediatrics-specific problems that would limit the usefulness of this medication in children are not expected.

**Geriatrics**
No information is available on the relationship of age to the effects of imiglucerase in geriatric patients.

**Medical considerations/Contraindications**
The medical considerations/contraindications included here have been selected on the basis of their potential clinical significance (reasons given in parentheses where appropriate)—not necessarily inclusive (» = major clinical significance).

*Except under special circumstances, this medication should not be used when the following medical problem exists:*
» Sensitivity to alglucerase or imiglucerase

**Patient monitoring**
The following may be especially important in patient monitoring (other tests may be warranted in some patients, depending on condition; » = major clinical significance):

Acid phosphatase, serum or
Angiotensin-converting enzymes, serum
    (determinations recommended every 2 to 3 months by some clinicians; values should decrease with imiglucerase treatment)

Alanine aminotransferase (ALT [SGPT]) and
Aspartate aminotransferase (AST [SGOT])
    (some clinicians recommend monitoring every 6 to 12 months; values should decrease during imiglucerase therapy)

Bilirubin concentrations, serum and
Calcium, serum and
Creatinine, serum and
Electrolyte concentrations, serum and
Phosphorus, serum
    (some clinicians recommend monitoring every 6 to 12 months)

Hemoglobin and
Platelet count
    (recommended monthly to assess effectiveness of imiglucerase therapy; if hemoglobin falls below 7 grams/dL [70 grams/L] and platelet count is under 50,000, monitoring at 2-week intervals may be recommended; both values should increase with treatment)

Liver volume and
Spleen volume
    (recommended every 6 months to assess effectiveness of therapy; liver and spleen should decrease in volume with imiglucerase treatment)

Magnetic resonance imaging (MRI) of long bones
    (some clinicians recommend monitoring every 1 to 2 years; skeletal response should improve with imiglucerase therapy)

## Side/Adverse Effects
The following side/adverse effects have been selected on the basis of their potential clinical significance (possible signs and symptoms in parentheses where appropriate)—not necessarily inclusive:

**Those indicating need for medical attention only if they continue or are bothersome**
Incidence less frequent
    *Abdominal discomfort; decrease in blood pressure; decrease in urinary frequency; dizziness; headache; nausea; pruritus* (itching); *rash*
    Note: *Decrease in blood pressure, nausea, pruritus,* and *rash* may be due to antibody formation, which occurs in approximately 10 to 16% of patients receiving imiglucerase. Antibody levels decrease in most patients with continuous therapy.

## Patient Consultation
As an aid to patient consultation, refer to *Advice for the Patient, Imiglucerase (Systemic)*.

In providing consultation, consider emphasizing the following selected information (» = major clinical significance):

**Before using this medication**
» Conditions affecting use, especially:
    Sensitivity to alglucerase or imiglucerase

**Proper use of this medication**
    Helps control and reverse problems caused by Gaucher's disease; possible need for lifelong therapy; serious consequences of untreated Gaucher's disease
» Proper dosing

**Precautions while using this medication**
    Importance of monitoring by the physician

## Parenteral Dosage Forms

### IMIGLUCERASE INJECTION

**Usual adult and adolescent dose**
Enzyme replenisher—
    Intravenous infusion, 15 to 60 Units per kg of body weight administered over one to two hours. The usual frequency of infusion is once every two weeks, but disease severity and patient convenience may dictate administration several times a week to once every two weeks. Dosage can be lowered depending on patient response. Dosage may be lowered at 6-month intervals, while monitoring response parameters.

**Usual pediatric dose**
See *Usual adult and adolescent dose.*

**Strength(s) usually available**
U.S.—
    200 Units per vial (Rx) [*Cerezyme*].
Canada—
    Not commercially available.

**Packaging and storage**
Store at 2 to 8 °C (36 to 46 °F).

**Preparation of dosage form**
On the day of use, the vial is reconstituted with 5.1 mL of Sterile Water for Injection USP to give a volume of 5.3 mL. Then, 5 mL is withdrawn from the vial and diluted with 0.9% Sodium Chloride Injection USP to a final volume of 100 to 200 mL.

**Stability**
Imiglucerase does not contain a preservative. The product information for imiglucerase states that when diluted to 50 mL and stored at 2 to 8 °C (36 to 46 °F), the reconstituted product is stable for up to 24 hours.

Developed: 06/16/95

---

# IMIPENEM AND CILASTATIN  Systemic

VA CLASSIFICATION (Primary): AM130

Note: For a listing of dosage forms and brand names by country availability, see *Dosage Forms* section(s). For a listing of brand names for the articles in this monograph, refer to the General Index.

## Category

Antibacterial (systemic).

## Indications

**General considerations**
Imipenem is the first of a class of beta-lactam antibiotics called carbapenems. It has a very wide spectrum of activity *in vitro*, including most gram-positive and gram-negative aerobic and anaerobic bacteria. It is also stable in the presence of bacterial beta-lactamases. Imipenem is administered with an equal amount of cilastatin, a renal dehydropeptidase inhibitor that blocks the renal metabolism of imipenem and increases its urinary recovery. Cilastatin has no antibacterial activity or effect on beta-lactamases, and does not potentiate or antagonize the effects of imipenem.
Imipenem has excellent *in vitro* activity against aerobic gram-positive organisms, including most strains of staphylococci, streptococci, and some enterococci. Exceptions to this include *Enterococcus faecium*, which is usually resistant, and an increasing number of strains of methicillin-resistant *Staphylococcus aureus* and coagulase-negative staphylococci.
Imipenem also has excellent *in vitro* activity against most species of Enterbacteriaceae, including *Escherichia coli*, *Klebsiella* species, *Citrobacter* sp., *Morganella morganii*, and *Enterobacter* sp. It is slightly less potent *in vitro* against *Serratia marcescens*, *Proteus mirabilis*, indole-positive *Proteus* sp., and *Providencia stuartii*. Most strains of *Pseudomonas aeruginosa* are susceptible; however, increasing resistance has been seen in patients receiving imipenem who have advanced, refractory infections. Many strains of *Ps. cepacia* and virtually all strains of *Xanthamonas maltophilia* are resistant.
Most anaerobic species are inhibited by imipenem, including *Bacteroides* sp., *Fusobacterium* sp., and *Clostridium* sp. However, *C. difficile* is only moderately susceptible. Other susceptible organisms *in vitro* include *Campylobacter* sp., *Haemophilus influenzae*, *Neisseria gonorrhoeae*, including penicillinase-producing strains, *Yersinia enterocolitica*, *Nocardia asteroides*, and *Legionella* sp. *Chlamydia trachomatis* is resistant to imipenem.

**Accepted**
Bone and joint infections (treatment)—Intravenous imipenem and cilastatin combination is indicated in the treatment of bone and joint infections caused by susceptible organisms.

Endocarditis, bacterial (treatment)—Intravenous imipenem and cilastatin combination is indicated in the treatment of bacterial endocarditis caused by susceptible organisms.

Intra-abdominal infections (treatment)—Intravenous and intramuscular imipenem and cilastatin combination is indicated in the treatment of intra-abdominal infections caused by susceptible organisms.

Pelvic infections, female (treatment)—Intravenous and intramuscular imipenem and cilastatin combination is indicated in the treatment of female pelvic infections caused by susceptible organisms.

Pneumonia, bacterial (treatment)—Intravenous and intramuscular imipenem and cilastatin combination is indicated in the treatment of bacterial pneumonia caused by susceptible organisms.

Septicemia, bacterial (treatment)—Intravenous imipenem and cilastatin combination is indicated in the treatment of bacterial septicemia caused by susceptible organisms.

Skin and soft tissue infections (treatment)—Intravenous and intramuscular imipenem and cilastatin combination is indicated in the treatment of skin and soft tissue infections caused by susceptible organisms.

Urinary tract infections, bacterial (treatment)—Intravenous imipenem and cilastatin combination is indicated in the treatment of bacterial urinary tract infections caused by susceptible organisms.

## Pharmacology/Pharmacokinetics

**Physicochemical characteristics**
Molecular weight—
    Imipenem: 317.36.
    Cilastatin sodium: 380.43.
pKa—pKa at 25 °C (77 °F):
    Imipenem—
        $pKa_1$—3.2
        $pKa_2$—9.9
    Cilastatin sodium (with aqueous sodium hydroxide)—
        $pKa_1$—2.0
        $pKa_2$—4.4
        $pKa_3$—9.2

**Mechanism of action/Effect**
Imipenem—Bactericidal; binds to penicillin-binding proteins (PBP) 1A, 1B, 2, 4, 5, and 6 of *E. coli* and to PBP 1A, 1B, 2, 4, and 5 of *Ps. aeruginosa*; this results in inhibition of bacterial cell wall synthesis; imipenem apparently has greatest affinity for PBP 1A, 1B, and 2, and the least affinity for PBP 3; imipenem's ability to bind to bacterial PBP 2 causes development of small spheres or ellipsoids without formation of filaments commonly seen with penicillins and cephalosporins, ultimately resulting in lysis and death; its lethal effect may also be related to binding to PBP 1A and 1B as well; imipenem is highly resistant to degradation by bacterial beta-lactamases and may demonstrate a "post-antibiotic" effect in some bacteria.
Cilastatin—A competitive, reversible, highly specific inhibitor of the renal dipeptidase, dehydropeptidase I (DHP I); cilastatin blocks tubular secretion of imipenem by competitive exclusion at its transport site, thereby preventing the renal metabolism of imipenem and resulting in significantly improved urinary recovery of imipenem; cilastatin may also prevent proximal renal tubular necrosis that occurs when imipenem is used alone; cilastatin does not inhibit bacterial beta-lactamases and has no intrinsic antibacterial activity.

## Absorption

Bioavailability—

Intramuscular:

Imipenem—95%.

Cilastatin—75%.

## Distribution

Imipenem rapidly and widely distributed to most tissues and fluids; distributed to sputum, pleural fluid, peritoneal fluid, interstitial fluid, bile, aqueous humor, reproductive organs, and bone; highest concentrations found in pleural fluid, interstitial fluid, peritoneal fluid, and reproductive organs; low concentrations have been detected in the cerebrospinal fluid (CSF).

$Vol_D$—

Neonates: 0.4 to 0.5 L/kg.

Children (2 to 12 years old): Approximately 0.7 L/kg.

Adults: 0.23 to 0.31 L/kg.

## Protein binding

Imipenem—Low (20%).

Cilastatin—Moderate (40%).

## Biotransformation

Imipenem—Renal; when given alone, imipenem is metabolized in the kidneys by hydrolysis of the beta-lactam ring caused by the renal dipeptidase, dehydropeptidase I (DHP I), resulting in low urinary concentrations; DHP I is an enzyme located on the brush border of the proximal renal tubular epithelium; DHP I acts only after imipenem has been cleared from the plasma by glomerular filtration or tubular secretion ("post-excretory" metabolism); metabolism occurs only in the tubular cell or glomerular filtrate; virtually all of the secreted fraction and approximately 75% of the filtered fraction are metabolized (a total of 60 to 95%).

Cilastatin—Metabolized to *N*-acetyl conjugate.

## Half-life

Adults—

Intravenous:

Normal renal function—

Imipenem: Approximately 1 hour.

Cilastatin: Approximately 1 hour.

Impaired renal function—

Imipenem: 2.9 to 4.0 hours.

Cilastatin: 13.3 to 17.1 hours.

Intramuscular:

Normal renal function—

Imipenem: 2 to 3 hours.

Neonates—

Intravenous:

Imipenem—1.7 to 2.4 hours.

Cilastatin—3.8 to 8.4 hours.

Children (2 to 12 years of age)—

Intravenous: 1 to 1.2 hours.

## Time to peak concentration

Intramuscular—

Imipenem: Within 2 hours.

Cilastatin: Within 1 hour.

## Peak serum concentration

Imipenem—

Intravenous: Approximately 14 to 24, 21 to 58, and 41 to 83 mcg per mL following a dose of 250 mg, 500 mg, and 1 gram, respectively, over 20 minutes.

Intramuscular: Approximately 10 and 12 mcg per mL following a dose of 500 mg and 750 mg, respectively.

Cilastatin—

Intravenous: Approximately 15 to 25, 31 to 49, and 56 to 80 mcg per mL following a dose of 250 mg, 500 mg, and 1 gram, respectively, over 20 minutes.

Intramuscular: Approximately 24 and 33 mcg per mL following a dose of 500 mg and 750 mg, respectively.

## Urine concentration

Imipenem—

>10 mcg per mL up to 8 hours following a 500 mg intravenous dose.

>10 mcg per mL for 12 hours following a 500 mg and 750 mg intramuscular dose.

## Elimination

Imipenem alone—

Renal; approximately 5 to 40% excreted in urine by both glomerular filtration and tubular secretion.

Cilastatin alone—

Renal; approximately 70 to 78% excreted in urine within 10 hours, by both glomerular filtration and tubular secretion.

Dialysis: Substantial amounts (approximately 40 to 82%) rapidly cleared from the blood by hemodialysis.

Imipenem with cilastatin—

Renal; approximately 70 to 76% excreted in urine within 10 hours, by both glomerular filtration and active tubular secretion (approximately two-thirds of that amount by glomerular filtration and one-third by tubular secretion); no further urinary excretion detectable.

Nonrenal; approximately 20 to 25% excreted by unknown nonrenal mechanism, possibly including up to 1 to 2% excreted via the bile in the feces.

Dialysis: Substantial amounts (approximately 73 to 90%) rapidly cleared from the blood by hemodialysis. A 3-hour session of intermittent hemofiltration has removed approximately 75% of a given dose.

# Precautions to Consider

## Cross-sensitivity and/or related problems

Patients allergic to other beta-lactam antibacterials (e.g., penicillins, cephalosporins) may be allergic to imipenem also.

Although imipenem has been administered without incident to some patients with rash-type penicillin allergy, caution is recommended when imipenem is administered to patients with a history of penicillin anaphylaxis because of cross-reactivity.

## Carcinogenicity/Mutagenicity

Gene toxicity studies such as the V79 mammalian cell mutation assay, Ames test, unscheduled DNA synthesis assay, and *in vivo* mouse cytogenicity test have shown no evidence of genetic damage with imipenem and cilastatin combination.

## Pregnancy/Reproduction

Pregnancy—Studies in humans have not been done.

Studies in mice, rats, and rabbits given doses ranging from the usual human dose up to 33 times the usual human dose have not shown that imipenem, cilastatin, or the combination causes adverse effects on the fetus. Studies in pregnant cynomolgus monkeys given intravenous bolus doses of 40 mg per kg of body weight (mg/kg) per day or 160 mg/kg per day subcutaneously resulted in maternal toxicity, including emesis, inappetence, weight loss, diarrhea, abortion, and death. No significant toxicity was observed when non-pregnant cynomolgus monkeys were given subcutaneous doses of up to 180 mg/kg per day. When doses of 100 mg/kg per day were administered to pregnant cynomolgus monkeys at an intravenous infusion rate which mimics human clinical use, there was minimal maternal intolerance (occasional emesis), no maternal deaths, no teratogenicity, but an increase in embryonic loss relative to the control groups.

FDA Pregnancy Category C.

## Breast-feeding

It is not known whether imipenem or cilastatin is distributed into breast milk. However, problems in humans have not been documented.

## Pediatrics

The half-life of imipenem in neonates is longer (1.7 to 2.4 hours) than that in adults with normal renal function (approximately 1 hour). The half-life in older pediatric patients (2 to 12 years of age) is 1 to 1.2 hours.

The half-life of cilastatin in neonates is longer (3.8 to 8.4 hours) than that in adults with normal renal function (approximately 1 hour).

Appropriate studies have not been performed in children up to 12 years of age.

## Geriatrics

No information is available on the relationship of age to the effects of imipenem and cilastatin combination in geriatric patients. However, elderly patients are more likely to have an age-related decrease in renal function, which may require a reduction of dosage in patients receiving imipenem and cilastatin.

## Dental

Imipenem and cilastatin may cause glossitis (inflammation of the tongue), tongue papillar hypertrophy, and increased salivation.

## Drug interactions and/or related problems

The following drug interactions and/or related problems have been selected on the basis of their potential clinical significance (possible mechanism in parentheses where appropriate)—not necessarily inclusive (» = major clinical significance):

Note: Combinations containing any of the following medications, depending on the amount present, may also interact with this medication.

Probenecid

(since concurrent use of probenecid results in only minimal increases in the serum concentrations and half-life of imipenem, concurrent use is not recommended where higher imipenem serum concentrations may be desirable)

## Laboratory value alterations

The following have been selected on the basis of their potential clinical significance (possible effect in parentheses where appropriate)—not necessarily inclusive (» = major clinical significance):

With diagnostic test results

Positive direct antiglobulin (Coombs') tests
(may occur during therapy)

With physiology/laboratory test values

» Alanine aminotransferase (ALT [SGPT]), serum and
» Alkaline phosphatase, serum and
» Aspartate aminotransferase (AST [SGOT]), serum and
Lactate dehydrogenase (LDH), serum
(values may be transiently increased)

Bilirubin, serum and
Blood urea nitrogen (BUN) concentrations and
Creatinine, serum
(concentrations may be transiently increased)

Hematocrit (HCT) and
Hemoglobin (Hb) concentrations
(may be decreased)

## Medical considerations/Contraindications

The medical considerations/contraindications included here have been selected on the basis of their potential clinical significance (reasons given in parentheses where appropriate)—not necessarily inclusive (» = major clinical significance).

*Risk-benefit should be considered when the following medical problems exist:*

» Allergy to imipenem, cilastatin, or other beta-lactams (penicillin, cephalosporins)

» Central nervous system (CNS) disorders (e.g., brain lesions or history of seizures)
(seizures are more likely to occur in patients receiving higher doses of imipenem, or in patients with CNS lesions, a history of seizure disorders, or renal function impairment)

» Renal function impairment
(because imipenem and cilastatin are primarily excreted through the kidneys, this medicine must be administered in a reduced dosage to patients with impaired renal function)

## Side/Adverse Effects

Note: The following side/adverse effects of imipenem and cilastatin combination are similar in nature and incidence to those of other beta-lactam antibacterials. However, the incidence of seizures is higher than that seen with other beta-lactam antibiotics; it is reported to be 1.5 to 2%. The risk of seizures increases in patients receiving more than 2 grams of imipenem per day, those with a pre-existing seizure disorder, and patients with decreased renal function.

The following side/adverse effects have been selected on the basis of their potential clinical significance (possible signs and symptoms in parentheses where appropriate)—not necessarily inclusive:

## Those indicating need for medical attention

Incidence more frequent
*Allergic reactions* (fever; hives; itching; skin rash; wheezing); *CNS toxicity* (confusion; dizziness; seizures; tremors); *thrombophlebitis* (pain at site of injection)

Incidence less frequent
*Infusion rate reaction* (dizziness; nausea and vomiting; sweating; unusual tiredness or weakness)—occurs with too rapid an infusion rate

Incidence rare
*Pseudomembranous colitis* (abdominal or stomach cramps and pain, severe; diarrhea, watery and severe, which may also be bloody; fever)

## Those indicating need for medical attention only if they continue or are bothersome

Incidence more frequent
*Gastrointestinal disturbances* (diarrhea; nausea and vomiting)

## Those indicating the need for medical attention if they occur after medication is discontinued

*Pseudomembranous colitis* (severe abdominal or stomach cramps and pain; watery and severe diarrhea, which may also be bloody; fever)

## Patient Consultation

As an aid to patient consultation, refer to *Advice for the Patient, Imipenem and Cilastatin (Systemic).*

In providing consultation, consider emphasizing the following selected information (» = major clinical significance):

## Before using this medication

» Conditions affecting use, especially:
Allergy to imipenem or cilastatin; patients allergic to other beta-lactams may also be allergic to imipenem
Dental—Imipenem and cilastatin may cause glossitis, tongue papillar hypertrophy, and increased salivation
Other medical problems, especially CNS disorders or renal function impairment

## Proper use of this medication

» Importance of receiving medication for full course of therapy and on regular schedule
» Proper dosing

## Precautions while using this medication

» Continuing anticonvulsant therapy in patients with a history of seizures
» For severe diarrhea, checking with physician before taking any antidiarrheals; for mild diarrhea, taking kaolin- or attapulgite-containing, but not other, antidiarrheals; checking with physician or pharmacist if mild diarrhea continues or worsens

## Side/adverse effects

Signs of potential side effects, especially allergic reactions, CNS toxicity, infusion rate reaction, pseudomembranous colitis, and thrombophlebitis

# General Dosing Information

Intravenous doses of 250 or 500 mg of imipenem should be given over a 20- to 30-minute period in adults. Doses of 1 gram should be given over a 40- to 60-minute period. In pediatric patients, imipenem may be administered over a 20- to 30-minute period.

Intramuscular imipenem and cilastatin combination should be administered by deep IM injection into a large muscle mass, such as the gluteal muscles or lateral part of the thigh.

In patients receiving more than 2 grams of imipenem per day, there is an increased risk of seizures.

If a dose of this medication is missed, give it as soon as possible. However, if it is almost time for the next dose, skip the missed dose and go back to the regular dosing schedule. Do not double doses.

## For treatment of adverse effects

Anticonvulsants should be continued in the treatment of patients receiving imipenem and cilastatin combination who have known seizure disorders. In patients who develop symptoms of CNS toxicity (e.g., focal tremors, myoclonus, or seizures) during treatment with imipenem, anticonvulsant therapy (e.g., phenytoin or benzodiazepines) should be initiated, and the dosage of imipenem should be reduced or the drug should be discontinued.

If an allergic reaction to imipenem and cilastatin combination occurs, the drug should be discontinued. Severe hypersensitivity reactions may require the administration of epinephrine or other emergency measures.

Some patients may develop nausea, vomiting, hypotension, dizziness, or sweating during administration of imipenem and cilastatin combination, especially after rapid infusion. If these symptoms develop, the rate of infusion should be slowed. If this is not effective, it may be necessary to discontinue the drug.

For antibiotic-associated pseudomembranous colitis (AAPMC)—

Some patients may develop AAPMC, caused by *Clostridium difficile* toxin, during or following administration of imipenem. Mild cases may respond to discontinuation of the drug alone. Moderate to severe cases may require fluid, electrolyte, and protein replacement.

In cases not responding to the above measures or in more severe cases, oral metronidazole, oral bacitracin, or oral vancomycin may be used. Oral vancomycin is effective in doses of 125 to 500 mg every 6 hours for 5 to 10 days. The dose of metronidazole is 250 to 500 mg every 8 hours for 5 to 10 days. Recurrences may be treated with a second course of these medications.

Cholestyramine and colestipol resins have been shown to bind *C. difficile* toxin *in vitro.* If cholestyramine or colestipol resin is administered in conjunction with oral vancomycin, the medications should be administered several hours apart since the resins have been shown to bind oral vancomycin also.

In addition, AAPMC may result in severe watery diarrhea which may occur during therapy or up to several weeks after therapy is discontinued. If diarrhea occurs, administration of antiperistaltic antidiarrheals is not recommended since they may delay the removal of toxins from the colon, thereby prolonging and/or worsening the diarrhea.

# Parenteral Dosage Forms

## IMIPENEM AND CILASTATIN FOR INJECTION USP

### Usual adult and adolescent dose
Antibacterial—
Intravenous infusion, based on anhydrous imipenem content:
Mild infections—250 to 500 mg every six hours.
Moderate infections—500 mg every six to eight hours to 1 gram every eight hours.
Severe, life-threatening infections—500 mg every six hours to 1 gram every six to eight hours.
Note: Lower doses are used in the treatment of infections caused by gram-positive organisms, anaerobes, and highly susceptible gram-negative organisms. Infections caused by other gram-negative organisms require higher doses.

Uncomplicated urinary tract infections: 250 mg every six hours.

Complicated urinary tract infections: 500 mg every six hours.

Adults with impaired renal function may require a reduction in dose as given below. Doses are based on an average body weight of 70 kg. Patients weighing less than 70 kg should receive a proportional reduction in dosage.

| Creatinine Clearance (mL/min/1.73 M²)/ (mL/sec) | Dose |
|---|---|
| >70/1.17 | See *Usual adult and adolescent dose* |
| 30–70/0.50–1.17 | 500 mg every 6 to 8 hours |
| 20–30/0.33–0.50 | 500 mg every 8 to 12 hours |
| 0–20/0–0.33 | 250 to 500 mg every 12 hours |
| Hemodialysis patients | Supplemental dose after hemodialysis, unless next dose scheduled within 4 hours |

### Usual adult prescribing limits
Up to a maximum of 50 mg (imipenem) per kg of body weight or 4 grams daily, whichever is lower.

### Usual pediatric dose
Antibacterial—
Infants and children up to 12 years of age: Dosage has not been established.
Children 12 years of age and older: See *Usual adult and adolescent dose.*

### Size(s) usually available
U.S.—
250 mg (anhydrous imipenem) and 250 mg (cilastatin) (Rx) [*Primaxin IV*].
500 mg (anhydrous imipenem) and 500 mg (cilastatin) (Rx) [*Primaxin IV*].
Canada—
250 mg (anhydrous imipenem) and 250 mg (cilastatin) (Rx) [*Primaxin*].
500 mg (anhydrous imipenem) and 500 mg (cilastatin) (Rx) [*Primaxin*].

### Packaging and storage
Prior to reconstitution, store below 30 °C (86 °F), unless otherwise specified by manufacturer.

### Preparation of dosage form
To prepare initial dilution for intravenous infusion, add approximately 10 mL of diluent (see manufacturer's package insert) to each 250- or 500-mg vial (13-mL) and shake well. The resulting suspension should be transferred to not less than 100 mL of suitable intravenous fluids. Do not administer the initially prepared suspension intravenously. Add an additional 10 mL of diluent to each previously reconstituted vial and shake well. Transfer the remaining contents of the vial to the infusion container. Shake the resulting mixture well until clear. Do not administer a cloudy solution.
For reconstitution of piggyback infusion bottles (120-mL), add 100 mL of diluent (see manufacturer's package insert) to each 250- or 500-mg infusion bottle. Shake the resulting mixture well until clear. Do not administer a cloudy solution.

### Stability
After reconstitution with sterile water for injection, solutions retain their potency for 8 hours at room temperature or for 48 hours if refrigerated at 4 °C (39 °F).

After reconstitution with 0.9% sodium chloride injection, solutions retain their potency for 10 hours at room temperature or for 48 hours if refrigerated at 4 °C (39 °F).
After reconstitution with other diluents, solutions retain their potency for 4 hours at room temperature or for 24 hours if refrigerated at 4 °C (39 °F).
Solutions of imipenem and cilastatin combination should not be frozen.
Solutions may vary from colorless to yellow in color; color changes within this range do not affect potency. Imipenem and cilastatin combination may become slightly discolored under strong ultraviolet (UV) light.

### Incompatibilities
Extemporaneous admixtures of beta-lactam antibacterials and aminoglycosides may result in substantial mutual inactivation. If they are administered concurrently, they should be administered in separate sites. Do not mix them in the same intravenous bag or bottle.

## IMIPENEM AND CILASTATIN FOR INJECTABLE SUSPENSION USP

### Usual adult and adolescent dose
Antibacterial—
Intramuscular, mild to moderate infections:
Female pelvic infections and
Pneumonia and
Skin and soft tissue infections—500 to 750 mg every twelve hours.
Intra-abdominal infections—750 mg every twelve hours.
Note: Safety and efficacy have not been studied in patients with a creatinine clearance of less than 20 mL/min.

### Usual adult prescribing limits
Up to 1500 mg daily.

### Usual pediatric dose
Antibacterial—
Infants and children up to 12 years of age: Dosage has not been established.
Children 12 years of age and older: See *Usual adult and adolescent dose.*

### Size(s) usually available
U.S.—
500 mg (anhydrous imipenem) and 500 mg (cilastatin) (Rx) [*Primaxin IM*].
750 mg (anhydrous imipenem) and 750 mg (cilastatin) (Rx) [*Primaxin IM*].
Canada—
Not commercially available.

### Packaging and storage
Prior to reconstitution, store below 30 °C (86 °F), unless otherwise specified by manufacturer.

### Preparation of dosage form
To prepare initial dilution for intramuscular use, add 2 mL of 1% lidocaine injection (without epinephrine) to each 500-mg vial, or 3 mL of 1% lidocaine injection (without epinephrine) to each 750-mg vial.

### Stability
After reconstitution with 1% lidocaine injection, the suspension should be used within one hour.
Suspensions are white to light tan in color; variations of color within this range do not affect the potency.

### Incompatibilities
Intramuscular imipenem and cilastatin combination should not be mixed with or physically added to other antibiotics. However, it may be administered concomitantly, but at separate sites, with other antibiotics.

Revised: 09/08/92
Interim revision: 04/01/94; 01/11/95; 06/20/95

# IMIPENEM-CONTAINING COMBINATIONS—
Imipenem and Cilastatin (Systemic)

# IMIPRAMINE—See *Antidepressants, Tricyclic (Systemic)*

# IMMUNE GLOBULIN INTRAVENOUS (HUMAN)  Systemic

VA CLASSIFICATION (Primary/Secondary): IM500/AM900; BL900; CV900; XX000

Other commonly used names are IGIV and IVIG.

Note: For a listing of dosage forms and brand names by country availability, see *Dosage Forms* section(s). For a listing of brand names for the articles in this monograph, refer to the General Index.

## Category

Immunizing agent (passive); platelet count stimulator (systemic); anti-Kawasaki disease (systemic); antibacterial (systemic); antiviral (systemic); antipolyneuropathy agent.

## Indications

Note: Bracketed information in the *Indications* section refers to uses that are not included in U.S. product labeling.

### Accepted

Immunodeficiency, primary (treatment)—Immune globulin intravenous (IGIV) is indicated for the treatment of patients with primary immunodeficiency syndromes, such as congenital agammaglobulinemia (x-linked agammaglobulinemia), hypogammaglobulinemia, common variable immunodeficiency, x-linked immunodeficiency with hyperimmunoglobulin M (IgM), severe combined immunodeficiency, and Wiskott-Aldrich syndrome, to replace or boost immunoglobulin G (IgG).

Although IGIV may be of benefit in severe combined immunodeficiency, the cellular immunodeficit in this disease will not be corrected.

IGIV may be the preferred form of immune globulin for treatment of patients who have bleeding disorders for which an intramuscular injection of immune globulin is not recommended, patients who need an immediate increase in intravascular immunoglobulin concentrations, or patients who have limited muscle mass.

Thrombocytopenic purpura, idiopathic (treatment)—IGIV is indicated for the treatment of idiopathic thrombocytopenic purpura (ITP) when a rapid rise in the platelet count is required, such as prior to surgery, to control excessive bleeding, or to defer or avoid splenectomy. Not all patients will respond however, and, if the rise does occur, it may be transient. This treatment should not be considered curative, although remissions have occurred.

[Kawasaki disease (treatment adjunct)][1]—IGIV along with aspirin is considered to be a standard treatment for Kawasaki disease to prevent the development of coronary artery abnormalities, such as dilation, aneurysm, or ectasia, which in turn could lead to myocardial infarction.

Leukemia, chronic lymphocytic (treatment adjunct)[1]—IGIV is indicated for the prevention of recurrent bacterial infections in patients with hypogammaglobulinemia associated with B-cell chronic lymphocytic leukemia (CLL).

[Immunodepression, iatrogenically induced or disease-associated (treatment or treatment adjunct)][1]—IGIV is used, either alone or in conjunction with appropriate anti-infective therapy, to prevent or modify acute bacterial or viral infections (e.g., cytomegalovirus infections) in patients with iatrogenically induced or disease-associated immunodepression who are undergoing major surgery, such as bone marrow or cardiac transplants, or who have hematologic malignancies, extensive burns, or collagen-vascular diseases.

[Immunodeficiency syndrome, acquired, (AIDS) (treatment)][1] or [Immunodeficiency syndrome–related complex, acquired, (ARC) (treatment)][1]—IGIV is used to control or prevent infections and improve immunologic conditions in infants and children who are immunosuppressed in association with AIDS or ARC.

[Neonates, high-risk, preterm, low-birthweight, infections in (prophylaxis and treatment adjunct)][1]—IGIV is used for the prophylaxis of, and as a treatment adjunct in, infections in some high-risk, preterm, low-birthweight neonates. Controlled studies to assess its efficacy in the prevention of infection are ongoing. Until these studies are completed, IGIV is not recommended as a standard prophylactic agent in low-birthweight infants. In addition, since trials have yielded mixed results, IGIV is not recommended for routine use as adjunctive therapy in neonatal infections.

[Polyneuropathies, chronic inflammatory demyelinating (treatment)][1]—IGIV is used in the treatment of chronic inflammatory demyelinating polyneuropathies. IGIV is used either alone or following therapeutic plasma exchange to prolong its effect. IGIV is considered easier to use than repeated therapeutic plasma exchange and to have fewer complications than long-term glucocorticoid therapy.

---

[1]Not included in Canadian product labeling.

## Pharmacology/Pharmacokinetics

### Physicochemical characteristics

Other characteristics—
The pH of the reconstituted solution of the lyophilized product is approximately 6.8
The pH of the sterile solution is 4.0 to 4.5

### Mechanism of action/Effect

Immune globulin intravenous (IGIV) is a sterile, highly purified preparation of intact, unmodified immunoglobulin (IgG). The immunoglobulin is isolated from large pools of human plasma. All IgG antibody activities present in the donor population are conserved. The distribution of IgG subclasses corresponds to that in normal human plasma.

Immunodeficiency—
IGIV is used to provide passive immunity against infection by increasing a person's antibody titer and antigen-antibody reaction potential.

IGIV supplies a broad spectrum of IgG antibodies against bacterial, viral, parasitic, and mycoplasmal antigens. These antibodies have retained full biological function for the prevention or attenuation of a wide variety of infectious diseases, including the abilities to promote opsonization, fix complement, and neutralize microbes and their toxins.

Idiopathic thrombocytopenic purpura (ITP)—
IGIV is used to induce a rapid increase in platelet counts in patients with ITP. The mechanism by which this occurs is not fully understood. In addition, it is not possible to predict which patients with ITP will respond to this therapy, although the increase in platelet counts seems to be greater in children than in adults.

Kawasaki disease—
IGIV has been shown to have a striking anti-inflammatory effect in Kawasaki disease. Reductions in fever, neutrophil counts, and acute phase reactants usually occur within a day or so of initiation of IGIV treatment. The mechanism by which this occurs is not known.

### Distribution

100% in the serum immediately following intravenous administration. During the first week, the distribution equilibrates to approximately 60% in the serum and approximately 40% in the extravascular space.

### Time to peak concentration

Essentially 100% of a dose of IGIV is immediately available in the patient's circulation. A relatively rapid fall in serum IgG level that occurs in the first week following IGIV administration is to be expected.

### Time to peak effect

Immediately following intravenous administration.

### Duration of action

ITP—The rise in platelets most often lasts from several days to several weeks. Rarely, the rise in platelets may last up to 1 year or longer.

## Precautions to Consider

### Cross-sensitivity and/or related problems

Patients allergic to other immune globulins, either intramuscular or intravenous, may be allergic to immune globulin intravenous (IGIV) also.

### Pregnancy/Reproduction

Fertility—It is not known whether IGIV affects fertility.

Pregnancy—IGIV crosses the placenta. IGIV should be administered to pregnant women only if clearly needed.

Past experience with immune globulin intramuscular has shown no adverse effect on the fetus; however, it is not known whether IGIV can cause harm to the fetus. Although studies specific for pregnancy have not been done in humans, other studies on the use of IGIV during pregnancy for treatment of disease have not shown IGIV to cause harm to the fetus.

Studies have not been done in animals.

FDA Pregnancy Category C.

### Breast-feeding

It is not known whether IGIV is distributed into breast milk. However, problems in humans have not been documented.

### Pediatrics

Appropriate studies on the relationship of age to the effects of IGIV have not been performed in the pediatric population. However, administration of high doses of IGIV to children with idiopathic thrombocytopenic purpura did not cause any pediatrics-specific problems.

### Geriatrics

Appropriate studies on the relationship of age to the effects of IGIV have not been performed in the geriatric population. However, no geriatrics-specific problems have been documented to date.

### Drug interactions and/or related problems

The following drug interactions and/or related problems have been selected on the basis of their potential clinical significance (possible mechanism in parentheses where appropriate)—not necessarily inclusive (» = major clinical significance):

Live virus vaccines
(antibodies contained in IGIV may interfere with the body's immune response to certain live virus vaccines; live virus vaccines, such as measles, mumps, and rubella, should be administered at least 14 days prior to, or at least 3 months after, administration of IGIV; however, there appears to be no interference between IGIV and oral polio vaccine [OPV], yellow fever vaccine, or diphtheria and tetanus toxoids and pertussis vaccine adsorbed [DTP])

### Medical considerations/Contraindications

The medical considerations/contraindications included here have been selected on the basis of their potential clinical significance (reasons given in parentheses where appropriate)—not necessarily inclusive (» = major clinical significance).

*Except under special circumstances, this medication should not be used when the following medical problems exist:*

» Allergic reaction to IGIV

» Immunoglobulin A (IgA) deficiencies, selective, in patients who have known antibody to IgA
(small amounts of IgA may be present in IGIV and may cause a severe allergic reaction in patients with antibody to IgA; IgA-sensitive patients may be more tolerant of *Gammagard* or *Polygam* brands of IGIV, since they are very low in IgA [not more than 10 mcg per mL])

*Risk-benefit should be considered when the following medical problems exist:*

Acid-base compensatory mechanisms, limited or compromised
(because of its pH [4.0 to 4.5], the effect of the additional acid load of *Gamimune N* brand of IGIV should be considered when it is administered to patients with limited or compromised acid-base compensatory mechanisms)

Agammaglobulinemia or
Hypogammaglobulinemia, extreme
(patients who have never received immune globulin substitution therapy or who were last treated more than 8 weeks ago may be at risk, if administered IGIV by rapid infusion, of developing inflammatory reactions, which may lead to shock)

» Cardiac function impairment in seriously ill patients
(these patients may be at increased risk of vasomotor or cardiac complications, such as elevated blood pressure and cardiac failure)

Sensitivity to maltose or sucrose
(these ingredients may be present in some IGIV products)

### Patient monitoring

The following may be especially important in patient monitoring (other tests may be warranted in some patients, depending on condition; » = major clinical significance):

Vital signs
(patients with agammaglobulinemia or severe hypogammaglobulinemia who have never received immune globulin substitution therapy or who were last treated more than 8 weeks ago may be at risk, if administered IGIV by rapid infusion, of developing inflammatory reactions, which may lead to shock; the patient's vital signs should be monitored continuously and the patient should be carefully observed throughout the infusion)

## Side/Adverse Effects

Note: Occasionally, immune globulin intravenous (IGIV) has caused a precipitous fall in blood pressure and signs of anaphylaxis. These reactions generally become evident within 30 to 60 minutes after the initiation of the infusion, and include fever, chills, nausea and vomiting, flushing, chest tightness, dizziness, sweating, and hypotension. Patients with agammaglobulinemia or extreme hypogammaglobulinemia who have never received immune globulin substitution therapy or who were last treated more than 8 weeks ago may be at increased risk of developing these reactions.

It appears that most side effects of IGIV are related to the rate of infusion, and may be relieved by decreasing the rate or temporarily stopping the infusion.

Backache, chills, flushing, headache, hypotension, myalgia, nausea, or pyrexia usually begins within 1 hour of the start of the infusion with IGIV. Symptoms usually subside within 30 minutes. Headache also may occur 3 to 24 hours after administration of IGIV.

IGIV appears to be safe with respect to the transmission of hepatitis B virus. Potential blood donors are screened, and studies have shown no evidence of the transmission of hepatitis B virus to patients who receive IGIV.

IGIV appears to be safe with respect to the transmission of the human immunodeficiency virus (HIV). Potential blood donors are screened for HIV. In addition, even when the donor plasma is deliberately spiked with HIV, tests of the final IGIV product do not show HIV in large enough quantities to be infective.

The following side/adverse effects have been selected on the basis of their potential clinical significance (possible signs and symptoms in parentheses where appropriate)—not necessarily inclusive:

**Those indicating need for medical attention**
Incidence more frequent
*Dyspnea* (troubled breathing); *tachycardia* (fast or pounding heartbeat)
Incidence less frequent
*Burning sensation in head; cyanosis* (bluish coloring of lips or nailbeds); *faintness or lightheadedness; fatigue* (unusual tiredness or weakness); *wheezing*

**Those indicating need for medical attention only if they continue or are bothersome**
Incidence more frequent
*Back ache or pain; headache; joint pain; malaise* (general feeling of discomfort or illness); *myalgia* (muscle pain)
Incidence less frequent
*Chest, back, or hip pain; erythema* (redness); *rash; or pain at injection site; leg cramps; urticaria* (hives)

## Overdose

For more information on the management of overdose or unintentional ingestion, **contact a Poison Control Center** (see *Poison Control Center Listing*).

### Clinical effects of overdose

Symptoms of overdose apparently may be caused by too-rapid infusion. The following effects have been selected on the basis of their potential clinical significance (possible signs and symptoms in parentheses where appropriate)—not necessarily inclusive:

Acute
*Chest tightness; chills; diaphoresis* (sweating); *dizziness; flushing* (redness of face); *hypotension* (unusual tiredness or weakness)—may become severe; *nausea; pyrexia* (fever); *vomiting*

## Patient Consultation

As an aid to patient consultation, refer to *Advice for the Patient, Immune Globulin Intravenous (Human) (Systemic)*.

In providing consultation, consider emphasizing the following selected information (» = major clinical significance):

### Before using this medication

» Conditions affecting use, especially:
Sensitivity to intramuscular or intravenous immune globulins
Other medical problems, especially allergic reaction to IGIV, selective IgA deficiencies, or cardiac function impairment in seriously ill patients

### Proper use of this medication

» Proper dosing

### Side/adverse effects

Signs of potential side effects, especially dyspnea, tachycardia, burning sensation in head, cyanosis, faintness or lightheadedness, fatigue, and wheezing

## General Dosing Information

Since there is individual patient variation in the half-life of immune globulin intravenous (IGIV), the frequency of administration of IGIV should be based on both the patient's immune globulin half-life and the dose of IGIV administered.

It is suggested that a patient's trough serum IgG concentration 4 weeks after a treatment be maintained at 400 to 500 mg per deciliter, which is a value close to the lower limit of the normal range. Although IGIV is usually administered every 4 weeks, the interval should be adjusted depending on the trough serum IgG concentration and the patient's clinical condition.

IGIV is recommended for intravenous administration only. The intramuscular and subcutaneous routes have not been evaluated for this medication and are not recommended.

The infusion of IGIV should be at approximately room temperature for administration.

Diluents are product-specific. Only the specific diluent indicated by each manufacturer should be used for its particular product.

### For treatment of adverse effects
Recommended treatment includes:
- For mild hypersensitivity reaction—Administering antihistamines and, if necessary, glucocorticoids.
- For severe hypersensitivity or anaphylactic reaction—Administering epinephrine. Antihistamines and/or glucocorticoids may also be administered as required.

## Parenteral Dosage Forms

Note: Bracketed uses in the *Dosage Forms* section refer to categories of use and/or indications that are not included in U.S. product labeling.

### IMMUNE GLOBULIN INTRAVENOUS (HUMAN) INJECTION

#### Usual adult and adolescent dose
Immunodeficiency—
Intravenous, 100 to 200 mg (2 to 4 mL) per kg of body weight once a month. If the patient's response is felt to be inadequate, the frequency of dosing may be increased to two times a month, or the dose may be increased to 400 mg (8 mL) per kg of body weight once a month.
Note: For immunodeficiency, the National Institutes of Health (NIH) 1990 consensus panel for IGIV states that dose ranges of 200 to 800 mg per kg of body weight per month have been effective.
Idiopathic thrombocytopenic purpura (ITP)—
Intravenous, 400 mg per kg of body weight per day for five consecutive days. If the patient's response to this five-day treatment period is inadequate, an additional 400 mg per kg of body weight may be administered as a single maintenance dose, repeated intermittently as needed.
Note: For ITP, the NIH 1990 consensus panel for IGIV states that doses of either 400 mg per kg of body weight per day for two to five days or 1 gram per kg of body weight per day for one or two days have been effective. Administration every ten to twenty-one days is usually required to maintain adequate platelet counts.
[Kawasaki disease][1]—
Intravenous, 400 mg per kg of body weight a day for four days; alternatively, a single dose of 2 grams per kg of body weight may be administered.
Note: For *Gamimune N,* the rate of infusion of the undiluted medication should be 0.01 to 0.02 mL per kg of body weight per minute for thirty minutes. If the patient does not experience any discomfort, the rate may be gradually increased up to a maximum of 0.08 mL per kg of body weight per minute.

#### Usual pediatric dose
See *Usual adult and adolescent dose.*

#### Size(s) usually available
U.S.—
500 mg protein in 10 mL solution (Rx) [*Gamimune N* (maltose 9 to 11%)].
2.5 grams protein in 50 mL solution (Rx) [*Gamimune N* (maltose 9 to 11%)].
5 grams protein in 100 mL solution (Rx) [*Gamimune N* (maltose 9 to 11%)].

12.5 grams protein in 250 mL solution (Rx) [*Gamimune N* (maltose 9 to 11%)].
Canada—
500 mg protein in 10 mL solution (Rx) [*Gamimune N* (maltose 9 to 11%)].
2.5 grams protein in 50 mL solution (Rx) [*Gamimune N* (maltose 9 to 11%)].
5 grams protein in 100 mL solution (Rx) [*Gamimune N* (maltose 9 to 11%)].
10 grams protein in 200 mL solution (Rx) [*Gamimune N* (maltose 9 to 11%)].
12.5 grams protein in 250 mL solution (Rx) [*Gamimune N* (maltose 9 to 11%)].
25 grams protein in 500 mL solution (Rx) [*Gamimune N* (maltose 9 to 11%)].
Note: Each mL contains approximately 50 mg of protein of which not less than 98% is gamma globulin (IgG). Not less than 90% of the IgG is monomer. Also present are traces of immune globulin A (IgA) and immune globulin M (IgM).

#### Packaging and storage
Store at 2 to 8 °C (35 to 45 °F), unless otherwise specified by manufacturer. Protect from freezing.
The Canadian product may be stored also at temperatures not exceeding 25 °C (77 °F) for 30 days, after which it must be discarded.

#### Preparation of dosage form
The medication may be diluted only with 5% dextrose in water.

#### Stability
A solution that has been frozen should be discarded.
The contents of any vial that has been entered should be used promptly. The solution should not be used if it is not clear and colorless. Partially used vials should be discarded.

#### Incompatibilities
Incompatibilities have not been evaluated. It is recommended that IGIV be administered through a separate line, by itself, and without mixing with other intravenous fluids (with the exception of 5% dextrose in water for this particular product) or medications.

### IMMUNE GLOBULIN INTRAVENOUS (HUMAN) FOR INJECTION

#### Usual adult and adolescent dose
Immunodeficiency—
*Gammagard* or *Polygam:* Intravenous, initially, 200 to 400 mg per kg of body weight once a month. Thereafter, monthly doses of at least 100 mg per kg of body weight may be adequate.
*Gammar-IV:* Intravenous, 100 to 200 mg per kg of body weight every three to four weeks. Initially, a loading dose of at least 200 mg per kg of body weight at more frequent intervals than every three weeks may be used.
*Iveegam:* Intravenous, 200 mg per kg of body weight once a month. If the patient's response is inadequate, the frequency of dosing may be increased, or the dose may be increased up to 800 mg per kg of body weight once a month.
*Sandoglobulin:* Intravenous, 200 mg per kg of body weight once a month. If the patient's response is inadequate, the frequency of dosing may be increased, or the dose may be increased to 300 mg per kg of body weight once a month.
*Venoglobulin-I:* Intravenous, 200 mg per kg of body weight once a month. If the patient's response is inadequate, the frequency of dosing may be increased, or the dose may be increased to 300 to 400 mg per kg of body weight once a month.
Note: For immunodeficiency, the NIH 1990 consensus panel for IGIV states that dose ranges of 200 to 800 mg per kg of body weight per month have been effective.
Idiopathic thrombocytopenic purpura (ITP)—
*Gammagard* or *Polygam:* Intravenous, 1 gram per kg of body weight as a single dose. If the patient's response is inadequate, 1 gram per kg of body weight may be administered on alternate days for up to three doses.
*Sandoglobulin:* Intravenous, 400 mg per kg of body weight per day for two to five consecutive days. If the patient's response is inadequate, 400 mg per kg of body weight may be administered as a single maintenance dose once every several weeks. In some patients, it may be necessary to increase the maintenance dose up to 800 mg or 1 gram per kg of body weight.
*Venoglobulin-I:* Intravenous, initially, up to 2 grams per kg of body weight per day for two to seven consecutive days. If the patient's response is inadequate, up to 2 grams per kg of body weight may be administered as a single maintenance dose every two weeks or more frequently as needed.

Note: For ITP, the NIH 1990 consensus panel for IGIV states that doses of either 400 mg per kg of body weight per day for two to five days or 1 gram per kg of body weight per day for one or two days have been effective. Administration every ten to twenty-one days is usually required to maintain adequate platelet counts.

Bacterial infections secondary to B-cell chronic lymphocytic leukemia (CLL)[1]—

*Gammagard* or *Polygam:* Intravenous, 400 mg per kg of body weight once every three to four weeks.

[Kawasaki disease][1]—

Intravenous, 400 mg per kg of body weight a day for four days; alternatively, a single dose of 2 grams per kg of body weight may be administered.

Note: *Gammagard* or *Polygam*—Initially, the 50-mg-per-mL solution should be administered at a rate of approximately 0.008 mL per kg of body weight per minute (0.5 mL per kg of body weight per hour). If the patient does not experience any discomfort, the rate may be gradually increased up to a maximum of approximately 0.066 mL per kg of body weight per minute (4 mL per kg of body weight per hour).

*Gammar-IV*—Initially, the 50-mg-per-mL solution should be administered at a rate of 0.01 mL per kg of body weight per minute (0.6 mL per kg of body weight per hour) for fifteen to thirty minutes. The rate may then be increased to 0.02 mL per kg of body weight per minute (1.2 mL per kg of body weight per hour). If the patient does not experience any discomfort, the rate may be gradually increased to 0.03 to 0.06 mL per kg of body weight per minute (1.8 to 3.6 mL per kg of body weight per hour).

*Iveegam*—The usual rate of administration for the 5% solution is 1 mL per minute up to a maximum of 2 mL per minute. In order to prevent adverse reactions, some previously untreated patients with severe immunodeficiency have had treatment initiated with lower doses that have been diluted with saline or 5% dextrose. The dosage was then gradually increased.

*Sandoglobulin*—Previously untreated patients with agammaglobulinemia or hypogammaglobulinemia should have their first infusion administered as a 3% solution. Initially the flow rate should be 10 to 20 drops (0.5 to 1 mL) per minute. After 15 to 30 minutes, the rate of infusion may be increased to 30 to 50 drops (1.5 to 2.5 mL) per minute. After the initial bottle of 3% solution is infused, and if the patient shows good tolerance, subsequent infusions may be administered at a higher concentration. Such increases should be made gradually, allowing fifteen to thirty minutes before each increment.

*Venoglobulin-I*—Initially, the 50-mg-per-mL solution should be administered at a rate of 0.01 to 0.02 mL per kg of body weight per minute (0.6 to 1.2 mL per kg of body weight per hour) for thirty minutes. If the patient does not experience any discomfort, the rate may be gradually increased to 0.04 mL per kg of body weight per minute (2.4 mL per kg of body weight per hour). If the patient tolerates the higher infusion rate, subsequent infusions may be administered at this higher rate.

**Usual pediatric dose**
See *Usual adult and adolescent dose.*

**Size(s) usually available**
U.S.—
  0.5 gram with 10 mL sterile water for injection as diluent (Rx) [*Gammagard* (sodium chloride 0.15 M; glucose 20 mg per mL; polyethylene glycol 2 mg per mL; glycine 0.3 M; human albumin 3 mg per mL); *Iveegam* (glucose 50 mg per mL; sodium chloride 3 mg per mL; polyethylene glycol < 0.5 gram per dL); *Polygam* (sodium chloride 0.15 M; glucose 20 mg per mL; polyethylene glycol 2 mg per mL; glycine 0.3 M; human albumin 3 mg per mL); *Venoglobulin-I* (D-mannitol 20 mg per mL; human albumin 10 mg per mL; sodium chloride 5 mg per mL; polyethylene glycol ≤ 6 mg per mL)].

  1 gram with 20 mL sterile water for injection as diluent (Rx) [*Gammar-IV* (human albumin 3%; sucrose 5%; sodium chloride 0.5%; citric acid; sodium carbonate); *Iveegam* (glucose 50 mg per mL; sodium chloride 3 mg per mL; polyethylene glycol < 0.5 gram per dL)].

  1 gram with 33 mL sodium chloride injection as diluent (Rx) [*Sandoglobulin*].

  2.5 grams with 50 mL sterile water for injection as diluent (Rx) [*Gammagard* (sodium chloride 0.15 M; glucose 20 mg per mL; polyethylene glycol 2 mg per mL; glycine 0.3 M; human albumin 3 mg per mL); *Gammar-IV* (human albumin 3%; sucrose 5%; sodium chloride 0.5%; citric acid; sodium carbonate); *Iveegam* (glucose 50 mg per mL; sodium chloride 3 mg per mL; polyethylene glycol < 0.5 gram per dL); *Polygam* (sodium chloride 0.15 M;

glucose 20 mg per mL; polyethylene glycol 2 mg per mL; glycine 0.3 M; human albumin 3 mg per mL)].

2.5 grams with or without 50 mL sterile water for injection as diluent (Rx) [*Venoglobulin-I* (D-mannitol 20 mg per mL; human albumin 10 mg per mL; sodium chloride 5 mg per mL; polyethylene glycol ≤ 6 mg per mL)].

3 grams with or without 100 mL sodium chloride injection as diluent (Rx) [*Sandoglobulin*].

5 grams with 100 mL sterile water for injection as diluent (Rx) [*Gammagard* (sodium chloride 0.15 M; glucose 20 mg per mL; polyethylene glycol 2 mg per mL; glycine 0.3 M; human albumin 3 mg per mL); *Gammar-IV* (human albumin 3%; sucrose 5%; sodium chloride 0.5%; citric acid; sodium carbonate); *Iveegam* (glucose 50 mg per mL; sodium chloride 3 mg per mL; polyethylene glycol < 0.5 gram per dL); *Polygam* (sodium chloride 0.15 M; glucose 20 mg per mL; polyethylene glycol 2 mg per mL; glycine 0.3 M; human albumin 3 mg per mL)].

5 grams with or without 100 mL sterile water for injection as diluent (Rx) [*Venoglobulin-I* (D-mannitol 20 mg per mL; human albumin 10 mg per mL; sodium chloride 5 mg per mL; polyethylene glycol ≤ 6 mg per mL)].

6 grams with or without 200 mL sodium chloride injection as diluent (Rx) [*Sandoglobulin*].

10 grams with 200 mL sterile water for injection as diluent (Rx) [*Gammagard* (sodium chloride 0.15 M; glucose 20 mg per mL; polyethylene glycol 2 mg per mL; glycine 0.3 M; human albumin 3 mg per mL); *Polygam* (sodium chloride 0.15 M; glucose 20 mg per mL; polyethylene glycol 2 mg per mL; glycine 0.3 M; human albumin 3 mg per mL)].

Note: When reconstituted according to directions, *Gammagard, Gammar-IV, Polygam,* and *Venoglobulin-I* contain approximately 50 mg of protein per mL, of which at least 90% is gamma globulin (IgG); *Iveegam* contains a 5% protein solution, which yields 50 mg ± 5 mg per mL of IgG; and *Sandoglobulin* contains either approximately 30 mg or 60 mg of protein per mL, of which at least 96% is IgG.

Also present are traces of IgA and IgM.

*Sandoglobulin* can be reconstituted with sterile water, 5% dextrose, or 0.9% saline to make solutions with protein concentrations of 3 to 12%.

Canada—
  0.5 gram with 10 mL sterile water for injection as diluent (Rx) [*Iveegam* (glucose 50 mg ± 5 mg per mL; sodium chloride 3 mg ± 1 mg per mL)].

  1 gram with 20 mL sterile water for injection as diluent (Rx) [*Iveegam* (glucose 50 mg ± 5 mg per mL; sodium chloride 3 mg ± 1 mg per mL)].

  2.5 grams with 50 mL sterile water for injection as diluent (Rx) [*Iveegam* (glucose 50 mg ± 5 mg per mL; sodium chloride 3 mg ± 1 mg per mL)].

  5 grams with 100 mL sterile water for injection as diluent (Rx) [*Iveegam* (glucose 50 mg ± 5 mg per mL; sodium chloride 3 mg ± 1 mg per mL)].

  7.5 grams with 150 mL sterile water for injection as diluent (Rx) [*Iveegam* (glucose 50 mg ± 5 mg per mL; sodium chloride 3 mg ± 1 mg per mL)].

  10 grams with 200 mL sterile water for injection as diluent (Rx) [*Iveegam* (glucose 50 mg ± 5 mg per mL; sodium chloride 3 mg ± 1 mg per mL)].

Note: When reconstituted according to directions, *Iveegam* contains 55 mg ± 5 mg of protein per mL, of which 50 mg ± 5 mg per mL is gamma globulin (IgG).

May also contain traces of IgA and IgM.

**Packaging and storage**
Store at temperatures not exceeding 25 °C (77 °F), unless otherwise specified by manufacturer. Protect the diluent from freezing.

**Preparation of dosage form**
The diluent and lyophilized product should be brought to room temperature prior to reconstitution. When the diluent is added, dissolution usually occurs within a few minutes, although in rare cases, or when the product and/or diluent are cold, dissolution may take up to 20 minutes. The reconstituted solution should not be shaken, since excessive shaking will cause foaming. Reconstituted solution should be at approximately room temperature at the time of administration.

**Stability**
Only the specific diluent that the product's manufacturer indicates for that particular product should be used. The solution should not be used if it is not clear and colorless to slightly straw colored, or if there is particulate matter present. Administration should begin promptly after

reconstitution, or within 2 or 3 hours, according to the individual manufacturer's instructions. Partially used vials should be discarded.

### Incompatibilities

Incompatibilities have not been evaluated. It is recommended that IGIV be administered through a separate line, by itself, and without mixing with other intravenous fluids (with the exception of the product's specified diluent) or medications. However, for *Iveegam*-Canada, if lower immune globulin concentrations are desired, the reconstituted 5% solution can be diluted using isotonic saline, isotonic glucose, or isotonic levulose solutions.

---

[1]Not included in Canadian product labeling.

### Selected Bibliography

Buckley RH, Schiff RI. The use of intravenous immune globulin in immunodeficiency diseases. N Engl J Med 1991 July 11; 325 (2): 110-17.

Intravenous immunoglobulin: prevention and treatment of disease. NIH Consens Dev Conf Consens Statement 1990 May 21-23; 8 (5).

ASHP Commission on Therapeutics. ASHP therapeutic guidelines for intravenous immune globulin. Clin Pharm 1992 Feb; 11: 117-36.

Revised: 06/21/93
Interim revision: 02/23/94

---

# INDAPAMIDE  Systemic

VA CLASSIFICATION (Primary/Secondary): CV701/CV490

Note: For a listing of dosage forms and brand names by country availability, see *Dosage Forms* section(s). For a listing of brand names for the articles in this monograph, refer to the General Index.

## Category

Antihypertensive; diuretic.

## Indications

### Accepted

Hypertension (treatment)—Indapamide is indicated, alone or in combination with other agents, for treatment of hypertension. Indapamide is effective in treating hypertension in patients with renal function impairment, although its diuretic effect is reduced.

For additional information on initial therapeutic guidelines related to the treatment of hypertension, see *Appendix III*.

Edema (treatment)—Indapamide is indicated for treatment of salt and fluid retention associated with congestive heart failure.

## Pharmacology/Pharmacokinetics

### Physicochemical characteristics

Molecular weight—365.83.
pKa—8.8.

### Mechanism of action/Effect

Antihypertensive—Not clearly understood, but may involve both renal and extrarenal effects. The diuretic effect (reduction of extracellular fluid and blood volume) probably contributes only minimally since indapamide decreases blood pressure at a dose well below the effective diuretic dose. The antihypertensive effect is thought to be the result of reduction in peripheral vascular resistance.

Diuretic—Indapamide inhibits reabsorption of water and electrolytes, primarily as a result of action on the cortical diluting segment of the distal tubule.

### Protein binding

High (71 to 79%), to plasma proteins. Also bound to elastin in vascular smooth muscle.

### Biotransformation

Hepatic (extensive).

### Half-life

In whole blood—Approximately 14 hours.

Terminal half-life of excretion of total radioactivity ([14]C-labeled indapamide)—26 hours.

### Onset of action

Antihypertensive—Multiple dose: 1 to 2 weeks.

### Time to peak concentration

Within 2 hours.

### Peak serum concentration

Approximately 260 nanograms per mL after oral administration of 5 mg.

### Time to peak effect

Antihypertensive—
Single dose: Approximately 24 hours.
Multiple doses: 8 to 12 weeks.

### Duration of action

Antihypertensive—Multiple doses: Up to 8 weeks.

### Elimination

Renal—60 to 70% (5 to 7% unchanged).
Fecal—20 to 23%.

## Precautions to Consider

### Cross-sensitivity and/or related problems

Patients sensitive to other sulfonamide-type medications may be sensitive to indapamide also.

### Carcinogenicity/Tumorigenicity

Studies in rats and mice found no evidence of carcinogenicity or tumorigenicity.

### Pregnancy/Reproduction

Fertility—Studies in animals have not shown that indapamide causes adverse effects on the fetus at up to 6250 times the therapeutic human dose.

Pregnancy—Adequate and well-controlled studies in humans have not been done. However, pregnant women should be advised to contact physician before taking this medication, since routine use of diuretics during normal pregnancy is inappropriate and exposes mother and fetus to unnecessary hazard.

Studies in animals have not shown that indapamide causes adverse effects on the fetus at up to 6250 times the therapeutic human dose.

FDA Pregnancy Category B.

### Breast-feeding

It is not known whether indapamide is excreted in breast milk. However, problems in humans have not been documented.

### Pediatrics

Appropriate studies on the relationship of age to the effects of indapamide have not been performed in the pediatric population. Safety and efficacy have not been established.

### Geriatrics

Although appropriate studies on the relationship of age to the effects of indapamide have not been performed in the geriatric population, the elderly may be more sensitive to the hypotensive and electrolyte effects. In addition, elderly patients are more likely to have age-related renal function impairment, which may require caution in patients receiving indapamide.

### Drug interactions and/or related problems

The following drug interactions and/or related problems have been selected on the basis of their potential clinical significance (possible mechanism in parentheses where appropriate)—not necessarily inclusive (» = major clinical significance):

Note: Combinations containing any of the following medications, depending on the amount present, may also interact with this medication.

Amiodarone
(concurrent use of indapamide with amiodarone may lead to an increased risk of arrhythmias associated with hypokalemia)

Anticoagulants, coumarin- or indandione-derivative
(effects may be decreased when these medications are used concurrently with indapamide, as a result of reduction of plasma volume leading to concentration of procoagulant factors in the blood; in addition, diuretic-induced improvement of hepatic congestion may lead to improved hepatic function resulting in increased procoagulant factor synthesis; dosage adjustments may be necessary)

» Digitalis glycosides
(concurrent use with indapamide may enhance the possibility of digitalis toxicity associated with hypokalemia)

Hypotension-producing medications, other (See *Appendix II*)
(antihypertensive and/or diuretic effects may be increased when
these medications are used concurrently with indapamide; although
some antihypertensive and/or diuretic combinations are used frequently for therapeutic advantage, dosage adjustment may be necessary during concurrent use)

» Lithium
(concurrent use with indapamide is not recommended, as it may
provoke lithium toxicity because of reduced renal clearance; in
addition, lithium has nephrotoxic effects)

Neuromuscular blocking agents, nondepolarizing
(indapamide may induce hypokalemia, which may enhance the
blockade of nondepolarizing neuromuscular blocking agents; serum potassium determinations may be necessary prior to administration of nondepolarizing neuromuscular blocking agents; careful postoperative monitoring of the patient may be necessary
following concurrent or sequential use, especially if there is a possibility of incomplete reversal of neuromuscular blockade)

Sympathomimetics
(antihypertensive effects of indapamide may be reduced when it is
used concurrently with sympathomimetics; the patient should be
carefully monitored to confirm that the desired effect is being
obtained)
(indapamide may decrease arterial responsiveness to norepinephrine, but does not usually significantly interfere with its clinical
effects)

**Laboratory value alterations**
The following have been selected on the basis of their potential clinical
significance (possible effect in parentheses where appropriate)—not
necessarily inclusive (» = major clinical significance):

With physiology/laboratory test values
Calcium and
Protein-bound iodine (PBI)
(serum concentrations may be slightly decreased)
Plasma renin activity (PRA)
(may be increased)
Potassium and
Sodium
(serum concentrations may be decreased but usually remain within
normal limits)
Uric acid
(serum concentrations may be increased but usually remain within
normal limits)

**Medical considerations/Contraindications**
The medical considerations/contraindications included here have been selected on the basis of their potential clinical significance (reasons given
in parentheses where appropriate)—not necessarily inclusive (» =
major clinical significance).

*Risk-benefit should be considered when the following medical problems
exist:*

» Anuria or severe renal function impairment
(diuretic effect reduced; may precipitate azotemia)
Diabetes mellitus
(possible impaired glucose tolerance)
Gout, history of or
Hyperuricemia
(serum uric acid concentrations may be elevated)
Hepatic function impairment
(risk of dehydration, which may precipitate hepatic coma and
death)
Sensitivity to indapamide or other sulfonamide-type medications
Sympathectomy
(antihypertensive effects may be enhanced)

**Patient monitoring**
The following may be especially important in patient monitoring (other
tests may be warranted in some patients, depending on condition;
» = major clinical significance):

Blood glucose concentration and
Blood urea nitrogen (BUN) concentration and
Uric acid concentration, serum
(determinations recommended prior to initiation of therapy and at
periodic intervals during therapy)
» Blood pressure measurements
(recommended at periodic intervals in patients being treated for
hypertension; selected patients may be trained to perform blood

pressure measurements at home and report the results at regular
physician visits)
Electrolyte concentrations, serum
(determinations recommended at periodic intervals for patients on
long-term therapy, especially if they are also taking cardiac glycosides or systemic steroids, or when severe cirrhosis is present)

## Side/Adverse Effects

The following side/adverse effects have been selected on the basis of their
potential clinical significance (possible signs and symptoms in parentheses where appropriate)—not necessarily inclusive:

### Those indicating need for medical attention
Incidence rare
*Allergic reaction* (skin rash, itching, or hives); *electrolyte imbalance,
specifically hyponatremia, hypochloremic alkalosis, or hypokalemia*
(dryness of mouth; increased thirst; irregular heartbeat; mood or mental changes; muscle cramps or pain; nausea or vomiting; unusual tiredness or weakness; weak pulse)

Note: *Electrolyte imbalance* is dose-related (*hypokalemia* occurs fairly
frequently) but is not usually symptomatic.

### Those indicating need for medical attention only if they continue
### or are bothersome
Incidence less frequent or rare
*Anorexia* (loss of appetite); *diarrhea; headache; orthostatic hypotension as a result of volume depletion* (dizziness or lightheadedness,
especially when getting up from a lying or sitting position); *trouble
in sleeping; stomach upset*

## Overdose

For more information on the management of overdose or unintentional
ingestion, **contact a Poison Control Center** (see *Poison Control Center Listing*).

### Treatment of overdose
Indapamide overdose should be treated by immediate evacuation of the
stomach followed by supportive, symptomatic treatment and monitoring of serum electrolyte concentrations and renal function.

## Patient Consultation

As an aid to patient consultation, refer to *Advice for the Patient,
Indapamide (Systemic).*

In providing consultation, consider emphasizing the following selected
information (» = major clinical significance):

### Before using this medication
» Conditions affecting use, especially:
Sensitivity to indapamide or other sulfonamide-type medications
Pregnancy—Routine use not recommended
Use in the elderly—Increased sensitivity to hypotensive and elec-
trolyte effects
Other medications, especially digitalis glycosides or lithium
Other medical problems, especially anuria or severe renal function
impairment

### Proper use of this medication
Diuretic effects of the medication and timing of doses to minimize
inconvenience of diuresis
Getting into habit of taking at same time each day to help increase
compliance
» Proper dosing
Missed dose: Taking as soon as possible; not taking if almost time for
next dose; not doubling doses
» Proper storage
*For use as an antihypertensive*
Possible need for control of weight and diet, especially sodium intake
» Patients may not experience symptoms of hypertension; importance of
taking medication even if feeling well
» Does not cure but helps control hypertension; possible need for life-
long therapy; checking with physician before discontinuing ther-
apy; serious consequences of untreated hypertension

### Precautions while using this medication
Regular visits to physician to check progress
» Possibility of hypokalemia; possible need for additional potassium in
diet; not changing diet without first checking with physician
To prevent dehydration, checking with physician if severe nausea,
vomiting, or diarrhea occurs and continues
*For use as an antihypertensive*
» Not taking other medications, especially nonprescription sympathom-
imetics, unless discussed with physician

## Side/adverse effects

Signs of potential side effects, especially allergic reaction and electrolyte imbalance

## General Dosing Information

The lowest effective dosage should be utilized to minimize potential electrolyte imbalance.

When used to promote diuresis, a single daily dose is preferably taken on arising in order to minimize the effect of increased frequency of urination on sleep. Intermittent dosage schedules (drug-free days) may reduce the possibility of electrolyte imbalance or hyperuricemia resulting from therapy.

Concurrent administration of potassium supplements or potassium-sparing diuretics may be indicated in patients considered to be at higher risk for developing hypokalemia. Caution in administering potassium supplements is recommended, however, since loss of potassium is not clinically significant in most patients, and supplementation leads to a risk of development of hyperkalemia.

Recent evidence suggests that withdrawal of antihypertensive therapy prior to surgery is not necessary, but that the anesthesiologist must be aware of such therapy.

## Oral Dosage Forms

### INDAPAMIDE TABLETS

#### Usual adult dose

Diuretic—

Oral, 2.5 mg once a day, adjusted according to response after one (for edema) to four (for hypertension) weeks up to 5 mg once a day.

Note: Geriatric patients may be more sensitive to the effects of the usual adult dose.

#### Usual pediatric dose

Safety and efficacy have not been established.

#### Strength(s) usually available

U.S.—

2.5 mg (Rx) [*Lozol* (lactose)].

Canada—

2.5 mg (Rx) [*Lozide*].

#### Packaging and storage

Store below 40 °C (104 °F), preferably between 15 and 30 °C (59 and 86 °F), in a well-closed container, unless otherwise specified by manufacturer. Protect from light.

#### Note

Check refill frequency to determine compliance in hypertensive patients.

### Selected Bibliography

Thomas JR. A review of 10 years of experience with indapamide as an antihypertensive agent. Hypertension 1985; 7 (Suppl 2): II–152-II–156.

The fifth report of the Joint National Committee on Detection, Evaluation, and Treatment of High Blood Pressure (JNC V). Arch Intern Med 1993; 153 (2): 154-83.

Revised: 01/20/93

---

# INDIUM In 111 OXYQUINOLINE   Systemic†

VA CLASSIFICATION (Primary): DX201

Note: For a listing of dosage forms and brand names by country availability, see *Dosage Forms* section(s). For a listing of brand names for the articles in this monograph, refer to the General Index.

†Not commercially available in Canada.

## Category

Diagnostic aid, radioactive (inflammatory lesions; thrombosis).

## Indications

Note: Bracketed information in the *Indications* section refers to uses that are not included in U.S. product labeling.

### Accepted

Leukocytes, labeling of:

Indium In 111 oxyquinoline is indicated for the labeling of autologous leukocytes. Indium In 111–labeled leukocytes are used for the following diagnostic studies:

Inflammatory lesions (diagnosis)—To locate inflammatory lesions such as abscesses. Indium In 111–labeled leukocytes are commonly used for the diagnosis of intra-abdominal abscesses, which may occur as complications of surgery, injuries, or inflammatory diseases of the gastrointestinal tract. Also, since labeled leukocytes localize in the inflamed gut mucosa, they are useful for demonstrating the presence, distribution, and extent of inflammatory bowel disease, including Crohn's disease and ulcerative colitis. In addition, labeled leukocytes are useful for demonstrating infections of prosthetic vascular grafts, and pyelonephritis and cystitis. Labeled leukocytes serve to evaluate acute and chronic osteomyelitis and are effective in demonstrating or excluding infection of orthopedic prostheses. The pattern of pulmonary uptake (diffuse vs. focal) of indium In 111–labeled leukocytes is used to rule out pulmonary or pleural infection, especially when chest x-rays are abnormal.

Indium In 111–labeled leukocyte scans have become useful as an adjunct to other diagnostic procedures in the detection of gastrointestinal and central nervous system (CNS) infections, such as focal encephalitis, cryptococcal meningitis, and cytomegalovirus encephalitis, in acquired immunodeficiency syndrome (AIDS) patients.

Ultrasound or computed tomography may be the preferred method for anatomical delineation of the infectious process when the location of the abscess is fairly well known. Indium In 111 oxy-quinoline–labeled leukocyte imaging is recommended when neither of those methods has been successful or when the results have been ambiguous.

[Platelets, labeling of]:

Indium In 111 oxyquinoline is used for the labeling of autologous platelets to be used for the following studies:

[Platelet survival studies]—For the evaluation of platelet kinetics in patients with thrombocytopenia of uncertain etiology (where accelerated platelet destruction may be a contributory mechanism).

[Thrombosis, cardiac (diagnosis)]; and

[Thrombosis, arterial and deep venous (diagnosis)]—For the scintigraphic localization of cardiac thrombi and arterial or deep venous thrombosis.

## Physical Properties

### Nuclear data

| Radionuclide (half-life) | Mode of decay | Principal photon emissions (keV) | Mean number of emissions/ disintegration |
|---|---|---|---|
| In 111 (2.83 days) | Electron capture | Gamma (171.3) Gamma (245.3) | 0.90 0.94 |

## Pharmacology/Pharmacokinetics

### Mechanism of action/Effect

Labeling of leukocytes—

When incubated with leukocytes, which have been isolated from whole blood, the indium-oxyquinoline complex, being lipid-soluble, penetrates the cell membrane of the leukocytes. Within the cell the radioactive indium dissociates from oxyquinoline and becomes firmly attached to cytoplasmic components, while the nonradioactive oxyquinoline is released by the cell.

Diagnosis of inflammatory lesions: The radioactive autologous leukocytes are subsequently reinjected to permit the detection of inflammatory lesions based on the normal physiological accumulation of leukocytes at such sites.

Labeling of platelets—

Diagnosis of thrombosis: The radiolabeled autologous platelets, when reinjected, deposit at sites of vascular endothelium injury as a normal hemostatic response. This permits detection of thrombi.

## Distribution

Indium In 111–labeled leukocytes—

Distribution of labeled leukocytes is dependent on the predominance of the cell types labeled and their condition.

Leukocytes tend to concentrate at sites of inflammation (50 to 75% of circulating cells). However, there is an initial accumulation of radioactivity in the lungs, half of which is cleared in 15 minutes and the remainder slowly (by 4 hours after injection there is no notable radioactivity in normal lungs). Twenty-five to 50% of the radioactivity is subsequently distributed in spleen, liver, and bone marrow. Cells with lowered viability give high levels of activity in the liver, while a preparation with higher viability but contaminated with red cells and lymphocytes results in high levels of radioactivity in the spleen.

Radioactivity in liver and spleen reaches a plateau at 2 to 48 hours after injection with no significant clearance observed at 72 hours.

Indium In 111–labeled platelets—

Some of the labeled platelets are rapidly taken up in the spleen and liver (about 30 and 10% of the injected dose, respectively). The remaining cells (60%) are cleared from the blood with a half-time of 4 to 5 days, and are distributed in red bone marrow, liver, spleen, and other tissues (about 25, 20, 5, and 10% of the injected dose, respectively).

## Half-life

Biological—

Clearance of indium In 111–labeled leukocytes from whole blood: 5 to 10 hours.

Clearance of indium In 111–labeled platelets from whole blood: 7 to 10 days.

## Time to radioactivity visualization

Images of indium In 111–labeled leukocyte (or platelet) localization at inflammatory sites may be obtained as early as 4 hours after injection, but optimal images are obtained at 18 to 24 hours following administration.

## Radiation dosimetry

| Organ | Estimated absorbed radiation dose* | | | |
| --- | --- | --- | --- | --- |
| | Indium-labeled leukocytes† | | Indium-labeled platelets | |
| | mGy/ MBq | rad/ MCi | mGy/ MBq | rad/ mCi |
| Spleen | 5.5 | 20.35 | 7.5 | 27.75 |
| Liver | 0.71 | 2.63 | 0.73 | 2.70 |
| Red marrow | 0.69 | 2.55 | 0.36 | 1.33 |
| Pancreas | 0.52 | 1.92 | 0.66 | 2.44 |
| Bone surfaces | 0.35 | 1.30 | 0.23 | 0.85 |
| Kidneys | 0.33 | 1.22 | 0.41 | 1.52 |
| Adrenals | 0.31 | 1.15 | 0.37 | 1.37 |
| Stomach wall | 0.28 | 1.04 | 0.35 | 1.30 |
| Heart | 0.17 | 0.63 | 0.39 | 1.44 |
| Small intestine | 0.16 | 0.59 | 0.14 | 0.52 |
| Large intestine (upper) | 0.16 | 0.59 | 0.14 | 0.52 |
| Lungs | 0.16 | 0.59 | 0.28 | 1.04 |
| Large intestine (lower) | 0.13 | 0.48 | 0.097 | 0.36 |
| Ovaries | 0.12 | 0.44 | 0.098 | 0.36 |
| Uterus | 0.12 | 0.44 | 0.095 | 0.35 |
| Breast | 0.090 | 0.33 | 0.10 | 0.37 |
| Bladder wall | 0.072 | 0.27 | 0.066 | 0.24 |
| Thyroid | 0.061 | 0.23 | 0.081 | 0.30 |
| Testes | 0.045 | 0.17 | 0.043 | 0.16 |
| Other tissue | 0.11 | 0.41 | 0.12 | 0.44 |

| Radionuclide and impurities | Effective dose* | | | |
| --- | --- | --- | --- | --- |
| | Indium-labeled leukocytes† | | Indium-labeled platelets | |
| | mSv/ MBq | rem/ MCi | mSv/ MBq | rem/ mCi |
| In 111 | 0.59 | 2.18 | 0.70 | 2.59 |
| In 114m‡ | 69 | 255 | 83 | 307 |

*For adults. Data based on the International Commission on Radiological Protection (ICRP) Publication 53—Radiation Dose to Patients from Radiopharmaceuticals.

†The actual leukocyte suspension used for labeling may also contain erythrocytes and thrombocytes, which become labeled at the same time.

There may also be some unbound activity. Radiation contributions from these other fractions of activity have to be considered.

‡Impurity. Radionuclidic impurity at calibration time is not greater then 0.037 MBq (1 microcurie) of indium In 114m per 37 MBq (1 millicurie) of indium In 111.

## Elimination

Renal and fecal. Negligible amount (less than 1%) of the injected dose eliminated in 24 hours.

# Precautions to Consider

## Carcinogenicity

Although earlier studies suggested oxyquinoline might have a carcinogenic potential, recent studies have not shown a carcinogenic effect in rats or mice given oxyquinoline in feed at concentrations of 1500 or 3000 parts per million for 103 weeks. In any case, the carcinogenic potential of oxyquinoline is of no real concern since the oxyquinoline that is released from the cell following radiolabeling is probably removed from the preparation by subsequent cell washings.

## Pregnancy/Reproduction

Pregnancy—The possibility of pregnancy should be assessed in women of child-bearing potential. Clinical situations exist where the benefit to the patient and fetus, from information derived from radiopharmaceutical use, outweighs the risks from fetal exposure to radiation. In these situations, the physician should use discretion and reduce the radiopharmaceutical dose to the lowest possible amount.

For indium In 111 oxyquinoline–labeled leukocytes—

Indium In 111 (injected as chloride) crosses the placenta. Studies have not been done in humans with indium In 111 oxyquinoline–labeled leukocytes.

Studies have not been done in animals.

FDA Pregnancy Category C.

## Breast-feeding

Indium In 111 is excreted in breast milk in small concentrations (0.09 Bq/mL per megabecquerel [0.09 nCi/mL per millicurie] injected). Because of the potential risk to the infant from radiation exposure, temporary discontinuation of nursing is recommended for a short period of time (e.g., 24 hours), at the end of which milk should be expressed and discarded.

## Pediatrics

Although indium In 111–labeled leukocytes (and platelets) are used in children, there have been no specific studies evaluating safety and efficacy of indium In 111 oxyquinoline in pediatric patients. When this radiopharmaceutical is used in children, the diagnostic benefit should be judged to outweigh the potential risk of radiation.

## Geriatrics

Appropriate studies on the relationship of age to the effects of indium In 111–labeled leukocytes (or platelets) have not been performed in the geriatric population. However, no geriatrics-specific problems have been documented to date.

## Drug interactions and/or related problems

See *Diagnostic interference*.

## Diagnostic interference

The following have been selected on the basis of their potential clinical significance (possible effect in parentheses where appropriate)—not necessarily inclusive (» = major clinical significance):

With results of *indium In 111–labeled leukocyte* studies

Cell clumping

(clumping of cells in final preparation may produce false positive results, especially if images are taken early after injection [approximately 4 hours] because of focal accumulation of radioactivity in lungs)

Contamination by red blood cells or platelets

(red blood cells or platelets in final preparation may produce cardiac blood pool activity)

Plasma contamination

(plasma contamination may impair labeling efficiency of leukocytes since transferrin in plasma competes for indium In 111 oxyquinoline)

*Due to other medications*

Antibiotics, long-term therapy, or

Corticosteroids or

Hyperalimentation or

Lidocaine, with higher-than-therapeutic concentrations or

Procainamide, with higher-than-therapeutic concentrations

(may produce false negative results because of decreased chemotaxis)

*Due to medical problems or conditions*

Aspiration or

Atelectasis or

Congestive heart failure or

Cystic fibrosis or

Embolism, pulmonary or
Metastases or
Post-cardiopulmonary resuscitation or
Post-radiation therapy or
Pulmonary hemorrhage or
Respiratory distress syndrome, adult or
Uremia or
Vasculitis or
Wegener's granulomatosis
   (may produce diffuse pulmonary uptake of indium In 111–labeled
   leukocytes)
Gastrointestinal bleeding
   (may produce false positive images because of localization in bowel)
Hematomas
   (may produce false positive images)
Infection, chronic
   (may produce false negative images)
Leukopenia
   (may decrease leukocyte labeling efficiency because of small number
   of available leukocytes; the use of donor cells may be considered in
   leukopenic patients)
Pneumonitis or
Respiratory infections, upper
   (swallowed purulent sputum may cause false positive images)
*Due to other diagnostic tests*
Gallium citrate Ga 67 scan, previous
   (background Ga 67 activity may preclude In 111–leukocyte study for
   at least 1 month)
With results of *indium In 111–labeled platelet* studies
Contamination by red blood cells
   (red blood cells in final preparation may produce cardiac blood pool
   activity)
*Due to other medications*
Heparin
   (although studies of the effect of heparin on In 111–labeled platelet
   accumulation on venous thrombi have yielded contradictory results,
   the possibility should be considered that false negative test results may
   occur in heparin-treated patients)
*Due to medical problems or conditions*
Hematoma
   (false positive images may result because of accumulation of indium
   In 111–labeled platelets at sites of bleeding [e.g., due to venipuncture])

### Medical considerations/Contraindications

The medical considerations/contraindications included here have been selected
on the basis of their potential clinical significance (reasons given in parentheses where appropriate)—not necessarily inclusive (» = major clinical significance).
See also *Diagnostic interference.*

*Risk-benefit should be considered when the following medical problem ex-
ists:*

Sensitivity to the radiopharmaceutical preparation

## Side/Adverse Effects

The following side/adverse effects have been selected on the basis of their
potential clinical significance (possible signs and symptoms in parentheses
where appropriate)—not necessarily inclusive:

### Those indicating need for medical attention

Incidence less frequent or rare
   *Allergic reaction* (skin rash, hives, or itching); *pyrogenic reaction from
   indium In 111–labeled leukocytes (or platelets)* (fever)—may also be clinical sign of abscess

## Patient Consultation

As an aid to patient consultation, refer to *Advice for the Patient,
Radiopharmaceuticals (Diagnostic).*

In providing consultation, consider emphasizing the following selected information (» = major clinical significance):

### Description of use

Action in the body: Concentration of radioactivity at sites of infection or
   thrombosis allows images to be obtained
Small amounts of radioactivity used in diagnosis; radiation received is low
   and considered safe

### Before having this test

» Conditions affecting use, especially:
   Pregnancy—Indium In 111 (administered as chloride) crosses the pla-
      centa; risk to fetus from radiation exposure as opposed to benefit
      derived from use should be considered
   Breast-feeding—Small concentration of radioactivity excreted in breast
      milk; temporary discontinuation of nursing recommended because
      of risk to infant from radiation exposure
   Use in children—Risk from radiation exposure as opposed to benefit
      derived from use should be considered

### Preparation for this test

Special preparatory instructions may apply; patient should inquire in
   advance

### Precautions after having this test

No special precautions

### Side/adverse effects

Signs of potential side effects, especially pyrogenic and allergic reactions

## General Dosing Information

Radiopharmaceuticals are to be administered only by or under the supervision
   of physicians who have had extensive training in the safe use and handling
   of radioactive materials and who are authorized by the appropriate Federal
   or State agency, if required, or, outside the U.S., the appropriate authority.
Indium In 111 oxyquinoline solution is *not* administered directly. It is intended
   only for use in the preparation of indium In 111–labeled leukocytes (or
   platelets).
The manufacturer's package insert or other appropriate literature should be
   consulted for the specific method of labeling leukocytes and for optimal
   times when imaging should be performed.

### Safety considerations for handling this radiopharmaceutical

Improper handling of this radiopharmaceutical may cause radioactive contamination. Guidelines for handling radioactive material have been prepared
   by scientific, professional, state, federal, and international bodies and are
   available to the specially qualified and authorized users who have access
   to radiopharmaceuticals.

## Parenteral Dosage Forms

Note: Bracketed uses in the *Dosage Forms* section refer to categories of use
   and/or indications that are not included in U.S. product labeling.

### INDIUM In 111 OXYQUINOLINE SOLUTION USP

#### Usual adult and adolescent administered activity

Diagnosis of inflammatory lesions—
   Intravenous, 7.4 to 18.5 megabecquerels (200 to 500 microcuries) of in-
      dium In 111 oxyquinoline–labeled leukocytes.
[Platelet survival studies]—
   Intravenous, 0.74 to 18.5 megabecquerels (20 to 500 microcuries) of in-
      dium In 111 oxyquinoline–labeled platelets.
[Diagnosis of thrombosis]—
   Intravenous, 18.5 megabecquerels (500 microcuries) of indium In 111
      oxyquinoline–labeled platelets.

#### Usual pediatric administered activity

Dosage has not been established.

Note: In the diagnosis of acute inflammatory conditions, in children and adolescents, dosages of 0.26 to 0.30 megabecquerel (7 to 8 microcuries)
   of indium In 111 oxyquinoline–labeled leukocytes per kg of body
   weight have been used. However, in most clinical studies a total dosage
   of 1.8 to 3.7 megabecquerels (50 to 100 microcuries) is recommended
   for optimal imaging quality.

#### Usual geriatric administered activity

See *Usual adult and adolescent administered activity.*

#### Strength(s) usually available

U.S.—
   37 megabecquerels (1 millicurie) per mL at calibration date (Rx)
      [GENERIC]

   Note: Indium In 111 oxyquinoline solution is *not* administered directly.
      It is intended only for use in the preparation of indium In 111
      oxyquinoline–labeled leukocytes (or platelets).

Canada—
   Not commercially available.

#### Packaging and storage

Store between 15 and 25 °C (59 and 77 °F), unless otherwise specified by
   manufacturer.

Note: The labeled leukocytes may be stored between 15 and 30 °C (59 and
   86 °F), for up to 3 hours.

**Stability**

Do not use if cell clumping is observed in final preparation.

Indium In 111 oxyquinoline solution should be used for labeling within 5 days after the calibration date.

Indium In 111 oxyquinoline–labeled leukocytes should preferably be administered within 1 hour of labeling. Administration of labeled leukocytes beyond 3 hours after preparation is not recommended since chemotaxis of granulocytes deteriorates during storage, causing false negative images.

**Note**

Caution—Radioactive material.

## Selected Bibliography

Gerzof SG, Oates ME. Imaging techniques for infections in the surgical patient. Surg Clin North Am 1988; 68 (1): 147-65.

Loken MK, Clay ME, Carpenter RT, et al. Clinical use of indium-111 labeled blood products. Clinical Nucl Med 1985; 10 (12): 902-11.

Datz FL. Physiologic imaging of radiolabeled leukocytes. Am J Physiol Imaging 1987; 2 (4): 196-207.

Datz FL. Radiolabeled leukocytes and platelets. Invest Radiol 1986; 21 (3): 191-200.

Intenzo CM, Desai AG, Thakur ML, et al. Comparison of leukocytes labeled with indium 111-2-mercaptopyridine-N-oxide and indium 111 oxine for abscess detection. J Nucl Med 1987; 28 (4): 438-41.

Revised: 01/18/93
Interim revision: 08/02/94

---

# INDIUM In 111 PENTETATE    Systemic†

VA CLASSIFICATION (Primary): DX201

Note: For a listing of dosage forms and brand names by country availability, see *Dosage Forms* section(s). For a listing of brand names for the articles in this monograph, refer to the General Index.

†Not commercially available in Canada.

## Category

Diagnostic aid, radioactive (cerebrospinal fluid flow disorders).

## Indications

### Accepted

Cisternography, radionuclide—Indium In 111 pentetate ($^{111}$In-DTPA) is indicated as an imaging agent in cisternography to study the flow of cerebrospinal fluid (CSF) in the brain, to diagnose abnormalities in CSF circulation, to assess and help localize the site of CSF leakage, and to test the patency of or localize blocks in CSF shunts.

Also, cisternography with $^{111}$In-DTPA is used in the diagnosis and classification of hydrocephalus, especially normal pressure hydrocephalus, and in the evaluation of obstructive hydrocephalus.

$^{111}$In-DTPA cisternography is useful to detect, localize, and quantify CSF rhinorrhea, especially when the CSF leaks are small, intermittent, or questionable.

In preterm infants with hydrocephalus, lumbar cisternography using $^{111}$In-DTPA helps to evaluate CSF dynamics and the patency of the cerebral ventricular system.

## Physical Properties

### Nuclear data

| Radionuclide (half-life) | Mode of decay | Principal photon emissions (keV) | Mean number of emissions/ disintegration |
|---|---|---|---|
| In 111 (2.83 days) | Electron capture | Gamma (171.3) | 0.90 |
|  |  | Gamma (245.4) | 0.94 |

## Pharmacology/Pharmacokinetics

### Mechanism of action/Effect

The use of indium In 111 pentetate ($^{111}$In-DTPA) in radionuclide cisternography is based on its distribution. When administered intrathecally, this agent diffuses to the basal, sylvian, and cerebral cisterns and subarachnoid space around the convexity of the brain; it is then absorbed via the subarachnoid granulations into the bloodstream. Since this transit can be followed by means of external imaging, any deviations from the normal pattern can be detected. Significant abnormalities may be manifest as delayed or non-appearance of the agent in the subarachnoid space around the convexity of the brain or as reflux of the agent into the cerebral ventricles. The site of CSF leakage may be identified by an abnormal collection of activity. When $^{111}$In-DTPA is used to test the patency of CSF shunts (e.g., ventriculoperitoneal), absent or markedly diminished accumulation in and transit through the shunt tubing is an indication of obstruction.

### Distribution

Diffuses to the basal, sylvian, and cerebral cisterns and subarachnoid space around the convexity of the brain, and is subsequently absorbed into the bloodstream.

### Time to radioactivity visualization

Basal cisterns—2 to 4 hours.

Subarachnoid space around the convexity of the brain—24 hours (in patients with no significant abnormalities).

### Radiation dosimetry

| Organ | Estimated absorbed radiation dose* | | | |
|---|---|---|---|---|
|  | Lumbar injection | | Cisternal injection | |
|  | mGy/ MBq | rad/ MCi | mGy/ MGq | rad/ mCi |
| Spinal cord | 0.95 | 3.51 | 0.57 | 2.10 |
| Red marrow | 0.24 | 0.88 | 0.14 | 0.52 |
| Bladder wall | 0.20 | 0.74 | 0.18 | 0.67 |
| Adrenals | 0.16 | 0.59 | 0.065 | 0.24 |
| Bone surfaces | 0.072 | 0.27 | 0.076 | 0.28 |
| Small intestine | 0.060 | 0.22 | 0.023 | 0.085 |
| Large intestine (upper) | 0.047 | 0.17 | 0.019 | 0.070 |
| Uterus | 0.044 | 0.16 | 0.029 | 0.11 |
| Spleen | 0.040 | 0.15 | 0.019 | 0.070 |
| Stomach wall | 0.040 | 0.15 | 0.027 | 0.10 |
| Ovaries | 0.039 | 0.14 | 0.020 | 0.074 |
| Liver | 0.036 | 0.13 | 0.017 | 0.063 |
| Lungs | 0.033 | 0.12 | 0.022 | 0.081 |
| Large intestine (lower) | 0.024 | 0.089 | 0.015 | 0.056 |
| Thyroid | 0.021 | 0.078 | 0.039 | 0.14 |
| Testes | 0.011 | 0.040 | 0.0085 | 0.031 |
| Breast | 0.010 | 0.037 | 0.0096 | 0.035 |
| Other tissue | 0.027 | 0.10 | 0.017 | 0.063 |

| Radionuclide and impurities | Effective dose* | | | |
|---|---|---|---|---|
|  | Lumbar injection | | Cisternal injection | |
|  | mSv/ MBq | rem/ mCi | mSv/ MBq | rem/ mCi |
| In 111 | 0.14 | 0.52 | 0.12 | 0.44 |
| In 114m† | 1.8 | 6.67 | 2.1 | 7.78 |

*For adults. Data based on the International Commission on Radiological Protection (ICRP) Publication 53—Radiation dose to patients from radiopharmaceuticals.

†Impurity. Radionuclidic purity at calibration time is at least 99.88% with less than 0.06% indium In 114m and 0.06% zinc Zn 65. The concentration of each radionuclidic contaminant changes with time.

### Elimination

Renal; about 65% of the injected activity eliminated within 24 hours in normal subjects.

## Precautions to Consider

### Carcinogenicity/Mutagenicity

Long-term animal studies to evaluate carcinogenic or mutagenic potential of indium In 111 pentetate ($^{111}$In-DTPA) have not been performed.

**Pregnancy/Reproduction**

Pregnancy—Indium In 111 crosses the placenta. However, studies have not been done in humans with [111]In-DTPA.

The possibility of pregnancy should be assessed in women of child-bearing potential. Clinical situations exist where the benefit to the patient and fetus, based on information derived from radiopharmaceutical use, outweighs the risks from fetal exposure to radiation. In these situations, the physician should use discretion and reduce the radiopharmaceutical dose to the lowest possible amount.

Studies have not been done in animals.

FDA Pregnancy Category C.

**Breast-feeding**

It is not known whether indium In 111 is distributed into breast milk. Because of the potential risk to the infant from radiation exposure, temporary discontinuation of nursing is recommended for a length of time that may be assessed by measuring the activity of breast milk and estimating the radiation exposure to the infant.

**Pediatrics**

Although [111]In-DTPA is used in children, there have been no specific studies evaluating safety and efficacy of [111]In-DTPA in pediatric patients. When this radiopharmaceutical is used in children, the diagnostic benefit should be judged to outweigh the potential risk of radiation.

**Geriatrics**

Appropriate studies on the relationship of age to the effects of [111]In-DTPA have not been performed in the geriatric population. However, no geriatrics-specific problems have been documented to date.

**Drug interactions and/or related problems**

The following drug interactions and/or related problems have been selected on the basis of their potential clinical significance (possible mechanism in parentheses where appropriate)—not necessarily inclusive (» = major clinical significance):

Note: Combinations containing any of the following medications, depending on the amount present, may also interfere with the diagnostic imaging.

Acetazolamide

(inhibition of carbonic anhydrase by acetazolamide may decrease the rate of cerebrospinal fluid [CSF] production by the choroid plexus, thus altering CSF kinetics; may result in a false-positive cisternogram)

**Medical considerations/Contraindications**

The medical considerations/contraindications included here have been selected on the basis of their potential clinical significance (reasons given in parentheses where appropriate)—not necessarily inclusive (» = major clinical significance).

*Risk-benefit should be considered when the following medical problems exist:*

Renal function impairment, severe
(elimination of the agent may be delayed or impaired)

Sensitivity to the radiopharmaceutical preparation

## Side/Adverse Effects

The following side/adverse effects have been selected on the basis of their potential clinical significance (possible signs and symptoms in parentheses where appropriate)—not necessarily inclusive:

**Those indicating need for medical attention**

Incidence rare

*Aseptic meningitis* (severe drowsiness; fever; severe headache; continuing loss of appetite; nausea; vomiting)

## Patient Consultation

As an aid to patient consultation, refer to *Advice for the Patient, Radiopharmaceuticals (Diagnostic)*.

In providing consultation, consider emphasizing the following selected information (» = major clinical significance):

**Description of use**

Action in the body: Distribution mimics that of cerebrospinal fluid

Transit of agent may be visualized by external imaging

Small amounts of radioactivity used in diagnosis; radiation received is low and considered safe

**Before having this test**

» Conditions affecting use, especially:

Sensitivity to the radiopharmaceutical preparation

Pregnancy—[111]In-DTPA may cross placenta; risk to fetus from radiation exposure as opposed to benefit derived from use should be considered

Breast-feeding—Not known if distributed into breast milk; temporary discontinuation of nursing recommended because of risk to infant from radiation exposure

Use in children—Risk from radiation exposure as opposed to benefit derived from use should be considered

**Preparation for this test**

Special preparatory instructions may be given; patient should inquire in advance

**Side/adverse effects**

Signs of potential side effects, especially aseptic meningitis

## General Dosing Information

Radiopharmaceuticals are to be administered only by or under the supervision of physicians who have had extensive training in the safe use and handling of radioactive materials and who are authorized by the the appropriate Federal or State agency, if required, or, outside the U.S., the appropriate authority.

**Safety considerations for handling this radiopharmaceutical**

Improper handling of this radiopharmaceutical may cause radioactive contamination. Guidelines for handling radioactive material have been prepared by scientific, professional, state, federal, and international bodies and are available to the specially qualified and authorized users who have access to radiopharmaceuticals.

## Parenteral Dosage Forms

### INDIUM In 111 PENTETATE INJECTION USP

**Usual adult and adolescent administered activity**

Cisternography—

Intrathecal, 18.5 megabecquerels (500 microcuries).

**Usual pediatric administered activity**

Dosage must be individualized by physician.

**Usual geriatric administered activity**

See *Usual adult and adolescent administered activity.*

**Strength(s) usually available**

U.S.—

37 megabecquerels (1 millicurie) per mL (total activity, 55.5 megabecquerels [1.5 millicuries] per single-dose vial) at calibration time (Rx) [*Indium DTPA In 111*].

Canada—

Not commercially available.

**Packaging and storage**

Store between 5 and 30 °C (41 and 86 °F), unless otherwise specified by manufacturer.

**Stability**

Do not use if contents are turbid.

Injection should be administered within 7 days after the calibration date. Discard after single use.

**Note**

Caution—Radioactive material.

## Selected Bibliography

Wolbers JG, van Halderen P, van Lingen A, et al. Quantitative radioisotope cisternography for the investigation of CSF circulation in the posterior fossa and basal cisterns—a preliminary report. Neurosurgery 1986; 9 (1–2): 125-8.

Maeda T, Ishida H, Matsuda H, et al. The utility of radionuclide myelography and cisternography in the progress of cerebrospinal fluid leaks. Eur J Nucl Med 1984; 9 (9): 416-8.

Revised: 04/30/96

# INDIUM In 111 PENTETREOTIDE     Systemic†

VA CLASSIFICATION (Primary): DX201

Note: For a listing of dosage forms and brand names by country availability, see *Dosage Forms* section(s). For a listing of brand names for the articles in this monograph, refer to the General Index.

†Not commercially available in Canada.

## Category

Diagnostic aid, radioactive (neuroendocrine tumors).

## Indications

### Accepted

Neuroendocrine tumors (diagnosis)—Indium In 111 pentetreotide is indicated for the scintigraphic localization of primary and metastatic neuroendocrine tumors bearing somatostatin receptors, mainly growth hormone–secreting pituitary tumors, endocrine pancreatic tumors, carcinoids, other neuroendocrine tumors with typical amine precursor uptake and decarboxylation (APUD) characteristics (e.g., paragangliomas, medullary thyroid carcinomas, some pheochromocytomas, and small cell lung carcinomas), neuroblastomas, brain tumors (e.g., meningiomas and glial tumors, especially astrocytomas), Merkel cell tumors, lymphomas, and certain breast carcinomas.

A drawback of indium In 111 pentetreotide for the localization of pheochromocytomas in the adrenal gland is its relatively high accumulation in the kidneys; therefore, I 123 or I 131 iobenguane ([123]I- or [131]I-mIBG) may be preferable for this use. However, indium In 111 pentetreotide and [123]I- or [131]I-mIBG appear to be similar and complementary, providing comparable information in many patients; each provides superior results in some patients.

## Physical Properties

### Nuclear data

| Radionuclide (half-life) | Mode of decay | Principal photon emissions (keV) | Mean number of emissions/disintegration |
|---|---|---|---|
| In 111 (2.83 days) | Electron capture | Gamma (171.3) | 0.90 |
|  |  | Gamma (245.4) | 0.94 |

## Pharmacology/Pharmacokinetics

### Mechanism of action/Effect

Pentetreotide, a diethylenetriaminopentaacetic (DTPA) conjugate of octreotide (an analog of somatostatin), binds to somatostatin receptors on cell surfaces throughout the body. Tumors containing a high density of somatostatin receptors concentrate indium In 111-labeled pentetreotide. After clearance of blood activity, visualization of somatostatin receptor-positive tissue is achieved with scintigraphic imaging techniques.

### Distribution

Within one hour of intravenous administration, indium In 111 pentetreotide is distributed from plasma to extravascular tissues and localizes in tumors as a function of the density of somatostatin receptors. Also, it localizes in the normal pituitary gland, thyroid gland, liver, spleen, urinary bladder, and to a lesser extent, in the bowel. Hepatic and biliary accumulation is 2% of the administered activity 4 hours after injection.

### Time to radioactivity visualization

Optimal diagnostic images (planar and SPECT)—24 hours.

Note: Early scintigraphic demonstration of carcinoid liver metastases has been observed at 30 minutes, of meningiomas at 2 hours, and of small cell lung carcinomas at 4 hours postinjection of indium In 111 pentetreotide.

Repeat scintigraphy may be indicated at 48 hours when the 24-hour scintigram shows accumulation of radioactivity in the abdomen, which can represent normal bowel elimination of the indium In 111 pentetreotide.

## Radiation dosimetry

| Organ | Estimated absorbed radiation dose* | |
|---|---|---|
|  | mGy/MBq | rad/mCi |
| Spleen | 0.66 | 2.46 |
| Kidneys | 0.49 | 1.80 |
| Bladder wall | 0.27 | 1.01 |
| Liver | 0.11 | 0.41 |
| Large intestine (lower) | 0.07 | 0.26 |
| Adrenals | 0.068 | 0.25 |
| Thyroid | 0.067 | 0.25 |
| Uterus | 0.057 | 0.21 |
| Large intestine (upper) | 0.052 | 0.19 |
| Stomach wall | 0.052 | 0.19 |
| Ovaries | 0.044 | 0.16 |
| Small intestine | 0.043 | 0.16 |
| Red marrow | 0.031 | 0.12 |
| Testes | 0.026 | 0.097 |

Effective dose: 0.12 mSv/MBq (0.43 rem/mCi)†

*For adults; intravenous injection. Includes correction for maximum 0.1% indium In 114m contaminant, at calibration. Assumes 4.8 hour voiding interval. Data based on calculations by Oak Ridge Associated Universities, Radiopharmaceutical Internal Dose Information Center.

†Data estimated according to International Commission on Radiological Protection (ICRP) Publication 53—Radiation dose to patients from radiopharmaceuticals.

### Elimination

Primarily renal. Fifty percent of the administered activity is excreted within 6 hours of injection, 85% within the first 24 hours, and over 90% by 2 days. During the first 4 hours after injection, indium In 111 pentetreotide appears predominantly in intact form (peptide-bound radioactivity) in the urine.

Less than 2% of the administered activity is found in the feces within 3 days after injection.

It is not known whether indium In 111 pentetreotide can be removed by dialysis.

## Precautions to Consider

### Carcinogenicity

Long-term animal studies to evaluate carcinogenic potential of indium In 111 pentetreotide have not been performed.

### Mutagenicity

No evidence of mutagenicity was found in an *in vitro* mouse lymphoma forward mutation assay and an *in vivo* mouse micronucleus assay.

### Pregnancy/Reproduction

Pregnancy—Indium In 111 administered as indium chloride crosses the placenta. Studies have not been done with indium In 111 pentetreotide in humans.

The possibility of pregnancy should be assessed in women of child-bearing potential. Clinical situations exist in which the benefit to the patient and fetus, based on information derived from radiopharmaceutical use, outweighs the risks from fetal exposure to radiation. In these situations, the physician should use discretion and reduce the radiopharmaceutical dose to the lowest possible amount.

Studies have not been done in animals.

FDA Pregnancy Category C.

### Breast-feeding

It is not known whether indium In 111 pentetreotide is distributed into breast milk. Because of the potential risk to the infant from radiation exposure, temporary discontinuation of nursing is recommended for a length of time that may be assessed by measuring the activity of breast milk and estimating the radiation exposure to the infant.

### Pediatrics

There have been no specific studies evaluating the safety and efficacy of indium In 111 pentetreotide in pediatric patients. When this radiopharmaceutical is used in children, the diagnostic benefit should be judged to outweigh the potential risk of radiation.

### Geriatrics

Diagnostic studies performed to date using indium In 111 pentetreotide have not demonstrated geriatrics-specific problems that would limit its usefulness in the elderly.

## Diagnostic interference

The following have been selected on the basis of their potential clinical significance (possible effect in parentheses where appropriate)—not necessarily inclusive (» = major clinical significance):

**With results of *this* test**

*Due to other medications*

Bleomycin
(may cause local pulmonary accumulation of indium In 111 pentetreotide)

Octreotide acetate
(concurrent administration of indium In 111 pentetreotide to patients receiving therapeutic doses of octreotide acetate may decrease the accumulation of radioactivity in the tumor; octreotide withdrawal for at least 12 hours is recommended)

Total parenteral nutrition (TPN) solutions
(administration of indium In 111 pentetreotide in TPN admixtures or into TPN intravenous lines may cause the formation of a complex glycosyl octreotide conjugate)

*Due to medical problems or conditions*

Cold/influenza
(may cause accumulation of radioactivity in the nasal region and lung hili)

Insulinomas
(administration of octreotide has produced severe hypoglycemia in patients with insulinomas; since pentetreotide is an analog of octreotide, an intravenous solution containing glucose should be administered before and during administration of indium In 111 pentetreotide to minimize the possibility of hypoglycemia)

Irradiation of lung, external
(may cause local pulmonary accumulation of indium In 111 pentetreotide)

Surgery, recent
(possible accumulation of radioactivity at sites of recent surgery)

## Medical considerations/Contraindications

The medical considerations/contraindications included here have been selected on the basis of their potential clinical significance (reasons given in parentheses where appropriate)—not necessarily inclusive (» = major clinical significance).

***Risk-benefit should be considered when the following medical problems exist:***

Renal function impairment
(excretion of indium In 111 pentetreotide may be decreased)

Sensitivity to the radiopharmaceutical preparation

## Side/Adverse Effects

The following side/adverse effects have been selected on the basis of their potential clinical significance (possible signs and symptoms in parentheses where appropriate)—not necessarily inclusive:

**Those indicating need for medical attention only if they continue or are bothersome**

Incidence less frequent or rare (less than 1%)
*Dizziness; fever; flushing of skin; headache; hypotension* (dizziness or lightheadedness); *increased sweating; joint pain; nausea; unusual weakness*

## Patient Consultation

As an aid to patient consultation, refer to *Advice for the Patient, Radiopharmaceuticals (Diagnostic)*.

In providing consultation, consider emphasizing the following selected information (» = major clinical significance):

**Description of use**

Action in the body: Localization at sites of tumor spread or growth
Tumor sites may be visualized by external imaging
Small amounts of radioactivity used in diagnosis; radiation received is relatively low and considered safe

**Before having this test**

» Conditions affecting use, especially:
Sensitivity to the radiopharmaceutical preparation
Pregnancy—Indium In 111 as indium chloride crosses placenta; risk to fetus from radiation exposure as opposed to benefit derived from use should be considered
Breast-feeding—Not known if distributed into breast milk; temporary discontinuation of nursing recommended because of risk to infant from radiation exposure
Use in children—Risk of radiation exposure as opposed to benefit derived from use should be considered

## Preparation for this test

Special preparatory instructions may be given; patient should inquire in advance
Adequate intake of fluids before and after administration of indium In 111 pentetreotide; voiding as often as possible for 24 hours after administration to promote urine flow and to minimize radiation to bladder
Possible administration of a laxative before imaging, to minimize imaging interference due to radioactivity localization in stool

## General Dosing Information

Radiopharmaceuticals are to be administered only by or under the supervision of physicians who have had extensive training in the safe use and handling of radioactive materials and who are authorized by the appropriate Federal or State agency, if required, or, outside the U.S., the appropriate authority.

Adequate hydration of the patient is recommended before and after administration of indium In 111 pentetreotide to promote urinary flow and blood pool clearance. Also, urination is recommended as often as possible for 24 hours after examination to promote urine flow, thereby minimizing radiation to the bladder.

Laxative administration prior to initial or follow-up images may be considered to minimize radioactivity, which may interfere with image interpretation, in bowel, due to excretion of radiopharmaceutical into stool.

### Safety considerations for handling this radiopharmaceutical

Improper handling of this radiopharmaceutical may cause radioactive contamination. Guidelines for handling radioactive material have been prepared by scientific, professional, state, federal, and international bodies and are available to the specially qualified and authorized users who have access to radiopharmaceuticals.

## Parenteral Dosage Forms

### INDIUM In 111 PENTETREOTIDE INJECTION

**Usual adult and adolescent administered activity**

For diagnosis of neuroendocrine tumors—
For planar imaging: Intravenous, 111 megabecquerels (3 millicuries).
For SPECT imaging: Intravenous, 222 megabecquerels (6 millicuries).

**Usual pediatric administered activity**

Safety and efficacy have not been established.

**Usual geriatric administered activity**

See *Usual adult and adolescent administered activity.*

**Strength(s) usually available**

U.S.—
10 micrograms of pentetreotide (DTPA-octreotide), 2 mg of gentisic acid, 4.9 mg of trisodium citrate (anhydrous), 0.37 mg of citric acid (anhydrous), and 10 mg of inositol, per 10-mL reaction vial; and in a separate 10-mL vial, 111 megabecquerels (3 millicuries) per mL of indium In 111 chloride sterile solution (Rx) [*OctreoScan*].

Canada—
Not commercially available.

**Packaging and storage**

Before radiolabeling, store between 2 and 8 °C (36 and 46 °F), unless otherwise specified by manufacturer.

Note: After radiolabeling, injection should be stored at or below 25 °C (77 °F) and administered within 6 hours.

**Preparation of dosage form**

To prepare injection, the sterile, pyrogen-free indium In 111 chloride solution is combined with the contents of the reaction vial. See manufacturer's package insert for complete instructions.

Immediately before injection, the indium In 111 pentetreotide solution may be diluted with 0.9% sodium chloride injection to a maximum volume of 3 mL.

**Stability**

Injection should be administered within 6 hours after radiolabeling.

**Note**

Caution—Radioactive material.

## Selected Bibliography

Krenning EP, Kwekkeboom DJ, Bakker WH, et al. Somatostatin receptor scintigraphy with [¹¹¹In-DTPA-D-Phe¹]- and [¹²³I-Tyr³]-octreotide: the Rotterdam experience with more than 1000 patients. Eur J Nucl Med 1993; 20 (8): 716-31.

Developed: 01/24/95

# INDIUM In 111 SATUMOMAB PENDETIDE    Systemic†

VA CLASSIFICATION (Primary): DX201

Note: For a listing of dosage forms and brand names by country availability, see *Dosage Forms* section(s). For a listing of brand names for the articles in this monograph, refer to the General Index.

---

†Not commercially available in Canada.

---

## Category

Diagnostic aid, radioactive (extrahepatic malignant disease).

## Indications

### Accepted

Extrahepatic malignant disease (diagnosis)—Indium In 111 satumomab pendetide is indicated for use in immunoscintigraphy in patients with known colorectal or ovarian cancer. Indium In 111 satumomab pendetide helps determine the extent and location of extrahepatic foci of disease, and can be helpful in the preoperative determination of the resectability of malignant lesions in these patients. It helps clarify equivocal results of, and serves to complement, other diagnostic evaluations.

Indium In 111 satumomab pendetide immunoscintigraphy, when combined with computed tomography (CT) scans results and carcinoembryonic antigen (CEA) or serum tumor marker levels, provides complementary information useful in the presurgical evaluation of colorectal or ovarian cancer patients.

### Unaccepted

Not indicated as a screening test for ovarian or colorectal cancer.

## Physical Properties

### Nuclear data

| Radionuclide (half-life) | Mode of decay | Principal photon emissions (keV) | Mean number of emissions/ disintegration |
|---|---|---|---|
| In 111 (2.83 days) | Electron capture | Gamma (171.3) | 0.90 |
| | | Gamma (245.4) | 0.94 |

## Pharmacology/Pharmacokinetics

### Mechanism of action/Effect

The murine monoclonal antibody of the immunoglobulin subclass $IgG_1$, satumomab (MAb B72.3), localizes or binds specifically to a tumor-associated glycoprotein (TAG-72), a cell surface antigen expressed at high levels on nearly all colorectal and ovarian adenocarcinomas. The monoclonal antibody B72.3 is site-specifically labeled with indium In 111 chloride using the linker-chelator, glycyl-tyrosyl- (N,epsilon-diethylenetriaminepentaacetic acid)-lysine or GYK-DTPA. The resultant radiolabeled monoclonal antibody conjugate, [111]In satumomab pendetide (CYT-103), retains the immunoreactivity of the unconjugated monoclonal antibody. Following intravenous administration, the indium In 111–labeled satumomab pendetide travels through the bloodstream until it encounters tumors bearing the TAG-72 antigen. The distribution of radioactivity is recorded by imaging.

### Distribution

Following intravenous administration, indium In 111 satumomab pendetide localizes rapidly in colorectal adenocarcinomas and common epithelial ovarian carcinomas. In *in vitro* immunohistologic studies indium In 111 satumomab pendetide has been reported to be reactive with the majority of breast, non–small cell lung, pancreatic, gastric, and esophageal carcinomas. Some non-antigen-dependent localization occurs, probably secondary to catabolism, in normal liver, spleen, and bone marrow. In some individuals, some radioactivity may localize in the bowel, blood pool, kidneys, urinary bladder, male genitalia, and breast nipples in women.

### Half-life

Elimination—$56 \pm 14$ hours (mean $\pm$ SD).

### Time to radioactivity visualization:

Optimal diagnostic images—48 to 72 hours.

Note: Variability occurs; diagnostic images have been obtained as early as 24 hours and as late as 120 hours after administration of the radiopharmaceutical. Delayed imaging allows clearance of the radiopharmaceutical from the cardiac and vascular pool, which improves image contrast.

### Radiation dosimetry

| Organ | Estimated absorbed radiation dose* | |
|---|---|---|
| | mGy/MBq | rad/mCi |
| Spleen | 0.86 | 3.2 |
| Liver | 0.81 | 3.0 |
| Red marrow | 0.65 | 2.41 |
| Kidney | 0.52 | 1.93 |
| Lungs | 0.26 | 0.96 |
| Adrenal | 0.24 | 0.89 |
| Pancreas | 0.20 | 0.74 |
| Bone | 0.18 | 0.67 |
| Heart wall | 0.17 | 0.63 |
| Stomach wall | 0.17 | 0.63 |
| Large intestine wall (upper) | 0.17 | 0.63 |
| Small intestine | 0.16 | 0.59 |
| Ovaries | 0.16 | 0.59 |
| Bladder | 0.15 | 0.56 |
| Uterus | 0.15 | 0.56 |
| Large intestine wall (lower) | 0.14 | 0.52 |
| Other tissues | 0.12 | 0.44 |
| Skin | 0.09 | 0.33 |
| Thyroid | 0.08 | 0.30 |
| Testes | 0.08 | 0.30 |
| Total body | 0.15 | 0.55 |

Effective dose: 0.32 mSv/MBq (1.2 rem/mCi)

---

*For adults; intravenous injection. Includes absorbed radiation doses from both the indium In 111 and the indium In 114 contaminant. The maximum permissible level (0.16% at expiration time) of indium In 114 was used for dose estimates.

### Elimination

Renal (10% of the administered activity excreted within 72 hours).

Note: The radioligand is excreted in the urine as a small molecular weight entity, which indicates that the indium In 111 has become catabolized from the immunoglobulin molecule.

## Precautions to Consider

### Cross-sensitivity and/or related problems

Patients sensitive to murine antibody–based products may be sensitive to indium In 111 satumomab pendetide also.

### Carcinogenicity/Mutagenicity

Long-term animal studies to evaluate carcinogenic or mutagenic potential of indium In 111 satumomab pendetide have not been performed.

### Pregnancy/Reproduction

Pregnancy—Indium In 111 crosses the placenta. Studies have not been done with indium In 111 satumomab pendetide in humans.

The possibility of pregnancy should be assessed in women of child-bearing potential. Clinical situations exist where the benefit to the patient and fetus, based on information derived from radiopharmaceutical use, outweighs the risks from fetal exposure to radiation. In these situations, the physician should use discretion and reduce the radiopharmaceutical dose to the lowest possible amount.

Studies have not been done in animals.

FDA Pregnancy Category C.

### Breast-feeding

In some women, indium In 111 satumomab pendetide has been found to localize in breast nipples. Because of the potential risk to the infant from radiation exposure, temporary discontinuation of nursing is recommended.

### Pediatrics

There have been no specific studies evaluating the safety and efficacy of indium In 111 satumomab pendetide in pediatric patients. When this radiopharmaceutical is used in children, the diagnostic benefit should be judged to outweigh the potential risk of radiation.

### Geriatrics

Diagnostic studies performed to date using indium In 111 satumomab pendetide have not demonstrated geriatrics-specific problems that would limit the usefulness of indium In 111 satumomab pendetide in the elderly.

**Laboratory value alterations**

The following have been selected on the basis of their potential clinical significance (possible effect in parentheses where appropriate)—not necessarily inclusive (» = major clinical significance):

With *other* diagnostic test results

Immunoassays, including carcinoembryonic antigen (CEA) and serum tumor marker (CA 125)

(human anti-murine antibodies [HAMAs] production may be induced by the administration of indium In 111 satumomab pendetide; HAMAs in serum may cause falsely elevated values of *in vitro* immunoassays; interference may persist for months; use of non-murine immunoassays, or HAMAs removal by adsorption, blocking, or heat inactivation is recommended to avoid interference)

**Diagnostic interference**

The following have been selected on the basis of their potential clinical significance (possible effect in parentheses where appropriate)—not necessarily inclusive (» = major clinical significance):

With results of *this* test

*Due to other medications*

Murine antibody–based products

(previous administration of murine antibody–based products, including this agent, may induce human anti-murine antibodies [HAMAs], which may alter the clearance and tissue biodistribution of indium In 111 satumomab pendetide; however, more studies are needed to establish the effects of circulating HAMAs on monoclonal antibody–based products)

*Due to medical problems or conditions*

Aneurysms, abdominal or
Bowel adhesions, postoperative or
Colostomy or
Inflammatory lesions, local or
Joint disease, degenerative or
Ovarian tumors, benign

(localization of indium In 111 satumomab pendetide may occur at these sites)

**Medical considerations/Contraindications**

The medical considerations/contraindications included here have been selected on the basis of their potential clinical significance (reasons given in parentheses where appropriate)—not necessarily inclusive (» = major clinical significance).

*Risk-benefit should be considered when the following medical problem exists:*

Sensitivity to murine antibody–based products or to the radiopharmaceutical preparation

## Side/Adverse Effects

The following side/adverse effects have been selected on the basis of their potential clinical significance (possible signs and symptoms in parentheses where appropriate)—not necessarily inclusive:

**Those indicating need for medical attention**

Incidence less frequent

*Fever*

Incidence rare

*Allergic reaction, including anaphylaxis; chest pain; confusion; hypertension; hypotension; hypothermia; skin rash*

**Those indicating need for medical attention only if they continue or are bothersome**

Incidence less frequent or rare

*Chills; diarrhea; dizziness; flushing of skin; headache; joint pain; nausea; nervousness*

## Patient Consultation

As an aid to patient consultation, refer to *Advice for the Patient, Radiopharmaceuticals (Diagnostic)*.

In providing consultation, consider emphasizing the following selected information (» = major clinical significance):

**Description of use**

Action in the body: Localization at sites of tumor spread or growth
Tumor sites may be visualized by external imaging
Small amounts of radioactivity used in diagnosis; radiation received is low and considered safe

**Before having this test**

» Conditions affecting use, especially:

Sensitivity to murine antibody–based products or to the radiopharmaceutical preparation

Pregnancy—Indium In 111 crosses placenta; risk to fetus from radiation exposure as opposed to benefit derived from use should be considered

Breast-feeding—Indium In 111 satumomab pendetide may be distributed into breast milk; temporary discontinuation of nursing recommended because of risk to infant from radiation exposure

Use in children—Risk of radiation exposure as opposed to benefit derived from use should be considered

**Preparation for this test**

Special preparatory instructions may be given; patient should inquire in advance

Administration of a laxative, before imaging, to minimize imaging interference due to radioactivity localization in stool

**Side/adverse effects**

Signs of potential side effects, especially allergic reactions including anaphylaxis, fever, chest pain, confusion, hypertension, hypotension, hypothermia, skin rash

## General Dosing Information

Radiopharmaceuticals are to be administered only by or under the supervision of physicians who have had extensive training in the safe use and handling of radioactive materials and who are authorized by the Nuclear Regulatory Commission (NRC) or the appropriate Agreement State agency, if required, or, outside the U.S., the appropriate authority.

Laxative administration prior to initial or follow-up images is recommended to minimize radioactivity in bowel, which is due to uptake of isotope in stool and which may interfere with image interpretation.

**Safety considerations for handling this radiopharmaceutical**

Improper handling of this radiopharmaceutical may cause radioactive contamination. Guidelines for handling radioactive material have been prepared by scientific, professional, state, federal, and international bodies and are available to the specially qualified and authorized users who have access to radiopharmaceuticals.

**For treatment of adverse effects**

Epinephrine, antihistamines, and corticosteroid agents should be available during the administration of indium In 111 satumomab pendetide because of the possibility of allergic reactions.

## Parenteral Dosage Forms

### INDIUM In 111 SATUMOMAB PENDETIDE INJECTION

**Usual adult and adolescent administered activity**

For diagnosis of extrahepatic disease—Intravenous, 1 mg of satumomab pendetide radiolabeled with 185 megabecquerels (5 millicuries) of indium In 111 chloride, administered over a period of five minutes.

**Usual pediatric administered activity**

Safety and efficacy have not been established.

**Usual geriatric administered activity**

See *Usual adult and adolescent administered activity*.

**Strength(s) usually available**

U.S.—

1 mg of satumomab pendetide per 2 mL-single-dose vial of sodium phosphate–buffered saline solution (Rx) [*OncoScint CR/OV*].

Canada—

Not commercially available.

**Packaging and storage**

Before radiolabeling, store between 2 and 8 °C (36 and 46 °F), unless otherwise specified by manufacturer.

Note: Product should be brought to room temperature before radiolabeling.

After radiolabeling, injection may be kept at room temperature, up to 8 hours, until administration.

**Preparation of dosage form**

To prepare injection, a sterile, pyrogen-free indium In 111 chloride solution is used. Isoptope solution must be buffered with sodium acetate before adding to the satumomab pendetide solution. See manufacturer's package insert for instructions.

**Stability**
Injection should be administered within 8 hours after radiolabeling.

**Note**
Caution—Radioactive material.

**Selected Bibliography**

Doerr RJ, Abdel-Nabi HH, Krag D, et al. Radiolabeled antibody imaging in the management of colorectal cancer. Ann Surg 1991; 214 (2): 118-24.

Harwood SJ, Carroll RG, Webster WB, et al. Human biodistribution of 111In-labeled B72.3 monoclonal antibody. Cancer Res 1990; (Suppl) 50: 932S-936S.

Revised: 06/14/93
Interim revision: 08/02/94

**INDOMETHACIN**—See *Anti-inflammatory Drugs, Nonsteroidal (Ophthalmic); Anti-inflammatory Drugs, Nonsteroidal (Systemic); Indomethacin—For Patent Ductus Arteriosus (Systemic)*

---

# INDOMETHACIN—For Patent Ductus Arteriosus   Systemic

INN: Indometacin

VA CLASSIFICATION (Primary/Secondary):
  Oral—MS102/MS400; CN850; CN105; CV900
  Parenteral—CV900

Note: For information pertaining to use of indomethacin for other indications, see *Anti-inflammatory Drugs, Nonsteroidal (Systemic)*.

Another commonly used name is indometacin.

Note: For a listing of dosage forms and brand names by country availability, see *Dosage Forms* section(s). For a listing of brand names for the articles in this monograph, refer to the General Index.

## Category

Ductus arteriosus, patent, closure adjunct.

## Indications

Note: Bracketed information in the *Indications* section refers to uses that are not included in U.S. product labeling.

**Accepted**

Ductus arteriosus, patent (treatment)—Intravenous indomethacin sodium is indicated to induce pharmacologic closure of a hemodynamically significant patent ductus arteriosus (PDA) in premature infants weighing 500 to 1750 grams. Evidence of a hemodynamically significant PDA (such as respiratory distress, continuous murmur, hyperactive precordium, enlarged heart, congestion in the lungs, and associated constitutional symptoms) should be present prior to therapy. In the U.S., indomethacin is FDA-approved for administration only if these signs and symptoms persist after 48 hours of conservative treatment, such as fluid restriction, diuretics, and respiratory support. [However, some neonatologists recommend that indomethacin therapy be instituted as soon as possible after identification of the PDA, especially if echocardiography shows the presence of a significant left-to-right shunt and/or the infant is being mechanically ventilated.][1]

Some investigators have not found successful closure to be associated with birth weight and postnatal age. However, others have reported the medication's efficacy to be decreased in infants >2 weeks of age (possibly because metabolism and/or clearance of indomethacin increases with neonatal age) and in infants weighing < 1000 grams (possibly because of insufficient muscular development in the ductal wall). Reopening of the ductus may occur following initial closure; although reclosure may occur spontaneously or in response to additional indomethacin, some infants may require surgery to achieve permanent closure.

[Indomethacin has also been administered orally (via a nasogastric tube) or rectally, as a suspension prepared from capsule contents, for this purpose.][1] However, intravenous administration is preferred because it produces more predictable indomethacin serum concentrations, leading to a higher closure rate (> 80%), than oral or rectal administration. Also, intravenous administration produces fewer gastrointestinal adverse effects than oral indomethacin.

[Indomethacin is not specifically approved by U.S. or Canadian regulatory agencies for administration to premature neonates without substantial evidence of a hemodynamically significant PDA. However, preliminary evidence suggests that administration at the first sign of a murmur (but no other symptoms) may prevent development of a symptomatic PDA in infants weighing < 1000 grams. These infants may be at greater risk of developing a symptomatic PDA than those with a murmur (but no other symptoms) weighing > 1000 grams.][1]

---

[1]Not included in Canadian product labeling.

## Pharmacology/Pharmacokinetics

**Physicochemical characteristics**
Molecular weight—Indomethacin: 357.79.
Indomethacin sodium (trihydrate): 433.80.
pKa—4.5.

**Mechanism of action/Effect**
Indomethacin inhibits the activity of the enzyme cyclo-oxygenase to decrease the formation of precursors of prostaglandins and thromboxanes from arachidonic acid. Inhibition of prostaglandin synthesis (and the consequent reduction of prostaglandin activity) permits constriction of the patent ductus arteriosus, which may be due to excessive production, and/or increased sensitivity of the premature ductus to the dilating effects, of prostaglandins of the E series.

**Other actions/effects**
Indomethacin reversibly inhibits platelet aggregation. However, its antiplatelet effect, unlike that of aspirin, is reversible.

**Absorption**
When administered via nasogastric tube—Poor and incomplete, possibly because of indomethacin's insolubility and/or abnormalities in gastric function (gastric acid secretion, gastric motility, etc.) or pH in premature neonates with a patent ductus arteriosus.

**Protein binding**
Has not been determined in the premature neonate. Very high (99%), to albumin, in adults.

**Biotransformation**
Hepatic; the rate of metabolism increases with neonatal age.

**Half-life**
Greatly prolonged as compared with that reported in adults; varies inversely with postnatal age and weight. The prolonged half-life may reflect extensive and/or repeated enterohepatic circulation and re-entry into plasma.

Infants <7 days of age—3 to 60 hours; average 20 hours.

Infants >7 days of age—4 to 38 hours; average 12 hours.

Infants <1000 grams—9 to 60 hours; average 21 hours.

Infants >1000 grams—2 to 52 hours; average 15 hours.

**Peak serum concentration**
Subject to wide individual variation when administered by any route but especially following oral administration.

**Elimination**
Renal and biliary excretion of metabolites and of unchanged indomethacin. In adults, 10 to 20% of a dose is excreted in the urine as unchanged indomethacin; the quantity excreted unchanged in the premature neonate has not been determined.
In dialysis—Indomethacin is not dialyzable.

## Precautions to Consider

**Drug interactions and/or related problems**
The following drug interactions and/or related problems have been selected on the basis of their potential clinical significance (possible mechanism in parentheses where appropriate)—not necessarily inclusive (» = major clinical significance):

Note: In addition to the interactions listed below, the possibility should be considered that additive or multiple effects leading to impaired blood clotting and/or increased risk of bleeding may occur if indomethacin is used concurrently with any medication having a significant potential for causing hypoprothrombinemia, thrombocytopenia, or gastrointestinal ulceration or hemorrhage.

» Aminoglycosides or
» Digitalis glycosides
(indomethacin may decrease renal clearance of aminoglycosides or digitalis glycosides, leading to increased plasma concentrations, elimination half-lives, and risk of aminoglycoside or digitalis toxicity; digitalis is not recommended for administration to a premature infant with an ''isolated'' patent ductus arteriosus; however, if digitalis administration should be required by an individual patient, it is recommended that digitalis dosage be reduced by 50% when indomethacin therapy is initiated and that further digitalis dose adjustment be based on monitoring of electrocardiogram (ECG) and digitalis concentration; dosage adjustment of aminoglycosides may also be required, based on evidence of toxicity and/or measurement of plasma concentration)

Nephrotoxic medications, other (See *Appendix II*)
(concurrent use with indomethacin may increase the risk and/or severity of adverse renal effects)

### Laboratory value alterations

The following have been selected on the basis of their potential clinical significance (possible effect in parentheses where appropriate)—not necessarily inclusive (» = major clinical significance):

With diagnostic test results
Urinary 5-hydroxyindoleacetic acid (5-HIAA) determinations
(false 5-HIAA concentration values may be measured via the Goldenberg modification of Undenfriend's method because indomethacin metabolites are structurally similar to 5-HIAA)

With physiology/laboratory test values
Bleeding time
(may be prolonged because of suppressed platelet aggregation; effects in the premature neonate may persist for several days after the medication is discontinued)

Blood glucose concentration
(may be decreased or, less frequently, increased)

Blood urea nitrogen (BUN) concentration and
Creatinine concentration, serum and
Glucose concentration, urine and
Potassium concentration, serum and
Protein (including albumin) concentrations, urine
(may be increased because indomethacin decreases glomerular filtration rate)

Chloride concentration, urine and
Creatinine clearance and
Free water clearance and
Glomerular filtration rate and
Osmolality, urine and
Potassium concentration, urine and
Sodium concentration, urine and
Sodium concentration, serum and
Urine volume
(may be decreased)

Note: Indomethacin may decrease both sodium and water excretion; however, water retention may exceed that of sodium so that the net effect is a reduction of serum sodium concentration (dilutional hyponatremia).

Leukocyte count and
Platelet count
(may be decreased)

Liver function tests, especially transaminase (AST [SGOT]; ALT [SGPT]) activity
(values may be increased; if significant abnormalities occur, clinical signs and symptoms consistent with liver disease develop, or systemic manifestations such as eosinophilia or rash occur, indomethacin should be discontinued)

Plasma renin activity (PRA)
(may be decreased; also, indomethacin may block the increase in PRA usually produced by bumetanide, furosemide, or indapamide)

### Medical considerations/Contraindications

The medical considerations/contraindications included here have been selected on the basis of their potential clinical significance (reasons given in parentheses where appropriate)—not necessarily inclusive (» = major clinical significance).

*Except under special circumstances, this medication should not be used when the following medical problems exist:*

» Bleeding, active, especially intracranial or gastrointestinal or
» Coagulation defects
(increased risk of severe hemorrhage because indomethacin inhibits platelet aggregation and may cause gastrointestinal bleeding)

» Enterocolitis, necrotizing, proven or suspected
(may be exacerbated)

» Heart disease, congenital, such as:
Coarctation of the aorta, severe
Pulmonary atresia
Tetralogy of Fallot, severe or
» Lesions, severely obstructive, left-sided, other
(patency of the ductus arteriosus may be required to provide satisfactory pulmonary or systemic blood flow; indomethacin should not be administered until the safety of inducing closure has been determined)

» Infection, untreated, confirmed or suspected
(symptoms of progression may be masked; also, sepsis may predispose the patient to renal insufficiency and increase the risk of renal impairment or failure; in addition, an unexpectedly high rate of treatment failure has been reported following indomethacin administration to infants with sepsis)

Jaundice, severe
(in patients with severe jaundice, indomethacin may cause displacement of bilirubin and increased risk of kernicterus, and should be used with caution)

» Renal function impairment, severe, as determined by serum creatinine concentration higher than 1.2 to 1.4 mg per dL (106-124 micromols/L) or other appropriate tests
(may be exacerbated)

*Risk-benefit should be considered when the following medical problems exist:*

Conditions predisposing to renal insufficiency, such as:
Congestive heart failure
Extracellular volume depletion
Hepatic function impairment
(increased risk of renal function impairment, including acute renal failure)

» Thrombocytopenia
(increased risk of severe hemorrhage because indomethacin inhibits platelet aggregation and may cause gastrointestinal bleeding; although platelets may be administered if necessary, indomethacin should be used only when the risk of surgery outweighs the risk of administering blood products)

### Patient monitoring

The following may be especially important in patient monitoring (other tests may be warranted in some patients, depending on condition; » = major clinical significance):

Electrolyte concentrations, serum and
Renal function tests
(monitoring recommended during and following indomethacin administration; if renal function impairment occurs [as shown by a serum creatinine concentration greater than 1.2 to 1.4 mg per dL (106-124 micromols/L) or other appropriate tests], therapy should be suspended until adequate renal function has been restored)

## Side/Adverse Effects

The following side/adverse effects have been selected on the basis of their potential clinical significance (possible signs and symptoms in parentheses where appropriate)—not necessarily inclusive:

### Those indicating need for medical attention
Incidence more frequent
*Gastrointestinal problems; renal function impairment*

Note: *Renal function impairment* (incidence >40%) is characterized by decreases in urine volume; free water clearance; urine osmolality; glomerular filtration rate; creatinine clearance; and excretion of sodium, potassium, and chloride. Corresponding increases in blood urea nitrogen (BUN), blood creatinine, and serum potassium occur. Water retention may be greater than sodium retention, leading to dilutional hyponatremia.

*Gastrointestinal problems* reported include bleeding (incidence 3 to 9%), vomiting, abdominal distention, ileus, and gastric perforation (incidences 1 to 3%). These effects have been reported more frequently with oral (via a nasogastric tube) than with intravenous administration.

Incidence less frequent
*Bleeding problems; hypoglycemia*

Note: *Bleeding problems* reported (in addition to gastrointestinal bleeding) include pulmonary hemorrhage, disseminated intravascular coagulopathy, microscopic hematuria, and oozing at needle puncture sites.

*Intracranial hemorrhage, necrotizing enterocolitis, and retrolental fibroplasia* have also been reported; however, the incidence in indomethacin-treated infants is not greater than that reported in other premature infants, who are known to be at risk for these complications.

Incidence rare
*Acidosis; alkalosis; apnea; bradycardia; exacerbation of pre-existing pulmonary infection*

## General Dosing Information

Sterile indomethacin sodium is to be administered intravenously only, over a 5- to 10-second period. Extravasation must be avoided because the solution is irritating to tissues.

Restriction of fluid intake (recommended for treatment of premature neonates with a patent ductus arteriosus) should be continued during indomethacin treatment.

Administration of 1 mg per kg of body weight (mg/kg) of furosemide immediately following indomethacin has been reported to prevent or reduce indomethacin-induced adverse renal effects without interfering with ductus arteriosus closure. However, furosemide administration is not a generally accepted measure for achieving this purpose. If a significant decrease in renal function occurs following a dose of indomethacin as indicated by a serum creatinine concentration greater than 1.2 to 1.4 mg per dL (106-124 micromols/L) or other appropriate tests, additional doses should be withheld until urine volume increases to normal levels (i.e., > 1 mL per kg of body weight per hour) and/or laboratory studies indicate return of normal renal function.

The medication should be discontinued if any severe adverse reaction, especially hepatic function impairment or disease, occurs.

If significant constriction or closure of the ductus arteriosus does not occur following 2 courses (3 doses per course) of indomethacin therapy, surgery may be required.

Reopening of the ductus arteriosus may occur following initial closure. Although spontaneous reclosure has occurred in many patients, additional indomethacin or surgery may be required.

### For treatment of adverse effects or overdose
Recommended treatment may include:
- Discontinuing or temporarily suspending administration.
- Monitoring the patient and treating observed symptoms. The possibility must be considered that gastrointestinal ulceration or hemorrhage may not occur until several days after administration.

Hemodialysis is not effective in removing indomethacin from the circulation.

## Oral Dosage Forms

Note: Bracketed uses in the *Dosage Forms* section refer to categories of use and/or indications that are not included in U.S. product labeling.

### INDOMETHACIN CAPSULES USP

#### Usual pediatric dose
[Patent ductus arteriosus closure adjunct][1]—
Infants up to 48 hours of age at time of first dose:
Oral, via nasogastric tube, 200 mcg (0.2 mg) of anhydrous indomethacin per kg of body weight initially. If necessary, one or two additional doses of 100 mcg (0.1 mg) of anhydrous indomethacin per kg of body weight may be given at twelve- to twenty-four-hour intervals.
Infants 2 to 7 days of age at time of first dose:
Oral, via nasogastric tube, 200 mcg (0.2 mg) of anhydrous indomethacin per kg of body weight initially. If necessary, one or two additional doses of 200 mcg (0.2 mg) of anhydrous indomethacin per kg of body weight may be given at twelve- to twenty-four-hour intervals.
Infants over 7 days of age at time of first dose:
Oral, via nasogastric tube, 200 mcg (0.2 mg) of anhydrous indomethacin per kg of body weight initially. If necessary, one or two additional doses of 250 mcg (0.25 mg) of anhydrous indomethacin per kg of body weight may be given at twelve- to twenty-four-hour intervals.

Note: Some investigators have used initial doses of 300 mcg (0.3 mg) per kg of body weight.

The recommended dose may also be administered rectally (as a suspension prepared from capsule contents); however, intravenous administration is preferred if available.

### Strength(s) usually available
U.S.—
25 mg (Rx) [*Indameth; Indocin;* GENERIC].
50 mg (Rx) [*Indameth; Indocin;* GENERIC].
Canada—
25 mg (Rx) [*Apo-Indomethacin; Indocid; Novomethacin*].
50 mg (Rx) [*Apo-Indomethacin; Indocid; Novomethacin*].

### Packaging and storage
Store below 40 °C (104 °F), preferably between 15 and 30 °C (59 and 86 °F). Store in a well-closed container.

## Parenteral Dosage Forms

### INDOMETHACIN SODIUM STERILE

#### Usual pediatric dose
Patent ductus arteriosus closure adjunct—
Infants up to 48 hours of age at time of first dose:
Intravenous, 200 mcg (0.2 mg) of anhydrous indomethacin per kg of body weight initially. If necessary, one or two additional doses of 100 mcg (0.1 mg) of anhydrous indomethacin per kg of body weight may be given at twelve- to twenty-four-hour intervals.
Infants 2 to 7 days of age at time of first dose:
Intravenous, 200 mcg (0.2 mg) of anhydrous indomethacin per kg of body weight initially. If necessary, one or two additional doses of 200 mcg (0.2 mg) of anhydrous indomethacin per kg of body weight may be given at twelve- to twenty-four-hour intervals.
Infants over 7 days of age at time of first dose:
Intravenous, 200 mcg (0.2 mg) of anhydrous indomethacin per kg of body weight initially. If necessary, one or two additional doses of 250 mcg (0.25 mg) of anhydrous indomethacin per kg of body weight may be given at twelve- to twenty-four-hour intervals.

Note: Some investigators have used initial doses of 300 mcg (0.3 mg) of anhydrous indomethacin per kg of body weight.

### Size(s) usually available
U.S.—
1 mg (anhydrous indomethacin) (Rx) [*Indocin I.V*].
Canada—
1 mg (anhydrous indomethacin) (Rx) [*Indocid PDA*].

### Packaging and storage
Store below 30 °C (86 °F), unless otherwise directed by manufacturer. Protect from light.

### Preparation of dosage form
Add 1 or 2 mL of preservative-free 0.9% sodium chloride injection or preservative-free sterile water for injection to the contents of the vial. A solution prepared using 1 mL of diluent contains 100 mcg (0.1 mg) of anhydrous indomethacin per 0.1 mL; a solution prepared using 2 mL of diluent contains 50 mcg (0.05 mg) of anhydrous indomethacin per 0.1 mL.

### Stability
Sterile indomethacin sodium contains no preservatives. Therefore, the medication should be reconstituted immediately prior to use and any unused solution should be discarded.

### Incompatibilities
Sterile indomethacin sodium contains no buffering agents. Further dilution of the reconstituted solution with intravenous infusion solutions is not recommended because free indomethacin may be precipitated if the pH of the solution is < 6.

---

[1]Not included in Canadian product labeling.

---

Revised: 03/10/93

# INFANT FORMULAS   Systemic

This monograph includes information on the following: Infant Formulas, Hypoallergenic; Infant Formulas, Milk-based; Infant Formulas, Soy-based.

VA CLASSIFICATION (Primary): TN200

Note: For a listing of dosage forms and brand names by country availability, see *Dosage Forms* section(s). For a listing of brand names for the articles in this monograph, refer to the General Index.

## Category
Nutritional replacement.

## Indications

### Accepted
Nutritional deficiency (prophylaxis and treatment)—Infant formulas are a type of enteral nutrition indicated as the sole or partial source of nutritional support in infants to sustain growth and activity. Under most circumstances, breast-feeding is the preferred method of providing nutritional support for the infant.

Hypoallergenic and soy-based formulas may also be used by older children and adults with allergies.

The Infant Formula Act of 1980 was set up by Congress to give the Food and Drug Administration (FDA) the authority to establish quality control procedures for commercial infant formula manufacturing, to establish recall procedures, to revise the list and levels of nutrients in infant formulas, and to require adequate labeling.

## Pharmacology/Pharmacokinetics

### Physicochemical characteristics
Hypoallergenic formulas are made from casein hydrolysate and supplemented with L-cystine, L-tyrosine, and L-tryptophan. Nonhypoallergenic formulas are made from nonfat milk, or nonfat milk and whey, or soy protein isolate and supplemented with L-methionine.

## Precautions to Consider

### Pediatrics
Side effects may occur if the selected infant formula is not prepared properly or is not used with appropriate medical supervision.

### Drug interactions and/or related problems
The following drug interactions and/or related problems have been selected on the basis of their potential clinical significance (possible mechanism in parentheses where appropriate)—not necessarily inclusive (» = major clinical significance):

Note: Combinations containing any of the following medications, depending on the amount present, may also interact with this infant formula.

Only specific interactions between enteral formulas and other oral medications have been identified in this monograph. However, enteral formulas that are administered continuously or at frequent intervals may reduce the rate and/or extent of absorption of medications that must be given on an empty stomach. Although these drug interactions and/or related problems have been reported only for adult enteral nutrition formulas, they may occur with infant enteral formulas.

Phenytoin, oral
    (enteral formulas have been found to decrease the absorption of phenytoin; if a nasogastric tube is used, it should be flushed 2 hours before and after administration of phenytoin; monitoring of phenytoin blood concentrations may be needed)

Sucralfate
    (concurrent use with enteral formulas in a nasogastric feeding tube has resulted in bezoar formation, due to the protein-binding properties of sucralfate)

Warfarin, oral
    (warfarin resistance has been reported with concurrent administration of enteral feedings, possibly due to the vitamin K found in some products; more frequent prothrombin time determinations may be needed)

### Laboratory value alterations
The following have been selected on the basis of their potential clinical significance (possible effect in parentheses where appropriate)—not necessarily inclusive (» = major clinical significance):

With physiology/laboratory test values
    Electrolytes, serum
        (concentrations may be increased or decreased)

### Medical considerations/Contraindications
The medical considerations/contraindications included here have been selected on the basis of their potential clinical significance (reasons given in parentheses where appropriate)—not necessarily inclusive (» = major clinical significance).

*Except under special circumstances, this infant formula should not be used when the following medical problems exist:*
»  Bowel obstruction, total or
»  Ileus, preventing nutrient absorption or
»  Perforated bowel
    (some patients may require postpyloric feeding to achieve enteral nutrition)

*Risk-benefit should be considered when the following medical problems exist:*
Note: Administration of infant formulas to infants with the following medical problems may be accomplished by careful selection of an infant formula or by changing the manner of administration.

Aspiration pneumonitis, especially in the presence of severe pulmonary disease
    (condition may be exacerbated by introduction of nasogastric tube)

Cardiac insufficiency
    (condition may be exacerbated, especially during initiation of feeding in severely malnourished patients; adjustment of intake may be required)

Dehydration
    (condition may be exacerbated, especially if supplementary fluids are not given; infants should be monitored for signs of dehydration and malabsorption of sugars such as lactose, sucrose, and glucose)

Diabetes mellitus or
Hyperglycemia
    (the carbohydrate content of many infant formulas may require adjustment of antidiabetic therapy or addition of insulin or other antidiabetic medications to the treatment regimen in patients with diabetes mellitus or hyperglycemia)

Diarrhea, severe
    (condition may be exacerbated by infant feedings; use of formulas with a low osmolality or altered carbohydrate content may decrease the risk of diarrhea; diarrhea may also be a sign of lactose intolerance)

Electrolyte abnormalities
    (electrolyte disturbances may occur with infant feedings; patient monitoring may be necessary)

»  Gastric function abnormalities
    (gastric emptying may be delayed with enteral feedings, which may lead to retention, nausea, and/or vomiting; switching to a formula with a low osmolality or to a modified or low-fat formula may be necessary)

Hepatic function impairment
    (enteral formulas have been reported to alter hepatic function)

Hyperlipidemia
    (the fat content of some infant formulas may exacerbate the condition)

Ketosis
    (may be caused or exacerbated by a formula that supplies more calories from fat than from protein and/or carbohydrate)

Lactose intolerance
    (some infant formulas contain lactose)

Pancreatic insufficiency with fat malabsorption
    (condition may be exacerbated; use of an infant formula with a low fat content or a formula that uses medium-chain triglycerides as part of fat may be necessary)

»  Phenylketonuria
    (infant formulas contain phenylalanine, which may exacerbate the condition)

Renal function impairment or underdeveloped renal function
(fluid, protein, electrolytes, vitamins, and minerals may need to be
restricted in patients with compromised renal function)

Respiratory difficulty
(condition may be exacerbated, especially with high carbohydrate
formulas, or regular type feeding in severely malnourished patients; adjustment of intake may be required)

» Vomiting, severe
(severe vomiting may be a sign of gastric outlet obstruction, protein allergy, or gastroesophageal reflux)

**Patient monitoring**

The following may be especially important in patient monitoring (other
tests may be warranted in some patients, depending on condition;
» = major clinical significance):

Note: For healthy infants receiving infant formulas, measuring and chart-
ing growth may be the only monitoring that is necessary. Any other
monitoring is at the discretion of the health care provider. For premature infants or those in poor health, patient monitoring may be
necessary.

Albumin, serum and
Transferrin, serum and
Urea nitrogen, 24-hour, urinary
(recommended periodically to assess protein status)

Anthropometric measurements
(recommended periodically as a measure of growth and changes
in lean body or adipose tissue mass)

Complete blood count and
Electrolytes, serum and
Glucose, serum and
Hepatic function determinations and
Mineral status and
Renal function determinations
(recommended periodically depending on patient condition; abnormal serum glucose may require an adjustment of insulin in diabetic patients; if a patient has abnormal renal function, there may
be a need to restrict fluids, electrolytes, vitamins, and/or trace
minerals)

Energy expenditure
(monitoring may be necessary to determine success of infant formula feedings)

## Side/Adverse Effects

The following side/adverse effects have been selected on the basis of their
potential clinical significance (possible signs and symptoms in parentheses where appropriate)—not necessarily inclusive:

**Those indicating need for medical attention**
Incidence more frequent
*Dehydration* (unusual thirst; unusual tiredness or weakness); *diarrhea*

Note: *Diarrhea* may produce severe dehydration, which may develop
quickly (within 24 hours). Diarrhea may result from improper
formula dilution.

Incidence less frequent
*Signs of milk allergy* (hives; wheezing)—estimated to occur in 0.4 to
7.5% of infants receiving formulas; *signs of milk intolerance* (abdominal distention; diarrhea; stomach cramps; vomiting)

## Patient Consultation

As an aid to patient consultation, refer to *Advice for the Patient, Infant
Formulas (Systemic)*.

In providing consultation, consider emphasizing the following selected
information (» = major clinical significance):

**Before using this infant formula**
» Conditions affecting use, especially:
Sensitivity to any ingredient in the infant formula

Other medical problems, especially bowel obstruction; gastric
function abnormalities; ileus, preventing nutrient absorption;
perforated bowel; phenylketonuria; or severe vomiting

**Proper use of this infant formula**
» Proper feeding
» Proper storage

**Side/adverse effects**
Dehydration, diarrhea, signs of milk allergy, signs of milk intolerance

## General Dosing Information
### General Feeding Information
Denser infant formulas are more likely to clog a feeding tube.

## Oral Dosage Forms
See *Table 1*, page 1651, *Table 2*, page 1652, and *Table 3*, page 1656.

**Use in adults and adolescents**
The administration of infant formula by continuous or intermittent feeding
and the amount are very individualized and are a decision of the prescribing physician.

**Use in pediatrics**
The administration of infant formula by continuous or intermittent feeding
and the amount are very individualized and are a decision of the prescribing physician.

**Packaging and storage**
The unopened product should be stored below 40 °C (104 °F), preferably
between 15 and 30 °C (59 and 86 °F), unless otherwise specified by
the manufacturer.

**Preparation of infant formula**
For formulas in the powder form—This product must be reconstituted
before administration. Follow carefully the directions for mixing on
the product container.
For formulas in the liquid concentrate form—This product must be diluted
before administration. Follow carefully the directions for mixing on
the product container.
For Enfamil Human Milk Fortifier—This product comes in a powder form
and is to be added to the mother's breast milk. Follow carefully the
directions for mixing on the product container.
For Similac Natural Care—This product is to be added to the mother's
breast milk or fed alternately with breast milk to low-birth-weight
infants as directed by a physician. Follow carefully the directions on
the product package.

**Stability**
For formulas in the ready-to-use form—Formulas should be refrigerated
after opening. Any unused portions should be discarded within 24 to
48 hours after opening.
For formulas in the powder or liquid concentrate form—Any unused solution should be refrigerated and used within 24 to 48 hours after
preparation, depending on the manufacturer's instructions.
For Enfamil Human Milk Fortifier—Any unused solution of fortifier plus
breast milk should be refrigerated and used within 24 hours.
For Similac Natural Care—Any unused solution of fortifier plus breast
milk should be refrigerated and used within 24 hours.

**Auxiliary labeling**
For ready-to-use liquids and/or liquid concentrates only—
• Shake container well before opening.

## Selected Bibliography
Am Pharmaceutical Assoc. Handbook of nonprescription drugs. 9th ed.
Washington DC 1990.
American Academy of Pediatrics Committee on Nutrition. Pediatric nu-
trition handbook. 3rd ed. Elk Grove Village, IL: American Academy
of Pediatrics; 1993.

Revised: 09/23/93
Interim revision: 08/03/95

## Table 1. Infant Formulas, Hypoallergenic

Note: For comparison purposes, the contents of breast milk are as follows:

| Brand name [availability] | KCal (kJoules) per mL | mOsm per kg water | Protein Grams per 100 mL | Protein Source; % KCal | Carbohydrates Grams per 100 mL | Carbohydrates Source; % KCal | Fat Grams per 100 mL | Fat Source; % KCal | Na+ mg (mEq) per 100 mL | K+ mg (mEq) per 100 mL | Ca++ mg (mEq) per 100 mL | Mg++ mg (mEq) per 100 mL | Phos mg per 100 mL | Iron (Fe) mg per 100 mL | Comment |
|---|---|---|---|---|---|---|---|---|---|---|---|---|---|---|---|
| Breast Milk (Mature) | 0.68 (2.8) | 290 | 1.05 | Casein, whey protein; 6 | 7.2 | Lactose; 42 | 3.9 | Milk fat; 52 | 18 (0.8) | 52.5 (1.3) | 28 (1.4) | 3.5 | 14 | 0.03 | |
| *Alimentum* Oral Solution [U.S./Canada] | 0.68 (2.8) | 370 | 1.9 | Casein hydrolysate, amino acids; 11 | 6.9 | Sucrose, modified tapioca starch; 41 | 3.8 | MCT* oil, safflower oil, soy oil; 48 | 30 (1.3) | 80 (2.1) | 71 (3.5) | 5.1 (0.4) | 51 | 1.2 | Lactose-free |
| *Nutramigen* Oral Concentrate [U.S.] Oral Solution [U.S.] for Oral Solution [U.S./Canada] | 0.68 (2.8) | 320 | 1.9 | Enzymatically hydrolyzed casein, amino acids; 11 | 7.4 | Corn syrup solids, modified cornstarch; 44 | 3.4 | Palm olein, soy oil, coconut oil, high oleic sunflower oil; 45 | 32 (1.39) | 74 (1.89) | 64 (3.2) | 7.4 (0.61) | 43 | 1.22 | Lactose-free |
| *Pregestimil* for Oral Solution [U.S./Canada] | 0.68 (2.8) | 320 | 1.9 | Enzymatically hydrolyzed casein, amino acids; 11 | 6.9 | Corn syrup solids, modified cornstarch, dextrose; 41 | 3.8 | Corn oil, MCT* oil (fractionated coconut oil), soy oil, high oleic safflower oil; 48 | 27 (1.17) | 74 (1.89) | 64 (3.2) | 7.4 (0.61) | 43 | 1.28 | Lactose-free |

*MCT=Medium-chain triglycerides

## Table 2. Infant Formulas, Milk-based

Note: For comparison purposes, the contents of breast milk are as follows:

| Brand name [availability] | KCal (kJoules) per mL | mOsm per kg water | Protein — Grams per 100 mL | Protein — Source; % KCal | Carbohydrates — Grams per 100 mL | Carbohydrates — Source; % KCal | Fat — Grams per 100 mL | Fat — Source; % KCal | Na+ mg (mEq) per 100 mL | K+ mg (mEq) per 100 mL | Ca++ mg (mEq) per 100 mL | Mg++ mg (mEq) per 100 mL | Phos mg per 100 mL | Iron (Fe) mg per 100 mL |
|---|---|---|---|---|---|---|---|---|---|---|---|---|---|---|
| Breast Milk (Mature) | 0.68 (2.8) | 290 | 1.05 | Casein, whey protein; 6 | 7.2 | Lactose; 42 | 3.9 | Milk fat; 52 | 18 (0.8) | 52.5 (1.3) | 28 (1.4) | 3.5 | 14 | 0.03 |

| Brand name [availability] | KCal (kJoules) per mL | mOsm per kg water | Protein — Grams per 100 mL | Protein — Source; % KCal | Carbohydrates — Grams per 100 mL | Carbohydrates — Source; % KCal | Fat — Grams per 100 mL | Fat — Source; % KCal | Na+ mg (mEq) per 100 mL | K+ mg (mEq) per 100 mL | Ca++ mg (mEq) per 100 mL | Mg++ mg (mEq) per 100 mL | Phos mg per 100 mL | Iron (Fe) mg per 100 mL | Comment |
|---|---|---|---|---|---|---|---|---|---|---|---|---|---|---|---|
| *Carnation Follow-Up Formula* Oral Concentrate [U.S.] Oral Solution [U.S.] for Oral Solution [U.S.] | 0.67 (2.8) | 326 | 1.8 | Nonfat milk; 10 | 8.9 | Corn syrup solids, lactose; 53 | 2.8 | Palm olein, soy oil, coconut oil, high oleic safflower oil; 37 | 26.4 (1.7) | 91.3 (2.3) | 91.3 (4.6) | 5.7 (0.5) | 60.9 (3.9) | 1.3 | |
| *Carnation Good Start* Oral Concentrate [U.S.] Oral Solution [U.S.] for Oral Solution [U.S.] | 0.67 (2.8) | 265 | 1.6 | Partially hydrolyzed whey; 9.7 | 7.4 | Lactose, maltodextrin; 44.2 | 3.4 | Palm olein, soy oil, coconut oil, high oleic safflower oil; 46.1 | 16.2 (0.7) | 66.3 (1.7) | 43.3 (2.2) | 4.5 (0.4) | 24.3 | 1 | |
| *Enfamil* Oral Concentrate [U.S.] Oral Solution [U.S.] for Oral Solution [U.S.] | 0.68 (2.8) | 300 | 1.45 | Whey protein, casein; 9 | 7.3 | Lactose; 43 | 3.6 | Palm olein, soy oil, coconut oil, high oleic sunflower oil; 48 | 18.3 (0.8) | 73 (1.87) | 53 (2.7) | 5.4 (0.45) | 36 | 0.47 | |
| *Enfamil Human Milk Fortifier* Oral Powder [U.S.] | 3.6 KCal per g | | 18 per 100 g | Whey protein, sodium caseinate | 71 per 100 g | Corn syrup solids, lactose | 1 per 100 g | | 181 (7.9) per 100 g | 400 (10.2) per 100 g | 2300 (115) per 100 g | 26 (2.1) per 100 g | 1170 per 100 g | N/A | |

Table 2. Infant Formulas, Milk-based (continued)

| Brand name [availability] | KCal (kJoules) per mL | mOsm per kg water | Protein Grams per 100 mL | Protein Source; % KCal | Carbohydrates Grams per 100 mL | Carbohydrates Source; % KCal | Fat Grams per 100 mL | Fat Source; %KCal | Na+ mg (mEq) per 100 mL | K+ mg (mEq) per 100 mL | Ca++ mg (mEq) per 100 mL | Mg++ mg (mEq) per 100 mL | Phos mg per 100 mL | Iron (Fe) mg per 100 mL | Comment |
|---|---|---|---|---|---|---|---|---|---|---|---|---|---|---|---|
| Enfamil with Iron Oral Concentrate [U.S.] Oral Solution [U.S.] for Oral Solution [U.S.] | 0.68 (2.8) | 300 | 1.45 | Whey protein, casein; 9 | 7.3 | Lactose; 43 | 3.6 | Palm olein, soy oil, coconut oil, high oleic sunflower oil; 48 | 18.3 (0.8) | 73 (1.87) | 53 (2.7) | 5.4 (0.45) | 36 | 1.22 | |
| Enfamil Premature Formula Formula Oral Solution [U.S.] | 0.68 (2.8) | 260 | 2 | Whey protein, casein; 12 | 7.5 | Corn syrup solids, lactose; 44 | 3.5 | MCT* oil, soy oil, coconut oil; 44 | 27 (1.17) | 70 (1.79) | 112 (5.6) | 4.6 (0.38) | 56 | 0.17 | |
|  | 0.81 (3.4) | 310 | 2.4 | Whey protein, casein; 12 | 9 | Corn syrup solids, lactose; 44 | 4.1 | MCT* oil, soy oil, coconut oil; 44 | 32 (1.39) | 83 (2.1) | 134 (6.7) | 5.5 (0.45) | 67 | 0.2 | |
| Enfamil Premature Formula with Iron Oral Solution [U.S.] | 0.68 (2.8) | 260 | 2 | Whey protein, casein; 12 | 7.5 | Corn syrup solids, lactose; 44 | 3.5 | MCT* oil, soy oil, coconut oil; 44 | 27 (1.17) | 70 (1.79) | 112 (5.6) | 4.6 (0.38) | 56 | 1.22 | |
|  | 0.81 (3.4) | 310 | 2.4 | Whey protein, casein; 12 | 9 | Corn syrup solids, lactose; 44 | 4.1 | MCT* oil, soy oil, coconut oil; 44 | 32 (1.39) | 83 (2.1) | 134 (6.7) | 5.5 (0.45) | 67 | 1.46 | |
| Gerber Baby Formula with Iron for Oral Solution [U.S.] | 0.68 (2.8) | 320 | 1.43 | Nonfat milk; 9 | 7.4 | Lactose; 43 | 3.6 | Palm olein, soy oil, coconut oil, high oleic sunflower oil; 48 | 20 (0.87) | 73 (1.87) | 53 (2.7) | 5.4 (0.45) | 36 | 1.22 | |
| Lactofree Oral Concentrate [U.S.] Oral Solution [U.S.] for Oral Solution [U.S.] | 0.68 (2.8) | 200 | 1.5 | Milk protein isolate; 9 | 7 | Corn syrup solids; 42 | 3.7 | Palm olein, soy oil, coconut oil, high oleic sunflower oil; 49 | 20 (0.87) | 74 (1.89) | 55 (2.8) | 5.4 (0.45) | 37 | 1.22 | |
| Preemie SMA 20 Oral Solution [U.S./Canada] | 0.68 (2.8) | 268 | 2 | Nonfat milk, de-mineralized whey; 11.9 | 7 | Maltodextrin, lactose; 41.5 | 3.5 | Coconut oil, oleic (safflower) oil, oleo and soybean oils, MCT* oil, soy lecithin; 46.7 | 32 (1.4) | 75 (1.9) | 75 (3.8) | 7 (0.6) | 38 | 0.3 | |

*MCT=Medium-chain triglycerides

Table 2. Infant Formulas, Milk-based *(continued)*

| Brand name [availability] | KCal (kJoules) per mL | mOsm per kg water | Protein | | Carbohydrates | | Fat | | Na+ mg (mEq) per 100 mL | K+ mg (mEq) per 100 mL | Ca++ mg (mEq) per 100 mL | Mg++ mg (mEq) per 100 mL | Phos mg per 100 mL | Iron (Fe) mg per 100 mL | Comment |
|---|---|---|---|---|---|---|---|---|---|---|---|---|---|---|---|
| | | | Grams per 100 mL | Source; % KCal | Grams per 100 mL | Source; % KCal | Grams per 100 mL | Source; %KCal | | | | | | | |
| *Preemie SMA 24* Oral Solution [U.S./Canada] | 0.8 (3.4) | 280 | 2 | Nonfat milk, demineralized whey; 9.6 | 8.6 | Maltodextrin, lactose; 41.9 | 4.4 | Coconut oil, oleic (safflower) oil, oleo and soybean oils, MCT* oil, soy lecithin; (48.5) | 32 (1.4) | 75 (1.9) | 75 (3.8) | 7 (0.6) | 40 | 0.3 | |
| *Similac 13* Oral Solution [U.S./Canada] | 0.44 (1.8) | 200 | 1.2 | Nonfat milk; 11 | 4.6 | Lactose; 42 | 2.3 | Soy oil, coconut oil, mono- and di-glycerides, soy lecithin; 47 | 15 (0.65) | 58 (1.5) | 40 (2) | 3.1 (0.25) | 31 | 0.1 | |
| *Similac 20* Oral Solution [U.S./Canada] | 0.68 (2.8) | 300 | 1.5 | Nonfat milk; 9 | 7.3 | Lactose; 43 | 3.7 | Soy oil, coconut oil, mono- and di-glycerides, soy lecithin; 48 | 18 (0.8) | 71 (1.8) | 49 (2.5) | 4.1 (0.34) | 38 | 0.15 | |
| *Similac 24* Oral Solution [U.S./Canada] | 0.81 (3.3) | 380 | 2.2 | Nonfat milk; 11 | 8.5 | Lactose; 42 | 4.3 | Soy oil, coconut oil, mono- and di-glycerides, soy lecithin; 47 | 28 (1.2) | 107 (2.7) | 73 (3.6) | 5.7 (0.47) | 57 | 0.18 | |
| *Similac 27* Oral Solution [U.S./Canada] | 0.91 (3.8) | 410 | 2.5 | Nonfat milk; 11 | 9.6 | Lactose; 42 | 4.8 | Soy oil, coconut oil, mono- and di-glycerides, soy lecithin; 47 | 31 (1.4) | 121 (3.1) | 82 (4.1) | 6.4 (0.53) | 64 | 0.2 | |
| *Similac with Iron 20* Oral Solution [U.S.] | 0.68 (2.8) | 300 | 1.5 | Nonfat milk; 9 | 7.3 | Lactose; 43 | 3.7 | Soy oil, coconut oil, mono- and di-glycerides, soy lecithin; 48 | 18 (0.8) | 71 (1.8) | 49 (2.5) | 4.1 (0.3) | 38 | 1.2 | |
| *Similac with Iron 24* Oral Solution [U.S.] | 0.81 (3.3) | 380 | 2.2 | Nonfat milk; 11 | 8.5 | Lactose; 42 | 4.3 | Soy oil, coconut oil, mono- and di-glycerides, soy lecithin; 47 | 28 (1.2) | 107 (2.7) | 73 (3.6) | 5.7 (0.4) | 57 | 1.5 | |
| *Similac Natural Care Human Milk Fortifier* Oral Solution [U.S.] | 0.81 (3.3) | 280 | 2.2 | Nonfat milk, whey protein concentrate; 11 | 8.6 | Lactose, hydrolyzed cornstarch; 42 | 4.4 | Soy oil, coconut oil, mono- and di-glycerides, soy lecithin; 47 | 35 (1.5) | 105 (2.7) | 171 (8.5) | 10 (0.8) | 85 | 0.3 | |
| *Similac PM 60/40* for Oral Solution [U.S./Canada] | 0.68 (2.8) | 280 | 1.6 | Whey protein concentrate, sodium caseinate; 9 | 6.9 | Lactose; 41 | 3.8 | Corn oil, coconut oil; 50 | 16 (0.7) | 58 (1.5) | 38 (1.9) | 4.1 (0.3) | 19 | 0.15 | |

Table 2. Infant Formulas, Milk-based *(continued)*

| Brand name [availability] | KCal (kJoules) per mL | mOsm per kg water | Protein Grams per 100 mL | Protein Source; % KCal | Carbohydrates Grams per 100 mL | Carbohydrates Source; % KCal | Fat Grams per 100 mL | Fat Source; % KCal | Na$^+$ mg (mEq) per 100 mL | K$^+$ mg (mEq) per 100 mL | Ca$^{++}$ mg (mEq) per 100 mL | Mg$^{++}$ mg (mEq) per 100 mL | Phos mg per 100 mL | Iron (Fe) mg per 100 mL | Comment |
|---|---|---|---|---|---|---|---|---|---|---|---|---|---|---|---|
| *Similac Special Care 20* Oral Solution [U.S./Canada] | 0.68 (2.8) | 235 | 1.8 | Nonfat milk, whey protein concentrate; 11 | 7.2 | Lactose, hydrolyzed cornstarch; 42 | 3.7 | Soy oil, coconut oil, mono- and di-glycerides, soy lecithin; 47 | 29 (1.3) | 87 (2.2) | 122 (6.1) | 8.1 (0.7) | 61 | 0.25 | |
| *Similac Special Care 24* Oral Solution [U.S./Canada] | 0.81 (3.3) | 280 | 2.2 | Nonfat milk, whey protein concentrate; 11 | 8.6 | Lactose, hydrolyzed cornstarch; 42 | 4.4 | Soy oil, coconut oil, mono- and di-glycerides, soy lecithin; 47 | 35 (1.5) | 105 (2.7) | 146 (7.3) | 10 (0.8) | 73 | 0.3 | |
| *Similac Special Care with Iron 24* Oral Solution [U.S.] | 0.81 (3.3) | 280 | 2.2 | Nonfat milk, whey protein concentrate; 11 | 8.6 | Lactose, hydrolyzed cornstarch; 42 | 4.4 | Soy oil, coconut oil, mono- and di-glycerides, soy lecithin; 47 | 35 (1.5) | 105 (2.7) | 146 (7.3) | 10 (0.8) | 73 | 1.5 | |
| *SMA 13* Oral Solution [U.S./Canada] | 0.44 (1.8) | 191 | 0.98 | Nonfat milk, demineralized whey; 8.9 | 4.7 | Lactose; 42.9 | 2.3 | Oleo, coconut oil, oleic (safflower or sunflower) oil, soybean oil, soy lecithin; 48.2 | 10 (0.4) | 36.4 (0.9) | 27.3 (1.38) | 3 (0.24) | 18 | 0.8 | |
| *SMA 20* Oral Solution [U.S./Canada] | 0.68 (2.8) | 300 | 1.5 | Nonfat milk, demineralized whey; 8.9 | 7.2 | Lactose; 42.9 | 3.6 | Oleo, coconut oil, oleic (safflower or sunflower) oil, soybean oil, soy lecithin; 48.2 | 15 (0.65) | 56 (1.4) | 42 (2.1) | 4.5 (0.36) | 28 | 1.2 | |
| *SMA 24* Oral Solution [U.S./Canada] | 0.8 (3.4) | 364 | 1.8 | Nonfat milk, demineralized whey; 8.9 | 8.6 | Lactose; 42.9 | 4.3 | Oleo, coconut oil, oleic (safflower or sunflower) oil, soybean oil, soy lecithin; 48.2 | 18 (0.78) | 67 (1.7) | 50.4 (2.5) | 5.4 (0.44) | 33.6 | 1.4 | |
| *SMA 27* Oral Solution [U.S./Canada] | 0.91 (3.8) | 416 | 2 | Nonfat milk, demineralized whey; 8.9 | 9.7 | Lactose; 42.9 | 4.9 | Oleo, coconut oil, oleic (safflower or sunflower) oil, soybean oil, soy lecithin; 48.2 | 20 (0.88) | 76 (1.9) | 57 (2.9) | 6 (0.5) | 38 | 1.6 | |
| *SMA Lo-Iron 13* Oral Solution [U.S./Canada] | 0.44 (1.8) | 191 | 0.98 | Nonfat milk, demineralized whey; 8.9 | 4.7 | Lactose; 42.9 | 2.3 | Oleo, coconut oil, oleic (safflower or sunflower) oil, soy oil, soy lecithin; 48.2 | 10 (0.4) | 36.4 (0.9) | 27.3 (1.38) | 3 (0.24) | 18 | 0.1 | |

*MCT=Medium-chain triglycerides

## Table 2. Infant Formulas, Milk-based (continued)

| Brand name [availability] | KCal (kJoules) per mL | mOsm per kg water | Protein Grams per 100 mL | Protein Source; % KCal | Carbohydrates Grams per 100 mL | Carbohydrates Source; % KCal | Fat Grams per 100 mL | Fat Source; % KCal | Na$^+$ mg (mEq) per 100 mL | K$^+$ mg (mEq) per 100 mL | Ca$^{++}$ mg (mEq) per 100 mL | Mg$^{++}$ mg (mEq) per 100 mL | Phos mg per 100 mL | Iron (Fe) mg per 100 mL | Comment |
|---|---|---|---|---|---|---|---|---|---|---|---|---|---|---|---|
| SMA Lo-Iron 20 Oral Solution [U.S./Canada] | 0.68 (2.8) | 300 | 1.5 | Nonfat milk, de-mineralized whey; 8.9 | 7.2 | Lactose; 42.9 | 3.6 | Oleo, coconut oil, oleic (safflower or sunflower) oil, soybean oil, soy lecithin; 48.2 | 15 (0.65) | 56 (1.4) | 42 (2.1) | 4.5 (0.36) | 28 | 0.15 | |
| SMA Lo-Iron 24 Oral Solution [U.S./Canada] | 0.8 (3.4) | 364 | 1.8 | Nonfat milk, de-mineralized whey; 8.9 | 8.6 | Lactose; 42.9 | 4.3 | Oleo, coconut oil, oleic (safflower or sunflower) oil, soybean oil, soy lecithin; 48.2 | 18 (0.78) | 67 (1.7) | 50.4 (2.5) | 5.4 (0.44) | 33.6 | 0.18 | |

*Medium-chain triglycerides.

## Table 3. Infant Formulas, Soy-based

Note: For comparison purposes, the contents of breast milk are as follows:

| | KCal (kJoules) per mL | mOsm per kg water | Protein Grams per 100 mL | Protein Source; % KCal | Carbohydrates Grams per 100 mL | Carbohydrates Source; % KCal | Fat Grams per 100 mL | Fat Source; % KCal | Na$^+$ mg (mEq) per 100 mL | K$^+$ mg (mEq) per 100 mL | Ca$^{++}$ mg (mEq) per 100 mL | Mg$^{++}$ mg (mEq) per 100 mL | Phos mg per 100 mL | Iron (Fe) mg per 100 mL |
|---|---|---|---|---|---|---|---|---|---|---|---|---|---|---|
| Breast Milk (Mature) | 0.68 (2.8) | 290 | 1.05 | Casein, whey protein; 6 | 7.2 | Lactose; 42 | 3.9 | Milk fat; 52 | 18 (0.8) | 52.5 (1.3) | 28 (1.4) | 3.5 | 14 | 0.03 |

| Brand name [availability] | KCal (kJoules) per mL | mOsm per kg water | Protein Grams per 100 mL | Protein Source; % KCal | Carbohydrates Grams per 100 mL | Carbohydrates Source; % KCal | Fat Grams per 100 mL | Fat Source; % KCal | Na$^+$ mg (mEq) per 100 mL | K$^+$ mg (mEq) per 100 mL | Ca$^{++}$ mg (mEq) per 100 mL | Mg$^{++}$ mg (mEq) per 100 mL | Phos mg per 100 mL | Iron (Fe) mg per 100 mL | Comment |
|---|---|---|---|---|---|---|---|---|---|---|---|---|---|---|---|
| Alsoy Oral Solution [U.S.] Oral Concentrate [U.S.] | 0.68 (2.8) | 270 | 2.1 | Soy isolate; 12 | 6.7 | Sucrose, tapioca, dextrin; 39 | 3.7 | Soy oil; 49 | 28.5 (1.3) | 80 2.1 | 68.3 (3.4) | 7.5 (0.6) | 47.9 | 1.3 | Lactose-free |
| Gerber Soy Formula Oral Solution [U.S.] Oral Concentrate [U.S.] | 0.68 (2.8) | 230 | 2 | Soy protein isolate, amino acids; 12 | 6.8 | Corn syrup solids, sucrose; 40 | 3.6 | Palm olein, soy oil, coconut oil, high oleic sunflower oil; 48 | 24 (1.04) | 81 (2.1) | 71 (3.6) | 7.4 (0.61) | 56 | 1.22 | Lactose-free |

Table 3. Infant Formulas, Soy-based (*continued*)

| Brand name [availability] | KCal (kJoules) per mL | mOsm per kg water | Protein Grams per 100 mL | Protein Source; % KCal | Carbohydrates Grams per 100 mL | Carbohydrates Source; % KCal | Fat Grams per 100 mL | Fat Source; % KCal | Na⁺ mg (mEq) per 100 mL | K⁺ mg (mEq) per 100 mL | Ca⁺⁺ mg (mEq) per 100 mL | Mg⁺⁺ mg (mEq) per 100 mL | Phos mg per 100 mL | Iron (Fe) mg per 100 mL | Comment |
|---|---|---|---|---|---|---|---|---|---|---|---|---|---|---|---|
| *Isomil* Oral Concentrate [U.S./Canada] Oral Solution [U.S./Canada] for Oral Solution [U.S./Canada] | 0.68 (2.8) | 240 | 1.7 | Soy protein isolate, amino acids; 10 | 7 | Corn syrup, sucrose; 41 | 3.7 | Soy oil, coconut oil, soy lecithin, mono- and diglycerides; 49 | 30 (1.3) | 73 (1.9) | 71 (3.5) | 5.1 (0.4) | 51 | 1.2 | Lactose-free |
| *Isomil SF* Oral Concentrate [U.S.] | 0.68 (2.8) | 180 | 1.8 | Soy protein isolate, amino acids; 11 | 6.8 | Hydrolyzed corn-starch; 40 | 3.7 | Soy oil, coconut oil, soy lecithin, mono- and diglycerides; 49 | 30 (1.3) | 73 (1.9) | 71 (3.5) | 5.1 (0.4) | 51 | 1.2 | Lactose-free; sugar-free |
| *Nursoy* Oral Solution [U.S./Canada] | 0.68 (2.8) | 296 | 1.8 | Soy protein isolate, L-methionine; 11 | 6.9 | Sucrose; 41 | 3.6 | Oleo, coconut oil, safflower oil, soy bean oil, soy lecithin; 48 | 20 (0.9) | 70 (1.8) | 60 (3.1) | 6.7 (0.5) | 42 | 1.2 | Lactose-free |
| for Oral Solution [U.S.] | 0.68 (2.8) | 296 | 1.8 | Soy protein isolate, L-methionine; 11 | 6.9 | Sucrose, corn syrup solids; 41 | 3.6 | Oleo, coconut oil, safflower oil, soy bean oil, soy lecithin; 48 | 20 (0.9) | 70 (1.8) | 60 (3.1) | 6.7 (0.5) | 42 | 1.2 | Lactose-free |
| *ProSobee* Oral Concentrate [U.S./Canada] Oral Solution [U.S./Canada] | 0.68 (2.8) | 200 | 2 | Soy protein isolate, amino acids; 12 | 6.8 | Corn syrup solids; 40 | 3.6 | Palm olein, soy oil, coconut oil, high oleic sunflower oil; 48 | 24 (1.04) | 81 (2.1) | 71 (3.6) | 7.4 (0.61) | 56 | 1.22 | Lactose-free; sucrose-free |
| *RCF* Oral Concentrate [U.S./Canada] | 0.41† (1.7) | 74 | 2 | Soy protein isolate, L-methionine; 20 | 0 | Selected by physician | 3.6 | Soy oil, coconut oil, mono- and di-glycerides, soy lecithin; 80 | 30 (1.3) | 73 (1.9) | 70 (3.5) | 5 (0.41) | 50 | 0.15 | Carbohydrate-free |
| *Soyalac* Oral Concentrate [U.S.] Oral Solution [U.S.] for Oral Solution [U.S.] | 0.68 (2.8) | 240 | 2.1 | Soybean solids; 12 | 6.7 | Sucrose, corn syrup solids, carbohydrates from soybean; 39 | 3.7 | Soy oil; 49 | 30 (1.3) | 80 (2.1) | 63 (3.1) | 8.2 (0.7) | 36.9 | 1.3 | Lactose-free |

*MCT=Medium-chain triglycerides.

†Values are for a 1:1 dilution with water. However, standard dilution is one part formula base to one part prescribed carbohydrate and water solution. If carbohydrate is not added to this product, a 1:1 dilution with water provides approximately 40.6 KCal/100 mL.

**INFANT FORMULAS, HYPOALLERGENIC**—See *Infant Formulas (Systemic)*

**INFANT FORMULAS, MILK-BASED**—See *Infant Formulas (Systemic)*

**INFANT FORMULAS, SOY-BASED**—See *Infant Formulas (Systemic)*

# INFLUENZA VIRUS VACCINE   Systemic

VA CLASSIFICATION (Primary): IM100

Note: This monograph refers to the Trivalent vaccine, Types A and B, 1996–97 formula. The components for the 1996–97 formula are A/Texas/36/91 antigen (H1N1), A/Nanchang/933/95 antigen (H3N2), and B/Harbin/07/94 antigen. Although A/Wuhan/359/95-like (H3N2) and B/Beijing/184/93-like antigens were chosen by the FDA's Vaccines and Related Biologicals Advisory Committee (VRBAC), the actual strains that are used by U.S. and Canadian manufacturers are A/Nanchang/933/95 (H3N2) and B/Harbin/07/94 antigens, respectively, which have better growth properties and are antigenically equivalent.

This vaccine has been selected for use during the 1996–97 season by the U.S. government and the Canadian government. The World Health Organization (WHO) is using other strains for the 1996–97 season.

Another commonly used name is flu vaccine.

Note: For a listing of dosage forms and brand names by country availability, see *Dosage Forms* section(s). For a listing of brand names for the articles in this monograph, refer to the General Index.

## Category
Immunizing agent (active).

## Indications

**Accepted**

Influenza (prophylaxis)—Influenza virus vaccine is indicated for immunization against certain strains of influenza virus. Based on epidemiological data gathered during the early months of each year, and after consultation with advisory groups and the World Health Organization (WHO), the U.S. government and the Canadian government each determine which virus strains will be included in their present year's influenza vaccine. Generally, the same viral strains are chosen by both countries, but this is not mandatory. Even though the present year's influenza vaccine may contain antigens used in a previous year's vaccine, revaccination on a yearly basis is necessary to provide optimal protection because immunity declines following immunization, possibly within 6 months. The single most important influenza-control measure is the administration of influenza vaccine to high-risk persons each year before the influenza season starts.

Unless otherwise contraindicated, annual influenza immunization should be considered for all infants 6 months of age and over, all children, and all adults, based on the following general guidelines for:

• Persons at increased medical risk of influenza-related complications:
—Adults and children who have chronic disorders of the cardiovascular or pulmonary systems, including asthma, that are severe enough to have required regular medical follow-up or hospitalization during the preceding year.
—Residents of nursing homes and other chronic-care facilities.
—Adults 65 years of age and older who are otherwise healthy.
—Adults and children who have chronic metabolic diseases (including diabetes mellitus), renal dysfunction, anemia, or immunosuppression that are severe enough to have required regular medical follow-up or hospitalization during the preceding year.
—Infants, children, and teenagers (6 months to 18 years of age) who receive long-term aspirin therapy and who, therefore, may be at risk of developing Reye's syndrome following an influenza infection.
• Persons potentially capable of nosocomial transmission of influenza to high-risk persons:
—Physicians, nurses, and other personnel who have extensive contact with high-risk patients.
—Providers of care to high-risk persons in the home setting. These include family members, visiting nurses, and volunteer workers.

—Members of households that include high-risk persons, whether or not such members are providers of care.
• Persons in the general population:
—Any person who wishes to reduce his/her chances of acquiring influenza infection.
—Persons who provide essential community services, such as employees of fire and police departments. Although these persons are not considered at increased occupational risk of serious influenza illness, they may be considered for vaccination programs designed to minimize the possible disruption of essential activities that may occur during severe epidemics.
—Persons infected with human immunodeficiency virus (HIV), whether they are asymptomatic or symptomatic. Although little information is available regarding the frequency and severity of influenza illness in HIV-infected persons, recent reports suggest that influenza symptoms may be prolonged and the risk of complications increased for these persons. Therefore, immunization with influenza vaccine is recommended and should result in protective antibody levels in many recipients. However, antibody response to the vaccine may be low in persons with advanced HIV illnesses, and a booster dose of vaccine has not improved the immune response of these persons.
—Travelers to foreign countries, especially the elderly and persons with high-risk medical conditions. The seasonal risk of influenza infection during foreign travel differs from that of the U.S. In the tropics, influenza can occur throughout the year. In the southern hemisphere, the period of greatest risk is April to September. Elderly and high-risk travelers should review their influenza immunization history before travel. Those not immunized the previous fall/winter season should receive the most currently available influenza vaccine before travel. If only the previous season's vaccine is available for administration before travel, the elderly and high-risk persons should be reimmunized in the fall/winter with the current vaccine.

## Pharmacology/Pharmacokinetics

**Physicochemical characteristics**

Source—Influenza vaccine is available as either a whole-virus or split-virus preparation. Split-virus preparations may be labeled as a split, subviron, or purified-surface-antigen type. The vaccine is prepared from highly purified, egg-grown influenza viruses that have been inactivated to yield a whole-virus preparation. The split and subviron types of the split-virus vaccine are produced by chemically treating a whole-virus preparation to cause inactivation and disruption of a significant proportion of the virus into smaller subunit particles called subvirons. The preparation is then refined to remove the unwanted substances. The purified-surface-antigen type of the split-virus vaccine is produced by chemically treating a whole-virus preparation. This removes most of the internal proteins and allows collection of the surface antigens, hemagglutinin and neuraminidase. The preparation is then refined to remove the unwanted substances.

Other characteristics—The viral antigen content of both the whole-virus vaccine and the split-virus (split, subviron, and purified-surface-antigen types) vaccine has been standardized by immunodiffusion tests, according to current U.S. Public Health Service requirements. Each 0.5-mL dose contains the proportions and not less than the microgram amounts of hemagglutinin antigens (mcg HA) representative of the specific components recommended for the present year's vaccine.

**Mechanism of action/Effect**

Following injection of influenza vaccine, the antigens prepared from the inactivated influenza virus stimulate the production of specific antibodies.

### Protective efficacy

Protection from influenza infection is afforded only against those strains of virus from which the vaccine is prepared or against closely related strains.

The degree of protection provided by immunization with the influenza vaccine may not be sufficient to prevent the disease if the exposure to the influenza virus strains is overwhelming or if the virus strains are not closely related antigenically to those used in the production of the vaccine.

Field studies of influenza vaccines conducted since the 1940s have shown marked yearly variation in efficacy, as measured by protection from disease, ranging from undemonstrable to 70 to 80% efficacy.

Elderly patients and patients with certain chronic diseases may develop lower antibody titers after immunization than healthy young adults and, therefore, may remain susceptible to influenza infection of the upper respiratory tract. Nonetheless, influenza vaccine may still be effective in preventing lower respiratory tract involvement or other complications of influenza among these high-risk persons.

### Time to protective efficacy

The development of an antibody response to immunization with influenza vaccine occurs after approximately 2 weeks.

### Duration of protective effect

Immunity declines following vaccination, possibly within 6 months.

## Precautions to Consider

### Cross-sensitivity and/or related problems

Patients sensitive to a previous year's influenza vaccine may be sensitive to this year's influenza vaccine also. Patients allergic to gentamicin sulfate, streptomycin sulfate, or other aminoglycosides may be allergic to influenza vaccines, since the vaccines may have been produced using these antibiotics.

Generally, a history of hypersensitivity reactions other than anaphylaxis, such as delayed-type allergic reaction (contact dermatitis), does not preclude immunization.

### Pregnancy/Reproduction

Pregnancy—Studies have not been done in humans. There is no evidence to suggest that influenza vaccine carries any maternal or fetal risk, and, being inactivated, the vaccine does not share any of the theoretical risks of live virus vaccines of causing infection of the fetus. To minimize any concern over the theoretical possibility of risk to the fetus, the vaccine should be given after the first trimester. However, it may be undesirable to delay immunizing a pregnant woman who has a high-risk condition and will still be in her first trimester of pregnancy when influenza activity usually begins.

Although pregnancy has not been demonstrated as a risk factor in the course of an influenza infection, except during the pandemics of 1918–19 and 1957–58, pregnant women with other medical conditions that increase their risk of complications from influenza infection should be immunized.

Studies have not been done in animals.

FDA Pregnancy Category C.

### Breast-feeding

Problems in humans have not been documented.

### Pediatrics

Side effects of influenza vaccine are common in infants and children because of their lack of previous exposure to influenza viruses comparable to the vaccine antigens.

For children 6 months to 4 years of age, only the split or subviron type of the split-virus vaccine should be used. For children 4 to 13 years of age, any of the split-virus vaccines (split, subviron, or purified-surface-antigen type) may be used. Split-virus vaccines have a lower potential for causing febrile adverse reactions than whole-virus vaccines.

Use of influenza virus vaccine is not recommended for infants up to 6 months of age.

### Geriatrics

Elderly patients may develop lower antibody titers after immunization than healthy younger adults and, therefore, may remain susceptible to influenza infection of the upper respiratory tract. Nonetheless, influenza vaccine may still be effective in preventing lower respiratory tract involvement or other complications of influenza.

### Drug interactions and/or related problems

The following drug interactions and/or related problems have been selected on the basis of their potential clinical significance (possible mechanism in parentheses where appropriate)—not necessarily inclusive (» = major clinical significance):

Note: Combinations containing any of the following medications, depending on the amount present, may also interact with this medication.

Aminopyrine or
Carbamazepine or
Phenobarbital or
Phenytoin or
Theophylline preparations or
Warfarin sodium
   (concurrent use of influenza vaccine with medications that are metabolized by the hepatic cytochrome *P*-450 has resulted in conflicting reports regarding enhanced drug effect or toxicity caused by changes in elimination of these drugs; however, although influenza vaccine may inhibit the clearance of these medications, studies have failed to show any adverse clinical effects attributable to the use of these medications in patients receiving influenza vaccine)

Immunosuppressive agents or
Radiation therapy
   (because normal defense mechanisms are suppressed, the patient's antibody response to influenza vaccine may be decreased. The precaution does not apply to corticosteroids used as replacement therapy, for short-term [less than 2 weeks] systemic therapy, or by other routes of administration that do not cause immunosuppression)

### Medical considerations/Contraindications

The medical considerations/contraindications included here have been selected on the basis of their potential clinical significance (reasons given in parentheses where appropriate)—not necessarily inclusive (» = major clinical significance).

*Except under special circumstances, this medication should not be used when the following medical problems exist:*

» Febrile illness, severe
   (to avoid confusing manifestations of illness with possible side/adverse effects of vaccine)

» Guillain-Barré syndrome (GBS), history of
   (to avoid the possibility of reactivating GBS)

» Respiratory disease, acute
   (influenza virus vaccine should not be administered until the acute symptoms of the patient's illness have abated, since the symptoms of the condition may be confused with the possible side effects of the vaccine)

*Risk-benefit should be considered when the following medical problems exist:*

» Allergy to eggs
   (patients allergic to eggs may be allergic to influenza vaccine, since it is produced in the allantoic fluids of chick embryos. Current influenza vaccines contain only a small quantity of egg protein; however, the vaccine is presumed capable of inducing immediate hypersensitivity reactions in persons with severe allergy to eggs. These persons should not be given influenza vaccine. This caution applies to persons who develop hives, swelling of the lips or tongue, or acute respiratory distress or circulatory collapse after eating eggs. It also applies to persons who have developed evidence of occupational asthma or other allergic responses from occupational exposure to egg protein or who have a documented IgE-mediated hypersensitivity reaction to eggs)

   (although there is a precaution regarding a history of hypersensitivity to eggs, no intolerance of a vaccine prepared in the allantoic fluids of chick embryos has been found in patients with a history of hypersensitivity to chicken, chicken feathers, or chicken dander)

Convulsions, febrile, history of
   (a febrile adverse reaction occurring following immunization with influenza vaccine may possibly precipitate a febrile convulsion)

Neurologic disorder, active
   (influenza vaccine should not be administered to a patient with an active neurologic disorder; the vaccine should be considered only after the disease process has been stabilized)

Sensitivity to influenza virus vaccine

Sensitivity to thimerosal
   (thimerosal may be used as a preservative in influenza vaccine)

## Side/Adverse Effects

Note: Side effects of influenza vaccine are generally minor in adults and occur infrequently, but, in infants and children, side effects may be particularly common. Severe side effects are uncommon in adults, and disabling side effects are very rare in any age group.

Generally, a history of hypersensitivity reactions other than anaphylaxis, such as delayed-type allergic reaction (contact dermatitis), does not preclude immunization.

There is a temporal association between neurologic disorders, including encephalopathy, and influenza immunization.

In 1976, Guillain-Barré syndrome (GBS) was associated with the administration of that year's influenza vaccine. It is hypothesized that the A/New Jersey/76 virus antigen (swine influenza vaccine) portion of the 1976 vaccine caused the problem, but this has not been proven. GBS is an uncommon illness characterized by ascending paralysis that is usually self-limiting and reversible. Although most persons with GBS recover without residual weakness, approximately 5% of the cases are fatal. Before 1976, there was no association of GBS with influenza vaccine. However, for the 10 weeks following immunization in 1976, the risk was found to be approximately 10 cases of GBS for every million recipients—an incidence 5 to 6 times higher than that in unimmunized persons. Younger persons (under 25 years) had a lower relative risk than others and also had a lower case-fatality rate. An active surveillance system for GBS was initiated in 1978, and data were collected for 3 years; however, a statistically significant excess risk of contracting GBS after receipt of the 1978–79, 1979–80, and 1980–81 influenza vaccine formulations could not be demonstrated. Unlike the 1976 swine influenza vaccine (containing A/New Jersey/8/76), subsequent vaccines, which have been prepared from other virus strains, have not been associated with an increased frequency of Guillain-Barré syndrome.

The following side/adverse effects have been selected on the basis of their potential clinical significance (possible signs and symptoms in parentheses where appropriate)—not necessarily inclusive:

**Those indicating need for medical attention**
Incidence rare
*Anaphylactic reaction, most likely to residual egg protein in the influenza vaccine* (difficulty in breathing or swallowing; hives; itching, especially of soles or palms; reddening of skin, especially around ears; swelling of eyes, face, or inside of nose; unusual tiredness or weakness, sudden and severe)

**Those indicating need for medical attention only if they continue or are bothersome**
Incidence more frequent
*Tenderness, redness, or induration at the site of injection, lasting 1 or 2 days* (tenderness, redness, or hard lump at place of injection)—incidence approximately 30%

Incidence less frequent
*Fever, malaise, and myalgia, starting 6 to 12 hours after administration and persisting 1 or 2 days* (general feeling of discomfort or illness; aches or pains in muscles)—usually attributed to the toxicity of the influenza virus itself (even though it is inactivated)
Note: *Fever, malaise, and myalgia* occur less frequently in adults and more frequently in children and others who have had no exposure to the influenza virus antigens in the vaccine

## Patient Consultation

As an aid to patient consultation, refer to *Advice for the Patient, Influenza Virus Vaccine (Systemic)*.

In providing consultation, consider emphasizing the following selected information (» = major clinical significance):

**Before using this medication**
» Conditions affecting use, especially:
Sensitivity to influenza vaccine or allergy to eggs, sodium bisulfite, thimerosal, gentamicin sulfate, streptomycin sulfate, or other aminoglycosides
Use in children—Use is not recommended for infants up to 6 months of age; for children 6 months to 4 years of age, only the split or subviron type of the split-virus vaccine should be used; for children 4 to 13 years of age, any of the split-virus vaccines (split, subviron, or purified-surface-antigen type) may be used; some side effects of vaccine, such as fever, unusual tiredness or weakness, or aches or pains in muscles, are more common in infants and children, who are usually more sensitive than adults to the effects of the vaccine
Use in the elderly—Elderly persons may develop lower antibody titers after immunization than healthy younger adults and, therefore, may remain susceptible to upper respiratory tract influenza infections; however, vaccine may still be effective in preventing lower respiratory tract involvement or other complications of influenza
Other medical problems, especially severe febrile illness, acute respiratory disease, or history of Guillain-Barré syndrome

**Proper use of this medication**
» Proper dosing

### Side/adverse effects
In 1976, approximately 10 persons out of every one million persons who received the swine flu vaccine that year developed Guillain-Barré syndrome (GBS). This was approximately 6 times the number of unimmunized persons who developed GBS. Persons under 25 years of age had a better chance of not getting GBS than did older persons. GBS causes paralysis that is usually self-limiting and reversible. Most persons with GBS recover completely; however, approximately 5% of persons die. Before 1976, there was no association between GBS and influenza vaccine. Since 1976, there has been no recurrence of GBS associated with influenza vaccination. It is hypothesized that the swine flu virus portion of the 1976 vaccine caused the problem, but this has not been proven. Since 1976, the swine flu virus has not been used in influenza vaccines

Fever, unusual tiredness or weakness, or aches or pains in muscles are more likely to occur in infants and children, who are usually more sensitive to the effects of influenza vaccine

Signs of potential side effects, especially anaphylactic reaction

## General Dosing Information

For children 6 months to 4 years of age, only the split or subviron type of the split-virus vaccine should be used. For children 4 to 13 years of age, any of the split-virus vaccines (split, subviron, or purified-surface-antigen type) may be used. Split-virus vaccines have a lower potential for causing febrile adverse reactions than whole-virus vaccines.

Two doses, 4 weeks apart, are recommended for maximum protection in children under 9 years of age who have not been previously vaccinated. Children who require 2 doses of vaccine should receive the second dose before December.

Adults and children 13 years of age and older experience similar immunogenicity and side effects from either the split-virus vaccines or the whole-virus vaccine.

Elderly patients may develop lower antibody titers after immunization than healthy young adults and, therefore, may remain susceptible to influenza infection of the upper respiratory tract. Nonetheless, influenza vaccine may still be effective in preventing lower respiratory tract involvement or other complications of influenza.

Influenza vaccine is administered by intramuscular injection, preferably into the deltoid muscle of adults and older children or into the anterolateral aspect of the thigh of infants and young children. It should not be injected intravenously. Because data on the immunogenicity and side effects of the influenza vaccine have been obtained primarily from administration of the vaccine by the deltoid route, high-risk adults and older children should be immunized using this route of administration whenever possible.

Before being immunized, persons suspected of having a hypersensitivity to egg protein should have a scratch test or an intradermal injection (0.05 to 0.1 mL) of vaccine diluted 1:100 in sterile saline or 1:100 in 0.03% Albumin Human USP. The resulting dilution is more stable when Albumin Human USP is used. Persons with a positive skin reaction should not receive immunization with the vaccine.

Based on epidemiological experience, for most of the U.S. November is the optimal time for administration of influenza vaccine through organized vaccination campaigns in chronic-care facilities, worksites, and other places where high-risk persons are routinely accessible. However, vaccination in September or October is desirable if warranted by regional experience (e.g., Alaska), upon hospital discharge of high-risk patients, or during routine medical visits in September or October if a return visit is unlikely. In addition, the prediction of an influenza epidemic should motivate health care providers to initiate immunization regardless of the time of year.

Influenza vaccine may be given right up to the time that influenza virus activity is documented in a region, and even thereafter. However, since the vaccine takes approximately 2 weeks to produce antibodies, chemoprophylaxis may be indicated also during this time for certain high-risk patients.

Influenza vaccine, either whole-virus vaccine or split-virus vaccines, may be administered concurrently with the following, using separate body sites, separate syringes, and the precautions that apply to each immunizing agent:
• Polysaccharide vaccines, such as haemophilus b polysaccharide vaccine, haemophilus b conjugate vaccine, meningococcal polysaccharide vaccine, or pneumococcal polyvalent vaccine.
• Diphtheria and/or tetanus toxoid.
• Diphtheria and tetanus toxoids and pertussis vaccine (DTaP or DTP).
• Live virus vaccines, such as measles, mumps, and/or rubella vaccines.

• Poliovirus vaccines (oral [OPV], inactivated [IPV], or enhanced-potency inactivated [enhanced-potency IPV]).
• Immune globulin and disease-specific immune globulins.
• Hepatitis B recombinant or plasma-derived vaccine, or other inactivated vaccines, except cholera, typhoid, and plague. It is recommended that cholera, typhoid, and plague vaccines be administered on separate occasions because of these vaccines' propensity to cause side/adverse effects.

**For treatment of adverse effects**
Recommended treatment includes:
• For mild hypersensitivity reaction—Administering antihistamines and, if necessary, corticosteroids.
• For severe hypersensitivity or anaphylactic reaction—Administering epinephrine. Antihistamines and/or corticosteroids may also be administered as required.

# Parenteral Dosage Forms

## INFLUENZA VIRUS VACCINE (Injection—Split virus [purified-surface-antigen type]) USP

**Usual adult and adolescent dose**
Influenza prophylaxis—
Adults and children 13 years of age and older: Intramuscular, 0.5 mL as a single dose of the split-virus vaccine.

**Usual pediatric dose**
Influenza prophylaxis—
Infants up to 6 months of age: Use is not recommended.
Infants 6 months to 4 years of age: Safety and efficacy have not been established.
Children 4 to 9 years of age: Intramuscular, 0.5 mL of the split-virus vaccine. Two doses of 0.5 mL each, 4 weeks apart, are recommended for maximum protection in persons under 9 years of age who have not been previously vaccinated.
Children 9 to 13 years of age: Intramuscular, 0.5 mL as a single dose of the split-virus vaccine.

**Usual geriatric dose**
See *Usual adult and adolescent dose.*

**Strength(s) usually available**
U.S.—
Each 0.5-mL dose contains the proportions, and not less than the microgram amounts, of hemagglutinin antigens (mcg HA) representative of the specific components recommended for the present year's vaccine (Rx) [*Fluvirin* (thimerosal 0.01%)].
Canada—
Not commercially available.

**Packaging and storage**
Store between 2 and 8 °C (35 and 46 °F), unless otherwise specified by manufacturer. Do not freeze.

**Stability**
Potency is destroyed by freezing; vaccine that has been frozen should not be used.

**Auxiliary labeling**
• Shake well.
• Do not freeze.

## INFLUENZA VIRUS VACCINE (Injection—Split virus [split or subviron type]) USP

**Usual adult and adolescent dose**
Influenza prophylaxis—
Adults and children 13 years of age and older: Intramuscular, 0.5 mL as a single dose of the split-virus vaccine.

**Usual pediatric dose**
Influenza prophylaxis—
Infants up to 6 months of age: Use is not recommended.
Infants 6 to 36 months of age: Intramuscular, 0.25 mL of the split-virus vaccine. Dose should be repeated in four or more weeks if the patient has not been previously vaccinated.
Children 3 to 9 years of age: Intramuscular, 0.5 mL of the split-virus vaccine. Two doses of 0.5 mL each, 4 weeks apart, are recommended for maximum protection in children under 9 years of age who have not been previously vaccinated.
Children 9 to 13 years of age: Intramuscular, 0.5 mL as a single dose of the split-virus vaccine.

**Usual geriatric dose**
See *Usual adult and adolescent dose.*

**Strength(s) usually available**
U.S.—
Each 0.5-mL dose contains the proportions, and not less than the microgram amounts, of hemagglutinin antigens (mcg HA) representative of the specific components recommended for the present year's vaccine (Rx) [*Fluogen* (streptomycin sulfate; sodium bisulfite; 1:10,000 thimerosal); *FluShield* (1:10,000 thimerosal; gentamicin sulfate); *Fluzone* (1:10,000 thimerosal); GENERIC (may contain gentamicin sulfate; 1:10,000 thimerosal)].
Canada—
Each 0.5-mL dose contains the proportions, and not less than the microgram amounts, of hemagglutinin antigens (mcg HA) representative of the specific components recommended for the present year's vaccine (Rx) [*Fluviral S/F* (thimerosal 0.01%); *Fluzone* (thimerosal)].
Note: Gentamicin sulfate, streptomycin sulfate, neomycin, polymyxin, and/or sodium bisulfite may be used in the production of influenza vaccine. By current assay procedures, concentrations of these products are not detectable in the final vaccine; however, they may still be able to cause hypersensitivity reactions in susceptible persons.

**Packaging and storage**
Store between 2 and 8 °C (35 and 46 °F), unless otherwise specified by manufacturer. Do not freeze.

**Stability**
Potency is destroyed by freezing; vaccine that has been frozen should not be used.

**Auxiliary labeling**
• Shake well.
• Do not freeze.

## INFLUENZA VIRUS VACCINE (Injection—Whole virus) USP

**Usual adult and adolescent dose**
Influenza prophylaxis—
Adults and children 13 years of age and older: Intramuscular, 0.5 mL as a single dose of the whole-virus vaccine.

**Usual pediatric dose**
Influenza prophylaxis—
Use is not recommended in children up to 13 years of age.
Note: Only split-virus influenza vaccines (split, subviron, or purified-surface-antigen type) should be used for children up to 13 years of age because of the vaccines' lower potential for causing febrile adverse reactions when compared to the whole-virus influenza vaccine. None of the influenza virus vaccines is recommended for infants up to 6 months of age.

**Usual geriatric dose**
See *Usual adult and adolescent dose.*

**Strength(s) usually available**
U.S.—
Each 0.5-mL dose contains the proportions, and not less than the microgram amounts, of hemagglutinin antigens (mcg HA) representative of the specific components recommended for the present year's vaccine (Rx) [*Fluzone* (1:10,000 thimerosal)].
Canada—
Each 0.5-mL dose contains the proportions, and not less than the microgram amounts, of hemagglutinin antigens (mcg HA) representative of the specific components recommended for the present year's vaccine (Rx) [*Fluviral* (thimerosal 0.01%); *Fluzone* (thimerosal)].

**Packaging and storage**
Store between 2 and 8 °C (35 and 46 °F), unless otherwise specified by manufacturer. Do not freeze.

**Stability**
Potency is destroyed by freezing; vaccine that has been frozen should not be used.

**Auxiliary labeling**
• Shake well.
• Do not freeze.

# Selected Bibliography

Centers for Disease Control and Prevention. Prevention and control of influenza: recommendations of the Advisory Committee on Immunization Practices (ACIP). MMWR 1996 May 3; 45 (No. RR-5): 1-24.
World Health Organization. WHO announces influenza vaccine formula for 1996/1997. 15 February 1996.

Revised: 07/12/94
Interim revision: 07/13/95; 07/09/96

# INSULIN    Systemic

This monograph includes information on the following: Buffered Insulin Human; Extended Insulin Zinc*; Extended Insulin Zinc, Human; Insulin; Insulin Human; Insulin Zinc; Insulin Zinc, Human; Isophane Insulin; Isophane Insulin, Human; Isophane Insulin, Human, and Insulin Human; Prompt Insulin Zinc*.

**INN:**

Extended Insulin Zinc Suspension—Insulin Zinc Suspension (Crystalline)

Insulin Human Injection—Insulin (Human)

Insulin Zinc Suspension—Insulin Zinc Suspension, Compound

Prompt Insulin Zinc Suspension—Insulin Zinc Suspension (Amorphous)

**BAN:**

Extended Insulin Zinc Suspension—Insulin Zinc Suspension (Crystalline)

Insulin Human Injection—Insulin (Human)

Insulin Zinc Suspension—Insulin Zinc

Isophane Insulin Suspension—Isophane Insulin

Prompt Insulin Zinc Suspension—Insulin Zinc Suspension (Amorphous)

**JAN:**

Extended Insulin Zinc Suspension—Crystalline Insulin Zinc Injection (Aqueous Suspension)

Insulin Human Injection—Insulin Human (Biosynthesis) and Insulin Human (Synthesis)

Isophane Insulin Suspension—Isophane Insulin Injection (Aqueous Suspension)

Insulin Zinc Suspension—Insulin Zinc Injection (Aqueous Suspension) and Insulin Zinc Purified Porcine (Suspension)

Prompt Insulin Zinc Suspension—Amorphous Insulin Zinc Injection (Aqueous Solution)

**VA CLASSIFICATION (Primary/Secondary): HS501/GA900; DX900**

Other commonly used names are: Lente insulin [Insulin Zinc], NPH insulin [Isophane Insulin], Regular insulin [Insulin], Semilente insulin [Prompt Insulin Zinc], Ultralente insulin [Extended Insulin Zinc]

Note: For a listing of dosage forms and brand names by country availability, see *Dosage Forms* section(s). For a listing of brand names for the articles in this monograph, refer to the General Index.

*Not commercially available in the U.S.

## Category

Antidiabetic agent; diagnostic aid (pituitary growth hormone reserve).

## Indications

Note: Bracketed information in the *Indications* section refers to uses that are not included in U.S. product labeling.

**Accepted**

Diabetes mellitus (treatment), including:

Diabetes mellitus, insulin-dependent (IDDM)—Insulin is indicated in the treatment of insulin-dependent diabetes mellitus (Type I diabetes; previously called ketosis-prone, brittle, or juvenile-onset diabetes), which occurs in individuals who produce little or no endogenous insulin. One of two regimens (conventional or intensive therapy) is commonly used to treat this condition. The intensive regimen provides more rigid control of blood glucose than the conventional regimen does, but requires more frequent monitoring and more frequent dosage adjustment, and, unless insulin is administered via an insulin pump, a larger number of injections.

Diabetes mellitus, non–insulin-dependent (NIDDM)—Insulin is indicated in the treatment of certain patients with NIDDM (Type II diabetes; previously known as adult-onset diabetes, maturity-onset diabetes, ketosis-resistant diabetes, or stable diabetes), which occurs in individuals who produce or secrete insufficient quantities of endogenous insulin or who have developed resistance to endogenous insulin. Insulin therapy in NIDDM is reserved for patients whose disease is not controlled by other measures (i.e., diet, exercise, oral antidiabetic agents) or who cannot tolerate oral antidiabetic agents.

Diabetes mellitus, gestational (GDM)

Diabetes mellitus, malnutrition-related or

Diabetes mellitus, other, associated with certain conditions or syndromes, such as:

• Pancreatic disease (congenital absence of the pancreatic islets, transient diabetes of the newborn, functional immaturity of insulin secretion in the neonate, or cystic fibrosis)

• Endocrine disease (endocrine overactivity due to Cushing's syndrome, hyperthyroidism, pheochromocytoma, somatostatinoma, or aldosteronoma; or endocrine underactivity due to hypoparathyroidism-hypocalcemia, type I isolated growth hormone deficiency, or multitropic pituitary deficiency) or

• Genetic syndromes, including inborn errors of metabolism, (glycogen-storage disease type I or insulin-resistant syndromes, such as muscular dystrophies, late onset proximal myopathy, and Huntington's chorea)—Insulin is indicated for the treatment of GDM and for the treatment of diabetes mellitus associated with certain conditions and syndromes uncontrolled by other treatment measures (diet, exercise, and oral antidiabetic agents). Insulin requirements increase eventually during pregnancy for all diabetics. Need for additional exogenous insulin usually stops postpartum for GDM patients due to hormonal and metabolic changes; however, some GDM patients progress to NIDDM or IDDM within 5 to 10 years. Insulin is also used to treat diabetes induced by hormones, medications, or chemicals. Insulin has been added to total parenteral nutrition or glucose solutions in order to facilitate glucose utilization in patients with poor glucose tolerance.

Insulin is also used to treat acute complications associated with diabetes, such as ketoacidosis, significant acidosis, ketosis, hyperglycemic hyperosmolar nonketotic coma, or diabetic coma. Also, temporary insulin dosing for diabetics not using insulin or an increased insulin dose for IDDM or insulin-requiring NIDDM patients may be warranted when these patients are subjected to physical stress (i.e., pregnancy, fever, severe infection, severe burns, major surgery, or other severe trauma).

Combination use of insulin and oral antidiabetic agents in IDDM patients is controversial because many studies have indicated that oral antidiabetic agents are not effective in the treatment of these patients. Some NIDDM patients resistant to sulfonylureas alone may benefit from the combination of low-dose insulin and oral sulfonylurea agents for diabetes; however, resultant weight gain and effects of hyperinsulinemia should be considered. In addition, the combination of metformin and sulfonylurea agents has been used successfully before discontinuation of oral agents and initiation of insulin therapy.

Concentrated insulin (500 USP Insulin Units) is used only to treat insulin-resistant patients needing a high dose (over 200 USP units) of insulin.

[Growth hormone deficiency (diagnosis)][1]—Intravenous regular insulin is used to assess the capacity of the pituitary gland to release growth hormone. Reliable results may require that more than one test using regular insulin be performed or that one additional test be conducted, such as one using arginine. Also, information regarding release of corticotropin from the pituitary can be assessed. A physician experienced in the use of the insulin tolerance test should be present because of the risk of hypoglycemia.

[1]Not included in Canadian product labeling.

## Pharmacology/Pharmacokinetics

**Physicochemical characteristics**

Source—

Bovine: Obtained from the pancreas of oxen; differs from human insulin by 2 amino acids at positions 8 and 10 on the A-chain and from porcine insulin by 1 amino acid at position 30 on the B-chain.

Human: Derived by enzymatic modification of the 1 different amino acid (threonine for alanine) in porcine insulin (semi-synthetic) or derived by microbial synthesis (recombinant DNA process involving genetically engineered *E. coli* or baker's yeast); identical to naturally occurring human insulin; contains 21 amino acids in the A-chain and 30 amino acids in the B-chain.

Porcine: Obtained from pork pancreas; differs from human insulin by 1 amino acid at position 30 on the B-chain.

Molecular weight—

Insulin (beef): 5733.61.

Insulin (pork): 5777.66.

Insulin Human (semisynthetic, biosynthetic): 5807.69.

## Mechanism of action/Effect

Insulin is a polypeptide hormone that controls the storage and metabolism of carbohydrates, proteins, and fats. This activity occurs primarily in the liver, in muscle, and in adipose tissues after binding of the insulin molecules to receptor sites on cellular plasma membranes. Although the mechanisms of insulin's molecular actions in the cellular area are still being explored, it is known that cell membrane transport characteristics, cellular growth, enzyme activation and inhibition, and alterations in protein and fat metabolism are all influenced by insulin. More specifically, insulin promotes uptake of carbohydrates, proteins, and fats in most tissues. Also, insulin influences carbohydrate, protein, and fat metabolism by stimulating protein and free fatty acid synthesis, and by inhibiting release of free fatty acid from adipose cells. Insulin increases active glucose transport through muscle and adipose cellular membranes, and promotes conversion of intracellular glucose and free fatty acid to the appropriate storage forms (glycogen and triglyceride, respectively). Although the liver does not require active glucose transport, insulin increases hepatic glucose conversion to glycogen and suppresses hepatic glucose output. Even though the actions of exogenous insulin are identical to those of endogenous insulin, the ability to negatively affect hepatic glucose output differs because a smaller quantity of exogenous insulin reaches the portal vein.

Antidiabetic—

    Administered insulin substitutes for the lack of endogenous insulin secretion and partially corrects the disordered metabolism and inappropriate hyperglycemia of diabetes mellitus, which are caused by either an absolute deficiency or a reduction in the biologic effectiveness of insulin, or possibly both. Maintenance of good blood glucose control by insulin, which is facilitated by increasing glucose uptake and use, may slow the progression of the serious long-term complications of diabetes.

Diagnostic aid, pituitary growth hormone reserve—

    Intravenous regular insulin stimulates growth hormone secretion by producing hypoglycemia; it is used to evaluate pituitary growth hormone reserve.

## Other actions/effects

Insulin increases the intracellular shift of potassium and magnesium and decreases renal excretion of sodium. Insulin decreases the synthesis of high density lipoprotein (HDL) cholesterol and increases the synthesis of very low density lipoprotein (VLDL) cholesterol in the liver. Insulin increases lipoprotein uptake and utilization in the lactating mammary gland. Also, insulin stimulates activity of and tissue response to the sympathetic nervous system. The growth-promoting action of insulin may contribute to an increase in peripheral vascular resistance through vascular hypertrophy.

| USP Insulin Type | Onset of action† (hrs) | Time to peak† (hrs) | Duration of action† (hrs) |
|---|---|---|---|
| Intravenous Insulin injection U-100 (regular insulin) mixed*, pork, purified pork, biosynthetic human semisynthetic human | $^1/_6$–$^1/_2$ | $^1/_4$–$^1/_2$ | $^1/_2$–1 |
| Subcutaneous Insulin injection U-100 (regular insulin) mixed*, pork, purified pork, biosynthetic human semisynthetic human | $^1/_2$–1 | 2–4 | 5–7 |
| Insulin injection U-500 (regular insulin) purified pork | | | 24‡ |
| Isophane insulin suspension U-100 (NPH insulin) mixed*, purified pork, biosynthetic human | 3–4 | 6–12 | 18–28 |
| Isophane insulin suspension (70%) and insulin injection (30%) U-100 biosynthetic human | $^1/_2$ | 4–8 | 24 |
| Insulin zinc suspension U-100 (lente insulin) mixed*, purified pork, biosynthetic human | 1–3 | 8–12 | 18–28 |

| USP Insulin Type | Onset of action† (hrs) | Time to peak† (hrs) | Duration of action† (hrs) |
|---|---|---|---|
| Extended insulin zinc suspension U-100 (ultralente) mixed*, biosynthetic human | 4–6 | 18–24 | 36 |
| Prompt insulin zinc suspension U-100 (semilente) mixed* | 1–3 | 2–8 | 12–16 |

*Mixed=Mixture of beef and pork insulins.
†Mean values; individual responses vary widely.
‡U-500 strength is absorbed slowly, resulting in a long duration of action.

## Absorption

Rate of subcutaneous and intramuscular insulin absorption is highly variable (up to 50% inter- and intraindividual variability) and is dependent on many factors including insulin formulation, injection site, injection technique, and route of injection. The addition of protamine or zinc to insulin produces a crystallized insulin in suspension that has a longer absorption phase (and a longer duration of action) than dissolved insulin does and is dependent on enzymatic degradation of the suspension at the injection site for absorption. Absorption of regular insulin, when mixed with equal or greater quantities of zinc insulin, may be slowed if the mixture is not injected immediately after preparation. Mixing regular insulin with isophane insulin does not alter the rate of absorption of either. Studies have shown that the absorption rate of human insulins is no different from, or only slightly higher than, the rate for animal insulins. The speed of injection and temperature of insulin do not alter absorption; however, capillary surface area and exercise do affect the intramuscular blood flow and can alter absorption. Exercising the limb into which the insulin was injected within 30 to 40 minutes postinjection may increase insulin absorption (delay of exercise may be warranted). Although longer-acting insulins have less pronounced variability in absorption among injection sites, the absorption rate for 12 USP Units of regular insulin given subcutaneously declined per region as follows: abdominal (87 minutes), deltoid (141 minutes), gluteal (155 minutes), and femoral (164 minutes). Finally, insulin absorption is faster with intramuscular injection than with subcutaneous injection, and is slower with very high insulin concentrations or high dose volumes.

A subcutaneous depot of insulin forms slowly at the injection site when a continuous subcutaneous infusion insulin pump is used, resulting in less variation in insulin availability and a smaller depot than occurs with use of subcutaneous injections. When injection sites are rotated, continued absorption from the first depot usually prevents plasma concentrations from decreasing to subtherapeutic values while another depot is forming.

## Distribution

Distributed into most cells.

## Biotransformation

Insulin—Hepatic and renal.

Isophane or zinc insulins—Split into protamine or zinc and insulin by subcutaneous enzymes prior to absorption.

## Half-life

Insulin—5 to 6 minutes; can be longer in some diabetics. Insulin antibodies, if present, bind to circulating plasma insulin and prolong its biologic half-life.

## Elimination

Renal, 30 to 80%; unchanged insulin is reabsorbed.

# Precautions to Consider

## Cross-sensitivity and/or related problems

Patients intolerant of beef or pork insulins may use the alternative single-source insulin under the direction of their physician. Intolerance of beef insulin is more common than intolerance of pork insulin. Intolerance is often reduced by the use of purified pork insulin, biosynthetic human insulin, or semisynthetic human insulin.

Patients hypersensitive to protamine sulfate also may be hypersensitive to protamine-containing insulins. Patients who have become sensitized to protamine through administration of a protamine-containing insulin are at risk for severe anaphylactoid reactions if protamine sulfate is subsequently administered for reversal of heparin effect.

## Pregnancy/Reproduction

Pregnancy—Insulin does not cross the placenta. However, maternal glucose and maternal insulin antibodies do cross the placenta and can cause fetal hyperinsulinemia and related problems, such as large-for-gestational-age infants and macrosomnia, possibly resulting in a need for early induced or cesarean delivery. Furthermore, high blood glucose concentrations occurring during early pregnancy (5 to 8 weeks gestation) have been associated with a higher incidence of major congenital abnormalities and, later in pregnancy, increased perinatal morbidity and mortality.

Diabetic women must be educated about the necessity of maintaining strict metabolic control before conception and throughout pregnancy, especially during early pregnancy, to significantly decrease the risk of maternal mortality, congenital anomalies, and perinatal morbidity and mortality. A study reported that initial hemoglobin $A_{1c}$ (a measurement of blood glucose control for the preceding 3 months) concentrations of 10% or more, 8 to 9.9%, and below 8% produced infant malformation rates of 35%, 12.9%, and 4.8%, respectively; the malformation rate in infants born to nondiabetic mothers is approximately 2%. Use of insulin rather than oral antidiabetic agents for the treatment of NIDDM and GDM permits maintenance of blood glucose at concentrations as close to normal as possible. Insulin requirements in pregnant diabetic patients are often decreased during the first trimester. Requirements are usually increased in the last 2 trimesters of pregnancy in response to the anti-insulin hormone activity associated with increased concentrations of human placental estrogen, progesterone, chorionic gonadotropin, and prolactin; peripheral insulin resistance due to increasing levels of fatty acids and triglycerides; and increased degradation of insulin by the placenta.

Postpartum—Insulin requirements drop quickly after childbirth, and GDM patients usually no longer need insulin. Inadequately controlled maternal blood glucose late in pregnancy may cause increased insulin production in the fetus resulting in neonatal hypoglycemia. Treatment may be necessary until euglycemic control is established by the neonate.

### Breast-feeding

Insulin is not distributed into breast milk. Problems in humans have not been documented. The insulin requirement in lactating women is reduced because of hormonal changes; in patients with IDDM, insulin requirements during lactation may be up to 27% lower than the patients' pre-pregnancy requirements. Daily monitoring for several months is important until insulin needs stabilize or until insulin is no longer needed.

### Pediatrics

Insulin therapy in pediatric patients is similar to that in other age groups. However, strict intensive insulin therapy is not generally used for this age group because noncompliance may be a problem and because this regimen may be less beneficial before puberty while risks of hypoglycemia may be higher due to higher insulin sensitivity.

### Adolescents

Insulin therapy in adolescents is similar to that in other age groups. Appropriate use of intensive insulin therapy may be beneficial when used cautiously. Diabetic patients have a transient increase in insulin requirement (by approximately 20 to 50%) at puberty during the growth spurt only. Adolescent females usually require more insulin than do adolescent males because of increased insulin resistance; this is thought to be due, in part, to an increased secretion of growth hormone, but not to an increased secretion of sex hormones. Increased growth hormone secretion also may require alteration of the timing of insulin doses to overcome the prominent *dawn phenomenon* of hyperglycemia in diabetic adolescents of both sexes.

### Geriatrics

Insulin therapy in older patients is similar to that in other age groups. However, strict intensive insulin therapy is not generally used. Also, dehydration, which may mask early signs of hypoglycemia and permit development of more severe symptoms; vision problems, which may lead to inaccurate dosage measurement and/or glucose monitoring; shakiness, which may interfere with measurement and self-administration of a dose; and lack of compliance with prescribed diet commonly occur in the elderly and may interfere with control of diabetes. Instructions may be needed to help the patient monitor urine or blood glucose if visual problems are present or early symptoms of hypoglycemia are missing or delayed, a particular problem in this age group. Special devices are available to help administer the insulin dose when help with visual clarity or steadiness is needed.

### Drug interactions and/or related problems

The following drug interactions and/or related problems have been selected on the basis of their potential clinical significance (possible mechanism in parentheses where appropriate)—not necessarily inclusive (» = major clinical significance):

Note: Combinations containing any of the following medications, depending on the amount present, may also interact with this medication.

If the need exists to administer any medications that may affect metabolic or glycemic control of diabetes mellitus, blood glucose concentrations should be monitored by the patient or health care professional. This is particularly important when any medication is added to or removed from an established drug regimen. Subsequent adjustments in diet or insulin dosage or both may be necessary; these adjustments may differ depending on the severity of the diabetes mellitus and other factors.

» Alcohol
   (consumption of moderate or large amounts of alcohol enhances insulin's hypoglycemic effect, increasing the risk of prolonged, severe hypoglycemia, especially under fasting conditions or when liver glycogen stores are low; small amounts of alcohol consumed with meals do not usually present problems)

Anabolic steroids, especially stanozolol, oxandrolone, and methandrostenolone or
Androgens
   (increased tissue sensitivity to insulin and increased tissue resistance to glucagon may occur, resulting in hypoglycemia, especially when insulin resistance is present; a decrease in insulin dose may be required)

Antidiabetic agents, oral, sulfonylurea or
Carbonic anhydrase inhibitors, especially acetazolamide
   (these medications chronically stimulate the pancreatic beta cell to release insulin and increase receptor and tissue sensitivity to insulin; although concurrent use of these medications with insulin may increase the hypoglycemic response, the effect may be unpredictable)

   (sulfonylurea antidiabetic agents have been used concurrently with insulin in treating a select group of NIDDM patients whose condition is not well-controlled with either agent alone; however, the long-term benefit of this use has not been established; many studies have shown there is generally no additional benefit from using sulfonylurea antidiabetic agents for the treatment of IDDM patients)

Anti-inflammatory drugs, nonsteroidal (NSAIDs) or
Salicylates, large doses
   (these medications inhibit synthesis of prostaglandin E [which inhibits endogenous insulin secretion], thereby increasing basal insulin secretion, the response to a glucose load, and the hypoglycemic effect of concurrently administered insulin; dosage adjustment of the NSAID or salicylate and/or insulin may be necessary, especially during and following chronic concurrent use)

» Beta-adrenergic blocking agents, including ophthalmics, if significant systemic absorption occurs
   (beta-adrenergic blocking agents may inhibit insulin secretion, modify carbohydrate metabolism, and increase peripheral insulin resistance, leading to hyperglycemia; however, they may also cause hypoglycemia and block the normal catecholamine-mediated response to hypoglycemia [glycogenolysis and mobilization of glucose], thereby prolonging the time it takes to achieve euglycemia and increasing the risk of a severe hypoglycemic reaction. Selective $beta_1$-adrenergic blocking agents [such as acebutolol, atenolol, betaxolol, bisoprolol, and metoprolol] exhibit the above actions to a lesser extent; however, any of these agents can blunt some of the symptoms of developing hypoglycemia, such as increased heart rate or blood pressure [increased sweating may not be altered], making detection of this complication more difficult)

Chloroquine or
Quinidine or
Quinine
   (concurrent use with insulin may increase the risk of hypoglycemia and increased blood insulin concentrations because of decreased insulin degradation)

» Corticosteroids
   (these agents antagonize insulin's effects by stimulating release of catecholamines, causing hyperglycemia; corticosteroid-induced diabetes can occur in up to 14% of the patients taking systemic corticosteroids for several weeks or with prolonged use of topical corticosteroids, but this condition rarely produces acidosis or ketonuria even with high glucose concentrations; reversal of effects may take several weeks or months; changes in insulin dose may be necessary for diabetics during and following concurrent use)

Diuretics, loop or
Diuretics, thiazide
   (concurrent use with insulin may increase the risk of hyperglycemia because the potassium-depleting effect of these diuretics may inhibit insulin secretion and decrease tissue sensitivity to insulin)

Guanethidine or

Monoamine oxidase (MAO) inhibitors, including furazolidone, procarbazine, and selegiline

(epinephrine release by these agents may cause hyperglycemia; however, chronic use results in hypoglycemia; the mechanism of the latter is unknown but may include stored catecholamine depletion and interference with the compensatory adrenergic response to a fall in blood glucose; a change in dose of insulin before, during, and after treatment with these agents may be necessary)

Hyperglycemia-causing agents, such as:
Calcium channel blockers
Clonidine
Danazol
Dextrothyroxine
Diazoxide, parenteral
Epinephrine
Estrogen
Estrogen-progestin–containing oral contraceptives
Glucagon
Growth hormone
Heparin
Histamine$_2$ receptor antagonists
Marijuana
Morphine
Nicotine
Phenytoin
Sulfinpyrazone
Thyroid hormones

(these medications may change metabolic control of glucose concentrations and, unless the changes can be controlled with diet, may necessitate an increase in the amount or a change in the timing of the insulin dose)

Hypoglycemia-causing agents, such as:
Angiotensin-converting enzyme inhibitors
Bromocriptine
Clofibrate
Ketoconazole
Lithium
Mebendazole
Pyridoxine
Sulfonamides
Theophylline

(these medications may change metabolic control of glucose concentrations and, unless the changes can be controlled with diet, may necessitate a decrease in the amount or a change in the timing of the insulin dose)

Octreotide

(octreotide can cause changes in the counterregulatory hormones secretion [insulin, glucagon, and growth hormone] and slow gastric emptying and gastrointestinal contractility resulting in delayed meal absorption and mild transient hypo- or hyperglycemia in normal and diabetic patients; insulin therapy may need to be reduced in diabetic patients following the initiation of octreotide and monitored for adjustments during and after octreotide treatment)

» Pentamidine

(pentamidine has a toxic effect on pancreatic beta cells resulting in a biphasic effect on glucose concentration, i.e., initial insulin release and hypoglycemia followed by hypoinsulinemia and hyperglycemia with continued use of pentamidine; initially, insulin dose should be reduced, then the dose should be increased with continued use of pentamidine)

Tetracycline

(a delayed onset of increased tissue sensitivity to insulin may occur in diabetic patients; reaction has not appeared in individuals with normal glucose tolerance)

Tobacco, smoking

(may antagonize insulin effects by stimulating release of catecholamines, causing hyperglycemia; also, smoking reduces subcutaneous insulin absorption; dosage reduction of insulin may be necessary when an insulin-dependent diabetic patient suddenly stops smoking)

## Medical considerations/Contraindications

The medical considerations/contraindications included here have been selected on the basis of their potential clinical significance (reasons given in parentheses where appropriate)—not necessarily inclusive (» = major clinical significance).

*Risk-benefit should be considered when the following medical problems exist:*

Note: The following medical problems may necessitate a change in insulin therapy and are not intended as contraindications.

» Diarrhea or
» Gastroparesis or
» Intestinal obstruction or
» Vomiting or
» Other conditions causing delayed food absorption or malabsorption

(vomiting or delayed stomach emptying may require a change in timing of the insulin dose to realign peak action to peak blood glucose concentrations)

Hepatic disease

(insulin requirements are complex, and an increase or decrease of dosage may be needed partly because of modifications in hepatic metabolism of insulin and alterations in hepatic and plasma glucose concentrations)

» Hyperglycemia-causing conditions, such as:
Female hormonal changes or
Fever, high or
Hyperadrenalism, not optimally controlled or
Infection, severe or
Psychological stress

(these conditions may increase blood glucose, increase or change the insulin requirement, and necessitate more frequent blood glucose monitoring)

(insulin requirements may be increased near or during a menstrual cycle and may return to normal after menstruation; also, a change to intravenous insulin administration may be needed during labor when close glucose control is needed)

Hyperthyroidism, not optimally controlled

(hyperthyroidism increases both the activity and the clearance of insulin, making glycemic control difficult until the patient is euthyroid)

» Hypoglycemia-causing conditions, such as:
Adrenal insufficiency, not optimally controlled or
Pituitary insufficiency, not optimally controlled

(these conditions, by reducing blood glucose concentrations, may decrease the insulin requirement and necessitate more frequent blood glucose monitoring)

(also, untreated or not optimally controlled adrenal or pituitary insufficiency may increase tissue sensitivity to insulin and reduce the patient's insulin requirement)

Renal disease

(insulin requirements are complex, and an increase or decrease of dosage may be needed due to modifications in renal clearance of insulin)

Surgery or
Trauma

(hypo- or hyperglycemia may occur depending on the surgery or trauma; a change to intravenous insulin administration may be needed when close glucose control is necessary)

## Patient monitoring

The following may be especially important in patient monitoring (other tests may be warranted in some patients, depending on condition; » = major clinical significance):

» Blood glucose determinations

(the concentration of blood or plasma glucose reflects the current degree of metabolic control and should be routinely monitored by the patient at home and by the physician [every 3 months and more often when patient is not stabilized] to confirm that blood glucose concentration is maintained within agreed upon targets by the selected diet and dosing regimen; particularly important during dosage adjustments. Self monitoring of blood glucose by patient may require testing at multiple times during the day for intensive insulin therapy or once to several times a week for conventional insulin therapy)

(caution in interpreting blood glucose concentrations is needed because normal whole blood glucose values are approximately 15% lower than plasma glucose values. Normal fasting whole blood glucose for adults of all ages is 65 to 95 mg/dL [3.6 to 5.3 mmol/L]. Normal fasting serum glucose is 70 to 105 mg/dL [3.9 to 5.8 mmol/L] for adults younger than 60 years of age and 80 to 115 mg/dL [4.4 to 6.4 mmol/L] for adults 60 years of age and older. For children, normal fasting serum glucose is less than 130 mg/dL [7.2 mmol/L] and fasting whole blood glucose is less than 115 mg/dL [5.6 mmol/L]. For pregnant diabetic women, normal fasting serum glucose is less than 105 mg/dL [5.8 mmol/L] and fasting whole blood glucose is less than 120 mg/dL [6.7 mmol/L]. Goals for intensive insulin therapy are to maintain fasting blood glucose between 60 and 120 mg/dL [3.3 and 6.7 mmol/L] and postprandial blood glucose at less than 180 mg/dL [10 mmol/L], while goals of conventional insulin therapy are based on the absence of symptoms of hyper- and hypoglycemia)

(capillary blood glucose measurement provides important information when done properly, but caution is warranted because of potential errors in technique and readings; it has been suggested that the values be relied upon only if the reported glucose concentration for stable diabetics is between 75 mg/dL and 325 mg/dL [4.12 mmol/L and 17.88 mmol/L, respectively])

Body weight determinations
(significant increase in body weight may require increase in insulin dosage)

Glucose, urine or
Ketones, urine
(if blood glucose concentrations exceed 200 mg/dL [11.1 mmol/L], it may be necessary to monitor urine for the presence of glucose and ketones; normalization of glucose in the urine generally lags quantitatively behind serum glucose concentrations; test methods are generally capable of detecting serum glucose concentrations greater than 180 mg/dL [10 mmol/L])

Glycosylated hemoglobin (hemoglobin $A_{1c}$) determinations
(hemoglobin $A_{1c}$ values [normal whole blood hemoglobin $A_{1c}$ is 4 to 6% of total hemoglobin; specific values are laboratory-dependent] reflect the metabolic control over the preceding 3 months, but assessment of this parameter does not eliminate the need for daily blood glucose monitoring. Hemoglobin $A_{1c}$ is falsely elevated in nonstabilized diabetics when the intermediate precursor is elevated [i.e., in alcoholism] and falsely lowered in conditions of shortened red blood cell lifespan [i.e., in anemia and acute or chronic blood loss] or in patients with hemoglobinopathies [i.e., sickle cell])

pH measurements, serum or
Potassium concentrations, serum
(determinations may be important if patient is hypoglycemic and ketoacidotic)

## Side/Adverse Effects

The following side/adverse effects have been selected on the basis of their potential clinical significance (possible signs and symptoms in parentheses where appropriate)—not necessarily inclusive:

**Those indicating need for medical attention**
Incidence more frequent
  *Hypoglycemia—mild, including nocturnal hypoglycemia* (anxiety; behavior change, similar to drunkenness; blurred vision; cold sweats; confusion; cool pale skin; difficulty in concentrating; drowsiness; excessive hunger; fast heartbeat; headache; nausea; nervousness; nightmares; restless sleep; shakiness; slurred speech; unusual tiredness or weakness); *hypoglycemia—severe* (convulsions or coma); *weight gain*

Note: The occurrence of a recent episode of *hypoglycemia* may lessen the symptoms of a second episode. In children and the elderly, *hypoglycemia* symptoms are variable and harder to identify. Furthermore, *nocturnal hypoglycemia* may be asymptomatic in 33% or more of affected patients. Also, rebound hyperglycemia may appear from $^{1}/_{2}$ to 24 hours after moderate to severe hypoglycemia (*Somogyi phenomenon*).

Hypoglycemic episodes, including severe hypoglycemic coma, occur 3 times more frequently with intensive insulin therapy than with conventional therapy.

*Weight gain* of 120% above ideal weight (mean of 4.6 kg after 5 years of treatment) is experienced by 12.7 patients per 100 patient-years during intensive insulin therapy and by 9.3 patients per 100 patient-years during conventional insulin therapy.

Incidence rare
  *Edema* (swelling of face, fingers, feet, or ankles); *lipoatrophy at injection site* (depression of the skin at the injection site); *lipohypertrophy at injection site* (thickening of skin tissues at the injection site)

Note: *Edema* due to sodium retention caused by insulin is reversible over several days to a week after euglycemic recovery from severe hyperglycemia or ketoacidosis.

The risk of *lipohypertrophy* may be decreased by rotating injection sites; risk of *lipoatrophy* may be reduced by injecting insulin into the periphery of the atrophic site in order to restore subcutaneous adipose tissue.

## Patient Consultation

As an aid to patient consultation, refer to *Advice for the Patient, Insulin (Systemic)*.

In providing consultation, consider emphasizing the following selected information (» = major clinical significance):

**Before using this medication**
» Conditions affecting use, especially:
    Allergy or local skin sensitivity to insulins
    Pregnancy—Importance of controlling and monitoring blood glucose to meet changing needs for insulin during and after pregnancy and to prevent maternal and fetal problems, including fetal macrosomnia, anomalies, and hyperglycemia; alerting physician to plans before becoming pregnant when possible
    Breast-feeding—Insulin is not distributed into breast milk; however, the maternal requirement for insulin is less during breast-feeding because of hormonal changes; checking blood glucose every day for several months to help determine variable insulin dosing needs
    Use in children—Use in children is similar to use in other age groups. However, prepubertal children have increased risk of hypoglycemia because they have greater sensitivity to insulin than do pubertal children
    Use in adolescents—Use in adolescents is similar to use in other age groups. However, insulin needs increase by 20–50% at puberty and decrease afterwards; girls may need higher insulin doses than boys
    Use in the elderly—Risk of hypoglycemia is increased in elderly patients. Special counseling with emphasis on hydration, diet, and exercise may be necessary because of the greater risk of hypoglycemia in this age group. Special training and equipment are available to help overcome these problems
    Other medications, especially alcohol, beta-adrenergic blocking agents, corticosteroids, or pentamidine
    Other medical problems, especially adrenal insufficiency, pituitary insufficiency, or other conditions causing hypoglycemia, diarrhea, gastroparesis, intestinal obstruction, vomiting, or other conditions causing delayed food absorption; female hormonal changes, high fever, hyperadrenalism, psychological distress, severe infection, or other conditions causing hyperglycemia

**Proper use of this medication**
» Understanding what is meant by source of insulin (beef and pork, pork, mixed insulins, and human) and only buying insulin derived from the source and of the type and strength that are prescribed; otherwise, consulting physician
» Selecting syringe of proper units of measure for insulin capacity; syringe should be made to measure insulin in units to facilitate accurate dose measurement; a $^{3}/_{10}$ cc syringe measures up to 30 USP Units, a $^{1}/_{2}$ cc syringe measures up to 50 USP Units, and a 1 cc syringe measures up to 100 USP Units
    Carefully selecting and rotating injection sites, following physician's recommendations
» Proper preparation of medication
    Washing hands with soap and water
    Measuring 1 type of insulin per dose
    Measuring and mixing 2 types of insulin per dose
» Proper administration technique
*Using various injection devices*
» Carefully reading patient instruction sheet contained in insulin or device package
» Disposing of syringes by separating needle from syringe, capping or clipping needle, and disposing in puncture-resistant container
    Understanding how to use insulin in insulin devices, such as automatic injector, continuous subcutaneous insulin infusion pump, disposable and nondisposable syringes, insulin pen devices, and insulin spray injector
» Compliance with therapy, including alternative dosing for changes in diet and exercise or sick day management
» Proper dosing
» Proper storage

**Precautions while using this medication**
» Regular visits to physician to check progress, especially during the first few weeks of treatment
» Carefully following special instructions of health care team:
    Discussing use of alcohol
    Discussing plans to stop chronic smoking of tobacco
    Not taking other medications unless discussed with physician
    Getting counseling for family to help assist diabetic; also, special counseling for pregnancy planning and contraception

> Discussing travel arrangements, including transporting insulin and carrying medical history and extra supplies of insulin and syringes

» Preparing for and knowing what to do in case of an emergency by carrying medical history and current drug list, wearing medical identification, and keeping nonexpired glucagon kit and needles, quick acting sugar, and having extra needed medical supplies nearby

» Recognizing symptoms of hypoglycemia

» Recognizing what brings on symptoms of hypoglycemia, such as delaying or missing a meal, exercising more than usual, drinking significant amounts of alcohol, taking certain medicines, using too much insulin, sickness including vomiting or diarrhea

» Knowing what to do if symptoms of hypoglycemia occur, such as using glucagon, eating glucose tablets or gel, corn syrup, honey, or sugar cubes, or drinking fruit juice, nondiet soft drink, or dissolved sugar in water; also, eating small snack, such as cheese and crackers, milk, or half sandwich when scheduled meal is longer than 1 hour away; not eating foods high in fat, such as chocolate, since fat slows gastric emptying

» Recognizing symptoms of hyperglycemia and ketoacidosis:

     Blurred vision
     Drowsiness
     Dry mouth
     Flushed, dry skin
     Fruit-like breath odor
     Increased urination (frequency and volume)
     Ketones in urine
     Loss of appetite
     Somnolence (sleepiness)
     Stomachache, nausea, or vomiting
     Tiredness
     Troubled breathing (rapid and deep)
     Unconsciousness
     Unusual thirst

» Recognizing what brings on symptoms of hyperglycemia, such as fever or infection; not taking enough insulin; skipping an insulin dose; exercising less than usual; taking certain medicines; overeating or not following meal plan

» Knowing what to do if symptoms of hyperglycemia occur, such as checking blood glucose and increasing the insulin dose (short term for supplementary or anticipatory doses) according to the individualized dosing schedule developed; contacting physician for more permanent dose changes; changing only 1 type of insulin dose (usually the first dose); anticipating how one change in an insulin dose affects other doses of the day; delaying a meal if blood glucose concentration exceeds 200 mg/dL (11.1 mmol/L); checking with physician when blood glucose concentration is above 240 mg/dL (13.3 mmol/L); not exercising when blood glucose concentration is above 240 mg/dL (13.3 mmol/L); or being hospitalized if ketoacidosis or coma occurs

### Side/adverse effects

Signs of potential side effects, especially mild hypoglycemia, including nocturnal; severe hypoglycemia; weight gain; edema; lipoatrophy or lipohypertrophy at injection site

## General Dosing Information

In the United States, the potency of insulin is expressed in terms of USP Insulin Units or USP Insulin Human Units. Bovine or porcine insulin contains not less than 26 USP Insulin Units per mg of insulin on the dried basis. Human insulin contains not less than 27.5 USP Insulin Human Units per mg of insulin on the dried basis. International Units cannot be compared directly to USP Units because the reference standards and the methodologies for manufacturing during are different.

It is generally not recommended that patients whose diabetes is well-controlled with animal insulins automatically be switched to human insulins. Human insulins may not offer any significant advantage over the highly purified pork insulins, with the exception of reduced antibody levels, which may be a consideration for some patients, especially children, young adults, patients who are pregnant or considering pregnancy, patients with allergies, or patients using insulin intermittantly. Patients should be informed of the possible need for dosage adjustment during the first 1 to 2 weeks following a change in the source (bovine and porcine, porcine, or human) of their insulin products and advised not to make such a change without first consulting their physicians.

Transferring patients from oral hypoglycemic agents to insulin can be immediate, although blood glucose concentrations should be evaluated for several days following the change and the prolonged effects of

chlorpropamide should be considered when determining the insulin dose.

The vial of insulin must not be shaken hard before being used. Frothing or bubble formation can cause an incorrect dose. Contents are mixed well by rolling the bottle slowly between the palms of the hands or by gently tipping the bottle over a few times. Insulin should not be used if it looks lumpy or grainy, or sticks to the bottle. Also, regular insulin should not be used if it becomes viscous or cloudy; only clear, colorless solutions should be used.

Dilution of insulin preparations generally should be avoided. However, some pediatric doses may be too small to measure accurately. If needed, diluting from U-100 to U-10 has been suggested to aid in accurate dosing for very small doses in pediatric patients. Such dilutions are stable for 2 months when stored at 4 °C (39 °F) or until the date of expiration of the insulin, whichever occurs first. Occasionally insulin must be diluted to avoid crystallization in the catheters when it is administered as a low-dose infusion via an insulin pump. In these rare cases, dilution should be performed aseptically in a laminar flow hood using diluents and mixing vials provided or recommended by the manufacturer. The differences in strength, dosage volume, and expiration date should be clearly labeled by the pharmacist and emphasized to the patient. If insulin needs to be diluted during an emergency and the diluents are not readily available, 0.9% sodium chloride injection without preservative may be used for dilution of small insulin doses. However, these solutions are not stable and should be used promptly. Stinging or burning at the site of injection may also occur due to the lower pH of these solutions.

Different types of insulin are sometimes mixed in the syringe in proportions ordered by the physician in order to achieve a more accurate matching of insulin availability to the patient's requirements in a single dose. If insulins are to be mixed, several factors should be considered:

• Each patient should always follow the same sequence of mixing the separate insulin preparations. As a general rule, regular insulin should be drawn first to avoid contamination and clouding of the vial of regular insulin by the other insulin. A mixture of regular insulin and another insulin will have a longer duration of action than does regular insulin alone.

• Insulin zinc, prompt insulin zinc, and extended insulin zinc may be mixed in any proportion without loss of the characteristics of the individual insulins. Such mixtures are stable for up to 18 months.

• Unbuffered regular insulin and isophane insulin may be mixed in any proportion in a syringe and stored upright if possible. The prefilled syringe can be used immediately, stored at room temperature and used within 14 days, or stored in a refrigerator for use within 3 weeks. Mixtures containing buffered regular insulin should be used immediately.

• Mixing unbuffered regular insulin and insulin zinc insulins (lente, semilente, and ultralente) is not recommended because the excess zinc in the insulin zinc insulin can form an extra zinc insulin complex with the regular insulin. This can lengthen the insulin's duration of action and give unpredictable clinical results. However, if these insulins are combined, it is recommended that the mixture be used immediately.

• Phosphate buffered regular insulin or isophane insulins should not be mixed with insulin zinc insulins. Zinc phosphate may precipitate from the mixture, which can shorten the expected duration of action and provide unpredictable clinical results.

• Phosphate buffered regular insulin should not be mixed with any other insulin when used in an external insulin infusion pump because of the potential problem of precipitation.

After receiving insulin at first diagnosis of IDDM, 20 to 30% of diabetics appear to normalize for a few weeks or months (called the honeymoon phase). Some clinicians continue insulin treatment in small doses of 0.2 to 0.5 USP Units per kg of body weight during this time.

Conventional and intensive insulin therapies are individualized insulin regimens that provide different levels of blood glucose control. Conventional therapy consists of 1 or 2 insulin injections a day and daily self-monitoring of urine or blood glucose, but not daily adjustments of insulin dose. Intensive insulin therapy provides tighter blood glucose control via administration of 3 or more injections a day or by use of an insulin pump. Also, adjustments of insulin dose according to the results of self-monitoring of blood glucose determinations are performed at least 4 times a day and before anticipated dietary intake and exercise. Close glucose control has been proven to delay the onset and slow the progression of diabetic retinopathy, nephropathy, and neuropathy. The dosage and the timing of administration of insulin can vary greatly and must therefore be determined for each individual patient by the attending physician. Matching the patient's specific insulin needs over a 24-hour period through the use of short-acting and longer-acting preparations may decrease long-term complications of diabetes mellitus.

If a pattern of metabolic noncontrol ensues (blood glucose concentrations changing for 3 days), the total daily insulin dose is usually adjusted by changing only 1 type of insulin and only 1 segment of the daily dose; the first preprandial dose is the one most commonly changed because it more prominently affects the other doses of the day.

Insulin requirements may change with diet or physical activity. Algorithms can be developed to aid a patient with supplemental or anticipatory insulin dosing needs based on the patient's sensitivity to insulin. Supplemental doses of regular insulin can be used to correct excessive preprandial blood glucose concentrations after the basic dose of insulin is established. Anticipatory insulin doses are based on anticipated dietary or physical activity changes. Patients should be cautioned against exercising if the blood glucose concentration exceeds 240 mg/dL (13.3 mmol/L), or when a condition exists that causes low glucagon stores, because of the increased risk of secondary hyperglycemia due to exercise.

Additional low doses of regular insulin (1 to 2 USP Units for each 30 to 40 mg/dL [1.7 to 2.2 mmol/L] incremental rise above the target blood glucose concentration) every 3 to 4 hours may be needed on sick days. Patients should be warned to inform the physician if the concentration remains above 240 mg/dL (13.3 mmol/L) after 3 supplementary insulin doses or if symptoms of ketoacidosis develop.

The patient should always use only one brand or type of syringe and should consult the physician before changing brands or syringe types. Among different brands or syringe types, the unmeasured volume between the needle point and the bottom calibration on the syringe barrel (called dead space) may differ enough to cause improper dosage.

The use of a disposable syringe and needle to administer more than one injection is controversial. Although USP medical advisory panels do not recommend this practice, it must be recognized that some patients reuse disposable syringes and needles because of economic constraints. Where this is occurring, it must be emphasized that the syringe and needle be used only for that particular patient, the needle should be wiped with alcohol, and the needle's cap replaced after each use. Also, the syringe and needle should be reused only for a limited number of injections. Disposable syringes and needles should not be reused on a continuing basis.

### For intravenous infusion
Regular insulin (Insulin Injection USP and Insulin Human Injection USP) in the 100-USP-Unit concentration is the only insulin type suitable for intravenous administration.

Insulin can be adsorbed to the surfaces of glass and plastic intravenous infusion containers (including PVC, ethylene vinyl acetate, and polyethylene). Adsorption is unpredictable and the clinical significance is uncertain. Recommendations for minimizing adsorption include adding 0.35% serum albumin human or approximately 5 mL of the patient's blood or using a syringe pump with a short cannula. For admixtures of insulin greater than 100 USP Units per 500 mL of intravenous solution, decant 50 mL of intravenous solution containing insulin through the administration apparatus and store for 30 minutes before using for optimal results. Afterwards, insulin dosage should be adjusted to meet patient's targeted blood glucose concentration. Regular insulin is compatible with dextrose in water, sodium chloride 0.9%, and combinations of these.

### For continuous subcutaneous insulin infusion pump
Generally, buffered regular insulin is used in insulin pumps, although unbuffered regular insulin has been used. The phosphate-buffered regular insulins are less likely to crystallize and block insulin pump catheters and are preferred over unbuffered regular insulin. Following insulin pump manufacturers' recommendations and suggested maintenance procedures is important to ensure optimal performance and to avoid problems, such as insulin adhesion or clogging. Consult individual manufacturer's package inserts.

When initiating a continuous subcutaneous insulin infusion with an insulin pump, a priming dose may be needed. Without an initial priming dose, the depot forms at a very slow rate. Pumps with a short pulse-rate interval have little superiority over pumps with a longer interval in relation to the depot formation. An additional priming dose is not necessary when the infusion site is changed. Absorption of insulin from the depot at the first site continues after discontinuation of the infusion, preventing insulin concentrations from decreasing to subtherapeutic values while another depot is forming at the new site.

### For treatment of adverse effects and/or overdose
Recommended treatment may include:
- For mild to moderate hypoglycemia—
  —Treating with immediate ingestion of a source of sugar, such as glucose gel, glucose tablets, fruit juice, corn syrup, non-diet soda, honey, sugar cubes, or table sugar dissolved in water. A frequently used source of sugar is a glassful of orange juice containing 2 or 3 teaspoonfuls of table sugar.
  —Documenting blood glucose and rechecking in 15 minutes.
  —Counseling patient to seek medical assistance promptly.
- For severe hypoglycemia or acute overdose, including coma—
  —Need for patient to obtain emergency medical assistance immediately.
  —Immediately treating with 50 mL of 50% dextrose given intravenously to stabilize, then administering a continuous infusion of 5 to 10% dextrose in water to maintain slight hyperglycemia (approximately 100 mg/dL blood glucose concentration) for up to 12 days. A nondiabetic adult usually exhibits a higher maximal hypoglycemic effect from insulin than does a diabetic adult. It is important to note that oral glucose cannot be relied upon to maintain euglycemia because 60% of an oral glucose dose is stored as hepatic glycogen with only 15% left for brain utilization and 15% for insulin-dependent tissues.
  —Glucagon, 1 to 2 mg intramuscular, is useful for fast onset of action to mobilize hepatic glucose stores but may be ineffective or variable in its effect if glycogen stores are depleted.
  —Monitoring vital signs, arterial blood gases, blood glucose, and serum electrolytes (especially calcium, potassium, and sodium) as required. Initially, blood glucose concentrations should be monitored as frequently as every 1 to 3 hours. Blood urea nitrogen and serum creatinine concentrations should also be obtained.
- Cerebral edema—Managed with mannitol and dexamethasone.
- Hypokalemia—Managed with potassium supplements.

Other supportive measures should also be employed as needed.

---

### BUFFERED INSULIN HUMAN

## Parenteral Dosage Forms
Note: Bracketed uses in the *Dosage Forms section* refer to categories of use and/or indications that are not included in U.S. product labeling.

### BUFFERED INSULIN HUMAN INJECTION
**Usual adult and adolescent dose**
Insulin-dependent diabetes mellitus (IDDM)—
  Initial:
    Subcutaneous or continuous subcutaneous insulin infusion, a total insulin dose, using one or more types of insulin, is 0.5 to 1.2 USP Insulin Human Units per kg of body weight a day in divided doses—taking body fat, blood glucose, and insulin sensitivity also under consideration. A few patients will require less than 0.5 USP Insulin Human Unit per kg of body weight a day. Dose titration to a targeted blood glucose goal is achieved over several days; a change in total daily insulin dose does not usually exceed 10% of the existing total daily insulin dose.
    When using a continuous subcutaneous insulin infusion pump, the basal insulin dose (usually forty to sixty percent of the total insulin daily dose) is divided into a dose that can be continuously infused subcutaneously over twenty-four hours. Also, a premeal injection (also, forty to sixty percent of total insulin dose) can be delivered preprogrammed or manually by the patient through the insulin pump.
    When using subcutaneous injections, regular human insulin is usually injected in low doses, e.g., less than 10 USP Insulin Human Units a dose.
    Both subcutaneous injections and premeal injections of regular human insulin using a continuous subcutaneous insulin infusion pump generally are given fifteen to thirty minutes before one or more meals and/or a bedtime snack.
  Maintenance:
    Subcutaneous or continuous subcutaneous insulin infusion, dosage must be determined by the physician, based on blood glucose concentrations.
Non–insulin-dependent diabetes mellitus (NIDDM)—
  Initial:
    Subcutaneous, a total insulin dose, using one or more types of insulin, may vary from 5 to 10 USP Insulin Human Units per day to 0.7 to 2.5 USP Insulin Human Units per kg of body weight a day in divided doses—taking body fat, blood glucose, and insulin sensitivity into consideration. Dose titration to a targeted blood glucose goal is achieved over several days with changes of no more than 2 to 6 USP Insulin Human Units a

day in the existing total daily insulin dose; again, with consideration of body weight. Very insulin-resistant patients using large doses, 200 USP Insulin Human Units or greater, may need to use a concentrated regular insulin (U-500) instead. Regular human insulin is usually given in low doses, i.e., often less than 10 USP Insulin Human Units a dose, fifteen or thirty minutes before one or more meals and/or a bedtime snack.

Maintenance:
Subcutaneous, dosage must be determined by the physician, based on blood glucose concentrations.

Gestational diabetes mellitus—
Subcutaneous, dosage must be determined by the physician, based on blood glucose concentrations and gestational duration.

Diabetes mellitus, other, associated with certain conditions or syndromes—
Subcutaneous, dosage must be determined by the physician, based on body weight and blood glucose concentrations.

Note: For treatment of diabetic ketoacidosis, an optional loading dose of 0.15 USP Insulin Human Unit per kg of body weight is given intravenously, followed by 0.1 USP Insulin Human Unit per kg of body weight per hour by continuous infusion. The rate of insulin infusion should be decreased when the plasma glucose concentration reaches 300 mg per dL. Infusion of 5% dextrose injection should be started separately from the insulin infusion when plasma glucose concentration reaches 250 mg per dL. Thirty minutes before discontinuing the insulin infusion, an appropriate dose of insulin should be injected subcutaneously; intermediate-acting insulin has been recommended. Alternatively, a loading dose of 0.5 USP Insulin Human Unit per kg of body weight is injected intramuscularly, followed by 0.1 USP Insulin Human Unit per kg of body weight injected intramuscularly every hour until the blood glucose concentration reaches 300 mg per dL. Then to maintain blood glucose concentration at 250 mg per dL, 0.1 USP Insulin Human Unit per kg of body weight is injected intramuscularly every 2 hours as needed. With either type of insulin administration, capillary blood glucose monitoring should be followed at least hourly and the insulin dose adjusted accordingly.

Insulin requirements may change during illness or events causing psychological or physical stress. Dosage changes for patients receiving conventional therapy should be determined by the physician, based on each patient's needs and insulin sensitivity. Patients receiving intensive therapy may adjust individual doses to compensate for anticipated changes in diet or exercise but should consult a physician if the permitted adjustments are inadequate and/or glucose monitoring indicates the need for a permanent change in the daily dose.

Some patients experience a honeymoon phase after initial therapy and lose their requirement for insulin altogether or require much less for a limited period of time (several months to several years).

Adolescents during puberty may require an increase in their total daily insulin dose.

[Diagnostic aid (pituitary growth hormone reserve)][1]—
Intravenous, 0.05 to 0.15 USP Insulin Human Unit per kg of body weight as a single rapid injection.

**Usual pediatric dose**
Antidiabetic—
Subcutaneous, dosage must be determined by the physician, based on body weight and blood glucose concentrations.

**Strength(s) usually available**
U.S.—
100 USP Insulin Human Units per mL (OTC) [*Velosulin BR* (semisynthetic; phosphate buffered)].
Canada—
100 USP Insulin Human Units per mL (OTC) [*Velosulin Human* (semisynthetic; phosphate buffered)].

**Packaging and storage**
Store between 2 and 8 °C (36 and 46 °F). Protect from freezing.

**Stability**
Do not use if cloudy, discolored, or unusually viscous.

**Auxiliary labeling**
• Refrigerate.
• Do not freeze.

**Note**
Patients should be advised not to mix phosphate buffered insulin with zinc-containing insulins.

Also, patients should be advised not to mix with any other insulin when using a continuous subcutaneous external insulin pump.

Buffered insulin human is the preferred regular insulin for use in continuous subcutaneous infusion insulin pumps, but may also be injected subcutaneously or intramuscularly with an insulin syringe, or used intravenously. When this insulin is used in a continuous subcutaneous infusion insulin pump, the catheter tubing and the insulin in the reservoir must be changed every 48 hours or the manufacturer's recommendations followed for specific external insulin pumps.

[1]Not included in Canadian product labeling.

## *EXTENDED INSULIN ZINC*

# Parenteral Dosage Forms
## EXTENDED INSULIN ZINC SUSPENSION (ULTRALENTE INSULIN) USP
**Usual adult and adolescent dose**
Insulin-dependent diabetes mellitus (IDDM)—
Initial: Subcutaneous, a total insulin dose is 0.5 to 0.8 USP Insulin Unit per kg of body weight sometimes as a single dose, depending on insulin type, or 0.5 to 1.2 USP Insulin Units per kg of body weight per day in divided doses. Body fat, blood glucose, and insulin sensitivity should also be considered. This total daily dose of insulin may be provided by one or more types of insulin. A few patients will require less than 0.5 USP Insulin Unit per kg of body weight per day. Dose titration to a targeted blood glucose goal is achieved over several days; a change in total daily insulin dose does not usually exceed 10% of the existing total daily insulin dose. Extended insulin zinc is given once or twice a day thirty to sixty minutes before a meal and/or a bedtime snack.
Maintenance: Subcutaneous, dosage must be determined by the physician, based on blood glucose concentrations.

Non–insulin-dependent diabetes mellitus (NIDDM)—
Initial: Subcutaneous, a total insulin dose may vary from 5 to 10 USP Insulin Units per day to 0.7 to 2.5 USP Insulin Units per kg of body weight per day—taking body fat, blood glucose, and insulin sensitivity also under consideration. This total daily dose of insulin may be provided by one or more types of insulin and, depending on insulin type, may be given as a single dose or as divided doses. Dose titration to a targeted blood glucose goal is achieved over several days with changes from the existing total daily insulin dose of no more than 2 to 6 USP Insulin Units a day; again, body weight should be considered. Very insulin-resistant patients using large doses, 200 USP Insulin Units or greater, may need to use a concentrated regular insulin (U-500) instead. Extended insulin zinc is given once or twice a day thirty or sixty minutes before a meal and/or a bedtime snack.
Maintenance: Subcutaneous, dosage must be determined by the physician, based on blood glucose concentrations.

Gestational diabetes mellitus—
Subcutaneous, dosage must be determined by the physician, based on blood glucose concentrations and gestational duration.

Diabetes mellitus, other, associated with certain conditions or syndromes—
Subcutaneous, dosage must be determined by the physician, based on body weight and blood glucose concentrations.

Note: Insulin requirements may change during illness or events causing psychological or physical stress. Dosage changes for patients receiving conventional therapy should be determined by the physician, based on each patient's needs and insulin sensitivity. Patients receiving intensive therapy may adjust individual doses to compensate for anticipated changes in diet or exercise but should consult a physician if the permitted adjustments are inadequate and/or glucose monitoring indicates the need for a permanent change in the daily dose.

Some patients experience a honeymoon phase after initial therapy and lose their requirement for insulin altogether or require much less for a limited period of time (several months to several years).

Adolescents during puberty may require an increase in their total daily insulin dose.

**Usual pediatric dose**
Antidiabetic—
Subcutaneous, dosage must be determined by the physician, based on body weight and blood glucose concentrations.

**Strength(s) usually available**
U.S.—
Not commercially available.

Canada—
100 USP Insulin Units per mL (OTC) [*Ultralente Insulin* (beef and pork)].

**Packaging and storage**
Store between 2 and 8 °C (36 and 46 °F). Protect from freezing.

**Stability**
Do not use if precipitate has become clumped or granular in appearance.

**Auxiliary labeling**
• Shake gently.
• Refrigerate.
• Do not freeze.

**Note**
Extended insulin zinc suspension is sometimes mixed with other insulin types as directed by physician.

---

### EXTENDED INSULIN ZINC, HUMAN

## Parenteral Dosage Forms

### EXTENDED INSULIN ZINC, HUMAN, SUSPENSION

**Usual adult and adolescent dose**
Insulin-dependent diabetes mellitus (IDDM)—
Initial: Subcutaneous, a total insulin dose is 0.5 to 0.8 USP Insulin Human Unit per kg of body weight as a single dose, depending on insulin type, or 0.5 to 1.2 USP Insulin Human Units per kg of body weight per day in divided doses. Body fat, blood glucose, and insulin sensitivity should also be considered. This total daily dose of insulin may be provided by one or more types of insulin. A few patients will require less than 0.5 USP Insulin Human Unit per kg of body weight per day. Dose titration to a targeted blood glucose goal is achieved over several days; a change in total daily insulin dose does not usually exceed 10% of the existing total daily insulin dose. Human extended insulin zinc is given once or twice a day thirty to sixty minutes before a meal and/or a bedtime snack.
Maintenance: Subcutaneous, dosage must be determined by the physician, based on blood glucose concentrations.
Non–insulin-dependent diabetes mellitus (NIDDM)—
Initial: Subcutaneous, a total insulin dose may vary from 5 to 10 USP Insulin Human Units per day to 0.7 to 2.5 USP Human Insulin Units per kg of body weight per day—taking body fat, blood glucose, and insulin sensitivity also under consideration. This total daily dose of insulin may be provided by one or more types of insulin and, depending on insulin type, may be given as a single dose or as divided doses. Dose titration to a targeted blood glucose goal is achieved over several days with changes from the existing total daily insulin dose of no more than 2 to 6 USP Insulin Human Units a day; again, body weight should be considered. Very insulin-resistant patients using large doses, 200 USP Insulin Human Units or greater, may need to use a concentrated regular insulin (U-500) instead. Human extended insulin zinc is given once or twice a day thirty to sixty minutes before a meal and/or a bedtime snack.
Maintenance: Subcutaneous, dosage must be determined by the physician, based on blood glucose concentrations.
Gestational diabetes mellitus—
Subcutaneous, dosage must be determined by the physician, based on blood glucose concentrations and gestational duration.
Diabetes mellitus, other, associated with certain conditions or syndromes—
Subcutaneous, dosage must be determined by the physician, based on body weight and blood glucose concentrations.
Note: Insulin requirements may change during illness or events causing psychological or physical stress. Dosage changes for patients receiving conventional therapy should be determined by the physician, based on each patient's needs and insulin sensitivity. Patients receiving intensive therapy may adjust individual doses to compensate for anticipated changes in diet or exercise but should consult a physician if the permitted adjustments are inadequate and/or glucose monitoring indicates the need for a permanent change in the daily dose.

Some patients experience a honeymoon phase after initial therapy and lose their requirement for insulin altogether or require much less for a limited period of time (several months to several years).

Adolescents during puberty may require an increase in their total daily insulin dose.

**Usual pediatric dose**
Antidiabetic—
Subcutaneous, dosage must be determined by the physician, based on body weight and blood glucose concentrations.

**Strength(s) usually available**
U.S.—
100 USP Insulin Human Units per mL (OTC) [*Humulin U Ultralente* (biosynthetic)].
Canada—
100 USP Insulin Human Units per mL (OTC) [*Humulin-U* (biosynthetic); *Novolin ge Ultralente* (biosynthetic)].

**Packaging and storage**
Store between 2 and 8 °C (36 and 46 °F). Protect from freezing.

**Stability**
Do not use if precipitate has become clumped or granular in appearance.

**Auxiliary labeling**
• Shake gently.
• Refrigerate.
• Do not freeze.

---

### INSULIN

## Parenteral Dosage Forms

Note: Bracketed uses in the *Dosage Forms section* refer to categories of use and/or indications that are not included in U.S. product labeling.

### INSULIN INJECTION (REGULAR INSULIN, CRYSTALLINE ZINC INSULIN) USP

**Usual adult and adolescent dose**
Insulin-dependent diabetes mellitus (IDDM)—
Initial:
Subcutaneous or continuous subcutaneous insulin infusion, a total insulin dose, using one or more types of insulin, is 0.5 to 1.2 USP Insulin Units per kg of body weight a day in divided doses—taking body fat, blood glucose, and insulin sensitivity also under consideration. A few patients will require less than 0.5 USP Insulin Unit per kg of body weight a day. Dose titration to a targeted blood glucose goal is achieved over several days; a change in total daily insulin dose does not usually exceed 10% of the existing total daily insulin dose.
When using a continuous subcutaneous insulin infusion pump, the basal insulin dose (usually forty to sixty percent of the total insulin daily dose) is divided into a dose that can be continuously infused subcutaneously over twenty-four hours. Also, a premeal injection (also, forty to sixty percent of total insulin dose) can be delivered preprogrammed or manually by the patient through the insulin pump.
When using subcutaneous injections, regular insulin is usually injected in low doses, i.e., often less than 10 USP Insulin Units a dose.
Both subcutaneous injections and premeal injections using a continuous subcutaneous insulin infusion pump of regular insulin generally are given fifteen to thirty minutes before one or more meals and/or a bedtime snack.
Maintenance:
Subcutaneous or continuous subcutaneous insulin infusion, dosage must be determined by the physician, based on blood glucose concentrations.
Non–insulin-dependent diabetes mellitus (NIDDM)—
Initial:
Subcutaneous, a total insulin dose, using one or more types of insulin, may vary from 5 to 10 USP Insulin Units per day to 0.7 to 2.5 USP Insulin Units per kg of body weight a day in divided doses—taking body fat, blood glucose, and insulin sensitivity into consideration. Dose titration to a targeted blood glucose goal is achieved over several days with changes from the existing total daily insulin dose of no more than 2 to 6 USP Insulin Units a day; again, with consideration of body weight. Very insulin-resistant patients using large doses, 200 USP Insulin Units or greater, may need to use a concentrated regular insulin (U-500) instead. Regular insulin is usually given in low doses, i.e., often less than 10 USP Insulin Units a dose, fifteen to thirty minutes before one or more meals and/or a bedtime snack.
Maintenance:
Subcutaneous, dosage must be determined by the physician, based on blood glucose concentrations.

Gestational diabetes mellitus—
   Subcutaneous, dosage must be determined by the physician, based on
      blood glucose concentrations and gestational duration.
Diabetes mellitus, other, associated with certain conditions or
   syndromes—
   Subcutaneous, dosage must be determined by the physician, based on
      body weight and blood glucose concentrations.
Note: For treatment of diabetic ketoacidosis, an optional loading dose of
   0.15 USP Insulin Unit per kg of body weight is given intravenously,
   followed by 0.1 USP Insulin Unit per kg of body weight per hour
   by continuous infusion. The rate of insulin infusion should be decreased when the plasma glucose concentration reaches 300 mg per
   dL. Infusion of 5% dextrose injection should be started separately
   from the insulin infusion when plasma glucose concentration
   reaches 250 mg per dL. Thirty minutes before discontinuing the
   insulin infusion, an appropriate dose of insulin should be injected
   subcutaneously; intermediate-acting insulin has been recommended.
   Alternatively, a loading dose of 0.5 USP Unit per kg of body weight
   is injected intramuscularly, followed by 0.1 USP Insulin Unit per
   kg of body weight injected intramuscularly every hour until the
   blood glucose concentration reaches 300 mg per dL. Then to maintain blood glucose concentration at 250 mg per dL, 0.1 USP Insulin
   Unit per kg of body weight is injected intramuscularly every 2
   hours as needed. With either type of insulin administration, capillary blood glucose monitoring should be followed at least hourly
   and the insulin dose adjusted accordingly.

Insulin requirements may change during illness or events causing
psychological or physical stress. Dosage changes for patients receiving conventional therapy should be determined by the physician, based on each patient's needs and insulin sensitivity. Patients
receiving intensive therapy may adjust individual doses to compensate for anticipated changes in diet or exercise but should consult
a physician if the permitted adjustments are inadequate and/or glucose monitoring indicates the need for a permanent change in the
daily dose.

Some patients experience a honeymoon phase after initial therapy
and lose their requirement for insulin altogether or require much
less for a limited period of time (several months to several years).

Adolescents during puberty may require an increase in their total
daily insulin dose.
[Diagnostic aid (pituitary growth hormone reserve)][1]—
   Intravenous, 0.05 to 0.15 USP Insulin Unit per kg of body weight as
      a single rapid injection.

## Usual pediatric dose
Antidiabetic—
   Subcutaneous, dosage must be determined by the physician, based on
      body weight and blood glucose concentrations.

## Strength(s) usually available
U.S.—
   100 USP Insulin Units per mL (OTC) [*Regular Iletin I* (beef and pork);
      *Regular Iletin II* (purified pork); *Regular Insulin* (pork); *Regular
      Insulin* (purified pork)].
   500 USP Insulin Units per mL (Rx) [*Regular (Concentrated) Iletin II,
      U-500* (purified pork)].
Canada—
   100 USP Insulin Units per mL (OTC) [*Insulin-Toronto* (beef and
      pork); *Regular Iletin* (beef and pork); *Regular Iletin II* (pork)].

## Packaging and storage
Store between 2 and 8 °C (36 and 46 °F). Protect from freezing.

## Stability
Do not use if cloudy, discolored, or unusually viscous.

## Auxiliary labeling
• Refrigerate.
• Do not freeze.

## Note
The 500-Unit strength is available only with a prescription and is used
   only for the treatment of insulin-resistant diabetic patients.

Insulin Injection USP is sometimes mixed with other insulin types as
   directed by physician.

Patient should be advised not to mix with any other insulin when using a
   continuous subcutaneous external insulin pump.

Regular insulin can be used in continuous subcutaneous infusion insulin
   pumps but may also be injected subcutaneously or intramuscularly
   with an insulin syringe or used intravenously. Phosphate-buffered insulin is preferred over nonphosphate-buffered insulin in insulin pumps.
   When this insulin is used in a continuous subcutaneous infusion insulin
   pump, the catheter tubing and the insulin in the reservoir must be

changed every 48 hours or the manufacturer's recommendations followed for specific external insulin pumps.

[1]Not included in Canadian product labeling.

## *INSULIN HUMAN*

# Parenteral Dosage Forms
Note: Bracketed uses in the *Dosage Forms section* refer to categories of
   use and/or indications that are not included in U.S. product labeling.

## INSULIN HUMAN INJECTION (REGULAR INSULIN HUMAN) USP

### Usual adult and adolescent dose
Insulin-dependent diabetes mellitus (IDDM)—
   Initial:
      Subcutaneous or continuous subcutaneous insulin infusion, a total
         insulin dose, using one or more types of insulin, is 0.5 to 1.2
         USP Insulin Human Units per kg of body weight a day in
         divided doses—taking body fat, blood glucose, and insulin sen-
         sitivity also under consideration. A few patients will require
         less than 0.5 USP Insulin Human Unit per kg of body weight
         a day. Dose titration to a targeted blood glucose goal is
         achieved over several days; a change in total daily insulin dose
         does not usually exceed 10% of the existing total daily insulin
         dose.
      When using a continuous subcutaneous insulin infusion pump, the
         basal insulin dose (usually forty to sixty percent of the total
         insulin daily dose) is divided into a dose that can be continu-
         ously infused subcutaneously over twenty-four hours. Also, a
         premeal injection (also, forty to sixty percent of total insulin
         dose) can be delivered preprogrammed or manually by the pa-
         tient through the insulin pump.
      When using subcutaneous injections, regular human insulin is usu-
         ally injected in low doses, i.e., often less than 10 USP Insulin
         Human Units a dose.
      Both subcutaneous injections and premeal injections of regular hu-
         man insulin using a continuous subcutaneous insulin infusion
         pump generally are given fifteen to thirty minutes before one
         or more meals and/or a bedtime snack.
   Maintenance:
      Subcutaneous or continuous subcutaneous insulin infusion, dosage
         must be determined by the physician, based on blood glucose
         concentrations.
Non–insulin-dependent diabetes mellitus (NIDDM)—
   Initial:
      Subcutaneous, a total insulin dose, using one or more types of
         insulin, may vary from 5 to 10 USP Insulin Human Units per
         day to 0.7 to 2.5 USP Insulin Human Units per kg of body
         weight a day in divided doses—taking body fat, blood glucose,
         and insulin sensitivity into consideration. Dose titration to a
         targeted blood glucose goal is achieved over several days with
         changes from the existing total daily insulin dose of no more
         than 2 to 6 USP Insulin Human Units a day; again, with con-
         sideration of body weight. Very insulin-resistant patients using
         large doses, 200 USP Insulin Human Units or greater, may
         need to use a concentrated regular insulin (U-500) instead.
         Regular human insulin is usually given in low doses, i.e., often
         less than 10 USP Insulin Human Units a dose, fifteen to thirty
         minutes before one or more meals and/or a bedtime snack.
   Maintenance:
      Subcutaneous, dosage must be determined by the physician, based
         on blood glucose concentrations.
Gestational diabetes mellitus—
   Subcutaneous, dosage must be determined by the physician, based on
      blood glucose concentrations and gestational duration.
Diabetes mellitus, other, associated with certain conditions or
   syndromes—
   Subcutaneous, dosage must be determined by the physician, based on
      body weight and blood glucose concentrations.
Note: For treatment of diabetic ketoacidosis, an optional loading dose of
   0.15 USP Insulin Human Unit per kg of body weight is given intravenously, followed by 0.1 USP Insulin Human Unit per kg of
   body weight per hour by continuous infusion. The rate of insulin
   infusion should be decreased when the plasma glucose concentration reaches 300 mg per dL. Infusion of 5% dextrose injection
   should be started separately from the insulin infusion when plasma
   glucose concentration reaches 250 mg per dL. Thirty minutes before discontinuing the insulin infusion, an appropriate dose of insulin should be injected subcutaneously; intermediate-acting insulin

has been recommended. Alternatively, a loading dose of 0.5 USP Insulin Human Unit per kg of body weight is injected intramuscularly, followed by 0.1 USP Insulin Human Unit per kg of body weight injected intramuscularly every hour until the blood glucose concentration reaches 300 mg per dL. Then, to maintain blood glucose concentration at 250 mg per dL, 0.1 USP Insulin Human Unit per kg of body weight is injected intramuscularly every 2 hours as needed. With either type of insulin administration, capillary blood glucose monitoring should be followed at least hourly and the insulin dose adjusted accordingly.

Insulin requirements may change during illness or events causing psychological or physical stress. Dosage changes for patients receiving conventional therapy should be determined by the physician, based on each patient's needs and insulin sensitivity. Patients receiving intensive therapy may adjust individual doses to compensate for anticipated changes in diet or exercise but should consult a physician if the permitted adjustments are inadequate and/or glucose monitoring indicates the need for a permanent change in the daily dose.

Some patients experience a honeymoon phase after initial therapy and lose their requirement for insulin altogether or require much less for a limited period of time (several months to several years).

Adolescents during puberty may require an increase in their total daily insulin dose.

[Diagnostic aid (pituitary growth hormone reserve)][1]—
   Intravenous, 0.05 to 0.15 USP Insulin Human Unit per kg of body weight as a single rapid injection.

**Usual pediatric dose**
Antidiabetic—
   Subcutaneous, dosage must be determined by the physician, based on body weight and blood glucose concentrations.

**Strength(s) usually available**
U.S.—
   100 USP Insulin Human Units per mL (OTC) [*Humulin R* (biosynthetic); *Novolin R* (biosynthetic); *Novolin R PenFill* (biosynthetic); *Novolin R Prefilled* (biosynthetic; prefilled single use syringe contains 150 USP Units in 1.5 mL)].

Canada—
   100 USP Insulin Human Units per mL (OTC) [*Humulin-R* (biosynthetic); *Novolin ge Toronto* (biosynthetic); *Novolin ge Toronto Penfill* (biosynthetic)].

**Packaging and storage**
Store between 2 and 8 °C (36 and 46 °F). Protect from freezing.

**Stability**
Do not use if cloudy, discolored, or unusually viscous.

**Auxiliary labeling**
• Refrigerate.
• Do not freeze.

**Note**
Insulin Human Injection USP is sometimes mixed with other insulin types as directed by physician.

Patient should be advised not to mix with any other insulin when using a continuous subcutaneous infusion insulin pump.

Insulin human may be used in continuous subcutaneous infusion insulin pumps but may also be injected subcutaneously or intramuscularly with an insulin syringe, or used intravenously. Phosphate-buffered insulin is preferred over nonphosphate-buffered insulin in insulin pumps. When this insulin is used in a continuous subcutaneous infusion insulin pump, the catheter tubing and the insulin in the reservoir must be changed every 48 hours or the manufacturer's recommendations followed for specific external insulin pumps.

[1]Not included in Canadian product labeling.

---

## INSULIN ZINC

# Parenteral Dosage Forms
## INSULIN ZINC SUSPENSION (LENTE INSULIN) USP

**Usual adult and adolescent dose**
Insulin-dependent diabetes mellitus (IDDM)—
   Initial: Subcutaneous, a total insulin dose is 0.5 to 0.8 USP Insulin Unit per kg of body weight as a single dose, depending on insulin type, or 0.5 to 1.2 USP Insulin Units per kg of body weight per day in divided doses. Body fat, blood glucose, and insulin sensitivity should also be considered. This total daily dose of insulin may be provided by one or more types of insulin. A few patients

will require less than 0.5 USP Insulin Unit per kg of body weight per day. Dose titration to a targeted blood glucose goal is achieved over several days; a change in total daily insulin dose does not usually exceed 10% of the existing total daily insulin dose. Insulin zinc is given thirty minutes before a meal and/or a bedtime snack.
Maintenance: Subcutaneous, dosage must be determined by the physician, based on blood glucose concentrations.
Non–insulin-dependent diabetes mellitus (NIDDM)—
   Initial: Subcutaneous, a total insulin dose may vary from 5 to 10 USP Insulin Units per day to 0.7 to 2.5 USP Insulin Units per kg of body weight per day—taking body fat, blood glucose, and insulin sensitivity also under consideration. This total daily dose of insulin may be provided by one or more types of insulin and, depending on insulin type, may be given as a single dose or as divided doses. Dose titration to a targeted blood glucose goal is achieved over several days with changes from the existing total daily insulin dose of no more than 2 to 6 USP Insulin Units a day; again, body weight should be considered. Very insulin-resistant patients using large doses, 200 USP Insulin Units or greater, may need to use a concentrated regular insulin (U-500) instead. Insulin zinc is given thirty minutes before a meal and/or a bedtime snack.
   Maintenance: Subcutaneous, dosage must be determined by the physician, based on blood glucose concentrations.
Gestational diabetes mellitus—
   Subcutaneous, dosage must be determined by the physician, based on blood glucose concentrations and gestational duration.
Diabetes mellitus, other, associated with certain conditions or syndromes—
   Subcutaneous, dosage must be determined by the physician, based on body weight and blood glucose concentrations.

Note: Insulin requirements may change during illness or events causing psychological or physical stress. Dosage changes for patients receiving conventional therapy should be determined by the physician, based on each patient's needs and insulin sensitivity. Patients receiving intensive therapy may adjust individual doses to compensate for anticipated changes in diet or exercise but should consult a physician if the permitted adjustments are inadequate and/or glucose monitoring indicates the need for a permanent change in the daily dose.

Some patients experience a honeymoon phase after initial therapy and lose their requirement for insulin altogether or require much less for a limited period of time (several months to several years).

Adolescents during puberty may require an increase in their total daily insulin dose.

**Usual pediatric dose**
Antidiabetic—
   Subcutaneous, dosage must be determined by the physician, based on body weight and blood glucose concentrations.

**Strength(s) usually available**
U.S.—
   100 USP Insulin Units per mL (OTC) [*Lente Iletin I* (beef and pork); *Lente Iletin II* (purified pork); *Lente L* (purified pork)].
Canada—
   100 USP Insulin Units per mL (OTC) [*Lente Iletin* (beef and pork); *Lente Iletin II* (pork); *Lente Insulin* (beef and pork)].

**Packaging and storage**
Store between 2 and 8 °C (36 and 46 °F). Protect from freezing.

**Stability**
Do not use if precipitate has become clumped or granular in appearance.

**Auxiliary labeling**
• Shake gently.
• Refrigerate.
• Do not freeze.

**Note**
Insulin zinc suspension is sometimes mixed with other insulin types as directed by physician.

---

## INSULIN ZINC, HUMAN

# Parenteral Dosage Forms
## INSULIN ZINC, HUMAN, SUSPENSION

**Usual adult and adolescent dose**
Insulin-dependent diabetes mellitus (IDDM)—
   Initial: Subcutaneous, a total insulin dose is 0.5 to 0.8 USP Insulin Human Unit per kg of body weight as a single dose, depending on insulin type, or 0.5 to 1.2 USP Insulin Human Units per kg of

body weight per day in divided doses. Body fat, blood glucose, and insulin sensitivity should also be considered. This total daily dose of insulin may be provided by one or more types of insulin. A few patients will require less than 0.5 USP Insulin Human Unit per kg of body weight per day. Dose titration to a targeted blood glucose goal is achieved over several days; a change in total daily insulin dose does not usually exceed 10% of the existing total daily insulin dose. Human insulin zinc is given thirty minutes before a meal and/or a bedtime snack.

Maintenance: Subcutaneous, dosage must be determined by the physician, based on blood glucose concentrations.

Non–insulin-dependent diabetes mellitus (NIDDM)—

Initial: Subcutaneous, a total insulin dose may vary from 5 to 10 USP Insulin Human Units per day to 0.7 to 2.5 USP Insulin Human Units per kg of body weight per day—taking body fat, blood glucose, and insulin sensitivity also under consideration. This total daily dose of insulin may be provided by one or more types of insulin and, depending on insulin type, may be given as a single dose or as divided doses. Dose titration to a targeted blood glucose goal is achieved over several days with changes from the existing total daily insulin dose of no more than 2 to 6 USP Insulin Human Units a day; again, body weight should be considered. Very insulin-resistant patients using large doses, 200 USP Insulin Human Units or greater, may need to use a concentrated regular insulin (U-500) instead. Human insulin zinc is given thirty minutes before a meal and/or a bedtime snack.

Maintenance: Subcutaneous, dosage must be determined by the physician, based on blood glucose concentrations.

Gestational diabetes mellitus—

Subcutaneous, dosage must be determined by the physician, based on blood glucose concentrations and gestational duration.

Diabetes mellitus, other, associated with certain conditions or syndromes—

Subcutaneous, dosage must be determined by the physician, based on body weight and blood glucose concentrations.

Note: Insulin requirements may change during illness or events causing psychological or physical stress. Dosage changes for patients receiving conventional therapy should be determined by the physician, based on each patient's needs and insulin sensitivity. Patients receiving intensive therapy may adjust individual doses to compensate for anticipated changes in diet or exercise but should consult a physician if the permitted adjustments are inadequate and/or glucose monitoring indicates the need for a permanent change in the daily dose.

Some patients experience a honeymoon phase after initial therapy and lose their requirement for insulin altogether or require much less for a limited period of time (several months to several years).

Adolescents during puberty may require an increase in their total daily insulin dose.

**Usual pediatric dose**

Antidiabetic—

Subcutaneous, dosage must be determined by the physician, based on body weight and blood glucose concentrations.

**Strength(s) usually available**

U.S.—

100 USP Insulin Human Units per mL (OTC) [*Humulin L* (biosynthetic); *Novolin L* (biosynthetic)].

Canada—

100 USP Insulin Human Units per mL (OTC) [*Humulin-L* (biosynthetic); *Novolin ge Lente* (biosynthetic)].

**Packaging and storage**

Store between 2 and 8 °C (36 and 46 °F). Protect from freezing.

**Stability**

Do not use if precipitate has become clumped or granular in appearance.

**Auxiliary labeling**

• Shake gently.
• Refrigerate.
• Do not freeze.

---

## *ISOPHANE INSULIN*

# Parenteral Dosage Forms

## ISOPHANE INSULIN SUSPENSION (NPH INSULIN) USP

**Usual adult and adolescent dose**

Insulin-dependent diabetes mellitus (IDDM)—

Initial: Subcutaneous, a total insulin dose is 0.5 to 0.8 USP Insulin Unit per kg of body weight as a single dose, depending on insulin

type, or 0.5 to 1.2 USP Insulin Units per kg of body weight per day in divided doses. Body fat, blood glucose, and insulin sensitivity should also be considered. This total daily dose of insulin may be provided by one or more types of insulin. A few patients will require less than 0.5 USP Insulin Unit per kg of body weight per day. Dose titration to a targeted blood glucose goal is achieved over several days; a change in total daily insulin dose does not usually exceed 10% of the existing total daily insulin dose. Isophane insulin is given thirty to sixty minutes before a meal and/or a bedtime snack.

Maintenance: Subcutaneous, dosage must be determined by the physician, based on blood glucose concentrations.

Non–insulin-dependent diabetes mellitus (NIDDM)—

Initial: Subcutaneous, a total insulin dose may vary from 5 to 10 USP Insulin Units per day to 0.7 to 2.5 USP Insulin Units per kg of body weight per day—taking body fat, blood glucose, and insulin sensitivity also under consideration. This total daily dose of insulin may be provided by one or more types of insulin and, depending on insulin type, may be given as a single dose or as divided doses. Dose titration to a targeted blood glucose goal is achieved over several days with changes from the existing total daily insulin dose of no more than 2 to 6 USP Insulin Units a day; again, body weight should be considered. Very insulin-resistant patients using large doses, 200 USP Insulin Units or greater, may need to use a concentrated regular insulin (U-500) instead. Isophane insulin is given thirty to sixty minutes before a meal and/or a bedtime snack.

Maintenance: Subcutaneous, dosage must be determined by the physician, based on blood glucose concentrations.

Non–insulin-dependent diabetes mellitus (NIDDM)—

Subcutaneous, dosage must be determined by the physician, based on blood glucose concentrations and gestational duration.

Diabetes mellitus, other, associated with certain conditions or syndromes—

Subcutaneous, dosage must be determined by the physician, based on body weight and blood glucose concentrations.

Note: Insulin requirements may change during illness or events causing psychological or physical stress. Dosage changes for patients receiving conventional therapy should be determined by the physician, based on each patient's needs and insulin sensitivity. Patients receiving intensive therapy may adjust individual doses to compensate for anticipated changes in diet or exercise but should consult a physician if the permitted adjustments are inadequate and/or glucose monitoring indicates the need for a permanent change in the daily dose.

Some patients experience a honeymoon phase after initial therapy and lose their requirement for insulin altogether or require much less for a limited period of time (several months to several years).

Adolescents during puberty may require an increase in their total daily insulin dose.

**Usual pediatric dose**

Antidiabetic—

Subcutaneous, dosage must be determined by the physician, based on body weight and blood glucose concentrations.

**Strength(s) usually available**

U.S.—

100 USP Insulin Units per mL (OTC) [*NPH Iletin I* (beef and pork); *NPH Iletin II* (purified pork); *NPH-N* (purified pork)].

Canada—

100 USP Insulin Units per mL (OTC) [*NPH Iletin* (beef and pork); *NPH Iletin II* (pork); *NPH Insulin* (beef and pork)].

**Packaging and storage**

Store between 2 and 8 °C (36 and 46 °F). Protect from freezing.

**Stability**

Do not use if precipitate has become clumped or granular in appearance or clings to sides of vial.

**Auxiliary labeling**

• Shake gently.
• Refrigerate.
• Do not freeze.

**Note**

Isophane insulin suspension is sometimes mixed with insulin injection as directed by physician.

---

### ISOPHANE INSULIN, HUMAN

## Parenteral Dosage Forms

### ISOPHANE INSULIN, HUMAN, SUSPENSION

**Usual adult and adolescent dose**
Insulin-dependent diabetes mellitus (IDDM)—
Initial: Subcutaneous, a total insulin dose is 0.5 to 0.8 USP Insulin Human Unit per kg of body weight as a single dose, depending on insulin type, or 0.5 to 1.2 USP Insulin Human Units per kg of body weight per day in divided doses. Body fat, blood glucose, and insulin sensitivity should also be considered. This total daily dose of insulin may be provided by one or more types of insulin. A few patients will require less than 0.5 USP Insulin Human Unit per kg of body weight per day. Dose titration to a targeted blood glucose goal is achieved over several days; a change in total daily insulin dose does not usually exceed 10% of the existing total daily insulin dose. Human isophane insulin is given thirty minutes before a meal and/or a bedtime snack.
Maintenance: Subcutaneous, dosage must be determined by the physician, based on blood glucose concentrations.
Non–insulin-dependent diabetes mellitus (NIDDM)—
Initial: Subcutaneous, a total insulin dose may vary from 5 to 10 USP Insulin Human Units per day to 0.7 to 2.5 USP Insulin Human Units per kg of body weight per day—taking body fat, blood glucose, and insulin sensitivity also under consideration. This total daily dose of insulin may be provided by one or more types of insulin and, depending on insulin type, may be given as a single dose or as divided doses. Dose titration to a targeted blood glucose goal is achieved over several days with changes from the existing total daily insulin dose of no more than 2 to 6 USP Insulin Human Units a day; again, body weight should be considered. Very insulin-resistant patients using large doses, 200 USP Insulin Human Units or greater, may need to use a concentrated regular insulin (U-500) instead. Human isophane insulin is given thirty minutes before a meal and/or a bedtime snack.
Maintenance: Subcutaneous, dosage must be determined by the physician, based on blood glucose concentrations.
Gestational diabetes mellitus—
Subcutaneous, dosage must be determined by the physician, based on blood glucose concentrations and gestational duration.
Diabetes mellitus, other, associated with certain conditions or syndromes—
Subcutaneous, dosage must be determined by the physician, based on body weight and blood glucose concentrations.
Note: Insulin requirements may change during illness or events causing psychological or physical stress. Dosage changes for patients receiving conventional therapy should be determined by the physician, based on each patient's needs and insulin sensitivity. Patients receiving intensive therapy may adjust individual doses to compensate for anticipated changes in diet or exercise but should consult a physician if the permitted adjustments are inadequate and/or glucose monitoring indicates the need for a permanent change in the daily dose.

Some patients experience a honeymoon phase after initial therapy and lose their requirement for insulin altogether or require much less for a limited period of time (several months to several years).

Adolescents during puberty may require an increase in their total daily insulin dose.

**Usual pediatric dose**
Antidiabetic—
Subcutaneous, dosage must be determined by the physician, based on body weight and blood glucose concentrations.

**Strength(s) usually available**
U.S.—
100 USP Insulin Human Units per mL (OTC) [*Humulin N* (biosynthetic); *Novolin N* (biosynthetic); *Novolin N PenFill* (biosynthetic); *Novolin N Prefilled* (biosynthetic; prefilled single-use syringe contains 150 USP Insulin Human Units in 1.5 mL)].
Canada—
100 USP Insulin Human Units per mL (OTC) [*Humulin-N* (biosynthetic); *Novolin ge NPH* (biosynthetic); *Novolin ge NPH Penfill* (biosynthetic)].

**Packaging and storage**
Store between 2 and 8 °C (36 and 46 °F). Protect from freezing.

**Stability**
Do not use if precipitate has become clumped or granular in appearance or clings to sides of vial.

**Auxiliary labeling**
• Shake gently.
• Gently rotate prefilled syringe up and down before injection.

---

• Refrigerate.
• Do not freeze.

---

### ISOPHANE INSULIN, HUMAN AND INSULIN HUMAN

## Parenteral Dosage Forms

### ISOPHANE INSULIN, HUMAN, SUSPENSION AND INSULIN HUMAN INJECTION

**Usual adult and adolescent dose**
Insulin-dependent diabetes mellitus (IDDM)—
Initial: Subcutaneous, a total insulin dose is 0.5 to 0.8 USP Insulin Human Unit per kg of body weight as a single dose, depending on insulin type, or 0.5 to 1.2 USP Insulin Human Units per kg of body weight per day in divided doses. Body fat, blood glucose, and insulin sensitivity should also be considered. This total daily dose of insulin may be provided by one or more types of insulin. A few patients will require less than 0.5 USP Insulin Human Unit per kg of body weight per day. Dose titration to a targeted blood glucose goal is achieved over several days; a change in total daily insulin dose does not usually exceed 10% of the existing total daily insulin dose. Human isophane insulin and human insulin is given fifteen or thirty minutes before a meal and/or a bedtime snack.
Maintenance: Subcutaneous, dosage must be determined by the physician, based on blood glucose concentrations.
Non–insulin-dependent diabetes mellitus (NIDDM)—
Initial: Subcutaneous, a total insulin dose may vary from 5 to 10 USP Insulin Human Units per day to 0.7 to 2.5 USP Insulin Human Units per kg of body weight per day—taking body fat, blood glucose, and insulin sensitivity also under consideration. This total daily dose of insulin may be provided by one or more types of insulin and, depending on insulin type, may be given as a single dose or as divided doses. Dose titration to a targeted blood glucose goal is achieved over several days with changes from the existing total daily insulin dose of no more than 2 to 6 USP Insulin Human Units a day; again, body weight should be considered. Very insulin-resistant patients using large doses, 200 USP Insulin Human Units or greater, may need to use a concentrated regular insulin (U-500) instead. Human isophane insulin and human insulin is given fifteen to thirty minutes before a meal and/or a bedtime snack.
Maintenance: Subcutaneous, dosage must be determined by the physician, based on blood glucose concentrations.
Gestational diabetes mellitus—
Subcutaneous, dosage must be determined by the physician, based on blood glucose concentrations and gestational duration.
Diabetes mellitus, other, associated with certain conditions or syndromes—
Subcutaneous, dosage must be determined by the physician, based on body weight and blood glucose concentrations.
Note: Insulin requirements may change during illness or events causing psychological or physical stress. Dosage changes for patients receiving conventional therapy should be determined by the physician, based on each patient's needs and insulin sensitivity. Patients receiving intensive therapy may adjust individual doses to compensate for anticipated changes in diet or exercise but should consult a physician if the permitted adjustments are inadequate and/or glucose monitoring indicates the need for a permanent change in the daily dose.

Some patients experience a honeymoon phase after initial therapy and lose their requirement for insulin altogether or require much less for a limited period of time (several months to several years).

Adolescents during puberty may require an increase in their total daily insulin dose.

**Usual pediatric dose**
Antidiabetic—
Subcutaneous, dosage must be determined by the physician, based on body weight and blood glucose concentrations.

**Strength(s) usually available**
U.S.—
100 USP Insulin Human Units per mL (50% isophane insulin, human, suspension and 50% insulin human injection) (OTC) [*Humulin 50/50* (biosynthetic)].
100 USP Insulin Human Units per mL (70% isophane insulin, human, suspension and 30% insulin human injection) (OTC) [*Humulin 70/30* (biosynthetic); *Novolin 70/30* (biosynthetic); *Novolin 70/30 PenFill* (biosynthetic); *Novolin 70/30 Prefilled* (biosynthetic; prefilled single-use syringe contains 150 USP Insulin Human Units in 1.5 mL)].
Canada—
100 USP Insulin Human Units per mL (10% insulin human injection and 90% isophane insulin, human) (OTC) [*Humulin 10/90* (biosynthetic); *Novolin ge 10/90 Penfill* (biosynthetic)].

100 USP Insulin Human Units per mL (20% insulin human injection and 80% isophane insulin, human) (OTC) [*Humulin 20/80* (biosynthetic); *Novolin ge 20/80 Penfill* (biosynthetic)].

100 USP Insulin Human Units per mL (30% insulin human injection and 70% isophane insulin, human) (OTC) [*Humulin 30/70* (biosynthetic); *Novolin ge 30/70* (biosynthetic); *Novolin ge 30/70 Penfill* (biosynthetic)].

100 USP Insulin Human Units per mL (40% insulin human injection and 60% isophane insulin, human) (OTC) [*Humulin 40/60* (biosynthetic); *Novolin ge 40/60 Penfill* (biosynthetic)].

100 USP Insulin Human Units per mL (50% insulin human injection and 50% isophane insulin, human) (OTC) [*Humulin 50/50* (biosynthetic); *Novolin ge 50/50 Penfill* (biosynthetic)].

**Packaging and storage**
Store between 2 and 8 °C (36 and 46 °F), unless otherwise specified by manufacturer. Protect from freezing.

**Stability**
Do not use if precipitate has become clumped or granular in appearance.

**Auxiliary labeling**
- Shake gently.
- Gently rotate prefilled syringe up and down before injection.
- Refrigerate.
- Do not freeze.

---

## PROMPT INSULIN ZINC

## Parenteral Dosage Forms

### PROMPT INSULIN ZINC SUSPENSION (SEMILENTE INSULIN) USP

**Usual adult and adolescent dose**
Insulin-dependent diabetes mellitus (IDDM)—
   Initial: Subcutaneous, a total insulin dose is 0.5 to 0.8 USP Insulin Unit per kg of body weight as a single dose, depending on insulin type, or 0.5 to 1.2 USP Insulin Units per kg of body weight per day in divided doses. Body fat, blood glucose, and insulin sensitivity should also be considered. This total daily dose of insulin may be provided by one or more types of insulin. A few patients will require less than 0.5 USP Insulin Unit per kg of body weight per day. Dose titration to a targeted blood glucose goal is achieved over several days; a change in total daily insulin dose does not usually exceed 10% of the existing total daily insulin dose. Prompt insulin zinc is given thirty to sixty minutes before a meal and/or a bedtime snack.
   Maintenance: Subcutaneous, dosage must be determined by the physician, based on blood glucose concentrations.
Non–insulin-dependent diabetes mellitus (NIDDM)—
   Initial: Subcutaneous, a total insulin dose may vary from 5 to 10 USP Insulin Units per day to 0.7 to 2.5 USP Insulin Units per kg of body weight per day—taking body fat, blood glucose, and insulin sensitivity also under consideration. This total daily dose of insulin may be provided by one or more types of insulin and, depending on insulin type, may be given as a single dose or as divided doses. Dose titration to a targeted blood glucose goal is achieved over several days with changes from the existing total daily insulin dose of no more than 2 to 6 USP Insulin Units a day; again, body weight should be considered. Very insulin-resistant patients using large doses, 200 USP Insulin Units or greater, may need to use a concentrated regular insulin (U-500) instead. Prompt insulin zinc is given thirty to sixty minutes before a meal and/or a bedtime snack.
   Maintenance: Subcutaneous, dosage must be determined by the physician, based on blood glucose concentrations.
Gestational diabetes mellitus—
   Subcutaneous, dosage must be determined by the physician, based on blood glucose concentrations and gestational duration.
Diabetes mellitus, other, associated with certain conditions or syndromes—
   Subcutaneous, dosage must be determined by the physician, based on body weight and blood glucose concentrations.
Note: Insulin requirements may change during illness or events causing psychological or physical stress. Dosage changes for patients receiving conventional therapy should be determined by the physician, based on each patient's needs and insulin sensitivity. Patients receiving intensive therapy may adjust individual doses to compensate for anticipated changes in diet or exercise but should consult a physician if the permitted adjustments are inadequate and/or glucose monitoring indicates the need for a permanent change in the daily dose.

   Some patients experience a honeymoon phase after initial therapy and lose their requirement for insulin altogether or require much less for a limited period of time (several months to several years).

Adolescents during puberty may require an increase in their total daily insulin dose.

**Usual pediatric dose**
Antidiabetic—
   Subcutaneous, dosage must be determined by the physician, based on body weight and blood glucose concentrations.

**Strength(s) usually available**
U.S.—
   Not commercially available.
Canada—
   100 USP Insulin Units per mL (OTC) [*Semilente Insulin* (beef and pork)].

**Packaging and storage**
Store between 2 and 8 °C (36 and 46 °F). Protect from freezing.

**Stability**
Do not use if precipitate has become clumped or granular in appearance.

**Auxiliary labeling**
- Shake gently.
- Refrigerate.
- Do not freeze.

**Note**
Prompt Insulin Zinc Suspension USP is sometimes mixed with other insulin types as directed by physician.

## Selected Bibliography
Koda-Kimble MA. Diabetes mellitus. In: Young LY, Koda-Kimble MA, editors. Applied therapeutics. The clinical use of drugs. 5th ed. Vancouver, WA: Applied Therapeutics, Inc., 1992: 72 (1)-72 (53).

The Diabetes Control and Complications Trial Research Group. The effect of intensive treatment of diabetes on the development and progression of long-term complications in insulin-dependent diabetes mellitus. N Engl J Med 1993; 329 (14): 977-86.

Revised: 07/26/95

---

**INSULIN HUMAN**—See *Insulin (Systemic)*

---

**INSULIN HUMAN, BUFFERED**—See *Insulin (Systemic)*

---

**INSULIN ZINC**—See *Insulin (Systemic)*

---

**INSULIN ZINC, EXTENDED**—See *Insulin (Systemic)*

---

**INSULIN ZINC, EXTENDED, HUMAN**—See *Insulin (Systemic)*

---

**INSULIN ZINC, HUMAN**—See *Insulin (Systemic)*

---

**INSULIN ZINC, PROMPT**—See *Insulin (Systemic)*

---

**INTERFERON ALFA-2A, RECOMBINANT**—See *Interferons, Alpha (Systemic)*

---

**INTERFERON ALFA-2B, RECOMBINANT**—See *Interferons, Alpha (Systemic)*

---

**INTERFERON ALFA-N1 (LNS)**—See *Interferons, Alpha (Systemic)*

---

**INTERFERON ALFA-N3**—See *Interferons, Alpha (Systemic)*

# INTERFERON, GAMMA    Systemic†

VA CLASSIFICATION (Primary): IM700

Note: For a listing of dosage forms and brand names by country availability, see *Dosage Forms* section(s). For a listing of brand names for the articles in this monograph, refer to the General Index.

†Not commercially available in Canada.

## Category

Biological response modifier; immunomodulator.

## Indications

### Accepted

Chronic granulomatous disease (treatment)—Interferon gamma-1b, recombinant, is indicated for reducing the frequency and severity of serious infections associated with chronic granulomatous disease (CGD). Interferon gamma-1b appears to be effective in all genetic types of CGD.

## Pharmacology/Pharmacokinetics

Note: Pharmacokinetic studies have been conducted in healthy male subjects only.

### Physicochemical characteristics

Source—Synthetic. Structurally identical to naturally occurring human gamma interferon. A protein chain of 140 amino acids produced by a recombinant DNA process involving genetically engineered *Escherichia coli*. Purification procedure involves conventional column chromatography.

Chemical group—Related to naturally occurring gamma interferon. Interferons are produced and secreted by cells in response to viral infections or various synthetic and biologic stimuli; gamma interferon is produced mainly by T-lymphyocytes.

### Mechanism of action/Effect

In general, interferons have antiviral, antiproliferative, and immunomodulatory activities.

Naturally occurring gamma interferon, which is secreted by antigen-stimulated T-lymphocytes (mainly CD4+ [helper] cells, plus CD8+ [suppressor] cells and natural killer [NK] cells), probably interacts with other lymphokines (cytokines) such as interleukin-2 in a complex immunoregulatory network. Gamma interferon induces activation of quiescent macrophages in blood monocytes to phagocytes, which have augmented antimicrobial and tumoricidal activity involving release of toxic oxygen metabolites. Macrophage activation is critical in the cellular immune response to intracellular and extracellular pathogens. Gamma interferon also enhances antibody-dependent cellular cytotoxicity and NK cell activity, histocompatibility class I and class II antigen expression, lymphocyte proliferation, and monocyte Fc receptor expression. Treatment with gamma interferon is associated with increased serum concentrations of beta-2 microglobulin and $H_2O_2$ secretion by peripheral blood monocytes, as well as a temporary increase in the T4/T8 cell ratio. Gamma interferon is also known as Type II interferon (based on interferon receptor types) and immune interferon.

In chronic granulomatous disease (CGD; an inherited disorder characterized by deficient phagocyte oxidative metabolism), gamma interferon enhances phagocytic function, resulting in an increase in superoxide anion production by granulocytes and monocytes; gamma interferon also enhances the oxygen-independent antimicrobial activity of monocytes from patients with classic X-linked CGD.

### Other actions/effects

May inhibit the hepatic microsomal cytochrome P450 system.

### Absorption

Intramuscular or subcutaneous—Slow; apparent fraction of dose absorbed is more than 89%.

### Biotransformation

Unknown.

### Half-life

Intramuscular—Mean: 2.9 hours

Intravenous—Mean: 38 minutes

Subcutaneous—Mean: 5.9 hours

### Time to peak plasma concentration

Intramuscular—4 hours.

Subcutaneous: 7 hours.

### Peak plasma concentration

After dose of 100 mcg per square meter of body surface—

Intramuscular: 1.5 nanograms per mL.

Subcutaneous: 0.6 nanograms per mL.

Note: Not related to blood monocyte activation capacity.

### Elimination

*In vitro* studies indicate that rabbit livers and kidneys are capable of clearing gamma interferon from perfusate; in nephrectomized mice and squirrel monkeys, clearance of gamma interferon from blood is reduced but elimination is not prevented.

## Precautions to Consider

### Cross-sensitivity and/or related problems

Patients sensitive to any *Escherichia coli* product may also be sensitive to gamma interferon.

### Carcinogenicity

Studies have not been done in either animals or humans.

### Mutagenicity

Results of Ames tests using five different tester strains of bacteria with and without metabolic activation showed no evidence of mutagenicity. No evidence of chromosomal damage was found in a micronucleus assay in bone marrow cells of mice following two intravenous doses of 20 mg per kg of body weight (mg/kg).

### Pregnancy/Reproduction

Fertility—In female cynomolgus monkeys, irregular menstrual cycles or absence of cyclicity occurred during treatment with daily subcutaneous doses of 150 mcg per kg of body weight (mcg/kg) (approximately 100 times the human dose), but not with doses of 3 or 30 mcg/kg.

Pregnancy—Adequate and well-controlled studies in humans have not been done.

Studies in primates at doses approximately 100 times the human dose found an increased incidence of abortions. No evidence of teratogenicity was found with intravenous doses of 2 to 100 times the human dose. Studies using recombinant murine gamma interferon in pregnant mice found increased incidences of uterine bleeding and abortifacient activity and decreased neonatal viability at maternally toxic doses; however, the clinical significance of this effect is unknown.

FDA Pregnancy Category C.

### Breast-feeding

It is not known whether gamma interferon is excreted in breast milk. However, because of the potential for serious adverse effects in nursing infants, avoidance of breast-feeding should be considered while gamma interferon is being administered.

### Pediatrics

Safety and efficacy in children less than 1 year of age have not been established. In one study, flu-like symptoms were twice as frequent in children 10 years of age or older as in those less than 10 years of age; the lowest incidence was in children 5 years of age or younger.

### Geriatrics

No information is available on the relationship of age to the effects of gamma interferon in geriatric patients.

### Drug interactions and/or related problems

The following drug interactions and/or related problems have been selected on the basis of their potential clinical significance (possible mechanism in parentheses where appropriate)—not necessarily inclusive (» = major clinical significance):

Note: Combinations containing any of the following medications, depending on the amount present, may also interact with this medication.

Blood dyscrasia–causing medications (See *Appendix II*)
(leukopenic and/or thrombocytopenic effects of gamma interferon, although usually not significant except at high doses, may be increased with concurrent or recent therapy if these medications cause the same effects; dosage adjustment of gamma interferon, if necessary, should be based on blood counts)

Bone marrow depressants, other (See *Appendix II*) or
Radiation therapy
(additive bone marrow depression may rarely occur; dosage reduction may be required when two or more bone marrow depressants, including radiation, are used concurrently or consecutively)

## Laboratory value alterations

The following have been selected on the basis of their potential clinical significance (possible effect in parentheses where appropriate)—not necessarily inclusive (» = major clinical significance):

With physiology/laboratory test values

Alanine aminotransferase (ALT [SGPT]) and
Alkaline phosphatase and
Aspartate aminotransferase (AST [SGOT]) and
Lactate dehydrogenase (LDH)
    (serum values may be slightly increased; dose related; reversible on withdrawal of gamma interferon)

Blood pressure
    (may be decreased)

Cortisol concentrations, plasma
    (may be increased; peak concentrations occur 2 to 4 hours after administration of gamma interferon)

Leukocyte counts (including neutrophils)
    (may be decreased; dose-related)

Platelet counts
    (may rarely be decreased)

Triglyceride concentrations, serum
    (may be increased; dose-related; resolve after treatment is withdrawn)

## Medical considerations/Contraindications

The medical considerations/contraindications included here have been selected on the basis of their potential clinical significance (reasons given in parentheses where appropriate)—not necessarily inclusive (» = major clinical significance).

*Risk-benefit should be considered when the following medical problems exist:*

Bone marrow depression
    (may be exacerbated)

» Cardiac disease, including symptoms of ischemia, congestive heart failure, or arrhythmia
    (may be exacerbated as a result of the stress of the fever and chills that occur in patients receiving gamma interferon; no direct cardiotoxic effect of gamma interferon has been demonstrated)

» CNS function, compromised or
» Seizure disorders
    (risk of CNS side effects)

» Multiple sclerosis or
» Systemic lupus erythematosus
    (there is some evidence that these may be exacerbated; however, there is also some evidence of a helpful effect of gamma interferon)

» Sensitivity to gamma interferon or *Escherichia coli*–derived products

    Caution should be used also in patients who have had previous cytotoxic drug therapy or radiation therapy.

## Patient monitoring

The following may be especially important in patient monitoring (other tests may be warranted in some patients, depending on condition; » = major clinical significance):

Alanine aminotransferase (ALT [SGPT]) values, serum and
Aspartate aminotransferase (AST [SGOT]) values, serum and
Bilirubin concentrations, serum and
Lactate dehydrogenase (LDH) values, serum
    (recommended prior to initiation of therapy and at periodic intervals during therapy)

» Leukocyte count, total and, if appropriate, differential and
» Platelet count
    (determinations recommended prior to initiation of therapy and at periodic intervals during therapy)

## Side/Adverse Effects

Note: Most side/adverse effects, except the flu-like syndrome, are dose-related.

    Development of neutralizing antibodies has not been reported with interferon gamma-1b, although it has been reported with interferon gamma-4a.

    Neutropenia and elevation of hepatic enzymes may occur at doses of 100 mcg per square meter of body surface per day and may be dose-limiting at doses above 250 mcg per square meter of body surface per day; they resolve after treatment is withdrawn. Thrombocytopenia and proteinuria are also rare.

The following side/adverse effects have been selected on the basis of their potential clinical significance (possible signs and symptoms in parentheses where appropriate)—not necessarily inclusive:

### Those indicating need for medical attention
Incidence more frequent
    *Leukopenia* (usually asymptomatic; rarely, fever or chills; cough or hoarseness; lower back or side pain; painful or difficult urination)
    Note: In *leukopenia*, neutrophil counts usually do not fall out of the normal range and usually recover within 2 to 5 days after a dose.

Incidence rare
    *Hypotension* (not symptomatic); *neurotoxicity* (confusion, parkinsonian symptoms [loss of balance control, mask-like face, shuffling walk, stiffness of arms or legs, trembling and shaking of hands and fingers, trouble in speaking or swallowing], trouble in thinking or concentrating, trouble in walking); *thrombocytopenia* (usually asymptomatic; rarely, unusual bleeding or bruising; black, tarry stools; blood in urine or stools; pinpoint red spots on skin)
    Note: *Neurotoxicity* is usually reversible after withdrawal.

### Those indicating need for medical attention only if they continue or are bothersome
Incidence more frequent
    *Diarrhea; flu-like syndrome* (aching muscles; fever and chills; general feeling of discomfort or illness; headache; less frequently, back pain; joint pain); *nausea or vomiting; skin rash; unusual tiredness*
    Note: The *flu-like syndrome* occurs in most patients; it may decrease in severity with continued treatment. Severity is dose-related.

Incidence less frequent
    *Dizziness; loss of appetite; weight loss*
    Note: *Dizziness* is a CNS effect.

## Patient Consultation

As an aid to patient consultation, refer to *Advice for the Patient, Interferon, Gamma (Systemic).*

In providing consultation, consider emphasizing the following selected information (» = major clinical significance):

### Before using this medication
» Conditions affecting use, especially:
    Sensitivity to gamma interferon
    Pregnancy—Abortifacient effects found in monkeys and mice
    Breast-feeding—Possible need to avoid during gamma interferon therapy because of risk of serious adverse effects
    Other medical problems, especially cardiac disease, compromised CNS function, multiple sclerosis, seizure disorders, and systemic lupus erythematosus

### Proper use of this medication
» Compliance with therapy
» Reading patient directions carefully with regard to:
    Preparation of the injection
    Use of disposable syringes
    Proper administration technique
    Stability of the injection
    Importance of ample fluid intake to reduce risk of hypotension
    Administration at bedtime to minimize flu-like symptoms
» Proper dosing
    Missed dose: Skipping missed dose and going back to regular schedule; not doubling doses; checking with physician
» Proper storage

### Precautions while using this medication
» Importance of close monitoring by physician
» Frequency of fever and flu-like symptoms; possible need for acetaminophen before and after a dose is given

### Side/adverse effects
    Signs of potential side effects, especially leukopenia, neurotoxicity, and thrombocytopenia

## General Dosing Information

Patients receiving gamma interferon should be under supervision of a physician experienced in immunomodulatory therapy.

The patient may be premedicated with acetaminophen at the time of gamma interferon dosing and the acetaminophen may be continued as needed to treat fever and headache.

If severe adverse effects occur, dosage reduction by 50% or temporary withdrawal of gamma interferon is recommended.

It is recommended that patients be well hydrated, especially during initial treatment with gamma interferon, to reduce the risk of hypotension associated with fluid depletion. Hypotension may require supportive treatment, including fluid replacement to maintain intravascular volume.

Patients who develop leukopenia should be observed carefully for signs of infection. Antibiotic support may be required. In neutropenic patients who develop fever, broad-spectrum antibiotic coverage should be initiated empirically, pending bacterial cultures and appropriate diagnostic tests. In some cases, it may be difficult to distinguish fever due to infection from fever associated with the flu-like syndrome.

Special precautions are recommended in patients who develop thrombocytopenia as a result of administration of gamma interferon. These may include extreme care in performing invasive procedures; regular inspection of intravenous sites, skin (including perirectal area), and mucous membrane surfaces for signs of bleeding or bruising; limiting frequency of venipuncture and avoiding intramuscular injections; testing urine, emesis, stool, and secretions for occult blood; care in use of regular toothbrushes, dental floss, toothpicks, safety razors, and fingernail and toenail cutters; avoiding constipation; and using caution to prevent falls and other injuries. Such patients should avoid alcohol and any aspirin intake because of the risk of gastrointestinal bleeding. Platelet transfusions may be required.

## Parenteral Dosage Forms

### INTERFERON GAMMA-1b, RECOMBINANT, INJECTION

#### Usual pediatric dose

Chronic granulomatous disease—
Body surface area greater than 0.5 square meter: Subcutaneous, 50 mcg (1.5 million Units) per square meter of body surface three times a week.
Body surface area less than or equal to 0.5 square meter: Subcutaneous, 1.5 mcg per kg of body weight three times a week.

Note: The optimum injection sites are the right and left deltoid and anterior thigh.

Either sterilized glass or plastic disposable syringes may be used for administration.

Safety and efficacy in children less than 1 year of age have not been established.

#### Strength(s) usually available

U.S.—
200 mcg per mL (100 mcg [3 million Units] per 0.5-mL vial) (Rx)
[*Actimmune* (mannitol; sodium succinate; polysorbate 20)].

Canada—
Not commercially available.

#### Packaging and storage

Store between 2 and 8 °C (36 and 46 °F), unless otherwise specified by manufacturer. Protect from freezing.

#### Stability

Contains no preservative; any unused portion should be discarded. Vials left at room temperature for a total time exceeding 12 hours should be discarded.

#### Note

Do not shake.

When dispensing for self-administration by the patient, make sure that patient instructions are included and that the patient understands how to prepare and administer the injection, including proper use of disposable syringes.

### Selected Bibliography

Ijzermans JNM, Marquet RL. Interferon-gamma: a review. Immunobiol 1989; 179: 456-73.
Murray HW. Interferon-gamma, the activated macrophage, and host defense against microbial challenge. Ann Intern Med 1988 Apr; 108: 595-608.

Revised: 06/04/92
Interim revision: 07/05/94

---

# INTERFERONS, ALPHA Systemic†

This monograph includes information on the following: Interferon Alfa-2a, Recombinant; Interferon Alfa-2b, Recombinant; Interferon Alfa-n1 (lns)*; Interferon Alfa-n3†.

VA CLASSIFICATION (Primary/Secondary): IM700/AN900

Note: For a listing of dosage forms and brand names by country availability, see *Dosage Forms* section(s). For a listing of brand names for the articles in this monograph, refer to the General Index.

*Not commercially available in the U.S.
†Not commercially available in Canada.

## Category

Biological response modifier; antineoplastic.

## Indications

Note: Bracketed information in the *Indications* section refers to uses that are not included in U.S. product labeling.

### Accepted

Leukemia, hairy cell (treatment)—Recombinant interferon alfa-2a, recombinant interferon alfa-2b, and interferon alfa-n1 (lns) are indicated for treatment of hairy cell leukemia, in splenectomized or nonsplenectomized patients. [Interferon alfa-n3] is also used for treatment of hairy cell leukemia.

Condylomata acuminata (treatment)—Recombinant interferon alfa-2b[1], interferon alfa-n1 (lns), and interferon alfa-n3 are indicated by intralesional injection for treatment of refractory or recurrent external condylomata acuminata (genital warts).

Hepatitis, chronic, active (treatment)—[Recombinant interferon alfa-2a][1], recombinant interferon alfa-2b, interferon alfa-n1 (lns)[1], and [interferon alfa-n3] are indicated for treatment of non-A, non-B/C hepatitis in patients 18 years of age or older with compensated liver disease who have a history of blood or blood product exposure and/or are HCV (hepatitis C virus) antibody positive. Safety and efficacy have not been established for treatment of patients with decompensated liver disease or for immune suppressed transplant recipients. Use is not recommended in patients with autoimmune hepatitis or a history of autoimmune disease.

Available data indicate that serum transaminase activity and markers of viral activity are reduced during alpha interferon treatment, although abnormalities may recur when treatment is withdrawn. Long-term effects of alpha interferon on development of chronic hepatitis are not established.

Kaposi's sarcoma, AIDS-associated (treatment)—Recombinant interferon alfa-2a and recombinant interferon alfa-2b are used for treatment of AIDS-associated Kaposi's sarcoma in selected patients 18 years of age and older. Interferon alfa-n1 (lns)[1] and [interferon alfa-n3] are also used for this indication.

Carcinoma, bladder (treatment)—[Recombinant interferon alfa-2a][1], [recombinant interferon alfa-2b][1], interferon alfa-n1 (lns)[1], and [interferon alfa-n3] are used to treat superficial bladder carcinoma (intravesically).

[Carcinoma, cervical (treatment)][1]—Recombinant interferon alfa-2b is being used for treatment of advanced cervical carcinoma.

Carcinoma, renal (treatment) or
Leukemia, chronic myelocytic (treatment)—[Recombinant interferon alfa-2a], [recombinant interferon alfa-2b][1], interferon alfa-n1 (lns)[1], and [interferon alfa-n3] are also used to treat renal carcinoma and chronic myelocytic leukemia.

Papillomatosis, laryngeal (treatment)—[Recombinant interferon alfa-2b][1], interferon alfa-n1 (lns), and [interferon alfa-n3] are indicated for treatment of laryngeal papillomatosis, including juvenile laryngeal papilloma.

Lymphomas, non-Hodgkin's (treatment) or
Malignant melanoma (treatment)
Multiple myeloma (treatment) or
Mycosis fungoides (treatment)—[Recombinant interferon alfa-2a][1], [recombinant interferon alfa-2b][1], interferon alfa-n1 (lns)[1], and [interferon alfa-n3] are used for treatment of non-Hodgkin's lymphomas, especially follicular small cleaved cell lymphoma (nodular poorly differentiated types), malignant melanoma, multiple myeloma, and mycosis fungoides.

Although efficacy of all alpha interferons for various indications appears to be similar, differences in relative efficacy for a particular indication may exist.

─────────────

[1]Not included in Canadian product labeling.

# Pharmacology/Pharmacokinetics

## Physicochemical characteristics
Source—
Interferon alfa-2a, recombinant: Synthetic. A protein chain of 165 amino acids produced by a recombinant DNA process involving genetically engineered *Escherichia coli*. Has a lysine group at position 23. Purification procedure includes affinity chromatography using a murine monoclonal antibody. Contains only a single alpha interferon subtype.
Interferon alfa-2b, recombinant: Synthetic. A protein chain of 165 amino acids produced by a recombinant DNA process involving genetically engineered *Escherichia coli*. Has an arginine group at position 23. Purification is done by proprietary methods. Contains only a single alpha interferon subtype.
Interferon alfa-n1 (lns): A highly purified blend of natural human alpha interferons, obtained from human lymphoblastoid cells following induction with Sendai virus. Is a mixture of natural alpha interferon subtypes, but in different proportions than in human leukocyte interferon.
Interferon alfa-n3: A highly purified mixture of up to 14 natural human alpha interferon subtypes. A protein chain of approximately 166 amino acids. Manufactured from pooled units of human leukocytes that have been induced by incomplete infection with an avian virus (Sendai virus) to produce interferon alfa-n3. The manufacturing process includes immunoaffinity chromatography with a murine monoclonal antibody, acidification (pH 2) for 5 days at 4 °C, and gel filtration chromatography.
Chemical group—
Interferon alfa-n1 and-n3: Naturally occurring alpha interferons.
Interferon alfa-2a and-2b, recombinant: Related to naturally occurring alpha interferons.
Interferons are produced and secreted by cells in response to viral infections or various synthetic and biologic inducers; alpha interferons are produced mainly by leukocytes.

## Mechanism of action/Effect
In general, interferons have antiviral, antiproliferative, and immunomodulatory activities. Antiviral and antiproliferative actions are thought to be related to alterations in synthesis of RNA, DNA, and cellular proteins, including oncogenes. The exact mechanism of antineoplastic activity is unknown, but may be related to any of these three actions.
Antiviral—Inhibit virus replication in virus-infected cells.
Antiproliferative—Suppress cell proliferation.
Immunomodulatory—Enhance phagocytic activity of macrophages and augment specific cytotoxicity of lymphocytes for target cells.

## Absorption
Intralesional—Plasma concentrations achieved are below detectable levels; however, systemic effects have been reported, indicating some systemic absorption.
Intramuscular and subcutaneous—Greater than 80%.

## Biotransformation
Renal, complete. Alpha interferons are totally filtered through the glomeruli and undergo rapid proteolytic degradation during tubular reabsorption.

## Half-life
Recombinant interferon alfa-2a—
Intramuscular: 6 to 8 hours.
Intravenous infusion: 3.7 to 8.5 (mean 5.1) hours.
Recombinant interferon alfa-2b—
Intramuscular or subcutaneous: 2 to 3 hours.
Interferon alfa-n1—
Intravenous infusion: About 8 hours.
Note: Accumulation may occur with daily intramuscular dosing.

## Onset of action
Hepatitis, chronic, active—Normalization of serum alanine aminotransferase (ALT) concentrations may occur as early as 2 weeks after initiation of treatment, although 6 months of treatment is usually recommended.

## Time to peak concentration
Recombinant interferon alfa-2a—Single dose:
Intramuscular—3.8 hours.
Subcutaneous—7.3 hours.

Recombinant interferon alfa-2b—Single dose:
Intramuscular or subcutaneous—3 to 12 hours.

## Time to peak effect
Condylomata acuminata—4 to 8 weeks after initiation of treatment.

## Elimination
With systemic use—Renal; metabolites almost completely reabsorbed in renal tubules, with only negligible amounts of unchanged alpha interferon reappearing in systemic circulation.

# Precautions to Consider

## Cross-sensitivity and/or related problems
Patients sensitive to any alpha interferon may also be sensitive to any other alpha interferon.
Patients sensitive to mouse immunoglobulin may also be sensitive to recombinant interferon alfa-2a.
Patients sensitive to mouse immunoglobulin, egg protein, or neomycin may also be sensitive to interferon alfa-n3.

## Carcinogenicity
Studies have not been done in either animals or humans.

## Mutagenicity
Results of Ames tests and *in vitro* treatment of human lymphocyte cultures with recombinant alpha interferon at noncytotoxic concentrations showed no evidence of mutagenicity. However, both genotoxicity and protection from chromosomal abnormalities produced by gamma rays have been reported in association with human leukocyte interferon *in vitro*.

## Pregnancy/Reproduction
Fertility—In humans, alpha interferon has been shown to affect the menstrual cycle and decrease serum estradiol and progesterone concentrations in adult females.
In Macaca mulatta (rhesus) monkeys given high doses (e.g., in the case of interferon alfa-n3, 326 times the average intralesional dose [120 times the maximum recommended dose]) intramuscularly daily, recombinant alpha interferon has been shown to cause menstrual cycle changes; normal menstrual rhythm returned when alpha interferon was withdrawn.
For interferon alfa-2a, recombinant: Has been shown to cause reversible menstrual irregularities, including prolonged or shortened menstrual periods and erratic bleeding with anovulation, in Macaca mulatta (rhesus) monkeys given 5 and 25 million Units per kg of body weight per day.
For interferon alfa-n3: No menstrual changes were reported in humans.
Pregnancy—Adequate and well-controlled studies in humans have not been done.
*For interferon alfa-2a, recombinant—*
Studies in rhesus monkeys at doses approximately 20 to 500 times the human dose found a significant increase in abortifacient activity but no evidence of teratogenic activity.
FDA Pregnancy Category C.
*For interferon alfa-2b, recombinant—*
Studies in Macaca mulatta (rhesus) monkeys at doses of 90 and 180 times the intramuscular or subcutaneous dose of 2 million Units per square meter of body surface found an abortifacient effect.
FDA Pregnancy Category C.
*For interferon alfa-n1 (lns)—*
Studies have not been done in animals.
*For interferon alfa-n3—*
Studies have not been done in animals.
FDA Pregnancy Category C.

## Breast-feeding
It is not known whether alpha interferon is excreted in human breast milk; in mice, mouse interferons are excreted in milk. However, because of the potential for serious adverse effects in nursing infants, avoidance of breast-feeding should be considered while alpha interferon is being administered.

## Pediatrics
Appropriate studies on the relationship of age to the effects of alpha interferons have not been performed in the pediatric population.

## Adolescents
Alpha interferons have been shown to affect the menstrual cycle in animals and decrease serum estradiol and progesterone concentrations in human females. These effects should be kept in mind when considering alpha interferon treatment in adolescent females.

**Geriatrics**

Although appropriate studies on the relationship of age to the effects of alpha interferons have not been performed in the geriatric population, neurotoxicity and cardiotoxicity may be more likely to occur in the elderly, who may have underlying central nervous system (CNS) and cardiac function impairment. In addition, elderly patients are more likely to have age-related renal function impairment, which may require caution in patients receiving alpha interferons.

**Dental**

The bone marrow depressant effects of alpha interferons may result in an increased incidence of microbial infection, delayed healing, and gingival bleeding. If leukopenia or thrombocytopenia occurs, dental work should be deferred until blood counts have returned to normal and patients should be instructed in proper oral hygiene, including caution in use of regular toothbrushes, dental floss, and toothpicks.

Interferon alfa-2a and alfa-2b may cause stomatitis and discomfort. Use of interferon alfa-2a or alfa-2b may decrease or inhibit salivary flow, thus contributing to the development of caries, periodontal disease, oral candidiasis, and discomfort.

**Drug interactions and/or related problems**

The following drug interactions and/or related problems have been selected on the basis of their potential clinical significance (possible mechanism in parentheses where appropriate)—not necessarily inclusive (» = major clinical significance):

Note: Combinations containing any of the following medications, depending on the amount present, may also interact with this medication.

The following information applies to systemic use.

Alcohol or
CNS depression–producing medications (See *Appendix II*)
(concurrent use may enhance the CNS depressant effects of either these medications or alpha interferon)

Blood dyscrasia–causing medications (See *Appendix II*)
(leukopenic and/or thrombocytopenic effects of interferon may be increased with concurrent or recent therapy if these medications cause the same effects; dosage adjustment of alpha interferon, if necessary, should be based on blood counts)

Bone marrow depressants, other (See *Appendix II*) or
Radiation therapy
(additive bone marrow depression may occur; dosage reduction may be required when two or more bone marrow depressants, including radiation, are used concurrently or consecutively)

**Laboratory value alterations**

The following have been selected on the basis of their potential clinical significance (possible effect in parentheses where appropriate)—not necessarily inclusive (» = major clinical significance):

With physiology/laboratory test values

Note: The following information applies to systemic use.

Alanine aminotransferase (ALT [SGPT]) and
Alkaline phosphatase and
Aspartate aminotransferase (AST [SGOT]) and
Lactate dehydrogenase
(serum values may be increased; dose related; reversible on withdrawal of alpha interferon)

Blood pressure
(mild and transient increase may occur; hypotension is more likely and may occur during administration or up to 2 days after administration)

Hemoglobin concentrations and
Hematocrit
(may be decreased)

Leukocyte counts (including neutrophils) and
Platelet counts
(may be decreased; dose-related)

Prothrombin time (PT) and
Partial thromboplastin time (PTT)
(may be increased by recombinant interferon alfa-2b; dose-related)

**Medical considerations/Contraindications**

The medical considerations/contraindications included here have been selected on the basis of their potential clinical significance (reasons given in parentheses where appropriate)—not necessarily inclusive (» = major clinical significance).

*Risk-benefit should be considered when the following medical problems exist:*

» Autoimmune disease, history of
(caution is recommended because alpha interferon may increase the activity of the immune system and thereby worsen the condition; use for treatment of non-A, non-B/C hepatitis is not recommended)

Bone marrow depression
(may be exacerbated)

» Cardiac disease, severe, including recent myocardial infarction or
» Diabetes mellitus prone to ketoacidosis or
» Pulmonary disease
(may be exacerbated as a result of the stress of the fever and chills that occur in most patients receiving alpha interferon)

(the risk of cardiotoxicity of alpha interferon may be increased in patients with a history of cardiac disease; myocardial infarction has been reported rarely)

» Chickenpox, existing or recent, including recent exposure or
» Herpes zoster
(risk of severe generalized disease)

» CNS function, compromised or
» Psychiatric conditions, severe, or history of or
» Seizure disorders
(risk of severe CNS side effects)

Hepatic disease, severe
(alpha interferons may elevate serum hepatic enzyme concentrations)

Herpes labialis, history of
(may be reactivated)

Renal disease, severe
(may be exacerbated by fever and dehydration caused by alpha interferon)

» Sensitivity to alpha interferon

Caution should be used also in patients who have had previous cytotoxic drug therapy or radiation therapy.

*For treatment of non-A, non-B/C hepatitis (in addition to the above)*
» Thyroid function impairment
(recombinant interferon alfa-2b has been reported to cause thyroid function abnormalities; serum thyroid-stimulating hormone [TSH] concentrations must be within normal limits before initiation of treatment)

*For recombinant interferon alfa-2b and interferon alfa-n3 only (in addition to the above)*
Coagulation disorders
(caution is recommended; recombinant interferon alfa-2b may prolong PT and PTT)

**Patient monitoring**

The following may be especially important in patient monitoring (other tests may be warranted in some patients, depending on condition; » = major clinical significance):

Note: The following information applies to systemic use.

Alanine aminotransferase (ALT [SGPT]) values and
Aspartate aminotransferase (AST [SGOT]) values and
Bilirubin concentrations, serum and
Lactate dehydrogenase (LDH) values
(recommended prior to initiation of therapy and at periodic intervals during therapy)

Blood pressure measurements
(recommended at periodic intervals)

Electrocardiogram (ECG)
(recommended prior to initiation of therapy and at periodic intervals during therapy in patients with cardiac disease or advanced malignancy)

» Hematocrit or hemoglobin and
» Platelet count and
» Total and, if appropriate, differential leukocyte count
(determinations recommended prior to initiation of therapy and at periodic intervals during therapy)

Liver biopsy
(recommended prior to discontinuing alpha interferon treatment when hepatic enzyme values return to normal)

Neuropsychiatric monitoring
(recommended especially in patients receiving high doses of alpha interferon)

Thyroid-stimulating hormone (TSH) concentrations, serum
(recommended prior to initiation of treatment for non-A, non-B/C
hepatitis and if symptoms of thyroid function impairment occur
during treatment)

## Side/Adverse Effects

See *Table 1*, page 1684.

## Patient Consultation

As an aid to patient consultation, refer to *Advice for the Patient,
Interferons, Alpha (Systemic)*.

In providing consultation, consider emphasizing the following selected
information (» = major clinical significance):

### Before using this medication
» Conditions affecting use, especially:
  Sensitivity to alpha interferons
  Pregnancy—Abortifacient effects found in rhesus monkeys
  Breast-feeding—Possible need to avoid during alpha interferon
  therapy because of risk of serious adverse effects
  Use in adolescents—Possible effects on menstrual cycle
  Use in the elderly—Risk of cardiotoxic and neurotoxic effects may
  be increased
  Other medical problems, especially history of autoimmune disease,
  severe cardiac disease, chicken pox, compromised CNS function, diabetes mellitus, herpes zoster, history of psychiatric disease, pulmonary disease, seizure disorders, and thyroid function impairment

### Proper use of this medication
» Compliance with therapy
» Reading patient directions carefully with regard to:
  —Preparation of the injection
  —Use of disposable syringes
  —Proper administration technique
  —Stability of the injection
  Importance of ample fluid intake to reduce risk of hypotension
  Administration at bedtime to minimize inconvenience of fatigue
» Proper dosing
  Missed dose: Skipping missed dose and going back to regular sched-
  ule; not doubling doses; checking with physician
» Proper storage

### Precautions while using this medication
» Importance of close monitoring by physician
» Not changing brands of interferon without consulting physician, be-
  cause of differences in dosage
» Caution in taking alcohol or other CNS depressants during therapy
» Caution when driving or doing anything else requiring alertness be-
  cause of possible fatigue and dizziness
» Frequency of fever and flu-like symptoms; possible need for acetaminophen before and after a dose is given
*Caution if bone marrow depression occurs:*
» Avoiding exposure to persons with bacterial infections, especially during periods of low blood counts; checking with physician immediately if fever or chills, cough or hoarseness, lower back or side
  pain, or painful or difficult urination occur
» Checking with physician immediately if unusual bleeding or bruising;
  black, tarry stools; blood in urine or stools; or pinpoint red spots
  on skin occur
  Caution in use of regular toothbrush, dental floss, or toothpick; physician, dentist, or nurse may suggest alternatives; checking with
  physician before having dental work done
  Not touching eyes or inside of nose unless hands washed immediately
  before
  Using caution to avoid accidental cuts with use of sharp objects such
  as safety razor or fingernail or toenail cutters
  Avoiding contact sports or other situations where bruising or injury
  could occur

### Side/adverse effects
Signs of potential side effects, especially cardiotoxicity, neurotoxicity,
peripheral neuropathy, leukopenia, and thrombocytopenia
Possibility of minor hair loss; hair should return after treatment has
ended

## General Dosing Information

Strengths and dosages of recombinant interferon alfa-2a and alfa-2b, interferon alfa-n1, and interferon alfa-n3 are expressed in terms of Units.
Units are determined by comparison of the antiviral activity of the
interferon with the activity of the international reference preparation

of human leukocyte interferon established by the World Health Organization (WHO).

Patients receiving alpha interferon should be under supervision of a physician experienced in immunomodulatory and/or cancer chemotherapy.

It is recommended that the patient be premedicated with acetaminophen
at the time of alpha interferon dosing and that the acetaminophen be
continued as needed to treat fever and headache. Dosage reduction of
alpha interferon may be necessary if headache persists.

Patients who develop leukopenia should be observed carefully for signs
of infection. Antibiotic support may be required. In neutropenic patients who develop fever, broad-spectrum antibiotic coverage should
be initiated empirically, pending bacterial cultures and appropriate diagnostic tests. In some cases, it may be difficult to distinguish fever
due to infection from fever associated with the flu-like syndrome.

Special precautions are recommended in patients who develop thrombocytopenia as a result of administration of alpha interferons. These may
include extreme care in performing invasive procedures; regular inspection of intravenous sites, skin (including perirectal area), and mucous membrane surfaces for signs of bleeding or bruising; limiting
frequency of venipuncture and avoiding intramuscular injections; testing urine, emesis, stool, and secretions for occult blood; care in use
of regular toothbrushes, dental floss, toothpicks, safety razors, and fingernail and toenail cutters; avoiding constipation; and using caution to
prevent falls and other injuries. Such patients should avoid alcohol and
any aspirin intake because of the risk of gastrointestinal bleeding.
Platelet transfusions may be required.

### For systemic use
The subcutaneous route of administration is recommended for patients
with thrombocytopenia or at risk for bleeding.

If severe adverse effects occur, dosage reduction by 50% or temporary
withdrawal of alpha interferon is recommended.

It is recommended that patients be well hydrated, especially during initial
treatment with alpha interferon, to reduce the risk of hypotension associated with fluid depletion. Hypotension may require supportive
treatment, including fluid replacement to maintain intravascular
volume.

---

### *INTERFERON ALFA-2a, RECOMBINANT*

## Summary of Differences

Pharmacology/pharmacokinetics:
  Source—Synthetic; produced by a recombinant DNA process. Purifi-
  cation procedure includes affinity chromatography using a murine
  monoclonal antibody. Single alpha interferon subtype.
  Half-life—
  Intramuscular: 6 to 8 hours.
  Intravenous infusion: 3.7 to 8.5 hours.
  Time to peak concentration—Single dose:
  Intramuscular—3.8 hours.
  Subcutaneous—7.3 hours.

## Parenteral Dosage Forms

### INTERFERON ALFA-2a, RECOMBINANT, INJECTION

**Usual adult dose**
Hairy cell leukemia—
  Induction: Intramuscular or subcutaneous, 3 million Units per day for
  sixteen to twenty-four weeks.
  Maintenance: Intramuscular or subcutaneous, 3 million Units three
  times per week.
Kaposi's sarcoma, AIDS-associated—
  Induction:
    Intramuscular or subcutaneous, 36 million Units (1 mL) per day
    for ten to twelve weeks, or
    Intramuscular or subcutaneous, 3 million Units per day on Days 1
    to 3, 9 million Units per day on Days 4 to 6, and 18 million
    Units per day on Days 7 to 9, followed by 36 million Units (1
    mL) per day for the remainder of the ten- to twelve-weeks
    induction period.
  Maintenance:
    Intramuscular or subcutaneous, 36 million Units (1 mL) three times
    per week.
Note: A variety of dosage schedules of interferon have been used for the
  unlabeled indications. Since these regimens are still largely investigational, the prescriber should consult the medical literature in
  choosing a specific dosage.

**Usual pediatric dose**
Dosage has not been established.

**Strength(s) usually available**

U.S.—

3 million Units per mL (Rx) [*Roferon-A* (sodium chloride; albumin; phenol)].

6 million Units per mL (18 million Units per vial) (Rx) [*Roferon-A* (sodium chloride; albumin; phenol)].

10 million Units per mL (9 million Units per 0.9-mL vial) (Rx) [*Roferon-A* (sodium chloride; albumin; phenol)].

36 million Units per mL (Rx) [*Roferon-A* (sodium chloride; albumin; phenol]

Note: The 10-million-Units-per-mL and 36-million-Units-per-mL strengths are for use for treatment of AIDS-associated Kaposi's sarcoma. They should *not* be used for treatment of hairy cell leukemia.

Canada—

3 million Units per mL (Rx) [*Roferon-A* (sodium chloride; albumin; phenol)].

6 million Units per mL (Rx) [*Roferon-A* (phenol)].

**Packaging and storage**

Store between 2 and 8 °C (36 and 46 °F), unless otherwise specified by manufacturer. Protect from freezing.

**Note**

Do not shake.

When dispensing for self-administration by the patient, make sure that patient instructions are included and that the patient understands how to prepare and administer the injection, including proper use of disposable syringes.

Interferon alfa-2a,-2b,-n1, and-n3 are not interchangeable.

## INTERFERON ALFA-2a, RECOMBINANT, FOR INJECTION

**Usual adult dose**

Hairy cell leukemia—

Induction: Intramuscular or subcutaneous, 3 million Units per day for sixteen to twenty-four weeks.

Maintenance: Intramuscular or subcutaneous, 3 million Units three times per week.

Note: A variety of dosage schedules of interferon have been used for the unlabeled indications. Since these regimens are still largely investigational, the prescriber should consult the medical literature in choosing a specific dosage.

**Usual pediatric dose**

Dosage has not been established.

**Size(s) usually available**

U.S.—

18 million Units (Rx) [*Roferon-A* (diluent contains sodium chloride, albumin, phenol)].

Canada—

18 million Units (Rx) [*Roferon-A* (diluent contains sodium chloride, albumin, phenol)].

**Packaging and storage**

Store between 2 and 8 °C (36 and 46 °F), unless otherwise specified by manufacturer. Protect from freezing.

**Preparation of dosage form**

Interferon alfa-2a, recombinant, for injection is prepared for parenteral use by adding 3 mL of diluent (containing sodium chloride, albumin, and phenol) provided by the manufacturer and swirling gently to dissolve, producing a solution containing 6 million Units per mL.

**Stability**

Reconstituted solution of interferon alfa-2a, recombinant, for injection should be used within 30 days and stored between 2 and 8 °C (36 and 46 °F).

**Note**

When dispensing for self-administration by the patient, make sure that patient instructions are included and that the patient understands how to prepare and administer the injection, including proper use of disposable syringes.

Interferon alfa-2a,-2b,-n1, and-n3 are not interchangeable.

## INTERFERON ALFA-2b, RECOMBINANT

## Summary of Differences

Pharmacology/pharmacokinetics:

Source—Synthetic; produced by a recombinant DNA process. Purification is done by proprietary methods. Single alpha interferon subtype.

Half-life—Intramuscular or subcutaneous: 2 to 3 hours.

Time to peak concentration—Intramuscular or subcutaneous: 3 to 12 hours.

Precautions:

Laboratory value alterations——

Nadir of leukocyte and platelet counts is at 3 to 5 days, with recovery within 3 to 5 days after withdrawal.

Prothrombin time (PT) and partial thromboplastin time (PTT) may be increased.

Medical considerations/contraindications—

Caution in coagulation disorders.

## Parenteral Dosage Forms

### INTERFERON ALFA-2b, RECOMBINANT, FOR INJECTION

**Usual adult dose**

Hairy cell leukemia—

Intramuscular or subcutaneous, 2 million Units per square meter of body surface three times per week.

Condylomata acuminata[1]—

Intralesional, 1 million units (using 10 million Units-per-mL strength) per wart (up to five warts) three times a week on alternate days for three weeks. If response is not satisfactory twelve to sixteen weeks after the initial treatment course, a second course may be given. Patients with six to ten warts may be given a second (sequential) course of treatment at the same dose to treat up to five additional warts per course; for patients with more than ten warts, additional courses may be given as needed with up to five additional warts per course.

Kaposi's sarcoma, AIDS-associated—

Intramuscular or subcutaneous, 30 million Units (using 50 million Units-per-mL strength) per square meter of body surface three times a week.

Hepatitis, chronic, active—

Non-A, non-B/C hepatitis: Intramuscular or subcutaneous, 3 million Units three times per week. Patients who relapse may be retreated with the same dose to which they had previously responded.

Note: A variety of dosage schedules of interferon have been used for the unlabeled indications. Since these regimens are still largely investigational, the prescriber should consult the medical literature in choosing a specific dosage.

**Usual pediatric dose**

Safety and efficacy have not been established.

**Size(s) usually available**

U.S.—

3 million Units (Rx) [*Intron A* (albumin)].

5 million Units (Rx) [*Intron A* (albumin)].

10 million Units (Rx) [*Intron A* (albumin)].

Note: The 10-million-Unit size is the only one that should be used for treatment of condylomata acuminata. Dilution of other sizes (3, 5, 25 million Units) that would be required for intralesional use would produce a hypertonic solution.

25 million Units (Rx) [*Intron A* (albumin)]

50 million Units (Rx) [*Intron A* (albumin)]

Note: The 50-million-Unit size is a special formulation for use for treatment of AIDS-associated Kaposi's sarcoma. It should *not* be used for treatment of hairy cell leukemia or condylomata acuminata.

Canada—

3 million Units (Rx) [*Intron A* (albumin)].

5 million Units (Rx) [*Intron A* (albumin)].

10 million Units (Rx) [*Intron A* (albumin)].

**Packaging and storage**

Store between 2 and 8 °C (36 and 46 °F), unless otherwise specified by manufacturer.

**Preparation of dosage form**

Interferon alfa-2b, recombinant, for injection is prepared for parenteral use by adding the appropriate amount of diluent (in the U.S., bacteriostatic water for injection provided by the manufacturer; in Canada, either sterile water for injection or bacteriostatic water for injection) and agitating gently to dissolve, producing a clear, colorless to light yellow solution:

| Size (Units) | Diluent (mL) | Final concentration (Units/mL) |
|---|---|---|
| U.S.— | | |
| *For treatment of hairy cell leukemia* | | |
| 3 million | 1 | 3 million |
| 5 million | 1 | 5 million |
| 10 million | 2 | 5 million |
| 25 million | 5 | 5 million |
| *For treatment of condylomata acuminata* | | |
| 10 million | 1 | 10 million |
| *For treatment of AIDS-associated Kaposi's sarcoma* | | |
| 50 million | 1 | 50 million |
| *For treatment of chronic active hepatitis* | | |
| 3 million | 1 | 3 million |
| Canada— | | |
| 3 million | 1 | 3 million |
| 5 million | 1 | 5 million |
| 10 million | 1 | 10 million |

**Stability**

Reconstituted solutions of interferon alfa-2b, recombinant, prepared with sterile water for injection are stable for 24 hours when stored between 2 and 8 °C (36 and 46 °F); solutions prepared with bacteriostatic water for injection are stable for 1 month when stored between 2 and 8 °C (36 and 46 °F).

**Note**

When dispensing for self-administration by the patient, make sure that patient instructions are included and that the patient understands how to prepare and administer the injection, including proper use of disposable syringes.

Interferon alfa-2a,-2b,-n1, and-n3 are not interchangeable.

¹Not included in Canadian product labeling.

---

## INTERFERON ALFA-n1 (LNS)

## Summary of Differences

Pharmacology/pharmacokinetics:
  Source—Obtained from pooled units of human lymphoblastoid cells following induction with Sendai virus. Mixture of natural alpha interferon subtypes, but in different proportions than in human leukocyte interferon.
  Half-life—Intravenous infusion: About 8 hours.

## Parenteral Dosage Forms

### INTERFERON ALFA-n1 (LNS) INJECTION

**Usual adult dose**

Hairy cell leukemia—
  Induction: Intramuscular or subcutaneous, 3 million Units per day for sixteen to twenty-four weeks.
  Maintenance: Intramuscular or subcutaneous, 3 million Units three times per week.
Condylomata acuminata—
  Intramuscular or subcutaneous, 1 to 3 million Units per square meter of body surface five times a week for two weeks, followed by three times a week for four weeks. The same dose is then continued every other day or three times a week for one month.

Note: As an adjunct to laser surgery or cryosurgery, the dose is 1 million Units per square meter of body surface intramuscularly or subcutaneously per day for seven days prior to and seven days following surgical resection of the lesions.

Note: A variety of dosage schedules of interferon have been used for the unlabeled indications. Since these regimens are still largely investigational, the prescriber should consult the medical literature in choosing a specific dosage.

**Usual pediatric dose**

Hairy cell leukemia or
Condylomata acuminata—
  Dosage has not been established.

Juvenile laryngeal papillomatosis—
  For children greater than 1 year of age:
    Body surface area less than 0.5 square meter—Intramuscular or subcutaneous, 1.5 million Units per day for twenty-eight days, followed by maintenance dosage three times a week for at least six months.
    Body surface area 0.5–1.0 square meter—Intramuscular or subcutaneous, 3 million Units per day for twenty-eight days, followed by maintenance dosage three times a week for at least six months.
    Body surface area greater than 1.0 square meter—Intramuscular or subcutaneous, 5 million Units per day for twenty-eight days, followed by maintenance dosage three times a week for at least six months.

**Size(s) usually available**

U.S.—
  Not commercially available.
Canada—
  3 million Units (Rx) [*Wellferon*].
  10 million Units (Rx) [*Wellferon*].

**Packaging and storage**

Store between 2 and 8 °C (36 and 46 °F), unless otherwise specified by manufacturer. Protect from light.

**Note**

Interferon alfa-2a,-2b,-n1, and-n3 are not interchangeable.

---

## INTERFERON ALFA-n3

## Summary of Differences

Pharmacology/pharmacokinetics:
  Source—Obtained from pooled units of human leukocytes that have been induced to produce interferon alfa-n3. Contains up to 14 natural alpha interferon subtypes. Human leukocyte interferon.
Precautions:
  Medical considerations/contraindications—Caution in coagulation disorders.

## Parenteral Dosage Forms

### INTERFERON ALFA-n3 INJECTION

**Usual adult dose**

Condylomata acuminata—
  Intralesional (at the base of the wart, preferably using a 30 gauge needle), 250,000 Units two times a week for up to eight weeks.

Note: For large warts, it may be injected at several points around the periphery of the wart, using a total dose of 250,000 Units.

  Safety and efficacy of more than one 8-week course have not been established.

  A variety of dosage schedules of interferon have been used for the unlabeled indications. Since these regimens are still largely investigational, the prescriber should consult the medical literature in choosing a specific dosage.

**Usual adult prescribing limits**

Up to 2.5 million Units per treatment session.

**Usual pediatric dose**

Dosage has not been established.

**Strength(s) usually available**

U.S.—
  5 million Units per mL (Rx) [*Alferon N* (phenol 3.3 mg per mL; human albumin 1 mg per mL)].
Canada—
  Not commercially available.

**Packaging and storage**

Store between 2 and 8 °C (36 and 46 °F), unless otherwise specified by manufacturer. Protect from freezing.

**Note**

Do not shake.

Interferon alfa-2a,-2b,-n1, and-n3 are not interchangeable.

---

Revised: 01/16/92
Interim revision: 04/17/93; 06/09/93; 07/05/94

## Table 1. Side/Adverse Effects

Note: Most side/adverse effects, except the flu-like syndrome, are dose-related. They are usually mild to moderate at systemic doses less than 10 million Units per day; hematologic and hepatic toxicities tend to be more frequent with doses above 10 million Units, and cardiovascular and neurologic toxicities tend to be more frequent with doses above 30 million Units. However, patient sensitivity varies.

Reduced blood pressure occurs frequently with systemic use but is rarely symptomatic; hypotension may occur during administration or up to two days after therapy, and may require supportive therapy including fluid replacement to maintain intravascular volume; hypertension may occur but is usually mild and transient.

Development of neutralizing antibodies has been reported. Relationship of the presence of neutralizing antibodies to loss of antitumor effects is controversial; a possible correlation with titer of neutralizing antibodies has been suggested but not confirmed. Differences in frequency of antibody formation have been reported among alpha interferons but relative frequency has not been studied prospectively. Differences may be related to the differences in the sensitivity of tests used in antibody detection, as well as to disease state, dose, schedule, and route of administration.

| The following side/adverse effects have been selected on the basis of their potential clinical significance (possible signs and symptoms in parentheses where appropriate)—not necessarily inclusive:* | Indication | | | | |
|---|---|---|---|---|---|
| | Hairy cell leukemia | Other malignancies | Condylomata acuminata | Kaposi's sarcoma | Hepatitis |
| **Those indicating need for medical attention** | | | | | |
| *Anemia* (usually asymptomatic) | N/A | M | L | M | M |
| *Cardiotoxicity* (chest pain, irregular heartbeat) <br> Note: Arrhythmias are usually supraventricular. | R | R | U | R | R |
| *Hepatotoxicity* (usually asymptomatic) | L | L | L | M | L |
| *Hyperthyroidism or hypothyroidism* (usually asymptomatic) | U | U | U | U | R |
| *Leukopenia* (usually asymptomatic; rarely, fever or chills, cough or hoarseness, lower back or side pain, painful or difficult urination) | N/A | M | M | M | M |
| *Neurotoxicity* (confusion, mental depression, nervousness, trouble in sleeping, trouble in thinking or concentrating) <br> Note: Usually reversible after withdrawal; in some patients, especially the elderly or those treated with high doses, stupor, obtundation, and coma have occurred. | L | L | L | L | L |
| *Peripheral neuropathy* (numbness or tingling of fingers, toes, or face) | L | L | L | L | R |
| *Thrombocytopenia* (usually asymptomatic; rarely, unusual bleeding or bruising; black, tarry stools; blood in urine or stools; pinpoint red spots on skin) | N/A | M | L | M | M |
| **Those indicating need for medical attention only if they continue or are bothersome** | | | | | |
| *Blurred vision* | L | L | L | L | L |
| *Change in taste or metallic taste* | M | M | R | M | R |
| *Cold sores or stomatitis* (sores in mouth and on lips) | L | L | R | R | R |
| *Diarrhea* | M | M | L | M | M |
| *Dizziness* <br> Note: Dizziness is a CNS effect. | M | M | L | M | L |
| *Dry mouth* | M | M | R | M | L |
| *Dry skin or itching* | L | L | L | L | L |
| *Flu-like syndrome* (aching muscles, fever and chills, headache, general feeling of discomfort or illness; less frequently, joint pain, back pain) <br> Note: Occurs in most patients; most pronounced in first week of treatment and gradually reduced, as a result of tachyphylaxis, within 2 to 4 weeks with continued treatment. | M | M | M | M | M |
| *Increased sweating* | L | L | L | L | L |
| *Leg cramps* | L | L | L | U | R |
| *Loss of appetite* <br> Note: Loss of appetite tends to become more prominent with continued treatment and may necessitate dosage reduction; usually resolves within 4 weeks after withdrawal of alpha interferon. | M | M | L | M | M |
| *Nausea or vomiting* <br> Note: Nausea or vomiting usually resolves within 3 to 5 days after withdrawal of alpha interferon. | M | M | M | M | M |
| *Skin rash* | M | M | L | M | L |

Table 1. Side/Adverse Effects *(continued)*

|  | Indication | | | | |
|---|---|---|---|---|---|
|  | Hairy cell leukemia | Other malignancies | Condylomata acuminata | Kaposi's sarcoma | Hepatitis |
| ***Unusual tiredness***<br>Note: Unusual tiredness tends to become more prominent with continued treatment and may necessitate dosage reduction; usually resolves several weeks after withdrawal of alpha interferon. | M | M | M | M | M |
| ***Weight loss*** | R | R | R | L | R |
| **Those not indicating need for medical attention**<br>Incidence less frequent<br>   *Loss of hair, partial*<br>   Note: Hair growth returns promptly after withdrawal of alpha interferon. | L | L | U | M | M |

*Differences in frequency of occurrence may reflect either lack of clinical-use data or actual pharmacologic distinctions among agents (although their pharmacologic similarity suggests that side effects occurring with one may occur with the others). M = more frequent; L = less frequent; R = rare; U = unknown; X = does not occur; N/A = Not applicable.

# INULIN   Systemic†

VA CLASSIFICATION (Primary): DX900
Note: For a listing of dosage forms and brand names by country availability, see *Dosage Forms* section(s). For a listing of brand names for the articles in this monograph, refer to the General Index.

†Not commercially available in Canada.

## Category
Diagnostic aid (renal function).

## Indications
### Accepted
Renal function studies—Inulin is indicated for evaluation of renal function as indicated by glomerular filtration rate (GFR).

Although inulin is considered to be ideal for measurement of GFR and gives the most accurate values, the test is cumbersome and suited more for research. In general, the inulin clearance test has been replaced in clinical situations by simpler (although less precise) tests such as creatinine clearance.

### Unaccepted
Use of inulin to estimate extracellular fluid (ECF) volume may not be reliable, especially during pregnancy, because the total ECF volume compartment is not measured.

## Pharmacology/Pharmacokinetics

### Mechanism of action/Effect
Inulin's usefulness as a diagnostic agent is based on the method of its elimination from the body. Inulin is not reabsorbed by the renal tubules and does not undergo tubular secretion, but is excreted almost entirely by glomerular filtration. Inulin clearance is considered to be identical to glomerular filtration rate (GFR).

### Other actions/effects
In extremely high doses, inulin has an osmotic diuretic effect.

### Protein binding
Minimal.

### Biotransformation
Not metabolized.

### Half-life
Neonates—10.5 hours.
Children over 1 year of age and adults—2 to 4 hours.

### Elimination
Renal (almost entirely by glomerular filtration); biliary (trace).

## Precautions to Consider

### Pregnancy/Reproduction
Pregnancy—Problems in humans have not been documented. However, when administered immediately prior to delivery, inulin has been found to appear in amniotic fluid, neonatal urine, and cord blood.
Glomerular filtration rate (GFR) increases significantly during the first trimester and throughout pregnancy (up to 50% above normal by the third trimester), but falls 15 to 30% after the 36th week and returns to normal immediately postpartum.

### Breast-feeding
Problems in humans have not been documented.

### Pediatrics
GFR is lower in children up to 1 year of age than in older children and adults.

### Geriatrics
GFR begins to decrease gradually in individuals over 40 years of age.

### Laboratory value alterations
The following have been selected on the basis of their potential clinical significance (possible effect in parentheses where appropriate)—not necessarily inclusive (» = major clinical significance):

With results of *this* test
 *Due to medical problems or conditions*
  Adrenal insufficiency or
  Conditions in which small vessel circulation is impaired, such as:
   Cirrhosis with ascitic accumulation
   Congestive heart failure
   Dehydration
   Shock or
  Hypothyroidism or
  Impeded urinary drainage or
  Renal function impairment
   (inulin clearance is reduced)

  Inulin clearance may also be reduced by severe exertion, and in patients over 40 years of age and neonates.

  Inulin clearance may be altered by normal diurnal variation or variations in hydration.

### Medical considerations/Contraindications
The medical considerations/contraindications included here have been selected on the basis of their potential clinical significance (reasons given in parentheses where appropriate)—not necessarily inclusive (» = major clinical significance).
See also *Laboratory value alterations.*

*Risk-benefit should be considered when the following medical problem exists:*
  Sensitivity to inulin

## Patient monitoring

The following may be especially important in patient monitoring (other tests may be warranted in some patients, depending on condition; » = major clinical significance):

Inulin, plasma and urinary concentrations
   (determinations recommended at appropriate intervals, according to the method being used to determine inulin clearance)

## Side/Adverse Effects

Inulin does not usually cause any side/adverse effects, although extremely large doses may cause osmotic diuresis.

## Patient Consultation

As an aid to patient consultation, refer to *Advice for the Patient, Inulin (Diagnostic)*.

In providing consultation, consider emphasizing the following selected information (» = major clinical significance):

### Description of use

Test procedure: Administered intravenously; blood and sometimes urine samples taken; possible use of catheter; measurement of medication in blood and/or urine
» Proper dosing

### Before having this test

» Conditions affecting use, especially:
   Sensitivity to inulin

### Preparation for this test

Special preparatory instructions may be given; patient should inquire in advance

## General Dosing Information

Inulin injection is administered by intravenous injection or intravenous infusion.

It is recommended that fluids be administered prior to and during the procedure to ensure adequate hydration and maintain an adequate urinary output.

Urine collection is usually accomplished by having the patient stand to void, but if there is any indication of obstruction or incomplete emptying, bladder catheterization may be necessary. Further accuracy can be achieved by using saline followed by air washes.

Normal inulin clearance is 130 mL per minute in adult males and 120 mL per minute in adult females (range, 100 to 150 mL per minute); it begins to decrease after 40 years of age. Clearance is 25 to 39 mL per minute per 1.73 square meters of body surface (mL/min/1.73m²) in neonates (up to 7 days of age) and 50 mL/min/1.73m² in older infants (1 month of age). Values approach normal adult values at a few months of age.

Values for inulin clearance may be corrected for differences in renal mass by multiplying clearance by 1.73/A (where 1.73 is the body surface area in square meters of the average adult and A is the body surface area of the patient).

There are several methods by which inulin clearance may be determined. One involves both urine and blood sample collections while another utilizes only blood samples. It is desirable in most methods to achieve a constant plasma concentration of inulin to maximize the accuracy of the results. Two commonly utilized test methods are briefly described below.

### Inulin renal clearance test—Method 1

The test is performed after the patient has rested and had a light breakfast (not including tea, coffee, or concentrated carbohydrates such as sugar, jelly, or jam).

A blood sample is drawn prior to administration of inulin, then centrifuged and refrigerated for use as a control.

Following inulin administration, the bladder is emptied and the fluid discarded. Then at timed intervals, additional urine collections are made and saved. A blood sample is drawn (and immediately centrifuged to separate the plasma), and the time recorded, at the midpoint in time between the initial discard and collection of the first urine specimen, and at the midpoint between urine collections thereafter.

Inulin clearance is calculated by analyzing urine collected over a specific period to determine the average concentration of inulin in the urine (U) in mg per mL and the average volume of urine collected (V) in mL per minute, and by analyzing blood samples drawn to determine the average concentration of inulin in plasma (P) in mg per mL, and then using these values to determine the number of mL of plasma that must have been filtered to account for the amount excreted per minute in urine.

Inulin clearance (and, therefore, glomerular filtration rate [GFR]) may be calculated using the following formula:

$$\text{Inulin clearance} = (U \times V) \div P$$

### Inulin plasma clearance test—Method 2

During inulin administration, blood samples are drawn at timed intervals and plasma inulin concentrations determined. This is continued until a constant (steady-state) plasma inulin concentration is achieved (usually within 4 hours); achievement of constant plasma inulin concentrations is critical to ensure the accuracy of results obtained by this method.

Inulin clearance is calculated by analyzing the plasma inulin concentration (P) in a blood sample obtained at steady-state, when the rate of elimination of inulin from the body ($U \times V$) is equal to the rate of administration ($I \times R$, where I is the concentration of inulin in the infusion and R is the rate of infusion).

Inulin clearance (and therefore GFR) may be calculated using the following formula:

$$\text{Inulin clearance} = (I \times R) \div P$$

## Parenteral Dosage Forms

### INULIN INJECTION

#### Usual adult and adolescent dose

Renal function studies—
   A loading dose, usually 50 mg per kg of body weight, is administered by intravenous injection (into the line of an intravenous infusion), followed by an intravenous infusion of inulin at a rate sufficient to achieve a stable plasma concentration of inulin. Most manufacturers recommend a sustaining dose of 18.8 mg per square meter of body surface per minute. Specific dosages may vary with the investigator or laboratory performing the test.

#### Usual pediatric dose

See *Usual adult and adolescent dose.*

#### Usual geriatric dose

See *Usual adult and adolescent dose.*

#### Strength(s) usually available

U.S.—
   100 mg per mL (Rx) [GENERIC].
Canada—
   Not commercially available.

#### Packaging and storage

Store below 40 °C (104 °F), preferably between 15 and 30 °C (59 and 86 °F), unless otherwise specified by manufacturer. Protect from freezing.

#### Preparation of dosage form

Inulin injection may be diluted in 0.9% sodium chloride injection for administration by intravenous infusion.

#### Stability

Crystals of inulin may form in the ampul. These must be dissolved by shaking the ampul, then heating in boiling water prior to administration. Inulin injection may be heated at 100 °C for up to 1 hour but *must be cooled to body temperature* for administration. If all crystals cannot be completely dissolved, the solution should not be used. In order to reduce crystallization, the solution should not be refrigerated.

## Selected Bibliography

Brenner BM, Ichikawa I, Deen WM. Glomerular filtration. In: Brenner BM, Rector FC, editors. The kidney, 2nd edition. Philadelphia: W.B. Saunders, 1981: 308-9.

Revised: 06/23/94

---

**IOBENGUANE I 123**—See *Iobenguane, Radioiodinated (Systemic—Diagnostic)*

---

**IOBENGUANE I 131**—See *Iobenguane, Radioiodinated (Systemic—Diagnostic)*

# IOBENGUANE, RADIOIODINATED  Systemic—Diagnostic†

VA CLASSIFICATION (Primary): DX201

A commonly used name for iobenguane is meta-iodobenzylguanidine or mIBG.

Note: For a listing of dosage forms and brand names by country availability, see *Dosage Forms* section(s). For a listing of brand names for the articles in this monograph, refer to the General Index.

†Not commercially available in Canada.

## Category

Diagnostic aid, radioactive (adrenomedullary disorders; neuroendocrine tumors).

## Indications

Note: Bracketed information in the *Indications* section refers to uses that are not included in U.S. product labeling. In addition, because iobenguane I 123 (123I-mIBG) injection is not commercially available in the U.S. or Canada, the bracketed information and the use of the superscript 1 in this monograph reflect the lack of labeled (approved) indications for this product.

### Accepted

Tumors, adrenal medulla (diagnosis)[1]—[123I]- and 131I-mIBG are used for diagnostic imaging of the adrenal medulla, for the evaluation and localization of intra- and extra-adrenal pheochromocytomas, paragangliomas, and neuroblastomas, as well as for localization of metastatic lesions from these tumors. [123I]- and 131I-mIBG can also be used for confirmation of diagnosis of pheochromocytoma when catecholamine determination tests are unclear.

[Tumors, carcinoid (diagnosis)][1]—123I- and 131I-mIBG scintigraphy are used as screening procedures for suspected carcinoid tumors, especially those of intestinal origin.

[Hyperplasia, adrenal medulla (diagnosis)][1]—123I- and 131I-mIBG are used in the evaluation of the adrenal medulla for disorders such as medullary hyperplasia in patients at risk of developing medullary disease (e.g., multiple endocrine neoplasia [MEN type 2, MEN type 3]).

[Carcinoma, thyroid (diagnosis)][1]—123I- and 131I-mIBG are used for diagnostic imaging of medullary thyroid carcinoma.

[1]Not included in Canadian product labeling.

## Physical Properties

### Nuclear data

| Radionuclide (half-life) | Decay constant | Mode of decay | Principal emissions (keV) | Mean number of emissions/ disintegration |
|---|---|---|---|---|
| I 123 (13.2 hr) | 0.0533 h⁻¹ | Electron capture | Gamma (159) | 0.83 |
| I 131 (8.08 days) | 0.00358 h⁻¹ | Beta | Beta (191.6) Gamma (364.5) | 0.90 0.81 |

## Pharmacology/Pharmacokinetics

### Mechanism of action/Effect

Iobenguane or meta-iodobenzylguanidine (mIBG) is a physiological analog of the guanidines, such as guanethidine and phenethylguanidine. In adrenergic nerves, guanidines are believed to share the same transport pathway as norepinephrine and to accumulate in, and displace norepinephrine from, intraneuronal storage granules. Similarly, 123I- and 131I-mIBG are concentrated in, stored in, and released from chromaffin granules. The retention of 123I- and 131I-mIBG in the adrenal medulla may be a result of their uptake in adrenergic neurons and subsequent sequestration into chromaffin storage granules. Due to their selective uptake mechanism, 123I- and 131I-mIBG allow specific detection and localization of neuroendocrine tumors and adrenal medullary hyperplasia. The gamma emissions given off by 123I- and 131I-mIBG allow detection of adrenergic tumors by scintigraphy.

Medullary thyroid carcinoma—Although the mechanism of 123I- and 131I-mIBG uptake by medullary thyroid carcinoma (MTC) is not completely understood, it has been found that MTC can produce catecholamines (epinephrine and norepinephrine). Therefore, 123I- and 131I-mIBG could be taken up and stored in catecholamine vesicles of MTC.

## Distribution

After intravenous administration, there is rapid uptake of mIBG mainly in the liver, and in lesser amounts in the lungs, heart, spleen, and salivary glands. Although the uptake in normal adrenal glands is very low, hyperplastic adrenals and tumors such as pheochromocytoma, neuroblastoma, and other tumors with neurosecretory granules have a relatively higher uptake.

Significant clearance of 131I-mIBG from the liver and the spleen occurs within 72 hours.

### Time to radioactivity visualization

123I-mIBG—In adrenal medullary tumors: Initial images may be obtained 2 to 3 hours after injection. Images may also be obtained at 18 to 24 hours, and as late as 48 hours post injection. Most pheochromocytomas are visualized at 24 hours. However, due to the short half-life of 123I-mIBG, images may not be possible at times when background (e.g., liver) activity is low and imaging would be optimal.

131I-mIBG—In adrenal medullary tumors: 48 hours. Early images at 24 hours after administration of 131I-mIBG are frequently positive in patients with pheochromocytoma. Decline in liver activity may permit optimal imaging at 48 or 72 hours.

### Radiation dosimetry

| Organ | Estimated absorbed radiation dose* | | | |
|---|---|---|---|---|
| | 123I-mIBG | | 131I-mIBG | |
| | mGy/ MBq | rad/ mCi | mGy/ MBq | rad/ mCi |
| Liver | 0.071 | 0.27 | 0.83 | 3.07 |
| Bladder wall | 0.070 | 0.30 | 0.59 | 2.18 |
| Spleen | 0.020 | 0.074 | 0.49 | 1.81 |
| Salivary glands | 0.017 | 0.063 | 0.23 | 0.85 |
| Lungs | 0.016 | 0.059 | 0.19 | 0.70 |
| Kidneys | 0.014 | 0.052 | 0.12 | 0.44 |
| Adrenals | 0.011 | 0.041 | 0.17 | 0.63 |
| Heart | 0.011 | 0.041 | 0.072 | 0.26 |
| Pancreas | 0.011 | 0.041 | 0.10 | 0.37 |
| Uterus | 0.011 | 0.041 | 0.080 | 0.29 |
| Red marrow | 0.0092 | 0.034 | 0.067 | 0.25 |
| Large intestine wall (upper) | 0.0089 | 0.033 | 0.080 | 0.29 |
| Small intestine | 0.0083 | 0.031 | 0.074 | 0.27 |
| Ovaries | 0.0080 | 0.030 | 0.066 | 0.24 |
| Stomach wall | 0.0078 | 0.029 | 0.077 | 0.28 |
| Large intestine wall (lower) | 0.0077 | 0.028 | 0.068 | 0.25 |
| Bone surfaces | 0.0076 | 0.028 | 0.061 | 0.23 |
| Breast | 0.0062 | 0.023 | 0.069 | 0.25 |
| Testes | 0.0054 | 0.020 | 0.059 | 0.22 |
| Thyroid (blocked)† | 0.0042 | 0.016 | 0.050 | 0.18 |
| Other tissue | 0.0065 | 0.024 | 0.062 | 0.23 |

| Radionuclide and impurities | Effective dose* | | | |
|---|---|---|---|---|
| | 123I-mIBG | | 131I-mIBG | |
| | mSv/ MBq | rem/ mCi | mSv/ MBq | rem/ mCi |
| I 123 | 0.018 | 0.067 | — | — |
| I 124 | 0.24 | 0.88 | — | — |
| I 125 | 0.049 | 0.18 | — | — |
| I 131 | — | — | 0.20 | 0.74 |

*For adults; intravenous injection. Data based on the International Commission on Radiological Protection (ICRP) Publication 53—Radiation dose to patients from radiopharmaceuticals.

†Thyroid dose listed assumes 0% thyroid uptake. However, uptakes ranging from 0.5 to 2% are more typical; consequently the absorbed radiation dose to the thyroid will be many times higher than listed.

### Elimination

Renal; about 40 to 50% of the injected activity is eliminated within 24 hours and about 70 to 90% within 4 days (mainly as unchanged drug with small amounts of 123I- or 131I-m-iodohippuric acid [123I- or 131I-mIHA], 123I or 131I iodide, and 123I- or 131I-m-iodobenzoic acid [123I- or 131I-mIBA]).

## Precautions to Consider

### Pregnancy/Reproduction

Pregnancy—The possibility of pregnancy should be assessed in women of child-bearing potential. Clinical situations exist where the benefit to the patient and fetus, based on information derived from radiopharmaceutical use, outweighs the risks from fetal exposure to radiation. In these situations, the physician should use discretion and reduce the administered activity to the lowest possible amount.

### Breast-feeding

It is not known whether [123]I- or [131]I-mIBG is distributed into breast milk. However, this preparation may be contaminated with free radioiodide, which may be distributed into breast milk. It has been recommended that, after administration of a radiopharmaceutical, nursing be resumed only after the infant's ingested effective dose equivalent (EDE) is below 1 mSv (100 mrem). A method to calculate the EDE has been proposed based on the effective half-life of the radionuclide, the activity administered to the mother, the fraction of administered activity ingested by the infant, and the total body effective dose to the newborn infant per unit of activity ingested. According to this method, it has been estimated that, for sodium iodide I 131, the time to reduce the EDE to the infant to below 1 mSv (100 mrem) is approximately 10 weeks after administration of 40 megabecquerels (1.08 millicuries) to the mother. For sodium iodide I 123, the time period required is 3 days with administration of an uncontaminated preparation, 40 days with a preparation contaminated with I 124, and 340 days for a product contaminated with I 125. Because of the difficulty of maintaining the maternal milk supply for such an extended period of time, complete cessation of nursing is usually recommended for all radioiodines, except for uncontaminated I 123.

### Pediatrics

[123]I- and [131]I-mIBG are used in children. When [123]I- or [131]I-mIBG is used in children, the diagnostic benefit should be judged to outweigh the potential risk of radiation.

### Geriatrics

Diagnostic studies performed to date using [123]I- or [131]I-mIBG have not demonstrated geriatrics-specific problems that would limit the usefulness of either agent in the elderly.

### Drug interactions and/or related problems

The following drug interactions and/or related problems have been selected on the basis of their potential clinical significance (possible mechanism in parentheses where appropriate)—not necessarily inclusive (» = major clinical significance):

- » Amphetamines or
- » Antidepressants, tricyclic or
- » Bretylium or
- » Calcium channel blocking agents or
- » Cocaine or
- » Guanethidine or
- » Haloperidol or
- » Labetalol or
- » Loxapine or
- » Metaraminol or
- » Phenothiazines or
- » Reserpine or
- » Sympathomimetics or
- » Thiothixene

  (these medications may interfere with the uptake of [123]I- or [131]I-mIBG; although the ideal time to stop treatment with potential interacting medicines is 1 week prior to administration of [123]I- or [131]I-mIBG, the following withdrawal periods are usually recommended based on the individual half-life of each medication: 24 hours for bretylium, cocaine, and metaraminol; 48 hours for amphetamines, calcium channel blocking agents, guanethidine, haloperidol, loxapine, tricyclic antidepressants, phenothiazines, sympathomimetics, and thiothixene; 72 hours for labetalol and reserpine)

- Phenoxybenzamine

  (although usual doses of phenoxybenzamine do not interfere with [123]I- or [131]I-mIBG uptake, when given in high doses necessary to control blood pressure in patients with pheochromocytomas or paragangliomas preparing for surgery, tumor uptake of [123]I- or [131]I-mIBG may be suppressed resulting in false-negative studies)

## Side/Adverse Effects

At present, there are no known side/adverse effects associated with the use of diagnostic dosages of [123]I- or [131]I-mIBG.

## Patient Consultation

As an aid to patient consultation, refer to *Advice for the Patient, Radiopharmaceuticals (Diagnostic)*.

In providing consultation, consider emphasizing the following selected information (» = major clinical significance):

### Description of use

Action in the body: Localization of [123]I- or [131]I-mIBG in adrenal medulla allows visualization of hyperactive adrenal medulla and neuroendocrine tumors

Small amounts of radioactivity used in diagnosis; radiation received is low and considered safe

### Before having this test

» Conditions affecting use, especially:

Pregnancy—Risk to fetus from radiation exposure as opposed to benefit derived from study should be considered

Breast-feeding—Not known if distributed into breast milk; however, free radioiodide, if present, may be distributed; cessation of nursing may be recommended to avoid any unnecessary absorbed radiation dose to the infant

Use in children—Diagnostic benefit should be judged to outweigh potential risk of radiation

Other medications, especially amphetamines, tricyclic antidepressants, bretylium, calcium channel blocking agents, cocaine, guanethidine, haloperidol, labetalol, loxapine, phenothiazines, reserpine, sympathomimetics, and thiothixene

### Preparation for this test

Special preparatory instructions may apply; patient should inquire in advance

Administration of potassium iodide or Lugol's solution one day before administration of [123]I- or [131]I-mIBG and for 6 days after administration to prevent or reduce thyroid uptake of radioiodide contaminant

## General Dosing Information

Radiopharmaceuticals are to be administered only by or under the supervision of physicians who have had extensive training in the safe use and handling of radioactive materials and who are authorized by the Nuclear Regulatory Commission (NRC) or the appropriate State agency, if required, or, outside the U.S., the appropriate authority.

To minimize uptake of radioactive iodine by the thyroid, potassium iodide (SSKI, 60 mg twice a day) or Lugol's solution (1 drop three times a day) may be used, beginning at least 24 hours before and continuing for 6 days after administration of [123]I- or [131]I-mIBG.

### Safety considerations for handling this radiopharmaceutical

Improper handling of this radiopharmaceutical may cause radioactive contamination. Guidelines for handling radioactive material have been prepared by scientific, professional, state, federal, and international bodies and are available to the specially qualified and authorized users who have access to radiopharmaceuticals.

## Parenteral Dosage Forms

Note: Bracketed information in the *Indications* section refers to uses that are not included in U.S. product labeling. In addition, because [123]I-mIBG sulfate injection is not commercially available in the U.S. or Canada, the bracketed information and the use of the superscript 1 in the *Dosage Forms* section reflect the lack of labeled (approved) indications for this product.

The dosing and strengths of both the [123]I- and [131]I-mIBG dosage forms are expressed in terms of the sulfate salt of iobenguane.

### IOBENGUANE I 123 INJECTION USP

#### Usual adult administered activity

[Diagnosis of tumors][1] or

[Diagnosis of medullary disease][1]—

Intravenous, 370 megabecquerels (10 millicuries) of [123]I-mIBG, with a specific activity of 740 megabecquerels to 1.3 gigabecquerels (20 to 35.6 millicuries) per mg (at time of calibration), administered over a period of fifteen to thirty seconds.

#### Usual pediatric administered activity

[Diagnosis of tumors][1] or

[Diagnosis of medullary disease][1]—

Children up to 18 years of age: Dosage must be individualized by physician.

#### Usual geriatric administered activity

See *Usual adult administered activity*.

**Strength(s) usually available**

U.S.—

    Not commercially available. In most cases, may be obtained from the University of Michigan Nuclear Pharmacy (UMNP) by physicians who have filed their own Investigational New Drug Application (IND).

Canada—

    Not commercially available. In most cases, may be obtained by physicians who have filed their own IND.

**Packaging and storage**

Store between −20 and −10 °C (−4 and −14 °F).

**Note**

Caution—Radioactive material.

## IOBENGUANE SULFATE I 131 INJECTION

**Usual adult administered activity**

Diagnosis of tumors[1] or

[Diagnosis of medullary disease][1]—

    Intravenous, 18.5 to 37 megabecquerels (0.5 to 1 millicurie) of [131]I-mIBG with a specific activity of 103.6 to 199 megabecquerels (2.8 to 5.38 millicuries) per mg (at time of calibration), administered over a period of fifteen seconds.

**Usual pediatric administered activity**

Diagnosis of tumors[1] or

[Diagnosis of medullary disease][1]—

    Children up to 18 years of age: Dosage must be individualized by physician.

    Note: In patients 1 year of age or older, the minimum dose necessary for a clinically acceptable study should not be less than 5 megabecquerels (0.135 millicuries).

**Usual geriatric administered activity**

See *Usual adult administered activity.*

**Strength(s) usually available**

U.S.—

    85.1 megabecquerels (2.3 millicuries) per mL (Rx) [GENERIC].

Canada—

    Not commercially available. In most cases, may be obtained by physicians who have filed their own IND.

**Packaging and storage**

Store between −20 and −10 °C (−4 and −14 °F), unless otherwise specified by manufacturer.

**Note**

Caution—Radioactive material.

    [1]Not included in Canadian product labeling.

## Selected Bibliography

McEwan AJ, Shapiro B, Sisson JC, et al. Radio-iodobenzylguanidine for the scintigraphic location and therapy of adrenergic tumors. Semin Nucl Med 1985; 15 (2): 132-53.

Solanki KK, Bomanji J, Moyes J, et al. A pharmacological guide to medicines which interfere with the biodistribution of radiolabelled meta-iodobenzylguanidine (MIBG). Nucl Med Commun 1992; 13: 513-21.

Revised: 05/05/93

Interim revision: 08/19/94; 04/25/95

---

# IOBENGUANE, RADIOIODINATED    Systemic—Therapeutic*†

VA CLASSIFICATION (Primary): AN600

A commonly used name for iobenguane is meta-iodobenzylguanidine or mIBG.

Note: For a listing of dosage forms and brand names by country availability, see *Dosage Forms* section(s). For a listing of brand names for the articles in this monograph, refer to the General Index.

    *Not commercially available in the U.S.

    †Not commercially available in Canada.

## Category

Antineoplastic.

## Indications

Note: Because I 131 iobenguane ([131]I-mIBG) sulfate injection is not commercially available in the U.S. or Canada, the bracketed information and the use of the superscript 1 in this monograph reflect the lack of labeled (approved) indications for this product.

**Accepted**

[Carcinoid syndrome (treatment)][1] or

[Pheochromocytoma (treatment)][1]—[131]I-mIBG is used in the treatment of pheochromocytoma and may be useful in other neuroendocrine tumors (e.g., carcinoid syndrome).

[Neuroblastoma (treatment)][1]—[131]I-mIBG is used in the treatment of neuroblastomas unresponsive to conventional chemotherapy. Although complete remissions have been achieved in only a few cases, partial remissions have occurred in nearly half the reported cases in which [131]I-mIBG has been used.

    [1]Not included in Canadian product labeling.

## Physical Properties

**Nuclear data:**

| Radionuclide (half-life) | Decay constant | Mode of decay | Principal emissions (keV) | Mean number of emissions/ disintegration |
|---|---|---|---|---|
| I 131 (8.08 days) | 0.00358 h⁻¹ | Beta (90%) | Beta (191.6) Gamma (364.5) | 0.90 0.81 |

## Pharmacology/Pharmacokinetics

**Mechanism of action/Effect**

Iobenguane or meta-iodobenzylguanidine (mIBG) is a physiological analog of the guanidines, such as guanethidine and phenethylguanidine. In adrenergic nerves, guanidines are believed to share the same transport pathway as norepinephrine and to accumulate in, and displace norepinephrine from, intraneuronal storage granules. Similarly, [131]I-mIBG is concentrated in, stored in, and released from chromaffin granules. The retention of [131]I-mIBG in the adrenal medulla may be a result of its uptake in adrenergic neurons and subsequent sequestration into chromaffin storage granules. Due to its selective uptake mechanism, when [131]I-mIBG is used at high levels of administered activity, the radionuclidic emissions can result in localized radiation therapy of tumor tissue.

**Distribution**

After intravenous administration, there is rapid uptake of mIBG mainly in the liver, and in lesser amounts in the lungs, heart, spleen, and salivary glands. Although the uptake in normal adrenal glands is very low, hyperplastic adrenals and tumors such as pheochromocytoma, neuroblastoma, and other tumors with neurosecretory granules have a relatively higher uptake.

**Onset of therapeutic action:**

In malignant pheochromocytoma—Variable (after 1 to 8 doses).

**Radiation dosimetry**

| Estimated absorbed radiation dose* | | |
|---|---|---|
| Organ | mGy/MBq | rad/mCi |
| Liver | 0.83 | 3.07 |
| Bladder wall | 0.59 | 2.18 |
| Spleen | 0.49 | 1.81 |
| Salivary glands | 0.23 | 0.85 |
| Lungs | 0.19 | 0.70 |
| Adrenals | 0.17 | 0.63 |
| Kidneys | 0.12 | 0.44 |
| Pancreas | 0.10 | 0.37 |
| Intestine wall (upper) | 0.080 | 0.29 |
| Uterus | 0.080 | 0.29 |

| Estimated absorbed radiation dose* | | |
|---|---|---|
| Organ | mGy/MBq | rad/mCi |
| Stomach wall | 0.077 | 0.28 |
| Small intestine | 0.074 | 0.27 |
| Heart | 0.072 | 0.26 |
| Breast | 0.069 | 0.25 |
| Intestine wall (lower) | 0.068 | 0.25 |
| Red marrow | 0.067 | 0.25 |
| Ovaries | 0.066 | 0.24 |
| Bone surface | 0.061 | 0.23 |
| Testes | 0.059 | 0.22 |
| Thyroid (blocked)† | 0.050 | 0.18 |
| Other tissue | 0.062 | 0.23 |

Effective dose: 0.20 mSv/MBq (0.74 rem/mCi)

*For adults; intravenous injection. Data based on the International Commission on Radiological Protection (ICRP) Publication 53—Radiation dose to patients from radiopharmaceuticals.

†Thyroid dose listed assumes 0% thyroid uptake. However, uptakes ranging from 0.5 to 2% are more typical; consequently the absorbed radiation dose to the thyroid will be many times higher than listed.

## Elimination

Renal; about 40 to 50% of the injected activity is eliminated within 24 hours and about 70 to 90% within 4 days (mainly as unchanged drug with small amounts of $^{131}$I-m-iodohippuric acid [$^{131}$I-mIHA], $^{131}$I iodide, and $^{131}$I-m-iodobenzoic acid [$^{131}$I-mIBA]).

## Precautions to Consider

### Pregnancy/Reproduction

Pregnancy—$^{131}$I-mIBG is not recommended for the treatment of disease during pregnancy.

To avoid the possibility of fetal exposure to radiation, in those circumstances where the patient's pregnancy status is uncertain a pregnancy test will help to prevent inadvertent administration of this preparation during pregnancy.

### Breast-feeding

It is not known whether $^{131}$I-mIBG is distributed into breast milk. However, this preparation may be contaminated with free radioiodide, which may be distributed into breast milk. In addition, free radioiodide will be produced during normal metabolism. In order to decrease the absorbed radiation dose to the breast and to avoid risk to the infant, complete cessation of nursing is recommended after $^{131}$I-mIBG is administered.

### Pediatrics

$^{131}$I-mIBG is used in children; however, the therapeutic benefit should be judged to outweigh the potential risk of radiation.

### Geriatrics

Treatment performed to date has not demonstrated geriatrics-specific problems that would limit the usefulness of $^{131}$I-mIBG in the elderly.

### Drug interactions and/or related problems

The following drug interactions and/or related problems have been selected on the basis of their potential clinical significance (possible mechanism in parentheses where appropriate)—not necessarily inclusive (» = major clinical significance):

» Amphetamines or
» Antidepressants, tricyclic, or
» Bretylium or
» Calcium channel blocking agents or
» Cocaine or
» Guanethidine or
» Haloperidol or
» Labetalol or
» Loxapine or
» Metaraminol or
» Phenothiazines or
» Reserpine or
» Sympathomimetics or
» Thiothixene

   (these medications may interfere with the uptake of $^{131}$I-mIBG; although the ideal amount of time to stop treatment with potential interacting medicines is 1 week prior to administration of $^{131}$I-mIBG, the following withdrawal periods are usually recommended based on the individual half-life of each medication: 24 hours for bretylium, cocaine, and metaraminol; 48 hours for amphetamines, calcium channel blocking agents, guanethidine, haloperidol, loxapine, tricyclic antidepressants, phenothiazines, sympathomimetics, and thiothixene; 72 hours for labetalol and reserpine)

Blood dyscrasia–causing medications (See *Appendix II*)

(leukopenic and/or thrombocytopenic effects of $^{131}$I-mIBG may be increased with concurrent or recent therapy with these medications)

Bone marrow depressants, other (See *Appendix II*)

   (concurrent use of bone marrow depressants with $^{131}$I-mIBG may increase leukopenic and/or thrombocytopenic effects)

Chemotherapy and/or

Radiation therapy

   (previous chemotherapy and/or radiotherapy may impair effectiveness of $^{131}$I-mIBG therapy)

### Laboratory value alterations

The following have been selected on the basis of their potential clinical significance (possible effect in parentheses where appropriate)—not necessarily inclusive (» = major clinical significance):

With physiology/laboratory test values

Alanine aminotransferase (ALT [SGPT]), serum and
Aspartate aminotransferase (AST [SGOT]), serum
   (concentrations may be increased)

Catecholamines, urinary
   (concentration may be increased transiently)

## Side/Adverse Effects

The following side/adverse effects have been selected on the basis of their potential clinical significance (possible signs and symptoms in parentheses where appropriate)—not necessarily inclusive:

### Those indicating need for medical attention

Incidence rare
   *Leukopenia and thrombocytopenia* (pale skin, sore throat and fever, unusual bleeding or bruising, unusual tiredness or weakness)

### Those indicating need for medical attention only if they continue or are bothersome

Incidence less frequent or rare
   *Flushing of skin; nausea; slight and transient increase in blood pressure*

## Patient Consultation

As an aid to patient consultation, refer to *Advice for the Patient, Iobenguane, Radioiodinated (Therapeutic)*.

In providing consultation, consider emphasizing the following selected information (» = major clinical significance):

### Description of use

Action in the body: Localization of $^{131}$I-mIBG in adrenal medulla and neuroendocrine tumors; large doses are used therapeutically to damage or destroy tissue in management of adrenal carcinoma, pheochromocytomas, and other neuroendocrine tumors

### Before using this medication

» Conditions affecting use, especially:
   Pregnancy—Use not recommended because of risk to fetus from radiation exposure
   Breast-feeding—Not known if distributed into breast milk; however, free radioiodide, if present, may be distributed; cessation of nursing is recommended because of risk to infant from radiation exposure
   Use in children—Benefit derived from treatment should be judged to outweigh potential risk of radiation
   Other medications, especially amphetamines, tricyclic antidepressants, bretylium, calcium channel blocking agents, cocaine, guanethidine, haloperidol, labetalol, loxapine, phenothiazines, reserpine, sympathomimetics, and thiothixene

### Proper use of this medication

Special preparatory instructions may apply; patient should inquire in advance

Administration of potassium iodide or Lugol's solution to block thyroid uptake of radioiodide contaminants before and for several weeks after treatment

### Side/adverse effects

Signs of potential side effects, especially leukopenia and thrombocytopenia

## General Dosing Information

Radiopharmaceuticals are to be administered only by or under the supervision of physicians who have had extensive training in the safe use and handling of radioactive materials and who are authorized by the Nuclear Regulatory Commission (NRC) or the appropriate Federal or

Agreement State agency, if required, or, outside the U.S., the appropriate authority.

To minimize uptake of radioactive iodine by the thyroid, potassium iodide (SSKI, 60 mg twice a day) or Lugol's solution (1 drop three times a day) may be used, beginning at least 24 hours before and continuing for at least 4 weeks after therapy with [131]I-mIBG.

When [131]I-mIBG is used for the treatment of pheochromocytoma, concurrent use of an alpha-adrenergic blocking agent, such as phenoxybenzamine is recommended to control episodes of hypertension.

Following administration of [131]I-mIBG the patient should be observed for possible reactions; competent personnel and emergency facilities should be available during this period.

**Safety considerations for handling this radiopharmaceutical**
Improper handling of this radiopharmaceutical may cause radioactive contamination. Guidelines for handling radioactive material have been prepared by scientific, professional, state, federal, and international bodies and are available to the specially qualified and authorized users who have access to radiopharmaceuticals.

## Parenteral Dosage Forms
Because I 131 iobenguane ([131]I-mIBG) sulfate injection is not commercially available in the U.S. or Canada, the bracketed information and the use of the superscript 1 in the *Dosage Forms* section reflect the lack of labeled (approved) indications for this product.

### I 131 IOBENGUANE SULFATE INJECTION

**Usual adult administered activity**
[Treatment of malignant pheochromocytoma][1]—
A safe and effective dosage has not been established. However, dosages in the range of 2.9 to 9.25 gigabecquerels (80 to 250 millicuries) of [131]I-mIBG, with a specific activity of 103.6 to 199 megabecquerels (2.8 to 5.38 millicuries) per mg (at time of calibration), administered by slow intravenous infusion over a 20- to 30-second period every three to six months, have been used.

**Usual pediatric administered activity**
[Treatment of neuroblastoma][1]—
A safe and effective dosage has not been established for children up to 18 years of age. However, dosages in the range of 2.6 to 6.8

gigabecquerels (70 to 184 millicuries), administered in two fractions by slow (four to eight hours) intravenous infusion at two- to four-day intervals have been used.

Note: Dosages ranging from 1.3 to 8 gigabecquerels (35 to 215 millicuries) have also been used.

**Usual geriatric administered activity**
See *Usual adult administered activity.*

**Strength(s) usually available**
U.S.—
Not commercially available for therapeutic use. In most cases, may be obtained from the University of Michigan Nuclear Pharmacy (UMNP) by physicians who have filed their own Investigational New Drug Application (IND).
Canada—
Not commercially available. In most cases, may be obtained by physicians who have filed their own IND.

**Packaging and storage**
Store between 2 and 8 °C (35.6 and 46.4 °F), but preferably between −20 and −10 °C (−4 and −14 °F), unless otherwise specified by manufacturer.

**Note**
Caution—Radioactive material.

[1]Not included in Canadian product labeling.

## Selected Bibliography
McEwan AJ, Shapiro B, Sisson JC, et al. Radio-iodobenzylguanidine for the scintigraphic location and therapy of adrenergic tumors. Semin Nucl Med 1985; 15(2): 132-53.

Revised: 05/05/93
Interim revision: 08/02/94

---

**IOCETAMIC ACID**—See *Cholecystographic Agents, Oral (Systemic)*

---

# IODINATED GLYCEROL   Systemic*†

VA CLASSIFICATION (Primary): RE400
Note: For a listing of dosage forms and brand names by country availability, see *Dosage Forms* section(s). For a listing of brand names for the articles in this monograph, refer to the General Index.

---

*Not commercially available in the U.S.
†Not commercially available in Canada.

---

## Category
Mucolytic-expectorant.

## Indications

**Unaccepted**
Iodinated glycerol has been used as a mucolytic-expectorant for adjunctive treatment in respiratory tract conditions such as bronchitis, bronchial asthma, pulmonary emphysema, cystic fibrosis, chronic sinusitis, or after surgery to help prevent atelectasis. However, its efficacy in these conditions has not been proven.

## Pharmacology/Pharmacokinetics

**Physicochemical characteristics**
Chemical group—An organic iodide; a mixture of several iodinated compounds formed by the reaction of iodine and glycerol. The major iodinated compounds are 3-iodo-1,2-propanediol and a mixture of diastereomers of 1,5,6-trihydroxy-2-iodomethyl-3-oxahexane. Iodinated glycerol contains virtually no free iodine and is stable in an acid medium
Molecular weight—258.06.

**Mechanism of action/Effect**
The mechanism of action of iodinated glycerol as a mucolytic is not completely understood; however, it appears to act by increasing respiratory tract secretions and thereby decreasing the viscosity of mucus. It is not known if the glycerol molecule contributes to the effects of iodinated glycerol.

**Absorption**
Readily absorbed from the gastrointestinal tract and concentrated primarily in the secretions of the respiratory tract.

**Biotransformation**
Unknown.

**Elimination**
Primarily renal.

## Precautions to Consider

**Cross-sensitivity and/or related problems**
Patients sensitive to inorganic iodides or iodine may be sensitive to this medication also.

**Carcinogenicity**
In 24-month carcinogenicity studies conducted by the National Toxicology Program (NTP) in rats and mice using doses of iodinated glycerol ranging between 13 and 52 times the recommended human dose, there was no evidence of carcinogenicity in female F344/N rats or in male B6C3F1 mice; however, there was some evidence in male F344/N rats, based on increased incidences of mononuclear cell leukemia and follicular cell carcinomas of the thyroid gland, and in female B6C3F1 mice, based on increased incidences of adenomas of the pituitary gland and neoplasms of the Harderian gland. There are no known human equivalents to mononuclear cell leukemia in the rat and Harderian gland neoplasms in the mouse; therefore, the relevance of these finding to humans is not known.

**Mutagenicity**
*In vitro* mutagenicity assays, conducted with or without microsomal activation, produced both positive and negative results with iodinated glycerol. In an *in vivo* study, the results were negative for genotoxic effects, in that no increase in micronucleated polychromatic erythrocytes was observed in the bone marrow of B6C3F1 mice after administration of either iodinated glycerol or 3-iodo-1,2-propanediol. The relevance of these findings to humans is not known.

**Pregnancy/Reproduction**

Fertility—No long-term animal studies on impairment of fertility have been performed with iodinated glycerol.

Pregnancy—Iodinated glycerol is not recommended for use during pregnancy. The human fetal thyroid begins to concentrate iodine in the twelfth to fourteenth week of gestation, and the use of inorganic iodides during this period of pregnancy and thereafter has been reported rarely to induce fetal goiter, with or without hypothyroidism, with the potential for airway obstruction.

FDA Pregnancy Category X.

**Breast-feeding**

Use of iodinated glycerol is not recommended in nursing mothers because it may cause skin rash and thyroid suppression in the infant.

**Pediatrics**

Children with cystic fibrosis appear to have an exaggerated susceptibility to the goitrogenic effect of iodides.

**Geriatrics**

No information is available on the relationship of age to the effects of iodinated glycerol in geriatric patients.

**Drug interactions and/or related problems**

The following drug interactions and/or related problems have been selected on the basis of their potential clinical significance (possible mechanism in parentheses where appropriate)—not necessarily inclusive (» = major clinical significance):

Note: Combinations containing any of the following medications, depending on the amount present, may also interact with this medication.

» Lithium or
» Other antithyroid agents
    (concurrent use may potentiate the hypothyroid and goitrogenic effects of either these medications or iodinated glycerol; baseline thyroid status should be determined at periodic intervals to detect changes in the thyroid-pituitary response)

**Laboratory value alterations**

The following have been selected on the basis of their potential clinical significance (possible effect in parentheses where appropriate)—not necessarily inclusive (» = major clinical significance):

With diagnostic test results
    Thyroid function tests
        (iodides may alter the results of these tests, and a high intake of inorganic iodides has also been shown to interfere with determination of protein bound iodine [PBI]; however, these effects have not been reported with iodinated glycerol in usual recommended doses, but they should be kept in mind for patients receiving prolonged therapy)

**Medical considerations/Contraindications**

The medical considerations/contraindications included here have been selected on the basis of their potential clinical significance (reasons given in parentheses where appropriate)—not necessarily inclusive (» = major clinical significance).

*Except under special circumstances, this medication should not be used when the following medical problem exists:*

» Previous allergic reaction to iodinated glycerol, inorganic iodides, or iodine

*Risk-benefit should be considered when the following medical problems exist:*

Acne, adolescent
    (condition may be exacerbated)

Cystic fibrosis, in children
    (possible exaggerated susceptibility to goitrogenic effect of iodides)

» Thyroid disease, or history of
    (iodine-induced goiter may occur in hyperthyroidism; prolonged use of iodides may result in hypothyroidism)

## Side/Adverse Effects

Note: Skin eruptions, which may be severe or fatal in rare instances, may occur following prolonged administration.
    The severity of the symptoms of chronic intoxication with iodide (iodism) is dose-related.

The following side/adverse effects have been selected on the basis of their potential clinical significance (possible signs and symptoms in parentheses where appropriate)—not necessarily inclusive:

**Those indicating need for medical attention**
Incidence rare
    *Allergic reaction* (fever; joint pain; skin rash, hives, or redness; swelling of face, lips, or eyelids); *parotitis, acute* (chills; continuing headache; loss of appetite; pain on chewing or swallowing; sore throat; tenderness or swelling below or in front of ear)

With prolonged use
    *Hypothyroidism* (dry skin; swelling around the eyes; unusual sensitivity to cold; unusual tiredness or weakness; unusual weight gain); *iodism* (burning of mouth and throat; severe headache; increased watering of the mouth; irritation of eyes or swelling of eyelids; metallic taste; runny nose, sneezing, and other symptoms of head cold; skin rash; soreness of teeth and gums); *thyroid gland enlargement* (swelling of neck)

**Those indicating need for medical attention only if they continue or are bothersome**
Incidence more frequent
    *Diarrhea; nausea or vomiting; stomach pain*

## Patient Consultation

As an aid to patient consultation, refer to *Advice for the Patient, Iodinated Glycerol (Systemic).*

In providing consultation, consider emphasizing the following selected information (» = major clinical significance):

**Before using this medication**
» Conditions affecting use, especially:
    Allergy to iodinated glycerol, inorganic iodides, or iodine
    Pregnancy—Use of iodinated glycerol is not recommended during pregnancy; because the human fetal thyroid begins to concentrate iodine in the twelfth to fourteenth week of gestation, use of inorganic iodides during this period of pregnancy and thereafter has been reported rarely to induce fetal goiter, with or without hypothyroidism, with the potential for airway obstruction
    Breast-feeding—Use of iodinated glycerol is not recommended in nursing mothers because of potential skin rash and thyroid suppression in the infant
    Use in children—Children with cystic fibrosis appear to have an exaggerated susceptibility to the goitrogenic effect of iodides
    Other medications, especially lithium or other antithyroid agents
    Other medical problems, especially thyroid disease (or history of)

**Proper use of this medication**
» Drinking a glass of water after each dose of medication to help thin and loosen mucus in lungs
» Importance of not taking more medication than the amount prescribed
» Proper dosing
    Missed dose: Taking as soon as possible; not taking if almost time for next dose; not doubling doses
» Proper storage
*For oral solution dosage form*
    Taking by mouth even if it comes in a dropper bottle
    Taking mixed in water or other liquid; drinking all of liquid to get full dose of medication

**Precautions while using this medication**
Regular visits to physician to check progress during therapy

**Side/adverse effects**
Signs of potential side effects, especially allergic reaction, acute parotitis, and, with prolonged use, hypothyroidism, iodism, and thyroid gland enlargement
Goiter or enlarged thyroid gland more likely to occur in children with cystic fibrosis

## General Dosing Information

Chronic use of iodinated glycerol should be avoided because of its effect on the thyroid gland.

If symptoms of iodism or rash or other evidence of hypersensitivity occurs, iodinated glycerol therapy should be discontinued.

**For treatment of adverse effects**
For hypothyroidism and thyroid gland enlargement: The medication should be discontinued or thyroid hormone may be administered.

For iodism: The medication should be withdrawn and appropriate supportive therapy administered. Symptoms of iodism disappear soon after administration is discontinued. Abundant fluid and sodium chloride intake aids in elimination of iodide.

# Oral Dosage Forms

## IODINATED GLYCEROL ELIXIR

### Usual adult dose
Oral, 60 mg four times a day.

### Usual pediatric dose
Oral, up to 30 mg four times a day (the dosage being based on body weight).

Note: Use is not recommended in neonates.

### Strength(s) usually available
U.S.—

   Not commercially available.

Canada—

   Not commercially available.

### Packaging and storage
Store below 40 °C (104 °F), preferably between 15 and 30 °C (59 and 86 °F), in a tight container, unless otherwise specified by manufacturer. Protect from freezing.

### Auxiliary labeling
• Keep container tightly closed.

## IODINATED GLYCEROL ORAL SOLUTION

### Usual adult dose
Oral, 60 mg four times a day, mixed with fruit juice or other liquid.

### Usual pediatric dose
Oral, up to 30 mg four times a day (the dosage being based on body weight), mixed with fruit juice or other liquid.

Note: Use is not recommended in neonates.

### Strength(s) usually available
U.S.—

   Not commercially available.

Canada—

   Not commercially available.

### Packaging and storage
Store below 40 °C (104 °F), preferably between 15 and 30 °C (59 and 86 °F), in a tight container, unless otherwise specified by manufacturer. Protect from freezing.

## IODINATED GLYCEROL TABLETS

### Usual adult dose
See *Iodinated Glycerol Elixir*.

### Usual pediatric dose
See *Iodinated Glycerol Elixir*.

### Strength(s) usually available
U.S.—

   Not commercially available.

Canada—

   Not commercially available.

### Packaging and storage
Store below 40 °C (104 °F), preferably between 15 and 30 °C (59 and 86 °F), in a tight container, unless otherwise specified by manufacturer.

Revised: 08/30/94

---

**IODINATED I 125 ALBUMIN**—See *Radioiodinated Albumin (Systemic)*

---

**IODINATED I 131 ALBUMIN**—See *Radioiodinated Albumin (Systemic)*

---

# IODINE    Topical†

VA CLASSIFICATION (Primary): DE100

Some commonly used names are iodine tincture and strong iodine tincture.

Note: For a listing of dosage forms and brand names by country availability, see *Dosage Forms* section(s). For a listing of brand names for the articles in this monograph, refer to the General Index.

†Not commercially available in Canada.

## Category
Antibacterial (topical).

## Indications

### Accepted
Skin infections, bacterial, minor (prophylaxis and treatment)—Iodine is indicated as an antiseptic and disinfectant in the topical prophylaxis and treatment of superficial skin infections caused by susceptible gram-positive and gram-negative bacteria in minor abrasions, burns, or cuts. It is the most effective disinfectant for intact skin and is used to disinfect the skin preoperatively or prior to obtaining blood cultures by venipuncture.

## Pharmacology/Pharmacokinetics

### Physicochemical characteristics
Molecular weight—126.9.

### Mechanism of action/Effect
Although the mechanism of action of topical iodine is not fully understood, it is thought that the medication's antimicrobial effects may be due to the presence of the diatomic elemental form of iodine (free iodine). It is believed that iodine precipitates the proteins of the microorganisms by forming salts via direct halogenation. Approximately 90% of the iodine absorbed by bacterial cells reappears as the iodide, thus confirming oxidative interaction as the major bactericidal mechanism of topical iodine.

Antimicrobial activity is significantly affected by pH and is greater under acidic conditions.

Solutions of iodine usually contain potassium or sodium iodide to enhance solubility of iodine through the formation of polyiodide ion.

### Other actions/effects
Iodine also possesses fungicidal, protozoacidal (e.g., trichomonicidal), cysticidal, virucidal, and some sporocidal activities.

### Absorption
Slightly absorbed as iodide when applied topically to intact skin. Absorption by damaged skin and mucous membranes may be extensive and may lead to $10^4$-fold increases in serum iodine concentrations compared to normal.

### Distribution
May be absorbed by the thyroid gland and may appear in saliva, sweat, and milk.

### Biotransformation
Undergoes minimal metabolism and is converted to the iodide.

### Elimination
Excreted unchanged in the urine.

## Precautions to Consider

### Pregnancy/Reproduction
Pregnancy—Iodine crosses the placenta; use is not recommended during pregnancy because of possible absorption and adverse effects on the fetus such as hypothyroidism and goiter.

Labor and delivery—Use may result in significant absorption both in the mother and the fetus; transient hypothyroidism has been found in infants exposed to topical iodine following vaginal or perineal use before delivery.

### Breast-feeding
Iodine applied topically may be distributed into breast milk; use is not recommended for nursing mothers because it may result in iodide overload and transient hypothyroidism in the nursing infants.

### Pediatrics
Use is not recommended for neonates because of their potential for increased absorption; topically applied iodine may result in skin hypersensitivity, iodide overload, and transient hypothyroidism.

### Geriatrics
Appropriate studies on the relationship of age to the effects of topical iodine have not been performed in the geriatric population. However, no geriatrics-specific problems have been documented to date.

## Dental

Iodine solution may be applied to the oral mucosa, teeth, or rubber dams for antibacterial purposes. However, it may cause irritation to the mucosa, resulting in a sensation of heat or itching, or blister formation. Iodine may also reversibly stain the oral mucosa, teeth, rubber dams, and acrylic, silicate, and porcelain restorations. These stains can be removed with alcohol.

## Medical considerations/Contraindications

The medical considerations/contraindications included here have been selected on the basis of their potential clinical significance (reasons given in parentheses where appropriate)—not necessarily inclusive (» = major clinical significance).

*Risk-benefit should be considered when the following medical problems exist:*

» Animal bites or
» Burns, severe or extensive or
» Puncture wounds, deep
    (risk of adverse effects associated with increased absorption and tissue irritation)
    Hypersensitivity to iodine

## Side/Adverse Effects

The following side/adverse effects have been selected on the basis of their potential clinical significance (possible signs and symptoms in parentheses where appropriate)—not necessarily inclusive:

### Those indicating need for medical attention

Incidence rare
    *Dermatitis* (blistering, crusting, irritation, itching, or reddening of skin)
Symptoms of overdose (when ingested)
    *Abdominal pain; anuria* (not passing urine); *diarrhea; excessive thirst; fever; nausea; vomiting*

## Patient Consultation

As an aid to patient consultation, refer to *Advice for the Patient, Iodine (Topical)*.

In providing consultation, consider emphasizing the following selected information (» = major clinical significance):

### Before using this medication

» Conditions affecting use, especially:
    Hypersensitivity to iodine
    Pregnancy—May cause thyroid problems in the newborn infant
    Breast-feeding—May cause thyroid problems in nursing babies
    Use in children—May cause skin and thyroid problems in infants
    Other medical problems, especially animal bites, deep wounds, or serious burns

### Proper use of this medication

Using only as directed
» Not swallowing medication
» Keeping medication away from the eyes; washing medication away with water if it accidentally gets in the eyes
» Not using on deep, puncture wounds, animal bites or serious burns
» Not using a tight dressing or bandage over the wound on which topical iodine was applied
» Proper dosing
    Using medication for full time of treatment
    Missed dose: Applying as soon as possible; not applying if almost time for next dose
» Proper storage

### Precautions while using this medication

Checking with doctor if skin problem becomes worse, or if constant irritation develops
May stain skin and clothing; removing stain on skin with alcohol; removing stain on clothing by washing and rinsing in dilute ammonia or with soap and water

### Side/adverse effects

Blistering, crusting, irritation, itching, or reddening of skin

## General Dosing Information

Topical iodine should not be used on wild or domestic animal bites. Instead, a physician should be consulted immediately for proper care.

Topical iodine should not be used on deep or puncture wounds, or serious burns, since these uses may increase absorption and tissue irritation.

Since iodine may cause burns on occluded skin, wounds treated with topical iodine should not be covered with a tight dressing or bandage.

For skin disinfection prior to medical procedures, such as venipuncture, lumbar puncture, or thoracentesis, topical iodine should be rubbed into the skin, working from the center of the area to be disinfected to the periphery in a concentric fashion. After application, the solution should be allowed to dry for at least 2 minutes (the amount of time needed for iodine to achieve its full effect) and then washed off with 70% alcohol to prevent any possibility of skin damage.

### For treatment of adverse effects and/or overdose

Recommended treatment consists of the following:
    • For severe skin reaction—Topical iodine should be removed promptly with 70% alcohol, or the skin washed with large amounts of water for 15 minutes.
    • For accidental ingestion—If the patient is conscious, milk may be given orally every 15 minutes to relieve gastric irritation; in addition, a starch solution, prepared by adding 15 mg of cornstarch or flour to 500 mL of water, may be administered to absorb the remaining iodine. Emesis and lavage should not be performed in the presence of esophageal injury.
    • Using other supportive measures to maintain vital functions, including administering oxygen to maintain respiration and administering antihistamines, epinephrine, or corticosteroids to treat anaphylaxis, especially if the patient is severely compromised.

## Topical Dosage Forms

### IODINE TINCTURE USP

#### Usual adult and adolescent dose

Antibacterial (topical)—
    Topical, to the affected area, as necessary.

Note: This medication should not be used for more than ten days.

#### Usual pediatric dose

Antibacterial (topical)—
    Children up to 1 month of age: Use is not recommended.
    Children 1 month of age and over—See *Usual adult and adolescent dose.*

#### Strength(s) usually available

U.S.—
    2% (OTC) [GENERIC (alcohol 47%; sodium iodide 2.4%)].
Canada—
    Not commercially available.

#### Packaging and storage

Store below 40 °C (104 °F), preferably between 15 and 30 °C (59 and 86 °F), in a tight container, unless otherwise specified by manufacturer.

#### Incompatibilities

Tincture of iodine is incompatible with ammonia; salts of iron, bismuth, copper, lead, and mercury; potassium chlorate and other oxidizing agents; mineral acids; strychnine hydrochloride; and quinine sulfate and other alkaloidal salts.

#### Auxiliary labeling

• For external use only.
• Keep out of reach of children.

### STRONG IODINE TINCTURE USP

#### Usual adult and adolescent dose

See *Iodine Tincture USP.*

#### Usual pediatric dose

See *Iodine Tincture USP.*

#### Strength(s) usually available

U.S.—
    7% (OTC) [GENERIC (alcohol 83%; potassium iodide 5%)].
Canada—
    Not commercially available.

#### Packaging and storage

Store below 40 °C (104 °F), preferably between 15 and 30 °C (59 and 86 °F), in a tight container, unless otherwise specified by manufacturer.

#### Incompatibilities

Strong tincture of iodine is incompatible with ammonia; salts of iron, bismuth, copper, lead, and mercury; potassium chlorate and other oxidizing agents; mineral acids; strychnine hydrochloride; and quinine sulfate and other alkaloidal salts.

#### Auxiliary labeling

• For external use only.
• Keep out of reach of children.

## Selected Bibliography

Kuipers JS, Van Weering HK. Skin disinfection with iodine compounds. Arch Chir Neerl 1973; 25 (1): 53-65.

L'Allemand D, Gruters A, Beyer P, Weber B. Iodine in contrast agents and skin disinfectants is the major cause for hypothyroidism in premature infants during intensive care. Horm Res 1987; 28 (1): 42-9.

Developed: 02/22/94

## IODINE-CONTAINING COMBINATIONS—

Chlorpheniramine, Phenylephrine, Codeine, and Potassium Iodide (Systemic)—See *Cough/Cold Combinations (Systemic)*

Codeine and Calcium Iodide (Systemic)—See *Cough/Cold Combinations (Systemic)*

Codeine and Iodinated Glycerol (Systemic)—See *Cough/Cold Combinations (Systemic)*

Dextromethorphan and Iodinated Glycerol (Systemic)—See *Cough/Cold Combinations (Systemic)*

Ephedrine and Potassium Iodide (Systemic)—See *Cough/Cold Combinations (Systemic)*

# IODINE, STRONG　Systemic

VA CLASSIFICATION (Primary/Secondary): HS852/AD900; TN499

Another commonly used name is Lugol's solution.

Note: For a listing of dosage forms and brand names by country availability, see *Dosage Forms* section(s). For a listing of brand names for the articles in this monograph, refer to the General Index.

## Category

Antihyperthyroid agent; radiation protectant (thyroid gland); iodine replenisher.

## Indications

Note: Bracketed information in the *Indications* section refers to uses that are not included in U.S. product labeling.

### Accepted

[Hyperthyroidism (treatment adjunct)][1]—Strong iodine is used as an adjunct in the treatment of hyperthyroidism.

[Radiation protection, thyroid gland][1]—Strong iodine is used as a radiation protectant (thyroid gland) prior to and following administration of radioactive isotopes of iodine or in radiation emergencies.

[Thyroid involution, preoperative (treatment adjunct)][1]—Strong iodine is used concurrently with an antithyroid agent to induce thyroid involution prior to thyroidectomy.

[Thyrotoxic crisis (treatment adjunct)][1]—Strong iodine is used as an adjunct in the treatment of thyrotoxic crisis.

[Iodine deficiency (treatment)]—Strong iodine is used in the treatment of iodine deficiency

[1]Not included in Canadian product labeling.

## Pharmacology/Pharmacokinetics

### Physicochemical characteristics

Molecular weight—Iodine: 126.90.
Potassium iodide: 166.00.

### Mechanism of action/Effect

Antihyperthyroid agent—In hyperthyroid patients, strong iodine produces rapid remission of symptoms by inhibiting the release of thyroid hormone into the circulation. The effects of strong iodine on the thyroid gland include reduction of vascularity, a firming of the glandular tissue, shrinkage of the size of individual cells, reaccumulation of colloid in the follicles, and increases in bound iodine. These actions may facilitate thyroidectomy when the medication is given prior to surgery.

Radiation protectant—Prior to and following administration of radioactive isotopes and in radiation emergencies, strong iodine protects the thyroid gland by blocking the thyroidal uptake of radioactive isotopes of iodine.

## Precautions to Consider

### Pregnancy/Reproduction

Iodides cross the placenta; use during pregnancy may result in abnormal thyroid function and/or goiter in the infant.

### Breast-feeding

Iodides are distributed into breast milk; use by nursing mothers may cause skin rash and thyroid suppression in the infant.

### Pediatrics

Iodides may cause skin rash and thyroid suppression in infants.

### Geriatrics

Appropriate studies on the relationship of age to the effects of strong iodine have not been performed in the geriatric population. However, geriatrics-specific problems that would limit the usefulness of this medication in the elderly are not expected.

### Dental

Strong iodine may cause salivary swelling or tenderness, burning of mouth or throat, metallic taste, soreness of teeth and gums, and unusual increase in salivation.

### Drug interactions and/or related problems

The following drug interactions and/or related problems have been selected on the basis of their potential clinical significance (possible mechanism in parentheses where appropriate)—not necessarily inclusive (» = major clinical significance):

Note: Combinations containing any of the following medications, depending on the amount present, may also interact with this medication.

» Antithyroid agents
　(concurrent use of these medications with strong iodine may potentiate the hypothyroid and goitrogenic effects of antithyroid agents or strong iodine; baseline thyroid status should be determined at periodic intervals to detect changes in the thyroid-pituitary response)

Captopril or
Enalapril or
Lisinopril
　(concurrent use of captopril, enalapril, or lisinopril with strong iodine may result in hyperkalemia; serum potassium concentrations should be monitored)

» Diuretics, potassium-sparing
　(concurrent use with strong iodine may increase the effects of potassium, possibly resulting in hyperkalemia and cardiac arrhythmias or cardiac arrest; serum potassium concentrations should be monitored)

» Lithium
　(concurrent use with strong iodine may potentiate the hypothyroid and goitrogenic effects of either medication; baseline thyroid status should be determined at periodic intervals to detect changes in the thyroid-pituitary response)

Sodium iodide I 131, therapeutic
　(strong iodine solution may decrease thyroidal uptake of I 131)

### Laboratory value alterations

The following have been selected on the basis of their potential clinical significance (possible effect in parentheses where appropriate)—not necessarily inclusive (» = major clinical significance):

With diagnostic test results
Thyroid function studies and
Thyroid imaging, radionuclide and
Thyroid uptake tests
　(strong iodine solution may decrease thyroidal uptake of I 131, I 123 and sodium pertechnetate Tc 99m)

### Medical considerations/Contraindications

The medical considerations/contraindications included here have been selected on the basis of their potential clinical significance (reasons given in parentheses where appropriate)—not necessarily inclusive (» = major clinical significance).

*Risk benefit should be considered when the following medical problems exist:*

» Bronchitis, acute or
» Edema, pulmonary or
Tuberculosis, pulmonary
　(may cause irritation and increase secretions)

» Hyperkalemia
　(condition may be exacerbated)

Hyperthyroidism—for use other than thyroid inhibitor
(prolonged use of iodine may cause thyroid gland hyperplasia, thyroid adenoma, goiter, or hypothyroidism)
» Renal function impairment
(may cause excessive serum potassium concentrations)
Sensitivity to iodine or potassium iodide

### Patient monitoring
The following may be especially important in patient monitoring (other tests may be warranted in some patients, depending on condition; » = major clinical significance):

Potassium, serum, concentrations
(determinations recommended at periodic intervals during therapy in patients with renal function impairment)

## Side/Adverse Effects
The following side/adverse effects have been selected on the basis of their potential clinical significance (possible signs and symptoms in parentheses where appropriate)—not necessarily inclusive:

### Those indicating need for medical attention
Incidence less frequent
*Allergic reactions, specifically angioedema* (swelling of the arms, face, legs, lips, tongue, and/or throat); *arthralgia* (joint pain); *eosinophilia; swelling of lymph nodes; urticaria* (hives)

With prolonged use
*Iodism* (burning of mouth or throat; gastric irritation; increased watering of mouth; metallic taste; severe headache; soreness of teeth and gums; symptoms of head cold); *potassium toxicity* (confusion; irregular heartbeat; numbness, tingling, pain, or weakness in hands or feet; unusual tiredness; weakness or heaviness of legs)

### Those indicating need for medical attention only if they continue or are bothersome
Incidence less frequent
*Diarrhea; nausea or vomiting; stomach pain*

## Patient Consultation
As an aid to patient consultation, refer to *Advice for the Patient, Strong Iodine (Systemic)*

In providing consultation, consider emphasizing the following selected information (» = major clinical significance):

### Before using this medication
» Conditions affecting use, especially:
Sensitivity to iodine or potassium iodide
Pregnancy—May cause thyroid problems or goiter in the newborn infant
Breast-feeding—May cause skin rash and thyroid problems in nursing babies
Use in children—May cause skin rash and thyroid problems in infants
Other medications, especially antithyroid agents, potassium-sparing diuretics, or lithium
Other medical problems, especially bronchitis, hyperkalemia, or renal function impairment

### Proper use of this medication
» Taking after meals or with food or milk to minimize gastrointestinal irritation
Proper administration technique for oral liquids
» Taking medication by mouth even if dispensed in a dropper bottle
Not using if solution turns brownish yellow
Taking medication in a full glass (240 mL) of water or in fruit juice, milk, or broth to improve taste and lessen gastric upset; drinking full dose
If crystals form in solution, warming closed container in warm water and gently shaking container
» Proper dosing
Missed dose: Taking as soon as possible; not taking if almost time for next dose; not doubling doses
» Proper storage

*For use as a radiation protectant (thyroid gland)*
Taking medication only upon instructions from state or local health authorities
» Taking medication daily for 10 days, unless otherwise instructed; not taking more medication or more often than instructed

### Precautions while using this medication
Regular visits to physician to check progress during therapy
» Caution in patients on potassium-restricted diet

### Side/adverse effects
» Signs of potential side effects, especially allergic reactions, iodism, or potassium toxicity

## General Dosing Information
The potassium content is 0.6 mEq (23.4 mg) per mL of strong iodine.

To protect against possible gastrointestinal injury, which has been associated with the oral ingestion of concentrated potassium salt preparations, and to improve the taste, it is recommended that the oral solution be administered in a full glass (240 mL) of water or in fruit juice, milk, or broth.

## Oral Dosage Forms
Note: Bracketed uses in the *Dosage Forms* section refer to categories of use and/or indications that are not included in U.S. product labeling.

### STRONG IODINE SOLUTION USP
**Usual adult and adolescent dose**
[Antihyperthyroid agent][1]—
Oral, 1 mL three times a day, the first dose being given at least one hour after the initial dose of antithyroid agent.
[Thyroid involution, preoperative][1]—
Prior to thyroidectomy: Oral, 3 to 5 drops (approximately 0.1 to 0.3 mL) three times a day for ten days before surgery, usually administered concurrently with an antithyroid agent.
[Radiation protectant (thyroid gland)][1]—
Oral, 130 mg a day for ten days.
[Iodine replenisher]—
Oral, 0.3 to 1 mL three or four times a day.

**Usual pediatric dose**
[Thyroid involution, preoperative][1]—
See *Usual adult and adolescent dose.*
[Radiation protectant (thyroid gland)][1]—
Oral, 65 mg per day for ten days.

**Strength(s) usually available**
U.S.—
50 mg of iodine and 100 mg of potassium iodide per mL (Rx)
[GENERIC].
Canada—
50 mg of iodine and 100 mg of potassium iodide per mL (OTC)
[GENERIC].

**Packaging and storage**
Store below 40 °C (104 °F), preferably between 15 and 30 °C (59 and 86 °F), unless otherwise specified by manufacturer. Store in a tight container. Protect from freezing.

**Stability**
Crystallization may occur under normal conditions of storage, especially if refrigerated; however, on warming and shaking, the crystals will redissolve.
Free iodine may be liberated by oxidation of the strong iodine, causing the solution to turn brownish yellow in color. If this occurs, the solution should be discarded.

**Auxiliary labeling**
• For oral use only.

---

[1]Not included in Canadian product labeling.

---

Revised: 04/15/92
Interim revision: 08/10/94

# IODIPAMIDE    Systemic

INN: Adipiodone

VA CLASSIFICATION (Primary): DX102

Note: For a listing of dosage forms and brand names by country availability, see *Dosage Forms* section(s). For a listing of brand names for the articles in this monograph, refer to the General Index.

## Category

Diagnostic aid, radiopaque (gallbladder disorders; biliary tract disorders).

Note: Iodipamide is an ionic radiopaque contrast agent.

## Indications

### Accepted

Cholangiography, intravenous and/or

Cholecystography, intravenous—Iodipamide is indicated for intravenous cholangiography and cholecystography for the visualization of the gallbladder and biliary ducts in acute abdominal conditions in which rapid diagnosis is required; for the visualization of the biliary ducts in patients with postcholecystectomy symptoms; for visualization of the gallbladder in patients unable to take oral contrast media or to absorb contrast media from the gastrointestinal tract. However, it should be noted that, because of the potential for systemic toxicity with intravenous cholangiography, sonography and hepatobiliary scintigraphy are usually the preferred methods for evaluation of the gallbladder and the bile ducts.

## Pharmacology/Pharmacokinetics

### Physicochemical characteristics

Molecular weight—1530.20.

### Mechanism of action/Effect

Organic iodine compounds block x-rays as they pass through the body, thereby allowing body structures containing iodine to be delineated in contrast to those structures that do not contain iodine. The degree of opacity produced by these iodinated organic compounds is directly proportional to the total amount (concentration and volume) of the iodinated contrast agent in the path of the x-rays. Iodipamide's primary excretion through the hepato-biliary system and concentration in bile allows visualization of the gallbladder and biliary ducts.

### Other actions/effects

Anticoagulant activity (inhibitory effect on platelet aggregation and blood clotting).

### Distribution

Rapidly distributed throughout extracellular fluid following intravascular administration.

### Protein binding

Very high, to plasma albumin.

### Biotransformation

Hepatic.

### Time to peak opacification

Biliary ducts—
With drip infusion: 40 to 80 minutes.
With intravenous injection: 20 to 30 minutes.

Gallbladder—
With drip infusion: 3 hours.
With intravenous injection: 2 hours (delayed opacification may occur in 24 hours).

### Elimination

Fecal—
Normal hepatic function: 80 to 95% of dose eliminated unchanged in 24 hours.

Renal—
Normal renal and hepatic function: 10 to 15% of dose eliminated unchanged within 24 hours.
Hepatic function impairment: Urinary elimination of iodipamide is increased.

## Precautions to Consider

### Cross-sensitivity and/or related problems

Patients sensitive to iodine or other iodinated contrast media may be sensitive to iodipamide also.

### Pregnancy/Reproduction

Pregnancy—Iodipamide crosses the placenta. Studies have not been done in humans. However, other organically bound iodine–containing preparations administered near term by intra-amniotic injection have caused hypothyroidism in some newborns.

Also, elective contrast radiography of the abdomen is usually not recommended during pregnancy because of the risks to the fetus from radiation exposure.

Studies have not been done in animals.

FDA Pregnancy Category C.

### Breast-feeding

Iodipamide is distributed unchanged into breast milk. Although problems in humans have not been documented, temporary discontinuation of breast-feeding is recommended for at least 24 hours following administration of iodipamide.

### Pediatrics

Dehydration may exacerbate uricosuric effects of iodipamide in infants and young children, especially those with polyuria, oliguria, diabetes, or pre-existing dehydration; adequate hydration is recommended before and following administration of iodipamide.

### Geriatrics

Dehydration may exacerbate uricosuric effects of iodipamide in geriatric patients, especially those with polyuria, oliguria, diabetes, or pre-existing dehydration; adequate hydration is recommended before and following administration of iodipamide.

The elderly may be more sensitive to the effects of iodipamide on thyroid function. Iodine-induced thyrotoxicosis may occur 4 to 12 weeks following contrast radiography. Thyroid function monitoring may be needed in geriatric patients.

### Drug interactions and/or related problems

The following drug interactions and/or related problems have been selected on the basis of their potential clinical significance (possible mechanism in parentheses where appropriate)—not necessarily inclusive (» = major clinical significance):

Note: Combinations containing any of the following medications, depending on the amount present, may also interact with this medication.

Cholecystographic agents, oral
(hepatic excretion of iodipamide may be blocked after administration of oral cholecystographic agents, increasing the risk of adverse effects; administration of cholecystographic agents is not recommended within 24 hours before or after iodipamide)

Interleukin-2
(incidence of delayed reactions to intravenous contrast media [e.g., hypersensitivity, fever, skin rash, flu-like symptoms, joint pain, flushing, pruritus, emesis, hypotension, dizziness occurring more than 1 hour after administration] may be increased in patients who have received interleukin-2; some symptoms may resemble a ''recall'' reaction to interleukin-2; supportive medical treatment may be necessary if symptoms are significant; there is some evidence that incidence is reduced if contrast media administration is delayed until 6 weeks after interleukin-2 administration)

Nephrotoxic medications, other (See *Appendix II*)
(concurrent intravascular administration of iodipamide with other nephrotoxic medications may increase the potential for nephrotoxicity)

Platelet aggregation inhibitors, other (See *Appendix II*)
(increased risk of bleeding may occur when these medications are used concurrently with iodipamide)

### Diagnostic interference

The following have been selected on the basis of their potential clinical significance (possible effect in parentheses where appropriate)—not necessarily inclusive (» = major clinical significance):

With results of *this* test

*Due to medical problems or conditions*

Hepatic or cystic duct obstruction
(visualization may be decreased)

Hepatic function impairment
(nonvisualization may result in patients whose sulfobromophthalein [BSP] retention is greater than 30 to 40%; bilirubin concentration of 3 mg per 100 mL caused by mechanical obstruction or hepatocellular damage may also result in nonvisualization)

With *other* diagnostic test results
  Blood pool imaging
    (imaging of blood pool may be impaired because of decreased tech-netium Tc 99m-labeling of red blood cells caused by the intravascular administration of iodipamide)
  Skeletal imaging
    (possible renal and hepatic uptake of technetium Tc 99m medronate, technetium Tc 99m oxidronate, technetium Tc 99m pyrophosphate, and technetium Tc 99m [pyro- and trimeta-] phosphates if iodipamide is administered intravenously immediately after one of these technetium Tc 99m-labeled agents)
  Phenolsulfonphthalein (PSP) excretion test
    (test results may be affected in patients given intravascular iodipamide, especially those patients with severely impaired renal function, because of decreased tubular excretion of PSP; concurrent use of intravascular iodipamide is not recommended in patients receiving a PSP excretion test)
  Thyroid function determinations and
  Thyroid imaging
    (prior administration of iodipamide may cause an increase of serum protein-bound iodine [PBI] and a decrease in radioactive iodine or pertechnetate ion uptake for a period varying from 1 week to several months; thyroid test should be performed prior to administration of iodipamide. Other thyroid function tests not based on measurement of iodine, such as resin triiodothyronine uptake, are not affected)
  Urinalysis
    (prior administration of iodipamide may produce abnormal results; urine should be collected prior to or at least 2 days after intravenous administration of iodipamide)
With physiology/laboratory test values
  Alanine aminotransferase (ALT [SGPT]) and
  Aspartate aminotransferase (AST [SGOT])
    (values may be increased)
  Bilirubin, serum and
  Blood urea nitrogen (BUN) and
  Creatinine, serum
    (concentrations may be increased)
  Platelet aggregation
    (may be decreased)
  Uric acid, serum and urinary
    (iodipamide may increase rate of excretion of uric acid resulting in decreased serum concentrations of uric acid and increased urinary excretion values for a few days)

## Medical considerations/Contraindications

The medical considerations/contraindications included here have been selected on the basis of their potential clinical significance (reasons given in parentheses where appropriate)—not necessarily inclusive (» = major clinical significance).

See also *Diagnostic interference.*

*Except under special circumstances, this medication should not be used when the following medical problem exists:*

» Hepatorenal disease, severe
    (elimination of iodipamide may be decreased; increased risk of nephrotoxicity)

*Risk-benefit should be considered when the following medical problems exist:*

» Allergic reaction (anaphylaxis) to penicillins or to skin allergens, previous
    (increased risk of anaphylactoid reaction)

» Allergies or asthma, history of
    (increased risk of idiosyncratic response or anaphylactoid reaction)

» Dehydration, especially associated with pre-existing renal or hepatic disease, advanced vascular disease, and diabetes mellitus, and in infants, young children, and elderly patients
    (dehydration may increase risk of renal tubular precipitation of iodipamide; also, uricosuric effects of iodipamide may increase risk of obstructive uric acid nephropathy; adequate hydration and alkalinization of urine is recommended)

  Hypertension, severe

  Hyperthyroidism
    (may precipitate thyroid storm)

  Pheochromocytoma
    (administration of iodipamide may precipitate severe hypertension; amount of iodipamide injected should be kept to a minimum and blood pressure should be monitored during the procedure)

» Sensitivity to iodinated contrast media
    (increased risk of anaphylactoid reaction in patients with history of prior reactions to contrast media)

Sickle cell disease
    (administration of contrast media may promote sickling in patients who are homozygous for sickle cell disease; although sickling has not been specifically reported for iodipamide, the possibility exists)

## Patient monitoring

The following may be especially important in patient monitoring (other tests may be warranted in some patients, depending on condition; » = major clinical significance):

Blood pressure determinations
    (may be required during examination, especially in patients with known or suspected pheochromocytoma)

# Side/Adverse Effects

Note: Adverse effects may vary directly with the concentration of the agent, the amount and technique used, and the underlying pathology. Increases in osmolality, volume, concentration, viscosity, and rate of administration of the solution may tend to increase the incidence and severity of adverse effects.

   Dehydration may exacerbate the uricosuric effects of iodipamide and increase the risk of obstructive uric acid nephropathy in infants and young children, and in geriatric, azotemic, and dehydrated or debilitated patients.

   Renal toxicity (proteinuria, crystalluria, renal tubular acidosis) may occur. Toxicity is dose-rate dependent.

The following side/adverse effects have been selected on the basis of their potential clinical significance (possible signs and symptoms in parentheses where appropriate)—not necessarily inclusive:

## Those indicating need for medical attention
Incidence less frequent or rare
  *Crystalluria* (blood in urine, lower back pain, pain or burning while urinating); *severe hepatotoxicity* (abdominal pain or tenderness, fever, nausea and vomiting); *transient hypotension* (severe unusual tiredness or weakness); *pseudo-allergic reaction* (skin rash or hives, swelling of face or skin, wheezing, tightness in chest, or troubled breathing)

  Note: *Pseudo-allergic reactions* are usually transient. However, they may be initial manifestations of more severe anaphylactoid reactions. The anaphylactoid reaction may progress to respiratory arrest and vasomotor collapse if appropriate treatment is not administered.

     *Hypotension* may be accompanied by dizziness, nausea, pallor, and, rarely, circulatory collapse.

## Those indicating need for medical attention only if they continue or are bothersome
Incidence more frequent
  *Vasodilation, arteriolar* (feeling of warmth and flushing of skin)
Incidence less frequent
  *Chills; dizziness or lightheadedness; headache; increased sweating; increased watering of mouth; nausea or vomiting*

  Note: The above are usually self-limited and of short duration; may occur with too rapid administration of iodipamide.

# Patient Consultation

As an aid to patient consultation, refer to *Advice for the Patient, Radiopaque Agents (Diagnostic).*

In providing consultation, consider emphasizing the following selected information (» = major clinical significance):

## Description of use
Action in the body: Concentrates in bile; visualization of bile ducts and gallbladder radiopacity possible with x-rays

## Before having this test
» Conditions affecting use, especially:
   Sensitivity to iodine or other iodinated contrast media
   Pregnancy—Iodipamide crosses the placenta; risk to the fetus from radiation exposure; possibility of causing hypothyroidism in the newborn
   Breast-feeding—Distributed into breast milk; temporary discontinuation of breast-feeding for at least 24 hours is recommended
   Use in children—Possible exacerbation of uricosuric effects of iodipamide in dehydrated children
   Use in the elderly—Possible exacerbation of uricosuric effects of iodipamide in dehydrated patients
   Other medical problems, especially allergies or asthma (history of), dehydration, previous allergic reaction to penicillins or to skin allergens, and severe hepatorenal disease

## Preparation for this test
Adequate intake of fluids to prevent dehydration

Special diet, use of laxative, and/or other preparatory instructions may apply; patient should inquire in advance

**Precautions after having this test**
Possible interference with future thyroid tests

**Side/adverse effects**
Signs of potential side effects, especially hepatotoxicity, hypotension, pseudo-allergic reaction, and renal toxicity

## General Dosing Information

Manufacturer's package insert or other appropriate literature should be consulted for specific techniques and procedures for administration of contrast media.

Sensitivity test doses are not usually recommended since severe or fatal reactions to contrast media are not predictable from a patient's history or a sensitivity test. On some occasions severe or fatal reactions have occurred with a test dose or with a full dose in patients who did not react to the test dose.

Pretreatment with corticosteroids or antihistamines has been used to minimize the incidence and severity of reactions in patients with a history of severe reactions to contrast media or with other high-risk conditions (e.g., asthma or history of allergies, positive allergy history to skin allergens or penicillin, dehydration, history of seizures, pheochromocytoma). In some studies, the additional use of ephedrine has been shown to be beneficial in preventing anaphylactoid reactions.

Adequate hydration is especially important in infants, young children, and geriatric or azotemic patients since dehydration may exacerbate uricosuric effects of the contrast medium.

Preparatory measures, such as a fat-free diet or fasting and use of laxatives, are recommended.

During and for at least 30 to 60 minutes after administration of contrast media, the patient should be observed for possible severe reactions, and competent personnel and emergency facilities should be available during this period.

## Parenteral Dosage Forms

### IODIPAMIDE MEGLUMINE INJECTION USP

**Usual adult and adolescent dose**
Cholangiography and
Cholecystography—
Intravenous drip infusion, 100 mL of a solution containing the equivalent of 51 mg of iodine per mL, administered slowly over a period of thirty to forty-five minutes.
Intravenous, 20 mL of a solution containing the equivalent of 260 mg of iodine per mL administered slowly over a period of ten minutes, not to be repeated for twenty-four hours.

**Usual pediatric dose**
Cholangiography and
Cholecystography—
Intravenous, 0.3 to 0.6 mL per kg of body weight, of a solution containing the equivalent of 260 mg of iodine per mL, not to exceed 20 mL.

**Usual geriatric dose**
See *Usual adult and adolescent dose.*

**Strength(s) usually available**
U.S.—
10.3% (103 mg per mL) of iodipamide meglumine with 5.1% (51 mg per mL) of iodine (Rx) [*Cholografin for Infusion* (0.32% sodium citrate and 0.04% sodium edetate)].
52% (520 mg per mL) of iodipamide meglumine with 26% (260 mg per mL) of iodine (Rx) [*Cholografin* (0.32% sodium citrate and 0.04% sodium edetate)].
Canada—
52% (520 mg per mL) of iodipamide meglumine with 26% (260 mg per mL) of iodine (Rx) [*Cholografin* (0.32% sodium citrate and 0.04% disodium edetate)].

**Packaging and storage**
Store below 40 °C (104 °F), preferably between 15 and 30 °C (59 and 86 °F), unless otherwise specified by manufacturer. Protect from light.

**Stability**
Crystals may form in the solution but are readily redissolved by immersing the container in a water bath at 40 to 50 °C (104 to 122 °F) and gently shaking it.
Any unused portion remaining in the container should be discarded.

**Incompatibilities**
Iodipamide Meglumine Injection USP is physically incompatible with diphenhydramine hydrochloride, chlorpheniramine maleate, brompheniramine maleate, gentamicin sulfate, and promethazine hydrochloride injection. A precipitate may form in the syringe or tubing if the antihistamine is mixed with iodipamide meglumine.

## Selected Bibliography

Patel JC, McInnes GC, Bagley JS, et al. The role of intravenous cholangiography in pre-operative assessment for laparoscopic cholecystectomy. Br J Radiol 1993 Dec; 66 (792): 1125-7.

Revised: 05/11/95

## IODIPAMIDE-CONTAINING COMBINATIONS—
Diatrizoate and Iodipamide (Local)

# IODOHIPPURATE SODIUM I 123  Systemic*

VA CLASSIFICATION (Primary): DX201
Note: For a listing of dosage forms and brand names by country availability, see *Dosage Forms* section(s). For a listing of brand names for the articles in this monograph, refer to the General Index.

*Not commercially available in the U.S.

## Category
Diagnostic aid, radioactive (renal disorders; urinary tract obstructions).

## Indications
**Accepted**
Renography—Iodohippurate sodium I 123 is indicated in renography to determine renal function, effective renal blood flow, and urinary tract obstruction.

Renal imaging, radionuclide—Iodohippurate sodium I 123 is indicated as a renal imaging agent to assess renal size, position, configuration, and function.

## Physical Properties
**Nuclear data**

| Radionuclide (half-life) | Mode of decay | Principal photon emissions (keV) | Mean number of emissions/ disintegration |
|---|---|---|---|
| I 123 (13.2 hr) | Electron capture | Gamma (159) | 0.83 |

## Pharmacology/Pharmacokinetics

**Mechanism of action/Effect**
Based on its elimination by both tubular secretion and glomerular filtration, which can be monitored or observed by appropriate imaging or detection equipment.

**Half-life**
For iodohippurate sodium (biological)—Approximately 20 to 30 minutes.

**Time to peak concentration**
Kidneys—Approximately 3 to 6 minutes.

## Radiation dosimetry

| Organ | Estimated absorbed radiation dose*† | | | |
|---|---|---|---|---|
| | With normal kidney function | | With impaired kidney function | |
| | mGy/ MBq | rad/mCi | mGy/ MBq | rad/mCi |
| Bladder wall | 0.20 | 0.74 | 0.11 | 0.41 |
| Uterus | 0.17 | 0.63 | 0.013 | 0.048 |
| Large intestine (lower) | 0.0075 | 0.028 | 0.0078 | 0.029 |
| Ovaries | 0.0073 | 0.027 | 0.0079 | 0.029 |
| Kidneys | 0.0064 | 0.024 | 0.027 | 0.099 |
| Testes | 0.0046 | 0.017 | 0.0053 | 0.020 |
| Small intestine | 0.0032 | 0.012 | 0.0060 | 0.022 |
| Large intestine (upper) | 0.0025 | 0.0093 | 0.0056 | 0.021 |
| Red marrow | 0.0025 | 0.0093 | 0.0064 | 0.024 |
| Bone surfaces | 0.0013 | 0.0048 | 0.0051 | 0.019 |
| Adrenals | 0.00092 | 0.0034 | 0.0053 | 0.020 |
| Pancreas | 0.00089 | 0.0033 | 0.0051 | 0.019 |
| Spleen | 0.00082 | 0.0030 | 0.0049 | 0.018 |
| Stomach wall | 0.00079 | 0.0029 | 0.0044 | 0.016 |
| Liver | 0.00072 | 0.0027 | 0.0059 | 0.022 |
| Lungs | 0.00048 | 0.0018 | 0.0038 | 0.014 |
| Breast | 0.00044 | 0.0016 | 0.0034 | 0.013 |
| Thyroid | 0.00037 | 0.0014 | 0.0030 | 0.011 |
| Other tissue | 0.0022 | 0.0081 | 0.0045 | 0.017 |
| Effective dose | 0.015 mSv/MBq | 0.056 rem/mCi | 0.013 mSv/MBq | 0.048 rem/mCi |

*For adults; intravenous administration.

†Data based on the International Commission on Radiological Protection (ICRP) Publication 53—Radiation Dose to Patients from Radiopharmaceuticals.

### Elimination

Renal, 50 to 75% within 25 minutes; 90 to 95% within 8 hours; primarily by tubular cell secretion, but also by glomerular filtration.

Iodide I 123 is excreted in breast milk, also.

## Precautions to Consider

### Carcinogenicity/Mutagenicity

Long-term animal studies to evaluate carcinogenic or mutagenic potential of iodohippurate sodium I 123 have not been performed.

### Pregnancy/Reproduction

Pregnancy—Studies have not been done in humans. Other radioiodines (e.g., iodide I 131) cross the placenta and may cause severe and irreversible hypothyroidism in the newborn and are not recommended for use during pregnancy.

The possibility of pregnancy should be assessed in women of child-bearing potential. Clinical situations exist where the benefit to the patient and fetus, based on information derived from radiopharmaceutical use, outweighs the risks from fetal exposure to radiation. In these situations, the physician should use discretion and reduce the radiopharmaceutical dose to the lowest possible amount.

Studies have not been done in animals.

FDA Pregnancy Category C.

### Breast-feeding

Iodide I 123 is excreted in breast milk. Because of the potential risk to the infant from radiation exposure, temporary discontinuation of nursing is recommended for approximately 3 days.

### Pediatrics

Although iodohippurate sodium I 123 is used in children, there have been no specific studies evaluating its safety and efficacy in pediatric patients. When this radiopharmaceutical is used in children, the diagnostic benefit should be judged to outweigh the potential risk of radiation.

### Geriatrics

Appropriate studies on the relationship of age to the effects of iodohippurate sodium I 123 have not been performed in the geriatric population. However, no geriatrics-specific problems have been documented to date.

### Drug interactions and/or related problems

See *Diagnostic interference.*

### Diagnostic interference

The following have been selected on the basis of their potential clinical significance (possible effect in parentheses where appropriate)—not necessarily inclusive (» = major clinical significance):

With results of *this* test

*Due to other medications*

Probenecid

(concurrent use may decrease kidney uptake of iodohippurate sodium I 123 due to a direct inhibition of the enzyme transport system in the proximal tubule by probenecid)

*Due to medical problems or conditions*

Dehydration

(may prolong renal transit time of iodohippurate sodium I 123, thus increasing the time required to reach peak radioactivity level in kidney)

*Due to other diagnostic tests*

Retrograde pyelogram

(may alter renogram curve; renogram should be performed before or at least 24 hours after this procedure)

With *other* diagnostic test results

Thyroid function determinations and

Thyroid imaging

(Lugol's solution used prior to the administration of iodohippurate sodium I 123 may cause a decrease in radioactive iodine or pertechnetate ion uptake for several weeks)

### Medical considerations/Contraindications

The medical considerations/contraindications included here have been selected on the basis of their potential clinical significance (reasons given in parentheses where appropriate)—not necessarily inclusive (» = major clinical significance).

See also *Diagnostic interference.*

*Risk-benefit should be considered when the following medical problem exists:*

Sensitivity to the radiopharmaceutical preparation

## Side/Adverse Effects

The following side/adverse effects have been selected on the basis of their potential clinical significance (possible signs and symptoms in parentheses where appropriate)—not necessarily inclusive:

**Those indicating need for medical attention**

Incidence rare

*Allergic reaction* (skin rash, hives, or itching); *fainting; nausea or vomiting*

## Patient Consultation

As an aid to patient consultation, refer to *Advice for the Patient, Radiopharmaceuticals (Diagnostic).*

In providing consultation, consider emphasizing the following selected information (» = major clinical significance):

**Description of use**

Action in the body: Elimination by tubular cell secretion and glomerular filtration

Appearance, concentration, and elimination of iodohippurate sodium I 123 in kidneys allows monitoring and visualization

Small amounts of radioactivity used in diagnosis; radiation received is low and considered safe

**Before having this test**

» Conditions affecting use, especially:

Sensitivity to the radiopharmaceutical preparation

Pregnancy—Risk to fetus from radiation exposure as opposed to benefit derived from use should be considered; possibility of hypothyroidism in newborn

Breast-feeding—Iodide I 123 excreted in breast milk; temporary discontinuation of nursing recommended because of risk to infant from radiation exposure

Use in children—Risk from radiation exposure as opposed to benefit derived from use should be considered

**Preparation for this test**

Special preparatory instructions may apply; patient should inquire in advance

**Precautions after having this test**

Possible interference with future thyroid tests

**Side/adverse effects**

Signs of potential side effects, especially allergic reaction, fainting, nausea or vomiting

# General Dosing Information

Radiopharmaceuticals are to be administered only by or under the supervision of physicians who have had extensive training in the safe use and handling of radioactive materials and who are authorized by the appropriate Federal or state agency, if required, or, outside the U.S., the appropriate authority.

To help minimize thyroidal uptake of free iodide I 123, a thyroid blocking agent such as a saturated solution of potassium iodide or potassium perchlorate should be given prior to administration of iodohippurate sodium I 123 and for several days afterwards.

To assure adequate urine flow, increased oral intake of fluids is recommended 1 hour prior to the diagnostic procedure, unless contraindicated because of the presence of edema or congestive heart failure.

Manufacturer's package insert or other appropriate literature should be consulted for optimal times when imaging should be performed. In general, imaging should be performed as close to time of calibration as possible since the quality of the image will degrade with time because of the increase in the proportion of radionuclidic contaminants (primarily I 124).

## Safety considerations for handling this radiopharmaceutical

Improper handling of this radiopharmaceutical may cause radioactive contamination. Guidelines for handling radioactive material have been prepared by scientific, professional, state, federal, and international bodies and are available to the specially qualified and authorized users who have access to radiopharmaceuticals.

# Parenteral Dosage Forms

## IODOHIPPURATE SODIUM I 123 INJECTION USP

### Usual adult and adolescent administered activity

Renography—
Intravenous, 3.7 to 14.8 megabecquerels (100 to 400 microcuries).

Renal imaging, radionuclide—
Intravenous, 37 megabecquerels (1 millicurie).

### Usual pediatric administered activity
Dosage must be individualized by physician.

### Usual geriatric administered activity
See *Usual adult and adolescent administered activity*.

### Strength(s) usually available
U.S.—
Not commercially available.
Canada—
37 megabecquerels (1 millicurie) of iodohippurate sodium I 123, at time of calibration, per vial (Rx) [*Nephropure*].
74 megabecquerels (2 millicuries) of iodohippurate sodium I 123, at time of calibration, per vial (Rx) [*Nephropure*].

### Packaging and storage
Store below 40 °C (104 °F), preferably between 15 and 30 °C (59 and 86 °F), unless otherwise specified by manufacturer. Protect from freezing.

### Note
Caution—Radioactive material.

# Selected Bibliography

Eshima D, Fritzber AR, Taylor A Jr. Tc 99m renal tubular function agents: current status. Sem Nuc Med 1990; 20 (1): 28-40.
Thrall JH, Koff SA, Keyes JW. Diuretic radionuclide renography and scintigraphy in the differential diagnosis of hydroureteronephrosis. Sem Nuc Med 1981; 11 (2): 89-104.

Revised: 02/01/93
Interim revision: 08/02/94

# IODOHIPPURATE SODIUM I 131   Systemic

VA CLASSIFICATION (Primary): DX201
Note: For a listing of dosage forms and brand names by country availability, see *Dosage Forms* section(s). For a listing of brand names for the articles in this monograph, refer to the General Index.

## Category
Diagnostic aid, radioactive (renal disorders; urinary tract obstructions).

## Indications

### Accepted
Renography—Iodohippurate sodium I 131 is indicated in renography to determine renal function, effective renal plasma flow, and urinary tract obstruction.

Renal imaging, radionuclide—Iodohippurate sodium I 131 is indicated as an imaging agent to assess renal size, position, configuration, and function.

## Physical Properties

### Nuclear data:

| Radionuclide (half-life) | Mode of decay | Principal photon emissions (keV) | Mean number of emissions/ disintegration |
|---|---|---|---|
| I 131 (8.08 days) | Beta | Beta (191.6) Gamma (364.4) | 0.90 0.81 |

## Pharmacology/Pharmacokinetics

### Mechanism of action/Effect
Based on its excretion by both tubular secretion and glomerular filtration, which can be observed by appropriate imaging or detection systems.

### Half-life
For iodohippurate sodium (biological)—Approximately 20 to 30 minutes.

### Time to peak concentration
Kidneys—Approximately 3 to 6 minutes.

## Radiation dosimetry

| Organ | Estimated absorbed radiation dose* | | | |
|---|---|---|---|---|
| | With normal kidney function | | With impaired kidney function | |
| | mGy/ MBq | rad/ mCi | mGy/ MBq | rad/ mCi |
| Bladder wall | 0.96 | 3.55 | 0.63 | 2.33 |
| Uterus | 0.35 | 1.30 | 0.039 | 0.14 |
| Kidneys | 0.30 | 1.11 | 0.15 | 0.56 |
| Large intestine (lower) | 0.17 | 0.63 | 0.027 | 0.099 |
| Ovaries | 0.17 | 0.63 | 0.026 | 0.096 |
| Testes | 0.12 | 0.44 | 0.022 | 0.081 |
| Small intestine | 0.0078 | 0.029 | 0.022 | 0.081 |
| Large intestine (upper) | 0.0069 | 0.026 | 0.021 | 0.078 |
| Red marrow | 0.0049 | 0.018 | 0.019 | 0.070 |
| Bone surfaces | 0.0030 | 0.011 | 0.017 | 0.063 |
| Adrenals | 0.0028 | 0.010 | 0.021 | 0.081 |
| Pancreas | 0.0026 | 0.0096 | 0.019 | 0.070 |
| Spleen | 0.0024 | 0.0089 | 0.019 | 0.070 |
| Stomach wall | 0.0025 | 0.0093 | 0.018 | 0.067 |
| Liver | 0.0023 | 0.0085 | 0.025 | 0.093 |
| Lungs | 0.0016 | 0.0059 | 0.015 | 0.056 |
| Thyroid | 0.0014 | 0.0052 | 0.014 | 0.052 |
| Other tissue | 0.0054 | 0.020 | 0.018 | 0.067 |
| Effective dose | 0.066 mSv/MBq | 0.24 rem/mCi | 0.065 mSv/MBq | 0.24 rem/mCi |

*For adults; intravenous administration.
†Data based on the International Commission on Radiological Protection (ICRP) Publication 53—Radiation dose to patients from radiopharmaceuticals.

### Elimination
Renal, 50 to 75% within 25 minutes and 90 to 95% within 8 hours (primarily by tubular cell secretion [80%], but also by glomerular filtration [20%]). Iodide I 131 is eliminated in breast milk, also.

# Precautions to Consider

## Pregnancy/Reproduction
Pregnancy—Studies have not been done in humans with iodohippurate sodium I 131. However, iodide I 131 crosses the placenta and may cause severe and irreversible hypothyroidism in the newborn. Iodohippurate sodium I 131 is not recommended for use during pregnancy.

The possibility of pregnancy should be assessed in women of child-bearing potential. Clinical situations exist where the benefit to the patient and fetus, based on information derived from radiopharmaceutical use, outweighs the risks from fetal exposure to radiation. In these situations, the physician should use discretion and reduce the radiopharmaceutical dose to the lowest possible amount.

Studies have not been done in animals.

FDA Pregnancy Category C.

## Breast-feeding
Iodide I 131 is excreted in breast milk. Because of the potential risk to the infant from radiation exposure, temporary discontinuation of nursing is recommended for approximately 5 days.

## Pediatrics
Although iodohippurate sodium I 131 is used in children, there have been no specific studies evaluating its safety and efficacy in children. When this radiopharmaceutical is used in children, the diagnostic benefit should be judged to outweigh the potential risk of radiation.

## Geriatrics
Appropriate studies on the relationship of age to the effects of iodohippurate sodium I 131 have not been performed in the geriatric population. However, no geriatrics-specific problems have been documented to date.

## Drug interactions and/or related problems
See *Diagnostic interference.*

## Diagnostic interference
The following have been selected on the basis of their potential clinical significance (possible effect in parentheses where appropriate)—not necessarily inclusive (» = major clinical significance):

With results of *this* test
*Due to other medications*
  Probenecid
    (concurrent use may decrease kidney uptake of iodohippurate sodium I 131 due to a direct inhibition of the enzyme transport system in the proximal tubule by probenecid)

*Due to medical problems or conditions*
  Dehydration
    (kidney uptake of iodohippurate sodium I 131 may be reduced and renal transit time may be prolonged)

*Due to other diagnostic tests*
  Retrograde pyelogram
    (may alter renogram curve; renogram should be performed before or at least 24 hours after this procedure)

With *other* diagnostic test results
  Thyroid function determinations and
  Thyroid imaging
    (Lugol's solution used prior to the administration of iodohippurate sodium I 131 may cause a decrease in radioactive iodine or pertechnetate ion uptake for several weeks)

## Medical considerations/Contraindications
The medical considerations/contraindications included here have been selected on the basis of their potential clinical significance (reasons given in parentheses where appropriate)—not necessarily inclusive (» = major clinical significance).

See also *Diagnostic interference.*

*Risk-benefit should be considered when the following medical problem exists:*
  Sensitivity to the radiopharmaceutical preparation

# Side/Adverse Effects
The following side/adverse effects have been selected on the basis of their potential clinical significance (possible signs and symptoms in parentheses where appropriate)—not necessarily inclusive:

## Those indicating need for medical attention
Incidence rare—not clearly related to iodohippurate sodium I 131
  *Fainting; nausea or vomiting*

# Patient Consultation
As an aid to patient consultation, refer to *Advice for the Patient, Radiopharmaceuticals (Diagnostic).*

In providing consultation, consider emphasizing the following selected information (» = major clinical significance):

## Description of use
  Action in the body: Elimination by tubular cell secretion and glomerular filtration
  Appearance, concentration, and elimination of iodohippurate sodium I 131 in kidneys allows monitoring and visualization
  Small amounts of radioactivity used in diagnosis; radiation received is low and considered safe

## Before having this test
» Conditions affecting use, especially:
    Sensitivity to the radiopharmaceutical preparation
    Pregnancy—Risk to fetus from radiation exposure as opposed to benefit derived from use should be considered; possibility of hypothyroidism in newborn
    Breast-feeding—Iodide I 131 excreted in breast milk; temporary discontinuation of nursing recommended because of risk to infant from radiation exposure
    Use in children—Risk from radiation exposure as opposed to benefit derived from use should be considered

## Preparation for this test
  Special preparatory instructions may apply; patient should inquire in advance

## Precautions after having this test
  Possible interference with future thyroid tests

## Side/adverse effects
  Signs of potential side effects, especially fainting, nausea, or vomiting

# General Dosing Information
Radiopharmaceuticals are to be administered only by or under the supervision of physicians who have had extensive training in the safe use and handling of radioactive materials and who are authorized by the Nuclear Regulatory Commission (NRC) or the appropriate Agreement State agency, if required, or, outside the U.S., the appropriate authority.

Approximately 25% of the free iodide content of iodohippurate sodium I 131 is taken up by the thyroid gland following intravenous administration. To help minimize thyroidal uptake of free iodide I 131, a thyroid blocking agent such as a saturated solution of potassium iodide or potassium perchlorate should be given prior to administration of iodohippurate sodium I 131 and for several days afterwards.

To assure adequate urine flow, increased oral intake of fluids is recommended 1 hour prior to the diagnostic procedure, unless contraindicated because of the presence of edema or congestive heart failure.

Iodohippurate Sodium I 131 Injection USP is not intended for intra-arterial use. Also, precautions should be taken to avoid extravasation during intravenous administration.

## Safety considerations for handling this radiopharmaceutical
Improper handling of this radiopharmaceutical may cause radioactive contamination. Guidelines for handling radioactive material have been prepared by scientific, professional, state, federal, and international bodies and are available to the specially qualified and authorized users who have access to radiopharmaceuticals.

# Parenteral Dosage Forms

## IODOHIPPURATE SODIUM I 131 INJECTION USP

### Usual adult and adolescent administered activity
Renography—
  Intravenous, 0.0185 megabecquerel (0.5 microcurie) per kg of body weight.
Renal imaging, radionuclide—
  Intravenous, 0.1 to 0.185 megabecquerel (3 to 5 microcuries) per kg of body weight.

### Usual pediatric administered activity
Dosage must be individualized by physician.

### Usual geriatric administered activity
See *Usual adult and adolescent administered activity.*

## Strength(s) usually available
U.S.—
    At time of calibration: Per multiple-dose vial—
        37 megabecquerels (1 millicurie) (Rx) [*Hippuran; Hipputope;* GENERIC].
        74 megabecquerels (2 millicuries) (Rx) [*Hipputope;* GENERIC].
Canada—
        Various concentrations as per manufacturer's labeling (Rx) [GENERIC].

## Packaging and storage
Store below 40 °C (104 °F), preferably between 15 and 30 °C (59 and 86 °F), unless otherwise specified by manufacturer. Protect from freezing.

## Note
Caution—Radioactive material.

## Selected Bibliography
Eshima D, Fritzber AR, Taylor A Jr. Tc 99m renal tubular function agents: current status. Semin Nucl Med 1990; 20 (1): 28-40.
Thrall JH, Koff SA, Keyes JW. Diuretic radionuclide renography and scintigraphy in the differential diagnosis of hydroureteronephrosis. Semin Nucl Med 1981; 11 (2): 89-104.

Revised: 02/01/93
Interim revision: 08/02/94

---

# IODOQUINOL    Oral-Local

INN: Diiodohydroxyquinoline
BAN: Diiodohydroxyquinoline
VA CLASSIFICATION (Primary): AP109
Other commonly used names are diiodohydroxyquin and diiodohydroxyquinoline.

Note: For a listing of dosage forms and brand names by country availability, see *Dosage Forms* section(s). For a listing of brand names for the articles in this monograph, refer to the General Index.

## Category
Antiprotozoal.

## Indications
Note: Bracketed information in the *Indications* section refers to uses that are not included in U.S. product labeling.

### Accepted
Amebiasis, intestinal (treatment)—Iodoquinol is indicated alone as a primary agent in the treatment of intestinal amebiasis in asymptomatic carriers (cyst passers) of *Entamoeba histolytica.*

[Amebiasis, extraintestinal (treatment)][1]—Iodoquinol is used concurrently or sequentially with metronidazole in the treatment of extraintestinal (invasive) amebiasis.

[Balantidiasis (treatment)][1]—Iodoquinol is used as a secondary agent in the treatment of balantidiasis caused by *Balantidium coli.*

Not all species or strains of a particular organism may be susceptible to iodoquinol.

### Unaccepted
Iodoquinol is not effective alone in the treatment of extraintestinal (invasive) amebiasis.

---

[1]Not included in Canadian product labeling.

## Pharmacology/Pharmacokinetics

### Physicochemical characteristics
Chemical group—Halogenated 8-hydroxyquinoline.
Molecular weight—396.95.

### Mechanism of action/Effect
The exact mechanism of action of iodoquinol is unknown. Iodoquinol acts against the trophozoites of *Entamoeba histolytica.* Iodoquinol produces its amebicidal effect at the site of infection, since it is poorly absorbed from the gastrointestinal tract and can reach high concentrations in the intestinal lumen.

### Absorption
Poorly absorbed after oral administration.

### Elimination
Fecal; less than 10% of the dose is recovered in the urine, mostly as glucuronides.

## Precautions to Consider

### Cross-sensitivity and/or related problems
Patients hypersensitive to chloroxine, iodine, pamaquine, pentaquine, primaquine, or other 8-hydroxyquinolines (e.g., clioquinol) may be hypersensitive to this medication also.

### Pregnancy/Reproduction
Problems in humans have not been documented.

### Breast-feeding
It is not known whether iodoquinol is distributed into breast milk. However, problems in humans have not been documented.

### Pediatrics
Children may be more susceptible to the side effects of 8-aminoquinolines, such as optic atrophy, optic neuritis, and peripheral neuropathy, especially with prolonged high-dose therapy.

### Geriatrics
No information is available on the relationship of age to the effects of iodoquinol in geriatric patients.

### Laboratory value alterations
The following have been selected on the basis of their potential clinical significance (possible effect in parentheses where appropriate)—not necessarily inclusive (» = major clinical significance):
With diagnostic test results
» Thyroid function tests
        (iodoquinol may increase protein-bound serum iodine concentrations, reflecting a decrease in $^{131}$I uptake; this effect may persist for as long as 6 months after discontinuation of therapy)

### Medical considerations/Contraindications
The medical considerations/contraindications included here have been selected on the basis of their potential clinical significance (reasons given in parentheses where appropriate)—not necessarily inclusive (» = major clinical significance).

*Risk-benefit should be considered when the following medical problems exist:*
» Hepatic disease
        (iodides should be used with caution in patients with hepatic disease)
Hypersensitivity to iodoquinol, chloroxine, iodine, pamaquine, pentaquine, primaquine, or other 8-hydroxyquinolines
Optic neuropathy, pre-existing
        (iodoquinol may cause optic neuritis when given in large doses and could worsen pre-existing optic neuropathy)
» Renal disease
        (iodides should be used with caution in patients with renal disease)
Thyroid disease
        (iodoquinol may interfere with thyroid function tests and may cause goiter)

## Side/Adverse Effects
The following side/adverse effects have been selected on the basis of their potential clinical significance (possible signs and symptoms in parentheses where appropriate)—not necessarily inclusive:

### Those indicating need for medical attention
Incidence less frequent
        *Fever or chills; hypersensitivity* (skin rash, hives, or itching); *thyroid gland enlargement* (swelling of neck)
With prolonged, high doses of 8-hydroxyquinolines—children may be more susceptible
        *Optic atrophy* (blurred vision or any change in vision); *optic neuritis* (decreased vision or eye pain); *peripheral neuropathy* (numbness, tingling, pain, or weakness in hands or feet); *subacute myelo-optic neu-*

*ropathy* (blurred vision or any change in vision, clumsiness or unsteadiness, increased weakness, or muscle pain)

**Those indicating need for medical attention only if they continue or are bothersome**
Incidence more frequent
  *Gastrointestinal disturbances* (diarrhea; nausea or vomiting; stomach pain)
Incidence less frequent
  *Headache; itching of the rectal area*

## Patient Consultation

As an aid to patient consultation, refer to *Advice for the Patient, Iodoquinol (Oral)*.

In providing consultation, consider emphasizing the following selected information (» = major clinical significance):

**Before using this medication**
» Conditions affecting use, especially:
    Hypersensitivity to iodoquinol, chloroxine, iodine, pamaquine, pentaquine, primaquine, or other 8-hydroxyquinolines
    Use in children—Children may be more likely to develop side effects, such as optic atrophy, optic neuritis, and peripheral neuropathy, especially with long-term, high-dose therapy
    Other medical problems, especially hepatic or renal disease

**Proper use of this medication**
» Taking after meals to minimize possible gastrointestinal irritation
  Crushing tablets and mixing with applesauce or chocolate syrup if unable to swallow tablets
» Compliance with full course of therapy
» Proper dosing
  Missed dose: Taking as soon as possible; not taking if almost time for next dose; not doubling doses
» Proper storage

**Precautions while using this medication**
» Caution if blurred vision or loss of vision occurs
» May interfere with thyroid function tests during and for 6 months following therapy

**Side/adverse effects**
  Signs of potential side effects, especially fever or chills, hypersensitivity, thyroid gland enlargement, optic atrophy, optic neuritis, peripheral neuropathy, and subacute myelo-optic neuropathy

## General Dosing Information

Iodoquinol should be taken after meals to minimize possible gastrointestinal irritation.

Prolonged high-dosage therapy with 8-hydroxyquinolines may cause optic neuritis, optic atrophy, peripheral neuropathy, or subacute myelo-optic neuropathy, especially in children.

The course of therapy may be repeated after a 2- to 3-week interval, if necessary.

## Oral Dosage Forms

Note: Bracketed uses in the *Dosage Forms* section refer to categories of use and/or indications that are not included in U.S. product labeling.

### IODOQUINOL TABLETS USP

**Usual adult and adolescent dose**
Amebiasis, intestinal; or
[Balantidiasis][1]—
  Oral, 630 or 650 mg three times a day for twenty days.

**Usual adult prescribing limits**
Up to 2 grams daily.

**Usual pediatric dose**
Amebiasis, intestinal; or
[Balantidiasis][1]—
  Oral, 10 to 13.3 mg per kg of body weight, or 333.3 mg per square meter of body surface, three times a day for twenty days. Dose should not exceed 1.95 grams in twenty-four hours.

**Strength(s) usually available**
U.S.—
  210 mg (Rx) [*Yodoxin*].
  650 mg (Rx) [*Diquinol; Yodoquinol; Yodoxin;* GENERIC].
Canada—
  210 mg (Rx) [*Diodoquin*].
  650 mg (Rx) [*Diodoquin* (scored)].

**Packaging and storage**
Store below 40 °C (104 °F), preferably between 15 and 30 °C (59 and 86 °F), unless otherwise specified by manufacturer. Store in a well-closed container.

**Auxiliary labeling**
• Continue medication for full time of treatment.
• Take after meals.

———

[1]Not included in Canadian product labeling.

Revised: 03/25/96

# IOFETAMINE I 123   Systemic

VA CLASSIFICATION (Primary): DX201
Note: For a listing of dosage forms and brand names by country availability, see *Dosage Forms* section(s). For a listing of brand names for the articles in this monograph, refer to the General Index.

## Category
Diagnostic aid, radioactive (cerebrovascular disease).

## Indications
Note: Bracketed information in the *Indications* section refers to uses that are not included in U.S. product labeling.

**Accepted**
Brain imaging, radionuclide—Iofetamine hydrochloride I 123 is indicated as a brain imaging agent in the localization and evaluation of nonlacunar stroke. It should be used within 96 hours of onset of focal neurological deficit.

[Seizures (diagnosis)][1]—Iofetamine hydrochloride I 123 is used in patients with partial complex seizures to establish the site of epileptogenic focus, which aids in the diagnosis and treatment of epilepsy.

[Dementia, Alzheimer-type (diagnosis)][1]—Iofetamine hydrochloride I 123 is used to study changes in regional cerebral blood flow in patients with senile dementia, which aids in the early diagnosis and classification of patients with senile dementia of the Alzheimer's type.

———

[1]Not included in Canadian product labeling.

## Physical Properties

### Nuclear data

| Radionuclide (half-life) | Decay constant | Mode of decay | Principal emissions (keV) | Mean number of emissions/ disintegration |
|---|---|---|---|---|
| I 123 (13.2 h) | 0.0533 h⁻¹ | Electron capture | 159 | 0.83 |

## Pharmacology/Pharmacokinetics

**Physicochemical characteristics**
Molecular weight—335.74.

**Mechanism of action/Effect**
Iofetamine I 123, due to its high lipid solubility, passes through the blood-brain barrier and is distributed within the brain as a function of relative cerebral perfusion. Although the mechanism by which it localizes in the brain is not fully understood, it is assumed that much of its retention within the brain is probably due to binding by relatively nonspecific, high-capacity binding sites.

**Distribution**
Rapidly distributed from the blood into body tissues. After 6 to 10 minutes, concentration in blood falls to about 3 to 8.5% of the administered dose; after 20 minutes, concentration falls to about 2.5%.

Most of the injected dose is sequestered in the lung, from which it is rapidly released. Brain uptake increases progressively for 30 minutes and remains stable after that until 60 minutes after administration. During this phase, the lungs act as a reservoir to supply additional activity as it is lost from the brain. The ratio of concentration in gray to white matter varies with time, being 2.4 at 15 minutes, 2.2 at 1 hour, 1.8 at 4 hours, and 0.6 at 24 hours. The percentages remaining in the brain, liver, and lungs, respectively, at 1, 5, and 22 hours post-injection are: 5.7, 4.1, 2.1; 12.5, 14.1, 5.5; and 16.8, 10.6, 6.1.

**Protein binding**
Low (<10%).

**Biotransformation**
First-pass extraction primarily by the brain and liver. The two major metabolites are p-iodoamphetamine and p-iodobenzoic acid; p-iodoamphetamine is further metabolized to p-iodobenzoic acid.

**Half-life**
Elimination—$1.6 \pm 1.2$ hours and $10.9 \pm 6.1$ hours.

**Time to radioactivity visualization**
10 minutes to 5 hours after administration of iofetamine I 123. However, since cerebral distribution of iofetamine I 123 changes over time, regional perfusion studies should be performed within 30 minutes after injection.

**Radiation dosimetry**

| Estimated absorbed radiation dose* | | |
|---|---|---|
| Organ | mGy/MBq | rad/mCi |
| Lungs | 0.12 | 0.44 |
| Liver | 0.11 | 0.41 |
| Bladder wall | 0.029 | 0.11 |
| Brain | 0.029 | 0.11 |
| Adrenals | 0.017 | 0.063 |
| Pancreas | 0.017 | 0.063 |
| Red marrow | 0.014 | 0.052 |
| Kidneys | 0.014 | 0.052 |
| Breast | 0.012 | 0.044 |
| Stomach wall | 0.012 | 0.044 |
| Bone surfaces | 0.011 | 0.041 |
| Spleen | 0.011 | 0.041 |
| Large intestine (upper) | 0.010 | 0.037 |
| Small intestine | 0.0087 | 0.032 |
| Uterus | 0.0082 | 0.030 |
| Ovaries | 0.0068 | 0.025 |
| Large intestine (lower) | 0.0064 | 0.024 |
| Thyroid | 0.0059 | 0.022 |
| Testes | 0.0045 | 0.017 |
| Other tissue | 0.0089 | 0.033 |

Effective dose: 0.032 mSv/MBq (0.12 rem/mCi)†

*For adults; intravenous injection.
†Effective dose of I 124 and I 125 impurities is 0.56 mSv/MBq (2.07 rem/mCi) and 0.094 mSv/MBq (0.027 rem/mCi), respectively.

**Elimination**
Renal, as p-iodohippuric acid—About 20% of dose eliminated after 1 day; about 40% after 2 days; and about 48% after 3 days.

# Precautions to Consider

## Cross-sensitivity and/or related problems
Patients sensitive to sympathomimetics (for example, albuterol, amphetamines, ephedrine, epinephrine, isoproterenol, metaproterenol, norepinephrine, phenylephrine, phenylpropanolamine, terbutaline) may be sensitive to this imaging agent also because of iofetamine's amphetamine-like structure.

## Carcinogenicity/Mutagenicity
Long-term animal studies to evaluate carcinogenic or mutagenic potential of iofetamine I 123 have not been performed.

## Pregnancy/Reproduction
Pregnancy—Well-controlled studies have not been done in humans with iofetamine I 123. However, risk-benefit must be considered since other radioiodines (e.g., iodide I 131) cross the placenta and have caused severe and irreversible hypothyroidism in the fetus.
The possibility of pregnancy should be assessed in women of child-bearing potential. Clinical situations exist where the benefit to the patient and fetus from information derived from radiopharmaceutical use outweighs the risks from fetal exposure to radiation. In this situation, the physician should use discretion and reduce the radiopharmaceutical dose to the lowest possible amount.

Studies have not been done in animals.
FDA Pregnancy Category C.

## Breast-feeding
Although it is currently unknown whether I 123 will appear in breast milk following intravenous administration of iofetamine I 123, it does appear when administered as sodium iodide I 123 and may reach concentrations equal to or greater than concentrations in maternal plasma. Because of the potential risk to the infant from radiation exposure, temporary discontinuation of nursing is recommended for a length of time that may be assessed by measuring the activity of breast milk and estimating the radiation exposure to the infant.

## Pediatrics
Although iofetamine I 123 is used in children, there have been no specific studies evaluating its safety and efficacy in children. When this radiopharmaceutical is used in children, the diagnostic benefit should be judged to outweigh the potential risk of radiation.

## Geriatrics
Appropriate studies on the relationship of age to the effects of iofetamine I 123 have not been performed in the geriatric population. However, no geriatric-specific problems have been documented to date.

## Drug interactions and/or related problems
The following drug interactions and/or related problems have been selected on the basis of their potential clinical significance (possible mechanism in parentheses where appropriate)—not necessarily inclusive (» = major clinical significance):
See also *Diagnostic interference.*
Note: Combinations containing any of the following medications, depending on the amount present, may also interact with this medication.

» Monoamine oxidase (MAO) inhibitors, including furazolidone, procarbazine, and selegiline
  (concurrent use may precipitate hypertensive crisis; iofetamine I 123 should not be administered during or within 14 days following the administration of an MAO inhibitor)

## Diagnostic interference
The following have been selected on the basis of their potential clinical significance (possible effect in parentheses where appropriate)—not necessarily inclusive (» = major clinical significance):

With results of *this* test
  *Due to other medications*
    Sympathomimetics
      (sympathomimetics when used concurrently with iofetamine I 123 may alter its biodistribution, therefore, affecting the image quality and usefulness)

## Medical considerations/Contraindications
The medical considerations/contraindications included here have been selected on the basis of their potential clinical significance (reasons given in parentheses where appropriate)—not necessarily inclusive (» = major clinical significance).

***Risk-benefit should be considered when the following medical problems exist:***
  Hypertension, history of
    (increased systolic blood pressure and dizziness with transient chest tightness may result [to date only one case has been reported in a patient with a history of hypertension])
  Respiratory tract infection
    (hearing loss may occur [to date only one case has been reported of transient unilateral hearing loss that occurred several hours after the administration of iofetamine I 123])

# Side/Adverse Effects
As with any organic iodine–containing preparation, allergic reactions are possible.

# Patient Consultation
As an aid to patient consultation, refer to *Advice for the Patient, Radiopharmaceuticals (Diagnostic).*

In providing consultation, consider emphasizing the following selected information (» = major clinical significance):

## Description of use
  Action in the body: Distribution of radioactive iofetamine in brain tissues as a function of respective blood flow
  Retention of radioactivity in brain tissues allows visualization
  Small amount of radioactivity used in diagnosis; radiation received is low and considered safe

**Before having this test**

» Conditions affecting use, especially:

Sensitivity to sympathomimetics

Pregnancy—Risk to fetus from radiation exposure as opposed to benefit derived from use should be considered; possibility of hypothyroidism in fetus

Breast-feeding—Risk to infant from radiation exposure

Use in children—Risk from radiation exposure as opposed to benefit derived from use should be considered

Other medications, especially MAO inhibitors

**Preparation for this test**

Special preparatory instructions may be given; patient should inquire in advance

**Precautions after having this test**

Increasing intake of fluids and voiding as often as possible after examination to minimize radiation exposure to bladder

**Side/adverse effects**

Allergic reactions are possible

## General Dosing Information

Radiopharmaceuticals are to be administered only by or under the supervision of physicians who have had extensive training in the safe use and handling of radioactive materials and who are authorized by the appropriate Federal or Agreement State agency, if required or, outside the U.S., the appropriate authority.

To help minimize thyroidal uptake of free iodide I 123, a thyroid blocking agent such as a saturated solution of potassium iodide or potassium perchlorate should be given $1/2$ to 1 hour prior to administration of iofetamine I 123.

Adequate hydration of the patient is recommended before and after examination to assure adequate urinary flow.

Urination is recommended as often as possible after the examination to reduce radiation exposure to the bladder.

Manufacturer's package insert or other appropriate literature should be consulted for optimal times when imaging should be performed.

**Safety considerations for handling this radiopharmaceutical**

Improper handling of this radiopharmaceutical may cause radioactive contamination. Guidelines for handling radioactive material have been prepared by scientific, professional, state, federal, and international

bodies and are available to the specially qualified and authorized users who have access to radiopharmaceuticals.

## Parenteral Dosage Forms

### IOFETAMINE HYDROCHLORIDE I 123 INJECTION

**Usual adult and adolescent administered activity**

Brain imaging—

Intravenous, 111 to 222 megabecquerels (3 to 6 millicuries).

**Usual pediatric administered activity**

Dosage has not been established.

**Strength(s) usually available**

U.S.—

At calibration time

37 megabecquerels (1 millicurie) of iofetamine hydrochloride I 123, per mL (Rx) [*Spectamine*].

Canada—

At calibration time

37 megabecquerels (1 millicurie) of iofetamine hydrochloride I 123, per mL (Rx) [*Spectamine*].

**Packaging and storage**

Store between 5 and 30 °C (41 and 86 °F). Protect from freezing.

**Stability**

Injection should be administered within 12 hours after calibration.

**Note**

Caution—Radioactive material.

## Selected Bibliography

Royal HD, Hill TC, Holman BL. Clinical brain imaging with Isopropyl-Iodoamphetamine and SPECT. Semin Nucl Med. 1985; 15 (4): 357-76.

Johnson KA et al. Cerebral perfusion imaging in Alzheimer's disease. Use of single-photon emission computed tomography and iofetamine hydrochloride I 123. Arch Neurol Feb 1987; 44 (2): 165-8.

Park CH et al. Iofetamine HCl I 123 Brain scanning in stroke: a comparison with transmission CT. Radiographics 1988; 8 (2): 305-26.

Revised: 09/28/92
Interim revision: 08/02/94

---

# IOHEXOL   Local

VA CLASSIFICATION (Primary): DX101

Note: For a listing of dosage forms and brand names by country availability, see *Dosage Forms* section(s). For a listing of brand names for the articles in this monograph, refer to the General Index.

## Category

Diagnostic aid, radiopaque (urinary tract disorders; uterus and fallopian tube disorders).

Note: Iohexol is a non-ionic radiopaque contrast agent.

## Indications

**Accepted**

Cystourethrography, retrograde[1]—Iohexol is indicated in retrograde cystourethrography to evaluate abnormalities of the urethra, bladder, and ureters; and to demonstrate the presence and extent of cystoureteric reflux.

Hysterosalpingography[1]—Iohexol is indicated for intrauterine instillation to determine the patency of the fallopian tubes and to visualize the uterine and tubal cavities for evaluation of abnormal conditions, such as tumors, of the uterus and fallopian tubes. Hysterosalpingography is used as a diagnostic tool in cases of infertility and other abnormal gynecological conditions; it serves as an adjunct to laparoscopy and ultrasound imaging in discovering subtle abnormalities, such as endometrial polyps and salpingitis isthmica nodosa.

Hysterosalpingography is *not* recommended during the menstrual period or when menstrual flow is imminent, during pregnancy, for at least 6 months after termination of pregnancy, or for 30 days after conization or curettage.

## Pharmacology/Pharmacokinetics

**Physicochemical characteristics**

Molecular weight—821.14.

Osmolality—Low. The osmolality of iohexol injection with iodine concentrations of 140, 180, 210, 240, 300, and 350 mg per mL is 322, 408, 460, 520, 672, and 844 mOsmol per kg of water, respectively.

**Mechanism of action/Effect**

Organic iodine compounds block x-rays as they pass through the body, thereby allowing body structures containing iodine to be delineated in contrast to those structures that do not contain iodine. The degree of opacity of these compounds is directly proportional to the total amount (concentration and volume) of the iodinated contrast agent in the path of the x-rays. The instillation of iohexol into the urinary bladder, kidneys, ureters, uterus, and fallopian tubes allows visualization of these areas.

**Absorption**

Intravesical instillation—Small amounts absorbed through the bladder.

Intrauterine instillation—Most of the medium within the uterine cavity is discharged into the vagina immediately upon termination of procedure. However, any medium retained in the uterine or peritoneal cavity is absorbed systemically within 60 minutes. May not be absorbed for up to 24 hours if tubes are obstructed and dilated.

**Protein binding**

Very low.

**Elimination**

Absorbed iohexol—Eliminated unchanged through the kidneys by glomerular filtration.

Unabsorbed iohexol—Expelled by spontaneous voiding or vaginally, depending on procedure.

---

[1]Not included in Canadian product labeling.

# Precautions to Consider

## Cross-sensitivity and/or related problems
Patients sensitive to iodine or other iodinated contrast media may be sensitive to iohexol also.

## Carcinogenicity/Mutagenicity
Long-term animal studies to evaluate carcinogenic or mutagenic potential of iohexol have not been performed.

## Pregnancy/Reproduction
Pregnancy—Adequate and well-controlled studies in humans have not been done. However, other organically bound iodine–containing preparations administered near term, by intra-amniotic injection, have caused hypothyroidism in some newborns. Also, elective contrast radiography of the abdomen is usually not recommended during pregnancy because of the risks to the fetus from radiation exposure.

Reproduction studies in rats and rabbits have not shown that iohexol, administered in doses up to 100 times the human dose, impairs fertility or causes harm to the fetus.

For intrauterine instillation: Intrauterine instillation is *not* recommended during pregnancy or for at least 6 months after the termination of pregnancy since the procedure may increase the risk of complications such as intrauterine infection.

FDA Pregnancy Category B.

## Breast-feeding
Although it is not known to what extent iohexol is distributed into milk, small amounts of this medium may be absorbed. Therefore, breast feeding is not recommended for at least 24 hours following administration of iohexol.

## Pediatrics
For intravesical instillation—Appropriate studies on the relationship of age to the effects of iohexol have not been performed in the pediatric population. However, no pediatrics-specific problems have been documented to date.

For intrauterine instillation—No information is available on the relationship of age to the effects of iohexol for intrauterine instillation in pediatric patients.

## Geriatrics
Appropriate studies on the relationship of age to the effects of iohexol for intrauterine or intravesical instillation have not been performed in geriatric patients. However, no geriatrics-specific problems have been documented to date.

## Diagnostic interference
The following have been selected on the basis of their potential clinical significance (possible effect in parentheses where appropriate)—not necessarily inclusive (» = major clinical significance):

With *other* diagnostic test results

Thyroid function determinations and

Thyroid imaging
(iohexol may cause an increase of serum protein–bound iodine [PBI] and a decrease in radioactive iodine or pertechnetate ion uptake for up to 2 weeks; thyroid test should be performed prior to administration of contrast medium; other thyroid function tests not based on measurement of iodine, such as resin triiodothyronine uptake, are not affected)

## Medical considerations/Contraindications
The medical considerations/contraindications included here have been selected on the basis of their potential clinical significance (reasons given in parentheses where appropriate)—not necessarily inclusive (» = major clinical significance).

*Except under special circumstances, this medication should not be used when the following medical problem exists:*

*For hysterosalpingography*
» Genital tract infection
(procedure may increase risk of complications)

*Risk-benefit should be considered when the following medical problems exist:*

Allergic reaction (anaphylaxis) to penicillins or to skin allergens, previous
(increased risk of anaphylactoid reaction)

Allergies or asthma, history of
(increased risk of idiosyncratic response or anaphylactoid reaction)

» Sensitivity to iodinated contrast media
(increased risk of anaphylactoid reaction in patients with a history of anaphylactoid reaction to iodinated contrast media)

*For hysterosalpingography*
» Pelvic inflammatory disease, acute
(condition may be aggravated)

Caution is also recommended just after cervical or uterine surgery to avoid the risk of complications.

# Side/Adverse Effects

Note: Adverse effects associated with the mechanics of retrograde genitourinary procedures include injury to the urethra, bladder, and ureter, and introduction of infection.

Systemic adverse effects, similar to those that occur with direct intravascular injection of iohexol may also occur with intravesical instillation as a result of inadvertent intravascular entry of the contrast solution due to either bladder absorption or pyelorenal backflow.

Systemic adverse effects, although rare, are possible with intrauterine instillation if medium is absorbed systemically after being retained in the uterine cavity or spilled into the peritoneal cavity.

The following side/adverse effects have been selected on the basis of their potential clinical significance (possible signs and symptoms in parentheses where appropriate)—not necessarily inclusive:

## Those indicating need for medical attention
Incidence less frequent
*Pyelorenal distention* (severe abdominal or stomach pain and discomfort, backache)—resulting from the instillation of an excess volume of contrast solution; renal colic and shock may follow

Incidence rare
*Pseudo-allergic reaction* (continuing chills, continuing fever, increased sweating, skin rash or hives, sneezing, swelling of face or skin, swelling of larynx, thickening of the tongue, wheezing, tightness in chest, or troubled breathing)—may be due to entry of medium into venous or lymphatic system

## Those indicating need for medical attention only if they continue or are bothersome
Incidence more frequent
*Abdominal or stomach pain and discomfort*

Note: *Abdominal pain and discomfort* may be associated with the insertion and positioning of the installation device. If occurring later during the procedure, may indicate spillage of contrast medium into the peritoneal cavity.

Incidence less frequent
*Drowsiness; fever; nausea and vomiting*

# Patient Consultation

As an aid to patient consultation, refer to *Advice for the Patient, Radiopaque Agents (Diagnostic, Local)*.

In providing consultation, consider emphasizing the following selected information (» = major clinical significance):

## Description of use
Instillation into bladder; visualization of radiopacity possible with x-rays

Instillation into uterus and fallopian tubes; visualization of radiopacity possible with x-rays

## Before having this test
» Conditions affecting use, especially:
Sensitivity to iodine or other iodinated contrast media
Pregnancy—Risk to the fetus from radiation exposure; intrauterine instillation contraindicated during pregnancy and for at least 6 months after delivery
Breast-feeding—Breast-feeding not recommended for 24 hours after test
Other medical problems, especially genital tract infection and acute pelvic inflammatory disease (for hysterosalpingography)

## Preparation for this test
Voiding before procedure
*For retrograde cystourethrography*
Special diet, use of laxative, and/or other preparatory instructions may apply; patient should inquire in advance
*For hysterosalpingography*
Enema, vaginal douche, and/or other preparatory instructions may apply; patient should inquire in advance

**Precautions after having this test**
Possible interference with future thyroid tests

**Side/adverse effects**
Signs of possible side effects, especially pyelorenal distention or pseudo-allergic reaction

# General Dosing Information

Manufacturer's package insert or other appropriate literature should be consulted for specific techniques and procedures for the administration of contrast media.

Sensitivity test doses are not usually recommended since severe or fatal reactions to contrast media are not predictable from a patient's history or a sensitivity test. On some occasions severe or fatal reactions have occurred with a test dose or with a full dose in patients who did not react to the test dose.

Pretreatment with corticosteroids and/or antihistamines is recommended to minimize the incidence and severity of reactions in patients with a history of severe reactions to contrast media or with other high-risk conditions (e.g., asthma or history of allergies, positive allergy history to skin allergens or penicillin). In some studies, the additional use of ephedrine has been shown to be beneficial in preventing anaphylactoid reactions (except in patients with a history of hypertension or cardiovascular disease). When considering the use of a contrast agent, the following protocols are recommended:

For high-risk patients
• Use of a high-osmolality contrast agent plus pretreatment with a corticosteroid (oral prednisone, 50 mg administered 13 hours, 7 hours, and 1 hour before the procedure) and an antihistamine (intramuscular, intravenous, or oral diphenhydramine, 50 mg administered 1 hour before the procedure) or
• Use of a low-osmolality contrast agent if pretreatment is not feasible or
• Use of a low-osmolality contrast agent plus corticosteroid pretreatment.

For low-risk patients
• Use of a high-osmolality contrast agent or
• Use of a high-osmolality contrast agent and corticosteroid pretreatment.

During and for at least 30 to 60 minutes after administration of contrast media, the patient should be observed for possible severe reactions; competent personnel and emergency facilities should be available during this period.

**For retrograde cystourethrography**
A low-residue diet the day before and a laxative the night before the procedure are generally recommended.

Iohexol labeled for retrograde cystourethrography is *not* for intravascular injection. It is to be instilled, after the bladder is emptied, directly into the bladder or ureter and renal pelvis by gravity flow, using an appropriate venoclysis set or syringe. Excessive pressure should be avoided with either method of administration.

Dosage and concentration of iohexol for intravesical instillation should be individualized and are usually in proportion to the age of the patient and the technique and equipment used.

**For hysterosalpingography**
An enema and a vaginal douche before the examination are optional. Patient should empty her bladder before the procedure.

Iohexol solution when used for hysterosalpingography is to be instilled directly into the uterus via a sterile syringe attached to a uterine cannula, or via a tubal insufflator with a salpingogram attachment. It is recommended that instillation into the uterine cavity be performed under controlled pressure with fluoroscopic monitoring. Excessive pressure and overfilling should be avoided.

Any unabsorbed contrast medium is expelled spontaneously upon removal of the cannula.

# Local Dosage Forms

## IOHEXOL INJECTION USP

**Usual adult and adolescent dose**
Cystourethrography, retrograde[1]—
Intravesical instillation, 50 to 300 mL of a solution containing the equivalent of 100 mg of iodine per mL or 50 to 600 mL of a solution containing the equivalent of 50 mg of iodine per mL, depending on age and bladder capacity.

Hysterosalpingography[1]—
Intrauterine instillation, 15 to 20 mL of a solution containing the equivalent of 240 mg or 300 mg of iodine per mL.

**Usual pediatric dose**
Cystourethrography, retrograde[1]—
See *Usual adult and adolescent dose.*
Hysterosalpingography[1]—
Dosage has not been established.

**Usual geriatric dose**
See *Usual adult and adolescent dose.*
Note: Geriatric patients may be more sensitive to the effects of the usual adult dose.

**Strength(s) usually available**
U.S.—
302 mg of iohexol with 140 mg of iodine per mL (Rx) [*Omnipaque 140*].
388.3 mg of iohexol with 180 mg of iodine per mL (Rx) [*Omnipaque 180*].
453 mg of iohexol with 210 mg of iodine per mL (Rx) [*Omnipaque 210*].
517.7 mg of iohexol with 240 mg of iodine per mL (Rx) [*Omnipaque 240*].
647.1 mg of iohexol with 300 mg of iodine per mL (Rx) [*Omnipaque 300*].
755 mg of iohexol with 350 mg of iodine per mL (Rx) [*Omnipaque 350*].
Canada—
302 mg of iohexol with 140 mg of iodine per mL (Rx) [*Omnipaque 140*].
388.3 mg of iohexol with 180 mg of iodine per mL (Rx) [*Omnipaque 180*].
453 mg of iohexol with 210 mg of iodine per mL (Rx) [*Omnipaque 210*].
517.7 mg of iohexol with 240 mg of iodine per mL (Rx) [*Omnipaque 240*].
647.1 mg of iohexol with 300 mg of iodine per mL (Rx) [*Omnipaque 300*].
755 mg of iohexol with 350 mg of iodine per mL (Rx) [*Omnipaque 350*].

Note: All formulations above contain 1.21 mg of tromethamine and 0.1 mg of edetate calcium disodium.

**Packaging and storage**
Store below 40 °C (104 °F), preferably between 15 and 30 °C (59 and 86 °F), unless otherwise specified by manufacturer. Store in a light-resistant container. Protect from freezing.

**Preparation of dosage form**

| Iohexol solution desired (mg I/mL) | Amount (mL) of sterile water for injection to add per 100 mL of a: | | |
|---|---|---|---|
| | 24%* solution | 30%* solution | 35%* solution |
| 100 | 140 | 200 | 250 |
| 90 | 167 | 233 | 289 |
| 80 | 200 | 275 | 338 |
| 70 | 243 | 330 | 400 |
| 60 | 300 | 400 | 483 |
| 50 | 380 | 500 | 600 |

*Iohexol solution 24% (240 mg of iodine per mL), 30% (300 mg of iodine per mL), and 35% (350 mg of iodine per mL).

**Stability**
Iohexol is a clear, colorless to pale yellow solution. Do not use if turbid or discolored.
Any unused portion remaining in the container should be discarded.

[1]Not included in Canadian product labeling.

# Selected Bibliography

Sauer MV. Investigation of the female pelvis. J Reprod Med 1993 Apr; 38 (4): 269-76.
Gutmann JN. Imaging in the evaluation of female infertility. J Reprod Med 1992 Jan; 37 (1): 54-61.

Revised: 05/18/95

# IOHEXOL    Systemic

VA CLASSIFICATION (Primary): DX101

Note: For a listing of dosage forms and brand names by country availability, see *Dosage Forms* section(s). For a listing of brand names for the articles in this monograph, refer to the General Index.

## Category

Note: Iohexol is a nonionic radiopaque contrast agent.

Diagnostic aid, radiopaque (central nervous system disorders); Diagnostic aid, radiopaque (cerebrospinal fluid disorders); Diagnostic aid, radiopaque (cardiac disease); Diagnostic aid, radiopaque (vascular disease); Diagnostic aid, radiopaque (urinary tract disorders); Diagnostic aid, radiopaque (peritoneal disorders); Diagnostic aid, radiopaque contrast enhancer in computed tomography; Diagnostic aid, radiopaque contrast enhancer adjunct in computed tomography; Diagnostic aid, radiopaque (biliary tract disorders); Diagnostic aid, radiopaque (joint disease); Diagnostic aid, radiopaque (gastrointestinal tract disorders).

## Indications

### Accepted
Intrathecal:

Myelography (lumbar, thoracic, cervical, total columnar)—Iohexol is indicated in adults and children for lumbar, thoracic, cervical, and total columnar myelography (standard or computed tomographic) to determine the presence of abnormalities in the spinal column, spinal canal, and the central nervous system (CNS).

Intravascular:

Angiocardiography—Iohexol is indicated in angiocardiography (selective coronary arteriography or ventriculography) to visualize lesions or malformations of the heart and obstructions or anomalies of the major thoracic vessels.

Angiography

Aortography

Arteriography or

Venography—Iohexol is indicated in aortography (aortic arch, ascending aorta, abdominal aorta and branches), arteriography (cerebral or peripheral), and in peripheral venography (phlebography) to visualize specific regions of the vascular system and blood flow in such areas to help in the diagnosis and evaluation of neoplasms (known or suspected) or vascular diseases (congenital or acquired) that may cause changes in normal vascular anatomy or physiology. Also, it is indicated in adults for intra-arterial and intravenous digital subtraction angiography of head, neck, abdominal, renal, and peripheral vessels.

In cerebral arteriography, iohexol is indicated to determine the presence and extent of certain neoplasms (e.g., gliomas, pituitary adenomas, metastatic lesions) and non-neoplastic lesions, such as cerebral infarctions, arteriovenous malformations, and aneurysms. In venography, it is used mainly for deep venous thrombosis.

Urography, excretory—Iohexol is indicated for excretion urography to evaluate abnormalities of the urinary tract such as urinary tract obstructions.

Herniography[1]—Iohexol is indicated in herniography in adults.

Brain imaging, computed tomographic—Iohexol is indicated for enhancement of computed tomographic images (CT of the brain) to determine the presence and extent of neoplasms or other lesions such as cerebral infarction or infection.

Body imaging, computed tomographic—Iohexol is indicated for enhancement of computed tomographic images (CT of the body) to detect and evaluate lesions in the liver, pancreas, kidneys, aorta, mediastinum, pelvis, abdominal cavity, and retroperitoneal space.

Intraductal:

Pancreatography, endoscopic retrograde[1] and

Cholangiopancreatography, endoscopic retrograde[1]—Iohexol is indicated in adults in endoscopic retrograde pancreatography and endoscopic retrograde cholangiopancreatography for visualization of all portions of the biliary tree.

Intrasynovial:

Arthrography—Iohexol is indicated for arthrography in the diagnosis of post-traumatic or degenerative joint diseases or synovial rupture, for visualization of communicating bursae or cysts, and in meniscography.

Oral:

Abdominal imaging, computed tomographic, adjunct[1]—Diluted iohexol administered orally is indicated for use in contrast enhanced computed tomography of the abdomen (CT of the abdomen) in conjunction with intravenous iohexol.

Radiography, gastrointestinal[1]—Undiluted iohexol is indicated for oral pass-through examination of the gastrointestinal tract.

---

[1]Not included in Canadian product labeling.

## Pharmacology/Pharmacokinetics

### Physicochemical characteristics
Molecular weight—821.14.

Osmolality—Low. The osmolality of the injection with iodine concentrations of 140, 180, 210, 240, 300, and 350 mg per mL is 322, 408, 460, 520, 672, and 844 mOsmol per kg of water, respectively

Note: Iohexol injection is hypertonic as compared to plasma and cerebrospinal fluid (approximately 285 and 301 mOsmol per kg of water, respectively).

### Mechanism of action/Effect
Organic iodine compounds block x-rays as they pass through the body, thereby allowing body structures containing iodine to be delineated in contrast to those structures that do not contain iodine. The degree of opacity produced by these compounds is directly proportional to the total amount (concentration and volume) of the iodinated contrast agent in the path of the x-rays. After intrathecal administration into the subarachnoid space, diffusion of iohexol in the CSF allows the visualization of the subarachnoid spaces of the head and spinal canal. After intravascular administration, iohexol makes opaque those vessels in its path of flow, allowing visualization of the internal structures until significant hemodilution occurs.

### Distribution
Intrathecal—Diffuses upward through the CSF; penetrates into nerve root sleeves, nerve rootlets, and narrow areas of the subarachnoid space. Also, enters extracellular fluid of the brain tissue and pial surface of cerebral and cerebellar tissue adjacent to subarachnoid areas. In patients with normal CSF dynamics, it is eliminated from CSF into the blood within several hours.

Intravascular—Rapidly distributed throughout extracellular fluid following intravenous administration. No significant deposition in tissues. Does not cross blood-brain barrier, but accumulates within the interstitial tissues of malignant tumors of the brain due to the break in the blood-brain barrier caused by the tumor.

### Protein binding
Very low.

### Half-life
Elimination—

Intrathecal: 3.4 hours (mean).

Intravascular: Approximately 2 hours (with normal renal function).

### Time to peak opacification:
Standard myelography—

Immediate and for up to 30 minutes.

CT myelography—

Thoracic region: 1 hour.

Cervical region: 2 hours.

Basal cisterns: 3 to 4 hours.

Ventricles and sulci: 5 to 6 hours.

Arteriography—

Immediate.

Urography—

5 to 15 minutes.

### Peak serum concentration:
Intrathecal—2 to 6 hours.

Intravascular—Immediate, but concentration falls rapidly as iohexol is distributed throughout the extravascular compartment.

### Elimination
Intrathecal—Primarily renal, mainly by glomerular filtration (88% of dose eliminated unchanged within 24 hours).

Intravascular—Primarily renal, mainly by glomerular filtration (80 to 90% of dose eliminated unchanged in 24 hours).

Intraductal or intrasynovial—Absorbed into the surrounding tissue and eliminated by the kidneys and bowel, as for intravascular administration.

Oral—Only 0.1 to 0.5% of the administered dose is excreted by the kidneys; renal elimination may increase in the presence of bowel perforation or obstruction.

Note: In patients with impaired renal function, the elimination of iohexol is prolonged depending upon the degree of impairment, thus, resulting in prolonged plasma iohexol levels. Excretion through the gallbladder and into the small intestine may increase.

## Precautions to Consider

### Cross-sensitivity and/or related problems
Patients sensitive to iodine or other iodinated contrast media may be sensitive to iohexol also.

### Carcinogenicity/Mutagenicity
Long-term animal studies to evaluate carcinogenic or mutagenic potential of iohexol have not been performed.

### Pregnancy/Reproduction
Pregnancy—Adequate and well-controlled studies in humans have not been done. However, other organically bound iodine–containing preparations administered near term by intra-amniotic injection have caused hypothyroidism in some neonates.

Also, elective contrast radiography of the abdomen is usually not recommended during pregnancy because of the risks to the fetus from radiation exposure.

Reproduction studies in rats and rabbits have not shown that iohexol, administered in doses up to 100 times the human dose, impairs fertility or causes harm to the fetus.

FDA Pregnancy Category B.

### Breast-feeding
Although it is not known to what extent iohexol is distributed into breast milk, breast-feeding is not recommended for at least 24 hours following administration of iohexol.

### Pediatrics
Appropriate studies on the relationship of age to the effects of iohexol have not been performed in pediatric patients. However, it is known that pediatric patients, especially those with asthma, allergies, congestive heart failure, or serum creatinine greater than 1.5 mg per dL or those less than 12 months of age, exhibit an increased risk of having severe adverse side effects to radiopaque contrast media.

Dehydration and/or the risk of renal failure may be exacerbated by iohexol in infants and young children, especially those with polyuria, oliguria, diabetes, or pre-existing dehydration; adequate hydration is recommended before and following intravascular administration of iohexol.

### Geriatrics
Diagnostic studies performed to date have not demonstrated geriatrics-specific problems that would limit the usefulness of iohexol in the elderly. However, elderly patients are more likely to have age-related renal function impairment, which may require lower dosage in patients receiving iohexol.

Dehydration and/or the risk of renal failure may be exacerbated by iohexol in geriatric patients, especially those with polyuria, oliguria, diabetes, or pre-existing dehydration; adequate hydration is recommended before and following administration of iohexol.

The elderly may be more sensitive to the effects of iohexol on thyroid function. Iodine-induced thyrotoxicosis may occur 4 to 12 weeks following contrast radiography. Thyroid function monitoring may be needed in geriatric patients.

### Drug interactions and/or related problems
The following drug interactions and/or related problems have been selected on the basis of their potential clinical significance (possible mechanism in parentheses where appropriate)—not necessarily inclusive (» = major clinical significance):

Note: Combinations containing any of the following medications, depending on the amount present, may also interact with this medication.

» Antidepressants, tricyclic or
CNS stimulation–producing medications (See *Appendix II*) or
Monoamine oxidase (MAO) inhibitors, including furazolidone, procarbazine, and selegiline or
» Phenothiazines or
» Trimeprazine
(although not specifically reported for iohexol, concurrent use of phenothiazines with intrathecal administration of metrizamide, another nonionic contrast agent, has been associated with occurrence of seizures because of lowered seizure threshold effect of these medications; until more conclusive evidence is available medications that lower the seizure threshold should be discontinued for at least 48 hours before and 24 hours after myelography)

Beta-adrenergic blocking agents
(concurrent intravascular administration of iohexol with beta-adrenergic blocking agents may increase the risk of moderate to severe anaphylactoid reaction; also, hypotensive effects may be exacerbated; discontinuation of the beta-adrenergic blocking agent

may be advisable before administration of contrast media in patients with other risk factors)

Cholecystographic agents, oral
(may increase the risk of renal toxicity when closely followed by intravascular iohexol, especially in patients with hepatic function impairment)

Hypotension-producing medications, other (See *Appendix II*)
(the risk of severe hypotension may be increased if iohexol is given concurrently with other medications that produce hypotension)

Interleukin-2
(incidence of delayed reactions to intravenous contrast media [e.g., hypersensitivity, fever, skin rash, flu-like symptoms, joint pain, flushing, pruritus, emesis, hypotension, dizziness occurring more than 1 hour after administration] may be increased in patients who have received interleukin-2; some symptoms may resemble a "recall" reaction to interleukin-2; supportive medical treatment may be necessary if symptoms are significant; delaying contrast media administration until 6 weeks after administration of interleukin-2 may reduce incidence of these reactions)

Nephrotoxic medications, other (See *Appendix II*)
(concurrent intrathecal or intravascular administration of iohexol with other nephrotoxic medications may increase the potential for nephrotoxicity)

### Diagnostic interference
The following have been selected on the basis of their potential clinical significance (possible effect in parentheses where appropriate)—not necessarily inclusive (» = major clinical significance):

With *other* diagnostic test results
Blood pool imaging
(intravascular administration of iohexol decreases technetium Tc 99m–labeling of red blood cells, which may impair blood pool imaging)

Leukocyte counts and
Red cell counts
(may be temporarily decreased)

Prothrombin time (PT) and
Thromboplastin time
(may be increased with iohexol since *in vitro* studies with animal blood have shown other nonionic contrast media to slightly inhibit all stages of coagulation)

Skeletal imaging
(intravenous administration of iohexol immediately after administration of Tc 99m medronate, technetium Tc 99m oxidronate, technetium Tc 99m pyrophosphate, and technetium Tc 99m [pyro- and trimeta-] phosphates may cause renal and hepatic uptake of these technetium Tc 99m–labeled agents)

Thyroid function determinations and
Thyroid imaging
(intravascular or intrathecal administration of iohexol may alter serum protein–bound iodine [PBI] concentrations and radioactive iodine or pertechnetate ion uptake for up to 2 weeks; thyroid test should be performed prior to administration of iohexol. Other thyroid function tests not based on measurement of iodine, such as resin triiodothyronine uptake, may not be affected)

Urinalysis
(iohexol may interfere with some chemical determinations made on urine, such as protein and specific gravity; urine should be collected prior to or at least 2 days after intravenous administration of iohexol)

With physiology/laboratory test values
Creatinine, serum
(concentration may be increased with iohexol)

### Medical considerations/Contraindications
The medical considerations/contraindications included here have been selected on the basis of their potential clinical significance (reasons given in parentheses where appropriate)—not necessarily inclusive (» = major clinical significance).

*Risk-benefit should be considered when the following medical problems exist:*

*For all procedures (especially those requiring intrathecal or intravascular administration)*
Allergic reaction (anaphylaxis) to penicillins or to skin allergens, previous
(although the risk of anaphylactoid reaction may be less with iohexol than with high-osmolality contrast agents, caution is recommended when administering iohexol to patients who have had a previous reaction to penicillins or to skin allergens)

Allergies or asthma, history of
    (although the risk of idiosyncratic response or anaphylactoid reaction may be less with iohexol than with high-osmolality contrast agents, caution is recommended when administering iohexol to patients with a history of allergies or asthma)

» Dehydration, especially associated with pre-existing renal disease, advanced vascular disease, or diabetes mellitus, or in pediatric and elderly patients
    (osmotic diuretic action of iohexol may exacerbate dehydration and increase risk of acute renal failure)

Renal function impairment, severe
    (elimination of iohexol may be delayed; although the risk of contrast-induced nephrotoxicity in the presence of renal insufficiency [serum creatinine ≥ 132.6 micromoles/L] may be less with iohexol than with high-osmolality contrast agents, caution is recommended)

» Sensitivity to iodinated contrast media
    (increased risk of anaphylactoid reaction in patients with history of prior reactions to contrast media)

*For intrathecal use*
Alcoholism, chronic
    (increased risk of side effects because of existing brain or liver damage)

Bleeding, subarachnoid
    (increased risk of meningeal irritation or arachnoiditis)

Epilepsy, history of
    (myelographic procedure may increase risk of seizures)

Infection, local or systemic, significant

Multiple sclerosis

*For intravascular use*
Hyperthyroidism
    (administration of iohexol may precipitate thyroid storm)

» Pheochromocytoma
    (use of iohexol may precipitate severe hypertension; amount of iohexol injected should be kept to a minimum and blood pressure should be monitored during the procedure; also, pretreatment with the alpha-adrenergic blocking agent phentolamine is recommended)

Sickle cell disease
    (iohexol may promote sickling in patients who are homozygous for sickle cell disease; however, sickling potential of iohexol is less than that of high-osmolality ionic agents)

*For angiocardiography*
Angina, unstable
    (increased risk of a severe cardiac reaction)

Cardiac failure, incipient
    (fluid overload, pressure changes, and expansion of blood volume may aggravate condition)

Pulmonary hypertension, severe
    (hypervolemic effect of iohexol may further increase pulmonary artery and venous pressures due to an increase in cardiac output and a rise in left ventricular end-diastolic and left atrial pressures)

*For cerebral arteriography*
Arteriosclerosis, advanced or
Cardiac decompensation or
Cerebral embolism, recent or
Hypertension, severe or
Migraine or
Senility or
Thrombosis, recent
    (increased risk of vessel occlusion)

» Homocystinuria
    (procedure may increase risk of thrombosis and embolism)

*For peripheral arteriography*
» Buerger's disease
    (procedure may induce severe arterial or venous spasm)

» Ischemia, severe, associated with ascending infection

*For excretory urography*
» Anuria or
» Diabetes mellitus
    (administration of iohexol may increase risk of acute renal failure)

*For arthrography*
» Infection in or near joint to be examined
    (procedure may increase risk of complications)

## Patient monitoring

The following may be especially important in patient monitoring (other tests may be warranted in some patients, depending on condition; » = major clinical significance):

*For intravascular use*
Blood pressure determinations
    (may be required during examination, especially in patients with known or suspected pheochromocytoma or hemodynamic compromise or instability)

Thyroid function determinations
    (iodine-induced thyrotoxicosis may occur 4 to 12 weeks following contrast radiography in geriatric patients; thyroid function monitoring may be needed)

# Side/Adverse Effects

Note: Adverse effects may vary directly with the concentration of the agent, the amount and technique used, and the underlying pathology. Increases in osmolality, volume, concentration, viscosity, and rate of administration of the solution may increase the incidence and severity of adverse effects.

Most of the adverse effects are usually self-limited and of short duration.

Overall incidence of adverse effects with nonionic contrast agents, such as iohexol, has been reported to be less than with ionic contrast agents.

Nonionic contrast media, such as iohexol, have been reported to produce fewer and less severe alterations in cardiac hemodynamics and electrocardiograms than standard ionic contrast agents during cardiac angiography.

Low-osmolality contrast agents, such as iohexol, are reported to cause less heat and pain on injection than high-osmolality agents, such as diatrizoates and iothalamate.

Thromboembolic events causing myocardial infarction and stroke have been reported during angiographic procedures with non-ionic contrast media; however, these events appear to be technique-related.

Headaches following intrathecal administration of iohexol may be more frequent and persistent in patients not adequately hydrated.

Dehydration may be exacerbated by the osmotic diuretic action of the hypertonic contrast solutions of iohexol, in some cases resulting in a shock-like state, following intravascular administration of iohexol in geriatric, azotemic, and dehydrated or debilitated patients.

Transient global amnesia has been reported in 2 patients after cerebral angiography, in which 20 mL of iohexol (containing the equivalent of 240 mg of iodine per mL) was administered into the ascending aorta.

The following side/adverse effects have been selected on the basis of their potential clinical significance (possible signs and symptoms in parentheses where appropriate)—not necessarily inclusive:

## Those indicating need for medical attention
Incidence rare
  *With all procedures*
    ***Pseudo-allergic reaction*** (skin rash or hives; stuffy nose; swelling of face or skin; swelling of the tongue; wheezing, tightness in chest or troubled breathing)
    Note: *Pseudo-allergic reactions* are usually transient. However, they may be initial manifestations of more severe anaphylactoid reactions. The anaphylactoid reaction may progress to respiratory arrest and vasomotor collapse if appropriate treatment is not administered.

  *With intrathecal or intravascular administration*
    ***Bronchospasm or pulmonary edema*** (severe wheezing or troubled breathing); ***severe hypotension*** (unusual tiredness or weakness)

  *With intravascular administration*
    ***Cardiotoxic effects, with ventricular tachycardia or fibrillation*** (fast or irregular heartbeat); ***seizures***
    Note: In angiocardiography, bradyarrhythmias occur far less commonly with low-osmolality contrast agents than with high-osmolality agents. For iohexol, bradycardia has been reported with an incidence of 1%.

## Those indicating need for medical attention only if they continue or are bothersome
Incidence more frequent
  *With intrathecal or intravascular administration*
    ***Mild to moderate headache; mild to moderate nausea and vomiting***

Note: *Headache, nausea, and vomiting* may occur 1 to 10 hours after intrathecal injection and last for a few hours, usually disappearing within 24 hours; or, less frequently after intravascular injection, may occur immediately and last for a few minutes.

*With intrathecal administration*
**Backache; dizziness; meningeal irritation** (stiffness of neck)

*With intrasynovial administration*
**Joint pain or exacerbation of existing pain; swelling at joint**

*With intraductal administration*
**Pain**

Note: *Pain* may be associated with injection pressure and volume injected.

*With oral administration*
**Mild, transient diarrhea**

Incidence less frequent or rare
*With intrathecal or intravascular administration*
**Mild unusual feeling of warmth**

*With intrathecal administration*
**CNS effects** (severe headache; ringing or buzzing in ears; unusual tiredness or weakness); **difficult urination; drowsiness; increased sensitivity of eyes to light; increased sweating; loss of appetite**

*With intravascular administration*
**Blurred vision or other changes in vision; drowsiness or light-headedness; metallic taste; pain or burning at injection site**

*With oral administration*
**Moderate diarrhea; nausea and vomiting**

## Patient Consultation

As an aid to patient consultation, refer to *Advice for the Patient, Radiopaque Agents (Diagnostic).*

In providing consultation, consider emphasizing the following selected information (» = major clinical significance):

**Description of use**
*Action in the body:*

Injection into spinal canal; visualization of radiopacity in head and spinal cord possible with x-rays

Injection into vein or artery; visualization of radiopacity in heart, blood vessels, and urinary tract possible with x-rays

Direct injection into region to be studied; visualization of joint spaces, peritoneal herniations, pancreatic and bile ducts

Oral administration; visualization of the gastrointestinal tract

**Before having this test**
» Conditions affecting use, especially:
   Sensitivity to iodine or other iodinated contrast media
   Pregnancy—Risk to the fetus from radiation exposure; may cause hypothyroidism in neonate
   Breast-feeding—Breast-feeding not recommended for 24 hours afterwards
   Use in children—Increased risk of severe adverse reactions, especially in children with other medical problems; possible exacerbation of dehydration
   Use in the elderly—Possible exacerbation of dehydration; increased risk of thyrotoxicosis
   Other medications, especially phenothiazines, tricyclic antidepressants, and trimeprazine (with intrathecal use)
   Other medical problems, especially anuria, dehydration, diabetes mellitus, and pheochromocytoma

**Preparation for this test**
Adequate intake of fluids to prevent dehydration
Special preparatory instructions may be given; patient should inquire in advance
*With intrathecal use*
Normal diet up to 2 hours before procedure; moderate amounts of clear liquids may be permitted up to time of procedure

**Precautions after having this test**
Possible interference with future thyroid tests
*With intrathecal use*
Avoiding movement during and for several hours after administration
Keeping head position as instructed during and after examination

**Side/adverse effects**
Signs of possible side effects, especially pseudo-allergic reaction and cardiac or pulmonary problems that may occur immediately or within minutes of administration

## General Dosing Information

Manufacturer's package insert or other appropriate literature should be consulted for specific techniques and procedures for the administration of contrast media.

Sensitivity test doses are not usually recommended since severe or fatal reactions to contrast media are not predictable from a patient's history or a sensitivity test. On some occasions, severe or fatal reactions have occurred with a test dose or with a full dose in patients who did not react to the test dose.

Pretreatment with corticosteroids and/or antihistamines may minimize the incidence and severity of reactions in patients with a history of severe reactions to contrast media or with other high-risk conditions (e.g., asthma or history of allergies, positive allergy history to skin allergens or penicillins, dehydration, history of seizures, pheochromocytoma). In some studies, the additional use of ephedrine has been shown to be beneficial in preventing anaphylactoid reactions (except in patients with a history of hypertension or cardiovascular disease). When the use of a contrast agent is being considered, the following protocols are recommended:
For high-risk patients
   • Use of a high-osmolality contrast agent plus pretreatment with a corticosteroid (oral prednisone 50 mg administered 13 hours, 7 hours, and 1 hour before procedure) and antihistamine (intramuscular, intravenous, or oral diphenhydramine, 50 mg administered 1 hour prior to procedure) or
   • Use of a low-osmolality contrast agent if pretreatment is not feasible or
   • Use of a low-osmolality contrast agent plus corticosteroid pretreatment.
For low-risk patients
   • Use of a high-osmolality contrast agent or
   • Use of a high-osmolality contrast agent and corticosteroid pretreatment.

Adequate hydration is recommended for all patients before and after the examination. Intravenous or oral intake of fluids may continue up to time of administration of iohexol.

During and for at least 30 to 60 minutes after intravascular injection of iohexol, and for at least 12 hours (up to 24 hours in some cases) after intrathecal administration, the patient should be observed for possible severe reactions; competent personnel and emergency facilities should be available during this period.

Dosage and concentration of iodine (as iohexol injection) are dependent upon the degree and extent of contrast needed in the areas under examination and on the equipment and technique used.

**For intrathecal use**
Pretreatment with barbiturates may be used in patients who have a history of seizures but are not on anticonvulsant therapy. Patients who are on anticonvulsant therapy should continue receiving their medication when receiving iohexol.

A normal diet may be ingested up to 2 hours prior to the administration of iohexol.

If inadvertent intracranial entry of a large or concentrated bolus of iohexol occurs, treatment with anticonvulsants may be used to minimize the risk of seizures.

Direct intracisternal or ventricular administration of iohexol for standard radiography is *not* recommended.

During and for several hours after the procedure the patient must remain inactive to minimize high cephalad dispersion of iohexol.

Information on patient management and positioning during and after procedure is included in the manufacturer's package insert.

**For intravascular use**
Nonionic contrast media, such as iohexol, inhibit blood coagulation *in vitro* less than ionic contrast media. Blood cell aggregation has been reported when blood remains in contact with syringes containing nonionic contrast media. Thus, thromboembolic events causing myocardial infarction and stroke, reported during angiographic procedures, may have resulted from aggregation of blood that had come in contact with the contrast agent outside the body. Risk factors for blood cell aggregation should be minimized by performing the procedure in the shortest time possible, using plastic rather than glass syringes, and flushing catheters with heparinized saline solutions.

During and immediately after administration of iohexol for digital subtraction angiography of neck and head, the patient must remain inactive and avoid swallowing. Otherwise, poor arterial visualization may result.

**For treatment of adverse effects**

Recommended treatment consists of the following:

- For major or life-threatening reactions, careful monitoring of vital signs and emergency therapy, including artificial respiration with oxygen, if needed for respiratory depression, and cardiac massage in the event of cardiac arrest.
- To restore blood pressure, administration of intravenous fluids and/or vasopressors. If hypotension necessitates the use of vasopressors, slow infusion of 0.008 to 0.012 mg per minute of norepinephrine or 0.1 to 0.18 mg per minute of phenylephrine, appropriately diluted. If hypotension is due to increased vagal activity (vasovagal reaction), intravenous administration of 1 mg of atropine, repeated in one to two hours if needed.
- Other specific treatment may include—

  Diphenhydramine: For minor allergic-like reactions—An antihistamine such as diphenhydramine hydrochloride (except in epileptic patients) may be administered intravenously.

  Epinephrine: For acute allergic-like or anaphylactoid reactions—Slow intravenous infusion of 0.1 mg of epinephrine (1:10,000).

  For mild to moderate bronchospasm—0.1 to 0.2 mg of epinephrine (1:1000) may be administered subcutaneously, except in hypotension. In extreme emergency, 0.1 mg of epinephrine (1:10,000) may be given slowly by intravenous route, followed by a continuous intravenous infusion at an initial rate of 0.001 mg per minute; the rate may be increased to 0.004 mg per minute if necessary. (Note: Patients on beta-adrenergic blocking agents should not receive epinephrine since they are at risk of unopposed alpha-adrenergic stimulation, which may result in hypertension, reflex bradycardia, and heart-block. In these patients, isoproterenol and norepinephrine are used instead of epinephrine to overcome bronchospasm and hypotension, respectively.)

  For cardiac arrest—0.1 to 1 mg of epinephrine may be administered by the intravenous route.

  Diazepam or phenobarbital: To control convulsions—5 to 10 mg of diazepam by slow, intravenous administration or phenobarbital sodium may be given intravenously or intramuscularly at a rate not to exceed 30 to 60 mg per minute.

# Parenteral Dosage Forms

## IOHEXOL INJECTION USP

**Usual adult and adolescent dose**

Intrathecal—

  Myelography:

    Lumbar myelography by lumbar injection—

      10 to 17 mL of a solution containing the equivalent of 180 mg of iodine per mL; or 7 to 12.5 mL of a solution containing the equivalent of 240 mg of iodine per mL.

    Thoracic myelography by lumbar or cervical injection—

      6 to 12.5 mL of a solution containing the equivalent of 240 mg of iodine per mL; or 6 to 10 mL of a solution containing the equivalent of 300 mg of iodine per mL.

    Cervical myelography by lumbar injection—

      6 to 12.5 mL of a solution containing the equivalent of 240 mg of iodine per mL; or 6 to 10 mL of a solution containing the equivalent of 300 mg of iodine per mL.

    Cervical myelography by C1/2 puncture—

      7 to 10 mL of a solution containing the equivalent of 180 mg of iodine per mL; 6 to 12.5 mL of a solution containing the equivalent of 240 mg of iodine per mL; or 4 to 10 mL of a solution containing the equivalent of 300 mg of iodine per mL.

    Total columnar myelography by lumbar injection—

      6 to 12.5 mL of a solution containing the equivalent of 240 mg of iodine per mL; or 6 to 10 mL of a solution containing the equivalent of 300 mg of iodine per mL.

Note: Injection should be made slowly over a period of 1 to 2 minutes to avoid excessive mixing with cerebrospinal fluid and resultant dilution of iohexol as well as premature cephalad dispersion.

Immediate repeat intrathecal administration is not recommended because of risk of overdose; 48 hours, or preferably 5 to 7 days, should elapse before repeat examination.

Intravascular—

  Angiocardiography:

    Aortic root and arch—Via catheter, 20 to 75 mL of a solution containing the equivalent of 350 mg of iodine per mL as a single dose.

    Ventriculography—Via catheter, 30 to 60 mL of a solution containing the equivalent of 350 mg of iodine per mL as a single dose, repeated as needed.

    Arteriography, selective coronary—Via catheter, 3 to 14 mL of a solution containing the equivalent of 350 mg of iodine per mL, administered into either artery.

  Angiography:

    Intra-arterial, by digital subtraction: Intra-arterial, as a solution containing the equivalent of 140 mg of iodine per mL, into the following vessels:

    Aorta: 20 to 45 mL injected at a rate of 8 to 20 mL per second.

    Carotid: 5 to 10 mL injected at a rate of 3 to 6 mL per second.

    Femoral: 9 to 20 mL injected at a rate of 3 to 6 mL per second.

    Vertebral: 4 to 10 mL injected at a rate of 2 to 8 mL per second.

    Renal: 6 to 12 mL injected at a rate of 3 to 6 mL per second.

    Other branches of the aorta: 8 to 25 mL injected at a rate of 3 to 10 mL per second.

  Angiography, peripheral:

    Arteriography, peripheral—Percutaneous or operative methods, 30 to 90 mL for aortofemoral runoffs or 10 to 60 mL for selective arteriograms, of a solution containing the equivalent of 300 mg of iodine per mL; or, 20 to 70 mL for aortofemoral runoffs or 10 to 30 mL for selective arteriograms, of a solution containing the equivalent of 350 mg of iodine per mL.

    Venography, peripheral—Percutaneous, 20 to 150 mL per leg, of a solution containing the equivalent of 240 mg of iodine per mL; or, 40 to 100 mL per leg, of a solution containing the equivalent of 300 mg of iodine per mL.

  Aortography:

    Via catheter, as a solution containing the equivalent of 300 mg or 350 mg of iodine per mL, as a single dose, repeated if needed, into the following vessels:

    Aorta: 50 to 80 mL.

    Major branches of the aorta: 30 to 60 mL.

    Renal arteries: 5 to 15 mL.

  Arteriography, cerebral:

    As a solution containing the equivalent of 300 mg of iodine per mL, by direct injection into the following vessels:

    Common carotid artery: 6 to 12 mL.

    External carotid artery: 6 to 9 mL.

    Internal carotid artery: 8 to 10 mL.

    Vertebral artery: 6 to 10 mL.

  Arteriography, digital, of the head and neck:

    Intravenous, 30 to 50 mL of a solution containing the equivalent of 350 mg of iodine per mL. Three or more injections may be needed.

  Urography, excretory:

    Intravenous, the equivalent of 200 to 350 mg of iodine per kg of body weight, of a solution containing the equivalent of 300 mg or 350 mg of iodine per mL.

  Herniography[1]:

    Intravenous, 50 mL of a solution containing the equivalent of 240 mg of iodine per mL.

  CT of the brain:

    Intravenous, by infusion, 120 to 250 mL of a solution containing the equivalent of 240 mg of iodine per mL; or, by rapid injection, 70 to 150 mL, of a solution containing the equivalent of 300 mg of iodine per mL; or, by rapid injection, 80 mL of a solution containing the equivalent of 350 mg of iodine per mL.

  CT of the body:

    Intravenous, by rapid injection or infusion, 50 to 200 mL, of a solution containing the equivalent of 300 mg of iodine per mL; or 60 to 100 mL of a solution containing the equivalent of 350 mg of iodine per mL.

Intraductal—

  Pancreatography, endoscopic retrograde[1] and

  Cholangiography, endoscopic retrograde[1]:

    Via catheter, 10 to 50 mL of a solution containing the equivalent of 240 mg of iodine per mL.

Intrasynovial—

  Arthrography:

    As a solution containing the equivalent of 210 mg of iodine per mL—Intra-articular, 3 mL into the shoulder joint.

    As a solution containing the equivalent of 240 mg of iodine per mL—Intra-articular:

    Knee joint—5 to 15 mL.

    Shoulder joint—3 mL.

    As a solution containing the equivalent of 300 mg of iodine per mL—Intra-articular:

    Knee joint—5 to 15 mL.

    Shoulder—10 mL.

    Temporomandibular—0.5 to 1 mL.

As a solution containing the equivalent of 350 mg of iodine per mL—Intra-articular, 5 to 10 mL into knee joint.

Oral—

CT of the abdomen, adjunct[1]:

500 to 1000 mL of a solution containing the equivalent of 6 to 9 mg of iodine per mL administered orally, in conjunction with the intravenous administration of 100 to 150 mL of a solution containing the equivalent of 300 mg of iodine per mL.

Note: Oral dose should be administered 20 to 40 minutes before the intravenous dose.

Gastrointestinal tract radiographic examination[1]:

For oral pass-through examination—50 to 100 mL of a solution containing the equivalent of 350 mg of iodine per mL.

## Usual adult prescribing limits

Intrathecal—Up to the equivalent of 3.06 grams of iodine.

Intravascular—For multiple or repeat procedures: Up to the equivalent of 87.5 grams of iodine or 250 mL of a solution containing the equivalent of 350 mg of iodine per mL.

## Usual pediatric dose

Intrathecal—Myelography: By lumbar injection—

As a solution containing the equivalent of 180 mg of iodine per mL:

Children up to 3 months of age—2 to 4 mL.
Children 3 months to 3 years of age—4 to 8 mL.
Children 3 to 7 years of age—5 to 10 mL.
Children 7 to 13 years of age—5 to 12 mL.
Children 13 to 18 years of age—6 to 15 mL.

As a solution containing the equivalent of 210 mg of iodine per mL:

Children up to 3 months of age—2 to 3 mL.
Children 3 months to 3 years of age—3 to 6 mL.
Children 3 to 7 years of age—5 to 8 mL.
Children 7 to 13 years of age—5 to 10 mL.
Children 13 to 18 years of age—6 to 14 mL.

Intravascular—

Angiocardiography:

Ventriculography—

Via catheter, 1.75 mL per kg of body weight, of a solution containing the equivalent of 300 mg of iodine per mL, up to a total volume of 291 mL; or, 1.25 mL per kg of body weight, of a solution containing the equivalent of 350 mg of iodine per mL, up to a total volume of 250 mL, as a single dose, repeated as needed but not to exceed 5 mL per kg of body weight.

Urography, excretory—

Intravenous, 1 to 1.5 mL per kg of body weight, of a solution containing the equivalent of 300 mg of iodine per mL, not to exceed a total dose of 3 mL per kg of body weight.

CT of the brain—

Intravenous, 1 to 2 mL per kg of body weight, of a solution containing the equivalent of 240 mg or 300 mg of iodine per mL.

Oral—

CT of the abdomen, adjunct[1]:

180 to 750 mL, of a solution containing the equivalent of 9 to 21 mg of iodine per mL, administered orally all at once or over a period of 30 to 45 minutes, in conjunction with the intravenous administration of 1 to 2 mL per kg of body weight of a solution containing the equivalent of 240 or 300 mg of iodine per mL.

Note: Oral dose should be administered 30 to 60 minutes before the intravenous dose.

Total oral dose should not exceed the equivalent of 5 grams of iodine for children up to 3 years of age, the equivalent of 10 grams of iodine for children 3 to 18 years of age.

Total intravenous dose should not exceed 3 mL per kg of body weight.

Gastrointestinal tract radiographic examination[1]: For oral pass-through examination—

Dosage must be individualized by physician in proportion to the size of the patient and the nature of the examination. The following guidelines are given for:

A solution containing the equivalent of 180 mg of iodine per mL—
Children up to 3 months of age: 5 to 30 mL.

A solution containing the equivalent of 180, 240, or 300 mg of iodine per mL—
Children 3 months to 3 years of age: Up to 60 mL.
Children 4 to 10 years of age: Up to 80 mL.
Children over 10 years of age: Up to 100 mL.

## Usual geriatric dose

See *Usual adult and adolescent dose.*

Note: Geriatric patients with renal function impairment may be more sensitive to the effects of the usual adult dose; lower doses are recommended.

## Strength(s) usually available

U.S.—

302 mg of iohexol with 140 mg of iodine per mL (Rx) [*Omnipaque 140*].

388.3 mg of iohexol with 180 mg of iodine per mL (Rx) [*Omnipaque 180*].

453 mg of iohexol with 210 mg of iodine per mL (Rx) [*Omnipaque 210*].

517.7 mg of iohexol with 240 mg of iodine per mL (Rx) [*Omnipaque 240*].

647.1 mg of iohexol with 300 mg of iodine per mL (Rx) [*Omnipaque 300*].

755 mg of iohexol with 350 mg of iodine per mL (Rx) [*Omnipaque 350*].

Canada—

302 mg of iohexol with 140 mg of iodine per mL (Rx) [*Omnipaque 140*].

388.3 mg of iohexol with 180 mg of iodine per mL (Rx) [*Omnipaque 180*].

453 mg of iohexol with 210 mg of iodine per mL (Rx) [*Omnipaque 210*].

517.7 mg of iohexol with 240 mg of iodine per mL (Rx) [*Omnipaque 240*].

647.1 mg of iohexol with 300 mg of iodine per mL (Rx) [*Omnipaque 300*].

755 mg of iohexol with 350 mg of iodine per mL (Rx) [*Omnipaque 350*].

Note: All formulations above contain 1.21 mg of tromethamine and 0.1 mg of edetate calcium disodium.

## Packaging and storage

Store below 40 °C (104 °F), preferably between 15 and 30 °C (59 and 86 °F), unless otherwise specified by manufacturer. Protect from light. Protect from freezing.

## Preparation of dosage form

| Final concentration of 1 liter of contrast solution (mg of iodine/mL) | Concentration of stock solution of iohexol (mg of iodine/mL) | Volume of stock solution (mL) | Amount of diluent (mL)* |
|---|---|---|---|
| 6 | 240 | 25 | 975 |
|  | 300 | 20 | 980 |
|  | 350 | 17 | 983 |
| 9 | 240 | 38 | 962 |
|  | 300 | 30 | 970 |
|  | 350 | 26 | 974 |
| 12 | 240 | 50 | 950 |
|  | 300 | 40 | 960 |
|  | 350 | 35 | 965 |
| 15 | 240 | 63 | 937 |
|  | 300 | 50 | 950 |
|  | 350 | 43 | 957 |
| 18 | 240 | 75 | 925 |
|  | 300 | 60 | 940 |
|  | 350 | 52 | 948 |
| 21 | 240 | 88 | 912 |
|  | 300 | 70 | 930 |
|  | 350 | 60 | 940 |

*Water, carbonated beverage, milk, or juice may be used as diluent.

## Stability

Iohexol is a clear, colorless to pale yellow solution. Do not use if turbid or discolored.

Any unused portion remaining in the container should be discarded.

[1]Not included in Canadian product labeling.

# Selected Bibliography

Kawada TK. Iohexol and iopamidol: second-generation nonionic radiographic contrast media. Drug Intell Clin Pharm 1985 Jul/Aug; 19: 525-9.

Spinler SA, Goldfarb S. Nephrotixicity of contrast media following cardiac angiography: pathogenesis, clinical course, and preventive measures, including the role of low-osmolality contrast media. Ann Pharmacother 1992 Jan; 26: 56-64.

Revised: 08/16/95

# IOPAMIDOL    Systemic

VA CLASSIFICATION (Primary): DX101
Note: For a listing of dosage forms and brand names by country availability, see *Dosage Forms* section(s). For a listing of brand names for the articles in this monograph, refer to the General Index.

## Category

Note: Iopamidol is a nonionic radiopaque contrast agent.

Diagnostic aid, radiopaque (brain disorders); Diagnostic aid, radiopaque (central nervous system disorders); Diagnostic aid, radiopaque (cerebrospinal fluid disorders); Diagnostic aid, radiopaque (cardiac disease); Diagnostic aid, radiopaque (vascular disease); Diagnostic aid, radiopaque contrast enhancer in computed tomography; Diagnostic aid, radiopaque (peritoneal disorders); Diagnostic aid, radiopaque (urinary tract disorders); Diagnostic aid, radiopaque (joint disease); Diagnostic aid, radiopaque (biliary tract disorders).

## Indications

Note: Bracketed information in the *Indications* section refers to uses that are not included in U.S. product labeling.

### Accepted
Intrathecal:
Myelography (lumbar, thoracic[1], cervical[1], total columnar[1])—Iopamidol is indicated for lumbar, thoracic, cervical, and total columnar myelography (standard or computed tomographic) to determine the presence of abnormalities in the spinal column, spinal canal, and the central nervous system (CNS).
Cisternography, computed tomographic (CT)[1]—Iopamidol is indicated in adults for computerized tomography of the intracranial subarachnoid spaces.

Intravascular:
Angiocardiography—Iopamidol is indicated for angiocardiography (selective coronary arteriography or ventriculography) to visualize lesions or malformations of the heart and obstructions or anomalies of the major thoracic vessels.
Angiography or
Aortography[1] or
Arteriography or
Venography—Iopamidol is indicated in adults to visualize specific regions of the vascular system and blood flow in such areas to help in the diagnosis and evaluation of neoplasms (known or suspected) or vascular diseases (congenital or acquired) that may cause changes in normal vascular anatomy or physiology. It is indicated for use in intra-arterial digital subtraction angiography; cerebral, peripheral, or selective visceral[1] arteriography; aortography; and peripheral venography (phlebography). In cerebral arteriography, iopamidol is indicated to determine the presence and extent of certain neoplasms (e.g., gliomas, pituitary adenomas, metastatic lesions) and non-neoplastic lesions, such as cerebral infarctions, arteriovenous malformations, and aneurysms[1].
Brain imaging, computed tomographic—Iopamidol is indicated for enhancement of computed tomographic images of the brain (CT of the brain) to determine the presence and extent of neoplasms or other lesions such as cerebral infarction or infection.
Body imaging, computed tomographic—Iopamidol is indicated for enhancement of computed tomographic images of the body (CT of the body) for detection and evaluation of lesions in the liver, pancreas, kidneys, aorta, mediastinum, abdominal cavity, pelvis, and retroperitoneal space.
Urography, excretory—Iopamidol is indicated in intravenous excretory urography to evaluate abnormalities of the urinary tract such as urinary tract obstruction.
[Herniography][1]—Iopamidol is used in herniography in adults.

Intraductal:
[Pancreatography, endoscopic retrograde][1] and
[Cholangiopancreatography, endoscopic retrograde][1]—Iopamidol is used in adults in endoscopic retrograde pancreatography and endoscopic retrograde cholangiopancreatography for visualization of all portions of the biliary tree.

Intrasynovial:
[Arthrography][1]—Iopamidol is used for arthrography in the diagnosis of post-traumatic or degenerative joint diseases or synovial rupture, for visualization of communicating bursae or cysts, and in meniscography.

---

[1]Not included in Canadian product labeling.

## Pharmacology/Pharmacokinetics

### Physicochemical characteristics
Molecular weight—777.09.
Osmolality—Low. The osmolalities of the injections of iopamidol with iodine concentrations of 200, 300, and 370 mg per mL are 413, 616, and 796 mOsmol per kg of water, respectively
Note: Iopamidol injection is hypertonic as compared to plasma and cerebrospinal fluid (approximately 265 and 301 mOsmol per kg of water, respectively).

### Mechanism of action/Effect
Organic iodine compounds block x-rays as they pass through the body, thereby allowing body structures containing iodine to be delineated in contrast to those structures that do not contain iodine. The degree of opacity produced by these compounds is directly proportional to the total amount (concentration and volume) of the iodinated contrast agent in the path of the x-rays. After intrathecal administration into the subarachnoid space, diffusion of iopamidol in the CSF allows the visualization of the subarachnoid spaces of the head and spinal canal. After intravascular administration, iopamidol makes opaque those vessels in its path of flow, allowing visualization of the internal structures until significant hemodilution occurs.

### Distribution
Intrathecal—Diffuses upward through the CSF; penetrates into nerve root sleeves, nerve rootlets, and narrow areas of the subarachnoid space. Also, enters extracellular fluid of the brain tissue and pial surface of cerebral and cerebellar tissue adjacent to subarachnoid areas. In patients with normal CSF dynamics, it is eliminated from CSF into the blood within 1 hour.
Intravascular—Rapidly distributed throughout circulating blood volume and diffused into extravascular space following intravenous administration. No significant deposition in tissues. Does not cross blood-brain barrier, but accumulates within the interstitial tissues of malignant tumors of the brain due to the break in the blood-brain barrier caused by the tumor.

### Protein binding
Very low.

### Half-life
Elimination—Intravascular: Approximately 2 hours (with normal renal function).

### Time to peak opacification:
Standard myelography—
Immediate and for up to 30 minutes.
CT myelography—
4 hours.
Intravascular—
5 to 40 minutes.
Urography: 5 to 15 minutes.

### Peak serum concentration:
Intravascular—Immediate, but concentration falls rapidly as iopamidol becomes distributed throughout the extravascular compartment.

### Elimination
Intrathecal—Primarily renal; 29 to 100% of administered dose excreted unchanged within 48 hours.
Intravascular—Primarily renal; 35 to 40% of administered dose excreted unchanged within 1 hour, and 80 to 90% in 8 hours.
Note: In patients with impaired renal function, the excretion of iopamidol is prolonged depending upon the degree of impairment.

## Precautions to Consider

### Cross-sensitivity and/or related problems
Patients sensitive to iodine or other iodinated contrast media may be sensitive to iopamidol also.

### Mutagenicity
Animal studies to evaluate mutagenic potential of iopamidol have not shown that iopamidol causes any increase in mutation rates.

### Pregnancy/Reproduction
Pregnancy—Adequate and well-controlled studies in humans have not been done. However, other organically bound iodine–containing preparations administered near term by intra-amniotic injection have caused hypothyroidism in some newborns.

Also, elective contrast radiography of the abdomen is usually not recommended during pregnancy because of the risks to the fetus from radiation exposure.

Teratology studies in animals have not shown that iopamidol causes harm to the fetus.

FDA Pregnancy Category B.

### Breast-feeding

It is not known whether iopamidol is distributed into breast milk. However, because other contrast media are distributed unchanged into breast milk, temporary discontinuation of breast-feeding is recommended for at least 24 hours following administration of iopamidol.

### Pediatrics

Appropriate studies on the relationship of age to the effects of iopamidol have not been performed in pediatric patients. However, it is known that pediatric patients, especially those with asthma, allergies, congestive heart failure, or serum creatinine greater than 1.5 mg per dL or those less than 12 months of age, exhibit an increased risk of having severe adverse effects to radiopaque contrast media.

Also, in infants and young children, especially those with polyuria, oliguria, diabetes, or pre-existing dehydration, dehydration and/or the risk of renal failure may be exacerbated by the radiopaque contrast media; adequate hydration is recommended before and following intravascular administration of iopamidol.

### Geriatrics

Diagnostic studies performed to date have not demonstrated geriatrics-specific problems that would limit the usefulness of iopamidol in the elderly. However, elderly patients are more likely to have age-related renal function impairment, which may require lower dosage in patients receiving iopamidol.

Dehydration and/or the risk of renal failure may be exacerbated in geriatric patients, especially those with polyuria, oliguria, diabetes, or pre-existing dehydration, by iopamidol; adequate hydration is recommended before and following administration of iopamidol.

The elderly may be more sensitive to the effects of iopamidol on thyroid function. Iodine-induced thyrotoxicosis may occur 4 to 12 weeks following contrast radiography. Thyroid function monitoring may be needed in geriatric patients.

### Drug interactions and/or related problems

The following drug interactions and/or related problems have been selected on the basis of their potential clinical significance (possible mechanism in parentheses where appropriate)—not necessarily inclusive (» = major clinical significance):

Note: Combinations containing any of the following medications, depending on the amount present, may also interact with this medication.

» Antidepressants, tricyclic or
CNS stimulation–producing medications (See *Appendix II*) or
Monoamine oxidase (MAO) inhibitors, including furazolidone, procarbazine, and selegiline or
» Phenothiazines or
» Trimeprazine
(although this effect has not been specifically reported for iopamidol, concurrent use with intrathecal administration of metrizamide, another nonionic contrast agent, has been associated with increased risk of seizures because of lowered seizure threshold effect of these medications; until more conclusive evidence is available, it is recommended that medications that lower the seizure threshold be discontinued for at least 48 hours before and 24 hours after myelography)

Beta-adrenergic blocking agents
(concurrent intravascular administration of iopamidol with beta-adrenergic blocking agents may increase the risk of moderate to severe anaphylactoid reaction; also, hypotensive effects may be exacerbated; discontinuation of the beta-adrenergic blocking agent before administration of contrast media may be advisable in patients with other risk factors)

Cholecystographic agents, oral
(may increase the risk of renal toxicity when closely followed by intravascular iopamidol, especially in patients with hepatic function impairment)

Hydralazine
(increased risk of systemic lupus erythematosus [SLE]–like syndrome if iopamidol is given to patients on hydralazine therapy)

Hypotension-producing medications, other (See *Appendix II*)
(the risk of severe hypotension may be increased if iopamidol is given concurrently with other medications that produce hypotension)

Interleukin-2
(incidence of delayed reactions to intravenous contrast media [e.g., hypersensitivity, fever, skin rash, flu-like symptoms, joint pain, flushing, pruritus, emesis, hypotension, dizziness occurring more than 1 hour after administration] may be increased in patients who have received interleukin-2; some symptoms may resemble a ''recall'' reaction to interleukin-2; supportive medical treatment may be necessary if symptoms are significant; there is some evidence that incidence is reduced if contrast media administration is delayed until 6 weeks after interleukin-2 administration)

Nephrotoxic medications, other (See *Appendix II*)
(concurrent intrathecal or intravascular administration of iopamidol with other nephrotoxic medications may increase the potential for nephrotoxicity)

### Diagnostic interference

The following have been selected on the basis of their potential clinical significance (possible effect in parentheses where appropriate)—not necessarily inclusive (» = major clinical significance):

With *other* diagnostic test results
Blood pool imaging
(imaging of blood pool may be impaired because of decreased technetium Tc 99m-labeling of red blood cells caused by the intravascular administration of iopamidol)

Leukocyte counts and
Red cell counts
(may be temporarily decreased)

Prothrombin time (PT) and
Thromboplastin time
(may be increased, since iopamidol has been shown to slightly inhibit all stages of coagulation in *in vitro* studies with animal blood)

Skeletal imaging
(possible renal and hepatic uptake of technetium Tc 99m medronate, technetium Tc 99m oxidronate, technetium Tc 99m pyrophosphate, or technetium Tc 99m [pyro- and trimeta-] phosphates if iopamidol is administered intravenously immediately after one of these technetium Tc 99m-labeled agents)

Thyroid function determinations and
Thyroid imaging
(intravascular or intrathecal administration of iopamidol may alter serum protein-bound iodine [PBI] concentrations and radioactive iodine or pertechnetate ion uptake for up to 2 weeks; thyroid test should be performed prior to administration of iopamidol. Other thyroid function tests not based on measurement of iodine, such as resin triiodothyronine uptake, may not be affected)

Urinalysis
(iopamidol may interfere with some chemical determinations made on urine, such as protein and specific gravity; urine should be collected prior to, or at least 2 days after, intravascular administration of iopamidol)

With physiology/laboratory test values
Creatinine, serum
(concentration may be increased temporarily with iopamidol)

Platelet aggregation
(may be decreased by high levels of plasma iopamidol)

### Medical considerations/Contraindications

The medical considerations/contraindications included here have been selected on the basis of their potential clinical significance (reasons given in parentheses where appropriate)—not necessarily inclusive (» = major clinical significance).

*Risk-benefit should be considered when the following medical problems exist:*

*For all procedures (especially those requiring intrathecal or intravascular administration)*
Allergic reaction (anaphylaxis) to penicillins or to skin allergens, previous
(although the risk of anaphylactoid reaction may be less with iopamidol than with high-osmolality contrast agents, caution is recommended when administering iopamidol to patients who have had a previous reaction to penicillins or to skin allergens)

Allergies or asthma, history of
(although the risk of idiosyncratic response or anaphylactoid reaction may be less with iopamidol than with high-osmolality contrast agents, caution is recommended when administering iopamidol to patients with a history of allergies or asthma)

» Dehydration, especially associated with pre-existing renal disease, advanced vascular disease, and diabetes mellitus, and in pediatric and elderly patients
  (intravascular administration may increase risk of acute renal failure)

Renal function impairment, severe
  (excretion of iopamidol may be delayed; although the risk of contrast-induced nephrotoxicity with intravascular use in the presence of renal insufficiency [serum creatinine ≥ 132.6 micromoles/L] may be less with iopamidol than with high-osmolality contrast agents, caution is recommended)

» Sensitivity to iodinated contrast media
  (increased risk of anaphylactoid reaction in patients with history of reactions to contrast media)

*For intrathecal use*
Alcoholism, chronic
  (increased risk of side effects because of possible brain or liver damage)

Bleeding, subarachnoid
  (increased risk of meningeal irritation or arachnoiditis)

Epilepsy, history of
  (myelographic procedure may increase risk of seizures)

Infection, local or systemic, significant

Multiple sclerosis

*For intravascular use*
Hyperthyroidism
  (administration of iopamidol may precipitate thyroid storm)

Pheochromocytoma
  (administration of iopamidol may precipitate severe hypertension; amount of iopamidol injected should be kept to a minimum and blood pressure should be monitored during the procedure; also, pretreatment with the alpha-adrenergic blocking agent, phentolamine, is recommended)

Sickle cell disease
  (administration of iopamidol may promote sickling in patients who are homozygous for sickle cell disease; however, sickling potential of iopamidol is less than that of high-osmolality ionic agents)

*For angiocardiography*
Angina, unstable
  (increased risk of severe cardiac reaction)

Cardiac disease
  (potential transitory increase in the circulatory osmotic load may aggravate condition)

Pulmonary hypertension, severe
  (hypervolemic effect of iopamidol may further increase pulmonary artery and venous pressures due to an increase in cardiac output and a rise in left ventricular end-diastolic and left atrial pressures)

*For cerebral arteriography*
Arteriosclerosis, advanced, or
Cardiac decompensation or
Cerebral embolism, recent or
Hypertension, severe or
Senility or
Thrombosis, recent
  (increased risk of vessel occlusion)

» Homocystinuria
  (procedure may increase risk of thrombosis and embolism)

*For peripheral arteriography*
» Buerger's disease
  (procedure may induce severe arterial or venous spasm)

» Ischemia, severe, associated with ascending infection

*For excretory urography*
» Anuria or
» Diabetes mellitus
  (administration of iopamidol may increase the risk of acute renal failure)

*For arthrography*
» Infection, in or near joint to be examined
  (procedure may increase risk of complications)

**Patient monitoring**
The following may be especially important in patient monitoring (other tests may be warranted in some patients, depending on condition; » = major clinical significance):

*For intravascular use*
Blood pressure determinations
  (may be required during examination, especially in patients with known or suspected pheochromocytoma or hemodynamic compromise or instability)

## Side/Adverse Effects

Note: Adverse effects may vary directly with the concentration of the agent, the amount and technique used, and the underlying pathology. Increases in osmolality, volume, concentration, viscosity, and rate of administration of the solution may increase the incidence and severity of adverse effects.

Most of the adverse effects occur soon after administration of contrast media and are usually self-limiting and of short duration. However, some adverse effects may be delayed and may be of a long-lasting nature.

Overall incidence of adverse effects with nonionic contrast agents, such as iopamidol, has been reported to be less than with ionic contrast agents.

Nonionic contrast media, such as iopamidol, have been reported to produce fewer and less severe alterations in cardiac hemodynamics and electrocardiograms than standard ionic contrast agents during cardiac angiography.

Low-osmolality contrast agents, such as iopamidol, are reported to cause less heat and pain on injection than high-osmolality agents, such as diatrizoates and iothalamate.

Thromboembolic events causing myocardial infarction and stroke have been reported during angiographic procedures with nonionic contrast media; however, these events appear to be technique-related.

Headaches following intrathecal administration of iopamidol may be more frequent and persistent in patients not adequately hydrated.

Dehydration and/or the risk of renal failure may be exacerbated by the hypertonic contrast solutions of iopamidol, and in some cases may cause a shock-like state, following intravascular administration of iopamidol in geriatric, azotemic, and dehydrated or debilitated patients.

Transient global amnesia has been reported in 2 patients after cerebral angiography in which 20 mL of another low-osmolality nonionic contrast agent (containing the equivalent of 240 mg of iodine per mL) was administered into the ascending aorta. The possibility that iopamidol may cause a similar response must be considered.

The following side/adverse effects have been selected on the basis of their potential clinical significance (possible signs and symptoms in parentheses where appropriate)—not necessarily inclusive:

**Those indicating need for medical attention**
Incidence rare
  *With all procedures*
    ***Pseudo-allergic reaction*** (skin rash or hives; stuffy nose; swelling of face or skin; wheezing, tightness in chest, or troubled breathing)
    Note: *Pseudo-allergic reactions* are usually transient. However, they may be an initial manifestations of a more severe anaphylactoid reaction. The anaphylactoid reaction may progress to respiratory arrest and vasomotor collapse if appropriate treatment is not administered.

  *With intrathecal or intravascular administration*
    ***Bronchospasm or pulmonary edema*** (severe wheezing or troubled breathing); ***hypotension*** (severe tiredness or weakness); ***seizures***

  *With intrathecal administration*
    ***Musculoskeletal effects*** (involuntary movements; paralysis of legs)

  *With intravascular administration*
    ***Cardiotoxic effects, with ventricular tachycardia or fibrillation*** (fast or irregular heartbeat)
    Note: In angiocardiography, bradyarrhythmias occur far less commonly with low-osmolality contrast agents than with high-osmolality agents. For iopamidol, *bradycardia* has been reported with an estimated incidence of 1.3%.

**Those indicating need for medical attention only if they continue or are bothersome**
Incidence more frequent
*With intrathecal or intravascular administration*
>   **Headache, mild to moderate; nausea and vomiting, mild to moderate**
>   Note: *Headache, nausea, and/or vomiting* may occur 1 to 10 hours after intrathecal injection and last for a few hours, usually disappearing within 24 hours; or, less frequently after intravascular injection, may occur immediately and last for a few minutes.

*With intrathecal administration*
>   **Backache; dizziness; leg pain or cramps; meningeal irritation** (stiffness of neck)

*With intravascular administration*
>   **Vasodilation, arteriolar** (hot flashes or sudden feeling of warmth; pain or burning at injection site, mild)

Incidence less frequent or rare
*With intrathecal administration*
>   **CNS effects** (severe headache, ringing or buzzing in ears, unusual tiredness or weakness); **difficult urination; drowsiness; increased sensitivity of eyes to light; increased sweating; loss of appetite**

*With intravascular administration*
>   **Blurred vision or other changes in vision; lightheadedness; unusual taste**

## Patient Consultation

As an aid to patient consultation, refer to *Advice for the Patient, Radiopaque Agents (Diagnostic)*.

In providing consultation, consider emphasizing the following selected information (» = major clinical significance):

**Description of use**
*Action in the body:*
>   Injection into spinal canal; visualization of radiopacity in head and spinal cord possible with x-rays

>   Injection into vein or artery; visualization of radiopacity in blood vessels, heart, brain, and other organs possible with x-rays

>   Direct injection into region to be studied; visualization of joint spaces, peritoneal herniations, pancreatic and bile ducts

**Before having this test**
» Conditions affecting use, especially:
>   Sensitivity to iodine or other iodinated contrast media
>   Pregnancy—Risk to the fetus from radiation exposure; may cause hypothyroidism in newborn
>   Breast-feeding—Not known if distributed into breast milk; temporary discontinuation of breast-feeding for at least 24 hours is recommended
>   Use in children—Increased risk of severe adverse reactions, especially in children with other medical problems; possible exacerbation of dehydration
>   Use in the elderly—Possible exacerbation of dehydration; increased risk of thyrotoxicosis
>   Other medications, especially phenothiazines, tricyclic antidepressants, and trimeprazine (with intrathecal administration of iopamidol)
>   Other medical problems, especially anuria, dehydration, and diabetes mellitus

**Preparation for this test**
>   Adequate intake of fluids to prevent dehydration
>   Special preparatory instructions may be given; patient should inquire in advance
*With intrathecal use*
>   Normal diet up to 2 hours before procedure; moderate amounts of clear liquids may be permitted up to time of procedure

**Precautions after having this test**
>   Possible interference with future thyroid tests
*With intrathecal use*
>   Avoiding movement during and for several hours after administration
>   Keeping head position as instructed during and after examination

**Side/adverse effects**
>   Signs of possible side effects, especially pseudo-allergic reaction and cardiac or pulmonary problems that may occur within minutes of administration

## General Dosing Information

Manufacturer's package insert or other appropriate literature should be consulted for specific techniques and procedures for the administration of contrast media.

Sensitivity test doses are not usually recommended since severe or fatal reactions to contrast media are not predictable from a patient's history or a sensitivity test. On some occasions, severe or fatal reactions have occurred with a test dose or with a full dose in patients who did not react to the test dose.

Pretreatment with corticosteroids and/or antihistamines may minimize the incidence and severity of reactions in patients with a history of severe reactions to contrast media or with other high-risk conditions (e.g., asthma or history of allergies, positive allergy history to skin allergens or penicillin, dehydration, history of seizures, pheochromocytoma). In some studies, the additional use of ephedrine has been shown to be beneficial in preventing anaphylactoid reactions (except in patients with a history of hypertension or cardiovascular disease). When considering the use of a contrast agent, the following protocols are recommended:
For high-risk patients
•   Use of a high-osmolality contrast agent plus pretreatment with a corticosteroid (oral prednisone, 50 mg administered 13 hours, 7 hours, and 1 hour before procedure) and an antihistamine (intramuscular, intravenous, or oral diphenhydramine, 50 mg administered one hour prior to procedure) or
•   Use of a low-osmolality agent if pretreatment is not feasible or
•   Use of a low-osmolality agent plus corticosteroid pretreatment.
For low-risk patients
•   Use of a high-osmolality contrast agent or
•   Use of a high-osmolality contrast agent and corticosteroid pretreatment.

Adequate hydration is recommended for all patients before and after the examination. Intravenous or oral intake of fluids may continue up to time of administration of iopamidol.

During and for at least 30 to 60 minutes after intravascular injection of iopamidol, and for at least 12 hours (up to 24 hours in some cases) after intrathecal administration, the patient should be observed for possible severe reactions; competent personnel and emergency facilities should be available during this period.

Dosage and concentration of iodine (as iopamidol injection) are dependent upon the degree and extent of contrast needed in the areas under examination and on the equipment and technique used.

**For intrathecal use**
Pretreatment with barbiturates may be used in patients who have a history of seizures but are not on anticonvulsant therapy. Patients who are on anticonvulsant therapy should continue receiving their medication when using iopamidol.

A normal diet may be ingested up to 2 hours prior to the administration of iopamidol.

If inadvertent intracranial entry of a large or concentrated bolus of iopamidol occurs, treatment with anticonvulsants may be used to minimize the risk of seizures.

Direct intracisternal or ventricular administration of iopamidol for standard radiography is *not* recommended.

During and for several hours after the procedure the patient must remain inactive to minimize high cephalad dispersion of iopamidol.

Information on patient management and positioning during and after procedure are included in the manufacturer's package insert.

**For intravascular use**
Nonionic contrast media such as iopamidol inhibit blood coagulation *in vitro* less than ionic contrast media. Blood cell aggregation has been reported when blood remains in contact with syringes containing nonionic contrast media. Thus, it is possible that thromboembolic events causing myocardial infarction and stroke, reported during angiographic procedures, may have resulted from coagulation of blood that had come in contact with the contrast agent outside the body. It is recommended that risk factors for aggregation be minimized by performing the procedure in the shortest time possible, using plastic rather than glass syringes, and flushing catheters with heparinized saline solutions.

**For treatment of adverse effects**
Recommended treatment consists of the following:
•   For major or life-threatening reactions, careful monitoring of vital signs and emergency therapy, including artificial respiration with oxygen, if needed for respiratory depression, and cardiac massage in the event of cardiac arrest.

- To restore blood pressure, administration of intravenous fluids and/or vasopressors. If hypotension necessitates the use of vasopressors, slow infusion of 0.008 to 0.012 mg per minute of norepinephrine or 0.1 to 0.18 mg per minute of phenylephrine, appropriately diluted. If hypotension is due to increased vagal activity (vasovagal reaction), intravenous administration of 1 mg of atropine, repeated in one to two hours if needed.
- Other specific treatment may include—

  *Diphenhydramine:* For minor allergic-like reactions—An antihistamine such as diphenhydramine hydrochloride (except in epileptic patients) may be administered intravenously.

  *Epinephrine or hydrocortisone:* For acute allergic-like or anaphylactoid reactions—Intravenous administration of 500 to 1000 mg of soluble hydrocortisone or slow intravenous infusion of 0.1 mg of epinephrine (1:10,000).

  For mild to moderate bronchospasm—0.1 to 0.2 mg of epinephrine (1:1000) may be administered subcutaneously, except in hypotension. In extreme emergency, 0.1 mg of epinephrine (1:10,000) may be given slowly by intravenous injection, followed by a continuous intravenous infusion at an initial rate of 0.001 mg per minute; the rate may be increased to 0.004 mg per minute if necessary.

  Patients on beta-adrenergic blocking agents should not receive epinephrine since they are at risk of excessive alpha-adrenergic stimulation, which may result in hypertension, reflex bradycardia, and heart block. In these patients, isoproterenol and norepinephrine are used instead of epinephrine to overcome bronchospasm and hypotension, respectively.

  For cardiac arrest—0.1 to 1 mg of epinephrine may be administered by the intravenous route.

  *Diazepam or phenobarbital:* To control convulsions—5 to 10 mg of diazepam by slow, intravenous administration or phenobarbital sodium intravenously or intramuscularly at a rate not to exceed 30 to 60 mg per minute may be given.

# Parenteral Dosage Forms

## IOPAMIDOL INJECTION USP

### Usual adult and adolescent dose

Intrathecal—

Myelography:

Lumbar and Thoracic myelography by lumbar injection[1]—
10 to 15 mL of a solution containing the equivalent of 200 mg of iodine per mL.

Cervical myelography by lumbar injection[1]—
10 to 15 mL of a solution containing the equivalent of 200 mg of iodine per mL; or 10 mL of a solution containing the equivalent of 300 mg of iodine per mL.

Cervical myelography by lateral cervical injection[1]—
10 mL of a solution containing the equivalent of 200 mg of iodine per mL.

Total columnar myelography by lumbar injection[1]—
10 mL of a solution containing the equivalent of 300 mg of iodine per mL.

CT cisternography by lumbar injection[1]:
4 to 6 mL of a solution containing the equivalent of 200 mg of iodine per mL.

Note: Injection should be administered slowly over a period of 1 to 2 minutes to avoid excessive mixing with cerebrospinal fluid and resultant dilution of iopamidol as well as premature cephalad dispersion.

Immediate repeat intrathecal administration is not recommended because of overdose risk; 48 hours, or preferably 5 to 7 days, should elapse before repeat examination.

Intravascular—

Angiography:

Intra-arterial, by digital subtraction—Via catheter, as a solution containing the equivalent of 128 mg of iodine per mL, into the following:

Carotid arteries—6 to 12 mL.
Vertebral arteries—4 to 10 mL.
Aortic arch—25 to 60 mL.
Renal arteries—6 to 15 mL.
Branches of the aorta—12 to 50 mL.
Abdominal aorta—25 to 60 mL.

Arteriography, cerebral:
Carotid puncture or transfemoral catheterization, 8 to 12 mL of a solution containing the equivalent of 300 mg of iodine per mL.

Arteriography, peripheral:
As a solution containing the equivalent of 300 mg of iodine per mL:
Direct injection into the femoral artery or subclavian artery, 5 to 40 mL.
Direct injection into the aorta for distal runoffs, 25 to 50 mL.

Arteriography, selective coronary:
Via catheter, 2 to 10 mL of a solution containing the equivalent of 370 mg of iodine per mL.

Arteriography, selective visceral[1]:
Via catheter, up to 50 mL into the larger vessels, such as the aorta or celiac artery, or up to 10 mL into the renal arteries of a solution containing the equivalent of 370 mg of iodine per mL.

Ventriculography:
Via catheter, 25 to 50 mL of a solution containing the equivalent of 370 mg of iodine per mL.

Venography, peripheral (phlebography):
Percutaneous, 25 to 150 mL of a solution containing the equivalent of 200 mg of iodine per mL per lower extremity.

CT of the brain:
Intravenous, 100 to 150 mL of a solution containing the equivalent of 250 mg of iodine per mL; or 50 to 100 mL of a solution containing the equivalent of 300 mg of iodine per mL; or 41 to 81 mL of a solution containing the equivalent of 370 mg of iodine per mL.

CT of the body:
Intravenous, 130 mL of a solution containing the equivalent of 250 mg of iodine per mL; or 50 to 100 mL of a solution containing the equivalent of 300 mg of iodine per mL; or 81 mL of a solution containing the equivalent of 370 mg of iodine per mL, by rapid administration.

Urography, excretory:
Intravenous, 50 to 100 mL of a solution containing the equivalent of 250 mg of iodine per mL; or 50 to 100 mL of a solution containing the equivalent of 300 mg of iodine per mL, by rapid administration.

### Usual adult prescribing limits

Intrathecal—
Up to 4.5 grams of iodine of a solution containing no more than the equivalent of 300 mg of iodine per mL.

Intravascular—
Intra-arterial digital subtraction angiography:
Up to 350 mL (total of multiple doses).

Cerebral arteriography:
Up to 90 mL (total of multiple doses) of a solution containing the equivalent of 300 mg of iodine per mL.

Peripheral arteriography:
Up to 250 mL of a solution containing the equivalent of 300 mg of iodine per mL.

Selective visceral arteriography and aortography:
Up to 225 mL (total of multiple doses) of a solution containing the equivalent of 370 mg of iodine per mL.

Coronary arteriography and ventriculography:
Up to 200 mL of a solution containing the equivalent of 370 mg of iodine per mL.

Venography:
Up to 350 mL (total of multiple doses).

### Usual pediatric dose

Intrathecal—Myelography—
Lumbar[1] and
Thoracic myelography by lumbar injection of a solution containing the equivalent of 200 mg of iodine per mL—
Children 2 to 7 years of age: 7 to 9 mL.
Children 8 to 12 years of age: 8 to 11 mL.
Children 13 to 18 years of age: 10 to 12 mL.

Intravascular—
Angiocardiography[1]:
By injection into a large peripheral vein or by direct catheterization of the heart as a solution containing the equivalent of 370 mg of iodine per mL:
Children up to 2 years of age: 10 to 15 mL administered as a single dose.
Children 2 to 9 years of age: 15 to 30 mL administered as a single dose.
Children 10 to 18 years of age: 20 to 50 mL administered as a single dose.

CT of the brain:
Intravenous, 1 to 3 mL per kg of body weight of a solution containing the equivalent of 300 mg of iodine per mL.

CT of the body:
Intravenous, 1.2 to 3.6 mL per kg of body weight of a solution containing the equivalent of 250 mg of iodine per mL; or 1 to 3 mL per kg of body weight of a solution containing the equivalent of 300 mg of iodine per mL.
Urography, excretory:
Intravenous, 1.2 to 3.6 mL per kg of body weight of a solution containing the equivalent of 250 mg of iodine per mL; or 1 to 3 mL per kg of body weight of a solution containing the equivalent of 300 mg of iodine per mL.

### Usual geriatric dose
See *Usual adult and adolescent dose*.

Note: Geriatric patients with renal function impairment may be more sensitive to the effects of the usual adult dose; lower dosages are recommended.

### Strength(s) usually available
U.S.—
261 mg of iopamidol with 128 mg of iodine per mL (Rx) [*Isovue-128* (tromethamine 1 mg, edetate calcium disodium 0.17 mg, sodium 0.001 mEq)].
408 mg of iopamidol with 200 mg of iodine per mL (Rx) [*Isovue-200* (tromethamine 1 mg, edetate calcium disodium 0.26 mg, sodium 0.001 mEq); *Isovue-M 200* (tromethamine 1 mg, edetate calcium disodium 0.26 mg, sodium 0.001 mEq)].
510 mg of iopamidol with 250 mg of iodine per mL (Rx) [*Isovue-250* (tromethamine 1 mg, edetate calcium disodium 0.33 mg, sodium 0.002 mEq)].
612 mg of iopamidol with 300 mg of iodine per mL (Rx) [*Isovue-300* (tromethamine 1 mg, edetate calcium disodium 0.39 mg, sodium 0.002 mEq); *Isovue-M 300* (tromethamine 1 mg, edetate calcium disodium 0.39 mg, sodium 0.002 mEq)].
755 mg of iopamidol with 370 mg of iodine per mL (Rx) [*Isovue-370* (tromethamine 1 mg, edetate calcium disodium 0.48 mg, sodium 0.002 mEq)].
Canada—
261 mg of iopamidol with 128 mg of iodine per mL (Rx) [*Isovue-128* (tromethamine 1 mg, edetate calcium disodium 0.17 mg, sodium 0.001 mEq)].

408 mg of iopamidol with 200 mg of iodine per mL (Rx) [*Isovue-200* (sodium 0.001 mEq)].
612 mg of iopamidol with 300 mg of iodine per mL (Rx) [*Isovue-300* (sodium 0.002 mEq)].
755 mg of iopamidol with 370 mg of iodine per mL (Rx) [*Isovue-370* (sodium 0.003 mEq)].

### Packaging and storage
Store between 15 and 30 °C (59 and 86 °F), unless otherwise specified by manufacturer. Protect from light. Protect from freezing.

### Stability
Iopamidol is a clear, colorless to pale yellow solution. Do not use if turbid or discolored.
Any unused portion remaining in the container should be discarded.
Crystals may form in the solution but are readily redissolved by immersing the container in hot water and gently shaking it.

### Incompatibilities
Iopamidol is physically incompatible with other medications. Other medications must *not* be mixed in the same syringe or IV administration set.

[1]Not included in Canadian product labeling.

## Selected Bibliography
Kawada TK. Iohexol and iopamidol: second-generation nonionic radiographic contrast media. Drug Intell Clin Pharm 1985 Jul/Aug; 19: 525-9.
Benotti JR. The comparative effects of ionic versus nonionic agents in cardiac catheterization. Invest Radiol 1988; 23 (Suppl 2): S366-S373.

Revised: 07/21/95

**IOPANOIC ACID**—See *Cholecystographic Agents, Oral (Systemic)*

# IOTHALAMATE    Local

VA CLASSIFICATION (Primary): DX102

Note: For a listing of dosage forms and brand names by country availability, see *Dosage Forms* section(s). For a listing of brand names for the articles in this monograph, refer to the General Index.

## Category
Diagnostic aid, radiopaque (urinary tract disorders).
Note: Iothalamate is an ionic radiopaque contrast agent.

## Indications

### Accepted
Cystography, retrograde and
Cystourethrography, retrograde—Iothalamate meglumine is indicated in retrograde cystography to evaluate abnormalities of the bladder and ureters. It is also indicated in retrograde cystourethrography to evaluate abnormalities of the urethra.
Pyelography, retrograde—Iothalamate meglumine is indicated in retrograde pyelography to evaluate abnormalities of the kidney and ureter.

## Pharmacology/Pharmacokinetics

### Physicochemical characteristics
Molecular weight—809.13.
Osmolality—High.

### Mechanism of action/Effect
Organic iodine compounds block x-rays as they pass through the body, thereby allowing body structures containing iodine to be delineated in contrast to those structures that do not contain iodine. The degree of opacity produced by these compounds is directly proportional to the total amount (concentration and volume) of the iodinated contrast agent in the path of the x-rays. The instillation of iothalamate into the urinary bladder, ureters, and kidneys allows visualization of these areas.

### Absorption
Intravesical instillation—Small amounts absorbed through the bladder.

### Elimination
Absorbed iothalamate—Primarily renal.
Unabsorbed iothalmate—Expelled by voiding.

## Precautions to Consider

### Cross-sensitivity and/or related problems
Patients sensitive to iodine or other iodinated contrast media may be sensitive to iothalamate also.

### Carcinogenicity/Mutagenicity
Long-term animal studies to evaluate carcinogenic or mutagenic potential of iothalamate have not been performed.

### Pregnancy/Reproduction
Pregnancy—Iothalamate crosses the placenta and is evenly distributed in fetal tissue. Adequate and well-controlled studies in humans have not been done. However, organically bound iodine–containing preparations administered near term by intra-amniotic injection have caused hypothyroidism in some newborns.
Also, elective contrast radiography of the abdomen is usually not recommended during pregnancy because of the risks to the fetus from radiation exposure.
Studies in animals have not shown that iothalamate causes teratogenic effects in the fetus.
FDA Pregnancy Category C.

### Breast-feeding
Problems in humans have not been documented. However, since small amounts of this medium may be absorbed and iothalamate is known to be distributed unchanged into breast milk when administered intravascularly, breast-feeding is not recommended for at least 24 hours following its administration.

## Pediatrics

Appropriate studies on the relationship of age to the effects of iothalamate have not been performed in pediatric patients. However, no pediatrics-specific problems have been documented to date.

## Geriatrics

Appropriate studies on the relationship of age to the effects of iothalamate have not been performed in geriatric patients. However, no geriatrics-specific problems have been documented to date.

## Drug interactions and/or related problems

See *Diagnostic interference*.

## Diagnostic interference

The following have been selected on the basis of their potential clinical significance (possible effect in parentheses where appropriate)—not necessarily inclusive (» = major clinical significance):

With results of *this* test
  *Due to other medications*
    Dyclonine
      (may interfere with visualization when used as local anesthetic in cystoscopic procedures following pyelography, because of possible reaction with the iodine in iothalamate, which may result in precipitation of iodine)
With *other* diagnostic test results
  Thyroid function determinations and
  Thyroid imaging
    (absorbed iothalamate may cause an increase of serum protein–bound iodine [PBI] and a decrease in radioactive iodine or pertechnetate ion uptake for up to 16 days; thyroid test should be performed prior to administration of contrast medium. Other thyroid function tests not based on measurement of iodine, such as resin triiodothyronine uptake, are not affected)

## Medical considerations/Contraindications

The medical considerations/contraindications included here have been selected on the basis of their potential clinical significance (reasons given in parentheses where appropriate)—not necessarily inclusive (» = major clinical significance).

*Except under special circumstances, this medication should not be used when the following medical problems exist:*

*For retrograde pyelography and retrograde urography*
» Obstruction to endoscopy or ureteral catheterization, such as in extensive urinary tuberculosis, bladder tumors, ureteral obstructions, and prostate enlargement
» Urinary tract infection, upper, acute
    (procedure may increase risk of complications)

*Risk-benefit should be considered when the following medical problems exist:*

  Allergic reaction (anaphylaxis) to penicillins or to skin allergens, previous
    (increased risk of anaphylactoid reaction)
  Allergies or asthma, history of
    (increased risk of idiosyncratic response or anaphylactoid reaction)
» Sensitivity to iodinated contrast media
    (increased risk of anaphylactoid reaction in patients with a history of anaphylactoid reaction to iodinated contrast media)
*For retrograde pyelography*
  Renal function impairment, severe
    (increased risk of oliguria or anuria)

## Side/Adverse Effects

Note: Adverse effects associated with the mechanics of the procedure include injury to the urethra, bladder, and ureter and introduction of infection.

  Systemic adverse effects, similar to those that occur with direct intravascular injection of the iothalamate salts, may also occur with intravesical or intraureteral instillation as a result of inadvertent intravascular entry of the contrast solution due to either bladder absorption or pyelorenal backflow.

  Cardiac arrest may occur due to accidental intravasation of iothalamate meglumine.

The following side/adverse effects have been selected on the basis of their potential clinical significance (possible signs and symptoms in parentheses where appropriate)—not necessarily inclusive:

Those indicating need for medical attention
  Incidence less frequent
    *Pyelorenal distention* (abdominal or stomach pain and discomfort, backache)—resulting from the instillation of an excess volume of contrast solution; renal colic and shock may follow
  Incidence rare
    *Pseudo-allergic reaction* (chills; fever; skin rash or hives; sneezing; sweating; swelling of face or skin; swelling of the larynx; wheezing, tightness in chest, or troubled breathing)—may be due to entry of medium into venous or lymphatic system

## Patient Consultation

As an aid to patient consultation, refer to *Advice for the Patient, Radiopaque Agents (Diagnostic, Local)*.

In providing consultation, consider emphasizing the following selected information (»= major clinical significance):

## Description of use

Instillation into bladder or ureters; visualization of radiopacity possible with x-rays

## Before having this test

» Conditions affecting use, especially:
    Sensitivity to iodine or other iodinated contrast media
    Pregnancy—Iothalamate crosses the placenta; risk to the fetus from radiation exposure
    Breast-feeding—May be distributed into breast milk; temporary discontinuation of breast-feeding for at least 24 hours is recommended
    Other medical problems, especially urinary tract obstruction or acute upper urinary tract infection

## Preparation for this test

Special diet, use of laxative, and/or other preparatory instructions may apply; patient should inquire in advance
Voiding before procedure

## Precautions after having this test

Possible interference with future thyroid tests
Voiding after procedure

## Side/adverse effects

Signs of potential side effects, especially pyelorenal distention and pseudo-allergic reaction

## General Dosing Information

Manufacturer's package insert and other appropriate literature should be consulted for specific techniques and procedures for the administration of contrast media.

Sensitivity test doses are not usually recommended since severe or fatal reactions to contrast media are not predictable from a patient's history or a sensitivity test. On some occasions severe or fatal reactions have occurred with a test dose or with a full dose in patients who did not react to the test dose.

Pretreatment with corticosteroids and/or antihistamines is recommended to minimize the incidence and severity of reactions in patients with a history of severe reactions to contrast media or with other high-risk conditions (e.g., asthma or history of allergies, or positive allergy history to skin allergens or penicillin). In some studies, the additional use of ephedrine has been shown to be beneficial in preventing anaphylactoid reactions (except in patients with a history of hypertension or cardiovascular disease). When considering the use of a contrast agent, the following protocols are recommended:
For high-risk patients—
  • Use of a high-osmolality contrast agent plus pretreatment with a corticosteroid (oral prednisone, 50 mg administered 13 hours, 7 hours, and 1 hour before procedure) and an antihistamine (intramuscular, intravenous, or oral diphenhydramine, 50 mg administered 1 hour before procedure) or
  • Use of a low-osmolality contrast agent if pretreatment is not feasible or
  • Use of a low-osmolality contrast agent plus corticosteroid pretreatment.
For low-risk patients—
  • Use of a high-osmolality contrast agent or
  • Use of a high-osmolality contrast agent and corticosteroid pretreatment.

Iothalamate meglumine sterile solution labeled for retrograde cystourethrography or retrograde pyelography is *not* for intravascular injection. It is to be instilled, after the bladder is emptied, directly into the bladder or ureter and renal pelvis by gravity flow, using an appropriate venoclysis set or syringe. Excessive pressure should be avoided with either method of administration.

A low-residue diet the day before and a laxative the night before the procedure are recommended.

Dosage and concentration of iothalamate meglumine for intravesical instillation should be individualized and are usually in proportion to the age of the patient and the technique and equipment used.

During and for at least 30 to 60 minutes after administration of contrast media, the patient should be observed for possible severe reactions; competent personnel and emergency facilities should be available during this period.

Bladder must be emptied at the completion of the procedure, since severe irritation of the urinary tract and hemorrhagic cystitis may occur as a result of prolonged exposure to the contrast media.

## Local Dosage Forms

### IOTHALAMATE MEGLUMINE INJECTION USP

**Usual adult and adolescent dose**
Cystography, retrograde and
Cystourethrography, retrograde—
  Intravesical instillation, 200 to 400 mL or more, depending on bladder capacity, of a solution containing the equivalent of 81 mg or 202 mg of iodine per mL.

Pyelography, retrograde—
  Intraureteral instillation, 15 or 25 mL of a solution containing the equivalent of 202 mg of iodine per mL for unilateral or bilateral pyelograms, respectively.

  Note: The solution containing the equivalent of 202 mg of iodine per mL may be diluted to a solution containing the equivalent of 81 mg of iodine per mL with sterile water for injection or sterile saline injection according to the manufacturer's instructions.

  In patients with reduced renal function, repeat retrograde pyelography is not recommended for at least 48 hours because of the possibility of temporary oliguria or anuria.

**Usual pediatric dose**
Cystography, retrograde, and
Cystourethrography, retrograde—
  Intravesical instillation, 30 to 300 mL, depending on bladder capacity, of a solution containing the equivalent of 81 mg or 202 mg of iodine per mL.

Pyelography, retrograde—
  Dosage must be individualized by physician according to size of child.

**Usual geriatric dose**
See *Usual adult and adolescent dose*.

**Strength(s) usually available**
U.S.—
  17.2% (172 mg per mL) of iothalamate meglumine with 8.1% (81 mg per mL) of iodine (Rx) [*Cysto-Conray II* (0.11 mg edetate calcium disodium per mL)].
  43% (430 mg per mL) of iothalamate meglumine with 20.2% (202 mg per mL) of iodine (Rx) [*Cysto-Conray* (0.11 mg edetate calcium disodium)].
Canada—
  17.2% (172 mg per mL) of iothalamate meglumine with 8.1% (81 mg per mL) of iodine (Rx) [*Cysto-Conray II* (0.11 mg edetate calcium disodium per mL)].
  43% (430 mg per mL) of iothalamate meglumine with 20.2% (202 mg per mL) of iodine (Rx) [*Cysto-Conray* (0.11 mg edetate calcium disodium per mL)].

**Packaging and storage**
Store below 30 °C (86 °F), unless otherwise specified by manufacturer. Protect from light. Protect from freezing.

**Stability**
Crystals may form in the solution at very cold temperatures but are readily redissolved by bringing the container of solution to room temperature and gently shaking it.
Any unused portion remaining in the container should be discarded.

## Selected Bibliography

Shehadi WH. Clinical problems and toxicity of contrast agents. Amer J Roentgen 1966; 97: 762.

Revised: 05/18/95

# IOTHALAMATE  Systemic

VA CLASSIFICATION (Primary): DX102
Note: For a listing of dosage forms and brand names by country availability, see *Dosage Forms* section(s). For a listing of brand names for the articles in this monograph, refer to the General Index.

## Category

Note: Iothalamate is an ionic radiopaque contrast agent.

Diagnostic aid, radiopaque (cardiac disease)—Iothalamate Meglumine and Iothalamate Sodium Injection; Iothalamate Sodium Injection.

Diagnostic aid, radiopaque (vascular disease)—Iothalamate Meglumine Injection; Iothalamate Meglumine and Iothalamate Sodium Injection; Iothalamate Sodium Injection.

Diagnostic aid, radiopaque (biliary tract disorders)—Iothalamate Meglumine Injection.

Diagnostic aid, radiopaque (pancreas disease)—Iothalamate Meglumine Injection.

Diagnostic aid, radiopaque (brain disorders)—Iothalamate Meglumine Injection; Iothalamate Meglumine and Iothalamate Sodium Injection; Iothalamate Sodium Injection.

Diagnostic aid, radiopaque contrast enhancer in computed tomography (CT)—Iothalamate Meglumine Injection; Iothalamate Meglumine and Iothalamate Sodium Injection; Iothalamate Sodium Injection.

Diagnostic aid, radiopaque (urinary tract disorders)—Iothalamate Meglumine Injection; Iothalamate Meglumine and Iothalamate Sodium Injection; Iothalamate Sodium Injection.

Diagnostic aid, radiopaque (joint disease)—Iothalamate Meglumine Injection.

## Indications

Note: Bracketed information in the *Indications* section refers to uses that are not included in U.S. product labeling.

**Accepted**
Intravascular:
  Angiocardiography—Iothalamate meglumine and iothalamate sodium injection and iothalamate sodium injection are indicated to visualize lesions or malformations of the heart and obstructions or anomalies of the major thoracic blood vessels.
  Angiography
  Arteriography or
  Venography—Iothalamate is indicated to visualize specific regions of the vascular system and blood flow in these areas to help in the diagnosis and evaluation of neoplasms (known or suspected) or vascular diseases (congenital or acquired) that may cause changes in normal vascular anatomy or physiology. Iothalamate meglumine injection is indicated for use in cerebral angiography, peripheral arteriography or venography, arterial digital subtraction angiography[1], and intravenous digital subtraction angiography. Iothalamate meglumine and iothalamate sodium injection is indicated for use in selective coronary arteriography, selective renal arteriography, and in intravenous digital subtraction angiography.
  The iothalamate meglumine and iothalamate sodium injection is *not* indicated for cerebral angiography by direct injection into the carotid or vertebral arteries because of its high concentration and viscosity.
  Aortography—Iothalamate meglumine and iothalamate sodium injection and iothalamate sodium injection are indicated to visualize the aorta and its major branches. However, the injection of iothalamate meglumine and iothalamate sodium is preferred because it generally causes less severe hemodynamic, neurotoxic, and cardiotoxic effects than the individual injection of iothalamate sodium.

Body imaging, computed tomographic—Iothalamate meglumine injection and iothalamate sodium injection are indicated for enhancement of computed tomographic scans of the body (CT of the body) performed for the detection and evaluation of lesions in the liver, pancreas, kidneys, abdominal aorta, mediastinum, abdominal cavity, and retroperitoneal space.

Brain imaging, computed tomographic—Iothalamate meglumine injection, iothalamate meglumine and iothalamate sodium injection, and iothalamate sodium injection are indicated for enhancement of computed tomographic scans of the brain (CT of the brain) to determine the presence and extent of neoplasms or other lesions such as cerebral infarction or infection.

Urography, excretory—Iothalamate meglumine injection, iothalamate meglumine and iothalamate sodium injection, and iothalamate sodium injection are indicated in excretion urography to evaluate abnormalities of the urinary tract such as urinary tract obstructions.

[Splenoportography][1]—Iothalamate is used for splenoportography to determine the site of the portal obstruction or to visualize collateral pathways of blood flow or esophageal varices in patients with portal hypertension or portal venous obstruction. It should be noted that splenoportography is being replaced by other procedures in which the portal system may be evaluated by late films of the celiac and superior mesenteric arterial systems (their venous phases). In other cases, it is being replaced by direct portography via the transhepatic route.

Intraductal:

Cholangiography, direct, operative—Iothalamate meglumine injection is indicated during surgery to visualize the biliary ducts and to evaluate the cause and location of biliary obstructions such as calculi or strictures, and after surgery to rule out the presence of retained calculi.

Cholangiography, direct, postoperative T-tube—Iothalamate meglumine injection is indicated to visualize, and thus ensure the patency of, the biliary ducts before removal of a surgically placed T-tube.

Cholangiography, percutaneous transhepatic—Iothalamate meglumine injection is indicated for percutaneous transhepatic cholangiography, which is used in *some* patients to determine the cause and site of biliary obstruction when other diagnostic examinations of the biliary system have not provided the needed information.

Cholangiopancreatography, endoscopic retrograde—Iothalamate meglumine injection is indicated in *some* patients with known or suspected pancreatic or biliary disease to visualize the pancreatic duct and/or common bile duct.

Intrasynovial:

Arthrography—Iothalamate meglumine injection is indicated for use in arthrography in the diagnosis of post-traumatic or degenerative joint disease or synovial rupture, for visualization of communicating bursae or cysts, and meniscography.

---

[1]Not included in Canadian product labeling.

## Pharmacology/Pharmacokinetics

### Physicochemical characteristics
Molecular weight—Iothalamate meglumine: 809.13.
Iothalamate sodium; 635.90.
Osmolality—High. The osmolality of iothalamate injections ranges from 600 to 2400 mOsmol per kg of water

### Mechanism of action/Effect
Organic iodine compounds block x-rays as they pass through the body, thereby allowing body structures containing iodine to be delineated in contrast to those structures that do not contain iodine. The degree of opacity produced by these compounds is directly proportional to the total amount (concentration and volume) of the iodinated contrast agent in the path of the x-rays. Iothalamate's distribution in and elimination from the body as iodinated ion allow the visualization of the internal structures in the path of its flow.

### Other actions/effects
Anticoagulant activity (inhibitory effect on platelet aggregation and blood clotting); vasodilating effects.

### Distribution
Intravascular—Rapidly distributed throughout extracellular fluid following intravascular administration.

### Protein binding
Low.
Iothalamate meglumine—1 to 4%.
Iothalamate sodium—8 to 27%.

### Half-life
Distribution (alpha phase)—10 minutes.
Elimination (beta phase)—90 minutes.

### Time to peak concentration
Immediate, after intravascular administration. Concentration falls rapidly as a result of flow-induced dilution within the vascular compartment.

### Time to peak opacification
Angiography—
Immediate, after intravascular administration.
Urography—
Renal parenchyma including the renal cortex: 1 minute following rapid injection of contrast media. Peak opacification is directly dependent on the peak plasma iodine concentration and the glomerular filtration rate of the patient's kidney.
Calyces, pelves, and ureters: 10 to 15 minutes after bolus injection of contrast media. Peak opacification is dependent on both the final urinary iodine concentration and the volume of urine within the respective regions of the urinary tract.

### Elimination
Renal—
Normal renal function: > 90% of intravascular dose eliminated within 24 hours via glomerular filtration.
Fecal—
Normal renal function: < 2% of intravascular dose.
Severe renal function impairment: Elimination in the feces via biliary tract may become a primary route.
In dialysis—
Removed by peritoneal dialysis or hemodialysis.

## Precautions to Consider

### Cross-sensitivity and/or related problems
Patients sensitive to iodine or other iodinated contrast media may be sensitive to iothalamate also.

### Carcinogenicity/Mutagenicity
Long-term animal studies to evaluate carcinogenic or mutagenic potential of iothalamate have not been performed.

### Pregnancy/Reproduction
Pregnancy—Iothalamate crosses the placenta and is evenly distributed in fetal tissue. Adequate and well-controlled studies in humans have not been done. However, risk-benefit must be considered since other organically bound–iodine containing preparations administered near term by intra-amniotic injection have caused hypothyroidism in some newborns.
Also, elective contrast radiography of the abdomen is usually not recommended during pregnancy because of the risks to the fetus from radiation exposure.
Studies in animals have not shown that iothalamate causes teratogenic effects in the fetus.
FDA Pregnancy Category B.

### Breast-feeding
Although problems in humans have not been documented, temporary discontinuation of breast-feeding is recommended for at least 24 hours following iothalamate administration since iothalamate is distributed unchanged into breast milk.

### Pediatrics
Convulsions are more likely to occur in infants than in other age groups with administration of iothalamate meglumine and iothalamate sodium injection, and iothalamate sodium injection for angiocardiography, especially after repeated administration.
Difficulty in breathing, unusually slow or irregular heartbeat, and unusual feeling of tiredness and depression are more likely to occur in cyanotic infants during angiocardiography with administration of iothalamate meglumine and iothalamate sodium injection and iothalamate sodium injection.
Dehydration and/or the risk of renal failure may be exacerbated by iothalamate in infants and young children, especially those with polyuria, oliguria, diabetes, or pre-existing dehydration; adequate hydration is recommended before and following intravascular administration of iothalamate.

### Geriatrics
Although overall prevalence of adverse effects has been reported to be less in patients 50 years of age and older, the severity of the reactions may be greater in this age group than in younger patients.
Dehydration and/or the risk of renal failure may be exacerbated by iothalamate in geriatric patients, especially those with polyuria, oliguria, diabetes, or pre-existing dehydration; adequate hydration is recom-

mended before and following intravascular administration of iothalamate.

The elderly may be more sensitive to the effects of iothalamate on thyroid function. Iodine-induced thyrotoxicosis may occur 4 to 12 weeks following contrast radiography. Thyroid function monitoring may be needed in geriatric patients.

## Drug interactions and/or related problems

The following drug interactions and/or related problems have been selected on the basis of their potential clinical significance (possible mechanism in parentheses where appropriate)—not necessarily inclusive (» = major clinical significance):

Note: Combinations containing any of the following medications, depending on the amount present, may also interact with this medication.

Beta-adrenergic blocking agents
(concurrent intravascular administration of iothalamate with beta-adrenergic blocking agents may increase the risk of moderate to severe anaphylactoid reaction; hypotensive effects may be exacerbated; discontinuation of the beta-adrenergic blocking agent may be advisable before administration of contrast media in patients with other risk factors)

Cholecystographic agents, oral
(may increase the risk of renal toxicity when followed by intravenous iothalamate, especially in patients with hepatic function impairment)

Hypotension-producing medications, other (See *Appendix II*)
(the risk of severe hypotension may be increased if iothalamate is given concurrently with other medications that produce hypotension)

Interleukin-2
(incidence of delayed reactions to intravenous contrast media [e.g., hypersensitivity, fever, skin rash, flu-like symptoms, joint pain, flushing, pruritus, emesis, hypotension, dizziness occurring more than 1 hour after administration] may be increased in patients who have received interleukin-2; some symptoms may resemble a "recall" reaction to interleukin-2; supportive medical treatment may be necessary if symptoms are significant; there is some evidence that incidence is reduced if contrast media administration is delayed until 6 weeks after interleukin-2 administration)

Nephrotoxic medications, other (See *Appendix II*)
(concurrent intravascular administration of iothalamate with other nephrotoxic medications may increase the potential for nephrotoxicity)

Platelet aggregation inhibitors, other (See *Appendix II*)
(increased risk of bleeding may occur when these medications are used concurrently with iothalamate)

Vasopressors (See *Appendix II*)
(neurologic effects, including paraplegia, of iothalamate may be increased during aortography when iothalamate is administered after hypertensive agents used to increase contrast, due to contraction of vessels in the splanchnic circulation forcing more of the contrast material into the vessels leading to the spine and spinal cord)

## Diagnostic interference

The following have been selected on the basis of their potential clinical significance (possible effects in parentheses where appropriate)—not necessarily inclusive (» = major clinical significance):

With *other* diagnostic test results
Blood pool imaging
(imaging of blood pool may be impaired because of decreased technetium Tc 99m labeling of red blood cells caused by the intravascular administration of iothalamate)

Leukocyte counts and
Red cell counts
(may be decreased)

Phenolsulfonphthalein (PSP) excretion test
(test results may be affected, especially in patients with severely impaired renal function who are also given intravascular iothalamate; although iothalamate is excreted by glomerular filtration, in patients with impaired renal function iothalamate may be secreted by the renal tubules, thus resulting in decreased tubular excretion of PSP; therefore, concurrent use of intravascular iothalamate is not recommended in patients receiving a PSP excretion test)

Prothrombin time (PT) and
Thromboplastin time
(may be increased since ionic contrast media have been shown to inhibit all stages of coagulation)

Skeletal imaging
(possible renal and hepatic uptake of technetium Tc 99m medronate, technetium Tc 99m oxidronate, technetium Tc 99m pyrophosphate, and technetium Tc 99m [pyro- and trimeta-] phosphates if iothalamate is administered intravenously immediately after one of these technetium Tc 99m-labeled agents)

Thyroid function determinations and
Thyroid imaging
(administration of iothalamate, especially for excretory urography or angiography, may cause an increase of serum protein–bound iodine [PBI] and a decrease in radioactive iodine or pertechnetate ion uptake for up to 16 days; thyroid test should be performed prior to administration of iothalamate. Other thyroid function tests not based on measurement of iodine, such as resin triiodothyronine uptake, are not affected)

Urinalysis
(may produce abnormal results; urine should be collected prior to or at least 2 days after intravenous administration of iothalamate)

With physiology/laboratory test values
Blood urea nitrogen (BUN)
Creatinine, serum
Glucose, plasma
(concentrations may be increased transiently following selective renal arteriography)

(peak rise in serum creatinine is usually delayed, occurring 3 to 5 days following contrast media administration and generally returning to baseline values in 7 to 10 days)

Platelet aggregation
(may be decreased)

Protein, urine
(may be increased; false positive results may occur with Lowry's and sulphosalicylic assays, or with protein reagent strips)

## Medical considerations/Contraindications

The medical considerations/contraindications included here have been selected on the basis of their potential clinical significance (reasons given in parentheses where appropriate)—not necessarily inclusive (» = major clinical significance).

### *Risk-benefit should be considered when the following medical problems exist:*

*For all procedures requiring intravascular administration of iothalamate*
» Allergic reaction (anaphylaxis) to penicillins or to skin allergens, previous
(increased risk of anaphylactoid reaction)

» Allergies or asthma, history of
(increased risk of idiosyncratic response or anaphylactoid reaction)

» Cardiovascular disease, severe
(increased risk of cardiac arrest; increased risk of anaphylactoid reaction)

» Dehydration, especially associated with diabetes mellitus, azotemia, or multiple myeloma
(osmotic diuretic action of iothalamate may exacerbate dehydration and increase risk of acute renal failure)

Hyperthyroidism
(intravascular administration of iothalamate may precipitate thyroid storm)

» Pheochromocytoma
(intravascular administration of iothalamate may precipitate severe hypertension; amount of medium injected should be kept to a minimum and blood pressure should be monitored during the procedure; also, pretreatment with the alpha-adrenergic blocking agent phentolamine is recommended)

» Renal function impairment
(intravascular administration of iothalamate may increase risk of acute renal failure in the presence of renal insufficiency [serum creatinine ≥ 132.6 micromoles/L]; preventive measures recommended to prevent contrast-associated nephropathy include reducing the dose or volume of contrast medium administered, lengthening the time between radiologic procedures, volume expansion with 0.9% sodium chloride, using drug therapy such as furosemide or mannitol or calcium antagonists, and administering low osmolality contrast media; however, validity of some of these recommendations remains controversial)

» Seizures, recent
(increased risk for reoccurrence)

» Sensitivity to iodinated contrast media
(increased risk of anaphylactoid reaction in patients with history of prior reactions to contrast media)

Sickle cell disease
(intravascular administration of iothalamate may promote sickling in patients who are homozygous for sickle cell disease)

*For angiocardiography*
Angina, unstable
(increased risk of severe cardiac reaction)

Aortic stenosis
(use of iothalamate may cause decreased coronary artery perfusion due to the systemic hypotension produced)

Cardiac failure, incipient
(fluid overload, pressure changes, and expansion of blood volume may aggravate condition)

Cyanosis, in infants
(use of iothalamate may increase risk of apnea, bradycardia, arrhythmias, acidosis, and central nervous system [CNS] effects in cyanotic infants)

Mitral stenosis
(increased blood flow may produce an increase in the mitral diastolic pressure gradient)

Myocardial ischemia
(systemic hypotension and resultant diminished cardiac perfusion may aggravate condition and precipitate heart failure)

» Pulmonary hypertension, severe
(hypervolemic effect of iothalamate may further increase pulmonary artery and venous pressures due to an increase in cardiac output and a rise in left ventricular end-diastolic and left atrial pressures)

*For cerebral angiography*
Arteriosclerosis, advanced or
Cardiac decompensation or
Cerebral embolism, recent or
Hemorrhage, subarachnoid or
Hypertension, severe or
Migraine or
Senility or
Thrombosis
(hemodynamic changes produced may result in decreased cerebral perfusion, which may cause CNS damage)

» Homocystinuria
(procedure may increase risk of thrombosis and embolism)

*For coronary arteriography*
» Myocardial infarction
(procedure done within 4 weeks may increase risk of cardiac complications; administration of iothalamate or manipulation of catheter may cause ventricular fibrillation)

*For peripheral arteriography*
» Buerger's disease or
» Ischemia, severe, associated with ascending infection
(procedure may induce severe arterial or venous spasm)

*For percutaneous transhepatic cholangiography*
» Coagulation disorders, such as prolonged prothrombin times
(procedure may increase risk of internal bleeding)

*For CT of the brain*
» Cerebral neoplasms, primary or metastatic
(use of iothalamate may precipitate convulsions)

Hemorrhage, cranial subarachnoid
(intravascular administration of contrast media has been associated with death in some patients; however, a causal relationship has not been established)

*For excretory urography*
» Anuria or
» Diabetes
(increased risk of acute renal failure)

» Congestive heart failure
(intravenous infusion may produce an increased osmotic load and may aggravate condition)

*For peripheral venography*
Infection, local or
Ischemia, severe or
Phlebitis or
Thrombosis or
Venous stasis or

Venous system obstruction
(procedure may increase risk of thrombophlebitis, syncope, and ischemic changes)

*For endoscopic retrograde cholangiopancreatography*
» Cholangitis, severe, or
» Pancreatitis, acute
(increased risk of adverse effects)

*For splenoportography*
» Coagulation defects, such as prolonged prothrombin times and significant thrombocytopenia or
Inflammation of spleen
(procedure may increase risk of rupture of the spleen)

*For arthrography*
» Infection in or near joint to be examined
(procedure may increase risk of complications)

**Patient monitoring**
The following may be especially important in patient monitoring (other tests may be warranted in some patients, depending on condition; » = major clinical significance):

Blood pressure determinations
(may be required during examination, especially in patients with known or suspected pheochromocytoma or hemodynamic compromise or instability; also recommended for approximately 10 minutes following intra-arterial administration of iothalamate)

Electrocardiogram (ECG)
(recommended for early detection of arrhythmias during coronary arteriography and angiocardiography)

Thyroid function determinations
(iodine-induced thyrotoxicosis may occur 4 to 12 weeks following contrast radiography in geriatric patients; thyroid function monitoring may be needed)

# Side/Adverse Effects

Note: Adverse effects may vary directly with the concentration of the agent, the amount and technique used, and the underlying pathology. Increases in osmolality, volume, concentration, viscosity, and rate of administration of the solution may tend to increase the incidence and severity of adverse effects.

Most of the adverse effects appear during or within a few minutes after intravascular administration of iothalamate.

Thromboembolic events causing myocardial infarction and stroke have been reported rarely during angiographic procedures with ionic contrast media.

Acute renal failure has been reported following intravascular administration of iothalamate, especially in patients with diabetic nephropathy and in susceptible nondiabetic patients. Also, a higher incidence of contrast-induced renal failure has been associated with severe congestive heart failure, in patients who have had multiple contrast studies within 72 hours, those receiving large volumes of contrast agent, and those with elevated uric acid levels. Renal function may also be slightly and temporarily impaired following intravascular administration of iothalamate during selective renal arteriography.

Convulsions are more likely to occur in infants than in other age groups with the administration of iothalamate meglumine and iothalamate sodium injection and iothalamate sodium injection, especially after repeated administration.

Difficulty in breathing, unusually slow or irregular heartbeat, unusual feeling of tiredness, and mental depression are more likely to occur in cyanotic infants during angiocardiography with the administration of iothalamate meglumine and iothalamate sodium injection or iothalamate sodium injection.

Dehydration and/or the risk of renal failure may be exacerbated by iothalamate and in some cases may cause a shock-like state in infants and young children, and in geriatric, azotemic, and dehydrated or debilitated patients.

Cortical blindness has been reported rarely after cardiac angiography; vision has returned within 24 to 48 hours.

Death has occurred rarely during injection or 5 to 10 minutes after, mainly due to cardiac arrest, especially in patients with cardiovascular disease.

The following side/adverse effects have been selected on the basis of their potential clinical significance (possible signs and symptoms in parentheses where appropriate)—not necessarily inclusive:

**Those indicating need for medical attention**
Incidence less frequent or rare
    *For all procedures*
        ***Pseudo-allergic reaction*** (skin rash or hives; swelling of face or skin; swelling of the larynx; wheezing, tightness in chest, or troubled breathing)
        Note: *Pseudo-allergic reactions* are usually transient. However, they may be initial manifestations of more severe anaphylactoid reactions. The anaphylactoid reaction may progress to respiratory arrest and vasomotor collapse if appropriate treatment is not administered.

    *With intravascular administration*
        ***Bronchospasm or pulmonary edema*** (severe wheezing or troubled breathing); ***cardiotoxic effects, with decreased contractile force and ventricular fibrillation*** (irregular heartbeat); ***convulsions, especially in patients with convulsive disorders; swelling of the larynx; severe swelling of salivary glands; vasovagal effects, with bradycardia and hypotension*** (slow heartbeat; severe unusual tiredness or weakness)

**Those indicating need for medical attention only if they continue or are bothersome**
Incidence more frequent
    *With intravascular administration*
        ***Redness, swelling, or pain at injection site; vasodilation, arteriolar*** (unusual warmth and flushing of skin)
    *With intrasynovial administration*
        ***Joint pain or exacerbation of existing pain***
Incidence less frequent or rare
    *With all procedures*
        ***Psychosomatic reaction*** (changes in vision, chills, CNS effects [numbness, tingling, pain, or weakness in hands or feet], confusion, dizziness or lightheadedness, headache, increased sweating, increased watering of the mouth, nausea or vomiting, unusual tiredness or weakness)
        Note: *Psychosomatic reactions* are associated with patient anxiety, fatigue, inadequate hydration, and poor nutrition; usually self-limited and of short duration; may also be initial manifestations of more severe reaction.

## Patient Consultation

As an aid to patient consultation, refer to *Advice for the Patient, Radiopaque Agents (Diagnostic)*.

In providing consultation, consider emphasizing the following selected information (» = major clinical significance):

**Description of use**
    Action in the body: Concentrates in particular area of the body; visualization of radiopacity possible with x-rays

**Before having this test**
»  Conditions affecting use, especially:
    Sensitivity to iodine or other iodinated contrast media
    Pregnancy—Iothalamate crosses the placenta; risk to the fetus from radiation exposure; possibility of causing hypothyroidism in the newborn
    Breast-feeding—Distributed into breast milk; temporary discontinuation of breast-feeding for at least 24 hours is recommended
    Use in children—Increased risk of severe adverse reactions, especially in children with other medical problems; possible exacerbation of dehydration
    Use in the elderly—Increased risk of severe adverse effects; possible exacerbation of dehydration; increased risk of thyrotoxicosis
    Other medical problems, especially allergies or asthma (history of), anuria, cardiovascular disease, dehydration, diabetes mellitus, pheochromocytoma, previous allergic reaction to penicillins or to skin allergens, renal function impairment, and seizures

**Preparation for this test**
    Adequate intake of fluids to prevent dehydration
    Special diet, use of laxative, and/or other preparatory instructions may apply (for excretory urography); patient should inquire in advance
    Omitting any food for several hours before examination to prevent possible aspiration of gastric contents; moderate amounts of clear liquids may be permitted

**Precautions after having this test**
    Possible interference with future thyroid tests

**Side/adverse effects**
    Signs of possible side effects, especially pseudo-allergic reaction, convulsions, and cardiac or pulmonary problems that may occur within minutes of administration

## General Dosing Information

The manufacturer's package insert or other appropriate literature should be consulted for specific techniques and procedures for the administration of contrast media.

Sensitivity test doses are not usually recommended since severe or fatal reactions to contrast media are not predictable from a patient's history or a sensitivity test. On some occasions severe or fatal reactions have occurred with a test dose or with a full dose in patients who did not react to the test dose.

Pretreatment with corticosteroids or antihistamines has been used to minimize the incidence and severity of reactions in patients with a history of severe reactions to contrast media or with other high-risk conditions (e.g., asthma or history of allergies, positive allergy history to skin allergens or penicillin, dehydration, history of seizures, pheochromocytoma). In some studies, the additional use of ephedrine has been shown to be beneficial in preventing anaphylactoid reactions. When considering the use of a contrast agent, the following protocols are recommended:
For high-risk patients
    • Use of a high-osmolality contrast agent plus pretreatment with a corticosteroid (oral prednisone, 50 mg administered 13 hours, 7 hours, and 1 hour before procedure) and an antihistamine (intramuscular, intravenous, or oral diphenhydramine, 50 mg administered one hour before procedure); or
    • Use of a low-osmolality contrast agent if pretreatment is not feasible; or
    • Use of a low-osmolality contrast agent plus corticosteroid pretreatment.
For low-risk patients
    • Use of a high-osmolality contrast agent; or
    • Use of a high-osmolality contrast agent and corticosteroid pretreatment.

Adequate hydration is especially important in infants, young children, and geriatric or azotemic patients receiving intravascular iothalamate since dehydration may be further increased by the contrast medium.

Preparatory partial dehydration has been used to increase the urinary concentration of, and contrast produced by, iothalamate. However, in general, dehydration is no longer recommended because, with modern contrast media and recommended doses, it is no longer necessary and may do harm. Dehydration is particularly contraindicated in patients with multiple myeloma since it may predispose to irreversible precipitation of myeloma protein in the renal tubules. In these patients fluids should be administered and urine should be made alkaline.

Dosage and concentration of iothalamate for intravascular administration should be individualized and are usually in proportion to the size of the specific region of the vascular system to be visualized and the anticipated degree of hemodilution in the region.

No food should be ingested for several hours before an examination to prevent aspiration of gastric contents if vomiting occurs. However, moderate amounts of clear liquids are permissible and even recommended by some clinicians to prevent dehydration.

During and for at least 30 to 60 minutes after administration of contrast medium, the patient should be observed for possible severe reactions; competent personnel and emergency facilities should be available during this period.

Thromboembolic events causing myocardial infarction and stroke, reported rarely during angiographic procedures, may have resulted from atherosclerotic lesions rather than from coagulation of blood that has come in contact with the contrast agent outside the body. Nonetheless, it is recommended that risk factors for blood cell aggregation be minimized by performing the procedure in the shortest time possible, using plastic rather than glass syringes, and flushing catheters with heparinized saline solutions.

*For excretory urography*
Administration of a laxative at bedtime the evening before the examination is recommended to eliminate gas from the intestine.

*For splenoportography*
Fasting is recommended for several hours before the examination, in case the patient may require surgery on an emergency basis. Also, a local anesthetic and a sedative may be given before the procedure.

### For treatment of adverse effects

Recommended treatment consists of the following:

• For major or life-threatening reactions, careful monitoring of vital signs and emergency therapy, including artificial respiration with oxygen if needed for respiratory depression, and cardiac massage in the event of cardiac arrest.

• To restore blood pressure, administration of intravenous fluids and/or vasopressors. If hypotension necessitates the use of vasopressors, slow infusion of 0.008 to 0.012 mg per minute of norepinephrine or 0.1 to 0.18 mg per minute of phenylephrine, appropriately diluted. If hypotension is due to increased vagal activity (vasovagal reaction), intravenous administration of 1 mg of atropine, repeated in one to two hours if needed.

• Other specific treatment may include—

*Diphenhydramine:* For minor allergic-like reactions—An antihistamine such as diphenhydramine hydrochloride (except in epileptic patients) may be administered intravenously.

*Epinephrine:* For acute allergic-like or anaphylactoid reactions—Slow intravenous infusion of 0.1 mg of epinephrine (1:10,000).

For mild to moderate bronchospasm—0.1 to 0.2 mg of epinephrine (1:1000) may be administered subcutaneously, except in hypotension. In extreme emergency, 0.1 mg of epinephrine (1:10,000) may be given slowly by intravenous route, followed by a continuous intravenous infusion at an initial rate of 0.001 mg per minute; the rate may be increased to 0.004 mg per minute if necessary.

Patients on beta-adrenergic blocking agents should not receive epinephrine since they are at risk of excessive alpha-adrenergic stimulation, which may result in hypertension, reflex bradycardia, and heart block. In these patients, isoproterenol and norepinephrine are used instead of epinephrine to overcome bronchospasm and hypotension, respectively.

For cardiac arrest—0.1 to 1 mg of epinephrine may be administered by the intravenous route.

*Diazepam or phenobarbital:* To control convulsions—5 to 10 mg of diazepam by slow, intravenous administration or phenobarbital sodium intravenously or intramuscularly at a rate not to exceed 30 to 60 mg per minute may be given.

## Parenteral Dosage Forms

### IOTHALAMATE MEGLUMINE INJECTION USP

#### Usual adult and adolescent dose

Intravascular—

Angiography, cerebral:

For carotid angiography—

Percutaneous or via catheter, 5 to 12 mL of a solution containing the equivalent of 282 mg of iodine per mL, repeated as needed.

For vertebral angiography—

Percutaneous or via catheter, 4 to 10 mL of a solution containing the equivalent of 282 mg of iodine per mL, repeated as needed.

For retrograde brachial cerebral angiography—

Percutaneous, 35 to 50 mL of a solution containing the equivalent of 282 mg of iodine per mL as a single dose, administered rapidly into the brachial artery.

Angiography, by digital subtraction:

Arterial[1]—

Via catheter, as a solution containing the equivalent of 141 mg of iodine per mL, repeated as needed, but not to exceed a total dose of 250 mL, into the following:

Abdominal aorta: 10 to 30 mL.

Aortic arch: 15 to 30 mL.

Carotid or vertebral arteries: 3 to 10 mL.

Major branches of the aorta: 5 to 30 mL.

Subclavian and brachial arteries: 5 to 15 mL.

Intravenous—

Via catheter, 20 to 40 mL of a solution containing the equivalent of 282 mg of iodine per mL, repeated as needed.

Arteriography, peripheral:

Percutaneous or operative methods, 20 to 40 mL of a solution containing the equivalent of 282 mg of iodine per mL as a single dose, administered rapidly into the brachial artery in the arm or the femoral artery in the leg.

Venography, peripheral:

Upper or lower extremity—

Percutaneous, 20 to 40 mL of a solution containing the equivalent of 282 mg of iodine per mL per extremity, administered rapidly into a superficial vein of the forearm or hand or lateral side of the foot.

Lower extremity—

Percutaneous, 30 to 125 mL of a solution containing the equivalent of 202 mg of iodine per mL administered rapidly into a superficial vein on the lateral side of the foot.

Body imaging, computed tomographic:

Intravenous, rapid intravenous infusion, or combination of bolus injection and infusion, 200 to 250 mL of a solution containing the equivalent of 202 mg of iodine per mL; or a bolus injection of 25 to 50 mL of a solution containing the equivalent of 282 mg of iodine per mL.

Note: When the combination bolus injection and infusion technique is used, 50 to 100 mL bolus injection is followed by a rapid infusion of 100 to 150 mL.

Brain imaging, computed tomographic:

Intravenous, 2 mL per kg of body weight of a solution containing the equivalent of 282 mg of iodine per mL, not to exceed 150 mL.

Intravenous infusion, 200 to 300 mL of a solution containing the equivalent of 141 mg of iodine per mL administered rapidly; or 3 mL per kg of body weight of a solution containing the equivalent of 202 mg of iodine per mL, not to exceed 200 mL.

Urography, excretory:

Intravenous infusion, 2 to 3 mL per kg of body weight of a solution containing the equivalent of 202 mg of iodine per mL, not to exceed 200 mL, administered at a rate of 40 to 50 mL per minute; or 2 to 4 mL of a solution containing the equivalent of 141 mg of iodine per mL per kg of body weight, not to exceed 300 mL, administered at a rate of 50 mL per minute.

Note: Geriatric patients or patients with cardiac disease may require a slower infusion rate.

Intravenous, rapid, 30 to 60 mL of a solution containing the equivalent of 282 mg of iodine per mL administered within 30 to 90 seconds.

Intraductal—

Cholangiography, direct:

Operative and postoperative—Intraductal, 10 to 25 mL of a solution containing the equivalent of 141 mg or 282 mg of iodine per mL into the cystic duct or common bile duct.

Pancreatitis, acute—Intraductal, 5 to 10 mL of a solution containing the equivalent of 282 mg of iodine per mL.

Percutaneous transhepatic cholangiography—Percutaneous, 20 to 40 mL of a solution containing the equivalent of 282 mg of iodine per mL administered slowly into the biliary ducts.

Cholangiopancreatography, endoscopic retrograde:

Via catheter, as a solution containing the equivalent of 282 mg of iodine per mL—

For visualization of the common bile duct: 10 to 100 mL.

For visualization of the pancreatic duct: 2 to 10 mL.

Intrasynovial—

Arthrography:

Intrasynovial, as a solution containing the equivalent of 282 mg of iodine per mL—Knee, shoulder, or hip joint: 5 to 15 mL.

Shoulder, ankle: 5 to 10 mL.

Other joints: 1 to 4 mL.

#### Usual pediatric dose

Intravascular—

Angiography, cerebral:

Dosage must be individualized by physician in proportion to body weight.

Arteriography, peripheral—

Dosage must be individualized by physician in proportion to body weight.

Venography, peripheral—

Dosage must be individualized by physician in proportion to body weight.

Cholangiography, direct—

Dosage must be individualized by physician in proportion to body weight.

Cholangiography, percutaneous transhepatic—

Dosage must be individualized by physician in proportion to body weight.

Body imaging, computed tomographic—

Dosage must be individualized by physician in proportion to body weight.

Brain imaging, computed tomographic—

Intravenous infusion, 4 mL per kg of body weight of a solution containing the equivalent of 141 mg of iodine per mL, administered rapidly.

Urography, excretory—
   Intravenous, as a solution containing the equivalent of
      282 mg of iodine per mL:
      Children up to 14 years of age: 0.5 to 1 mL per kg
         of body weight.
      Children 14 years of age and over: See *Usual adult
         and adolescent dose.*
   Intravenous infusion, as a solution containing the equiv-
      alent of 202 mg of iodine per mL:
      Children up to 12 years of age: See *Usual adult and
         adolescent dose.*

Intrasynovial—
   Arthrography:
      Dosage must be individualized by physician in proportion to body
         weight.

## Usual geriatric dose
See *Usual adult and adolescent dose.*
Note: Geriatric patients may be more sensitive to the effects of the usual
   adult dose.

   In excretory urography, geriatric patients may require a slower infusion rate.

## Strength(s) usually available
U.S.—
   30% (300 mg per mL) of iothalamate meglumine with 14.1% (141 mg
      per mL) of iodine (Rx) [*Conray-30* (0.11 mg of edetate calcium
      disodium per mL)].
   43% (430 mg per mL) of iothalamate meglumine with 20.2% (202 mg
      per mL) of iodine (Rx) [*Conray-43* (0.11 mg of edetate calcium
      disodium per mL)].
   60% (600 mg per mL) of iothalamate meglumine with 28.2% (282 mg
      per mL) of iodine (Rx) [*Conray* (0.09 mg of edetate calcium di-
      sodium per mL)].
Canada—
   30% (300 mg per mL) of iothalamate meglumine with 14.1% (141 mg
      per mL) of iodine (Rx) [*Conray-30* (0.11 mg of edetate calcium
      disodium per mL)].
   43% (430 mg per mL) of iothalamate meglumine with 20.2% (202 mg
      per mL) of iodine (Rx) [*Conray-43* (0.11 mg of edetate calcium
      disodium per mL)].
   60% (600 mg per mL) of iothalamate meglumine with 28.2% (282 mg
      per mL) of iodine (Rx) [*Conray-60* (0.09 mg of edetate calcium
      disodium per mL)].

## Packaging and storage
Store below 30 °C (86 °F), unless otherwise specified by manufacturer.
Protect from light. Protect from freezing.

## Preparation of dosage form
A 30% solution (containing the equivalent of 141 mg of iodine per mL)
may be prepared from a 60% solution (containing the equivalent of
282 mg of iodine per mL) by dilution with 0.9% sodium chloride
injection.

## Stability
Crystals may form in the solution at very cold temperatures but are readily
redissolved by bringing the container of solution to room temperature
and gently shaking it.
Any unused portion remaining in the container should be discarded.

## Incompatibilities
Iothalamate meglumine injection is physically incompatible with promethazine hydrochloride injection.

# IOTHALAMATE MEGLUMINE AND IOTHALAMATE
# SODIUM INJECTION USP

## Usual adult and adolescent dose
Intravascular—
   Angiocardiography:
      Via catheter, 40 to 50 mL as a single dose, administered rapidly,
         within one to two seconds, into the chambers of the heart or
         associated blood vessels.
      Intravenous, 50 to 100 mL administered rapidly into a large pe-
         ripheral vein. Dose may be divided and administered bilaterally
         into the antecubital veins by simultaneous pressure injection.
   Angiography, by digital subtraction:
      Intravenous—
         Via catheter, 20 to 60 mL, may be repeated as necessary.
      Note: For central catheter injections, a power injector with an
         injection rate between 10 and 30 mL per second is usu-
         ally used.

         For peripheral injections, rates of 12 to 20 mL per sec-
         ond should be used, depending on size of vein.

Flushing of arm vein is recommended immediately fol-
   lowing injection using 20 to 25 mL of 5% dextrose in
   water or normal saline.
Arteriography:
   Nonselective coronary arteriography—
      Via catheter, 30 to 50 mL. One-half of the usual dose may be
         administered at the sinus of Valsalva on either side.
   Selective coronary arteriography—
      Via catheter, 4 to 7 mL injected into a coronary artery; may
         be administered into each coronary artery and repeated.
   Renal arteriography—
      Selective: Via catheter, 4 to 8 mL administered into the renal
         artery; may be repeated.
      By aortography: Via catheter, 10 to 25 mL administered into
         the aorta above the renal arteries.
Aortography:
   Retrograde or antegrade catheter method, 20 to 50 mL.
   Intravenous, 1 mL per kg of body weight. Dose may be divided
      equally for simultaneous bilateral injection.
   Translumbar, 15 to 30 mL.
Brain imaging, computed tomographic:
   Intravenous, 1.5 mL per kg of body weight, not to exceed 100 mL,
      administered rapidly.
Urography, excretory:
   Intravenous, 25 to 50 mL administered rapidly over a period of 30
      to 90 seconds.
   Note: In patients with reduced renal function, repeat urography is
      not recommended for at least 48 hours because of the pos-
      sibility of temporary oliguria or anuria.

## Usual pediatric dose
Intravascular—
   Angiocardiography:
      Children up to 14 years of age: Via catheter, 0.5 to 1 mL per kg
         of body weight as a single dose, administered rapidly, within
         one to two seconds, into a large peripheral vein or into the
         chambers of the heart or associated blood vessels.
      Note: In infants up to 2 months of age, the total dose administered
         should not exceed 3 mL per kg of body weight.

         In infants weighing less than 7 kg, especially in those with
         right-heart strain or failure and with decreased or nonfunc-
         tional pulmonary vascular beds, repeated injections are not
         recommended.
   Arteriography:
      Dosage must be individualized by physician in proportion to body
         weight.
   Aortography:
      Retrograde or antegrade catheter method—See *Usual adult and
         adolescent dose.*
      Intravenous—See *Usual adult and adolescent dose.*
      Translumbar—Dosage must be individualized by physician in pro-
         portion to body weight.
   Brain imaging, computed tomographic:
      See *Usual adult and adolescent dose.*
   Urography, excretory:
      Intravenous, 0.5 mL per kg of body weight administered rapidly.

## Usual geriatric dose
See *Usual adult and adolescent dose.*
Note: Geriatric patients may be more sensitive to the effects of the usual
   adult dose.

## Strength(s) usually available
U.S.—
   52% (520 mg per mL) of iothalamate meglumine and 26% (260 mg
      per mL) of iothalamate sodium with 40% (400 mg per mL) of
      iodine (Rx) [*Vascoray* (0.11 mg of edetate calcium disodium per
      mL)].
Canada—
   Not commercially available.

## Packaging and storage
Store below 40 °C (104 °F), preferably between 15 and 30 °C (59 and 86
°F), unless otherwise specified by manufacturer. Protect from light.
Protect from freezing.

## Stability
Crystals may form in the solution at very cold temperatures but are readily
redissolved by bringing the container of solution to room temperature
and gently shaking it.
Any unused portion remaining in the container should be discarded.

**Incompatibilities**

Iothalamate meglumine and iothalamate sodium injection is physically incompatible with promethazine hydrochloride injection.

## IOTHALAMATE SODIUM INJECTION USP

**Usual adult and adolescent dose**

Intravascular—

Angiocardiography:

Via catheter, 40 to 50 mL of a solution containing the equivalent of 400 mg or 480 mg of iodine per mL as a single dose, administered rapidly, within one to two seconds, into the chambers of the heart or associated blood vessels.

Intravenous, 50 to 100 mL of a solution containing the equivalent of 400 mg or 480 mg of iodine per mL administered rapidly, within one to two seconds, into a large peripheral vein. Dose may be divided and administered bilaterally into the antecubital veins by simultaneous pressure injection.

Arteriography, renal, by aortography:

Via catheter, 10 to 25 mL of the solution containing the equivalent of 400 mg or 480 mg of iodine per mL.

Aortography: As a solution containing the equivalent of 400 mg or 480 mg of iodine per mL:

Retrograde or antegrade catheter method, 20 to 50 mL as a single dose.

Intravenous, 1 mL per kg of body weight. Dose may be divided equally for simultaneous bilateral injection.

Translumbar, 20 mL.

Body imaging, computed tomographic:

Intravenous, rapid bolus injection, 25 to 60 mL of a solution containing the equivalent of 400 mg of iodine per mL.

Brain imaging, computed tomographic:

Intravenous, 1.5 mL per kg of body weight of a solution containing the equivalent of 400 mg of iodine per mL, not to exceed 100 mL, administered rapidly.

Urography, excretory:

Intravenous, 30 to 60 mL of a solution containing the equivalent of 325 mg of iodine per mL or 25 to 50 mL of a solution containing the equivalent of 400 mg of iodine per mL, administered rapidly.

Note: In patients with reduced renal function, repeat urography is not recommended for at least 48 hours because of the possibility of temporary oliguria or anuria.

**Usual pediatric dose**

Intravascular—

Angiocardiography:

Via catheter, 0.5 to 1 mL per kg of body weight of a solution containing the equivalent of 400 mg or 480 mg of iodine per mL, as a single dose, administered rapidly, within one to two seconds, into a large peripheral vein or into the chambers of the heart or associated blood vessels.

Note: In infants up to 2 months of age, the total dose administered should not exceed 3 mL per kg of body weight.

In infants weighing less than 7 kg, especially in those with right-heart strain or failure and with decreased or nonfunctional pulmonary vascular beds, repeated injections are not recommended.

Arteriography, renal, by aortography:

Dosage must be individualized by physician in proportion to body weight.

Aortography: As a solution containing the equivalent of 400 mg or 480 mg of iodine per mL:

Retrograde or antegrade catheter method: Dosage must be individualized by physician in proportion to body weight.

Intravenous: 1 mL per kg of body weight.

Translumbar: Dosage must be individualized by physician in proportion to body weight.

Body imaging, computed tomographic:

Dosage must be individualized by physician in proportion to body weight.

Brain imaging, computed tomographic:

Intravenous, 1.5 mL per kg of body weight of a solution containing the equivalent of 400 mg of iodine per mL, not to exceed 100 mL, administered rapidly.

Urography, excretory:

Intravenous, 0.5 mL per kg of body weight of a solution containing the equivalent of 325 mg or 400 mg of iodine per mL, administered rapidly.

**Usual geriatric dose**

See *Usual adult and adolescent dose.*

Note: Geriatric patients may be more sensitive to the effects of the usual adult dose.

**Strength(s) usually available**

U.S.—

54.3% (543 mg per mL) of iothalamate sodium with 32.5% (325 mg per mL) of iodine (Rx) [*Conray-325* (0.135 mg of edetate calcium disodium per mL)].

66.8% (668 mg per mL) of iothalamate sodium with 40% (400 mg per mL) of iodine (Rx) [*Conray-400*].

80% (800 mg per mL) of iothalamate sodium with 48% (480 mg per mL) of iodine (Rx) [*Angio-Conray* (0.11 mg of edetate calcium disodium per mL)].

Canada—

54.3% (543 mg per mL) of iothalamate sodium with 32.5% (325 mg per mL) of iodine (Rx) [*Conray-325* (0.11 mg of edetate calcium disodium per mL)].

**Packaging and storage**

Store below 40 °C (104 °F), preferably between 15 and 30 °C (59 and 86 °F), unless otherwise specified by manufacturer. Protect from light. Protect from freezing.

**Stability**

Crystals may form in the solution at very cold temperatures but are readily redissolved by bringing the container of solution to room temperature and gently shaking it.

Any unused portion remaining in the container should be discarded.

**Incompatibilities**

Iothalamate sodium injection is physically incompatible with promethazine hydrochloride injection.

---

[1]Not included in Canadian product labeling.

## Selected Bibliography

Almén T. Contrast media: the relation of chemical structure, animal toxicity and adverse clinical effects. Am J Cardiol 1990; 66: 2F-8F.

Brinker JA. Selection of a contrast agent in the cardiac catheterization laboratory. Am J Cardiol 1990; 66: 26F-33F.

---

Revised: 06/29/95

---

# IOVERSOL   Systemic

---

VA CLASSIFICATION (Primary): DX101

Note: For a listing of dosage forms and brand names by country availability, see *Dosage Forms* section(s). For a listing of brand names for the articles in this monograph, refer to the General Index.

## Category

Note: Ioversol is a nonionic radiopaque contrast agent.

Diagnostic aid, radiopaque (cardiac disease); Diagnostic aid, radiopaque (vascular disease); Diagnostic aid, radiopaque (urinary tract disorders); Diagnostic aid, radiopaque contrast enhancer in computed tomography; Diagnostic aid, radiopaque (peritoneal disorders); Diagnostic aid, radiopaque (biliary tract disorders); Diagnostic aid, radiopaque (joint disease).

## Indications

Note: Bracketed information in the *Indications* section refers to uses that are not included in U.S. product labeling.

**Accepted**

Intravascular:

Angiocardiography—Ioversol is indicated in angiocardiography (coronary arteriography and left ventriculography) to visualize lesions or malformations of the heart and obstructions or anomalies of the major thoracic vessels.

Angiography

Aortography

Arteriography or

Venography—Ioversol is indicated in aortography, arteriography (cerebral, peripheral, visceral, renal), peripheral venography (phlebography), and intra-arterial and intravenous digital subtraction angiography to visualize specific regions of the vascular system and blood flow in such areas to help in the diagnosis and evaluation of neoplasms (known or suspected) or vascular diseases (congenital or acquired) that may cause changes in normal vascular anatomy or physiology.

Urography, excretory—Ioversol is indicated for excretion urography to evaluate abnormalities of the urinary tract such as urinary tract obstructions.

Brain imaging, computed tomographic—Ioversol is indicated for enhancement of computed tomographic images (CT of the brain) to determine the presence and extent of neoplasms, such as gliomas, glioblastomas, astrocytomas, oligodendrogliomas, ependymomas, medulloblastomas, meningiomas, neuromas, pinealomas, pituitary adenomas, craniopharyngiomas, germinomas, and metastatic lesions, or nonneoplastic lesions such as cerebral infarction or infection. Also, depending on the iodine content of the circulating blood pool, arteriovenous malformations and aneurysms may show contrast enhancement.

Body imaging, computed tomographic—Ioversol is indicated for enhancement of computed tomographic images (CT of the body) to detect and evaluate lesions in the liver, pancreas, kidneys, aorta, mediastinum, pelvis, abdominal cavity, and retroperitoneal space.

[Herniography][1]—Ioversol is used in herniography in adults.

Intraductal:

[Pancreatography, endoscopic retrograde][1] and
[Cholangiopancreatography, endoscopic retrograde][1]—Ioversol is used in adults in endoscopic retrograde pancreatography and endoscopic retrograde cholangiopancreatography for visualization of all portions of the biliary tree.

Intrasynovial:

[Arthrography][1]—Ioversol is used for arthrography in the diagnosis of post-traumatic or degenerative joint diseases or synovial rupture, for visualization of communicating bursae or cysts, and in meniscography.

---

[1]Not included in Canadian product labeling.

## Pharmacology/Pharmacokinetics

### Physicochemical characteristics

Molecular weight—807.12.

Osmolality—Low. The osmolalities of the injections with iodine concentrations of 160, 240, 300, 320, and 350 mg per mL are 355, 502, 651, 702, and 792 mOsmol per kg of water, respectively

Note: Ioversol injection is hypertonic as compared to plasma (approximately 1.2 to 2.5 times the osmolality of plasma).

### Mechanism of action/Effect

Organic iodine compounds block x-rays as they pass through the body, thereby allowing body structures containing iodine to be delineated in contrast to those structures that do not contain iodine. The degree of opacity produced by these compounds is directly proportional to the total amount (concentration and volume) of the iodinated contrast agent in the path of the x-rays. After intravascular administration, ioversol makes opaque those vessels in its path of flow, allowing visualization of the internal structures until significant hemodilution occurs.

### Distribution

Rapidly distributed throughout extracellular fluid following intravenous administration. No significant deposition in tissues. Does not cross blood-brain barrier, but accumulates within the interstitial tissues of malignant tumors and other lesions of the brain due to alterations in blood-brain barrier permeability caused by the tumor or lesions.

### Protein binding

Low (9 to 13%).

### Half-life

Elimination—Approximately 2 hours (with normal renal function).

### Time to peak serum concentration:

Immediate, but concentration falls rapidly within 5 to 10 minutes as ioversol is distributed throughout the extravascular compartment.

### Time to peak opacification:

Renal calyces and pelves—5 to 15 minutes (with normal renal function).
CT scan (dynamic)—30 to 90 seconds.

### Elimination

Renal—More than 95% of dose is eliminated unchanged in 24 hours. In patients with impaired renal function, the elimination of ioversol is prolonged depending upon the degree of impairment.

Fecal—3 to 9%.

## Precautions to Consider

### Cross-sensitivity and/or related problems

Patients sensitive to iodine or other iodinated contrast media may be sensitive to ioversol also.

### Carcinogenicity/Mutagenicity

Long-term animal studies to evaluate carcinogenic or mutagenic potential of ioversol have not been performed.

### Pregnancy/Reproduction

Pregnancy—Adequate and well-controlled studies in humans have not been done. However, other organically bound iodine–containing preparations administered near term, by intra-amniotic injection, have caused hypothyroidism in some neonates.

Also, elective contrast radiography of the abdomen is usually not recommended during pregnancy because of the risks to the fetus from radiation exposure.

Studies in animals have not shown that ioversol causes harm to the fetus.

FDA Pregnancy Category B.

### Breast-feeding

Although it is not known whether ioversol is distributed into breast milk, temporary discontinuation of breast-feeding is recommended for at least 24 hours following administration of ioversol.

### Pediatrics

Appropriate studies on the relationship of age to the effects of ioversol have not been performed in pediatric patients. However, it is known that pediatric patients, especially those with asthma, allergies, congestive heart failure, or serum creatinine greater than 1.5 mg per dL or those up to 12 months of age, exhibit an increased risk of having severe adverse reactions to radiopaque contrast media.

Dehydration and/or the risk of renal failure may be exacerbated by ioversol in infants and young children, especially those with polyuria, oliguria, diabetes, or pre-existing dehydration; adequate hydration is recommended before and following administration of ioversol.

### Geriatrics

Diagnostic studies performed to date have not demonstrated geriatrics-specific problems that would limit the usefulness of ioversol in the elderly. However, elderly patients are more likely to have age-related renal function impairment, which may require lower dosage in patients receiving ioversol.

Dehydration and/or the risk of renal failure may be exacerbated by ioversol in geriatric patients, especially those with polyuria, oliguria, diabetes, or pre-existing dehydration; adequate hydration is recommended before and following administration of ioversol.

Elderly patients may be more sensitive to the effects of ioversol on thyroid function. Iodine-induced thyrotoxicosis may occur 4 to 12 weeks following contrast radiography. Thyroid function monitoring may be needed in geriatric patients.

### Drug interactions and/or related problems

The following drug interactions and/or related problems have been selected on the basis of their potential clinical significance (possible mechanism in parentheses where appropriate)—not necessarily inclusive (» = major clinical significance):

Note: Combinations containing any of the following medications, depending on the amount present, may also interact with this medication.

Beta-adrenergic blocking agents

(concurrent intravascular administration of ioversol with beta-adrenergic blocking agents may increase the risk of moderate to severe anaphylactoid reaction and may exacerbate hypotensive effects; discontinuation of the beta-adrenergic blocking agent before administration of contrast media may be advisable in patients with other risk factors)

Cholecystographic agents, oral

(may increase the risk of renal toxicity when closely followed by intravascular ioversol, especially in patients with hepatic function impairment)

Interleukin-2

(incidence of delayed reactions to intravenous contrast media [e.g., hypersensitivity, fever, skin rash, flu-like symptoms, joint pain, flushing, pruritus, emesis, hypotension, dizziness occurring more than 1 hour after administration] may be increased in patients who have received interleukin-2; some symptoms may resemble a "recall" reaction to interleukin-2; supportive medical treatment may be necessary if symptoms are significant; delaying contrast media administration until 6 weeks after administration of interleukin-2 may reduce incidence of these reactions)

Hypotension-producing medications, other (See *Appendix II*)
(the risk of severe hypotension may be increased if ioversol is given concurrently with other medications that produce hypotension)

Nephrotoxic medications, other (See *Appendix II*)
(concurrent intravascular administration of ioversol with other nephrotoxic medications may increase the potential for nephrotoxicity)

Vasopressors
(increased risk of neurologic effects when followed by arterial injection of ioversol)

**Diagnostic interference**

The following have been selected on the basis of their potential clinical significance (possible effect in parentheses where appropriate)—not necessarily inclusive (» = major clinical significance):

With *other* diagnostic test results

Blood pool imaging
(intravascular administration of ioversol decreases technetium Tc 99m–labeling of red blood cells, which may impair blood pool imaging)

Prothrombin time (PT) and
Thromboplastin time
(may be increased with ioversol since *in vitro* studies with animal blood have shown other nonionic contrast media to slightly inhibit all stages of coagulation)

Skeletal imaging
(intravenous administration of ioversol immediately after administration of technetium Tc 99m medronate, technetium Tc 99m oxidronate, technetium Tc 99m pyrophosphate, and technetium Tc 99m [pyro- and trimeta-] phosphates may cause renal and hepatic uptake of these technetium Tc 99m–labeled agents)

Thyroid function determinations and
Thyroid imaging
(intravascular or intrathecal administration of ioversol may alter serum protein–bound iodine [PBI] concentrations and radioactive iodine or pertechnetate ion uptake for up to 2 weeks; thyroid test should be performed prior to administration of ioversol. Other thyroid function tests not based on measurement of iodine, such as resin triiodothyronine uptake, may not be affected)

With physiology/laboratory test values

Creatinine, serum
(concentration may be increased with ioversol since temporary increases of serum creatinine have occurred with other nonionic contrast media)

**Medical considerations/Contraindications**

The medical considerations/contraindications included here have been selected on the basis of their potential clinical significance (reasons given in parentheses where appropriate)—not necessarily inclusive (» = major clinical significance).

***Risk-benefit should be considered when the following medical problems exist:***

*For all procedures (especially those requiring intravascular administration)*

Allergic reaction (anaphylaxis) to penicillins or to skin allergens, previous
(although the risk of anaphylactoid reaction may be less with ioversol than with high-osmolality contrast agents, caution is recommended when administering ioversol to patients who have had a previous reaction to penicillins or to skin allergens)

Allergies or asthma, history of
(although the risk of idiosyncratic response or anaphylactoid reaction may be less with ioversol than with high-osmolality contrast agents, caution is recommended when administering ioversol to patients with a history of allergies or asthma)

» Dehydration, especially associated with pre-existing renal disease, advanced vascular disease, or diabetes mellitus, or in pediatric and elderly patients
(osmotic diuretic action of ioversol may exacerbate dehydration and increase risk of acute renal failure)

Hyperthyroidism
(administration of ioversol may precipitate thyroid storm)

» Pheochromocytoma
(use of ioversol may precipitate severe hypertension; amount of ioversol injected should be kept to a minimum and blood pressure should be monitored during the procedure; also, pretreatment with the alpha-adrenergic blocking agent phentolamine is recommended)

Renal function impairment, severe
(elimination of ioversol may be delayed; although the risk of contrast-induced nephrotoxicity in the presence of renal insufficiency [serum creatinine ≥ 132.6 micromoles/L] may be less with ioversol than with high-osmolality contrast agents, caution is recommended)

» Sensitivity to iodinated contrast media
(increased risk of anaphylactoid reaction in patients with history of prior reaction to contrast media)

Sickle cell disease
(ioversol may promote sickling in patients who are homozygous for sickle cell disease; however, sickling potential of ioversol is less than that of high-osmolality ionic agents)

*For angiocardiography*

Angina, unstable
(increased risk of a severe cardiac reaction)

Cardiac failure, incipient
(fluid overload, pressure changes, and expansion of blood volume may aggravate condition)

Pulmonary hypertension, severe
(hypervolemic effect of ioversol may further increase pulmonary artery and venous pressures due to an increase in cardiac output and a rise in left ventricular end-diastolic and left atrial pressures)

*For aortography*

Abdominal compression or
Hypertension or
Hypotension or
Obstruction, aortoiliac and/or femoral artery
(increased risk of serious neurological complications, including paraplegia)

*For cerebral arteriography*

Arteriosclerosis, advanced or
Cardiac decompensation or
Cerebral embolism, recent or
Hypertension, severe or
Migraine or
Senility or
Thrombosis, recent
(increased risk of vessel occlusion)

» Homocystinuria
(procedure may increase risk of thrombosis and embolism)

*For peripheral arteriography*

» Buerger's disease
(procedure may induce severe arterial or venous spasms)

» Ischemia, severe, associated with ascending infection

*For venography*

Infection, local or
Ischemia, severe or
Phlebitis or
Thrombosis or
Venous stasis or
Venous system obstruction
(procedure may cause venous inflammatory changes, thrombosis, or gangrene; irrigation with normal saline is recommended following the procedure to decrease the risk of thrombosis)

*For excretory urography*

» Anuria or
» Diabetes mellitus
(administration of ioversol may increase risk of acute renal failure)

*For arthrography*

» Infection in or near joint to be examined
(procedure may increase risk of complications)

**Patient monitoring**

The following may be especially important in patient monitoring (other tests may be warranted in some patients, depending on condition; » = major clinical significance):

Blood pressure determinations
(may be required during procedure, especially in patients with known or suspected pheochromocytoma or hemodynamic compromise or instability)

Thyroid function determinations
(iodine-induced thyrotoxicosis may occur 4 to 12 weeks following contrast radiography in geriatric patients; thyroid function monitoring may be needed)

# Side/Adverse Effects

Note: Adverse effects may vary directly with the concentration of the agent, the amount and technique used, and the underlying pathology. Increases in osmolality, volume, concentration, viscosity, and rate of administration of the solution may increase the incidence and severity of adverse effects.

Most of the adverse effects are usually self-limited and of short duration.

Overall incidence of adverse effects with nonionic contrast agents, such as ioversol, has been reported to be less than with ionic contrast agents.

Nonionic contrast media, such as ioversol, have been reported to produce fewer and less severe alterations in cardiac hemodynamics and electrocardiograms than standard ionic contrast agents during cardiac angiography.

Low-osmolality contrast agents, such as ioversol, are reported to cause less heat and pain on injection than high-osmolality agents, such as diatrizoates and iothalamate.

Thromboembolic events causing myocardial infarction and stroke have been reported during angiographic procedures with nonionic contrast media; however, these events appear to be technique-related.

Dehydration may be exacerbated by the osmotic diuretic action of the hypertonic contrast solutions of ioversol, in some cases resulting in a shock-like state, following intravascular administration of ioversol in geriatric, azotemic, and dehydrated or debilitated patients.

Transient global amnesia has been reported in 2 patients after cerebral angiography, in which 20 mL of another low-osmolality nonionic contrast agent (containing the equivalent of 240 mg of iodine per mL) was administered into the ascending aorta. The possibility that ioversol may cause a similar response must be considered.

The following side/adverse effects have been selected on the basis of their potential clinical significance (possible signs and symptoms in parentheses where appropriate)—not necessarily inclusive:

## Those indicating need for medical attention
Incidence rare
*With all procedures*
    **Pseudo-allergic reaction** (skin rash or hives, stuffy nose, swelling of face or skin, thickening of the tongue, wheezing, tightness in chest, or troubled breathing)
    Note: *Pseudo-allergic reactions* are usually transient. However, they may be initial manifestations of more severe anaphylactic reactions. The anaphylactoid reaction may progress to respiratory arrest and vasomotor collapse if appropriate treatment is not administered.

*With intravascular administration*
    **Angina pectoris** (chest pain); **arrhythmia, transient, and/or bradycardia** (slow or irregular heartbeat); **CNS effects** (confusion, hallucinations); **hypertension; hypotension** (severe and unusual tiredness or weakness); **infarct, cerebral** (severe headache, blurred vision)

## Those indicating need for medical attention only if they continue or are bothersome
Incidence less frequent or rare
*With intravascular administration*
    **Blurred vision or other changes in vision; dizziness or lightheadedness; headache, mild to moderate; nausea and vomiting, mild to moderate; respiratory problems** (coughing, sneezing, stuffy nose); **unusual feeling of warmth**

*With intrasynovial administration*
    **Joint pain or exacerbation of existing pain; swelling at joint**

# Patient Consultation

As an aid to patient consultation, refer to *Advice for the Patient, Radiopaque Agents (Diagnostic).*

In providing consultation, consider emphasizing the following selected information (» = major clinical significance):

## Description of use
*Action in the body:*
    Injection into vein or artery; visualization of radiopacity in brain, heart, blood vessels, and urinary tract possible with x-rays
    Direct injection into region to be studied; visualization of joint spaces, pancreatic and bile ducts

## Before having this test
» Conditions affecting use, especially:
    Sensitivity to iodine or other iodinated contrast media

    Pregnancy—Risk to the fetus from radiation exposure; may cause hypothyroidism in neonate
    Breast-feeding—Temporary discontinuation of breast-feeding for at least 24 hours
    Use in children—Increased risk of severe adverse reactions, especially in children with other medical problems; possible exacerbation of dehydration
    Use in the elderly—Increased risk of side effects; possible exacerbation of dehydration; increased risk of thyrotoxicosis
    Other medical problems, especially anuria, dehydration, diabetes mellitus, and pheochromocytoma

## Preparation for this test
Adequate intake of fluids to prevent dehydration
Special preparatory instructions may be given; patient should inquire in advance

## Precautions after having this test
Possible interference with future thyroid tests

## Side/adverse effects
Signs of possible side effects, especially pseudo-allergic reaction, cardiovascular problems, and CNS effects

# General Dosing Information

Manufacturer's package insert or other appropriate literature should be consulted for specific techniques and procedures for the administration of contrast media.

Sensitivity test doses are not usually recommended since severe or fatal reactions to contrast media are not predictable from a patient's history or a sensitivity test. On some occasions, severe or fatal reactions have occurred with a test dose or with a full dose in patients who did not react to the test dose.

Pretreatment with corticosteroids and/or antihistamines may minimize the incidence and severity of reactions in patients with a history of severe reactions to contrast media or other high-risk conditions (e.g., asthma or history of allergies, positive allergy history to skin allergens or penicillins, dehydration, history of seizures, pheochromocytoma). In some studies, the additional use of ephedrine has been shown to be beneficial in preventing anaphylactoid reactions (except in patients with a history of hypertension or cardiovascular disease). When the use of a contrast agent is being considered, the following protocols are recommended:
For high-risk patients
    • Use of a high-osmolality contrast agent plus pretreatment with a corticosteroid (oral prednisone 50 mg administered 13 hours, 7 hours, and 1 hour before procedure) and an antihistamine (intramuscular, intravenous, or oral diphenhydramine, 50 mg administered one hour prior to procedure) or
    • Use of a low-osmolality contrast agent if pretreatment is not feasible or
    • Use of a low-osmolality contrast agent plus corticosteroid pretreatment.
For low-risk patients
    • Use of a high-osmolality contrast agent or
    • Use of a high-osmolality contrast agent and corticosteroid pretreatment.

Adequate hydration is recommended for all patients before and after the procedure. Intravenous or oral intake of fluids may continue up to time of administration of ioversol.

During and for at least 30 to 60 minutes after intravascular injection of ioversol, the patient should be observed for possible severe reactions; competent personnel and emergency facilities should be available during this period.

Nonionic contrast media, such as ioversol, inhibit blood coagulation *in vitro* less than ionic contrast media. Blood cell aggregation has been reported when blood remains in contact with syringes containing nonionic contrast media. Thus, thromboembolic events causing myocardial infarction and stroke, reported during angiographic procedures, may have resulted from aggregation of blood that had come in contact with the contrast agent outside the body. It is recommended that risk factors for aggregation be minimized by performing the procedure in the shortest time possible, using plastic rather than glass syringes, and flushing catheters with heparinized saline solutions.

Dosage and concentration of iodine (as ioversol injection) are dependent upon the degree and extent of contrast needed in the areas under examination and on the equipment and technique used.

## For treatment of adverse effects
Recommended treatment consists of the following:
    • For major or life-threatening reactions, careful monitoring of vital signs and emergency therapy, including artificial respiration

with oxygen, if needed for respiratory depression, and cardiac massage in the event of cardiac arrest.

• To restore blood pressure, administration of intravenous fluids and/or vasopressors. If hypotension necessitates the use of vasopressors, slow infusion of 0.008 to 0.012 mg per minute of norepinephrine or 0.1 to 0.18 mg per minute of phenylephrine, appropriately diluted. If hypotension is due to increased vagal activity (vasovagal reaction), intravenous administration of 1 mg of atropine, repeated in one to two hours if needed.

• Other specific treatment may include—

Diphenhydramine: For minor allergic-like reactions—An antihistamine such as diphenhydramine hydrochloride (except in epileptic patients) may be administered intravenously.

Epinephrine: For acute allergic-like or anaphylactoid reactions—Slow intravenous infusion of 0.1 mg of epinephrine (1:10,000).

For mild to moderate bronchospasm—0.1 to 0.2 mg of epinephrine (1:1000) may be administered subcutaneously, except in patients with hypotension. In extreme emergency, 0.1 mg of epinephrine (1:10,000) may be given slowly by intravenous route, followed by a continuous intravenous infusion at an initial rate of 0.001 mg per minute; the rate may be increased to 0.004 mg per minute if necessary. (Note: Patients on beta-adrenergic blocking agents should not receive epinephrine since they are at risk of unopposed alpha-adrenergic stimulation, which may result in hypertension, reflex bradycardia, and heart-block. In these patients, isoproterenol and norepinephrine are used instead of epinephrine to overcome bronchospasm and hypotension, respectively.)

For cardiac arrest—0.1 to 1 mg of epinephrine may be administered by the intravenous route.

Diazepam or phenobarbital: To control convulsions—5 to 10 mg of diazepam by slow, intravenous administration or phenobarbital sodium may be given intravenously or intramuscularly at a rate not to exceed 30 to 60 mg per minute.

# Parenteral Dosage Forms

Note: Bracketed uses in the *Dosage Forms* section refer to categories of use and/or indications that are not included in U.S. product labeling.

## IOVERSOL INJECTION

### Usual adult and adolescent dose

Angiography—

Intra-arterial, by digital subtraction:

Intra-arterial, as a solution containing the equivalent of 160 mg of iodine per mL, injected at a rate approximately equal to the flow rate of the blood vessel and repeated, as necessary, into the following vessels:

Carotid arteries, 6 to 10 mL.

Vertebral arteries, 4 to 8 mL.

Aorta, 20 to 50 mL.

Subclavian or brachial arteries, 2 to 10 mL.

Major branches of the abdominal aorta, 2 to 20 mL.

Intravenous, by digital subtraction:

Via catheter, 30 to 50 mL of a solution containing the equivalent of 350 mg of iodine per mL, repeated as needed.

Arteriography, cerebral—

Via catheter, as a solution containing the equivalent of 240 mg, 300 mg, or 320 mg of iodine per mL, into the following vessels:

Carotid or vertebral arteries, 2 to 12 mL, repeated as necessary.

Aortic arch, 20 to 50 mL for simultaneous four-vessel study.

Venography, peripheral—

Percutaneous, 50 to 100 mL per extremity of a solution containing the equivalent of 240 mg or 350 mg of iodine per mL.

Note: Following venography, the venous system should be flushed with 0.9% sodium chloride injection or 5% dextrose in water. Massage and elevation of the extremities are also recommended to help clear the contrast medium from the extremities.

Aortography and

Arteriography, visceral and renal—

Via catheter, as a solution containing the equivalent of 320 mg of iodine per mL, repeated as necessary, into the following arteries:

Aorta, 45 mL (range, 10 to 80 mL).

Celiac, 45 mL (range, 12 to 60 mL).

Superior mesenteric, 45 mL (range, 15 to 60 mL).

Renal or inferior mesenteric, 9 mL (range, 6 to 15 mL).

Arteriography, coronary and

Ventriculography, left—

Via catheter, as a solution containing the equivalent of 320 mg or 350 mg of iodine per mL, repeated as necessary, into the following vessels:

Left coronary, 8 mL (range, 2 to 10 mL).

Right coronary, 6 mL (range, 1 to 10 mL).

Left ventricle, 40 mL (range, 30 to 50 mL).

Arteriography, peripheral—

Percutaneous or operative methods, as a solution containing the equivalent of 300 mg or 320 mg of iodine per mL, repeated as necessary, into the following arteries:

Aortoiliac runoff, 60 mL (range, 20 to 90 mL).

Common iliac and femoral, 40 mL (range, 10 to 50 mL).

Subclavian, brachial, 20 mL (range, 15 to 30 mL).

Urography, excretory—

Intravenous, 75 to 100 mL of a solution containing the equivalent of 240 mg of iodine per mL; or 50 to 75 mL of a solution containing the equivalent of 300 mg, 320 mg, or 350 mg of iodine per mL.

Note: In patients with impaired renal function, poor visualization is anticipated; therefore, doses of 2 mL per kg of body weight of a solution containing the equivalent of 240 mg of iodine per mL (maximum 200 mL); or 1.6 mL per kg of body weight of a solution containing the equivalent of 300 mg of iodine per mL (maximum 150 mL); or 1.5 to 2 mL per kg of body weight of a solution containing the equivalent of 320 mg of iodine per mL (maximum 150 mL); or 1.4 mL per kg of body weight of a solution containing the equivalent of 350 mg of iodine per mL (maximum 140 mL), may be indicated for urography.

CT of the brain—

Intravenous, 100 to 250 mL of a solution containing the equivalent of 240 mg of iodine per mL; or 50 to 150 mL of a solution containing the equivalent of 300 mg or 320 mg of iodine per mL.

CT of the body—

Intravenous, 35 to 100 mL by bolus injection, or 70 to 200 mL by infusion of a solution containing the equivalent of 240 mg of iodine per mL; or 25 to 75 mL by bolus injection, or 50 to 150 mL by infusion of a solution containing the equivalent of 300 mg, 320 mg, or 350 mg of iodine per mL.

### Usual adult prescribing limits

Angiography, intra-arterial, by digital subtraction and

Aortography and

Arteriography, peripheral and

Arteriography, visceral and renal and

Venography, peripheral—Up to 250 mL.

Arteriography, cerebral—Up to 200 mL.

Arteriography, coronary and

Ventriculography, left—Up to 250 mL for combined procedures.

CT of the brain and

CT of the body—Up to 250 mL of a solution containing the equivalent of 240 mg of iodine per mL; or up to 150 mL of a solution containing the equivalent of 300 mg or 320 mg of iodine per mL.

### Usual pediatric dose

Angiocardiography—

By single injection, 1.25 mL per kg of body weight, with a range of 1 to 1.5 mL per kg of body weight of a solution containing the equivalent of 320 mg or 350 mg of iodine per mL.

Note: When multiple injections are given, the total administered dose should not exceed 5 mL per kg of body weight, up to a total volume of 250 mL.

[Angiography]—

Intra-arterial, by digital subtraction: Intra-arterial 1 to 3 mL per kg of body weight of a solution containing the equivalent of 300 mg of iodine per mL.

[Arteriography, coronary] and

[Ventriculography, left]—

Via catheter, 1.25 mL per kg of body weight, with a range of 1 to 1.5 mL per kg of body weight of a solution containing the equivalent of 320 mg of iodine per mL.

Urography, excretory—

Intravenous, 0.5 to 3 mL per kg of body weight of a solution containing the equivalent of 300 mg or 320 mg of iodine per mL.

CT of the brain and

CT of the body—

Intravenous, 1 to 3 mL per kg of body weight of a solution containing the equivalent of 320 mg of iodine per mL.

### Usual geriatric dose

See *Usual adult and adolescent dose*.

Note: Geriatric patients with renal function impairment may be more sensitive to the effects of the usual adult dose; lower dosages are recommended.

For excretory urography, poor visualization is anticipated in elderly patients; therefore, doses of 2 mL per kg of body weight of a solution containing the equivalent of 240 mg of iodine per mL (maximum 200 mL); or 1.6 mL per kg of body weight of a solution containing the equivalent of 300 mg of iodine per mL (maximum 150 mL); or 1.5 to 2 mL per kg of body weight of a solution containing the equivalent of 320 mg of iodine per mL (maximum 150 mL); or 1.4 mL per kg of body weight of a solution containing the equivalent of 350 mg of iodine per mL (maximum 140 mL) may be indicated.

### Strength(s) usually available

U.S.—

339 mg of ioversol with 160 mg of iodine per mL (Rx) [*Optiray 160*].
509 mg of ioversol with 240 mg of iodine per mL (Rx) [*Optiray 240*].
636 mg of ioversol with 300 mg of iodine per mL (Rx) [*Optiray 300*].
678 mg of ioversol with 320 mg of iodine per mL (Rx) [*Optiray 320*].
741 mg of ioversol with 350 mg of iodine per mL (Rx) [*Optiray 350*].

Canada—

339 mg of ioversol with 160 mg of iodine per mL (Rx) [*Optiray 160*].
509 mg of ioversol with 240 mg of iodine per mL (Rx) [*Optiray 240*].
636 mg of ioversol with 300 mg of iodine per mL (Rx) [*Optiray 300*].
678 mg of ioversol with 320 mg of iodine per mL (Rx) [*Optiray 320*].

741 mg of ioversol with 350 mg of iodine per mL (Rx) [*Optiray 350*].

Note:  All formulations above contain 3.6 mg of tromethamine per mL as a buffer and 0.2 mg of edetate calcium disodium per mL as a stabilizer.

### Packaging and storage
Store between 15 and 30 °C (59 and 86 °F), in a light-resistant container, unless otherwise specified by manufacturer. Protect from freezing.

### Stability
Ioversol is a clear, colorless to pale yellow solution. Do not use if turbid or discolored.

Any unused portion remaining in the container should be discarded.

## Selected Bibliography

Piao ZE, Murdock DK, Hwang MH, et al. Hemodynamic effects of contrast media during coronary angiography: a comparison of three non-ionic agents to Hypaque-76. Cathet Cadiovasc Diagn 1988; 14 (1): 53-8.

Dawson P. Cardiovascular effects of contrast agents. Am J Cardiol 1989; 64: 2E-9E.

Revised: 08/16/95

---

# IOXAGLATE    Local

VA CLASSIFICATION (Primary): DX102

Note:  For a listing of dosage forms and brand names by country availability, see *Dosage Forms* section(s). For a listing of brand names for the articles in this monograph, refer to the General Index.

## Category
Diagnostic aid, radiopaque (uterus and fallopian tube disorders)

Note: Ioxaglate is an ionic radiopaque contrast agent.

## Indications

### Accepted
Hysterosalpingography—Ioxaglate meglumine and ioxaglate sodium injection is indicated for hysterosalpingography, by which the patency of the fallopian tubes may be determined and uterine and tubal cavities may be visualized for the evaluation of abnormal conditions, such as tumors, of the uterus and fallopian tubes. Hysterosalpingography is used as a diagnostic tool in cases of infertility and other abnormal gynecological conditions; it serves as an adjunct to laparoscopy and ultrasound imaging in discovering subtle abnormalities, such as endometrial polyps and salpingitis isthmica nodosa.

Hysterosalpingography is *not* recommended during the menstrual period or when menstrual flow is imminent, when infection is present in any portion of the genital tract, during pregnancy or for 6 months after termination of pregnancy, or for 30 days after conization or curettage.

## Pharmacology/Pharmacokinetics

### Physicochemical characteristics
Molecular weight—
Ioxaglate meglumine: 1464.10.
Ioxaglate sodium: 1290.87.
Osmolality—Low (approximately 600 mOsmol per kg of water for a solution containing 320 mg of iodine per mL)

### Mechanism of action/Effect
Organic iodine compounds block x-rays as they pass through the body, thereby allowing body structures containing iodine to be delineated in contrast to those structures that do not contain iodine. The degree of opacity produced by these compounds is directly proportional to the total amount (concentration and volume) of the iodinated contrast agent in the path of the x-rays. Instillation of ioxaglate meglumine and ioxaglate sodium solution into the uterus and fallopian tubes allows visualization of these areas.

### Absorption
Intrauterine instillation—Most of the medium within the uterine cavity is discharged into the vagina immediately upon termination of procedure. However, any medium retained in the uterine cavity is absorbed systemically.

### Protein binding
Very low.

### Elimination
Absorbed medium—Primarily renal.
Unabsorbed medium—Expelled vaginally, following the procedure.

## Precautions to Consider

### Cross-sensitivity and/or related problems
Patients sensitive to iodine or other iodinated contrast media may be sensitive to ioxaglate also.

### Pregnancy/Reproduction
Pregnancy—Ioxaglate meglumine and ioxaglate sodium injection for intrauterine instillation is not recommended during pregnancy since ioxaglate may cross the placenta, or for at least 6 months after the termination of pregnancy since the procedure may increase the risk of complications such as intrauterine infection.

Also, other organically bound iodine–containing preparations administered near term by intra-amniotic injection have caused hypothyroidism in some newborns. In addition, elective contrast radiography of the abdomen is usually not recommended during pregnancy because of the risks to the fetus from radiation exposure.

### Breast-feeding
Problems in humans have not been documented. However, since small amounts of this medium may be absorbed and ioxaglate is known to be distributed unchanged into breast milk when administered intravascularly, breast-feeding is not recommended for at least 24 hours following its administration.

### Pediatrics
No information is available on the use of ioxaglate for hysterosalpingography in pediatric patients.

### Geriatrics
Appropriate studies on the relationship of age to the effects of ioxaglate for intrauterine instillation have not been performed in geriatric patients. However, no geriatrics-specific problems have been documented to date.

### Diagnostic interference
The following have been selected on the basis of their potential clinical significance (possible effect in parentheses where appropriate)—not necessarily inclusive (» = major clinical significance):

With *other* diagnostic test results
Thyroid function determinations and
Thyroid imaging
(absorbed ioxaglate may cause an increase of serum protein–bound iodine [PBI] and a decrease in radioactive iodine or pertechnetate ion uptake for a period varying from 1 week to several months; thyroid test should be performed prior to administration of contrast medium. Other thyroid function tests not based on measurement of iodine, such as resin triiodothyronine uptake, are not affected)

**Medical considerations/Contraindications**

The medical considerations/contraindications included here have been selected on the basis of their potential clinical significance (reasons given
in parentheses where appropriate)—not necessarily inclusive (» =
major clinical significance).

*Except under special circumstances, this medication should not be used
when the following medical problem exists:*

» Genital tract infection
    (procedure may increase risk of complications)

*Risk-benefit should be considered when the following medical problems
exist:*

Allergic reaction (anaphylaxis) to penicillins or to skin allergens,
    previous
    (increased risk of anaphylactoid reaction)

Allergies or asthma, history of
    (increased risk of idiosyncratic response or anaphylactoid reaction)

» Pelvic inflammatory disease, acute
    (condition may be aggravated)

» Sensitivity to iodinated contrast media
    (increased risk of anaphylactoid reaction in patients with a history
    of anaphylactoid reaction to iodinated contrast media)

Caution is also recommended just after cervical or uterine surgery to
    avoid the risk of complications.

## Side/Adverse Effects

Note: Systemic adverse effects, although rare, are possible with intrau-
    terine instillation if medium is absorbed systemically after being
    retained in the uterine cavity or spilled into the peritoneal cavity.

The following side/adverse effects have been selected on the basis of their
    potential clinical significance (possible signs and symptoms in paren-
    theses where appropriate)—not necessarily inclusive:

**Those indicating need for medical attention**
Incidence rare
    *Pseudo-allergic reaction* (increased sweating; skin rash or hives;
    sneezing; stuffy nose; swelling of face or skin; swelling of the larynx;
    thickening of the tongue; wheezing, tightness in chest, or troubled
    breathing)—may be due to entry of medium into venous or lymphatic
    system
    Note: *Pseudo-allergic reactions* are usually transient. However, they
        may be initial manifestations of more severe anaphylactoid re-
        actions. The anaphylactoid reaction may progress to respiratory
        arrest and vasomotor collapse if appropriate treatment is not
        administered.

**Those indicating need for medical attention only if they continue
or are bothersome**
Incidence more frequent
    *Abdominal or stomach pain and discomfort*
    Note: *Abdominal pain and discomfort* may be associated with the in-
        sertion and positioning of the instillation device. If occurring
        later during the procedure, may indicate spillage of contrast
        medium into the peritoneal cavity.

Incidence less frequent
    *Fever*

## Patient Consultation

As an aid to patient consultation, refer to *Advice for the Patient,
Radiopaque Agents (Diagnostic, Local)*.

In providing consultation, consider emphasizing the following selected
information (» = major clinical significance):

**Description of use**
    Instillation into uterus and fallopian tubes; visualization of radiopacity
    possible with x-rays

**Before having this test**
» Conditions affecting use, especially:
    Sensitivity to iodine or other iodinated contrast media
    Pregnancy—Risk to the fetus from radiation exposure; intrauterine
        instillation contraindicated during pregnancy and for at least 6
        months after delivery
    Breast-feeding—May be distributed into breast milk; breast-feed-
        ing not recommended for 24 hours after use
    Other medical problems, especially acute pelvic inflammatory dis-
        ease or genital tract infection

**Preparation for this test**
    Enema, vaginal douche, and/or other special preparatory instructions
        may be given; patient should inquire in advance
    Voiding before procedure

**Precautions after having this test**
    Possible interference with future thyroid tests

**Side/adverse effects**
    Signs of possible side effects, especially pseudo-allergic reaction

# General Dosing Information

Manufacturer's package insert or other appropriate literature should be
    consulted for specific techniques and procedures for the administration
    of contrast media.

Sensitivity test doses are not usually recommended since severe or fatal
    reactions to contrast media are not predictable from a patient's history
    or a sensitivity test. On some occasions severe or fatal reactions have
    occurred with a test dose or with a full dose in patients who did not
    react to the test dose.

Pretreatment with corticosteroids and/or antihistamines is recommended
    to minimize the incidence and severity of reactions in patients with a
    history of severe reactions to contrast media or with other high-risk
    conditions (e.g., asthma or history of allergies, positive allergy history
    to skin allergens or penicillin). In some studies, the additional use of
    ephedrine has been shown to be beneficial in preventing anaphylactoid
    reactions (except in patients with a history of hypertension or cardi-
    ovascular disease). When considering the use of a contrast agent, the
    following protocols are recommended:
For high-risk patients
    • Use of a high-osmolality contrast agent plus pretreatment with a
    corticosteroid (oral prednisone, 50 mg administered 13 hours, 7 hours,
    and 1 hour before procedure) and antihistamine (intramuscular, intra-
    venous, or oral diphenhydramine, 50 mg administered 1 hour before
    procedure) or
    • Use of a low-osmolality contrast agent if pretreatment is not feasible
    or
    • Use of a low-osmolality contrast agent plus corticosteroid
    pretreatment.
For low-risk patients
    • Use of a high-osmolality contrast agent or
    • Use of a high-osmolality contrast agent and corticosteroid
    pretreatment.

An enema and vaginal douche before the examination are optional. Patient
    should empty her bladder before the procedure.

Ioxaglate meglumine and ioxaglate sodium injection for intrauterine in-
    stillation is to be instilled directly into the uterus via a sterile syringe
    attached to a uterine cannula, or via a tubal insufflator with a salpin-
    gogram attachment. It is recommended that instillation into the uterine
    cavity be performed under controlled pressure with fluoroscopic mon-
    itoring. Excessive pressure and overfilling should be avoided.

During and for at least 30 to 60 minutes after administration of contrast
    media, the patient should be observed for possible severe reactions;
    competent personnel and emergency facilities should be available dur-
    ing this period.

Any unabsorbed contrast medium is expelled spontaneously upon removal
    of the cannula.

# Local Dosage Forms

## IOXAGLATE MEGLUMINE AND IOXAGLATE SODIUM
## INJECTION

**Usual adult and adolescent dose**
Hysterosalpingography—
    Intrauterine instillation, 5 to 15 mL of a solution containing the equiv-
        alent of 320 mg of iodine per mL administered slowly in fractional
        doses of 1 to 2 mL and without undue pressure.

**Usual pediatric dose**
Dosage has not been established.

**Usual geriatric dose**
See *Usual adult and adolescent dose*.

**Strength(s) usually available**
U.S.—
    39.3% (393 mg per mL) of ioxaglate meglumine and 19.6% (196 mg
        per mL) of ioxaglate sodium with 32% (320 mg per mL) of iodine
        (Rx) [*Hexabrix* (0.10 mg of edetate calcium disodium; 3.48 mg or
        0.15 mEq of sodium, per mL)].
Canada—
    39.3% (393 mg per mL) of ioxaglate meglumine and 19.6% (196 mg
        per mL) of ioxaglate sodium with 32% (320 mg per mL) of iodine
        (Rx) [*Hexabrix-320* (0.10 mg of edetate calcium disodium; 3.48
        mg or 0.15 mEq of sodium, per mL)].

**Packaging and storage**
Store below 30 °C (86 °F), unless otherwise specified by manufacturer. Protect from light. Protect from freezing.

**Stability**
Ioxaglate meglumine and ioxaglate sodium injection is a clear, colorless to pale yellow solution. Do not use if turbid or discolored.
Crystals may form in the solution at very cold temperatures but are readily redissolved by bringing the container of solution to room temperature and gently shaking it.
Any unused portion remaining in the container should be discarded.

**Selected Bibliography**
Sauer MV. Investigation of the female pelvis. J Reprod Med 1993 Apr; 38 (4): 269-76.
Gutmann JN. Imaging in the evaluation of female infertility. J Reprod Med 1992 Jan; 37 (1): 54-61.

Revised: 06/01/95

# IOXAGLATE   Systemic

VA CLASSIFICATION (Primary): DX102
Note: For a listing of dosage forms and brand names by country availability, see *Dosage Forms* section(s). For a listing of brand names for the articles in this monograph, refer to the General Index.

## Category

Diagnostic aid, radiopaque (cardiac disease; vascular disease; joint disease; urinary tract disorders; brain disorders); Diagnostic aid, radiopaque contrast enhancer in computed tomography.
Note: Ioxaglate is an ionic radiopaque contrast agent.

## Indications

**Accepted**
Intravascular:
  Angiocardiography—Ioxaglate meglumine and ioxaglate sodium injection is indicated for pediatric angiocardiography to visualize lesions or malformations of the heart and obstructions or anomalies of the major thoracic blood vessels.
  Angiography
  Aortography or
  Arteriography—Ioxaglate meglumine and ioxaglate sodium injection is used to visualize specific regions of the vascular system and blood flow in these areas. It is indicated in cerebral angiography, intra-arterial digital subtraction angiography; intravenous digital subtraction angiography; aortography; peripheral arteriography; selective visceral arteriography[1]; and coronary selective arteriography (with or without left ventriculography).
  Venography—Ioxaglate meglumine and ioxaglate sodium injection is indicated in peripheral venography (phlebography) to visualize the peripheral venous circulation.
  Urography, excretory—Ioxaglate meglumine and ioxaglate sodium injection is indicated in excretion urography to evaluate abnormalities of the urinary tract such as urinary tract obstructions.
  Brain imaging, computed tomographic—Ioxaglate meglumine and ioxaglate sodium injection is indicated for enhancement of computed tomographic scans of the brain (CT of the brain) to determine the presence and extent of primary and metastatic malignancies of the head or other non-neoplastic lesions such as cerebral infarction or infection.
  Body imaging, computed tomographic—Ioxaglate meglumine and ioxaglate sodium injection is indicated for enhancement of computed tomographic scans of the body (CT of the body) performed for the detection and evaluation of lesions in the liver, pancreas, kidneys, abdominal aorta, mediastinum, abdominal cavity, and retroperitoneal space.
Intrasynovial:
  Arthrography—Ioxaglate meglumine and ioxaglate sodium injection is indicated for arthrography in diagnosis of post-traumatic or degenerative joint diseases or synovial rupture, for visualization of communicating bursae or cysts, and in meniscography.

[1]Not included in Canadian product labeling.

## Pharmacology/Pharmacokinetics

**Physicochemical characteristics**
Molecular weight—Ioxaglate meglumine: 1464.10.
Ioxaglate sodium: 1290.87.
Osmolality—Low. The osmolalities of the injections of ioxaglate with iodine concentrations of 200 and 320 mg per mL are 356 and 600 mOsmol per kg of water, respectively

**Mechanism of action/Effect**
Organic iodine compounds block x-rays as they pass through the body, thereby allowing body structures containing iodine to be delineated in contrast to those structures that do not contain iodine. The degree of opacity produced by these compounds is directly proportional to the total amount (concentration and volume) of the iodinated contrast agent in the path of the x-rays. Ioxaglate's distribution in and elimination from the body as iodinated ion allow the visualization of the internal structures in the path of its flow.

**Other actions/effects**
Anticoagulant activity; vasodilating effects.

**Distribution**
Rapidly distributed throughout the extracellular fluid following intravascular administration.

**Protein binding**
Very low.

**Half-life**
With normal renal function—
  Distribution (alpha phase): 12 (range, 4 to 17) minutes.
  Elimination (beta phase): 92 (range, 61 to 140) minutes.

**Time to peak concentration**
2 (range, 1 to 3) minutes, in plasma, following intravenous administration of 50 mL of a solution containing the equivalent of 320 mg of iodine per mL.

**Time to peak opacification**
CT scanning (dynamic)—30 to 90 seconds after bolus administration.

**Peak serum concentration**
2.1 (range, 1.8 to 2.8) mg per mL, following intravenous administration of 50 mL of a solution containing the equivalent of 320 mg of iodine per mL.

**Elimination**
Normal renal function—Primarily renal (by glomerular filtration, but some tubular reabsorption may occur); approximately 50% of intravascular dose eliminated unchanged within 2 hours, and 90% eliminated unchanged within 24 hours.
Severe renal function impairment—Elimination in the feces via biliary tract may become a primary route.
In dialysis—Removed by peritoneal dialysis or hemodialysis.

## Precautions to Consider

**Cross-sensitivity and/or related problems**
Patients sensitive to iodine or other iodinated contrast media may be sensitive to ioxaglate also.

**Carcinogenicity**
Long-term animal studies to evaluate carcinogenic potential of ioxaglate have not been performed.

**Mutagenicity**
Ioxaglate has not been shown to have mutagenic potential in animal studies.

**Pregnancy/Reproduction**
Pregnancy—Ioxaglate crosses the placenta. Adequate and well-controlled studies in humans have not been done. However, risk-benefit must be considered since other organically bound iodine–containing preparations administered near term by intra-amniotic injection have caused hypothyroidism in some newborns.
Also, elective contrast radiography of the abdomen is usually not recommended during pregnancy because of the risks to the fetus from radiation exposure.

Studies in rats and rabbits, at doses up to two times the maximum adult human dose, have not shown that ioxaglate causes adverse effects on the fetus.

FDA Pregnancy Category B.

## Breast-feeding

Ioxaglate is distributed unchanged into breast milk. Breast-feeding is not recommended for 24 hours following the administration of ioxaglate.

## Pediatrics

Dehydration and/or the risk of renal failure may be exacerbated in infants and young children, especially those with polyuria, oliguria, diabetes, or pre-existing dehydration, by ioxaglate; adequate hydration is recommended before and following intravascular administration of ioxaglate.

Convulsions are more likely to occur in infants than in other age groups with the administration of ioxaglate, especially after repeated administration.

Difficulty in breathing, slow or irregular heartbeat, unusual feeling of tiredness, and mental depression are more likely to occur in cyanotic infants during angiocardiography with the administration of ioxaglate.

## Geriatrics

Although overall prevalence of adverse effects has been reported to be less in patients 50 years of age and older, the severity of the reactions may be greater in this age group than in younger patients.

Dehydration and/or the risk of renal failure may be exacerbated in geriatric patients, especially those with polyuria, oliguria, diabetes, or pre-existing dehydration, by ioxaglate; adequate hydration is recommended before and following intravascular administration of ioxaglate.

The elderly may be more sensitive to the effects of ioxaglate on thyroid function. Iodine-induced thyrotoxicosis may occur 4 to 12 weeks following contrast radiography. Thyroid function monitoring may be needed in geriatric patients.

## Drug interactions and/or related problems

The following drug interactions and/or related problems have been selected on the basis of their potential clinical significance (possible mechanism in parentheses where appropriate)—not necessarily inclusive (» = major clinical significance):

Note: Combinations containing any of the following medications, depending on the amount present, may also interact with this medication.

Beta-adrenergic blocking agents
(concurrent intravascular administration of ioxaglate with beta-adrenergic blocking agents may increase the risk of moderate to severe anaphylactoid reaction; also, hypotensive effects may be exacerbated; discontinuation of the beta-adrenergic blocking agent may be advisable before administration of contrast media in patients with other risk factors)

Cholecystographic agents, oral
(may increase the risk of renal toxicity when followed by intravenous ioxaglate, especially in patients with hepatic function impairment)

Hypotension-producing medications, other (See *Appendix II*)
(the risk of severe hypotension may be increased if ioxaglate is given concurrently with other medications that produce hypotension)

Interleukin-2
(the incidence of delayed reactions to intravenous contrast media [e.g., hypersensitivity, fever, skin rash, flu-like symptoms, joint pain, flushing, pruritus, emesis, hypotension, dizziness occurring more than 1 hour after administration] may be increased in patients who have received interleukin-2; some symptoms may resemble a "recall" reaction to interleukin-2; supportive medical treatment may be necessary if symptoms are significant; there is some evidence that the incidence is reduced if contrast media administration is delayed until 6 weeks after interleukin-2 administration)

Nephrotoxic medications, other (See *Appendix II*)
(concurrent intravascular administration of ioxaglate with other nephrotoxic medications may increase the potential for nephrotoxicity)

Vasopressors (See *Appendix II*)
(neurologic effects, including permanent paralysis, of ioxaglate may be increased during cerebral arteriography, selective spinal arteriography, and arteriography of vessels supplying the spinal cord, when ioxaglate is administered after hypertensive agents used to increase contrast; this increase in neurologic effects is due to contraction of vessels in the splanchnic circulation, which forces more of the contrast material into the vessels leading to the spine and spinal cord)

## Diagnostic interference

The following have been selected on the basis of their potential clinical significance (possible effect in parentheses where appropriate)—not necessarily inclusive (» = major clinical significance):

With *other* diagnostic test results
Blood pool imaging
(imaging of blood pool may be impaired because of decreased technetium Tc 99m-labeling of red blood cells caused by the intravascular administration of ioxaglate)

Leukocyte counts and
Red cell counts
(may be decreased)

Phenolsulfonphthalein (PSP) excretion test
(test results may be affected, especially in patients with severely impaired renal function who are also given intravascular ioxaglate; some of the ioxaglate is secreted by the renal tubules, resulting in decreased tubular excretion of PSP; therefore, concurrent use of intravascular ioxaglate is not recommended in patients receiving a PSP excretion test)

Prothrombin time (PT) and
Thromboplastin time
(may be increased with ioxaglate since ionic contrast media have been shown to inhibit all stages of coagulation)

Skeletal imaging
(possible renal and hepatic uptake of technetium Tc 99m medronate, technetium Tc 99m oxidronate, technetium Tc 99m pyrophosphate, or technetium Tc 99m [pyro- and trimeta-] phosphates if ioxaglate is administered intravenously immediately after one of these technetium Tc 99m-labeled agents)

Thyroid function determinations and
Thyroid imaging
(intravascular or intrathecal administration of ioxaglate may alter serum protein-bound iodine [PBI] concentrations and radioactive iodine or pertechnetate ion uptake for up to 2 weeks; thyroid test should be performed prior to administration of ioxaglate. Other thyroid function tests not based on measurement of iodine, such as resin triiodothyronine uptake, may not be affected)

Urinalysis
(may produce abnormal results; urine should be collected prior to, or at least 2 days after, intravascular administration of ioxaglate)

With physiology/laboratory test values
Creatinine, serum
(may be increased temporarily)

Platelet aggregation
(may be decreased by high levels of plasma ioxaglate)

## Medical considerations/Contraindications

The medical considerations/contraindications included here have been selected on the basis of their potential clinical significance (reasons given in parentheses where appropriate)—not necessarily inclusive (» = major clinical significance).

*Risk-benefit should be considered when the following medical problems exist:*

*For all procedures*
Allergic reaction (anaphylaxis) to penicillins or to skin allergens, previous
(although the risk of anaphylactoid reaction may be less with ioxaglate than with high-osmolality contrast agents, caution is recommended when administering ioxaglate to patients who have had a previous reaction to penicillins or to skin allergens)

Allergies or asthma, history of
(although the risk of idiosyncratic response or anaphylactoid reaction may be less with ioxaglate than with high-osmolality contrast agents, caution is recommended when administering ioxaglate to patients with a history of allergies or asthma)

Cardiovascular disease, severe
(increased risk of cardiac arrest)

» Dehydration, especially associated with diabetes mellitus, azotemia, or multiple myeloma
(osmotic diuretic action of ioxaglate may exacerbate dehydration and increase the risk of acute renal failure)

» Hemorrhage, cranial subarachnoid
(intravascular administration may cause convulsions and death)

Hepatic function impairment, severe
(increased risk of renal toxicity and damage)

Hypertension, severe

Hyperthyroidism
(intravascular administration of ioxaglate may precipitate thyroid storm)

» Pheochromocytoma
(intravascular administration of ioxaglate may precipitate severe hypertension; amount of medium injected should be kept to a minimum and blood pressure should be monitored during the procedure; also, pretreatment with the alpha-adrenergic blocking agent phentolamine is recommended)

Renal function impairment
(although the risk of acute renal failure in the presence of renal insufficiency [serum creatinine ≥ 132.6 micromoles/L] may be less with ioxaglate than with high-osmolality contrast agents, caution is recommended)

» Seizures, recent
(increased risk for reoccurrence)

» Sensitivity to iodinated contrast media
(increased risk of anaphylactoid reaction in patients with history of prior reactions to contrast media)

Sickle cell disease
(intravascular administration of ioxaglate may promote sickling in patients who are homozygous for sickle cell disease; fluid restriction is not recommended in these patients)

Caution is also recommended in recent kidney transplant patients since excretion of ioxaglate may be impaired.

*For angiocardiography*
Angina, unstable
(increased risk of severe cardiac reaction)

Cardiac failure, incipient
(fluid overload, pressure changes, and expansion of blood volume may aggravate condition)

Cyanosis, in infants
(use of ioxaglate may increase risk of apnea, bradycardia, arrhythmias, acidosis, and central nervous system [CNS] effects in cyanotic infants)

» Pulmonary hypertension, severe
(hypervolemic effect of ioxaglate may further increase pulmonary artery and venous pressures due to an increase in cardiac output and a rise in left ventricular end-diastolic and left atrial pressures)

*For cerebral angiography*
Arteriosclerosis, advanced, or
Cardiac decompensation or
Cerebral embolism, recent or
Hemorrhage, subarachnoid or
Migraine or
Senility or
Thrombosis, recent
(hemodynamic changes produced by ioxaglate may result in decreased cerebral perfusion, which may cause CNS damage)

» Homocystinuria
(procedure may increase risk of thrombosis and embolism)

*For peripheral arteriography*
Buerger's disease or
Ischemia, severe, associated with ascending infection
(procedure may induce severe arterial or venous spasm)

*For coronary arteriography*
» Myocardial infarction
(procedure done within 2 weeks may increase risk of cardiac complications)

*For selective coronary arteriography*
Cardiac failure, incipient
(increased risk of aggravating condition)

Hypotension
(may result in serious arrhythmias)

*For peripheral venography*
Infection, local or
Ischemia, severe or
Phlebitis or
Thrombosis or
Venous stasis or
Venous system obstruction
(procedure may increase risk of thrombophlebitis, syncope, and gangrene)

*For excretory urography*
» Anuria or
» Diabetes mellitus
(increased risk of acute renal failure)

» Congestive heart failure
(intravenous infusion may produce an increased osmotic load and may aggravate condition)

*For arthrography*
» Infection, in or near joint to be examined
(procedure may increase risk of complications)

**Patient monitoring**
The following may be especially important in patient monitoring (other tests may be warranted in some patients, depending on condition; » = major clinical significance):

Blood pressure determinations
(recommended for approximately 10 minutes following intra-arterial administration of ioxaglate; may be required during examination in patients with known or suspected pheochromocytoma or hemodynamic compromise or instability)

Electrocardiogram (ECG)
(recommended for early detection of arrhythmias during coronary arteriography)

## Side/Adverse Effects

Note: Adverse effects may vary directly with the concentration of the agent, the amount and technique used, and the underlying pathology. Increases in osmolality, volume, concentration, viscosity, and rate of administration of the solution may tend to increase the incidence and severity of adverse effects.

Most of the adverse effects appear during or within a few minutes after intravascular administration of ioxaglate; however, severe delayed reactions may also occur.

Low-osmolality contrast agents, such as ioxaglate, are reported to cause less heat and pain on injection than high-osmolality agents, such as diatrizoates and iothalamate.

Acute renal failure has been reported following intravascular administration of iodinated contrast agents during excretory urography, especially in patients with diabetic nephropathy and in susceptible nondiabetic patients. Also, a higher incidence of contrast-induced renal failure has been associated with severe congestive heart failure, in patients who have had multiple contrast studies within 72 hours, those receiving large volumes of contrast agent, and those with elevated uric acid levels. Renal function may also be slightly and temporarily impaired following intravascular administration of ioxaglate during selective renal arteriography.

Thromboembolic events causing myocardial infarction and stroke have been reported rarely during angiographic procedures with ionic contrast media.

Convulsions are more likely to occur in infants than in other age groups with the administration of ioxaglate, especially after repeated administration.

Difficulty in breathing, slow or irregular heartbeat, unusual feeling of tiredness, and mental depression are more likely to occur in cyanotic infants during angiocardiography with the administration of ioxaglate.

Dehydration and/or the risk of renal failure may be exacerbated by the hypertonic contrast solutions of ioxaglate, and in some cases may cause a shock-like state in infants; young children; and geriatric, azotemic, dehydrated, or debilitated patients.

Hypotensive collapse and shock have been reported rarely following urography.

In addition to those side/adverse effects listed below as needing medical attention, other severe reactions, such as loss of consciousness, shock, and cardiac arrest, may occur rarely during or a few minutes after intravascular administration of ioxaglate.

Death has occurred rarely during or a few minutes after injection, mainly due to cardiac arrest, especially in patients with cardiovascular disease. Disseminated intravascular coagulation has also resulted in death in extremely rare cases.

Transient global amnesia has been reported in 2 patients after cerebral angiography, in which 20 mL of a low-osmolality nonionic contrast agent (containing the equivalent of 240 mg of iodine per mL) was administered into the ascending aorta. The possibility that ioxaglate may cause a similar response must be considered.

The following side/adverse effects have been selected on the basis of their potential clinical significance (possible signs and symptoms in parentheses where appropriate)—not necessarily inclusive:

**Those indicating need for medical attention**

Incidence less frequent or rare

*For all procedures*

**Pseudo-allergic reaction** (coughing or choking; nasal congestion; skin rash or hives; stuffy nose; swelling of face or skin; thickening of the tongue; wheezing, tightness in chest, or troubled breathing)

Note: *Pseudo-allergic reactions* are usually transient. However, they may be an initial manifestation of a more severe anaphylactoid reaction. The anaphylactoid reaction may progress to respiratory arrest and vasomotor collapse if appropriate treatment is not administered.

*With intravascular administration*

**Bronchospasm or pulmonary edema** (severe wheezing or troubled breathing); **cardiotoxic effects, with decreased contractile force and ventricular fibrillation** (irregular heartbeat); **convulsions; swelling of larynx; vasovagal effects, with bradycardia and hypotension** (slow heartbeat; severe tiredness or weakness)

Note: Compared to high-osmolality agents, there is a decreased incidence of significant *bradycardia, ventricular tachyarrhythmias,* and *hypotension* associated with low-osmolality agents, such as ioxaglate.

**Those indicating need for medical attention only if they continue or are bothersome**

Incidence more frequent

*With intravascular administration*

**Nausea or vomiting; unusual warmth and flushing of skin**

*With intrasynovial administration*

**Joint pain or exacerbation of existing pain**

Incidence less frequent or rare

*With intravascular administration*

**Changes in vision; chest pain; chills; dizziness or lightheadedness; headache; increased sweating; numbness, tingling, pain, or weakness in hands or feet; redness, swelling, or pain at injection site; trembling; unusual tiredness or weakness**

Note: These effects are usually self-limiting and of short duration.

## Patient Consultation

As an aid to patient consultation, refer to *Advice for the Patient, Radiopaque Agents (Diagnostic).*

In providing consultation, consider emphasizing the following selected information (» = major clinical significance):

**Description of use**

Action in the body: Concentrates in particular area of the body; visualization of radiopacity possible with x-rays

**Before having this test**

» Conditions affecting use, especially:

Sensitivity to iodine or other iodinated contrast media

Pregnancy—Crosses the placenta; risk to the fetus from radiation exposure; may cause hypothyroidism in newborn

Breast-feeding—Distributed into breast milk; discontinuation of breast-feeding for 24 hours recommended

Use in children—Increased risk of severe adverse reactions, especially in children with other medical problems; possible exacerbation of dehydration

Use in the elderly—Increased risk of severe adverse effects; possible exacerbation of dehydration; increased risk of thyrotoxicosis

Other medical problems, especially anuria, dehydration, diabetes mellitus, pheochromocytoma, and seizures

**Preparation for this test**

Adequate intake of fluids to prevent dehydration

Special preparatory instructions may apply; patient should inquire in advance

Not eating for several hours before examination to prevent possible aspiration of gastric contents; moderate amounts of clear liquids may be permitted

**Precautions after having this test**

Possible interference with future thyroid tests

**Side/adverse effects**

Signs of potential side effects, especially pseudo-allergic reaction, convulsions, and cardiac or pulmonary problems that may occur immediately or within minutes of administration

## General Dosing Information

The manufacturer's package insert or other appropriate literature should be consulted for specific techniques and procedures for the administration of ioxaglate.

Sensitivity test doses are not usually recommended since severe or fatal reactions to contrast media are not predictable from a patient's history or a sensitivity test. On some occasions severe or fatal reactions have occurred with a test dose or with a full dose in patients who did not react to the test dose.

Pretreatment with corticosteroids and/or antihistamines has been used to minimize the incidence and severity of reactions in patients with a history of severe reactions to contrast media and other high-risk conditions (e.g., asthma or history of allergies, positive allergy history to skin allergens or penicillins, dehydration, history of seizures, pheochromocytoma). In some studies, the additional use of ephedrine has been shown to be beneficial in preventing anaphylactoid reactions. When considering the use of a contrast agent, the following protocols are recommended:

For high-risk patients

• Use of a high-osmolality contrast agent plus pretreatment with a corticosteroid (oral prednisone, 50 mg administered 13 hours, 7 hours, and 1 hour before procedure) and an antihistamine (intramuscular, intravenous, or oral diphenhydramine, 50 mg administered one hour prior to procedure) or

• Use of a low-osmolality agent if pretreatment is not feasible or

• Use of a low-osmolality agent plus corticosteroid pretreatment.

For low-risk patients

• Use of a high-osmolality contrast agent or

• Use of a high-osmolality contrast agent and corticosteroid pretreatment.

Adequate hydration is especially important in infants, young children, and geriatric or azotemic patients receiving intravascular ioxaglate since dehydration may be further increased by the osmotic diuretic effect of the contrast medium. Although preparatory partial dehydration has been used to increase the urinary concentration of and contrast produced by contrast agents, it is no longer recommended with modern contrast media because it is no longer necessary and may do harm. Dehydration is particularly contraindicated in patients with multiple myeloma since it may predispose to irreversible precipitation of myeloma protein in the renal tubules. In these patients fluids should be administered and urine should be made alkaline.

No food should be ingested for several hours before an examination to prevent aspiration of gastric contents if vomiting occurs. However, moderate amounts of clear liquids are permissible and even recommended by some clinicians to prevent dehydration.

Dosage of ioxaglate for intravascular administration should be individualized and is usually in proportion to the size of the specific region of the vascular system to be visualized and the anticipated degree of hemodilution in that region.

During and for at least 30 to 60 minutes after administration of ioxaglate, the patient should be observed for possible severe reactions; competent personnel and emergency facilities should be available during this period.

Thromboembolic events causing myocardial infarction and stroke, reported rarely during angiographic procedures, may have resulted from atherosclerotic lesions rather than from coagulation of blood that had come in contact with the contrast agent outside the body. Nonetheless, it is recommended that risk factors for blood cell aggregation be minimized by performing the procedure in the shortest time possible, using plastic rather than glass syringes, and flushing catheters with heparinized saline solutions.

**For treatment of adverse effects**

Recommended treatment consists of the following:

• For major or life-threatening reactions, careful monitoring of vital signs and emergency therapy, including artificial respiration with oxygen, if needed for respiratory depression, and cardiac massage in the event of cardiac arrest.

• To restore blood pressure, administration of intravenous fluids and/or vasopressors. If hypotension necessitates the use of vasopressors, slow infusion of 0.008 to 0.012 mg per minute of norepinephrine or 0.1 to 0.18 mg per minute of phenylephrine, appropriately diluted. If hypotension is due to increased vagal activity (vasovagal reaction), intravenous administration of 1 mg of atropine, repeated in one to two hours if needed.

• Other specific treatment may include—

*Diphenhydramine:* For minor allergic-like reactions—An antihistamine such as diphenhydramine hydrochloride (except in epileptic patients) may be administered intravenously.

*Epinephrine:* For acute allergic-like or anaphylactoid reactions—Slow intravenous infusion of 0.1 mg of epinephrine (1:10,000).

For mild to moderate bronchospasm—0.1 to 0.2 mg of epinephrine (1:1000) may be administered subcutaneously, except in hypotension. In extreme emergency, 0.1 mg of epinephrine (1:10,000) may be given slowly by intravenous route, followed by a continuous intravenous infusion at an initial rate of 0.001 mg per minute; the rate may be increased to 0.004 mg per minute if necessary.

Patients on beta-adrenergic blocking agents should not receive epinephrine since they are at risk of unopposed alpha-adrenergic stimulation, which may result in hypertension, reflex bradycardia, and heart block. In these patients, isoproterenol and norepinephrine are used instead of epinephrine to overcome bronchospasm and hypotension, respectively.

For cardiac arrest—0.1 to 1 mg of epinephrine may be administered by the intravenous route.

*Diazepam or phenobarbital:* To control convulsions—5 to 10 mg of diazepam by slow, intravenous administration or phenobarbital sodium intravenously or intramuscularly at a rate not to exceed 30 to 60 mg per minute may be given.

# Parenteral Dosage Forms

## IOXAGLATE MEGLUMINE AND IOXAGLATE SODIUM INJECTION

### Usual adult and adolescent dose
Intravascular—
Angiography, cerebral:
  Carotid angiography—
    Percutaneous or via catheter, 9 mL (range, 6 to 12 mL) of a solution containing the equivalent of 320 mg of iodine per mL, repeated as needed.
  Vertebral angiography—
    Percutaneous or via catheter, 8 mL (range, 5 to 12 mL) of a solution containing the equivalent of 320 mg of iodine per mL, repeated as needed.
  Aortic arch in conjunction with cerebral angiography—
    Percutaneous or via catheter, 40 mL (range, 30 to 50 mL) of a solution containing the equivalent of 320 mg of iodine per mL.
Angiography, intra-arterial, by digital subtraction:
  Via catheter, as a solution containing the equivalent of 200 mg or 320 mg of iodine per mL, repeated as needed, as follows:
  Carotid arteries—6 to 10 mL.
  Vertebral arteries—4 to 8 mL.
  Aorta—25 to 50 mL.
  Subclavian or brachial arteries—2 to 10 mL.
  Major branches of the abdominal aorta—2 to 20 mL.
  Note: For intra-arterial digital subtraction angiography, a 1:1 dilution of ioxaglate meglumine and ioxaglate sodium injection with Sterile Water for Injection USP is used.
Angiography, intravenous, by digital subtraction:
  Via catheter, 30 to 50 mL of a solution containing the equivalent of 320 mg of iodine per mL, as a single dose; may be repeated as needed.
  Note: Injection rates vary depending on the site of catheter placement and vessel size. Central catheter injections are usually made at a rate between 10 and 30 mL per second. Peripheral injections are usually made at a rate between 12 and 20 mL per second.

  Flushing the vein with 20 to 25 mL of 5% dextrose in water or normal saline, immediately after the injection, is recommended since the injected medium could otherwise remain in the arm vein for an extended period of time.
Arteriography:
  Coronary arteriography—
    As a solution containing the equivalent of 320 mg of iodine per mL:
    Left coronary arteriography—Via catheter, 8 mL (range, 2 to 14 mL), repeated as needed.
    Right coronary arteriography—Via catheter, 5 mL (range, 1 to 10 mL), repeated as needed.
    Left ventriculography—Via catheter, 45 mL (range, 35 to 45 mL), as a single dose, repeated as needed.
  Peripheral arteriography—
    As a solution containing the equivalent of 320 mg of iodine per mL:

Aorto-iliac runoff studies—Percutaneous or operative methods, 45 mL (range, 20 to 80 mL) as a single dose, repeated as needed.
Common iliac, external iliac, and femoral arteries—Percutaneous or operative methods, 30 mL (range, 10 to 50 mL) as a single dose, repeated as needed.
Upper limb—Percutaneous or operative methods, 20 mL (range, 15 to 30 mL) as a single dose, repeated as needed.
Aortography:
  Via catheter, 25 to 50 mL of a solution containing the equivalent of 320 mg of iodine per mL administered into the aorta as a single dose; may be repeated as needed.
Visceral arteriography, selective[1]:
  Via catheter, as a solution containing the equivalent of 320 mg of iodine per mL, administered into the appropriate visceral artery, and repeated as needed, as follows:
  Aorta—25 to 50 mL.
  Superior mesenteric artery—20 to 40 mL.
  Inferior mesenteric artery—8 to 15 mL.
  Celiac artery—40 mL.
Venography, peripheral:
  Intravenous injection or intravenous infusion, 50 to 100 mL for the lower extremity and 15 to 30 mL for an upper extremity of a solution containing the equivalent of 200 mg of iodine per mL; or, 40 to 60 mL per lower extremity and 10 to 20 mL for an upper extremity, of a solution containing the equivalent of 320 mg of iodine per mL.
  Note: Flushing the venous system with 5% Dextrose Injection USP, normal saline, or Water for Injection USP is recommended immediately after the procedure, to clear the contrast agent from the extremity.
Urography, excretory:
  Intravenous, 50 to 75 mL of a solution containing the equivalent of 320 mg of iodine per mL administered within 30 to 90 seconds.
  Note: Patients in whom poor visualization is anticipated (e.g., obese patients, patients with impaired renal function) may require a dose of 100 to 150 mL (1.5 to 2 mL per kg of body weight).
CT of the brain:
  As a solution containing the equivalent of 320 mg of iodine per mL:
  Adults weighing up to 70 kg—Intravenous, 2 mL per kg of body weight.
  Adults weighing 70 kg and over—Intravenous, 135 mL, not to exceed 150 mL.
CT of the body:
  Intravenous injection, 60 mL of a solution containing the equivalent of 200 mg of iodine per mL; or, by intravenous bolus injection, rapid infusion, or combination of bolus injection and infusion, 0.9 to 2 mL per kg of body weight of a solution containing the equivalent of 320 mg of iodine per mL.
  Note: When prolonged enhancement is required, up to 200 mL of a solution containing the equivalent of 200 mg of iodine per mL may be used, of which 40 to 80 mL should be administered as a bolus injection and the remainder as an infusion. Or, up to 150 mL of a solution containing the equivalent of 320 mg of iodine per mL may be used, of which 25 to 50 mL is administered as a bolus injection and the remainder as an infusion.
Intrasynovial—Arthrography: Intrasynovial, as a solution containing the equivalent of 320 mg of iodine per mL as follows—
  Knee, hip: 5 to 15 mL.
  Shoulder, ankle: 5 to 20 mL.
  Temporomandibular: 0.5 to 0.7 mL.

### Usual adult prescribing limits
Intravascular—
  Cerebral angiography: Up to 150 mL of a solution containing the equivalent of 320 mg of iodine per mL.
  Intravenous digital subtraction angiography: Up to 250 mL of a solution containing the equivalent of 320 mg of iodine per mL.
  Coronary arteriography: Up to 150 mL of a solution containing the equivalent of 320 mg of iodine per mL.
  Combined selective coronary arteriography and left ventriculography: Up to 250 mL of a solution containing the equivalent of 320 mg of iodine per mL.
  Peripheral arteriography: Up to 250 mL of a solution containing the equivalent of 320 mg of iodine per mL.
  Aortography: Up to 250 mL of a solution containing the equivalent of 320 mg of iodine per mL.

Selective visceral arteriography[1]: Up to 250 mL of a solution containing the equivalent of 320 mg of iodine per mL.
CT of the brain: Up to 150 mL of a solution containing the equivalent of 320 mg of iodine per mL.
CT of the body: Up to 200 mL of a solution containing the equivalent of 200 mg of iodine per mL; or up to 150 mL of a solution containing the equivalent of 320 mg of iodine per mL.

**Usual pediatric dose**
For all procedures, dosage must be individualized by physician according to body weight. However, doses should not exceed 3 to 5 mL per kg of body weight of a solution containing the equivalent of 320 mg of iodine per mL.
Angiocardiography:
Via catheter, 1.5 mL (range, 1 to 2 mL) per kg of body weight, of a solution containing the equivalent of 320 mg of iodine per mL, as a single dose administered rapidly within one to two seconds. For older children, single doses of 30 to 45 mL are administered.
Urography, excretory[1]:
Intravenous, as follows: Of a solution containing the equivalent of 320 mg of iodine per mL—Children up to 6 months of age: 3 mL per kg of body weight.
Children 6 months of age and older: 2 mL per kg of body weight.

**Usual geriatric dose**
See *Usual adult and adolescent dose.*

Note: Geriatric patients, in whom poor visualization is anticipated, may require a dose of 100 to 150 mL (1.5 to 2 mL per kg of body weight) of a solution containing the equivalent of 320 mg of iodine per mL for excretory urography.

**Strength(s) usually available**
U.S.—
39.3% (393 mg per mL) of ioxaglate meglumine and 19.6% (196 mg per mL) of ioxaglate sodium with 32% (320 mg per mL) of iodine

(Rx) [*Hexabrix* (0.10 mg of edetate calcium disodium; 3.48 mg or 0.15 mEq of sodium, per mL)].
Canada—
24.6% (246 mg per mL) of ioxaglate meglumine and 12.3% (123 mg per mL) of ioxaglate sodium with 20% (200 mg per mL) of iodine (Rx) [*Hexabrix-200* (0.10 mg of edetate calcium disodium; 3.48 mg or 0.15 mEq of sodium, per mL)].
39.3% (393 mg per mL) of ioxaglate meglumine and 19.6% (196 mg per mL) of ioxaglate sodium with 32% (320 mg per mL) of iodine (Rx) [*Hexabrix-320* (0.10 mg of edetate calcium disodium; 3.48 mg or 0.15 mEq of sodium, per mL)].

**Packaging and storage**
Store below 30 °C (86 °F), unless otherwise specified by manufacturer. Protect from light. Protect from freezing.

**Stability**
Ioxaglate meglumine and ioxaglate sodium injection is a clear, colorless to pale yellow solution. Do not use if turbid or discolored.
Crystals may form in the solution at very cold temperatures but are readily redissolved by bringing the container of solution to room temperature and gently shaking it.
Any unused portion remaining in the container should be discarded.

**Incompatibilities**
Ioxaglate meglumine and ioxaglate sodium injection is physically incompatible with other medications and must *not* be mixed in the same syringe or IV administration set.

[1]Not included in Canadian product labeling.

## Selected Bibliography
Almén T. Contrast media: the relation of chemical structure, animal toxicity and adverse clinical effects. Am J Cardiol 1990; 66: 2F-8F.

Revised: 07/24/95

---

# IPECAC Oral-Local

VA CLASSIFICATION (Primary): GA600
Note: For a listing of dosage forms and brand names by country availability, see *Dosage Forms* section(s). For a listing of brand names for the articles in this monograph, refer to the General Index.

## Category
Emetic.

## Indications
**Accepted**
Toxicity, nonspecific (treatment)—Ipecac syrup is indicated as an emetic for emergency use in the treatment of drug overdose and in some cases of poisoning. Ipecac should not be used if strychnine or corrosives such as alkalies (lye) or strong acids have been ingested. Use in strychnine poisoning may precipitate seizures, and use in corrosive poisoning may cause additional injury to the esophagus.

Also, ipecac should not be used in semiconscious or unconscious persons since there is an increased risk that the vomited material may enter the lungs and cause pneumonia.

In addition, ipecac is usually not used in patients who have ingested petroleum distillates such as kerosene, gasoline, coal oil, fuel oil, paint thinner, or cleaning fluid because of the high risk of pulmonary aspiration, possibly resulting in pneumonia; however, this is controversial. The benefits of ipecac may outweigh the risks of aspiration or toxic reactions from the petroleum distillate, depending on the amount ingested and the relative toxicity of the petroleum distillate or the chemical dissolved in it.

## Pharmacology/Pharmacokinetics
**Mechanism of action/Effect**
The actions of ipecac are mainly those of its major alkaloids, emetine and cephaeline. They act locally by irritating the gastric mucosa and centrally by stimulating the medullary chemoreceptor trigger zone to induce vomiting.

**Onset of action**
20 to 30 minutes.

**Duration of action**
20 to 25 minutes.

**Elimination**
Emetine—Eliminated from body very slowly; may be detected in urine up to 60 days after ipecac use.

## Precautions to Consider
**Pregnancy/Reproduction**
Pregnancy—Studies have not been done in humans.
Studies have not been done in animals.
FDA Pregnancy Category C.

**Breast-feeding**
It is not known whether ipecac is distributed into breast milk. However, problems in humans have not been documented.

**Pediatrics**
In children under 1 year of age, there is an increased risk of aspiration of vomitus. Medical advice and/or supervision on proper positioning to avoid aspiration is important in this age group.

**Geriatrics**
Appropriate studies performed to date have not demonstrated geriatrics-specific problems that would limit the usefulness of ipecac in the elderly.

**Drug interactions and/or related problems**
The following drug interactions and/or related problems have been selected on the basis of their potential clinical significance (possible mechanism in parentheses where appropriate)—not necessarily inclusive (» = major clinical significance):
Note: Combinations containing any of the following medications, depending on the amount present, may also interact with this medication.

Antiemetics
(prior ingestion of these medications may decrease the emetic response to ipecac)

Beverages, carbonated
(concurrent use with ipecac is not recommended since these beverages may cause distention of the stomach)

Charcoal, activated
  (if both ipecac and activated charcoal are to be used in the treatment of poisoning, it is generally recommended that activated charcoal be administered only after vomiting has been induced and completed; however, in some clinical trials in which activated charcoal was administered pre-emesis 10 minutes after high doses of ipecac, the emetic properties of ipecac were not inhibited)

Milk or milk products
  (concurrent use is not recommended since milk has been reported to decrease the effectiveness of ipecac)

### Medical considerations/Contraindications
The medical considerations/contraindications included here have been selected on the basis of their potential clinical significance (reasons given in parentheses where appropriate)—not necessarily inclusive (» = major clinical significance).

*Except under special circumstances, this medication should not be used when the following medical problems exist:*
»  Any condition in which there is an increased risk of aspiration of vomitus, such as:
»  Decreased patient alertness or
»  Depressed gag reflex or
»  Seizures or history of or
»  Shock or
»  Unconsciousness
       (risk of aspiration pneumonia)
»  Ingestion of corrosive materials, such as alkalies (lye) or strong acids
       (vomiting may cause additional injury to the esophagus)

*Risk-benefit should be considered when the following medical problems exist:*
Heart disease
   (increased risk of tachycardia, hypotension, precordial chest pain, dyspnea, and electrocardiogram (ECG) abnormalities if ipecac is not vomited)
»  Ingestion of petroleum distillates, such as kerosene, gasoline, coal oil, fuel oil, paint thinner, or cleaning fluid
       (risk of aspiration pneumonia)
Strychnine poisoning
   (increased risk of seizures)

## Side/Adverse Effects

Note: Toxic myopathy, cardiac toxicity, and several deaths have been reported as a result of the chronic use of ipecac among young women with anorexia nervosa, bulimia, and related eating disorders. These patients used ipecac as a means of inducing emesis to lose weight.

## Overdose

For more information on the management of overdose or unintentional ingestion, **contact a Poison Control Center** (see *Poison Control Center Listing*).

### Clinical effects of overdose
The following effects have been selected on the basis of their potential clinical significance (possible signs and symptoms in parentheses where appropriate)—not necessarily inclusive (may also be symptoms of chronic abuse):

*Diarrhea; fast or irregular heartbeat; nausea or vomiting, continuing more than 30 minutes; stomach cramps or pain; troubled breathing; unusual tiredness or weakness; weakness, aching, and stiffness of muscles, especially those of the neck, arms, and legs*
Note: *Cardiac and muscle disorders* are related to emetine toxicity.

## Patient Consultation

As an aid to patient consultation, refer to *Advice for the Patient, Ipecac (Oral)*.

In providing consultation, consider emphasizing the following selected information (» = major clinical significance):

### Before using this medication
»  Calling physician, poison control center, or emergency room before taking medication
»  Conditions affecting use, especially:
       Use in children—Increased risk of aspiration of vomitus in children under 1 year of age
       Other medical problems, especially any condition in which there is an increased risk of aspiration of vomitus, and ingestion of corrosive materials or petroleum distillates

### Proper use of this medication
»  Importance of not taking more medication than recommended on the label or otherwise directed
»  Not giving medication to semiconscious or unconscious persons
    Importance of drinking water immediately after taking medication
»  Avoiding concurrent use with milk or carbonated beverages
    Getting medical attention immediately if vomiting does not occur within 20 minutes after second dose
»  Taking activated charcoal only after vomiting has been induced by this medication and completed, if both are to be used
»  Proper dosing
»  Proper storage

### Side/adverse effects
    Signs of potential side effects, especially cardiac and muscle disorders related to emetine toxicity (with chronic abuse)

## General Dosing Information

To increase the emetic action of ipecac, it is recommended that adults drink 1 full glass (240 mL) of water and children drink ½ to 1 full glass (120 to 240 mL) of water immediately after taking the ipecac syrup. In young and frightened children, water may be given before the ipecac syrup if necessary.

No more than 2 doses of ipecac syrup should be taken since ipecac can be cardiotoxic.

## Oral Dosage Forms
### IPECAC SYRUP USP

Note: *Ipecac Fluidextract* and *Ipecac Tincture* have been replaced by *Ipecac Syrup*, the preferred dosage form. *Ipecac Fluidextract* is 14 times more concentrated than *Ipecac Syrup*, and is not recommended for use because of its high potency and toxicity.

### Usual adult and adolescent dose
Emetic—
   Oral, 15 to 30 mL, followed immediately by one full glass (240 mL) of water. Dose may be repeated after twenty to thirty minutes if emesis does not occur. If emesis does not occur after the second dose, gastric lavage should be performed.

### Usual pediatric dose
Emetic—
   Children up to 6 months of age: Ipecac syrup should be administered only under the supervision of a physician.
   Children 6 months to 1 year of age: Oral, 5 to 10 mL, preceded or followed by one-half to one full glass (120 to 240 mL) of water.
   Children 1 to 12 years of age: Oral, 15 mL, preceded or followed by one-half to one full glass (120 to 240 mL) of water.

Note: Doses may be repeated after twenty to thirty minutes if emesis does not occur. If emesis does not occur after the second dose, gastric lavage should be performed.

   For children 6 months to 1 year of age, professional advice on proper positioning to avoid aspiration of vomitus is important.

### Strength(s) usually available
U.S.—
   15 mL (OTC) [GENERIC].
   30 mL (OTC) [GENERIC].
Canada—
   15 mL (OTC) [GENERIC].
   30 mL (OTC) [GENERIC].

Note: Each mL of ipecac syrup contains 1.23 to 1.57 mg of the total ether-soluble alkaloids of ipecac.

   Alcohol content ranges from 1 to 2%.

**Packaging and storage**
Store preferably at a temperature below 25 °C (77 °F), in a tight container.
Note: Containers intended for sale to the public without prescription contain not more than 30 mL of ipecac syrup.

**Note**
If ipecac syrup is to be used as an emetic for emergency use in poisoning, consider providing on the label the telephone number for physician, poison control center, or emergency room.

## Selected Bibliography
Manno BR, Manno JE. Toxicology of ipecac: a review. Clin Toxicol 1977; 10: 221-42.

Revised: 08/04/94

---

**IPECAC-CONTAINING COMBINATIONS—**
Chlorpheniramine, Ephedrine, Phenylephrine, Dextromethorphan, Ammonium Chloride, and Ipecac (Systemic)—See *Cough/Cold Combinations (Systemic)*

---

**IPODATE**—See *Cholecystographic Agents, Oral (Systemic)*

---

# IPRATROPIUM   Inhalation-Local

VA CLASSIFICATION (Primary): RE105
Note: For a listing of dosage forms and brand names by country availability, see *Dosage Forms* section(s). For a listing of brand names for the articles in this monograph, refer to the General Index.

## Category
Bronchodilator.

## Indications
Note: Bracketed information in the *Indications* section refers to uses that are not included in U.S. product labeling.

**Accepted**
Bronchitis (treatment) or
Emphysema, pulmonary (treatment) or
Pulmonary disease, chronic obstructive, other (treatment)—Ipratropium is indicated for maintenance treatment of bronchospasm associated with chronic obstructive pulmonary disease, including chronic bronchitis and pulmonary emphysema. Regular use of ipratropium results in at least as great an increase in airflow as that with use of other bronchodilators and fewer adverse effects. If additional bronchodilation is needed in these patients, an adrenergic bronchodilator may be used as an adjunct to ipratropium.

[Ipratropium is indicated as an adjunct to adrenergic bronchodilators for treatment of acute exacerbations of chronic obstructive pulmonary disease.]

[Asthma (treatment adjunct)]—Ipratropium is used as an adjunct to anti-inflammatory therapy or bronchodilators to prevent[1] exacerbations of asthma in patients who respond poorly to therapy or as an alternative to other bronchodilators in patients who develop significant side effects with these medications.

Ipratropium is used as an adjunct to adrenergic bronchodilators for the treatment of acute exacerbations of asthma. It is not used alone because it has a relatively slower onset of action and time to peak effect as compared with adrenergic bronchodilators.

[1]Not included in Canadian product labeling.

## Pharmacology/Pharmacokinetics

**Physicochemical characteristics**
Source—A synthetic quaternary ammonium compound, chemically related to atropine
Molecular weight—430.38.
Other characteristics—Fairly stable in neutral solutions and in acid solutions; rapidly hydrolyzed in alkaline solutions

**Mechanism of action/Effect**
The bronchodilation produced by ipratropium is primarily a local, site-specific effect rather than a systemic effect. Ipratropium appears to produce bronchodilation by competitive inhibition of cholinergic receptors on bronchial smooth muscle. This effect antagonizes the action of acetylcholine at its membrane-bound receptor site and thereby blocks the bronchoconstrictor action of vagal efferent impulses.

**Absorption**
Systemic absorption is minimal following inhalation. Blood concentration and renal and fecal excretion studies have shown that ipratropium is poorly absorbed into the systemic circulation from both the surface of the lung and the gastrointestinal tract. At a dose of 14 times the recommended therapeutic inhalation dose, the peak plasma concentration is 0.06 nanograms/mL. Plasma concentrations after inhalation of usual doses are about 1000 times lower than equipotent oral or intravenous doses (15 and 0.15 mg, respectively).

**Distribution**
Studies in rats have shown that ipratropium does not penetrate the blood-brain barrier.

**Biotransformation**
Hepatic, for the small amount of ipratropium systemically absorbed; metabolites have little or no anticholinergic activity.

**Onset of action**
Within 5 to 15 minutes.

**Time to peak effect**
About 90 minutes (range, 1 to 2 hours).

**Duration of action**
About 3 to 4 hours in the majority of patients, but up to 6 to 8 hours in some patients.

**Elimination**
Primarily fecal; up to 90% of inhaled dose is swallowed and eliminated as unchanged drug. Absorbed portion of dose is excreted primarily in the urine.

## Precautions to Consider

**Cross-sensitivity and/or related problems**
Patients sensitive to belladonna alkaloids may be sensitive to ipratropium also, since ipratropium is chemically related to atropine. Although rare, allergic reactions to ipratropium metered-dose inhaler have been reported; however, the causative component has not been identified. Therefore, patients allergic to soybean protein or other legumes, such as peanuts, may be allergic to soya lecithin contained in the metered-dose inhaler as a suspending agent.

**Carcinogenicity/Tumorigenicity**
Two-year carcinogenicity studies in mice and rats have shown that ipratropium, at oral doses up to 1250 times the maximum recommended human daily dose, has no carcinogenic potential. Also, studies in mice and rats have shown that ipratropium, at oral doses up to 6 mg per kg of body weight (mg/kg), does not have a carcinogenic or tumorigenic effect.

**Mutagenicity**
Various studies in mice and hamsters have shown that ipratropium is not mutagenic.

**Pregnancy/Reproduction**
Fertility—Although studies in male and female rats have shown that ipratropium, at oral doses up to approximately 10,000 times the maximum recommended human daily dose, does not affect fertility, ipratropium has been shown to increase resorption and decrease conception rates when the medication was administered at doses above 18,000 times the maximum recommended human daily dose.

Pregnancy—Although adequate and well-controlled studies in humans have not been done, no increased risk of congenital malformation has been reported.

Reproduction studies with ipratropium in mice, rats, and rabbits given oral doses of 10, 100, and 125 mg per kg of body weight (mg/kg), respectively, and in rats and rabbits given inhalation doses of 1.5 and

1.8 mg/kg (or approximately 38 and 45 times the recommended human daily dose), respectively, have shown no evidence of teratogenic effects.

FDA Pregnancy Category B.

**Breast-feeding**

It is not known whether ipratropium is distributed into breast milk. However, problems in humans have not been documented. Although lipid-insoluble quaternary bases, such as ipratropium, are distributed into breast milk, it is unlikely that inhaled ipratropium would reach significant concentrations in maternal serum, and the concentration in breast milk would probably be undetectable.

**Pediatrics**

Appropriate studies performed to date have not demonstrated pediatrics-specific problems that would limit the usefulness of ipratropium in children.

**Geriatrics**

Studies performed to date on patients over 65 years of age have not demonstrated geriatrics-specific problems that would limit the usefulness of ipratropium inhalation in the elderly.

**Drug interactions and/or related problems**

The following drug interactions and/or related problems have been selected on the basis of their potential clinical significance (possible mechanism in parentheses where appropriate)—not necessarily inclusive (» = major clinical significance):

Note: Combinations containing any of the following medications, depending on the amount present, may also interact with this medication.

Anticholinergics, other, or other medications with anticholinergic activity (see *Appendix II*)
(concurrent use of other anticholinergics, including ophthalmic preparations, or other medications with anticholinergic action with ipratropium may result in additive effects)

Tacrine
(because tacrine is thought to act by increasing effective acetylcholine concentrations, concurrent use may decrease the effects of either ipratropium or tacrine)

**Medical considerations/Contraindications**

The medical considerations/contraindications included here have been selected on the basis of their potential clinical significance (reasons given in parentheses where appropriate)—not necessarily inclusive (» = major clinical significance).

*Risk-benefit should be considered when the following medical problems exist:*

» Glaucoma, angle-closure
(an acute attack may be precipitated or condition may be exacerbated if ipratropium inhalation aerosol is sprayed directly into the eyes or if a poorly fitting face mask is used with nebulized ipratropium inhalation solution, alone or in combination with an adrenergic bronchodilator)

Sensitivity to ipratropium or belladonna alkaloids; also, allergy to soya lecithin, soybean protein, or other legumes such as peanuts for patients using the metered-dose inhaler

Urinary retention
(rarely, condition may be aggravated)

## Side/Adverse Effects

Note: Usual therapeutic doses of ipratropium generally do not cause systemic side/adverse effects because of the low blood concentrations achieved with the inhalation; however, the potential for systemic side/adverse effects exists.

Although rare, cases of precipitation or worsening of narrow-angle glaucoma and acute eye pain have been reported following use of ipratropium aerosol, and inhalation solution alone or in combination with an adrenergic bronchodilator, when the spray came into contact with the eyes.

Acute overdose of ipratropium by inhalation is unlikely since the medication is not well absorbed systemically.

The following side/adverse effects have been selected on the basis of their potential clinical significance (possible signs and symptoms in parentheses where appropriate)—not necessarily inclusive:

**Those indicating need for medical attention**
Incidence rare
*Bronchospasm, increased* (increased wheezing; tightness in chest; difficulty in breathing); *dermatitis, hypersensitivity-induced; angioedema* (swelling of face, lips, or eyelids); *skin rash; urticaria* (hives);

*eye pain, acute; paralytic ileus* (continuing constipation; lower abdominal pain or distention)—especially in patients with cystic fibrosis

Note: *Increased bronchospasm* may be due to sensitivity to benzalkonium chloride and edetate disodium present in the multiple-dose container of inhalation solution.

**Those indicating need for medical attention only if they continue or are bothersome**
Incidence more frequent
*Cough; dryness of mouth; unpleasant taste*
Incidence rare
*Blurred vision or other changes in vision; burning eyes; dizziness; headache; nausea; nervousness; palpitations* (pounding heartbeat); *sweating; trembling; urinary retention* (difficult urination)

**Treatment of overdose**
Cholinesterase inhibitors may be used for serious anticholinergic toxicity.

## Patient Consultation

As an aid to patient consultation, refer to *Advice for the Patient, Ipratropium (Inhalation).*

In providing consultation, consider emphasizing the following selected information (» = major clinical significance):

**Before using this medication**
» Conditions affecting use, especially:
Sensitivity to ipratropium or belladonna alkaloids; also, allergy to soya lecithin, soybean protein, or peanuts for patients using metered-dose inhaler
Other medical problems, especially angle-closure glaucoma

**Proper use of this medication**
» Helps control symptoms of lung disease; inhalation solution used only with other bronchodilators when treating acute asthma attacks
» Importance of not using more medication than the amount prescribed
» Avoiding contact with the eyes; closing eyes if necessary when inhaling; if accidentally sprayed into the eyes or if nebulized solution escapes into the eyes, irritation or blurring of vision may occur; rinsing eyes with cool water if necessary
Reading patient instructions carefully before using
» If using regularly, importance of using every day at regularly spaced times.
» Proper dosing
Missed dose: If used regularly, using as soon as possible; using any remaining doses for that day at regularly spaced intervals
» Proper storage
*For inhalation aerosol dosage form*
Checking periodically with health care professional for proper use of inhaler to prevent improper technique and incorrect dosage
Testing or priming inhaler before using first time or first time in a while
Proper administration technique without spacer device
Proper administration technique with spacer device
Proper cleaning procedure for inhaler

*For inhalation solution dosage form*
Using only in nebulizer as instructed by physician
Preparing solution for nebulizer
Proper administration technique: Using in a power-operated nebulizer with an adequate flow rate and equipped with a face mask or mouthpiece

**Precautions while using this medication**
» Checking with physician immediately if symptoms do not improve within 30 minutes after using this medication or if condition becomes worse
*For patients using ipratropium inhalation solution*
» If also using cromolyn inhalation solution, not mixing cromolyn inhalation solution with ipratropium inhalation solution containing the preservative benzalkonium chloride for use in a nebulizer

**Side/adverse effects**
Signs of potential side effects, especially increased bronchospasm, hypersensitivity-induced dermatitis, acute eye pain, and paralytic ileus

## General Dosing Information

For nebulization of ipratropium bromide inhalation solution, a gas flow (oxygen or compressed air) of 6 to 10 liters per minute should be used. Nebulizers with either a face mask or mouthpiece have been used, although a mouthpiece may be preferable to a face mask because it reduces the risk of solution entering the eyes.

Patients should be advised to contact their physician immediately if they do not respond to the usual dose of ipratropium because this may be a sign of seriously worsening airflow obstruction or the development of concurrent illness requiring reassessment of therapy.

The contents of metered dose inhalers should generally not be floated in water to assess the contents since this method may not reliably predict the amount of medication remaining in the canister. A record should be kept of the number of inhalations used.

## Inhalation Dosage Forms

Note: Bracketed uses in the *Dosage Forms* section refers to indications that are not included in U.S. product labeling.

### IPRATROPIUM BROMIDE INHALATION AEROSOL

**Usual adult and adolescent dose**
Bronchitis (treatment)
Emphysema, pulmonary (treatment) or
Pulmonary disease, chronic obstructive, other (treatment)—
    Oral inhalation, 2 to 4 inhalations (36 to 72 mcg) three or four times a day. Some patients may require up to 6 to 8 inhalations (108 to 144 mcg) three times a day. For severe exacerbations, 6 to 8 inhalations may be administered, using a spacer device, every three to four hours.
[Asthma (treatment adjunct)][1]—
    Oral inhalation, 1 to 4 inhalations (18 to 72 mcg) four times a day as necessary.

**Usual pediatric dose**
[Asthma (treatment adjunct)][1]—
    Children up to 12 years of age: Oral inhalation, 1 to 2 inhalations (18 to 36 mcg) every six to eight hours as necessary.

**Strength(s) usually available**
U.S.—
    18 mcg per metered spray (Rx) [*Atrovent* (dichlorodifluoromethane; dichlorotetrafluoroethane; trichloromonofluoromethane; soya lecithin)].
Canada—
    20 mcg per metered spray (Rx) [*Atrovent* (dichlorodifluoromethane; dichlorotetrafluoroethane; trichloromonofluoromethane; soya lecithin)].

Note: In Canada, metered dose inhalers are labeled according to the amount of ipratropium delivered at the valve; in the U.S., metered dose inhalers are labeled according to the amount of ipratropium delivered at the mouthpiece or actuator. Therefore, 20 mcg of ipratropium delivered at the valve is equivalent to 18 mcg delivered at the mouthpiece.

**Packaging and storage**
Store between 15 and 30 °C (59 and 86 °F), unless otherwise specified by manufacturer.

**Auxiliary labeling**
• For oral inhalation only.
• Shake well before using.
• Store away from heat and direct sunlight.

**Note**
Include patient instructions when dispensing.
Demonstrate inhalation technique to patient when dispensing.

**Additional information**
Each canister contains medication for about 200 inhalations.

### IPRATROPIUM BROMIDE INHALATION SOLUTION

**Usual adult and adolescent dose**
Bronchitis (treatment)
Emphysema, pulmonary (treatment) or
Pulmonary disease, chronic obstructive, other (treatment)—
    Oral inhalation, 250 to 500 mcg (0.25 to 0.5 mg), diluted, if necessary; dose is administered via nebulization three or four times a day, every six to eight hours. For severe exacerbations of COPD, 500 mcg may be administered every four to eight hours.

[Asthma (treatment adjunct)][1]—
    Oral inhalation, 500 mcg (0.5 mg), diluted, if necessary; dose is administered via nebulization three or four times a day, every six to eight hours as necessary.

**Usual pediatric dose**
[Asthma (treatment adjunct)][1]—
    Children up to 5 years of age: Safety and efficacy have not been established.
    Children 5 to 12 years of age: Oral inhalation, 125 to 250 mcg (0.125 to 0.25 mg), diluted, if necessary, to three to five mL with preservative-free sterile sodium chloride inhalation solution 0.9%; dose is administered via nebulization every four to six hours as necessary.

**Strength(s) usually available**
U.S.—
    Single-dose vial
        0.02% (200 mcg per mL [2.5 mL]) (Rx) [*Atrovent*; GENERIC].
Canada—
    Single-dose vial
        0.0125% (125 mcg per mL [2 mL]) (Rx) [*Atrovent*].
        0.025% (250 mcg per mL [1 or 2 mL]) (Rx) [*Atrovent*].
    Multiple-dose vial
        0.025% (250 mcg per mL) (Rx) [*Apo-Ipravent* (benzalkonium chloride; EDTA-disodium); *Atrovent* (benzalkonium chloride; EDTA-disodium); *Kendral-Ipratropium*].

**Packaging and storage**
Prior to opening container, store between 15 and 30 °C (59 and 86 °F), unless otherwise specified by manufacturer. Protect from freezing. Protect from light.

**Preparation of dosage form**
Ipratropium inhalation solution can be diluted with preservative-free sterile 0.9% sodium chloride.

**Stability**
Solutions of ipratropium containing the preservative benzalkonium chloride may be diluted with preservative-free sterile sodium chloride inhalation solution 0.9%. The solution should be used within twenty-four hours from time of dilution when stored at room temperature and within forty-eight hours when stored in the refrigerator.
Preservative-free albuterol inhalation solution can be mixed in the nebulizer with ipratropium inhalation solution, if used within one hour.
Preservative-free ipratropium inhalation solution is recommended when combining ipratropium with cromolyn inhalation solution. This combination is compatible for up to one hour. Mixing ipratropium inhalation solution containing the preservative benzalkonium chloride with cromolyn in a nebulizer results in cloudiness of the solution, which is due to complexation between cromolyn sodium and benzalkonium chloride. No precipitation or significant decrease in the concentration of cromolyn or ipratropium occurs.

**Auxiliary labeling**
• For oral inhalation only.

**Note**
Include patient instructions for preparation of solution when dispensing.

---

[1]Not included in Canadian product labeling.

## Selected Bibliography

Gross NJ. Ipratropium bromide. N Engl J Med 1988; 319: 486-94.
Spector SL, Nicklas RA, editors. Practice parameters for the diagnosis and treatment of asthma. J Allergy Clin Immunol 1995; 96: 786-9.
American Thoracic Society. Standards for the diagnosis and care of patients with chronic obstructive pulmonary disease. Am J Respir Crit Care Med 1995; 152 Suppl: 77S-120S.

---

Revised: 06/21/96

---

# IPRATROPIUM    Nasal*

VA CLASSIFICATION (Primary): NT900
Note: For a listing of dosage forms and brand names by country availability, see *Dosage Forms* section(s). For a listing of brand names for the articles in this monograph, refer to the General Index.

*Not commercially available in the U.S.

## Category
Anticholinergic (nasal).

## Indications

### Accepted
Rhinorrhea (treatment)—Ipratropium nasal aerosol is indicated for the symptomatic treatment of rhinorrhea associated with vasomotor rhinitis. Ipratropium nasal aerosol has not been shown to control rhinitis symptoms other than rhinorrea; it has little or no effect on sneezing, itching, or nasal congestion caused by vasodilation.

## Pharmacology/Pharmacokinetics

### Physicochemical characteristics
Source—A synthetic quaternary ammonium compound, chemically related to atropine.

### Mechanism of action/Effect
Ipratropium antagonizes the actions of acetylcholine at parasympathetic, postganglionic, effector-cell junctions by competing with acetylcholine for receptor sites. When administered intranasally, ipratropium has a localized parasympathetic blocking action, which reduces watery hypersecretion from mucosal glands in the nose.

### Absorption
Systemic absorption from the nasal mucosa is rapid but minimal following nasal administration.

### Biotransformation
Hepatic, for the small amount of nasal ipratropium systemically absorbed; metabolites have little or no anticholinergic activity.

### Half-life
Elimination—About 3.5 hours (range, 1.5 to 4 hours).

### Onset of action
Within 5 minutes.

### Time to peak effect
1 to 4 hours.

### Duration of action
About 4 to 8 hours.

### Elimination
Absorbed portion of dose is excreted primarily in the urine; also excreted in the bile.

## Precautions to Consider

### Cross-sensitivity and/or related problems
Patients sensitive to belladonna alkaloids may be sensitive to ipratropium also, since ipratropium is chemically related to atropine.

### Carcinogenicity/Tumorigenicity
Studies of several weeks duration in mice and rats have shown that ipratropium, at oral doses of up to 6 mg/kg of body weight, does not have a carcinogenic or tumorigenic effect.

### Mutagenicity
Although several studies have shown that ipratropium is not mutagenic, one study has shown a dose-related increase in the number of chromatoid gaps; however, the significance of this finding is not known.

### Pregnancy/Reproduction
Fertility—A fertility study in rats given oral doses of 5, 50, and 500 mg of ipratropium per kg of body weight for 60 days before and during early gestation showed that fertility was delayed in 8 of 20 females; the conception rate was decreased in 75% of females given the 500 mg/kg dose.

Pregnancy—Adequate and well-controlled studies in humans have not been done.

Reproduction studies in mice, rats, and rabbits given ipratropium at oral doses of approximately 2, 10, and 20 mg/kg, and reproduction studies in rabbits given ipratropium at inhalation doses of 0.3, 0.9, and 1.8 mg/kg, have shown no evidence of embryotoxic or teratogenic effects.

### Breast-feeding
It is not known whether ipratropium is distributed into breast milk. Problems in humans have not been documented.

### Pediatrics
Appropriate studies on the relationship of age to the effects of ipratropium nasal aerosol have not been performed in children up to 12 years of age. However, no pediatrics-specific problems have been documented to date.

### Geriatrics
No information is available on the relationship of age to the effects of ipratropium nasal aerosol in geriatric patients.

### Dental
Higher doses and prolonged use of ipratropium nasal aerosol may decrease or inhibit salivary flow, thus contributing to the development of caries, periodontal disease, oral candidiasis, and discomfort.

### Drug interactions and/or related problems
The following drug interactions and/or related problems have been selected on the basis of their potential clinical significance (possible mechanism in parentheses where appropriate)—not necessarily inclusive (» = major clinical significance):

Note: Combinations containing any of the following medications, depending on the amount present, may also interact with this medication.

Anticholinergics, other, or other medications with anticholinergic activity (See *Appendix II*)
(concurrent use of other anticholinergics, including ophthalmic preparations, or other medications with anticholinergic action with ipratropium nasal aerosol may result in additive effects)

### Medical considerations/Contraindications
The medical considerations/contraindications included here have been selected on the basis of their potential clinical significance (reasons given in parentheses where appropriate)—not necessarily inclusive (» = major clinical significance).

*Risk-benefit should be considered when the following medical problems exist:*

Glaucoma, angle-closure
(an acute attack may be precipitated or condition may be exacerbated if ipratropium nasal aerosol is sprayed directly into the eyes)

Sensitivity to ipratropium or belladonna alkaloids

## Side/Adverse Effects

Note: Usual therapeutic doses of ipratropium given intranasally generally do not cause systemic side/adverse effects because of the low blood concentrations achieved with nasal administration; however, the potential for systemic side/adverse effects exists.

In addition, acute overdose of ipratropium nasal aerosol is unlikely, since the medication is not well absorbed systemically.

The following side/adverse effects have been selected on the basis of their potential clinical significance (possible signs and symptoms in parentheses where appropriate)—not necessarily inclusive:

### Those indicating need for medical attention
Incidence rare
*Blurred vision or other changes in vision; bronchospasm* (wheezing, tightness in chest, or difficulty in breathing); *difficult or painful urination; difficulty in swallowing; eye pain, severe; fast or irregular heartbeat; skin rash or hives; stomatitis* (sores in mouth and on lips); *swelling of tongue or lips*

### Those indicating need for medical attention only if they continue or are bothersome
Incidence more frequent
*Dryness of nose or mouth; headache; irritation and crusting in nose*
Incidence less frequent or rare
*Bleeding or burning in nose; diarrhea or constipation; dryness of throat; nausea; nervousness; stomach pain; stuffy nose*

## Patient Consultation

As an aid to patient consultation, refer to *Advice for the Patient, Ipratropium (Nasal)*.

In providing consultation, consider emphasizing the following selected information (» = major clinical significance):

### Before using this medication
» Conditions affecting use, especially:
Sensitivity to ipratropium or belladonna alkaloids

### Proper use of this medication
» Compliance with therapy; importance of not using more medication than the amount prescribed
» Avoiding contact with the eyes; if accidentally sprayed into the eyes, irritation or blurring of vision may occur; rinsing eyes with cool water if necessary
Reading patient instructions carefully before using; clearing nasal passages before each use
Checking with health care professional for proper use of aerosol spray device to prevent incorrect dosage
Testing aerosol spray device before using first time
Proper administration technique
Proper cleaning procedure for aerosol spray device

» Proper dosing
  Missed dose: Using as soon as possible; not using if almost time for next dose; using any remaining doses for that day at regularly spaced intervals
» Proper storage

**Precautions while using this medication**
» Checking with physician if symptoms do not improve within 1 or 2 weeks or if condition becomes worse
  Possible dryness of mouth or throat; using sugarless candy or gum, ice, or saliva substitute for relief; checking with physician or dentist if dryness of mouth continues for more than 2 weeks

**Side/adverse effects**
Signs of potential side effects, especially severe eye pain, blurred vision or other changes in vision, bronchospasm, difficult or painful urination, difficulty in swallowing, fast or irregular heartbeat, skin rash or hives, stomatitis, and swelling of tongue or lips

## General Dosing Information

The smallest dose required to control symptoms should be used as a maintenance dose after the desired clinical response is achieved.

Prior to administration of ipratropium nasal aerosol, the nasal passages should be carefully cleared. During administration, patient should not breathe in so the medication will be deposited only on nasal mucosa. The patient may sniff gently, but not deeply inhale, to distribute the medication into the nose.

## Intranasal Dosage Form

### IPRATROPIUM BROMIDE NASAL AEROSOL

**Usual adult and adolescent dose**
Anticholinergic—
  Intranasal, 40 mcg (0.04 mg—2 metered sprays) into each nostril two times a day.

Note: The dosage frequency may be increased to three or four times a day as needed; however, administration should not be more frequent than every six hours.

**Usual adult prescribing limits**
320 mcg (0.32 mg—16 metered sprays) per twenty-four hours.

**Usual pediatric dose**
Children up to 12 years of age—Use is not recommended.

**Strength(s) usually available**
U.S.—
  Not commercially available.
Canada—
  20 mcg (0.02 mg) per metered spray (Rx) [*Atrovent* (dichlorodifluoromethane; dichlorotetrafluoroethane; trichloromonofluoromethane; soya lecithin)].

**Packaging and storage**
Store below 30 °C (86 °F), unless otherwise specified by manufacturer. Protect from freezing.

**Auxiliary labeling**
• For the nose.
• Shake well before using.
• Store away from heat and direct sunlight.

**Note**
Include patient instructions when dispensing.

Demonstrate nasal administration technique to patient.

**Additional information**
Each 10-mL canister contains medication for approximately 200 metered sprays.

## Selected Bibliography

Borts MR, Druce HM. The use of intranasal anticholinergic agents in the treatment of nonallergic perennial rhinitis. J Allergy Clin Immunol 1992; 90: 1065-70.

Meltzer EO. Intranasal anticholinergic therapy of rhinorrhea. J Allergy Clin Immunol 1992; 90: 1055-64.

Developed: 08/09/94

---

**IRON DEXTRAN**—See *Iron Supplements (Systemic)*

---

**IRON-POLYSACCHARIDE**—See *Iron Supplements (Systemic)*

---

**IRON SORBITOL**—See *Iron Supplements (Systemic)*

---

# IRON SUPPLEMENTS   Systemic

This monograph includes information on the following: Ferrous Fumarate; Ferrous Gluconate; Ferrous Sulfate; Iron Dextran†; Iron-Polysaccharide†; Iron Sorbitol*.

VA CLASSIFICATION (Primary): TN401

Another commonly used name for dried ferrous sulfate is ferrous sulfate exsiccated.

Note: For a listing of dosage forms and brand names by country availability, see *Dosage Forms* section(s). For a listing of brand names for the articles in this monograph, refer to the General Index.

---

*Not commercially available in the U.S.
†Not commercially available in Canada.

---

## Category
Antianemic; nutritional supplement (mineral).

## Indications

**Accepted**

Iron deficiency anemia (prophylaxis and treatment)—Iron supplements are indicated in the prevention and treatment of iron deficiency anemia, which may result from inadequate diet, malabsorption, pregnancy, rapid growth during childhood, and/or blood loss.

  Iron dextran and iron sorbitol are recommended for patients in whom iron deficiency has been determined, only after the cause has been corrected, if possible, and only when oral administration has been found unsatisfactory or impossible.

Note: The cause of iron deficiency states should always be determined, as it may relate to a serious condition.

Deficiency of iron may lead to fatigue, shortness of breath, decreased physical performance, impaired learning in children and adults, altered body temperature, and altered immune function.

Requirements may be increased and/or supplementation may be necessary in the following persons or conditions (based on documented iron deficiency):
  Achlorhydria
  Blood loss, excessive
  Burns
  Gastrectomy
  Hemodialysis
  Hemorrhage
  Infants—full-term infants after 4 months of age and preterm infants after 2 months of age, especially those receiving breast milk or low-iron formulas
  Intestinal diseases—celiac, Crohn's, diarrhea, inflammatory bowel disease, malabsorption

In addition, individuals with conditions that cause chronic blood loss (e.g., peptic ulcer, hemorrhoids, hookworms) may be at risk for iron deficiency anemia.

Some unusual diets (e.g., reducing diets that drastically restrict food selection) may not supply minimum daily requirements of iron. Supplementation may be necessary in patients receiving total parenteral nutrition (TPN) or undergoing rapid weight loss or in those with malnutrition, because of inadequate dietary intake.

Recommended intakes for all vitamins and most minerals are increased during pregnancy. Many physicians recommend that pregnant women receive multivitamin and mineral supplements, especially those pregnant women who do not consume an adequate diet and those in high-risk categories (i.e., women carrying more than one fetus, heavy cigarette smokers, and alcohol and drug abusers). However, taking excessive amounts of multivitamin and mineral supplements may be harmful to the mother and/or fetus and should be avoided.

Recommended intakes for all vitamins and most minerals are increased during breast-feeding.

Recommended intakes may be increased by the following medications: Antacids, calcium supplements, epoetin, penicillamine, trientine, zinc supplements, and any medications that cause bleeding from the gastrointestinal tract.

## Pharmacology/Pharmacokinetics

### Physicochemical characteristics
Molecular weight—
Ferrous fumarate: 169.91.
Ferrous gluconate: 482.18.
Ferrous sulfate: 278.02.
Ferrous sulfate, dried: 151.91.

### Mechanism of action/Effect
Iron is an essential component in the physiological formation of hemoglobin, adequate amounts of which are necessary for effective erythropoiesis and the resultant oxygen transport capacity of the blood. A similar function is provided by iron in myoglobin production. Iron also serves as a cofactor of several essential enzymes, including cytochromes that are involved in electron transport. Iron is necessary for catecholamine metabolism and the proper functioning of neutrophils.

### Absorption
Absorption is increased when iron stores are depleted or red blood cell production is increased. Conversely, high iron blood concentrations decrease absorption.
Oral dosage forms—
When taken orally, in food or as a supplement, iron passes through the mucosal cells in the ferrous state and is bound with the protein transferrin.
Iron-deficient individuals: 10 to 30% is absorbed, the amount being approximately proportional to the degree of deficiency.
Non–iron-deficient individuals: Approximately 5 to 15% of ingested iron is absorbed.
Absorption occurs principally in the duodenum and proximal jejunum.
Absorption is most efficient when iron is ingested in its ferrous rather than its ferric form, on an empty stomach. Gastric acid increases absorption by maintaining ferric iron in a soluble form.
Twenty to 30% of heme iron is absorbed from the diet. Two to 10% of nonheme iron is absorbed from the diet, and its absorption is affected by other foods ingested. Ascorbic acid, as a supplement or in foods, reduces ferric salts to the ferrous form and thus enhances the absorption of nonheme iron. Meat and other animal tissues also enhance the absorption of nonheme iron. Certain foods and supplements, such as coffee, tea, milk, eggs, calcium, whole grains, and phosphorus, may inhibit nonheme iron absorption.
Parenteral dosage forms—
Iron dextran: Iron dextran is absorbed from the injection site into the capillaries and lymphatic system. The majority of the intramuscular injection is absorbed within 72 hours. The remaining iron is absorbed in the following 3 to 4 weeks. Evidence of a therapeutic response is observed in a few days as an increase in reticulocyte count. The intravenous dose is available much more rapidly.
Iron sorbitol: Iron sorbitol is absorbed directly into the bloodstream as well as via the lymphatic system. Sixty-six percent of the intramuscular injection is absorbed within 3 hours.

### Distribution
Oral dosage forms—Iron is transported in the body to bone marrow for red blood cell production in the iron-transferrin complex form.
Iron dextran—Iron dextran is removed from the plasma by cells of the reticuloendothelial system and dissociated into iron and dextran. The released iron is immediately bound to protein moieties to form hemosiderin or ferritin or, to a lesser extent, transferrin. The protein-bound iron eventually replenishes the depleted iron stores and is incorporated into hemoglobin.

### Protein binding
Very high (90% or more).
Hemoglobin—High.
Myoglobin, enzymes, and transferrin—Low.
Ferritin and hemosiderin—Low.

### Storage
Iron is stored as ferritin or hemosiderin, primarily in hepatocytes and in the reticuloendothelial system, with some storage in muscle.

### Half-life
Ferrous sulfate—6 hours.
Iron dextran, intravenously administered—5 to more than 20 hours. However, half-life values do not represent clearance of iron from the body.

### Time to peak concentration
Iron sorbitol—2 hours.

### Elimination
No physiological system of elimination exists for iron, and it can accumulate in the body to toxic amounts; however, small amounts are lost daily in the shedding of skin, hair, and nails; and in feces, perspiration, breast milk (0.5 to 1 mg per day), menstrual blood, and urine.
Average daily loss of iron for healthy adults is—
Males: 1 mg per day.
Postmenopausal females: 1 mg per day.
Healthy premenopausal adult females: 1.5 to 2 mg per day.
Iron sorbitol—
30% of dose excreted in urine in 24 hours.

## Precautions to Consider

### Carcinogenicity/Tumorigenicity
For iron dextran—Tumors at the injection site have been reported in humans who had previously received intramuscular injections of iron-carbohydrate complexes. However, the actual risk of such tumors is unknown because of the long latency period between injection and appearance of a tumor. Animal studies have shown the production of sarcoma in rodents injected repeatedly at the same site with large doses of iron-carbohydrate complexes. However, the rodent tumors were a different type than those reported in humans.
For iron sorbitol—There was no evidence of lymphatic obstruction or tumors at the injection site in mice receiving iron sorbitol subcutaneously at doses of 1 mg a week for seven months.

### Pregnancy/Reproduction
Pregnancy—
*For ferrous fumarate, ferrous gluconate, ferrous sulfate, and iron-polysaccharide—*
In the first trimester of pregnancy, adequate iron intake is usually obtained from a proper diet; however, in the second and third trimesters, when iron deficiency is more prevalent because of greatly increased requirements, iron supplements may be recommended. However, some clinicians prefer to evaluate the patient before giving routine iron supplementation.
Studies in humans have not been done, and problems in humans have not been documented with intake of normal daily recommended amounts.
Studies in animals have not been done.
*For iron dextran—*
Iron dextran crosses the placenta. Studies in humans have not been done.
Iron dextran has been shown to be teratogenic and embryocidal in mice, rats, rabbits, dogs, and monkeys when given in doses three times the maximum human dose.

FDA Pregnancy Category C.
*For iron sorbitol—*
Although no adequate and well-controlled studies have been done in humans, there have been a few reports of abortion after use of iron sorbitol in early pregnancy. Use is not recommended in the first 3 to 4 months of pregnancy.
Studies in animals have not been done.

### Breast-feeding
*For ferrous fumarate, ferrous gluconate, ferrous sulfate, and iron-polysaccharide—*
Problems in humans have not been documented with intake of normal daily recommended amounts.
*For iron dextran—*
Only traces of unmetabolized iron dextran are distributed into breast milk.

### Pediatrics
The American Academy of Pediatrics recommends that iron supplementation (as iron-fortified formula or cereal or as iron-containing drops) be given to preterm infants after 2 months of age and to full-term infants after 4 months of age, whether breast or formula fed.
Problems in pediatrics have not been documented with intake of normal daily recommended amounts. Iron dextran is not normally given to infants under 4 months of age. There have been reports from other countries of increased gram-negative sepsis in neonates given iron dextran, probably due to *Escherichia coli*, after intramuscular injection.

## Geriatrics

Problems in geriatrics have not been documented with intake of normal daily recommended amounts. Some geriatric patients may require a larger than usual daily ingestion of bioavailable iron to correct an iron deficiency, because their ability to absorb iron has been diminished by reduced gastric secretions and achlorhydria.

## Drug interactions and/or related problems

The following drug interactions and/or related problems have been selected on the basis of their potential clinical significance (possible mechanism in parentheses where appropriate)—not necessarily inclusive (» = major clinical significance):

Note: Combinations containing any of the following, depending on the amount present, may also interact with this iron supplement.

» Acetohydroxamic acid
(iron, and possibly other heavy metals, when taken orally, are chelated by acetohydroxamic acid; this may result in reduced intestinal absorption of both acetohydroxamic acid and oral iron supplements; if iron therapy is indicated during treatment with acetohydroxamic acid, parenteral administration of iron is recommended)

Alcohol
(concurrent use with ferric iron for a prolonged period may result in toxicity since absorption and hepatic storage of iron are increased, especially if alcohol usage is high)

» Antacids or
Calcium supplements (calcium carbonate or phosphate) or
Coffee or
Eggs or
Foods or medications containing bicarbonates, carbonates, oxalates, or phosphates or
Milk or milk products or
Tea containing tannic acid or
Whole-grain breads and cereals (contain phytic acid) and dietary fiber
(concurrent use with iron may decrease iron absorption because of the formation of less soluble or insoluble complexes; iron supplements should not be taken within 1 hour before or 2 hours after ingestion of any of the above)

Cimetidine
(the decrease in gastric acid caused by cimetidine may decrease the absorption of nonheme iron; concurrent use with iron supplements is not recommended; iron supplements should be taken at least 2 hours before or after cimetidine)

Deferoxamine, and possibly other chelating agents
(deferoxamine chelates iron and is used in the treatment of iron overdose and other iron overload conditions; iron may be necessary in patients receiving other chelating agents; however, it should be given at least 2 hours after the chelating agent)

» Dimercaprol
(concurrent administration of medicinal iron with dimercaprol results in the formation of a toxic complex; if iron deficiency is present, its treatment should be postponed until therapy with dimercaprol has been discontinued for at least 24 hours; severe iron deficiency anemia occurring during dimercaprol therapy should be managed with blood transfusion)

» Etidronate
(concurrent use may prevent absorption of oral etidronate; patients should be advised to avoid using iron supplements within 2 hours of etidronate)

» Fluoroquinolones
(iron may reduce absorption of fluoroquinolones by chelation, resulting in lower serum and urine concentrations of fluoroquinolones; fluoroquinolones should be taken at least 2 hours before or 2 hours after iron supplements)

Pancreatin or
Pancrelipase
(concurrent use of these medications with iron supplements may decrease iron absorption)

Penicillamine or
Trientine
(concurrent use with iron supplements may decrease the therapeutic effects of these medications; if necessary, iron may be administered in short courses, but a period of 2 hours should elapse between administration of penicillamine or trientine and iron)

» Tetracyclines, oral
(concurrent use with iron reduces absorbability and resultant therapeutic effects of oral tetracyclines; patients should be advised to take iron supplements 2 hours after tetracycline)

Zinc supplements, oral
(large doses of iron supplements have been found to inhibit the intestinal absorption of zinc; this may be a problem in individuals taking commercial multivitamin-mineral preparations or infant formulas that have a high iron-to-zinc ratio; however, most firms in the U.S. have reformulated their products; zinc supplements should be taken at least 2 hours after iron supplements)

## Laboratory value alterations

The following have been selected on the basis of their potential clinical significance (possible effect in parentheses where appropriate)—not necessarily inclusive (» = major clinical significance):

With diagnostic test results

*For all iron supplements*
Iron concentrations, serum
(caution in interpretation of serum iron values in blood samples drawn within 1 to 2 weeks of administration of large doses of iron dextran and within 4 hours of oral iron)

Orthotolidine test
(presence of iron may give false-positive results)

Technetium Tc 99m–labeled phosphates and phosphonates
(iron supplements may cause a decrease in bone uptake of technetium Tc 99m-labeled phosphates and phosphonates because of iron overload; bone scans with Tc 99m diphosphonate, taken 1 to 6 days after intramuscular iron dextran administration, may show dense areas of activity in the buttock, following the contour of the iliac crest)

Tumor and/or abscess imaging with Ga-67 gallium citrate
(iron supplements may cause a decrease in tumor and/or abscess uptake of Ga-67 gallium citrate due to competition for the same binding sites)

*For ferrous sulfate only (in addition to those laboratory value alterations listed above)*
Glucose oxidase tests
(presence of ferrous sulfate may give false-negative results)

With physiology/laboratory test values
Occult blood in stools
(may be obscured by black coloration of iron in stool)

Serum discoloration
(large doses of iron dextran have been reported to impart a brown color to serum in blood drawn 4 hours after intravenous administration)

## Medical considerations/Contraindications

The medical considerations/contraindications included here have been selected on the basis of their potential clinical significance (reasons given in parentheses where appropriate)—not necessarily inclusive (» = major clinical significance).

*Except under special circumstances, this medication should not be used when the following medical problems exist:*

» Hemochromatosis or
» Hemosiderosis
(existing iron overload may be increased)

» Other anemic conditions, unless accompanied by iron deficiency (some conditions, such as hemolytic anemia or thalassemia, may cause excess storage of iron)

» Porphyria cutanea tarda
(may be caused by hepatic accumulation of iron, as in iron overload)

*Risk-benefit should be considered when the following medical problems exist:*

Alcoholism, active or in remission
(alcohol may increase absorption and hepatic storage of iron and increase iron toxicity)

Allergies or
Asthma
(increased risk of hypersensitivity reactions with parenteral administration)

Cardiovascular disease
(may be exacerbated by possible adverse reactions caused by administration of iron dextran)

Hepatitis or hepatic function impairment or
Kidney disease, acute, infectious
(may cause an accumulation of iron)

Intestinal tract inflammatory conditions, such as enteritis, colitis, diverticulitis, and ulcerative colitis or
Peptic ulcer
(may be exacerbated with oral iron dosage forms)

Rheumatoid arthritis
(acute exacerbation of joint pain and swelling following intravenous administration of parenteral iron)

Sensitivity to iron

» Caution is recommended also in patients receiving repeated blood transfusions because the addition of high erythrocytic iron content may produce iron overload.

## Patient monitoring

The following may be especially important in patient monitoring (other tests may be warranted in some patients, depending on condition; » = major clinical significance):

Ferritin concentrations, serum and
Iron concentrations, serum
(determinations are recommended when deemed necessary to recognize and prevent hemosiderosis and progressive accumulation of iron in patients with chronic renal failure, Hodgkin's disease, or rheumatoid arthritis, or in patients receiving large doses of iron dextran; patients on chronic renal dialysis may not show a valid correlation of serum iron ferritin with body iron stores while receiving iron dextran)

Hemoglobin and hematocrit determinations and
Reticulocyte counts
(suggested at 3-week intervals for the first 2 months of therapy; recommended a few days after parenteral administration to determine therapeutic response; if there has not been at least a 1-gram-per-100-mL rise in hemoglobin within 2 weeks of initiation of iron dextran therapy, a review of the diagnosis of iron deficiency anemia may be necessary)

Total iron binding capacity (TIBC) or
Transferrin, percentage saturation of
(some clinicians recommend monthly determinations during parenteral iron administration; however, while transferrin saturation may reflect a depletion of stored iron, it is less sensitive to changes in iron stores than serum ferritin; some clinicians recommend that TIBC and/or transferrin be monitored only in the case of suspected iron overload)

## Side/Adverse Effects

Note: Stools commonly become dark green or black when iron preparations are taken orally. This is caused by the presence of unabsorbed iron and is harmless. However, bleeding in the gastrointestinal tract may also cause black stools of a sticky consistency, often accompanied by other symptoms such as red streaks in the stool, cramping, soreness, or sharp pains in the stomach or abdominal region. Medical attention is needed for proper evaluation of the cause.

The parenteral administration of iron has resulted in anaphylactic reactions that, on rare occasions, have been fatal. Such reactions occur within the first several minutes of administration and have been characterized by sudden onset of respiratory difficulties and/or cardiovascular collapse. Therefore, epinephrine should be kept near the patient in case of emergency.

The following effects have been selected on the basis of their potential clinical significance (possible signs and symptoms in parentheses where appropriate)—not necessarily inclusive:

### Those indicating need for medical attention

Incidence more frequent
*Oral use only*
**Abdominal or stomach pain, cramping, or soreness**
*Parenteral use only*
**Allergic reaction** (skin rash or hives; trouble in breathing); *backache or muscle pain; chills; dizziness; fever with increased sweating; headache; metallic taste; nausea or vomiting; numbness, pain, or tingling of hands or feet; chest pain; hypotension* (dizziness or fainting); *fast heartbeat; flushing or redness of skin*—with excessive rate of intravenous administration; *pain and redness or sores at intramuscular injection site; redness at intravenous injection site*

Note: *Backache or muscle pain, chills, dizziness, fever with increased sweating, headache, metallic taste, nausea or vomiting,* or *numbness, pain, or tingling of hands or feet* due to delayed reaction, with recommended doses; onset may be in 24 to 48 hours after administration and subsides in 3 to 7 days.

Incidence less frequent or rare
*Oral use only*
**Contact irritation** (chest or throat pain, especially when swallowing; stools containing fresh or digested blood)

Note: *Contact irritation* due to contact with ulcerous areas or high concentration of iron in one area resulting from improper release from dosage form or delayed passage of dosage form through alimentary tract.

### Those indicating need for medical attention only if they continue or are bothersome

Incidence more frequent
*Oral use only*
**Constipation; diarrhea; nausea; vomiting**
*Parenteral use only*
**Brown discoloration of skin**—usually fading within several weeks or months
Incidence less frequent
*Oral use only*
**Darkened urine** (iron sulfide formation following large doses); *heartburn; staining of teeth*—with liquid dosage forms

## Overdose

Note: Acute toxicity, with symptoms ranging from vomiting to coma, has been reported with ingestion of 200 to 250 mg per kg of body weight (mg/kg) of ferrous sulfate in adults and 20 mg/kg of elemental iron in children. There have been no reports of chronic iron toxicity in individuals who do not have genetic defects that increase iron absorption.

For specific information on the agents used in the management of iron overdose, see
• *Deferoxamine (Systemic)* monograph
• *Ipecac (Oral-Local)* monograph; and/or
• *Sodium Bicarbonate (Systemic)* monograph.

For more information on the management of overdose or unintentional ingestion, **contact a Poison Control Center** (see *Poison Control Center Listing*).

### Clinical effects of overdose

The following effects have been selected on the basis of their potential clinical significance (possible signs and symptoms in parentheses where appropriate)—not necessaarily inclusive:

Acute effects
Early symptoms of acute iron toxicity
Oral use only
**Diarrhea, sometimes containing blood; fever; nausea, severe; stomach pain or cramping, sharp; vomiting, severe, sometimes containing blood**

Note: Early symptoms may not be evident for up to 60 minutes or longer; if overdose is suspected, emergency room treatment should not be delayed for evidence of symptoms, but should begin immediately.

Early signs may also include increased blood glucose and leukocytosis.

A latency period lasting from 2 to about 48 hours after ingestion may occur between the 2 symptomatic phases. During this time, the patient may appear to improve clinically.

Late symptoms of acute iron toxicity
Oral use only
**Bluish-colored lips, fingernails, palms of hands; drowsiness; pale, clammy skin; seizures; unusual tiredness or weakness; weak and fast heartbeat**

Note: Late signs may also include metabolic acidosis, hypotension, hypoglycemia, hepatic injury or failure, cardiovascular collapse, and gastrointestinal scarring.

### For treatment of acute overdose

**Overdose of ingested iron can be fatal, especially in small children. Immediate treatment is essential.** Serious poisoning may result in small children from ingestion of 3 or 4 ferrous sulfate tablets (200 mg of elemental iron).

Acute overdose of iron requires immediate medical treatment that should be completed as soon as possible following ingestion.

After one hour, excessive systemic absorption of iron and possible erosion of stomach and intestinal tissues complicate evacuative and supportive procedures.

Transport of patient to emergency room should not be delayed. If syrup of ipecac has been administered, emesis may require up to 30 minutes or even a repeat dose. However, patient transport must not wait for emetic effect.

Overdose symptoms may be delayed (10 to 60 minutes or longer) because of many intervening factors such as the iron salt taken, amount of food in stomach, and size of dose.

To decrease absorption—
    Inducing emesis with syrup of ipecac or lavaging with sodium bicarbonate if patient is comatose or having convulsions may be used, depending on the patient's condition.
    If intact radiopaque tablets are visualized on x-ray, repeating lavage may be necessary.

Monitoring—
    Laboratory studies on heparinized blood should include serum iron, hemoglobin, hematocrit, electrolytes, blood gases and blood glucose, total iron-binding capacity (TIBC), complete blood count, blood type, and cross-match.
    Serum iron determinations should be repeated. Serum drawn early (within 2 hours of ingestion) may have artificially high concentrations of iron. Peak serum concentrations are reached about 6 hours after ingestion. However, achievement of peak serum concentrations is delayed if the iron was in extended-release form, if the patient had a significant amount of food in his/her stomach, and if the dose of iron was large.

Specific treatment—
    Fluid and electrolyte balance must be maintained. Acidosis may be corrected with intravenous sodium bicarbonate.
    Antidote—Deferoxamine, administered slowly, intravenously or intramuscularly, is used in more severe iron toxicity, when symptoms are other than minimal vomiting or diarrhea. Deferoxamine chelates iron to form a red soluble ferric complex (ferrioxamine) that is excreted in the urine. Children with a history of ingesting >40 mg of elemental iron per kg of body weight, or if serum iron determinations and TIBC are not available, should receive an intramuscular test dose of deferoxamine, regardless of symptoms. If the urine turns an orange-rose (vin rosé) color, deferoxamine should be continued intravenously. However, a negative test dose does not rule out iron toxicity, since false negative tests have been reported with deferoxamine. When results of serum iron determinations and TIBC are available, dosing should continue, if necessary.
    Avoid deferoxamine in patients who have developed renal failure.
    Dialysis is of no value in removing serum iron alone, but may be used to increase excretion of the iron-deferoxamine complex, and is indicated in the presence of anuria or oliguria.
    Exchange transfusion may be successful.
    Whole bowel irrigation is being used by some clinicians, but is not standard practice.

Supportive care—
    Patient must be observed for a minimum of 24 hours after becoming asymptomatic. Delayed effects may include shock and severe gastrointestinal bleeding (24 to 48 hours), and gastrointestinal obstruction (weeks to months). Residual damage may be ruled out with liver and upper gastrointestinal studies.
    Patients in whom intentional overdose is confirmed or suspected should be referred for psychiatric consultation.

## Patient Consultation

As an aid to patient consultation, refer to *Advice for the Patient, Iron Supplements (Systemic)*.

In providing consultation, consider emphasizing the following selected information (» = major clinical significance):

**Description of use**
    Description should include function in body, signs of deficiency, and conditions that may cause deficiency

**Importance of diet**
    Importance of proper nutrition; supplement may be needed because of inadequate dietary intake
    Best dietary sources of iron
    Recommended daily intake for iron

**Before using this dietary supplement**
» Conditions affecting use, especially:
    Sensitivity to iron
    Other medications, especially acetohydroxamic acid, antacids, dimercaprol, etidronate, fluoroquinolones, or oral tetracyclines
    Other medical problems, especially hemochromatosis, hemosiderosis, other anemic conditions, or prophyria cutanea tarda

**Proper use of this dietary supplement**
» Proper dosing
    Taking on empty stomach 1 hour before or 2 hours after meals; or with food to lessen possibility of stomach upset
    Taking with water or fruit juice, a full glass (240 mL) for adults, 1/2 glass (120 mL) for children
    Following health care professional's directions if dietary supplement was prescribed

Following manufacturer's package directions on nonprescription (OTC) iron

*For preventing, reducing, or removing iron stains on teeth:*
    Diluting liquid forms in water or fruit juice
    Using drinking tube or straw
    Placing dropper doses well back on tongue
    Brushing teeth with baking soda or hydrogen peroxide 3%

    Missed dose: Skipping missed dose; going back to regular schedule; not doubling doses
» Proper storage

**Precautions while using this dietary supplement**
    Taking iron supplements 1 hour before or 2 hours after eating dairy products, eggs, coffee, tea, whole-grain breads and cereals, antacids, or calcium supplements
    Not taking iron supplements orally if receiving iron by injection
    Avoiding regular use of large amounts of iron supplements several times daily for more than 6 months unless approved by health care professional
    Extended-release dosage forms may not release iron properly; checking with health care professional if stools are not black during therapy
    Keeping iron preparations out of the reach of children. Keeping syrup of ipecac readily available in case ordered for emergency
    Keeping telephone numbers of poison control center, nearest hospital emergency room, and doctor readily available
» Suspected overdose: Immediately contacting physician, poison control center, or emergency room; following any instructions given on phone; not delaying emergency treatment; taking container of iron medicine to emergency room

**Side/adverse effects**
    Iron supplements cause black stools, which may be alarming to patient although medically insignificant; checking with physician if black stools occur with other symptoms of internal blood loss
    Signs of potential side effects, especially abdominal pain or contact irritation in alimentary tract

## General Dosing Information

The elemental iron content of iron salts is as follows:

| Iron Salt | % Elemental Iron |
| --- | --- |
| Ferrous fumarate | Ferrous 33 |
| Ferrous gluconate | Ferrous 11.6 |
| Ferrous sulfate | Ferrous 20 |
| Ferrous sulfate, dried | Ferrous ≈30 |
| Iron dextran | Ferric* |
| Iron-polysaccharide | Ferric* |

*Variable, depending on product.

Noncompliance is a major factor in slow therapeutic results, especially in patients requiring prolonged treatment.

In healthy adult males, there are approximately 50 mg per kg of body weight (mg/kg) of iron and 14 to 18 grams of hemoglobin per 100 mL of whole blood.

In healthy adult females, there are approximately 35 mg/kg of iron and 12 to 16 grams of hemoglobin per 100 mL of whole blood.

The hemoglobin concentration of an iron-deficient patient usually reaches normal parameters after iron therapy of 1 or 2 months, but the plasma iron concentration often requires 3 to 6 months of therapy to reflect the normalization of body iron stores.

The American Academy of Pediatrics recommends that breast-fed preterm infants 2 months of age and older receive 2 to 3 mg/kg a day of elemental iron in the form of ferrous sulfate. Full-term infants 4 months of age and older should receive 1 mg/kg a day of elemental iron, preferably from iron-fortified formula or cereal.

Concurrent use of ascorbic acid with iron in proper ratio is thought to enhance iron absorption by maintaining ferrous salts in the reduced state and by reducing ferric salts to the more absorbable ferrous form; the suggested ratio is over 200 mg of ascorbic acid to 30 mg of elemental iron.

**Diet/Nutrition**

Absorption of iron is most effective when the iron is ingested on an empty stomach; taking it with food will lessen absorption but will also lessen the chance of gastrointestinal irritation.

Taking iron supplements 1 hour before or 2 hours after eating dairy products, eggs, coffee, tea, or whole-grain breads and cereals will prevent the formation of less soluble or insoluble complexes, which decrease iron absorption.

Recommended dietary intakes for iron are defined differently worldwide. For U.S.—

The Recommended Dietary Allowances (RDAs) for vitamins and minerals are determined by the Food and Nutrition Board of the National Research Council and are intended to provide adequate nutrition in most healthy persons under usual environmental stresses. In addition, a different designation may be used by the FDA for food and dietary supplement labeling purposes, such as Daily Value (DV). DVs replace the previous labeling terminology United States Recommended Daily Allowances (USRDAs).

For Canada—

Recommended Nutrient Intakes (RNIs) for vitamins, minerals, and protein are determined by Health and Welfare Canada and provide recommended amounts of a specific nutrient while minimizing the risk of chronic diseases.

Daily recommended intakes for elemental iron are generally defined as follows:

| Persons | U.S. (mg) | Canada (mg) |
|---|---|---|
| Infants and children | | |
| Birth to 3 years of age | 6–10 | 0.3–6 |
| 4 to 6 years of age | 10 | 8 |
| 7 to 10 years of age | 10 | 8–10 |
| Adolescent and adult males | 10 | 8–10 |
| Adolescent and adult females | 10–15 | 8–13 |
| Pregnant females | 30 | 17–22 |
| Breast-feeding females | 15 | 8–13 |

The best dietary source of iron is lean red meat. Chicken, turkey, and fish are less important sources of iron. Foods rich in vitamin C (e.g., citrus fruits and fresh vegetables) and heme iron–containing foods (such as found in meats) enhance nonheme iron absorption from cereals, beans, and other vegetables. Foods containing phytates, oxalates, fiber, and calcium may inhibit the absorption of nonheme iron. In food preparation, additional iron may be added through cooking in iron pots.

**For treatment of allergic reaction**
Treatment may include the following:
• Administering epinephrine subcutaneously or intramuscularly. The usual adult dose for acute allergic (anaphylactic) reactions is 0.5 mL of a 1:1000 (1 mg/mL) solution (500 mcg of epinephrine base).
• Isoproterenol or similar beta-agonists may be required in patients taking beta-blockers because of an inadequate response to epinephrine.

---

### *FERROUS FUMARATE*

## Summary of Differences

General dosing information: Contains 33% elemental ferrous iron.

## Oral Dosage Forms
### FERROUS FUMARATE CAPSULES

**Usual adult and adolescent dose**
Deficiency (prophylaxis)—
Oral, amount based on normal daily recommended intakes of elemental iron:

| Persons | U.S. (mg) | Canada (mg) |
|---|---|---|
| Adolescent and adult males | 10 | 8–10 |
| Adolescent and adult females | 10–15 | 8–13 |
| Pregnant females | 30 | 17–22 |
| Breast-feeding females | 15 | 8–13 |

Deficiency (treatment)—
Treatment dose is individualized by prescriber based on severity of deficiency.

**Usual pediatric dose**
Dosage form is not recommended for use in children.

**Strength(s) usually available**
U.S.—
Not commercially available.
Canada—
300 mg (100 mg of elemental iron) (OTC) [*Neo-Fer; Palafer*].
Note: The strength of these iron preparations may exceed the dosage range recommended by USP DI Advisory Panels based on the amount necessary to meet normal nutritional needs.

**Packaging and storage**
Store below 40 °C (104 °F), preferably between 15 and 30 °C (59 and 86 °F), in a tight container, unless otherwise specified by manufacturer.

**Auxiliary labeling**
• Keep out of reach of children.

**Note**
Caution patients about toxic effects of accidental overdose, especially in children, and need for immediate medical aid.

### FERROUS FUMARATE EXTENDED-RELEASE CAPSULES

**Usual adult and adolescent dose**
See *Ferrous Fumarate Capsules.*

**Usual pediatric dose**
Dosage form is not recommended for use in children.

**Strength(s) usually available**
U.S.—
325 mg (106 mg of elemental iron) (OTC) [*Span-FF* (sucrose)].
Canada—
Not commercially available.
Note: The strength of this iron preparation may exceed the dosage range recommended by USP DI Advisory Panels based on the amount necessary to meet normal nutritional needs.

**Packaging and storage**
Store below 40 °C (104 °F), preferably between 15 and 30 °C (59 and 86 °F), in a well-closed container, unless otherwise specified by manufacturer.

**Auxiliary labeling**
• Swallow capsules whole.
• Keep out of reach of children.

**Note**
Caution patients about toxic effects of accidental overdose, especially in children, and need for immediate medical aid.

### FERROUS FUMARATE ORAL SOLUTION

**Usual adult and adolescent dose**
See *Ferrous Fumarate Capsules.*

**Usual pediatric dose**
Deficiency (prophylaxis)—
Oral, amount based on normal daily recommended intakes of elemental iron:

| Persons | U.S. (mg) | Canada (mg) |
|---|---|---|
| Infants and children | | |
| Birth to 3 years of age | 6–10 | 0.3–6 |
| 4 to 6 years of age | 10 | 8 |
| 7 to 10 years of age | 10 | 8–10 |

Deficiency (treatment)—
Treatment dose is individualized by prescriber based on severity of deficiency.

**Strength(s) usually available**
U.S.—
45 mg (15 mg of elemental iron) per 0.6 mL (OTC) [*Feostat Drops*].
Canada—
Not commercially available.
Note: The strength of this iron preparation may exceed the dosage range recommended by USP DI Advisory Panels based on the amount necessary to meet normal nutritional needs.

**Packaging and storage**
Store below 40 °C (104 °F), preferably between 15 and 30 °C (59 and 86 °F), in a tight container, unless otherwise specified by manufacturer. Protect from freezing.

**Auxiliary labeling**
• Protect from freezing.
• Keep out of reach of children.

**Note**
Explain dosage measurement; provide dropper or other dose-measuring device if indicated.

Explain dilution requirements.

Caution patients about toxic effects of overdose, especially in children, and need for immediate medical aid.

### FERROUS FUMARATE ORAL SUSPENSION

**Usual adult and adolescent dose**
See *Ferrous Fumarate Capsules.*

**Usual pediatric dose**

See *Ferrous Fumarate Oral Solution.*

**Strength(s) usually available**

U.S.—

100 mg (33 mg of elemental iron) per 5 mL (OTC) [*Feostat*].

Canada—

300 mg (100 mg of elemental iron) per 5 mL (OTC) [*Palafer*].

Note: The strength of these iron preparations may exceed the dosage range recommended by USP DI Advisory Panels based on the amount necessary to meet normal nutritional needs.

**Packaging and storage**

Store below 40 °C (104 °F), preferably between 15 and 30 °C (59 and 86 °F), in a tight container, unless otherwise specified by manufacturer. Protect from freezing.

**Auxiliary labeling**

• Shake well before using.
• Protect from freezing.
• Keep out of reach of children.

**Note**

Explain dosage measurement; provide dropper or other dose-measuring device if indicated.

Explain dilution requirements.

Caution patients about toxic effects of overdose, especially in children, and need for immediate medical aid.

## FERROUS FUMARATE TABLETS USP

**Usual adult and adolescent dose**

See *Ferrous Fumarate Capsules.*

**Usual pediatric dose**

See *Ferrous Fumarate Oral Solution.*

**Strength(s) usually available**

U.S.—

63 mg (20 mg of elemental iron) (OTC) [*Femiron*].
195 mg (64 mg of elemental iron) (OTC) [*Fumerin*].
200 mg (66 mg of elemental iron) (OTC) [*Fumasorb; Ircon*].
300 mg (99 mg of elemental iron) (OTC) [GENERIC].
325 mg (106 mg of elemental iron) (OTC) [*Hemocyte;* GENERIC].
350 mg (115 mg of elemental iron) (OTC) [*Nephro-Fer*].

Canada—

200 mg (66 mg of elemental iron) (OTC) [*Novofumar* (sucrose)].

Note: The strength of these iron preparations may exceed the dosage range recommended by USP DI Advisory Panels based on the amount necessary to meet normal nutritional needs.

**Packaging and storage**

Store below 40 °C (104 °F), preferably between 15 and 30 °C (59 and 86 °F), unless otherwise specified by manufacturer. Store in a tight container.

**Auxiliary labeling**

• Keep out of reach of children.

**Note**

Caution patients about toxic effects of accidental overdose, especially in children, and need for immediate medical aid.

## FERROUS FUMARATE CHEWABLE TABLETS

**Usual adult and adolescent dose**

See *Ferrous Fumarate Capsules.*

**Usual pediatric dose**

See *Ferrous Fumarate Oral Solution.*

**Strength(s) usually available**

U.S.—

100 mg (33 mg of elemental iron) (OTC) [*Feostat*].

Canada—

Not commercially available.

Note: The strength of this iron preparation may exceed the dosage range recommended by USP DI Advisory Panels based on the amount necessary to meet normal nutritional needs.

**Packaging and storage**

Store below 40 °C (104 °F), preferably between 15 and 30 °C (59 and 86 °F), in a tight container, unless otherwise specified by manufacturer.

**Auxiliary labeling**

• Chew well before swallowing.
• Keep out of reach of children.

**Note**

Caution patients about toxic effects of accidental overdose, especially in children, and need for immediate medical aid.

---

## *FERROUS GLUCONATE*

## Summary of Differences

General dosing information: Contains 11.6% elemental ferrous iron.

## Oral Dosage Forms

### FERROUS GLUCONATE CAPSULES USP

**Usual adult and adolescent dose**

Deficiency (prophylaxis)—
Oral, amount based on normal daily recommended intakes of elemental iron:

| Persons | U.S. (mg) | Canada (mg) |
|---|---|---|
| Adolescent and adult males | 10 | 8–10 |
| Adolescent and adult females | 10–15 | 8–13 |
| Pregnant females | 30 | 17–22 |
| Breast-feeding females | 15 | 8–13 |

Deficiency (treatment)—
Treatment dose is individualized by prescriber based on severity of deficiency.

**Usual pediatric dose**

Deficiency (prophylaxis)—
Oral, amount based on normal daily recommended intakes of elemental iron:

| Persons | U.S. (mg) | Canada (mg) |
|---|---|---|
| Infants and children | | |
| Birth to 3 years of age | 6–10 | 0.3–6 |
| 4 to 6 years of age | 10 | 8 |
| 7 to 10 years of age | 10 | 8–10 |

Deficiency (treatment)—
Treatment dose is individualized by prescriber based on severity of deficiency.

**Strength(s) usually available**

U.S.—

86 mg (10 mg of elemental iron) (OTC) [*Simron* (not USP)].

Canada—

Not commercially available.

Note: The strength of this iron preparation may exceed the dosage range recommended by USP DI Advisory Panels based on the amount necessary to meet normal nutritional needs.

**Packaging and storage**

Store below 40 °C (104 °F), preferably between 15 and 30 °C (59 and 86 °F), unless otherwise specified by manufacturer. Store in a tight container.

**Auxiliary labeling**

• Keep out of reach of children.

**Note**

Caution patients about toxic effects of overdose, especially in children, and need for immediate medical aid.

### FERROUS GLUCONATE ELIXIR USP

**Usual adult and adolescent dose**

See *Ferrous Gluconate Capsules USP.*

**Usual pediatric dose**

See *Ferrous Gluconate Capsules USP.*

**Strength(s) usually available**

U.S.—

300 mg (34 mg of elemental iron) per 5 mL (OTC) [*Fergon* (alcohol 7%); GENERIC].

Canada—

Not commercially available.

Note: The strength of these iron preparations may exceed the dosage range recommended by USP DI Advisory Panels based on the amount necessary to meet normal nutritional needs.

**Packaging and storage**

Store below 40 °C (104 °F), preferably between 15 and 30 °C (59 and 86 °F), unless otherwise specified by manufacturer. Store in a tight, light-resistant container. Protect from freezing.

**Auxiliary labeling**

• Keep out of reach of children.

**Note**

Caution patients about toxic effects of overdose, especially in children, and need for immediate medical aid.

## FERROUS GLUCONATE SYRUP

**Usual adult and adolescent dose**

See *Ferrous Gluconate Capsules USP.*

**Usual pediatric dose**

See *Ferrous Gluconate Capsules USP.*

**Strength(s) usually available**

U.S.—

Not commercially available.

Canada—

300 mg (35 mg of elemental iron) per 5 mL (OTC) [*Fertinic*].

Note: The strength of this iron preparation may exceed the dosage range recommended by USP DI Advisory Panels based on the amount necessary to meet normal nutritional needs.

**Packaging and storage**

Store below 40 °C (104 °F), preferably between 15 and 30 °C (59 and 86 °F), in a tight container, unless otherwise specified by manufacturer. Protect from light. Protect from freezing.

**Auxiliary labeling**

• Keep out of reach of children.

**Note**

Caution patients about toxic effects of overdose, especially in children, and need for immediate medical aid.

## FERROUS GLUCONATE TABLETS USP

**Usual adult and adolescent dose**

See *Ferrous Gluconate Capsules USP.*

**Usual pediatric dose**

See *Ferrous Gluconate Capsules USP.*

**Strength(s) usually available**

U.S.—

300 mg (34 mg of elemental iron) (OTC) [GENERIC].

320 mg (37 mg of elemental iron) (OTC) [*Fergon* (not USP); *Ferralet*].

325 mg (38 mg of elemental iron) (OTC) [GENERIC].

Canada—

300 mg (35 mg of elemental iron) (OTC) [*Apo-Ferrous Gluconate; Fertinic; Novoferrogluc;* GENERIC].

Note: The strength of these iron preparations may exceed the dosage range recommended by USP DI Advisory Panels based on the amount necessary to meet normal nutritional needs.

**Packaging and storage**

Store below 40 °C (104 °F), preferably between 15 and 30 °C (59 and 86 °F), unless otherwise specified by manufacturer. Store in a tight container.

**Auxiliary labeling**

• Keep out of reach of children.

**Note**

Caution patients about toxic effects of overdose, especially in children, and need for immediate medical aid.

## FERROUS GLUCONATE EXTENDED-RELEASE TABLETS

**Usual adult and adolescent dose**

See *Ferrous Gluconate Capsules USP.*

**Usual pediatric dose**

Dosage form is not recommended for use in children.

**Strength(s) usually available**

U.S.—

320 mg (37 mg of elemental iron) (OTC) [*Ferralet Slow Release*].

Canada—

Not commercially available.

Note: The strength of this iron preparation may exceed the dosage range recommended by USP DI Advisory Panels based on the amount necessary to meet normal nutritional needs.

**Packaging and storage**

Store below 40 °C (104 °F), preferably between 15 and 30 °C (59 and 86 °F), unless otherwise specified by manufacturer.

**Auxiliary labeling**

• Keep out of reach of children.

**Note**

Caution patients about toxic effects of overdose, especially in children, and need for immediate medical aid.

---

## FERROUS SULFATE

## Summary of Differences

Precautions: Laboratory value alterations—Ferrous sulfate may give false-negative results for glucose oxidase tests.

General dosing information: Contains 20% of elemental ferrous iron (dried ferrous sulfate contains approximately 32% of elemental iron).

## Oral Dosage Forms

### FERROUS SULFATE CAPSULES

**Usual adult and adolescent dose**

Deficiency (prophylaxis)—

Oral, amount based on normal daily recommended intakes of elemental iron:

| Persons | U.S. (mg) | Canada (mg) |
|---|---|---|
| Adolescent and adult males | 10 | 8–10 |
| Adolescent and adult females | 10–15 | 8–13 |
| Pregnant females | 30 | 17–22 |
| Breast-feeding females | 15 | 8–13 |

Deficiency (treatment)—

Treatment dose is individualized by prescriber based on severity of deficiency.

**Usual pediatric dose**

Deficiency (prophylaxis)—

Oral, amount based on normal daily recommended intakes of elemental iron:

| Persons | U.S. (mg) | Canada (mg) |
|---|---|---|
| Infants and children | | |
| Birth to 3 years of age | 6–10 | 0.3–6 |
| 4 to 6 years of age | 10 | 8 |
| 7 to 10 years of age | 10 | 8–10 |

Deficiency (treatment)—

Treatment dose is individualized by prescriber based on severity of deficiency.

**Strength(s) usually available**

U.S.—

250 mg (50 mg of elemental iron) (OTC) [*Ferospace;* GENERIC].

Canada—

Not commercially available.

Note: The strength of these iron preparations may exceed the dosage range recommended by USP DI Advisory Panels based on the amount necessary to meet normal nutritional needs.

**Packaging and storage**

Store below 40 °C (104 °F), preferably between 15 and 30 °C (59 and 86 °F), in a tight container, unless otherwise specified by manufacturer.

**Auxiliary labeling**

• Keep out of reach of children.

**Note**

Caution patients about toxic effects of overdose, especially in children, and need for immediate medical aid.

### FERROUS SULFATE (DRIED) CAPSULES

**Usual adult and adolescent dose**

See *Ferrous Sulfate Capsules.*

**Usual pediatric dose**

See *Ferrous Sulfate Capsules.*

**Strength(s) usually available**

U.S.—

190 mg, dried (60 mg of elemental iron) (OTC) [*Fer-In-Sol Capsules* (lecithin)].

Canada—

Not commercially available.

Note: The strength of this iron preparation may exceed the dosage range recommended by USP DI Advisory Panels based on the amount necessary to meet normal nutritional needs.

**Packaging and storage**
Store below 40 °C (104 °F), preferably between 15 and 30 °C (59 and 86 °F), in a tight container, unless otherwise specified by manufacturer.

**Auxiliary labeling**
• Swallow capsules whole.
• Keep out of reach of children.

**Note**
Caution patients about toxic effects of overdose, especially in children, and need for immediate medical aid.

## FERROUS SULFATE (DRIED) EXTENDED-RELEASE CAPSULES

**Usual adult and adolescent dose**
See *Ferrous Sulfate Capsules.*

**Usual pediatric dose**
Dosage form is not recommended for use in children.

**Strength(s) usually available**
U.S.—
     150 mg (30 mg of elemental iron) (OTC) [GENERIC].
     159 mg (50 mg of elemental iron) (OTC) [*Feosol* (sucrose)].
     250 mg (50 mg of elemental iron) (OTC) [*Ferralyn Lanacaps; Ferra-TD;* GENERIC].
Canada—
     Not commercially available.
Note: The strength of these iron preparations may exceed the dosage range recommended by USP DI Advisory Panels based on the amount necessary to meet normal nutritional needs.

**Packaging and storage**
Store below 40 °C (104 °F), preferably between 15 and 30 °C (59 and 86 °F), in a well-closed container, unless otherwise specified by manufacturer.

**Auxiliary labeling**
• Swallow capsules whole.
• Keep out of reach of children.

**Note**
Caution patients about toxic effects of overdose, especially in children, and need for immediate medical aid.

## FERROUS SULFATE ELIXIR

**Usual adult and adolescent dose**
See *Ferrous Sulfate Capsules.*

**Usual pediatric dose**
See *Ferrous Sulfate Capsules.*

**Strength(s) usually available**
U.S.—
     220 mg (44 mg of elemental iron) per 5 mL (OTC) [*Feosol* (alcohol 5%); GENERIC].
Canada—
     Not commercially available.
Note: The strength of these iron preparations may exceed the dosage range recommended by USP DI Advisory Panels based on the amount necessary to meet normal nutritional needs.

**Packaging and storage**
Store below 40 °C (104 °F), preferably between 15 and 30 °C (59 and 86 °F), in a tight container, unless otherwise specified by manufacturer. Protect from freezing.

**Auxiliary labeling**
• Keep out of reach of children.

**Note**
Caution patients about toxic effects of overdose, especially in children, and need for immediate medical aid.

## FERROUS SULFATE ORAL SOLUTION USP

Note: The oral solution is sometimes known as concentrate, drops, or syrup.

**Usual adult and adolescent dose**
See *Ferrous Sulfate Capsules.*

**Usual pediatric dose**
See *Ferrous Sulfate Capsules.*

**Strength(s) usually available**
U.S.—
     75 mg (15 mg of elemental iron) per 0.6 mL (OTC) [*Fer-gen-sol* (alcohol 0.2%); *Fer-In-Sol Drops* (alcohol 0.2% v/v); GENERIC].
     90 mg (18 mg of elemental iron) per 5 mL (OTC) [*Fer-In-Sol Syrup* (alcohol 5%)].

     125 mg (25 mg of elemental iron) per mL (OTC) [*Fer-Iron Drops;* GENERIC].
     300 mg (60 mg elemental iron) per 5 mL [GENERIC].
Canada—
     75 mg (15 mg of elemental iron) per 0.6 mL (OTC) [*Fer-In-Sol Drops* (alcohol 0.2%); *PMS-Ferrous Sulfate*].
     150 mg (30 mg of elemental iron) per 5 mL (OTC) [*Fer-In-Sol Syrup; PMS-Ferrous Sulfate*].
Note: The strength of these iron preparations may exceed the dosage range recommended by USP DI Advisory Panels based on the amount necessary to meet normal nutritional needs.

**Packaging and storage**
Store below 40 °C (104 °F), preferably between 15 and 30 °C (59 and 86 °F), unless otherwise specified by manufacturer. Store in a tight container. Protect from light. Protect from freezing.

**Auxiliary labeling**
• Keep out of reach of children.

**Note**
Caution patients about toxic effects of overdose, especially in children, and need for immediate medical aid.

## FERROUS SULFATE TABLETS USP

**Usual adult and adolescent dose**
See *Ferrous Sulfate Capsules.*

**Usual pediatric dose**
See *Ferrous Sulfate Capsules.*

**Strength(s) usually available**
U.S.—
     195 mg (39 mg of elemental iron) (OTC) [*Mol-Iron* (sucrose)].
     300 mg (60 mg of elemental iron) (OTC) [*Feratab;* GENERIC].
     325 mg (65 mg of elemental iron) (OTC) [GENERIC].
Canada—
     300 mg (60 mg of elemental iron) (OTC) [*Apo-Ferrous Sulfate; No-voferrosulfa; PMS-Ferrous Sulfate*].
Note: The strength of these iron preparations may exceed the dosage range recommended by USP DI Advisory Panels based on the amount necessary to meet normal nutritional needs.

**Packaging and storage**
Store below 40 °C (104 °F), preferably between 15 and 30 °C (59 and 86 °F), unless otherwise specified by manufacturer. Store in a tight container.

**Auxiliary labeling**
• Swallow tablets whole.
• Keep out of reach of children.

**Note**
Caution patients about toxic effects of overdose, especially in children, and need for immediate medical aid.

## FERROUS SULFATE TABLETS (DRIED) USP

**Usual adult and adolescent dose**
See *Ferrous Sulfate Capsules.*

**Usual pediatric dose**
See *Ferrous Sulfate Capsules.*

**Strength(s) usually available**
U.S.—
     200 mg, dried (65 mg of elemental iron) (OTC) [*Feosol* (glucose)].
Canada—
     Not commercially available.
Note: The strength of this iron preparation may exceed the dosage range recommended by USP DI Advisory Panels based on the amount necessary to meet normal nutritional needs.

**Packaging and storage**
Store below 40 °C (104 °F), preferably between 15 and 30 °C (59 and 86 °F), unless otherwise specified by manufacturer. Store in a tight container.

**Auxiliary labeling**
• Swallow tablets whole.
• Keep out of reach of children.

**Note**
Caution patients about toxic effects of overdose, especially in children, and need for immediate medical aid.

## FERROUS SULFATE ENTERIC-COATED TABLETS

**Usual adult and adolescent dose**
See *Ferrous Sulfate Capsules.*

**Usual pediatric dose**

Dosage form is not recommended for use in children.

**Strength(s) usually available**

U.S.—

325 mg (approximately 65 mg of elemental iron) (OTC) [GENERIC].

Canada—

300 mg (60 mg of elemental iron) (OTC) [*Apo-Ferrous Sulfate; No-voferrosulfa;* GENERIC].

Note: The strength of these iron preparations may exceed the dosage range recommended by USP DI Advisory Panels based on the amount necessary to meet normal nutritional needs.

**Packaging and storage**

Store below 40 °C (104 °F), preferably between 15 and 30 °C (59 and 86 °F), in a tight container, unless otherwise specified by manufacturer.

**Auxiliary labeling**

• Swallow tablets whole.
• Keep out of reach of children.

**Note**

Caution patients about toxic effects of overdose, especially in children, and need for immediate medical aid.

## FERROUS SULFATE EXTENDED-RELEASE TABLETS

**Usual adult and adolescent dose**

See *Ferrous Sulfate Capsules.*

**Usual pediatric dose**

Dosage form is not recommended for use in children.

**Strength(s) usually available**

U.S.—

325 mg (65 mg elemental iron) (OTC) [GENERIC].
525 mg (105 mg of elemental iron) (OTC) [*Fero-Gradumet*].

Canada—

525 mg (105 mg of elemental iron) (OTC) [*Fero-Grad*].

Note: The strength of these iron preparations may exceed the dosage range recommended by USP DI Advisory Panels based on the amount necessary to meet normal nutritional needs.

**Packaging and storage**

Store below 40 °C (104 °F), preferably between 15 and 30 °C (59 and 86 °F), in a tight container, unless otherwise specified by manufacturer.

**Auxiliary labeling**

• Swallow tablets whole.
• Keep out of reach of children.

**Note**

Caution patients about toxic effects of overdose, especially in children, and need for immediate medical aid.

**Additional information**

Products utilize a plastic matrix that may appear intact in the stool.

## FERROUS SULFATE (DRIED) EXTENDED-RELEASE TABLETS

**Usual adult and adolescent dose**

See *Ferrous Sulfate Capsules.*

**Usual pediatric dose**

Dosage form is not recommended for use in children.

**Strength(s) usually available**

U.S.—

160 mg, dried (50 mg of elemental iron) (OTC) [*Slow Fe* (lactose; wax matrix)].

Canada—

160 mg, dried (50 mg of elemental iron) (OTC) [*Slow Fe* (lactose; wax matrix)].

Note: The strength of these iron preparations may exceed the dosage range recommended by USP DI Advisory Panels based on the amount necessary to meet normal nutritional needs.

**Packaging and storage**

Store below 40 °C (104 °F), preferably between 15 and 30 °C (59 and 86 °F), in a tight container, unless otherwise specified by manufacturer.

**Auxiliary labeling**

• Swallow tablets whole.
• Keep out of reach of children.

**Note**

Caution patients about toxic effects of overdose, especially in children, and need for immediate medical aid.

**Additional information**

Products utilize a porous wax matrix that may appear intact in the stool.

---

## IRON DEXTRAN

## Summary of Differences

General dosing information: Contains elemental ferric form of iron.

## Additional Dosing Information

Oral iron must be discontinued before the administration of parenteral iron.

Epinephrine should be immediately available during injection of iron dextran, especially in patients with allergies or asthma.

Overdose with iron dextran produces no acute toxicity. However, excessive doses beyond the amounts required for restoration of hemoglobin and replenishment of iron stores may result in hemosiderosis. Excess iron may also increase a patient's susceptibility to infection, especially *Yersinia enterocolitica*.

Factors contributing to the formula for determining dosages for patients with iron deficiency include:

Blood volume—7.0% of body weight

Normal hemoglobin (males and females)—

15 kg (33 lb) or less: 12 grams/deciliter (dL)

Over 15 kg (33 lb): 14.8 grams/dL

Iron content of hemoglobin—0.34%

Body weight

Serum ferritin peaks approximately 7 to 9 days after an intravenous dose of iron dextran, and returns to baseline after about 3 weeks.

*For intravenous injection*

Iron dextran is administered undiluted and injected slowly at a rate not exceeding 1 mL per minute. However, some clinicians recommend that the calculated dose of iron dextran for the patient be added to 500 mL of dextrose 5% and infused over 4 to 5 hours, after a test infusion of 10 drops per minute for 10 minutes.

The manufacturer does not recommend that iron dextran be mixed with other medications or added to parenteral nutrition solutions for intravenous infusion; however, iron dextran is added to total parenteral nutrition solutions in current medical practice. Iron dextran should not be added to total nutrient admixtures (TNA) because it has been reported to affect lipid emulsion stability.

*For intramuscular injection*

• Iron dextran should be injected only into the muscle mass of the upper outer quadrant of the buttock. It should *never* be injected into the arm or other exposed areas.

• Deep injection with a 2- to 3-inch, 19- or 20-gauge needle is recommended.

• If the patient is standing during administration of iron dextran, body weight should be on the leg opposite to the injection site.

• If the patient is lying down during administration of iron dextran, he/she should be in a lateral position with injection site uppermost.

• A Z-track technique (displacement of the skin laterally prior to injection) is recommended to avoid injection or leakage into subcutaneous tissue.

Test dose—An intramuscular or intravenous test dose of 25 mg (elemental iron) should be given to all patients before receiving their first therapeutic dose. Although anaphylactic reactions may be evident within the first few minutes after injection, one hour or longer should elapse before the initial therapeutic dose. The intramuscular test dose should be administered in the same injection site and by the same technique as the therapeutic dose.

If no adverse reactions are observed after the test dose, the daily dose of iron dextran may be given according to the following schedule until the total calculated amount has been reached:

For infants up to 5 kg of body weight—25 mg (elemental iron)

For children under 10 kg—50 mg (elemental iron)

Other patients—100 mg (elemental iron)

## Parenteral Dosage Forms

### IRON DEXTRAN INJECTION USP

**Usual adult and adolescent dose**

Deficiency (treatment)—

To restore hemoglobin and replenish iron stores: Intravenous or intramuscular, the dosage being determined by the following dosage table:

| Patient Weight | | Total Iron Dextran Requirement (mL)* | | | | | | | |
|---|---|---|---|---|---|---|---|---|---|
| | | Based on Observed Hemoglobin (grams/dL) of: | | | | | | | |
| lb | kg | 3 | 4 | 5 | 6 | 7 | 8 | 9 | 10 |
| 11 | 5 | 3 | 3 | 3 | 3 | 2 | 2 | 2 | 2 |
| 22 | 10 | 7 | 6 | 6 | 5 | 5 | 4 | 4 | 3 |
| 33 | 15 | 10 | 9 | 9 | 8 | 7 | 7 | 6 | 5 |
| 44 | 20 | 16 | 15 | 14 | 13 | 12 | 11 | 10 | 9 |
| 55 | 25 | 20 | 18 | 17 | 16 | 15 | 14 | 13 | 12 |
| 66 | 30 | 23 | 22 | 21 | 19 | 18 | 17 | 15 | 14 |
| 77 | 35 | 27 | 26 | 24 | 23 | 21 | 20 | 18 | 17 |
| 88 | 40 | 31 | 29 | 28 | 26 | 24 | 22 | 21 | 19 |
| 99 | 45 | 35 | 33 | 31 | 29 | 27 | 25 | 23 | 21 |
| 110 | 50 | 39 | 37 | 35 | 32 | 30 | 28 | 26 | 24 |
| 121 | 55 | 43 | 41 | 38 | 36 | 33 | 31 | 28 | 26 |
| 132 | 60 | 47 | 44 | 42 | 39 | 36 | 34 | 31 | 28 |
| 143 | 65 | 51 | 48 | 45 | 42 | 39 | 36 | 34 | 31 |
| 154 | 70 | 55 | 52 | 49 | 45 | 42 | 39 | 36 | 33 |
| 165 | 75 | 59 | 55 | 52 | 49 | 45 | 42 | 39 | 35 |
| 176 | 80 | 63 | 59 | 55 | 52 | 48 | 45 | 41 | 38 |
| 187 | 85 | 66 | 63 | 59 | 55 | 51 | 48 | 44 | 40 |
| 198 | 90 | 70 | 66 | 62 | 58 | 54 | 50 | 46 | 42 |
| 209 | 95 | 74 | 70 | 66 | 62 | 57 | 53 | 49 | 45 |
| 220 | 100 | 78 | 74 | 69 | 65 | 60 | 56 | 52 | 47 |
| 231 | 105 | 82 | 77 | 73 | 68 | 63 | 59 | 54 | 50 |
| 242 | 110 | 86 | 81 | 76 | 71 | 67 | 62 | 57 | 52 |
| 253 | 115 | 90 | 85 | 80 | 75 | 70 | 64 | 59 | 54 |
| 264 | 120 | 94 | 88 | 83 | 78 | 73 | 67 | 62 | 57 |

*Dosage calculations based on a normal adult hemoglobin of 14.8 grams per dL for patients weighing more than 15 kg (33 pounds) and on hemoglobin of 12 grams/dL for patients weighing 15 kg (33 pounds) or less than or equal to 15 kg (33 pounds).

To calculate the total amount of iron dextran (mL) required to restore hemoglobin and to replenish iron stores in adults and children weighing over 15 kg (33 pounds), when LBW=lean body weight in kg and H=hemoglobin in grams/ dL:
• Iron dextran (mL)=0.0442 (Desired H- Observed H) × LBW + (0.26 × LBW)
• The dosage table above is *not* to be used for simple iron replacement from periodic blood loss in patients with hemorrhagic diatheses (familial telangiectasia; hemophilia; gastrointestinal bleeding) or patients on renal hemodialysis.

To replace the equivalent amount of iron represented in blood loss (based on the approximation that 1 mL of normocytic, normochromic red cells contains 1 mg of elemental iron)—Intramuscular or intravenous, the total iron requirement to be determined as follows:
• Replacement iron (mg) = Blood loss (mL) × hematocrit.
• To calculate dose in mL of iron dextran injection, divide result by 50.

**Usual pediatric dose**
Deficiency (treatment)—
   To restore hemoglobin and replenish iron stores: Intravenous or intramuscular, the dosage being determined by the following dosage table:

| Patient Weight | | Total Iron Dextran Requirement (mL)* | | | | | | | |
|---|---|---|---|---|---|---|---|---|---|
| | | Based on Observed Hemoglobin (grams/dL) of: | | | | | | | |
| lb | kg | 3 | 4 | 5 | 6 | 7 | 8 | 9 | 10 |
| 11 | 5 | 3 | 3 | 3 | 3 | 2 | 2 | 2 | 2 |
| 22 | 10 | 7 | 6 | 6 | 5 | 5 | 4 | 4 | 3 |
| 33 | 15 | 10 | 9 | 9 | 8 | 7 | 7 | 6 | 5 |
| 44 | 20 | 16 | 15 | 14 | 13 | 12 | 11 | 10 | 9 |
| 55 | 25 | 20 | 18 | 17 | 16 | 15 | 14 | 13 | 12 |
| 66 | 30 | 23 | 22 | 21 | 19 | 18 | 17 | 15 | 14 |
| 77 | 35 | 27 | 26 | 24 | 23 | 21 | 20 | 18 | 17 |
| 88 | 40 | 31 | 29 | 28 | 26 | 24 | 22 | 21 | 19 |
| 99 | 45 | 35 | 33 | 31 | 29 | 27 | 25 | 23 | 21 |
| 110 | 50 | 39 | 37 | 35 | 32 | 30 | 28 | 26 | 24 |
| 121 | 55 | 43 | 41 | 38 | 36 | 33 | 31 | 28 | 26 |
| 132 | 60 | 47 | 44 | 42 | 39 | 36 | 34 | 31 | 28 |
| 143 | 65 | 51 | 48 | 45 | 42 | 39 | 36 | 34 | 31 |
| 154 | 70 | 55 | 52 | 49 | 45 | 42 | 39 | 36 | 33 |
| 165 | 75 | 59 | 55 | 52 | 49 | 45 | 42 | 39 | 35 |
| 176 | 80 | 63 | 59 | 55 | 52 | 48 | 45 | 41 | 38 |
| 187 | 85 | 66 | 63 | 59 | 55 | 51 | 48 | 44 | 40 |
| 198 | 90 | 70 | 66 | 62 | 58 | 54 | 50 | 46 | 42 |
| 209 | 95 | 74 | 70 | 66 | 62 | 57 | 53 | 49 | 45 |
| 220 | 100 | 78 | 74 | 69 | 65 | 60 | 56 | 52 | 47 |
| 231 | 105 | 82 | 77 | 73 | 68 | 63 | 59 | 54 | 50 |

| Patient Weight | | Total Iron Dextran Requirement (mL)* | | | | | | | |
|---|---|---|---|---|---|---|---|---|---|
| | | Based on Observed Hemoglobin (grams/dL) of: | | | | | | | |
| lb | kg | 3 | 4 | 5 | 6 | 7 | 8 | 9 | 10 |
| 242 | 110 | 86 | 81 | 76 | 71 | 67 | 62 | 57 | 52 |
| 253 | 115 | 90 | 85 | 80 | 75 | 70 | 64 | 59 | 54 |
| 264 | 120 | 94 | 88 | 83 | 78 | 73 | 67 | 62 | 57 |

*Dosage calculations based on a normal adult hemoglobin of 14.8 grams per dL for patients weighing more than 15 kg (33 pounds) and on hemoglobin of 12 grams/dL for patients weighing less than or equal to 15 kg.

Note: To calculate the total amount of iron dextran (mL) required to restore hemoglobin and to replenish iron stores in children weighing between 5 and 15 kg (11 and 33 pounds), when W=body weight in kg and H=hemoglobin in grams/dL:
   • Iron dextran (mL)=0.0442 (Desired H − Observed H) × W + (0.26 × W)
   • The dosage table above is *not* to be used for simple iron replacement from periodic blood loss in patients with hemorrhagic diatheses (familial telangiectasia; hemophilia; gastrointestinal bleeding) or patients on renal hemodialysis.

**Strength(s) usually available**
U.S.—
   50 mg (elemental ferric iron) per mL (Rx) [*InFeD*].
Canada—
   Not commercially available.

**Packaging and storage**
Store below 40 °C (104 °F), preferably between 15 and 30 °C (59 and 86 °F), unless otherwise specified by manufacturer. Protect from freezing.

**Incompatibilities**
Addition of iron dextran to blood for transfusion is not recommended. Iron dextran has been reported to affect lipid emulsion stability in certain total nutrient admixture (TNA) formulations.

**Additional information**
Vehicle in iron dextran injection is 0.9% sodium chloride injection.

---

### *IRON-POLYSACCHARIDE*

## Summary of Differences
General dosing information: Contains elemental ferric form of iron.

## Additional Dosing Information
Strengths of products expressed in terms of elemental iron content only.

## Oral Dosage Forms
### IRON-POLYSACCHARIDE CAPSULES
**Usual adult and adolescent dose**
Deficiency (prophylaxis)—
   Oral, amount based on normal daily recommended intakes of elemental iron:

| Persons | U.S. (mg) | Canada (mg) |
|---|---|---|
| Adolescent and adult males | 10 | 8–10 |
| Adolescent and adult females | 10–15 | 8–13 |
| Pregnant females | 30 | 17–22 |
| Breast-feeding females | 15 | 8–13 |

Deficiency (treatment)—
   Treatment dose is individualized based on severity of deficiency.

**Usual pediatric dose**
Dosage form is not recommended for use in children.

**Strength(s) usually available**
U.S.—
   150 mg (elemental ferric iron) (OTC) [*Hytinic; Niferex-150; Nu-Iron 150*].
Canada—
   Not commercially available.

Note: The strength of these iron preparations may exceed the dosage range recommended by USP DI Advisory Panels based on the amount necessary to meet normal nutritional needs.

**Packaging and storage**
Store below 40 °C (104 °F), preferably between 15 and 30 °C (59 and 86 °F), unless otherwise specified by manufacturer. Store in a tight container.

**Auxiliary labeling**
• Keep out of reach of children.

**Note**
Caution patients about toxic effects of overdose, especially in children, and need for immediate medical aid.

## IRON-POLYSACCHARIDE ELIXIR

**Usual adult and adolescent dose**
See *Iron-Polysaccharide Capsules.*

**Usual pediatric dose**
Deficiency (prophylaxis)—
Oral, amount based on normal daily recommended intakes of elemental iron:

| Persons | U.S. (mg) | Canada (mg) |
|---|---|---|
| Infants and children | | |
| Birth to 3 years of age | 6–10 | 0.3–6 |
| 4 to 6 years of age | 10 | 8 |
| 7 to 10 years of age | 10 | 8–10 |

Deficiency (treatment)—
Treatment dose is individualized by prescriber based on severity of deficiency.

**Strength(s) usually available**
U.S.—
100 mg (elemental ferric iron) per 5 mL (OTC) [*Niferex* (alcohol 10%); *Nu-Iron* (alcohol 10%)].
Canada—
Not commercially available.
Note: The strength of these iron preparations may exceed the dosage range recommended by USP DI Advisory Panels based on the amount necessary to meet normal nutritional needs.

**Packaging and storage**
Store below 40 °C (104 °F), preferably between 15 and 30 °C (59 and 86 °F), unless otherwise specified by manufacturer. Store in a tight container. Protect from freezing.

**Auxiliary labeling**
• Keep out of reach of children.

**Note**
Caution patients about toxic effects of overdose, especially in children, and need for immediate medical aid.
When indicated by dosage, include a calibrated liquid-measuring device and explain use.

## IRON-POLYSACCHARIDE TABLETS

**Usual adult and adolescent dose**
See *Iron-Polysaccharide Capsules.*

**Usual pediatric dose**
See *Iron-Polysaccharide Elixir.*

**Strength(s) usually available**
U.S.—
50 mg (elemental ferric iron) (OTC) [*Niferex*].
Canada—
Not commercially available.
Note: The strength of this iron preparation may exceed the dosage range recommended by USP DI Advisory Panels based on the amount necessary to meet normal nutritional needs.

**Packaging and storage**
Store below 40 °C (104 °F), preferably between 15 and 30 °C (59 and 86 °F), unless otherwise specified by manufacturer. Store in a tight container.

**Auxiliary labeling**
• Keep out of reach of children.

**Note**
Caution patients about toxic effects of overdose, especially in children, and need for immediate medical aid.

---

### IRON SORBITOL

## Summary of Differences

General dosing information: Contains elemental ferric form of iron.

## Additional Dosing Information

Oral iron must be discontinued before the administration of parenteral iron.

*For intramuscular injection*
• Iron sorbitol should be injected only into the muscle mass of the upper outer quadrant of the buttock. It should *never* be injected into the arm or other exposed areas.
• Deep injection with a 2- to 3-inch, 19- or 20-gauge needle is recommended.
• If the patient is standing during administration of iron sorbitol, body weight should be on the leg opposite to the injection site.
• If the patient is lying down during administration of iron sorbitol, he/she should be in a lateral position with injection site uppermost.
• A Z-track technique (displacement of the skin laterally prior to injection) is recommended to avoid injection or leakage into subcutaneous tissue.

## Parenteral Dosage Forms

### IRON SORBITOL INJECTION

**Usual adult and adolescent dose**
Deficiency (treatment)—
To restore hemoglobin and replenish iron stores: Intramuscular, the daily dosage is determined based on 1.5 mg of elemental iron per kg of body weight. The calculated daily dose may be administered daily or every other day until hemoglobin values are normal.
To increase hemoglobin by 1 gram per 100 mL: Intramuscular administration of 200 mg elemental iron for women and 250 mg for men is necessary. To replenish iron stores, an additional 250 to 1000 mg of elemental iron is needed.
Note: Some clinicians recommend that iron sorbitol injection be given in divided doses of 50 mg per week because larger doses are painful to the patient.

**Usual adult prescribing limits**
100 mg per day.

**Usual pediatric dose**
Deficiency (treatment)—
To restore hemoglobin and replenish iron stores: Intramuscular, the daily dosage is determined based on 1.5 mg of elemental iron per kg of body weight. The calculated daily dose may be administered daily or every other day until hemoglobin values are normal.
Note: Some clinicians recommend that iron sorbitol injection be given in doses of 50 mg per week because larger doses are painful to the patient.

**Strength(s) usually available**
U.S.—
Not commercially available.
Canada—
50 mg (elemental ferric iron) per mL (Rx) [*Jectofer*].

**Packaging and storage**
Store below 40 °C (104 °F), preferably between 15 and 30 °C (59 and 86 °F), unless otherwise specified by manufacturer.

---

Revised: 04/16/92
Interim revision: 06/29/92; 06/19/95

---

## ISOCARBOXAZID—See *Antidepressants, Monoamine Oxidase (MAO) Inhibitor (Systemic)*

---

## ISOETHARINE—See *Bronchodilators, Adrenergic (Systemic)*

**ISOFLURANE**—See *Anesthetics, Inhalation (Systemic)*

**ISOFLUROPHATE**—See *Antiglaucoma Agents, Cholinergic, Long-acting (Ophthalmic)*

**ISOMETHEPTENE-CONTAINING COMBINATIONS**—
Isometheptene, Dichloralphenazone, and Acetaminophen (Systemic)

---

# ISOMETHEPTENE, DICHLORALPHENAZONE, AND ACETAMINOPHEN   Systemic

INN: Acetaminophen—Paracetamol

VA CLASSIFICATION (Primary/Secondary): CN103/CN105

Note: For a listing of dosage forms and brand names by country availability, see *Dosage Forms* section(s). For a listing of brand names for the articles in this monograph, refer to the General Index.

## Category

Vascular headache suppressant (migraine).

Note: Some headache specialists question the validity of the term "vascular headache" because a correlation between dilatation of cerebral blood vessels and symptoms of migraine has not been demonstrated conclusively.

## Indications

### Accepted

Headache, migraine (treatment) and

Headache, tension-type (treatment)—Isometheptene, dichloralphenazone, and acetaminophen combination is indicated to relieve occasional migraine headaches (with or without aura) and coexisting migraine and tension-type headaches ("mixed" headache syndrome). However, the U.S. FDA has classified this combination as being "possibly" effective in the treatment of migraine headaches. This classification requires the submission of adequate and well-controlled studies in order to provide substantial evidence of effectiveness.

Note: Some headache specialists question the value of this formulation in pure tension-type headaches. However, the distinction between vascular, tension-type, and "mixed" headaches is often difficult or uncertain, and the medication may relieve some headaches characterized as tension-type.

Because frequent use of headache-aborting medications by headache-prone individuals may lead to tolerance and dependence, this medication is not recommended for regular use by patients who experience frequent, especially daily, headaches.

To reduce analgesic use, underlying problems that may contribute to tension-type headaches, such as inflammation or structural abnormalities in the cervical or temporomandibular areas, should be identified and treated. In some patients, application of heat, muscle relaxants, and/or physical therapy may be helpful. Other medications having the potential to cause habituation (e.g., benzodiazepines used as muscle relaxants) should be used as infrequently as possible.

Chronic tension-type headaches and severe migraines that occur more frequently than twice a month may require additional prophylactic treatment to reduce the frequency, severity, and/or duration of the headaches. The prophylactic agents most commonly used for tension-type headaches are tricyclic antidepressants, especially amitriptyline, and/or beta-adrenergic blocking agents, especially propranolol. For migraines, beta-adrenergic blocking agents, calcium channel blocking agents, tricyclic antidepressants, monoamine oxidase inhibitors, methysergide, pizotyline (not commercially available in the U.S.), and sometimes cyproheptadine (especially in children) are used as prophylaxis. The combination of amitriptyline plus propranolol has been found superior to either agent used alone as prophylaxis against "mixed" headaches.

Identification and avoidance of precipitating factors is also important in the overall management of the patient with migraine headaches. Relaxation and/or biofeedback techniques may also be helpful in controlling some types of headache, and may reduce the need for medication.

## Pharmacology/Pharmacokinetics

### Physicochemical characteristics

Molecular weight—
Isometheptene mucate: 492.7.
Dichloralphenazone: 519.04.
Acetaminophen: 151.16.

### Mechanism of action/Effect

Isometheptene—The mechanism of action has not been established. Isometheptene is an indirect-acting sympathomimetic agent with vaso-constricting activity. It has been proposed that constriction of cerebral blood vessels reduces the pulsation in cerebral arteries that may be responsible for the pain of migraine headaches. However, studies have not consistently shown a significant correlation between dilatation of cerebral blood vessels and pain or other symptoms of migraine headaches, or between a vasoconstrictive action and relief of migraine.

Dichloralphenazone—A complex of chloral hydrate and antipyrine (INN: phenazone). It is present in this formulation as a mild sedative and relaxant.

Acetaminophen—The mechanism of analgesic action has not been fully determined. Acetaminophen may act predominantly by inhibiting prostaglandin synthesis in the central nervous system (CNS) and, to a lesser extent, through a peripheral action by blocking pain-impulse generation. The peripheral action may also be due to inhibition of prostaglandin synthesis or to inhibition of the synthesis or actions of other substances that sensitize pain receptors to mechanical or chemical stimulation.

### Absorption

Acetaminophen—Rapid and almost complete; may be decreased if taken following a high-carbohydrate meal.

### Distribution

In breast milk—Acetaminophen: Peak concentrations of 10 to 15 mcg per mL (66.2 to 99.3 micromoles/L) have been measured 1 to 2 hours following maternal ingestion of a single 650-mg dose.

### Biotransformation

Dichloralphenazone—Hydrolyzed to the active compounds chloral hydrate and antipyrine. Chloral hydrate is metabolized in the liver and erythrocytes to the active metabolite trichloroethanol, which may be further metabolized to inactive metabolites. It is also metabolized in the liver and kidneys to inactive metabolites.

Acetaminophen—Approximately 90 to 95% of a dose is metabolized in the liver, primarily by conjugation with glucuronic acid, sulfuric acid, and cysteine. An intermediate metabolite, which may accumulate in overdosage after the primary metabolic pathways become saturated, is hepatotoxic and possibly nephrotoxic.

### Half-life

Acetaminophen—
1 to 4 hours; does not change with renal failure but may be prolonged in acute overdosage, in some forms of hepatic disease, and in the elderly; may be somewhat shortened in children.
In breast milk: 1.35 to 3.5 hours.

### Time to peak concentration

Acetaminophen—0.5 to 2 hours.

### Peak plasma concentration

Acetaminophen—5 to 20 mcg per mL (with doses up to 650 mg).

### Time to peak effect

Acetaminophen—1 to 3 hours.

### Duration of action

Acetaminophen—3 to 4 hours.

### Elimination

Acetaminophen—Renal, as metabolites, primarily conjugates; 3% of a dose may be excreted unchanged.

In dialysis:
>    Hemodialysis: 120 mL per minute (for unmetabolized drug); me-
>        tabolites are also cleared rapidly.
>    Hemoperfusion: 200 mL per minute.
>    Peritoneal dialysis: <10 mL per minute.

## Precautions to Consider

Note: The quantity of dichloralphenazone in this combination formulation
    does not provide full therapeutic doses of its active components
    chloral hydrate and antipyrine (phenazone). However, the possibil-
    ity should be considered that precautions applying to chloral hy-
    drate (see *Chloral Hydrate [Systemic]*) and to antipyrine may apply
    to ingestion of an overdose or to overuse of this combination
    medication.

### Cross-sensitivity and/or related problems

Patients sensitive to aspirin are usually not sensitive to acetaminophen;
however, acetaminophen has caused mild bronchospastic reactions in
some aspirin-sensitive asthmatics (less than 5% of those tested).

### Pregnancy/Reproduction

Fertility—Chronic toxicity studies in animals have shown that high doses
of acetaminophen cause testicular atrophy and inhibition of spermatogenesis; the relevance of this finding to use in humans is not known.

Pregnancy—Acetaminophen crosses the placenta. However, problems in
humans have not been documented.

### Breast-feeding

Problems in humans have not been documented. Although peak concentrations of 10 to 15 mcg per mL (66.2 to 99.3 micromoles/L) of acetaminophen have been measured in breast milk 1 to 2 hours following
maternal ingestion of a single 650-mg dose, neither acetaminophen
nor its metabolites were detected in the urine of the nursing infants.
The half-life in breast milk is 1.35 to 3.5 hours.

### Pediatrics

No published information is available on the relationship of age to the
effects of this combination medication in pediatric patients.

### Geriatrics

No published information is available on the relationship of age to the
effects of this combination medication in geriatric patients. Geriatric
patients are more likely to have peripheral vascular disease, and are
therefore more likely to be adversely affected by peripheral vasoconstriction, than are younger adults. However, isometheptene may be
safer for elderly patients than the ergot derivatives used to abort acute
vascular headaches. Also, elderly patients are more likely to have age-
related renal function impairment, which may require caution in patients receiving acetaminophen and isometheptene.

### Drug interactions and/or related problems

The following drug interactions and/or related problems have been selected on the basis of their potential clinical significance (possible
mechanism in parentheses where appropriate)—not necessarily inclusive (» = major clinical significance):

Note: Combinations containing any of the following medications, de-
    pending on the amount present, may also interact with this
    medication.

Alcohol or
CNS depressants
>    (concurrent use with dichloralphenazone may cause additive
>    sedation)

Alcohol, especially chronic abuse of or
Hepatic enzyme inducers (See *Appendix II*) or
Hepatotoxic medications, other (See *Appendix II*)
>    (risk of hepatotoxicity with single toxic doses of acetaminophen
>    may be increased in alcoholics or in patients regularly taking other
>    hepatotoxic medications or hepatic enzyme–inducing agents)

>    (chronic use of barbiturates [except butalbital] or primidone has
>    been reported to decrease the therapeutic effects of acetaminophen,
>    probably because of increased metabolism resulting from induction
>    of hepatic microsomal enzyme activity; the possibility should be
>    considered that similar effects may occur with other hepatic en-
>    zyme inducers)

» Monoamine oxidase (MAO) inhibitors
>    (concurrent use with an indirect-acting sympathomimetic such as
>    isometheptene may cause sudden and severe hypertension and hy-
>    perpyrexia, which can reach crisis levels)

### Laboratory value alterations

The following have been selected on the basis of their potential clinical
significance (possible effect in parentheses where appropriate)—not
necessarily inclusive (» = major clinical significance):

With diagnostic test results
Glucose, blood, determinations
>    (acetaminophen may cause values to be falsely decreased when
>    measured by the glucose oxidase/peroxidase method but probably
>    not when measured by the hexokinase [glucose-6-phosphate de-
>    hydrogenase (G6PD)] method)

5-Hydroxyindoleacetic acid (5-HIAA), serum, determinations
>    (acetaminophen may cause false-positive results with qualitative
>    screening tests using nitrosonaphthol reagent; the quantitative test
>    is unaffected)

Pancreatic function test using bentiromide
>    (administration of acetaminophen prior to the bentiromide test will
>    invalidate test results because acetaminophen is also metabolized
>    to an arylamine and will thus increase the apparent quantity of
>    para-aminobenzoic acid [PABA] recovered; it is recommended that
>    acetaminophen be discontinued at least 3 days prior to administra-
>    tion of bentiromide)

Uric acid, serum, determinations
>    (acetaminophen may cause falsely increased values when the phos-
>    photungstate uric acid test method is used)

With physiology/laboratory test values
Bilirubin, serum and
Lactate dehydrogenase (LDH), serum and
Prothrombin time and
Transaminase, serum
>    (values may be increased indicating acetaminophen-induced hep-
>    atotoxicity, especially in alcoholics, patients taking other hepatic
>    enzyme inducers, or patients with pre-existing hepatic disease,
>    when single toxic doses [>8 to 10 grams] are taken)

### Medical considerations/Contraindications

The medical considerations/contraindications included here have been selected on the basis of their potential clinical significance (reasons given
in parentheses where appropriate)—not necessarily inclusive (» =
major clinical significance).

***Risk-benefit should be considered when the following medical problems
exist:***

» Alcoholism, active or
» Hepatic function impairment or
» Viral hepatitis
>    (increased risk of acetaminophen-induced hepatotoxicity)

Any condition in which the vasoconstrictive or other sympathomimetic
    effects of isometheptene may be hazardous, such as:
Cardiovascular or cerebrovascular insufficiency, including recent my-
    ocardial infarction or stroke
» Glaucoma, not optimally controlled
» Hypertension, not optimally controlled
» Organic heart disease
Peripheral vascular disease

» Renal function impairment, severe
Sensitivity to acetaminophen or to isometheptene, history of

## Side/Adverse Effects

Note: The quantity of dichloralphenazone in this combination formulation
    does not provide full therapeutic doses of its active metabolites
    chloral hydrate and antipyrine (phenazone). However, the possibil-
    ity should be considered that ingestion of an overdose or overuse
    of this combination medication may induce side effects character-
    istic of chloral hydrate (see *Chloral Hydrate [Systemic]*) and/or
    antipyrine.

The following side/adverse effects have been selected on the basis of their
potential clinical significance (possible signs and symptoms in parentheses where appropriate)—not necessarily inclusive:

### Those indicating need for medical attention

Incidence less frequent
>    *Anemia or methemoglobinemia* (unusual tiredness or weakness)

Incidence rare
>    *Agranulocytosis* (unexplained sore throat and fever); *anemia* (unusual
>    tiredness or weakness); *dermatitis, allergic* (skin rash, hives, or itch-
>    ing); *hepatitis* (yellow eyes or skin); *thrombocytopenia* (usually
>    asymptomatic; rarely, unusual bleeding or bruising; black, tarry stools;
>    blood in urine or stools; pinpoint red spots on skin)

Symptoms of tolerance and/or dependence—with overuse
   *Headaches*—more frequent, severe, and difficult to treat than previously

**Those indicating need for medical attention only if they continue or are bothersome**
Incidence more frequent
   *Drowsiness*

Incidence less frequent or rare—dose-related
   *Dizziness; fast or irregular heartbeat*

## Overdose

For specific information on the agents used in the management of isometheptene, dichloralphenazone, and acetaminophen overdose, see:
• *Acetylcysteine (Systemic)* monograph.

For more information on the management of overdose or unintentional ingestion, **contact a Poison Control Center** (see *Poison Control Center Listing*).

**Clinical effects of overdose**
The following effects have been selected on the basis of their potential clinical significance (possible signs and symptoms in parentheses where appropriate)—not necessarily inclusive:

Acute
   *Gastrointestinal upset* (diarrhea; loss of appetite; nausea or vomiting; stomach cramps or pain); *increased sweating*

   Note: Early signs and symptoms of acetaminophen overdose, i.e., *gastrointestinal upset* and *increased sweating* often do not occur. However, when they do occur, they usually appear within 6 to 14 hours after ingestion of an overdose and persist for about 24 hours.

Chronic
   *Hepatotoxicity* (pain, tenderness, and/or swelling in upper abdominal area)

   Note: The first indications of overdosage may be signs and symptoms of possible *liver damage* and abnormalities in liver function tests, which may not occur until 2 to 4 days after ingestion of the overdose. Maximal changes in liver function tests usually occur 3 to 5 days after ingestion of the overdose.

   Overt *hepatic disease or failure* may occur 4 to 6 days after ingestion of the overdose. *Hepatic encephalopathy* (with mental changes, confusion, agitation, or stupor), *convulsions, respiratory depression, coma, cerebral edema, coagulation defects, gastrointestinal bleeding, disseminated intravascular coagulation, hypoglycemia, metabolic acidosis, cardiac arrhythmias, and cardiovascular collapse* may occur.

   *Renal tubular necrosis* leading to *renal failure* (signs may include bloody or cloudy urine and sudden decrease in amount of urine) has also been reported in acetaminophen overdose, usually, but not exclusively, in conjunction with acetaminophen-induced *hepatotoxicity*.

**Treatment of overdose**
For acetaminophen—
   To decrease absorption—Emptying the stomach via induction of emesis or gastric lavage.
   Removing activated charcoal (if used) by gastric lavage may be advisable. Although activated charcoal is recommended in cases of mixed drug overdose, it may interfere with absorption of orally administered acetylcysteine (antidote used to protect against acetaminophen-induced hepatotoxicity) and decrease its efficacy.
   To enhance elimination—Instituting hemodialysis or hemoperfusion to remove acetaminophen from the circulation may be beneficial if acetylcysteine administration cannot be instituted within 24 hours following ingestion of a massive acetaminophen overdose. However, the efficacy of such treatment in preventing acetaminophen-induced hepatotoxicity is not known.
   Specific treatment—Use of acetylcysteine. *It is recommended that acetylcysteine administration be instituted as soon as possible after ingestion of an overdose has been reported,* without waiting for the results of plasma acetaminophen determinations or other laboratory tests. Acetylcysteine is most effective if treatment is started within 10 to 12 hours after ingestion of the overdose; however, it may be of some benefit if treatment is started within 24 hours. See the package insert or *Acetylcysteine (Systemic)* monograph for specific dosing guidelines for use of this product.
   Monitoring—Determining plasma acetaminophen concentration at least 4 hours following ingestion of the overdose. Determinations performed prior to this time are not reliable for assessing potential hepatotoxicity. Initial plasma concentrations above 150 mcg per mL (mcg/mL [993 micromoles/L]) at 4 hours, 100 mcg/mL (662

micromoles/L) at 6 hours, 70 mcg/mL (463.4 micromoles/L) at 8 hours, 50 mcg/mL (331 micromoles/L) at 10 hours, 20 mcg/mL (132.4 micromoles/L) at 15 hours, 8 mcg/mL (53 micromoles/L) at 20 hours, or 3.5 mcg/mL (23.2 micromoles/L) at 24 hours postingestion indicate possible hepatotoxicity and the need for completing the full course of acetylcysteine treatment. If the initial determination indicates a plasma concentration below those listed at the times indicated, cessation of acetylcysteine therapy can be considered. However, some clinicians advise that more than one determination should be performed to ascertain peak absorption and half-life of acetaminophen prior to considering discontinuation of acetylcysteine.
   Monitoring renal and cardiac function and administering appropriate therapy as required.
   Performing liver function tests (serum aspartate aminotransferase [AST; SGOT], serum alanine aminotransferase [ALT; SGPT], prothrombin time, and bilirubin) at 24-hour intervals for at least 96 hours postingestion if the plasma acetaminophen concentration indicates potential hepatotoxicity. If no abnormalities are detected within 96 hours, further determinations are not needed.
   Supportive care—May include maintaining fluid and electrolyte balance, correcting hypoglycemia, and administering vitamin $K_1$ (if prothrombin time ratio exceeds 1.5) and fresh frozen plasma or clotting factor concentrate (if prothrombin time ratio exceeds 3.0).
For dichloralphenazone—
   To decrease absorption—May include gastric lavage (endotracheal tube with inflated cuff should be in place to prevent aspiration of vomitus).
   To enhance elimination—Hemodialysis may be effective in promoting the clearance of the active metabolite trichloroethanol.
   Specific treatment—May include providing artificial respiration with oxygen.
   Monitoring—Continuous cardiac monitoring is important, especially in patients with predisposing cardiac disease.
   Supportive care— May include maintaining normal body temperature, maintaining appropriate fluid and electrolyte therapy and urinary output, and supporting respiration and circulation. Patients in whom intentional overdose is known or suspected should be referred for psychiatric consultation.
For isometheptene—
   To decrease absorption—Emptying the stomach by induction of emesis or gastric lavage.
   Monitoring—May include monitoring the patient, especially for signs and symptoms of excessive sympathetic stimulation or vasoconstriction, and treating observed symptoms as necessary.

## Patient Consultation

As an aid to patient consultation, refer to *Advice for the Patient, Isometheptene, Dichloralphenazone, and Acetaminophen (Systemic)*.

In providing consultation, consider emphasizing the following selected information (» = major clinical significance):

**Before using this medication**
» Conditions affecting use, especially:
   Allergic reaction to acetaminophen or to this combination medication, history of
   Pregnancy—Acetaminophen crosses the placenta
   Breast-feeding—Acetaminophen is excreted in breast milk
   Other medications, especially monoamine oxidase inhibitors
   Other medical problems, especially alcoholism (active), glaucoma, hypertension, heart disease, hepatic disease or viral hepatitis, and severe renal function impairment

**Proper use of this medication**
» Importance of not taking more medication than the amount prescribed; risk of tolerance and dependence with too frequent use; also, acetaminophen may cause liver damage with long-term use or greater than recommended doses
» Most effective when taken as soon as headache appears or at first sign of migraine attack (prodromal stage)
» Lying down in a quiet, dark room after taking initial dose
» Compliance with prophylactic therapy, if prescribed
» Proper dosing
» Proper storage

**Precautions while using this medication**
» Checking with physician if usual dose fails to relieve headaches, or if frequency and/or severity of headaches increases; possibility that tolerance to the medication has developed and/or withdrawal (rebound) or chronic, daily headaches are occurring
» Caution if other medications containing acetaminophen are used

» Caution when driving or doing jobs requiring alertness because of possible drowsiness or dizziness, especially if also taking a CNS depressant.

» Avoiding use of alcohol, which increases the risk of liver toxicity with high doses of acetaminophen, especially in alcoholics; also, alcohol may aggravate or induce headache

**Side/adverse effects**

Signs of potential side effects, especially allergic dermatitis, blood dyscrasias, hepatotoxicity, and methemoglobinemia

## General Dosing Information

Therapy is most effective when initiated at the first symptoms of a headache (during the prodrome, for migraine with aura).

After the first dose has been administered, it is recommended that the patient lie down and relax in a quiet, darkened room, because this contributes to relief of headaches.

In headache-prone individuals, frequent use of headache relievers may cause tolerance, leading to an increased dosage requirement, and to physical dependence, leading to both medication abuse and chronic (daily or near-daily) headaches. Patients who experience frequent headaches may also be dependent on a variety of other medications, including opioid analgesics, barbiturate-containing analgesic combinations, simple analgesics such as acetaminophen or aspirin, ergotamine, and antianxiety agents or sedatives.

Chronic headaches resulting from overmedication may be difficult to relieve, especially if the patient continues to take headache suppressants and/or analgesics. It is recommended that all such medications be discontinued. In-patient treatment may be necessary during detoxification. Naproxen, alone or together with amitriptyline, may reduce the severity of the headaches. Repetitive intravenous administration of dihydroergotamine (in conjunction with metoclopramide [to control dihydroergotamine-induced nausea and vomiting]) is recommended by some headache specialists to relieve chronic, intractable headaches associated with dependency on headache-aborting medications. Appropriate treatment for symptoms of withdrawal from other substances frequently used or abused by chronic headache patients may also be needed. In addition, appropriate prophylactic treatment should be initiated or adjusted to reduce the frequency and/or severity of future headaches.

## Oral Dosage Forms

### ISOMETHEPTENE MUCATE, DICHLORALPHENAZONE, AND ACETAMINOPHEN CAPSULES USP

**Usual adult dose**

Tension-type headache—
Oral, 1 or 2 capsules every four hours as needed, up to 8 capsules a day.

Vascular headache suppressant (migraine)—
Oral, 2 capsules at the start of the attack (during the prodrome, for migraine with aura), followed by 1 capsule every hour as needed, up to 5 capsules in twelve hours.

**Usual pediatric dose**

Dosage has not been established.

**Strength(s) usually available**

U.S.—

65 mg of isometheptene mucate, 100 mg of dichloralphenazone, and 325 mg of acetaminophen (Rx) [*Amidrine; I.D.A; Iso-Acetazone; Isocom; Midchlor; Midrin; Migrapap; Migquin; Migratine; Migrazone; Migrend; Migrex; Mitride*].

**Packaging and storage**

Store below 40 °C (104 °F), preferably between 15 and 30 °C (59 and 86 °F). Store in a well-closed container.

## Selected Bibliography

Kunkel RS. Diagnosis and treatment of muscle contraction (tension-type) headaches. Med Clin N Amer 1991; 75: 595-603.

Anthony M. The treatment of migraine and other headaches. Curr Opin Neurol Neurosurg 1991; 4: 245-52.

Diamond S. Migraine headache. Med Clin N Amer 1991; 75: 545-66.

Revised: 08/18/92
Interim revision: 05/17/95

# ISONIAZID   Systemic

VA CLASSIFICATION (Primary): AM500
Another commonly used name is INH.

Note: For a listing of dosage forms and brand names by country availability, see *Dosage Forms* section(s). For a listing of brand names for the articles in this monograph, refer to the General Index.

## Category

Antibacterial (antimycobacterial).

## Indications

Note: Bracketed information in the *Indications* section refers to uses that are not included in U.S. product labeling.

**Accepted**

Tuberculosis (prophylaxis)—Isoniazid is indicated alone in the prophylaxis of all forms of tuberculosis in the following persons:

• Household members and other close contacts of patients with recently diagnosed tuberculosis who have a positive tuberculin skin test (PPD) of ≥ 5-mm; [tuberculin-negative children and adolescents who have been close contacts of infectious persons within the past 3 months are also candidates for preventative therapy until a repeat PPD is done 12 weeks after contact with the infectious source][1];

• [Human immunodeficiency virus (HIV)–infected persons of any age with a positive PPD of ≥ 5-mm or a past history of a positive PPD; also, persons with risk factors for HIV infection whose HIV status is unknown but who are suspected of having HIV infection][1];

• Positive PPD reactors of ≥ 5-mm with chest x-ray findings consistent with nonprogressive tuberculosis in whom there are neither positive bacteriologic findings nor a history of adequate chemotherapy for tuberculosis;

• [Children with a positive PPD of ≥ 5-mm who have an immunosuppressive condition, including HIV infection or immunosuppression due to corticosteroids][1];

• Adults with positive PPD reactions of ≥ 10-mm who are receiving immunosuppressives or prolonged therapy with corticosteroids, who have certain hematologic and reticuloendothelial diseases such as leukemia or Hodgkin's disease, who have diabetes mellitus or silicosis, or who have undergone gastrectomy;

• Children less than 4 years of age with a positive PPD of ≥ 10-mm who are at increased risk of dissemination because of their young age[1];

• [Children with a positive PPD of ≥ 10-mm who are at increased risk of dissemination because of medical risk factors other than immunosuppression due to corticosteroid therapy or HIV infection, such as Hodgkin's disease, lymphoma, diabetes mellitus, chronic renal failure, and malnutrition][1];

• [Positive PPD reactors with a PPD of ≥ 10-mm among intravenous drug abusers (IVDA) known to be HIV-negative, alcoholics, or homeless persons of any age, and children frequently exposed to these persons][1];

• [Positive PPD reactions of ≥ 10-mm in foreign-born persons up to 35 years of age, or children whose parents are from high-prevalence areas, such as Asia, Africa, or Latin America][1];

• [Positive PPD reactions of ≥ 10-mm in residents of long-term care facilities, prisons, nursing homes, and mental institutions, and children frequently exposed to these persons][1];

• [Positive PPD reactions of ≥ 10-mm in medically underserved low-income populations, up to 35 years of age, including high-risk racial or ethnic minority populations, especially blacks, Hispanics, and Native Americans][1]; or

• Recent converters, as indicated by a PPD increase of ≥ 10-mm within 2 years for those up to 35 years of age, and a PPD increase of ≥15-mm for those 35 years of age and older; [also children 4 years of age and older with a PPD of ≥ 15-mm without any risk factors][1].

Tuberculosis (treatment)—Isoniazid is indicated, in combination with other antituberculars, in the treatment of all forms of tuberculosis, including tuberculous meningitis.

Resistance to isoniazid is a rapidly increasing problem. The primary cause of drug-resistance to antitubercular medications is inadequate therapy due to patient noncompliance. To try to avoid this continuing trend, administration of 4-drug therapy that is directly observed is currently recommended. (See *General Dosing Information*.)

Not all species or strains of a particular organism may be susceptible to isoniazid.

### Unaccepted

Isoniazid is not recommended for use in the treatment of atypical mycobacterial infections, such as *Mycobacterium avium* complex (MAC), because isoniazid has weak activity against MAC compared to other antimycobacterial agents.

¹Not included in Canadian product labeling.

## Pharmacology/Pharmacokinetics

### Physicochemical characteristics
Molecular weight—137.14.

### Mechanism of action/Effect
Isoniazid (INH) is a synthetic, bactericidal antitubercular agent, which is active against many mycobacteria, primarily those that are actively dividing. Its exact mechanism of action is not known, but it may relate to inhibition of mycolic acid synthesis and disruption of the cell wall in susceptible organisms.

### Absorption
Readily absorbed following oral administration; however, may undergo significant first pass metabolism. Absorption and bioavailability are reduced when isoniazid is administered with food.

### Distribution
Widely distributed to all fluids and tissues, including cerebrospinal fluid (CSF), pleural and ascitic fluids, skin, sputum, saliva, lungs, muscle, and caseous tissue. Crosses the placenta and is distributed into breast milk.

$Vol_D$ =0.57 to 0.76 L per kg.

### Protein binding
Very low (0–10%).

### Biotransformation
Hepatic; isoniazid is acetylated by *N*-acetyl transferase to *N*-acetylisoniazid; it is then biotransformed to isonicotinic acid and monoacetylhydrazine. Monoacetylhydrazine is associated with hepatotoxicity via formation of a reactive intermediate metabolite when *N*-hydroxylated by the cytochrome P-450 mixed oxidase system. The rate of acetylation is genetically determined; slow acetylators are characterized by a relative lack of hepatic *N*-acetyl transferase.

### Half-life
Adults (including elderly patients)—
    Fast acetylators: 0.5 to 1.6 hours.
    Slow acetylators: 2 to 5 hours.
    Acute and chronic liver disease: May be prolonged (6.7 hours vs 3.2 hours in controls).
Children (age 1.5 to 15 years)—
    2.3 to 4.9 hours.
Neonates—
    7.8 and 19.8 hours in 2 newborns who received isoniazid transplacentally. The long half-life may be due to the limited acetylation capacity of neonates.

### Time to peak serum concentration:
1 to 2 hours.

### Peak serum concentration:
3 to 7 mcg per mL after a single 300-mg oral dose.

### Elimination
Renal; approximately 75–95% excreted by the kidneys within 24 hours, primarily as the inactive metabolites, *N*-acetylisoniazid and isonicotinic acid; of this amount, 93% of the isoniazid excreted in the urine may occur as the acetylated form in fast acetylators and 63% in slow acetylators, with the remainder, in both cases, occurring as the free or conjugated form.
Small amounts are excreted in feces.
In dialysis—
    Significant amounts of isoniazid are removed from the blood by hemodialysis. A single 5-hour hemodialysis period has removed up to 73% of the isoniazid in the blood.
    Peritoneal dialysis is of limited benefit.

## Precautions to Consider

### Cross-sensitivity and/or related problems
Patients hypersensitive to ethionamide, pyrazinamide, niacin (nicotinic acid), or other chemically related medications may be hypersensitive to this medication also.

### Carcinogenicity/Tumorigenicity
Isoniazid has been shown to cause pulmonary tumors in a number of strains of mice. However, isoniazid has not been shown to be carcinogenic or tumorigenic in humans.

### Pregnancy/Reproduction
Pregnancy—Isoniazid crosses the placenta, resulting in fetal serum concentrations that may exceed maternal serum concentrations. Problems in humans have not been documented. It is recommended that pregnant women with tuberculosis be treated for a minimum of 9 months with multi-drug therapy, including isoniazid.
Studies in rats and rabbits have shown that isoniazid may be embryocidal. However, isoniazid has not been shown to be teratogenic in mice, rats, or rabbits.

FDA Pregnancy Category C.

### Breast-feeding
Isoniazid is distributed into breast milk. An estimated 0.75 to 2.3% of the daily adult dose could be ingested by the infant. Problems in nursing newborns have not been documented and breast-feeding should not be discouraged. However, because isoniazid concentrations are so low in breast milk, breast-feeding cannot be relied upon for adequate tuberculosis prophylaxis or therapy for nursing infants.

### Pediatrics
Studies performed in children have not demonstrated pediatrics-specific problems that would limit the usefulness of isoniazid in children. However, newborn infants may have a limited acetylation capacity, prolonging the elimination half-life of isoniazid.
Children do not require routine hepatic function determinations unless they have pre-existing hepatic disease.
Pyridoxine supplementation is not usually required in children if dietary intake is adequate.

### Geriatrics
Patients over 50 years of age have the highest incidence of hepatitis.

### Drug interactions and/or related problems
The following drug interactions and/or related problems have been selected on the basis of their potential clinical significance (possible mechanism in parentheses where appropriate)—not necessarily inclusive (» = major clinical significance):
Note: Combinations containing any of the following medications, depending on the amount present, may also interact with this medication.

Acetaminophen
    (concurrent use of acetaminophen with isoniazid may increase the potential for hepatotoxicity and, possibly, nephrotoxicity; isoniazid is thought to induce cytochrome P-450, resulting in a greater proportion of acetaminophen being converted to toxic metabolite)

» Alcohol
    (concurrent daily use of alcohol may result in increased incidence of isoniazid-induced hepatotoxicity and increased metabolism of isoniazid; dosage adjustments of isoniazid may be necessary; patients should be monitored closely for signs of hepatotoxicity and should be advised to restrict intake of alcoholic beverages)

» Alfentanil
    (chronic preoperative or perioperative use of isoniazid, a hepatic enzyme inhibitor, may decrease the plasma clearance and prolong the duration of action of alfentanil)

Antacids, especially aluminum-containing
    (antacids may delay and decrease absorption and serum concentrations of orally administered isoniazid; concurrent use should be avoided, or patients should be advised to take oral isoniazid at least 1 hour before aluminum-containing antacids)

Anticoagulants, coumarin- or indandione-derivative
    (concurrent use with isoniazid may result in increased anticoagulant effect because of the inhibition of enzymatic metabolism of anticoagulants)

Benzodiazepines
    (isoniazid may decrease the hepatic metabolism of benzodiazepines, such as diazepam, chlordiazepoxide, flurazepam, and prazepam, that are metabolized by phase I reactions [*N*-demethylation and hydroxylation]; it may also impair the oxidation of triazolam, increasing plasma benzodiazepine concentrations; isoniazid may decrease first-pass metabolism and elimination of midazolam in the

liver, probably by competitive inhibition at the cytochrome P-450 binding sites, increasing steady-state plasma concentrations of midazolam)

» Carbamazepine
(concurrent use with isoniazid increases serum carbamazepine levels and toxicity, probably through inhibition of carbamazepine metabolism; also, carbamazepine may induce microsomal metabolism of isoniazid, increasing formation of an INH-reactive intermediate metabolite, which may lead to hepatotoxicity)

Cheese, such as Swiss or Cheshire, or
Fish, such as tuna, skipjack, or Sardinella
(concurrent ingestion with isoniazid may result in redness or itching of the skin, hot feeling, rapid or pounding heartbeat, sweating, chills or clammy feeling, headache, or lightheadedness; this is thought to be due to the inhibition of plasma monoamine oxidase and diamine oxidase by isoniazid, interfering with the metabolism of tyramine and histamine found in fish and cheese)

Corticosteroids, glucocorticoid
(concurrent use of prednisolone, and probably other related corticosteroids, with isoniazid may increase hepatic metabolism and/or excretion of isoniazid, leading to decreased plasma concentrations and effectiveness of isoniazid, especially in patients who are rapid acetylators; isoniazid dosage adjustments may be required)

Cycloserine
(concurrent use may result in increased incidence of central nervous system [CNS] effects such as dizziness or drowsiness; dosage adjustments may be necessary and patients should be monitored closely for signs of CNS toxicity)

» Disulfiram
(concurrent use in alcoholics may result in increased incidence of CNS effects such as dizziness, incoordination, irritability, or insomnia; reduced dosage or discontinuation of disulfiram may be necessary)

Enflurane
(isoniazid may increase formation of the potentially nephrotoxic inorganic fluoride metabolite when used concurrently with enflurane)

» Hepatotoxic medications, other (See *Appendix II*)
(concurrent use of other hepatotoxic medications with isoniazid may increase the potential for hepatotoxicity and should be avoided)

» Ketoconazole
(concurrent use of ketoconazole with isoniazid has been reported to decrease serum concentrations of ketoconazole; isoniazid should be used with caution when given concurrently with ketoconazole)

Neurotoxic medications, other (See *Appendix II*)
(concurrent use of other neurotoxic medications with isoniazid may produce additive neurotoxicity)

» Phenytoin
(concurrent use with isoniazid inhibits the metabolism of phenytoin, resulting in increased phenytoin serum concentrations and toxicity; phenytoin dosage adjustments may be necessary during and after isoniazid therapy, especially in slow acetylators of isoniazid)

Pyridoxine
(isoniazid may cause peripheral neuritis by acting as a pyridoxine antagonist or increasing renal excretion of pyridoxine; requirements for pyridoxine may be increased in patients receiving isoniazid concurrently)

» Rifampin
(concurrent use of rifampin with isoniazid may increase the risk of hepatotoxicity, especially in patients with pre-existing hepatic impairment and/or in fast acetylators of isoniazid; patients receiving rifampin and isoniazid concurrently should be monitored closely for signs of hepatotoxicity during the first 3 months of therapy)

Theophylline
(concurrent use may reduce the metabolism of theophylline, increasing theophylline plasma concentrations)

**Laboratory value alterations**
The following have been selected on the basis of their potential clinical significance (possible effect in parentheses where appropriate)—not necessarily inclusive (» = major clinical significance):
With diagnostic test results
Glucose, urine
(isoniazid may cause hyperglycemia with a secondary glycosuria, giving a positive response to copper sulfate tests; glucose enzymatic tests are not affected)

With physiology/laboratory test values
Alanine aminotransferase (ALT [SGPT]) and
Aspartate aminotransferase (AST [SGOT]) and
Bilirubin, serum
(values may be transiently, and asymptomatically increased in approximately 10 to 20% of patients tested)

**Medical considerations/Contraindications**
The medical considerations/contraindications included here have been selected on the basis of their potential clinical significance (reasons given in parentheses where appropriate)—not necessarily inclusive (» = major clinical significance).

*Risk-benefit should be considered when the following medical problems exist:*
» Alcoholism, active or in remission, or
» Hepatic function impairment
(increased risk of hepatitis with daily consumption of alcohol or hepatic function impairment)
» Hypersensitivity to isoniazid, ethionamide, pyrazinamide, niacin (nicotinic acid), or other chemically related medications
Renal failure, severe
(there may be an increased risk of toxicity in patients who have both severe renal failure [creatinine clearance <10 mL/min])
Seizure disorders
(isoniazid may be neurotoxic and cause seizures)

**Patient monitoring**
The following may be especially important in patient monitoring (other tests may be warranted in some patients, depending on condition; » = major clinical significance):
Hepatic function determinations
(AST [SGOT], ALT [SGPT], and serum bilirubin determinations may be required prior to and monthly or more frequently during treatment; however, elevated serum enzyme values may not be predictive of clinical hepatitis and values may return to normal despite continued treatment; therefore, routine measurement of hepatic function is generally not recommended unless there is pre-existing hepatic disease; patients should be instructed to report promptly any prodromal symptoms of hepatitis; if signs and symptoms of hepatotoxicity occur, isoniazid should be promptly discontinued; if isoniazid therapy must be reinstituted, very small and gradually increasing doses should be used, and then only after signs and symptoms of hepatotoxicity have cleared; isoniazid should be withdrawn immediately if any further evidence of hepatotoxicity occurs)
» Ophthalmologic examinations
(if symptoms of optic neuritis occur in either adults or children during treatment, ophthalmologic examinations may be required immediately and periodically thereafter; ophthalmologic examinations are not recommended in asymptomatic patients)

# Side/Adverse Effects

Note: Isoniazid has been reported to cause severe, and sometimes fatal, age-related hepatitis. If signs and symptoms of hepatotoxicity occur, isoniazid should be promptly discontinued. The incidence of clinical hepatitis in young, healthy adults is 0.3%, but can increase to 2.6% for those who drink alcohol daily, have chronic liver disease, or are elderly.

Patients with advanced HIV disease have been reported to have an increased incidence of adverse reactions to antitubercular medications. This was not found in HIV-seropositive patients being treated for tuberculosis.

Peripheral neuritis is usually preventable by administering 10 to 25 mg of pyridoxine per day. It is recommended for patients at risk of neuritis, including those over 65 years of age, pregnant women, patients with diabetes mellitus, chronic renal failure, alcoholism, malnutrition, and those taking anticonvulsant medications.

The following side/adverse effects have been selected on the basis of their potential clinical significance (possible signs and symptoms in parentheses where appropriate)—not necessarily inclusive:

**Those indicating need for medical attention**
Incidence more frequent
*Hepatitis* (dark urine, yellow eyes or skin); *hepatitis prodromal symptoms* (loss of appetite, nausea or vomiting, unusual tiredness or weakness); *peripheral neuritis* (clumsiness or unsteadiness; numbness, tingling, burning, or pain in hands and feet)
Incidence rare
*Blood dyscrasias* (fever and sore throat, unusual bleeding and bruising, unusual tiredness or weakness); *hypersensitivity* (fever, joint pain, skin

rash); *neurotoxicity* (seizures, mental depression, mood or other mental changes); *optic neuritis* (blurred vision or loss of vision, with or without eye pain)

**Those indicating need for medical attention only if they continue or are bothersome**

Incidence more frequent

*Gastrointestinal disturbances* (diarrhea, nausea and vomiting, stomach pain)

Incidence not reported

*Local irritation at the site of intramuscular injections*

## Overdose

For specific information on the agents used in the management of isoniazid overdose, see

- *Pyridoxine (Systemic)* monograph;
- *Diazepam* in *Benzodiazepines (Systemic)* monograph; and/or
- *Thiopental* in *Barbiturates (Systemic)* monograph.

For more information on the management of overdose or unintentional ingestion, **contact a Poison Control Center** (see *Poison Control Center Listing*).

The information below applies to the clinical effects and treatment of isoniazid overdose.

**Clinical effects of isoniazid overdose**

The following effects have been selected on the basis of their potential clinical significance (possible signs and symptoms in parentheses where appropriate)—not necessarily inclusive:

Acute and chronic effects

*Gastrointestinal disturbances* (severe nausea and vomiting); *neurotoxicity* (dizziness; slurred speech; lethargy; disorientation; hyperreflexia; seizures; coma)

Note: Patients may be asymptomatic for 30 minutes to 2 hours after an acute overdose. Early symptoms include *nausea and vomiting, dizziness, slurred speech, lethargy, disorientation,* and *hyperreflexia. Seizures* usually occur within 1 to 3 hours after ingestion, and are often repetitive and refractory to treatment with usual anticonvulsants. Lactic acid accumulation produces an anion-gap metabolic acidosis within a few hours, which is often severe and refractory to treatment with sodium bicarbonate. Hyperglycemia, glycosuria, and ketonuria have also been reported.

**Treatment of isoniazid overdose**

To decrease absorption—

Because seizures may occur soon after ingestion, induction of emesis with ipecac is not recommended. Gastric lavage may be performed within 2 to 3 hours of ingestion, and activated charcoal and a cathartic may be administered if the patient's seizures are controlled and the airway protected.

Specific treatment—

Administering intravenous pyridoxine in a gram-for-gram dose, equivalent to the amount of isoniazid ingested; dose should be administered as a 5 or 10% solution in water for injection over 30 to 60 minutes. If the amount of isoniazid ingested is unknown, administering 5-gram doses of pyridoxine every 5 to 30 minutes until seizures stop or consciousness is regained.

Controlling seizures with diazepam, which acts synergistically with pyridoxine. Phenytoin should be used with caution, if at all, since isoniazid inhibits phenytoin metabolism. Thiopental has been effective in treating refractory seizures.

Carefully administering sodium bicarbonate if pyridoxine and diazepam do not control seizure activity. Use caution against overcorrection and watch for hypokalemia or hyperkalemia.

Supportive care—

Supportive measures such as establishing intravenous lines, hydration, correction of electrolyte imbalance, oxygenation, and support of ventilatory function are essential for maintaining the vital functions of the patient. Patients in whom intentional overdose is confirmed or suspected should be referred for psychiatric consultation.

## Patient Consultation

As an aid to patient consultation, refer to *Advice for the Patient, Isoniazid (Systemic)*.

In providing consultation, consider emphasizing the following selected information (» = major clinical significance):

**Before using this medication**

» Conditions affecting use, especially:

Hypersensitivity to isoniazid, ethionamide, pyrazinamide, niacin (nicotinic acid), or other chemically related medications

Pregnancy—Isoniazid crosses the placenta; fetal serum concentrations may exceed maternal serum concentrations

Breast-feeding—Isoniazid is distributed into breast milk

Use in children—Children may be less susceptible to pyridoxine deficiency and hepatotoxicity than adults, unless they have preexisting hepatic disease; newborn infants may have prolonged elimination

Use in the elderly—Patients over the age of 50 have the highest incidence of hepatitis

Other medicines, especially daily alcohol use, alfentanil, carbamazepine, disulfiram, other hepatotoxic medications, ketoconazole, phenytoin, or rifampin

Other medical problems, especially alcoholism, active or in remission, or hepatic function impairment

**Proper use of this medication**

Taking this medication with food or antacids, but not within 1 hour of aluminum-containing antacids, if gastrointestinal irritation occurs (oral only)

Proper administration technique for oral liquids

» Compliance with full course of therapy, which may take 6 months to 2 years

» Taking pyridoxine concurrently to prevent or minimize symptoms of peripheral neuritis; not usually required in children if dietary intake is adequate

» Proper dosing

Missed dose: Taking as soon as possible; not taking if almost time for next dose; not doubling doses

» Proper storage

**Precautions while using this medication**

» Regular visits to physician to check progress, as well as ophthalmologic examinations if signs of optic neuritis occur in either adults or children

Checking with physician if vascular reactions occur following concurrent ingestion of cheese or fish with isoniazid

Checking with physician if no improvement within 2 to 3 weeks

» Avoiding alcoholic beverages while taking this medication

» Need to report to physician promptly prodromal signs of hepatitis or peripheral neuritis

» Diabetics: False-positive reactions with copper sulfate urine glucose tests may occur

**Side/adverse effects**

Hepatitis may be more likely to occur in patients over 50 years of age

Signs of potential side effects, especially hepatitis, peripheral neuritis, blood dyscrasias, hypersensitivity, neurotoxicity, and optic neuritis

## General Dosing Information

All patients may be divided into 2 groups: slow and fast acetylators of isoniazid. Patients who are slow acetylators may be more prone to development of adverse effects, especially peripheral neuritis, and may require lower-than-usual doses. Fast acetylators do not generally require higher doses, nor is isoniazid less effective in these patients. Eskimo, Oriental, and American Indian populations have the lowest prevalence of slow acetylators, while Egyptian, Israeli, Scandinavian, other Caucasian, and black populations have the highest prevalence of slow acetylators.

Tuberculosis therapy must be continued for 6 months to 2 years, depending on the treatment regimen. Uncomplicated pulmonary tuberculosis is often successfully treated within 6 to 12 months. Several different treatment regimens are currently recommended.

- The Infectious Diseases Society of America recommends standard triple-drug therapy for patients born in the United States who have never been treated, do not reside in communities with a known high prevalence of drug-resistant *Mycobacterium* strains, and have no risk factors for drug-resistant tuberculosis.

—Isoniazid, rifampin, and, usually, pyrazinamide are given together daily for the first 2 months, then isoniazid and rifampin are continued daily or twice a week for the remainder of the treatment period. Directly observed therapy is recommended for patients suspected of being noncompliant. If a patient is at risk of being infected with drug-resistant organisms, 4-drug therapy, consisting of isoniazid, rifampin, pyrazinamide, and ethambutol, is recommended.

- The Centers for Disease Control recommend 3 other treatment regimen options available for non–HIV-infected patients:

—In geographic areas where the isoniazid resistance rate is documented to be ≥ 4%, an initial 4-drug regimen of isoniazid, rifampin, pyrazinamide, and streptomycin or ethambutol, taken under direct observation, is recommended. This should be administered for 8 weeks. After that time and provided that the organism is found to be susceptible, isoniazid and rifampin are administered daily, or 2 or 3 times a week, under direct observation, for 16 weeks. When results of susceptibility tests for these medications become available, the regimen should be altered as appropriate.

—Isoniazid, rifampin, pyrazinamide, and streptomycin or ethambutol taken daily under direct observation for 2 weeks, followed by twice-weekly administration of all 4 medications for 6 weeks, under direct observation. This is then followed by twice-weekly administration, directly observed, of isoniazid and rifampin for 16 weeks.

—Isoniazid, rifampin, pyrazinamide, and streptomycin or ethambutol taken 3 times a week under direct observation for 6 months.

HIV-infected patients may use any of the 3 options recommended by the CDC; however, treatment regimens should continue for a total of 9 months and at least 6 months beyond culture conversion.

Healthcare or correctional institutions experiencing outbreaks of tuberculosis that are resistant to isoniazid and rifampin, or that are resuming therapy for a patient with a prior history of antitubercular therapy, may need to begin 5- or 6-drug regimens as initial therapy. These regimens should include the 4-drug regimen and at least 3 medications to which the suspected multi–drug-resistant strain may be susceptible.

The regimen for treating pulmonary tuberculosis should be effective in treating extrapulmonary tuberculosis. Some experts recommend extending the duration of therapy to 9 months in patients with disseminated disease, miliary tuberculosis, disease involving bones or joints, or tuberculosis lymphadenitis. Adjunctive therapies, such as surgery and corticosteroids, may be beneficial.

The clinical presentation of tuberculosis in HIV-infected patients may be hard to distinguish from other pulmonary complications in AIDS patients, making diagnosis difficult. Many patients with advanced HIV disease are anergic and will not react to a PPD skin test. A PPD reaction of ≥ 5-mm induration should be cause for evaluation in HIV-infected patients. Extrapulmonary tuberculosis occurs in 25 to 70% of HIV-associated TB cases. The most frequent extrapulmonary sites of disease include the lymph nodes, blood, bone marrow, the CNS, and urinary tract. A chest x-ray may not be consistent with the usual TB picture, being more diffuse and less cavitary in patients with AIDS. However, it should be noted that HIV-seropositive tuberculosis patients have the same incidence of pulmonary TB as do HIV-seronegative patients, and 50 to 80% of HIV-seronegative patients with TB will also react to a PPD test. Compared to AIDS patients, HIV-seropositive patients have chest x-rays more like those seen in seronegative patients. Specimens should be obtained for culture from various sites, especially in patients with advanced HIV disease. However, the inability to demonstrate acid-fast bacilli does not exclude the diagnosis of tuberculosis.

Prophylactic therapy with daily isoniazid should continue for at least 1 year in HIV-infected patients; however, some clinicians favor lifelong chemoprophylaxis in this population.

Patients with impaired renal function do not generally require a reduction in dose if the plasma creatinine concentration is less than 6 mg per 100 mL. If renal impairment is more severe or if patients are slow acetylators, a reduction in dose and/or serum determinations may be required. Slow acetylators may require dosage adjustments to ensure isoniazid serum concentrations of less than 1 mcg per mL measured 24 hours after the preceding dose. In anuric patients, one-half the usual maintenance dose is recommended.

**For oral dosage forms only**

Isoniazid may be taken with meals if gastrointestinal irritation occurs. Antacids may also be taken. However, isoniazid should be taken at least 1 hour before aluminum-containing antacids.

Oral absorption may be decreased if isoniazid is taken with food or antacids.

## Oral Dosage Forms

### ISONIAZID SYRUP USP

**Usual adult and adolescent dose**
Tuberculosis—
Prophylaxis: Oral, 300 mg once a day.
Treatment: In combination with other antituberculosis medications—
Oral, 300 mg of isoniazid once a day for the entire treatment period; or 15 mg per kg of body weight, up to 900 mg, two or three times a week, as specified by the treatment regimen.

**Usual adult prescribing limits**
300 mg daily.

**Usual pediatric dose**
Tuberculosis—
Prophylaxis: Oral, 10 mg per kg of body weight, up to 300 mg, once a day.
Treatment: In combination with other antituberculosis medications—
Oral, 10 to 20 mg of isoniazid per kg of body weight, up to 300 mg, once a day; or 20 to 40 mg per kg of body weight, up to 900 mg, two or three times a week, as specified by the treatment regimen.

**Strength(s) usually available**
U.S.—
50 mg per 5 mL (Rx) [*Laniazid;* GENERIC].
Canada—
50 mg per 5 mL (Rx) [*Isotamine; PMS Isoniazid*].

**Packaging and storage**
Store below 40 °C (104 °F), preferably between 15 and 30 °C (59 and 86 °F), unless otherwise specified by manufacturer. Store in a tight, light-resistant container. Protect from freezing.

**Auxiliary labeling**
• Continue medicine for full time of treatment.
• Avoid alcoholic beverages.

**Note**
When dispensing, include a calibrated liquid-measuring device.

### ISONIAZID TABLETS USP

**Usual adult and adolescent dose**
See *Isoniazid Syrup USP.*

**Usual adult prescribing limits**
See *Isoniazid Syrup USP.*

**Usual pediatric dose**
See *Isoniazid Syrup USP.*

**Strength(s) usually available**
U.S.—
50 mg (Rx) [*Laniazid;* GENERIC].
100 mg (Rx) [*Laniazid;* GENERIC].
300 mg (Rx) [*Laniazid;* GENERIC].
Canada—
50 mg (Rx) [*PMS Isoniazid*].
100 mg (Rx) [*PMS Isoniazid*].
300 mg (Rx) [*PMS Isoniazid*].

**Packaging and storage**
Store below 40 °C (104 °F), preferably between 15 and 30 °C (59 and 86 °F), unless otherwise specified by manufacturer. Store in a well-closed, light-resistant container.

**Auxiliary labeling**
• Continue medicine for full time of treatment.
• Avoid alcoholic beverages.

## Parenteral Dosage Forms

### ISONIAZID INJECTION USP

**Usual adult and adolescent dose**
Tuberculosis—
Prophylaxis: Intramuscular, 300 mg once a day.
Treatment: In combination with other antituberculosis medications—
Intramuscular, 5 mg of isoniazid per kg of body weight, up to 300 mg, once a day for the entire treatment period; or 15 mg per kg of body weight, up to 900 mg, two or three times a week, as specified by the treatment regimen.

**Usual adult prescribing limits**
300 mg daily.

**Usual pediatric dose**
Tuberculosis—
Prophylaxis: Intramuscular, 10 mg per kg of body weight, up to 300 mg, once a day.
Treatment: In combination with other antituberculosis medications—
Intramuscular, 10 to 20 mg of isoniazid per kg of body weight, up to 300 mg, once a day; or 20 to 40 mg per kg of body weight, up to 900 mg, two or three times a week, as specified by the treatment regimen.

**Strength(s) usually available**
U.S.—
100 mg per mL (Rx) [*Nydrazid*].
Canada—
Not commercially available.

### Packaging and storage

Store below 40 °C (104 °F), preferably between 15 and 30 °C (59 and 86 °F), unless otherwise specified by manufacturer. Protect from light. Protect from freezing.

Note: Crystallization may occur at low temperatures. Upon warming to room temperature, the crystals will redissolve.

### Selected Bibliography

Committee on Infectious Diseases, American Academy of Pediatrics. Chemotherapy for tuberculosis in infants and children. Pediatrics 1992; 89 (1): 161-5.

Centers for Disease Control. Initial therapy for tuberculosis in the era of multidrug resistance: recommendations of the advisory council for the elimination of tuberculosis. MMWR 1993; 42 (RR-7): 1-8.

Revised: 06/22/94

---

## ISONIAZID-CONTAINING COMBINATIONS—

Isoniazid and Thiacetazone (Systemic)
Rifampin and Isoniazid (Systemic)
Rifampin, Isoniazid, and Pyrazinamide (Systemic)

---

## ISONIAZID AND THIACETAZONE—Since Isoniazid and Thiacetazone is not commercially available in the U.S. or Canada, the

*Isoniazid and Thiacetazone (Systemic)* monograph is not included in this published version of the USP DI database. Copies of the monograph are available on request from the USP Division of Information Development, 12601 Twinbrook Parkway, Rockville, MD 20852; telephone (301) 816-8351; telefax (301) 816-8374.

---

## ISOPHANE INSULIN—See *Insulin (Systemic)*

---

## ISOPHANE INSULIN, HUMAN—See *Insulin (Systemic)*

---

## ISOPHANE INSULIN, HUMAN, AND INSULIN HUMAN (SYSTEMIC)—See *Insulin (Systemic)*

---

## ISOPROTERENOL—See *Bronchodilators, Adrenergic (Systemic)*; *Sympathomimetic Agents—Cardiovascular Use (Parenteral-Systemic)*

---

## ISOPROTERENOL-CONTAINING COMBINATIONS—

Isoproterenol and Phenylephrine (Systemic)

---

# ISOPROTERENOL AND PHENYLEPHRINE   Systemic

VA CLASSIFICATION (Primary): RE109

Note: For a listing of dosage forms and brand names by country availability, see *Dosage Forms* section(s). For a listing of brand names for the articles in this monograph, refer to the General Index.

## Category

Bronchodilator-decongestant.

## Indications

### Accepted

Asthma, bronchial (treatment)
Bronchiectasis (treatment)
Bronchitis (treatment)
Emphysema, pulmonary (treatment) or
Pulmonary disease, chronic obstructive, other (treatment)—Isoproterenol and phenylephrine combination is indicated for the treatment of bronchospasm associated with acute and chronic bronchial asthma, pulmonary emphysema, bronchitis, bronchiectasis, and other chronic obstructive pulmonary disease.

## Pharmacology/Pharmacokinetics

### Physicochemical characteristics

Molecular weight—Isoproterenol hydrochloride: 247.72.
Phenylephrine hydrochloride: 203.67.

### Mechanism of action/Effect

Isoproterenol—Isoproterenol is a direct-acting sympathomimetic amine that acts predominantly on beta-adrenergic receptors. It relaxes bronchial smooth muscle by acting on beta-2-adrenergic receptors, thereby relieving bronchospasm, increasing vital capacity, reducing residual volume in the lungs, and facilitating passage of pulmonary secretions. It may also inhibit antigen-induced release of histamine.

Phenylephrine—Phenylephrine is both a direct-acting and an indirect-acting sympathomimetic amine. It acts on alpha-adrenergic receptors of the bronchiolar vascular beds to produce vasoconstriction, thereby reducing bronchiolar blood flow, shrinking swollen membranes, relieving congestion and edema, and prolonging the duration of action of the isoproterenol by slowing systemic absorption of the medication.

### Absorption

Isoproterenol—Inhalation: Rapidly absorbed.

### Biotransformation

Isoproterenol—Hepatic; also metabolized in the lungs and other tissues.
Phenylephrine—Gastrointestinal and hepatic.

### Half-life

Isoproterenol—Inhalation: 5 minutes.

### Onset of action

Within a few minutes.

### Duration of action

Up to 3 hours.

### Elimination

Primarily renal.

## Precautions to Consider

### Cross-sensitivity and/or related problems

Patients sensitive to other sympathomimetics may be sensitive to this medication also.

### Carcinogenicity/Mutagenicity

Long-term studies in animals have not been done to evaluate the carcinogenic or mutagenic potential of isoproterenol or phenylephrine.

### Pregnancy/Reproduction

Pregnancy—Studies on teratogenic effects with isoproterenol or phenylephrine have not been done in humans.

Use of phenylephrine during late pregnancy or during labor may cause fetal anoxia and bradycardia by increasing contractility of the uterus and decreasing uterine blood flow.

Studies on teratogenic effects with isoproterenol or phenylephrine have not been done in animals.

FDA Pregnancy Category C.

### Breast-feeding

It is not known whether isoproterenol or phenylephrine is distributed into breast milk. However, problems in humans have not been documented.

### Pediatrics

Appropriate studies on the relationship of age to the effects of isoproterenol and phenylephrine combination have not been performed in children up to 12 years of age.

### Geriatrics

No information is available on the relationship of age to the effects of isoproterenol and phenylephrine combination in geriatric patients.

### Drug interactions and/or related problems

The following drug interactions and/or related problems have been selected on the basis of their potential clinical significance (possible mechanism in parentheses where appropriate)—not necessarily inclusive (» = major clinical significance):

Note: Combinations containing any of the following medications, depending on the amount present, may also interact with this medication.

Anesthetics, hydrocarbon inhalation, such as:
Chloroform
Cyclopropane
Enflurane
Halothane
Isoflurane
Methoxyflurane
Trichloroethylene
(administration of high doses of isoproterenol and phenylephrine combination prior to or shortly after anesthesia with chloroform, cyclopropane, halothane, or trichloroethylene may increase the risk of severe ventricular arrhythmias, especially in patients with pre-existing heart disease, because these anesthetics greatly sensitize the myocardium to the effects of sympathomimetics)

(enflurane, isoflurane, or methoxyflurane may also cause some sensitization of the myocardium to the effects of sympathomimetics; caution is recommended during concurrent use with the sympathomimetic)

» Antidepressants, tricyclic or
» Maprotiline
(concurrent use may potentiate cardiovascular effects of isoproterenol and phenylephrine, possibly resulting in arrhythmias, tachycardia, or severe hypertension or hyperpyrexia)

Antihypertensives or
Diuretics used as antihypertensives
(antihypertensive effects may be reduced when these medications are used concurrently with isoproterenol and phenylephrine; the patient should be carefully monitored to confirm that the desired effect is being obtained)

» Beta-adrenergic blocking agents
(concurrent use with isoproterenol may result in mutual inhibition of therapeutic effects; beta-blockade may antagonize beta-2-adrenergic bronchodilating effects of isoproterenol; use of a cardioselective beta-2-adrenergic blocker, such as acebutolol, atenolol, or metoprolol, at low doses may reduce antagonism of the bronchodilating effect)

Central nervous system (CNS) stimulation–producing medications, other (see *Appendix II*)
(concurrent use with isoproterenol may result in additive CNS stimulation to excessive levels, which may cause unwanted effects such as nervousness, irritability, insomnia, or possibly convulsions or cardiac arrhythmias; close observation is recommended)

» Cocaine, mucosal-local
(in addition to increasing CNS stimulation, concurrent use with phenylephrine may increase the cardiovascular effects of either or both medications and the risk of adverse effects)

» Digitalis glycosides
(concurrent use with isoproterenol and phenylephrine may increase the risk of cardiac arrhythmias; caution and electrocardiographic monitoring are very important if concurrent use is necessary)

Dihydroergotamine
» Ergoloid mesylates
Ergonovine
» Ergotamine
Methylergonovine
Methysergide or
Oxytocin
(concurrent use of dihydroergotamine, ergonovine, methylergonovine, or methysergide with phenylephrine may result in enhanced vasoconstriction; dosage adjustments may be necessary)

(concurrent use of ergoloid mesylates or ergotamine with phenylephrine may produce peripheral vascular ischemia and gangrene and is not recommended)

(concurrent use of ergonovine, ergotamine, methylergonovine, or oxytocin with phenylephrine may potentiate the pressor effect of phenylephrine with possible severe hypertension and rupture of cerebral blood vessels)

Guanadrel or
Guanethidine
(in addition to possibly decreasing the hypotensive effect of guanadrel or guanethidine, concurrent use may potentiate the pressor effect of phenylephrine; these actions are a result of inhibition of sympathomimetic uptake by adrenergic neurons and may lead to hypertension and cardiac arrhythmias)

Levodopa
(concurrent use with isoproterenol and phenylephrine may increase the possibility of cardiac arrhythmias; dosage reduction of the sympathomimetic is recommended)

Mazindol or
Methylphenidate
(concurrent use may potentiate the pressor effect of phenylephrine)

Mecamylamine or
» Methyldopa or
Trimethaphan
(in addition to possibly decreasing the hypotensive effects of these medications, concurrent use may enhance the pressor response to phenylephrine)

» Monoamine oxidase (MAO) inhibitors, including furazolidone and procarbazine
(concurrent use may prolong and intensify cardiac stimulant and vasopressor effects of phenylephrine because of release of catecholamines that accumulate in intraneuronal storage sites during MAO inhibitor therapy, resulting in headache, cardiac arrhythmias, vomiting, or sudden and severe hypertensive and/or hyperpyretic crises; phenylephrine should not be administered during or within 14 days following administration of MAO inhibitors)

Nitrates
(concurrent use with isoproterenol and phenylephrine may reduce the antianginal effects of these medications)

Rauwolfia alkaloids
(in addition to possibly decreasing the hypotensive effects of rauwolfia alkaloids, concurrent use may theoretically prolong the action of direct-acting sympathomimetics, such as phenylephrine, by preventing uptake into storage granules; a "denervation supersensitivity" response is also possible; although concurrent use with systemic phenylephrine is not known to produce severe adverse effects, a significant increase in blood pressure has been documented when phenylephrine ophthalmic drops have been administered to patients taking reserpine, and caution and close observation are recommended)

Sympathomimetics, other
(concurrent use may increase the cardiovascular effects of either the other sympathomimetics or isoproterenol and phenylephrine and the potential for side effects)

Thyroid hormones
(concurrent use may increase the effects of either these medications or isoproterenol and phenylephrine; thyroid hormones enhance risk of coronary insufficiency when sympathomimetic agents are administered to patients with coronary artery disease; dosage adjustment is recommended, although problem is reduced in euthyroid patients)

Xanthines, such as:
Aminophylline
Caffeine
Dyphylline
Oxtriphylline
Theophylline
(in addition to possibly increasing CNS stimulation, concurrent use with isoproterenol may result in other additive toxic effects)

**Medical considerations/Contraindications**
The medical considerations/contraindications included here have been selected on the basis of their potential clinical significance (reasons given in parentheses where appropriate)—not necessarily inclusive (» = major clinical significance).

*Risk-benefit should be considered when the following medical problems exist:*

» Cardiac arrhythmias associated with tachycardia, pre-existing, or
Cardiovascular disorders, including coronary insufficiency, or
Hypertension
(condition may be exacerbated due to drug-induced cardiovascular effects)

Diabetes mellitus
Hyperthyroidism
(adverse reactions more likely to occur)

Sensitivity to isoproterenol, phenylephrine, or other sympathomimetics

# Side/Adverse Effects

The following side/adverse effects have been selected on the basis of their potential clinical significance (possible signs and symptoms in parentheses where appropriate)—not necessarily inclusive:

**Those indicating need for medical attention**
Incidence rare
  *Angina* (chest pain); *cardiac arrhythmias* (irregular heartbeat)

**Those indicating need for medical attention only if they continue or are bothersome**
Incidence more frequent
  *Insomnia* (trouble in sleeping); *nervousness; restlessness*
Incidence less frequent
  *Dizziness or lightheadedness; flushing or redness of face or skin; headache; increased sweating; nausea or vomiting; palpitations* (pounding heartbeat); *tachycardia* (fast heartbeat); *trembling; weakness*

**Those not indicating need for medical attention**
  *Pinkish to red coloration of saliva*

# Overdose

For specific information on the agents used in the management of isoproterenol and phenylephrine overdose, see
  • *Barbiturates (Systemic)* monograph;
  • *Beta-adrenergic Blocking Agents (Systemic)* monograph; or
  • Phentolamine in *Sympathomimetic Agents—Cardiovascular Use (Parenteral-systemic)* monograph.

For more information on the management of overdose or unintentional ingestion, **contact a Poison Control Center** (see *Poison Control Center Listing*).

**Symptoms of overdose**
The following effects have been selected on the basis of their potential clinical significance (possible signs and symptoms in parentheses where appropriate)—not necessarily inclusive:

  *Angina, continuing or severe* (chest pain); *bradycardia, continuing* (slow heartbeat); *cardiac arrhythmias, continuing or severe* (irregular heartbeat); *dizziness or lightheadedness, continuing or severe; headache, continuing or severe; increase in blood pressure; nausea or vomiting, continuing or severe; palpitations* (pounding heartbeat); *sensation of fullness in head; tachycardia, continuing* (fast heartbeat); *tingling in hands or feet; trembling, severe; unusual anxiety, nervousness, or restlessness; weakness, severe*

**Treatment of overdose**
Discontinuation of medication.
  Specific treatment—
    For CNS stimulation induced by isoproterenol, administering sedatives, such as barbiturates.
    For tachycardia and arrhythmias induced by isoproterenol, administering a beta-adrenergic blocker, such as propranolol; however, it should not be given to asthmatics since bronchospasm may be increased. A cardioselective beta-adrenergic blocker, such as acebutolol, atenolol, or metoprolol, may be indicated in asthmatics; however, it should be used with caution since an asthmatic attack could be induced by the beta-blocker.
    For excessive hypertensive effect induced by phenylephrine, administering an alpha-adrenergic blocker, such as phentolamine.
  Supportive care—
    General supportive measures.

# Patient Consultation

As an aid to patient consultation, refer to *Advice for the Patient, Isoproterenol and Phenylephrine (Systemic).*

In providing consultation, consider emphasizing the following selected information (» = major clinical significance):

**Before using this medication**
» Conditions affecting use, especially:
    Sensitivity to isoproterenol, phenylephrine, or other sympathomimetics
    Pregnancy—Use of phenylephrine during late pregnancy or during labor may cause fetal anoxia and bradycardia by increasing contractility of the uterus and decreasing uterine blood flow
    Other medications, especially antidepressants, beta-adrenergic blocking agents, cocaine (mucosal-local), digitalis glycosides, ergoloid mesylates, ergotamine, or methyldopa
    Other medical problems, especially pre-existing cardiac arrhythmias associated with tachycardia

**Proper use of this medication**
  Proper administration: Reading patient instructions carefully before using
  Avoiding contact with the eyes
» Taking no more than 2 inhalations at one time with interval of 1 to 5 minutes between inhalations
  Saving applicator; refill units may be available
» Importance of not using more medication than the amount prescribed
» Proper dosing
» Proper storage

**Precautions while using this medication**
» Checking with physician immediately if difficulty in breathing persists after using this medication or if condition becomes worse
*For patients also using a corticosteroid or ipratropium inhalation aerosol*
» Using isoproterenol and phenylephrine inhalation aerosol 5 minutes prior to the corticosteroid or ipratropium inhalation aerosol, unless otherwise directed by physician

**Side/adverse effects**
  Signs of potential side effects, especially chest pain and irregular heartbeat
  Pinkish to red coloration of saliva caused by oxidation of isoproterenol in mouth may be alarming to patient although medically insignificant

# General Dosing Information

Excessive use may result in loss of effectiveness. If this occurs, discontinuation of the medication and use of alternative therapy are recommended.

Repeated excessive use may result in severe paradoxical airway resistance.

Isoproterenol and epinephrine may be used alternately, but not concurrently, provided that enough time has elapsed for the effects of one medication to subside before the alternate medication is administered.

When used in conjunction with a corticosteroid or ipratropium oral inhalation aerosol, isoproterenol and phenylephrine inhalation aerosol should be administered 5 minutes prior to the corticosteroid or ipratropium inhalation aerosol. This interval allows for bronchodilation to occur and increased deposition of the corticosteroid or ipratropium within the bronchi.

# Inhalation Dosage Forms

## ISOPROTERENOL HYDROCHLORIDE AND PHENYLEPHRINE BITARTRATE INHALATION AEROSOL USP

**Usual adult and adolescent dose**
Asthma, bronchial
Bronchiectasis
Bronchitis
Emphysema, pulmonary, or
Other chronic obstructive pulmonary disease—
  Oral inhalation, 1 inhalation, repeated after two to five minutes if necessary, four to six times a day.

**Usual pediatric dose**
Children up to 12 years of age: Dosage has not been established.
Children 12 years of age and over: See *Usual adult and adolescent dose.*

**Strength(s) usually available**
U.S.—
  160 mcg (0.16 mg) of isoproterenol hydrochloride (equivalent to 137 mcg [0.137 mg] of isoproterenol) and 240 mcg (0.24 mg) of phenylephrine bitartrate (equivalent to 126 mcg [0.126 mg] of phenylephrine) per metered spray (Rx) [*Duo-Medihaler* (cetylpyridinium chloride, dichlorodifluoromethane, dichlorotetrafluoroethane, trichloromonogluoromethane, sorbitran trioleate)].
Canada—
  160 mcg (0.16 mg) of isoproterenol hydrochloride (equivalent to 137 mcg [0.137 mg] of isoproterenol) and 240 mcg (0.24 mg) of phenylephrine bitartrate (equivalent to 126 mcg [0.126 mg] of phenylephrine) per metered spray (Rx) [*Duo-Medihaler* (cetylpyridinium chloride, fluorochlorohydrocarbons, sorbitran trioleate)].

**Packaging and storage**
Store below 40 °C (104 °F), preferably between 15 and 30 °C (59 and 86 °F), unless otherwise specified by manufacturer. Store in a light-resistant container. Protect from freezing.

**Auxiliary labeling**
• For oral inhalation only.
• Shake well.
• Store away from heat and direct sunlight.

**Note**
Include patient instructions when dispensing.

Revised: August 1990
Interim revision: 09/02/94

---

**ISOTRETINOIN** Systemic

VA CLASSIFICATION (Primary): DE751/DE890
Note: For a listing of dosage forms and brand names by country availability, see *Dosage Forms* section(s). For a listing of brand names for the articles in this monograph, refer to the General Index.

## Category
Antiacne agent (systemic); antirosacea agent (systemic); keratinization stabilizer.

## Indications
Note: Bracketed information in the *Indications* section refers to uses that are not included in U.S. product labeling.

**Accepted**
NOTE: FOR WOMEN OF CHILD-BEARING POTENTIAL, SEE THE *PREGNANCY/REPRODUCTION* SECTION OF *PRECAUTIONS TO CONSIDER* FOR RESTRICTIONS ON THE USE OF ISOTRETINOIN.
Acne vulgaris (treatment)—Isotretinoin is indicated only for the treatment of severe recalcitrant nodular acne.

In most patients, a single course of therapy may result in complete and prolonged remission of severe cystic acne. However, if a second course of therapy is necessary, it should not be initiated for at least 8 weeks after completion of the first course, because improvement in the condition may continue following discontinuation of isotretinoin.

[Isotretinoin is also indicated for severe acne and conglobate acne.]

Because of its potential adverse effects, isotretinoin should be reserved for patients who are unresponsive to or intolerant of conventional therapy, including antibiotics.

[Folliculitis, gram-negative (treatment)][1] or
[Rosacea, severe (treatment)][1]—Isotretinoin is used in the treatment of severe rosacea and gram-negative folliculitis.

[Hidradenitis suppurativa (treatment)][1]—Isotretinoin is used in the treatment of hidradenitis suppurativa.

Isotretinoin may also be effective in correcting severe keratinization disorders, such as—[Erythroderma, congenital ichthyosiform][1]

[Ichthyosis, lamellar, and other ichthyoses][1]
[Keratosis follicularis (Darier's disease)][1]
[Keratosis palmaris et plantaris][1]
[Pityriasis rubra pilaris (PRP)][1]

However, longer periods of isotretinoin therapy may be required for keratinization disorders than for acne vulgaris, thus increasing the risk of side effects, including skeletal changes and cardiovascular complications.

**Unaccepted**
Isotretinoin should not be used in the treatment of mild to moderate acne vulgaris.

[1]Not included in Canadian product labeling.

## Pharmacology/Pharmacokinetics

**Physicochemical characteristics**
Chemical group—Vitamin A derivative (retinoid).
Molecular weight—300.44.
Chemical name—Retinoic acid, 13-*cis*-.

**Mechanism of action/Effect**
The exact mechanism of action is not known. However, isotretinoin reduces sebaceous gland size and inhibits sebaceous gland activity, thereby decreasing sebum secretion. This action is probably responsible for the rapid initial clinical improvement in cystic acne. Isotre-

tinoin has also been shown to decrease the number of *Propionibacterium acnes* organisms within the follicle. However, since isotretinoin has no effect on *P. acnes in vitro*, this action is probably a secondary effect due to decreased sebum secretion and the resulting decrease in nutrients and not a direct effect of isotretinoin. In addition, isotretinoin has been shown to have anti-keratinizing and anti-inflammatory actions. The exact role of these actions in clinical improvement of cystic acne is not known, especially with respect to prolonged remissions.

**Absorption**
Rapidly absorbed from the gastrointestinal tract.

**Protein binding**
Very high (99.9%), almost exclusively to albumin.

**Biotransformation**
Metabolized in liver and possibly in the gut wall. The major identified metabolite in blood and urine is 4-oxo-isotretinoin; other identified metabolites are tretinoin and 4-oxo-tretinoin.

**Half-life**
10 to 20 hours.
Note: The apparent half-life of the major metabolite, 4-oxo-isotretinoin, is similar to isotretinoin, since its terminal elimination is formation-rate limited.

**Time to peak plasma concentration**
Approximately 3 hours following an 80-mg dose.
Note: Maximum concentration of the major metabolite occurs at 6 to 20 hours, with the blood concentration of the metabolite generally exceeding that of isotretinoin after 6 hours.

**Peak plasma concentration**
98 to 535 nanograms per mL (mean 262 nanograms per mL) in cystic acne patients following an 80-mg dose.
Note: Peak plasma concentration of major metabolite 4-oxo-isotretinoin is 87 to 399 nanograms per mL.

**Steady-state blood concentration**
$160 \pm 19$ nanograms per mL following doses of 40 mg twice a day.

**Elimination**
Biliary; renal.

## Precautions to Consider

Note: Patients receiving isotretinoin should not donate blood during or for 30 days after therapy, because of the risk to the developing fetus of a pregnant patient who may receive such blood.

**Cross-sensitivity and/or related problems**
Patients sensitive to etretinate, tretinoin, or vitamin A derivatives may be sensitive to this medication also, since isotretinoin is related to both retinoic acid and retinol (vitamin A).

**Carcinogenicity/Tumorigenicity**
Studies in Fischer 344 rats have shown that isotretinoin administered at doses of 8 or 32 mg per kg of body weight (mg/kg) per day for more than 18 months increased the incidence of pheochromocytoma; the incidence of adrenal medullary hyperplasia was also increased at the higher dosage. However, pheochromocytoma is known to occur with a relatively high frequency in the species of animals tested. On the other hand, a decreased incidence of hepatic adenomas and angiomas and leukemia was observed at doses of 8 and 32 mg/kg per day.

**Mutagenicity**
*In vitro* tests have not shown isotretinoin to be mutagenic.

**Pregnancy/Reproduction**
Pregnancy—**Isotretinoin is contraindicated during pregnancy**, since it has caused major human fetal abnormalities including hydrocephalus, microcephalus, abnormalities of the external ear (micropinna, small or

---

**ISOSORBIDE DINITRATE**—See *Nitrates (Systemic)*

---

**ISOSORBIDE MONONITRATE**—See *Nitrates (Systemic)*

absent external auditory canals), microphthalmia, and cardiovascular abnormalities.

**In addition, isotretinoin is contraindicated in women of childbearing potential, unless all of the following criteria have been met:**
- Patient has severe, disfiguring, recalcitrant cystic acne or one of the accepted unlabeled indications above.
- Patient is reliable in understanding and carrying out instructions.
- Patient is capable of complying with the mandatory contraceptive measures. An effective form of contraception should be used for at least 1 month before therapy, during therapy, and for 1 month following discontinuation of therapy.
- Patient has received both oral and written warnings of the hazards of pregnancy, and has indicated her understanding and acceptance of these warnings in writing.
- Pregnancy has been definitely excluded through a negative pregnancy test and appropriate history and physical examination. The pregnancy test should be performed within 2 weeks prior to isotretinoin therapy. Isotretinoin therapy should then be initiated on the second or third day of the next normal menstrual period. In addition, it is recommended that pregnancy testing and contraception counseling be repeated on a monthly basis.

Reproduction studies in male and female rats receiving isotretinoin in doses of 2, 8, or 32 mg/kg have shown no evidence of adverse effects on gonadal function, fertility, conception rate, gestation, or parturition. However, reproduction studies in male dogs receiving isotretinoin in doses of 20 or 60 mg/kg for approximately 30 weeks showed testicular atrophy and microscopic evidence of depression of spermatogenesis. Studies in humans have shown no clinically significant changes in the number or motility of spermatozoa in the ejaculate of human males receiving isotretinoin for the treatment of cystic acne.

FDA Pregnancy Category X.

### Breast-feeding
It is not known whether isotretinoin is distributed into breast milk and problems in humans have not been documented. However, use is not recommended during breast-feeding, because of the potential for adverse effects in infants of mothers taking this medication.

### Pediatrics
Although appropriate studies on the relationship of age to the effects of isotretinoin have not been performed in the pediatric population, use is not recommended, because children may be more sensitive to the effects of isotretinoin.

During clinical trials of disorders of keratinization using a mean dose of 2.24 mg of isotretinoin per kg of body weight a day, 2 children showed x-ray changes suggestive of premature epiphyseal closure. It is not known whether these adverse effects occur more commonly in children, but they may be more significant because of the growth process.

### Geriatrics
No information is available on the relationship of age to the effects of isotretinoin in geriatric patients.

### Drug interactions and/or related problems
The following drug interactions and/or related problems have been selected on the basis of their potential clinical significance (possible mechanism in parentheses where appropriate)—not necessarily inclusive (» = major clinical significance):

Note: Combinations containing any of the following medications, depending on the amount present, may also interact with this medication.

Abrasive or medicated soaps or cleansers or
Acne preparations or preparations containing a peeling agent such as
  Benzoyl peroxide
  Resorcinol
  Salicylic acid
  Sulfur
  Tretinoin or
Acne preparations, topical, other or
Alcohol-containing preparations, topical such as
  After-shave lotions
  Astringents
  Perfumed toiletries
  Shaving creams or lotions or
Cosmetics or soaps with a strong drying effect or
Medicated cosmetics or "cover-ups"
  (concurrent use with isotretinoin may cause a cumulative irritant or drying effect, especially with the application of peeling, desquamating, or abrasive agents, resulting in excessive irritation of the skin)

Alcohol, oral
  (high alcohol consumption during isotretinoin therapy may result in hypertriglyceridemia, since both alcohol and isotretinoin may increase plasma triglycerides concentration)
» Etretinate or
» Tretinoin or
» Vitamin A
  (concurrent use with isotretinoin may result in additive toxic effects)

Photosensitizing medications, other
  (concurrent use of isotretinoin with these medications may cause additive photosensitizing effects)
» Tetracyclines
  (concurrent use with isotretinoin may increase the potential for development of pseudotumor cerebri)

### Laboratory value alterations
The following have been selected on the basis of their potential clinical significance (possible effect in parentheses where appropriate)—not necessarily inclusive (» = major clinical significance):

With physiology/laboratory test values
Alanine aminotransferase (ALT [SGPT]) and
Alkaline phosphatase and
Aspartate aminotransferase (AST [SGOT]) and
Lactate dehydrogenase (LDH)
  (increases in serum values have occurred in about 10 to 20% of patients)
Creatine phosphokinase (CPK) concentration and
Fasting blood sugar concentration and
Uric acid concentration
  (increases have occurred in less than 1% of patients; elevated CPK concentrations have occurred in some patients engaging in vigorous physical activity)
High-density lipoprotein (HDL)
  (decreases in serum HDL concentrations have occurred in about 16% of patients; reversible upon discontinuation of medication)
Liver enzyme concentrations
  (during clinical trials, mild to moderate elevations of liver enzymes have been observed in approximately 15% of patients; some of these concentrations returned to normal levels with dosage reduction or continued administration of isotretinoin; if normalization does not readily occur or if hepatitis is suspected, isotretinoin should be discontinued)
Platelet counts and
Sedimentation rate, erythrocyte
  (elevated sedimentation rates have been reported in about 40% of patients; increases in platelet counts have occurred in about 10 to 20% of patients)
Red blood cell parameters and
White blood cell counts
  (decreases have occurred in about 10 to 20% of patients)
Triglyceride concentrations, plasma and
Cholesterol concentrations, serum
  (elevated plasma triglyceride concentration occurs in about 25% of patients and is dose-related; elevation of serum triglycerides to concentrations in excess of 800 mg per dL has been associated with acute pancreatitis; minimal increase in serum cholesterol concentration has occurred in about 7% of patients; these effects are reversible upon discontinuation of medication)

### Medical considerations/Contraindications
The medical considerations/contraindications included here have been selected on the basis of their potential clinical significance (reasons given in parentheses where appropriate)—not necessarily inclusive (» = major clinical significance).

*Risk-benefit should be considered when the following medical problems exist:*
Conditions predisposing to hypertriglyceridemia, such as
  High alcohol intake, or history of
Hypertriglyceridemia, family history of
Obesity
  (isotretinoin may increase plasma triglyceride concentration, possibly increasing patient's cardiovascular risk status)
Diabetes mellitus, or family history of
  (possibility of alteration in blood sugar concentration; isotretinoin may increase plasma triglyceride concentration in patients with diabetes mellitus, possibly increasing their cardiovascular risk status)
Sensitivity to isotretinoin

**Patient monitoring**

The following may be especially important in patient monitoring (other tests may be warranted in some patients, depending on condition; » = major clinical significance):

Blood count, complete (CBC) and

12-channel biochemical profile (sequential multiple analysis [SMA-12])

(baseline determinations of both prior to therapy are recommended; SMA-12 is also recommended after 4 to 6 weeks of therapy)

Blood lipid determinations

(recommended under fasting conditions prior to therapy, then repeated at 1- or 2-week intervals until the lipid response to isotretinoin is established, which usually occurs within 1 month. After 1 month, the test is repeated only if there are significant increases in blood lipid concentration, or if the patient has associated risk factors. Following consumption of alcohol, 36 hours should elapse before blood lipid determination)

Blood sugar determinations

(recommended during therapy in known or suspected diabetics because some patients have experienced problems in controlling their blood sugar)

Hepatic function determinations

(recommended prior to therapy; after 1 month of therapy; and then repeated only if there are liver function abnormalities at 1 month, especially in patients with a history of liver disease because transient abnormalities of liver function have been reported)

## Side/Adverse Effects

Note: Most side/adverse reactions in cystic acne patients have been reversible upon discontinuation of therapy.

Corneal opacities and diffuse interstitial skeletal hyperostosis have occurred in patients receiving isotretinoin for acne. Corneal opacities occurred more frequently when higher doses were used, such as in patients with keratinization disorders. Also, studies in patients with keratinization disorders have shown that prolonged isotretinoin therapy causes skeletal abnormalities, including more extensive hyperostosis in adults and premature closure of the epiphyses in children.

Proteinuria, red blood cells in urine, and hyperuricemia have occurred in less than 1% of patients receiving isotretinoin. White cells in the urine have occurred in about 10 to 20% of patients.

An exaggerated healing response, characterized by exuberant granulation tissue with crusting, has been reported occasionally.

Decreased night vision has occurred in a number of patients undergoing isotretinoin therapy. In some patients, the onset was sudden.

Studies in animals have shown that prolonged isotretinoin therapy increased the incidence of focal calcification; fibrosis and inflammation of the myocardium; calcification of coronary, pulmonary, and mesenteric arteries; and metastatic calcification of the gastric mucosa. Also, long bone fractures have been reported in rats given isotretinoin at a dosage of 32 mg per kg of body weight (mg/kg) per day for 15 weeks.

The following side/adverse effects have been selected on the basis of their potential clinical significance (possible signs and symptoms in parentheses where appropriate)—not necessarily inclusive:

**Those indicating need for medical attention**

Incidence more frequent

*Burning, redness, itching, or other sign of inflammation of eye*—about 40%; *nosebleeds*—up to 80% in cystic acne patients; *scaling, redness, burning, pain, or other sign of inflammation of lips*—90%

Incidence less frequent

*Mental depression; skin infection*—about 5%; *skin rash*—<10%

Incidence rare

*Bleeding or inflammation of gums; cataracts, corneal opacities, or pseudotumor cerebri* (blurred vision or other changes in vision; pseudotumor cerebri can also cause severe or continuing headache or nausea and vomiting); *hepatitis* (yellow eyes or skin); *inflammatory bowel disease or regional ileitis* (severe abdominal or stomach pain; rectal bleeding; severe diarrhea); *mood changes; optic neuritis* (pain or tenderness of eyes)

Note: If symptoms of *inflammatory bowel disease, visual disturbances,* or signs or symptoms of *pseudotumor cerebri* occur, isotretinoin should be discontinued. Patients with signs or symptoms of pseudotumor cerebri should be referred to a neurologist for further diagnosis and care.

**Those indicating need for medical attention only if they continue or are bothersome**

Incidence more frequent

*Dryness of mouth or nose; dryness or itching of skin*

Note: *Dryness of mouth or nose* or *dryness or itching of skin* may occur in up to 80% of cystic acne patients.

Incidence less frequent

*Dryness of eyes; headache, mild*—about 5%; *increased sensitivity of skin to sunlight*—about 5%; *pain, tenderness, or stiffness in muscles, bones, or joints*—about 16%; *peeling of skin on palms of hands or soles of feet*—about 5%; *stomach upset*—about 5%; *thinning of hair*—less than 10%; *unusual tiredness*—about 5%

## Patient Consultation

As an aid to patient consultation, refer to *Advice for the Patient, Isotretinoin (Systemic).*

In providing consultation, consider emphasizing the following selected information (» = major clinical significance):

**Before using this medication**

» Conditions affecting use, especially:

Sensitivity to isotretinoin, etretinate, tretinoin, or vitamin A derivatives

Pregnancy—Not taking isotretinoin during pregnancy, because it causes birth defects in humans. In addition, not taking if there is a chance that pregnancy may occur during treatment or within one month following treatment. Not taking isotretinoin unless an effective form of contraception (birth control) is used for at least 1 month before beginning treatment. Contraception must be continued during treatment and for one month after isotretinoin is stopped

Breast-feeding—Although it is not known whether isotretinoin passes into the breast milk, medication is not recommended during breast-feeding, because it may cause unwanted effects in nursing babies

Use in children—Use is not recommended, because children may be more sensitive to the effects of isotretinoin

Other medications, especially etretinate, tretinoin, vitamin A, or tetracyclines

**Proper use of this medication**

» Importance of not taking more medication than the amount prescribed

» Proper dosing

Missed dose: Taking as soon as possible; not taking if almost time for next dose; not doubling doses

» Proper storage

**Precautions while using this medication**

Regular visits to physician to check progress during therapy

» Stopping medication immediately and checking with physician if pregnancy is suspected, since isotretinoin causes birth defects in humans

» Not donating blood to a blood bank during or for 30 days after therapy has been completed to prevent possibility of a pregnant patient receiving the blood

» Avoiding concurrent use of vitamin A and vitamin supplements containing vitamin A, unless prescribed by physician

» Not drinking, or at least reducing consumption of, alcoholic beverages, because of possible hypertriglyceridemia and consequent cardiovascular risks

Diabetics: May alter blood sugar concentrations

» Caution if decrease in night vision, which may be sudden, occurs; not driving, using machines, or doing other things that could be dangerous if unable to see well; checking with physician if this occurs

Possible dryness of eyes; may decrease tolerance to contact lenses during therapy and for up to about 2 weeks after discontinuation of therapy; checking with physician about using ocular lubricant to relieve dryness of eyes or if inflammation occurs

Possible photosensitivity; avoiding unprotected exposure to sunlight or use of sunlamp

Possible dryness of mouth and nose; for mouth dryness, using sugarless candy or gum, ice, or saliva substitute for relief; checking with physician or dentist if dry mouth continues for more than 2 weeks

*For patients with acne*

Possibility that acne may appear to worsen during initial therapy; checking with physician if irritation or other symptoms of condition become severe

**Side/adverse effects**

Signs of potential side effects, especially bleeding or inflammation of gums; burning, redness, itching, or other sign of inflammation of eye; cataracts; corneal opacities; hepatitis; inflammatory bowel disease; mental depression; mood changes; optic neuritis; nosebleeds; pseudotumor cerebri; regional ileitis; scaling, redness, burning, pain, or other sign of inflammation of lips; skin infection; or skin rash

## General Dosing Information

Generally, the initial dosage of isotretinoin should be individualized according to the patient's weight and the severity and location of the disease.

### For use as an antiacne agent

Higher doses of isotretinoin (i.e., up to 2 mg per kg of body weight [mg/kg] per day) may be required in patients whose disease is very severe or is primarily located on the chest and back instead of on the face.

During the initial period of isotretinoin therapy, transient exacerbation of acne may occur; concomitant adrenocorticoid therapy may be required.

Following 4 or more weeks of therapy, dosage adjustment should be based on response of the disease to isotretinoin and the occurrence of side effects.

Improvement in cystic acne may occur after 1 to 2 months, but marked improvement may require 4 to 5 months of therapy. Also, improvement may continue after discontinuation of isotretinoin.

If a second course of therapy is necessary, it should not be initiated for at least 8 weeks following completion of the first course, since improvement in condition may continue after isotretinoin is discontinued.

## Oral Dosage Forms

Note: Bracketed uses in the *Dosage Forms* section refer to categories of use and/or indications that are not included in U.S. product labeling.

### ISOTRETINOIN CAPSULES

**Usual adult and adolescent dose**
Severe recalcitrant cystic acne—
 Oral, 0.5 to 1 mg per kg of body weight per day (in two divided doses) for fifteen to twenty weeks; the maximum recommended dose is 2 mg per kg of body weight per day.

[Severe acne and conglobate acne]—
 Oral, 0.5 to 1 mg per kg of body weight per day (in two divided doses) for fifteen to twenty weeks; the maximum recommended dose is 2 mg per kg of body weight per day.
[Folliculitis, gram-negative][1] or
[Rosacea, severe][1]—
 Oral, 0.5 to 1 mg per kg of body weight per day in two divided doses.
[Keratinization disorders][1]—
 Oral, up to 4 mg per kg of body weight per day, the dosage depending on the specific disease and its severity.

**Usual pediatric dose**
Use is not recommended.

**Strength(s) usually available**
U.S.—
 10 mg (Rx) [*Accutane* (edetate disodium; methylparaben; propylparaben)].
 20 mg (Rx) [*Accutane* (edetate disodium; methylparaben; propylparaben)].
 40 mg (Rx) [*Accutane* (edetate disodium; methylparaben; propylparaben)].
Canada—
 10 mg (Rx) [*Accutane Roche* (parabens)].
 40 mg (Rx) [*Accutane Roche* (parabens)].

**Packaging and storage**
Store between 15 and 30 °C (59 and 86 °F), in a tight, light-resistant container, unless otherwise specified by manufacturer.

---

[1]Not included in Canadian product labeling.

Revised: June 1990
Interim revision: 07/14/94

---

# ISOXSUPRINE  Systemic

VA CLASSIFICATION (Primary/Secondary): CV500/GU900
Note: For a listing of dosage forms and brand names by country availability, see *Dosage Forms* section(s). For a listing of brand names for the articles in this monograph, refer to the General Index.

## Category

Vasospastic therapy adjunct; senility symptoms treatment adjunct; labor (premature) inhibitor; antidysmenorrheal.

## Indications

Note: Bracketed information in the *Indications* section refers to uses that are not included in U.S. product labeling.

### Accepted

Cerebrovascular insufficiency (treatment) or
Vascular disease, peripheral (treatment)[1]—FDA has classified isoxsuprine as being possibly effective for its labeled indications, which include relief of symptoms associated with cerebrovascular insufficiency and peripheral vascular disease, i.e., arteriosclerosis obliterans, thromboangiitis obliterans (Buerger's disease), and Raynaud's disease. This classification requires the submission of adequate and well-controlled studies in order to provide substantial evidence of effectiveness.

[Labor, premature (prophylaxis and treatment)]—Isoxsuprine is also used for management of threatened premature labor in pregnancies of 20 or more weeks' gestation. Use is not recommended prior to the 20th week of pregnancy. In order for isoxsuprine to be most effective, it is recommended that therapy be started as soon as the diagnosis of preterm labor is confirmed. Efficacy in advanced labor has not been established. Use in patients with ruptured membranes must be weighed against the risk of intrauterine infection.

[Dysmenorrhea (treatment)][1]—Isoxsuprine has been used in the treatment of dysmenorrhea.

---

[1]Not included in Canadian product labeling.

## Pharmacology/Pharmacokinetics

**Physicochemical characteristics**
Molecular weight—337.85.

**Mechanism of action/Effect**
Vasospastic therapy adjunct and senility symptoms treatment adjunct—Isoxsuprine produces peripheral vasodilation by a direct effect on vascular smooth muscle, primarily within skeletal muscle with little effect on cutaneous blood flow. Its effects were once thought to be due to beta-adrenergic receptor stimulation but are not reversed by beta-adrenergic blocking agents.
Labor (premature) inhibitor and antidysmenorrheal—Isoxsuprine produces uterine relaxation through a direct effect on smooth muscles.

**Other actions/effects**
Isoxsuprine-induced cardiac stimulation leads to increases in heart rate and cardiac output.
Isoxsuprine-induced peripheral vasodilation leads to decreased peripheral vascular resistance.

**Absorption**
Isoxsuprine is well absorbed from the gastrointestinal tract.

**Biotransformation**
Partially conjugated in the blood.

**Half-life**
Adults—
 Approximately 1.25 hours.
Neonates (following maternal administration [to inhibit premature labor])—
 Near term: 1.5 to 3 hours.
 Less mature: 6 to 8 hours.

**Onset of action**
Oral—1 hour.
Intravenous—10 minutes.

**Elimination**
Primarily in the urine; fecal excretion insignificant.

# Precautions to Consider

## Pregnancy/Reproduction

Pregnancy—Isoxsuprine crosses the placenta. Maternal isoxsuprine administration for prevention of premature labor has been associated with tachycardia, hypoglycemia, hypocalcemia, ileus, and hypotension in the neonate. Incidence of toxicity is related directly to neonatal blood concentrations of isoxsuprine, which are affected by both gestational age and the interval between administration of isoxsuprine and delivery (with regard to rate of elimination of the drug).

## Breast-feeding

Problems in humans have not been documented.

## Geriatrics

No information is available on the relationship of age to the effects of isoxsuprine in geriatric patients. However, the risk of isoxsuprine-induced hypothermia may be increased in elderly patients.

## Drug interactions and/or related problems

The following drug interactions and/or related problems have been selected on the basis of their potential clinical significance (possible mechanism in parentheses where appropriate)—not necessarily inclusive (» = major clinical significance):

Smoking, tobacco
   (concurrent heavy use may interfere with the therapeutic effects of isoxsuprine because nicotine constricts blood vessels)

## Laboratory value alterations

The following have been selected on the basis of their potential clinical significance (possible effect in parentheses where appropriate)—not necessarily inclusive (» = major clinical significance):

With physiology/laboratory test values
Free fatty acids, serum and
Glucose, blood and
Insulin, serum
   (concentrations may be transiently increased during intravenous infusion but usually return to pretreatment values within 24 to 72 hours, even with continued infusion)

Potassium, serum
   (concentrations may be decreased during intravenous infusion; related to changes in glucose and insulin)

## Medical considerations/Contraindications

The medical considerations/contraindications included here have been selected on the basis of their potential clinical significance (reasons given in parentheses where appropriate)—not necessarily inclusive (» = major clinical significance):

*Except under special circumstances, this medication should not be used immediately postpartum or when the following medical problems exist:*

*For use in management of premature labor only*
» Cardiac disorders, especially those associated with arrhythmias, or
» Hyperthyroidism, maternal
      (isoxsuprine may precipitate arrhythmias or heart failure; occult cardiac disease may be unmasked)
» Chorioamnionitis (intrauterine infection) or
» Hemorrhage or
» Intrauterine fetal death or known abnormality
      (immediate delivery required)
» Eclampsia (toxemia) and severe pre-eclampsia
» Pulmonary hypertension

*Risk-benefit should be considered when the following medical problems exist:*

*For all indications*
   Bleeding disorders
» Cerebrovascular disease, severe, or
   Myocardial infarction, recent, or
» Obliterative coronary artery disease, severe
      (a "steal effect" may occur, since isoxsuprine has a greater effect on peripheral than on cerebral and coronary vessels, leading to a further decrease in flow to ischemic areas)
   Glaucoma
» Hypotension—for parenteral administration only; intravenous administration not recommended
   Sensitivity to isoxsuprine
» Tachycardia—for parenteral administration only; intravenous administration not recommended

*For use in management of premature labor only (in addition to the above)*
   Asthma being treated with beta-adrenergic stimulants and/or steroids

» Diabetes mellitus
      (may be aggravated)
   Hypertension
» Pre-eclampsia, mild to moderate

## Patient monitoring

The following may be especially important in patient monitoring (other tests may be warranted in some patients, depending on condition; » = major clinical significance):

*For all indications*
   Blood pressure measurement in lying, sitting, and standing positions
      (recommended at periodic intervals to detect hypotension in patients receiving isoxsuprine)

*For use in premature labor only*
» Blood glucose concentrations and
» Fluid and electrolyte status
      (should be monitored carefully during prolonged intravenous administration, especially in diabetic patients or those receiving adrenocorticoids, potassium-depleting diuretics, or digitalis glycosides)
   Fetal heart rate and
   Maternal heart rate and blood pressure and
   Uterine activity
      (should be monitored frequently during intravenous administration)

# Side/Adverse Effects

Note: A potentially serious maternal pulmonary edema has occurred with intravenous administration of isoxsuprine for premature labor. Although the exact cause is unknown, it may be related to fluid overload and has sometimes occurred with concurrent corticosteroid administration.

The following side/adverse effects have been selected on the basis of their potential clinical significance (possible signs and symptoms in parentheses where appropriate)—not necessarily inclusive:

## Those indicating need for medical attention

Incidence rare
   *Allergic reaction* (skin rash); *chest pain; hypotension* (dizziness; fainting)—low blood pressure; *pulmonary edema* (shortness of breath); *tachycardia* (fast heartbeat)

Note: Incidence of *hypotension* and *tachycardia* may be increased with higher doses and with parenteral administration, and may occur in both mother and baby during use for delay of premature labor.

## Those indicating need for medical attention only if they continue or are bothersome

Incidence less frequent
   *Nausea or vomiting*

Note: *Nausea or vomiting* may occur more frequently with parenteral administration.

# Patient Consultation

As an aid to patient consultation, refer to *Advice for the Patient, Isoxsuprine (Systemic)*.

In providing consultation, consider emphasizing the following selected information (» = major clinical significance):

## Before using this medication
» Conditions affecting use, especially:
      Sensitivity to isoxsuprine
      Pregnancy—Risk of tachycardia, hypoglycemia, hypocalcemia, ileus, and hypotension in the neonate
      Use in the elderly—Increased risk of isoxsuprine-induced hypothermia
      Other medical problems, especially cerebrovascular disease, coronary artery disease, diabetes mellitus (for use in premature labor), hyperthyroidism (for use in premature labor), or other cardiac disease (for use in premature labor)

## Proper use of this medication
» Taking with meals, milk, or antacids to reduce gastrointestinal irritation
» Proper dosing
   Missed dose: Taking as soon as possible; not taking if almost time for next dose; not doubling doses
» Proper storage

## Precautions while using this medication
   Checking with physician before discontinuing medication since it may take some time to work

Avoiding smoking (nicotine constricts blood vessels)

» Caution when getting up from a lying or sitting position, when climbing stairs, or if dizziness occurs

*For use in premature labor*

» Checking with physician immediately if contractions begin again or water breaks

### Side/adverse effects

Signs of potential side effects, especially allergic reaction, chest pain, pulmonary edema, hypotension, and tachycardia

## General Dosing Information

It is recommended that isoxsuprine therapy be discontinued if skin rash occurs.

Isoxsuprine may be administered with meals, milk, or antacids to reduce gastrointestinal irritation.

### For use in premature labor

For inhibition of premature labor, isoxsuprine has been administered by intravenous infusion at an initial rate of 200 mcg (0.2 mg) to 1 mg per minute followed by 100 to 300 mcg (0.1 to 0.3 mg) per minute until 1 to 1.5 hours after contractions have been abolished. This is usually followed by oral administration of 5 to 20 mg every 3 to 6 hours until term.

In order to prevent toxicity in the neonate, isoxsuprine should be discontinued when it becomes apparent that delivery is imminent.

## Oral Dosage Forms

### ISOXSUPRINE HYDROCHLORIDE TABLETS USP

#### Usual adult dose

Vasospastic therapy adjunct—
Oral, 10 to 20 mg three or four times a day.

#### Strength(s) usually available

U.S.—

10 mg (Rx) [*Vasodilan;* GENERIC].

20 mg (Rx) [*Vasodilan;* GENERIC].

Canada—

10 mg (Rx) [*Vasodilan*].

20 mg (Rx) [*Vasodilan*].

#### Packaging and storage

Store below 40 °C (104 °F), preferably between 15 and 30 °C (59 and 86 °F), unless otherwise specified by manufacturer. Store in a tight container.

## Parenteral Dosage Forms

### ISOXSUPRINE HYDROCHLORIDE INJECTION USP

#### Usual adult dose

Labor (premature) inhibitor—
Intramuscular, 5 to 10 mg two or three times a day.

### Usual adult prescribing limits

Because of the risk of hypotension and tachycardia, single intramuscular doses greater than 10 mg are not recommended, although repeated administration of 5 to 10 mg at suitable intervals is considered acceptable.

### Strength(s) usually available

U.S.—

Not commercially available.

Canada—

5 mg per mL (Rx) [*Vasodilan*].

### Packaging and storage

Store below 40 °C (104 °F), preferably between 15 and 30 °C (59 and 86 °F), unless otherwise specified by manufacturer. Protect from freezing.

### Preparation of dosage form

An intravenous infusion is prepared by dilution of the injection in an appropriate quantity of 5% dextrose injection, 5% dextrose in 0.45% sodium chloride injection, or 5% dextrose in 0.23% sodium chloride injection. Dilution in 0.9% sodium chloride injection is not recommended because of the risk of pulmonary edema.

## Selected Bibliography

Caritis SN, Edelstone DI, Mueller-Heubach E. Pharmacologic inhibition of preterm labor. Am J Obstet Gynecol 1979; 133: 557-78.

Revised: 07/06/92
Interim revision: 07/15/94

---

**ISRADIPINE**—See *Calcium Channel Blocking Agents (Systemic)*

---

**ITRACONAZOLE**—See *Antifungals, Azole (Systemic)*

---

**IVERMECTIN**—Since Ivermectin is not commercially available in the U.S. or Canada, the *Ivermectin (Systemic)* monograph is not included in this published version of the USP DI database. Copies of the monograph are available on request from the USP Division of Information Development, 12601 Twinbrook Parkway, Rockville, MD 20852; telephone (301) 816-8351; telefax (301) 816-8374.

# JAPANESE ENCEPHALITIS VIRUS VACCINE    Systemic

VA CLASSIFICATION (Primary): IM100

Note: For a listing of dosage forms and brand names by country availability, see *Dosage Forms* section(s). For a listing of brand names for the articles in this monograph, refer to the General Index.

## Category

Immunizing agent (active).

## Indications

### Accepted

Japanese encephalitis (prophylaxis)—Japanese encephalitis virus vaccine (JE vaccine) is indicated for immunization against Japanese encephalitis (JE).

Immunization with JE vaccine should be considered for adults and children one year of age and older who plan to reside in or travel to areas where JE is endemic or epidemic during a transmission season. JE vaccine is not recommended for all persons traveling to or residing in Asia. The incidence of JE in the location of intended stay, the conditions of housing, the nature of activities, the duration of stay, and the possibility of unexpected travel to high-risk areas are factors that should be considered in the decision to administer JE vaccine. In general, JE vaccine should be considered for use in persons spending a month or longer in epidemic or endemic areas during the transmission season, especially if travel will include rural areas. Depending on the epidemic circumstances, JE vaccine should also be considered for persons spending less than 30 days if their activities, such as extensive outdoor activities in rural areas, place them at particularly high risk for exposure. Immunization with JE vaccine is not intended to take the place of the usual precautions to reduce exposure to mosquito bites.

Immunization with JE vaccine also is recommended for all laboratory workers who may be exposed to infectious JE virus.

## Pharmacology/Pharmacokinetics

### Mechanism of action/Effect

Following subcutaneous administration, JE vaccine induces the formation of protective neutralizing antibodies.

### Protective effect

The precise relationship between antibody level and efficacy has not been established.

In a U.S. Army study using 538 volunteers, 100% of recipients demonstrated neutralizing antibodies 2 months after immunization with 3 doses of JE vaccine. In another study, substantial neutralizing antibody titers were elicited by 3 doses of JE vaccine in more than 90% of U.S. travelers without a history of prior JE immunization or prior exposure to JE. However, less than 80% of U.S. travelers receiving 2 doses of JE vaccine demonstrated neutralizing antibodies, and the neutralizing antibody levels declined substantially in most of these recipients within 6 months.

### Time to protective effect

An immune response is thought to occur within 10 days.

### Duration of protective effect

At least 2 years in persons receiving 3 doses of JE vaccine. Protection for longer than 2 years has not yet been determined.

## Precautions to Consider

### Cross-sensitivity and/or related problems

Patients sensitive to thimerosal, formaldehyde, gelatin, or rodent protein or neural products may be sensitive to JE vaccine also, since these products are used in the production of JE vaccine.

### Carcinogenicity/Mutagenicity

No studies have been performed.

### Pregnancy/Reproduction

Pregnancy—Studies have not been done in humans. It is not known whether JE vaccine can cause fetal harm when administered to a pregnant woman. However, JE infection acquired during the first or second trimester of pregnancy may cause intrauterine infection and miscarriage. JE infection acquired during the third trimester of pregnancy has not been associated with adverse effects in neonates. Pregnant women who must travel to an area where the risk of JE infection is high should be immunized only when the risk of infection outweighs the unknown risks to the fetus of immunization with JE vaccine.

Studies have not been done in animals.

FDA Pregnancy Category C.

### Breast-feeding

It is not known whether JE vaccine is distributed into breast milk.

### Pediatrics

Appropriate studies on the relationship of age to the effects of JE vaccine have not been performed in infants up to 1 year of age. Safety and efficacy have not been established.

### Geriatrics

No information is available on the relationship of age to the effects of JE vaccine in geriatric patients; however, advanced age may be a risk factor for the development of symptomatic illness following infection with JE.

### Medical considerations/Contraindications

The medical considerations/contraindications included here have been selected on the basis of their potential clinical significance (reasons given in parentheses where appropriate)—not necessarily inclusive (» = major clinical significance).

*Except under special circumstances, this medication should not be used when the following medical problems exist:*

» Hypersensitivity to rodent protein or neural products
    (JE vaccine is produced from infected mouse brains)

» Hypersensitivity to thimerosal

*Risk-benefit should be considered when the following medical problem exists:*

» Urticaria, history of
    (persons with this condition appear to have a greater risk of adverse reactions following immunization with JE vaccine and should be cautioned and monitored appropriately)

## Side/Adverse Effects

Note: Adverse reactions to JE vaccine manifesting as generalized urticaria or angioedema may occur within minutes following immunization. A possibly related reaction has occurred as late as 17 days after immunization. Most reactions occur within 10 days after immunization with the majority occurring within 48 hours. There is no increase in the number or severity of adverse reactions after 1, 2, or 3 doses of JE vaccine. Continued use of this medication is contraindicated when angioedema or generalized urticaria occurs following a dose of JE vaccine.

The following serious adverse events have been reported following immunization with JE vaccine; however the etiology of these adverse events is unknown:
• One case of Guillain-Barré syndrome has been reported in the U.S. since 1984; however, the patient was diagnosed as having mononucleosis 3 weeks before the onset of weakness.
• One case of urticaria, hepatitis, and respiratory failure occurred one week after dose 2 (the patient had eosinophilia and showed effusion and infiltrates on the chest x-ray).
• One case of respiratory and renal failure occurred 1 week after a dose of JE vaccine (the patient, a 26-month-old male, had infiltrates on chest x-ray and acid-fast bacilli in sputum).
• One case of newly diagnosed hypertension occurred in a young adult male presenting with headache several hours after receiving the first dose.
• Sudden death occurred in a 21-year-old U.S. military person approximately 60 hours after the person received the first dose of JE vaccine. The person had a history of recurrent hypersensitivity and a previous episode of possible anaphylaxis. The person also had received the third dose of plague vaccine approximately 12 to 15 hours prior to death. There was no evidence of urticaria or angioedema. The cause of death was not established during autopsy. Because of the severity of some of the adverse reactions to JE vaccine, patients should be encouraged to seek medical attention immediately upon onset of any adverse reaction.

The following side/adverse effects have been selected on the basis of their potential clinical significance (possible signs and symptoms in parentheses where appropriate)—not necessarily inclusive:

### Those indicating need for medical attention
Incidence rare
    *angioedema of the face (especially lips), oropharynx, or extremities* (swelling of face, lips, eyelids, throat, tongue, hands, or feet); *hypo-*

*tension, severe* (severe, unusual tiredness or weakness); *urticaria* (hives); *wheezing or troubled breathing*

**Those indicating need for medical attention only if they continue or are bothersome**
Incidence more frequent
*tenderness, soreness, redness, or swelling at injection site*
Incidence less frequent
*abdominal pain; chills; dizziness; fever; headache; itching or skin rash; malaise* (general feeling of discomfort or illness); *myalgia* (aches or pains in muscles); *nausea or vomiting*
Incidence rare
*erythema multiforme* (skin rash); *erythema nodosum* (skin rash); *joint swelling*

## Patient Consultation

As an aid to patient consultation, refer to *Advice for the Patient, Japanese Encephalitis Virus Vaccine (Systemic)*.

In providing consultation, consider emphasizing the following selected information (» = major clinical significance):

**Before using this vaccine**
» Conditions affecting use, especially:
   Sensitivity to thimerosal, formaldehyde, gelatin, or rodent protein or neural products
   Use in children—Not recommended for use in infants under 1 year of age
   Other medical problems, especially a history of urticaria

**Proper use of this vaccine**
» Importance of receiving all 3 doses of vaccine
» Importance of not traveling out of the country for at least 10 days following the last dose of vaccine
» Proper dosing

**Precautions after receiving this vaccine**
» Importance of using precautions against mosquito bites

**Side/adverse effects**
Patients are encouraged to seek medical attention for any side effect that occurs, since a mild-appearing side effect may portend a more serious one
Importance of telling physician about any side effect that occurs after a dose of vaccine; may mean that patient should not receive any more doses of vaccine
Signs of potential side effects, especially angioedema of the face (especially lips), oropharynx, or extremities; severe hypotension; urticaria; or wheezing or troubled breathing

## General Dosing Information

Patients should be observed for 30 minutes after immunization with JE vaccine and warned about the possibility of delayed generalized urticaria, often in a generalized distribution, or angioedema of the face (especially lips), oropharynx, or extremities.

Continued use of JE vaccine is contraindicated if angioedema or generalized urticaria occurs following a dose.

The final dose of the immunization series should be administered at least 10 days before international travel, to ensure an adequate immune response and access to medical care in the event of delayed adverse reactions. In addition, patients should be advised to remain in areas where they have ready access to medical care for 10 days after receiving a dose of JE vaccine. Patients should be instructed to seek medical attention immediately upon onset of any reaction.

When time constraints prevent the use of one of the recommended 3-dose schedules, 2 doses, administered 1 week apart, may be used. However, a 2-dose regimen will induce antibody formation in only approximately 80% of recipients, and therefore this regimen should be used only under unusual circumstances.

There are no data supporting the efficacy of prophylactic antihistamines or steroids in preventing JE vaccine–related allergic reactions.

The decision to administer JE vaccine should take into consideration the chance of exposure to the virus and of developing illness, the availability and acceptability of repellents and other alternative protective measures, and the side effects of immunization.

Limited data suggest that diphtheria and tetanus toxoids and pertussis vaccine (DTP and DTaP) may be administered concurrently with JE vac-

cine. There are no data on the effect of concurrent administration of other vaccines, medications (e.g., chloroquine, mefloquine), or biologicals on the safety and immunogenicity of JE vaccine. In the event that JE vaccine and other vaccines are given concurrently, separate syringes and separate sites should be used.

**For treatment of adverse effects**
Recommended treatment includes
• For mild hypersensitivity reaction—Administering antihistamines and, if necessary, glucocorticoids.
• For severe hypersensitivity or anaphylactic reaction—Administering epinephrine. Antihistamines and/or glucocorticoids may also be administered as required.

## Parenteral Dosage Forms
### JAPANESE ENCEPHALITIS VIRUS VACCINE INACTIVATED (FOR INJECTION)

**Usual adult and adolescent dose**
Japanese encephalitis (prophylaxis)—
   Subcutaneous, 1 mL, administered on days zero, seven, and thirty. If there are time constraints, an abbreviated schedule of days zero, seven, and fourteen may be used instead. A booster dose of 1 mL may be administered two years after the initial immunization series.

**Usual pediatric dose**
Japanese encephalitis (prophylaxis)—
   Infants up to 1 year of age: Safety and efficacy have not been established.
   Children 1 to 3 years of age: Subcutaneous, 0.5 mL, administered on days zero, seven, and thirty. If there are time constraints, an abbreviated schedule of days zero, seven, and fourteen may be used instead. A booster dose of 0.5 mL may be administered two years after the initial immunization series.
   Children 3 years of age and over: See *Usual adult and adolescent dose*.

**Strength(s) usually available**
U.S.—
   Less than 50 nanograms of mouse serum protein per 1-mL dose (Rx)
   [*Je-Vax* (thimerosal 0.007%, formaldehyde 100 mcg)].
Canada—
   Less than 50 nanograms of mouse serum protein per 1-mL dose (Rx)
   [*Je-Vax* (thimerosal 0.007%, formaldehyde 100 mcg)].

**Packaging and storage**
Store the lyophilized form of the vaccine and the reconstituted form of the vaccine between 2 and 8 °C (36 and 46 °F), unless otherwise specified by manufacturer. Protect from freezing.

**Preparation of dosage form**
To reconstitute, use only the diluent provided by the manufacturer.
The entire volume of diluent should be withdrawn into the syringe. All the diluent in the syringe should be injected into the vial of lyophilized vaccine and the vial should be shaken thoroughly. Immediately before withdrawing each dose, the vial should be shaken thoroughly.

**Stability**
The reconstituted vaccine should be used within 8 hours.

**Auxiliary labeling**
• Store in refrigerator.
• Protect from freezing.
• Discard reconstituted solution if not used within 8 hours.

**Note**
The date and time of reconstitution should be indicated on the vial if the reconstituted vaccine is not used at once.

## Selected Bibliography
Centers for Disease Control and Prevention. Inactivated Japanese encephalitis virus vaccine. Recommendations of the advisory committee on immunization practices (ACIP). MMWR 1993 Jan 8; 42 (RR-1): 1-15.

Revised: 06/21/93
Interim revision: 06/27/95

**KANAMYCIN**—See *Aminoglycosides (Systemic)*; *Kanamycin (Oral-Local)*

---

# KANAMYCIN    Oral-Local†

VA CLASSIFICATION (Primary/Secondary): AM300/GA900

Note: For a listing of dosage forms and brand names by country availability, see *Dosage Forms* section(s). For a listing of brand names for the articles in this monograph, refer to the General Index.

†Not commercially available in Canada.

---

## Category

Hepatic encephalopathy therapy adjunct; bowel preparation (preoperative) adjunct.

## Indications

### Accepted

Bowel preparation, preoperative—Oral-local kanamycin is indicated in preoperative bowel preparation for the prophylaxis of infections.

Hepatic coma (treatment)—Oral-local kanamycin has been used as adjunctive treatment of hepatic coma; however, it generally has been replaced by safer and more effective agents.

Not all species or strains of a particular organism may be susceptible to kanamycin.

### Unaccepted

Oral kanamycin is not indicated in the treatment of systemic infections.

## Pharmacology/Pharmacokinetics

### Physicochemical characteristics

Molecular weight—582.58.

### Mechanism of action/Effect

Aminoglycoside; actively transported across the bacterial cell membrane, binds to a specific receptor protein on the 30 S subunit of bacterial ribosomes, and interferes with an initiation complex between mRNA (messenger RNA) and the 30 S subunit, inhibiting protein synthesis. DNA may be misread, thus producing nonfunctional proteins; polyribosomes are split apart and are unable to synthesize protein.

Note: Aminoglycosides are bactericidal, while most other antibiotics that interfere with protein synthesis are bacteriostatic.

Oral nonabsorbable antibiotics suppress the growth of bacteria in the bowel, including those which produce ammonia.

### Absorption

Although only negligible amounts (approximately 1%) of kanamycin are absorbed through intact intestinal mucosa, significant amounts may be absorbed through ulcerated or denuded mucosa or if inflammation is present.

### Elimination

Fecal.

## Precautions to Consider

### Cross-sensitivity and/or related problems

Patients hypersensitive to one aminoglycoside may be hypersensitive to other aminoglycosides also.

### Pregnancy/Reproduction

Problems in humans have not been documented.

### Breast-feeding

It is not known whether oral-local kanamycin is excreted in breast milk. However, problems in humans have not been documented.

### Pediatrics

Appropriate studies on the relationship of age to the effects of oral-local kanamycin have not been performed in the pediatric population. However, no pediatrics-specific problems have been documented to date.

### Geriatrics

No information is available on the relationship of age to the effects of oral kanamycin in geriatric patients.

### Drug interactions and/or related problems

Because of minimal absorption of oral kanamycin, serum concentrations are not usually high enough to interact systemically with other medications, even in severe renal failure. For systemic drug interactions with parenteral kanamycin, see *Aminoglycosides (Systemic)*.

### Medical considerations/Contraindications

The medical considerations/contraindications included here have been selected on the basis of their potential clinical significance (reasons given in parentheses where appropriate)—not necessarily inclusive (» = major clinical significance).

*Except under special circumstances, this medication should not be used when the following medical problem exists:*
» Intestinal obstruction

*Risk-benefit should be considered when the following medical problems exist:*
» Eighth-cranial-nerve impairment
   (patients who receive prolonged kanamycin therapy may be at increased risk of ototoxicity)

     Hypersensitivity to kanamycin or other aminoglycosides
» Renal function impairment
   (patients receiving prolonged, high-dose therapy may require a reduction of dosage due to potential renal toxicity)
» Ulcerative lesions of the bowel
   (ulcerative lesions of the bowel may increase the systemic absorption of kanamycin, increasing the risk of toxicity)

## Side/Adverse Effects

The following side/adverse effects have been selected on the basis of their potential clinical significance (possible signs and symptoms in parentheses where appropriate)—not necessarily inclusive:

### Those indicating need for medical attention

Incidence rare—with prolonged, high-dose therapy
   *Nephrotoxicity* (greatly decreased frequency of urination or amount of urine; increased thirst); *auditory ototoxicity* (any loss of hearing; ringing or buzzing; a feeling of fullness in the ears); *vestibular ototoxicity* (clumsiness; dizziness; unsteadiness)

### Those indicating need for medical attention only if they continue or are bothersome

Incidence more frequent
   *Gastrointestinal disturbances* (diarrhea; nausea or vomiting)

Incidence rare—with prolonged therapy
   *Malabsorption syndrome* (diarrhea; increased amount of gas; light-colored, frothy, fatty-appearing stools)

## Patient Consultation

As an aid to patient consultation, refer to *Advice for the Patient, Kanamycin (Oral)*.

In providing consultation, consider emphasizing the following selected information (» = major clinical significance):

### Before using this medication

» Conditions affecting use, especially:
   Hypersensitivity to kanamycin or other aminoglycosides
   Other medical problems, especially eighth-cranial-nerve impairment, intestinal obstruction, renal function impairment, or ulcerative lesions of the bowel

### Proper use of this medication

     Taking on a full or empty stomach
» Compliance with full course of therapy
» Proper dosing
» Proper storage
*For use as a preoperative bowel preparation*
Missed dose: Taking as soon as possible; not taking if almost time for next dose; not doubling doses

### Side/adverse effects

     Signs of potential side effects, especially nephrotoxicity, auditory ototoxicity, and vestibular ototoxicity

## General Dosing Information

Kanamycin may be taken on a full or empty stomach.

## Oral Dosage Forms

Note: The dosing and strengths of the dosage forms available are expressed in terms of kanamycin base (not the sulfate salt).

### KANAMYCIN SULFATE CAPSULES USP

**Usual adult and adolescent dose**
Hepatic encephalopathy therapy adjunct—
  Oral, 2 to 3 grams (base) every six hours.
Bowel preparation (preoperative) adjunct—
  Oral, 1 gram (base) every hour for four hours, then 1 gram every six hours for thirty-six to seventy-two hours.

**Usual pediatric dose**
Hepatic encephalopathy therapy adjunct—See *Usual adult and adolescent dose.*
Bowel preparation (preoperative) adjunct—See *Usual adult and adolescent dose.*

**Strength(s) usually available**
U.S.—
  500 mg (base) (Rx) [*Kantrex* (lactose)].

Canada—
  Not commercially available.

**Packaging and storage**
Store below 40 °C (104 °F), preferably between 15 and 30 °C (59 and 86 °F), unless otherwise specified by manufacturer. Store in a tight container.

**Auxiliary labeling**
• Continue medicine for full time of treatment.

Revised: 09/08/92
Interim revision: 03/17/94

---

## KAOLIN-CONTAINING COMBINATIONS—

Kaolin and Pectin (Oral-Local)
Kaolin, Pectin, Hyoscyamine, Atropine, and Scopolamine (Systemic)—
  See *Kaolin, Pectin, and Belladonna Alkaloids (Systemic)*
Kaolin, Pectin, and Paregoric (Systemic)

---

# KAOLIN AND PECTIN  Oral-Local

**VA CLASSIFICATION (Primary): GA400**
Note: For a listing of dosage forms and brand names by country availability, see *Dosage Forms* section(s). For a listing of brand names for the articles in this monograph, refer to the General Index.

## Category

Antidiarrheal (adsorbent).

## Indications

Note: The efficacy of any antidiarrheal medication for treatment of most cases of nonspecific diarrhea is questionable, especially in children. **Preferred treatment for acute, nonspecific diarrhea consists of fluid and electrolyte replacement, nutritional therapy, and, if possible, elimination of the underlying cause of the diarrhea.**

**Accepted**
Diarrhea (treatment)—Kaolin and pectin may be indicated as an adjunct to rest, fluids, and an appropriate diet in the symptomatic treatment of mild to moderately acute diarrhea. Use is recommended in chronic diarrhea only as temporary symptomatic treatment until the etiology is determined. Kaolin and pectin combination should not be used if diarrhea is accompanied by fever or if there is blood or mucus in the stool.

## Pharmacology/Pharmacokinetics

**Mechanism of action/Effect**
Adsorbent and protectant. Kaolin is a natural hydrated aluminum silicate that is believed to adsorb large numbers of bacteria and toxins and reduce water loss. Pectin is a polyuronic polymer for which the mechanism of action is unknown. Pectin consists of purified carbohydrate extracted from citrus fruit or apple pomace. Studies have shown no decrease in stool frequency or fecal weight and water content with this combination even though stools appeared more formed.

**Absorption**
Not absorbed (up to 90% of pectin is decomposed in gastrointestinal tract).

## Precautions to Consider

**Pregnancy/Reproduction**
Pregnancy—Problems in humans have not been documented. Kaolin and pectin combination is poorly absorbed after oral administration.

**Breast-feeding**
Problems in humans have not been documented. Kaolin and pectin combination is poorly absorbed after oral administration.

**Pediatrics**
In infants and children up to 3 years of age with diarrhea, use is not recommended unless directed by a physician because of the risk of fluid and electrolyte loss. Oral rehydration therapy is recommended in children with diarrhea to prevent loss of fluids and electrolytes.

**Geriatrics**
In geriatric patients with diarrhea, caution is recommended because of the risk of fluid and electrolyte loss; these patients should be referred to a physician.

**Drug interactions and/or related problems**
The following drug interactions and/or related problems have been selected on the basis of their potential clinical significance (possible mechanism in parentheses where appropriate)—not necessarily inclusive (» = major clinical significance):

Note: Combinations containing any of the following medications, depending on the amount present, may also interact with this medication.

Anticholinergics or other medications with anticholinergic activity (See *Appendix II*), or
Antidyskinetics or
Digitalis glycosides or
Lincomycins or
Loxapine or
Phenothiazines or
Thioxanthenes
  (concurrent use with kaolin and pectin combination may impair absorption of these medications when it is administered orally, resulting in decreased therapeutic effectiveness; it is recommended that kaolin and pectin combination be administered not less than 2 hours before or 3 to 4 hours after oral lincomycins; patients receiving digitalis should be monitored closely for evidence of altered effect)

Oral medications, other
  (prolonged use of adsorbents may interfere with absorption of other oral agents administered concurrently; it is recommended that kaolin and pectin combination be administered at least 2 to 3 hours before or after other oral medications)

**Medical considerations/Contraindications**
The medical considerations/contraindications included here have been selected on the basis of their potential clinical significance (reasons given in parentheses where appropriate)—not necessarily inclusive (» = major clinical significance).

*Risk-benefit should be considered when the following medical problems exist:*
» Dehydration
    (although adsorbent antidiarrheals may increase the consistency of feces and decrease the frequency of evacuation, they do not reduce the amount of fluid loss, but only mask its extent; rehydration therapy is essential if signs or symptoms of dehydration, such as dryness of mouth, excessive thirst, wrinkled skin, decreased urination, and dizziness or lightheadedness are present; fluid loss may have serious consequences, such as circulatory collapse and renal failure, especially in young children)

Diarrhea, parasite-associated, suspected
    (use of adsorbent antidiarrheals may make recognition of parasitic causes of diarrhea more difficult; if parasitic agents are suspected

pathogens, appropriate stool analyses should be performed prior to therapy with adsorbents)
» Dysentery, acute, characterized by bloody stools and elevated temperature
(sole treatment with adsorbent antidiarrheals may be inadequate; antibiotic therapy may be required)

## Side/Adverse Effects

The following side/adverse effects have been selected on the basis of their potential clinical significance (possible signs and symptoms in parentheses where appropriate)—not necessarily inclusive:

**Those indicating need for medical attention only if they continue or are bothersome**
Incidence dose-related
*Constipation*—usually mild and transient, but may rarely lead to fecal impaction

## Patient Consultation

As an aid to patient consultation, refer to *Advice for the Patient, Kaolin and Pectin (Oral)*.

In providing consultation, consider emphasizing the following selected information (» = major clinical significance):

**Before using this medication**
» Conditions affecting use, especially:
Use in children—Not using in infants and children up to 3 years of age unless prescribed by a physician because of risk of dehydration associated with diarrhea; oral rehydration therapy recommended in children with diarrhea
Use in the elderly—Risk of dehydration associated with diarrhea
Other medical problems, especially dehydration and acute dysentery

**Proper use of this medication**
» Not using if diarrhea is accompanied by fever or by blood or mucus in the stool; contacting physician
Taking after each loose bowel movement until diarrhea is controlled
» Importance of maintaining adequate hydration and proper diet
» Proper dosing
» Proper storage

**Precautions while using this medication**
» Checking with physician if diarrhea is not controlled within 48 hours and/or fever develops
Taking doses of other oral medications 2 to 3 hours before or after doses of kaolin and pectin combination

## Oral Dosage Forms

### KAOLIN AND PECTIN ORAL SUSPENSION

**Usual adult dose**
Antidiarrheal—
Oral, 60 to 120 mL after each loose bowel movement.

**Usual pediatric dose**
Antidiarrheal—
Children up to 3 years of age: Use is not recommended unless directed by a physician.
Children 3 to 6 years of age: Oral, 15 to 30 mL after each loose bowel movement.
Children 6 to 12 years of age: Oral, 30 to 60 mL after each loose bowel movement.
Children 12 years of age and over: Oral, 45 to 60 mL after each loose bowel movement.
Note: In general, dietary treatment of diarrhea in children is preferred whenever possible.

**Strength(s) usually available**
U.S.—
5.2 grams of kaolin and 260 mg of pectin per 30 mL (OTC) [*Kao-Spen; K-P*].
5.85 grams of kaolin and 130 mg of pectin per 30 mL (OTC) [*Kapectolin;* GENERIC].
Canada—
6 grams of kaolin and 143 mg of pectin per 30 mL (OTC) [*Donnagel-MB* (alcohol 3.8%)].

**Packaging and storage**
Store below 40 °C (104 °F), preferably between 15 and 30 °C (59 and 86 °F), in a well-closed container, unless otherwise specified by manufacturer. Protect from freezing.

**Auxiliary labeling**
• Shake well.

**Note**
Refer patients with recurrent or persistent diarrhea to a physician.

## Selected Bibliography

Brownlee HJ. Family practitioner's guide to patient self-treatment of acute diarrhea. Am J Med 1990; 88 (6A Suppl): 27S-29S.

Revised: 08/04/94

---

# KAOLIN, PECTIN, AND BELLADONNA ALKALOIDS  Systemic

VA CLASSIFICATION (Primary): GA400

**NOTE:** The *Kaolin, Pectin, and Belladonna Alkaloids (Systemic)* monograph is maintained on the USP DI electronic data base. For a printed copy of the most recent revision of the complete monograph, contact the USP Division of Information Development, 12601 Twinbrook Parkway, Rockville, MD 20852.

For information on the specific components of this combination, see the *USP DI* monographs for *Anticholinergics/Antispasmodics (Systemic)* and *Kaolin and Pectin (Oral-Local)*.

The information that follows is selectively abstracted from the complete monograph and is provided to facilitate drug use review and patient counseling.

Note: For a listing of dosage forms and brand names by country availability, see *Dosage Forms* section(s). For a listing of brand names for the articles in this monograph, refer to the General Index.

## Category
Antidiarrheal (adsorbent).

## Indications

Note: The efficacy of any antidiarrheal medication for treatment of most cases of nonspecific diarrhea is questionable, especially in children. **Preferred treatment for acute, nonspecific diarrhea consists of fluid and electrolyte replacement, nutritional therapy, and, if possible, elimination of the underlying cause of the diarrhea.**

**Unaccepted**
The U.S. Food and Drug Administration (FDA) has banned the inclusion of belladonna alkaloids in antidiarrheal preparations because of lack of proof of their effectiveness. FDA has requested that manufacturers wishing to obtain the agency's approval for inclusion of these ingredients in their product provide FDA with evidence that the ingredients are safe and effective for their intended use. This medication has been replaced by equally or more effective, and safer, agents for the treatment of diarrhea.

## Patient Consultation

As an aid to patient consultation, refer to *Advice for the Patient, Kaolin, Pectin, and Belladonna Alkaloids (Systemic)*.

In providing consultation, consider emphasizing the following selected information (» = major clinical significance):

**Before using this medication**
» Conditions affecting use, especially:
Sensitivity to any of the belladonna alkaloids
Pregnancy—Belladonna alkaloids cross the placenta
Breast-feeding—Belladonna alkaloids are distributed into breast milk
Use in children—Not using in infants and children up to 6 years of age because use does not preclude, and may aggravate, risk of dehydration associated with diarrhea; oral rehydration therapy recommended in children with diarrhea; increased susceptibility to side/adverse effects of belladonna alkaloids
Use in the elderly—Risk of dehydration associated with diarrhea; increased sensitivity to effects of belladonna alkaloids

Dental—Possible development of dental problems because of decreased salivary flow

Other medications, especially CNS depressants, ketoconazole, MAO inhibitors, or potassium chloride

Other medical problems, especially acute dysentery, asthma or respiratory disease, dehydration, diarrhea caused by poisoning, glaucoma, hepatic and/or renal function impairment, prostatic hyperplasia or urinary retention, or severe colitis

### Proper use of this medication

Taking with food or meals if gastric irritation occurs
» Importance of not taking more medication than the amount prescribed
Proper administration technique
» Importance of maintaining adequate hydration and proper diet
» Proper dosing
» Proper storage

### Precautions while using this medication

» Consulting physician if diarrhea is not controlled within 48 hours and/or fever develops
Possible interference with laboratory values
» Avoiding use of alcohol or other CNS depressants
» Caution if drowsiness occurs
Possible increased sensitivity of eyes to light
» Caution during exercise and hot weather; overheating may result in heatstroke
Possible dryness of mouth, nose, and throat; using sugarless candy or gum, ice, or saliva substitute for relief; checking with physician or dentist if dry mouth continues for more than 2 weeks

### Side/adverse effects

Signs of potential side effects, especially allergic reaction, CNS depression, hallucinations, increased intraocular pressure, paralytic ileus or toxic megacolon, or slow heartbeat

## Oral Dosage Forms

### KAOLIN, PECTIN, HYOSCYAMINE SULFATE, ATROPINE SULFATE, AND SCOPOLAMINE HYDROBROMIDE ORAL SUSPENSION

### Usual adult and adolescent dose

Oral, 30 mL every three hours as needed to control diarrhea.

### Usual adult prescribing limits

Four doses in twenty-four hours.

### Usual pediatric dose

Children up to 6 years of age: Use is not recommended unless directed by a physician.

Children over 6 years of age: Oral, 5 to 10 mL every three hours as needed to control diarrhea, up to four doses in twenty-four hours.

Note: In general, oral rehydration therapy and dietary treatment of diarrhea in children are preferred whenever possible.

### Usual geriatric dose

See *Usual adult and adolescent dose*.

Note: Geriatric patients may be more sensitive to the effects of the usual adult dose.

### Strength(s) usually available

U.S.—

Not commercially available.

Canada—

6 grams of kaolin, 142.8 mg of pectin, 104 mcg (0.104 mg) of hyoscyamine sulfate, 19 mcg (0.019 mg) of atropine sulfate, and 7 mcg (0.007 mg) of scopolamine hydrobromide per 30 mL (Rx) [*Donnagel* (alcohol 3.8%; sodium <2.6 mg per 5 mL; sugar)].

### Auxiliary labeling

• May cause drowsiness.
• Avoid alcoholic beverages.
• Do not take other medicines without your doctor's advice.
• Keep out of reach of children.
• Shake well before using.

Revised: 04/27/95

# KAOLIN, PECTIN, AND PAREGORIC  Systemic

VA CLASSIFICATION (Primary): GA400

NOTE: The *Kaolin, Pectin, and Paregoric (Systemic)* monograph is maintained on the USP DI electronic data base. For a printed copy of the most recent revision of the complete monograph, contact the USP Division of Information Development, 12601 Twinbrook Parkway, Rockville, MD 20852.

For information on the specific components of this combination, see the *USP DI* monographs for *Kaolin and Pectin (Oral-Local)* and *Paregoric (Systemic)*.

The information that follows is selectively abstracted from the complete monograph and is provided to facilitate drug use review and patient counseling.

Note: For a listing of dosage forms and brand names by country availability, see *Dosage Forms* section(s). For a listing of brand names for the articles in this monograph, refer to the General Index.

## Category

Antidiarrheal (adsorbent).

## Indications

Note: The efficacy of any antidiarrheal medication for treatment of most cases of nonspecific diarrhea is questionable, especially in children. **Preferred treatment for acute, nonspecific diarrhea consists of fluid and electrolyte replacement, nutritional therapy, and, if possible, elimination of the underlying cause of the diarrhea.**

### Unaccepted

The U.S. Food and Drug Administration (FDA) has banned the inclusion of paregoric in antidiarrheal preparations because of lack of proof of its effectiveness. FDA has requested that manufacturers wishing to obtain the agency's approval for inclusion of this ingredient in their product provide FDA with evidence that the ingredient is safe and effective for its intended use. Paregoric-containing medications have

been replaced by equally or more effective, and safer, agents for the treatment of diarrhea.

## Patient Consultation

As an aid to patient consultation, refer to *Advice for the Patient, Kaolin, Pectin, and Paregoric (Systemic)*.

In providing consultation, consider emphasizing the following selected information (» = major clinical significance):

### Before using this medication

» Conditions affecting use, especially:
Sensitivity to paregoric or other opiates
Pregnancy—Opium alkaloids cross placenta; possible fetal dependence with regular use late in pregnancy
Breast-feeding—Opium alkaloids distributed into breast milk
Use in children—Not using in infants and children up to 2 years of age because of risk of dehydration associated with diarrhea; oral rehydration therapy recommended in children with diarrhea; increased sensitivity to opiate effects
Use in the elderly—Risk of dehydration associated with diarrhea; increased sensitivity to opiate effects
Other medications, especially antiperistaltic antidiarrheals, CNS depressants, naloxone, and naltrexone; spacing doses of other oral medications 2 to 3 hours before or after doses of kaolin and pectin–containing medication is recommended
Other medical problems, especially acute dysentery, acute respiratory depression, asthma or respiratory disease, dehydration, diarrhea associated with *C. difficile* or caused by poisoning, and severe inflammatory bowel disease

### Proper use of this medication

Taking with food or meals if gastric irritation occurs
» Importance of not taking more medication than the amount prescribed because of habit-forming potential
Using specially marked spoon or measuring device
» Importance of maintaining adequate hydration and proper diet

» Proper dosing
» Proper storage

**Precautions while using this medication**
» Consulting physician if diarrhea is not controlled within 48 hours and/ or fever develops
» Caution if taking alcohol or other central nervous system (CNS) depressants
» Caution if drowsiness occurs

**Side/adverse effects**
Signs of potential side effects, especially allergic reaction, histamine-release related effects, mental depression, and toxic megacolon

## Oral Dosage Forms

### KAOLIN, PECTIN, AND PAREGORIC ORAL SUSPENSION

**Usual adult and adolescent dose**
Antidiarrheal—Oral, 30 mL after each loose bowel movement.

**Usual adult prescribing limits**
Four doses within twelve hours.

**Usual pediatric dose**
Antidiarrheal—
Children up to 2 years of age:
Use is not recommended.
Children 2 years of age and over:
Children up to 4.5 kg of body weight—Dosage must be individualized by physician.

Children 4.5 to 9 kg of body weight—Oral, 2.5 mL after each loose bowel movement.
Children 9 to 13.5 kg of body weight—Oral, 5 mL after each loose bowel movement.
Children 13.5 kg of body weight and over—Oral, 5 to 10 mL after each loose bowel movement.

Note: No more than 4 doses should be administered within twelve hours.
In general, oral rehydration therapy and dietary treatment of diarrhea in children are preferred whenever possible.

**Usual geriatric dose**
See *Usual adult and adolescent dose.*

Note: Geriatric patients may be more sensitive to the effects of the usual adult dose.

**Strength(s) usually available**
U.S.—
Not commercially available.
Canada—
6 grams of kaolin, 142.8 mg of pectin, and 6 mL of paregoric, per 30 mL (N) [*Donnagel-PG* (alcohol 5%; sodium <1 mmol per 5 mL)].

**Auxiliary labeling**
• May cause drowsiness.
• Avoid alcoholic beverages.
• Do not take other medicines without your doctor's advice.
• Keep out of reach of children.
• May be habit-forming.
• Shake well before using.

Revised: 04/26/95

---

# KETAMINE  Systemic

**VA CLASSIFICATION (Primary/Secondary): CN203/CN205**
Note: For a listing of dosage forms and brand names by country availability, see *Dosage Forms* section(s). For a listing of brand names for the articles in this monograph, refer to the General Index.

## Category
Anesthetic (general).

## Indications
Note: Bracketed information in the *Indications* section refers to uses that are not included in U.S. product labeling.

**Accepted**
Anesthesia, general—Ketamine is indicated to provide anesthesia for short diagnostic and surgical procedures that do not require skeletal muscle relaxation. It is also indicated to induce anesthesia prior to administration of other general anesthetics.

[Ketamine is used to provide obstetrical anesthesia.][1]

Anesthesia, general, adjunct—Ketamine is indicated to supplement low-potency anesthetics such as nitrous oxide.

[Anesthesia, local, adjunct][1]—Ketamine is used as a supplement to local and regional anesthesia.

Caution is recommended when ketamine is considered for use in surgical procedures of the pharynx, larynx, or trachea because it increases salivary and tracheal-bronchial secretions and does not reliably suppress pharyngeal and laryngeal reflexes.

In subhypnotic doses, ketamine produces a dissociative state. The patient does not appear to be asleep and experiences a feeling of being dissociated from the environment.

[1]Not included in Canadian product labeling.

## Pharmacology/Pharmacokinetics

**Physicochemical characteristics**
Molecular weight—274.19.

**Mechanism of action/Effect**
The precise mechanism of action is unknown. Ketamine has been shown to block afferent impulses associated with the affective-emotional component of pain perception within the medial medullary reticular formation, to suppress spinal cord activity, and to interact with several central nervous system (CNS) transmitter systems.

**Absorption**
Rapid.

**Distribution**
Rapidly distributed into highly perfused tissues including the brain. Animal studies have shown ketamine to be highly concentrated in body fat, liver, and lung.

**Biotransformation**
Hepatic. However, termination of anesthetic effects may be caused by redistribution from the brain to other tissues.

**Half-life**
Distribution—Approximately 7 to 11 minutes.
Elimination—Approximately 2 to 3 hours.

**Time to induction of anesthesia**
Intravenous (following a dose of 1 to 2 mg per kg of body weight [mg/kg])—
Sensation of dissociation: 15 seconds.
Anesthesia: 30 seconds.
Intramuscular (following a dose of 5 to 10 mg/kg)—
Anesthesia: 3 to 4 minutes.

**Duration of anesthesia**
Intravenous (following a dose of 2 mg/kg)—5 to 10 minutes.
Intramuscular (following a dose of 10 mg/kg)—12 to 25 minutes.

**Time to recovery**
Rapid.

**Elimination**
Renal, 90%; about 4% as unchanged ketamine.
Fecal, up to 5%.

## Precautions to Consider

**Pregnancy/Reproduction**
Studies in animals have not shown that ketamine causes birth defects; however, it crosses the placenta. Also, in one study in rats, ketamine produced histologic changes in the heart, liver, and kidneys of the offspring, including focal nuclear hypochromatosis, interfibrillary edema, parenchymal cell degeneration, proximal convoluted tubule degeneration, and diffuse hematopoietic cell infiltration. The degenerative effects were dependent on both dosage and duration of administration. Ketamine is used in low doses to provide obstetrical anesthesia. It has not been shown to cause adverse effects.

**Breast-feeding**
Problems in humans have not been documented.

**Pediatrics**

Appropriate studies performed to date have not demonstrated pediatrics-specific problems that would limit the usefulness of ketamine in children.

**Geriatrics**

Appropriate studies performed to date have not demonstrated geriatrics-specific problems that would limit the use of ketamine in the elderly.

**Drug interactions and/or related problems**

The following drug interactions and/or related problems have been selected on the basis of their potential clinical significance (possible mechanism in parentheses where appropriate)—not necessarily inclusive (» = major clinical significance):

Note: Combinations containing any of the following medications, depending on the amount present, may also interact with this medication.

Anesthetics, halogenated hydrocarbon inhalation, such as:
   Enflurane
   Halothane
   Isoflurane
   Methoxyflurane
      (halogen hydrocarbon inhalation anesthetics may prolong the elimination half-life of ketamine; recovery from anesthesia may be prolonged following concurrent use)

Antihypertensives or

CNS depression–producing medications, including those commonly used as preanesthetic medication or for induction, supplementation, or maintenance of anesthesia (See *Appendix II*)
   (concurrent use with ketamine, especially high-dose or rapidly administered ketamine, may increase the risk of hypotension and/or respiratory depression)

Thyroid hormones
   (ketamine should be administered with caution to patients receiving thyroid hormones because of the increased risk of hypertension and tachycardia)

**Laboratory value alterations**

The following have been selected on the basis of their potential clinical significance (possible effect in parentheses where appropriate)—not necessarily inclusive (» = major clinical significance):

With physiology/laboratory test values
   Cerebrospinal fluid (CSF) pressure, or
   Intraocular pressure
      (may be increased)

**Medical considerations/Contraindications**

The medical considerations/contraindications included here have been selected on the basis of their potential clinical significance (reasons given in parentheses where appropriate)—not necessarily inclusive (» = major clinical significance).

*Except under special circumstances, this medication should not be used when the following medical problems exist:*

» Any condition in which a significant elevation of blood pressure would be hazardous, such as:
» Cardiovascular disease, severe
» Heart failure
» Hypertension, severe or poorly controlled
» Myocardial infarction, recent
» Stroke, history of
» Cerebral trauma
» Intracerebral mass or hemorrhage

*Risk-benefit should be considered when the following medical problems exist:*

Alcohol abuse (or history of)

Alcohol intoxication, acute

Congestive heart failure or
Hypertension, mild, uncomplicated or
Myocardial ischemia or
Tachyarrhythmias
   (may be exacerbated)

» Eye injury, open globe

» Increased cerebrospinal fluid (CSF) pressure
   (ketamine may further elevate CSF pressure)

» Increased intraocular pressure
   (ketamine may further elevate intraocular pressure)

» Psychiatric disorders such as schizophrenia or acute psychosis

Sensitivity to ketamine

» Thyrotoxic states
   (increased risk of hypertension and tachycardia)

**Patient monitoring**

The following may be especially important in patient monitoring (other tests may be warranted in some patients, depending on condition; » = major clinical significance):

Cardiac function
   (monitoring throughout the procedure is recommended, especially in patients with congestive heart failure, hypertension, myocardial ischemia, or tachyarrhythmias)

## Side/Adverse Effects

The following side/adverse effects have been selected on the basis of their potential clinical significance (possible signs and symptoms in parentheses where appropriate)—not necessarily inclusive:

**Those indicating need for medical attention**

Incidence more frequent
   *Increased blood pressure*—may reach hypertensive levels; *tachycardia; tonic and clonic muscle movements*—may resemble seizures; *tremor; vocalization*

Incidence less frequent
   *Bradycardia; hypotension; respiratory depression*—may lead to apnea; *vomiting*—following administration

Incidence rare
   *Cardiac arrhythmias; laryngospasm or other forms of airway obstruction*

**Those indicating need for medical attention only if they continue or are bothersome**

Incidence more frequent in patients between 15 and 45 years of age; less frequent in other age groups
   *Emergence reaction* (alterations in mood or body image; delirium; dissociative or floating sensations; *vivid dreams or illusions; visual hallucinations*

   Note: Although *vivid dreams* and/or *hallucinations* usually disappear upon wakening, some patients may experience flashbacks several weeks postoperatively.

Incidence less frequent or rare
   *Double vision; loss of appetite; nausea with or without vomiting; nystagmus* (wandering or back-and-forth eye movements); *pain at injection site; reddened skin or skin rash*

## Patient Consultation

As an aid to patient consultation, refer to *Advice for the Patient, Anesthetics, General (Systemic)*.

In providing consultation, consider emphasizing the following selected information (» = major clinical significance):

**Before receiving this medication**

» Conditions affecting use, especially:
   Sensitivity to ketamine
   Pregnancy—Ketamine crosses the placenta
   Any other medication, including use of "street" drugs
   Other medical problems, especially cardiac or cardiovascular disease, glaucoma, hypertension, hyperthyroidism, psychiatric disorders, and stroke

**Proper use of this medication**

Proper dosing

**Precautions after receiving this medication**

» Possibility of psychomotor impairment following anesthesia; using caution in driving or performing other tasks requiring alertness for about 24 hours postanesthesia

» Avoiding alcohol or other CNS depressants within 24 hours following anesthesia unless prescribed or otherwise approved by physician or dentist

**Side/adverse effects**

Signs of potential delayed side effects, especially mood or mental changes, nightmares or unusual dreams, and blurred vision

## General Dosing Information

The usual adult dosages are intended as a guideline. Actual dosage must be individualized to meet the needs of each patient.

Ketamine may cause vomiting following administration. To prevent possible aspiration of vomitus, ketamine should be administered to the patient on an empty stomach.

Because ketamine increases salivary and tracheal-bronchial mucous gland secretions, use of atropine, scopolamine, or another drying agent is recommended prior to induction of anesthesia. The fact that atropine has been shown to increase the frequency of unpleasant dreams should be kept in mind.

Ketamine may be administered intramuscularly or intravenously. Intravenous administration produces anesthesia more rapidly than intramuscular administration.

Administration of an overdose, or administering ketamine at too rapid a rate, may produce respiratory depression, apnea, and hypertension. Intravenous ketamine should be administered over a period of 60 seconds unless a rapid-sequence induction technique is indicated.

Tolerance to the effects of ketamine has been reported following repeated administration.

A state of confusion (emergence delirium) may occur during recovery. Although it has been suggested that minimizing verbal, tactile, and visual stimulation during recovery may reduce the incidence of emergence reactions, the efficacy of such measures has not been documented. Administration of a benzodiazepine prior to or concurrently with ketamine, or just prior to termination of surgery, may decrease the incidence of emergence delirium.

### For treatment of adverse effects
Recommended treatment may include
- For respiratory depression or apnea—Assisting respiration mechanically may be preferred over administration of analeptics.
- For severe emergence reaction—Administering a short- or ultrashort-acting barbiturate.

## Parenteral Dosage Forms

Note: Bracketed uses in the *Dosage Forms* section refer to categories of use and/or indications that are not included in U.S. product labeling.

### KETAMINE HYDROCHLORIDE INJECTION USP

#### Usual adult and adolescent dose
Anesthetic (general)—
  Induction:
    Intravenous, 1 to 2 mg (base) per kg of body weight, administered as a single dose or by intravenous infusion at a rate of 500 mcg (0.5 mg) (base) per kg of body weight per minute; or
    Intramuscular, 5 to 10 mg (base) per kg of body weight.
  Maintenance:
    Intravenous, 10 to 50 mcg (0.01 to 0.05 mg) (base) per kg of body weight by continuous infusion at a rate of 1 to 2 mg per minute.
    Note: Maintenance dosage must be adjusted as determined by the patient's anesthetic requirements and concurrent use of an additional anesthetic agent.

    Tonic-clonic movements that may appear during anesthesia are not indicative of the need for additional ketamine.
[Anesthesia, local, adjunct][1]—
    Intravenous, 5 to 30 mg (base), prior to administration of the local anesthetic. May be repeated if necessary.
[Sedation and analgesia][1]—
    Intravenous: 200 to 750 mcg (0.2 to 0.75 mg) (base) per kg of body weight administered over 2 to 3 minutes initially, followed by 5 to 20 mcg (0.005 to 0.02 mg) (base) per kg of body weight per minute as a continuous intravenous infusion.
    Intramuscular: 2 to 4 mg (base) per kg of body weight initially, followed by 5 to 20 mcg (0.005 to 0.02 mg) (base) per kg of body weight per minute as a continuous intravenous infusion.

### Usual adult prescribing limits
Anesthesia, general, induction—
  Intravenous: Up to 4.5 mg (base) per kg of body weight.
  Intramuscular: Up to 13 mg (base) per kg of body weight.
[Anesthesia, local, adjunct][1]—
  Intravenous, up to 30 mg (base).

### Usual pediatric dose
See *Usual adult and adolescent dose.*

### Usual geriatric dose
See *Usual adult and adolescent dose.*

### Strength(s) usually available
U.S.—
  10 mg (base) per mL (Rx) [*Ketalar;* GENERIC (benzethonium chloride)].
  50 mg (base) per mL (Rx) [*Ketalar;* GENERIC (benzethonium chloride)].
  100 mg (base) per mL (Rx) [*Ketalar;* GENERIC (benzethonium chloride)].
Canada—
  10 mg (base) per mL (Rx) [*Ketalar*].
  50 mg (base) per mL (Rx) [*Ketalar*].
U.K.—
  10 mg (base) per mL (Rx) [*Ketalar*].
  50 mg (base) per mL (Rx) [*Ketalar*].
  100 mg (base) per mL (Rx) [*Ketalar*].

### Packaging and storage
Store below 40 °C (104 °F), preferably between 15 and 30 °C (59 and 86 °F), unless otherwise specified by manufacturer. Protect from light and heat. Protect from freezing.

### Preparation of dosage form
For direct intravenous administration—The 100-mg-per-mL concentration of ketamine must be diluted with an equal volume of sterile water for injection, 0.9% sodium chloride injection, or 5% dextrose injection prior to injection.
For intravenous infusion—Add 10 mL of the 50-mg-per-mL concentration, or 5 mL of the 100-mg-per-mL concentration, of ketamine (base) to 500 mL of 5% dextrose injection or 0.9% sodium chloride injection and mix well. The resultant solution will contain 1 mg of ketamine (base) per mL. If fluid restriction is necessary, 250 mL of the diluent may be used to provide a solution containing 2 mg of ketamine (base) per mL.

### Incompatibilities
Ketamine and barbiturates should not be injected from the same syringe because they will form a precipitate.
If diazepam is administered concurrently with ketamine, the two medications should be given separately. The two medications should not be mixed together in a syringe or added to the same intravenous infusion solution.

---

[1]Not included in Canadian product labeling.

---

Revised: 06/21/90
Interim revision: 08/23/94

---

### KETAZOLAM—See *Benzodiazepines (Systemic)*

---

### KETOCONAZOLE—See *Antifungals, Azole (Systemic)*

---

# KETOCONAZOLE   Topical

VA CLASSIFICATION (Primary): DE102

Note: For a listing of dosage forms and brand names by country availability, see *Dosage Forms* section(s). For a listing of brand names for the articles in this monograph, refer to the General Index.

## Category
Antifungal (topical).

## Indications
Note: Bracketed information in the *Indications* section refers to uses that are not included in U.S. product labeling.

### Accepted
Tinea corporis (treatment) or
Tinea cruris (treatment)—Ketoconazole cream is indicated as a primary agent in the topical treatment of tinea corporis (ringworm of the body) and tinea cruris (ringworm of the groin; jock itch) caused by *Trichophyton rubrum, T. mentagrophytes,* and *Epidermophyton floccosum* (*Acrothesium floccosum*).
Tinea pedis (treatment)—Ketoconazole cream is indicated as a primary agent in the topical treatment of tinea pedis (athlete's foot).
Pityriasis versicolor (treatment)—Ketoconazole cream is indicated as a primary agent in the topical treatment of pityriasis versicolor (tinea

versicolor; "sun fungus") caused by *Malassezia furfur (Pityrosporon orbiculare)*.

Candidiasis, cutaneous (treatment)[1]—Ketoconazole cream is indicated as a primary agent in the topical treatment of cutaneous candidiasis caused by *Candida* species.

Dermatitis, seborrheic (treatment)—Ketoconazole cream is indicated in the treatment of seborrheic dermatitis.

Dandruff (treatment)—Ketoconazole shampoo is indicated for the reduction of scaling due to dandruff.

[Paronychia (treatment)][1]
[Tinea barbae (treatment)][1] or
[Tinea capitis (treatment)][1]—Ketoconazole cream is used as a primary agent in the topical treatment of paronychia. Ketoconazole cream is used as a secondary agent in the topical treatment of tinea barbae and tinea capitis.

Not all species or strains of a particular organism may be susceptible to ketoconazole.

---

[1]Not included in Canadian product labeling.

## Pharmacology/Pharmacokinetics

### Physicochemical characteristics
Chemical group—Imidazoles.
Molecular weight—531.44.

### Mechanism of action/Effect
Fungistatic; may be fungicidal, depending on concentration; inhibits biosynthesis of ergosterol or other sterols, damaging the fungal cell membrane and altering its permeability; as a result, loss of essential intracellular elements may occur; also inhibits biosynthesis of triglycerides and phospholipids by fungi; in addition, inhibits oxidative and peroxidative enzyme activity, resulting in intracellular buildup of toxic concentrations of hydrogen peroxide, which may contribute to deterioration of subcellular organelles and cellular necrosis. In the treatment of *Candida albicans*, inhibits transformation of blastospores into invasive mycelial form.

### Absorption
No systemic absorption detected at a sensitivity level of 5 nanograms per mL in the blood over a 72-hour period following a single topical application to the chest, back, and arms of normal volunteers.

## Precautions to Consider

### Cross-sensitivity and/or related problems
Persons sensitive to miconazole or other imidazoles may be sensitive to ketoconazole also.

### Carcinogenicity
A long-term feeding study in Swiss albino mice and Wistar rats has shown no evidence of carcinogenicity.

### Mutagenicity
The dominant lethal mutation test in male and female mice, given single oral doses of ketoconazole as high as 80 mg per kg of body weight (mg/kg), has shown no mutations at any stage of germ cell development. The Ames *Salmonella* microsomal activator assay has also shown negative results.

### Pregnancy/Reproduction
Pregnancy—Ketoconazole crosses the placenta. Adequate and well-controlled studies in humans have not been done.
Studies in rats, given oral doses of 80 mg/kg per day (10 times the maximum recommended human dose [MRHD]), have shown ketoconazole to be teratogenic, causing syndactyly and oligodactyly.

FDA Pregnancy Category C.

### Breast-feeding
It is not known whether ketoconazole, applied topically on a regular basis, is absorbed systemically in sufficient amounts to be distributed into breast milk in detectable quantities. However, no systemic absorption was detected following a single application to the chest, back, and arms of healthy volunteers. Therefore, topical ketoconazole is unlikely to be distributed into breast milk in significant amounts or to cause adverse effects in the nursing infant.

### Pediatrics
No information is available on the relationship of age to the effects of this medicine in pediatric patients. Safety and efficacy have not been established.

### Geriatrics
No information is available on the relationship of age to the effects of this medicine in geriatric patients.

### Medical considerations/Contraindications
The medical considerations/contraindications included here have been selected on the basis of their potential clinical significance (reasons given in parentheses where appropriate)—not necessarily inclusive (» = major clinical significance).

*Risk-benefit should be considered when the following medical problem exists:*
Sensitivity to topical ketoconazole

## Side/Adverse Effects
The following side/adverse effects have been selected on the basis of their potential clinical significance (possible signs and symptoms in parentheses where appropriate)—not necessarily inclusive:

**Those indicating need for medical attention**
Incidence more frequent
*Itching, stinging, or irritation not present before therapy*

## Patient Consultation
As an aid to patient consultation, refer to *Advice for the Patient, Ketoconazole (Topical)*.

In providing consultation, consider emphasizing the following selected information (» = major clinical significance):

**Before using this medication**
» Conditions affecting use, especially:
  Sensitivity to topical ketoconazole
  Pregnancy—Ketoconazole crosses the placenta; studies in animals found ketoconazole to be teratogenic

**Proper use of this medication**
» Avoiding contact with the eyes
» Proper dosing
  Missed dose: Applying as soon as possible; not applying if almost time for next dose
» Proper storage
*For the cream form*
  Applying sufficient medication to cover affected and surrounding areas, and rubbing in gently
» Compliance with full course of therapy; fungal infections may require prolonged therapy
*For the shampoo form*
  Wetting hair and scalp with water
  Applying adequate shampoo for lather and massaging in for approximately 1 minute
  Rinsing and repeating application
  Leaving shampoo on an additional 3 minutes
  Rinsing thoroughly and drying hair

**Precautions while using this medication**
*For the cream form*
  Checking with physician if no improvement within 2 to 4 weeks
» Using hygienic measures to cure infection and prevent reinfection
*For tinea pedis*
  Carefully drying feet, especially between toes, after bathing
  Not wearing socks made from wool or synthetic materials; wearing clean, cotton socks and changing them daily or more often if feet perspire excessively
  Wearing sandals or well-ventilated shoes
  Using a bland, absorbent powder or an antifungal powder between toes, on feet, and in socks and shoes liberally once or twice daily; using the powder between administration times for the cream
*For tinea cruris*
  Not wearing underwear that is tight-fitting or made from synthetic materials; wearing loose-fitting cotton underwear instead
  Using a bland, absorbent powder or an antifungal powder on the skin between administration times for the cream

**Side/adverse effects**
  Signs of potential side effects, especially itching, stinging, or irritation

## General Dosing Information
Prolonged use of topical ketoconazole may rarely lead to skin sensitization, resulting in hypersensitivity reactions with subsequent topical or systemic use of the medication.

### For cream dosage form
To reduce the possibility of recurrence of infection, candida, tinea corporis, tinea cruris, and pityriasis versicolor should be treated for at least 2 weeks. Seborrheic dermatitis should be treated for at least 4

weeks or until clinical clearing. Tinea pedis should be treated for approximately 6 weeks.

## Topical Dosage Forms

Note: Bracketed uses in the *Dosage Forms* section refer to categories of use and/or indications that are not included in U.S. product labeling.

### KETOCONAZOLE CREAM

#### Usual adult and adolescent dose
Tinea corporis or
Tinea cruris or
Tinea pedis or
Pityriasis versicolor—
    Topical, to the affected skin and surrounding areas, once a day.
Candidiasis, cutaneous—
    Topical, to the affected skin and surrounding areas, once a day.
Seborrheic dermatitis—
    Topical, to the affected skin and surrounding areas, two times a day.
[Paronychia][1] or
[Tinea barbae][1] or
[Tinea capitis][1]—
    Topical, to the affected skin and surrounding areas, two or three times a day.

#### Usual pediatric dose
Safety and efficacy have not been established.

#### Strength(s) usually available
U.S.—
    2% (Rx) [*Nizoral Cream* (stearyl alcohol; cetyl alcohol; sodium sulfite anhydrous)].

Canada—
    2% (Rx) [*Nizoral Cream*].

### Packaging and storage
Store below 30 °C (86 °F), in a well-closed container, unless otherwise specified by manufacturer. Protect from freezing.

### Auxiliary labeling
• For external use only.
• Continue medicine for full time of treatment.

### KETOCONAZOLE SHAMPOO

#### Usual adult and adolescent dose
Dandruff—
    Topical, as a shampoo, every four days for four weeks, then once every one or two weeks.

#### Usual pediatric dose
Safety and efficacy have not been established.

#### Strength(s) usually available
U.S.—
    2% (Rx) [*Nizoral Shampoo*].
Canada—
    2% (Rx) [*Nizoral Shampoo*].

    [1]Not included in Canadian product labeling.

Revised: 06/21/93

---

**KETOPROFEN—**See *Anti-inflammatory Drugs, Nonsteroidal (Systemic)*

---

# KETOROLAC   Ophthalmic

VA CLASSIFICATION (Primary/Secondary): OP300/OP900

Note: For a listing of dosage forms and brand names by country availability, see *Dosage Forms* section(s). For a listing of brand names for the articles in this monograph, refer to the General Index.

## Category
Anti-inflammatory, nonsteroidal (ophthalmic); antipruritic (ophthalmic).

## Indications
Note: Bracketed information in the *Indications* section refers to uses that are not included in U.S. product labeling.

### Accepted
Conjunctivitis, allergic (treatment)[1]—Ketorolac ophthalmic is indicated for the treatment of ocular itching caused by seasonal allergic conjunctivitis.

[Inflammation, ocular (prophylaxis and treatment)]—Ketorolac ophthalmic is indicated for the prophylaxis and treatment of postoperative ocular inflammation in patients undergoing cataract extraction with or without implantation of an intraocular lens.

    [1]Not included in Canadian product labeling.

## Pharmacology/Pharmacokinetics

### Physicochemical characteristics
Molecular weight—Ketorolac tromethamine: 376.41.
Osmolality—290 mOsmol per kg.
pKa—3.5.
pH—7.4.

### Mechanism of action/Effect
Ketorolac is a nonsteroidal anti-inflammatory drug (NSAID) that is chemically related to indomethacin and tolmetin. Ocular administration of ketorolac reduces prostaglandin $E_2$ levels in aqueous humor, secondary to inhibition of prostaglandin biosynthesis.

### Other actions/effects
Ketorolac ophthalmic has no significant effect on intraocular pressure.

### Absorption
Negligible.

### Distribution
Plasma—In a study where 26 subjects were administered 1 drop of 0.5% ketorolac ophthalmic solution in 1 eye 3 times a day for 21 days, 5 of 26 subjects had detectable (greater than 10 nanograms per mL) plasma levels of 11 to 22 nanograms per mL of ketorolac when they were tested 15 minutes after the first dose on day 10. When the subjects were tested on day 24, none had detectable plasma levels. In comparison, 10 mg of systemic ketorolac administered every 6 hours results in a steady state plasma level of approximately 960 nanograms per mL.
Aqueous humor—Eight of 9 patients administered 2 drops of 0.5% ketorolac ophthalmic solution in each eye 12 hours and 1 hour prior to cataract extraction had detectable (greater than or equal to 40 nanograms per mL) levels of 40 to 170 nanograms per mL (mean concentration 95 nanograms per mL) of ketorolac in the aqueous humor.

## Precautions to Consider

### Cross-sensitivity and/or related problems
Patients sensitive to aspirin; phenylacetic acid derivatives, such as diclofenac; or other systemic or ophthalmic nonsteroidal anti-inflammatory drugs (NSAIDs) may be sensitive to ketorolac also.

### Tumorigenicity
No evidence of tumorigenicity was found in an 18-month study in mice given oral doses of ketorolac equivalent to the parenteral maximum recommended human dose (MRHD) and a 24-month study in rats given oral doses of ketorolac equivalent to 2.5 times the parenteral MRHD.

### Mutagenicity
Ketorolac was not mutagenic in the Ames test, the unscheduled DNA synthesis and repair test, and in forward mutation assays. In addition, ketorolac did not cause chromosome breakage in the *in vivo* mouse micronucleus assay. However, at 1590 mcg per mL and higher concentrations of ketorolac, there was an increased incidence of chromosomal aberrations in Chinese hamster ovarian cells.

### Pregnancy/Reproduction
Fertility—Male and female rats given ketorolac at oral doses of 9 mg per kg of body weight (mg/kg) and 16 mg/kg, respectively, did not show impairment of fertility.

Pregnancy—Adequate and well-controlled studies in humans have not been done.
Studies in rabbits and rats given ketorolac at oral doses of 3.6 mg/kg a day and 10 mg/kg a day, respectively, during organogenesis did not

show evidence of teratogenicity. However, rats given oral doses of 1.5 mg/kg after gestation day 17 had a higher pup mortality rate.

FDA Pregnancy Category C.

Labor—Rats given oral doses of 1.5 mg/kg of ketorolac after gestation day 17 developed dystocia.

### Breast-feeding
Problems in humans have not been documented.

### Pediatrics
Appropriate studies on the relationship of age to the effects of ophthalmic ketorolac have not been performed in the pediatric population. Safety and efficacy have not been established.

### Geriatrics
Appropriate studies on the relationship of age to the effects of ophthalmic ketorolac have not been performed in the geriatric population. However, no geriatrics-specific problems have been documented to date.

### Drug interactions and/or related problems
The following drug interactions and/or related problems have been selected on the basis of their potential clinical significance (possible mechanism in parentheses where appropriate)—not necessarily inclusive (» = major clinical significance):

Note: Combinations containing any of the following medications, depending on the amount present, may also interact with this medication.

Any medication that may interfere with blood clotting or prolong bleeding time, such as:
Anticoagulants, coumarin- or indandione-derivative, or
Heparin or
Platelet aggregation inhibitors
(ophthalmic NSAIDs, such as ketorolac, may also increase the tendency to bleed; concurrent use may increase the risk of postoperative ocular bleeding)

### Medical considerations/Contraindications
The medical considerations/contraindications included here have been selected on the basis of their potential clinical significance (reasons given in parentheses where appropriate)—not necessarily inclusive (» = major clinical significance).

*Risk-benefit should be considered when the following medical problems exist:*

Hemophilia or other bleeding problems or coagulation defects or
Prolonged bleeding time
(increased risk of bleeding following ocular surgery)
Sensitivity to ophthalmic ketorolac

## Side/Adverse Effects
The following side/adverse effects have been selected on the basis of their potential clinical significance (possible signs and symptoms in parentheses where appropriate)—not necessarily inclusive:

### Those indicating need for medical attention
Incidence less frequent or rare
*Hypersensitivity* (itching, rash, redness, swelling, or other sign of irritation not present before therapy); *keratitis, superficial* (redness of the clear part of the eye); *ocular irritation* (itching, redness, tearing, or other sign of eye irritation not present before use of this medicine or becoming worse during use)

### Those indicating need for medical attention only if they continue or are bothersome
Incidence more frequent
*Stinging or burning upon instillation of medication*

## Patient Consultation
As an aid to patient consultation, refer to *Advice for the Patient, Ketorolac (Ophthalmic).*

In providing consultation, consider emphasizing the following selected information (» = major clinical significance):

### Before using this medication
» Conditions affecting use, especially:
Sensitivity to ophthalmic or systemic ketorolac; aspirin; phenylacetic acid derivatives, such as diclofenac; or other systemic or ophthalmic nonsteroidal anti-inflammatory drugs (NSAIDs)

### Proper use of this medication
Proper administration; using a second drop if necessary; not touching applicator tip to any surface; keeping container tightly closed
» Proper dosing
Missed dose: Using as soon as possible; not using if almost time for next dose; using next dose at regularly scheduled time; not doubling doses
» Proper storage

### Precautions while using this medication
Checking with doctor if symptoms do not improve or if they become worse
Expecting stinging or burning of eye upon administration of medication

### Side/adverse effects
Signs of potential side effects, especially hypersensitivity; keratitis, superficial; or ocular irritation

## General Dosing Information
The manufacturer recommends that patients not wear soft contact lenses during treatment with ketorolac ophthalmic solution. However, medical experts do not believe this precaution is necessary unless the patient has corneal epithelial problems and the medication is to be used more often than once every 1 to 2 hours. No significant problems have been documented with ophthalmic solutions that contain 0.03% or less of benzalkonium chloride as a preservative and are used as eye drops in patients with no significant corneal surface problems.

Ketorolac ophthalmic may be administered in conjunction with other ophthalmic medications, such as antibiotics, beta-adrenergic blocking agents, carbonic anhydrase inhibitors, cycloplegics, and mydriatics.

## Ophthalmic Dosage Forms
Note: Bracketed uses in the *Dosage Forms* section refer to categories of use and/or indications that are not included in U.S. product labeling.

### KETOROLAC TROMETHAMINE OPHTHALMIC SOLUTION

#### Usual adult and adolescent dose
Conjunctivitis, allergic (treatment)[1]—
Topical, to the conjunctiva, 1 drop in each eye four times a day.
[Inflammation, ocular (prophylaxis and treatment)]—
Topical, to the conjunctiva, 1 drop in each eye every six to eight hours beginning twenty-four hours before surgery and continuing for three to four weeks.

#### Usual pediatric dose
Safety and efficacy have not been established.

#### Strength(s) usually available
U.S.—
0.5% (Rx) [*Acular* (benzalkonium chloride 0.01%)].
Canada—
0.5% (Rx) [*Acular* (benzalkonium chloride)].

#### Packaging and storage
Store between 15 and 30 °C (59 and 86 °F), unless otherwise specified by manufacturer. Protect from light.

#### Auxiliary labeling
• For the eye.

---

[1]Not included in Canadian product labeling.

## Selected Bibliography
Ketorolac for seasonal allergic conjunctivitis. Med Lett Drugs Ther 1993 Sep 17; 35 (905): 88-9.

Tinkelman DG, Rupp G, Kaufman H, et al. Double-masked, paired-comparison clinical study of ketorolac tromethamine 0.5% ophthalmic solution compared with placebo eyedrops in the treatment of seasonal allergic conjunctivitis. Surv Ophthalmol 1993 Jul-Aug; 38 suppl: 133-40.

Ballas Z, Blumenthal M, Tinkelman DG, et al. Clinical evaluation of ketorolac tromethamine 0.5% ophthalmic solution for the treatment of seasonal allergic conjunctivitis. Surv Ophthalmol 1993 Jul-Aug; 38 suppl: 141-8.

---

Developed: 08/11/94

# KETOROLAC Systemic

VA CLASSIFICATION (Primary):

Note: For a listing of dosage forms and brand names by country availability, see *Dosage Forms* section(s). For a listing of brand names for the articles in this monograph, refer to the General Index.

## Category

Analgesic.

## Indications

Note: Ketorolac, like other nonsteroidal anti-inflammatory drugs (NSAIDs), has antipyretic and anti-inflammatory, as well as analgesic actions. However, indications for specific NSAIDs may vary because of lack of specific testing and/or clinical-use data as well as the toxicity of the individual agent.

### Accepted

Pain (treatment)—Ketorolac is indicated for the short-term management of moderately severe acute pain that would otherwise require treatment with an opioid analgesic. It is most commonly used to relieve postoperative pain. The oral dosage form is indicated only for continuation of therapy following initial parenteral administration. Because the risk of gastrointestinal bleeding and other severe adverse effects increases with the duration of treatment, **ketorolac should not be administered by any route or combination of routes for longer than 5 days**.

Before ketorolac is used perioperatively, its platelet aggregation–inhibiting activity, which increases the risk of bleeding, must be considered. Postoperative hematomas and other signs of wound bleeding have been reported in ketorolac-treated patients. Therefore, **ketorolac should not be given prior to major surgery to prevent postoperative pain; nor should it be administered intraoperatively when control of bleeding is critical**. Also, ketorolac lacks the sedative and anti-anxiety activity usually desired in a preoperative medication.

### Unaccepted

Although ketorolac may be used for short-term (up to 5 days) treatment of moderately severe acute arthritic pain in patients who are not receiving chronic treatment with other NSAIDs, it is not recommended for the long-term treatment of chronic rheumatic disease.

Ketorolac is not recommended for treatment of mild pain or for long-term treatment of chronic pain.

Ketorolac is not recommended for obstetrical analgesia because its safety has not been studied adequately. Inhibition of prostaglandin synthesis by NSAIDs such as ketorolac may decrease uterine contractility, increase the risk of intrauterine bleeding, and/or cause premature constriction of the fetal ductus arteriosus.

## Pharmacology/Pharmacokinetics

### Physicochemical characteristics

Molecular weight—376.41.

$pKa$—3.5.

### Mechanism of action/Effect

Ketorolac is a nonsteroidal anti-inflammatory drug (NSAID) chemically related to indomethacin and tolmetin. Currently available NSAIDs inhibit the activity of the enzyme cyclo-oxygenase, leading to decreased formation of precursors of prostaglandins and thromboxanes from arachidonic acid. The resultant reduction in prostaglandin synthesis and activity may be at least partially responsible for many of the adverse, as well as the therapeutic, effects of these medications. Analgesia is probably produced via a peripheral action in which blockade of pain impulse generation results from decreased prostaglandin activity. However, inhibition of the synthesis or actions of other substances that sensitize pain receptors to mechanical or chemical stimulation may also contribute to the analgesic effect.

### Other actions/effects

Ketorolac has anti-inflammatory and antipyretic actions that, together with its analgesic effects, may mask the onset and/or progression of an infection.

Ketorolac inhibits platelet aggregation. This effect is reversible (unlike aspirin-induced platelet inhibition, which persists for the life of the exposed platelets). Recovery of platelet function usually occurs within 24 to 48 hours following discontinuation of ketorolac.

Like other NSAIDs, ketorolac may cause gastrointestinal ulceration and bleeding. These effects probably result from ketorolac-induced reduction of the synthesis and activity of prostaglandins that exert a protective effect on the gastrointestinal mucosa; they may occur after parenteral as well as after oral administration. However, when administered orally, this acidic medication probably also exerts a direct irritant or erosive effect on the mucosa.

Like other NSAIDs, ketorolac may cause renal toxicity (i.e., sodium and fluid retention, decreased renal perfusion, and decreased renal function), probably by inhibiting the synthesis and activity of renal prostaglandins, which are directly involved in the maintenance of renal hemodynamics and sodium and fluid balance. Renal prostaglandins are especially important in maintaining renal function in the presence of generalized vasoconstriction or volume depletion.

### Absorption

Intramuscular—Rapid and complete.

Oral—Rapid (more rapid than after intramuscular administration in some individuals) and complete. The rate, but not the extent, of absorption is decreased when the medication is taken with a high fat meal. Absorption is not altered by concurrent administration with an antacid.

### Distribution

The volume of distribution ($Vol_D$) of racemic ketorolac in patients with normal renal function is 0.15 to 0.33 L per kg of body weight. In patients with renal function impairment, the $Vol_D$ of the active S-enantiomer of ketorolac is twice as large as in individuals with normal renal function, and the $Vol_D$ of the inactive R-enantiomer is approximately 20% larger. Penetration of ketorolac across the blood-brain barrier is poor; concentrations in cerebrospinal fluid are 0.2%, or less, of those achieved in plasma.

In breast milk—Maximum concentrations of 7.3 nanograms per mL (0.019 micromoles/L) 2 hours after the first dose and 7.9 nanograms per mL (0.021 micromoles/L) 2 hours after the fifth dose were measured in the breast milk of women receiving 10 mg of ketorolac, orally, 4 times a day. However, in 40% of the subjects tested, the concentration in breast milk did not reach the lowest detection limit of 5 nanograms per mL (0.013 micromoles/L).

### Protein binding

Very high (> 99%).

### Biotransformation

Primarily hepatic. Less than 50% of a dose is metabolized. The major metabolites are a glucuronide conjugate, which may also be formed in the kidney, and *p*-hydroxy ketorolac. Neither metabolite has significant analgesic activity.

### Half-life

Terminal—

Individuals with normal renal function—

About 5.3 hours in healthy young adults (ranges, 3.5 to 9.2 hours after 30 mg intramuscularly, 4 to 7.2 hours after 30 mg intravenously, and 2.4 to 9.0 hours after 10 mg orally). Mean values are higher in healthy geriatric subjects, but remain within the same ranges reported for younger adults. Hepatic function impairment does not significantly prolong the half-life.

Patients with renal function impairment—

About 10.3 to 10.8 hours in patients with a serum creatinine of 1.9 to 5 mg per 100 mL (168 to 442 micromoles/L) (ranges, 5.9 to 19.2 hours after 30 mg intramuscularly and 3.4 to 18.9 hours after 10 mg orally). Values are even higher in patients receiving renal dialysis (13.6 [range, 8 to 39.1] hours after 30 mg intramuscularly).

Note: The above values apply to racemic ketorolac. In patients with normal renal function, terminal half-life values for the active S-enantiomer and the inactive R-enantiomer are approximately 2.5 hours and 5 hours, respectively.

### Onset of action

Dose-dependent; generally within 30 minutes to 1 hour.

### Time to peak plasma concentration

Intramuscular—

Single dose of up to 60 mg—30 to 60 minutes.

Intravenous—

Single 15-mg dose: 1.1 ± 0.7 minutes.

Single 30-mg dose: 2.9 ± 1.8 minutes.

Oral—

Single 10-mg dose—44 ± 34 minutes.

### Time to steady-state plasma concentration

Intramuscular or oral—About 24 hours, when the medication is administered at 6-hour intervals.

## Steady-state plasma concentration

With administration 4 times a day at 6-hour intervals—

Intramuscular—

   15 mg—Average, 0.94 ± 0.29 mcg/mL (2.5 ± 0.77 micromoles/L).
   30 mg—Average, 1.88 ± 0.59 mcg/mL (5 ± 1.57 micromoles/L).

Intravenous—

   15 mg—Average, 1.09 ± 0.3 mcg/mL (2.89 ± 0.8 micromoles/L).
   30 mg—Average, 2.17 ± 0.59 mcg/mL (5.77 ± 1.57 micromoles/L).

Oral—

   10 mg—Average, 0.59 ± 0.2 mcg/mL (1.57 ± 0.53 micromoles/L).

Note: Determination of minimum (trough) concentrations for each of the above routes of administration has shown that ketorolac concentrations do not decrease to subtherapeutic levels between doses.

## Peak plasma concentration

Following administration of a single dose—

| Route* | Dose (mg) | Concentration | |
|---|---|---|---|
| | | mcg/mL | micromoles/L |
| IM | 15 | 1.14 ± 0.32 | 3.03 ± 0.85 |
| | 30 | 2.42 ± 0.68 | 6.44 ± 1.81 |
| | 60 | 4.5 ± 1.27 | 11.97 ± 3.38 |
| IV | 15 | 2.47 ± 0.51 | 6.57 ± 1.36 |
| | 30 | 4.65 ± 0.96 | 12.37 ± 2.55 |
| PO | 10 | 0.87 ± 0.22 | 2.31 ± 0.58 |

*IM = intramuscular; IV = intravenous; PO = oral.

## Therapeutic plasma concentration

0.3 mcg/mL (0.8 micromoles/L), at steady-state.

## Time to peak effect

Intramuscular or intravenous—1 to 2 hours.
Oral—2 to 3 hours.

## Duration of action

Intramuscular—

   6 hours or longer in approximately 50% of patients receiving a single 10-mg dose and in approximately 60% of patients receiving a single 30-mg dose in clinical studies.

Oral—

   Approximately 4 hours in 75 to 80% of patients and 6 hours or longer in about 65% of patients receiving a single 10-mg dose in clinical studies.

## Elimination

91% renal; approximately 6% biliary/fecal. The active S-enantiomer is cleared approximately twice as rapidly as the inactive R-enantiomer. Average total clearance rates following administration of a single dose—

Healthy young adults:

   Intramuscular, 30 mg—0.023 (range, 0.01 to 0.046) liters per hour per kg of body weight (L/hr/kg).
   Intravenous, 30 mg—0.03 (range, 0.017 to 0.051) L/hr/kg.
   Oral, 10 mg—0.025 (range, 0.013 to 0.05) L/hr/kg.

Elderly adults:

   Intramuscular, 30 mg—0.019 (range, 0.013 to 0.034) L/hr/kg.
   Oral, 10 mg—0.024 (range, 0.018 to 0.034) L/hr/kg.

Patients with hepatic function impairment:

   Intramuscular, 30 mg—0.029 (range, 0.13 to 0.066) L/hr/kg.
   Oral, 10 mg—0.033 (range, 0.019 to 0.051) L/hr/kg.

Patients with renal function impairment:

   Serum creatinine 1.9 to 5 mg/100 mL (168 to 442 micromoles/L)—

      Intramuscular, 30 mg: 0.015 (range, 0.005 to 0.043) L/hr/kg.
      Oral, 10 mg: 0.016 (range, 0.007 to 0.052) L/hr/kg.

   Renal dialysis patients:

      Intravenous, 30 mg: 0.016 (range, 0.003 to 0.036) L/hr/kg.

In dialysis—

   Hemodialysis does not remove significant quantities of ketorolac from the body.

# Precautions to Consider

## Cross-sensitivity and/or related problems

Patients sensitive to aspirin or other nonsteroidal anti-inflammatory drugs (NSAIDs) may be sensitive to ketorolac also. Severe asthmatic and anaphylactoid reactions have occurred in such patients.

## Tumorigenicity

No evidence of tumorigenicity was found in an 18-month study in mice receiving up to 2 mg per kg of body weight (mg/kg) per day or a 24-month study in rats receiving up to 5 mg/kg per day orally. These doses are considered, on the basis of area under the concentration-time curve (AUC) comparisons, to be equivalent to 0.9 and 0.5 times, respectively, the human exposure resulting from intramuscular or intravenous administration of 30 mg 4 times a day.

## Mutagenicity

No evidence of mutagenicity was found in the Ames test, unscheduled DNA synthesis and repair, and forward mutation assays. Also, ketorolac did not cause chromosome breakage in the *in vivo* mouse micronucleus assay. However, in a concentration of 1590 mcg per mL (mcg/mL) (approximately 1000 times average human plasma concentrations), ketorolac increased the occurrence of chromosomal aberrations in Chinese hamster ovarian cells.

## Pregnancy/Reproduction

Fertility—No impairment of fertility was observed in male rats given 9 mg/kg per day or female rats given 16 mg/kg per day, orally (53.1 and 50 mg per square meter of body surface area [mg/m$^2$] per day). These doses are equivalent to 0.9 and 1.6 times, respectively, the human exposure resulting from intramuscular or intravenous administration of 30 mg 4 times a day, based on AUC comparisons.

Pregnancy—

*First trimester—*

   Adequate and well-controlled studies have not been done in pregnant women.
   No teratogenicity occurred in offspring of rabbits receiving oral doses of up to 3.6 mg/kg per day (42.35 mg/m$^2$ per day; equivalent to 0.37 times the human exposure resulting from intramuscular or intravenous administration of 30 mg 4 times a day, based on AUC comparisons) or rats receiving up to 10 mg/kg per day (59 mg/m$^2$ per day; equivalent to the human exposure, based on AUC comparisons).

*Second and third trimesters—*

   Although studies in pregnant women have not been done with ketorolac, chronic use of any NSAID during the second half of pregnancy is not recommended because of possible adverse effects in the fetus, such as premature closure of the ductus arteriosus, which may lead to persistent pulmonary hypertension in the newborn. Such effects have been documented in animal studies with other NSAIDs.
   Chronic administration of 1.5 mg/kg per day (8.8 mg/m$^2$ per day) of ketorolac to rats after Day 17 of gestation caused dystocia and higher pup mortality. This dose is equivalent to 0.14 times the human exposure resulting from intramuscular or intravenous administration of 30 mg 4 times a day, based on AUC comparisons. Higher doses (9 mg/kg or more per day, administered to rats from Day 15 of gestation) significantly increased the length of gestation, in addition to increasing the incidence of maternal deaths associated with dystocia and decreasing birth weights and survival rates in the offspring.

   FDA Pregnancy Category C.

Labor and delivery—Although a few studies have investigated the use of ketorolac in obstetrics, it is not recommended for obstetrical preoperative medication or obstetrical analgesia. When administered during labor, ketorolac crosses the placenta and inhibits platelet aggregation in the neonate. Also, potential adverse effects on uterine contractility and the fetal ductus arteriosus, resulting in a risk of increased uterine bleeding and fetal circulatory disturbances, respectively, must be considered.

## Breast-feeding

Because of potential adverse effects in the nursing infant, use of ketorolac by nursing mothers is not recommended. Ketorolac is distributed into breast milk in small quantities. Maximum concentrations of 7.3 nanograms per mL (nanograms/mL) (0.019 micromoles/L) 2 hours after the first dose and 7.9 nanograms/mL (0.021 micromoles/L) 2 hours after the fifth dose were measured in the breast milk of women receiving 10 mg of ketorolac, orally, 4 times a day, although the concentration in breast milk failed to reach the lowest detection limit of 5 nanograms/mL (0.013 micromoles/L) in 40% of the subjects tested. Milk-to-plasma concentration ratios of 0.037 and 0.025 have been calculated after administration of a single dose and at steady-state, respectively.

## Pediatrics

No information is available on the relationship of age to the effects of ketorolac in pediatric patients. Safety and efficacy in patients younger than 16 years of age have not been established.

## Geriatrics

Studies have shown that clearance of ketorolac is reduced in healthy individuals 65 years of age or older, leading to significant prolongation of the elimination half-life. Also, geriatric patients are more likely to have age-related renal function impairment, which may further reduce ketorolac clearance and increase the risk of NSAID-induced renal or hepatic toxicity. The risk of gastrointestinal ulceration, bleeding, and perforation is higher in elderly patients receiving ketorolac than in younger adults. Also, ketorolac-induced gastrointestinal ulceration and/or bleeding is more likely to cause serious consequences, including fatalities, in geriatric patients. It is recommended that ketorolac be used with caution, in the lower of the recommended dosage regimens, and with careful monitoring of the patient.

### Drug interactions and/or related problems

The following drug interactions and/or related problems have been selected on the basis of their potential clinical significance (possible mechanism in parentheses where appropriate)—not necessarily inclusive (» = major clinical significance):

Note: Combinations containing any of the following medications, depending on the amount present, may also interact with this medication.

All of the interactions listed below have not been documented with ketorolac. However, they have been reported with other NSAIDs and should be considered potential precautions to the use of ketorolac also.

In addition to the interactions listed below, the possibility should be considered that additive or multiple effects leading to impaired blood clotting and/or increased risk of bleeding may occur if any NSAID is used concurrently with any medication having a significant potential for causing hypoprothrombinemia, thrombocytopenia, or gastrointestinal ulceration or hemorrhage.

Acetaminophen
(prolonged concurrent use of acetaminophen with an NSAID may increase the risk of adverse renal effects; it is recommended that patients be under close medical supervision while receiving such combined therapy)

Alcohol or
Corticosteroids, glucocorticoid or
Corticotropin (chronic therapeutic use) or
Potassium supplements
(concurrent use with an NSAID may increase the risk of gastrointestinal side effects, including ulceration or hemorrhage)

» Anticoagulants, coumarin- or indandione-derivative or
» Heparin or
» Thrombolytic agents, such as:
Alteplase
Anistreplase
Streptokinase
Urokinase
(ketorolac has not been shown to alter the pharmacokinetic or pharmacodynamic properties of warfarin or heparin; however, inhibition of platelet aggregation by ketorolac, and the potential occurrence of ketorolac-induced gastrointestinal ulceration or bleeding, may be hazardous to patients receiving anticoagulant or thrombolytic therapy; caution and careful monitoring of the patient are recommended, as there is evidence that administration of ketorolac to patients receiving an anticoagulant, possibly including low [prophylactic] doses of heparin [2500 to 5000 Units every 12 hours], increases the risk of bleeding and intramuscular hematoma formation)

Antihypertensives or
Diuretics
(increased monitoring of the response to any antihypertensive agent may be advisable when ketorolac is used concurrently because several other NSAIDs have been shown to reduce or reverse the effects of many antihypertensives, possibly by inhibiting renal prostaglandin synthesis and/or by causing sodium and fluid retention)

(NSAIDs may decrease the diuretic and natriuretic, as well as the antihypertensive, effects of diuretics, probably by inhibiting renal prostaglandin synthesis; ketorolac inhibited the diuretic effect of furosemide, decreasing sodium and urine output by about 20%, in a study in normovolemic healthy subjects)

(concurrent use of an NSAID and a diuretic may also increase the risk of renal failure secondary to a decrease in renal blood flow caused by inhibition of renal prostaglandin synthesis)

(concurrent use of ketorolac with an angiotensin-converting enzyme [ACE] inhibitor may also increase the risk of renal function impairment, especially in hypovolemic patients)

» Aspirin or other salicylates or
» Other NSAIDs
(concurrent use of aspirin or other salicylates or NSAIDs with ketorolac is not recommended because of the potential for additive toxicity)

(concurrent use of ketorolac with antirheumatic doses of salicylates other than aspirin should be undertaken with caution and in reduced doses because therapeutic plasma concentrations of salicylate [30 mg per 100 mL (2.17 mmol per L)] decrease the protein binding of ketorolac sufficiently to potentially double the plasma concentration of free [unbound] ketorolac)

» Cefamandole or
» Cefoperazone or
» Cefotetan or
» Plicamycin or
» Valproic acid
(these medications may cause hypoprothrombinemia; in addition, plicamycin or valproic acid may inhibit platelet aggregation; concurrent use with an NSAID may increase the risk of bleeding because of additive interferences with blood clotting and/or the potential occurrence of gastrointestinal ulceration or hemorrhage during NSAID therapy)

Gold compounds
(although other NSAIDs are commonly used concurrently with gold compounds in the treatment of arthritis, the possibility should be considered that concurrent use of a gold compound with any NSAID, including ketorolac, may increase the risk of adverse renal effects)

» Lithium
(although the effect of ketorolac on lithium plasma concentration has not been studied, increases in lithium concentration have been reported during concomitant administration of ketorolac; increased monitoring of lithium plasma concentrations is recommended during and following concurrent use so that lithium dosage can be adjusted if necessary)

» Methotrexate
(the effect of ketorolac on methotrexate concentrations and/or toxicity has not been studied; however, administration of moderate- or high-dose methotrexate infusions to patients receiving other NSAIDs has resulted in severe, sometimes fatal, methotrexate toxicity, possibly because NSAIDs may reduce renal function, thereby decreasing methotrexate excretion; it is recommended that ketorolac not be administered for 24 hours prior to, and for at least 12 hours [or until the methotrexate plasma concentration has decreased to a nontoxic level] following, a high-dose methotrexate infusion)

(severe, sometimes fatal, methotrexate toxicity has also been reported with the relatively low to moderate doses of methotrexate used in the treatment of rheumatoid arthritis or psoriasis when an NSAID was given concurrently; it is recommended that concurrent use of ketorolac with low to moderate doses of methotrexate also be undertaken with caution, with methotrexate dosage being adjusted as determined by monitoring plasma methotrexate concentration and/or adequacy of the patient's renal function)

Nephrotoxic medications, other (See *Appendix II*)
(concurrent use with an NSAID may increase the risk and/or severity of adverse renal effects)

Platelet aggregation inhibitors, other (See *Appendix II*)
(concurrent use of any of these medications with an NSAID, including ketorolac, may increase the risk of bleeding because of additive inhibition of platelet aggregation as well as the potential occurrence of gastrointestinal ulceration or hemorrhage during NSAID therapy)

» Probenecid
(concurrent use with ketorolac is not recommended because probenecid decreases elimination of ketorolac, resulting in significantly increased ketorolac plasma concentrations [the area under the concentration-time curve (AUC) being increased about 3-fold, from 5.4 to 17.8 mcg per hour per mL] and half-life [which is more than doubled, to about 15 hours])

### Laboratory value alterations

The following have been selected on the basis of their potential clinical significance (possible effect in parentheses where appropriate)—not necessarily inclusive (» = major clinical significance):

With physiology/laboratory test values
Bleeding time
(may be prolonged because ketorolac inhibits platelet aggregation; effects may persist for 24 to 48 hours after discontinuation of therapy)

Blood urea nitrogen (BUN) or
Creatinine, serum, or
Potassium, serum
(may be increased)

Liver function tests, especially serum transaminase activity
(although borderline elevations in test values may occur in up to 15% of patients receiving ketorolac, significant elevations [3 times the upper limit] of serum transaminases have occurred in fewer than 1%; ketorolac therapy should be discontinued if significant abnormalities occur)

**Medical considerations/Contraindications**
The medical considerations/contraindications included here have been selected on the basis of their potential clinical significance (reasons given in parentheses where appropriate)—not necessarily inclusive (» = major clinical significance).

*Except under special circumstances, this medication should not be used when the following medical problems exist:*
» Cerebrovascular bleeding, suspected or confirmed or
» Hemophilia or other bleeding problems including coagulation or platelet function disorders
(increased risk of bleeding because ketorolac inhibits platelet aggregation and may also cause gastrointestinal ulceration or hemorrhage)
» Gastrointestinal bleeding, active, recent, or history of or
» Gastrointestinal perforation, recent or
» Peptic ulceration, ulcerative colitis, or other ulcerative gastrointestinal disease, active or history of
(increased risk of gastrointestinal ulceration, perforation, and/or hemorrhage)
» Nasal polyps associated with bronchospasm, aspirin-induced, or angioedema, anaphylaxis, or other severe allergic reaction induced by aspirin, ketorolac, or other NSAIDs, history of
(high risk of severe allergic reactions because of cross-sensitivity)
» Renal function impairment, severe
(increased risk of renal failure)

*Risk-benefit should be considered when the following medical problems exist:*
» Allergic reaction, mild, such as allergic rhinitis, urticaria, or skin rash, induced by aspirin, ketorolac, or other NSAIDs, history of
(possibility of cross-sensitivity)
Asthma
(may be exacerbated)
Cholestasis or
Hepatitis, active
(although other forms of hepatic function impairment apparently do not alter the clearance of ketorolac, studies to assess the possible effect of cholestasis or active hepatitis on the pharmacokinetics of the medication have not been done)
Conditions predisposing to gastrointestinal toxicity, such as:
Alcoholism, active or
» Inflammatory bowel disease or
Tobacco use, or recent history of
(caution and close supervision are recommended for patients in whom there is a significant risk of gastrointestinal toxicity; misoprostol or sucralfate should be considered as prophylaxis for those at high risk)
Conditions predisposing to and/or exacerbated by fluid retention, such as:
Compromised cardiac function or
Congestive heart disease or
Edema, pre-existing or
Hypertension
(ketorolac may cause fluid retention and edema)
Congestive heart failure or
Diabetes mellitus or
Edema, pre-existing or
Hepatic function impairment or
» Hypovolemia or
Sepsis
(increased risk of renal failure; caution and monitoring of urine output, serum urea, and serum creatinine are advised; hypovolemia should be corrected before ketorolac therapy is initiated)
(hepatotoxicity, as indicated by significant abnormalities in liver function tests, is more likely to occur in patients with pre-existing hepatic function impairment)
» Renal function impairment, mild to moderate
(ketorolac and its metabolites are excreted primarily via the kidney, which may also be a site of ketorolac metabolism; a substantial reduction in ketorolac clearance, leading to significant prolongation of its half-life, has been demonstrated in patients with renal function impairment; a reduction in dosage is recommended for patients with moderate elevations of serum creatinine)

(caution and careful monitoring of the patient are also recommended because of possible patient predisposition toward development of NSAID-induced adverse renal effects, including acute renal failure)
Systemic lupus erythematosus (SLE)
(increased risk of renal function impairment)

# Side/Adverse Effects

Note: Ketorolac shares the risks associated with other nonsteroidal anti-inflammatory drugs (NSAIDs), including gastrointestinal and/or renal toxicity.

The risk of adverse effects increases with the duration of treatment as well as with the total daily dose of ketorolac. Also, side effects are more frequent when plasma concentrations of ketorolac exceed 5 mcg per mL (13.3 micromoles/L). In a long-term study in patients with chronic pain, oral administration of 10 mg 4 times a day of ketorolac caused more gastrointestinal toxicity than 650 mg 4 times a day of aspirin; the frequency of occurrence of gastrointestinal ulceration or bleeding was 0.69% after 3 months and 1.59% after 6 months in patients receiving ketorolac and 0% after 3 months and 0.73% after 6 months in patients receiving aspirin. An unusually large number of cases of upper gastrointestinal bleeding (20% of which were fatal) has been reported with ketorolac, mostly in elderly patients.

Studies have shown that there is also a substantial risk of gastrointestinal bleeding during short-term parenteral administration of ketorolac (a maximum of 20 doses, administered over 5 days), especially in patients older than 65 years of age and/or patients with a history of gastrointestinal perforation, ulcer, or bleeding (PUB). The following percentages of patients experienced clinically significant gastrointestinal bleeding in these studies:

| Patient | | Total dose/day (mg) | | | |
|---|---|---|---|---|---|
| Age (yr) | PUB History | ≤60 | >60– 90 | >90– 120 | >120 |
| <65 | No | 0.4% | 0.4% | 0.9% | 4.6% |
| | Yes | 2.1% | 4.6% | 7.8% | 15.4% |
| ≥65 | No | 1.2% | 2.8% | 2.2% | 7.7% |
| | Yes | 4.7% | 3.7% | 2.8% | 25% |

The following side/adverse effects have been selected on the basis of their potential clinical significance (possible signs and symptoms in parentheses where appropriate)—not necessarily inclusive:

**Those indicating need for medical attention**
Incidence more frequent (4%)
*Edema* (swelling of face, fingers, lower legs, ankles, and/or feet; unusual weight gain)
Incidence less frequent (1 to 3%)
*Hypertension* (high blood pressure); *purpura* (small, red spots on skin; bruising); *skin rash*—rarely including maculopapular rash, or itching; *stomatitis* (sores, ulcers, or white spots on lips or in mouth)
Incidence rare (< 1%)
*Anaphylaxis or anaphylactoid reaction* (changes in facial skin color; skin rash, hives, and/or itching; fast or irregular breathing; puffiness or swelling of the eyelids or around the eyes; shortness of breath, troubled breathing, tightness in chest, and/or wheezing); *anemia* (unusual tiredness or weakness); *aseptic meningitis* (fever; severe headache; drowsiness; confusion; stiff neck and/or back; general feeling of illness; nausea); *asthma, bronchospasm, or dyspnea* (shortness of breath, troubled breathing, tightness in chest, and/or wheezing); *bleeding from wound, postoperatively; bloody stools; blurred vision or other vision change; cholestatic jaundice* (dark urine; fever; itching; light-colored stools; pain, tenderness, and/or swelling in upper abdominal area; skin rash; swollen glands; yellow eyes or skin); *convulsions; edema of tongue; eosinophilia; exfoliative dermatitis* (fever with or without chills; red, thickened, or scaly skin; swollen and/or painful glands; unusual bruising); *fainting; fever; flank pain, with or without hematuria and/or azotemia* (pain in lower back and/or side; bloody or cloudy urine); *gastrointestinal, usually peptic, ulceration, possibly with perforation and/or bleeding* (abdominal pain, cramping, or burning, severe; bloody or black, tarry stools; vomiting of blood or material that looks like coffee grounds; nausea, heartburn, and/or indigestion, severe and continuing); *hallucinations; hearing loss; hemolytic uremic syndrome; hepatitis* (loss of appetite; nausea; vomiting; yellow eyes or skin; swelling in upper abdominal area); *hives; hyperactivity* (restlessness, severe); *hypotension* (low blood pressure); *increase in frequency of urination; increased urine volume; laryngeal edema* (shortness of breath or troubled breathing); *leukopenia* (rarely, fever or chills; cough or hoarseness; lower back or side pain; painful or

difficult urination)—usually asymptomatic; *mental depression; nephritis* (bloody or cloudy urine; increased blood pressure; sudden decrease in amount of urine; swelling of face, fingers, feet, and/or lower legs; rapid weight gain); *nosebleeds; oliguria* (decrease in amount of urine); *pancreatitis, acute* (abdominal pain; fever with or without chills; swelling and/or tenderness in upper abdominal or stomach area); *psychosis* (mood changes; unusual behavior); *pulmonary edema* (difficult, fast, noisy breathing, sometimes with wheezing; blue lips and fingernails; pale skin; increased sweating); *rectal bleeding; renal failure, acute* (increased blood pressure; shortness of breath; troubled breathing, tightness in chest, and/or wheezing; sudden decrease in amount of urine; swelling of face, fingers, feet, and/or lower legs; continuing thirst; unusual tiredness or weakness; weight gain); *rhinitis* (runny nose); *Stevens-Johnson syndrome* (bleeding or crusting sores on lips; chest pain; fever with or without chills; muscle cramps or pain; skin rash; sores, ulcers, or white spots in mouth; sore throat); *thrombocytopenia* (rarely, unusual bleeding or bruising; black, tarry stools; blood in urine or stools; pinpoint red spots on skin)—usually asymptomatic; *tinnitus* (ringing or buzzing in ears); *toxic epidermal necrolysis [Lyell's syndrome]* (redness, tenderness, itching, burning, or peeling of skin; sore throat; fever with or without chills)

Note: *Hemolytic uremic syndrome* is characterized by hemolytic *anemia, renal failure, thrombocytopenia,* and *purpura.* These adverse effects may also occur independently of hemolytic uremic syndrome and are listed separately above.

**Those indicating need for medical attention only if they continue or are bothersome**
Incidence more frequent (> 3%)
*Abdominal pain*—[13%]; *bruising at injection site; diarrhea*—[7%]; *dizziness*—[7%]; *drowsiness*—[6%]; *headache*—[17%]; *indigestion*—[12%]; *nausea*—[12%]

Incidence less frequent (1 to 3%)
*Bloated feeling or gas; burning or pain at injection site; constipation; feeling of fullness in gastrointestinal tract; increased sweating; vomiting*

## Overdose

For specific information on the agents used in the management of ketorolac overdose, see:
• *Antacids (Oral-Local)* monograph;
• *Charcoal, Activated (Oral-Local)* monograph;
• *Histamine H₂-receptor Antagonists (Systemic)* monograph;
• *Misoprostol (Systemic)* monograph;
• *Omeprazole (Systemic)* monograph;
and/or
• *Sucralfate (Oral-Local)* monograph.

For more information on the management of overdose or unintentional ingestion, **contact a Poison Control Center** (see *Poison Control Center Listing*).

Factors that are associated with an increased risk of ketorolac toxicity (in addition to total daily dosage and duration of treatment) include hypovolemia; renal insufficiency; a patient history of gastrointestinal perforation, ulceration, or bleeding; and patient age of 65 years or older.

**Clinical effects of overdose**
The following effects have been selected on the basis of their potential clinical significance (possible signs and symptoms in parentheses where appropriate)—not necessarily inclusive:
*Abdominal pain; gastrointestinal ulceration and bleeding; metabolic acidosis*

**Treatment of overdose**
To decrease absorption—
Administering activated charcoal (if the medication was ingested orally). The initial dose of charcoal may be followed by a cathartic, such as magnesium citrate, if the charcoal is not pre-mixed with sorbitol. Gastric lavage may also be performed.
Induction of emesis may also be helpful.
To enhance elimination—Hemodialysis does not remove significant quantities of ketorolac from the body.
Specific treatment—
For treatment of abdominal pain: Administering an antacid. See the product label or *Antacids (Oral-Local)* for specific dosing guidelines.
For treatment of gastrointestinal ulceration or bleeding: Discontinuing ketorolac therapy immediately. Depending on the site and severity of the ulcer, administering antacids, histamine H₂-receptor antagonists (cimetidine, famotidine, nizatidine, ranitidine), misoprostol, omeprazole, and/or sucralfate. See the package inserts or *Antacids (Oral-Local), Histamine H₂-receptor Antagonists (Systemic), Misoprostol (Systemic), Omeprazole (Systemic),* or *Sucralfate (Oral-Local)* for specific dosing guidelines for these products.

Supportive care—Supportive measures, such as establishing intravenous lines, hydration, administration of plasma volume expanders, and support of ventilatory function, should be instituted as needed. Patients in whom intentional overdose is confirmed or suspected should be referred for psychiatric consultation.

## Patient Consultation

As an aid to patient consultation, refer to *Advice for the Patient, Ketorolac (Systemic).*

In providing consultation, consider emphasizing the following selected information (» = major clinical significance):

**Before using this medication**
» Conditions affecting use, especially:
Sensitivity to ketorolac, aspirin, or any other nonsteroidal anti-inflammatory drug (NSAID)
Pregnancy—Crosses the placenta; use during second half of pregnancy may cause adverse effects on fetal or neonatal blood flow
Breast-feeding—Not recommended because of potential adverse effects in the infant; ketorolac is distributed into breast milk
Use in the elderly—Higher risk of gastrointestinal and/or renal toxicity, possibly because of reduced clearance in addition to increased sensitivity
Other medications, especially anticoagulants, aspirin or other salicylates, other NSAIDs, those cephalosporins that may adversely affect blood clotting, lithium, methotrexate, plicamycin, probenecid, and valproic acid
Other medical problems, especially bleeding (active, history of, or predisposition to), peptic ulcer or other ulcerative or inflammatory gastrointestinal tract disease (active or history of), and renal function impairment

**Proper use of this medication**
Proper administration:
*For oral dosage form*
Taking with food (a meal or snack) to reduce gastrointestinal irritation, or with an antacid
Taking with a full glass of water, then remaining in an upright position for at least 15 to 30 minutes, to reduce risk of esophageal irritation
*For injection*
Proper injection technique (if self-medicating at home)
» Not using more medication than prescribed or using for longer than 5 days
Not saving unused medication for the future, and not sharing it with others
» Proper dosing
Missed dose (scheduled dosing): Using as soon as possible; not using if almost time for next dose; not doubling doses
» Proper storage

**Precautions while using this medication**
» Not using acetaminophen concurrently for more than a few days, and not using aspirin, other salicylates, or other NSAIDs concurrently, unless combination therapy prescribed and monitored by physician or dentist
» Caution if dizziness or drowsiness occurs; not driving, using machines, or doing anything else that requires alertness

**Side/adverse effects**
Signs of potential side effects, especially edema; hypertension; purpura; skin rash or itching; stomatitis; anaphylaxis or anaphylactoid reaction; aseptic meningitis; asthma, bronchospasm, or dyspnea; anemia; aseptic meningitis; bloody stools; blurred vision or other vision change; cholestatic jaundice; convulsions; edema of tongue; exfoliative dermatitis; fainting; fever; flank pain; gastrointestinal ulceration or bleeding; hallucinations; hearing loss; hemolytic uremic syndrome; hepatitis; hives; hyperactivity; hypotension; increase in frequency or volume of urination; laryngeal edema; leukopenia; mental depression; nephritis; nosebleeds; oliguria; pancreatitis, acute; psychosis; pulmonary edema; rectal bleeding; renal failure; rhinitis; Stevens-Johnson syndrome; thrombocytopenia; tinnitus; or toxic epidermal necrolysis

## General Dosing Information

Ketorolac may be administered on a scheduled or on an as-needed basis, depending on the type and severity of pain.

Ketorolac may be administered intramuscularly, intravenously, or orally. An intravenous dose should be given over at least 15 seconds. An intramuscular injection should be given slowly, deep into the muscle. Ketorolac injection contains alcohol and should not be administered intrathecally or epidurally.

Because of the risk of anaphylaxis or other severe allergic reactions, equipment and medications to treat these complications should be available for immediate use when the first dose of ketorolac is administered.

Hypovolemia increases the risk of adverse renal effects and should be corrected before ketorolac therapy is instituted.

Ketorolac therapy should be initiated with parenteral administration, after which additional doses may be given parenterally or orally. However, the duration of treatment by any route or combination of routes is not to exceed 5 days. The patient should be transferred to another analgesic as quickly as possible.

Concurrent use of ketorolac with an opioid analgesic provides additive analgesia and may permit lower doses of both medications to be utilized. Breakthrough pain that occurs during ketorolac treatment may be treated with an opioid analgesic (unless contraindicated); increasing the dose or the frequency of administration of ketorolac is not recommended.

### For treatment of adverse effects

For abdominal pain—Administering an antacid. See the product label or *Antacids (Oral-Local)* for specific dosing guidelines for these products.

For gastrointestinal ulceration or bleeding—Discontinuing ketorolac therapy immediately. Depending on the site and severity of the ulcer, administering antacids, histamine H$_2$-receptor antagonists (cimetidine, famotidine, nizatidine, ranitidine), misoprostol, omeprazole, and/or sucralfate. See the package inserts or *Antacids (Oral-Local), Histamine H$_2$-receptor Antagonists (Systemic), Misoprostol (Systemic), Omeprazole (Systemic),* or *Sucralfate (Oral-Local)* for specific dosing guidelines for these products.

For severe hypersensitivity reactions (e.g., anaphylaxis or anaphylactoid reaction or laryngeal edema)—Depending on the nature and severity of the symptoms, administering epinephrine and corticosteroids, and, in some cases, antihistamines. See the package inserts or *Antihistamines (Systemic), Corticosteroids/Corticotropin—Glucocorticoid Effects (Systemic),* or *Sympathomimetic Agents—Cardiovascular Use (Parenteral)* for specific dosing guidelines for individual agents.

For renal failure—Dialysis may be needed. However, dialysis is not likely to assist in removing ketorolac from the body after an overdose; decreased clearance and prolongation of half-life have been reported in patients receiving dialysis.

## Oral Dosage Forms

### KETOROLAC TROMETHAMINE TABLETS USP

**Usual adult dose**
Analgesic—
Oral, as a continuation of initial parenteral therapy
Patients 16 to 64 years of age who weigh at least 50 kg and have normal renal function—
20 mg initially, followed by 10 mg up to four times a day at four- to six-hour intervals as needed.
Patients weighing less than 50 kg; and/or
Patients with renal function impairment—
10 mg up to four times a day, at four- to six-hour intervals as needed.
Note: The recommended doses and frequency of administration should not be increased if pain relief is inadequate or breakthrough pain occurs between doses. Supplemental doses of opioid analgesic may be used, if not contraindicated, to provide additional analgesia.

**Usual adult prescribing limits**
Oral, 40 mg per day. The duration of treatment (parenteral followed by oral administration) is not to exceed five days.

**Usual pediatric dose**
Patients up to 16 years of age— Safety and efficacy have not been established.

**Usual geriatric dose**
Analgesic—
Oral, as a continuation of initial parenteral therapy: 10 mg up to four times a day at four- to six-hour intervals as needed.
Note: The recommended doses and frequency of administration should not be increased if pain relief is inadequate or breakthrough pain occurs between doses. Supplemental doses of opioid analgesic may be used, if not contraindicated, to provide additional analgesia.

**Usual geriatric prescribing limits**
Oral, 40 mg per day. The duration of treatment (parenteral followed by oral administration) is not to exceed five days.

**Strength(s) usually available**
U.S.—
10 mg (Rx) [*Toradol* (lactose)].
Canada—
10 mg (Rx) [*Toradol* (lactose)].

**Packaging and storage**
Store between 15 and 30 °C (59 and 86 °F), unless otherwise specified by manufacturer. Protect from light and excessive humidity.

## Parenteral Dosage Forms

### KETOROLAC TROMETHAMINE INJECTION USP

**Usual adult dose**
Analgesic—
Patients 16 to 64 years of age who weigh at least 50 kg and have normal renal function—
Intramuscular, a single dose of 60 mg followed, if necessary, by oral ketorolac (See *Ketorolac Tromethamine Tablets USP*) or by other analgesic therapy, or
Intramuscular, 30 mg every six hours, up to a maximum of twenty doses given over five days, or
Intravenous, 30 mg as a single dose or as multiple doses administered every six hours, up to a maximum of twenty doses given over five days.
Patients weighing less than 50 kg; and/or
Patients with renal function impairment—
Intramuscular, a single dose of 30 mg followed, if necessary, by oral ketorolac (See *Ketorolac Tromethamine Tablets USP*) or by other analgesic therapy, or
Intramuscular, 15 mg every six hours, up to a maximum of twenty doses given over five days, or
Intravenous, 15 mg as a single dose or as multiple doses administered every six hours, up to a maximum of twenty doses given over five days.
Note: The recommended doses and frequency of administration should not be increased if pain relief is inadequate or breakthrough pain occurs between doses. Supplemental doses of opioid analgesic may be used, if not contraindicated, to provide additional analgesia.

**Usual adult prescribing limits**
Patients 16 to 64 years of age who weigh at least 50 kg and have normal renal function—
Intramuscular or intravenous, 120 mg per day. The duration of therapy is not to exceed five days.
Patients weighing less than 50 kg; and/or
Patients with renal function impairment—
Intramuscular or intravenous, 60 mg per day. The duration of therapy is not to exceed five days.

**Usual pediatric dose**
Patients up to 16 years of age—Safety and efficacy have not been established.

**Usual geriatric dose**
Analgesic—
Intramuscular, a single dose of 30 mg, followed, if necessary, by oral ketorolac (See *Ketorolac Tromethamine Tablets USP*) or by other analgesic therapy, or
Intramuscular, 15 mg every six hours, up to a maximum of twenty doses administered over five days, or
Intravenous, 15 mg as a single dose or as multiple doses administered every six hours, up to a maximum of twenty doses administered over five days.
Note: The recommended doses and frequency of administration should not be increased if pain relief is inadequate or breakthrough pain occurs between doses. Supplemental doses of opioid analgesic may be used, if not contraindicated, to provide additional analgesia.

**Usual geriatric prescribing limits**
Intramuscular or intravenous, 60 mg per day. The duration of therapy is not to exceed five days.

**Strength(s) usually available**
U.S.—
1.5% (15 mg per mL) (Rx) [*Toradol* (alcohol 10%)].
3% (30 mg per mL; 60 mg per 2 mL) (Rx) [*Toradol* (alcohol 10%)].
Canada—
1% (10 mg per mL) (Rx) [*Toradol* (alcohol 10%)].
1.5% (15 mg per mL) (Rx) [*Toradol* (alcohol 10%)].
3% (30 mg per mL; 60 mg per 2 mL) (Rx) [*Toradol* (alcohol 10%)].

Note: The product containing 60 mg in 2 mL is not recommended for intravenous administration.

**Packaging and storage**

Store between 15 and 30 °C (59 and 86 °F), unless otherwise specified by manufacturer. Protect from light.

## Selected Bibliography

O'Hara DA, Fragen RJ, Kinzer M, Pemberton D. Ketorolac tromethamine as compared with morphine sulfate for treatment of postoperative pain. Clin Pharmacol Ther 1987 May; 41: 556-61.

Revised: 07/24/95

---

# KRYPTON Kr 81m    Systemic

VA CLASSIFICATION (Primary): DX201

Note: For a listing of dosage forms and brand names by country availability, see *Dosage Forms* section(s). For a listing of brand names for the articles in this monograph, refer to the General Index.

## Category

Diagnostic aid, radioactive (pulmonary disease; pulmonary emboli).

## Indications

Note: Bracketed information in the *Indications* section refers to uses that are not included in U.S. product labeling.

**Accepted**

Pulmonary function studies—Krypton Kr 81m for inhalation is indicated in pulmonary ventilation studies to assess and evaluate regional pulmonary function in lung diseases.

[Embolism, pulmonary (diagnosis)]—Krypton Kr 81m is used to complement lung perfusion studies to detect pulmonary emboli.

## Physical Properties

**Nuclear data**

| Radionuclide (half-life) | Mode of decay | Principal photon emissions (keV) | Mean number of emissions/ disintegration |
|---|---|---|---|
| Kr 81m (13.1 seconds) | Isomeric transition | Gamma (191) | 0.66 |
| Kr 81* (2.1 × 10^5 years) | | | |

\*Decay product.

## Pharmacology/Pharmacokinetics

**Mechanism of action/Effect**

Krypton Kr 81m diffuses easily, passing through cell membranes and exchanging freely between blood and tissue. It is distributed in the lungs in a manner similar to air, thus representing the regions of the lung that are aerated. The gamma photons of krypton Kr 81m can then be employed to obtain counts per minute per lung or region of the lung, or to display their distribution as a scan.

**Distribution**

When inhaled, krypton Kr 81m enters the alveolar wall and passes to the pulmonary venous circulation via capillaries. Most of it that enters the circulation from a single breath returns to the lungs and is exhaled after a single pass through the peripheral circulation.

**Radiation dosimetry**

| Estimated absorbed radiation dose* | | |
|---|---|---|
| Organ | mGy/MBq | mrad/mCi |
| Lungs | 0.00021 | 0.78 |
| Breast | 0.0000046 | 0.017 |
| Pancreas | 0.0000035 | 0.013 |
| Adrenals | 0.0000034 | 0.013 |
| Liver | 0.0000034 | 0.013 |
| Spleen | 0.0000031 | 0.011 |
| Stomach wall | 0.0000025 | 0.0093 |
| Red marrow | 0.0000021 | 0.0078 |
| Bone surfaces | 0.0000017 | 0.0063 |
| Kidneys | 0.0000012 | 0.0044 |
| Large intestine (upper) | 0.00000032 | 0.0012 |
| Small intestine | 0.00000027 | 0.0010 |
| Ovaries | 0.00000017 | 0.00063 |
| Large intestine (lower) | 0.00000014 | 0.00052 |
| Uterus | 0.00000013 | 0.00048 |

| Estimated absorbed radiation dose* | | |
|---|---|---|
| Organ | mGy/MBq | mrad/mCi |
| Bladder wall | 0.000000068 | 0.00025 |
| Testes | 0.000000017 | 0.000063 |
| Other tissue | 0.0000018 | 0.0067 |

Effective dose: 0.000027 mSv/MBq (0.0001 rem/mCi)

\*For adults; by continuous inhalation. Data based on the International Commission on Radiological Protection (ICRP) Publication 53—Radiation dose to patients from radiopharmaceuticals.

**Elimination**

Eliminated via lungs.

## Precautions to Consider

**Carcinogenicity/Mutagenicity**

Long-term animal studies to evaluate carcinogenic or mutagenic potential of krypton Kr 81m have not been performed.

**Pregnancy/Reproduction**

Pregnancy—Studies have not been done in humans. The possibility of pregnancy should be assessed in women of child-bearing potential. Clinical situations exist where the benefit to the patient and fetus from information derived from radiopharmaceutical use outweighs the risks of fetal exposure to radiation. In these situations, the physician should use discretion and reduce the radiopharmaceutical dose to the lowest possible amount.

Studies have not been done in animals.

FDA Pregnancy Category C.

**Breast-feeding**

It is not known whether krypton Kr 81m is distributed into breast milk. However, risk to the infant from radiation exposure is considered negligible because of the short half-life of krypton Kr 81m. Also, most of the amount that passes into the venous circulation returns to the lungs to be exhaled.

**Pediatrics**

Because of the potential risk of radiation exposure, risk-benefit must be considered. Although krypton Kr 81m is used in children, there have been no specific studies evaluating its safety and efficacy in children. When this radiopharmaceutical is used in children, the diagnostic benefit should be judged to outweigh the potential risk of radiation.

**Geriatrics**

Appropriate studies on the relationship of age to the effects of krypton Kr 81m have not been performed in the geriatric population. However, geriatrics-specific problems that would limit the usefulness of this radiopharmaceutical in the elderly are not expected.

## Side/Adverse Effects

At the present time, there are no known side/adverse effects associated with diagnostic doses of krypton Kr 81m.

## Patient Consultation

As an aid to patient consultation, refer to *Advice for the Patient, Radiopharmaceuticals (Diagnostic)*.

In providing consultation, consider emphasizing the following selected information (» = major clinical significance):

**Description of use**

Action in the body: Accumulation of radioactivity in lungs during continuous breathing

Radioactivity retained in lungs during continuous breathing allows visualization

Small amounts of radioactivity used in diagnosis; radiation exposure is low and considered safe

**Before having this test**

» Conditions affecting use, especially:

Pregnancy—Risk to fetus from radiation exposure as opposed to benefit derived from use should be considered

Breast-feeding—Not known if krypton Kr 81m is distributed into breast milk; however, based on the short half-life of krypton Kr 81m, discontinuation of nursing is not necessary

Use in children—Risk from radiation exposure as opposed to benefit derived from use should be considered

**Preparation for this test**

Special preparatory instructions may be given; patient should inquire in advance

**Precautions after having this test**

No special precautions when used for diagnosis

## General Dosing Information

Radiopharmaceuticals are to be administered only by or under the supervision of physicians who have had extensive training in the safe use and handling of radioactive materials and who are authorized by the Nuclear Regulatory Commission (NRC) or the appropriate Federal or Agreement State agency, if required or, outside the U.S., the appropriate authority.

The manufacturer's package insert or other appropriate literature should be consulted for optimal times when imaging should be performed.

### Safety considerations for handling this radiopharmaceutical

Improper handling of this radiopharmaceutical may cause radioactive contamination. Guidelines for handling radioactive material have been prepared by scientific, professional, state, federal, and international bodies and are available to the specially qualified and authorized users who have access to radiopharmaceuticals.

## Inhalation Dosage Forms

### KRYPTON Kr 81m USP

**Usual adult and adolescent administered activity**

Pulmonary function studies—

Inhalation (continuous), 37 to 370 megabecquerels (1 to 10 millicuries) of krypton Kr 81m, not to exceed 3.7 gigabecquerel-minutes (100 millicurie-minutes).

**Usual pediatric administered activity**

Dosage must be individualized by physician.

**Usual geriatric administered activity**

See *Usual adult and adolescent administered activity*.

**Strength(s) usually available**

U.S.—

At calibration time

As rubidium Rb 81, with an activity of 74 to 370 megabecquerels (2 to 10 millicuries) (Rx) [*Krypton Kr 81m Gas Generator*].

Canada—

At calibration time

As rubidium Rb 81, with an activity of 74 to 370 megabecquerels (2 to 10 millicuries) (Rx) [*Krypton Kr 81m Gas Generator*].

Note: Thirty-seven megabecquerels (one millicurie) of rubidium Rb 81 yields 35.5 megabecquerels (0.96 millicurie) of krypton Kr 81m at equilibrium.

**Packaging and storage**

Store below 40 °C (104 °F), preferably between 15 and 30 °C (59 and 86 °F), unless otherwise specified by manufacturer.

**Stability**

Gas generator expires 12 hours after date and time of calibration.

**Note**

Caution—Radioactive material.

Revised: 04/30/96

# LAMIVUDINE   Systemic

**VA CLASSIFICATION (Primary): AM800**

Note: For a listing of dosage forms and brand names by country availability, see *Dosage Forms* section(s). For a listing of brand names for the articles in this monograph, refer to the General Index.

## Category

Antiviral (systemic).

## Indications

Note: Bracketed information in the *Indications* section refers to uses that are not included in U.S. product labeling.

### General considerations

Lamivudine is the negative enantiomer of 2'-deoxy-3'-thiacytidine. Both the positive and negative enantiomers have *in vitro* activity against human immunodeficiency virus (HIV), but the negative enantiomer has greater activity and less toxicity. *In vitro* inhibition of DNA polymerase gamma, which is thought to be associated with peripheral neuropathy, is minimal.

Lamivudine has *in vitro* activity against HIV-1 and HIV-2, including zidovudine-resistant isolates, as well as hepatitis B virus. Lamivudine is indicated in combination with zidovudine for the treatment of HIV infection. Lamivudine and zidovudine have been found to act synergistically *in vitro*. This is thought to produce better efficacy than either medication alone. Resistance to lamivudine is associated with a mutation at codon 184 in HIV-1 reverse transcriptase; this can suppress the expression of pre-existing resistance to zidovudine in a number of different HIV isolates. Strains of HIV-1 resistant to both lamivudine and zidovudine have been isolated.

### Accepted

Human immunodeficiency virus (HIV) infection (treatment) or

Immunodeficiency syndrome, acquired (AIDS) (treatment)—Lamivudine is indicated, in combination with zidovudine, in the treatment of HIV infection or AIDS when therapy is warranted based on clinical and/or immunological evidence of disease progression.

[Human immunodeficiency virus (HIV) infection, occupational exposure (prophylaxis)][1]—Lamivudine may be used prophylactically in health care workers at risk of acquiring HIV infection after occupational exposure to the virus. It is being used in combination with zidovudine and, in some cases, a protease inhibitor.

### Acceptance not established

Lamivudine is being studied for the treatment of *chronic hepatitis B infection*. However, reactivation of hepatitis B virus infection has been reported after lamivudine therapy was discontinued.

[1]Not included in Canadian product labeling.

## Pharmacology/Pharmacokinetics

### Physicochemical characteristics

Molecular weight—229.26.

### Mechanism of action/Effect

Lamivudine is metabolized intracellularly to its active 5'–triphosphate metabolite, lamivudine triphosphate (L-TP), which inhibits human immunodeficiency virus (HIV) reverse transcription via viral DNA chain termination.

### Other actions/effects

Lamivudine also potently inhibits the replication of hepatitis B virus by interfering with reverse transcriptase activity.

### Absorption

Rapidly absorbed; bioavailability in adults and adolescents is 80 to 88% and in children is approximately 66 to 68%. Food delays the peak serum concentration and the time to peak serum concentration; however, there is no significant difference in bioavailability. Therefore, lamivudine may be administered with or without food.

### Distribution

Lamivudine is widely distributed. Lamivudine crosses the blood-brain barrier and is distributed into the cerebrospinal fluid (CSF) to a limited extent. In children, CSF concentrations ranged from 10 to 17% of the corresponding, non–steady-state serum concentration. Lamivudine crosses the placenta in rats, rabbits, and humans.

Apparent Vol $_D$ =Approximately 1.3 liters per kg.

### Protein binding

Low (36%).

### Biotransformation

Trans-sulfoxide is the only known metabolite of lamivudine; serum concentrations of this metabolite have not been determined.

### Half-life

Intracellular lamivudine triphosphate—

11 to 15 hours.

Lamivudine (serum)—

Adults: 2 to 11 hours.

Children (4 months to 14 years of age): 1.7 to 2 hours.

Renal function impairment—

Creatinine clearance, 10 to 40 mL per min (mL/min) (0.17 to 0.67 mL per sec [mL/sec])—Approximately 13.6 hours.

Creatinine clearance, less than 10 mL/min (0.17 mL/sec)—Approximately 19.4 hours.

### Time to peak concentration

With food—

Approximately 3.2 hours.

Fasting—

Approximately 1 hour.

### Peak serum concentration

Adults and adolescents—

2 mg per kg of body weight (mg/kg): 1.5 micrograms per mL (mcg/mL) (6.5 micromoles per liter).

Children—

8 mg/kg: 1.1 mcg/mL (4.8 micromoles per liter).

### Elimination

Renal; the majority of lamivudine is eliminated unchanged in the urine (68 to 71%); approximately 5.2% of the trans-sulfoxide metabolite is excreted in the urine within 12 hours. The renal clearance of lamivudine is greater than the glomerular filtration rate, implying active secretion into the renal tubules.

In dialysis—

It is not known whether lamivudine is removed by peritoneal dialysis or hemodialysis.

## Precautions to Consider

### Carcinogenicity

Long-term carcinogenicity studies in animals have not been completed.

### Mutagenicity

Lamivudine was not active in a microbial mutagenicity screen or in an *in vitro* cell transformation assay. It showed weak *in vitro* mutagenic activity in a cytogenic assay using cultured human lymphocytes and in the mouse lymphoma assay. However, lamivudine showed no evidence of *in vivo* genotoxic activity in rats at oral doses of up to 2000 mg per kg of body weight (mg/kg), which is approximately 65 times the recommended human dose based on body surface area.

### Pregnancy/Reproduction

Fertility—Rats given doses of lamivudine up to 130 times the usual adult dose based on body surface area revealed no evidence of impaired fertility.

Pregnancy—Adequate and well-controlled studies have not been done in humans. However, lamivudine has been found to cross the placenta in humans.

Lamivudine crosses the placenta in rats and rabbits. Studies have been done in rats and rabbits administered doses up to approximately 130 to 60 times the usual adult dose, respectively. Some evidence of embryolethality in rabbits, but not in rats, at doses similar to the usual adult dose or higher has been seen.

FDA Pregnancy Category C.

### Breast-feeding

It is not known whether lamivudine is distributed into human breast milk. Lamivudine is distributed into the milk of lactating rats in concentrations that are slightly higher than those in the plasma.

### Pediatrics

In one study, pancreatitis was reported in 14 of 97 (14%) and paresthesias and peripheral neuropathies were seen in 13 of 97 (13%) of pediatric patients receiving lamivudine monotherapy. However, the patients who developed these complications had advanced HIV disease and a prior history of pancreatitis, most commonly associated with the use of didanosine. The combination of lamivudine and zidovudine should be used with caution in children with advanced HIV disease and/or a history of pancreatitis. In addition, an increase in serum transaminases (greater than 10 times the upper limits of normal) was observed in 3 of 89 (3%) of pediatric patients receiving lamivudine monotherapy.

The pharmacokinetics of lamivudine have not been studied in combination with zidovudine in children. Pharmacokinetic properties of lamivudine monotherapy were assessed in 57 children (ages 4.8 months to 16 years). The absolute bioavailability was 66 to 68%, which is less than the 86% seen in adults and adolescents. The mechanism for this diminished bioavailability in infants and children is unknown. The area under the serum concentration–time curve (AUC) was comparable for pediatric patients receiving a dose of 8 mg/kg per day and adults receiving a dose of 4 mg/kg per day.

### Geriatrics

No information is available on the relationship of age to the effects of lamivudine in geriatric patients. However, elderly patients are more likely to have age-related renal function impairment, which may require a dosage adjustment in patients receiving lamivudine.

Lamivudine pharmacokinetics have not been studied in patients over 65 years of age.

### Drug interactions and/or related problems

The following drug interactions and/or related problems have been selected on the basis of their potential clinical significance (possible mechanism in parentheses where appropriate)—not necessarily inclusive (» = major clinical significance):

Note: Combinations containing any of the following medications, depending on the amount present, may also interact with this medication.

Drugs associated with pancreatitis, such as alcohol, didanosine, intravenous pentamidine, sulfonamides, or zalcitabine
(pancreatitis was seen in 14% (14 of 97) of pediatric patients receiving lamivudine monotherapy; this population had advanced HIV disease and a history of pancreatitis; although no interactions have been documented to date, concurrent use of lamivudine with medications associated with the development of pancreatitis should be avoided or, if concurrent use is necessary, used with caution)

Drugs associated with peripheral neuropathy, such as dapsone, didanosine, isoniazid, stavudine, or zalcitabine
(paresthesias and peripheral neuropathy were seen in 13% (13 of 97) of pediatric patients with advanced HIV disease receiving lamivudine monotherapy; although no interactions have been documented to date, other medications associated with the development of neuropathy should be avoided or, if concurrent use is necessary, used with caution)

Indinavir
(concurrent administration of lamivudine 150 mg twice a day, indinavir 800 mg every eight hours, and zidovudine 200 mg every eight hours resulted in a 6% decrease in the AUC of lamivudine, no change in AUC of indinavir, and a 36% increase in the AUC of zidovudine; no adjustment in dose is necessary)

Sulfamethoxazole and trimethoprim combination
(in one small study, concurrent administration of sulfamethoxazole and trimethoprim combination resulted in a 44% increase in lamivudine AUC and a 30% decrease in lamivudine renal clearance; the pharmacokinetic properties of sulfamethoxazole and trimethoprim were not altered by concurrent administration of lamivudine; no adjustment in dose is necessary unless the patient has renal function impairment)

Zidovudine
(in one small study, concurrent administration of lamivudine resulted in a 39% increase in the peak plasma concentration of zidovudine; although statistically significant, this increase is not thought to be significant to patient safety; no significant changes were observed in the AUC or total clearance of lamivudine or zidovudine)

### Laboratory value alterations

The following have been selected on the basis of their potential clinical significance (possible effect in parentheses where appropriate)—not necessarily inclusive (» = major clinical significance):

With physiology/laboratory test values
Alanine aminotransferase (ALT [SGPT]) and
Aspartate aminotransferase (AST [SGOT])
(an increase in serum transaminases [greater than 10 times the upper limits of normal] was observed in 3 of 89 (3%) of pediatric patients receiving lamivudine monotherapy)

Amylase, serum
(values may be increased)

Hemoglobin concentration and
Neutrophil count
(values may be decreased)

### Medical considerations/Contraindications

The medical considerations/contraindications included here have been selected on the basis of their potential clinical significance (reasons given in parentheses where appropriate)—not necessarily inclusive (» = major clinical significance).

*Risk-benefit should be considered when the following medical problems exist:*

Hypersensitivity to lamivudine

Pancreatitis, or history of
(pancreatitis occurred in 14% (14 of 97) of pediatric patients receiving lamivudine monotherapy; these patients had advanced HIV disease and a history of pancreatitis; pancreatitis has been reported rarely in adults; lamivudine should be used with extreme caution in patients who have pancreatitis or a history of pancreatitis)

Peripheral neuropathy, or history of
(peripheral neuropathy occurred in approximately 13% (13 of 97) of pediatric patients receiving lamivudine monotherapy; these patients had advanced HIV disease; it has also been reported rarely in adults; lamivudine should be used with caution in patients who have peripheral neuropathy or a history of peripheral neuropathy)

» Renal function impairment
(decreased renal function has been found to result in an increase in the peak plasma concentration and elimination half-life of lamivudine; dosage modification is recommended in patients with a creatinine clearance of < 50 mL/min [0.83 mL/sec])

### Patient monitoring

The following may be especially important in patient monitoring (other tests may be warranted in some patients, depending on condition; » = major clinical significance):

Alanine aminotransferase (ALT [SGPT]) and
Aspartate aminotransferase (AST [SGOT])
(an increase in serum transaminases [greater than 10 times the upper limits of normal] was observed in 3 of 89 (3%) of pediatric patients receiving lamivudine monotherapy)

» Amylase, serum, and
» Lipase, serum, and
Triglycerides, serum
(lamivudine administration has been associated with pancreatitis in approximately 14% of pediatric patients; patients should be monitored for laboratory changes consistent with pancreatitis, such as elevated amylase, lipase, and triglyceride concentrations)

» Blood urea nitrogen (BUN) and
» Creatinine, serum
(blood urea nitrogen and serum creatinine concentrations should be monitored in patients with renal function impairment; an adjustment in dosage or dosage interval may be required)

## Side/Adverse Effects

Note: Lamivudine is given in combination with zidovudine, and, in some cases, it may also be given with other antiretroviral agents. Some side effects, such as pancreatitis, peripheral neuropathy, and hematologic abnormalities, may be seen with other antiretroviral agents, such as zidovudine, and/or severe human immunodeficiency virus (HIV) disease; therefore, differentiation between the side effects of lamivudine and other medications or the complications of HIV disease may be difficult.

In one study, 14 of 97 pediatric patients (14%) being treated with lamivudine monotherapy developed pancreatitis; in a second pediatric study, 7 of 47 patients (15%) receiving lamivudine in combination therapy with other antiretroviral agents developed pancreatitis. Pancreatitis was most commonly seen in patients who had advanced HIV disease, as well as a prior history of pancreatitis, most commonly associated with the use of didanosine. The combination of lamivudine and zidovudine therapy should be used with caution in pediatric patients with a history of pancreatitis or other risk factors for pancreatitis. Pancreatitis was seen in only 3 of 656 adult patients (< 0.5%) who received lamivudine. Lamivudine should be discontinued immediately if any signs or symptoms of pancreatitis occur. In addition, an increase in serum transaminases (greater than 10 times the upper limits of normal) was observed in 3 of 89 (3%) of pediatric patients receiving lamivudine monotherapy.

Paresthesias and peripheral neuropathy were reported in 13% of pediatric patients and have been reported rarely in adults.

The following side/adverse effects have been selected on the basis of their potential clinical significance (possible signs and symptoms in parentheses where appropriate)—not necessarily inclusive:

**Those indicating need for medical attention**
Incidence more frequent
*Pancreatitis* (nausea; vomiting; severe abdominal or stomach pain)— more frequent in children; *paresthesias and peripheral neuropathy* (tingling, burning, numbness, or pain in the hands, arms, feet, or legs)—more frequent in children

Incidence rare
*Anemia* (unusual tiredness or weakness); *neutropenia* (fever, chills, or sore throat); *skin rash*

**Those indicating need for medical attention only if they continue or are bothersome**
Incidence less frequent
*Cough; dizziness; fatigue* (unusual tiredness or weakness); *gastrointestinal distress* (abdominal or stomach pain; diarrhea; nausea; vomiting); *headache; insomnia* (trouble in sleeping)

Incidence rare
*Hair loss*

## Overdose

There is no known antidote for lamivudine. There is one reported case in which an adult ingested 6 grams of lamivudine; no clinical signs and symptoms were noted and hematologic tests remained normal. It is not known whether lamivudine is removed by peritoneal dialysis or hemodialysis.

For more information on the management of overdose or unintentional ingestion, **contact a Poison Control Center** (see *Poison Control Center Listing*).

## Patient Consultation

As an aid to patient consultation, refer to *Advice for the Patient, Lamivudine (Systemic)*.

In providing consultation, consider emphasizing the following selected information (» = major clinical significance):

**Before using this medication**
» Conditions affecting use, especially:
 Hypersensitivity to lamivudine
 Pregnancy—Lamivudine has caused embryolethality in rabbits at doses similar to the usual adult dose or higher
 Use in children—Lamivudine monotherapy has resulted in the development of pancreatitis in 14% (14 of 97) of children with advanced HIV disease and a prior history of pancreatitis, and paresthesias and peripheral neuropathies in 13% (13 of 97) of pediatric patients with advanced HIV disease; in addition, an increase in serum transaminases (greater than 10 times the upper limits of normal) was observed in 3 of 89 (3%) of pediatric patients receiving lamivudine monotherapy; the absolute bioavailability is 66 to 68% in children, less than the 86% seen in adults and adolescents
 Other medical problems, especially renal function impairment

**Proper use of this medication**
» Importance of not taking more medication than prescribed; importance of not discontinuing lamivudine or zidovudine without checking with physician
» Compliance with full course of therapy
» Importance of not missing doses and of taking at evenly spaced times
 Proper administration technique for oral liquids
 Not sharing medication with others
» Proper dosing
 Missed dose: Taking as soon as possible; not taking if almost time for next dose; not doubling doses
» Proper storage

**Precautions while using this medication**
» Regular visits to physician for blood tests
» Importance of not taking other medications concurrently without checking with physician

**Side/adverse effects**
Signs of potential side effects, especially pancreatitis, paresthesias, peripheral neuropathy, anemia, neutropenia, or skin rash

## General Dosing Information

Lamivudine may be taken on a full or empty stomach.

Patients 16 years of age and older with renal function impairment require a reduction in dose as follows:

| Creatinine Clearance (mL/min)/ (mL/sec) | Dose |
|---|---|
| ≥50/0.83 | 150 mg twice a day |
| 30–49/0.50–0.82 | 150 mg once a day |
| 15–29/0.25–0.48 | 150 mg first dose, then 100 mg once a day |
| 5–14/0.08–0.23 | 150 mg first dose, then 50 mg once a day |
| <5/<0.08 | 50 mg first dose, then 25 mg once a day |

## Oral Dosage Forms

Note: Bracketed uses in the *Dosage Forms* section refer to categories of use and/or indications that are not included in U.S. product labeling.

### LAMIVUDINE ORAL SOLUTION

**Usual adult and adolescent dose**
Human immunodeficiency virus (HIV) infection (treatment) or Immunodeficiency syndrome, acquired (AIDS) (treatment)—
 Adults and adolescents weighing 50 kg (110 pounds) or more: Oral, 150 mg of lamivudine twice a day in combination with zidovudine 200 mg three times a day.
 Adults weighing less than 50 kg (110 pounds): Oral, 2 mg per kg of body weight of lamivudine twice a day in combination with zidovudine 200 mg three times a day.
[Human immunodeficiency virus (HIV) infection, occupational exposure (prophylaxis)][1]—
 Oral, 150 mg of lamivudine twice a day, in combination with zidovudine 200 mg three times a day, for four weeks. In certain cases, a protease inhibitor may also be added to the regimen.

**Usual pediatric dose**
Children 3 months to 12 years of age—Oral, 4 mg per kg of body weight of lamivudine, up to a 150-mg dose, twice a day in combination with 180 mg per square meter of body surface of zidovudine every six hours.

**Strength(s) usually available**
U.S.—
 10 mg per mL (Rx) [*Epivir* (ethanol 6% v/v; methylparaben; propylparaben; sucrose)].
Canada—
 10 mg per mL (Rx) [*3TC* (ethanol 6% v/v; methylparaben; propylparaben; sucrose)].

**Packaging and storage**
Store between 2 and 25 °C (36 and 77 °F) in a tight container.

**Auxiliary labeling**
• Continue medicine for full time of treatment.

**Note**
When dispensing, include a calibrated liquid-measuring device.

### LAMIVUDINE TABLETS

**Usual adult and adolescent dose**
See *Lamivudine Oral Solution*.

**Usual pediatric dose**
See *Lamivudine Oral Solution*.

**Strength(s) usually available**
U.S.—
 150 mg (Rx) [*Epivir*].
Canada—
 150 mg (Rx) [*3TC*].

**Packaging and storage**
Store between 2 and 30 °C (36 and 86 °F) in a tight container.

**Auxiliary labeling**
• Continue medicine for full time of treatment.

[1]Not included in Canadian product labeling.

Developed: 08/08/96

# LAMOTRIGINE   Systemic

VA CLASSIFICATION (Primary): CN400

Another commonly used name is LTG.

Note: For a listing of dosage forms and brand names by country availability, see *Dosage Forms* section(s). For a listing of brand names for the articles in this monograph, refer to the General Index.

## Category

Anticonvulsant.

## Indications

### Accepted

Epilepsy (treatment adjunct)—Lamotrigine is indicated as an adjunct to other anticonvulsant medications in the treatment of partial seizures in adults 16 years of age and older with epilepsy.

### Acceptance not established

Additional data are required to confirm the safety and effectiveness of lamotrigine use in children, as monotherapy, in the treatment of *secondary generalized seizures*, in the treatment of *primary generalized seizures* including *absence seizures*, and in the treatment of *Lennox-Gastaut syndrome*.

Note: Although lamotrigine is approved in some countries for use in children, as monotherapy, and in the treatment of both primary and secondary generalized seizures, the USP DI Advisory Panels believe that currently there is insufficient evidence to support the safety and effectiveness of lamotrigine for use in these indications.

## Pharmacology/Pharmacokinetics

### Physicochemical characteristics

Chemical group—Phenyltriazine. Structurally unrelated to existing anticonvulsant medications.

Molecular weight—256.09.

pKa—5.7.

### Mechanism of action/Effect

The exact mechanism of action is unknown. *In vitro* studies suggest that lamotrigine blocks voltage-sensitive sodium channels, thereby stabilizing neuronal membranes and inhibiting the presynaptic release of neurotransmitters, principally glutamate. Lamotrigine may also directly inhibit high-frequency sustained repetitive firing of sodium-dependent action potentials.

### Other actions/effects

Lamotrigine is a weak dihydrofolate reductase inhibitor *in vitro* and in animal studies. No effect on folate concentrations has been noted in clinical studies. However, complete inhibition of erythropoiesis occurred in one patient with heterozygous beta-thalassemia, possibly due to inhibition of dihydrofolate reductase by lamotrigine.

Animal studies have shown that lamotrigine binds to melanin-containing tissues, such as eye tissues and pigmented skin. The long-term effects of this binding are not known, but no effects have been seen in humans.

The 2-*N*-methyl metabolite of lamotrigine causes cardiac conduction disturbances in dogs in a dose-dependent manner. This metabolite is present in trace amounts in the urine of people taking lamotrigine, but the clinical significance of its presence is unknown.

### Absorption

Rapid. Bioavailability of lamotrigine is approximately 98% and is unaffected by food.

### Distribution

Volume of distribution (Vol$_D$) is approximately 1.2 liters per kg (L/kg). In a 10-year-old patient undergoing topectomy 4 hours post-dose, lamotrigine concentration in brain tissue was greater than unbound lamotrigine concentration in plasma. Lamotrigine is distributed into breast milk.

### Protein binding

Moderate (55%).

### Biotransformation

Hepatic glucuronic acid conjugation. Evidence of autoinduction has been seen in some studies but not in others. Further evaluation of possible lamotrigine autoinduction is needed. The 2-*N*-methyl metabolite of lamotrigine is present in trace amounts in the urine of people taking lamotrigine, but the clinical significance of its presence is unknown.

### Half-life

Elimination—

With no other medication: $25 \pm 10$ hours.

With enzyme-inducing anticonvulsants only: $14 \pm 6$ hours.

With valproic acid only: Approximately 59 hours.

With enzyme-inducing anticonvulsants and valproic acid: Approximately 28 hours.

### Time to peak concentration

1.4 to 4.8 hours. A second peak may be seen 4 to 6 hours after oral or intravenous administration; this peak may reflect enterohepatic recirculation.

### Therapeutic serum concentration

The therapeutic concentration range for lamotrigine has not been determined. Over a range of 50 to 400 mg given as a single dose, peak plasma concentrations increased linearly from 0.58 to 4.63 mg/L in healthy subjects. In 2 small studies of patients with epilepsy, plasma concentrations increased linearly with doses of 50 to 350 mg given 2 times a day. Titration of dosage is based on clinical response.

### Elimination

Renal—Approximately 73% (about 10% unchanged, 80 to 90% as glucuronide conjugates, less than 5% as other metabolites, and trace amounts as the 2-*N*-methyl metabolite).

Fecal—Approximately 2%.

In dialysis—In 6 patients, $17 \pm 10\%$ of the lamotrigine in the body was removed in 4 hours of hemodialysis.

## Precautions to Consider

### Carcinogenicity

In 2-year studies, at plasma concentrations equal to those seen in humans receiving 300 to 500 mg of lamotrigine a day, rats and mice showed no evidence of carcinogenicity.

### Mutagenicity

No evidence of mutagenicity was found in appropriate *in vitro* and *in vivo* testing.

### Pregnancy/Reproduction

Fertility—No adverse effect on fertility was seen in rats given up to 0.4 times an equivalent human dose of 500 mg per day (mg/day) on a mg per square meter of body surface area (mg/m$^2$) basis.

Pregnancy—Lamotrigine should be used during pregnancy only if the potential benefit justifies the potential risk to the fetus.

Folic acid supplementation should be considered for all women of childbearing potential who are taking lamotrigine.

Studies have not been done in humans.

Studies in rats and rabbits indicate that lamotrigine crosses the placenta, yielding placental and fetal concentrations comparable to concentrations in maternal plasma. No teratogenic effects were seen in animal studies employing up to 1.2 times an equivalent human dose of 500 mg per day on a mg/m$^2$ basis. However, rats receiving up to 0.5 times an equivalent human dose of 500 mg per day on a mg/m$^2$ basis produced offspring with decreased fetal folate concentrations, an effect known to be associated with teratogenicity in humans and animals. In addition, stillbirths and postnatal deaths were increased among offspring of rats receiving lamotrigine in doses less than half of an equivalent human dose of 500 mg per day on a mg/m$^2$ basis, probably due to *in utero* exposure to lamotrigine. The clinical significance of these effects is unknown.

FDA Pregnancy Category C.

Labor and delivery—The effect of lamotrigine on labor and delivery is not known.

### Breast-feeding

Lamotrigine is distributed into breast milk. However, the effects on the nursing infant are unknown.

### Pediatrics

Uncontrolled studies performed in a limited number of pediatric epilepsy patients 2 to 16 years of age have not demonstrated pediatrics-specific problems that would limit the usefulness of lamotrigine in children. Pharmacokinetic data from these studies indicate that lamotrigine elimination half-life may be shorter, and clearance may be more rapid, in children than in adults. However, data from controlled trials are still needed to establish safety and efficacy in children.

### Geriatrics

Appropriate studies on the relationship of age to the effects of lamotrigine have not been performed in the geriatric population. However, one single-dose pharmacokinetic study comparing 12 healthy volunteers 65 to 76 years of age and 12 healthy volunteers 26 to 38 years of age found that lamotrigine clearance was 37% lower, area under the concentration-time curve (AUC) was 55% higher, peak plasma concentration was 27% higher, and elimination half-life was 6 hours longer in the older group. In addition, elderly patients are more likely to have age-related renal function impairment, which may require dosage adjustment. It is recommended that elderly patients receive dosages at the low end of the normal range.

### Drug interactions and/or related problems

The following drug interactions and/or related problems have been selected on the basis of their potential clinical significance (possible mechanism in parentheses where appropriate)—not necessarily inclusive (» = major clinical significance):

Note: Combinations containing any of the following medications, depending on the amount present, may also interact with this medication.

Possible interactions between lamotrigine and hepatic enzyme inducers or inhibitors not listed below should be considered.

Acetaminophen
(half-life and area under the concentration-time curve of lamotrigine may be reduced slightly by chronic, high-dose acetaminophen use)

Alcohol or central nervous system (CNS) depression–producing medications, other (See *Appendix II*)
(lamotrigine may enhance the CNS depressant effects of these medications or alcohol)

» Carbamazepine or
» Phenobarbital or
» Phenytoin or
» Primidone
(clearance of lamotrigine is increased; clearance may be expected to decrease when concomitant enzyme-inducing therapy is discontinued; initial lamotrigine dosage and rate of lamotrigine dosage escalation should be based on concomitant anticonvulsant therapy; monitoring of plasma concentrations of lamotrigine and other anticonvulsant medications should be considered, especially during dosage adjustments)

(an increased incidence of CNS adverse effects, including ataxia, blurred vision, diplopia, dizziness, or increased excitation, may occur with concomitant carbamazepine use; reduction of dosage of either lamotrigine or carbamazepine may reduce these effects)

Folate antagonists, other (See *Appendix II*)
(lamotrigine inhibits dihydrofolate reductase, and should be used with caution with other folate antagonists)

» Valproic acid
(half-life and plasma concentrations of lamotrigine are increased, probably due to competition for hepatic glucuronidation; half-life and plasma concentrations may be expected to decrease when valproic acid is discontinued; initial lamotrigine dosage, and rate of lamotrigine dosage escalation, should be based on concomitant anticonvulsant therapy; monitoring of plasma concentrations of lamotrigine and valproic acid should be considered, especially during dosage adjustments)

(disabling tremor and an increased incidence of rash, including severe rash, have occurred with concomitant valproic acid use)

(there is some evidence that the combination of lamotrigine and valproic acid may improve seizure control in patients who are refractory to either agent used alone, but controlled studies have not been done)

### Medical considerations/Contraindications

The medical considerations/contraindications included here have been selected on the basis of their potential clinical significance (reasons given in parentheses where appropriate)—not necessarily inclusive (» = major clinical significance).

*Except under special circumstances, this medication should not be used when the following medical problem exists:*

» Hypersensitivity to lamotrigine

*Risk-benefit should be considered when the following medical problems exist:*

Cardiac conduction abnormalities
(in one clinical trial, minor electrocardiogram [ECG] changes were seen in some patients with normal cardiac function who were taking lamotrigine; there is no experience with lamotrigine treatment in patients with cardiac conduction disturbances)

Hepatic function impairment
(lamotrigine metabolism may be decreased)

» Renal function impairment
(large interindividual differences in lamotrigine plasma concentration were seen in uremic patients, and elimination half-life is prolonged in patients with significant renal function impairment; patients with renal function impairment may require reduced maintenance doses)

» Thalassemia
(erythropoiesis may be decreased significantly)

## Side/Adverse Effects

Note: Disseminated intravascular coagulation and multi-organ failure have occurred very rarely in patients taking lamotrigine. Most cases have been in association with other serious medical events, such as status epilepticus and overwhelming sepsis, and it is uncertain whether these effects were related to lamotrigine use.

An increased incidence of CNS adverse effects, including ataxia, blurred vision, diplopia, dizziness, or increased excitation, may occur with concomitant carbamazepine use; reduction of dosage of either lamotrigine or carbamazepine may reduce these effects.

Lamotrigine may be less sedating than other anticonvulsant medications.

The following side/adverse effects have been selected on the basis of their potential clinical significance (possible signs and symptoms in parentheses where appropriate)—not necessarily inclusive:

### Those indicating need for medical attention
Incidence more frequent

*Ataxia* (clumsiness or unsteadiness); *skin rash; vision abnormalities, including blurred vision; and diplopia* (double vision)

Note: The incidence of *skin rash* is highly dependent upon the initial rate of lamotrigine dosage escalation. Higher incidence of *skin rash* is seen with concurrent valproic acid therapy, higher lamotrigine starting doses, or rapid lamotrigine dosage escalation. Rash is usually maculopapular and/or erythematous and occurs within the first 4 to 6 weeks of treatment. Rash usually resolves when lamotrigine is discontinued. A mild rash may subside even with continuation of lamotrigine therapy; however, close monitoring is essential. Some patients have been successfully rechallenged with lamotrigine after discontinuation due to mild rash. Rarely, more severe rashes with systemic involvement may occur. It is recommended that any patient who acutely develops any combination of unexplained rash, fever, flu-like symptoms, or worsening of seizure control should discontinue lamotrigine and should be closely monitored; monitoring should include determinations of hepatic and renal function, and clotting parameters.

Incidence less frequent

*CNS toxicity, specifically anxiety; confusion; depression; irritability; or other mood or mental changes; increased seizures; or nystagmus* (continuous, uncontrolled back and forth and/or rolling eye movements)

Incidence rare

*Angioedema* (trouble in breathing; swelling of face, mouth, hands, or feet); *blood dyscrasias, including anemia; eosinophilia; leukopenia; or thrombocytopenia* (fever and sore throat; unusual bleeding or bruising; unusual tiredness or weakness); *erythema multiforme, Stevens-Johnson syndrome, or toxic epidermal necrolysis* (blistering, peeling, or loosening of skin; muscle cramps, pain, or weakness; red or irritated eyes; skin rash or itching; sore throat, fever, and chills; sores, ulcers, or white spots in mouth or on lips); *fever; hypersensitivity syndrome* (dark-colored urine; fever; flu-like symptoms; skin rash; facial swelling; swollen lymph nodes; unusual tiredness or weakness; yellow eyes or skin); *petechia* (small red or purple spots on skin)

### Those indicating need for medical attention only if they continue or are bothersome
Incidence more frequent

*CNS effects, specifically dizziness; drowsiness; or headache; gastrointestinal effects, specifically nausea or vomiting*

Note: A higher incidence of *dizziness* is seen in females than in males.

Incidence less frequent or rare

*Asthenia* (loss of strength); *dysarthria* (slurred speech); *dyspepsia* (indigestion); *insomnia* (trouble in sleeping); *rhinitis* (runny nose); *tremor* (trembling or shaking)

# Overdose

For specific information on the agents used in the management of lamotrigine overdose, see:
- *Charcoal, Activated (Oral-Local)* monograph.

For more information on the management of overdose or unintentional ingestion, **contact a Poison Control Center** (see *Poison Control Center Listing*).

## Clinical effects of overdose

The following effects have been selected on the basis of their potential clinical significance (possible signs and symptoms in parentheses where appropriate)—not necessarily inclusive:

Acute effects

*CNS toxicity, specifically ataxia, severe* (clumsiness or unsteadiness); *coma; dizziness, severe; drowsiness, severe; dysarthria, severe* (slurred speech); *or nystagmus, severe* (continuous, uncontrolled back and forth and/or rolling eye movements); *dryness of mouth; electrocardiogram (ECG) changes, specifically prolonged QRS interval; increased heart rate*

Note: Experience with lamotrigine overdose is very limited. Overdoses with lamotrigine have ranged from 1350 to over 4000 milligrams. Some of these clinical effects have occurred in only one patient, and general applicability to lamotrigine overdose is unknown.

## Treatment of overdose

To decrease absorption—Emesis may be induced or gastric lavage may be performed, if indicated, with precautions taken to protect the airway, keeping in mind the rapid absorption of lamotrigine. Activated charcoal also may be administered. These procedures may need to be repeated several times. The use of a cathartic to accelerate elimination of charcoal and medication from the lower gastrointestinal tract should be considered.

To enhance elimination—Hemodialysis is of questionable efficacy. The extraction ratio of lamotrigine in 6 patients with renal failure was $17 \pm 10\%$ in 4 hours of hemodialysis.

Specific treatment—There is no known antidote to lamotrigine overdose.

Monitoring—Patient should be observed closely, with frequent monitoring of vital signs. Close electrocardiogram (ECG) monitoring may be advisable in patients showing QRS interval prolongation.

Supportive care—General supportive care is the basis of lamotrigine overdose treatment. Patients in whom intentional overdose is confirmed or suspected should be referred for psychiatric consultation.

# Patient Consultation

As an aid to patient consultation, refer to *Advice for the Patient, Lamotrigine (Systemic)*.

In providing consultation, consider emphasizing the following selected information (» = major clinical significance):

## Before using this medication
» Conditions affecting use, especially:
    Hypersensitivity to lamotrigine
    Pregnancy—Crossed the placenta in animal studies; increased stillbirths and postnatal deaths among offspring of rats receiving less than maximum human dose
    Breast-feeding—Distributed into breast milk; effect on nursing infant is unknown
    Other medications, especially carbamazepine, phenobarbital, phenytoin, primidone, or valproic acid
    Other medical problems, especially renal function impairment or thalassemia

## Proper use of this medication
» Compliance with therapy; not taking more or less medicine than prescribed; not missing any doses
    Taking with or without food or on a full or empty stomach, as directed by physician
» Proper dosing
    Missed dose: Taking as soon as possible; if almost time for next dose, skipping missed dose and returning to regular dosing schedule; not doubling doses
» Proper storage

## Precautions while using this medication
» Regular visits to physician to check progress of therapy
    Discussing alcohol use and use of other CNS depressants with physician
» Possible blurred or double vision, dizziness, drowsiness, impairment of motor skills; caution when driving or doing jobs requiring alertness, coordination, or clear vision

» Immediately notifying physician if skin rash or increase in seizures occurs
» Not discontinuing lamotrigine abruptly; consulting physician about gradually reducing dosage

## Side/adverse effects
Signs of potential side effects, especially ataxia; skin rash; vision abnormalities; anxiety, confusion, depression, irritability, or other mood or mental changes; increased seizures; nystagmus; angioedema; blood dyscrasias; erythema multiforme, Stevens-Johnson syndrome, or toxic epidermal necrolysis; fever; hypersensitivity syndrome; or petechia

# General Dosing Information

Lamotrigine should be initiated at a low dose, and dosage escalation should proceed slowly, to minimize the occurrence of skin rash. The incidence of skin rash is highly dependent upon the initial rate of lamotrigine dosage escalation.

Physician should be notified immediately if an acute worsening of seizure control or a skin rash occurs.

Anticonvulsant medications should not be discontinued abruptly because of the possibility of increased seizures. Lamotrigine dosage may be decreased by 25 to 33% every 2 weeks. If more rapid discontinuation is required, the dosage should be tapered over at least 2 weeks, if possible, with the dose decreased by 50% each week.

# Oral Dosage Forms

## LAMOTRIGINE TABLETS

Note: Lamotrigine therapy should be initiated at a low dose, and dosage escalation should proceed slowly to minimize the occurrence of skin rash, including severe skin rash.

### Usual adult dose
Anticonvulsant—
    With enzyme-inducing anticonvulsants only: Oral, 50 mg once a day for two weeks, then 100 mg a day, divided into two doses, for two weeks. The dosage may be increased by 100 mg a day every week based on clinical response.
    With enzyme-inducing anticonvulsants and valproic acid: Oral, 25 mg once every other day for two weeks, then 25 mg once a day for two weeks. The dosage may be increased by 25 to 50 mg a day every one or two weeks based on clinical response.

Note: Lamotrigine dosing in patients receiving only valproic acid concurrently has not been firmly established. However, lamotrigine dosing identical to that used in patients receiving lamotrigine with valproic acid and enzyme-inducing anticonvulsants has been used in some patients and is the recommended dosing in the United Kingdom. Lamotrigine plasma concentrations in patients receiving only valproic acid concurrently may be up to two times those seen in patients who are also receiving enzyme-inducing anticonvulsants.

Lamotrigine is approved for use as monotherapy in some countries. Monotherapy dosage being used for patients over 12 years of age is 25 mg per day for the first two weeks then 50 mg per day for the second two weeks. The dosage may be increased, based on clinical response, up to 200 mg per day given in one dose or two divided doses.

### Usual adult prescribing limits
With enzyme-inducing anticonvulsants only—500 mg a day in two divided doses.
With enzyme-inducing anticonvulsants and valproic acid—200 mg a day in two divided doses.

### Usual pediatric dose
Safety and efficacy have not been established.

### Strength(s) usually available
U.S.—
    25 mg (Rx) [*Lamictal* (scored; lactose; magnesium stearate; microcrystalline cellulose; povidone; sodium starch glycolate)].
    100 mg (Rx) [*Lamictal* (scored; FD&C Yellow No. 6 Lake; lactose; magnesium stearate; microcrystalline cellulose; povidone; sodium starch glycolate)].
    150 mg (Rx) [*Lamictal* (scored; ferric oxide yellow; lactose; magnesium stearate; microcrystalline cellulose; povidone; sodium starch glycolate)].
    200 mg (Rx) [*Lamictal* (scored; FD&C Blue No. 2 Lake; lactose; magnesium stearate; microcrystalline cellulose; povidone; sodium starch glycolate)].
Canada—
    25 mg (Rx) [*Lamictal* (scored; cellulose; lactose; magnesium stearate; povidone; sodium starch glycolate)].

50 mg (Rx) [*Lamictal* (scored; cellulose; ferric oxide red; lactose; magnesium stearate; povidone; sodium starch glycolate)].

100 mg (Rx) [*Lamictal* (scored; cellulose; lactose; magnesium stearate; povidone; sodium starch glycolate; Sunset Yellow FCF Lake)].

150 mg (Rx) [*Lamictal* (scored; cellulose; ferric oxide yellow; lactose; magnesium stearate; povidone; sodium starch glycolate)].

200 mg (Rx) [*Lamictal* (scored; cellulose; Indigotine Lake; lactose; magnesium stearate; povidone; sodium starch glycolate)].

250 mg (Rx) [*Lamictal* (scored; cellulose; lactose; magnesium stearate; povidone; sodium starch glycolate)].

**Packaging and storage**

Store between 15 and 25 °C (59 and 77 °F), in a well-closed container, unless otherwise specified by manufacturer. Protect from light and moisture.

**Auxiliary labeling**

- May cause blurred vision.
- May cause dizziness.
- May cause drowsiness. Alcohol may intensify this effect.

**Selected Bibliography**

Gilman JT. Lamotrigine: An antiepileptic agent for the treatment of partial seizures. Ann Pharmacother 1995 Feb; 29: 144-51.

Burstein AH. Lamotrigine. Pharmacotherapy 1995; 15 (2): 129-43.

Fitton A, Goa KL. Lamotrigine: An update of its pharmacology and therapeutic use in epilepsy. Drugs 1995; 50 (4): 691-713.

Developed: 05/23/96

---

# LANSOPRAZOLE   Systemic

VA CLASSIFICATION (Primary/Secondary): GA900/GA309

Note: For a listing of dosage forms and brand names by country availability, see *Dosage Forms* section(s). For a listing of brand names for the articles in this monograph, refer to the General Index.

## Category

Gastric acid pump inhibitor; antiulcer agent.

## Indications

**Accepted**

Ulcer, duodenal (treatment)—Lansoprazole is indicated for short-term (up to 4 weeks) treatment for symptom relief and healing in patients with active duodenal ulcer.

Esophagitis, erosive (treatment)—Lansoprazole is indicated for short-term (up to 8 weeks) treatment for symptom relief and healing of all grades of erosive esophagitis associated with gastroesophageal reflux disease (GERD). Lansoprazole may be indicated for an additional 8 weeks of treatment in patients in whom healing has not occurred. If erosive esophagitis recurs, an additional course of lansoprazole treatment may be considered.

Hypersecretory conditions, gastric (treatment)—Lansoprazole is indicated for the long-term treatment of pathological hypersecretory conditions, including Zollinger-Ellison syndrome.

[Ulcer, gastric (treatment)]—Lansoprazole is indicated for short-term (up to 8 weeks) treatment in patients with active gastric ulcer.

**Acceptance not established**

There are insufficient data to date to establish the safety and appropriateness of use of lansoprazole for maintenance treatment of *duodenal* or *gastric ulcer*.

## Pharmacology/Pharmacokinetics

Note: A wide range of intersubject variability has been observed in the pharmacokinetic parameters of lansoprazole.

**Physicochemical characteristics**

Note: Lansoprazole is chemically and pharmacologically related to omeprazole.

Chemical group—Substituted benzimidazole.

Molecular weight—369.37.

pKa—8.5.

**Mechanism of action/Effect**

Lansoprazole is a selective and irreversible proton pump inhibitor. In the acidic environment of the gastric parietal cell, lansoprazole is converted to active sulphenamide derivatives that bind to the sulfhydryl group of $(H^+, K^+)$-adenosine triphosphatase [ $(H^+, K^+)$-ATPase], also known as the proton pump. $(H^+, K^+)$-ATPase catalyzes the final step in the gastric acid secretion pathway. Lansoprazole's inhibition of $(H^+, K^+)$-ATPase results in inhibition of both centrally and peripherally mediated gastric acid secretion. The inhibitory effect is dose-related. Lansoprazole inhibits both basal and stimulated gastric acid secretion regardless of the stimulus.

Following oral administration, lansoprazole significantly decreases basal acid output and significantly increases the mean gastric pH and percent of time the gastric pH remains above 3 and 4. It also significantly reduces meal-stimulated gastric acid output and secretion volume, as well as pentagastrin-stimulated acid output. In addition, lansoprazole

inhibits the normal increases in secretion volume, acidity, and acid output induced by insulin.

Lansoprazole does not have anticholinergic or histamine $H_2$-receptor antagonist properties.

**Other actions/effects**

Due to the normal physiologic effects caused by the inhibition of gastric acid secretion, blood flow in the antrum, pylorus, and duodenal bulb is decreased by about 17%; however, mucosal blood flow in the fundus of the stomach is not significantly affected by lansoprazole. Gastric emptying of digestible solids following intake of lansoprazole is significantly slowed. Lansoprazole increases serum pepsinogen levels and decreases pepsin activity under basal conditions and in response to meal stimulation or insulin injection. As with other agents that elevate intragastric pH, lansoprazole may cause an increase in the number of nitrate-reducing bacteria and an elevation in the nitrate concentration of gastric secretions in patients with gastric ulcer; however, significantly elevated nitrosamine levels have not been reported to date, suggesting no risk of carcinogenesis by this mechanism.

Lansoprazole and its active metabolites have demonstrated antimicrobial activity *in vitro* against *Helicobacter pylori*, a gram-negative bacilli strongly associated with peptic ulcers. Lansoprazole may influence the mucosal immune response to *H. pylori*. Mucosal *H. pylori*–specific IgA response is significantly enhanced after short-term treatment with lansoprazole, strongly suggesting that the secretory immune system is actively involved in host defense against *H. pylori*, and that the efficacy of such a system at the gastric mucosal level is crucial for complete eradication of *H. pylori*. Although lansoprazole alone has a relatively low clearance effect on *H. pylori*, it may enhance the ability of other agents to eradicate the organism; lansoprazole's activity as an antisecretory agent may be the more important factor explaining its effectiveness.

Lansoprazole has the ability to inhibit the hepatic cytochrome P450 enzyme system.

**Absorption**

Since lansoprazole is acid-labile, it is administered as a capsule containing enteric-coated granules to prevent gastric decomposition and to increase bioavailability. Once lansoprazole has left the stomach, absorption is rapid and relatively complete, with absolute bioavailability over 80%. Bioavailability may be decreased if lansoprazole is administered within 30 minutes of food intake as compared to that of a fasting state. Absorption may be delayed in patients with hepatic cirrhosis.

**Distribution**

Distributed in tissue, particularly gastric parietal cells. Apparent oral volume of distribution following administration of 30 mg of lansoprazole is about 0.5 liters per kilogram (L/kg).

**Protein binding**

Very high (around 97%); protein binding remains constant over the concentration range of 0.05 to 5 mcg per mL. In patients with renal function impairment, protein binding may be decreased by 1 to 1.5%.

**Biotransformation**

Lansoprazole is extensively metabolized in the liver to two main excretory metabolites that are inactive. In the acidic environment of the gastric parietal cell, lansoprazole is converted to two active compounds that inhibit acid secretion by $(H+, K+)$-ATPase within the parietal cell canaliculus, but that are not present in the systemic circulation.

## Half-life

Elimination—

Normal renal function: Approximately 1.5 hours.

Renal function impairment: Shortened elimination half-life.

Elderly patients: 1.9 to 2.9 hours.

Hepatic function impairment: 3.2 to 7.2 hours.

## Onset of action

An increase in gastric pH is seen within 2 to 3 hours following a single 15-mg dose, 1 to 2 hours following a single 30-mg dose or a 15-mg multiple-dose regimen, and 1 hour following a 30-mg multiple-dose regimen.

## Time to peak concentration

Approximately 1 to 2 hours. Time to peak concentration ($t_{max}$) is shorter when lansoprazole is administered in the morning as opposed to the evening.

## Peak serum concentration

Mean peak serum concentrations ($C_{max}$) ranged from 0.75 to 1.15 milligrams per Liter (mg/L) following administration of a single oral 30-mg dose of lansoprazole to volunteers. Although there is no correlation with serum concentrations of lansoprazole per se, inhibition of gastric secretion appears to be dose-proportional. Serum concentrations after morning dosing may be increased by twofold or more as compared to evening dosing regimens. Both $C_{max}$ and the area under the plasma concentration–time curve (AUC) decrease by about 50% when lansoprazole is administered within 30 minutes of food intake as opposed to fasting conditions. The concentration of lansoprazole and its active metabolites within the gastric parietal cell is the main determining factor of antisecretory efficacy.

## Duration of action

More than 24 hours. Following discontinuation of lansoprazole, gastric acid levels do not increase to half the basal output until 39 hours have elapsed. No rebound gastric acidity has been observed following discontinuation of lansoprazole. In patients with Zollinger-Ellison syndrome, the duration of action of lansoprazole is prolonged.

## Elimination

Renal—Approximately 14 to 25% of a dose of lansoprazole is excreted in the urine, as conjugated and unconjugated hydroxylated metabolites. Less than 1% of unchanged lansoprazole is detectable in the urine.

Biliary/fecal—Approximately two-thirds of a dose of lansoprazole is detected as metabolites in the feces.

In dialysis—Lansoprazole and its metabolites are not significantly dialyzed; no appreciable fraction is removed by hemodialysis.

Note: Elimination is prolonged in healthy elderly subjects, in adult and elderly patients with mild renal impairment, and in patients with severe liver disease.

# Precautions to Consider

## Carcinogenicity

In 2-year studies in rats receiving up to 40 times the recommended human dose, lansoprazole produced dose-related gastric enterochromaffin-like (ECL) cell hyperplasia and ECL cell carcinoids in both male and female rats. Lansoprazole also increased the incidence of intestinal metaplasia of the gastric epithelium, and produced dose-related increases in the incidence of testicular interstitial adenomas. In a 1-year toxicity study in rats receiving 13 times the recommended human dose, testicular interstitial cell adenoma also occurred in 1 of 30 rats. In a 2-year study in mice receiving up to 80 times the recommended human dose, lansoprazole produced an increased incidence of liver tumors (hepatocellular adenomas and carcinomas), a dose-related increase in the incidence of gastric ECL cell hyperplasia, and adenomas of the rete testis in males.

## Mutagenicity

Lansoprazole was not genotoxic in the Ames test, the *ex vivo* rat hepatocyte unscheduled DNA synthesis (UDS) test, the *in vivo* mouse micronucleus test, or the rat bone marrow cell chromosomal aberration test. It was positive in *in vitro* human lymphocyte chromosomal aberration assays.

## Pregnancy/Reproduction

Fertility—Reproduction studies in rats and rabbits have shown no evidence of impaired fertility.

Pregnancy—Adequate and well-controlled studies in humans have not been done.

Reproductive studies in rats and rabbits at doses 40 times the recommended human dose have not shown that lansoprazole causes adverse effects in the fetus.

FDA Pregnancy Category B.

## Breast-feeding

It is not known whether lansoprazole is distributed into breast milk. However, lansoprazole or its metabolites are distributed into the milk of rats. Because lansoprazole has been shown to cause tumorigenic effects in animals, a decision should be made as to whether nursing should be discontinued or the medication withdrawn, taking into account the importance of lansoprazole to the mother.

## Pediatrics

No information is available on the relationship of age to the effects of lansoprazole in pediatric patients up to 18 years of age. Safety and efficacy have not been established.

## Geriatrics

Studies in elderly patients indicate that the clearance of lansoprazole is decreased in the elderly, resulting in a 50 to 100% increase in the elimination half-life. Because the mean half-life in the elderly remains between 1.9 and 2.9 hours, repeated once-daily dosing does not result in accumulation of lansoprazole. However, subsequent doses higher than 30 mg a day should not be administered unless additional gastric acid suppression is necessary.

## Drug interactions and/or related problems

The following drug interactions and/or related problems have been selected on the basis of their potential clinical significance (possible mechanism in parentheses where appropriate)—not necessarily inclusive ($\gg$ = major clinical significance):

Note: Only specific interactions between lansoprazole and other medications have been identified in this monograph. However, lansoprazole, by decreasing gastric pH, has the potential to affect the bioavailability of any medication whose absorption is pH-dependent. Also, lansoprazole may prevent the degradation of acid-labile drugs.

Possible interactions of lansoprazole with medications known to be metabolized by the hepatic cytochrome P450 enzyme system should be considered. To date, however, lansoprazole appears to interact minimally with other agents, and no clinically relevant interactions have been reported with antipyrine; diazepam; ibuprofen, indomethacin, or other nonsteroidal anti-inflammatory drugs (NSAIDs); oral contraceptives; phenytoin; prednisone or prednisolone; propranolol; or warfarin.

Combinations containing any of the following medications, depending on the amount present, may also interact with this medication.

Ampicillin esters or

Digoxin or

Iron salts or

Ketoconazole

(lansoprazole causes prolonged inhibition of gastric acid secretion, and thereby may interfere with the absorption of these medications and others for which bioavailability is determined by gastric pH)

Cyanocobalamin

(lansoprazole appears to produce a dose-dependent decrease in the absorption of cyanocobalamin; this may be due to lansoprazole-induced hypochlorhydria or achlorhydria)

$\gg$ Sucralfate

(lansoprazole absorption is delayed and bioavailability is decreased; lansoprazole should be taken at least 30 minutes prior to sucralfate)

Theophylline

(minor increases in the clearance of theophylline may occur, but the interaction is unlikely to be clinically significant; however, some patients may require adjustment of theophylline dosage when initiating or stopping lansoprazole therapy to maintain clinically effective concentrations of theophylline)

## Laboratory value alterations

The following have been selected on the basis of their potential clinical significance (possible effect in parentheses where appropriate)—not necessarily inclusive ($\gg$ = major clinical significance):

Note: Although abnormalities in test values reported to date have generally not been of substantial clinical significance, the following have been selected on the basis of their *potential* clinical significance.

With physiology/laboratory test values

Alanine aminotransferase (ALT [SGPT]) and

Alkaline phosphatase and

Aspartate aminotransferase (AST [SGOT]) and

Bilirubin and

Gamma-glutamyltransferase (GGT) and

Globulins and

Lactate dehydrogenase (LDH)
  (serum values may be increased)
Albumin/globulin (AG) ratio
  (may be abnormal)
Cholesterol and
Electrolytes
  (serum concentrations may be increased or decreased)
Creatinine, serum and
Glucocorticoids and
Triglycerides, serum and
Uric acid
  (concentrations may be increased)
Gastrin, serum
  (concentrations may be increased; median fasting gastrin concentrations may increase 50 to 100% from baseline but remain in the normal range following treatment with lansoprazole at doses of 15 to 60 mg; observations in over 2100 patients showed that elevations reached a plateau after 2 months of therapy and returned to baseline after treatment was discontinued)
Hematocrit and
Hemoglobin
  (levels may be increased)
Platelet count and
Red blood cell (RBC) count and
White blood cell (WBC) count
  (may be increased or decreased, and abnormalities may be present)

**Medical considerations/Contraindications**
The medical considerations/contraindications included here have been selected on the basis of their potential clinical significance (reasons given in parentheses where appropriate)—not necessarily inclusive (» = major clinical significance).

*Risk-benefit should be considered when the following medical problems exist:*
Hepatic function impairment
  (dosage reduction may be required in patients with severe hepatic disease because of the prolonged plasma half-life of lansoprazole)
Sensitivity to lansoprazole

## Side/Adverse Effects

The following side/adverse effects have been selected on the basis of their potential clinical significance (possible signs and symptoms in parentheses where appropriate)—not necessarily inclusive:

**Those indicating need for medical attention**
Incidence more frequent
  *Diarrhea; skin rash or itching*
Incidence less frequent
  *Abdominal or stomach pain; increased or decreased appetite; nausea*
Incidence rare
  *Anxiety; constipation; flu syndrome* (flu-like symptoms); *increased cough; mental depression; myalgia* (muscle pain); *thrombocytopenia* (unusual bleeding or bruising); *ulcerative colitis* (diarrhea, abdominal pain, rectal bleeding); *upper respiratory tract inflammation or infection* (cold symptoms)

**Those indicating need for medical attention only if they continue or are bothersome**
Incidence more frequent
  *Dizziness; headache*

## Overdose

For information on the management of overdose or unintentional ingestion, **contact a Poison Control Center** (see *Poison Control Center Listing*).

**Clinical effects of overdose**
Experience with lansoprazole overdose is limited. In one case in which a patient consumed 600 mg of lansoprazole, no adverse reaction was noted.

**Treatment of overdose**
There is no specific antidote for lansoprazole. Treatment is essentially symptomatic and supportive. Hemodialysis does not remove an appreciable fraction of the total quantity of lansoprazole or its metabolites.

Patients in whom intentional overdose is confirmed or suspected should be referred for psychiatric consultation.

## Patient Consultation

As an aid to patient consultation, refer to *Advice for the Patient, Lansoprazole (Systemic).*

In providing consultation, consider emphasizing the following selected information (» = major clinical significance):

**Before using this medication**
» Conditions affecting use, especially:
    Sensitivity to lansoprazole
    Breast-feeding—Distributed into milk in rat studies; may cause potentially serious adverse effects in nursing infants
    Use in children—Safety and efficacy not established in children up to 18 years of age
    Other medications, especially sucralfate

**Proper use of this medication**
» Importance of taking before a meal, preferably in the morning
» Swallowing capsule whole without crushing, breaking, or chewing; however, if patient cannot swallow whole, capsule may be opened and intact granules sprinkled on one tablespoon of applesauce and swallowed immediately; granules should not be chewed or crushed
» Compliance with therapy
» Proper dosing
» Missed dose: Taking as soon as possible; not taking if almost time for next dose; not doubling doses
» Proper storage

**Precautions while using this medication**
» Regular visits to physician to check progress

**Side/adverse effects**
Signs of potential side effects, especially diarrhea, skin rash or itching, abdominal or stomach pain, increased or decreased appetite, nausea, anxiety, constipation, flu syndrome, increased cough, mental depression, myalgia, thrombocytopenia, ulcerative colitis, upper respiratory tract inflammation or infection

## General Dosing Information

Since lansoprazole is acid-labile, it is administered as a capsule containing enteric-coated granules to prevent gastric decomposition and to increase bioavailability. Capsules should be swallowed whole, and not chewed or crushed. However, if the patient has difficulty swallowing capsules, the capsule may be opened and the intact granules may be sprinkled on one tablespoon of applesauce and swallowed immediately; granules should not be chewed or crushed.

Symptomatic response to therapy does not preclude the presence of gastric malignancy.

In patients with hypersecretory conditions such as Zollinger-Ellison syndrome, dosing should be adjusted according to individual needs and should continue for as long as clinically indicated. In general, treatment goals are to maintain basal acid output below 10 mEq per hour (<10 mmol/hr). Doses up to 90 mg two times a day have been administered, in some cases for as long as four years.

## Oral Dosage Forms

Note: Bracketed uses in the *Dosage Forms* section refer to categories of use and/or indications that are not included in U.S. product labeling.

### LANSOPRAZOLE DELAYED-RELEASE CAPSULES

**Usual adult dose**
Ulcer, duodenal (treatment)—
  Oral, 15 to 30 mg once a day, preferably in the morning before a meal, for up to four weeks.
Esophagitis, erosive (treatment)—
  Oral, 30 mg once a day, preferably in the morning before a meal, for up to eight weeks. An additional eight-week course may be helpful for patients who do not heal in the first eight weeks. For recurrence of erosive esophagitis, a third eight-week course of treatment may be considered.
Hypersecretory conditions, gastric, including Zollinger-Ellison syndrome (treatment)—
  Oral, initially 60 mg once a day, preferably in the morning before a meal, the dosage being increased as needed. Some patients have received doses as high as 90 mg two times a day for as long as four years.
[Ulcer, gastric (treatment)]—
  Oral, 15 to 30 mg once a day, preferably in the morning before breakfast for four to eight weeks.
Note: Daily dosages greater than 120 mg should be administered in divided doses.

  Dosage reduction should be considered in patients with severe hepatic function impairment; the dose generally should not exceed 30 mg a day in these patients.

**Usual adult prescribing limits**
For duodenal and gastric ulcers—
    30 mg a day.
For hypersecretory conditions—
    180 mg a day.

**Usual pediatric dose**
Safety and efficacy in children up to 18 years of age have not been established.

**Usual geriatric dose**
See *Usual adult dose.*

**Usual geriatric prescribing limits**
30 mg a day.

**Strength(s) usually available**
U.S.—
    15 mg (Rx) [*Prevacid*].
    30 mg (Rx) [*Prevacid*].
Canada—
    15 mg (Rx) [*Prevacid*].
    30 mg (Rx) [*Prevacid*].

**Packaging and storage**
Store below 40 °C (104 °F), preferably between 15 and 30 °C (59 and 86 °F), unless otherwise specified by manufacturer. Store in a tight container.

**Auxiliary labeling**
• Take before a meal.

Developed: 05/29/96

---

# LAXATIVES   Local

This monograph includes information on the following: Bisacodyl; Bisacodyl and Docusate*; Casanthranol†; Casanthranol and Docusate; Cascara Sagrada; Cascara Sagrada and Aloe†; Cascara Sagrada and Phenolphthalein; Castor Oil; Danthron and Docusate*; Dehydrocholic Acid†; Dehydrocholic Acid and Docusate†; Dehydrocholic Acid, Docusate, and Phenolphthalein†; Docusate; Glycerin; Lactulose; Magnesium Citrate; Magnesium Hydroxide‡; Magnesium Hydroxide and Cascara Sagrada†; Magnesium Hydroxide and Mineral Oil; Magnesium Oxide‡†; Magnesium Sulfate†; Malt Soup Extract†; Malt Soup Extract and Psyllium†; Methylcellulose†; Mineral Oil; Mineral Oil and Glycerin*; Mineral Oil, Glycerin, and Phenolphthalein*; Mineral Oil and Phenolphthalein†; Phenolphthalein; Phenolphthalein and Docusate; Phenolphthalein and Senna*; Poloxamer 188†; Polycarbophil; Potassium Bitartrate and Sodium Bicarbonate†; Psyllium; Psyllium and Senna†; Psyllium Hydrophilic Mucilloid; Psyllium Hydrophilic Mucilloid and Carboxymethylcellulose†; Psyllium Hydrophilic Mucilloid and Senna*; Psyllium Hydrophilic Mucilloid and Sennosides†; Senna; Sennosides; Sennosides and Docusate; Sodium Phosphate.

**VA CLASSIFICATION (Primary/Secondary):**
Bisacodyl
    Oral—GA204
    Rectal—RS300
Bisacodyl and Docusate
    Oral—GA209
Casanthranol
    Oral—GA204
Casanthranol and Docusate
    Oral—GA209
Cascara Sagrada
    Oral—GA204
Cascara Sagrada and Aloe
    Oral—GA204
Cascara Sagrada and Phenolphthalein
    Oral—GA204
Castor Oil
    Oral—GA204
Danthron and Docusate
    Oral—GA209
Dehydrocholic Acid
    Oral—GA204/GA900
Dehydrocholic Acid and Docusate
    Oral—GA209
Dehydrocholic Acid, Docusate, and Phenolphthalein
    Oral—GA209
Docusate [Sodium Dioctyl Sulfosuccinate for Docusate Sodium]
    Oral—GA205
    Rectal—RS300
Glycerin [Glycerol]
    Rectal—RS300
Lactulose
    Oral—GA202/GA900
Magnesium Citrate
    Oral—GA202
Magnesium Hydroxide
    Oral—GA202/GA108

Magnesium Hydroxide and Cascara Sagrada
    Oral—GA209
Magnesium Hydroxide and Mineral Oil
    Oral—GA209
Magnesium Oxide
    Oral—GA202/GA108
Magnesium Sulfate
    Oral—GA202
Malt Soup Extract
    Oral—GA201
Malt Soup Extract and Psyllium
    Oral—GA201
Methylcellulose
    Oral—GA201
Mineral Oil
    Oral—GA203
    Rectal—RS300
Mineral Oil and Glycerin
    Oral—GA209
Mineral Oil, Glycerin, and Phenolphthalein
    Oral—GA209
Mineral Oil and Phenolphthalein
    Oral—GA209
Phenolphthalein
    Oral—GA204
Phenolphthalein and Docusate
    Oral—GA209
Phenolphthalein and Senna
    Oral—GA204
Poloxamer 188 [Poloxalkol]
    Oral—GA205
Polycarbophil
    Oral—GA201/GA400
Potassium Bitartrate and Sodium Bicarbonate
    Rectal—RS300
Psyllium
    Oral—GA201
Psyllium Hydrophilic Mucilloid
    Oral—GA201/GA400; CV350
Psyllium Hydrophilic Mucilloid and Carboxymethylcellulose
    Oral—GA201
Psyllium Hydrophilic Mucilloid and Senna
    Oral—GA209
Psyllium Hydrophilic Mucilloid and Sennosides
    Oral—GA209
Psyllium and Senna
    Oral—GA209
Senna
    Oral—GA204
    Rectal—RS300
Sennosides
    Oral—GA204
Sennosides and Docusate
    Oral—GA209
Sodium Phosphate
    Oral—GA202
    Rectal—RS300

Note: For a listing of dosage forms and brand names by country availability, see *Dosage Forms* section(s). For a listing of brand names for the articles in this monograph, refer to the General Index.

---

\*Not commercially available in the U.S.

†Not commercially available in Canada.

‡See *Antacids (Oral-Local)* for antacid use of magnesium hydroxide and magnesium oxide

---

# Category

Note: The term "laxative" includes the historically used terms "cathartic," "drastic," and "purgative."

Laxative—
> Bulk-forming—Malt Soup Extract; Malt Soup Extract and Psyllium; Methylcellulose; Polycarbophil; Psyllium; Psyllium Hydrophilic Mucilloid; Psyllium Hydrophilic Mucilloid and Carboxymethylcellulose.
> Bulk-forming and stimulant—Psyllium Hydrophilic Mucilloid and Senna; Psyllium Hydrophilic Mucilloid and Sennosides; Psyllium and Senna.
> Carbon dioxide–releasing—Potassium Bitartrate and Sodium Bicarbonate.
> Hyperosmotic—Glycerin; Lactulose.
> Hyperosmotic, saline—Magnesium Citrate; Magnesium Hydroxide; Magnesium Oxide; Magnesium Sulfate; Sodium Phosphate.
> Hyperosmotic and lubricant—Magnesium Hydroxide and Mineral Oil; Mineral Oil and Glycerin.
> Hyperosmotic, lubricant, and stimulant—Mineral Oil, Glycerin, and Phenolphthalein.
> Hyperosmotic and stimulant—Magnesium Hydroxide and Cascara Sagrada.
> Lubricant—Mineral Oil.
> Lubricant and stimulant—Mineral Oil and Phenolphthalein.
> Stimulant or contact—Bisacodyl; Casanthranol; Cascara Sagrada; Cascara Sagrada and Aloe; Cascara Sagrada and Phenolphthalein; Castor Oil; Dehydrocholic Acid; Phenolphthalein (White or Yellow); Phenolphthalein and Senna; Senna; Sennosides.
> Stimulant and stool softener—Bisacodyl and Docusate; Casanthranol and Docusate; Danthron and Docusate; Dehydrocholic Acid and Docusate; Dehydrocholic Acid, Docusate, and Phenolphthalein; Phenolphthalein and Docusate; Sennosides and Docusate.
> Stool softener or emollient—Docusate; Poloxamer 188 (poloxalkol).

Antacid—Magnesium Hydroxide; Magnesium Oxide.

Antihyperammonemic—Lactulose.

Hydrocholeretic—Dehydrocholic Acid.

Antidiarrheal—Polycarbophil; Psyllium Hydrophilic Mucilloid.

Antihyperlipidemic—Psyllium Hydrophilic Mucilloid.

# Indications

Note: Bracketed information in the *Indications* section refers to uses that are not included in U.S. product labeling.

> In the treatment of constipation or in the evacuation of the bowel, or in any other conditions in which a laxative is indicated, the advantage of using certain laxative combinations rather than a single laxative preparation has not been established. In some instances, just as with the selection of a single entity laxative, the improper selection of a laxative combination may turn constipation into a more serious condition. FDA's tentative final monograph for laxative drug products for OTC use has listed specific active laxative ingredients to be included in bulk-forming, bulk-forming and lubricant, bulk-forming and stimulant, lubricant and stimulant, lubricant and saline, saline and stimulant, and stimulant combinations.

> Some of the laxative combinations contain other active ingredients that have no laxative properties. For example, atropine has been added for its antispasmodic properties probably as an adjunct to relieve constipation-induced cramping. However, a fixed combination of a laxative with any other medication is generally considered irrational and may be unsafe in some combinations.

**Accepted**

Constipation (prophylaxis)—Oral bulk-forming, lubricant, and stool softener laxatives are indicated prophylactically in patients who should not strain during defecation, such as those with an episiotomy wound, painful thrombosed hemorrhoids, fissures or perianal abscesses, body wall and diaphragmatic hernias, anorectal stenosis, or postmyocardial infarction.

Constipation (treatment)—Oral laxatives are indicated for the short-term relief of constipation. Oral bulk-forming laxatives, stimulant laxatives, and carbon dioxide–releasing suppositories are indicated to facilitate defecation in geriatric patients with diminished colonic motor re-

sponse. Oral bulk-forming laxatives and stool softener laxatives are preferred to treat constipation that may occur during pregnancy and postpartum to help re-establish normal bowel function or to avoid straining if hemorrhoids are present.

In severe cases of constipation, such as with fecal impaction, mineral oil and stool softener laxatives administered orally or rectally are indicated to soften the impacted feces. To help complete the evacuation of the impacted colon, a rectal stimulant or saline laxative may follow.

Bowel evacuation—Pre- and postpartum: Carbon dioxide–releasing suppositories are indicated to evacuate the colon in preparation for delivery and for a few days after to help re-establish normal bowel function.

Preoperative and

Pre-radiography: Oral or rectal stimulant and oral saline laxatives, rectal preparations of glycerin, and carbon dioxide–releasing suppositories are also indicated to evacuate the colon in preparation for rectal and bowel examinations, and elective colon surgery.

Parasites, intestinal (treatment adjunct): Oral saline laxatives are indicated to accelerate excretion of various parasites including nematodes, after anthelmintic therapy.

Toxicity, nonspecific (treatment adjunct): Oral saline laxatives are also indicated to hasten excretion of poisonous substances (except acids or alkalies) from the gastrointestinal tract.

Laxative dependency (treatment)—Glycerin suppositories are indicated temporarily to re-establish normal bowel function in laxative-dependent patients.

Hyperacidity (treatment)—See Magnesium Hydroxide and Magnesium Oxide, in *Antacids (Oral-Local)*.

Hyperammonemia (prophylaxis and treatment)—Lactulose is indicated for the prevention and treatment of portal-systemic encephalopathy, including the stages of hepatic pre-coma and coma.

Biliary tract disorders (treatment)—Dehydrocholic acid is indicated as an adjunct in conditions involving the biliary tract.

Diarrhea (treatment)—Polycarbophil is indicated in the treatment of diarrhea associated with irritable bowel syndrome and diverticulosis, and acute nonspecific diarrhea. [Psyllium hydrophilic mucilloid is used in the treatment of choleretic diarrhea and diarrhea caused by vagotomy, small bowel resection, or disease of the terminal ileum.]

Bowel syndrome, irritable (treatment adjunct)—Polycarbophil is indicated [and other bulk-forming laxatives are used] to relieve constipation associated with irritable or spastic bowel.

[Hyperlipidemia (treatment)]—Psyllium hydrophilic mucilloid is used as an adjunct to diet in the treatment of mild to moderate hypercholesterolemia.

# Pharmacology/Pharmacokinetics

See *Table 1*, page 1811.

**Physicochemical characteristics**

Molecular weight—
> Bisacodyl: 361.40.
> Danthron: 240.21.
> Dehydrocholic acid: 402.53.
> Docusate calcium: 883.22.
> Docusate potassium: 460.67.
> Docusate sodium: 444.56.
> Glycerin: 92.09.
> Lactulose: 342.30.
> Magnesium citrate: 451.12.
> Magnesium hydroxide: 58.32.
> Magnesium sulfate: 246.47.
> Phenolphthalein: 318.33.
> Poloxamer: The average molecular weight is 8400.
> Sodium phosphate, dibasic: 268.07.

**Mechanism of action/Effect**

Bulk-forming—
> Absorb water and expand to provide increased bulk and moisture content to the stool. The increased bulk encourages normal peristalsis and bowel motility.

Carbon dioxide–releasing—
> Carbon dioxide released from combined potassium bitartrate and sodium bicarbonate induces gentle pressure in the rectum, thus promoting bowel movement.

Hyperosmotic—
> Glycerin: Attracts water into the stool thereby stimulating rectal contraction; also, lubricates and softens inspissated fecal mass.
> Lactulose: Produces osmotic effect in colon resulting from biodegradation by colonic bacterial flora into lactic, formic, and acetic

acids. Fluid accumulation produces distention, which in turn promotes increased peristalsis and bowel evacuation.

Saline: Produces osmotic effect primarily in small intestine by drawing water into the intestinal lumen. Fluid accumulation produces distention, which in turn promotes increased peristalsis and bowel evacuation. During the use of saline laxatives, the release of cholecystokinin from the intestinal mucosa may enhance the laxative effect.

Lubricant—
Increase water retention in the stool by coating surfaces of stool and intestines with a water-immiscible film. Lubricant effect eases passage of contents through intestines. Emulsification of lubricant tends to enhance its ability to soften stool mass.

Stool softener—
Reduce surface film tension of interfacing liquid contents of the bowel, promoting permeation of additional liquid into the stool to form a softer mass.

Stimulant—
Precise mechanism of action is unknown. Thought to increase peristalsis by a direct effect on the smooth intestinal musculature by stimulation of intramural nerve plexi. Also have been shown to promote fluid and ion accumulation in the colon (castor oil and phenolphthalein act on the small intestine) to increase the laxative effect.

Antihyperammonemic—
Lactulose decreases blood ammonia concentrations probably as a result of its bacterial degradation, in the colon, into low molecular weight organic acids that decrease the pH of the colonic contents. Acidification of colonic contents results in the retention of ammonia in the colon as the ammonium ion. The osmotic laxative action of the metabolites of lactulose expels the trapped ammonium from the colon.

Hydrocholeretic—
Dehydrocholic acid has no effect on the production of bile salts; however, it increases bile volume and flow by increasing water output, thus producing bile of relatively low specific gravity, viscosity, and total solid content.

Antidiarrheal—
Psyllium hydrophilic mucilloid and polycarbophil's water and bile salt binding capacity may result in fewer and bulkier stools.

Antihyperlipidemic—
Psyllium hydrophilic mucilloid has an antihyperlipidemic effect. It decreases serum total cholesterol, low-density lipoprotein (LDL) cholesterol, and the ratio of LDL cholesterol to high-density lipoprotein (HDL) cholesterol. Although exact mechanism of psyllium's antihyperlipidemic effect is not known, it is believed that psyllium increases bile acid secretion, thus draining cholesterol products from the body.

Note: Knowledge of many specifics of the mechanisms of action is limited. The determination of influence of factors such as cyclic-AMP, electrolyte transportation, hormones, and enzymes may change such currently accepted mechanisms.

# Precautions to Consider

## Carcinogenicity/Tumorigenicity
Chronic administration of high doses of danthron to mice and rats has resulted in the development of intestinal and liver tumors. Danthron toxicity in humans has not been demonstrated; however, in the U.S., because of the potential risk to humans, the FDA has banned all manufacturing, relabeling, repackaging, and further distribution of human drug products containing danthron.

## Pregnancy/Reproduction
Hyperosmotic—Saline: Sodium-containing preparations may promote sodium retention with resultant edema.

Lubricant—Repeated oral use of mineral oil may decrease absorption of foods, fat-soluble vitamins, and some oral medications. Hypoprothrombinemia and hemorrhagic disease of the neonate have occurred following chronic use during pregnancy.

Stimulant—Castor oil is contraindicated since its use often results in pelvic area engorgement, which may initiate reflex stimulation of the gravid uterus.

## Breast-feeding
Stimulant—Cascara sagrada and danthron preparations may be distributed into breast milk. The amounts are reportedly large enough to produce loose stools in the infant, although this still remains controversial. Phenolphthalein in laxative products is also distributed into breast milk but with no reported ill effects.

## Pediatrics
*For all laxatives—*
Laxatives should not be given to young children (up to 6 years of age) unless prescribed by a physician. Since children are not usually able to describe their symptoms precisely, proper diagnosis should precede the use of a laxative. This will avoid the complication of an existing condition (e.g., appendicitis) or the appearance of more severe side effects.

*For lubricant—*
Oral mineral oil is not recommended for children up to 6 years of age since patients in this age group are more prone to aspiration of oil droplets, which may produce lipid pneumonia.

*For stimulant—*
Bisacodyl enteric-coated tablets are not recommended for children up to 6 years of age since patients in this age group may have difficulty swallowing the tablet without chewing it. Gastric irritation may occur if the enteric coating is destroyed by chewing.

*For rectal solutions—*
Weakness, excessive perspiration, shock, seizures, and/or coma may occur in children with the use of rectal solutions due to water intoxication or dilutional hyponatremia.

Seizures with hypocalcemia may occur as a result of absorption of large amounts of phosphate in children receiving sodium phosphates rectal solution.

## Geriatrics
*For lubricant—*
Oral mineral oil is not recommended for bedridden elderly patients since they are more prone to aspiration of oil droplets, which may produce lipid pneumonia.

*For stimulant—*
Weakness, incoordination, and orthostatic hypotension may be exacerbated in elderly patients as a result of significant electrolyte loss when stimulant laxatives are used repeatedly to evacuate the colon.

*For rectal solutions—*
Weakness, excessive perspiration, shock, seizures, and/or coma may occur in elderly patients with the use of rectal solutions due to water intoxication or dilutional hyponatremia.

## Drug interactions and/or related problems
The following drug interactions and/or related problems have been selected on the basis of their potential clinical significance (possible mechanism in parentheses where appropriate)—not necessarily inclusive (» = major clinical significance):

Note: Combinations containing any of the following medications, depending on the amount present, may also interact with this medication.

*For all classes*
Diuretics, potassium-sparing, or
Potassium supplements
(chronic use or overuse of laxatives may reduce serum potassium concentrations by promoting excessive potassium loss from the intestinal tract; may interfere with potassium-retaining effects of potassium-sparing diuretics)

*For bulk-forming*
Anticoagulants, oral or
Digitalis glycosides or
Salicylates
(concurrent use with cellulose bulk-forming laxatives may reduce the desired effect because of physical binding or other absorptive hindrance; a 2-hour interval between dosage with such medication and laxative dosage is recommended)

» Tetracyclines, oral
(concurrent use with calcium polycarbophil may decrease absorption because of possible formation of nonabsorbable complexes with free calcium released after ingestion; patients should be advised not to take calcium polycarbophil laxative within 1 to 2 hours of tetracyclines)

*For hyperosmotic-saline, magnesium-containing*
» Anticoagulants, coumarin- or indandione-derivative, oral or
» Digitalis glycosides or
Phenothiazines, especially chlorpromazine
(these medications have been shown to have reduced effectiveness in the presence of aluminum- and magnesium-containing antacids; pending further studies, their concurrent administration with magnesium-containing saline hyperosmotic laxatives is best avoided)

» Ciprofloxacin
(magnesium-containing laxatives may reduce absorption by chelation of ciprofloxacin, resulting in lower serum and urine concentrations of the antibiotic; therefore, concurrent use is not recommended)

» Etidronate

(concurrent use may prevent absorption of oral etidronate; patients should be advised to avoid using magnesium-containing laxatives within 2 hours of etidronate)

» Sodium polystyrene sulfonate

(sodium polystyrene sulfonate may bind with magnesium, preventing neutralization of bicarbonate ions and leading to systemic alkalosis, which may be severe; concurrent use is not recommended, although the risk may be less with rectal administration of the resin)

» Tetracyclines, oral

(concurrent use with magnesium-containing laxatives may result in formation of nonabsorbable complexes; patients should be advised not to take these laxatives within 1 to 2 hours of tetracyclines)

*For lubricant*

Anticoagulants, coumarin- or indandione-derivative, oral or
Contraceptives, oral or
Digitalis glycosides or
Vitamins, fat-soluble, such as A, D, E, and K

(concurrent use with mineral oil may interfere with the proper absorption of these or other medications and reduce their effectiveness)

(in addition to interfering with absorption of oral anticoagulants, mineral oil also decreases absorption of vitamin K, which may lead to increased anticoagulant effects)

Stool softener laxatives

(concurrent use may cause increased absorption of mineral oil and result in the formation of tumor-like deposits in tissues)

*For stimulant*

Antacids or
Histamine $H_2$-receptor antagonists, such as:
    Cimetidine
    Famotidine
    Nizatidine
    Ranitidine or
Milk

(administration within one hour of bisacodyl tablets may cause the enteric coating to dissolve too rapidly, resulting in gastric or duodenal irritation)

*For stool softener*

Danthron or
Mineral oil or
Phenolphthalein

(concurrent use with a stool softener laxative may enhance the systemic absorption of these agents. Although such combinations are intentionally used in some "fixed-dose" laxative preparations, the propensity for toxic effects is greatly increased. Liver injury has been reported with the danthron combination following repeated dosage)

**Laboratory value alterations**

The following have been selected on the basis of their potential clinical significance (possible effect in parentheses where appropriate)—not necessarily inclusive (» = major clinical significance):

With diagnostic test results

*For stimulant*

Phenolsulfonphthalein (PSP) test

(cascara, danthron, and senna may color urine pink to red, red to violet, or red to brown, and phenolphthalein may color it pink to red in event of alkalinity and also may increase the rate of excretion of PSP)

With physiology/laboratory test values

*For all classes*

Blood glucose concentrations

(may be elevated, usually after extended use)

Potassium concentrations, serum

(may be decreased; hypokalemia has occurred with extended use)

**Medical considerations/Contraindications**

The medical considerations/contraindications included here have been selected on the basis of their potential clinical significance (reasons given in parentheses where appropriate)—not necessarily inclusive (» = major clinical significance).

***Except under special circumstances, this medication should not be used when the following medical problems exist:***

*For all classes*

» Appendicitis, or symptoms of

» Bleeding, rectal, undiagnosed

» Congestive heart failure or

» Hypertension

Note: Applies to those preparations containing sodium; an alternative sodium-free laxative may usually be used. Preparations containing less than 5 mg of sodium per dose unit are utilized in many cases.

» Diabetes mellitus

Note: Applies to those preparations containing substantial amounts of dextrose, galactose, and/or sucrose; bulk-forming and liquid dosage forms of laxatives cause most concern.

» Intestinal obstruction

» Sensitivity to the class of laxative being used

*For bulk-forming*

» Dysphagia

(esophageal obstruction may occur)

*For hyperosmotic—saline*

» Dehydration

(may be aggravated by repeated use of saline laxatives)

» Renal function impairment

(hyperkalemia and hypermagnesemia may result, especially with preparations containing magnesium and potassium salts; tetany with hypocalcemia and hyperphosphatemia may occur with the use of phosphate salts)

*For hyperosmotic—saline and lubricant*

» Colostomy or

» Ileostomy

(increased risk of electrolyte or fluid imbalance)

*For lubricant*

» Dysphagia

(oral mineral oil may be aspirated and cause lipid pneumonitis)

» Caution is also recommended with bedridden patients, who may develop lipid pneumonia from aspiration of mineral oil.

## Side/Adverse Effects

Note: Steatorrhea, proteinuria, hematuria and anuria, and a systemic lupus-like syndrome have been reported rarely with phenolphthalein.

The following side/adverse effects have been selected on the basis of their potential clinical significance (possible signs and symptoms in parentheses where appropriate)—not necessarily inclusive:

**Those indicating need for medical attention**

Incidence less frequent

*For rectal solutions—more frequent with sodium phosphates*

*Rectal irritation* (rectal bleeding, blistering, burning, itching, or pain)

Incidence rare

*For bulk-forming*

*Allergies to some vegetable components* (difficulty breathing; skin rash or itching); *esophageal blockage or intestinal impaction*

Note: Usually *esophageal blockage or intestinal impaction* occurs because of insufficient fluid intake

*For hyperosmotic—saline*

*Electrolyte imbalance* (confusion; irregular heartbeat; muscle cramps; unusual tiredness or weakness)—due to acute overdosage or chronic misuse; *magnesium accumulation in presence of renal function impairment* (dizziness or lightheadedness)

*For stimulant*

*Allergic reaction to dehydrocholic acid or phenolphthalein* (skin rash); *electrolyte imbalance* (confusion; irregular heartbeat; muscle cramps; unusual tiredness or weakness)—due to acute overdosage or chronic misuse; *pink to red discoloration of alkaline urine and feces*—with phenolphthalein only; *pink to red, red to violet, or red to brown discoloration of alkaline urine*—with cascara, danthron, and/or senna only; *yellow to brown discoloration of acid urine*—with cascara, phenolphthalein, and/or senna only

*For stool softeners*

*Allergies, undetermined* (skin rash)

**Those indicating need for medical attention only if they continue or are bothersome**

Incidence less frequent

*For hyperosmotic—glycerin*

*Skin irritation surrounding rectal area*

*For hyperosmotic—lactulose or saline*

*Cramping; diarrhea; gas formation; increased thirst*

*For lubricant*
**Skin irritation surrounding rectal area**

*For stimulant*
**Belching; cramping**—more frequent with aloe and certain senna preparations; **diarrhea; nausea; rectal irritation** (skin irritation surrounding rectal area)—with suppository dosage form

*For stool softeners*
**Stomach and/or intestinal cramping; throat irritation**—with liquid forms

## Patient Consultation

As an aid to patient consultation, refer to *Advice for the Patient, Laxatives (Oral)* and *Laxatives (Rectal)*.

In providing consultation, consider emphasizing the following selected information (» = major clinical significance):

**Before using this medication**
Importance of diet, fluids, and exercise
» Conditions affecting use, especially:
   Sensitivity to a particular class of laxative
   Pregnancy—
      For saline: May promote sodium retention resulting in edema
      For lubricant: Mineral oil may decrease absorption of foods, fat-soluble vitamins, and medications; possibility of hypoprothrombinemia and hemorrhage in neonate
      For stimulant: Castor oil not recommended; pelvic engorgement may stimulate uterus
   Breast-feeding—For stimulant: May be distributed into breast milk and may produce loose stools in nursing infant
   Use in children—Proper diagnosis recommended before using laxatives
      For lubricant: Risk of pneumonia due to aspiration of mineral oil droplets
      For stimulant: Bisacodyl enteric-coated tablets not recommended because of risk of gastric irritation if chewed
      For rectal solutions: Risk of water intoxication or dilutional hyponatremia; risk of seizures if large amounts of phosphate absorbed (for sodium phosphates)
   Use in the elderly—
      For lubricant: Risk of pneumonia in bedridden patients due to aspiration of mineral oil droplets
      For stimulant: Possible exacerbation of weakness, incoordination, and hypotension due to electrolyte loss with repeated use
      For rectal solutions: Risk of water intoxication or dilutional hyponatremia
   Other medications, especially anticoagulants, ciprofloxacin, digitalis glycosides, etidronate, sodium polystyrene sulfonate (with magnesium-containing), or oral tetracyclines (with bulk-forming and magnesium-containing)
   Other medical problems, especially appendicitis, intestinal obstruction, or rectal bleeding; congestive heart failure or hypertension (with sodium-containing); diabetes (with dextrose-, galactose-, or sucrose-containing); dysphagia (with bulk-forming or lubricant); dehydration or renal function impairment (with hyperosmotic, saline); colostomy or ileostomy (with hyperosmotic [saline] or lubricant)

**Proper use of this medication**
*For all classes*
   Following physician's directions on prescribed laxative
   Following manufacturer's package directions on nonprescription (OTC) laxative
» Proper dosing
» Proper storage
*For oral dosage forms*
   Drinking at least 6 to 8 full glasses (240 mL each) of liquids each day when using any laxative, to aid stool softening
*For rectal dosage forms*
   Proper administration technique; reading patient directions carefully
   Lubrication of anus with petroleum jelly before insertion of enema applicator and careful insertion to prevent damage to rectal wall
   Moistening suppository with water by placing either under water tap for 30 seconds or in a cup of water for at least 10 seconds, before rectal insertion
*For bulk-forming*
   Not swallowing in dry form; taking with liquid
   Drinking a full glass (240 mL) or more of liquid with each dose plus additional liquid during the day
   Results obtained in 12 hours to 3 days

*For carbon dioxide–releasing*
   Results usually obtained in 5 to 30 minutes
*For hyperosmotic—glycerin*
   Results usually obtained in 15 minutes to 1 hour
*For hyperosmotic—lactulose*
   Drinking a full glass (240 mL) of liquid or more with each dose for best results
   Flavor improved by following dose with fruit juice or citrus-flavored carbonated beverage
   May require 24 to 48 hours for results
*For hyperosmotic—saline*
*Oral dosage forms only*
   Drinking a full glass (240 mL) of liquid or more with each dose to prevent dehydration
   Flavor improved by following dose with fruit juice or citrus-flavored carbonated beverage
   Results obtained within $1/2$ to 3 hours; not taking late in day unless at bedtime with food
   Faster effect when taken on empty stomach, with a full glass (240 mL) of liquid or more
*Rectal dosage forms only*
   Results usually obtained in 2 to 5 minutes with sodium phosphates enema
*For lubricant*
*Oral dosage forms only*
   Not taking within 2 hours of meals; may interfere with absorption of food nutrients and vitamins
   Usually taken at bedtime, but not while reclining; results obtained in about 6 to 8 hours
*Rectal dosage forms only*
   Results usually obtained in 2 to 15 minutes
*For stimulant*
*Oral dosage forms only*
   Taking on empty stomach for faster results
   Preparations of this group (except castor oil) are sometimes taken at bedtime for morning results (some require up to 24 hours)
   Bisacodyl only:
      —not chewing or crushing tablets; swallowing whole because of enteric coating; not taking with milk or antacids
   Castor oil only:
      —not taking late in day; results within 2 to 6 hours
      —chilling and mixing in cold orange juice to improve taste; emulsion available
   Phenolphthalein only:
      —may cause laxative effect for up to 3 days in some individuals
*Rectal dosage forms only*
   Results usually obtained in 15 minutes to 1 hour with bisacodyl; or in 30 minutes to 2 hours with senna
*For stool softeners*
*Oral dosage forms only*
   Flavor of liquid forms improved in milk or fruit juice
   Results obtained in 1 to 2 days after first dose; may require 3 to 5 days
*Rectal dosage forms only*
   Results usually obtained in 2 to 15 minutes

**Precautions while using this medication**
*For all classes*
» Not using laxatives:
      —if symptoms of appendicitis are present
      —more often than recommended
      —unnecessarily (for example, for cold, as tonic, to clean system)
      —because bowel movement is missed 1 or 2 days
» Checking with physician if sudden change in bowel habit persists beyond 2 weeks
   Avoiding laxative habit; overuse or extended use may cause dependence for bowel function
*For oral laxatives*
» Not taking:
      —longer than 1 week unless by physician's order
      —within 2 hours of other medicine
» Checking with physician if skin rash develops while taking
*For rectal laxatives*
» Checking with physician if signs of rectal irritation or infection occur with the use of rectal solutions
   Not lubricating suppository with mineral oil or petroleum jelly

*For bulk-forming*

Diabetics and patients on sodium-restricted diet—Some products are high in sugar and/or sodium content

*For hyperosmotic (oral dosage forms only)*

Diabetics and patients on sodium-restricted diet—Some products contain sugar and/or sodium

*For lubricant (oral dosage forms only)*

Not to be taken repeatedly for prolonged time—Some absorption may cause problems; may interfere with absorption of food nutrients and vitamins A, D, E, and K

Need for protection of clothing, since large doses may cause oil leakage from rectum

Inhalation of oil droplets may cause a form of pneumonia, especially in children and bedridden elderly

Not taking mineral oil within 2 hours of a stool softener; absorption of mineral oil may be increased

*For stimulant (oral dosage forms only)*

Often associated with:
—laxative habit
—skin rash
—cramping, especially on empty stomach
—potassium loss

Diabetics and patients on sodium-restricted diet—Some products contain sugar and/or sodium

### Side/adverse effects

Signs of potential side effects, especially rectal irritation (with rectal solutions); allergic reactions; esophageal blockage or intestinal impaction (with bulk-forming); electrolyte imbalance (with hyperosmotic [saline] or stimulant); magnesium accumulation (with hyperosmotic [saline]); discoloration of urine and feces (with cascara, danthron, phenolphthalein, senna)

## General Dosing Information

### For bulk-forming

Bulk-forming laxatives are suitable for long-term therapy, if necessary.

For polycarbophil when used as antidiarrheal—

Polycarbophil is available as chewable tablets that absorb up to 60 times their weight in water. They are sometimes utilized to control diarrheal conditions by administering less fluid with each dose.

The usual oral adult dose of calcium polycarbophil when used as antidiarrheal is 1 gram one to four times a day.

The usual oral pediatric dose for children 3 to 6 years of age is 500 mg two times a day; for children 6 to 12 years of age the dose may be given three times a day, but not to exceed 3 grams a day.

For psyllium hydrophilic mucilloid when used as antihyperlipidemic—

Reduced values for serum total cholesterol, low density lipoprotein (LDL), and for the ratio of LDL cholesterol to high density lipoprotein (HDL) cholesterol have been achieved with three 3.4-gram doses of psyllium per day.

### For hyperosmotic—lactulose and saline

For lactulose—

Has no effect on small intestine; lowers pH of colon.

Use with caution in diabetics—Contains up to 1.2 grams of lactose and up to 2.2 grams of galactose per 15 mL.

Dose may be mixed with milk or fruit juice to improve flavor.

For lactulose when used as an antihyperammonemic—

The usual oral adult dose of lactulose when used as antihyperammonemic is 20 to 30 grams (30 to 45 mL) three or four times a day. This dose may be adjusted every day or two to produce two to three soft stools daily. In the initial phase of therapy 20 to 30 grams (30 to 45 mL) may be given every hour to induce rapid laxation.

Concurrent use of other laxatives during initial phase of therapy for portal-systemic encephalopathy may result in loose stools and falsely suggest adequate lactulose dosage has been obtained.

For saline—

Solid forms must be completely dissolved before swallowing.

Because of relatively short response time, saline laxatives are not usually given at bedtime or late in the day unless the dose is relatively small and given with food.

This type of laxative may contain large amounts of sodium (up to 1 gram or more per dose in some preparations).

### For lubricant

Commonly administered at bedtime, when slower peristalsis allows longer transit time to improve laxative effect. If administered at bedtime, patient should not be reclining to avoid aspiration of oil droplets.

Because mineral oil may interfere with absorption of oil-soluble nutrients and/or medications, this type of laxative is not administered within 2 hours of meals or other medications.

To avoid oil leakage through the anal sphincter, the dose of mineral oil may be reduced or divided, or a stable emulsion may be used instead.

### For stimulant

Many preparations of this group are administered at bedtime with a snack to produce results in the morning—*except* castor oil. Because of its shorter response time, castor oil is not usually taken at bedtime or late in the day.

Bisacodyl tannex (bisacodyl and tannic acid complex) should not be used if multiple enemas are required. If absorbed in sufficient amounts, tannic acid is hepatotoxic.

Phenolphthalein discolors alkaline feces and urine pink to red and acid urine yellow to brown.

Cascara, danthron, and/or senna preparations may discolor alkaline urine pink to red, red to violet, or red to brown. Acid urine may be discolored yellow to brown with cascara and/or senna preparations.

For dehydrocholic acid when used as hydrocholeretic—

The usual oral adult dose of dehydrocholic acid when used as hydrocholeretic is 244 to 500 mg three times a day after meals.

### For stool softeners

Because stool softener laxatives may increase absorption of other laxatives, including mineral oil, they are not given within 2 hours of such preparations. Patients should be informed.

The bitter taste of some liquid preparations of this type of laxative may be improved by diluting each dose in milk or fruit juice.

### For oral dosage forms

With the possible exception of bulk-forming laxatives, more rapid results are obtained when laxatives are taken on an empty stomach. When taken with food and/or at bedtime, results tend to be delayed.

Intake of at least 6 to 8 full glasses (240 mL each) of fluid per day is necessary to aid in producing a soft stool and to protect the patient against dehydration when large volumes of water are lost with passage of the stool.

### For rectal dosage forms

Lubrication of anus with petroleum jelly is recommended to prevent rectal abrasion and/or laceration produced by the insertion of a hard enema tip.

Lubrication of suppositories with mineral oil or petrolatum is not recommended since it may interfere with the action of the suppository. Instead, the suppository should be moistened with water by placing under a water tap for 30 seconds or in a cup of water for at least 10 seconds, before rectal insertion.

### Oral Dosage Forms

See *Table 2*, page 1812.

### Rectal Dosage Forms

See *Table 3*, page 1851.

## Selected Bibliography

Shafik A. Constipation: pathogenesis and management. Drugs 1993; (45)4: 528-40.

Revised: 06/25/93
Interim revision: 08/01/95; 07/31/96

## Table 1. Pharmacology/Pharmacokinetics

| Type of Laxative | Absorption | | Onset of action | | Type of stool formed | Elimination (of absorbed doses) |
|---|---|---|---|---|---|---|
| | Oral | Rectal | Oral | Rectal | | |
| Bulk-forming | Not absorbed | | 12–24 hrs (up to 3 days) | | Soft formed stool | |
| Carbon dioxide–releasing | | | | 5–30 min | | |
| Stool softener or emollient | Unknown amount | Unknown amount | 24–48 hrs (up to 3–5 days) | 2–15 min | Soft formed stool | Fecal |
| Hyperosmotic Glycerin | | Poor | | $^{1}/_{4}$–1 hr | | |
| Lactulose | Minimal (<3% dose) | | 24–48 hrs | | Soft formed stool | Renal |
| Saline | Up to 20% dose | | $^{1}/_{2}$–3 hrs | 2–5 min | Watery stool (with high doses) | Renal |
| Lubricant | Minimal* | Minimal | 6–8 hrs | 2–15 min | | |
| Stimulant Anthraquinone derivatives | Minimal | | 6–8 hrs† | $^{1}/_{2}$–2 hrs | Soft or formed stool | Fecal and/or renal |
| Bisacodyl | Minimal | Minimal | | $^{1}/_{4}$–1 hr | | Renal |
| Castor oil | Unknown amount‡ | | 2–6 hrs | | Watery stool | |
| Danthron | Significant amount | | | | Soft or formed stool | Fecal and/or renal |
| Dehydrocholic acid | Significant amount | | | | | Fecal |
| Phenolphthalein | 15% | | | | Semifluid stool | Renal and fecal |

*Emulsified mineral oil may be absorbed 30 to 60%.
†Action may be prolonged up to 3–4 days.
‡Ricinoleic acid, the active principle of castor oil produced by hydrolization, is absorbed to a small extent and metabolized like other fatty acids.

Table 2. Oral Dosage Forms
Note: Content per capsule, caramel, packet, tablet, wafer, or 5 mL, unless otherwise stated.

| Brand or generic name [availability] | Bulk-forming | Stool softener or emollient | Hyper-osmotic | Lubricant | Stimulant | Other content information as per product label | Usual adult and adolescent dose* (maximum recommended daily dose) | Usual pediatric dose* | Packaging and storage§ | Auxiliary labeling§ |
|---|---|---|---|---|---|---|---|---|---|---|
| *Acilac* Solution USP (Rx) [Canada] | | | Lactulose 3.3 grams | | | Galactose <0.7 gram Lactose <0.4 gram | 15–60 mL | | c, e, f, h | l, m |
| *Afko-Lube* Capsules USP (OTC) [U.S.] | | Docusate sodium 100 mg | | | | | 2 caps | >6 yrs: 1 cap | d, e, g | l, m |
| *Afko-Lube Lax* Capsules (OTC) [U.S.] | | Docusate sodium 100 mg | | | Casanthranol 30 mg | | 1–2 caps | >6 yrs: 1 cap | d, e, g | l, m, r |
| *Agarol Plain* Emulsion (OTC) [Canada] | | | Glycerin 800 mg | Mineral oil 1.6 mL | | Sodium 0.33 mEq Agar Sugar free | 10–20 mL; repeat in am 2 hrs after breakfast | >6 yrs: 2.5 mL hs; repeat in am 2 hrs after breakfast | d | l, m, n |
| *Agarol Marshmallow* Emulsion (OTC) [U.S.] | | | | Mineral oil 4.2 grams | Phenolphthalein 0.2 gram | Sugar free | 7.5–15 mL hs | >6 yrs: 2.5–3.75 mL hs | d | n |
| *Agarol Raspberry* Emulsion (OTC) [U.S.] | | | | Mineral oil 4.2 grams | Phenolphthalein 0.2 gram | Sugar free | 7.5–15 mL hs | >6 yrs: 2.5–3.75 mL hs | d | n |
| *Agarol Strawberry* Emulsion (OTC) [Canada] | | | Glycerin 200 mg | Mineral oil 1.6 mL | Phenolphthalein 65 mg | Sodium 0.39 mEq Agar Sugar free | 10–20 mL hs; repeat in am 2 hrs after breakfast | >6 yrs: 2.5 mL hs; repeat in am 2 hrs after breakfast | d | l, m, n, r |
| *Agarol Vanilla* Emulsion (OTC) [Canada] | | | Glycerin 200 mg | Mineral oil 1.6 mL | Phenolphthalein 65 mg | Sodium 0.37 mEq Agar Sugar free | 10–20 mL hs; repeat in am 2 hrs after breakfast | >6 yrs: 2.5 mL hs; repeat in am 2 hrs after breakfast | d | l, m, n, r |
| *Alaxin* Capsules (OTC) [U.S.] | | Poloxamer 188 240 mg | | | | | 2 caps | >6 yrs: 1–2 caps | d, e | m |
| *Albert Docusate* Capsules USP (OTC) [Canada] | | Docusate calcium 240 mg | | | | | 1 cap | | d, e, g | l, m |
| *Alophen* Tablets USP (OTC) [U.S.] | | | | | Phenolphthalein 60 mg | | 1–2 tabs 1–2 times/day | | d | |

## Table 2. Oral Dosage Forms (continued)

Note: Content per capsule, caramel, packet, tablet, wafer, or 5 mL, unless otherwise stated.

| Brand or generic name [availability] | Bulk-forming | Stool softener or emollient | Hyper-osmotic | Lubricant | Stimulant | Other content information as per product label | Usual adult and adolescent dose* (maximum recommended daily dose) | Usual pediatric dose* | Packaging and storage§ | Auxiliary labeling§ |
|---|---|---|---|---|---|---|---|---|---|---|
| *Alphamul* Emulsion USP (OTC) [U.S.] | | | | | Castor oil 60% w/v | | 15–45 mL | <2 yrs: 1–5 mL >2 yrs: 5–15 mL | a, e, h | l, n, o |
| *Alramucil Orange* Effervescent Powder (OTC) [U.S.] | Psyllium hydrophilic mucilloid 3.6 grams/ packet | | | | | | 1 packet in 240 mL water or other liquid 1–3 times/day | | c, g | l, m, p |
| *Alramucil Regular* Effervescent Powder (OTC) [U.S.] | Psyllium hydrophilic mucilloid 3.6 grams/ packet | | | | | | 1 packet in 240 mL water or other liquid 1–3 times/day | | c, g | l, m, p |
| *Apo-Bisacodyl* Tablets USP (OTC) [Canada] | | | | | Bisacodyl 5 mg | Enteric-coated Sodium free | 2–3 tabs | | c | i, k, l, m |
| *Bicholate Lilas* Tablets (OTC) [Canada] | | | | | Phenolphthalein 100 mg Cascara sagrada 30 mg | Aloin 12 mg Bile salts 60 mg | 1–2 tabs | >6 yrs: 1 tab | a | l, m, r |

*Generally taken as a single daily dose at bedtime, unless otherwise stated.

†Products containing more than 5 mEq (115 mg) sodium in the maximum recommended daily dose are not recommended for patients on low salt diet. Products containing more than 50 mEq (600 mg) magnesium or more than 25 mEq (975 mg) of potassium in the maximum recommended daily dose are not recommended for patients with kidney disease.

§For appropriate *Packaging and storage* and *Auxiliary labeling* information refer to designated letters as follows:

a—Store below 40 °C (104 °F), preferably between 15 and 30 °C (59 and 86 °F), unless otherwise specified by manufacturer.
b—Store below 40 °C (104 °F), preferably between 15 and 30 °C (59 and 86 °F), unless otherwise specified by manufacturer.
c—Store below 30 °C (86 °F), unless otherwise specified by manufacturer.
d—Store between 15 and 30 °C (59 and 86 °F), in a well-closed container, unless otherwise specified by manufacturer.
e—Store in a tight container.
f—Store in a light-resistant container.
g—Store in a dry place.
h—Protect from freezing.
i—Auxiliary labeling: • Do not chew.
j—Auxiliary labeling: • Chew well before swallowing.
k—Auxiliary labeling: • Do not take within 1 hour of antacids or milk.
l—Auxiliary labeling: • Drink increased fluids.
m—Auxiliary labeling: • Take each dose with a full glass of water or other liquid.
n—Auxiliary labeling: • Shake well.
o—Auxiliary labeling: • Chill in refrigerator before taking.
p—Auxiliary labeling: • Dissolve or mix in water or other liquid before taking.
q—Auxiliary labeling: • Store in a cool place.
r—Auxiliary labeling: • May discolor urine and/or stools.

## Table 2. Oral Dosage Forms (continued)

Note: Content per capsule, caramel, packet, tablet, wafer, or 5 mL, unless otherwise stated.

| Brand or generic name [availability] | Bulk-forming | Stool softener or emollient | Hyper-osmotic | Lubricant | Stimulant | Other content information as per product label | Usual adult and adolescent dose* (maximum recommended daily dose) | Usual pediatric dose* | Packaging and storage§ | Auxiliary labeling§ |
|---|---|---|---|---|---|---|---|---|---|---|
| Bilagog Tablets (Rx) [U.S.] | | | Magnesium sulfate 300 mg | | | Atropine sulfate 0.12 mg Ox bile (desiccated) Enteric-coated | 1–2 tabs | | b | l, m |
| Bilax Capsules (OTC) [U.S.] | | Docusate sodium 100 mg | | | Dehydrocholic acid 50 mg | | 1–2 caps | Pediatric strength not available | d | l, m |
| Bisac-Evac Tablets USP (OTC) [U.S.] | | | | | Bisacodyl 5 mg | Enteric-coated Sodium free | 2–3 tabs | <6 yrs: Not recommended 6–12 yrs: 1 tab | c | i, k, l, m |
| Bisacodyl Tablets USP (OTC) [U.S./Canada] | | | | | Bisacodyl 5 mg | Enteric-coated | 2–3 tabs (6 tabs) | <6 yrs: Not recommended >6 yrs: 1 tab | b | i, k, l, m |
| Bisacolax Tablets USP (OTC) [Canada] | | | | | Bisacodyl 5 mg | Sodium <0.2 mEq Enteric-coated | 2–3 tabs (6 tabs) | <6 yrs: Not recommended >6 yrs: 1 tab | b | i, k, l, m |
| Black-Draught Syrup (OTC) [U.S.] | | | | | Casanthranol 30 mg | Alcohol 5% Tartrazine | 5–15 mL (30 mL) | <2 yrs: 1.25–3.75 mL 2–12 yrs: 2.5–7.5 mL | c, e, f, h | l, m, r |
| Black-Draught Lax-Senna Granules (OTC) [U.S.] | | | | | Senna equivalent 1.65 grams/ ½ tsp | Tartrazine | ¼–½ tsp | Not established | b | l, p, r |
| Tablets (OTC) [U.S.] | | | | | Senna equivalent 600 mg | | 2 tabs (3 tabs) | >6 yrs: 1 tab (2 tabs) | b | l, m, r |
| Caroid Tablets (OTC) [Canada] | | | | | Phenolphthalein 32.4 mg Cascara sagrada 48.6 mg | Ox bile extract 36.5 mg | 2 tabs 2 hr after breakfast and hs | | a | l, m, r |

## Table 2. Oral Dosage Forms (continued)

Note: Content per capsule, caramel, packet, tablet, wafer, or 5 mL, unless otherwise stated.

| Brand or generic name [availability] | Bulk-forming | Stool softener or emollient | Hyper-osmotic | Lubricant | Stimulant | Other content information as per product label | Usual adult and adolescent dose* (maximum recommended daily dose) | Usual pediatric dose* | Packaging and storage§ | Auxiliary labeling§ |
|---|---|---|---|---|---|---|---|---|---|---|
| *Carter's Little Pills* Tablets USP (OTC) [U.S.] | | | | | Bisacodyl 5 mg | Enteric-coated | 1–3 tabs | <6 yrs: Not recommended; 6–12 yrs: 1 tab | c | i, k, l, m |
| Tablets (OTC) [Canada] | | | | | Phenolphthalein 16 mg Aloin 8 mg | | 1–3 tabs | | c | l, m, r |
| Cascara Tablets USP (OTC) [U.S./Canada] | | | | | Cascara sagrada 325 mg | | 1–2 tabs | Pediatric strength not available | b (if coated) | l, m, r |
| Cascara, Aromatic Fluidextract USP (OTC) [U.S.] | | | | | Cascara sagrada 1 gram/mL | Alcohol 18–20% | 5 mL (15 mL) | >2 yrs: 1–3 mL | a, e, f | l, m, n, r |
| Fluidextract USP (OTC) [Canada] | | | | | Total hydroxy-anthracene derivatives from Cascara sagrada extract | Alcohol | 2.5–5 mL 1–3 times/day | | a, e, f | l, m, r |
| Cascara Sagrada Fluidextract (OTC) [U.S.] | | | | | Cascara sagrada 1 gram/mL | Alcohol 19% | 1 mL | | a, e, f | l, m, n, r |
| Castor Oil Oil USP (OTC) [U.S./Canada] | | | | | Castor oil | | 15–60 mL | <2 yrs: 1–5 mL; >2 yrs: 5–15 mL | a, e, h | l, m, o |

*Generally taken as a single daily dose at bedtime, unless otherwise stated.

†Products containing more than 5 mEq (115 mg) sodium in the maximum recommended daily dose are not recommended for patients on low salt diet. Products containing more than 50 mEq (600 mg) magnesium or more than 25 mEq (975 mg) of potassium in the maximum recommended daily dose are not recommended for patients with kidney disease.

§For appropriate *Packaging and storage* and *Auxiliary labeling* information refer to designated letters as follows:

a—Store below 40 °C (104 °F), preferably between 15 and 30 °C (59 and 86 °F), unless otherwise specified by manufacturer.

b—Store below 40 °C (104 °F), preferably between 15 and 30 °C (59 and 86 °F), in a well-closed container, unless otherwise specified by manufacturer.

c—Store below 30 °C (86 °F), unless otherwise specified by manufacturer.

d—Store between 15 and 30 °C (59 and 86 °F), unless otherwise specified by manufacturer.

e—Store in a tight container.

f—Store in a light-resistant container.

g—Store in a dry place.

h—Protect from freezing.

i—Auxiliary labeling: • Do not chew.

j—Auxiliary labeling: • Chew well before swallowing.

k—Auxiliary labeling: • Do not take within 1 hour of antacids or milk.

l—Auxiliary labeling: • Drink increased fluids.

m—Auxiliary labeling: • Take each dose with a full glass of water or other liquid.

n—Auxiliary labeling: • Shake well.

o—Auxiliary labeling: • Chill in refrigerator before taking.

p—Auxiliary labeling: • Dissolve or mix in water or other liquid before taking.

q—Auxiliary labeling: • Store in a cool place.

r—Auxiliary labeling: • May discolor urine and/or stools.

Table 2. Oral Dosage Forms (continued)

Note: Content per capsule, caramel, packet, tablet, wafer, or 5 mL, unless otherwise stated.

| Brand or generic name [availability] | Bulk-forming | Stool softener or emollient | Hyperosmotic | Lubricant | Stimulant | Other content information as per product label | Usual adult and adolescent dose* (maximum recommended daily dose) | Usual pediatric dose* | Packaging and storage§ | Auxiliary labeling§ |
|---|---|---|---|---|---|---|---|---|---|---|
| *Cholac* Solution USP (Rx) [U.S.] | | | Lactulose 3.3 gram | | | | 15–30 mL (60 mL) | Not established | c, e, f, h | l, m |
| *Chronulac* Solution USP (Rx) [U.S.] | | | Lactulose 3.3 grams | | | Galactose <0.7 gram Lactose <0.4 gram Other sugars <0.4 gram | 15–60 mL (60 mL) | Not established | c, e, f, h | l, m |
| Solution USP (OTC) [Canada] | | | | | | | | | | |
| *Cillium* Powder (OTC) [U.S.] | Psyllium 4.94 grams/ full tsp | | | | | | 1 full tsp in 240 mL water or other liquid 1–3 times/day | >6 yrs: ¹/₂ tsp in 120 mL water or other liquid | c, g | l, m, p |
| *Citroma* Oral Solution USP (OTC) [U.S.] | | | See Magnesium Citrate Oral Solution | | | See Magnesium Citrate Oral Solution | 240 mL | 2–6 yrs: 4–12 mL 6–12 yrs: 50–100 mL | d, e, h | l, m, o, q |
| *Citro-Mag* Oral Solution USP (OTC) [Canada] | | | Magnesium citrate (anhydrous) 0.25 gram (15 grams/ 300 mL.) | | | Sodium 0.5 mEq (0.31 mEq/ 300 mL)† | 75–150 mL | 6–12 yrs: 30–60 mL | d, e, h | l, m, o, q |
| *Citrucel Orange Flavor* Granules (OTC) [U.S.] | Methyl-cellulose 2 grams/ heaping tbsp or 19-gram packet | | | | | | 1 heaping tbsp or 1 19-gram packet in 240 mL water 1–3 times/day | >6 yrs: ¹/₂ tbsp in 240 mL water 1–3 times/ day | c, e, g | l, p |
| *Citrucel Sugar-Free Orange Flavor* Granules (OTC) [U.S.] | Methyl-cellulose 2 grams/ full tbsp | | | | | Aspartame | 1 full tbsp in 240 mL water 1–3 times/day | >6 yrs: ¹/₂ tbsp in 240 mL water 1–3 times/ day | c, g | l, p |
| *Colace* Capsules USP (OTC) [U.S.] | | Docusate sodium 50 mg | | | | Sodium 0.11 mEq† | 1–4 caps | >6 yrs: 1–2 caps | d, e, g | l, m |
| Capsules USP (OTC) [U.S./Canada] | | Docusate sodium 100 mg | | | | | 1–2 caps | >6 yrs: 1 cap | d, e, g | l, m |

## Table 2. Oral Dosage Forms (continued)

Note: Content per capsule, caramel, packet, tablet, wafer, or 5 mL, unless otherwise stated.

| Brand or generic name [availability] | Bulk-forming | Stool softener or emollient | Hyper-osmotic | Lubricant | Stimulant | Other content information as per product label | Usual adult and adolescent dose* (maximum recommended daily dose) | Usual pediatric dose* | Packaging and storage§ | Auxiliary labeling§ |
|---|---|---|---|---|---|---|---|---|---|---|
| *Colace (continued)* Solution USP (Oral) (OTC) [U.S./Canada] | | Docusate sodium 50 mg (10 mg/mL) | | | | | Intended for pediatric use. See *Colace* Syrup. | <3 yrs: 1–2 mL, 3–6 yrs: 2 mL, 1–3 times/day 6–12 yrs: See *Colace* Syrup | d, e, f, h | l, m |
| Syrup USP (OTC) [U.S./Canada] | | Docusate sodium 20 mg | | | | Alcohol <1% | 15–45 mL | 3–6 yrs: 5–15 mL/day 6–12 yrs: 10 mL 1–3 times/day | d, e, f, h | l, m |
| *Colax* Tablets (OTC) [U.S.] | | Docusate sodium 100 mg | | | Phenolphthalein (yellow) 65 mg | | 1–2 tabs | >6 yrs: 1 tab | a | l, m, r |
| *Cologel* Oral Solution USP (OTC) [U.S.] | Methyl-cellulose 450 mg | | | | | Alcohol 5% Sugar free | 5–20 mL 3 times/day | >6 yrs: 5 mL 2 times/day | a, e, f, h | l, m, n, p |
| *Constilac* Solution USP (Rx) [U.S.] | | | Lactulose 3.3 gram | | | | 15–30 mL (60 mL) | Not established | c, e, f, h | l, m |
| *Constulose* Solution USP (Rx) [U.S.] | | | Lactulose 3.3 grams | | | Galactose <0.7 gram Lactose <0.4 gram Other sugars ≤0.4 gram | 15–30 mL (60 mL) | Not established | c, e, f, h | l, m |

*Generally taken as a single daily dose at bedtime, unless otherwise stated.

†Products containing more than 5 mEq (115 mg) sodium in the maximum recommended daily dose are not recommended for patients on low salt diet. Products containing more than 50 mEq (600 mg) magnesium or more than 25 mEq (975 mg) of potassium in the maximum recommended daily dose are not recommended for patients with kidney disease.

§For appropriate *Packaging and storage* and *Auxiliary labeling* information refer to designated letters as follows:

a—Store below 40 °C (104 °F), preferably between 15 and 30 °C (59 and 86 °F), unless otherwise specified by manufacturer.
b—Store below 40 °C (104 °F), preferably between 15 and 30 °C (59 and 86 °F), in a well-closed container, unless otherwise specified by manufacturer.
c—Store below 30 °C (86 °F), unless otherwise specified by manufacturer.
d—Store between 15 and 30 °C (59 and 86 °F), unless otherwise specified by manufacturer.
e—Store in a tight container.
f—Store in a light-resistant container.
g—Store in a dry place.
h—Protect from freezing.
i—Auxiliary labeling: • Do not chew.
j—Auxiliary labeling: • Chew well before swallowing.
k—Auxiliary labeling: • Do not take within 1 hour of antacids or milk.

l—Auxiliary labeling: • Drink increased fluids.
m—Auxiliary labeling: • Take each dose with a full glass of water or other liquid.
n—Auxiliary labeling: • Shake well.
o—Auxiliary labeling: • Chill in refrigerator before taking.
p—Auxiliary labeling: • Dissolve or mix in water or other liquid before taking.
q—Auxiliary labeling: • Store in a cool place.
r—Auxiliary labeling: • May discolor urine and/or stools.

Table 2. Oral Dosage Forms (continued)

Note: Content per capsule, caramel, packet, tablet, wafer, or 5 mL, unless otherwise stated.

| Brand or generic name [availability] | Bulk-forming | Stool softener or emollient | Hyper-osmotic | Lubricant | Stimulant | Other content information as per product label | Usual adult and adolescent dose* (maximum recommended daily dose) | Usual pediatric dose* | Packaging and storage§ | Auxiliary labeling§ |
|---|---|---|---|---|---|---|---|---|---|---|
| *Correctol* Tablets USP (OTC) [U.S.] | | | | | Bisacodyl 5 mg | | 1–3 tabs | 6–12 yrs: 1 tab | c | i, k, l, m |
| Tablets (OTC) [Canada] | | | | | Bisacodyl 5 mg | | 1–3 tabs | >6 yrs: 1 tab am or hs | b | l, m, r |
| *Correctol Caplets* Tablets USP (OTC) [U.S.] | | | | | Bisacodyl 5 mg | | 1–3 tabs | 6–12 yrs: 1 tab | c | i, k, l, m |
| *Correctol Herbal Tea* for Oral Solution (OTC) [U.S.] | | | | | Senna (30 mg total sennosides/bag) | | 1 tea bag in 6 oz boiling water (3 bags) | | c, g | l, m, r |
| *Correctol Stool Softener Soft Gels* Capsules USP (OTC) [U.S./Canada] | | Docusate sodium 100 mg | | | | | 2 caps | 6–12 yrs: 1 cap | c, h | m |
| *Ducodyl* Tablets USP (OTC) [U.S.] | | | | | Bisacodyl 5 mg | Enteric-coated | 2–3 tabs (6 tabs) | <6 yrs: Not recommended >6 yrs: 1 tab | c | i, k, l, m |
| *DC Softgels* Capsules USP (OTC) [U.S.] | | Docusate calcium 240 mg | | | | | 1 cap | | d, e, g | l, m |
| *Decholin* Tablets USP (OTC) [U.S.] | | | | | Dehydrocholic acid 250 mg | | 1–2 tabs 3 times/day (6 tabs) | Not established | d | l, m |
| *Deficol* Tablets USP (OTC) [U.S.] | | | | | Bisacodyl 5 mg | Enteric-coated | 2–3 tabs | < 6 yrs: Not recommended > 6 yrs: 1 tab | c, e, f, g | i, k, l, m |
| *Dehydrocholic Acid* Tablets USP (Rx) [U.S.] | | | | | Dehydrocholic acid 250 mg | | 1–2 tabs 3 times/day (6 tabs) | Not established | d | l, m |
| *Dialose* Tablets USP (OTC) [U.S.] | | Docusate sodium 100 mg | | | | | 1 tab 1–3 times/day | >6 yrs: 1 tab | d | l, m |
| *Dialose Plus* Tablets (OTC) [U.S.] | | Docusate sodium 100 mg | | | Phenolphthalein (yellow) 65 mg | | 1–2 tabs 2 times/day | >6 yrs: 1 tab | d | l, m, r |

Table 2. Oral Dosage Forms (continued)

Note: Content per capsule, caramel, packet, tablet, wafer, or 5 mL, unless otherwise stated.

| Brand or generic name [availability] | Bulk-forming | Stool softener or emollient | Hyper-osmotic | Lubricant | Stimulant | Other content information as per product label | Usual adult and adolescent dose* (maximum recommended daily dose) | Usual pediatric dose* | Packaging and storage§ | Auxiliary labeling§ |
|---|---|---|---|---|---|---|---|---|---|---|
| *Diocto* Solution USP (Oral) (OTC) [U.S.] | | Docusate sodium 50 mg | | | | | 5–20 mL | <3 yrs: 1–2 mL, 3–6 yrs: 2–6 mL, 6–12 yrs: 4–12 mL, 1–3 times/day | d, e, h | l, m, n |
| Syrup USP (OTC) [U.S.] | | Docusate sodium 20 mg | | | | | 15–45 mL | 3–6 yrs: 5–15 mL/day 6–12 yrs: 10 mL 1–3 times/day | d, e, f, h | l, m |
| *Diocto-C* Syrup (OTC) [U.S.] | | Docusate sodium 20 mg | | | Casanthranol 10 mg | Alcohol 10% | 15–30 mL | >6 yrs: 5–15 mL | a, e, f | l, m, n, r |
| *Diocto-K* Capsules USP (OTC) [U.S.] | | Docusate potassium 100 mg | | | | | 1 cap 3 times/day | >6 yrs: 1 cap | d, e | l, m |
| *Diocto-K Plus* Capsules (OTC) [U.S.] | | Docusate potassium 100 mg | | | Casanthranol 30 mg | | 1 cap 2 times/day | >6 yrs: 1 cap | d, e | l, m |
| *Dioctolose Plus* Capsules (OTC) [U.S.] | | Docusate potassium 100 mg | | | Casanthranol 30 mg | | 1 cap 2 times/day | | d, e | l, m |
| *Dioeze* Capsules USP (OTC) [U.S.] | | Docusate sodium 250 mg | | | | | 1 cap | Not recommended | d, e | l, m |

*Generally taken as a single daily dose at bedtime, unless otherwise stated.

†Products containing more than 5 mEq (115 mg) sodium in the maximum recommended daily dose are not recommended for patients on low salt diet. Products containing more than 50 mEq (600 mg) magnesium or more than 25 mEq (975 mg) of potassium in the maximum recommended daily dose are not recommended for patients with kidney disease.

§For appropriate *Packaging and storage* and *Auxiliary labeling* information refer to designated letters as follows:

a—Store below 40 °C (104 °F), preferably between 15 and 30 °C (59 and 86 °F), unless otherwise specified by manufacturer.
b—Store below 40 °C (104 °F), preferably between 15 and 30 °C (59 and 86 °F), unless otherwise specified by manufacturer.
c—Store below 30 °C (86 °F), unless otherwise specified by manufacturer.
d—Store between 15 and 30 °C (59 and 86 °F), unless otherwise specified by manufacturer.
e—Store in a tight container.
f—Store in a light-resistant container.
g—Store in a dry place.
h—Protect from freezing.
i—Auxiliary labeling: • Do not chew.
j—Auxiliary labeling: • Chew well before swallowing.
k—Auxiliary labeling: • Do not take within 1 hour of antacids or milk.
l—Auxiliary labeling: • Drink increased fluids.
m—Auxiliary labeling: • Take each dose with a full glass of water or other liquid.
n—Auxiliary labeling: • Shake well.
o—Auxiliary labeling: • Chill in refrigerator before taking.
p—Auxiliary labeling: • Dissolve or mix in water or other liquid before taking.
q—Auxiliary labeling: • Store in a cool place.
r—Auxiliary labeling: • May discolor urine and/or stools.

## Table 2. Oral Dosage Forms (continued)

Note: Content per capsule, caramel, packet, tablet, wafer, or 5 mL, unless otherwise stated.

| Brand or generic name [availability] | Bulk-forming | Stool softener or emollient | Hyper-osmotic | Lubricant | Stimulant | Other content information as per product label | Usual adult and adolescent dose* (maximum recommended daily dose) | Usual pediatric dose* | Packaging and storage§ | Auxiliary labeling§ |
|---|---|---|---|---|---|---|---|---|---|---|
| Diosuccin Capsules USP (OTC) [U.S.] | | Docusate sodium 100 mg | | | | | 1–2 caps | >6 yrs: 1 cap | d, e | l, m |
| | | Docusate sodium 250 mg | | | | | 1 cap | Not recommended | | |
| Di-Sosul Tablets USP (OTC) [U.S.] | | Docusate sodium 50 mg | | | | | 1–4 tabs | >6 yrs: 1–2 tabs | b | l, m |
| Di-Sosul Forte Tablets (OTC) [U.S.] | | Docusate sodium 100 mg | | | Casanthranol 30 mg | | 1–2 tabs | >6 yrs: 1 tab | b | l, m |
| Docucal-P Capsules (OTC) [U.S.] | | Docusate calcium 60 mg | | | Phenolphthalein 65 mg | | 1–2 caps | >6 yrs: 1 cap | d, e, g | l, m, r |
| Docu-K Plus Capsules (OTC) [U.S.] | | Docusate potassium 100 mg | | | Casanthranol 30 mg | | 1 cap | > 6 yrs: 1 cap 2 times/day | d, g, | l, m |
| Docusate calcium Capsules USP (OTC) [U.S./Canada] | | Docusate calcium 240 mg | | | | | 1 cap | Pediatric strength not available | d, e, g | l, m |
| Docusate calcium w/ Phenolphthalein Capsules (OTC) [U.S.] | | Docusate calcium 60 mg | | | Phenolphthalein 65 mg | | 1–2 caps | >6 yrs: 1 cap | d, e, g | l, m, r |
| Docusate potassium w/ Casanthranol Capsules (OTC) [U.S.] | | Docusate potassium 100 mg | | | Casanthranol 30 mg | | 1 cap 2 times/day | >6 yrs: 1 cap | d, e, g | l, m |
| Docusate sodium Capsules USP (OTC) [U.S./Canada] | | Docusate sodium 50 mg | | | | | 1–4 caps | >6 yrs: 1–2 caps | d, e, g | l, m |
| | | Docusate sodium 100 mg | | | | | 1–2 caps | >6 yrs: 1 cap | | |
| | | Docusate sodium 240 mg | | | | | 1 cap | Not recommended | | |
| | | Docusate sodium 250 mg | | | | | | | | |

Table 2. Oral Dosage Forms (*continued*)

Note: Content per capsule, caramel, packet, tablet, wafer, or 5 mL, unless otherwise stated.

| Brand or generic name [availability] | Bulk-forming | Stool softener or emollient | Hyper-osmotic | Lubricant | Stimulant | Other content information as per product label | Usual adult and adolescent dose* (maximum recommended daily dose) | Usual pediatric dose* | Packaging and storage§ | Auxiliary labeling§ |
|---|---|---|---|---|---|---|---|---|---|---|
| Docusate sodium (*continued*) Solution USP (Oral) (OTC) [U.S./Canada] | | Docusate sodium 50 mg | | | | | 5–20 mL | <3 yrs: 1–2 mL, 3–6 yrs: 2–6 mL, 6–12 yrs: 4–12 mL | d, e, h | l, m |
| Syrup USP (OTC) [U.S.] | | Docusate sodium 16.7 mg | | | | | 15–45 mL | 3–6 yrs: 5–10 mL/day 7–12 yrs: 10 mL 2–3 times/day | d, e, f, h | l, m |
| Syrup USP (OTC) [U.S./Canada] | | Docusate sodium 20 mg | | | | May contain alcohol | 15–45 mL | 3–6 yrs: 5–10 mL/day 7–12 yrs: 10 mL 2–3 times/day | d, e, f, h | l, m |
| Docusate sodium w/ Casanthranol Capsules (OTC) [U.S.] | | Docusate sodium 100 mg | | | Casanthranol 30 mg | | 1–2 caps | >6 yrs: 1 cap | d, g | l, m |
| Syrup (OTC) [U.S.] | | Docusate sodium 20 mg | | | Casanthranol 10 mg | | 15–30 mL | >6 yrs: 5–15 mL | d, h | l, m, n |
| *DOK* Syrup USP (OTC) [U.S.] | | Docusate sodium 20 mg | | | | | 15–45 mL/day | 3–6 yrs: 5–15 mL/day 6–12 yrs: 10 mL 1–3 times/day | d, e, f, h | l, m |

*Generally taken as a single daily dose at bedtime, unless otherwise stated.

†Products containing more than 5 mEq (115 mg) sodium in the maximum recommended daily dose are not recommended for patients on low salt diet. Products containing more than 50 mEq (600 mg) magnesium or more than 25 mEq (975 mg) of potassium in the maximum recommended daily dose are not recommended for patients with kidney disease.

§For appropriate *Packaging and storage* and *Auxiliary labeling* information refer to designated letters as follows:

a—Store below 40 °C (104 °F), preferably between 15 and 30 °C (59 and 86 °F), unless otherwise specified by manufacturer.
b—Store below 40 °C (104 °F), preferably between 15 and 30 °C (59 and 86 °F), unless otherwise specified by manufacturer.
c—Store below 30 °C (86 °F), unless otherwise specified by manufacturer.
d—Store between 15 and 30 °C (59 and 86 °F), unless otherwise specified by manufacturer.
e—Store in a tight container.
f—Store in a light-resistant container.
g—Store in a dry place.
h—Protect from freezing.
i—Auxiliary labeling: • Do not chew.
j—Auxiliary labeling: • Chew well before swallowing.
k—Auxiliary labeling: • Do not take within 1 hour of antacids or milk.
l—Auxiliary labeling: • Drink increased fluids.
m—Auxiliary labeling: • Take each dose with a full glass of water or other liquid.
n—Auxiliary labeling: • Shake well.
o—Auxiliary labeling: • Chill in refrigerator before taking.
p—Auxiliary labeling: • Dissolve or mix in water or other liquid before taking.
q—Auxiliary labeling: • Store in a cool place.
r—Auxiliary labeling: • May discolor urine and/or stools.

## Table 2. Oral Dosage Forms (continued)

Note: Content per capsule, caramel, packet, tablet, wafer, or 5 mL, unless otherwise stated.

| Brand or generic name [availability] | Bulk-forming | Stool softener or emollient | Hyper-osmotic | Lubricant | Stimulant | Other content information as per product label | Usual adult and adolescent dose* (maximum recommended daily dose) | Usual pediatric dose* | Packaging and storage§ | Auxiliary labeling§ |
|---|---|---|---|---|---|---|---|---|---|---|
| DOK Softgels Capsules USP (OTC) [U.S.] | | Docusate sodium 100 mg | | | | | 1–2 caps | | d, e, g | l, m |
| | | Docusate sodium 250 mg | | | | | 1 cap | | | |
| D.O.S. Softgels Capsules USP (OTC) [U.S.] | | Docusate sodium 250 mg | | | | | 1 cap | | d, e | l, m |
| Dosaflex Syrup USP (OTC) [U.S.] | | | | | Standardized extract of senna fruit | Alcohol 7% Sugar 3.5 grams | 10–15 mL (15 mL 2 times/day) | 1 mos–1 yr: 1.25–2.5 mL (2.5 mL 2 times/day) 1–5 yrs: 2.5–5 mL (5 mL 2 times/day) >5 yrs: 5–10 mL (10 mL 2 times/day) | d, e, f, h | l, m, r |
| Doss Tablets (OTC) [Canada] | | Docusate sodium 60 mg | | | Danthron 50 mg | Sodium 0.13 mEq† Sugar coated Tartrazine | 1–2 tabs hs | Not recommended | a | l, m, r |
| Doxidan Capsules (OTC) [Canada] | | Docusate calcium 60 mg | | | Phenolphthalein (yellow) 65 mg | | 1–2 caps | | d, e, g | l, m, r |
| Doxidan Liqui-Gels Capsules (OTC) [U.S.] | | Docusate sodium 100 mg | | | Casanthranol 30 mg | Alcohol <1.5% | 1–2 caps | >6 yrs: 1 cap | d, e, g | l, m, r |
| Dr. Caldwell Senna Laxative Oral Solution (OTC) [U.S.] | | | | | Senna concentrate 166.5 mg | Alcohol 4.9% | 15–30 mL | 2–5 yrs: 5–10 mL; >6 yrs: 10–15 mL, hs | a | n |
| DSMC Plus Capsules (OTC) [U.S.] | | Docusate potassium 100 mg | | | Casanthranol 30 mg | Sodium free | 1–3 caps | >6 yrs: 1 cap | d, g | l, m |
| D-S-S Capsules USP (OTC) [U.S.] | | Docusate sodium 100 mg | | | | | 1–3 caps | 6–12 yrs: 1 cap | d, e, g | l, m |

Table 2. Oral Dosage Forms (continued)

Note: Content per capsule, caramel, packet, tablet, wafer, or 5 mL, unless otherwise stated.

| Brand or generic name [availability] | Bulk-forming | Stool softener or emollient | Hyper-osmotic | Lubricant | Stimulant | Other content information as per product label | Usual adult and adolescent dose* (maximum recommended daily dose) | Usual pediatric dose* | Packaging and storage§ | Auxiliary labeling§ |
|---|---|---|---|---|---|---|---|---|---|---|
| D-S-S plus Capsules (OTC) [U.S.] | | Docusate sodium 100 mg | | | Casanthranol 30 mg | | 1–3 caps | >6 yrs: 1 cap | d, g | l, m |
| Dulcodos Tablets (OTC) [Canada] | | Docusate sodium 100 mg | | | Bisacodyl 5 mg | Enteric-coated | 1–2 tabs | <6 yrs: Not recommended; >6 yrs: 1 tab | c | i, l, m |
| Dulcolax Tablets USP (OTC) [U.S./Canada] | | | | | Bisacodyl 5 mg | Enteric-coated; Tartrazine (Canada) | 2–3 tabs am or hs (3 tabs) | <6 yrs: Not recommended; >6 yrs: 1 tab | c, g | i, k, l, m |
| Duosol Capsules USP (OTC) [U.S.] | | Docusate sodium 100 mg | | | | | 2 caps | >6 yrs: 1 cap | d, e, g | l, m |
| | | Docusate sodium 250 mg | | | | | 1 cap | Not recommended | | |
| Duphalac Solution USP (Rx) [U.S.] | | | Lactulose 3.3 grams | | | Galactose <0.6 gram; Lactose <0.4 gram; Other sugars ≤0.4 gram | 15–30 mL (60 mL) | Not established | d, e, f, h | l, m |

*Generally taken as a single daily dose at bedtime, unless otherwise stated.

†Products containing more than 5 mEq (115 mg) sodium in the maximum recommended daily dose are not recommended for patients on low salt diet. Products containing more than 50 mEq (600 mg) magnesium or more than 25 mEq (975 mg) of potassium in the maximum recommended daily dose are not recommended for patients with kidney disease.

§For appropriate Packaging and storage and Auxiliary labeling information refer to designated letters as follows:

a—Store below 40 °C (104 °F), preferably between 15 and 30 °C (59 and 86 °F), unless otherwise specified by manufacturer.

b—Store below 40 °C (104 °F), preferably between 15 and 30 °C (59 and 86 °F), in a well-closed container, unless otherwise specified by manufacturer.

c—Store below 30 °C (86 °F), unless otherwise specified by manufacturer.

d—Store between 15 and 30 °C (59 and 86 °F), unless otherwise specified by manufacturer.

e—Store in a tight container.

f—Store in a light-resistant container.

g—Store in a dry place.

h—Protect from freezing.

i—Auxiliary labeling: • Do not chew.

j—Auxiliary labeling: • Chew well before swallowing.

k—Auxiliary labeling: • Do not take within 1 hour of antacids or milk.

l—Auxiliary labeling: • Drink increased fluids.

m—Auxiliary labeling: • Take each dose with a full glass of water or other liquid.

n—Auxiliary labeling: • Shake well.

o—Auxiliary labeling: • Chill in refrigerator before taking.

p—Auxiliary labeling: • Dissolve or mix in water or other liquid before taking.

q—Auxiliary labeling: • Store in a cool place.

r—Auxiliary labeling: • May discolor urine and/or stools.

Table 2. Oral Dosage Forms (continued)

Note: Content per capsule, caramel, packet, tablet, wafer, or 5 mL, unless otherwise stated.

| Brand or generic name [availability] | Bulk-forming | Stool softener or emollient | Hyper-osmotic | Lubricant | Stimulant | Other content information as per product label | Usual adult and adolescent dose* (maximum recommended daily dose) | Usual pediatric dose* | Packaging and storage§ | Auxiliary labeling§ |
|---|---|---|---|---|---|---|---|---|---|---|
| *Effer-syllium* Effervescent Powder (OTC) [U.S.] | Psyllium hydrophilic mucilloid 3 grams/full tsp or 7-gram packet | | | | | | 1 full tsp or 1 7-gram packet in 240 mL water 1–3 times/day | >6 yrs: 1 level tsp or 1/2 packet in 120 mL water | a, e, g | l, m, p |
| *Emulsoil* Emulsion USP (OTC) [U.S.] | | | | | Castor oil 95% w/v | Sodium free Sugar free | 15–60 mL in 120–240 mL of water or other liquid | <2 yrs: 1–5 mL 2–12 yrs: 5–15 mL | a, e, h | l, m, n, o |
| *Enulose* Solution USP (Rx) [U.S.] | | | Lactulose 3.3 grams | | | Galactose <0.7 gram Lactose <0.4 gram Other sugars ≤0.4 gram | 15–30 mL (60 mL) | Not established | c, e, f, h | l, m |
| *Equalactin* Chewable Tablets (OTC) [U.S.] | Calcium polycarbophil 500 mg (base) | | | | | | 2 tabs 1–4 times/day (8 tabs) | 3–6 yrs: 1 tab 1–2 times/day 6–12 yrs: 1 tab 1–4 times/day | d | j, l, m |
| *Evac-U-Gen* Tablets USP (Chewable) (OTC) [U.S.] | | | | | Phenolphthalein (yellow) 97.2 mg | Sodium 0.004 mEq† Scored | 1–2 tabs | >6 yrs: 1/2 tab | a, e | j, l, m, r |
| *Evac-U-Lax* Tablets USP (Chewable) (OTC) [U.S.] | | | | | Phenolphthalein (yellow) 80 mg | | 1–2 tabs (3 tabs) | >6 yrs: 1/2–1 tab | a, e | j, l, m, r |
| *Evalose* Solution USP (Rx) [U.S.] | | | Lactulose 3.3 grams | | | Galactose <0.5 gram Lactose <0.4 gram Other sugars ≤0.4 gram | 15–30 mL (60 mL) | | c, e, f, h | l, m |
| *Ex-Lax* Tablets USP (Chewable) (OTC) [U.S.] | | | | | Phenolphthalein (yellow) 90 mg | Flavored (chocolate) | 1–2 tabs | >6 yrs: 1/2 tab | d | j |

## Table 2. Oral Dosage Forms (continued)

Note: Content per capsule, caramel, packet, tablet, wafer, or 5 mL, unless otherwise stated.

| Brand or generic name [availability] | Bulk-forming | Stool softener or emollient | Hyper-osmotic | Lubricant | Stimulant | Other content information as per product label | Usual adult and adolescent dose* (maximum recommended daily dose) | Usual pediatric dose* | Packaging and storage§ | Auxiliary labeling§ |
|---|---|---|---|---|---|---|---|---|---|---|
| *Ex-Lax (continued)* Tablets USP (Chewable) (OTC) [Canada] | | | | | Phenolphthalein (yellow) 95 mg | Flavored (chocolate) | 1–2 tabs | 6–12 yrs: ½ tab | d | j, l, m, r |
| *Ex-Lax Gentle Nature Pills* Tablets USP (OTC) [U.S.] | | | | | Sennosides 20 mg | | 1–2 tabs | >6 yrs: 1 tab | d | m |
| *Ex-Lax Light Formula* Tablets (OTC) [Canada] | | Docusate sodium 75 mg | | | Phenolphthalein (yellow) 65 mg | | 1–2 tabs | | d | l, m, r |
| *Ex-Lax Maximum Relief Formula* Tablets USP (OTC) [U.S.] | | | | | Phenolphthalein (yellow) 135 mg | | 1–2 tabs | | d | m |
| *Ex-Lax Pills* Tablets USP (OTC) [U.S.] | | | | | Phenolphthalein (yellow) 90 mg | | 1–2 tabs | | d | m |
| Tablets USP (OTC) [Canada] | | | | | Phenolphthalein (yellow) 95 mg | | 1–2 tabs | | d | l, m, r |
| *Extra Gentle Ex-Lax* Tablets (OTC) [U.S.] | | Docusate sodium 75 mg | | | Phenolphthalein (yellow) 65 mg | | 1–2 tabs | | d | m |

*Generally taken as a single daily dose at bedtime, unless otherwise stated.

†Products containing more than 5 mEq (115 mg) sodium in the maximum recommended daily dose are not recommended for patients on low salt diet. Products containing more than 50 mEq (600 mg) magnesium or more than 25 mEq (975 mg) of potassium in the maximum recommended daily dose are not recommended for patients with kidney disease.

§For appropriate *Packaging and storage* and *Auxiliary labeling* information refer to designated letters as follows:

a—Store below 40 °C (104 °F), preferably between 15 and 30 °C (59 and 86 °F), unless otherwise specified by manufacturer.
b—Store below 40 °C (104 °F), preferably between 15 and 30 °C (59 and 86 °F), in a well-closed container, unless otherwise specified by manufacturer.
c—Store below 30 °C (86 °F), unless otherwise specified by manufacturer.
d—Store between 15 and 30 °C (59 and 86 °F), unless otherwise specified by manufacturer.
e—Store in a tight container.
f—Store in a light-resistant container.
g—Store in a dry place.
h—Protect from freezing.
i—Auxiliary labeling: • Do not chew.
j—Auxiliary labeling: • Chew well before swallowing.
k—Auxiliary labeling: • Do not take within 1 hour of antacids or milk.
l—Auxiliary labeling: • Drink increased fluids.
m—Auxiliary labeling: • Take each dose with a full glass of water or other liquid.
n—Auxiliary labeling: • Shake well.
o—Auxiliary labeling: • Chill in refrigerator before taking.
p—Auxiliary labeling: • Dissolve or mix in water or other liquid before taking.
q—Auxiliary labeling: • Store in a cool place.
r—Auxiliary labeling: • May discolor urine and/or stools.

## Table 2. Oral Dosage Forms (continued)

Note: Content per capsule, caramel, packet, tablet, wafer, or 5 mL, unless otherwise stated.

| Brand or generic name [availability] | Bulk-forming | Stool softener or emollient | Hyper-osmotic | Lubricant | Stimulant | Other content information as per product label | Usual adult and adolescent dose* (maximum recommended daily dose) | Usual pediatric dose* | Packaging and storage§ | Auxiliary labeling§ |
|---|---|---|---|---|---|---|---|---|---|---|
| *Feen-a-mint* Tablets (OTC) [U.S.] | | | | | Bisacodyl 5 mg | | 1–3 tabs | 6–12 yrs: 1 tab | b | i, k, l, m |
| *Feen-a-Mint Pills* Tablets USP (OTC) [Canada] | | | | | Bisacodyl 5 mg | Tartrazine | 1–3 tabs | >6 yrs: 1 tab | a, e | k |
| *FemiLax* Tablets (OTC) [U.S.] | | Docusate sodium 100 mg | | | Phenolphthalein (yellow) 65 mg | | 1–2 tabs | >6 yrs: 1 tab | a | l, m, r |
| *Fiberall* Powder (OTC) [U.S.] | Psyllium hydrophilic mucilloid 3.4 grams/ full tsp | | | | | Sodium 0.4 mEq†, Potassium 1.6 mEq†, per full tsp Sugar free | 1 full tsp in 240 mL water or other liquid 1–3 times/day | >6 yrs: 1/2 tsp in 240 mL water or other liquid 1–3 times/day | a, g | l, m, p |
| *Fibercon Caplets* Tablets (OTC) [U.S.] | Calcium polycarbophil 625 mg | | | | | Film coated Scored Sodium free | 2 tabs 1–4 times/day | | a, g | l, m |
| *Fiber-Lax* Tablets (OTC) [U.S.] | Calcium polycarbophil 625 mg | | | | | | 2 tabs 1–4 times/day (8 tabs) | 6–12 yrs: 1 tab 1–3 times/day (3 tabs) | a, g | l, m |
| *FiberNorm* Tablets (OTC) [U.S.] | Calcium polycarbophil 625 mg | | | | | | 2 tabs 1–4 times/day | | a | l, m |
| *Fibrepur* For Oral Suspension USP (OTC) [Canada] | Psyllium hydrophilic mucilloid 6 grams/ full tsp | | | | | Sodium <0.2 mEq† per full tsp Sugar free | 1 full tsp in 250 mL water or other liquid 1–3 times/day | >6 yrs: 1/2 tsp 120 mL water or other liquid 1–3 times/day | a, e, g | l, m, p |
| *Fleet Laxative* Tablets USP (OTC) [U.S.] | | | | | Bisacodyl 5 mg | Enteric-coated | 2 tabs (6 tabs) | <6 yrs: Not recommended >6 yrs: 1 tab | c | i, k, l, m |
| *Fleet Mineral Oil* Emulsion USP (OTC) [U.S.] | | | | Mineral oil | | | 15–45 mL | 6–12 yrs: 5–15 mL | d, e, f | l, m |

## Table 2. Oral Dosage Forms (continued)

Note: Content per capsule, caramel, packet, tablet, wafer, or 5 mL, unless otherwise stated.

| Brand or generic name [availability] | Bulk-forming | Stool softener or emollient | Hyper-osmotic | Lubricant | Stimulant | Other content information as per product label | Usual adult and adolescent dose* (maximum recommended daily dose) | Usual pediatric dose* | Packaging and storage§ | Auxiliary labeling§ |
|---|---|---|---|---|---|---|---|---|---|---|
| Fleet Phospho-Soda Oral Solution USP (OTC) [U.S.] | | | Dibasic sodium phosphate 0.9 grams, Monobasic sodium phosphate 2.4 grams | | | Sodium 24.1 mEq† Sugar free | 20 mL (for laxative effect) or 45 mL (for purgative effect) diluted in 120 mL water | 5–10 yrs: 5 mL, >10 yrs: 10 mL, diluted in 120 mL water | a, e | l, m, p |
| Fleet Sof lax Gelcaps Tablets (OTC) [U.S.] | | Docusate sodium 100 mg | | | | | 1–2 tabs | 6–12 yrs: 1 tab | d, e, g | l, m |
| Fleet Softlax Overnight Gelcaps Tablets (OTC) [U.S.] | | Docusate sodium 100 mg | | | Casanthranol 30 mg | | 1–2 tabs | 6–12 yrs: 1 tab | d, e, g | l, m |
| Fletcher's Castoria Oral Solution (OTC) [U.S.] | | | | | Senna 675 mg (135 mg/mL) | Alcohol 3.5% Sodium 0.15 mEq (0.03 mEq/mL)† | Intended for pediatric use | 1–6 mos: 0.125–2.5 mL, 7–12 mos: 2.5–5 mL, 1–5 yrs: 5–10 mL, 6–12 yrs: 10–15 mL | a, h | n |
| Oral Solution (OTC) [Canada] | | | | | Sennosides A & B 350 mL | Alcohol | Intended for pediatric use | 6–12 yrs: 10–15 mL | a, h | n |

*Generally taken as a single daily dose at bedtime, unless otherwise stated.

†Products containing more than 5 mEq (115 mg) sodium in the maximum recommended daily dose are not recommended for patients on low salt diet. Products containing more than 50 mEq (600 mg) magnesium or more than 25 mEq (975 mg) of potassium in the maximum recommended daily dose are not recommended for patients with kidney disease.

§For appropriate *Packaging and storage* and *Auxiliary labeling* information refer to designated letters as follows:

a—Store below 40 °C (104 °F), preferably between 15 and 30 °C (59 and 86 °F), unless otherwise specified by manufacturer.
b—Store below 40 °C (104 °F), preferably between 15 and 30 °C (59 and 86 °F), unless otherwise specified by manufacturer.
c—Store below 30 °C (86 °F), unless otherwise specified by manufacturer.
d—Store between 15 and 30 °C (59 and 86 °F), in a well-closed container, unless otherwise specified by manufacturer.
e—Store in a tight container.
f—Store in a light-resistant container.
g—Store in a dry place.
h—Protect from freezing.
i—Auxiliary labeling: • Do not chew.
j—Auxiliary labeling: • Chew well before swallowing.
k—Auxiliary labeling: • Do not take within 1 hour of antacids or milk.

l—Auxiliary labeling: • Drink increased fluids.
m—Auxiliary labeling: • Take each dose with a full glass of water or other liquid.
n—Auxiliary labeling: • Shake well.
o—Auxiliary labeling: • Chill in refrigerator before taking.
p—Auxiliary labeling: • Dissolve or mix in water or other liquid before taking.
q—Auxiliary labeling: • Store in a cool place.
r—Auxiliary labeling: • May discolor urine and/or stools.

Table 2. Oral Dosage Forms (continued)

Note: Content per capsule, caramel, packet, tablet, wafer, or 5 mL, unless otherwise stated.

| Brand or generic name [availability] | Bulk-forming | Stool softener or emollient | Hyper-osmotic | Lubricant | Stimulant | Other content information as per product label | Usual adult and adolescent dose* (maximum recommended daily dose) | Usual pediatric dose* | Packaging and storage§ | Auxiliary labeling§ |
|---|---|---|---|---|---|---|---|---|---|---|
| Genasoft Plus Softgels Capsules (OTC) [U.S.] | | Docusate sodium 100 mg | | | Casanthranol 30 mg | | 1–2 caps | | d, g | l, m |
| Gentle Laxative Tablets USP (OTC) [U.S.] | | | | | Bisacodyl 5 mg | Enteric-coated | 2–3 tabs | 6–12 yrs: 1 tab | c | i, k, l, m |
| Glysennid Tablets USP (OTC) [Canada] | | | | | Sennosides 8.6 mg | | 2–3 tabs | 6–12 yrs: 1–2 tabs | d | l, m |
| | | | | | Sennosides 12 mg | Tartrazine | 1–2 tabs | 6–12 yrs: 1 tab | | |
| Haley's M-O Emulsion (OTC) [U.S.] | | | Milk of Magnesia 3.75 mL (Magnesium hydroxide 300 mg) | Mineral oil 1.25 mL | | Sugar free | 15–30 mL | 3–6 yrs: 5–10 mL 6–12 yrs: 10–20 mL | a, h | l, m, n |
| Hepahydrin Tablets USP (OTC) [U.S.] | | | | | Dehydrocholic acid 244 mg | | 1–2 tabs 3 times/day (6 tabs) | Not established | d | l, m |
| Heptalac Solution USP (Rx) [U.S.] | | | Lactulose 3.3 grams | | | Galactose <0.5 gram Lactose <0.4 gram Other sugars ≤0.4 gram | 30–45 mL 3–4 times/day | | c, e, f, h | l, m |
| Herbal Laxative Tablets USP (OTC) [U.S.] | | | | | Sennosides 4 mg | | 6 tabs hs | | b | l, m |
| Tablets (OTC) [Canada] | | | | | Senna leaf powder 175 mg | | 2–3 tabs hs | | a | l, m |
| Hydrocil Instant Powder (OTC) [U.S.] | Psyllium hydrophilic mucilloid 3.5 grams/ 3.7-gram scoop or packet | | | | | Sodium <0.4 mEq†/ 3.7-gram scoop or packet Sugar free | 1 3.7-gram scoop or packet in 240 mL water or other liquid 1–2 times/day | ½ scoop or packet in 120 mL water or other liquid 1–2 times/day | a, e, g | l, m, p |

## Table 2. Oral Dosage Forms (continued)

Note: Content per capsule, caramel, packet, tablet, wafer, or 5 mL, unless otherwise stated.

| Brand or generic name [availability] | Bulk-forming | Stool softener or emollient | Hyper-osmotic | Lubricant | Stimulant | Other content information as per product label | Usual adult and adolescent dose* (maximum recommended daily dose) | Usual pediatric dose* | Packaging and storage§ | Auxiliary labeling§ |
|---|---|---|---|---|---|---|---|---|---|---|
| Karacil Powder (OTC) [Canada] | Psyllium hydrophilic mucilloid 3.5 grams/full tsp | | | | | Dextrose 3.5 grams/full tsp | 1 full tsp in 240 mL water or other liquid 1-3 times/day | >6 yrs: 1/2 tsp in 120 mL water or other liquid 1-3 times/days | c, g | l, p |
| Kasof Capsules USP (OTC) [U.S.] | | Docusate potassium 240 mg | | | | Sodium free | 1 cap | Not recommended | d, e | l, m |
| Kellogg's Castor Oil USP (OTC) [U.S.] | | | | | Castor oil 100% | Sodium free Sugar free | 30-60 mL | <2 yrs: 1-5 mL >2 yrs: 5-15 mL | a, e | l, m, o |
| Kondremul Emulsion USP (OTC) [Canada] | | | | Mineral oil (heavy) 2.75 mL | | | 15-30 mL | >6 yrs: 5-10 mL | a, e, h | l, m, n |
| Kondremul Plain Emulsion USP (OTC) [U.S.] | | | | Mineral oil (heavy) 2.75 mL | | Irish moss Sugar free | 15-30 mL | >6 yrs: 5-10 mL | a, e, h | l, m, n |
| Konsyl Powder (OTC) [U.S.] | Psyllium 100% | | | | | Sodium free Sugar free | 1 full tsp or 6-gram packet in 240 mL water or other liquid 1-3 times/day | >6 yrs: 1/2 tsp or packet in 240 mL water or other liquid 1-3 times/day | c, g | l, p |

*Generally taken as a single daily dose at bedtime, unless otherwise stated.

†Products containing more than 5 mEq (115 mg) sodium in the maximum recommended daily dose are not recommended for patients on low salt diet. Products containing more than 50 mEq (600 mg) magnesium or more than 25 mEq (975 mg) of potassium in the maximum recommended daily dose are not recommended for patients with kidney disease.

§For appropriate *Packaging and storage* and *Auxiliary labeling* information refer to designated letters as follows:

a—Store below 40 °C (104 °F), preferably between 15 and 30 °C (59 and 86 °F), unless otherwise specified by manufacturer.
b—Store below 40 °C (104 °F), preferably between 15 and 30 °C (59 and 86 °F), in a well-closed container, unless otherwise specified by manufacturer.
c—Store below 30 °C (86 °F), unless otherwise specified by manufacturer.
d—Store between 15 and 30 °C (59 and 86 °F), unless otherwise specified by manufacturer.
e—Store in a tight container.
f—Store in a light-resistant container.
g—Store in a dry place.
h—Protect from freezing.
i—Auxiliary labeling: • Do not chew.
j—Auxiliary labeling: • Chew well before swallowing.
k—Auxiliary labeling: • Do not take within 1 hour of antacids or milk.
l—Auxiliary labeling: • Drink increased fluids.
m—Auxiliary labeling: • Take each dose with a full glass of water or other liquid.
n—Auxiliary labeling: • Shake well.
o—Auxiliary labeling: • Chill in refrigerator before taking.
p—Auxiliary labeling: • Dissolve or mix in water or other liquid before taking.
q—Auxiliary labeling: • Store in a cool place.
r—Auxiliary labeling: • May discolor urine and/or stools.

Table 2. Oral Dosage Forms *(continued)*

Note: Content per capsule, caramel, packet, tablet, wafer, or 5 mL, unless otherwise stated.

| Brand or generic name [availability] | Bulk-forming | Stool softener or emollient | Hyper-osmotic | Lubricant | Stimulant | Other content information as per product label | Usual adult and adolescent dose* (maximum recommended daily dose) | Usual pediatric dose* | Packaging and storage§ | Auxiliary labeling§ |
|---|---|---|---|---|---|---|---|---|---|---|
| *Konsyl (continued)* Tablets (OTC) [U.S.] | Calcium polycarbophil 625 mg | | | | | | 2 tabs 1–4 times/day | >6 yrs: 1 tab 1–3 times/day | d, g | i, l, m |
| *Konsyl-D* Powder (OTC) [U.S.] | Psyllium hydrophilic mucilloid 3.4 grams/ full tsp or 6.5-gram packet | | | | | Sodium free Dextrose 3.5 grams, per full tsp or 6.5-gram packet | 1 full tsp or 6.5-gram packet in 240 mL water or other liquid 1–3 times/day | >6 yrs: ½ tsp or packet in 240 mL water or other liquid 1–3 times/day | c, e, g | l, p |
| *Konsyl-Orange* Powder (OTC) [U.S.] | Psyllium hydrophilic mucilloid 3.4 grams/ full tbsp or 12-gram packet | | | | | | 1 full tbsp or 12-gram packet in 240 mL water or other liquid 1–3 times/day | >6 yrs: ½ tbsp or packet in 240 mL water or other liquid 1–3 times/day | c, e, g | l, p |
| *Konsyl-Orange Sugar Free* Powder (OTC) [U.S.] | Psyllium hydrophilic mucilloid 3.4 grams/ full tsp | | | | | Phenylalanine 21 mg/full tsp | 1 full tsp in 240 mL water or other liquid 1–3 times/day | >6 yrs: ½ tsp in 240 mL water or other liquid 1–3 times/day | c, e, g | l, p |
| *Lactulax* Solution USP (OTC) [Canada] | | | Lactulose 3.3 grams | | | Galactose <0.7 gram | 15–30 mL (60 mL) | Not established | c, e, f, h | l, m |
| Lactulose Solution USP (Rx) [U.S.] | | | Lactulose 3.3 grams | | | Galactose <0.7 gram Lactose <0.4 gram Other sugars ≤0.4 gram | 15–30 mL (60 mL) | Not established | c, e, f, h | l, m |
| Solution USP (OTC) [Canada] | | | Lactulose 3.3 grams | | | | 15–60 mL | | d, e, h | l, m |
| *Lansoyl* Gel (OTC) [Canada] | | | | Mineral oil 78% | | | 15–60 mL hs | >6 yrs: 5–20 mL hs | a, h | l |
| *Lansoyl Sugar Free* Gel (OTC) [Canada] | | | | Mineral oil 78% | | | 15–45 mL hs | >6 yrs: 5–15 mL hs | a, h | l |

Table 2. Oral Dosage Forms (continued)

Note: Content per capsule, caramel, packet, tablet, wafer, or 5 mL, unless otherwise stated.

| Brand or generic name [availability] | Bulk-forming | Stool softener or emollient | Hyper-osmotic | Lubricant | Stimulant | Other content information as per product label | Usual adult and adolescent dose* (maximum recommended daily dose) | Usual pediatric dose* | Packaging and storage§ | Auxiliary labeling§ |
|---|---|---|---|---|---|---|---|---|---|---|
| Laxavite Tablets (OTC) [Canada] | | | | | Phenolphthalein 100 mg Cascara sagrada 30 mg | Aloin 12 mg Bile salts 60 mg | 1–2 tabs | | a | l, m, r |
| Laxilose Solution USP (Rx) [Canada] | | | Lactulose 3.3 gram | | | | 15–60 mL (60 mL) | | c, e, f, h | l, m |
| Laxinate 100 Capsules USP (OTC) [U.S.] | | Docusate sodium 100 mg | | | | | 1–2 caps | 6–12 yrs: 1 cap | d, e, g | l, m |
| Laxit Tablets USP (OTC) [Canada] | | | | | Bisacodyl 5 mg | Enteric-coated | 2–3 tabs (6 tabs) | <6 yrs: Not recommended >6 yrs: 1 tab | c, e | i, k, l, m |
| Lax-Pills Tablets USP (OTC) [U.S.] | | | | | Phenolphthalein (yellow) 90 mg | | 1–2 tabs | >6 yrs: 1 tab | c, e | l, r |
| Liqui-Doss Emulsion (OTC) [U.S.] | | | | Mineral oil | | Alcohol free Sugar free | 15–30 mL | >6 yrs: 5–10 mL | a, h | l, m, n |
| Magnesia Tablets USP (OTC) [Canada] | | | Magnesium hydroxide 385 mg | | | Sugar free | 6–8 tabs hs | >7 yrs: 2–4 tabs hs | b | l, m |

*Generally taken as a single daily dose at bedtime, unless otherwise stated.

†Products containing more than 5 mEq (115 mg) sodium in the maximum recommended daily dose are not recommended for patients on low salt diet. Products containing more than 50 mEq (600 mg) magnesium or more than 25 mEq (975 mg) of potassium in the maximum recommended daily dose are not recommended for patients with kidney disease.

§For appropriate *Packaging and storage* and *Auxiliary labeling* information refer to designated letters as follows:

a—Store below 40 °C (104 °F), preferably between 15 and 30 °C (59 and 86 °F), unless otherwise specified by manufacturer.
b—Store below 40 °C (104 °F), preferably between 15 and 30 °C (59 and 86 °F), unless otherwise specified by manufacturer.
c—Store below 30 °C (86 °F), unless otherwise specified by manufacturer.
d—Store between 15 and 30 °C (59 and 86 °F), in a well-closed container, unless otherwise specified by manufacturer.
e—Store in a tight container.
f—Store in a light-resistant container.
g—Store in a dry place.
h—Protect from freezing.
i—Auxiliary labeling: • Do not chew.
j—Auxiliary labeling: • Chew well before swallowing.
k—Auxiliary labeling: • Do not take within 1 hour of antacids or milk.

l—Auxiliary labeling: • Drink increased fluids.
m—Auxiliary labeling: • Take each dose with a full glass of water or other liquid.
n—Auxiliary labeling: • Shake well.
o—Auxiliary labeling: • Chill in refrigerator before taking.
p—Auxiliary labeling: • Dissolve or mix in water or other liquid before taking.
q—Auxiliary labeling: • Store in a cool place.
r—Auxiliary labeling: • May discolor urine and/or stools.

## Table 2. Oral Dosage Forms (continued)

Note: Content per capsule, caramel, packet, tablet, wafer, or 5 mL, unless otherwise stated.

| Brand or generic name [availability] | Bulk-forming | Stool softener or emollient | Hyper-osmotic | Lubricant | Stimulant | Other content information as per product label | Usual adult and adolescent dose* (maximum recommended daily dose) | Usual pediatric dose* | Packaging and storage§ | Auxiliary labeling§ |
|---|---|---|---|---|---|---|---|---|---|---|
| Milk of Magnesia USP (OTC) [U.S.] | | | Magnesium hydroxide 400 mg | | | † | 30–60 mL | <1 yr: 5 mL; 1–12 yrs: 7.5–30 mL | c, e, h | l, m, n |
| Milk of Magnesia USP (OTC) [Canada] | | | Magnesium hydroxide 440 mg | | | Sugar free | 30–45 mL | 6–12 yrs: 15–30 mL | c, e, h | l, m, n |
| Triple Strength Milk of Magnesia USP (Rx) [U.S.] | | | Magnesium hydroxide 1200 mg | | | | 10–20 mL | | c, e, h | l, m, n |
| Concentrated Milk of Magnesia-Cascara Oral Suspension (OTC) [U.S.] | | | Milk of Magnesia (Magnesium hydroxide) 2.34 g/15 mL | | Aromatic cascara fluidextract 5 mL/15 mL | Alcohol 7% Sugar free | 15 mL | | c, e, h | l, m, n |
| Magnesium Citrate Oral Solution USP (OTC) [U.S./Canada] | | | Magnesium citrate (equivalent to Magnesium oxide 1.55–1.9 grams per 100 mL), Citric acid (anhydrous) 7.59 grams, per 100 mL | | | † | 240 mL | 2–6 yrs: 4–12 mL; 6–12 yrs: 50–100 mL | d, e, h | l, m, o, q |
| Magnesium Sulfate (Epsom salts) Crystals (OTC) [U.S./Canada] | | | Magnesium sulfate | | | † | 15 grams dissolved in 240 mL water | >6 yrs: 5–10 grams dissolved in 120 mL water | b | l, m, p |
| Magnolax Emulsion (OTC) [Canada] | | | Magnesium hydroxide 300 mg | Mineral oil 1.25 mL | | Alcohol free | 7.5–15 mL | 6–12 yrs: 1.25–10 mL | a, h | l, m, n |
| Mag-Ox 400 Tablets USP (OTC) [U.S.] | | | Magnesium oxide 400 mg | | | † | 5–10 tabs | Not established | b | l, m |

Table 2. Oral Dosage Forms (*continued*)

Note: Content per capsule, caramel, packet, tablet, wafer, or 5 mL, unless otherwise stated.

| Brand or generic name [availability] | Bulk-forming | Stool softener or emollient | Hyper-osmotic | Lubricant | Stimulant | Other content information as per product label | Usual adult and adolescent dose* (maximum recommended daily dose) | Usual pediatric dose* | Packaging and storage§ | Auxiliary labeling§ |
|---|---|---|---|---|---|---|---|---|---|---|
| *Maltsupex* Powder (OTC) [U.S.] | Malt soup extract 16 grams/ full tbsp | | | | | Potassium 3.1–5.5 mEq/ full tbsp† | 2 full tbsp 2 times/day for 3–4 days, then 1–2 tbsp hs | 1 mos–2 yrs: Bottle-fed— 1–2 tsp/feeding Breast-fed— 1–2 tsp in 2–4 ounces water or fruit juice 1–2 times/day >2 yrs: 1–2 tbsp in 8 ounces liquid 1–2 times/day | b | l, m, p |
| Oral Solution (OTC) [U.S.] | Malt soup extract 5.3 grams (16 grams/ 15 mL) | | | | | Potassium 1–1.8 mEq (3.1–5.5 mEq/15 mL)† | 30 mL 2 times/day for 3–4 days, then 15–30 mL hs | 1 mos–2 yrs: Bottle-fed— 5–10 mL/feeding (up to 30mL/day) Breast-fed— 5–10 mL in 2–4 ounces water or fruit juice 1–2 times/day >2 yrs: 15–30 mL in 8 ounces liquid 1–2 times/day | a, e, h | l, m, n, p |
| Tablets (OTC) [U.S.] | Malt soup extract 750 mg | | | | | Potassium 0.15–0.25 mEq† | 4 tabs 4 times/day, then 2–4 tabs hs | See *Maltsupex* Powder or Oral Solution. | b | l, m |

*Generally taken as a single daily dose at bedtime, unless otherwise stated.

†Products containing more than 5 mEq (115 mg) sodium in the maximum recommended daily dose are not recommended for patients on low salt diet. Products containing more than 50 mEq (600 mg) magnesium or more than 25 mEq (975 mg) of potassium in the maximum recommended daily dose are not recommended for patients with kidney disease.

§For appropriate *Packaging and storage* and *Auxiliary labeling* information refer to designated letters as follows:

a—Store below 40 °C (104 °F), preferably between 15 and 30 °C (59 and 86 °F), unless otherwise specified by manufacturer.

b—Store below 40 °C (104 °F), preferably between 15 and 30 °C (59 and 86 °F), in a well-closed container, unless otherwise specified by manufacturer.

c—Store below 30 °C (86 °F), unless otherwise specified by manufacturer.

d—Store between 15 and 30 °C (59 and 86 °F), unless otherwise specified by manufacturer.

e—Store in a tight container.

f—Store in a light-resistant container.

g—Store in a dry place.

h—Protect from freezing.

i—Auxiliary labeling: • Do not chew.

j—Auxiliary labeling: • Chew well before swallowing.

k—Auxiliary labeling: • Do not take within 1 hour of antacids or milk.

l—Auxiliary labeling: • Drink increased fluids.

m—Auxiliary labeling: • Take each dose with a full glass of water or other liquid.

n—Auxiliary labeling: • Shake well.

o—Auxiliary labeling: • Chill in refrigerator before taking.

p—Auxiliary labeling: • Dissolve or mix in water or other liquid before taking.

q—Auxiliary labeling: • Store in a cool place.

r—Auxiliary labeling: • May discolor urine and/or stools.

## Table 2. Oral Dosage Forms (continued)

Note: Content per capsule, caramel, packet, tablet, wafer, or 5 mL, unless otherwise stated.

| Brand or generic name [availability] | Bulk-forming | Stool softener or emollient | Hyper-osmotic | Lubricant | Stimulant | Other content information as per product label | Usual adult and adolescent dose* (maximum recommended daily dose) | Usual pediatric dose* | Packaging and storage§ | Auxiliary labeling§ |
|---|---|---|---|---|---|---|---|---|---|---|
| *Maax 420* Tablets USP (OTC) [U.S.] | | | Magnesium oxide 420 mg | | | † | 5–10 tabs | Not established | b | l, m |
| *Medilax* Tablets USP (OTC) [U.S.] | | | | | Phenolphthalein 120 mg | Aspartame | ¼–2 tabs | Not recommended | c, e | l, r |
| *Metamucil* Powder (OTC) [U.S./Canada] | Psyllium hydrophilic mucilloid 3.4 grams/ full tsp | | | | | Sodium 0.1 mEq, Dextrose 3.5 grams, Potassium 0.09 mEq†, per full tsp | 1 full tsp in 240 mL water or other liquid 1–3 times/day | >6 yrs: ½ tsp in 240 mL water or other liquid 1–3 times/day | a, e | l, p |
| *Metamucil Apple Crisp Fiber Wafers* (OTC) [U.S.] | Psyllium hydrophilic mucilloid 3.4 grams/ 2 wafers | | | | | Sodium 0.9 mEq†, Potassium 1.3 mEq†, per 2 wafers | 2 wafers 1–3 times/day | >6 yrs: 1 wafer 1–3 times/day | a | j, l, m |
| *Metamucil Cinnamon Spice Fiber Wafers* (OTC) [U.S.] | Psyllium hydrophilic mucilloid 3.4 grams/ 2 wafers | | | | | Sodium 0.7 mEq Potassium 1.3 mEq†, per 2 wafers | 2 wafers 1–3 times/day | >6 yrs: 1 wafer 1–3 times/day | a | j, l, m |
| *Metamucil Orange Flavor* Powder (OTC) [U.S./Canada] | Psyllium hydrophilic mucilloid 3.4 grams/ full tbsp | | | | | Sodium 0.05 mEq†, Potassium 0.09 mEq†, Sucrose 7.1 grams, per full tbsp | 1 full tbsp in 240 mL cool water 1–3 times/day | >6 yrs: ½ tbsp in 120 mL cool water 1–3 times/day | a, e, g | l, p |
| *Metamucil Smooth, Citrus Flavor* Powder (OTC) [U.S.] | Psyllium hydrophilic mucilloid 3.4 grams/ full tbsp or 12-gram packet | | | | | Sodium 0.2 mEq†, Potassium 1 mEq†, per full tbsp | 1 full tbsp or 12-gram packet in 240 mL water or other liquid 1–3 times/day | >6 yrs: ½ tbsp in 240 mL water or other liquid 1–3 times/day | a, e, g | l, p |

Table 2. Oral Dosage Forms (continued)

Note: Content per capsule, caramel, packet, tablet, wafer, or 5 mL, unless otherwise stated.

| Brand or generic name [availability] | Bulk-forming | Stool softener or emollient | Hyper-osmotic | Lubricant | Stimulant | Other content information as per product label | Usual adult and adolescent dose* (maximum recommended daily dose) | Usual pediatric dose* | Packaging and storage§ | Auxiliary labeling§ |
|---|---|---|---|---|---|---|---|---|---|---|
| *Metamucil Smooth, Orange Flavor* Powder (OTC) [U.S.] | Psyllium hydrophilic mucilloid 3.4 grams/ full tbsp or 12-gram packet | | | | | Sodium 0.2 mEq†, Potassium 0.8 mEq†, per full tbsp | 1 full tbsp or 12-gram packet in 240 mL water or other liquid 1–3 times/day | >6 yrs: ½ tbsp in 240 mL water or other liquid 1–3 times/day | a, e, g | l, p |
| *Metamucil Smooth Sugar-Free, Citrus Flavor* Powder (OTC) [U.S.] | Psyllium hydrophilic mucilloid 3.4 grams/ full tsp or 5.8-gram packet | | | | | Sodium 0.2 mEq†, Potassium 0.8 mEq†, per full tsp Phenylalanine 25 mg | 1 full tsp or 5.8-gram packet in 240 mL water or other liquid 1–3 times/day | >6 yrs: ½ tsp in 240 mL water or other liquid 1–3 times/day | a, e, g | l, p |
| *Metamucil Smooth Sugar-Free, Orange Flavor* Powder (OTC) [U.S.] | Psyllium hydrophilic mucilloid 3.4 grams/ full tsp or 5.8-gram packet | | | | | Sodium 0.2 mEq†, Potassium 0.8 mEq†, per full tsp Phenylalanine 25 mg | 1 full tsp or 5.8-gram packet in 240 mL water or other liquid 1–3 times/day | >6 yrs: ½ tsp in 240 mL water or other liquid 1–3 times/day | a, e, g | l, p |
| *Metamucil Smooth Sugar-Free, Regular Flavor* Powder (OTC) [U.S.] | Psyllium hydrophilic mucilloid 3.4 grams/ full tsp | | | | | Sodium 0.2 mEq†, Potassium 0.8 mEq†, per full tsp | 1 full tsp in 240 mL water or other liquid 1–3 times/day | >6 yrs: ½ tsp in 240 mL water or other liquid 1–3 times/day | a, e, g | l, p |

*Generally taken as a single daily dose at bedtime, unless otherwise stated.

†Products containing more than 5 mEq (115 mg) sodium in the maximum recommended daily dose are not recommended for patients on low salt diet. Products containing more than 50 mEq (600 mg) magnesium or more than 25 mEq (975 mg) of potassium in the maximum recommended daily dose are not recommended for patients with kidney disease.

§For appropriate *Packaging and storage* and *Auxiliary labeling* information refer to designated letters as follows:

a—Store below 40 °C (104 °F), preferably between 15 and 30 °C (59 and 86 °F), unless otherwise specified by manufacturer.
b—Store below 40 °C (104 °F), preferably between 15 and 30 °C (59 and 86 °F), in a well-closed container, unless otherwise specified by manufacturer.
c—Store below 30 °C (86 °F), unless otherwise specified by manufacturer.
d—Store between 15 and 30 °C (59 and 86 °F), unless otherwise specified by manufacturer.
e—Store in a tight container.
f—Store in a light-resistant container.
g—Store in a dry place.
h—Protect from freezing.
i—Auxiliary labeling: • Do not chew.
j—Auxiliary labeling: • Chew well before swallowing.
k—Auxiliary labeling: • Do not take within 1 hour of antacids or milk.
l—Auxiliary labeling: • Drink increased fluids.
m—Auxiliary labeling: • Take each dose with a full glass of water or other liquid.
n—Auxiliary labeling: • Shake well.
o—Auxiliary labeling: • Chill in refrigerator before taking.
p—Auxiliary labeling: • Dissolve or mix in water or other liquid before taking.
q—Auxiliary labeling: • Store in a cool place.
r—Auxiliary labeling: • May discolor urine and/or stools.

## Table 2. Oral Dosage Forms (continued)

Note: Content per capsule, caramel, packet, tablet, wafer, or 5 mL, unless otherwise stated.

| Brand or generic name [availability] | Bulk-forming | Stool softener or emollient | Hyper-osmotic | Lubricant | Stimulant | Other content information as per product label | Usual adult and adolescent dose* (maximum recommended daily dose) | Usual pediatric dose* | Packaging and storage§ | Auxiliary labeling§ |
|---|---|---|---|---|---|---|---|---|---|---|
| *Metamucil Sugar Free Powder* (OTC) [Canada] | Psyllium hydrophilic mucilloid 3.4 grams/full tsp | | | | | Sodium <0.5 mEq† full tsp | 1 full tsp in 240 mL water 1–3 times/day | >6 yrs: ½ tsp in 120 mL water 1–3 times/day | a, e, g | l, p |
| *Metamucil Sugar-Free, Lemon-Lime Flavor Effervescent Powder* (OTC) [U.S.] | Psyllium hydrophilic mucilloid 3.4 grams/ 5.4-gram packet | | | | | Sodium 0.4 mEq†, Potassium 7 mEq†, per 5.4-gram packet Phenylalanine 30 mg | 1 5.4-gram packet in 240 mL cool water 1–3 times/day | >6 yrs: ½ packet in 240 mL cool water 1–3 times/day | a, e, g | l, p |
| *Metamucil Sugar-Free, Orange Flavor Powder* (OTC) [Canada] | Psyllium hydrophilic mucilloid 3.4 grams/full tsp | | | | | Sodium 0.2 mEq†, Potassium 7 mEq†, Phenylalanine 25 mg, per full tsp | 1 full tsp in 240 mL cool water 1–3 times/day | >6 yrs: ½ tsp in 240 mL cool water 1–3 times/day | a, e, g | l, p |
| *Effervescent Powder* (OTC) [U.S.] | Psyllium hydrophilic mucilloid 3.4 grams/ 5.2-gram packet | | | | | Sodium 0.2 mEq†, Potassium 7 mEq†, Phenylalanine 28 mg, per 5.2-gram packet | 1 5.2-gram packet in 240 mL cool water 1–3 times/day | >6 yrs: ½ packet in 240 mL cool water 1–3 times/day | a, e, g | l, p |
| Methylcellulose* Capsules (OTC) [U.S.] | Methyl-cellulose 500 mg | | | | | | 2–3 caps 3 times/day | >6 yrs: 1–2 caps 2 times/day | b | l, m |
| Powder (OTC) [U.S.] | Methyl-cellulose USP | | | | | | 1–1.5 grams 3 times/day | 1–1.5 grams/day | b | l, m |
| Tablets USP (OTC) [U.S.] | Methyl-cellulose 500 mg | | | | | | 2–3 tabs 3 times/day | >6 yrs: 1–2 tabs 2 times/day | b | l, m |

## Table 2. Oral Dosage Forms (continued)

Note: Content per capsule, caramel, packet, tablet, wafer, or 5 mL, unless otherwise stated.

| Brand or generic name [availability] | Bulk-forming | Stool softener or emollient | Hyper-osmotic | Lubricant | Stimulant | Other content information as per product label | Usual adult and adolescent dose* (maximum recommended daily dose) | Usual pediatric dose* | Packaging and storage§ | Auxiliary labeling§ |
|---|---|---|---|---|---|---|---|---|---|---|
| *Milkinol* Emulsion USP (OTC) [U.S.] | | | | Mineral oil 4.75 mL (approx.) | | Sugar free | 15–45 mL in 60 mL water or other liquid hs | 6–12 yrs: 5–15 mL hs | d, h | l, n |
| *Mineral Oil\** Oil USP (OTC) [U.S./Canada] | | | | Mineral oil | | | 15–45 mL | >6 yrs: 5–15 mL | d, e, h | l, m, n |
| *Mitrolan* Chewable Tablets (OTC) [U.S./Canada] | Calcium polycarbophil USP 500 mg (base) | | | | | Sodium <0.02 mEq | 2 tabs 4 times/day (12 tabs) | 3–6 yrs: 1 tab 2 times/day (3 tabs) 6–12 yrs: 1 tab 3 times/day (6 tabs) | d | j, l, m |
| *Modane* Tablets USP (OTC) [U.S.] | | | | | Phenolphthalein 130 mg | | 1–2 tabs | Not recommended | c, e | l, r |
| *Modane Bulk* Powder (OTC) [U.S.] | Psyllium hydrophilic mucilloid 3.4 grams/full tsp | | | | | Dextrose 3.5 grams/full tsp Citric acid | 1 full tsp in 240 mL water or other liquid 1–3 times/day | >6 yrs: ½ tsp in 240 mL water or other liquid 1–3 times/day | a, e, g | l, p |
| *Modane Plus* Tablets (OTC) [U.S.] | | Docusate sodium 100 mg | | | Phenolphthalein 65 mg | | 1–3 tabs | Not recommended | b | l, m, r |

*Generally taken as a single daily dose at bedtime, unless otherwise stated.

†Products containing more than 5 mEq (115 mg) sodium in the maximum recommended daily dose are not recommended for patients on low salt diet. Products containing more than 50 mEq (600 mg) magnesium or more than 25 mEq (975 mg) of potassium in the maximum recommended daily dose are not recommended for patients with kidney disease.

§For appropriate *Packaging and storage* and *Auxiliary labeling* information refer to designated letters as follows:

a—Store below 40 °C (104 °F), preferably between 15 and 30 °C (59 and 86 °F), unless otherwise specified by manufacturer.
b—Store below 40 °C (104 °F), preferably between 15 and 30 °C (59 and 86 °F), in a well-closed container, unless otherwise specified by manufacturer.
c—Store below 30 °C (86 °F), unless otherwise specified by manufacturer.
d—Store between 15 and 30 °C (59 and 86 °F), unless otherwise specified by manufacturer.
e—Store in a tight container.
f—Store in a light-resistant container.
g—Store in a dry place.
h—Protect from freezing.
i—Auxiliary labeling: • Do not chew.
j—Auxiliary labeling: • Chew well before swallowing.
k—Auxiliary labeling: • Do not take within 1 hour of antacids or milk.
l—Auxiliary labeling: • Drink increased fluids.
m—Auxiliary labeling: • Take each dose with a full glass of water or other liquid.
n—Auxiliary labeling: • Shake well.
o—Auxiliary labeling: • Chill in refrigerator before taking.
p—Auxiliary labeling: • Dissolve or mix in water or other liquid before taking.
q—Auxiliary labeling: • Store in a cool place.
r—Auxiliary labeling: • May discolor urine and/or stools.

## Table 2. Oral Dosage Forms (continued)

Note: Content per capsule, caramel, packet, tablet, wafer, or 5 mL, unless otherwise stated.

| Brand or generic name [availability] | Bulk-forming | Stool softener or emollient | Hyper-osmotic | Lubricant | Stimulant | Other content information as per product label | Usual adult and adolescent dose* (maximum recommended daily dose) | Usual pediatric dose* | Packaging and storage§ | Auxiliary labeling§ |
|---|---|---|---|---|---|---|---|---|---|---|
| Modane Soft Capsules USP (OTC) [U.S.] | | Docusate sodium 100 mg | | | | | 1–3 caps | >2 yrs: 1 cap | d, e, g | l, m |
| Molatoc Tablets USP (OTC) [U.S.] | | Docusate sodium 100 mg | | | | | 2 tabs | 6–12 yrs: 1 tab | d | l, m |
| Molatoc-CST Tablets (OTC) [U.S.] | | Docusate sodium 100 mg | | | Casanthranol 30 mg | | 1–2 tabs | >6 yrs: 1 tab | d | l, m |
| Mucinum Tablets (OTC) [Canada] | | | | | Phenolphthalein 75 mg Leaves of senna 40 mg | | 1–2 tabs | | a | l, r |
| Mylanta Natural Fiber Supplement Powder (OTC) [U.S.] | Psyllium hydrophilic mucilloid 3.4 grams/ full tbsp | | | | | Sucrose | 1 full tbsp in 240 mL water or other liquid 1–3 times/day | 6–12 yrs: ¹/₂ tbsp in 240 mL water or other liquid 1–3 times/day | a, g | m, p |
| Mylanta Sugar Free Natural Fiber Supplement Powder (OTC) [U.S.] | Psyllium hydrophilic mucilloid 3.4 grams/ full tsp | | | | | Phenylalanine 30 mg/full tsp | 1 full tsp in 240 mL water or other liquid 1–3 times/day | 6–12 yrs: ¹/₂ tsp in 240 mL water or other liquid 1–3 times/day | a, g | m, p |
| Naturacil Caramels (OTC) [U.S.] | Psyllium seed husks 1.7 grams | | | | | Sodium 0.3 mEq† | 2 caramels 1–3 times/day | >6 yrs: 1 caramel 1–3 times/day | a | j, l, m |
| Natural Source Fibre Laxative Powder (OTC) [Canada] | Psyllium hydrophilic mucilloid 3 grams/ full tsp | | | | | Dextrose | 1 full tsp in 240 mL water or other liquid 1–3 times/day | >6 yrs: ¹/₂ tsp in 240 mL water or other liquid 1–3 times/day | c, e, g | l, p |
| Nature's Remedy Tablets (OTC) [U.S.] | | | | | Aloe 100 mg Cascara sagrada 150 mg | Film coated | 2 tabs | >8 yrs: 1 tab | a | l, m, r |

## Table 2. Oral Dosage Forms (continued)

Note: Content per capsule, caramel, packet, tablet, wafer, or 5 mL, unless otherwise stated.

| Brand or generic name [availability] | Bulk-forming | Stool softener or emollient | Hyper-osmotic | Lubricant | Stimulant | Other content information as per product label | Usual adult and adolescent dose* (maximum recommended daily dose) | Usual pediatric dose* | Packaging and storage§ | Auxiliary labeling§ |
|---|---|---|---|---|---|---|---|---|---|---|
| Nature's Remedy (continued) Tablets (OTC) [Canada] | | | | | Aloe 100 mg Cascara sagrada 150 mg | | 1–2 tabs | >8 yrs: 1 tab | a | l, m, r |
| Neolax Tablets (Rx) [U.S.] | | Docusate sodium 50 mg | | | Dehydrocholic acid 240 mg | | 1–2 tabs 3 times/day | Not established | d | l, m |
| Neoloid Emulsion USP (OTC) [U.S.] | | | | | Castor oil 36.4% | | 30–60 mL | <2 yrs: 1–5 mL >2 yrs: 5–15 mL | a, e, h | l, m, n, o |
| Nujol Oil USP (OTC) [Canada] | | | | Mineral oil (extra heavy) | | Sugar free | 15–45 mL | >6 yrs: 5–15 mL | a, e, h | |
| Nytilax Tablets USP (OTC) [U.S.] | | | | | Sennosides 12 mg | | 1–3 tabs | >6 yrs: 1 tab (2 tabs) | b | l, m |
| Perdiem Granules (OTC) [U.S.] | Psyllium 3.25 grams/ full tsp or 6-gram packet | | | | Senna 0.74 grams/ full tsp or 6-gram packet | Sodium 0.08 mEq†, Potassium 0.91 mEq†, per full tsp or 6-gram packet Dye free | 1–2 full tsp or 6-gram packet 1–2 times/day (2 full tsp q 6 hr) | >7 yrs: 1 full tsp or ½ packet 1–2 times/day | a, g | i, l, m |

*Generally taken as a single daily dose at bedtime, unless otherwise stated.

†Products containing more than 5 mEq (115 mg) sodium in the maximum recommended daily dose are not recommended for patients on low salt diet. Products containing more than 50 mEq (600 mg) magnesium or more than 25 mEq (975 mg) of potassium in the maximum recommended daily dose are not recommended for patients with kidney disease.

§For appropriate *Packaging and storage* and *Auxiliary labeling* information refer to designated letters as follows:

a—Store below 40 °C (104 °F), preferably between 15 and 30 °C (59 and 86 °F), unless otherwise specified by manufacturer.
b—Store below 40 °C (104 °F), preferably between 15 and 30 °C (59 and 86 °F), in a well-closed container, unless otherwise specified by manufacturer.
c—Store below 30 °C (86 °F), unless otherwise specified by manufacturer.
d—Store between 15 and 30 °C (59 and 86 °F), unless otherwise specified by manufacturer.
e—Store in a tight container.
f—Store in a light-resistant container.
g—Store in a dry place.
h—Protect from freezing.
i—Auxiliary labeling: • Do not chew.
j—Auxiliary labeling: • Chew well before swallowing.
k—Auxiliary labeling: • Do not take within 1 hour of antacids or milk.
l—Auxiliary labeling: • Drink increased fluids.
m—Auxiliary labeling: • Take each dose with a full glass of water or other liquid.
n—Auxiliary labeling: • Shake well.
o—Auxiliary labeling: • Chill in refrigerator before taking.
p—Auxiliary labeling: • Dissolve or mix in water or other liquid before taking.
q—Auxiliary labeling: • Store in a cool place.
r—Auxiliary labeling: • May discolor urine and/or stools.

Table 2. Oral Dosage Forms *(continued)*

Note: Content per capsule, caramel, packet, tablet, wafer, or 5 mL, unless otherwise stated.

| Brand or generic name [availability] | Bulk-forming | Stool softener or emollient | Hyper-osmotic | Lubricant | Stimulant | Other content information as per product label | Usual adult and adolescent dose* (maximum recommended daily dose) | Usual pediatric dose* | Packaging and storage§ | Auxiliary labeling§ |
|---|---|---|---|---|---|---|---|---|---|---|
| *Perdiem Fiber Granules* (OTC) [U.S.] | Psyllium 4.03 grams/ full tsp | | | | | Sodium 0.08 mEq†, Potassium 0.93 mEq†, per full tsp Dye free | 1–2 full tsp 1–2 times/day (2 full tsp q 6 hr) | >7 yrs: 1 full tsp 1–2 times/day | a, g | i, l, m |
| *Peri-Colace* Capsules (OTC) [U.S./Canada] | | Docusate sodium 100 mg | | | Casanthranol 30 mg | | 1–2 caps | <6 yrs: See *Peri-Colace* Syrup >6 yrs: 1 cap | d, h | l, m |
| Syrup (OTC) [U.S.] | | Docusate sodium 20 mg | | | Casanthranol 10 mg | Alcohol 10% | 15–30 mL | >3 yrs: 5–15 mL | d, h | l, m |
| *Peri-Dos Softgels* Capsules (OTC) [U.S.] | | Docusate sodium 100 mg | | | Casanthranol 30 mg | | 1–2 caps | | d, g | l, m |
| *Petrogalar Plain* Oral Suspension (OTC) [U.S.] | | | | Mineral oil 3.25 mL | | Sugar free | 15 mL | >6 yrs: 5 mL | d, e, h | l, m, n |
| *Phenolphthalein Petrogalar* Oral Suspension (OTC) [U.S.] | | | | Mineral oil 3.25 mL | Phenolphthalein 15 mg | Sugar free | 15 mL | >6 yrs: 5 mL | d, h | l, m, n |
| *Phillips' Chewable* Magnesia Tablets USP (OTC) [U.S.] | | | Magnesium hydroxide 311 mg | | | | 6–8 tabs | 2–5 yrs: 1–2 tabs, 6–11 yrs: 3–4 tabs | b | l, m |
| *Phillips' Concentrated Double Strength* Milk of Magnesia USP (OTC) [U.S.] | | | Magnesium hydroxide 800 mg | | | | 15–30 mL | 2–5 yrs: 2.5–7.5 mL, 6–11 yrs: 7.5–15 mL | c, e, h | l, m, n |
| *Phillips' Gelcaps* Capsules (OTC) [U.S.] | | Docusate sodium 83 mg | | | Phenolphthalein 90 mg | | 1–2 caps | Pediatric strength not available | d, e, g | l, m, r |
| *Phillips' LaxCaps* Capsules (OTC) [U.S.] | | Docusate sodium 83 mg | | | Phenolphthalein 90 mg | | 1–2 caps | Pediatric strength not available | d, e, g | l, m, r |

Table 2. Oral Dosage Forms *(continued)*

Note: Content per capsule, caramel, packet, tablet, wafer, or 5 mL, unless otherwise stated.

| Brand or generic name [availability] | Bulk-forming | Stool softener or emollient | Hyper-osmotic | Lubricant | Stimulant | Other content information as per product label | Usual adult and adolescent dose* (maximum recommended daily dose) | Usual pediatric dose* | Packaging and storage§ | Auxiliary labeling§ |
|---|---|---|---|---|---|---|---|---|---|---|
| *Phillips' Magnesia Tablets* Tablets USP (OTC) [Canada] | | | Magnesium hydroxide 311 mg | | | Sucrose 195 mg | 6–8 tabs | >7 yrs: 2–4 tabs | b | l, m |
| *Phillips' Milk of Magnesia* Milk of Magnesia USP (OTC) [U.S.] | | | Magnesium hydroxide 400 mg (approx.) | | | | 30–60 mL | 2–5 yrs: 5–15 mL >6 yrs: 15–30 mL | c, e, h | l, m, n |
| *Phillips' Milk of Magnesia* Milk of Magnesia USP [Canada] | | | Magnesium hydroxide 400 mg (approx.) | | | Sugar free | 30–60 mL | 7–30 mL | c, e, h | l, m, n |
| *PMS-Bisacodyl* Tablets USP (OTC) [Canada] | | | | | Bisacodyl 5 mg | Enteric-coated | 2–3 tabs | <6 yrs: Not recommended >6 yrs: 1 tab | c | i, k, l, m |
| *PMS-Docusate Calcium* Capsules USP (OTC) [Canada] | | Docusate calcium 240 mg | | | | | 1 cap | | d, e, g | l, m |
| *PMS-Docusate Sodium* Capsules USP (OTC) [Canada] | | Docusate sodium 100 mg | | | | | 1 cap | | d, e, g | l, m |
| | | Docusate sodium 200 mg | | | | | 1 cap | | | |
| Oral Solution USP (OTC) [Canada] | | Docusate sodium 10 mg/mL | | | | | | 3–6 yrs: 2 mL 1–2 times/day | d, e | p |

*Generally taken as a single daily dose at bedtime, unless otherwise stated.

†Products containing more than 5 mEq (115 mg) sodium in the maximum recommended daily dose are not recommended for patients on low salt diet. Products containing more than 50 mEq (600 mg) magnesium or more than 25 mEq (975 mg) of potassium in the maximum recommended daily dose are not recommended for patients with kidney disease.

§For appropriate *Packaging and storage* and *Auxiliary labeling* information refer to designated letters as follows:

a—Store below 40 °C (104 °F), preferably between 15 and 30 °C (59 and 86 °F), unless otherwise specified by manufacturer.

b—Store below 40 °C (104 °F), preferably between 15 and 30 °C (59 and 86 °F), in a well-closed container, unless otherwise specified by manufacturer.

c—Store below 30 °C (86 °F), unless otherwise specified by manufacturer.

d—Store between 15 and 30 °C (59 and 86 °F), unless otherwise specified by manufacturer.

e—Store in a tight container.

f—Store in a light-resistant container.

g—Store in a dry place.

h—Protect from freezing.

i—Auxiliary labeling: • Do not chew.

j—Auxiliary labeling: • Chew well before swallowing.

k—Auxiliary labeling: • Do not take within 1 hour of antacids or milk.

l—Auxiliary labeling: • Drink increased fluids.

m—Auxiliary labeling: • Take each dose with a full glass of water or other liquid.

n—Auxiliary labeling: • Shake well.

o—Auxiliary labeling: • Chill in refrigerator before taking.

p—Auxiliary labeling: • Dissolve or mix in water or other liquid before taking.

q—Auxiliary labeling: • Store in a cool place.

r—Auxiliary labeling: • May discolor urine and/or stools.

## Table 2. Oral Dosage Forms (continued)

Note: Content per capsule, caramel, packet, tablet, wafer, or 5 mL, unless otherwise stated.

| Brand or generic name [availability] | Bulk-forming | Stool softener or emollient | Hyper-osmotic | Lubricant | Stimulant | Other content information as per product label | Usual adult and adolescent dose* (maximum recommended daily dose) | Usual pediatric dose* | Packaging and storage§ | Auxiliary labeling§ |
|---|---|---|---|---|---|---|---|---|---|---|
| *PMS-Docusate Sodium* (continued) Syrup USP (OTC) [Canada] | | Docusate sodium 20 mg | | | | Ethyl alcohol 0.03 mL Sodium 0.16 mEq | 15–45 mL | 6–12 yrs: 10–30 mL in divided doses 1–3 times/day | d, e, f, h | l, m, n |
| | | Docusate sodium 250 mg | | | | Alcohol 5% Sodium 0.23 mEq | 2.5–5 mL | 1–2 mL | | |
| *PMS-Lactulose* Solution USP (OTC) [Canada] | | | Lactulose 3.3 grams | | | Galactose <0.7 gram Lactose <0.4 gram Other sugars <0.4 gram | 15–60 mL | | c, e, f, h | l, m |
| *PMS-Phosphates* Oral Solution USP (OTC) [Canada] | | Dibasic sodium phosphate 0.9 gram Monobasic sodium phosphate 2.4 grams | | | | Sodium 24.1 mEq | 20 mL (for laxative effect) or 45 mL (for purgative effect) diluted in 120 mL water | 6–9 yrs: 5 mL, >10 yrs: 10 mL, diluted in 120 mL water | a, e | l, m, p |
| *PMS-Sennosides* Tablets USP (OTC) [Canada] | | | | | Sennosides 8.6 mg | | 2 tabs hs | 1 tab hs | b | l, m |
| | | | | | Sennosides 12 mg | | 2 tabs hs | 1 tab hs | | |
| *Portulac* Solution USP (Rx) [U.S.] | | | Lactulose 3.3 grams | | | | 15–30 mL (60 mL) | Not established | c, e, f, h | l, m |
| *Pro-Cal-Sof* Capsules USP (OTC) [U.S.] | | Docusate calcium 240 mg | | | | | 1 cap | Not recommended | d, e, g | l, m |

Table 2. Oral Dosage Forms (continued)

Note: Content per capsule, caramel, packet, tablet, wafer, or 5 mL, unless otherwise stated.

| Brand or generic name [availability] | Bulk-forming | Stool softener or emollient | Hyper-osmotic | Lubricant | Stimulant | Other content information as per product label | Usual adult and adolescent dose* (maximum recommended daily dose) | Usual pediatric dose* | Packaging and storage§ | Auxiliary labeling§ |
|---|---|---|---|---|---|---|---|---|---|---|
| *Prodiem Plain* Granules (OTC) [Canada] | Psyllium hydrophilic mucilloid 3.25 grams/ level tsp | | | | | Sodium 0.06 mEq†, Potassium 0.77 mEq†, per level tsp Dye free | 1 level tsp placed in mouth and swallowed unchewed with 240 mL water or other liquid | >6 yrs: ½ adult dose | a, g | i, l, m |
| *Prodiem Plus* Granules (OTC) [Canada] | Psyllium hydrophilic mucilloid 2.71 grams/ level tsp | | | | Senna pod 0.62 gram/ level tsp | Sodium 0.06 mEq†, Potassium 0.77 mEq†, per level tsp Dye free | 1 level tsp placed in mouth and swallowed unchewed with 240 mL water or other liquid | >6 yrs: ½ adult dose | a, g | i, l, m, r |
| *Pro-Lax* Powder (OTC) [U.S.] | Psyllium hydrophilic mucilloid 3.4 grams/ full tsp | | | | | Dextrose 3.5 grams/ full tsp | 1 full tsp in 240 mL water or other liquid 1–3 times/day | >6 yrs: ½ tsp in 120 mL water or other liquid 1–3 times/day | a, g | l, m, p |
| *Prompt* Powder (OTC) [U.S.] | Psyllium hydrophilic mucilloid 3.5 grams/ full tsp or 7-gram packet | | | | Sennosides 12.4 mg/ full tsp or 7-gram packet | Sucrose | 1–2 full tsp or packet in water or juice | >6 yrs: ½ tsp or packet in water or juice | a, g | l, m, p |

*Generally taken as a single daily dose at bedtime, unless otherwise stated.

†Products containing more than 5 mEq (115 mg) sodium in the maximum recommended daily dose are not recommended for patients on low salt diet. Products containing more than 50 mEq (600 mg) magnesium or more than 25 mEq (975 mg) of potassium in the maximum recommended daily dose are not recommended for patients with kidney disease.

§For appropriate *Packaging and storage* and *Auxiliary labeling* information refer to designated letters as follows:

a—Store below 40 °C (104 °F), preferably between 15 and 30 °C (59 and 86 °F), unless otherwise specified by manufacturer.
b—Store below 40 °C (104 °F), preferably between 15 and 30 °C (59 and 86 °F), unless otherwise specified by manufacturer.
c—Store below 30 °C (86 °F), unless otherwise specified by manufacturer.
d—Store between 15 and 30 °C (59 and 86 °F), unless otherwise specified by manufacturer.
e—Store in a tight container.
f—Store in a light-resistant container.
g—Store in a dry place.
h—Protect from freezing.
i—Auxiliary labeling: • Do not chew.
j—Auxiliary labeling: • Chew well before swallowing.
k—Auxiliary labeling: • Do not take within 1 hour of antacids or milk.
l—Auxiliary labeling: • Drink increased fluids.
m—Auxiliary labeling: • Take each dose with a full glass of water or other liquid.
n—Auxiliary labeling: • Shake well.
o—Auxiliary labeling: • Chill in refrigerator before taking.
p—Auxiliary labeling: • Dissolve or mix in water or other liquid before taking.
q—Auxiliary labeling: • Store in a cool place.
r—Auxiliary labeling: • May discolor urine and/or stools.

## Table 2. Oral Dosage Forms (continued)

Note: Content per capsule, caramel, packet, tablet, wafer, or 5 mL, unless otherwise stated.

| Brand or generic name [availability] | Bulk-forming | Stool softener or emollient | Hyper-osmotic | Lubricant | Stimulant | Other content information as per product label | Usual adult and adolescent dose* (maximum recommended daily dose) | Usual pediatric dose* | Packaging and storage§ | Auxiliary labeling§ |
|---|---|---|---|---|---|---|---|---|---|---|
| Pro-Sof Capsules USP (OTC) [U.S.] | | Docusate sodium 100 mg | | | | | 1–2 caps | | d, e, g | l, m |
| | | Docusate sodium 250 mg | | | | | 1 cap | Not recommended | | |
| Pro-Sof Plus Capsules (OTC) [U.S.] | | Docusate sodium 100 mg | | | Casanthranol 30 mg | | 1–2 caps | | d, g | l, m |
| Prulet Tablets USP (OTC) [U.S.] | | | | | Phenolphthalein (white) 60 mg | Scored | ½–4½ tabs | 2–6 yrs: ¼–½ tab<br>>6 yrs: ½–1 tab | d, e | l, m |
| Purge Oil USP (OTC) [U.S.] | | | | | Castor Oil 95% | | 15–60 mL | <2 yrs: Consult physician<br>>2 yrs: 5–15 mL | a, e | n |
| Regulace Capsules (OTC) [U.S.] | | Docusate sodium 100 mg | | | Casanthranol 30 mg | | 1–2 caps | >6 yrs: 1 cap | d, g | l, m |
| Regulax SS Capsules USP (OTC) [U.S.] | | Docusate sodium 100 mg | | | | | 1–2 caps | >6 yrs: 1 cap | d, e, g | l, m |
| | | Docusate sodium 250 mg | | | | | 1–2 caps | Not recommended | | |
| Regulex Capsules USP (OTC) [Canada] | | Docusate sodium 100 mg | | | | Sodium 0.24 mEq† | 1–2 caps hs | >6 yrs: 1 cap hs | d, e, g | l, m |
| Regulex-D Capsules (OTC) [Canada] | | Docusate sodium 60 mg | | | Danthron 50 mg | Sodium 0.19 mEq† | 1–2 caps hs | >6 yrs: 1 cap hs | a | l, m, r |
| Reguloid Natural Powder (OTC) [U.S.] | Psyllium hydrophilic mucilloid 3.4 grams/full tsp | | | | | Dextrose 3.5 grams/full tsp | 1 full tsp in 240 mL cold water or other liquid 1–3 times/day | >6 yrs: ½ tsp in 240 mL cold water or other liquid 1–3 times/day | c, e, g | l, m, p |

Table 2. Oral Dosage Forms (continued)

Note: Content per capsule, caramel, packet, tablet, wafer, or 5 mL, unless otherwise stated.

| Brand or generic name [availability] | Bulk-forming | Stool softener or emollient | Hyper-osmotic | Lubricant | Stimulant | Other content information as per product label | Usual adult and adolescent dose* (maximum recommended daily dose) | Usual pediatric dose* | Packaging and storage§ | Auxiliary labeling§ |
|---|---|---|---|---|---|---|---|---|---|---|
| Reguloid Natural Sugar Free Powder (OTC) [U.S.] | Psyllium hydrophilic mucilloid 3.4 grams/full tsp | | | | | Phenylalanine 6 mg/full tsp | 1 full tsp in 240 mL cold water or other liquid 1-3 times/day | >6 yrs: ½ tsp in 240 mL cold water or other liquid 1-3 times/day | c, e, g | l, m, p |
| Reguloid Orange Powder (OTC) [U.S.] | Psyllium hydrophilic mucilloid 3.4 grams/full tbsp | | | | | Sucrose 7.7 grams/full tbsp | 1 full tbsp in 240 mL cold water or other liquid 1-3 times/day | >6 yrs: ½ tbsp in 240 mL cold water or other liquid 1-3 times/day | c, e, g | l, m, p |
| Reguloid Orange Sugar Free Powder (OTC) [U.S.] | Psyllium hydrophilic mucilloid 3.4 grams/full tbsp | | | | | Phenylalanine 30 mg/full tsp | 1 full tsp in 240 mL cold water or other liquid 1-3 times/day | >6 yrs: ½ tbsp in 240 mL cold water or other liquid 1-3 times/day | c, e, g | l, m, p |
| Senexon Tablets (OTC) [U.S.] | | | | | Senna concentrate 187 mg | | 2 tabs (4 tabs 2 times/day) | >6 yrs: 1 tab (2 tabs 2 times/day) | b | l, m, r |
| Senna-Gen Tablets (OTC) [U.S.] | | | | | Senna concentrate 187 mg | | 2-4 tabs 1-2 times/day | 2-6 yrs: ½-2 tabs, 6-12 yrs: 1-2 tabs, 1-2 times/day | d, e | l, m, r |

*Generally taken as a single daily dose at bedtime, unless otherwise stated.

†Products containing more than 5 mEq (115 mg) sodium in the maximum recommended daily dose are not recommended for patients on low salt diet. Products containing more than 50 mEq (600 mg) magnesium or more than 25 mEq (975 mg) of potassium in the maximum recommended daily dose are not recommended for patients with kidney disease.

§For appropriate Packaging and storage and Auxiliary labeling information refer to designated letters as follows:

a—Store below 40 °C (104 °F), preferably between 15 and 30 °C (59 and 86 °F), unless otherwise specified by manufacturer.
b—Store below 40 °C (104 °F), preferably between 15 and 30 °C (59 and 86 °F), in a well-closed container, unless otherwise specified by manufacturer.
c—Store below 30 °C (86 °F), unless otherwise specified by manufacturer.
d—Store between 15 and 30 °C (59 and 86 °F), unless otherwise specified by manufacturer.
e—Store in a tight container.
f—Store in a light-resistant container.
g—Store in a dry place.
h—Protect from freezing.
i—Auxiliary labeling: • Do not chew.
j—Auxiliary labeling: • Chew well before swallowing.
k—Auxiliary labeling: • Do not take within 1 hour of antacids or milk.

l—Auxiliary labeling: • Drink increased fluids.
m—Auxiliary labeling: • Take each dose with a full glass of water or other liquid.
n—Auxiliary labeling: • Shake well.
o—Auxiliary labeling: • Chill in refrigerator before taking.
p—Auxiliary labeling: • Dissolve or mix in water or other liquid before taking.
q—Auxiliary labeling: • Store in a cool place.
r—Auxiliary labeling: • May discolor urine and/or stools.

Table 2. Oral Dosage Forms (*continued*)

Note: Content per capsule, caramel, packet, tablet, wafer, or 5 mL, unless otherwise stated.

| Brand or generic name [availability] | Bulk-forming | Stool softener or emollient | Hyper-osmotic | Lubricant | Stimulant | Other content information as per product label | Usual adult and adolescent dose* (maximum recommended daily dose) | Usual pediatric dose* | Packaging and storage§ | Auxiliary labeling§ |
|---|---|---|---|---|---|---|---|---|---|---|
| Sennosides Tablets USP (OTC) [Canada] | | | | | Sennosides A & B 8.6 mg | | 2–3 tabs | 6–12 yrs: 1–2 tabs | b | l, m |
| | | | | | Sennosides A & B 12 mg | | 1–2 tabs | 6–12 yrs: 1 tab | | |
| *Senokot* Granules (OTC) [U.S./Canada] | | | | | Sennosides 15 mg/ level tsp | Sodium 0.06 mEq†/ level tsp Sucrose 2 grams/ level tsp | 1 level tsp (4 tsp) | 2–6 yrs: ¼ tsp (1 tsp) 6–12 yrs: ½ tsp (2 tsp) | b | l, m, p, r |
| Syrup USP (OTC) [U.S./Canada] | | | | | Sennosides 8.8 mg | Alcohol 7% Sucrose 3 grams | 10–15 mL (30 mL) | | d, e, f, h | l, m, r |
| Tablets (OTC) [U.S./Canada] | | | | | Sennosides 8.6 mg | Sugar free | 2 tabs (8 tabs) | 2–6 yrs: ½ tab (2 tabs) 6–12 yrs: 1 tab (4 tabs) | b | l, m, r |
| *Senokot Children's* Syrup (OTC) [U.S.] | | | | | Sennosides 8.8 mg | Alcohol free Sucrose 3 grams | Intended for pediatric use. See *Senokot* Syrup. | 2–6 yrs: 2.5 mL (7.5 mL) 6–12 yrs: 5 mL (15 mL) | d, e, f, h | l, m, r |
| *Senokot-S* Tablets (OTC) [U.S./Canada] | | Docusate sodium 50 mg | | | Sennosides 8.6 mg | Sugar free Sodium 0.1 mEq† | 2 tabs (8 tabs) | 2–6 yrs: ½ tab (2 tabs) 6–12 yrs: 1 tab (4 tabs) | a | l, m, r |
| *SenokotXTRA* Tablets (OTC) [U.S./Canada] | | | | | Sennosides 17.2 mg | Sugar free | 1 tab (4 tabs) | >6 yrs: ½ tab (2 tabs) | b | l, m, r |
| *Senolax* Tablets (OTC) [U.S.] | | | | | Senna concentrate 187 mg | | 2 tabs (8 tabs) | >6 yrs: 1 tab (4 tabs) | b | l, m, r |
| *Serutan* Powder (OTC) [U.S.] | Psyllium hydrophilic mucilloid 3.2 grams/ full tsp | | | | | | 1 full tsp in 240 mL water 1–3 times/day | >6 yrs: ½ tsp in 120 mL water 1–3 times/day | a, g | l, m, p |

## Table 2. Oral Dosage Forms (continued)

Note: Content per capsule, caramel, packet, tablet, wafer, or 5 mL, unless otherwise stated.

| Brand or generic name [availability] | Bulk-forming | Stool softener or emollient | Hyper-osmotic | Lubricant | Stimulant | Other content information as per product label | Usual adult and adolescent dose* (maximum recommended daily dose) | Usual pediatric dose* | Packaging and storage§ | Auxiliary labeling§ |
|---|---|---|---|---|---|---|---|---|---|---|
| *Serutan Toasted Granules* Granules (OTC) [U.S.] | Psyllium hydrophilic mucilloid 2.7 grams/full tsp; Carboxymethyl-cellulose sodium 266 mg/full tsp | | | | | | 1 full tsp sprinkled on food 1–3 times/day | >6 yrs: ½ tsp sprinkled on food 1–3 times/day | a, g | l, m |
| *Silace* Syrup USP (OTC) [U.S.] | | Docusate sodium 20 mg | | | | Alcohol <1% | 15–45 mL | 6–12 yrs: 10 mL 1–3 times/day | d, e | l, m, p |
| Syrup USP (OTC) [Canada] | | Docusate sodium 20 mg | | | | Alcohol <1% | 15–45 mL | 3–6 yrs: 5–10 mL/day 6–12 yrs: 12.5 mL 1–3 times/day | d, e, f | p |
| *Silace-C* Syrup (OTC) [U.S.] | | Docusate sodium 20 mg | | | Casanthranol 10 mg | Alcohol 10% | 15–30 mL hs or 30 mL 2 times/day | | d, e | l, m, r |

*Generally taken as a single daily dose at bedtime, unless otherwise stated.

†Products containing more than 5 mEq (115 mg) sodium in the maximum recommended daily dose are not recommended for patients on low salt diet. Products containing more than 50 mEq (600 mg) magnesium or more than 25 mEq (975 mg) of potassium in the maximum recommended daily dose are not recommended for patients with kidney disease.

§For appropriate *Packaging and storage* and *Auxiliary labeling* information refer to designated letters as follows:

a—Store below 40 °C (104 °F), preferably between 15 and 30 °C (59 and 86 °F), unless otherwise specified by manufacturer.
b—Store below 40 °C (104 °F), preferably between 15 and 30 °C (59 and 86 °F), in a well-closed container, unless otherwise specified by manufacturer.
c—Store below 30 °C (86 °F), unless otherwise specified by manufacturer.
d—Store between 15 and 30 °C (59 and 86 °F), unless otherwise specified by manufacturer.
e—Store in a tight container.
f—Store in a light-resistant container.
g—Store in a dry place.
h—Protect from freezing.
i—Auxiliary labeling: • Do not chew.
j—Auxiliary labeling: • Chew well before swallowing.
k—Auxiliary labeling: • Do not take within 1 hour of antacids or milk.
l—Auxiliary labeling: • Drink increased fluids.
m—Auxiliary labeling: • Take each dose with a full glass of water or other liquid.
n—Auxiliary labeling: • Shake well.
o—Auxiliary labeling: • Chill in refrigerator before taking.
p—Auxiliary labeling: • Dissolve or mix in water or other liquid before taking.
q—Auxiliary labeling: • Store in a cool place.
r—Auxiliary labeling: • May discolor urine and/or stools.

## Table 2. Oral Dosage Forms (continued)

Note: Content per capsule, caramel, packet, tablet, wafer, or 5 mL, unless otherwise stated.

| Brand or generic name [availability] | Bulk-forming | Stool softener or emollient | Hyper-osmotic | Lubricant | Stimulant | Other content information as per product label | Usual adult and adolescent dose* (maximum recommended daily dose) | Usual pediatric dose* | Packaging and storage§ | Auxiliary labeling§ |
|---|---|---|---|---|---|---|---|---|---|---|
| Sodium Phosphate Effervescent Powder (OTC) [U.S.] | | | Sodium phosphate (dibasic) 2 grams/10 grams | | | † | 10–20 grams in 240 mL or more of water | 5–10 yrs: 1.12–5.05 grams, >10 yrs: 2.25–10.1 grams, in 240 mL water | a, e | l, m |
| Sodium Phosphates Oral Solution USP (OTC) [U.S.] | | | Sodium biphosphate 2.4 grams Sodium phosphate 0.9 grams | | | Sodium 24.1 mEq† | 10–40 mL dissolved in 120 mL water | 5–10 yrs: 2.5–5 mL dissolved in 120 mL water | a, e, h | l, p |
| Softlax Capsules USP (OTC) [Canada] | | Docusate sodium 100 mg | | | | | 1 cap | | d, g | l, m |
| Softlax Drops Solution USP (Oral) (OTC) [Canada] | | Docusate sodium 10 mg/mL | | | | | | 3–6 yrs: 2 mL 1–2 times/day | d, e, h | l, m |
| Stulex Tablets USP (OTC) [U.S.] | | Docusate sodium 100 mg | | | | | 1–2 tabs | >6 yrs: 1 tab | b | l, m |
| Sulfolax Capsules USP (OTC) [U.S.] | | Docusate calcium 240 mg | | | | | 1 cap | | d, e, g | l, m |
| Surfak Capsules USP (OTC) [U.S./Canada] | | Docusate calcium 50 mg | | | | | 2–3 caps | >6 yrs: 1–3 caps | d, e | l, m |
| | | Docusate calcium 240 mg | | | | | 1 cap | Not recommended | | |
| Syllact Powder (OTC) [U.S.] | Psyllium seed husks 3.3 grams/full tsp | | | | | Dextrose 3.3 grams/full tsp | 1 full tsp in 240 mL water or other liquid 1–3 times/day (9 full tsp) | >6 yrs: ½ tsp in 240 mL water or other liquid 1–3 times/day | c, g | l, p |

## Table 2. Oral Dosage Forms (*continued*)

Note: Content per capsule, caramel, packet, tablet, wafer, or 5 mL, unless otherwise stated.

| Brand or generic name [availability] | Bulk-forming | Stool softener or emollient | Hyper-osmotic | Lubricant | Stimulant | Other content information as per product label | Usual adult and adolescent dose* (maximum recommended daily dose) | Usual pediatric dose* | Packaging and storage§ | Auxiliary labeling§ |
|---|---|---|---|---|---|---|---|---|---|---|
| *Syllamalt* Powder (OTC) [U.S.] | Malt soup extract 4 grams, Psyllium seed husks 3 grams, per tsp | | | | | | 1–2 tsp in 240 mL water 1–3 times/day | >6 yrs: ½ tsp in 240 mL water 1–3 times/day | c, g | l, p |
| *Trilax* Capsules (OTC) [U.S.] | | Docusate sodium 200 mg | | | Dehydrocholic acid 20 mg Phenolphthalein 30 mg | | 1–2 caps | Pediatric strength not available | a | l, m, r |
| *Unilax* Capsules (OTC) [U.S.] | | Docusate sodium 230 mg | | | Phenolphthalein (yellow) 130 mg | | 1 cap hs | Not recommended | a | l, m, r |
| *Veracolate* Tablets (OTC) [U.S.] | | | | | Phenolphthalein 32.4 mg, Cascara sagrada extract 75 mg, Oleoresin capsicum 0.05 min | | 1 tab 3 times/day or 2 tabs hs | Not recommended | a | l, m |

*Generally taken as a single daily dose at bedtime, unless otherwise stated.

†Products containing more than 5 mEq (115 mg) sodium in the maximum recommended daily dose are not recommended for patients on low salt diet. Products containing more than 50 mEq (600 mg) magnesium or more than 25 mEq (975 mg) of potassium in the maximum recommended daily dose are not recommended for patients with kidney disease.

§For appropriate *Packaging and storage* and *Auxiliary labeling* information refer to designated letters as follows:

a—Store below 40 °C (104 °F), preferably between 15 and 30 °C (59 and 86 °F), unless otherwise specified by manufacturer.
b—Store below 40 °C (104 °F), preferably between 15 and 30 °C (59 and 86 °F), in a well-closed container, unless otherwise specified by manufacturer.
c—Store below 30 °C (86 °F), unless otherwise specified by manufacturer.
d—Store between 15 and 30 °C (59 and 86 °F), unless otherwise specified by manufacturer.
e—Store in a tight container.
f—Store in a light-resistant container.
g—Store in a dry place.
h—Protect from freezing.
i—Auxiliary labeling: • Do not chew.
j—Auxiliary labeling: • Chew well before swallowing.
k—Auxiliary labeling: • Do not take within 1 hour of antacids or milk.
l—Auxiliary labeling: • Drink increased fluids.
m—Auxiliary labeling: • Take each dose with a full glass of water or other liquid.
n—Auxiliary labeling: • Shake well.
o—Auxiliary labeling: • Chill in refrigerator before taking.
p—Auxiliary labeling: • Dissolve or mix in water or other liquid before taking.
q—Auxiliary labeling: • Store in a cool place.
r—Auxiliary labeling: • May discolor urine and/or stools.

Table 2. Oral Dosage Forms (continued)

Note: Content per capsule, caramel, packet, tablet, wafer, or 5 mL, unless otherwise stated.

| Brand or generic name [availability] | Bulk-forming | Stool softener or emollient | Hyper-osmotic | Lubricant | Stimulant | Other content information as per product label | Usual adult and adolescent dose* (maximum recommended daily dose) | Usual pediatric dose* | Packaging and storage§ | Auxiliary labeling§ |
|---|---|---|---|---|---|---|---|---|---|---|
| *Vitalax Super Smooth Sugar Free Orange Flavor* For Oral Suspension USP (OTC) [Canada] | Psyllium hydrophilic mucilloid 3.5 grams/ full tsp | | | | | Sugar free | 1 full tsp in 240 mL water or other liquid 1–3 times/day | | d, e, g | l, p |
| *Vitalax Unflavored* For Oral Suspension USP (OTC) [Canada] | Psyllium hydrophilic mucilloid 3.5 grams/ full tsp | | | | | Sugar 3.5 grams/ full tsp | 1 full tsp in 240 mL water or other liquid 1–3 times/day | | d, e, g | l, p |
| *V-Lax* Powder (OTC) [U.S.] | Psyllium hydrophilic mucilloid 3.5 grams/ full tsp | | | | | Dextrose 3.5 grams/ full tsp | 1 full tsp in 240 mL water or other liquid 1–3 times/day | >6 yrs: $1/2$ tsp in 120 mL water or other liquid 1–3 times/day | d, g | l, p |
| *X-Prep Liquid* Oral Solution (OTC) [U.S.] | | | | | Standardized extract of senna fruit | Alcohol 7% Sugar 675 mg/mL | 74 mL—entire contents of bottle at 2–4 pm on day prior to diagnostic procedure | | d, e, f, h | l, m, r |
| *Zymenol* Emulsion USP (OTC) [U.S.] | | | | Mineral oil 2.5 mL | | Sugar free | 15–45 mL | >6 yrs: 5–15 mL | d, e, h | m, n |

*Generally taken as a single daily dose at bedtime, unless otherwise stated.

†Products containing more than 5 mEq (115 mg) sodium in the maximum recommended daily dose are not recommended for patients on low salt diet. Products containing more than 50 mEq (600 mg) magnesium or more than 25 mEq (975 mg) of potassium in the maximum recommended daily dose are not recommended for patients with kidney disease.

§For appropriate *Packaging and storage* and *Auxiliary labeling* information refer to designated letters as follows:

a—Store below 40 °C (104 °F), preferably between 15 and 30 °C (59 and 86 °F), unless otherwise specified by manufacturer.
b—Store below 40 °C (104 °F), preferably between 15 and 30 °C (59 and 86 °F), in a well-closed container, unless otherwise specified by manufacturer.
c—Store below 30 °C (86 °F), unless otherwise specified by manufacturer.
d—Store between 15 and 30 °C (59 and 86 °F), unless otherwise specified by manufacturer.
e—Store in a tight container.
f—Store in a light-resistant container.
g—Store in a dry place.
h—Protect from freezing.
i—Auxiliary labeling: • Do not chew.
j—Auxiliary labeling: • Chew well before swallowing.
k—Auxiliary labeling: • Do not take within 1 hour of antacids or milk.

l—Auxiliary labeling: • Drink increased fluids.
m—Auxiliary labeling: • Take each dose with a full glass of water or other liquid.
n—Auxiliary labeling: • Shake well.
o—Auxiliary labeling: • Chill in refrigerator before taking.
p—Auxiliary labeling: • Dissolve or mix in water or other liquid before taking.
q—Auxiliary labeling: • Store in a cool place.
r—Auxiliary labeling: • May discolor urine and/or stools.

Table 3. Rectal Dosage Forms

Note: Content per rectal solution administration unit or suppository, unless otherwise stated.

| Brand or generic name [availability] | Stool softener or emollient | Carbon dioxide-releasing | Hyper-osmotic | Lubricant | Stimulant | Other content information as per product label | Usual adult and adolescent dose* | Usual pediatric dose* | Packaging and storage† | Auxiliary labeling† |
|---|---|---|---|---|---|---|---|---|---|---|
| *Apo-Bisacodyl* Suppositories USP (OTC) [Canada] | | | | | Bisacodyl 10 mg | | 1 supp | | c, e | h |
| *Bisacodyl* Suppositories USP (OTC) [U.S./Canada] | | | | | Bisacodyl 10 mg | | 1 supp | >6 yrs: ½ supp | b, e | h |
| *Bisacolax* Suppositories USP (OTC) [Canada] | | | | | Bisacodyl 10 mg | | 1 supp | <2 yrs: ½ supp >2 yrs: 1 supp | b, e | h |
| *Bisco-Lax* Suppositories USP (OTC) [U.S.] | | | | | Bisacodyl 10 mg | | 1 supp | >6 yrs: ½ supp | b, e | h |
| *Ceo-Two* Suppositories (OTC) [U.S.] | | Potassium bitartrate and Sodium bicarbonate | | | | | 1–2 supp | Not recommended | b, g | h |
| *Dacodyl* Suppositories USP (OTC) [U.S.] | | | | | Bisacodyl 10 mg | | 1 supp | <2 yrs: ½ supp >2 yrs: 1 supp | b, e | h |
| *Deficol* Suppositories USP (OTC) [U.S.] | | | | | Bisacodyl 10 mg | | 1 supp | <2 yrs: ½ supp >2 yrs: 1 supp | b, e | h |
| *Dulcolax* Rectal Solution (OTC) [Canada] | | | | | Bisacodyl 10 mg/5 mL | | 1 5-mL enema 1–2 hrs before procedure | >6 yrs: ½ enema | b | h |
| Suppositories USP (OTC) [U.S./Canada] | | | | | Bisacodyl 5 mg (Canada only) Bisacodyl 10 mg | | Intended for pediatric use 1 supp | >6 yrs: 1 supp >6 yrs: ½ supp | b, e, g | h |

*Generally used at time bowel movement is required, unless otherwise stated.

†For appropriate *Packaging and storage* and *Auxiliary labeling* information refer to designated letters as follows:

a—Store below 40 °C (104 °F), preferably between 15 and 30 °C (59 and 86 °F), unless otherwise specified by manufacturer.

b—Store below 30 °C (86 °F), unless otherwise specified by manufacturer.

c—Store between 15 and 30 °C (59 and 86 °F), unless otherwise specified by manufacturer.

d—Store in a tight container.

e—Store in a well-closed container.

f—Protect from freezing.

g—Store in a dry place.

h—Auxiliary labeling: • For rectal use only.

i—Auxiliary labeling: • Shake well.

Table 3. Rectal Dosage Forms (continued)

Note: Content per rectal solution administration unit or suppository, unless otherwise stated.

| Brand or generic name [availability] | Carbon dioxide–releasing | Stool softener or emollient | Hyper-osmotic | Lubricant | Stimulant | Other content information as per product label | Usual adult and adolescent dose* | Usual pediatric dose* | Packaging and storage† | Auxiliary labeling† |
|---|---|---|---|---|---|---|---|---|---|---|
| *Enemol* Enema USP (OTC) [Canada] | | | Dibasic sodium phosphate 6 grams, Monobasic sodium phosphate 16 grams, per 100 mL | | | | 120 mL (delivered dose/130-mL bottle) | Not recommended | a, e | h |
| *Fleet Babylax* Rectal Solution (OTC) [U.S.] | | | Glycerin 80% v/v | | | | Intended for pediatric use | 2–6 yrs: entire contents of applicator | a, e | h |
| *Fleet Bisacodyl* Enema (OTC) [U.S.] | | | | | Bisacodyl 10 mg/30 mL | | 30 mL (delivered dose/bottle) | <2 yrs: Not recommended 6–12 yrs: 15 mL (¹/₂ bottle) | b | h, i |
| *Fleet Enema* Enema (OTC) [U.S.] | | | Dibasic sodium phosphate 7 grams, Monobasic sodium phosphate 19 grams, per 118 mL | | | Sodium 4.4 grams/118 mL | 118 mL (delivered dose/133-mL bottle) | Not recommended | a, e | h |
| Enema (OTC) [Canada] | | | Dibasic sodium phosphate 6 grams, Monobasic sodium phosphate 16 grams, per 100 mL | | | | 120 mL (delivered dose/130-mL bottle) | 14 kg: 30 mL 27 kg: 60 mL 40 kg: 90 mL | a, e | h |
| *Fleet Enema for Children* Enema (OTC) [U.S.] | | | Monobasic sodium phosphate 9.5 grams, Dibasic sodium phosphate 3.5 grams, per 59 mL | | | Sodium 2.2 grams/59 mL | Intended for pediatric use | >2 yrs: 59 mL (delivered dose/66.5-mL bottle) | a, e | h |

## Table 3. Rectal Dosage Forms (continued)

Note: Content per rectal solution administration unit or suppository, unless otherwise stated.

| Brand or generic name [availability] | Carbon dioxide–releasing | Stool softener or emollient | Hyper-osmotic | Lubricant | Stimulant | Other content information as per product label | Usual adult and adolescent dose* | Usual pediatric dose* | Packaging and storage† | Auxiliary labeling† |
|---|---|---|---|---|---|---|---|---|---|---|
| *Fleet Enema Mineral Oil* Enema USP (OTC) [U.S.] | | | | Mineral oil | | | 118 mL (delivered dose/133-mL bottle) | >2 yrs: 59 mL (½ 133-mL bottle) | a, d | h |
| Enema USP (OTC) [Canada] | | | | Mineral oil | | | 120 mL (delivered dose/130-mL bottle) | >2 yrs: 30–60 mL | a, d | h |
| *Fleet Glycerin Laxative* Rectal Solution (OTC) [U.S.] | | | Glycerin | | | | Entire contents of applicator | >6 yrs: entire contents of applicator | a, e | h |
| *Fleet Laxative* Suppositories USP (OTC) [U.S.] | | | | | Bisacodyl 10 mg | | 1 supp | >6 yrs: ½ supp | b, e | h |
| *Fleet Pediatric Enema* Enema (OTC) [Canada] | | | Monobasic sodium phosphate 16 grams, Dibasic sodium phosphate 6 grams, per 100 mL | | | Sodium 2.2 grams/ 59 mL | Intended for pediatric use | >2 yrs: 60 mL (delivered dose/ 65-mL bottle) | a, e | h |
| *Gent-L-Tip* Enema (OTC) [Canada] | | | Sodium biphosphate 16 grams, Sodium phosphate 6 grams, per 100 mL | | | Sodium 4.4 grams/ 118 mL | 118 mL (delivered dose/ 133-mL bottle) | >2 yrs: 59 mL (½ bottle) | a, e | h |
| *Glycerin* Suppositories USP (OTC) [U.S./Canada] | | | Glycerin | | | | 1 adult-size supp | <6 yrs: 1 pediatric-size supp; >6 yrs: 1 adult-size supp | b, e | h |
| *Laxit* Suppositories USP (OTC) [Canada] | | | | | Bisacodyl 10 mg | | 1 supp | <2 yrs: ½ supp; >2 yrs: 1 supp | b, e | h |

*Generally used at time bowel movement is required, unless otherwise stated.

†For appropriate *Packaging and storage* and *Auxiliary labeling* information refer to designated letters as follows:

a—Store below 40 °C (104 °F), preferably between 15 and 30 °C (59 and 86 °F), unless otherwise specified by manufacturer.
b—Store below 30 °C (86 °F), unless otherwise specified by manufacturer.
c—Store between 15 and 30 °C (59 and 86 °F), unless otherwise specified by manufacturer.
d—Store in a tight container.
e—Store in a well-closed container.
f—Protect from freezing.
g—Store in a dry place.
h—Auxiliary labeling: • For rectal use only.
i—Auxiliary labeling: • Shake well.

## Table 3. Rectal Dosage Forms (continued)

Note: Content per rectal solution administration unit or suppository, unless otherwise stated.

| Brand or generic name [availability] | Carbon dioxide-releasing | Stool softener or emollient | Hyper-osmotic | Lubricant | Stimulant | Other content information as per product label | Usual adult and adolescent dose* | Usual pediatric dose* | Packaging and storage† | Auxiliary labeling† |
|---|---|---|---|---|---|---|---|---|---|---|
| *PMS-Bisacodyl* Suppositories USP (OTC) [Canada] | | | | | Bisacodyl 10 mg | | 1 supp | | c, e | h |
| *Sani-Supp* Suppositories USP (OTC) [U.S.] | | | Glycerin | | | | 1 adult-size supp | <6 yrs: 1 pediatric-size supp >6 yrs: 1 adult-size supp | b, e | h |
| *Senokot* Suppositories (OTC) [U.S./Canada] | | | | | Senna concentrate 625 mg | | 1 supp after meals | >6 yrs: ½ supp after meals | c | h |
| *Theralax* Suppositories USP (OTC) [U.S.] | | | | | Bisacodyl 10 mg | | 1 supp | <2 yrs: ½ supp >2 yrs: 1 supp | b, e | h |
| *Therevac Plus* Rectal Solution (OTC) [U.S.] | | Docusate sodium 283 mg/4-mL unit | | | | Benzocaine 20 mg/4-mL unit | 1 unit | 1 unit | c, f | h |
| *Therevac-SB* Rectal Solution (OTC) [U.S.] | | Docusate sodium 283 mg/4-mL unit | | | | | 1 unit | 1 unit | c, f | h |

*Generally used at time bowel movement is required, unless otherwise stated.

†For appropriate *Packaging and storage* and *Auxiliary labeling* information refer to designated letters as follows:
a—Store below 40 °C (104 °F), preferably between 15 and 30 °C (59 and 86 °F), unless otherwise specified by manufacturer.
b—Store below 30 °C (86 °F), unless otherwise specified by manufacturer.
c—Store between 15 and 30 °C (59 and 86 °F), unless otherwise specified by manufacturer.
d—Store in a tight container.
e—Store in a well-closed container.
f—Protect from freezing.
g—Store in a dry place.
h—Auxiliary labeling: • For rectal use only.
i—Auxiliary labeling: • Shake well.

# LEUCOVORIN   Systemic

VA CLASSIFICATION (Primary/Secondary): VT102/AD900; BL400; AN400

Other commonly used names are citrovorum factor and folinic acid.

Note: For a listing of dosage forms and brand names by country availability, see *Dosage Forms* section(s). For a listing of brand names for the articles in this monograph, refer to the General Index.

## Category

Antidote (to folic acid antagonists); antianemic; antineoplastic adjunct.

## Indications

Note: Bracketed information in the *Indications* section refers to uses that are not included in U.S. product labeling.

### Accepted

Methotrexate toxicity (prophylaxis and treatment)

Pyrimethamine toxicity (prophylaxis and treatment) or

Trimethoprim toxicity (prophylaxis and treatment)—Leucovorin is indicated as an antidote to the toxic effects of folic acid antagonists such as methotrexate, pyrimethamine, or trimethoprim.

Leucovorin is indicated as a rescue after high-dose methotrexate therapy in osteosarcoma[1].

Leucovorin is indicated to prevent severe toxicity due to overdose of methotrexate or high-dose[1] methotrexate therapy, to treat severe reactions to low or moderate doses of methotrexate, and [as a part of chemotherapeutic treatment programs in the management of several forms of cancer][1].

Anemia, megaloblastic (treatment)—Leucovorin is indicated to treat megaloblastic anemias associated with sprue, nutritional deficiency, pregnancy, and infancy when oral folic acid therapy is not feasible.

Leucovorin is not recommended for use in the treatment of pernicious anemia or other megaloblastic anemias secondary to lack of vitamin $B_{12}$, since it may produce a hematologic remission while neurologic manifestations continue to progress.

Carcinoma, colorectal (treatment adjunct)—Leucovorin is indicated for use in combination with fluorouracil to prolong survival in the palliative treatment of patients with advanced colorectal cancer.

---

[1]Not included in Canadian product labeling.

## Pharmacology/Pharmacokinetics

### Physicochemical characteristics

Molecular weight—601.58.

pKa—3.1, 4.8, and 10.4.

### Mechanism of action/Effect

Antidote (to folic acid antagonists)—Leucovorin is a reduced form of folic acid, which is readily converted to other reduced folic acid derivatives (e.g., tetrahydrofolate). Because it does not require reduction by dihydrofolate reductase as does folic acid, leucovorin is not affected by blockage of this enzyme by folic acid antagonists (dihydrofolate reductase inhibitors). This allows purine and thymidine synthesis, and thus DNA, RNA, and protein synthesis, to occur. Leucovorin may limit methotrexate action on normal cells by competing with methotrexate for the same transport processes into the cell. Leucovorin given at the appropriate time rescues bone marrow and gastrointestinal cells from methotrexate but has no apparent effect on pre-existing methotrexate nephrotoxicity.

### Absorption

Rapidly absorbed after oral administration; bioavailability is approximately 97% for a 25-mg dose, 75% for a 50-mg dose, and 37% for a 100-mg dose.

### Distribution

Crosses blood-brain barrier in moderate amounts; largely concentrated in liver.

### Biotransformation

Hepatic and intestinal mucosal, mainly to 5-methyltetrahydrofolate (active). After oral administration, leucovorin is substantially (greater than 90%) and rapidly (within 30 minutes) metabolized. Metabolism is less extensive (about 66% after intravenous and 72% after intramuscular administration) and slower with parenteral administration.

### Half-life

Serum total reduced folate half-disappearance time—Intramuscular, intravenous, or oral: 6.2 hours.

### Onset of action

Oral—20 to 30 minutes.

Intramuscular—10 to 20 minutes.

Intravenous—Less than 5 minutes.

### Time to peak serum reduced folate concentration

Oral—$1.72 \pm 0.8$ hours.

Intramuscular—$0.71 \pm 0.09$ hour.

### Peak serum reduced folate concentration

After 15 mg dose—

    Oral: $268 \pm 18$ nanograms per mL (approximately 1 micromolar [$1 \times 10^{-6}$ $M$ ]).

    Intramuscular: $241 \pm 17$ nanograms per mL (approximately 1 micromolar [$1 \times 10^{-6}$ $M$ ]).

### Duration of action

All routes—3 to 6 hours.

### Elimination

Renal—80 to 90%.

Fecal—5 to 8%.

## Precautions to Consider

### Pregnancy/Reproduction

Pregnancy—Studies have not been done in either animals or humans.

FDA Pregnancy Category C.

Recommended for treatment of megaloblastic anemia caused by pregnancy.

### Breast-feeding

It is not known whether leucovorin is distributed into breast milk. However, problems in humans have not been documented.

### Pediatrics

Leucovorin may increase the frequency of seizures in susceptible children by counteracting the anticonvulsant effects of barbiturates, hydantoin anticonvulsants, and primidone.

### Geriatrics

No information is available on the relationship of age to the effects of leucovorin in geriatric patients. However, elderly patients are more likely to have age-related renal function impairment, which may require adjustment of dosage in patients receiving leucovorin as a rescue from the effects of high-dose methotrexate.

### Drug interactions and/or related problems

The following drug interactions and/or related problems have been selected on the basis of their potential clinical significance (possible mechanism in parentheses where appropriate)—not necessarily inclusive ($\gg$ = major clinical significance):

Note: Combinations containing any of the following medications, depending on the amount present, may also interact with this medication.

Anticonvulsants, barbiturate or

Anticonvulsants, hydantoin or

Primidone

    (large doses of leucovorin may counteract the anticonvulsant effects of these medications)

Central nervous system (CNS) depression–producing medications (See *Appendix II*)

    (should be used with caution in patients receiving leucovorin calcium oral solution, because of its high alcohol content)

Fluorouracil

    (concurrent use of leucovorin may increase the therapeutic and toxic effects of fluorouracil; although the two medications may be used together for therapeutic advantage, caution is necessary)

### Medical considerations/Contraindications

The medical considerations/contraindications included here have been selected on the basis of their potential clinical significance (reasons given in parentheses where appropriate)—not necessarily inclusive ($\gg$ = major clinical significance):

*Except under special circumstances, this medication should not be used when the following medical problems exist:*

*For treatment of anemia (as the sole agent)*

$\gg$ Pernicious anemia or

$\gg$ Vitamin $B_{12}$ deficiency

    (may produce a partial hematologic response while neurologic manifestations continue to progress)

*This medication should be used with caution when the following medical problems exist:*

Sensitivity to leucovorin

*As a rescue from the effects of high-dose methotrexate*

Aciduria (urine pH less than 7) or
Ascites or
Dehydration or
Gastrointestinal obstruction or
Pleural or peritoneal effusions or
» Renal function impairment

(risk of methotrexate toxicity is increased because elimination of methotrexate may be impaired and accumulation may occur; even small doses of methotrexate may lead to severe myelosuppression and mucositis; larger doses and/or increased duration of leucovorin treatment may be necessary, along with careful monitoring of methotrexate concentrations)

Nausea and vomiting

(absorption of leucovorin may be impaired; parenteral administration recommended; inadequate hydration secondary to severe nausea and vomiting may also result in increased methotrexate toxicity)

**Patient monitoring**

The following may be especially important in patient monitoring (other tests may be warranted in some patients, depending on condition; » = major clinical significance):

*For patients receiving high-dose methotrexate*

» Creatinine clearance determinations

(recommended prior to initiation of high-dose methotrexate with leucovorin rescue therapy or if serum creatinine concentrations increase by 50% or more)

» Creatinine concentrations, serum

(recommended prior to and every 24 hours after each methotrexate dose, until plasma or serum methotrexate concentrations are less than $5 \times 10^{-8}$ *M*, to detect developing renal function impairment and predict methotrexate toxicity. An increase of greater than 50% over the pretreatment concentration at 24 hours is associated with severe renal toxicity)

» Methotrexate concentrations, plasma or serum

(recommended by some clinicians every 12 to 24 hours after high-dose methotrexate administration to determine dose and duration of leucovorin treatment needed to maintain rescue. May aid in identifying patients with delayed methotrexate clearance; toxicity appears to be related at least as much to the length of time that methotrexate concentrations are elevated as to the peak concentrations achieved. In general, monitoring should continue until concentrations are less than $5 \times 10^{-8}$ *M*)

» pH determinations, urine

(recommended prior to each dose of high-dose methotrexate therapy and about every 6 hours throughout leucovorin rescue, until plasma or serum methotrexate concentrations are less than $5 \times 10^{-8}$ *M*, to ensure that pH remains greater than 7.0 so as to minimize the risk of methotrexate nephropathy from precipitation of methotrexate or metabolites in urine)

## Side/Adverse Effects

The following side/adverse effects have been selected on the basis of their potential clinical significance (possible signs and symptoms in parentheses where appropriate)—not necessarily inclusive:

**Those indicating need for medical attention**

Incidence rare

*Allergic reaction* (skin rash, hives, or itching; wheezing); *seizures*—reported with use in cancer chemotherapy

## Patient Consultation

As an aid to patient consultation, refer to *Advice for the Patient, Leucovorin (Systemic).*

In providing consultation, consider emphasizing the following selected information (» = major clinical significance):

**Before using this medication**

» Conditions affecting use, especially:

Sensitivity to leucovorin
Use in children—May increase frequency of seizures in susceptible children
Other medical problems, especially renal function impairment

**Proper use of this medication**

» Importance of taking as directed and not missing doses; taking at evenly spaced times

» Checking with physician before discontinuing medication or if vomiting occurs shortly after dose is taken
» Proper dosing
» Missed dose: Checking with physician right away; possible need for additional leucovorin; importance of not increasing dose unless directed by physician
» Proper storage

**Side/adverse effects**

Signs of potential side effects, especially allergic reaction

## General Dosing Information

A 15-mg dose produces a serum reduced folate concentration of approximately 1 micromolar ($1 \times 10^{-6}$ *M*).

**For use as an antidote to folic acid antagonists**

Patients receiving leucovorin as a "rescue" from the toxic effects of methotrexate should be under supervision of a physician experienced in high-dose methotrexate therapy.

Parenteral administration of leucovorin is recommended if it appears that absorption may be impaired as a result of nausea and vomiting.

Methotrexate administration should not be initiated unless creatinine clearance and serum creatinine concentrations are normal. If renal function impairment develops during therapy, methotrexate should be withdrawn until renal function becomes acceptable.

*High-dose methotrexate administration should not be initiated unless leucovorin is physically present and ready to be administered, since rescue is critical.*

A variety of dosage schedules of leucovorin in combination with high-dose methotrexate have been used. Since this regimen is still largely investigational, the prescriber should consult the medical literature in choosing a specific dosage. Alkalinization of urine (with bicarbonate and/or acetazolamide) and intravenous hydration (1000 mL per square meter of body surface over six hours prior to beginning the methotrexate infusion and 3000 mL per square meter of body surface per day during the methotrexate infusion and for two days after the infusion is completed) are also important to prevent renal toxicity caused by methotrexate and/or its metabolites.

Administration of leucovorin should be consecutive to rather than simultaneous with methotrexate administration so as not to interfere with methotrexate's antineoplastic effects. However, leucovorin has been administered simultaneously with pyrimethamine and trimethoprim in oral or intramuscular doses ranging from 400 mcg (0.4 mg) to 5 mg to prevent megaloblastic anemia due to high doses of these medications.

In general, it is recommended that the first dose of leucovorin be administered within the first 24 to 42 hours of starting a high-dose methotrexate infusion (within 1 hour of an overdose), in a dosage to produce blood concentrations equal to or greater than methotrexate blood concentrations (leucovorin in a dose of 15 mg produces peak plasma concentrations of approximately 1 micromolar [$1 \times 10^{-6}$ *M* ]). Duration of leucovorin administration varies with the dosage of methotrexate and plasma concentrations achieved (including rate of elimination); in general, leucovorin administration is continued until methotrexate concentrations fall to less than $5 \times 10^{-8}$ *M*.

A larger dose and/or longer duration of leucovorin treatment may be required in patients with aciduria, ascites, dehydration, gastrointestinal obstruction, renal function impairment, or pleural or peritoneal effusions because excretion of methotrexate is slowed and the length of time for plasma methotrexate concentrations to decrease to nontoxic levels ($<5 \times 10^{-8}$ *M*) is increased. It is recommended that duration of leucovorin administration in these patients be based on determination of plasma methotrexate concentrations.

**For use as an adjunct to fluorouracil for colorectal carcinoma**

Patients receiving leucovorin in combination with fluorouracil should be under supervision of a physician experienced in cancer chemotherapy.

## Oral Dosage Forms

Note: The dosing and strengths of the dosage forms available are expressed in terms of leucovorin base (not the calcium salt).

### LEUCOVORIN CALCIUM TABLETS USP

**Usual adult and adolescent dose**

Antidote (to folic acid antagonists)—

To methotrexate:

Oral, 10 mg (base) per square meter of body surface every six hours until methotrexate blood concentrations fall to less than $5 \times 10^{-8}$ *M*.

To pyrimethamine or trimethoprim:
> Prevention—Oral, 400 mcg (0.4 mg) to 5 mg (base) with each dose of the folic acid antagonist.
> Treatment—Oral, 5 to 15 mg (base) per day.

Megaloblastic anemia, secondary to folate deficiency—
> Oral, up to 1 mg (base) per day.

Note: Doses higher than 25 mg should be given parenterally because oral absorption is saturable at doses above 25 mg.

### Usual pediatric dose
See *Usual adult and adolescent dose.*

### Strength(s) usually available
U.S.—
> 5 mg (base) (Rx) [*Wellcovorin* (scored); GENERIC (Lederle—scored)].
> 10 mg (base) (Rx) [GENERIC (Lederle—scored)].
> 15 mg (base) (Rx) [GENERIC (Lederle—scored)].
> 25 mg (base) (Rx) [*Wellcovorin* (scored)].

Canada—
> 5 mg (base) (Rx) [GENERIC (scored)].

### Packaging and storage
Store below 40 °C (104 °F), preferably between 15 and 30 °C (59 and 86 °F), in a well-closed container. Protect from light.

## Parenteral Dosage Forms
Note: The dosing and strengths of the dosage forms available are expressed in terms of leucovorin base (not the calcium salt).

### LEUCOVORIN CALCIUM INJECTION USP

#### Usual adult and adolescent dose
Antidote (to folic acid antagonists)—
> To methotrexate (inadvertent overdose):
>> Intramuscular or intravenous, 10 mg (base) per square meter of body surface every six hours until methotrexate blood concentrations fall to less than $5 \times 10^{-8}$ M.
>>
>> Note: If, at 24 hours following methotrexate administration, the serum creatinine is increased by 50% or greater over baseline or serum methotrexate is greater than $5 \times 10^{-6}$ M, the dose of leucovorin should be 100 mg (base) per square meter of body surface every three hours intravenously until methotrexate concentrations are reduced to appropriate levels. *Leucovorin calcium injection containing benzyl alcohol should not be used for doses greater than 10 mg per square meter of body surface.*

To pyrimethamine or trimethoprim:
> Prevention—Intramuscular, 400 mcg (0.4 mg) to 5 mg (base) with each dose of the folic acid antagonist.
> Treatment—Intramuscular, 5 to 15 mg (base) per day.

Megaloblastic anemia, secondary to folate deficiency—
> Intramuscular, up to 1 mg (base) per day.

#### Usual pediatric dose
See *Usual adult and adolescent dose.*

#### Strength(s) usually available
U.S.—
> 3 mg (base) per mL (Rx) [GENERIC (with preservative)].
> 5 mg (base) per mL (Rx) [*Wellcovorin* (with preservative); GENERIC (with or without preservative)].

Canada—
> 3 mg (base) per mL (Rx) [GENERIC (with preservative)].

#### Packaging and storage
Store below 40 °C (104 °F), preferably between 15 and 30 °C (59 and 86 °F). Protect from freezing.

#### Stability
Intravenous solutions containing leucovorin calcium in 10% dextrose injection, 10% dextrose in 0.9% sodium chloride injection, lactated Ringer's injection, or Ringer's injection have been found to maintain at least 90% of labeled potency when used within twenty-four hours.

Note: This product should *not* be used for doses greater than 10 mg per square meter of body surface.

### LEUCOVORIN CALCIUM FOR INJECTION

#### Usual adult and adolescent dose
Antidote (to folic acid antagonists)—
> To methotrexate (inadvertent overdose):
>> Intramuscular or intravenous, 10 mg (base) per square meter of body surface every six hours until methotrexate blood concentrations fall to less than $5 \times 10^{-8}$ M.

Note: If, at 24 hours following methotrexate administration, the serum creatinine is increased 50% over baseline or serum methotrexate is greater than $5 \times 10^{-6}$ M, the dose of leucovorin should be 100 mg (base) per square meter of body surface every three hours intravenously until methotrexate concentrations are reduced to appropriate levels. *Only solutions prepared with sterile water for injection (i.e., without benzyl alcohol) should be used for doses greater than 10 mg per square meter of body surface.*

To pyrimethamine or trimethoprim:
> Prevention—Intramuscular, 400 mcg (0.4 mg) to 5 mg (base) with each dose of the folic acid antagonist.
> Treatment—Intramuscular, 5 to 15 mg (base) per day.

Megaloblastic anemia, secondary to folate deficiency—
> Intramuscular, up to 1 mg (base) per day.

Carcinoma, colorectal (treatment adjunct)—
> Intravenous, 200 mg per square meter of body surface over a minimum of three minutes, followed by fluorouracil 370 mg per square meter of body surface intravenously, or
> Intravenous, 20 mg per square meter of body surface, followed by fluorouracil 425 mg per square meter of body surface intravenously.
> Either regimen is given daily for five days, and the course may be repeated at four-week intervals for two courses and then at four- to five-week intervals, as determined by toxicity to the previous course.

Note: Only solutions prepared with sterile water for injection (i.e., without benzyl alcohol) should be used, since the dose is greater than 10 mg per square meter of body surface.

#### Usual pediatric dose
Antidote (to folic acid antagonists) or
Megaloblastic anemia—See *Usual adult and adolescent dose.*
Carcinoma, colorectal (treatment adjunct)—Dosage has not been established.

#### Size(s) usually available
U.S.—
> 50 mg (base) (Rx) [GENERIC (without preservative)].
> 100 mg (base) (Rx) [*Wellcovorin* (without preservative); GENERIC (without preservative)].
> 350 mg (base) (Rx) [GENERIC (without preservative)].

Canada—
> 50 mg (base) (Rx) [GENERIC (without preservative)].
> 350 mg (base) (Rx) [GENERIC (without preservative)].

#### Packaging and storage
Prior to reconstitution, store below 40 °C (104 °F), preferably between 15 and 30 °C (59 and 86 °F), unless otherwise specified by manufacturer. Protect from light.

#### Preparation of dosage form
Leucovorin calcium for injection is prepared for parenteral use by adding 5 or 10 mL of bacteriostatic water for injection (preserved with benzyl alcohol) to the vial containing 50 or 100 mg (base), respectively, producing a solution containing 10 mg per mL. If doses greater than 10 mg per square meter of body surface are to be used, sterile water for injection should be used for reconstitution and the resulting solution used immediately.

Caution: Use of diluents containing benzyl alcohol is not recommended for preparation of medications for use in neonates. A fatal toxic syndrome consisting of metabolic acidosis, CNS depression, respiratory problems, renal failure, hypotension, and possibly seizures and intracranial hemorrhages has been associated with this use.

#### Stability
Reconstituted solutions prepared with bacteriostatic water for injection (preserved with benzyl alcohol) should be used within 7 days. Intravenous solutions containing leucovorin calcium in 10% dextrose injection, 10% dextrose in 0.9% sodium chloride injection, lactated Ringer's injection, or Ringer's injection have been found to maintain at least 90% of labeled potency when used within twenty-four hours.

---

Revised: 07/23/92
Interim revision: 11/17/93; 07/05/94; 04/11/95

# LEUPROLIDE   Systemic

VA CLASSIFICATION (Primary/Secondary): HS100/AN500
Another commonly used name is leuprorelin.

Note: For a listing of dosage forms and brand names by country availability, see *Dosage Forms* section(s). For a listing of brand names for the articles in this monograph, refer to the General Index.

## Category

Gonadotropin-releasing hormone (GnRH) agonist; antineoplastic.

## Indications

### Accepted

Carcinoma, prostatic (treatment)—Leuprolide is indicated for the palliative treatment of advanced prostatic cancer, especially as an alternative to orchiectomy or estrogen administration.

Endometriosis (treatment)—Leuprolide is indicated for management of endometriosis, including pain relief and reduction of endometriotic lesions.

## Pharmacology/Pharmacokinetics

### Physicochemical characteristics

Source—Synthetic gonadotropin-releasing hormone (GnRH) analog.
Molecular weight—1269.47.

### Mechanism of action/Effect

Like naturally occurring luteinizing hormone–releasing hormone (LHRH), initial or intermittent administration of leuprolide stimulates release of luteinizing hormone (LH) and follicle-stimulating hormone (FSH) from the anterior pituitary.

Prostatic carcinoma—LH and FSH release from the anterior pituitary transiently increases testosterone concentrations in males. However, continuous administration of leuprolide in the treatment of prostatic carcinoma suppresses secretion of gonadotropin-releasing hormone, with a resultant fall in testosterone concentrations and a "medical castration."

Endometriosis—Initial stimulation of gonadotropins from the anterior pituitary is followed by prolonged suppression. Gonadotropin release from the anterior pituitary transiently increases estrone and estradiol concentrations in females. However, continuous administration of leuprolide in the treatment of endometriosis produces a fall in estrogens to postmenopausal levels. As a consequence of suppression of ovarian function, both normal and ectopic endometrial tissues become inactive and atrophic. As a result, amenorrhea occurs.

### Other actions/effects

Leuprolide also has some androgenic effects in females.

### Absorption

Bioavailability after intramuscular injection of the depot formulation is estimated to be about 90%.

### Protein binding

Moderate (46%).

### Onset of action

Testosterone concentrations—Transient increase occurs within first week of therapy, but decline to castrate levels occurs within 2 to 4 weeks.

### Time to peak effect

Amenorrhea—Usually occurs after 1 to 2 months of therapy.

### Duration of action

Pituitary-gonadal system—Normal function is usually restored within 4 to 12 weeks after therapy is withdrawn.

Amenorrhea—Cyclic bleeding usually returns within 60 to 90 days after therapy is withdrawn.

## Precautions to Consider

### Cross-sensitivity and/or related problems

Patients sensitive to other synthetic GnRH analogs may also be sensitive to leuprolide.

### Carcinogenicity

Studies in rats and mice for two years at daily subcutaneous doses of 0.6 to 4 mg per kg of body weight (mg/kg) and up to 60 mg/kg, respectively, found only an increased incidence of benign pituitary hyperplasia and benign pituitary adenomas at 24 months in the rats.

### Mutagenicity

Mutagenicity studies in bacterial and mammalian systems found no evidence of mutagenic effects.

### Pregnancy/Reproduction

Fertility—In males: Suppression of testosterone secretion results in impairment of fertility. Although it is not known whether fertility is restored after leuprolide is withdrawn, reversal of fertility suppression does occur after withdrawal of similar analogs.

Pregnancy—Leuprolide is not recommended during pregnancy.

Because the effects on fetal mortality would logically result from the hormonal effects of leuprolide, it can be concluded that there is a risk of spontaneous abortion if leuprolide is administered during pregnancy.

Use of nonhormonal contraception is recommended during treatment.

Studies in rabbits at doses of 0.00024, 0.0024, and 0.024 mg/kg (1/600 to 1/6 the human dose) on day 6 of pregnancy found a dose-related increase in major fetal abnormalities; these effects did not occur at similar doses in rats. The two higher doses in rabbits and the highest dose in rats were associated with increased fetal mortality and decreased fetal weights.

FDA Pregnancy Category X.

### Breast-feeding

It is not known whether leuprolide passes into breast milk. However, because of potential adverse effects in the infant, breast-feeding is usually not recommended during treatment with leuprolide.

### Geriatrics

Appropriate studies on the relationship of age to the effects of leuprolide have not been performed in the geriatric population. However, this medication is frequently used in elderly patients, especially for treatment of prostatic carcinoma, and geriatrics-specific problems that would limit the usefulness of this medication in the elderly are not expected.

### Laboratory value alterations

The following have been selected on the basis of their potential clinical significance (possible effect in parentheses where appropriate)—not necessarily inclusive (» = major clinical significance):

With physiology/laboratory test values

  Acid phosphatase
    (transient increases in serum concentrations may occur early in treatment of prostatic carcinoma, but usually decrease to or near baseline by the fourth week)

  Estrogen
    (serum concentrations are usually increased during the first weeks of therapy for endometriosis but then decrease to postmenopausal levels)

  Testosterone
    (serum concentrations are usually increased during the first week of therapy for prostatic carcinoma but then decrease; castrate levels are reached within 2 to 4 weeks)

### Medical considerations/Contraindications

The medical considerations/contraindications included here have been selected on the basis of their potential clinical significance (reasons given in parentheses where appropriate)—not necessarily inclusive (» = major clinical significance).

*Risk-benefit should be considered when the following medical problems exist:*

Sensitivity to leuprolide or other GnRH analogs

*For treatment of endometriosis*

Osteoporosis, history of
  (risk of loss of bone density may be increased)

» Vaginal bleeding, undiagnosed abnormal

*For treatment of prostatic carcinoma*

» Metastatic vertebral lesions
    (worsening of symptoms during first few weeks of leuprolide therapy, with risk of neurologic problems, including paralysis)

» Urinary tract obstruction
    (worsening of symptoms during first few weeks of leuprolide therapy)

**Patient monitoring**

The following may be especially important in patient monitoring (other tests may be warranted in some patients, depending on condition; » = major clinical significance):

*For treatment of endometriosis*
Pregnancy test
(recommended if treatment is not started during menstruation or in patients with irregular cycles)

*For treatment of prostatic carcinoma*
Acid phosphatase concentrations, serum and/or

Prostate-specific antigen (PSA) concentrations, serum and/or

Testosterone concentrations, serum
(recommended at periodic intervals to monitor response)

## Side/Adverse Effects

Note: Many of the side/adverse effects of leuprolide are related to hypoestrogenism in females and hypotestosteronism in males.

There is a risk of increased loss of vertebral trabecular bone density during treatment for endometriosis, some of which may be irreversible. However, the loss usually is small over the usual 6-month treatment period, except in patients with existing risk factors (e.g., history of osteoporosis).

The following side/adverse effects have been selected on the basis of their potential clinical significance (possible signs and symptoms in parentheses where appropriate)—not necessarily inclusive:

**Those indicating need for medical attention**
Incidence less frequent
*In both females and males*
*Cardiac arrhythmias or palpitations* (fast or irregular heartbeat)
*In females only*
*Androgenic effects* (deepening of voice; increased hair growth)
*In males only*
*Angina* (chest pain)
Incidence rare
*In males only*
*Myocardial infarction* (pains in chest); *pulmonary embolism* (sudden shortness of breath); *thrombophlebitis* (pains in groin or legs, especially calves of legs)

**Those indicating need for medical attention only if they continue or are bothersome**
Incidence more frequent—above 50%
*In both females and males*
*Hot flashes* (sudden sweating and feelings of warmth)
*In females only*
*Amenorrhea* (stopping of menstrual periods); *or spotting* (light, irregular vaginal bleeding)
Incidence less frequent
*In both females and males*
*Blurred vision; dizziness; edema* (swelling of feet or lower legs); *headache; injection site reaction* (burning, itching, redness, or swelling at site of injection); *nausea or vomiting; paresthesias* (numbness or tingling of hands or feet); *trouble in sleeping; weight gain*
*In females only*
*Decreased libido* (decreased interest in sex); *disease flare, transient* (pelvic pain); *increased tenderness of breasts; mood changes; vaginitis* (burning, dryness, or itching of vagina)
Note: A *disease flare*, with a transient increase in symptoms (pelvic pain, dysmenorrhea, dyspareunia, pelvic tenderness, induration), may occur shortly after initiation of therapy for endometriosis, as a result of the temporary increase in serum estradiol.

*In males only*
*Constipation; decreased size of testicles; disease flare, transient* (bone pain); *gynecomastia* (swelling and increased tenderness of breasts); *impotence or decreased libido* (inability to have or keep an erection; decreased interest in sex); *loss of appetite*
Note: A *disease flare*, with a transient, sometimes severe, increase in bone or tumor pain, may occur shortly after initiation of therapy for prostatic carcinoma, usually associated with the increase in serum testosterone, but usually subsides with continued leuprolide treatment. Analgesics may be required during this time. Other signs and symptoms of prostatic carcinoma, including difficult urination and spinal compression, may also worsen transiently. In addition, worsening of neurologic signs and symptoms in patients with vertebral

metastases may result in temporary weakness and paresthesias of the lower extremities; paralysis, with or without fatal complications, is possible; initiation of leuprolide therapy with daily administration for the first 2 weeks to facilitate withdrawal of treatment may be necessary in patients at risk.

## Patient Consultation

As an aid to patient consultation, refer to *Advice for the Patient, Leuprolide (Systemic).*

In providing consultation, consider emphasizing the following selected information (» = major clinical significance):

**Before using this medication**
» Conditions affecting use, especially:
Sensitivity to leuprolide or other GnRH agonists
Pregnancy—Pregnancy/reproduction—
For males: May cause sterility
For females: Not recommended during pregnancy; causes birth defects in animals; may cause spontaneous abortion
Other medical problems, especially undiagnosed abnormal vaginal bleeding (for endometriosis) or urinary tract obstruction (for prostatic carcinoma)

**Proper use of this medication**
» Carefully reading patient instruction sheet contained in package
Using disposable syringes provided in kit
» Importance of not using more or less medication than the amount prescribed
» Importance of continuing medication despite side effects
» Proper dosing
Missed dose: For daily dosing—Using as soon as remembered; not using if not remembered until next day; not doubling doses
» Proper storage

**Precautions while using this medication**
» Importance of close monitoring by the physician
*For treatment of endometriosis*
Possibility of amenorrhea or irregular menstrual periods; checking with physician if regular menstruation does not occur within 60 to 90 days after discontinuation of medication
Advisability of using nonhormonal forms of contraception during therapy; not using oral contraceptives
» Stopping medication and checking with physician if pregnancy is suspected

**Side/adverse effects**
Signs of potential side effects, especially cardiac arrhythmias or palpitations, androgenic effects in females, angina in males, pulmonary embolism in males, thrombophlebitis in males, and myocardial infarction in males

## General Dosing Information

It is recommended that the intramuscular depot injection be administered by the physician.

Leuprolide has approximately 15 to 50 times the activity of naturally occurring luteinizing hormone–releasing hormone (LHRH), and 80 to 100 times that of synthetic LHRH (gonadorelin).

**For use in treatment of endometriosis**
It is recommended that therapy begin with the first day of the menstrual cycle after pregnancy has been ruled out.

Development of amenorrhea is usually evidence of a clinical response, although spotting or bleeding from the atrophic endometrium can still occur.

Therapy should be continued uninterrupted for 6 months.

**For use in treatment of prostatic carcinoma**
Patients receiving leuprolide should be under supervision of a physician experienced in cancer chemotherapy.

## Parenteral Dosage Forms

### LEUPROLIDE ACETATE INJECTION

**Usual adult dose**
Prostatic carcinoma—
Subcutaneous, 1 mg per day.

**Strength(s) usually available**
U.S.—
5 mg per mL (Rx) [*Lupron* (benzyl alcohol)].
Canada—
5 mg per mL (Rx) [*Lupron* (benzyl alcohol)].

**Packaging and storage**
Store between 2 and 8 °C (36 and 46 °F) before dispensing and between 15 and 30 °C (59 and 86 °F) after dispensing, unless otherwise specified by manufacturer. Protect from freezing. Protect from light.

**Auxiliary labeling**
• Do not freeze.

## LEUPROLIDE ACETATE FOR INJECTION

**Usual adult dose**
Prostatic carcinoma—
Intramuscular, 7.5 mg once a month.
Endometriosis—
Intramuscular, 3.75 mg once a month.

**Strength(s) usually available**
U.S.—
3.75 mg, with 1 ampul special diluent (Rx) [*Lupron Depot* (D-mannitol 6.6 mg; purified gelatin; DL-lactic and glycolic acids copolymer; diluent contains carboxymethylcellulose sodium 7.5 mg, D-mannitol 75 mg, polysorbate 80 1.5 mg, and acetic acid)].
7.5 mg, with 1 ampul special diluent (Rx) [*Lupron Depot* (D-mannitol 13.2 mg; purified gelatin; DL-lactic and glycolic acids copolymer; diluent contains carboxymethylcellulose sodium 7.5 mg, D-mannitol 75 mg, polysorbate 80 1.5 mg, and acetic acid)].
Canada—
3.75 mg, with 1 ampul special diluent (Rx) [*Lupron Depot*].
7.5 mg, with 1 ampul special diluent (Rx) [*Lupron Depot* (D-mannitol; diluent contains carboxymethylcellulose sodium 5 mg, D-mannitol 50 mg, and polysorbate 80 1 mg)].

**Packaging and storage**
Store between 15 and 30 °C (59 and 86 °F), unless otherwise specified by manufacturer. Protect from freezing.

**Preparation of dosage form**
Leuprolide acetate for injection is reconstituted with 1 mL of diluent provided by the manufacturer, shaking the suspension thoroughly to evenly disperse particles.

**Stability**
Since leuprolide for injection and the diluent contain no preservatives, the reconstituted suspension should be used immediately after preparation and any unused portion should be discarded.

**Auxiliary labeling**
• Do not freeze.

## Selected Bibliography

Wojciechowski NJ, Carter CA, Skoutakis VA, et al. Leuprolide: a gonadotropin-releasing hormone analog for the palliative treatment of prostatic cancer. Drug Intell Clin Pharm 1986 Oct; 20: 746-51.

The management of clinically localized prostate cancer. National Institutes of Health Consensus Development Conference Statement 1987 June 15-17; 6 (10).

Revised: 08/06/93

# LEVAMISOLE   Systemic

VA CLASSIFICATION (Primary/Secondary): IM700/AN400
Note: For a listing of dosage forms and brand names by country availability, see *Dosage Forms* section(s). For a listing of brand names for the articles in this monograph, refer to the General Index.

## Category
Biological response modifier; antineoplastic adjunct.

## Indications
Note: Bracketed information in the *Indications* section refers to uses that are not included in U.S. product labeling.

**Accepted**
Carcinoma, colorectal (treatment adjunct)—Levamisole is indicated, in combination with fluorouracil, for treatment of Dukes C adenocarcinoma of the colon (i.e., with regional lymph node involvement) after complete resection of primary tumor, with no gross or microscopic evidence of residual disease and no evidence of distant metastases or remaining local metastases that could not be removed en bloc with the primary resection. It is not useful for therapy of advanced and metastatic disease.

[Melanoma, malignant (treatment)]—Levamisole is used for treatment of malignant melanoma with poor prognosis, following surgical excision and exclusion of metastatic disease.

## Pharmacology/Pharmacokinetics

**Physicochemical characteristics**
Molecular weight—240.75.

**Mechanism of action/Effect**
Not precisely known. Levamisole appears to act as an immunorestorative agent in the presence of immunosuppression resulting from recent surgery and chemotherapy, but does not stimulate the immune response to above normal levels. May be related to T-cell activation and proliferation, augmentation of monocyte and macrophage activity (including phagocytosis and chemotaxis), and an increase in neutrophil mobility, adherence, and chemotaxis. Does not have cytotoxic effects.

**Other actions/effects**
Anthelmintic. Also has cholinergic, mood-elevating, and, at high doses, convulsant effects. Inhibits alkaline phosphatase in animals.

**Absorption**
Rapidly absorbed from gastrointestinal tract.

**Biotransformation**
Hepatic, extensive.

**Half-life**
Levamisole—3 to 4 hours.
Metabolites—16 hours.

**Time to peak plasma concentration**
1.5 to 2 hours.

**Elimination**
Renal, 70% over 3 days (less than 5% unchanged); fecal, 5% (less than 0.2% unchanged).

## Precautions to Consider

**Carcinogenicity**
Adequate studies in animals have not been done. Studies at doses of 5, 20, and 80 mg per kg of body weight (mg/kg) per day for up to 18 months in mice and up to 24 months in rats found no evidence of carcinogenicity; however, these studies were not conducted at the maximum tolerated dose, and there is a possibility that the animals may not have been exposed to a reasonable drug challenge. Chronic administration of high doses (25 mg/kg) in New Zealand Black mice increased the rate and intensity of spontaneous lymphomas. No carcinogenic effect was found in 12- to 18-month studies in dogs.

**Mutagenicity**
Levamisole was not found to be mutagenic in dominant lethal studies in male and female mice, in an Ames test, and in a study to detect chromosomal aberrations in cultured peripheral human lymphocytes.

**Pregnancy/Reproduction**
Fertility—Administration through 3 generations of rats and rabbits did not affect fertility. No adverse effects on male or female fertility were noted in rats given oral doses of 2.5, 10, 40, and 160 mg/kg. In a rat gavage study at doses of 20, 60, and 180 mg/kg, the copulation period was increased, the duration of pregnancy was slightly increased, and fertility, pup viability and weight, lactation index, and number of fetuses were decreased at a dose of 60 mg/kg. No adverse reproductive effects occurred when the offspring were allowed to mate and litter.

Pregnancy—Adequate and well-controlled studies in humans have not been done.

Studies in rats and rabbits at oral doses up to 180 mg/kg found no evidence of fetal malformations. Embryotoxicity occurred at doses of 160 mg/kg in rats and was significant in rabbits at doses of 180 mg/kg.

FDA Pregnancy Category C.

**Breast-feeding**
It is not known whether levamisole is excreted in human breast milk; however, it is excreted in cows' milk.

**Pediatrics**

No information is available on the relationship of age to the effects of levamisole in pediatric patients. Safety and efficacy have not been established.

**Geriatrics**

Appropriate studies on the relationship of age to the effects of levamisole have not been performed in the geriatric population. However, clinical trials were conducted in older patients and geriatrics-specific problems that would limit the usefulness of this medication in the elderly are not expected.

**Dental**

The leukopenic effects of levamisole may result in an increased incidence of microbial infection, delayed healing, and gingival bleeding. If leukopenia occurs, dental work should be deferred until blood counts have returned to normal and patients should be instructed in proper oral hygiene, including caution in use of regular toothbrushes, dental floss, and toothpicks.

Levamisole may also cause mild stomatitis associated with discomfort (severe stomatitis may occur during combination therapy with fluorouracil).

**Drug interactions and/or related problems**

The following drug interactions and/or related problems have been selected on the basis of their potential clinical significance (possible mechanism in parentheses where appropriate)—not necessarily inclusive (» = major clinical significance):

Note: Combinations containing any of the following medications, depending on the amount present, may also interact with this medication.

Anticoagulants, coumarin
(there have been reports of prolongation of the prothrombin time beyond the therapeutic range with concurrent use; monitoring of prothrombin time and adjustment of anticoagulant dose, if necessary, are recommended)

Bone marrow depressants (See *Appendix II*) or
Radiation therapy
(leukopenic and/or thrombocytopenic effects of bone marrow depressants or radiation may be increased with concurrent or recent therapy if levamisole causes the same effects; dosage adjustment of the bone marrow depressant, if necessary, should be based on blood counts)

**Medical considerations/Contraindications**

The medical considerations/contraindications included here have been selected on the basis of their potential clinical significance (reasons given in parentheses where appropriate)—not necessarily inclusive (» = major clinical significance).

*Risk-benefit should be considered when the following medical problems exist:*

» Bone marrow depression
(may be increased)

» Infection
(may be worsened because of bone marrow depression)

Seizure disorder
(incidence of seizures associated with levamisole therapy may be increased)

» Sensitivity to levamisole

**Patient monitoring**

The following may be especially important in patient monitoring (other tests may be warranted in some patients, depending on condition; » = major clinical significance):

*For use in adjuvant treatment of colorectal carcinoma*
Alanine aminotransferase (ALT [SGPT]) values, serum and
Alkaline phosphatase values, serum, and
Aspartate aminotransferase (AST [SGOT]) values, serum and
Bilirubin values, serum
(recommended prior to initiation of therapy and at 3, 6, 9, and 12 months after initiation of therapy)

» Complete blood counts, including differential and platelets
(recommended prior to initiation of therapy and before each dose of fluorouracil; although leukopenia is not an indication for withdrawal of levamisole, it is an indication for delaying administration of fluorouracil)

Electrolyte concentrations, serum
(recommended prior to initiation of therapy and 3, 6, 9, and 12 months after initiation of therapy)

Monitoring for tumor recurrence or second primary, which may include:
Carcinoembryonic antigen (CEA)
Chest x-ray
Computed tomographic (CT) scan of abdomen and pelvis
» Colonoscopy or double contrast barium enema x-ray
» History and physical examination
Proctosigmoidoscopy
(prior to initiation of therapy and at periodic intervals during therapy)

# Side/Adverse Effects

Note: Frequency of side effects listed is for levamisole alone. Side effects are usually mild. Incidence of most side effects, especially hematological and gastrointestinal effects, is more frequent with combination treatment with fluorouracil, although not more frequent than would be expected with fluorouracil alone.

The following side/adverse effects have been selected on the basis of their potential clinical significance (possible signs and symptoms in parentheses where appropriate)—not necessarily inclusive:

**Those indicating need for medical attention**
Incidence less frequent
*Blood dyscrasias, including agranulocytosis or leukopenia* (usually mild and asymptomatic; rarely, fever or chills; cough or hoarseness; lower back or side pain; painful or difficult urination); *or thrombocytopenia* (usually asymptomatic; rarely, unusual bleeding or bruising; black, tarry stools; blood in urine or stools; pinpoint red spots on skin); *flu-like syndrome* (fever; chills; unusual feeling of discomfort or weakness); *mild stomatitis* (sores in mouth and on lips)—more frequent with combination treatment with fluorouracil

Note: *Agranulocytosis* is an idiosyncratic-allergic effect. Sudden onset; commonly preceded by and associated with flu-like syndrome, but may be asymptomatic. Reversible, usually within 7 to 10 days, after levamisole therapy is withdrawn. Sometimes fatal.

*Leukopenia* is not associated with bone marrow function impairment. Usually does not develop into agranulocytosis and leukocyte counts usually recover even with continued levamisole therapy (does not apply to combination therapy with fluorouracil).

The *flu-like syndrome* is commonly associated with agranulocytosis and may be an early sign of agranulocytosis, but may also occur in the absence of agranulocytosis; also an allergic-type reaction; usually occurs within hours of a dose; may be mild and transient or severe and progressive.

Incidence rare
*Central nervous system toxicity, specifically ataxia* (trouble in walking); *blurred vision; confusion; paranoia; paresthesias* (numbness, tingling, or pain in face, hands, or feet); *seizures; tardive dyskinesia* (lip smacking or puckering; puffing of cheeks; rapid or worm-like movements of tongue; uncontrolled movements of arms and legs); *or tremors; cerebrospinal fluid (CSF) pleiocytosis* (blurred vision; fever); *hepatotoxicity* (not symptomatic)

**Those indicating need for medical attention only if they continue or are bothersome**
Incidence more frequent
*Diarrhea; metallic taste; nausea*

Incidence less frequent
*Arthralgia or myalgia* (pain in joints or muscles); *central nervous system (CNS) effects, specifically anxiety or nervousness; dizziness; headache; insomnia; mental depression; nightmares; or unusual tiredness or sleepiness; dermatitis* (skin rash or itching); *vomiting*

Note: A life-threatening *exfoliative dermatitis* has been reported.

**Those not indicating need for medical attention**
Incidence less frequent
*Alopecia* (loss of hair)

# Overdose

For more information on the management of overdose or unintentional ingestion, **contact a Poison Control Center** (see *Poison Control Center Listing*).

**Treatment of overdose**
Recommended treatment of overdose includes gastric lavage with symptomatic and supportive treatment.

## Patient Consultation

As an aid to patient consultation, refer to *Advice for the Patient, Levamisole (Systemic)*.

In providing consultation, consider emphasizing the following selected information (» = major clinical significance):

**Before using this medication**
» Conditions affecting use, especially:
   Sensitivity to levamisole
   Other medical problems, especially infection

**Proper use of this medication**
» Importance of not taking more or less medication than the amount prescribed
   Checking with physician if vomiting occurs shortly after dose is taken
» Proper dosing
   Missed dose: Not taking at all; not doubling doses; checking with physician
» Proper storage

**Precautions while using this medication**
» Importance of close monitoring by the physician

**Side/adverse effects**
   Signs of potential side effects, especially leukopenia, agranulocytosis, flu-like syndrome, stomatitis, and thrombocytopenia
   Physician or nurse can help in dealing with side effects

## General Dosing Information

Patients receiving levamisole should be under supervision of a physician experienced in cancer therapy.

If agranulocytosis occurs in patients receiving levamisole alone, it is recommended that levamisole be discontinued. However, if leukopenia (leukocyte count of 2500–3500) occurs, single-agent levamisole therapy may be continued with careful monitoring.

Patients who develop leukopenia should be observed carefully for signs of infection. Antibiotic support may be required. In neutropenic patients who develop fever, broad-spectrum antibiotic coverage should be initiated empirically, pending bacterial cultures and appropriate diagnostic tests.

Special precautions are recommended in patients who develop thrombocytopenia as a result of administration of levamisole. These may include extreme care in performing invasive procedures; regular inspection of intravenous sites, skin (including perirectal area), and mucous membrane surfaces for signs of bleeding or bruising; limiting frequency of venipuncture and avoiding intramuscular injections; testing urine, emesis, stool, and secretions for occult blood; care in use of regular toothbrushes, dental floss, toothpicks, safety razors, and fingernail and toenail cutters; avoiding constipation; and using caution to prevent falls and other injuries. Such patients should avoid alcohol and aspirin intake because of the risk of gastrointestinal bleeding. Platelet transfusions may be required.

**For use in combination with fluorouracil for colorectal carcinoma**
Fluorouracil therapy should be discontinued promptly if the patient develops stomatitis or diarrhea. If stomatitis or diarrhea develops during weekly therapy, the next dose of fluorouracil should be withheld until it has resolved. If these effects are moderate to severe, a 20% reduction in dosage is recommended when fluorouracil therapy is resumed.

If leukopenia occurs, the following adjustments in fluorouracil therapy are recommended:
• If the leukocyte count is 2500–3500, the fluorouracil dose should be withheld until the count exceeds 3500.
• If the leukocyte count is less than 2500, the fluorouracil dose should be withheld until the count exceeds 3500, then resumed with a dosage reduction of 20%. If the leukocyte count remains below 2500 for over 10 days despite withholding of fluorouracil, administration of both levamisole and fluorouracil should be discontinued.

If thrombocytopenia occurs, it is recommended that both levamisole and fluorouracil be withheld until platelet counts exceed 100,000.

## Oral Dosage Forms

Note: Bracketed uses in the *Dosage Forms* section refer to categories of use and/or indications that are not included in U.S. product labeling.

### LEVAMISOLE HYDROCHLORIDE TABLETS

Note: The dosing and strengths are expressed in terms of levamisole base.

**Usual adult dose**
Colorectal carcinoma—
   Oral, beginning seven to thirty days after surgery, 50 mg (base) every eight hours for three days, repeated every two weeks for one year. It is given in combination with fluorouracil 450 mg per square meter of body surface by rapid intravenous push once a day for five days concomitant with a three-day course of levamisole, followed by 450 mg per square meter of body surface once a week beginning twenty-eight days after initiation of the five-day course and continued for a total treatment time of one year. Fluorouracil therapy should be initiated between twenty-one and thirty-five days after surgery. If levamisole treatment is initiated from seven to twenty days after surgery, fluorouracil should be initiated with the second course of levamisole (i.e., at twenty-one to thirty-four days). If levamisole is initiated from twenty-one to thirty days after surgery, fluorouracil should be initiated with the first course of levamisole.

Note: Although fluorouracil dosages are based on the patient's actual weight, use of estimated lean body mass (dry weight) is recommended in obese patients or those with weight gain due to edema, ascites, or other abnormal fluid retention.

[Malignant melanoma]—
   Oral, 2.5 mg per kg of body weight once a day, for two consecutive days every week.

**Usual pediatric dose**
Safety and efficacy have not been established.

**Strength(s) usually available**
U.S.—
   50 mg (base) (Rx) [*Ergamisol* (lactose)].
Canada—
   50 mg (base) (Rx) [*Ergamisol* (lactose)].

**Packaging and storage**
Store below 40 °C (104 °F), preferably between 15 and 30 °C (59 and 86 °F), unless otherwise specified by manufacturer.

## Selected Bibliography

Laurie JA, Moertel C, Fleming TR. Surgical adjuvant therapy of large-bowel carcinoma: an evaluation of levamisole and the combination of levamisole and fluorouracil. J Clin Oncol 1989 Oct; 7: 1447-56.

Spreafico F. Use of levamisole in cancer patients. Drugs 1980; 19: 105-16.

Moertel CG, Fleming TR, Macdonald JS, et al. Levamisole and fluorouracil for adjuvant therapy of resected colon carcinoma. New Engl J Med 1990 Feb 8; 322: 352-8.

Grem JL. Levamisole as a therapeutic agent for colorectal carcinoma. Cancer Cells 1990: 131-7.

Revised: 08/12/92
Interim revision: 07/08/94

---

**LEVOBUNOLOL**—See  *Beta-adrenergic   Blocking   Agents (Ophthalmic)*

---

# LEVOCABASTINE   Ophthalmic

VA CLASSIFICATION (Primary): OP900

Note: For a listing of dosage forms and brand names by country availability, see *Dosage Forms* section(s). For a listing of brand names for the articles in this monograph, refer to the General Index.

## Category

Antihistaminic (H$_1$-receptor) (ophthalmic); antiallergic (ophthalmic).

## Indications

**Accepted**
Conjunctivitis, seasonal allergic (treatment)—Levocabastine is indicated in the treatment of seasonal allergic conjunctivitis.

## Pharmacology/Pharmacokinetics

### Physicochemical characteristics
Chemical group—Levocabastine is a cyclohexylpiperidine derivative that has no structural relationship to other antihistamines.
Molecular weight—456.99.
pH—Ophthalmic suspension: 6 to 8.

### Mechanism of action/Effect
Levocabastine is a potent, selective histamine $H_1$-receptor antagonist. It works by competing with histamine for $H_1$-receptor sites on effector cells. It thereby prevents, but does not reverse, responses mediated by histamine alone. Levocabastine does not block histamine release, but rather prevents histamine binding and activity.

### Absorption
Low; following ophthalmic administration of 0.05% levocabastine, mean plasma concentrations reached 1 to 2 nanograms per mL.

### Biotransformation
Oral administration—10 to 20% is metabolized to the acylglucuronide of levocabastine.

### Onset of action
Ophthalmic administration—Within 10 to 15 minutes.

### Duration of action
Ophthalmic administration—At least 2 to 4 hours.

### Elimination
Oral administration—
    Renal, 70% (unchanged), 10 to 20% (as acylglucuronide).
    Fecal, 10 to 20%.

## Precautions to Consider

### Carcinogenicity
Levocabastine was not carcinogenic when administered daily for up to 24 months in the diet of female mice, male mice, female rats, and male rats, in doses of up to 3.2 mg per kg of body weight (mg/kg), 49 mg/kg, 34 mg/kg, and 24 mg/kg, respectively, per day. However, female mice administered oral doses of 12.9 mg/kg per day of levocabastine (5,000 times the maximum human ophthalmic dose), showed an increased incidence of pituitary gland adenoma and mammary gland adenocarcinoma. The increased incidence of these tumors was possibly related to the associated increase in prolactin levels.

### Mutagenicity
Levocabastine was not mutagenic when tested in Ames' Salmonella Reversion test, *Escherichia coli* test, *Drosophila melanogaster* test, mouse Dominant Lethal Assay test, or rat Micronucleus test.

### Pregnancy/Reproduction
Fertility—Rats given oral doses of 20 mg/kg per day of levocabastine showed no evidence of impaired fertility.

Pregnancy—Adequate and well-controlled studies have not been done in humans.

Oral doses of levocabastine equivalent to 16,500 times the maximum human ophthalmic dose were shown to be teratogenic (causing polydactyly) in rats. Oral doses of levocabastine equivalent to 66,000 times the maximum human ophthalmic dose were shown to be teratogenic (causing polydactyly, hydrocephaly, and brachygnathia), embryotoxic, and maternotoxic in rats.

FDA Pregnancy Category C.

### Breast-feeding
Levocabastine is distributed into breast milk. A study of a breast-feeding woman receiving the usual dose of ophthalmic levocabastine showed that the infant received a daily dose of 0.5 mcg of levocabastine.

### Pediatrics
Appropriate studies on the relationship of age to the effects of levocabastine have not been performed in the pediatric population. Safety and efficacy have not been established for children up to 12 years of age.

### Geriatrics
No information is available on the relationship of age to the effects of levocabastine in geriatric patients.

### Medical considerations/Contraindications
The medical considerations/contraindications included here have been selected on the basis of their potential clinical significance (reasons given in parentheses where appropriate)—not necessarily inclusive (» = major clinical significance).

*Risk-benefit should be considered when the following medical problem exists:*
    Sensitivity to levocabastine

## Side/Adverse Effects

Note: Ophthalmic levocabastine does not produce CNS depressive effects or clinically significant systemic antihistaminic effects in patients.

The following side/adverse effects have been selected on the basis of their potential clinical significance (possible signs and symptoms in parentheses where appropriate)—not necessarily inclusive:

### Those indicating need for medical attention
Incidence less frequent
    *Headache*
Incidence rare
    *Cough; dyspnea* (troubled breathing); *eyelid edema* (swelling of eyelids); *eye pain; fatigue* (unusual tiredness or weakness); *nausea; pharyngitis* (sore throat); *redness, tearing, discharge, or other eye irritation not present before therapy or becoming worse during therapy; skin rash; visual disturbances* (change in vision or trouble in seeing)

### Those indicating need for medical attention only if they continue or are bothersome
Incidence more frequent
    *Burning or stinging, transient, upon administration of medication*
Incidence less frequent
    *Dry eyes; dry mouth; somnolence* (feeling sleepy)

## Patient Consultation

As an aid to patient consultation, refer to *Advice for the Patient, Levocabastine (Ophthalmic)*.

In providing consultation, consider emphasizing the following selected information (» = major clinical significance):

### Before using this medication
» Conditions affecting use, especially:
    Sensitivity to levocabastine
    Carcinogenicity—Levocabastine is carcinogenic in female mice, but not in male mice or male or female rats
    Pregnancy—Levocabastine is teratogenic in rats
    Breast-feeding—Ophthalmic levocabastine is distributed into breast milk
    Use in children—Safety and efficacy have not been established for children up to 12 years of age

### Proper use of this medication
    Proper administration technique; not touching applicator tip to any surface; keeping container tightly closed
» Compliance with therapy; symptomatic response usually occurs within a few days
» Proper dosing
    Missed dose: Using as soon as possible
» Proper storage

### Precautions while using this medication
» Checking with physician if symptoms do not improve within 3 days or if condition becomes worse
    After application, occasional stinging or burning may occur

### Side/adverse effects
    Signs of potential side effects, especially headache; cough; dyspnea; eye pain; eyelid edema; fatigue; nausea; pharyngitis; redness, tearing, discharge, or other eye irritation not present before therapy or becoming worse during therapy; skin rash; or visual disturbances.

## General Dosing Information

The manufacturer recommends that patients not wear soft contact lenses during treatment with levocabastine ophthalmic suspension. However, medical experts do not believe this precaution is necessary unless the patient has corneal epithelial problems and the medication is to be used more often than once every 1 to 2 hours. No significant problems have been documented with the use of ophthalmic solutions containing 0.03% or less of benzalkonium chloride as a preservative in patients with no significant corneal surface problems.

If there is no improvement in the condition after 3 days of therapy, the medication should be withdrawn, since further therapy will not be useful.

Clinical studies to support the continuous treatment with levocabastine for longer than 16 weeks have not been done.

## Ophthalmic Dosage Forms

### LEVOCABASTINE HYDROCHLORIDE OPHTHALMIC SUSPENSION

**Usual adult and adolescent dose**
Antiallergic (ophthalmic) or
Antihistaminic (H₁-receptor) (ophthalmic)—
Topical, to the conjunctiva, 1 drop four times a day for up to two weeks.

Note: In Canada, the initial dose is 1 drop two times a day, the dose being increased to 1 drop three or four times a day if needed.

**Usual pediatric dose**
Antiallergic (ophthalmic) or
Antihistaminic (H₁-receptor) (ophthalmic)—
Children up to 12 years of age: Safety and efficacy have not been established.
Children 12 years of age and over: See *Usual adult and adolescent dose.*

**Strength(s) usually available**
U.S.—
0.05% (Rx) [*Livostin* (benzalkonium chloride 0.15 mg)].
Canada—
0.05% (Rx) [*Livostin* (benzalkonium chloride 0.15 mg)].

**Packaging and storage**
Store between 15 and 30 °C (59 and 86 °F), unless otherwise specified by manufacturer. Protect from freezing.

**Stability**
The medication should be discarded 1 month after the applicator bottle is first opened.
The medication should be discarded if it has become discolored.

**Auxiliary labeling**
• For the eye.
• Shake well.

### Selected Bibliography

Janssens M. Efficacy of levocabastine in conjunctival provocation studies. Doc Ophthalmol 1992; 82 (4): 341-51.

Estelle F, Simons R, Simons KJ. Pharmacokinetic optimization of histamine H1-receptor antagonist therapy. Clin Pharmacokinet 1991 Nov; 21 (5): 372-93.

Dechant KL, Goa KL. Levocabastine. A review of its pharmacological properties and therapeutic potential as a topical antihistamine in allergic rhinitis and conjunctivitis. Drugs 1991 Feb; 41 (2): 202-24.

Developed: 08/11/94

---

# LEVOCARNITINE    Systemic

VA CLASSIFICATION (Primary): TN900
Another commonly used name is L-Carnitine.
Note: For a listing of dosage forms and brand names by country availability, see *Dosage Forms* section(s). For a listing of brand names for the articles in this monograph, refer to the General Index.

## Category
Carnitine deficiency therapy agent.

## Indications
Note: Bracketed information in the *Indications* section refers to uses that are not included in U.S. product labeling.

**Accepted**
Carnitine deficiency (treatment)—Levocarnitine is indicated for treatment of primary systemic carnitine deficiency, a genetic impairment of normal biosynthesis or utilization of levocarnitine from dietary sources. It is also used for the treatment of secondary carnitine deficiency that accompanies several organic acidurias.

Deficiency of levocarnitine may lead to elevated triglyceride and free fatty acid concentrations, reduced ketogenesis, and lipid infiltration of liver and muscle. Severe, chronic deficiency may lead to hypoglycemia, progressive myasthenia, hypotonia, lethargy, hepatomegaly, hepatic encephalopathy, hepatic coma, cardiomegaly, congestive heart failure, cardiac arrest, neurologic disturbances, and impaired infant growth and development.

[Carnitine deficiency, secondary to valproic acid toxicity (prophylaxis and treatment)][1]—Levocarnitine oral solution is used for the prevention and treatment of carnitine deficiency secondary to valproic acid toxicity.

**Unaccepted**
Levocarnitine has not been proven effective for treatment of abnormal plasma lipoprotein patterns or cardiac conditions unrelated to systemic carnitine deficiency. It has also not been proven effective for improvement of athletic performance.

[1]Not included in Canadian product labeling.

## Pharmacology/Pharmacokinetics

**Physicochemical characteristics**
Molecular weight—161.20.

**Mechanism of action/Effect**
Levocarnitine is necessary for normal mammalian fat utilization and energy metabolism. It facilitates entry of long-chain fatty acids into cellular mitochondria, where they are used during oxidation and energy production. It also exports acyl groups from subcellular organelles and from cells to urine before they accumulate to toxic concentrations.

Only the L isomer of carnitine (sometimes called vitamin B_T) affects lipid metabolism. The "vitamin B_T" form actually contains D,L-carnitine, which competitively inhibits levocarnitine and can cause deficiency.

**Elimination**
Renal/fecal—Plasma carnitine concentrations may be increased in patients with renal failure.
In dialysis—Removable by hemodialysis; deficiency may occur.

## Precautions to Consider

**Carcinogenicity**
Studies have not been done in either animals or humans.

**Mutagenicity**
Studies in *Salmonella typhimurium*, *Saccharomyces cerevisiae*, and *Schizosaccharomyces pombe* found no evidence of mutagenicity.

**Pregnancy/Reproduction**
Pregnancy—Adequate and well-controlled studies have not been done in humans.
Studies in rats and rabbits at parenteral doses equivalent on a mg per kg of body weight (mg/kg) basis to the usual adult dose have not shown that levocarnitine causes adverse effects on the fetus.
FDA Pregnancy Category B.

**Breast-feeding**
It is not known whether levocarnitine is distributed into breast milk. Problems in humans have not been documented. Carnitine occurs naturally in human milk.

**Pediatrics**
Appropriate studies on the relationship of age to the effects of levocarnitine have not been performed in the pediatric population. However, pediatrics-specific problems that would limit the usefulness of this medicine in children are not expected.

**Geriatrics**
Appropriate studies on the relationship of age to the effects of levocarnitine have not been performed in the geriatric population. However, geriatrics-specific problems that would limit the usefulness of this medication in the elderly are not expected.

**Drug interactions and/or related problems**
The following drug interactions and/or related problems have been selected on the basis of their potential clinical significance (possible mechanism in parentheses where appropriate)—not necessarily inclusive (» = major clinical significance):
Valproic acid
(requirements for carnitine may be increased in patients receiving valproic acid)

**Patient monitoring**

The following may be especially important in patient monitoring (other tests may be warranted in some patients, depending on condition; » = major clinical significance):

Carnitine concentrations and
Free fatty acid concentrations and
Triglyceride concentrations
   (plasma determinations recommended at periodic intervals to assess efficacy of levocarnitine)

## Side/Adverse Effects

Note: Side/adverse effects are dose-related and may be reduced by decreasing the dose of levocarnitine.

The following side/adverse effects have been selected on the basis of their potential clinical significance (possible signs and symptoms in parenthesis where appropriate)—not necessarily inclusive:

**Those indicating need for medical attention only if they continue or are bothersome**
Incidence more frequent
   *Body odor; diarrhea or stomach cramps; nausea or vomiting*

## Patient Consultation

As an aid to patient consultation, refer to *Advice for the Patient, Levocarnitine (Systemic)*.

In providing consultation, consider emphasizing the following selected information (» = major clinical significance):

**Description of use**
   Description should include caution against confusion with the D,L-carnitine form

**Proper use of this medication**
   Taking during or immediately following meals and consuming slowly to reduce gastrointestinal upset
   Taking at evenly spaced times throughout day (every 3 or 4 hours)
» Proper dosing
   Missed dose: Not taking at all and not doubling doses
» Proper storage

**Precautions while using this medication**
   Not changing brands or dosage forms of levocarnitine without checking with physician

## General Dosing Information

Even spacing of doses throughout the day (every 3 or 4 hours) will help increase tolerance of levocarnitine.

**Diet/Nutrition**
Levocarnitine oral solution may be given alone. However, to reduce gastrointestinal side effects caused by overly rapid ingestion, it is recommended that the solution be dissolved in drinks or other liquid foods and that no more than 10 mL (1 gram) be taken at each dose.

Levocarnitine tablets should be taken with meals to minimize gastrointestinal upset.

**Bioequivalence information**
There are no data showing the therapeutic equivalence of those levocarnitine products approved for drug use and those products sold as food supplements.

## Oral Dosage Forms

### LEVOCARNITINE ORAL SOLUTION USP

**Usual adult and adolescent dose**
Carnitine deficiency—
   Oral/enteral, initially 1 gram once a day with food, the dosage being increased slowly as needed and tolerated. For a 50-kg patient, the usual dose is 1 gram one to three times a day with meals.

**Usual pediatric dose**
Carnitine deficiency—
   Oral/enteral, initially 50 mg per kg of body weight a day with food, the dosage being increased slowly as needed and tolerated. The usual dose is 50 to 100 mg per kg of body weight a day with meals (maximum 3 grams a day).

**Strength(s) usually available**
U.S.—
   100 mg per mL (Rx) [*Carnitor*].
Canada—
   100 mg per mL (Rx) [*Carnitor*].

**Packaging and storage**
Store below 40 °C (104 °F), preferably between 15 and 30 °C (59 and 86 °F), unless otherwise specified by manufacturer. Store in a tight container. Protect from freezing.

**Stability**
Should be used immediately after opening. Any unused portion should be discarded.

**Auxiliary labeling**
• Take with meals.

**Note**
Not for parenteral use.

### LEVOCARNITINE TABLETS USP

Note: Certain levocarnitine tablets are labeled and sold as food supplements only. These products have not been approved as drugs by the Food and Drug Administration for use in the treatment of carnitine deficiency. When used on prescription, one levocarnitine product should not be substituted for another unless otherwise directed by the patient's physician. There are no data showing the therapeutic equivalence of those products approved for drug use and those products sold as food supplements.

**Usual adult and adolescent dose**
Carnitine deficiency—
   Oral, 1 gram two or three times a day with meals.

**Usual pediatric dose**
Carnitine deficiency—
   Oral, initially 50 mg per kg of body weight a day with food, the dosage being increased slowly as needed and tolerated. The usual dose is 50 to 100 mg per kg of body weight a day with meals (maximum 3 grams a day).

**Strength(s) usually available**
U.S.—
   330 mg (Rx) [*Carnitor*].
Canada—
   330 mg (Rx) [*Carnitor*].

**Packaging and storage**
Store below 40 °C (104 °F), preferably between 15 and 30 °C (59 and 86 °F), in a well-closed container, unless otherwise specified by manufacturer.

**Auxiliary labeling**
• Take with meals.

## Parenteral Dosage Forms

### LEVOCARNITINE INJECTION

**Usual adult dose**
Carnitine deficiency—
   Intravenous, 50 mg per kg (mg/kg) of body weight a day.
For severe metabolic crisis—
   Intravenous, loading dose of 50 mg/kg of body weight, followed by a total of 50 mg/kg every 3 or 4 hours for one day, then 50 mg/kg a day.

**Pediatric dose—**
   See *Usual adult dose*.

**Strength(s) usually available**
U.S.—
   200 mg per mL (Rx) [*Carnitor*].
Canada—
   200 mg per mL (Rx) [*Carnitor*].

**Packaging and storage**
Store at 25 °C (77 °F). Keep ampuls in original container and protect from light.

Revised: 03/04/92
Interim revision: 08/10/92; 05/28/93; 08/29/94; 08/07/95

# LEVODOPA   Systemic

VA CLASSIFICATION (Primary): CN500

Note: For a listing of dosage forms and brand names by country availability, see *Dosage Forms* section(s). For a listing of brand names for the articles in this monograph, refer to the General Index.

## Category

Antidyskinetic.

## Indications

### Accepted

Parkinsonism (treatment)—Levodopa is indicated to alleviate symptoms and allow more normal body movements with improved muscular control in the treatment of idiopathic Parkinson's disease (paralysis agitans), postencephalitic parkinsonism, or symptomatic parkinsonism that may follow injury to the nervous system by carbon monoxide intoxication or manganese intoxication. It is also indicated in parkinsonism associated with cerebral arteriosclerosis.

## Pharmacology/Pharmacokinetics

### Physicochemical characteristics

Molecular weight—197.19.

### Mechanism of action/Effect

The precise mechanism of action has not been established. It is believed that the small percentage of each dose crossing the blood-brain barrier is decarboxylated to dopamine. The dopamine then stimulates dopaminergic receptors in the basal ganglia to improve the balance between cholinergic and dopaminergic activity, resulting in the improved modulation of voluntary nerve impulses transmitted to the motor cortex.

### Other actions/effects

Levodopa's metabolite, dopamine, stimulates beta-adrenergic cardiac receptors, interacts with chemoreceptors in the medullary emetic center, and promotes release of pituitary growth hormone.

### Absorption

Rapidly absorbed from the small intestine by an active amino acid transport system, with 30 to 50% reaching general circulation. High gastric acidity, delayed stomach emptying time, and the presence of certain other amino acids, such as those that occur after digestion of a protein meal, may delay absorption of levodopa.

### Distribution

Widely distributed to most body tissues, but not to the central nervous system (CNS), which receives less than 1% of the dose because of extensive metabolism in the periphery.

### Biotransformation

95% converted to dopamine by L-aromatic amino acid decarboxylase enzyme in the lumen of the stomach and intestines and on first pass through liver.

### Half-life

1 to 3 hours.

### Onset of action

Significant improvement may occur in 2 to 3 weeks. Some patients may require up to 6 months of continuous levodopa therapy to obtain optimal therapeutic benefit.

### Time to peak concentration

1 to 3 hours (may be longer when taken with food).

### Duration of action

Up to 5 hours per dose.

### Elimination

Renal; 80% of dose eliminated within 24 hours as dopamine metabolites, mainly dihydroxyphenylacetic acid (DOPAC) and homovanillic acid (HVA). Some of the eliminated metabolites may color the urine red.

## Precautions to Consider

### Pregnancy/Reproduction

Pregnancy—Studies in humans have not been done.

Reproduction studies in rodents have shown that levodopa, when given in doses in excess of 200 mg per kg of body weight (mg/kg) per day, depresses fetal and postnatal growth and viability. Also, studies in rabbits have shown that levodopa alone or in combination with carbidopa causes visceral and skeletal malformations.

### Breast-feeding

Levodopa is distributed into breast milk. Although problems in humans have not been documented, breast-feeding is not recommended because of the potential for side effects in the infant.

Also, levodopa may inhibit lactation.

### Pediatrics

Appropriate studies on the relationship of age to the effects of levodopa have not been performed in children up to 12 years of age. Safety and efficacy have not been established.

### Geriatrics

Smaller doses may be required in geriatric patients since they may have a reduced tolerance to the effects of levodopa. Also, peripheral dopa decarboxylase, the enzyme responsible for decarboxylation, decreases with age, thus making large doses unnecessary.

Geriatric patients, especially those with osteoporosis, responsive to antiparkinsonian therapy should resume normal activity gradually and with caution because increased mobility may increase risk of fractures.

Psychic side effects, such as anxiety, confusion, or nervousness, occur more frequently in geriatric patients receiving other antiparkinsonian medications, especially anticholinergics.

Geriatric patients, especially those with pre-existing coronary disease, are more susceptible to levodopa's cardiac effects, such as arrhythmias. These cardiac effects are minimized or eliminated when levodopa is combined with carbidopa.

### Dental

Involuntary movements of jaws may result in poor retention of full dentures; dosage reduction may be required.

### Drug interactions and/or related problems

The following drug interactions and/or related problems have been selected on the basis of their potential clinical significance (possible mechanism in parentheses where appropriate)—not necessarily inclusive (» = major clinical significance):

Note: Combinations containing any of the following medications, depending on the amount present, may also interact with this medication.

Amantadine or
Benztropine or
Procyclidine or
Trihexyphenidyl
   (concurrent use may result in increased efficacy of levodopa; however, concurrent use is not recommended if there is a history of psychosis)

» Anesthetics, hydrocarbon inhalation
   (concurrent administration may result in cardiac arrhythmias because of increased endogenous dopamine concentration; levodopa should be discontinued 6 to 8 hours before administration of anesthetics, especially halothane)

» Anticonvulsants, hydantoin or
Benzodiazepines or
Droperidol or
» Haloperidol or
Loxapine or
Metyrosine or
Papaverine or
» Phenothiazines or
Rauwolfia alkaloids or
Thioxanthenes
   (concurrent use may decrease the therapeutic effects of levodopa; hydantoin anticonvulsants increase the metabolism of levodopa when used concurrently, thus decreasing its effect; since droperidol, haloperidol, loxapine, papaverine, phenothiazines, and the thioxanthenes block the dopamine receptors in the brain, they may induce extrapyramidal symptoms, thus aggravating parkinsonism and antagonizing the effects of levodopa; the rauwolfia alkaloids cause dopamine depletion in the brain, thus opposing the effects of levodopa)

Bromocriptine
   (may produce additive effects, allowing reduction in levodopa dosage)

» Cocaine
   (concurrent use with levodopa may increase the risk of cardiac arrhythmias; if use of cocaine is necessary in patients receiving levodopa, it is recommended that cocaine be administered with caution, in reduced dosage, and in conjunction with electrocardiographic monitoring)

Foods, especially high-protein
(concurrent or previous ingestion of food may decrease the absorption of levodopa from the gastrointestinal tract, consequently delaying its effect; in addition, proteins in food may be degraded into the amino acids that compete with levodopa for transport to the brain, thus decreasing and/or making erratic the response to levodopa; however, rather than cutting down on daily protein intake to avoid this effect on levodopa, it is recommended that the intake of proteins be distributed equally throughout the day)

Hypotension-producing medications, other (See *Appendix II*)
(concurrent use with levodopa may result in an increased hypotensive effect)

Methyldopa
(concurrent use with levodopa may alter the antiparkinsonian effects of levodopa and may also produce additive toxic CNS effects such as psychosis)

Metoclopramide
(gastric emptying of levodopa may be accelerated with concurrent use of metoclopramide, thus possibly increasing levodopa's rate and extent of absorption from the small intestine; the clinical significance of this interaction has not been determined)

Molindone
(concurrent use may inhibit antiparkinsonian effects of levodopa by blocking dopamine receptor in the brain; also, levodopa may counteract the antipsychotic effects of molindone)

» Monoamine oxidase (MAO) inhibitors, including furazolidone and procarbazine
(concurrent use with levodopa is not recommended as the combination may result in a hypertensive crisis; it is recommended that MAO inhibitors be discontinued for 2 to 4 weeks prior to initiation of levodopa therapy)

» Pyridoxine
(concurrent use with levodopa is not recommended since levodopa's antiparkinsonian effects are reversed by as little as 10 mg of orally administered pyridoxine)

» Selegiline
(although sometimes used in conjunction with levodopa or with carbidopa and levodopa combination, selegiline may enhance levodopa-induced dyskinesias, nausea, orthostatic hypotension, confusion, and hallucinations; levodopa dosage should be reduced within 2 to 3 days after the initiation of selegiline therapy)

Sympathomimetics
(concurrent use with levodopa may increase the possibility of cardiac arrhythmias; dosage reduction of the sympathomimetic is recommended; the administration of carbidopa with levodopa reduces the tendency of sympathomimetics to cause dopamine-induced cardiac arrhythmias)

## Laboratory value alterations
The following have been selected on the basis of their potential clinical significance (possible effect in parentheses where appropriate)—not necessarily inclusive (» = major clinical significance):

With diagnostic test results
Coombs' (antiglobulin) test
(occasionally becomes positive after long-term levodopa therapy)

Glucose, urine
(tests using copper reduction methods may cause false-positive results; tests using glucose oxidase methods may cause false-negative results)

Gonadorelin test
(levodopa may elevate serum gonadotropin concentrations)

Ketones, urine
(tests using dipstick methods may cause false-positive results)

Norepinephrine, urine
(test shows false-positive results)

Pancreas imaging
(in animal studies, levodopa decreased pancreatic uptake of selenomethionine Se 75, probably because of levodopa-induced stimulation of growth hormone release by the pituitary; human data are not available)

Protein, urine
(use of the Lowery test may cause false-positive results)

Thyroid function determinations
(chronic use of levodopa may inhibit the TSH response to protirelin)

Uric acid, serum and urine
(tests may show high concentrations with colorimetric measurements, but not with uricase)

With physiology/laboratory test values
Alanine aminotransferase (ALT [SGPT]) and
Alkaline phosphatase and
Aspartate aminotransferase (AST [SGOT]) and
Bilirubin and
Lactate dehydrogenase (LDH) and
Protein-bound iodine (PBI)
(serum concentrations may be increased)

Blood urea nitrogen (BUN)
(concentrations may be increased)

## Medical considerations/Contraindications
The medical considerations/contraindications included here have been selected on the basis of their potential clinical significance (reasons given in parentheses where appropriate)—not necessarily inclusive (» = major clinical significance).

### Risk-benefit should be considered when the following medical problems exist:

» Bronchial asthma, emphysema, and other severe pulmonary diseases
(respiratory effects of levodopa may aggravate condition)

» Cardiovascular disease, severe
(increased risk of cardiac arrhythmias)

Convulsive disorders, history of
(use of levodopa may precipitate seizures)

Diabetes mellitus
(use of levodopa may adversely affect control of glucose in blood)

Endocrine diseases
(use of levodopa may adversely affect hypothalamus or pituitary function)

» Glaucoma, angle-closure, or predisposition to
(mydriatic effect resulting in increased intraocular pressure may precipitate an acute attack of angle-closure glaucoma)

Glaucoma, open-angle, chronic
(mydriatic effect may cause a slight increase in intraocular pressure; glaucoma therapy may need to be adjusted)

Hepatic function impairment

» Melanoma, history of or suspected
(use of levodopa may activate a malignant melanoma)

» Myocardial infarction, history of, with residual arrhythmias
(use of levodopa may precipitate or aggravate condition)

» Peptic ulcer, history of
(increased risk of upper gastrointestinal hemorrhage)

» Psychotic states
(increased risk of developing depression and suicidal tendencies)

» Renal function impairment
(use of levodopa may lead to urinary retention)

Sensitivity to levodopa

» Urinary retention
(use of levodopa may precipitate or aggravate condition)

## Patient monitoring
The following may be especially important in patient monitoring (other tests may be warranted in some patients, depending on condition; » = major clinical significance):

Blood cell counts and
Hemoglobin determinations and
Hepatic function determinations and
Ophthalmologic examinations for glaucoma and monitoring of intraocular pressure in patients with open-angle glaucoma and
Renal function determinations
(recommended at periodic intervals for patients on long-term levodopa therapy; also, blood cell counts and hepatic and renal function determinations are recommended after withdrawal of levodopa therapy as part of the evaluation of a patient with suspected neuroleptic malignant–like syndrome)

Cardiovascular monitoring for detection of arrhythmias or orthostatic hypotensive tendencies
(recommended during the period of initial dosage adjustment)

Creatine phosphokinase concentrations
(serum determinations recommended after discontinuation of levodopa therapy, especially if fever is present; an elevated serum creatine phosphokinase level may be an early indication of the presence of neuroleptic malignant–like syndrome)

# Side/Adverse Effects

Note: Patients receiving this medication for one to several years may experience sudden, unexpected akinesia, tremor, and rigidity, such as the "on-off" phenomenon. Emotional stress may precipitate akinesia paradoxica or "start hesitation" in these patients.

A syndrome resembling neuroleptic malignant syndrome, which includes intermittent dystonia alternating with substantial agitation, hyperthermia, and mental changes, has been reported after the abrupt discontinuation of levodopa therapy.

Convulsions have been reported but a causal relationship to the use of levodopa has not been established.

The following side/adverse effects have been selected on the basis of their potential clinical significance (possible signs and symptoms in parentheses where appropriate)—not necessarily inclusive:

**Those indicating need for medical attention**
Incidence more frequent
*Difficult urination; irregular heartbeat; mental depression; mood or mental changes, such as aggressive behavior; nausea or vomiting, severe or continuing; orthostatic hypotension* (dizziness or lightheadedness when getting up from a lying or sitting position); *unusual and uncontrolled movements of the body, including the face, tongue, arms, hands, head, and upper body*—may indicate excessive concentration of dopamine in the striatum

Note: *Orthostatic hypotension* occurs in about 30% of patients at the initiation of levodopa therapy.

*Nausea and vomiting* occur in nearly 80% of patients in early levodopa therapy with tolerance being gradually achieved during continued use.

*Difficult urination, dizziness or lightheadedness, irregular heartbeat,* and *nausea and vomiting* may become less frequent when levodopa is combined with carbidopa because of the reduced dose requirements and unavailability of peripheral dopamine.

*Choreiform and other involuntary movements* occur in 50 to 80% of patients and are usually dose-related.

Incidence less frequent
*Spasm or closing of eyelids*—possible early sign of overdose
Incidence rare
*Duodenal ulcer* (stomach pain); *hemolytic anemia* (unusual tiredness or weakness); *hypertension* (high blood pressure)

**Those indicating need for medical attention only if they continue or are bothersome**
Incidence more frequent
*Anxiety, confusion, or nervousness*—especially in elderly patients receiving other antiparkinsonian medication; *constipation; nightmares*

Note: *Constipation* and *nightmares* may become less frequent when levodopa is combined with carbidopa because of the reduced dose requirements and unavailability of peripheral dopamine.

Incidence less frequent
*Anorexia* (loss of appetite); *diarrhea; dryness of mouth; flushing of skin; headache; insomnia* (trouble in sleeping); *muscle twitching; unusual tiredness or weakness*

**Those not indicating need for medical attention**
Incidence less frequent
*Darkening in color of urine or sweat*

## Overdose

For more information on the management of overdose or unintentional ingestion, **contact a Poison Control Center** (see *Poison Control Center Listing*).

### Clinical effects of overdose

The following effects have been selected on the basis of their potential clinical significance (possible signs and symptoms in parentheses where appropriate)–not necessarily inclusive:

*Spasm or closing of eyelids*—possible early sign of overdose

### Treatment of overdose

Since there is no specific antidote for acute overdose with levodopa, treatment is symptomatic and supportive, with possible utilization of the following:
• To decrease absorption—Immediate gastric lavage.
The value of dialysis in the treatment of overdose is not known.
• Specific treatment—Antiarrhythmic medication, if necessary.
• Pyridoxine in oral doses of 10 to 25 mg has been reported to reverse toxic and therapeutic effects of levodopa; however, in the treatment of acute overdosage, its usefulness has not been established.
• Supportive care—Patients in whom intentional overdose is confirmed or suspected should be referred for psychiatric consultation.

## Patient Consultation

As an aid to patient consultation, refer to *Advice for the Patient, Levodopa (Systemic)*.

In providing consultation, consider emphasizing the following selected information (» = major clinical significance):

**Before using this medication**
» Conditions affecting use, especially:
Sensitivity to levodopa
Pregnancy—No studies in humans; depressed growth and malformations in animal studies
Breast-feeding—Distributed into breast milk; may inhibit lactation
Use in the elderly—Reduced tolerance to effects of levodopa; caution in resuming normal activity, especially in patients with osteoporosis
Dental—Possible difficulty in retention of full dentures
Other medications, especially haloperidol, hydantoin anticonvulsants, hydrocarbon inhalation anesthetics, phenothiazines, cocaine, MAO inhibitors, pyridoxine, and selegiline
Other medical problems, especially severe cardiovascular disease, severe pulmonary diseases, glaucoma, melanoma (history of or suspected), peptic ulcer (history of), psychosis, renal function impairment, or urinary retention

**Proper use of this medication**
» Taking food shortly after taking medication to relieve gastric irritation; taking food before or concurrently may retard levodopa's effect
» Compliance with therapy; taking medication only as directed; not stopping medication unless ordered by physician
» Maximum effectiveness of medication may not occur for several weeks or months after therapy is initiated
» Proper dosing
Missed dose: Taking as soon as possible; skipping dose if next scheduled dose is within 2 hours; not doubling doses
» Proper storage

**Precautions while using this medication**
Caution if any kind of surgery (including dental surgery) or emergency treatment is required
Diabetics: May interfere with urine tests for sugar and ketones
» Caution if drowsiness occurs
» Caution when getting up suddenly from lying or sitting position; dizziness and fainting may occur
» Avoiding foods or vitamin products containing pyridoxine (vitamin $B_6$); diminished levodopa effect when used with pyridoxine
» Caution in resuming normal physical activities when condition has improved, especially for geriatric patients
Possibility of "on-off" phenomenon

**Side/adverse effects**
Signs of potential side effects, especially difficult urination, duodenal ulcer, hemolytic anemia, hypertension, irregular heartbeat, mental depression, mood or mental changes, severe nausea or vomiting, orthostatic hypotension, spasm or closing of eyelids, uncontrolled movements of body
Occasional darkening of urine or sweat may be alarming to patient although medically insignificant

## General Dosing Information

Titrated dosage is necessary to achieve the individual therapeutic blood concentration requirements and to minimize side effects. This is especially important for geriatric patients and patients receiving other medications.

Postencephalitic and geriatric patients often require and tolerate lower dosage levels than other parkinsonism patients.

The concurrent administration of carbidopa may permit the dose of levodopa to be reduced by up to 75% and yet achieve equal therapeutic results. Carbidopa also reduces the adverse effect of pyridoxine on levodopa.

Amantadine or anticholinergic medications are often used concurrently with levodopa in the more advanced cases of parkinsonism or when response to levodopa decreases. Gradual dosage reduction of these medications is recommended during initiation of therapy with levodopa and after optimum dosage is reached to maintain proper control of the patient's condition.

When levodopa is to be discontinued, dosage should be reduced gradually to prevent the occurrence of a syndrome that resembles the neuroleptic malignant syndrome. Careful patient monitoring after withdrawal of levodopa will allow early diagnosis and treatment of neuroleptic malignant-like syndrome.

**Diet/Nutrition**

Food should be eaten shortly after levodopa is taken to relieve gastric irritation; taking food before or concurrently may retard levodopa's effects.

High protein diets should be avoided, because amino acid degradation products compete with levodopa for transport to the brain, resulting in a decreased or erratic response to levodopa. It is recommended that intake of normal amounts of protein be distributed equally throughout the day.

In addition, pyridoxine (vitamin B₆) reverses the effects of levodopa. Vitamin products containing pyridoxine should be avoided; intake of foods containing large amounts of pyridoxine (such as avocado, bacon, beans, beef liver, dry skim milk, oatmeal, peas, pork, sweet potato, tuna, and certain health foods) may need to be limited.

**For treatment of adverse effects**

Immediate relief of nausea and vomiting may sometimes be obtained by reducing the daily dose, giving smaller individual doses at more frequent intervals, giving smaller doses concurrently with carbidopa, or having patient take food shortly after each dose; however, high-protein foods should be avoided since they may decrease levodopa's effect as well (see *Absorption; Drug interactions and/or related problems*). Since the nausea results primarily from the CNS effects of levodopa, non-phenothiazine antiemetics are sometimes successfully used. Phenothiazine antiemetics may be more effective but should not be used because of their tendency to negate levodopa's therapeutic effect.

The appearance of choreiform and other involuntary movements may require a reduction in dosage since tolerance usually does not develop.

Serious psychiatric disturbances, such as severe mental depression, with or without suicidal tendencies, may require reduction in dosage or complete withdrawal of levodopa.

Orthostatic hypotension may be controlled by the use of elastic hosiery and an increase in sodium intake. However, use of the carbidopa and levodopa combination reduces the incidence of this side effect.

The temporary withdrawal of levodopa has been used to prevent some of the complications of long-term therapy. Also, it has been used to enhance the efficacy of levodopa when therapy is reinstated since drug withdrawal presumably allows resensitization of the striatal dopamine receptors. However, full withdrawal of levodopa involves certain risks, such as worsening of parkinsonian symptoms, immobility, depression, pulmonary embolism, and thrombophlebitis. The patient, in most cases, will require nursing care and daily physical therapy during the temporary withdrawal.

After discontinuation of levodopa therapy, dantrolene and/or bromocriptine may be used in patients with evidence of neuroleptic malignant–like syndrome, to help reduce fever and thus avoid a potentially lethal complication.

## Oral Dosage Forms

### LEVODOPA CAPSULES USP

**Usual adult and adolescent dose**

Antidyskinetic—

Oral, 250 mg two to four times a day initially, the dosage per day being increased by an additional 100 to 750 mg at three- to seven-day intervals as tolerated until the desired response is obtained.

Note: Postencephalitic patients may be more sensitive to the effects of the usual adult dose.

**Usual adult prescribing limits**

Up to 8 grams daily.

**Usual pediatric dose**

Children up to 12 years of age: Safety and efficacy have not been established.

Children 12 years of age and over: See *Usual adult and adolescent dose.*

**Usual geriatric dose**

See *Usual adult and adolescent dose.*

Note: Geriatric patients may be more sensitive to the effects of the usual adult dose.

**Strength(s) usually available**

U.S.—

    100 mg (Rx) [*Dopar; Larodopa*].

    250 mg (Rx) [*Dopar; Larodopa*].

    500 mg (Rx) [*Dopar; Larodopa*].

Canada—

    Not commercially available.

**Packaging and storage**

Store between 15 and 30 °C (59 and 86 °F), unless otherwise specified by manufacturer. Store in a tight, light-resistant container.

**Auxiliary labeling**

• May darken urine or sweat.

### LEVODOPA TABLETS USP

**Usual adult and adolescent dose**

See *Levodopa Capsules USP.*

**Usual adult prescribing limits**

See *Levodopa Capsules USP.*

**Usual pediatric dose**

See *Levodopa Capsules USP.*

**Usual geriatric dose**

See *Levodopa Capsules USP.*

**Strength(s) usually available**

U.S.—

    100 mg (Rx) [*Larodopa*].

    250 mg (Rx) [*Larodopa*].

    500 mg (Rx) [*Larodopa*].

Canada—

    250 mg (Rx) [*Larodopa* (scored)].

**Packaging and storage**

Store between 15 and 30 °C (59 and 86 °F), unless otherwise specified by manufacturer. Store in a tight, light-resistant container.

**Auxiliary labeling**

• May darken urine or sweat.

Revised: 08/18/92
Interim revision: 08/17/94

## LEVODOPA-CONTAINING COMBINATIONS—

Carbidopa and Levodopa (Systemic)

# LEVOMETHADYL    Systemic†

INN: Levomethadyl acetate—Levacetylmethadol.

VA CLASSIFICATION (Primary): CN101

Note: Controlled substance in the U.S.—II.

Other commonly used names are LAAM, LAM, levacetylmethadol, levo-alpha-acetylmethadol, levomethadyl acetate, and MK790.

Note: For a listing of dosage forms and brand names by country availability, see *Dosage Forms* section(s). For a listing of brand names for the articles in this monograph, refer to the General Index.

†Not commercially available in Canada.

## Category

Opioid (narcotic) abuse therapy adjunct.

Note: Levomethadyl is an opioid (narcotic) analgesic, but is not used for relief of pain.

## Indications

### General considerations

In the U.S., levomethadyl is permitted to be dispensed only through opioid addiction treatment programs approved by the Food and Drug Administration (FDA), Drug Enforcement Administration (DEA), and designated state authorities. Use of levomethadyl in such programs is subject to treatment requirements stipulated in Federal regulations.

### Accepted

Opioid (narcotic) drug use, illicit (treatment adjunct)—Levomethadyl is indicated as an adjunct to other measures, which may include psychological and social counseling and medical and rehabilitative services, in the treatment of opioid dependence. It may be used in detoxification programs (to assist withdrawal from illicit opioids) and in maintenance programs (to discourage illicit use of other opioids). Appropriate evaluation, planning, counseling, and follow-up are essential components of successful treatment. There is no evidence that administration of an opioid alone is effective treatment for opioid addiction.

Note: In the U.S., Federal regulations permit specific opioids (levomethadyl and methadone) to be used in approved detoxification and interim or comprehensive maintenance treatment programs. Levomethadyl is administered only 3 times a week and may be particularly useful for patients who do not require daily visits to the clinic, whereas methadone must be administered every day and may be more useful for patients who benefit from the support of daily clinic visits. Also, because some patients experience effects perceived as aversive during treatment with one opioid or the other, the selection of a particular opioid may depend on patient acceptance.

Short-term (up to 30 days) or long-term (up to 180 days) detoxification programs use an opioid to alleviate adverse physiological or psychological consequences of withdrawal from illicit opioids, with dosage gradually being decreased until a drug-free state is achieved. After 180 days, patients who have not achieved a drug-free state are considered to be receiving maintenance treatment. Patients may also be enrolled directly into a maintenance program without first attempting detoxification. In maintenance treatment programs, relatively stable doses of opioid are given on a continuing basis as a substitute for illicit opioids.

Detoxification and comprehensive maintenance programs must include a full range of medical and rehabilitative services in addition to opioid administration. However, patients who are awaiting admission to a comprehensive maintenance program may receive up to 120 days of interim maintenance treatment, which consists only of opioid administration and needed medical services.

## Pharmacology/Pharmacokinetics

### Physicochemical characteristics

Chemical group—Opioid analgesic; chemically related to both oxymorphone and naloxone.

Molecular weight—Levomethadyl acetate hydrochloride: 389.97.

Octanol:water partition coefficient—405:1.

### Mechanism of action/Effect

Levomethadyl is a mu-receptor opioid agonist. It substitutes for opioids of the morphine type, thereby suppressing withdrawal symptoms in individuals who are addicted to such agents. With chronic use, levomethadyl produces cross-tolerance to the effects of other mu-receptor agonists, including the subjective "high" they produce, and decreases the addict's desire for such drugs.

### Other actions/effects

Levomethadyl produces effects characteristic of mu-receptor opioid analgesics, including analgesia, respiratory depression, sedation, pupillary constriction, and physical dependence.

### Absorption

Rapid.

### Distribution

Extensive. The volume of distribution is about 20 L per kg of body weight (L/kg).

### Protein binding

High (approximately 80%); primarily to an alpha globulin. Studies in heroin addicts have demonstrated that levomethadyl, levomethadyl's active metabolites, and methadone bind to, compete for, and displace each other from the same protein-binding sites.

### Biotransformation

Levomethadyl undergoes extensive first-pass metabolism to the active demethylated metabolite nor-levomethadyl (nor-LAAM), which is further demethylated to a second active metabolite, dinor-levomethadyl (dinor-LAAM). Smaller quantities of levomethadyl are also deacetylated to methadol, nor-methadol, and dinor-methadol. The rate of biotransformation is subject to interindividual variability. Although biotransformation to nor-LAAM generally occurs more slowly in males than in females, the differences are not as great as the interindividual differences.

### Half-life

Distribution—

Levomethadyl: Approximately 6 hours.

Elimination—

Levomethadyl: Approximately 2.6 days.

nor-LAAM: Approximately 2 days.

dinor-LAAM: Approximately 4 days.

### Onset of action

Although some opioid analgesic effects are apparent 2 to 4 hours after an oral dose, suppression of opioid withdrawal symptoms occurs after a delay of at least several days, during which levomethadyl's active metabolites are forming and accumulating.

### Time to peak concentration

Levomethadyl—Usually 1.5 to 2 hours, but up to 4 hours in some studies.

nor-LAAM—Usually 4 to 7 hours, but up to 10 hours in some individuals.

dinor-LAAM—Usually 5 to 7 hours, but 24 to 48 hours in some individuals.

### Peak serum concentration

One study in 12 patients reported substantial interindividual variability in the peak concentrations of levomethadyl and its active metabolites after single and multiple doses. Plasma concentrations of levomethadyl, nor-LAAM, and dinor-LAAM were higher after multiple doses than after single doses, but the concentrations of the metabolites, especially dinor-LAAM, were increased to a greater extent than those of levomethadyl.

Studies of peak and trough steady-state concentrations showed that there is great interindividual variability in levomethadyl concentrations over a 72-hour dosing interval. Also, although the concentration of levomethadyl itself decreased considerably during the 72-hour interval, the concentrations of the active metabolites, especially dinor-LAAM, decreased to a much lesser extent.

### Time to steady state

Three-times-per-week dosing schedule—1 to 2 weeks (approximately 9, 8, and 12.5 days for levomethadyl, nor-LAAM, and dinor-LAAM, respectively).

### Time to peak effect

Suppression of opioid withdrawal symptoms—Approximately 7 to 10 days after initiation of treatment.

### Duration of action

Suppression of opioid withdrawal symptoms—
Single 30- to 60-mg dose: 24 to 48 hours.
Single 80-mg or higher dose: 48 to 72 hours.

### Elimination

Approximately 27% of a dose is eliminated in the urine as levomethadyl and various metabolites (nor-LAAM, dinor-LAAM, methadol, nor-methadol, and dinor-methadol). The disposition of the remainder of the dose has not been determined in humans, but extensive biliary elimination has been demonstrated in animal studies.

## Precautions to Consider

### Carcinogenicity

Levomethadyl was not carcinogenic in 2-year studies in rats given 13 mg per kg of body weight (mg/kg) (77 mg per square meter of body surface area [mg/m$^2$]) or in mice given 30 mg/kg (90 mg/m$^2$).

### Mutagenicity

Levomethadyl was not mutagenic in the Ames test, the unscheduled DNA synthesis and repair test, *in vitro* mouse lymphoma cell studies, or *in vivo* rat chromosomal aberration tests. However, levomethadyl exhibited mutagenic activity in the ad-3 forward mutation assay in *N. crassa* in concentrations of 150 mcg per mL (mcg/mL) *in vitro* and in the heritable translocation assay in mice receiving 21 mg/kg (63 mg/m$^2$). The significance of these findings to clinical use in humans is not known.

### Pregnancy/Reproduction

Pregnancy—Methadone is the agent of choice for pregnant women in comprehensive maintenance treatment programs. There are no clinical data on the safety of levomethadyl during pregnancy. Levomethadyl administration should not be started or continued during pregnancy except by the written order of a physician who determines levomethadyl to be the best choice of therapy for an individual patient. In the U.S., Federal regulations require that women of childbearing potential receive a pregnancy test prior to initiation of, and monthly during, levomethadyl maintenance treatment.

Animal reproduction studies have not been completed. However, in one study administration of 0.2 or 2 mg/kg per day to rats prior to and throughout gestation caused opioid dependence in both the dams and pups. The larger dose also produced high incidences of premature delivery, stillbirths, and decreased pup weights. However, there were no differences in the rates of implantation, resorption, or morphological abnormalities between treated and control groups.

FDA Pregnancy Category C.

Labor and delivery—The effects of levomethadyl on labor and delivery are not known.

Postpartum—Use of levomethadyl during pregnancy may result in respiratory depression and/or physical dependence with delayed emergence of withdrawal symptoms in the neonate.

**Breast-feeding**

It is not known whether levomethadyl is distributed into breast milk in quantities sufficient to affect the nursing infant.

**Pediatrics**

In the U.S., Federal regulations prohibit use of levomethadyl in addicts younger than 18 years of age.

**Geriatrics**

No information is available on the relationship of age to the effects of levomethadyl in geriatric patients.

**Dental**

Opioid analgesics may decrease or inhibit salivary flow, thus contributing to the development of caries, periodontal disease, oral candidiasis, and discomfort.

**Drug interactions and/or related problems**

The following drug interactions and/or related problems have been selected on the basis of their potential clinical significance (possible mechanism in parentheses where appropriate)—not necessarily inclusive (» = major clinical significance):

Note: Combinations containing any of the following medications, depending on the amount present, may also interact with this medication.

» Alcohol or
» CNS depression–producing medications, other (See *Appendix II*)
    (concurrent use may increase the CNS depressant, respiratory depressant, and hypotensive effects of these medications and/or levomethadyl; a reduction in dosage of levomethadyl and/or other prescribed CNS depressants may be required if concurrent use is necessary; also, opioid addicts should be warned of the risk of additive effects and potential for serious toxicity if they abuse alcohol or other CNS depressants while receiving levomethadyl)

» Enzyme inducers, hepatic, cytochrome P450 (see *Appendix II*)
    (induction of the hepatic cytochrome P450 enzyme system may increase the rate of levomethadyl metabolism to its active metabolites and enhance its peak effectiveness, but may also shorten its duration of action)

» Enzyme inhibitors, hepatic (see *Appendix II*)
    (inhibition of hepatic enzymes may slow the onset, lower the peak activity, and/or increase the duration of action of levomethadyl; adjustment of levomethadyl dosage and/or the interval between doses may be required)

» Opioid analgesics, mixed agonist/antagonist, such as:
    Butorphanol
    Nalbuphine
    Pentazocine
» Opioid analgesics, partial mu-receptor agonist, such as:
    Buprenorphine
    Dezocine or
» Opioid antagonists, such as:
    Naloxone
    Naltrexone
    (these medications may precipitate withdrawal symptoms if administered to a patient receiving levomethadyl therapy; the severity of withdrawal symptoms will depend on the potency and dose of the antagonist or partial agonist and on the degree to which physical dependence is present)

    (opioid analgesics such as levomethadyl will be ineffective if treatment is initiated in a patient receiving naltrexone, which blocks the therapeutic effects of opioids)

» Opioid analgesics, mu-receptor agonist, other, such as:
    Alfentanil
    Anileridine
    Codeine
    Fentanyl
    Heroin
    Hydrocodone
    Hydromorphone
    Levorphanol
    Meperidine
    Methadone
    Morphine
    Opium
    Oxycodone
    Oxymorphone

    Propoxyphene
    Sufentanil
    (chronic use of levomethadyl produces cross-tolerance to the therapeutic effects, but not necessarily to the toxic effects, of other mu-receptor opioid agonists, leading to a considerably higher-than-normal dosage requirement for other mu-receptor agonists and a substantial risk of additive toxicity; deaths have occurred early in levomethadyl treatment in opioid addicts who continued to use illicit opioids during the 1- to 2-week delay in levomethadyl's onset of action. Administration of a mu-receptor opioid analgesic to levomethadyl-treated patients, if necessary for therapeutic purposes, requires extreme caution and careful monitoring. Opioid agonists that are *N*-demethylated to long-acting, excitatory metabolites [e.g., meperidine, propoxyphene] should not be used because the high dosage requirement also leads to an unacceptably high risk of metabolite-induced toxicity)

**Laboratory value alterations**

The following have been selected on the basis of their potential clinical significance (possible effect in parentheses where appropriate)—not necessarily inclusive (» = major clinical significance):

Note: The following laboratory value alterations have not been documented with levomethadyl. However, they are commonly produced by other mu-receptor opioid agonists and should be considered potential effects of levomethadyl also.

    Because of the long half-life of levomethadyl and its active metabolites, effects on laboratory values may persist for several days after treatment has been discontinued.

With diagnostic test results
    Gastric emptying studies
      (opioid analgesics may delay gastric emptying, thereby invalidating test results)

    Hepatobiliary imaging using technetium Tc 99m disofenin
      (delivery of technetium Tc 99m disofenin to the small bowel may be prevented because of opioid analgesic–induced constriction of the sphincter of Oddi and increased biliary tract pressure; these actions result in delayed visualization and thus resemble obstruction of the common bile duct)

With physiology/laboratory test values
    Amylase, plasma and
    Lipase, plasma
      (values may be increased because opioid analgesics can cause contractions of the sphincter of Oddi and increased biliary tract pressure)

    Cerebrospinal fluid (CSF) pressure
      (may be increased; effect is secondary to respiratory depression–induced carbon dioxide retention)

**Medical considerations/Contraindications**

The medical considerations/contraindications included here have been selected on the basis of their potential clinical significance (reasons given in parentheses where appropriate)—not necessarily inclusive (» = major clinical significance).

*Risk-benefit should be considered when the following medical problems exist:*

    Abdominal conditions, acute
      (diagnosis or clinical course may be obscured)
» Asthma, acute attack or
» Respiratory depression, acute or
» Respiratory impairment or disease, chronic
      (risk of apnea because opioids decrease respiratory drive and increase airway resistance)
    Cardiac dysrhythmias
      (levomethadyl may cause QT interval prolongation; careful monitoring is recommended during therapy)
    Dependence on or abuse of nonopioid medications, history of, including alcoholism or
    Emotional instability or
    Suicidal ideation or attempts
      (addicts often attempt suicide using combinations of opioids and other drugs of abuse. Patients who continue to use illicit opioids or other CNS-active medications despite adequate levomethadyl therapy require individualized evaluation and treatment planning; hospitalization may be necessary)
    Diagnostic, surgical, or other procedure requiring general anesthesia or sedation
      (levomethadyl-induced alterations in patient response to medications that may be used in conjunction with general anesthesia or sedation [e.g., tolerance to the therapeutic effects of mu-receptor opioid agonists; increased risk of severe CNS and/or respiratory

depression with anesthetics, sedatives, and opioid analgesics] and
the risk of precipitating withdrawal via use of opioid antagonists,
mixed agonists/antagonists, or partial mu-receptor agonists must
be taken into consideration when selecting medications and dosages to be administered)

Diarrhea associated with pseudomembranous colitis caused by antibiotics or

Diarrhea caused by poisoning
(opioids may slow the elimination of toxic material, and it is generally recommended that they not be administered until after toxins
have been cleared from the gastrointestinal tract; however, levomethadyl administration should not be interrupted if these conditions occur during treatment)

Gallbladder disease or gallstones
(opioids may cause biliary colic)

Gastrointestinal tract surgery, recent
(opioids may alter gastrointestinal motility)

Head injury or
Increased intracranial pressure, pre-existing or
Intracranial lesions
(increased risk of respiratory depression and further elevation of
cerebrospinal fluid pressure; also, opioids may cause sedation and
pupillary changes that may obscure the clinical course of head
injury)

Hepatic function impairment or
Renal function impairment
(although studies have not been done in patients with clinically
significant hepatic or renal function impairment, the possibility
must be considered that formation of levomethadyl's active metabolites and/or elimination of levomethadyl and its active metabolites may be substantially altered; because of its less complex
metabolic profile, methadone may be preferable for such patients)

Hypothyroidism
(risk of respiratory depression and prolonged CNS depression is
greatly increased)

» Inflammatory bowel disease, severe
(risk of toxic megacolon may be increased)

Prostatic hypertrophy or obstruction or
Urethral stricture or
Urinary tract surgery, recent
(increased risk of urinary retention, which may be induced by these
conditions as well as by opioids)

Sensitivity to levomethadyl, history of

**Patient monitoring**
The following may be especially important in patient monitoring (other
tests may be warranted in some patients, depending on condition;
» = major clinical significance):

» Drug screen
(in the U.S., Federal regulations mandate screening for drugs of
abuse [amphetamines, barbiturates, cocaine, other opioids, and any
other agents known to be abused in the program's locality] at the
time a prospective patient first appears at the treatment center.
Further testing is not required for patients undergoing detoxification from opioid drugs. Patients receiving interim maintenance
treatment must be tested at least twice during a 120-day interim
program, and patients receiving comprehensive maintenance treatment must be tested at least 8 times at random intervals during the
first year of treatment and at least quarterly thereafter)

» Pregnancy test
(in the U.S., Federal regulations require that women of childbearing potential receive a pregnancy test prior to initiation of, and
monthly during, levomethadyl maintenance therapybecause levomethadyl administration should not be started or continued during
pregnancy except by the written order of a physician who determines levomethadyl to be the best choice of therapy for an individual patient)

## Side/Adverse Effects

Note: Many symptoms typical of opioid withdrawal (listed below) occur
during levomethadyl treatment. Early in treatment, while levomethadyl's active metabolites are forming and accumulating, such
symptoms probably indicate withdrawal from illicit opioid analgesics. However, they may continue to occur many weeks after treatment has begun, especially on the days between doses. Adjustment
of levomethadyl dosage, supplemental low doses of methadone,
and/or a suppressant such as clonidine or guanabenz may be
needed.

In addition to the side/adverse effects listed below, the following
have been reported in patients receiving levomethadyl (although a
causal relationship has not been established): Amenorrhea; electrocardiographic irregularities, including prolongation of the QT interval and nonspecific ST-T wave changes; hepatitis; liver function
test abnormalities; and pyuria.

The following side/adverse effects have been selected on the basis of their
potential clinical significance (possible signs and symptoms in parentheses where appropriate)—not necessarily inclusive:

**Those indicating need for medical attention**
Incidence less frequent (1 to 3%)
*Edema* (swelling of face, fingers, feet, and/or lower legs; weight gain);
*mental depression; skin rash*

**Those indicating need for medical attention only if they continue
or are bothersome**
Incidence more frequent (3% or higher)
*Abdominal pain; constipation; general feeling of discomfort or ill-
ness; joint pain; nervousness; sexual problems in males; sweating;
trouble in sleeping; weakness*
Incidence less frequent (1 to 3%)
*Back pain; blurred vision; chills; CNS symptoms* (anxiety; decreased
sensitivity to stimulation; drowsiness; false sense of well-being; headache; unusual dreams); *coughing; decreased desire for sex; diarrhea;
dry mouth; flu-like syndrome; hot flashes; nausea and vomiting;
runny nose; yawning*

Note: In some clinical trials, a significant number of patients experienced symptoms of stimulation, such as anxiety and nervousness, on the day of administration. Some patients continued to
experience these symptoms on the days between doses, whereas
others experienced symptoms such as lack of energy, dysphoria,
and depression.
Patients should be advised to report severe *drowsiness* or stimulation (e.g., feeling ''wired'') at the next visit to the clinic,
because dosage adjustment may be needed.

Incidence less than 1%
*Hypotension, postural* (dizziness, lightheadedness, or feeling faint
when rising from a lying or sitting position); *muscle pain; watery eyes*

**Those indicating possible withdrawal and/or the need for dosage
adjustment or other treatment if they occur during therapy or
after medication is discontinued**
*Body aches; diarrhea; fast heartbeat; gooseflesh; increased sweat-
ing; loss of appetite; nausea or vomiting; nervousness, restlessness,
or irritability; runny nose; shivering or trembling; sneezing; stomach
cramps; trouble in sleeping; unexplained fever; unusually large pupils of eyes; weakness; yawning*

## Overdose

For specific information on the agents used in the management of
levomethadyl overdose, see:
• *Naloxone (Systemic)* monograph; and/or
• *Charcoal, Activated (Oral-Local)* monograph.

For more information on the management of overdose, **contact a Poison
Control Center** (see *Poison Control Center Listing*).

Levomethadyl toxicity is more likely to develop when therapy is started
in patients who have not developed tolerance to the effects of opioids.
In nontolerant patients, initial doses of 20 to 40 mg may cause somnolence, and larger initial doses may cause serious toxicity. Opioid-
tolerant individuals may also experience symptoms, but at higher initial doses.

Although overdose with levomethadyl alone has been reported rarely, as
a result of too-frequent (daily) administration, most overdoses have
involved ingestion of other opioids in addition to levomethadyl. Deaths
have occurred when patients continued to use illicit opioids after initiation of levomethadyl treatment.

**Clinical effects of overdose**
The following effects have been selected on the basis of their potential
clinical significance (possible signs and symptoms in parentheses
where appropriate)—not necessarily inclusive:
*Cold, clammy skin; confusion; low blood pressure; pinpoint pupils
of eyes; respiratory depression* (blue lips, fingernails, or skin; slow or
troubled breathing); *severe dizziness, drowsiness, muscle weakness,
nervousness, or restlessness; slow heartbeat; unconsciousness*

Note: In severe overdosage, extreme CNS and respiratory depression
may result in apnea, shock, pulmonary edema, cardiac arrest,
and death.

## Treatment of overdose

Primary importance should be given to maintaining adequate ventilation. Assessing the patient's respiratory status and, if necessary, administering oxygen or otherwise assisting respiration are essential. Provision of an artificial airway may be necessary.

To decrease absorption—Emptying the stomach by inducing emesis and/or administering activated charcoal. The initial dose of charcoal should be followed by a cathartic, such as magnesium citrate, if the charcoal is not pre-mixed with sorbitol. Gastric lavage may also be performed. During these procedures, care should be taken to protect the airway of any patient who is not fully alert. However, treatment of respiratory depression or other life-threatening complications must take precedence.

To enhance elimination—Forced diuresis, peritoneal dialysis, hemoperfusion, and hemodialysis are not likely to be effective for removal of levomethadyl because of its lipophilicity and large volume of distribution.

Specific treatment—Administering naloxone, keeping in mind that rapid reversal of opioid effects may precipitate severe withdrawal symptoms, which may rarely lead to cardiac instability, in this patient population. Administration of several doses of naloxone, starting with considerably lower-than-usual quantities that may be increased gradually, if necessary, until the desired effect has been achieved is preferable to administration of large, single doses. Prolonged naloxone treatment, via repeated injections or continuous intravenous infusion, is likely to be necessary because of levomethadyl's long duration of action. Oral administration of the long-acting opioid antagonist naltrexone may precipitate prolonged withdrawal symptoms and is not recommended. See the package insert or *Naloxone (Systemic)* for specific dosing guidelines for use of this product.

Monitoring—

Respiration, oxygenation, patient alertness, and vital signs should be monitored. Because of levomethadyl's long duration of action, prolonged observation will be needed..

A screen for other medications, especially other drugs of abuse, should be performed and additional treatment instituted as required.

Supportive care—

Supportive measures include establishing intravenous lines, hydration, and administering vasopressors if necessary.

## Patient Consultation

As an aid to patient consultation, refer to *Advice for the Patient, Levomethadyl (Systemic)*.

In providing consultation, consider emphasizing the following selected information (» = major clinical significance):

**Before using this medication**
» Conditions affecting use, especially:

Sensitivity to levomethadyl

Pregnancy—Not starting levomethadyl during pregnancy; methadone is preferred medication for treating pregnant opioid addicts

Use in children—Use in patients up to 18 years of age not permitted by U.S. Federal regulations

Other medications, especially alcohol or other CNS depressants, hepatic enzyme inducers or inhibitors, other opioid analgesics, and opioid antagonists

Other medical problems, especially diarrhea caused by antibiotics or by poisoning, asthma or other respiratory problems, and severe inflammatory bowel disease

**Proper use of this medication**
» Medication must be taken at clinic, usually 3 times per week
» Proper dosing

**Precautions while using this medication**
» Importance of compliance with other measures necessary for rehabilitation, e.g., counseling, attending support group meetings, making lifestyle changes
» Avoiding use of alcoholic beverages and illicit opioids or other CNS depressants during therapy, even if experiencing withdrawal symptoms and cravings, because of the risk of potentially fatal additive toxicity or overdose
» Caution if severe drowsiness occurs, especially when treatment initiated or dosage adjusted
» Getting up slowly from a lying or sitting position; lying down for a while may relieve symptoms associated with postural hypotension, such as dizziness, lightheadedness, or feeling faint
» Need to inform physicians and dentists of levomethadyl use, particularly if any kind of surgery (including dental surgery) or emergency treatment is required

Possible need for regimen to prevent severe constipation

Possible dryness of mouth; using sugarless gum or candy, ice, or saliva substitute for relief; checking with dentist if dry mouth continues for more than 2 weeks
» Female patients only: Not becoming pregnant during treatment; discussing planned pregnancy with counselor ahead of time; informing counselor if pregnancy suspected
» If transferring to methadone: Not taking first dose of methadone for at least 48 hours after last dose of levomethadyl
» Suspected overdose: Getting emergency help at once; need to inform emergency practitioners that the patient is physically dependent on a long-acting opioid, naloxone is likely to precipitate withdrawal, and prolonged observation and monitoring are needed

**Side/adverse effects**

Getting emergency help immediately if respiratory depression or other symptoms of overdose occur

Signs and symptoms of other potential side effects, especially edema, mental depression, and skin rash

Informing counselor at clinic if severe drowsiness, severe stimulation, or withdrawal symptoms occurred after previous dose

# General Dosing Information

In the U.S., levomethadyl is available only through treatment programs that have been approved by the Food and Drug Administration, Drug Enforcement Agency, and designated state authorities.

Levomethadyl is given only by the oral route. The commercially available oral solution must be diluted before being administered to the patient. Treatment centers that dispense both levomethadyl and methadone (which must also be dispensed as a dilute liquid) should use liquids of different colors for preparing each medication, so that they can be distinguished from each other readily.

Levomethadyl is to be ingested by the patient at the treatment center. Take-home doses are not permitted.

Levomethadyl treatment should be initiated using a dose that suppresses withdrawal symptoms and decreases craving for illicit opioids without inducing excessive opioid effects. Interpatient variability in levomethadyl kinetics and each patient's level of tolerance to opioids must be taken into account when selecting initial dosage. However, because of levomethadyl's slow onset of action and the risk of toxicity if dosage is increased too rapidly, elimination of withdrawal symptoms and craving may not be possible during the first 1 or 2 weeks of therapy. Patients may need extra counseling and support and/or administration of a withdrawal suppressant, preferably a nonopioid such as clonidine or guanabenz, during this time. Alternatively, treatment may be initiated with methadone (especially if the patient's degree of tolerance to opioids is not known), since effective dosage can be achieved more rapidly, and the patient transferred to levomethadyl after a few weeks. The changeover from methadone to levomethadyl may be accomplished in a single dose.

Levomethadyl is usually administered 3 times a week (on Monday, Wednesday, and Friday or on Tuesday, Thursday, and Saturday), but some patients experience withdrawal symptoms during the 72-hour Friday-to-Monday or Saturday-to-Tuesday interval. Administration of a higher dose on Friday or Saturday prevents or minimizes this problem in most patients. However, in a clinical trial patients receiving such a regimen reported feeling overmedicated on the day that the higher dose was given and undermedicated after the next (lower) dose. For some patients, use of a withdrawal suppressant such as clonidine or guanabenz; provision of a low take-home dose of methadone (if the patient meets the criteria specified in U.S. Federal regulations for take-home methadone); arranging the patient's schedule so that the 72-hour interval occurs during the week, so that a small dose of methadone can be administered to the patient at the clinic if necessary; or administration of levomethadyl on an every-other-day basis may be necessary. **Levomethadyl should not be administered daily** because rapid accumulation of the medication and its active metabolites may lead to an overdose.

Patients receiving levomethadyl may be transferred directly to methadone, although some patients may experience mild withdrawal symptoms during the first 1 or 2 weeks. The initial dose of methadone, which should be taken at least 48 hours after the last dose of levomethadyl, should be 80% of the patient's lower levomethadyl dose. For example, a patient receiving three-times-a week treatment with 80, 80, and 100 mg of levomethadyl would be given 64 mg of methadone per day, initially. The daily dose of methadone may be increased or decreased by 5 or 10 mg if symptoms of withdrawal or opioid excess occur. This regimen may also be used, provided that the regulations and requirements for take-home methadone are met, when a levomethadyl-treated patient who is unable to attend the clinic regularly for a period of time (for example, because of illness or travel) requires a temporary transfer to take-home methadone. The risk of the methadone's being diverted to illicit use must be considered. The number of take-home methadone doses should be 2 fewer than the number of days of expected absence, but must not exceed the maximum number of take-home doses specified in U.S. Federal regulations. When the patient returns to the clinic levomethadyl may be resumed, following the same dosage regimen as before the temporary change in treatment. However, if the last methadone dose was taken more than 48 hours previously, levomethadyl should be reintroduced at a dose based on clinical and/or toxicological evaluation of the patient.

Patients who miss a single dose of levomethadyl and who arrive at the clinic the next day should receive their usual dose on an every-other-day basis for the remainder of the week, then resume their normal dosing schedule the following week. For example, a missed Monday dose would be administered on Tuesday, after which the remaining doses for the week would be given on Thursday and Saturday and the normal Monday, Wednesday, and Friday schedule resumed the following Monday. Although most patients who miss a single dose and return to the clinic on their next regularly scheduled day should be able to tolerate the usual dose of levomethadyl, some individuals may require a reduced dose. After 2 doses have been missed, treatment should be restarted using only one-half to three-fourths of the previous maintenance dose for the first dose and increasing each subsequent dose by 5 or 10 mg until the previous maintenance dose is reached. After a lapse of 3 doses (1 week) or more, therapy should be reinstituted with induction doses.

Discontinuation of levomethadyl maintenance therapy may be considered after the patient has achieved behavioral objectives outlined in the patient's comprehensive treatment plan, i.e., stopped using illicit drugs, reached social and occupational goals, and changed his or her lifestyle to decrease the risk of relapse. Treatment should not be stopped prematurely, and appropriate nonpharmacological support should be provided to reduce further the risk of relapse. Stable long-term treatment is preferable to cycles of discontinuation of therapy followed by recidivism. Treatment has been successfully discontinued by abrupt withdrawal or by reducing dosage gradually (by 5 to 10% per week). One study comparing both methods of detoxification found that withdrawal symptoms were not more severe, and a significantly higher number of patients were successfully withdrawn from maintenance treatment without returning to illicit opioid use, when levomethadyl was stopped abruptly.

### Safety considerations for handling this medication

Because of the risk of diversion of this potent opioid, security measures stipulated in the U.S. Federal Code of Regulations should be taken to safeguard supplies of the medication.

There are no known hazards associated with dermal or aerosol exposure to levomethadyl. However, if the medication is spilled onto an individual, contaminated clothing should be removed and the exposed skin rinsed with cool water.

## Oral Dosage Forms

### LEVOMETHADYL ACETATE HYDROCHLORIDE ORAL SOLUTION

#### Usual adult dose
Opioid (narcotic) abuse therapy adjunct—
  Induction:
    Patients not receiving prior methadone maintenance treatment—Oral, 20 to 40 mg for the first dose. Subsequent doses, given at forty-eight- or seventy-two-hour intervals, may be increased by 5 to 10 mg until the desired effects (absence of withdrawal symptoms and decreased craving for illicit opioids) have been achieved or decreased by the same amount if undue sedation or other symptoms of opioid excess occur.
    Patients transferred from methadone maintenance treatment—Oral, a quantity of levomethadyl equivalent to 1.2 to 1.3 times the patient's daily methadone dose, up to a maximum of 120 mg, for the first dose. Subsequent doses, administered at forty-eight- or seventy-two-hour intervals, should be adjusted according to the response of the individual patient, using caution not to increase the dose too rapidly because of the risk of toxicity. Dosage is generally increased by 5 to 10 mg every second or third dose.
  Maintenance:
    Dosage must be individualized according to the patient's tolerance and response. Most patients can be stabilized on 60 to 80 mg, administered three times a week at forty-eight- or seventy-two-

hour intervals. However, maintenance doses as low as 10 mg and as high as 140 mg, administered three times a week, have been used in clinical trials. If necessary to prevent withdrawal over a seventy-two-hour interdose interval, the dose prior to this interval may be increased, in 6- to 10-mg increments, to up to forty percent higher than the doses given prior to a forty-eight-hour interval. At least two weeks are required to achieve a new clinical plateau after each adjustment of levomethadyl dosage.

Note: U.S. Federal regulations require that single doses of 140 mg or more be justified in the patient's record.

#### Usual adult prescribing limits
Initial induction dose—40 mg (if the patient's level of opioid tolerance is unknown) or 120 mg (if the patient's level of tolerance, based on methadone dosage requirements, is known).
Maintenance—Dosage should not exceed 140 mg three times a week or every other day, or two 130-mg doses and one 180-mg dose per week.

#### Usual pediatric dose
U.S. Federal regulations prohibit use of levomethadyl in patients younger than 18 years of age.

#### Usual geriatric dose
See *Usual adult dose.*

#### Strength(s) usually available
U.S.—
    10 mg per mL (Rx) [*Orlaam* (methylparaben 1.8 mg; and propylparaben 0.2 mg per mL)].
Canada—
    Not commercially available.

#### Packaging and storage
Store between 15 and 30 °C (59 and 86 °F), protected from freezing, unless otherwise specified by manufacturer.

#### Preparation of dosage form
U.S. Federal regulations stipulate that the oral solution must be diluted before being administered to the patient. The liquid used for dilution should be colored differently than a liquid used to prepare methadone solutions in the same clinic.

### Selected Bibliography

Tennant FS, Rawson RA, Pumphrey E, et al. Clinical experiences with 959 opioid-dependent patients treated with levo-alpha-acetylmethadol (LAAM). J Subst Abuse Treat 1986; 3: 195-202.

Ling W, Blakis M, Holmes ED, et al. Restabilization with methadone after methadyl acetate maintenance. Arch Gen Psychiatry 1980; 37: 194-6.

Judson BA, Goldstein A, Inturrisi CE. Methadyl acetate (LAAM) in the treatment of heroin addicts. II. Double-blind comparison of graduated and abrupt detoxification. Arch Gen Psychiatry 1983; 40: 834-40.

Developed: 08/11/95

## LEVONORDEFRIN-CONTAINING COMBINATIONS—

Mepivacaine and Levonordefrin (Parenteral-Local)—See *Anesthetics (Parenteral-Local)*
Propoxycaine, Procaine, and Levonordefrin (Parenteral-Local)—See *Anesthetics (Parenteral-Local)*

## LEVONORGESTROL—See *Progestins (Systemic)*

## LEVORPHANOL—See *Opioid (Narcotic) Analgesics (Systemic)*

## LEVOTHYROXINE—See *Thyroid Hormones (Systemic)*

## LIDOCAINE—See *Anesthetics (Mucosal-Local); Anesthetics (Parenteral-Local); Anesthetics (Topical); Lidocaine (Systemic)*

# LIDOCAINE   Systemic

VA CLASSIFICATION (Primary): CV300

Note: For a listing of dosage forms and brand names by country availability, see *Dosage Forms* section(s). For a listing of brand names for the articles in this monograph, refer to the General Index.

## Category

Antiarrhythmic.

## Indications

### Accepted

Arrhythmias, ventricular (treatment)—Lidocaine (systemic) is indicated and is the drug of choice in the acute management of ventricular arrhythmias, such as those resulting from acute myocardial infarction, digitalis toxicity, cardiac surgery, or cardiac catheterization.

## Pharmacology/Pharmacokinetics

### Physicochemical characteristics

pKa—7.86.

### Mechanism of action/Effect

Antiarrhythmic—Lidocaine decreases the depolarization, automaticity, and excitability in the ventricles during the diastolic phase by a direct action on the tissues, especially the Purkinje network, without involvement of the autonomic system. Neither contractility, systolic arterial blood pressure, atrioventricular (AV) conduction velocity, nor absolute refractory period is altered by usual therapeutic doses. In the Vaughan Williams classification of antiarrhythmics, lidocaine is considered to be a class IB agent.

### Absorption

Nearly complete following intramuscular injection.

### Distribution

Rapid; distribution volume about 1 L/kg of body weight (but reduced in heart failure patients).

### Protein binding

Moderate to high (60 to 80%; dependent on drug concentration).

### Biotransformation

90% hepatic; active metabolites, monoethylglycinexylidide and glycinexylidide, may contribute to therapeutic and toxic effects especially after infusions lasting 24 hours or more.

### Half-life

1 to 2 hours (average about 100 minutes); dose-dependent (tends to be biphasic with the distribution phase of 7 to 9 minutes causing the short duration of action following an intravenous loading dose); increased to 3 hours or longer during prolonged intravenous infusions (longer than 24 hours).

### Onset of action

Intravenous—Immediate (45 to 90 seconds).
Intramuscular—5 to 15 minutes.

### Time to steady-state plasma concentration

Continuous intravenous infusion—3 to 4 hours (8 to 10 hours in patients with acute myocardial infarction).

### Therapeutic plasma concentration

1.5 to 5 mcg/mL (concentrations exceeding 5 mcg/mL are considered to be in the toxic range).

### Duration of action

Intravenous—10 to 20 minutes.
Intramuscular—60 to 90 minutes.

### Elimination

Renal, 10% unchanged.
In dialysis—Very little removable by dialysis.

## Precautions to Consider

### Cross-sensitivity and/or related problems

Patients sensitive to other amide-type anesthetics or flecainide or tocainide may be sensitive to lidocaine also. Cross-sensitivity with procainamide or quinidine has not been reported.

### Carcinogenicity/Mutagenicity

Long term animal studies evaluating the carcinogenic or mutagenic potential of lidocaine have not been done.

### Pregnancy/Reproduction

Pregnancy—Lidocaine crosses the placenta. Adequate and well-controlled studies in humans have not been done.

Studies in rats at doses up to 6.6 times the maximum human dose have not shown that lidocaine causes adverse effects in the fetus. However, lidocaine has been shown to constrict uterine arteries in sheep and in experimentally isolated uterine artery segments. Furthermore, studies in sheep have shown that lidocaine causes significant increases in fetal blood pressure and increases or decreases in fetal heart rate related to the rate of lidocaine infusion.

FDA Pregnancy Category B.

### Breast-feeding

It is not known whether lidocaine is excreted in human breast milk. However, problems in humans have not been documented.

### Pediatrics

Appropriate studies on the relationship of age to the effects of lidocaine have not been performed in the pediatric population. However, no pediatrics-specific problems have been documented to date.

### Geriatrics

Elderly patients are more prone to the adverse effects of lidocaine. In patients over 65 years of age, dose and rate of infusion should be reduced by one-half and adjusted slowly as needed and tolerated. In addition, elderly patients are more likely to have age-related renal function impairment, which may require dosage adjustment.

### Drug interactions and/or related problems

The following drug interactions and/or related problems have been selected on the basis of their potential clinical significance (possible mechanism in parentheses where appropriate)—not necessarily inclusive (» = major clinical significance):

Note: Combinations containing any of the following medications, depending on the amount present, may also interact with this medication.

Antiarrhythmics, other
(although some antiarrhythmic agents may be used in combination for therapeutic advantage, combined use may sometimes potentiate risk of adverse cardiac effects)

» Anticonvulsants, hydantoin
(concurrent use with lidocaine may have additive cardiac depressant effects; hydantoin anticonvulsants may also promote increased hepatic metabolism of lidocaine and thus reduce its intravenous concentration)

Beta-adrenergic blocking agents, systemic and ophthalmic (if systemic absorption occurs)
(concurrent use may slow hepatic metabolism and increase the risk of toxicity of lidocaine because of reduced hepatic blood flow)

Cimetidine
(concurrent administration with lidocaine may result in reduced hepatic clearance of lidocaine, possibly resulting in delayed elimination and increased blood concentrations; monitoring of blood concentrations and clinical parameters as a guide to dosage is recommended)

Neuromuscular blocking agents
(effects may be potentiated when used concurrently with large doses [such as those over 5 mg per kg] of intravenous lidocaine)

### Laboratory value alterations

The following have been selected on the basis of their potential clinical significance (possible effect in parentheses where appropriate)—not necessarily inclusive (» = major clinical significance):

With diagnostic test results
Bentiromide
(concurrent administration of lidocaine during a bentiromide test period will invalidate test results since lidocaine is also metabolized to arylamines and will thus increase the percent of PABA recovered; discontinuation of lidocaine at least 3 days prior to the administration of bentiromide is recommended)

With physiology/laboratory test values
Creatine kinase (CK)
(serum concentration may be increased by intramuscular administration of lidocaine; serum concentration of this enzyme without isoenzyme separation is an unreliable diagnostic test for acute myocardial infarction)

## Medical considerations/Contraindications

The medical considerations/contraindications included here have been selected on the basis of their potential clinical significance (reasons given in parentheses where appropriate)—not necessarily inclusive (» = major clinical significance).

*Except under special circumstances, this medication should not be used when the following medical problems exist:*

» Adams-Stokes syndrome or
» Severe heart block, including atrioventricular, intraventricular, or sinoatrial blocks
    (heart block may be worsened)

*Risk-benefit should be considered when the following medical problems exist:*

» Congestive heart failure or
    Hepatic function impairment or
» Reduced hepatic blood flow or
    Renal function impairment
    (accumulation may occur; dose and rate of infusion should be reduced by one-half)

» Hypovolemia and shock or
» Incomplete heart block or
» Sinus bradycardia or
» Wolff-Parkinson-White syndrome
    (may be aggravated)
    Sensitivity to lidocaine

## Patient monitoring

The following may be especially important in patient monitoring (other tests may be warranted in some patients, depending on condition; » = major clinical significance):

Blood pressure determinations and
» Electrocardiograph (ECG) determinations
    (recommended throughout therapy to help adjust dosage and detect toxicity; intravenous infusion of lidocaine should be promptly discontinued if ECG determinations show a prolonged PR interval and QRS complex or if arrhythmias occur or become worse)

Electrolyte concentrations, serum
    (periodic to allow imbalance corrections during prolonged infusions)

Lidocaine concentrations, serum
    (useful to avoid toxicity during prolonged or high-dose infusions or in patients receiving drugs that alter lidocaine clearance)

## Side/Adverse Effects

Note: Adverse effects are dose- and age-related; incidence is increased in patients over 65 years of age.

Adverse cardiovascular effects at therapeutic doses are rare, except in patients with existing compromised ventricular function. Cardiac conduction disturbances are extremely rare. High plasma lidocaine concentrations may lead to hypotension, arrhythmias, heart block, and respiratory and cardiac arrest.

The following side/adverse effects have been selected on the basis of their potential clinical significance (possible signs and symptoms in parentheses where appropriate)—not necessarily inclusive:

**Those indicating need for medical attention**
Incidence rare
    *Allergic reaction* (difficulty in breathing; itching; skin rash; swelling of skin)

**Those indicating need for medical attention only if they continue or are bothersome**
Incidence less frequent or rare
    *Pain at site of injection*—with intramuscular or prolonged intravenous use

Incidence dose-related
    *With serum lidocaine concentrations of 1.5 to 6 mcg/mL*
        *Anxiety or nervousness; dizziness; drowsiness; feelings of coldness, heat, or numbness*

## Overdose

For more information on the management of overdose or unintentional ingestion, **contact a Poison Control Center** (see *Poison Control Center Listing*).

## Clinical effects of overdose

The following effects have been selected on the basis of their potential clinical significance (possible signs and symptoms in parentheses where appropriate)—not necessarily inclusive:

With serum lidocaine concentrations of 6 to 8 mcg/mL
    *Blurred or double vision; nausea or vomiting; ringing in ears; tremors or twitching*

With serum lidocaine concentrations of >8 mcg/mL
    *Difficulty in breathing; dizziness, severe, or fainting; seizures; slow heartbeat*

## Treatment of overdose (for severe reactions)

Stopping administration of lidocaine; monitoring patient closely.
Maintenance of airway and administration of oxygen.
    Specific treatment—
        For circulatory depression—Administration of a vasopressor (such as ephedrine or metaraminol) and intravenous fluids if necessary.
        For seizures—If no satisfactory response to respiratory support is obtained, diazepam in 2.5-mg increments, or an ultra-short-acting barbiturate (such as thiopental or thiamylal) in 50- to 100-mg increments, is often beneficial. Caution must be maintained because of possible additive circulatory depression. If patient is under anesthesia, a short-acting muscle relaxant (such as succinylcholine) administered intravenously is sometimes helpful. When such relaxants are used, artificial respiration capability is mandatory.

# Patient Consultation

As an aid to patient consultation, refer to *Advice for the Patient, Lidocaine—for Self-Injection (Systemic)*.

In providing consultation, consider emphasizing the following selected information (» = major clinical significance):

**Before using this medication**
» Conditions affecting use, especially:
    Sensitivity to lidocaine, other amide-type anesthetics, or flecainide or tocainide
    Pregnancy—May reduce blood supply to fetus
    Use in the elderly—Increased sensitivity to effects
    Other medications, especially hydantoin anticonvulsants
    Other medical problems, especially congestive heart failure or other heart problems or hepatic function impairment

**Proper use of this medication**
    Making sure medication is easily accessible and not outdated
» Telephoning physician immediately if symptoms of heart attack occur
» Reading patient directions carefully before medication is needed, to become familiar with procedure
    Proper administration:
    Removing the safety cap
    Placing black end on thickest part of thigh and pressing hard; feeling needle prick
    Holding in place 10 seconds, then massaging area for 10 seconds
» Proper dosing
» Proper storage

**Precautions while using this medication**
» Not administering unless specifically instructed by physician
» Not driving after administering medication unless absolutely necessary

**Side/adverse effects**
    Signs of potential side effects, especially allergic reaction

# General Dosing Information

See also *Patient monitoring*.

Dosage should be adjusted to meet the individual requirements of each patient, on the basis of clinical response.

The use of lidocaine necessitates concurrent ECG monitoring and the availability of oxygen, resuscitative equipment, and emergency medications for management of possible adverse reactions involving the cardiovascular system and/or central nervous system (CNS) and/or those of an allergic nature.

**For intramuscular administration**

Intramuscular injection of lidocaine is recommended only when ECG monitoring equipment is not available and the physician believes the benefits outweigh the risks, when used by paramedical personnel in a mobile coronary care unit under a physician's direction, or when used by specially selected and trained patients under a physician's direction.

Intramuscular injections of lidocaine are preferably administered in the deltoid muscle, which provides more rapid and complete systemic availability of the medication than do other large muscle tissues. The thigh muscle is used for the self-injection dosage form for ease of administration.

To avoid possible intravascular injection, frequent aspirations should be made during intramuscular injection (except with the self-injection dosage form).

**For intravenous administration**

Lidocaine for intravenous administration must *not* contain preservatives or other medications such as epinephrine.

The preferred diluent for lidocaine infusion is 5% dextrose injection.

Lidocaine must *not* be added to blood transfusions.

To achieve optimal control of lidocaine dosage and rate of administration, it is recommended that lidocaine be administered intravenously by means of an infusion pump, a micro-drip regulator, or a similar device that allows precise adjustment of the flow rate.

A loading dose of lidocaine is commonly administered for the initial intravenous dose to partially compensate for its rapid perfusion and distribution, which tend to delay attainment of a therapeutic serum concentration. If the initial loading dose does not provide the desired effect within 5 minutes, a second loading dose reduced to one-half to one-third of the first dose may be given.

Dosage reduction may be required with prolonged intravenous infusions (longer than 24 hours) because of the risk of accumulation.

## Parenteral Dosage Forms

### LIDOCAINE HYDROCHLORIDE INJECTION (FOR CONTINUOUS INTRAVENOUS INFUSION) USP

**Usual adult dose**

Antiarrhythmic—

Continuous intravenous infusion (usually following a loading dose), 20 to 50 mcg (0.02 to 0.05 mg) per kg of body weight at a rate of 1 to 4 mg per minute.

Note: Geriatric patients may be more sensitive to the effects of the usual adult dose.

**Usual adult prescribing limits**

Up to 300 mg (about 4.5 mg per kg of body weight) in any one-hour period.

**Usual pediatric dose**

Antiarrhythmic—

Continuous intravenous infusion (usually following a loading dose), 30 mcg (range, 20 to 50 mcg) (0.03 mg; range, 0.02 to 0.05 mg) per kg of body weight per minute.

**Strength(s) usually available**

U.S.—

4% w/v (40 mg per mL [1 gram per 25 mL or 2 grams per 50 mL]) (Rx) [*Xylocaine* (preservative-free); GENERIC (may contain methylparaben)].

10% w/v (100 mg per mL [1 gram per 10 mL]) (Rx) [GENERIC (may contain methylparaben)].

20% w/v (200 mg per mL [1 gram per 5 mL or 2 grams per 10 mL]) (Rx) [*Xylocaine* (preservative-free); GENERIC (may contain methylparaben)].

Canada—

2% (20 mg per mL [1 gram per 50 mL]) (Rx) [*Xylocard*].

20% (200 mg per mL [1 gram per 5 mL]) (Rx) [*Xylocard*].

**Packaging and storage**

Store below 40 °C (104 °F), preferably between 15 and 30 °C (59 and 86 °F), unless otherwise specified by manufacturer. Protect from freezing.

**Preparation of dosage form**

To prepare solution for intravenous infusion, add 1 gram of lidocaine hydrochloride (25 mL of 4% or 5 mL of 20% Lidocaine Hydrochloride Injection USP) to 1 liter of 5% dextrose injection; the resultant concentration will be 1 mg per mL. Check manufacturer's package insert for additional dilution information.

**Stability**

After dilution in the appropriate intravenous solution for infusion, lidocaine hydrochloride is stable for at least 24 hours.

**Auxiliary labeling**

Following dilution, a label stating the concentration of the lidocaine hydrochloride contents with time and date of dilution should be placed on the infusion solution container.

### LIDOCAINE HYDROCHLORIDE INJECTION (FOR DIRECT INTRAVENOUS INJECTION) USP

**Usual adult dose**

Antiarrhythmic—

Direct intravenous injection, 1 mg per kg of body weight (usually 50 to 100 mg) as a loading dose at a rate of about 25 to 50 mg per minute, the dose being repeated after five minutes if necessary; usually followed by continuous intravenous infusion of lidocaine to maintain antiarrhythmic effects.

Note: Geriatric patients may be more sensitive to the effects of the usual adult dose.

**Usual adult prescribing limits**

Up to 300 mg (about 4.5 mg per kg of body weight) in any one-hour period.

**Usual pediatric dose**

Antiarrhythmic—

Direct intravenous injection, 1 mg per kg of body weight as a loading dose at a rate of about 25 to 50 mg per minute, the dose being repeated after five minutes if necessary but not exceeding a total dose of 3 mg per kg; usually followed by continuous intravenous infusion of lidocaine to maintain antiarrhythmic effects.

**Strength(s) usually available**

U.S.—

1% w/v (10 mg per mL [50 mg per 5 mL or 100 mg per 10 mL]) (Rx) [*Xylocaine* (preservative-free); GENERIC (may contain methylparaben)].

2% w/v (20 mg per mL [100 mg per 5 mL]) (Rx) [*Xylocaine* (preservative-free); GENERIC (may contain methylparaben)].

Canada—

2% w/v (20 mg per mL [100 mg per 5 mL]) (Rx) [*Xylocard*; GENERIC].

**Packaging and storage**

Store below 40 °C (104 °F), preferably between 15 and 30 °C (59 and 86 °F), unless otherwise specified by manufacturer. Protect from freezing.

**Stability**

When dilution is required, it should be done immediately prior to direct intravenous administration.

### LIDOCAINE HYDROCHLORIDE INJECTION (FOR INTRAMUSCULAR INJECTION) USP

**Usual adult dose**

Antiarrhythmic—

Intramuscular, 4.3 mg per kg of body weight (approximately 300 mg for a 70-kg adult), the dosage being repeated after sixty to ninety minutes if necessary.

Note: Geriatric patients may be more sensitive to the effects of the usual adult dose.

**Usual adult prescribing limits**

Up to 300 mg (about 4.5 mg per kg of body weight) in any one-hour period.

Note: A single dose of 300 mg may be administered by a patient using the self-injection dosage form.

**Usual pediatric dose**

Dosage has not been established.

Note: Use of the self-injection dosage form is not recommended in children weighing less than 50 kg.

**Strength(s) usually available**

U.S.—

10% w/v (100 mg per mL [300 mg per self-injection dosage form]) (Rx) [*LidoPen* (methylparaben; disodium edetate); *Xylocaine* (preservative-free)].

Canada—

Not commercially available.

**Packaging and storage**

Store below 40 °C (104 °F), preferably between 15 and 30 °C (59 and 86 °F), unless otherwise specified by manufacturer. Protect from freezing.

**Stability**

When dilution is required, it should be done immediately prior to intramuscular administration.

**Note**

When dispensing for self-administration by the patient, make sure that patient instructions are included and that the patient understands how to prepare and administer the injection, including proper use of disposable syringes.

## STERILE LIDOCAINE HYDROCHLORIDE USP

**Usual adult dose**
Antiarrhythmic—
Continuous intravenous infusion (usually following a loading dose), 20 to 50 mcg (0.02 to 0.05 mg) per kg of body weight at a rate of 1 to 4 mg per minute.

Note: Geriatric patients may be more sensitive to the effects of the usual adult dose.

**Usual adult prescribing limits**
Up to 300 mg (about 4.5 mg per kg of body weight) in any one-hour period.

**Usual pediatric dose**
Antiarrhythmic—
Continuous intravenous infusion (usually following a loading dose), 30 mcg (0.03 mg) (range, 20 to 50 mcg) per kg of body weight per minute.

**Size(s) usually available**
U.S.—
1 gram (Rx) [GENERIC].
2 grams (Rx) [GENERIC].
Canada—
Not commercially available.

**Packaging and storage**
Store below 40 °C (104 °F), preferably between 15 and 30 °C (59 and 86 °F), unless otherwise specified by manufacturer.

**Preparation of dosage form**
Sterile Lidocaine Hydrochloride USP is prepared for continuous intravenous infusion by adding 1 or 2 grams to 1000 mL of 5% dextrose injection, producing a solution containing 1 or 2 mg of lidocaine hydrochloride per mL, respectively. Check manufacturer's package insert for additional dilution information.

**Stability**
After dilution in the appropriate intravenous solution for infusion, lidocaine hydrochloride is stable for at least 24 hours.

**Auxiliary labeling**
Following dilution, a label stating the concentration of the lidocaine hydrochloride contents with time and date of dilution should be placed on the infusion solution container.

## LIDOCAINE HYDROCHLORIDE AND DEXTROSE INJECTION (FOR CONTINUOUS INTRAVENOUS INFUSION) USP

**Usual adult dose**
Antiarrhythmic—
Continuous intravenous infusion (usually following a loading dose), 20 to 50 mcg (0.02 to 0.05 mg) of lidocaine hydrochloride per kg of body weight at a rate of 1 to 4 mg per minute.

Note: Geriatric patients may be more sensitive to the effects of the usual adult dose.

**Usual adult prescribing limits**
Up to 300 mg (about 4.5 mg per kg of body weight) in any one-hour period.

**Usual pediatric dose**
Antiarrhythmic—
Continuous intravenous infusion (usually following a loading dose), 30 mcg (range, 20 to 50 mcg) (0.03 mg; range, 0.02 to 0.05 mg) of lidocaine hydrochloride per kg of body weight per minute at a rate of 1 to 4 mg per minute.

**Strength(s) usually available**
U.S.—
Lidocaine Hydrochloride
0.1% w/v (1 mg per mL [250 mg per 250 mL, 500 mg per 500 mL, or 1 gram per 1000 mL]) (Rx) [GENERIC].
0.2% w/v (2 mg per mL [500 mg per 250 mL, 1 gram per 500 mL or 2 grams per 1000 mL]) (Rx) [GENERIC].
0.4% w/v (4 mg per mL [1 gram per 250 mL, 2 grams per 500 mL, or 4 grams per 1000 mL]) (Rx) [GENERIC].
0.8% w/v (8 mg per mL [2 grams per 250 mL, 4 grams per 500 mL, 8 grams per 1000 mL]) (Rx) [GENERIC].
Canada—
Lidocaine Hydrochloride
0.1% w/v (1 mg per mL [250 mg per 250 mL, 500 mg per 500 mL, or 1 gram per 1000 mL]) (Rx) [GENERIC].
0.2% w/v (2 mg per mL [500 mg per 250 mL, 1 gram per 500 mL, or 2 grams per 1000 mL]) (Rx) [GENERIC].
0.4% w/v (4 mg per mL [1 gram per 250 mL, 2 grams per 500 mL, or 4 grams per 1000 mL]) (Rx) [GENERIC].
0.8% w/v (8 mg per mL [2 grams per 250 mL or 4 grams per 500 mL]) (Rx) [GENERIC].

**Packaging and storage**
Store below 40 °C (104 °F), preferably between 15 and 30 °C (59 and 86 °F), unless otherwise specified by manufacturer. Protect from freezing.

## Selected Bibliography

Anderson JL. Current understanding of lidocaine as an antiarrhythmic agent: a review. Clin Ther 1984; 1986 (2): 125-44.
Harrison DC. Current classification of antiarrhythmic drugs as a guide to their rational clinical use. Drugs 1986; 31: 93-5.
Perry RS, Illsky SS. Basic cardiac electrophysiology and mechanisms of antiarrhythmic agents. Am J Hosp Pharm 1986 Apr; 43: 957-74.

Revised: 10/21/92
Interim revision: 10/27/93

## LIDOCAINE-CONTAINING COMBINATIONS—

Lidocaine and Epinephrine (Parenteral-Local)—See *Anesthetics (Parenteral-Local)*
Lidocaine and Prilocaine (Topical)

# LIDOCAINE AND PRILOCAINE    Topical

BAN: Lidocaine—Lignocaine
VA CLASSIFICATION (Primary): DE700
Another commonly used name for lidocaine is lignocaine.

Note: For a listing of dosage forms and brand names by country availability, see *Dosage Forms* section(s). For a listing of brand names for the articles in this monograph, refer to the General Index.

## Category
Anesthetic, local.

## Indications

Note: Bracketed information in the *Indications* section refers to uses that are not included in U.S. product labeling.

**Accepted**
Anesthesia, local—Indicated for application to normal, intact skin, to provide topical anesthesia prior to procedures such as insertion of an intravascular cannula, venipuncture or other needle insertion; skin graft harvesting; minor dermal procedures, such as laser treatment of port-wine stains and removal of mollusca, warts, or tattoos; lumbar puncture; and diathermy.

[This topical anesthetic is also applied to the genital mucosa, to provide anesthesia for surgical removal of localized lesions (e.g., removal of condolymata via carbon dioxide laser or thermocautery). It is used for this purpose only in adults; application to the mucosa of children is *not* recommended.][1]

**Unaccepted**
Application of this medication to mucous membranes other than the genital mucosa of adults, especially application to the gums or other oral mucosa, is not recommended.

[1]Not included in Canadian product labeling.

## Pharmacology/Pharmacokinetics

Note: Information reported below on various pharmacokinetic parameters and on the onset of action, time to peak effect, and duration of action after application to the skin was obtained in studies in Caucasians. Preliminary evidence from a study in a limited number of subjects indicates that the rate and extent of absorption are decreased, the onset of action and time to peak effect are increased, and the overall efficacy of the medication is reduced, after application to black skin.

## Physicochemical characteristics

Chemical group—Both lidocaine and prilocaine are amide-type local anesthetics.

Molecular weight—
Lidocaine: 234.34.
Prilocaine: 220.31.

Octanol-to-aqueous buffer solution (pH 7.4) partition ratio—
Lidocaine: 43
Prilocaine: 25

## Mechanism of action/Effect

Local anesthetics block both the initiation and conduction of nerve impulses by decreasing the neuronal membrane's permeability to sodium ions. This reversibly stabilizes the membrane and inhibits depolarization, resulting in the failure of a propagated action potential and subsequent conduction blockade.

The base (nonionized) form of a local anesthetic is able to diffuse across neuronal membranes to produce local anesthesia much more readily than a salt (ionized) form of the agent. However, penetration through intact skin of effective concentrations of the highly lipophilic base form of an anesthetic is generally not achieved after application of topical formulations that contain single anesthetics. This lidocaine- and prilocaine-containing formulation is an oil-in-water emulsion in which the oil phase is a eutectic mixture formed by combining equal parts by weight of lidocaine and prilocaine bases. Because the eutectic mixture is a liquid, the anesthetics need not be dissolved in oil before being incorporated into the water phase of the formulation; this increases the concentration of active substance in droplets of the emulsion and permits larger quantities of anesthetic to penetrate to the nerve endings in deeper skin layers.

The depth at which anesthesia is present after application to intact, healthy skin, as determined by needle insertion, increases with the length of time that the medication remains on the skin, about 3 mm after a 60-minute application, 4 mm after a 90-minute application, and 5 mm after a 120-minute application. However, when the medication remains on the skin for less than 120 minutes, the depth at which anesthesia is present may continue to increase for an additional 30 to 60 minutes after the anesthetic is removed, depending on the location at which the medication is applied.

## Other actions/effects

This medication may produce vascular responses, i.e., vasoconstriction (manifested by blanching of the skin) and/or vasodilatation (manifested by erythema). In a study in which the medication was applied to normal skin, maximal blanching occurred after a 90-minute application, and erythema occurred only after a much longer application time (more than 3 hours). In another study in a limited number of patients, a product twice as strong as the formulation now commercially available in the U.S. and Canada produced vascular responses much more rapidly in skin affected by atopic dermatitis or eczema than in normal skin. In patients with atopic dermatitis or eczema, blanching and erythema occurred after application times of only 5 to 15 minutes and 30 to 60 minutes, respectively, whereas in individuals with normal skin, blanching and erythema occurred after application times of 30 to 60 minutes and 2 to 4 hours, respectively.

## Absorption

Application to the skin—The rate and extent of systemic absorption are dependent on the the thickness of the skin and the size of the area to which the medication is applied as well as the duration of application. In general, mean absorption rates in children and adults are $45 \pm 16$ mcg per square centimeter of skin area (mcg/cm$^2$) per hour and $77 \pm 36$ mcg/cm$^2$ per hour for lidocaine and prilocaine, respectively. Absorption may be increased when the formulation is applied to broken or inflamed skin or to areas 2000 cm$^2$ or larger in size. Also, absorption is more rapid when the cream is applied to the skin of patients with atopic dermatitis and generalized eczema or other patients with damaged or thin skin.

Application to genital mucosa—The rate and extent of absorption are significantly greater than after application to normal, intact skin.

## Distribution

Both lidocaine and prilocaine cross the blood-brain barrier and the placenta.

Note: The mean volumes of distribution at steady state, determined after intravenous administration, are $1.5 \pm 0.3$ liters per kg of body weight (L/kg) for lidocaine and $2.6 \pm 1.3$ L/kg for prilocaine.

## Protein binding

Lidocaine—High (70%), primarily to alpha-1-acid glycoprotein, at plasma concentrations produced by application of this topical formulation. At much higher concentrations ($> 1$ mcg per mL [mcg/mL] [4.3 micromoles/L]), binding is dependent on the concentration.

Prilocaine—Moderate (40%)

## Biotransformation

Lidocaine—Hepatic; rapid. One metabolite is active, but a less potent local anesthetic than the parent compound; another metabolite has no local anesthetic activity, but may be more toxic than lidocaine itself. Whether metabolism occurs in the skin after topical application has not been determined.

Prilocaine—Hepatic, by amidases; metabolism in renal tissues has also been demonstrated *in vitro*. One or more of the metabolic products is toxic (causing methemoglobinemia). Whether metabolism occurs in the skin after topical application has not been determined.

## Half-life

Elimination (mean values)—
Lidocaine—$110 \pm 24$ minutes (determined after intravenous administration of lidocaine hydrochloride); may be increased in patients with cardiac or hepatic function impairment.
Prilocaine—$70 \pm 48$ minutes; may be increased in patients with hepatic or renal function impairment.

## Onset of action

Application to the skin—Dependent on the epidermal and dermal thickness at the location to which the medication is applied; about 1 hour after application to intact skin, but much more rapid (less than 15 minutes) after application to skin areas affected by atopic dermatitis or eczema.

## Time to peak serum concentration

Application to normal, intact skin—Dependent on the area to which the medication is applied and subject to interpatient variability; about 4 hours (range, 2 to 6 hours) when 60 grams is applied to a 400-cm$^2$ area of the thigh and allowed to remain, under an occlusive dressing, for 3 hours and 1.5 to 3 hours when 10 grams is applied to a 100-cm$^2$ area of the face and allowed to remain for 2 hours.

## Peak serum concentration

Application to intact skin—
Lidocaine: The highest concentration measured after application of about 150 grams of the lidocaine and prilocaine formulation to up to 1300 cm$^2$ of intact skin for up to 3 hours is 1.1 mcg/mL (4.73 micromoles/L).
Prilocaine: The highest concentration measured after application of about 150 grams of the lidocaine and prilocaine formulation to up to 1300 cm$^2$ of intact skin for up to 3 hours is 0.2 mcg/mL (0.87 micromoles/L).

Note: The total quantity of prilocaine absorbed over a given time is greater than that of lidocaine, even though equal quantities of each are present in the formulation. However, prilocaine's larger volume of distribution and more rapid clearance result in lower plasma concentrations.

## Time to peak effect

Application to intact skin—About 2 to 3 hours. In general, 1 hour of application under occlusion produces sufficient anesthesia for procedures such as intravascular catheter placement or venipuncture; 2 hours of application under occlusion produces sufficient anesthesia for procedures such as split skin graft harvesting. However, one study showed that 2 hours of application under occlusion may be required to provide sufficient anesthesia for venipuncture in children with black skin.

Application to genital mucosa—Sufficient anesthesia for removal of localized lesions occurs about 5 to 7 minutes after application; efficacy begins to decrease as soon as 10 to 15 minutes after application.

## Duration of action

Application to intact skin—Effective anesthesia following a 1- or 2-hour application generally persists for an additional 1 or 2 hours after the medication is removed. However, the duration of anesthesia is dependent on the blood flow in the underlying tissue; efficacy may decline more rapidly in highly perfused areas, such as the face. One study demonstrated that a relatively short duration follows a rapid onset and a more prolonged duration follows a delayed onset.

## Elimination

Lidocaine—More than 98% of the quantity absorbed is eliminated in the urine; less than 3% as unchanged lidocaine and the remainder as metabolites. Mean systemic clearance is $13 \pm 3$ mL per minute per kg of body weight (mL/min/kg).

Prilocaine—Renal; less than 3% as unchanged prilocaine. Mean systemic clearance is $38 \pm 15$ mL/min/kg.

# Precautions to Consider

Note: In the animal studies reported in the *Carcinogenicity*, *Mutagenicity*, and *Pregnancy/Reproduction* sections below, the doses administered to, or blood concentrations achieved in, the animals are compared to the equivalent in humans of a Single Dermal Administration (SDA), defined as a single application of 60 grams of the local anesthetic formulation over 400 square centimeters ($cm^2$) of the skin area of a 50-kg person for 3 hours.

**Cross-sensitivity and/or related problems**
Patients sensitive to other amide-type local anesthetics may rarely be sensitive to lidocaine and/or prilocaine also.

**Carcinogenicity**
*Lidocaine—*
   A 2-year study showed the metabolite 2,6-xylidine to be carcinogenic, causing carcinomas, adenomas, and rhabdomyosarcomas in the nasal cavities of both male and female rats; subcutaneous fibromas and/or fibrosarcomas in both male and female rats; and neoplastic nodules of the liver in female rats when given in daily oral doses of 150 mg per kg of body weight (mg/kg) per day (900 mg per square meter of body surface area [mg/m$^2$] [60 times the SDA] per day). Statistically significant increases in nasal carcinomas and/or adenomas in male and female rats did not occur with oral doses of 50 mg/kg per day (300 mg/m$^2$ [30 times the SDA] per day), and no nasal tumors occurred with oral doses of 15 mg/kg per day (90 mg/m$^2$ [6 times the SDA] per day).

*Prilocaine—*
   The metabolite ortho-toluidine, given chronically to mice in oral doses of 150 to 2400 mg/kg per day (900 to 14,400 mg/m$^2$ [60 to 90 times the SDA] per day) or to rats in oral doses of 150 to 800 mg/kg per day (900 to 4800 mg/m$^2$ [60 to 320 times the SDA] per day), was carcinogenic in both species at all dosage levels tested. Tumors included hepatocarcinomas and adenomas in female mice; hemangiosarcomas and hemangiomas in male and female mice; sarcomas of multiple organs and transitional-cell carcinomas and papillomas of the urinary bladder in both sexes of rats; subcutaneous fibromas, fibrosarcomas, and mesotheliomas in male rats; and mammary gland fibroadenomas and adenomas in female rats.

**Mutagenicity**
*Lidocaine—*
   No evidence of mutagenicity was shown with lidocaine hydrochloride in the Ames *Salmonella*/mammalian microsome test or analysis of structural chromosome aberrations in human lymphocytes *in vitro*, or in the mouse micronucleus test *in vivo*. The metabolite 2,6-xylidine was weakly mutagenic in the Ames test only under metabolic activation conditions. The metabolite was also mutagenic at the thymidine kinase locus, with or without activation, and induced chromosome aberrations and sister chromatid exchanges at concentrations at which the substance precipitated out of solution (1.2 mg/mL). No evidence of genotoxicity was found in the *in vivo* assays measuring unscheduled DNA synthesis in rat hepatocytes, chromosome damage in polychromatic erythrocytes, or preferential killing of DNA repair-deficient bacteria in liver, lung, kidney, testes, and blood extracts from mice. However, covalent binding studies of DNA from liver and ethmoid turbinates in rats indicate that the metabolite may be genotoxic under certain conditions *in vivo*.

*Prilocaine—*
   The metabolite ortho-toluidine produced positive results in *Escherichia coli* DNA repair and phage-induction assays in a concentration of 0.5 mcg/mL. Urine concentrates from rats given the metabolite (300 mg/kg orally [300 times the SDA]) were mutagenic for *Salmonella typhimurium* with metabolic activation. Several other tests on the metabolite, including reverse mutations in five different *Salmonella typhimurium* strains with or without activation and with single strand breaks in DNA of V79 Chinese hamster cells, were negative.

**Pregnancy/Reproduction**
Fertility—
   *Prilocaine—*
      Studies in rats given 300 mg/kg intramuscularly as the hydrochloride salt (188 times the SDA) have not shown evidence of impaired fertility.

Pregnancy—
   *Lidocaine and prilocaine mixture—*
      Adequate and well-controlled studies have not been done in humans.
      Studies in rats given subcutaneous injections of an aqueous mixture of the hydrochloride salts of lidocaine and prilocaine (40 mg/kg of each [equivalent to 29 times the SDA for lidocaine and 25 times the SDA for prilocaine] per day) have not shown evidence of teratogenicity, embryotoxicity, or fetotoxicity. Also, studies in rats with the individual anesthetics (30 mg/kg subcutaneously [22 times the SDA] of lidocaine hydrochloride

or 300 mg/kg intramuscularly [188 times the SDA] of prilocaine hydrochloride) have not shown evidence of harm to the fetus.

FDA Pregnancy Category B.

**Breast-feeding**
Lidocaine is, and prilocaine probably is, distributed into breast milk in small quantities. The risk of adverse effects in nursing infants is considered to be minimal.

**Pediatrics**
*Infants up to 3 months of age—*
   Use in this age group is not recommended because of the especially high risk of methemoglobinemia.
*Older infants and children—*
   **Application to the mucosa of pediatric patients is not recommended.**
   Methemoglobin concentrations are increased in infants and children after application of this medication. Although the concentrations generally do not reach clinically significant levels, overt methemoglobinemia developed after use of the anesthetic mixture in a 3-month-old infant who was also receiving other medication known to cause methemoglobinemia. It is recommended that the anesthetic formulation not be used for infants up to 12 months of age who are receiving such medications. Also, a study in children 1 to 6 years of age found that methemoglobin concentrations remain elevated for 24 hours after a 2-hour application of 5 grams of the medication. The possibility of cumulative effects on methemoglobin concentrations should be considered if the medication is needed on a daily basis.
   Studies have shown that, because of fearfulness in children younger than 7 years of age, this medication provides less overall benefit (as determined by reaction to needle insertion) to these patients than it does to older children and adults. Use of this product does not eliminate the need for emotional and psychological support for young children who are undergoing medical or surgical procedures.

**Geriatrics**
No information is available on the relationship of age to the effects of this lidocaine and prilocaine topical formulation in geriatric patients. However, experience with other local anesthetic formulations has shown that geriatric patients are more likely than younger adults to develop local anesthetic–induced systemic toxicity after the medications are administered by injection or applied to mucous membranes.

**Drug interactions and/or related problems**
The following drug interactions and/or related problems have been selected on the basis of their potential clinical significance (possible mechanism in parentheses where appropriate)—not necessarily inclusive (» = major clinical significance):

Note: Combinations containing any of the following medications, depending on the amount present, may also interact with this medication.

Anesthetics, general
   (symptoms of local anesthetic–induced CNS toxicity, which may occur if excessive quantities of the medication are absorbed, may be masked if the local anesthetic is used in conjunction with a general anesthetic)

Anesthetics, local, other or
Structurally related medications, such as mexiletine or tocainide
   (the risk of systemic toxicity may be increased, especially if large quantities of the lidocaine and prilocaine topical formulation are used concurrently with any of these medications)

Methemoglobinemia-inducing medications, other, especially:
Acetaminophen, chronic use of
Chloroquine
Dapsone
Nitrates or nitrites, including nitrofurantoin, nitroglycerin, and nitroprusside
Para-aminosalicylic acid
Phenacetin—not commercially available in the U.S. or Canada
Phenobarbital
Phenytoin
Primaquine
» Sulfonamides, including mafenide
   (concurrent use with the lidocaine and prilocaine topical formulation may increase the risk of overt methemoglobinemia, especially in infants; concurrent use in infants younger than 12 months of age is not recommended)

**Laboratory value alterations**

The following have been selected on the basis of their potential clinical significance (possible effect in parentheses where appropriate)—not necessarily inclusive (» = major clinical significance):

With diagnostic test results

Skin tests, intradermal or epicutaneous

(application of the lidocaine- and prilocaine-containing topical anesthetic prior to skin testing may reduce flare induced by injection of histamine [often used as a positive control for these tests]; false-negative interpretation of weakly positive tests may result)

**Medical considerations/Contraindications**

The medical considerations/contraindications included here have been selected on the basis of their potential clinical significance (reasons given in parentheses where appropriate)—not necessarily inclusive (» = major clinical significance).

*Risk-benefit should be considered when the following medical problems exist:*

» Any situation in which absorption may be increased, such as:

Application to open wounds, burns, or broken or inflamed skin or

Atopic dermatitis or

Eczema

(the rate and extent of anesthetic absorption may be increased, leading to a higher risk of systemic toxicity; application to open wounds is not recommended)

(in burn patients, the presence of a pre-existing hemoglobin abnormality [carboxyhemoglobin] may also increase the risk of systemic toxicity)

(a study in a limited number of patients has shown that, after the medication is applied to skin affected by atopic dermatitis or eczema, the onset of action is more rapid than after application to healthy skin; a shorter application time may be appropriate for patients with these conditions, but additional clinical experience is needed before guidelines for use in these patients can be established)

Connective tissue disease, Ehlers Danlos Type III

(a study in a limited number of patients has shown that the topical lidocaine and prilocaine formulation does not provide adequate anesthesia in individuals with this condition)

» Glucose-6-phosphate dehydrogenase (G6PD) deficiency or other predisposition to methemoglobinemia or

» Methemoglobinemia, congenital or idiopathic

(medication may induce, or exacerbate pre-existing, methemoglobinemia)

Hepatic function impairment, severe

(capacity for metabolizing the anesthetics is reduced, which increases the risk of systemic effects)

» Sensitivity to lidocaine, prilocaine, or other amide-type local anesthetics, history of

(increased risk of allergic reaction)

Caution is also recommended in geriatric, acutely ill, or debilitated patients, who may be predisposed to local anesthetic–induced systemic toxicity

## Side/Adverse Effects

Note: Like other local anesthetics, lidocaine and prilocaine (individually) have rarely caused allergic and anaphylactoid reactions, including angioedema, bronchospasm, urticaria, and shock.

Systemic effects are unlikely when recommended guidelines for use of this medication are followed, but central nervous system (CNS) toxicity and/or cardiovascular depression may occur if sufficiently high plasma concentrations of the anesthetics are produced. Early signs of cardiovascular depression include bradycardia and hypotension. If treatment is not initiated promptly, decreases in cardiac output, total peripheral resistance, and mean arterial pressure may occur and may progress to hypoxia, acidosis, heart block, and cardiac arrest.

CNS toxicity induced by local anesthetics consists of CNS stimulation and/or CNS depression. CNS stimulation (signs and symptoms may include apprehension, nervousness, or euphoria; confusion; dizziness, light-headedness, or drowsiness; blurred or double vision; nausea and vomiting; ringing or buzzing in the ears; sensations of heat, cold, or numbness; and twitching, tremors, or convulsions) often occurs first, followed by CNS depression, characterized by drowsiness, unconsciousness, and respiratory depression and arrest. However, CNS excitation may be transient or absent, so that drowsiness may be the first sign of CNS toxicity in some patients, especially children.

The following side/adverse effects have been selected on the basis of their potential clinical significance (possible signs and symptoms in parentheses where appropriate)—not necessarily inclusive:

**Those indicating need for medical attention**

Incidence rare

*Methemoglobinemia* (blue or blue-purple color of lips, fingernails, or skin; fatigue; weakness; breathing problems; rapid heartbeat; headache; dizziness; collapse; altered mental status; dark urine)

Note: If *methemoglobinemia* is relatively mild, cyanosis may be the only sign. The other signs and symptoms occur when *methemoglobinemia* is severe and/or the patient cannot tolerate the reduced oxygen-carrying capacity of the blood.

**Those indicating need for medical attention only if they continue or are bothersome**

Incidence more frequent

*Localized skin reactions* (burning feeling, swelling, itching, or skin rash at place of application); *vasoconstriction* (very white skin at place of application); *vasodilatation* (red skin at place of application)

Note: *Localized skin reactions* generally resolve spontaneously within 1 or 2 hours. The adhesive in the occlusive dressing may also cause localized *sensitivity reactions* manifested by skin rash, itching, and/or redness.

*Vasoconstriction-induced blanching* generally occurs first and may be followed, depending on the application time, by *vasodilatation-induced erythema.*

## Overdose

For specific information on the agents used in the management of lidocaine and prilocaine overdose, see:

- *Ascorbic Acid (Systemic)* monograph;
- *Benzodiazepines (Systemic)* monograph;
- *Methylene Blue (Systemic)* monograph; and/or
- *Sympathomimetic Agents—Cardiovascular Use (Parenteral-Systemic)* monograph.

For more information on the management of overdose or unintentional ingestion, **contact a Poison Control Center** (see *Poison Control Center Listing*).

**Clinical effects of overdose**

The following effects have been selected on the basis of their potential clinical significance (possible signs and symptoms in parentheses where appropriate)—not necessarily inclusive:

Acute and chronic

*Circulatory depression; convulsions; methemoglobinemia*

**Treatment of overdose**

To decrease absorption—

For systemic reactions caused by excessive absorption—Removing any remaining medication from the skin surface.

Specific treatment—

For circulatory depression—Administering a vasopressor and intravenous fluids.

For convulsions—Administering an anticonvulsant. Benzodiazepines are most commonly used, such as diazepam (for adults: 5 to 10 mg by slow intravenous injection, repeated as needed up to a total dose of 30 mg, or 150 to 500 mcg per kg of body weight, administered rectally, up to a maximum of 20 mg per dose; for children: 200 to 500 mcg by slow intravenous injection, repeated as needed up to a total dose of 5 mg for children up to 5 years of age, or 1 mg by slow intravenous injection, repeated as needed up to a total dose of 10 mg for children 5 years of age or older, or 200 to 500 mcg per kg of body weight, administered rectally) or lorazepam (50 mcg per kg of body weight, intravenously, repeated as needed up to a total dose of 4 mg [for adults] or 2 mg [for children]). Because intravenously administered benzodiazepines may cause respiratory and circulatory depression, especially when administered rapidly, medications and equipment needed for support of respiration and for resuscitation must be immediately available.

For methemoglobinemia—Administering methylene blue (1 to 2 mg per kg of body weight, intravenously) and/or ascorbic acid (100 to 200 mg orally).

Supportive care—

Securing and maintaining a patent airway, administering 100% oxygen, and instituting assisted or controlled respiration as needed. In some patients, endotracheal intubation may be required.

## Patient Consultation

As an aid to patient consultation, refer to *Advice for the Patient, Lidocaine and Prilocaine (Topical).*

In providing consultation, consider emphasizing the following selected information (» = major clinical significance):

**Before using this medication**
» Conditions affecting use, especially:
  Sensitivity to lidocaine, prilocaine, or other amide-type local anesthetics
  Use in children—Increased risk of adverse effect (methemoglobinemia) in infants younger than 1 year of age; use of medication does not eliminate need for comforting frightened children
  Use in the elderly—Possibility of increased risk of systemic effects, based on experience with local anesthetics administered by other routes
  Other medications, especially sulfonamides
  Other medical problems, especially conditions that may increase absorption and methemoglobinemia or predisposition to (e.g., glucose-6-phosphate dehydrogenase deficiency)

**Proper use of this medication**
» Using only for appropriate indications, as directed by physician or nurse
» Not applying to open wounds, burns, or broken or inflamed skin, unless otherwise directed by physician or nurse
» Avoiding contact with eyes; if inadvertent contact does occur, not touching eyes and contacting physician immediately
» Avoiding contact with lips or mouth
» Following instructions provided by physician or nurse and/or patient information provided by manufacturer
» Contacting health care provider if any questions about method, site, or time of application
» Proper application technique:
  Applying a thick layer of medication to specified area or areas; not spreading the medication
  Covering the medication with an occlusive dressing; sealing tightly, making sure a thick layer remains under the dressing; not disturbing the dressing
  If directed to do so, removing the bandage after 1 or 2 hours, wiping off the medication, then cleaning the area with antiseptic solution; if not directed to do so, keeping medication and bandage in place until removed by physician or nurse
» Proper dosing
» Proper storage

**Precautions while using this medication**
» Monitoring small children after administration, to make sure they do not disturb the dressing and/or ingest any medication
» Caution that injury may occur undetected while numbness persists in the affected area; using care to prevent injury (e.g., not scratching, rubbing, or exposing the affected area to extreme hot or cold temperatures) until sensation has returned

**Side/adverse effects**
Possibility of allergic reactions (anaphylactoid reactions, angioedema, bronchospasm, urticaria) and systemic effects (cardiovascular and/or CNS toxicity); obtaining medical assistance immediately if signs and/or symptoms occur
Signs and symptoms of other potential adverse effects, especially methemoglobinemia

## General Dosing Information

Contact with the eyes should be avoided, because the medication may cause severe corneal irritation. Also, the anesthetic effect results in loss of protective reflexes, which may allow damage to the eye. If contact with an eye occurs, the eye should be washed with water or 0.9% sodium chloride solution and protected against injury until sensation returns.

The medication should not be applied to open wounds.

Although application of the medication to small sites (approximately 20 to 25 square centimeters [2 inches square]) may take place at home, before the patient travels to a medical appointment, it is recommended that the medication be applied to larger sites only under the supervision of medical personnel (e.g., in the office, clinic, or hospital).

The optimal application time may depend on the thickness and structure of the surface to which the medication is applied as well as the procedure being performed.

Prior to the procedure, the dressing should be removed, the medication wiped off, and the entire skin area cleaned with an antiseptic solution.

## Topical Dosage Forms

Note: Bracketed uses in the *Dosage Forms* section refer to categories of use and/or indications that are not included in U.S. product labeling.

## LIDOCAINE AND PRILOCAINE CREAM

**Usual adult dose**
Anesthesia, topical—
  Dermal procedures:
    Topical, to intact skin, a thick layer to be applied and covered with an occlusive dressing.
    For minor procedures involving a small area (e.g., intravascular cannulation, venipuncture)—2.5 grams, applied over twenty to twenty-five square centimeters of skin surface area and allowed to remain in contact with the skin surface for at least one hour. A second site may be prepared, to be used if a technical problem with cannulation or needle insertion should arise at the first site.
    For major dermal procedures involving larger areas (e.g., split thickness skin graft harvesting)—2 grams per ten square centimeters of skin surface area. The medication should be allowed to remain in contact with the skin surface for at least two hours.
    For laser treatment (removal of warts, tattoos, etc.)—1 to 2 grams per ten square centimeters of skin surface area.
    Note: A study performed in children has shown that application of smaller quantities of medication in a thin layer over a given surface area is not as effective as the recommended thick layer.
      Longer application times may be needed after application to black skin.
  [Genital mucosal procedures (e.g., removal of condylomata or other localized lesions)][1]:
    Topical, to the mucosa, up to 10 grams. The medication should be allowed to remain in contact with the mucosa for 5 to 10 minutes, after which the procedure should be started immediately.

**Usual adult prescribing limits**
Dermal procedures—
  The maximum recommended duration of exposure is four to five hours. Leaving the medication on the skin for longer than five hours is not likely to provide additional benefit, and may actually result in decreased anesthetic efficacy as well as an increased risk of systemic toxicity.

**Usual pediatric dose**
Anesthesia, topical—
  Infants up to 3 months of age:
    Use is not recommended.
  Infants and children older than 3 months of age:
    Dermal procedures—See *Usual adult dose*.
  [Genital mucosal procedures][1]: Use in children for this indication is not recommended.

**Usual pediatric prescribing limits**
Dermal procedures—
  The maximum recommended area of application in pediatric patients of various weights is:
    Up to 10 kg—100 square centimeters.
    10 to 20 kg—600 square centimeters.
    More than 20 kg—2000 square centimeters.

**Usual geriatric dose**
See *Usual adult dose*.

**Strength(s) usually available**
U.S.—
  5% (2.5% [25 mg per gram] of each anesthetic) (Rx) [*EMLA*].
Canada—
  5% (2.5% [25 mg per gram] of each anesthetic) (OTC) [*EMLA*].

**Packaging and storage**
Store between 15 and 30 °C (59 and 86 °F), unless otherwise specified by manufacturer. Protect from freezing.

**Auxiliary labeling**
• For topical use only.
• Keep away from eyes.
• Keep away from mouth.

[1]Not included in Canadian product labeling.

## Selected Bibliography

Halperin DL, Koren G, Attias D, Pellegrini E, Greenberg ML, Wyss M. Topical skin anesthesia for venous, subcutaneous drug reservoir and lumbar punctures in children. Pediatrics 1989; 84: 281-4.
Steward DJ, editor. Management of childhood pain: New approaches to procedure-related pain. J Pediatrics 1993; 122 (5, Part 2): S1-S46.

Revised: 08/18/93

# LINCOMYCIN Systemic

VA CLASSIFICATION (Primary): AM350

Note: For a listing of dosage forms and brand names by country availability, see *Dosage Forms* section(s). For a listing of brand names for the articles in this monograph, refer to the General Index.

## Category

Antibacterial (systemic).

## Indications

### Accepted

Lincomycin has been used in the treatment of serious infections caused by susceptible strains of streptococci, pneumococci, and staphylococci. However, lincomycin generally has been replaced by safer and more effective agents.

Not all species or strains of a particular organism may be susceptible to lincomycin.

## Pharmacology/Pharmacokinetics

### Physicochemical characteristics

Molecular weight—461.01.

### Mechanism of action/Effect

Antibacterial (systemic)—Lincomycin inhibits protein synthesis in susceptible bacteria by binding to the 50 S subunits of bacterial ribosomes and preventing peptide bond formation. It is usually considered bacteriostatic, but may be bactericidal in high concentrations or when used against highly susceptible organisms.

### Absorption

Rapidly absorbed from the gastrointestinal tract following oral administration. Approximately 20 to 30% absorbed orally in fasting state; absorption decreased when taken with food.

### Distribution

Widely and rapidly distributed to most fluids and tissues, except cerebrospinal fluid (CSF); high concentrations in bone, bile, and urine; lincomycin may reach significant concentrations in the eye following parenteral administration.

Readily crosses the placenta. Up to 25% of maternal serum concentrations. Also distributed into breast milk.

### Protein binding

Protein binding decreases with increased plasma concentrations. Range, 28 to 86% (average, 70 to 75%). Albumin is not thought to be the primary binding component.

### Biotransformation

Presumed to be hepatic; metabolites have not been fully characterized.

### Half-life

Normal renal function—5.4 hours (range, 4 to 6 hours).
End-stage renal disease—10 to 20 hours.
Impaired hepatic function—Half-life almost doubled.

### Time to peak serum concentration

Oral: 2 to 4 hours.
Intramuscular: 0.5 hour.
Intravenous: End of infusion.

### Elimination

Renal, biliary. Mean urinary recovery of unchanged drug over a 24-hour period ranges from 10–47% after an intramuscular dose, 13–72% after an intravenous dose, and 3–13% after a fasting oral dose. Approximately 30–40% of an oral dose is excreted unchanged in the feces within 72 hours.

In dialysis—Not removed from the blood by hemodialysis or peritoneal dialysis.

## Precautions to Consider

### Cross-sensitivity and/or related problems

Patients hypersensitive to clindamycin may be hypersensitive to lincomycin also. A case of apparent cross-sensitivity has also been reported with doxorubicin.

### Pregnancy/Reproduction

Lincomycin crosses the placenta and may be concentrated in the fetal liver. However, problems in humans have not been documented.

### Breast-feeding

Lincomycin is distributed into breast milk; reported concentrations range from 0.5 to 2.4 mcg per mL. However, problems in humans have not been documented.

### Pediatrics

Lincomycin hydrochloride injection contains benzyl alcohol, which has been associated with a fatal gasping syndrome in premature infants.

### Geriatrics

No information is available on the relationship of age to the effects of lincomycin in geriatric patients.

### Drug interactions and/or related problems

The following drug interactions and/or related problems have been selected on the basis of their potential clinical significance (possible mechanism in parentheses where appropriate)—not necessarily inclusive (» = major clinical significance):

Note: Combinations containing any of the following medications, depending on the amount present, may also interact with this medication.

» Anesthetics, hydrocarbon inhalation, such as:
   Chloroform
   Cyclopropane
   Enflurane
   Halothane
   Isoflurane
   Methoxyflurane
   Trichloroethylene or
» Neuromuscular blocking agents
   (concurrent use of these medications with lincomycin, if necessary, should be carefully monitored since neuromuscular blockade may be enhanced, resulting in skeletal muscle weakness and respiratory depression or paralysis [apnea]; caution is also recommended when these medications are used concurrently with lincomycin during surgery or in the postoperative period; treatment with anticholinesterase agents or calcium salts may help reverse the blockade)

» Antidiarrheals, adsorbent
   (concurrent use of kaolin- or attapulgite-containing antidiarrheals with oral lincomycin may significantly decrease absorption of oral lincomycin; concurrent use should be avoided or patients should be advised to take adsorbent antidiarrheals not less than 2 hours before or 3 to 4 hours after oral lincomycin)

» Antidiarrheals, antiperistaltic
   (antiperistaltic agents, such as opiates, difenoxin, diphenoxylate, or loperamide, may prolong or worsen pseudomembranous colitis by delaying toxin elimination)

Antimyasthenics
   (concurrent use of medications with neuromuscular blocking action may antagonize the effect of antimyasthenics on skeletal muscle; temporary dosage adjustments of antimyasthenics may be necessary to control symptoms of myasthenia gravis during and following concurrent use)

» Chloramphenicol or
» Erythromycins
   (may displace lincomycin from or prevent its binding to 50 S subunits of bacterial ribosomes, thus antagonizing the effects of lincomycin; concurrent use is not recommended)

Opioid (narcotic) analgesics
   (respiratory depressant effects of drugs with neuromuscular blocking activity may be additive to central respiratory depressant effects of opioid analgesics, possibly leading to increased or prolonged respiratory depression or paralysis [apnea]; caution and careful monitoring of the patient are recommended)

### Laboratory value alterations

The following have been selected on the basis of their potential clinical significance (possible effect in parentheses where appropriate)—not necessarily inclusive (» = major clinical significance):

With physiology/laboratory test values
   Alanine aminotransferase (ALT [SGPT]), serum and
   Alkaline phosphatase, serum and
   Aspartate aminotransferase (ALT [SGOT]), serum
      (values may be increased)

### Medical considerations/Contraindications

The medical considerations/contraindications included here have been selected on the basis of their potential clinical significance (reasons given in parentheses where appropriate)—not necessarily inclusive (» = major clinical significance).

*Risk-benefit should be considered when the following medical problems exist:*

» Gastrointestinal disease, history of, especially ulcerative colitis, regional enteritis, or antibiotic-associated colitis
(lincomycin may cause pseudomembranous colitis)

» Hepatic function impairment, severe
(the half-life of lincomycin is prolonged in patients with severe hepatic function impairment; this may require an adjustment in dosage)

Hypersensitivity to lincomycins or doxorubicin

» Renal function impairment, severe
(patients with impaired renal function do not generally require a reduction in dose unless the impairment is severe; patients receiving lincomycin with severely impai-red renal function should receive 25 to 30% of the usual dose of patients with normal renal function)

### Patient monitoring

The following may be especially important in patient monitoring (other tests may be warranted in some patients, depending on condition; » = major clinical significance):

*For antibiotic-associated pseudomembranous colitis (AAPMC)*
Proctosigmoidoscopy and/or
Colonoscopy
(proctosigmoidoscopy and/or colonoscopy may be required in selected, severely ill patients with persistant symptoms of AAPMC to document the presence of pseudomembranes; it is no longer recommended as a routine monitoring parameter)

Stool examinations
(cytotoxin assays of stool samples for the presence of *Clostridium difficile* and its cytotoxin, neutralizable by *C. sordellii* antitoxin, may be required prior to treatment in patients with AAPMC to document the presence of *C. difficile* and/or its cytotoxin; however, *C. difficile* and its cytotoxin may persist following treatment with oral vancomycin despite clinical improvement; follow-up cytotoxin assays are generally not recommended with complete clinical improvement)

## Side/Adverse Effects

The following side/adverse effects have been selected on the basis of their potential clinical significance (possible signs and symptoms in parentheses where appropriate)—not necessarily inclusive:

**Those indicating need for medical attention**
Incidence more frequent
*Pseudomembranous colitis* (abdominal or stomach cramps and pain, severe; abdominal tenderness; diarrhea, watery and severe, which may also be bloody; fever)

Incidence less frequent
*Hypersensitivity* (skin rash, redness, and itching); *neutropenia* (sore throat and fever); *thrombocytopenic purpura* (unusual bleeding or bruising)

**Those indicating need for medical attention only if they continue or are bothersome**
Incidence more frequent
*Gastrointestinal disturbances* (abdominal pain; diarrhea; nausea and vomiting)

Incidence less frequent
*Fungal overgrowth* (itching of rectal or genital areas)

**Those indicating possible pseudomembranous colitis and the need for medical attention if they occur after medication is discontinued**
*Abdominal or stomach cramps and pain, severe; abdominal tenderness; diarrhea, watery and severe, which may also be bloody; fever*

## Patient Consultation

As an aid to patient consultation, refer to *Advice for the Patient, Lincomycin (Systemic).*

In providing consultation, consider emphasizing the following selected information (» = major clinical significance):

**Before using this medication**
» Conditions affecting use, especially:
Hypersensitivity to lincomycin, clindamycin, or doxorubicin
Pregnancy—Lincomycin crosses the placenta
Breast-feeding—Lincomycin is distributed into breast milk
Use in children—Lincomycin is not recommended in infants up to 1 month of age; lincomycin injection contains benzyl alcohol, which has been associated with a fatal gasping syndrome in premature infants

Other medications, especially hydrocarbon inhalation anesthetics, neuromuscular blocking agents, antiperistaltic and adsorbent antidiarrheals, chloramphenicol, or erythromycins
Other medical problems, especially a history of gastrointestinal disease, particularly ulcerative colitis, severe renal function impairment, or severe hepatic function impairment

### Proper use of this medication
» Taking on an empty stomach with an 8 ounce glass of water
» Compliance with full course of therapy, especially in streptococcal infections
» Importance of not missing doses and taking at evenly spaced times
» Proper dosing
Missed dose: Taking as soon as possible; not taking if almost time for next dose; not doubling doses
» Proper storage

### Precautions while using this medication
Regular visits to physician to check progress
Checking with physician if no improvement within a few days
» For severe diarrhea, checking with physician before taking any antidiarrheals; for mild diarrhea, taking kaolin- or attapulgite-containing antidiarrheals at least 2 hours before or 3 to 4 hours after taking oral lincomycin; other antidiarrheals may worsen or prolong the diarrhea; checking with physician or pharmacist if mild diarrhea continues or worsens
Caution if surgery with general anesthesia is required

### Side/adverse effects
Signs of potential side effects, especially hypersensitivity, neutropenia, thrombocytopenic purpura, and pseudomembranous colitis

## General Dosing Information

Therapy should be continued for at least 10 days in group A beta-hemolytic streptococcal infections to help prevent the occurrence of acute rheumatic fever.

### For oral dosage forms only
Lincomycin should preferably be taken with a full glass (240 mL) of water on an empty stomach (either 1 hour before or 2 hours after meals) to obtain optimum serum concentrations.

### For intravenous administration
Lincomycin should be infused over a period of at least one hour. Rare instances of cardiopulmonary arrest and hypotension have been reported after administration at greater-than-recommended concentration and rate.

### For treatment of adverse effects
For antibiotic-associated pseudomembranous colitis (AAPMC)
• Some patients may develop AAPMC, caused by *Clostridium difficile* toxin, during or following administration of lincomycins. Mild cases may respond to discontinuation of the drug alone. Moderate to severe cases may require fluid, electrolyte, and protein replacement.
• In cases not responding to the above measures or in more severe cases, oral doses of metronidazole, bacitracin, cholestyramine, or vancomycin may be used. Oral vancomycin is effective in doses of 125 to 500 mg every 6 hours for 5 to 10 days. The dose of metronidazole is 250 to 500 mg every 8 hours; cholestyramine, 4 grams four times a day; and bacitracin, 25,000 units, orally, four times a day. Recurrences may be treated with a second course of these medications.
• Cholestyramine and colestipol resins have been shown to bind *C. difficile* toxin *in vitro*. If cholestyramine or colestipol resin is administered in conjunction with oral vancomycin, the medications should be administered several hours apart since the resins have been shown to bind oral vancomycin also.
• In addition, antibiotic-associated pseudomembranous colitis may result in severe watery diarrhea, which may occur during therapy or up to several weeks after therapy is discontinued. If diarrhea occurs, administration of antiperistaltic antidiarrheals (e.g., opiates, diphenoxylate and atropine combination, loperamide) is not recommended since they may delay the removal of toxins from the colon, thereby prolonging and/or worsening the condition.

## Oral Dosage Forms

Note: The dosing and strengths of the dosage forms available are expressed in terms of lincomycin base (not the hydrochloride salt).

## LINCOMYCIN HYDROCHLORIDE CAPSULES USP

**Usual adult and adolescent dose**
Antibacterial—
Oral, 500 mg (base) every six to eight hours.

**Usual pediatric dose**
Antibacterial—
Infants up to 1 month of age: Use is not recommended.
Infants 1 month of age and over: Oral, 7.5 to 15 mg (base) per kg of body weight every six hours; or 10 to 20 mg per kg of body weight every eight hours.

**Strength(s) usually available**
U.S.—
250 mg (base) (Rx) [*Lincocin*].
500 mg (base) (Rx) [*Lincocin*].
Canada—
500 mg (Rx) [*Lincocin*].

**Packaging and storage**
Store below 40 °C (104 °F), preferably between 15 and 30 °C (59 and 86 °F), unless otherwise specified by manufacturer. Store in a tight container.

**Auxiliary labeling**
• Take on empty stomach.
• Continue medicine for full time of treatment.

## Parenteral Dosage Forms

Note: The dosing and strengths of the dosage forms available are expressed in terms of lincomycin base (not the hydrochloride salt).

## LINCOMYCIN HYDROCHLORIDE INJECTION USP

**Usual adult and adolescent dose**
Antibacterial—
Intramuscular, 600 mg (base) every twelve to twenty-four hours.
Intravenous, 600 mg to 1 gram (base), administered over at least one hour, every eight to twelve hours.
Subconjunctival, 75 mg (base).

**Usual adult prescribing limits**
Intravenous, up to 8 grams (base) daily.

**Usual pediatric dose**
Antibacterial—
Infants up to 1 month of age:
Use is not recommended.

Infants 1 month of age and over:
Intramuscular, 10 mg (base) per kg of body weight every twelve to twenty-four hours.
Intravenous, administered over at least one hour: 3.3 to 6.7 mg (base) per kg of body weight every eight hours; or 5 to 10 mg per kg of body weight every twelve hours.

**Strength(s) usually available**
U.S.—
600 mg (base) in 2 mL (Rx) [*Lincocin* (benzyl alcohol 9.45 mg per mL)].
3000 mg (base) in 10 mL (Rx) [*Lincorex*].
Canada—
600 mg (base) in 2 mL (Rx) [*Lincocin* (benzyl alcohol 9.45 mg per mL)].

**Packaging and storage**
Store below 40 °C (104 °F), preferably between 15 and 30 °C (59 and 86 °F), unless otherwise specified by manufacturer. Protect from freezing.

**Preparation of dosage form**
To prepare initial dilution for intravenous use, each dose must be diluted as follows:

| Dose (grams) | Diluent (mL) | Duration of Administration (hr) |
| --- | --- | --- |
| ≤1 | 125 | 1 |
| 2 | 200 | 2 |
| 3 | 300 | 3 |
| 4 | 400 | 4 |

**Stability**
Lincomycin is physically compatible for 4 hours at room temperature with intravenous solutions containing penicillin G sodium or colistimethate.
Lincomycin is physically compatible for 24 hours at room temperature with 5 and 10% dextrose injection, 5 or 10% dextrose and 0.9% sodium chloride injection, Ringer's injection, M/6 sodium lactate injection, 6% dextran and 0.9% sodium chloride injection, or 10% invert sugar and electrolytes injection, and with intravenous solutions containing vitamin B complex, vitamin B complex and ascorbic acid, cephalothin, cephoranide, tetracycline hydrochloride, ampicillin, methicillin, chloramphenicol, or polymyxin B sulfate.

**Incompatibilities**
Lincomycin is physically incompatible with novobiocin and kanamycin.

Revised: 10/06/92
Interim revision: 03/24/94

# LINDANE   Topical

VA CLASSIFICATION (Primary/Secondary): AP300/AP900
[Former name—Gamma Benzene Hexachloride]
Another commonly used name is gamma benzene hexachloride.

Note: For a listing of dosage forms and brand names by country availability, see *Dosage Forms* section(s). For a listing of brand names for the articles in this monograph, refer to the General Index.

## Category

Pediculicide—Lindane Shampoo; Lindane Cream; Lindane Lotion.
Scabicide—Lindane Cream; Lindane Lotion.

## Indications

Note: Bracketed information in the *Indications* section refers to uses that are not included in U.S. product labeling.

**Accepted**
Pediculosis capitis (treatment) or
Pediculosis pubis (treatment)—Lindane shampoo, [cream], and [lotion] are indicated for the treatment of pediculosis (lice) infestations caused by *Pediculus humanus* var. *capitis* (head louse) and *Phthirus pubis* (pubic or crab louse) and their ova.
Scabies (treatment)—Lindane cream and lotion are indicated for the treatment of scabies infestation caused by *Sarcoptes scabiei*.

**Unaccepted**
In the U.S., lindane cream and lotion are no longer indicated for the treatment of pediculosis capitis (head lice) or pediculosis pubis (pubic or crab lice).

## Pharmacology/Pharmacokinetics

**Physicochemical characteristics**
Molecular weight—290.83.

**Mechanism of action/Effect**
Lindane is a central nervous system (CNS) stimulant when absorbed systemically. Following absorption through the chitinous exoskeleton of arthropods, lindane is presumed to stimulate the nervous system, resulting in convulsions and death.

**Absorption**
Lindane is absorbed significantly through the skin.
Lotion—In one study, a mean peak blood concentration of 28 nanograms per mL occurred in infants and children 6 hours after total body application of lindane lotion for scabies.
Shampoo—In one study, a mean peak blood concentration of 3 nanograms per mL occurred in persons 6 hours after topical use of lindane shampoo.

**Half-life**
In one study, the half-life of lindane was 18 hours in infants and children treated for scabies using total body application of lindane lotion.

## Precautions to Consider

**Carcinogenicity**
Studies in animals have not shown lindane to have carcinogenic properties.

**Tumorigenicity**
In one study, despite the high incidence of tumors in the control group, lindane was thought to be associated with a significant increase in the incidence of hepatoma.

**Mutagenicity**
Studies have not shown lindane to have mutagenic properties.

**Pregnancy/Reproduction**
Pregnancy—Adequate and well-controlled studies in humans have not been done. Because lindane is absorbed through the skin and has the potential for causing CNS toxicity, some clinicians do not recommend the use of lindane during pregnancy. If lindane is used, however, the recommended dosage should not be exceeded in pregnant women, and these women should not be treated more than twice during pregnancy.
Studies in animals have not shown that lindane causes adverse effects on the fetus.

FDA Pregnancy Category B.

**Breast-feeding**
Problems in humans have not been documented; however, lindane is systemically absorbed and is distributed into breast milk. Although the concentrations found in human blood following topical application of lindane make it unlikely that breast milk will contain amounts of lindane sufficient to cause toxicity, an alternate method of feeding the infant should be used for 2 days.

**Pediatrics**
Caution is recommended in infants and children, since studies have shown that the potential for toxic effects of topically applied lindane is greater in the young than in adults.
Lindane is not recommended for use in premature neonates, because their skin is likely to be more permeable than that of full-term neonates and their liver enzymes may not be sufficiently developed to metabolize the medication.

**Geriatrics**
Although appropriate studies on the relationship of age to the effects of lindane have not been performed in the geriatric population, no geriatrics-specific problems have been documented to date. However, some experts believe that absorption of lindane may be increased in the elderly because of possible increased permeability of their skin. In addition, elderly patients with a history of seizure activity may be especially sensitive to the CNS toxicity effects of lindane.

**Drug interactions and/or related problems**
The following drug interactions and/or related problems have been selected on the basis of their potential clinical significance (possible mechanism in parentheses where appropriate)—not necessarily inclusive (» = major clinical significance):

Skin, scalp, or hair preparations, other, such as creams, lotions, ointments, or oils
   (simultaneous application may increase the percutaneous absorption of lindane)

**Medical considerations/Contraindications**
The medical considerations/contraindications included here have been selected on the basis of their potential clinical significance (reasons given in parentheses where appropriate)—not necessarily inclusive (» = major clinical significance).

*Risk-benefit should be considered when the following medical problems exist:*
Convulsive disorders
   (sufficient systemic absorption of lindane may induce seizures)
Sensitivity to lindane
Skin rash or raw or broken skin
   (possible increased absorption of lindane)

## Side/Adverse Effects

Note: Lindane is absorbed through the skin and has the potential for CNS toxicity, especially in infants, children, and possibly the elderly.

The following side/adverse effects have been selected on the basis of their potential clinical significance (possible signs and symptoms in parentheses where appropriate)—not necessarily inclusive:

**Those indicating need for medical attention**
Incidence rare
   *Skin irritation not present before therapy*—if lindane is applied incorrectly or repeatedly, the incidence of skin irritation is increased; *skin rash*

Symptoms of CNS toxicity
   *Convulsions; dizziness, clumsiness, or unsteadiness; fast heartbeat; muscle cramps; nervousness, restlessness, or irritability; vomiting*

**Those indicating need for medical attention if they occur and continue or are bothersome after medication is discontinued**
   *Itching of skin*—acquired sensitivity to mites and their products; may continue for one to several weeks

## Patient Consultation

As an aid to patient consultation, refer to *Advice for the Patient, Lindane (Topical).*

In providing consultation, consider emphasizing the following selected information (» = major clinical significance):

**Before using this medication**
» Conditions affecting use, especially:
   Sensitivity to lindane
   Pregnancy—Lindane is absorbed through the skin and has the potential for causing toxic effects in the CNS of the fetus; not increasing the amount, frequency, or length of therapy that physician ordered; not being treated more than twice during a pregnancy
   Breast-feeding—Lindane is distributed into breast milk; another method of feeding infant should be used for 2 days after use of lindane
   Use in children—Caution is recommended, since infants and children are especially sensitive to the effects of lindane; in addition, use is not recommended in premature infants
   Use in the elderly—Absorption may be increased in the elderly because of increased permeability of their skin; elderly patients with a history of seizure activity may be especially sensitive to the CNS toxicity effects of lindane

**Proper use of this medication**
» Poison; importance of keeping away from mouth
» Importance of not using more lindane than the amount prescribed
» Avoiding contact with the eyes
» Not using on open wounds, such as cuts or sores on skin or scalp, to minimize systemic absorption
   When applying lindane to another person: Wearing plastic disposable or rubber gloves to prevent systemic absorption, especially if you are pregnant or are breast-feeding
   Proper administration: Reading patient directions carefully before using
   If necessary, treating sexual partner or partners, especially, and all members of household, since infestation may spread to persons in close contact; checking with doctor if these persons have not been checked or if there are any questions
*For cream or lotion dosage form*
   For scabies—
      Washing, rinsing, and drying skin well before using lindane if skin has any cream, lotion, ointment, or oil on it
      Drying skin well if warm bath or shower is taken before using lindane
      Applying enough lindane to dry skin to cover entire skin surface from neck down; rubbing in well
      Leaving lindane on skin for 8 hours
      Removing lindane by washing thoroughly

*For shampoo dosage form*
   For lice—
      Shampooing, rinsing, and drying hair and scalp well before using lindane if hair or scalp has any cream, lotion, ointment, or oil-based product on it
» If applying shampoo in the shower or in the bathtub, making sure shampoo does not run down on other parts of body; also, not applying shampoo in a bathtub where shampoo may run into bath water in which patient is sitting; this minimizes systemic absorption; when rinsing out the shampoo, thoroughly rinsing entire body to remove any shampoo that may have gotten on it
      Applying enough to dry hair (1 ounce or less for short hair, 1½ ounces for medium length hair and 2 ounces or less for long hair) to thoroughly wet the hair and skin or scalp of affected and surrounding hairy areas
      Rubbing thoroughly into hair and skin or scalp; allowing to remain in place for 4 minutes
      Using just enough water to work up a good lather
      Rinsing thoroughly; drying with clean towel
      When hair is dry, combing with fine-toothed comb to remove any remaining nits or nit shells
» Not using as a regular shampoo

» Proper dosing
» Proper storage

**Precautions while using this medication**

To help prevent reinfestation or spreading of the infestation to other persons:

For scabies—Washing in very hot water or dry-cleaning all recently worn underwear and pajamas and used sheets, pillowcases, and towels

For lice—Washing in very hot water or dry-cleaning all recently worn clothing and used bed linens and towels

**Side/adverse effects**

Risk of systemic absorption greater in infants and children than in adults; use not recommended in premature neonates, because risk of systemic absorption greater than in older infants

Signs of potential side effects, especially skin irritation or rash not present before therapy or CNS toxicity

## General Dosing Information

Since lindane has no continuing effect after treatment, it is not effective as a prophylaxis against possible future infestation.

**For scabies (using the cream or lotion)**

Sexual partners and persons living in the same household should receive prophylactic treatment for scabies, since the signs of scabies can appear as late as 1 to 2 months after exposure and scabies can be transmitted during this period of time.

Although a total body application is considered to be from the neck down including the soles of the feet, scabies may also affect the heads of infants (scabies rarely affects the heads of children or adults). Consideration should be given to treating the head also if the patient is an infant.

If the skin has any cream, lotion, ointment, or oil on it, the skin should be washed, rinsed, and dried well before application of the medication.

If a warm bath or shower is taken before the cream or lotion is used, the skin should be well dried prior to application. The cream or lotion should be applied to dry skin in an amount sufficient to cover the entire body surface from the neck down including the soles of the feet (usually 1 to 2 ounces for an adult). The medication should be left on for 8 hours, then removed by thorough washing.

To help prevent reinfestation or spreading of the infestation, all recently worn underwear and pajamas and used sheets, pillowcases, and towels should be washed in very hot water or dry-cleaned.

**For pediculosis (using the shampoo)**

Sexual partners and other persons in close contact or living in the same household should be checked for infestation and treated if necessary, since the infestation may spread to persons in close contact.

If the hair or scalp has any cream, lotion, ointment, or oil-based product on it, shampoo, rinse, and dry hair and scalp well before the application of lindane.

A sufficient amount of shampoo should be used on dry hair (1 ounce or less for short hair, 1½ ounces for medium length hair, and 2 ounces or less for long hair) to thoroughly wet the hair and skin or scalp of the affected and surrounding hairy areas. The shampoo should be rubbed thoroughly into the hair and skin or scalp and allowed to remain in place for 4 minutes. Then, just enough water should be used to work up a good lather. The hair and skin or scalp should be rinsed thoroughly and dried with a clean towel. When the hair is dry, patient should use a fine-toothed comb to remove any remaining nits or nit shells.

Lindane shampoo should not be used as a regular shampoo.

For treatment of eyelashes, petroleum jelly can be applied 3 times a day for 1 week.

To help prevent reinfestation or spreading of the infestation, all recently worn clothing and used bed linens and towels should be washed in very hot water or dry-cleaned.

**For treatment of toxicity**

Recommended treatment includes

• If accidental ingestion occurs, it may be life threatening and prompt gastric lavage is recommended.

• Since oils favor absorption, saline cathartics should be administered rather than oily cathartics for intestinal evacuation.

• If CNS manifestations occur, they may be treated by the administration of pentobarbital, phenobarbital, or diazepam.

## Topical Dosage Forms

Note: Bracketed uses in the *Dosage Forms* section refer to categories of use and/or indications that are not included in U.S. product labeling.

### LINDANE CREAM USP

**Usual adult and adolescent dose**

[Pediculicide] or
Scabicide—

Topical, to the skin, as a 1% cream for one application.

**Usual pediatric dose**

[Pediculicide] or
Scabicide—

Premature neonates: Use is not recommended.
Infants and children: See *Usual adult and adolescent dose.*

**Strength(s) usually available**

U.S.—

1% (Rx) [*Kwell*].

Canada—

1% (Rx) [*Kwellada*].

**Packaging and storage**

Store below 40 °C (104 °F), preferably between 15 and 30 °C (59 and 86 °F), unless otherwise specified by manufacturer. Store in a tight container. Protect from freezing.

**Auxiliary labeling**

• Poison.
• For external use only.

**Note**

When dispensing, include patient instructions.

### LINDANE LOTION USP

**Usual adult and adolescent dose**

[Pediculicide] or
Scabicide—

Topical, to the skin, as a 1% lotion for one application.

**Usual pediatric dose**

[Pediculicide] or
Scabicide—

Premature neonates: Use is not recommended.
Infants and children: See *Usual adult and adolescent dose.*

**Strength(s) usually available**

U.S.—

1% (Rx) [*Bio-Well; G-well; Kildane; Kwell; Kwildane; Scabene; Thionex;* GENERIC].

Canada—

1% (Rx) [*GBH; Kwellada; PMS Lindane;* GENERIC].

**Packaging and storage**

Store below 40 °C (104 °F), preferably between 15 and 30 °C (59 and 86 °F), unless otherwise specified by manufacturer. Store in a tight container. Protect from freezing.

**Auxiliary labeling**

• Poison.
• For external use only.
• Shake well.

**Note**

When dispensing, include patient instructions.

### LINDANE SHAMPOO USP

**Usual adult and adolescent dose**

Pediculicide—

Topical, to the scalp or skin, as a 1% shampoo for one application, repeated after seven days if necessary.

**Usual pediatric dose**

Pediculicide—

Premature neonates: Use is not recommended.
Infants and children: See *Usual adult and adolescent dose.*

**Strength(s) usually available**

U.S.—

1% (Rx) [*Bio-Well; GBH; G-well; Kildane; Kwell; Kwildane; Scabene;* GENERIC].

Canada—

1% (Rx) [*GBH; Hexit; Kwellada; PMS Lindane;* GENERIC].

**Packaging and storage**
Store below 40 °C (104 °F), preferably between 15 and 30 °C (59 and 86 °F), unless otherwise specified by manufacturer. Store in a tight container. Protect from freezing.

**Auxiliary labeling**
• Poison.
• For external use only.
• Shake well.

**Note**
When dispensing, include patient instructions.

Revised: 08/15/94

---

**LIOTHYRONINE**—See *Thyroid Hormones (Systemic)*

---

**LIOTRIX**—See *Thyroid Hormones (Systemic)*

---

**LISADIMATE-CONTAINING COMBINATIONS—**
Lisadimate, Oxybenzone, and Padimate O (Topical)—See *Sunscreen Agents (Topical)*
Lisadimate and Padimate O (Topical)—See *Sunscreen Agents (Topical)*

---

**LISINOPRIL**—See *Angiotensin-converting Enzyme (ACE) Inhibitors (Systemic)*

---

**LISINOPRIL-CONTAINING COMBINATIONS—**
Lisinopril and Hydrochlorothiazide (Systemic)—See *Angiotensin-converting Enzyme (ACE) Inhibitors and Hydrochlorothiazide (Systemic)*

---

# LITHIUM    Systemic

VA CLASSIFICATION (Primary/Secondary): CN750/CN900; BL400
Note: For a listing of dosage forms and brand names by country availability, see *Dosage Forms* section(s). For a listing of brand names for the articles in this monograph, refer to the General Index.

## Category
Antimanic; antidepressant therapy adjunct; granulopoietic; vascular headache prophylactic.

## Indications
Note: Bracketed information in the *Indications* section refers to uses that are not included in U.S. product labeling.

**Accepted**
Bipolar disorder (treatment)—Lithium is indicated as the primary agent in the treatment of acute manic and hypomanic episodes in bipolar disorder, and for maintenance therapy to help diminish the intensity and frequency of subsequent manic episodes in patients with a history of mania.

Lithium is used in some patients as the agent of choice in the prevention of bipolar depression. Clinicians have observed a diminished intensity and frequency of severe depressive episodes.

[Depression, mental (treatment)]¹—Lithium is used alone for maintenance therapy in unipolar depression, and for acute and maintenance therapy in schizoaffective disorder. It is also used to augment the antidepressant effect of tricyclic or monoamine oxidase (MAO) inhibitor antidepressants in the treatment of major unipolar depression in patients not responsive to antidepressants alone.

[Headache, vascular (prophylaxis)]¹—Lithium is used to reduce the frequency of the occurrence of episodic and chronic cluster headaches.

[Neutropenia (treatment)]¹—Lithium is used to reduce the incidence of infection in patients with chemotherapy-induced neutropenia and in patients with chronic or acquired neutropenia.

---

¹Not included in Canadian product labeling.

## Pharmacology/Pharmacokinetics

**Physicochemical characteristics**
Molecular weight—
Lithium carbonate: 73.89.
Lithium citrate: 282.00.
Other characteristics—A monovalent cation easily assayed in biological fluids; salts share some chemical characteristics with salts of sodium and potassium

**Mechanism of action/Effect**
Antimanic—Has not been established. The mood-stabilizing effect has been postulated to relate to a reduction of catecholamine neurotransmitter concentration, possibly mediated by lithium ion ($Li^+$) effect on $Na^+K^+$ adenosine triphosphatase ($Na^+K^+ATPase$) to produce improved transneuronal membrane transport of sodium ion. An alternate postulate is that lithium may decrease cyclic adenosine monophosphate (cyclic AMP) concentrations, which would result in decreased sensitivity of hormonal-sensitive adenylcyclase receptors. Another hypoth-

esis is the "second messenger" theory of lithium's interference with lipid inositol metabolism. This theory postulates that a group of improperly regulated neurons may be the underlying cause of manic symptoms. A phospholipase C-type enzyme hydrolyzes the plasma membrane–located lipid, phosphatidylinositol biphosphate, to diacylglycerol and inositol triphosphate, postsynaptic second messengers that contribute to chronic cell stimulation by altering electrical activity in the neuron. Inositol formed during this process is recycled by the inositol phospholipid–synthesizing enzymes in the CNS. There is evidence that cells in the CNS do not have access to plasma sources of inositol but, instead, depend on the synthesis of inositol for the transduction of neuronal signals. Lithium, in therapeutic concentrations, blocks the activity of the enzyme, inositol-1-phosphatase, resulting in a depletion of neuronal inositol and ultimately a decrease in the levels of phosphatidylinositol biphosphate. The lipid will no longer be able to stimulate the formation of adequate quantities of the second messengers or alter electrical activity. Subsequent cells in the CNS become relatively insensitive to the agonist stimulation, and clinical improvement results.
Granulopoietic—The exact mechanism of action has not been established; however, studies have shown that lithium stimulates granulopoiesis, enhances marrow proliferation, elevates neutrophil production, and increases the granulocyte pool.
Vascular headache prophylactic—Specific mechanism has not been established. It has been postulated that the action of lithium in cluster headaches may be directly related to changes in platelet serotonin and histamine concentrations.
Antidepressant—Has not been established. However, the mechanism may involve enhancement of serotonergic activity and downregulation of beta-receptors.

**Absorption**
Rapid; complete within 6 to 8 hours. Absorption rate of slow-release capsules is slower and the total amount of lithium absorbed is lower than with other dosage forms.

**Protein binding**
Not bound to plasma proteins.

**Biotransformation**
None.

**Half-life (average)**
Elimination—
Adults: 24 hours.
Adolescents: 18 hours.
Elderly patients: Up to 36 hours.
Note: When therapy is initiated, the serum concentration decreases rapidly during the initial 5 or 6 hours, followed by a more gradual decline over the next 24 hours.

**Time to peak serum concentration**
Syrup—0.5 hours.
Capsules or tablets—1 to 3 hours.
Extended-release tablets—4 hours.
Slow-release capsules—3 hours.
Steady-state serum concentrations—4 days.

Thyroid function determinations
(serum thyroxine and thyroxine-stimulating hormone [TSH] should be evaluated at baseline before lithium therapy is initiated and at 6-month intervals during therapy; patient should be monitored for symptoms of hypothyroidism; maintenance of adequate thyroid function is important in children to maintain a satisfactory growth rate)

» White blood cell count, total and differential
(recommended prior to therapy and repeated if signs of unusual tiredness or weakness develop because of possible rare leukemia that may develop during lithium therapy; however, the association of lithium with leukemia is controversial; benign leukocytosis may be reversible on discontinuation of therapy)

## Side/Adverse Effects

The following side/adverse effects have been selected on the basis of their potential clinical significance (possible signs and symptoms in parentheses where appropriate)—not necessarily inclusive:

### Those indicating need for medical attention
Incidence less frequent
*Cardiovascular problems* (fainting; fast or slow heartbeat; irregular pulse; troubled breathing [dyspnea] on exertion); *leukocytosis* (unusual tiredness or weakness); *weight gain*

Note: *Sinus node function impairment, sinoatrial block,* or *ventricular irritability* may occur at therapeutic serum lithium concentrations; possibly reversible when lithium is discontinued.

*Leukocytosis* is usually reversible upon discontinuation of lithium, but a rare leukemia may develop during lithium therapy.

Incidence rare
*Blue color and pain in fingers and toes; coldness of arms and legs; pseudotumor cerebri* (dizziness; eye pain; headache; nausea or vomiting; noises in ears; vision problems)

Note: If undetected, *pseudotumor cerebri* may result in enlargement of blind spot, constriction of visual fields, and eventual blindness, due to optic atrophy.

Symptoms of hypothyroidism
*Dry, rough skin; hair loss; hoarseness; mania* (unusual excitement); *mental depression; sensitivity to cold; swelling of feet or lower legs; swelling of neck*

### Those indicating need for medical attention only if they continue or are bothersome
Incidence more frequent
*Diarrhea; increased thirst; nausea, mild; stress incontinence or urinary urgency* (increased frequency of urination; loss of bladder control); *trembling of hands, slight*

Note: *Stress incontinence* or *urinary urgency* is dose-related; more common in women; usually begins 2 to 7 years after start of treatment with lithium.

Incidence less frequent
*Acne or skin rash; bloated feeling or pressure in the stomach; muscle twitching, slight*

## Overdose

For specific information on the agents used in the management of lithium overdose, see:
- *Acetazolamide* in *Carbonic Anhydrase Inhibitors (Systemic)* monograph; and/or
- *Mannitol (Systemic)* monograph.

For more information on the management of overdose or unintentional ingestion, **contact a Poison Control Center** (see *Poison Control Center Listing*).

### Clinical effects of overdose
The following effects have been selected on the basis of their potential clinical significance (possible signs and symptoms in parentheses where appropriate)—not necessarily inclusive:

Early symptoms of toxicity
*Diarrhea; drowsiness; loss of appetite; muscle weakness; nausea or vomiting; slurred speech; trembling*

Late symptoms of toxicity
*Blurred vision; clumsiness or unsteadiness; confusion; convulsions; dizziness; increase in amount of urine; trembling, severe*

### Treatment of overdose
No specific antidote is available. Early toxic symptoms can usually be treated by reducing or stopping administration of lithium and resuming treatment at a lower dosage after 24 to 48 hours.

Treatment of more severe toxicity or acute overdose may include the following:
To decrease absorption—
Inducing vomiting or using small volume (100 mL) gastric lavage (in acute overdose).
To enhance elimination—
Utilizing intermittent hemodialysis if plasma lithium does not drop more than 10% every 3 hours or half-life is greater than 36 hours. Since plasma lithium determinations immediately after dialysis do not take into account the rebound increase that occurs as lithium redistributes from tissue to blood, determinations must be obtained 6 hours later.
Possibly increasing lithium excretion with single dose of intravenous acetazolamide or using mannitol as an osmotic diuretic.
Monitoring—
Measuring plasma lithium concentrations every 3 hours until lithium is less than 1.0 mEq per liter.
Monitoring patient closely.
Supportive care—
Maintaining electrolyte balance and body fluids.
Regulating kidney function.
Maintaining adequate respiration.
Preventing infection.
Patients in whom intentional overdose is known or suspected should be referred for psychiatric consultation.

## Patient Consultation

As an aid to patient consultation, refer to *Advice for the Patient, Lithium (Systemic).*

In providing consultation, consider emphasizing the following selected information (» = major clinical significance):

### Before using this medication
» Conditions affecting use, especially:
Sensitivity to lithium
Pregnancy—Lithium crosses placenta; contraindicated in first trimester because of possible neonatal goiter and cardiovascular malformations; at delivery, hypotonia, lethargy, and cyanosis in newborns of mothers taking lithium at term
Breast-feeding—Excreted in breast milk; may cause hypotonia, hypothermia, cyanosis, and ECG changes in some babies
Use in children—May decrease bone formation or density
Use in the elderly—Elderly more prone to develop CNS toxicity, hypothyroidism and goiter; lower doses and more frequent monitoring required
Other medications, especially iodine-containing preparations, nonsteroidal anti-inflammatory drugs, chlorpromazine (and possibly other phenothiazines), diuretics, haloperidol, or molindone
Other medical problems, especially history of leukemia, cardiovascular disease, epilepsy, parkinsonism, severe dehydration, renal insufficiency, urinary retention, or severe infections with prolonged sweating, vomiting, or diarrhea

### Proper use of this medication
Taking after a meal or snack to prevent laxative action and to decrease the severity of stomach upset, tremors, or weakness by slowing absorption rate
» Importance of adequate fluid (2.5 to 3 liters each day) and sodium intake
» Importance of not taking more medication than the amount prescribed
» Compliance with therapy; improvement in condition may require 1 to 3 weeks; importance of maintaining adequate blood levels even though symptoms improved
» Proper dosing
Missed dose: Taking as soon as possible, unless within 4 hours (6 hours for extended-release tablets or slow-release capsules) of next scheduled dose; not doubling doses
» Proper storage
*For extended-release or slow-release dosage form*
Swallowing tablet or capsule whole
Not breaking, crushing, or chewing
*For syrup dosage form*
Diluting dose with fruit juice or other flavored beverage before taking

### Precautions while using this medication
» Regular visits to physician to check progress during therapy; importance of serum lithium monitoring
Caution in drinking large amounts of coffee, tea, or colas because of diuretic effect
» Possible drowsiness or dizziness; caution if driving or doing jobs requiring alertness
» Caution during exercise, saunas, and hot weather

» Caution during illnesses that cause high fevers with profuse sweating, vomiting, or diarrhea
» Caution on self-imposed dieting
» Importance of patient and family knowing early symptoms of overdose or toxicity
*For slow-release dosage form*
» Not using interchangeably with any other dosage form

### Side/adverse effects
» Early symptoms of lithium overdose or toxicity:
    Diarrhea
    Drowsiness
    Loss of appetite
    Muscle weakness
    Nausea or vomiting
    Slurred speech
    Trembling
    Side effects are more likely to occur in the elderly
    Signs of potential side effects, especially cardiovascular problems, leukocytosis, weight gain, blue color and pain in fingers and toes, coldness of arms and legs, pseudotumor cerebri, symptoms of hypothyroidism

## General Dosing Information

Warning—Lithium toxicity can occur with doses at or near therapeutic serum concentrations. Facilities for prompt and accurate serum lithium determinations must be available during therapy. Accurate patient evaluation requires both clinical and laboratory analysis.

During the acute manic phase, the patient may have a greater ability to tolerate lithium. This tolerance decreases as the manic symptoms subside and often necessitates a corresponding dosage adjustment.

During the acute manic phase, lithium administration of 300 (8 mEq) to 600 mg three times a day should usually produce effective serum concentrations ranging from 0.8 to 1.2 mEq per liter, with weekly adjustments based on plasma lithium concentrations. An increase of 8 mEq a day will increase plasma concentrations by $0.3 \pm 0.1$ mEq per liter. The maintenance dose of 300 mg three or four times a day usually produces effective serum concentrations ranging from 0.5 to 1.0 mEq per liter.

If a satisfactory therapeutic response to lithium at the highest tolerated serum concentrations within the therapeutic range is not achieved within 3 weeks, lithium therapy should be discontinued.

Slow-release lithium carbonate capsules and tablets are not bioequivalent to other lithium dosage forms and should not be used interchangeably with them.

### Diet/Nutrition
Since lithium decreases sodium reabsorption by the renal tubules, a normal diet with an average consumption of salt and adequate fluid intake, 2.5 to 3 liters of fluid per day, is essential to prevent sodium depletion leading to lithium toxicity.

This medication may be taken with food, juice, or milk, if necessary, to lessen laxative action, stomach irritation, tremors, or weakness, by slowing absorption of lithium. The syrup must be diluted in juice or other flavored beverage before administration.

### For treatment of adverse effects
Early side effects—If slight hand tremor, mild nausea or diarrhea, unusual drowsiness, or acne do not subside with continued treatment, a reduction in lithium dosage may be necessary. If hand tremor is especially bothersome, shifting a majority of the dose to bedtime, decreasing caffeine intake, or adding a beta-blocker such as propranolol may be helpful.

Suppression of thyroid activity—May necessitate thyroid hormone replacement therapy.

Urinary incontinence—Lowering dose of lithium whenever possible, adding an anticholinergic agent or an antidepressant with anticholinergic properties, or switching to another medication for treatment of bipolar disorder.

Polyuria—Lowering dose of lithium alone, whenever possible. If the lower plasma lithium concentration is inadequate to maintain a response, adding a thiazide diuretic and reducing the lithium dose by 50%, then readjusting it to reproduce the original plasma lithium concentration, may be effective. Alternatively, extended-release or slow-release lithium products can improve the patient's renal concentrating ability.

Weight gain—May be safely and effectively treated by limiting calorie intake with emphasis on adequate fluid and sodium intake.

## Oral Dosage Forms
### LITHIUM CARBONATE CAPSULES USP

**Usual adult and adolescent dose**
Antimanic—
    Acute mania: Oral, initially 300 to 600 mg (8 to 16 mEq) three times a day, the dosage being adjusted as needed and tolerated at weekly intervals.
    Maintenance: Oral, 300 mg three or four times a day, the dosage being adjusted as needed and tolerated.

Note: Geriatric or debilitated patients usually require a lower dosage.

**Usual adult prescribing limits**
Up to 2.4 grams a day.

**Usual pediatric dose**
Antimanic—
    Children up to 12 years of age: Oral, initially 15 to 20 mg (0.4 to 0.5 mEq) per kg of body weight a day in two or three divided doses, the dosage being adjusted at weekly intervals, based on plasma lithium concentrations.
    Children 12 to 18 years of age: See *Usual adult and adolescent dose*.

**Strength(s) usually available**
U.S.—
    150 mg (Rx) [GENERIC].
    300 mg (Rx) [*Eskalith; Lithonate;* GENERIC].
    600 mg (Rx) [GENERIC].
Canada—
    150 mg (Rx) [*Carbolith*].
    300 mg (Rx) [*Carbolith; Lithane*].

**Packaging and storage**
Store below 40 °C (104 °F), preferably between 15 and 30 °C (59 and 86 °F), unless otherwise specified by manufacturer. Store in a well-closed container.

**Auxiliary labeling**
• May cause drowsiness.
• Take after a meal or snack.

### LITHIUM CARBONATE SLOW-RELEASE CAPSULES

**Usual adult and adolescent dose**
Antimanic—
    Acute mania: Oral, initially 600 to 900 mg a day on the first day, the dosage being increased, thereafter, to 1200 to 1800 mg a day in three divided doses, as needed and tolerated.
    Maintenance: Oral, 900 to 1200 mg a day in three divided doses, the dosage being adjusted as needed and tolerated.

**Usual adult prescribing limits**
Up to 2.4 grams a day.

**Usual pediatric dose**
Antimanic—
    Children up to 12 years of age: Dosage has not been established.
    Children 12 to 18 years of age: See *Usual adult and adolescent dose*.

**Usual geriatric dose**
Antimanic—
    Oral, 600 to 1200 mg a day in three divided doses.

**Strength(s) usually available**
U.S.—
    Not commercially available.
Canada—
    150 mg (Rx) [*Lithizine*].
    300 mg (Rx) [*Lithizine*].

Note: Not bioequivalent to other lithium dosage forms and should not be used interchangeably with them.

**Packaging and storage**
Store below 40 °C (104 °F), preferably between 15 and 30 °C (59 and 86 °F), unless otherwise specified by manufacturer. Store in a well-closed container.

**Auxiliary labeling**
• Swallow whole.
• May cause drowsiness.

### LITHIUM CARBONATE TABLETS USP

**Usual adult and adolescent dose**
See *Lithium Carbonate Capsules USP*.

**Usual adult prescribing limits**
See *Lithium Carbonate Capsules USP*.

**Usual pediatric dose**
See *Lithium Carbonate Capsules USP*.

**Strength(s) usually available**

U.S.—

300 mg (Rx) [*Eskalith* (scored); *Lithane* (tartrazine); *Lithotabs;* GENERIC].

Canada—

300 mg (Rx) [*Lithane*].

**Packaging and storage**

Store below 40 °C (104 °F), preferably between 15 and 30 °C (59 and 86 °F), unless otherwise specified by manufacturer. Store in a well-closed container.

**Auxiliary labeling**

• May cause drowsiness.
• Take after a meal or snack.

## LITHIUM CARBONATE EXTENDED-RELEASE TABLETS

**Usual adult and adolescent dose**

Antimanic—

Acute mania: Oral, 450 to 900 mg two times a day or 300 to 600 mg three times a day, the dosage being adjusted as needed and tolerated.

Maintenance: Oral, 450 mg two times a day or 300 mg three times a day, the dosage being adjusted as needed and tolerated.

Note: Geriatric or debilitated patients usually require a lower dosage.

**Usual adult prescribing limits**

Up to 2.4 grams a day.

**Usual pediatric dose**

Antimanic—

Children up to 12 years of age: Dosage has not been established.
Children 12 to 18 years of age: See *Usual adult and adolescent dose.*

**Strength(s) usually available**

U.S.—

300 mg (Rx) [*Lithobid*].
450 mg (Rx) [*Eskalith CR* (scored)].

Canada—

300 mg (Rx) [*Duralith* (scored)].

**Packaging and storage**

Store below 40 °C (104 °F), preferably between 15 and 30 °C (59 and 86 °F), in a well-closed container, unless otherwise specified by manufacturer.

**Auxiliary labeling**

• Swallow whole.
• May cause drowsiness.
• Take after a meal or snack.

## LITHIUM CITRATE SYRUP USP

**Usual adult and adolescent dose**

Antimanic—

Acute mania: Oral, the equivalent of 300 to 600 mg (8 to 16 mEq) of lithium carbonate three times a day, the dosage being adjusted as needed and tolerated.

Maintenance: Oral, the equivalent of 300 mg of lithium carbonate three or four times a day, the dosage being adjusted as needed and tolerated.

Note: Geriatric or debilitated patients usually require a lower dosage.

**Usual adult prescribing limits**

Up to the equivalent of 2.4 grams of lithium carbonate a day.

**Usual pediatric dose**

Antimanic—

Children up to 12 years of age: Oral, initially the equivalent of 15 to 20 mg (0.4 to 0.5 mEq) of lithium carbonate per kg of body weight a day in two or three divided doses, the dosage being adjusted at weekly intervals, based on plasma lithium concentrations.

Children 12 to 18 years of age: See *Usual adult and adolescent dose.*

**Strength(s) usually available**

U.S.—

8 mEq of lithium ion (equivalent to approximately 300 mg of lithium carbonate) per 5 mL (Rx) [*Cibalith-S;* GENERIC].

Canada—

Not commercially available.

**Packaging and storage**

Store between 15 and 30 °C (59 and 86 °F), unless otherwise specified by manufacturer. Store in a tight container. Protect from freezing.

**Incompatibilities**

Lithium citrate syrup should not be mixed with or administered at the same time as other medication, solid or liquid, that contains a basic form, such as chlorpromazine concentrate, haloperidol, thioridazine, or trifluoperazine, and tricyclic antidepressants.

**Auxiliary labeling**

• May cause drowsiness.
• Take after a meal or snack.
• Dilute with juice or other beverage before taking.

Revised: 03/09/93

# LODOXAMIDE   Ophthalmic†

BAN: Lodoxamide trometamol

VA CLASSIFICATION (Primary): OP900

Note: For a listing of dosage forms and brand names by country availability, see *Dosage Forms* section(s). For a listing of brand names for the articles in this monograph, refer to the General Index.

†Not commercially available in Canada.

## Category

Mast cell stabilizer (ophthalmic); antiallergic (ophthalmic).

## Indications

**Accepted**

Conjunctivitis, vernal (treatment)
Keratitis, vernal (treatment) or
Keratoconjunctivitis, vernal (treatment)—Lodoxamide is indicated in the treatment of certain ocular disorders, specifically, vernal conjunctivitis, vernal keratitis, and vernal keratoconjunctivitis.

## Pharmacology/Pharmacokinetics

**Physicochemical characteristics**

Molecular weight—Lodoxamide tromethamine: 553.91.

**Mechanism of action/Effect**

Lodoxamide is a mast cell stabilizer that inhibits the Type I immediate hypersensitivity reaction by preventing the antigen-stimulated release of histamine. Lodoxamide also prevents the release of SRS-A (slow-reacting substances of anaphylaxis, also known as pepido-leukotrienes) and inhibits eosinophil chemotaxis. Lodoxamide's precise mechanism of action is unknown; however, it has been reported to prevent calcium transport into mast cells during antigen stimulation.

**Absorption**

Using a minimum detection limit of 2.5 nanograms per mL, one drop of lodoxamide 0.1% administered in each eye 4 times a day for 10 days to 12 volunteers was not detectable in the plasma.

**Half-life**

Elimination—For $^{14}$C-lodoxamide administered orally: 8.5 hours in urine.

**Elimination**

Primarily in urine.

## Precautions to Consider

**Carcinogenicity**

A 2-year study in rats administered lodoxamide orally showed no neoplastic effects at doses of 100 mg per kg of body weight (mg/kg) per day.

**Tumorigenicity**

A 2-year study in rats administered lodoxamide orally showed no tumorigenic effects at doses of 100 mg/kg per day.

**Mutagenicity**

No evidence of genetic damage was shown in various genotoxicity assays. However, in a mammalian cell transformation assay, some increase in the number of transformed foci were seen at concentrations of lodox-amide that were greater than 4 mg per mL.

**Pregnancy/Reproduction**
Fertility—No evidence of impairment of reproductive function was shown in laboratory animal studies.

Pregnancy—Adequate and well-controlled studies in humans have not been done.

Reproductive studies in rats and rabbits administered lodoxamide orally in doses of 100 mg/kg per day did not show any evidence of devel-opmental toxicity.

FDA Pregnancy Category B.

**Breast-feeding**
It is not known whether lodoxamide is distributed into breast milk. How-ever, problems in humans have not been documented. Ophthalmic lo-doxamide was not detectable in plasma using a minimum detection limit of 2.5 nanograms per mL and the medication would be expected to reach even lower concentrations in breast milk.

**Pediatrics**
Appropriate studies on the relationship of age to the effects of ophthalmic lodoxamide have not been performed in children up to 2 years of age. Safety and efficacy have not been established. In older children, no pediatrics-specific problems have been documented to date.

**Geriatrics**
No information is available on the relationship of age to the effects of lodoxamide in geriatric patients.

**Medical considerations/Contraindications**
The medical considerations/contraindications included here have been se-lected on the basis of their potential clinical significance (reasons given in parentheses where appropriate)—not necessarily inclusive (» = major clinical significance).

*Risk-benefit should be considered when the following medical problem exists:*
Sensitivity to lodoxamide

## Side/Adverse Effects

The following side/adverse effects have been selected on the basis of their potential clinical significance (possible signs and symptoms in paren-theses where appropriate)—not necessarily inclusive:

**Those indicating need for medical attention**
Incidence less frequent
*Blurred vision; foreign body sensation* (feeling of something in eye); *hyperemia* (redness of eye); *discomfort; pruritus* (itching of eye); *tearing or discharge; or other eye irritation not present before ther-apy or becoming worse during therapy*

Incidence rare
*Anterior chamber cells* (sensitivity of eyes to light, eye discomfort, eye redness); *blepharitis* (eyelid irritation or redness); *chemosis* (swelling of the membrane covering the white part of the eye); *corneal abrasion* (eye irritation or redness); *corneal erosion or ulcer* (eye irritation or redness); *edema* (swelling of eye surface or eyelid); *mucus from eye; or eye pain not present before therapy or becoming worse during therapy; dizziness; headache; keratitis or keratopathy* (eye irritation or redness); *skin rash*

**Those indicating need for medical attention only if they continue or are bothersome**
Incidence more frequent
*Burning or stinging, transient, upon administration of medication*
Incidence less frequent or rare
*Aching eyes; crystalline deposits* (crusting in corner of eye or on eye-lid); *dryness of nose or eyes; heat sensation on body; nausea or stomach discomfort; ocular fatigue* (tired eyes); *ocular warming sen-sation* (feeling of heat in eye); *scales on eyelid or eyelash; sneezing; somnolence* (drowsiness or sleepiness); *sticky feeling of eyes*

## Patient Consultation

As an aid to patient consultation, refer to *Advice for the Patient, Lodoxamide (Ophthalmic)*.

In providing consultation, consider emphasizing the following selected information (» = major clinical significance):

**Before using this medication**
» Conditions affecting use, especially:
Sensitivity to lodoxamide
Use in children—Safety and efficacy have not been established in children up to 2 years of age

**Proper use of this medication**
Proper administration technique; not touching applicator tip to any surface; keeping container tightly closed
Compliance with therapy
» Proper dosing
Missed dose: Using as soon as possible
» Proper storage

**Precautions while using this medication**
» Checking with physician if symptoms do not improve or if condition becomes worse

**Side/adverse effects**
Signs of potential side effects, especially blurred vision; foreign body sensation; hyperemia; discomfort, pruritus, tearing or discharge, or other eye irritation not present before therapy or becoming worse during therapy; anterior chamber cells; blepharitis; chemosis; cor-neal abrasion; corneal erosion or ulcer, edema, mucus from eye, or eye pain not present before therapy or becoming worse during therapy; dizziness; headache; keratitis or keratopathy; or skin rash

## General Dosing Information

Symptomatic response to therapy (decreased itching, redness, and tearing) usually occurs within a week; however, an extended period of treat-ment may be required.

The manufacturer recommends that patients not wear soft contact lenses during treatment with lodoxamide ophthalmic solution. However, medical experts do not believe this precaution is necessary unless the patient has corneal epithelial problems and the medication is to be used more often than once every 1 to 2 hours. No significant problems have been documented with ophthalmic solutions containing 0.03% or less of benzalkonium chloride as a preservative, and used as eye drops in patients with no significant corneal surface problems.

## Ophthalmic Dosage Forms
### LODOXAMIDE TROMETHAMINE OPHTHALMIC SOLUTION

**Usual adult and adolescent dose**
Conjunctivitis, vernal (treatment)
Keratitis, vernal (treatment) or
Keratoconjunctivitis, vernal (treatment)—
Topical, to the conjunctiva, 1 drop four times a day for up to 3 months.

**Usual pediatric dose**
Conjunctivitis, vernal (treatment)
Keratitis, vernal (treatment) or
Keratoconjunctivitis, vernal (treatment)—
Children up to 2 years of age: Safety and efficacy have not been established.
Children 2 years of age and older: See *Usual adult and adolescent dose.*

**Strength(s) usually available**
U.S.—
0.1% (Rx) [*Alomide* (benzalkonium chloride 0.007%; edetate disodium)].
Canada—
Not commercially available.
Note: 1.78 mg of lodoxamide tromethamine is equivalent to 1 mg lodoxamide.

**Packaging and storage**
Store between 15 and 27 °C (59 and 80 °F), unless otherwise specified by manufacturer.

**Auxiliary labeling**
• For the eye.

## Selected Bibliography
Abelson MB, Schaefer K. Conjunctivitis of allergic origin: Immunologic mechanisms and current approaches to therapy. Surv Ophthalmol 1993; 38 (Suppl): 115-32.
Allansmith MR, Ross RN. Ocular allergy and mast cell stabilizers. Surv Ophthalmol 1986 Jan-Feb; 30 (4): 229-44.

Developed: 03/29/94

**LOMEFLOXACIN**—See *Fluoroquinolones (Systemic)*

# LOMUSTINE   Systemic

VA CLASSIFICATION (Primary): AN100

Another commonly used name is CCNU.

Note: For a listing of dosage forms and brand names by country availability, see *Dosage Forms* section(s). For a listing of brand names for the articles in this monograph, refer to the General Index.

## Category
Antineoplastic.

## Indications

Note: Bracketed information in the *Indications* section refers to uses that are not included in U.S. product labeling.

**Accepted**

Tumors, brain, primary (treatment)
[Carcinoma, gastrointestinal (treatment)][1]
[Carcinoma, lung (treatment)]
[Carcinoma, renal (treatment)] or
[Carcinoma, breast (treatment)]—Lomustine is indicated for treatment of both primary and metastatic brain tumors, in patients who have already received appropriate surgical and/or radiotherapeutic procedures. It is also used for treatment of gastrointestinal carcinoma, lung carcinoma (squamous cell, anaplastic large cell, and adenocarcinoma), renal carcinoma, and advanced breast carcinoma after conventional therapy has failed.

Lymphomas, Hodgkin's (treatment)—Lomustine is indicated for treatment of Hodgkin's disease, as secondary therapy in combination with other drugs in patients who relapse while being treated with primary therapy or in patients who fail to respond to primary therapy.

[Multiple myeloma (treatment)][1]—Lomustine is also used for treatment of multiple myeloma.

[Melanoma, malignant (treatment)]—Lomustine is used for treatment of malignant melanoma, alone or in combination with other drugs.

---

[1]Not included in Canadian product labeling.

## Pharmacology/Pharmacokinetics

**Physicochemical characteristics**

Molecular weight—233.70.

**Mechanism of action/Effect**

Lomustine is an alkylating agent of the nitrosourea type. Lomustine (and/or its metabolites) interferes with the function of DNA and RNA. It is cell cycle–phase nonspecific. Lomustine also acts to inhibit DNA synthesis by inhibiting key enzymatic processes.

**Absorption**

Well and rapidly absorbed from the gastrointestinal tract.

**Distribution**

Crosses the blood-brain barrier.

**Protein binding**

Moderate (50%; metabolites).

**Biotransformation**

Hepatic; rapid and complete (active metabolites).

**Half-life**

Biologic—Approximately 94 minutes.

Chemical—Approximately 15 minutes.

Metabolites—Prolonged; 16 to 48 hours.

**Elimination**

Renal (totally as metabolites); some enterohepatic circulation is believed to occur.

Fecal (less than 5%).

Respiratory (10%).

## Precautions to Consider

**Carcinogenicity/Mutagenicity**

Secondary malignancies are potential delayed effects of many antineoplastic agents, although it is not clear whether the effect is related to their mutagenic or immunosuppressive action. The effect of dose and duration of therapy is also unknown, although risk seems to increase with long-term use. Although information is limited, available data seem to indicate that the carcinogenic risk is greatest with the alkylating agents.

Long-term use of nitrosoureas in humans has been reported to be possibly associated with development of secondary malignancies (acute leukemia) and bone marrow dysplasias.

Lomustine is carcinogenic in rats and mice at the approximate clinical dose and, like other alkylating agents, is probably carcinogenic in humans.

**Pregnancy/Reproduction**

Fertility—Gonadal suppression, resulting in amenorrhea or azoospermia, may occur in patients taking antineoplastic therapy, especially with the alkylating agents. In general, these effects appear to be related to dose and length of therapy and may be irreversible. Prediction of the degree of testicular or ovarian function impairment is complicated by the common use of combinations of several antineoplastics, which makes it difficult to assess the effects of individual agents.

Lomustine suppresses gonadal function in male rats (at higher than the human dose) and in humans.

Pregnancy—Adequate and well-controlled studies in humans have not been done.

First trimester: It is usually recommended that use of antineoplastics, especially combination chemotherapy, be avoided whenever possible, especially during the first trimester. Although information is limited because of the relatively few instances of antineoplastic administration during pregnancy, the mutagenic, teratogenic, and carcinogenic potential of these medications must be considered.

Other hazards to the fetus include adverse reactions seen in adults.

In general, use of a contraceptive is recommended during cytotoxic drug therapy.

Lomustine is embryotoxic in rats and rabbits and teratogenic in rats at doses approximately equivalent to the human dose.

FDA Pregnancy Category D.

**Breast-feeding**

Lomustine is excreted in breast milk. Breast-feeding is not recommended during chemotherapy because of the risks to the infant (adverse effects, mutagenicity, carcinogenicity).

**Pediatrics**

Appropriate studies on the relationship of age to the effects of lomustine have not been performed in the pediatric population. However, pediatrics-specific problems that would limit the usefulness of this medication in children are not expected.

**Geriatrics**

No information is available on the relationship of age to the effects of lomustine in geriatric patients. However, elderly patients are more likely to have age-related renal function impairment, which may require caution in patients receiving lomustine.

**Dental**

The bone marrow depressant effects of lomustine may result in an increased incidence of microbial infection, delayed healing, and gingival bleeding. Dental work, whenever possible, should be completed prior to initiation of therapy or deferred until blood counts have returned to normal. Patients should be instructed in proper oral hygiene during treatment, including caution in use of regular toothbrushes, dental floss, and toothpicks.

Lomustine may also cause stomatitis associated with considerable discomfort.

**Drug interactions and/or related problems**

The following drug interactions and/or related problems have been selected on the basis of their potential clinical significance (possible mechanism in parentheses where appropriate)—not necessarily inclusive ( » = major clinical significance):

Blood dyscrasia–causing medications (See *Appendix II*)
(leukopenic and/or thrombocytopenic effects of lomustine may be increased with concurrent or recent therapy if these medications cause the same effects; dosage adjustment of lomustine, if necessary, should be based on blood counts)

» Bone marrow depressants, other (See *Appendix II*) or
Radiation therapy
(additive bone marrow depression may occur; dosage reduction may be required when two or more bone marrow depressants, including radiation, are used concurrently or consecutively)

Vaccines, killed virus
(because normal defense mechanisms may be suppressed by lomustine therapy, the patient's antibody response to the vaccine may be decreased. The interval between discontinuation of medications that cause immunosuppression and restoration of the pa-

tient's ability to respond to the vaccine depends on the intensity and type of immunosuppression-causing medication used, the underlying disease, and other factors; estimates vary from 3 months to 1 year)

» Vaccines, live virus

(because normal defense mechanisms may be suppressed by lomustine therapy, concurrent use with a live virus vaccine may potentiate the replication of the vaccine virus, may increase the side/ adverse effects of the vaccine virus, and/or may decrease the patient's antibody response to the vaccine; immunization of these patients should be undertaken only with extreme caution after careful review of the patient's hematologic status and only with the knowledge and consent of the physician managing the lomustine therapy. The interval between discontinuation of medications that cause immunosuppression and restoration of the patient's ability to respond to the vaccine depends on the intensity and type of immunosuppression-causing medication used, the underlying disease, and other factors; estimates vary from 3 months to 1 year. Patients with leukemia in remission should not receive live virus vaccine until at least 3 months after their last chemotherapy. Immunization with oral poliovirus vaccine should also be postponed in persons in close contact with the patient, especially family members)

**Laboratory value alterations**

The following have been selected on the basis of their potential clinical significance (possible effect in parentheses where appropriate)—not necessarily inclusive (» = major clinical significance):

With physiology/laboratory test values
  Hepatic function tests
    (may be elevated transiently and reversibly)

**Medical considerations/Contraindications**

The medical considerations/contraindications included here have been selected on the basis of their potential clinical significance (reasons given in parentheses where appropriate)—not necessarily inclusive (» = major clinical significance).

*Risk-benefit should be considered when the following medical problems exist:*

» Bone marrow depression

» Chickenpox, existing or recent (including recent exposure) or

» Herpes zoster
    (risk of severe generalized disease)

» Infection

» Pulmonary function impairment, especially with a baseline below 70% of the forced vital capacity (FVC) or carbon monoxide diffusion capacity (DL$_{CO}$)
    (increased risk of pulmonary toxicity)

» Renal function impairment

» Sensitivity to lomustine

» Caution should be used also in patients who have had previous cytotoxic drug therapy and radiation therapy.

**Patient monitoring**

The following are especially important in patient monitoring (other tests may be warranted in some patients, depending on condition; » = major clinical significance):

Alanine aminotransferase (ALT [SGPT]) values, serum and
Aspartate aminotransferase (AST [SGOT]) values, serum and
Bilirubin values, serum and
Lactate dehydrogenase (LDH) values, serum
    (recommended prior to initiation of therapy and at periodic intervals during therapy; frequency varies according to clinical state, agent, dose, and other agents being used concurrently)

» Blood urea nitrogen (BUN) concentrations and

» Creatinine concentrations, serum
    (recommended prior to initiation of therapy and at periodic intervals during therapy; frequency varies according to clinical state, agent, dose, and other agents being used concurrently)

» Hematocrit or hemoglobin and

» Leukocyte count, total and, if appropriate, differential and

» Platelet count
    (determinations recommended prior to initiation of therapy and at periodic intervals during and after therapy; frequency varies according to clinical state, agent, dose, and other agents being used concurrently)

Pulmonary function tests
    (recommended prior to initiation of therapy and at periodic intervals during therapy)

## Side/Adverse Effects

Note:  Many "side effects" of antineoplastic therapy are unavoidable and represent the medication's pharmacologic action. Some of these (for example, leukopenia and thrombocytopenia) are actually used as parameters to aid in individual dosage titration.

The following side/adverse effects have been selected on the basis of their potential clinical significance (possible signs and symptoms in parentheses where appropriate)—not necessarily inclusive:

**Those indicating need for medical attention**
Incidence more frequent
  *Immunosuppression or leukopenia or infection* (usually asymptomatic; less frequently, fever or chills; cough or hoarseness; lower back or side pain; painful or difficult urination); *thrombocytopenia* (usually asymptomatic; less frequently, unusual bleeding or bruising; black, tarry stools; blood in urine or stools; pinpoint red spots on skin)

  Note: Maximum *thrombocytopenia* occurs about 4 weeks after a dose and persists for 1 to 2 weeks. Maximum *leukopenia* occurs about 4 to 6 weeks after a dose and persists for 1 to 2 weeks. Recovery usually occurs within 6 to 7 weeks after administration. Severity of bone marrow depression varies and determines subsequent dosage of lomustine.

Incidence less frequent
  *Anemia* (unusual tiredness or weakness); *neurotoxicity* (awkwardness; confusion; slurred speech; unusual tiredness)—not definitely attributed to medication; *renal toxicity and failure* (decrease in urination; swelling of feet or lower legs)—especially with long-term therapy; *stomatitis* (sores in mouth and on lips)

Incidence rare
  *Hepatotoxicity* (usually not symptomatic); *pulmonary infiltrates and/ or fibrosis* (cough; shortness of breath)

  Note: *Pulmonary toxicity* has occurred after cumulative doses ranging from 600 to 1240 mg or therapy of 6 months or more.

**Those indicating need for medical attention only if they continue or are bothersome**
Incidence more frequent
  *Loss of appetite; nausea and vomiting*

  Note: *Loss of appetite* may persist for 2 to 3 days after a dose.
    *Nausea and vomiting* occur 3 to 6 hours after a dose and usually persist less than 24 hours.

Incidence less frequent
  *Darkening of skin; diarrhea; skin rash and itching*

**Those not indicating need for medical attention**
Incidence less frequent
  *Loss of hair*

**Those indicating the need for medical attention if they occur after medication is discontinued**
  *Bone marrow depression* (black, tarry stools; blood in urine or stools; cough or hoarseness; fever or chills; lower back or side pain; painful or difficult urination; pinpoint red spots on skin; unusual bleeding or bruising)

  Note: Cumulative *myelosuppression* may occur with repeated doses.

## Patient Consultation

As an aid to patient consultation, refer to *Advice for the Patient, Lomustine (Systemic)*.

In providing consultation, consider emphasizing the following selected information (» = major clinical significance):

**Before using this medication**
» Conditions affecting use, especially:
    Sensitivity to lomustine
    Pregnancy—Use not recommended because of mutagenic, teratogenic, and carcinogenic potential; advisability of using contraception; telling physician immediately if pregnancy is suspected
    Breast-feeding—Not recommended because of risk of serious side effects
    Other medications, especially other bone marrow depressants or previous cytotoxic drug or radiation therapy
    Other medical problems, especially chickenpox, herpes zoster, infection, pulmonary function impairment, or renal function impairment

**Proper use of this medication**
» Importance of not taking more or less medication than the amount prescribed

Explanation of different kinds of capsules included in one container

Caution in taking combination therapy; taking each medication at the right time

Frequency of nausea and vomiting, which usually lasts less than 24 hours; taking on an empty stomach to reduce nausea

Checking with physician if vomiting occurs shortly after dose is taken

» Proper dosing

**Precautions while using this medication**

» Importance of close monitoring by the physician

» Avoiding immunizations unless approved by physician; other persons in patient's household should avoid immunizations with oral poliovirus vaccine; avoiding other persons who have taken oral poliovirus vaccine or wearing a protective mask that covers nose and mouth

*Caution if bone marrow depression occurs:*

» Avoiding exposure to persons with bacterial infections, especially during periods of low blood counts; checking with physician immediately if fever or chills, cough or hoarseness, lower back or side pain, or painful or difficult urination occur

» Checking with physician immediately if unusual bleeding or bruising; black, tarry stools; blood in urine or stools; or pinpoint red spots on skin occur

Caution in use of regular toothbrush, dental floss, or toothpick; physician, dentist, or nurse may suggest alternatives; checking with physician before having dental work done

Not touching eyes or inside of nose unless hands washed immediately before

Using caution to avoid accidental cuts with use of sharp objects such as safety razor or fingernail or toenail cutters

Avoiding contact sports or other situations where bruising or injury could occur

**Side/adverse effects**

May cause adverse effects such as blood problems, loss of hair, and cancer; importance of discussing possible effects with physician

Signs of potential side effects, especially immunosuppression, leukopenia, infection, thrombocytopenia, anemia, neurotoxicity, renal toxicity, stomatitis, hepatotoxicity, and pulmonary infiltrates and/or fibrosis

Physician or nurse can help in dealing with side effects

# General Dosing Information

Patients receiving lomustine should be under supervision of a physician experienced in cancer chemotherapy.

A variety of dosage schedules and regimens of lomustine, alone or in combination with other antitumor agents, are used. The prescriber may consult the medical literature as well as the manufacturer's literature in choosing a specific dosage.

Treatment with lomustine is continued as long as the medication is effective. If no response occurs after 1 or 2 courses, a response is unlikely.

Some cross-resistance has been reported between lomustine and carmustine.

Frequency and duration of nausea and vomiting may be reduced in some patients by administration of antiemetics prior to dosing and by administration of lomustine to fasting patients.

Dosage subsequent to the initial dose should be adjusted to meet the individual requirements of each patient based on the hematological response of the patient to the previous dose. An additional course of lomustine should be given only after circulating blood elements have returned to acceptable levels (leukocytes above 4000 per cubic millimeter and platelets above 100,000 per cubic millimeter).

Because of the delayed and cumulative bone marrow suppression caused by lomustine, the medication should be given no more frequently than every 6 weeks.

Special precautions are recommended in patients who develop thrombocytopenia as a result of administration of lomustine. These may include extreme care in performing invasive procedures; regular inspection of intravenous sites, skin (including perirectal area), and mucous membrane surfaces for signs of bleeding or bruising; limiting frequency of venipuncture and avoiding intramuscular injections; testing urine, emesis, stool, and secretions for occult blood; care in use of regular toothbrushes, dental floss, toothpicks, safety razors, and fingernail and toenail cutters; avoiding constipation; and using caution to prevent falls and other injuries. Such patients should avoid alcohol and any aspirin intake because of the risk of gastrointestinal bleeding. Platelet transfusions may be required.

Patients who develop leukopenia should be observed carefully for signs of infection. Antibiotic support may be required. In neutropenic patients who develop fever, broad-spectrum antibiotic coverage should be initiated empirically, pending bacterial cultures and appropriate diagnostic tests.

**Combination chemotherapy**

Lomustine may be used in combination with other agents in various regimens. As a result, incidence and/or severity of side effects may be altered and different dosages (usually reduced) may be used. For example, lomustine is part of the following chemotherapeutic combinations (some commonly used acronyms are in parentheses):

—lomustine, doxorubicin, and vinblastine (CAVe).

—cyclophosphamide, methotrexate, and lomustine (CMC-High dose).

—methotrexate, doxorubicin, cyclophosphamide, and lomustine (MACC).

—procarbazine, vincristine, cyclophosphamide, and lomustine (POCC).

For specific dosages and schedules, consult the literature. For information regarding each agent, consult the individual monographs.

# Oral Dosage Forms

Note: Bracketed uses in the *Dosage Forms* section refer to categories of use and/or indications that are not included in U.S. product labeling.

## LOMUSTINE CAPSULES

**Usual adult and adolescent dose**

Tumors, brain, primary or

[Carcinoma, gastrointestinal][1] or

[Carcinoma, lung] or

[Carcinoma, renal] or

[Carcinoma, breast] or

Lymphomas, Hodgkin's or

[Multiple myeloma] or

[Melanoma, malignant]—

Initial: As a single agent—Oral, 100 to 130 mg per square meter of body surface as a single dose, repeated every six weeks. A lower dose is used when lomustine is combined with other agents.

Note: In patients with suppressed bone marrow function, dosage is reduced to 100 mg per square meter of body surface as a single dose, repeated every six weeks.

A suggested dosage adjustment schedule for subsequent doses is:

| Nadir after Prior Dose (cells per cubic millimeter) | | Prior Dose To Be Given (%) |
|---|---|---|
| Leukocytes | Platelets | |
| >4000 | >100,000 | 100 |
| 3000–3999 | 75,000–99,999 | 75 |
| 2000–2999 | 25,000–74,999 | 50 |
| <2000 | <25,000 | 0 |

**Usual pediatric dose**

See *Usual adult and adolescent dose.*

**Strength(s) usually available**

U.S.—

10 mg (Rx) [*CeeNU* (mannitol)].

40 mg (Rx) [*CeeNU* (mannitol)].

100 mg (Rx) [*CeeNU* (mannitol)].

Canada—

10 mg (Rx) [*CeeNU* (mannitol)].

40 mg (Rx) [*CeeNU* (mannitol)].

100 mg (Rx) [*CeeNU* (mannitol)].

**Packaging and storage**

Store below 40 °C (104 °F), preferably between 15 and 30 °C (59 and 86 °F), in a well-closed container, unless otherwise specified by manufacturer.

**Auxiliary labeling**

• There may be two or more different types of capsules in this container. This is not an error. It is important that you take all of the capsules so that you receive the right dose of the medicine.

• Take on an empty stomach.

**Note**
The total dosage (to within 10 mg) is obtained by placing the appropriate number of each capsule strength in a single container.

A patient information label should be attached, explaining the difference in appearance of the capsules and advising the patient that all of the capsules together constitute one dose.

No more than one dose should be dispensed at a time and refills supplied only after direct verbal or written order by the physician.

**Selected Bibliography**
Weiss RB, Issell BF. The nitrosoureas: carmustine (BCNU) and lomustine (CCNU). Cancer Treat Rev 1982; 9: 313-30.

[1]Not included in Canadian product labeling.

Revised: 08/09/92
Interim revision: 06/21/94

---

# LOPERAMIDE    Oral-Local

VA CLASSIFICATION (Primary): GA400
Note: For a listing of dosage forms and brand names by country availability, see *Dosage Forms* section(s). For a listing of brand names for the articles in this monograph, refer to the General Index.

## Category
Antidiarrheal.

## Indications
Note: Bracketed information in the *Indications* section refers to uses that not included in U.S. product labeling.
Note: The efficacy of any antidiarrheal medication for treatment of most cases of nonspecific diarrhea is questionable. **Preferred treatment consists of fluid and electrolyte replacement, nutritional therapy, and, if possible, elimination of the underlying cause of the diarrhea.**

**Accepted**
Diarrhea (treatment)—Loperamide is indicated in adults for the control and symptomatic relief of acute nonspecific diarrhea and of chronic diarrhea associated with inflammatory bowel disease. Loperamide is also indicated to reduce the volume of discharge from ileostomies, colostomies, and other intestinal resections.

[Loperamide may be used in children to treat diarrhea caused by rapid transit when the anatomy of the bowel has been altered by disease or by surgical procedures.][1]

Traveler's diarrhea (treatment)—Loperamide is indicated for symptomatic relief of secretory diarrhea produced by bacteria, viruses, and parasites.

**Unaccepted**
Loperamide is not recommended for use in children up to 6 years of age unless directed by a physician. Loperamide is also not recommended for routine use or as the first line of therapy for treatment of diarrhea resulting from infection or food allergy in otherwise healthy, older children.

Loperamide should not be used if diarrhea is accompanied by fever or if there is blood or mucus in the stool.

[1]Not included in Canadian product labeling.

## Pharmacology/Pharmacokinetics

**Physicochemical characteristics**
Molecular weight—513.51.
pKa—8.6.

**Mechanism of action/Effect**
Loperamide acts on receptors along the small intestine to increase circular and longitudinal muscle activity. Loperamide exerts its antidiarrheal action by slowing intestinal transit and increasing contact time, and perhaps also by directly inhibiting fluid and electrolyte secretion and/or stimulating salt and water absorption.

**Other actions/effects**
High doses may inhibit gastric acid secretion.

**Absorption**
Not well absorbed from gastrointestinal tract.

**Protein binding**
Very high (97%).

**Biotransformation**
Hepatic.

**Half-life**
9.1 to 14.4 (average 10.8) hours.

**Time to peak concentration**
Capsules—5 hours.
Oral solution—2.5 hours.

**Duration of action**
Up to 24 hours.

**Elimination**
Fecal/renal.

## Precautions to Consider

**Carcinogenicity**
Carcinogenic potential was not documented in a study using rats administered doses up to 133 times the maximum human dose.

**Pregnancy/Reproduction**
Fertility—Reproduction studies in rats and rabbits have shown that loperamide administered in doses up to 30 times the human therapeutic dose does not interfere with fertility.

Pregnancy—Adequate and well-controlled studies have not been done in humans.

Reproduction studies in rats and rabbits have shown that loperamide administered in doses up to 30 times the human therapeutic dose did not cause harm to the offspring, or produce teratogenic effects. Higher doses, however, impaired maternal and neonate survival.

FDA Pregnancy Category B.

**Breast-feeding**
It is not known whether loperamide is distributed into breast milk. However, in a pre- and post-natal study, loperamide administered to female nursing rats at a dose of 40 mg per kg of body weight caused a decrease in pup survival.

**Pediatrics**
Loperamide is not recommended for use in children up to 6 years of age unless directed by a physician, or for routine use or as initial therapy in children older than 6 years of age.

Oral rehydration therapy is the preferred treatment for children with diarrhea because loperamide may mask dehydration and depletion of electrolytes. Dehydration may further increase the variability in the response to loperamide.

Children, especially those under 3 years of age, are more susceptible to the opiate-like effects (CNS effects) of loperamide.

**Geriatrics**
In geriatric patients with diarrhea, caution is recommended because loperamide may mask dehydration and depletion of electrolytes. Dehydration may further increase the variability in the response to loperamide.

**Drug interactions and/or related problems**
The following drug interactions and/or related problems have been selected on the basis of their potential clinical significance (possible mechanism in parentheses where appropriate)—not necessarily inclusive (» = major clinical significance):

» Opioid (narcotic) analgesics
   (concurrent use of loperamide with an opioid analgesic may increase the risk of severe constipation)

**Medical considerations/Contraindications**
The medical considerations/contraindications included here have been selected on the basis of their potential clinical significance (reasons given in parentheses where appropriate)—not necessarily inclusive (» = major clinical significance).

*Except under special circumstances, this medication should not be used when the following medical problems exist:*

» Colitis, severe
   (patient may develop toxic megacolon)

Loracarbef has *in vitro* activity against most pathogens responsible for upper respiratory tract infections. It is active *in vitro* against *Streptococcus pneumoniae*, as well as beta-lactamase positive and negative *Haemophilus influenzae* and *Moraxella catarrhalis*. Loracarbef may not be active against bacteria such as penicillin-resistant *S. pneumoniae* and nonbeta-lactamase–producing ampicillin-resistant *H. influenzae*. Loracarbef has good activity *in vitro* against *S. pyogenes* (group A streptococci), and groups B, C, and G streptococci. *Enterococcus* species (group D streptococci) are resistant. Most strains of *Staphylococcus aureus* are susceptible to loracarbef; however, beta-lactamase–producing strains may be less susceptible and methicillin-resistant staphylococci are resistant.

Some gram-negative bacteria have *in vitro* susceptibility to loracarbef, including *Escherichia coli*, *Salmonella* species, *Klebsiella pneumoniae*, *Proteus mirabilis*, and *Citrobacter diversus*. However, strains of *E. coli* and *K. pneumoniae* with high production of beta-lactamase may be resistant. *Citrobacter freundii*, *Proteus vulgaris*, *Klebsiella oxytoca*, *Serratia marcescens*, *Morganella morganii*, *Enterobacter* species, *Providencia* species, and *Pseudomonas* species are all resistant to loracarbef.

### Accepted

Bronchitis, bacterial exacerbation of (treatment)—Loracarbef is indicated in the treatment of bacterial exacerbations of bronchitis caused by susceptible organisms.

Otitis media (treatment)—Loracarbef is indicated in the treatment of otitis media caused by susceptible organisms.

Pharyngitis, streptococcal (treatment)—Loracarbef is indicated in the treatment of streptococcal pharyngitis caused by susceptible organisms.

Pneumonia (treatment)—Loracarbef is indicated in the treatment of pneumonia caused by susceptible organisms.

Sinusitis (treatment)—Loracarbef is indicated in the treatment of sinusitis caused by susceptible organisms.

Skin and soft tissue infections (treatment)—Loracarbef is indicated in the treatment of skin and soft tissue infections caused by susceptible organisms.

Urinary tract infections, bacterial (treatment)—Loracarbef is indicated in the treatment of bacterial urinary tract infections caused by susceptible organisms.

## Pharmacology/Pharmacokinetics

### Physicochemical characteristics
Chemical group—Carbacephems are chemically similar to cephalosporins
Molecular weight—367.8.

### Mechanism of action/Effect
Bactericidal; binds to essential target proteins of the bacterial cell wall, leading to inhibition of cell wall synthesis and cellular lysis.

### Absorption
Well absorbed (90%) from the gastrointestinal tract. When administered with food, the peak plasma concentration ($C_{max}$) decreases by 50 to 60%, and the time to peak plasma concentration ($T_{max}$) increases by 30 to 60 minutes; however, the total absorption remains unchanged.

### Distribution
Concentrations in middle ear fluid, skin-blister fluid, and tonsillar tissue are approximately 40 to 50% of the simultaneous plasma concentration. Concentration in urine is still in the therapeutic range for most organisms 6 to 12 hours after administration. Cerebrospinal fluid (CSF) levels are not available.

### Protein binding
Approximately 25%.

### Biotransformation
There is no evidence of metabolism in humans.

### Half-life
Single dose—
  Normal renal function:
    Approximately 1 hour.
  Creatinine clearance:
    10 to 50 mL/min (0.17 to 0.83 mL/sec)—Approximately 5.6 hours.
    <10 mL/min (0.17 mL/sec)—Approximately 32 hours.

### Time to peak concentration
Capsules—Approximately 1.2 hours.
Suspension—0.5 to 0.8 hour.

### Peak serum concentration
Single dose—
  Capsule:
    200 mg—Approximately 8 mcg/mL.
    400 mg—Approximately 14 mcg/mL.
  Suspension:
    400 mg—Approximately 17 mcg/mL.
    7.5 mg/kg—Approximately 13 mcg/mL.
    15 mg/kg—Approximately 19 mcg/mL.

### Elimination
Renal; virtually all of loracarbef (87 to 97%) is excreted unchanged in the urine.
In dialysis—Hemodialysis reduces the half-life of loracarbef to approximately 4 hours.

## Precautions to Consider

### Cross-sensitivity and/or related problems
Patients allergic to cephalosporins or penicillins may be allergic to loracarbef. Loracarbef should be administered with caution to penicillin-allergic patients since the cross-reactivity among beta-lactam antibiotics is approximately 10%.

### Carcinogenicity
Lifetime carcinogenic studies in animals have not been performed.

### Mutagenicity
No mutagenic potential was found in bacterial mutation tests or in *in vitro* and *in vivo* mammalian systems.

### Pregnancy/Reproduction
Fertility—Fertility and reproductive performance were not affected in rats given doses of loracarbef up to 33 times the maximum human exposure in mg per kg of body weight (mg/kg).

Pregnancy—Adequate and well-controlled studies in humans have not been done.

Studies in mice, rats, and rabbits given doses up to 33 times the maximum human exposure of loracarbef in mg/kg have revealed no evidence of harm to the fetus.

FDA Pregnancy Category B.

### Breast-feeding
It is not known whether loracarbef is distributed into breast milk.

### Pediatrics
Appropriate studies on the relationship of age to the effects of loracarbef have not been performed in children up to 6 months of age. The pharmacokinetics and clinical response to loracarbef in children 6 months to 17 years of age are very similar to those in adults.

### Geriatrics
Appropriate studies performed to date have not demonstrated geriatrics-specific problems that would limit the usefulness of loracarbef in the elderly. However, elderly patients are more likely to have age-related renal function impairment, which may require a dosage adjustment in patients receiving loracarbef.

### Drug interactions and/or related problems
The following drug interactions and/or related problems have been selected on the basis of their potential clinical significance (possible mechanism in parentheses where appropriate)—not necessarily inclusive (» = major clinical significance):

Note: Combinations containing any of the following medications, depending on the amount present, may also interact with this medication.

» Probenecid
    (probenecid decreases the renal tubular secretion of loracarbef, increasing the area-under-the-curve [AUC] by approximately 80% and the half-life from 1 hour to 1.5 hours)

### Laboratory value alterations
The following have been selected on the basis of their potential clinical significance (possible effect in parentheses where appropriate)—not necessarily inclusive (» = major clinical significance):

With physiology/laboratory test values
  Alanine aminotransferase (ALT [SGPT]), serum or
  Alkaline phosphatase, serum or
  Aspartate aminotransferase (AST [SGOT]), serum
    (values may be increased transiently)

  Blood urea nitrogen (BUN) or
  Creatinine, serum
    (concentrations may be increased transiently)

Leukocyte count and
Platelet count
  (may be decreased; transient leukopenia, thrombocytopenia, eosinophilia have been seen on rare occasion)

## Medical considerations/Contraindications

The medical considerations/contraindications included here have been selected on the basis of their potential clinical significance (reasons given
in parentheses where appropriate)—not necessarily inclusive (» =
major clinical significance).

*Except under special circumstances, this medication should not be used
when the following medical problem exists:*

» Previous allergic reaction (anaphylaxis) to penicillins or cephalosporins

*Risk-benefit should be considered when the following medical problem
exists:*

» Renal function impairment
  (loracarbef is excreted renally; patients with renal function impairment may require a reduced dosage)

## Side/Adverse Effects

The following side/adverse effects have been selected on the basis of their
potential clinical significance (possible signs and symptoms in parentheses where appropriate)—not necessarily inclusive:

### Those indicating need for medical attention

Incidence less frequent
  *Hypersensitivity* (itching; skin rash)

### Those indicating need for medical attention only if they continue or are bothersome

Incidence more frequent
  *Gastrointestinal disturbances* (abdominal pain; anorexia; diarrhea;
  nausea and vomiting)
Incidence rare
  *Central nervous system disturbances* (dizziness; headache; drowsi-
  ness; insomnia; nervousness); *vaginitis* (vaginal itching and discharge)

## Patient Consultation

As an aid to patient consultation, refer to *Advice for the Patient,
Loracarbef (Systemic).*

In providing consultation, consider emphasizing the following selected
information (» = major clinical significance):

### Before using this medication
» Conditions affecting use, especially:
  Allergy to penicillins or cephalosporins
  Other medications, especially probenecid
  Other medical problems, especially renal function impairment

### Proper use of this medication
  Taking at least 1 hour before or 2 hours after meals
» Compliance with full course of therapy, especially in streptococcal
  infections
» Importance of not missing doses and taking at evenly spaced times
» Proper dosing
  Missed dose: Taking as soon as possible; not taking if almost time for
  next dose; not doubling doses
» Proper storage

### Precautions while using this medication
  Checking with physician if no improvement within a few days
» May cause diarrhea—
  For severe diarrhea, checking with physician before taking any
  antidiarrheals
  For mild diarrhea, kaolin- or attapulgite-containing, but not other, an-
  tidiarrheals may be tried
  Checking with physician or pharmacist if mild diarrhea continues or
  worsens

### Side/adverse effects
  Signs of potential side effects, especially hypersensitivity reactions

## General Dosing Information

Therapy should be continued for at least 10 days in group A beta-hemolytic streptococcal infections to prevent acute rheumatic fever or
glomerulonephritis.

Because loracarbef has a high degree of chemical stability, refrigeration
of the reconstituted oral suspension is not required.

Adults and children with renal function impairment require a reduction in
dose as follows:

| Creatinine Clearance (mL/min)/ (mL/sec) | Dose |
|---|---|
| ≥50/0.83 | See *Usual adult and adolescent dose* |
| 10–49/0.17–0.82 | One-half the *Usual adult and adolescent dose* or administer the *Usual adult and adolescent dose* at twice the regular dosing interval |
| <10/0.17 | *Usual adult and adolescent dose* given every 3 to 5 days |
| Hemodialysis patients | Administer after hemodialysis |

### Diet/Nutrition

Loracarbef should be taken on an empty stomach (1 hour before or 2
hours after meals).

## Oral Dosage Forms

### LORACARBEF CAPSULES

**Usual adult and adolescent dose**
Bronchitis, bacterial exacerbations—
  Oral, 200 to 400 mg every twelve hours for seven days.
Pharyngitis, streptococcal—
  Oral, 200 mg every twelve hours for ten days.
Pneumonia, caused by *S. pneumoniae* or *H. influenzae*—
  Oral, 400 mg every twelve hours for fourteen days.
Sinusitis—
  Oral, 400 mg every twelve hours for ten days.
Skin and soft tissue infections—
  Oral, 200 mg every twelve hours for seven days.
Urinary tract infections—
  Uncomplicated cystitis—Oral, 200 mg every twenty-four hours for
    seven days.
  Uncomplicated pyelonephritis—Oral, 400 mg every twelve hours for
    fourteen days.

**Usual pediatric dose**
Otitis media—
  Oral, 15 mg per kg of body weight every twelve hours for ten days.
Pharyngitis, streptococcal: Oral, 7.5 mg per kg of body weight every
    twelve hours for ten days.
Skin and soft tissue infections—
  Oral, 7.5 mg per kg of body weight every twelve hours for seven days.

**Strength(s) usually available**
U.S.—
  200 mg (Rx) [*Lorabid*].
  400 mg (Rx) [*Lorabid*].
Canada—
  Not commercially available.

**Packaging and storage**
Store below 40 °C (104 °F), preferably between 15 and 30 °C (59 and 86
  °F), unless otherwise specified by manufacturer. Store in a tight
  container.

**Auxiliary labeling**
• Continue medicine for full time of treatment.
• Take on an empty stomach.

### LORACARBEF FOR ORAL SUSPENSION

**Usual adult and adolescent dose**
See *Loracarbef Capsules.*

**Usual pediatric dose**
See *Loracarbef Capsules.*

**Strength(s) usually available**
U.S.—
  100 mg per 5 mL (when reconstituted according to the manufacturer's
    instructions) (Rx) [*Lorabid*].
  200 mg per 5 mL (when reconstituted according to the manufacturer's
    instructions) (Rx) [*Lorabid*].
Canada—
  Not commercially available.

**Packaging and storage**
Store below 40 °C (104 °F), preferably between 15 and 30 °C (59 and 86 °F), unless otherwise specified by manufacturer. Store in a tight container. Discard reconstituted suspension after 14 days.

**Auxiliary labeling**
• Continue medicine for full time of treatment.
• Shake well.
• Take on an empty stomach.

Revised: 08/18/93
Interim revision: 06/09/94; 06/20/95

---

**LORATADINE**—See *Antihistamines (Systemic)*

---

**LORATADINE-CONTAINING COMBINATIONS**—
Loratadine and Pseudoephedrine (Systemic)—See *Antihistamines and Decongestants (Systemic)*

---

**LORAZEPAM**—See *Benzodiazepines (Systemic)*

---

# LOSARTAN   Systemic†

VA CLASSIFICATION (Primary/Secondary): CV490/CV805
Other commonly used names are DuP 753 and MK594.
Note: For a listing of dosage forms and brand names by country availability, see *Dosage Forms* section(s). For a listing of brand names for the articles in this monograph, refer to the General Index.

†Not commercially available in Canada.

## Category

Antihypertensive; angiotensin II receptor antagonist.

## Indications

**Accepted**
Hypertension—Losartan is indicated for the treatment of hypertension. It may be used alone or in combination with other antihypertensive agents.

For additional information on initial therapeutic guidelines related to the treatment of hypertension, see *Appendix III*.

## Pharmacology/Pharmacokinetics

**Physicochemical characteristics**
Molecular weight—Losartan potassium: 461.01.

**Mechanism of action/Effect**
Losartan is a nonpeptide angiotensin II receptor antagonist with high affinity and selectivity for the $AT_1$ receptor. Losartan blocks the vasoconstrictor and aldosterone-secreting effects of angiotensin II by inhibiting the binding of angiotensin II to the $AT_1$ receptor. $AT_1$ receptor blockade results in an increase in plasma renin activity (PRA) followed by increases in plasma angiotensin II concentration. The potential clinical consequences of these increases are not clear. Angiotensin II agonist effects have not been demonstrated.

**Other actions/effects**
*In vitro* platelet aggregometry shows that losartan appears to be a weak antagonist to human platelet thromboxane $A_2$/prostaglandin $H_2$ (TP) receptors. The clinical relevance of this effect is presently unclear. Losartan also appears to have a uricosuric effect. However, the clinical significance of this effect has not been delineated.

**Absorption**
Well-absorbed following oral administration. Bioavailability is approximately 33%.

**Protein binding**
Losartan—Very high (98.7%).
Carboxylic acid metabolite—Very high (99.8%).

**Biotransformation**
Losartan undergoes substantial first-pass metabolism by the cytochrome P450 system. Biotransformation results in a major active carboxylic acid metabolite that is 10 to 40 times more potent than the parent compound and is responsible for most of the pharmacologic activity. In addition, there are 5 minor metabolites that are much less active than the parent compound.

**Half-life**
Elimination—
Losartan: Approximately 2 hours.
Carboxylic acid metabolite: Approximately 6 to 9 hours.

**Time to peak concentration**
Losartan—Approximately 1 hour.
Carboxylic acid metabolite—Approximately 2 to 4 hours.

**Time to peak effect**
Approximately 6 hours.

**Duration of action**
Single dose—24 hours or more.

**Elimination**
Renal—Approximately 35% (4% of dose as parent and 6% of dose as active metabolite).
Fecal (biliary)—Approximately 60%.
In dialysis—Losartan and its carboxylic acid metabolite are not removable by hemodialysis.

## Precautions to Consider

**Carcinogenicity**
Losartan was not carcinogenic in rats and mice given maximally tolerated doses of 270 mg per kg of body weight (mg/kg) per day and 200 mg/kg per day, respectively, for 105 and 92 weeks, respectively. However, female rats had a slightly higher incidence of pancreatic acinar adenoma. The maximally tolerated doses of losartan provided systemic exposures of up to 160 times (rats) and 30 times (mice) the exposure of a 50 kg human given 100 mg per day.

**Mutagenicity**
Losartan was not mutagenic in a number of *in vitro* and *in vivo* assays.

**Pregnancy/Reproduction**
Fertility—Studies in male rats given oral doses of up to 150 mg/kg per day did not reveal adverse effects on fertility or reproductive performance. However, toxic doses of 300 and 200 mg/kg per day given to females resulted in significant decreases in the number of corpora lutea, implants, and live fetuses. The relationship of these findings to losartan is uncertain.

Pregnancy—Medications affecting the renin-angiotensin system, such as losartan, can cause fetal and neonatal morbidity and mortality when administered to pregnant women. Losartan should be discontinued as soon as possible when pregnancy is detected.

Fetal exposure to medications affecting the renin-angiotensin system during the second and third trimesters of pregnancy have been associated with hypotension, neonatal skull hypoplasia, anuria, renal failure, and even death in the newborn. Maternal oligohydramnios has also been reported, probably reflecting decreasing fetal renal function. Oligohydramnios in this setting has been associated with fetal limb contractures, craniofacial deformation, and hypoplastic lung development. Prematurity, intrauterine growth retardation, and patent ductus arteriosus also have been reported. However, it is not clear that these occurrences were related to drug exposure.

It is recommended that infants exposed *in utero* to losartan be closely observed for hypotension, oliguria, and hyperkalemia. Oliguria should be treated with support of blood pressure and renal perfusion. If oligohydramnios is observed, losartan should be discontinued unless it is considered lifesaving for the mother. Oligohydramnios, however, may not appear until after the fetus has sustained irreversible damage.

Losartan exposure during late gestation at doses approximately 3 times the maximum recommended human dose on a mg per square meter of body surface area basis produced adverse effects in rat fetuses and neonates, including decreased body weight, delayed physical and behavioral development, mortality, and renal toxicity.

FDA Pregnancy Category C (first trimester) and D (second and third trimesters).

**Breast-feeding**
It is not known whether losartan is distributed into breast milk. However, significant concentrations of losartan and its active metabolite are present in the milk of rats.

**Pediatrics**

No information is available on the relationship of age to the effects of losartan in pediatric patients. Safety and efficacy have not been established.

**Geriatrics**

Use of losartan in a limited number of patients 65 years of age and over has not demonstrated geriatrics-specific problems that would limit the usefulness of losartan in the elderly.

**Drug interactions and/or related problems**

The following drug interactions and/or related problems have been selected on the basis of their potential clinical significance (possible mechanism in parentheses where appropriate)—not necessarily inclusive (» = major clinical significance):

Note: Combinations containing any of the following medications, depending on the amount present, may also interact with this medication.

Anti-inflammatory drugs, nonsteroidal (NSAIDs), especially indomethacin
(NSAIDs may antagonize the antihypertensive effect of losartan by inhibiting renal prostaglandin synthesis and/or causing sodium and fluid retention; the patient should be carefully monitored to confirm that the desired effect is being obtained)

Blood from blood bank (may contain up to 30 mEq [mmol] of potassium per L of plasma or up to 65 mEq [mmol] per L of whole blood when stored for more than 10 days) or

Cyclosporine or

Diuretics, potassium-sparing or

Low-salt milk (may contain up to 60 mEq [mmol] of potassium per liter) or

Potassium-containing medications or

Potassium supplements or substances containing high concentrations of potassium or

Salt substitutes (most contain substantial amounts of potassium)
(concurrent administration with losartan may result in hyperkalemia since reduction of aldosterone production induced by losartan may lead to elevation of serum potassium; determination of serum potassium concentrations is recommended if concurrent use of these agents is necessary)

» Diuretics
(symptomatic hypotension may occur after initiation of losartan therapy in patients taking a diuretic; caution and a lower starting dose are recommended)

Hypotension-producing medications, other (See *Appendix II*)
(concurrent use with losartan may produce additive hypotensive effects)

Sympathomimetics
(concurrent use of these agents may reduce the antihypertensive effects of losartan; the patient should be carefully monitored to confirm that the desired effect is being obtained)

**Laboratory value alterations**

The following have been selected on the basis of their potential clinical significance (possible effect in parentheses where appropriate)—not necessarily inclusive (» = major clinical significance):

With physiology/laboratory test values
Alanine aminotransferase (ALT) and
Aspartate aminotransferase (AST)
(transient increases have been reported rarely; these increases were infrequently greater than 2 or 3 times the upper limit of normal)

Bilirubin, serum
(concentrations may be increased)

Hemoglobin and
Hematocrit
(small increases occur frequently, but are rarely of clinical significance)

Potassium, serum
(concentrations may be slightly increased as a result of reduced aldosterone concentrations)

Uric acid, serum
(concentrations may be decreased, reflecting losartan's uricosuric effect)

Uric acid, urine
(concentrations may be increased; losartan appears to significantly increase uric acid excretion; this effect appears to be related to the parent compound, losartan, and not the carboxylic acid metabolite)

**Medical considerations/Contraindications**

The medical considerations/contraindications included here have been selected on the basis of their potential clinical significance (reasons given in parentheses where appropriate)—not necessarily inclusive (» = major clinical significance).

*Risk-benefit should be considered when the following medical problems exist:*

» Hepatic function impairment
(increased plasma concentrations may occur; total plasma clearance of losartan may be 50% lower and oral bioavailability about 2 times higher than in individuals with normal hepatic function; lower dosages are recommended)

» Renal artery stenosis, bilateral or in a solitary kidney
(increased risk of renal function impairment)

Renal function impairment, moderate to severe
(losartan area under the curve [AUC] may be increased by approximately 50%; however, dosage adjustments are not necessary unless patient is volume-depleted)
(in patients whose renal function is dependent on the renin-angiotensin-aldosterone system, especially those with congestive heart failure, there may be a risk of losartan–induced renal failure)

Sensitivity to losartan

» Caution is recommended in patients who are sodium- or volume-depleted. Symptomatic hypotension may occur following initiation of losartan therapy. Sodium- or volume-depletion should be corrected or a lower starting dose is recommended in these patients.

**Patient monitoring**

The following may be especially important in patient monitoring (other tests may be warranted in some patients, depending on condition; » = major clinical significance):

» Blood pressure measurements
(recommended at periodic intervals; selected patients may be taught to monitor their blood pressure at home and report the results at regular physician visits)

Renal function determinations
(recommended at periodic intervals, especially in patients who are sodium- and volume-depleted as a result of diuretic therapy or who have severe congestive heart failure)

## Side/Adverse Effects

Note: A case of angioedema has been reported in a patient being treated with losartan.

The following side/adverse effects have been selected on the basis of their potential clinical significance (possible signs and symptoms in parentheses where appropriate)—not necessarily inclusive:

**Those indicating need for medical attention**

Incidence less frequent
*Dizziness; upper respiratory infection* (cough, fever, or sore throat)

**Those indicating need for medical attention only if they continue or are bothersome**

Incidence more frequent
*Headache*

Incidence less frequent
*Back pain; diarrhea; fatigue; nasal congestion*

Incidence rare
*Cough, dry; insomnia* (trouble in sleeping); *leg pain; muscle cramps or pain; sinus problems*

## Overdose

For more information on the management of overdose or unintentional ingestion, **contact a Poison Control Center** (see *Poison Control Center Listing*).

**Clinical effects of overdose**

The following effects have been selected on the basis of their potential clinical significance (possible signs and symptoms in parentheses where appropriate)—not necessarily inclusive:
*Bradycardia due to vagal stimulation; hypotension; tachycardia*

**Treatment of overdose**

Symptomatic and supportive.

## Patient Consultation

As an aid to patient consultation, refer to *Advice for the Patient, Losartan (Systemic).*

In providing consultation, consider emphasizing the following selected information (» = major clinical significance):

**Before using this medication**

» Conditions affecting use, especially:
Sensitivity to losartan

Pregnancy—Can cause fetal and neonatal morbidity and mortality; not recommended for use during pregnancy

Other medications, especially diuretics

Other medical problems, especially hepatic and renal function impairment, renal artery stenosis, or sodium or volume depletion

### Proper use of this medication

Getting into the habit of taking at same time each day to help increase compliance

Possible need for control of weight and diet, especially sodium intake; risks associated with sodium depletion; not taking salt substitutes or using low-salt milk unless approved by physician

» Patient may not experience symptoms of hypertension; importance of taking medication even if feeling well

» Does not cure, but helps control hypertension; possible need for lifelong therapy; checking with physician before discontinuing medication; serious consequences of untreated hypertension

May be taken with or without food

» Proper dosing

Missed dose: Taking as soon as possible; not taking if almost time for next dose; not doubling doses

» Proper storage

### Precautions while using this medication

» Notifying physician immediately if pregnancy is suspected

Regular visits to physician to check progress

» Not taking other medications, especially nonprescription sympathomimetics, unless discussed with physician

Caution when driving or doing other things requiring alertness, because of possible dizziness, especially after initial dose of losartan in patients taking diuretics

To prevent dehydration and hypotension, checking with physician if severe nausea, vomiting, or diarrhea occurs and continues

Caution when exercising or during hot weather because of the risk of dehydration and hypotension due to reduced fluid volume

» Caution in using alcohol because of the risk of dehydration and hypotension due to reduced fluid volume

### Side/adverse effects

Signs of potential side effects, especially dizziness or upper respiratory infection

## General Dosing Information

Dosage must be adjusted to meet the individual requirements of each patient, on the basis of clinical response.

Although there does not appear to be a rebound effect after abrupt withdrawal of losartan, gradual dosage reduction is recommended to minimize any risk of a rebound effect.

Recent evidence suggests that withdrawal of antihypertensive therapy prior to surgery may be undesirable. However, the anesthesiologist must be aware of such therapy.

### Diet/Nutrition

Losartan may be taken with or without food.

## Oral Dosage Forms
### LOSARTAN POTASSIUM TABLETS

**Usual adult dose**

Antihypertensive—

    Initial:

        Oral, 50 mg once a day.

        Note: In patients with possible volume depletion and patients with a history of hepatic function impairment an initial dose of 25 mg once a day is recommended.

    Maintenance:

        Oral, 25 to 100 mg a day. Dose may be given once a day or divided into two doses.

Note: If adequate blood pressure control is not achieved by losartan alone, a low dose of a diuretic may be added for an additive effect.

**Usual pediatric dose**

Safety and efficacy have not been established.

**Strength(s) usually available**

U.S.—

    25 (Rx) [*Cozaar* (potassium 2.12 mg [0.054 mEq])].

    50 (Rx) [*Cozaar* (potassium 4.24 mg [0.108 mEq])].

Canada—

    Not commercially available.

**Packaging and storage**

Store below 40 °C (104 °F), preferably between 15 and 30 °C (59 and 86 °F), in a tightly closed container. Protect from light.

**Auxiliary labeling**

• Do not take other medicines without your doctor's advice.

## Selected Bibliography

Goldberg AI, Dunlay MC, Sweet CS. Safety and tolerability of losartan potassium, an angiotensin II receptor antagonist, compared with hydrochlorothiazide, atenolol, felodipine ER, and angiotensin-converting enzyme inhibitors for the treatment of systemic hypertension. Am J Cardiol 1995; 75: 793-5.

Developed: 08/15/95
Interim revision: 09/21/95

---

**LOVASTATIN**—See *HMG-CoA Reductase Inhibitors (Systemic)*

---

# LOXAPINE Systemic

VA CLASSIFICATION (Primary/Secondary): CN709/CN900

Note: For a listing of dosage forms and brand names by country availability, see *Dosage Forms* section(s). For a listing of brand names for the articles in this monograph, refer to the General Index.

## Category

Antipsychotic; antianxiety agent–antidepressant.

## Indications

Note: Bracketed information in the *Indications* section refers to uses that are not included in U.S. product labeling.

### Accepted

Psychotic disorders (treatment)—Loxapine is indicated for the management of symptoms and characteristics of psychotic conditions.

[Anxiety associated with mental depression (treatment)][1]—Loxapine has been used to treat anxiety neurosis with depression.

[1]Not included in Canadian product labeling.

## Pharmacology/Pharmacokinetics

Note: The pharmacological effects of loxapine are similar to those of phenothiazines.

### Physicochemical characteristics

Chemical group—A tricyclic dibenzoxazepine derivative.

Molecular weight—

    Loxapine: 327.81.

    Loxapine succinate: 445.90.

pKa—6.6.

### Mechanism of action/Effect

Although the exact mechanism of action has not been completely established, loxapine is thought to improve psychotic conditions by blocking dopamine at postsynaptic receptor sites in the brain.

### Other actions/effects

Antiemetic—Inhibits the medullary chemoreceptor trigger zone.

Sedative—May cause indirect reduction of stimuli to the brain reticular activating system.

### Biotransformation

Hepatic. Major active metabolites are 8-hydroxyloxapine, 7-hydroxyloxapine, and 8-hydroxyamoxapine.

### Half-life

Oral—3 to 4 hours.

Intramuscular—12 hours.

### Onset of action

30 minutes.

**Time to peak effect**
$1^{1}/_{2}$ to 3 hours.

**Duration of action**
Up to 12 hours.

**Elimination**
Biliary, as unconjugated metabolites. Renal, as conjugated metabolites.

## Precautions to Consider

### Cross-sensitivity and/or related problems
Patients sensitive to amoxapine (a dibenzoxazepine derivative) may be sensitive to loxapine also.

### Carcinogenicity/Tumorigenicity
Most neuroleptic medications have been found to cause increased serum prolactin concentrations. Although the clinical significance of this increase is not known for most patients, *in vitro* studies have shown approximately $^{1}/_{3}$ of human breast cancers to be prolactin dependent. Additionally, an increase in mammary neoplasms has been found in rodents after chronic administration of neuroleptics. However, a definite association between the chronic administration of these medications and mammary tumorigenesis is considered inconclusive because of limited evidence available.

### Pregnancy/Reproduction
Pregnancy—Problems in humans have not been documented.
Fetotoxic effects, such as increased fetal resorptions and decreased fetal weight, were seen in rats and mice given doses within the range of the human therapeutic dose.
FDA Pregnancy Category C.

### Breast-feeding
It is not known whether loxapine is excreted in breast milk. However, loxapine and its metabolites have been found in the milk of lactating dogs.

### Pediatrics
Appropriate studies on the relationship of age to the effects of loxapine have not been performed in the pediatric population. Safety and efficacy have not been established.

### Geriatrics
Geriatric patients tend to develop higher plasma concentrations of loxapine because of changes in distribution due to decreases in lean body mass, total body water, and albumin, and often an increase in total body fat composition. These patients usually require lower initial dosage and a more gradual titration of dose.
Elderly patients also appear to be more prone to orthostatic hypotension and exhibit an increased sensitivity to the anticholinergic and sedative effects of loxapine. In addition, they are more prone to develop extrapyramidal side effects, such as tardive dyskinesia and parkinsonism. The signs of tardive dyskinesia are persistent, difficult to control, and, in some patients, appear to be irreversible. There is no known effective treatment. The symptoms may be masked during long treatment but may appear if loxapine is discontinued. Careful observation during treatment for early signs of tardive dyskinesia and reduction of dosage or discontinuation of medication may prevent a more severe manifestation of the syndrome.

### Dental
The peripheral anticholinergic effects of loxapine may decrease or inhibit salivary flow, especially in middle-aged or elderly patients, thus contributing to the development of caries, periodontal disease, oral candidiasis, and discomfort.
Extrapyramidal reactions induced by loxapine will result in increased motor activity of the head, face, and neck. Occlusal adjustments, bite registrations, and treatment for bruxism may be made less reliable.
The leukopenic and thrombocytopenic effects of loxapine may result in an increased incidence of microbial infection, delayed healing, and gingival bleeding. Although the occurrence is rare with loxapine, if leukopenia or thrombocytopenia occurs, dental work should be deferred until blood counts have returned to normal. Patients should be instructed in proper oral hygiene, including caution in use of regular toothbrushes, dental floss, and toothpicks.

### Drug interactions and/or related problems
The following drug interactions and/or related problems have been selected on the basis of their potential clinical significance (possible mechanism in parentheses where appropriate)—not necessarily inclusive (» = major clinical significance):

Note: Combinations containing any of the following medications, depending on the amount present, may also interact with this medication.

Although not all of the following interactions have been documented specifically for loxapine, a potential exists for their occurrence because of loxapine's close pharmacological similarity to phenothiazine medications.

» Alcohol or
» Central nervous system (CNS) depression–producing medications, other, especially anesthetics, barbiturates, and opioid (narcotic) analgesics (See *Appendix II*)
(concurrent use may potentiate and prolong the CNS depressant effects of either these medications or loxapine; dosage adjustments to approximately $^{1}/_{2}$ to $^{1}/_{4}$ of the usual dose may be necessary)

Amphetamines
(concurrent use may decrease the effects of amphetamines since loxapine produces alpha-adrenergic blockade)

Antacids or
Antidiarrheals, adsorbent
(concurrent use may inhibit the absorption of orally administered loxapine)

Anticholinergics or other medications with anticholinergic activity (See *Appendix II*) or
Antidyskinetic agents
(concurrent use with loxapine may intensify anticholinergic effects of both medications; patients should be advised to report gastrointestinal problems since paralytic ileus may occur; antidyskinetic agents should not be used for prophylaxis of pseudoparkinsonism during therapy with loxapine)

Anticonvulsants
(loxapine may lower the seizure threshold; dosage adjustment of anticonvulsant medications may be necessary; potentiation of anticonvulsant effects does not occur)

Antidepressants, tricyclic or
Monoamine oxidase (MAO) inhibitors, including furazolidone, procarbazine, and more than 10 mg of selegiline a day
(concurrent use may prolong and intensify the sedative and anticholinergic effects of either these medications or loxapine; serum concentrations of the antidepressant may be increased when it is administered concomitantly with loxapine; dosage reduction of antidepressant may be necessary)

Bromocriptine
(concurrent use with loxapine may antagonize effects of bromocriptine on serum prolactin activity; dosage adjustment of bromocriptine may be necessary)

Carbamazepine
(in addition to enhancement of CNS depressant effects and lowering of seizure threshold, the concurrent use of carbamazepine with loxapine, and possibly other neuroleptics, may decrease plasma concentrations of the neuroleptic; patient should be observed for clinical signs of ineffectiveness of loxapine and dosage adjusted accordingly)

Dopamine
(when dopamine is used concurrently with loxapine, alpha-adrenergic blocking action of loxapine may antagonize peripheral vasoconstriction produced by high doses of dopamine)

Ephedrine
(when used concurrently with loxapine, alpha-adrenergic blocking action of loxapine may decrease the pressor response to ephedrine)

Epinephrine
(alpha-adrenergic effects of epinephrine may be blocked when epinephrine is used concurrently with loxapine, possibly resulting in severe hypotension and tachycardia)

» Extrapyramidal reaction–causing medications, other (See *Appendix II*)
(concurrent use with loxapine may increase the severity and frequency of extrapyramidal effects)

» Guanadrel or
» Guanethidine
(concurrent use with loxapine may decrease the hypotensive effects of these agents because of their displacement from and inhibition of uptake by adrenergic neurons)

Levodopa
(concurrent use may inhibit the antiparkinsonian effects of levodopa by blocking dopamine receptors in the brain)

Metaraminol
(concurrent use usually decreases, but does not reverse or completely block, the pressor effect of metaraminol)

Methoxamine
(prior administration of alpha-adrenergic blocking agents such as loxapine may block the pressor effect and decrease the duration of action of methoxamine)

Ototoxic medications, especially ototoxic antibiotics
(concurrent use with loxapine may mask the symptoms of ototoxicity such as tinnitus, dizziness, or vertigo)

Phenylephrine or
Norepinephrine
(prior administration of loxapine may decrease the pressor response to phenylephrine or norepinephrine because of the alpha-adrenergic blocking action of loxapine, but severe hypotension associated with overdosage of loxapine would be expected to respond to either agent)

## Medical considerations/Contraindications
The medical considerations/contraindications included here have been selected on the basis of their potential clinical significance (reasons given in parentheses where appropriate)—not necessarily inclusive (» = major clinical significance).

*Except under special circumstances, this medication should not be used when the following medical problems exist:*
» CNS depression, drug-induced, severe or
» Comatose states
(may be exacerbated)

*Risk-benefit should be considered when the following medical problems exist:*
» Alcoholism, active
(CNS depression may be potentiated)
Cardiovascular disease
(increased risk of arrhythmias and hypotension)
Glaucoma, or predisposition to or
Parkinson's disease or
Urinary retention
(may be exacerbated)
» Hepatic function impairment
(metabolism may be altered)
Prostatic hypertrophy, symptomatic
(risk of urinary retention)
Seizure disorders
(seizure threshold may be lowered)
Sensitivity to amoxapine or loxapine

## Patient monitoring
The following may be especially important in patient monitoring (other tests may be warranted in some patients, depending on condition; » = major clinical significance):
Blood cell counts
(may be required at periodic intervals during high-dose or prolonged therapy)
Careful observation for early symptoms of tardive dyskinesia
(recommended at periodic intervals, especially in the elderly and patients on high or extended maintenance dosage; loxapine should be discontinued if early symptoms of tardive dyskinesia appear, since there is no known effective treatment)
Hepatic function determinations and
Urine tests for bilirubin and bile
(may be required if jaundice or grippe-like symptoms occur)
Ophthalmologic examination
(may be advisable at periodic intervals during high-dose or prolonged therapy since deposition of particulate matter in the lens and cornea has occurred with some other antipsychotic medications)

# Side/Adverse Effects
The following side/adverse effects have been selected on the basis of their potential clinical significance (possible signs and symptoms in parentheses where appropriate)—not necessarily inclusive:

## Those indicating need for medical attention
Incidence more frequent
*Akathisia* (restlessness or need to keep moving); *extrapyramidal effects, parkinsonian* (difficulty in speaking or swallowing; loss of balance control; mask-like face; shuffling walk; slowed movements; stiffness of arms and legs; trembling and shaking of fingers and hands); *tardive dyskinesia, persistent* (lip smacking or puckering; puffing of cheeks; rapid or worm-like movements of tongue; uncontrolled movements of the arms and legs; uncontrolled chewing movements)
Note: *Parkinsonian extrapyramidal effects* are more common during first few days of treatment or following dosage increases.
*Tardive dyskinesia* is initially dose related, but may increase with long-term treatment and total cumulative dose; may persist after discontinuation of loxapine.

Incidence less frequent
*Allergic reaction* (skin rash); *anticholinergic effect* (difficult urination); *constipation, severe*—may lead to paralytic ileus; *extrapyramidal effects, dystonic* (difficulty in swallowing; inability to move eyes; muscle spasms, especially of the neck and back; twisting movements of body)—may be severe
Incidence rare
*Agranulocytosis* (sore throat and fever; unusual bleeding or bruising); *jaundice, obstructive* (yellow eyes or skin); *neuroleptic malignant syndrome [NMS]* (convulsions; difficult or unusually fast breathing; fast heartbeat or irregular pulse; high fever; high or low [irregular] blood pressure; increased sweating; loss of bladder control; severe muscle stiffness or rigidity; unusual tiredness or weakness; unusually pale skin); *tardive dystonia* (increased blinking or spasms of eyelid; unusual facial expressions or body positions; uncontrolled twisting movements of neck, trunk, arms, or legs)
Note: *NMS* may occur at any time during neuroleptic therapy, but is more commonly seen soon after start of therapy, or after patient has switched from one neuroleptic to another, during combined therapy with another psychotropic medication, or after a dosage increase. Along with the overt signs of skeletal muscle rigidity, hyperthermia, autonomic dysfunction, and altered consciousness, differential diagnosis may reveal leukocytosis (9500 to 26,000 cells per cubic millimeter), elevated liver function tests, and elevated creatine phosphokinase (CPK).

## Those indicating need for medical attention only if they continue or are bothersome
Incidence more frequent
*Blurred vision; confusion; drowsiness; dryness of mouth; hypotension, orthostatic* (dizziness, lightheadedness, or fainting)
Incidence less frequent
*Constipation, mild; decreased sexual ability; enlargement of breasts, in males and females; headache; increased sensitivity of skin to sun; missing menstrual periods; nausea or vomiting; trouble in sleeping; unusual secretion of milk; weight gain*

## Those indicating the need for medical attention if they occur after the medication is discontinued
*Dizziness; dyskinesia, withdrawal emergent* (uncontrolled, repetitive movements of mouth, tongue, and jaw); *nausea and vomiting; stomach upset or pain; trembling of fingers and hands*

# Overdose
For specific information on the agents used in the management of loxapine overdose, see:
• *Norepinephrine* and *Phenylephrine* in *Sympathomimetic Agents—Cardiovascular Use (Parenteral-Systemic)* monograph.
For more information on the management of overdose or unintentional ingestion, **contact a Poison Control Center** (see *Poison Control Center Listing*).

## Clinical effects of overdose
The following effects have been selected on the basis of their potential clinical significance (possible signs and symptoms in parentheses where appropriate)—not necessarily inclusive:
*Dizziness; drowsiness, severe, or comatose state; muscle trembling, jerking, stiffness, or uncontrolled movements, severe; troubled breathing, severe; unusual tiredness or weakness, severe*

## Treatment of overdose
No specific antidote for loxapine is available. Treatment is symptomatic and supportive.
Specific treatment—
In event of severe hypotension, epinephrine should not be used, since it may further lower blood pressure in presence of partial adrenergic blockade. Norepinephrine or phenylephrine may be effective.
Supportive care—
Oxygen, intravenous fluids, anticonvulsant therapy, and anticholinergic agents may be indicated.
Patients in whom intentional overdose is known or suspected should be referred for psychiatric consultation.
Note: Because of the antiemetic effect of loxapine, centrally acting emetics, such as syrup of ipecac, may have little effect.

# Patient Consultation
As an aid to patient consultation, refer to *Advice for the Patient, Loxapine (Systemic)*.

In providing consultation, consider emphasizing the following selected information (» = major clinical significance):

**Before using this medication**
» Conditions affecting use, especially:
    Sensitivity to loxapine or amoxapine
    Pregnancy—Studies in rats showed an increased number of fetal resorptions and decreased fetal weight
    Use in the elderly—Elderly patients are more likely to develop extrapyramidal, anticholinergic, hypotensive, and sedative effects; reduced dosage recommended
    Dental—Loxapine-induced blood dyscrasias may result in infections, delayed healing, and bleeding; dry mouth may cause caries and candidiasis; increased motor activity of face, head, and neck may interfere with some dental procedures
    Other medications, especially alcohol, other CNS depression–producing medications, other extrapyramidal reaction–producing medications, guanadrel, or guanethidine
    Other medical problems, especially severe CNS depression, active alcoholism, or hepatic function impairment

**Proper use of this medication**
    Taking with food, milk, or water to reduce stomach irritation
    Measuring oral solution only with dropper provided by manufacturer
    Mixing oral solution with orange or grapefruit juice just before each dose
» Compliance with therapy; not taking more or less medicine, nor taking more often, than directed
» Proper dosing
    Missed dose: Taking as soon as possible; not taking if within 1 hour of next dose; returning to regular dosing schedule; not doubling doses
» Proper storage

**Precautions while using this medication**
    Regular visits to physician to check progress of therapy
» Checking with physician before discontinuing medication; gradual dosage reduction may be needed
» Avoiding use of alcoholic beverages or other CNS depressants during therapy
    Avoiding use of antacids or antidiarrheal medication within 2 hours of taking loxapine
» Possible drowsiness; caution when driving, using machines, or doing other things requiring alertness while taking loxapine
    Possible dizziness or lightheadedness; caution when getting up suddenly from a lying or sitting position
    Possible skin photosensitivity; avoiding unprotected exposure to sun; using protective clothing; using a sun block product that includes protection against both UVA-caused photosensitivity reactions and UVB-caused sunburn reactions; avoiding use of sunlamp, tanning bed, or tanning booth
    Possible dryness of the mouth: using sugarless gum or candy, ice, or saliva substitute for relief; checking with physician or dentist if dry mouth continues for more than 2 weeks
» Caution if any kind of surgery, dental treatment, or emergency treatment is required

**Side/adverse effects**
    Side effects are more likely to occur in the elderly
    Signs of potential side effects, especially tardive dyskinesia, akathisia, dystonias, parkinsonism effects, anticholinergic effects, allergic skin reactions, agranulocytosis, obstructive jaundice, neuroleptic malignant syndrome (NMS), constipation (severe)
» Stopping medication and notifying physician immediately if symptoms of NMS appear, especially muscle rigidity, fever, difficult or fast breathing, seizures, fast heartbeat, increased sweating, loss of bladder control, unusually pale skin, unusual tiredness or weakness
» Notifying physician immediately if early symptoms of tardive dyskinesia appear, such as fine worm-like movements of the tongue or other uncontrolled movements of the mouth, tongue, jaw, or arms and legs; dosage adjustment or discontinuation may be needed to prevent irreversibility
    Possibility of withdrawal symptoms

## General Dosing Information

Dosage must be individualized by titration from the lower dose range over the first 7 to 10 days of therapy until effective control of psychotic symptoms is obtained. After such control is established, the dosage is gradually decreased to the lowest level that will maintain an adequate clinical response.

Loxapine has an antiemetic effect that may mask signs of overdose of other medication or may obscure diagnosis of conditions whose main symptoms include nausea. However, since the antiemetic effect of lox-apine is central, nausea is not affected when it results from vestibular stimulation or local gastrointestinal irritation.

Upon cessation of extended maintenance therapy, a gradual reduction in loxapine dosage is recommended since abrupt withdrawal may cause some patients to experience transient dyskinetic signs, nausea, vomiting, gastritis, trembling, and dizziness.

**For oral dosage forms only**
The oral solution should be measured only with the dropper provided by the manufacturer and diluted with orange or grapefruit juice just before each dose.

**For parenteral dosage form only**
Because hypotension is a possible side effect of loxapine, intramuscular administration is used for bedfast patients or for appropriate acute ambulatory patients who can be closely monitored. Patients should remain lying down for at least $1/2$ hour after the injection to avoid possible acute orthostatic hypotensive effects.

**Diet/Nutrition**
This medication may be taken with food or a full glass (240 mL) of water or milk if necessary to lessen stomach irritation.

**For treatment of adverse effects**
Neuroleptic malignant syndrome—
    Treatment is essentially symptomatic and supportive and includes the following
    • *Discontinuing loxapine immediately*.
    • Hyperthermia—Administering antipyretics (aspirin or acetaminophen); using cooling blanket.
    • Dehydration—Restoring fluids and electrolytes.
    • Cardiovascular instability—Monitoring blood pressure and cardiac rhythm closely.
    • Hypoxia—Administering oxygen; consider airway insertion and assisted ventilation.
    • Muscle rigidity—Dantrolene sodium may be administered (100 to 300 mg a day in divided doses; 1.25 to 1.5 mg per kg of body weight intravenously). Bromocriptine (5 to 7.5 mg every eight hours) has been used to reverse hyperpyrexia and muscle rigidity.
Parkinsonism—
    Many authorities advise that the only appropriate treatment of extrapyramidal symptoms is reduction of the antipsychotic dosage, if possible. Oral antidyskinetic agents such as trihexyphenidyl, 2 mg three times a day, or benztropine, may be effective in treating more severe parkinsonism and acute motor restlessness but should be used sparingly, only when side effects appear, and then usually for no longer than 3 months. Milder effects may be treated by adjusting dosage. In the elderly patient, the use of amantadine, 100 to 200 mg at bedtime, minimizes severe anticholinergic effects that may occur with other antidyskinetics.
Akathisia—
    May respond to antiparkinsonian drugs or propranolol (30 to 80 mg a day); nadolol (40 mg a day); pindolol (5 to 60 mg a day), lorazepam (1 or 2 mg two or three times a day), or diazepam (2 mg two or three times a day), but often requires dosage reduction of loxapine.
Dystonia—
    Acute dystonic postures or oculogyric crisis may be relieved by parenteral administration of benztropine (2 mg intramuscularly); diphenhydramine (50 mg intramuscularly); or diazepam (5 to 7.5 mg intravenously), to be followed by oral antidyskinetic medication for one or two days to prevent recurrent dystonic episodes. Dosage adjustments of loxapine may control these effects, and discontinuation of loxapine may reverse severe symptoms.
Tardive dyskinesia or tardive dystonia—
    No known effective treatment. Dosage of loxapine should be lowered or medication discontinued, if clinically feasible, at earliest signs of tardive dyskinesia or tardive dystonia, to prevent irreversible effects.

## Oral Dosage Forms

Note: The dosing and strengths of the dosage forms available are expressed in terms of loxapine base.

### LOXAPINE HYDROCHLORIDE ORAL SOLUTION

**Usual adult dose**
Antipsychotic—
    Initial: Oral, 10 mg (base) two times a day, the dosage being increased gradually during the first seven to ten days as needed for symptomatic control and as tolerated.
    Maintenance: Oral, 15 to 25 mg (base) two to four times a day.

Note: This dosage form is intended primarily for institutional use.

Dose to be measured only with calibrated dropper provided by manufacturer.

Severely disturbed patients—Initial: Oral, 10 to 25 mg (base) two times a day.

**Usual adult prescribing limits**
Up to 250 mg (base) a day.

**Usual pediatric dose**
Children up to 16 years of age—Safety and efficacy have not been established.

**Usual geriatric dose**
Initial, oral, 3 to 5 mg (base) two times a day.

**Strength(s) usually available**
U.S.—
    25 mg (base) per mL (Rx) [*Loxitane C* (propylene glycol)].
Canada—
    25 mg (base) per mL (Rx) [*Loxapac*].

**Packaging and storage**
Store below 40 °C (104 °F), preferably between 15 and 30 °C (59 and 86 °F), in a well-closed container, unless otherwise specified by manufacturer. Protect from freezing.

**Auxiliary labeling**
- Take by mouth.
- May cause drowsiness.
- Avoid alcoholic beverages.
- Must be diluted before use.

**Note**
When dispensing, include the manufacturer-provided graduated dropper for dose measuring.

Explain administration technique and the necessary dilution in orange or grapefruit juice.

## LOXAPINE SUCCINATE CAPSULES

**Usual adult dose**
See *Loxapine Hydrochloride Oral Solution.*

**Usual pediatric dose**
See *Loxapine Hydrochloride Oral Solution.*

**Strength(s) usually available**
U.S.—
    5 mg (base) (Rx) [*Loxitane;* GENERIC].
    10 mg (base) (Rx) [*Loxitane;* GENERIC].
    25 mg (base) (Rx) [*Loxitane;* GENERIC].
    50 mg (base) (Rx) [*Loxitane;* GENERIC].
Canada—
    Not commercially available.

**Packaging and storage**
Store below 40 °C (104 °F), preferably between 15 and 30 °C (59 and 86 °F), in a well-closed container, unless otherwise specified by manufacturer.

**Auxiliary labeling**
- May cause drowsiness.
- Avoid alcoholic beverages.

## LOXAPINE SUCCINATE TABLETS

**Usual adult dose**
See *Loxapine Hydrochloride Oral Solution.*

**Usual pediatric dose**
See *Loxapine Hydrochloride Oral Solution.*

**Strength(s) usually available**
U.S.—
    Not commercially available.
Canada—
    5 mg (base) (Rx) [*Loxapac*].
    10 mg (base) (Rx) [*Loxapac*].
    25 mg (base) (Rx) [*Loxapac*].
    50 mg (base) (Rx) [*Loxapac*].

**Packaging and storage**
Store below 40 °C (104 °F), preferably between 15 and 30 °C (59 and 86 °F), in a well-closed container, unless otherwise specified by manufacturer.

**Auxiliary labeling**
- May cause drowsiness.
- Avoid alcoholic beverages.

## Parenteral Dosage Forms

Note: The dosing and strengths of the dosage forms available are expressed in terms of loxapine base.

### LOXAPINE HYDROCHLORIDE INJECTION

**Usual adult dose**
Intramuscular, 12.5 to 50 mg (base) every four to six hours as needed and tolerated.

Note: For intramuscular administration only. Not for intravenous use.

**Usual adult prescribing limits**
Up to 250 mg (base) a day.

**Usual pediatric dose**
Children up to 16 years of age—Safety and efficacy have not been established.

**Strength(s) usually available**
U.S.—
    50 mg (base) per mL (Rx) [*Loxitane IM* (polysorbate 80 [5% w/v]; propylene glycol [70% v/v])].
Canada—
    50 mg (base) per mL (Rx) [*Loxapac*].

**Packaging and storage**
Store below 40 °C (104 °F), preferably between 15 and 30 °C (59 and 86 °F), unless otherwise specified by manufacturer. Protect from light. Protect from freezing.

**Stability**
A darkening of the solution to a light amber will not alter potency or effectiveness. Do not use if markedly discolored or if a precipitate is present.

**Note**
Advise patient to remain lying down for ½ hour following administration to avoid severe orthostatic hypotension.

Revised: 01/29/93

# LYPRESSIN   Systemic

VA CLASSIFICATION (Primary/Secondary): HS702/CV900

Note: For a listing of dosage forms and brand names by country availability, see *Dosage Forms* section(s). For a listing of brand names for the articles in this monograph, refer to the General Index.

## Category

Antidiuretic (central diabetes insipidus).

## Indications

**Accepted**

Diabetes insipidus, central (treatment)—Lypressin is indicated for the prevention or control of polydipsia, polyuria, and dehydration associated with central diabetes insipidus caused by insufficient antidiuretic hormone.

Lypressin may be useful in patients who are unresponsive to other forms of therapy or who have shown various adverse reactions to other preparations of antidiuretic hormone of animal origin.

Lypressin is ineffective in the treatment of polyuria associated with nephrogenic or psychogenic diabetes insipidus, renal disease, hypokalemia, hypercalcemia, or the administration of demeclocycline or lithium.

## Pharmacology/Pharmacokinetics

**Physicochemical characteristics**
Source—Lypressin is a synthetic vasopressin analog.
Molecular weight—1056.22.

## Mechanism of action/Effect

Increases water reabsorption in the kidney by increasing the cellular permeability of the collecting ducts, resulting in an increase in urine osmolality with a concurrent decrease in urine output.

### Other actions/effects

Little pressor activity.

### Absorption

Rapid from nasal mucosa.

### Biotransformation

Renal and hepatic.

### Half-life

Approximately 15 minutes.

### Onset of action

Within 1 hour.

### Time to peak effect

30 to 120 minutes.

### Duration of action

3 to 4 hours.

### Elimination

Renal, a small amount unchanged.

## Precautions to Consider

### Cross-sensitivity and/or related problems

Patients sensitive to vasopressin may also be sensitive to lypressin.

### Carcinogenicity

Studies have not been done.

### Pregnancy/Reproduction

Pregnancy—Studies have not been done in either animals or humans.
FDA Pregnancy Category C.

### Breast-feeding

It is not known whether lypressin is distributed into breast milk. However, problems in humans have not been documented.

### Pediatrics

Appropriate studies on the relationship of age to the effects of lypressin have not been performed in the pediatric population. However, pediatrics-specific problems that would limit the usefulness of this medication in children are not expected.

### Geriatrics

No information is available on the relationship of age to the effects of lypressin in geriatric patients.

### Drug interactions and/or related problems

The following drug interactions and/or related problems have been selected on the basis of their potential clinical significance (possible mechanism in parentheses where appropriate)—not necessarily inclusive (» = major clinical significance):

Note: Combinations containing any of the following medications, depending on the amount present, may also interact with this medication.

Carbamazepine or
Chlorpropamide or
Clofibrate
    (may potentiate the antidiuretic effect of lypressin when used concurrently)

Demeclocycline or
Lithium or
Norepinephrine
    (may decrease the antidiuretic effect of lypressin when used concurrently)

### Medical considerations/Contraindications

The medical considerations/contraindications included here have been selected on the basis of their potential clinical significance (reasons given in parentheses where appropriate)—not necessarily inclusive (» = major clinical significance).

*Risk-benefit should be considered when the following medical problems exist:*

Allergic rhinitis or
Nasal congestion or
Upper respiratory infection
    (may interfere with absorption of lypressin through the nasal mucosa)

Hypertensive cardiovascular disease
    (although pressor effects of lypressin are minimal)
Sensitivity to lypressin

## Side/Adverse Effects

The following side/adverse effects have been selected on the basis of their potential clinical significance (possible signs and symptoms in parentheses where appropriate)—not necessarily inclusive:

### Those indicating need for medical attention

Incidence rare
    *Inadvertent inhalation* (continuing cough; feeling of tightness in chest; shortness of breath; troubled breathing); *water intoxication and overdose* (coma; confusion; continuing headache; drowsiness; problems with urination; seizures; weight gain)

### Those indicating need for medical attention only if they continue or are bothersome

Incidence less frequent or rare
    *Abdominal or stomach cramps; excessive administration with drippage into pharynx* (heartburn); *headache; increased bowel movements; irritation or pain in the eye; itching, irritation, or sores inside nose; runny or stuffy nose*

## Overdose

For specific information on the agents used in the management of lypressin overdose, see *Furosemide* in *Diuretics, Loop (Systemic)* monograph.

For more information on the management of overdose or unintentional ingestion, **contact a Poison Control Center** (see *Poison Control Center Listing*).

### Treatment of overdose

To enhance elimination—Diuresis with furosemide and hypertonic saline if there is a risk of congestive heart failure.

Supportive care—Withdrawal of lypressin and restriction of fluid intake. Correction of electrolyte imbalance. Patients in whom intentional overdose is known or suspected should be referred for psychiatric consultation.

## Patient Consultation

As an aid to patient consultation, refer to *Advice for the Patient, Lypressin (Systemic)*.

In providing consultation, consider emphasizing the following selected information (» = major clinical significance):

### Before using this medication

» Conditions affecting use, especially:
    Allergies to lypressin or vasopressin

### Proper use of this medication

» Importance of not using more medication than the amount prescribed
Proper administration technique
» Proper dosing
    Missed dose: Using as soon as possible; not using at all if almost time for next dose; not doubling doses
» Proper storage

### Side/adverse effects

Signs of potential side effects, especially inadvertent inhalation or water intoxication

## General Dosing Information

Lypressin is administered intranasally; it should not be inhaled.

Patients with nasal congestion, allergic rhinitis, and upper respiratory infections may experience decreased efficacy because of a decrease in absorption through the nasal mucosa. Larger doses of lypressin or adjunctive therapy may be required in such patients.

Since more than 2 or 3 sprays per nostril usually results in wastage, it is recommended that the time interval between sprays be reduced rather than increasing the number of sprays if a patient requires more than 3 sprays.

## Nasal Dosage Forms

### LYPRESSIN NASAL SOLUTION USP

#### Usual adult and adolescent dose

Antidiuretic—
    Intranasal, 1 or 2 sprays in each nostril four times a day.
Note: Whenever the frequency of urination increases or increased thirst develops, the patient may administer 1 or 2 sprays to control these symptoms.

If the regular daily dosage of lypressin does not control nocturia, an additional dose may be given at bedtime.

The dosage has ranged from 1 spray per day at bedtime to 10 sprays in each nostril every three to four hours.

## Usual pediatric dose

Children up to 6 weeks of age—Safety and efficacy have not been established in children less than 6 weeks of age.

Children 6 weeks of age and over— See *Usual adult and adolescent dose.*

## Strength(s) usually available

U.S.—

0.185 mg (equivalent to 50 USP Posterior Pituitary Units) per mL; or approximately 0.007 mg (equivalent to 2 Posterior Pituitary Units) per spray (Rx) [*Diapid* (methylparaben; propylparaben)].

## Packaging and storage

Store below 40 °C (104 °F), preferably between 15 and 30 °C (59 and 86 °F), unless otherwise specified by manufacturer. Protect from freezing.

## Auxiliary labeling

• For the nose.

## Note

Instruct patient to assume a vertical position with head upright and to hold bottle upright when administering the spray.

Revised: 07/01/93

# MAFENIDE    Topical†

VA CLASSIFICATION (Primary/Secondary): DE101/DE102

Note: For a listing of dosage forms and brand names by country availability, see *Dosage Forms* section(s). For a listing of brand names for the articles in this monograph, refer to the General Index.

†Not commercially available in Canada.

## Category

Antibacterial (topical); antifungal (topical).

Note: Mafenide is a broad-spectrum antibacterial agent having an antibacterial spectrum similar to that of silver sulfadiazine.

## Indications

Note: Bracketed information in the *Indications* section refers to uses that are not included in U.S. product labeling.

**Accepted**

Burn wound infections (prophylaxis and treatment)—Mafenide is indicated [as a primary agent] in the topical prophylaxis and treatment of burn wound infections caused by *Candida albicans (Monilia albicans)*, *Citrobacter* species, *Enterobacter* species (including *E. cloacae*), enterococci, *Escherichia coli*, *Klebsiella* species, *Mima-Herellea* species, *Morganella morganii (Proteus morganii)*, *P. mirabilis*, *P. vulgaris*, *Providencia rettgeri (Proteus rettgeri)*, *Pseudomonas aeruginosa*, *Serratia* species, *Staphylococcus aureus*, *S. epidermidis*, and beta-hemolytic streptococci in patients with second- and third-degree burns.

[Mafenide is also indicated as a primary agent in the treatment of burn wound infections in patients having a thick eschar (e.g., in electrical burns).]

Not all species or strains of a particular organism may be susceptible to mafenide.

## Pharmacology/Pharmacokinetics

**Physicochemical characteristics**

Chemical group—Methylated sulfonamide

Molecular weight—246.28.

Other characteristics—Sulfonamides have certain chemical similarities to some goitrogens, diuretics (acetazolamide and thiazides), and oral antidiabetic agents.

**Mechanism of action/Effect**

Bacteriostatic for many gram-negative and gram-positive organisms, including *Pseudomonas aeruginosa* and certain strains of anaerobes. Unlike most sulfonamides, mafenide is not inhibited by aminobenzoates (PABA), blood, serum, or pus. Its activity is not altered by changes in acidity. Mafenide is highly soluble and diffuses into and through eschar.

Topical mafenide produces a marked reduction in number of bacteria present, even in avascular tissue of second- and third-degree burns. Reduction in bacterial growth has been reported to result in spontaneous healing of deep partial-thickness burns, thus preventing their conversion to full-thickness burns. However, delayed eschar separation has occurred in some patients.

**Other actions/effects**

Mafenide and its metabolite also inhibit carbonic anhydrase activity, which may result in metabolic acidosis. However, hyperventilation usually compensates for the acidosis in normal persons.

**Absorption**

Mafenide is absorbed through devascularized areas into the systemic circulation following topical administration.

**Biotransformation**

Rapidly metabolized to a nontoxic metabolite, *p*-carboxybenzenesulfonamide, which has no antibacterial activity.

**Time to peak concentration**

24 hours following initial application in patients with second- and third-degree burns covering approximately 35 to 70% of the total body surface.

**Elimination**

Renal—Metabolite rapidly excreted in urine in high concentrations; however, the parent compound has not been detected in urine.

## Precautions to Consider

**Cross-sensitivity and/or related problems**

Patients sensitive to other sulfonamides, furosemide, thiazide diuretics, sulfonylureas, or carbonic anhydrase inhibitors may be sensitive to this medication also.

**Carcinogenicity/Mutagenicity**

Long-term studies in animals have not been performed to evaluate mafenide's carcinogenic or mutagenic potential.

**Pregnancy/Reproduction**

Fertility—Long-term studies in animals or humans have not been performed to evaluate mafenide's effect on fertility.

Pregnancy—Studies have not been done in humans. However, use is not recommended in women of child-bearing potential unless the burn area covers more than 20% of the total body surface. In addition, absorbed sulfonamides may displace bilirubin from protein-binding sites in the fetal plasma, thus increasing the possibility of kernicterus in the neonate. Therefore, mafenide should not be used at term.

Studies have not been done in animals.

FDA Pregnancy Category C.

**Breast-feeding**

It is not known whether mafenide, applied topically, is distributed into breast milk. However, mafenide is absorbed systemically following topical application. Caution is recommended in nursing women, since systemically administered sulfonamides are distributed into breast milk and may cause kernicterus in nursing infants. Also, sulfonamides may cause hemolytic anemia in glucose-6-phosphate dehydrogenase (G6PD)-deficient infants.

**Pediatrics**

Use is not recommended in premature or newborn infants up to 2 months of age, since sulfonamides may cause kernicterus in these neonates.

**Geriatrics**

Appropriate studies on the relationship of age to the effects of mafenide have not been performed in the geriatric population. However, no geriatrics-specific problems have been documented to date.

**Medical considerations/Contraindications**

The medical considerations/contraindications included here have been selected on the basis of their potential clinical significance (reasons given in parentheses where appropriate)—not necessarily inclusive (» = major clinical significance).

*Risk-benefit should be considered when the following medical problems exist:*

Blood dyscrasias
(sulfonamides may cause or contribute to blood dyscrasias)

Glucose-6-phosphate dehydrogenase (G6PD) deficiency
(sulfonamides may cause hemolytic anemia in G6PD-deficient patients)

Metabolic acidosis or
Pulmonary function impairment or
Renal function impairment
(mafenide and its metabolite may inhibit carbonic anhydrase activity, causing or contributing to metabolic acidosis; pulmonary or renal function impairment may increase this risk)

Sensitivity to mafenide

**Patient monitoring**

The following may be especially important in patient monitoring (other tests may be warranted in some patients, depending on condition; » = major clinical significance):

»  Acid-base balance
(mafenide and its metabolite inhibit carbonic anhydrase activity, which may result in metabolic acidosis; close monitoring of acid-base balance is recommended during therapy with mafenide, especially in patients with extensive second-degree or partial-thickness burns and in patients with pulmonary or renal function impairment)

## Side/Adverse Effects

Note: If significant absorption occurs, side/adverse effects (e.g., Stevens-Johnson syndrome, Lyell's syndrome, blood dyscrasias, crystalluria) usually seen with systemic sulfonamides may occur with mafenide therapy, although few have been reported.

Fatal hemolytic anemia, accompanied by disseminated intravascular coagulation, has been reported with mafenide therapy.

The following side/adverse effects have been selected on the basis of their potential clinical significance (possible signs and symptoms in parentheses where appropriate)—not necessarily inclusive:

**Those indicating need for medical attention**
Incidence less frequent
   *Allergic reaction* (itching, skin rash or redness, swelling of face or skin; wheezing or troubled breathing)
Incidence rare
   *Bleeding or oozing of skin; metabolic acidosis* (drowsiness; nausea; rapid, deep breathing)—hyperventilation may compensate for the acidosis

**Those indicating need for medical attention only if they continue or are bothersome**
Incidence more frequent
   *Pain or burning feeling on treated area(s)*

## Patient Consultation

As an aid to patient consultation, refer to *Advice for the Patient, Mafenide (Topical)*.

In providing consultation, consider emphasizing the following selected information (» = major clinical significance):

**Before using this medication**
» Conditions affecting use, especially:
   Sensitivity to mafenide, other sulfonamides, furosemide, thiazide diuretics, sulfonylureas, or carbonic anhydrase inhibitors
   Pregnancy—Use is not recommended in women of child-bearing potential unless burn area covers more than 20% of total body surface; absorbed sulfonamides may increase the possibility of kernicterus in the neonate; do not use at term
   Breast-feeding—May cause kernicterus in nursing infants; may cause hemolytic anemia in G6PD-deficient infants
   Use in children—Not recommended in premature or newborn infants up to 2 months of age; may cause kernicterus

**Proper use of this medication**
*To use:*
   Before applying, cleansing affected area(s); removing necrotic or burned skin and other debris
   Wearing a sterile glove to apply the medication; applying a thin layer (approximately 1.5 mm) to affected area(s); keeping affected area(s) covered with the medication at all times
   Reapplying mafenide that has been removed by patient activity or washed off by bathing, showering, or use of a whirlpool bath
   After applying, covering treated area(s) with a dressing or leaving treated area(s) uncovered as desired
» Compliance with full course of therapy; continuing medication until burn has healed or is ready for skin grafting
» Proper dosing
   Missed dose: Applying as soon as possible; not applying if almost time for next dose
» Proper storage

**Precautions while using this medication**
   Regular visits to physician to check progress
   Checking with physician if no improvement within a few days or weeks (for more serious burns or burns over more extensive areas)

**Side/adverse effects**
   Signs of potential side effects, especially allergic reaction, bleeding or oozing of skin, or metabolic acidosis

## General Dosing Information

Mafenide may be used concurrently with sutilains ointment without loss of enzyme activity.

Before application of mafenide, burn wounds should be cleansed and debrided following control of shock and pain. A sterile glove should be worn to apply the medication. A thin layer (approximately 1.5 mm) of mafenide should then be applied to the affected area(s). A thicker layer is not recommended. The burn areas should be kept covered with mafenide at all times. When necessary, the medication should be reapplied to any areas from which it has been removed by patient activity or washed off by bathing, showering, or use of a whirlpool bath.

Dressings, although not required, may be applied if necessary.

Treatment with mafenide should be continued until satisfactory healing has occurred or until the burn site is ready for skin grafting. Therapy should not be discontinued while the possibility of infection exists, unless significant toxicity occurs.

Burn patients should be bathed daily, if feasible, to aid in debridement of the burned area(s). Whirlpool baths are particularly helpful, although burn patients may be bathed in bed or in a shower. Following this, mafenide should be reapplied.

**For treatment of adverse effects**
Recommended treatment consists of the following
   • Administering antihistamines for allergic reaction.
   • Discontinuing mafenide therapy for 24 to 48 hours, continuing fluid therapy, administering sodium bicarbonate parenterally, and using assisted ventilation, if necessary, to restore acid-base balance.

## Topical Dosage Forms
### MAFENIDE ACETATE CREAM USP

**Usual adult and adolescent dose**
Antibacterial or
Antifungal—
   Topical, to the affected area(s), one or two times a day, applied to a thickness of approximately 1.5 mm.

**Usual pediatric dose**
Antibacterial or
Antifungal—
   Premature and newborn infants up to 2 months of age: Use is not recommended, since sulfonamides may cause kernicterus in these neonates.
   Infants and children 2 months of age and over: See *Usual adult and adolescent dose.*

**Strength(s) usually available**
U.S.—
   85 mg (base) per gram (Rx) [*Sulfamylon* (sodium metabisulfite; methylparaben; propylparaben; edetate disodium)].
Canada—
   Not commercially available.

**Packaging and storage**
Store below 40 °C (104 °F), in a tight, light-resistant container. Protect from freezing.

**Auxiliary labeling**
   • For external use only.
   • Continue medicine for full time of treatment.

**Additional information**
Mafenide acetate cream is available in a nonstaining, water-miscible base. It can be readily washed off with water.

Revised: 04/22/94

---

## MAGALDRATE—See *Antacids (Oral-Local)*

---

## MAGALDRATE-CONTAINING COMBINATIONS—
Magaldrate and Simethicone (Oral-Local)—See *Antacids (Oral-Local)*

---

## MAGNESIA-CONTAINING COMBINATIONS—

Alumina and Magnesia (Oral-Local)—See *Antacids (Oral-Local)*
Alumina, Magnesia, and Calcium Carbonate (Oral-Local)—See *Antacids (Oral-Local)*
Alumina, Magnesia, Calcium Carbonate, and Simethicone (Oral-Local)—See *Antacids (Oral-Local)*
Alumina, Magnesia, and Simethicone (Oral-Local)—See *Antacids (Oral-Local)*
Aspirin, Buffered (Systemic)—See *Salicylates (Systemic)*
Aspirin and Codeine, Buffered (Systemic)—See *Opioid (Narcotic) Analgesics and Aspirin (Systemic)*
Calcium Carbonate and Magnesia (Oral-Local)—See *Antacids (Oral-Local)*
Calcium Carbonate, Magnesia, and Simethicone (Oral-Local)—See *Antacids (Oral-Local)*
Magnesium Hydroxide and Cascara Sagrada (Oral-Local)—See *Laxatives (Local)*
Magnesium Hydroxide and Mineral Oil (Oral-Local)—See *Laxatives (Local)*
Simethicone, Alumina, Magnesium Carbonate, and Magnesia (Oral-Local)—See *Antacids (Oral-Local)*

# MAGNESIUM CARBONATE–CONTAINING COMBINATIONS—

Alumina and Magnesium Carbonate (Oral-Local)—See *Antacids (Oral-Local)*

Calcium and Magnesium Carbonates (Oral-Local)—See *Antacids (Oral-Local)*

Calcium and Magnesium Carbonates and Magnesium Oxide (Oral-Local)—See *Antacids (Oral-Local)*

Magnesium Carbonate and Sodium Bicarbonate (Oral-Local)—See *Antacids (Oral-Local)*

Simethicone, Alumina, Magnesium Carbonate, and Magnesia (Oral-Local)—See *Antacids (Oral-Local)*

# MAGNESIUM CHLORIDE—See *Magnesium Supplements (Systemic)*

# MAGNESIUM CITRATE—See *Laxatives (Local)*; *Magnesium Supplements (Systemic)*

# MAGNESIUM GLUCEPTATE—See *Magnesium Supplements (Systemic)*

# MAGNESIUM GLUCONATE—See *Magnesium Supplements (Systemic)*

# MAGNESIUM HYDROXIDE—See *Antacids (Oral-Local)*; *Laxatives (Local)*; *Magnesium Supplements (Systemic)*

# MAGNESIUM LACTATE—See *Magnesium Supplements (Systemic)*

# MAGNESIUM OXIDE—See *Antacids (Oral-Local)*; *Laxatives (Local)*; *Magnesium Supplements (Systemic)*

# MAGNESIUM OXIDE–CONTAINING COMBINATIONS—

Aspirin, Buffered (Systemic)—See *Salicylates (Systemic)*

Calcium and Magnesium Carbonates and Magnesium Oxide (Oral-Local)—See *Antacids (Oral-Local)*

# MAGNESIUM PIDOLATE—See *Magnesium Supplements (Systemic)*

# MAGNESIUM SALICYLATE—See *Salicylates (Systemic)*

# MAGNESIUM SALICYLATE–CONTAINING COMBINATIONS—

Choline and Magnesium Salicylates (Systemic)—See *Salicylates (Systemic)*

# MAGNESIUM SULFATE—See *Laxatives (Local)*; *Magnesium Sulfate (Systemic)*; *Magnesium Supplements (Systemic)*

# MAGNESIUM SULFATE    Systemic

VA CLASSIFICATION (Primary): TN406/CN400; GU900; CV300

Note: For a listing of dosage forms and brand names by country availability, see *Dosage Forms* section(s). For a listing of brand names for the articles in this monograph, refer to the General Index.

## Category

Anticonvulsant; electrolyte replenisher; tocolytic; antiarrhythmic.

## Indications

Note: Bracketed information in the *Indications* section refers to uses that are not included in U.S. product labeling.

**Accepted**

Seizures, in toxemia of pregnancy (prophylaxis and treatment)—Intravenous magnesium sulfate is indicated for the prevention and immediate control of life-threatening seizures in the treatment of severe toxemias (pre-eclampsia and eclampsia) of pregnancy.

Hypomagnesemia (prophylaxis and treatment)—Magnesium sulfate is indicated for replacement therapy in magnesium deficiency, especially in acute hypomagnesemia accompanied by signs of tetany similar to those of hypocalcemia.

In patients receiving total parenteral nutrition, magnesium sulfate is added to the nutrient admixture to prevent or treat magnesium deficiency.

[Premature labor (treatment)][1]—Magnesium sulfate may be used as a tocolytic agent in the management of premature labor.

[Tachycardia, ventricular, polymorphous (treatment)][1]—Magnesium sulfate is used in the treatment of torsades de pointes. It is not effective in congenital QT interval prolongation syndromes.

**Acceptance not established**

Early studies seemed to show that intravenous magnesium sulfate administered in the setting of *acute myocardial infarction* reduced the mortality rate. Pooled data from 8 randomized controlled trials showed that intravenous magnesium administered within 24 to 48 hours after onset of symptoms decreased ventricular tachycardia and fibrillation by 49% and the incidence of cardiac arrest by 58% in patients who had not been treated with thrombolytic agents. Intravenous magnesium also reduced the early mortality rate in patients with suspected myocardial infarction in the second Leicester Intravenous Magnesium Intervention Trial (LIMIT-2). Magnesium's efficacy appeared to be independent of that of thrombolytic or antiplatelet therapy. In this study, little effect was seen on arrhythmic events, but the incidence of left ventricular failure was reduced in the treatment group.

However, recent data from the large randomized controlled trial, the Fourth International Study of Infarct Survival (ISIS-4), seems to challenge these earlier studies. ISIS-4 showed that intravenous magnesium was ineffective in significantly reducing mortality, independent of thrombolytic or antiplatelet therapy, in patients with suspected acute myocardial infarction. There was no significant evidence that magnesium had any effect on 5-week mortality and follow-up at one year did not indicate any beneficial effect. In direct contrast to the results of some earlier studies, administration of intravenous magnesium was associated with small but significant increases in heart failure, cardiogenic shock, and in deaths attributed to cardiogenic shock.

Differences in study design, particularly between ISIS-4 and LIMIT-2, may explain the conflicting results. Intravenous magnesium was administered later in the course of myocardial infarction in ISIS-4, as compared to LIMIT-2. The ISIS-4 study was not designed to detect a highly time-dependent effect of magnesium on reperfusion injury. Therefore, there is conflicting evidence that the **routine** use of intravenous magnesium sulfate in the setting of acute myocardial infarction is beneficial.

[1]Not included in Canadian product labeling.

# Pharmacology/Pharmacokinetics

## Physicochemical characteristics
Molecular weight—246.47.

Other characteristics—Magnesium sulfate, as the hydrated salt, contains approximately 10% of the labeled weight as magnesium and 49% as anhydrous magnesium sulfate. Doses are calculated based on the hydrate weight unless otherwise stated. One gram of magnesium sulfate heptahydrate ($MgSO_4 \cdot 7H_2O$) is equivalent to 8.12 mEq of magnesium.

## Mechanism of action/Effect
Anticonvulsant—Exact mechanism is not clearly understood. Magnesium may decrease the amount of acetylcholine released at the myoneuronal junction, resulting in depression of neuromuscular transmission. Magnesium also may have a direct depressant effect on smooth muscle and may cause central nervous system (CNS) depression.

Antiarrhythmic—The exact mechanism of magnesium's antiarrhythmic effect is not clear. Magnesium may decrease myocardial cell excitability by contributing to the re-establishment of ionic equilibrium and stabilizing cell membranes. Magnesium also appears to modulate the sodium current, the slow inward calcium current, and at least one potassium current.

Myocardial infarction—Possible mechanisms include antiarrhythmic action or direct cardioprotection. Magnesium's cardioprotective action may involve coronary vasodilation, reduction in peripheral vascular resistance, platelet aggregation inhibition, and an effect on the calcium current.

Tocolytic—The exact mechanism is not known. It is speculated that magnesium may decrease myometrial contractility by altering calcium uptake, binding, and distribution in smooth muscle cells. Magnesium has been shown to increase uterine blood flow secondary to vasodilation of uterine vessels.

## Onset of action
Intramuscular—About 1 hour.
Intravenous—Nearly immediate.

## Therapeutic serum concentrations
Anticonvulsant—4 to 7 mEq per L (2 to 3.5 mmol per L).

## Duration of action
Intramuscular—3 to 4 hours.
Intravenous—About 30 minutes.

## Elimination
Renal, at a rate proportional to the plasma concentration and glomerular filtration rate.

# Precautions to Consider

## Pregnancy/Reproduction
Pregnancy—Parenteral magnesium sulfate has been administered to pregnant women in the treatment of pre-eclampsia and eclampsia (toxemia) of pregnancy and as a tocolytic agent. It readily crosses the placenta and rapidly attains fetal serum concentrations that approximate those in the mother. Magnesium's effects in the neonate may be similar to those in the mother and may include hypotonia, drowsiness, and respiratory depression. Bony abnormalities and congenital rickets have been reported in neonates born to mothers treated with parenteral magnesium sulfate for prolonged periods of time (4 to 13 weeks' duration).

FDA Pregnancy Category A.

## Breast-feeding
Magnesium sulfate is distributed into breast milk. Milk concentrations are approximately twice those in maternal serum.

## Pediatrics
Appropriate studies on the relationship of age to the effects of magnesium sulfate have not been performed in the pediatric population. However, no pediatrics-specific problems have been documented to date.

## Geriatrics
Appropriate studies on the relationship of age to the effects of magnesium sulfate have not been performed in the geriatric population. However, elderly patients are more likely to have age-related renal function impairment, which may require dosage reduction in patients receiving magnesium sulfate.

## Drug interactions and/or related problems
The following drug interactions and/or related problems have been selected on the basis of their potential clinical significance (possible mechanism in parentheses where appropriate)—not necessarily inclusive (» = major clinical significance):

Note: Combinations containing any of the following medications, depending on the amount present, may also interact with this medication.

Calcium (intravenous salts)
(concurrent use may neutralize effects of parenteral magnesium sulfate; calcium gluconate and calcium gluceptate are used to antagonize the toxic effects of hypermagnesemia; also, calcium sulfate may precipitate when a calcium salt is admixed with magnesium sulfate in the same intravenous solution; however, calcium salts and magnesium sulfate may be administered concurrently through separate intravenous lines if required in post-parathyroidectomy "hungry bones" syndrome or tetany associated with hypocalcemia and hypomagnesemia)

CNS depression–producing medications, other (see *Appendix II*)
(CNS depressant effects may be potentiated when these medications are used concurrently with parenteral magnesium sulfate)

Digitalis glycosides
(parenteral magnesium sulfate must be administered with extreme caution in digitalized patients, especially if intravenous calcium salts are also employed; cardiac conduction changes and heart block may occur)

Neuromuscular blocking agents or
Nifedipine
(concurrent use with parenteral magnesium sulfate may result in severe and unpredictable potentiation of neuromuscular blockade)
(concurrent use of parenteral magnesium sulfate with nifedipine may produce an exaggerated hypotensive response)

## Laboratory value alterations
The following have been selected on the basis of their potential clinical significance (possible effect in parentheses where appropriate)—not necessarily inclusive (» = major clinical significance):

With diagnostic test results
Reticuloendothelial cell imaging
(parenteral magnesium sulfate may impair reticuloendothelial cell imaging with technetium Tc 99m sulfur colloid by causing clumping of colloidal particles with subsequent entrapment in the vasculature of the lungs rather than in the liver, spleen, and bone marrow)

## Medical considerations/Contraindications
The medical considerations/contraindications included here have been selected on the basis of their potential clinical significance (reasons given in parentheses where appropriate)—not necessarily inclusive (» = major clinical significance).

*Except under special circumstances, this medication should not be used when the following medical problems exist:*

» Heart block
(magnesium may exacerbate this condition)

» Renal failure (creatinine clearance <20 mL per minute)
(clearance of magnesium decreased; risk of magnesium toxicity)

*Risk-benefit should be considered when the following medical problems exist:*

Myasthenia gravis
(magnesium sulfate may precipitate an acute myasthenic crisis by decreasing the sensitivity of the motor endplate to acetylcholine)

» Renal function impairment, severe
(risk of developing hypermagnesemia and magnesium toxicity; patients with severely impaired renal function should receive no more than 20 grams of magnesium sulfate [162 mEq of magnesium] within a 48-hour period; caution is recommended against administering intravenous magnesium too rapidly in patients with oliguria or severe renal failure; close monitoring of serum magnesium concentration is recommended)

Respiratory disease
(increased risk of respiratory depression)

Sensitivity to magnesium sulfate

## Patient monitoring
The following may be especially important in patient monitoring (other tests may be warranted in some patients, depending on condition; » = major clinical significance):

Blood pressure monitoring
(recommended at periodic intervals)

Cardiac function monitoring (ECG) and
Magnesium concentrations, serum
(recommended at periodic intervals during therapy as indicated by the clinical situation; normal average serum magnesium concentrations are 1.6 to 2.6 mEq per L [0.8 to 1.2 mmol per L])

Deep tendon reflexes, especially patellar reflex or knee jerk determinations
(used as an indication of CNS depression prior to administration of repeated doses; suppression of reflex may be related to impend-

ing respiratory arrest. The patellar reflex should be tested before each dose and, if the reflex is absent, no additional doses should be given until a positive response is obtained. The disappearance of the reflex is a useful sign for detecting excessive magnesium serum concentrations)

Renal function determinations, especially urine output
(recommended at periodic intervals; urine output should be at least 100 mL per 4 hours)

Respiration rate determination
(rate should be at least 16 per minute prior to each parenteral dose of magnesium sulfate, since respiratory depression is the most critical side effect of this medication, rapidly proceeding to fatal respiratory paralysis)

## Side/Adverse Effects

The following side/adverse effects have been selected on the basis of their potential clinical significance (possible signs and symptoms in parentheses where appropriate)—not necessarily inclusive:

Note: Although the side/adverse effects are stratified according to serum magnesium concentrations and early signs and symptoms of hypermagnesemia, these effects may occur early or late in the course of hypermagnesemia and may not always correlate with serum magnesium concentrations.

### Those indicating need for prompt medical attention
*Signs of hypermagnesemia*—in order of increasing serum magnesium concentrations:

| Effect | Serum magnesium concentration (mEq per L) |
|---|---|
| *Deep tendon reflexes present, but possibly hypoactive* | 4 to 7 |
| *Prolonged PQ interval; widened QRS interval on ECG* | 5 to 10 |
| *Loss of deep tendon reflexes* | 8 to 10 |
| *Respiratory paralysis* | 10 to 13 |
| *Altered cardiac conduction* | 15 |
| *Cardiac arrest* | 25 |

Early signs and symptoms of hypermagnesemia
*Bradycardia; diplopia; flushing; headache; hypotension; nausea; shortness of breath; slurred speech; vomiting; weakness*

## Overdose

For more information on the management of overdose or unintentional ingestion, **contact a Poison Control Center** (see *Poison Control Center Listing*).

### Treatment of overdose
Blood pressure and respiratory support; artificial respiration is often required.

Slow injection of intravenous calcium gluconate, 5 to 10 mEq of calcium or 10 to 20 mL of a 10% solution (diluted if desirable with 0.9% sodium chloride injection) to reverse heart block or respiratory depression.

Subcutaneous administration of physostigmine (0.5 to 1 mg) may be helpful; however, routine use is not recommended because of its toxicity.

Dialysis may be required to remove magnesium sulfate if renal function is reduced.

## General Dosing Information

Magnesium sulfate injection 50% must be diluted to a concentration of 20% or less prior to intravenous infusion.

The rate of intravenous injection should generally not exceed 150 mg per minute, except in severe eclampsia with seizures.

## Parenteral Dosage Forms

Note: Bracketed uses in the *Dosage Forms* section refer to categories of use and/or indications that are not included in U.S. product labeling.

### MAGNESIUM SULFATE INJECTION USP

#### Usual adult and adolescent dose
Seizures, in toxemia of pregnancy—
Intravenous, 4 to 5 grams (32 to 40 mEq [16 to 20 mmol] of magnesium) in 250 mL of 5% dextrose injection USP or 0.9% sodium chloride infused over thirty minutes. Simultaneously, intramuscular doses of up to 10 grams (5 grams or 10 mL of undiluted 50% solution in each buttock) are given. Alternatively, the initial intravenous dose of 4 grams may be given by diluting the 50% solution to a 10 or 20% concentration; the diluted fluid (40 mL of a 10%

solution or 20 mL of a 20% solution) may then be injected intravenously over a period of three to four minutes. Subsequently, 4 to 5 grams are injected intramuscularly into alternate buttocks every four hours as needed. Alternatively, after the initial intravenous dose, some clinicians administer 1 or 2 grams per hour as an intravenous infusion.

Hypomagnesemia—
Severe deficiency:
Intramuscular, 250 mg (2 mEq [1 mmol] of magnesium) per kg of body weight administered within a four-hour period.
Intravenous infusion, 5 grams (40 mEq [20 mmol] of magnesium) in 1 L of 5% dextrose injection or 0.9% sodium chloride injection, administered slowly over a three-hour period.
Mild deficiency:
Intramuscular, 1 gram (8 mEq [4 mmol] of magnesium) as a 50% solution, administered every six hours for four doses (a total of 32.5 mEq of magnesium) per twenty-four hours.

Total parenteral nutrition (TPN)—
Intravenous infusion, 1 to 3 grams (8 to 24 mEq [4 to 12 mmol] of magnesium) a day.
Note: Up to 6 grams a day may be necessary in selected patients, such as in patients with short bowel syndrome.

[Ventricular tachycardia, polymorphous][1]—
Intravenous, 2 grams (16 mEq [8 mmol] of magnesium) given over one to two minutes; the dose may be repeated if the arrhythmia is not controlled after five to fifteen minutes. Additionally, an intravenous infusion of 3 to 20 mg per minute may be needed.

[Premature labor][1]—
Initial: Intravenous, 4 to 6 grams (32 to 48 mEq [16 to 24 mmol] of magnesium) infused over twenty to thirty minutes.
Maintenance: Intravenous infusion, 1 to 3 grams (8 to 24 mEq [4 to 12 mmol] of magnesium) per hour until contractions abate.

Note: Extreme care must be used in the parenteral administration of magnesium sulfate in order to avoid toxic serum concentrations.

Geriatric patients often require lower dosages because of reduced renal function.

An intravenous preparation of a calcium salt (e.g., 10% calcium gluconate or gluceptate) should be readily available when magnesium sulfate is administered.

### Usual adult prescribing limits
Up to 40 grams (320 mEq [160 mmol] of magnesium) a day.

### Usual pediatric dose
Total parenteral nutrition (TPN)—
Intravenous infusion, 0.25 to 1.25 grams (2 to 10 mEq [1 to 5 mmol] of magnesium) a day.

### Strength(s) usually available
U.S.—
10% w/v (1 gram [8 mEq of magnesium] per 10 mL) (Rx) [GENERIC].
12.5% w/v (1.25 grams [10 mEq of magnesium] per 10 mL) (Rx) [GENERIC].
50% w/v (5 grams [40 mEq of magnesium] per 10 mL) (Rx) [GENERIC].

Canada—
20% w/v (2 grams [16 mEq of magnesium] per 10 mL) (Rx) [GENERIC].
50% w/v (5 grams [40 mEq of magnesium] per 10 mL) (Rx) [GENERIC].

### Packaging and storage
Store below 40 °C (104 °F), preferably between 15 and 30 °C (59 and 86 °F), unless otherwise specified by manufacturer. Protect from freezing.

### Incompatibilities
Formation of a precipitate may result when magnesium sulfate is mixed with solutions containing:
Alcohol (in high concentrations)
Alkali carbonates and bicarbonates
Alkali hydroxides
Arsenates
Barium
Calcium
Clindamycin phosphate
Heavy metals
Hydrocortisone sodium succinate
Phosphates
Polymyxin B sulfate
Procaine hydrochloride
Salicylates
Strontium
Tartrates

The potential for incompatibility will often be influenced by changes in the concentration of reactants and the pH of the solutions.

Separation of intravenous fat emulsions may occur with concentrations of magnesium greater than 20 mEq per mL in total parenteral nutrition admixtures.

It has been reported that magnesium may reduce the antibiotic activity of streptomycin, tetracycline, and tobramycin when given together.

----

¹Not included in Canadian product labeling.

## Selected Bibliography

Chau AC, Gabert HA, Miller JM. A prospective comparison of terbutaline and magnesium for tocolysis. Obstet Gynecol 1992; 80: 847-51.

Sibai BM. Magnesium sulfate is the ideal anticonvulsant in preeclampsia-eclampsia. Am J Obstet Gynecol 1990; 162: 1141-5.

----

Revised: 08/03/94
Interim revision: 08/15/95

# MAGNESIUM SUPPLEMENTS   Systemic

This monograph includes information on the following: Magnesium Chloride†; Magnesium Citrate§; Magnesium Gluceptate*; Magnesium Gluconate; Magnesium Hydroxide‡§; Magnesium Lactate†; Magnesium Oxide‡§; Magnesium Pidolate*; Magnesium Sulfur#.

INN:

Magnesium gluceptate—Magnesium glucoheptonate
Magnesium pidolate—Magnesium pyroglutamate

VA CLASSIFICATION (Primary): TN406

Note: For a listing of dosage forms and brand names by country availability, see Dosage Forms section(s). For a listing of brand names for the articles in this monograph, refer to the General Index.

----

*Not commercially available in the U.S.
†Not commercially available in Canada.
‡See Antacids (Oral-Local) for antacid use of magnesium hydroxide and magnesium oxide.
§See Laxatives (Local) for laxative use of magnesium citrate, magnesium hydroxide, magnesium oxide, and magnesium sulfate.
#See Magnesium Sulfate (Systemic) for use in seizures and uterine tetany.

----

## Category

Antihypomagnesemic—Magnesium Chloride; Magnesium Citrate; Magnesium Gluceptate; Magnesium Gluconate; Magnesium Hydroxide; Magnesium Lactate; Magnesium Oxide; Magnesium Pidolate; Magnesium Sulfate.

Electrolyte replenisher—Magnesium Chloride Injection; Magnesium Sulfate.

Nutritional supplement (mineral)—Magnesium Chloride; Magnesium Citrate; Magnesium Gluceptate; Magnesium Gluconate; Magnesium Hydroxide; Magnesium Lactate; Magnesium Oxide; Magnesium Pidolate; Magnesium Sulfate.

## Indications

Note: Bracketed information in the Indications section refers to uses that are not included in U.S. product labeling.

### Accepted

Electrolyte depletion (treatment)—Parenteral magnesium chloride and magnesium sulfate are used in conditions that require an increase in magnesium ions for electrolyte adjustment.

Hypomagnesemia (prophylaxis and treatment)—Magnesium supplements are indicated for correction of hypomagnesemia in patients with low or restricted oral intake or conditions in which requirements for magnesium are increased, such as chronic alcoholism, diabetic ketoacidosis, gastrointestinal disease (chronic diarrhea, Crohn's, ulcerative colitis), hyperaldosteronism, hypercalcemia, hypomagnesemic hypocalcemia, hypomagnesemic hypokalemia, hyperparathyroidism, hyperthyroidism, pancreatic insufficiency, renal tubular acidosis, stress, or possibly patients who are receiving thiazide or loop diuretics, cisplatin, amphotericin B therapy, cyclosporine, gentamicin, or digitalis glycosides, or are on total parenteral nutrition (TPN) therapy. For prophylaxis of magnesium deficiency, dietary improvement, rather than supplementation, is advisable. For treatment of magnesium deficiency, supplementation is preferred.

Deficiency of magnesium may lead to irritability, mental derangement, muscle weakness, tetany, and cardiac arrhythmias.

Recommended intakes for all vitamins and most minerals are increased during pregnancy. Many physicians recommend that pregnant women receive multivitamin and mineral supplements, especially those pregnant women who do not consume an adequate diet and those in high-risk categories (i.e., women carrying more than one fetus, heavy cigarette smokers, and alcohol and drug abusers). Taking excessive amounts of a multivitamin and mineral supplement may be harmful to the mother and/or fetus and should be avoided.

Recommended intakes for all vitamins and most minerals are increased during breast-feeding.

Antacid—See Antacids (Oral-Local).

Laxative—See Laxatives (Local).

Seizures (treatment)—See Magnesium Sulfate (Systemic).

[Tachycardia, ventricular, atypical (treatment)]—See Magnesium Sulfate (Systemic).

Tetany, uterine (treatment)—See Magnesium Sulfate (Systemic).

## Pharmacology/Pharmacokinetics

### Physicochemical characteristics

Molecular weight—

Elemental magnesium: 24.3.
Magnesium chloride: 203.3.
Magnesium citrate: 451.1.
Magnesium gluceptate: 474.7.
Magnesium gluconate: 450.6.
Magnesium hydroxide: 58.3.
Magnesium lactate: 202.4.
Magnesium oxide: 40.3.
Magnesium pidolate: 280.5.
Magnesium sulfate: 246.47.

### Mechanism of action/Effect

Magnesium is necessary for the proper functioning of over 300 enzymes, including several in glycolysis and the Krebs cycle, adenyl cyclase, which forms cyclic-AMP, and various phosphatase reactions in protein and nucleic acid synthesis. Magnesium is also necessary for neuromuscular transmission and activity, bone mineralization, and parathyroid hormone function.

### Other effects

Calcium homeostasis is dependent on magnesium, with hypomagnesemia often being accompanied by hypocalcemia. Magnesium is necessary for secretion of parathyroid hormone (PTH) and also for the action of PTH at the site of its target organs. High doses of magnesium have been found to inhibit calcium absorption due to suppression of PTH secretion. Hypokalemia is frequently found with hypomagnesemia, possibly due to magnesium deficiency enhancing renal excretion of potassium or magnesium deficiency effecting the sodium-potassium pump.

### Absorption

Approximately 35 to 40% of dietary magnesium is absorbed through the jejunum and ileum. Some magnesium is reabsorbed from bile and pancreatic and intestinal juices. High fat diets or fat malabsorption syndromes have been found to interfere with magnesium absorption.

### Protein binding

Approximately 30% of magnesium is bound intracellularly to protein and energy-rich phosphates.

### Storage

Primarily bone, skeletal muscle, kidney, liver, and heart; small amounts found in extracellular fluid and erythrocytes.

### Time to peak concentration

Oral—4 hours.

### Duration of action

Oral—4 to 6 hours.

### Elimination

Parenteral magnesium is eliminated renally. Oral magnesium is eliminated renally and fecally.

# Precautions to Consider

## Pregnancy/Reproduction

Pregnancy—
> *Parenteral magnesium sulfate—*
>> When magnesium sulfate is parenterally administered in the treatment of eclampsias (toxemias) of pregnancy, it readily crosses the placenta and rapidly attains fetal serum concentrations that approximate those of the mother. The effects of magnesium on the neonate are similar to those on the mother and may include hypotonia, hyporeflexia, hypotension, and respiratory depression when the mother has received magnesium sulfate prior to delivery. It is therefore usually not administered to the mother during the 2 hours preceding delivery unless it is the only therapy available to prevent eclamptic seizures. Magnesium sulfate can be administered continuously by intravenous drip at a rate of 1 to 2 grams every hour, provided the patient is closely monitored for magnesium plasma concentrations, blood pressure, respiratory rate, and deep tendon reflexes.

>> FDA Pregnancy Category D.
> *Other magnesium salts and oral magnesium sulfate—*
>> Problems in humans have not been documented with intake of normal daily recommended amounts.
>> FDA pregnancy categories have not been assigned.

## Breast-feeding
Problems in humans have not been documented with intake of normal daily recommended amounts.

## Pediatrics
Problems in pediatrics have not been documented with intake of normal daily recommended amounts.

Magnesium chloride injection that contains benzyl alcohol as a preservative should not be used in newborn and immature infants. The use of benzyl alcohol in neonates has been associated with a fatal toxic syndrome consisting of metabolic acidosis and CNS, respiratory, circulatory, and renal function impairment.

## Geriatrics
Problems in geriatrics have not been documented with intake of normal daily recommended amounts.

The elderly may be at risk of developing a magnesium deficiency due to poor food selection, decreased absorption, diseases that cause magnesium depletion, or medications that may increase urinary loss of magnesium.

## Drug interactions and/or related problems
The following drug interactions and/or related problems have been selected on the basis of their potential clinical significance (possible mechanism in parentheses where appropriate)—not necessarily inclusive (» = major clinical significance):

Note: Combinations containing any of the following medications, depending on the amount present, may also interact with magnesium supplements.

Alcohol or
Glucose
> (high alcohol or glucose intake has been found to increase urinary excretion of magnesium)

Amphotericin B or
Cisplatin or
Cyclosporine or
Gentamicin
> (magnesium requirements may be increased in patients receiving these nephrotoxic medications due to renal magnesium wasting)

Calcium (intravenous salts)
> (concurrent use may neutralize effects of parenteral magnesium sulfate; however, calcium gluconate and calcium gluceptate are used to antagonize the toxic effects of hypermagnesemia, also, calcium sulfate may precipitate when a calcium salt is admixed with magnesium sulfate in the same intravenous solution; calcium salts and magnesium sulfate may be administered through separate intravenous lines if required in post-parathyroidectomy "hungry bones" syndrome or tetany associated with hypocalcemia and hypomagnesemia)

Calcium-containing medications, oral
> (concurrent use with magnesium supplements may increase serum calcium or magnesium concentrations in susceptible patients, primarily patients with renal insufficiency)

» Cellulose sodium phosphate

Edetate disodium
> (concurrent use with magnesium supplements may result in binding of magnesium; patients should be advised not to take magnesium supplements within 1 hour of cellulose sodium phosphate or edetate disodium)

CNS depression–producing medications, other (See *Appendix II*)
> (CNS depressant effects may be potentiated when these medications are used concurrently with parenteral magnesium)

Digitalis glycosides
> (hypomagnesemia has been reported in patients receiving digitalis glycosides and may lead to digitalis toxicity; therefore, serum magnesium concentrations should be monitored in patients receiving digitalis glycosides, as magnesium supplements may be necessary)
> (concurrent use with magnesium supplements may inhibit absorption, possibly decreasing plasma concentrations of digitalis glycosides; magnesium salts in digitalized patients must be administered with extreme caution, especially if intravenous calcium salts are also employed; cardiac conduction changes and heart block may occur)

Diuretics, loop or
Diuretics, thiazide
> (long-term use of loop or thiazide diuretics may impair the magnesium-conserving ability of the kidneys and lead to hypomagnesemia; serum magnesium levels should be monitored in patients receiving thiazide or loop diuretics)

Diuretics, potassium-sparing
> (long-term use of potassium-sparing diuretics has been found to increase renal tubular reabsorption of magnesium; use with magnesium supplements may cause hypermagnesemia, especially in patients with renal insufficiency)

Etidronate, oral
> (concurrent use with oral magnesium supplements may prevent absorption of oral etidronate; patients should be advised to avoid using magnesium supplements within 2 hours of etidronate)

» Magnesium-containing preparations, other, such as:
Antacids
Laxatives
> (concurrent use with magnesium supplements may cause magnesium toxicity, especially in patients with renal insufficiency)

Misoprostol
> (concurrent use with magnesium supplements may aggravate misoprostol-induced diarrhea)

Neuromuscular blocking agents
> (concurrent use with parenteral magnesium may result in severe and unpredictable potentiation of neuromuscular blockade)

» Sodium polystyrene sulfonate
> (sodium polystyrene sulfonate may bind with oral magnesium supplements; concurrent use is not recommended, although the risk may be less with rectal administration of sodium polystyrene sulfonate)

» Tetracyclines, oral
> (concurrent use with magnesium supplements may decrease absorption of tetracyclines because of possible formation of nonabsorbable complexes; patients should be advised not to take magnesium supplements within 1 to 3 hours of taking an oral tetracycline)

## Medical considerations/Contraindications
The medical considerations/contraindications included here have been selected on the basis of their potential clinical significance (reasons given in parentheses where appropriate)—not necessarily inclusive (» = major clinical significance).

*Risk-benefit should be considered when the following medical problems exist:*

Heart block or
Myocardial damage
> (conditions may be exacerbated; magnesium should be infused at a slower rate with careful monitoring of serum magnesium concentrations)

Renal function impairment, severe
> (may cause high levels of magnesium; reduction of magnesium supplement dosage may be necessary)

Sensitivity to parenteral magnesium
> (sensitivity has been reported with use of parenteral magnesium in higher doses; sensitivity to oral magnesium supplements in recommended doses has not been reported)

## Patient monitoring
The following may be especially important in patient monitoring (other tests may be warranted in some patients, depending on condition; » = major clinical significance):

Magnesium concentrations, serum and urinary
(recommended daily for severe deficiency and monthly for chronic
deficiency to determine status; magnesium equilibrates slowly with
the intracellular compartment; thus serum magnesium concentrations may not be reliable indicators of normal tissue levels)

## Side/Adverse Effects

The following side/adverse effects have been selected on the basis of their
potential clinical significance (possible signs and symptoms in parentheses where appropriate)—not necessarily inclusive:

**Those indicating need for medical attention**
Incidence rare (with parenteral magnesium only)
*Flushing; hypotension* (dizziness or fainting); *irritation and pain at
injection site*—for intramuscular administration only; *muscle paralysis; respiratory depression* (troubled breathing)

**Those indicating need for medical attention only if they continue
or are bothersome**
Incidence less frequent (with oral magnesium)
*Diarrhea*

## Overdose

For specific information on the agents used in the management of magnesium overdose, see
• *Calcium Gluconate* in *Calcium Supplements* monograph.

For more information on the management of overdose or unintentional
ingestion, **contact a Poison Control Center** (see *Poison Control Center Listing*).

**Clinical effects of overdose**
The following effects have been selected on the basis of their potential
clinical significance (possible signs and symptoms in parentheses
where appropriate)—not necessarily inclusive:

Symptoms of overdose (rare in patients with normal renal function)
*Asystole; bradycardia* (slow heartbeat); *CNS depression* (severe
drowsiness); *coma; hypotension* (dizziness or fainting); *muscle paralysis; renal failure* (blurred or double vision; increased or decreased
urination); *respiratory failure* (troubled breathing)

**Treatment of overdose**
Discontinue magnesium-containing preparations.
Supportive care—
Maintain respiration.
Specific treatment—
If serum magnesium levels exceed 5 mEq per liter and adult patient
is symptomatic, giving 10 mL of 10% calcium gluconate over sev-
eral minutes. The dose may be repeated one time.

## Patient Consultation

As an aid to patient consultation, refer to *Advice for the Patient,
Magnesium Supplements (Systemic)*.

In providing consultation, consider emphasizing the following selected
information (» = major clinical significance):

**Description of use**
Description should include function in the body; signs of deficiency

**Importance of diet**
Importance of proper nutrition; supplement may be needed because of
inadequate dietary intake
Food sources of magnesium; effects of processing
Recommended daily intake for magnesium

**Before using this medication**
» Conditions affecting use, especially:
Sensitivity to magnesium
Use in the elderly—More likely to develop magnesium deficiency
Other medications, especially cellulose sodium phosphate, oral tet-
racyclines, other magnesium-containing preparations, or so-
dium polystyrene sulfonate
Other medical problems, especially heart block, renal function im-
pairment, hypotension, or respiratory depression

**Proper use of this medication**
» Proper dosing
Taking with meals to prevent diarrhea
*Proper administration technique*
Not crushing or chewing extended-release dosage forms, unless oth-
erwise directed
Proper mixing for powder form
Missed dose: No cause for concern because of length of time necessary
for depletion; remembering to take as directed
» Proper storage

## Side/adverse effects
Signs of potential side effects, especially dizziness or fainting; flushing, irritation and pain at injection site for intramuscular injection
only, muscle paralysis, or troubled breathing (with injection)

## General Dosing Information

Magnesium supplements should be taken with meals because taking them
on an empty stomach may cause diarrhea.

The action of magnesium supplements depends upon their content of magnesium ion. There are 12.2 mg of elemental magnesium per 1 mEq
elemental magnesium. The various magnesium salts contain the following amounts of elemental magnesium:

| Magnesium salt | Magnesium (mg/gram) | Magnesium (mEq/gram) | Magnesium (mM/gram) | % Magnesium |
|---|---|---|---|---|
| Magnesium chlo-ride (hydrous) | 120 | 9.8 | 4.9 | 12 |
| Magnesium citrate (anhydrous) | 162 | 4.4 | 2.2 | 16.2 |
| Magnesium glu-ceptate (anhydrous) | 51.3 | 4.2 | 2.1 | 5.1 |
| Magnesium glu-conate (hydrous) | 54 | 4.4 | 2.2 | 5.4 |
| Magnesium hy-droxide (anhydrous) | 417 | 34.3 | 17.2 | 41.7 |
| Magnesium lactate (anhydrous) | 120 | 9.8 | 4.9 | 12 |
| Magnesium oxide (anhydrous) | 603 | 49.6 | 24.8 | 60.3 |
| Magnesium pido-late (anhydrous) | 87 | 7.2 | 3.6 | 8.7 |
| Magnesium sulfate (hydrous) | 99 | 8.1 | 4.1 | 9.9 |

**For parenteral dosage forms only**
In most cases, parenteral administration is indicated only when oral administration is not acceptable (for example, in nausea, vomiting, preoperative and postoperative conditions) or possible (for example, in
malabsorption syndromes or following gastric resection).

**Diet/Nutrition**
Recommended dietary intakes for magnesium are defined differently
worldwide.
For U.S.—
The Recommended Dietary Allowances (RDAs) for vitamins and min-
erals are determined by the Food and Nutrition Board of the Na-
tional Research Council and are intended to provide adequate nu-
trition in most healthy persons under usual environmental stresses.
In addition, a different designation may be used by the FDA for
food and dietary supplement labeling purposes, as with Daily
Value (DV). DVs replace the previous labeling terminology United
States Recommended Daily Allowances (USRDAs).
For Canada—
Recommended Nutrient Intakes (RNIs) for vitamins, minerals, and
protein are determined by Health and Welfare Canada and provide
recommended amounts of a specific nutrient while minimizing the
risk of chronic diseases.
Daily recommended intakes for elemental magnesium are generally defined as follows:

| Persons | U.S. (mg) | Canada (mg) |
|---|---|---|
| Infants and children | | |
| Birth to 3 years of age | 40–80 | 20–50 |
| 4 to 6 years of age | 120 | 65 |
| 7 to 10 years of age | 170 | 100–135 |
| Adolescent and adult males | 270–400 | 130–250 |
| Adolescent and adult females | 280–300 | 135–210 |
| Pregnant females | 320 | 195–245 |
| Breast-feeding females | 340–355 | 245–265 |

The best dietary sources of magnesium include green leafy vegetables,
nuts, legumes, and cereal grains in which the germ or outer layers
have not been removed. Hard water has a higher concentration of
magnesium than soft water. The magnesium content of food is reduced
by refining and cooking.

---

### *MAGNESIUM CHLORIDE*

---

## Summary of Differences

Category: Injection may also be used as an electrolyte replenisher.

Precautions: Drug interactions and/or related problems—Possible additive effects when parenteral calcium chloride given with CNS depression–producing medications and neuromuscular blocking agents.

## Oral Dosage Forms

### MAGNESIUM CHLORIDE TABLETS

**Usual adult and adolescent dose**

Hypomagnesemia (prophylaxis)—
  Oral, amount based on normal daily recommended intakes of elemental magnesium:

| Persons | U.S. (mg) | Canada (mg) |
|---|---|---|
| Adolescent and adult males | 270–400 | 130–250 |
| Adolescent and adult females | 280–300 | 135–210 |
| Pregnant females | 320 | 195–245 |
| Breast-feeding females | 340–355 | 245–265 |

Hypomagnesemia (treatment)—
  Treatment dose is individualized by prescriber based on severity of deficiency

**Usual pediatric dose**

Hypomagnesemia (prophylaxis)—
  Oral, amount based on normal daily recommended intakes of elemental magnesium:

| Persons | U.S. (mg) | Canada (mg) |
|---|---|---|
| Infants and children | | |
| Birth to 3 years of age | 40–80 | 20–50 |
| 4 to 6 years of age | 120 | 65 |
| 7 to 10 years of age | 170 | 100–135 |

Hypomagnesemia (treatment)—
  Treatment dose is individualized by prescriber based on severity of deficiency.

**Strength(s) usually available**

U.S.—
  64 mg elemental magnesium (OTC) [*Slow-Mag*].

Canada—
  Not commercially available.

Note: The strength of this magnesium preparation may exceed the dosage range recommended by USP DI Advisory Panels based on the amount necessary to meet normal nutritional needs.

**Packaging and storage**

Store below 40 °C (104 °F), preferably between 15 and 30 °C (59 and 86 °F), unless otherwise specified by manufacturer.

### MAGNESIUM CHLORIDE ENTERIC-COATED TABLETS

**Usual adult and adolescent dose**

See *Magnesium Chloride Tablets*.

**Usual pediatric dose**

Dosage form not appropriate for use in children.

**Strength(s) usually available**

U.S.—
  100 mg elemental magnesium (833 mg magnesium chloride) (OTC) [*Mag-L-100*].

Canada—
  Not commercially available.

Note: The strength of this magnesium preparation may exceed the dosage range recommended by USP DI Advisory Panels based on the amount necessary to meet normal nutritional needs.

**Packaging and storage**

Store below 40 °C (104 °F), preferably between 15 and 30 °C (59 and 86 °F), unless otherwise specified by manufacturer.

### MAGNESIUM CHLORIDE EXTENDED-RELEASE TABLETS

**Usual adult and adolescent dose**

See *Magnesium Chloride Tablets*.

**Usual pediatric dose**

Dosage form not appropriate for use in children.

**Strength(s) usually available**

U.S.—
  64 mg elemental magnesium (535 mg magnesium chloride) (OTC) [*Slow-Mag*].

Canada—
  Not commercially available.

Note: The strength of this magnesium preparation may exceed the dosage range recommended by USP DI Advisory Panels based on the amount necessary to meet normal nutritional needs.

**Packaging and storage**

Store below 40 °C (104 °F), preferably between 15 and 30 °C (59 and 86 °F), unless otherwise specified by manufacturer.

## Parenteral Dosage Forms

### MAGNESIUM CHLORIDE INJECTION

**Usual adult and adolescent dose**

Electrolyte replenisher—
  For intravenous infusion, 4 grams of magnesium chloride (39.2 mEq of elemental magnesium) diluted in 250 mL of dextrose 5% and infused at a rate not to exceed 3 mL per minute.

Hypomagnesemia (prophylaxis)—
  Intravenous infusion, as part of total parenteral nutrition solution, the specific amount determined by individual patient need.

**Usual adult prescribing limits**

40 grams a day.

**Usual pediatric dose**

Hypomagnesemia (prophylaxis)—
  Intravenous infusion, as part of total parenteral nutrition solution, the specific amount determined by individual patient need.

Note: Magnesium chloride injection that contains benzyl alcohol as a preservative should not be used in newborn and immature infants. The use of benzyl alcohol in neonates has been associated with a fatal toxic syndrome consisting of metabolic acidosis and CNS, respiratory, circulatory, and renal function impairment.

**Strength(s) usually available**

U.S.—
  200 mg magnesium chloride per mL (Rx) [*Chloromag*; GENERIC].

Canada—
  Not commercially available.

**Packaging and storage**

Store below 40 °C (104 °F), preferably between 15 and 30 °C (59 and 86 °F), unless otherwise specified by manufacturer.

---

### *MAGNESIUM CITRATE*

---

## Oral Dosage Forms

### MAGNESIUM CITRATE ORAL SOLUTION USP

**Usual adult dose**

Hypomagnesemia (prophylaxis)—
  Oral, amount based on normal daily recommended intakes of elemental magnesium:

| Persons | U.S. (mg) | Canada (mg) |
|---|---|---|
| Adolescent and adult males | 270–400 | 130–250 |
| Adolescent and adult females | 280–300 | 135–210 |
| Pregnant females | 320 | 195–245 |
| Breast-feeding females | 340–355 | 245–265 |

Hypomagnesemia (treatment)—
  Treatment dose is individualized by prescriber based on severity of deficiency.

**Usual pediatric dose**

Hypomagnesemia (prophylaxis)—
  Oral, amount based on normal daily recommended intakes of elemental magnesium:

| Persons | U.S. (mg) | Canada (mg) |
|---|---|---|
| Infants and children | | |
| Birth to 3 years of age | 40–80 | 20–50 |
| 4 to 6 years of age | 120 | 65 |
| 7 to 10 years of age | 170 | 100–135 |

Hypomagnesemia (treatment)—
  Treatment dose is individualized by prescriber based on severity of deficiency.

**Strength(s) usually available**

U.S.—

   47 mg elemental magnesium (290 mg magnesium citrate) per 5 mL (OTC) [*Citroma;* GENERIC].

Canada—

   40.5 mg elemental magnesium (250 mg magnesium citrate) per 5 mL (OTC) [*Citro-Mag*].

Note: Some strengths of these magnesium preparations may exceed the dosage range recommended by USP DI Advisory Panels based on the amount necessary to meet normal nutritional needs.

**Packaging and storage**

Store below 40 °C (104 °F), preferably between 15 and 30 °C (59 and 86 °F), unless otherwise specified by manufacturer.

---

## *MAGNESIUM GLUCEPTATE*

# Oral Dosage Forms

## MAGNESIUM GLUCEPTATE ORAL SOLUTION

**Usual adult and adolescent dose**

Hypomagnesemia (prophylaxis)—

   Oral, amount based on normal daily recommended intakes of elemental magnesium:

| Persons | U.S. (mg) | Canada (mg) |
|---|---|---|
| Adolescent and adult males | 270–400 | 130–250 |
| Adolescent and adult females | 280–300 | 135–210 |
| Pregnant females | 320 | 195–245 |
| Breast-feeding females | 340–355 | 245–265 |

Hypomagnesemia (treatment)—

   Treatment dose is individualized by prescriber based on severity of deficiency.

**Usual pediatric dose**

Hypomagnesemia (prophylaxis)—

   Oral, amount based on normal daily recommended intakes of elemental magnesium:

| Persons | U.S. (mg) | Canada (mg) |
|---|---|---|
| Infants and children | | |
| Birth to 3 years of age | 40–80 | 20–50 |
| 4 to 6 years of age | 120 | 65 |
| 7 to 10 years of age | 170 | 100–135 |

Hypomagnesemia (treatment)—

   Treatment dose is individualized by prescriber based on severity of deficiency.

**Strength(s) usually available**

U.S.—

   Not commercially available.

Canada—

   25 mg elemental magnesium (500 mg magnesium gluceptate) per 5 mL (OTC) [*Magnesium-Rougier*].

Note: The strength of this magnesium preparation may exceed the dosage range recommended by USP DI Advisory Panels based on the amount necessary to meet normal nutritional needs.

**Packaging and storage**

Store below 40 °C (104 °F), preferably between 15 and 30 °C (59 and 86 °F), unless otherwise specified by manufacturer.

---

## *MAGNESIUM GLUCONATE*

# Oral Dosage Forms

## MAGNESIUM GLUCONATE ORAL SOLUTION

**Usual adult and adolescent dose**

Deficiency (prophylaxis)—

   Oral, amount based on normal daily recommended intakes of elemental magnesium:

| Persons | U.S. (mg) | Canada (mg) |
|---|---|---|
| Adolescent and adult males | 270–400 | 130–250 |
| Adolescent and adult females | 280–300 | 135–210 |
| Pregnant females | 320 | 195–245 |
| Breast-feeding females | 340–355 | 245–265 |

Deficiency (treatment)—

   Treatment dose is individualized by prescriber based on severity of deficiency.

**Usual pediatric dose**

Deficiency (prophylaxis)—

   Oral, amount based on normal daily recommended intakes of elemental magnesium:

| Persons | U.S. (mg) | Canada (mg) |
|---|---|---|
| Infants and children | | |
| Birth to 3 years of age | 40–80 | 20–50 |
| 4 to 6 years of age | 120 | 65 |
| 7 to 10 years of age | 170 | 100–135 |

Deficiency (treatment)—

   Treatment dose is individualized by prescriber based on severity of deficiency.

**Strength(s) usually available**

U.S.—

   54 mg elemental magnesium (1 gram magnesium gluconate) per 5 mL (OTC) [*Magonate*].

Canada—

   Not commercially available.

Note: The strength of this magnesium preparation may exceed the dosage range recommended by USP DI Advisory Panels based on the amount necessary to meet normal nutritional needs.

## MAGNESIUM GLUCONATE TABLETS USP

**Usual adult and adolescent dose**

See *Magnesium Gluconate Oral Solution.*

**Usual pediatric dose**

See *Magnesium Gluconate Oral Solution.*

**Strength(s) usually available**

U.S.—

   27 mg elemental magnesium (500 mg magnesium gluconate) [*Almora* (OTC); *Magonate* (OTC); *Magtrate* (OTC); *MGP* (Rx); GENERIC (Rx/OTC)].

   29 mg elemental magnesium (550 mg magnesium gluconate) (Rx) [GENERIC].

Canada—

   29.3 mg elemental magnesium (500 mg magnesium gluconate) (OTC) [*Maglucate*].

Note: Some strengths of these magnesium preparations may exceed the dosage range recommended by USP DI Advisory Panels based on the amount necessary to meet normal nutritional needs.

**Packaging and storage**

Store below 40 °C (104 °F), preferably between 15 and 30 °C (59 and 86 °F), unless otherwise specified by manufacturer.

---

## *MAGNESIUM HYDROXIDE*

# Oral Dosage Forms

## MAGNESIA TABLETS USP

**Usual adult and adolescent dose**

Hypomagnesemia (prophylaxis)—

   Oral, amount based on normal daily recommended intakes of elemental magnesium:

| Persons | U.S. (mg) | Canada (mg) |
|---|---|---|
| Adolescent and adult males | 270–400 | 130–250 |
| Adolescent and adult females | 280–300 | 135–210 |
| Pregnant females | 320 | 195–245 |
| Breast-feeding females | 340–355 | 245–265 |

Hypomagnesemia (treatment)—

   Treatment dose is individualized by prescriber based on severity of deficiency.

**Usual pediatric dose**

Hypomagnesemia (prophylaxis)—
Oral, amount based on intake of normal daily recommended intakes of elemental magnesium:

| Persons | U.S. (mg) | Canada (mg) |
|---|---|---|
| Infants and children | | |
| Birth to 3 years of age | 40–80 | 20–50 |
| 4 to 6 years of age | 120 | 65 |
| 7 to 10 years of age | 170 | 100–135 |

Hypomagnesemia (treatment)—
Treatment dose is individualized by prescriber based on severity of deficiency.

**Strength(s) usually available**

U.S.—
135 mg elemental magnesium (325 mg magnesium hydroxide) (OTC) [GENERIC].

Canada—
Not commercially available.

Note: Some strengths of these magnesium preparations may exceed the dosage range recommended by USP DI Advisory Panels based on the amount necessary to meet normal nutritional needs.

**Packaging and storage**

Store below 40 °C (104 °F), preferably between 15 and 30 °C (59 and 86 °F), unless otherwise specified by manufacturer.

## MAGNESIA TABLETS (CHEWABLE) USP

**Usual adult and adolescent dose**

See *Magnesium Tablets USP*.

**Usual pediatric dose**

See *Magnesia Tablets USP*.

**Strength(s) usually available**

U.S.—
130 mg elemental magnesium (311 mg magnesium hydroxide) (OTC) [*Phillips' Chewable Tablets*].

Canada—
129 mg elemental magnesium (310 mg magnesium hydroxide) (OTC) [*Phillips' Magnesia Tablets*].

Note: Some strengths of these magnesium preparations may exceed the dosage range recommended by USP DI Advisory Panels based on the amount necessary to meet normal nutritional needs.

**Packaging and storage**

Store below 40 °C (104 °F), preferably between 15 and 30 °C (59 and 86 °F), unless otherwise specified by manufacturer.

## MILK OF MAGNESIA USP

**Usual adult and adolescent dose**

See *Magnesia Tablets USP*.

**Usual pediatric dose**

See *Magnesia Tablets USP*.

**Strength(s) usually available**

U.S.—
164 mg elemental magnesium (400 mg magnesium hydroxide) per 5 mL (OTC) [*Phillips' Milk of Magnesia;* GENERIC].
328 mg elemental magnesium (800 mg magnesium hydroxide) per 5 mL (OTC) [*Concentrated Phillips' Milk of Magnesia*].

Canada—
170 mg elemental magnesium (408 mg magnesium hydroxide) per 5 mL (OTC) [*Phillips' Milk of Magnesia*].

Note: Some strengths of these magnesium preparations may exceed the dosage range recommended by USP DI Advisory Panels based on the amount necessary to meet normal nutritional needs.

**Packaging and storage**

Store below 40 °C (104 °F), preferably between 15 and 30 °C (59 and 86 °F), unless otherwise specified by manufacturer.

---

### *MAGNESIUM LACTATE*

## Oral Dosage Forms

### MAGNESIUM LACTATE EXTENDED-RELEASE TABLETS

**Usual adult and adolescent dose**

Hypomagnesemia (prophylaxis)—
Oral, amount based on normal daily recommended intakes of elemental magnesium:

| Persons | U.S. (mg) | Canada (mg) |
|---|---|---|
| Adolescent and adult males | 270–400 | 130–250 |
| Adolescent and adult females | 280–300 | 135–210 |
| Pregnant females | 320 | 195–245 |
| Breast-feeding females | 340–355 | 245–265 |

Hypomagnesemia (treatment)—
Treatment dose is individualized by prescriber based on severity of deficiency.

**Usual pediatric dose**

Dosage form not appropriate for use in children.

**Strength(s) usually available**

U.S.—
84 mg elemental magnesium (840 mg magnesium lactate) (OTC) [*Mag-Tab SR*].

Canada—
Not commercially available.

Note: The strength of this magnesium preparation may exceed the dosage range recommended by USP DI Advisory Panels based on the amount necessary to meet normal nutritional needs.

**Packaging and storage**

Store below 40 °C (104 °F), preferably between 15 and 30 °C (59 and 86 °F), unless otherwise specified by manufacturer.

---

### *MAGNESIUM OXIDE*

## Oral Dosage Forms

### MAGNESIUM OXIDE CAPSULES USP

**Usual adult and adolescent dose**

Hypomagnesemia (prophylaxis)—
Oral, amount based on normal daily recommended intakes of elemental magnesium:

| Persons | U.S. (mg) | Canada (mg) |
|---|---|---|
| Adolescent and adult males | 270–400 | 130–250 |
| Adolescent and adult females | 280–300 | 135–210 |
| Pregnant females | 320 | 195–245 |
| Breast-feeding females | 340–355 | 245–265 |

Hypomagnesemia (treatment)—
Treatment dose is individualized by prescriber based on severity of deficiency.

**Usual pediatric dose**

Hypomagnesemia (prophylaxis)—
Oral, amount based on normal daily recommended intakes of elemental magnesium:

| Persons | U.S. (mg) | Canada (mg) |
|---|---|---|
| Infants and children | | |
| Birth to 3 years of age | 40–80 | 20–50 |
| 4 to 6 years of age | 120 | 65 |
| 7 to 10 years of age | 170 | 100–135 |

Hypomagnesemia (treatment)—
Treatment dose is individualized by prescriber based on severity of deficiency.

**Strength(s) usually available**

U.S.—
84.5 mg elemental magnesium (140 mg magnesium oxide) (OTC) [*Uro-Mag;* GENERIC].

Canada—
Not commercially available.

Note: The strengths of these magnesium preparations may exceed the dosage range recommended by USP DI Advisory Panels based on the amount necessary to meet normal nutritional needs.

**Packaging and storage**

Store below 40 °C (104 °F), preferably between 15 and 30 °C (59 and 86 °F), unless otherwise specified by manufacturer.

### MAGNESIUM OXIDE TABLETS USP

**Usual adult and adolescent dose**

See *Magnesium Oxide Capsules USP*.

**Usual pediatric dose**

See *Magnesium Oxide Capsules USP*.

**Strength(s) usually available**

U.S.—

    200 mg elemental magnesium (332 mg magnesium oxide) [*Mag-200*].

    241.3 mg elemental magnesium (400 mg magnesium oxide) (OTC) [*Mag-Ox 400* (scored); GENERIC].

    250 mg elemental magnesium (420 mg magnesium oxide) (OTC) [*Maox* (tartrazine); GENERIC].

    302 mg elemental magnesium (500 mg magnesium oxide) (OTC) [GENERIC].

Canada—

    50 mg elemental magnesium (OTC) [GENERIC].

Note: Some strengths of these magnesium preparations may exceed the dosage range recommended by USP DI Advisory Panels based on the amount necessary to meet normal nutritional needs.

**Packaging and storage**

Store below 40 °C (104 °F), preferably between 15 and 30 °C (59 and 86 °F), unless otherwise specified by manufacturer.

---

## MAGNESIUM PIDOLATE

# Oral Dosage Forms

## MAGNESIUM PIDOLATE FOR ORAL SOLUTION

**Usual adult and adolescent dose**

Hypomagnesemia (prophylaxis)—

    Oral, amount based on normal daily recommended intakes of elemental magnesium:

| Persons | U.S. (mg) | Canada (mg) |
|---|---|---|
| Adolescent and adult males | 270–400 | 130–250 |
| Adolescent and adult females | 280–300 | 135–210 |
| Pregnant females | 320 | 195–245 |
| Breast-feeding females | 340–355 | 245–265 |

Hypomagnesemia (treatment)—

    Treatment dose is individualized by prescriber based on severity of deficiency.

**Usual pediatric dose**

Hypomagnesemia (prophylaxis)—

    Oral, amount based on normal daily recommended intakes of elemental magnesium:

| Persons | U.S. (mg) | Canada (mg) |
|---|---|---|
| Infants and children | | |
|   Birth to 3 years of age | 40–80 | 20–50 |
|   4 to 6 years of age | 120 | 65 |
|   7 to 10 years of age | 170 | 100–135 |

Hypomagnesemia (treatment)—

    Treatment dose is individualized by prescriber based on severity of deficiency.

**Strength(s) usually available**

U.S.—

    Not commercially available.

Canada—

    122 mg elemental magnesium (1500 mg magnesium pidolate) per 4 grams (OTC) [*Mag 2*].

Note: The strength of this magnesium preparation may exceed the dosage range recommended by USP DI Advisory Panels based on the amount necessary to meet normal nutritional needs.

**Packaging and storage**

Store below 40 °C (104 °F), preferably between 15 and 30 °C (59 and 86 °F), unless otherwise specified by manufacturer.

**Preparation of dosage form**

Pour contents of one pouch into a glass, add some water and stir quickly.

**Auxiliary labeling**

• Take before meals.

---

## MAGNESIUM SULFATE

# Summary of Differences

Category: Injection may also be used as an electrolyte replenisher.

Precautions: Drug interactions and/or related problems—Parenteral magnesium sulfate may form a precipitate when mixed with calcium salts.

Possible additive effects when given with CNS depression–producing medications and neuromuscular blocking agents.

# Oral Dosage Forms

## MAGNESIUM SULFATE CRYSTALS

**Usual adult and adolescent dose**

Hypomagnesemia (prophylaxis)—

    Oral, amount based on normal daily recommended intakes of elemental magnesium:

| Persons | U.S. (mg) | Canada (mg) |
|---|---|---|
| Adolescent and adult males | 270–400 | 130–250 |
| Adolescent and adult females | 280–300 | 135–210 |
| Pregnant females | 320 | 195–245 |
| Breast-feeding females | 340–355 | 245–265 |

Hypomagnesemia (treatment)—

    Treatment dose is individualized by prescriber based on severity of deficiency.

**Usual pediatric dose**

Hypomagnesemia (prophylaxis)—

    Oral, amount based on normal daily recommended intakes of elemental magnesium:

| Persons | U.S. (mg) | Canada (mg) |
|---|---|---|
| Infants and children | | |
|   Birth to 3 years of age | 40–80 | 20–50 |
|   4 to 6 years of age | 120 | 65 |
|   7 to 10 years of age | 170 | 100–135 |

Hypomagnesemia (treatment)—

    Treatment dose is individualized by prescriber based on severity of deficiency.

**Strength(s) usually available**

U.S.—

    40 mEq per 5 mg (OTC) [GENERIC].

Canada—

    Not commercially available.

Note: The strength of this magnesium preparation may exceed the dosage range recommended by USP DI Advisory Panels based on the amount necessary to meet normal nutritional needs.

**Packaging and storage**

Store below 40 °C (104 °F), preferably between 15 and 30 °C (59 and 86 °F), unless otherwise specified by manufacturer.

# Parenteral Dosage Forms

## MAGNESIUM SULFATE INJECTION USP

**Usual adult and adolescent dose**

Antihypomagnesemic or

Electrolyte replenisher—

    Intramuscular, 1 to 2 grams of a 50% solution (8.1 to 16.2 mEq elemental magnesium) four times a day until serum magnesium is within normal limits.

    Intravenous infusion, 5 grams (40.5 mEq elemental magnesium) in 1000 mL of dextrose 5% or sodium chloride 0.9% infused over 3 hours.

Hypomagnesemia (prophylaxis)—

    Intravenous infusion, as part of total parenteral nutrition solution, the specific amount determined by individual patient need.

**Usual pediatric dose**

Antihypomagnesemic or

Electrolyte replenisher—

    Intramuscular, 20 to 40 mg (0.16 to 0.32 mEq elemental magnesium) per kg of body weight in a 20% solution, repeated as necessary.

Hypomagnesemia (prophylaxis)—Intravenous infusion, as part of total parenteral nutrition solutions, the specific amount determined by individual patient need.

**Strength(s) usually available**

U.S.—

    10% w/v (100 mg, 0.8 mEq, 0.8 mOsm per mL) (Rx) [GENERIC].

    12.5% w/v (125 mg, 1 mEq, 1 mOsm per mL) (Rx) [GENERIC].

    25% w/v (250 mg, 2 mEq per mL) (Rx) [GENERIC].

    50% w/v (500 mg, 4 mEq, 4 mOsm per mL) (Rx) [GENERIC].

Canada—

    50% w/v (500 mg per mL) (Rx) [GENERIC].

**Packaging and storage**
Store below 40 °C (104 °F), preferably between 15 and 30 °C (59 and 86 °F), unless otherwise specified by manufacturer.

**Incompatibilities**
Magnesium sulfate in solution may form a precipitate when mixed with solutions containing:

| | |
|---|---|
| Alcohol (in high concentrations) | Heavy metals |
| | Hydrocortisone sodium |
| Alkali carbonates and bicarbonates | succinate |
| | Phosphates |
| Alkali hydroxides | Polymyxin B sulfate |
| Arsenates | Procaine hydrochloride |
| Barium | Salicylates |
| Calcium | Sodium bicarbonate |
| Clindamycin phosphate | Strontium |
| Dobutamine | Tartrates |
| Fat emulsions | |

The potential incompatibility will often be influenced by changes in the concentration of reactants and the pH of the solution.

It has been reported that magnesium may reduce the antibiotic activity of streptomycin, tetracycline, and tobramycin when any of those medicines and magnesium are given together.

## Selected Bibliography

Gums J. Clinical significance of magnesium: a review. DICP 1987; 21: 240-6.

Wester P. Magnesium. Am J Clin Nutr 1987; 45: 1305-12.

Revised: 12/03/92
Interim revision: 03/28/93; 08/23/94; 07/11/95

## MAGNESIUM TRISILICATE–CONTAINING COMBINATIONS—

Alumina and Magnesium Trisilicate (Oral-Local)—See *Antacids (Oral-Local)*

Alumina, Magnesium Trisilicate, and Sodium Bicarbonate (Oral-Local)—See *Antacids (Oral-Local)*

---

# MALATHION    Topical†

VA CLASSIFICATION (Primary): AP300

Note:    For a listing of dosage forms and brand names by country availability, see *Dosage Forms* section(s). For a listing of brand names for the articles in this monograph, refer to the General Index.

†Not commercially available in Canada.

## Category

Pediculicide.

Note:    Malathion is an organophosphate cholinesterase inhibitor generally used as an insecticide.

## Indications

**Accepted**

Pediculosis capitis (treatment)—Malathion is indicated for the treatment of infestation caused by *Pediculus humanus* var. *capitis* (head louse) and its ova.

## Pharmacology/Pharmacokinetics

**Physicochemical characteristics**

Molecular weight—330.4.

**Mechanism of action**

Malathion acts via cholinesterase inhibition. It exerts both lousicidal and ovicidal actions *in vitro*.

**Absorption**

Malathion in an acetone vehicle has been reported to be absorbed through normal human skin only to the extent of 8% of the applied dose. Percutaneous absorption of malathion in alcohol has not been studied; malathion lotion contains 78% isopropyl alcohol. Absorption may be increased when malathion is applied to damaged skin.

## Precautions to Consider

Note:    Although topical malathion used in recommended dosage has not been reported to cause cholinesterase inhibition, the possibility exists.

**Carcinogenicity**

Carcinogenicity studies with topical malathion have not been done. However, studies in animals have not shown that malathion is carcinogenic in either male or female F344 rats fed for 2 years with up to 4000 ppm (0.4%) of malathion.

**Tumorigenicity**

Studies in animals have not shown that malathion is tumorigenic in either Osborn-Mendel rats or B6C3F1 mice after feeding for 80 weeks with 8000 ppm (0.8%) and 16,000 ppm (1.6%) of malathion, respectively.

**Mutagenicity**

Studies on the mutagenic effects of malathion have not been done.

**Pregnancy/Reproduction**

Pregnancy—Studies in humans have not been done. However, malathion in an acetone vehicle has been shown to be systemically absorbed.

Studies in animals have not shown that malathion causes adverse effects in the fetus.

FDA Pregnancy Category B.

**Breast-feeding**

It is not known whether malathion is distributed into breast milk. Problems in humans have not been documented; however, malathion in an acetone vehicle has been shown to be systemically absorbed.

**Pediatrics**

Infants and children up to 2 years of age—No information is available on the relationship of age to the effects of malathion in infants and children up to 2 years of age. Safety and efficacy have not been established.

Children 2 years of age and older—Appropriate studies performed to date have not demonstrated pediatrics-specific problems that would limit the usefulness of malathion in children 2 years of age and older.

**Geriatrics**

Appropriate studies on the relationship of age to the effects of malathion have not been performed in the geriatric population. However, no geriatrics-specific problems have been documented to date.

**Drug interactions and/or related problems**

The following drug interactions and/or related problems have been selected on the basis of their potential clinical significance (possible mechanism in parentheses where appropriate)—not necessarily inclusive (» = major clinical significance):

Note:    Combinations containing any of the following medications, depending on the amount present, may also interact with this medication.

Aminoglycosides, parenteral
(if significant systemic absorption of topical malathion occurs, concurrent use may result in additive respiratory depression because of the neuromuscular blocking action of parenteral aminoglycosides)

Anesthetics, mucosal-local, ester-derivative, such as benzocaine, butacaine, butamben, and tetracaine
(if significant systemic absorption of topical malathion occurs, concurrent use may inhibit the metabolism of ester-derivative local anesthetics, including those topically applied and absorbed in significant amounts, leading to increased risk of systemic toxicity)

» Antimyasthenics or
» Cholinesterase inhibitors, other
(if significant systemic absorption of topical malathion occurs, concurrent use of antimyasthenics or other cholinesterase inhibitors [including ophthalmic cholinesterase inhibitors] with topical malathion may result in additive toxicity)

Carbamate- or organophosphate-type insecticides or pesticides
(if systemic absorption of topical malathion occurs, exposure to these preparations may increase the possibility of systemic effects due to absorption of the insecticide or pesticide through the respiratory tract or skin; patients should be advised to protect them-

selves from contact with such insecticides or pesticides during therapy with malathion)

Cocaine

(if significant systemic absorption of topical malathion occurs, the resulting inhibition of cholinesterase activity reduces or slows cocaine metabolism, thereby increasing and/or prolonging cocaine's effects and increasing the risk of toxicity)

Edrophonium

(since systemic absorption of topical malathion may occur, caution is recommended in administering edrophonium to patients with symptoms of myasthenic weakness who are also using topical malathion because symptoms of cholinergic crisis [overdosage] may be similar to symptoms occurring with myasthenic crisis [underdosage] and the patient's condition may be worsened by use of edrophonium)

» Succinylcholine

(if significant systemic absorption of topical malathion occurs, plasma concentrations or activity of pseudocholinesterase, the enzyme that metabolizes succinylcholine, may be decreased, thereby enhancing the neuromuscular blockade of succinylcholine when the two medications are used concurrently; increased or prolonged respiratory depression or paralysis [apnea] may occur but is of minor clinical significance while the patient is being mechanically ventilated; however, caution and careful monitoring of the patient are recommended following sequential use)

### Medical considerations/Contraindications

The medical considerations/contraindications included here have been selected on the basis of their potential clinical significance (reasons given in parentheses where appropriate)—not necessarily inclusive (» = major clinical significance).

*Risk-benefit should be considered when the following medical problems exist:*

Asthma, bronchial

(significant systemic absorption of malathion may precipitate an asthmatic attack)

Bradycardia and hypotension, pronounced or
Gastrointestinal disturbances, spastic or
Myocardial infarction, recent or
Parkinsonism or
Peptic ulcer or
Vagotonia, severe

(significant systemic absorption of malathion may exacerbate condition due to vagotonic effects of malathion)

Brain surgery, recent

(significant systemic absorption of malathion may cause central nervous system [CNS] toxicity, including seizures)

Conditions in which low concentrations of plasma cholinesterase may exist, such as:

Anemia, severe
Dehydration
Exposure to neurotoxic insecticides
Hepatic disease, severe or cirrhosis
Malnutrition
Recessive hereditary trait

(significant systemic absorption of malathion may result in additive respiratory depression)

Neuromuscular disease, such as myasthenia gravis

(significant systemic absorption of malathion may exacerbate condition)

Seizure disorders

(significant systemic absorption of malathion may precipitate seizures)

Sensitivity to malathion

## Side/Adverse Effects

Note: Although topical malathion used in recommended dosage has not been reported to cause systemic toxicity, the possibility exists.

Malathion is considered to be one of the least toxic organophosphorus insecticides because it is hydrolyzed and detoxified much more rapidly in mammals than in insects. The estimated lethal dose of malathion in mammals is 1 gram per kg of body weight. Daily application of 10% malathion dust to adult human skin for 3 weeks has been shown to produce little or no inhibition of blood cholinesterase.

The following side/adverse effects have been selected on the basis of their potential clinical significance (possible signs and symptoms in parentheses where appropriate)—not necessarily inclusive:

**Those indicating need for medical attention**
Incidence rare
*Allergic contact dermatitis* (skin rash)

Symptoms of systemic toxicity—may be delayed for up to 12 hours
*Abdominal cramps; anxiety or restlessness; clumsiness or unsteadiness; confusion or mental depression; diarrhea; dizziness; drowsiness; increased sweating; increased watering of mouth or eyes; loss of bowel or bladder control; muscle twitching of eyelids, face, and neck; pinpoint pupils; respiratory distress* (difficult or labored breathing); *seizures; slow heartbeat; trembling; unusual weakness*

**Those indicating need for medical attention only if they continue or are bothersome**
Incidence less frequent or rare
*Stinging or irritation of scalp*

## Patient Consultation

As an aid to patient consultation, refer to *Advice for the Patient, Malathion (Topical).*

In providing consultation, consider emphasizing the following selected information (» = major clinical significance):

**Before using this medication**
» Conditions affecting use, especially:
Sensitivity to malathion
Other medications, especially antimyasthenics or other cholinesterase inhibitors

**Proper use of this medication**
» Poison; importance of keeping away from mouth
» Importance of not using more medication than the amount prescribed
*Proper administration technique*
Applying by sprinkling on dry hair; rubbing in until hair and scalp thoroughly moistened
Washing hands immediately after using medication
Allowing hair to dry naturally; using no heat and leaving hair uncovered
Leaving medication on hair and scalp for 8 to 12 hours
» Washing hair with nonmedicated shampoo and rinsing thoroughly
Using fine-toothed comb to remove dead lice and eggs from hair
» Avoiding contact with the eyes
Medication is flammable; not using near heat, near open flame, or while smoking
» Importance of household family members being examined for infestation, and treated if infested
» Proper dosing
» Proper storage

**Precautions while using this medication**
*Using hygienic measures to control reinfestation or spread of infestation*
Washing all clothing, bedding, towels, and washcloths in very hot water or dry-cleaning them
Washing hairbrushes and combs in very hot soapy water; not sharing them with other people
Cleaning house or room by thorough vacuuming

Caution in exposure to carbamate- or organophosphate-type insecticides or pesticides during therapy

**Side/adverse effects**
Signs of potential side effects, especially skin rash or symptoms of systemic toxicity

## General Dosing Information

Malathion lotion contains 78% of isopropyl alcohol.

**For treatment of systemic toxicity**
Recommended treatment includes
• *Ingested* malathion should be removed immediately by inducing vomiting or by gastric lavage with 5% sodium bicarbonate solution.
• Artificial respiration and other supportive measures, such as removal of secretions and maintenance of an adequate airway, may be required.
• Atropine should be administered intravenously to counteract the symptoms of cholinesterase depletion. The usual initial dose of atropine is 1 to 4 mg, with supplemental doses administered as needed.

• Intravenous pralidoxime chloride may be used as an adjunct to atropine and supportive measures to reverse muscle paralysis. It appears to be most effective if administered within a few hours after poisoning occurs; it is usually not effective if initially administered after 48 hours have elapsed.

• A short-acting barbiturate may be given to control seizures.

• The patient should be observed for signs of deterioration due to delayed absorption.

• Repeat analyses of serum and red blood cell (RBC) cholinesterase may be used to establish diagnosis.

## Topical Dosage Forms

### MALATHION LOTION USP

**Usual adult and adolescent dose**
Pediculosis capitis—
Topical, to the hair and scalp, as a 0.5% lotion for one application, repeated after seven to nine days, if necessary.

**Usual pediatric dose**
Infants and children up to 2 years of age—Safety and efficacy have not been established.
Children 2 years of age and older—See *Usual adult and adolescent dose*.

**Strength(s) usually available**
U.S.—
0.5% (Rx) [*Ovide* (isopropyl alcohol 78%)].
Canada—
Not commercially available.
Other countries—
0.5% [*Derbac-M; Suleo-M*].

**Packaging and storage**
Store below 40 °C (104 °F), preferably between 15 and 30 °C (59 and 86 °F), unless otherwise specified by manufacturer. Store in a tight container. Protect from freezing.

**Auxiliary labeling**
• For external use only.

Revised: 07/25/94

---

## MALT SOUP EXTRACT—See *Laxatives (Local)*

---

## MALT SOUP EXTRACT–CONTAINING COMBINATIONS—

Malt Soup Extract and Psyllium (Oral-Local)—See *Laxatives (Local)*

---

## MANGANESE CHLORIDE—See *Manganese Supplements (Systemic)*

---

## MANGANESE SULFATE—See *Manganese Supplements (Systemic)*

---

# MANGANESE SUPPLEMENTS   Systemic†

This monograph includes information on the following: Manganese Chloride; Manganese Sulfate†.

VA CLASSIFICATION (Primary): TN499

Note: For a listing of dosage forms and brand names by country availability, see *Dosage Forms* section(s). For a listing of brand names for the articles in this monograph, refer to the General Index.

†Not commercially available in Canada.

## Category

Nutritional supplement (mineral).

## Indications

**Accepted**
Manganese deficiency (prophylaxis and treatment)—Manganese supplements are indicated in the prevention and treatment of manganese deficiency, which may result from inadequate nutrition or intestinal malabsorption but does not occur in healthy individuals receiving an adequate balanced diet. For prophylaxis of manganese deficiency, dietary improvement, rather than supplementation, is advisable. For treatment of manganese deficiency, supplementation is preferred.

Although deficiency in humans has not been documented, deficiency of manganese in animals may lead to poor reproductive performance, growth retardation, congenital malformations in the offspring, abnormal formation of bone and cartilage, dermatitis, and impaired glucose tolerance.

Some unusual diets (e.g., reducing diets that drastically restrict food selection) may not supply minimum daily requirements of manganese. Supplementation may be necessary in patients receiving total parenteral nutrition (TPN) or undergoing rapid weight loss or in those with malnutrition, because of inadequate dietary intake.

## Pharmacology/Pharmacokinetics

**Physicochemical characteristics**
Molecular weight—
Manganese chloride: 203.3.
Manganese sulfate: 169.01.
Elemental manganese: 54.9.

**Mechanism of action/Effect**
Manganese is an activator for enzymes such as polysaccharide polymerase, liver arginase, cholinesterase, and pyruvate carboxylase. It may also be a cofactor in lipid, protein, and carbohydrate metabolism.

**Absorption**
Variable, ranging from 3 to 50%. Manganese does undergo enterohepatic circulation.

**Protein binding**
Bound to a specific transport protein, transmanganin, a beta-1-globulin.

**Storage**
Manganese is concentrated in mitochondria-rich tissues such as brain, kidney, pancreas, and liver.

**Elimination**
Primarily through bile, but may be eliminated in pancreatic juice or returned to the lumen of duodenum, jejunum, or ileum in the event of biliary obstruction. Urinary excretion is negligible.

## Precautions to Consider

**Pregnancy/Reproduction**
Pregnancy—Studies have not been done in humans and problems in humans have not been documented with intake of normal daily recommended amounts.
Studies have not been done in animals.
FDA Pregnancy Category C (parenteral manganese).

**Breast-feeding**
Problems in humans have not been documented with intake of normal daily recommended amounts.

**Pediatrics**
Problems in pediatrics have not been documented with intake of normal daily recommended amounts.
Manganese sulfate injection that contains benzyl alcohol as a preservative should not be used in newborn and immature infants. The use of benzyl alcohol in neonates has been associated with a fatal toxic syndrome consisting of metabolic acidosis and CNS, respiratory, circulatory, and renal function impairment.

**Geriatrics**
Problems in geriatrics have not been documented with intake of normal daily recommended amounts.

**Medical considerations/Contraindications**
The medical considerations/contraindications included here have been selected on the basis of their potential clinical significance (reasons given in parentheses where appropriate)—not necessarily inclusive (» = major clinical significance).

*Risk-benefit should be considered when the following medical problems exist:*
Biliary tract dysfunction or
Hepatic dysfunction
(increased manganese blood concentrations may result because manganese is excreted in the bile)

### Patient monitoring

The following may be especially important in patient monitoring (other tests may be warranted in some patients, depending on condition; » = major clinical significance):

Manganese concentrations, plasma
(determinations may be recommended at monthly intervals; however, some clinicians do not recommend monitoring manganese concentrations because deficiency is rare)

## Side/Adverse Effects

There have been no reports of toxicity or side effects from oral manganese supplements.

## Patient Consultation

As an aid to patient consultation, refer to *Advice for the Patient, Manganese Supplements (Systemic).*

In providing consultation, consider emphasizing the following selected information (» = major clinical significance):

### Description of use
Description should include function in the body, signs of deficiency

### Importance of diet
Importance of proper nutrition; supplement may be needed because of inadequate dietary intake
Food sources of manganese
Recommended daily intake for manganese

### Proper use of this dietary supplement
» Proper dosing
Missed dose: No cause for concern because of length of time necessary for depletion; remembering to take as directed
» Proper storage

## General Dosing Information

Because of the infrequency of manganese deficiency occurring alone, combinations of several vitamins and/or minerals are commonly administered. Many commercial vitamin-mineral complexes are available.

### For parenteral dosage forms only
In most cases, parenteral administration is indicated only when oral administration is not acceptable (for example, in nausea, vomiting, preoperative and postoperative conditions) or possible (for example, in malabsorption syndromes or following gastric resection).

### Diet/Nutrition
Recommended dietary intakes for manganese are defined differently worldwide.
For U.S.—
The Recommended Dietary Allowances (RDAs) for vitamins and minerals are determined by the Food and Nutrition Board of the National Research Council and are intended to provide adequate nutrition in most healthy persons under usual environmental stresses. In addition, a different designation may be used by the FDA for food and dietary supplement labeling purposes, as with Daily Value (DV). DVs replace the previous labeling terminology United States Recommended Daily Allowances (USRDAs).
For Canada—
Recommended Nutrient Intakes (RNIs) for vitamins, minerals, and protein are determined by Health and Welfare Canada and provide recommended amounts of a specific nutrient while minimizing the risk of chronic diseases.

There is no RDA or RNI established for manganese. The following daily intakes are considered adequate for all individuals:
Infants and children:
Birth to 3 years of age: 0.3 to 1.5 mg.
4 to 6 years of age: 1.5 to 2 mg.
7 to 10 years of age: 2 to 3 mg.
Adolescents and adults:
2 to 5 mg.
The best dietary sources of manganese include whole grains, cereal products, lettuce, dry beans, and peas.

---

### *MANGANESE CHLORIDE*

## Parenteral Dosage Forms
### MANGANESE CHLORIDE INJECTION USP

**Usual adult and adolescent dose**
Deficiency (prophylaxis and treatment)—
Intravenous, 200 mcg (0.2 mg) of elemental manganese a day, added to total parenteral nutrition (TPN).

**Usual pediatric dose**
Deficiency (prophylaxis and treatment)—
Intravenous, 2 to 10 mcg (0.002 to 0.01 mg) of elemental manganese a day, added to total parenteral nutrition (TPN).

**Strength(s) usually available**
U.S.—
360 mcg (0.36 mg) (0.1 mg elemental manganese) per mL (Rx)
[GENERIC].
Canada—
Not commercially available.

**Packaging and storage**
Store below 40 °C (104 °F), preferably between 15 and 30 °C (59 and 86 °F), unless otherwise specified by manufacturer.

---

### *MANGANESE SULFATE*

## Parenteral Dosage Forms
### MANGANESE SULFATE INJECTION USP

**Usual adult and adolescent dose**
See *Manganese Chloride Injection USP.*

**Usual pediatric dose**
See *Manganese Chloride Injection USP.*

Note: Injection that contains benzyl alcohol as a preservative should not be used in newborn and immature infants. The use of benzyl alcohol in neonates has been associated with a fatal toxic syndrome consisting of metabolic acidosis and CNS, respiratory, circulatory, and renal function impairment.

**Strength(s) usually available**
U.S.—
308 mcg (0.308 mg) (0.1 mg elemental manganese) per mL (Rx)
[GENERIC].
Canada—
Not commercially available.

**Packaging and storage**
Store below 40 °C (104 °F), preferably between 15 and 30 °C (59 and 86 °F), unless otherwise specified by manufacturer.

**Preparation of dosage form**
Manganese sulfate is compatible with amino acids, dextrose, electrolytes, and vitamins usually used for total parenteral nutrition (TPN).

---

Revised: 02/01/92
Interim revision: 08/07/92; 08/15/94; 04/25/95

# MANNITOL Systemic

VA CLASSIFICATION (Primary/Secondary): CV709/OP106

Note: For a listing of dosage forms and brand names by country availability, see *Dosage Forms* section(s). For a listing of brand names for the articles in this monograph, refer to the General Index.

## Category

Diuretic; antiglaucoma agent (systemic); antihemolytic.

## Indications

Note: Bracketed information in the *Indications* section refers to uses that are not included in U.S. product labeling.

### Accepted

Edema (treatment)—Mannitol is indicated as an adjunct to other measures such as fluid replacement to prevent acute tubular necrosis or treat oliguria in acute renal failure due to various causes, and for symptomatic relief of edema.

Edema, cerebral (treatment)—Mannitol is indicated to treat cerebral edema and reduce brain mass and intracranial pressure.

Hypertension, ocular (treatment)—Mannitol is indicated to reduce elevated intraocular pressure after other methods have failed or in preparation for intraocular surgery.

Toxicity, nonspecific (treatment)—Mannitol is indicated to promote urinary excretion of and prevent renal damage due to toxic substances (for example, salicylates, barbiturates, bromides, lithium).

Hemolysis (prophylaxis)—Mannitol also is indicated as an irrigating solution to prevent hemolysis and hemoglobin buildup during transurethral prostatic resection. [It has also been used to prevent hemolysis during cardiopulmonary bypass procedures.][1]

### Unaccepted

Mannitol is indicated to measure glomerular filtration rate (GFR) in acute oliguria but has generally been replaced by more accurate tests.

---

[1]Not included in Canadian product labeling.

## Pharmacology/Pharmacokinetics

### Physicochemical characteristics

Molecular weight—182.17.

### Mechanism of action/Effect

Mannitol is an osmotic diuretic.

Osmotic agent (systemic)—
Elevates blood plasma osmolality, resulting in enhanced flow of water from tissues, including the brain and cerebrospinal fluid, into interstitial fluid and plasma. As a result, cerebral edema, elevated intracranial pressure, and cerebrospinal fluid volume and pressure may be reduced.

Diuretic—
Induces diuresis because mannitol is not reabsorbed in the renal tubule, thereby increasing the osmolality of the glomerular filtrate, facilitating excretion of water, and inhibiting the renal tubular reabsorption of sodium, chloride, and other solutes. It may, therefore, promote the urinary excretion of toxic materials and protect against nephrotoxicity by preventing the concentration of toxic substances in the tubular fluid.

Antiglaucoma agent—
Elevates blood plasma osmolarity, resulting in enhanced flow of water from the eye into plasma and a consequent reduction in intraocular pressure.

Antihemolytic—
When used as an irrigating solution in transurethral prostatic resection, dilute solutions of mannitol may minimize the hemolytic effect of water used alone. The entrance of hemolyzed blood into the circulation and the resultant hemoglobinemia may also be reduced.

Diagnostic aid (renal function)—
Mannitol is freely filtered by the glomeruli with less than 10% tubular reabsorption. Therefore, its urinary excretion rate may serve as a measurement of glomerular filtration rate (GFR).

### Absorption

Intravascular absorption during irrigation for transurethral prostatic resection is variable.

### Distribution

Mannitol remains in the extracellular compartment. If very high concentrations of mannitol are present in the plasma or the patient has acidosis, then mannitol may cross the blood-brain barrier and cause a rebound increase in intracranial pressure.

### Biotransformation

Mannitol is metabolized only slightly, if at all, to glycogen in the liver.

### Half-life

Approximately 100 minutes (may be increased to 36 hours in acute renal failure).

### Onset of action

Diuresis—1 to 3 hours.
Reduction in cerebrospinal and intraocular fluid pressure—Within 15 minutes after start of infusion.

### Time to peak effect

Reduction in intraocular pressure—30 to 60 minutes after injection.

### Duration of action

Reduction in cerebrospinal fluid pressure—persists for 3 to 8 hours after infusion is discontinued.
Reduction in intraocular pressure—persists for 4 to 8 hours.

### Elimination

Renal; 80% of a 100-gram intravenous dose appears in the urine within 3 hours.

## Precautions to Consider

### Carcinogenicity

An early study with 1, 5, and 10% mannitol given for 94 weeks to Wistar rats found a low incidence of benign thymomas in females. However, a subsequent lifetime study at similar doses in Sprague-Dawley, Fischer, and Wistar rats found no evidence of carcinogenicity.

### Mutagenicity

*In vivo* and *in vitro* mutagenicity studies were negative.

### Pregnancy/Reproduction

Pregnancy—Adequate and well-controlled studies have not been done in humans.
Studies in mice, rats, and rabbits at oral doses up to 1600 mg per kg of body weight (mg/kg) did not find adverse effects on the fetus.
FDA Pregnancy Category B.

### Breast-feeding

It is not known whether mannitol is excreted in breast milk. However, problems in humans have not been documented.

### Pediatrics

Studies performed to date have not demonstrated pediatrics-specific problems that would limit the usefulness of mannitol in children.

### Geriatrics

No information is available on the relationship of age to the effects of mannitol in geriatric patients. However, elderly patients are more likely to have age-related renal function impairment, which may require caution in patients receiving mannitol.

### Drug interactions and/or related problems

The following drug interactions and/or related problems have been selected on the basis of their potential clinical significance (possible mechanism in parentheses where appropriate)—not necessarily inclusive (» = major clinical significance):

Note: Combinations containing any of the following medications, depending on the amount present, may also interact with this medication.

» Digitalis glycosides
   (concurrent use with mannitol may enhance the possibility of digitalis toxicity associated with hypokalemia)

Diuretics, other, including carbonic anhydrase inhibitors
   (diuretic and intraocular pressure–reducing effects may be potentiated when these medications are used concurrently with mannitol; dosage adjustments may be necessary)

### Laboratory value alterations

The following have been selected on the basis of their potential clinical significance (possible effect in parentheses where appropriate)—not necessarily inclusive (» = major clinical significance):

With physiology/laboratory test values
   Phosphate or
   Potassium or
   Sodium
      (serum concentrations may be decreased by excessive and prolonged use)

## Medical considerations/Contraindications

The medical considerations/contraindications included here have been selected on the basis of their potential clinical significance (reasons given in parentheses where appropriate)—not necessarily inclusive (» = major clinical significance).

*Except under special circumstances, this medication should not be used when the following medical problems exist:*

» Anuria, with well-established acute tubular necrosis due to severe renal disease
(if patients do not respond to test dose; accumulation may lead to overexpansion of extracellular fluid and circulatory overload)

» Dehydration, severe
(may be exacerbated by fluid loss caused by mannitol; may result in serious electrolyte imbalances)

» Intracranial bleeding, active, except during craniotomy
(mannitol may increase bleeding by increasing cerebral blood flow)

» Pulmonary congestion or pulmonary edema, severe

*Risk-benefit should be considered when the following medical problems exist:*

» Cardiopulmonary function impairment, significant
(sudden expansion of extracellular fluid may lead to congestive heart failure)

Hyperkalemia or
Hyponatremia
(may be aggravated by changes in electrolyte balance)

Hypovolemia
(may be masked and intensified)

» Renal function impairment, significant
(accumulation of mannitol may lead to overexpansion of extracellular fluid and circulatory overload)

Sensitivity to mannitol

## Patient monitoring

The following may be especially important in patient monitoring (other tests may be warranted in some patients, depending on condition; » = major clinical significance):

Blood pressure measurements and

» Electrolyte measurements, serum, including potassium and sodium, and

» Renal function determinations and

» Urine output determinations
(recommended during administration of mannitol, especially with large or repeated doses)

## Side/Adverse Effects

Note: The most serious side/adverse effect of mannitol is fluid and electrolyte imbalance.

Rapid administration of large doses may lead to accumulation of mannitol, overexpansion of extracellular fluid, dilutional hyponatremia and occasional hyperkalemia, and circulatory overload, especially in patients with acute or chronic renal failure.

Inadequate hydration or hypovolemia may be obscured by the diuresis produced by mannitol, which may lead to tissue dehydration, promotion of oliguria, and intensification of pre-existing hemoconcentration.

Extravasation of mannitol may result in edema and skin necrosis.

The following side/adverse effects have been selected on the basis of their potential clinical significance (possible signs and symptoms in parentheses where appropriate)—not necessarily inclusive:

**Those indicating need for medical attention**
Incidence rare
*Chest pain or fast heartbeat; chills or fever; difficult urination; electrolyte imbalance* (confusion; irregular heartbeat; muscle cramps or pain; numbness, tingling, pain, or weakness in hands or feet; seizures; trembling; unusual tiredness or weakness; weakness and heaviness of legs); *pulmonary congestion* (coughing; troubled breathing; wheezing); *renal failure* (sudden decrease in amount of urine; swelling of face, feet, or lower legs; skin rash; unusual weight gain; shortness of breath; troubled breathing; wheezing; tightness in chest; increase in blood pressure; unusual thirst); *swelling of feet or lower legs; thrombophlebitis* (redness, swelling, or pain at injection site)

**Those indicating need for medical attention only if they continue or are bothersome**
Incidence more frequent
*Dryness of mouth or increased thirst; headache; increased urination; nausea or vomiting*

Incidence less frequent
*Blurred vision; dizziness; skin rash or hives*

Note: In some cases, *headache, nausea* or *vomiting, blurred vision,* and *dizziness* may be symptoms of subdural or subarachnoid hemorrhage as a result of dehydration of the brain.

## General Dosing Information

One gram of mannitol is equivalent to approximately 5.5 mOsm.

The number of mOsm of mannitol per liter of sterile water for injection is as follows:

| Mannitol (%) | mOsm/liter (approx) |
|---|---|
| 5 | 275 |
| 10 | 550 |
| 15 | 825 |
| 20 | 1100 |
| 25 | 1375 |

Mannitol must be administered by intravenous infusion.

The administration set should include a filter when mannitol solutions with concentrations of 15% or above are infused, since these solutions have a greater tendency to crystallize when exposed to low temperatures.

The dose and concentration of mannitol used to produce diuresis depend on the fluid status of the patient.

The risk of dehydration and electrolyte depletion may be reduced by using lower mannitol concentrations and solutions containing sodium chloride. Adequate hydration and electrolyte therapy are important.

A test dose of mannitol is recommended prior to therapy in patients with marked oliguria or possible inadequate renal function. The test dose is given as an intravenous infusion, 200 mg per kg of body weight (mg/kg) as a 15 to 25% solution, administered over a period of three to five minutes. In children the dose is 200 mg/kg or 6 grams per square meter of body surface as a 15 to 25% solution, administered over a period of three to five minutes. If urine flow does not increase to at least 30 to 50 mL per hour for two to three hours after this or a second test dose, mannitol should be withheld until the patient is re-evaluated.

Withdrawal of mannitol therapy may be necessary if renal failure, heart failure, or pulmonary congestion continues to progress.

Alkalinization of the urine with sodium bicarbonate may be necessary to aid in treatment of salicylate or barbiturate poisonings.

## Parenteral Dosage Forms

### MANNITOL INJECTION USP

**Usual adult dose**
Diuretic—
Intravenous infusion, 50 to 100 grams as a 5 to 25% solution, administered at a rate adjusted to maintain a urine flow of at least 30 to 50 mL per hour.

Cerebral edema or
Elevated intracranial pressure or
Glaucoma—
Intravenous infusion, 0.25 to 2 grams per kg of body weight as a 15 to 25% solution, administered over a period of thirty to sixty minutes.

Note: In small or debilitated patients, a dose of 500 mg per kg of body weight may be sufficient.

Toxicity, nonspecific—
Intravenous infusion, 50 to 200 grams as a 5 to 25% solution, administered at a rate adjusted to maintain a urine flow of 100 to 500 mL per hour.

Antihemolytic—
Mannitol may be used as a 2.5% irrigating solution for the bladder during transurethral prostatic resection or other transurethral surgical procedures.

**Usual adult prescribing limits**
Up to 6 grams per kg of body weight per twenty-four hours.

**Usual pediatric dose**
Diuretic—
Intravenous infusion, 0.25 to 2 grams per kg of body weight or 60 grams per square meter of body surface as a 15 to 20% solution, administered over a period of two to six hours.

Cerebral edema or
Elevated intracranial pressure or

Glaucoma—
Intravenous infusion, 1 to 2 grams per kg of body weight or 30 to 60 grams per square meter of body surface as a 15 to 20% solution, administered over a period of thirty to sixty minutes.
Note: In small or debilitated patients, a dose of 500 mg per kg of body weight may be sufficient.
Toxicity, nonspecific—
Intravenous infusion, up to 2 grams per kg of body weight or 60 grams per square meter of body surface as a 5 to 10% solution.

### Strength(s) usually available
U.S.—
5% (Rx) [*Osmitrol;* GENERIC].
10% (Rx) [*Osmitrol;* GENERIC].
15% (Rx) [*Osmitrol;* GENERIC].
20% (Rx) [*Osmitrol;* GENERIC].
25% (Rx) [*Osmitrol;* GENERIC].
Canada—
5% (Rx) [*Osmitrol*].
10% (Rx) [*Osmitrol*].
15% (Rx) [*Osmitrol*].
20% (Rx) [*Osmitrol*].
25% (Rx) [GENERIC].

### Packaging and storage
Store below 40 °C (104 °F), preferably between 15 and 30 °C (59 and 86 °F), unless otherwise specified by manufacturer. Protect from freezing.

### Preparation of dosage form
To prepare a 2.5% irrigating solution, add the contents of two 50-mL ampuls of 25% Mannitol Injection USP to 900 mL of sterile water for injection.

### Stability
Solutions of mannitol may crystallize, especially if chilled. To dissolve crystals, see manufacturer's package insert for directions. If all crystals cannot be completely dissolved, the solution should not be used.
The contents of opened containers should be used promptly. Unused contents should be discarded.

### Incompatibilities
Electrolyte-free mannitol solutions should not be given conjointly with blood. If blood must be administered simultaneously with mannitol, at least 20 mEq (mmol) of sodium chloride should be added to each liter of mannitol solution to prevent pseudoagglutination.

### Selected Bibliography
Nissenson AR, Weston RE, Kleeman CR. Mannitol. West J Med 1979 Oct; 131: 277-84.
Warren SE, Blantz RC. Mannitol. Arch Intern Med 1981 Mar; 141: 493-7.

Revised: 01/20/93

---

# MAPROTILINE  Systemic

VA CLASSIFICATION (Primary/Secondary): CN609/CN103
Note: For a listing of dosage forms and brand names by country availability, see *Dosage Forms* section(s). For a listing of brand names for the articles in this monograph, refer to the General Index.

## Category
Antidepressant; antineuralgic.

## Indications
Note: Bracketed information in the *Indications* section refers to uses that are not included in U.S. product labeling.

### Accepted
Depression, mental (treatment)—Maprotiline is indicated in the treatment of patients with major depressive disorder (unipolar depression); dysthymia (depressive neurosis); and bipolar disorder, depressed type.

Anxiety associated with mental depression (treatment)—Maprotiline is also indicated for the management of anxiety associated with mental depression.

[Pain, neurogenic (treatment)][1]—Maprotiline is used to treat some types of chronic pain.

[1]Not included in Canadian product labeling.

## Pharmacology/Pharmacokinetics

### Physicochemical characteristics
Molecular weight—313.87.

### Mechanism of action/Effect
A tetracyclic antidepressant, maprotiline is thought to increase the synaptic concentration of norepinephrine in the central nervous system (CNS) by blocking its re-uptake by the presynaptic neuronal membrane. No effect on serotonin re-uptake has been observed. Recent research has suggested that after long-term treatment with antidepressants, changes in postsynaptic beta-adrenergic receptor sensitivity and enhancement of response to alpha-adrenergic and serotonergic stimulation may contribute to the mechanism of antidepressant action. Antidepressants may produce a downregulation (desensitization) of presynaptic $alpha_2$ receptors, equilibrating the noradrenergic system, and thus correcting the dysregulated output of depressed patients.

### Absorption
Completely absorbed following oral administration.

### Protein binding
High (88%).

### Biotransformation
Hepatic.

### Half-life
Elimination—27 to 58 hours (average 43 hours).
Active metabolite—60 to 90 hours.

### Onset of action
For desired therapeutic effect, up to 2 or 3 weeks, but sometimes within 7 days.

### Time to peak concentration
12 hours.

### Elimination
Biliary—About 30%, in feces.
Renal—About 65%, mostly as glucuronide metabolites.

## Precautions to Consider
Note: The similarity of pharmacological effects of maprotiline and tricyclic antidepressants suggests that the same considerations and precautions be observed in the use of both medications. Therefore, until additional specific clinical information on maprotiline is available, certain precautionary guidelines for tricyclic antidepressants are included for consideration.

### Carcinogenicity
No evidence of carcinogenicity was found in studies of animals given large daily doses of maprotiline for up to 1 year.

### Mutagenicity
No evidence of mutagenicity was found in offspring of female mice mated with male mice treated with up to 60 times the maximum daily human dose.

### Pregnancy/Reproduction
Pregnancy—Adequate and well-controlled studies in humans have not been done.
Studies in animals have not shown that maprotiline causes adverse effects on the fetus.
FDA Pregnancy Category B.

### Breast-feeding
Maprotiline is distributed into breast milk in the same concentration as in blood.

### Pediatrics
Appropriate studies on the relationship of age to the effects of maprotiline have not been performed in children up to 18 years of age. Safety and efficacy have not been established.

### Geriatrics
Elderly patients are more likely to exhibit increased dose sensitivity to the anticholinergic, sedative, and hypotensive effects of maprotiline; therefore, a lower initial dose should usually be used and the dosage maintained at the lowest effective level. Careful monitoring is necessary to maintain optimum therapeutic serum concentrations in the elderly. Or-

thostatic hypotension, although rare, may occur in elderly patients and caution must be observed to prevent falls.

### Dental

The peripheral anticholinergic effects of maprotiline may decrease or inhibit salivary flow, especially in middle-aged or elderly patients, thus contributing to the development of caries, periodontal disease, oral candidiasis, and discomfort.

Although rarely reported, the blood dyscrasia–causing effects of maprotiline may result in an increased incidence of microbial infection, delayed healing, and gingival bleeding. If agranulocytosis, eosinophilia, purpura, or thrombocytopenia occurs, dental work should be deferred until blood counts have returned to normal. Patient instruction in proper oral hygiene should include caution in use of regular toothbrushes, dental floss, and toothpicks.

### Drug interactions and/or related problems

The following drug interactions and/or related problems have been selected on the basis of their potential clinical significance (possible mechanism in parentheses where appropriate)—not necessarily inclusive (» = major clinical significance):

Note: Combinations containing any of the following medications, depending on the amount present, may also interact with this medication.

Although not all of the following interactions have been documented to pertain specifically to maprotiline, a potential exists for their occurrence because of the close similarity of maprotiline's pharmacological effects to those of tricyclic antidepressants.

» Alcohol or
» CNS depression–producing medications, other (See *Appendix II*)
   (concurrent use with maprotiline may result in serious potentiation of CNS depressant effects)

Anticholinergics or other medications with anticholinergic activity (See *Appendix II* ) or
Antihistamines
   (concurrent use may potentiate the anticholinergic effects of either these medications or maprotiline; dosage adjustments may be necessary)

Anticonvulsants
   (maprotiline may enhance CNS depression, lower the seizure threshold, and decrease the effects of the anticonvulsant medication)

Antidepressants, tricyclic or
Bupropion or
Clozapine or
Haloperidol or
Loxapine or
Molindone or
Phenothiazines or
Pimozide or
Thioxanthenes or
Trazodone
   (concurrent use may prolong and intensify the anticholinergic and sedative effects of either these medications or maprotiline; in addition, these medications may increase the risk of seizures by lowering the seizure threshold, and should be added or withdrawn with caution)

Cimetidine
   (concurrent use may increase plasma concentrations of maprotiline; dosage adjustment of maprotiline may be necessary when cimetidine therapy is initiated or discontinued)

Clonidine or
Guanadrel or
Guanethidine
   (antihypertensive effects may be decreased when these medications are used concurrently with maprotiline)
   (concurrent use of clonidine with maprotiline may result in serious potentiation of CNS depressant effects)

Contraceptives, oral, estrogen-containing or
Estrogens
   (concurrent use of large doses of estrogens with tricyclic antidepressants may potentiate antidepressant side effects and reduce the therapeutic effects of the tricyclic antidepressants; although not documented, similar effects may occur with maprotiline, a tetracyclic antidepressant)

Fluoxetine
   (plasma concentrations of tricyclic antidepressants may be increased twofold or more when fluoxetine is used concurrently; although not documented, similar increases may occur with maprotiline, a tetracyclic antidepressant; some clinicians recommend dosage reductions of maprotiline of 50% or greater if used concomitantly with fluoxetine)

» Monoamine oxidase (MAO) inhibitors, including furazolidone, procarbazine, and selegiline
   (concurrent use with maprotiline is generally not recommended, especially on an outpatient basis, as hyperpyretic episodes, severe convulsions, hypertensive crises, and death have resulted in a small number of patients from concurrent use with tricyclic antidepressants; a minimum of 14 days should elapse between discontinuing MAO inhibitors and initiating maprotiline therapy)

Naphazoline, ophthalmic or
Oxymetazoline, nasal or
Phenylephrine, nasal or ophthalmic or
Xylometazoline, nasal
   (if significant systemic absorption occurs, concurrent use with maprotiline may potentiate pressor effects of these medications)

» Sympathomimetics
   (concurrent use with maprotiline may potentiate cardiovascular effects, possibly resulting in arrhythmias, tachycardia, or severe hypertension or hyperpyrexia; phentolamine can control the adverse reaction)
   (significant systemic absorption of ophthalmic epinephrine may also potentiate cardiovascular effects; also, local anesthetics with vasoconstrictors should be avoided or a minimal amount of the vasoconstrictor should be used with the local anesthetic)
   (concurrent use with maprotiline may decrease the pressor effects of ephedrine and mephentermine)

Thyroid hormones
   (concurrent use with maprotiline may enhance the possibility of cardiac arrhythmias; dosage adjustments may be necessary)

### Medical considerations/Contraindications

The medical considerations/contraindications included here have been selected on the basis of their potential clinical significance (reasons given in parentheses where appropriate)—not necessarily inclusive (» = major clinical significance).

*Except under special circumstances, this medication should not be used when the following medical problems exist:*

» Myocardial infarction, during the acute recovery period
» Seizure disorders, including epilepsy, or history of seizures
   (risk of seizures is increased)

*Risk-benefit should be considered when the following medical problems exist:*

» Alcoholism, active
   (increased risk of seizures and CNS depression)
» Asthma or
» Blood disorders or
» Glaucoma, angle-closure or
» Increased intraocular pressure or
» Urinary retention, or history of
   (may be exacerbated)
» Bipolar disorder
   (swing to hypomanic or manic phase may be accelerated and rapid cycling between mania and depression may be induced by maprotiline)
» Cardiovascular disorders
   (increased risk of conduction defects, arrhythmias, myocardial infarction, strokes, and tachycardia)
Gastrointestinal disorders
   (risk of paralytic ileus)
» Hepatic function impairment
   (metabolism may be altered)
» Hyperthyroidism
   (increased risk of cardiovascular toxicity)
» Myocardial infarction, history of
   (increased risk of recurrence)
Prostatic hypertrophy
   (risk of urinary retention)
» Schizophrenia
   (psychosis may be aggravated)
Sensitivity to maprotiline or tricyclic antidepressants

**Patient monitoring**

The following may be especially important in patient monitoring (other tests may be warranted in some patients, depending on condition; » = major clinical significance):

Blood cell counts

(may be required at periodic intervals during long-term therapy; in patients with sore throat and fever, leukocyte and differential counts may be necessary; maprotiline should be discontinued if there is evidence of pathologic neutrophil depression)

Blood pressure determinations and
Cardiac function monitoring and
Hepatic function determinations

(may be required at periodic intervals during therapy to detect development of adverse effects that may not be evident to the patient)

Careful observation for possibility of drug-induced acceleration to hypomania or mania

(recommended periodically although most patients respond favorably to maprotiline when it is used to treat the depressed phase of bipolar disorder)

Careful observation for possibility of suicide attempt

(suicidal tendencies may persist in some severely depressed patients during the early phases of therapy until significant remission of depression occurs)

## Side/Adverse Effects

Note: Although not all of the following side effects have been attributed specifically to maprotiline, a potential exists for their occurrence as with the tricyclic antidepressants.

The following side/adverse effects have been selected on the basis of their potential clinical significance (possible signs and symptoms in parentheses where appropriate)—not necessarily inclusive:

**Those indicating need for medical attention**
Incidence more frequent
*Skin rash, redness, swelling, or itching*

Incidence less frequent
*Constipation, severe*—may lead to paralytic ileus; *nausea or vomiting; seizures; shakiness or trembling; unusual excitement; weight loss*

Note: *Seizures* may occur in patients with or without a history of seizures, usually with doses above 200 mg a day. The lowest effective maintenance dose is recommended to reduce further risk. Drugs that alter seizure threshold should be added to or withdrawn from maprotiline regimen with caution.

Incidence rare
*Agranulocytosis* (sore throat and fever)—rarely reported for maprotiline, but has occurred with tricyclic antidepressants; *anticholinergic effect* (difficulty in urinating); *breast enlargement*—in males and females; *confusion*—especially in elderly; *hallucinations; hypotension* (fainting); *inappropriate secretion of milk*—in females; *irregular heartbeat; jaundice, cholestatic* (yellow eyes or skin); *swelling of testicles*

**Those indicating need for medical attention only if they continue or are bothersome**
Incidence more frequent
*Blurred vision; dizziness or lightheadedness*—especially in the elderly; *drowsiness; dryness of mouth; headache; impotence* (decreased sexual ability); *increased or decreased sexual drive; tiredness or weakness*

Incidence less frequent
*Constipation, mild; diarrhea; heartburn; increased appetite and weight gain*—related to carbohydrate craving; *increased sensitivity of skin to sunlight; increased sweating; insomnia* (trouble in sleeping); *weight loss*

## Overdose

For specific information on the agents used in the management of maprotiline overdose, see:
- *Barbiturates (Systemic)* monograph;
- *Benzodiazepines (Systemic)* monograph;
- *Charcoal, Activated (Oral-Local)* monograph;
- *Corticosteroids—Glucocorticoid Effects (Systemic)* monograph;
- *Digitalis Glycosides (Systemic)* monograph;
- *Phenytoin* in *Anticonvulsants, Hydantoin (Systemic)* monograph;
- *Propranolol* in *Beta-adrenergic Blocking Agents (Systemic)* monograph; and/or
- *Sodium Bicarbonate (Systemic)* monograph.

For more information on the management of overdose or unintentional ingestion, **contact a Poison Control Center** (see *Poison Control Center Listing*).

**Clinical effects of overdose**
The following effects have been selected on the basis of their potential clinical significance (possible signs and symptoms in parentheses where appropriate)—not necessarily inclusive:

*Coma; convulsions; dizziness, severe; drowsiness, severe; fast or irregular heartbeat; fever; muscle stiffness or weakness, severe; restlessness or agitation; trouble in breathing; vomiting*

Note: Risk of *seizures, respiratory complications,* and *cardiotoxicity* is greater with maprotiline than with tricyclic antidepressants, and duration of comatose state and QRS complex is longer.

**Treatment of overdose**
There is no specific antidote for maprotiline overdose. The following steps of supportive and symptomatic treatment may be considered:
To decrease absorption—
Emptying stomach with emetic and/or lavage.
Administering activated charcoal slurry followed by a stimulant cathartic.

Specific treatment—
For circulatory collapse—Administering intravenous fluids, oxygen, and corticosteroids.
For congestive heart failure—Digitalizing rapidly.
For cardiac arrhythmias—Alkalinizing blood with sodium bicarbonate. Arrhythmias refractory to sodium bicarbonate may be treated with phenytoin. Propranolol may be used with caution.
For seizures and hyperirritability—Administering carefully titrated parenteral benzodiazepines or barbiturates. However, barbiturates should not be used if monoamine oxidase inhibitors have been used in recent therapy. Also, barbiturates may cause respiratory depression, especially in children. Equipment should be available to provide artificial ventilation and resuscitation. Administration of physostigmine salicylate is not recommended because of an increase in the risk of seizures.

Supportive care—
Controlling hyperpyrexia by any available means, including ice packs if necessary.
Patients in whom intentional overdose is known or suspected should be referred for psychiatric consultation.

Note: Dialysis of maprotiline has not been successful because of its high protein binding.

## Patient Consultation

As an aid to patient consultation, refer to *Advice for the Patient, Maprotiline (Systemic).*

In providing consultation, consider emphasizing the following selected information (» = major clinical significance):

**Before using this medication**
» Conditions affecting use, especially:
Sensitivity to maprotiline or tricyclic antidepressants
Use in the elderly—Elderly patients may be more prone to develop anticholinergic, sedative, and hypotensive effects
Dental—Dry mouth may cause caries, oral candidiasis, periodontal disease, and discomfort; rare blood dyscrasias may result in increased incidence of microbial infection, delayed healing, and gingival bleeding
Other medications, especially alcohol or other CNS depression–producing medications, MAO inhibitors, or sympathomimetics
Other medical problems, especially active alcoholism, asthma, bipolar disorder, blood disorders, cardiovascular disorders, glaucoma, hepatic function impairment, hyperthyroidism, increased intraocular pressure, schizophrenia, seizure disorders, or urinary retention

**Proper use of this medication**
» Compliance with therapy
» May require up to 2 to 3 weeks of therapy to obtain optimal antidepressant effects
» Proper dosing
Missed dose: If dosing schedule is:
More than one dose a day—Taking as soon as possible; if almost time for next dose, skipping missed dose; going back to regular dosing schedule; not doubling doses
One dose a day at bedtime—Not taking missed dose following morning; checking with doctor
» Proper storage

**Precautions while using this medication**
Regular visits to physician to check progress during therapy

» Avoiding the use of alcohol or other CNS depressants during maprotiline therapy
» Possible drowsiness; caution when driving, using machines, or doing other things requiring alertness
» Possible dizziness or lightheadedness; caution when getting up suddenly from a lying or sitting position
» Possible dryness of mouth; using sugarless gum or candy, ice, or saliva substitute for relief; checking with physician or dentist if dry mouth continues for more than 2 weeks
» Caution if any kind of surgery, dental treatment, or emergency treatment is required
» Checking with physician before discontinuing medication; gradual dosage reduction may be needed

**Side/adverse effects**
Anticholinergic, sedative, and hypotensive effects more likely to occur in the elderly
Precautions followed for 3 to 7 days after discontinuing medication
Signs of potential side effects, especially skin rash, redness, swelling, or itching; severe constipation; convulsions; nausea or vomiting; shakiness or trembling; unusual excitement; weight loss; agranulocytosis; anticholinergic effect; breast enlargement; confusion; hallucinations; hypotension; inappropriate secretion of milk; irregular heartbeat; jaundice; or swelling of testicles

## General Dosing Information

Dosage of maprotiline must be individualized for each patient by titration.

Correlations between plasma concentration, clinical response, side effects, and toxicity have not been established.

Some clinicians recommend that for maintenance therapy, the optimal daily dose may be reduced somewhat, sometimes given as a single dose at bedtime, and often continued for 6 months to 1 year. (A divided dose may be preferred for geriatric, adolescent, or cardiovascular patients.) In patients with recurrent depression, however, continuation of the full treatment dose during maintenance therapy may be optimal.

The single daily dose at bedtime is useful when side effects such as excessive drowsiness or dizziness might be bothersome or dangerous during working hours.

A gradual reduction in dosage is recommended when this medication is to be discontinued.

Potentially suicidal patients should not have access to large quantities of this medication since depressed patients, particularly those who may use alcohol excessively, may continue to exhibit suicidal tendencies until significant improvement occurs. Some clinicians recommend that the patient be supplied with the least amount of medication necessary for satisfactory patient management.

## Oral Dosage Forms

### MAPROTILINE HYDROCHLORIDE TABLETS USP

**Usual adult and adolescent dose**
Antidepressant—
Oral, initially 25 to 75 mg a day, in divided doses, for at least two weeks, the dosage being adjusted gradually by 25 mg a day as needed and tolerated
Note: The effective maintenance dose is usually about 150 mg a day, often given once a day at bedtime.

**Usual adult prescribing limits**
Outpatients: Up to 150 mg a day.
Hospitalized patients: Up to 225 mg a day.

**Usual pediatric dose**
Children up to 18 years of age: Safety and efficacy have not been established.

**Usual geriatric dose**
Initial: Oral, 25 mg a day.
Maintenance: Oral, 50 to 75 mg a day.

**Strength(s) usually available**
U.S.—
25 mg (Rx) [*Ludiomil* (lactose); GENERIC].
50 mg (Rx) [*Ludiomil* (lactose); GENERIC].
75 mg (Rx) [*Ludiomil* (lactose); GENERIC].
Canada—
10 mg (Rx) [*Ludiomil* (lactose)].
25 mg (Rx) [*Ludiomil* (lactose; tartrazine)].
50 mg (Rx) [*Ludiomil* (lactose)].
75 mg (Rx) [*Ludiomil* (scored; lactose)].

**Packaging and storage**
Store below 40 °C (104 °F), preferably between 15 and 30 °C (59 and 86 °F), unless otherwise specified by manufacturer. Store in a well-closed container.

**Auxiliary labeling**
• May cause drowsiness.
• Avoid alcoholic beverages.

Revised: 08/29/94

---

# MASOPROCOL   Topical†

VA CLASSIFICATION (Primary): DE600
Note: For a listing of dosage forms and brand names by country availability, see *Dosage Forms* section(s). For a listing of brand names for the articles in this monograph, refer to the General Index.

†Not commercially available in Canada.

## Category
Antineoplastic (topical).

## Indications
**Accepted**
Actinic keratoses, multiple (treatment)—Topical masoprocol is indicated for treatment of actinic (solar) keratoses.

## Pharmacology/Pharmacokinetics

**Physicochemical characteristics**
Molecular weight—302.37.

**Mechanism of action/Effect**
Unknown. Masoprocol is a potent 5-lipoxygenase inhibitor and has antiproliferative activity against keratinocytes in tissue culture, but the relationship between this activity and its effectiveness in actinic keratoses is unknown.

**Absorption**
Less than 2%.

## Precautions to Consider

**Cross-sensitivity and/or related problems**
Patients sensitive to sulfites may be sensitive to topical masoprocol because of the sulfite preservatives present.

**Carcinogenicity**
Studies in animals have not been done.

**Mutagenicity**
Masoprocol was mutagenic in the Ames assay (negative in three strains of *Salmonella* and positive in one). In an *in vivo* mouse estrogenic activity assay, a subcutaneous dose of 2 mg of masoprocol per kg of body weight (mg/kg) per day for 4 days produced no more estrogenic activity than did vehicle controls.

**Pregnancy/Reproduction**
Fertility—Studies in animals have not been done.
Pregnancy—Adequate and well-controlled studies in humans have not been done.
Studies in rabbits and rats at doses up to 6 and 16 times the human dose (on a mg per square meter of body surface basis), respectively, found no evidence of teratogenicity.
FDA Pregnancy Category B.

**Breast-feeding**
It is not known whether masoprocol is distributed into breast milk. However, because some systemic absorption occurs, caution is recommended while topical masoprocol is being administered.

**Pediatrics**
Appropriate studies on the relationship of age to the effects of topical masoprocol have not been performed in the pediatric population.

**Geriatrics**

Appropriate studies on the relationship of age to the effects of topical masoprocol have not been performed in the geriatric population.

**Medical considerations/Contraindications**

The medical considerations/contraindications included here have been selected on the basis of their potential clinical significance (reasons given in parentheses where appropriate)—not necessarily inclusive (» = major clinical significance).

*Risk-benefit should be considered when the following medical problem exists:*

» Sensitivity to masoprocol

**Patient monitoring**

The following may be especially important in patient monitoring (other tests may be warranted in some patients, depending on condition; » = major clinical significance):

Biopsy

(may be recommended to confirm diagnosis if solar keratoses do not respond or if they recur after treatment)

## Side/Adverse Effects

Note: Local skin reactions usually resolve within two weeks after withdrawal of masoprocol.

The following side/adverse effects have been selected on the basis of their potential clinical significance (possible signs and symptoms in parentheses where appropriate)—not necessarily inclusive:

**Those indicating need for medical attention**

Incidence more frequent

*Contact dermatitis* (redness and swelling of normal skin; redness, soreness, swelling, itching, dryness, and flaking of skin where medication is applied)

Note: Allergic *contact dermatitis*, confirmed by patch testing, has been reported in up to 10% of patients, usually within 3 weeks after initiation of treatment. In patients rechallenged with masoprocol cream, both frequency and severity of reactions increased.

Incidence less frequent

*Blistering or oozing at site of application*

Signs and symptoms of allergic reaction to sulfites

*Bluish coloration of skin; dizziness, severe, or feeling faint; wheezing or trouble in breathing*

**Those indicating need for medical attention only if they continue or are bothersome**

Incidence more frequent

*Burning feeling at site of application*

Incidence less frequent

*Leathery feeling to skin; skin roughness; wrinkles*

## Patient Consultation

As an aid to patient consultation, refer to *Advice for the Patient, Masoprocol (Topical)*.

In providing consultation, consider emphasizing the following selected information (» = major clinical significance):

**Before using this medication**

» Conditions affecting use, especially:

Sensitivity to masoprocol or sulfite preservatives

Pregnancy—Caution recommended; some systemic absorption occurs

Breast-feeding—Caution recommended; some systemic absorption occurs

**Proper use of this medication**

» Compliance with therapy; applying enough medication to cover affected areas

Washing area to be treated with mild soap and water and drying thoroughly; using fingertips to apply

» Washing hands immediately after application to prevent accidental transfer of medication from fingertips to eyes or mouth

Possible unsightly reaction during and for about 2 weeks after therapy is completed; checking with physician before discontinuing medication

» Proper dosing

Missed dose: Applying as soon as remembered; not applying if not remembered within a few hours; checking with physician if more than one dose is missed

» Proper storage

**Precautions while using this medication**

» Importance of close monitoring by physician

» Caution in applying medication; avoiding eyes, nose, and mouth

» Possibility of allergic reaction to sulfites contained in the preparation; checking with physician immediately if signs of allergic reaction occur

**Side/adverse effects**

Signs of potential side effects, especially contact dermatitis

## General Dosing Information

Patients using topical masoprocol should be under supervision of a physician experienced in use of the medication.

Masoprocol has not been shown to produce necrosis, scarring, or ulceration during the initial course of therapy. Therapeutic efficacy does not rely on production of a local inflammatory skin reaction.

Use of occlusive dressings is not recommended.

It is recommended that treatment with masoprocol be discontinued if contact dermatitis occurs or if an excessive inflammatory response occurs on normal skin.

## Topical Dosage Forms

### MASOPROCOL CREAM

**Usual adult dose**

Actinic (solar) keratoses—

Topical, to the skin, as a 10% cream twice a day in a sufficient amount to cover the lesions.

**Usual pediatric dose**

Safety and efficacy have not been established.

**Strength(s) usually available**

U.S.—

10% (Rx) [*Actinex* (methylparaben; propylparaben; sodium metabisulfite)].

Canada—

Not commercially available.

**Packaging and storage**

Store between 15 and 30 °C (59 and 86 °F), unless otherwise specified by manufacturer.

**Auxiliary labeling**

• For the skin.

• Continue medicine for full course of treatment.

## Selected Bibliography

Olsen EA, Abernethy ML, Kulp-Shorten C, et al. A double-blind, vehicle-controlled study evaluating masoprocol cream in the treatment of actinic keratoses on the head and neck. J Am Acad Dermatol 1991 May; 24 (5 Pt 1): 738-43.

Developed: 07/31/95

---

**MAZINDOL**—See *Appetite Suppressants (Systemic)*

# MEASLES VIRUS VACCINE LIVE   Systemic

VA CLASSIFICATION (Primary): IM100

Note: This monograph is specific for the measles vaccine (Moraten) prepared from a more attenuated line of measles virus derived from the Enders' attenuated Edmonston strain.

In the U.S., the usual age to initiate immunization with measles vaccine is 15 months of age.

In Canada, the usual age to initiate immunization with measles vaccine is 12 months of age.

Note: For a listing of dosage forms and brand names by country availability, see *Dosage Forms* section(s). For a listing of brand names for the articles in this monograph, refer to the General Index.

## Category

Immunizing agent (active).

## Indications

### Accepted

Measles (prophylaxis)—Measles virus vaccine live is indicated for immunization against measles (rubeola; morbilli; coughing, hard, red, or ten-day measles). The main objective of measles immunization is to prevent the severe complications, such as pneumonia, ear infections, sinusitis, encephalitis, subacute sclerosing panencephalitis, and death, which may arise from a measles infection. The risk of serious complications and death from a natural measles infection is greater for adults and infants than for children and adolescents.

Unless otherwise contraindicated, all susceptible persons born in or after 1957 (persons born before 1957 are presumed to be immune because of past natural infection) should be immunized against measles, including
- Children 15 months of age and older, including those with chronic diseases, such as cystic fibrosis, heart disease, and asthma and other chronic pulmonary diseases, and children with inactive tuberculosis or active tuberculosis under treatment.
- Children 12 to 15 months of age in high-risk areas. Even though immunization before the age of 15 months results in a slightly lower efficacy of the vaccine, the benefits of preventing measles infection in these children are considered to outweigh the slightly lower efficacy.
- Persons who were previously vaccinated with measles vaccine before their first birthday. Measles vaccine administered before a person's first birthday should not be considered part of the immunization schedule against measles.
- School-age children through college-age students, who were not previously fully immunized with 2 doses of vaccine.
- Medical personnel and employees in medical facilities, since they are at increased risk of contracting measles from, or transmitting measles to, patients. Those born in or after 1957 should receive the usual 2 doses of vaccine; those born before 1957 should receive at least 1 dose of vaccine, in case they have escaped natural infection or have been inadequately immunized with an earlier available vaccine.
- Persons 12 months of age or older who have been exposed to measles. If measles vaccine is administered within 72 hours of exposure, the measles infection may be prevented or ameliorated because the onset of action of the vaccine is shorter than the incubation period of the natural measles infection. Unless otherwise contraindicated, if exposure to measles has occurred within 72 hours, administration of measles vaccine is preferable to the use of immune globulin. In addition, since a single exposure may not cause infection, post-exposure vaccination provides future protection. Immune globulin may be administered to persons exposed to measles more than 3 days, but less than 6 days, before, especially if these persons are at high risk of complications, as are infants under 12 months of age, pregnant women, and immunocompromised persons. Three months after administration of immune globulin (or when the person is 15 months of age, whichever is later) the person should receive measles vaccine unless it is otherwise contraindicated.
- Persons traveling outside the U.S., since measles is endemic in many countries. Approximately 50% of imported cases of measles occur in returning U.S. citizens who were not immunized against measles. In addition, because measles vaccine is not 100% effective and the risk of exposure to measles abroad may be substan-

tially greater than in the U.S., and because the risk of serious complications and death is greater for adults than for children, a second dose of measles vaccine is recommended for previously immunized persons born in 1957 or later who have not yet received their second dose and who do not have evidence of measles immunity. No additional dose is recommended for travelers born before 1957. Children from 12 to 15 months of age should receive their first dose of measles vaccine (preferably as the measles, mumps, and rubella combination vaccine [MMR]) before departure. The second dose should be administered as usual, normally when the child enters school. Children from 6 to 12 months of age should receive a dose of the single-antigen measles vaccine (preferred) or MMR before departure. Subsequently these children should receive 2 doses of MMR, the first dose as early as 12 months of age if the child stays in a high-risk area, even though the optimal age for the first revaccination dose is 15 months. The second revaccination dose should be administered as usual, normally when the child enters school. Immunization is not required for children up to 6 months of age, since they are protected by maternally derived antibodies.
- Persons previously vaccinated with inactivated (killed) measles vaccine (available in the U.S. from 1963 to 1967 and in Canada until 1970), alone or followed by live measles vaccine within 3 months, or persons vaccinated with an unknown type of measles vaccine during these years, since they may have received the inactivated measles vaccine. Some of these individuals have developed severe atypical measles syndrome when exposed to natural measles virus and, of these individuals, some developed serious complications requiring hospitalization. Although the incidence and the severity of side/adverse effects are increased in persons previously vaccinated with inactivated measles vaccine and revaccinated with live measles vaccine, the severity of a possible infection with natural measles virus outweighs these risks.
- Females of child-bearing potential, if they are not pregnant and if they are counseled not to become pregnant for 3 months following vaccination.
- Postpartum women who do not plan to breast-feed, preferably before discharge from the hospital. Although problems in humans have not been documented, postpartum women who plan to breast-feed should consult with their physician to consider the risk-benefit before receiving immunization with measles vaccine.
- Household contacts of susceptible pregnant women or of other persons with medical contraindications to measles vaccination, to reduce the risk to persons unable to receive measles vaccine.
- Persons born between 1957 and 1972 who received measles vaccine before they were 13 months of age, since many of these individuals have significantly lower antibody titers against measles infection than those born in 1972 or later because of the type of vaccine administered.
- Persons previously vaccinated with live attenuated Edmonston B vaccine, which was distributed from 1963 to 1975. Since the vaccine had a greater incidence of adverse effects, it was the practice to administer immune globulin or measles immune globulin in a separate syringe simultaneously with the vaccine to reduce the severity of the adverse effects. If the vaccine was administered on or after the first birthday, it is acceptable as an effective first dose.
- Persons previously vaccinated with further attenuated live measles vaccine (e.g., Schwartz or Moraten) or an unknown type of live measles vaccine, if either was accompanied by immune globulin or measles immune globulin. Immune globulin or measles immune globulin administered simultaneously with a further attenuated measles vaccine may weaken or prevent the immune response. These persons should be reimmunized with 2 doses of measles vaccine.
- Persons who lack adequate documentation of immunity, even though they may be immune to measles. There is no evidence of increased risk of adverse effects when persons already immune to measles are revaccinated.

Persons born in or after 1957 should be considered immune to measles only if they have:
- Documentation of immunization with 2 doses of live measles vaccine that were initiated on or after their first birthday, spaced at least 1 month apart, and preferably administered as MMR.
- Physician's diagnosis of previous measles infection.
- Laboratory evidence of measles immunity.

# Pharmacology/Pharmacokinetics

## Mechanism of action/Effect
Following subcutaneous injection, measles vaccine induces the formation of protective antibodies in susceptible individuals. This produces a modified, noncommunicable measles infection and provides active immunity to measles.

## Protective effect
Immunity to measles occurs in at least 95% of susceptible individuals vaccinated at 15 months of age or older. However, immunity to measles occurs in only 80 to 95% of susceptible individuals vaccinated between 12 and 15 months of age, presumably because transplacental maternal antibody persists in some children and interferes with the response to the vaccine.

## Time to protective effect
Effective immunity occurs within 7 to 10 days.
Measles antibody levels are detectable on the 12th through the 31st day following vaccination.

## Duration of protective effect
At least 13 to 16 years and probably lifetime immunity in the great majority of immunized persons.

# Precautions to Consider

## Cross-sensitivity and/or related problems
Patients allergic to neomycin or streptomycin may be allergic to the measles virus vaccine live available in the U.S. and Canada because it may contain a small amount of neomycin and/or streptomycin. The antibiotics are used in the production of the vaccine to prevent bacterial overgrowth in the viral culture. A history of hypersensitivity reactions other than anaphylaxis, such as delayed-type allergic reaction (contact dermatitis), generally does not preclude immunization.

## Pregnancy/Reproduction
Pregnancy—Although adequate studies have not been done in humans, use in pregnant women is not recommended, because increased rates of spontaneous abortion, premature births, low birth-weight neonates, and possibly congenital defects have been observed with natural measles infection during pregnancy, and the possibility exists that measles vaccine may cause similar effects. In addition, it is recommended that pregnancy be avoided for 3 months following vaccination.
Studies have not been done in animals.
FDA Pregnancy Category C.

## Breast-feeding
It is not known whether this vaccine is distributed into breast milk. However, problems in humans have not been documented.

## Pediatrics
Children who were vaccinated when younger than 12 months of age should be revaccinated.
In the U.S., immunization is not generally recommended for infants younger than 15 months of age, since maternal measles-neutralizing antibodies may interfere with the immune response. However, if exposure to measles infection has occurred less than 72 hours previously or is imminent, children between 6 and 15 months of age can be vaccinated, provided that those vaccinated before their first birthday are revaccinated at 15 months of age.
In Canada, immunization is recommended for infants 12 months of age.

## Drug interactions and/or related problems
The following drug interactions and/or related problems have been selected on the basis of their potential clinical significance (possible mechanism in parentheses where appropriate)—not necessarily inclusive (» = major clinical significance):

Note: Combinations containing any of the following medications, depending on the amount present, may also interact with this medication.

Blood products or
Immune globulins
(concurrent administration with measles vaccine may interfere with the patient's immune response to the virus because of the possibility of antibodies to measles virus in these products. Measles vaccine should be administered at least 14 days before, or more than 3 months after, administration of blood products or immune globulins)
» Immunosuppressive agents or
» Radiation therapy
(because normal defense mechanisms are suppressed, concurrent use with measles vaccine may potentiate the replication of the vaccine virus, may increase the side/adverse effects of the vaccine virus, and/or may decrease the patient's antibody response to mea-

sles vaccine. The interaction may be severe enough to cause death. The interval between discontinuing medications that cause immunosuppression and regaining the ability to respond to measles vaccine depends on the intensity and type of immunosuppressive medication used, the underlying disease, and other factors; estimates vary from 3 months to 1 year. Patients with leukemia in remission should not receive measles vaccine until at least 3 months after their last chemotherapy. The precaution does not apply to corticosteroids used as replacement therapy, for short-term [less than 2 weeks] systemic therapy, or by other routes of administration that do not cause immunosuppression)

Live virus vaccines, other
(although data are lacking on impairment of antibody responses to rubella, measles, mumps, or oral polio vaccine when these vaccines are administered on different days within 1 month of each other, the chance exists that the immune responses may be impaired when live virus vaccines are administered in this manner; therefore, when feasible, live virus vaccines not administered on the same day should be given at least 1 month apart)

## Laboratory value alterations
The following have been selected on the basis of their potential clinical significance (possible effect in parentheses where appropriate)—not necessarily inclusive (» = major clinical significance):
With diagnostic test results
» Tuberculin skin test
(short-term suppression lasting several weeks may occur, starting 4 to 7 days after vaccination, and may result in false-negative tests; if required, tuberculin skin tests should be done before, simultaneously with, or at least 4 to 6 weeks after administration of measles vaccine)

Skin tests, other
(decreased responsiveness to skin test antigens may occur because of vaccine-induced transient suppression of delayed-type hypersensitivity; the period of time for which responsiveness is decreased depends upon the particular skin test used)

## Medical considerations/Contraindications
The medical considerations/contraindications included here have been selected on the basis of their potential clinical significance (reasons given in parentheses where appropriate)—not necessarily inclusive (» = major clinical significance).

*Except under special circumstances, this medication should not be used when the following medical problems exist:*
» Febrile illness, severe
(to avoid confusing manifestations of illness with possible side/adverse effects of vaccine; minor illnesses, such as upper respiratory infection, do not preclude administration of vaccine)
» Immune deficiency conditions, congenital or hereditary, family history of, or
» Immune deficiency conditions, primary or acquired
(because of reduced or suppressed defense mechanisms, the use of live virus vaccines, including measles vaccine, may potentiate the replication of the vaccine virus, may increase the side/adverse effects of the vaccine virus, and/or may decrease the patient's antibody response to measles)
(persons with leukemia in remission may receive live virus vaccines if at least 3 months have passed since their last chemotherapy treatment)
(persons infected with human immunodeficiency virus [HIV] may receive measles vaccine if they are asymptomatic; in addition, immunization with measles vaccine should be considered for persons with symptomatic HIV infection)
(when there is a family history of congenital or hereditary immune deficiency conditions, the patient should not be vaccinated until his/her immune competence is demonstrated)

*Risk-benefit should be considered when the following medical problems exist:*
Allergy to eggs
(patients allergic to eggs may be allergic to the measles virus vaccine live available in the U.S. and Canada, since it is produced in chick embryo cell cultures. A history of hypersensitivity reactions other than anaphylaxis generally does not preclude immunization. In addition, no allergy to measles vaccine has been found in patients allergic to chicken or chicken feathers)

Conditions requiring avoidance of fever, such as cerebral injury or history of febrile seizures
(because of possible vaccine-induced fever)

Sensitivity to measles vaccine

Tuberculosis, active, untreated

(tuberculosis may be exacerbated by natural measles infection, although there is no evidence that measles vaccine exacerbates tuberculosis. In addition, persons under treatment for tuberculosis have not experienced exacerbation when vaccinated with measles vaccine. However, since measles vaccine suppresses the tuberculin skin test for several weeks, patients thought to have tuberculosis or to be at risk for tuberculosis should be tested before, or simultaneously with, administration of measles vaccine [See also *Laboratory value alterations.*])

### Patient monitoring

The following may be especially important in patient monitoring (other tests may be warranted in some patients, depending on condition; » = major clinical significance):

Seroconversion test

(may be performed 4 or more weeks following vaccination in patients in whom immunity is considered crucial [e.g., persons traveling outside the U.S. or women in high-risk areas who intend to become pregnant], since vaccination with measles vaccine may not result in seroconversion in all susceptible patients)

## Side/Adverse Effects

Note: Fever or skin rash may occur from 5 to 12 days after immunization and usually lasts several days.

A history of hypersensitivity reactions other than anaphylaxis, such as delayed-type allergic reaction (contact dermatitis), generally does not preclude immunization.

Encephalitis and encephalopathy have been temporally related to measles vaccine administration and occur once per million doses administered. However, no causal relationship has been established. The incidence of these diseases after a natural measles infection is one per thousand persons.

Although there is a temporal relationship, no definite causal relationship has been established between the isolated reports of the occurrence of Guillain-Barré syndrome or ocular palsies following the administration of measles vaccine.

It is not known whether some of the cases of subacute sclerosing panencephalitis (SSPE) attributed to the measles vaccine were actually from unrecognized natural measles infection during the first year of life. However, the use of the measles vaccine has reduced the incidence of SSPE from 5 to 10 cases per million cases of natural measles infection to 1 case per million doses of measles vaccine.

The incidence of side/adverse effects does not appear to be age-related.

Persons who are immune to measles because of past vaccination or infection are not at increased risk of adverse effects from the vaccine.

There have been no reports of transmission of the measles virus from immunized persons to susceptible contacts.

The following side/adverse effects have been selected on the basis of their potential clinical significance (possible signs and symptoms in parentheses where appropriate)—not necessarily inclusive:

### Those indicating need for medical attention

Incidence more frequent—5 to 15%
  *Fever over 39.4 °C (103 °F)*

Incidence rare
  *Anaphylactic reaction* (difficulty in breathing or swallowing; hives; itching, especially of soles or palms; reddening of skin, especially around ears; swelling of eyes, face, or inside of nose; sudden and severe unusual tiredness or weakness); *convulsions, encephalitis, or meningoencephalitis* (confusion, severe or continuing headache, irritability, stiff neck, or vomiting); *ocular palsies* (double vision); *thrombocytopenic purpura* (bruising or purple spots on skin)

### Additional side/adverse effects that may occur because of a previous vaccination with inactivated (killed) measles virus vaccine and indicating need for medical attention

Incidence rare
  *Fever over 39.4 °C (103 °F), prolonged; lymphadenopathy* (swelling of glands in neck); *swelling, blistering, edema, or pain at injection site, severe and extensive*

Note: Some of these side/adverse effects may be severe enough to necessitate hospitalization.

### Those indicating need for medical attention only if they continue or are bothersome

Incidence more frequent
  *Burning or stinging at injection site*—due to acid pH of vaccine; *fever of 37.7 °C (100 °F) or less*

Incidence less frequent
  *Allergic reaction, delayed-type, cell-mediated* (itching, swelling, redness, tenderness, or hard lump at injection site); *fever between 37.7 and 39.4 °C (100 and 103 °F); skin rash*

## Patient Consultation

As an aid to patient consultation, refer to *Advice for the Patient, Measles Virus Vaccine Live (Systemic).*

In providing consultation, consider emphasizing the following selected information (» = major clinical significance):

### Before receiving this vaccine

» Conditions affecting use, especially:

Sensitivity to measles vaccine or allergy to eggs, neomycin, or streptomycin

Pregnancy—Use of measles vaccine during pregnancy or pregnancy within 3 months of immunization is not recommended, since the natural measles infection has been shown to increase the chance of birth defects and there is a possibility that the live virus vaccine might cause similar problems

Use in children—In the U.S., use is usually not recommended for infants up to 15 months of age. In Canada, use is not recommended for infants up to 12 months of age

Other medications, especially immunosuppressive agents or radiation therapy

Other medical problems, especially severe febrile illness, primary or acquired immune deficiency conditions, or family history of congenital or hereditary immune deficiency conditions

### Proper use of this vaccine

» Proper dosing

*Precautions after receiving this vaccine*

» Not becoming pregnant for 3 months without first checking with physician, because of theoretical risk of birth defects

Checking with physician before receiving:

Blood transfusions or other blood products within 2 weeks of this vaccine

Gamma globulin or other globulins within 2 weeks of this vaccine

Any other live-virus vaccines within 1 month of this vaccine

Tuberculin skin test within 6 weeks of this vaccine, since the results of the test may be affected by measles vaccine

### Side/adverse effects

Fever and skin rash may occur from 5 to 12 days after vaccination and usually last 1 or 2 days

Signs of potential side effects, especially fever over 39.4 °C (103 °F), anaphylactic reaction, convulsions, encephalitis, meningoencephalitis, ocular palsies, or thrombocytopenic purpura

## General Dosing Information

Persons who have received 2 doses of measles virus vaccine live, at least 1 month apart, on or after their first birthday should be considered fully immunized against measles. These persons require no further doses.

It is recommended that both doses of measles vaccine be administered as the measles, mumps, and rubella combination vaccine (MMR) to assure immunity to all 3 viruses. Mumps reimmunization is especially important, since recent studies have shown that mumps can occur among persons with prior vaccination with mumps vaccine.

The dosage of measles vaccine is the same for all persons: infants, children, and adults.

When sterilizing syringes and skin before vaccination, care should be taken to avoid preservatives, antiseptics, detergents, and disinfectants, since the vaccine virus is easily inactivated by these substances.

To prevent inactivation of the vaccine, it is recommended that only the diluent provided by the manufacturer be used for vaccine reconstitution.

A 25-gauge, 5/8th-inch needle is recommended for administration of the vaccine.

Measles vaccine is administered subcutaneously. It should not be injected intravenously.

Immune globulin should not be given with the measles vaccine currently in use in the U.S. and Canada, because it may inactivate the vaccine virus.

Although measles, mumps, and rubella vaccines are commercially available as a combination vaccine (MMR) and, as such, are administered as a single injection, the commercially available individual vaccines should not be mixed in the same syringe or administered at the same body site.

Although the fourth dose of DTP and the third dose of OPV have traditionally been administered in the U.S. to children 18 months of age and MMR has traditionally been administered in the U.S. to children 15 months of age, it is now recommended in the U.S. that DTP, OPV, and MMR be administered concurrently to children 15 months of age. MMR should not be postponed in order to administer these vaccines concurrently at 18 months of age. In addition, the traditional method is still an acceptable alternative.

Measles vaccine, a live virus vaccine, may be administered concurrently with the following, using separate body sites, separate syringes, and the precautions that apply to each immunizing agent
- Polysaccharide vaccines, such as haemophilus b polysaccharide vaccine, haemophilus b conjugate vaccine, meningococcal polysaccharide vaccine, or pneumococcal polyvalent vaccine.
- Influenza vaccine, whole or split virus.
- Diphtheria toxoid, tetanus toxoid, and/or pertussis vaccine.
- Live virus vaccines, other, such as mumps, rubella, or oral polio vaccine (OPV), but only if the vaccines are administered on the same day; otherwise they should be administered at least 1 month apart.
- Inactivated poliovirus vaccine (IPV) or enhanced-potency inactivated poliovirus vaccine (enhanced-potency IPV).
- Hepatitis B recombinant or plasma-derived vaccine.
- Inactivated vaccines, other, except cholera, typhoid, and plague. It is recommended that cholera, typhoid, and plague vaccines be administered on separate occasions because of these vaccines' propensity to cause side/adverse effects.

### For treatment of adverse effects
Recommended treatment includes
- For mild hypersensitivity reaction—Administering antihistamines, and, if necessary, corticosteroids.
- For severe hypersensitivity or anaphylactic reaction—Administering epinephrine. Antihistamines or corticosteroids may also be administered as required.

## Parenteral Dosage Forms

### MEASLES VIRUS VACCINE LIVE (FOR INJECTION) USP

#### Usual adult and adolescent dose
Immunizing agent (active)—
Subcutaneous, 0.5 mL, preferably into the outer aspect of the upper arm:
First dose—At initial visit.
Second dose—At least one month after the first dose.

#### Usual pediatric dose
Immunizing agent (active)—
U.S.:
Infants up to 6 months of age—Use is not recommended, since maternal measles-neutralizing antibodies may interfere with the immune response.
Infants 6 to 12 months of age traveling outside the U.S.—Subcutaneous, 0.5 mL, preferably into the outer aspect of the upper arm. However, this dose should not be counted as one of the two regular doses of measles vaccine. The first regular dose should be given as early as 12 months of age if the child stays in a high-risk area; otherwise, as usual at 15 months of age.
Infants 12 to 15 months of age in high-risk areas or traveling outside the U.S.—Subcutaneous, 0.5 mL, preferably into the outer aspect of the upper arm. This dose should be counted as the first regular dose.
Infants and children 15 months of age and older— See *Usual adult and adolescent dose.*

Note: Since the recommendation for a second dose of measles vaccine is relatively new, at present the timing of the second dose is based primarily on the decision of the jurisdiction in which the child resides.

The Immunization Practices Advisory Committee (ACIP) recommends that the second dose be administered at 4 to 6 years of age (i.e., entry to kindergarten or first grade), which coincides with the current schedule for administration of other childhood immunizing agents.

The American Academy of Pediatrics (AAP) recommends that the second dose be administered at the time of entrance to middle school or junior high school (i.e., at approximately 11 to 12 years of age)

Canada:
Infants up to 12 months of age—Use is not recommended.
Infants and children 12 months of age and older—Subcutaneous, 0.5 mL, preferably into the outer aspect of the upper arm, for one dose.

### Strength(s) usually available
U.S.—
Not less than the equivalent of 1000 $TCID_{50}$ (quantity of virus estimated to infect 50% of inoculated cultures times 1000) of the U.S. Reference Measles Virus in each 0.5 mL dose (Rx) [*Attenuvax* (neomycin approximately 25 mcg)].
Canada—
Not less than the equivalent of 1000 $TCID_{50}$ (quantity of virus estimated to infect 50% of inoculated cultures times 1000) of a reference measles virus in each 0.5 mL dose (Rx) [GENERIC (may contain neomycin, streptomycin)].

### Packaging and storage
Store the lyophilized form of the vaccine, the diluent, and the reconstituted form of the vaccine between 2 and 8 °C (36 and 46 °F), unless otherwise specified by manufacturer.
Alternatively, the diluent for the single-dose vials may be stored between 15 and 30 °C (59 and 86 °F).
Protect both the lyophilized form and the reconstituted form of the vaccine from light.

### Preparation of dosage form
To reconstitute, use only the diluent provided by the manufacturer, since it is free of preservatives and other substances that might inactivate the vaccine.
Withdraw the entire volume of diluent (approximately 0.5 mL) into the syringe. Inject all the diluent in the syringe into the vial of lyophilized vaccine and agitate to mix thoroughly. Withdraw the entire contents into the syringe and inject the total volume of restored vaccine subcutaneously.

### Stability
Both the lyophilized and the reconstituted vaccine should be protected from light, which may inactivate the virus.
Use the reconstituted vaccine as soon as possible. Discard unused reconstituted vaccine after 8 hours.
The reconstituted vaccine is clear yellow. It should not be used if it is discolored.

### Incompatibilities
Preservatives or other substances may inactivate the vaccine; therefore, only the diluent supplied by the manufacturer should be used for reconstitution.
Also, a sterile syringe free of preservatives, antiseptics, and detergents should be used for each injection and/or reconstitution of the vaccine because these substances may inactivate the live virus vaccine.

### Auxiliary labeling
- Protect from light.
- Store in refrigerator.
- Discard reconstituted vaccine if not used within 8 hours.

### Note
The date and time of reconstitution should be indicated on the vial if the reconstituted vaccine is not used at once.

Revised: 07/12/94

# MEBENDAZOLE Systemic

VA CLASSIFICATION (Primary): AP200

Note: For a listing of dosage forms and brand names by country availability, see *Dosage Forms* section(s). For a listing of brand names for the articles in this monograph, refer to the General Index.

## Category

Anthelmintic (systemic).

## Indications

Note: Bracketed information in the *Indications* section refers to uses that are not included in U.S. product labeling.

### Accepted

Ascariasis (treatment)—Mebendazole is indicated as a primary agent for ascariasis caused by *Ascaris lumbricoides* (common roundworm).

Enterobiasis (treatment)—Mebendazole is indicated as a primary agent for enterobiasis caused by *Enterobius vermicularis* (pinworm).

Hookworm infection (treatment)—Mebendazole is indicated as a primary agent for hookworm disease caused by *Ancylostoma duodenale* (common hookworm; Old World hookworm) and *Necator americanus* (American hookworm; New World hookworm).

Intestinal roundworm, multiple (treatment)—Mebendazole is indicated in the treatment of multiple intestinal roundworm infections.

Trichuriasis (treatment)—Mebendazole is indicated as a primary agent for trichuriasis caused by *Trichuris trichiura* (whipworm).

[Capillariasis (treatment)][1]—Mebendazole is used in the treatment of capillariasis caused by *Capillaria philippinensis*.

[Gnathostomiasis (treatment)][1]—Mebendazole is used in the treatment of gnathostomiasis caused by *Gnathostoma spinigerum*.

[Hydatid disease, alveolar (treatment)][1]—Mebendazole is used in the treatment of alveolar hydatid disease caused by *Echinococcus multilocularis (E. alveolaris)*.

[Hydatid disease, unilocular (treatment)][1]—Mebendazole is used in the treatment of unilocular hydatid disease caused by *E. granulosus*. Mebendazole is used as a secondary agent in patients in whom surgery is contraindicated or has failed, in after-spill during surgery, or in recurrences. Very high doses may be effective.

[Trichinosis (treatment)][1]—Mebendazole is used as a secondary agent in the treatment of trichinosis (trichinellosis) caused by *Trichinella spiralis* (pork worm). Systemic corticosteroids are used concurrently, especially in patients with severe symptoms, to minimize inflammatory reactions to *Trichinella* larvae.

Not all species or strains of a particular helminth may be susceptible to mebendazole. In addition, efficacy varies with respect to pre-existing diarrhea, gastrointestinal transit time, and degree of infection.

---

[1]Not included in Canadian product labeling.

## Pharmacology/Pharmacokinetics

### Physicochemical characteristics
Molecular weight—295.30.

### Mechanism of action/Effect
Vermicidal; may also be ovicidal for ova of most helminths; mebendazole causes degeneration of parasite's cytoplasmic microtubules and thereby selectively and irreversibly blocks glucose uptake in susceptible adult intestine-dwelling helminths and their tissue-dwelling larvae; inhibition of glucose uptake apparently results in depletion of the parasite's glycogen stores; this, in turn, results in reduced formation of adenosine triphosphate (ATP) required for survival and reproduction of the helminth; corresponding energy levels are gradually reduced until death of the parasite ensues; mebendazole does not appear to affect serum glucose concentrations in humans, however.

### Absorption
Poorly absorbed (approximately 5 to 10%) from gastrointestinal tract; absorption may be increased when taken with food, especially fatty food.

### Distribution
Distributed to serum, cyst fluid, liver, omental fat, and pelvic, pulmonary, and hepatic cysts; highest concentrations found in liver; relatively high concentrations also found in muscle-encysted *Trichinella spiralis* larvae; also crosses the placenta.

### Protein binding
High to very high (90–95%).

### Biotransformation
Primarily hepatic; metabolized to inactive amino, hydroxy, and hydroxy-amino metabolites; primary metabolite is 2-amino-5-benzoyl-benzimidazole.

### Half-life
Normal hepatic function—2.5 to 5.5 hours (range: 2.5 to 9 hours).

Impaired hepatic function (cholestasis)—Approximately 35 hours.

### Time to peak serum concentration
2 to 5 hours (range—0.5 to 7 hours).

### Peak serum concentration
Following a dose of 100 mg twice a day for 3 days—
    Mebendazole: Not more than 0.03 mcg per mL.
    2-Amino metabolite: Not more than 0.09 mcg per mL.
Serum concentrations up to 0.5 mcg per mL have been reported in chronic, high-dose therapy.

### Elimination
Fecal—Approximately 95% excreted unchanged or as the primary metabolite (2-amino derivative) in feces.
Renal—Approximately 2 to 5% excreted unchanged or as the primary metabolite in urine.

## Precautions to Consider

### Carcinogenicity
Carcinogenicity studies in mice and rats given doses as high as 40 mg per kg of body weight (mg/kg) daily for over two years have not shown mebendazole to be carcinogenic.

### Mutagenicity
Dominant lethal mutation studies in mice given single doses as high as 640 mg/kg have not shown that mebendazole is mutagenic. The spermatocyte test, the $F_1$ translocation test, and the Ames test produced negative results.

### Pregnancy/Reproduction
Fertility—Studies in mice given doses of up to 40 mg/kg for 60 days prior to gestation in males and 14 days in females have not shown that mebendazole causes adverse effects on the fetus or offspring. However, mebendazole has been shown to cause slight maternal toxicity at this dose.

Pregnancy—Mebendazole crosses the placenta. A post-marketing survey in pregnant women who inadvertently took mebendazole during the first trimester has not shown an incidence of spontaneous abortion or malformation greater than that of the general population. In a total of 170 deliveries at term, mebendazole has not been shown to be teratogenic in humans.

Studies in rats given single oral doses as low as 10 mg/kg have shown that mebendazole is teratogenic and embryotoxic.

FDA Pregnancy Category C.

### Breast-feeding
It is not known whether mebendazole is distributed into breast milk. However, problems in humans have not been documented.

### Pediatrics
Appropriate studies on the relationship of age to the effects of mebendazole have not been performed in children up to 2 years of age. However, no pediatrics-specific problems have been documented to date in children over the age of 2.

### Geriatrics
No information is available on the relationship of age to the effects of mebendazole in geriatric patients.

### Drug interactions and/or related problems
The following drug interactions and/or related problems have been selected on the basis of their potential clinical significance (possible mechanism in parentheses where appropriate)—not necessarily inclusive (» = major clinical significance):

Note: Combinations containing any of the following medications, depending on the amount present, may also interact with this medication.

Carbamazepine
    (in patients receiving high doses of mebendazole for treatment of tissue-dwelling organisms such as *Echinococcus multilocularis* or *E. granulosus* [hydatid disease], carbamazepine has been shown to lower mebendazole plasma concentrations by induction of hepatic microsomal enzymes and to impair the therapeutic response; if carbamazepine is being used for seizures, replacement with val-

proic acid is recommended; treatment of intestinal helminths such as whipworms or hookworms does not appear to be affected by the rate of hepatic metabolism of mebendazole)

### Laboratory value alterations

The following have been selected on the basis of their potential clinical significance (possible effect in parentheses where appropriate)—not necessarily inclusive (» = major clinical significance):

With physiology/laboratory test values
- » Alanine aminotransferase (ALT [SGPT]), serum, and
- » Alkaline phosphatase, serum, and
- » Aspartate aminotransferase (AST [SGOT]), serum, and
  Blood urea nitrogen (BUN)
  (values may be transiently increased)

  Hemoglobin, serum
  (concentration may be decreased)

### Medical considerations/Contraindications

The medical considerations/contraindications included here have been selected on the basis of their potential clinical significance (reasons given in parentheses where appropriate)—not necessarily inclusive (» = major clinical significance).

*Risk-benefit should be considered when the following medical problems exist:*

Crohn's ileitis or
Ulcerative colitis
(may increase absorption and toxicity of mebendazole, especially in high-dose therapy)
- » Hepatic function impairment
  (mebendazole is metabolized primarily in liver; prolonged half-life and drug accumulation may occur, with an increased incidence of side effects; dosage may need to be decreased)

  Hypersensitivity to mebendazole

### Patient monitoring

The following may be especially important in patient monitoring (other tests may be warranted in some patients, depending on condition; » = major clinical significance):

*For pinworms*
- » Perianal examinations
  (cellophane tape swabs of the perianal area to detect the presence of eggs may be required prior to and starting 1 week following treatment with mebendazole, especially in patients with persisting symptoms; swabs should be taken every morning prior to defecation and bathing for at least 3 days to determine efficacy or proof of cure; perianal examinations may also be required to detect the presence of adult worms in the perianal area; no patient should be considered cured unless perianal swabs have been negative for 7 consecutive days)

*For roundworms, whipworms, and capillariasis*
- » Stool examinations
  (may be required prior to and approximately 1 to 3 weeks following treatment with mebendazole to determine efficacy or proof of cure; because of colonic mixing, eggs may persist in the stool for up to 1 week following cure)

*For patients on high-dose therapy*
- » Complete blood counts (CBCs)
  (may be required prior to and periodically during the first month of treatment with mebendazole since high-dose mebendazole may cause granulocytopenia, neutropenia, and/or leukopenia; CBC's performed two or three times a week from day 10 through day 25, and weekly thereafter, are recommended)

## Side/Adverse Effects

The following side/adverse effects have been selected on the basis of their potential clinical significance (possible signs and symptoms in parentheses where appropriate)—not necessarily inclusive:

**Those indicating need for medical attention**
Incidence rare
  *Hypersensitivity* (fever; skin rash or itching); *neutropenia* (sore throat and fever; unusual tiredness and weakness)—with high doses, reversible

**Those indicating need for medical attention only if they continue or are bothersome**
Incidence less frequent
  *Gastrointestinal disturbances* (abdominal pain or upset; diarrhea; nausea or vomiting)
Incidence rare
  *Alopecia* (hair loss)—with high doses; *dizziness; headache*

## Overdose

For more information on the management of overdose or unintentional ingestion, **contact a Poison Control Center** (see *Poison Control Center Listing*).

In accidental overdose, gastrointestinal symptoms may occur and may last up to a few hours.

### Treatment of overdose

Supportive care—
  Supportive therapy necessary to maintain the vital functions of the patient may be administered.

## Patient Consultation

As an aid to patient consultation, refer to *Advice for the Patient, Mebendazole (Systemic)*.

In providing consultation, consider emphasizing the following selected information (» = major clinical significance):

### Before using this medication
- » Conditions affecting use, especially:
    Hypersensitivity to mebendazole
    Pregnancy—Mebendazole crosses the placenta
    Other medical problems, especially hepatic function impairment

### Proper use of this medication
Reading patient instructions before taking medication
No special preparations or other measures (e.g., dietary restrictions or fasting, concurrent medications, purging, or cleansing enemas) required before, during, or immediately after therapy
Chewing tablets, swallowing whole, or crushing tablets and mixing with food
- » Compliance with full course of therapy; second course may be required in some infections
- » Proper dosing
  Missed dose: Taking as soon as possible; not taking if almost time for next dose; not doubling doses
- » Proper storage
*For pinworms*
  Treating all household members concurrently; treating again in 2 to 3 weeks
*For patients on high-dose therapy*
- » Taking with meals, especially fatty ones, to increase absorption; checking with physician if on low-fat diet

### Precautions while using this medication
Regular visits to physician to check progress, especially in high-dose therapy
Checking with physician if no improvement within a few days
*For hookworms or whipworms*
  Importance of taking iron supplements daily during treatment and for up to 6 months following treatment if patient is anemic at the time of therapy
*For pinworms*
  Washing (not shaking) all bedding and nightclothes after treatment to prevent reinfection
  Other measures may be recommended by some physicians

### Side/adverse effects
Signs of potential side effects, especially hypersensitivity and neutropenia

## General Dosing Information

No special preparations (e.g., dietary restrictions or fasting, concurrent medications, purging, or cleansing enemas) are required before, during, or immediately after treatment with mebendazole.

Mebendazole tablets may be chewed, swallowed whole, or crushed and mixed with food.

Patients who are heavily infected with helminths may require more prolonged treatment.

**For high-dose therapy**
In the treatment of tissue-dwelling helminth infections, the administration of much higher doses of mebendazole may be necessary because of poor absorption.

Mebendazole should preferably be taken with meals, especially fatty ones. This increases the bioavailability, absorption, and serum concentrations of mebendazole.

**For hookworms and whipworms**
In the treatment of hookworms and whipworms, especially in patients who are heavily infected or who have inadequate dietary intake of iron, concurrent iron therapy may be required if anemia is present. Iron

therapy may need to be continued for up to 6 months to replenish iron stores.

### For pinworms

Because of the high probability of transfer of pinworms, it is usually recommended that all members of the household be treated concurrently. Retreatment is recommended 2 to 3 weeks following initial treatment.

## Oral Dosage Forms

Note: Bracketed uses in the *Dosage Forms* section refer to categories of use and/or indications that are not included in U.S. product labeling.

### MEBENDAZOLE TABLETS (CHEWABLE) USP

#### Usual adult and adolescent dose

Ascariasis; or
Trichuriasis; or
Hookworm—
    Oral, 100 mg two times a day, morning and evening, for three days. May be repeated in two to three weeks if required.
Enterobiasis—
    Oral, 100 mg as a single dose. Repeat in two to three weeks.
Intestinal roundworm, multiple—
    Oral, 100 mg two times a day, morning and evening, for three days.
[Capillariasis]¹—
    Oral, 200 mg two times a day for twenty days.
[Gnathostomiasis]¹—
    Oral, 200 mg every three hours for six days.
[Hydatid disease]¹—
    Oral, 13.3 to 16.7 mg per kg of body weight three times a day for up to three to six months.
[Trichinosis]¹—
    Oral, 200 to 400 mg three times a day for three days, then 400 to 500 mg three times a day for ten days.

#### Usual adult prescribing limits

[Hydatid disease]¹—Doses up to 200 mg per kg of body weight daily have been used.

#### Usual pediatric dose

Children up to 2 years of age—Dosage has not been established.
Children 2 years of age and over—Ascariasis, [capillariasis]¹, enterobiasis, intestinal roundworm infections, trichuriasis, and uncinariasis: See *Usual adult and adolescent dose.*

Note: In the treatment of infections caused by tissue-dwelling organisms in which high doses are required, dosage should be based on the patient's body weight.

#### Strength(s) usually available

U.S.—
    100 mg (Rx) [*Vermox;* GENERIC].
Canada—
    100 mg (Rx) [*Vermox* (scored)].

#### Packaging and storage

Store below 40 °C (104 °F), preferably between 15 and 30 °C (59 and 86 °F), unless otherwise specified by manufacturer. Store in a well-closed container.

#### Auxiliary labeling

• May be chewed, crushed, or swallowed whole.
• Take with meals (high-dose therapy).
• Continue medication for full time of treatment.

¹Not included in Canadian product labeling.

Revised: 08/01/95

---

# MECAMYLAMINE    Systemic†

VA CLASSIFICATION (Primary): CV490

Note: For a listing of dosage forms and brand names by country availability, see *Dosage Forms* section(s). For a listing of brand names for the articles in this monograph, refer to the General Index.

†Not commercially available in Canada.

## Category

Antihypertensive.

## Indications

### Accepted

Hypertension (treatment)—Mecamylamine is indicated in the treatment of moderately severe to severe hypertension and uncomplicated malignant hypertension. It is not considered to be a primary agent in the treatment of hypertension. Use has declined because of the numerous side effects.

Nonpharmacologic management (especially sodium restriction, weight reduction and exercise, and moderation of alcohol consumption) is recommended first for some patients, including those with mild hypertension, and is recommended as an adjunct to all pharmacologic hypertensive therapy.

## Pharmacology/Pharmacokinetics

### Physicochemical characteristics

Molecular weight—203.75.
pKa—11.2.

### Mechanism of action/Effect

Ganglionic blocker; prevents stimulation of postsynaptic receptors by acetylcholine released from presynaptic nerve endings; hypotensive effect is due to reduction in sympathetic tone, vasodilation, and reduced cardiac output, and is primarily postural.

### Absorption

Almost completely absorbed from the gastrointestinal tract.

### Onset of action

30 minutes to 2 hours.

### Duration of action

6 to 12 hours or more.

### Elimination

Renal, unchanged; excretion increased in acidic urine and reduced in alkaline urine.

## Precautions to Consider

### Carcinogenicity/Mutagenicity

Studies have not been done.

### Pregnancy/Reproduction

Pregnancy—Mecamylamine crosses the placenta. Studies in humans have not been done. However, use in pregnancy is not recommended since mecamylamine's ganglionic blocking effects may decrease gastrointestinal motility in the fetus, resulting in meconium ileus. In addition, maternal sensitivity to the hypotensive effects is increased during pregnancy.

FDA Pregnancy Category C.

### Breast-feeding

It is not known whether mecamylamine is excreted in breast milk. However, problems in humans have not been documented.

### Pediatrics

No information is available on the relationship of age to the effects of mecamylamine in pediatric patients. Safety and efficacy have not been established.

### Geriatrics

Although appropriate studies on the relationship of age to the effects of mecamylamine have not been performed in the geriatric population, the elderly may be more sensitive to the hypotensive effects. In addition, elderly patients are more likely to have age-related renal function impairment, which may require caution in patients receiving mecamylamine.

### Dental

Use of mecamylamine may decrease or inhibit salivary flow, thus contributing to the development of caries, periodontal disease, oral candidiasis, and discomfort.

### Drug interactions and/or related problems

The following drug interactions and/or related problems have been selected on the basis of their potential clinical significance (possible mechanism in parentheses where appropriate)—not necessarily inclusive (» = major clinical significance):

Note: Combinations containing any of the following medications, depending on the amount present, may also interact with this medication.

» Alkalizers, urinary, especially carbonic anhydrase inhibitors, antacids, or sodium bicarbonate
(alkalinization of urine by these agents slows excretion and prolongs the effects of mecamylamine; concurrent use is not recommended)

Allopurinol or
Colchicine or
Probenecid or
Sulfinpyrazone
(mecamylamine may raise the concentration of blood uric acid; dosage adjustment of antigout medications may be necessary to control hyperuricemia and gout)

» Ambenonium or
» Neostigmine or
» Pyridostigmine
(concurrent use may interfere with the antimyasthenic effect of ambenonium, neostigmine, or pyridostigmine, leading to weakness and sudden inability to swallow)

» Antibiotics or
» Sulfonamides
(patients with chronic pyelonephritis being treated with these medications should not be treated with ganglionic blockers)

Anti-inflammatory drugs, nonsteroidal (NSAIDs), especially indomethacin
(antihypertensive effects of mecamylamine may be reduced when it is used concurrently with these agents; indomethacin, and possibly other NSAIDs, may antagonize the antihypertensive effect by inhibiting renal prostaglandin synthesis and/or by causing sodium and fluid retention; the patient should be carefully monitored to confirm that the desired effect is being obtained)

Estrogens
(estrogen-induced fluid retention may lead to increased blood pressure)

Hypotension-producing medications, other (see *Appendix II*)
(antihypertensive effects may be potentiated when these medications are used concurrently with mecamylamine; although some combinations are frequently used for therapeutic advantage, dosage adjustments may be necessary during concurrent use; if mecamylamine is given with a thiazide diuretic, the dose of mecamylamine, not the diuretic, should be reduced)

Preanesthetic and anesthetic agents used in surgery, especially spinal anesthetics
(may potentiate the hypotensive response, with increased risk of severe hypotension, shock, and cardiovascular collapse during surgery)

Sympathomimetics
(mecamylamine may enhance the pressor response to sympathomimetic pressor amines, and the hypotensive effect of mecamylamine may be decreased or reversed by all sympathomimetics)

**Medical considerations/Contraindications**
The medical considerations/contraindications included here have been selected on the basis of their potential clinical significance (reasons given in parentheses where appropriate)—not necessarily inclusive (» = major clinical significance).

*Risk-benefit should be considered when the following medical problems exist:*

Bladder neck obstruction or
Prostatic hypertrophy or
Urethral stricture
(because of possible urinary retention)

» Cardiovascular insufficiency, including coronary insufficiency, or Cerebrovascular insufficiency or
» Myocardial infarction, recent
(ischemia may be aggravated by hypotension)

Fever or
Hemorrhage or
Infection or
Salt depletion as a result of diminished intake or nausea and vomiting, diarrhea, excessive sweating, or use of diuretics
(hypotensive effects may be potentiated)

» Glaucoma, predisposition to
(high doses may increase intraocular pressure)

» Organic pyloric stenosis
(may increase risk of ileus)

Renal function impairment or
» Uremia
(increased effects due to reduced excretion)
Sensitivity to mecamylamine

**Patient monitoring**
The following may be especially important in patient monitoring (other tests may be warranted in some patients, depending on condition; » = major clinical significance):

» Blood pressure measurements
(recommended at periodic intervals in patients being treated for hypertension; selected patients may be trained to perform blood pressure measurements at home and report the results at regular physician visits)

» Cardiovascular and renal function determinations

## Side/Adverse Effects

Note: Most side effects are dose-related.

The following side/adverse effects have been selected on the basis of their potential clinical significance (possible signs and symptoms in parentheses where appropriate)—not necessarily inclusive:

**Those indicating need for medical attention**
Incidence more frequent—dose-related
*Hypotension, postural* (dizziness or lightheadedness, especially when getting up from a lying or sitting position)
Incidence less frequent—dose-related
*Parasympathetic blockade* (difficult urination)
Incidence rare
*Central nervous system (CNS) stimulation, specifically choreiform movements* (uncontrolled movements of face, hands, arms, or legs) *convulsions; mental changes* (confusion or excitement, mental depression); *tremors* (trembling); *interstitial pulmonary edema and fibrosis* (shortness of breath); *paralytic ileus* (bloating; frequent loose stools followed by severe constipation)

**Those indicating need for medical attention only if they continue or are bothersome**
Incidence more frequent—dose-related
*Drowsiness; parasympathetic blockade* (blurred vision, less frequently or rarely; constipation; decreased sexual ability; dryness of mouth; enlarged pupils; weakness); *unusual tiredness*
Note: *Constipation* may be preceded by small, frequent liquid stools and may rarely lead to paralytic ileus.

Incidence less frequent or rare—dose-related
*Decreased sexual ability or interest in sex; loss of appetite; nausea and vomiting*

## Overdose

For more information on the management of overdose or unintentional ingestion, **contact a Poison Control Center** (see *Poison Control Center Listing*).

**Treatment of overdose**
Overdose may be treated by administration of pressor amines with caution, keeping in mind the possibility of increased sensitivity to their effects.

## Patient Consultation

As an aid to patient consultation, refer to *Advice for the Patient, Mecamylamine (Systemic)*.

In providing patient consultation, consider emphasizing the following selected information (» = major clinical significance):

**Before using this medication**
» Conditions affecting use, especially:
Sensitivity to mecamylamine
Pregnancy—Use not recommended because of risk of decreased gastrointestinal motility in fetus and increased maternal sensitivity to hypotensive effects
Breast-feeding—May be excreted in breast milk
Use in the elderly—Increased sensitivity to hypotensive effects
Other medications, especially urinary alkalizers, antimyasthenics, antibiotics, or sulfonamides
Other medical problems, especially cardiovascular insufficiency, recent myocardial infarction, glaucoma, organic pyloric stenosis, or uremia

**Proper use of this medication**
Possible need for control of weight and diet, especially sodium intake

» Patient may not experience symptoms of hypertension; importance of taking medication even if feeling well

» Does not cure, but helps control hypertension; possible need for life-long therapy; checking with physician before discontinuing medication; serious consequences of untreated hypertension

Getting into habit of taking at same time each day to help increase compliance

» Proper dosing

» Missed dose: Taking as soon as possible; checking with physician if two or more doses in a row are missed; possible severe reaction if stopped abruptly

» Proper storage

### Precautions while using this medication

Regular visits to physician to check progress

» Checking with physician before discontinuing medication; gradual dosage reduction may be necessary to avoid serious rebound hypertension

» Having enough medication on hand to get through weekends, holidays, and vacations; possibly carrying second prescription for emergency use

» Not taking other medications, especially nonprescription sympathomimetics, unless discussed with physician

» Caution when getting up suddenly from a lying or sitting position, especially in the morning

» Caution in using alcohol, while standing for long periods or exercising, and during hot weather because of enhanced orthostatic hypotensive effects

Caution in taking antacids, especially those containing sodium bicarbonate

Reporting fever or infection to physician; dosage adjustment may be required

Possible dryness of mouth; using sugarless candy or gum, ice, or saliva substitute for relief; checking with physician or dentist if dry mouth continues for more than 2 weeks

Caution if any kind of surgery (including dental surgery) or emergency treatment is required

### Side/adverse effects

Signs of potential side effects, especially convulsions, mental changes, tremors, postural hypotension, parasympathetic blockade, CNS stimulation, interstitial pulmonary edema and fibrosis, and paralytic ileus

### General Dosing Information

Because of wide individual variation in response to mecamylamine, dosage must be adjusted to meet the individual requirements of each patient on the basis of clinical response.

The optimal dosage of mecamylamine is at or just under that which produces dizziness or faintness in the standing position.

The hypotensive effect of mecamylamine is especially pronounced when the patient is standing. If feasible, blood pressure readings should be taken in the supine position, after standing for 10 minutes, and immediately after exercise. Dosage increases should be made only if there has been no decrease in the standing blood pressure from previous levels.

Hospitalized patients should not be discharged until the effect of mecamylamine on their standing blood pressure has been determined.

Incidence and severity of side effects may be reduced by initiating therapy at a low dose and increasing gradually to the minimum effective dose.

It is recommended that dosage increments be made no more frequently than every 2 days.

It is recommended that a morning dose, if given at all, be the smallest dose of the day since an increased hypotensive response may occur in the morning.

More frequent daily doses may be given to patients in whom smooth control is difficult to obtain.

Recent evidence suggests that withdrawal of antihypertensive therapy prior to surgery is not necessary but that the anesthesiologist must be aware of such therapy.

With continuing use, limited tolerance to the antihypertensive effects of mecamylamine may develop as a result of fluid retention and expanded plasma volume.

The abrupt interruption of mecamylamine therapy, including several consecutive missed doses, may result in severe rebound hypertension, especially in patients being treated for malignant hypertension. This may lead to cerebrovascular accidents or acute congestive heart failure. Gradual withdrawal is recommended when mecamylamine is discontinued, and substitution of other antihypertensive therapy may be necessary.

### Diet/Nutrition

It is recommended that mecamylamine be administered at consistent times in relationship to meals, since hypotension may occur after a meal because of dilation of splanchnic blood vessels. Administration after meals may be preferable to administration on an empty stomach, resulting in more gradual absorption and smoother control of high blood pressure.

## Oral Dosage Forms

### MECAMYLAMINE HYDROCHLORIDE TABLETS USP

**Usual adult dose**
Antihypertensive—
Initial: Oral, 2.5 mg two times a day, the dosage being increased in increments of 2.5 mg every two or more days until the optimal response is achieved.
Maintenance: Oral, 25 mg a day in three divided doses.
Note: Geriatric patients may be more sensitive to the effects of the usual adult dose.

**Usual pediatric dose**
Safety and efficacy have not been established.

**Strength(s) usually available**
U.S.—
2.5 mg (Rx) [*Inversine* (scored; lactose)].
Canada—
Not commercially available.

**Packaging and storage**
Store below 40 °C (104 °F), preferably between 15 and 30 °C (59 and 86 °F), unless otherwise specified by manufacturer. Store in a well-closed container.

**Auxiliary labeling**
• Do not take other medicines without your doctor's advice.

**Note**
Check refill frequency to determine compliance in hypertensive patients.

Revised: 01/20/93

---

# MECHLORETHAMINE   Systemic

INN: Chlormethine
VA CLASSIFICATION (Primary/Secondary): AN100/DE600
Other commonly used names are chlormethine and nitrogen mustard.
Note: For a listing of dosage forms and brand names by country availability, see *Dosage Forms* section(s). For a listing of brand names for the articles in this monograph, refer to the General Index.

## Category

Antineoplastic.

## Indications

### Accepted

Carcinoma, lung (treatment)—Mechlorethamine is indicated for treatment of bronchogenic carcinoma.

Leukemia, chronic lymphocytic (treatment) or
Leukemia, chronic myelocytic (treatment)—Mechlorethamine is indicated for treatment of chronic lymphocytic and chronic myelocytic leukemia.

Lymphomas, Hodgkin's (treatment) or
Lymphomas, non-Hodgkin's (treatment)—Mechlorethamine is indicated

for the palliative treatment of Hodgkin's disease (Stages III and IV) and for treatment of some non-Hodgkin's lymphomas, including lymphosarcoma.

Malignant effusions, pericardial (treatment)

Malignant effusions, peritoneal (treatment) or

Malignant effusions, pleural (treatment)—Mechlorethamine is indicated by intracavitary administration for palliative treatment of metastatic carcinoma resulting in effusion.

Mycosis fungoides (treatment)—Mechlorethamine is indicated for treatment of mycosis fungoides.

Polycythemia vera (treatment)—Mechlorethamine is indicated for treatment of polycythemia vera.

## Pharmacology/Pharmacokinetics

### Physicochemical characteristics
Molecular weight—192.52.
pKa—6.1.

### Mechanism of action/Effect
Mechlorethamine is a bifunctional alkylating agent and is cell cycle–phase nonspecific. Activity occurs as a result of formation of an unstable ethylenimmonium ion, which alkylates or binds with many intracellular molecular structures, including nucleic acids. Its cytotoxic action is primarily due to cross-linking of strands of DNA and RNA, as well as inhibition of protein synthesis. With intracavitary use, mechlorethamine causes sclerosis and an inflammatory reaction on serous membranes, leading to adherence of serosal surfaces.

### Other actions/effects
Has weak immunosuppressive activity.

### Absorption
Mechlorethamine is incompletely absorbed following intracavitary administration, probably because of rapid deactivation by body fluids.

### Biotransformation
Rapidly deactivated in body fluids and tissues.

### Onset of action
Effects occur within a few seconds or minutes.

### Elimination
Apparently renal (less than 0.01% unchanged).

## Precautions to Consider

### Carcinogenicity/Mutagenicity
Secondary malignancies are potential delayed effects of many antineoplastic agents, although it is not clear whether the effect is related to their mutagenic or immunosuppressive action. The effect of dose and duration of therapy is also unknown, although risk seems to increase with long-term use. Although information is limited, available data seem to indicate that the carcinogenic risk is greatest with the alkylating agents.

Mechlorethamine has been associated with an increased risk of development of secondary carcinomas in animals and humans.

### Pregnancy/Reproduction
Fertility—Gonadal suppression, resulting in amenorrhea or azoospermia, may occur in patients taking antineoplastic therapy, especially with the alkylating agents. In general, these effects appear to be related to dose and length of therapy and may be irreversible. Prediction of the degree of testicular or ovarian function impairment is complicated by the common use of combinations of several antineoplastics, which makes it difficult to assess the effects of individual agents.

Mechlorethamine causes testicular atrophy and interferes with spermatogenesis.

Pregnancy—Although several successful pregnancies have been reported, there is evidence that mechlorethamine is teratogenic, especially when administered early in pregnancy.

First trimester: It is usually recommended that use of antineoplastics, especially combination chemotherapy, be avoided whenever possible, especially during the first trimester. Although information is limited because of the relatively few instances of antineoplastic administration during pregnancy, the mutagenic, teratogenic, and carcinogenic potential of these medications must be considered.

Other hazards to the fetus include adverse reactions seen in adults.

In general, use of a contraceptive is recommended during cytotoxic drug therapy.

FDA Pregnancy Category D.

### Breast-feeding
Although very little information is available regarding distribution of antineoplastic agents into breast milk, breast-feeding is not recommended while mechlorethamine is being administered because of the risks to the infant (adverse effects, mutagenicity, carcinogenicity). It is not known whether mechlorethamine is distributed into breast milk.

### Pediatrics
Appropriate studies on the relationship of age to the effects of mechlorethamine have not been performed in the pediatric population. However, pediatrics-specific problems that would limit the usefulness of this medication in children are not expected.

### Geriatrics
No information is available on the relationship of age to the effects of mechlorethamine in geriatric patients.

### Dental
The bone marrow depressant effects of mechlorethamine may result in an increased incidence of microbial infection, delayed healing, and gingival bleeding. Dental work, whenever possible, should be completed prior to initiation of therapy or deferred until blood counts have returned to normal. Patients should be instructed in proper oral hygiene during treatment, including caution in use of regular toothbrushes, dental floss, and toothpicks.

Mechlorethamine may also rarely cause stomatitis associated with considerable discomfort.

### Drug interactions and/or related problems
The following drug interactions and/or related problems have been selected on the basis of their potential clinical significance (possible mechanism in parentheses where appropriate)—not necessarily inclusive (» = major clinical significance):

Note: Combinations containing any of the following medications, depending on the amount present, may also interact with this medication.

Allopurinol or
Colchicine or
» Probenecid or
» Sulfinpyrazone
(mechlorethamine may raise the concentration of blood uric acid; dosage adjustment of antigout agents may be necessary to control hyperuricemia and gout; allopurinol may be preferred to prevent or reverse mechlorethamine-induced hyperuricemia because of risk of uric acid nephropathy with uricosuric antigout agents)

Blood dyscrasia–causing medications (See *Appendix II*)
(leukopenic and/or thrombocytopenic effects of mechlorethamine may be increased with concurrent or recent therapy if these medications cause the same effects; dosage adjustment of mechlorethamine, if necessary, should be based on blood counts)

» Bone marrow depressants, other (See *Appendix II*) or
Radiation therapy
(additive bone marrow depression may occur; dosage reduction may be required when two or more bone marrow depressants, including radiation, are used concurrently or consecutively)

Vaccines, killed virus
(because normal defense mechanisms may be suppressed by mechlorethamine therapy, the patient's antibody response to the vaccine may be decreased. The interval between discontinuation of medications that cause immunosuppression and restoration of the patient's ability to respond to the vaccine depends on the intensity and type of immunosuppression-causing medication used, the underlying disease, and other factors; estimates vary from 3 months to 1 year)

» Vaccines, live virus
(because normal defense mechanisms may be suppressed by mechlorethamine therapy, concurrent use with a live virus vaccine may potentiate the replication of the vaccine virus, may increase the side/adverse effects of the vaccine virus, and/or may decrease the patient's antibody response to the vaccine; immunization of these patients should be undertaken only with extreme caution after careful review of the patient's hematologic status and only with the knowledge and consent of the physician managing the mechlorethamine therapy. The interval between discontinuation of medications that cause immunosuppression and restoration of the patient's ability to respond to the vaccine depends on the intensity and type of immunosuppression-causing medication used, the underlying disease, and other factors; estimates vary from 3 months to 1 year. Patients with leukemia in remission should not receive live virus vaccine until at least 3 months after their last chemotherapy. Immunization with oral poliovirus vaccine should also be postponed in persons in close contact with the patient, especially family members)

**Laboratory value alterations**

The following have been selected on the basis of their potential clinical significance (possible effect in parentheses where appropriate)—not necessarily inclusive (» = major clinical significance):

With physiology/laboratory test values

Isocitric acid dehydrogenase (ICD)
(concentrations may be increased, indicating hepatotoxicity)

Cholinesterase
(plasma concentrations may be decreased)

Uric acid
(concentrations in blood and urine may be increased)

**Medical considerations/Contraindications**

The medical considerations/contraindications included here have been selected on the basis of their potential clinical significance (reasons given in parentheses where appropriate)—not necessarily inclusive (» = major clinical significance).

*Risk-benefit should be considered when the following medical problems exist:*

» Bone marrow depression

» Chickenpox, existing or recent (including recent exposure) or

» Herpes zoster
(risk of severe generalized disease)

Gout, history of or
Urate renal stones, history of
(risk of hyperuricemia)

» Infection

Sensitivity to mechlorethamine

» Tumor cell infiltration of bone marrow

» Caution should be used also in patients who have had previous cytotoxic drug therapy and radiation therapy.

**Patient monitoring**

The following are especially important in patient monitoring (other tests may be warranted in some patients, depending on condition; » = major clinical significance):

Alanine aminotransferase (ALT [SGPT]) values, serum and
Aspartate aminotransferase (AST [SGOT]) values, serum and
Bilirubin values, serum and
Lactate dehydrogenase (LDH) values, serum
(recommended prior to initiation of therapy and at periodic intervals during therapy; frequency varies according to clinical state, agent, dose, and other agents being used concurrently)

» Audiometric testing
(may be recommended at periodic intervals in patients receiving high doses)

» Hematocrit or hemoglobin and

» Leukocyte count, total and, if appropriate, differential and

» Platelet count
(determinations recommended prior to initiation of therapy and at periodic intervals during therapy; frequency varies according to clinical state, agent, dose, and other agents being used concurrently)

Uric acid concentrations, serum
(recommended prior to initiation of therapy and at periodic intervals during therapy; frequency varies according to clinical state, agent, dose, and other agents being used concurrently)

X-ray examination
(recommended after intracavitary administration to detect reaccumulation of fluid)

## Side/Adverse Effects

Note: Many "side effects" of antineoplastic therapy are unavoidable and represent the medication's pharmacologic action. Some of these (for example, leukopenia and thrombocytopenia) are actually used as parameters to aid in individual dosage titration.

Systemic effects are unpredictable following intracavitary administration.

Pain after intracavitary administration and nausea, vomiting, and diarrhea after intraperitoneal injection occur frequently and may persist for 2 or 3 days.

The following side/adverse effects have been selected on the basis of their potential clinical significance (possible cause in parentheses where appropriate)—not necessarily inclusive:

**Those indicating need for medical attention**

Incidence more frequent

*Gonadal suppression* (missing menstrual periods); *idiosyncratic reaction or precipitation of herpes zoster* (painful rash); *leukopenia, immunosuppression, or infection* (usually asymptomatic; less frequently, fever or chills, cough or hoarseness, lower back or side pain, painful or difficult urination); *thrombocytopenia* (usually asymptomatic; less frequently, unusual bleeding or bruising; black, tarry stools; blood in urine or stools; pinpoint red spots on skin)

Note: *Lymphocytopenia* usually occurs within 24 hours after the first dose. Significant granulocytopenia usually occurs within 6 to 8 days and lasts 10 days to 3 weeks.

Incidence more frequent with high doses or regional perfusion

*Ototoxicity* (dizziness; ringing in the ears; loss of hearing)

Incidence less frequent

*Hyperuricemia or uric acid nephropathy* (joint pain; lower back or side pain; swelling of feet or lower legs); *thrombosis, thrombophlebitis, or extravasation* (pain or redness at the site of injection)

Note: *Hyperuricemia or uric acid nephropathy* occurs most commonly during initial treatment of patients with leukemia or lymphoma, as a result of rapid cell breakdown which leads to elevated serum uric acid concentrations.

*Pain or redness at the site of injection* may persist for 4 to 6 weeks.

Incidence rare

*Allergic reaction* (shortness of breath, itching, wheezing); *hepatotoxicity* (yellow eyes or skin); *peptic ulcer* (black, tarry stools); *peripheral neuropathy* (numbness, tingling, or burning of fingers, toes, or face)

Note: An *allergic reaction* may also occur in patients previously treated with topical mechlorethamine.

**Those indicating need for medical attention only if they continue or are bothersome**

Incidence more frequent

*Nausea and vomiting*

Note: *Nausea and vomiting* occur in 90% of patients, usually within 1 to 3 hours of a dose; vomiting usually subsides within 8 hours, while nausea may persist for 24 hours.

Incidence less frequent

*Diarrhea; loss of appetite; metallic taste; neurotoxicity* (confusion; drowsiness; headache)—especially with high doses; *weakness*

**Those not indicating need for medical attention**

Incidence less frequent

*Loss of hair*

**Those indicating the need for medical attention if they occur after medication is discontinued**

*Bone marrow depression* (black, tarry stools; blood in urine or stools; cough or hoarseness; fever or chills; lower back or side pain; painful or difficult urination; pinpoint red spots on skin; unusual bleeding or bruising)

## Patient Consultation

As an aid to patient consultation, refer to *Advice for the Patient, Mechlorethamine (Systemic)*.

In providing consultation, consider emphasizing the following selected information (» = major clinical significance):

**Before using this medication**

» Conditions affecting use, especially:

Sensitivity to mechlorethamine

Pregnancy—Use not recommended because of mutagenic, teratogenic, and carcinogenic potential; advisability of using contraception; telling physician immediately if pregnancy is suspected

Breast-feeding—Not recommended because of risk of serious side effects

Other medications, especially other bone marrow depressants, probenecid, or sulfinpyrazone

Other medical problems, especially chickenpox, herpes zoster, or infection

**Proper use of this medication**

Caution in taking combination therapy; taking each medication at the right time

Importance of ample fluid intake and subsequent increase in urine output to aid in excretion of uric acid

Frequency of nausea, vomiting, and loss of appetite; importance of continuing medication despite stomach upset
» Proper dosing

**Precautions while using this medication**
» Importance of close monitoring by the physician
» Avoiding immunizations unless approved by physician; other persons in patient's household should avoid immunizations with oral poliovirus vaccine; avoiding persons who have taken oral poliovirus vaccine or wearing a protective mask that covers nose and mouth
*Caution if bone marrow depression occurs:*
» Avoiding exposure to persons with bacterial infections, especially during periods of low blood counts; checking with physician immediately if fever or chills, cough or hoarseness, lower back or side pain, or painful or difficult urination occur
» Checking with physician immediately if unusual bleeding or bruising; black, tarry stools; blood in urine or stools; or pinpoint red spots on skin occur
Caution in use of regular toothbrush, dental floss, or toothpick; physician, dentist, or nurse may suggest alternatives; checking with physician before having dental work done
Not touching eyes or inside of nose unless hands washed immediately before
Using caution to avoid accidental cuts with use of sharp objects such as safety razor or fingernail or toenail cutters
Avoiding contact sports or other situations where bruising or injury could occur
» Possibility of local tissue injury and scarring if infiltration of intravenous solution occurs; telling doctor or nurse right away about redness, pain, or swelling at injection site

**Side/adverse effects**
Importance of discussing possible effects, including cancer, with physician
Signs of potential side effects, especially gonadal suppression, idiosyncratic reaction, precipitation of herpes zoster, leukopenia, immunosuppression, infection, thrombocytopenia, ototoxicity, hyperuricemia, uric acid nephropathy, thrombosis, thrombophlebitis, extravasation, allergic reaction, hepatotoxicity, peptic ulcer, and peripheral neuropathy
Physician or nurse can help in dealing with side effects
Possibility of hair loss; should return after treatment has ended

# General Dosing Information

**For intravenous and intracavitary use**
Patients receiving mechlorethamine should be under supervision of a physician experienced in cancer chemotherapy or immunosuppressive therapy.

A variety of dosage schedules, regimens, and routes of administration of mechlorethamine, alone or in combination with other antitumor agents, are used. The prescriber may consult the medical literature as well as the manufacturer's literature in choosing a specific dosage.

Dosage must be adjusted to meet the individual requirements of each patient, based on clinical response and appearance or severity of toxicity.

Although dosages are based on the patient's actual weight, use of estimated lean body mass (dry weight) is recommended in obese patients or those with weight gain due to edema, ascites, or other abnormal fluid retention.

Because mechlorethamine may contribute to the development of amyloidosis, it is recommended that the medication be used only if foci of acute and chronic suppurative inflammation are absent.

Severity of nausea and vomiting may be reduced in some patients by administration of antiemetics, in addition to sedatives such as barbiturates or chlorpromazine, prior to dosing.

Administration of mechlorethamine at night is recommended if sedation for side effects is required.

Development of uric acid nephropathy in patients with leukemia or lymphoma may be prevented by adequate oral hydration and, in some cases, administration of allopurinol. Alkalinization of urine may be necessary if serum uric acid concentrations are elevated.

It is recommended that mechlorethamine therapy be withdrawn if leukocyte (particularly granulocyte) or platelet levels fall markedly. Therapy may be resumed at a lower dosage when leukocyte and platelet counts return to satisfactory levels.

Special precautions are recommended in patients who develop thrombocytopenia as a result of administration of mechlorethamine. These may include extreme care in performing invasive procedures; regular inspection of intravenous sites, skin (including perirectal area), and mucous membrane surfaces for signs of bleeding or bruising; limiting frequency of venipuncture and avoiding intramuscular injections; testing urine, emesis, stool, and secretions for occult blood; care in use of regular toothbrushes, dental floss, toothpicks, safety razors, and fingernail and toenail cutters; avoiding constipation; and using caution to prevent falls and other injuries. Such patients should avoid alcohol and aspirin intake because of the risk of gastrointestinal bleeding. Platelet transfusions may be required.

Patients who develop leukopenia should be observed carefully for signs of infection. Antibiotic support may be required. In neutropenic patients who develop fever, broad-spectrum antibiotic coverage should be initiated empirically, pending bacterial cultures and appropriate diagnostic tests.

**For intravenous use only**
Mechlorethamine may be administered by intravenous push, although injection into the tubing of a running intravenous infusion is preferred to reduce the risk of local toxicity. Administration by intravenous infusion is not recommended because of deactivation of the medication by the solution. The injection should be completed within a few minutes.

Avoid high concentration and prolonged contact with the medication, especially in cases of elevated pressure in the antebrachial vein.

If extravasation occurs, the reaction may be minimized by prompt infiltration of the area with sterile isotonic sodium thiosulfate (0.125 *M*) or 1% lidocaine and application of an ice compress for 6 to 12 hours.

**For intracavitary use only**
Administration of mechlorethamine by the intracavitary route is not recommended in patients receiving other systemic bone marrow depressants concurrently.

Prior removal of excess fluid (paracentesis) improves contact of the medication with the peritoneal and pleural linings.

Prior administration of analgesics usually is required to offset pain of treatment.

For intrapleural or intrapericardial injection, a thoracentesis needle is used. For intraperitoneal injection, mechlorethamine is given through a rubber catheter inserted into the trocar used for paracentesis or through an 18-gauge needle inserted at another site. Slow injection with frequent aspiration is recommended to prevent or detect extravasation and to ensure adequate dissemination of the medication.

Changing the position of the patient (prone, supine, right side, left side, knee-chest) every 5 to 10 minutes for an hour ensures uniform distribution of the medication in the serous cavity.

Remaining fluid is removed by paracentesis 24 to 36 hours later.

Intrapleural administration may produce increased pleural fluid as a result of pleural irritation by mechlorethamine.

**Safety considerations for handling this medication**
There is limited but increasing evidence and concern that personnel involved in preparation and administration of parenteral antineoplastics may be at some risk because of the potential mutagenicity, teratogenicity, and/or carcinogenicity of these agents, although the actual risk is unknown. USP advisory panels recommend cautious handling both in preparation and disposal of antineoplastic agents. Precautions that have been suggested include:
• Use of a biological containment cabinet during reconstitution and dilution of parenteral medications and wearing of disposable surgical gloves and masks.
• Use of proper technique to prevent contamination of the medication, work area, and operator during transfer between containers (including proper training of personnel in this technique).
• Cautious and proper disposal of needles, syringes, vials, ampuls, and unused medication.
A number of medical centers have developed detailed guidelines for handling of antineoplastic agents.

**Combination chemotherapy**
Mechlorethamine may be used in combination with other agents in various regimens. As a result, incidence and/or severity of side effects may be altered and different dosages (usually reduced) may be used. For example, mechlorethamine is part of the following chemotherapeutic combinations (some commonly used acronyms are in parentheses):
—mechlorethamine, vincristine, procarbazine, and prednisone (MOPP).
—mechlorethamine, vincristine, procarbazine, prednisone, and bleomycin (MOPP-LO BLEO).
For specific dosages and schedules, consult the literature. For information regarding each agent, consult the individual monographs.

## Parenteral Dosage Forms

### MECHLORETHAMINE HYDROCHLORIDE FOR INJECTION USP

**Usual adult and adolescent dose**
Carcinoma, lung or
Leukemia, chronic lymphocytic or
Leukemia, chronic myelocytic or
Lymphomas, Hodgkin's or
Lymphomas, non-Hodgkin's or
Mycosis fungoides or
Polycythemia vera—
  Intravenous, total dose of 400 mcg (0.4 mg) per kg of body weight as a single dose or divided into two or four successive daily doses.
Malignant effusions, pericardial or
Malignant effusions, peritoneal or
Malignant effusions, pleural—
  Intracavitary, 400 mcg (0.4 mg) per kg of body weight, or 200 mcg (0.2 mg) per kg of body weight by intrapericardial route.
Note: Total dosage in patients who have received prior cytotoxic drug therapy or radiation therapy should not exceed 200 to 300 mcg (0.2 to 0.3 mg) per kg of body weight.

**Usual adult prescribing limits**
Total intravenous dose exceeding 400 mcg (0.4 mg) per kg of body weight may result in severe bone marrow depression, bleeding, sepsis, and death, although 800 mcg (0.8 mg) of mechlorethamine per kg of body weight, as a single agent, is tolerated in some patients.

**Usual pediatric dose**
See *Usual adult and adolescent dose.*

**Strength(s) usually available**
U.S.—
  10 mg (Rx) [*Mustargen*].
Canada—
  10 mg (Rx) [*Mustargen*].

**Packaging and storage**
Store below 40 °C (104 °F), preferably between 15 and 30 °C (59 and 86 °F), unless otherwise specified by manufacturer.

**Preparation of dosage form**
Mechlorethamine Hydrochloride for Injection USP is reconstituted for intravenous use by adding 10 mL of sterile water for injection or 0.9% sodium chloride injection to the vial and, with the needle still in the rubber stopper, shaking to dissolve, producing a clear, colorless solution containing 1 mg of mechlorethamine hydrochloride per mL.
Mechlorethamine Hydrochloride for Injection USP is reconstituted for intracavitary use by adding 10 mL of sterile water for injection or 0.9% sodium chloride injection to the vial (50 to 100 mL of 0.9% sodium chloride injection has also been used) and shaking to dissolve.

**Stability**
Solution should be freshly reconstituted immediately (less than 15 minutes) prior to each dose. Any unused portion should be discarded.

**Note**
Do not use if solution is discolored or if droplets of water appear in the vial.

Avoid inhalation of powder or vapors. If accidental contact with skin or mucous membranes occurs, immediately and thoroughly irrigate the affected part with a large volume of water for at least 15 minutes, followed by 2% sodium thiosulfate solution; if eye contact occurs, irrigation is performed with 0.9% sodium chloride solution or a balanced salt ophthalmic irrigating solution.

Any equipment used for administration of mechlorethamine (rubber gloves, tubing, glassware, etc.) should be neutralized immediately after use by soaking in an aqueous solution containing equal volumes of 5% sodium thiosulfate and 5% sodium bicarbonate for 45 minutes, washing away excess reagents and reaction products with water. Unused solution is neutralized by adding an equal volume of the sodium thiosulfate–bicarbonate solution and allowing the mixture to stand for 45 minutes. Vials that have contained mechlorethamine should be treated in the same way before disposal.

### Selected Bibliography

Dorr RT, Fritz WL. Cancer chemotherapy handbook. New York: Elsevier, 1980: 498-506.

Revised: August 1990
Interim revision: 07/29/93; 12/15/93; 06/21/94

---

# MECHLORETHAMINE   Topical*†

INN: Chlormethine
VA CLASSIFICATION (Primary): DE600
Other commonly used names are chlormethine and nitrogen mustard.
Note: For a listing of dosage forms and brand names by country availability, see *Dosage Forms* section(s). For a listing of brand names for the articles in this monograph, refer to the General Index.

  *Not commercially available in the U.S.
  †Not commercially available in Canada.

## Category
Antineoplastic, topical.

## Indications

**Accepted**
Mycosis fungoides (treatment)—Mechlorethamine has been used topically, without occlusive dressings, in the treatment of cutaneous manifestations of mycosis fungoides.

## Pharmacology/Pharmacokinetics

**Physicochemical characteristics**
Molecular weight—192.52.
pKa—6.1.

**Mechanism of action/Effect**
Mechlorethamine is a bifunctional alkylating agent and is cell cycle–phase nonspecific. Activity occurs as a result of formation of an unstable ethylenimmonium ion, which alkylates or binds with many intracellular molecular structures, including nucleic acids. Its cytotoxic action is primarily due to cross-linking of strands of DNA and RNA, as well as inhibition of protein synthesis. Topical mechlorethamine destroys rapidly proliferating cells.

## Precautions to Consider

### Carcinogenicity/Mutagenicity
Long-term topical use is associated with development of malignancies of the skin, including squamous cell carcinomas, keratoacanthomas, basal cell carcinomas, and actinic keratoses, mostly on sun-exposed areas and genital skin.

### Pregnancy/Reproduction
Problems in humans have not been documented; however, some systemic absorption may occur, and the fact that all antineoplastics affect cell kinetics and can theoretically cause mutagenicity or teratogenicity must be considered. Systemic mechlorethamine may be teratogenic.

### Breast-feeding
Problems in humans have not been documented. However, since some systemic absorption may occur and potential adverse effects are very serious, breast-feeding is not recommended while mechlorethamine is being used.

### Pediatrics
Appropriate studies have not been performed in the pediatric population.

### Geriatrics
No geriatrics-specific information is available on the use of topical mechlorethamine in geriatric patients.

## Side/Adverse Effects

Note: Systemic toxicity does not occur with topical use.

The following side/adverse effects have been selected on the basis of their potential clinical significance (possible signs and symptoms in parentheses where appropriate)—not necessarily inclusive:

**Those indicating need for medical attention**
Incidence more frequent
*Allergy, contact* (skin rash or itching; sore, reddened skin)
Note: *Contact allergy* occurs in approximately 50% of patients using the solution and 25% of patients using the ointment, usually within 2 weeks to 12 months after the onset of therapy; cutaneous irritation or nonallergic dermatitis occurs in about 10% of patients.

Incidence rare
*Allergic reaction, immediate* (hives; sudden shortness of breath)
Note: An *immediate allergic reaction* may be life-threatening; it usually occurs within 5 minutes after application and may not occur until after several doses.

**Those indicating need for medical attention only if they continue or are bothersome**
Incidence more frequent
*Darkening of skin; dry skin*—less frequent with the ointment

## Patient Consultation

As an aid to patient consultation, refer to *Advice for the Patient, Mechlorethamine (Topical).*

Consider advising the patient on the following (» = major clinical significance):

**Before using this medication**
See *Precautions to Consider.*

**Proper use of this medication**
» For patients using the solution: Mixing according to physician's instructions
» *When preparing solution:*
   Not using if solution is discolored or droplets appear in vial
   Avoiding inhaling powder or vapors; if accidental skin contact occurs, flushing area with water for at least 15 minutes; using irrigating solution for accidental eye contact; additional instructions from physician
   Neutralizing equipment according to physician's instructions
   Showering and rinsing carefully before each treatment unless otherwise instructed by physician; drying thoroughly before applying ointment; not showering until next treatment
   Applying over entire body; using rubber or plastic gloves or, for solution, a 2-inch-wide soft brush or gauze; allowing to dry
   Applying more lightly to groin, armpits, inside bends of elbows, and backs of knees because of increased risk of dermatitis
   Avoiding contact with eyes, nose, or mouth
   Treatment usually done once a day; following physician's instructions; possible need for months or years of treatment
» Proper dosing
   Missed dose: Skipping dose and checking with physician; not changing amount used
» Proper storage

**Precautions while using this medication**
» Importance of close monitoring by the physician

**Side/adverse effects**
May cause skin cancer with prolonged use; importance of discussing possible effects with physician
No known systemic side effects; possibility of allergic reaction, dermatitis

## General Dosing Information

Patients using topical mechlorethamine should be under supervision of a physician experienced in use of the medication.

Use of occlusive dressings may result in increased incidence of inflammatory reactions and is not recommended.

It is recommended that treatment with mechlorethamine be discontinued if an excessive inflammatory response or allergic reaction occurs. If an immediate allergic reaction (e.g., urticaria) occurs, mechlorethamine therapy should not be restarted. However, if a delayed contact allergic reaction occurs, mechlorethamine therapy may be reinstituted after a desensitization procedure.

**Safety considerations for handling this medication**
There is limited but increasing evidence and concern that personnel involved in handling of antineoplastics may be at some risk because of the potential mutagenicity, teratogenicity, and/or carcinogenicity of these agents, although the actual risk is unknown. USP advisory panels recommend cautious handling both in preparation and disposal of antineoplastic agents. Precautions that have been suggested include:
• Use of a biological containment cabinet during reconstitution and dilution of parenteral medications and wearing of disposable surgical gloves and masks.
• Use of proper technique to prevent contamination of the medication, work area, and operator during transfer between containers (including proper training of personnel in this technique).
• Cautious and proper disposal of needles, syringes, vials, ampuls, and unused medication.
A number of medical centers have developed detailed guidelines for handling of antineoplastic agents.

## Topical Dosage Forms

### MECHLORETHAMINE HYDROCHLORIDE OINTMENT

Note: Mechlorethamine hydrochloride ointment is not commercially available in the U.S. or Canada.

**Usual adult dose**
Mycosis fungoides—
Topical, as a 0.01 to 0.04% ointment, applied to the entire skin surface once a day (up to four times a day in severe cases) until six to twelve months after a complete response is obtained, followed by maintenance treatments one to several times a week for three years after the response occurs.

**Usual pediatric dose**
Dosage has not been established.

**Strength(s) usually available**
U.S.—
Dosage form not commercially available. Compounding required for prescription.

**Packaging and storage**
Store below 40 °C (104 °F), preferably between 15 and 30 °C (59 and 86 °F). Protect from freezing.

**Preparation of dosage form**
There is no official formula or method for compounding mechlorethamine ointment. Whichever one is used, it is critical that the physician and the pharmacist participate in its development. One commonly used formulation is prepared as follows:
• Mechlorethamine Hydrochloride for Injection USP (90 mg) is mixed with 10 mL of absolute alcohol; a precipitate of sodium chloride forms immediately.
• The solution and precipitate are blended into a sufficient quantity of Aquaphor to make 900 grams of an ointment in a strength of 0.01%.

**Auxiliary labeling**
• For the skin.
• Continue medicine for full course of treatment.

**Note**
Do not use if droplets of water appear in the vial.

Avoid inhalation of powder or vapors. If accidental contact with skin or mucous membranes occurs, immediately and thoroughly irrigate the affected part with a large volume of water for at least 15 minutes, followed by 2% sodium thiosulfate solution; if eye contact occurs, irrigation is performed with 0.9% sodium chloride solution or a balanced salt ophthalmic irrigating solution.

Any equipment used for preparation or administration of mechlorethamine (rubber gloves, tubing, glassware, etc.) should be neutralized immediately after use by soaking in an aqueous solution containing equal volumes of 5% sodium thiosulfate and 5% sodium bicarbonate for 45 minutes, washing away excess reagents and reaction products with water. Unused solution is neutralized by adding an equal volume of the sodium thiosulfate–bicarbonate solution and allowing the mixture to stand for 45 minutes. Vials that have contained mechlorethamine should be treated in the same way before disposal.

### MECHLORETHAMINE HYDROCHLORIDE TOPICAL SOLUTION

Note: Mechlorethamine hydrochloride topical solution is not commercially available in the U.S. or Canada.

**Usual adult dose**
Mycosis fungoides—
Topical, in the appropriate strength (usually 10 mg per 50 mL) applied to the entire skin surface once a day until six to twelve months after a complete response is obtained, followed by maintenance treatments one to several times a week for three years after the response occurs.

**Usual pediatric dose**
Dosage has not been established.

**Strength(s) usually available**

U.S.—

Dosage form not commercially available. Compounding required for prescription.

**Packaging and storage**

Should not be stored after reconstitution. Mechlorethamine Hydrochloride for Injection USP—Store below 40 °C (104 °F), preferably between 15 and 30 °C (59 and 86 °F).

**Preparation of dosage form**

The solution should be freshly prepared just prior to use; 10 mg of Mechlorethamine Hydrochloride for Injection USP is dissolved in 5 to 10 mL of normal saline, then diluted with water to the desired strength.

**Stability**

Solution should be freshly reconstituted immediately (less than 15 minutes) prior to each dose. Any unused portion should be discarded.

**Auxiliary labeling**

• For the skin.
• Continue medicine for full course of treatment.

**Note**

Do not use if droplets of water appear in the vial.

Avoid inhalation of powder or vapors. If accidental contact with skin or mucous membranes occurs, immediately and thoroughly irrigate the affected part with a large volume of water for at least 15 minutes, followed by 2% sodium thiosulfate solution; if eye contact occurs, irrigation is performed with 0.9% sodium chloride solution or a balanced salt ophthalmic irrigating solution.

Any equipment used for preparation or administration of mechlorethamine (rubber gloves, tubing, glassware, etc.) should be neutralized immediately after use by soaking in an aqueous solution containing equal volumes of 5% sodium thiosulfate and 5% sodium bicarbonate for 45 minutes, washing away excess reagents and reaction products with water. Unused solution is neutralized by adding an equal volume of the sodium thiosulfate–bicarbonate solution and allowing the mixture to stand for 45 minutes. Vials that have contained mechlorethamine should be treated in the same way before disposal.

## Selected Bibliography

Vonderheid EC. Topical mechlorethamine chemotherapy. Considerations on its use in mycosis fungoides. Int J Dermatol 1984 Apr; 23 (3): 180-6.

Revised: 08/90
Interim revision: 07/12/94

---

# MECLIZINE    Systemic

INN: Meclozine
BAN: Meclozine
VA CLASSIFICATION (Primary/Secondary): GA700/CN550

Note: For a listing of dosage forms and brand names by country availability, see *Dosage Forms* section(s). For a listing of brand names for the articles in this monograph, refer to the General Index.

## Category

Antiemetic; antivertigo agent.

## Indications

Note: Bracketed information in the *Indications* section refers to uses that are not included in U.S. product labeling.

**Accepted**

Motion sickness (prophylaxis and treatment)—Meclizine is indicated for the prophylaxis and treatment of nausea, vomiting, and dizziness associated with motion sickness or radiotherapy.

Vertigo (prophylaxis and treatment)—The U.S. Food and Drug Administration (FDA) has classified meclizine as possibly effective in the management of vertigo associated with diseases affecting the vestibular system, such as labyrinthitis and Meniere's disease. This classification requires the submission of adequate and well-controlled studies to provide substantial evidence of effectiveness.

[Nausea and vomiting, radiotherapy-induced (prophylaxis and treatment)]—Meclizine is indicated for the prophylaxis and treatment of nausea, vomiting, and dizziness associated with radiotherapy.

## Pharmacology/Pharmacokinetics

**Physicochemical characteristics**

Molecular weight—481.90.

**Mechanism of action/Effect**

Antiemetic; antivertigo agent—The mechanism by which meclizine exerts its antiemetic, antimotion sickness, and antivertigo effects is not precisely known but may be related to its central anticholinergic actions. It diminishes vestibular stimulation and depresses labyrinthine function. An action on the medullary chemoreceptive trigger zone may also be involved in the antiemetic effect.

**Other actions/effects**

Meclizine also has antihistaminic, anticholinergic, central nervous system (CNS) depressant, and local anesthetic effects.

**Half-life**

6 hours.

**Onset of action**

1 hour.

**Duration of action**

8 to 24 hours.

## Precautions to Consider

**Pregnancy/Reproduction**

Pregnancy—Epidemiological studies in pregnant women have not shown that meclizine causes an increase in the risk of fetal abnormalities.

Studies in rats have shown that meclizine causes cleft palate when given in doses corresponding to 25 to 50 times the recommended human dose.

FDA Pregnancy Category B.

**Breast-feeding**

Meclizine may be distributed into breast milk. However, problems in humans have not been documented.

Because of its anticholinergic actions, meclizine may inhibit lactation.

**Pediatrics**

No information is available on the relationship of age to the effects of meclizine in pediatric patients. However, it is known that pediatric patients exhibit increased sensitivity to anticholinergics, which are related pharmacologically to meclizine.

**Geriatrics**

No information is available on the relationship of age to the effects of meclizine in geriatric patients. However, it is known that geriatric patients exhibit increased sensitivity to anticholinergics, which are related pharmacologically to meclizine. Therefore, constipation, dryness of mouth, and urinary retention (especially in males) are more likely to occur in the elderly.

**Drug interactions and/or related problems**

The following drug interactions and/or related problems have been selected on the basis of their potential clinical significance (possible mechanism in parentheses where appropriate)—not necessarily inclusive (» = major clinical significance):

Note: Combinations containing any of the following medications, depending on the amount present, may also interact with this medication.

» Alcohol or
» CNS depression–producing medications, other (See *Appendix II*)
(concurrent use may potentiate the CNS depressant effects of either these medications or meclizine)

Anticholinergics or other medications with anticholinergic activity (See *Appendix II*)
(concurrent use with meclizine may potentiate anticholinergic effects)

Apomorphine
(prior administration of meclizine may decrease the emetic response to apomorphine)

## Laboratory value alterations

The following have been selected on the basis of their potential clinical significance (possible effect in parentheses where appropriate)—not necessarily inclusive (» = major clinical significance):

With diagnostic test results
Skin tests using allergen extracts
(may inhibit the cutaneous histamine response, thus producing false-negative results; it is recommended that meclizine be discontinued at least 72 hours before testing begins)

## Medical considerations/Contraindications

The medical considerations/contraindications included here have been selected on the basis of their potential clinical significance (reasons given in parentheses where appropriate)—not necessarily inclusive (» = major clinical significance).

*Risk-benefit should be considered when the following medical problems exist:*

Bladder neck obstruction or
Prostatic hyperplasia, symptomatic
(anticholinergic effects of meclizine may precipitate urinary retention)
Gastroduodenal obstruction
(decrease in motility and tone may occur, aggravating obstruction and gastric retention)
Glaucoma, angle-closure, predisposition to
(increased intraocular pressure may precipitate an acute attack of angle-closure glaucoma)
Pulmonary disease, chronic obstructive
(reduction in bronchial secretion may cause inspissation and formation of bronchial plugs)
Sensitivity to meclizine

## Side/Adverse Effects

The following side/adverse effects have been selected on the basis of their potential clinical significance (possible signs and symptoms in parentheses where appropriate)—not necessarily inclusive:

**Those indicating need for medical attention only if they continue or are bothersome**
Incidence more frequent
*Drowsiness*
Incidence less frequent or rare
*Blurred vision; dryness of mouth, nose, and throat*

## Patient Consultation

As an aid to patient consultation, refer to *Advice for the Patient, Meclizine/Buclizine/Cyclizine (Systemic).*

In providing consultation, consider emphasizing the following selected information (» = major clinical significance):

**Before using this medication**
» Conditions affecting use, especially:
Sensitivity to meclizine
Pregnancy—No increase in fetal abnormalities in human studies; animal studies have shown meclizine to cause cleft palate at doses above recommended human dose
Breast-feeding—May be distributed into breast milk; may inhibit lactation due to anticholinergic effects
Use in children—Possible increased susceptibility to anticholinergic side effects
Use in the elderly—Possible increased susceptibility to anticholinergic side effects
Other medications, especially other CNS depressants

**Proper use of this medication**
Not taking more medication than the amount recommended
» Proper dosing
Missed dose (if on a regular dosing regimen): Taking as soon as possible; not taking if almost time for next dose; not doubling doses
» Proper storage

**Precautions while using this medication**
Possible interference with skin tests using allergens; need to inform physician of use of this medication
» Avoiding use of alcohol or other CNS depressants
» Caution if drowsiness occurs
Possible dryness of mouth; using sugarless candy or gum, ice, or saliva substitute for relief; checking with physician or dentist if dry mouth continues for more than 2 weeks

## General Dosing Information

For prophylaxis of motion sickness, this medication should be taken at least 1 hour before exposure to conditions that may precipitate motion sickness.

## Oral Dosage Forms

Note: Bracketed uses in the *Dosage Forms* section refer to categories of use and/or indications that are not included in U.S. product labeling.

### MECLIZINE HYDROCHLORIDE CAPSULES

**Usual adult and adolescent dose**
Motion sickness (prophylaxis and treatment)—Oral, 25 to 50 mg one hour before travel. Dose may be repeated every twenty-four hours as needed.
Vertigo (prophylaxis and treatment)—Oral, 25 to 100 mg a day as needed, in divided doses.
[Nausea and vomiting, radiotherapy-induced (prophylaxis and treatment)]—Oral, 50 mg two to twelve hours prior to radiotherapy.

**Usual pediatric dose**
Antiemetic or
Antivertigo agent—
Children up to 12 years of age: Use is not recommended unless directed by a physician.
Children 12 years of age or older: See *Usual adult and adolescent dose.*

**Usual geriatric dose**
See *Usual adult and adolescent dose.*
Note: Geriatric patients may be more sensitive to the effects of the usual adult dose.

**Strength(s) usually available**
U.S.—
15 mg (OTC) [*D-Vert 15*].
25 mg (Rx) [*Meni-D*].
30 mg (OTC) [*D-Vert 30*].
Canada—
Not commercially available.

**Packaging and storage**
Store below 40 °C (104 °F), preferably between 15 and 30 °C (59 and 86 °F), in a well-closed container, unless otherwise specified by manufacturer.

**Auxiliary labeling**
• May cause drowsiness.
• Avoid alcoholic beverages.

### MECLIZINE HYDROCHLORIDE TABLETS USP

**Usual adult and adolescent dose**
See *Meclizine Hydrochloride Capsules.*

**Usual pediatric dose**
See *Meclizine Hydrochloride Capsules.*

**Usual geriatric dose**
See *Meclizine Hydrochloride Capsules.*

**Strength(s) usually available**
U.S.—
12.5 mg (Rx) [*Antivert;* GENERIC].
25 mg [*Antivert/25* (Rx); *Dramamine II* (OTC); GENERIC (Rx/OTC)].
50 mg (Rx) [*Antivert/50* (scored); GENERIC].
Canada—
Not commercially available.

**Packaging and storage**
Store below 40 °C (104 °F), preferably between 15 and 30 °C (59 and 86 °F), unless otherwise specified by manufacturer. Store in a well-closed container.

**Auxiliary labeling**
• May cause drowsiness.
• Avoid alcoholic beverages.

### MECLIZINE HYDROCHLORIDE TABLETS (CHEWABLE) USP

**Usual adult and adolescent dose**
See *Meclizine Hydrochloride Capsules.*

**Usual pediatric dose**
See *Meclizine Hydrochloride Capsules.*

**Usual geriatric dose**
See *Meclizine Hydrochloride Capsules.*

**Strength(s) usually available**

U.S.—

25 mg [*Bonine* (OTC); GENERIC (Rx/OTC)].

Canada—

25 mg (Rx) [*Bonamine* (scored)].

**Packaging and storage**

Store between 15 and 30 °C (59 and 86 °F), unless otherwise specified by manufacturer. Store in a well-closed container.

**Auxiliary labeling**

• May cause drowsiness.

• Avoid alcoholic beverages.

• May be chewed or swallowed whole.

Revised: 01/03/96

---

**MECLOCYCLINE**—See *Tetracyclines (Topical)*

---

**MECLOFENAMATE**—See *Anti-inflammatory Drugs, Nonsteroidal (Systemic)*

---

**MEDROGESTONE**—See *Progestins (Systemic)*

---

**MEDROXYPROGESTERONE**—See *Progestins (Systemic)*

---

**MEDRYSONE**—See *Corticosteroids (Ophthalmic)*

---

**MEFENAMIC ACID**—See *Anti-inflammatory Drugs, Nonsteroidal (Systemic)*

---

# MEFLOQUINE   Systemic†

VA CLASSIFICATION (Primary): AP101

Note: For a listing of dosage forms and brand names by country availability, see *Dosage Forms* section(s). For a listing of brand names for the articles in this monograph, refer to the General Index.

†Not commercially available in Canada.

## Category

Antimalarial.

## Indications

### Accepted

Malaria (prophylaxis)—Mefloquine is indicated for the prophylaxis of malaria caused by chloroquine-resistant and multiple drug–resistant (including sulfadoxine and pyrimethamine–resistant) strains of *Plasmodium falciparum*. It is also effective as a prophylactic agent against malaria caused by *P. vivax*, *P. ovale*, and *P. malariae*.

Malaria (treatment)—Mefloquine is indicated for the treatment of chloroquine-resistant strains of *P. falciparum* malaria, usually as an alternative agent to quinine. It is also used for malaria caused by multiple drug–resistant (including sulfadoxine and pyrimethamine–resistant) strains of *P. falciparum*.

Since mefloquine does not eliminate the exoerythrocytic (intrahepatic) stages of *P. vivax* or *P. ovale* infection, subsequent treatment with primaquine is recommended to effect a radical cure and to avoid a relapse.

Not all species or strains of a particular organism may be susceptible to mefloquine.

### Unaccepted

Because of the potentially serious side effects caused by sulfadoxine and pyrimethamine combination, its use is not recommended concurrently with mefloquine for the prophylaxis of chloroquine-resistant *P. falciparum* malaria.

## Pharmacology/Pharmacokinetics

### Physicochemical characteristics

Chemical group—A 4-quinolinemethanol chemical structural analog of quinine.

Molecular weight—414.78.

### Mechanism of action/Effect

Exact mechanism of action unknown. However, mefloquine has been shown to act as a blood schizonticide. Inhibits replication of asexual erythrocytic parasites; has no effect on the gametocytes of *P. falciparum*. May bind weakly to DNA, resulting in inhibition of nucleic acid synthesis and protein synthesis. May also act as a weak base, raising the intravesicular pH of acid vesicles of the parasite and thus inhibiting parasitic growth. In addition, may have non–weak base effects on vesicular pH by means of a specific interaction between mefloquine and parasitic acid vesicles, resulting in swelling of secondary lysosomes (food vacuoles) of the parasite. Mefloquine does not eliminate the exoerythrocytic (intrahepatic) stages of *P. vivax* or *P. ovale* infection.

### Absorption

Well absorbed from the gastrointestinal tract; bioavailability greater than 85%. Rate of absorption is usually relatively rapid, but may be prolonged in some patients. Absorption may be incomplete in seriously ill patients, such as patients with cerebral malaria.

### Distribution

Distributed to blood, urine, cerebrospinal fluid (CSF), and tissues; concentrated in erythrocytes; also distributed to breast milk in low concentrations (approximately 3 to 4% of the ingested dose).

Apparent $Vol_D$ =9 to 29 L/kg (median 20 L/kg).

### Protein binding

Very high (98 to 99%).

### Biotransformation

Hepatic (partial); metabolized primarily to the carboxylic acid metabolite.

### Half-life

Absorption—1 to 4 hours.

Elimination—13 to 33 days (median 20 days); may be shorter in seriously ill patients, such as patients with acute malaria.

### Time to peak concentration

7 to 24 hours (median 17 hours).

### Peak plasma concentration

Approximately 290 to 340 nanograms per mL following a single 250-mg dose.

Approximately 540 to 1240 nanograms per mL following a single 1-gram dose.

Mean steady state concentrations may vary from 560 to 1250 nanograms per mL in healthy adults following a 250-mg dose once a week for up to 21 weeks. Steady state concentrations may be significantly lower in pregnant women.

### Elimination

Biliary/fecal; eliminated very slowly, primarily through bile into the feces. Subtherapeutic concentrations may persist in the blood for up to several months or more.

Renal; approximately 5% of the oral dose is excreted unchanged in the urine.

## Precautions to Consider

### Cross-sensitivity and/or related problems

Patients hypersensitive to quinidine, quinine, or related medications may be hypersensitive to this medication also.

### Carcinogenicity

Two-year feeding studies in rats and mice, fed doses of up to 30 mg per kg of body weight (mg/kg) daily, have not shown that mefloquine is carcinogenic.

### Mutagenicity

Mefloquine has not been shown to be mutagenic in the Ames test, host-mediated assays in mice, fluctuation tests, and mouse micronucleus assays, with or without prior metabolic activation. In addition, mefloquine has not been shown to be mutagenic in modified Ames tests utilizing *Salmonella typhimurium* strains, with or without microsomal activation.

## Pregnancy/Reproduction

Fertility—Studies in adult human males, at doses of 250 mg once a week for 22 weeks, have not shown that mefloquine causes any adverse effects on spermatozoa.

However, studies in rats given doses of 5, 20, and 50 mg/kg daily have shown that mefloquine causes adverse effects on fertility in males at doses of 50 mg/kg daily and in females at doses of 20 and 50 mg/kg daily. In addition, degenerative lesions in the epididymides of male rats have been reported at doses of 20 and 50 mg/kg daily for 13 weeks.

Pregnancy—Adequate and well-controlled studies in humans have not been done. However, malaria in pregnant women may be more severe than in nonpregnant women and may result in maternal death. The risk of adverse pregnancy outcomes, including premature births, still-births, and abortion, may be increased. Although mefloquine is not recommended for use during pregnancy and its safety has not been proven, it has been used in women at high risk from falciparum malaria during the second and third trimester of pregnancy with no complications, and no adverse effects in development of their children to date.

If possible, pregnant women should avoid traveling to areas where chloroquine-resistant falciparum malaria is endemic. If travel to the malarious area and mefloquine chemoprophylaxis are considered necessary, women of child-bearing potential should be warned to take reliable contraceptive precautions while taking mefloquine and for 2 months after the last dose.

Studies in rats given doses of 5, 20, and 50 mg/kg daily have shown that mefloquine causes reduced litter size and reduced growth of offspring at the two higher dosage levels. Mefloquine also has been shown to cause an increased incidence of externally visible soft tissue and skeletal abnormalities in rats given doses of 100 mg/kg daily from day 6 to 15 of gestation. Studies utilizing similar doses in mice have shown that mefloquine causes reduced fetal growth and cleft palate. Other studies in rats and mice given doses of 100 mg/kg daily have shown that mefloquine is teratogenic. Studies in rabbits have shown that mefloquine is teratogenic at doses of 80 mg/kg daily and is both embryotoxic and teratogenic at doses of 160 mg/kg daily.

FDA Pregnancy Category C.

## Breast-feeding

Mefloquine is distributed into breast milk in low concentrations (approximately 3 to 4%) following administration of a 250-mg dose. Although the effects of mefloquine distribution into breast milk in nursing infants have not been studied, and the amount the infant is exposed to is small, caution should be exercised.

## Pediatrics

Although the safety and efficacy of mefloquine have not been well studied, it has been effective in preventing and treating malaria caused by *P. falciparum* in children. As in adults, nausea, vomiting, and dizziness have been the reported side effects of mefloquine use in children living in endemic malarious areas. Use is not recommended in infants and children up to 2 years of age or less than 15 kg of body weight.

## Geriatrics

No information is available on the relationship of age to the effects of mefloquine in geriatric patients.

## Drug interactions and/or related problems

The following drug interactions and/or related problems have been selected on the basis of their potential clinical significance (possible mechanism in parentheses where appropriate)—not necessarily inclusive (» = major clinical significance):

Note: Combinations containing any of the following medications, depending on the amount present, may also interact with this medication.

» Beta-adrenergic blocking agents or
» Calcium channel blocking agents or
» Quinidine or
» Quinine
    (concurrent use of these agents with mefloquine may result in sinus bradycardia, prolonged QT intervals, or cardiac arrest; the risk of seizures may also be increased with quinine; concurrent use should be avoided; if concurrent use is necessary, close monitoring of patient response is recommended; in addition, patients should be advised to take mefloquine at least 12 hours after the last dose of quinidine or quinine)

» Chloroquine
    (concurrent use of chloroquine with mefloquine may increase the risk of seizures)

» Divalproex or
» Valproic acid
    (concurrent use of divalproex or valproic acid with mefloquine may result in low valproic acid serum concentrations and loss of seizure control; monitoring of valproic acid serum concentrations is recommended and dosage adjustments may be necessary during and after therapy with mefloquine)

Typhoid vaccine, oral
    (concurrent use of the oral typhoid vaccine with mefloquine may decrease the effectiveness of the oral typhoid vaccine; doses of the two medications should be separated by 7 to 10 days)

## Laboratory value alterations

The following have been selected on the basis of their potential clinical significance (possible effect in parentheses where appropriate)—not necessarily inclusive (» = major clinical significance):

With physiology/laboratory test values
    Alanine aminotransferase (ALT [SGPT]), serum, and
    Aspartate aminotransferase (AST [SGOT]), serum
        (values may be transiently increased in patients taking mefloquine)

## Medical considerations/Contraindications

The medical considerations/contraindications included here have been selected on the basis of their potential clinical significance (reasons given in parentheses where appropriate)—not necessarily inclusive (» = major clinical significance).

*Risk-benefit should be considered when the following medical problems exist:*

Epilepsy or
Seizure disorder, history of
    (mefloquine may rarely cause seizures)
» Heart block, first or second degree
» Psychiatric disorders, history of
    (mefloquine may cause psychosis, hallucinations, confusion, anxiety, or mental depression)

Sensitivity to mefloquine, quinidine, quinine, or related medications
» Caution is also required in any patient whose occupation requires fine coordination and spatial discrimination, such as airline pilots or neurosurgeons

# Side/Adverse Effects

Note: Some side/adverse effects of mefloquine may be difficult to distinguish from the symptoms of acute malaria infection. However, side effects are thought to be dose-related and may occur more frequently in therapeutic regimens (greater than 15 mg per kg of body weight [mg/kg]) than in prophylactic regimens. In therapeutic regimens, vomiting of doses has resulted in low plasma mefloquine concentrations and treatment failure. The incidence of vomiting may be reduced by dividing the dose into parts to be given at 8 to 24 hour intervals.

The following side/adverse effects have been selected on the basis of their potential clinical significance (possible signs and symptoms in parentheses where appropriate)—not necessarily inclusive:

### Those indicating need for medical attention
Incidence rare
    *Bradycardia* (slow heartbeat); *neuropsychiatric toxicity* (anxiety confusion, seizures, hallucinations, mental depression, psychosis, or restlessness)

### Those indicating need for medical attention only if they continue or are bothersome
Incidence more frequent
    *CNS toxicity* (difficulty concentrating; dizziness; headache; insomnia; lightheadedness; vertigo); *gastrointestinal disturbances* (abdominal or stomach pain, diarrhea, loss of appetite, or nausea or vomiting; *visual disturbances*

# Overdose

For more information on the management of overdose or unintentional ingestion, **contact a Poison Control Center** (see *Poison Control Center Listing*).

### Treatment of overdose
Since there is no known specific antidote, treatment of mefloquine overdose should include the following:
    To decrease absorption—
        Standard gastric decontamination procedures.
    Specific treatment—
        Symptomatic treatment may be given.

Supportive care—
Supportive measures such as maintaining an open airway, respiration, and circulation may be necessary. Patients in whom intentional overdose is known or suspected should be referred for psychiatric consultation.

## Patient Consultation

As an aid to patient consultation, refer to *Advice for the Patient, Mefloquine (Systemic)*.

In providing consultation, consider emphasizing the following selected information (» = major clinical significance):

### Before using this medication
» Conditions affecting use, especially:
Allergies to mefloquine, quinidine, quinine, or related medications
Pregnancy—Not recommended for use during pregnancy; however, the risk of maternal and fetal morbidity and mortality from malaria must be considered for women who are at high risk from falciparum malaria
Breast-feeding—Distributed into breast milk in low concentrations
Use in children—Not recommended for use in infants and children up to 2 years of age or less than 15 kg of body weight
Other medications, especially beta-adrenergic blocking agents, calcium channel blocking agents, chloroquine, divalproex, quinidine, quinine, or valproic acid
Other medical problems, especially a history of psychiatric disorders or heart block

### Proper use of this medication
» Not giving to infants and children up to 2 years of age or less than 15 kg of body weight
Taking with full glass (240 mL) of water and with food
» Proper storage
*For suppression of malaria symptoms*
Starting medication 1 week before entering malarious area to ascertain response and allow time to substitute another medication if reactions occur
» Continuing medication while staying in area and for 4 weeks after leaving area
» Checking with physician immediately if fever or "flu-like" symptoms develop while traveling in, or within several months after departure from, endemic area
» Importance of not missing doses and taking medication on a regular schedule
» Proper dosing
Missed dose: Taking as soon as possible; not taking if almost time for next dose; not doubling doses
*For treatment of malaria*
» Compliance with therapy

### Precautions while using this medication
» Caution if visual disturbances, dizziness, lightheadedness, or hallucinations occur
Mosquito-control measures to help prevent malaria:
Sleeping under mosquito netting
Wearing long-sleeved shirts or blouses and long trousers to protect arms and legs when mosquitoes are out
Applying mosquito repellant to uncovered areas of skin when mosquitoes are out
Using a pyrethrum-containing flying insect spray to kill mosquitoes
» Taking mefloquine at least 12 hours after the last dose of quinidine or quinine
*For treatment of malaria*
Checking with physician if no improvement within a few days

### Side/adverse effects
Signs of potential side effects, especially bradycardia and neuropsychiatric toxicity

## General Dosing Information

Malaria prophylaxis should be started 1 week before the patient enters a malarious area, while in the malarious area, and for 4 weeks after the patient leaves the area. Starting the medication in advance will help to determine the patient's tolerance to the medication and allow time to substitute other antimalarials if the patient develops allergies to the medication or other adverse effects.

Mefloquine is also available in combination with sulfadoxine and pyrimethamine as a tablet, but because of toxicity, its use is not recommended. These medications were combined to try to prevent the development of mefloquine resistance to *P. falciparum*; however, in some countries, such as Thailand, *P. falciparum* is already resistant to

sulfadoxine and pyrimethamine. *In vitro* mefloquine resistance has also been reported in Thailand, and may be related to the routine use of quinine.

In the treatment of serious, overwhelming, or life-threatening *P. falciparum* malaria, patients should be given intravenous antimalarial agents during the acute phase. Following this, oral mefloquine may be given to complete the course of therapy. Allow at least 12 hours between the last dose of quinine or quinidine and the start of mefloquine.

In the treatment of acute *P. vivax* or *P. ovale* malaria, it is recommended that mefloquine therapy be followed by treatment with primaquine to effect a radical cure and avoid a relapse since mefloquine does not eliminate the exoerythrocytic (intrahepatic) stages of *P. vivax* or *P. ovale* infection.

The *salt/base equivalence* of mefloquine products differs between the U.S. product and that of other countries. In the U.S., a 250 mg Larium tablet contains 250 mg of mefloquine salt, which is equivalent to 228 mg of mefloquine base. In Canada and other countries, a 250 mg Larium tablet contains 250 mg of mefloquine base, which is equivalent to 274 mg of mefloquine salt. This should be considered when dosing a patient with mefloquine.

Patients with impaired renal function do not generally require a reduction in dose since the urinary clearance of mefloquine is very low.

### Diet/Nutrition
Mefloquine should preferably be taken with a full glass (240 mL) of water and with food.

## Oral Dosage Forms

### MEFLOQUINE HYDROCHLORIDE TABLETS

Note:  The dosing below is based on the product available in the U.S., in which a 250 mg tablet is equivalent to 228 mg of mefloquine base. The product available in Canada and other countries is 250 mg of mefloquine base, equivalent to 274 mg of mefloquine hydrochloride.

### Usual adult and adolescent dose
Antimalarial—
Prophylaxis: Oral, 250 mg (228 mg base) once a week, starting one week before travel, then weekly during travel in malarious areas and for four weeks after leaving endemic areas.
Therapeutic: Chloroquine-resistant *P. falciparum* malaria: Oral, 1250 mg (1140 mg base) as a single dose, or 16.5 mg (15 mg base) per kg of body weight as a single dose.

### Usual pediatric dose
Antimalarial—
Prophylaxis:
Infants and children up to 15 kg of body weight—Use is not recommended.
Children 15 to 19 kg of body weight—Oral, 62.5 mg (57 mg base) (¹/₄ tablet) once a week, starting one week before travel, then weekly during travel in malarious areas and for four weeks after leaving endemic areas.
Children 20 to 30 kg of body weight—Oral, 125 mg (114 mg base) (¹/₂ tablet) once a week, starting one week before travel, then weekly during travel in malarious areas and for four weeks after leaving endemic areas.
Children 31 to 45 kg of body weight—Oral, 187.5 mg (171 mg base) (³/₄ tablet) once a week, starting one week before travel, then weekly during travel in malarious areas and for four weeks after leaving endemic areas.
Children over 45 kg of body weight—See *Usual adult and adolescent dose* .
Therapeutic:
Oral, 16.5 mg (15 mg base) per kg of body weight as a single dose.

### Usual pediatric prescribing limits
Prophylaxis—Up to 250 mg (228 mg base) once a week.

### Usual geriatric dose
See *Usual adult and adolescent dose.*

### Strength(s) usually available
U.S.—
250 mg (228 mg base) (Rx) [*Lariam* (scored; lactose)].
Canada—
Not commercially available; however, those who wish to prescribe mefloquine should contact the medical department of Hoffmann-LaRoche to obtain the name of the nearest principal investigator to arrange to become a co-investigator and for a supply of the drug.

**Packaging and storage**
Store between 15 and 30 °C (59 and 86 °F), unless otherwise specified by manufacturer.

**Auxiliary labeling**
• Take with food and full glass of water.
• May cause dizziness or vision problems.
• Continue medication for full time of treatment.

## Selected Bibliography

Krogstad DJ, Herwaldt BL, Schlesinger PH. Antimalarial agents: specific treatment regimens. Antimicrob Agents Chemother 1988; 32: 957-61.
Keystone JS. Prevention of malaria. Drugs 1990; 39 (3): 337-54.
Panisko DM, Keystone JS. Treatment of malaria-1990. Drugs 1990; 39 (2): 160-89.
Anonymous. Change of dosing regimen for malaria prophylaxis with mefloquine. JAMA 91; 265 (7): 849.
Lobel HO, et al. Effectiveness and tolerance of long-term malaria prophylaxis with mefloquine. JAMA 1991; 265 (3): 361-4.

Revised: 10/06/92
Interim revision: 08/26/94

---

**MEGESTROL**—See *Progestins (Systemic)*

---

**MEGLUMINE ANTIMONIATE**—Since Meglumine Antimoniate is not commercially available in the U.S. or Canada, the *Meglumine Antimoniate (Systemic)* monograph is not included in this published version of the USP DI database. Copies of the monograph are available on request from the USP Division of Information Development, 12601 Twinbrook Parkway, Rockville, MD 20852; telephone (301) 816-8351; telefax (301) 816-8374.

---

**MELARSOPROL**—Since Melarsoprol is not commercially available in the U.S. or Canada, the *Melarsoprol (Systemic)* monograph is not included in this published version of the USP DI database. Copies of the monograph are available on request from the USP Division of Information Development, 12601 Twinbrook Parkway, Rockville, MD 20852; telephone (301) 816-8351; telefax (301) 816-8374.

---

# MELPHALAN    Systemic

VA CLASSIFICATION (Primary): AN100

Other commonly used names are L-PAM and phenylalanine mustard.

Note: For a listing of dosage forms and brand names by country availability, see *Dosage Forms* section(s). For a listing of brand names for the articles in this monograph, refer to the General Index.

## Category

Antineoplastic.

## Indications

Note: Bracketed information in the *Indications* section refers to uses that are not included in U.S. product labeling.

**Accepted**
Carcinoma, ovarian (treatment)
[Carcinoma, breast (treatment)][1] or
[Carcinoma, testicular (treatment)][1]—Melphalan is indicated for the palliative treatment of nonresectable epithelial carcinoma of the ovary. It is also used for treatment of breast carcinoma and testicular carcinoma.

Multiple myeloma (treatment)—Melphalan is indicated for the palliative treatment of multiple myeloma.

[1]Not included in Canadian product labeling.

## Pharmacology/Pharmacokinetics

**Physicochemical characteristics**
Molecular weight—305.20.

**Mechanism of action/Effect**
Melphalan is an alkylating agent of the nitrogen mustard type. Melphalan is a bifunctional alkylating agent and is cell cycle–phase nonspecific. Activity occurs as a result of formation of an unstable ethylenimmonium ion, which alkylates or binds with many intracellular molecular structures including nucleic acids. Its cytotoxic action is primarily due to cross-linking of strands of DNA and RNA, as well as inhibition of protein synthesis.

**Other actions/effects**
Has some immunosuppressant activity.

**Absorption**
Variably and incompletely absorbed from the gastrointestinal tract.

**Protein binding**
Low (30% or less).

**Biotransformation**
Deactivated in body fluids and tissues; remains active in blood for approximately 6 hours.

**Half-life**
Terminal—Approximately 90 minutes.

**Elimination**
Renal—50% (10 to 15% unchanged).
Fecal—20 to 50%.
In dialysis—Not removable by hemodialysis.

## Precautions to Consider

**Cross-sensitivity and/or related problems**
Patients sensitive to chlorambucil may also be sensitive (in form of skin rash) to melphalan.

**Carcinogenicity/Mutagenicity**
Secondary malignancies are potential delayed effects of many antineoplastic agents, although it is not clear whether the effect is related to their mutagenic or immunosuppressive action. The effect of dose and duration of therapy is also unknown, although risk seems to increase with long-term use. Although information is limited, available data seem to indicate that the carcinogenic risk is greatest with the alkylating agents.
Melphalan has been associated with an increased risk of development of secondary carcinomas, especially leukemia or myeloproliferative syndrome, in humans. Melphalan treatment in the pregnant or lactating mother may increase the risk of development of leukemia in the child.
Melphalan produces chromosomal aberrations in human cells both *in vitro* and *in vivo*.

**Pregnancy/Reproduction**
Fertility—Gonadal suppression, resulting in amenorrhea or azoospermia, may occur in patients taking antineoplastic therapy, especially with the alkylating agents. In general, these effects appear to be related to dose and length of therapy and may be irreversible. Prediction of the degree of testicular or ovarian function impairment is complicated by the common use of combinations of several antineoplastics, which makes it difficult to assess the effects of individual agents. Melphalan causes gonadal suppression in humans.
Pregnancy—First trimester: It is usually recommended that use of antineoplastics, especially combination chemotherapy, be avoided whenever possible, especially during the first trimester. Although information is limited because of the relatively few instances of antineoplastic administration during pregnancy, the mutagenic, teratogenic, and carcinogenic potential of these medications must be considered.
FDA Pregnancy Category D.
Other hazards to the fetus include adverse reactions seen in adults.
In general, use of a contraceptive is recommended during cytotoxic drug therapy.

**Breast-feeding**
Although very little information is available regarding excretion of antineoplastic agents in breast milk, breast-feeding is not recommended while melphalan is being administered because of the risks to the infant (adverse effects, mutagenicity, carcinogenicity). It is not known whether melphalan is excreted in breast milk.

**Pediatrics**
Appropriate studies have not been performed in the pediatric population.

**Geriatrics**

No geriatrics-specific information is available on the use of melphalan in geriatric patients. However, elderly patients are more likely to have age-related renal function impairment, which may require caution in patients receiving melphalan.

**Dental**

The bone marrow depressant effects of melphalan may result in an increased incidence of microbial infection, delayed healing, and gingival bleeding. Dental work, whenever possible, should be completed prior to initiation of therapy or deferred until blood counts have returned to normal. Patients should be instructed in proper oral hygiene during treatment, including caution in use of regular toothbrushes, dental floss, and toothpicks.

Melphalan may also rarely cause stomatitis associated with considerable discomfort.

**Drug interactions and/or related problems**

The following drug interactions and/or related problems have been selected on the basis of their potential clinical significance (possible mechanism in parentheses where appropriate)—not necessarily inclusive (» = major clinical significance):

Note: Combinations containing any of the following medications, depending on the amount present, may also interact with this medication.

Allopurinol or
Colchicine or
» Probenecid or
» Sulfinpyrazone

(melphalan may raise the concentration of blood uric acid; dosage adjustment of antigout agents may be necessary to control hyperuricemia and gout; allopurinol may be preferred to prevent or reverse melphalan-induced hyperuricemia because of risk of uric acid nephropathy with uricosuric antigout agents)

Blood dyscrasia–causing medications (See *Appendix II*)

(leukopenic and/or thrombocytopenic effects of melphalan may be increased with concurrent or recent therapy if these medications cause the same effects; dosage adjustment of melphalan, if necessary, should be based on blood counts)

» Bone marrow depressants, other (See *Appendix II*) or
Radiation therapy

(additive bone marrow depression may occur; dosage reduction may be required when two or more bone marrow depressants, including radiation, are used concurrently or consecutively)

Vaccines, killed virus

(because normal defense mechanisms may be suppressed by melphalan therapy, the patient's antibody response to the vaccine may be decreased. The interval between discontinuation of medications that cause immunosuppression and restoration of the patient's ability to respond to the vaccine depends on the intensity and type of immunosuppression-causing medication used, the underlying disease, and other factors; estimates vary from 3 months to 1 year)

» Vaccines, live virus

(because normal defense mechanisms may be suppressed by melphalan therapy, concurrent use with a live virus vaccine may potentiate the replication of the vaccine virus, may increase the side/ adverse effects of the vaccine virus, and/or may decrease the patient's antibody response to the vaccine; immunization of these patients should be undertaken only with extreme caution after careful review of the patient's hematologic status and only with the knowledge and consent of the physician managing the melphalan therapy. The interval between discontinuation of medications that cause immunosuppression and restoration of the patient's ability to respond to the vaccine depends on the intensity and type of immunosuppression-causing medication used, the underlying disease, and other factors; estimates vary from 3 months to 1 year. Patients with leukemia in remission should not receive live virus vaccine until at least 3 months after their last chemotherapy. Immunization with oral poliovirus vaccine should also be postponed in persons in close contact with the patient, especially family members)

**Laboratory value alterations**

The following have been selected on the basis of their potential clinical significance (possible effect in parentheses where appropriate)—not necessarily inclusive (» = major clinical significance):

With physiology/laboratory test values
Uric acid concentrations in blood and urine
(may be increased)

Urinary 5-hydroxyindoleacetic acid (5-HIAA) concentrations
(may be increased, possibly as a result of tumor cell destruction with accompanying release of metabolites)

**Medical considerations/Contraindications**

The medical considerations/contraindications included here have been selected on the basis of their potential clinical significance (reasons given in parentheses where appropriate)—not necessarily inclusive (» = major clinical significance).

*Risk-benefit should be considered when the following medical problems exist:*

» Bone marrow depression
» Chickenpox, existing or recent (including recent exposure) or
» Herpes zoster
(risk of severe generalized disease)

Gout, history of or
Urate renal stones, history of
(risk of hyperuricemia)

» Infection
» Renal function impairment
(effect on toxicity difficult to predict)

Sensitivity to melphalan

» Tumor cell infiltration of bone marrow
» Caution should be used also in patients who have had previous cytotoxic drug therapy and radiation therapy within 3 to 4 weeks.

**Patient monitoring**

The following are especially important in patient monitoring (other tests may be warranted in some patients, depending on condition; » = major clinical significance):

Blood urea nitrogen (BUN) concentrations and
Serum creatinine concentrations
(recommended prior to initiation of therapy and at periodic intervals during therapy; frequency varies according to clinical state, agent, dose, and other agents being used concurrently)

» Hematocrit or hemoglobin and
» Platelet count and
» Total and, if appropriate, differential leukocyte count
(determinations recommended prior to initiation of therapy and at periodic intervals during therapy; frequency varies according to clinical state, agent, dose, and other agents being used concurrently)

Serum uric acid concentrations
(recommended prior to initiation of therapy and at periodic intervals during therapy; frequency varies according to clinical state, agent, dose, and other agents being used concurrently)

# Side/Adverse Effects

Note: Many "side effects" of antineoplastic therapy are unavoidable and represent the medication's pharmacologic action. Some of these (for example, leukopenia and thrombocytopenia) are actually used as parameters to aid in individual dosage titration.

A severe recurrent vasculitis and pulmonary fibrosis occurring with prolonged melphalan therapy have been reported.

The following side/adverse effects have been selected on the basis of their potential clinical significance (possible cause in parentheses where appropriate)—not necessarily inclusive:

**Those indicating need for medical attention**

Incidence more frequent—dose-related

*Neutropenia or infection* (usually asymptomatic; less frequently, fever or chills; cough or hoarseness; lower back or side pain; painful or difficult urination); *thrombocytopenia* (usually asymptomatic; less frequently, unusual bleeding or bruising; black, tarry stools; blood in urine or stools; pinpoint red spots on skin)

Note: *Myelosuppression* usually occurs within 2 to 3 weeks of initiation of therapy, although leukopenia may occur within 5 days in a few patients. The nadir of leukocyte and platelet counts usually occurs within 3 to 5 weeks, and leukocyte and platelet counts usually return to normal within 4 to 8 weeks.

Incidence less frequent or rare

*Allergic reaction* (sudden skin rash or itching); *hyperuricemia or uric acid nephropathy* (joint pain; lower back or side pain; swelling of feet or lower legs); *stomatitis* (sores in mouth and on lips)

Note: *Hyperuricemia or uric acid nephropathy* occurs most commonly during initial treatment of patients with leukemia or lymphoma, as a result of rapid cell breakdown which leads to elevated serum uric acid concentrations.

**Those indicating need for medical attention only if they continue or are bothersome**
Incidence less frequent
  *Nausea and vomiting*—dose-related

**Those indicating the need for medical attention if they occur after medication is discontinued**
  *Bone marrow depression* (black, tarry stools; blood in urine or stools; cough or hoarseness; fever or chills; lower back or side pain; painful or difficult urination; pinpoint red spots on skin; unusual bleeding or bruising)
  Note: Cumulative *myelosuppression* may occur with repeated dosing.

## Patient Consultation

As an aid to patient consultation, refer to *Advice for the Patient, Melphalan (Systemic).*

Consider advising the patient on the following (» = major clinical significance):

**Before using this medication**
» Conditions affecting use, especially:
   Pregnancy—Advisability of using contraception; telling physician immediately if pregnancy is suspected
  See also *Precautions to Consider.*

**Proper use of this medication**
» Importance of not taking more or less medication than the amount prescribed
  Caution in taking combination therapy; taking each medication at the right time
  Importance of ample fluid intake and subsequent increase in urine output to aid in excretion of uric acid
» Frequency of nausea and vomiting; importance of continuing medication despite stomach upset
  Checking with physician if vomiting occurs shortly after dose is taken
» Proper dosing
  Missed dose: Not taking at all; not doubling doses
» Proper storage

**Precautions while using this medication**
» Importance of close monitoring by the physician
» Avoiding immunizations unless approved by physician; other persons in patient's household should avoid immunizations with oral poliovirus vaccine; avoiding other persons who have taken oral poliovirus vaccine or wearing a protective mask that covers nose and mouth
  *Caution if bone marrow depression occurs:*
» Avoiding exposure to persons with bacterial infections, especially during periods of low blood counts; checking with physician immediately if fever or chills, cough or hoarseness, lower back or side pain, or painful or difficult urination occur
» Checking with physician immediately if unusual bleeding or bruising; black, tarry stools; blood in urine or stools; or pinpoint red spots on skin occur
  Caution in use of regular toothbrush, dental floss, or toothpick; physician, dentist, or nurse may suggest alternatives; checking with physician before having dental work done
  Not touching eyes or inside of nose unless hands washed immediately before
  Using caution to avoid accidental cuts with use of sharp objects such as safety razor or fingernail or toenail cutters
  Avoiding contact sports or other situations where bruising or injury could occur

**Side/adverse effects**
  May cause adverse effects such as blood problems and cancer; importance of discussing possible effects with physician
  Physician or nurse can help in dealing with side effects
  See also *Side/Adverse Effects.*

## General Dosing Information

Patients receiving melphalan should be under supervision of a physician experienced in cancer chemotherapy.

A variety of dosage schedules and regimens of melphalan, alone or in combination with other antitumor agents, are used. The prescriber may consult the medical literature as well as the manufacturer's literature in choosing a specific dosage.

Dosage must be adjusted to meet the individual requirements of each patient, based on clinical response and degree of bone marrow depression. This is especially important because of unreliable absorption of orally administered melphalan.

Development of uric acid nephropathy in patients with leukemia or lymphoma may be prevented by adequate oral hydration and, in some cases, administration of allopurinol. Alkalinization of urine may be necessary if serum uric acid concentrations are elevated.

It is recommended that melphalan therapy be discontinued if marked leukopenia (particularly granulocytopenia) or thrombocytopenia occurs. Therapy may be resumed at a lower dosage when the clinical and laboratory examinations are satisfactory.

Special precautions are recommended in patients who develop thrombocytopenia as a result of administration of melphalan. These may include extreme care in performing invasive procedures; regular inspection of intravenous sites, skin (including perirectal area), and mucous membrane surfaces for signs of bleeding or bruising; limiting frequency of venipuncture and avoiding intramuscular injections; testing urine, emesis, stool, and secretions for occult blood; care in use of regular toothbrushes, dental floss, toothpicks, safety razors, and fingernail and toenail cutters; avoiding constipation; and using caution to prevent falls and other injuries. Such patients should avoid alcohol and any aspirin intake because of the risk of gastrointestinal bleeding. Platelet transfusions may be required.

Patients who develop leukopenia should be observed carefully for signs of infection. Antibiotic support may be required. In neutropenic patients who develop fever, broad-spectrum antibiotic coverage should be initiated empirically, pending bacterial cultures and appropriate diagnostic tests.

**Combination chemotherapy**
Melphalan may be used in combination with other agents in various regimens. As a result, incidence and/or severity of side effects may be altered and different dosages (usually reduced) may be used. For example, melphalan is part of the following chemotherapeutic combinations (some commonly used acronyms are in parentheses):
  —vincristine, carmustine, cyclophosphamide, melphalan, and prednisone (M-2 Protocol).
  —melphalan and prednisone (MPL + PRED, MP).
For specific dosages and schedules, consult the literature. For information regarding each agent, consult the individual monographs.

## Oral Dosage Forms
### MELPHALAN TABLETS USP

**Usual adult dose**
Multiple myeloma—
  Oral, 150 mcg (0.15 mg) per kg of body weight per day for seven days, followed by a rest period of at least three weeks, during which time the leukocyte count will fall. When white cell and platelet counts are rising, a maintenance dose of 50 mcg (0.05 mg) per kg of body weight per day may be instituted, or
  Oral, 100 to 150 mcg (0.1 to 0.15 mg) per kg of body weight per day for two to three weeks, or 250 mcg (0.25 mg) per kg of body weight per day for four days, followed by a rest period of two to four weeks. When leukocyte counts rise above 3000 to 4000 per cubic millimeter and platelet counts above 100,000 per cubic millimeter, a maintenance dose of 2 to 4 mg per day may be instituted, or
  Oral, 7 mg per square meter of body surface or 250 mcg (0.25 mg) per kg of body weight per day for five days every five to six weeks, adjusted to produce mild leukopenia and thrombocytopenia.
Ovarian carcinoma—
  Oral, 200 mcg (0.2 mg) per kg of body weight per day for five days, repeated every four to five weeks if blood counts return to normal.

**Usual pediatric dose**
Children up to 12 years of age—Dosage has not been established.

**Strength(s) usually available**
U.S.—
  2 mg (Rx) [*Alkeran* (scored; lactose; sucrose)].
Canada—
  2 mg (Rx) [*Alkeran* (scored)].

**Packaging and storage**
Store below 40 °C (104 °F), preferably between 15 and 30 °C (59 and 86 °F), unless otherwise directed by manufacturer. Store in a well-closed, light-resistant container.

**Note**
Dispense in a glass container.

## Selected Bibliography

Dorr RT, Fritz WL. Cancer chemotherapy handbook. New York: Elsevier, 1980: 507-12.

Revised: 08/90
Interim revision: 07/29/93; 07/11/94

**MENADIOL**—See *Vitamin K (Systemic)*

# MENINGOCOCCAL POLYSACCHARIDE VACCINE   Systemic

VA CLASSIFICATION (Primary): IM100

Note: This monograph refers to the vaccine containing the polysaccharides from *Neisseria meningitidis* serogroups A, C, Y, and W-135.

Note: For a listing of dosage forms and brand names by country availability, see *Dosage Forms* section(s). For a listing of brand names for the articles in this monograph, refer to the General Index.

## Category

Immunizing agent (active).

## Indications

**Accepted**

Meningitis, meningococcal (prophylaxis)—Meningococcal polysaccharide vaccine consists of purified bacterial capsular polysaccharides and contains no viable components. It is indicated for immunization against meningococcal disease caused by *Neisseria meningitidis*, Group A, Group C, Group Y, or Group W-135. *N. meningitidis* is the second most common cause of bacterial meningitis in the U.S., affecting approximately 3000 to 4000 persons each year. The serogroups protected against by this vaccine are responsible for approximately 50% of these cases. The fatality rate from disease caused by all serogroups of *N. meningitidis* is approximately 10% for persons with meningococcal meningitis and 30% for persons with meningococcemia, despite appropriate treatment with antimicrobial agents. The incidence of endemic meningococcal disease peaks in late winter to early spring in the U.S.

Meningococcal polysaccharide vaccine is indicated primarily for persons 2 years of age and older at risk in epidemic or highly endemic areas, including:
• Military recruits. Before the advent of routine administration of meningococcal vaccine to military personnel in 1971, military recruits were at high risk, especially from the serogroup C disease.
• Persons with anatomic or functional asplenia. Asplenic persons seem to be at increased risk of developing meningococcal disease and experience particularly severe infections. Persons who have had their spleens removed because of trauma or non-lymphoid tumors have acceptable antibody responses to the vaccine, although clinical efficacy has not been documented.

In addition, immunization should be considered for:
• Household or institutional contacts of persons with meningococcal disease as an adjunct to antibiotic chemoprophylaxis.
• Medical and laboratory personnel at risk of exposure to meningococcal disease.
• Travelers to countries having epidemic meningococcal disease, particularly travelers who will have prolonged contact with the local populace. One area of the world recognized as having recurrent epidemics of meningococcal disease is the part of sub-Saharan Africa that extends from Mauritania in the west to Ethiopia in the east.
• Immunosuppressed persons. It is uncertain whether persons with diseases associated with immunosuppression (other than asplenia listed above) are at higher risk of acquiring meningococcal disease, as they are of acquiring disease caused by other encapsulated bacteria.

Revaccination may be indicated for persons in the above high risk categories, particularly children at high-risk who were first immunized when under 4 years of age; such children should be considered for revaccination after 2 or 3 years if they remain at high risk. The purpose of this revaccination is to reinstate the primary immune response of the vaccine if it has declined; the revaccination will not evoke a booster response.

**Unaccepted**

Because this vaccine protects against only *Neisseria meningitidis* serogroups A, C, Y, and W-135, protection against other serogroups, such as serogroup B, is not an indication for immunization with this vaccine.

## Pharmacology/Pharmacokinetics

**Mechanism of action/Effect**

Meningococcal bacteria are surrounded by polysaccharide capsules, which make the bacteria resistant to attack by white blood cells. However, human blood serum contains antibodies, which render the bacteria vulnerable to attack. The vaccine, which is composed of the purified capsular polysaccharides from bacterial cells, stimulates production of these antibodies and provides active immunity to the 4 serogroups of *N. meningitidis* bacteria represented in the vaccine.

The vaccine will not stimulate protection against infections caused by organisms other than those in Groups A, C, Y, and W-135.

**Protective effect**

The antibody response to each of the 4 polysaccharides in the vaccine is independent of the antibody responses to the other polysaccharides.

In a study of children 2 to 12 years of age, seroconversion rates as measured by bactericidal antibody were 72% for Group A, 58% for Group C, 90% for Group Y, and 82% for Group W-135. In the same study, seroconversion rates as measured by solid phase radioimmunoassay were 99% for Group A, 99% for Group C, 97% for Group Y, and 89% for Group W-135.

**Time to protective effect**

Adequate antibody titers are achieved within 10 to 14 days after vaccination.

**Duration of protective effect**

Antibodies against Group A and C polysaccharides decline markedly over the first 3 years following a single dose of vaccine. This antibody decline is more rapid in infants and young children than in adults. One study, conducted with Group A vaccine in children who were under 4 years of age at the time of vaccination, showed a decline in efficacy from greater than 90% to less than 10% within 3 years; in older children, efficacy was 67% 3 years after vaccination. Vaccine-induced clinical protection probably persists in school children and adults for at least 3 years.

## Precautions to Consider

**Cross-sensitivity and/or related problems**

Patients allergic to thimerosal or lactose may be allergic to the meningococcal polysaccharide vaccine available in the U.S. and Canada because it may contain a small amount of thimerosal and lactose.

**Pregnancy/Reproduction**

Pregnancy—Adequate and well-controlled studies have not been done in humans. Even though there is no convincing evidence of risk to the fetus from immunization of pregnant women using bacterial vaccines, it is recommended that the vaccine not be used in pregnant women, unless there is a substantial risk of infection. Evaluation of meningococcal polysaccharide vaccine used in pregnant women during an epidemic in Brazil demonstrated no adverse effects. In addition, antibody studies in these women showed good antibody levels in maternal and cord blood following vaccination during any given trimester. Furthermore, antibody titers in the neonates declined over the first few months and did not affect their subsequent response to immunization.

Studies have not been done in animals.

FDA Pregnancy Category C.

**Breast-feeding**

Problems in humans have not been documented.

**Pediatrics**

Meningococcal polysaccharide vaccine is not recommended for use in children up to 2 years of age, because children in this age group are unlikely to have an adequate antibody response to the vaccine.

Revaccination may be indicated for children at high risk who were first immunized when under 4 years of age; such children should be considered for revaccination after 2 or 3 years if they remain at high risk. The purpose of this revaccination is to reinstate the primary immune response of the vaccine if it has declined; the revaccination will not evoke a booster response.

**Geriatrics**
Appropriate studies on the relationship of age to the effects of this vaccine have not been performed in the geriatric population. However, no geriatrics-specific problems have been documented to date.

**Drug interactions and/or related problems**
The following drug interactions and/or related problems have been selected on the basis of their potential clinical significance (possible mechanism in parentheses where appropriate)—not necessarily inclusive (» = major clinical significance):

Note: Combinations containing any of the following medications, depending on the amount present, may also interact with this medication.

Immunosuppressive agents or
Radiation therapy
(because normal defense mechanisms are suppressed, the patient's antibody response to the meningococcal polysaccharide vaccine may be decreased. The precaution does not apply to corticosteroids used as replacement therapy, for short-term [less than 2 weeks] systemic therapy, or by other routes of adminisration that do not cause immunosuppression)

**Medical considerations/Contraindications**
The medical considerations/contraindications included here have been selected on the basis of their potential clinical significance (reasons given in parentheses where appropriate)—not necessarily inclusive (» = major clinical significance).

*Risk-benefit should be considered when the following medical problems exist:*
Febrile illness, severe
(to avoid confusing manifestations of illness with possible side/adverse effects of vaccine; minor illnesses, such as upper respiratory infection, do not preclude administration of vaccine)
Sensitivity to meningococcal polysaccharide vaccine

## Side/Adverse Effects

The following side/adverse effects have been selected on the basis of their potential clinical significance (possible signs and symptoms in parentheses where appropriate)—not necessarily inclusive:

**Those indicating need for medical attention**
Incidence rare
*Anaphylactic reaction* (difficulty in breathing or swallowing; hives; itching, especially of soles or palms; reddening of skin, especially around ears; swelling of eyes, face, or inside of nose; unusual tiredness or weakness, sudden and severe)

**Those indicating need for medical attention only if they continue or are bothersome**
Incidence more frequent
*Erythema at injection site* (redness)—lasting 1 or 2 days; *tenderness, soreness, or pain at injection site*
Incidence less frequent
*Chills; fatigue* (tiredness or weakness); *fever over 37.8 °C (100 °F)* (over 38.3° C [101° F])—rare; *headache; induration at injection site* (hard lump); *malaise* (general feeling of discomfort or illness)

## Patient Consultation

As an aid to patient consultation, refer to *Advice for the Patient, Meningococcal Polysaccharide Vaccine (Systemic).*

In providing consultation, consider emphasizing the following selected information (» = major clinical significance):

**Before receiving this vaccine**
» Conditions affecting use, especially:
Sensitivity to meningococcal vaccine, thimerosal, or lactose; the vaccine contains thimerosal and lactose
Use in children—Not recommended for use in children up to 2 years of age

**Proper use of this vaccine**
» Proper dosing

**Side/adverse effects**
Signs of potential side effects, especially anaphylactic reaction

## General Dosing Information

The dosage of meningococcal polysaccharide vaccine is the same for all persons—children and adults.

Meningococcal polysaccharide vaccine is administered by subcutaneous injection. The vaccine should not be administered intramuscularly, intradermally, or intravenously.

Meningococcal polysaccharide vaccine may be administered concurrently with the following, using separate body sites, separate syringes, and the precautions that apply to each immunizing agent:
• Polysaccharide vaccines, other, such as haemophilus b conjugate, haemophilus b polysaccharide, and pneumococcal polyvalent vaccines.
• Influenza vaccine, whole or split virus.
• Diphtheria toxoid, tetanus toxoid, and/or pertussis vaccine.
• Live virus vaccines, such as measles, mumps, or rubella vaccines.
• Poliovirus vaccines (oral [OPV], inactivated [IPV], or enhanced-potency inactivated [enhanced-potency IPV]).
• Hepatitis B recombinant or plasma-derived vaccine.
• Immune globulin and disease-specific immune globulins.
• Inactivated vaccines, except cholera, typhoid, and plague. It is recommended that cholera, typhoid, and plague vaccines be administered on separate occasions because of these vaccines' propensity to cause side/adverse effects.

Revaccination may be indicated for persons at high risk of infection, particularly children at high risk who were first immunized when under 4 years of age; such children should be considered for revaccination after 2 or 3 years if they remain at high risk.

In the U.S. and Canada, the vaccine is available in a 10-dose vial for use with either a needle and syringe or a jet injector and in a 50-dose vial for use only with a jet injector. However, although the manufacturer gives instructions and cautions for using a jet injector to administer the immunizing agent, it is recommended that jet injectors not be used to administer any medication until there is clarification of the risk of transmission of hepatitis B virus, human immunodeficiency virus (HIV), or other infectious agents by jet injectors.

**For treatment of adverse effects**
Recommended treatment includes
• For mild hypersensitivity reaction—Administering antihistamines, and, if necessary, corticosteroids.
• For severe hypersensitivity or anaphylactic reaction—Administering epinephrine. Antihistamines or corticosteroids may also be administered as required.

## Parenteral Dosage Forms

### MENINGOCOCCAL POLYSACCHARIDE VACCINE FOR INJECTION

**Usual adult and adolescent dose**
Immunizing agent (active)—
Subcutaneous, 0.5 mL.

**Usual pediatric dose**
Immunizing agent (active)—
Children up to 2 years of age: Use is not recommended.
Children 2 years of age and older: See *Usual adult and adolescent dose.*

**Strength(s) usually available**
U.S.—
50 mcg of polysaccharide from each of the 4 serogroups of meningococci represented in the vaccine in each 0.5 mL dose (Rx) [*Menomune* (thimerosal 1:10,000; lactose 2.5 to 5 mg)].
Canada—
50 mcg of polysaccharide from each of the 4 serogroups of meningococci represented in the vaccine in each 0.5 mL dose (Rx) [*Menomune* (thimerosal 1:10,000; lactose 2.5 to 5 mg)].

**Packaging and storage**
Store both the freeze-dried and the reconstituted vaccine between 2 and 8 °C (35 and 46 °F), unless otherwise specified by manufacturer. Protect from freezing.

**Preparation of dosage form**
• Reconstitute the vaccine using only the diluent supplied by the manufacturer.
• Draw up the appropriate amount of diluent into a suitably sized syringe and inject the diluent into the vial containing the vaccine.
• Shake the vial until the vaccine is dissolved.

**Stability**
Solution should not be used if there is extraneous particulate matter and/or discoloration prior to administration.
The date of reconstitution should be recorded on the label of the vaccine vial.
Single-dose vials of vaccine should be used within 24 hours of reconstitution.
Multidose vials of vaccine that have been reconstituted for administration by syringe should be discarded after 5 days.

Multidose vials of vaccine that have been reconstituted for administration by jet injector should be administered promptly. Partially used vials of vaccine should be discarded immediately.

## Selected Bibliography

Centers for Disease Control and Prevention. ACIP: Meningococcal vaccines: recommendation of the ACIP. MMWR 1985 May 10: 255-9.

Menomune-A/C/Y/W-135 package insert (Connaught—US), Rev 1/83, Rec 6/90.

Cadoz M, et al. Tetravalent (A, C, Y, W 135) meningococcal vaccine in children: immunogenicity and safety. Vaccine 1985 Sep; 3: 340-2.

Revised: 07/12/94

---

# MENOTROPINS   Systemic

VA CLASSIFICATION (Primary/Secondary): HS400/HS900

Note: Controlled substance in some states in the U.S.—Schedule IV.

Another commonly used name is human menopausal gonadotropins (HMG).

Note: For a listing of dosage forms and brand names by country availability, see *Dosage Forms* section(s). For a listing of brand names for the articles in this monograph, refer to the General Index.

## Category

Gonadotropin; infertility therapy adjunct.

## Indications

**Accepted**

Infertility, female (treatment)—Menotropins are indicated, in conjunction with chorionic gonadotropin, for stimulation of ovulation and pregnancy in patients with ovulatory dysfunction not due to primary ovarian failure. In general, menotropins are the treatment of choice for induction of ovulation in patients with hypothalamic hypogonadism or those who do not respond to clomiphene.

Reproductive technologies, assisted[1]—Menotropins are indicated, in conjunction with chorionic gonadotropin (hCG), to stimulate the development of multiple oocytes in ovulatory patients who are attempting to conceive by means of assisted reproductive technologies, such as gamete intrafallopian transfer (GIFT) or *in vitro* fertilization (IVF).

Infertility, male (treatment)—Menotropins are also indicated in combination with chorionic gonadotropin for stimulation of spermatogenesis in men with primary or secondary hypogonadotropic hypogonadism.

---

[1]Not included in Canadian product labeling.

## Pharmacology/Pharmacokinetics

**Physicochemical characteristics**

Source—Extracted from urine of postmenopausal women.

**Mechanism of action/Effect**

Menotropins contain follicle-stimulating hormone (FSH) and luteinizing hormone (LH).

For induction of ovulation and assisted reproductive technologies (ART)—

Menotropins prepare the ovarian follicle for ovulation. The combination of FSH and LH stimulates follicular growth and maturation. Chorionic gonadotropin, whose actions are nearly identical to those of LH, is administered following menotropins to mimic the naturally occurring surge of LH that triggers ovulation.

For treatment of male infertility—

Following administration of chorionic gonadotropin to increase testosterone concentrations in men with hypogonadotropic hypogonadism, administration of menotropins induces spermatogenesis.

**Elimination**

Renal, 8% unchanged.

## Precautions to Consider

**Carcinogenicity**

Long-term studies have not been done in animals to evaluate the carcinogenic potential of menotropins.

**Pregnancy/Reproduction**

Fertility—Use of menotropins to induce ovulation is associated with a high incidence of multiple gestations and multiple births. As a result, this may increase the risk of neonatal prematurity, as well as other complications associated with multiple gestations.

Pregnancy—Although problems in humans have not been documented, use of menotropins during pregnancy is unnecessary.

Ovarian hyperstimulation syndrome (OHS), which may be induced by menotropins therapy, is more common, more severe, and protracted in patients who conceive.

FDA Pregnancy Category X.

**Breast-feeding**

It is not known whether menotropins are distributed into breast milk. However, menotropins are not indicated during the course of breast-feeding.

**Medical considerations/Contraindications**

The medical considerations/contraindications included here have been selected on the basis of their potential clinical significance (reasons given in parentheses where appropriate)—not necessarily inclusive (» = major clinical significance).

*Except under special circumstances, this medication should not be used when the following medical problems exist:*

*For females only*

» Abnormal vaginal bleeding, undiagnosed

(may indicate the presence of endometrial hyperplasia or carcinoma, which may be exacerbated by menotropins-induced increases in estrogen serum concentrations; other possible endocrinopathies should also be ruled out)

» Ovarian cyst or enlargement not associated with polycystic ovarian syndrome

(risk of further enlargement)

**Patient monitoring**

The following may be especially important in patient monitoring (other tests may be warranted in some patients, depending on condition; » = major clinical significance):

*For females only*

» Estradiol

(measurement of serum concentrations is recommended as needed, continuing through the day of chorionic gonadotropin administration; recommended to determine optimal dose and to lessen the risk of ovarian hyperstimulation)

» Ultrasound examination

(recommended during menotropins therapy and prior to administration of chorionic gonadotropin to provide information on the number and size of mature follicles, to follow follicular development, and to lessen the risk of ovarian hyperstimulation syndrome and multiple gestation)

Daily basal body temperature

(can be used in ovulation induction to determine if ovulation has occurred; if basal body temperature following a cycle of treatment is biphasic and is not followed by menses, a pregnancy test is recommended)

Progesterone

(measurement of serum or urine concentrations can be used prior to menotropins therapy to confirm anovulation; serum concentrations can be used after therapy to detect luteinized ovarian follicles)

*For males only*

Sperm count and determinations of sperm motility

(to evaluate success of treatment)

Testosterone

(measurement of baseline serum concentrations recommended prior to therapy, to rule out other causes of infertility and following therapy to evaluate success of treatment; should increase)

## Side/Adverse Effects

Note: Arterial thromboembolism has been reported in patients who have received menotropins and chorionic gonadotropin, both in association with and separate from ovarian hyperstimulation syndrome. Complications resulting from thromboembolism have included venous thrombophlebitis, pulmonary embolism, pulmonary infarction, stroke, arterial occlusion necessitating limb amputation, and (rarely) death.

Serious respiratory complications have occurred with menotropins therapy. These conditions included atelectasis and acute respiratory distress syndrome. Rarely, death has resulted.

The following side/adverse effects have been selected on the basis of their potential clinical significance (possible signs and symptoms in parentheses where appropriate)—not necessarily inclusive:

**Those indicating need for medical attention**
Incidence more frequent—about 20%
*For females only*
  *Uncomplicated, mild to moderate, ovarian enlargement or ovarian cysts* (mild bloating, abdominal or pelvic pain)—usually mild to moderate and abate within 7 to 10 days; *pain, swelling, or irritation at injection site; rash at injection site or on body*

Incidence less frequent or rare
*For females only*
  *Severe ovarian hyperstimulation syndrome* (severe abdominal or stomach pain; feeling of indigestion; moderate to severe bloating; decreased amount of urine; continuing or severe nausea, vomiting, or diarrhea; severe pelvic pain; rapid weight gain; swelling of lower legs; shortness of breath)

  Note: In clinical trials, *ovarian hyperstimulation syndrome (OHS)* occurred in 0.4% of patients treated with 150 Units or less each of FSH and LH and in 1.3% of patients treated with higher doses of menotropins. OHS may often occur 7 to 10 days after ovulation or completion of therapy. OHS differs from uncomplicated ovarian enlargement and can rapidly progress to cause serious medical problems. With OHS, a marked increase in vascular permeability results in rapid accumulation of fluid in the peritoneal, pleural, and pericardial cavities (third-spacing of fluids). Medical complications ultimately arising from this increased vascular permeability may include hypovolemia, hemoconcentration, electrolyte imbalance, ascites, hemoperitoneum, pleural effusions, hydrothorax, acute pulmonary distress, and thromboembolic events. OHS is more common, more severe, and protracted in patients who conceive.

*For males only*
  *Erythrocytosis* (shortness of breath; irregular heartbeat; dizziness; loss of appetite; headache; fainting; more frequent nosebleeds)—has been reported in one patient

**Those indicating need for medical attention only if they continue or are bothersome**
Incidence less frequent
*For males only*
  *Gynecomastia* (enlargement of breasts)

## Patient Consultation

As an aid to patient consultation, refer to *Advice for the Patient, Menotropins (Systemic)*.

In providing consultation, consider emphasizing the following selected information (» = major clinical significance):

**Before using this medication**
» Conditions affecting use, especially:
    Sensitivity to menotropins or gonadotropins
    Other medical problems, especially abnormal vaginal bleeding or ovarian cyst or enlargement

**Proper use of this medication**
» Proper dosing

**Precautions while using this medication**
» Importance of close monitoring by physician
*For females only*
» Importance of recording of basal body temperature and timing of intercourse, when recommended by physician

**Side/adverse effects**
  Signs of potential side effects, especially ovarian cysts, enlargement, or hyperstimulation syndrome or skin reactions (for ovulation induction) and erythrocytosis (for males)

## General Dosing Information

Patients receiving menotropins should be under supervision of a physician experienced in the treatment of gynecologic or endocrine disorders.

**For females only**
Dosage varies considerably and must be adjusted to meet the individual requirements of each patient, on the basis of clinical response.

Conception should be attempted within 48 hours of ovulation. It is recommended that the couple have intercourse or insemination performed daily beginning the day after chorionic gonadotropin is administered until ovulation is thought to have occurred.

If ovulation does not occur after any cycle of therapy, the therapeutic regimen employed should be reevaluated. If ovulation does not occur after 3 cycles of menotropins therapy, the appropriateness of continuing use of menotropins for ovulation induction should be reconsidered.

**For treatment of adverse effects**
Ovarian enlargement or ovarian cyst formation
  • Discontinuing therapy until ovarian size has returned to baseline. Human chorionic gonadotropin should also be withheld for that cycle
  • Prohibiting intercourse until ovarian size has returned to baseline to prevent cyst rupture.
  • Reducing dosage in next course of therapy.
Ovarian hyperstimulation syndrome (OHS)—
  Acute phase:
  • Discontinuing therapy.
  • Prohibiting intercourse until ovarian size has returned to baseline to prevent cyst rupture.
  • Most cases of OHS will spontaneously resolve when menses begins. In selected cases, hospitalization of the patient with bed rest may be necessary.
  • Utilizing therapy to prevent hemoconcentration and minimize risk of thromboembolism and renal injury.
  • Correcting (cautiously) electrolyte imbalance while maintaining acceptable intravascular volume; in the acute phase, intravascular volume deficit cannot be completely corrected without increasing third space fluid volume.
  • Monitoring fluid intake and output, body weight, hematocrit, serum and urine electrolytes, urine specific gravity, blood urea nitrogen (BUN), creatinine, and abdominal girth daily or as often as required.
  • Monitoring serum potassium concentrations for development of hyperkalemia.
  • Limiting performance of pelvic examinations since they may result in rupture of ovarian cysts and hemoperitoneum.
  • Administering intravenous fluids, electrolytes, and human serum albumin as needed to maintain adequate urine output and to avoid hemoconcentration.
  • Administering analgesics as needed.
  • Avoiding diuretic use since it reduces intravascular volume further.
  • Removing ascitic, pleural, or pericardial fluid *only* if it is imperative for relief of symptoms such as respiratory distress or cardiac tamponade; to do so may increase risk of injury to the ovary.
  • In patients who require surgery to control bleeding from ovarian cyst rupture, employing surgical measures which also maximally conserve ovarian tissue.
  Intermediate phase:
  • Once patient is stabilized, minimizing third spacing of fluids by cautiously replacing potassium, sodium, and fluids as required, based on monitoring of serum electrolyte concentrations.
  • Avoiding diuretic use.
  Resolution phase:
  • The third space fluid shifts to intravascular compartment, resulting in decreased hematocrit value and increased urinary output.
  • Peripheral and/or pulmonary edema may result if third space fluid volume mobilized exceeds renal output.
  • Administering diuretics when required, to manage pulmonary edema.

## Parenteral Dosage Forms

### MENOTROPINS FOR INJECTION USP

**Usual adult dose**
Induction of ovulation—
  Intramuscular, 75 Units of FSH and 75 Units of LH activity once a day for usually seven or more days, followed by 5000 to 10,000 Units of chorionic gonadotropin one day after the last dose of menotropins. If necessary, the dose of menotropins may be increased by 75 to 150 Units FSH and 75 to 150 Units LH every four or five days. Up to 450 Units FSH and 450 Units LH a day may be required.
Assisted reproductive technologies[1]—
  Intramuscular, 150 Units of FSH and 150 Units of LH activity once a day for usually seven or more days, followed by 5000 to 10,000 Units of chorionic gonadotropin one day after the last dose of menotropins. If necessary, the dose of menotropins may be in-

creased by 75 to 150 Units FSH and 75 to 150 Units LH every four or five days.

Note: Dosage regimen may vary according to physician preference or patient response.

If the ovaries are abnormally enlarged or the serum estradiol concentration is excessively elevated on the last day of menotropins therapy, human chorionic gonadotropin should not be given for that cycle.

Male infertility (hypogonadotropic hypogonadism)

Intramuscular, 75 Units of FSH and 75 Units of LH activity three times a week (plus chorionic gonadotropin 2000 Units twice a week) for at least four months following pretreatment with chorionic gonadotropin (5000 Units three times a week for up to four to six months). If an increase in spermatogenesis has not occurred after four months, the dose may be increased to 150 Units FSH and 150 Units LH three times a week (with no change in dose of chorionic gonadotropin).

**Size(s) usually available**

U.S.—

75 Units of FSH and 75 Units of LH activity (Rx) [*Pergonal*].

150 Units of FSH and 150 Units of LH activity (Rx) [*Pergonal*].

Canada—

75 Units of FSH and 75 Units of LH activity (Rx) [*Pergonal*].

**Packaging and storage**

Store below 40 °C (104 °F), preferably between 15 and 30 °C (59 and 86 °F), unless otherwise specified by manufacturer.

**Preparation of dosage form**

Using standard aseptic technique, reconstitute by adding 1 to 2 mL of 0.9% sodium chloride injection to each ampul of menotropins.

**Stability**

Use immediately after reconstitution; discard any unused portion.

[1]Not included in Canadian product labeling.

Revised: 07/07/92
Interim revision: 06/30/94

---

## MENTHYL ANTHRANILATE—See *Sunscreen Agents (Topical)*

---

## MENTHYL ANTHRANILATE-CONTAINING COMBINATIONS—

Homosalate, Menthyl Anthranilate, and Octyl Methoxycinnamate (Topical)—See *Sunscreen Agents (Topical)*

Homosalate, Menthyl Anthranilate, Octyl Methoxycinnamate, and Octyl Salicylate (Topical)—See *Sunscreen Agents (Topical)*

Homosalate, Menthyl Anthranilate, Octyl Methoxycinnamate, Octyl Salicylate, and Oxybenzone (Topical)—See *Sunscreen Agents (Topical)*

Homosalate, Menthyl Anthranilate, Octyl Methoxycinnamate, and Oxybenzone (Topical)—See *Sunscreen Agents (Topical)*

Menthyl Anthranilate, Octocrylene, and Octyl Methoxycinnamate (Topical)—See *Sunscreen Agents (Topical)*

Menthyl Anthranilate, Octocrylene, Octyl Methoxycinnamate, and Oxybenzone (Topical)—See *Sunscreen Agents (Topical)*

Menthyl Anthranilate and Octyl Methoxycinnamate (Topical)—See *Sunscreen Agents (Topical)*

Menthyl Anthranilate, Octyl Methoxycinnamate, and Octyl Salicylate (Topical)—See *Sunscreen Agents (Topical)*

Menthyl Anthranilate, Octyl Methoxycinnamate, Octyl Salicylate, and Oxybenzone (Topical)—See *Sunscreen Agents (Topical)*

Menthyl Anthranilate, Octyl Methoxycinnamate, and Oxybenzone (Topical)—See *Sunscreen Agents (Topical)*

Menthyl Anthranilate and Padimate O (Topical)—See *Sunscreen Agents (Topical)*

Menthyl Anthranilate and Titanium Dioxide (Topical)—See *Sunscreen Agents (Topical)*

---

## MEPENZOLATE—See *Anticholinergics/Antispasmodics (Systemic)*

---

## MEPERIDINE—See *Opioid (Narcotic) Analgesics (Systemic)*

---

## MEPHENTERMINE—See *Sympathomimetic Agents—Cardiovascular Use (Parenteral-Systemic)*

---

## MEPHENYTOIN—See *Anticonvulsants, Hydantoin (Systemic)*

---

## MEPHOBARBITAL—See *Barbiturates (Systemic)*

---

## MEPIVACAINE—See *Anesthetics (Parenteral-Local)*

---

## MEPIVACAINE-CONTAINING COMBINATIONS—

Mepivacaine and Levonordefrin (Parenteral-Local)—See *Anesthetics (Parenteral-Local)*

---

# MEPROBAMATE   Systemic

VA CLASSIFICATION (Primary): CN309

Note: Controlled substance in the U.S.—Schedule IV.

Note: For a listing of dosage forms and brand names by country availability, see *Dosage Forms* section(s). For a listing of brand names for the articles in this monograph, refer to the General Index.

## Category

Antianxiety agent.

## Indications

**Accepted**

Anxiety (treatment)—Meprobamate is indicated for the management of anxiety disorders or for the short-term relief of the symptoms of anxiety. Meprobamate is usually not indicated for the treatment of anxiety or tension associated with everyday life. Effectiveness of this medication for long-term (more than 4 months) management of anxiety has not been assessed by systematic clinical studies. The medication's efficacy should be reassessed at periodic intervals.

## Pharmacology/Pharmacokinetics

**Physicochemical characteristics**

Chemical group—A carbamate derivative.

Molecular weight—218.25.

**Mechanism of action/Effect**

The mechanism of action of meprobamate is not known. It appears to act at multiple sites in the central nervous system (CNS), including the thalamus and limbic system.

**Absorption**

Well absorbed from the gastrointestinal tract.

**Biotransformation**

Hepatic.

**Half-life**

Plasma half-life is about 10 hours.

**Elimination**

Renal. About 8 to 19% of drug is excreted unchanged.

# Precautions to Consider

### Cross-sensitivity and/or related problems
Patients sensitive to other carbamate derivatives (for example, carbromal, carisoprodol, mebutamate, or tybamate) may be sensitive to this medication also.

### Pregnancy/Reproduction
Pregnancy—Meprobamate crosses the placenta. This medication has been reported to increase the risk of congenital malformations when used during the first trimester of pregnancy. Risk-benefit must be considered. However, since use of meprobamate is rarely a matter of urgency, its use during pregnancy, especially during the first trimester, should generally be avoided.

### Breast-feeding
Meprobamate is excreted in breast milk in a concentration of 2 to 4 times maternal plasma concentrations; use by nursing mothers may cause sedation in the infant.

### Pediatrics
Appropriate studies on the relationship of age to the effects of meprobamate have not been performed in the pediatric population. However, no pediatrics-specific problems have been documented to date.

### Geriatrics
Elderly patients may be more sensitive to the effects of meprobamate. The lowest effective dose should be administered to these patients to avoid oversedation. In addition, elderly patients are more likely to have age-related renal function impairment, which may require reduction of dosage in patients receiving meprobamate.

### Dental
Prolonged use of meprobamate may decrease or inhibit salivary flow, thus contributing to the development of caries, periodontal disease, oral candidiasis, and discomfort.

### Drug interactions and/or related problems
The following drug interactions and/or related problems have been selected on the basis of their potential clinical significance (possible mechanism in parentheses where appropriate)—not necessarily inclusive (» = major clinical significance):

Note: Combinations containing any of the following medications, depending on the amount present, may also interact with this medication.

Addictive medications, other, especially central nervous system (CNS) depressants with habituating potential
(prolonged concurrent use may increase the risk of habituation; caution is recommended)
» Alcohol or
» CNS depression–producing medications, other (See *Appendix II*)
(concurrent use may increase the CNS depressant effects of either these medications or meprobamate; caution is recommended and dosage of one or both agents should be reduced)

### Laboratory value alterations
The following have been selected on the basis of their potential clinical significance (possible effect in parentheses where appropriate)—not necessarily inclusive (» = major clinical significance):

With diagnostic test results
Metyrapone test
(response to metyrapone may be decreased)
Phentolamine test
(meprobamate may cause false-positive phentolamine test; it is recommended that all medications be withdrawn at least 24 hours, preferably 48 to 72 hours, prior to a phentolamine test)
Urinary steroid determinations
(meprobamate may falsely increase 17-ketosteroid and 17-ketogenicsteroid concentrations in the Zimmerman reaction and 17-hydroxycorticosteroid concentrations in the modified Glenn-Nelson technique)

### Medical considerations/Contraindications
The medical considerations/contraindications included here have been selected on the basis of their potential clinical significance (reasons given in parentheses where appropriate)—not necessarily inclusive (» = major clinical significance).

*Risk-benefit should be considered when the following medical problems exist:*

» Alcoholism, active or in remission or
» Drug abuse or dependence, history of
(predisposition of patients to habituation and dependence)
Epilepsy
(seizures may be precipitated)

Hepatic function impairment
(meprobamate metabolized in liver)
» Porphyria, acute intermittent
(condition may be exacerbated)
Renal function impairment
(meprobamate excreted via kidneys)
Sensitivity to meprobamate or other carbamate derivatives, such as carbromal, carisoprodol, mebutamate, or tybamate

### Patient monitoring
The following may be especially important in patient monitoring (other tests may be warranted in some patients, depending on condition; » = major clinical significance):

Reassessment of medication's efficacy
(recommended at periodic intervals since the effectiveness of meprobamate in long-term use, more than 4 months, has not been assessed by systematic clinical studies)

# Side/Adverse Effects
The following side/adverse effects have been selected on the basis of their potential clinical significance (possible signs and symptoms in parentheses where appropriate)—not necessarily inclusive:

### Those indicating need for medical attention
Incidence less frequent
*Allergic reaction* (skin rash, hives, or itching; wheezing, shortness of breath, or troubled breathing [rare])
Incidence rare
*Fast, pounding, or irregular heartbeat; intolerance to meprobamate* (confusion); *leukopenia* (sore throat and fever); *paradoxical reaction* (unusual excitement); *thrombocytopenia* (unusual bleeding or bruising)

### Those indicating need for medical attention only if they continue or are bothersome
Incidence more frequent
*Clumsiness or unsteadiness; drowsiness*
Incidence less frequent
*Blurred vision or change in near or distant vision; diarrhea; dizziness or lightheadedness; false sense of well-being; headache; nausea or vomiting; unusual tiredness or weakness*

### Those indicating possible withdrawal and the need for medical attention if they occur (usually within 2 days) after medication is discontinued
*Clumsiness or unsteadiness; confusion; convulsions; hallucinations; increased dreaming; insomnia* (trouble in sleeping); *muscle twitching; nausea or vomiting; nervousness or restlessness; nightmares; trembling*

# Overdose
For specific information on the agents used in the management of meprobamate overdose, see:
• *Mannitol (Systemic)* monograph.

For more information on the management of overdose or unintentional ingestion, **contact a Poison Control Center** (see *Poison Control Center Listing*).

### Clinical effects of overdose
The following effects have been selected on the basis of their potential clinical significance (possible signs and symptoms in parentheses where appropriate)—not necessarily inclusive:

Acute
*Confusion, severe; drowsiness, severe; shortness of breath or slow or troubled breathing; slow heartbeat; weakness, severe*
Chronic
*Dizziness or lightheadedness, continuing; slurred speech; staggering*

### Treatment of overdose
Recommended treatment of meprobamate overdose includes the following:
To decrease absorption—
Removing meprobamate from the stomach.
To enhance elimination—
Diuresis, osmotic (mannitol) diuresis, peritoneal dialysis, and hemodialysis have been effectively used.
Monitoring—
Monitoring urinary output; however, caution should be used to avoid overhydration, since it may produce pulmonary edema.
Supportive care—
Administering symptomatic treatment.

If respiration or blood pressure becomes compromised, cautiously administering respiratory assistance and pressor agents as indicated.

Patients in whom intentional overdose is known or suspected should be referred for psychiatric consultation.

## Patient Consultation

As an aid to patient consultation, refer to *Advice for the Patient, Meprobamate (Systemic)*.

In providing consultation, consider emphasizing the following selected information (» = major clinical significance):

**Before using this medication**
» Conditions affecting use, especially:

Sensitivity to meprobamate or other carbamate derivatives, such as carbromal, carisoprodol, mebutamate, or tybamate

Pregnancy—Meprobamate crosses placenta; risk of congenital malformations may be increased when medication used during first trimester of pregnancy

Breast-feeding—Excreted in breast milk in concentration of 2 to 4 times maternal plasma concentrations; use by nursing mothers may cause sedation in infant

Use in the elderly—Elderly patients may be more sensitive to effects of meprobamate; lowest effective dose should be administered to avoid oversedation

Dental—Prolonged use of meprobamate may decrease or inhibit salivary flow, which may contribute to development of caries, periodontal disease, oral candidiasis, and discomfort

Other medications, especially alcohol or other CNS depression–producing medications

Other medical problems, especially alcohol or drug abuse or dependence, or acute intermittent porphyria

**Proper use of this medication**
» Importance of not using more medication than the amount prescribed because of habit-forming potential
» Proper dosing

Missed dose: Taking right away if remembered within an hour or so; not taking if remembered later; not doubling doses
» Proper storage

**Precautions while using this medication**

Regular visits to physician to check progress during prolonged therapy

Checking with physician before discontinuing medication after prolonged use; gradual dosage reduction may be necessary to avoid possibility of withdrawal symptoms
» Avoiding use of alcohol or other CNS depressants

Caution if any laboratory tests required; possible interference with results of metyrapone or phentolamine tests
» Suspected overdose: Getting emergency help at once
» Caution if dizziness, lightheadedness, or drowsiness occurs

Possible dryness of mouth; using sugarless gum or candy, ice, or saliva substitute for relief; checking with dentist if dry mouth continues for more than 2 weeks

**Side/adverse effects**

Signs of potential side effects, especially allergic reaction; fast, pounding, or irregular heartbeat; intolerance to meprobamate; leukopenia; paradoxical reaction; and thrombocytopenia

## General Dosing Information

Prolonged use in larger than usual therapeutic doses may result in psychological or physical dependence.

Following prolonged administration, meprobamate should be withdrawn gradually in order to avoid the possibility of precipitating withdrawal symptoms.

**For treatment of dependence**

Dosage of meprobamate should be reduced gradually over a period of 1 to 2 weeks. Alternatively, a barbiturate such as phenobarbital may be substituted, then gradually reduced.

## Oral Dosage Forms

### MEPROBAMATE EXTENDED-RELEASE CAPSULES

**Usual adult dose**

Antianxiety agent—

Oral, 400 to 800 mg two times a day, in the morning and at bedtime.

Note: Geriatric or debilitated patients may be more sensitive to the effects of the usual adult dose.

**Usual adult prescribing limits**

Up to 2.4 grams daily.

**Usual pediatric dose**

Antianxiety agent—

Children up to 6 years of age: Dosage has not been established.

Children 6 to 12 years of age: Oral, 200 mg two times a day, in the morning and at bedtime.

**Strength(s) usually available**

U.S.—

200 mg (Rx) [*Meprospan 200* (corn starch; FD&C Blue No. 1; FD&C Yellow No. 6; gelatin; sucrose)].

400 mg (Rx) [*Meprospan 400* (corn starch; FD&C Yellow No. 6; gelatin; sucrose)].

Canada—

400 mg (Rx) [*Meprospan-400*].

**Packaging and storage**

Store below 40 °C (104 °F), preferably between 15 and 30 °C (59 and 86 °F), in a well-closed container, unless otherwise specified by manufacturer.

**Auxiliary labeling**
• Avoid alcoholic beverages.
• May cause drowsiness.

**Note**

Controlled substance in the U.S.

### MEPROBAMATE TABLETS USP

**Usual adult dose**

Antianxiety agent—

Oral, 400 mg three or four times a day; or 600 mg two times a day.

Note: Geriatric or debilitated patients may be more sensitive to the effects of the usual adult dose.

**Usual adult prescribing limits**

Up to 2.4 grams daily.

**Usual pediatric dose**

Antianxiety agent—

Children up to 6 years of age: Dosage has not been established.

Children 6 to 12 years of age: Oral, 100 to 200 mg two or three times a day.

Note: The 600-mg tablet is not recommended for use in children.

**Strength(s) usually available**

U.S.—

200 mg (Rx) [*Equanil*; *'Miltown'-200*; *Trancot*; GENERIC].

400 mg (Rx) [*Equanil* (scored); *'Miltown'-400* (scored); *Probate*; *Trancot*; GENERIC].

600 mg (Rx) [*'Miltown'-600*].

Canada—

400 mg (Rx) [*Apo-Meprobamate* (scored); *Equanil* (scored); *Miltown* (scored)].

**Packaging and storage**

Store below 40 °C (104 °F), preferably between 15 and 30 °C (59 and 86 °F), unless otherwise specified by manufacturer. Store in a well-closed container.

**Auxiliary labeling**
• Avoid alcoholic beverages.
• May cause drowsiness.

**Note**

Controlled substance in the U.S.

Revised: 01/13/93

# MEPROBAMATE AND ASPIRIN Systemic

VA CLASSIFICATION (Primary): CN103

**NOTE:** The *Meprobamate and Aspirin (Systemic)* monograph is maintained on the USP DI electronic data base. For a printed copy of the most recent revision of the complete monograph, contact the USP Division of Information Development, 12601 Twinbrook Parkway, Rockville, MD 20852.

For information on the specific components of this combination, see the *USP DI* monographs for *Meprobamate (Systemic)* and *Salicylates (Systemic)*.

The information that follows is selectively abstracted from the complete monograph and is provided to facilitate drug use review and patient counseling.

Note: For a listing of dosage forms and brand names by country availability, see *Dosage Forms* section(s). For a listing of brand names for the articles in this monograph, refer to the General Index.

## Category

Analgesic.

## Indications

### Accepted

Pain, with anxiety and tension (treatment) or

Headache, tension (treatment)—Meprobamate and aspirin combination is indicated as an adjunct in the short-term treatment of pain accompanied by tension and/or anxiety in patients with musculoskeletal disease or tension headache. It appears to provide greater relief of pain in these conditions than when aspirin is used alone. Effectiveness of this medication for long-term (more than 4 months) management of anxiety has not been assessed by systematic clinical studies. The medication's efficacy should be reassessed at periodic intervals.

## Patient Consultation

As an aid to patient consultation, refer to *Advice for the Patient, Meprobamate and Aspirin (Systemic)*.

In providing consultation, consider emphasizing the following selected information (» = major clinical significance):

### Before using this medication

» Conditions affecting use, especially:

Sensitivity to meprobamate or other carbamate derivatives, such as carbromal, carisoprodol, mebutamate, or tybamate, or to aspirin or other salicylates including methyl salicylate (oil of wintergreen) or other nonsteroidal anti-inflammatory drugs or related analgesics

Pregnancy—

Meprobamate crosses placenta; risk of congenital malformations may be increased when meprobamate is used during first trimester

Aspirin and its salicylate metabolite readily cross placenta; studies in animals have shown that aspirin increases fetal resorptions and birth defects; use of aspirin during pregnancy reported to increase risk of birth defects in humans, but controlled studies using usual therapeutic doses have not shown proof of teratogenicity; chronic, high-dose aspirin therapy may prolong gestation, increase risk of postmaturity syndrome, and increase risk of maternal antenatal hemorrhage; ingestion of aspirin during last 2 weeks of pregnancy may increase risk of fetal or neonatal hemorrhage; regular use of aspirin during late pregnancy may result in constriction or premature closure of fetal ductus arteriosus, possibly leading to persistent pulmonary hypertension and heart failure in the neonate; overuse or abuse of aspirin late in pregnancy reported to reduce birthweight and to increase risk of stillbirth or neonatal death, possibly because of hemorrhage or premature ductus arteriosus closure

Labor and delivery—Chronic, high-dose aspirin therapy late in pregnancy may result in prolonged labor, complicated deliveries, and increased risk of maternal or fetal hemorrhage

Breast-feeding—

Meprobamate excreted in breast milk in concentration of 2 to 4 times maternal plasma concentrations; use by nursing mothers may cause sedation in infant

Salicylate excreted in breast milk

Use in children and teenagers—Checking with physician before giving medication to children or teenagers with symptoms of acute febrile illness, especially influenza or varicella, because of the risk of Reye's syndrome; also, pediatric patients, especially those with fever and dehydration, may be more susceptible to toxic effects of aspirin

Use in the elderly—Elderly patients may be more sensitive to effects of meprobamate; also, they may be more susceptible to toxic effects of aspirin

Dental—Prolonged use of meprobamate may decrease or inhibit salivary flow, which may contribute to development of caries, periodontal disease, oral candidiasis, and discomfort

Other medications, especially alcohol or other CNS depression–producing medications, anticoagulants, antidiabetic agents (oral), cefamandole, cefoperazone, cefotetan, heparin, methotrexate, moxalactam, nonsteroidal anti-inflammatory drugs (other), platelet aggregation inhibitors, plicamycin, probenecid, sulfinpyrazone, thrombolytic agents, urinary alkalizers, valproic acid, or vancomycin

Other medical problems, especially asthma, allergies, and nasal polyps; bleeding ulcers or other hemorrhagic states; erosive gastritis; peptic ulcer; coagulation or platelet function disorders; history of alcohol or drug abuse or dependence; or acute intermittent porphyria

### Proper use of this medication

» Taking with food or a full glass (240 mL) of water to minimize gastrointestinal irritation

» Not taking medication if it has a strong vinegar-like odor

» Not giving to children or teenagers with symptoms of influenza or varicella without first checking with physician because of risk of Reye's syndrome

» Importance of not taking more medication than the amount prescribed; meprobamate is potentially habit-forming and too much aspirin may cause stomach problems or result in overdose

» Proper dosing

» Proper storage

### Precautions while using this medication

Regular visits to physician to check progress during prolonged therapy

Checking with physician before discontinuing medication after prolonged use; gradual dosage reduction may be necessary to avoid possibility of meprobamate withdrawal symptoms

» Caution if other medications containing aspirin or other salicylates (including bismuth subsalicylate) are used

» Avoiding use of alcohol or other CNS depressants

Alcohol consumption may increase risk of salicylate-induced gastrointestinal toxicity

Not using a nonsteroidal anti-inflammatory drug together with this medication on a regular basis, unless otherwise directed by physician or dentist

Not taking a cellulose-containing laxative within 2 hours of this combination containing aspirin

Diabetics: Aspirin present in combination may cause false urine sugar test results with prolonged use of 8 or more 325-mg (5-grain) doses per day

Caution if any laboratory tests required; possible interference with results of metyrapone and phentolamine tests

Caution if any kind of surgery is required; aspirin should be discontinued 5 days prior to surgery unless otherwise directed by physician

» Suspected overdose: Getting emergency help at once

» Caution if dizziness, lightheadedness, or drowsiness occurs

Possible dryness of mouth; using sugarless gum or candy, ice, or saliva substitute for relief; checking with dentist if dry mouth continues for more than 2 weeks

### Side/adverse effects

Signs of potential side effects, especially aspirin-induced gastrointestinal bleeding or ulceration, intolerance to meprobamate, allergic reactions, blood dyscrasias due to meprobamate

## Oral Dosage Forms

### MEPROBAMATE AND ASPIRIN TABLETS

**Usual adult dose**

Analgesic—

Oral, 1 or 2 tablets three or four times a day as needed.

Note: Geriatric or debilitated patients may be more sensitive to the effects of the usual adult dose.

**Usual pediatric dose**
Analgesic—
    Children up to 12 years of age: Use is not recommended.

**Strength(s) usually available**
U.S.—
    200 mg of meprobamate and 325 mg of aspirin (Rx) [*Epromate-M; Equagesic; Heptogesic; Meprogesic; Meprogesic Q; Micrainin;* GENERIC].
Canada—
    200 mg of meprobamate, 75 mg of ethoheptazine citrate, and 250 mg of aspirin (Rx) [*Equagesic*].

**Auxiliary labeling**
• Avoid alcoholic beverages.
• May cause drowsiness.

Revised: 01/13/93

## MEPROBAMATE-CONTAINING COMBINATIONS—
Meprobamate and Aspirin (Systemic)

# MERCAPTOPURINE   Systemic

VA CLASSIFICATION (Primary/Secondary): AN300/IM600; MS105; GA900

Another commonly used name is 6-MP.

Note: For a listing of dosage forms and brand names by country availability, see *Dosage Forms* section(s). For a listing of brand names for the articles in this monograph, refer to the General Index.

## Category
Antineoplastic; immunosuppressant.

## Indications
Note: Bracketed information in the *Indications* section refers to uses that are not included in U.S. product labeling.

**Accepted**
Leukemia, acute lymphocytic (treatment)
Leukemia, acute myelocytic (treatment) or
Leukemia, acute myelomonocytic (treatment)—Mercaptopurine is indicated for remission induction and maintenance therapy of acute lymphocytic, acute myelocytic, and acute myelomonocytic leukemia.
[Leukemia, chronic myelocytic (treatment)]—Mercaptopurine is used for treatment of chronic myelocytic leukemia.
[Lymphomas, non-Hodgkin's (treatment)][1]—Mercaptopurine is used for treatment of some pediatric non-Hodgkin's lymphomas.
[Polycythemia vera (treatment)][1]—Mercaptopurine is used for treatment of polycythemia vera.
[Bowel disease, inflammatory (treatment)][1]—Mercaptopurine is also being used in the treatment of regional enteritis (Crohn's disease) and ulcerative colitis.
[Arthritis, psoriatic (treatment)][1]—Mercaptopurine is being used in the treatment of selected cases of severe psoriatic arthritis.

Extreme caution is recommended in use of mercaptopurine for non-neoplastic conditions because of potential carcinogenicity with long-term use of this agent.

[1]Not included in Canadian product labeling.

## Pharmacology/Pharmacokinetics

**Physicochemical characteristics**
Molecular weight—170.19.
pKa—7.6.

**Mechanism of action/Effect**
Mercaptopurine is an antimetabolite of the purine analog type. Mercaptopurine is cell cycle–specific for the S phase of cell division. Activity occurs as the result of activation in the tissues and may include inhibition of DNA synthesis with a lesser effect on RNA synthesis.

**Absorption**
Variably and incompletely (up to 50%) absorbed from the gastrointestinal tract.

**Distribution**
Crosses the blood-brain barrier, but in insufficient amounts to treat meningeal leukemia.

**Protein binding**
Low (20%).

**Biotransformation**
Hepatic (activation and catabolism); degradation primarily by xanthine oxidase.

**Half-life**
Triphasic—45 minutes, 2.5 hours, and 10 hours.

**Elimination**
Renal (7 to 39% unchanged).
In dialysis—Removable by dialysis.

## Precautions to Consider

**Carcinogenicity/Mutagenicity**
Secondary malignancies are potential delayed effects of many antineoplastic agents, although it is not clear whether the effect is related to their mutagenic or immunosuppressive action. The effect of dose and duration of therapy is also unknown, although risk seems to increase with long-term use. Although information is limited, available data seem to indicate that the carcinogenic risk is greatest with the alkylating agents.
Antimetabolites have been shown to be carcinogenic in animals and may be associated with an increased risk of development of secondary carcinomas in humans, although the risk appears to be less than with alkylating agents.
Mercaptopurine causes chromosome abnormalities in animals and humans and dominant-lethal mutations in male mice.

**Pregnancy/Reproduction**
Fertility—Gonadal suppression, resulting in amenorrhea or azoospermia, may occur in patients taking antineoplastic therapy, especially with the alkylating agents. In general, these effects appear to be related to dose and length of therapy and may be irreversible. Prediction of the degree of testicular or ovarian function impairment is complicated by the common use of combinations of several antineoplastics, which makes it difficult to assess the effects of individual agents.
Pregnancy—Mercaptopurine is not recommended during pregnancy.
First trimester: It is usually recommended that use of antineoplastics, especially combination chemotherapy, be avoided whenever possible, especially during the first trimester. Although information is limited because of the relatively few instances of antineoplastic administration during pregnancy, the mutagenic, teratogenic, and carcinogenic potential of these medications must be considered.
Other hazards to the fetus include adverse reactions seen in adults.
In general, use of a contraceptive is recommended during cytotoxic drug therapy.
Mercaptopurine is embryopathic in rats and has been associated with an increased risk of abortion or premature births in humans; the risk of teratogenicity in surviving offspring has not been studied.
FDA Pregnancy Category D.

**Breast-feeding**
Although very little information is available regarding distribution of antineoplastic agents into breast milk, breast-feeding is not recommended while mercaptopurine is being administered because of the risks to the infant (adverse effects, mutagenicity, carcinogenicity). It is not known whether mercaptopurine is distributed into breast milk.

**Pediatrics**
Appropriate studies on the relationship of age to the effects of mercaptopurine have not been performed in the pediatric population. However, pediatrics-specific problems that would limit the usefulness of this medication in children are not expected.

**Geriatrics**
No information is available on the relationship of age to the effects of mercaptopurine in geriatric patients. However, elderly patients are more likely to have age-related renal function impairment, which may require dosage reduction in patients receiving mercaptopurine.

**Dental**

The bone marrow depressant effects of mercaptopurine may result in an increased incidence of microbial infection, delayed healing, and gingival bleeding. Dental work, whenever possible, should be completed prior to initiation of therapy or deferred until blood counts have returned to normal. Patients should be instructed in proper oral hygiene during treatment, including caution in use of regular toothbrushes, dental floss, and toothpicks.

Mercaptopurine may also cause stomatitis associated with considerable discomfort.

**Drug interactions and/or related problems**

The following drug interactions and/or related problems have been selected on the basis of their potential clinical significance (possible mechanism in parentheses where appropriate)—not necessarily inclusive (» = major clinical significance):

Note: Combinations containing any of the following medications, depending on the amount present, may also interact with this medication.

» Allopurinol or
   Colchicine or
» Probenecid or
» Sulfinpyrazone
   (concurrent use with allopurinol may result in greatly increased mercaptopurine activity and toxicity because of inhibition of metabolism; careful monitoring is recommended. It is recommended that mercaptopurine dosage be reduced to one-third to one-fourth of the usual dosage in patients receiving 300 to 600 mg of allopurinol a day concurrently to reduce or prevent hyperuricemia or to slow the metabolism of mercaptopurine. In addition, mercaptopurine may raise the concentration of blood uric acid; dosage adjustment of antigout agents may be necessary to control hyperuricemia and gout; concurrent use of uricosuric antigout agents should be avoided because of the risk of uric acid nephropathy)

Anticoagulants, coumarin- or indandione-derivative
   (mercaptopurine may increase anticoagulant activity and/or increase the risk of hemorrhage as a result of decreased hepatic synthesis of procoagulant factors and interference with platelet formation or may reduce anticoagulant activity by means of increased prothrombin synthesis or activation)

Blood dyscrasia–causing medications (See *Appendix II*)
   (leukopenic and/or thrombocytopenic effects of mercaptopurine may be increased with concurrent or recent therapy if these medications cause the same effects; dosage adjustment of mercaptopurine, if necessary, should be based on blood counts)

» Bone marrow depressants, other (See *Appendix II*) or
   Radiation therapy
   (additive bone marrow depression may occur; dosage reduction may be required when two or more bone marrow depressants, including radiation, are used concurrently or consecutively)

» Hepatotoxic medications, other (See *Appendix II* )
   (concurrent use may increase the risk of hepatotoxicity and should be avoided)

» Immunosuppressants, other, such as:
   Azathioprine
   Chlorambucil
   Corticosteroids, glucocorticoid
   Corticotropin (ACTH)
   Cyclophosphamide
   Cyclosporine
   Muromonab-CD3
   (concurrent use with mercaptopurine may increase the risk of infection and development of neoplasms)

Vaccines, killed virus
   (because normal defense mechanisms may be suppressed by mercaptopurine therapy, the patient's antibody response to the vaccine may be decreased. The interval between discontinuation of medications that cause immunosuppression and restoration of the patient's ability to respond to the vaccine depends on the intensity and type of immunosuppression-causing medication used, the underlying disease, and other factors; estimates vary from 3 months to 1 year)

» Vaccines, live virus
   (because normal defense mechanisms may be suppressed by mercaptopurine therapy, concurrent use with a live virus vaccine may potentiate the replication of the vaccine virus, may increase the side/adverse effects of the vaccine virus, and/or may decrease the patient's antibody response to the vaccine; immunization of these patients should be undertaken only with extreme caution after careful review of the patient's hematologic status and only with the knowledge and consent of the physician managing the mercaptopurine therapy. The interval between discontinuation of medications that cause immunosuppression and restoration of the patient's ability to respond to the vaccine depends on the intensity and type of immunosuppression-causing medication used, the underlying disease, and other factors; estimates vary from 3 months to 1 year. Patients with leukemia in remission should not receive live virus vaccine until at least 3 months after their last chemotherapy. Immunization with oral poliovirus vaccine should also be postponed in persons in close contact with the patient, especially family members)

**Laboratory value alterations**

The following have been selected on the basis of their potential clinical significance (possible effect in parentheses where appropriate)—not necessarily inclusive (» = major clinical significance):

With diagnostic test results
   Glucose and
   Uric acid
      (serum concentrations may be falsely increased when the sequential multiple analyzer [SMA] is used)

With physiology/laboratory test values
   Uric acid
      (concentrations in blood and urine may be increased)

**Medical considerations/Contraindications**

The medical considerations/contraindications included here have been selected on the basis of their potential clinical significance (reasons given in parentheses where appropriate)—not necessarily inclusive (» = major clinical significance).

***Risk-benefit should be considered when the following medical problems exist:***

» Bone marrow depression
» Chickenpox, existing or recent (including recent exposure) or
» Herpes zoster
      (risk of severe generalized disease)

   Gout, history of or
   Urate renal stones, history of
      (risk of hyperuricemia)

» Hepatic function impairment
      (lower dosage recommended)

» Infection

» Renal function impairment
      (lower dosage recommended)

   Sensitivity to mercaptopurine

» Caution should be used also in patients who have had previous cytotoxic drug therapy and radiation therapy.

**Patient monitoring**

The following are especially important in patient monitoring (other tests may be warranted in some patients, depending on condition; » = major clinical significance):

» Alanine aminotransferase (ALT [SGPT]) values, serum and
» Aspartate aminotransferase (AST [SGOT]) values, serum and
» Bilirubin values, serum and
» Lactate dehydrogenase (LDH) values, serum
      (recommended prior to initiation of therapy and at periodic intervals during therapy; frequency varies according to clinical state, agent, dose, and other agents being used concurrently)

   Blood urea nitrogen (BUN) concentrations and
   Creatinine concentrations, serum
      (recommended prior to initiation of therapy and at periodic intervals during therapy; frequency varies according to clinical state, agent, dose, and other agents being used concurrently)

» Hematocrit or hemoglobin and
» Leukocyte count, total and, if appropriate, differential and
» Platelet count
      (determinations recommended prior to initiation of therapy and at periodic intervals during therapy; frequency varies according to clinical state, agent, dose, and other agents being used concurrently)

   Uric acid concentrations, serum
      (recommended prior to initiation of therapy and at periodic intervals during therapy; frequency varies according to clinical state, agent, dose, and other agents being used concurrently)

Note: In patients with acute leukemia and high total leukocyte counts, a rapid fall in leukocyte count may occur with mercaptopurine therapy. Daily blood counts are recommended in these patients.

# Side/Adverse Effects

Note: Many "side effects" of antineoplastic therapy are unavoidable and represent the medication's pharmacologic action. Some of these (for example, leukopenia and thrombocytopenia) are actually used as parameters to aid in individual dosage titration.

The following side/adverse effects have been selected on the basis of their potential clinical significance (possible signs and symptoms in parentheses where appropriate)—not necessarily inclusive:

## Those indicating need for medical attention
Incidence more frequent
*Anemia* (unusual tiredness or weakness); *hepatotoxicity or biliary stasis* (yellow eyes or skin); *immunosuppression, leukopenia, or infection* (usually asymptomatic; less frequently, fever or chills; cough or hoarseness; lower back or side pain; painful or difficult urination); *thrombocytopenia* (usually asymptomatic; less frequently, unusual bleeding or bruising; black, tarry stools; blood in urine or stools; pinpoint red spots on skin)

Note: *Anemia* occurs with high doses.

*Leukopenia* and *thrombocytopenia* (usually mild) may begin 5 to 6 days after initiation of therapy and persist about 7 days after withdrawal.

Incidence less frequent
*Hyperuricemia or uric acid nephropathy* (joint pain; lower back or side pain; swelling of feet or lower legs); *loss of appetite or nausea and vomiting*

Note: *Hyperuricemia* and *uric acid nephropathy* occur most commonly during initial treatment of patients with leukemia or lymphoma, as a result of rapid cell breakdown which leads to elevated serum uric acid concentrations.

Crystals of mercaptopurine have been found in urine of children receiving high dosage (1000 mg per square meter of body surface daily).

*Loss of appetite* or *nausea and vomiting* may be symptoms of overdosage.

Incidence rare
*Gastrointestinal ulceration* (black, tarry stools; stomach pain); *stomatitis* (sores in mouth and on lips)

Note: *Stomatitis* is common with large doses.

## Those indicating need for medical attention only if they continue or are bothersome
Incidence less frequent
*Darkening of skin; diarrhea; headache; skin rash and itching; weakness*

## Those indicating need for medical attention if they occur after medication is discontinued
*Bone marrow depression* (black, tarry stools; blood in urine or stools; cough or hoarseness; fever or chills; lower back or side pain; painful or difficult urination; pinpoint red spots on skin; unusual bleeding or bruising); *hepatotoxicity* (yellow eyes or skin)

# Patient Consultation

As an aid to patient consultation, refer to *Advice for the Patient, Mercaptopurine (Systemic)*.

In providing consultation, consider emphasizing the following selected information (» = major clinical significance):

## Before using this medication
» Conditions affecting use, especially:
   Sensitivity to mercaptopurine
   Pregnancy—Use not recommended because of mutagenic, teratogenic, and carcinogenic potential; advisability of using contraception; telling physician immediately if pregnancy is suspected
   Breast-feeding—Not recommended because of risk of serious side effects
   Other medications, especially allopurinol, other bone marrow depressants, other hepatotoxic medications, other immunosuppressants, probenecid, or sulfinpyrazone
   Other medical problems, especially chickenpox, herpes zoster, hepatic function impairment, infection, or renal function impairment

## Proper use of this medication
» Importance of not taking more or less medication than the amount prescribed
   Caution in taking combination therapy; taking each medication at the right time

Importance of ample fluid intake and subsequent increase in urine output to aid in excretion of uric acid
Checking with physician if vomiting occurs shortly after dose is taken
» Proper dosing
   Missed dose: Not taking at all; not doubling doses
» Proper storage

## Precautions while using this medication
» Importance of close monitoring by the physician
» Possibility of increased toxicity if alcohol is ingested
» Avoiding immunizations unless approved by physician; other persons in patient's household should avoid immunizations with oral poliovirus vaccine; avoiding persons who have taken oral poliovirus vaccine or wearing a protective mask that covers nose and mouth
*Caution if bone marrow depression occurs:*
» Avoiding exposure to persons with bacterial infections, especially during periods of low blood counts; checking with physician immediately if fever or chills, cough or hoarseness, lower back or side pain, or painful or difficult urination occur
» Checking with physician immediately if unusual bleeding or bruising; black, tarry stools; blood in urine or stools; or pinpoint red spots on skin occur
   Caution in use of regular toothbrush, dental floss, or toothpick; physician, dentist, or nurse may suggest alternatives; checking with physician before having dental work done
   Not touching eyes or inside of nose unless hands washed immediately before
   Using caution to avoid accidental cuts with use of sharp objects such as safety razor or fingernail or toenail cutters
   Avoiding contact sports or other situations where bruising or injury could occur

   Caution if any laboratory tests required; possible interference with serum glucose and uric acid values measured by sequential multiple analyzer (SMA)

## Side/adverse effects
   Importance of discussing possible effects, including cancer, with physician
   Signs of potential side effects, especially anemia, hepatotoxicity, biliary stasis, immunosuppression, leukopenia, infection, thrombocytopenia, hyperuricemia, uric acid nephropathy, loss of appetite, nausea and vomiting, gastrointestinal ulceration, and stomatitis
   Physician or nurse can help in dealing with side effects

# General Dosing Information

Patients receiving mercaptopurine should be under supervision of a physician experienced in immunosuppressive and antimetabolite chemotherapy.

A variety of dosage schedules and regimens of mercaptopurine, alone or in combination with other antitumor agents, are used. The prescriber may consult the medical literature as well as the manufacturer's literature in choosing a specific dosage.

Dosage must be adjusted to meet the individual requirements of each patient, based on clinical response and appearance or severity of toxicity.

Development of uric acid nephropathy in patients with leukemia or lymphoma may be prevented by adequate oral hydration. Alkalinization of urine may be necessary if serum uric acid concentrations are elevated. Allopurinol should be administered with caution and only if uric acid concentrations are unacceptably high.

It is recommended that mercaptopurine dosage be reduced to one-third to one-fourth of the usual dosage in patients receiving 300 to 600 mg of allopurinol a day concurrently to reduce or prevent hyperuricemia or to slow the metabolism of mercaptopurine.

Because the actions of mercaptopurine may be delayed, it is recommended that mercaptopurine therapy be discontinued promptly at the first sign of marked leukopenia (particularly granulocytopenia) or thrombocytopenia, hemorrhage or bleeding tendencies, or jaundice. Therapy may be resumed at one-half the previous dosage when the leukocyte count remains constant for 2 or 3 days, or rises.

In acute leukemia, mercaptopurine may be administered despite the presence of thrombocytopenia and bleeding; stoppage of bleeding and increase in platelet count have occurred during treatment in some cases and platelet transfusions may be useful in others.

Special precautions are recommended in patients who develop thrombocytopenia as a result of administration of mercaptopurine. These may include extreme care in performing invasive procedures; regular inspection of intravenous sites, skin (including perirectal area), and mucous membrane surfaces for signs of bleeding or bruising; limiting frequency of venipuncture and avoiding intramuscular injections; testing urine, emesis, stool, and secretions for occult blood; care in use of regular toothbrushes, dental floss, toothpicks, safety razors, and fingernail and toenail cutters; avoiding constipation; and using caution to prevent falls and other injuries. Such patients should avoid alcohol and aspirin intake because of the risk of gastrointestinal bleeding. Platelet transfusions may be required.

Patients who develop leukopenia should be observed carefully for signs of infection. Antibiotic support may be required. In neutropenic patients who develop fever, broad-spectrum antibiotic coverage should be initiated empirically, pending bacterial cultures and appropriate diagnostic tests.

**Combination chemotherapy**

Mercaptopurine may be used in combination with other agents in various regimens. As a result, incidence and/or severity of side effects may be altered and different dosages (usually reduced) may be used. For example, mercaptopurine is part of the following chemotherapeutic combinations (some commonly used acronyms are in parentheses):
—daunorubicin, cytarabine, prednisolone, and mercaptopurine (Ara-C + DNR + PRED + MP).
—methotrexate and mercaptopurine (MTX + MP).
—methotrexate, mercaptopurine, and cyclophosphamide (MTX + MP + CTX).

For specific dosages and schedules, consult the literature. For information regarding each agent, consult the individual monographs.

## Oral Dosage Forms

Note: Bracketed uses in the *Dosage Forms* section refer to categories of use and/or indications that are not included in U.S. product labeling.

### MERCAPTOPURINE TABLETS USP

**Usual adult dose**

Leukemia, acute lymphocytic or
Leukemia, acute myelocytic or
Leukemia, acute myelomonocytic—
    Initial: Oral, 2.5 mg per kg of body weight or 80 to 100 mg per square meter of body surface (to the nearest 25 mg) a day in single or

divided doses. If there is no clinical improvement and no leukocyte depression after four weeks at this dosage, an increase in dosage to 5 mg per kg of body weight a day may be attempted.
    Maintenance: Oral, 1.5 to 2.5 mg per kg of body weight or 50 to 100 mg per square meter of body surface a day.
[Inflammatory bowel disease][1]—
    Oral, 1.5 mg per kg of body weight per day, the dosage being adjusted as necessary. If there is no clinical improvement and no leukocyte depression after two to three months at this dosage, a gradual increase in dosage to 2.5 mg per kg of body weight per day may be attempted.

**Usual pediatric dose**

Leukemia, acute lymphocytic or
Leukemia, acute myelocytic or
Leukemia, acute myelomonocytic—
    Oral, 2.5 mg per kg of body weight or 75 mg per square meter of body surface (to the nearest 25 mg) a day in single or divided doses.

**Strength(s) usually available**

U.S.—
    50 mg (Rx) [*Purinethol* (scored; lactose)].
Canada—
    50 mg (Rx) [*Purinethol* (scored)].

**Packaging and storage**

Store below 40 °C (104 °F), preferably between 15 and 30 °C (59 and 86 °F), unless otherwise specified by manufacturer. Store in a well-closed container.

---

[1]Not included in Canadian product labeling.

---

Revised: 8/90
Interim revision: 07/29/93; 12/10/93; 06/21/94

---

# MESALAMINE   Oral-Local

INN: Mesalazine.
BAN: Mesalazine.
VA CLASSIFICATION (Primary): GA900
Other commonly used names are 5-aminosalicylic acid and 5-ASA.
Note: For a listing of dosage forms and brand names by country availability, see *Dosage Forms* section(s). For a listing of brand names for the articles in this monograph, refer to the General Index.

## Category

Bowel disease (inflammatory) suppressant.

## Indications

Note: Bracketed information in the *Indications* section refers to uses that are not included in U.S. product labeling.

**Accepted**

Bowel disease, inflammatory (prophylaxis and treatment)—Mesalamine is indicated to treat and to maintain remission of mild to moderate ulcerative colitis or [Crohn's disease].

## Pharmacology/Pharmacokinetics

**Physicochemical characteristics**
Molecular weight—153.14.

**Mechanism of action/Effect**
Bowel disease (inflammatory) suppressant—
    Uncertain. Mucosal production of arachidonic acid metabolites, both through the cyclooxygenase and lipoxygenase pathways, is increased in patients with inflammatory bowel disease. Mesalamine appears to diminish inflammation by inhibiting cyclooxygenase and lipoxygenase, thereby decreasing the production of prostaglandins, and leukotrienes and hydroxyeicosatetraenoic acids (HETEs), respectively.
    It is also believed that mesalamine acts as a scavenger of oxygen-derived free radicals, which are produced in greater numbers in patients with inflammatory bowel disease.

**Absorption**
20 to 30% absorbed following oral administration. The site of mesalamine release and absorption within the gastrointestinal tract varies among the different formulations.
*Asacol*—Coated with an acrylic-based resin, Eudragit S, which dissolves at pH 7 or greater, releasing mesalamine into the distal ileum and the colon.
*Mesasal* and *Salofalk*—Coated with an acrylic-based resin, Eudragit L, which dissolves at pH 6 or greater, releasing mesalamine into the distal ileum and the colon.
*Pentasa*—Microgranules of mesalamine individually coated with ethylcellulose, which allows continuous release of mesalamine into the small (jejunum and ileum) and large (colon) bowel, independent of luminal pH.

**Biotransformation**
Absorbed mesalamine is rapidly acetylated to *N*-acetyl-5-aminosalicylic acid (Ac-5-ASA) in the intestinal mucosal wall and the liver.

**Half-life**
Elimination—
    Asacol:
        Mesalamine—3 hours.
        Ac-5-ASA—10 hours.
    Pentasa:
        Because of the continuous release and absorption of mesalamine throughout the gastrointestinal tract, the true elimination half-life cannot be determined following oral administration.
    Salofalk:
        Ac-5-ASA—5 to 10 hours.

**Time to peak concentration**
*Asacol*—4 to 12 hours.
*Mesasal*—6.5 to 7 hours.
*Pentasa*—3 hours.

**Peak serum concentration**
Mesasal—
    Mesalamine: 1.2 mcg per mL following a single 500-mg oral dose.
    Ac-5-ASA: 1.9 mcg per mL following a single 500-mg oral dose.

Pentasa—
    Mesalamine: 1 mcg per mL following a single 1-gram oral dose.
    Ac-5-ASA: 1.8 mcg per mL following a single 1-gram oral dose.

### Elimination
Fecal—
    *Asacol:* Approximately 80% of an administered dose is recovered in
        the feces.
    *Pentasa:* Approximately 13% of an administered dose is recovered in
        the feces.
    *Salofalk:* Partially recovered unchanged in the feces.
Renal—
    Excreted in the urine as the Ac-5-ASA metabolite.

## Precautions to Consider

### Cross-sensitivity and/or related problems
Patients sensitive to olsalazine, sulfasalazine, or salicylates may be sensitive to mesalamine also.

### Carcinogenicity
Long-term studies in animals have not been performed to evaluate the
carcinogenic potential of mesalamine.

### Mutagenicity
No evidence of mutagenicity was observed in an *in vitro* Ames test or in
an *in vivo* mouse micronucleus test.

### Pregnancy/Reproduction
Fertility—Oligospermia and infertility in men, which have been reported
    in association with sulfasalazine, have not been seen with mesalamine.
Mesalamine was found to have no effect on the fertility and reproductive
    performance of male and female rats when given orally at a dose
    corresponding to 7 times the maximum human dose.
Pregnancy—Mesalamine crosses the placenta. Adequate and well-con-
    trolled studies have not been done in humans.
Studies in pregnant rats and rabbits given doses of 1000 and 800 mg per
    kg of body weight (mg/kg) per day, respectively, have not shown that
    mesalamine causes adverse effects in the fetus.
FDA Pregnancy Category B.

### Breast-feeding
Mesalamine and its metabolite, *N*-acetyl-5-aminosalicylic acid, are distributed into breast milk. However, problems in humans have not been
documented.

### Pediatrics
Appropriate studies on the relationship of age to the effects of mesalamine
have not been performed in the pediatric population. Safety and efficacy have not been established.

### Geriatrics
No information is available on the relationship of age to the effects of
mesalamine in geriatric patients. However, elderly patients are more
likely to have age-related renal function impairment, which may require caution in patients receiving mesalamine.

### Drug interactions and/or related problems
The following drug interactions and/or related problems have been se-
    lected on the basis of their potential clinical significance (possible
    mechanism in parentheses where appropriate)—not necessarily inclu-
    sive (» = major clinical significance):

Note: Combinations containing any of the following medications, de-
    pending on the amount present, may also interact with this
    medication.

Lactulose
    (acidification of the colonic lumen by lactulose may impair release
    of mesalamine from delayed- or extended-release formulations)

Omeprazole
    (omeprazole may increase gastrointestinal pH; concurrent use may
    result in an increase in the absorption of mesalamine)

### Laboratory value alterations
The following have been selected on the basis of their potential clinical
    significance (possible effect in parentheses where appropriate)—not
    necessarily inclusive (» = major clinical significance):

With physiology/laboratory test values
Alanine aminotransferase (ALT [SGPT]) and
Alkaline phosphatase and
Aspartate aminotransferase (AST [SGOT])
    (values may be increased, but return to normal with either contin-
    uation or discontinuation of therapy)
Bilirubin, serum
    (concentration may be increased, but returns to normal with either
    continuation or discontinuation of therapy)

### Medical considerations/Contraindications
The medical considerations/contraindications included here have been se-
    lected on the basis of their potential clinical significance (reasons given
    in parentheses where appropriate)—not necessarily inclusive (» =
    major clinical significance).

*Risk-benefit should be considered when the following medical problems
    exist:*
Renal function impairment
    (increased risk of interstitial nephritis and nephrotic syndrome)
Sensitivity to mesalamine, olsalazine, sulfasalazine, or salicylates
Stenosis, pyloric
    (prolonged gastric retention may delay release of mesalamine)

### Patient monitoring
The following may be especially important in patient monitoring (other
    tests may be warranted in some patients, depending on condition;
    » = major clinical significance):
Blood urea nitrogen (BUN) and
Creatinine, serum and
Urinalysis
    (determinations recommended prior to, and periodically during,
    therapy)

## Side/Adverse Effects
The following side/adverse effects have been selected on the basis of their
    potential clinical significance (possible signs and symptoms in paren-
    theses where appropriate)—not necessarily inclusive:

### Those indicating need for medical attention
Incidence less frequent
    *Acute intolerance syndrome* (abdominal or stomach cramps or pain,
        severe; bloody diarrhea; fever; headache, severe; skin rash and itching)
    Note: Prompt withdrawal of mesalamine is recommended at the first
        signs of *acute intolerance syndrome.*

Incidence rare
    *Hepatitis* (yellow eyes or skin); *pancreatitis* (back or stomach pain,
        severe; fast heartbeat; fever; nausea or vomiting; swelling of the stom-
        ach); *pericarditis* (anxiety; blue or pale skin; chest pain, possibly mov-
        ing to the left arm, neck, or shoulder; chills; shortness of breath;
        unusual tiredness or weakness)

### Those indicating need for medical attention only if they continue
or are bothersome
Incidence more frequent
    *Abdominal or stomach cramps or pain, mild; diarrhea, mild; dizzi-
    ness; headache, mild; nausea or vomiting; rhinitis* (runny or stuffy
    nose or sneezing); *unusual tiredness or weakness*

Incidence less frequent or rare
    *Acne; alopecia* (loss of hair); *anorexia* (loss of appetite); *back or joint
    pain; dyspepsia* (indigestion); *gas or flatulence*

## Overdose
For specific information on the agents used in the management of
    mesalamine overdose, see:
    • *Charcoal, Activated (Oral-Local)* monograph;
    • *Ipecac (Oral-Local)* monograph; and/or
    • *Salicylates (Systemic)* monograph.

For more information on the management of overdose or unintentional
    ingestion, **contact a Poison Control Center** (see *Poison Control Cen-
    ter Listing*).

### Clinical effects of overdose
The following effects have been selected on the basis of their potential
    clinical significance (possible signs and symptoms in parentheses
    where appropriate)—not necessarily inclusive:

Acute effects
    *Confusion; diarrhea, severe or continuing; dizziness or lighthead-
    edness; drowsiness, severe; fast or deep breathing; headache, severe
    or continuing; hearing loss or ringing or buzzing in ears, continuing;
    nausea or vomiting, continuing*

### Treatment of overdose
There has been no clinical experience with mesalamine overdosage. How-
    ever, because mesalamine is an aminosalicylate, the symptoms of
    overdose may mimic the symptoms of salicylate overdose; therefore,
    measures used to treat salicylate overdose may be applied to mesalam-
    ine overdose.

To decrease absorption—The stomach may be emptied by induction of
    emesis with ipecac syrup (with care being taken to guard against as-
    piration) or by gastric lavage. Activated charcoal may also be
    administered.

Supportive care—Fluid and electrolyte imbalance should be corrected by the administration of appropriate intravenous therapy. Vital functions should be monitored and supported. Patients in whom intentional overdose is confirmed or suspected should be referred for psychiatric consultation.

## Patient Consultation

As an aid to patient consultation, refer to *Advice for the Patient, Mesalamine (Oral)*.

In providing consultation, consider emphasizing the following selected information (» = major clinical significance):

**Before using this medication**
»   Conditions affecting use, especially:
        Sensitivity to mesalamine, olsalazine, sulfasalazine, or salicylates
        Pregnancy—Crosses the placenta
        Breast-feeding—Distributed into breast milk

**Proper use of this medication**
        Swallowing capsules or tablets whole without breaking, crushing, or chewing
        Taking medicine before meals and at bedtime with a full glass (8 ounces) of water
»   Compliance with full course of therapy
»   Not switching brands without consulting physician
»   Proper dosing
        Missed dose: Taking as soon as possible; not taking if almost time for next dose; not doubling doses
»   Proper storage

**Precautions while using this medication**
        Regular visits to physician to check progress
        Patient may notice small beads or empty tablet in stool left over after medication is absorbed

**Side/adverse effects**
        Signs of potential side effects, especially acute intolerance syndrome, hepatitis, pancreatitis, and pericarditis

## General Dosing Information

Mesalamine should be taken before meals and at bedtime with a full glass (8 ounces) of water.

## Oral Dosage Forms

Note: Bracketed uses in the *Dosage Forms* section refer to categories of use and/or indications that are not included in U.S. product labeling.

### MESALAMINE EXTENDED-RELEASE CAPSULES

**Usual adult dose**
Ulcerative colitis; or
[Crohn's disease]—
        1 gram four times a day for up to eight weeks.

**Usual pediatric dose**
Safety and efficacy have not been established.

**Usual geriatric dose**
See *Usual adult dose*.

**Strength(s) usually available**
U.S.—
    250 mg (Rx) [*Pentasa* (acetylated monoglyceride; castor oil; colloidal silicon dioxide; ethylcellulose; hydroxypropyl methylcellulose; starch; stearic acid; sugar; talc; white wax)].
Canada—
    250 mg (Rx) [*Pentasa*].

**Packaging and storage**
Store at controlled room temperature between 15 and 30 °C (59 and 86 °F).

**Auxiliary labeling**
• Take with a full glass (8 ounces) of water.

### MESALAMINE DELAYED-RELEASE TABLETS

Note: There are differences in the rate and site of absorption among the various brands of mesalamine delayed-release tablets; therefore, these preparations are not bioequivalent, and one brand should not be substituted for another unless otherwise directed by the patient's physician.

**Usual adult dose**
Ulcerative colitis; or
[Crohn's disease]—
    *Asacol*: 800 mg three times a day for six weeks.
    *Mesasal*: 1.5 to 3 grams daily in divided doses.
    *Salofalk*: 1 gram three or four times a day.

**Usual pediatric dose**
Safety and efficacy have not been established.

**Usual geriatric dose**
See *Usual adult dose*.

**Strength(s) usually available**
U.S.—
    400 mg (Rx) [*Asacol* (Eudragit S)].
Canada—
    250 mg (Rx) [*Salofalk* (Eudragit L)].
    400 mg (Rx) [*Asacol* (Eudragit S)].
    500 mg (Rx) [*Mesasal* (Eudragit L); *Salofalk* (Eudragit L)].

**Packaging and storage**
Store at controlled room temperature between 15 and 30 °C (59 and 86 °F).

**Auxiliary labeling**
• Take with a full glass (8 ounces) of water.

### MESALAMINE EXTENDED-RELEASE TABLETS

**Usual adult dose**
See *Mesalamine Extended-release Capsules*.

**Usual pediatric dose**
Safety and efficacy have not been established.

**Usual geriatric dose**
See *Mesalamine Extended-release Capsules*.

**Strength(s) usually available**
U.S.—
    Not commercially available.
Canada—
    250 mg (Rx) [*Pentasa*].
    500 mg (Rx) [*Pentasa*].

**Packaging and storage**
Store at controlled room temperature between 15 and 30 °C (59 and 86 °F).

**Auxiliary labeling**
• Take with a full glass (8 ounces) of water.

## Selected Bibliography

Thomson ABR. Review article: new developments in the use of 5-aminosalicylic acid in patients with inflammatory bowel disease. Aliment Pharmacol Ther 1991; 5: 449-70.

Developed: 03/17/95

# MESALAMINE   Rectal-Local

INN: Mesalazine

BAN: Mesalazine

VA CLASSIFICATION (Primary): RS100

Other commonly used names are 5-aminosalicylic acid and 5-ASA.

Note: For a listing of dosage forms and brand names by country availability, see *Dosage Forms* section(s). For a listing of brand names for the articles in this monograph, refer to the General Index.

## Category

Bowel disease (inflammatory) suppressant.

## Indications

Note: Bracketed information in the *Indications* section refers to uses that are not included in U.S. product labeling.

### Accepted

Bowel disease, inflammatory (treatment)—Mesalamine is indicated for the treatment of mild to moderate distal ulcerative colitis, proctosigmoiditis, and proctitis.

[Bowel disease, inflammatory (prophylaxis)]—Mesalamine rectal suspension is indicated to help maintain remission of distal ulcerative colitis.

## Pharmacology/Pharmacokinetics

### Physicochemical characteristics

Molecular weight—153.14.

pKa—5.8.

### Mechanism of action/Effect

Bowel disease (inflammatory) suppressant—

Uncertain. Mucosal production of arachidonic acid metabolites, both through the cyclooxygenase and lipoxygenase pathways, is increased in patients with inflammatory bowel disease. Mesalamine appears to diminish inflammation by inhibiting cyclooxygenase and lipoxygenase, thereby decreasing the production of prostaglandins, and leukotrienes and hydroxyeicosatetraenoic acids (HETEs), respectively.

It is also believed that mesalamine acts as a scavenger of oxygen-derived free radicals, which are produced in greater numbers in patients with inflammatory bowel disease.

### Absorption

Ten to 35% absorbed from the colon; extent of absorption is determined by the length of time the drug is retained in the colon.

### Distribution

The distribution of absorbed mesalamine is not known.

### Biotransformation

Absorbed mesalamine is acetylated to *N*-acetyl-5-ASA (Ac-5-ASA); however, it is not known whether acetylation takes place at colonic or systemic sites. Ac-5-ASA is further acetylated (deactivated) in at least 2 sites, the colonic epithelium and the liver.

### Half-life

Elimination—

Mesalamine: 0.5 to 1.5 hours.

Ac-5-ASA: 5 to 10 hours.

### Elimination

Unabsorbed—Fecal.

Absorbed—Renal; 10 to 30% of administered dose is excreted in the urine within 24 hours as the Ac-5-ASA metabolite.

## Precautions to Consider

### Cross-sensitivity and/or related problems

Patients sensitive to olsalazine, sulfasalazine, or salicylates may be sensitive to mesalamine also.

### Carcinogenicity/Tumorigenicity

In a 2-year study in rats given mesalamine orally in doses up to 320 mg per kg of body weight (mg/kg) per day, no increase in the incidence of neoplastic lesions was found.

### Mutagenicity

No evidence of mutagenicity was observed in an Ames mutagen test using *Salmonella typhimurium*. In addition, there was neither evidence of reverse mutations in an assay using an *Escherichia coli* strain, nor evidence of adverse chromosomal effects in an *in vivo* mouse micro-

nucleus assay in doses of 600 mg/kg or in an *in vivo* sister chromatid exchange test in doses up to 610 mg/kg.

### Pregnancy/Reproduction

Fertility—Oligospermia and infertility in men, which have been reported in association with sulfasalazine, have not been seen with mesalamine. Mesalamine was found to have no effect on the fertility of rats when given orally in doses up to 320 mg/kg per day.

Pregnancy—Adequate and well-controlled studies in humans have not been done.

Studies in rats and rabbits at oral doses 5 to 8 times the maximum recommended human dose, respectively, have not shown that mesalamine causes adverse effects in the embryo or the fetus.

FDA Pregnancy Category B.

### Breast-feeding

It is not known whether rectally administered mesalamine or its metabolites are distributed into breast milk. Orally administered mesalamine and its metabolite, *N*-acetyl-5-aminosalicylic acid, are distributed into breast milk.

### Pediatrics

Appropriate studies on the relationship of age to the effects of mesalamine have not been performed in the pediatric population. Safety and efficacy have not been established.

### Geriatrics

No information is available on the relationship of age to the effects of mesalamine in geriatric patients. However, elderly patients are more likely to have age-related renal function impairment, which may require caution in patients receiving mesalamine.

### Medical considerations/Contraindications

The medical considerations/contraindications included here have been selected on the basis of their potential clinical significance (reasons given in parentheses where appropriate)—not necessarily inclusive ( » = major clinical significance).

**Risk-benefit should be considered when the following medical problems exist:**

Renal function impairment

(although absorption of mesalamine is limited, the possibility of increased risk of renal damage should be considered)

Sensitivity to mesalamine, olsalazine, sulfasalazine, or salicylates

### Patient monitoring

The following may be especially important in patient monitoring (other tests may be warranted in some patients, depending on condition; » = major clinical significance):

Blood urea nitrogen (BUN) and

Creatinine, serum and

Urinalysis

(determinations may be required in patients with renal function impairment and in patients concurrently using oral medications, such as sulfasalazine, that liberate mesalamine)

## Side/Adverse Effects

The following side/adverse effects have been selected on the basis of their potential clinical significance (possible signs and symptoms in parentheses where appropriate)—not necessarily inclusive:

### Those indicating need for medical attention

Incidence rare

*Acute intolerance syndrome* (abdominal or stomach cramps or pain, severe; bloody diarrhea; fever; headache, severe; skin rash); *anal irritation; hepatitis* (yellow eyes or skin); *pancreatitis* (back or stomach pain, severe; fast heartbeat; fever; nausea or vomiting; swelling of the stomach); *pericarditis* (anxiety; blue or pale skin; chest pain, possibly moving to the left arm, neck, or shoulder; chills; shortness of breath; unusual tiredness or weakness)

Note: Prompt withdrawal of mesalamine is recommended at the first signs of the *acute intolerance syndrome*, particularly in patients with a known allergy to sulfasalazine.

### Those indicating need for medical attention only if they continue or are bothersome

Incidence more frequent

*Abdominal or stomach cramps or pain, mild; gas or flatulence; headache, mild; nausea*

Incidence less frequent or rare

*Alopecia* (loss of hair)

## Patient Consultation

As an aid to patient consultation, refer to *Advice for the Patient, Mesalamine (Rectal)*.

In providing consultation, consider emphasizing the following selected information (» = major clinical significance):

**Before using this medication**
» Conditions affecting use, especially:
   Sensitivity to mesalamine, olsalazine, sulfasalazine, or salicylates

**Proper use of this medication**
   Carefully reading and following patient directions for enema or suppository dosage forms
   Emptying bowel immediately prior to enema or suppository, for best results
» Compliance with full course of therapy
» Proper dosing
   Missed dose:
      Mesalamine enema—Using as soon as possible if remembered same night; using next dose at regularly scheduled time; not doubling doses
      Mesalamine suppository—Using as soon as possible unless almost time for next dose; not doubling doses
» Proper storage

**Precautions while using this medication**
   Regular visits to physician to check progress
   Checking with physician if signs of rectal irritation occur
   Enema may stain clothing, fabrics, painted surfaces, marble, granite, vinyl, or other surfaces with which it comes into contact

**Side/adverse effects**
   Signs of potential side effects, especially acute intolerance syndrome, anal irritation, hepatitis, pancreatitis, and pericarditis

## General Dosing Information

The mesalamine enema should be used at bedtime with the objective of retaining the rectal suspension for at least 8 hours. The mesalamine suppository should be used two to three times a day with the objective of retaining it for at least 3 hours.

For best results, bowel should be emptied immediately prior to the rectal administration of mesalamine.

Response to therapy with mesalamine may occur within 3 to 21 days; however, the usual course of therapy is from 3 to 6 weeks depending on symptoms and sigmoidoscopic examinations.

After remission, some patients may be maintained on mesalamine enema on a less than nightly schedule; however, the possibility of relapse increases as the frequency of mesalamine enema administration is decreased.

Studies to date have not determined if mesalamine suppositories modify the relapse rate after remission; however, it is recommended that abrupt discontinuation be avoided.

## Rectal Dosage Forms

Note: Bracketed uses in the *Dosage Forms* section refer to categories of use and/or indications that are not included in U.S. product labeling.

### MESALAMINE RECTAL SUSPENSION

**Usual adult and adolescent dose**
Bowel disease, inflammatory (treatment)—
   Rectal, 4 grams as a retention enema each night for three to six weeks.

[Bowel disease, inflammatory (prophylaxis)]—
   Rectal, 2 grams as a retention enema each night. Alternatively, 4 grams every other, or every third night.

**Usual pediatric dose**
Safety and efficacy have not been established.

**Usual geriatric dose**
See *Usual adult and adolescent dose*.

**Strength(s) usually available**
U.S.—
   4 grams per 60-mL unit (Rx) [*Rowasa* (potassium metabisulfite; carbomer 943P; edetate disodium; potassium acetate; water; xanthan gum; sodium benzoate)].
Canada—
   2 grams per 60-mL unit (Rx) [*Salofalk* (potassium metabisulfite; sodium benzoate)].
   4 grams per 60-mL unit (Rx) [*Salofalk* (potassium metabisulfite; sodium benzoate)].

**Packaging and storage**
Store between 15 and 30 °C (59 and 86 °F), unless otherwise specified by manufacturer.

**Stability**
Mesalamine rectal suspension may darken with time. Slight darkening will not affect potency; however, enemas with a dark brown color should be discarded.

**Auxiliary labeling**
• For rectal use.
• Shake well.

## MESALAMINE SUPPOSITORIES

**Usual adult and adolescent dose**
Bowel disease, inflammatory (treatment)—
   Rectal, 500 mg two or three times a day for three to six weeks. For best results, suppositories should be retained for at least 3 hours.

**Usual pediatric dose**
Safety and efficacy have not been established.

**Usual geriatric dose**
See *Usual adult and adolescent dose*.

**Strength(s) usually available**
U.S.—
   500 mg (Rx) [*Rowasa* (hard fat)].
Canada—
   250 mg (Rx) [*Salofalk* (hard fat)].
   500 mg (Rx) [*Salofalk* (hard fat)].

**Packaging and storage**
Store between 19 and 26 °C (66 and 79 °F).

**Auxiliary labeling**
• For rectal use.

## Selected Bibliography

Biddle WL, Greenberger NJ, Swan JT, et al. 5-Aminosalicylic acid enemas: effective agent in maintaining remission in left-sided ulcerative colitis. Gastroenterology 1988; 94: 1075-9.
Guarino J, Chatzinoff M, Berk T, et al. 5-Aminosalicylic acid enemas in refractory distal ulcerative colitis: long-term results. Am J Gastroenterol 1987; 82: 732-7.

Revised: 01/30/96

---

# MESNA    Systemic

VA CLASSIFICATION (Primary): AD900
Note: For a listing of dosage forms and brand names by country availability, see *Dosage Forms* section(s). For a listing of brand names for the articles in this monograph, refer to the General Index.

## Category

Hemorrhagic cystitis prophylactic.

## Indications

Note: Bracketed information in the *Indications* section refers to uses that are not included in U.S. product labeling.

**Accepted**
Hemorrhagic cystitis, oxazaphosphorine-induced (prophylaxis)—Mesna is indicated to reduce the incidence of ifosfamide-induced or [cyclophosphamide-induced] hemorrhagic cystitis. Mesna is not effective in preventing hematuria due to other pathological conditions such as thrombocytopenia and does not affect other toxicities of oxazaphosphorines.

## Pharmacology/Pharmacokinetics

**Physicochemical characteristics**
Molecular weight—164.17.
Other characteristics—Mesna injection: pH is 6.5–8.5.

**Mechanism of action/Effect**

Mesna disulfide, which is physically inert, is reduced in the kidney (in the renal tubular epithelium) to mesna, which binds to and detoxifies urotoxic metabolites of oxazophosphorines (for ifosfamide, 4-hydroxyifosfamide and acrolein).

**Distribution**

Volume of distribution—0.652 liter per kg.

**Biotransformation**

Rapid, by oxidation to one metabolite, mesna disulfide (dimesna).

**Half-life**

Mesna—0.36 hours

Dimesna—1.17 hours

**Elimination**

Renal, rapid, by glomerular filtration; 32% as mesna and 33% as dimesna.

## Precautions to Consider

**Carcinogenicity**

Studies have not been done.

**Mutagenicity**

Mesna was not found to be mutagenic in the Ames *Salmonella typhimurium* test, mouse micronucleus assay, and frequency of sister chromatid exchange and chromosomal aberrations in PHA stimulated lymphocytes *in vitro* assays.

**Pregnancy/Reproduction**

Pregnancy—Studies in humans have not been done.

Studies in rats and rabbits at oral doses up to 1000 mg per kg of body weight (mg/kg) have not shown that mesna causes adverse effects on the fetus.

FDA Pregnancy Category B.

**Breast-feeding**

It is not known whether mesna is excreted in breast milk. However, problems in humans have not been documented.

**Pediatrics**

Appropriate studies on the relationship of age to the effects of mesna have not been performed in the pediatric population. However, no pediatrics-specific problems have been documented to date.

**Geriatrics**

No information is available on the relationship of age to the effects of mesna in geriatric patients.

**Laboratory value alterations**

The following have been selected on the basis of their potential clinical significance (possible effect in parentheses where appropriate)—not necessarily inclusive (» = major clinical significance):

With physiology/laboratory test values

Ketones, urinary

(false-positive results may be produced; in this test, a red-violet color develops, which returns to violet with the addition of glacial acetic acid)

**Medical considerations/Contraindications**

The medical considerations/contraindications included here have been selected on the basis of their potential clinical significance (reasons given in parentheses where appropriate)—not necessarily inclusive (» = major clinical significance).

*Risk-benefit should be considered when the following medical problem exists:*

Sensitivity to mesna

**Patient monitoring**

The following may be especially important in patient monitoring (other tests may be warranted in some patients, depending on condition; » = major clinical significance):

Examination of urine for microscopic hematuria

(recommended prior to administration of each dose of ifosfamide or cyclophosphamide and mesna)

## Side/Adverse Effects

The following side/adverse effects have been selected on the basis of their potential clinical significance (possible signs and symptoms in parentheses where appropriate)—not necessarily inclusive:

**Those indicating need for medical attention**

Incidence rare

*Allergic reaction* (skin rash or itching)

**Those indicating need for medical attention only if they continue or are bothersome**

Incidence less frequent

*Diarrhea; nausea or vomiting; unpleasant taste*

## Patient Consultation

As an aid to patient consultation, refer to *Advice for the Patient, Mesna (Systemic)*.

In providing consultation, consider emphasizing the following selected information (» = major clinical significance):

**Before using this medication**

» Conditions affecting use, especially:

Sensitivity to mesna

**Proper use of this medication**

» Proper dosing

**Side/adverse effects**

Signs of potential side effects, especially allergic reaction

## General Dosing Information

Patients receiving mesna should be under supervision of a physician experienced in cancer chemotherapy.

## Parenteral Dosage Forms

**MESNA INJECTION**

**Usual adult and adolescent dose**

Prophylaxis of ifosfamide-induced hemorrhagic cystitis—

Intravenous injection, rapid, in a dosage equal to 20% of the ifosfamide dosage (w/w) at the time of ifosfamide administration and four and eight hours after each dose of ifosfamide (i.e., the total daily dose of mesna is equal to 60% of the total daily dose of ifosfamide) each day that ifosfamide is administered. For example, patients receiving a daily ifosfamide dose of 1.2 grams per square meter of body surface should receive 240 mg of mesna per square meter of body surface at zero, four, and eight hours after administration of each dose of ifosfamide.

Note: If the dose of ifosfamide is adjusted, the dose of mesna should be adjusted accordingly.

**Usual pediatric dose**

Dosage has not been established.

**Strength(s) usually available**

U.S.—

100 mg per mL (Rx) [*MESNEX*].

Canada—

100 mg per mL (Rx) [*Uromitexan*].

**Packaging and storage**

Store below 40 °C (104 °F), preferably between 15 and 30 °C (59 and 86 °F), unless otherwise specified by manufacturer.

**Preparation of dosage form**

Mesna injection is prepared for intravenous administration by adding it to a sufficient quantity of 5% dextrose injection, 5% dextrose and sodium chloride injection, 0.9% sodium chloride injection, or lactated Ringer's injection to produce a solution containing 20 mg of mesna per mL.

**Stability**

Diluted solutions of mesna are chemically and physically stable for 24 hours at 25 °C (77 °F). However, it is recommended that diluted solutions be refrigerated and used within 6 hours. Because exposure to oxygen causes mesna to be oxidized to dimesna, any unused portion of an ampul should be discarded.

**Incompatibilities**

Mesna injection is incompatible with cisplatin injection.

## Selected Bibliography

Zalupski M, Baker LH. Ifosfamide. J Natl Cancer Inst 1988 Jun 15; 80 (8): 556-66.

Shaw IC, Graham MI. Mesna—A short review. Cancer Treat Rev 1987 Jun; 14 (2):67-86.

Burkert H. Clinical overview of mesna. Cancer Treat Rev 1983; 10 (Suppl A): 175-81.

Revised: 08/09/92

Interim revision: 07/06/94

**MESORIDAZINE**—See *Phenothiazines (Systemic)*

**MESTRANOL-CONTAINING COMBINATIONS—**
Norethindrone and Mestrandol (Systemic)—See *Estrogens and Progestins (Systemic)*

**METAPROTERENOL—**See *Bronchodilators, Adrenergic (Systemic)*

**METARAMINOL—**See *Sympathomimetic Agents—Cardiovascular Use (Parenteral-Systemic)*

**METAXALONE—**See *Skeletal Muscle Relaxants (Systemic)*

# METFORMIN Systemic

JAN: Metformin Hydrochloride
VA CLASSIFICATION (Primary): HS502
Note: For a listing of dosage forms and brand names by country availability, see *Dosage Forms* section(s). For a listing of brand names for the articles in this monograph, refer to the General Index.

## Category
Antihyperglycemic agent.

## Indications

### Accepted
Non–insulin-dependent diabetes mellitus (NIDDM) (treatment)—Metformin is indicated in NIDDM patients to control hyperglycemia that cannot be controlled by diet management, exercise, or weight reduction, or when insulin therapy is not required or feasible. It is used as monotherapy or as an adjunct to sulfonylureas when the sulfonylurea alone does not achieve adequate glycemic control. It can be tried if primary or secondary failure of sulfonylureas occurs. Caution and clinical judgment should be used when combining metformin with maximum doses of sulfonylureas for treating non-obese NIDDM patients who clearly are not responding to the sulfonylureas when insulin may be the preferred treatment.

## Pharmacology/Pharmacokinetics

### Physicochemical characteristics
Chemical group—Biguanide.
Molecular weight—165.63.
pKa—2.8 and 11.5.

### Mechanism of action/Effect
Metformin potentiates the effect of insulin by mechanisms not fully understood. Metformin does not stimulate pancreatic beta cells to increase secretion of insulin; insulin secretion must be present for metformin to work properly. It is postulated that metformin decreases hepatic glucose production and improves insulin sensitivity by increasing peripheral glucose uptake and utilization.
Specifically, it is thought that metformin may increase the number and/or affinity of insulin receptors on cell surface membranes, especially at peripheral receptor sites, and help to correct down regulation of the insulin receptor. This effect increases the sensitivity to insulin at receptor and postreceptor binding sites and increases glucose uptake peripherally. Insulin concentrations remain unchanged or are slightly reduced as glucose metabolism improves. At therapeutic doses, metformin does not cause hypoglycemia in diabetic or nondiabetic individuals. In addition, metformin's metabolic effects increase hepatic glycogen stores in diabetic patients (but not in nondiabetic patients), may decrease intestinal glucose absorption, and reduce fatty acid oxidation and acetyl coenzyme A formation. Glucose uptake or free fatty acid oxidation are effects considered to be caused by non–insulin-mediated mechanisms. Some studies have shown lipid-lowering effects in both diabetics and nondiabetics, while others have shown no clear evidence that metformin decreases lipid concentrations in all diabetics. These effects could manifest as weight reduction with nominal disturbance of the metabolic rate.

### Other actions/effects
Metformin interferes with the absorption of vitamin $B_{12}$ by competitive inhibition of calcium-dependent binding of the intrinsic factor-vitamin $B_{12}$ complex to its receptor; anemia in predisposed individuals may be possible.

### Absorption
Absorbed over 6 hours; bioavailability is 50 to 60% under fasting conditions. Food delays absorption (lowers peak concentration by 40%)

and decreases the extent absorbed (lowers area under the concentration-time curve [AUC] by 25%).

### Distribution
Apparent volume of distribution is $654 \pm 358$ L. Main sites of concentration without accumulation are the intestinal mucosa and the salivary glands; also, the erythrocyte mass may be a compartment of distribution.

### Protein binding
Negligible.

### Biotransformation
Metformin is not metabolized.

### Half-life
Plasma elimination—6.2 hours, mean, based on an initial elimination of 1.7 to 3 hours and terminal elimination of 9 to 17 hours.

### Time to peak concentration
$2.25 \pm 0.44$ hours.

### Peak serum concentration
At steady-state—Approximately 1 to 2 mcg/mL (6.04 to 12.08 mmol/L).

### Elimination
Renal—Up to 90% of a dose, eliminated unchanged. The renal clearance is 450 to 513 mL/min.
Feces—Up to 30% of a dose.
In dialysis—Hemodialysis with clearance of 170 mL per minute prevents accumulation of metformin.

## Precautions to Consider

### Carcinogenicity
A study in rats and in mice for 104 weeks and 91 weeks, respectively, at 3 times the recommended human daily dose showed no evidence of carcinogenicity.

### Tumorigenicity
A study in male rats showed no evidence of tumorigenicity; however, female rats given 3 times the recommended human daily dose on a mg/kg weight basis, or 900 mg a day, had an increased incidence of benign stromal uterine polyps.

### Mutagenicity
Metformin was not found to be mutagenic in the Ames test, gene mutation test (mouse lymphoma cells), chromosome aberration test (human lymphocytes), or *in vivo* micronuclei formation test (mouse bone marrow).

### Pregnancy/Reproduction
Fertility—Problems in humans have not been documented.
No evidence of impairment of fertility was found in male or female rats given twice the recommended human daily dose of metformin.

Pregnancy—Adequate and well-controlled studies in humans have not been done. Control of blood glucose during pregnancy with diet alone or a combination of diet and insulin is recommended, while use of all oral antidiabetic agents is discouraged. Use of insulin rather than metformin for the treatment of NIDDM and gestational diabetes mellitus (GDM) permits maintenance of blood glucose at concentrations as close to normal as possible. High blood glucose concentrations have been associated with a higher incidence of major congenital abnormalities early in pregnancy (5 to 8 weeks gestation) and high perinatal morbidity and mortality later in pregnancy. A study reported infant malformation rates of 35, 12.9 and 4.8% when initial hemoglobin $A_{1c}$ (an indicator of blood glucose control for the preceding 3 months) was 10% or more, 8 to 9.9%, and below 8%, respectively. The malformation rate in infants born to nondiabetic mothers is approximately 2%.
Teratological studies in albino rats found no abnormalities.
FDA Pregnancy Category B.

## Breast-feeding

Problems in humans have not been documented. Metformin is distributed into breast milk.

## Pediatrics

No information is available on the relationship of age to the effects of metformin in pediatric patients. Safety and efficacy have not been established.

## Adolescents

No information is available on the relationship of age to the effects of metformin in adolescent patients. Safety and efficacy have not been established.

## Geriatrics

Appropriate studies performed to date have not demonstrated geriatrics-specific problems that would limit the usefulness of metformin in the elderly. However, because of possible gastrointestinal intolerance, it is recommended that treatment be initiated with low doses that are adjusted gradually, according to renal clearance. Maximum doses should not be used. Elderly patients are more likely to have age-related renal function impairment or peripheral vascular disease, which may require adjustment of dosage or dosage interval, or discontinuation of treatment when appropriate.

## Drug interactions and/or related problems

The following drug interactions and/or related problems have been selected on the basis of their potential clinical significance (possible mechanism in parentheses where appropriate)—not necessarily inclusive (» = major clinical significance):

Note: Combinations containing any of the following medications, depending on the amount present, may also interact with this medication.

Administration of any medication that may affect metabolic or glycemic control of diabetes mellitus requires careful monitoring of blood glucose concentrations by the patient or health care professional. This is particularly important when any medication is added to or removed from an established treatment regimen. Subsequent adjustments in diet or in dose of antidiabetic agent or both may be necessary; these adjustments may differ depending on the severity of the diabetes.

» Alcohol, acute or chronic ingestion of
(excessive intake may elevate blood lactate concentrations or increase the risk of developing hypoglycemia, especially when alcohol is ingested without meals)

» Cimetidine or
» Other cationic medications excreted by renal tubular transport, such as:
   Amiloride
   Calcium channel blocking agents, especially nifedipine
   Digoxin
   Morphine
   Procainamide
   Quinidine
   Quinine
   Ranitidine
   Triamterene
   Trimethoprim
   Vancomycin
(cimetidine inhibits the renal tubular secretion of metformin, decreases renal clearance of metformin by 27% over 24 hours, and can significantly increase plasma concentrations of metformin by 60% for up to 6 hours when cimetidine and metformin are taken together; clinical significance is not known, but dosage reduction of metformin potentially may be needed)

(nifedipine increased absorption of metformin in a single-dose study, resulting in a 9% increase of area under the concentration-time curve [AUC] and a 20% increase in peak serum concentration with no change in half-life and urinary excretion; clinical significance is not known; it is not known whether similar effects are produced by other calcium channel blocking agents)

(other cationic medications excreted by renal tubular transport have the potential to increase metformin's plasma concentration or interfere with renal clearance; careful monitoring of blood glucose would be especially appropriate when these medications are given concurrently with metformin)

» Furosemide
(in one study, furosemide increased metformin's AUC by 15% in normal healthy volunteers; renal clearance was not affected; clinical significance is not known, but dosage reduction of metformin potentially may be needed)

Hyperglycemia-causing medications, such as:
   Contraceptives, estrogen-containing, oral
   Corticosteroids
   Diuretics, thiazide
   Estrogens
   Isoniazid
   Nicotinic acid
   Phenothiazines, especially chlorpromazine
   Phenytoin
   Sympathomimetics
   Thyroid hormones
(these medications may contribute to hyperglycemia; an increased dose of metformin or a change to another antidiabetic agent may be needed)

Hypoglycemia-causing medications, such as:
   Clofibrate
   Monoamine oxidase inhibitors
   Probenecid
   Propranolol
   Rifabutin
   Rifampin
   Salicylates
   Sulfonamides, long-acting
   Sulfonylureas
(these medications may cause hypoglycemia and decrease the dosage of metformin needed; although studies with many of these agents in combination with metformin have not been done, it is expected that those medications that are highly protein-bound will cause fewer problems when used with metformin than when used with some of the sulfonylurea antidiabetic agents)

## Laboratory value alterations

The following have been selected on the basis of their potential clinical significance (possible effect in parentheses where appropriate)—not necessarily inclusive (» = major clinical significance):

With diagnostic test results
   Ketones, urine
   (may produce false positive tests)

With physiology/laboratory test values
   Cholesterol, total, serum or
   Low-density lipoproteins (LDL), serum or
   Triglycerides, serum
(the effects of metformin on these lipid subfractions in NIDDM patients are inconsistent and may depend on weight control; further studies are needed to fully characterize these effects. Generally, concentrations of cholesterol, low-density lipoproteins, or triglycerides may be lowered or unchanged in metformin users. This is thought to be independent of metformin's glucose lowering effect; it may involve suppression of free fatty acid oxidation and lipid oxidation or reduction in the triglyceride content of the LDL and VLDL fractions by metformin)

Lactate, fasting, serum
(may increase to the upper range of normal, 2 mEq/L [2 mmol/L], or show no change with therapeutic doses; although the source is unknown, any small increase is thought to be due to glucose metabolism in the splanchnic beds, not in skeletal muscle)

Lipoproteins, high-density (HDL), serum
(may be slightly increased or unchanged)

## Medical considerations/Contraindications

The medical considerations/contraindications included here have been selected on the basis of their potential clinical significance (reasons given in parentheses where appropriate)—not necessarily inclusive (» = major clinical significance).

### Except under special circumstances, this medication should not be used when the following medical problems exist:

» Any condition needing close blood glucose control, such as:
   Burns, severe
   Dehydration
   Diabetic coma
   Diabetic ketoacidosis
   Hyperosmolar nonketotic coma
   Infection, severe
   Surgery, major
   Trauma, severe
(risks of side effects related to uncontrolled blood glucose or lactic acidosis may be increased, and metformin should be discontinued; insulin controls blood glucose best in patients with these conditions; also, metformin should be discontinued 2 days prior to surgery)

» Conditions associated with hypoxemia, such as:
    Cardiorespiratory insufficiency
    Cardiovascular collapse
    Congestive heart failure
    Myocardial infarction, acute or
» Hepatic disease, severe, acute, or chronic or
» Lactic acidosis, active or history of or
» Renal function impairment or renal disease
    (lactic acidosis is associated with these conditions and the risk is further increased when metformin is given concurrently)
    (risk of lactic acidosis increases with the degree of renal dysfunction, impairment of renal clearance, and age of patient; patients who have demonstrated fasting serum lactate values above the upper limit of normal should not receive metformin)
» Diagnostic or medical examinations using contrast media such as:
    Angiography
    Pyelography
    (metformin should be discontinued 2 days prior to medical or diagnostic examinations requiring use of contrast media that can cause functional oliguria because of the increased risk of lactic acidosis; metformin therapy should not be reinstated until after renal function evaluation)
» Hypersensitivity to metformin

**Risk-benefit should be considered when the following medical problems exist:**
» Diarrhea or
» Gastroparesis or
» Intestinal obstruction or
» Vomiting or
» Other conditions causing delayed food absorption
    (conditions that decrease or delay stomach emptying may require a modification of metformin dose or a change to insulin)
» Hyperglycemia-causing conditions, such as:
    Female hormonal changes
    Fever, high
    Hypercortisolism, not optimally treated
    Psychological stress
    (these conditions, by increasing blood glucose, may increase the need for more frequent glucose monitoring and increase the need for a temporary or permanent dose increase of metformin or a change to insulin if blood glucose is uncontrolled)
» Hyperthyroidism, not optimally controlled
    (hyperthyroidism aggravates diabetes mellitus by increasing plasma glucose concentrations and glucose absorption and impairing glucose tolerance; thyroid hormone has dose-dependent biphasic effects on glycogenolysis and glycogeneogenesis, which can make glycemic control difficult until the patient is euthyroid; patients with hyperthyroidism may require an increased dose of metformin until euthyroidism is achieved)
» Hypoglycemia-causing conditions, such as:
    Adrenal insufficiency, not optimally controlled
    Debilitated physical condition
    Malnutrition
    Pituitary insufficiency, not optimally controlled
    (these conditions, which inherently predispose patients to the risk of developing hypoglycemia, increase the patient's risk of developing severe hypoglycemia during metformin treatment; reduction of metformin dose or more frequent blood glucose monitoring may be required)
» Hypothyroidism, not optimally controlled
    (this condition is associated with reduced glucose absorption and altered glucose and lipoprotein metabolism; lower-than-normal doses of metformin may be needed when hypothyroid conditions exist, although an increase in metformin dose may be required when initiating thyroid treatment; glucose control may be difficult until the patient is euthyroid)

**Patient monitoring**
The following may be especially important in patient monitoring (other tests may be warranted in some patients, depending on condition; » = major clinical significance):

Folic acid concentrations, serum and
Vitamin $B_{12}$ concentrations, serum
    (recommended every 1 or 2 years during long-term metformin therapy because metformin may interfere with their absorption)
» Glucose concentration, blood or serum
    (blood or serum glucose reflects the current degree of metabolic control and should be routinely self-monitored by the patient at home and by the physician [every 3 months or more often when patient is not stabilized] to confirm that blood glucose concentra-

tion is maintained within agreed upon targets by the selected diet and dosing regimen; this is particularly important during dosage adjustments. Self-monitoring of blood glucose by the patient may require testing several times a day or once to several times a week)
    (caution in interpreting blood glucose concentrations is needed because normal whole blood glucose values are approximately 15% lower than serum glucose values; it is also laboratory- and method-specific. Normal fasting whole blood glucose for adults of all ages is 65 to 95 mg/dL [3.6 to 5.3 mmol/L]. Normal fasting serum glucose is 70 to 105 mg/dL [3.9 to 5.8 mmol/L] for adults younger than 60 years of age and 80 to 115 mg/dL [4.4 to 6.4 mmol/L] for adults 60 years of age and older. For pregnant diabetic women, a normal fasting serum glucose is less than 105 mg/dL [5.8 mmol/L] and a fasting whole blood glucose is less than 120 mg/dL [6.7 mmol/L].)
    (capillary blood glucose measurement provides important information when done properly, but caution is warranted because of potential errors in technique and readings; it has been suggested that the values be relied upon only if the reported glucose concentration for stable diabetics is between 75 mg/dL and 325 mg/dL [4.12 mmol/L and 17.88 mmol/L, respectively])

Glucose concentrations, urine and
Ketone concentrations, urine
    (if blood glucose concentrations exceed 200 mg/dL [11.1 mmol/L], monitoring of urine for the presence of glucose and ketones may be necessary; normalization of glucose in the urine generally lags quantitatively behind serum glucose concentrations; test methods are generally capable of detecting glucose concentrations in the urine greater than 180 mg/dL [10 mmol/L])
» Glycosylated hemoglobin (hemoglobin $A_{1c}$) determinations
    (monitoring should be done every 3 months or as often as necessary; assessment of this parameter does not eliminate the need for daily blood glucose monitoring. Hemoglobin $A_{1c}$ values reflect the blood glucose control over the preceding 3 months. Normal whole blood hemoglobin $A_{1c}$ is approximately 4 to 6% of total hemoglobin; specific values are laboratory-dependent. Hemoglobin $A_{1c}$ is falsely elevated in unstable diabetics when the intermediate precursor is elevated [i.e., in alcoholism] and falsely lowered in conditions of shortened red blood cell lifespan [i.e., in anemia and acute or chronic blood loss] or in patients with hemoglobinopathies [i.e., sickle cell])

Physical examinations
    (regular examinations as often as necessary to reassess appropriateness of continuation of metformin therapy)
» Renal function assessment
    (recommended annually, more often for at-risk patients)

## Side/Adverse Effects

The following side/adverse effects have been selected on the basis of their potential clinical significance (possible signs and symptoms in parentheses where appropriate)—not necessarily inclusive:

**Those indicating need for medical attention**
Incidence rare
    *Anemia, megaloblastic* (tiredness; weakness); *hypoglycemia* (anxiousness; cold sweats; concentration difficulties; confusion; cool, pale skin; drowsiness; excessive hunger; headache; nausea; nervousness; rapid pulse; shakiness; unusual tiredness or weakness; vision changes); *lactic acidosis* (diarrhea; fast, shallow breathing; muscle pain or cramping; sleepiness; unusual tiredness or weakness)

Note: *Hypoglycemia* does not usually occur with use of metformin unless predisposing conditions or factors are present, such as unusual fasting, concurrent use of other antidiabetic agents, or toxic doses of metformin. Metformin, in combination with sulfonylureas, has been reported to lower basal glucose concentrations typically by at least 20% more than do sulfonylureas used alone.

*Lactic acidosis* is a potentially fatal complication. Twenty-eight cases have been reported in 600,000 users of metformin worldwide, and in each case a contraindication existed; otherwise, the risk is minimal with use of metformin. Patients usually presented not with symptoms of lactic acidosis but rather with acute symptoms of other problems that resulted in metformin accumulation because of renal function impairment or failure in conditions, such as myocardial infarction or renal or hepatic disease.

**Those indicating need for medical attention only if they continue or are bothersome**

Incidence more frequent

*Anorexia; dyspepsia* (stomachache); *flatulence* (gas in stomach or intestines); *headache; metallic taste; nausea; vomiting; weight loss*

Note: *Nausea, dyspepsia,* and *diarrhea* are less frequent when small doses are used initially and, along with *metallic taste* and *headache,* are transient. If *diarrhea* occurs after several months of metformin therapy, lactic acidosis should be considered.

## Overdose

For more information on the management of overdose or unintentional ingestion, **contact a Poison Control Center** (see *Poison Control Center Listing*).

**Clinical effects of overdose**

The following effects have been selected on the basis of their potential clinical significance (possible signs and symptoms in parentheses where appropriate)—not necessarily inclusive:

*Hypoglycemia; lactic acidosis*

## Patient Consultation

As an aid to patient consultation, refer to *Advice for the Patient, Metformin (Systemic).*

In providing consultation, consider emphasizing the following selected information (» = major clinical significance):

**Before using this medication**
» Conditions affecting use, especially:
    Hypersensitivity to metformin
    Pregnancy—Use of any oral antidiabetic medicine is discouraged during pregnancy, while diet or diet/insulin is recommended to prevent maternal and fetal problems; importance of controlling and monitoring blood glucose during pregnancy; alerting physician to plans before becoming pregnant when possible
    Breast-feeding—Metformin is distributed into breast milk
    Use in the elderly—Age-related renal function impairment or peripheral vascular disease may require discontinuation of metformin treatment or special precautions in the elderly
    Other medications, especially alcohol, amiloride, calcium channel blocking agents, cimetidine, digoxin, furosemide, morphine, procainamide, quinidine, quinine, ranitidine, triamterene, trimethoprim, vancomycin, or any other cationic medication excreted by renal transport
    Other medical problems, especially hepatic disease (severe, acute, or chronic); hyper- or hypothyroidism (not optimally controlled); lactic acidosis (active or history of); renal function impairment or renal disease; conditions associated with hypoxemia; conditions causing delayed food absorption (e.g., diarrhea, gastroparesis, intestinal obstruction, or vomiting); conditions causing hyper- or hypoglycemia; or conditions needing close blood glucose control

**Proper use of this medication**
» Compliance with therapy, including not taking more or less medication than directed; alternative dosing or therapy changes for modifications in blood glucose testing, diet, exercise, fluid replacement, and sick day management
» Proper dosing
    Missed dose: Taking as soon as possible; not taking if almost time for next dose; not doubling doses
» Proper storage

**Precautions while using this medication**
» Regular visits to physician to check progress
» Carefully following special instructions of health care team:
    Discussing use of alcohol
    Not taking other medications unless discussed with physician
    Getting counseling for family to help assist diabetic; also, special counseling for pregnancy planning and contraception
    Travel considerations
» Preparing for and understanding what to do in case of an emergency; having or wearing medical identification and keeping a glucagon kit and needles and quick-acting source of sugar close by
» Informing physician when medical examinations that require administration of contrast media or when surgery are scheduled; metformin should be discontinued 2 days before surgery or appropriate medical tests
» Recognizing symptoms of lactic acidosis, such as diarrhea, severe muscle pain or cramping, shallow and fast breathing, unusual tiredness and weakness, unusual sleepiness

» Knowing what to do if symptoms of lactic acidosis occur, such as checking blood glucose and getting immediate emergency medical help
» Checking with physician if vomiting occurs
» Recognizing what brings on symptoms of hypoglycemia, such as delaying or missing a meal, exercising more than usual, drinking significant amounts of alcohol, taking certain medicines, using too much antidiabetic medication (insulin or a sulfonylurea), illness, especially with vomiting or diarrhea
» Knowing what to do if symptoms of hypoglycemia occur, such as using glucagon, eating glucose tablets or gel, corn syrup, honey, or sugar cubes, or drinking fruit juice, nondiet soft drink, or dissolved sugar in water; also, eating small snack, such as crackers or half sandwich, when scheduled meal is longer than 1 hour away; not eating foods high in fat, such as chocolate, since fat slows gastric emptying
» Recognizing symptoms of hyperglycemia and ketoacidosis, such as blurred vision; drowsiness; dry mouth; flushed, dry skin; fruit-like breath odor; increased urination (frequency and volume); ketones in urine; loss of appetite; nausea or vomiting; stomachache; tiredness; somnolence (sleepiness); troubled breathing (rapid and deep); unconsciousness; unusual thirst
» Recognizing what brings on symptoms of hyperglycemia, such as fever or infection; not taking enough or missing a dose of antidiabetic medication; exercising less than usual; taking certain medicines; overeating or not following meal plan
» Knowing what to do if symptoms of hyperglycemia occur, such as checking blood glucose and contacting a member of the health care team

**Side/adverse effects**
Signs and symptoms of potential side effects, especially megaloblastic anemia, hypoglycemia, or lactic acidosis

## General Dosing Information

Individual determination of the minimum dose of metformin that lowers blood glucose adequately is recommended. Short-term treatment during periods of transient loss of glucose control may be sufficient for some patients. Some clinicians recommend that metformin be discontinued annually or semi-annually to assess its continued contribution to the control of blood glucose concentrations, especially if there are progressive signs of secondary failure. Metformin should be discontinued if it is not significantly contributing to disease management.

Metformin should be withdrawn or the dose reduced temporarily if vomiting occurs. Treatment may be resumed cautiously after the possibility of lactic acidosis has been excluded.

When transferring a patient from a sulfonylurea to metformin, no transition period is necessary, except when chlorpropamide has been used for treatment. Chlorpropamide's prolonged action requires more frequent monitoring for hypoglycemia during the first 2 weeks following the transition.

When adding a sulfonylurea to maximum doses of metformin or metformin to maximum doses of a sulfonylurea, even if primary or secondary failure of a sulfonylurea has occurred, the new medication should be added gradually and titrated to the lowest effective dose. Both agents should be discontinued and insulin should be initiated if the patient does not respond to maximum doses within 3 months (or less, depending on clinician's decision).

**Diet/Nutrition**
Metformin should be taken with food to reduce nausea or diarrhea.

**For treatment of adverse effects and/or overdose**
Recommended treatment consists of the following:
    For treatment of lactic acidosis
        • Hemodialysis with sodium bicarbonate has been used but is controversial because there is a lack of published information concerning outcome and lack of cases of metformin-induced lactic acidosis; peritoneal dialysis also has been used, but hemodialysis is thought to be the preferred method when dialysis is needed, such as in patients with shock syndrome. Dialysis is probably not necessary when renal function can be restored because of metformin's rapid renal elimination. Dialysis solutions commonly contain lactate as the buffering agent and these should not be used in cases of metformin-induced lactic acidosis.
    For mild to moderate hypoglycemia
        • Treating with immediate ingestion of a source of glucose, such as glucose gel, glucose tablets, fruit juice, corn syrup, non-diet soft drinks, honey, sugar cubes, or table sugar dissolved in water. A frequently used source of glucose is a glassful of orange juice containing 2 or 3 teaspoonfuls of table sugar.
        • Documenting blood glucose and rechecking in 15 minutes.

• Counseling patient to seek medical assistance promptly.
• Possible adjustment of metformin dosage.
• Possible adjustment of meal pattern.

For severe hypoglycemia or acute overdose, including coma

Note: Dextrose administration is the basis for treatment of hypoglycemia; however, an exposure to sudden hyperglycemia caused by a rapid injection of hypertonic dextrose injection may further stimulate the sulfonylurea-primed pancreas when sulfonylureas are used with metformin to release more insulin, worsening the hypoglycemia.

• Counseling patient to obtain emergency medical assistance immediately.
• Immediately treating with 50 mL of 50% dextrose given intravenously to stabilize the patient. Then, administering a continuous infusion of 5 to 10% dextrose in water to maintain slight hyperglycemia (approximately 100 mg/dL [5.55 mmol/L] blood glucose concentration) for up to 12 days. Intravenous dextrose therapy should not be terminated suddenly. Oral dextrose cannot be relied upon to maintain euglycemia because 60% of an oral dextrose dose is stored as hepatic glycogen with only 15% left for brain utilization and 15% for insulin-dependent tissues.
• Glucagon, 1 to 2 mg administered intramuscularly, is useful for fast onset of action to mobilize hepatic glucose stores but may be ineffective or variable in its effect if glycogen stores are depleted. Therefore, glucagon should be administered after dextrose administration.
• Diazoxide (200 mg orally every 4 hours or 300 mg intravenously over a 30-minute period every 4 hours) can be used for nonresponders to dextrose therapy or for patients in a coma as an aid to dextrose infusion to reduce hypoglycemia; patient must be monitored for sodium concentration and hypotension.
• Emesis can be induced with ipecac syrup if the metformin overdose is recent (within the past 30 minutes) and if the patient is alert, has an intact gag reflex, and is not obtunded or convulsing. Otherwise, gastric lavage after endotracheal tube placement is required.
• Gastric decontamination by administration of repeated doses of oral activated charcoal with appropriate cathartic may be attempted, although the usefulness of this has not been established.
• Monitoring vital signs, arterial blood gases, blood glucose, and serum electrolytes (especially calcium, potassium, and sodium) as required. Initially, blood glucose concentrations should be monitored as frequently as every 1 to 3 hours. Blood urea nitrogen and serum creatinine concentrations should also be obtained.
• Cerebral edema—Managing with mannitol and dexamethasone.
• Hypokalemia—Managing with potassium supplements.

• Hospitalization for 6 to 91 hours (mean, 24 hours), because the hypoglycemia may be recurrent and prolonged.
• Other supportive measures should also be employed as needed.

## Oral Dosage Forms

### METFORMIN HYDROCHLORIDE TABLETS

**Usual adult dose**
Antihyperglycemic agent—
   Initial: Oral, 500 mg two times a day, taken with morning and evening meals. The daily dose may be increased by 500 mg at weekly intervals as needed. An alternative dose is 850 mg a day, taken with the morning meal. The daily dose may be increased by 850 mg at fourteen-day intervals.
   Maintenance: Oral, 500 or 850 mg two to three times a day, taken with meals.

**Usual adult prescribing limits**
2550 mg a day.

**Usual pediatric dose**
Safety and efficacy have not been established.

**Usual geriatric dose**
See *Usual adult dose.* For some sensitive individuals, lower initial doses may be needed. Maximum doses are not advised for use in the elderly.

**Strength(s) usually available**
U.S.—
   500 mg (Rx) [*Glucophage* (scored)].
   850 mg (Rx) [*Glucophage* (scored)].
Canada—
   500 mg (Rx) [*Glucophage* (scored); *Novo-Metformin* (scored)].

**Packaging and storage**
Store below 40 °C (104 °F), preferably between 15 and 30 °C (59 and 86 °F), unless otherwise specified by manufacturer.

**Auxiliary labeling**
• Take with food.
• Do not drink alcohol.

## Selected Bibliography

Watkins PJ. Guidelines for good practice in the diagnosis and treatment of non-insulin–dependent diabetes mellitus. Report of a joint working party of the British Diabetic Association, the Research Unit of the Royal College of Physicians, and the Royal College of General Practitioners. J R Coll Physicians Lond 1993 Jul; 27 (3): 259-66.

Aguilar C. Reza A, Garcia JE, et al. Biguanide related lactic acidosis: incidence and risk factors. Arch Med Res 1992 Spring; 23 (1): 19-24.

Developed: 07/26/95

---

# METHACHOLINE   Inhalation-Local†

VA CLASSIFICATION (Primary): DX900

Note: For a listing of dosage forms and brand names by country availability, see *Dosage Forms* section(s). For a listing of brand names for the articles in this monograph, refer to the General Index.

†Not commercially available in Canada.

## Category

Diagnostic aid (bronchial airway hyperreactivity).

## Indications

### Accepted

Asthma (diagnosis) or

Bronchial airway hyperreactivity (diagnosis)—Methacholine for inhalation is indicated for the diagnosis of bronchial airway hyperreactivity, including asthma, in individuals who do not have clinically apparent asthma.

   Because of the potential for severe bronchoconstriction, methacholine challenge should not be performed in any patient with clinically apparent asthma, wheezing, or very low baseline pulmonary function tests (e.g., forced expiratory volume in 1 second [FEV₁] less than 1 to 1.5 liters or less than 70% of the predicted values).

## Pharmacology/Pharmacokinetics

### Physicochemical characteristics

Source—Methacholine chloride is the beta-methyl homolog of acetylcholine.
Molecular weight—195.69.

### Mechanism of action/Effect

Methacholine is a parasympathomimetic (cholinergic) bronchoconstrictor. It is the beta-methyl homolog of acetylcholine and differs from acetylcholine primarily in its greater duration and selectivity of action.

Bronchial smooth muscle contains significant parasympathetic (cholinergic) innervation, and bronchoconstriction occurs when the vagus nerve is stimulated and acetylcholine is released from the nerve endings. Because acetylcholine is rapidly inactivated by acetylcholinesterase, muscle constriction is confined primarily to the local site of release. Methacholine is more slowly hydrolyzed by acetylcholinesterase than acetylcholine and is almost completely resistant to inactivation by nonspecific cholinesterase or pseudocholinesterase. When methacholine (in a sodium chloride solution) is inhaled, patients with asthma are significantly more sensitive to methacholine-induced bronchoconstriction than are healthy individuals. This difference in response is the basis for the diagnosis of asthma.

# Precautions to Consider

### Cross-sensitivity and/or related problems
Patients sensitive to other parasympathomimetics (cholinergics) may be sensitive to this medication also.

### Carcinogenicity/Mutagenicity
Studies have not been done to determine the carcinogenic or mutagenic potential of methacholine.

### Pregnancy/Reproduction
Fertility—Studies have not been done to determine the effects of methacholine on fertility.

Pregnancy—Studies have not been done in humans.

In females of childbearing potential, the manufacturer recommends that methacholine inhalation challenge be performed either within 10 days following the onset of menses or within 2 weeks of a negative pregnancy test because it is not known whether methacholine causes fetal harm when administered to a pregnant patient or affects reproductive capacity.

Studies have not been done in animals.

FDA Pregnancy Category C.

### Breast-feeding
It is not known whether methacholine is distributed into breast milk.

### Pediatrics
Appropriate studies on the relationship of age to the effects of methacholine have not been performed in children up to 5 years of age. However, no pediatrics-specific problems have been documented to date.

### Geriatrics
No information is available on the relationship of age to the effects of methacholine in geriatric patients.

### Drug interactions and/or related problems
The following drug interactions and/or related problems have been selected on the basis of their potential clinical significance (possible mechanism in parentheses where appropriate)—not necessarily inclusive (» = major clinical significance):

See also *Laboratory value alterations.*

Note: Combinations containing any of the following medications, depending on the amount present, may also interact with this medication.

» Beta-adrenergic blocking agents
(methacholine inhalation challenge should not be performed in patients receiving beta-adrenergic blocking agents, since the reaction to methacholine in these patients may be exaggerated or prolonged and may not respond as rapidly to treatment with bronchodilators)

### Laboratory value alterations
The following have been selected on the basis of their potential clinical significance (possible effect in parentheses where appropriate)—not necessarily inclusive (» = major clinical significance):

With results of *this* test
 *Due to other medications*
» Anticholinergics or other medications with anticholinergic activity or
» Bronchodilators
(may cause false-negative test results; extended-release capsule or tablet dosage form of aminophylline, oxtriphylline, or theophylline should be discontinued 24 hours before methacholine challenge; any other bronchodilators or anticholinergics or other medications with anticholinergic action should be discontinued 12 hours before methacholine challenge)

Corticosteroids or
Cromolyn
(may decrease slightly, but inconsistently, the response to methacholine challenge; however, these medications generally do not cause false-negative tests)

Smoking
(may cause false-positive test results)

 *Due to medical problems or conditions*
Lung disease, chronic (cystic fibrosis, sarcoidosis, tuberculosis, chronic obstructive pulmonary disease) or
Respiratory illness, viral, or
Rhinitis, allergic
(may cause false-positive test results)

Note: Also, approximately 18% of nonatopic family members or siblings of asthmatics have a false-positive reaction to methacholine challenge.

### Medical considerations/Contraindications
The medical considerations/contraindications included here have been selected on the basis of their potential clinical significance (reasons given in parentheses where appropriate)—not necessarily inclusive (» = major clinical significance).

See also *Laboratory value alterations.*

***Risk-benefit should be considered when the following medical problems exist:***
» Asthma, clinically apparent or
» Hay fever or
» Wheezing
(potential for severe bronchoconstriction with methacholine)

Cardiovascular disease accompanied by bradycardia or
Epilepsy or
Peptic ulcer disease or
Thyroid disease or
Urinary tract obstruction or
Vagotonia
(condition may be exacerbated by cholinergic action of methacholine)

» Sensitivity to methacholine or other cholinergics

### Patient monitoring
The following may be especially important in patient monitoring (other tests may be warranted in some patients, depending on condition; » = major clinical significance):

» Pulmonary function tests
(baseline pulmonary function tests recommended before methacholine challenge is initiated; patient must have a forced expiratory volume in 1 second [$FEV_1$] of at least 70% of the predicted value; the target level for a positive challenge is a 20% reduction in the $FEV_1$, compared with the baseline value after inhalation of the control sodium chloride solution; the target value should be calculated and recorded before the challenge is begun)

(FEV$_1$ values are to be determined within 3 to 5 minutes following administration of each serial concentration of methacholine)

# Side/Adverse Effects

Note: When methacholine is administered orally or parenterally, it is reported to cause nausea, vomiting, substernal pain or pressure, hypotension, fainting, and complete heart block; however, these side/adverse effects have not been reported with methacholine administered by inhalation.

Also, overdosage of oral or parenteral methacholine can result in a syncopal reaction with cardiac arrest and loss of consciousness.

The following side/adverse effects have been selected on the basis of their potential clinical significance (possible signs and symptoms in parentheses where appropriate)—not necessarily inclusive:

**Those indicating need for medical attention**
 *Wheezing, tightness in chest, or difficulty in breathing, continuing or severe*

**Those indicating need for medical attention only if they continue or are bothersome**
Incidence less frequent or rare
 *Headache or lightheadedness; irritation of throat; itching*

# Overdose

For more information on the management of overdose or unintentional ingestion, **contact a Poison Control Center** (see *Poison Control Center Listing*).

### Specific treatment
Intramuscular or intravenous administration of 500 mcg (0.5 mg) to 1 mg of atropine sulfate.

For severe cardiovascular or bronchoconstrictor responses—Subcutaneous administration of 100 mcg (0.1 mg) to 1 mg of epinephrine may be useful to treat severe cardiovascular or bronchoconstrictor responses.

# Patient Consultation

As an aid to patient consultation, refer to *Advice for the Patient, Methacholine (Inhalation).*

In providing consultation, consider emphasizing the following selected information (» = major clinical significance):

### Description of use
Test procedure: Pulmonary function determination prior to test; 5 oral inhalations of each ascending concentration administered via nebulizer; pulmonary function determined 3 to 5 minutes after administration of each concentration; wheezing and difficulty in breathing may occur; physician may prescribe bronchodilator inhalation for relief of effects

**Before having this test**

» Conditions affecting use, especially:

Sensitivity to methacholine or other cholinergics

Pregnancy—In females of childbearing potential, manufacturer recommends that methacholine inhalation challenge be performed either within 10 days following onset of menses or within 2 weeks of negative pregnancy test because it is not known whether methacholine causes fetal harm when administered during pregnancy or affects reproductive capacity

Other medications, especially beta-adrenergic blocking agents

Other medical problems, especially asthma clinically (apparent), hay fever, or wheezing

**Preparation for this test**

» Not taking any extended-release capsule or tablet dosage form of aminophylline, oxtriphylline, or theophylline for 24 hours before the test; not using any other medicine, especially anticholinergics or medicine for breathing problems, sinus problems, or hay fever or other allergies (including nose drops or sprays), for 12 hours before the test; test results may be altered by these medications

**Side/adverse effects**

Signs of potential side effects, especially wheezing, tightness in chest, or difficulty in breathing (continuing)

# General Dosing Information

**Methacholine inhalation challenge should be performed only under the supervision of a physician trained in and thoroughly familiar with all aspects of the technique of methacholine challenge and the management of respiratory distress.**

Emergency equipment and medication (e.g., parenteral bronchodilators, such as epinephrine and aminophylline) should be immediately available to treat acute respiratory distress.

Methacholine should be administered only by inhalation. Oral or intravenous administration can cause cardiac arrest.

Severe bronchoconstriction and reduction in respiratory function can result from the administration of methacholine inhalation; patients with severe hyperreactivity of the airways can experience bronchoconstriction at a dosage as low as 0.025 mg per mL (0.125 cumulative units).

The methacholine challenge is performed by administering ascending serial concentrations of methacholine via a nebulizer that permits intermittent delivery time of 0.6 seconds by either a Y-tube or a breath-actuated timing device (dosimeter). At each of the 5 oral inhalations of a serial concentration, the patient begins at functional residual capacity (FRC) and should slowly and completely inhale the dose delivered. Within 3 to 5 minutes after the administration of each serial concentration, $FEV_1$ values should be determined. The procedure is completed either when there is a 20% or greater reduction in the $FEV_1$ compared with the baseline sodium chloride solution value (i.e., a positive response) or when 188.88 total cumulative units have been administered and $FEV_1$ has been reduced by $\leq 14\%$ (i.e., a negative response). If there is a reduction of 15 to 19% in the $FEV_1$ compared with the baseline value, either the challenge at that concentration may be repeated or a higher concentration may be given. The dosage administered should not exceed 188.88 total cumulative units.

Following the methacholine challenge, a beta-agonist inhalation may be administered to help return the $FEV_1$ to baseline and to relieve patient discomfort. Normal pulmonary function usually returns within 5 minutes following administration of a bronchodilator or within 30 to 45 minutes without any bronchodilator.

Repeated administration of the methacholine challenge test on the same day is not recommended. Methacholine challenges done repeatedly at daily intervals do not alter airway responsiveness to methacholine.

**For treatment of adverse effects**

Recommended treatment for severe bronchospasm—Administering a rapid-acting bronchodilator (beta-agonist) by inhalation to immediately reverse the bronchoconstriction.

# Inhalation Dosage Forms

## METHACHOLINE CHLORIDE FOR INHALATION

**Usual adult and adolescent dose**

Diagnostic aid (bronchial airway hyperreactivity)—

Oral inhalation, in ascending serial concentrations (beginning with 25 mcg [0.025 mg] per mL and ending with 25 mg per mL)—At each concentration, 5 inhalations administered via a nebulizer that permits intermittent delivery time of 0.6 seconds by either a Y-tube or a breath-actuated timing device (dosimeter). The recommended administration schedule for methacholine challenge is as follows:

| Serial Concentration (mg/mL) | Number of Inhalations | Cumulative Units per Concentration* | Total Cumulative Units† |
|---|---|---|---|
| 0.025 | 5 | 0.125 | 0.125 |
| 0.25 | 5 | 1.25 | 1.375 |
| 2.5 | 5 | 12.5 | 13.88 |
| 10.0 | 5 | 50.0 | 63.88 |
| 25.0 | 5 | 125.0 | 188.88‡ |

*Cumulative units are calculated by multiplying the number of inhalations by the concentration administered.

†Total cumulative units is the sum of cumulative units for each concentration administered.

‡Dosage should not exceed 188.88 total cumulative units.

**Usual pediatric dose**

Diagnostic aid (bronchial airway hyperreactivity)—

Children up to 5 years of age: Safety and efficacy have not been established.

Children 5 years of age and over: See *Usual adult and adolescent dose*.

**Size(s) usually available**

U.S.—

100 mg per 5-mL vial (Rx) [*Provocholine*].

Canada—

Not commercially available.

**Packaging and storage**

Prior to reconstitution, store the powder between 15 and 30 °C (59 and 86 °F), unless otherwise specified by manufacturer.

After reconstitution, store the solution between 8 and 15 °C (36 and 46 °F), unless otherwise specified by manufacturer.

**Preparation of dosage form**

Do not inhale the powder. Also, do not handle the medication if you have asthma or hay fever, unless the following protective measures are used—

• Use of a biological containment cabinet during reconstitution and dilution of methacholine for inhalation and wearing of disposable mask.

• Use of proper technique to prevent contamination of work area during transfer between vials.

• Cautious and proper disposal of needles, syringes, vials, and unused medication.

All dilutions should be made with 0.9% sodium chloride injection containing 0.4% phenol (pH 7.0) as follows—

Vial A: Add 4 mL of 0.9% sodium chloride injection to the 5-mL vial containing 100 mg of methacholine chloride to prepare a concentration of 25 mg per mL.

Vial B: Remove 3 mL from vial A (25 mg per mL solution), transfer to another vial, and add 4.5 mL of 0.9% sodium chloride injection to prepare a concentration of 10 mg per mL. Another method of preparing vial B is to remove 1 mL from vial A and add 1.5 mL of 0.9% sodium chloride injection (for single patient testing).

Vial C: Remove 1 mL from vial A (25 mg per mL solution), transfer to another vial, and add 9 mL of 0.9% sodium chloride injection to prepare a concentration of 2.5 mg per mL.

Vial D: Remove 1 mL from vial C (2.5 mg per mL solution), transfer to another vial, and add 9 mL of 0.9% sodium chloride injection to prepare a concentration of 250 mcg (0.25 mg) per mL.

Vial E: Remove 1 mL from vial D (250 mcg [0.25 mg] per mL solution), transfer to another vial, and add 9 mL of 0.9% sodium chloride injection to prepare a concentration of 25 mcg (0.025 mg) per mL.

After adding the sodium chloride solution, shake each vial to obtain a clear solution.

**Stability**

After reconstitution, dilutions A through D retain their potency for up to 2 weeks if refrigerated. After this time, the dilutions should be discarded and new dilutions prepared. Freezing does not affect the stability of dilutions A through D.

Vial E must be prepared on the day of the challenge test.

A bacterial-retentive filter (porosity 0.22 microns) should be used when transferring a solution from each vial to a nebulizer.

Revised: 08/09/94

**METHADONE**—See *Opioid (Narcotic) Analgesics (Systemic)*

**METHAMPHETAMINE**—See *Amphetamines (Systemic)*

**METHANTHELINE**—See *Anticholinergics/Antispasmodics (Systemic)*

**METHARBITAL**—See *Barbiturates (Systemic)*

**METHAZOLAMIDE**—See *Carbonic Anhydrase Inhibitors (Systemic)*

**METHDILAZINE**—See *Antihistamines, Phenothiazine-derivative (Systemic)*

# METHENAMINE  Systemic

VA CLASSIFICATION (Primary): AM550
Note: For a listing of dosage forms and brand names by country availability, see *Dosage Forms* section(s). For a listing of brand names for the articles in this monograph, refer to the General Index.

## Category
Antibacterial (systemic).

## Indications
### Accepted
Urinary tract infections, bacterial (prophylaxis) or
Urinary tract infections, bacterial (treatment)—Methenamine is indicated in the prophylaxis of urinary tract infections in patients with sterile urine after the eradication of urinary tract infections by other antibacterials.

Methenamine is indicated in the treatment of uncomplicated lower urinary tract infections and in the suppressive treatment of urinary tract infections in patients with neurogenic bladder or in patients being catheterized intermittently.

Virtually all bacteria and fungi are susceptible to the nonspecific action of free formaldehyde produced by the hydrolysis of methenamine.

### Unaccepted
Methenamine is not recommended when urine acidification to a pH of 5.5 or below is contraindicated or unattainable.

Methenamine is not effective in patients with indwelling urinary catheters.

## Pharmacology/Pharmacokinetics
### Physicochemical characteristics
Molecular weight—Methenamine: 140.19.
Methenamine hippurate: 319.36.
Methenamine mandelate: 292.34.

### Mechanism of action/Effect
Methenamine, an inactive weak base, slowly hydrolyzes in acidic urine to ammonia and the nonspecific antibacterial, formaldehyde. Formaldehyde is thought to act by denaturation of protein. Urinary formaldehyde concentrations may be bactericidal or bacteriostatic, depending on urine pH (which controls the amount of formaldehyde released), volume, and flow rate. Most organisms are susceptible and resistance does not develop. Acids that dissociate from the hippurate or mandelate salt may contribute to maintenance of acidic urinary pH and liberation of formaldehyde.

### Absorption
Methenamine—Rapid, but 30 to 60% hydrolyzed by gastric acid if not enteric-coated.
Methenamine hippurate—Rapid, from the gastrointestinal tract.
Methenamine mandelate (enteric-coated tablets)—Absorption slightly delayed; total absorption essentially unaffected.

### Distribution
Freely distributed to body tissues and fluids, but not clinically significant because methenamine does not hydrolyze at pH greater than 6.8.
$Vol_D$ =Approximately 0.56 L/kg.

### Protein binding
Some formaldehyde is bound to substances in the urine and the surrounding tissues.

### Half-life
Approximately 4.3 hours.

### Time to peak urinary formaldehyde concentration (pH 5.6)
Methenamine—0.5 to 1.5 hours.
Methenamine hippurate—2 hours.
Methenamine mandelate (enteric-coated tablets)—3 to 8 hours.

### Elimination
Renal; rapid.
Methenamine—
  Almost completely (90%) excreted within 24 hours; of this amount at pH 5, approximately 20% is formaldehyde.
  Note: Methenamine may accumulate in patients with impaired renal function. However, it does not hydrolyze in the blood (pH 7.4) and is not considered toxic. Urinary formaldehyde concentrations may be inadequate in these patients.

Hippuric acid and mandelic acid—
  40% excreted unchanged within 8 hours by glomerular filtration and tubular secretion; can accumulate in patients with severely impaired renal function and may be toxic.

## Precautions to Consider
### Pregnancy/Reproduction
Pregnancy—Methenamine crosses the placenta. Adequate and well-controlled studies have not been done in either humans or animals. However, published reports on the use of methenamine in pregnant women have not shown an increased risk of fetal abnormalities during pregnancy.
FDA Pregnancy Category C.

### Breast-feeding
Methenamine is distributed into breast milk. However, problems in humans have not been documented.

### Pediatrics
Appropriate studies on the relationship of age to the effects of methenamine have not been performed in the pediatric population. However, no pediatrics-specific problems have been documented to date.

### Geriatrics
No information is available on the relationship of age to the effects of methenamine in geriatric patients.

### Drug interactions and/or related problems
The following drug interactions and/or related problems have been selected on the basis of their potential clinical significance (possible mechanism in parentheses where appropriate)—not necessarily inclusive (» = major clinical significance):

Note: Combinations containing any of the following medications, depending on the amount present, may also interact with this medication.

» Alkalizers, urinary, such as:
  Antacids, calcium- and/or magnesium-containing
  Carbonic anhydrase inhibitors
  Citrates
  Sodium bicarbonate, or
» Diuretics, thiazide
  (may cause the urine to become alkaline, thereby reducing the effectiveness of methenamine by inhibiting its conversion to formaldehyde; concurrent use is not recommended)

  Sulfamethizole
  (in acid urine methenamine breaks down into formaldehyde, which may form an insoluble precipitate with sulfamethizole, and may also increase the danger of crystalluria; concurrent use is not recommended)

**Laboratory value alterations**

The following have been selected on the basis of their potential clinical significance (possible effect in parentheses where appropriate)—not necessarily inclusive (» = major clinical significance):

With diagnostic test results

Catecholamine, urinary and
17-hydroxycorticosteroid (17-OHCS), urinary, and
Vanillylmandelic acid (VMA), urinary
(concentrations may be falsely increased)

Estriol, urinary, and
5-hydroxyindoleacetic acid (5-HIAA), urinary
(concentrations may be falsely decreased)

**Medical considerations/Contraindications**

The medical considerations/contraindications included here have been selected on the basis of their potential clinical significance (reasons given in parentheses where appropriate)—not necessarily inclusive (» = major clinical significance).

*Risk-benefit should be considered when the following medical problems exist:*

Dehydration, severe, or
» Renal function impairment, severe
(salts of methenamine may precipitate, causing crystalluria, in patients with a low urine output)
» Hepatic function impairment, severe
(because methenamine is hydrolyzed to ammonia, it should not be given to patients with severe hepatic impairment)
Hypersensitivity to methenamine

## Side/Adverse Effects

Note: Large doses of methenamine (8 grams daily for 3 to 4 weeks) have been reported to cause bladder irritation, painful and frequent urination, and gross hematuria.

The following side/adverse effects have been selected on the basis of their potential clinical significance (possible signs and symptoms in parentheses where appropriate)—not necessarily inclusive:

**Those indicating need for medical attention**

Incidence less frequent
*Skin rash*

Incidence rare
*Crystalluria or hematuria* (blood in urine; lower back pain; pain or burning while urinating)

**Those indicating need for medical attention only if they continue or are bothersome**

Incidence less frequent
*Gastrointestinal disturbance* (nausea and vomiting)

## Patient Consultation

As an aid to patient consultation, refer to *Advice for the Patient, Methenamine (Systemic)*.

In providing consultation, consider emphasizing the following selected information (» = major clinical significance):

**Before using this medication**

» Conditions affecting use, especially:
Hypersensitivity to methenamine
Pregnancy—Methenamine crosses the placenta
Breast-feeding—Methenamine is excreted in breast milk
Other medications, especially urinary alkalinizers or thiazide diuretics
Other medical problems, especially severe hepatic function impairment or severe renal function impairment

**Proper use of this medication**

» Using phenaphthazine paper or other test and dietary measures to measure and appropriately adjust urine pH; importance of maintaining acidic urine (pH 5.5 or below)
Taking after meals and at bedtime if nausea or gastrointestinal irritation occurs
Proper administration technique for dry granules, oral liquids, and enteric-coated tablets
» Compliance with full course of therapy
» Proper dosing
Missed dose: Taking as soon as possible; not taking if almost time for next dose; not doubling doses
» Proper storage

**Precautions while using this medication**

Checking with physician if no improvement within a few days

**Side/adverse effects**

Signs of potential side effects, especially crystalluria, hematuria, and skin rash

## General Dosing Information

Urine pH should be monitored before starting and throughout therapy since the effectiveness of methenamine is increased if a pH of 5.5 or below is maintained. To check urine pH, phenaphthazine paper, which has a pH range of 4.5 to 7.5, may be used.

To maintain a urine pH of 5.5 or below, most fruits (especially citrus fruits and juices), milk and other dairy products, and other alkalinizing foods should be avoided. A protein-rich diet with liberal amounts of cranberries (especially ascorbic acid–enriched cranberry juice), plums, or prunes may be helpful. If these measures do not produce a sufficiently acid urine, they may be supplemented with large doses of ascorbic acid (4 grams or more per day), arginine hydrochloride, or methionine. However, some brands of ascorbic acid may contain varying amounts of ascorbate sodium and may actually alkalinize the urine. Alternatively, ammonium chloride or sodium biphosphate may be given (caution—large doses of ammonium chloride may cause metabolic acidosis in patients with impaired renal function and may be contraindicated in patients with hepatic insufficiency).

Methenamine may be taken after meals and at bedtime to help minimize nausea or gastrointestinal irritation.

Urea-splitting organisms (e.g., *Proteus mirabilis* and some strains of *Pseudomonas* and *Enterobacter*) may cause an increase in urine pH and thereby decrease the effectiveness of methenamine. Care should be taken to ensure urine acidification.

If recurrent urinary tract infections are prevented by 4 grams of methenamine mandelate daily, the dose may be reduced to a maintenance level of 1 gram of the mandelate 2 times a day. However, close observation of the patient is recommended to ensure the continued effectiveness of the lower dose of medication.

Methenamine may cause dysuria, which may be controlled by reducing the dose and the urinary acidification.

## Oral Dosage Forms

### METHENAMINE HIPPURATE TABLETS USP

**Usual adult and adolescent dose**

Antibacterial—
Oral, 1 gram two times a day, morning and evening.

**Usual adult prescribing limits**

Up to 4 grams daily.

**Usual pediatric dose**

Antibacterial—
Children 6 to 12 years of age: 500 mg to 1 gram two times a day, morning and evening.
Children 12 years of age and over: See *Usual adult and adolescent dose.*

**Strength(s) usually available**

U.S.—
1 gram (Rx) [*Hiprex* (scored; tartrazine); *Urex* (scored)].
Canada—
1 gram (Rx) [*Hip-Rex* (scored)].

**Packaging and storage**

Store below 40 °C (104 °F), preferably between 15 and 30 °C (59 and 86 °F), unless otherwise specified by manufacturer. Store in a well-closed container.

**Auxiliary labeling**

· Maintain acid urine.
· Continue medicine for full time of treatment.

### METHENAMINE MANDELATE FOR ORAL SOLUTION (Granules) USP

**Usual adult and adolescent dose**

Antibacterial—
Oral, 1 gram four times a day, after meals and at bedtime.

**Usual adult prescribing limits**

Up to 12 grams daily.

**Usual pediatric dose**

Antibacterial—
Children up to 6 years of age: Oral, 18.3 mg per kg of body weight four times a day, after meals and at bedtime.
Children 6 to 12 years of age: Oral, 500 mg four times a day, after meals and at bedtime.

Children 12 years of age and over: See *Usual adult and adolescent dose.*

**Size(s) usually available**

U.S.—

1 gram (Rx) [*Mandelamine* (sucrose)].

Canada—

Not commercially available.

**Packaging and storage**

Prior to reconstitution, store below 40 °C (104 °F), preferably between 15 and 30 °C (59 and 86 °F), unless otherwise specified by manufacturer. Store in a well-closed container.

**Preparation of dosage form**

Contents of each packet of granules should be dissolved in 60 to 120 mL of cold water immediately prior to administration.

**Auxiliary labeling**

• Maintain acid urine.

• Dissolve in water before taking.

• Continue medicine for full time of treatment.

**Note**

Explain administration technique.

Available as dry granules for reconstitution.

## METHENAMINE MANDELATE ORAL SUSPENSION USP

**Usual adult and adolescent dose**

See *Methenamine Mandelate for Oral Solution USP (Granules).*

**Usual adult prescribing limits**

See *Methenamine Mandelate for Oral Solution USP (Granules)* .

**Usual pediatric dose**

See *Methenamine Mandelate for Oral Solution USP (Granules).*

**Strength(s) usually available**

U.S.—

250 mg per 5 mL (Rx) [*Mandelamine* (parabens)].

500 mg per 5 mL (Rx) [*Mandelamine* (parabens); GENERIC].

Canada—

Not commercially available.

**Packaging and storage**

Store below 40 °C (104 °F), preferably between 15 and 30 °C (59 and 86 °F), unless otherwise specified by manufacturer. Store in a tight container. Protect from freezing.

**Auxiliary labeling**

• Maintain acid urine.

• Shake well.

• Continue medicine for full time of treatment.

**Note**

When dispensing, include a calibrated liquid-measuring device.

## METHENAMINE MANDELATE TABLETS (ENTERIC-COATED) USP

**Usual adult and adolescent dose**

See *Methenamine Mandelate for Oral Solution USP (Granules).*

**Usual adult prescribing limits**

See *Methenamine Mandelate for Oral Solution USP (Granules).*

**Usual pediatric dose**

See *Methenamine Mandelate for Oral Solution USP (Granules).*

**Strength(s) usually available**

U.S.—

500 mg (Rx) [GENERIC].

1 gram (Rx) [GENERIC].

Canada—

Not commercially available.

**Packaging and storage**

Store below 40 °C (104 °F), preferably between 15 and 30 °C (59 and 86 °F), unless otherwise specified by manufacturer. Store in a well-closed container.

**Auxiliary labeling**

• Maintain acid urine.

• Swallow tablets whole.

• Continue medicine for full time of treatment.

## METHENAMINE MANDELATE TABLETS USP

**Usual adult and adolescent dose**

See *Methenamine Mandelate for Oral Solution USP (Granules).*

**Usual adult prescribing limits**

See *Methenamine Mandelate for Oral Solution USP (Granules).*

**Usual pediatric dose**

See *Methenamine Mandelate for Oral Solution USP (Granules)* .

**Strength(s) usually available**

U.S.—

500 mg (Rx) [*Mandelamine;* GENERIC].

1 gram (Rx) [*Mandelamine;* GENERIC].

Canada—

500 mg (Rx) [*Mandelamine*].

1 gram (Rx) [*Mandelamine*].

**Packaging and storage**

Store below 40 °C (104 °F), preferably between 15 and 30 °C (59 and 86 °F), unless otherwise specified by manufacturer. Store in a well-closed container.

**Auxiliary labeling**

• Maintain acid urine.

• Swallow tablets whole.

• Continue medicine for full time of treatment.

Revised: 10/20/92

Interim revision: 03/17/94

## METHENAMINE-CONTAINING COMBINATIONS—

Atropine, Hyoscyamine, Methenamine, Methylene Blue, Phenyl Salicylate, and Benzoic Acid (Systemic)

## METHICILLIN—See *Penicillins (Systemic)*

## METHIMAZOLE—See *Antithyroid Agents (Systemic)*

## METHOCARBAMOL—See *Skeletal Muscle Relaxants (Systemic)*

## METHOHEXITAL—See *Anesthetics, Barbiturate (Systemic)*

# METHOTREXATE—For Cancer   Systemic

VA CLASSIFICATION (Primary): AN300

Another commonly used name is amethopterin.

Note: For a listing of dosage forms and brand names by country availability, see *Dosage Forms* section(s). For a listing of brand names for the articles in this monograph, refer to the General Index.

## Category

Antineoplastic.

## Indications

Note: Bracketed information in the *Indications* section refers to uses that are not included in U.S. product labeling.

**Accepted**

Carcinoma, breast (treatment)[1]

Carcinoma, head and neck (treatment)[1]

Carcinoma, lung (treatment)[1]

Tumors, trophoblastic (treatment)

[Carcinoma, cervical (treatment)][1]

[Carcinoma, ovarian (treatment)][1]

[Carcinoma, bladder (treatment)][1]

[Carcinoma, renal (treatment)][1]
[Carcinoma, prostatic (treatment)][1] or
[Carcinoma, testicular (treatment)][1]—Methotrexate is indicated for treatment of breast carcinoma, head and neck cancers (epidermoid), lung carcinoma (especially squamous cell and small cell types), trophoblastic tumors (gestational choriocarcinoma, chorioadenoma destruens, hydatidiform mole), cervical carcinoma, ovarian carcinoma, bladder carcinoma, renal carcinoma, prostatic carcinoma, and testicular carcinoma.

Leukemia, acute lymphocytic (treatment)
Leukemia, meningeal (prophylaxis and treatment) or
[Leukemia, acute myelocytic (treatment)][1]—Methotrexate is indicated for treatment of acute lymphocytic leukemia, prophylaxis and treatment of meningeal leukemia, and treatment of acute myelocytic leukemia.

Lymphomas, non-Hodgkin's (treatment)—Methotrexate is indicated for treatment of non-Hodgkin's lymphomas, including advanced cases of lymphosarcoma (particularly in children).

Mycosis fungoides (treatment)—Methotrexate is indicated for treatment of advanced cases of mycosis fungoides.

Osteosarcoma (treatment)[1]—Methotrexate is indicated in high doses along with leucovorin rescue, in combination with other agents, for treatment of nonmetastatic osteosarcoma in patients who have undergone primary surgical treatment.

[Multiple myeloma (treatment)][1]—Methotrexate is used for treatment of multiple myeloma.

---

[1]Not included in Canadian product labeling.

## Pharmacology/Pharmacokinetics

### Physicochemical characteristics
Molecular weight—454.44.

### Mechanism of action/Effect
Methotrexate is an antimetabolite of the folic acid analog type. Methotrexate is cell cycle–specific for the S phase of cell division. Activity is due to inhibition of DNA, RNA, thymidylate, and protein synthesis as a result of relatively irreversible binding with dihydrofolate reductase, which prevents reduction of dihydrofolate to the active tetrahydrofolate. Growth of rapidly proliferating cells (malignant cells, bone marrow, fetal cells, buccal and intestinal mucosa, cells of the urinary bladder, spermatogonia) is affected more than growth of most normal tissues and skin.

### Other actions/effects
Also has mild immunosuppressant activity.

### Absorption
Widely variable.

### Distribution
Crosses the blood-brain barrier (from blood to central nervous system [CNS]) in only limited amounts (dose-related); however, passes significantly into systemic circulation after intrathecal administration.

### Protein binding
Moderate (approximately 50%), primarily to albumin.

### Biotransformation
Hepatic; intracellular (to polyglutamates, which are retained in the cells).

### Half-life
Terminal—
    Low doses: 3 to 10 hours.
    High doses: 8 to 15 hours.
    Note: There is wide interindividual variation in clearance rates. Small amounts of methotrexate and metabolites are bound and may remain in tissues (kidneys, liver) for weeks to months; the presence of fluids such as ascites or pleural effusion will also delay clearance.

### Time to peak serum concentration:
Oral—1 to 2 hours.
Intramuscular—30 to 60 minutes.

### Elimination
Single dose—
    Renal (unchanged), 80 to 90% in the first 24 hours; some accumulation of polyglutamates in tissues occurs with repeated doses.
    Biliary, 10% or less.

## Precautions to Consider

### Carcinogenicity/Mutagenicity
Secondary malignancies are potential delayed effects of many antineoplastic agents, although it is not clear whether the effect is related to their mutagenic or immunosuppressive action. The effect of dose and duration of therapy is also unknown, although risk seems to increase with long-term use. Although information is limited, available data seem to indicate that the carcinogenic risk is greatest with the alkylating agents.
Antimetabolites have been shown to be carcinogenic in animals, and may be associated with an increased risk of development of secondary carcinomas in humans, although the risk appears to be less than with alkylating agents.
Carcinogenicity studies with methotrexate in animals have been inconclusive. However, there is evidence that methotrexate causes chromosomal damage to animal somatic cells and human bone marrow cells.

### Pregnancy/Reproduction
Fertility—Gonadal suppression, resulting in amenorrhea or azoospermia, may occur in patients taking antineoplastic therapy, especially with the alkylating agents. In general, these effects appear to be related to dose and length of therapy and may be irreversible. Prediction of the degree of testicular or ovarian function impairment is complicated by the common use of combinations of several antineoplastics, which makes it difficult to assess the effects of individual agents. Methotrexate appears to have only a slight effect on gonadal function; however, reversible impairment of fertility, defective oogenesis and spermatogenesis, and menstrual function impairment have been reported.

Pregnancy—Methotrexate crosses the placenta and has been shown to cause adverse effects on the fetus. Methotrexate is a potent abortifacient.

First trimester: It is usually recommended that use of antineoplastics, especially combination chemotherapy, be avoided whenever possible, especially during the first trimester. Although information is limited because of the relatively few instances of antineoplastic administration during pregnancy, the mutagenic, teratogenic, and carcinogenic potential of these medications must be considered.

Other hazards to the fetus include adverse reactions seen in adults.

In general, use of a contraceptive is recommended during cytotoxic drug therapy.

FDA Pregnancy Category X.

### Breast-feeding
Methotrexate is excreted in breast milk; breast-feeding is not recommended while methotrexate is being administered because of the risks to the infant (adverse effects, mutagenicity, carcinogenicity).

### Pediatrics
Caution should be used in neonates and infants because of reduced renal and hepatic function.

### Geriatrics
Although appropriate studies with methotrexate have not been performed in the geriatric population, caution should be used in the elderly because of possible reduced renal and hepatic function and reduced folate stores. Dosage adjustment, especially on the basis of renal function, may be necessary.

### Dental
The bone marrow depressant effects of methotrexate may result in an increased incidence of microbial infection, delayed healing, and gingival bleeding. Dental work, whenever possible, should be completed prior to initiation of therapy or deferred until blood counts have returned to normal. Patients should be instructed in proper oral hygiene during treatment, including caution in use of regular toothbrushes, dental floss, and toothpicks.
Methotrexate also commonly causes ulcerative stomatitits, gingivitis, and pharyngitis associated with considerable discomfort.

### Drug interactions and/or related problems
The following drug interactions and/or related problems have been selected on the basis of their potential clinical significance (possible mechanism in parentheses where appropriate)—not necessarily inclusive (» = major clinical significance):

Note: Combinations containing any of the following medications, depending on the amount present, may also interact with this medication.

» Acyclovir, parenteral
    (concurrent administration of intrathecal methotrexate with acyclovir may result in neurological abnormalities; use with caution)

» Alcohol or
» Hepatotoxic medications, other (See *Appendix II*)
    (concurrent use may increase the risk of hepatotoxicity)

Allopurinol or
Colchicine or

» Probenecid or
» Sulfinpyrazone
(methotrexate may raise the concentration of blood uric acid; dosage adjustment of antigout agents may be necessary to control hyperuricemia and gout; allopurinol may be preferred to prevent or reverse methotrexate-induced hyperuricemia because of risk of uric acid nephropathy with uricosuric antigout agents)

Anticoagulants, coumarin- or indandione-derivative
(methotrexate may increase anticoagulant activity and/or increase the risk of hemorrhage as a result of decreased hepatic synthesis of procoagulant factors and interference with platelet formation)

» Anti-inflammatory analgesics, nonsteroidal (NSAIAs)
(concurrent use of phenylbutazone with methotrexate may increase the risk of agranulocytosis or bone marrow depression and is not recommended; also, phenylbutazone may displace methotrexate from its protein-binding sites and decrease its renal clearance, leading to increased methotrexate plasma concentration and risk of toxicity, especially during high-dose methotrexate infusion therapy. If concurrent use with phenylbutazone cannot be avoided, especially careful monitoring of the patient for plasma methotrexate concentrations or signs of methotrexate toxicity and/or adequacy of renal function is recommended; also, phenylbutazone therapy should be discontinued for 7 to 12 days prior to, and for at least 12 hours [depending on plasma methotrexate concentrations] following, administration of a high-dose methotrexate infusion)

(administration of high-dose methotrexate infusions to patients receiving diflunisal or ketoprofen has resulted in severe and [with ketoprofen] sometimes fatal methotrexate toxicity; a few fatalities have also occurred in patients receiving intermediate-dose methotrexate infusions concurrently with indomethacin, possibly because of decreased methotrexate excretion leading to increased and prolonged methotrexate plasma concentration; however, severe methotrexate toxicity did not occur when ketoprofen was administered 12 hours following completion of the methotrexate infusion. It is recommended that NSAIA therapy be discontinued for 24 to 48 hours [for diflunisal] or 12 to 24 hours [for ketoprofen] prior to, and for at least 12 hours [depending on plasma methotrexate concentrations] following, a high-dose methotrexate infusion and that indomethacin be discontinued for 24 to 48 hours prior to, and for at least 12 hours [depending on plasma methotrexate concentrations] following, administration of an intermediate- or high-dose methotrexate infusion)

(although not well documented, the possibility exists that other NSAIAs may also decrease methotrexate excretion and increase its plasma concentration to potentially toxic levels; it is recommended that NSAIA therapy be discontinued for 12 to 24 hours [for NSAIAs with a short elimination half-life] to up to 10 days [for piroxicam] prior to, and for at least 12 hours [depending on plasma methotrexate concentrations] following, administration of a high-dose methotrexate infusion)

(severe, sometimes fatal, methotrexate toxicity has also been reported with low to moderate doses in patients receiving diclofenac, indomethacin, naproxen, or phenylbutazone; it is recommended that use of NSAIAs with low to moderate doses of methotrexate be undertaken with caution, with methotrexate dosage being adjusted by monitoring plasma methotrexate concentrations and/or adequacy of renal function)

» Asparaginase
(concurrent use may block the effects of methotrexate by inhibiting cell replication; this inhibition of methotrexate's action appears to correlate with suppression of asparagine concentrations. Some studies indicate that administration of asparaginase 9 to 10 days before or within 24 hours after methotrexate does not produce this inhibition of antineoplastic effect and may reduce the gastrointestinal and hematological effects of methotrexate)

Blood dyscrasia–causing medications (See *Appendix II*)
(leukopenic and/or thrombocytopenic effects of methotrexate may be increased with concurrent or recent therapy if these medications cause the same effects; dosage adjustment of methotrexate, if necessary, should be based on blood counts)

» Bone marrow depressants, other (See *Appendix II*) or
Radiation therapy
(additive bone marrow depression may occur; dosage reduction may be required when two or more bone marrow depressants, including radiation, are used concurrently or consecutively)

(leukoencephalopathy has been reported following intravenous methotrexate administration to patients who have received craniospinal irradiation)

Cytarabine
(administration of cytarabine 48 hours before or 10 minutes after initiation of methotrexate therapy may result in a synergistic cytotoxic effect; however, evidence is inconclusive and dosage adjustment based on routine hematologic monitoring is recommended)

Folic acid
(may interfere with the antifolate effects of methotrexate)

Neomycin, oral
(may decrease absorption of oral methotrexate)

» Probenecid
(concurrent use may inhibit renal excretion of methotrexate and result in toxic plasma concentrations; if used concurrently with probenecid, methotrexate dosage should be decreased, the patient observed for signs of toxicity, and/or plasma methotrexate concentrations monitored)

Pyrimethamine or
Triamterene or
Trimethoprim
(concurrent use may rarely increase the toxic effects of methotrexate because of similar folic acid antagonist actions)

» Salicylates and other weak organic acids
(concurrent use may inhibit renal tubular secretion of methotrexate and result in toxic plasma concentrations; salicylates may also increase plasma concentrations by displacing methotrexate from binding sites; if methotrexate is used concurrently with these medications, the patient should be observed for signs of toxicity and/or methotrexate plasma concentration monitored. In addition, it is recommended that salicylate therapy be discontinued for 24 to 48 hours prior to, and for at least 12 hours [depending on plasma methotrexate concentrations] following, administration of a high-dose methotrexate infusion)

Sulfonamides
(in addition to increased risk of hepatotoxicity that may occur when sulfonamides are used concurrently with other hepatotoxic medications, medications that cause displacement from plasma protein binding may theoretically produce toxic plasma concentrations of methotrexate when used concurrently, although clinical significance has not been established)

Vaccines, killed virus
(because normal defense mechanisms may be suppressed by methotrexate therapy, the patient's antibody response to the vaccine may be decreased. The interval between discontinuation of medications that cause immunosuppression and restoration of the patient's ability to respond to the vaccine depends on the intensity and type of immunosuppression-causing medication used, the underlying disease, and other factors; estimates vary from 3 months to 1 year)

» Vaccines, live virus
(because normal defense mechanisms may be suppressed by methotrexate therapy, concurrent use with a live virus vaccine may potentiate the replication of the vaccine virus, may increase the side/adverse effects of the vaccine virus, and/or may decrease the patient's antibody response to the vaccine; immunization of these patients should be undertaken only with extreme caution after careful review of the patient's hematologic status and only with the knowledge and consent of the physician managing the methotrexate therapy. The interval between discontinuation of medications that cause immunosuppression and restoration of the patient's ability to respond to the vaccine depends on the intensity and type of immunosuppression-causing medication used, the underlying disease, and other factors; estimates vary from 3 months to 1 year. Patients with leukemia in remission should not receive live virus vaccine until at least 3 months after their last chemotherapy. Immunization with oral poliovirus vaccine should also be postponed in persons in close contact with the patient, especially family members)

## Laboratory value alterations
The following have been selected on the basis of their potential clinical significance (possible effect in parentheses where appropriate)—not necessarily inclusive (» = major clinical significance):

With diagnostic test results
Assay for folate
(methotrexate may inhibit the organism used in the assay and interfere with detection of folic acid deficiency)

With physiology/laboratory test values
Isocitric acid dehydrogenase (ICD) concentrations
(may be increased, indicating hepatotoxicity)

Serum aspartate aminotransferase (AST [SGOT]) concentrations
(may be increased transiently during high-dose therapy)

Uric acid concentrations in blood and urine
(may be increased)

### Medical considerations/Contraindications

The medical considerations/contraindications included here have been selected on the basis of their potential clinical significance (reasons given
in parentheses where appropriate)—not necessarily inclusive (» =
major clinical significance).

*Except under special circumstances, this medication should not be used
when the following medical problem exists:*

» Immunodeficiency

*Risk-benefit should be considered when the following medical problems
exist:*

Aciduria (urine pH less than 7) or
» Ascites or
Dehydration or
Gastrointestinal obstruction or
» Pleural or peritoneal effusions or
» Renal function impairment
(risk of methotrexate toxicity is increased because elimination of
methotrexate may be impaired and accumulation may occur; even
small doses may lead to severe myelosuppression and mucositis;
larger doses and/or increased duration of leucovorin treatment, if
used, may be necessary, along with careful monitoring of methotrexate concentrations)

(a lower dosage of methotrexate and careful monitoring of plasma
or serum methotrexate concentrations are recommended for patients with impaired renal function)

» Bone marrow depression
» Chickenpox, existing or recent (including recent exposure) or
» Herpes zoster
(risk of severe generalized disease)
Gout, history of or
Urate renal stones, history of
(risk of hyperuricemia)
» Hepatic function impairment
» Infection
» Mucositis, oral
Nausea and vomiting
(inadequate hydration secondary to severe nausea and vomiting
may result in increased methotrexate toxicity)
» Peptic ulcer
Sensitivity to methotrexate
» Ulcerative colitis
» Caution should be used also in patients who have had previous cyto-
toxic drug therapy and radiation therapy, and in cases of general
debility.

### Patient monitoring

The following are especially important in patient monitoring (other tests
may be warranted in some patients, depending on condition; » =
major clinical significance):

» Blood urea nitrogen (BUN) concentrations and
Creatinine clearance and/or
» Serum creatinine concentrations
(recommended prior to initiation of therapy and at periodic intervals during therapy; frequency varies according to clinical state,
agent, dose, and other agents being used concurrently)

Bone marrow aspiration studies and
Liver biopsy
(may be useful during high-dose or long-term therapy or if hematologic or hepatic function test results are abnormal; also recommended in patients who have received a cumulative dose of
1500 mg)

Examination of patient's mouth for ulceration
(recommended before administration of each dose)

» Hematocrit or hemoglobin and
» Platelet count and
» Total and, if appropriate, differential leukocyte count
(determinations recommended prior to initiation of therapy and at
periodic intervals during therapy; frequency varies according to
clinical state, agent, dose, and other agents being used
concurrently)

» Serum alanine aminotransferase (ALT [SGPT]) concentrations and
» Serum aspartate aminotransferase (AST [SGOT]) concentrations and

» Serum bilirubin concentrations and
» Serum lactate dehydrogenase (LDH) concentrations
(recommended prior to initiation of therapy and at periodic intervals during therapy; frequency varies according to clinical state,
agent, dose, and other agents being used concurrently)

Serum uric acid concentrations
(recommended prior to initiation of therapy and at periodic intervals during therapy; frequency varies according to clinical state,
agent, dose, and other agents being used concurrently)

*For patients receiving high-dose methotrexate*

» Creatinine clearance determinations
(recommended prior to initiation of high-dose methotrexate with
leucovorin rescue therapy or if serum creatinine concentrations increase by 50% or more)

» Plasma or serum methotrexate concentrations
(recommended by some clinicians every 12 to 24 hours after high-
dose methotrexate administration to determine dose and duration
of leucovorin treatment needed to maintain rescue. May aid in
identifying patients with delayed methotrexate clearance; toxicity
appears to be related at least as much to the length of time that
methotrexate concentrations are elevated as to the peak concentrations achieved. In general, monitoring should continue until concentrations are less than $5 \times 10^{-8}$ *M*)

» Serum creatinine concentrations
(recommended prior to and every 24 hours after each methotrexate
dose, until plasma or serum methotrexate concentrations are less
than $5 \times 10^{-8} M$, to detect developing renal function impairment and
predict methotrexate toxicity. An increase of greater than 50% over
the pretreatment concentration at 24 hours is associated with severe
renal toxicity)

» Urine pH determinations
(recommended prior to each dose of high-dose methotrexate therapy
and about every 6 hours throughout leucovorin rescue, until plasma
or serum methotrexate concentrations are less than $5 \times 10^{-8} M$, to ensure
that pH remains greater than 7.0 so as to minimize the risk of methotrexate nephropathy from precipitation of methotrexate or metabolites
in the urine)

## Side/Adverse Effects

Note: Many "side effects" of antineoplastic therapy are unavoidable and
represent the medication's pharmacologic action. Some of these (for
example, leukopenia and thrombocytopenia) are actually used as
parameters to aid in individual dosage titration.

Incidence and severity of side effects, particularly hepatotoxicity,
appear to be related to dosage frequency and duration of methotrexate therapy. Toxicity tends to occur less frequently and be less
severe with a total dose administered as intermittent weekly dosage
than with prolonged daily dosage.

The following side/adverse effects have been selected on the basis of their
potential clinical significance (possible signs and symptoms in parentheses where appropriate)—not necessarily inclusive:

### Those indicating need for medical attention
Incidence more frequent
*Gastrointestinal ulceration and bleeding, enteritis, or intestinal per-
foration, which may be fatal* (black, tarry stools; bloody vomit; diarrhea; stomach pain); *leukopenia, bacterial infection, or septicemia*
(usually asymptomatic; less frequently, fever or chills; cough or
hoarseness; lower back or side pain; painful or difficult urination);
*thrombocytopenia* (usually asymptomatic; less frequently, unusual
bleeding or bruising; black, tarry stools; blood in urine or stools; pinpoint red spots on skin); *stomatitis, ulcerative, gingivitis, or pharyngitis* (sores in mouth and on lips)

Note: With *leukopenia* and *thrombocytopenia* the nadir of the leukocyte and platelet counts occurs after 7 to 10 days, with recovery
7 days later.

Incidence more frequent (with high-dose therapy)
*Renal failure, azotemia, hyperuricemia, or severe nephropathy*
(blood in urine; joint pain; swelling of feet or lower legs); *severe acute
methotrexate toxicity, cutaneous vasculitis, or reactivation of sunburn or increased erythematous response to ultraviolet therapy* (reddening of skin)

Note: *Hyperuricemia* and *uric acid nephropathy* occur most commonly during initial treatment of patients with leukemia or lymphoma, as a result of rapid cell breakdown which leads to elevated serum uric acid concentrations. With high-dose

methotrexate therapy, symptoms resembling uric acid nephropathy may also be due to renal tubular damage resulting from precipitation of methotrexate or metabolites in the urine.

Incidence less frequent, more frequent with prolonged daily therapy
*Hepatotoxicity, including liver atrophy, necrosis, cirrhosis, fatty changes, periportal fibrosis* (dark urine; yellow eyes or skin); *pneumonitis, potentially fatal, or pulmonary fibrosis* (cough; shortness of breath)

Incidence less frequent, more frequent with intrathecal or prolonged high-dose administration
*Central nervous system (CNS) effects, increased cerebrospinal fluid pressure, leukoencephalopathy, demyelination, or chemical arachnoiditis* (back pain; blurred vision; confusion; convulsions; dizziness; drowsiness; fever; headache; unusual tiredness or weakness)

**Those indicating need for medical attention only if they continue or are bothersome**
Incidence more frequent
*Loss of appetite; nausea or vomiting*

Incidence less frequent
*Acne; boils; pale skin; skin rash or itching*

**Those not indicating need for medical attention**
Incidence less frequent
*Loss of hair*

**Those indicating need for medical attention if they occur after medication is discontinued**
*CNS toxicity (encephalopathy, especially after intrathecal administration, or CNS leukemia)* (back pain; blurred vision; confusion; convulsions; dizziness; drowsiness; fever; headache; unusual tiredness or weakness)

## Patient Consultation

As an aid to patient consultation, refer to *Advice for the Patient, Methotrexate—For Cancer (Systemic)*.

In providing consultation, consider emphasizing the following selected information (» = major clinical significance):

**Before using this medication**
» Conditions affecting use, especially:
    Sensitivity to methotrexate
    Pregnancy—Use not recommended because of mutagenic, teratogenic, and carcinogenic potential; advisability of using contraception; telling physician immediately if pregnancy is suspected
    Breast-feeding—Not recommended because of risk of serious side effects
    Use in children—Newborns and other infants may be more sensitive to effects
    Use in the elderly—Side/adverse effects may be more frequent
    Other medications, especially alcohol or other hepatotoxic medications, probenecid, sulfinpyrazone, nonsteroidal anti-inflammatory drugs (NSAIDs), other bone marrow depressants, salicylates, or previous cytotoxic drug therapy or radiation therapy
    Other medical problems, especially chickenpox, herpes zoster, hepatic function impairment, renal function impairment, infection, oral mucositis, peptic ulcer, or ulcerative colitis

**Proper use of this medication**
» Importance of not taking more or less medication than the amount prescribed
    Caution in taking combination therapy; taking each medication at the right time
    Importance of ample fluid intake and subsequent increase in urine output to prevent nephrotoxicity and aid in excretion of uric acid
» Frequency of nausea and vomiting; importance of continuing medication despite stomach upset
    Checking with physician if vomiting occurs shortly after dose is taken
» Proper dosing
    Missed dose: Not taking at all; not doubling doses
» Proper storage

**Precautions while using this medication**
» Importance of close monitoring by physician
» Avoiding alcoholic beverages, which may increase hepatotoxicity
    Possible photosensitivity reactions; avoiding too much unprotected exposure to sun or overuse of sunlamp
» Avoiding salicylate-containing products and NSAIDs, which may increase toxicity
» Avoiding immunizations unless approved by physician; other persons in patient's household should avoid immunizations with oral poliovirus vaccine; avoiding other persons who have taken oral po-

liovirus vaccine or wearing a protective mask that covers nose and mouth

*Caution if bone marrow depression occurs:*
» Avoiding exposure to persons with bacterial infections, especially during periods of low blood counts; checking with physician immediately if fever or chills, cough or hoarseness, lower back or side pain, or painful or difficult urination occurs
» Checking with physician immediately if unusual bleeding or bruising; black, tarry stools; blood in urine or stools; or pinpoint red spots on skin occur
    Caution in use of regular toothbrush, dental floss, or toothpick; physician, dentist, or nurse may suggest alternatives; checking with physician before having dental work done
    Not touching eyes or inside of nose unless hands washed immediately before
    Using caution to avoid accidental cuts with use of sharp objects such as safety razor or fingernail or toenail cutters
    Avoiding contact sports or other situations where bruising or injury could occur

**Side/adverse effects**
    May cause adverse effects such as blood problems; stomach, kidney, or liver problems; loss of hair; or cancer; importance of discussing possible effects with physician
    Signs of potential side effects, especially gastrointestinal ulceration and bleeding, enteritis, intestinal perforation, leukopenia, bacterial infection, septicemia, thrombocytopenia, ulcerative stomatitis, gingivitis, pharyngitis, renal failure, azotemia, hyperuricemia, severe nephropathy, severe acute methotrexate toxicity, cutaneous vasculitis, reactivation of sunburn or reaction to ultraviolet light, hepatotoxicity, pneumonitis, pulmonary fibrosis, and CNS effects
    Physician or nurse can help in dealing with side effects
    Possibility of hair loss; should return after treatment has ended

## General Dosing Information

Patients receiving methotrexate should be under supervision of a physician experienced in antineoplastic chemotherapy.

A variety of dosage schedules and regimens of methotrexate, alone or in combination with other antitumor agents, are used. The prescriber may consult the medical literature as well as the manufacturer's literature in choosing a specific dosage.

Dosage must be adjusted to meet the individual requirements of each patient, based on clinical response and appearance or severity of toxicity.

In general, use of intermittent courses of methotrexate is associated with less risk of serious toxicity than prolonged daily dosage.

A significant amount of methotrexate passes into systemic circulation after intrathecal administration and may produce toxic levels in patients also receiving systemic methotrexate therapy; an adjustment in systemic dosage may be necessary.

Development of uric acid nephropathy in patients with leukemia or lymphoma may be prevented by adequate oral hydration and, in some cases, administration of allopurinol. Alkalinization of urine may be necessary if serum uric acid concentrations are elevated.

If severe bone marrow depression occurs, withdrawal of methotrexate may be necessary. However, in some patients with acute leukemia, methotrexate may be administered despite the presence of thrombocytopenia and bleeding; stoppage of bleeding and increase in platelet count have occurred during treatment in some cases and platelet transfusions may be useful in others.

Special precautions are recommended in patients who develop thrombocytopenia as a result of administration of methotrexate. These may include extreme care in performing invasive procedures; regular inspection of intravenous sites, skin (including perirectal area), and mucous membrane surfaces for signs of bleeding or bruising; limiting frequency of venipuncture and avoiding intramuscular injections; testing urine, emesis, stool, and secretions for occult blood; care in use of regular toothbrushes, dental floss, toothpicks, safety razors, and fingernail and toenail cutters; avoiding constipation; and using caution to prevent falls and other injuries. Such patients should avoid alcohol and any aspirin intake because of the risk of gastrointestinal bleeding. Platelet transfusions may be required.

Patients who develop leukopenia should be observed carefully for signs of infection. Antibiotic support may be required. In neutropenic patients who develop fever, broad-spectrum antibiotic coverage should be initiated empirically, pending bacterial cultures and appropriate diagnostic tests.

It is recommended that methotrexate therapy be interrupted if diarrhea or ulcerative stomatitis occurs, because of the risk of hemorrhagic enteritis and fatal intestinal perforation.

It is recommended that methotrexate therapy be interrupted if pulmonary symptoms (especially a dry, unproductive cough) occur, because of the risk of potentially irreversible pulmonary toxicity.

**For use in high-dose methotrexate therapy**

Because of its ability to bypass the effects of methotrexate, leucovorin calcium (folinic acid, citrovorum factor) is administered as a "rescue" from the hematologic and gastrointestinal effects of high-dosage methotrexate.

*High-dose methotrexate administration should not be initiated unless leucovorin is physically present and ready to be administered, since rescue is critical.*

Methotrexate administration should not be initiated unless creatinine clearance and serum creatinine concentrations are normal. If renal function impairment develops during therapy, methotrexate should be withdrawn until renal function becomes acceptable.

A variety of dosage schedules of leucovorin in combination with high-dose methotrexate have been used. The prescriber should consult the medical literature in choosing a specific dosage. Alkalinization of urine (with bicarbonate and/or acetazolamide) and intravenous hydration (1000 mL per square meter of body surface over six hours prior to beginning the methotrexate infusion and 3000 mL per square meter of body surface per day during the methotrexate infusion and for two days after the infusion is completed) are also important to prevent renal toxicity caused by methotrexate and/or its metabolites.

Administration of leucovorin should be consecutive to rather than simultaneous with methotrexate administration so as not to interfere with methotrexate's antineoplastic effects.

In general, it is recommended that the first dose of leucovorin be administered within the first 24 to 42 hours of starting a high-dose methotrexate infusion (within 1 hour of an overdose), in a dosage to produce blood concentrations equal to or greater than methotrexate blood concentrations (leucovorin in a dose of 15 to 25 mg per square meter of body surface produces peak plasma concentrations of approximately 1 micromolar or $1 \times 10^{-6}$ *M*). Duration of leucovorin administration varies with the dosage of methotrexate and plasma concentrations achieved (including rate of elimination); in general, leucovorin administration is continued until methotrexate concentrations fall to less than $5 \times 10^{-8}$ *M*.

A larger dose and/or longer duration of leucovorin treatment may be required in patients with aciduria, ascites, dehydration, gastrointestinal obstruction, pleural or peritoneal effusions, renal function impairment, or pleural or peritoneal effusions because excretion of methotrexate is slowed and the length of time for plasma methotrexate concentrations to decrease to nontoxic levels ($<5 \times 10^{-8}$ *M*) is increased. It is recommended that duration of leucovorin administration in these patients be based on determination of plasma methotrexate concentrations.

**For parenteral use**

Methotrexate may be administered intramuscularly, intravenously (rapid or continuous infusion), intrathecally, intra-arterially, or intraventricularly.

Caution is recommended in making sure that the appropriate diluent for the intended route of administration is used when preparing methotrexate for administration.

**Safety considerations for handling this medication**

There is limited but increasing evidence and concern that personnel involved in preparation and administration of parenteral antineoplastics may be at some risk because of the potential mutagenicity, teratogenicity, and/or carcinogenicity of these agents, although the actual risk is unknown. USP advisory panels recommend cautious handling both in preparation and disposal of antineoplastic agents. Precautions that have been suggested include:

• Use of a biological containment cabinet during reconstitution and dilution of parenteral medications and wearing of disposable surgical gloves and masks.

• Use of proper technique to prevent contamination of the medication, work area, and operator during transfer between containers (including proper training of personnel in this technique).

• Cautious and proper disposal of needles, syringes, vials, ampuls, and unused medication.

A number of medical centers have developed detailed guidelines for handling of antineoplastic agents.

**Combination chemotherapy**

Methotrexate may be used in combination with other agents in various regimens. As a result, incidence and/or severity of side effects may be altered and different dosages (usually reduced) may be used. For

example, methotrexate is part of the following chemotherapeutic combinations (some commonly used acronyms are in parentheses):

—cyclophosphamide, doxorubicin, methotrexate, and procarbazine (CAMP).

—cyclophosphamide, methotrexate, and lomustine (CMC-High dose).

—cyclophosphamide, methotrexate, and fluorouracil (CMF).

—cyclophosphamide, methotrexate, fluorouracil, and prednisone (CMFP).

—cyclophosphamide, methotrexate, fluorouracil, vincristine, and prednisone (CMFVP, Cooper's Regimen).

—methotrexate, doxorubicin, cyclophosphamide, and lomustine (MACC).

—methotrexate and mercaptopurine (MTX + MP).

—methotrexate, mercaptopurine, and cyclophosphamide (MTX + MP + CTX).

—methotrexate and fluorouracil.

For specific dosages and schedules, consult the literature. For information regarding each agent, consult the individual monographs.

# Oral Dosage Forms

## METHOTREXATE TABLETS USP

**Usual adult dose**

Choriocarcinoma or

Chorioadenoma destruens or

Hydatidiform mole—

Oral, 15 to 30 mg per day for five days, the course being repeated three to five times with one to two weeks between courses. Usually, one or two courses are given after normalization of urinary human chorionic gonadotropin (HCG) concentrations.

Acute lymphocytic leukemia—

Induction: Oral, 3.3 mg per square meter of body surface per day in combination with prednisone or other agents.

Maintenance: Oral, 30 mg per square meter of body surface per week.

Burkitt's lymphoma—

Stages I–II: Oral, 10 to 25 mg per day for four to eight days, the course being repeated several times with seven to ten days between courses.

Stage III: Oral, as for Stage I–II, in combination with other agents.

Lymphosarcoma (Stage III)—

Oral, 625 mcg (0.625 mg) to 2.5 mg per kg of body weight per day.

Mycosis fungoides—

Oral, 2.5 to 10 mg a day for weeks or months.

**Usual pediatric dose**

Antineoplastic—

Oral, 20 to 40 mg per square meter of body surface, once a week.

**Strength(s) usually available**

U.S.—

2.5 mg (Rx) [GENERIC].

Canada—

2.5 mg (Rx) [GENERIC].

**Packaging and storage**

Store below 40 °C (104 °F), preferably between 15 and 30 °C (59 and 86 °F), unless otherwise specified by manufacturer. Store in a well-closed container.

**Auxiliary labeling**

• Avoid alcoholic beverages.

• Do not take other medicines without advice from your doctor.

• Avoid overexposure to sun.

# Parenteral Dosage Forms

## METHOTREXATE SODIUM INJECTION USP

**Usual adult dose**

Choriocarcinoma or

Chorioadenoma destruens or

Hydatidiform mole—

Intramuscular, 15 to 30 mg (base) per day for five days, the course being repeated three to five times with one to two weeks between courses. Usually, one or two courses are given after normalization of urinary human chorionic gonadotropin (HCG) concentrations.

Acute lymphocytic leukemia—

Induction:

Intramuscular, 3.3 mg (base) per square meter of body surface per day in combination with prednisone or other agents.

Maintenance:

Intramuscular, 30 mg (base) per square meter of body surface per week; or

Intravenous, 2.5 mg (base) per kg of body weight every fourteen days.

Osteosarcoma—
  Intravenous infusion (over four hours), 12 grams (base) per square meter of body surface, followed by leucovorin rescue (usually 15 mg orally every six hours for ten doses starting at twenty-four hours after the methotrexate infusion is started), on weeks 4, 5, 6, 7, 11, 12, 15, 16, 29, 30, 44, and 45 after surgery on a combination chemotherapy schedule that also includes doxorubicin, cisplatin, bleomycin, cyclophosphamide, and dactinomycin. The dose may be increased, if necessary, to 15 grams (base) per square meter of body surface to achieve a peak serum methotrexate concentration of $1 \times 10^{-3}$ *M* per liter.

Note: *High-dose methotrexate administration should not be initiated unless leucovorin is physically present and ready to be administered, since rescue is critical.*

  If the patient is vomiting or cannot take oral medication, leucovorin may be administered intravenously or intramuscularly in the same dose as the oral dose.
Mycosis fungoides—
  Intramuscular, 50 mg (base) once a week or 25 mg (base) two times a week.

### Usual pediatric dose
Antineoplastic—
  Intramuscular, 20 to 40 mg (base) per square meter of body surface, once a week.

### Strength(s) usually available
U.S.—
  2.5 mg (base) per mL (Rx) [GENERIC (with preservative)].
  25 mg (base) per mL (Rx) [*Folex PFS* (without preservative); *Mexate-AQ* (with or without preservative); GENERIC (with and without preservative)].
Canada—
  2.5 mg (base) per mL (Rx) [GENERIC (with and without preservative)].
  10 mg (base) per mL (Rx) [GENERIC (without preservative)].
  25 mg (base) per mL (Rx) [GENERIC (with and without preservative)].

### Packaging and storage
Store below 40 °C (104 °F), preferably between 15 and 30 °C (59 and 86 °F), unless otherwise specified by manufacturer. Protect from light.

### Preparation of dosage form
Methotrexate Sodium Injection USP may be further diluted with an appropriate preservative-free medium such as 0.9% sodium chloride injection or 5% dextrose injection.

### Stability
If stored for 24 hours at a temperature of 21 to 25 °C (70 to 77 °F), a diluted solution of methotrexate sodium injection maintains 90% of its labeled potency. However, preservative-free solutions should be diluted immediately prior to use and any unused portion discarded.

## METHOTREXATE SODIUM FOR INJECTION USP

### Usual adult dose
Meningeal leukemia—
  Induction: Intrathecal, 12 mg (base) every two to five days until the cell count of the cerebrospinal fluid (CSF) returns to normal.
  Prophylaxis: Intrathecal, 12 mg (base) at an interval determined by consultation of the medical literature.
Choriocarcinoma or
Chorioadenoma destruens or
Hydatidiform mole—
  Intramuscular, 15 to 30 mg (base) per day for five days, the course being repeated three to five times with one to two weeks between courses. Usually, one or two courses are given after normalization of urinary human chorionic gonadotropin (HCG) concentrations.
Acute lymphocytic leukemia—
  Induction:
    Intramuscular, 3.3 mg (base) per square meter of body surface per day in combination with prednisone or other agents.
  Maintenance:
    Intramuscular, 30 mg (base) per square meter of body surface per week; or
    Intravenous, 2.5 mg (base) per kg of body weight every fourteen days.

Osteosarcoma—
  Intravenous infusion (over four hours), 12 grams (base) per square meter of body surface, followed by leucovorin rescue (usually 15 mg orally every six hours for ten doses starting at twenty-four hours after the methotrexate infusion is started), on weeks 4, 5, 6, 7, 11, 12, 15, 16, 29, 30, 44, and 45 after surgery on a combination chemotherapy schedule that also includes doxorubicin, cisplatin, bleomycin, cyclophosphamide, and dactinomycin. The dose may be increased, if necessary, to 15 grams (base) per square meter of body surface to achieve a peak serum methotrexate concentration of $1 \times 10^{-3}$ *M* per liter.

Note: *High-dose methotrexate administration should not be initiated unless leucovorin is physically present and ready to be administered, since rescue is critical.*

  If the patient is vomiting or cannot take oral medication, leucovorin may be administered intravenously or intramuscularly in the same dose as the oral dose.
Mycosis fungoides—
  Intramuscular, 50 mg (base) once a week or 25 mg (base) two times a week.

### Usual pediatric dose
Meningeal leukemia—
  For children up to 1 year of age: Intrathecal, 6 mg (base) every two to five days until the cell count of the CSF returns to normal.
  For children 1 year of age: Intrathecal, 8 mg (base) every two to five days until the cell count of the CSF returns to normal.
  For children 2 years of age: Intrathecal, 10 mg (base) every two to five days until the cell count of the CSF returns to normal.
  For children 3 years of age and over: Intrathecal, 12 mg (base) every two to five days until the cell count of the CSF returns to normal.
Antineoplastic, other—
  Intramuscular, 20 to 40 mg (base) per square meter of body surface, once a week.

### Size(s) usually available
U.S.—
  20 mg (base) (Rx) [*Mexate;* GENERIC (without preservative)].
  25 mg (base) (Rx) [*Folex* (without preservative)].
  50 mg (base) (Rx) [*Folex* (without preservative); *Mexate;* GENERIC (without preservative)].
  100 mg (base) (Rx) [*Folex* (without preservative); *Mexate;* GENERIC (without preservative)].
  250 mg (base) (Rx) [*Folex* (without preservative); *Mexate;* GENERIC (without preservative)].
  1 gram (base) (Rx) [GENERIC (without preservative)].
Canada—
  20 mg (base) (Rx) [GENERIC (without preservative)].

### Packaging and storage
Store below 40 °C (104 °F), preferably between 15 and 30 °C (59 and 86 °F), unless otherwise specified by manufacturer. Protect from light.

### Preparation of dosage form
For intrathecal use, methotrexate sodium for injection (containing no preservative) is recommended. It must be reconstituted immediately prior to use with an appropriate volume of a sterile, preservative-free medium such as 0.9% sodium chloride injection or Elliott's B solution to yield a solution containing 1 mg (base) per mL.
For intravenous or intramuscular use, methotrexate sodium for injection is diluted with 2 to 25 mL (depending on route of administration) of 0.9% sodium chloride injection (for *Folex*) or with 2 to 10 mL of sterile water for injection, 0.9% sodium chloride injection, or bacteriostatic water for injection with parabens or benzyl alcohol (for *Mexate*).

### Stability
Solutions without preservative should be freshly reconstituted immediately prior to each dose; any unused portion should be discarded. Solutions (for *Mexate*) prepared with Bacteriostatic Water for Injection USP with parabens or benzyl alcohol are stable for 4 weeks at 25 °C (77 °F) or for 3 months at 4 °C (39 °F) or −15 °C (5 °F).

---

Revised: 8/90
Interim revision: 07/08/93; 06/21/94

# METHOTREXATE—For Noncancerous Conditions  Systemic

VA CLASSIFICATION (Primary/Secondary): DE801/MS105

Another commonly used name is amethopterin.

Note: For a listing of dosage forms and brand names by country availability, see *Dosage Forms* section(s). For a listing of brand names for the articles in this monograph, refer to the General Index.

## Category

Antipsoriatic (systemic); antirheumatic (disease-modifying).

## Indications

Note: Bracketed information in the *Indications* section refers to uses that are not included in U.S. product labeling.

### Accepted

Psoriasis (treatment)—Methotrexate is indicated only for treatment of severe, recalcitrant, disabling psoriasis not adequately responsive to other forms of therapy, as confirmed by biopsy and/or dermatologic consultation. Methotrexate is contraindicated in pregnant psoriatic patients and those with existing severe renal or hepatic disease or pre-existing blood dyscrasias.

Arthritis, rheumatoid (treatment)—Methotrexate tablets are indicated [and the parenteral dosage forms are used][1] in the treatment of selected cases of severe rheumatoid arthritis not adequately responsive to other forms of therapy, as confirmed by rheumatologic consultation. Methotrexate is contraindicated in pregnant rheumatoid arthritis patients and those with existing renal or hepatic disease or pre-existing blood dyscrasias.

[Arthritis, psoriatic (treatment)][1]—Methotrexate is being used in the treatment of selected cases of active severe psoriatic arthritis.

[Dermatomyositis, systemic (treatment)][1]—Methotrexate is used for treatment of systemic dermatomyositis (polymyositis).

Caution is recommended in use of methotrexate for non-neoplastic conditions because of potential toxicity with long-term use of this agent.

[1]Not included in Canadian product labeling.

## Pharmacology/Pharmacokinetics

### Physicochemical characteristics
Molecular weight—454.44.

### Mechanism of action/Effect
Methotrexate is an antimetabolite of the folic acid analog type. Methotrexate is cell cycle–specific for the S phase of cell division. Activity is due to inhibition of DNA, RNA, thymidylate, and protein synthesis as a result of relatively irreversible binding with dihydrofolate reductase, which prevents reduction of dihydrofolate to the active tetrahydrofolate. Growth of rapidly proliferating cells (epithelial cells in psoriasis, bone marrow, fetal cells, buccal and intestinal mucosa, cells of the urinary bladder, spermatogonia) is affected more than growth of most normal tissues and skin.

### Other actions/effects
Also has mild immunosuppressant activity.

### Absorption
Widely variable.

### Distribution
Crosses the blood-brain barrier (from blood to central nervous system [CNS]) in only limited amounts (dose-related); however, passes significantly into systemic circulation after intrathecal administration.

### Protein binding
Moderate (approximately 50%), primarily to albumin.

### Biotransformation
Hepatic; intracellular (to polyglutamates, which are retained in the cells).

### Half-life
Terminal—
    Low doses: 3 to 10 hours.
    High doses: 8 to 15 hours.
    Note: There is wide interindividual variation in clearance rates. Small amounts of methotrexate and metabolites are bound and may remain in tissues (kidneys, liver) for weeks to months; the presence of fluids such as ascites or pleural effusion will also delay clearance.

### Time to peak serum concentration
Oral—1 to 2 hours.
Intramuscular—30 to 60 minutes.

### Elimination
Single dose—
    Renal (unchanged), 80 to 90% in the first 24 hours; some accumulation of polyglutamates in tissues occurs with repeated doses.
    Biliary, 10% or less.

## Precautions to Consider

### Carcinogenicity/Mutagenicity
Secondary malignancies are potential delayed effects of many antineoplastic agents, although it is not clear whether the effect is related to their mutagenic or immunosuppressive action. The effect of dose and duration of therapy is also unknown, although risk seems to increase with long-term use. Although information is limited, available data seem to indicate that the carcinogenic risk is greatest with the alkylating agents.

Antimetabolites have been shown to be carcinogenic in animals, and may be associated with an increased risk of development of secondary carcinomas in humans, although the risk appears to be less than with alkylating agents.

Carcinogenicity studies with methotrexate in animals have been inconclusive. However, there is evidence that methotrexate causes chromosomal damage to animal somatic cells and human bone marrow cells.

### Pregnancy/Reproduction
Fertility—Methotrexate appears to have only a slight effect on gonadal function; however, reversible impairment of fertility, defective oogenesis and spermatogenesis, and menstrual function impairment have been reported.

Pregnancy—Methotrexate crosses the placenta and has been shown to cause adverse effects on the fetus. Methotrexate is a potent abortifacient.

Use as an antipsoriatic or antiarthritic agent is contraindicated in pregnant women.

FDA Pregnancy Category X.

### Breast-feeding
Methotrexate is excreted in breast milk; breast-feeding is not recommended while methotrexate is being administered because of the risks to the infant (adverse effects, mutagenicity, carcinogenicity).

### Pediatrics
Caution should be used in neonates and infants because of reduced renal and hepatic function.

### Geriatrics
Although appropriate studies with methotrexate have not been performed in the geriatric population, caution should be used in the elderly because of possible reduced renal and hepatic function and reduced folate stores. Dosage adjustment, especially on the basis of renal function, may be necessary.

### Dental
The bone marrow depressant effects of methotrexate may result in an increased incidence of microbial infection, delayed healing, and gingival bleeding. Dental work, whenever possible, should be completed prior to initiation of therapy or deferred until blood counts have returned to normal. Patients should be instructed in proper oral hygiene during treatment, including caution in use of regular toothbrushes, dental floss, and toothpicks.

Methotrexate also commonly causes ulcerative stomatitits, gingivitis, and pharyngitis associated with considerable discomfort.

### Drug interactions and/or related problems
The following drug interactions and/or related problems have been selected on the basis of their potential clinical significance (possible mechanism in parentheses where appropriate)—not necessarily inclusive (» = major clinical significance):

Note: Combinations containing any of the following medications, depending on the amount present, may also interact with this medication.

» Alcohol or
» Hepatotoxic medications, other (See *Appendix II* )
    (concurrent use may increase the risk of hepatotoxicity)

Anticoagulants, coumarin- or indandione-derivative
(methotrexate may increase anticoagulant activity and/or increase the risk of hemorrhage as a result of decreased hepatic synthesis of procoagulant factors and interference with platelet formation)

» Anti-inflammatory analgesics, nonsteroidal (NSAIAs)
(concurrent use of phenylbutazone with methotrexate may increase the risk of agranulocytosis or bone marrow depression and is not recommended; also, phenylbutazone may displace methotrexate from its protein-binding sites and decrease its renal clearance, leading to increased methotrexate plasma concentration and risk of toxicity. If concurrent use with phenylbutazone cannot be avoided, especially careful monitoring of the patient for plasma methotrexate concentrations or signs of methotrexate toxicity and/or adequacy of renal function is recommended)

(although not well documented, the possibility exists that other NSAIAs may also decrease methotrexate excretion and increase its plasma concentration to potentially toxic levels)

(severe, sometimes fatal, methotrexate toxicity has also been reported with low to moderate doses in patients receiving diclofenac, indomethacin, naproxen, or phenylbutazone; it is recommended that use of NSAIAs with low to moderate doses of methotrexate be undertaken with caution, with methotrexate dosage being adjusted by monitoring plasma methotrexate concentrations and/or adequacy of renal function)

Blood dyscrasia–causing medications (See *Appendix II*)
(leukopenic and/or thrombocytopenic effects of methotrexate may be increased with concurrent or recent therapy if these medications cause the same effects; dosage adjustment of methotrexate, if necessary, should be based on blood counts)

» Bone marrow depressants, other (See *Appendix II*) or
Radiation therapy
(additive bone marrow depression may occur; dosage reduction may be required when two or more bone marrow depressants, including radiation, are used concurrently or consecutively)

Folic acid
(may interfere with the antifolate effects of methotrexate)

Neomycin, oral
(may decrease absorption of oral methotrexate)

» Probenecid
(concurrent use may inhibit renal excretion of methotrexate and result in toxic plasma concentrations; if used concurrently with probenecid, methotrexate dosage should be decreased, the patient observed for signs of toxicity, and/or plasma methotrexate concentrations monitored)

Pyrimethamine or
Triamterene or
Trimethoprim
(concurrent use may rarely increase the toxic effects of methotrexate because of similar folic acid antagonist actions)

» Salicylates and other weak organic acids
(concurrent use may inhibit renal tubular secretion of methotrexate and result in toxic plasma concentrations; salicylates may also increase plasma concentrations by displacing methotrexate from binding sites; if methotrexate is used concurrently with these medications, the patient should be observed for signs of toxicity and/or methotrexate plasma concentration monitored)

Sulfonamides
(in addition to increased risk of hepatotoxicity that may occur when sulfonamides are used concurrently with other hepatotoxic medications, medications that cause displacement from plasma protein binding may theoretically produce toxic plasma concentrations of methotrexate when used concurrently, although clinical significance has not been established)

Vaccines, killed virus
(because normal defense mechanisms may be suppressed by methotrexate therapy, the patient's antibody response to the vaccine may be decreased. The interval between discontinuation of medications that cause immunosuppression and restoration of the patient's ability to respond to the vaccine depends on the intensity and type of immunosuppression-causing medication used, the underlying disease, and other factors; estimates vary from 3 months to 1 year)

» Vaccines, live virus
(because normal defense mechanisms may be suppressed by methotrexate therapy, concurrent use with a live virus vaccine may potentiate the replication of the vaccine virus, may increase the side/adverse effects of the vaccine virus, and/or may decrease the patient's antibody response to the vaccine; immunization of these patients should be undertaken only with extreme caution after careful review of the patient's hematologic status and only with the knowledge and consent of the physician managing the methotrexate therapy. The interval between discontinuation of medications that cause immunosuppression and restoration of the patient's ability to respond to the vaccine depends on the intensity and type of immunosuppression-causing medication used, the underlying disease, and other factors; estimates vary from 3 months to 1 year. Immunization with oral poliovirus vaccine should also be postponed in persons in close contact with the patient, especially family members)

### Laboratory value alterations
The following have been selected on the basis of their potential clinical significance (possible effect in parentheses where appropriate)—not necessarily inclusive (» = major clinical significance):

With diagnostic test results
Assay for folate
(methotrexate may inhibit the organism used in the assay and interfere with detection of folic acid deficiency)

With physiology/laboratory test values
Isocitric acid dehydrogenase (ICD) concentrations
(may be increased, indicating hepatotoxicity)

### Medical considerations/Contraindications
The medical considerations/contraindications included here have been selected on the basis of their potential clinical significance (reasons given in parentheses where appropriate)—not necessarily inclusive (» = major clinical significance).

*Except under special circumstances, this medication should not be used when the following medical problems exist:*

» Bone marrow depression

» Hepatic function impairment, severe

» Immunodeficiency

» Renal function impairment, severe

*Risk-benefit should be considered when the following medical problems exist:*

» Ascites or
Gastrointestinal obstruction or

» Pleural or peritoneal effusions or

» Renal function impairment
(risk of methotrexate toxicity is increased because elimination of methotrexate may be impaired and accumulation may occur; even small doses may lead to severe myelosuppression and mucositis)

(a lower dosage of methotrexate and careful monitoring of plasma or serum methotrexate concentrations are recommended for patients with impaired renal function)

» Chickenpox, existing or recent (including recent exposure) or

» Herpes zoster
(risk of severe generalized disease)

» Hepatic function impairment

» Infection

» Mucositis, oral

Nausea and vomiting
(inadequate hydration secondary to severe nausea and vomiting may result in increased methotrexate toxicity)

» Peptic ulcer

Sensitivity to methotrexate

» Ulcerative colitis

» Caution should be used also in patients who have had previous cytotoxic drug therapy and radiation therapy, and in cases of general debility.

### Patient monitoring
The following are especially important in patient monitoring (other tests may be warranted in some patients, depending on condition; » = major clinical significance):

Blood urea nitrogen (BUN) concentrations and
Creatinine clearance and/or
Serum creatinine concentrations
(recommended prior to initiation of therapy and at periodic intervals during therapy; frequency varies according to clinical state, agent, dose, and other agents being used concurrently)

Examination of patient's mouth for ulceration
(recommended before administration of each dose)

» Hematocrit or hemoglobin and
» Platelet count and
» Total and, if appropriate, differential leukocyte count
   (determinations recommended prior to initiation of therapy and at periodic intervals during therapy; frequency varies according to clinical state, agent, dose, and other agents being used concurrently)

Liver biopsy
   (may be useful during long-term therapy or if hepatic function test results are abnormal; also recommended in patients who have received a cumulative dose of 1500 mg)

» Serum alanine aminotransferase (ALT [SGPT]) concentrations and
» Serum aspartate aminotransferase (AST [SGOT]) concentrations and
» Serum bilirubin concentrations and
» Serum lactate dehydrogenase (LDH) concentrations
   (recommended prior to initiation of therapy and at periodic intervals during therapy; frequency varies according to clinical state, agent, dose, and other agents being used concurrently)

## Side/Adverse Effects

Note: Incidence and severity of side effects, particularly hepatotoxicity, appear to be related to dosage frequency and duration of methotrexate therapy. Toxicity tends to occur less frequently and be less severe with a total dose administered as intermittent weekly dosage than with prolonged daily dosage.

The following side/adverse effects have been selected on the basis of their potential clinical significance (possible signs and symptoms in parentheses where appropriate)—not necessarily inclusive:

### Those indicating need for medical attention
Incidence less frequent
   *Gastrointestinal ulceration and bleeding, enteritis, or intestinal perforation, which may be fatal* (diarrhea; stomach pain); *leukopenia, bacterial infection, or septicemia* (usually asymptomatic; rarely, fever or chills; cough or hoarseness; lower back or side pain; painful or difficult urination); *thrombocytopenia* (usually asymptomatic; rarely, unusual bleeding or bruising; black, tarry stools; blood in urine or stools; pinpoint red spots on skin); *severe acute methotrexate toxicity, cutaneous vasculitis, or reactivation of sunburn or increased erythematous response to ultraviolet therapy* (reddening of skin); *ulcerative stomatitis, gingivitis, or pharyngitis* (sores in mouth and on lips)

   Note: With *leukopenia* and *thrombocytopenia*, the nadir of the leukocyte and platelet counts occurs after 7 to 10 days, with recovery 7 days later.

Incidence rare—dose-related
   *Central nervous system (CNS) effects, increased cerebrospinal fluid pressure, leukoencephalopathy, demyelination, or chemical arachnoiditis* (back pain; blurred vision; convulsions; dizziness; drowsiness; fever; headache; unusual tiredness or weakness); *hepatotoxicity, including liver atrophy; necrosis; cirrhosis; fatty changes; periportal fibrosis* (yellow eyes or skin); *pneumonitis, potentially fatal, or pulmonary fibrosis* (cough; shortness of breath)

### Those indicating need for medical attention only if they continue or are bothersome
Incidence less frequent or rare
   *Acne; boils; loss of appetite; nausea; pale skin; skin rash or itching; vomiting*

### Those not indicating need for medical attention
Incidence less frequent or rare
   *Loss of hair*

## Patient Consultation

As an aid to patient consultation, refer to *Advice for the Patient, Methotrexate—For Noncancerous Conditions (Systemic)*.

In providing consultation, consider emphasizing the following selected information (» = major clinical significance):

### Before using this medication
» Conditions affecting use, especially:
   Sensitivity to methotrexate
   Pregnancy—Use not recommended because of teratogenic, abortifacient, and carcinogenic potential; advisability of using contraception; telling physician immediately if pregnancy is suspected
   Breast-feeding—Not recommended because of risk of serious side effects
   Use in children—Newborns and other infants may be more sensitive to effects
   Use in the elderly—Side/adverse effects may be more frequent

Other medications, especially alcohol or other hepatotoxic medications, nonsteroidal anti-inflammatory drugs (NSAIDs), other bone marrow depressants, probenecid, salicylates, or previous cytotoxic drug therapy or radiation therapy
Other medical problems, especially hepatic function impairment, renal function impairment, chickenpox, herpes zoster, infection, oral mucositis, peptic ulcer, or ulcerative colitis

### Proper use of this medication
» Importance of not taking more or less medication than the amount prescribed
» Frequency of nausea; importance of continuing medication despite stomach upset; checking with physician if vomiting occurs
   Checking with physician if vomiting occurs shortly after dose is taken
» Proper dosing
   Missed dose: Not taking at all; not doubling doses
» Proper storage

### Precautions while using this medication
» Importance of close monitoring by the physician
» Avoiding alcoholic beverages, which may increase hepatotoxicity
   Possible photosensitivity reactions; avoiding too much unprotected exposure to sun or overuse of sunlamp
» Avoiding salicylate-containing products and NSAIDs, which may increase toxicity
» Avoiding immunizations unless approved by physician; other persons in patient's household should avoid immunizations with oral poliovirus vaccine; avoiding other persons who have taken oral poliovirus vaccine or wearing a protective mask that covers nose and mouth
*Caution if bone marrow depression occurs*
» Avoiding exposure to persons with bacterial infections, especially during periods of low blood counts; checking with physician immediately if fever or chills, cough or hoarseness, lower back or side pain, or painful or difficult urination occurs
» Checking with physician immediately if unusual bleeding or bruising; black, tarry stools; blood in urine or stools; or pinpoint red spots on skin occur
   Caution in use of regular toothbrush, dental floss, or toothpick; physician, dentist, or nurse may suggest alternatives; checking with physician before having dental work done
   Not touching eyes or inside of nose unless hands washed immediately before
   Using caution to avoid accidental cuts with use of sharp objects such as safety razor or fingernail or toenail cutters
   Avoiding contact sports or other situations where bruising or injury could occur

### Side/adverse effects
   May cause adverse effects such as blood problems; stomach, kidney, or liver problems; loss of hair; or cancer; importance of discussing possible effects with physician
   Signs of potential side effects, especially gastrointestinal ulceration and bleeding, enteritis, intestinal perforation, leukopenia, bacterial infection, septicemia, thrombocytopenia, severe acute methotrexate toxicity, cutaneous vasculitis, reactivation of sunburn or reaction to ultraviolet light, ulcerative stomatitis, gingivitis, pharyngitis, CNS effects, hepatotoxicity, pneumonitis, and pulmonary fibrosis
   Physician or nurse can help in dealing with side effects
   Possibility of hair loss; should return after treatment has ended

## General Dosing Information

Patients receiving methotrexate should be under supervision of a physician experienced in antimetabolite chemotherapy.

In general, use of intermittent courses of methotrexate is associated with less risk of serious toxicity than prolonged daily dosage.

It is recommended that methotrexate therapy be interrupted if diarrhea or ulcerative stomatitis occurs, because of the risk of hemorrhagic enteritis and fatal intestinal perforation.

It is recommended that methotrexate therapy be interrupted if pulmonary symptoms (especially a dry, unproductive cough) occur, because of the risk of potentially irreversible pulmonary toxicity.

If bone marrow depression occurs, withdrawal of methotrexate is recommended. The following precautions may also be useful:
• Special precautions are recommended in patients who develop thrombocytopenia as a result of administration of methotrexate. These may include extreme care in performing invasive procedures; regular inspection of intravenous sites, skin (including perirectal area), and mucous membrane surfaces for signs of bleeding or bruising; limiting frequency of venipuncture and avoiding intramuscular injections; testing urine, emesis, stool, and secretions for occult blood; care in use of regular toothbrushes, dental floss, toothpicks, safety razors, and fin-

gernail and toenail cutters; avoiding constipation; and using caution to prevent falls and other injuries. Such patients should avoid alcohol and any aspirin intake because of the risk of gastrointestinal bleeding. Platelet transfusions may be required.
• Patients who develop leukopenia should be observed carefully for signs of infection. Antibiotic support may be required. In neutropenic patients who develop fever, broad-spectrum antibiotic coverage should be initiated empirically, pending bacterial cultures and appropriate diagnostic tests.

### For use as an antipsoriatic
After a favorable response is obtained, it is recommended that the dosage be decreased gradually to the lowest dosage and longest rest period that will maintain an adequate clinical response. To reduce the methotrexate requirement, it is recommended that an attempt be made to return to conventional therapy or to concomitant topical conventional therapy as soon as possible.

### For use as an antirheumatic
Methotrexate appears to be effective by the oral, intramuscular, or intravenous route; however, oral administration is associated with less toxicity.

### For parenteral use
Methotrexate may be administered intramuscularly or intravenously (rapid or continuous infusion).

### Safety considerations for handling this medication
There is limited but increasing evidence and concern that personnel involved in preparation and administration of parenteral cytotoxic agents may be at some risk because of the potential mutagenicity, teratogenicity, and/or carcinogenicity of these agents, although the actual risk is unknown. USP advisory panels recommend cautious handling both in preparation and disposal of antineoplastic agents. Precautions that have been suggested include:
• Use of a biological containment cabinet during reconstitution and dilution of parenteral medications and wearing of disposable surgical gloves and masks.
• Use of proper technique to prevent contamination of the medication, work area, and operator during transfer between containers (including proper training of personnel in this technique).
• Cautious and proper disposal of needles, syringes, vials, ampuls, and unused medication.
A number of medical centers have developed detailed guidelines for handling of antineoplastic agents.

## Oral Dosage Forms
Note: Bracketed uses in the *Dosage Forms* section refer to categories of use and/or indications that are not included in U.S. product labeling.

### METHOTREXATE TABLETS USP
**Usual adult dose**
Psoriasis or
Rheumatoid arthritis or
[Psoriatic arthritis][1]—
  Oral, initially 2.5 to 5 mg every twelve hours for three doses once a week, the dosage being increased as necessary in increments of 2.5 mg per week up to a maximum of 20 mg per week; or
  Oral, initially 10 mg once a week, the dosage being increased as necessary up to 25 mg once a week.
Note: Some clinicians recommend an initial test dose at the lowest dosage level because of interindividual variation in sensitivity to methotrexate.

**Usual pediatric dose**
Dosage has not been established.

**Strength(s) usually available**
U.S.—
  2.5 mg (Rx) [*Rheumatrex;* GENERIC].
Canada—
  2.5 mg (Rx) [*Rheumatrex;* GENERIC].

**Packaging and storage**
Store below 40 °C (104 °F), preferably between 15 and 30 °C (59 and 86 °F), unless otherwise specified by manufacturer. Store in a well-closed container.

**Auxiliary labeling**
• Avoid alcoholic beverages.
• Do not take other medicines without advice from your doctor.
• Avoid overexposure to sun.

## Parenteral Dosage Forms
### METHOTREXATE SODIUM INJECTION USP
**Usual adult dose**
Psoriasis or
[Rheumatoid arthritis][1]—Intramuscular or intravenous, initially 10 mg (base) once a week, the dosage being increased as necessary up to 25 mg (base) once a week.
Note: Some clinicians recommend an initial test dose of 10 mg because of interindividual variation in sensitivity to methotrexate.

**Usual pediatric dose**
Dosage has not been established.

**Strength(s) usually available**
U.S.—
  2.5 mg (base) per mL (Rx) [GENERIC (with preservative)].
  25 mg (base) per mL (Rx) [*Folex PFS* (without preservative); *Mexate-AQ* (with or without preservative); GENERIC (with and without preservative)].
Canada—
  2.5 mg (base) per mL (Rx) [GENERIC (with and without preservative)].
  10 mg (base) per mL (Rx) [GENERIC (without preservative)].
  25 mg (base) per mL (Rx) [GENERIC (with and without preservative)].

**Packaging and storage**
Store below 40 °C (104 °F), preferably between 15 and 30 °C (59 and 86 °F), unless otherwise specified by manufacturer. Protect from light.

**Preparation of dosage form**
Methotrexate Sodium Injection USP may be further diluted with an appropriate preservative-free medium such as 0.9% sodium chloride injection or 5% dextrose injection.

**Stability**
If stored for 24 hours at a temperature of 21 to 25 °C (70 to 77 °F), a diluted solution of methotrexate sodium injection maintains 90% of its labeled potency. However, preservative-free solutions should be diluted immediately prior to use and any unused portion discarded.

### METHOTREXATE SODIUM FOR INJECTION USP
**Usual adult dose**
Psoriasis or
[Rheumatoid arthritis][1]—Intramuscular or intravenous, initially 10 mg (base) once a week, the dosage being increased as necessary up to 25 mg (base) once a week.
Note: Some clinicians recommend an initial test dose of 10 mg because of interindividual variation in sensitivity to methotrexate.

**Usual pediatric dose**
Dosage has not been established.

**Size(s) usually available**
U.S.—
  20 mg (base) (Rx) [*Mexate;* GENERIC (without preservative)].
  25 mg (base) (Rx) [*Folex* (without preservative)].
  50 mg (base) (Rx) [*Folex* (without preservative); *Mexate;* GENERIC (without preservative)].
  100 mg (base) (Rx) [*Folex* (without preservative); *Mexate;* GENERIC (without preservative)].
  250 mg (base) (Rx) [*Folex* (without preservative); *Mexate;* GENERIC (without preservative)].
  1 gram (base) [GENERIC (without preservative)].
Canada—
  20 mg (base) (Rx) [GENERIC (without preservative)].

**Packaging and storage**
Store below 40 °C (104 °F), preferably between 15 and 30 °C (59 and 86 °F), unless otherwise specified by manufacturer. Protect from light.

**Preparation of dosage form**
For intravenous or intramuscular use, methotrexate sodium for injection is diluted with 2 to 25 mL (depending on route of administration) of 0.9% sodium chloride injection (for *Folex*) or with 2 to 10 mL of sterile water for injection, 0.9% sodium chloride injection, or bacteriostatic water for injection with parabens or benzyl alcohol (for *Mexate*).

**Stability**
Solutions without preservative should be freshly reconstituted immediately prior to each dose; any unused portion should be discarded. Solutions (for *Mexate*) prepared with Bacteriostatic Water for Injection USP with parabens or benzyl alcohol are stable for 4 weeks at 25 °C (77 °F) or for 3 months at 4 °C (39 °F) or −15 °C (5 °F).

[1]Not included in Canadian product labeling.

Revised: 08/90
Interim revision: 07/08/93; 07/05/94

---

**METHOTRIMEPRAZINE—**See *Phenothiazines (Systemic)*

---

**METHOXAMINE—**See *Sympathomimetic Agents—Cardiovascular Use (Parenteral-Systemic)*

---

# METHOXSALEN  Systemic

VA CLASSIFICATION (Primary/Secondary): DE801/DE890; AN900

Note: **Methoxsalen soft gelatin capsules should not be used interchangeably with the hard gelatin capsules, since the soft gelatin capsule dosage form exhibits significantly greater bioavailability and earlier photosensitization onset time than does the hard gelatin capsule dosage form.**

Note: For a listing of dosage forms and brand names by country availability, see *Dosage Forms* section(s). For a listing of brand names for the articles in this monograph, refer to the General Index.

## Category

Repigmenting agent (systemic); antipsoriatic (systemic); antineoplastic; hair growth stimulant, alopecia areata (systemic).

Note: Methoxsalen is used in conjunction with ultraviolet light A (UVA). This mode of treatment is known as PUVA (psoralen plus ultraviolet light A).

**Methoxsalen soft gelatin capsules should not be used interchangeably with the hard gelatin capsules,** since the soft gelatin capsule dosage form exhibits significantly greater bioavailability and earlier photosensitization onset time than does the hard gelatin capsule dosage form.

## Indications

Note: Bracketed information in the *Indications* section refers to uses that are not included in U.S. product labeling.

**Accepted**

Psoriasis (treatment)—PUVA, using methoxsalen hard gelatin capsules or soft gelatin capsules, is indicated in the treatment of severe, refractory, disabling psoriasis that has not responded to other therapy.

Vitiligo (treatment)—PUVA, using methoxsalen hard gelatin capsules [or soft gelatin capsules], is indicated for repigmentation in the treatment of vitiligo. PUVA is not effective in producing pigmentation in leukoderma of infectious origin or in albinism.

Mycosis fungoides (treatment)[1]—Photopheresis (using methoxsalen hard gelatin capsules [or soft gelatin capsules] with ultraviolet radiation of white blood cells) is indicated for use with the UVAR System in the palliative treatment of the skin manifestations of mycosis fungoides (also known as cutaneous T-cell lymphoma) in persons who have not been responsive to other forms of treatment. [PUVA is also used in the treatment of mycosis fungoides.][1]

[Alopecia areata (treatment)][1]
[Atopic dermatitis (treatment)]
[Dermatoses, inflammatory (treatment)][1]
[Eczema (treatment)][1]
[Lichen planus (treatment)][1] or
[Skin, increased tolerance to sunlight][1]—PUVA is also used in the treatment of alopecia areata, atopic dermatitis, inflammatory dermatoses, eczema, and lichen planus. PUVA is also used to increase skin tolerance to sunlight.

**Unaccepted**

The unsupervised use of methoxsalen to promote tanning is dangerous and should be discouraged.

[1]Not included in Canadian product labeling.

## Pharmacology/Pharmacokinetics

**Physicochemical characteristics**
Molecular weight—216.19.

**Mechanism of action/Effect**
Methoxsalen is a psoralen derivative with photosensitizing activity. Exact mechanism of erythemogenic, melanogenic, and cytotoxic response in the epidermis is unknown, but may involve increased tyrosinase activity in melanin-producing cells, as well as inhibition of DNA synthesis, cell division, and epidermal turnover. Successful pigmentation requires the presence of functioning melanocytes.

**Absorption**
Methoxsalen is variably (approximately 95%) absorbed from the gastrointestinal tract. It has been postulated that poor response in some patients may be due to poor absorption.

**Protein binding**
High.

**Biotransformation**
Activated by long-wavelength UVA in the range of 320 to 400 nanometers (nm). Further metabolism: hepatic.

**Half-life**
Hard gelatin capsule—1.1 hours.
Soft gelatin capsule—Approximately 2 hours.

**Onset of action**
Vitiligo—Up to 6 months or longer.
Psoriasis—30 treatments (10 weeks or longer).
For increased sensitivity of skin to sunlight—1 hour.
Tanning—Within a few days.

**Time to peak photosensitivity**
Hard gelatin capsule—3.9 to 4.25 hours.
Soft gelatin capsule—1.5 to 2.1 hours.

**Mean minimal erythema dose (MED)**
Substantially fewer Joules per square cm are required with the soft gelatin capsule dosage form than with the hard gelatin capsule dosage form.

**Peak serum concentration**
Hard gelatin capsule—1.5 to 6 hours (mean of 3 hours), when administered with 8 ounces of milk.
Soft gelatin capsule—0.5 to 4 hours (mean of 1.8 hours), when administered with 8 ounces of milk.

**Duration of action**
Increased sensitivity of skin to sunlight—Approximately 8 hours.

**Elimination**
Renal —As metabolites (80 to 90% in 8 hours; 95% in 24 hours).
Fecal—4 to 10%.

## Precautions to Consider

**Carcinogenicity**
Psoralens have been found to augment UVA-induced carcinogenicity in laboratory animals. In addition, studies in humans treated with systemic methoxsalen plus UVA have shown an increase in the risk of squamous cell carcinoma. The possibility of increased risk may exist also for topical methoxsalen and systemic trioxsalen. This risk appears to be greatest in patients with predisposing risk factors, such as fair skin or a hypersensitivity to sunlight; a history of skin cancer, exposure to ionizing radiation, or excessive exposure to sunlight; or a history of treatment with tar and UVB (prolonged), arsenicals, or topical nitrogen mustard.

**Pregnancy/Reproduction**
Pregnancy—Studies have not been done in humans.
Studies have not been done in animals.

FDA Pregnancy Category C.

**Breast-feeding**
It is not known whether methoxsalen is distributed into breast milk. However, problems in humans have not been documented.

**Pediatrics**
Children up to 12 years of age—Appropriate studies on the relationship of age to the effects of methoxsalen have not been performed; however, some side effects are more likely to occur in children up to 12 years of age, since these children may be more sensitive to the effects of methoxsalen.

Children 12 years of age and over—Appropriate studies on the relationship of age to the effects of methoxsalen have not been performed in this age group. However, no problems specific to this age group have been documented to date.

**Geriatrics**
Although appropriate studies on the relationship of age to the effects of methoxsalen have not been performed in the geriatric population, no geriatrics-specific problems have been documented to date.

**Drug interactions and/or related problems**
The following drug interactions and/or related problems have been selected on the basis of their potential clinical significance (possible mechanism in parentheses where appropriate)—not necessarily inclusive (» = major clinical significance):

Note: Combinations containing any of the following medications, depending on the amount present, may also interact with this medication.

Furocoumarin-containing foods, such as limes, figs, parsley, parsnips, mustard, carrots, and celery
(although there have been no reports of serious reactions, caution and avoidance of these foods are recommended because of the risk of additive phototoxicity)

Photosensitizing medications, other
(concurrent use of methoxsalen with these medications, systemic or topical, may cause additive photosensitizing effects; concurrent use with coal tar or coal tar derivatives or with trioxsalen is not recommended)

(concurrent use of systemic methoxsalen with phenothiazines may potentiate intraocular photochemical damage to the choroid, retina, and lens)

» Caution should be used also in evaluating for treatment and subsequently treating patients with a history of having taken arsenicals or having received x-rays, cytotoxic therapy, or coal tar and ultraviolet light B (UVB) therapy because of the increased risk of skin cancer

**Laboratory value alterations**
The following have been selected on the basis of their potential clinical significance (possible effect in parentheses where appropriate)—not necessarily inclusive (» = major clinical significance):

With physiology/laboratory test values
Hepatic function tests
(abnormal hepatic function tests have been reported, but the relationship to the medication is not clear)

**Medical considerations/Contraindications**
The medical considerations/contraindications included here have been selected on the basis of their potential clinical significance (reasons given in parentheses where appropriate)—not necessarily inclusive (» = major clinical significance).

*Risk-benefit should be considered when the following medical problems exist:*
» Albinism or
» Hydroa or
» Leukoderma of infectious origin or
» Lupus erythematosus, acute or
Polymorphic light eruptions or
» Porphyria or
» Xeroderma pigmentosum
(these conditions are associated with photosensitization)
» Aphakia
(increased risk of retinal damage due to lack of lenses)
Cardiovascular disease, severe
(because of the potential heat stress or the prolonged standing associated with each UVA treatment, patients with this problem should be carefully monitored and, if possible, not treated in a vertical UVA chamber)
» Cataracts
Gastrointestinal diseases

Hepatic function impairment
(metabolism may be impaired)
Infection, chronic
Sensitivity to methoxsalen
» Skin cancer, history of
Sunlight allergy, or family history of
(PUVA may cause photoallergic contact dermatitis or precipitate sunlight allergy)
» Caution should be used also in evaluating for treatment and subsequently treating patients with a history of having taken arsenicals or having received x-rays, cytotoxic therapy, or coal tar and ultraviolet light B (UVB) therapy because of the increased risk of skin cancer

**Patient monitoring**
The following may be especially important in patient monitoring (other tests may be warranted in some patients, depending on condition; » = major clinical significance):

Antinuclear antibodies test and
Complete blood count and
Hepatic function tests and
Renal function tests
(recommended prior to initiation of therapy)

Monitoring for melanoma and other skin carcinomas
(recommended in patients receiving methoxsalen for prolonged periods, since long-term safety has not been established)

Ophthalmic examination
(recommended prior to initiation of therapy and yearly thereafter during therapy)

## Side/Adverse Effects

Note: Cataracts have been reported with psoralen use; however, risk is very low in patients who wear UVA-absorbing, wraparound sunglasses when exposed to sunlight or ultraviolet light during the 24 hours after taking methoxsalen.

There is an increased risk of skin cancer with psoralen use. This risk appears to be greatest in patients with predisposing risk factors, such as fair skin or a hypersensitivity to sunlight; a history of skin cancer, exposure to ionizing radiation, or excessive exposure to sunlight; or a history of treatment with tar and UVB (prolonged), arsenicals, or topical nitrogen mustard.

Premature aging of the skin may occur as a result of prolonged PUVA therapy. This effect is permanent and is similar to the results of excessive exposure to sunlight.

Toxic hepatitis has been reported in patients treated with methoxsalen, but the relationship to the medication is not clear.

The following side/adverse effects have been selected on the basis of their potential clinical significance (possible signs and symptoms in parentheses where appropriate)—not necessarily inclusive:

**Those indicating need for medical attention**
Symptoms of overdose or overexposure to ultraviolet light
*Blistering and peeling of skin; reddened, sore skin; swelling, especially in feet or lower legs*

**Those indicating need for medical attention only if they continue or are bothersome**
Incidence more frequent
*Itching of skin; nausea*
Incidence less frequent
*Dizziness; headache; mental depression; nervousness; trouble in sleeping*

## Overdose

For more information on the management of overdose or unintentional ingestion, **contact a Poison Control Center** (see *Poison Control Center Listing*).

**Clinical effects of overdose**
The following effects have been selected on the basis of their potential clinical significance (possible signs and symptoms in parentheses where appropriate)—not necessarily inclusive:

*Blistering and peeling of skin; reddened, sore skin; swelling, especially in feet or lower legs*

**Treatment of overdose**
To decrease absorption—
Inducing emesis, if it can be accomplished within the first 2 to 3 hours after ingestion, since maximum blood levels are reached by that time.

Specific treatment—
    For overdosage of methoxsalen: Keeping patient in a darkened room for at least 24 hours following methoxsalen ingestion to prevent the possibility of sun exposure and subsequent burn injury.
    For overexposure to sunlight or ultraviolet light: Keeping patient in a darkened room for at least 24 hours following ingestion of methoxsalen to prevent the possibility of further sun exposure and subsequent burn injury while assessment of the extent of damage is made.

Monitoring—
    Observing patient for erythema greater than Grade 2 (Grade 2 being marked erythema with no edema) occurring within 24 hours, which may signal the beginning of a potentially serious burn, since peak erythemal reaction to PUVA usually occurs approximately 48 hours following methoxsalen ingestion.

Supportive Care—
    Treating patient symptomatically for burns, depending on their extent and severity.

## Patient Consultation

As an aid to patient consultation, refer to *Advice for the Patient, Methoxsalen (Systemic).*

In providing consultation, consider emphasizing the following selected information (» = major clinical significance):

**Before using this medication**
» Conditions affecting use, especially:
    Sensitivity to methoxsalen
    Diet—Avoiding eating furocoumarin-containing foods (limes, figs, parsley, parsnips, mustard, carrots, celery)
    Other medical problems, especially acute lupus erythematosus; albinism; aphakia; cataracts; hydroa; leukoderma of infectious origin; porphyria; xeroderma pigmentosum; history of skin cancer; history of having taken arsenicals; history of having received x-rays, cytotoxic therapy, or coal tar and ultraviolet light B (UVB) therapy
    Not using for suntanning purposes

**Proper use of this medication**
    Usually comes with patient instructions; reading carefully before using medication
» May take 6 to 8 weeks to work; importance of not increasing the dosage of medication or exposure to ultraviolet light because of the risk of serious burns
    The hard capsule dosage form may be taken with food or milk (the soft capsule dosage form may be taken with low fat food or low fat milk) to reduce gastrointestinal irritation
» Proper dosing
    Late or missed dose: Notifying physician for rescheduling of light treatment
» Proper storage

**Precautions while using this medication**
    Importance of regular visits to physician to have progress checked, including eye examinations
» Protecting skin from sunlight, even through window glass or on cloudy days, for at least 24 hours before and 8 hours following treatment; protecting lips with sun block lipstick that has a skin protection factor (SPF) of at least 15
    Possibility of continued skin sensitivity to sunlight because of medication; using extra precautions for at least 48 hours following each treatment; not sunbathing anytime during course of treatment
» Wearing special sunglasses during daylight hours (even in indirect light, such as through window glass or on cloudy days) for 24 hours following each dose of medication
» Possibility of dry skin or itching; checking with physician before treating
» Possible long-term effects (cataracts, premature skin aging, carcinogenesis)

**Side/adverse effects**
    Slight reddening of skin 24 to 48 hours after treatment is normal response to therapy
    There is an increased risk of developing skin cancer. The body should be examined regularly and the physician shown skin sores that do not heal, new skin growths, and skin growths that have changed in appearance or feel
    Premature aging of the skin may occur as a result of prolonged PUVA therapy. This effect is permanent and is similar to the results of excessive exposure to sunlight

    Signs of potential side effects, especially blistering and peeling of skin; reddened, sore skin; swelling, especially in feet or lower legs
Note: Some side effects are more likely to occur in children.

## General Dosing Information

Methoxsalen soft gelatin capsules should not be used interchangeably with the hard gelatin capsules, since the soft gelatin capsule dosage form exhibits significantly greater bioavailability and earlier photosensitization onset time than does the hard gelatin capsule dosage form.

Patients receiving methoxsalen should be under the supervision of a physician experienced in PUVA therapy.

Methoxsalen hard gelatin capsules may be taken with food or milk (the soft gelatin capsules may be taken with low fat food or low fat milk) to reduce gastrointestinal irritation, or the dose may be split in two and the two halves taken one-half hour apart.

Dosage of methoxsalen should not be increased, although some clinicians recommend an increased dose in the treatment of psoriasis if there is no response after 15 treatments at the recommended dose. A lower-than-recommended dose will produce the same effect, but it will occur more slowly.

Although dosage of methoxsalen is generally based on body weight, usually no change in dose is necessary if the patient's weight changes. However, if the physician believes the weight change to be significant enough to warrant an alteration, adjustment of UVA exposure time should be made instead of adjustment of methoxsalen dosage.

When used to increase skin tolerance to sunlight, treatment should be limited to fourteen days, since adequate pigment will have been formed by that time.

Exposure to sunlight or ultraviolet light should be carefully controlled and adjusted on an individual basis according to skin type and tolerance. Exposure time to sunlight should be reduced at high altitudes or at midday.

Patients with pre-existing erythrodermic psoriasis require special care because the erythema may obscure a possible treatment-related phototoxic erythema. These patients should be treated the same as sun-sensitive skin types.

Skin should be protected from sunlight, even through window glass or on a cloudy day, for at least 24 hours before and 8 hours following oral PUVA treatment by protective clothing, such as long-sleeved shirts, full-length slacks, wide-brimmed hat, and gloves and by using a sun block product that has a skin protection factor of at least 15 on body areas that cannot be covered by clothing. In addition, lips should be protected with a sun block lipstick that has a skin protection factor of at least 15. Also, since the skin continues to be sensitive to sunlight for some time after treatment, the patient should avoid overexposure to sunlight for 48 hours following administration of methoxsalen. In addition, the patient should not sunbathe anytime during the course of treatment.

If a scheduled treatment is missed, the dose of UVA at the next treatment should not be increased; if more than one treatment is missed, the subsequent dose of UVA should be reduced in proportion to the number of treatments missed to reduce the risk of painful erythema.

Repigmentation occurs most rapidly on fleshy areas (face, abdomen, buttocks) and more slowly on the extremities and bony areas (hands and feet).

Tolerance to the effects of methoxsalen may occur when pigmentation precedes erythema by a long period of time. Hyperpigmentation reduces subsequent responsiveness.

Lack of response in psoriasis may be caused by a general phototoxic reaction; this may be confirmed by temporary withdrawal for 2 weeks, with subsequent improvement in the condition. If improvement does not occur, treatment with methoxsalen is considered to be a failure.

Use of psoralen derivatives to promote suntanning has resulted in serious reactions, including acute generalized dermatitis, blistering, and edema; residual edema of the legs and cutaneous damage have been reported.

Temporary withdrawal of therapy is recommended if burning or blistering of skin occurs.

Reduction in dosage or withdrawal of methoxsalen therapy is recommended if signs of hepatic function impairment occur.

## Oral Dosage Forms

Note: Bracketed uses in the *Dosage Forms* section refer to categories of use and/or indications that are not included in U.S. product labeling.

## METHOXSALEN CAPSULES (XXI) (HARD GELATIN) USP

**Usual adult and adolescent dose**

Vitiligo—

Oral, 20 mg a day, two to four hours before measured periods of UVA exposure, two or three times a week (at least forty-eight hours apart).

Sunlight—Initial exposure time should not exceed fifteen minutes for light skin colors, twenty minutes for medium skin colors, or twenty-five minutes for dark skin colors; may subsequently be increased five minutes each treatment, based on erythema and tenderness.

Artificial light—Initial exposure time should not exceed one-half of that producing erythema after sunlight exposure, or should be based on the minimal phototoxic dose (MPD) and manufacturer's directions for the specific light source being used. The MPD can be determined by irradiating several areas of skin 2 cm in diameter; a range of light exposure times is used and the time that produces erythema at seventy-two hours after exposure is the MPD.

Psoriasis or

[Mycosis fungoides, use of PUVA in][1]—

Oral, 600 mcg (0.6 mg) per kg of body weight, two hours before measured periods of high-intensity UVA exposure, two or three times a week (at least forty-eight hours apart). Exposure time should be based on skin type and response to therapy, according to the manufacturer's directions for the specific light source being used. Frequency of exposure may be gradually reduced for maintenance treatment; UVA exposure may be adjusted according to response.

Note: A commonly used dosage schedule according to weight is:

| Weight (kg) | Dose (mg) |
|---|---|
| <30 | 10 |
| 30–50 | 20 |
| 51–65 | 30 |
| 66–80 | 40 |
| 81–90 | 50 |
| 91–115 | 60 |
| >115 | 70 |

**Usual pediatric dose**

Children up to 12 years of age—Dosage has not been established.
Children 12 years of age and over—See *Usual adult and adolescent dose.*

**Strength(s) usually available**

U.S.—

10 mg (Rx) [*8-MOP* (tartrazine)].

Canada—

10 mg (Rx) [*Oxsoralen*].

**Packaging and storage**

Store below 40 °C (104 °F), preferably between 15 and 30 °C (59 and 86 °F) unless otherwise specified by manufacturer. Store in a tight, light-resistant container.

**Auxiliary labeling**

• Take with food or milk.

**Note**

Methoxsalen soft gelatin capsules should not be used interchangeably with the hard gelatin capsules.

## METHOXSALEN CAPSULES (XXII) (SOFT GELATIN) USP

**Usual adult and adolescent dose**

Psoriasis—

Oral, 400 mcg (0.4 mg) per kg of body weight, one and one-half to two hours before measured periods of high-intensity UVA exposure, two or three times a week (at least forty-eight hours apart). Exposure time should be based on skin type and response to therapy, according to the manufacturer's directions for the specific light source being used. Frequency of exposure may be gradually reduced for maintenance treatment; UVA exposure may be adjusted according to response.

Note: **The soft capsule dosage form exhibits significantly greater bioavailability and earlier photosensitization onset time than the hard capsule dosage form.** When this dosage form is used, the patient's minimum phototoxic dose (MPD) and phototoxic peak time after drug administration should be determined prior to initiation of photochemotherapy. The manufacturer's directions should be consulted for full information concerning dosage and administration.

**Usual pediatric dose**

Children up to 12 years of age—Dosage has not been established.
Children 12 years of age and over—See *Usual adult and adolescent dose.*

**Strength(s) usually available**

U.S.—

10 mg (Rx) [*Oxsoralen-Ultra*].

Canada—

10 mg (Rx) [*Ultra MOP*].

**Packaging and storage**

Store below 40 °C (104 °F), preferably between 15 and 30 °C (59 and 86 °F), in a tight container, unless otherwise specified by manufacturer. Protect from light.

**Auxiliary labeling**

• Take with low fat food or milk.

**Note**

Methoxsalen soft gelatin capsules should not be used interchangeably with the hard gelatin capsules.

[1]Not included in Canadian product labeling.

Revised: 06/24/94

# METHOXSALEN    Topical

VA CLASSIFICATION (Primary/Secondary): DE900/DE802

Note: For a listing of dosage forms and brand names by country availability, see *Dosage Forms* section(s). For a listing of brand names for the articles in this monograph, refer to the General Index.

## Category

Repigmenting agent (topical); hair growth stimulant, alopecia areata (topical); antipsoriatic (topical).

Note: Methoxsalen is used in conjunction with ultraviolet light A (UVA). This mode of treatment is known as PUVA (psoralen plus ultraviolet light A).

## Indications

Note: Bracketed information in the *Indications* section refers to uses that are not included in U.S. product labeling.

**Accepted**

Vitiligo (treatment)—PUVA is indicated for repigmentation in the treatment of vitiligo. It is not effective in producing pigmentation in leukoderma of infectious origin or in albinism.

[Skin, increased tolerance to sunlight][1]—PUVA has been used to increase skin tolerance to sunlight.

[Psoriasis (treatment)]—PUVA has been used in the treatment of severe psoriasis that has not responded to other therapy.

[Mycosis fungoides (treatment)][1]—PUVA is used in the treatment of mycosis fungoides.

[Alopecia areata (treatment)][1]
[Dermatoses, inflammatory (treatment)][1]
[Eczema (treatment)][1] or
[Lichen planus (treatment)][1]—PUVA is used in the treatment of alopecia areata, inflammatory dermatoses, eczema, and lichen planus.

**Unaccepted**

The unsupervised use of methoxsalen to promote tanning is dangerous and should be discouraged.

[1]Not included in Canadian product labeling.

## Pharmacology/Pharmacokinetics

### Physicochemical characteristics
Chemical group—Psoralen derivative.
Molecular weight—216.19.

### Mechanism of action/Effect
Exact mechanism of erythemogenic, melanogenic, and cytotoxic response in the epidermis is unknown, but may involve increased tyrosinase activity in melanin-producing cells, as well as inhibition of DNA synthesis, cell division, and epidermal turnover. Successful pigmentation requires the presence of functioning melanocytes.

### Absorption
Extent of systemic absorption is unknown.

### Biotransformation
Activated by long-wavelength UVA in the range of 320 to 400 (maximal effect at 365) nanometers (nm).

### Onset of action
Vitiligo—Up to 6 months.
For increased sensitivity of skin to sunlight—1 hour.
Tanning—Within a few days.

### Time to peak effect
Increased sensitivity of skin to sunlight—2 hours (peak erythematous response may not occur for 2 days).

### Duration of action
Increased sensitivity of skin to sunlight—Several days.

## Precautions to Consider

### Carcinogenicity
Psoralens have been found to augment UVA-induced carcinogenicity in laboratory animals. In addition, studies in humans treated with systemic methoxsalen plus UVA have shown an increase in the risk of squamous cell carcinoma. The possibility of increased risk may exist also for topical methoxsalen and systemic trioxsalen. This risk appears to be greatest in patients with predisposing risk factors, such as fair skin or a hypersensitivity to sunlight; a history of skin cancer, exposure to ionizing radiation, or excessive exposure to sunlight; or a history of treatment with tar and UVB (prolonged), arsenicals, or topical nitrogen mustard.

### Pregnancy/Reproduction
Pregnancy—Studies have not been done in humans.
Studies have not been done in animals.

FDA Pregnancy Category C.

### Breast-feeding
It is not known whether topical methoxsalen is distributed into breast milk. However, problems in humans have not been documented.

### Pediatrics
Appropriate studies on the relationship of age to the effects of topical methoxsalen have not been performed in children up to 12 years of age. Safety and efficacy have not been established.

### Geriatrics
Appropriate studies on the relationship of age to the effects of topical methoxsalen have not been performed in the geriatric population. However, no geriatrics-specific problems have been documented to date.

### Drug interactions and/or related problems
The following drug interactions and/or related problems have been selected on the basis of their potential clinical significance (possible mechanism in parentheses where appropriate)—not necessarily inclusive (» = major clinical significance):

Note: Combinations containing any of the following medications, depending on the amount present, may also interact with this medication.

Furocoumarin-containing foods, such as limes, figs, parsley, parsnips, mustard, carrots, and celery
(although there have been no reports of serious reactions, caution and avoidance of these foods are recommended because of the risk of additive phototoxicity)

Photosensitizing medications, other
(concurrent use of methoxsalen with other photosensitizing medications, systemic or topical, may cause additive photosensitizing effects; concurrent use with coal tar or coal tar derivatives or with trioxsalen is not recommended)

### Laboratory value alterations
The following have been selected on the basis of their potential clinical significance (possible effect in parentheses where appropriate)—not necessarily inclusive (» = major clinical significance):

With physiology/laboratory test values
Liver function tests
(Abnormal liver function tests have been reported, but the relationship to the medication is not clear)

### Medical considerations/Contraindications
The medical considerations/contraindications included here have been selected on the basis of their potential clinical significance (reasons given in parentheses where appropriate)—not necessarily inclusive (» = major clinical significance).

*Risk-benefit should be considered when the following medical problems exist:*
» Albinism or
» Hydroa or
» Leukoderma of infectious origin or
» Lupus erythematosus, acute or
» Polymorphic light eruptions or
» Porphyria or
» Xeroderma pigmentosum
(these conditions are associated with photosensitization)

Cardiovascular disease, severe
(because of the potential heat stress or the prolonged standing associated with each UVA treatment, patients with severe cardiovascular disease should be carefully monitored and if possible not be treated in a vertical UVA chamber)

Infection, chronic

Sensitivity to methoxsalen

» Skin cancer, history of

Sunlight allergy, or family history of
(PUVA may cause photoallergic contact dermatitis or precipitate sunlight allergy)

» Caution should be used in evaluating for treatment and subsequently treating patients with a history of having taken arsenicals or having received x-rays, cytotoxic therapy, or coal tar and ultraviolet light B (UVB) therapy because of the increased risk of skin cancer.

### Patient monitoring
The following may be especially important in patient monitoring (other tests may be warranted in some patients, depending on condition; » = major clinical significance):

Monitoring for melanoma and other skin carcinomas
(recommended in patients receiving methoxsalen for prolonged periods, since long-term safety has not been established)

## Side/Adverse Effects

Note: There is an increased risk of skin cancer with systemic methoxsalen plus UVA. The possibility of increased risk may exist also with topical methoxsalen. This risk appears to be greatest in patients with predisposing risk factors, such as fair skin or a hypersensitivity to sunlight; a history of skin cancer, exposure to ionizing radiation, or excessive exposure to sunlight; or a history of treatment with tar and UVB (prolonged), arsenicals, or topical nitrogen mustard.

Premature aging of the skin may occur as a result of prolonged treatment with systemic methoxsalen plus UVA. The possibility of risk may exist also with topical methoxsalen. This effect is permanent and is similar to the results of excessive exposure to sunlight.

The following effects have been selected on the basis of their potential clinical significance (possible signs and symptoms in parentheses where appropriate)—not necessarily inclusive:

### Those indicating need for medical attention
Symptoms of overdose or overexposure to ultraviolet light
*Blistering and peeling of skin; reddened, sore skin; swelling, especially in feet or lower legs*

## Overdose

For more information on the management of overdose or unintentional ingestion, **contact a Poison Control Center** (see *Poison Control Center Listing*).

## Clinical effects of overdose

The following effects have been selected on the basis of their potential clinical significance (possible signs and symptoms in parentheses where appropriate)—not necessarily inclusive:

*Blistering and peeling of skin; reddened, sore skin; swelling, especially in feet or lower legs*

## Treatment of overdose

To decrease absorption—
  Inducing emesis.
Specific treatment—
  For ingestion of topical methoxsalen solution: Keeping patient in a darkened room for at least 24 hours following methoxsalen ingestion to prevent the possibility of sun exposure and subsequent burn injury.
  For overexposure to sunlight or ultraviolet light: Keeping patient in a darkened room for at least 24 hours following ingestion of methoxsalen to prevent the possibility of further sun exposure and subsequent burn injury while assessment of the extent of damage is made. With topical methoxsalen, erythema may not begin for several hours following overexposure and may not peak for 2 or 3 days or longer.
Supportive care—
  Treating patient symptomatically for burns, depending on their extent and severity. Patients in whom intentional overdose is known or suspected should be referred for psychiatric consultation.

## Patient Consultation

As an aid to patient consultation, refer to *Advice for the Patient, Methoxsalen (Topical).*

In providing consultation, consider emphasizing the following selected information (» = major clinical significance):

### Before using this medication

» Conditions affecting use, especially:
    Sensitivity to methoxsalen
    Carcinogenicity—Possibility of increased risk of squamous cell carcinoma, especially in patients with predisposing risk factors such as fair skin and those with increased sensitivity to sunlight
    Use in children—Not recommended for use in children up to 12 years of age
    Diet—Avoiding eating furocoumarin-containing foods (limes, figs, parsley, parsnips, mustard, carrots, celery)
    Other medical problems, especially acute lupus erythematosus; albinism; hydroa; leukoderma of infectious origin; polymorphic light eruptions; porphyria; xeroderma pigmentosum; history of skin cancer; history of having taken arsenicals; history of having received x-rays, cytotoxic therapy, or coal tar and ultraviolet light B (UVB) therapy

### Proper use of this medication

    Using medication only under the direct supervision of the physician
» Proper dosing

### Precautions while using this medication

    Importance of regular visits to physician for treatments and to have progress checked
» Protecting skin from sunlight, even through window glass or on a cloudy day, for at least 12 to 48 hours following treatment; washing treated areas after light treatment
    Possibility of continued skin sensitivity to sunlight because of medication; using extra precautions for at least 72 hours following each treatment; not sunbathing anytime during course of treatment
» Possibility of dry skin or itching; checking with physician before treating

### Side/adverse effects

    There is an increased risk of developing skin cancer when treated with systemic methoxsalen. The possibility of increased risk may exist also with topical methoxsalen. The treated areas should be examined regularly and the physician shown skin sores that do not heal, new skin growths, and skin growths that have changed in appearance or feel.
    Premature aging of the skin may occur as a result of prolonged treatment with systemic methoxsalen. The possibility of risk may exist also with topical methoxsalen. This effect is permanent and is similar to the results of excessive exposure to sunlight.
    Signs of potential side effects, especially symptoms of overdose or overexposure to ultraviolet light

## General Dosing Information

Topical application should be performed only by or under the direct supervision of a physician familiar with the use of PUVA therapy.

Topical application causes a greater and less predictable photosensitizing response than does oral administration.

It is recommended that methoxsalen be applied only to small, well-defined lesions (less than 10 square cm) and that it be removed from the skin following exposure to sunlight or ultraviolet light.

Exposure to sunlight or ultraviolet light should be carefully controlled and adjusted on an individual basis according to skin type and tolerance. Exposure time to sunlight should be reduced at high altitudes or at midday.

Because topical application results in a higher concentration of methoxsalen in the epidermis than does oral administration, the dose of UVA is generally lower with topical application.

Following topical administration of methoxsalen, the treated skin should be protected from sunlight, even through window glass or on a cloudy day, for at least 12 to 48 hours by protective clothing or a sun block product that has a protection factor of at least 15. Furthermore, since the treated skin continues to be sensitive to sunlight for some time after treatment, the patient should avoid overexposure to sunlight for 72 hours following application of methoxsalen. In addition, the patient should not sunbathe anytime during the course of treatment.

Pigmentation may begin after a few weeks of treatment, but significant repigmentation may require 6 to 9 months. Periodic retreatment may be necessary to retain all of the new pigment. Repigmentation occurs most rapidly and is more predictable on fleshy areas (face, abdomen, buttocks) and occurs more slowly and is less effective on the extremities and bony areas (hands and feet).

Tolerance to the effects of methoxsalen may occur when pigmentation precedes erythema by a long period of time. Hyperpigmentation reduces subsequent responsiveness.

Use of psoralen derivatives to promote suntanning has resulted in serious reactions, including acute generalized dermatitis, blistering, and edema; residual edema of the legs and cutaneous damage have been reported.

Temporary withdrawal of therapy is recommended if burning or blistering of skin occurs.

Dilution to a strength of 1:1000 or 1:10,000 is sometimes necessary to avoid serious reactions.

## Topical Dosage Forms

### METHOXSALEN TOPICAL SOLUTION USP

#### Usual adult and adolescent dose

Repigmenting agent (topical)—
    The topical solution should be applied to a small, well-defined vitiliginous lesion, allowed to dry for one to two minutes, then reapplied. This is done two to two and one-half hours before measured periods of UVA exposure. Following exposure, the lesions should be washed with soap and water and protected with an opaque sunscreen.
    Sunlight—Initial exposure time should not exceed one minute and should be increased subsequently with caution.
    Artificial light—Initial exposure time should not exceed one-half of the time that produces erythema after sunlight exposure, or should be based on the minimal phototoxic dose (MPD) and manufacturer's directions for the specific light source being used. The MPD can be determined by irradiating several areas of skin 2 cm in diameter; a range of light-exposure times is used and the time that produces erythema at seventy-two hours after exposure is the MPD.

Note: The manufacturer recommends once-weekly treatment; however, some clinicians recommend treatment every three to five days.

#### Usual pediatric dose

Repigmenting agent (topical)—
    Children up to 12 years of age: Dosage has not been established.
    Children 12 years of age and over: See *Usual adult and adolescent dose.*

#### Strength(s) usually available

U.S.—
    1% (Rx) [*Oxsoralen Lotion* (alcohol 71%; acetone)].
Canada—
    1% (Rx) [*Oxsoralen Lotion; UltraMOP Lotion*].

**Packaging and storage**
Store below 40 °C (104 °F), preferably between 15 and 30 °C (59 and 86
°F), unless otherwise specified by manufacturer. Store in a tight, light-
resistant container. Protect from freezing.

**Note**
Do not dispense to the patient for use at home.

Revised: 05/26/94

**METHOXYFLURANE**—See *Anesthetics, Inhalation (Systemic)*

**METHSCOPOLAMINE**—See *Anticholinergics/Antispasmodics (Systemic)*

**METHSCOPOLAMINE-CONTAINING COMBINATIONS**—
Chlorpheniramine, Phenylephrine, and Methscopolamine (Systemic)—See
*Antihistamines, Decongestants, and Anticholinergics (Systemic)*

Chlorpheniramine, Phenylpropanolamine, and Methscopolamine (Systemic)—See *Antihistamines, Decongestants, and Anticholinergics (Systemic)*

**METHSUXIMIDE**—See *Anticonvulsants, Succinimide (Systemic)*

**METHYCLOTHIAZIDE**—See *Diuretics, Thiazide (Systemic)*

**METHYCLOTHIAZIDE-CONTAINING COMBINATIONS**—
Deserpidine and Methyclothiazide (Systemic)—See *Rauwolfia Alkaloids and Thiazide Diuretics (Systemic)*
Reserpine and Methyclothiazide (Systemic)—See *Rauwolfia Alkaloids and Thiazide Diuretics (Systemic)*

**METHYLCELLULOSE**—See *Laxatives (Local)*

# METHYLDOPA    Systemic

VA CLASSIFICATION (Primary): CV490
Note: For a listing of dosage forms and brand names by country availability, see *Dosage Forms* section(s). For a listing of brand names
for the articles in this monograph, refer to the General Index.

## Category
Antihypertensive.

## Indications
**Accepted**
Hypertension (treatment)—Methyldopa is indicated in the treatment of
moderate to severe hypertension, including that complicated by renal
disease.
For additional information on initial therapeutic guidelines related to
the treatment of hypertension, see *Appendix III.*
Methyldopate may be used intravenously in the treatment of hypertensive crises. However, because of its slow onset of action, methyldopate is generally not recommended as sole initial therapy in hypertensive crises.

## Pharmacology/Pharmacokinetics
**Physicochemical characteristics**
Molecular weight—Methyldopa: 238.24.
Methyldopate hydrochloride: 275.73.

**Mechanism of action/Effect**
The exact mechanism of antihypertensive action has not been conclusively
demonstrated. However, the major antihypertensive effect appears to
result from conversion to alpha-methylnorepinephrine, a potent alpha-
2 adrenergic agonist. Alpha-methylnorepinephrine acts centrally to
stimulate alpha receptors. This results in a decrease in sympathetic
outflow and decreased blood pressure.

**Absorption**
Absorption of methyldopa from the gastrointestinal tract is variable but
averages approximately 50%.

**Protein binding**
Methyldopa—Low (less than 20%).
Sulfate conjugate—Moderate.

**Biotransformation**
Extensive.
Converted to alpha-methylnorepinephrine in central adrenergic neurons;
methyldopate hydrochloride is hydrolyzed to methyldopa.
Hepatic; sulfate conjugation occurs to a greater extent after oral than after
intravenous administration.

**Half-life**
Normal—Alpha: 1.7 hours.
Anuric—Alpha: 3.6 hours.

**Time to peak effect**
Single dose—4 to 6 hours.
Multiple doses—2 to 3 days.

**Duration of action**
Variable.
Oral—
Single dose—12 to 24 hours.
Multiple doses—24 to 48 hours.
Intravenous—
10 to 16 hours.

**Elimination**
Renal; approximately 70% of absorbed drug is excreted in urine as methyldopa and its mono-0-sulfate metabolite. Unabsorbed oral methyldopa
is excreted unchanged in the feces.
In dialysis—Methyldopa is removable by both hemodialysis and peritoneal dialysis.

## Precautions to Consider
**Cross-sensitivity and/or related problems**
Patients sensitive to sulfites may be sensitive to some methyldopa products
because of the sulfite preservatives present.

**Tumorigenicity**
No evidence of a tumorigenic effect was seen in mice given doses up to
1800 mg per kg of body weight (mg/kg) per day (30 times the maximum recommended human dose) for 2 years or in rats given doses
up to 240 mg/kg per day (4 times the maximum recommended human
dose) for 2 years.

**Mutagenicity**
Methyldopa was not mutagenic in the Ames test with or without metabolic
activation. There was no increase in chromosomal aberration or sister
chromatid exchanges in Chinese hamster ovary cells.

**Pregnancy/Reproduction**
Fertility—Methyldopa did not affect fertility in male and female rats given
doses of 100 mg/kg per day (1.7 times the maximum daily human
dose). However, at doses of 200 mg/kg and 400 mg/kg per day (3.3
and 6.7 times the maximum daily human dose) methyldopa decreased
sperm count, sperm motility, the number of late spermatids, and the
male fertility index.

Pregnancy—Methyldopa crosses the placenta. Adequate and well-controlled studies of methyldopa use in pregnant women during the first
and second trimesters have not been done. Studies of methyldopa use
in pregnant women during the third trimester have not been associated
with adverse effects.
Studies in rabbits at doses of 200 mg/kg per day (3.3 times the maximum
daily human dose), mice at doses of 1000 mg/kg per day (16.6 times
the maximum daily human dose), and rats at doses of 100 mg/kg per
day (1.7 times the maximum daily human dose) showed no adverse
effects.

FDA Pregnancy Category B.

**Breast-feeding**

Methyldopa is distributed into breast milk. However, problems in humans have not been documented.

**Pediatrics**

Appropriate studies on the relationship of age to the effects of methyldopa have not been performed in the pediatric population. However, pediatrics-specific problems that would limit the usefulness of this medication in children are not expected.

**Geriatrics**

Although appropriate studies on the relationship of age to the effects of methyldopa have not been performed in the geriatric population, the elderly may be more sensitive to the hypotensive and sedative effects. In addition, elderly patients are more likely to have age-related renal function impairment, which may require lower doses in patients receiving methyldopa.

**Dental**

Use of methyldopa may decrease or inhibit salivary flow, thus contributing to the development of caries, periodontal disease, oral candidiasis, and discomfort.

**Drug interactions and/or related problems**

The following drug interactions and/or related problems have been selected on the basis of their potential clinical significance (possible mechanism in parentheses where appropriate)—not necessarily inclusive (» = major clinical significance):

Note: Combinations containing any of the following medications, depending on the amount present, may also interact with this medication.

Alcohol or
Central nervous system (CNS) depression–producing medications (See *Appendix II*)
(concurrent use may enhance the CNS depressant effects of either these medications or methyldopa)

Anticoagulants, coumarin- or indandione-derivative
(concurrent use with methyldopa may increase the anticoagulant effect of these medications; adjustment of anticoagulant dosage based on prothrombin-time determinations is recommended)

Antidepressants, tricyclic
(may reduce antihypertensive effects of methyldopa; the patient should be carefully monitored to confirm that the desired effect is being obtained)

Anti-inflammatory drugs, nonsteroidal (NSAIDs), especially indomethacin
(antihypertensive effects of methyldopa may be reduced when it is used concurrently with these medications; indomethacin, and possibly other NSAIDs, may antagonize the antihypertensive effect by inhibiting renal prostaglandin synthesis and/or by causing sodium and fluid retention; the patient should be carefully monitored to confirm that the desired effect is being obtained)

Appetite suppressants, with the exception of fenfluramine
(concurrent use may decrease the hypotensive effects of methyldopa)

Bromocriptine
(methyldopa may increase serum prolactin concentrations and interfere with effects of bromocriptine; dosage adjustment of bromocriptine may be necessary)

Estrogens
(estrogen-induced fluid retention tends to increase blood pressure)

Fenfluramine
(concurrent use may increase the hypotensive effects of methyldopa)

Haloperidol
(concurrent use of haloperidol with methyldopa may cause unwanted mental effects such as disorientation and slowed or difficult thought process)

Hypotension-producing medications, other (See *Appendix II*)
(hypotensive effects may be potentiated when these medications are used concurrently with methyldopa; although some antihypertensive and/or diuretic combinations are frequently used for therapeutic advantage, dosage adjustments may be necessary during concurrent use)

Levodopa
(concurrent use with methyldopa may alter the antiparkinsonian effects of levodopa and may also produce additive toxic CNS effects such as psychosis)

Lithium
(concurrent use with methyldopa may increase the risk of lithium toxicity, even though serum lithium concentrations remain within the recommended therapeutic range)

» Monoamine oxidase (MAO) inhibitors, including furazolidone, procarbazine, and selegiline
(methyldopa may cause hyperexcitability in patients receiving MAO inhibitors; headache, severe hypertension, and hallucinations have been reported)

Sympathomimetics, such as:
»   Cocaine
     Dobutamine
     Dopamine
     Ephedrine
     Epinephrine
     Mephentermine
     Metaraminol
     Methoxamine
»   Norepinephrine
»   Phenylephrine or
     Phenylpropanolamine
(concurrent use with sympathomimetic pressor amines may decrease the hypotensive effect of methyldopa and potentiate the pressor effect of these medications; if concurrent use of cocaine, norepinephrine, or phenylephrine is indicated, caution is required, and only very small initial doses should be administered)

**Laboratory value alterations**

The following have been selected on the basis of their potential clinical significance (possible effect in parentheses where appropriate)—not necessarily inclusive (» = major clinical significance):

With diagnostic test results
Aspartate aminotransferase (AST [SGOT]) measurement, serum, using colorimetric methods
(methyldopa may interfere with measurement of AST)

Creatinine measurement, serum, using the alkaline picrate method
(methyldopa may interfere with measurement of serum creatinine)

Urinary catecholamine measurement
(methyldopa may produce falsely elevated results since it causes fluorescence at the same wavelengths as catecholamines; methyldopa does not interfere with urinary vanillylmandelic acid [VMA] determinations)

Urinary uric acid measurement, using the phosphotungstate method
(methyldopa may interfere with measurement of urinary uric acid)

With physiology/laboratory test values
Alanine aminotransferase (ALT [SGPT]) and
Alkaline phosphatase and
Aspartate aminotransferase (AST [SGOT]) and
Bilirubin
(serum concentrations may be increased, indicating possible hepatotoxicity)

Blood urea nitrogen (BUN) and
Potassium and sodium, serum and
Prolactin, serum and
Uric acid, serum
(concentrations may be increased)

Positive direct antiglobulin (Coombs') tests
(may be produced in 10 to 20% of patients on prolonged methyldopa therapy and usually occur after 6 to 12 months of therapy; rarely, these are associated with hemolytic anemia; the positive Coombs' test may not revert to normal until weeks or months after methyldopa is discontinued; less frequently, a positive indirect Coombs' test may occur, which may interfere with crossmatching of blood; lowest incidence is with daily doses of 1 gram or less)

Prothrombin time
(may be prolonged indicating possible hepatotoxicity)

**Medical considerations/Contraindications**

The medi' considerations/contraindications included here have been selected on the basis of their potential clinical significance (reasons given in parentheses where appropriate)—not necessarily inclusive (» = major clinical significance):

*Except under special circumstances, this medication should not be used when the following medical problem exists:*

» Hepatic disease, active, such as acute hepatitis and active cirrhosis

*Risk-benefit should be considered when the following medical problems exist:*

Cerebrovascular disease, severe bilateral
(rarely, involuntary choreoathetotic movements have been observed during methyldopa therapy)

Coronary insufficiency, including angina pectoris
    (may be aggravated)
» Hemolytic anemia, autoimmune, history of
» Hepatic disease, history of, in conjunction with past use of methyldopa
Hepatic function impairment
    (reduced biotransformation; lower doses may be required)
Mental depression, history of
Parkinson's disease
    (may be exacerbated)
» Pheochromocytoma
    (interference with tests for catecholamines; in addition, pressor responses have been reported)
Renal function impairment
    (increased sensitivity to effects of methyldopa, possibly due to accumulation of the sulfate conjugate; lower doses may be required)
Sensitivity to methyldopa

## Patient monitoring

The following may be especially important in patient monitoring (other tests may be warranted in some patients, depending on condition; » = major clinical significance):

Antinuclear antibody (ANA) titer and
Complete blood counts and
Lupus erythematosus cell preparations
    (may be indicated if patient develops arthralgia, continued malaise, or other symptoms of systemic lupus erythematosus (SLE)–like syndrome)
Blood cell counts, including hematocrit, hemoglobin, or red cell count
    (recommended prior to initiation of therapy to establish a baseline for determination of development of hemolytic anemia; may also be required at periodic intervals during therapy)
» Blood pressure measurements
    (recommended at periodic intervals in patients being treated for hypertension; selected patients may be trained to perform blood pressure measurements at home and report the results at regular physician visits)
Direct Coombs' test
    (recommended before initiation of treatment and after 6 and 12 months of treatment)
Hepatic function determinations
    (recommended at baseline and at periodic intervals during therapy, especially during the first 6 to 12 weeks of therapy or whenever an unexplained fever occurs)

## Side/Adverse Effects

Note: Darkening of urine on exposure to air, caused by breakdown of methyldopa or its metabolites, may occur rarely.

The following side/adverse effects have been selected on the basis of their potential clinical significance (possible signs and symptoms in parentheses where appropriate)—not necessarily inclusive:

### Those indicating need for medical attention
Incidence more frequent
    *Edema, peripheral* (swelling of feet or lower legs)
Incidence less frequent
    *Drug fever* (fever, shortly after onset of therapy); *mental status changes* (mental depression or anxiety, nightmares or unusually vivid dreams)
    Note: *Drug fever* usually occurs within the first 3 months of therapy and is sometimes accompanied by eosinophilia or hepatic function test changes. The hepatic reaction to methyldopa appears to be immunologic or hypersensitive in nature.

Incidence rare
    *Cholestasis or hepatitis and hepatocellular injury* (dark or amber urine; pale stools; yellow eyes or skin); *colitis* (severe or continuing diarrhea or stomach cramps); *hemolytic anemia, autoimmune* (continuing tiredness or weakness after having taken this medication for several weeks); *leukopenia, reversible, or granulocytopenia, reversible; myocarditis* (fever, chills, troubled breathing, and fast heartbeat); *pancreatitis* (severe stomach pain with nausea and vomiting); *systemic lupus erythematosus (SLE)–like syndrome* (general feeling of discomfort or illness or weakness; joint pain; skin rash or itching); *thrombocytopenia*
    Note: *Hemolytic anemia* occurs in less than 5% of patients showing a positive Coombs' test.
        Rarely, fatal *hepatic necrosis* has been reported.

### Those indicating need for medical attention only if they continue or are bothersome
Incidence more frequent—more than 5%
    *Drowsiness; dryness of mouth; headache*
    Note: *Drowsiness* is especially likely to occur at initiation of therapy and after dosage increases.
Incidence less frequent or rare
    *Decreased sexual ability or interest in sex*—more common in men than in women; *diarrhea; hyperprolactinemia* (swelling of breasts or unusual milk production); *nausea or vomiting; orthostatic hypotension* (dizziness or lightheadedness when getting up from a lying or sitting position); *paresthesias* (numbness, tingling, pain, or weakness in hands or feet); *sinus bradycardia* (slow heartbeat); *stuffy nose*

## Overdose

For more information on the management of overdose or unintentional ingestion, **contact a Poison Control Center** (See *Poison Control Center Listing*).

### Clinical effects of overdose
The following effects have been selected on the basis of their potential clinical significance (possible signs and symptoms in parentheses where appropriate)—not necessarily inclusive:
    *Bradycardia; constipation; diarrhea; dizziness; flatus; gastric distention; hypotension, acute; lightheadedness; nausea; sedation, excessive; vomiting; weakness*

### Treatment of overdose
To decrease absorption—
    If clinically indicated and ingestion is recent, gastric lavage or emesis may reduce absorption.
Specific treatment—
    Management is mostly symptomatic and supportive. This includes particular attention to heart rate and cardiac output, blood volume, electrolyte balance, paralytic ileus, urinary function, and cerebral activity. Sympathomimetic agents may be indicated.

## Patient Consultation

As an aid to patient consultation, refer to *Advice for the Patient, Methyldopa (Systemic)*.

In providing consultation, consider emphasizing the following selected information (» = major clinical significance):

### Before using this medication
» Conditions affecting use, especially:
    Sensitivity to methyldopa
    Breast-feeding—Distributed into breast milk
    Use in the elderly—Increased sensitivity to hypotensive and sedative effects
    Other medications, especially MAO inhibitors
    Other medical problems, especially active hepatic disease, history of hepatic disease associated with methyldopa, history of autoimmune hemolytic anemia, or pheochromocytoma

### Proper use of this medication
Possible need for control of weight and diet, especially sodium intake
» Patient may not experience symptoms of hypertension; importance of taking medication even if feeling well
» Does not cure, but helps control hypertension; possible need for lifelong therapy; checking with physician before discontinuing medication; serious consequences of untreated hypertension
Getting into habit of taking at same time each day to help increase compliance
» Proper dosing
Missed dose: Taking as soon as possible; not taking if almost time for next dose; not doubling doses
» Proper storage

### Precautions while using this medication
Regular visits to physician to check progress
» Not using other medications, especially nonprescription sympathomimetics, unless ordered by physician
» Reporting fever to physician
Caution if any kind of surgery (including dental surgery) or emergency treatment is required
» Caution when driving or doing things requiring alertness, because of possible drowsiness
Caution when getting up suddenly from a lying or sitting position
Possible dryness of mouth; using sugarless candy or gum, ice, or saliva substitute for relief; checking with physician or dentist if dry mouth continues for more than 2 weeks

Caution if any laboratory tests required; possible interference with test results

### Side/adverse effects

Signs of potential side effects, especially edema, drug fever, mental status changes, cholestasis, hepatitis, hepatocellular injury, colitis, hemolytic anemia, leukopenia, granulocytopenia, myocarditis, pancreatitis, SLE-like syndrome, and thrombocytopenia

# General Dosing Information

If methyldopa is added to a thiazide diuretic regimen, the dosage of the thiazide need not be changed. If methyldopa is to be given with other antihypertensives, the initial dosage of methyldopa for an adult should be limited to 500 mg daily.

Any increase in dosage should be initiated with the evening dose of methyldopa to minimize the effects of sedation.

Tolerance to methyldopa may develop within 2 or 3 months after initiation of therapy as a result of fluid retention and expanded plasma volume. Adding a diuretic or increasing the dosage of methyldopa may restore control. Addition of thiazide diuretics to the regimen is recommended if therapy has not been started with a thiazide or if a daily dose of 2 grams of methyldopa does not maintain control.

If orthostatic hypotension occurs, dosage reduction is recommended.

Recent evidence suggests that withdrawal of antihypertensive therapy prior to surgery is not necessary, but that the anesthesiologist must be aware of such therapy.

It is recommended that methyldopa be discontinued if Coombs' positive hemolytic anemia occurs. Although the anemia usually remits promptly, corticosteroids may be administered if necessary. If this effect is shown to be due to methyldopa, therapy with the drug should not be reinstituted.

If a blood transfusion is needed in a patient receiving methyldopa, both a direct and indirect Coombs' test are recommended. If hemolytic anemia is not present, usually only the direct Coombs' test will be positive, which will not interfere with typing or positive crossmatching. However, a positive indirect Coombs' test may interfere with the major crossmatch, and a hematologist or transfusion expert will be needed.

It is recommended that methyldopa be withdrawn if fever, abnormal liver function tests, or jaundice occurs. If these effects are shown to be due to methyldopa, therapy with the drug should not be reinstituted.

### For parenteral dosage forms only

Intramuscular or subcutaneous administration is not recommended because of unreliable absorption.

Following stabilization of blood pressure using intravenous methyldopate, the patient should be transferred to methyldopa tablets at the same dosage as was used parenterally.

# Oral Dosage Forms

## METHYLDOPA ORAL SUSPENSION USP

### Usual adult dose

Antihypertensive—

Initial: Oral, 250 mg two or three times a day for two days, the dosage then being adjusted, preferably at intervals of not less than two days, until the desired response is obtained.

Maintenance: Oral, 500 mg to 2 grams a day, divided into two to four doses.

Note: Geriatric patients may be more sensitive to the effects of the usual adult dose and may require a lower dose to prevent syncope.

### Usual adult prescribing limits

Up to 3 grams a day.

### Usual pediatric dose

Antihypertensive—

Oral, initially 10 mg per kg of body weight or 300 mg per square meter of body surface, divided into two to four doses, the dosage then being adjusted, preferably at intervals of not less than two days, until the desired response is obtained, but not exceeding 65 mg per kg of body weight or 3 grams daily, whichever is less.

### Strength(s) usually available

U.S.—

50 mg per mL (Rx) [Aldomet (alcohol 1%; benzoic acid; sodium bisulfite; sugar; polysorbate)].

Canada—

Not commercially available.

### Packaging and storage

Store below 26 °C (79 °F), unless otherwise specified by manufacturer. Store in a tight, light-resistant container. Protect from freezing.

### Auxiliary labeling

• Shake well before using.
• May cause drowsiness.
• Do not take other medicines without your doctor's advice.

### Note

Check refill frequency to determine compliance in hypertensive patients.

## METHYLDOPA TABLETS USP

### Usual adult dose

Antihypertensive—

Initial: Oral, 250 mg two or three times a day for two days, the dosage then being adjusted, preferably at intervals of not less than two days, until the desired response is obtained.

Maintenance: Oral, 500 mg to 2 grams a day, divided into two to four doses.

Note: Geriatric patients may be more sensitive to the effects of the usual adult dose and may require a lower dose to prevent syncope.

### Usual adult prescribing limits

Up to 3 grams a day.

### Usual pediatric dose

Antihypertensive—

Oral, initially 10 mg per kg of body weight or 300 mg per square meter of body surface, divided into two to four doses, the dosage then being adjusted, preferably at intervals of not less than two days, until the desired response is obtained, but not exceeding 65 mg per kg of body weight or 3 grams daily, whichever is less.

### Strength(s) usually available

U.S.—

125 mg (Rx) [Aldomet (without sodium metabisulfite preservative); GENERIC (with or without sodium metabisulfite preservative)].

250 mg (Rx) [Aldomet (without sodium metabisulfite preservative); GENERIC (with or without sodium metabisulfite preservative)].

500 mg (Rx) [Aldomet (without sodium metabisulfite preservative); GENERIC (with or without sodium metabisulfite preservative)].

Canada—

125 mg (Rx) [Aldomet; Apo-Methyldopa; Dopamet; Novomedopa; Nu-Medopa].

250 mg (Rx) [Aldomet; Apo-Methyldopa; Dopamet; Novomedopa; Nu-Medopa].

500 mg (Rx) [Aldomet; Apo-Methyldopa; Dopamet; Novomedopa; Nu-Medopa].

### Packaging and storage

Store below 40 °C (104 °F), preferably between 15 and 30 °C (59 and 86 °F), unless otherwise specified by manufacturer. Store in a well-closed container.

### Auxiliary labeling

• May cause drowsiness.
• Do not take other medicines without your doctor's advice.

### Note

Check refill frequency to determine compliance in hypertensive patients.

# Parenteral Dosage Forms

## METHYLDOPATE HYDROCHLORIDE INJECTION USP

### Usual adult dose

Antihypertensive—

Intravenous infusion, 250 to 500 mg in 100 mL of 5% dextrose injection, administered slowly over a thirty- to sixty-minute period, every six hours if necessary.

Note: Geriatric patients may be more sensitive to the effects of the usual adult dose and may require a lower dose to prevent syncope.

### Usual adult prescribing limits

Up to 1 gram every 6 hours.

### Usual pediatric dose

Antihypertensive—

Intravenous infusion, 20 to 40 mg per kg of body weight in 5% dextrose injection, administered slowly over a thirty- to sixty-minute period, every six hours if necessary, but not exceeding 65 mg per kg of body weight or 3 grams daily, whichever is less.

### Strength(s) usually available

U.S.—

50 mg per mL (Rx) [Aldomet (sodium bisulfite; methylparaben; propylparaben); GENERIC (may contain sodium metabisulfite, methylparaben, propylparaben)].

Canada—

50 mg per mL (Rx) [Aldomet (sodium bisulfite; methylparaben; propylparaben)].

## Packaging and storage

Store below 40 °C (104 °F), preferably between 15 and 30 °C (59 and 86 °F), unless otherwise specified by manufacturer. Protect from freezing.

## Selected Bibliography

The fifth report of the Joint National Committee on Detection, Evaluation, and Treatment of High Blood Pressure (JNC V). Arch Intern Med 1993; 153 (2): 154-83.

Revised: 07/22/96

## METHYLDOPA-CONTAINING COMBINATIONS—

Methyldopa and Chlorothiazide (Systemic)—See *Methyldopa and Thiazide Diuretics (Systemic)*

Methyldopa and Hydrochlorothiazide (Systemic)—See *Methyldopa and Thiazide Diuretics (Systemic)*

---

# METHYLDOPA AND THIAZIDE DIURETICS   Systemic

This monograph includes information on the following: Methyldopa and Chlorothiazide; Methyldopa and Hydrochlorothiazide.

VA CLASSIFICATION (Primary): CV400

**NOTE:** The *Methyldopa and Thiazide Diuretics (Systemic)* monograph is maintained on the USP DI electronic data base. For a printed copy of the most recent revision of the complete monograph, contact the USP Division of Information Development, 12601 Twinbrook Parkway, Rockville, MD 20852.

For information on the specific components of this combination, see the *USP DI* monographs for) *Diuretics, Thiazide (Systemic)* and *Methyldopa (Systemic)*.

The information that follows is selectively abstracted from the complete monograph and is provided to facilitate drug use review and patient counseling.

Note: For a listing of dosage forms and brand names by country availability, see *Dosage Forms* section(s). For a listing of brand names for the articles in this monograph, refer to the General Index.

## Category

Antihypertensive.

## Indications

### Accepted

Hypertension (treatment)—This combination is indicated for treatment of hypertension.

Fixed-dosage combinations are generally not recommended for initial therapy and are useful for subsequent therapy only when the proportion of the component agents corresponds to the dose of the individual agents, as determined by titration.

For additional information on initial therapeutic guidelines related to the treatment of hypertension, see *Appendix III*.

## Patient Consultation

As an aid to patient consultation, refer to *Advice for the Patient, Methyldopa and Thiazide Diuretics (Systemic)*.

In providing consultation, consider emphasizing the following selected information (» = major clinical significance):

### Before using this medication
» Conditions affecting use, especially:
   Sensitivity to methyldopa, thiazide diuretics, other sulfonamide-type medications, bumetanide, furosemide, or carbonic anhydrase inhibitors
   Pregnancy—Thiazide diuretics not recommended for routine use; may cause jaundice, thrombocytopenia, hypokalemia in infant
   Breast-feeding—Excreted in breast milk; recommended that nursing mothers avoid thiazides during first month of breast-feeding because of reports of suppression of lactation
   Use in the elderly—Increased sensitivity to hypotensive, sedative, and electrolyte effects
   Other medications, especially MAO inhibitors, digitalis glycosides, or lithium
   Other medical problems, especially cerebrovascular disease, active hepatic disease, history of hemolytic anemia, history of hepatic disease associated with methyldopa, pheochromocytoma, or anuria or severe renal function impairment

### Proper use of this medication
   Possible need for control of weight and diet, especially sodium intake
» Patient may not experience symptoms of hypertension; importance of taking medication even if feeling well

» Does not cure, but helps control hypertension; possible need for life-long therapy; checking with physician before discontinuing medication; serious consequences of untreated hypertension
   Diuretic effects of the medication and timing of doses to minimize inconvenience of diuresis
   Getting into habit of taking at same time each day to help increase compliance
» Proper dosing
   Missed dose: Taking as soon as possible; not taking if almost time for next dose; not doubling doses
» Proper storage

### Precautions while using this medication
   Regular visits to physician to check progress
» Not using other medications, especially nonprescription sympathomimetics, unless ordered by physician
» Possibility of hypokalemia; possible need for additional potassium in diet; not changing diet without first checking with physician
   To prevent dehydration, checking with physician if severe nausea, vomiting, or diarrhea occurs and continues
   Caution if any kind of surgery (including dental surgery) or emergency treatment is required
» Reporting fever to physician
» Caution when driving or doing things requiring alertness because of possible drowsiness
   Caution when getting up suddenly from a lying or sitting position
» Caution in using alcohol, while standing for long periods or exercising, and during hot weather because of enhanced orthostatic hypotensive effects
   Diabetics: May increase blood sugar levels
   Possible dryness of mouth; using sugarless candy or gum, ice, or saliva substitute for relief; checking with physician or dentist if dry mouth continues for more than 2 weeks
» Possible photosensitivity; avoiding unprotected exposure to sun; using protective clothing and sun block product; avoiding use of sunlamp, tanning bed, or tanning booth
   Caution if any laboratory tests required; possible interference with test results

### Side/adverse effects
   Signs of potential side effects, especially drug fever, hypokalemia, mental changes, agranulocytosis, leukopenia, granulocytopenia, allergic reaction, cholestasis, hepatitis, cholecystitis, pancreatitis, colitis, hemolytic anemia, hyperuricemia, gout, myocarditis, SLE-like syndrome, and thrombocytopenia

## Oral Dosage Forms

### METHYLDOPA AND CHLOROTHIAZIDE TABLETS USP

**Usual adult dose**
Antihypertensive—
   Oral, 2 to 4 tablets a day in single or divided daily doses, as determined by individual titration with the component agents.

Note: Geriatric patients may be more sensitive to the effects of the usual adult dose and may require a lower dose to prevent syncope.

**Usual pediatric dose**
Oral, as determined by individual titration with the component agents.

**Strength(s) usually available**
U.S.—
   250 mg of methyldopa and 150 mg of chlorothiazide (Rx) [*Aldoclor;* GENERIC].
   250 mg of methyldopa and 250 mg of chlorothiazide (Rx) [*Aldoclor;* GENERIC].

**Strength(s) usually available**
U.S.—

   250 mg of methyldopa and 150 mg of chlorothiazide (Rx) [*Aldoclor;*
   GENERIC].
   250 mg of methyldopa and 250 mg of chlorothiazide (Rx) [*Aldoclor;*
   GENERIC].
Canada—
   250 mg of methyldopa and 150 mg of chlorothiazide (Rx) [*Supres*].
   250 mg of methyldopa and 250 mg of chlorothiazide (Rx) [*Supres*].

**Auxiliary labeling**
• May cause drowsiness.
• Do not take other medicines without your doctor's advice.

## METHYLDOPA AND HYDROCHLOROTHIAZIDE TABLETS USP

**Usual adult dose**
Antihypertensive—
   Oral, 2 to 4 tablets a day in single or divided daily doses, as deter-
   mined by individual titration with the component agents.

Note: Geriatric patients may be more sensitive to the effects of the usual
   adult dose and may require a lower dose to prevent syncope.

**Usual pediatric dose**
Oral, as determined by individual titration with the component agents.

**Strength(s) usually available**
U.S.—

   250 mg of methyldopa and 15 mg of hydrochlorothiazide (Rx) [*Aldoril;*
   GENERIC].
   250 mg of methyldopa and 25 mg of hydrochlorothiazide (Rx) [*Aldoril;*
   GENERIC].
   500 mg of methyldopa and 30 mg of hydrochlorothiazide (Rx) [*Aldoril;*
   GENERIC].
   500 mg of methyldopa and 50 mg of hydrochlorothiazide (Rx) [*Aldoril;*
   GENERIC].
Canada—
   250 mg of methyldopa and 15 mg of hydrochlorothiazide (Rx) [*Aldoril;*
   *Novodoparil; PMS Dopazide*].
   250 mg of methyldopa and 25 mg of hydrochlorothiazide (Rx) [*Aldoril;*
   *Novodoparil; PMS Dopazide*].

**Auxiliary labeling**
• May cause drowsiness.
• Do not take other medicines without your doctor's advice.

Revised: 04/13/93

# METHYLENE BLUE   Systemic

INN: Methylthioninium chloride

VA CLASSIFICATION (Primary/Secondary): AD900/DX900

Other commonly used names are aniline violet, methylthionine chloride,
   and tetrametylthionine chloride.

Note: For a listing of dosage forms and brand names by country availability, see *Dosage Forms* section(s). For a listing of brand names
   for the articles in this monograph, refer to the General Index.

# Category
Antimethemoglobinemic; diagnostic aid (tissue dye).

# Indications

**Accepted**
Methemoglobinemia, acquired (treatment) and
Methemoglobinemia, idiopathic (treatment)—Methylene blue is indicated
   in the treatment of acquired and idiopathic methemoglobinemia.

Tissue dye in diagnostic procedures—Methylene blue is used as a bacte-
   riological stain, as a dye in diagnostic procedures, such as fistula detection, and for the selective staining of certain body tissues during
   surgery. Methylene blue is also used intraamniotically to diagnose premature rupture of fetal membranes and to identify separate amniotic
   sacs in twin pregnancies.

**Unaccepted**
Methylene blue has been used to produce methemoglobinemia in the treatment of cyanide poisoning; however, sodium nitrite is considered to
   be a safer, more effective alternative.

Methylene blue has been used as a urinary tract antibacterial agent; however, this medication has been replaced by more effective agents.

# Pharmacology/Pharmacokinetics

**Physicochemical characteristics**
Molecular weight—373.90.
pH—3 to 4.5

**Mechanism of action/Effect**
Methemoglobinemia—Methylene blue, in low concentrations, acts as a
   cofactor to accelerate the conversion of methemoglobin to hemoglobin
   in erythrocytes. Methylene blue combines with nicotinamide adenine
   dinucleotide phosphate reduced (NADPH), in the presence of
   NADPH-methemoglobin reductase, to produce leukomethylene blue;
   leukomethylene blue then reduces methemoglobin to hemoglobin.
Tissue dye—Methylene blue's usefulness as a diagnostic aid is based on
   its ability to stain tissue.

**Other actions/effects**
In high concentrations, methylene blue oxidizes the ferrous iron of hemoglobin to the ferric state, facilitating the conversion of hemoglobin
   to methemoglobin.

Methylene blue has mild antiseptic activity that may inhibit bacterial
   proliferation.

**Absorption**
Poorly absorbed from the gastrointestinal tract after oral administration.

**Biotransformation**
Rapidly reduced to leukomethylene blue.

**Elimination**
Excreted in the urine and bile, primarily as leukomethylene blue. Some
   unchanged drug is also excreted in the urine.

# Precautions to Consider

**Pregnancy/Reproduction**
Pregnancy—Studies have not been done in humans.
Studies have not been done in animals.
FDA Pregnancy Category C.

**Breast-feeding**
It is not known whether methylene blue is distributed into breast milk.
   However, problems in humans have not been documented.

**Pediatrics**
Extreme caution should be exercised when administering methylene blue
   to infants. During the first 4 months of life, infants have lower concentrations of the enzymes necessary for reducing methemoglobin to
   hemoglobin, making these infants more susceptible to methemoglobinemia produced by high doses of methylene blue.
Intraamniotic injection of methylene blue has resulted in hemolytic anemia, hyperbilirubinemia, methemoglobinemia, and deep blue staining
   of the newborn.

**Geriatrics**
Appropriate studies on the relationship of age to the effects of methylene
   blue have not been performed in the geriatric population. However,
   no geriatrics-specific problems have been documented to date.

**Laboratory value alterations**
The following have been selected on the basis of their potential clinical
   significance (possible effect in parentheses where appropriate)—not
   necessarily inclusive (» = major clinical significance):

With diagnostic test results
» Phenolsulfonphthalein (PSP) excretion test
      (methylene blue may cause a false positive test result)
   Urinary free formaldehyde and
   Urine pH
      (methylene blue may interfere with analysis)

**Medical considerations/Contraindications**
The medical considerations/contraindications included here have been selected on the basis of their potential clinical significance (reasons given
   in parentheses where appropriate)—not necessarily inclusive (» =
   major clinical significance).

*Except under special circumstances, this medication should not be used when the following medical problems exist:*

» Glucose-6-phosphate dehydrogenase (G6PD) deficiency
   (use of methylene blue may aggravate methemoglobinemia and precipitate hemolytic anemia)

» Methemoglobinemia, to treat cyanide toxicity
   (methylene blue increases release of cyanide from methemoglobin, increasing the concentration of cyanide in the blood)

*Risk-benefit should be considered when the following medical problems exist:*

Renal function impairment
   (elimination may be reduced; dosage reduction may be required)

Sensitivity to methylene blue

### Patient monitoring

The following may be especially important in patient monitoring (other tests may be warranted in some patients, depending on condition; » = major clinical significance):

Complete blood counts and
» Reticulocyte counts
   (recommended following methylene blue therapy to assure that hemolysis has not occurred)

» Methemoglobin concentrations
   (recommended 1 to 2 hours following administration of methylene blue to assess the effectiveness of therapy)

## Side/Adverse Effects

The following side/adverse effects have been selected on the basis of their potential clinical significance (possible signs and symptoms in parentheses where appropriate)—not necessarily inclusive:

**Those indicating need for medical attention only if they continue or are bothersome**
Incidence more frequent
   *Greenish blue to blue discoloration of urine and feces*
Incidence less frequent
   *Diarrhea; nausea and vomiting; painful urination or increased urinary frequency*—with oral administration

## Overdose

For more information on the management of overdose or unintentional ingestion, **contact a Poison Control Center** (see *Poison Control Center Listing*).

### Clinical effects of overdose

The following side/adverse effects have been selected on the basis of their potential clinical significance (possible signs and symptoms in parentheses where appropriate)—not necessarily inclusive:

   *Abdominal pain; anxiety; chest pain; confusion; electrocardiographic changes* (diminished or inverted T wave amplitude; diminished R wave amplitude); *hemolytic anemia* (abdominal, back, or leg pain; chills); *methemoglobinemia* (bluish fingernails, lips, or skin; difficulty in breathing; dizziness; headache; unusual tiredness or weakness); *nausea and vomiting; severe sweating; tremors*

## Patient Consultation

As an aid to patient consultation, refer to *Advice for the Patient, Methylene Blue (Systemic)*.

In providing consultation, consider emphasizing the following selected information (» = major clinical significance):

**Before using this medication**
» Conditions affecting use, especially:
   Sensitivity to methylene blue
   Use in children—Cautious use in infants up to 4 months of age because they have lower concentrations of enzymes that reduce methemoglobin to hemoglobin; intraamniotic injection may cause hemolytic anemia, hyperbilirubinemia, methemoglobinemia, or deep blue staining of newborn
   Other medical problems, especially glucose-6-phosphate dehydrogenase (G6PD) deficiency and methemoglobinemia to treat cyanide toxicity

**Proper use of this medication**
   Taking tablets after meals with a full glass (240 mL) of water
» Proper dosing
   Missed dose
» Proper storage

**Precautions while using this medication**
   Possible interference with laboratory values

### Side/adverse effects

Greenish blue to blue discoloration of urine and feces may be alarming to patient although medically insignificant

## General Dosing Information

Treatment of acquired methemoglobinemia should be initiated with general supportive care and removal of the toxic agent, which, depending on the severity of the poisoning, may include administering 100% oxygen, and removing the toxic agent from the body. This can be done by removing contaminated clothing and rinsing the skin with water, inducing emesis, instituting gastric lavage, administering activated charcoal and cathartic, or instituting hemodialysis. In most cases of methemoglobinemia, these treatment measures stabilize the patient.

Specific antidotal therapy with methylene blue should be reserved for cases of methemoglobinemia in which the methemoglobin concentration is greater than 30% or in which there are clinical signs of hypoxia.

If adequate methylene blue therapy fails and toxic concentrations of methemoglobin persist, the possibility of glucose-6-phosphate dehydrogenase (G6PD) deficiency, nicotinamide adenine dinucleotide phosphate reduced (NADPH) methemoglobin reductase deficiency, hemoglobin M, or sulfhemoglobinemia should be considered. In these cases, exchange transfusion may be required. Hyperbaric oxygen has also been recommended, but its efficacy in this setting has been questioned and there is little experience with its use.

Chronic, idiopathic methemoglobinemia usually requires treatment only for cosmetic purposes. Administration of ascorbic acid, orally or intravenously, 100 to 500 mg two or three times a day is a non-toxic alternative to methylene blue. Ascorbic acid usually maintains the methemoglobin concentration below the level that causes cyanosis, preventing a cyanotic appearance. However, ascorbic acid reduces methemoglobin to hemoglobin too slowly to be of benefit in the treatment of acquired methemoglobinemia.

**For oral dosage forms only**
Methylene blue tablets should be taken after meals with a full glass (240 mL) of water.

**For parenteral dosage forms only**
Methylene blue should be administered by intravenous injection. Subcutaneous or intrathecal injection may result in tissue necrosis or neural damage, respectively.

## Oral Dosage Forms
### METHYLENE BLUE TABLETS

**Usual adult and adolescent dose**
Methemoglobinemia, idiopathic—
   Oral, 100 to 300 mg per day.

**Usual adult prescribing limits**
7 mg per kg of body weight.

**Strength(s) usually available**
U.S.—
   65 mg (Rx) [*Urolene Blue;* GENERIC].
Canada—
   Not commercially available.

**Packaging and storage**
Store below 40 °C (104 °F), preferably between 15 and 30 °C (59 and 86 °F), unless otherwise specified by manufacturer. Protect from light.

**Auxiliary labeling**
• Take after meals with a full glass (240 mL) of water.
• May discolor urine and/or stools.

## Parenteral Dosage Forms
### METHYLENE BLUE INJECTION USP

**Usual adult and adolescent dose**
Methemoglobinemia—
   Intravenous, 1 to 2 mg per kg of body weight or 25 to 50 mg per square meter of body surface area, administered over five minutes. The dose may be repeated after one hour if needed.

Note: For treatment of methemoglobinemia following overdose of agents in which there is prolonged or continuous methemoglobin formation (e.g., dapsone), methylene blue may be administered by continuous intravenous infusion at a rate of 0.1 to 0.15 mg per kg of body weight per hour, following an initial dose of 1 to 2 mg per kg of body weight.

**Usual adult prescribing limits**
7 mg per kg of body weight.

**Usual pediatric dose**
See *Usual adult and adolescent dose*.

**Strength(s) usually available**
U.S.—
   10 mg per mL (Rx) [GENERIC].
Canada—
   10 mg per mL (Rx) [GENERIC].

**Packaging and storage**
Store below 40 °C (104 °F), preferably between 15 and 30 °C (59 and 86 °F), unless otherwise specified by manufacturer. Protect from light.

**Preparation of dosage form**
For continuous intravenous infusion, methylene blue should be admixed with a compatible solution, such as 0.9% sodium chloride injection, to a final concentration of 0.05%.

**Auxiliary labeling**
• May discolor urine and/or stools.

## Selected Bibliography
Curry S. Methemoglobinemia. Ann Emerg Med 1982; 11: 214-21.

Developed: 05/27/94

---

# METHYLERGONOVINE   Systemic†

INN: Methylergometrine
VA CLASSIFICATION (Primary): GU600
Another commonly used name is methylergometrine.
Note: For a listing of dosage forms and brand names by country availability, see *Dosage Forms* section(s). For a listing of brand names for the articles in this monograph, refer to the General Index.

   †Not commercially available in Canada.

## Category
Uterine stimulant.

## Indications
Note: Bracketed information in the *Indications* section refers to uses that are not included in U.S. product labeling.

**Accepted**
Hemorrhage, postpartum and postabortal (prophylaxis and treatment)—Methylergonovine is indicated in the prevention or treatment of postpartum or postabortal uterine bleeding due to uterine atony or subinvolution. Its use is not recommended prior to delivery of the placenta since placental entrapment may occur.

[Abortion, incomplete (treatment)]—In cases of incomplete abortion, methylergonovine may be used to hasten expulsion of uterine contents.

**Unaccepted**
Methylergonovine is not as effective in treatment of migraine as other ergot alkaloids and use is not recommended.

Methylergonovine is not indicated for induction or augmentation of labor, to induce abortion, or in cases of threatened spontaneous abortion because of its propensity to produce nonphysiologic, tetanic contractions and its long duration of action.

## Pharmacology/Pharmacokinetics

**Physicochemical characteristics**
Chemical group—Amine ergot alkaloid.
Molecular weight—455.51.

**Mechanism of action/Effect**
Uterine stimulant—
   Methylergonovine directly stimulates the uterine muscle to increase force and frequency of contractions. When usual doses of methylergonovine are used, these contractions precede periods of relaxation; when larger doses are used, basal uterine tone is elevated and these relaxation periods will be decreased. Contraction of the uterine wall around bleeding vessels at the placental site produces hemostasis. The sensitivity of the uterus to the oxytocic effect is much greater toward the end of pregnancy. The oxytocic actions of methylergonovine are greater than its vascular effects.
Vasoconstriction—
   Methylergonovine, like other ergot alkaloids, produces arterial vasoconstriction by stimulation of alpha-adrenergic and serotonin receptors and inhibition of endothelial-derived relaxation factor release. It is a less potent vasoconstrictor than ergotamine.

**Other actions/effects**
Methylergonovine has minor actions on the central nervous system (CNS). In the CNS, methylergonovine is a partial agonist and partial antagonist at some serotonin and dopamine receptors. Methylergonovine also possesses weak dopaminergic antagonist actions in certain blood vessels and partial agonist actions at serotonin receptors in umbilical and placental blood vessels. It does not possess significant alpha-adrenergic blocking activity.

**Absorption**
Absorption is rapid after oral (60%) and intramuscular (78%) administration.

**Distribution**
Rapidly, primarily to plasma and extracellular fluid following intravenous administration; distribution to tissues also occurs rapidly.
In a study in women who had received 125 mcg of methylergonovine orally 3 times a day for 5 days, concentrations in breast milk ranged from less than 0.5 (limit of detection) to 1.3 nanograms per mL at 1 hour after a 250 mcg oral dose and from 0 to 1.2 nanograms per mL at 8 hours.

**Biotransformation**
Likely hepatic, with extensive first-pass metabolism.

**Half-life**
Intravenous—
   2 to 3 minutes or less (alpha phase).
   20 to 30 minutes or longer (beta phase).

**Onset of action**
Contraction of uterus, postpartum—
   Oral: 5 to 10 minutes.
   Intramuscular: 2 to 5 minutes.
   Intravenous: Immediate.

**Time to peak concentration**
In a study in postpartum patients, peak plasma concentrations occurred at 3 hours after a 250 mcg oral dose. In a study in healthy fasting males, peak plasma concentrations occurred at 30 minutes.

**Peak serum concentration**
In a study in postpartum patients, peak plasma concentrations were 3 nanograms per mL after a 250 mcg oral dose. In a study in healthy fasting males, similar concentrations were achieved. Women given 125 mcg by mouth 3 times a day for 5 days had plasma concentrations within the range of 0.6 to 4.4 nanograms per mL at 1 hour after a 250 mcg oral dose and from 0 to 0.6 nanograms per mL at 8 hours.

**Duration of action**
Contraction of uterus, postpartum—
   Oral: Approximately 3 hours.
   Intramuscular: Approximately 3 hours.
   Intravenous: 45 minutes (although rhythmic contractions may persist for up to 3 hours).

**Elimination**
Primarily renal excretion of metabolites; some fecal. Renal elimination of unchanged drug is responsible for less than 5% of total elimination. Methylergonovine does not appear to accumulate after multiple doses.

## Precautions to Consider

**Cross-sensitivity and/or related problems**
Patients sensitive to other ergot derivatives may be sensitive to this medication also, although there is some degree of variation among ergot alkaloids in their ability to elicit oxytocic, CNS, or vasoconstrictive effects.

**Pregnancy/Reproduction**
Pregnancy—Methylergonovine is contraindicated during pregnancy. Tetanic contractions may result in decreased uterine blood flow and fetal distress.

Labor and delivery—High doses of methylergonovine administered prior to delivery may cause uterine tetany and fetal distress. Methylergonovine should *not* be administered prior to delivery of the placenta. Administration prior to delivery of the placenta may cause captivation of the placenta or missed diagnosis of twin gestation, due to excessive uterine contraction.

### Breast-feeding
Problems in humans have not been documented. Ergot alkaloids are excreted in breast milk. However, very little passes into breast milk in humans. In a study in women who had received 125 mcg of methylergonovine orally 3 times a day for 5 days, concentrations in breast milk ranged from less than 0.5 (limit of detection) to 1.3 nanograms per mL at 1 hour after a 250 mcg oral dose and from 0 to 1.2 nanograms per mL at 8 hours.

Inhibition of lactation has not been reported for methylergonovine. However, studies have shown that methylergonovine may interfere with the secretion of prolactin (to a lesser degree than bromocriptine) in the immediate postpartum period. This could result in delayed or diminished lactation with prolonged use.

Ergot alkaloids have the potential to cause chronic ergot poisoning in the infant only if used in the mother in higher-than-recommended doses or if used for a longer period of time than is generally recommended.

### Pediatrics
In newborns, elimination of methylergonovine may be prolonged. Neonates inadvertently administered ergonovine in overdose amounts have developed respiratory depression, myoclonic movements, purpuric symptoms, mild jaundice, and severe peripheral vasoconstriction.

### Geriatrics
No information is available on the effects of methylergonovine in geriatric patients.

### Drug interactions and/or related problems
The following drug interactions and/or related problems have been selected on the basis of their potential clinical significance (possible mechanism in parentheses where appropriate)—not necessarily inclusive (» = major clinical significance):

Note: Combinations containing any of the following medications, depending on the amount present, may also interact with this medication.

Anesthetics, general, especially halothane
(peripheral vasoconstriction may be potentiated by the concurrent use of general anesthetics with methylergonovine)

(concurrent use of halothane in concentrations greater than 1% may interfere with the oxytocic actions of methylergonovine, resulting in severe uterine hemorrhage)

Bromocriptine or
Ergot alkaloids, other
(the incidence of rare cases of hypertension, strokes, seizures, and myocardial infarction associated with the postpartum use of bromocriptine or other ergot alkaloids may be increased with the use of ergot alkaloids)

Nicotine or
Smoking, tobacco
(nicotine absorption from heavy smoking may result in enhanced vasoconstriction)

Nitroglycerin or
Antianginal agents, other
(ergot alkaloids may induce coronary vasospasm, lowering the efficacy of nitroglycerin or other antianginal agents; increased doses of nitroglycerin or antianginal agents and/or use of intracoronary nitroglycerin may be necessary)

Vasoconstrictors, other, including those present in local anesthetics or
Vasopressors
(concurrent use may result in enhanced vasoconstriction; dosage adjustments may be necessary)

(the pressor effect of sympathomimetic pressor amines may be potentiated, resulting in potentially severe hypertension, headache, and rupture of cerebral blood vessels; gangrene developed in a patient receiving both dopamine and ergonovine infusions)

### Laboratory value alterations
The following have been selected on the basis of their potential clinical significance (possible effect in parentheses where appropriate)—not necessarily inclusive (» = major clinical significance):

With physiology/laboratory test values
Blood pressure or
Central venous pressure
(may be elevated due to peripheral vasoconstriction primarily of postcapillary vessels; less likely with methylergonovine than er-

gonovine; has sometimes been associated with preeclampsia, history of hypertension, intravenous administration of methylergonovine, or concurrent use of local anesthetics containing vasoconstrictors; hypotension has also been reported)

Heart rate
(may be decreased due primarily to an increase in vagal tone, and possibly to decreased central sympathetic activity and direct depression of the myocardium)

Prolactin
(serum concentrations may be decreased)

### Medical considerations/Contraindications
The medical considerations/contraindications included here have been selected on the basis of their potential clinical significance (reasons given in parentheses where appropriate)—not necessarily inclusive (» = major clinical significance).

*Except under special circumstances, this medication should not be used when the following medical problems exist:*

»  Angina pectoris, unstable or
»  Myocardial infarction, recent
(vasospasm caused by methylergonovine may precipitate angina or myocardial infarction)

»  Cardiovascular disease or
»  Coronary artery disease
(patients may be more susceptible to angina or myocardial infarction caused by methylergonovine-induced vasospasm)

»  Cerebrovascular accident, history of or
»  Transient ischemic attack, history of
(patients may be susceptible to recurrence due to increases in blood pressure)

»  Eclampsia or
»  Preeclampsia
(may be exacerbated; patients may be more likely to develop methylergonovine-induced hypertension; headaches, severe cardiac arrhythmias, seizures, and cerebrovascular accidents have occurred)

»  Hypertension, severe, or history of
(may be exacerbated)

»  Occlusive peripheral vascular disease or
»  Raynaud's phenomenon, severe
(may be exacerbated; a patient with Raynaud's phenomenon developed impalpable arterial pulses with use of ergonovine)

*Risk-benefit should be considered when the following medical problems exist:*

Allergy or sensitivity to methylergonovine or other ergot alkaloids
»  Hepatic function impairment
(impaired metabolism of methylergonovine may result in ergot overdose)

Hypocalcemia
(oxytocic response to methylergonovine may be reduced; cautious use of intravenous calcium gluconate may restore oxytocic response to methylergonovine)

»  Mitral valve stenosis or
»  Venoatrial shunts
(vasospasm caused by methylergonovine may precipitate angina or myocardial infarction)

»  Renal function impairment
»  Sepsis
(possible increased sensitivity to effects of methylergonovine)

### Patient monitoring
The following may be especially important in patient monitoring (other tests may be warranted in some patients, depending on condition; » = major clinical significance):

Blood pressure determinations and
Pulse rate determinations and
Uterine response
(recommended at frequent intervals after parenteral therapy to monitor for adverse reactions; especially important with intravenous administration or before repeating doses)

## Side/Adverse Effects

Note: Because the duration of therapy with methylergonovine is generally short, many of the side effects seen with other ergot alkaloids do not occur.

The following side/adverse effects have been selected on the basis of their potential clinical significance (possible signs and symptoms in parentheses where appropriate)—not necessarily inclusive:

**Those indicating need for medical attention**
Incidence less frequent
   *Bradycardia* (slow heartbeat); *coronary vasospasm* (chest pain)
Incidence rare
   *Allergic reaction, including shock; cardiac arrest or ventricular arrhythmias, including fibrillation and tachycardia* (irregular heartbeat); *dyspnea* (unexplained shortness of breath); *hypertension, sudden and severe* (sudden, severe headache; blurred vision; seizures); *myocardial infarction* (crushing chest pain; unexplained shortness of breath)—has occurred with the use of ergot preparations in the postpartum period; *peripheral vasospasm* (itching of skin; pain in arms, legs, or lower back; pale or cold hands or feet; weakness in legs)—dose-related

**Those indicating need for medical attention only if they continue or are bothersome**
Incidence more frequent
   *Nausea*—especially after intravenous use; *uterine cramping; vomiting*—especially after intravenous use
   Note: *Uterine cramping* will occur to some degree in all patients and is indicative of efficacy. However, dosage reduction may be required in occasional patients with severe or intolerable uterine cramps.
Incidence less frequent
   *Abdominal or stomach pain; diarrhea; dizziness; sweating; tinnitus* (ringing in the ears)

## Overdose

For specific information on the agents used in the management of methylergonovine overdose, see:
   • *Charcoal, Activated (Oral-Local)* monograph;
   • *Chlorpromazine* in *Phenothiazines (Systemic)* monograph;
   • *Diazepam* in *Benzodiazepines (Systemic)* monograph;
   • *Hydralazine (Systemic)* monograph;
   • *Laxatives (Local)* monograph;
   • *Nitroglycerin* in *Nitrates (Systemic)* monograph;
   • *Nitroprusside (Systemic)* monograph;
   • *Phentolamine (Systemic)* monograph;
   • *Phenytoin* in *Anticonvulsants, Hydantoin (Systemic)* monograph; and/or
   • *Tolazoline (Parenteral-Systemic)* monograph.

For more information on the management of overdose or unintentional ingestion, **contact a Poison Control Center** (see *Poison Control Center Listing*).

### Clinical effects of overdose
The following effects have been selected on the basis of their potential clinical significance (possible signs and symptoms in parentheses where appropriate)—not necessarily inclusive:
Acute
   *Angina* (chest pain); *bradycardia* (slow heartbeat); *confusion; drowsiness; fast, weak pulse; miosis* (small pupils); *peripheral vasoconstriction, severe* (coolness, paleness, or numbness of arms or legs; muscle pain; weak or absent arterial pulse in arms or legs; tingling, itching, and coolness of skin); *respiratory depression* (decreased breathing rate or trouble in breathing; bluish color of skin or inside of nose or mouth); *seizures; tachycardia* (fast heartbeat); *unconsciousness; unusual thirst; uterine tetany* (severe cramping of the uterus)
Chronic
   *Formication* (false feeling of insects crawling on the skin); *gangrene* (dry, shriveled appearance of skin on hands, lower legs, or feet); *hemiplegia* (paralysis of one side of the body); *thrombophlebitis* (pain and redness in an arm or leg)
   Note: Chronic overdose symptoms are unlikely with proper use since treatment is of short duration.

### Treatment of overdose
Immediate discontinuation of methylergonovine. Since there is no specific antidote for the management of methylergonovine overdose, treatment is primarily supportive and symptomatic and may include the following:
To decrease absorption—
   Gastrointestinal decontamination for oral overdose, preferably with multiple doses of activated charcoal and an appropriate cathartic. Gastric lavage may also be considered.
Specific treatment—
   Use of nitroglycerin for treatment of myocardial ischemia. Intracoronary nitroglycerin may be necessary.
   Use of diazepam or phenytoin for treatment of seizures.

Use of sodium nitroprusside, tolazoline, or phentolamine for treatment of peripheral ischemia.
   Use of sodium nitroprusside, chlorpromazine 15 mg, or hydralazine for treatment of severe hypertension.
Monitoring—
   Frequent monitoring of vital signs, arterial blood gases, and electrolytes. Electrocardiogram monitoring to assess cardiac function and perfusion. Monitoring of serum methylergonovine levels is not predictive of the outcome of overdose.
Supportive care—
   May include maintaining an open airway and breathing, maintaining proper fluid and electrolyte balance, correcting hypertension, and controlling seizures. Patients in whom intentional overdose is known or suspected should be referred for psychiatric consultation.

## Patient Consultation

As an aid to patient consultation, refer to *Advice for the Patient, Ergonovine/Methylergonovine (Systemic)*.

In providing consultation, consider emphasizing the following selected information (» = major clinical significance):

**Before using this medication**
» Conditions affecting use, especially:
      Allergies or sensitivity to methylergonovine or other ergot alkaloids
      Pregnancy—Should not be used prior to delivery or delivery of the placenta
      Breast-feeding—Ergot alkaloids are excreted in breast milk
      Other medical problems, especially cardiac or vascular disease, hepatic function impairment, severe hypertension or history of hypertension, renal function impairment, and sepsis

**Proper use of this medication**
» Importance of not using more medication or using for longer than prescribed; risk of ergotism and gangrene with prolonged use
» Proper dosing
   Missed dose: Not taking missed dose; not doubling doses
» Proper storage

**Precautions while using this medication**
   Notifying physician if infection develops, since infection may cause increased sensitivity to medication

**Side/adverse effects**
   Signs of potential side effects, especially allergic reaction, coronary vasospasm or other cardiovascular complications, dyspnea, severe hypertension, or peripheral vasospasm

## General Dosing Information

Antiemetic medications such as prochlorperazine may be administered prior to use of methylergonovine.

**For parenteral dosage forms only**
Because the risk of severe adverse effects is increased with intravenous use of methylergonovine, such use is recommended only for emergencies such as excessive uterine bleeding.

If intravenous use is warranted, administration must be done slowly, over a period of at least 1 minute; some clinicians recommend dilution of the solution with normal saline before administration.

In some patients who do not respond to methylergonovine because of hypocalcemia, cautious intravenous administration of calcium gluconate (provided the patient is not receiving digitalis) may restore the oxytocic action.

## Oral Dosage Forms

### METHYLERGONOVINE MALEATE TABLETS USP

**Usual adult and adolescent dose**
Uterine stimulant—
   Oral, 200 to 400 mcg (0.2 to 0.4 mg) two to four times a day (every six to twelve hours) until the danger of uterine atony and hemorrhage has passed.
Note: Generally, a treatment course of 48 hours is sufficient. However, in some patients, treatment for up to 7 days may be necessary, especially when used for treatment of incomplete abortion. Oral administration usually follows an initial parenteral dose.

**Strength(s) usually available**
U.S.—
   200 mcg (0.2 mg) (Rx) [*Methergine*].
Canada—
   Not commercially available.

## Packaging and storage
Store below 40 °C (104 °F), preferably between 15 and 30 °C (59 and 86 °F), unless otherwise specified by manufacturer. Store in a tight container. Protect from light.

## Parenteral Dosage Forms
### METHYLERGONOVINE MALEATE INJECTION USP

**Usual adult and adolescent dose**
Uterine stimulant—
Intramuscular or intravenous, 200 mcg (0.2 mg), repeated in two to four hours if necessary, up to five doses.

**Strength(s) usually available**
U.S.—
200 mcg (0.2 mg) per mL (Rx) [*Methergine*].

Canada—
Not commercially available.

## Packaging and storage
Store below 40 °C (104 °F), preferably between 15 and 30 °C (59 and 86 °F), unless otherwise specified by manufacturer. Protect from light. Protect from freezing.

## Stability
Discolored solutions or solutions containing visible particles should not be used.

Revised: 06/07/93

---

# METHYLPHENIDATE   Systemic

VA CLASSIFICATION (Primary): CN802

Note: Controlled substance in the U.S. and Canada.

Note: For a listing of dosage forms and brand names by country availability, see *Dosage Forms* section(s). For a listing of brand names for the articles in this monograph, refer to the General Index.

## Category
Central nervous system stimulant.

## Indications
Note: Bracketed information in the *Indications* section refers to uses that are not included in U.S. product labeling.

**Accepted**
Attention-deficit hyperactivity disorder (treatment)—Methylphenidate is used as the primary agent in a total treatment program that includes other remedial measures (psychological, educational, and social) to stabilize some children [and adults] with attention-deficit hyperactivity disorder (ADHD). This complex behavioral syndrome has been known in the past as hyperkinetic child syndrome, minimal brain damage, minimal cerebral dysfunction, or minor cerebral dysfunction.

Narcolepsy (treatment)—Methylphenidate is indicated in the management of the symptoms of narcolepsy.

[Depression, mental, secondary to medical illness (treatment)][1]—Methylphenidate may be useful in selected patients whose medical condition complicates treatment with conventional antidepressants.

**Unaccepted**
Methylphenidate is *not* recommended for the treatment of mental depression amenable to treatment with conventional antidepressants, for the prevention or treatment of normal fatigue states, or for children who exhibit symptoms secondary to environmental factors and/or psychiatric disorders, including psychosis.

[1]Not included in Canadian product labeling.

## Pharmacology/Pharmacokinetics

**Physicochemical characteristics**
Molecular weight—269.77.

**Mechanism of action/Effect**
Central nervous system (CNS) stimulant—Although the primary mechanism is largely unknown, the effects of methylphenidate appear to be mediated by blockage of the reuptake mechanism of dopaminergic neurons. In children with attention deficit disorder, methylphenidate decreases motor restlessness and enhances the ability to pay attention. In narcolepsy, methylphenidate appears to act at the cerebral cortex and subcortical structures, including the thalamus, to produce CNS stimulation, resulting in increased motor activity, increased mental alertness, diminished sense of fatigue, brighter spirits, and mild euphoria.

**Time to peak serum concentration**
Extended-release tablets—
4.7 hours (range, 1.3 to 8.2 hours) in children.
Tablets—
1.9 hours (range, 0.3 to 4.4 hours) in children.

**Elimination**
Renal—
An average of 67% of the methylphenidate in an extended-release tablet is excreted by children (as compared to 86% by adults).

## Precautions to Consider

**Carcinogenicity/Tumorigenicity**
In a lifetime carcinogenicity study in a mouse strain that is sensitive to the development of hepatic tumors (B6C3F1 mice), methylphenidate caused an increase in hepatocellular adenomas (benign tumors) at a dose of approximately 60 mg per kg of body weight (mg/kg) a day, or approximately 2.5 times a human dose of 60 mg a day on a mg per square meter of body surface area (mg/m$^2$) basis. In the same study, male mice showed an increase in hepatoblastomas (rare malignant tumors). There was no increase in total malignant hepatic tumors. A similar study in F344 rats showed no increase in tumors. The significance of these findings to humans is unknown.

**Mutagenicity**
No mutagenic potential was found in the Ames reverse mutation assay or in the *in vitro* mouse lymphoma cell forward mutation assay. A weak clastogenic response was found in an *in vitro* assay in cultured Chinese Hamster Ovary cells. *In vivo* assays of genotoxic potential of methylphenidate have not been performed. The significance of these findings to humans is unknown.

**Pregnancy/Reproduction**
Pregnancy—Studies have not been done in humans.
Studies have not been done in animals.

**Breast-feeding**
It is not known whether methylphenidate is distributed into breast milk.

**Pediatrics**
Long-term effects of methylphenidate in children are not well established. Children are more prone than adults to develop anorexia, insomnia, stomach pain, tachycardia, and weight loss. Monitoring of growth (both height and weight gain) has been recommended during long-term therapy since chronic administration of methylphenidate may be associated with growth inhibition, although data are inadequate to determine this conclusively. Some clinicians may recommend medication-free periods during methylphenidate treatment to evaluate the need for continued therapy.

**Geriatrics**
No information is available on the relationship of age to the effects of methylphenidate in geriatric patients.

**Drug interactions and/or related problems**
The following drug interactions and/or related problems have been selected on the basis of their potential clinical significance (possible mechanism in parentheses where appropriate)—not necessarily inclusive (» = major clinical significance):

Note: Combinations containing any of the following medications, depending on the amount present, may also interact with this medication.

Anticholinergics or other medications with anticholinergic activity (See *Appendix II*)
(concurrent use may intensify anticholinergic effects because of secondary anticholinergic effects of methylphenidate)

Anticonvulsants, especially phenytoin, phenobarbital, and primidone or
Anticoagulants, coumarin- or indandione-derivative or
Phenylbutazone
(serum concentrations may be increased when these medications are used concurrently with methylphenidate because of metabolism inhibition, possibly resulting in toxicity; dosage adjustments may be necessary)

Antidepressants, tricyclic, especially desipramine and imipramine
(serum concentrations may be increased when these medications are used concurrently with methylphenidate because of inhibition of metabolism; also, concurrent use may antagonize the effects of methylphenidate)

Antihypertensives or
Diuretics used as antihypertensives
(hypotensive effects may be reduced when these medications are used concurrently with methylphenidate; the patient should be carefully monitored to confirm that the desired effect is being obtained)

» CNS stimulation–producing medications, other (See *Appendix II*)
(concurrent use with methylphenidate may result in additive CNS stimulation to excessive levels, causing nervousness, irritability, insomnia, or possibly seizures or cardiac arrhythmias; close observation is recommended)

» Monoamine oxidase (MAO) inhibitors, including furazolidone, procarbazine, and selegiline
(concurrent use may potentiate the effects of methylphenidate, possibly resulting in a hypertensive crisis; methylphenidate should not be administered during or within 14 days following the administration of MAO inhibitors)

» Pimozide
(concurrent use with methylphenidate may mask the cause of tics since methylphenidate itself may provoke tics; before therapy with pimozide is initiated, methylphenidate should be withdrawn)

Vasopressors
(pressor effects may be potentiated when vasopressors are used concurrently with methylphenidate)

## Medical considerations/Contraindications
The medical considerations/contraindications included here have been selected on the basis of their potential clinical significance (reasons given in parentheses where appropriate)—not necessarily inclusive (» = major clinical significance).

*Except under special circumstances, this medication should not be used when the following medical problems exist:*
» Anxiety, tension, or agitation, severe or
» Depression, mental, which is amenable to treatment with conventional antidepressants or
» Glaucoma or
» Motor tics other than Tourette's disorder
(may be exacerbated)

*Risk-benefit should be considered when the following medical problems exist:*
Emotional instability, including history of drug dependence or alcoholism
(increased potential for addiction or abuse)
Epilepsy or other seizure disorders
(seizure threshold may be lowered)
» Gilles de la Tourette's syndrome, family history or diagnosis of
(motor and vocal tics may be exacerbated; however, some patients, under close supervision, may benefit from cautious trials)
» Hypertension
(may be exacerbated)
Psychosis
(symptoms of behavior disturbance and thought disorder may be exacerbated in psychotic children)
Sensitivity to methylphenidate

## Patient monitoring
The following may be especially important in patient monitoring (other tests may be warranted in some patients, depending on condition; » = major clinical significance):
Assessment of amount and frequency of medication use
(recommended at periodic intervals to detect signs of dependence or abuse during long-term therapy)
Blood pressure determinations
(recommended at periodic intervals during therapy, especially for patients with hypertension)

Complete blood cell, differential, and platelet counts
(recommended at periodic intervals for patients on prolonged therapy)
Monitoring of growth, both height and weight gain, in children
(recommended during long-term therapy, since data are inadequate to determine whether chronic administration of methylphenidate may be associated with growth inhibition)
Reassessment of need for therapy for behavioral syndrome in children
(interruption of therapy at periodic intervals is recommended to determine if a recurrence of behavioral symptoms is sufficient to continue therapy; tapering of dose may be necessary to prevent withdrawal symptoms)

# Side/Adverse Effects
The following side/adverse effects have been selected on the basis of their potential clinical significance (possible signs and symptoms in parentheses where appropriate)—not necessarily inclusive:

### Those indicating need for medical attention
Incidence more frequent
*Hypertension* (increased blood pressure); *tachycardia* (fast heartbeat)—especially with doses greater than 0.5 mg per kg of body weight (mg/kg)
Incidence less frequent
*Angina* (chest pain); *arthralgia* (joint pain); *dyskinesia* (uncontrolled movements of the body); *fever; skin rash or hives; thrombocytopenic purpura* (rarely, unusual bleeding or bruising; black tarry stools; blood in urine or stools; pinpoint red spots on skin)—usually asymptomatic
Note: *Arthralgia, fever, skin rash or hives, and thrombocytopenic purpura* may be indicative of a hypersensitivity reaction to methylphenidate.

Incidence rare
*Blurred vision or any change in vision; Tourette's syndrome* (uncontrolled vocal outbursts and tics [uncontrolled repeated body movements])
With prolonged use or at high doses
*Psychosis, toxic* (mood or mental changes); *weight loss*—possibly more frequent in children

### Those indicating need for medical attention only if they continue or are bothersome
Incidence more frequent
*Anorexia* (loss of appetite)—possibly more frequent in children; *CNS stimulation* (nervousness; trouble in sleeping)—possibly more frequent in children
Incidence less frequent
*Dizziness; drowsiness; headache; nausea; stomach pain*—possibly more frequent in children

### Those indicating possible withdrawal and the need for medical attention if they occur after medication is discontinued
*Mental depression, severe; unusual behavior; unusual tiredness or weakness*

# Overdose
For specific information on the agents used in the management of methylphenidate overdose, see:
• *Barbiturates (Systemic)* monograph.
For more information on the management of overdose or unintentional ingestion, **contact a Poison Control Center** (see *Poison Control Center Listing*).

### Clinical effects of overdose
The following effects have been selected on the basis of their potential clinical significance (possible signs and symptoms in parentheses where appropriate)–not necessarily inclusive:

*Agitation; cardiac arrhythmias* (fast or irregular heartbeat); *confusion; delirium* (extreme confusion); *dryness of mouth or mucous membranes; euphoria* (false sense of well-being); *fever; hallucinations* (seeing, hearing, or feeling things that are not there); *headache, severe; hyperreflexia* (overactive reflexes); *increased blood pressure; increased sweating; muscle twitching; mydriasis* (large pupils); *palpitations* (fast, pounding, or irregular heartbeat); *seizures*—may be followed by coma; *tachycardia* (fast heartbeat); *trembling or tremors; vomiting*

### Treatment of overdose

Since there is no specific antidote for overdose with methylphenidate, treatment is symptomatic and supportive with possible utilization of the following:

To decrease absorption—
Emptying stomach by emesis or gastric lavage.

Specific treatment—
For severe overdose, administering a short-acting barbiturate using carefully titrated dosage.

Supportive care—
Maintaining quiet, protective surroundings.
Maintaining adequate circulatory and respiratory function.
Using external cooling procedures for hyperpyrexia.
Patients in whom intentional overdose is known or suspected should be referred for psychiatric consultation.

Note: Usefulness of peritoneal dialysis or extracorporeal hemodialysis has not been established.

## Patient Consultation

As an aid to patient consultation, refer to *Advice for the Patient, Methylphenidate (Systemic)*.

In providing consultation, consider emphasizing the following selected information (» = major clinical significance):

### Before using this medication
» Conditions affecting use, especially:
Sensitivity to methylphenidate
Use in children—In attention-deficit hyperactivity disorder (ADHD), drug-free periods may be recommended during treatment; monitoring of height and weight recommended; children more likely to develop stomach pain, trouble in sleeping, and loss of appetite and weight
Other medications, especially other CNS stimulation–producing medications, MAO inhibitors, or pimozide
Other medical problems, especially severe anxiety, tension, or agitation; depression amenable to conventional treatment; glaucoma; hypertension; motor tics; or Tourette's syndrome

### Proper use of this medication
» Importance of not using more medication than the amount prescribed because of possible habit-forming potential
Taking with or after a meal or snack
Taking the last dose of the short-acting tablets for each day before 6 p.m. to minimize the possibility of insomnia
Not increasing dose if medication seems less effective after a few weeks; checking with physician
Proper administration for extended-release dosage form: Swallowing whole; not breaking, crushing, or chewing
» Proper dosing
Missed dose: Taking as soon as possible; taking any remaining doses for that day at regularly spaced intervals; not doubling doses
» Proper storage

### Precautions while using this medication
Regular visits to physician to check progress during therapy
» Checking with physician before discontinuing medication after long-term and high-dose therapy; gradual dosage reduction may be necessary to avoid possibility of withdrawal symptoms
» Suspected psychological or physical dependence; checking with physician

### Side/adverse effects
Possibility of withdrawal effects
Signs of potential side effects, especially hypertension, tachycardia, angina, arthralgia, dyskinesia, fever, skin rash or hives, thrombocytopenic purpura, blurred vision or any change in vision, Tourette's syndrome, toxic psychosis, or weight loss

## General Dosing Information

To reduce the possibility of insomnia, the last dose of methylphenidate tablets for each day should be administered before 6 p.m.

When symptoms of attention-deficit hyperactivity disorder are controlled in children, dosage reduction or interruption in therapy may be possible during the summer months and at other times when the child is under less stress; medication may be given on each of the 5 school days during the week, with medication-free weekends and school holidays. However, some children may require daily dosing and summer use.

Prolonged use of methylphenidate may result in psychological or physical dependence.

When the medication is to be discontinued following high-dose and long-term administration, the dosage should be reduced gradually in order to avoid the possibility of withdrawal symptoms.

### Diet/Nutrition
Methylphenidate should be taken with or after a meal or snack.

## Oral Dosage Forms
### METHYLPHENIDATE HYDROCHLORIDE TABLETS USP

#### Usual adult and adolescent dose
For narcolepsy or attention-deficit hyperactivity disorder—
Oral, 5 to 20 mg two or three times a day, preferably with or after meals.

#### Usual adult prescribing limits
90 mg a day.

#### Usual pediatric dose
Attention-deficit hyperactivity disorder—
Children up to 6 years of age: Dosage has not been established.
Children 6 years of age and over: Oral, 5 mg two times a day, with or after breakfast and lunch, the dosage being increased as needed and tolerated by 5 to 10 mg at one-week intervals up to a maximum of 60 mg a day.

Note: If improvement in condition does not occur after appropriate dosage adjustment over a one-month period, it is recommended that the medication be discontinued.

#### Strength(s) usually available
U.S.—
5 mg (Rx) [*Ritalin;* GENERIC].
10 mg (Rx) [*Ritalin* (scored); GENERIC].
20 mg (Rx) [*Ritalin* (scored); GENERIC].
Canada—
10 mg (Rx) [*PMS-Methylphenidate* (scored); *Ritalin* (scored)].
20 mg (Rx) [*PMS-Methylphenidate* (scored); *Ritalin* (scored)].

#### Packaging and storage
Store below 30 °C (86 °F), preferably between 15 and 30 °C (59 and 86 °F), protected from light, unless otherwise specified by manufacturer. Store in a tight container.

#### Note
Controlled substance in the U.S. and Canada.

### METHYLPHENIDATE HYDROCHLORIDE EXTENDED-RELEASE TABLETS USP

Note: Extended-release tablets have a duration of action of 8 hours, and may be used in place of the conventional tablets when the 8-hour dosage of the extended-release tablets corresponds to the titrated 8-hour dosage of the tablets.

#### Usual adult and adolescent dose
For narcolepsy or attention-deficit hyperactivity disorder—
Oral, 20 mg one to three times a day at eight-hour intervals.

#### Usual pediatric dose
Attention-deficit hyperactivity disorder—
Children up to 6 years of age: Dosage has not been established.
Children 6 years of age and over: Oral, 20 mg one to three times a day at eight-hour intervals.

#### Strength(s) usually available
U.S.—
20 mg (Rx) [*Ritalin-SR;* GENERIC].
Canada—
20 mg (Rx) [*Ritalin SR*].

#### Packaging and storage
Store below 30 °C (86 °F), preferably between 15 and 30 °C (59 and 86 °F), protected from light, unless otherwise specified by manufacturer. Store in a tight container.

#### Auxiliary labeling
• Swallow tablets whole.

#### Note
Controlled substance in the U.S. and Canada.

Revised: 08/15/95
Interim revision: 06/26/96

**METHYLPREDNISOLONE**—See *Corticosteroids—Glucocorticoid Effects (Systemic)*

**METHYLTESTOSTERONE**—See *Androgens (Systemic)*

**METHYLTESTOSTERONE-CONTAINING COMBINATIONS**—

Conjugated Estrogens and Methyltestosterone (Systemic)—See *Androgens and Estrogens (Systemic)*

Diethylstilbestrol and Methyltestosterone (Systemic)—See *Androgens and Estrogens (Systemic)*

Esterified Estrogens and Methyltestosterone (Systemic)—See *Androgens and Estrogens (Systemic)*

**METHYPRYLON**—Since Methyprylon is not commercially available in the U.S. or Canada, the *Methyprylon (Systemic)* monograph is not included in this published version of the USP DI database. Copies of the monograph are available on request from the USP Division of Information Development, 12601 Twinbrook Parkway, Rockville, MD 20852; telephone (301) 816-8351; telefax (301) 816-8374.

# METHYSERGIDE    Systemic

VA CLASSIFICATION (Primary): CN105

Note: For a listing of dosage forms and brand names by country availability, see *Dosage Forms* section(s). For a listing of brand names for the articles in this monograph, refer to the General Index.

## Category
Vascular headache prophylactic.

## Indications

**Accepted**

Headache vascular (prophylaxis)—Methysergide is indicated for prevention of vascular headaches such as migraine and cluster headaches in patients with frequent and/or disabling headaches not responsive to other treatment.

**Unaccepted**

Methysergide is not recommended for treatment of acute attacks or tension headaches.

## Pharmacology/Pharmacokinetics

**Physicochemical characteristics**
Molecular weight—469.54.

**Mechanism of action/Effect**
Antiserotonin; actions on central nervous system (CNS); direct stimulation of smooth muscle leading to vasoconstriction. Little alpha-adrenergic blocking activity. The exact mechanism of action in preventing migraine is unknown, although it may be related to the antiserotonin effect.

**Absorption**
Rapid after oral administration.

**Biotransformation**
Probably hepatic.

**Onset of action**
1 to 2 days.

**Duration of action**
1 to 2 days.

**Elimination**
Renal, 56%, as unchanged drug and metabolites.

## Precautions to Consider

**Cross-sensitivity and/or related problems**
Patients sensitive to other ergot derivatives may be sensitive to this medication also.

**Pregnancy/Reproduction**
Problems in humans have not been documented.

**Breast-feeding**
Problems in humans have not been documented; however, ergot alkaloids are excreted in breast milk. Ergot alkaloids inhibit lactation and may cause ergotism (vomiting, diarrhea, weak pulse, unstable blood pressure, seizures) in the infant.

**Pediatrics**
Because of the hazards of long-term use of this medication, use in pediatric patients is not recommended.

**Geriatrics**
Caution is recommended in the elderly, who are more likely to have occlusive peripheral vascular disease, and are therefore more likely to be adversely affected by peripheral vasoconstriction, than are younger adults. This increases the risk of hypothermia and other ischemic complications. Elderly patients are also more likely to have age-related renal function impairment, which requires caution in patients receiving methysergide.

**Drug interactions and/or related problems**
The following drug interactions and/or related problems have been selected on the basis of their potential clinical significance (possible mechanism in parentheses where appropriate)—not necessarily inclusive (» = major clinical significance):

Note: Combinations containing any of the following medications, depending on the amount present, may also interact with this medication.

Ergot alkaloids, other or
Vasoconstrictors, systemic, other, such as:
  Cocaine
  Epinephrine, parenteral
  Metaraminol
  Methoxamine
  Norepinephrine
  Phenylephrine, parenteral or
Vasoconstrictor-containing local anesthetic solutions
  (concurrent use with methysergide may result in enhanced vasoconstriction; a reduced dosage of ergot alkaloids may be necessary when they are used to treat an acute attack)

Smoking, tobacco
  (administration of methysergide to patients who smoke heavily may increase the risk of peripheral vascular ischemia because nicotine also constricts blood vessels)

**Laboratory value alterations**
The following have been selected on the basis of their potential clinical significance (possible effect in parentheses where appropriate)—not necessarily inclusive (» = major clinical significance):

With physiology/laboratory test values
Blood urea nitrogen (BUN)
  (may be increased, indicating renal failure, if retroperitoneal fibrosis occurs)

**Medical considerations/Contraindications**
The medical considerations/contraindications included here have been selected on the basis of their potential clinical significance (reasons given in parentheses where appropriate)—not necessarily inclusive (» = major clinical significance).

*Risk-benefit should be considered when the following medical problems exist:*
» Coronary artery disease, especially:
»   Angina, unstable or vasospastic
      (vasospasm may aggravate existing angina, or cause angina or myocardial infarction)
» Hepatic function impairment
      (impaired metabolism may result in ergot poisoning)
» Hypertension, severe
      (may be aggravated)

Peptic ulcer
   (methysergide may elevate gastric hydrochloric acid concentrations)
» Peripheral vascular disease, occlusive or
» Pruritus, severe, especially when associated with hepatic disease or
» Sepsis or other severe infection
   (sensitivity to vascular effects may be increased)
» Pulmonary disease or
» Rheumatoid arthritis or other collagen diseases or
» Valvular heart disease
   (risk of retroperitoneal, pleuropulmonary, or cardiac fibrosis)
» Renal function impairment
   Sensitivity to methysergide or other ergot alkaloids, history of

### Patient monitoring

The following may be especially important in patient monitoring (other tests may be warranted in some patients, depending on condition; » = major clinical significance):

Retroperitoneal imaging
   (recommended prior to initiation of anticipated long-term therapy and at 6- to 12-month intervals during therapy to detect early signs of retroperitoneal fibrosis; may also be indicated if signs of urinary obstruction occur)

## Side/Adverse Effects

Note: Most side effects are dose-related and are usually relieved by a reduction in dosage or withdrawal of the medication.

The following side/adverse effects have been selected on the basis of their potential clinical significance (possible signs and symptoms in parentheses where appropriate)—not necessarily inclusive:

### Those indicating need for medical attention
Incidence more frequent
   *Ischemia, peripheral vasospasm–induced* (abdominal pain; chest pain; itching of skin; numbness and tingling of fingers, toes, or face; pain in arms, legs, or lower back; pale or cold hands or feet; weakness in legs)—specific symptoms are dependent on the blood vessel(s) involved, and may also rarely be caused by vascular insufficiency

Incidence less frequent or rare—dose-related
   *Changes in vision; clumsiness or unsteadiness; CNS stimulation, mild* (excitement or difficulty in thinking; feeling of being outside the body; hallucinations; nightmares); *edema, peripheral* (swelling of hands, ankles, feet, or lower legs); *fast or slow heartbeat; leukopenia* (rarely, fever or chills; cough or hoarseness; lower back or side pain; painful or difficult urination)—usually asymptomatic; *mental depression; redness or flushing of face; skin rash; telangiectasia* (raised red spots on skin)
   Note: Although methysergide is chemically related to the hallucinogen lysergic acid diethylamide (LSD), some of the listed CNS symptoms may be associated with vascular headaches rather than an effect of the medication.

Incidence rare—dependent on duration of therapy
   *Fibrosis* (chest pain; difficult or painful urination; fever; large increase or decrease in amount of urine; leg cramps; loss of appetite; lower back, side, or groin pain; shortness of breath or difficult breathing; swelling of hands, ankles, feet, or lower legs; tightness in chest; weight loss)—fibrosis may occur in cardiac, penile, pleuropulmonary, and/or retroperitoneal tissues; specific symptoms depend on the site involved and the occurrence of associated complications, such as ureteral obstruction and vascular insufficiency

### Those indicating need for medical attention only if they continue or are bothersome
Incidence more frequent
   *CNS effect or hypotension, orthostatic* (dizziness or lightheadedness, especially when getting up from a lying or sitting position); *diarrhea; drowsiness; nausea, vomiting, or stomach pain*

Incidence less frequent or rare
   *Constipation; heartburn; trouble in sleeping*

### Those indicating possible withdrawal and the need for medical attention if they occur after medication is discontinued
   *Headache*

## Overdose

For specific information on the agents used in the management of methysergide overdose, see:
   • *Thiopental* in *Anesthetics, Barbiturates (Systemic)* monograph;
   • *Diazepam* in *Benzodiazepines (Systemic)* monograph; and/or
   • *Neuromuscular Blocking Agents (Systemic)*.

For more information on the management of overdose or unintentional ingestion, **contact a Poison Control Center** (see *Poison Control Center Listing*).

### Clinical effects of overdose
The following effects have been selected on the basis of their potential clinical significance (possible signs and symptoms in parentheses where appropriate)—not necessarily inclusive:
Acute and chronic
   *Cold and pale hands or feet; dizziness, severe; excitement*

### Treatment of overdose
Discontinuing methysergide administration.

To decrease absorption—Gastric lavage.

Specific Treatment—
   For treatment of convulsions:
      If convulsions do not respond to respiratory support, administration of a benzodiazepine such as diazepam or an ultrashort-acting barbiturate such as thiopental or thiamylal is recommended. The fact that these agents, especially the barbiturates, may cause circulatory depression when administered intravenously must be kept in mind. Administration of a neuromuscular blocking agent has also been recommended to decrease the muscular manifestations of persistent convulsions; artificial respiration is mandatory if such an agent is used. See the package inserts or *Diazepam Benzodiazepines (Systemic), Anesthetics, Barbiturate (Systemic)* or *Neuromuscular Blocking Agents (Systemic)* for specific dosing guidelines for use of these products.
   Peripheral vasospasm:
      Treat by applying warmth (but avoiding excessive heat) to ischemic extremities and, in some cases, by use of prazosin or sodium nitroprusside (the risk of hypotension being kept in mind). Also, careful nursing technique designed to prevent tissue damage should be instituted.

Monitoring—Prolonged and careful monitoring.

Supportive care—Support of respiration. Patients in whom intentional overdose is known or suspected should be referred for psychiatric consultation.

## Patient Consultation

As an aid to patient consultation, refer to *Advice for the Patient, Methysergide (Systemic)*.

In providing consultation, consider emphasizing the following selected information (» = major clinical significance):

### Before using this medication
» Conditions affecting use, especially:
   Sensitivity to ergot derivatives
   Breast-feeding—Ergot alkaloids inhibit lactation; also, they are excreted in breast milk and may cause ergotism in the infant
   Use in children—Use is not recommended, because of the hazards associated with long-term use of methysergide
   Use in the elderly—Increased risk of hypothermia and other adverse effects associated with peripheral vasoconstriction
   Other medical problems, especially cardiovascular disease, hepatic function impairment, hypertension, peripheral vascular disease, severe pruritus (especially when associated with hepatic disease), severe infection, pulmonary disease, rheumatoid arthritis, valvular heart disease, and renal function impairment

### Proper use of this medication
» Importance of not using more medication than the amount prescribed; risk of ergotism and gangrene with overdosage
» Taking with meals or milk to reduce gastrointestinal irritation
   Missed dose: Not taking at all; not doubling doses
» Proper dosing
» Proper storage

### Precautions while using this medication
» Checking with physician before discontinuing medication; withdrawal headache may occur
» Not taking for longer than 6 months at a time
» Caution in driving or doing jobs requiring alertness because of possible dizziness, lightheadedness, or drowsiness
   Caution when getting up suddenly from a lying or sitting position
   Avoiding alcohol, which aggravates headache
   Avoiding smoking since nicotine constricts blood vessels
   Avoiding exposure to excessive cold, which may aggravate peripheral vasoconstriction
   Notifying physician if infection develops, since infection may cause increased sensitivity to medication

**Side/adverse effects**

    Signs of potential side effects, especially CNS stimulation, fibrosis, ischemia, peripheral edema, and leukopenia

## General Dosing Information

Methysergide is not as potent a vasoconstrictor as ergotamine.

Because of the risk of fibrosis, methysergide should be administered for no longer than 6 months, with a drug-free interval of 3 to 4 weeks between each course.

Incidence and severity of some of the side effects may be minimized if the dosage is increased slowly to its therapeutic concentration and methysergide is given with meals.

If a response has not occurred after 3 weeks of treatment, further treatment is unlikely to produce an effect.

Gradual withdrawal of methysergide over 2 to 3 weeks is recommended to prevent rebound headache.

It is recommended that methysergide be withdrawn immediately and diagnostic tests performed if signs of retroperitoneal, pleuropulmonary, or cardiac fibrosis occur. Partial to complete regression may occur after the medication is discontinued, although surgery may be necessary in some patients.

Methysergide should be withdrawn at the first sign of vascular insufficiency.

## Oral Dosage Forms

### METHYSERGIDE MALEATE TABLETS USP

**Usual adult dose**
Oral, 4 to 6 mg a day in divided doses.

**Strength(s) usually available**
U.S.—
    2 mg (Rx) [*Sansert* (lactose; tartrazine)].
Canada—
    2 mg (Rx) [*Sansert* (lactose; tartrazine)].

**Packaging and storage**
Store below 40 °C (104 °F), preferably between 15 and 30 °C (59 and 86 °F), unless otherwise specified by manufacturer. Store in a tight container.

**Auxiliary labeling**
• Take with meals or milk.

Revised: July 1990
Interim revision: 08/17/94

---

**METIPRANOLOL**—See *Beta-adrenergic Blocking Agents (Ophthalmic)*

---

# METOCLOPRAMIDE    Systemic

VA CLASSIFICATION (Primary/Secondary): AU300/GA700
Note: For a listing of dosage forms and brand names by country availability, see *Dosage Forms* section(s). For a listing of brand names for the articles in this monograph, refer to the General Index.

## Category

Dopaminergic blocking agent; gastrointestinal emptying (delayed) adjunct; peristaltic stimulant; antiemetic.

## Indications

Note: Bracketed information in the *Indications* section refers to uses that are not included in U.S. product labeling.

**Accepted**
Radiography, gastrointestinal, adjunct and
Intubation, intestinal—Metoclopramide injection is indicated to facilitate intestinal intubation in adults and children, and to stimulate gastric emptying and intestinal transit of barium in cases where delayed emptying interferes with radiological examinations of stomach or small intestine.

Gastroparesis (treatment)[1]—Metoclopramide is indicated for the relief of symptoms of acute and recurrent diabetic gastroparesis.

Nausea and vomiting, cancer chemotherapy–induced (prophylaxis)—Metoclopramide injection is indicated in high doses for the prevention of nausea and vomiting associated with emetogenic cancer chemotherapy.

    Some clinicians may prefer ondansetron to high-dose metoclopramide for prophylaxis of cancer chemotherapy–induced nausea and vomiting because ondansetron is less toxic, and in some studies, has been proven more effective than high-dose metoclopramide.

Nausea and vomiting, postoperative (prophylaxis)—Metoclopramide is indicated for the prophylaxis of postoperative nausea and vomiting in cases where nasogastric suction is undesirable.

Reflux, gastroesophageal (treatment)[1]—Oral metoclopramide is indicated in adults for the symptomatic short-term treatment of heartburn and reflux esophagitis due to delayed gastric emptying. [In infants, it is used in the treatment of chronic vomiting and recurrent bronchopulmonary manifestations associated with gastroesophageal reflux.]

[Nausea and vomiting, postoperative, drug-related (treatment)]—Metoclopramide is used in the treatment of drug-related postoperative nausea and vomiting.

[Gastric emptying, slow (treatment)] or
[Gastric stasis, in preterm infants (treatment)]—Metoclopramide is used for correcting the slow gastric emptying in postvagotomy stasis, in idiopathic stasis, and in various collagen diseases such as scleroderma. In addition, it is used for persistent functional feeding intolerance and gastric stasis in preterm infants.

[Pneumonitis, aspiration (prophylaxis)][1]—Metoclopramide is used prior to general anesthesia to promote gastric emptying and reduce the risk of aspiration, especially in emergency surgery, cesarean sections, or delivery.

[Headache, vascular (treatment adjunct)][1]—Metoclopramide is used to counteract the gastric stasis and nausea associated with migraine, and to promote the absorption of orally administered analgesics given in the treatment of migraine.

[Hiccups, persistent (treatment)][1]—Metoclopramide is used in the control of persistent hiccups.

[Metoclopramide has been used in the treatment of lactation deficiency; however, it has generally been replaced by more effective medications.]

---

[1]Not included in Canadian product labeling.

## Pharmacology/Pharmacokinetics

**Physicochemical characteristics**
pKa—0.6 and 9.3.

**Mechanism of action/Effect**
Dopaminergic blocking agents—Gastrointestinal emptying (delayed) adjunct; peristaltic stimulant: Exact mechanism of action is unknown; however, it is believed that metoclopramide inhibits gastric smooth muscle relaxation produced by dopamine, thus enhancing cholinergic responses of the gastrointestinal smooth muscle. Accelerates intestinal transit and gastric emptying by preventing relaxation of gastric body and increasing the phasic activity of antrum. At the same time, this action is accompanied by relaxation of the upper small intestine, resulting in an improved coordination between the body and antrum of the stomach and the upper small intestine. Decreases reflux into the esophagus by increasing the resting pressure of the lower esophageal sphincter and improves acid clearance from the esophagus by increasing amplitude of esophageal peristaltic contractions.
Antiemetic—Dopamine antagonist action raises the threshold of activity in the chemoreceptor trigger zone and decreases the input from afferent visceral nerves. High doses of metoclopramide have been found to antagonize 5-hydroxytryptamine (5-HT) receptors in the peripheral nervous system in animals.

**Other actions/effects**
Metoclopramide stimulates prolactin secretion and causes a transient increase in circulating aldosterone levels, which may be associated with transient fluid retention.

**Absorption**
Rapid.

**Protein binding**
Approximately 30%.

**Biotransformation**
Hepatic.

**Half-life**
4 to 6 hours.

**Onset of action**
Intramuscular—10 to 15 minutes.
Intravenous—1 to 3 minutes.
Oral—30 to 60 minutes.

**Time to peak serum concentrations**
1 to 2 hours after a single oral dose.

**Duration of action**
1 to 2 hours.

**Elimination**
Renal; approximately 85% of an oral dose appears in the urine within 72 hours as unchanged drug and sulfate and glucuronide conjugates.

## Precautions to Consider

### Cross-sensitivity and/or related problems
Patients sensitive to procaine and procainamide may be sensitive to this medication also.

### Pregnancy/Reproduction
Fertility—Studies in rats, mice, and rabbits at doses from 12 to 250 times the human dose have shown that metoclopramide does not impair fertility.

Pregnancy—Extensive studies in humans have not been done.
Studies in animals have not shown that metoclopramide causes adverse effects in the fetus.

FDA Pregnancy Category B.

### Breast-feeding
Problems in humans have not been documented; however, risk-benefit must be considered since metoclopramide is distributed into breast milk.

### Pediatrics
Extrapyramidal effects, especially dystonic reactions, of metoclopramide are more likely to occur in children shortly after initiation of therapy, and usually with doses higher than 0.5 mg per kg of body weight (mg/kg) per day. Methemoglobinemia has been reported in premature and full-term neonates receiving metoclopramide intramuscularly at a dose of 1 to 2 mg/kg a day for 3 days or more.

### Geriatrics
Extrapyramidal effects, especially parkinsonism and tardive dyskinesia, of metoclopramide are more likely to occur in elderly patients following usual or high doses over a long period of time.

### Drug interactions and/or related problems
The following drug interactions and/or related problems have been selected on the basis of their potential clinical significance (possible mechanism in parentheses where appropriate)—not necessarily inclusive (» = major clinical significance):

Note: Combinations containing any of the following medications, depending on the amount present, may also interact with this medication.

   Only specific interactions between metoclopramide and other oral medications have been identified in this monograph. However, because of increased gastrointestinal motility and decreased gastric emptying time caused by metoclopramide, absorption of oral medications from the stomach may be decreased, while absorption from the small intestine may be enhanced.

» Alcohol
   (concurrent use may increase the central nervous system [CNS] depressant effects of either alcohol or metoclopramide; concurrent use also may accelerate gastric emptying of alcohol, thus possibly increasing its rate and extent of absorption from the small intestine)

Anticholinergics or other medications with anticholinergic activity (See *Appendix II*) or
Opioid-containing medications
   (concurrent use may antagonize the effects of metoclopramide on gastrointestinal motility)

Apomorphine
   (prior administration of metoclopramide may decrease the emetic response to apomorphine; also, concurrent use may potentiate the CNS depressant effects of either apomorphine or metoclopramide)

Bromocriptine
   (metoclopramide may increase serum prolactin concentrations and interfere with effects of bromocriptine; dosage adjustment of bromocriptine may be necessary)

Cimetidine
   (concurrent use may decrease the effect of cimetidine due to decreased absorption)

» CNS depression–producing medications, other (See *Appendix II*)
   (concurrent use may increase the sedative effects of either these medications or metoclopramide)

Cyclosporine
   (the decrease in gastric emptying time caused by metoclopramide may increase the bioavailability of cyclosporine; monitoring of cyclosporine concentrations may be necessary)

Digoxin
   (concurrent use may decrease absorption of digoxin from stomach; dosage adjustment of digoxin may be necessary)

Extrapyramidal reaction–causing medications (See *Appendix II*)
   (concurrent use with metoclopramide may increase the frequency and severity of extrapyramidal effects)

Hepatotoxic medications (See *Appendix II*)
   (concurrent use with metoclopramide may increase the risk of hepatotoxicity)

Levodopa
   (metoclopramide has been reported to decrease the effectiveness of levodopa with concurrent use)

Mexiletine
   (concurrent use with metoclopramide may accelerate absorption of mexiletine)

Monoamine oxidase (MAO) inhibitors, including furazolidine and procarbazine
   (metoclopramide releases catecholamines in patients with essential hypertension and should be used cautiously in patients receiving MAO inhibitors)

Pergolide
   (dopamine antagonists such as metoclopramide may decrease the effectiveness of pergolide)

Succinylcholine
   (metoclopramide has been reported to prolong succinylcholine block; dosage reduction of succinylcholine may be necessary with concurrent use)

### Laboratory value alterations
The following have been selected on the basis of their potential clinical significance (possible effect in parentheses where appropriate)—not necessarily inclusive (» = major clinical significance):

With diagnostic test results
   Gonadorelin test
      (concurrent use with metoclopramide may blunt the response to gonadorelin by increasing serum prolactin concentrations)

   Hepatic function test
      (results may be altered)

With physiology/laboratory test values
   Aldosterone and
   Prolactin, serum
      (concentrations may be increased)

### Medical considerations/Contraindications
The medical considerations/contraindications included here have been selected on the basis of their potential clinical significance (reasons given in parentheses where appropriate)—not necessarily inclusive (» = major clinical significance).

*Except under special circumstances, this medication should not be used when the following medical problems exist:*

» Epilepsy
   (severity and frequency of seizures may be increased)

» Gastrointestinal hemorrhage, mechanical obstruction, or perforation
   (stimulation of gastrointestinal motility may aggravate condition)

» Pheochromocytoma
   (may cause hypertensive crisis)

*Risk-benefit should be considered when the following medical problems exist:*

Asthma
   (administration of metoclopramide may increase risk of bronchospasm)

Hypertension
   (administration of intravenous metoclopramide may worsen condition due to release of catecholamines)

Liver failure
   (risk of increased adverse effects because of increased accumulation of the drug due to impaired clearance; reduced dosage is recommended)

Parkinson's disease
(symptoms may be exacerbated)
» Renal failure, severe, chronic
(risk of extrapyramidal effects may be increased; reduced dosage
is recommended)
Sensitivity to metoclopramide, procaine, or procainamide

## Side/Adverse Effects

Note: Methemoglobinemia has been reported in premature and full-term
neonates receiving metoclopramide intramuscularly at a dose of 1
to 2 mg per kg of body weight (mg/kg) a day for 3 days or more.

The following side/adverse effects have been selected on the basis of their
potential clinical significance (possible signs and symptoms in parentheses where appropriate)—not necessarily inclusive:

### Those indicating need for medical attention
Incidence rare
*Agranulocytosis* (chills; fever; sore throat; general feeling of tiredness
or weakness); *cardiovascular effects, specifically hypotension* (dizziness or fainting); *hypertension* (dizziness; severe or continuing headaches; increase in blood pressure); *tachycardia* (fast or irregular heartbeat); *extrapyramidal effects, parkinsonian* (difficulty in speaking or
swallowing; loss of balance control; mask-like face; shuffling walk;
stiffness of arms or legs; trembling and shaking of hands and fingers);
*tardive dyskinesia* (lip smacking or puckering; puffing of cheeks; rapid
or worm-like movements of tongue; uncontrolled chewing movements;
uncontrolled movements of arms and legs)—usually occurs after at
least one year of continuous treatment and may persist after discontinuation of metoclopramide

Note: *Extrapyramidal effects* may occur at therapeutic doses in any
age group. However, they occur more frequently in children and
young adults, and at the higher doses used in prophylaxis of
vomiting due to cancer chemotherapy. Dystonic reactions may
start within minutes after start of intravenous therapy, and disappear within 24 hours after discontinuation of metoclopramide.
Onset of *parkinsonian* symptoms may vary from a few weeks
to several months after initiation of therapy and are reversible
upon discontinuation of metoclopramide.

With high doses
*Agitation* (unusual nervousness, restlessness, or irritability); *panic-like
sensation; restless legs syndrome* (aching or discomfort in lower legs
or sensation of crawling in legs)

Note: The onset may occur within minutes of receiving high doses of
metoclopramide and may last for 2 to 24 hours.

### Those indicating need for medical attention only if they continue
### or are bothersome
Incidence more frequent
*Diarrhea*—with high doses; *drowsiness*—about 10%; *restlessness*—
about 10%; *unusual tiredness or weakness*—about 10%
Incidence less frequent or rare
*Breast tenderness and swelling; changes in menstruation; constipa-
tion; depression; dizziness; headache; prolactin stimulation* (increased flow of breast milk); *nausea; skin rash; trouble in sleeping;
unusual dryness of mouth; unusual irritability*

## Overdose

For specific information on the agents used in the management of meto-
clopramide overdose, see:
• *Diphenhydramine* in *Antihistamines (Systemic)* monograph; and/or
• *Methylene Blue (Systemic)* monograph.

For more information on the management of overdose or unintentional
ingestion, **contact a Poison Control Center** (see *Poison Control Center Listing*).

### Clinical effects of overdose
The following have been selected on the basis of their potential clinical
significance (possible signs and symptoms in parentheses where appropriate)—not necessarily inclusive:
*Confusion; drowsiness, severe*

### Treatment of overdose
Specific treatment—
Anticholinergic or antiparkinson drugs or antihistamines with anticholinergic properties (50 mg of diphenhydramine administered intramuscularly in adults and 1 mg per kg of body weight [mg/kg]
intramuscularly or intravenously in infants and children) to help in
controlling the extrapyramidal reactions.
Methylene blue (1 to 2 mg/kg of a 1% solution injected intravenously
over a 5-minute period) is used to reverse methemoglobinemia

resulting from metoclopramide administration in premature and
full-term infants.
Supportive care—
Patients in whom intentional overdose is confirmed or suspected
should be referred for psychiatric consultation.

## Patient Consultation

As an aid to patient consultation, refer to *Advice for the Patient,
Metoclopramide (Systemic)*.

In providing consultation, consider emphasizing the following selected
information (» = major clinical significance):

### Before using this medication
» Conditions affecting use, especially:
Sensitivity to metoclopramide, procaine, or procainamide
Breast-feeding—Distributed into breast milk
Use in children—Extrapyramidal effects more likely; increased
risk of methemoglobinemia in premature and full-term infants
Use in the elderly—Extrapyramidal effects more likely
Other medications, especially alcohol and CNS depressants
Other medical problems, especially epilepsy; gastrointestinal
bleeding, mechanical obstruction, or perforation; or severe re-
nal function impairment

### Proper use of this medication
» Taking 30 minutes before meals and at bedtime (for oral dosage forms)
» Not taking more medication than the amount prescribed
» Proper dosing
Missed dose: Using as soon as possible; not using if almost time for
next dose
» Proper storage

### Precautions while using this medication
» Avoiding use of alcohol or other CNS depressants
» Caution if drowsiness occurs

### Side/adverse effects
Signs of potential side effects, especially agranulocytosis, extrapyramidal effects, and tardive dyskinesia

## General Dosing Information

In patients with hepatic or severe renal function impairment, the normally
prescribed dose should be reduced by 50%, since adverse effects are
more likely to be exacerbated.

### For parenteral dosage forms only
Intravenous injections of metoclopramide should be made *slowly* over a
1- to 2-minute period, since a transient but intense feeling of anxiety
and restlessness followed by drowsiness may occur with rapid
administration.
Intravenous infusion should be made *slowly* over a period of not less than
15 minutes. Metoclopramide injection may be diluted for intravenous
infusion with 50 mL of 5% dextrose in water, sodium chloride injection, 5% dextrose in 0.45% sodium chloride, Ringer's injection, or
lactated Ringer's injection.

### For treatment of adverse effects and/or overdose
Recommended treatment for metoclopramide's adverse effects and/or
overdose includes:
• Anticholinergic or antiparkinson drugs or antihistamines with anticholinergic properties (50 mg of diphenhydramine administered intramuscularly in adults and 1 mg per kg of body weight [mg/kg] intramuscularly or intravenously in infants and children) to help in
controlling the extrapyramidal reactions.
• Methylene blue (1 to 2 mg/kg of a 1% solution injected intravenously over a 5-minute period) is used to reverse methemoglobinemia
resulting from metoclopramide administration in premature and full-
term infants.

## Oral Dosage Forms

Note: Bracketed uses in the *Dosage Forms* section refer to categories of
use and/or indications that are not included in U.S. product labeling.

Note: The dosing and strengths of the dosage forms available are expressed in terms of metoclopramide base.

### METOCLOPRAMIDE TABLETS USP

**Usual adult and adolescent dose**
Treatment of diabetic gastroparesis[1]—
Oral, 10 mg thirty minutes before symptoms are likely to occur or
before each meal and at bedtime, up to four times a day.

Note: In the initial treatment of diabetic gastroparesis, the parenteral
route of administration is recommended if severe symptoms are
present. Therapy may begin at 10 mg administered intramus-

cularly or intravenously three or four times a day, the dose adjusted as needed.

Treatment of gastroesophageal reflux[1]—

Oral, 10 to 15 mg thirty minutes before symptoms are likely to occur or before each meal and at bedtime, up to four times a day.

Note: Intermittent symptoms may be treated by taking 20 mg of metoclopramide prior to the provoking situation.

[Treatment of hiccups][1]—

Oral, 10 to 20 mg four times a day for seven days. An initial dose of 10 mg intramuscularly may be given if necessary.

### Usual adult and adolescent prescribing limits

Up to 500 mcg (0.5 mg) per kg of body weight per day.

### Usual pediatric dose

Gastrointestinal emptying (delayed) adjunct or
Peristaltic stimulant—

Children 5 to 14 years of age: Oral, 2.5 to 5 mg three times a day thirty minutes before meals and at bedtime.

### Usual geriatric dose

See *Usual adult and adolescent dose.*

Note: Geriatric patients may be more sensitive to the usual adult dose.

### Strength(s) usually available

U.S.—

5 mg (Rx) [*Clopra*].

10 mg (Rx) [*Clopra* (scored); *Octamide; Reclomide; Reglan* (scored); GENERIC].

Canada—

5 mg (Rx) [*Apo-Metoclop; Maxeran; Reglan*].

10 mg (Rx) [*Apo-Metoclop; Emex; Maxeran* (scored); *Reglan*].

### Packaging and storage

Store below 40 °C (104 °F), preferably between 15 and 30 °C (59 and 86 °F), unless otherwise specified by manufacturer. Store in a tight, light-resistant container.

### Auxiliary labeling

• May cause drowsiness.
• Avoid alcoholic beverages.

## METOCLOPRAMIDE HYDROCHLORIDE SYRUP

### Usual adult and adolescent dose

Treatment of diabetic gastroparesis[1]—

Oral, 10 mg (base) thirty minutes before symptoms are likely to occur or before each meal and at bedtime, up to four times a day.

Note: In the initial treatment of diabetic gastroparesis, the parenteral route of administration is recommended if severe symptoms are present. Therapy may begin at 10 mg (base) administered intramuscularly or intravenously three or four times a day, the dose adjusted as needed.

Treatment of gastroesophageal reflux[1]—

Oral, 10 to 15 mg (base) thirty minutes before symptoms are likely to occur or before each meal and at bedtime, up to four times a day.

Note: Intermittent symptoms may be treated by taking 20 mg of metoclopramide prior to the provoking situation.

[Treatment of hiccups][1]—

Oral, 10 to 20 mg (base) four times a day for seven days.

Note: An initial dose of 10 mg intramuscularly may be given if necessary.

### Usual adult and adolescent prescribing limits

Up to 500 mcg (0.5 mg) per kg of body weight per day.

### Usual pediatric dose

Gastrointestinal emptying (delayed) adjunct or
Peristaltic stimulant—

Oral, 0.1 to 0.2 mg per kg of body weight per dose, given thirty minutes before meals and at bedtime.

### Strength(s) usually available

U.S.—

5 mg (base) per 5 mL (Rx) [*Reglan;* GENERIC].

Canada—

5 mg (base) per 5 mL (Rx) [*Maxeran; Reglan*].

### Packaging and storage

Store below 40 °C (104 °F), preferably between 15 and 30 °C (59 and 86 °F), in a tight container, unless otherwise specified by manufacturer. Protect from freezing.

### Auxiliary labeling

• May cause drowsiness.
• Avoid alcoholic beverages.

# Parenteral Dosage Forms

Note: Bracketed uses in the *Dosage Forms* section refer to categories of use and/or indications that are not included in U.S. product labeling.

## METOCLOPRAMIDE INJECTION USP

### Usual adult and adolescent dose

Gastrointestinal emptying (delayed) adjunct or
Peristaltic stimulant—

Intravenous, 10 mg as a single dose.

[Treatment of hiccups][1]—

Intramuscular, 10 mg initially, followed by oral metoclopramide at a dose of 10 to 20 mg four times a day for seven days.

Antiemetic: For prevention of cancer chemotherapy–induced emesis—

Intravenous infusion, 2 mg per kg of body weight, administered thirty minutes before cisplatin or other highly emetogenic chemotherapeutic agent; may be repeated as needed every two or three hours.

Note: For prevention of emesis induced by chemotherapeutic agents with low emetic potential—Intravenous infusion, 1 mg per kg of body weight.

Continuous intravenous infusion, 3 mg per kg of body weight before chemotherapy, followed by 0.5 mg per kg of body weight per hour for eight hours.

Antiemetic: For prevention of postoperative emesis—

Intramuscular, 10 to 20 mg near the end of surgery.

### Usual pediatric dose

Antiemetic—For prevention of cancer chemotherapy–induced emesis
Gastrointestinal emptying (delayed) adjunct or
Peristaltic stimulant—

Intravenous, 1 mg per kg of body weight as a single dose. May be repeated one time after sixty minutes.

Note: To reduce the chance of increased adverse reactions, dosages should not exceed 2 mg per kg of body weight. Some clinicians recommend concurrent therapy with diphenhydramine at an intravenous dose of 1 mg per kg of body weight 15 minutes prior to metoclopramide infusion to limit side effects that may occur with doses of less than 2 mg per kg of body weight.

### Strength(s) usually available

U.S.—

5 mg per mL (Rx) [*Octamide PFS; Reglan;* GENERIC].

Canada—

5 mg per mL (Rx) [*Maxeran; Reglan*].

### Packaging and storage

Store between 15 and 30 °C (59 and 86 °F), unless otherwise specified by manufacturer. Protect from light (if injection does not contain an antioxidant).

### Preparation of dosage form

Doses of Metoclopramide Injection USP in excess of 10 mg may be mixed with 50 mL of 0.9% sodium chloride injection, 5% dextrose injection, 5% dextrose in 0.45% sodium chloride injection, Ringer's injection, or lactated Ringer's injection.

### Stability

Unused portion should be discarded.

Dilutions of metoclopramide injection may be stored for up to 48 hours after preparation if protected from light.

Dilutions of metoclopramide and 0.9% sodium chloride may be stored frozen for up to 4 weeks after preparation.

### Incompatibilities

Metoclopramide injection is incompatible with calcium gluconate, cephalothin sodium, chloramphenicol sodium, cisplatin, erythromycin lactobionate, furosemide, methotrexate, penicillin G potassium, and sodium bicarbonate.

---

[1]Not included in Canadian product labeling.

---

Revised: 05/20/92
Interim revision: 08/16/94

---

**METOCURINE**—See *Neuromuscular Blocking Agents (Systemic)*

---

**METOLAZONE**—See *Diuretics, Thiazide (Systemic)*

**METOPROLOL**—See *Beta-adrenergic Blocking Agents (Systemic)*

**METOPROLOL-CONTAINING COMBINATIONS**—
Metoprolol and Hydrochlorothiazide (Systemic)—See *Beta-adrenergic Blocking Agents and Thiazide Diuretics (Systemic)*

# METRIZAMIDE    Systemic†

VA CLASSIFICATION (Primary): DX101

Note: For a listing of dosage forms and brand names by country availability, see *Dosage Forms* section(s). For a listing of brand names for the articles in this monograph, refer to the General Index.

†Not commercially available in Canada.

## Category

Note: Metrizamide is a nonionic radiopaque contrast agent.

Diagnostic aid, radiopaque (central nervous system disorders); Diagnostic aid, radiopaque (cerebrospinal fluid disorders); Diagnostic aid, radiopaque (brain disorders); Diagnostic aid, radiopaque (cardiac disease); Diagnostic aid, radiopaque (vascular disease); Diagnostic aid, radiopaque (urinary tract disorders).

## Indications

### Accepted
Intrathecal:

Myelography (lumbar, thoracic, cervical, total columnar)—Metrizamide is indicated in adults and pediatric patients for lumbar, thoracic, cervical, and total columnar myelography to determine the presence of abnormalities in the spinal column, spinal canal, and central nervous system (CNS).

Cisternography—Metrizamide is indicated in pediatric patients for cisternography by direct injection using standard radiologic techniques to visualize the basal cistern of the brain.

Cisternography, computed tomographic—Metrizamide is indicated in adults and pediatric patients for computerized tomography (CT) of the intracranial subarachnoid spaces.

Ventriculography—Metrizamide is indicated in pediatric patients for ventriculography by direct injection using standard radiologic techniques to visualize the cerebral ventricles.

Intravascular:

Angiocardiography—Metrizamide is indicated in pediatric angiocardiography to visualize lesions or malformations of the heart and obstructions or anomalies of the major thoracic vessels.

Arteriography—Metrizamide is indicated in adult peripheral arteriography to visualize specific regions of the vascular system and blood flow in such areas to help in the diagnosis and evaluation of neoplasms (known or suspected) or vascular diseases (congenital or acquired) that may cause changes in normal vascular anatomy or physiology. Metrizamide is also indicated in adults for intravenous digital arteriography of head and neck.

## Pharmacology/Pharmacokinetics

### Physicochemical characteristics
Molecular weight—789.10.
Osmolality—Low. The osmolalities of the injections with iodine concentrations of 170 and 300 mg per mL are 300 and 484 mOsmol per kg of water, respectively.
Note: Metrizamide is isotonic with the cerebrospinal fluid (CSF) at an approximate concentration of 170 mg of iodine per mL of solution.

### Mechanism of action/Effect
Organic iodine compounds block x-rays as they pass through the body, thereby allowing body structures containing iodine to be delineated in contrast to those structures that do not contain iodine. The degree of opacity produced by these compounds is directly proportional to the total amount (concentration and volume) of the iodinated contrast agent in the path of the x-rays. After intrathecal administration into the subarachnoid space, diffusion of metrizamide in the CSF allows the visualization of the subarachnoid spaces of the head and spinal canal. After intravascular administration, metrizamide makes opaque those vessels in its path of flow, allowing visualization of the internal structures until significant hemodilution occurs.

### Other actions/effects
Competitive inhibitor of the glucose site of brain hexokinase.

### Absorption
Oral/Rectal—Absorption from gastrointestinal tract is negligible.

### Distribution
Intrathecal—Diffuses upward through the CSF; rapidly penetrates into nerve root sleeves, nerve rootlets, and narrow areas of the subarachnoid space. Also, enters extracellular fluid of the brain tissue and pial surface of cerebral and cerebellar tissue adjacent to subarachnoid areas. In patients with normal CSF dynamics, it is eliminated from CSF into the blood within several hours.
Intravascular—Rapidly distributed throughout extracellular fluid following intravenous administration.

### Time to peak opacification
Standard myelography—
Immediate and for up to 30 minutes.
CT myelography—
Lumbar region: Immediate.
Thoracic region: 1 hour.
Cervical region: 2 hours.
Basal cisterns: 3 to 4 hours.

### Peak serum concentration
Intrathecal—1 to 3 hours after lumbar subarachnoid injection.
Intravascular—Immediate, but concentration falls rapidly as metrizamide becomes distributed throughout the extravascular compartment.

### Elimination
Intrathecal—
Normal renal function: Primarily renal (60% of dose excreted unchanged within 48 hours).
Severe renal function impairment or renal failure: Fecal elimination via biliary tract becomes primary route of elimination.
Intravascular—
Renal: 94% of dose is excreted unchanged in 24 hours.
Fecal: 5% of dose.

## Precautions to Consider

### Cross-sensitivity and/or related problems
Patients sensitive to iodine or other iodinated contrast media may be sensitive to metrizamide also.

### Pregnancy/Reproduction
Pregnancy—Adequate and well-controlled studies in humans have not been done. However, other organically bound iodine–containing preparations administered near term by intra-amniotic injection have caused hypothyroidism in some newborns.
Also, elective contrast radiography of the abdomen is usually not recommended during pregnancy because of the risks to the fetus from radiation exposure.
Reproduction studies in rats and rabbits have not shown that metrizamide, administered in doses up to 70 times the human dose, impairs fertility or causes harm to the fetus.
FDA Pregnancy Category B.

### Breast-feeding
Up to 1 mg of the injected myelographic dose of metrizamide is distributed into the breast milk over 2 days.

### Pediatrics
*For intravascular use—*
Dehydration and/or the risk of renal failure may be exacerbated in infants and young children, especially those with polyuria, oliguria, diabetes, or pre-existing dehydration, by the the contrast media; adequate hydration is recommended before and following administration of metrizamide.

### Geriatrics
*For all procedures—*
Elderly patients may be more sensitive to the effects of metrizamide on thyroid function. Iodine-induced thyrotoxicosis may occur 4 to 12 weeks following contrast radiography. Thyroid function monitoring may be needed in geriatric patients.

*For intravascular use—*
Diagnostic studies performed to date have not demonstrated geriatrics-specific problems that would limit the usefulness of metrizamide in the elderly. However, elderly patients are more likely to have age-related renal function impairment, which may require lower dosage in patients receiving metrizamide.

Dehydration and/or the risk of renal failure may be exacerbated in geriatric patients, especially those with polyuria, oliguria, diabetes, or pre-existing dehydration, by the contrast media; adequate hydration is recommended before and following administration of metrizamide.

*For intrathecal use—*
Geriatric patients may be prone to develop mental confusion with the intrathecal administration of metrizamide.

### Drug interactions and/or related problems
The following drug interactions and/or related problems have been selected on the basis of their potential clinical significance (possible mechanism in parentheses where appropriate)—not necessarily inclusive (» = major clinical significance):

Note: Combinations containing any of the following medications, depending on the amount present, may also interact with this medication.

» Antidepressants, tricyclic or
   CNS stimulation–producing medications (See *Appendix II*) or
   Monoamine oxidase (MAO) inhibitors, including furazolidone, procarbazine, and selegiline or
» Phenothiazines or
» Trimeprazine
   (concurrent use with intrathecal administration of metrizamide may increase risk of seizures because of lowered seizure threshold effect of these medications; it is recommended that these medications be discontinued for at least 48 hours before and 24 hours after myelography)

Beta-adrenergic blocking agents
   (concurrent intravascular administration of metrizamide with beta-adrenergic blocking agents may increase the risk of moderate to severe anaphylactoid reaction and may exacerbate hypotensive effects; discontinuation of the beta-adrenergic blocking agent before administration of contrast media may be advisable in patients with other risk factors)

Cholecystographic agents, oral
   (the risk of renal toxicity may be increased if an oral cholecystographic agent is given before the intravascular administration of metrizamide, especially in patients with hepatic function impairment)

Glucocorticoids, intrathecal
   (concurrent intrathecal administration of metrizamide with intrathecal administration of glucocorticoids may increase risk of arachnoiditis)

Hypotension-producing medications, other (See *Appendix II*)
   (the risk of severe hypotension may be increased if metrizamide is given concurrently with other medications that produce hypotension)

Interleukin-2
   (incidence of delayed reactions to intravenous contrast media [e.g., hypersensitivity, fever, skin rash, flu-like symptoms, joint pain, flushing, pruritus, emesis, hypotension, dizziness occurring more than 1 hour after administration] may be increased in patients who have received interleukin-2; some symptoms may resemble a ''recall'' reaction to interleukin-2; supportive medical treatment may be necessary if symptoms are significant; delaying contrast media administration until 6 weeks after administration of interleukin-2 may reduce incidence of these reactions)

Nephrotoxic medications, other (See *Appendix II*)
   (concurrent intrathecal or intravascular administration of metrizamide with other nephrotoxic medications may increase the potential for nephrotoxicity)

### Diagnostic interference
The following have been selected on the basis of their potential clinical significance (possible effect in parentheses where appropriate)—not necessarily inclusive (» = major clinical significance):

With *other* diagnostic test results
Electroencephalogram (EEG) readings
   (intrathecal administration of metrizamide may cause transient increases in slow wave activity; pre-existing EEG changes may also be exacerbated in some patients)

Leukocyte counts and
Red cell counts
   (may be temporarily decreased)

Prothrombin time (PT) and
Thromboplastin time
   (may be increased with metrizamide since *in vitro* studies with animal blood have shown other nonionic contrast media to slightly inhibit all stages of coagulation)

Thyroid function determinations and
Thyroid imaging
   (intravascular or intrathecal administration of metrizamide may cause an alteration of serum protein–bound iodine [PBI] concentrations and radioactive iodine and pertechnetate ion uptake for up to 16 days; thyroid test should be performed prior to administration of metrizamide. Other thyroid function tests not based on measurement of iodine, such as resin triiodothyronine uptake, may not be affected)

Urinalysis
   (metrizamide may interfere with some chemical determinations made on urine, such as protein and specific gravity; urine should be collected prior to or at least 2 days after intravenous administration of metrizamide)

With physiology/laboratory test values
Cerebrospinal fluid (CSF) leukocyte count and
CSF protein count
   (may be increased transiently following intrathecal administration of metrizamide)

Creatinine, serum
   (concentration may be increased with metrizamide since temporary increases of serum creatinine have occurred with other nonionic contrast media)

### Medical considerations/Contraindications
The medical considerations/contraindications included here have been selected on the basis of their potential clinical significance (reasons given in parentheses where appropriate)—not necessarily inclusive (» = major clinical significance).

*Risk-benefit should be considered when the following medical problems exist:*

*For all procedures*
Allergic reaction (anaphylaxis) to penicillins or to skin allergens, previous
   (although the risk of anaphylactoid reaction may be less with metrizamide than with high-osmolality contrast agents, caution is recommended when administering metrizamide to patients who have had a previous reaction to penicillins or to skin allergens)

Allergies or asthma, history of
   (although the risk of idiosyncratic response or anaphylactoid reaction may be less with metrizamide than with high-osmolality contrast agents, caution is recommended when administering metrizamide to patients with a history of allergies or asthma)

» Dehydration, especially associated with pre-existing renal disease, advanced vascular disease, or diabetes mellitus; or in infants, young children, and elderly patients
   (intravascular administration may increase risk of acute renal failure; incidence and severity of headaches may be increased with intrathecal administration)

» Hepatorenal disease
   (elimination of metrizamide may be delayed or impaired)

Renal function impairment, severe
   (elimination of metrizamide may be delayed; because of the risk of inducing temporary oliguria, an interval of 48 hours should elapse before repeat examination)

» Sensitivity to iodinated contrast media
   (increased risk of anaphylactoid reaction in patients with history of prior reactions to contrast media)

*For intrathecal use*
Alcoholism, chronic
   (increased risk of side effects because of possible brain or liver damage)

Bleeding, subarachnoid
   (increased risk of meningeal irritation or arachnoiditis)

Epilepsy, history of
   (increased risk of seizures)

Infection, local or systemic, significant

Multiple sclerosis

*For intravascular use*
Hyperthyroidism
   (administration of metrizamide may precipitate thyroid storm)

» Pheochromocytoma

(administration of metrizamide may precipitate severe hypertension; amount of metrizamide injected should be kept to a minimum and blood pressure should be monitored during the procedure; pretreatment with the alpha-adrenergic blocking agent, phentolamine, is recommended)

Sickle cell disease

(metrizamide may promote sickling in patients who are homozygous for sickle cell disease; however, sickling potential of metrizamide is less compared to high-osmolality ionic agents)

**Patient monitoring**

The following may be especially important in patient monitoring (other tests may be warranted in some patients, depending on condition; » = major clinical significance):

*For intravascular use*

Blood pressure determinations

(may be required during examination, especially in patients with known or suspected pheochromocytoma or hemodynamic compromise or instability)

Thyroid function determinations

(iodine-induced thyrotoxicosis may occur 4 to 12 weeks following contrast radiography in geriatric patients; thyroid function monitoring may be needed)

## Side/Adverse Effects

Note: Adverse effects may vary directly with the concentration of the contrast agent, the amount and technique used, and the underlying pathology. Increases in osmolality, volume, concentration, viscosity, and rate of administration of the solution may increase the incidence and severity of adverse effects.

Most of the adverse effects are usually self-limited and of short duration.

Overall incidence of adverse effects with nonionic contrast agents, such as metrizamide, has been reported to be less than with ionic contrast agents.

Nonionic contrast media, such as metrizamide, have been reported to produce fewer and less severe alterations in cardiac hemodynamics (e.g., bradycardia, hypotension) and electrocardiograms than standard ionic contrast agents during cardiac angiography.

Low-osmolality agents, such as metrizamide, are reported to cause less heat and pain on injection than high-osmolality agents, such as diatrizoates and iothalamate.

Thromboembolic events causing myocardial infarction and stroke have been reported during angiographic procedures with nonionic contrast media; however, these events appear to be technique-related.

Major motor seizures have occurred rarely with intrathecal administration of metrizamide in patients with a history of epilepsy, with overdosage, with inadvertent intracranial entry of a large or concentrated bolus dose, with concurrent administration of neuroleptic medications or phenothiazine antiemetics, and with excessive patient movement or failure to maintain proper head elevation.

Severe mental disturbances have rarely been reported following intrathecal administration of metrizamide. These usually have an onset of 8 to 10 hours and may last 24 hours. They are more prevalent following cervical myelography and may be related to metrizamide's competitive inhibition for the glucose site of brain hexokinase; they may also be dose-related.

Headaches following intrathecal administration of metrizamide may be more frequent, severe, and persistent in those patients not adequately hydrated.

Dehydration may be exacerbated by the osmotic diuretic action of the hypertonic contrast solutions of metrizamide and in some cases cause a shock-like state, following intravascular administration of metrizamide in infants and young children and in geriatric, azotemic, and dehydrated or debilitated patients.

Cardiac arrest and shock have also been reported rarely during or a few minutes after administration of metrizamide.

Transient global amnesia has been reported in 2 patients after cerebral angiography, in which 20 mL of another low-osmolality nonionic contrast agent (containing the equivalent of 240 mg of iodine per mL) was administered into the ascending aorta. The possibility that metrizamide may cause a similar response must be considered.

The following side/adverse effects have been selected on the basis of their potential clinical significance (possible signs and symptoms in parentheses where appropriate)—not necessarily inclusive:

**Those indicating need for medical attention**

Incidence less frequent or rare

*With all procedures*

**Cardiotoxic effects, with ventricular tachycardia or fibrillation** (fast or irregular heartbeat); *hypotension* (severe tiredness or weakness); *pseudo-allergic reaction* (skin rash or hives; stuffy nose; swelling of face or skin; swelling of the tongue, wheezing, tightness in chest, or troubled breathing); *pulmonary edema* (severe wheezing or troubled breathing)

Note: *Pseudo-allergic reactions* are usually transient. However, they may be initial manifestations of more severe anaphylactoid reactions. The anaphylactoid reaction may progress to respiratory arrest and vasomotor collapse if appropriate treatment is not administered.

Incidence rare

*With intrathecal administration*

**CNS effects** (paralysis of one side of body or of legs and arms); *hallucinations; severe nausea and vomiting; seizures, focal or generalized grand mal*

Note: In case of *severe vomiting*, the use of phenothiazine antiemetics may increase the risk of seizures; however, risk-benefit must be considered.

*Seizures* usually occur 4 to 12 hours following injection of metrizamide. May be dose-related. Seizures that occur within 2 hours of administration may indicate early substantial intracranial entry.

**Those indicating need for medical attention only if they continue or are bothersome**

Incidence more frequent

*With all procedures*

**Nausea and vomiting, mild to moderate; restlessness; trembling**

Note: *Nausea and vomiting* may occur 3 to 8 hours after intrathecal injection and last for a few hours, usually disappearing within 24 hours; or, after intravascular injection, may occur immediately and last for a few minutes.

*With intrathecal administration*

**Mild to moderate headache**

Note: *Mild to moderate headache* may occur 3 to 8 hours after injection and last for a few hours, usually disappearing within 24 hours. Often accompanied by nausea and/or less frequently by vomiting.

Incidence less frequent or rare

*With intrathecal administration*

**Backache; chills; CNS effects** (blurred or double vision or other changes in vision; confusion, especially in the elderly; dizziness; severe headache; ringing or buzzing in ears; speech difficulty; unusual tiredness or weakness); *fever*—more frequent in children; *increased sweating; meningeal irritation* (stiffness of neck)

*With intravascular administration*

**Increase in amount of urine; unusual warmth and flushing of skin**

## Overdose

**Treatment of overdose**

Specific treatment—Intravenous diazepam or administration of phenobarbital sodium, for the control of seizures.

## Patient Consultation

As an aid to patient consultation, refer to *Advice for the Patient, Radiopaque Agents (Diagnostic)*.

In providing consultation, consider emphasizing the following selected information (» = major clinical significance):

**Description of use**

Action in the body:

Injection into spinal canal; visualization of radiopacity in head and spinal cord possible with x-rays

Injection into vein or artery; visualization of radiopacity in heart and blood vessels possible with x-rays

Direct injection into region to be studied; visualization of radiopacity in joint spaces

**Before having this test**

» Conditions affecting use, especially:

Sensitivity to iodine or other iodinated contrast media

Pregnancy—Risk to the fetus from radiation exposure; possible risk of hypothyroidism in newborn

Breast-feeding—Distributed into breast milk

Use in children—Possible exacerbation of dehydration (with intravascular use)

Use in the elderly—Possible exacerbation of dehydration; increased risk of thyrotoxicosis

Other medications, especially phenothiazines, tricyclic antidepressants, and trimeprazine (with intrathecal use)

Other medical problems, especially dehydration, hepatorenal disease, and pheochromocytoma

### Preparation for this test

Adequate intake of fluids to prevent dehydration

Special preparatory instructions may be given; patient should inquire in advance

*With intrathecal use*

Normal diet up to 2 hours before procedure; moderate amounts of clear fluids may continue up to time of procedure

### Precautions after having this test

Possible interference with future thyroid tests

*With intrathecal use*

Avoiding movement during and for several hours after administration

Keeping head position as instructed during and after examination

*With intravascular use*

For digital arteriography of head and neck: Not moving or swallowing during and immediately after administration

### Side/adverse effects

Signs of possible side effects, especially pseudo-allergic reaction or cardiac effects; hallucinations, severe nausea and vomiting, paralysis of one side of body or of arm(s) or leg(s), and seizures (with intrathecal use), severe tiredness or weakness, severe wheezing, or troubled breathing

## General Dosing Information

Manufacturer's package insert or other appropriate literature should be consulted for specific techniques and procedures for the administration of contrast media.

Sensitivity test doses are not usually recommended since severe or fatal reactions to contrast media are not predictable from a patient's history or a sensitivity test. On some occasions, severe or fatal reactions have occurred with a test dose or with a full dose in patients who did not react to the test dose.

Pretreatment with corticosteroids and/or antihistamines has been used to minimize the incidence and severity of reactions in patients with a history of severe reactions to contrast media or with other high-risk conditions (e.g., asthma or history of allergies, positive allergy history to skin allergens or penicillins, dehydration, history of seizures, pheochromocytoma). In some studies, the additional use of ephedrine has been shown to be beneficial in preventing anaphylactoid reactions (except in patients with a history of hypertension or cardiovascular disease). When the use of a contrast agent is being considered, the following protocols are recommended:

For high-risk patients—
• Use of a high-osmolality contrast agent plus pretreatment with a corticosteroid (oral prednisone 50 mg administered 13 hours, 7 hours, and 1 hour before procedure) and an antihistamine (intramuscular, intravenous, or oral diphenhydramine, 50 mg administered 1 hour prior to procedure) or
• Use of a low-osmolality contrast agent if pretreatment is not feasible or
• Use of a low-osmolality contrast agent plus corticosteroid pretreatment.

For low-risk patients—
• Use of a high-osmolality contrast agent or
• Use of a high-osmolality contrast agent and corticosteroid pretreatment.

Adequate hydration is recommended for all patients. Intravenous or oral intake of fluids may continue up to time of administration of metrizamide.

During and for at least 30 to 60 minutes after intravascular injection, and for at least 12 hours (up to 24 hours in some cases) after intrathecal administration, of contrast media the patient should be observed for possible severe reactions; competent personnel and emergency facilities should be available during this period.

Dosage of metrizamide is expressed in terms of iodine.

Dosage and concentration of iodine as metrizamide injection are dependent upon the degree and extent of contrast needed in the areas under examination and on the equipment and technique used.

### For intrathecal use

Pretreatment with barbiturates or phenytoin may be used in patients who have a history of seizures but who are not on anticonvulsant therapy. Patients who are on anticonvulsant therapy should continue receiving their medication when using metrizamide.

A normal diet may be ingested up to 2 hours prior to the administration of metrizamide. Moderate amounts of clear liquids are permissible and even recommended by some clinicians to prevent dehydration.

To minimize the risk of seizures, treatment with anticonvulsants may be used if inadvertent intracranial entry of a large or concentrated bolus of metrizamide occurs.

Direct intracisternal or ventricular administration of metrizamide for standard radiography is *not* recommended.

During and for several hours after the procedure the patient must remain inactive to minimize high cephalad dispersion of metrizamide.

Information on patient management and positioning during and after procedure is included in the manufacturer's package insert.

### For intravascular use

Nonionic contrast media, such as metrizamide, inhibit blood coagulation, *in vitro*, less than ionic contrast media. Blood cell aggregation has been reported when blood remains in contact with syringes containing nonionic contrast media. Thus, thromboembolic events causing myocardial infarction and stroke, reported during angiographic procedures, may have resulted from aggregation of blood that had come in contact with the contrast agent outside the body. Risk factors for aggregation should be minimized by performing the procedure in the shortest time possible, using plastic rather than glass syringes, and flushing catheters with heparinized saline solutions.

During and immediately after administration of metrizamide for intravenous digital arteriography of neck and head, the patient must remain inactive. Otherwise, poor arterial visualization may result. Swallowing must also be avoided during and after the injection of metrizamide for carotid-cerebral arteriography.

### For treatment of adverse effects

Recommended treatment consists of the following:
• For major or life-threatening reactions, careful monitoring of vital signs and emergency therapy, including artificial respiration with oxygen, if needed for respiratory depression, and cardiac massage in the event of cardiac arrest.
• To restore blood pressure, administration of intravenous fluids and/or vasopressors. If hypotension necessitates the use of vasopressors, slow infusion of 0.008 to 0.012 mg per minute of norepinephrine or 0.1 to 0.18 mg per minute of phenylephrine, appropriately diluted. If hypotension is due to increased vagal activity (vasovagal reaction), intravenous administration of 1 mg of atropine, repeated in 1 to 2 hours if needed.
• Other specific treatment may include—
   Diphenhydramine: For minor allergic-like reactions—An antihistamine such as diphenhydramine hydrochloride (except in epileptic patients) may be administered intravenously.
   Epinephrine: For acute allergic-like or anaphylactoid reactions—Slow intravenous infusion of 0.1 mg of epinephrine (1:10,000).
   For mild to moderate bronchospasm—0.1 to 0.2 mg of epinephrine (1:1000) may be administered subcutaneously, except in hypotension. In extreme emergency, 0.1 mg of epinephrine (1:10,000) may be given slowly by intravenous route, followed by a continuous intravenous infusion at an initial rate of 0.001 mg per minute, the rate may be increased to 0.004 mg per minute if necessary. (Note: Patients on beta-adrenergic blocking agents should not receive epinephrine since they are at risk of unopposed alpha-adrenergic stimulation, which may result in hypertension, reflex bradycardia, and heart-block. In these patients, isoproterenol and norepinephrine are used instead of epinephrine to overcome bronchospasm and hypotension, respectively.)
   For cardiac arrest—0.1 to 1 mg of epinephrine may be administered by the intravenous route.
   Diazepam or phenobarbital: To control convulsions—5 to 10 mg of diazepam by slow, intravenous administration or phenobarbital sodium may be given intravenously or intramuscularly at a rate not to exceed 30 to 60 mg per minute.

# Parenteral Dosage Forms

## METRIZAMIDE FOR INJECTION

### Usual adult and adolescent dose

Intrathecal—

Myelography:

Lumbar myelography by lumbar injection—10 to 15 mL of a solution containing the equivalent of 170 to 190 mg of iodine per mL.

Thoracic myelography by lumbar injection—12 mL of a solution containing the equivalent of 220 mg of iodine per mL.

Cervical myelography by lumbar injection—10 mL of a solution containing the equivalent of 250 to 300 mg of iodine per mL.

Cervical myelography by lateral cervical injection—10 mL of a solution containing the equivalent of 220 mg of iodine per mL.

Total columnar myelography by lumbar injection—10 mL of a solution containing the equivalent of 250 to 280 mg of iodine per mL.

CT cisternography by lumbar injection:

4 to 6 mL of a solution containing the equivalent of 170 to 190 mg of iodine per mL.

Note: Injection should be given slowly over a period of 1 to 2 minutes.

Immediate repeat intrathecal administration is not recommended because of risk of overdose; 48 hours, or preferably 5 to 7 days, should elapse before repeat examination.

Intravascular—As a solution containing the equivalent of 370 mg of iodine per mL—

Arteriography, peripheral:

Via catheter, 25 to 65 mL into the femoral artery, or advanced to the level of the renal artery if necessary. Two or more injections may be needed.

Digital arteriography of the head and neck:

Intravenous, 30 to 60 mL. Three injections may be needed, up to a total volume of 120 mL.

### Usual adult prescribing limits

Intrathecal—Up to the equivalent of 3 grams of iodine.

Intravascular—Up to the equivalent of 87.5 grams of iodine.

### Usual pediatric dose

Intrathecal—

Myelography:

Lumbar and

Thoracic myelography by lumbar injection—

The following amounts of a solution containing the equivalent of 170 to 190 mg of iodine per mL:

Children up to 2 months of age—2 to 3 mL.

Children 2 months to 2 years of age—2 to 4 mL.

Children 3 to 7 years of age—4 to 8 mL.

Children 8 to 12 years of age—7 to 9 mL.

Children 13 to 18 years of age—8 to 10 mL.

Cervical myelography by lumbar injection—

Children up to 2 months of age—2 to 3 mL of a solution containing the equivalent of 170 to 210 mg of iodine per mL.

Children 2 months to 2 years of age—2 to 4 mL of a solution containing the equivalent of 170 to 200 mg of iodine per mL.

Children 3 to 7 years of age—4 to 8 mL of a solution containing the equivalent of 170 to 210 mg of iodine per mL.

Children 8 to 12 years of age—7 to 9 mL of a solution containing the equivalent of 170 to 230 mg of iodine per mL.

Children 13 to 18 years of age—8 to 10 mL of a solution containing the equivalent of 170 to 230 mg of iodine per mL.

Cervical myelography by lateral cervical injection—

Children up to 8 years of age—Dosage must be individualized by the physician.

Children 8 to 18 years of age—3 to 5 mL of a solution containing the equivalent of 200 to 220 mg of iodine per mL.

Cisternography by direct injection[1]:

Children up to 2 months of age—2 to 3 mL of a solution containing the equivalent of 170 to 220 mg of iodine per mL.

Children 2 months to 8 years of age—Dosage must be individualized by the physician.

Children 8 to 18 years of age—2 to 5 mL of a solution containing the equivalent of 170 to 220 mg of iodine per mL.

Cisternography by lumbar injection:

Children 2 months to 2 years of age—2 to 3 mL of a solution containing the equivalent of 170 to 220 mg of iodine per mL.

Children 3 to 7 years of age—3 to 5 mL of a solution containing the equivalent of 170 to 190 mg of iodine per mL.

Children 8 to 12 years of age—5 to 6 mL of a solution containing the equivalent of 170 to 190 mg of iodine per mL.

CT cisternography by lumbar injection:

Children up to 3 years of age—Dosage must be individualized by physician.

Children 3 to 18 years of age—3 to 5 mL of a solution containing the equivalent of 170 to 190 mg of iodine per mL.

Ventriculography by direct injection:

Children up to 2 years of age—2 to 3 mL of a solution containing the equivalent of 170 to 220 mg of iodine per mL.

Children 3 to 12 years of age—2 to 4 mL of a solution containing the equivalent of 170 to 220 mg of iodine per mL.

Children 13 to 18 years of age—2 to 5 mL of a solution containing the equivalent of 190 to 220 mg of iodine per mL.

Ventriculography by lumbar injection:

Children up to 2 years of age—2 to 3 mL of a solution containing the equivalent of 170 to 220 mg of iodine per mL.

CT ventriculography by direct injection of a solution containing the equivalent of 170 to 220 mg of iodine per mL:

Children up to 2 years of age—2 mL.

Children 3 to 7 years of age—3 mL.

CT ventriculography by lumbar injection:

Children 3 to 7 years of age—3 mL of a solution containing the equivalent of 170 to 220 mg of iodine per mL.

Intravascular—

Angiocardiography: 1.5 mL of a solution containing the equivalent of 370 mg of iodine per mL per kg of body weight.

### Usual geriatric dose

See *Usual adult and adolescent dose.*

Note: Geriatric patients with renal function impairment may be more sensitive to the effects of the usual adult dose; lower dosages are recommended.

### Strength(s) usually available

U.S.—

3.75 grams of metrizamide with 1.81 grams of iodine, per 20-mL vial (Rx) [*Amipaque* (1.2 mg edetate calcium disodium)].

6.75 grams of metrizamide with 3.26 grams of iodine, per 50-mL vial (Rx) [*Amipaque* (2.16 mg edetate calcium disodium)].

Canada—

Not commercially available.

### Packaging and storage

Store below 40 °C (104 °F), preferably between 15 and 30 °C (59 and 86 °F), in a light-resistant container, unless otherwise specified by manufacturer.

### Preparation of dosage form

Metrizamide for injection is reconstituted to the specific iodine concentration by adding the appropriate volume of diluent (0.005% sodium bicarbonate injection) provided by the manufacturer. See maufacturer's package insert for preparation of solutions.

### Stability

After reconstitution, solution must be used immediately. The diluent provided by the manufacturer contains no preservative.

Any unused portion remaining in the container should be discarded.

---

[1]Not included in Canadian product labeling.

## Selected Bibliography

Benotti JR. The comparative effects of ionic versus nonionic agents in cardiac catheterization. Invest Radiol 1988; 23 (Suppl 2): S366–S373.

---

Revised: 08/16/95

# METRONIDAZOLE   Systemic

VA CLASSIFICATION (Primary/Secondary): AM900/AP109; AP200; GA900

Note: For a listing of dosage forms and brand names by country availability, see *Dosage Forms* section(s). For a listing of brand names for the articles in this monograph, refer to the General Index.

## Category

Antibacterial (systemic); antiprotozoal; bowel disease (inflammatory) suppressant; anthelmintic (systemic).

## Indications

Note: Bracketed information in the *Indications* section refers to uses that are not included in U.S. product labeling.

**Accepted**

Amebiasis, extraintestinal (treatment)—Metronidazole is indicated in the treatment of extraintestinal amebiasis, including amebic liver abscess, caused by *Entamoeba histolytica*. When used in the treatment of invasive amebiasis, metronidazole should be administered concurrently or sequentially with a luminal amebicide (e.g., iodoquinol, paromomycin, tetracycline, diloxanide furoate).

Amebiasis, intestinal (treatment)—Oral metronidazole is indicated in the treatment of acute intestinal amebiasis caused by *Entamoeba histolytica*. Metronidazole may not eradicate intestinal amebic infections, requiring treatment with a luminal amebicide.

Bone and joint infections (treatment)—Metronidazole is indicated in the treatment of bone and joint infections caused by *Bacteroides* species, including the *B. fragilis* group (*B. fragilis, B. distasonis, B. ovatus, B. thetaiotaomicron, B. vulgatus*).

Brain abscess (treatment)—Metronidazole is indicated in the treatment of brain abscess caused by *Bacteroides* species, including the *B. fragilis* group.

Central nervous system (CNS) infections (treatment)—Metronidazole is indicated in the treatment of CNS infections, including meningitis, caused by *Bacteroides* species, including the *B. fragilis* group.

Endocarditis, bacterial (treatment)—Metronidazole is indicated in the treatment of endocarditis caused by *Bacteroides* species, including the *B. fragilis* group.

Intra-abdominal infections (treatment)—Metronidazole is indicated in the treatment of intra-abdominal infections, including peritonitis, intra-abdominal abscess, and liver abscess, caused by *Bacteroides* species, including the *B. fragilis* group, *Clostridium* species, *Eubacterium* species, *Peptococcus* species, and *Peptostreptococcus* species.

Pelvic infections, female (treatment)—Metronidazole is indicated in the treatment of female pelvic infections, including endometritis, endomyometritis, tubo-ovarian abscess, and postsurgical vaginal cuff infections, caused by *Bacteroides* species, including the *B. fragilis* group, *Clostridium* species, *Peptococcus* species, and *Peptostreptococcus* species.

Perioperative infections, colorectal (prophylaxis)—Intravenous metronidazole is indicated for the prophylaxis of perioperative infections during colorectal surgery.

Pneumonia, *Bacteroides* species (treatment)—Metronidazole is indicated in the treatment of lower respiratory tract infections, including pneumonia, empyema, and lung abscess, caused by *Bacteroides* species, including the *B. fragilis* group.

Septicemia, bacterial (treatment)—Metronidazole is indicated in the treatment of bacterial septicemia caused by *Bacteroides* species, including the *B. fragilis* group, and *Clostridium* species.

Skin and soft tissue infections (treatment)—Metronidazole is indicated in the treatment of skin and soft tissue infections caused by *Bacteroides* species, including the *B. fragilis* group, *Clostridium* species, *Fusobacterium* species, *Peptococcus* species, and *Peptostreptococcus* species.

Trichomoniasis (treatment)—Oral metronidazole is indicated in the treatment of symptomatic and asymptomatic trichomoniasis, in males and females, caused by *Trichomonas vaginalis*.

[Balantidiasis (treatment)][1]—Metronidazole is used in the treatment of *Balantidium coli* infection.

[Bowel disease, inflammatory (treatment)][1]—Metronidazole is used in the treatment of inflammatory bowel disease.

[Colitis, antibiotic-associated (treatment)][1]—Metronidazole is used in the treatment of antibiotic-associated diarrhea and colitis caused by *C. difficile*.

[Dracunculiasis (treatment)][1]—Metronidazole is used in the treatment of dracunculiasis (guinea worm infection) caused by *Dracunculus medinensis*. It decreases the inflammation around the ulcer, increasing the ease of removing the worm.

[Gastritis, *Helicobacter pylori*–associated (treatment adjunct)][1] or

[Ulcer, duodenal, *Helicobacter pylori*–associated (treatment adjunct)][1]—Some studies indicate that metronidazole may be effective, in combination with bismuth subsalicylate or colloidal bismuth subcitrate, and other oral antibiotic therapy, such as ampicillin or amoxicillin, in the treatment of *Helicobacter pylori*–associated gastritis and duodenal ulcer. However, metronidazole resistance may occur, especially in patients who have been previously exposed to metronidazole.

[Giardiasis (treatment)][1]—Oral metronidazole is used in the treatment of giardiasis caused by *Giardia lamblia*.

[Periodontal infections (treatment)][1]—Metronidazole is used in the treatment of periodontal infections caused by *Bacteroides* species.

[Vaginosis, bacterial (treatment)][1]—Oral metronidazole is used in the treatment of bacterial vaginosis caused by *Gardnerella vaginalis*.

Not all species or strains of a particular organism may be equally susceptible to metronidazole.

**Unaccepted**

Metronidazole is not effective against facultative anaerobes, obligate aerobes, *Propionibacterium acnes*, *Actinomyces* species, or *Candida albicans*.

---

[1]Not included in Canadian product labeling.

## Pharmacology/Pharmacokinetics

**Physicochemical characteristics**
Molecular weight—Metronidazole: 171.16.
Metronidazole hydrochloride: 207.62.

**Mechanism of action/Effect**
Antibacterial (systemic); antiprotozoal—Microbicidal; active against most obligate anaerobic bacteria and protozoa by undergoing intracellular chemical reduction via mechanisms unique to anaerobic metabolism. Reduced metronidazole, which is cytotoxic but short-lived, interacts with DNA to cause a loss of helical structure, strand breakage, and resultant inhibition of nucleic acid synthesis and cell death.

**Absorption**
Well absorbed orally; bioavailability at least 80%.

**Distribution**
Distributed to saliva, bile, seminal fluid, breast milk, bone, liver and liver abscesses, lungs, and vaginal secretions; crosses the placenta and blood-brain barrier, also.
$Vol_D$—
    In adults: Approximately 0.55 L/kg.
    In neonates: 0.54–0.81 L/kg.

**Protein binding**
Low (<20%).

**Biotransformation**
Hepatic; metabolized primarily by side-chain oxidation and glucuronide conjugation to 2-hydroxymethyl (also active) and other metabolites.

**Half-life**
In adults—
    Normal liver function: 8 hours (range, 6 to 12 hours).
    Alcoholic liver disease: 18 hours (range, 10 to 29 hours).
In neonates—
    28 to 30 weeks gestational age: Approximately 75 hours.
    32 to 35 weeks gestational age: Approximately 35 hours.
    36 to 40 weeks gestational age: Approximately 25 hours.

**Time to peak serum concentration**
1 to 2 hours (oral).

**Peak serum concentration**
Peak serum concentrations following a 250-mg, 500-mg, and 2-gram oral dose are approximately 6, 12, and 40 mcg/mL, respectively.
At recommended intravenous doses, peak steady-state serum concentrations are approximately 25 mcg/mL; trough concentrations are approximately 18 mcg/mL.

**Elimination**
Renal—60 to 80%; of this amount, approximately 20% excreted unchanged in urine. Renal clearance approximately 10 mL/min/1.73 $M^2$.
Fecal—6 to 15%; inactive metabolites also present in feces.

In dialysis—
    Hemodialysis: Metronidazole and primary metabolites rapidly removed from the blood by hemodialysis (half-life shortened to approximately 2.6 hours).
    Peritoneal dialysis: Metronidazole is not significantly removed by peritoneal dialysis.

# Precautions to Consider

## Carcinogenicity/Tumorigenicity
Metronidazole has been shown to be carcinogenic in a number of studies in mice. Pulmonary tumorigenesis has been reported in six studies in mice, including one study in which the animals were dosed on an intermittent schedule (every four weeks). Malignant hepatic tumors have also been reported in male mice given very high doses (approximately 500 mg/kg/day). Malignant lymphomas have been reported in one lifetime feeding study in mice.
Metronidazole has also been shown to be carcinogenic in rats. Several long-term, oral-dosing studies in rats have shown that metronidazole causes a statistically significant increase in the incidence of various neoplasms, especially mammary and hepatic tumors, in female rats.
Two lifetime tumorigenicity studies in hamsters have given negative results.
Metronidazole has not been shown to be carcinogenic or tumorigenic in humans.

## Mutagenicity
Studies have shown that metronidazole is mutagenic in bacteria and fungi, although this has not been confirmed in mammals.

## Pregnancy/Reproduction
Fertility; pregnancy—
Metronidazole crosses the placenta and enters the fetal circulation rapidly. Adequate and well-controlled studies in humans have not been done. Studies in rats, given doses of up to 5 times the human dose, have not shown that metronidazole causes impaired fertility or birth defects in the fetus. Metronidazole, administered intraperitoneally to pregnant mice at approximately the human dose, has been shown to cause fetotoxicity. When administered orally, no fetotoxicity was seen in pregnant mice. However, the use of metronidazole in the treatment of trichomoniasis is not recommended during the first trimester. If metronidazole is used during the second and third trimesters for trichomoniasis, it is recommended that its use be limited to those patients whose symptoms are not controlled by local palliative treatment. Also, the 1-day course of therapy should not be used since this results in higher maternal and fetal serum concentrations.
Studies in rats given doses of up to 5 times the usual human dose have not shown that metronidazole causes impaired fertility or birth defects in the fetus. Metronidazole, administered intraperitoneally to pregnant mice at approximately the human dose, has been shown to cause fetotoxicity. When metronidazole was administered orally, no fetotoxicity was seen in pregnant mice.

FDA Pregnancy Category B.

## Breast-feeding
Metronidazole is distributed into breast milk; concentrations are similar to those found in the maternal plasma. Use is not recommended in nursing mothers since some studies in rats and mice have shown that metronidazole is carcinogenic and may cause adverse effects in the infant. However, use in the treatment of anaerobic bacterial infections or a short course of treatment with metronidazole for amebiasis, severe periodontal infections, or trichomoniasis may be necessary in nursing mothers. During treatment with metronidazole, the breast milk should be expressed and discarded. Breast-feeding may be resumed 24 to 48 hours after treatment is completed.

## Pediatrics
When used for the treatment of anaerobic infections and amebiasis, metronidazole has not demonstrated any pediatrics-specific problems that would limit its usefulness in children.

## Geriatrics
No information is available on the relationship of age to the effects of metronidazole in geriatric patients. However, elderly patients are more likely to have an age-related decrease in hepatic function, which may require an adjustment in dosage in patients receiving metronidazole.

## Dental
Metronidazole may cause dry mouth, an unpleasant or sharp metallic taste, and alteration of taste sensation. Dry mouth may contribute to the development of caries, periodontal disease, oral candidiasis, and discomfort.

## Drug interactions and/or related problems
The following drug interactions and/or related problems have been selected on the basis of their potential clinical significance (possible mechanism in parentheses where appropriate)—not necessarily inclusive (» = major clinical significance):
Note: Combinations containing any of the following medications, depending on the amount present, may also interact with this medication.

» Alcohol
    (it is recommended that metronidazole not be used concurrently with, or for at least 1 day following, ingestion of alcohol; accumulation of acetaldehyde by interference with the oxidation of alcohol may occur, resulting in disulfiram-like effects such as abdominal cramps, nausea, vomiting, headache, or flushing; in addition, modifications in the taste of alcoholic beverages have been reported during concurrent use)

» Anticoagulants, coumarin- or indandione-derivative
    (effects may be potentiated when these agents are used concurrently with metronidazole, because of inhibition of enzymatic metabolism of anticoagulants; periodic prothrombin time determinations may be required during therapy to determine if dosage adjustments of anticoagulants are necessary)

Cimetidine
    (hepatic metabolism of metronidazole may be decreased when metronidazole and cimetidine are used concurrently, possibly resulting in delayed elimination and increased serum metronidazole concentrations; monitoring of serum concentrations as a guide to dosage is recommended since dosage adjustments of metronidazole may be necessary during and after cimetidine therapy)

» Disulfiram
    (it is recommended that metronidazole not be used concurrently with, or for 2 weeks following, disulfiram in alcoholic patients; such use may result in confusion and psychotic reactions because of combined toxicity)

Neurotoxic medications, other (See *Appendix II*)
    (concurrent use of metronidazole with other neurotoxic medications may increase the potential for neurotoxicity)

Phenobarbital
    (phenobarbital may induce microsomal liver enzymes, increasing metronidazole's metabolism and resulting in a decrease in half-life and plasma concentration)

Phenytoin
    (metronidazole may impair the clearance of phenytoin, increasing phenytoin's plasma concentration)

## Laboratory value alterations
The following have been selected on the basis of their potential clinical significance (possible effect in parentheses where appropriate)—not necessarily inclusive (» = major clinical significance):
With diagnostic test results
Alanine aminotransferase (ALT [SGPT]), serum and
Aspartate aminotransferase (AST [SGOT]), serum and
Lactate dehydrogenase (LDH)
    (metronidazole has a high absorbance at the wavelength at which nicotinamide-adenine dinucleotide [NADH] is determined; therefore, elevated liver enzyme concentrations may appear to be suppressed by metronidazole when measured by continuous-flow methods based on endpoint decrease in reduced NADH; unusually low liver enzyme concentrations, including zero values, have been reported)

## Medical considerations/Contraindications
The medical considerations/contraindications included here have been selected on the basis of their potential clinical significance (reasons given in parentheses where appropriate)—not necessarily inclusive (» = major clinical significance).

### Risk-benefit should be considered when the following medical problems exist:
» Active organic disease of the CNS, including epilepsy
    (metronidazole may cause CNS toxicity, including seizures with high doses, and peripheral neuropathy)

» Blood dyscrasias, or history of
    (metronidazole may cause leukopenia)

Cardiac function impairment
    (parenteral dosage forms—because of sodium content)

» Hepatic function impairment, severe
    (metabolized in the liver; hepatic dysfunction may lead to decreased plasma clearance and accumulation of metronidazole and

its metabolites; dosage may need to be reduced with severe hepatic function impairment)

Hypersensitivity to metronidazole

### Patient monitoring

The following may be especially important in patient monitoring (other tests may be warranted in some patients, depending on condition; » = major clinical significance):

*For giardiasis*
» Stool examinations
(3 stool examinations, taken several days apart, beginning 3 to 4 weeks following treatment are recommended if symptoms persist; however, in some successfully treated patients, the lactose intolerance brought on by the infection may persist for a period of some weeks or months, mimicking the symptoms of giardiasis; in cases of treatment failure, alternate drugs may be used)

## Side/Adverse Effects

The following side/adverse effects have been selected on the basis of their potential clinical significance (possible signs and symptoms in parentheses where appropriate)—not necessarily inclusive;

### Those indicating need for medical attention
Incidence less frequent
*Peripheral neuropathy* (numbness, tingling, pain, or weakness in hands or feet)—usually with high doses or prolonged use; *seizures*—usually with high doses
Incidence rare
*CNS toxicity* (ataxia—clumsiness or unsteadiness; encephalopathy—mood or other mental changes); *hypersensitivity* (skin rash, hives, redness, or itching); *leukopenia* (sore throat and fever); *pancreatitis* (severe abdominal and back pain; anorexia; nausea and vomiting); *thrombophlebitis* (pain, tenderness, redness, or swelling at site of injection); *vaginal candidiasis* (any vaginal irritation, discharge, or dryness not present before therapy)

### Those indicating need for medical attention only if they continue or are bothersome
Incidence more frequent
*CNS effects* (dizziness or lightheadedness; headache); *gastrointestinal disturbance* (diarrhea; loss of appetite; nausea or vomiting; stomach pain or cramps)
Incidence less frequent or rare
*Change in taste sensation; dryness of mouth; unpleasant or sharp metallic taste*

### Those not indicating need for medical attention
Incidence less frequent or rare
*Dark urine*

## Overdose

For more information on the management of overdose or unintentional ingestion, **contact a Poison Control Center** (see *Poison Control Center Listing*).

### Treatment of overdose
Since there is no specific antidote, treatment for metronidazole overdose should be symptomatic and supportive.

## Patient Consultation

As an aid to patient consultation, refer to *Advice for the Patient, Metronidazole (Systemic)*.

In providing consultation, consider emphasizing the following selected information (» = major clinical significance):

### Before using this medication
» Conditions affecting use, especially:
Hypersensitivity to metronidazole
Pregnancy—Metronidazole crosses the placenta; use is not recommended during the first trimester of pregnancy
Breast-feeding—Metronidazole is distributed into breast milk; metronidazole is not recommended during breast-feeding
Dental—Metronidazole may cause dry mouth, an unpleasant or sharp metallic taste, and alteration of taste sensation
Other medications, especially alcohol, coumarin- or indandione-derivative anticoagulants, or disulfiram
Other medical problems, especially active organic disease of the CNS, a history of blood dyscrasias, or severe hepatic function impairment

### Proper use of this medication
Taking with meals or a snack to minimize gastrointestinal irritation
» Compliance with full course of therapy

» Importance of not missing doses and taking at evenly spaced times
» Proper dosing
Missed dose: Taking as soon as possible; not taking if almost time for next dose; not doubling doses
» Proper storage

### Precautions while using this medication
Follow-up visit to physician after treatment for giardiasis to ensure that infection has been eradicated.
Checking with physician if no improvement within a few days
» Avoiding use of alcoholic beverages or other alcohol-containing preparations while taking and for at least 1 day after discontinuing this medication
Possible dryness of mouth; using sugarless candy or gum, ice, or saliva substitute for relief; checking with dentist if dry mouth continues for more than 2 weeks
» Caution if dizziness or lightheadedness occurs
Prevention of reinfection in trichomoniasis; possible need for concurrent treatment of male sexual partner and use of a condom

### Side/adverse effects
Signs of potential side effects, especially CNS toxicity, hypersensitivity, leukopenia, pancreatitis, seizures, peripheral neuropathy, vaginal candidiasis, and thrombophlebitis
Dark urine may be alarming to patient although medically insignificant

## General Dosing Information

Patients with severely impaired hepatic function metabolize metronidazole slowly. Close monitoring for toxicity, as well as reduction in dose, may be required.

Anuric patients do not generally require a reduction in dose since metabolites of metronidazole may be rapidly removed by hemodialysis. Also, reduced renal function does not significantly affect single-dose pharmacokinetics of metronidazole.

### For oral dosage forms only
Metronidazole may be taken with meals or a snack to lessen gastrointestinal irritation.

When metronidazole is used in the treatment of trichomoniasis, sexual partners should receive concurrent therapy since asymptomatic trichomoniasis in the male partner is a frequent source of reinfection in the female. The male partner should be advised to use a condom for the duration of treatment.

### For parenteral dosage forms only
Parenteral metronidazole should be administered by slow intravenous infusion only, either continuously or intermittently over a 1-hour period.

If metronidazole is administered concurrently with a primary intravenous solution, the primary solution should be discontinued while metronidazole is being infused.

## Oral Dosage Forms

Note: Bracketed uses in the *Dosage Forms* section refer to categories of use and/or indications that are not included in U.S. product labeling.

### METRONIDAZOLE CAPSULES

#### Usual adult and adolescent dose
Antibacterial (systemic)—
Anaerobic infections: Oral, 7.5 mg (base) per kg of body weight, up to a maximum of 1 gram, every six hours for seven days or longer.
[Bowel disease, inflammatory][1]: Oral, 500 mg (base) four times a day.
[Colitis, antibiotic-associated][1]: Oral, 500 mg (base) three or four times a day.
[Gastritis, *Helicobacter pylori*–associated (treatment adjunct)][1] or
[Ulcer, duodenal, *Helicobacter pylori*–associated (treatment adjunct)][1]—Oral, 500 mg (base) three times a day, in conjunction with bismuth subsalicylate or colloidal bismuth subcitrate and other oral antibiotic therapy, such as ampicillin or amoxicillin, for one to two weeks.
[Vaginosis, bacterial][1]: Oral, 500 mg (base) two times a day for seven days.
Antiprotozoal—
Amebiasis: Oral, 500 to 750 mg (base) three times a day for five to ten days.
[Balantidiasis][1]: Oral, 750 mg (base) three times a day for five or six days.
[Giardiasis][1]: Oral, 2 grams (base) once a day for three days; or 250 mg three times a day for five to seven days.
Trichomoniasis: Oral, 2 grams (base) as a single dose; 1 gram two times a day for one day; or 250 mg three times a day for seven days.
Anthelmintic (systemic)—
[Dracunculiasis][1]: Oral, 250 mg (base) three times a day for ten days.

**Usual adult prescribing limits**

Antibacterial (systemic)—

Up to a maximum of 4 grams (base) daily.

**Usual pediatric dose**

Antibacterial (systemic)—

Anaerobic infections[1]: Oral, 7.5 mg (base) per kg of body weight every six hours, or 10 mg per kg of body weight every eight hours.

Antiprotozoal—

Amebiasis: Oral, 11.6 to 16.7 mg (base) per kg of body weight three times a day for ten days.

[Balantidiasis][1]: Oral, 11.6 to 16.7 mg (base) per kg of body weight three times a day for five days.

[Giardiasis][1]: Oral, 5 mg (base) per kg of body weight three times a day for five to seven days.

Trichomoniasis: Oral, 5 mg (base) per kg of body weight three times a day for seven days.

Anthelmintic (systemic)—

[Dracunculiasis][1]: Oral, 8.3 mg (base) per kg of body weight, up to a maximum of 250 mg, three times a day for ten days.

**Strength(s) usually available**

U.S.—

Not commercially available.

Canada—

500 mg (base) (Rx) [*Flagyl* (sodium 5.47 mg); *Trikacide*].

**Packaging and storage**

Store below 40 °C (104 °F), preferably between 15 and 30 °C (59 and 86 °F), in a well-closed container, unless otherwise specified by manufacturer. Store in a light-resistant container.

**Auxiliary labeling**

• Avoid alcoholic beverages.

• May cause dizziness.

• Continue medicine for full time of treatment.

## METRONIDAZOLE TABLETS USP

**Usual adult and adolescent dose**

See *Metronidazole Capsules*.

**Usual adult prescribing limits**

See *Metronidazole Capsules*.

**Usual pediatric dose**

See *Metronidazole Capsules*.

**Strength(s) usually available**

U.S.—

250 mg (base) (Rx) [*Flagyl; Metric 21; Protostat* (scored; lactose); GENERIC].

500 mg (base) (Rx) [*Flagyl; Protostat* (scored; lactose); GENERIC].

Canada—

250 mg (base) (Rx) [*Apo-Metronidazole; Flagyl* (sodium 3.1 mg); *Novonidazol* (scored; sodium 2.2 mg); *Trikacide*].

**Packaging and storage**

Store below 40 °C (104 °F), preferably between 15 and 30 °C (59 and 86 °F), unless otherwise specified by manufacturer. Store in a well-closed, light-resistant container.

**Preparation of dosage form**

For patients who cannot take oral solids—According to the primary manufacturer, the tablets may be crushed and suspended in Cherry Syrup NF to prepare a pediatric dosage form. The recommended concentration per 5 mL is the dose calculated for a particular pediatric patient. The suspension is stable for 30 days if stored at ambient room temperature or refrigerated. Dispense with ''shake well'' instructions.

**Auxiliary labeling**

• Avoid alcoholic beverages.

• May cause dizziness.

• Continue medicine for full time of treatment.

## Parenteral Dosage Forms

Note: Bracketed uses in the *Dosage Forms* section refer to categories of use and/or indications that are not included in U.S. product labeling.

Note: The dosing and dosage forms available are expressed in terms of metronidazole base.

## METRONIDAZOLE INJECTION USP

**Usual adult and adolescent dose**

Antibacterial (systemic)—

Anaerobic infections: Intravenous infusion, 15 mg (base) per kg of body weight initially, then 7.5 mg per kg of body weight, up to a maximum of 1 gram, every six hours for seven days or longer.

Perioperative infections, colonic (prophylaxis): Intravenous infusion, 15 mg (base) per kg of body weight one hour prior to the start of surgery; and 7.5 mg per kg of body weight six and twelve hours after the initial dose.

[Antiprotozoal—Amebiasis][1]—

Intravenous infusion, 500 to 750 mg (base) every eight hours for five to ten days.

**Usual adult prescribing limits**

Antibacterial (systemic)—

Up to a maximum of 4 grams (base) daily.

**Usual pediatric dose**

Antibacterial (systemic)—Anaerobic infections:

Preterm infants—Intravenous infusion, 15 mg per kg of body weight (base) as an initial dose, then 7.5 mg per kg of body weight every twelve hours starting 48 hours after the initial dose.Term infants—Intravenous infusion, 15 mg (base) per kg of body weight as an initial dose, then 7.5 mg per kg of body weight every twelve hours starting 24 hours after the initial dose.Infants greater than 7 days of age and children—Intravenous infusion, 15 mg (base) per kg of body weight as an initial dose, then 7.5 mg per kg of body weight every six hours.

**Strength(s) usually available**

U.S.—

500 mg in 100 mL (base) (Rx) [*Flagyl I.V. RTU* (sodium 14 mEq); *Metro I.V.* (sodium 13.5 mEq); GENERIC].

Canada—

500 mg in 100 mL (base) (Rx) [*Flagyl;* GENERIC].

**Packaging and storage**

Store below 40 °C (104 °F), preferably between 15 and 30 °C (59 and 86 °F), unless otherwise specified by manufacturer. Protect from light during storage. Protect from freezing.

**Incompatibilities**

Intravenous admixtures of metronidazole and other medications are not recommended.

**Additional information**

Metronidazole Injection USP is an isotonic (297 to 310 mOsm per liter), ready-to-use solution, requiring no dilution or buffering prior to administration.

Metronidazole Injection USP in prefilled plastic minibags should not be used in series connections. This may result in air embolism because of residual air (approximately 15 mL), which may be drawn from the primary plastic bag before administration of the infusion from the secondary plastic bag is completed.

## METRONIDAZOLE HYDROCHLORIDE FOR INJECTION

**Usual adult and adolescent dose**

See *Metronidazole Injection USP*.

**Usual adult prescribing limits**

See *Metronidazole Injection USP*.

**Usual pediatric dose**

See *Metronidazole Injection USP*.

**Size(s) usually available**

U.S.—

500 mg (base) (Rx) [*Flagyl I.V.* (sodium 5 mEq)].

Canada—

Not commercially available.

**Packaging and storage**

Prior to reconstitution, store below 30 °C (86 °F), in a light-resistant container, unless otherwise specified by manufacturer.

**Preparation of dosage form**

Metronidazole hydrochloride for injection must not be given by direct intravenous injection since the initial dilution has an extremely low pH (0.5 to 2.0). It must be diluted further and neutralized prior to administration.

To prepare initial dilution for intravenous infusion, add 4.4 mL of sterile water for injection, bacteriostatic water for injection, 0.9% sodium chloride injection, or bacteriostatic sodium chloride injection to each 500-mg vial to provide a concentration of 100 mg per mL (pH 0.5 to 2.0). The resulting solution should be further diluted in 100 mL of 0.9% sodium chloride injection, 5% dextrose injection, or lactated Ringer's injection. The final dilution must be neutralized with approximately 5 mEq of sodium bicarbonate injection per 500 mg of metronidazole (final pH 6 to 7). Since carbon dioxide gas is produced during neutralization, it may be necessary to relieve the pressure in the final container. The final concentration should not exceed 8 mg per mL since neutralization decreases the solubility of metronidazole and precipitation may occur.

**Stability**
After reconstitution, solutions retain their potency for 96 hours if stored below 30 °C (86 °F) in room light. Diluted and neutralized solutions retain their potency for 24 hours.
Do not refrigerate neutralized solutions since precipitation may occur.

**Incompatibilities**
Do not use with aluminum needles or hubs.
Intravenous admixtures of metronidazole with other medications are not recommended.

---

[1]Not included in Canadian product labeling.

---

Revised: 10/20/92
Interim revision: 03/24/94

---

# METRONIDAZOLE  Topical

VA CLASSIFICATION (Primary): DE752
Note: For a listing of dosage forms and brand names by country availability, see *Dosage Forms* section(s). For a listing of brand names for the articles in this monograph, refer to the General Index.

## Category
Antirosacea agent (topical).

## Indications
Note: Bracketed information in the *Indications* section refers to uses that are not included in U.S. product labeling.

**Accepted**
Rosacea (treatment)—Topical metronidazole is indicated [as a primary agent] in the treatment of the inflammatory papules, pustules, and erythema of rosacea (acne rosacea; "adult acne") [in adults].

**Unaccepted**
Topical metronidazole is not effective against the accompanying telangiectasias seen in rosacea patients.

## Pharmacology/Pharmacokinetics

**Physicochemical characteristics**
Chemical group—Nitroimidazole
Molecular weight—171.16.

**Mechanism of action/Effect**
Unknown, but apparently not due to an antiparasitic effect on the mite *Demodex folliculorum*, found in hair follicles and sebaceous secretions, or to any effect on sebum production. Topical metronidazole may have an antioxidant effect. It has been shown to significantly reduce the concentrations of neutrophil-generated reactive oxygen species, hydroxyl radicals and hydrogen peroxide, which are potent oxidants capable of causing tissue injury at the site of inflammation. Topical metronidazole may also have an effect on neutrophil cellular functions, which is partly attributable to its direct anti-inflammatory effect.

**Absorption**
Minimal; only trace amounts found in the serum following topical application of a 0.75% gel.

**Distribution**
Absorbed metronidazole crosses the placenta and the blood-brain barrier.

**Peak serum concentration**
Minimal; up to 66 nanograms per mL following application of 1 gram of gel (equivalent to 7.5 mg of metronidazole) to the face of rosacea patients. Serum concentrations were reported to be undetectable in some patients.

## Precautions to Consider

**Cross-sensitivity and/or related problems**
Patients sensitive to parabens may be sensitive to metronidazole topical gel also since it contains methyl- and propylparabens.

**Carcinogenicity/Tumorigenicity**
Carcinogenicity studies have not been done using topical formulations of metronidazole.
A number of studies using chronic, oral administration of metronidazole in mice and rats have shown that metronidazole is carcinogenic and tumorigenic. However, metronidazole has not been shown to be carcinogenic or tumorigenic in humans (See *Metronidazole [Systemic]*).

**Mutagenicity**
Studies have shown that metronidazole is mutagenic in bacteria and fungi, although this has not been confirmed in mammals.

**Pregnancy/Reproduction**
Fertility—Adequate and well-controlled studies using topical metronidazole in humans have not been done. However, studies using oral metronidazole in rats or mice have not shown that metronidazole causes impaired fertility.
Pregnancy—Absorbed metronidazole crosses the placenta and enters the fetal circulation rapidly. Adequate and well-controlled studies using topical metronidazole in humans have not been done.
Studies using oral metronidazole in rats and mice have not shown that metronidazole causes adverse effects on the fetus.
FDA Pregnancy Category B.

**Breast-feeding**
Metronidazole, applied topically, is minimally absorbed. Only trace amounts appear in the serum following topical application. Therefore, topical metronidazole is unlikely to be distributed into breast milk in significant amounts since the topical dose is small. In addition, it is unlikely that the nursing infant would absorb significant amounts of metronidazole or that it would cause serious problems in the nursing infant.

**Pediatrics**
Safety and efficacy have not been established. Since rosacea is considered primarily an adult-onset disease, topical metronidazole is not indicated in the treatment of pediatric patients.

**Geriatrics**
No information is available on the relationship of age to the effects of topical metronidazole in geriatric patients.

**Medical considerations/Contraindications**
The medical considerations/contraindications included here have been selected on the basis of their potential clinical significance (reasons given in parentheses where appropriate)—not necessarily inclusive (» = major clinical significance).

*Risk-benefit should be considered when the following medical problem exists:*
Sensitivity to topical metronidazole

## Side/Adverse Effects

Note: Because metronidazole is minimally absorbed, with only trace amounts appearing in the serum following topical application, those side/adverse effects reported with systemic use of metronidazole have not been reported with topical use of the medication.

If local irritation occurs, metronidazole topical gel should be applied less frequently or discontinued.

The following side/adverse effects have been selected on the basis of their potential clinical significance (possible signs and symptoms in parentheses where appropriate)—not necessarily inclusive:

**Those indicating need for medical attention only if they continue or are bothersome**
Incidence less frequent
*Dry skin; redness or other signs of skin irritation not present before therapy; stinging or burning of the skin; watering of eyes*

## Patient Consultation

As an aid to patient consultation, refer to *Advice for the Patient, Metronidazole (Topical)*.

In providing consultation, consider emphasizing the following selected information (» = major clinical significance):

**Before using this medication**
» Conditions affecting use, especially:
     Sensitivity to topical metronidazole or to methyl- and propylparabens

Pregnancy—Absorbed metronidazole crosses the placenta and enters fetal circulation rapidly

### Proper use of this medication

» Not using medication in or near the eyes; tearing may occur

Washing eyes out immediately with large amounts of cool tap water if medication gets into eyes; checking with physician if eyes continue to burn or are painful

Before applying, thoroughly washing affected area(s) with a mild, non-irritating cleanser, rinsing well, and gently patting dry

*To use*

After washing affected area(s), applying medication with fingertips; washing medication off hands afterward

» Importance of applying medication to entire affected area

» Compliance with full course of therapy, which may take 9 weeks or longer

» Proper dosing

Missed dose: Applying as soon as possible; not applying if almost time for next dose

» Proper storage

### Precautions while using this medication

Checking with physician if no improvement within 3 weeks; may take up to 9 weeks before full therapeutic benefit is seen

Possibility of stinging or burning of the skin after application; checking with physician if irritation continues

Using only ''oil-free'' cosmetics to avoid worsening rosacea

## General Dosing Information

Topical metronidazole has also been used as a 1% cream formulation in the treatment of rosacea.

Before this medication is applied, the affected area(s) should be washed thoroughly with a mild, nonirritating cleanser, rinsed well, and gently patted dry.

After washing the affected area(s), a thin film of the gel should be applied and rubbed into the entire affected area.

Metronidazole topical gel should not be used in or near the eyes. Tearing has been reported when the gel is applied too close to the eyes.

If local irritation occurs, metronidazole topical gel should be applied less frequently or discontinued.

## Topical Dosage Forms
### METRONIDAZOLE TOPICAL GEL

### Usual adult dose
Rosacea—

Topical, to the affected area(s) two times a day, morning and evening, for nine weeks.

### Usual pediatric dose
Safety and efficacy have not been established. Since rosacea is considered primarily an adult-onset disease, topical metronidazole is not needed in the treatment of pediatric patients.

### Strength(s) usually available
U.S.—

0.75% (Rx) [*MetroGel* (methylparaben; propylparaben; propylene glycol; edetate disodium)].

Canada—

0.75% (Rx) [*MetroGel* (methylparaben; propylparaben)].

### Packaging and storage
Store between 15 and 30 °C (59 and 86 °F), in a well-closed container, unless otherwise specified by manufacturer. Protect from freezing.

### Auxiliary labeling
• For external use only.
• Continue medication for full time of treatment.

### Additional information
Metronidazole topical gel is an aqueous, nongreasy, invisible, and nonstaining preparation.

## Selected Bibliography

Bleicher PA, Charles HJ, Sober AJ. Topical metronidazole therapy for rosacea. Arch Dermatol 1987 May; 123: 609-14.

Aronson IK, Rumsfield JA, West DP, Alexander J, Fischer JH, Paloucek FP. Evaluation of topical metronidazole gel in acne rosacea. Drug Intell Clin Pharm 1987 Apr; 21: 348-51.

Nielsen PG. Metronidazole treatment in rosacea. Int J Dermatol 1988 Jan-Feb; 27: 1-5.

Revised: 06/24/94

---

# METRONIDAZOLE   Vaginal

VA CLASSIFICATION (Primary): GU300

Note: For a listing of dosage forms and brand names by country availability, see *Dosage Forms* section(s). For a listing of brand names for the articles in this monograph, refer to the General Index.

## Category
Anti-infective (vaginal).

## Indications

Note: Bracketed information in the *Indications* section refers to uses that are not included in U.S. product labeling.

### Accepted

Vaginosis, bacterial (treatment)—Vaginal metronidazole is indicated in the local treatment of bacterial vaginosis (previously known as *Haemophilus* vaginitis, *Gardnerella* vaginitis, nonspecific vaginitis, *Corynebacterium* vaginitis, or anaerobic vaginosis).

Because of the limited clinical data regarding metronidazole gel's efficacy in treating bacterial vaginosis, the Centers for Disease Control (CDC) recommends vaginal metronidazole gel only as alternative therapy to oral metronidazole.

[Trichomoniasis (treatment)]—Metronidazole vaginal inserts and vaginal cream are indicated in the local treatment of trichomoniasis.

Not all species or strains of a particular organism may be equally susceptible to metronidazole.

### Unaccepted

Vaginal metronidazole is not effective against aerobic or facultative anaerobic bacteria, or in the treatment of vulvovaginitis caused by *Chlamydia trachomatis*, *Neisseria gonorrhoeae*, *Candida albicans*, or *Herpes simplex* virus. Metronidazole vaginal gel has not been proven to be clinically effective in the treatment of *Trichomonas vaginalis*.

## Pharmacology/Pharmacokinetics

### Physicochemical characteristics
Chemical group—Imidazole.
Molecular weight—171.16.

### Mechanism of action/Effect
The exact mechanism of action has not been completely established. Metronidazole is thought to be microbicidal against most obligate anaerobic bacteria and protozoa. To be active, it must undergo intracellular chemical reduction via mechanisms unique to anaerobic metabolism. The short-lived reduced forms are cytotoxic and interact with DNA to cause a loss of helical structure and strand breakage resulting in inhibition of nucleic acid synthesis and cell death.

Note: Metronidazole permits natural vaginal flora recovery because it has little effect on *Lactobacillus sp.*

### Other actions/effects
Metronidazole may produce a local antioxidant and anti-inflammatory effect on inflamed tissue by affecting neutrophil function.

### Absorption
Vaginal cream or

Vaginal insert—Approximately 20% of the administered dose of metronidazole (500 mg) is absorbed systemically, producing plasma concentrations approximately 12% of that resulting from a single 500-mg oral dose. The rate of absorption is less predictable with the insert than with the cream.

Vaginal gel—Approximately 56% of the administered dose of metronidazole (37.5 mg) is absorbed systemically, producing plasma concentrations approximately 2% of that resulting from a single 500-mg oral dose.

### Distribution
Systemically absorbed metronidazole may be distributed into breast milk and to most tissues. It crosses the blood-brain barrier and placenta.

**Protein binding**
Low (<20%).

**Biotransformation**
Systemically absorbed metronidazole is metabolized primarily by side-chain oxidation by the hepatic cytochrome P-450 enzyme system to 2 active metabolites, 1-[2-hydroxyethyl]-2-hydroxymethyl-5-nitroimidazole and 1-acetic acid-2-methyl-5-nitroimidazole. The hydroxylated metabolite is approximately 30% as potent as the parent compound while the acetic acid metabolite is 5% as potent. Small amounts of other metabolites (including glucuronide and sulfide conjugates) are also formed.

**Half-life**
Elimination (determined with systemic administration)—Normal hepatic function: 8 hours (range, 6 to 12 hours) for unchanged metronidazole.

**Time to peak serum concentration**
Vaginal cream—11 hours.
Vaginal gel—6 to 12 hours.
Vaginal insert—20 hours.

**Peak serum concentration**
Vaginal cream—1.86 mg per liter (mg/L) (10.87 micromole/L).
Vaginal gel—0.152 to 0.368 mg/L (0.89 to 2.15 micromole/L).
Vaginal insert—1.89 mg/L (11.04 micromole/L).

**Elimination**
Renal—60 to 80% of a systemic dose; of this amount, approximately 20% is excreted unchanged.
Fecal—6 to 15% of a systemic dose.

# Precautions to Consider

Note:   Some of the following information relates to the oral formulation. Depending on the vaginal product's strength and formulation, the vaginal administration of metronidazole may yield 2 to 12% of the blood concentrations achieved after a single 500-mg oral dose. The possibility of systemic effects may need to be considered until further studies quantify the degree of clinical significance.

**Carcinogenicity**
Carcinogenicity studies have not been done using vaginal formulations of metronidazole. Systemic metronidazole has not been shown to be carcinogenic in humans.
Systemic metronidazole has been shown to be carcinogenic in a number of studies in mice and rats, including a study in which it produced malignant lymphomas in mice.

**Tumorigenicity**
Tumorigenicity studies have not been done using vaginal formulations of metronidazole. Systemic metronidazole has not been shown to be tumorigenic in humans.
Pulmonary tumorigenesis has been reported in 6 studies in mice, including a study in which the animals were dosed every 4 weeks. Malignant hepatic tumors have also been reported in male mice given very high doses (approximately 500 mg per kg of body weight [mg/kg] per day). Several long-term oral-dose studies in rats have shown that metronidazole causes a statistically significant increase in the incidence of various neoplasms, especially mammary and hepatic tumors in female rats. Two lifetime tumorigenicity studies in hamsters using oral formulations have given negative results.

**Mutagenicity**
Studies have shown that metronidazole is mutagenic in bacteria and fungi, although this has not been confirmed in mammals.

**Pregnancy/Reproduction**
Fertility—No evidence of impaired fertility was found in mice.
Pregnancy—Metronidazole crosses the placenta, entering the fetal circulation rapidly. Adequate and well-controlled studies in humans have not been done.
Tumorigenicity has been demonstrated in animal studies, which may suggest that metronidazole should be withheld during pregnancy or at least during the first trimester and used with caution in the last 2 trimesters. Metronidazole has been used in pregnant women with no reports of adverse effects.
A small study reported that intrauterine deaths resulted when metronidazole was administered intraperitoneally to pregnant mice in doses comparable to the oral human dose. No fetotoxicity or teratogenicity occurred with orally administered metronidazole.
FDA Pregnancy Category B.

**Breast-feeding**
Metronidazole is distributed into breast milk; concentrations are similar to those found in the maternal plasma. Use in nursing mothers is not recommended. The theoretical risk is based on tumorigenicity studies

in animals; human data have not supported this. Also, metronidazole may change the taste of the breast milk. If a nursing mother is treated with metronidazole, the breast milk may be expressed and discarded and breast-feeding resumed 24 to 48 hours after treatment is completed.

**Pediatrics**
No information is available on the relationship of age to the effects of vaginal metronidazole in pediatric patients.

**Geriatrics**
No information is available on the relationship of age to the effects of vaginal metronidazole in geriatric patients. However, elderly patients are more likely to have an age-related decrease in hepatic function, which may affect metronidazole elimination.

**Drug interactions and/or related problems**
The following drug interactions and/or related problems have been selected on the basis of their potential clinical significance (possible mechanism in parentheses where appropriate)—not necessarily inclusive (» = major clinical significance):

Note:   Combinations containing any of the following medications, depending on the amount present, may also interact with this medication.

»   Alcohol
(caution in concurrent use with vaginal metronidazole and for at least one day following completion of treatment is advisable because systemic metronidazole may interfere with the oxidation of alcohol; such use may result in disulfiram-like effects such as abdominal cramps, nausea, vomiting, headache, or flushing of the face from acetaldehyde accumulation; changes in the taste of alcoholic beverages have also been reported during concurrent use)

»   Anticoagulants, coumarin- or indandione-derivative
(anticoagulant effects may be potentiated when these agents are used concurrently with metronidazole, because of inhibition of enzymatic metabolism of anticoagulants; periodic prothrombin time determinations may be required during and following concurrent therapy to determine if dosage adjustments of anticoagulants are necessary)

Cimetidine
(hepatic metabolism of metronidazole may be decreased when metronidazole and cimetidine are used concurrently, possibly resulting in delayed elimination and increased serum metronidazole concentrations)

»   Disulfiram
(it is recommended that metronidazole not be used concurrently with, or for 2 weeks following, disulfiram in alcoholic patients; such use may result in confusion and psychotic reactions because of combined toxicity)

Lithium
(concurrent use of systemic metronidazole with lithium has resulted in decreased renal clearance of lithium and lithium toxicity; adjustments of lithium dosage may be required)

Neurotoxic medications, other (See *Appendix II*)
(concurrent use of systemic metronidazole with other neurotoxic medications may increase the potential for neurotoxicity)

Phenytoin
(systemic metronidazole may impair the metabolism of phenytoin by inhibiting microsomal enzymes and increasing phenytoin's plasma concentration; the extent to which intravaginal metronidazole affects phenytoin is not presently known)

**Laboratory value alterations**
The following have been selected on the basis of their potential clinical significance (possible effect in parentheses where appropriate)—not necessarily inclusive (» = major clinical significance):

With diagnostic test results
Alanine aminotransferase (ALT [SGPT]) and
Aspartate aminotransferase (AST [SGOT]) and
Hexokinase glucose and
Lactate dehydrogenase (LDH) and
Triglycerides
(metronidazole has a high absorbance at the wavelength at which nicotinamide-adenine dinucleotide [NADH] is determined; therefore, falsely low values may occur when these substances are measured by continuous-flow methods based on endpoint decrease in reduced NADH)

White blood cell count
(may be increased or decreased)

## Medical considerations/Contraindications

The medical considerations/contraindications included here have been selected on the basis of their potential clinical significance (reasons given in parentheses where appropriate)—not necessarily inclusive (» = major clinical significance).

*Risk-benefit should be considered when the following medical problems exist:*

» Epilepsy or
» Other neurologic disease
      (systemic metronidazole has caused CNS toxicity, including seizures and peripheral neuropathy)

» Hepatic function impairment, severe
      (metronidazole is metabolized in the liver; hepatic function impairment may lead to decreased plasma clearance and accumulation of metronidazole and its metabolites and increased risk of side effects; dosage may need to be reduced in patients with severe hepatic function impairment)

Hypersensitivity to metronidazole

Leukopenia, or history of
      (oral metronidazole has caused leukopenia; the possibility should be considered that vaginal metronidazole may induce or exacerbate leukopenia, especially with prolonged or multiple courses of therapy)

### Patient monitoring

The following may be especially important in patient monitoring (other tests may be warranted in some patients, depending on condition; » = major clinical significance):

Leukocyte count, total and differential
      (determinations recommended when metronidazole is used for longer than 10 days or if a second course of therapy is needed)

## Side/Adverse Effects

Note: Convulsions, peripheral neuropathy, and ataxia have been reported rarely with systemic administration of metronidazole. The possibility should be considered that these effects may also occur with vaginal administration, especially with the higher-potency formulations available in Canada or with prolonged use. If neurological symptoms occur, the medication should be discontinued. Severe symptoms may require immediate medical attention.

The incidences of side effects listed below are those reported in studies with the 0.75% gel. Although specific information about the incidence of side effects with the vaginal insert or vaginal cream is not available, it is possible that some adverse effects could occur more frequently with these higher-potency formulations than with the gel. Also, the possibility of systemic effects may need to be considered since vaginal administration of metronidazole may yield 2 to 12% of the blood concentrations achieved after a single oral 500-mg dose.

The following side/adverse effects have been selected on the basis of their potential clinical significance (possible signs and symptoms in parentheses where appropriate)—not necessarily inclusive:

**Those indicating need for medical attention**
Incidence more frequent
      *Candida cervicitis or vaginitis* (itching in the vagina; pain during sexual intercourse; thick, white vaginal discharge without odor or with mild odor)—incidence 6 to 15%
Incidence less frequent
      *Abdominal cramping or pain*—incidence 3.4%; *burning or irritation of penis of sexual partner; burning or increased frequency of urination; vulvitis* (itching, stinging or redness of genital area)

**Those indicating need for medical attention only if they continue or are bothersome**
Incidence less frequent
      *Altered taste sensation including metallic taste; CNS effects* (dizziness or lightheadedness; headache); *dryness of mouth; furry tongue; gastrointestinal disturbances* (diarrhea, nausea or vomiting); *loss of appetite*

**Those not indicating need for medical attention**
Incidence less frequent
      *Dark urine*

**Those indicating possible need for medical attention if they occur after medication is discontinued**
      *Vaginal candidiasis* (itching of the vagina or outside genitals; pain during sexual intercourse; thick, white vaginal discharge without odor or with mild odor)

## Patient Consultation

As an aid to patient consultation, refer to *Advice for the Patient, Metronidazole (Vaginal)*.

In providing consultation, consider emphasizing the following selected information (» = major clinical significance):

### Before using this medication
» Conditions affecting use, especially:
      Sensitivity to metronidazole
      Pregnancy—Metronidazole crosses the placenta; use cautiously during pregnancy, possibly withholding its use in the first trimester
      Breast-feeding—Metronidazole is distributed into breast milk and is not recommended during breast-feeding
      Other medications, especially alcohol, coumarin- or indandione-derivative anticoagulants, or disulfiram
      Other medical problems, especially epilepsy or other neurologic disease or severe hepatic function impairment

### Proper use of this medication
      Washing hands immediately before and after vaginal administration
      Avoiding getting medication into the eyes; washing with large amounts of cool tap water immediately if medication does get into eyes; checking with physician if eyes continue to be painful
      Reading patient directions carefully before use
*Proper administration technique*
      Following directions regarding filling the applicator, insertion technique, and cleaning the applicator after each use
*For cream or gel dosage forms*
      Puncturing metal tamper-resistant seal on tube with top of cap
*For insert dosage form*
      Placing insert into the applicator, immersing exposed insert in tap water for a few seconds before vaginal insertion to facilitate disintegration

» Compliance with full course of therapy, even during menstruation
» Proper dosing
      Missed dose: Inserting as soon as possible; not inserting if almost time for next dose
» Proper storage

### Precautions while using this medication
      Checking with physician if no improvement within a few days
      Follow-up visit to physician after treatment for bacterial vaginosis to ensure that infection has been eradicated
» Avoiding use of alcoholic beverages or other alcohol-containing preparations while using and for at least 1 day after discontinuing this medication
» Caution if dizziness or lightheadedness occurs
      Protecting clothing because of possible soiling with vaginal metronidazole; avoiding use of tampons
» Using hygienic measures to cure infection and prevent reinfection, e.g., wearing freshly washed cotton panties instead of synthetic panties
» Sexual abstinence is recommended during treatment to prevent cross-infection, reinfection, or dilution of the dose
*For trichomoniasis*
» Using condoms to prevent reinfection with trichomoniasis after treatment; possible need for concurrent treatment of male partner for trichomoniasis

### Side/adverse effects
      Signs of potential side effects, especially candida cervicitis or vaginitis, abdominal cramping or pain, burning or irritation of penis of sexual partner, increased frequency of urination, vulvitis, altered taste sensation, CNS effects, dryness of mouth, furry tongue, gastrointestinal disturbances, loss of appetite
      Dark urine may be alarming to patient although medically insignificant
      Possibility of vaginal candidiasis occurring after medication has been discontinued

## General Dosing Information

If sensitization or irritation occurs, treatment with vaginal metronidazole should be discontinued.

The cream and the insert (but not the gel) may contain oils that may damage latex contraceptive devices, such as cervical caps, condoms, or diaphragms and reduce their efficacy.

Vaginal applicators should be used with caution after the sixth month of pregnancy.

If there is no response to therapy, the presence of pathogens unresponsive to metronidazole should be ruled out by potassium hydroxide (KOH) smears and cultures before a second course of therapy is initiated.

In treating bacterial vaginosis, concurrent treatment of the male partner generally is unnecessary.

In treating trichomoniasis, both sexual partners should receive metronidazole therapy concurrently since asymptomatic trichomoniasis in the male partner is a frequent source of reinfection in the female.

## Vaginal Dosage Forms

Note: Bracketed uses in the *Dosage Forms* section refer to categories of use and/or indications that are not included in U.S. product labeling.

### METRONIDAZOLE VAGINAL CREAM

**Usual adult and adolescent dose**

Bacterial vaginosis or

[Trichomoniasis]—

Intravaginal, 500 mg (one applicatorful) one or two times a day for ten or twenty consecutive days.

**Usual pediatric dose**

Safety and efficacy have not been established.

**Strength(s) usually available**

U.S.—

Not commercially available.

Canada—

10% w/w (Rx) [*Flagyl* (methylparaben; propylparaben)].

**Packaging and storage**

Store below 40 °C (104 °F), preferably between 15 and 30 °C (59 and 86 °F), unless otherwise specified by manufacturer. Protect from freezing.

**Auxiliary labeling**
• May cause dizziness.
• Continue medicine for full time of treatment.
• For vaginal use only.
• Avoid alcoholic beverages.

**Note**

Include patient package insert (PPI) when dispensing.

### METRONIDAZOLE VAGINAL GEL

**Usual adult and adolescent dose**

Bacterial vaginosis—

Intravaginal, 37.5 mg (one applicatorful) two times a day, once in the morning and once in the evening, for five days.

**Usual pediatric dose**

Safety and efficacy have not been established.

**Strength(s) usually available**

U.S.—

0.75% (Rx) [*MetroGel-Vaginal* (EDTA; methylparaben; propylparaben; propylene glycol)].

Canada—

Not commercially available.

**Packaging and storage**

Store below 40 °C (104 °F), preferably between 15 and 30 °C (59 and 86 °F), unless otherwise specified by manufacturer. Protect from freezing. Keep out of reach of children.

**Auxiliary labeling**
• May cause dizziness.
• Continue medicine for full time of treatment.
• For vaginal use only.
• Avoid alcoholic beverages.

**Note**

Include patient package insert (PPI) when dispensing.

### METRONIDAZOLE VAGINAL INSERTS

**Usual adult and adolescent dose**

Bacterial vaginosis or

[Trichomoniasis]—

Intravaginal, 500 mg placed high into the vagina every night for ten or twenty consecutive days.

**Usual pediatric dose**

Safety and efficacy have not been established.

**Strength(s) usually available**

U.S.—

Not commercially available.

Canada—

500 mg (Rx) [*Flagyl*].

**Packaging and storage**

Store below 40 °C (104 °F), preferably between 15 and 30 °C (59 and 86 °F), unless otherwise specified by manufacturer. Protect from light.

**Auxiliary labeling**
• May cause dizziness.
• Continue medicine for full time of treatment.
• For vaginal use only.
• Avoid alcoholic beverages.

**Note**

Include patient package insert (PPI) when dispensing.

Patient should be instructed on technique for placement including immersing the insert (in applicator) in tap water for a few seconds before insertion to facilitate disintegration.

## Selected Bibliography

Alper MM, Barwin N, McLean WM, McGilveray IJ, Sved S. Systemic absorption of metronidazole by the vaginal route. Obstet Gynecol 1985 Jun; 65 (6): 781-4.

Hillier SL, Lipinski C, Briseldene A, Eschenbach DA. Efficacy of intravaginal 0.75% metronidazole gel for the treatment of bacterial vaginosis. Obstet Gynecol 1993 June; 81 (6): 963-7.

Developed: 05/16/94

---

# METYRAPONE    Systemic

VA CLASSIFICATION (Primary/Secondary): DX900/HS900

Note: For a listing of dosage forms and brand names by country availability, see *Dosage Forms* section(s). For a listing of brand names for the articles in this monograph, refer to the General Index.

## Category

Diagnostic aid (pituitary function); antiadrenal.

## Indications

Note: Bracketed information in the *Indications* section refers to uses that are not included in U.S. product labeling.

**Accepted**

Adrenocortical insufficiency, secondary (diagnosis)—Metyrapone is indicated in the diagnosis of adrenocortical insufficiency resulting from panhypopituitarism or partial hypopituitarism (limited pituitary reserve). Metyrapone testing is infrequently performed because plasma corticotropin (ACTH) can be measured directly and the results of metyrapone testing are less specific than such direct measurements. Therefore, metyrapone testing is generally performed only in patients in whom insulin hypoglycemia testing is contraindicated.

[Cushing's syndrome (treatment)][1]—Metyrapone is used as short-term treatment for Cushing's syndrome, irrespective of etiology. However, because of the significant expense of therapy and the incidence of side effects, it is generally recommended as adjunctive therapy. Metyrapone is most frequently used concurrently with aminoglutethimide in the treatment of pituitary-dependent Cushing's disease. Metyrapone was used concurrently with sodium valproate in one patient to therapeutic advantage to suppress pituitary release of ACTH in response to decreased serum cortisol concentrations. Metyrapone has also been used in patients with Cushing's disease during radiation therapy to control symptoms in the interim before pituitary irradiation becomes effective. Metyrapone may also be used to stabilize Cushing's syndrome patients prior to surgery. Long-term metyrapone therapy has been used as primary therapy for Cushing's disease. Metyrapone may only be temporarily effective in treating certain other types of Cushing's syndrome.

[Cushing's syndrome (diagnosis)][1]—Metyrapone is used in the differential diagnosis of Cushing's syndrome caused by adrenal adenoma, ectopic ACTH/CRH syndrome, Cushing's disease, and adrenal hyperplasia.

**Unaccepted**

Metyrapone has been used to treat resistant edema caused by increased aldosterone production in patients with cirrhosis, nephrosis, and congestive heart failure. However, this use of metyrapone has generally declined with the availability of more effective diuretic agents.

Metyrapone has been used to decrease plasma cholesterol concentrations associated with familial hypercholesterolemia type II. However, there are currently insufficient data to establish the safety and efficacy of the use of metyrapone for this indication.

---

[^1]Not included in Canadian product labeling.

## Pharmacology/Pharmacokinetics

### Mechanism of action/Effect

Metyrapone inhibits enzymatic 11-beta hydroxylation of desoxycorticosterone (DOC) to corticosterone, 11-deoxycortisol (Compound S) to cortisol (hydrocortisone), and other aldosterone precursors to aldosterone. Consequently, serum concentrations of these products are decreased. DOC and 11-deoxycortisol have no significant inhibitory effect on the secretion of corticotropin-releasing hormone (CRH) by the hypothalamus and ACTH (corticotropin) by the pituitary. In a normally functioning pituitary gland, a compensatory increase in release of CRH and ACTH occurs in response to lowered serum cortisol concentrations. The continued block of 11-beta hydroxylase then results in greatly increased adrenal production of 11-desoxycortisol, DOC, and aldosterone precursors. A corresponding increase occurs in the urinary excretion of the metabolites of these products (tetrahydro-11-desoxycortisol [THS], 17-hydroxycorticosteroids [17-OHCS], and 17-ketogenic steroids [17-KGS]). Normal increases in urinary excretion of 17-OHCS and 17-KGS after administration of metyrapone are 2 to 4 times baseline value and 2 times baseline value, respectively.

For diagnosis of secondary adrenocortical insufficiency—

Patients with secondary adrenocortical insufficiency do not exhibit a compensatory increase in pituitary ACTH release, plasma DOC and 11-desoxycortisol, and urine THS, 17-OHCS, or 17-KGS after metyrapone administration. When functional ACTH-secreting mechanisms are present but a limited pituitary-adrenal reserve exists, the pituitary does not respond to metyrapone because it is already maximally secreting ACTH to meet basal requirements. Creating additional physiological stress or decreasing cortisol levels via administration of metyrapone does not result in additional performance from this exhausted or limited reserve. If previous ACTH testing rules out adrenal insufficiency, a subnormal response to metyrapone is related to malfunctioning of the CNS-pituitary mechanism of ACTH secretion. Alternatively, measurement of baseline and post-metyrapone ACTH serum concentrations eliminates the need for ACTH testing to separate primary from secondary adrenal insufficiency. Patients with primary adrenal insufficiency will have elevated baseline serum ACTH concentrations, which do not increase in response to metyrapone administration. In contrast, patients with secondary adrenocortical insufficiency generally have normal baseline ACTH serum concentrations, which also do not increase in response to metyrapone block.

Patients with partial hypopituitarism or limited pituitary reserve do not exhibit clinical or chemical signs of disease, respond normally to ACTH testing, and have normal baseline organ functions. However, a subnormal increase in urine corticosteroids (<2-fold increase in 17-OHCS after longer metyrapone test) or in plasma 11-deoxycortisol (0800-hour value of <7 micrograms per deciliter after the short metyrapone test) will occur in response to metyrapone testing.

In patients with panhypopituitarism, clinical and chemical signs of hypogonadism, hypothyroidism, and hypoadrenocorticism are already evident, baseline urine steroid levels are generally low, and adrenal atrophy may also result in a decreased ACTH testing response. Though metyrapone is not critical in diagnosing panhypopituitarism, a minimal increase in urine corticosteroids or plasma 11-desoxycortisol will occur after metyrapone testing.

For treatment of Cushing's syndrome—

Metyrapone decreases the serum concentration of cortisol by inhibiting beta-hydroxylation of 11-desoxycortisol, the final step in cortisol formation.

For diagnosis of Cushing's syndrome—

An exaggerated response to metyrapone (>35 mg of urine 17-OHCS or 17-KGS per 24 hours after longer metyrapone test) occurs in patients with Cushing's syndrome caused by excessive production of ACTH by the pituitary (Cushing's disease), which results in adrenal hyperplasia. These patients also exhibit elevated baseline urine corticosteroid concentrations and excessive response to ACTH testing.

A subnormal response to metyrapone in patients with Cushing's syndrome may indicate the presence of autonomous adrenal tumors

that suppress pituitary ACTH release or of nonendocrine tumors that secrete CRH or ACTH (ectopic CRH or ACTH syndrome). In ectopic ACTH syndrome, patients have a subnormal response to metyrapone and low pituitary ACTH concentrations. In contrast, patients with ectopic CRH syndrome may respond to metyrapone and have very high plasma ACTH concentrations. However, some patients with adrenal adenomas (approximately 50%), adrenal carcinomas (approximately 25%), and ectopic ACTH syndrome caused by bronchial carcinoid tumors will also respond to metyrapone.

### Other actions/effects

Metyrapone also inhibits 18-, 19-, and 21-hydroxylases, but to a lesser extent.

### Absorption

Rapidly and well-absorbed from the gastrointestinal tract.

### Biotransformation

Hepatic, by rapid reduction of ketone to an active alcohol (metyrapol) and the glucuronidation of metyrapone and its reduced metabolite.

### Half-life

20 to 26 minutes (elimination).

### Time to peak concentration

1 hour (approximately).

### Peak serum concentration

0.5 to 1 mcg/mL (plasma). In one study, average plasma levels of 3.7 mcg/mL were achieved after a 750 mg oral dose. Plasma levels decline to a mean concentration of 0.5 mcg/mL 4 hours following 6 oral doses of 750 mg given every 4 hours.

### Time to peak diagnostic effect

Peak steroid excretion occurs in the 24-hour period following completion of dosing.

### Duration of action

Inhibition of 11-beta hydroxylase declines rapidly within 4 hours of oral metyrapone administration.

### Elimination

Renal; within 2 days of completion of dosing (750 mg every 4 hours for 6 doses), approximately 0.5% is excreted in the urine unchanged, 3% as metyrapol, and 37% as glucuronides of metyrapone and its metabolites. Within 72 hours of the first 750-mg dose of a 6-dose series, 5.3% of the total dose was excreted unchanged in the urine (9.2% free and 90.8% as glucuronide) and 38.5% as metyrapol (8.1% free and 91.9% as glucuronide).

## Precautions to Consider

### Carcinogenicity/Mutagenicity

Long-term studies have not been performed in animals.

### Pregnancy/Reproduction

Pregnancy—Adequate and well-controlled studies in humans have not been done. One case of clinical improvement of severe Cushing's syndrome due to adrenal tumor and the subsequent delivery of a normal fetus has been reported with metyrapone treatment in weeks 23 to delivery at 37 weeks. However, maternal urinary estrogen concentrations became undetectable from weeks 27 to 31 and remained subnormal until delivery. This effect was presumably due to the inhibition of $C_{19}$ hydroxylation of estriol synthesis in the placenta. In one study in 20 women in the second and third trimester, the fetal pituitary responded to enzymatic blockade during metyrapone testing. Metyrapone can impair the synthesis of fetal adrenocorticoids. Because the safety of the use of metyrapone during pregnancy has not been clearly established, risk-benefit should be carefully considered.

FDA Pregnancy Category C.

### Breast-feeding

It is not known whether metyrapone is distributed into breast milk. However, breast-feeding is not recommended during the use of metyrapone because the potential exists for neonatal pituitary response to enzymatic block.

### Pediatrics

Appropriate studies performed to date have not demonstrated pediatrics-specific problems that would limit the usefulness of metyrapone in children and adolescents. One death has been reported in a 6 year old female who received an overdose of 2 2-gram doses of metyrapone.

### Geriatrics

On the basis of clinical usage information, no geriatrics-specific problems are expected in the use of metyrapone. However, because the rate of elimination of adrenal steroids may be decreased in geriatric patients, urine 17-ketogenic steroid concentrations may be decreased after metyrapone testing. This effect has not been seen with the measurement of plasma 11-deoxycortisol concentrations. Therefore, measurement of plasma 11-deoxycortisol may result in false negative results in patients with moderate adrenal insufficiency.

### Drug interactions and/or related problems
The following drug interactions and/or related problems have been selected on the basis of their potential clinical significance (possible mechanism in parentheses where appropriate)—not necessarily inclusive (» = major clinical significance):

Note: Combinations containing any of the following medications, depending on the amount present, may also interact with this medication.

> See also *Laboratory value alterations.*

Antidiabetic agents, sulfonylurea or
Insulin
> (symptoms of metyrapone overdose may be worsened or altered)

Hydrocortisone
> (metyrapone increases the metabolic clearance rate of hydrocortisone by approximately 2-fold and increases its volume of distribution)

### Laboratory value alterations
The following have been selected on the basis of their potential clinical significance (possible effect in parentheses where appropriate)—not necessarily inclusive (» = major clinical significance):

With results of *this* test
 *Due to other medications*
Acetazolamide or
Chlordiazepoxide or
Chlorothiazide or
Cloxacillin or
Dexamphetamine or
Glutethimide or
Hydralazine or
Nalidixic acid or
Paraldehyde or
Phenazopyridine or
Prochlorperazine or
Quinine
> (presence of these medications may interfere with the assay for urine 17-ketosteroids or 17-ketogenic steroids)

Amitriptyline or
Carisoprodol or
Chlordiazepoxide or
Chlorpromazine or
Meprobamate
> (response to metyrapone may be decreased)

Antithyroid agents
> (drug-induced hypothyroidism may cause a delayed or absent response to metyrapone)

» Corticosteroids, systemic, glucocorticoid or mineralocorticoid
> (should be discontinued 24 to 48 hours before and during testing because a variable response to ACTH testing may occur and response to metyrapone will be decreased)

» Estrogens or
» Oral contraceptives, combined estrogen and progestin
> (urine 11-hydroxycorticosteroid concentrations may be decreased by enhanced cortisol protein binding due to an estrogen-induced increase in cortisol-binding globulin concentrations)

» Hepatic enzyme inducers (See *Appendix II*)
> (increased metabolism of metyrapone by any hepatic enzyme inducer may decrease the response to metyrapone)

> (phenytoin accelerates biotransformation of metyrapone in patients taking phenytoin within 2 weeks of testing, resulting in falsely low urine adrenocorticoid levels; increasing the metyrapone dose by 2-fold to 750 mg every 2 hours for 12 doses may counteract this effect)

 *Due to medical problems or conditions*
Breast cancer, metastatic or
Congestive heart failure or
Diabetes mellitus or
Hypoglycemia, reactive
> (response to metyrapone may be elevated)

Hepatic cirrhosis or
Hepatic function impairment
> (delayed response may occur due to a delay in the metabolism of cortisol)

Hyperthyroidism or
Thyrotoxicosis
> (response to metyrapone may be decreased)

Hypothyroidism
> (delayed or absent response to metyrapone may occur)

Obesity
> (response to metyrapone may be falsely elevated because 50% of obese patients with Cushing's syndrome exhibit elevated cortisol secretion rates and urine 17-OHCS concentrations)

Pregnancy
> (response to metyrapone may be decreased due to the presence of high estrogen levels)

With physiology/laboratory test values
Adrenocorticotropic hormone (ACTH), plasma and/or
Cortisol, plasma and/or
Urinary free cortisol
> (in healthy subjects, ACTH concentrations will be elevated and cortisol will be decreased)

Blood pressure
> (may be elevated with long-term use of metyrapone in treatment of Cushing's syndrome due to excessive production of the mineralocorticoid, 11-desoxycorticosterone; rarely decreased during short-term use)

Chloride or
Sodium
> (serum concentrations may be decreased in overdose)

Dehydroepiandosterone or
Testosterone
> (serum concentrations may be increased during treatment for Cushing's syndrome)

Potassium
> (serum concentrations may be increased in overdose)

White blood cell count
> (rarely, values have been decreased)

### Medical considerations/Contraindications
The medical considerations/contraindications included here have been selected on the basis of their potential clinical significance (reasons given in parentheses where appropriate)—not necessarily inclusive (» = major clinical significance).

*Except under special circumstances, this medication should not be used when the following medical problems exist:*
*For all indications*
» Adrenal cortical insufficiency
> (metyrapone may precipitate acute adrenal insufficiency; risk is greater with use of longer metyrapone testing method and concurrent use of other agents that inhibit adrenal steroid synthesis, such as aminoglutethimide; an ACTH test should be performed prior to metyrapone testing to demonstrate adrenal responsiveness)

*For use in the treatment of Cushing's syndrome*
» Hypopituitarism
> (metyrapone should not be used in the presence of hypopituitarism, for the treatment of Cushing's syndrome)

Preeclampsia or
Significant risk of hypertensive crisis
> (long-term use of metyrapone may precipitate hypertensive crisis)

*Risk-benefit should be considered when the following medical problems exist:*
Allergy to metyrapone
Hirsutism
> (may be worsened during long-term use due to an increase in production of adrenal androgens)

» Hypopituitarism, severe
> (possibility of precipitating acute adrenal insufficiency or hypoglycemia with seizures)

» Porphyria, acute
> (metyrapone has been shown to be porphyrinogenic *in vitro* and in animal studies)

### Patient monitoring
The following may be especially important in patient monitoring (other tests may be warranted in some patients, depending on condition; » = major clinical significance):

Adrenocorticotropic hormone (ACTH), plasma and/or
Cortisol, plasma and/or
Urinary free cortisol
> (determinations may be used in the management of symptoms of Cushing's syndrome to titrate dose and to confirm continued effectiveness)

Blood pressure and
Electrolyte concentrations, serum
(recommended during long-term use)

## Side/Adverse Effects

The following side/adverse effects have been selected on the basis of their potential clinical significance (possible signs and symptoms in parentheses where appropriate)—not necessarily inclusive:

**Those indicating need for medical attention**
Incidence less frequent
*Allergic reaction* (skin rash)

Incidence rare
*Bone marrow depression* (sore throat or fever; unusual bleeding or bruising; unusual tiredness or weakness); *edema* (swelling of feet or lower legs; rapid weight gain)—has been reported with long-term and high-dose therapy; *enlargement of clitoris*—has been reported in one patient during treatment of Cushing's disease; *hypokalemic alkalosis* (irregular heartbeat; muscle cramps or pain; severe weakness of extremities and trunk)—may occur during long-term therapy

**Those indicating need for medical attention only if they continue or are bothersome**
Incidence more frequent
*Dizziness or lightheadedness; drowsiness; headache; nausea*
Incidence rare
*Alopecia* (greater-than-normal loss of scalp hair)—has been reported in treatment of Cushing's syndrome; *anorexia* (loss of appetite); *confusion or mental slowing; epigastric pain* (upper abdominal or stomach pain); *hirsutism* (excessive hair growth); *increased sweating; vomiting; worsening of acne*—has been reported in treatment of Cushing's syndrome

## Overdose

For specific information on the agents used in the management of metyrapone overdose, see:
• *Charcoal, Activated (Oral-Local)* monograph; and/or
• *Hydrocortisone* in *Corticosteroids/Corticotropin—Glucocorticoid Effects (Systemic)* monograph.

For more information on the management of overdose or unintentional ingestion, **contact a Poison Control Center** (see *Poison Control Center Listing*).

**Clinical effects of overdose**
The following effects have been selected on the basis of their potential clinical significance (possible signs and symptoms in parentheses where appropriate)—not necessarily inclusive:
*Gastrointestinal effects* (severe nausea, vomiting, diarrhea, and abdominal or stomach pain); *acute adrenal insufficiency, including symptoms such as nervousness, confusion, or sudden weakness; dehydration* (unusual thirst); *decrease in consciousness; cardiac arrhythmias* (irregular heartbeat)

**Treatment of overdose**
Recommended treatment is primarily symptomatic and supportive.

To decrease absorption—Using standard methods such as gastric lavage or oral activated charcoal.

Specific treatment—Administering a large hydrocortisone dose immediately.

Monitoring—Monitoring blood pressure and fluid and electrolyte status for several days.

Supportive care—Simultaneously infusing intravenous saline and glucose. Patients in whom intentional overdose is confirmed or suspected should be referred for psychiatric consultation.

## Patient Consultation

As an aid to patient consultation, refer to *Advice for the Patient, Metyrapone (Systemic).*

In providing consultation, consider emphasizing the following selected information (» = major clinical significance):

**Description of use**
Test procedure: Administered orally; blood and/or urine samples taken; possible use of catheter; measurement of hormones in blood and/or urine

**Before using this medication**
» Conditions affecting use, especially:
Allergy to metyrapone
Pregnancy—Risk-benefit must be carefully considered because fetal pituitary and adrenal glands may respond to metyrapone

Breast-feeding—Not recommended during use of metyrapone because of potential for response to metyrapone in infant
Other medications, especially corticosteroids, estrogen-containing products, or hepatic enzyme inducers
Other medical problems, especially adrenal or pituitary insufficiency or acute porphyria

**Proper use of this medication**
Taking medication with milk or food
Caution if any laboratory tests required; possible interference with test results
» Proper dosing
Missed dose:
For treatment of Cushing's syndrome—Taking as soon as possible; not taking if almost time for next dose; not doubling doses
For diagnostic procedures—Contacting physician in event of missed dose
» Proper storage

**Precautions while using this medication**
Caution if drowsiness, dizziness, or lightheadedness occurs

**Side/adverse effects**
Signs of potential side effects, especially bone marrow depression, edema, and hypokalemic alkalosis

## General Dosing Information

**For pituitary function testing**
Short metyrapone test—
Day 1: Oral metyrapone is administered at 2300 hours.
Day 2: Blood sample is collected at 0800 hours for measurement of plasma 11-deoxycortisol concentration and/or corticotropin (ACTH) concentration.
6-Day metyrapone test—
Day 1: 24-hour urine sample is collected to determine baseline values of 17-hydroxycorticosteroids (17-OHCS) or 17-ketogenic steroids (17-KGS). A normal range for 17-OHCS is 3 to 12 mg excreted per 24 hours.
Day 2: ACTH test is performed to demonstrate adrenal gland responsiveness. In patients with normal adrenal gland function, ACTH 50 Units infused over 8 hours should result in 24-hour 17-OHCS excretion of 15 to 45 mg. If ACTH testing demonstrates adrenal cortex responsiveness, metyrapone testing may be continued.
Days 3 and 4: 48-hour rest period should follow completion of ACTH testing.
Day 5: Oral metyrapone is administered.
Day 6: 24-hour urine sample is collected for measurement of excretion of 17-OHCS or 17-KGS.

**Diet/Nutrition**
Administration of dose with milk or food may lessen gastrointestinal effects.

## Oral Dosage Forms

Note: Bracketed uses in the *Dosage Forms* section refer to categories of use and/or indications that are not included in U.S. product labeling.

### METYRAPONE TABLETS USP

**Usual adult dose**
Adrenal insufficiency, secondary (diagnosis) or
[Cushing's syndrome (diagnosis)][1]—
Oral, 750 mg (approximately 10 to 15 mg per kg of body weight) every four hours for six doses or
2 to 3 grams (2 grams in patients weighing <70 kg, 2.5 grams in patients weighing 70 to 90 kg, and 3 grams if body weight >90 kg), administered at 2300 hours (short metyrapone test).
[Cushing's syndrome (treatment)][1]—
Oral, 250 mg to 6 grams per day, divided in up to six doses.

**Usual pediatric dose**
Adrenal insufficiency, secondary (diagnosis)—
Oral, 300 mg per square meter of body surface area or 15 mg per kg of body weight (minimum 250 mg per dose) every four hours for six doses.

**Strength(s) usually available**
U.S.—
250 mg (Rx) [*Metopirone* (scored)].
Canada—
250 mg (Rx) [*Metopirone* (scored)].

**Packaging and storage**
Store below 40 °C (104 °F), preferably between 15 and 30 °C (59 and 86 °F), unless otherwise specified by manufacturer. Store in a tight, light-resistant container.

**Auxiliary labeling**
• Take with milk or food.

¹Not included in Canadian product labeling.

## Selected Bibliography

Dickstein G, et al. Primary therapy for Cushing's disease with metyrapone. JAMA 1986; 255 (9): 1167-9.

Schteingart DE. Cushing's syndrome. Endocrinol Metab Clin North Am 1989; 18 (2): 311-38.
Spiger M, et al. Single-dose metyrapone test: a review of a four-year experience. Arch Intern Med 1975; 135: 668-70.
Jeffcoate WJ, et al. Metyrapone in long-term management of Cushing's disease. Brit Med J 1977; 2: 215-7.

Revised: 07/08/92
Interim revision: 06/30/94

# METYROSINE  Systemic†

VA CLASSIFICATION (Primary): CV490
Note: For a listing of dosage forms and brand names by country availability, see *Dosage Forms* section(s). For a listing of brand names for the articles in this monograph, refer to the General Index.

†Not commercially available in Canada.

## Category

Antihypertensive (pheochromocytoma).

## Indications

**Accepted**
Pheochromocytoma (treatment)—Metyrosine is indicated in the treatment of pheochromocytoma as preoperative preparation for surgery, management of patients when surgery is contraindicated, and chronic management of patients with malignant pheochromocytoma.

**Unaccepted**
Metyrosine is not as useful as other agents in the treatment of essential hypertension.

## Pharmacology/Pharmacokinetics

**Physicochemical characteristics**
Molecular weight—195.22.
pKa—2.7 and 10.1.

**Mechanism of action/Effect**
Reduces catecholamine biosynthesis up to 80% by blocking tyrosine hydroxylase activity in converting tyrosine to dihydroxyphenylalanine (DOPA), which is the initial and rate-limiting step. Endogenous levels and urinary excretion of catecholamines and their metabolites are decreased in patients with pheochromocytoma, resulting in reduced blood pressure.

**Absorption**
Well absorbed from gastrointestinal tract.

**Biotransformation**
Minimal (catechol metabolites account for less than 1% of a dose).

**Half-life**
3.4 to 3.7 hours.

**Time to peak effect**
Reduction of urinary catecholamines—2 to 3 days (with multiple doses).
Reduction of blood pressure—Blood pressure usually decreases progressively during the first 2 days after initiation of therapy.

**Duration of action**
Reduction of urinary catecholamines—The return to pretreatment levels usually occurs within 3 to 4 days after withdrawal of the medication.
Reduction of blood pressure—Blood pressure increases gradually to pretreatment levels within 2 to 3 days after withdrawal.

**Elimination**
Renal, 53 to 88% (mean 69%) unchanged; less than 1% of a dose is excreted as catechol metabolites, but this quantity is sufficient to interfere with determination of urinary catecholamines by routine techniques.

## Precautions to Consider

**Carcinogenicity/Mutagenicity**
Studies have not been done.

**Pregnancy/Reproduction**
Pregnancy—Studies have not been done in humans.
Studies have not been done in animals.
FDA Pregnancy Category C.

**Breast-feeding**
It is not known whether metyrosine is excreted in breast milk. However, problems in humans have not been documented.

**Pediatrics**
Appropriate studies on the relationship of age to the effects of metyrosine have not been performed in the pediatric population. Safety and efficacy have not been established in children up to 12 years of age.

**Geriatrics**
Appropriate studies on the relationship of age to the effects of metyrosine have not been performed in the geriatric population. However, elderly patients are more likely to have age-related renal function impairment, which may require caution in patients receiving metyrosine.

**Drug interactions and/or related problems**
The following drug interactions and/or related problems have been selected on the basis of their potential clinical significance (possible mechanism in parentheses where appropriate)—not necessarily inclusive (» = major clinical significance):
Note: Combinations containing any of the following medications, depending on the amount present, may also interact with this medication.

Alcohol or
Antidepressants, tricyclic or
Central nervous system (CNS) depression–producing medications, other (see *Appendix II*)
    (concurrent use may increase the sedative effects of either these medications or metyrosine)

Haloperidol or
Metoclopramide or
Molindone or
Phenothiazines
    (concurrent use with metyrosine may potentiate the extrapyramidal effects of these medications)

Levodopa
    (effects of levodopa may be reduced because of extrapyramidal effects of metyrosine; dosage adjustment of either or both medications may be required)

**Laboratory value alterations**
The following have been selected on the basis of their potential clinical significance (possible effect in parentheses where appropriate)—not necessarily inclusive (» = major clinical significance):

With diagnostic test results
Catecholamine measurements, urinary
    (falsely increased because of presence of very small amounts of catechol metabolites of metyrosine)

With physiology/laboratory test values
Aspartate aminotransferase (AST [SGOT]) concentrations, serum and
Eosinophil count
    (may be increased)

**Medical considerations/Contraindications**
The medical considerations/contraindications included here have been selected on the basis of their potential clinical significance (reasons given in parentheses where appropriate)—not necessarily inclusive (» = major clinical significance).

*Risk-benefit should be considered when the following medical problems exist:*

    Hepatic function impairment or
    Renal function impairment
        (may impair metyrosine elimination)

    Mental depression, or history of or
    Parkinson's disease
        (metyrosine may aggravate these conditions)

    Sensitivity to metyrosine

**Patient monitoring**

The following may be especially important in patient monitoring (other tests may be warranted in some patients, depending on condition; » = major clinical significance):

» Blood pressure and
» Electrocardiogram (ECG)
    (continuous monitoring recommended during surgery for pheochromocytoma to detect hypertensive crises or arrhythmias)

» Catecholamine measurements, urinary
    (recommended at periodic intervals during initial therapy to determine maximal dose)

    Hepatic function tests
    (recommended at periodic intervals in patients on long-term therapy)

## Side/Adverse Effects

Note: Life-threatening arrhythmias may occur during anesthesia and surgery, which may necessitate treatment with a beta-adrenergic blocking agent or lidocaine. In addition, use of metyrosine preoperatively does not completely eliminate the risk of hypertensive crises or arrhythmias during surgery, which may require administration of phentolamine.

The following side/adverse effects have been selected on the basis of their potential clinical significance (possible signs and symptoms in parentheses where appropriate)—not necessarily inclusive:

**Those indicating need for medical attention**
Incidence approximately 10%
  *Diarrhea, possibly severe; extrapyramidal effects* (drooling; trembling and shaking of hands and fingers; trouble in speaking)
  Note: *Extrapyramidal effects* are occasionally accompanied by trismus and frank parkinsonism.

Incidence rare
  *Allergic reaction, such as urticaria* (itching; skin rash); *pharyngeal edema* (shortness of breath); *hematologic effects, specifically anemia,* (unusual tiredness or weakness); *eosinophilia; thrombocytopenia* (unusual bleeding or bruising; black, tarry stools; blood in urine or stools; pinpoint red spots on skin); *thrombocytosis; parkinsonism, frank* (restlessness; shuffling walk; tic-like [jerky] movements of head, face, mouth, and neck); *swelling of feet or lower legs; trismus* (muscle spasm, especially of neck and back); *urinary problems, specifically dysuria caused by crystalluria or urolithiasis* (painful urination); *hematuria* (blood in urine)

Incidence dose-related
  *CNS effects* (anxiety; confusion; hallucinations; mental depression)

**Those indicating need for medical attention only if they continue or are bothersome**
Incidence more frequent—occurs in almost all patients
  *Drowsiness, moderate to severe*
  Note: *Sedative effects* usually occur within the first 24 hours, are maximal within 2 to 3 days, and diminish within the first week, although they may persist with doses greater than 2 grams a day.

Incidence less frequent
  *Decreased salivation* (dryness of mouth); *galactorrhea* (unusual milk production); *impotence or trouble in ejaculating; nausea, vomiting, or stomach pain; stuffy nose; swelling of breasts*

After abrupt discontinuation of medication
  *Increased energy; trouble in sleeping*—lasting 2 or 3 days

**Those indicating possible gastrointestinal irritation and the need for medical attention if they occur after medication is discontinued**
  *Diarrhea*

## Patient Consultation

As an aid to patient consultation, refer to *Advice for the Patient, Metyrosine (Systemic).*

In providing consultation, consider emphasizing the following selected information (» = major clinical significance):

**Before using this medication**
» Conditions affecting use, especially:
    Sensitivity to metyrosine
    Use in children—Safety and efficacy not established in children up to 12 years of age

**Proper use of this medication**
» Importance of not taking more or less medication than the amount prescribed
    Getting into the habit of taking at same times each day
» Proper dosing
    Missed dose: Taking as soon as possible; not taking if almost time for next dose; not doubling doses
» Proper storage

**Precautions while using this medication**
    Regular visits to physician to check progress
» Importance of ample fluid intake and subsequent frequent urination to prevent crystalluria
» Caution in taking alcohol or other CNS depressants
» Caution if any kind of surgery (including dental surgery) or emergency treatment is required
» Caution when driving or doing things requiring alertness because of possible drowsiness

**Side/adverse effects**
    Signs of potential side effects, especially diarrhea, extrapyramidal effects, allergic reaction, hematologic effects, frank parkinsonism or trismus, swelling of feet or lower legs, urinary problems, and CNS effects

## General Dosing Information

Dosage must be adjusted to meet the individual requirements of each patient on the basis of clinical response and urinary catecholamine determinations.

To minimize the risk of crystalluria, it is recommended that patients maintain sufficient fluid intake to achieve a daily urine volume of at least 2000 mL, especially when they are taking more than 2 grams of metyrosine a day. Metyrosine crystallization will appear on examination as needles or rods in urine. If crystalluria occurs, fluid intake may be increased, but if it persists, reduction in dosage or withdrawal of the medication is recommended.

When metyrosine, alone or in combination with alpha-adrenergic blocking agents, is used in the preoperative treatment of patients with pheochromocytoma, it is important to maintain fluid volume both during and after surgery to prevent problems due to vasodilation and hypotension.

## Oral Dosage Forms

### METYROSINE CAPSULES USP

**Usual adult and adolescent dose**
Antihypertensive (pheochromocytoma)—
    Initial: Oral, 250 mg four times a day, the dosage being increased by increments of 250 to 500 mg a day to the maximally effective dose.
    Maintenance: Oral, 2 to 3 grams a day in four divided doses.
Note: When used for preoperative preparation, therapy for at least 5 to 7 days at the maximal dose is recommended.

**Usual adult prescribing limits**
Up to 4 grams a day.

**Usual pediatric dose**
Children up to 12 years of age—Safety and efficacy have not been established.
Children 12 years of age and over—See *Usual adult and adolescent dose.*

**Strength(s) usually available**
U.S.—
    250 mg (Rx) [*Demser*].
Canada—
    Not commercially available.

**Packaging and storage**
Store below 40 °C (104 °F), preferably between 15 and 30 °C (59 and 86 °F), unless otherwise specified by manufacturer. Store in a well-closed container.

**Selected Bibliography**
Brogden RN, Heel RC, Speight TM, et al. α-Methyl-*p*-tyrosine: a review of its pharmacology and clinical use. Drugs 1981; 21: 81-9.

Revised: 01/20/93

# MEXILETINE    Systemic

VA CLASSIFICATION (Primary): CV300
Note: For a listing of dosage forms and brand names by country availability, see *Dosage Forms* section(s). For a listing of brand names for the articles in this monograph, refer to the General Index.

## Category
Antiarrhythmic.

## Indications
### Accepted
Arrhythmias, ventricular (treatment)—Mexiletine is indicated for the treatment of documented, life-threatening ventricular arrhythmias, such as ventricular tachycardia.

### Unaccepted
Mexiletine is not recommended for use in the treatment of lesser arrhythmias, such as asymptomatic premature ventricular contractions following an acute myocardial infarction. Although the Cardiac Arrhythmias Suppression Trial (CAST) showed that treatment of asymptomatic, non–life-threatening arrhythmias following an acute myocardial infarction with encainide or flecainide was deleterious, the extrapolation of these results to other patient populations or antiarrhythmic agents remains uncertain.

## Pharmacology/Pharmacokinetics

### Physicochemical characteristics
Molecular weight—215.72.
pKa—8.4.

### Mechanism of action/Effect
Blocks the fast sodium channel in cardiac tissues, especially the Purkinje network, without involvement of the autonomic system. Reduces the rate of rise and amplitude of the action potential and decreases automaticity (increases the threshold of excitability) in the Purkinje fibers. Shortens the action potential duration and, to a lesser extent, decreases the effective refractory period in the Purkinje fibers. Does not usually alter conduction velocity, although it may slow conduction in patients with pre-existing conduction abnormalities. Does not significantly affect resting membrane potential or sinus node automaticity, left ventricular function, systolic arterial blood pressure, atrioventricular (AV) conduction velocity, or QRS or QT intervals. In the Vaughan Williams classification of antiarrhythmics, mexiletine is considered to be a class IB agent.

### Other actions/effects
Also has local anesthetic and anticonvulsant properties.

### Absorption
Well absorbed (approximately 90%) from upper intestinal section of gastrointestinal tract; low first-pass metabolism. Rate of absorption, but not bioavailability, is reduced in conditions in which gastric emptying time is increased (e.g., acute myocardial infarction) or with concurrent use of narcotics, atropine, or alumina and magnesia; metoclopramide may accelerate absorption.

### Protein binding
Moderate (60 to 75%).

### Biotransformation
Hepatic, approximately 85%, to inactive metabolites.

### Half-life
Normal—
    10 to 12 hours.
In moderate to severe hepatic disease—
    25 hours.
In severely reduced cardiac output—
    25 hours.
In renal disease—
    Creatinine clearance less than 10 mL per minute: 15.7 hours.
    Creatinine clearance 11 to 40 mL per minute: 13.4 hours.

In acute myocardial infarction—
    15 to 17 hours.

### Onset of action
30 minutes to 2 hours.

### Time to peak concentration
2 to 3 hours.

### Therapeutic plasma concentration
0.5 to 2 mcg per mL; however, toxicity may occur even at therapeutic plasma concentrations.

### Elimination
Biliary.
Renal, approximately 10%, unchanged; excretion is accelerated in markedly acid urine and retarded in markedly alkaline urine.
Mexiletine is excreted in breast milk in concentrations similar to maternal plasma concentrations.
In dialysis—May be removable by hemodialysis; supplementary dose may be required on day of dialysis. Not removable by peritoneal dialysis.

## Precautions to Consider

### Cross-sensitivity and/or related problems
Patients sensitive to other amide-type anesthetics (e.g., lidocaine) may be sensitive to mexiletine also.

### Tumorigenicity
Studies in rats and mice for 24 months and 18 months, respectively, found no evidence of tumorigenicity.

### Mutagenicity
Results of mutagenicity studies using the Ames test were negative.

### Pregnancy/Reproduction
Fertility—Studies in rats, mice, and rabbits at doses up to 4 times the maximum human oral dose found no impairment of fertility.
Pregnancy—Adequate and well-controlled studies have not been done in humans.
Studies in rats, mice, and rabbits at doses up to 4 times the maximum human oral dose found an increased incidence of fetal resorption but not teratogenicity.
FDA Pregnancy Category C.

### Breast-feeding
Mexiletine is distributed into human breast milk in concentrations similar to maternal plasma concentrations. Because of the potential for serious adverse effects in nursing infants, breast-feeding is generally not recommended while mexiletine is being administered.

### Pediatrics
Appropriate studies on the relationship of age to the effects of mexiletine have not been performed in the pediatric population. Safety and efficacy have not been established.

### Geriatrics
No information is available on the relationship of age to the effects of mexiletine in geriatric patients.

### Drug interactions and/or related problems
The following drug interactions and/or related problems have been selected on the basis of their potential clinical significance (possible mechanism in parentheses where appropriate)—not necessarily inclusive (» = major clinical significance):
Note: Combinations containing any of the following medications, depending on the amount present, may also interact with this medication.

    Acidifiers, urinary, such as:
      Ammonium chloride
      Ascorbic acid
      Potassium or sodium phosphates
        (marked acidification of urine may accelerate renal excretion of mexiletine)

Alkalizers, urinary, such as:
  Antacids, calcium- and/or magnesium-containing
  Carbonic anhydrase inhibitors
  Citrates
  Sodium bicarbonate
    (marked alkalinization of urine may retard renal excretion of
    mexiletine)
Antiarrhythmics, other
    (concurrent use with mexiletine may produce additive cardiac ef-
    fects; although some combinations are used for therapeutic advan-
    tage, when used concurrently dosage adjustments may be
    necessary)
Hepatic enzyme inducers (see *Appendix II*)
    (may accelerate metabolism and result in decreased plasma con-
    centrations of mexiletine; plasma concentrations of mexiletine
    should be monitored during concurrent use to ensure that efficacy
    is maintained)
Metoclopramide
    (may accelerate absorption of mexiletine)
Smoking, tobacco
    (may induce hepatic metabolism and reduce the half-life of
    mexiletine)
Theophylline
    (concurrent use may decrease theophylline clearance, resulting in
    prolonged elimination half-life, increased serum theophylline con-
    centrations, and increased risk of theophylline-related CNS toxic-
    ity; serum theophylline concentrations should be monitored and
    dosage adjustments may be required)

**Laboratory value alterations**
The following have been selected on the basis of their potential clinical
    significance (possible effect in parentheses where appropriate)—not
    necessarily inclusive (» = major clinical significance):

With physiology/laboratory test values
  Antinuclear antibody (ANA) titers
    (positive test results may occur infrequently)
  Aspartate aminotransferase (AST [SGOT]), serum
    (values may be increased to as much as 3 times or greater the
    upper limit of normal in 1 to 2% of patients; usually asymptomatic
    and transient)

**Medical considerations/Contraindications**
The medical considerations/contraindications included here have been se-
    lected on the basis of their potential clinical significance (reasons given
    in parentheses where appropriate)—not necessarily inclusive (» =
    major clinical significance).

*Risk-benefit should be considered when the following medical problems
    exist:*
» Atrioventricular (AV) block, pre-existing 2nd or 3rd degree, without
        pacemaker
        (risk of complete heart block)
» Cardiogenic shock
        (risk of further reduction of blood pressure)
  Congestive heart failure, severe or
  Myocardial infarction, acute
        (may reduce hepatic metabolism and result in prolongation of
        effect)
        (congestive heart failure may be aggravated by mexiletine)
  Hepatic function impairment
        (possible prolongation of effect)
  Hypotension
        (may be exacerbated)
  Intraventricular conduction abnormalities or
  Sinus node function impairment
        (use of mexiletine has been reported to result in depression of sinus
        rate, prolongation of sinus node recovery time, decreased conduc-
        tion velocity, and increased effective refractory period of the in-
        traventricular conduction system)
  Seizure disorders
        (mexiletine may precipitate seizures)
  Sensitivity to mexiletine

**Patient monitoring**
The following may be especially important in patient monitoring (other
    tests may be warranted in some patients, depending on condition;
    » = major clinical significance):

Aspartate aminotransferase (AST [SGOT]) values, serum
    (recommended prior to initiation of therapy and at periodic inter-
    vals during therapy; if persistent or worsening elevation occurs,
    withdrawal of mexiletine may be necessary)
» Electrocardiogram (ECG)
    (recommended continuously via Holter monitoring during therapy
    to assess efficacy and aid in dosage adjustment; intermittent chest
    x-rays may also be useful)
  Mexiletine concentrations, plasma
    (may be useful in some cases to aid in dosage adjustment)

## Side/Adverse Effects

Note: In the National Heart, Lung and Blood Institute's Cardiac Arrhyth-
    mias Suppression Trial (CAST), treatment with encainide or fle-
    cainide was found to be associated with excessive mortality or in-
    creased nonfatal cardiac arrest rate, as compared with placebo, in
    patients with asymptomatic, non–life-threatening arrhythmias who
    had a recent myocardial infarction. The implications of these results
    for other patient populations or other antiarrhythmic agents are
    uncertain.

    Incidence of side effects, especially some central nervous system
    (CNS) side effects, is related to plasma mexiletine concentrations
    and is greatest at concentrations exceeding 2 mcg per mL.

    Exacerbation of ventricular arrhythmias, including torsade de poin-
    tes, may occur.

    Hepatic necrosis has occurred rarely.

    A fatal overdose caused gastrointestinal disturbances, respiratory
    failure, and asystole.

    Pulmonary changes, including pulmonary fibrosis, have been re-
    ported in patients receiving other medications or having other con-
    ditions known to result in pulmonary toxicity; therefore, the rela-
    tionship to mexiletine is unknown.

The following side/adverse effects have been selected on the basis of their
    potential clinical significance (possible signs and symptoms in paren-
    theses where appropriate)—not necessarily inclusive:

**Those indicating need for medical attention**
Incidence less frequent
    *Chest pain; premature ventricular contractions* (fast or irregular
    heartbeat); *shortness of breath*
Incidence rare
    *Leukopenia or agranulocytosis* (fever or chills); *or thrombocytopenia*
    (unusual bleeding or bruising); *seizures*
    Note: *Thrombocytopenia* occurs within a few days after initiation of
        therapy, and blood counts usually return to normal within 1
        month after withdrawal of mexiletine.

**Those indicating need for medical attention only if they continue
or are bothersome**
Incidence more frequent
    *CNS effects* (dizziness or lightheadedness, nervousness; trembling or
    shaking of hands; unsteadiness or trouble in walking); *heartburn; nau-
    sea and vomiting*
    Note: *Nausea* and *vomiting* usually occur within 2 hours after a dose
        and tend to lessen with continued treatment.

Incidence less frequent
    *Blurred vision; confusion; constipation or diarrhea; headache;
    numbness or tingling of fingers and toes; ringing in the ears; skin
    rash; slurred speech; trouble in sleeping; unusual tiredness or
    weakness*

## Overdose

For more information on the management of overdose or unintentional
    ingestion, **contact a Poison Control Center** (see *Poison Control Cen-
    ter Listing*).

**Treatment of overdose**
Treatment is primarily supportive and symptomatic and may include acid-
    ification of urine to accelerate excretion of mexiletine. Administration
    of atropine may be indicated if hypotension or bradycardia occurs.

## Patient Consultation

As an aid to patient consultation, refer to *Advice for the Patient, Mexiletine
    (Systemic)*.

In providing consultation, consider emphasizing the following selected information (» = major clinical significance):

**Before using this medication**
» Conditions affecting use, especially:
    Sensitivity to amide-type anesthetics
    Pregnancy—Increased incidence of fetal resorptions in animals
    Breast-feeding—Distributed into breast milk
    Medical problems, especially atrioventricular (AV) block, pre-existing 2nd or 3rd degree, without pacemaker or cardiogenic shock

**Proper use of this medication**
» Compliance with therapy; taking as directed even if feeling well
    Taking with food, milk, or an antacid to reduce stomach upset
» Importance of not missing doses and taking at evenly spaced intervals
» Proper dosing
    Missed dose: Taking as soon as possible if remembered within 4 hours; not taking if remembered later; not doubling doses
» Proper storage

**Precautions while using the medication**
    Regular visits to physician to check progress
    Carrying medical identification card or bracelet
» Caution if any kind of surgery (including dental surgery) or emergency treatment is required
» Caution when driving or doing things requiring alertness, because of possible dizziness

**Side/adverse effects**
    Signs of adverse effects, especially chest pain, premature ventricular contractions, shortness of breath, leukopenia, agranulocytosis, thrombocytopenia, and seizures

## General Dosing Information

When mexiletine is replacing other antiarrhythmic therapy, the first dose may be given 6 to 12 hours after the last dose of quinidine sulfate or disopyramide, 3 to 6 hours after the last dose of procainamide, or 8 to 12 hours after the last dose of tocainide. In patients being transferred from parenteral lidocaine to oral mexiletine, substantial reduction of dose or withdrawal of lidocaine is recommended 1 to 2 hours after initiation of mexiletine therapy; lower initial doses of mexiletine (e.g., 100 to 200 mg every eight hours) may also be appropriate. In patients at risk of life-threatening arrhythmias, transfer to mexiletine therapy should take place in the hospital.

Mexiletine should be taken with food, milk, or antacid to reduce gastrointestinal irritation.

Patients with impaired hepatic function or severe congestive heart failure may require lower or less frequent doses of mexiletine.

It is recommended that dosage adjustments be made no more frequently than every 2 to 3 days.

It is recommended that the patient be evaluated carefully and mexiletine therapy may need to be withdrawn if significant leukopenia or thrombocytopenia occurs.

## Oral Dosage Forms

### MEXILETINE HYDROCHLORIDE CAPSULES USP

**Usual adult dose**
Arrhythmias, ventricular (treatment)—
    Oral, initially 200 mg every eight hours, the dosage being increased or decreased in increments or decrements of 50 to 100 mg per dose every two to three days as needed and tolerated.

Note: For rapid control of ventricular arrhythmias, a loading dose of 400 mg may be administered, followed by a 200-mg dose eight hours later.

    Some patients may tolerate twice-a-day dosing. For patients adequately maintained on a dose of 300 mg or less every eight hours, the total daily dose may be given in divided doses every twelve hours.

    Patients not adequately controlled by dosing every eight hours (i.e., those experiencing breakthrough ectopy two hours before the next dose) may respond to dosing four times a day.

**Usual adult prescribing limits**
Up to 1200 mg per day when given every eight hours (i.e., 400 mg per dose) or 900 mg per day when given every twelve hours (i.e., 450 mg per dose).

**Usual pediatric dose**
Safety and efficacy have not been established.

**Strength(s) usually available**
U.S.—
    150 mg (Rx) [*Mexitil*].
    200 mg (Rx) [*Mexitil*].
    250 mg (Rx) [*Mexitil*].
Canada—
    100 mg (Rx) [*Mexitil*].
    200 mg (Rx) [*Mexitil*].

**Packaging and storage**
Store below 40 °C (104 °F), preferably between 15 and 30 °C (59 and 86 °F), unless otherwise specified by manufacturer. Store in a tight container.

**Auxiliary labeling**
• Take with food, milk, or antacid.

## Selected Bibliography

Schrader BJ, Bauman JL. Mexiletine: a new type I antiarrhythmic agent. Drug Intell Clin Pharm 1986 Apr; 20: 255-60.
Fenster PE, Comess KA. Pharmacology and clinical use of mexiletine. Pharmacother 1986 Jan/Feb; 6: 1-9.

Revised: 10/06/92
Interim revision: 07/14/94

---

**MEZLOCILLIN**—See *Penicillins (Systemic)*

---

**MICONAZOLE**—See *Antifungals, Azole (Systemic)*; *Antifungals, Azole (Vaginal)*; *Miconazole (Systemic)*; *Miconazole (Topical)*

---

# MICONAZOLE  Topical

VA CLASSIFICATION (Primary): DE102
Note: For a listing of dosage forms and brand names by country availability, see *Dosage Forms* section(s). For a listing of brand names for the articles in this monograph, refer to the General Index.

## Category

Antifungal (topical).

## Indications

Note: Bracketed information in the *Indications* section refers to uses that are not included in U.S. product labeling.

**Accepted**
Candidiasis, cutaneous (treatment)—Miconazole is indicated in the topical treatment of cutaneous candidiasis caused by *Candida albicans*.

Tinea corporis (treatment)
Tinea cruris (treatment) or
Tinea pedis (treatment)—Miconazole is indicated in the topical treatment of tinea corporis (ringworm of the body), tinea cruris (ringworm of the groin; jock itch), and tinea pedis (ringworm of the foot; athlete's foot) caused by *Trichophyton rubrum*, *T. mentagrophytes*, and *Epidermophyton floccosum*.

Tinea versicolor (treatment)—Miconazole is indicated in the topical treatment of tinea versicolor (pityriasis versicolor; ''sun fungus'') caused by *Malassezia furfur (Pityrosporon orbiculare)*.

[Paronychia (treatment)]
[Tinea barbae (treatment)] or

[Tinea capitis (treatment)]—Miconazole is used in the topical treatment of paronychia, tinea barbae, and tinea capitis.

Not all species or strains of a particular organism may be susceptible to miconazole.

## Pharmacology/Pharmacokinetics

### Physicochemical characteristics
Molecular weight—479.15.

### Mechanism of action/Effect
Fungistatic; may be fungicidal, depending on concentration; inhibits biosynthesis of ergosterol or other sterols, damaging the fungal cell wall membrane and altering its permeability; as a result, loss of essential intracellular elements may occur; also inhibits biosynthesis of triglycerides and phospholipids by fungi; in addition, inhibits oxidative and peroxidative enzyme activity, resulting in intracellular buildup of toxic concentrations of hydrogen peroxide, which may contribute to deterioration of subcellular organelles and cellular necrosis. In *Candida albicans*, inhibits transformation of blastospores into invasive mycelial form.

## Precautions to Consider

### Pregnancy/Reproduction
Problems in humans have not been documented.

### Breast-feeding
Problems in humans have not been documented.

### Pediatrics
Appropriate studies on the relationship of age to the effects of topical miconazole have not been performed in the pediatric population. However, no pediatrics-specific problems have been documented to date.

### Geriatrics
Appropriate studies on the relationship of age to the effects of topical miconazole have not been performed in the geriatric population. However, no geriatrics-specific problems have been documented to date.

### Medical considerations/Contraindications
The medical considerations/contraindications included here have been selected on the basis of their potential clinical significance (reasons given in parentheses where appropriate)—not necessarily inclusive (» = major clinical significance).

*Risk-benefit should be considered when the following medical problem exists:*
Sensitivity to topical miconazole

## Side/Adverse Effects

The following side/adverse effects have been selected on the basis of their potential clinical significance (possible signs and symptoms in parentheses where appropriate)—not necessarily inclusive:

### Those indicating need for medical attention
*Blistering, burning, redness, skin rash, or other sign of skin irritation not present before therapy*

## Patient Consultation

As an aid to patient consultation, refer to *Advice for the Patient, Miconazole (Topical)*.

In providing consultation, consider emphasizing the following selected information (» = major clinical significance):

### Before using this medication
» Conditions affecting use, especially:
    Sensitivity to topical miconazole

### Proper use of this medication
» Avoiding contact with the eyes
    Applying sufficient medication to cover affected area, and rubbing in gently
    Proper administration technique for topical aerosol powder, topical powder, and topical aerosol solution
» Not applying occlusive dressing over this medication unless directed to do so by physician
» Compliance with full course of therapy
» Proper dosing
    Missed dose: Applying as soon as possible; not applying if almost time for next dose
» Proper storage

### Precautions while using this medication
Checking with physician or pharmacist if no improvement within 4 weeks

### Side/adverse effects
Signs of potential side effects, especially blistering, burning, redness, skin rash, or other sign of skin irritation not present before therapy

## General Dosing Information

Use of topical antifungals may lead to skin sensitization, resulting in hypersensitivity reactions with subsequent topical or systemic use of the medication.

The lotion is preferred for use on intertriginous areas; if the cream is used, it should be used sparingly and massaged in well to avoid maceration effects.

When this medication is used in the treatment of candidiasis, occlusive dressings should be avoided since they provide conditions that favor growth of yeast and release of its irritating endotoxin.

To reduce the possibility of recurrence, *Candida* infections, tinea cruris, and tinea corporis should be treated for 2 weeks and tinea pedis for 1 month.

## Topical Dosage Forms

### MICONAZOLE NITRATE TOPICAL AEROSOL POWDER

#### Usual adult and adolescent dose
Tinea corporis or
Tinea cruris or
Tinea pedis—
    Topical, to the skin, two times a day, morning and evening.

#### Usual pediatric dose
See *Usual adult and adolescent dose*.

#### Strength(s) usually available
U.S.—
    2% (OTC) [*Micatin* (alcohol 10%)].
Canada—
    Not commercially available.

#### Packaging and storage
Store below 40 °C (104 °F), preferably between 15 and 30 °C (59 and 86 °F), unless otherwise specified by manufacturer.

#### Auxiliary labeling
• Shake well.
• For external use only.
• Continue medication for full time of treatment.
• Store away from heat and direct sunlight.

### MICONAZOLE NITRATE TOPICAL AEROSOL SOLUTION

#### Usual adult and adolescent dose
See *Miconazole Nitrate Topical Aerosol Powder*.

#### Usual pediatric dose
See *Miconazole Nitrate Topical Aerosol Powder*.

#### Strength(s) usually available
U.S.—
    2% (OTC) [*Micatin* (alcohol 17%)].
Canada—
    Not commercially available.

#### Packaging and storage
Store below 40 °C (104 °F), preferably between 15 and 30 °C (59 and 86 °F), unless otherwise specified by manufacturer. Protect from freezing.

#### Auxiliary labeling
• Shake well.
• For external use only.
• Continue medication for full time of treatment.
• Store away from heat and direct sunlight.

### MICONAZOLE NITRATE CREAM USP

#### Usual adult and adolescent dose
Candidiasis, cutaneous or
Tinea corporis or
Tinea cruris or
Tinea pedis—
    Topical, to the skin, two times a day, morning and evening.
Tinea versicolor—
    Topical, to the skin, once a day.

#### Usual pediatric dose
See *Usual adult and adolescent dose*.

## Strength(s) usually available
U.S.—
    2% (Rx/OTC) [*Micatin; Monistat-Derm;* GENERIC].
Canada—
    2% (Rx) [*Micatin; Monistat-Derm*].

## Packaging and storage
Store below 40 °C (104 °F), preferably between 15 and 30 °C (59 and 86 °F), unless otherwise specified by manufacturer. Store in a collapsible tube or tight container. Protect from freezing.

## Auxiliary labeling
• For external use only.
• Continue medication for full time of treatment.

# MICONAZOLE NITRATE LOTION

## Usual adult and adolescent dose
See *Miconazole Nitrate Cream USP*.

## Usual pediatric dose
See *Miconazole Nitrate Cream USP*.

## Strength(s) usually available
U.S.—
    2% (Rx) [*Monistat-Derm*].
Canada—
    2% (Rx) [*Micatin*].

## Packaging and storage
Store between 15 and 30 °C (59 and 86 °F), in a well-closed container, unless otherwise specified by manufacturer. Protect from freezing.

## Auxiliary labeling
• Shake well.
• For external use only.
• Continue medication for full time of treatment.

# MICONAZOLE NITRATE TOPICAL POWDER USP

## Usual adult and adolescent dose
Tinea corporis or
Tinea cruris or
Tinea pedis—
    See *Miconazole Nitrate Topical Aerosol Powder*.

## Usual pediatric dose
See *Miconazole Nitrate Topical Aerosol Powder*.

## Strength(s) usually available
U.S.—
    2% (OTC) [*Micatin; Zeasorb-AF*].
Canada—
    Not commercially available.

## Packaging and storage
Store below 40 °C (104 °F), preferably between 15 and 30 °C (59 and 86 °F), unless otherwise specified by manufacturer.

## Auxiliary labeling
• For external use only.
• Continue medication for full time of treatment.
• Keep container tightly closed.
• Keep in a dry place.

Revised: 07/25/94

# MIDAZOLAM    Systemic

VA CLASSIFICATION (Primary/Secondary): CN302/CN205
Note: Controlled substance in the U.S.—Schedule IV.
Note: For a listing of dosage forms and brand names by country availability, see *Dosage Forms* section(s). For a listing of brand names for the articles in this monograph, refer to the General Index.

## Category
Sedative-hypnotic; anesthetic, general, adjunct; anesthetic, local, adjunct.

## Indications
Note: Bracketed information in the *Indications* section refers to uses that are not included in U.S. product labeling.

**WARNING: Intravenous midazolam should be used only in hospital or ambulatory care settings, including physicians' and dentists' offices, that provide for continuous monitoring of respiratory and cardiac function; also, resuscitative drugs and equipment, and personnel trained in their use, should be immediately available.** Midazolam administered intravenously has been associated with respiratory depression and respiratory arrest, especially when used concomitantly with opioid analgesics for conscious sedation or when rapidly administered; in some cases, death or hypoxic encephalopathy has occurred.

### Accepted
Sedation and amnesia—Midazolam, used intramuscularly, is indicated for preoperative sedation (induction of sleepiness or drowsiness and relief of apprehension) and to impair memory of perioperative events.

Sedation, conscious—Midazolam, used intravenously either alone or in conjunction with a narcotic, is indicated to produce conscious sedation prior to short diagnostic procedures or endoscopic procedures, such as bronchoscopy, gastroscopy, cystoscopy, coronary angiography, and cardiac catheterization.

[Midazolam is also being used intravenously for conscious sedation prior to certain dental and minor surgical procedures. This medication may be preferable to diazepam for intravenous sedation because of its faster onset of action, more consistent anterograde amnesia, and virtual lack of venous complications.][1]

Anesthesia, general, adjunct—Midazolam, used intravenously, is indicated for induction of general anesthesia prior to administration of other anesthetic agents. It may be used in conjunction with narcotic premedication, thereby achieving induction of anesthesia within a relatively narrow dose range and in a short period of time. It may also be used for intravenous supplementation of nitrous oxide and oxygen (balanced anesthesia) for short surgical procedures; however, the recovery time may be prolonged compared to that of thiopental. The use of midazolam in longer surgical procedures has not been studied.

[Anesthesia, local, adjunct][1]—Midazolam, administered intravenously, has been shown to be useful as an adjunct to local or regional anesthesia for some diagnostic and therapeutic procedures. It may be used for sedation of healthy patients receiving subarachnoid or epidural anesthesia.

[1]Not included in Canadian product labeling.

## Pharmacology/Pharmacokinetics

### Physicochemical characteristics
Molecular weight—362.23.
pKa—Midazolam base: 6.0.

### Mechanism of action/Effect
Midazolam is a relatively short-acting benzodiazepine central nervous system (CNS) depressant. Its effects on the CNS are dependent on the dose administered, the route of administration, and whether it is used concomitantly with other medications.

Midazolam has anxiolytic, hypnotic, anticonvulsant, muscle relaxant, and anterograde amnesic effects, which are characteristic of benzodiazepines. The mechanism of action of midazolam is not clearly understood; however, it is probably similar to that of other benzodiazepines.

Although the exact mechanisms of the actions of benzodiazepines have not been completely established, it has been postulated that the actions of benzodiazepines are mediated through the inhibitory neurotransmitter gamma-aminobutyric acid (GABA), which is one of the major inhibitory neurotransmitters in the brain. Benzodiazepines are believed to increase the activity of GABA, thereby calming the patient, relaxing skeletal muscles, and, in high doses, producing sleep.

Benzodiazepines reportedly act as agonists at the benzodiazepine receptors, which have been shown to form a component of the benzodiazepine-GABA receptor-chloride ionophore complex. Most anxiolytics appear to act through at least one component of this complex to enhance the inhibitory action of GABA. Other actions of benzodiazepines, such as sedative, anticonvulsant, and muscle relaxant effects, may be mediated through a similar mechanism, although different receptor subtypes may be involved.

The hypnotic effect of midazolam appears to be related to GABA accumulation and occupation of the benzodiazepine receptor. Midazolam has a relatively high affinity (about twice that of diazepam) for the benzodiazepine receptor. It is believed that there are separate benzodiazepine and GABA receptors coupled to a common ionophore (chloride) channel, and that occupation of both receptors produces membrane hyperpolarization and neuronal inhibition. Midazolam reportedly interferes with reuptake of GABA, thereby causing accumulation of GABA. Also, it is postulated that the action of midazolam in induction of anesthesia involves excess GABA at neuronal synapses.

The site and mechanism of the amnestic action of midazolam are not known; however, the degree of amnesia usually, but not always, parallels the degree of drowsiness produced by midazolam.

**Other actions/effects**

Midazolam causes a moderate decrease in cerebrospinal fluid pressure (lumbar puncture measurements), similar to that produced by thiopental, when it is used for induction of anesthesia in patients without intracranial lesions.

In intracranial surgical patients with normal intracranial pressure but decreased compliance (subarachnoid screw measurements), midazolam attenuates the increase in intracranial pressure due to intubation to a degree comparable to that of thiopental.

Studies have shown that intraocular pressure is lowered moderately when midazolam is used for induction of anesthesia in patients without eye disease; studies have not been done in patients with glaucoma.

Respiratory depression is produced; however, the respiratory depressant effect of midazolam is dose-related.

The cardiovascular effects of midazolam appear to be minimal. Cardiac hemodynamic studies have shown midazolam to cause a slight to moderate decrease in mean arterial pressure, cardiac output, stroke volume, and systemic vascular resistance when used for induction of anesthesia. Midazolam may cause slow heart rates (less than 65 per minute) to rise slightly, especially in patients taking propranolol for angina; it may cause faster heart rates (e.g., 85 per minute) to slow slightly.

**Absorption**

Mean absolute bioavailability of midazolam following intramuscular administration is greater than 90%.

**Distribution**

Widely distributed in body, including the cerebrospinal fluid and brain. The volume of distribution (vol$_D$) usually averages between 1 and 2.5 (range, 0.95 to 6.6) liters per kg of body weight in the majority of patients.

Note: In patients with congestive heart failure—A 2- to 3-fold increase in vol$_D$ has been shown in a small group of patients, following a single intravenous dose of 5 mg.

In obese patients—Significant increase in vol$_D$ because of greatly enhanced distribution of midazolam into peripheral adipose tissue.

**Protein binding**

Plasma—Very high, 97% in healthy individuals and 93.5% in patients with renal failure.

**Biotransformation**

Rapidly metabolized to 1-hydroxymethyl midazolam and 4-hydroxymidazolam. These metabolites may have some pharmacologic activity but less than that of the parent compound. Hydroxylation is by hepatic microsomal oxidative mechanisms.

**Half-life**

Distribution—
15 minutes
Elimination—
Midazolam: Approximately 2.5 (range, 1 to 5; rarely up to 12.3) hours in healthy patients.

Note: In patients with congestive heart failure—A 2- to 3-fold increase in elimination half-life has been shown in a small group of patients; however, total body clearance appeared to remain unchanged.

In patients with chronic renal failure—Elimination half-life does not appear to be significantly altered.

In obese patients—Because of greatly enhanced distribution of midazolam into peripheral adipose tissue, elimination half-life is prolonged but there is no change in total body clearance.

1-Hydroxymethyl midazolam and 4-hydroxymidazolam: Elimination half-life is similar to that of midazolam.

**Onset of action**

Sedation—
Intramuscular: Within 15 minutes.
Intravenous: Within 1.5 to 5 minutes.
Anesthesia, induction—
Intravenous: With narcotic premedication—Approximately 0.75 to 1.5 minutes.
Without narcotic premedication—1.5 to 3 minutes.

Amnesia—
Intramuscular: In one study—30 minutes after administration, no recall shown in 73% of patients; 60 minutes after administration, no recall shown in 40% of patients.
Intravenous: For sedation in endoscopy studies—71% of patients had no recall of introduction of endoscope and 82% of patients had no recall of withdrawal of endoscope.
Note: Time of onset is affected by total dose administered and whether narcotic premedication is used concurrently.
Rapid onset of action after intravenous administration is due to the high lipophilicity of midazolam at physiologic pH.

**Time to peak effect**

Intramuscular—15 to 60 minutes

**Duration of action**

The relatively short duration of action of midazolam is due in part to its very high metabolic clearance and rapid rate of elimination. The termination of action after single doses is caused by both distribution into peripheral tissues and metabolic transformation.

The duration of the amnestic action appears to be directly dose-related.

**Time to recovery**

Usually within 2 hours, but may take up to 6 hours.

Note: Patients who receive midazolam usually recover at a slower rate than patients who receive thiopental.

**Elimination**

Renal; following intravenous administration, less than 0.03% of dose is excreted in urine as unchanged drug; 1-hydroxymethyl midazolam and 4-hydroxymidazolam metabolites are excreted in the urine as glucuronide conjugates.

Note: Elimination following intramuscular administration is comparable to that following intravenous administration.

# Precautions to Consider

**Cross-sensitivity and/or related problems**

Patients sensitive to other benzodiazepines may be sensitive to this medication also.

**Carcinogenicity/Tumorigenicity**

In two-year studies in mice, midazolam was administered with the diet in doses of 1, 9, and 80 mg per kg of body weight (mg/kg) per day. At doses of 80 mg/kg per day, midazolam greatly increased the incidence of hepatic tumors in female mice and caused a small but significant increase in benign thyroid follicular cell tumors in male mice. These tumors occurred after chronic administration of midazolam, whereas only a single or several doses are usually used in humans. When midazolam was administered at doses of 9 mg/kg per day (25 times a human dose of 0.35 mg/kg per day), there was no increase in the incidence of tumors.

**Mutagenicity**

Midazolam was shown to have no mutagenic activity in *Salmonella typhimurium* (5 bacterial strains), Chinese hamster lung cells (V79), human lymphocytes, or in the micronucleus test in mice.

**Pregnancy/Reproduction**

Fertility—A reproduction study in male and female rats did not show midazolam to cause any impairment of fertility when given at doses up to 10 times the human intravenous dose of 0.35 mg/kg.

Pregnancy—Midazolam crosses the placenta. Since chlordiazepoxide and diazepam have been reported to increase the risk of congenital malformations when used during the first trimester of pregnancy, midazolam may be associated with this increased risk also. Risk-benefit must be carefully considered.

Segment II teratology studies in rabbits and rats did not show midazolam to cause teratogenic effects when the medication was administered in doses 5 to 10 times the human dose of 0.35 mg/kg. In addition, studies in rats did not show midazolam to cause any adverse effects during gestation and lactation when administered at doses approximately 10 times the human dose of 0.35 mg/kg.

FDA Pregnancy Category D.

Labor and delivery—In humans, measurable concentrations of midazolam have been found in maternal venous serum, umbilical venous and arterial serum, and amniotic fluid, indicating placental transfer of the medication. Following intramuscular administration of 0.05 mg/kg of midazolam, both the venous and umbilical arterial serum concentrations were lower than maternal concentrations.

Clinical studies on the use of midazolam in obstetrics have not been done. However, midazolam is usually not recommended for induction of anesthesia prior to Cesarean section because of the secondary CNS depressant effects on the neonate. Administration of other benzodiazepines during the last weeks of pregnancy has caused neonatal CNS depression.

Also, use of benzodiazepines just prior to or during labor may cause neonatal flaccidity.

**Breast-feeding**
It is not known whether midazolam is excreted in breast milk. However, problems in humans have not been documented.

**Pediatrics**
Appropriate studies on the relationship of age to the effects of midazolam have not been performed in children up to 18 years of age. However, no pediatrics-specific problems have been documented to date.

**Geriatrics**
When midazolam is used intravenously for conscious sedation in patients who are 60 years of age and over, debilitated, and/or chronically ill, dosage increments should be smaller and the rate of injection slower than in younger adults because the risk of underventilation or apnea is greater in older patients. Also, if concomitant CNS depressant premedication is used, dosage of midazolam should be reduced by at least 50%.

When midazolam is used for induction of anesthesia, patients over 55 years of age, whether premedicated or not, usually require lower doses.

Also, time to complete recovery after midazolam administration for the induction of anesthesia may be prolonged in the elderly.

In addition, elderly patients are more likely to have age-related chronic renal failure, which may require reduction of dosage in patients receiving midazolam.

**Drug interactions and/or related problems**
The following drug interactions and/or related problems have been selected on the basis of their potential clinical significance (possible mechanism in parentheses where appropriate)—not necessarily inclusive (» = major clinical significance):

Note: Combinations containing any of the following medications, depending on the amount present, may also interact with this medication.

» Alcohol or
» CNS depression–producing medications, other, including those commonly used for preanesthetic medication or induction or supplementation of anesthesia (See *Appendix II*)
    (concurrent use may increase the CNS depressant, respiratory depressant, and hypotensive effects of either these medications or midazolam; decrease dosage requirements of either these medications or midazolam; and prolong recovery from anesthesia)

    (when midazolam is used as an intramuscular premedication prior to use of thiopental as an induction agent, a reduction in thiopental dosage of about 15% may be required)

Cimetidine or
Ranitidine
    (inhibition of the cytochrome P-450 enzyme system by cimetidine, and possibly by ranitidine, may cause a decrease in the hepatic metabolism of midazolam, which may result in delayed elimination and increased blood concentration)

Hypotension-producing medications, other (See *Appendix II*)
    (hypotensive effects may be potentiated when these medications are used concurrently with midazolam; patients should be monitored for excessive fall in blood pressure during and following concurrent use)

**Medical considerations/Contraindications**
The medical considerations/contraindications included here have been selected on the basis of their potential clinical significance (reasons given in parentheses where appropriate)—not necessarily inclusive (» = major clinical significance).

*Risk-benefit should be considered when the following medical problems exist:*

Alcohol intoxication, acute, with depressed vital signs
    (potential additive CNS depression)

Coma or
Shock
    (hypnotic or hypotensive effects may be intensified or prolonged)

Congestive heart failure
    (possible 2- to 3-fold increase in elimination half-life and volume of distribution)

Hepatic function impairment
    (midazolam metabolized by liver)

» Myasthenia gravis or
Neuromuscular disorders, other, such as muscular dystrophies and myotonias
    (condition may be exacerbated)

Obesity
    (midazolam's elimination half-life may be prolonged and volume of distribution may be increased)

» Pulmonary disease, obstructive, chronic, severe or
» Pulmonary insufficiency, acute
    (midazolam has respiratory depressant effect; sedation and respiratory depression may be prolonged)

Renal failure, chronic
    (peak concentration of midazolam may be higher in these patients than in healthy patients; induction of anesthesia may occur more rapidly, and recovery may be prolonged)

Sensitivity to midazolam or other benzodiazepines

Caution is also recommended in geriatric or debilitated patients and in higher risk surgical patients, whether premedicated or not, because they may require lower doses for induction of anesthesia. In addition, caution should be used when intravenous midazolam is administered to patients with uncompensated acute illnesses, such as electrolyte disturbances.

Also, caution should be used in ophthalmology patients during surgery because some patients may be confused or disoriented if they awaken during the procedure. This is especially important in patients with an open globe for cataract surgery or in patients where movement might be critical.

## Side/Adverse Effects

Note: The most frequent side/adverse effects of midazolam during anesthesia and surgery include decreased tidal volume and/or respiratory rate (in 23.3% of patients following intravenous administration and in 10.8% of patients following intramuscular administration) and apnea (in 15.4% of patients following intravenous administration). In addition, variations in blood pressure and pulse rate may occur.

**Serious cardiorespiratory side/adverse effects have occurred primarily in older, chronically ill patients, with concomitant administration of other cardiorespiratory depressants (such as opioid [narcotic] analgesics), and with rapid administration of midazolam; these side/adverse effects have included respiratory depression, apnea, respiratory arrest, and/or cardiac arrest, sometimes resulting in death.**

**Midazolam administered intravenously has been associated with respiratory depression and respiratory arrest, especially when used concomitantly with opioid analgesics for conscious sedation or when rapidly administered; in some cases, death or hypoxic encephalopathy has occurred.**

Impairment of psychomotor skills may occur following midazolam sedation or anesthesia and may persist for varying lengths of time, depending upon the combination of medications and total dosages administered. Possible adverse effects on the patient's ability to drive or perform other tasks requiring alertness and coordination should be kept in mind when midazolam is administered for an outpatient procedure. It is recommended that patients not operate hazardous machinery or a motor vehicle until the effects of midazolam, such as drowsiness and amnesia, have subsided or until the day after anesthesia and surgery, whichever is longer.

The following side/adverse effects have been selected on the basis of their potential clinical significance (possible signs and symptoms in parentheses where appropriate)—not necessarily inclusive:

**Those indicating need for medical attention**
*Muscle tremor; uncontrolled or jerky movements of body; unusual excitement, irritability, or restlessness*

Note: The above side/adverse effects are possibly due to inadequate or excessive dosing or improper administration of medication; also, the possibility of cerebral hypoxia or paradoxical reaction should be considered.

Incidence more frequent
    *Hypotension*—especially in patients premedicated with narcotic

Incidence rare—< 1%, primarily following intravenous administration
    *Emergence delirium* (confusion; disorientation; hallucinations; unusual anxiety, excitement, nervousness, or restlessness); *hyperventilation* (fast breathing); *irregular or fast heartbeat; phlebitis* (redness, pain, swelling, and warmth at intravenous injection site); *skin rash, hives, or itching; wheezing or difficulty in breathing*

**Those indicating need for medical attention only if they continue or are bothersome**
Incidence more frequent
    *Hiccups; pain at intramuscular injection site; pain during intravenous injection; tenderness at intravenous injection site*

Incidence less frequent or rare
> *Blurred vision or other changes in vision; coughing; dizziness, light-headedness, or feeling faint; drowsiness, prolonged; headache; lumps or hardness at injection site; muscle stiffness at intramuscular injection site; nausea; numbness, tingling, pain, or weakness in hands or feet; redness at injection site; vomiting*

## Overdose

For specific information on the agents used in the management of mida-zolam overdose, see:

- *Flumazenil (Systemic)* monograph; and/or
- *Sympathomimetic Agents—Cardiovascular Use (Parenteral-Systemic)* monograph.

For more information on the management of overdose or unintentional ingestion, **contact a Poison Control Center** (see *Poison Control Center Listing*).

### Clinical effects of overdose

The following effects have been selected on the basis of their potential clinical significance (possible signs and symptoms in parentheses where appropriate)—not necessarily inclusive:

Acute
    *Cardiovascular depression; respiratory depression*

### Treatment of overdose

To enhance elimination—
    It is not known if peritoneal dialysis, forced diuresis, or hemodialysis is useful in the treatment of midazolam overdose.

Specific treatment—
    Administering flumazenil. See the package insert or the *Flumazenil (Systemic)* monograph for specific dosing guidelines for the use of this product.
    For hypotension—treatment may include intravenous fluid therapy, repositioning, vasopressors (if indicated), and other appropriate countermeasures.

Monitoring—
    Monitoring of respiration, pulse rate, and blood pressure.

Supportive care—
    General supportive measures.
    Maintenance of a patent airway and support of ventilation.

## Patient Consultation

As an aid to patient consultation, refer to *Advice for the Patient, Midazolam (Systemic)*.

In providing consultation, consider emphasizing the following selected information (» = major clinical significance):

### Before receiving this medication
» Conditions affecting use, especially:
    Sensitivity to midazolam or other benzodiazepines
    Carcinogenicity/tumorigenicity—In two-year studies in mice, chronic administration of midazolam at doses of 80 mg per kg of body weight (mg/kg) per day greatly increased incidence of hepatic tumors in female mice and caused a small but significant increase in benign thyroid follicular cell tumors in male mice
    Pregnancy—Risk of congenital malformations may be increased when midazolam is used during first trimester
    Labor and delivery—Midazolam is usually not recommended for induction of anesthesia prior to Cesarean section because of secondary CNS depressant effects on neonate; use of benzodiazepines just prior to or during labor may cause neonatal flaccidity
    Use in the elderly—Use in the elderly—When midazolam is used intravenously for conscious sedation in patients 60 years of age and over, dosage increments should be smaller and rate of injection slower than in younger adults because risk of underventilation or apnea is greater in older patients; if concomitant CNS depressant premedication is used, dosage of midazolam should be reduced by at least 50%; time to complete recovery after midazolam administration for induction of anesthesia may be prolonged in the elderly
    Other medications, especially alcohol or other CNS depression–producing medications
    Other medical problems, especially myasthenia gravis, severe chronic obstructive pulmonary disease, or acute pulmonary insufficiency

### Proper use of this medication
» Proper dosing

### Precautions after receiving this medication
» Possibility of psychomotor impairment following use of midazolam; using caution in driving or performing other tasks requiring alertness and coordination until the effects of midazolam have subsided or until the day after receiving midazolam, whichever is longer
» Avoiding use of alcohol or other CNS depressants within 24 hours after receiving midazolam, except as directed by doctor

### Side/adverse effects
Signs of potential side effects, especially emergence delirium; hyperventilation; hypotension; irregular or fast hearbeat; muscle tremor; phlebitis; skin rash, hives, or itching; uncontrolled or jerky movements of body; unusual excitement, irritability, or restlessness; and wheezing or difficulty in breathing

## General Dosing Information

Midazolam has been shown to be three to four times as potent per mg as diazepam.

**Dosage of midazolam must be individualized for each patient.** Lower doses are usually required for elderly, debilitated, or higher risk surgical patients. The dosage of intravenously administered midazolam should be adjusted according to the type and amount of premedication used.

**Intravenous midazolam should be used only in hospital or ambulatory care settings, including physicians' and dentists' offices,** that provide for continuous monitoring of respiratory and cardiac function.

**Prior to intravenous administration of midazolam in any dose, appropriate resuscitative equipment, oxygen, and skilled personnel for the maintenance of a patent airway and support of ventilation must be immediately available.**

**Midazolam should be administered intravenously as an induction agent only by a person trained in general anesthesia and should be used for conscious sedation only when a person skilled in maintaining a patent airway and supporting ventilation is present,** because of possible respiratory depression.

**When midazolam is administered intravenously for conscious sedation, it should be injected slowly; it should not be administered by rapid or single bolus intravenous injection** because of respiratory depression and/or arrest, especially in elderly or debilitated patients.

To facilitate slower intravenous injection of midazolam, the 1 mg-per-mL solution or dilution of the 1 mg-per-mL or 5 mg-per-mL solution is recommended.

During intravenous administration of midazolam, patients should be monitored continuously for early signs of underventilation or apnea, which can lead to hypoxia/cardiac arrest unless effective countermeasures are immediately taken. Also, monitoring of vital signs should be continued during the recovery period.

Caution should be taken to avoid intra-arterial injection because adverse effects of intra-arterial administration of intravenous midazolam in humans are not known. Extravasation should also be avoided.

When midazolam is administered intramuscularly, it is recommended that the medication be injected deep into a large muscle mass.

When midazolam is used for peroral endoscopic procedures, a topical anesthetic agent and the availability of necessary countermeasures are recommended because an increase in cough reflex and laryngospasm may occur.

When midazolam is used for bronchoscopic procedures, a narcotic premedication is recommended.

When midazolam is administered intravenously, it usually produces partial or complete impairment of recall for up to several hours, depending on the dose.

### For treatment of adverse effects
Recommended treatment for adverse effects of midazolam includes the following:
- Monitoring of respiration, pulse rate, and blood pressure.
- General supportive measures.
- Maintenance of a patent airway and support of ventilation.
- For hypotension, treatment may include intravenous fluid therapy, repositioning, vasopressors (if indicated), and other appropriate countermeasures.

## Parenteral Dosage Forms

Note: Bracketed uses in the *Dosage Forms* section refer to categories of use and/or indications that are not included in U.S. product labeling. The dosing and dosage forms are expressed in terms of midazolam base.

# MIDAZOLAM HYDROCHLORIDE INJECTION

## Usual adult dose

Sedation, preoperative, and amnesia—

Dosage must be individualized; however, as a general guideline: Intramuscular, 70 to 80 mcg (0.07 to 0.08 mg) (base) per kg of body weight, approximately thirty to sixty minutes before surgery.

Note: Lower doses may be sufficient in elderly or debilitated patients.

Midazolam may be administered concurrently with atropine or scopolamine hydrochloride and reduced doses of narcotics.

Sedation, conscious (endoscopic or cardiovascular procedures)—

Patients up to 60 years of age: Unpremedicated—Dosage must be individualized; however, as a general guideline: Intravenous, initially no more than 2.5 mg (base), administered slowly over a period of at least two minutes, immediately prior to procedure; after an additional two or more minutes to allow for clinical effect, dosage may be further titrated in small increments of the initial dose (with intervals of two or more minutes being allowed after each increment) to the desired effect. A total dose of more than 5 mg is not usually necessary. Additional maintenance doses may be administered, if necessary, in increments of 25% of initial dose to maintain desired level of sedation.

Note: When midazolam is administered concomitantly with narcotic analgesics or other CNS depressants, the dosage of midazolam should be reduced by approximately 30%.

Patients 60 years of age and over, and debilitated or chronically ill patients: Unpremedicated—Dosage must be individualized; however, as a general guideline: Intravenous, initially no more than 1.5 mg (base), administered slowly over a period of at least two minutes, immediately prior to procedure; after an additional two or more minutes to allow for clinical effect, dosage may be further titrated, if necessary, but the rate of administration should not exceed 1 mg over a two-minute period (intervals of two or more minutes should be allowed each time). A total dose of more than 3.5 mg is not usually necessary. Additional maintenance doses may be administered, if necessary, in increments of 25% of initial dose to maintain desired level of sedation.

Note: When midazolam is administered concomitantly with narcotic analgesics or other CNS depressants, the dosage of midazolam should be reduced by 50%.

Also, dosage increments should be smaller and the rate of injection slower because the danger of underventilation or apnea is greater in elderly patients and patients with chronic disease states or decreased pulmonary reserve; also, it may take longer to achieve the peak effect in these patients.

Note: The desired endpoint for conscious sedation can usually be attained within 3 to 6 minutes, depending on the total dose administered and whether or not narcotic premedication is used concomitantly.

The therapeutic dosage range between sedation and unconsciousness or disorientation appears to be narrower than for other benzodiazepines (e.g., diazepam, lorazepam).

Anesthesia, general, adjunct (prior to administration of other general anesthetics)—

Unpremedicated patients:

Up to 55 years of age—Dosage must be individualized; however, as a general guideline: Intravenous, initially 200 to 350 mcg (0.2 to 0.35 mg) (base) per kg of body weight, administered over a period of five to thirty seconds and allowing two minutes for effect.

Note: If necessary to complete induction, additional doses may be given in increments of about 25% of initial dose, or inhalation general anesthetics may be used.

Up to 600 mcg (0.6 mg) (base) per kg of body weight as a total dose may be used for induction, if necessary; however, larger doses may prolong recovery.

55 years of age and over—ASA I or II (good risk surgical patients): Dosage must be individualized; however, as a general guideline—Intravenous, initially 150 to 300 mcg (0.15 to 0.3 mg) (base) per kg of body weight, administered over a period of twenty to thirty seconds.

ASA III or IV (patients with severe systemic disease or debilitation): Dosage must be individualized; however, as a general guideline—Intravenous, initially 150 to 250 mcg (0.15 to 0.25 mg) (base) per kg of body weight, administered over a period of twenty to thirty seconds.

Premedicated (sedative or narcotic) patients:

Up to 55 years of age—Dosage must be individualized; however, as a general guideline: Intravenous, 150 to 350 mcg (0.15 to 0.35 mg) (base) per kg of body weight, administered over a period of twenty to thirty seconds and allowing two minutes for effect. A dose of 250 mcg (0.25 mg) per kg of body weight is usually sufficient.

55 years of age and over—ASA I or II: Dosage must be individualized; however, as a general guideline—Intravenous, initially 200 mcg (0.2 mg) (base) per kg of body weight.

ASA III or IV: Dosage must be individualized; however, as a general guideline—Intravenous, 150 mcg (0.15 mg) (base) per kg of body weight may be sufficient.

Note: When sedative or, especially, narcotic premedication has been administered, the recommended dose range of midazolam is 150 to 250 mcg (0.15 to 0.25 mg) (base) per kg of body weight.

Additional doses may be given in increments of about 25% of induction dose in response to signs of lightening anesthesia, repeated as necessary.

The endpoint for induction of anesthesia does not appear to be as clearly defined with midazolam as it is with thiopental.

Narcotic premedications frequently used include: fentanyl (1.5 to 2 mcg [0.0015 to 0.002 mg] per kg of body weight intravenously five minutes before induction); morphine (up to 150 mcg [0.15 mg] per kg of body weight intramuscularly, the dosage being individualized); meperidine (up to 1 mg per kg of body weight intramuscularly, the dosage being individualized); and fentanyl citrate and droperidol combination (0.02 mL per kg of body weight intramuscularly).

Sedative premedications frequently used include: hydroxyzine pamoate (100 mg orally) and secobarbital sodium (200 mg orally).

Premedications should be administered at least thirty to sixty minutes prior to midazolam induction, with the exception of narcotic analgesics (e.g., fentanyl) which should be administered two to five minutes before induction.

[Anesthetic, local, adjunct (epidural or axillary block)][1]—

Dosage must be individualized; however, as a general guideline: Intravenous, 30 to 60 mcg (0.03 to 0.06 mg) (base) per kg of body weight, the dosage being slowly titrated.

## Usual pediatric dose

Sedation, preoperative, and amnesia—

Dosage must be individualized; however, as a general guideline: Intramuscular, 80 to 200 mcg (0.08 to 0.2 mg) (base) per kg of body weight.

Sedation, conscious (endoscopic or cardiovascular procedures)—

Dosage must be individualized by physician.

Anesthesia, general, adjunct (prior to administration of other general anesthetics)—

Dosage must be individualized; however, as a general guideline: Intravenous, 50 to 200 mcg (0.05 to 0.2 mg) (base) per kg of body weight.

## Strength(s) usually available

U.S.—

1 mg (base) per mL (Rx) [*Versed* (benzyl alcohol 1%; disodium edetate 0.01%; sodium chloride 0.8%)].

5 mg (base) per mL (Rx) [*Versed* (benzyl alcohol 1%; disodium edetate 0.01%; sodium chloride 0.8%)].

Canada—

5 mg (base) per mL (Rx) [*Versed* (benzyl alcohol 10.45 mg; disodium edetate 0.1 mg; sodium chloride 8 mg)].

## Packaging and storage

Store between 15 and 30 °C (59 and 86 °F), unless otherwise specified by manufacturer. Protect from freezing.

**Preparation of dosage form**
Midazolam injection is compatible with 5% dextrose in water, 0.9% sodium chloride, and lactated Ringer's solution.
Midazolam injection may be mixed in same syringe with frequently used premedications, such as morphine sulfate, meperidine hydrochloride, atropine sulfate, or scopolamine hydrobromide.

**Stability**
Midazolam injection should not be used if it contains a precipitate or is discolored.
When midazolam injection is mixed in the same syringe with frequently used premedicants, such as morphine sulfate, meperidine hydrochloride, atropine sulfate, or scopolamine hydrobromide, the solution is stable for 30 minutes.

When midazolam injection is diluted in 5% dextrose in water or 0.9% sodium chloride, the solution is stable for 24 hours; if mixed with lactated Ringer's solution (Hartmann's solution), the solution should be used within 4 hours.

**Note**
Controlled substance in the U.S.

---

[1]Not included in Canadian product labeling.

---

Revised: 11/11/91
Interim revision: 08/17/94

## MILK-BASED ENTERAL NUTRITION FORMULAS—See *Enteral Nutrition Formulas (Systemic)*

---

# MILRINONE Systemic†

VA CLASSIFICATION (Primary): CV900
Note: For a listing of dosage forms and brand names by country availability, see *Dosage Forms* section(s). For a listing of brand names for the articles in this monograph, refer to the General Index.

---

†Not commercially available in Canada.

---

## Category
Cardiotonic.

## Indications

**Accepted**
Congestive heart failure (treatment)—Milrinone is indicated for the short-term management of congestive heart failure. Milrinone has been used primarily in patients concurrently receiving digoxin and diuretics.

## Pharmacology/Pharmacokinetics

**Physicochemical characteristics**
Molecular weight—211.22.

**Mechanism of action/Effect**
Milrinone is a direct positive inotropic agent with vasodilatory effects. Milrinone relaxes both arterial and venous smooth muscle, thereby reducing both preload and afterload. These effects are mediated by an increase in cytoplasmic cyclic adenosine monophosphate (cAMP) resulting from phosphodiesterase III inhibition in cardiac and smooth muscle.

**Other actions/effects**
Slightly increases atrioventricular (AV) conduction velocity. Milrinone may also have a favorable effect on ventricular diastolic function.

**Protein binding**
High (70%).

**Half-life**
Elimination—2.3 to 2.7 hours.

**Duration of action**
3 to 6 hours.

**Elimination**
Renal.

## Precautions to Consider

**Cross-sensitivity and/or related problems**
Patients sensitive to amrinone may also be sensitive to milrinone.

**Carcinogenicity**
Twenty-four-month oral administration of milrinone to mice at doses of up to 40 mg per kg of body weight (mg/kg) per day (50 times the human oral therapeutic dose in a 50 kg patient) or to rats at doses of up to 5 mg/kg per day (about 6 times the human oral therapeutic dose) did not reveal carcinogenic potential.

**Mutagenicity**
Positive results were observed in the presence of a metabolic activation system with the Chinese hamster ovary chromosome aberration assay. However, negative results were observed in the Ames test, mouse lymphoma assay, micronucleus test, and the *in vivo* rat bone marrow metaphase analysis.

**Pregnancy/Reproduction**
Fertility—No effect on male or female fertility was observed when milrinone was studied in rats at oral doses of up to 32 mg/kg per day.

Pregnancy—Adequate and well-controlled studies have not been done in humans.

Studies in pregnant rats and rabbits given milrinone during organogenesis revealed no evidence of teratogenicity at oral doses of up to 40 mg/kg per day and 12 mg/kg per day, respectively. Lack of teratogenic effect was also observed in rats or rabbits given milrinone intravenously at doses of up to 3 mg/kg per day and 12 mg/kg per day, respectively. However, an increased resorption rate was observed in rabbits at doses at or above 8 mg/kg per day.

FDA Pregnancy Category C.

**Breast-feeding**
It is not known whether milrinone is distributed into breast milk.

**Pediatrics**
No information is available on the relationship of age to the effects of milrinone in pediatric patients. Safety and efficacy have not been established.

**Geriatrics**
Although appropriate studies on the relationship of age to the effects of milrinone have not been performed in the geriatric population, patients given milrinone in clinical trials included patients up to 80 years of age (mean age 57 to 61). These trials have not demonstrated geriatrics-specific problems that would limit the usefulness of milrinone in the elderly. However, elderly patients are more likely to have age-related renal function impairment, which may require adjustment of dosage in patients receiving milrinone.

**Drug interactions and/or related problems**
The following drug interactions and/or related problems have been selected on the basis of their potential clinical significance (possible mechanism in parentheses where appropriate)—not necessarily inclusive (» = major clinical significance):
Note: Combinations containing any of the following medications, depending on the amount present, may also interact with this medication.

Hypotension-producing medications (see *Appendix II*)
(concurrent use with milrinone may produce additive hypotensive effects)

**Laboratory value alterations**
The following have been selected on the basis of their potential clinical significance (possible effect in parentheses where appropriate)—not necessarily inclusive (» = major clinical significance):

With physiology/laboratory test values
Blood pressure
(may be decreased)
Potassium concentrations, serum
(milrinone-induced improvement in cardiac output with resultant diuresis may predispose patients to hypokalemia)

**Medical considerations/Contraindications**
The medical considerations/contraindications included here have been selected on the basis of their potential clinical significance (reasons given in parentheses where appropriate)—not necessarily inclusive (» = major clinical significance).

*Except under special circumstances, this medication should not be used when the following medical problem exists:*
» Aortic or pulmonic valvular disease, severe
(surgical relief of obstruction required)

*Risk-benefit should be considered when the following medical problems exist:*
Hypertrophic subaortic stenosis
(milrinone may aggravate outflow tract obstruction)
» Myocardial infarction, acute
(no experience with use of milrinone in this setting)
Renal function impairment
(milrinone elimination reduced; dosage adjustment may be necessary)

**Patient monitoring**
The following may be especially important in patient monitoring (other tests may be warranted in some patients, depending on condition; » = major clinical significance):
» Blood pressure and
» Heart rate
(determinations recommended at periodic intervals; milrinone infusion should be slowed or stopped in patients who develop an excessive fall in blood pressure)
Body weight/fluid status and
Cardiac index and
Central venous pressure and
Pulmonary capillary wedge pressure
(determinations recommended at periodic intervals to confirm efficacy of milrinone)
Electrocardiogram (ECG), continuous
(recommended throughout infusion period to monitor for potential arrhythmias)
Platelet counts
(recommended prior to initiation of therapy and at periodic intervals during milrinone therapy)
Renal function determinations and
Electrolyte, especially potassium, concentrations, serum
(recommended at periodic intervals; hypokalemia secondary to improved cardiac output and resultant diuresis may contribute to risk of arrhythmias)

## Side/Adverse Effects

The following side/adverse effects have been selected on the basis of their potential clinical significance (possible signs and symptoms in parentheses where appropriate)—not necessarily inclusive:

**Those indicating need for medical attention**
Incidence less frequent
*Arrhythmias; hypotension*
Incidence rare
*Angina; thrombocytopenia*
Note: *Thrombocytopenia* has been reported in approximately 0.4% of patients; in some cases decreases in platelet counts were judged to be only possibly related to milrinone therapy.

**Those indicating need for medical attention only if they continue or are bothersome**
Incidence less frequent
*Headache*

## Overdose

For more information on the management of overdose or unintentional ingestion, **contact a Poison Control Center** (see *Poison Control Center Listing*).

**Clinical effects of overdose**
The following effects have been selected on the basis of their potential clinical significance (possible signs and symptoms in parentheses where appropriate)—not necessarily inclusive:
*Hypotension*

**Treatment of overdose**
Treatment of overdose consists of general measures for circulatory support.

## General Dosing Information

Pretreatment with digitalis is recommended in patients with atrial flutter/fibrillation since milrinone's slight enhancement of atrioventricular (AV) conduction may increase ventricular response rates.

Patients who have received vigorous diuretic therapy may need cautiously liberalized fluid and electrolyte intake to ensure an adequate cardiac filling pressure for response to milrinone.

Caution is recommended to avoid extravasation of milrinone infusion.

## Parenteral Dosage Forms

Note: The available dosage form contains milrinone lactate, but dosages and strengths are expressed in terms of the base.

### MILRINONE INJECTION

**Usual adult dose**
Congestive heart failure—
Initial: Intravenous, 50 mcg (0.05 mg) (base) per kg of body weight, administered slowly over ten minutes.
Maintenance: Intravenous infusion, 0.375 to 0.75 mcg (0.000375 to 0.00075 mg) (base) per kg of body weight per minute, the dosage being adjusted according to clinical response. Patients have been maintained on milrinone infusions for up to 5 days.
Note: Rates of infusion for concentrations of 100, 150, and 200 mcg per mL:

| Milrinone delivery rate (mcg/kg/min) | Infusion delivery rate | | |
|---|---|---|---|
| | 100 mcg/mL* (mL/kg/hr) | 150 mcg/mL† (mL/kg/hr) | 200 mcg/mL‡ (mL/kg/hr) |
| 0.375 | 0.22 | 0.15 | 0.11 |
| 0.400 | 0.24 | 0.16 | 0.12 |
| 0.500 | 0.30 | 0.20 | 0.15 |
| 0.600 | 0.36 | 0.24 | 0.18 |
| 0.700 | 0.42 | 0.28 | 0.21 |
| 0.750 | 0.45 | 0.30 | 0.22 |

*180 mL of diluent per 20-mg vial of milrinone.
†113 mL of diluent per 20-mg vial of milrinone.
‡80 mL of diluent per 20-mg vial of milrinone.

Reduction in infusion rate may be necessary in patients with renal function impairment. The following is recommended:

| Creatinine Clearance (mL/min/1.73m²) | Infusion Rate (mcg/kg/min) |
|---|---|
| 5 | 0.20 |
| 10 | 0.23 |
| 20 | 0.28 |
| 30 | 0.33 |
| 40 | 0.38 |
| 50 | 0.43 |

**Usual adult prescribing limits**
Up to 1.13 mg (base) per kg of body weight per day.

**Usual pediatric dose**
Safety and efficacy have not been established.

**Strength(s) usually available**
U.S.—
1 mg (base [as the lactate]) per mL (Rx) [*Primacor*].
Canada—
Not commercially available.

**Packaging and storage**
Store below 40 °C (104 °F), preferably between 15 and 30 °C (59 and 86 °F), unless otherwise specified by manufacturer. Protect from freezing.

**Preparation of dosage form**
For administration by intravenous infusion, milrinone injection may be diluted with 0.45% or 0.9% sodium chloride injection or 5% dextrose injection.

**Incompatibilities**
Milrinone should not be administered in intravenous lines containing furosemide, since an immediate precipitate is formed.

## Selected Bibliography

Hilleman DE, Forbes WP. Role of milrinone in the management of congestive heart failure. DICP, Ann Pharmacother 1989; 23: 357-62.

Young RA, Ward A. Milrinone. A preliminary review of its pharmacological properties and therapeutic use. Drugs 1988; 36: 158-92.

Revised: 07/19/93

---

**MINERAL OIL**—See *Laxatives (Local)*

---

## MINERAL OIL–CONTAINING COMBINATIONS—

Magnesium Hydroxide and Mineral Oil (Oral-Local)—See *Laxatives (Local)*

Mineral Oil and Cascara Sagrada (Oral-Local)—See *Laxatives (Local)*

Mineral Oil and Glycerin (Oral-Local)—See *Laxatives (Local)*

Mineral Oil, Glycerin, and Phenolphthalein (Oral-Local)—See *Laxatives (Local)*

Mineral Oil and Phenolphthalein (Oral-Local)—See *Laxatives (Local)*

---

**MINOCYCLINE**—See *Tetracyclines (Systemic)*

---

# MINOXIDIL Systemic

VA CLASSIFICATION (Primary): CV490

Note: For a listing of dosage forms and brand names by country availability, see *Dosage Forms* section(s). For a listing of brand names for the articles in this monograph, refer to the General Index.

## Category

Antihypertensive.

## Indications

**Accepted**

Hypertension (treatment)—Minoxidil is indicated for treatment of hypertension.

Because of its serious side effects, minoxidil is not considered to be a primary agent in the treatment of essential hypertension. It is recommended for use only in patients with symptomatic or organ-damaging hypertension not responsive to other treatment.

For additional information on initial therapeutic guidelines related to the treatment of hypertension, see *Appendix III*.

**Unaccepted**

Use of extemporaneous topical preparations from minoxidil oral tablets is not recommended for treatment of male pattern baldness because there is lack of data on the best formulation and the risks associated with possible systemic absorption. A topical product is commercially available for this indication.

## Pharmacology/Pharmacokinetics

**Physicochemical characteristics**
Molecular weight—209.25.
pKa—Approximately 4.6.

**Mechanism of action/Effect**
The exact cellular mechanism of antihypertensive action is unknown. The predominant effect of minoxidil is direct vasodilation of arterioles with little effect on veins. It reduces peripheral resistance and causes a reflex increase in heart rate and cardiac output.

**Absorption**
At least 90% absorbed from the gastrointestinal tract.

**Biotransformation**
Hepatic, at least 90%; metabolites have much less pharmacologic activity than minoxidil.

**Half-life**
Drug and metabolites—4.2 hours; not altered in impaired renal function.

**Onset of action**
30 minutes.

**Time to peak concentration**
1 hour.

**Time to peak effect**
Single dose—2 to 3 hours.
Multiple doses—Maximum blood pressure response with continued use usually occurs within 3 to 7 days (patients receiving the largest doses respond in the shortest period of time and vice versa).

**Duration of action**
Usually 24 to 48 hours; up to 75 hours in some patients.

**Elimination**
Fecal—3% (may be increased to up to 20% in severe renal function impairment).
Renal—97%, mostly as metabolites.
In dialysis—Removable by hemodialysis; however, this does not rapidly reverse the pharmacologic effect.

## Precautions to Consider

**Carcinogenicity**
Twenty-two-month studies in rats at doses 15 times the human dose revealed no evidence of tumorigenicity.

**Mutagenicity**
In Ames test, no evidence of mutagenicity was found.

**Pregnancy/Reproduction**
Fertility—A reduction in conception rate occurred in rats receiving minoxidil at doses 5 times the human dose.

Pregnancy—Minoxidil crosses the placenta. Studies in humans have not been done. However, hypertrichosis has been reported in newborns following maternal minoxidil administration.

Studies in rats and rabbits did not reveal teratogenic effects; however, there was an increased incidence of fetal resorptions in rabbits given minoxidil at 5 times the human dose.

FDA Pregnancy Category C.

**Breast-feeding**
Minoxidil passes into breast milk. However, problems in humans have not been documented.

**Pediatrics**
Appropriate studies on the relationship of age to the effects of minoxidil have not been performed in the pediatric population. However, pediatrics-specific problems that would limit the usefulness of this medication in children are not expected.

**Geriatrics**
Although appropriate studies on the relationship of age to the effects of minoxidil have not been performed in the geriatric population, the elderly may be more sensitive to the hypotensive effects. In addition, the risk of minoxidil-induced hypothermia may be increased in elderly patients. Elderly patients are also more likely to have age-related renal function impairment, which may require reduction of dosage in patients receiving minoxidil.

**Drug interactions and/or related problems**
The following drug interactions and/or related problems have been selected on the basis of their potential clinical significance (possible mechanism in parentheses where appropriate)—not necessarily inclusive (» = major clinical significance):

Note: Combinations containing any of the following medications, depending on the amount present, may also interact with this medication.

» Antihypertensives, potent parenteral, such as diazoxide or nitroprusside or
» Guanethidine or
» Nitrates
(concurrent use with minoxidil may result in a severe, additive hypotensive effect; patients should be continuously observed for excessive fall in blood pressure for several hours after concurrent administration of potent peripheral antihypertensives or nitrates; concurrent use with guanethidine is not recommended)

Anti-inflammatory drugs, nonsteroidal (NSAIDs), especially indomethacin
> (may reduce antihypertensive effects of minoxidil; indomethacin, and possibly other NSAIDs, may antagonize the antihypertensive effect by inhibiting renal prostaglandin synthesis and/or by causing sodium and fluid retention; the patient should be carefully monitored to confirm that the desired effect is being obtained)

Estrogens
> (estrogen-induced fluid retention may increase blood pressure)

Hypotension-producing medications, other (see *Appendix II*)
> (hypotensive effects may be potentiated when these medications are used concurrently with minoxidil)
>
> (although some antihypertensive and/or diuretic combinations are used for therapeutic advantage, dosage adjustments may be necessary during concurrent use)

Sympathomimetics
> (may reduce antihypertensive effects of minoxidil; the patient should be carefully monitored to confirm that the desired effect is being obtained)

**Laboratory value alterations**

The following have been selected on the basis of their potential clinical significance (possible effect in parentheses where appropriate)—not necessarily inclusive (» = major clinical significance):

With physiology/laboratory test values
Alkaline phosphatase concentrations, serum and
Plasma renin activity (PRA) and
Sodium concentrations, serum
> (may be increased)

Blood urea nitrogen (BUN) and
Creatinine
> (serum concentrations may be increased initially, but decline to pretreatment levels with continued treatment)

Erythrocyte count and
Hematocrit and
Hemoglobin concentrations
> (may be decreased as a result of hemodilution; usually recover to pretreatment levels with continued treatment)

**Medical considerations/Contraindications**

The medical considerations/contraindications included here have been selected on the basis of their potential clinical significance (reasons given in parentheses where appropriate)—not necessarily inclusive (» = major clinical significance).

*Risk-benefit should be considered when the following medical problems exist:*

Cerebrovascular disease or accident or
Myocardial infarction
> (a reduction in arterial pressure caused by minoxidil may further limit blood flow to the ischemic area)

» Congestive heart failure not due to hypertension
> (may be exacerbated secondary to fluid retention caused by minoxidil)

» Coronary insufficiency, including angina pectoris
> (may be exacerbated)

» Pericardial effusion
> (minoxidil may aggravate this condition)

» Pheochromocytoma
> (use may stimulate release of catecholamines from the tumor)

» Renal function impairment
> (reduced elimination; lower doses may be required)

Sensitivity to minoxidil

**Patient monitoring**

The following may be especially important in patient monitoring (other tests may be warranted in some patients, depending on condition; » = major clinical significance):

» Blood pressure measurements
> (recommended at periodic intervals in patients being treated for hypertension; selected patients may be trained to perform blood pressure measurements at home and report the results at regular physician visits)

» Weight measurements
> (daily weight measurements by the patient are recommended to detect excessive sodium and water retention)

## Side/Adverse Effects

Note: Minoxidil has been shown to cause severe myocardial toxicity in dogs. However, this effect has not been observed in other animals

or in humans at this time, although nonspecific electrocardiogram (ECG) changes are commonly seen, pericardial effusion (sometimes progressing to cardiac tamponade) occurs in about 3% of patients, and pericarditis has been reported.

The following side/adverse effects have been selected on the basis of their potential clinical significance (possible signs and symptoms in parentheses where appropriate)—not necessarily inclusive:

**Those indicating need for medical attention**
Incidence more frequent
> *Reflex sympathetic activation* (fast or irregular heartbeat; flushing or redness of skin); *sodium and water retention* (bloating; swelling of feet or lower legs; rapid weight gain of more than 5 pounds [2 kg] in adults or 2 pounds [1 kg] in children)

Incidence less frequent
> *Angina, new or exacerbated, or pericarditis* (chest pain)

Incidence rare
> *Allergic reaction or Stevens-Johnson syndrome* (skin rash and itching)

With long-term use
> *Paresthesia* (numbness or tingling of hands, feet, or face); *pericardial effusion or pulmonary hypertension* (shortness of breath)

**Those indicating need for medical attention only if they continue or are bothersome**
Incidence more frequent—occurs in most patients
> *Hypertrichosis* (excessive hair growth, usually on face, arms, and back)
>
> Note: *Hypertrichosis* usually develops within 3 to 6 weeks after initiation of minoxidil therapy, and return to pretreatment appearance occurs approximately 1 to 6 months after the medication is withdrawn. The increased hair growth may be extensive and may be especially disturbing to women and children; various depilatory methods may help.

Incidence less frequent or rare
> *Breast tenderness in males and females; vasodilation* (headache)

## Overdose

For more information on the management of overdose or unintentional ingestion, **contact a Poison Control Center** (see *Poison Control Center Listing*).

**Treatment of overdose**

Administration of intravenous sodium chloride injection is recommended to maintain blood pressure and facilitate urine formation.

Sympathomimetics such as norepinephrine or epinephrine should be avoided because of the risk of excessive cardiac stimulation.

Hypotension may be treated with phenylephrine, vasopressin, or dopamine, but they are recommended only if lack of perfusion of a vital organ occurs.

## Patient Consultation

As an aid to patient consultation, refer to *Advice for the Patient, Minoxidil (Systemic).*

In providing consultation, consider emphasizing the following selected information (» = major clinical significance):

**Before using this medication**
» Conditions affecting use, especially:
> Sensitivity to minoxidil
> Pregnancy—Decreased conception and increased resorption in animals; hypertrichosis reported in newborns
> Breast-feeding—Passes into breast milk
> Other medications, especially guanethidine or nitrates
> Other medical problems, especially congestive heart failure, coronary insufficiency, pericardial effusion, pheochromocytoma, or renal function impairment

**Proper use of this medication**
Possible need for control of weight and diet, especially sodium intake
» Patient may not experience symptoms of hypertension; importance of taking medication even if feeling well
» Does not cure, but helps control hypertension; possible need for life-long therapy; serious consequences of untreated hypertension
> Getting into the habit of taking at same time each day to help increase compliance
> Caution in taking combination therapy; taking each drug at the right time

» Proper dosing
   Missed dose: Taking as soon as remembered if within a few hours; not taking if forgotten until next day; not doubling doses
» Proper storage

**Precautions while using this medication**
   Regular visits to physician to check progress
» Checking resting pulse as directed; checking with physician if an increase of 20 or more beats per minute above normal occurs
» Checking weight daily; weight gain of 2 to 3 lb (approximately 1 kg) in adults is normal and is usually lost with continued treatment; checking with physician if rapid weight gain of more than 5 lb (2 lb in children) or signs of fluid retention occur
» Not taking other medications, especially nonprescription sympathomimetics, unless discussed with physician

**Side/adverse effects**
   Probability of hypertrichosis, which is reversible when medication is withdrawn
   Signs of potential side effects, especially sodium and water retention, reflex sympathetic activation, angina, pericarditis, allergic reaction, Stevens-Johnson syndrome, paresthesia, and pulmonary hypertension

## General Dosing Information

Sodium and water retention occurs rapidly in almost all patients receiving minoxidil and is difficult to control. Concomitant use of a diuretic (usually a loop diuretic) is recommended to prevent serious fluid accumulation and possible development of tolerance due to expansion of plasma volume.

Reflex tachycardia also occurs very commonly and may be less pronounced if a beta-adrenergic blocking agent or other sympathetic nervous system suppressant is used concurrently. The usual dose of beta-adrenergic blocker recommended is the equivalent of 80 to 160 mg of propranolol a day in divided doses. If beta-adrenergic blocking agents cannot be used, methyldopa in a dose of 250 to 750 mg twice a day may be substituted. Some investigators have used clonidine in a dose of 100 to 200 mcg (0.1 to 0.2 mg) twice a day.

If pericardial effusion occurs and does not respond to therapeutic measures, it is recommended that minoxidil therapy be withdrawn.

Because a few cases of rebound hypertension have been reported following abrupt withdrawal of minoxidil, caution is recommended when discontinuing the medication.

## Oral Dosage Forms

### MINOXIDIL TABLETS USP

**Usual adult and adolescent dose**
Antihypertensive—
   Initial: Oral, 5 mg a day as a single dose or as two divided doses, the dosage being adjusted in 100% increments as required (i.e., up to 10, 20, 40 mg, etc.).
   Maintenance: Oral, 10 to 40 mg a day, as a single dose or in divided daily doses.

Note: It is recommended that an interval of at least three days be allowed between each dosage adjustment, in order for the full effect of each dose to be obtained. In some patients, dosage adjustment may be made every six hours with careful monitoring.

   Geriatric patients may be more sensitive to effects of the usual adult dose.

**Usual adult prescribing limits**
Up to 100 mg a day.

**Usual pediatric dose**
Antihypertensive—

#### Children up to 12 years of age
Initial—Oral, 200 mcg (0.2 mg) per kg of body weight a day as a single dose or as two divided doses, the dosage being adjusted as required (i.e., in increments of 100, 150, 200 mcg per kg of body weight, etc.), up to 50 mg a day.
Maintenance—Oral, 250 mcg (0.25 mg) to 1 mg per kg of body weight a day, as a single dose or in divided daily doses, up to 50 mg a day.

#### Children over 12 years of age
See *Usual adult and adolescent dose.*

Note: It is recommended that an interval of at least three days be allowed between each dosage adjustment, in order for the full effect of each dose to be obtained. When more rapid control of blood pressure is required, dosage adjustment may be made every six hours with careful monitoring.

**Strength(s) usually available**
U.S.—
   2.5 mg (Rx) [*Loniten* (scored); GENERIC (scored)].
   10 mg (Rx) [*Loniten* (scored); GENERIC (scored)].
Canada—
   2.5 mg (Rx) [*Loniten* (scored)].
   10 mg (Rx) [*Loniten* (scored)].

**Packaging and storage**
Store below 40 °C (104 °F), preferably between 15 and 30 °C (59 and 86 °F) unless otherwise specified by manufacturer. Store in a tight container.

**Auxiliary labeling**
• Do not take other medicines without your doctor's advice.

**Note**
Check refill frequency to determine compliance in hypertensive patients.

## Selected Bibliography
The fifth report of the Joint National Committee on Detection, Evaluation, and Treatment of High Blood Pressure (JNC V). Arch Intern Med 1993; 153 (2): 154-83.

Revised: 05/26/93

---

# MINOXIDIL    Topical

VA CLASSIFICATION (Primary): DE900
Note: For a listing of dosage forms and brand names by country availability, see *Dosage Forms* section(s). For a listing of brand names for the articles in this monograph, refer to the General Index.

## Category
Hair growth stimulant, alopecia androgenetica, topical.

## Indications

**Accepted**
Alopecia androgenetica (treatment)—Minoxidil topical solution is indicated for treatment of alopecia androgenetica (also called male pattern baldness in men) in both males and females. Alopecia androgenetica is expressed in males as baldness of the vertex of the scalp and/or as frontal hair recession. In females, it is expressed as diffuse hair loss or thinning of the frontoparietal areas. Topical minoxidil is less likely to be effective in men with predominantly frontal hair loss than in patients with the other forms of alopecia androgenetica.

**Acceptance not established**
There are *insufficient data* to show minoxidil to be effective in the treatment of alopecia areata.

## Pharmacology/Pharmacokinetics

**Physicochemical characteristics**
Molecular weight—209.25.
pKa—4.6.

**Mechanism of action/Effect**
Topical minoxidil stimulates hair growth in some persons with androgenetic alopecia. The mechanism by which minoxidil stimulates hair growth is not established, but possible mechanisms include increased cutaneous blood flow as a result of vasodilation, stimulation of resting hair follicles (telogen phase) into active growth (anagen phase), and stimulation of hair follicle cells.

**Other actions/effects**
Systemically absorbed minoxidil may cause peripheral arterial vasodilation, reduced peripheral resistance, a reflex increase in heart rate and cardiac output, and fluid retention.

**Absorption**
Average 1.4% (range 0.3 to 4.5%) of the total applied dose; may be increased if applied to inflamed skin.

**Onset of action**
At least 4 months with twice daily applications; further growth continues through 1 year.

**Duration of action**
In one study with continuous treatment using topical minoxidil, hair regrowth tended to peak at one year with a slow decline in regrowth over subsequent years. Even so, after 4¹/₂ to 5 years of treatment, there were still more nonvellus hairs than there were at the beginning of the treatment.
New hair growth achieved during therapy may be expected to be lost 3 to 4 months after withdrawal of minoxidil, and progressive hair loss will resume.

**Elimination**
Renal—Approximately 95% of systemically absorbed minoxidil is eliminated within 4 days.

## Precautions to Consider

**Carcinogenicity**
A 1-year study of minoxidil applied topically in rats and rabbits found no evidence of carcinogenicity.

**Mutagenicity**
Minoxidil was not found to be mutagenic in the Salmonella (Ames) test, the DNA damage/alkaline elution assay, or the rat micronucleus test.

**Pregnancy/Reproduction**
Fertility—There was a dose-dependent decreased conception rate in male and female rats given 1 or 5 times the maximum recommended oral antihypertensive human dose.
Pregnancy—If pregnancy is desired, it is recommended that topical minoxidil be discontinued at least one month before birth control measures are discontinued.
Adequate and well-controlled studies in humans have not been done.
With oral administration of minoxidil, no teratogenic effects occurred in rats or rabbits, but there was evidence of increased fetal resorption in rabbits (but not rats) at 5 times the maximum recommended antihypertensive human dose.
FDA Pregnancy Category C.
Labor and delivery—The effects of minoxidil on labor or delivery are unknown.

**Breast-feeding**
One woman treated with 10 mg daily of oral minoxidil distributed minoxidil into her breast milk. It is not known whether topical minoxidil is distributed into breast milk. However, because of the potential for adverse effects, topical minoxidil should not be administered to women who are breast-feeding.

**Geriatrics**
No information is available on the relationship of age to the effects of this medication in geriatric patients.

**Drug interactions and/or related problems**
The following drug interactions and/or related problems have been selected on the basis of their potential clinical significance (possible mechanism in parentheses where appropriate)—not necessarily inclusive (» = major clinical significance):
Note: Combinations containing any of the following medications, depending on the amount present, may also interact with this medication.

» Corticosteroids, topical or
» Petrolatum, topical or
» Retinoids, topical
    (concurrent use may enhance cutaneous absorption of topical minoxidil because of increased stratum corneum permeability and is not recommended)

Guanethidine
    (concurrent use may increase the chance of orthostatic hypotension)

» Minoxidil, systemic
    (if topical minoxidil is systemically absorbed, concurrent use with systemic minoxidil may increase the risk of toxicity)

**Medical considerations/Contraindications**
The medical considerations/contraindications included here have been selected on the basis of their potential clinical significance (reasons given in parentheses where appropriate)—not necessarily inclusive (» = major clinical significance).

*Risk-benefit should be considered when the following medical problems exist:*
Cardiovascular disease or
Hypertension
    (possible adverse systemic effects if significant absorption occurs)
Intolerance to minoxidil
Skin irritation or abrasion, including scalp psoriasis or severe sunburn (systemic absorption may be increased)

**Patient monitoring**
The following may be especially important in patient monitoring (other tests may be warranted in some patients, depending on condition; » = major clinical significance):
Blood pressure and
Heart rate and
Weight
    (if a patient's history indicates a potential problem, determinations are recommended prior to initiation of therapy and at periodic intervals during therapy to check for possible systemic effects; if systemic effects occur, it is recommended that minoxidil be discontinued)

## Side/Adverse Effects

Note: Sudden death has been reported in several patients treated with topical minoxidil, but a causal relationship has not been established.

The following side/adverse effects have been selected on the basis of their potential clinical significance (possible signs and symptoms in parentheses where appropriate)—not necessarily inclusive:

**Those indicating need for medical attention**
Incidence less frequent
    *Dermatitis* (itching or skin rash)
Incidence rare
    *Allergic reaction* (skin rash; swelling of face); *alopecia, increased* (increased hair loss); *burning of scalp; dizziness; eczema* (skin rash); *folliculitis* (soreness at root of hair); *headache; lightheadedness; sexual dysfunction* (decrease of sexual ability or desire); *visual disturbances, including decreased visual acuity* (blurred vision or other change in vision)
Signs and symptoms of systemic absorption—Rare
    *Chest pain; fast or irregular heartbeat; hypotension*—usually not symptomatic; *neuritis* (numbness or tingling of hands, feet, or face); *sodium and water retention* (swelling of face, hands, feet, or lower legs; rapid weight gain); *vasodilation* (flushing; headache)
    Note: Signs and symptoms of toxicity resulting from systemic absorption may occur if minoxidil is applied too frequently, if it is applied to large surface areas, or if it is applied to scalps that have higher than normal permeability (e.g., from skin irritation).

**Those indicating need for medical attention only if they continue or are bothersome**
Incidence less frequent
    *Dry or flaking skin; erythema* (reddened skin); *pruritus* (itching)

## Overdose

For specific information on the agents used in the management of minoxidil overdose, see:
    • *Phenylephrine* or *Dopamine* in *Sympathomimetic Agents—Cardiovascular Use (Parenteral-Systemic)* monograph; and/or
    • *Vasopressin (Systemic)* monograph.
For more information on the management of overdose or unintentional ingestion, **contact a Poison Control Center** (see *Poison Control Center Listing*).

**Clinical effects of overdose**
The following effects have been selected on the basis of their potential clinical significance (possible signs and symptoms in parentheses where appropriate)—not necessarily inclusive:
    *Chest pain; fast or irregular heartbeat; hypotension*—usually not symptomatic; *neuritis* (numbness or tingling of hands, feet, or face); *sodium and water retention* (swelling of face, hands, feet, or lower legs; rapid weight gain); *vasodilation* (flushing; headache)

**Treatment of overdose**
If systemic toxicity occurs as a result of accidental ingestion or deliberate overdose, treatment may include the following:
To enhance elimination—Hemodialysis. Minoxidil and its metabolites are hemodialyzable.
Specific treatment—Hypotension may be treated with phenylephrine, angiotensin II, vasopressin, or dopamine, but these medications are rec-

ommended only if lack of perfusion of a vital organ occurs. Sympathomimetics, such as norepinephrine or epinephrine, should be avoided because of the risk of excessive cardiac stimulation.

Supportive Care—Administration of intravenous sodium chloride injection is recommended to maintain blood pressure and facilitate urine formation. Patients in whom intentional overdose is known or suspected should be referred for psychiatric consultation.

## Patient Consultation

As an aid to patient consultation, refer to *Advice for the Patient, Minoxidil (Topical)*.

In providing consultation, consider emphasizing the following selected information (» = major clinical significance):

**Before using this medication**
» Conditions affecting use, especially:
  Sensitivity to minoxidil
  Pregnancy—Animal studies have shown problems during pregnancy, but not birth defects
  Breast-feeding—Not recommended, since medication may cause problems in nursing babies
  Other medications, especially topical corticosteroids, minoxidil (systemic), petrolatum, or retinoids

**Proper use of this medication**
  Reading patient instructions carefully
» Not using more medication or more frequently than prescribed; not applying to other parts of body; risk of adverse systemic effects with excessive use
» Not using other skin products on treated skin
  Proper administration technique
    Shampooing hair each morning, before first daily application; applying to affected area of dry scalp, beginning at the center of the balding area
    Method of application depends on applicator used (spray, extended spray tip, dropper, and/or rub-on assembly)
    Washing hands immediately after application to remove any medication that may be on them
    Not using hairdryer to speed drying
    Not going to bed until at least 30 minutes after application, to minimize transfer onto pillowcase
  Checking with physician before applying to abraded, irritated, or sunburned scalp
» Avoiding contact with eyes, nose, or mouth; flushing area with large amounts of cool tap water if accidental contact occurs; avoiding inhalation of pump spray
» Proper dosing
  Missed dose: Using as soon as remembered if within a few hours; not using if almost time for next dose; not doubling amount used
» Proper storage

**Precautions while using this medication**
  Regular visits to physician to check progress
  Telling physician if itching, burning, or redness occur after application; if reaction is severe, washing minoxidil off and checking with physician before using again

**Side/adverse effects**
  Signs of potential side effects, especially dermatitis, allergic reaction, burning of scalp, folliculitis, increased alopecia, dizziness, eczema, lightheadedness, headache, sexual dysfunction, visual disturbances (including decreased visual acuity), and systemic absorption (chest pain, fast or irregular heartbeat, hypotension, neuritis, sodium and water retention, and vasodilation)

## General Dosing Information

If systemic effects occur, topical minoxidil should be discontinued and the patient seen by a physician. Fluid retention may be managed with a diuretic and a sodium-restricted diet. Angina or tachycardia may be controlled by use of a beta-adrenergic blocker or other sympathetic nervous system suppressant. Hypotension may be treated with intravenous normal saline.

If dermatologic reactions occur, it is recommended that discontinuation of topical minoxidil therapy be considered.

## Topical Dosage Forms
### MINOXIDIL TOPICAL SOLUTION

**Usual adult dose**
Hair growth stimulant—
  Topical, to the scalp, 1 mL of a 2% solution two times a day.
  Note: The same dose is used regardless of the size of the area being treated.

**Usual adult prescribing limits**
Up to 2 mL of a 2% solution per day.

**Strength(s) usually available**
U.S.—
  2% (20 mg per mL) (OTC) [*Rogaine For Men* (alcohol 60% v/v); *Rogaine For Women* (alcohol 60% v/v); GENERIC].
Canada—
  2% (20 mg per mL) (Rx) [*Apo-Gain* (alcohol 63%); *Gen-Minoxidil; Minoxigaine* (alcohol 63%); *Rogaine* (alcohol 63%)].
Note: Packaging may include spray, extended spray, dropper, and/or rub-on tips for application.

**Packaging and storage**
Store between 15 and 30 °C (59 and 86 °F), unless otherwise specified by manufacturer. Store in a tight container. Protect from light. Protect from freezing.

**Auxiliary labeling**
• For external use only.

## Selected Bibliography
Rumsfield JA, West DP, Fiedler-Weiss VC, et al. Topical minoxidil therapy for hair regrowth. Clin Pharm 1987 May; 6 (5): 386-92.
Clissold SP, Heel RC. Topical minoxidil. A preliminary review of its pharmacodynamic properties and therapeutic efficacy in alopecia areata and alopecia androgenetica [review]. Drugs 1987 Feb; 33 (2): 107-22.
Kvedar JC, Baden HP. Topical minoxidil in the treatment of male pattern alopecia [review]. Pharmacotherapy 1987; 7 (6): 191-7.

Revised: 04/14/92
Interim revision: 07/14/94; 7/15/96

---

# MISOPROSTOL   Systemic

VA CLASSIFICATION (Primary): HS875
Note: For a listing of dosage forms and brand names by country availability, see *Dosage Forms* section(s). For a listing of brand names for the articles in this monograph, refer to the General Index.

## Category
Gastric mucosa protectant; antiulcer agent.

## Indications
Note: Bracketed information in the *Indications* section refers to uses that are not included in U.S. product labeling.

**Accepted**
Ulcer, gastric, nonsteroidal anti-inflammatory drug–induced (prophylaxis)—Misoprostol is indicated for the prevention of gastric ulcer associated with the use of nonsteroidal anti-inflammatory drugs (NSAIDs), including aspirin, in patients at high risk of complications from gastric ulcer, such as the elderly, and in patients with concomitant disease or patients at high risk of developing gastric ulceration, such as those with a history of ulcer.

[Ulcer, duodenal (treatment)]—Misoprostol is indicated in the short-term treatment of duodenal ulcer.

## Pharmacology/Pharmacokinetics

**Physicochemical characteristics**
Molecular weight—382.54.

**Mechanism of action/Effect**
Cytoprotective—Misoprostol enhances natural gastromucosal defense mechanisms and healing in acid-related disorders, probably by increasing production of gastric mucus and mucosal secretion of bicarbonate.

**Antisecretory**—Misoprostol inhibits basal and nocturnal gastric acid secretion by direct action on the parietal cells; also inhibits gastric acid secretion stimulated by food, histamine, and pentagastrin. It decreases pepsin secretion under basal, but not histamine stimulation. Misoprostol has no significant effect on fasting or postprandial gastrin or intrinsic factor output.

**Absorption**
Rapidly absorbed following oral administration.

**Protein binding**
High (approximately 85%).

**Biotransformation**
Rapidly de-esterified to misoprostol acid (primary biologically active metabolite). The de-esterified metabolite undergoes further metabolism by beta and omega oxidation, which can take place in various tissues in the body.

**Half-life**
Terminal—20–40 minutes.

**Time to peak concentration**
12 ± 3 minutes.

**Peak serum concentration**
<1 mcg (0.001 mg) per liter.

**Duration of action**
3–6 hours.

**Elimination**
Renal (64 to 73% of the oral dose excreted within the first 24 hours). Fecal (15% of the oral dose).

## Precautions to Consider

### Cross-sensitivity and/or related problems
Patients sensitive to other prostaglandins or prostaglandin analogs may be sensitive to misoprostol also.

### Carcinogenicity/Mutagenicity
Animal studies have not shown misoprostol to be carcinogenic or mutagenic.

### Pregnancy/Reproduction
Pregnancy—**Misoprostol is contraindicated during pregnancy**. Studies in humans have shown that misoprostol causes an increase in the frequency and intensity of uterine contractions. Misoprostol administration has also been associated with a higher incidence of uterine bleeding and expulsion of uterine contents. Miscarriages caused by misoprostol are likely to be incomplete, resulting in very serious medical complications, sometimes requiring hospitalization and surgery, and possibly causing infertility.

FDA Pregnancy Category X.

Patients of childbearing potential may use misoprostol if nonsteroidal anti-inflammatory drug (NSAID) therapy is required and patient is at high risk of complications from gastric ulcers associated with the use of NSAIDs, or is at high risk of developing gastric ulceration. Such patients must comply with effective contraceptive measures, must have had a negative serum pregnancy test within 2 weeks prior to initiation of therapy, and must start misoprostol therapy only on the second or third day of the next normal menstrual period.

### Breast-feeding
It is unlikely that misoprostol is distributed into breast milk since it is rapidly metabolized throughout the body. However, it is not known if the active metabolite, misoprostol acid, is distributed into breast milk. Therefore, administration of misoprostol to nursing women is not recommended because of the potential distribution of misoprostol acid, which could cause significant diarrhea in the nursing infant.

### Pediatrics
Appropriate studies on the relationship of age to the effects of misoprostol have not been performed in patients up to 18 years of age.

### Geriatrics
Studies performed in approximately 500 ulcer patients 65 years of age or older have not demonstrated geriatrics-specific problems that would limit the usefulness of misoprostol in the elderly.

### Drug interactions and/or related problems
The following drug interactions and/or related problems have been selected on the basis of their potential clinical significance (possible mechanism in parentheses where appropriate)—not necessarily inclusive (» = major clinical significance):

Note: Combinations containing any of the following medications, depending on the amount present, may also interact with this medication.

Magnesium-containing antacids
   (concurrent use with misoprostol may aggravate misoprostol-induced diarrhea)

**Medical considerations/Contraindications**
The medical considerations/contraindications included here have been selected on the basis of their potential clinical significance (reasons given in parentheses where appropriate)—not necessarily inclusive (» = major clinical significance).

*Risk-benefit should be considered when the following medical problems exist:*
Cerebral vascular disease or
Coronary artery disease
   (although the effect has not been reported with misoprostol, prostaglandins and prostaglandin analogs have been reported to cause hypotension, thus increasing the risk of severe complications in these conditions)
Epilepsy
   (although the effect has not been reported with misoprostol, prostaglandins and prostaglandin analogs have been reported to cause epileptic seizures when given by routes other than oral; it is recommended that misoprostol be used in epileptics only when their condition is adequately controlled)
Sensitivity to prostaglandins or prostaglandin analogs

## Side/Adverse Effects

The following side/adverse effects have been selected on the basis of their potential clinical significance (possible signs and symptoms in parentheses where appropriate)—not necessarily inclusive:

**Those indicating need for medical attention only if they continue or are bothersome**
Incidence more frequent
   *Abdominal or stomach pain, mild; diarrhea*—13 to 40%
   Note: *Diarrhea* is dose-related; usually developing early in the course of therapy. Self-limiting, often resolving after 8 days. However, some patients (<2%) have required discontinuation of misoprostol because of continuing severe diarrhea.

Incidence less frequent or rare
   *Constipation*—1.1%; *flatulence*—2.9%; *headache*—2.4%; *nausea and/or vomiting; uterine stimulation* (cramps in lower abdomen or stomach area); *vaginal bleeding*

## Patient Consultation

As an aid to patient consultation, refer to *Advice for the Patient, Misoprostol (Systemic)*.

In providing consultation, consider emphasizing the following selected information (» = major clinical significance):

**Before using this medication**
» Conditions affecting use, especially:
   Sensitivity to prostaglandins or prostaglandin analogs
   Pregnancy—Contraindicated during pregnancy because of risk of miscarriage; patients of childbearing potential must take measures to assure they are not pregnant prior to therapy and to prevent pregnancy during therapy
   Breast-feeding—Not recommended because of possibility of causing diarrhea in nursing infant

**Proper use of this medication**
   Taking with or after meals and at bedtime
» Proper dosing
   Missed dose: Taking as soon as possible; not taking if almost time for next dose; not doubling doses
» Proper storage
*For use in the treatment of duodenal ulcer*
   Taking antacids for relief of ulcer pain; not taking magnesium-containing antacids
   Compliance with full course of therapy and keeping appointments for check-ups
» Not taking for more than 4 weeks unless otherwise directed by physician

**Precautions while using this medication**
   Stopping medication and checking with physician immediately if pregnancy is suspected
   Consulting physician if diarrhea develops and continues for more than a week

**Side/adverse effects**
   Signs of potential side effects, especially continuing and severe diarrhea

## General Dosing Information

Misoprostol therapy should be started at the onset of treatment with non-steroidal anti-inflammatory drugs (NSAIDs).

Misoprostol should be taken with or after meals and at bedtime, for maximum effectiveness.

### For treatment of duodenal ulcer

If required, antacids may be administered before or after misoprostol for the relief of pain. However, magnesium-containing antacids are not recommended since they may aggravate the misoprostol-induced diarrhea.

Therapy with misoprostol should continue for a total of 4 weeks unless healing has been documented by endoscopic examination. If necessary, treatment may continue for an additional 4 weeks if ulcers have not fully healed after the initial 4 weeks.

## Oral Dosage Forms

Note: Bracketed uses in the *Dosage forms* section refer to categories of use and/or indications that are not included in U.S. product labeling.

### MISOPROSTOL TABLETS

#### Usual adult dose

Prevention of nonsteroidal anti-inflammatory drug–induced gastric ulcer
or
[Treatment of duodenal ulcer]—
　　Oral, 200 mcg (0.2 mg) four times a day with or after meals and at bedtime; or 400 mcg (0.4 mg) two times a day with the last dose taken at bedtime.

Note: Dose may be reduced to 100 mcg (0.1 mg) in those patients sensitive to higher doses.

#### Usual pediatric and adolescent dose

Dosage has not been established.

#### Usual geriatric dose

See *Usual adult dose.*

#### Strength(s) usually available

U.S.—
　　0.1 mg (Rx) [*Cytotec* (scored)].
　　0.2 mg (Rx) [*Cytotec* (scored)].
Canada—
　　0.1 mg (Rx) [*Cytotec* (scored)].
　　0.2 mg (Rx) [*Cytotec* (scored)].

#### Packaging and storage

Store below 30 °C (86 °F), in a well-closed container, unless otherwise specified by manufacturer.

#### Stability

Misoprostol tablets have an expiration date of 18 months following the date of manufacture.

#### Auxiliary labeling

• Continue medicine for full time of treatment.
• Do not give medication to any other persons.

## Selected Bibliography

Jones J, Baily R. Misoprostol: a prostaglandin E₁ analog with antisecretory and cytoprotective properties. DICP 1989; 23: 276-281.
Knodell RG, et.al. Stress-related mucosal damage: critical evaluation of potential new therapeutic agents. Pharmacotherapy 1987; 7 (6 Pt 2): 104S-9S.
Garris RE, Kirkwood CF. Misoprostol: a prostaglandin E₁ analogue. Clin Pharm 1989; 8: 627–41.

Revised: 04/14/92
Interim revision: 08/10/94

---

# MITOMYCIN　Systemic

VA CLASSIFICATION (Primary/Secondary): AN200/DE600

Note: For a listing of dosage forms and brand names by country availability, see *Dosage Forms* section(s). For a listing of brand names for the articles in this monograph, refer to the General Index.

## Category

Antineoplastic.

## Indications

Note: Bracketed information in the *Indications* section refers to uses that are not included in U.S. product labeling.

### Accepted

Carcinoma, gastric (treatment)
Carcinoma, pancreatic (treatment)
[Carcinoma, colorectal (treatment)]
[Carcinoma, breast (treatment)][1]
[Carcinoma, head and neck (treatment)][1]
[Carcinoma, biliary (treatment)][1]
[Carcinoma, lung (treatment)][1]
[Carcinoma, cervical (treatment)][1]—Mitomycin is indicated, in combination with other agents, for palliative treatment of adenocarcinoma of the stomach or pancreas unresponsive to surgery and/or radiotherapy. Mitomycin is also used for treatment of adenocarcinoma of the colon or breast; some head and neck tumors; and advanced biliary, lung, and cervical squamous cell carcinomas.

[Carcinoma, bladder (treatment)]—Mitomycin is used for topical treatment of superficial transitional cell carcinoma of the urinary bladder.

[Leukemia, chronic myelocytic (treatment)][1]—Mitomycin is used for treatment of chronic myelocytic leukemia.

---

[1]Not included in Canadian product labeling.

## Pharmacology/Pharmacokinetics

### Physicochemical characteristics

Molecular weight—334.33.

### Mechanism of action/Effect

Mitomycin is classified as an antibiotic but is not useful as an antimicrobial agent because of its toxicity. Mitomycin is cell cycle–phase non-specific, although it is most active in the G and S phases of cell division. After enzyme activation in the tissues, it functions as a bifunctional or trifunctional alkylating agent. Mitomycin causes cross-linking of DNA and inhibits DNA synthesis and, to a lesser extent, also inhibits RNA and protein synthesis.

### Distribution

Does not cross the blood-brain barrier.

### Biotransformation

Hepatic (primarily); some in other tissues, including the kidney.

### Half-life

Initial—5 to 15 minutes.
Terminal—About 50 minutes.

### Elimination

Renal (10% unchanged); small amounts in bile and feces.

## Precautions to Consider

### Carcinogenicity/Mutagenicity

Secondary malignancies are potential delayed effects of many antineoplastic agents, although it is not clear whether the effect is related to their mutagenic or immunosuppressive action. The effect of dose and duration of therapy is also unknown, although risk seems to increase with long-term use. Although information is limited, available data seem to indicate that the carcinogenic risk is greatest with the alkylating agents.
Mitomycin is carcinogenic in rats.

### Pregnancy/Reproduction

Fertility—Gonadal suppression, resulting in amenorrhea or azoospermia, may occur in patients taking antineoplastic therapy, especially with the alkylating agents. In general, these effects appear to be related to dose and length of therapy and may be irreversible. Prediction of the degree of testicular or ovarian function impairment is complicated by the common use of combinations of several antineoplastics, which makes it difficult to assess the effects of individual agents.

Pregnancy—First trimester: It is usually recommended that use of antineoplastics, especially combination chemotherapy, be avoided whenever possible, especially during the first trimester. Although information is limited because of the relatively few instances of antineoplastic administration during pregnancy, the mutagenic, teratogenic, and carcinogenic potential of these medications must be considered.

Other hazards to the fetus include adverse reactions seen in adults.

In general, use of a contraceptive is recommended during cytotoxic drug therapy.

Mitomycin is reported to cause teratogenicity in animals.

### Breast-feeding

Although very little information is available regarding distribution of antineoplastic agents into breast milk, breast-feeding is not recommended while mitomycin is being administered because of the risks to the infant (adverse effects, mutagenicity, carcinogenicity).

### Pediatrics

Appropriate studies on the relationship of age to the effects of mitomycin have not been performed in the pediatric population. However, pediatric-specific problems that would limit the usefulness of this medication in children are not expected.

### Geriatrics

No information is available on the relationship of age to the effects of mitomycin in geriatric patients. However, elderly patients are more likely to have age-related renal function impairment, which may require caution in patients receiving mitomycin.

### Dental

The bone marrow depressant effects of mitomycin may result in an increased incidence of microbial infection, delayed healing, and gingival bleeding. Dental work, whenever possible, should be completed prior to initiation of therapy or deferred until blood counts have returned to normal. Patients should be instructed in proper oral hygiene during treatment, including caution in use of regular toothbrushes, dental floss, and toothpicks.

Mitomycin may also cause stomatitis associated with considerable discomfort.

### Drug interactions and/or related problems

The following drug interactions and/or related problems have been selected on the basis of their potential clinical significance (possible mechanism in parentheses where appropriate)—not necessarily inclusive (» = major clinical significance):

Note: Combinations containing any of the following medications, depending on the amount present, may also interact with this medication.

Blood dyscrasia–causing medications (See *Appendix II*)
(leukopenic and/or thrombocytopenic effects of mitomycin may be increased with concurrent or recent therapy if these medications cause the same effects; dosage adjustment of mitomycin, if necessary, should be based on blood counts)

» Bone marrow depressants, other (See *Appendix II*) or
Radiation therapy
(additive bone marrow depression may occur; dosage reduction may be required when two or more bone marrow depressants, including radiation, are used concurrently or consecutively)

Doxorubicin
(concurrent use may result in increased cardiotoxicity; it is recommended that the total dose of doxorubicin not exceed 450 mg per square meter of body surface)

Vaccines, killed virus
(because normal defense mechanisms may be suppressed by mitomycin therapy, the patient's antibody response to the vaccine may be decreased. The interval between discontinuation of medications that cause immunosuppression and restoration of the patient's ability to respond to the vaccine depends on the intensity and type of immunosuppression-causing medication used, the underlying disease, and other factors; estimates vary from 3 months to 1 year)

» Vaccines, live virus
(because normal defense mechanisms may be suppressed by mitomycin therapy, concurrent use with a live virus vaccine may potentiate the replication of the vaccine virus, may increase the side/adverse effects of the vaccine virus, and/or may decrease the patient's antibody response to the vaccine; immunization of these patients should be undertaken only with extreme caution after careful review of the patient's hematologic status and only with the knowledge and consent of the physician managing the mitomycin therapy. The interval between discontinuation of medications that cause immunosuppression and restoration of the patient's ability to respond to the vaccine depends on the intensity and type of immunosuppression-causing medication used, the underlying disease, and other factors; estimates vary from 3 months to 1 year. Patients with leukemia in remission should not receive live virus vaccine until at least 3 months after their last chemotherapy. Immunization with oral poliovirus vaccine should also be postponed

in persons in close contact with the patient, especially family members)

### Laboratory value alterations

The following have been selected on the basis of their potential clinical significance (possible effect in parentheses where appropriate)—not necessarily inclusive (» = major clinical significance):

With physiology/laboratory test values
Blood urea nitrogen (BUN) and
Creatinine, serum
(concentrations may be increased, indicating renal toxicity)

### Medical considerations/Contraindications

The medical considerations/contraindications included here have been selected on the basis of their potential clinical significance (reasons given in parentheses where appropriate)—not necessarily inclusive (» = major clinical significance):

*Risk-benefit should be considered when the following medical problems exist:*

» Bone marrow depression
» Chickenpox, existing or recent (including recent exposure) or
» Herpes zoster
(risk of severe generalized disease)
» Coagulation disorders
» Infection
» Renal function impairment
(use is not recommended in patients with a serum creatinine greater than 1.7 mg per 100 mL)
Sensitivity to mitomycin
» Caution should be used also in patients who have received previous cytotoxic drug therapy or radiation therapy.

### Patient monitoring

The following are especially important in patient monitoring (other tests may be warranted in some patients, depending on condition; » = major clinical significance):

» Blood urea nitrogen (BUN) concentrations and
» Creatinine concentrations, serum
(recommended prior to initiation of therapy and at periodic intervals during therapy; frequency varies according to clinical state, agent, dose, and other agents being used concurrently)
» Hematocrit or hemoglobin and
» Leukocyte count, total and, if appropriate, differential and
» Observation for fragmented red blood cells on peripheral blood smears and
» Platelet count
(determinations recommended prior to initiation of therapy and at periodic intervals during therapy; frequency varies according to clinical state, agent, dose, and other agents being used concurrently)
Note: It is recommended that renal and hematologic function be followed during and for several months after mitomycin therapy, especially in patients receiving doses of 60 mg or more to detect possible hemolytic-uremic syndrome.

## Side/Adverse Effects

Note: Many "side effects" of antineoplastic therapy are unavoidable and represent the medication's pharmacologic action. Some of these (for example, leukopenia and thrombocytopenia) are actually used as parameters to aid in individual dosage titration.

The following side/adverse effects have been selected on the basis of their potential clinical significance (possible signs and symptoms in parentheses where appropriate)—not necessarily inclusive:

### Those indicating need for medical attention

Incidence more frequent
*Leukopenia or infection* (usually asymptomatic; less frequently, fever or chills; cough or hoarseness; lower back or side pain; painful or difficult urination); *thrombocytopenia* (usually asymptomatic; less frequently, unusual bleeding or bruising; black, tarry stools; blood in urine or stools; pinpoint red spots on skin)
Note: *Leukopenia* and *thrombocytopenia* occur within 3 to 8 weeks of initiation of therapy, and counts return to normal within 10 weeks after therapy is stopped, although in about 25% of episodes counts do not recover. Duration of myelosuppression appears to be inversely related to the initial counts. Severity of bone marrow depression varies and determines subsequent dosage of mitomycin.

Incidence less frequent

*Pneumopathy* (cough; shortness of breath); *renal toxicity* (blood in urine; decreased urination; shortness of breath; swelling of feet or lower legs); *stomatitis* (sores in mouth and on lips)

Note: *Pneumopathy* usually occurs after several doses; it can be severe and may be life-threatening.

*Renal toxicity* has included a hemolytic-uremic syndrome (consisting of microangiopathic hemolytic anemia [hematocrit 25% or less], irreversible renal failure, thrombocytopenia [platelet count less than 100,000], and less frequently, pulmonary hypertension, neurologic abnormalities, and hypertension), which is fatal in greater than 50% of cases. Renal failure without hemolysis has also been reported. The syndrome may occur at any time during therapy with mitomycin, alone or in combination with other chemotherapy. Use of blood product transfusions may exacerbate the symptoms in some patients. Incidence appears to be greatest in patients receiving doses of mitomycin of 60 mg or greater.

Incidence rare

*Bloody vomit; thrombophlebitis, cellulitis, or extravasation* (redness or pain, especially at site of injection)

Note: *Extravasation* may also occur without accompanying burning or stinging. Delayed erythema and ulceration have occurred weeks to months after mitomycin administration, at or distant from the injection site.

**Those indicating need for medical attention only if they continue or are bothersome**
Incidence more frequent

*Loss of appetite; nausea and vomiting*

Note: *Nausea and vomiting* usually occur within 1 to 2 hours; vomiting usually stops in 3 to 4 hours, while nausea may persist for 2 or 3 days.

Incidence less frequent

*Numbness or tingling in fingers and toes; purple-colored bands on nails*—occur with repeated doses; *skin rash; unusual tiredness or weakness*—may last several days to 3 weeks

**Those not indicating need for medical attention**
Incidence less frequent

*Loss of hair*

**Those indicating the need for medical attention if they occur after medication is discontinued**

*Bone marrow depression* (black, tarry stools; blood in urine or stools; cough or hoarseness; fever or chills; lower back or side pain; painful or difficult urination; pinpoint red spots on skin; unusual bleeding or bruising); *possible hemolytic-uremic syndrome* (blood in urine, decreased urination, shortness of breath, swelling of feet or lower legs); *delayed skin reaction* (red or painful skin)

Note: Cumulative *myelosuppression* may occur with repeated doses.

## Patient Consultation

As an aid to patient consultation, refer to *Advice for the Patient, Mitomycin (Systemic)*.

As an aid to patient consultation, consider emphasizing the following selected information (» = major clinical significance):

**Before using this medication**
» Conditions affecting use, especially:

Sensitivity to mitomycin

Pregnancy—Use not recommended because of mutagenic, teratogenic, and carcinogenic potential; advisability of using contraception; telling physician immediately if pregnancy is suspected

Breast-feeding—Not recommended because of risk of serious side effects

Other medications, especially other bone marrow depressants

Other medical problems, especially chickenpox, coagulation disorders, herpes zoster, infection, or renal function impairment

**Proper use of this medication**
Caution in taking combination therapy; taking each medication at the right time

Frequency of nausea and vomiting; importance of continuing medication despite stomach upset

» Proper dosing

**Precautions while using this medication**
» Importance of close monitoring by physician
» Avoiding immunizations unless approved by physician; other persons in patient's household should avoid immunizations with oral po-

liovirus vaccine; avoiding persons who have taken oral poliovirus vaccine or wearing a protective mask that covers nose and mouth

*Caution if bone marrow depression occurs:*

» Avoiding exposure to persons with bacterial infections, especially during periods of low blood counts; checking with physician immediately if fever or chills, cough or hoarseness, lower back or side pain, or painful or difficult urination occur

» Checking with physician immediately if unusual bleeding or bruising; black, tarry stools; blood in urine or stools; or pinpoint red spots on skin occur

Caution in use of regular toothbrush, dental floss, or toothpick; physician, dentist, or nurse may suggest alternatives; checking with physician before having dental work done

Not touching eyes or inside of nose unless hands washed immediately before

Using caution to avoid accidental cuts with use of sharp objects such as safety razor or fingernail or toenail cutters

Avoiding contact sports or other situations where bruising or injury could occur

» Possibility of local tissue injury and scarring if infiltration of intravenous solution occurs or as delayed reaction; telling doctor or nurse right away about redness, pain, or swelling at injection or any other site

**Side/adverse effects**
Importance of discussing possible effects, including cancer, with physician

Signs of potential side effects, especially leukopenia, infection, thrombocytopenia, pneumopathy, renal toxicity, stomatitis, bloody vomit, thrombophlebitis, cellulitis, and extravasation

Physician or nurse can help in dealing with side effects

Possibility of hair loss; should return after treatment has ended

## General Dosing Information

Patients receiving mitomycin should be under supervision of a physician experienced in cancer chemotherapy.

A variety of dosage schedules and regimens of mitomycin in combination with other antitumor agents are used. The prescriber may consult the medical literature as well as the manufacturer's literature in choosing a specific dosage.

Mitomycin is usually administered intravenously via a functioning intravenous catheter.

Care must be taken to avoid extravasation during intravenous administration because of the risk of severe ulceration and necrosis.

If extravasation of mitomycin occurs during intravenous administration, as indicated by local burning or stinging (although it may also occur without stinging or burning sensation), the injection should be stopped immediately and resumed in another vein to complete the dose. Surgical excision of the involved area may be needed.

Mitomycin must not be administered intramuscularly or subcutaneously because it will cause local tissue necrosis.

Mitomycin has also been administered intra-arterially (for example, into hepatic artery) for treatment of some tumors.

Dosage of mitomycin subsequent to the initial course should be adjusted to meet the individual requirements of each patient, on the basis of hematological response of the patient to the previous dose. An additional course of mitomycin should be given only after circulating blood elements have returned to acceptable levels (leukocytes above 3000 per cubic millimeter and platelets above 75,000 per cubic millimeter).

Patients who have not responded after 2 courses of mitomycin are unlikely to show a response.

Because of the delayed and cumulative bone marrow suppression caused by mitomycin, the medication should be given no more frequently than every 6 weeks.

If leukocyte (particularly granulocyte) or platelet counts fall markedly, or a progressive decline occurs in either, it is recommended that mitomycin therapy be withdrawn temporarily until the values recover.

Special precautions are recommended in patients who develop thrombocytopenia as a result of administration of mitomycin. These may include extreme care in performing invasive procedures; regular inspection of intravenous sites, skin (including perirectal area), and mucous membrane surfaces for signs of bleeding or bruising; limiting frequency of venipuncture and avoiding intramuscular injections; testing urine, emesis, stool, and secretions for occult blood; care in use of regular toothbrushes, dental floss, toothpicks, safety razors, and fingernail and toenail cutters; avoiding constipation; and using caution to prevent falls and other injuries. Such patients should avoid alcohol and any aspirin intake because of the risk of gastrointestinal bleeding. Platelet transfusions may be required.

Patients who develop leukopenia should be observed carefully for signs of infection. Antibiotic support may be required. In neutropenic patients who develop fever, broad-spectrum antibiotic coverage should be initiated empirically, pending bacterial cultures and appropriate diagnostic tests.

Topical bladder instillations with 20 to 40 mg of mitomycin in a strength of 1 mg per mL in distilled water, which is retained for as long as possible (usually 2 to 3 hours), are used once weekly for 8 procedures per course in the treatment of small bladder papillomas.

### Safety considerations for handling this medication
There is limited but increasing evidence and concern that personnel involved in preparation and administration of parenteral antineoplastics may be at some risk because of the potential mutagenicity, teratogenicity, and/or carcinogenicity of these agents, although the actual risk is unknown. USP advisory panels recommend cautious handling both in preparation and disposal of antineoplastic agents. Precautions that have been suggested include:

• Use of a biological containment cabinet during reconstitution and dilution of parenteral medications and wearing of disposable surgical gloves and masks.
• Use of proper technique to prevent contamination of the medication, work area, and operator during transfer between containers (including proper training of personnel in this technique).
• Cautious and proper disposal of needles, syringes, vials, ampuls, and unused medication.

A number of medical centers have developed detailed guidelines for handling of antineoplastic agents.

### Combination chemotherapy
Mitomycin may be used in combination with other agents in various regimens. As a result, incidence and/or severity of side effects may be altered and different dosages (usually reduced) may be used. For example, mitomycin is part of the following chemotherapeutic combination (a commonly used acronym is in parentheses):
—fluorouracil, doxorubicin, and mitomycin (FAM).
For specific dosages and schedules, consult the literature. For information regarding each agent, consult the individual monographs.

## Parenteral Dosage Forms

Note: Bracketed uses in the *Dosage Forms* section refer to categories of use and/or indications that are not included in U.S. product labeling.

### MITOMYCIN FOR INJECTION USP

#### Usual adult and adolescent dose
Carcinoma, gastric or
Carcinoma, pancreatic or
[Carcinoma, colorectal]—
    Intravenous, 10 to 20 mg per square meter of body surface as a single dose repeated every six to eight weeks.
    A suggested dosage adjustment schedule for subsequent doses is:

| Nadir after Prior Dose (cells per cubic millimeter) | | Percentage of Prior Dose to Be Given |
|---|---|---|
| Leukocytes | Platelets | |
| >4000 | >100,000 | 100 |
| 3000–3999 | 75,000–99,999 | 100 |
| 2000–2999 | 25,000–74,999 | 70 |
| <2000 | <25,000 | 50 |

#### Usual adult prescribing limits
Doses greater than 20 mg per square meter of body surface appear to be no more effective than lower doses and increase the risk of toxicity.

#### Usual pediatric dose
See *Usual adult and adolescent dose.*

#### Size(s) usually available
U.S.—
    5 mg (Rx) [*Mutamycin* (mannitol 10 mg)].
    20 mg (Rx) [*Mutamycin* (mannitol 20 mg)].
    40 mg (Rx) [*Mutamycin* (mannitol 40 mg)].
Canada—
    5 mg (Rx) [*Mutamycin* (mannitol 10 mg)].
    20 mg (Rx) [*Mutamycin* (mannitol 20 mg)].

#### Packaging and storage
Store below 40 °C (104 °F), preferably between 15 and 30 °C (59 and 86 °F), unless otherwise specified by manufacturer. Protect from light.

#### Preparation of dosage form
Mitomycin for Injection USP is reconstituted for intravenous use by adding 10 mL (5-mg vial), 40 mL (10-mg vial), or 80 mL (40-mg vial) of sterile water for injection to the vial and shaking to dissolve, allowing to stand at room temperature if necessary until solution occurs; a blue-gray solution is produced.
Reconstituted solutions may be further diluted with 5% dextrose injection, 0.9% sodium chloride injection, or sodium lactate injection for administration by intravenous infusion.

#### Stability
Reconstituted solutions of mitomycin are stable for 14 days refrigerated or 7 days at room temperature, when protected from light. When further diluted for administration by intravenous infusion, reconstituted solutions are stable for 3 hours in 5% dextrose injection, 12 hours in 0.9% sodium chloride injection, or 24 hours in sodium lactate injection at room temperature.

### Selected Bibliography
Dorr RT, Fritz WL. Cancer chemotherapy handbook. New York: Elsevier, 1980: 548-55.

Revised: 06/90
Interim revision: 07/30/93; 12/13/93; 07/05/94

---

# MITOTANE   Systemic

VA CLASSIFICATION (Primary/Secondary): AN900/HS900
Another commonly used name is o,p'-DDD.

Note: For a listing of dosage forms and brand names by country availability, see *Dosage Forms* section(s). For a listing of brand names for the articles in this monograph, refer to the General Index.

## Category
Antineoplastic; antiadrenal.

## Indications
Note: Bracketed information in the *Indications* section refers to uses that are not included in U.S. product labeling.

### Accepted
Carcinoma, adrenal cortex (treatment)—Mitotane is indicated in the treatment of inoperable functional and nonfunctional adrenocortical carcinoma.

[Cushing's syndrome (treatment)][1]—Mitotane is also used in the treatment of Cushing's syndrome.

---
[1]Not included in Canadian product labeling.

## Pharmacology/Pharmacokinetics

### Physicochemical characteristics
Molecular weight—320.05.

### Mechanism of action/Effect
Mitotane apparently suppresses the activity of the adrenal cortex. Mechanism of cytotoxic action is unknown, but may be related to adrenal suppression.

### Absorption
Approximately 35 to 40% absorbed from the gastrointestinal tract.

### Distribution
To all body tissues; stored in fat; small amount (as metabolite) crosses blood-brain barrier.

### Biotransformation
Hepatic and renal to water-soluble metabolite.

### Half-life
18 to 159 days.

### Onset of action
Reduced concentrations of 17-hydroxycorticosteroid usually occur within 2 or 3 days after initiation of therapy; tumor response may occur within 6 weeks.

**Time to peak plasma concentration:**
3 to 5 hours.

**Elimination**
Renal, 10 to 25% (as metabolite); bile, 1 to 17% (as metabolite). Measurable plasma concentrations persist for 6 to 9 weeks after withdrawal of mitotane.

## Precautions to Consider

### Carcinogenicity/Mutagenicity
Studies have not been done.

### Pregnancy/Reproduction
Pregnancy—Studies have not been done in either animals or humans (FDA Pregnancy Category C). Problems in humans have not been documented. However, caution is recommended, especially during the first trimester.

### Breast-feeding
It is not known whether mitotane is excreted in breast milk. However, problems in humans have not been documented.

### Pediatrics
Appropriate studies with mitotane have not been performed in the pediatric population. However, pediatrics-specific problems that would limit the usefulness of this medication in children are not expected.

### Geriatrics
No geriatrics-specific information is available on the use of mitotane in geriatric patients.

### Drug interactions and/or related problems
The following drug interactions and/or related problems have been selected on the basis of their potential clinical significance (possible mechanism in parentheses where appropriate)—not necessarily inclusive (» = major clinical significance):

Note: Combinations containing any of the following medications, depending on the amount present, may also interact with this medication.

Adrenocorticoids, glucocorticoid and mineralocorticoid
(higher dosage may be required to treat adrenal insufficiency since mitotane alters metabolism)

» Central nervous system (CNS) depression–producing medications (See *Appendix II*)
(concurrent use may produce additive CNS depressant effects)

Corticotropin (ACTH)
(mitotane may inhibit the adrenal response to ACTH; this may interfere with the therapeutic response to ACTH)

### Laboratory value alterations
The following have been selected on the basis of their potential clinical significance (possible effect in parentheses where appropriate)—not necessarily inclusive (» = major clinical significance):

With physiology/laboratory test values
Plasma cortisol concentrations and
Urinary 17-hydroxycorticosteroid concentrations
(may be decreased as a result of adrenocortical inhibition)

Protein-bound iodine (PBI) concentrations
(may be decreased as a result of mitotane binding to thyroid-binding globulin)

Serum uric acid concentrations
(may be decreased)

### Medical considerations/Contraindications
The medical considerations/contraindications included here have been selected on the basis of their potential clinical significance (reasons given in parentheses where appropriate)—not necessarily inclusive (» = major clinical significance).

*Risk-benefit should be considered when the following medical problems exist:*

» Hepatic function impairment other than metastatic lesion of the adrenal cortex
(reduced metabolism and possible accumulation; reduction in dosage may be required)

» Infection
Sensitivity to mitotane

### Patient monitoring
The following are especially important in patient monitoring (other tests may be warranted in some patients, depending on condition; » = major clinical significance):

Neurological assessments
(recommended at periodic intervals in patients receiving mitotane for longer than 2 years)

» 8 a.m. plasma cortisol concentrations or

» 24-hour urinary 17-hydroxycorticosteroid concentrations
(recommended at periodic intervals to aid in assessing clinical response and to determine if steroid supplement therapy is necessary)

## Side/Adverse Effects

The following side/adverse effects have been selected on the basis of their potential clinical significance (possible signs and symptoms in parentheses where appropriate)—not necessarily inclusive:

**Those indicating need for medical attention**
Incidence more frequent—40 to 80%
*Adrenocortical insufficiency* (darkening of skin; diarrhea; dizziness; drowsiness; loss of appetite; mental depression; nausea and vomiting; skin rash; unusual tiredness)
Incidence less frequent
*Double vision; hemorrhagic cystitis* (blood in urine); *lens opacity or toxic retinopathy* (blurred vision)
Incidence rare
*Allergic reaction* (shortness of breath; wheezing)

**Those indicating need for medical attention only if they continue or are bothersome**
Incidence less frequent
*Aching muscles; fever; flushing or redness of skin; muscle twitching; orthostatic hypotension* (dizziness or lightheadedness when getting up from a lying or sitting position)

## Patient Consultation

As an aid to patient consultation, refer to *Advice for the Patient, Mitotane (Systemic)*.

Consider advising the patient on the following (» = major clinical significance):

**Before using this medication**
See *Precautions to Consider*.

**Proper use of this medication**
» Importance of not taking more or less medication than the amount prescribed

» Checking with physician before discontinuing medication because of risk of adrenal suppression

» Proper dosing
Missed dose: Taking as soon as possible; not taking if almost time for next dose; not doubling doses; checking with physician

» Proper storage

**Precautions while using this medication**
» Importance of close monitoring by the physician
Carrying medical identification card

» Caution in taking alcohol or other CNS depressants

» Caution if dizziness or drowsiness occurs, especially if driving, using machines, or doing other things that require alertness

» Checking with physician immediately if injury, infection, or other illness occurs, because of the risk of adrenal insufficiency; physician may prescribe steroid supplement

**Side/adverse effects**
Signs of potential side effects, especially adrenocortical insufficiency, double vision, hemorrhagic cystitis, lens opacity, toxic retinopathy, and allergic reaction

## General Dosing Information

Patients receiving mitotane should be under supervision of a physician experienced in cancer chemotherapy.

Initial treatment often occurs in the hospital until dosage is stabilized.

Dosage must be adjusted to the maximum dose tolerated to meet the individual requirements of each patient, based on appearance of adverse reactions and improvement in clinical response.

Glucocorticoid therapy is usually required in patients being treated with mitotane; mineralocorticoid therapy may also be required, especially with prolonged therapy. Because metabolism of exogenous adrenocorticoids may be altered in patients receiving mitotane, higher than normal replacement doses may be required. Steroid therapy may have to be continued after mitotane is withdrawn, until adrenocortical function returns to normal.

Continuous treatment with the maximum tolerated dosage of mitotane appears to be more effective than intermittent courses.

Duration of treatment depends on clinical response. Only 10% of patients showing no response after 3 months of treatment at the maximum tolerated dosage will show a response to continued therapy.

It is recommended that mitotane be temporarily withdrawn immediately following shock or severe trauma and that steroids be administered, because adrenal suppression may prevent the normal response to stress.

## Oral Dosage Forms

Note: Bracketed uses in the *Dosage Forms* section refer to categories of use and/or indications that are not included in U.S. product labeling.

### MITOTANE TABLETS USP

**Usual adult dose**
Carcinoma, adrenal cortex—
Initial: Oral, 8 to 10 grams per day in three or four divided doses; the dosage may be increased until adverse reactions occur.
Note: The maximum tolerated dosage may vary from 2 to 16 grams per day, with an average dosage of 8 to 10 grams per day.
[Cushing's syndrome][1]—
Initial: Oral, 3 to 6 grams per day in three or four divided doses.

Maintenance: Oral, 500 mcg (0.5 mg) two times a week to 2 grams per day.

**Usual pediatric dose**
Carcinoma, adrenal cortex—
Oral, 100 to 500 mcg (0.1 to 0.5 mg) per kg of body weight; or initially, 1 to 2 grams per day in divided doses, the dosage being gradually increased to 5 to 7 grams per day.

**Strength(s) usually available**
U.S.—
500 mg (Rx) [*Lysodren* (scored)].
Canada—
500 mg (Rx) [*Lysodren* (scored)].

**Packaging and storage**
Store below 40 °C (104 °F), preferably between 15 and 30 °C (59 and 86 °F), unless otherwise specified by manufacturer. Store in a tight, light-resistant container.

**Auxiliary labeling**
• May cause drowsiness.

[1]Not included in Canadian product labeling.

## Selected Bibliography

Dorr RT, Fritz WL. Cancer chemotherapy handbook. New York: Elsevier, 1980: 556-60.

Revised: 08/90
Interim revision: 06/30/94

# MITOXANTRONE  Systemic

VA CLASSIFICATION (Primary): AN900

Note: For a listing of dosage forms and brand names by country availability, see *Dosage Forms* section(s). For a listing of brand names for the articles in this monograph, refer to the General Index.

## Category
Antineoplastic.

## Indications

Note: Bracketed information in the *Indications* section refers to uses that are not included in U.S. product labeling.

**Accepted**
Leukemia, acute myelocytic (treatment)
Leukemia, acute promyelocytic (treatment)
Leukemia, acute monocytic (treatment) or
Leukemia, acute erythroid (treatment)—Mitoxantrone is indicated, in combination with other agents, for the treatment of acute nonlymphocytic (including myelocytic, promyelocytic, monocytic, and erythroid) leukemia in adults.

[Carcinoma, breast (treatment)]—Mitoxantrone is indicated, alone or in combination with other agents, for treatment of breast carcinoma, including locally advanced and metastatic disease.

[Carcinoma, hepatic (treatment)] or
[Lymphomas, non-Hodgkin's (treatment)]—Mitoxantrone is indicated for treatment of hepatoma and non-Hodgkin's lymphomas.

## Pharmacology/Pharmacokinetics

**Physicochemical characteristics**
Molecular weight—517.41.

**Mechanism of action/Effect**
Mitoxantrone appears to be most active in the late S phase of cell division, but is not cycle phase–specific. Although the exact mechanism of action is unknown, evidence seems to indicate involvement of two effects—binding to DNA by intercalation between base pairs, and a nonintercalative electrostatic interaction—resulting in inhibition of DNA and RNA synthesis.

**Other actions/effects**
Also has antiviral, antibacterial, antiprotozoal, and immunosuppressant effects.

**Distribution**
Rapid and extensive; largest concentrations are in the thyroid, liver, heart, and red blood cells.

**Protein binding**
High (78%).

**Biotransformation**
Hepatic.

**Half-life**
Mean, 5.8 days (range, 2.3–13.0 days).

**Elimination**
Biliary/fecal, up to 25% in 5 days.
Renal, 6-11% (65% unchanged).
Extensive tissue uptake and binding accounts for most of a dose, which is then thought to be gradually released.
In dialysis—Because of extensive tissue binding, unlikely to be significantly removed by hemodialysis or peritoneal dialysis.

## Precautions to Consider

**Carcinogenicity**
Secondary malignancies are potential delayed effects of many antineoplastic agents, although it is not clear whether the effect is related to their mutagenic or immunosuppressive action. The effect of dose and duration of therapy is also unknown, although the risk seems to increase with long-term use. Although information is limited, available data seem to indicate that the carcinogenic risk is greatest with the alkylating agents.

**Mutagenicity**
Mitoxantrone may cause chromosomal aberrations in animals and is mutagenic in bacterial systems. It has been reported to cause DNA damage and sister chromatid exchanges *in vitro*.

**Pregnancy/Reproduction**
Fertility—Gonadal suppression, resulting in amenorrhea or azoospermia, may occur in patients taking antineoplastic therapy, especially with the alkylating agents. In general, these effects appear to be related to dose and length of therapy and may be irreversible. Prediction of the degree of testicular or ovarian function impairment is complicated by the common use of combinations of several antineoplastics, which makes it difficult to assess the effects of individual agents.

Pregnancy—Adequate and well-controlled studies in humans have not been done.

First trimester: It is usually recommended that use of antineoplastics, especially combination chemotherapy, be avoided whenever possible, especially during the first trimester. Although information is limited because of the relatively few instances of antineoplastic administration during pregnancy, the mutagenic, teratogenic, and carcinogenic potential of these medications must be considered.

Other hazards to the fetus include adverse reactions seen in adults.

In general, use of a contraceptive is recommended during cytotoxic drug therapy.

Studies in rats found an increased incidence of low fetal birth weight and retarded development of the fetal kidney, and studies in rabbits found an increased incidence of premature delivery. Mitoxantrone was not found to be teratogenic in rabbits.

FDA Pregnancy Category D.

### Breast-feeding

Although very little information is available regarding distribution of antineoplastic agents into breast milk, breast-feeding is not recommended while mitoxantrone is being administered because of the risks to the infant (adverse effects, mutagenicity, carcinogenicity). It is not known whether mitoxantrone is distributed into breast milk.

### Pediatrics

Appropriate studies on the relationship of age to the effects of mitoxantrone have not been performed in the pediatric population.

### Geriatrics

Appropriate studies on the relationship of age to the effects of mitoxantrone have not been performed in the geriatric population. However, no geriatrics-specific problems have been documented to date.

### Dental

The bone marrow depressant effects of mitoxantrone may result in an increased incidence of microbial infection, delayed healing, and gingival bleeding. Dental work, whenever possible, should be completed prior to initiation of therapy or deferred until blood counts have returned to normal. Patients should be instructed in proper oral hygiene during treatment, including caution in use of regular toothbrushes, dental floss, and toothpicks.

Mitoxantrone also causes stomatitis/mucositis, which may be associated with considerable discomfort.

### Drug interactions and/or related problems

The following drug interactions and/or related problems have been selected on the basis of their potential clinical significance (possible mechanism in parentheses where appropriate)—not necessarily inclusive (» = major clinical significance):

Note: Combinations containing any of the following medications, depending on the amount present, may also interact with this medication.

Allopurinol or
Colchicine or
» Probenecid or
» Sulfinpyrazone
    (mitoxantrone may raise the concentration of blood uric acid; dosage adjustment of antigout medications may be necessary to control hyperuricemia and gout; allopurinol may be preferred to prevent or reverse mitoxantrone-induced hyperuricemia because of risk of uric acid nephropathy with uricosuric antigout agents)

Blood dyscrasia–causing medications (See *Appendix II*)
    (leukopenic and/or thrombocytopenic effects of mitoxantrone may be increased with concurrent or recent therapy if these medications cause the same effects; dosage adjustment of mitoxantrone, if necessary, should be based on blood counts)

» Bone marrow depressants, other (See *Appendix II*) or
Radiation therapy
    (additive bone marrow depression may occur; dosage reduction may be required when two or more bone marrow depressants, including radiation, are used concurrently or consecutively)

Daunorubicin or
Doxorubicin or
Radiation therapy to mediastinal area
    (use of mitoxantrone in a patient who has previously received any of these increases the risk of cardiotoxicity)

Vaccines, killed virus
    (because normal defense mechanisms may be suppressed by mitoxantrone therapy, the patient's antibody response to the vaccine may be decreased. The interval between discontinuation of medications that cause immunosuppression and restoration of the patient's ability to respond to the vaccine depends on the intensity and type of immunosuppression-causing medication used, the underlying disease, and other factors; estimates vary from 3 months to 1 year)

» Vaccines, live virus
    (because normal defense mechanisms may be suppressed by mitoxantrone therapy, concurrent use with a live virus vaccine may potentiate the replication of the vaccine virus, may increase the side/adverse effects of the vaccine virus, and/or may decrease the patient's antibody response to the vaccine; immunization of these patients should be undertaken only with extreme caution after careful review of the patient's hematologic status and only with the knowledge and consent of the physician managing the mitoxantrone therapy. The interval between discontinuation of medications that cause immunosuppression and restoration of the patient's ability to respond to the vaccine depends on the intensity and type of immunosuppression-causing medication used, the underlying disease, and other factors; estimates vary from 3 months to 1 year. Patients with leukemia in remission should not receive live virus vaccine until at least 3 months after their last chemotherapy. Immunization with oral poliovirus vaccine should also be postponed in persons in close contact with the patient, especially family members)

### Laboratory value alterations

The following have been selected on the basis of their potential clinical significance (possible effect in parentheses where appropriate)—not necessarily inclusive (» = major clinical significance):

With physiology/laboratory test values
    Alanine aminotransferase (ALT [SGPT]) values, serum and
    Aspartate aminotransferase (AST [SGOT]) values, serum and
    Bilirubin concentrations, serum
        (may be increased, indicating hepatotoxicity)

    Uric acid
        (concentrations in blood and urine may be increased)

### Medical considerations/Contraindications

The medical considerations/contraindications included here have been selected on the basis of their potential clinical significance (reasons given in parentheses where appropriate)—not necessarily inclusive (» = major clinical significance).

*Risk-benefit should be considered when the following medical problems exist:*

» Bone marrow depression

» Chickenpox, existing or recent (including recent exposure) or
» Herpes zoster
    (risk of severe generalized disease)

Gout, history of or
Urate renal stones, history of
    (risk of hyperuricemia)

» Heart disease
    (increased risk of cardiotoxicity)

Hepatic function impairment, severe
    (mitoxantrone clearance may be reduced; dosage adjustment may be necessary)

» Infection

Sensitivity to mitoxantrone

» Caution should be used also in patients with inadequate bone marrow reserves due to previous cytotoxic drug or radiation therapy.

### Patient monitoring

The following may be especially important in patient monitoring (other tests may be warranted in some patients, depending on condition; » = major clinical significance):

Alanine aminotransferase (ALT [SGPT]) values, serum and
Aspartate aminotransferase (AST [SGOT]) values, serum and
Bilirubin concentrations, serum and
Lactate dehydrogenase (LDH) values, serum
    (recommended prior to initiation of therapy and at periodic intervals during therapy; frequency varies according to clinical state, agent, dose, and other agents being used concurrently)

» Chest x-ray and
» Echocardiography and
Electrocardiogram (ECG) studies and
» Radionuclide angiography determination of ejection fraction
    (recommended prior to initiation of therapy and at periodic intervals during therapy)

» Hematocrit or hemoglobin and
» Leukocyte count, total and, if appropriate, differential and
» Platelet count
    (determinations recommended prior to initiation of therapy and at periodic intervals during therapy; frequency varies according to clinical state, agent, dose, and other agents being used concurrently)

Uric acid concentrations, serum
(recommended prior to initiation of therapy and at periodic intervals during therapy)

## Side/Adverse Effects

Note: Many "side effects" of antineoplastic therapy are unavoidable and represent the medication's pharmacologic action. Some of these (for example, leukopenia and thrombocytopenia) are actually used as parameters to aid in individual dosage titration.

Cardiotoxicity has been reported, including decreased left ventricular ejection fraction, congestive heart failure, ECG changes, arrhythmias such as tachycardia, and, rarely, myocardial infarction. The risk of cardiotoxicity seems to be increased at cumulative mitoxantrone doses exceeding 140 mg per square meter of body surface (100 mg per square meter of body surface in patients with risk factors such as previous treatment with anthracyclines or mediastinal radiation or existing heart disease).

The following side/adverse effects have been selected on the basis of their potential clinical significance (possible signs and symptoms in parentheses where appropriate)—not necessarily inclusive:

### Those indicating need for medical attention
Incidence more frequent
*Cough or shortness of breath; gastrointestinal bleeding* (black, tarry stools); *leukopenia or infection* (usually asymptomatic; less frequently, fever or chills; cough or hoarseness; lower back or side pain; painful or difficult urination); *stomach pain; stomatitis or mucositis* (sores in mouth and on lips)

Note: *Cough or shortness of breath* may be associated with congestive heart failure.

In *leukopenia*, the nadir of the leukocyte count usually occurs within 10 days and usually recovers within 21 days.

*Stomatitis or mucositis* usually occurs within 1 week after the start of treatment.

Incidence less frequent
*Arrhythmias* (fast or irregular heartbeat); *congestive heart failure* (swelling of feet and lower legs); *conjunctivitis* (sore, red eyes); *jaundice* (yellow eyes or skin); *renal failure* (decrease in urination); *seizures; thrombocytopenia* (usually asymptomatic; rarely, unusual bleeding or bruising; black, tarry stools; blood in urine or stools; pinpoint red spots on skin)

Incidence rare
*Allergic reaction, possible* (skin rash); *extravasation* (blue skin at site of injection, pain or redness at site of injection); *local irritation or phlebitis* (pain or redness at site of injection)

Note: Tissue necrosis has been reported in only a few cases after *extravasation*.

### Those indicating need for medical attention only if they continue or are bothersome
Incidence more frequent
*Diarrhea; headache; nausea and vomiting*

Note: *Nausea and vomiting* are usually mild to moderate.

### Those not indicating need for medical attention
Incidence more frequent
*Blue-green urine; loss of hair*

Incidence less frequent
*Blue color in whites of eyes*

## Patient Consultation

As an aid to patient consultation, refer to *Advice for the Patient, Mitoxantrone (Systemic).*

In providing consultation, consider emphasizing the following selected information (» = major clinical significance):

### Before using this medication
» Conditions affecting use, especially:
Sensitivity to mitoxantrone
Pregnancy—Use not recommended because of mutagenic, teratogenic, and carcinogenic potential; advisability of using contraception; telling physician immediately if pregnancy is suspected
Breast-feeding—Not recommended because of risk of serious side effects
Other medications, especially other bone marrow depressants, probenecid, or sulfinpyrazone
Other medical problems, especially chickenpox, herpes zoster, heart disease, or infection

### Proper use of this medication
Caution in taking combination therapy; taking each medication at the right time
Importance of ample fluid intake and subsequent increase in urine output to aid in excretion of uric acid
Frequency of nausea and vomiting; importance of continuing medication despite stomach upset
» Proper dosing

### Precautions while using this medication
» Importance of close monitoring by the physician
» Avoiding immunizations unless approved by physician; other persons in patient's household should avoid immunizations with oral poliovirus vaccine; avoiding persons who have taken oral poliovirus vaccine or wearing a protective mask that covers nose and mouth
*Caution if bone marrow depression occurs:*
» Avoiding exposure to persons with bacterial infections, especially during periods of low blood counts; checking with physician immediately if fever or chills, cough or hoarseness, lower back or side pain, or painful or difficult urination occurs
» Checking with physician immediately if unusual bleeding or bruising; black, tarry stools; blood in urine or stools; or pinpoint red spots on skin occur
Caution in use of regular toothbrush, dental floss, or toothpick; physician, dentist, or nurse may suggest alternatives; checking with physician before having dental work done
Not touching eyes or inside of nose unless hands washed immediately before
Using caution to avoid accidental cuts with use of sharp objects such as safety razor or fingernail or toenail cutters
Avoiding contact sports or other situations where bruising or injury could occur

### Side/adverse effects
Importance of discussing possible effects with physician
Signs of potential side effects, especially cough, shortness of breath, gastrointestinal bleeding, leukopenia, infection, stomach pain, stomatitis, mucositis, arrhythmias, congestive heart failure, conjunctivitis, jaundice, renal failure, seizures, thrombocytopenia, allergic reaction, extravasation, local irritation, and phlebitis
Physician or nurse can help in dealing with side effects
Urine may have blue-green color and whites of eyes may have a blue color during treatment
Possibility of hair loss; normal hair growth should return after treatment has ended

## General Dosing Information

Patients receiving mitoxantrone should be under supervision of a physician experienced in cancer chemotherapy.

A variety of dosage schedules of mitoxantrone, alone or in combination with other antitumor agents, are used. The prescriber may consult the medical literature as well as the manufacturer's literature in choosing a specific dosage.

Dosage must be adjusted to meet the individual requirements of each patient, on the basis of clinical response and appearance or severity of toxicity.

Mitoxantrone hydrochloride injection should not be administered intrathecally; paralysis has occurred after administration by this route. Safety of administration by any route other than the intravenous route has not been established.

*Mitoxantrone hydrochloride concentrate for injection must be diluted prior to intravenous administration.*

An additional course of mitoxantrone should be given only after toxic hematological effects from the first course have subsided.

Although mitoxantrone is nonvesicant and does not usually cause a severe local reaction, if extravasation occurs during intravenous administration, the injection and infusion should be stopped immediately and resumed, completing the dose, in another vein.

Development of uric acid nephropathy in patients with leukemia or lymphoma may be prevented by adequate oral hydration and, in some cases, administration of allopurinol. Alkalinization of urine may be necessary if serum uric acid concentrations are elevated.

Special precautions are recommended in patients who develop thrombocytopenia as a result of administration of mitoxantrone. These may include extreme care in performing invasive procedures; regular inspection of intravenous sites, skin (including perirectal area), and mucous membrane surfaces for signs of bleeding or bruising; limiting frequency of venipuncture and avoiding intramuscular injections; testing urine, emesis, stool, and secretions for occult blood; care in use of regular toothbrushes, dental floss, toothpicks, safety razors, and fingernail and toenail cutters; avoiding constipation; and using caution to prevent falls and other injuries. Such patients should avoid alcohol and any aspirin intake because of the risk of gastrointestinal bleeding. Platelet transfusions may be required.

Patients who develop leukopenia should be observed carefully for signs of infection. Antibiotic support may be required. In neutropenic patients who develop fever, broad-spectrum antibiotic coverage should be initiated empirically, pending bacterial cultures and appropriate diagnostic tests.

### Safety considerations for handling this medication

There is limited but increasing evidence and concern that personnel involved in preparation and administration of parenteral antineoplastics may be at some risk because of the potential mutagenicity, teratogenicity, and/or carcinogenicity of these agents, although the actual risk is unknown. USP advisory panels recommend cautious handling both in preparation and disposal of antineoplastic agents. Precautions that have been suggested include:

• Use of a biological containment cabinet during reconstitution and dilution of parenteral medications and wearing of disposable surgical gloves and masks.

• Use of proper technique to prevent contamination of the medication, work area, and operator during transfer between containers (including proper training of personnel in this technique).

• Cautious and proper disposal of needles, syringes, vials, ampuls, and unused medication.

A number of medical centers have developed detailed guidelines for handling of antineoplastic agents.

## Parenteral Dosage Forms

Note: Bracketed uses in the *Dosage Forms* section refer to categories of use and/or indications that are not included in U.S. product labeling.

### MITOXANTRONE FOR INJECTION CONCENTRATE USP

Note: Although Mitoxantrone for Injection Concentrate USP is available as the hydrochloride salt, dosing and strengths are expressed in terms of the base.

### Usual adult dose

Leukemia, acute myelocytic or
Leukemia, acute promyelocytic or
Leukemia, acute monocytic or
Leukemia, acute erythroid—
  Initial:
    Intravenous infusion (introduced slowly into the tubing of a freely running intravenous infusion of 0.9% sodium chloride injection or 5% dextrose injection over a period of not less than 3 minutes), 12 mg (base) per square meter of body surface daily on Days 1 to 3, in combination with 100 mg of cytarabine (cytosine arabinoside) per square meter of body surface daily given as a continuous 24-hour intravenous infusion on Days 1 to 7.
    Note: If response to the initial course is inadequate, a second induction course at the same dosage may be given.

      If severe or life-threatening nonhematologic toxicity occurs during the first induction course, it is recommended that the second course not be administered until the toxicity has resolved.
  Maintenance:
    Intravenous infusion (introduced slowly into the tubing of a freely running intravenous infusion of 0.9% sodium chloride injection or 5% dextrose injection over a period of not less than 3 minutes), 12 mg (base) per square meter of body surface daily on Days 1 and 2, in combination with 100 mg of cytarabine (cytosine arabinoside) per square meter of body surface daily

given as a continuous 24-hour intravenous infusion on Days 1 to 5.
    Note: The maintenance or consolidation course should not be initiated until leukocyte and platelet counts have returned to pretreatment levels. The maintenance course is usually given approximately six weeks after the first induction course. A second consolidation course may be given four weeks after the first.

[Carcinoma, breast] or
[Carcinoma, hepatic] or
[Lymphomas, non-Hodgkin's]—
  Intravenous infusion (introduced slowly into the tubing of a freely running intravenous infusion of 0.9% sodium chloride injection or 5% dextrose injection over a period of not less than 3 minutes), 14 mg (base) per square meter of body surface every twenty-one days.
  Note: A lower initial dose (12 mg [base] per square meter of body surface) is recommended in patients with inadequate bone marrow reserves. Each subsequent dose should not be given until leukocyte and platelet counts have recovered after the previous dose; dosage reduction may be necessary if severe bone marrow depression occurs.

### Usual pediatric dose

Dosage has not been established.

### Strength(s) usually available

U.S.—
  2 mg (base) per mL (5-, 10-, 12.5-, and 15-mL vials) (Rx) [*Novantrone*].
Canada—
  2 mg (base) per mL (10- and 12.5-mL vials) (Rx) [*Novantrone*].

### Packaging and storage

Store between 15 and 25 °C (59 and 77 °F). Protect from freezing.

### Preparation of dosage form

Mitoxantrone for Injection Concentrate USP must be diluted for administration by intravenous infusion. The dose of mitoxantrone for injection concentrate should be diluted to at least 50 mL in 0.9% sodium chloride injection or 5% dextrose injection.

### Stability

Mitoxantrone for Injection Concentrate USP contains no preservative. Unused portions of solution prepared for intravenous infusion should be discarded. After penetration of the stopper, remaining portions of undiluted mitoxantrone for injection concentrate may be stored for no longer than 7 days at room temperature (15 to 25 °C [59 to 77 °F]) or 14 days in the refrigerator.

### Incompatibilities

Mitoxantrone should not be mixed with heparin, since a precipitate may form.

### Note

Any mitoxantrone solution that comes in contact with the skin or mucosae should be washed off thoroughly with warm water.

## Selected Bibliography

Koeller J, Eble M. Mitoxantrone: a novel anthracycline derivative. Clin Pharm 1988 Aug; 7: 574-81.

Shenkenberg TD, Von Hoff DD. Mitoxantrone: a new anticancer drug with significant clinical activity. Ann Intern Med 1986 Jul; 105: 67-81.

Faulds D, Balfour JA, Chrisp P, et al. Mitoxantrone. A review of its pharmacodynamic and pharmacokinetic properties, and therapeutic potential in the chemotherapy of cancer. Drugs 1991; 41: 400-49.

Revised: 03/16/95

# MIVACURIUM   Systemic†

**VA CLASSIFICATION (Primary): MS300**
Note: For a listing of dosage forms and brand names by country availability, see *Dosage Forms* section(s). For a listing of brand names for the articles in this monograph, refer to the General Index.

†Not commercially available in Canada.

## Category

Neuromuscular blocking agent.

Note: Mivacurium is a nondepolarizing neuromuscular blocking agent with a short duration of action.

## Indications

**Accepted**

Muscle (skeletal) relaxation, for surgery—Mivacurium is indicated as an adjunct to anesthesia to facilitate endotracheal intubation and to induce skeletal muscle relaxation in the surgical field.

**Unaccepted**

Mivacurium has not been adequately studied for facilitating prolonged mechanical ventilation in intensive care patients.

## Pharmacology/Pharmacokinetics

**Physicochemical characteristics**

Source—Synthetic.
Chemical group—bis-Benzylisoquinolinium diester compound.
Molecular weight—1100.18.

Note: Mivacurium is a mixture of 3 stereoisomers, the trans-trans, cis-trans, and cis-cis diesters. The mixture contains about 57% of the trans-trans diester and about 36% of the cis-trans diester. These stereoisomers have neuromuscular blocking activities that are approximately equal to each other and to the mixture as a whole. In animals, the cis-cis diester is approximately one-tenth as potent as the other stereoisomers. Interconversion of the isomers does not occur *in vivo*.

**Mechanism of action/Effect**

Mivacurium is a nondepolarizing (competitive) neuromuscular blocking agent. Nondepolarizing neuromuscular blocking agents inhibit neuromuscular transmission by competing with acetylcholine for the cholinergic receptors of the motor end plate, thereby reducing the response of the end plate to acetylcholine. This type of neuromuscular block is usually antagonized by anticholinesterase agents. Because mivacurium is hydrolyzed by plasma cholinesterase, the possibility that anticholinesterase agents might prolong, rather than reverse, the effects of mivacurium has been considered. However, both neostigmine and edrophonium have been shown to reverse the effects of mivacurium.

Neuromuscular blocking agents have no clinically significant effect on consciousness or the pain threshold.

**Other actions/effects**

Mivacurium may cause histamine release, especially when relatively large doses are administered rapidly, leading to a decrease in blood pressure and an increase in heart rate.

**Distribution**

Volume of distribution—0.15 (range, 0.06 to 0.24), 0.27 (range, 0.08 to 0.56), and 0.31 (range, 0.18 to 0.46) L per kg of body weight, for the trans-trans, cis-trans, and cis-cis diesters, respectively.

**Biotransformation**

Extensive and rapid; via enzymatic hydrolysis catalyzed by plasma cholinesterase. Biotransformation may be significantly slowed in patients with abnormal or decreased plasma cholinesterase activity, especially individuals with a homozygous atypical cholinesterase gene abnormality.

**Half-life**

Elimination—5 to 10 minutes, estimated using the premise that doubling the dose of a medication prolongs the duration of action by the length of its elimination half-life. Half-life values of 2.3 (range, 1.4 to 3.6) and 2.1 (range, 0.8 to 4.8) minutes have been reported for the trans-trans and cis-trans stereoisomers, respectively. A value of 55 (range, 32 to 102) minutes has been reported for the cis-cis diester, but this isomer is not likely to contribute significantly to the effects of the mixture. The half-life is not significantly prolonged in geriatric patients.

**Onset of action**

Time to achieve intubating conditions—
150 mcg per kg of body weight (mcg/kg): About 2.5 minutes.
200 or 250 mcg/kg: About 2 minutes.

**Time to peak effect**

Note: The time to maximal suppression of the twitch response to peripheral nerve stimulation is dependent on dosage and the age of the patient. Also, administration of a volatile inhalation agent (specified below when applicable) may produce a dose-dependent decrease in the time to peak effect.

Children 2 to 12 years of age—
110 to 120 mcg/kg: 2.8 (range, 1.2 to 4.6) minutes.
200 mcg/kg: 1.9 (range, 1.3 to 3.3) minutes.
250 mcg/kg: 1.6 (range, 1.0 to 2.2) minutes.
Nongeriatric adults with normal hepatic and renal function—
70 to 100 mcg/kg: 4.9 (range, 2.0 to 7.6) minutes.
150 mcg/kg: 3.3 (range, 1.5 to 8.8) minutes.
200 mcg/kg: 2.5 (range, 1.2 to 6.0) minutes.
250 mcg/kg: 2.3 (range, 1.0 to 4.8) minutes.
Nongeriatric adults with end-stage renal failure undergoing renal transplantation—
150 mcg/kg (isoflurane/nitrous oxide/oxygen anesthesia): 2.6 (range, 1.0 to 4.5) minutes.
Nongeriatric adults with end-stage hepatic disease undergoing hepatic transplantation—
150 mcg/kg (isoflurane/oxygen anesthesia): 2.1 (range, 1 to 4) minutes.
Geriatric adults 68 to 77 years of age—
100 mcg/kg (isoflurane/nitrous oxide/oxygen anesthesia): 4.8 (range, 3 to 7) minutes; about 1.5 minutes longer than for nongeriatric adults receiving this dose under the same anesthetic regimen.

**Duration of action**

Note: Mivacurium's duration of action is dependent on the patient's age and plasma cholinesterase activity. In addition, the duration of action is more prolonged during anesthesia with a volatile inhalation anesthetic (specified below when applicable) than during other types of anesthesia. Although studies in a limited number of individuals have shown prolonged effects in patients with impaired hepatic or renal function, the contribution of these medical problems to the prolongation of effect, independent of decreased plasma cholinesterase activity and/or the anesthesia given, has not been ascertained.

The duration of mivacurium's clinical effect (time to 25% spontaneous recovery) is influenced by the dose to a significantly lesser extent than that of other nondepolarizing neuromuscular blocking agents. In children, increasing the dose from 110 to 200 mcg/kg, or from 120 to 250 mcg/kg, extends the duration of clinical effect by only 2 to 4 minutes. In adults, the duration of clinical effect of a 200 mcg/kg dose is about 25% longer, and that of a 300 mcg/kg dose is about 50% longer, than that of a 100 mcg/kg dose. In clinical studies, cumulative effects on the duration or depth of neuromuscular blockade did not occur when single supplemental doses were injected after 25% recovery from the previous dose or after cessation of a continuous infusion that was administered at a rate titrated to maintain 95% inhibition of the twitch response to peripheral stimulation.

Duration of clinical effect (time for spontaneous recovery of a single-twitch response to peripheral nerve stimulation to 25% of the control value [$T_{25}$])—
Children 2 to 12 years of age:
110 to 120 mcg/kg—7 (range, 4 to 10) minutes.
200 mcg/kg—10 (range, 6 to 15) minutes.
250 mcg/kg—9 (range, 5 to 12) minutes.
Nongeriatric adults with normal hepatic and renal function:
70 to 100 mcg/kg—13 (range, 8 to 24) minutes.
150 mcg/kg—16 (range, 9 to 38) minutes.
200 mcg/kg—20 (range, 10 to 36) minutes.
250 mcg/kg—23 (range, 14 to 38) minutes.
Nongeriatric adults with end-stage renal disease undergoing renal transplantation:
150 mcg/kg (isoflurane/nitrous oxide/oxygen anesthesia)—30 (range, 19 to 58) minutes.
Nongeriatric adults with end-stage hepatic disease undergoing hepatic transplantation:
150 mcg/kg (isoflurane/oxygen anesthesia)—57 (range, 29 to 80) minutes.

Geriatric adults 68 to 77 years of age:
    100 mcg/kg (isoflurane/nitrous oxide/oxygen anesthesia)—20 (range, 14 to 28) minutes; about 3 minutes longer than for nongeriatric adults receiving this dose under the same anesthetic regimen.
Recovery index (time for the twitch response to peripheral stimulation to increase spontaneously from 25 to 75% of the control value [$T_{25-75}$])—
  Children 2 to 10 years of age:
    200 mcg/kg—About 5 minutes.
  Nongeriatric adults with normal hepatic and renal function:
    150 mcg/kg—About 6 minutes.
    200 or 250 mcg/kg—About 7 to 8 minutes.
Time to spontaneous 95% recovery of the twitch response to peripheral stimulation ($T_{95}$)—
  Children 2 to 12 years of age:
    110 mcg/kg—About 8 minutes.
    200 mcg/kg—19 (range, 14 to 26) minutes.
  Nongeriatric adults with normal hepatic and renal function:
    70 to 100 mcg/kg—21 (range, 10 to 36) minutes.
    150 mcg/kg—26 (range, 16 to 41) minutes.
    200 mcg/kg—31 (range, 15 to 51) minutes.
    250 mcg/kg—34 (range, 22 to 64) minutes.
  Geriatric adults 65 to 80 years of age:
    100 mcg/kg (isoflurane/nitrous oxide/oxygen anesthesia)—Approximately 37 minutes; about 5 minutes longer than for nongeriatric adults receiving this dose under the same anesthetic regimen.
Time to spontaneous recovery of the $T_4:T_1$ ratio (train-of-four stimulation) to 0.75—
  Children 2 to 12 years of age:
    200 mcg/kg—16 (range, 12 to 23) minutes.
  Nongeriatric adults with normal hepatic and renal function:
    70 to 100 mcg/kg—21 (range, 10 to 36) minutes.
    150 mcg/kg—26 (range, 15 to 45) minutes.
    200 mcg/kg—34 (range, 19 to 56) minutes.
    250 mcg/kg—43 (range, 26 to 75) minutes.

**Elimination**
Renal and biliary, as inactive metabolites, following biotransformation (enzymatic hydrolysis catalyzed by plasma cholinesterase). Plasma clearances of the 3 stereoisomers are 53 (range, 32 to 105), 99 (range, 52 to 230), and 4.2 (range, 2.4 to 5.4) mL per kg of body weight per minute for the trans-trans, cis-trans, and cis-cis diesters, respectively.

# Precautions to Consider

## Carcinogenicity
Studies in animals have not been done.

## Mutagenicity
Mivacurium displayed no mutagenicity in the Ames *Salmonella* assay, the mouse lymphoma assay, the human lymphocyte assay, or the *in vivo* rat bone marrow cytogenetic assay.

## Pregnancy/Reproduction
Pregnancy—Adequate and well-controlled studies have not been done in pregnant women. However, the possibility of a prolonged response should be considered, because plasma cholinesterase activity may be reduced during pregnancy.
In animal studies, no maternal or fetal toxicity or teratogenicity occurred with subcutaneous administration of maximal subparalyzing doses to nonventilated pregnant rats or mice.
FDA Pregnancy Category C.
Labor and delivery—Use of mivacurium during labor, vaginal delivery, or cesarean section has not been studied. Whether administration during labor and delivery has any effects in the fetus has not been determined.
In animal studies, administration of 80 or 200 mcg per kg of body weight (mcg/kg) of mivacurium to female beagles undergoing cesarean section produced negligible concentrations of mivacurium in neonatal umbilical vessel blood. No deleterious effects on the puppies were observed.

## Breast-feeding
It is not known whether mivacurium is distributed into human breast milk.

## Pediatrics
Infants and children younger than 2 years of age—Appropriate studies on the relationship of age to the effects of mivacurium have not been performed in patients up to 2 years of age.
Children 2 to 12 years of age—Appropriate studies performed to date have not shown that mivacurium causes different, or more severe, adverse effects than have been reported in adults, or that the risk of adverse effects is increased in children. However, the $ED_{95}$ of mivacurium (dose required to produce 95% suppression of the adductor pollicis

muscle twitch response to ulnar nerve stimulation) and the average infusion rate required to maintain a given degree of neuromuscular blockade are higher in children than in adults. The inverse relationship between mivacurium dosage requirement and the patient's age is significant among children of different ages (as well as between children and adults) when dosage is calculated on an mcg/kg basis, but not when it is calculated on an mcg per square meter of body surface area basis. Also, the onset of action of mivacurium is more rapid, and its duration of action is shorter, in children than in adults. Recovery after administration of a reversal agent also occurs more rapidly in children than in adults.

## Geriatrics
Mivacurium has been studied in geriatric patients, some of whom had significant cardiovascular disease. No geriatrics-specific problems have been documented to date. Although the duration of effect may be about 15 to 20% longer in elderly patients than in younger adults, studies have not shown significant variability in the pharmacokinetics of mivacurium (e.g., elimination half-life or clearance rate) that would account for the observed differences.

## Drug interactions and/or related problems
The following drug interactions and/or related problems have been selected on the basis of their potential clinical significance (possible mechanism in parentheses where appropriate)—not necessarily inclusive (» = major clinical significance):
Note:  Combinations containing any of the following medications, depending on the amount present, may also interact with this medication.

    Some of the following interactions have not been documented with mivacurium. However, because they have been reported to occur with other nondepolarizing neuromuscular blocking agents, the possibility of a significant interaction with mivacurium must be considered.

    Interactions reported below that may lead to enhanced neuromuscular blockade may result in prolonged paralysis, prolonged respiratory insufficiency, and/or difficulty in reversal. These interactions are of minimal clinical significance while the patient is being mechanically ventilated. With the exception of medications that can reduce the concentration or activity of plasma cholinesterase, these interactions may be less significant with a short-acting neuromuscular blocking agent such as mivacurium than with longer-acting agents. However, caution and careful monitoring of the patient are recommended during and following concurrent or sequential use of mivacurium with a medication that may significantly potentiate its effects, especially if there is a possibility of incomplete reversal of neuromuscular blockade postoperatively.

»  Aminoglycosides, possibly including oral neomycin (if significant quantities are absorbed by patients with renal function impairment) or
    Anesthetics, parenteral-local (large doses leading to significant plasma concentrations) or
    Bacitracin or
»  Capreomycin or
»  Citrate-anticoagulated blood (massive transfusions) or
»  Clindamycin or
    Colistin or
    Colistimethate sodium or
    Lidocaine (systemic use, with intravenous doses > 5 mg/kg) or
»  Lincomycin or
»  Polymyxins or
    Procaine (systemic use) or
    Tetracyclines or
    Trimethaphan (large doses)
      (neuromuscular blocking activity of these medications may be additive to that of neuromuscular blocking agents; reversal agents have sometimes been ineffective in reversing neuromuscular blockade potentiated by aminoglycosides, clindamycin, lincomycin, or polymyxins)
    Analgesics, opioid (narcotic), especially those commonly used as adjuncts to anesthesia
      (central respiratory depressant effects of opioid analgesics may be additive to the respiratory insufficiency induced by neuromuscular blocking agents)
      (concurrent use of a neuromuscular blocking agent prevents or reverses muscle rigidity induced by sufficiently high doses of most opioid analgesics, especially alfentanil, fentanyl, or sufentanil)
    Anesthetics, hydrocarbon inhalation, such as:
      Chloroform
      Cyclopropane
      Desflurane

Enflurane
Ether
Halothane
Isoflurane
Methoxyflurane
Trichloroethylene
(neuromuscular blocking activity of inhalation hydrocarbon anesthetics, especially desflurane, enflurane, or isoflurane, may be additive to that of nondepolarizing neuromuscular blocking agents, with the degree of potentiation being increased as the concentration of the anesthetic is increased; a reduction of mivacurium dosage may be necessary when it is given after steady-state anesthesia with one of these anesthetics has been established; with enflurane or isoflurane anesthesia, it is recommended that mivacurium dosage be decreased by about 25% for initial single doses and about 35 to 40% for administration by continuous infusion; although specific recommendations for altering mivacurium dosage during desflurane anesthesia are not currently available, desflurane has been shown to decrease the ED$_{95}$ of other nondepolarizing neuromuscular blocking agents [specifically, atracurium and pancuronium] by approximately 50%)

(halothane potentiates the effects of mivacurium to a lesser extent than enflurane or isoflurane; prior halothane administration may not decrease initial mivacurium dosage requirements, but halothane may decrease maintenance dose [infusion rate] requirements by about 20%, decrease mivacurium's onset of action, and prolong mivacurium's duration of action)

Antihypertensives or other hypotension-inducing medications or
Bradycardia-inducing medications
(although histamine release induced by rapid injection of large doses of mivacurium may increase heart rate, this effect is generally of brief duration, so that mivacurium should not significantly counteract bradycardia induced by other medications or vagal stimulation; however, mivacurium-induced histamine release may cause a temporary decrease in blood pressure, and it is possible that the risk of severe hypotension may be increased in patients receiving other hypotension-inducing medications; therefore, the incidence and/or severity of these effects may be higher with mivacurium than with a neuromuscular blocking agent that has significant vagolytic activity, especially in patients with compromised cardiac function and in patients receiving 2 or more medications that may decrease heart rate and/or blood pressure [e.g., benzodiazepines, beta-adrenergic blocking agents, calcium channel blocking agents, opioid analgesics] prior to and/or during surgery)

Antimyasthenics or
Edrophonium
(these agents antagonize the effects of nondepolarizing neuromuscular blocking agents; parenteral neostigmine, pyridostigmine, or edrophonium are indicated to reverse neuromuscular blockade following surgery, if necessary)

(neuromuscular blocking agents may antagonize the effects of antimyasthenics on skeletal muscle; temporary dosage adjustment may be required to control symptoms of myasthenia gravis following surgery)

Any medication that may reduce plasma cholinesterase concentrations or activity, such as:
Cytotoxic antineoplastic agents
» Demecarium
» Echothiophate
» Insecticides, neurotoxic, recent exposure to, possibly including large quantities of topical malathion
» Isoflurophate
Metoclopramide
Phenelzine
Procaine (systemic)
(reduction of plasma concentrations or activity of cholinesterase, the enzyme that catalyzes hydrolysis of mivacurium, to 50% or less of normal, may enhance and prolong mivacurium's effects; reduction of plasma cholinesterase activity may persist for weeks or months after therapy with demecarium, echothiophate, or isoflurophate has been discontinued)

Calcium channel blocking agents
(although an interaction with mivacurium has not been documented, verapamil and nifedipine have been shown to potentiate the effects of several other neuromuscular blocking agents; also, difficulty in reversing verapamil-potentiated neuromuscular blockade with a single dose of neostigmine has been reported)

Calcium salts
(calcium salts may reverse the effects of nondepolarizing neuromuscular blocking agents)

Carbamazepine and/or
Phenytoin
(although an interaction with mivacurium has not been documented, resistance to the effects of other nondepolarizing neuromuscular agents has occurred in patients receiving chronic carbamazepine and/or phenytoin therapy, leading to a lengthening of the time needed to achieve adequate skeletal muscle relaxation and to significantly accelerated recovery from an initial or supplemental dose)

Dantrolene or
Furosemide or
Lithium or
Magnesium salts, parenteral, or
» Procainamide or
» Quinidine
(these medications may enhance and/or prolong the effects of neuromuscular blocking agents)

Neuromuscular blocking agents, other
(prior administration of succinylcholine [for endotracheal intubation] has caused potentiation of some of the other nondepolarizing neuromuscular blocking agents; although the effect of succinylcholine administration on subsequent administration of mivacurium has not been studied, it is recommended that mivacurium not be administered until after spontaneous recovery from succinylcholine has begun)

(use of subparalyzing doses of mivacurium prior to succinylcholine, to attenuate some of succinylcholine's adverse effects, has not been studied)

(administration of mivacurium in conjunction with other nondepolarizing neuromuscular blocking agents has not been studied)

**Medical considerations/Contraindications**
The medical considerations/contraindications included here have been selected on the basis of their potential clinical significance (reasons given in parentheses where appropriate)—not necessarily inclusive (» = major clinical significance).

Note: Medical problems that may lead to enhanced neuromuscular blockade may result in prolonged paralysis, prolonged respiratory impairment, and/or difficulty in reversal. With the exception of medical conditions associated with a reduction of the concentration or activity of plasma cholinesterase, such medical problems may be less troublesome with a short-acting neuromuscular blocking agent such as mivacurium than with longer-acting agents. However, some patients may require unexpectedly prolonged monitoring and ventilatory assistance postoperatively.

*Except under special circumstances, this medication should not be used when the following medical problem exists:*
» Genetic abnormality, homozygous for atypical cholinesterase gene
(patients with homozygous atypical cholinesterase gene abnormality are extremely sensitive to the effects of mivacurium; in 3 such patients, a dose of only 30 mcg/kg produced complete neuromuscular block lasting from 26 to 128 minutes, although administration of conventional doses of neostigmine after spontaneous recovery began effectively antagonized the remaining block; in a fourth patient, a dose of 180 mcg/kg produced complete neuromuscular block for about 4 hours, and the patient was not extubated until 8 hours after administration [reversal was not attempted]; it is recommended that an alternative nondepolarizing neuromuscular blocking agent be used instead)

*Risk-benefit should be considered when the following medical problems exist:*
Allergy, including asthma, or other conditions predisposing to complications associated with histamine release or
Cardiovascular disease or other conditions in which histamine release–induced hypotension or tachycardia would be particularly hazardous
(it is recommended that initial dosage of mivacurium not exceed 150 mcg/kg, administered over 60 seconds, to decrease the risk of histamine release–related adverse effects)

Burns
(although resistance to the effects of nondepolarizing neuromuscular blocking agents has been reported in burn patients, the reduction in plasma cholinesterase activity that may occur in burn patients may prolong the effect of mivacurium; because the effect of mivacurium in these patients may be unpredictable, it is recommended that the response to a test dose of 15 to 20 mcg/kg, as determined via peripheral nerve stimulation, be used as a guide to appropriate dosage)

Carcinoma, bronchogenic, or other malignancy
>> (the duration of action of nondepolarizing neuromuscular agents may be prolonged in patients with bronchogenic carcinoma; also, the reduction in plasma cholinesterase activity that may occur in patients with malignancy may prolong the effect of mivacurium)

Dehydration or
Electrolyte or acid-base imbalance, especially:
Hypokalemia
(action of neuromuscular blocking agents may be altered; neuromuscular blockade is usually counteracted by alkalosis and enhanced by acidosis, but mixed imbalances may be present, leading to unpredictable responses; also, the reduction in plasma cholinesterase activity that may occur in dehydrated patients may prolong the effect of mivacurium)

(serum potassium determinations may be advisable prior to administration of a nondepolarizing neuromuscular blocking agent, because hypokalemia tends to enhance the blockade produced by these medications; adjustment of dosage of the neuromuscular blocking agent, or correction of potassium concentration prior to administration, may be needed)

» Familial periodic paralysis, hypokalemic or hyperkalemic, or
» Muscular dystrophy or
» Myasthenia gravis or
» Myasthenic syndrome (Eaton-Lambert syndrome) or
» Other neuromuscular disease leading to muscle weakness
(risk of severe and prolonged muscle paralysis or weakness is increased; neuromuscular blocking agents are best avoided in patients with familial periodic paralysis or myasthenia gravis [and may not be needed in patients with myasthenia gravis if a volatile anesthetic with potent relaxant properties, such as enflurane or isoflurane, is administered in sufficient quantities]; if a neuromuscular blocking agent is needed for these patients, mivacurium may be preferable to longer-acting agents, but caution is recommended; patient response to a test dose of 15 to 20 mcg/kg, as determined via peripheral nerve stimulation, should be used as a guide to appropriate dosage)

» Genetic abnormality, heterozygous for atypical cholinesterase gene, or
Other conditions in which plasma cholinesterase activity may be substantially reduced, such as:
Anemia, severe
Exposure to neurotoxic insecticides or other cholinesterase inhibitors
Hepatic disease, severe or chronic, including hepatic cirrhosis
Malnutrition
Pregnancy
(effects of mivacurium may be enhanced and/or prolonged, especially when plasma cholinesterase activity is reduced to 50% or less of normal; in most patients, the time to 25% recovery of the twitch response to peripheral stimulation [$T_{25}$] is prolonged [by 8 to 11 minutes following doses of 100 to 200 mcg/kg in patients with heterozygous gene abnormality, compared with genotypically normal patients], but not the time from 25% to 75% recovery [$T_{25-75}$]; although mivacurium has been used safely in patients with reduced plasma cholinesterase activity, it is recommended that the response to a test dose of 15 to 20 mcg/kg, as determined via peripheral nerve stimulation, be used as a guide to appropriate dosage)

Hypothermia
(intensity and duration of action of nondepolarizing neuromuscular blocking agents may be increased)

Obesity
(the risk of a > 30% decrease in mean arterial blood pressure is increased in obese patients receiving doses calculated on the basis of actual body weight; it is recommended that dosage for these patients be calculated on the basis of ideal body weight)

Pulmonary function impairment or
Respiratory depression
(risk of additive respiratory depression or impairment)

Sensitivity to mivacurium

## Side/Adverse Effects

Note: Mivacurium failed to trigger malignant hyperthermia in a study in malignant hyperthermia–susceptible swine. Whether mivacurium may precipitate malignant hyperthermia in susceptible humans has not been assessed.

Bradycardia may occur during mivacurium-assisted anesthesia, but is not likely to be a direct effect of the medication. Because mivacurium (unlike gallium and pancuronium) does not have vagolytic activity, it does not counteract bradycardia induced by other medications (e.g., anesthetics, opioid analgesics) or vagal stimulation.

The following side/adverse effects have been selected on the basis of their potential clinical significance (possible signs and symptoms in parentheses where appropriate)—not necessarily inclusive:

**Those indicating need for medical attention**
Incidence less frequent
*Hypotension*

Incidence rare (1% or less)
*Bronchospasm; cardiac arrhythmia; erythema; hypoxemia; injection site reaction; phlebitis; skin rash; tachycardia; urticaria; wheezing*

Note: *Hypotension, tachycardia, bronchospasm,* and/or *wheezing* may result from mivacurium-induced histamine release, which may occur when large initial doses of the medication are administered rapidly. In most patients, these effects last only a few minutes and do not require treatment. In clinical trials, *hypotension* requiring treatment occurred in 1 to 2% of patients receiving > 200 mcg per kg of body weight (mcg/kg) of mivacurium over 5 to 15 seconds, and 2 to 4% of cardiac surgery patients receiving > 200 mcg/kg over 60 seconds, but did not occur with doses of 150 mcg/kg or less.

*Hypotension* may also occur during mivacurium-assisted surgery because mivacurium does not counteract the hypotensive effects of other medications or vagal stimulation.

**Those indicating need for medical attention only if they continue or are bothersome**
Incidence less frequent or rare
*Dizziness; muscle spasm*

**Those not indicating need for medical attention**
Incidence more frequent
*Flushing*—incidence 15 to 20%

Note: *Flushing* occurs mostly when initial doses of 150 mcg/kg or higher are administered over 5 to 15 seconds. It usually appears within 1 to 2 minutes after administration and persists for 3 to 5 minutes.

## Overdose

For specific information on the agents used in the management of mivacurium overdose, see:
• *Atropine* in *Anticholinergics/Antispasmodics (Systemic)* monograph;
• *Edrophonium (Systemic)* monograph;
• *Glycopyrrolate* in *Anticholinergics/Antispasmodics (Systemic)* monograph; and/or
• *Neostigmine* in *Antimyasthenics (Systemic)* monograph.

For more information on the management of overdose or unintentional ingestion, **contact a Poison Control Center** (see *Poison Control Center Listing*).

**For treatment of overdose**
Specific treatment—
Because of mivacurium's short duration of action, administration of a reversal agent may not be necessary, or may not speed recovery to a clinically significant extent. However, an anticholinesterase agent, e.g., neostigmine or edrophonium, may be administered if needed. Use of an antagonist is an adjunct to, and not a substitute for, measures to ensure adequate ventilation. Ventilatory assistance must be continued until the patient can maintain an adequate ventilatory exchange unassisted. A suitable antimuscarinic agent (e.g., atropine, glycopyrrolate) should be administered prior to or concurrently with the antagonist to counteract its muscarinic side effects. It is recommended that reversal agents be administered only after some spontaneous recovery, as demonstrated using a peripheral nerve stimulator, has taken place. In adults, doses of 30 to 64 mcg/kg of neostigmine or 500 mcg/kg of edrophonium, administered at 10% recovery from neuromuscular block, generally produce 95% recovery of the single twitch response, and 75% recovery of the $T_4$:$T_1$ ratio (train-of-four stimulation), in about 10 minutes. In children younger than 12 years of age, 300 mcg/kg of edrophonium, administered at 11% or more recovery, produces 95% recovery of the single twitch response in less than 4 minutes. However, recovery may be delayed if the reversal agent is administered in the presence of medications or medical conditions that tend to prolong the effects of mivacurium.

Monitoring—
Determining the degree of the neuromuscular blockade with a peripheral nerve stimulator.

Supportive care—
For hypotension or other adverse hemodynamic effects—Cardiovascular support, e.g., fluid administration, proper positioning of the patient, and/or administration of a vasopressor may be needed.

For apnea or prolonged paralysis—Maintaining an adequate airway and assisting or controlling ventilation. If prolonged paralysis occurs, checking the patient's plasma cholinesterase activity (via determination of dibucaine number and activity). If the patient's cholinesterase activity is found to be significantly reduced, continued respiratory support, rather than administration of a reversal agent, is recommended.

## General Dosing Information

Neuromuscular blocking agents have no clinically significant effect on consciousness or the pain threshold; therefore, when used as an adjunct to surgery, they should always be used with adequate anesthesia or sedation.

Because neuromuscular blocking agents suppress respiration, they should be used only by individuals experienced in tracheal intubation, artificial respiration, and the administration of oxygen under positive pressure; facilities for these procedures should be immediately available.

Mivacurium is intended for intravenous administration only.

The stated doses are intended as a guideline. Actual dosage must be individualized. It is recommended that a peripheral nerve stimulator be used to monitor response, need for additional doses, and reversal.

The ED$_{95}$ (dose required to produce maximum [95%] suppression of the adductor pollicis muscle twitch response to ulnar nerve stimulation) is about 70 (range, 60 to 90) mcg per kg of body weight (mcg/kg) in adults and about 100 to 110 mcg/kg in children 2 to 12 years of age (opioid/nitrous oxide/oxygen anesthesia).

A reduction in initial and maintenance doses of a nondepolarizing neuromuscular blocking agent may be required when it is administered after steady-state anesthesia has been established with a volatile (hydrocarbon) inhalation anesthetic. Halothane may cause less potentiation of mivacurium than desflurane, enflurane, or isoflurane.

A reduction of initial dosage may be advisable for patients in whom histamine release may be hazardous; patients with decreased plasma cholinesterase activity, hepatic or renal disease, burns, severe electrolyte abnormalities, or neuromuscular disease; and other patients in whom there is a risk of potentiation of neuromuscular blockade or difficulty with reversal. Supplemental doses should be titrated according to patient response. A slower rate of administration (i.e., administration of initial doses over 30 to 60 seconds) and/or pretreatment with antihistamines (both H$_1$- and H$_2$-receptor blockers) may also decrease the risk to patients who may be harmed by histamine release.

For obese patients (> 30% above ideal body weight for height), dosage of mivacurium should be calculated on the basis of ideal body weight.

## Parenteral Dosage Forms

### MIVACURIUM INJECTION

Note: Mivacurium injection contains mivacurium chloride, but the dosing and strengths are expressed in terms of mivacurium base.

**Usual adult dose**
Neuromuscular blocking agent—
Initial (for endotracheal intubation and surgical relaxation):
Intravenous, 150 to 200 mcg (0.15 to 0.2 mg) per kg of body weight, administered over five to fifteen seconds, to provide intubating conditions in about two to two and one-half minutes and about fifteen to twenty minutes of clinically effective neuromuscular block (opioid/nitrous oxide/oxygen anesthesia).

Note: Satisfactory intubating conditions are attained more slowly when initial doses lower than 150 mcg per kg of body weight are administered.

For patients with cardiovascular disease or other patients who may be especially sensitive to histamine release, it is recommended that initial doses of 150 mcg per kg of body weight, or lower, be administered over at least sixty seconds. In most other patients, higher initial doses may be administered when a more rapid onset of action is needed, although the risk of inducing hypotension in some patients must be kept in mind. However, administration of higher initial doses may not reduce the onset of action sufficiently to permit emergency intubation. Initial doses higher than 250 mcg (0.25 mg) per kg of body weight are not recommended.

Initial dosage may be decreased by 25% or more when mivacurium is administered after anesthesia with enflurane or isoflurane has been established. The need for a reduction in initial dosage should also be anticipated after anesthesia with desflurane has been established, but studies to determine the extent to which dosage should be reduced have

not been done. A reduction in the initial mivacurium dose may not be needed after anesthesia with halothane has been established.

Maintenance:
Intravenous, to be administered after the twitch response to a previous dose has returned to about 10 to 25% of the control value, or after reappearance of the second twitch response to train-of-four stimulation—About 100 mcg (0.1 mg) per kg of body weight, to provide about fifteen additional minutes of clinically effective block (opioid/nitrous oxide/oxygen anesthesia). Smaller or larger doses may be given as needed to provide shorter or longer durations of action.

Note: Maintenance dosage requirements may be reduced by 25% or more when enflurane or isoflurane is being administered, and by a smaller amount when halothane is being administered. The need for a reduction in maintenance dosage should also be anticipated when desflurane is being administered, but studies to determine the extent to which dosage should be reduced have not been done.

Maintenance doses of mivacurium injection may also be given by intravenous infusion. See *Mivacurium in dextrose injection* for recommended doses. The manufacturer's prescribing information contains a table showing infusion delivery rate requirements (in mL per hour) for administration of various doses (in mcg per kg of body weight per minute) to patients of different weights.

**Usual pediatric dose**
Neuromuscular blocking agent—
Children up to 2 years of age:
Dosage has not been established.
Children 2 to 12 years of age:
Initial—Intravenous, 200 to 250 mcg (0.2 to 0.25 mg) per kg of body weight, administered over fifteen seconds, to provide maximum blockade in about two minutes and about ten minutes of clinically effective block (opioid/nitrous oxide/oxygen anesthesia).

Maintenance—Intravenous, as required by clinical circumstances and the desired duration of clinically effective block. Additional doses may be required more frequently than in adults.

Note: No information is available about the effect of desflurane, enflurane, or isoflurane anesthesia on dosage requirements and/or the duration of clinical effect of mivacurium in pediatric patients. However, in two studies, the duration of clinical effect with nitrous oxide/halothane/oxygen anesthesia was not significantly different from that produced by the same dose under nitrous oxide/opioid/oxygen anesthesia.

Maintenance doses of mivacurium injection may also be given by intravenous infusion. See *Mivacurium in dextrose injection* for recommended doses. The manufacturer's prescribing information contains a table showing infusion delivery rate requirements (in mL per hour) for administration of various doses (in mcg per kg of body weight per minute) to patients of different weights.

**Strength(s) usually available**
U.S.—
2 mg per mL (Rx) [*Mivacron*].
Canada—
Not commercially available.

**Packaging and storage**
Store between 15 and 25 °C (59 and 77 °F), protected from exposure to direct ultraviolet light and from freezing, unless otherwise specified by manufacturer.

**Stability**
Mivacurium injection is physically and chemically stable for up to 24 hours when diluted to 500 mcg (0.5 mg) per mL with 5% dextrose injection, 5% dextrose and 0.9% sodium chloride injection, 0.9% sodium chloride injection, lactated Ringer's injection, or 5% dextrose in lactated Ringer's injection and stored in polyvinyl chloride bags at 5 to 25 °C (4 to 77 °F). After preparation, the diluted solution should be used within 24 hours. Also, the solution should be used for one patient only, and unused portions discarded.

**Incompatibilities**
Mivacurium injection should not be admixed with other medications (except for preparation of an infusion solution using a diluent listed under *Stability*, above). Mivacurium injection is acidic (pH 3.5 to 5.0) and may not be compatible with alkaline solutions (pH > 8.5), such as barbiturate solutions.

## MIVACURIUM IN DEXTROSE INJECTION

Note: Mivacurium in dextrose injection contains mivacurium chloride, but the dosing and strengths are expressed in terms of mivacurium base.

**Usual adult dose**
Neuromuscular blocking agent—
  Maintenance: Intravenous infusion, started after some evidence of recovery from an initial dose—Initially 9 to 10 mcg (0.009 to 0.01 mg) per kg of body weight per minute (opioid/nitrous oxide/oxygen anesthesia), then adjusted according to clinical conditions and response to peripheral nerve stimulation. Infusion rate requirements are generally significantly higher during the first fifteen minutes of infusion, after which an average dose of 6 to 7 mcg (0.006 to 0.007) per kg of body weight per minute is usually sufficient. Although infusion rate requirements are subject to wide interindividual variability (ranging from 1 to 15 mcg [0.001 to 0.015 mg] per kg of body weight per minute), dosage requirements for an individual patient, after the first fifteen-minute adjustment period, remain fairly stable.

Note: A lower initial infusion rate, e.g., 4 mcg (0.004 mg) per kg of body weight per minute, is recommended when an intravenous infusion is started simultaneously with administration of an initial dose.

Infusion rate requirements are reduced after anesthesia with a volatile hydrocarbon anesthetic has been established. Enflurane or isoflurane, depending on the concentration being administered, may reduce the infusion rate requirement by 35 to 40% or more. Halothane may reduce the infusion rate requirement by about 20%.

The manufacturer's prescribing information contains a table showing infusion delivery rate requirements (in mL per hour) for administration of various doses (in mcg per kg of body weight per minute) to patients of different weights.

**Usual pediatric dose**
Neuromuscular blocking agent—
  Maintenance: Infants and children up to 2 years of age—Dosage has not been established.
  Children 2 to 12 years of age—Intravenous infusion, about 14 mcg (0.014 mg) per kg of body weight per minute (average for opioid/nitrous oxide/oxygen anesthesia) or as required. In general, higher infusion rates are required for pediatric patients than for adults.

Note: The manufacturer's prescribing information contains a table showing infusion delivery rate requirements (in mL per hour) for administration of various doses (in mcg per kg of body weight per minute) to patients of different weights.

**Strength(s) usually available**
U.S.—
  500 mcg (0.5 mg) of mivacurium and 5% of dextrose per mL (Rx) [*Mivacron*].
Canada—
  Not commercially available.

**Packaging and storage**
Store between 15 and 25 °C (59 and 77 °F), protected from exposure to direct ultraviolet light and from freezing, unless otherwise specified by manufacturer.

**Stability**
Mivacurium in dextrose injection is intended for single-patient use only. Unused portions of the solution should be discarded.
For Y-site administration, mivacurium in dextrose injection is compatible with 5% dextrose injection, 0.9% sodium chloride injection, 5% dextrose and 0.9% sodium chloride injection, lactated Ringer's injection, 5% dextrose in lactated Ringer's injection, and, when the following are diluted for intravenous injection as directed, with alfentanil hydrochloride injection, fentanyl citrate injection, midazolam hydrochloride injection, and droperidol injection.

**Incompatibilities**
Mivacurium in dextrose injection is acidic (pH 3.5 to 5.0) and may not be compatible with alkaline solutions (pH > 8.5), such as barbiturate solutions.
Mivacurium in dextrose injection should not be admixed with other medications or used in series connections with other medications.

## Selected Bibliography

Savarese JJ, Ali HH, Basta SJ, et al. The clinical neuromuscular pharmacology of mivacurium chloride (BW B1090U). Anesthesiology 1988; 68: 723-32.
Sarner JB, Brandom BW, Woelfel SK, et al. Clinical pharmacology of mivacurium chloride (BW B1090U) in children during nitrous oxide–halothane and nitrous oxide–narcotic anesthesia. Anesth Analg 1989; 68: 116-21.
Choi WW, Mehta MP, Murray DJ, et al. Neuromuscular and cardiovascular effects of mivacurium chloride in surgical patients receiving nitrous oxide–narcotic or nitrous oxide–isoflurane anaesthesia. Can J Anaesth 1989; 36: 641-50.

Revised: 01/18/93

## MODULAR ENTERAL NUTRITION FORMULAS—
See *Enteral Nutrition Formulas (Systemic)*

# MOLINDONE   Systemic†

VA CLASSIFICATION (Primary): CN709
Note: For a listing of dosage forms and brand names by country availability, see *Dosage Forms* section(s). For a listing of brand names for the articles in this monograph, refer to the General Index.

†Not commercially available in Canada.

## Category
Antipsychotic.

## Indications

**Accepted**
Psychotic disorders (treatment)—Molindone is indicated for the management of the manifestations of psychotic conditions, especially in patients with chronic schizophrenia, brief reactive psychosis, or schizophreniform disorders.

**Unaccepted**
Molindone is *not* recommended for management of behavioral complications in mentally retarded patients.

## Pharmacology/Pharmacokinetics

**Physicochemical characteristics**
Molecular weight—312.84.
pKa—6.94.

**Mechanism of action/Effect**
The exact mechanism has not been established; however, based on electroencephalogram (EEG) studies, molindone is thought to act by occupying dopamine ($D_2$) receptor sites in the reticular activating and limbic systems in the brain, thus decreasing dopamine activity.

**Other actions/effects**
Causes changes in resting and sleeping EEG readings.
May decrease the duration of sleep.
May have an antiemetic effect.

**Absorption**
Rapidly absorbed from the gastrointestinal tract after oral administration.

**Biotransformation**
Probably hepatic; 36 recognized metabolites, some of which may be active.

**Time to peak serum concentration**
1.5 hours.

**Duration of action**
24 to 36 hours.

**Elimination**
More than 90% of a single dose is excreted as metabolites in urine and feces within 24 hours. Less than 2 to 3% is excreted unchanged. Small amount excreted via lungs as carbon dioxide.

# Precautions to Consider

### Cross-sensitivity and/or related problems
Patients sensitive to other antipsychotic agents, such as phenothiazines, thioxanthenes, haloperidol, and loxapine, may be sensitive to this medication also.

### Carcinogenicity/Tumorigenicity
Most antipsychotic medications have been found to cause increased serum prolactin concentrations. Although the clinical significance of this increase is not known for most patients, *in vitro* studies have shown approximately $1/3$ of human breast cancers to be prolactin-dependent. In addition, an increase in mammary neoplasms has been found in rodents after chronic administration of antipsychotics. However, a definite association between the chronic administration of these medications and mammary tumorigenesis has not been established, because of limited evidence currently available.

### Pregnancy/Reproduction
Pregnancy—Adequate and well-controlled studies in humans have not been done.

Studies in animals have not shown that molindone causes birth defects. Studies in mice have shown that molindone at oral doses of 20 and 40 mg per kg of body weight (mg/kg) per day for 10 days caused a slight increase in resorptions.

### Breast-feeding
It is not known if molindone is excreted in breast milk. However, problems in humans have not been documented.

### Pediatrics
Appropriate studies on the relationship of age to the effects of molindone have not been performed in children up to 12 years of age. Safety and efficacy have not been established.

### Geriatrics
Geriatric patients tend to develop higher plasma concentrations of molindone because of changes in distribution due to decreases in lean body mass, total body water, and albumin, and often an increase in total body fat composition. Therefore, these patients usually require lower initial dosage and a more gradual titration of dose.

Elderly patients appear to be more prone to orthostatic hypotension and exhibit an increased sensitivity to the anticholinergic and sedative effects of molindone. In addition, they are more prone to develop extrapyramidal side effects, such as tardive dyskinesia and parkinsonism. The symptoms of tardive dyskinesia are persistent, difficult to control, and, in some patients, appear to be irreversible. There is no known effective treatment. Careful observation during treatment for early signs of tardive dyskinesia and reduction of dosage or discontinuation of medication may prevent a more severe manifestation of the syndrome.

It has been suggested that elderly patients should receive half the usual adult dose. A periodic attempt should be made to discontinue medication as soon as the patient improves.

### Dental
The peripheral anticholinergic effects of molindone may decrease or inhibit salivary flow, especially in middle-aged or elderly patients, thus contributing to the development of caries, periodontal disease, candidiasis, or discomfort.

Extrapyramidal reactions induced by molindone will result in increased motor activity of the head, face, and neck. Occlusal adjustments, bite registrations, and treatment for bruxism may be made less reliable.

### Drug interactions and/or related problems
The following drug interactions and/or related problems have been selected on the basis of their potential clinical significance (possible mechanism in parentheses where appropriate)—not necessarily inclusive (» = major clinical significance):

Note: Combinations containing any of the following medications, depending on the amount present, may also interact with this medication.

Although not all of the following interactions have been documented specifically for molindone, a potential exists for their occurrence because of the close similarity of molindone's pharmacological effects to those of phenothiazines and other antipsychotic medications.

» Alcohol or
» Central nervous system (CNS) depression–producing medications, other, especially anesthetics, barbiturates, benzodiazepines, and opioid (narcotic) analgesics (See *Appendix II*)
    (concurrent use may potentiate and prolong the CNS depressant effects of either these medications or molindone)

Amphetamines
    (concurrent use with molindone may antagonize the stimulant effects of amphetamines and counteract the antipsychotic effects of molindone)

Antacids or
Antidiarrheals, adsorbent
    (concurrent use may inhibit the absorption of molindone; these medications should not be taken within 1 to 2 hours of molindone)

Anticholinergics or other medications with anticholinergic activity (See *Appendix II*) or
Antidyskinetic agents or
Antihistamines
    (concurrent use with molindone may potentiate anticholinergic effects, such as urinary retention, blurred vision, dry mouth, and constipation)

Antidepressants, tricyclic or
Maprotiline or
Monoamine oxidase (MAO) inhibitors, including furazolidone and procarbazine or
Trazodone
    (concurrent use may prolong and intensify the sedative or anticholinergic effects of these medications or molindone)

Antidiabetic agents, oral or
Insulin
    (high doses of molindone, when added to an existing antidiabetic regimen, may increase plasma glucose concentrations, leading to loss of control of diabetes)

Beta-adrenergic blocking agents, especially metoprolol or propranolol
    (concurrent use may increase the effects of beta-blockers by decreasing first-pass metabolism; reduction in dosage of beta-blocking agent may be required)

Bromocriptine
    (molindone may increase serum prolactin concentrations and interfere with therapeutic effects of bromocriptine; dosage increase of bromocriptine may be necessary)

» Extrapyramidal reaction–causing medications, other (See *Appendix II*)
    (concurrent use with molindone may increase the severity and frequency of extrapyramidal effects)

Levodopa
    (concurrent use may inhibit antiparkinsonian effects of levodopa by blocking dopamine receptors in the brain and may counteract the antipsychotic effects of molindone)

» Lithium
    (concurrent use with molindone may produce neurotoxic symptoms, such as confusion, delirium, seizures, somnambulism, or abnormal EEG changes; extrapyramidal symptoms may be increased; also, antiemetic effect of molindone may mask nausea and vomiting, which are early signs of lithium toxicity)

Phenytoin or
Tetracycline
    (calcium ions from the excipient in molindone may interfere with the absorption of these medications)

### Laboratory value alterations
The following have been selected on the basis of their potential clinical significance (possible effect in parentheses where appropriate)—not necessarily inclusive (» = major clinical significance):

With physiology/laboratory test values
Blood urea nitrogen (BUN) and
Glucose, serum and
Red blood cell counts
    (alterations may occur but are not considered clinically significant)

Electrocardiogram (ECG) readings
    (rare, transient, nonspecific T-wave changes have been reported)

Prolactin
    (serum concentrations may be persistently elevated during chronic administration)

White blood cell counts
    (may be increased or decreased, but molindone therapy may be continued if clinical symptoms of leukopenia or leukocytosis are absent; however, it has been suggested that if the white blood cell count is below 4000 without clinical symptoms, molindone should be discontinued until white blood cell counts increase; then therapy should be re-evaluated)

## Medical considerations/Contraindications

The medical considerations/contraindications included here have been selected on the basis of their potential clinical significance (reasons given in parentheses where appropriate)—not necessarily inclusive (» = major clinical significance):

*Except under special circumstances, this medication should not be used when the following medical problems exist:*

» CNS depression, severe, drug-induced

» Comatose states

*Risk-benefit should be considered when the following medical problems exist:*

Brain tumor or
Intestinal obstruction
 (antiemetic effect of molindone may mask early signs of brain tumor or intestinal obstruction and interfere with diagnosis)

Glaucoma or
Hepatic function impairment or
Prostatic hypertrophy or
Urinary retention
 (may be aggravated)

Parkinson's disease
 (potentiation of extrapyramidal effects)

Sensitivity to molindone or other antipsychotic medications

### Patient monitoring

The following may be especially important in patient monitoring (other tests may be warranted in some patients, depending on condition; » = major clinical significance):

Careful observation for early symptoms of tardive dyskinesia
 (recommended at periodic intervals, especially in the elderly and those patients on high or extended maintenance dosage, although symptoms may appear when doses are small and treatment periods brief; since there is no known effective treatment if syndrome should develop, molindone should be discontinued, if clinically feasible, at the appearance of early symptoms, such as unusual tongue and mouth movements)

Careful observation for early symptoms of tardive dystonia
 (recommended at periodic intervals; since there is no known effective treatment if syndrome should develop, molindone should be discontinued, if clinically feasible, at the earliest signs)

Liver function tests
 (may be required periodically during therapy)

Ophthalmologic examinations
 (may be required at periodic intervals during high-dose or prolonged therapy since deposition of particulate matter in the lens and cornea has occurred with some phenothiazines, although not reported with molindone)

# Side/Adverse Effects

The following side/adverse effects have been selected on the basis of their potential clinical significance (possible signs and symptoms in parentheses where appropriate)—not necessarily inclusive:

### Those indicating need for medical attention

Incidence more frequent

*Akathisia* (severe restlessness or need to keep moving)—may be more frequent in elderly patients; *extrapyramidal effects, dystonic* (muscle spasms of face, neck, and back; tic-like or twitching movements; twisting movements of body; inability to move eyes; weakness of arms and legs); *extrapyramidal effects, parkinsonian* (difficulty in talking; loss of balance control; mask-like face; shuffling walk; stiffness of arms and legs; trembling and shaking of hands); *tardive dyskinesia, persistent* (lip smacking or puckering; puffing of cheeks; rapid or worm-like movements of tongue; uncontrolled movements of arms and legs; uncontrolled chewing movements)

Note: *Akathisia* or *dystonic extrapyramidal effects* may occur within 24 to 48 hours of first dose; more frequent in young and male patients.

*Parkinsonian extrapyramidal effects* may appear in the first few days of treatment; frequency usually increases with increase of dosage; may be more frequent in elderly patients.

*Tardive dyskinesia* occurs more frequently in elderly females; initially dose-related, but may appear when doses are small and treatment periods are brief; may increase with long-term treatment and total cumulative dose; may be masked when dosage is increased or treatment reinitiated, or may persist after molindone is discontinued.

Incidence less frequent
 *Mental depression*

Incidence rare

*Allergic reaction* (skin rash); *heat stroke* (hot, dry skin; inability to sweat; muscle weakness; confusion); *hepatitis or jaundice, cholestatic* (yellow eyes or skin); *neuroleptic malignant syndrome (NMS)* (convulsions; fast heartbeat; fever; high or low [irregular] blood pressure; increased sweating; loss of bladder control; severe muscle stiffness; troubled breathing; unusually pale skin; unusual tiredness); *tardive dystonia* (increased blinking or spasms of eyelid; unusual facial expressions or body positions; uncontrolled twisting movements of neck, trunk, arms, or legs)

Note: *Heat stroke* may occur in environmental conditions of high heat and high humidity; caused by molindone-induced suppression of central and peripheral temperature regulation in the hypothalamus. The effectiveness of sweating as a cooling mechanism may be reduced by humid conditions and by the anticholinergic effects of molindone or its combination with other anticholinergic medications such as nonprescription cold medications or antihistamines. Adequate interior temperature control (air conditioning) must be maintained for institutionalized patients during hot weather because of the increased risk of heat stroke and NMS. Patients should be advised to avoid exertion, stay in cool areas, and avoid dehydration and other anticholinergic medications.

*NMS* may occur at any time during neuroleptic therapy, but is more commonly seen soon after start of therapy, or after patient has switched from another neuroleptic to another, during combined therapy with another psychotropic medication, or after a dosage increase. Along with the overt signs of skeletal muscle rigidity, hyperthermia, autonomic dysfunction, and altered consciousness, differential diagnosis may reveal leukocytosis (9500 to 26,000 cells per cubic millimeter), elevated liver function tests, and elevated creatine phosphokinase (CPK).

### Those indicating need for medical attention only if they continue or are bothersome

Incidence more frequent

*Blurred vision; constipation; decreased sweating; difficult urination; drowsiness; dryness of mouth; headache; hypotension, orthostatic* (dizziness or lightheadedness, especially when getting up suddenly from a lying or sitting position); *nausea; stuffy nose*

Incidence less frequent

*Changes in menstrual periods; decreased sexual ability; false sense of well-being; swelling of breasts; unusual secretion of milk*

### Those indicating the need for medical attention if they occur after medication is discontinued

*Tardive dyskinesia, withdrawal emergent* (lip smacking or puckering; puffing of cheeks; rapid or worm-like movements of tongue; uncontrolled chewing movements; uncontrolled movements of arms and legs)

# Patient Consultation

As an aid to patient consultation, refer to *Advice for the Patient, Molindone (Systemic).*

In providing consultation, consider emphasizing the following selected information (» = major clinical significance):

### Before using this medication

» Conditions affecting use, especially:

Sensitivity to molindone or other antipsychotic medications

Pregnancy—Studies in mice have shown a slight increase in resorptions

Use in the elderly—Elderly patients are more likely to develop extrapyramidal, anticholinergic, hypotensive, and sedative effects; reduced dosage recommended

Dental—Dry mouth may cause caries, candidiasis, periodontal disease, and discomfort; increased motor activity of face, head, and neck may interfere with some dental procedures

Other medications, especially alcohol, other CNS depression–producing medications, other extrapyramidal reaction–producing medications, or lithium

Other medical problems, especially severe drug-induced CNS depression

## Proper use of this medication

Taking with food or a full glass (8 ounces) of water or milk to reduce gastric irritation

Taking liquid form of medicine undiluted or mixed with water, milk, fruit juice, or carbonated beverage

» Compliance with therapy: importance of not taking more or less medication than the amount prescribed

» May require several weeks of therapy to obtain optimal effects

» Proper dosing

Missed dose: Taking as soon as possible; not taking if within 2 hours of next scheduled dose; resuming regular schedule; not doubling doses

» Proper storage

## Precautions while using this medication

Regular visits to physician to check progress of therapy

» Checking with physician before discontinuing medication; gradual dosage reduction may be needed

» Avoiding use of antacids or antidiarrheal medication within 2 hours of taking molindone

» Avoiding use of alcoholic beverages or other CNS depressants during therapy

Avoiding the use of over-the-counter medications for colds or allergies, to prevent increased anticholinergic effects and risk of heat stroke

» Possible drowsiness; caution when driving, using machinery, or doing other things that require alertness

» Possible dizziness or lightheadedness; caution when getting up suddenly from a lying or sitting position

» Possible heat stroke: caution during exercise, hot weather, or hot baths or saunas

Possible dryness of mouth; using sugarless gum or candy, ice, or saliva substitute for relief; checking with physician or dentist if dry mouth continues for more than 2 weeks

## Side/adverse effects

» Stopping medication and notifying physician immediately if symptoms of neuroleptic malignant syndrome (NMS) appear

» Notifying physician as soon as possible if early signs of tardive dyskinesia appear

Possibility of withdrawal emergent dyskinesia

Signs of potential side effects, especially akathisia, dystonias, parkinsonism, tardive dyskinesia, mental depression, allergic reaction, heat stroke, cholestatic jaundice or hepatitis, neuroleptic malignant syndrome (NMS), or tardive dystonia

# General Dosing Information

## Diet/Nutrition

Molindone should be taken with food or a full glass (8 ounces) of water or milk to reduce gastric irritation.

## For treatment of adverse effects

Neuroleptic malignant syndrome—

Treatment is essentially symptomatic and supportive and includes the following:

• *Discontinuing molindone immediately.*
• Hyperthermia—Administering antipyretics (aspirin or acetaminophen); using cooling blanket.
• Dehydration—Restoring fluids and electrolytes.
• Cardiovascular instability—Monitoring blood pressure and cardiac rhythm closely.
• Hypoxia—Administering oxygen; consider airway insertion and assisted ventilation.
• Muscle rigidity—Dantrolene sodium may be administered (100 to 300 mg per day in divided doses; 1.25 to 1.5 mg per kg, intravenously). Bromocriptine (5 to 7.5 mg every eight hours) has also been used.

Parkinsonism, severe—

Many authorities advise that the only appropriate treatment of extrapyramidal symptoms is reduction of the antipsychotic dosage, if possible. Oral antidyskinetics such as trihexyphenidyl, 2 mg three times per day, benztropine, or diphenhydramine may be effective in treating more severe parkinsonism and acute motor restlessness but should be used sparingly, only when side effects appear, and then usually for no longer than 3 months. In the elderly patient, the use of amantadine, 100 to 200 mg at bedtime, minimizes severe anticholinergic effects that may occur with other antidyskinetics.

Akathisia—

May respond to antiparkinsonian medications, or propranolol (30 to 120 mg per day), nadolol (40 mg per day), pindolol (5 to 60 mg per day), lorazepam (1 or 2 mg two or three times a day), or diazepam (2 mg two or three times a day), but often requires dosage reduction of molindone.

Dystonia—

Acute dystonic postures or oculogyric crisis may be relieved by parenteral administration of benztropine, 2 mg intramuscularly; diphenhydramine, 50 mg intramuscularly; or diazepam, 5 to 7.5 mg intravenously, to be followed by oral antidyskinetic medication for one or two days to prevent recurrent dystonic episodes. Dosage adjustments of molindone may control these effects, and discontinuation of molindone may reverse severe symptoms in weeks to months.

Tardive dyskinesia or tardive dystonia—

No known effective treatment. Dosage of molindone should be lowered or medication discontinued, if clinically feasible, at earliest signs of tardive dyskinesia or tardive dystonia, to prevent irreversible effects.

# Oral Dosage Forms

## MOLINDONE HYDROCHLORIDE ORAL SOLUTION

### Usual adult dose

Antipsychotic—

Initial:

Oral, 50 to 75 mg a day, in three or four divided doses, the dose being increased to 100 mg a day in three to four days as needed and tolerated.

Maintenance:

Mild psychosis—Oral, 5 to 15 mg three or four times a day.
Moderate psychosis—Oral, 10 to 25 mg three or four times a day.
Severe psychosis—Oral, 225 mg a day in divided doses.

Note: Elderly or debilitated patients usually require a lower initial dose, the dose being adjusted gradually as needed and tolerated.

### Usual adult prescribing limits

225 mg a day.

### Usual pediatric dose

Children up to 12 years of age—Safety and efficacy have not been established.

### Strength(s) usually available

U.S.—

20 mg per mL (Rx) [*Moban Concentrate* (alcohol; artificial cherry flavor; artificial cover flavor; edetate sodium; glycerin; liquid sugar; methylparaben; propylparaben; sodium metabisulfite; sorbitol solution; hydrochloric acid)].

Canada—

Not commercially available.

### Packaging and storage

Store below 40 °C (104 °F), preferably between 15 and 30 °C (59 and 86 °F), in a tight container, unless otherwise specified by manufacturer. Protect from freezing.

### Auxiliary labeling

• May cause drowsiness.
• Avoid alcoholic beverages.

### Additional information

Studies have shown that oral doses of the tablet and solution are equivalent in bioavailability.

## MOLINDONE HYDROCHLORIDE TABLETS

### Usual adult dose

See *Molindone Hydrochloride Oral Solution.*

### Usual adult prescribing limits

See *Molindone Hydrochloride Oral Solution.*

### Usual pediatric dose

See *Molindone Hydrochloride Oral Solution.*

**Strength(s) usually available**
U.S.—
    5 mg (Rx) [*Moban* (calcium sulfate; lactose; magnesium stearate; microcrystalline cellulose; povidone; alginic acid; colloidal silicon dioxide; FD&C Yellow No. 6)].
    10 mg (Rx) [*Moban* (calcium sulfate; lactose; magnesium stearate; microcrystalline cellulose; povidone; alginic acid; colloidal silicon dioxide; FD&C Blue No. 2; FD&C Red No. 40)].
    25 mg (Rx) [*Moban* (calcium sulfate; lactose; magnesium stearate; microcrystalline cellulose; povidone; alginic acid; colloidal silicon dioxide; FD&C Blue No. 2; FD&C Yellow No. 6; D&C Yellow No. 10)].
    50 mg (Rx) [*Moban* (calcium sulfate; lactose; magnesium stearate; microcrystalline cellulose; povidone; FD&C Blue No. 2; starch)].
    100 mg (Rx) [*Moban* (calcium sulfate; lactose; magnesium stearate; microcrystalline cellulose; povidone; FD&C Blue No. 2; FD&C Yellow No. 6; sodium starch glycolate)].

Canada—
    Not commercially available.

**Packaging and storage**
Store below 40 °C (104 °F), preferably between 15 and 30 °C (59 and 86 °F), in a tight container, unless otherwise specified by manufacturer. Protect from light.

**Auxiliary labeling**
• May cause drowsiness.
• Avoid alcoholic beverages.

**Additional information**
Studies have shown that oral doses of the tablet and solution are equivalent in bioavailability.

Revised: 03/19/93

---

# MOLYBDENUM SUPPLEMENTS   Systemic†

VA CLASSIFICATION (Primary): TN499
Note: For a listing of dosage forms and brand names by country availability, see *Dosage Forms* section(s). For a listing of brand names for the articles in this monograph, refer to the General Index.

    †Not commercially available in Canada.

## Category
Nutritional supplement (mineral).

## Indications
### Accepted
Molybdenum deficiency (prophylaxis and treatment)—Molybdenum is indicated in the prevention and treatment of molybdenum deficiency, which is rare but may result from inadequate nutrition or intestinal malabsorption. Molybdenum deficiency does not occur in healthy individuals receiving an adequate balanced diet. For prophylaxis of molybdenum deficiency, dietary improvement, rather than supplementation, is advisable. For treatment of molybdenum deficiency supplementation is preferred.

Deficiency of molybdenum is rare, but when it occurs it may lead to an intolerance of sulfur-containing amino acids.

Some unusual diets (e.g., reducing diets that drastically restrict food selection) may not supply minimum daily requirements of molybdenum. Supplementation may be necessary in patients receiving total parenteral nutrition (TPN) or undergoing rapid weight loss or in those with malnutrition, because of inadequate dietary intake.

## Pharmacology/Pharmacokinetics
### Physicochemical characteristics
Molecular weight—Ammonium molybdate: 1235.86.
Elemental molybdenum: 95.94.

### Mechanism of action/Effect
Molybdenum is a component of the enzymes xanthine oxidase, sulfite oxidase, and aldehyde oxidase. These enzymes are responsible for conversion of xanthine and hypoxanthine to uric acid, conversion of sulfite to sulfate, and detoxification of several harmful organic molecules, respectively.

### Absorption
Dietary molybdenum is well absorbed in the gastrointestinal tract.

### Storage
Molybdenum is stored in the liver, kidneys, spleen, lung, brain, and muscles.

### Elimination
Primarily in urine, with small amounts excreted in bile.

## Precautions to Consider
### Pregnancy/Reproduction
Pregnancy—Studies have not been done in humans and problems have not been documented with intake of normal daily recommended amounts.
Studies have not been done in animals.
FDA Pregnancy Category C (parenteral molybdenum).

### Breast-feeding
Problems in humans have not been documented with intake of normal daily recommended amounts.

### Pediatrics
Problems in pediatrics have not been documented with intake of normal daily recommended amounts.

### Geriatrics
Problems in geriatrics have not been documented with intake of normal daily recommended amounts.

### Drug interactions and/or related problems
The following drug interactions and/or related problems have been selected on the basis of their potential clinical significance (possible mechanism in parentheses where appropriate)—not necessarily inclusive (» = major clinical significance):

Note: Combinations containing any of the following medications, depending on the amount present, may also interact with this medication.

Copper supplements
    (excessive amounts of molybdenum may mobilize copper from tissue and increase urinary excretion of copper; copper supplements may be recommended with molybdenum therapy)

### Medical considerations/Contraindications
The medical considerations/contraindications included here have been selected on the basis of their potential clinical significance (reasons given in parentheses where appropriate)—not necessarily inclusive (» = major clinical significance).

*Risk-benefit should be considered when the following medical problems exist:*

Biliary obstruction or
Renal dysfunction
    (may cause an accumulation of molybdenum, since molybdenum is normally eliminated in bile and urine; a reduction in molybdenum dosage may be necessary)

Copper deficiency
    (condition may be exacerbated due to the mobilization of tissue copper and increased urinary excretion of copper by thiomolybdate)

### Patient monitoring
The following may be especially important in patient monitoring (other tests may be warranted in some patients, depending on condition; » = major clinical significance):

Copper
    (serum copper concentrations may be decreased by thiomolybdate; monitoring of copper every six months may be required with long-term use of molybdenum)

Molybdenum, blood or urinary
    (monitoring every six months by atomic absorption spectrophotometric method may be recommended by some clinicians to determine molybdenum status if deficiency or toxicity of molybdenum is suspected)

Purine and sulfur metabolic profiles
    (monitoring every six months may be recommended by some clinicians if deficiency or toxicity of molybdenum is suspected)

## Side/Adverse Effects

No side effects have been reported with molybdenum with recommended dosages.

## Overdose

For information on the management of overdose or unintentional ingestion, **contact a Poison Control Center** (see *Poison Control Center Listing*).

### Clinical effects of overdose

The following effects have been selected on the basis of their potential clinical significance (possible signs and symptoms in parentheses where appropriate)—not necessarily inclusive:

*Hyperuricemia* (joint pain; side, lower back, or stomach pain; swelling of feet or lower legs)—rarely has been reported from consumption of foods grown in molybdeniferous soil

## Patient Consultation

As an aid to patient consultation, refer to *Advice for the Patient, Molybdenum Supplements (Systemic)*.

In providing consultation, consider emphasizing the following selected information (» = major clinical significance):

### Description of use

Description should include function in the body, signs of deficiency

### Importance of diet

Importance of proper nutrition; supplement may be needed because of inadequate dietary intake

Food sources of molybdenum

Recommended daily intake for molybdenum

### Proper use of this dietary supplement

» Proper dosing

Missed dose: No cause for concern because of length of time necessary for depletion; remembering to take as directed

» Proper storage

### Precautions while taking this dietary supplement

Importance of taking copper supplement

## General Dosing Information

Because of the infrequency of molybdenum deficiency alone, combinations of several vitamins and/or minerals are commonly administered. In the oral form, molybdenum is available only as a vitamin/mineral combination.

### For parenteral dosage forms only

In most cases, parenteral administration is indicated only when oral administration is not acceptable (for example, in nausea, vomiting, preoperative and postoperative conditions) or possible (for example, in malabsorption syndromes or following gastric resection).

### Diet/Nutrition

Recommended dietary intakes for molybdenum are defined differently worldwide.

For U.S.—

The Recommended Dietary Allowances (RDAs) for vitamins and minerals are determined by the Food and Nutrition Board of the National Research Council and are intended to provide adequate nutrition in most healthy persons under usual environmental stresses. In addition, a different designation may be used by the FDA for food and dietary supplement labeling purposes, as with Daily Value (DV). DVs replace the previous labeling terminology United States Recommended Daily Allowances (USRDAs).

For Canada—

Recommended Nutrient Intakes (RNIs) for vitamins, minerals, and protein are determined by Health and Welfare in Canada and provide recommended amounts of a specific nutrient while minimizing the risk of chronic diseases.

There is no RDA or RNI established for molybdenum. The following daily intakes are considered adequate for all individuals—

Infants and children:

Birth to 3 years of age: 15 to 50 mcg.

4 to 6 years of age: 30 to 75 mcg.

7 to 10 years of age: 50 to 150 mcg.

Adolescents and adults:

75 to 250 mcg.

The amount of molybdenum in foods varies, depending on the environment in which the food is grown. Legumes, grain products, leafy vegetables, and low-fat milk are good sources of molybdenum.

## Parenteral Dosage Forms

### AMMONIUM MOLYBDATE INJECTION USP

#### Usual adult and adolescent dose

Deficiency (treatment)—

Intravenous, 163 mcg (0.163 mg) elemental molybdenum a day, added to total parenteral nutrition (TPN).

Deficiency (prophylaxis)—

Intravenous, 20 to 120 mcg (0.02 to 0.12 mg) elemental molybdenum a day, added to total parenteral nutrition (TPN).

#### Strength(s) usually available

U.S.—

46 mcg (0.046 mg) (25 mcg elemental molybdenum) per mL (Rx)

[*Molypen;* GENERIC].

Canada—

Not commercially available.

#### Packaging and storage

Store below 40 °C (104 °F), preferably between 15 and 30 °C (59 and 86 °F), unless otherwise specified by manufacturer.

#### Preparation of dosage form

Ammonium molybdate is physically compatible with amino acid solutions, dextrose solutions, electrolytes, and other trace elements.

Revised: 03/02/92

Interim revision: 07/31/92; 08/10/94; 04/25/95

---

**MOMETASONE**—See *Corticosteroids (Topical)*

---

# MONOCTANOIN    Local†

VA CLASSIFICATION (Primary): GA900

Another commonly used name is monooctanoin.

Note: For a listing of dosage forms and brand names by country availability, see *Dosage Forms* section(s). For a listing of brand names for the articles in this monograph, refer to the General Index.

---

†Not commercially available in Canada.

---

## Category

Cholelitholytic; solubilizing agent (cholesterol).

## Indications

### Accepted

Gallstone disease (treatment)—Monoctanoin is indicated for the dissolution of cholesterol gallstones retained in the bile duct following cholecystectomy, when mechanical removal has been unsuccessful or is impossible.

Monoctanoin therapy is more likely to be effective if the stones are radiolucent. Bilirubinate stones or stones containing less than 20% cholesterol do not appreciably dissolve in monoctanoin.

Complete stone dissolution is much more likely in cases involving a single stone than in those involving multiple stones.

## Pharmacology/Pharmacokinetics

### Physicochemical characteristics

Molecular weight—Component A: 218.29.

Component B: 246.35.

Component C: 344.49.

Component D: 92.10.

### Mechanism of action/Effect

Cholelitholytic; solubilizing agent (cholesterol)—Physical dissolution of cholesterol stones.

### Absorption
Hydrolysis products of monoctanoin are readily absorbed by the portal vein.

### Biotransformation
Rapidly hydrolyzed by pancreatic and other lipases to fatty acids and glycerol. Octanoic acid, a hydrolyzation product, is metabolized to carbon dioxide in the liver.

## Precautions to Consider

### Cross-sensitivity and/or related problems
Patients sensitive to vegetable oils may be sensitive to monoctanoin.

### Carcinogenicity/Mutagenicity
Studies have not been done to evaluate the carcinogenic or mutagenic potential of monoctanoin.

### Pregnancy/Reproduction
Pregnancy—Studies have not been done in humans.
Studies have not been done in animals.

FDA Pregnancy Category C.

### Breast-feeding
It is not known whether monoctanoin is distributed into breast milk. However, problems in humans have not been documented.

### Pediatrics
Appropriate studies on the relationship of age to the effects of monoctanoin have not been performed in the pediatric population. Safety and efficacy have not been established.

### Geriatrics
No information is available on the relationship of age to the effects of monoctanoin in geriatric patients.

### Laboratory value alterations
The following have been selected on the basis of their potential clinical significance (possible effect in parentheses where appropriate)—not necessarily inclusive ($\gg$ = major clinical significance):

With physiology/laboratory test values
   Amylase
      (serum concentrations may be increased)

### Medical considerations/Contraindications
The medical considerations/contraindications included here have been selected on the basis of their potential clinical significance (reasons given in parentheses where appropriate)—not necessarily inclusive ($\gg$ = major clinical significance).

*Except under special circumstances, this medication should not be used when the following medical problems exist:*
$\gg$ Biliary tract infection, severe or
$\gg$ Jaundice, obstructive or
$\gg$ Pancreatitis
   (use of monoctanoin may aggravate condition)
$\gg$ Hepatic function impairment, severe
   (hepatic metabolism of fatty acids generated from monoctanoin hydrolysis may be impaired, resulting in adverse effects)
$\gg$ Jejunitis or
$\gg$ Ulcer, duodenal, recent
   (use of monoctanoin may aggravate condition or increase risk of ulceration and hemorrhage)

*Risk-benefit should be considered when the following medical problems exist:*
$\gg$ Bile duct obstruction
   (possible systemic absorption of monoctanoin may increase risk of adverse effects; ascending cholangitis may also occur; if monoctanoin is used, intermittent instillation and aspiration is recommended to avoid increased pressure in the bile duct system)
   Sensitivity to monoctanoin or vegetable oils

### Patient monitoring
The following may be especially important in patient monitoring (other tests may be warranted in some patients, depending on condition; $\gg$ = major clinical significance):

Blood pressure and
Pulse rate and
Temperature
   (monitoring recommended every 4 to 6 hours during perfusion with monoctanoin)
Cholangiogram
   (recommended every 3 days during treatment with monoctanoin for monitoring stone dissolution)

Hepatic function determinations
   (recommended during perfusion with monoctanoin, especially in patients with impaired hepatic function because metabolic acidosis may result)

## Side/Adverse Effects

Note: Reversible irritation of the duodenal mucosa has been observed by endoscopy; it usually disappears within 2 to 7 days after completion of therapy.

The following side/adverse effects have been selected on the basis of their potential clinical significance (possible signs and symptoms in parentheses where appropriate)—not necessarily inclusive:

### Those indicating need for medical attention
Incidence less frequent or rare
   *Acidosis* (drowsiness, severe; nausea, continuing; shortness of breath, severe)—possibly due to systemic absorption of monoctanoin and more likely in patients with impaired hepatic function; *gastrointestinal effects* (abdominal or stomach pain, severe; back pain, severe)—usually result from increased pressure and distention in the biliary tract caused by the infusion; *leukopenia* (chills, fever, or sore throat)

### Those indicating need for medical attention only if they continue or are bothersome
Incidence more frequent
   *Abdominal or stomach pain, mild, or burning sensation*
Incidence less frequent
   *Diarrhea*—due to hygroscopic effect of monoctanoin; *loss of appetite; nausea or vomiting*
Incidence rare
   *Back pain, mild; flushing or redness of face; metallic taste*

## Patient Consultation

As an aid to patient consultation, refer to *Advice for the Patient, Monoctanoin (Local)*.

In providing consultation, consider emphasizing the following selected information ($\gg$ = major clinical significance):

### Before using this medication
$\gg$ Conditions affecting use, especially:
   Sensitivity to monoctanoin or vegetable oils
   Other medical problems, especially bile duct obstruction, jejunitis, obstructive jaundice, pancreatitis, recent duodenal ulcer, severe biliary tract infection, or severe hepatic function impairment

### Proper use of this medication
$\gg$ Proper dosing

### Side/adverse effects
   Signs of potential side effects, especially acidosis, gastrointestinal effects, or leukopenia

## General Dosing Information

Monoctanoin solution should *not* be used for intravenous or intramuscular administration.

Monoctanoin therapy should be preceded by an analysis of the surgically removed gallstone (saved from previous cholecystectomy and kept dry without preservatives) to determine its composition and solubility. Therapy with monoctanoin should not be instituted if analysis of the stone shows its composition to be less than 20% cholesterol or if no dissolution is observed after 6 hours of *in vitro* incubation in a stirred ether solution.

Monoctanoin is administered as a continuous perfusion through a catheter inserted directly into the common bile duct generally by a T-tube or nasobiliary tube placed by endoscopy.

An infusion pump is used to regulate perfusion of monoctanoin into the bile duct. An overflow manometer must also be included in the administration system to ensure that biliary pressure does not exceed 20 cm of water.

Careful monitoring and control of perfusion pressures are recommended to minimize gastrointestinal and/or biliary tract irritation and systemic absorption of monoctanoin.

Perfusion of monoctanoin may be stopped for 1 to 2 hours at meal times to decrease the likelihood of gastrointestinal side effects.

The duration of monoctanoin perfusion necessary for complete stone dissolution is variable, ranging from 2 to 10 days.

Monoctanoin therapy is unlikely to be effective and should be discontinued if, after 10 days, endoscopy or x-ray examination does not show a significant decrease in stone size or complete stone dissolution.

## For treatment of adverse effects
Gastrointestinal effects, such as severe abdominal or back pain, may result from increased pressure and distention in the biliary tract. Recommended treatment includes:
- Decreasing the perfusion rate or stopping the infusion.
- Hourly aspiration of bile (may be needed in some patients).

## Local Dosage Forms

### MONOCTANOIN IRRIGATION

**Usual adult and adolescent dose**
Cholelitholytic; solubilizing agent (cholesterol)—
Via catheter, continuous perfusion for 2 to 10 days at a rate of 3 to 5 mL per hour at a pressure of 10 cm of water.

**Usual pediatric dose**
Safety and efficacy have not been established.

**Size(s) usually available**
U.S.—
120 mL (Rx) [*Moctanin*].
Canada—
Not commercially available.

**Packaging and storage**
Store between 15 and 30 °C (59 and 86 °F).

## Preparation of dosage form
Thirteen mL of sterile water for injection may be added to each 120 mL vial of monoctanoin (10% dilution) to reduce viscosity and enhance bathing of the stone.
Prior to administration, monoctanoin should be warmed to 37 °C (98.6 °F). This temperature should be maintained for the duration of the perfusion.

## Stability
When stored at temperatures below 15 °C (59 °F), monoctanoin may form a semi-solid, which may be reliquified by warming to 21 °C (70 °F).

## Selected Bibliography
Abate MA, Moore TL. Monooctanoin use for gallstone dissolution. Drug Intell Clin Pharm 1985; 19: 708-13.
Talamini MA, Gadacz TR. Gallstone dissolution. Surg Clin North Am 1990; 70: 1217-30.

Revised: 07/20/95

## MONOMERIC (ELEMENTAL) ENTERAL NUTRITION FORMULAS—See *Enteral Nutrition Formulas (Systemic)*

# MORICIZINE    Systemic†

INN: Moracizine
VA CLASSIFICATION (Primary): CV300
Note: For a listing of dosage forms and brand names by country availability, see *Dosage Forms* section(s). For a listing of brand names for the articles in this monograph, refer to the General Index.

†Not commercially available in Canada.

## Category
Antiarrhythmic.

## Indications

### Accepted
Arrhythmias, ventricular (treatment)—Moricizine is indicated for suppression of documented life-threatening ventricular arrhythmias, including sustained ventricular tachycardia.

### Unaccepted
Use of moricizine is not accepted for treatment of less severe arrhythmias such as nonsustained ventricular tachycardias or frequent premature ventricular contractions, even if patients are symptomatic. In these cases, there is a possibility that proarrhythmic potential may outweigh any beneficial effect. In the National Heart, Lung and Blood Institute's Cardiac Arrhythmia Suppression Trial (CAST), encainide or flecainide treatment was associated with excessive mortality or increased non-fatal cardiac arrest rate as compared with placebo in patients with asymptomatic, non–life-threatening arrhythmias who had a recent myocardial infarction; and, therefore, the encainide and flecainide arms of CAST were prematurely terminated. The CAST protocol was modified and continued as CAST-II with the moricizine arm compared to placebo. However, CAST-II was subsequently terminated prematurely because of excessive cardiac mortality during the first 2 weeks of moricizine exposure as compared to placebo. Furthermore, it appeared unlikely that moricizine would improve long-term survival.

## Pharmacology/Pharmacokinetics

### Physicochemical characteristics
Source—Phenothiazine derivative
Molecular weight—Moricizine hydrochloride: 427.52.
pKa—6.4.

### Mechanism of action/Effect
Inhibits the rapid inward sodium current across myocardial cell membranes. Has potent local anesthetic activity and membrane stabilizing effect. Decreases excitability, conduction velocity, and automaticity as a result of slowed atrioventricular (AV) nodal and His-Purkinje conduction. Decreases the action potential duration (APD) in Purkinje fibers; also decreases the effective refractory period (ERP) but to a lesser extent than the APD, so the ERP/APD ratio is increased. Decreases the maximum rate of Phase 0 depolarization ($V_{max}$), but does not affect action potential amplitude or maximum diastolic potential. Does not affect atrial, AV nodal, or left ventricular refractory periods and has minimal effect on ventricular repolarization (evidenced by the overall decrease in JT interval). Has no effect on sinoatrial (SA) nodal or intra-atrial conduction and only minimal effect on sinus cycle length and sinus node recovery time. In the Vaughan Williams classification of antiarrhythmics, moricizine is considered to be a class I agent. It has properties of class IA, IB, and IC agents but does not clearly belong to any of the three subclasses. It has less effect on the slope of phase 0 and a greater effect on action potential duration and effective refractory period than class IC agents.

### Other actions/effects
Causes a small but consistent increase in resting blood pressure and heart rate. May inhibit platelet aggregation. May have anticholinergic effects.

### Absorption
Well absorbed; absorption is complete within 2 to 3 hours. Significant first-pass metabolism results in an absolute bioavailability of approximately 38%. Administration within 30 minutes after a meal slows the rate, but does not affect the extent, of absorption, although peak plasma concentrations are reduced.

### Protein binding
Very high (approximately 95%).

### Biotransformation
Hepatic, extensive, to at least 26 metabolites, none accounting for as much as 1% of the administered dose. Two metabolites may be pharmacologically active but are present in extremely small quantities.
Moricizine induces its own metabolism (it induces hepatic cytochrome P-450 activity). Average plasma concentrations decline with continued dosing, but the clinical effect does not appear to be altered.

### Half-life
1.5 to 3.5 (usually 2) hours. Duration of action is longer than would be predicted on the basis of this figure.

### Onset of action
Prolongation of PR interval—Occurs promptly but normalization occurs within 2 hours.
Effect on ventricular premature depolarization (VPD) rates—Within 2 hours.

### Time to peak concentration
0.5 to 2 hours; plasma concentration is directly dose-related.

### Time to peak effect
Shortening of JT interval—6 hours.
Effect on VPD rates—10 to 14 hours.

### Duration of action
Shortening of JT interval—At least 10 hours.
Effect on VPD rates—In full for more than 10 hours and continues to be significant at 24 hours.

### Elimination
Biliary/fecal, 56%; renal, 39%. Less than 1% of a dose is excreted unchanged. Some enterohepatic recycling occurs.
In dialysis—Not significantly removable by hemodialysis.

# Precautions to Consider

## Carcinogenicity

A 24-month study in mice at oral doses up to 320 mg per kg of body weight (mg/kg) per day produced a borderline statistically significant incidence of ovarian tubular adenomas and granulosa cell tumors. A 24-month study in rats at oral doses of 25, 50, and 100 mg/kg per day produced a Zymbal's gland carcinoma in one mid-dose and two high-dose males. A dose-related increase in hepatocellular cholangioma (also described as bile ductile cystadenoma or cystic hyperplasia), along with fatty metamorphosis, possibly due to disruption of hepatic choline utilization for phospholipid biosynthesis, also occurred in rats of both sexes (the rat is uniquely sensitive to alteration in choline metabolism).

## Mutagenicity

Moricizine was not found to be mutagenic in *in vitro* bacterial (Ames test) and mammalian (Chinese hamster ovary/hypoxanthine-guanine phosphoribosyl transferase and sister chromatid exchange) cell systems or in *in vivo* mammalian systems (rat bone cytogenicity and mouse micronucleus).

## Pregnancy/Reproduction

Fertility—Studies in male and female rats at doses of up to 6.7 times the maximum recommended human dose found no evidence of impaired fertility.

Pregnancy—Adequate and well-controlled studies in humans have not been done.

Teratogenicity studies in rats and rabbits at doses of up to 6.7 and 4.7 times the maximum recommended human dose, respectively, have not shown that moricizine causes adverse effects in the fetus.

A study in rats at doses of 3.4 and 6.7 times the maximum recommended human dose given prior to mating, during mating, and throughout gestation found a dose-related decrease in both pup and maternal weight gain, possibly related to a larger litter size; a study in which doses of 6.7 times the maximum recommended human dose were begun on Day 15 of gestation found retardation of maternal weight gain but no effect on pup growth.

FDA Pregnancy Category B.

## Breast-feeding

Moricizine has been reported to be present in human breast milk and is distributed into the milk of laboratory animals.

## Pediatrics

Appropriate studies on the relationship of age to the effects of moricizine have not been performed in the pediatric population. However, moricizine was used in 12 children with atrial ectopic tachycardia and did not demonstrate pediatrics-specific problems that would limit the usefulness of moricizine in children.

## Geriatrics

One study found a decreased incidence of neurological side/adverse effects in patients over 65 years of age; there were no other age-related differences in incidence of side/adverse effects. In addition, elderly patients are more likely to have age-related renal function impairment, which, when significant, may require dosage reduction in patients receiving moricizine.

## Drug interactions and/or related problems

The following drug interactions and/or related problems have been selected on the basis of their potential clinical significance (possible mechanism in parentheses where appropriate)—not necessarily inclusive (» = major clinical significance):

Antiarrhythmics, other
(although some antiarrhythmic agents may be used in combination for therapeutic advantage, combined use may potentiate risk of adverse cardiac effects)

Cimetidine
(concurrent use of cimetidine has been reported to decrease clearance of moricizine by about 49% and increase plasma concentrations 1.4 fold; although clinical effects of moricizine do not appear to be changed, caution is recommended if concurrent use with cimetidine is necessary)

Theophylline
(concurrent use with moricizine significantly increases clearance and decreases half-life of theophylline, with a resultant decrease in plasma theophylline concentrations, possibly as a result of hepatic microsomal enzyme induction; monitoring of plasma theophylline concentrations is recommended when moricizine therapy is initiated or discontinued)

## Laboratory value alterations

The following have been selected on the basis of their potential clinical significance (possible effect in parentheses where appropriate)—not necessarily inclusive (» = major clinical significance):

With physiology/laboratory test values

*Electrocardiogram (ECG) changes such as:*
JT interval
(slight shortening occurs)

QRS widening and
PR prolongation
(occur in most patients; dose-related)
(PR interval prolongation occurs promptly after single doses, but the interval returns to normal within 2 hours)

QT prolongation
(may occur secondary to QRS widening, but usually is not significant)
Note: ECG changes produced by moricizine do not necessarily indicate efficacy, toxicity, or overdose.

## Medical considerations/Contraindications

The medical considerations/contraindications included here have been selected on the basis of their potential clinical significance (reasons given in parentheses where appropriate)—not necessarily inclusive (» = major clinical significance).

*Except under special circumstances, this medication should not be used when the following medical problems exist:*

» Atrioventricular (AV) block, pre-existing second or third degree without pacemaker, or

» Right bundle branch block associated with a left hemiblock (bifascicular block) without pacemaker
(risk of complete heart block)

*Risk-benefit should be considered when the following medical problems exist:*

» Cardiogenic shock

Cardiomegaly
(incidence of moricizine-induced arrhythmias is increased; the possibility of proarrhythmic effects should be kept in mind during moricizine therapy)

Congestive heart failure, severe
(worsening has been reported; incidence of moricizine-induced arrhythmias is increased; absorption, half-life, and clearance of moricizine are not affected)

Coronary artery disease
(incidence of moricizine-induced arrhythmias is increased; the possibility of proarrhythmic effects should be kept in mind during moricizine therapy)

Hepatic function impairment
(reduced clearance and increased half-life of moricizine; lower doses of moricizine and close monitoring are recommended)

Hypokalemia or hyperkalemia or
Hypomagnesemia
(effects of moricizine may be altered; any electrolyte imbalance should be corrected prior to beginning therapy with moricizine)

Myocardial infarction, history of
(incidence of moricizine-induced arrhythmias is increased; the possibility of proarrhythmic effects should be kept in mind during moricizine therapy)

Renal function impairment
(reduced elimination; if significant, dosage reduction and close monitoring are recommended)

» Sensitivity to moricizine

» Sick sinus syndrome
(sinus node recovery time prolonged; sinus bradycardia, sinus pause, or sinus arrest may occur)

Caution is also recommended in patients with existing pacemakers because the risk of moricizine-induced arrhythmias may be increased; the effect of moricizine on endocardial pacing thresholds has not been studied.

## Patient monitoring

The following may be especially important in patient monitoring (other tests may be warranted in some patients, depending on condition; » = major clinical significance):

» ECG, 24-hour Holter monitoring and

» Exercise testing and/or

Programmed electrical stimulation
(may be recommended prior to initiation of therapy and at periodic intervals during therapy to help assess efficacy and detect possible proarrhythmic effects)

## Side/Adverse Effects

Note: In the National Heart, Lung and Blood Institute's Cardiac Arrhythmia Suppression Trial (CAST), encainide or flecainide treatment was found to be associated with excessive mortality or increased nonfatal cardiac arrest rate as compared with placebo in patients with asymptomatic, non–life-threatening arrhythmias who had a recent myocardial infarction. CAST-II comparing moricizine to placebo was discontinued because of excessive cardiac mortality during the first 2 weeks of moricizine exposure as compared to placebo. Furthermore, it appeared unlikely that moricizine would improve long-term survival.

Adverse cardiac effects reported with moricizine administration include new or exacerbated ventricular arrhythmias in about 3.7% of patients and, in 1% or less of patients, new or exacerbated congestive heart failure, second or third degree atrioventricular (AV) block, sinus bradycardia, sinus pause, or sinus arrest.

Side/adverse effects are usually mild and transient. However, deaths have been reported from overdosage of moricizine.

The following side/adverse effects have been selected on the basis of their potential clinical significance (possible signs and symptoms in parentheses where appropriate)—not necessarily inclusive:

**Those indicating need for medical attention**
Incidence less frequent
*Chest pain; congestive heart failure* (shortness of breath; swelling of feet or lower legs); *ventricular tachyarrhythmias* (fast or irregular heartbeat)

Note: *Ventricular tachyarrhythmias* are potentially fatal; incidence is increased in patients with coronary artery disease, sustained ventricular tachycardia, cardiomegaly, congestive heart failure, or history of myocardial infarction. Proarrhythmic effects usually occur during the first week of therapy and are not dose-related.

Incidence rare
*Drug fever* (sudden high fever); *hepatotoxicity* (not symptomatic)

**Those indicating need for medical attention only if they continue or are bothersome**
Incidence more frequent
*Dizziness*—dose-related
Incidence less frequent
*Blurred vision; diarrhea; dryness of mouth; headache; hypesthesias or paresthesias* (numbness or tingling in arms or legs or around mouth); *nausea or vomiting; nervousness; pain in arms or legs; stomach pain; trouble in sleeping; unusual tiredness or weakness*

## Overdose

For more information on the management of overdose or unintentional ingestion, **contact a Poison Control Center** (see *Poison Control Center Listing*).

**Clinical effects of overdose**
The following effects have been selected on the basis of their potential clinical significance (possible signs and symptoms in parentheses where appropriate)—not necessarily inclusive:
*Conduction disturbances; hypotension; exacerbation of congestive heart failure; myocardial infarction; sinus arrest; arrhythmias* (including junctional bradycardia, ventricular tachycardia, ventricular fibrillation, and asystole); *emesis; lethargy; coma; syncope; respiratory failure*

**Treatment of overdose**
Treatment is primarily supportive and symptomatic and includes immediate evacuation of the stomach, with special care to avoid aspiration; cardiac, respiratory, and CNS monitoring.

## Patient Consultation

As an aid to patient consultation, refer to *Advice for the Patient, Moricizine (Systemic).*

In providing consultation, consider emphasizing the following selected information (» = major clinical significance):

**Before using this medication**
» Conditions affecting use, especially:
Sensitivity to moricizine
Other medical problems, especially second or third degree atrioventricular (AV) block, right bundle branch block associated with a left hemiblock, cardiogenic shock, or sick sinus syndrome

**Proper use of this medication**
» Compliance with therapy; taking as directed even if feeling well
» Importance of not missing doses and taking at evenly spaced intervals
» Proper dosing
Missed dose: Taking as soon as possible if remembered within 4 hours; not taking if remembered later; not doubling doses
» Proper storage

**Precautions while using this medication**
Regular visits to physician to check progress
Carrying medical identification card or bracelet
» Caution if any kind of surgery (including dental surgery) or emergency treatment is required
Caution when driving or doing things requiring alertness because of possible dizziness

**Side/adverse effects**
Signs of potential side effects, especially chest pain, congestive heart failure, ventricular tachyarrhythmias, and drug fever

## General Dosing Information

It is recommended that treatment be initiated in the hospital because of the risk of proarrhythmic effects associated with moricizine administration.

In general, it is recommended that previous antiarrhythmic therapy be withdrawn 1 to 2 plasma half-lives before initiation of moricizine therapy. However, individual circumstances must be taken into consideration.

If second- or third-degree AV block occurs, moricizine therapy should be withdrawn unless a ventricular pacemaker is in place.

## Oral Dosage Forms
### MORICIZINE HYDROCHLORIDE TABLETS

**Usual adult dose**
Antiarrhythmic—
Oral, 600 to 900 mg per day in three divided doses given every eight hours, the dosage being increased, if necessary, in increments of 150 mg per day at three-day intervals up to a total dose of 900 mg per day.

Note: In patients with hepatic function impairment or significant renal function impairment, an initial dose of 600 mg per day or less is recommended with close monitoring, including ECG intervals, before dosage adjustment.

Some patients whose arrhythmias are well-controlled may be changed to every-twelve-hour dosing if necessary to aid in compliance. Incidence of dizziness and nausea may be increased with higher doses.

**Usual pediatric dose**
Safety and efficacy have not been established.

Note: One study involving 12 pediatric patients used a daily dose of 200 mg per square meter of body surface divided into three equal doses, increased as necessary up to a maximum of 600 mg per square meter of body surface per day.

**Strength(s) usually available**
U.S.—
200 mg (Rx) [*Ethmozine* (lactose)].
250 mg (Rx) [*Ethmozine* (lactose)].
300 mg (Rx) [*Ethmozine* (lactose)].
Canada—
Not commercially available.

**Packaging and storage**
Store between 15 and 30 °C (59 and 86 °F), unless otherwise specified by manufacturer. Store in a tight container. Protect from light.

## Selected Bibliography

Carnes CA, Coyle JD. Moricizine: a novel antiarrhythmic agent. DICP 1990 Jul/Aug; 24: 745-53.

Fitton A, Buckley MM. Moricizine: A review of its pharmacological properties, and therapeutic efficacy in cardiac arrhythmias. Drugs 1990; 40 (1): 138-67.

Morganroth J, Bigger JT, editors. A symposium: pharmacologic management of ventricular arrhythmias—current status in the role of moricizine HCl. Am J Cardiol 1990; 65 (8): 1D-71D.

Revised: 09/27/92
Interim revision: 06/30/94

**MORPHINE**—See *Opioid (Narcotic) Analgesics (Systemic)*

# MUMPS VIRUS VACCINE LIVE   Systemic

VA CLASSIFICATION (Primary): IM100

Note: This monograph is specific for the Jeryl Lynn strain of mumps virus vaccine live.

Note: For a listing of dosage forms and brand names by country availability, see *Dosage Forms* section(s). For a listing of brand names for the articles in this monograph, refer to the General Index.

## Category
Immunizing agent (active).

## Indications

### Accepted
Mumps (prophylaxis)—Mumps virus vaccine live is indicated for immunization against mumps. The main objective of mumps immunization is to prevent complications, such as orchitis, which may occur in up to 20% of postpubescent and adult males infected with mumps virus, and meningoencephalitis, which may occur in up to 15% of persons infected with mumps virus. In addition, mumps infection during the first trimester of pregnancy may increase the rate of spontaneous abortion.

Unless otherwise contraindicated, all susceptible children, adolescents, and adults should be immunized against mumps, including
• Persons born between 1967 and 1977. There has been an increase in recent years in cases of mumps infection in persons born between 1967 and 1977. This has been attributed to the relatively large number of persons born during this period who were not immunized, but were nonetheless afforded protection against exposure because of the immunization of their contemporaries.
• Children 12 months of age and older, including school-age children and children in day-care centers and custodial institutions. Children vaccinated before their first birthday should be revaccinated.
• Prepubescent and postpubescent males, including adult males; the incidence of orchitis resulting from a natural mumps infection is greater in postpubescent and adult males.
• Females of child-bearing potential, if they are not pregnant and if they are counseled not to become pregnant for 3 months following vaccination.
• Household contacts of susceptible pregnant women or other persons with medical contraindications to mumps vaccination, to reduce the risk to persons unable to receive mumps vaccine. Vaccinated persons do not transmit mumps vaccine virus.
• Persons who have been exposed to mumps, since a single exposure may not cause infection and post-exposure vaccination provides future protection. There is no evidence that vaccinating an individual incubating mumps is harmful, but neither will it prevent illness.
• Persons previously vaccinated with inactivated (killed) mumps vaccine, since the immunity induced by this vaccine is transient. The killed vaccine was available in the U.S. from 1950 through 1978; however, in 1967, the live vaccine became available and the killed vaccine was in limited use thereafter.
• Persons traveling outside the U.S., since mumps is endemic in many countries.
• Persons who lack adequate documentation of immunity, even though they may be immune to mumps. There is no evidence of adverse effects when patients already immune to mumps are revaccinated. In addition, skin tests and serologic tests for mumps immunity are either unreliable, such as the mumps skin test and the complement-fixation antibody test, or not readily available, such as the neutralization, enzyme immunoassay, and radial hemolysis antibody tests.

Although the mumps vaccine currently available in the U.S. contains approximately 25 mcg of neomycin in each 0.5-mL dose and is produced in chick embryo cell cultures, a history of hypersensitivity reactions, other than anaphylaxis, to neomycin or to eggs generally does not preclude immunization with mumps vaccine.

Persons should be considered immune to mumps only if they have
• Documentation of immunization with live mumps vaccine on or after their first birthday.
• Physician's diagnosis of previous mumps infection.
• Laboratory evidence of immunity.

The measles, mumps, and rubella combination vaccine (MMR) should be used for vaccinating individuals who are likely to be susceptible to more than one of these viruses, unless otherwise contraindicated. Vaccines containing measles antigen should be administered to persons 15 months of age or older under routine conditions. Most individuals born before 1957 can generally be considered immune to measles and mumps because of probable previous infection, even though, in the case of mumps, they may not have had clinically recognizable disease.

## Pharmacology/Pharmacokinetics

### Mechanism of action/Effect
Following subcutaneous injection, mumps vaccine produces a modified, noncommunicable mumps infection and provides active immunity to mumps.

Mumps vaccine induces a number of antibody and cell-mediated immunity (CMI) responses, but it is not certain which of these is responsible for protection.

### Protective effect
Immunity to mumps occurs in approximately 95% of susceptible vaccinated individuals.

### Time to protective effect
A serologic response occurs within 2 to 3 weeks.

### Duration of protective effect
At least 20 years and probably lifetime immunity.

## Precautions to Consider

### Cross-sensitivity and/or related problems
Patients allergic to systemic or topical neomycin may be allergic to the mumps virus vaccine live available in the U.S. and Canada because it may contain a small amount of neomycin, which is used in the production of the vaccine to prevent bacterial overgrowth in the viral culture. A history of allergic reactions other than anaphylaxis, such as delayed-type allergic reaction (contact dermatitis), generally does not preclude immunization.

### Pregnancy/Reproduction
Pregnancy—Studies have not been done in humans. However, use in pregnant women is not recommended, because mumps vaccine virus may infect the placenta, although the vaccine virus has not been isolated from electively aborted fetuses from women who were vaccinated during pregnancy. In addition, it is recommended that pregnancy be avoided for 3 months following vaccination.

Natural mumps infection can infect the placenta and fetus, but there is no evidence that natural mumps infection during pregnancy causes congenital malformations. Therefore, there is no reason to suspect or evidence to indicate that mumps vaccine would cause congenital malformations.

Studies have not been done in animals.

FDA Pregnancy Category C.

### Breast-feeding
It is not known whether mumps vaccine is distributed into breast milk. However, problems in humans have not been documented.

### Pediatrics
*Infants up to 12 months of age—*
Immunization is not recommended for infants younger than 12 months of age, since maternal mumps-neutralizing antibodies may interfere with the immune response.
Children who were vaccinated when younger than 12 months of age should be revaccinated.

*Infants and children 12 months of age and older—*
Appropriate studies have not been performed in the pediatric population. However, no pediatrics-specific problems have been documented to date.
When mumps vaccine is part of a combination vaccination that includes measles vaccine, the minimum age for vaccination is 15 months in order to maximize measles seroconversion.

**Drug interactions and/or related problems**

The following drug interactions and/or related problems have been selected on the basis of their potential clinical significance (possible mechanism in parentheses where appropriate)—not necessarily inclusive (» = major clinical significance):

Note: Combinations containing any of the following medications, depending on the amount present, may also interact with this medication.

Blood products or
Immune globulins
    (concurrent administration with mumps vaccine may interfere with the patient's immune response to the virus because of the possibility of antibodies to mumps virus in these products. Mumps vaccine should be administered at least 14 days before, or more than 3 months after, administration of blood products or immune globulins)

» Immunosuppressive agents or
» Radiation therapy
    (because normal defense mechanisms are suppressed, concurrent use with mumps vaccine may potentiate the replication of the vaccine virus, may increase the side/adverse effects of the vaccine virus, and/or may decrease the patient's antibody response to mumps vaccine. The interval between discontinuation of medications that cause immunosuppression and restoration of the patient's ability to respond to mumps vaccine depends on the intensity and type of immunosuppression-causing medication used, the underlying disease, and other factors; estimates vary from 3 months to 1 year. Patients with leukemia in remission should not receive mumps vaccine until at least 3 months after their last chemotherapy. The precaution does not apply to corticosteroids used as replacement therapy, for short-term [less than 2 weeks] systemic therapy, or by other routes of administration that do not cause immunosuppression)

Live virus vaccines, other
    (although data are lacking on impairment of antibody responses to rubella, measles, mumps, or oral polio vaccine when these vaccines are administered on different days within 1 month of each other, the chance exists that the immune responses may be impaired when live virus vaccines are administered in this manner; therefore, when feasible, live virus vaccines not administered on the same day should be given at least 1 month apart)

**Laboratory value alterations**

The following have been selected on the basis of their potential clinical significance (possible effect in parentheses where appropriate)—not necessarily inclusive (» = major clinical significance):

With diagnostic test results
Tuberculin skin test
    (short-term suppression of 4 weeks or longer may occur and may result in false-negative tests; if required, tuberculin skin tests should be done before, simultaneously with, or at least 6 weeks after administration of mumps vaccine)

**Medical considerations/Contraindications**

The medical considerations/contraindications included here have been selected on the basis of their potential clinical significance (reasons given in parentheses where appropriate)—not necessarily inclusive (» = major clinical significance).

*Except under special circumstances, this medication should not be used when the following medical problems exist:*

» Febrile illness, severe
    (to avoid confusing manifestations of illness with possible side/adverse effects of vaccine. Minor illnesses, such as upper respiratory infection, do not preclude administration of vaccine)

» Immune deficiency conditions, congenital or hereditary, family history of, or

» Immune deficiency conditions, primary or acquired
    (because of reduced or suppressed defense mechanisms, the use of live virus vaccines, including mumps vaccine, may potentiate the replication of the vaccine virus, may increase the side/adverse effects of the vaccine virus, and/or may decrease the patient's antibody response to mumps)
    (persons with leukemia in remission may receive live virus vaccines if at least 3 months have passed since their last chemotherapy treatment)
    (persons infected with human immunodeficiency virus [HIV] may receive this vaccine if they are asymptomatic; in addition, immunization with this vaccine should be considered for persons with symptomatic HIV infection; in either case, the measles, mumps, and rubella combination vaccine [MMR] is generally preferred)

(when there is a family history of congenital or hereditary immune deficiency conditions, the patient should not be vaccinated until his/her immune competence is demonstrated)

*Risk-benefit should be considered when the following medical problems exist:*

Allergy to eggs
    (patients allergic to eggs may be allergic to the mumps virus vaccine live available in the U.S. and Canada, since it is produced in chick embryo cell cultures. A history of hypersensitivity reactions other than anaphylaxis generally does not preclude immunization. In addition, no allergy to mumps vaccine has been found in patients allergic to chicken or chicken feathers)

Sensitivity to mumps vaccine

Tuberculosis, active, untreated
    (since mumps vaccine may suppress the tuberculin skin test for 4 or more weeks, patients thought to have tuberculosis or to be at risk for tuberculosis should be tested before, or simultaneously with, administration of mumps vaccine. Otherwise the tuberculin skin test should be done at least 6 weeks after administration of mumps vaccine [See also *Laboratory value alterations.*])

## Side/Adverse Effects

Note: A history of allergic reactions other than anaphylaxis, such as delayed-type allergic reaction (contact dermatitis), generally does not preclude immunization.

Encephalitis and other central nervous system (CNS) reactions have been temporally related to mumps vaccine administration; however, no causal relationship has been established. In addition, the incidence of these disorders in patients vaccinated with mumps vaccine is no more frequent than the incidence found in the general population.

Persons previously vaccinated with inactivated (killed) mumps vaccine and revaccinated with live mumps vaccine are at no increased risk of side/adverse effects.

There is no proven association between administration of mumps vaccine and pancreatic damage or subsequent diabetes mellitus.

The following side/adverse effects have been selected on the basis of their potential clinical significance (possible signs and symptoms in parentheses where appropriate)—not necessarily inclusive:

**Those indicating need for medical attention**

Incidence rare
    *Anaphylactic reaction* (difficulty in breathing or swallowing; hives; itching, especially of soles or palms; reddening of skin, especially around ears; swelling of eyes, face, or inside of nose; unusual tiredness or weakness, sudden and severe); *convulsions, encephalitis, or meningoencephalitis* (confusion; severe or continuing headache; irritability; stiff neck; or vomiting); *fever over 39.4 °C (103 °F); orchitis in postpubescent and adult males* (pain, tenderness, or swelling in testicles and scrotum); *thrombocytopenic purpura* (bruising or purple spots on skin)

**Those indicating need for medical attention only if they continue or are bothersome**

Incidence more frequent
    *Burning or stinging at injection site*—due to acid pH of vaccine

Incidence less frequent or rare
    *Delayed-type, cell-mediated, allergic reaction* (itching, swelling, redness, tenderness, or hard lump at injection site); *fever of 37.7 °C (100 °F) or less; parotitis* (swollen glands on side of face or neck); *skin rash*

## Patient Consultation

As an aid to patient consultation, refer to *Advice for the Patient, Mumps Virus Vaccine Live (Systemic).*

In providing consultation, consider emphasizing the following selected information (» = major clinical significance):

**Before receiving this vaccine**

» Conditions affecting use, especially:
    Sensitivity to mumps vaccine or allergy to eggs or neomycin
    Pregnancy—Mumps vaccine may infect the placenta, although the vaccine has not been shown to infect the fetus or to cause birth defects
    Use in children—Use is not recommended for infants up to 12 months of age
    Other medications, especially immunosuppressive agents or radiation therapy

Other medical problems, especially severe febrile illness; primary
or acquired immune deficiency conditions; or family history of
congenital or hereditary immune deficiency conditions

### Proper use of this vaccine
» Proper dosing

*Precautions after receiving this vaccine*
» Not becoming pregnant for 3 months without first checking with phy-
sician, because of possible problems during pregnancy
Checking with physician before receiving:
Blood transfusions or other blood products within 2 weeks of this
vaccine
Gamma globulin or other globulins within 2 weeks of this vaccine
Any other live virus vaccines within 1 month of this vaccine
Tuberculin skin test within 6 weeks of this vaccine, since the results
of the test may be affected by mumps vaccine

### Side/adverse effects
Signs of potential side effects, especially anaphylactic reaction, convulsions, encephalitis, meningoencephalitis, fever over 39.4 °C, orchitis in postpubescent and adult males, or thrombocytopenic
purpura

## General Dosing Information

The dosage of mumps vaccine is the same for all persons: infants, children, and adults.

When sterilizing syringes before vaccination, care should be taken to
avoid preservatives, antiseptics, detergents, and disinfectants, since the
vaccine virus is easily inactivated by these substances.

To prevent inactivation of the vaccine, it is recommended that only the
diluent provided by the manufacturer be used.

A 25-gauge, 5/8th-inch needle is recommended for administration of the
vaccine.

Mumps vaccine is administered subcutaneously. While not routinely recommended, intramuscular administration is considered effective and
safe also. The vaccine should not be injected intravenously.

Although measles, mumps, and rubella vaccines are commercially available as a combination vaccine (MMR) and, as such, are administered
as a single injection, the commercially available individual vaccines
should not be mixed in the same syringe or administered at the same
body site.

Mumps vaccine, a live virus vaccine, can be administered concurrently
with the following, using separate body sites, separate syringes,
and the precautions that apply to each immunizing agent:
• Polysaccharide vaccines, such as haemophilus b polysaccharide
vaccine, haemophilus b conjugate vaccine, meningococcal polysaccharide vaccine, or pneumococcal polyvalent vaccine.
• Influenza vaccine, whole or split virus.
• Diphtheria toxoid, tetanus toxoid, and/or pertussis vaccine.
• Live virus vaccines, other, such as measles, rubella, or oral polio
vaccine (OPV), but only if the vaccines are administered on the
same day; otherwise they should be administered at least 1 month
apart.
• Inactivated poliovirus vaccine (IPV) or enhanced-potency inactivated vaccine (enhanced-potency IPV).
• Hepatitis B recombinant or plasma-derived vaccine.
• Inactivated vaccines, other, except cholera, typhoid, and plague.
It is recommended that cholera, typhoid, and plague vaccines be
administered on separate occasions because of the propensity of
these vaccines to cause side/adverse effects.

Although the fourth dose of DTP and the third dose of OPV have traditionally been administered to children 18 months of age and MMR
has traditionally been administered to children 15 months of age, it is
now recommended that DTP, OPV, and MMR be administered concurrently to children 15 months of age. MMR should not be postponed
in order to administer these vaccines concurrently at 18 months of age.
In addition, the traditional method is still an acceptable alternative.

Additional doses of mumps vaccine are not required for persons known
to have been vaccinated at 12 months of age or older. However, if
there is doubt that the original vaccination was effective, the patient
should be revaccinated, since studies have indicated that there are no
adverse effects when patients already immune to mumps are
revaccinated.

### For treatment of adverse effects
Recommended treatment includes:
• For mild hypersensitivity reaction—Administering antihistamines, and, if necessary, corticosteroids.
• For severe hypersensitivity or anaphylactic reaction—Administering epinephrine. Antihistamines or corticosteroids may also be
administered as required.

## Parenteral Dosage Forms

### MUMPS VIRUS VACCINE LIVE (FOR INJECTION) USP

#### Usual adult and adolescent dose
Immunizing agent (active)—
Subcutaneous, 0.5 mL, preferably into the outer aspect of the upper
arm.

#### Usual pediatric dose
Immunizing agent (active)—
Infants up to 12 months of age: Use is not recommended, since maternal mumps-neutralizing antibodies may interfere with the immune response.
Infants and children 12 months of age and older: See *Usual adult and
adolescent dose.*

#### Strength(s) usually available
U.S.—
Not less than the equivalent of 20,000 TCID$_{50}$ (quantity of virus es-
timated to infect 50% of inoculated cultures times 20,000) of the
U.S. Reference Mumps Virus in each 0.5 mL dose (Rx) [*Mumps-
vax* (neomycin 25 mcg)].
Canada—
Not less than the equivalent of 5000 TCID$_{50}$ (quantity of virus esti-
mated to infect 50% of inoculated cultures times 5000) of the U.S.
Reference Mumps Virus in each 0.5 mL dose (Rx) [*Mumpsvax*
(neomycin 17.5 mcg)].

#### Packaging and storage
Store the lyophilized form of the vaccine, the diluent, and the reconstituted
form of the vaccine between 2 and 8 °C (36 and 46 °F), unless otherwise specified by manufacturer.
Alternatively, the diluent for the single-dose vials only may be stored
between 15 and 30 °C (59 and 86 °F).
Protect both the lyophilized form and the reconstituted form of the vaccine
from light.

#### Preparation of dosage form
To reconstitute, use only the diluent provided by the manufacturer, since
it is free of preservatives or other substances that might inactivate the
vaccine.
Single-dose vial—Withdraw the entire volume of diluent (approximately
0.5 mL) into the syringe. Inject all the diluent in the syringe into the
vial of lyophilized vaccine and agitate to mix thoroughly. Withdraw
the entire contents into the syringe and inject the total volume of restored vaccine subcutaneously.
10-dose vial (in U.S., available only to government agencies/institutions)—
Withdraw the entire contents (7 mL) of the diluent vial into the syringe
to be used for reconstitution. Inject all of the diluent in the syringe
into the 10-dose vial of lyophilized vaccine and agitate to mix thoroughly. The 10-dose container can be used with either syringes or jet
injector. Since the vaccine and diluent do not contain preservatives,
special care should be taken to prevent contamination of the multiple-
dose vial of vaccine. In addition, the vial should be stored properly
until the reconstituted vaccine is used. Discard unused vaccine after 8
hours.
50-dose vial (in U.S., available only to government agencies/institutions)—
Withdraw the entire contents (30 mL) of the diluent vial into the syringe to be used for reconstitution. Inject all of the diluent in the
syringe into the 50-dose vial of lyophilized vaccine and agitate to mix
thoroughly. The 50-dose container is designed to be used only with a
jet injector. Since the vaccine and diluent do not contain preservatives,
special care should be taken to prevent contamination of the multiple-
dose vial of vaccine. In addition, the vial should be stored properly
until the reconstituted vaccine is used. Discard unused vaccine after 8
hours.

#### Stability
Both the lyophilized and reconstituted vaccine should be stored between
2 and 8 °C (36 and 46 °F) and protected from light. Improper storage
and protection may inactivate the virus.
Use the reconstituted vaccine as soon as possible. Discard unused reconstituted vaccine after 8 hours.
The reconstituted vaccine is clear yellow. It should not be used if it is
discolored.

#### Incompatibilities
Preservatives or other substances may inactivate the vaccine; therefore,
only the diluent supplied by the manufacturer should be used for
reconstitution.
A sterile syringe free of preservatives, antiseptics, disinfectants, and detergents should be used for each injection and/or reconstitution of the
vaccine because these substances may inactivate the live virus vaccine.

**Auxiliary labeling**
- Protect from light.
- Store in refrigerator.
- Discard reconstituted vaccine if not used within 8 hours.

**Note**
The date and time of reconstitution should be indicated on the vial if the reconstituted vaccine is not used at once.

Revised: 07/12/94

---

# MUPIROCIN    Topical

VA CLASSIFICATION (Primary): DE101
Another commonly used name is pseudomonic acid.

Note: For a listing of dosage forms and brand names by country availability, see *Dosage Forms* section(s). For a listing of brand names for the articles in this monograph, refer to the General Index.

## Category
Antibacterial (topical).

## Indications
Note: Bracketed information in the *Indications* section refers to uses that are not included in U.S. product labeling.

**Accepted**
Impetigo (treatment)—Mupirocin is indicated [alone as a primary agent] in the topical treatment of [localized] impetigo caused by *Staphylococcus aureus* and beta-hemolytic streptococci, including *Streptococcus pyogenes*.

[However, some USP medical experts prefer systemic antibacterials in the treatment of most cases of impetigo.]

[Eczema, infected (treatment)] or
[Folliculitis (treatment)][1]—Mupirocin is used as a primary agent in the topical treatment of localized infected eczema and folliculitis caused by *S. aureus*.

[Skin infections, bacterial, minor (prophylaxis)]—Mupirocin is used in the topical prophylaxis of minor bacterial skin infections.

Not all species or strains of a particular organism may be susceptible to mupirocin.

**Unaccepted**
Mupirocin is not effective against *Enterobacteriaceae*, *Pseudomonas aeruginosa*, or fungi.

[1]Not included in Canadian product labeling.

## Pharmacology/Pharmacokinetics

**Physicochemical characteristics**
Source—Produced by fermentation of *Pseudomonas fluorescens*.
Chemical group—Structurally unrelated to other systemic or topical antibacterials.
Molecular weight—500.63.

**Mechanism of action/Effect**
The mechanism of action is not completely understood. Mupirocin is bacteriostatic at low concentrations and bactericidal at high concentrations. This agent reversibly and specifically binds to bacterial isoleucyl transfer RNA synthetase, thereby inhibiting bacterial protein and RNA synthesis. DNA synthesis and cell wall formation are affected to a lesser extent.

**Absorption**
Virtually no systemic absorption (< 1.1 nanograms per mL of whole blood) following application to lower arm of normal males with occlusion for 24 hours.

## Precautions to Consider

**Pregnancy/Reproduction**
Fertility—Adequate and well-controlled studies in humans have not been done.
Studies in rats and rabbits given oral, subcutaneous, and intramuscular doses of up to 100 times the human topical dose, have not shown that mupirocin causes impaired fertility.

Pregnancy—Adequate and well-controlled studies in humans have not been done.
Studies in rats and rabbits given oral, subcutaneous, and intramuscular doses of up to 100 times the human topical dose, have not shown that mupirocin causes adverse effects in the fetus.

FDA Pregnancy Category B.

**Breast-feeding**
It is not known whether mupirocin is distributed into breast milk. However, problems in humans have not been documented. Mupirocin is unlikely to be distributed into breast milk in significant amounts since virtually no systemic absorption occurs following topical administration.

**Pediatrics**
No information is available on the relationship of age to the effects of mupirocin in pediatric patients. Safety and efficacy have not been established.

**Geriatrics**
No information is available on the relationship of age to the effects of mupirocin in geriatric patients.

**Medical considerations/Contraindications**
The medical considerations/contraindications included here have been selected on the basis of their potential clinical significance (reasons given in parentheses where appropriate)—not necessarily inclusive (» = major clinical significance).

*Risk-benefit should be considered when the following medical problem exists:*
Sensitivity to mupirocin

## Side/Adverse Effects
Note: The polyethylene glycol vehicle in mupirocin ointment may irritate broken skin or mucous membranes.

When mupirocin ointment is applied to extensive open wounds or burns, the possibility of absorption of the polyethylene glycol vehicle, resulting in serious renal toxicity, should be considered.

Mupirocin ointment has not been reported to cause contact sensitization or photosensitivity reactions.

The following side/adverse effects have been selected on the basis of their potential clinical significance (possible signs and symptoms in parentheses where appropriate)—not necessarily inclusive:

**Those indicating need for medical attention only if they continue or are bothersome**
Incidence less frequent
*Dry skin; skin burning, itching, pain, rash, redness, stinging, or swelling*

## Patient Consultation
As an aid to patient consultation, refer to *Advice for the Patient, Mupirocin (Topical)*.

In providing consultation, consider emphasizing the following selected information (» = major clinical significance):

**Proper use of this medication**
» Not for ophthalmic use
*To use*
Before applying, washing affected area(s) with soap and water and drying thoroughly; applying small amount and rubbing in gently
After applying, covering treated area(s) with gauze dressing if desired
» Compliance with full course of therapy
» Proper dosing
Missed dose: Applying as soon as possible; not applying if almost time for next dose
» Proper storage

**Precautions while using this medication**
Checking with physician or pharmacist if no improvement within 3 to 5 days

## General Dosing Information
Topical mupirocin is not for ophthalmic use.

The treated area(s) may be covered with a gauze dressing if desired.

When mupirocin ointment is applied to extensive open wounds or burns, the possibility of absorption of the polyethylene glycol vehicle, resulting in serious renal toxicity, should be considered.

If skin irritation or hypersensitivity develops, treatment with mupirocin ointment should be discontinued.

## Topical Dosage Forms

Note: Bracketed uses in the *Dosage Forms* section refer to categories of use and/or indications that are not included in U.S. product labeling.

### MUPIROCIN OINTMENT USP

**Usual adult and adolescent dose**
Impetigo or
[Eczema, infected] or
[Folliculitis][1]—
     Topical, to the affected area(s), three times a day.

**Usual pediatric dose**
See *Usual adult and adolescent dose.*

**Strength(s) usually available**
U.S.—
     2% (Rx) [*Bactroban* (polyethylene glycol [PEG] 400; PEG 3350)].

Canada—
     2% (OTC) [*Bactroban* (polyethylene glycol [PEG] 400; PEG 3350)].

**Packaging and storage**
Store between 15 and 30 °C (59 and 86 °F), in a well-closed container, unless otherwise specified by manufacturer. Protect from freezing.

**Auxiliary labeling**
• For external use only.
• Continue medicine for full time of treatment.

**Note**
Mupirocin ointment is available in a bland, water-miscible ointment base.

[1]Not included in Canadian product labeling.

## Selected Bibliography

Rumsfield J. West DP, Aronson IK. Topical mupirocin in the treatment of bacterial skin infections. Drug Intell Clin Pharm 1988 Dec; 20: 943-8.
Parenti MA, Hartfield SM, Leyden JJ. Mupirocin: a topical antibiotic with a unique structure and mechanism of action. Clin Pharm 1987 Oct; 6: 761-70.

Revised: 06/24/94

---

# MUROMONAB-CD3    Systemic

VA CLASSIFICATION (Primary): IM600
Note: For a listing of dosage forms and brand names by country availability, see *Dosage Forms* section(s). For a listing of brand names for the articles in this monograph, refer to the General Index.

## Category
Monoclonal antibody; immunosuppressant.

## Indications

### Accepted
Transplant rejection, organ (treatment)—Muromonab-CD3 is indicated, usually in combination with azathioprine, cyclosporine, and/or corticosteroids, for treatment of acute rejection of renal transplants (allografts). It is also indicated for treatment of steroid-resistant acute rejection of hepatic and cardiac transplants.

## Pharmacology/Pharmacokinetics

### Mechanism of action/Effect
Muromonab-CD3, a murine monoclonal antibody, reacts with a T3 (CD3) molecule that is linked to an antigen receptor on the surface membrane of human T-lymphocytes and thereby blocks both the generation and function of the T-cells in response to antigenic challenge. Initially, binding of muromonab-CD3 to T-lymphocytes leads to early activation of T-cells and subsequent cytokine release; however, ultimately, T-cell functions are blocked. Muromonab-CD3 does not cause myelosuppression.

### Onset of action
Number of circulating CD3 positive T-cells is reduced within minutes after administration.

### Time to steady-state serum trough concentration
3 days.

### Steady-state trough serum concentration
With dose of 5 mg per day—0.9 mcg per mL.

### Duration of action
Number of circulating CD3 positive T-cells returns to pretreatment levels, and T-cell function returns to normal, within 1 week after muromonab-CD3 is withdrawn.

## Precautions to Consider

### Cross-sensitivity and/or related problems
Patients sensitive to any product of murine (mouse) origin may also be sensitive to muromonab-CD3. Muromonab-CD3 may induce human anti-mouse antibody production and hypersensitivity in patients.

### Carcinogenicity
Studies have not been done in either animals or humans; however, suppression of cell-mediated immunity in organ transplant patients is associated with an increased risk of benign and malignant lymphopro-

liferative disorders, lymphomas, and skin cancers. Lymphomas have developed in humans treated with muromonab-CD3, although a definite causal relationship has not been established. Other infrequently reported neoplasms have included multiple myeloma, leukemia, breast carcinoma, adenocarcinoma, cholangiocarcinoma, and recurrences of pre-existing hepatoma and renal cell carcinoma.

### Pregnancy/Reproduction
Pregnancy—Studies have not been done in humans. However, muromonab-CD3 is an immunoglobulin G (IgG) antibody that may cross the human placenta; the effect of cytokine release and immunosuppression on the fetus is unknown.
Studies have not been done in animals.
FDA Pregnancy Category C.

### Breast-feeding
Problems in humans have not been documented. However, breast-feeding is generally not recommended while muromonab-CD3 is being administered because of the potential risks to the infant (adverse effects, carcinogenicity). It is not known whether muromonab-CD3 is distributed into breast milk.

### Pediatrics
Appropriate studies on the relationship of age to the effects of muromonab-CD3 have not been performed in the pediatric population. Muromonab-CD3 has been used in children, with appropriate dosage adjustments. Small children may be at increased risk of dehydration as a result of gastrointestinal fluid loss from diarrhea and/or vomiting with the cytokine release syndrome. The risk of long-term adverse sequelae to high fever, seizures, central nervous system (CNS) infections, aseptic meningitis, etc., is unknown.

### Geriatrics
No information is available on the relationship of age to the effects of muromonab-CD3 in geriatric patients.

### Dental
The immunosuppressant effects of muromonab-CD3 may result in an increased incidence of microbial infection and delayed healing. Dental work, whenever possible, should be completed prior to initiation of therapy and undertaken only with great caution during therapy. Patients should be instructed in proper oral hygiene during treatment, including caution in use of regular toothbrushes, dental floss, and toothpicks.

### Drug interactions and/or related problems
The following drug interactions and/or related problems have been selected on the basis of their potential clinical significance (possible mechanism in parentheses where appropriate)—not necessarily inclusive (» = major clinical significance):
» Immunosuppressant agents, other, such as:
     Azathioprine
     Chlorambucil
     Corticosteroids, glucocorticoid
     Cyclophosphamide
     Cyclosporine

Cytarabine
Mercaptopurine
(although muromonab-CD3 is often administered in conjunction
with azathioprine, cyclosporine, and/or corticosteroids, concurrent
use may increase the risk of infection and development of lymphoproliferative disorders; reduced dosage of corticosteroids and
azathioprine is recommended when muromonab-CD3 therapy is
begun; continued use of cyclosporine is recommended only with
extreme caution and in reduced dosage)

(concurrent use of other immunosuppressant agents with muro-
monab-CD3 has been shown to alter the time course of anti-mouse
antibody development as well as the specificity [idiotypic, isotypic,
allotypic] of the antibodies formed)

Vaccines, killed virus
(because normal defense mechanisms may be suppressed by mu-
romonab-CD3 therapy, the patient's antibody response to the vaccine may be decreased. The interval between discontinuation of
medications that cause immunosuppression and restoration of the
patient's ability to respond to the vaccine depends on the intensity
and type of immunosuppression-causing medication used, the underlying disease, and other factors; estimates vary from 3 months
to 1 year)

» Vaccines, live virus
(because normal defense mechanisms may be suppressed by mu-
romonab-CD3 therapy, concurrent use with a live virus vaccine
may potentiate the replication of the vaccine virus, may increase
the side/adverse effects of the vaccine virus, and/or may decrease
the patient's antibody response to the vaccine; immunization of
these patients should be undertaken only with extreme caution after
careful review of the patient's immunologic status and only with
the knowledge and consent of the physician managing the muro-
monab-CD3 therapy. The interval between discontinuation of medications that cause immunosuppression and restoration of the patient's ability to respond to the vaccine depends on the intensity
and type of immunosuppression-causing medication used, the underlying disease, and other factors; estimates vary from 3 months
to 1 year. Immunization with oral poliovirus vaccine should also
be postponed in persons in close contact with the patient, especially family members)

**Laboratory value alterations**
The following have been selected on the basis of their potential clinical
significance (possible effect in parentheses where appropriate)—not
necessarily inclusive (» = major clinical significance):
With physiology/laboratory test values
Hepatic transaminase
(serum values may be increased transiently after the first few doses
of muromonab-CD3)

**Medical considerations/Contraindications**
The medical considerations/contraindications included here have been selected on the basis of their potential clinical significance (reasons given
in parentheses where appropriate)—not necessarily inclusive (» =
major clinical significance).

*Except under special circumstances, this medication should not be used
when the following medical problems exist:*
» Anti-mouse antibody titre of 1:1000 or more
(increased risk of hypersensitivity to muromonab-CD3)
» Fever greater than 37.8 °C (100 °F)
(should be lowered by antipyretics, after infection has been ruled
out, before administration of muromonab-CD3)
» Fluid overload, as seen on chest x-ray or as a weight gain of greater
than 3% within 1 week before administration is planned or
» Heart failure, uncompensated
(risk of severe and potentially fatal pulmonary edema)

*Risk-benefit should be considered when the following medical problems
exist:*
» Angina, unstable or
» Cerebrovascular disease or
» Chronic obstructive pulmonary disease or
» Heart failure of any etiology or
» Intravascular volume overload or depletion of any etiology (e.g., ex-
cessive dialysis, recent intensive diuresis, blood loss, etc.) or
» Ischemic heart disease, symptomatic or
» Myocardial infarction, recent or
» Neuropathy, advanced symptomatic or
» Pulmonary edema of any etiology or
» Seizures, history of or
» Septic shock or

» Vascular disease, advanced symptomatic
(increased risk of serious complications from cytokine release syndrome; condition should be corrected or stabilized prior to initiation of muromonab-CD3 therapy)
» Chickenpox, existing or recent (including recent exposure) or
» Herpes zoster
(risk of severe generalized disease)
» Infection
Sensitivity to muromonab-CD3
Thrombosis, history of
(arterial or venous thromboses of allografts and other vascular beds
[e.g., heart, lungs, brain, bowel] have been reported in patients
treated with muromonab-CD3)

**Patient monitoring**
The following may be especially important in patient monitoring (other
tests may be warranted in some patients, depending on condition;
» = major clinical significance):
» Assay for circulating T-cells expressing the CD3 antigen or
» Muromonab-CD3 concentrations, plasma, as determined by enzyme-
linked immunosorbent assay (ELISA)
(recommended at periodic intervals during therapy to assess
efficacy)
Note: Recommended targets are fewer than 25 CD3-positive T-
cells per cubic millimeter or muromonab-CD3 concentrations of 800 nanograms per mL (ng/mL) or more.

Blood counts, complete, including differential and leukocytes and
Platelet counts
(recommended at periodic intervals during therapy)
» Body temperature determinations
(recommended prior to administration and at frequent intervals for
several hours after administration, especially with the first two
doses)
Hepatic function determinations, including serum transaminase and alkaline phosphatase values and bilirubin concentrations and
Renal function determinations, including blood urea nitrogen and serum creatinine concentrations
(recommended at periodic intervals during therapy)

# Side/Adverse Effects

Note: Neutralizing antibodies, primarily of the IgG class, have been detected in most patients during or following the second week of
muromonab-CD3 therapy and may potentially reduce subsequent
effectiveness by blocking the ability of muromonab-CD3 to bind
to the CD3 antigen on T-lymphocytes. Development of neutralizing
antibodies has been linked to reappearance of CD3 positive T-cells
prior to withdrawal of muromonab-CD3.

The following side/adverse effects have been selected on the basis of their
potential clinical significance (possible signs and symptoms in parentheses where appropriate)—not necessarily inclusive:

**Those indicating need for medical attention**
Incidence more frequent
*Cytokine release syndrome, mild* (diarrhea; dizziness or faintness; fever [often spiking and up to 42 °C or 107 °F] and chills; headache;
malaise; muscle or joint pain; nausea and vomiting)
Note: Symptoms of the *cytokine release syndrome* occur in most patients, usually 30 minutes to 48 hours after the first dose, and
last several hours; both frequency and severity seem to decrease
with each subsequent dose; fever and chills occurring later may
be due to infection; cytokine release syndrome may also occur
with dosage increases or resumption of dosing after a period of
withdrawal.

Incidence less frequent
*Anaphylaxis* (rapid or irregular heartbeat; shortness of breath or
wheezing; swelling of face or throat); *or hypersensitivity* (itching or
tingling; skin rash); *cytokine release syndrome, severe* (chest pain;
rapid or irregular heartbeat; shortness of breath or wheezing; trembling
and shaking of hands; weakness); *neuropsychiatric reactions, including seizures; encephalopathy* (confusion; hallucinations; unusual
tiredness; coma); *cerebral edema; aseptic meningitis syndrome* (fever;
headache; stiff neck; unusual sensitivity of eyes to light; rarely,
seizures); *and headache*
Note: *Anaphylactic reactions*, which are serious and occasionally fatal, usually occur within 10 minutes after a dose, and may be
difficult to differentiate from the cytokine release syndrome.
Such reactions may include cardiovascular collapse, cardiorespiratory arrest, loss of consciousness, hypotension/shock, tach-

ycardia, tingling, angioedema (including laryngeal, pharyngeal, or facial edema), airway obstruction, bronchospasm, dyspnea, urticaria, and pruritus.

Symptoms of the *cytokine release syndrome* occur in most patients, usually 30 minutes to 48 hours after the first dose, and last several hours; both frequency and severity seem to decrease with each subsequent dose; fever and chills occurring later may be due to infection; cytokine release syndrome may also occur with dosage increases or resumption of dosing after a period of withdrawal.

Cardiorespiratory findings with the *cytokine release syndrome* may include tachypnea; respiratory distress, failure, or arrest; cardiovascular collapse; cardiac arrest; myocardial infarction; tachycardia; hypertension; hemodynamic instability; hypotension including profound shock; heart failure; cardiogenic and noncardiogenic pulmonary edema; adult respiratory distress syndrome; hypoxemia; apnea; and arrhythmias. Of these, severe, potentially fatal pulmonary edema is the most serious.

An acute and transient decline in the glomerular filtration rate and diminished urine output, manifested as an increase in the serum creatinine concentration, may occur as a result of *cytokine release*, and may lead to reversible renal function impairment.

*Neuropsychiatric reactions* may be caused partly by T-cell activation resulting in systemic release of cytokines.

*Neurologic* signs and symptoms are usually reversible, even with continued treatment, but are sometimes irreversible.

Symptoms of *aseptic meningitis syndrome* usually occur within the first 3 days of therapy. Examination of cerebrospinal fluid may show leukocytosis, elevated protein, or reduced glucose concentrations.

Other *neurologic events* that have been reported occasionally include impaired vision, irreversible blindness, para- or quadriparesis/plegia, cerebrovascular accident [hemiparesis/plegia], aphasia, transient ischemic attack, subarachnoid hemorrhage, palsy of the VI cranial nerve, and hearing loss.

**Those indicating possible need for medical attention if they occur after medication is discontinued**
    *Infection* (fever and chills)

## Patient Consultation

As an aid to patient consultation, refer to *Advice for the Patient, Muromonab-CD3 (Systemic)*.

In providing consultation, consider emphasizing the following selected information (» = major clinical significance):

**Before using this medication**
» Conditions affecting use, especially:
    Sensitivity to muromonab-CD3
    Pregnancy—May cross placenta; risk of adverse effects unknown
    Breast-feeding—Not recommended because of risk of serious side effects
    Use in children—Possible increased risk of dehydration as a result of diarrhea and/or vomiting associated with cytokine release syndrome
    Other medications, especially other immunosuppressants
    Other medical problems, especially unstable angina, cerebrovascular disease, chickenpox, chronic obstructive pulmonary disease, fever, heart failure, herpes zoster, infection, symptomatic ischemic heart disease, recent myocardial infarction, advanced symptomatic neuropathy, pulmonary edema, history of seizures, septic shock, or advanced symptomatic vascular disease

**Proper use of this medication**
» Proper dosing

**Precautions while using this medication**
» Importance of close monitoring by physician
» Avoiding immunizations unless approved by physician; other persons in patient's household should avoid immunizations with oral poliovirus vaccine; avoiding persons who have taken oral poliovirus vaccine or wearing a protective mask that covers nose and mouth
    Avoiding exposure to persons with bacterial infections; telling physician if signs of bacterial infection occur
» Possible cytokine release syndrome, which should be reduced after second and subsequent doses; telling doctor or nurse immediately if symptoms of angioedema, cardiac effects, or pulmonary edema occur

**Side/adverse effects**
    Signs of potential side effects, especially cytokine release syndrome, anaphylaxis or hypersensitivity, and neuropsychiatric reactions

## General Dosing Information

Patients receiving muromonab-CD3 should be under supervision of a physician experienced in immunosuppressive therapy.

It is recommended that equipment and medications necessary for cardiopulmonary resuscitation be immediately available during administration of each dose of muromonab-CD3.

Muromonab-CD3 should be administered by intravenous push over a period of less than 1 minute.

Acetaminophen and antihistamines may be used to reduce or treat early reactions. Patient temperature should be maintained below 37.8 °C (100 °F) at administration of each dose.

Dosage reduction of other immunosuppressive therapy is recommended when muromonab-CD3 therapy is begun. Dosage should be returned to maintenance levels approximately 3 days before muromonab-CD3 therapy is completed.

Initiation of anti-infective prophylaxis may be warranted in patients at high risk for infection or viral-induced lymphoproliferative disorders. If an infection develops, it must be treated promptly; withdrawal of muromonab-CD3 may be necessary.

**For treatment of adverse effects**
Intensive treatment with oxygen, intravenous fluids, corticosteroids, pressor amines, antihistamines, intubation, etc., may be required for serious manifestations of the cytokine release syndrome.
Subcutaneous aqueous epinephrine (0.3 to 0.5 mL of the 1:1000 dilution), along with other resuscitative measures, may be required for severe anaphylaxis.

## Parenteral Dosage Forms
### MUROMONAB-CD3 INJECTION

**Usual adult and adolescent dose**
Immunosuppressant—
    Intravenous (rapid), 5 mg per day for ten to fourteen days.
    Note: Intravenous administration of methylprednisolone sodium succinate (8 mg per kg of body weight) one to four hours prior to the first dose of muromonab-CD3 is recommended to reduce the incidence and severity of the cytokine release syndrome.

**Usual pediatric dose**
Immunosuppressant—
    Children less than 12 years of age: Intravenous (rapid), 100 mcg (0.1 mg) per kg of body weight per day for ten to fourteen days.

**Strength(s) usually available**
U.S.—
    1 mg per mL (Rx) [*Orthoclone OKT3* (polysorbate 80)].
Canada—
    1 mg per mL (Rx) [*Orthoclone OKT3*].

**Packaging and storage**
Store between 2 and 8 °C (36 and 46 °F), unless otherwise specified by manufacturer. Protect from freezing.

**Preparation of dosage form**
Sterile muromonab-CD3 is prepared for intravenous administration by drawing the solution into a syringe through a low protein–binding 0.2 or 0.22 micrometer filter, then discarding the filter and attaching an appropriate needle.

**Stability**
Because the product contains no bacteriostatic agent, muromonab-CD3 injection should be used immediately after the ampule is opened and any unused portion should be discarded. In addition, muromonab-CD3 injection, like other protein solutions, may develop a few fine translucent particles, which have not been shown to affect potency.

**Incompatibilities**
Muromonab-CD3 should not be administered by intravenous infusion or in conjunction with other drug solutions.

**Auxiliary labeling**
• Do not shake.

Revised: 08/08/95

# NABILONE  Systemic*

VA CLASSIFICATION (Primary): GA700

Note: Controlled substance in Canada—N.

Note: For a listing of dosage forms and brand names by country availability, see *Dosage Forms* section(s). For a listing of brand names for the articles in this monograph, refer to the General Index.

---

*Not commercially available in the U.S.

---

## Category
Antiemetic.

## Indications
### Accepted
Nausea and vomiting, cancer chemotherapy–induced (prophylaxis)—Nabilone is indicated in selected patients for the prevention of nausea and vomiting associated with emetogenic cancer chemotherapy when other antiemetic medications are not effective.

## Pharmacology/Pharmacokinetics
### Physicochemical characteristics
Chemical group—Synthetic 9-ketocannabinoid; resembles the cannabinols but is not a tetrahydrocannabinol
Molecular weight—372.55.

### Mechanism of action/Effect
The exact mechanism of nabilone's antiemetic action is not known. However, animal studies with other cannabinoids suggest it may be due to inhibition of the vomiting control mechanism in the medulla oblongata.

### Other actions/effects
Central nervous system (CNS) depression and stimulation; may increase supine and standing heart rates (dose-dependent); may inhibit prolactin release.

### Absorption
Rapidly absorbed from the gastrointestinal tract after oral administration.

### Biotransformation
Hepatic.

### Half-life
Elimination—
   Terminal phase:
      Nabilone—2 hours.
      Other metabolites—35 hours.

### Time to peak concentration
2 hours.

### Elimination
Primarily fecal (biliary); approximately 65% of an oral dose appears in the feces and 20% in the urine.

## Precautions to Consider
### Cross-sensitivity and/or related problems
Patients sensitive to other marijuana products may be sensitive to this preparation also.

### Carcinogenicity
Studies to evaluate the carcinogenic potential of nabilone have not been performed.

### Pregnancy/Reproduction
Pregnancy—Adequate and well-controlled studies in humans have not been done.
Studies in rats and rabbits at doses 150 and 40 times, respectively, the usual human adult dose have shown that nabilone decreases litter size, and increases the incidence of fetal resorptions and stillborn pups.

### Breast-feeding
It is not known whether nabilone is distributed into breast milk. However, use of nabilone in nursing mothers is not recommended since dronabinol, another synthetic cannabinoid closely related to nabilone, is concentrated and distributed into breast milk.

### Pediatrics
Appropriate studies on the relationship of age to the effects of nabilone have not been performed in children up to 18 years of age. Safety and efficacy have not been established.

### Geriatrics
Although appropriate studies on the relationship of age to the effects of nabilone have not been performed in the geriatric population, the elderly may be more sensitive to the cardiac effects and orthostatic hypotension produced by nabilone.
Also, because of this medication's psychoactive effects and potential for dependence, therapy could be more troublesome in the elderly and should be used with caution, after less toxic alternatives have been considered and found ineffective. Recommended doses should not be exceeded, and the elderly patient should be carefully monitored during therapy.

### Drug interactions and/or related problems
The following drug interactions and/or related problems have been selected on the basis of their potential clinical significance (possible mechanism in parentheses where appropriate)—not necessarily inclusive (» = major clinical significance):

Note: Combinations containing any of the following medications, depending on the amount present, may also interact with this medication.

» Alcohol or
» CNS depression–producing medications, other (See *Appendix II*)
   (concurrent use may potentiate the CNS depressant effects of either these medications or nabilone)

Apomorphine
   (prior administration of nabilone may decrease the emetic response to apomorphine; also, concurrent use may potentiate the CNS depressant effects of either apomorphine or nabilone)

### Medical considerations/Contraindications
The medical considerations/contraindications included here have been selected on the basis of their potential clinical significance (reasons given in parentheses where appropriate)—not necessarily inclusive (» = major clinical significance).

*Risk-benefit should be considered when the following medical problems exist:*
Cardiac disorders
   (nabilone may elevate supine and standing heart rates)
Drug abuse or dependence, history of, including active or treated alcoholism
   (increased risk of nabilone abuse and dependence)
Hepatic function impairment, severe
   (increased risk of toxic effects because of decreased metabolism of nabilone)
Hypertension
   (hypertensive effects of nabilone may cause an increase in blood pressure)
Hypotension
   (hypotensive effects of nabilone may further decrease blood pressure)
» Manic or depressive states or
» Schizophrenia
   (symptoms may be exacerbated)
Sensitivity to nabilone or other marijuana products

### Patient monitoring
The following may be especially important in patient monitoring (other tests may be warranted in some patients, depending on condition; » = major clinical significance):

Blood pressure determinations and
Cardiac function monitoring
   (recommended for early detection of tachycardia and changes in blood pressure, especially in patients with hypertension or cardiac disease)

## Side/Adverse Effects
Note: Overdose may occur either with therapeutic doses or at higher, non-therapeutic doses.

The following side/adverse effects have been selected on the basis of their potential clinical significance (possible signs and symptoms in parentheses where appropriate)—not necessarily inclusive:

### Those indicating need for medical attention
*Psychiatric effects* (changes in mood; confusion, possibly including delusions and feelings of depersonalization or unreality; hallucinations; mental depression; nervousness or anxiety); *difficulty in*

*breathing; hypotension* (severe dizziness or fainting); *fast, slow, irregular, or pounding heartbeat; increase in blood pressure; unusual tiredness or weakness, severe*

Note: *Psychiatric effects* usually resolve by themselves within 72 hours after discontinuation of nabilone.

### Those indicating need for medical attention only if they continue or are bothersome

Incidence more frequent
> *Clumsiness or unsteadiness; difficulty concentrating; dizziness; drowsiness; dryness of mouth; false sense of well-being; headache*

Incidence less frequent or rare
> *Blurred vision or any changes in vision; dizziness or lightheadedness, especially when getting up from a lying or sitting position* (orthostatic hypotension)—more frequent with high doses; *loss of appetite; muscle pain or weakness*

## Overdose

Note: Overdose may occur either with therapeutic doses or at higher, nontherapeutic, doses.

For more information on the management of overdose or unintentional ingestion, **contact a Poison Control Center** (see *Poison Control Center Listing*).

### Clinical effects of overdose

The following effects have been selected on the basis of their potential clinical significance (possible signs and symptoms in parentheses where appropriate)–not necessarily inclusive:

> *Psychiatric effects* (changes in mood; confusion, possibly including delusions and feelings of depersonalization or unreality; hallucinations; mental depression; nervousness or anxiety); *difficulty in breathing; hypotension* (severe dizziness or fainting); *fast, slow, irregular, or pounding heartbeat; increase in blood pressure; unusual tiredness or weakness, severe*

Note: *Psychiatric effects* usually resolve by themselves within 72 hours after discontinuation of nabilone.

### Treatment of overdose

Specific treatment—Observation of patient in a quiet environment. Verbal support and comforting if psychotic episodes occur; in severe cases, antipsychotic drugs may be used with careful attention being paid to possible CNS-depressant additive effects. Treatment of hypertension or hypotension, if necessary.

Monitoring—Continuous blood pressure monitoring; cardiac monitoring.

Supportive care—Supportive therapy. Patients in whom intentional overdose is confirmed or suspected should be referred for psychiatric consultation.

## Patient Consultation

As an aid to patient consultation, refer to *Advice for the Patient, Nabilone (Systemic)*.

In providing consultation, consider emphasizing the following selected information (» = major clinical significance):

### Before using this medication
» Conditions affecting use, especially:
> Sensitivity to nabilone or other marijuana products
> Pregnancy—No studies in humans; increased risk of fetal resorptions and stillbirths in animal studies with doses many times the usual human dose
> Breast-feeding—Use not recommended; although not known if distributed into breast milk, possibility exists
> Use in the elderly—Increased sensitivity to cardiac effects and orthostatic hypotension; caution recommended because of psychoactive effects and potential for dependence
> Other medications, especially CNS depressants
> Other medical problems, especially manic depression and schizophrenia

### Proper use of this medication
» Importance of not taking more medication than the amount prescribed because of danger of overdose
» Proper dosing
» Missed dose: Taking as soon as possible; not taking if almost time for next dose; not doubling doses
» Proper storage

### Precautions while using this medication
» Avoiding use of alcohol or other CNS depressants during therapy

» Suspected overdose: Getting emergency help at once
» Caution if dizziness, drowsiness, lightheadedness, or false sense of well-being occurs
> Caution when getting up suddenly from a lying or sitting position
> Possible dryness of mouth; using sugarless candy or gum, ice, or saliva substitute for relief

### Side/adverse effects
Signs of potential side effects, especially psychiatric effects, difficulty in breathing, hypotension, tachycardia, hypertension, and unusual tiredness or weakness

## General Dosing Information

Amount of nabilone dispensed should be limited to the amount necessary for a single cycle of chemotherapy.

Patients on nabilone therapy should be closely observed, if possible within an inpatient setting. Since response and tolerance to the effects of nabilone vary with each patient, the period of patient supervision required should be determined by the physician on an individual basis.

Adequate and well-controlled studies have not been done to determine whether psychological and physical dependence will develop with chronic administration of nabilone. However, like other similar cannabinoids, nabilone has a high potential for abuse and for production of psychological dependence.

### For treatment of adverse effects
Recommended treatment includes
> • Observation of patient in a quiet environment.
> • Verbal support and comforting if psychotic episodes occur; in severe cases, antipsychotic drugs may be used with careful attention being paid to possible CNS depressant additive effects.
> • Supportive therapy.
> • Continuous blood pressure monitoring.
> • Cardiac monitoring.
> • Treatment of hypertension or hypotension, if necessary.

## Oral Dosage Forms

### NABILONE CAPSULES

#### Usual adult and adolescent dose
Antiemetic—
> Oral, 1 or 2 mg two times a day. A dose of 1 or 2 mg may be given the night before chemotherapy is initiated. On the day of chemotherapy, the initial dose of nabilone should be given one to three hours before the chemotherapeutic agent. The dose of nabilone may be administered two or three times a day during the course of chemotherapy and, if needed, for forty-eight hours after the last dose of the chemotherapeutic cycle.

Note: The lower starting dose should be used to minimize side effects. Dosage may be increased as necessary if side effects are not significant.

#### Usual adult prescribing limits
Up to 6 mg daily, in divided doses three times a day.

#### Usual pediatric dose
Safety and efficacy have not been established.

#### Usual geriatric dose
See *Usual adult and adolescent dose*.

Note: Geriatric patients may be more sensitive to the effects of the usual adult dose.

#### Strength(s) usually available
U.S.—
> Not commercially available.

Canada—
> 1 mg (Rx) [*Cesamet*].

#### Packaging and storage
Store between 15 and 30 °C (59 and 86 °F), unless otherwise specified by manufacturer.

#### Auxiliary labeling
• May cause drowsiness.
• Avoid alcoholic beverages.

#### Note
Controlled substance in Canada.

Revised: 06/17/93

**NABUMETONE**—See *Anti-inflammatory Drugs, Nonsteroidal (Systemic)*

**NADOLOL**—See *Beta-adrenergic Blocking Agents (Systemic)*

**NADOLOL-CONTAINING COMBINATIONS**—
Nadolol and Bendroflumethiazide (Systemic)—See *Beta-adrenergic Blocking Agents and Thiazide Diuretics (Systemic)*

# NAFARELIN  Systemic

INN: Nafarelin

VA CLASSIFICATION (Primary): HS900

Note: For a listing of dosage forms and brand names by country availability, see *Dosage Forms* section(s). For a listing of brand names for the articles in this monograph, refer to the General Index.

## Category
Gonadotropin-releasing hormone analog; gonadotropin inhibitor; antiendometriotic agent.

## Indications

### Accepted
Endometriosis (treatment)—Nafarelin is indicated for the management of endometriosis, including treatment of pelvic pain associated with all stages of endometriosis and reduction in the size and number of implants. Nafarelin may also have a modest effect on infertility in those patients with moderate endometriosis. Preoperative use of nafarelin in infertile patients with severe endometriosis may also facilitate the surgical procedure.

Nafarelin has been shown to be as effective as danazol in decreasing the size and extent of endometrial implants, as well as in reducing clinical symptoms of endometriosis.

Generally, the use of nafarelin or other gonadotropin-releasing hormone (GnRH) analogs for the treatment of endometriosis is limited to short-term, single courses of therapy of 6 months and to those patients who cannot tolerate the androgenic side effects of danazol or who are not candidates for surgery, because its use is associated with significant, but largely reversible, decreases in bone mass. The long-term, clinical significance and safety of these changes in bone mass are unknown.

## Pharmacology/Pharmacokinetics

### Physicochemical characteristics
Chemical group—Nafarelin acetate is a decapeptide, which is an agonistic analog of the hypothalamic hormone, gonadotropin-releasing hormone (GnRH). Substitution of a naphthylalanine group for glycine at the 6th amino acid position results in higher affinity for the GnRH receptor in the pituitary gland (approximately 200 times greater than GnRH), resistance to degradation by endopeptidases, and increased lipophilicity.

Molecular weight—1322.51 (anhydrous free decapeptide).

### Mechanism of action/Effect
Like GnRH, initial or intermittent administration of nafarelin acetate stimulates release of the gonadotropins luteinizing hormone (LH) and follicle-stimulating hormone (FSH) from the pituitary gland, which in turn transiently increases production of estradiol in females and testosterone in both sexes. However, with continuous daily administration, nafarelin continuously occupies the GnRH receptor. A reversible down-regulation of the GnRH receptors in the pituitary gland and desensitization of the pituitary gonadotropes occurs. This causes a significant and sustained decline in the production of LH and FSH. A decline in gonadotropin production and release causes a dramatic reversible decrease in synthesis of estradiol, progesterone, and testosterone by the ovaries or testes.

Like normal endometrium, endometriotic implants contain estrogen receptors. Estrogen stimulates the growth of endometrium. Use of nafarelin induces anovulation and amenorrhea and decreases serum concentrations of estradiol to the postmenopausal range, which induces atrophy of endometrial implants. Nafarelin does not abolish the underlying pathophysiology of endometriosis, however. After nafarelin therapy is discontinued, pituitary and ovarian function normalize and estradiol serum concentrations increase to pre-treatment levels. Recurrences of endometriosis are frequent after cessation of any hormonal therapy or surgery that leaves the ovaries and/or uterus intact.

### Absorption
Rapidly absorbed across nasal mucosa.

Bioavailability—2.8% (average, relative; range, 1.2 to 5.6%) after a 400 mcg dose.

### Protein binding
78 to 84% (*in vitro* estimation), primarily to albumin.

### Biotransformation
Enzymatic hydrolysis.

### Half-life
Elimination—3 hours (range, 2 to 4 hours).

### Onset of action
Within approximately 4 weeks, complete suppression of gonadal steroids occurs.

### Time to peak concentration
10 to 40 minutes.

### Peak serum concentration
200 mcg dose—0.6 nanograms per mL (average).
400 mcg dose—1.8 nanograms per mL.

### Time to peak effect
Maximal suppression of estradiol serum concentrations—20 days, with use of 400 to 800 mcg per day.

### Duration of action
Relief of symptoms may persist for up to 3 to 6 months after discontinuance of nafarelin therapy.

### Elimination
In one study in 3 males given a single subcutaneous dose of radiolabeled nafarelin, 44 to 55% of the radiolabel appeared in urine and 19 to 44% appeared in stool over 7 days following administration. Most of the radioactivity was recovered within the first 48 hours. Approximately 3% appears in the urine unchanged.

## Precautions to Consider

### Carcinogenicity/Tumorigenicity/Mutagenicity
In studies conducted in rats and mice, use of nafarelin at proportionately high doses and for prolonged periods induced hyperplasia and/or neoplasia of endocrine organs. Increases in pancreatic islet cell adenomas, benign adrenal medullary tumors, Harderian gland tumors, benign testicular and ovarian tumors, pituitary adenomas and carcinomas were noted in some animal treatment groups. No metastases of these tumors were observed. Generally, tumorigenicity in rodents is particularly sensitive to hormonal stimulation.

No evidence of tumorigenicity has been reported in monkeys or humans.

No evidence of mutagenic potential was seen in mutagenicity studies conducted in bacterial, yeast, and mammalian systems.

### Pregnancy/Reproduction
Fertility—Nafarelin usually induces anovulation and amenorrhea in most patients. This effect is reversible and the average time to return of menses after discontinuance of therapy is about 45 days. A nonhormonal contraceptive method should be used during nafarelin therapy. If an inadequate dose is used or successive doses are missed, breakthrough bleeding or ovulation may occur.

In one study, ovulation was detected (by monitoring of serum progesterone concentrations) in less than 18% of menstrual cycles over 3 to 6 months of dosing with 100 or 200 mcg per day. At a dose of 500 mcg twice a day, ovulation was completely suppressed.

Pregnancy—Nafarelin should not be given during the course of pregnancy. It is not known what effects nafarelin may have on the embryo if administered during pregnancy. The pre-existence of a pregnancy should be ruled out prior to it use. A nonhormonal contraceptive method should be used during nafarelin therapy.

Major fetal abnormalities were observed in one study in rats, but not in mice or rabbits after administration of nafarelin throughout gestation. A similar, repeat study in rats failed to show an increase in fetal abnormalities. A dose-related increase in fetal mortality and a decrease in fetal weight occurred in rabbits and rats. The effects on rat fetal mortality were expected results of the changes in gonadal steroid levels induced by nafarelin.

FDA Pregnancy Category X.

**Breast-feeding**
It is not known whether nafarelin is distributed into breast milk.

**Drug interactions and/or related problems**
The following drug interactions and/or related problems have been selected on the basis of their potential clinical significance (possible mechanism in parentheses where appropriate)—not necessarily inclusive (» = major clinical significance):

Note: Combinations containing any of the following medications, depending on the amount present, may also interact with this medication.

    Decongestants, nasal, topical
        (it is not known whether use of topical nasal decongestants will interfere with the absorption of nafarelin; it is recommended that patients allow 30 minutes to pass after the use of nafarelin before applying a topical nasal decongestant if needed)

**Laboratory value alterations**
The following have been selected on the basis of their potential clinical significance (possible effect in parentheses where appropriate)—not necessarily inclusive (» = major clinical significance):

With diagnostic test results
» Pituitary gonadotropic function testing and
» Gonadal function testing
    (therapeutic doses of nafarelin suppress the pituitary–gonadal system; baseline function is usually restored within 4 to 8 weeks of discontinuance of nafarelin)

With physiology/laboratory test values
    Alkaline phosphatase, serum and
    Calcium-to-creatinine ratio, urine and
    Hydroxyproline-to-creatinine ratio, urine and
    Phosphate, serum and
    Phosphorous, plasma
        (values are increased to postmenopausal levels during use of nafarelin, indicating increased bone remodeling; generally reversible within 3 to 6 months of discontinuation of nafarelin therapy)

    Androstenedione and
» Estradiol and
    Follicle-stimulating hormone and
    Luteinizing hormone and
» Progesterone and
    Sex-hormone binding globulin and
» Testosterone, total and free
        (serum concentrations are transiently increased at the onset of therapy; with continued use, serum concentrations will be suppressed; estradiol serum concentrations will decline to postmenopausal levels; effects are reversible upon discontinuation of nafarelin)

» Bone mineral content
    (hypoestrogenism-induced loss of bone mineral content occurs in most patients during use of nafarelin, which is especially evident in those skeletal regions that are composed mostly of trabecular bone, such as the spinal vertebrae; bone mineral content decreases reported range from 0 to 2% for the forearm [mostly cortical bone] and from 6 to 11% for the spinal vertebrae, after 6 months of therapy; in the 6 months following discontinuance of therapy, this effect has been reported to be largely reversible, with a net overall loss of approximately 1 to 1$^1$/$_2$%; the long-term, clinical significance of these changes in bone mass are unknown, and their importance in the selection of therapy is controversial)

    Calcium
        (serum concentrations are decreased during nafarelin therapy)

    Eosinophil count
        (asymptomatic eosinophilia has occurred in approximately 10 to 15% of patients during nafarelin therapy in clinical trials)

    White blood cell count
        (asymptomatic leukopenia has occurred in approximately 10 to 15% of patients during nafarelin therapy in clinical trials)

**Medical considerations/Contraindications**
The medical considerations/contraindications included here have been selected on the basis of their potential clinical significance (reasons given in parentheses where appropriate)—not necessarily inclusive (» = major clinical significance).

*Risk-benefit should be considered when the following medical problems exist:*
    Allergy to nafarelin acetate
    Significant risk factors for low bone mineral content
        (nafarelin may additionally increase the risk for development of osteopenia or osteoporosis; repeat courses of therapy with gonadotropin-releasing hormone analogs are not advisable)

## Side/Adverse Effects

The following side/adverse effects have been selected on the basis of their potential clinical significance (possible signs and symptoms in parentheses where appropriate)—not necessarily inclusive:

**Those indicating need for medical attention**
Incidence more frequent
    *Breakthrough bleeding* (vaginal bleeding between regular menstrual periods, which may require the use of a pad or tampon); *menorrhagia* (longer or heavier menstrual periods); *spotting* (light vaginal bleeding between regular menstrual periods, which does not require the use of a pad or tampon)

    Note: In the first two months after beginning nafarelin therapy, most women experience changes in vaginal bleeding patterns. However, the continuing occurrence of irregular vaginal bleeding may indicate noncompliance with the prescribed therapeutic regimen or the need for an increase in dose. Menorrhagia has been reported during the use of low doses (≤ 200 mcg per day).

Incidence rare
    *Arthralgia* (joint pain); *galactorrhea* (unexpected or excess milk flow); *hypersensitivity, immediate* (shortness of breath; chest pain; hives)—0.2% in clinical trials; *ovarian cysts; ovarian enlargement or; ovarian hyperstimulation, mild* (pelvic bloating or tenderness)

    Note: *Ovarian cysts, enlargement, or hyperstimulation* have been reported during use of low doses (≤200 mcg per day) or in the first 2 months of therapy. Ovarian cysts have primarily occurred in patients with polycystic ovary disease. Most ovarian cysts resolve spontaneously, within 4 to 6 weeks of therapy, but some cases may require discontinuation of nafarelin and/or surgery.

**Those indicating need for medical attention only if they continue or are bothersome**
Incidence more frequent
    *Amenorrhea* (stopping of menstrual periods); *hypoestrogenism* (acne; hot flashes; decreased libido; dyspareunia; reduced breast size; vaginal dryness; palpitations; oily skin)—occurs in nearly all patients
Incidence less frequent or rare
    *Emotional lability* (mood swings); *headache, mild and transient; maculopapular rash* (skin rash); *mastalgia* (breast pain); *mental depression, mild and transient; rhinitis* (irritated or runny nose)—about 10% incidence; *weight changes*

## Patient Consultation

As an aid to patient consultation, refer to *Advice for the Patient, Nafarelin (Systemic).*

In providing consultation, consider emphasizing the following selected information (» = major clinical significance):

**Before using this medication**
» Conditions affecting use, especially:
    Pregnancy—Pregnancy should be ruled out prior to use of nafarelin; nonhormonal contraceptive should be used during therapy
    Other medications, especially topical nasal decongestants; waiting 30 minutes after use of nafarelin to apply nasal decongestant
    Other medical conditions, especially significant risk factors for low bone mineral content

**Proper use of this medication**
    Using nasal spray correctly
» Proper dosing
» Proper storage

**Precautions while using this medication**
    Importance of regular follow-up visits to monitor progress
    Use of vaginal lubricants if needed

**Side/adverse effects**
    Signs of potential side effects, especially arthralgia, galactorrhea, irregular vaginal bleeding or ovarian enlargement or hyperstimulation

## General Dosing Information

### Diet/Nutrition
Supplementation with calcium has not been shown to help to prevent the loss of bone mineral content associated with the use of GnRH analogs.

## Nasal Dosage Forms
Note: The dosing and strengths of the dosage forms available are expressed in terms of nafarelin base (not the acetate).

### NAFARELIN ACETATE NASAL SOLUTION

#### Usual adult and adolescent dose
Endometriosis—
   Intranasal, 200 mcg (base) into one nostril in the morning and 200 mcg into the other nostril in the evening (total daily dose of 400 mcg). The usual recommended duration of therapy is six months. Treatment should begin between days 2 and 4 of the menstrual cycle.

   In an occasional patient, a total daily dose of 400 mcg does not produce amenorrhea. If regular menstrual cycles persist after 2 months of therapy, the total daily dose may be increased to 800 mcg, administered by applying 200 mcg into each nostril in the morning and 200 mcg into each nostril in the evening.

#### Strength(s) usually available
U.S.—
   200 mcg per metered spray (Rx) [*Synarel*].

Canada—
   200 mcg per metered spray (Rx) [*Synarel*].

### Packaging and storage
Store bottle upright, at temperatures below 40 °C (104 °F), preferably between 15 and 30 °C (59 and 86 °F), unless otherwise specified by manufacturer.

### Auxiliary labeling
• For nasal use only.

## Selected Bibliography
Henzl MR, et al. Administration of nasal nafarelin as compared with oral danazol for endometriosis: a multicenter double-blind comparative clinical trial. N Engl J Med 1988; 318 (8): 485-9.

Barbieri RL. Endometriosis 1990: current treatment approaches [review]. Drugs 1990; 39 (4): 502-10.

Letassy NA, et al. Nafarelin acetate: a gonadotropin-releasing hormone agonist for the treatment of endometriosis [review]. DICP 1990; 24: 1204-9.

Revised: 10/26/92
Interim revision: 07/05/94

**NAFCILLIN—**See *Penicillins (Systemic)*

---

# NAFTIFINE   Topical

VA CLASSIFICATION (Primary): DE102.

Note: For a listing of dosage forms and brand names by country availability, see *Dosage Forms* section(s). For a listing of brand names for the articles in this monograph, refer to the General Index.

## Category
Antifungal (topical).
Note: Naftifine is a broad-spectrum antifungal.

## Indications
Note: Bracketed information in the *Indications* section refers to uses that are not included in U.S. product labeling.

### Accepted
Tinea corporis (treatment)
Tinea cruris (treatment) or
Tinea pedis (treatment)—Naftifine hydrochloride is indicated [as a primary agent] in the topical treatment of tinea corporis (ringworm of the body), tinea cruris (jock itch; ringworm of the groin), and tinea pedis (athlete's foot; ringworm of the foot) caused by *Epidermophyton floccosum*, *Microsporum canis*, *Trichophyton rubrum*, and *T. mentagrophytes*.

[Tinea barbae (treatment)] or
[Tinea capitis (treatment)]—Naftifine is used in combination with griseofulvin or systemic ketoconazole (for griseofulvin-resistant cases) in the topical treatment of tinea barbae (ringworm of the beard) and tinea capitis (ringworm of the scalp).

[Tinea versicolor (treatment)]—Naftifine is used as a primary agent in the topical treatment of tinea versicolor (pityriasis versicolor; "sun fungus") caused by *Pityrosporon orbiculare (Malassezia furfur)*.

Not all species or strains of a particular organism may be susceptible to naftifine.

## Pharmacology/Pharmacokinetics

### Physicochemical characteristics
Chemical group—Allylamine derivative.
Molecular weight—323.86.

### Mechanism of action/Effect
Fungicidal to dermatophytes at low concentrations and fungistatic to yeasts at somewhat higher concentrations. Exact mechanism unknown. Appears to selectively inhibit the enzyme squalene 2,3-epoxidase, resulting in inhibition of sterol biosynthesis. This results in decreased amounts of sterols, especially ergosterol (the primary fungal membrane sterol), and a corresponding accumulation of squalene in fungal cells.

### Absorption
Following a single application to the skin of healthy patients, approximately 6% of the applied dose of 1% cream, and approximately 4.2% of the applied dose of 1% gel, is absorbed systemically.

### Half-life
Approximately 2 to 3 days.

### Elimination
Renal and fecal; naftifine and/or metabolites excreted in the urine and feces.

## Precautions to Consider

### Cross-sensitivity and/or related problems
Patients sensitive to benzoates may be sensitive to naftifine hydrochloride cream also since it may contain benzyl alcohol as a preservative.

### Carcinogenicity
Long-term studies in animals to evaluate the carcinogenic potential of naftifine have not been done.

### Mutagenicity
*In vitro* and animal studies have not shown that naftifine is mutagenic.

### Pregnancy/Reproduction
Fertility—Adequate and well-controlled studies in humans have not been done.

Studies in rats and rabbits given oral doses of 150 or more times the topical dose have not shown that naftifine causes impaired fertility.

Pregnancy—Adequate and well-controlled studies in humans have not been done.

Studies in rats and rabbits given oral doses of 150 or more times the topical dose have not shown that naftifine causes adverse effects on the fetus.

FDA Pregnancy Category B.

### Breast-feeding
Approximately 4.2 and 6%, respectively, of the applied dose of 1% naftifine hydrochloride gel and cream is absorbed systemically following a single application to the skin of healthy patients. In addition, naftifine has a long half-life (2 to 3 days) in the body. Therefore, it may be necessary to discontinue breast-feeding or discontinue the medication. However, it is not known whether naftifine is distributed into human breast milk and problems in humans have not been documented.

### Pediatrics
Appropriate studies on the relationship of age to the effects of naftifine have not been performed in the pediatric population. Safety and efficacy have not been established.

### Geriatrics

Appropriate studies on the relationship of age to the effects of naftifine have not been performed in the geriatric population. However, no geriatrics-specific problems have been documented to date.

### Medical considerations/Contraindications

The medical considerations/contraindications included here have been selected on the basis of their potential clinical significance (reasons given in parentheses where appropriate)—not necessarily inclusive (» = major clinical significance).

*Risk-benefit should be considered when the following medical problem exists:*

Sensitivity to naftifine or benzoates

## Side/Adverse Effects

The following side/adverse effects have been selected on the basis of their potential clinical significance (possible signs and symptoms in parentheses where appropriate)—not necessarily inclusive:

**Those indicating need for medical attention only if they continue or are bothersome**
Incidence more frequent
   *Burning or stinging feeling on treated area(s)*
Incidence less frequent
   *Dry skin; itching, redness, or other sign of skin irritation not present before therapy*

## Patient Consultation

As an aid to patient consultation, refer to *Advice for the Patient, Naftifine (Topical)*.

In providing consultation, consider emphasizing the following selected information (» = major clinical significance):

### Before using this medication
» Conditions affecting use, especially:
   Sensitivity to naftifine or benzoates
   Breast-feeding—Approximately 4.2 and 6%, respectively, of applied dose of naftifine hydrochloride gel and cream absorbed systemically; also naftifine has long half-life; may be necessary to discontinue breast-feeding or discontinue medication

### Proper use of this medication
» Avoiding contact with the eyes and mucous membranes such as the inside of the nose, mouth, or vagina
» Avoiding use of occlusive dressings on the area being treated unless otherwise directed by physician
*To use*
» Applying sufficient medication to cover affected skin and surrounding areas, and rubbing in gently
   Washing hands after application to remove any residual medication
» Compliance with full course of therapy; continuing therapy for 1 to 2 weeks after symptoms have subsided
» Proper dosing
   Missed dose: Applying as soon as possible; not applying if almost time for next dose
» Proper storage

### Precautions while using this medication
Checking with physician if no improvement within 4 weeks
» Using hygienic measures to help cure infection and to help prevent reinfection:
*For tinea pedis*
   Carefully drying feet, especially between toes, after bathing
   Not wearing socks made from wool or synthetic materials; wearing clean, cotton socks and changing them daily or more often if feet perspire excessively
   Wearing well-ventilated shoes or sandals
   Using a bland, absorbent powder or an antifungal powder liberally between toes, on feet, and in socks and shoes once or twice daily; using the powder after naftifine has been applied and has disappeared into the skin; not using the powder as the only therapy for your fungal infection
*For tinea cruris*
   Carefully drying inguinal area after bathing
   Not wearing underwear that is tight-fitting or made from synthetic materials; wearing loose-fitting cotton underwear instead

   Using a bland, absorbent powder or an antifungal powder liberally once or twice daily; using the powder after naftifine has been applied and has disappeared into the skin; not using the powder as the only therapy for your fungal infection
*For tinea corporis*
   Carefully drying the body after bathing
   Avoiding excess heat and humidity if possible; keeping moisture from accumulating on affected areas of the body
   Wearing well-ventilated clothing
   Using a bland, absorbent powder or an antifungal powder liberally once or twice daily; using the powder after naftifine has been applied and has disappeared into the skin; not using the powder as the only therapy for your fungal infection

## General Dosing Information

Naftifine hydrochloride should not be used in the eyes and on mucous membranes such as the inside of the nose, mouth, or vagina.

A sufficient quantity of naftifine hydrochloride cream should be gently massaged into the affected skin and surrounding areas once a day. Naftifine hydrochloride gel should be applied two times a day, morning and evening. The hands should be washed after application to remove any residual medication.

Use of topical antifungals may lead to skin sensitization, resulting in hypersensitivity reactions with subsequent topical use of the medication. If skin irritation or hypersensitivity develops, treatment with naftifine hydrochloride should be discontinued.

To reduce the possibility of recurrence of infection, treatment should be continued for 1 to 2 weeks after symptoms have subsided.

## Topical Dosage Forms

### NAFTIFINE HYDROCHLORIDE CREAM

**Usual adult and adolescent dose**
Tinea corporis or
Tinea cruris or
Tinea pedis—
   Topical, to the affected skin and surrounding areas, once a day.

**Usual pediatric dose**
Safety and efficacy have not been established.

**Strength(s) usually available**
U.S.—
   1% (Rx) [Naftin].
Canada—
   1% (OTC) [Naftin].

**Packaging and storage**
Store below 30 °C (86 °F), in a well-closed container, unless otherwise specified by manufacturer. Protect from freezing.

**Auxiliary labeling**
• For external use only.
• Continue medication for full time of treatment.

### NAFTIFINE HYDROCHLORIDE GEL

**Usual adult and adolescent dose**
Tinea corporis or
Tinea cruris or
Tinea pedis—
   Topical, to the affected skin and surrounding areas, two times a day, morning and evening.

**Usual pediatric dose**
Safety and efficacy have not been established.

**Strength(s) usually available**
U.S.—
   1% (Rx) [Naftin].
Canada—
   1% (OTC) [Naftin].

**Packaging and storage**
Store below 30 °C (86 °F), in a well-closed container, unless otherwise specified by manufacturer. Protect from freezing.

**Auxiliary labeling**
• For external use only.
• Continue medication for full time of treatment.

## Selected Bibliography

Millikan LE, Galen WK, Gewirtzman GB, Horwitz SN, Landow RK, Nesbitt LT, et al. Naftifine cream 1% versus econazole cream 1% in the treatment of tinea cruris and tinea corporis. J Am Acad Dermatol 1988; 18: 52-6.

Revised: 07/25/94

---

**NALBUPHINE**—See *Opioid (Narcotic) Analgesics (Systemic)*

---

# NALIDIXIC ACID   Systemic

VA CLASSIFICATION (Primary): AM900

Note: For a listing of dosage forms and brand names by country availability, see *Dosage Forms* section(s). For a listing of brand names for the articles in this monograph, refer to the General Index.

## Category

Antibacterial (systemic).

Note: Nalidixic acid is a synthetic narrow-spectrum antibacterial. It is bacteriostatic or bactericidal depending on the concentration. At urine concentrations normally found clinically, it is bactericidal against most gram-negative bacilli (except *Pseudomonas* species) that commonly cause urinary tract infections.

## Indications

### Accepted

Urinary tract infections, bacterial (treatment)—Nalidixic acid is indicated in the treatment of urinary tract infections caused by susceptible strains of gram-negative organisms, including *Proteus* species, *Klebsiella* species, *Enterobacter* species, and *Escherichia coli*.

Since nalidixic acid achieves only low concentrations in the serum and is concentrated in the urine, it is indicated only in the treatment of urinary tract infections.

Not all species or strains of a particular organism may be susceptible to nalidixic acid.

## Pharmacology/Pharmacokinetics

### Physicochemical characteristics

Molecular weight—232.24.

### Mechanism of action/Effect

Nalidixic acid appears to act by inhibiting bacterial DNA synthesis, probably by interfering with DNA polymerization. Resistance may develop rapidly during treatment.

### Absorption

Rapidly and almost completely absorbed from the gastrointestinal tract; bioavailability is approximately 96%. Absorption may be delayed if taken with antacids.

### Distribution

Parent drug and active metabolite are distributed to most tissues, especially to the kidneys and to urine; serum concentrations are low; traces of drug cross the placenta. Excreted in breast milk, also. Drug does not penetrate into prostatic fluid.

### Protein binding

Nalidixic acid—Very high (93%).
Hydroxynalidixic acid—Moderate (63%)

### Biotransformation

Hepatic; 30% metabolized to the active metabolite, hydroxynalidixic acid; rapid conjugation of parent drug and active metabolite to inactive metabolites. Metabolism may vary widely among individuals. In the urine, hydroxynalidixic acid represents 80 to 85% of the antibacterial activity.

### Half-life

Serum—
  Adults:
    Normal renal function—1.1 to 2.5 hours.
    Impaired renal function—Up to 21 hours.
  Elderly (n=6, 70 to 89 years old):
    11.5 hours (6.9 to 25.6 hours).
Urine—
  6 hours.

### Time to peak serum concentration

1 to 2 hours (normal renal function).

### Time to peak urine concentration

3 to 4 hours.

### Elimination

Renal—2 to 3% excreted unchanged, 13% as active metabolite and more than 80% as inactive metabolites; rapidly and almost completely excreted within 24 hours; active drug does not accumulate in patients with impaired renal function, but inactive metabolites accumulate and may be toxic.
Fecal—Approximately 4%.

## Precautions to Consider

### Cross-sensitivity and/or related problems

Since nalidixic acid is closely related chemically to other quinolone derivatives (e.g., cinoxacin and fluoroquinolones), patients hypersensitive to other quinolones may also be hypersensitive to this medication.

### Pregnancy/Reproduction

Pregnancy—Nalidixic acid crosses the placenta. Adequate and well-controlled studies in humans have not been done. However, since nalidixic acid and other related compounds have been shown to cause arthropathy in immature animals, use is not recommended in pregnancy.

### Breast-feeding

Nalidixic acid is excreted in breast milk. The milk:plasma ratio has been reported to be 0.08 to 0.13. One case of hemolytic anemia occurred in a nursing infant with glucose-6-phosphate dehydrogenase deficiency; however, nalidixic acid is considered to be compatible with breast-feeding.

### Pediatrics

Nalidixic acid causes lameness in immature dogs due to permanent lesions of the cartilage of weight-bearing joints. In addition, related drugs (e.g., cinoxacin, fluoroquinolones) have been reported to cause similar lesions, as well as other signs of arthropathy in immature animals of various species. Therefore, use is not recommended in infants up to 3 months of age.

### Geriatrics

Studies performed to date have not demonstrated geriatrics-specific problems that would limit the usefulness of nalidixic acid in the elderly. However, elderly patients are more likely to have age-related decrease in renal function, resulting in a prolonged half-life and decreased drug clearance.

### Drug interactions and/or related problems

The following drug interactions and/or related problems have been selected on the basis of their potential clinical significance (possible mechanism in parentheses where appropriate)—not necessarily inclusive (» = major clinical significance):

Note: Combinations containing any of the following medications, depending on the amount present, may also interact with this medication.

» Anticoagulants, coumarin- or indandione-derivative
    (coumarin- or indandione-derivative anticoagulants, especially warfarin and dicumarol, may be displaced from protein-binding sites by nalidixic acid, resulting in increased anticoagulant effect; dosage adjustments may be necessary during and after nalidixic acid therapy)

Nitrofurantoin
    (nitrofurantoin interferes with the therapeutic effects of nalidixic acid)

## Laboratory value alterations

The following have been selected on the basis of their potential clinical significance (possible effect in parentheses where appropriate)—not necessarily inclusive (» = major clinical significance):

With diagnostic test results

Glucose determinations, urine

(may give false-positive test results with copper sulfate tests, such as *Benedict's* or *Fehling's* solutions because of liberation of glucuronic acid, a reducing agent; glucose enzymatic tests, such as *Clinistix* Reagent Strips or *Tes-Tape*, are not affected)

17-ketogenic steroid (17-KGS), urine and

17-ketosteroid (17-KS), urine

(false increase in concentration may occur because of interaction between nalidixic acid and *m-* dinitrobenzene; use Porter-Silber method for 17-hydroxycorticosteroid [17-OHCS] determinations)

Metyrapone

(nalidixic acid may interfere with the assay for urine 17-ketosteroids or 17-ketogenic steroids)

## Medical considerations/Contraindications

The medical considerations/contraindications included here have been selected on the basis of their potential clinical significance (reasons given in parentheses where appropriate)—not necessarily inclusive (» = major clinical significance).

***Risk-benefit should be considered when the following medical problems exist:***

Cerebral arteriosclerosis, severe or

» Seizure disorders, history of

(patients with severe cerebral arteriosclerosis or a history of seizure disorders may be at increased risk of toxicity)

Glucose-6-phosphate dehydrogenase (G6PD) deficiency

(hemolytic anemia may occur)

» Hepatic function impairment

(patients with hepatic function impairment may be at increased risk of toxicity)

Hypersensitivity to nalidixic acid or other quinolone derivatives (cinoxacin, fluoroquinolones)

Renal function impairment, severe

(patients with severe renal function impairment [creatinine clearance of <10 mL/min (0.17 mL/second)] may be at increased risk of toxicity)

## Patient monitoring

The following may be especially important in patient monitoring (other tests may be warranted in some patients, depending on condition; » = major clinical significance):

Complete blood counts (CBCs) and

Hepatic function determinations and

Renal function determinations

(may be required periodically during therapy if nalidixic acid is continued for more than 2 weeks; patients with impaired renal function do not generally require a reduction in dose unless the impairment is severe [creatinine clearance of <10 mL/min])

Glucose-6-phosphate dehydrogenase (G6PD) concentration

(determination recommended in patients at high risk prior to treatment; if a deficiency is found, nalidixic acid should be given with extreme caution since hemolytic effects may be exaggerated)

## Side/Adverse Effects

The following side/adverse effects have been selected on the basis of their potential clinical significance (possible signs and symptoms in parentheses where appropriate)—not necessarily inclusive:

### Those indicating need for medical attention

Incidence less frequent

*Visual disturbances* (blurred or decreased vision; change in color vision; double vision; halos around lights; overbright appearance of lights)

Incidence rare

*Blood dyscrasias* (pale skin; sore throat and fever; unusual bleeding or bruising; unusual tiredness or weakness); *cholestatic jaundice* (dark or amber urine; pale stools; stomach pain, severe; yellow eyes or skin); *CNS toxicity, specifically hallucinations, mood or other mental changes, increased intracranial pressure* (bulging anterior fontanel; papilledema; headache); *hypersensitivity* (skin rash, redness, itching); *seizures*—usually with excessive doses

### Those indicating need for medical attention only if they continue or are bothersome

Incidence more frequent

*CNS toxicity* (dizziness; drowsiness; headache); *gastrointestinal disturbance* (abdominal pain; diarrhea; nausea; vomiting)

Incidence less frequent

*Photosensitivity* (increased sensitivity of skin to sunlight)

## Overdose

For more information on the management of overdose or unintentional ingestion, **contact a Poison Control Center** (see *Poison Control Center Listing*).

**Treatment of overdose**

Recommended treatment consists of the following:

To decrease absorption—Performing gastric lavage if overdose is noted early.

Specific treatment—Administering anticonvulsants if needed for seizures.

Supportive care—Administering fluids and supportive measures such as oxygen and artificial respiration if absorption has occurred. Patients in whom intentional overdose is known or suspected should be referred for psychiatric consultation.

## Patient Consultation

As an aid to patient consultation, refer to *Advice for the Patient, Nalidixic Acid (Systemic)*.

In providing consultation, consider emphasizing the following selected information (» = major clinical significance):

**Before using this medication**

» Conditions affecting use, especially:

Hypersensitivity to nalidixic acid or other quinolone derivatives (cinoxacin, fluoroquinolones)

Pregnancy—Nalidixic acid crosses the placenta and is not recommended during pregnancy

Breast-feeding—Nalidixic acid is excreted in breast milk

Use in children—Nalidixic acid is not recommended in infants up to 3 months of age since it has been found to cause arthropathy in young animals

Other medications, especially coumarin- and indandione-derivative anticoagulants

Other medical problems, especially a history of seizure disorders or severe hepatic impairment

**Proper use of this medication**

» Not giving to infants up to 3 months of age; has caused arthropathy in immature animals

Taking on an empty stomach, or with food or milk if gastrointestinal irritation occurs

Proper administration technique for oral liquids

» Compliance with full course of therapy

» Proper dosing

Missed dose: Taking as soon as possible; not taking if almost time for next dose; not doubling doses

» Proper storage

**Precautions while using this medication**

Regular visits to physician to check progress if therapy lasts longer than 2 weeks

Checking with physician if no improvement within 2 days

» Caution if blurred vision or other vision problems, dizziness, or drowsiness occurs

» Possible skin photosensitivity; avoiding unprotected exposure to sun; using protective clothing; using a sun block product that includes protection against both UVA-caused photosensitivity reactions and UVB-caused sunburn reactions; avoiding use of sunlamp, tanning bed, or tanning booth

» Diabetics: False-positive reactions with copper sulfate urine glucose tests may occur

**Side/adverse effects**

Signs of potential side effects, especially visual disturbances, blood dyscrasias, cholestatic jaundice, CNS toxicity, and hypersensitivity

## General Dosing Information

Nalidixic acid should preferably be taken with a full glass (240 mL) of water on an empty stomach (either 1 hour before or 2 hours after meals) to obtain optimum urine concentrations. However, if gastrointestinal irritation occurs, this medication may be taken with food or milk.

# Oral Dosage Forms

## NALIDIXIC ACID ORAL SUSPENSION USP

### Usual adult and adolescent dose
Antibacterial—
    Initial: Oral, 1 gram every six hours for one to two weeks.
    Maintenance: Oral, 500 mg every six hours.

### Usual adult prescribing limits
Up to 4 grams daily.

Note: Doses up to 6 grams daily have been used in severe urinary tract
    infections, although side effects may be increased at high dosage.

### Usual pediatric dose
Antibacterial—
    Infants up to 3 months of age: Use is not recommended in infants up
        to 3 months of age since nalidixic acid causes arthropathy in im-
        mature animals.
    Children 3 months to 12 years of age: Oral, 55 mg per kg of body
        weight per day in four equally divided doses for one to two weeks
        initially, followed by a maintenance dose of 33 mg per kg of body
        weight per day in four equally divided doses.
    Children 12 years of age and over: See *Usual adult and adolescent
        dose.*

### Strength(s) usually available
U.S.—
    250 mg per 5 mL (Rx) [*NegGram* (parabens; sorbitol)].
Canada—
    Not commercially available.

### Packaging and storage
Store below 40 °C (104 °F), preferably between 15 and 30 °C (59 and 86
    °F), unless otherwise specified by manufacturer. Store in a tight con-
    tainer. Protect from freezing.

### Auxiliary labeling
• Shake well.
• May cause blurred vision, dizziness, or drowsiness.
• Avoid too much sun or use of sunlamp.
• Continue medicine for full time of treatment.

### Note
When dispensing, include a calibrated liquid-measuring device.

## NALIDIXIC ACID TABLETS USP

### Usual adult and adolescent dose
See *Nalidixic Acid Oral Suspension USP.*

### Usual adult prescribing limits
See *Nalidixic Acid Oral Suspension USP.*

### Usual pediatric dose
See *Nalidixic Acid Oral Suspension USP.*

### Strength(s) usually available
U.S.—
    250 mg (Rx) [*NegGram* (scored); GENERIC].
    500 mg (Rx) [*NegGram* (scored); GENERIC].
    1 gram (Rx) [*NegGram* (scored); GENERIC].
Canada—
    500 mg (Rx) [*NegGram* (scored)].

### Packaging and storage
Store below 40 °C (104 °F), preferably between 15 and 30 °C (59 and 86
    °F), unless otherwise specified by manufacturer. Store in a tight
    container.

### Auxiliary labeling
• May cause blurred vision, dizziness, or drowsiness.
• Avoid too much sun or use of sunlamp.
• Continue medicine for full time of treatment.

Revised: 05/14/93

---

# NALOXONE  Systemic

VA CLASSIFICATION (Primary): CN102

Note: For a listing of dosage forms and brand names by country availa-
    bility, see *Dosage Forms* section(s). For a listing of brand names
    for the articles in this monograph, refer to the General Index.

## Category
Opioid (narcotic) antagonist.

## Indications

Note: Bracketed information in the *Indications* section refers to uses that
    are not included in U.S. product labeling.

### Accepted
Respiratory depression, opioid (narcotic)-induced (treatment)
Respiratory depression, opioid (narcotic)-induced, post-anesthesia (treat-
    ment) or
Toxicity, opioid (narcotic) (diagnosis and treatment)—Naloxone is con-
    sidered the drug of choice to reverse respiratory depression caused by
    opioid drugs, including those with mixed agonist/antagonist activity
    such as buprenorphine (although the effects of buprenorphine are es-
    pecially resistant to reversal by naloxone), butorphanol, nalbuphine,
    and pentazocine, and other effects due to known or suspected opioid
    overdose, including sedation, coma, excitation, or convulsions. Nal-
    oxone will not increase respiratory depression caused by nonopioid
    medications or disease processes and may therefore be used when the
    cause is unknown. A satisfactory response to naloxone confirms the
    diagnosis of opioid toxicity.

Naloxone is also indicated to reverse respiratory depression in neo-
    nates caused by opioids given to the mother during labor and delivery.

When naloxone is given to reverse postoperative opioid depression,
    dosage must be carefully titrated so as not to interfere with control of
    postoperative pain or cause other adverse effects.

[Opioid drug use, illicit (diagnosis)][1]—Naloxone is used to diagnose
    opioid dependence or suspected illicit opioid use because it precipi-
    tates withdrawal symptoms in patients who are physically dependent
    on opioids (except for buprenorphine). Use of laboratory methods to
    detect an opioid drug in the urine of the suspected addict may be
    preferable. However, a naloxone challenge test is recommended to
    detect possible opioid use or dependence prior to initiation of naltrex-

one therapy in opioid addicts who have completed a detoxification
regimen.

[1]Not included in Canadian product labeling.

## Pharmacology/Pharmacokinetics

### Physicochemical characteristics
Molecular weight—363.84.

### Mechanism of action/Effect
The precise mechanism by which naloxone reverses most of the effects
    of opioid analgesics has not been fully determined. It has been pro-
    posed that there are multiple subtypes of opioid receptors within the
    central nervous system (CNS), each mediating different therapeutic
    and/or side effects of opioid drugs. At least two of these types of
    receptors (mu and kappa) mediate analgesia as well as side effects. A
    third type of receptor (sigma) may not mediate analgesia; actions at
    this receptor may produce the subjective and psychotomimetic effects
    characteristic of several opioids having mixed agonist/antagonist ac-
    tivity (i.e., butorphanol, nalbuphine, and pentazocine). Naloxone ap-
    parently displaces previously administered opioid analgesics from all
    of these types of receptors and competitively inhibits their actions.
    Antagonism of opioid actions may precipitate withdrawal symptoms
    in patients who are physically dependent on opioid drugs (except for
    buprenorphine). Naloxone has no opioid agonist activity of its own.

### Biotransformation
Hepatic.

### Half-life
60 to 100 minutes.

### Onset of action
Intravenous: 1 or 2 minutes.
Intramuscular: 2 to 5 minutes.

### Time to peak effect
5 to 15 minutes.

### Duration of action
Dose- and route-dependent. In one study, effects persisted for 45 minutes
    following a 400-mcg (0.4 mg) intravenous dose. Intramuscular admin-
    istration provides a more prolonged duration of action.

**Elimination**
Renal; about 70% of a dose is excreted within 72 hours.

## Precautions to Consider

### Pregnancy/Reproduction
Fertility—Reproduction studies in mice and rats receiving up to 1000 times the human dose have not shown that naloxone impairs fertility.

Pregnancy—Although problems in humans have not been documented, adequate and well-controlled studies have not been done. Studies in rats and mice receiving up to 1000 times the human dose have not shown teratogenic or other harmful effects on the fetus

FDA Pregnancy Category B.

Risk-benefit must be considered before naloxone is administered to a pregnant woman who is known or suspected to be opioid-dependent because maternal dependence leads to fetal dependence. Naloxone crosses the placenta and may precipitate withdrawal in the fetus as well as in the mother.

### Breast-feeding
Problems in humans have not been documented.

### Pediatrics
Studies performed to date have not demonstrated pediatrics-specific problems that would limit the usefulness of naloxone in children.

### Geriatrics
Appropriate studies with naloxone have not been performed in the geriatric population. However, geriatrics-specific problems that would limit the usefulness of this medication in the elderly are not expected.

### Drug interactions and/or related problems
The following drug interactions and/or related problems have been selected on the basis of their potential clinical significance (possible mechanism in parentheses where appropriate)—not necessarily inclusive (» = major clinical significance):

Note: Combinations containing any of the following medications, depending on the amount present, may also interact with this medication.

Butorphanol or
Nalbuphine or
Pentazocine
   (naloxone reverses the analgesic and side effects of these opioid agonist/antagonist analgesics and may precipitate withdrawal symptoms in physically dependent patients)

Opioid agonist analgesics, including alfentanil, fentanyl, and sufentanil
   (naloxone reverses the analgesic and side effects of opioid agonist analgesics and may precipitate withdrawal symptoms in physically dependent patients, including patients being treated for opioid dependence with methadone)

   (when naloxone is used to reverse the effects of opioid agonists used as anesthesia adjuncts, dosage of the antagonist must be carefully titrated in order to achieve the desired effect without interfering with control of postoperative pain or causing other adverse effects)

### Medical considerations/Contraindications
The medical considerations/contraindications included here have been selected on the basis of their potential clinical significance (reasons given in parentheses where appropriate)—not necessarily inclusive (» = major clinical significance).

*Risk-benefit should be considered when the following medical problems exist:*

Allergic reaction to naloxone, history of

Cardiac irritability
   (may be exacerbated)

Opioid dependence or addiction, current
   (naloxone may precipitate withdrawal)

## Side/Adverse Effects

Note: Convulsions have been reported to occur infrequently following naloxone administration. Also, ventricular tachycardia or fibrillation has been reported in a few patients with preexisting ventricular irritability who received naloxone following cardiopulmonary bypass procedures. However, a direct causal relationship has not been established.

The following side/adverse effects have been selected on the basis of their potential clinical significance (possible signs and symptoms in parentheses where appropriate)—not necessarily inclusive:

**Those indicating need for medical attention**
   *Fast or irregular heartbeat; increased or decreased blood pressure*

Note: In some cardiac patients receiving naloxone, *hypertension* and *tachycardia* may result in left ventricular failure and pulmonary edema.

**Those indicating need for medical attention only if they continue or are bothersome**
   *Increased sweating; nausea or vomiting; nervousness, restlessness, excitement, or irritability; trembling*

**Those indicating possible precipitation of withdrawal in a patient physically dependent on opioids**
   *Body aches; diarrhea; fast heartbeat; fever, runny nose, or sneezing; gooseflesh; increased sweating; increased yawning; nausea or vomiting; nervousness, restlessness, or irritability; shivering or trembling; stomach cramps; weakness*

Note: A degree of physical dependence may occur during prolonged administration of an opioid analgesic as an adjunct to anesthesia. It has been proposed that adverse effects (such as tachycardia, hypertension, hyperpnea, hyperalgesia, nausea, and vomiting) occurring (rarely) after naloxone is administered for reversal of opioid effects following lengthy surgical procedures may be manifestations of an induced abstinence syndrome in acutely dependent individuals. However, other symptoms more commonly associated with an opioid withdrawal syndrome have not been reported.

In the neonate
   *Convulsions; diarrhea; excessive crying; fever; hyperactive reflexes; sneezing; tremors; unusual irritability; vomiting; yawning*

## General Dosing Information

When naloxone is used to antagonize the effects of buprenorphine, butorphanol, nalbuphine, or pentazocine, larger doses may be needed than are required to antagonize the effects of most opioids having only agonist activity. Propoxyphene overdose may also require larger doses of naloxone.

Use of naloxone should be supplemented by other resuscitative procedures, such as administration of oxygen and/or vasopressors, artificial respiration, mechanical ventilation, and/or cardiac massage.

Lack of significant improvement of CNS depression and/or respiratory depression following administration of an adequate dose (10 mg) of naloxone usually indicates that the condition is due to a nonopioid CNS depressant that is not affected by the antagonist or to disease processes. However, the effects of buprenorphine (a partial mu-receptor opioid agonist with high affinity for the mu receptor) are especially resistant to reversal by naloxone; doses of naloxone as high as 16 mg have been ineffective. The respiratory stimulant doxapram and/or prolonged mechanical ventilation may also be required to treat buprenorphine-induced respiratory depression.

When naloxone is administered to a patient known or suspected to be physically dependent on an opioid analgesic, dosage should be carefully titrated. Withdrawal symptoms may occur within a few minutes and may last up to 2 hours. The duration and severity of the abstinence syndrome depend upon the dose of antagonist, the specific opioid involved, and the degree to which dependence has developed. However, naloxone does not precipitate withdrawal symptoms in buprenorphine-dependent individuals.

The naloxone challenge test (recommended prior to initiation of naltrexone therapy in detoxified opioid addicts) should *not* be administered if withdrawal symptoms are present or the patient's urine contains opioids. Naloxone may be administered intravenously or subcutaneously. If the intravenous route is used, one-fourth of the total dose should be administered and the patient observed for 30 seconds for withdrawal symptoms; if none occurs, the remainder of the dose should be administered and the patient observed for 20 minutes. If the subcutaneous route is used, the full dose should be administered and the patient observed for 45 minutes for withdrawal symptoms. If withdrawal symptoms occur, the naloxone challenge should be repeated at suitable intervals until absence of opioid dependence is confirmed.

## Parenteral Dosage Forms

Note: Bracketed uses in the *Dosage Forms* section refer to categories of use and/or indications that are not included in U.S. product labeling.

## NALOXONE HYDROCHLORIDE INJECTION USP

**Usual adult and adolescent dose**
Opioid (narcotic) antagonist—
    Opioid toxicity:

        Intravenous (preferred in emergencies), intramuscular, or subcutaneous, 400 mcg (0.4 mg) to 2 mg as a single dose. The intravenous dose may be repeated at two- to three-minute intervals as needed.

        Note: Dosage must be individualized.

            If the patient is suspected of being physically dependent on an opioid medication and is not in immediate danger, the dose may be reduced to 100 to 200 mcg (0.1 to 0.2 mg). This dose may be repeated at two- to three-minute intervals as needed.

            Continued monitoring of the patient is necessary, especially if the duration of action of the opioid being antagonized exceeds that of naloxone, to detect re-emergence of opioid toxicity following initial reversal. Additional single doses of naloxone may be administered intravenously as needed. However, longer-lasting effects may be obtained if supplemental doses are administered via the intramuscular route. Also, initial treatment may be followed by continuous intravenous infusion of naloxone, with the rate of infusion being adjusted according to patient response.

    Postoperative opioid depression:

        Intravenous, 100 to 200 mcg (0.1 to 0.2 mg) every two to three minutes until adequate ventilation and alertness without significant pain are obtained. If necessary, dosage may be repeated at one- or two-hour intervals.

        Note: Dosage must be carefully titrated to avoid interference with control of postoperative pain; initial doses as low as 0.5 mcg (0.0005 mg) per kg of body weight have been recommended.

    [Opioid dependence diagnosis][1]:

        Intravenous, 200 mcg (0.2 mg) initially, followed by 600 mcg (0.6 mg) thirty seconds later if withdrawal symptoms are not apparent; or

        Subcutaneous, 800 mcg (0.8 mg).

        Note: If necessary to confirm that the patient is not opioid-dependent, a rechallenge using 1.6 mg of naloxone intravenously may be performed.

**Usual pediatric dose**
Neonates—
    Opioid-induced depression: Intravenous via the umbilical vein (preferred), intramuscular, or subcutaneous, 10 mcg (0.01 mg) per kg of body weight. The intravenous dose may be repeated at two- to three-minute intervals until the desired response is obtained.
Children—
    Opioid toxicity: Intravenous (preferred in emergencies), intramuscular, or subcutaneous, 10 mcg (0.01 mg) per kg of body weight. The intravenous dose may be repeated at two- to three-minute intervals for one or two additional doses.

Postoperative opioid depression: Intravenous, 5 to 10 mcg (0.005 to 0.01 mg) every two to three minutes until adequate ventilation and alertness without significant pain are obtained. If necessary, dosage may be repeated at one- or two-hour intervals.

Note: Dosage must be individualized according to the requirements and response of the patient. Doses much higher than those listed above have been used to treat opioid toxicity.

The medication may be diluted with sterile water for injection.

Naloxone should be administered cautiously to neonates of mothers who are physically dependent on opioids.

**Strength(s) usually available**
U.S.—
    With preservatives (methylparaben and propylparaben)
        20 mcg (0.02 mg) per mL (Rx) [*Narcan;* GENERIC].
        400 mcg (0.4 mg) per mL (Rx) [*Narcan;* GENERIC].
        1 mg per mL (Rx) [*Narcan;* GENERIC].
    Without preservative
        20 mcg (0.02 mg) per mL (Rx) [*Narcan;* GENERIC].
        400 mcg (0.4 mg) per mL (Rx) [*Narcan;* GENERIC].
        1 mg per mL (Rx) [*Narcan;* GENERIC].
Canada—
    With preservatives (methylparaben and propylparaben)
        20 mcg (0.02 mg) per mL (Rx) [*Narcan*].
        400 mcg (0.4 mg) per mL (Rx) [*Narcan*].

**Packaging and storage**
Store below 40 °C (104 °F), preferably between 15 and 30 °C (59 and 86 °F), unless otherwise specified by manufacturer. Protect from light. Protect from freezing.

**Preparation of dosage form**
For continuous intravenous infusion—Add 2 mg (5 mL of solution containing 400 mcg [0.4 mg] per mL or 2 mL of solution containing 1 mg per mL) of naloxone hydrochloride to 500 mL of 0.9% sodium chloride injection or 5% dextrose injection to prepare a solution containing 4 mcg (0.004 mg) per mL.

**Stability**
After dilution for intravenous infusion, the solution should be used within 24 hours. Any unused solution should be discarded after 24 hours.
It is recommended that naloxone not be mixed with any medicinal or chemical agent unless the chemical and physical stability of the mixture has first been established. In particular, naloxone should not be mixed with any preparation containing bisulfite, metabisulfite, or long-chain or high molecular weight anions, or with any solution having an alkaline pH.

---

[1]Not included in Canadian product labeling.

Revised: June 1990

---

## NALOXONE-CONTAINING COMBINATIONS—

Pentazocine and Naloxone (Systemic)—See *Opioid (Narcotic) Analgesics (Systemic)*

---

# NALTREXONE   Systemic

VA CLASSIFICATION (Primary): CN102
Note: For a listing of dosage forms and brand names by country availability, see *Dosage Forms* section(s). For a listing of brand names for the articles in this monograph, refer to the General Index.

## Category

Opioid (narcotic) antagonist; opioid (narcotic) abuse therapy adjunct.

## Indications

**Accepted**
Opioid (narcotic) drug use, illicit (treatment adjunct)—Naltrexone is indicated as an adjunct to other measures, including psychological and social counseling, in the treatment of detoxified, formerly opioid-dependent individuals. Naltrexone assists in maintaining an opioid-free state in these individuals; however, an unequivocally beneficial effect on recidivism rates has not been demonstrated.

**Unaccepted**
Naltrexone is *not* effective in treating dependency on substances other than opioid drugs.

## Pharmacology/Pharmacokinetics

**Physicochemical characteristics**
Molecular weight—377.87.

**Mechanism of action/Effect**
Although the precise mechanism of action is not completely understood, naltrexone apparently binds to opioid receptors in the central nervous system (CNS) and competitively inhibits the actions of opioid drugs (both pure agonists and agonist/antagonists). Naltrexone markedly attenuates or completely blocks opioid-induced euphoria and physical dependence; with continued use it may therefore reduce the patient's desire for such drugs. Naltrexone may be more effective in blocking the subjective effects (such as euphoria) than the objective effects (such as respiratory depression or miosis) of opioids.

**Other actions/effects**

Naltrexone precipitates withdrawal symptoms in individuals who are physically dependent on opioid drugs (with the probable exception of buprenorphine). It also blocks the therapeutic (e.g., analgesic, antidiarrheal, and antitussive) actions of opioids. Although naltrexone has few if any actions other than opioid blockade, it produces some pupillary constriction via an unknown mechanism.

**Absorption**

Rapid and almost complete.

**Protein binding**

Low (21%).

**Biotransformation**

Hepatic; approximately 95% of a dose is metabolized. Naltrexone is subject to extensive first-pass hepatic metabolism. The major metabolite, 6-beta-naltrexol, has opioid antagonist activity and may contribute to the therapeutic effect.

**Half-life (elimination)**

Naltrexone—Approximately 4 hours; independent of dose.
6-Beta-naltrexol—Approximately 13 hours; independent of dose.

**Time to peak concentration**

For both naltrexone and 6-beta-naltrexol—1 hour; independent of dose.

**Peak serum concentration**

Following a single 50-mg dose—
    Naltrexone: 8.6 nanograms per mL.
    6-Beta-naltrexol: 99.3 nanograms per mL.

Note: Naltrexone does not accumulate with chronic dosing; however, the peak serum concentration of 6-beta-naltrexol may increase to approximately 140 nanograms per mL during chronic administration.

**Duration of action**

Dose-dependent; as determined by blockade of the effects of 25 mg of intravenously administered heroin—
    50-mg dose: 24 hours.
    100-mg dose: 48 hours.
    150-mg dose: 72 hours.

**Elimination**

Primarily renal; 60% of a dose is excreted in the urine within 48 hours. Less than 1% of a dose is excreted in the urine as unchanged naltrexone; about 38% of a dose is excreted as unchanged or conjugated 6-beta-naltrexol. Up to 5% of a dose may also be excreted in the feces.

# Precautions to Consider

**Carcinogenicity/Tumorigenicity**

Studies in rats have shown that naltrexone caused small increases in the numbers of mesotheliomas in males and tumors of vascular origin in both sexes. However, only the incidence of vascular tumors in females (4%) exceeded the maximum (2%) reported in historical control groups.

**Mutagenicity**

Naltrexone produced weakly positive findings in the Drosophila recessive lethal assay and in nonspecific DNA repair tests with *E. coli*. However, no positive findings were reported in twenty other tests using bacterial, mammalian, and tissue culture systems. The significance of these findings is not known.

**Pregnancy/Reproduction**

Fertility—Studies in rats given doses of 100 mg per kg (approximately 140 times the human therapeutic dose) have shown that naltrexone causes a significant increase in pseudopregnancy and a decrease in the pregnancy rate of mated females. The relevance of these findings to humans is not known.

Pregnancy—Adequate and well-controlled studies in humans have not been done.

Naltrexone has been shown to be embryocidal in rats (doses of 100 mg per kg prior to and throughout gestation) and rabbits (doses of 60 mg per kg during the period of organogenesis).

FDA Pregnancy Category C.

**Breast-feeding**

It is not known whether naltrexone is excreted in breast milk. However, problems in humans have not been documented.

**Pediatrics**

Appropriate studies have not been performed in patients up to 18 years of age.

**Geriatrics**

No published geriatrics-specific information is available.

**Drug interactions and/or related problems**

The following drug interactions and/or related problems have been selected on the basis of their potential clinical significance (possible mechanism in parentheses where appropriate)—not necessarily inclusive ($\gg$ = major clinical significance):

Note: Combinations containing any of the following medications also interact with this medication.

$\gg$ Opioid (narcotic) medications
    (administration of naltrexone to a patient physically dependent on opioid drugs [probably excepting buprenorphine] will precipitate withdrawal symptoms; symptoms may appear within 5 minutes of naltrexone administration, persist for up to 48 hours, and be difficult to reverse)
    (naltrexone blocks the therapeutic effects of opioids [i.e., analgesic, antidiarrheal, and antitussive]; naltrexone therapy should not be initiated in patients receiving these agents for therapeutic purposes; also, patients receiving naltrexone should be advised to use alternative medications when necessary)
    (administration of increased doses of opioids to override naltrexone-induced blockade of opioid receptors may result in increased and more prolonged respiratory depression and/or circulatory collapse)
    (naltrexone should be discontinued several days prior to elective surgery if administration of an opioid medication prior to, during, or following surgery is unavoidable)
    (the efficacy of naltrexone in antagonizing opioid effects not mediated via opioid receptors [i.e., those which may be caused by histamine release, such as facial swelling, itching, generalized erythema, hives, and, to some extent, hypotension] has not been fully determined; naltrexone may not antagonize these effects completely)

**Laboratory value alterations**

The following have been selected on the basis of their potential clinical significance (possible effect in parentheses where appropriate)—not necessarily inclusive ($\gg$ = major clinical significance):

With physiology/laboratory test values
    Serum transaminase (ALT [SGPT]; AST [SGOT]) activity
    (elevation of serum transaminase activity may occur; although mild abnormalities occur frequently in drug addicts and are not necessarily related to naltrexone-induced hepatotoxicity, significant abnormalities indicative of the medication's hepatotoxic potential have occurred in subjects receiving up to five times the recommended daily dose; the abnormalities were reversible upon discontinuation of naltrexone, and symptomatic hepatotoxicity with clinical use has not been reported)

**Medical considerations/Contraindications**

The medical considerations/contraindications included here have been selected on the basis of their potential clinical significance (reasons given in parentheses where appropriate)—not necessarily inclusive ($\gg$ = major clinical significance).

*Except under special circumstances, this medication should not be used when the following medical problems exist:*

$\gg$ Dependence on opioid drugs (probably excepting buprenorphine), current, as demonstrated by presence of withdrawal symptoms, detection of opioid drugs in urine, or failure to pass naloxone challenge test
    (naltrexone will precipitate or exacerbate withdrawal symptoms)

$\gg$ Hepatic failure or
$\gg$ Hepatitis, acute
    (increased risk of hepatotoxicity)

*Risk-benefit should be considered when the following medical problems exist:*

    Allergic reaction to naltrexone, history of

$\gg$ Hepatic disease, current or recent history of, excluding mild liver function abnormalities known to be associated with opioid addiction
    (increased risk of hepatotoxicity)

**Patient monitoring**

The following may be especially important in patient monitoring (other tests may be warranted in some patients, depending on condition; $\gg$ = major clinical significance):

$\gg$ Hepatic function tests
    (recommended prior to initiation of therapy to detect hepatic injury and/or to determine baseline values, then monthly during the first six months of therapy and periodically thereafter; naltrexone should be discontinued if significant abnormalities occur)

## Side/Adverse Effects

The following side/adverse effects have been selected on the basis of their potential clinical significance (possible signs and symptoms in parentheses where appropriate)—not necessarily inclusive:

**Those indicating need for medical attention**

Incidence 1–10%
*Skin rash*

Incidence <1%
*Blurred vision or aching, burning, or swollen eyes; confusion; discomfort while urinating and/or frequent urination; earache; edema* (swelling of face, fingers, feet, or lower legs; weight gain); *fever; gastrointestinal ulceration* (abdominal or stomach pain, severe); *hallucinations; increased blood pressure; itching; mental depression or other mood or mental changes; nosebleeds, unexplained; phlebitis* (pain, tenderness, or color changes in legs or feet); *ringing or buzzing in ears; shortness of breath; swollen glands*

**Those indicating need for medical attention only if they continue or are bothersome**

Incidence >10%
*Abdominal cramping or pain, mild to moderate; anxiety, nervousness, restlessness, and/or trouble in sleeping; headache; joint or muscle pain; nausea or vomiting; unusual tiredness*

Incidence up to 10%
*Chills; constipation; cough, hoarseness, runny or stuffy nose, sinus problems, sneezing, and/or sore throat; diarrhea; dizziness; fast or pounding heartbeat; increased thirst; irritability; loss of appetite; sexual problems in males*

Note: In some individuals, *loss of appetite* has led to substantial weight loss requiring discontinuation of therapy.

Some of the above-listed side/adverse effects are identical to symptoms of *opioid withdrawal* (see list below). Several of them, such as *body aches, abdominal pain, nausea or vomiting, lassitude, and anxiety,* may lessen or disappear during continued use. It has been suggested that such effects may in fact be mild withdrawal symptoms in some patients.

**Those indicating possible withdrawal in patients physically dependent on opioid drugs**—may occur within 5 minutes after administration of naltrexone and persist for up to 48 hours

*Anxiety, nervousness, restlessness, or irritability; body aches; diarrhea; fast heartbeat; fever, continuing runny nose, or sneezing; gooseflesh; increased sweating; increased yawning; loss of appetite; nausea or vomiting; shivering or trembling; stomach cramps; trouble in sleeping; weakness*

## Overdose

For more information on the management of overdose or unintentional ingestion, **contact a Poison Control Center** (see *Poison Control Center Listing*).

**Treatment of overdose**

Clinical experience with overdose is lacking. It is recommended that the patient be closely monitored and the observed symptoms treated as required.

## Patient Consultation

As an aid to patient consultation, refer to *Advice for the Patient, Naltrexone (Systemic)*.

In providing consultation, consider emphasizing the following selected information (» = major clinical significance):

**Before using this medication**
» Conditions affecting use, especially:
  Allergic reaction to naltrexone, history of
  Other medications, especially opioids
  Other medical problems, especially hepatitis or other hepatic disease

**Proper use of this medication**
» Importance of taking each dose as scheduled
» Proper dosing
  Missed dose: If dosing schedule is—
    One tablet every day—
      Taking as soon as possible; not taking if not remembered until next day; not doubling next day's dose
    One tablet every weekday and two tablets on Saturday—
      If weekday dose missed—Following missed dose directions as for one tablet every day
      If Saturday dose missed—Taking two tablets as soon as possible if remembered same day or taking one tablet if not

remembered until Sunday, then returning to regular dosing schedule on Monday
    Two tablets every other day—
      Taking two tablets as soon as remembered, skipping a day, then continuing every other day; or
      Taking two tablets as soon as possible if remembered same day or taking one tablet if not remembered until next day, then returning to regular dosing schedule
    Two tablets on Monday and Wednesday and three tablets on Friday—
      If Monday or Wednesday dose missed—Taking two tablets as soon as possible if remembered same day or taking one tablet if not remembered until next day, then returning to regular dosing schedule
      If Friday dose missed—Taking three tablets as soon as possible if remembered same day; taking two tablets if not remembered until Saturday or one tablet if not remembered until Sunday; returning to regular dosing schedule on Monday
    Three tablets every three days—
      Taking three tablets as soon as remembered, skipping two days, then continuing every three days; or
      Taking three tablets as soon as possible if remembered same day; taking two tablets if not remembered until next day or one tablet if not remembered until following day, then returning to regular dosing schedule
» Proper storage

**Precautions while using this medication**
» Regular visits to physician or clinic; blood tests may be needed to detect possible hepatotoxicity
» Importance of compliance with other treatments, including attending counseling sessions and/or support group meetings; naltrexone intended only as an aid to other forms of therapy in discouraging return to opioid use
» Not attempting to overcome effects of medication by taking large doses of opioids; such attempts may lead to coma or death
» Not using opioid medications to relieve pain, diarrhea, or cough because medication also prevents therapeutic effects of opioids
» Never sharing medication with friends, including those dependent on opioids
» Notifying all physicians, dentists, and pharmacists of use of medication
» Carrying identification card indicating use of medication

**Side/adverse effects**
Signs of potential side effects, especially aching, burning, or swollen eyes; blurred vision; CNS effects; earache; edema; fever; gastrointestinal ulceration; nosebleeds; phlebitis; ringing or buzzing in ears; shortness of breath; skin rash or itching; swollen glands; and uncomfortable or frequent urination

## General Dosing Information

*Naltrexone therapy should not be initiated until the patient has been completely detoxified,* is free of withdrawal symptoms, and has remained opioid-free for 7 to 10 days (following use of a relatively short-acting opioid such as heroin) or longer (following use of a longer-acting opioid such as methadone). Abstinence should be verified by examination of the urine for opioids and/or a naloxone challenge test.

Clonidine or methadone may be used to prevent or attenuate withdrawal symptoms during detoxification; however, if methadone is used, initiation of naltrexone therapy must be delayed until there is no risk of precipitating withdrawal symptoms.

The naloxone challenge test should *not* be administered if withdrawal symptoms are present or the patient's urine contains opioids. Naloxone may be administered intravenously or subcutaneously. If the intravenous route is used, an initial dose of 200 mcg (0.2 mg) should be administered and the patient observed for 30 seconds for withdrawal symptoms; if none occurs, an additional 600 mcg (0.6 mg) of naloxone should be administered and the patient observed for 20 minutes. If the subcutaneous route is used, 800 mcg (0.8 mg) of naloxone should be administered and the patient observed for 45 minutes for withdrawal symptoms. If necessary to confirm that the patient is not opioid-dependent, a rechallenge using 1.6 mg of naloxone intravenously may be performed. If withdrawal symptoms occur, the naloxone challenge should be repeated at suitable intervals until absence of opioid dependence is confirmed.

It is recommended that naltrexone therapy be initiated with low doses, which should be gradually increased as tolerated. As an alternative to daily administration, several maintenance dosing regimens permitting administration of higher doses every second or third day on an occasional (especially over weekends) or regular basis have been utilized.

It has been suggested that less frequent dosing, scheduled to suit the individual patient, may improve compliance.

Compliance may also be improved if the medication is administered by someone other than the patient, e.g., family member, physician or nurse, etc.

In emergency situations requiring an opioid analgesic, the effects of naltrexone can be overcome by administration of sufficiently high doses of analgesic. It is recommended that a rapidly acting analgesic with minimal potential for respiratory depression be administered in doses carefully titrated according to the needs of the patient. Because high doses of analgesic are required, the risk of adverse effects, including severe, prolonged respiratory depression and circulatory collapse, is greatly increased. Therefore, such treatment must be carried out in a hospital setting with the patient being carefully monitored by trained personnel.

Naltrexone does not cause physical or psychological dependence.

Tolerance to the opioid-blocking action of naltrexone has not been reported.

### For treatment of adverse effects

Precipitation of withdrawal symptoms in physically dependent patients: Symptoms may be very difficult to reverse. Monitoring the patient closely and treating observed symptoms as required are recommended.

## Oral Dosage Forms

### NALTREXONE HYDROCHLORIDE TABLETS

**Usual adult dose**
Initial:
Oral, 25 mg for the first dose; an additional 25 mg may be given one hour later if no withdrawal symptoms occur.

Maintenance:
Oral, 50 mg every twenty-four hours. Alternatively, the weekly dose of 350 mg may be administered using an intermittent dosing schedule, such as:
Oral, 50 mg every twenty-four hours on weekdays and 100 mg on Saturday; or
Oral, 100 mg every forty-eight hours; or
Oral, 100 mg every Monday and Wednesday and 150 mg on Friday; or
Oral, 150 mg every seventy-two hours.

**Usual pediatric dose**
Dosage in patients up to 18 years of age has not been established.

**Strength(s) usually available**
U.S.—
50 mg (Rx) [*Trexan* (scored)].

**Packaging and storage**
Store below 40 °C (104 °F), preferably between 15 and 30 °C (59 and 86 °F), in a tight, light-resistant container, unless otherwise specified by manufacturer.

Revised: June 1990
Interim revision: 08/16/94

---

**NANDROLONE**—See *Anabolic Steroids (Systemic)*

---

# NAPHAZOLINE   Ophthalmic

VA CLASSIFICATION (Primary): OP800
Note: For a listing of dosage forms and brand names by country availability, see *Dosage Forms* section(s). For a listing of brand names for the articles in this monograph, refer to the General Index.

## Category
Decongestant (ophthalmic).

## Indications

**Accepted**
Ocular redness (treatment)—Naphazoline is indicated for the temporary relief of redness associated with minor irritations of the eye, such as those caused by pollen-related allergies, colds, dust, smog, wind, swimming, or wearing contact lenses.

## Pharmacology/Pharmacokinetics

**Physicochemical characteristics**
Molecular weight—246.74.

**Mechanism of action/Effect**
A direct-acting sympathomimetic amine. Acts on alpha-adrenergic receptors in the arterioles of the conjunctiva to produce vasoconstriction, resulting in decreased conjunctival congestion.

**Onset of action**
Within 10 minutes.

**Duration of action**
2 to 6 hours.

## Precautions to Consider

**Cross-sensitivity and/or related problems**
Patients sensitive to other ophthalmic sympathomimetics may be sensitive to this medication also.

**Pregnancy/Reproduction**
Pregnancy—Naphazoline may be systemically absorbed.
Studies have not been done in either animals or humans.
FDA Pregnancy Category C.

**Breast-feeding**
It is not known whether naphazoline is distributed into breast milk and problems in humans have not been documented; however, naphazoline may be systemically absorbed.

**Pediatrics**
Use in infants and children is not recommended, since central nervous system (CNS) depression leading to coma and severe reduction in body temperature may result.

**Geriatrics**
Appropriate studies on the relationship of age to the effects of ophthalmic naphazoline have not been performed in the geriatric population. However, no geriatrics-specific problems have been documented to date.

**Drug interactions and/or related problems**
The following drug interactions and/or related problems have been selected on the basis of their potential clinical significance (possible mechanism in parentheses where appropriate)—not necessarily inclusive (» = major clinical significance):

Note: Combinations containing any of the following medications, depending on the amount present, may also interact with this medication.

Antidepressants, tricyclic or
Maprotiline
(if significant systemic absorption of ophthalmic naphazoline occurs, concurrent use of maprotiline or tricyclic antidepressants may potentiate the pressor effect of naphazoline)

**Medical considerations/Contraindications**
The medical considerations/contraindications included here have been selected on the basis of their potential clinical significance (reasons given in parentheses where appropriate)—not necessarily inclusive (» = major clinical significance).

*Except under special circumstances, this medication should not be used when the following medical problem exists:*
» Glaucoma, narrow-angle, or predisposition to
(naphazoline may cause significant mydriasis, which may precipitate an acute attack of narrow-angle glaucoma)

*Risk-benefit should be considered when the following medical problems exist:*
Cardiovascular disease
(systemic absorption of naphazoline may cause cardiac irregularities)

Diabetes mellitus
(systemic absorption of naphazoline may cause minimal hyperglycemia)
Eye disease, serious, or infection or injury
Hypertension
(systemic absorption of naphazoline may cause hypertension)
Hyperthyroidism
Sensitivity to naphazoline

## Side/Adverse Effects

Note: Serious side/adverse effects occur rarely with ophthalmic naphazoline. However, excessive dosage and/or prolonged use may cause increased irritation of the conjunctiva and systemic side effects.

Prolonged use may cause reactive hyperemia, which may result in overuse of the medication.

This medication may cause liberation of pigment granules, presumably from the iris, especially when high concentrations are used in elderly patients.

The following side/adverse effects have been selected on the basis of their potential clinical significance (possible signs and symptoms in parentheses where appropriate)—not necessarily inclusive:

**Those indicating need for medical attention**
With excessive dosage and/or prolonged use
*Hyperemia, reactive* (increase in eye irritation)
Symptoms of systemic absorption
*Dizziness; headache; increased sweating; nausea; nervousness; weakness*

**Those indicating need for medical attention only if they continue or are bothersome**
Incidence less frequent or rare
*Blurred vision; large pupils*

## Overdose

For more information on the management of overdose or unintentional ingestion, **contact a Poison Control Center** (see *Poison Control Center Listing*).

**Clinical effects of overdose**
The following effects have been selected on the basis of their potential clinical significance (possible signs and symptoms in parentheses where appropriate)—not necessarily inclusive:

Acute and chronic
*Decrease in body temperature; drowsiness; slow heartbeat; weakness, severe*

## Patient Consultation

As an aid to patient consultation, refer to *Advice for the Patient, Naphazoline (Ophthalmic)*.

In providing consultation, consider emphasizing the following selected information (» = major clinical significance):

**Before using this medication**
» Conditions affecting use, especially:
Sensitivity to naphazoline
Use in children—Use in infants and children is not recommended
Other medical problems, especially narrow-angle glaucoma or predisposition to narrow-angle glaucoma

**Proper use of this medication**
Not using if solution becomes cloudy or changes color
» Not using in infants and children
» Importance of not using more medication than the amount recommended; or using for more than 72 hours, unless otherwise directed by physician
Proper administration technique
Preventing contamination: Not touching applicator tip to any surface and keeping container tightly closed

» Proper dosing
» Proper storage

**Precautions while using this medication**
» Stopping medication and checking with physician if eye pain or change in vision occurs or if redness or irritation continues, gets worse, or lasts for more than 72 hours

**Side/adverse effects**
Signs of potential side effects, especially reactive hyperemia or systemic absorption

## General Dosing Information

Treatment should not be continued for more than 72 hours, unless otherwise directed by physician.

Although some of the manufacturers recommend that patients not wear soft contact lenses during treatment with naphazoline ophthalmic solution, USP medical experts do not believe this precaution is necessary, unless the patient has corneal epithelial problems and the medication is to be used more often than once every 1 to 2 hours. No significant problems have been documented with ophthalmic solutions containing 0.03% or less of benzalkonium chloride as a preservative when they are used as eyedrops in patients with no significant corneal surface problem.

## Ophthalmic Dosage Forms

### NAPHAZOLINE HYDROCHLORIDE OPHTHALMIC SOLUTION USP

**Usual adult and adolescent dose**
Ophthalmic decongestant—
Topical, to the conjunctiva, 1 drop of a 0.012% solution up to four times a day as needed, or 1 drop of a 0.1% solution every three to four hours as needed.

**Usual pediatric dose**
Use is not recommended.

**Strength(s) usually available**
U.S.—
0.012% (OTC) [*Allerest; Allergy Drops; Clear Eyes Lubricating Eye Redness Reliever; Degest 2; Estivin II; Naphcon*].
0.02% (OTC) [*VasoClear; VasoClear A*].
0.025% (OTC) [GENERIC].
0.03% (OTC) [*Comfort Eye Drops*].
0.1% (Rx) [*Ak-Con* (benzalkonium chloride 0.01%); *Albalon* (polyvinyl alcohol 1.4%; benzalkonium chloride 0.004%); *I-Naphline; Muro's Opcon; Nafazair; Naphcon Forte* (benzalkonium chloride 0.01%); *Ocu-Zoline Sterile Ophthalmic Solution; Vasocon Regular*; GENERIC].
Canada—
0.1% (OTC) [*Ak-Con* (polyvinyl alcohol); *Albalon Liquifilm* (polyvinyl alcohol 1.4%); *Naphcon Forte; Vasocon* (polyvinyl alcohol)].

**Packaging and storage**
Store below 40 °C (104 °F), preferably between 15 and 30 °C (59 and 86 °F), unless otherwise specified by manufacturer. Store in a tight container. Protect from freezing.

**Stability**
Do not use if solution contains a precipitate or changes color.

**Auxiliary labeling**
• For the eye.
• Keep container tightly closed.

Revised: 05/14/92
Interim revision: 02/24/94

---

**NAPROXEN**—See *Anti-inflammatory Drugs, Nonsteroidal (Systemic)*

# NATAMYCIN  Ophthalmic†

VA CLASSIFICATION (Primary): OP202

Another commonly used name is pimaricin.

Note: For a listing of dosage forms and brand names by country availability, see *Dosage Forms* section(s). For a listing of brand names for the articles in this monograph, refer to the General Index.

---

†Not commercially available in Canada.

---

## Category
Antifungal (ophthalmic).

## Indications

### Accepted
Blepharitis, fungal (treatment) or

Conjunctivitis, fungal (treatment)—Ophthalmic natamycin is indicated in the treatment of fungal blepharitis and fungal conjunctivitis caused by susceptible organisms.

Keratitis, fungal (treatment)—Ophthalmic natamycin is indicated in the treatment of fungal keratitis caused by susceptible organisms, including *Fusarium solani*.

Note: Not all species or strains of a particular organism may be susceptible to natamycin.

## Pharmacology/Pharmacokinetics

### Physicochemical characteristics
Chemical group—Tetraene polyene antifungal.
Molecular weight—665.73.
Chemical name—Pimaricin.
pH—5.0 to 7.5.

### Mechanism of action/Effect
Natamycin probably exerts its antifungal effects by binding to sterols in the fungal cell membrane to produce a change in membrane permeability that allows loss of essential cellular constituents. Following topical application, natamycin is retained in the conjunctival fornices and attains effective concentrations within the corneal stroma. Significant drug concentration is usually not attained in the intraocular fluid.

## Precautions to Consider

### Carcinogenicity/Mutagenicity
Studies have not been done.

### Pregnancy/Reproduction
Fertility—Studies have not been done.

Pregnancy—Studies have not been done in humans.
Studies have not been done in animals.

FDA Pregnancy Category C.

### Breast-feeding
It is not known whether natamycin is distributed into breast milk. However, problems in humans have not been documented.

### Pediatrics
Appropriate studies on the relationship of age to the effects of natamycin have not been performed in the pediatric population. Safety and efficacy have not been established.

### Geriatrics
Appropriate studies on the relationship of age to the effects of natamycin have not been performed in the geriatric population. However, no geriatrics-specific problems have been documented to date.

### Medical considerations/Contraindications
The medical considerations/contraindications included here have been selected on the basis of their potential clinical significance (reasons given in parentheses where appropriate)—not necessarily inclusive (» = major clinical significance).

*Except under special circumstances, this medication should not be used when the following medical problem exists:*
» Sensitivity to natamycin

### Patient monitoring
The following may be especially important in patient monitoring (other tests may be warranted in some patients, depending on condition; » = major clinical significance):

Monitoring of tolerance to medication
(recommended at least twice a week when natamycin is used in the treatment of fungal keratitis)

## Side/Adverse Effects
The following side/adverse effects have been selected on the basis of their potential clinical significance (possible signs and symptoms in parentheses where appropriate)—not necessarily inclusive:

### Those indicating need for medical attention
*Conjunctival chemosis or hyperemia* (eye irritation, redness, or swelling not present before therapy)

## Patient Consultation
As an aid to patient consultation, refer to *Advice for the Patient, Natamycin (Ophthalmic).*

In providing consultation, consider emphasizing the following selected information (» = major clinical significance):

### Before using this medication
» Conditions affecting use, especially:
Sensitivity to natamycin

### Proper use of this medication
Proper administration technique for ophthalmic suspension
» Compliance with full course of therapy
» Proper dosing
Missed dose: Applying as soon as possible
» Proper storage

### Precautions while using this medication
Regular visits to physician to check progress during therapy
Checking with physician if no improvement within 7 to 10 days

### Side/adverse effects
Signs of potential side effects, especially conjunctival chemosis or hyperemia

## General Dosing Information
Although some manufacturers recommend a dose of 2 drops of an ophthalmic solution at appropriate intervals, the conjunctival sac will usually hold only 1 drop.

In fungal keratitis, therapy should be continued for 14 to 21 days or until the active keratitis is resolved; however, if there is no improvement after 7 to 10 days of natamycin therapy, re-evaluation of the condition is recommended.

## Ophthalmic Dosage Forms

### NATAMYCIN OPHTHALMIC SUSPENSION USP

#### Usual adult and adolescent dose
Blepharitis, fungal or
Conjunctivitis, fungal—
Topical, to the conjunctiva, 1 drop every four to six hours initially.
Keratitis, fungal—
Topical, to the conjunctiva, 1 drop every one or two hours for the first three or four days, the dosage being reduced to 1 drop six to eight times a day thereafter.

#### Usual pediatric dose
Safety and efficacy have not been established.

#### Strength(s) usually available
U.S.—
5% (Rx) [*Natacyn* (benzalkonium chloride 0.02%)].
Canada—
Not commercially available.

#### Packaging and storage
Store below 40 °C (104 °F), preferably between 15 and 30 °C (59 and 86 °F), unless otherwise specified by manufacturer. Store in a tight, light-resistant container. Protect from freezing.

#### Auxiliary labeling
• For the eye.
• Shake well.
• Keep container tightly closed.
• Continue medicine for full time of treatment.

---

Revised: 05/16/94

# NEDOCROMIL    Inhalation-Local

VA CLASSIFICATION (Primary/Secondary): RE101/RE109

Note: For a listing of dosage forms and brand names by country availability, see *Dosage Forms* section(s). For a listing of brand names for the articles in this monograph, refer to the General Index.

## Category

Anti-inflammatory, nonsteroid (inhalation); asthma prophylactic; antiallergic (inhalation).

## Indications

Note: Bracketed information in the *Indications* section refers to indications that are not included in U.S. product labeling.

### Accepted

Asthma, bronchial (prophylaxis)—Nedocromil is indicated for prevention of airway inflammation and bronchoconstriction in patients with bronchial asthma who require daily therapy. It may be used alone as primary therapy or with other asthma medications, such as bronchodilators and/or corticosteroids. In mild or moderate asthma, nedocromil may be used instead of corticosteroids, inhaled or systemic.

[Bronchospasm (prophylaxis)]—Nedocromil is indicated for prevention of bronchospasm in patients with reversible obstructive airways disease. It may be used regularly or occasionally just prior to an anticipated exposure to such provocation as inhaled allergens, exercise, cold air, or atmospheric pollutants.

### Unaccepted

Nedocromil is not a bronchodilator and, therefore, is not indicated for the reversal or relief of acute bronchospasm, especially in status asthmaticus.

## Pharmacology/Pharmacokinetics

### Physicochemical characteristics

Chemical group—Pyranoquinoline.
Molecular weight—415.31.
pKa—2.

### Mechanism of action/Effect

Nedocromil inhibits activation and release of inflammatory mediators from a variety of cell types in the lumen and mucosa of the bronchial tree. These mediators, which include the leukotrienes, histamine, and prostaglandins, are preformed or derived from arachidonic acid metabolism through the lipoxygenase and cyclo-oxygenase pathways. A range of human cells associated with asthma, such as eosinophils, neutrophils, macrophages, monocytes, mast cells, and platelets, may be involved. Nedocromil exhibits specific anti-inflammatory properties when administered directly to the bronchial mucosa. It has demonstrated a significant inhibitory effect on allergen-induced early and late asthmatic reactions and on bronchial hyperresponsiveness. Nedocromil may also affect sensory nerves in the lung. The mechanism of action of nedocromil may be due partly to inhibition of axon reflexes and release of sensory neuropeptides, such as substance P, neurokinin A, and calcitonin-gene–related peptides. The result is inhibition of bradykinin-induced bronchoconstriction.

### Absorption

The extent of absorption is about 7 to 9% of a single inhaled dose of 3.5 to 4 mg and 17% of multiple inhaled doses, with absorption largely from the respiratory tract.

Gastrointestinal tract—Although most of an inhaled dose of nedocromil is subsequently swallowed, only 2 to 3% of it is absorbed from the gastrointestinal tract.

Respiratory tract—5 to 6% of an inhaled dose of nedocromil is absorbed slowly from the respiratory tract.

### Distribution

Distributed into plasma. With repeated dosing, nedocromil seems to exert a residual effect that allows for twice-a-day dosing for some patients.

### Protein binding

Approximately 89% is reversibly bound to plasma proteins when plasma concentrations range between 0.5 and 50 mcg/mL.

### Biotransformation

Nedocromil is not metabolized.

### Half-life

Approximately 1.5 to 3.3 hours.

### Onset of action

Nedocromil has been shown to prevent bronchospasm when administered up to 30 minutes before exposure to a chemical irritant, an allergen, or exercise.

When nedocromil is used as maintenance therapy, clinical improvement in symptoms and lung function usually occurs within 2 to 4 weeks of the beginning of treatment. In some patients, improvement of symptoms can occur within a few days.

### Time to peak concentration

Following single-dose or multiple-dose inhalation—In asthmatic patients: 5 to 90 minutes.

### Peak serum concentration:

Following single-dose or multiple-dose inhalation—In asthmatic patients: 2.8 nanograms per mL.

### Duration of action

When a single dose is administered prior to an allergen challenge, nedocromil inhibits the late reactions of bronchoconstriction occurring 6 to 12 hours after provocation.

### Elimination

Rapidly excreted as unchanged drug, in the bile and urine.

## Precautions to Consider

### Cross-sensitivity and/or related problems

Patients sensitive to fluorocarbons may be sensitive to the fluorocarbons, dichlorotetrafluoroethane and dichlorodifluoromethane, contained in this preparation.

### Carcinogenicity/Mutagenicity

Various animal studies and *in vitro* studies using human cells showed no evidence of mutagenic or carcinogenic potential.

### Pregnancy/Reproduction

Pregnancy—Adequate and well controlled studies in humans have not been done.

In reproduction studies in rats and mice, small amounts of nedocromil crossed the placenta but did not cause teratogenic or embryotoxic effects.

FDA Pregnancy Category B.

### Breast-feeding

It is not known whether nedocromil is distributed into human breast milk. However, problems in humans have not been documented. In animal studies, small amounts of nedocromil were distributed into milk but did not cause adverse effects.

### Pediatrics

Appropriate studies have been performed in children 6 years of age and older, although data regarding use of nedocromil in treatment of childhood asthma remain limited to date. These studies have not demonstrated pediatrics-specific problems that would limit the usefulness of nedocromil in children.

### Geriatrics

No information is available on the relationship of age to the effects of nedocromil in geriatric patients.

### Medical considerations/Contraindications

The medical considerations/contraindications included here have been selected on the basis of their potential clinical significance (reasons given in parentheses where appropriate)—not necessarily inclusive (» = major clinical significance).

*Risk-benefit should be considered when the following medical problem exists:*
Sensitivity to nedocromil

## Side/Adverse Effects

The following side/adverse effects have been selected on the basis of their potential clinical significance (possible signs and symptoms in parentheses where appropriate)—not necessarily inclusive:

**Those indicating need for medical attention**
Incidence less frequent (about 5%)
    *Bronchospasm, increased* (increased wheezing, tightness in chest, or difficulty in breathing)—may be due to sensitivity to nedocromil or fluorocarbon propellants

**Those indicating need for medical attention only if they continue or are bothersome**
Incidence less frequent (about 4 to 7%)
    *Cough; headache; nausea; rhinitis* (runny or stuffy nose); *throat irritation*

**Those not indicating need for medical attention**
Incidence more frequent (about 12% or more)
    *Unpleasant taste after inhalation*

## Patient Consultation

As an aid to patient consultation, refer to *Advice for the Patient, Nedocromil (Inhalation)*.

In providing consultation, consider emphasizing the following selected information (» = major clinical significance):

**Before using this medication**
» Conditions affecting use, especially:
    Sensitivity to nedocromil

**Proper use of this medication**
» Helps prevent, but does not relieve, acute attacks of asthma or bronchospasm
    Reading patient instructions carefully before using
    Using metered dose inhaler; checking periodically with doctor, nurse, or pharmacist for proper use of inhaler to prevent incorrect dosage
    Testing inhaler before using first time or if not used for a while
    Proper administration technique
    Proper administration technique if spacer device used
    Proper cleaning procedure for inhaler
» Proper dosing
» Proper storage
    Missed dose: If used regularly, using as soon as possible; using any remaining doses for that day at regularly spaced intervals
*For patients on scheduled dosing regimen*
» Compliance with therapy; 2 to 4 weeks usually required for maximum therapeutic benefit after the beginning of nedocromil therapy

**Precautions while using this medication**
» Checking with physician if symptoms do not improve within 2 to 4 weeks; checking with physician immediately if condition becomes worse
» Importance of not discontinuing any concurrent antiasthmatic medication without physician's advice
    Gargling or rinsing mouth after inhalation to relieve throat irritation and unpleasant taste

**Side/adverse effects**
    Signs of potential side effects, especially increased bronchospasm

## General Dosing Information

In maintenance therapy, nedocromil must be used regularly, even during symptom-free periods, to achieve benefit.

It is essential that patients be properly instructed in the use of the inhaler, and that the correct method be reinforced periodically.

A decrease in severity of clinical symptoms or in the need for concomitant therapy is a sign of improvement that usually will be evident in the first 2 to 4 weeks of therapy if patient responds to nedocromil therapy.

After a patient becomes stabilized on nedocromil, the frequency of administration may be slowly decreased to a frequency that maintains freedom from exacerbations of asthma. The frequency of administration is usually no less than twice a day.

When nedocromil is added to an existing regimen of bronchodilators and/or inhaled or systemic corticosteroids, a reduction in dosage of the corticosteroid or bronchodilator may be achieved in some patients. However, the reduction should be gradual and under close medical supervision to avoid an exacerbation of asthma, since nedocromil has a very limited capacity to effectively substitute for inhaled or systemic corticosteroids.

## Inhalation Dosage Forms

Note: Bracketed uses in the *Dosage Forms* section refer to categories of use and/or indications that are not included in U.S. product labeling.

### NEDOCROMIL INHALATION AEROSOL

**Usual adult and adolescent dose**
Asthma, bronchial (prophylaxis)—
    Oral inhalation, 3.5 or 4 mg (2 inhalations) four times a day at regular intervals. Dosage frequency may be reduced to three times a day and then two times a day when patient's asthma is under good control.
[Bronchospasm (prophylaxis)]—
    Oral inhalation, 4 mg (2 inhalations) as a single dose up to thirty minutes before exercise or exposure to any precipitating factor.

**Usual adult prescribing limits**
Up to 16 mg of nedocromil per twenty-four hours.

**Usual pediatric dose**
Children up to 12 years of age: Safety and efficacy have not been established.
    Children 12 years of age and older: See *Usual adult and adolescent dose*.

**Usual geriatric dose**
See *Usual adult and adolescent dose*.

**Strength(s) usually available**
U.S.—
    1.75 mg per metered spray (Rx) [*Tilade*].
Canada—
    2 mg per metered spray (Rx) [*Tilade*].
Note: In Canada, metered dose inhalers are labeled according to the amount of nedocromil delivered at the valve; in the U.S., metered dose inhalers are labeled according to the amount of nedocromil delivered at the mouthpiece or actuator. Therefore, 2 mg of nedocromil delivered at the valve is equivalent to 1.75 mg delivered at the mouthpiece.

**Packaging and storage**
Store between 15 and 30 °C (59 and 86 °F), unless otherwise specified by manufacturer. Protect from freezing.

**Auxiliary labeling**
• For oral inhalation only.
• Shake well before using.
• Store away from heat and direct sunlight.
• Do not use with other mouthpieces.

**Note**
Include patient instructions when dispensing.
Demonstrate inhalation technique to patient when dispensing.

**Additional information**
This product contains dichlorotetrafluoroethane and dichlorodifluoromethane, substances that harm public health and the environment by destroying ozone in the upper atmosphere.

## Selected Bibliography

Parish RC, Miller LJ. Nedocromil sodium. Ann Pharmacother 1993; 27: 599-606.

Brogden RN, Sorkin EM. Nedocromil sodium. An updated review of its pharmacological properties and therapeutic efficacy in asthma. Drugs 1993; 45 (5): 693-715.

Revised: 08/09/94

---

**NEOMYCIN**—See *Aminoglycosides (Systemic)*; *Neomycin (Ophthalmic)*; *Neomycin (Oral-Local)*; *Neomycin (Topical)*

# NEOMYCIN    Ophthalmic*†

VA CLASSIFICATION (Primary): OP201

Note: For a listing of dosage forms and brand names by country availability, see *Dosage Forms* section(s). For a listing of brand names for the articles in this monograph, refer to the General Index.

*Not commercially available in the U.S.
†Not commercially available in Canada.

## Category
Antibacterial (ophthalmic).

## Indications

### Accepted
Ocular infections (treatment)—Ophthalmic neomycin is indicated in the treatment of superficial ocular infections, involving the conjunctiva and/or cornea, caused by susceptible organisms.

Blepharitis, bacterial (treatment)
Blepharoconjunctivitis (treatment)
Conjunctivitis, bacterial (treatment)
Keratitis, bacterial (treatment) or
Keratoconjunctivitis, bacterial (treatment)—Ophthalmic neomycin is used in the treatment of bacterial blepharitis, blepharoconjunctivitis, bacterial conjunctivitis, bacterial keratitis, and bacterial keratoconjunctivitis.

Note: Not all species or strains of a particular organism may be susceptible to neomycin.

### Unaccepted
Neomycin is not effective against *Pseudomonas aeruginosa*.

## Pharmacology/Pharmacokinetics

### Physicochemical characteristics
Family—Aminoglycosides.

### Mechanism of action/Effect
Aminoglycoside; actively transported across the bacterial cell membrane, binds to a specific receptor protein on the 30 S subunit of bacterial ribosomes, and interferes with an initiation complex between mRNA (messenger RNA) and the 30 S subunit, inhibiting protein synthesis. DNA may be misread, thus producing nonfunctional proteins; polyribosomes are split apart and are unable to synthesize protein.

Note: Aminoglycosides are bactericidal, while most other antibiotics that interfere with protein synthesis are bacteriostatic.

### Absorption
May be absorbed following topical application to the eye if tissue damage is present.

## Precautions to Consider

### Cross-sensitivity and/or related problems
Patients sensitive to one aminoglycoside may be sensitive to other aminoglycosides also.

### Pregnancy/Reproduction
Pregnancy—Problems in humans have not been documented.

### Breast-feeding
Problems in humans have not been documented.

### Pediatrics
Appropriate studies on the relationship of age to the effects of neomycin have not been performed in the pediatric population. However, no pediatrics-specific problems have been documented to date.

### Geriatrics
Appropriate studies on the relationship of age to the effects of neomycin have not been performed in the geriatric population. However, no geriatrics-specific problems have been documented to date.

### Medical considerations/Contraindications
The medical considerations/contraindications included here have been selected on the basis of their potential clinical significance (reasons given in parentheses where appropriate)—not necessarily inclusive (» = major clinical significance).

*Risk-benefit should be considered when the following medical problem exists:*
Sensitivity to neomycin

## Side/Adverse Effects
The following side/adverse effects have been selected on the basis of their potential clinical significance (possible signs and symptoms in parentheses where appropriate)—not necessarily inclusive:

### Those indicating need for medical attention
Incidence more frequent
*Hypersensitivity* (itching, rash, redness, swelling, or other sign of irritation not present before therapy)

### Those indicating need for medical attention only if they continue or are bothersome
Incidence less frequent
*Burning or stinging*

### Those not indicating need for medical attention
*Blurred vision*

## Patient Consultation
As an aid to patient consultation, refer to *Advice for the Patient, Neomycin (Ophthalmic).*

In providing consultation, consider emphasizing the following selected information (» = major clinical significance):

### Before using this medication
» Conditions affecting use, especially:
    Sensitivity to neomycin or to any related antibiotic, such as amikacin, gentamicin, kanamycin, netilmicin, streptomycin, or tobramycin

### Proper use of this medication
Proper administration technique for ophthalmic ointment
» Compliance with full course of therapy
» Proper dosing
    Missed dose: Applying as soon as possible; not applying if almost time for next dose
» Proper storage

### Precautions while using this medication
Checking with physician if no improvement within a few days

### Side/adverse effects
Blurred vision may occur for a few minutes after application of ophthalmic ointments
Signs of potential side effects, especially hypersensitivity

## Ophthalmic Dosage Forms

### NEOMYCIN SULFATE OPHTHALMIC OINTMENT USP

#### Usual adult and adolescent dose
Antibacterial, ophthalmic—
    Topical, to the conjunctiva, a thin strip (approximately 1 cm) of ointment every eight to twenty-four hours.

#### Usual pediatric dose
See *Usual adult and adolescent dose.*

#### Strength(s) usually available
U.S.—
    Not commercially available.
Canada—
    Not commercially available.
Note: Compounding is required. Each gram of ophthalmic ointment should contain 5 mg of neomycin sulfate, equivalent to 3.5 mg of neomycin base.

#### Packaging and storage
Store below 40 °C (104 °F) preferably between 15 and 30 °C (59 and 86 °F), unless otherwise specified by manufacturer. Protect from freezing. Preserve in collapsible ophthalmic ointment tubes.

#### Auxiliary labeling
• For the eye.
• Continue medicine for full time of treatment.

Revised: 05/16/94

# NEOMYCIN   Oral-Local

VA CLASSIFICATION (Primary/Secondary): AM300/GA900

Note: For a listing of dosage forms and brand names by country availability, see *Dosage Forms* section(s). For a listing of brand names for the articles in this monograph, refer to the General Index.

## Category

Hepatic encephalopathy therapy adjunct; bowel preparation (preoperative) adjunct.

## Indications

### Accepted

Bowel preparation, preoperative—Oral-local neomycin is indicated concurrently with enteric-coated erythromycin base as part of an adjunctive regimen for the suppression of normal bacterial flora in the preoperative preparation of the bowel.

Hepatic encephalopathy (treatment adjunct)—Oral-local neomycin is indicated in the adjunctive treatment of hepatic encephalopathy.

Not all species or strains of a particular organism may be susceptible to neomycin.

### Unaccepted

Oral neomycin is not indicated in the treatment of systemic infections because it is poorly absorbed. It is not effective against *Pseudomonas aeruginosa*.

Oral neomycin has been used in the treatment of hyperlipidemia; however, its use is not recommended because other available medications have a more favorable benefit/risk ratio.

## Pharmacology/Pharmacokinetics

### Mechanism of action/Effect

Antibacterial (oral-local)—Aminoglycoside; actively transported across the bacterial cell membrane, binds to a specific receptor protein on the 30 S subunit of bacterial ribosomes, and interferes with an initiation complex between mRNA (messenger RNA) and the 30 S subunit, inhibiting protein synthesis. DNA may be misread, thus producing nonfunctional proteins; polyribosomes are split apart and are unable to synthesize protein.

Oral nonabsorbable antibiotics suppress the growth of bacteria in the bowel. Oral neomycin is thought to reduce the production of ammonia in the intestine by inhibiting urease-producing bacteria responsible for catalyzing ammonia synthesis.

### Absorption

Although only approximately 3% of neomycin is absorbed through intact intestinal mucosa, significant amounts may be absorbed through ulcerated or denuded mucosa or if inflammation is present.

### Peak plasma concentrations

Single oral dose of 3 grams—1 to 4 mcg per mL.

### Elimination

Absorbed drug (approximately 3%)—Renal.
Unabsorbed drug (approximately 97%)—Fecal.

## Precautions to Consider

### Cross-sensitivity and/or related problems

Patients hypersensitive to one aminoglycoside may be hypersensitive to other aminoglycosides also.

### Carcinogenicity/Mutagenicity

Long-term studies in animals have not been done to evaluate the carcinogenic or mutagenic potential of oral neomycin.

### Pregnancy/Reproduction

Fertility—Long-term studies in animals have not been done to evaluate the effect of oral neomycin on fertility.

Pregnancy—Neomycin crosses the placenta and may be nephrotoxic in the human fetus. In addition, some aminoglycosides (e.g., streptomycin, tobramycin) have been reported to cause total irreversible, bilateral congenital deafness in children whose mothers received aminoglycosides during pregnancy.

FDA Pregnancy Category D.

### Breast-feeding

It is not known whether neomycin, taken orally, is excreted in breast milk. However, aminoglycosides are poorly absorbed from the gastrointestinal tract, and problems in humans have not been documented.

### Pediatrics

Acute aminoglycoside-induced toxicity is more likely to occur in premature infants and neonates.

### Geriatrics

Since geriatric patients may be at greater risk of aminoglycoside-induced toxicity because of an age-related decrease in renal function, monitoring of renal function during therapy with aminoglycosides is recommended in these patients. Recommended doses should not be exceeded.

### Dental

Oral-local neomycin may cause irritation or soreness of the mouth.

### Drug interactions and/or related problems

The following drug interactions and/or related problems have been selected on the basis of their potential clinical significance (possible mechanism in parentheses where appropriate)—not necessarily inclusive (» = major clinical significance):

Note: Combinations containing any of the following medications, depending on the amount present, may also interact with this medication.

Aminoglycosides, other or
Capreomycin
(if significant systemic absorption of oral neomycin occurs, concurrent systemic use of these medications, especially in patients with renal insufficiency, may increase the potential for ototoxicity, nephrotoxicity, and neuromuscular blockade; hearing loss may occur and may progress to deafness even after discontinuation of the drug and is usually permanent; neuromuscular blockade may result in skeletal muscle weakness and respiratory depression or paralysis; treatment with anticholinesterase agents or calcium salts may help reverse the blockade)

Anesthetics, halogenated hydrocarbon inhalation or
Citrate-anticoagulated blood, massive transfusions or
Neuromuscular blocking agents
(if significant systemic absorption of oral neomycin occurs, concurrent use of these medications, especially in patients with renal insufficiency, may enhance neuromuscular blockade, resulting in skeletal muscle weakness and respiratory depression or paralysis; treatment with anticholinesterase agents or calcium salts may help reverse the blockade)

Chenodiol
(effectiveness of chenodiol may be decreased when used concurrently with antihyperlipidemics since they tend to increase cholesterol saturation of bile)

Digitalis glycosides, oral or
Fluorouracil (5-FU) or
Methotrexate, oral or
Penicillin V or
Vitamin A, oral or
Vitamin B₁₂, oral
(oral neomycin may impair absorption of these medications, resulting in decreased therapeutic effect; serum digoxin concentrations should be monitored and patients should be watched closely for evidence of altered digitalis effect)
(requirements for vitamin B₁₂, especially when used in combination with colchicine, and vitamin A may be increased in patients receiving oral neomycin concurrently)

Nephrotoxic medications, other (See *Appendix II*) or
Ototoxic medications, other (See *Appendix II*)
(if significant systemic absorption of oral neomycin occurs, concurrent systemic use of these medications, especially in patients with renal insufficiency, may increase the potential for ototoxicity and nephrotoxicity; hearing loss may occur and may progress to deafness even after discontinuation of the drug and may be permanent)

Polymyxins, parenteral
(if significant systemic absorption of oral neomycin occurs, concurrent systemic use of these medications, especially in patients with renal insufficiency, may increase the potential for nephrotoxicity and neuromuscular blockade; neuromuscular blockade may result in skeletal muscle weakness and respiratory depression or paralysis; treatment with anticholinesterase agents or calcium salts may help reverse the blockade)

Warfarin
(oral neomycin may enhance the effect of warfarin by altering vitamin K gut flora production, thereby decreasing vitamin K avail-

ability; it is not thought to have an effect on blood levels of prothrombin)

**Medical considerations/Contraindications**

The medical considerations/contraindications included here have been selected on the basis of their potential clinical significance (reasons given in parentheses where appropriate)—not necessarily inclusive (» = major clinical significance).

*Except under special circumstances, this medication should not be used when the following medical problems exist:*

» Hypersensitivity to aminoglycosides
» Intestinal obstruction

*Risk-benefit should be considered when the following medical problems exist:*

» Eighth-cranial-nerve impairment
 (if significant systemic absorption of oral neomycin occurs, it may cause auditory and vestibular toxicity)
» Myasthenia gravis or
» Parkinson's disease
 (if significant systemic absorption of oral neomycin occurs, it may cause neuromuscular blockade, resulting in further skeletal muscle weakness)
» Renal function impairment
 (patients with impaired renal function may require a reduction in dose or discontinuation of oral neomycin)
» Ulcerative lesions of the bowel
 (significant amounts of oral neomycin may be absorbed through ulcerated or denuded mucosa of the bowel or if inflammation is present)

**Patient monitoring**

The following may be especially important in patient monitoring (other tests may be warranted in some patients, depending on condition; » = major clinical significance):

Audiograms and
Renal function determinations
 (may be required prior to and during treatment in patients with preexisting renal or eighth-cranial-nerve impairment or on long-term therapy; patients with impaired renal or eighth-cranial-nerve function may require a reduction in dose)

## Side/Adverse Effects

The following side/adverse effects have been selected on the basis of their potential clinical significance (possible signs and symptoms in parentheses where appropriate)—not necessarily inclusive:

**Those indicating need for medical attention**

Incidence rare
 *Malabsorption syndrome* (diarrhea; increased amount of gas; light-colored, frothy, fatty-appearing stools); *nephrotoxicity* (greatly decreased frequency of urination or amount of urine; increased thirst); *neuromuscular blockade* (difficulty in breathing; drowsiness; weakness); *ototoxicity*—auditory (any loss of hearing, ringing or buzzing or a feeling of fullness in the ears); *ototoxicity*—vestibular (clumsiness, dizziness, unsteadiness); *skin rash*

**Those indicating need for medical attention only if they continue or are bothersome**

Incidence more frequent
 *Gastrointestinal disturbance* (diarrhea; nausea; vomiting); *irritation or soreness of the mouth or rectal area*

## Overdose

For more information on the management of overdose or unintentional ingestion, **contact a Poison Control Center** (see *Poison Control Center Listing*).

**Treatment of overdose**

Recommended treatment consists of the following:

To decrease absorption—Administering activated charcoal.

Specific treatment—Hemodialysis to remove absorbed neomycin from the blood in severe cases.

Supportive care—Maintaining urine output. Patients in whom intentional overdose is known or suspected should be referred for psychiatric consultation.

## Patient Consultation

As an aid to patient consultation, refer to *Advice for the Patient, Neomycin (Oral).*

In providing consultation, consider emphasizing the following selected information (» = major clinical significance):

**Before using this medication**

» Conditions affecting use, especially:
 Hypersensitivity to aminoglycosides
 Pregnancy—Neomycin crosses the placenta and may be nephrotoxic to the fetus
 Use in children—Aminoglycoside-induced toxicity is more likely to occur in premature infants and neonates
 Use in the elderly—Geriatric patients are at greater risk of aminoglycoside-induced toxicity
 Dental—Neomycin may cause irritation or soreness of the mouth
 Other medical problems, especially eighth-cranial-nerve impairment, intestinal obstruction, myasthenia gravis, Parkinson's disease, renal function impairment, or ulcerative lesions of the bowel

**Proper use of this medication**

 Taking on a full or empty stomach
 Proper administration technique for oral solution
» Compliance with full course of therapy
» Proper dosing
 Missed dose: Taking as soon as possible; not taking if almost time for next dose; not doubling doses
» Proper storage

**Side/adverse effects**

 Side effects are more likely to occur in elderly patients and in premature and newborn infants
 Signs of potential side effects, especially malabsorption syndrome, nephrotoxicity, neuromuscular blockage, auditory ototoxicity, vestibular ototoxicity, and skin rash

## General Dosing Information

Neomycin may be taken on a full or empty stomach.

Chronic hepatic insufficiency (hepatic encephalopathy) may require 2 to 4 grams daily for an extended period. Risks for the development of neomycin-induced toxicity progressively increase when treatment is prolonged for longer than 3 weeks.

If patients are unable to take neomycin orally in the treatment of hepatic encephalopathy, a 1% solution prepared from sterile neomycin sulfate powder may be administered as a retention enema.

## Oral Dosage Forms

### NEOMYCIN SULFATE ORAL SOLUTION USP

**Usual adult and adolescent dose**

Hepatic encephalopathy therapy adjunct—
 Oral, 1 to 3 grams every six hours for five or six days.
Bowel preparation (preoperative) adjunct—
 Oral, 1 gram every hour for four hours, then 1 gram every four hours for the balance of twenty-four hours; or 1 gram at nineteen hours, eighteen hours, and nine hours before the start of surgery.

**Usual adult prescribing limits**

Hepatic encephalopathy therapy adjunct—
 Up to 12 grams daily.

**Usual pediatric dose**

Hepatic encephalopathy therapy adjunct—
 Oral, 625 mg to 1.75 grams per square meter of body surface every six hours for five or six days.
Bowel preparation (preoperative) adjunct—
 Oral, 14.7 mg per kg of body weight or 417 mg per square meter of body surface every four hours for three days.

**Strength(s) usually available**

U.S.—
 125 mg per 5 mL (Rx) [*Mycifradin* (methylparaben; propylparaben); GENERIC].
Canada—
 125 mg per 5 mL (Rx) [*Mycifradin* (methylparaben; propylparaben)].

**Packaging and storage**

Store preferably between 15 and 30 °C (59 and 86 °F), unless otherwise specified by manufacturer. Store in a tight, light-resistant container. Protect from freezing.

**Auxiliary labeling**

• Continue medicine for full time of treatment.

**Note**

When dispensing, include a calibrated liquid-measuring device.

## NEOMYCIN SULFATE TABLETS USP

**Usual adult and adolescent dose**
See *Neomycin Sulfate Oral Solution USP*.

**Usual adult prescribing limits**
See *Neomycin Sulfate Oral Solution USP*.

**Usual pediatric dose**
See *Neomycin Sulfate Oral Solution USP*.

**Strength(s) usually available**
U.S.—
500 mg (Rx) [GENERIC].
Canada—
500 mg (Rx) [*Mycifradin*].

**Packaging and storage**
Store below 40 °C (104 °F), preferably between 15 and 30 °C (59 and 86 °F), unless otherwise specified by manufacturer. Store in a tight container.

**Stability**
Tablets may vary in color; this variation does not affect their potency.

**Auxiliary labeling**
• Continue medicine for full time of treatment.

**Note**
Dispense in a glass bottle, unless otherwise specified by manufacturer.

Revised: 10/20/92
Interim revision: 03/17/94

---

# NEOMYCIN    Topical

VA CLASSIFICATION (Primary): DE101

Note: For a listing of dosage forms and brand names by country availability, see *Dosage Forms* section(s). For a listing of brand names for the articles in this monograph, refer to the General Index.

## Category

Antibacterial (topical).

## Indications

Note: Bracketed information in the *Indications* section refers to uses that are not included in U.S. product labeling.

**Accepted**
Skin infections, bacterial, minor (prophylaxis)—Topical neomycin is indicated in the prophylaxis of superficial infections in minor abrasions, burns, and cuts.
[Skin infections, bacterial, minor (treatment)] or
[Ulcer, dermal (treatment)]—Topical neomycin is used in the treatment of minor bacterial skin infections and dermal ulcer.

Not all species or strains of a particular organism may be susceptible to neomycin.

**Unaccepted**
Neomycin is not effective against *Pseudomonas aeruginosa*.

## Pharmacology/Pharmacokinetics

**Physicochemical characteristics**
Chemical group—Aminoglycosides

**Mechanism of action/Effect**
Actively transported across the bacterial cell membrane, binds to a specific receptor protein on the 30 S subunit of bacterial ribosomes, and interferes with an initiation complex between mRNA (messenger RNA) and the 30 S subunit, inhibiting protein synthesis. DNA may be misread, thus producing nonfunctional proteins; polyribosomes are split apart and are unable to synthesize protein.
Note: Aminoglycosides are bactericidal, while most other antibiotics that interfere with protein synthesis are bacteriostatic.

**Absorption**
Although not absorbed through intact skin, topical neomycin is readily absorbed from large denuded, burned, or granulating areas. Greater and more rapid absorption occurs with neomycin cream than with the ointment.

## Precautions to Consider

**Cross-sensitivity and/or related problems**
Patients sensitive to one aminoglycoside may be sensitive to other aminoglycosides also.

**Pregnancy/Reproduction**
Pregnancy—Problems in humans have not been documented.

**Breast-feeding**
It is not known whether topical neomycin is distributed into breast milk. However, problems in humans have not been documented.

**Pediatrics**
No information is available on the relationship of age to the effects of topical neomycin in pediatric patients.

**Geriatrics**
No information is available on the relationship of age to the effects of topical neomycin in geriatric patients.

**Drug interactions and/or related problems**
The following drug interactions and/or related problems have been selected on the basis of their potential clinical significance (possible mechanism in parentheses where appropriate)—not necessarily inclusive (» = major clinical significance):
Note: Combinations containing any of the following medications, depending on the amount present, may also interact with this medication.

Aminoglycosides, other
(concurrent topical and systemic use of neomycin or related drugs is not recommended since hypersensitivity reactions may occur more frequently during concurrent use; if significant systemic absorption occurs, hearing loss may also result; this may progress to deafness even after discontinuation of the drug, and may be permanent)

**Medical considerations/Contraindications**
The medical considerations/contraindications included here have been selected on the basis of their potential clinical significance (reasons given in parentheses where appropriate)—not necessarily inclusive (» = major clinical significance).

*Risk-benefit should be considered when the following medical problem exists:*
Sensitivity to aminoglycosides

## Side/Adverse Effects

The following side/adverse effects have been selected on the basis of their potential clinical significance (possible signs and symptoms in parentheses where appropriate)—not necessarily inclusive:

**Those indicating need for medical attention**
Incidence more frequent
*Contact dermatitis* (itching, rash, redness, swelling, or other sign of skin irritation not present before therapy)
Incidence rare
*Ototoxicity* (any loss of hearing)

## Patient Consultation

As an aid to patient consultation, refer to *Advice for the Patient, Neomycin (Topical)*.

In providing consultation, consider emphasizing the following selected information (» = major clinical significance):

**Before using this medication**
» Conditions affecting use, especially:
Sensitivity to aminoglycosides

**Proper use of this medication**
Not using on deep or puncture wounds, serious burns, or raw areas unless directed by physician
Not for ophthalmic use
Before applying, washing affected area with soap and water, and drying thoroughly
Proper administration technique for cream and ointment
After applying, covering treated area with gauze dressing if desired
» Compliance with full course of therapy
» Proper dosing

Missed dose: Applying as soon as possible; not applying if almost time for next dose

» Proper storage

**Precautions while using this medication**

Checking with physician or pharmacist if no improvement within 1 week

**Side/adverse effects**

Signs of potential side effects, especially contact dermatitis and auditory ototoxicity

## General Dosing Information

Use of topical antibacterials may lead to skin sensitization, resulting in hypersensitivity reactions with subsequent topical or systemic use of the medication.

The treated area(s) may be covered with a gauze dressing if desired.

Nephrotoxicity and moderate to severe ototoxicity may occur, especially if renal function is impaired and systemic nephrotoxic and/or ototoxic drugs are given concurrently.

## Topical Dosage Forms

### NEOMYCIN SULFATE CREAM USP

**Usual adult and adolescent dose**

Antibacterial—
Topical, to the skin, one to three times a day.

Note: May be applied up to five times daily.

**Usual pediatric dose**

See *Usual adult and adolescent dose.*

**Strength(s) usually available**

U.S.—
0.5% (OTC) [*Myciguent*].

Canada—
Not commercially available.

**Packaging and storage**

Store preferably between 15 and 30 °C (59 and 86 °F), unless otherwise specified by manufacturer. Store in a well-closed container. Protect from freezing.

**Auxiliary labeling**

• For external use only.
• Continue medication for full time of treatment.

### NEOMYCIN SULFATE OINTMENT USP

**Usual adult and adolescent dose**

See *Neomycin Sulfate Cream USP.*

Note: May be applied up to five times daily.

**Usual pediatric dose**

See *Neomycin Sulfate Cream USP.*

**Strength(s) usually available**

U.S.—
0.5% (OTC) [*Myciguent;* GENERIC].

Canada—
0.5% (Rx) [*Myciguent*].

Note: Each gram of ointment contains 5 mg of neomycin sulfate, equivalent to 3.5 mg of neomycin base.

**Packaging and storage**

Store preferably between 15 and 30 °C (59 and 86 °F), unless otherwise specified by manufacturer. Store in a well-closed container. Protect from freezing.

**Auxiliary labeling**

• For external use only.
• Continue medication for full time of treatment.

Revised: 08/15/94

## NEOMYCIN-CONTAINING COMBINATIONS—

Colistin, Neomycin, and Hydrocortisone (Otic)
Neomycin and Polymyxin B (Topical)
Neomycin, Polymyxin B, and Bacitracin (Ophthalmic)
Neomycin, Polymyxin B, and Bacitracin (Topical)
Neomycin, Polymyxin B, and Gramicidin (Ophthalmic)
Neomycin, Polymyxin B, and Hydrocortisone (Ophthalmic)
Neomycin, Polymyxin B, and Hydrocortisone (Otic)

# NEOMYCIN AND POLYMYXIN B    Topical†

VA CLASSIFICATION (Primary): DE101

Note: For a listing of dosage forms and brand names by country availability, see *Dosage Forms* section(s). For a listing of brand names for the articles in this monograph, refer to the General Index.

†Not commercially available in Canada.

## Category

Antibacterial (topical).

## Indications

Note: Bracketed information in the *Indications* section refers to uses that are not included in U.S. product labeling.

**Accepted**

Skin infections, bacterial, minor (prophylaxis)—Neomycin and polymyxin B combination is indicated in the topical prophylaxis of superficial skin infections caused by susceptible organisms in minor abrasions, burns, and cuts.

[Ulcer, dermal (treatment)]—Neomycin and polymyxin B combination is used in the topical treatment of dermal ulcer.

Not all species or strains of a particular organism may be susceptible to neomycin and polymyxin B combination.

## Pharmacology/Pharmacokinetics

**Physicochemical characteristics**

Source—Neomycin: Derived from *Streptomyces fradiae.*
Polymyxin B: Derived from polymyxin $B_1$ and polymyxin $B_2$, which are produced by the growth of *Bacillus polymyxa.*
Chemical group—Neomycin: Aminoglycoside.
Polymyxin B: Polypeptide.

**Mechanism of action/Effect**

Neomycin—Actively transported across the bacterial cell membrane, binds to a specific receptor protein on the 30 S subunit of bacterial ribosomes, and interferes with an initiation complex between messenger RNA (mRNA) and the 30 S subunit, inhibiting protein synthesis. RNA may be misread, thus producing nonfunctional proteins. Polyribosomes are split apart and are unable to synthesize protein.

Note: Aminoglycosides are bactericidal, while most other antibiotics that interfere with protein synthesis are bacteriostatic.

Polymyxin B—Bactericidal; active against *Pseudomonas aeruginosa* and other gram-negative bacteria. It is a surface-active basic polypeptide that binds to anionic phospholipid sites in bacterial cytoplasmic membranes, disrupts membrane structure, and alters membrane permeability to allow leakage of intracellular contents.

**Absorption**

Neomycin—Although not absorbed through intact skin, topical neomycin is readily absorbed through large denuded, burned, or granulating areas.

Polymyxin B—Does not appear to be significantly absorbed following topical application to intact or damaged skin or to mucous membranes.

## Precautions to Consider

**Cross-sensitivity and/or related problems**

Patients sensitive to other aminoglycosides or polymyxins may be sensitive to this medication also.

**Pregnancy/Reproduction**

Pregnancy—Problems in humans have not been documented.

**Breast-feeding**

Problems in humans have not been documented.

**Pediatrics**
Appropriate studies on the relationship of age to the effects of neomycin and polymyxin B combination have not been performed in the pediatric population. However, no pediatrics-specific problems have been documented to date.

**Geriatrics**
No information is available on the relationship of age to the effects of neomycin and polymyxin B combination in geriatric patients.

**Drug interactions and/or related problems**
The following drug interactions and/or related problems have been selected on the basis of their potential clinical significance (possible mechanism in parentheses where appropriate)—not necessarily inclusive (» = major clinical significance):

Note: Combinations containing any of the following medications, depending on the amount present, may also interact with this medication.

Aminoglycosides, other
(concurrent topical and systemic use with neomycin or related drugs is not recommended since hypersensitivity reactions may occur more frequently; if significant systemic absorption occurs, hearing loss may also result, may progress to deafness even after discontinuation of the drug, and may be permanent)

**Medical considerations/Contraindications**
The medical considerations/contraindications included here have been selected on the basis of their potential clinical significance (reasons given in parentheses where appropriate)—not necessarily inclusive (» = major clinical significance).

*Risk-benefit should be considered when the following medical problem exists:*

Sensitivity to neomycin, polymyxin B, other aminoglycosides or polymyxins, or parabens

## Side/Adverse Effects

Note: Since ototoxicity and nephrotoxicity have been reported, neomycin and polymyxin B combination should not be used on large areas of the body or for a prolonged period of time. In addition, toxicity may be increased when this medication is used in the treatment of leg ulcers, decubitus ulcers, and otitis externa.

Neomycin-containing preparations commonly cause contact dermatitis. In addition, prolonged use increases the possibility of allergic reactions.

If redness, irritation, swelling, or pain occurs, treatment with neomycin and polymyxin B combination should be discontinued.

The following side/adverse effects have been selected on the basis of their potential clinical significance (possible signs and symptoms in parentheses where appropriate)—not necessarily inclusive:

**Those indicating need for medical attention**
Incidence more frequent
*Hypersensitivity* (itching, pain, skin rash, swelling, redness, or other sign of skin irritation not present before therapy)
Incidence rare
*Ototoxicity* (loss of hearing)

## Patient Consultation

As an aid to patient consultation, refer to *Advice for the Patient, Neomycin and Polymyxin B (Topical).*

In providing consultation, consider emphasizing the following selected information (» = major clinical significance):

**Before using this medication**
» Conditions affecting use, especially:
Sensitivity to aminoglycosides, polymyxins, or parabens

**Proper use of this medication**
» Not using on deep wounds, puncture wounds, animal bites, serious burns, or raw areas without checking with physician or pharmacist
» Not for ophthalmic use
*To use*
Before applying, washing affected area(s) with soap and water, and drying thoroughly
Applying small amount of medication to affected area(s) and rubbing in gently

After applying, covering treated area(s) with gauze dressing if desired
» Not using for longer than 1 week or on extensive areas of the body unless directed by physician; may increase the possibility of side effects
» Compliance with full course of therapy
» Proper dosing
Missed dose: Applying as soon as possible; not applying if almost time for next dose
» Proper storage

**Precautions while using this medication**
Checking with physician or pharmacist if no improvement within 1 week

**Side/adverse effects**
Signs of potential side effects, especially hypersensitivity and ototoxicity

## General Dosing Information

Neomycin and polymyxin B combination should not be used in the eyes.

This medication should not be used on extensive areas of the body or for more than 1 week unless directed by physician. Ototoxicity and nephrotoxicity have been reported. Toxicity may also be increased when this medication is used in the treatment of leg ulcers, decubitus ulcers, and otitis externa.

This medication should not be used on deep wounds, puncture wounds, animal bites, serious burns, or raw areas without checking with physician or pharmacist.

Prolonged use of neomycin-containing preparations increases the possibility of allergic reactions.

If redness, irritation, swelling, or pain occurs, treatment with neomycin and polymyxin B combination should be discontinued.

The treated area(s) may be covered with a gauze dressing if desired.

Use of topical antibacterials may lead to skin sensitization, resulting in hypersensitivity reactions with subsequent topical or systemic use of the medication.

## Topical Dosage Forms

### NEOMYCIN AND POLYMYXIN B SULFATES CREAM USP

**Usual adult and adolescent dose**
Skin infections, bacterial, minor (prophylaxis)—
Topical, to the affected area(s), one to three times a day.

**Usual pediatric dose**
Skin infections, bacterial, minor (prophylaxis)—
Children up to 2 years of age: Dosage has not been established.
Children 2 years of age and over: See *Usual adult and adolescent dose.*

**Strength(s) usually available**
U.S.—
3.5 mg of neomycin (base) and 10,000 Units of polymyxin B (base) per gram (OTC) [*Neosporin Cream* (methylparaben 0.25%; propylene glycol)].
Canada—
Not commercially available.
Note: In Canada, *Neosporin* cream also contains gramicidin.

**Packaging and storage**
Store below 40 °C (104 °F), preferably between 15 and 30 °C (59 and 86 °F), in a well-closed container. Protect from freezing.

**Incompatibilities**
The action of polymyxin B is antagonized by calcium and magnesium ions.

**Auxiliary labeling**
• For external use only.
• Continue medication for full time of treatment.

**Additional information**
Neomycin and polymyxin B sulfates cream is available in a nongreasy, nonstaining, water-washable base.

Revised: 06/09/94

# NEOMYCIN, POLYMYXIN B, AND BACITRACIN    Ophthalmic

VA CLASSIFICATION (Primary): OP201

Note: For a listing of dosage forms and brand names by country availability, see *Dosage Forms* section(s). For a listing of brand names for the articles in this monograph, refer to the General Index.

## Category

Antibacterial (ophthalmic).

## Indications

Note: Bracketed information in the *Indications* section refers to uses that are not included in U.S. product labeling.

### Accepted

Ocular infections (treatment)—Ophthalmic neomycin, polymyxin B, and bacitracin combination is indicated in the short-term treatment of superficial external ocular infections caused by susceptible organisms.

[Blepharitis, bacterial (treatment)]
[Blepharoconjunctivitis (treatment)]
[Conjunctivitis, bacterial (treatment)]
[Keratitis, bacterial (treatment)] or
[Keratoconjunctivitis, bacterial (treatment)]—Ophthalmic neomycin, polymyxin B, and bacitracin combination is used in the treatment of bacterial blepharitis, blepharoconjunctivitis, bacterial conjunctivitis, bacterial keratitis, and bacterial keratoconjunctivitis.

Note: Long-term treatment with this medication is rarely indicated.

Not all species or strains of a particular organism may be susceptible to neomycin, polymyxin B, and bacitracin combination.

## Pharmacology/Pharmacokinetics

### Physicochemical characteristics

Source—
Neomycin: Derived from *Streptomyces fradiae*.
Polymyxin B: Derived from polymyxin $B_1$ and polymyxin $B_2$, which are produced by the growth of *Bacillus polymyxa*.
Bacitracin: Derived from a mixture of related antibiotics (mainly bacitracin A), which are produced by the growth of *Bacillus subtilis* ssp. *licheniformis*.
Chemical group—
Neomycin: Aminoglycosides.
Polymyxin B: Polypeptides.
Bacitracin: Cyclic polypeptides.

### Mechanism of action/Effect

Neomycin—See *Neomycin (Ophthalmic)*.
Polymyxin B is bactericidal and active against *Pseudomonas aeruginosa* and other gram-negative bacteria. It is a surface-active basic polypeptide that binds to anionic phospholipid sites in bacterial cytoplasmic membranes, disrupts membrane structure, and alters membrane permeability to allow leakage of intracellular contents. Its action is antagonized by calcium and magnesium.
Bacitracin, a polypeptide antibiotic, is usually bactericidal against gram-positive organisms. It acts within the bacterial cell membrane and interferes with bacterial cell wall synthesis by binding to and inhibiting the dephosphorylation of a membrane-bound lipid pyrophosphate. Pyrophosphate is the precursor of a carrier molecule, undecaprenyl phosphate, which is involved in peptidoglycan polymerization.

### Absorption

Neomycin and polymyxin B—May be absorbed following topical application to the eye if tissue damage is present.
Bacitracin—Not significantly absorbed.

## Precautions to Consider

### Cross-sensitivity and/or related problems

Patients sensitive to one aminoglycoside or polymyxin may be sensitive to other aminoglycosides or polymyxins also.

### Pregnancy/Reproduction

Pregnancy—Problems in humans have not been documented.

### Breast-feeding

Problems in humans have not been documented.

### Pediatrics

Appropriate studies on the relationship of age to the effects of neomycin, polymyxin B, and bacitracin combination have not been performed in the pediatric population. However, no pediatrics-specific problems have been documented to date.

### Geriatrics

Appropriate studies on the relationship of age to the effects of neomycin, polymyxin B, and bacitracin combination have not been performed in the geriatric population. However, no geriatrics-specific problems have been documented to date.

### Medical considerations/Contraindications

The medical considerations/contraindications included here have been selected on the basis of their potential clinical significance (reasons given in parentheses where appropriate)—not necessarily inclusive (» = major clinical significance).

*Risk-benefit should be considered when the following medical problem exists:*

Sensitivity to neomycin, polymyxin B, or bacitracin

## Side/Adverse Effects

The following side/adverse effects have been selected on the basis of their potential clinical significance (possible signs and symptoms in parentheses where appropriate)—not necessarily inclusive:

### Those indicating need for medical attention

Incidence more frequent
*Hypersensitivity* (itching, rash, redness, swelling, or other sign of irritation not present before therapy)

### Those not indicating need for medical attention

*Blurred vision, from the ointment*

## Patient Consultation

As an aid to patient consultation, refer to *Advice for the Patient, Neomycin, Polymyxin B, and Bacitracin (Ophthalmic)*.

In providing consultation, consider emphasizing the following selected information (» = major clinical significance):

### Before using this medication

» Conditions affecting use, especially:
Sensitivity to neomycin, polymyxin B, or bacitracin or to any related antibiotic, such as amikacin, colistimethate, colistin, gentamicin, kanamycin, netilmicin, paromomycin, streptomycin, or tobramycin

### Proper use of this medication

Proper administration technique for ophthalmic ointment
» Compliance with full course of therapy
» Proper dosing
Missed dose: Applying as soon as possible; not applying if almost time for next dose
» Proper storage

### Precautions while using this medication

Checking with physician if no improvement within a few days

### Side/adverse effects

Blurred vision may occur for a few minutes after application of ophthalmic ointments
Signs of potential side effects, especially hypersensitivity

## Ophthalmic Dosage Forms

### NEOMYCIN AND POLYMYXIN B SULFATES AND BACITRACIN ZINC OPHTHALMIC OINTMENT USP

#### Usual adult and adolescent dose

Ophthalmic antibacterial—Topical, to the conjunctiva, a thin strip (approximately 1 cm) of ointment every three to four hours for seven to ten days.

#### Usual pediatric dose

See *Usual adult and adolescent dose*.

#### Strength(s) usually available

U.S.—
3.5 mg of neomycin (base), 5,000 Units of polymyxin B (base), and 400 Units of bacitracin zinc per gram (Rx) [*Neotal; Triple Antibiotic*].
3.5 mg of neomycin (base), 10,000 Units of polymyxin B (base), and 400 Units of bacitracin zinc per gram (Rx) [*Ak-Spore Ophthalmic Ointment; Neocidin Ophthalmic Ointment; Neosporin Ophthalmic Ointment; Ocu-Spor-B; Ocusporin; Ocutricin Ophthalmic Ointment; Ophthalmic; Spectro-Sporin;* GENERIC].

Canada—
　3.5 mg of neomycin (base), 10,000 Units of polymyxin B (base), and 400 Units of bacitracin zinc per gram (Rx) [*Neosporin Ophthalmic Ointment*].

## Packaging and storage
Store below 40 °C (104 °F), preferably between 15 and 30 °C (59 and 86 °F), unless otherwise specified by manufacturer. Store in a collapsible ophthalmic ointment tube. Protect from freezing.

## Auxiliary labeling
• For the eye.
• Continue medicine for full time of treatment.

Revised: 05/16/94
Interim revision: 05/24/95

---

# NEOMYCIN, POLYMYXIN B, AND BACITRACIN　　Topical

VA CLASSIFICATION (Primary): DE101

Note: For a listing of dosage forms and brand names by country availability, see *Dosage Forms* section(s). For a listing of brand names for the articles in this monograph, refer to the General Index.

## Category
Antibacterial (topical).

## Indications
Note: Bracketed information in the *Indications* section refers to uses that are not included in U.S. product labeling.

### Accepted
Skin infections, bacterial, minor (prophylaxis)—Topical neomycin, polymyxin B, and bacitracin combination is indicated in the prophylaxis of superficial skin infections caused by susceptible organisms in minor abrasions, burns, and cuts.

[Skin infections, bacterial, minor (treatment)] or
[Ulcer, dermal (treatment)]—Topical neomycin, polymyxin B, and bacitracin combination is used in the treatment of minor bacterial skin infections and dermal ulcer.

Not all species or strains of a particular organism may be susceptible to neomycin, polymyxin B, and bacitracin combination.

### Unaccepted
Neomycin is not effective against *Pseudomonas aeruginosa*.

## Pharmacology/Pharmacokinetics

### Physicochemical characteristics
Source—
　Neomycin: Derived from *Streptomyces fradiae*.
　Polymyxin B: Derived from polymyxin B₁ and polymyxin B₂, which are produced by the growth of *Bacillus polymyxa*.
　Bacitracin: Derived from a mixture of related antibiotics (mainly bacitracin A), which are produced by the growth of *Bacillus subtilis* ssp *licheniformis*.
Chemical group—
　Neomycin: Aminoglycosides.
　Polymyxin B: Polypeptides.
　Bacitracin: Cyclic polypeptides.

### Mechanism of action/Effect
Neomycin—See *Neomycin (Topical)*.
Polymyxin B; bacitracin—See *Neomycin, Polymyxin B, and Bacitracin (Ophthalmic)*.

### Absorption
Neomycin—Although not absorbed through intact skin, topical neomycin is readily absorbed through large denuded, burned, or granulating areas.
Polymyxin B; bacitracin—Neither polymyxin B nor bacitracin appears to be significantly absorbed following topical application to intact or damaged skin or to mucous membranes.

## Precautions to Consider

### Cross-sensitivity and/or related problems
Patients sensitive to one aminoglycoside or polymyxin may be sensitive to other aminoglycosides or polymyxins also.

### Pregnancy/Reproduction
Pregnancy—Problems in humans have not been documented.

### Breast-feeding
It is not known whether topical neomycin, polymyxin B, and bacitracin are distributed into breast milk. However, problems in humans have not been documented.

### Pediatrics
No pediatrics-specific information is available on the relationship of age to the effects of topical neomycin, polymyxin B, and bacitracin in pediatric patients.

### Geriatrics
No geriatrics-specific information is available on the relationship of age to the effects of topical neomycin, polymyxin B, and bacitracin in geriatric patients.

### Drug interactions and/or related problems
The following drug interactions and/or related problems have been selected on the basis of their potential clinical significance (possible mechanism in parentheses where appropriate)—not necessarily inclusive (» = major clinical significance):

Note: Combinations containing any of the following medications, depending on the amount present, may also interact with this medication.

Aminoglycosides, other
　(concurrent topical and systemic use with neomycin or related drugs is not recommended since hypersensitivity reactions may occur more frequently during concurrent use; if significant systemic absorption occurs, hearing loss may also result, may progress to deafness even after discontinuation of the drug, and may be permanent)

### Medical considerations/Contraindications
The medical considerations/contraindications included here have been selected on the basis of their potential clinical significance (reasons given in parentheses where appropriate)—not necessarily inclusive (» = major clinical significance).

*Risk-benefit should be considered when the following medical problem exists:*
　Sensitivity to aminoglycosides or polymyxins

## Side/Adverse Effects
The following side/adverse effects have been selected on the basis of their potential clinical significance (possible signs and symptoms in parentheses where appropriate)—not necessarily inclusive:

### Those indicating need for medical attention
Incidence more frequent
　*Hypersensitivity* (itching, skin rash, redness, swelling, or other sign of irritation not present before therapy)
Incidence rare
　*Ototoxicity* (any loss of hearing)

## Patient Consultation
As an aid to patient consultation, refer to *Advice for the Patient, Neomycin, Polymyxin B, and Bacitracin (Topical)*.

In providing consultation, consider emphasizing the following selected information (» = major clinical significance):

### Before using this medication
» Conditions affecting use, especially:
　　Sensitivity to aminoglycosides or polymyxins

### Proper use of this medication
　Not using on deep or puncture wounds, serious burns, or raw areas unless directed by physician
　Not for ophthalmic use
　Before applying, washing affected area with soap and water, and drying thoroughly
　After applying, covering treated area with gauze dressing if desired
» Compliance with full course of therapy
» Proper dosing
　　Missed dose: Applying as soon as possible; not applying if almost time for next dose

» Proper storage

**Precautions while using this medication**
Checking with physician or pharmacist if no improvement within 1 week

**Side/adverse effects**
Signs of side effects, especially hypersensitivity and ototoxicity

## General Dosing Information

Use of topical antibacterials may lead to skin sensitization, resulting in hypersensitivity reactions with subsequent topical or systemic use of the medication.

The treated area(s) may be covered with a gauze dressing if desired.

Nephrotoxicity and moderate to severe ototoxicity may occur, especially if renal function is impaired and systemic nephrotoxic and/or ototoxic drugs are given concurrently.

Neomycin, polymyxin B, and bacitracin ointment is available in a petrolatum base that helps retain moisture and may be useful in treating infections on dry or scaling skin. It is also available in a base containing polyethylene glycols, liquid and white petrolatum, and glyceride wax that is miscible with tissue exudates and skin oils and waxes and may be used on weeping, exudative lesions.

## Topical Dosage Forms

### NEOMYCIN AND POLYMYXIN B SULFATES AND BACITRACIN OINTMENT USP

**Usual adult and adolescent dose**
Antibacterial—
Topical, to the skin, two to five times a day.

**Usual pediatric dose**
See *Usual adult and adolescent dose.*

**Strength(s) usually available**
U.S.—
3.5 mg of neomycin (base), 5000 Units of polymyxin B (base), and 400 Units of bacitracin per gram (OTC) [GENERIC].
3.5 mg of neomycin (base), 5000 Units of polymyxin B (base), and 500 Units of bacitracin per gram (OTC) [*Bactine First Aid Antibiotic; Foille; Mycitracin;* GENERIC].

Canada—
Not commercially available.

**Packaging and storage**
Store preferably between 15 and 30 °C (59 and 86 °F), unless otherwise specified by manufacturer. Store in a tight, light-resistant container. Protect from freezing.

**Auxiliary labeling**
• For external use only.
• Continue medication for full time of treatment.

### NEOMYCIN AND POLYMYXIN B SULFATES AND BACITRACIN ZINC OINTMENT USP

**Usual adult and adolescent dose**
See *Neomycin and Polymyxin B Sulfates and Bacitracin Ointment USP.*

**Usual pediatric dose**
See *Neomycin and Polymyxin B Sulfates and Bacitracin Ointment USP.*

**Strength(s) usually available**
U.S.—
3.5 mg of neomycin (base), 5000 Units of polymyxin B (base), and 400 Units of bacitracin zinc per gram (OTC) [*Neosporin Ointment; Topisporin;* GENERIC].
3.5 mg of neomycin (base), 10,000 Units of polymyxin B (base), and 500 Units of bacitracin zinc per gram (OTC) [*Neosporin Maximum Strength Ointment*].

Canada—
3.5 mg of neomycin (base), 5000 Units of polymyxin B (base), and 400 Units of bacitracin zinc per gram (Rx) [GENERIC].

**Packaging and storage**
Store preferably between 15 and 30 °C (59 and 86 °F), unless otherwise specified by manufacturer. Store in a well-closed container. Protect from freezing.

**Auxiliary labeling**
• For external use only.
• Continue medication for full time of treatment.

Revised: 07/25/94

# NEOMYCIN, POLYMYXIN B, AND GRAMICIDIN    Ophthalmic

VA CLASSIFICATION (Primary): OP201
Note: For a listing of dosage forms and brand names by country availability, see *Dosage Forms* section(s). For a listing of brand names for the articles in this monograph, refer to the General Index.

## Category
Antibacterial (ophthalmic).

## Indications
Note: Bracketed information in the *Indications* section refers to uses that are not included in U.S. product labeling.

**Accepted**
Ocular infections (treatment)—Ophthalmic neomycin, polymyxin B, and gramicidin combination is indicated in the treatment of short-term superficial external ocular infections caused by susceptible organisms.
[Blepharitis, bacterial (treatment)]
[Blepharoconjunctivitis (treatment)]
[Conjunctivitis, bacterial (treatment)]
[Keratitis, bacterial (treatment)] or
[Keratoconjunctivitis, bacterial (treatment)]—Ophthalmic neomycin, polymyxin B, and gramicidin combination is used in the treatment of bacterial blepharitis, blepharoconjunctivitis, bacterial conjunctivitis, bacterial keratitis, and bacterial keratoconjunctivitis.

Note: Not all species or strains of a particular organism may be susceptible to neomycin, polymyxin B, and gramicidin combination.

## Pharmacology/Pharmacokinetics

**Physicochemical characteristics**
Source—
Neomycin: Derived from *Streptomyces fradiae.*

Polymyxin B: Derived from polymyxin B₁ and polymyxin B₂, which are produced by the growth of *Bacillus polymyxa.*
Gramicidin: Mixture of three pairs of antibacterial substances (gramicidin A, B, and C), which are produced by the growth of *Bacillus brevis.*
Chemical group—
Neomycin: Aminoglycosides.
Polymyxin B: Polypeptides.
Gramicidin: Polypeptides.

**Mechanism of action/Effect**
Neomycin—See *Neomycin (Ophthalmic).*
Polymyxin B—See *Neomycin, Polymyxin B, and Bacitracin (Ophthalmic).*
Gramicidin acts as a cationic detergent by altering the permeability of bacterial cytoplasmic membranes, with resultant changes in the intracellular cation content, especially potassium.

Note: Gramicidin, which has activity against gram-positive cocci and some *Neisseria,* is considered to be bactericidal, but may be bacteriostatic depending on the susceptibility of the organism. It is inactivated by serum and body fluids and is only effective topically. It should not be used systemically since it is very toxic and is a potent hemolytic.

**Absorption**
Neomycin; polymyxin B—May be absorbed following topical application to the eye if tissue damage is present.
Gramicidin—Not significantly absorbed.

## Precautions to Consider

**Cross-sensitivity and/or related problems**
Patients sensitive to one aminoglycoside or polymyxin may be sensitive to other aminoglycosides or polymyxins also.

**Pregnancy/Reproduction**
Pregnancy—Problems in humans have not been documented.

**Breast-feeding**
Problems in humans have not been documented.

**Pediatrics**
Appropriate studies on the relationship of age to the effects of neomycin, polymyxin B, and gramicidin combination have not been performed in the pediatric population. However, no pediatrics-specific problems have been documented to date.

**Geriatrics**
Appropriate studies on the relationship of age to the effects of neomycin, polymyxin B, and gramicidin combination have not been performed in the geriatric population. However, no geriatrics-specific problems have been documented to date.

**Medical considerations/Contraindications**
The medical considerations/contraindications included here have been selected on the basis of their potential clinical significance (reasons given in parentheses where appropriate)—not necessarily inclusive (» = major clinical significance).

*Risk-benefit should be considered when the following medical problem exists:*
Sensitivity to neomycin, polymyxin B, or gramicidin

## Side/Adverse Effects

The following side/adverse effects have been selected on the basis of their potential clinical significance (possible signs and symptoms in parentheses where appropriate)—not necessarily inclusive:

**Those indicating need for medical attention**
Incidence more frequent
*Hypersensitivity* (itching, rash, redness, swelling, or other sign of irritation in or around the eye not present before therapy)

**Those indicating need for medical attention only if they continue or are bothersome**
Incidence less frequent
*Burning or stinging of the eye*

## Patient Consultation

As an aid to patient consultation, refer to *Advice for the Patient, Neomycin, Polymyxin B, and Gramicidin (Ophthalmic).*

In providing consultation, consider emphasizing the following selected information (» = major clinical significance):

**Before using this medication**
» Conditions affecting use, especially:
    Sensitivity to neomycin, polymyxin B, or gramicidin or to any related antibiotic, such as amikacin, colistimethate, colistin, gentamicin, kanamycin, netilmicin, paromomycin, streptomycin, or tobramycin

**Proper use of this medication**
    Proper administration technique for ophthalmic solution
» Compliance with full course of therapy

» Proper dosing
    Missed dose: Applying as soon as possible; not applying if almost time for next dose
» Proper storage

**Precautions while using this medication**
Checking with physician if no improvement within a few days

**Side/adverse effects**
Signs of potential side effects, especially hypersensitivity

## General Dosing Information

Although some manufacturers recommend a dose of 2 drops of an ophthalmic solution at appropriate intervals, the conjunctival sac will usually hold only 1 drop.

## Ophthalmic Dosage Forms

### NEOMYCIN AND POLYMYXIN B SULFATES AND GRAMICIDIN OPHTHALMIC SOLUTION USP

**Usual adult and adolescent dose**
Antibacterial, ophthalmic—
    Acute infections: Topical, to the conjunctiva, 1 drop every 15 to 30 minutes initially, the frequency being reduced gradually depending on patient response.
    Other infections: Topical, to the conjunctiva, 1 drop two to four times a day, or more frequently, for seven to ten days.

**Usual pediatric dose**
See *Usual adult and adolescent dose.*

**Strength(s) usually available**
U.S.—
    1.75 mg of neomycin (base), 10,000 Units of polymyxin B (base), and 25 mcg (0.025 mg) of gramicidin per mL (Rx) [*Ak-Spore Ophthalmic Solution* (alcohol 0.5%; thimerosal 0.001%); *Neocidin Ophthalmic Solution; Neosporin Ophthalmic Solution* (alcohol 0.5%; thimerosal 0.001%); *Ocu-Spor-G; Ocutricin Ophthalmic Solution; P.N. Ophthalmic; Tribiotic; Tri-Ophthalmic;* GENERIC].
Canada—
    1.75 mg of neomycin (base), 10,000 Units of polymyxin B (base), and 25 mcg (0.025 mg) of gramicidin per mL (Rx) [*Neosporin Ophthalmic Solution* (alcohol 0.5%, benzalkonium chloride)].

**Packaging and storage**
Store below 40 °C (104 °F), preferably between 15 and 30 °C (59 and 86 °F), unless otherwise specified by manufacturer. Store in a tight container. Protect from freezing.

**Auxiliary labeling**
• For the eye.
• Continue medicine for full time of treatment.

Revised: 06/21/94

---

# NEOMYCIN, POLYMYXIN B, AND HYDROCORTISONE   Ophthalmic

VA CLASSIFICATION (Primary): OP350
Note: For a listing of dosage forms and brand names by country availability, see *Dosage Forms* section(s). For a listing of brand names for the articles in this monograph, refer to the General Index.

## Category
Antibacterial-corticosteroid (ophthalmic).

## Indications

**Accepted**
Ocular infections (treatment)—Ophthalmic neomycin, polymyxin B, and hydrocortisone combination is indicated in the treatment of ocular infections, accompanied by inflammation, caused by *Staphylococcus aureus, Escherichia coli, Haemophilus influenzae, Klebsiella* species, *Enterobacter (Aerobacter)* species, and *Neisseria* species.

Note: Not all species or strains of a particular organism may be susceptible to neomycin and polymyxin B.

**Unaccepted**
Neomycin alone is not effective against *Pseudomonas aeruginosa.* Neomycin, polymyxin B, and hydrocortisone combination is not effective against *Serratia marcescens* or streptococci.

## Pharmacology/Pharmacokinetics

**Physicochemical characteristics**
Source—
    Neomycin: Derived from *Streptomyces fradiae.*
    Polymyxin B: Derived from polymyxin $B_1$ and polymyxin $B_2$, which are produced by the growth of *Bacillus polymyxa.*
Chemical group—
    Neomycin: Aminoglycosides.
    Polymyxin B: Polypeptides.
    Hydrocortisone: Corticosteroids.
Molecular weight—Hydrocortisone: 362.47.

**Mechanism of action/Effect**
Neomycin—See *Neomycin (Ophthalmic).*
Polymyxin B—See *Neomycin, Polymyxin B, and Bacitracin (Ophthalmic).*
Hydrocortisone—See *Corticosteroids (Ophthalmic).*

## Absorption

Neomycin; polymyxin B—May be absorbed following topical application to the eye if tissue damage is present.

Hydrocortisone—May be absorbed following topical application to the eye.

## Precautions to Consider

### Cross-sensitivity and/or related problems

Patients sensitive to one aminoglycoside or polymyxin may be sensitive to other aminoglycosides or polymyxins also.

### Pregnancy/Reproduction

Pregnancy—Adequate and well-controlled studies in humans have not been done for ophthalmic neomycin, polymyxin B, and hydrocortisone combination.

Topical corticosteroids have been shown to be teratogenic in rabbits at concentrations of 0.5% on days 6-18 of gestation, and in mice at a concentration of 15% on days 10-13 of gestation.

FDA Pregnancy Category C.

### Breast-feeding

Problems in humans have not been documented.

### Pediatrics

Appropriate studies on the relationship of age to the effects of ophthalmic neomycin, polymyxin B, and hydrocortisone combination have not been performed in the pediatric population. However, no pediatrics-specific problems have been documented to date.

### Geriatrics

Appropriate studies on the relationship of age to the effects of ophthalmic neomycin, polymyxin B, and hydrocortisone combination have not been performed in the geriatric population. However, no geriatrics-specific problems have been documented to date.

### Medical considerations/Contraindications

The medical considerations/contraindications included here have been selected on the basis of their potential clinical significance (reasons given in parentheses where appropriate)—not necessarily inclusive (» = major clinical significance).

*Risk-benefit should be considered when the following medical problems exist:*

*For hydrocortisone*
» Dendritic keratitis
» Herpes simplex keratitis
» Tubercular or fungal infections of the eye
» Vaccinia, varicella, or other viral disease of the cornea or conjunctiva

*For neomycin and/or polymyxin B*
Blepharitis, acute, purulent
Conjunctivitis, acute, purulent

*For neomycin, polymyxin B, and/or hydrocortisone*
Sensitivity to the medication

### Patient monitoring

The following may be especially important in patient monitoring (other tests may be warranted in some patients, depending on condition; » = major clinical significance):

Ophthalmologic examinations
(may be required at periodic intervals for patients on long-term therapy [more than 6 weeks], since chronic therapy may cause posterior subcapsular cataracts, especially in children; may cause increased intraocular pressure and glaucoma; and may enhance the establishment of secondary ocular infections)

## Side/Adverse Effects

The following side/adverse effects have been selected on the basis of their potential clinical significance (possible signs and symptoms in parentheses where appropriate)—not necessarily inclusive:

### Those indicating need for medical attention

Incidence more frequent
*Hypersensitivity* (itching, rash, redness, swelling, or other sign of irritation not present before therapy)

### Those indicating need for medical attention only if they continue or are bothersome

Incidence less frequent
*Burning or stinging*

## Patient Consultation

As an aid to patient consultation, refer to *Advice for the Patient, Neomycin, Polymyxin B, and Hydrocortisone (Ophthalmic)*.

In providing consultation, consider emphasizing the following selected information (» = major clinical significance):

### Before using this medication
» Conditions affecting use, especially:
Sensitivity to neomycin, polymyxin B, or hydrocortisone or to any related antibiotic, such as amikacin, colistimethate, colistin, gentamicin, kanamycin, netilmicin, paromomycin, streptomycin, or tobramycin
Other medical problems, especially dendritic keratitis; herpes simplex keratitis; tubercular or fungal infections of the eye; or vaccinia, varicella, or other viral disease of the cornea or conjunctiva

### Proper use of this medication

Proper administration technique for ophthalmic suspension
» Compliance with full course of therapy
» Proper dosing
Missed dose: Applying as soon as possible; not applying if almost time for next dose
» Checking with physician before using leftover medication on other eye problems
» Proper storage

### Precautions while using this medication

Need for ophthalmologic examinations at regular intervals during long-term therapy (more than 6 weeks)
Checking with physician if no improvement within a few days

### Side/adverse effects

Signs of potential side effects, especially hypersensitivity

## General Dosing Information

Although some manufacturers recommend a dose of 2 drops of an ophthalmic solution at appropriate intervals, the conjunctival sac will usually hold only 1 drop.

## Ophthalmic Dosage Forms

### NEOMYCIN AND POLYMYXIN B SULFATES AND HYDROCORTISONE OPHTHALMIC SUSPENSION USP

Note: The dosing and strengths of the dosage forms available are expressed in terms of neomycin base.

**Usual adult and adolescent dose**
Ocular infections—
Topical, to the conjunctiva, 1 drop every three to four hours. The medication may be used more frequently if necessary.

**Usual pediatric dose**
See *Usual adult and adolescent dose*.

**Strength(s) usually available**
U.S.—
3.5 mg of neomycin (base), 10,000 Units of polymyxin B (base), and 10 mg of hydrocortisone per mL (Rx) [*Ak-Spore H.C; Bacticort; Cobiron; Cortisporin Ophthalmic Suspension; Cortomycin; Hydromycin; I-Neocort; Ocutricin HC; Triple-Gen;* GENERIC].

Canada—
3.5 mg of neomycin (base), 10,000 Units of polymyxin B sulfate, and 10 mg of hydrocortisone per mL (Rx) [*Cortisporin Ophthalmic Suspension* (benzalkonium chloride 0.01%)].

**Packaging and storage**
Store below 40 °C (104 °F), preferably between 15 and 30 °C (59 and 86 °F), unless otherwise specified by manufacturer. Store in a tight container. Protect from freezing.

**Auxiliary labeling**
• For the eye.
• Shake well.
• Continue medicine for full time of treatment.

Revised: 07/01/93

# NEOMYCIN, POLYMYXIN B, AND HYDROCORTISONE    Otic

VA CLASSIFICATION (Primary): OT250

Note: For a listing of dosage forms and brand names by country availability, see *Dosage Forms* section(s). For a listing of brand names for the articles in this monograph, refer to the General Index.

## Category

Antibacterial-corticosteroid (otic).

## Indications

Note: Bracketed information in the *Indications* section refers to uses that are not included in U.S. product labeling.

### Accepted

Ear canal infections, external (treatment) or

Mastoidectomy cavity infections (treatment)—Otic neomycin, polymyxin B, and hydrocortisone combination is indicated in the treatment of external ear canal infections and mastoidectomy cavity infections caused by susceptible organisms.

[Otitis media, chronic suppurative (treatment)][1]—Otic neomycin, polymyxin B, and hydrocortisone combination is used in the treatment of chronic suppurative otitis media.

Not all species or strains of a particular organism may be susceptible to neomycin and polymyxin B.

---

[1]Not included in Canadian product labeling.

## Pharmacology/Pharmacokinetics

### Physicochemical characteristics
Source—
 Neomycin: Derived from *Streptomyces fradiae*.
 Polymyxin B: Derived from polymyxin $B_1$ and polymyxin $B_2$, which are produced by the growth of *Bacillus polymyxa*.
Chemical group—
 Neomycin: Aminoglycosides.
 Polymyxin B: Polypeptides.
 Hydrocortisone: Corticosteroids.
Molecular weight—Hydrocortisone: 362.47.

### Mechanism of action/Effect
Neomycin—See *Neomycin (Ophthalmic)*.
Polymyxin B—See *Neomycin, Polymyxin B, and Bacitracin (Ophthalmic)*.
Hydrocortisone—See *Corticosteroids (Otic)*.

### Absorption
Neomycin; polymyxin B; hydrocortisone—May be absorbed following topical application to the ear if the eardrum is perforated or tissue damage is present.

## Precautions to Consider

### Cross-sensitivity and/or related problems
Patients sensitive to one aminoglycoside or polymyxin may be sensitive to other aminoglycosides or polymyxins also.

### Carcinogenicity
Long-term studies in animals (rats, rabbits, mice) given oral corticosteroids showed no carcinogenicity.

### Pregnancy/Reproduction
Pregnancy—Adequate and well-controlled studies in humans have not been done for otic neomycin, polymyxin B, and hydrocortisone combination.

Topical corticosteroids have been shown to be teratogenic in rabbits when applied at concentrations of 0.5% on days 6 to 18 of gestation and in mice when applied at a concentration of 15% on days 10 to 13 of gestation.

FDA Pregnancy Category C.

### Breast-feeding
Oral hydrocortisone is distributed into breast milk. It is not known if otic neomycin, polymyxin B, and hydrocortisone combination is distributed into breast milk. However, problems in humans have not been documented.

### Pediatrics
Appropriate studies on the relationship of age to the effects of otic neomycin, polymyxin B, and hydrocortisone combination have not been performed in the pediatric population. However, no pediatrics-specific problems have been documented to date.

### Geriatrics
Appropriate studies on the relationship of age to the effects of otic neomycin, polymyxin B, and hydrocortisone combination have not been performed in the geriatric population. However, no geriatrics-specific problems have been documented to date.

### Medical considerations/Contraindications
The medical considerations/contraindications included here have been selected on the basis of their potential clinical significance (reasons given in parentheses where appropriate)—not necessarily inclusive (» = major clinical significance).

***Risk-benefit should be considered when the following medical problems exist:***
 Sensitivity to aminoglycosides, polymyxins, or sulfites
*For hydrocortisone*
» Bullous myringitis
» Herpes simplex
» Herpes zoster oticus
» Tubercular or fungal infections of the ear
» Vaccinia, varicella, or other viral disease of the ear

*For neomycin and/or polymyxin B*
 Otitis media, chronic or
 Perforated eardrum
  (possibility of ototoxicity)

## Side/Adverse Effects

The following side/adverse effects have been selected on the basis of their potential clinical significance (possible signs and symptoms in parentheses where appropriate)—not necessarily inclusive:

### Those indicating need for medical attention
Incidence more frequent
 *Hypersensitivity* (itching, skin rash, redness, swelling, or other sign of irritation in or around the ear not present before therapy)

## Patient Consultation

As an aid to patient consultation, refer to *Advice for the Patient, Neomycin, Polymyxin B, and Hydrocortisone (Otic)*.

In providing consultation, consider emphasizing the following selected information (» = major clinical significance):

### Before using this medication
» Conditions affecting use, especially:
  Sensitivity to aminoglycosides, polymyxins, or sulfites
  Pregnancy—Topical corticosteroids have been shown to be teratogenic in rabbits and mice

### Proper use of this medication
Proper administration technique for otic solution and suspension
» Compliance with full course of therapy
» Proper dosing
  Missed dose: Applying as soon as possible; not applying if almost time for next dose
» Not using longer than 10 days unless otherwise directed by physician
» Proper storage

### Precautions while using this medication
Checking with physician if no improvement within 1 week

### Side/adverse effects
Signs of potential side effects, especially hypersensitivity

## General Dosing Information

This medication may be warmed, but not above body temperature, prior to administration.

A cotton wick may be placed in the ear canal and then saturated with the suspension. The wick should be kept moist by adding suspension every 4 to 8 hours and it should be replaced at least once daily.

Therapy should not be continued for more than 10 days.

If infection has not improved within 1 week, condition should be re-evaluated.

## Otic Dosage Forms

Note: Bracketed uses in the *Dosage Forms* section refer to categories of use and/or indications that are not included in U.S. product labeling.

## NEOMYCIN AND POLYMYXIN B SULFATES AND HYDROCORTISONE OTIC SOLUTION USP

**Usual adult and adolescent dose**
Ear canal infections, external—
     Topical, to the ear canal, 4 drops three or four times a day.
Mastoidectomy cavity infections or
[Otitis media, chronic suppurative][1]—
     Topical, to the mastoidectomy cavity or ear canal, 4 to 10 drops every six to eight hours.
Note: In the treatment of mastoidectomy cavity infections, the dose depends on the size of the mastoidectomy cavity. Some cavities may require up to 1 or 2 dropperfuls of otic solution or suspension in adults.

**Usual pediatric dose**
Ear canal infections, external—
     Topical, to the ear canal, 3 drops three or four times a day.
Mastoidectomy cavity infections—
     Topical, to the mastoidectomy cavity, 4 or 5 drops every six to eight hours.
Note: In the treatment of mastoidectomy cavity infections, the dose depends on the size of the mastoidectomy cavity.
[Otitis media, chronic suppurative][1]—
     Topical, to the ear canal, 2 to 5 drops every six to eight hours.

**Strength(s) usually available**
U.S.—
     3.5 mg of neomycin (base), 10,000 Units of polymyxin B (base), and 10 mg of hydrocortisone per mL (Rx) [*AK-Spore HC Otic* (potassium metabisulfite; propylene glycol; glycerin); *Antibiotic Ear; Cortatrigen Modified Ear Drops* (potassium metabisulfite; propylene glycol; glycerin); *Cort-Biotic; Cortisporin* (potassium metabisulfite 0.1%; cupric sulfate; glycerin; hydrochloric acid; propylene glycol); *Drotic* (potassium metabisulfite; propylene glycol; glycerin); *Ear-Eze* (potassium metabisulfite; propylene glycol; glycerin); *LazerSporin-C; Masporin Otic; Octicair* (potassium metabisulfite; propylene glycol; glycerin); *Octigen; Otic-Care* (glycerin; hydrochloric acid; propylene glycol; potassium metabisulfite); *Otic-Care Ear* (glycerin; hydrochloric acid; propylene glycol; potassium metabisulfite); *Otimar; Otocidin; Otocort;* GENERIC].
Canada—
     3.5 mg of neomycin (base), 10,000 Units of polymyxin B (base), and 10 mg of hydrocortisone per mL (Rx) [*Cortisporin* (benzalkonium chloride)].

**Packaging and storage**
Store below 40 °C (104 °F), preferably between 15 and 30 °C (59 and 86 °F), unless otherwise specified by manufacturer. Store in a tight, light-resistant container. Protect from freezing.

**Auxiliary labeling**
• For the ear.
• Continue medicine for full time of treatment.

## NEOMYCIN AND POLYMYXIN B SULFATES AND HYDROCORTISONE OTIC SUSPENSION USP

**Usual adult and adolescent dose**
Ear canal infections, external—
     Topical, to the ear canal, 4 drops three or four times a day.

Mastoidectomy cavity infections; or
[Otitis media, chronic suppurative][1]—
     Topical, to the mastoidectomy cavity or ear canal, 4 to 10 drops every six to eight hours.
Note: In the treatment of mastoidectomy cavity infections, the dose depends on the size of the mastoidectomy cavity. Some cavities may require up to 1 or 2 dropperfuls of otic solution or suspension in adults.

**Usual pediatric dose**
Ear canal infections, external—
     Topical, to the ear canal, 3 drops three or four times a day.
Mastoidectomy cavity infections—
     Topical, to the mastoidectomy cavity, 4 or 5 drops every six to eight hours.
Note: In the treatment of mastoidectomy cavity infections, the dose depends on the size of the mastoidectomy cavity.
[Otitis media, chronic suppurative][1]—
     Topical, to the ear canal, 2 to 5 drops every six to eight hours.

**Strength(s) usually available**
U.S.—
     3.5 mg of neomycin (base), 10,000 Units of polymyxin B (base), and 10 mg of hydrocortisone per mL (Rx) [*AK-Spore HC Otic* (cetyl alcohol; propylene glycol; polysorbate 80; thimerosal); *Antibiotic Ear; Cortatrigen Ear* (cetyl alcohol; propylene glycol; polysorbate 80; thimerosal); *Cort-Biotic; Cortisporin* (thimerosal 0.01%; cetyl alcohol; propylene glycol; polysorbate 80); *Cortomycin; Masporin Otic; Octigen; Otic-Care* (cetyl alcohol; polyoxyl 40 stearate; polysorbate 80; propylene glycol; sulfuric acid; benzalkonium chloride); *Otic-Care Ear* (cetyl alcohol; propylene glycol; polysorbate 80; thimerosal); *Otimar; Otisan; Otocort; Pediotic* (thimerosal 0.001%; cetyl alcohol; glyceryl monostearate; mineral oil; polyoxyl 40 stearate; propylene glycol); *UAD Otic;* GENERIC].
Canada—
     3.5 mg of neomycin (base), 10,000 Units of polymyxin B (base), and 10 mg of hydrocortisone per mL (Rx) [*Cortisporin* (benzalkonium chloride)].

**Packaging and storage**
Store below 40 °C (104 °F), preferably between 15 and 30 °C (59 and 86 °F), unless otherwise specified by manufacturer. Store in a tight, light-resistant container. Protect from freezing.

**Auxiliary labeling**
• Shake well.
• For the ear.
• Continue medicine for full time of treatment.

---

[1]Not included in Canadian product labeling.

---

Revised: 06/21/94
Interim revision: 06/02/95

---

## NEOSTIGMINE—See *Antimyasthenics (Systemic)*

---

## NETILMICIN—See *Aminoglycosides (Systemic)*

---

# NEUROMUSCULAR BLOCKING AGENTS    Systemic

This monograph includes information on the following: Atracurium Besylate; Gallamine; Metocurine; Pancuronium; Succinylcholine; Tubocurarine; Vecuronium.
Note: See also the individual *Doxacurium (Systemic), Mivacurium (Systemic),* and *Pipecuronium (Systemic)* monographs.
INN:
     Atracurium Besylate—Atracurium besilate
     Succinylcholine—Suxamethonium
VA CLASSIFICATION (Primary/Secondary):
     Atracurium—MS300
     Gallamine—MS300
     Metocurine—MS300
     Pancuronium—MS300
     Succinylcholine—MS300
     Tubocurarine—MS300/DX900
     Vecuronium—MS300

Other commonly used names are: Atracurium besilate [Atracurium Besylate], Curare [Tubocurarine], Suxamethonium [Succinylcholine].
Note: For a listing of dosage forms and brand names by country availability, see *Dosage Forms* section(s). For a listing of brand names for the articles in this monograph, refer to the General Index.

## Category

Neuromuscular blocking agent.
Note: Depolarizing neuromuscular blocking agent—Succinylcholine.
     Nondepolarizing neuromuscular blocking agent—Atracurium, Gallamine, Metocurine, Pancuronium, Tubocurarine, Vecuronium.

# Indications

Note: Bracketed information in the *Indications* section refers to uses that are not included in U.S. product labeling.

## Accepted

Muscle (skeletal) relaxation, for surgery—The neuromuscular blocking agents are indicated as adjuncts to anesthesia to induce skeletal muscle relaxation and to facilitate the management of patients undergoing mechanical ventilation.

Generally, a relatively short-acting nondepolarizing neuromuscular blocking agent or a single dose of the depolarizing neuromuscular blocking agent succinylcholine is used to facilitate endotracheal intubation. Continuous infusion of succinylcholine may be used for short surgical procedures requiring muscle relaxation. Nondepolarizing neuromuscular blocking agents, or, less commonly, succinylcholine administered by continuous infusion, are used for surgical procedures requiring an intermediate or prolonged duration of muscle relaxant action and to facilitate controlled ventilation.

Convulsions (treatment)—[Atracurium][1], [gallamine], metocurine, [pancuronium][1], [succinylcholine], tubocurarine, and [vecuronium][1] are indicated to reduce the intensity of muscle contractions of pharmacologically or electrically induced convulsions. Succinylcholine is generally preferred because of its short duration of action.

[Neuromuscular blocking agents are also used to decrease the muscular manifestations of persistent convulsions associated with toxic reactions to other medications.][1]

Myasthenia gravis (diagnosis)—Tubocurarine is indicated as a diagnostic aid for myasthenia gravis when the results of tests with neostigmine or edrophonium are inconclusive.

---

[1]Not included in Canadian product labeling.

# Pharmacology/Pharmacokinetics

See *Table 1*, page 2125 and *Table 2*, page 2125.

## Physicochemical characteristics

Molecular weight—
Atracurium besylate: 1243.49.
Gallamine triethiodide: 891.54.
Metocurine iodide: 906.64.
Pancuronium bromide: 732.68.
Succinylcholine chloride: 397.34 (dihydrate); 361.31 (anhydrous).
Tubocurarine chloride: 771.73 (pentahydrate); 681.65 (anhydrous).
Vecuronium bromide: 637.74.

## Mechanism of action/Effect

Neuromuscular blocking agents produce skeletal muscle paralysis by blocking neural transmission at the myoneural junction. The paralysis is selective initially and usually appears in the following muscles consecutively: levator muscles of eyelids, muscles of mastication, limb muscles, abdominal muscles, muscles of the glottis, and finally, the intercostal muscles and the diaphragm. Neuromuscular blocking agents have no known effect on consciousness or the pain threshold.

*Depolarizing neuromuscular blocking agents* compete with acetylcholine for the cholinergic receptors of the motor end plate and, like acetylcholine, combine with these receptors to produce depolarization; however, because of their high affinity for the cholinergic receptors and their resistance to acetylcholinesterase, they produce a more prolonged depolarization than does acetylcholine. This results initially in transient muscle contractions, usually visible as fasciculations, followed by inhibition of neuromuscular transmission. This type of neuromuscular block is not antagonized, and may even be enhanced, by anticholinesterase agents.

With prolonged or repeated use of depolarizing neuromuscular blocking agents, neuromuscular blockade resembling a nondepolarization block may be produced, resulting in prolonged respiratory depression or apnea.

*Nondepolarizing neuromuscular blocking agents* inhibit neuromuscular transmission by competing with acetylcholine for the cholinergic receptors of the motor end plate, thereby reducing the response of the end plate to acetylcholine. This type of neuromuscular block is usually antagonized by anticholinesterase agents.

## Other actions/effects

Tubocurarine and, to a lesser extent, atracurium, metocurine, and succinylcholine may cause histamine release. Gallamine, pancuronium, and vecuronium are least likely to cause histamine release.

Gallamine and pancuronium also have vagolytic activity.

# Precautions to Consider

## Cross-sensitivity and/or related problems

Patients sensitive to bromides may be sensitive to the bromide salts of pancuronium or vecuronium also.

Patients sensitive to iodine or iodides may be sensitive to the iodide salts of gallamine or metocurine also.

## Mutagenicity

*For atracurium*—Mutagenic activity was observed in the mouse lymphoma assay under conditions in which more than 80% of the treated cells were killed, i.e., a relatively strong effect with concentrations of 80 and 100 mcg per mL in the absence of metabolic activation and a much weaker effect with concentrations of 1.2 mg per mL or higher in the presence of metabolic activation. However, mutagenic activity has not been demonstrated in the Ames test or in a rat bone marrow cytogenicity assay.

## Pregnancy/Reproduction

Pregnancy—*For atracurium:* Adequate and well-controlled studies have not been done in humans. However, studies in rabbits (doses of 0.15 mg per kg of body weight (mg/kg) once a day or 0.1 mg/kg twice a day on Day 6 through Day 18 of gestation) have shown that atracurium causes visceral and skeletal anomalies. Also, postimplantation losses were greater in the group given 0.15 mg/kg once daily than in controls.

FDA Pregnancy Category C.

*For gallamine:* Problems in humans have not been documented. However, it has been determined that gallamine crosses the placenta.

*For metocurine:* Adequate and well-controlled studies have not been done in humans. However, it has been determined that metocurine crosses the placenta. Six minutes after intravenous injection in the mother, the fetal plasma concentration is approximately one-tenth of that in the mother.

FDA Pregnancy Category C.

*For pancuronium:* Studies have not been done in either animals or humans. However, problems in humans have not been documented.

FDA Pregnancy Category C.

*For succinylcholine:* Studies have not been done in humans. However, succinylcholine has been shown to cause intrauterine growth retardation and limb deformities resembling clubfoot when administered to the rat fetus between the 16th and 19th days of gestation or when injected in chick embryos from the 5th to 15th days of incubation.

*For tubocurarine:* Although adequate and well-controlled studies have not been done in humans, it has been determined that tubocurarine crosses the placenta. In animal studies, intramuscular injection of tubocurarine into the intercapsular region of the rat fetus on the 16th and 19th days of gestation caused growth retardation (incidence 21–23%) and limb deformity (incidence 7–8%), respectively. Tubocurarine has also caused growth retardation and limb deformities when injected into chick embryos from the 5th to the 15th day of incubation.

FDA Pregnancy Category C.

Tubocurarine may cause congenital fetal contractures if large and repeated doses are administered during the early months of pregnancy, possibly by immobilizing the fetus at the time of joint formation.

*For vecuronium:* Vecuronium crosses the placenta. Studies have not been done in either animals or humans.

FDA Pregnancy Category C.

Labor and delivery—Atracurium has been shown to cross the placenta in small quantities following administration to pregnant women for delivery by cesarean section. Although no adverse effects in the neonates were reported with atracurium, tubocurarine has been reported to cause diminished skeletal muscle activity leading to respiratory difficulty in the newborn when large and repeated doses are given near delivery. The possibility of neonatal respiratory depression or reduced skeletal muscle activity should be considered when any of these agents is used near delivery.

## Breast-feeding

Problems in humans have not been documented.

## Pediatrics

Specific products that contain benzyl alcohol, or that are diluted with bacteriostatic water for injection (which contains benzyl alcohol), should not be administered to premature neonates because the preservative has been associated with a fatal "gasping syndrome" in these patients.

*For atracurium, gallamine, metocurine, pancuronium, and tubocurarine*—Neonates up to 1 month of age may be more sensitive to the effects of nondepolarizing neuromuscular blocking agents. However, studies with atracurium have not been done in this age group.

No other pediatrics-specific problems have been documented in studies done to date.

*For succinylcholine—*
Pediatric patients may be especially susceptible to succinylcholine–induced myoglobinemia, myoglobinuria, and cardiac effects such as transient bradycardia, hypotension, cardiac arrhythmias, and/or sinus arrest.

*For vecuronium—*
Pediatric patients 7 weeks to 1 year of age are more sensitive to the effects of vecuronium (on a mg-per-kg basis) than are adults. Recovery time may be $1^{1}/_{2}$ times that of adults.

## Geriatrics

Although appropriate studies with neuromuscular blocking agents have not been performed in the geriatric population, geriatrics-specific problems that would limit the usefulness of these medications in the elderly are not expected. However, elderly patients are more likely to have age-related renal function impairment, which may decrease the rate of clearance of gallamine, metocurine, pancuronium, succinylcholine, or tubocurarine from the body and thereby prolong their effects.

## Drug interactions and/or related problems

The following drug interactions and/or related problems have been selected on the basis of their potential clinical significance (possible mechanism in parentheses where appropriate)—not necessarily inclusive (» = major clinical significance):

See *Table 3,* page 2126.

## Laboratory value alterations

The following have been selected on the basis of their potential clinical significance (possible effect in parentheses where appropriate)—not necessarily inclusive (» = major clinical significance):

With physiology/laboratory test values

*For succinylcholine*
Serum potassium concentrations
(may be increased; increase may cause cardiac arrest or arrhythmias in patients with severe trauma, burns, or neurologic disorders; this effect may persist for several weeks or months after the initial trauma)

## Medical considerations/Contraindications

The medical considerations/contraindications included here have been selected on the basis of their potential clinical significance (reasons given in parentheses where appropriate)—not necessarily inclusive (» = major clinical significance).

See *Table 4,* page 2130.

## Side/Adverse Effects

See *Table 5,* page 2131.

Note: Overdose of the neuromuscular blocking agents may result in prolonged respiratory depression or apnea and cardiovascular collapse.

## Overdose

For specific information on the agents used in the management of a neuromuscular blocking agent overdose, see:
- *Atropine* in *Anticholinergics/Antispasmodics (Systemic)* monograph;
- *Edrophonium (Systemic)* monograph;
- *Neostigmine* in *Antimyasthenics (Systemic)* monograph; and/or
- *Pyridostigmine* in *Antimyasthenics (Systemic)* monograph.

For more information on the management of overdose or unintentional ingestion, **contact a Poison Control Center** (see *Poison Control Center Listing*).

## Clinical effects of overdose

The following effects have been selected on the basis of their potential clinical significance (possible signs and symptoms in parentheses where appropriate)—not necessarily inclusive:

Acute

*Apnea; hypotension, severe; paralysis, prolonged; shock*

## Treatment of overdose

Specific treatment—
Administering anticholinesterase agents, such as edrophonium, neostigmine, or pyridostigmine, to antagonize the action of the nondepolarizing neuromuscular blocking agents. It is recommended that atropine or another suitable anticholinergic agent be administered prior to or concurrently with the antagonist to counteract its cholinergic side effects.

The depolarization block produced by succinylcholine is not antagonized by anticholinesterase agents such as edrophonium, neostigmine, and pyridostigmine. However, if succinylcholine has been administered over a prolonged period of time and the characteristic depolarization block has gradually changed to a nondepolarization block, as determined with a peripheral nerve stimulator, small

doses of the anticholinesterase agent may be tried as an antagonist. If an anticholinesterase agent is used as an antagonist, it is recommended that atropine be administered prior to or concurrently with the antagonist to counteract its cholinergic side effects. Patients should be closely observed for at least 1 hour after reversal of nondepolarization block for possible return of muscle relaxation. The antagonists are merely adjuncts to, and are not to be substituted for, the institution of measures to ensure adequate ventilation. Ventilatory assistance must be continued until the patient can maintain an adequate ventilatory exchange unassisted.

Monitoring—
Determining the nature and degree of the neuromuscular blockade, using a peripheral nerve stimulator.

Supportive care—
For apnea or prolonged paralysis—maintaining an adequate airway and administering manual or mechanical ventilation. Artificial respiration should be continued until complete recovery of normal respiration is assured.
For severe hypotension or shock—administering fluids and vasopressors as needed to treat

## General Dosing Information

Neuromuscular blocking agents have no known effect on consciousness or the pain threshold; therefore, when used as an adjunct to surgery, the neuromuscular blocking agent should always be used with adequate anesthesia.

Since neuromuscular blocking agents may cause respiratory depression, they should be used only by those individuals experienced in the techniques of tracheal intubation, artificial respiration, and the administration of oxygen under positive pressure; facilities for these procedures should be immediately available.

The stated doses are intended as a guideline. Actual dosage must be individualized. To minimize the risk of overdosage, it is recommended that a peripheral nerve stimulator be used to monitor response to the neuromuscular blocking agents.

When nondepolarizing neuromuscular blocking agents are administered concurrently with potent general anesthetics such as enflurane, ether, isoflurane, methoxyflurane, or cyclopropane, the dosage of vecuronium should be decreased by 15%, and that of the other neuromuscular blocking agents should be reduced by 33 to 50%, or as determined with a peripheral nerve stimulator. Halothane causes less potentiation of neuromuscular blockade than either enflurane or isoflurane; therefore, a smaller reduction in the dosage of the neuromuscular blocking agent may be considered.

---

## *ATRACURIUM*

## Summary of Differences

Pharmacology/pharmacokinetics:
Mechanism of action/effect—
A nondepolarizing neuromuscular blocking agent.
Action is usually antagonized by anticholinesterase agents.
Other actions/effects—
May cause histamine release.
Protein-binding—
High.
Biotransformation—
In plasma, by ester hydrolysis and by Hofmann elimination; independent of hepatic or renal function or plasma pseudocholinesterase activity.
Half-life—
Distribution: 2–3.4 minutes.
Elimination: 20 minutes.
Onset of action—
Initial effect within 2 minutes; intubation conditions in 2–2.5 minutes.
Time to peak effect—
1.7–10 (average 3–5) minutes.
Duration of peak effect—
20–35 minutes (balanced anesthesia); not changed by repeated dosing, provided that recovery from the prior dose begins before subsequent doses are given.
Time to recovery—
From time of injection (balanced anesthesia):
25% of twitch response achieved in 35–45 minutes and 95% of twitch response achieved in 60–70 minutes.

From beginning of recovery:
>Balanced anesthesia—95% of twitch response achieved in 30 minutes.
>Inhalation anesthesia—95% of twitch response achieved in 40 minutes.

Elimination—
>Renal and biliary; less than 10% of the quantity excreted via the biliary route as unchanged atracurium.

Precautions:
Pregnancy—
>Teratogenic and embryotoxic effects have been demonstrated in rabbits.
>Has been shown to cross the human placenta.

Drug interactions and/or related problems—
>May increase incidence and severity of bradycardia and hypotension when used together with opioid analgesics; also, histamine release may be additive to that induced by many opioids.
>Use with digitalis glycosides not reported to cause cardiac arrhythmias or other undesirable cardiac effects.
>Effects may be enhanced or prolonged in patients receiving chronic lithium therapy.
>Effects not prolonged by cholinesterase inhibitors or hexafluorenium.
>Serious side effects with concurrent use of methotrimeprazine have not been reported.
>Additive effects with physostigmine have not been reported.

Medical considerations/Contraindications—
>Lower risk of problems than with gallamine or pancuronium if used in patients with cardiac conditions in which tachycardia would be undesirable.
>Efficacy not reduced by hepatic function impairment.
>Caution required in patients with pre-existing hypotension.
>Effects not prolonged in patients with renal function impairment or shock.

Side/adverse effects:
>Moderate risk of side effects associated with histamine release.
>More likely than other neuromuscular blocking agents to cause flushing of skin.
>Hives and laryngospasm have been reported.

## Additional Dosing Information

See also *General Dosing Information.*

Atracurium must be administered intravenously because intramuscular injection may cause tissue irritation and because there are no clinical data to support intramuscular administration.

A reduction in dosage and rate of administration is recommended for patients in whom histamine release may be hazardous. Also, patients with neuromuscular disease, severe electrolyte disorders, or carcinomatosis should receive lower doses because of potential enhancement of neuromuscular blockade or difficulties with reversal.

Bradycardia occurring during atracurium administration may be treated by intravenous administration of atropine.

## Parenteral Dosage Forms

### ATRACURIUM BESYLATE INJECTION

**Usual adult and adolescent dose**
Initial—
>Intravenous, 400 to 500 mcg (0.4 to 0.5 mg) per kg of body weight;
>or
>For patients in whom histamine release might be hazardous:
>>Intravenous, 300 to 400 mcg (0.3 to 0.4 mg) per kg of body weight, administered slowly or in divided doses over a period of one minute.

For administration after steady-state enflurane or isoflurane anesthesia has been established:
>Intravenous, 250 to 350 mcg (0.25 to 0.35 mg) per kg of body weight, or approximately one-third less than the usual initial dose. Halothane causes less potentiation of neuromuscular blockade; therefore, a smaller reduction in atracurium dosage may be considered.

After succinylcholine-assisted endotracheal intubation under balanced anesthesia:
>Intravenous, 300 to 400 mcg (0.3 to 0.4 mg) per kg of body weight. If a potent inhalation anesthetic is being administered, even lower doses may be required. The effects of succinylcholine, as determined using a peripheral nerve stimulator, should be permitted to subside prior to administration of atracurium.

Supplemental—
>Intravenous, 80 to 100 mcg (0.08 to 0.1 mg) per kg of body weight twenty to forty-five minutes following the initial dose, then every fifteen to twenty-five minutes or as required by clinical conditions; or
>Intravenous infusion (initiated after recovery from the effects of an initial intravenous dose of 300 to 500 mcg [0.3 to 0.5 mg])
>Balanced anesthesia—
>>9 to 10 mcg (0.009 to 0.01 mg) per kg of body weight per minute until the desired degree of neuromuscular blockade is re-established, after which the rate of infusion may be adjusted according to clinical requirements and patient response. Most patients require 5 to 9 mcg (0.005 to 0.009 mg) per kg of body weight per minute, although some may require as little as 2 mcg (0.002 mg) per kg of body weight per minute and others may require as much as 15 mcg (0.015 mg) per kg of body weight per minute.

After steady-state enflurane or isoflurane anesthesia has been established—
>The required rate of infusion may be reduced by approximately 33%. A smaller reduction in the rate of infusion may be considered for patients anesthetized with halothane.

For cardiopulmonary bypass procedures in which hypothermia is induced—
>The required rate of infusion may be reduced by approximately 50%.

**Usual pediatric dose**
Neonates up to 1 month of age—
>Dosage has not been established.

Children 1 month to 2 years of age (under halothane anesthesia)—
>Intravenous, 300 to 400 mcg (0.3 to 0.4 mg) per kg of body weight, initially.

Children 2 years of age and over—
>See *Usual adult and adolescent dose.*

Note: Maintenance doses may be required somewhat more frequently than in adults.

**Strength(s) usually available**
U.S.—
>10 mg per mL (Rx) [*Tracrium* (benzyl alcohol [multiple-dose vials only])].

Canada—
>10 mg per mL (Rx) [*Tracrium*].

**Packaging and storage**
Store between 2 and 8 °C (36 and 46 °F), unless otherwise specified by manufacturer. Protect from freezing.

**Preparation of dosage form**
For intravenous infusion—Atracurium besylate injection may be diluted with 0.9% sodium chloride injection, 5% dextrose injection, or 5% dextrose in 0.9% sodium chloride injection. Lactated Ringer's injection should *not* be used (see *Incompatibilities,* below). A solution prepared by adding 2 mL of atracurium besylate injection (10 mg per mL) to 98 mL of diluent contains 200 mcg (0.2 mg) of atracurium besylate per mL; a solution prepared by adding 5 mL of atracurium besylate injection (10 mg per mL) to 95 mL of diluent contains 500 mcg (0.5 mg) per mL.

**Stability**
Intravenous infusion solutions prepared with 5% dextrose injection, 0.9% sodium chloride injection, or 5% dextrose in 0.9% sodium chloride injection may be stored in a refrigerator or at room temperature for up to 24 hours without significant loss of potency. Unused portions of such solutions should be discarded after 24 hours.

Atracurium besylate injection should be used within 14 days if stored at room temperature (25 °C [77 °F]), even if later refrigerated.

**Incompatibilities**
Alkaline solutions such as barbiturate injections should not be mixed in the same syringe, or administered simultaneously through the same intravenous needle, with atracurium. Alkaline solutions may change the pH of the acidic atracurium solution, resulting in inactivation of atracurium or precipitation of a free acid.

Spontaneous degradation of atracurium has been shown to occur more rapidly when the medication is diluted with lactated Ringer's injection than when the medication is diluted with 0.9% sodium chloride injection. Therefore, it is recommended that lactated Ringer's injection not be used to prepare intravenous infusion solutions containing atracurium.

## GALLAMINE

## Summary of Differences

Pharmacology/pharmacokinetics:
 Mechanism of action/effect—
  A nondepolarizing neuromuscular blocking agent.
  Action is usually antagonized by anticholinesterase agents.
 Other actions/effects—
  Has vagolytic activity.
  Less likely than most other neuromuscular blocking agents to cause histamine release.
 Biotransformation—
  Essentially none.
 Half-life—
  Distribution: 16 minutes.
  Elimination: 150 minutes.
 Onset of action—
  Initial effect within 1–2 minutes.
 Time to peak effect—
  3–5 minutes.
 Duration of peak effect—
  15–30 minutes; increased by repeated dosing.
 Elimination—
  Renal, almost completely as unchanged gallamine.
Precautions:
 Cross-sensitivity and/or related problems—
  Cross-sensitivity may occur in patients sensitive to iodine or iodides.
 Drug interactions and/or related problems—
  Vagolytic activity may decrease risk of opioid analgesic–induced bradycardia and/or hypotension, but may increase risk of tachycardia and/or hypertension in some patients.
  Use with digitalis glycosides not reported to cause cardiac arrhythmias or other undesirable cardiac effects.
  Effects may be enhanced or prolonged by beta-adrenergic blocking agents.
 Medical considerations/Contraindications—
  More likely than most other neuromuscular blocking agents to cause problems in patients with cardiac conditions in which tachycardia would be undesirable.
  Less likely than other neuromuscular blocking agents to cause problems in patients for whom histamine release would be hazardous.
  Caution required in patients with pre-existing hypertension.
  Prolongation of effects in patients with renal function impairment or shock more likely and/or more severe than with other neuromuscular blocking agents.
Side/adverse effects:
 Side effects caused by histamine release have not been reported.
 More likely than other neuromuscular blocking agents to cause hypertension and/or tachycardia.

## Additional Dosing Information

See also *General Dosing Information*.

In usual doses, gallamine has a slightly shorter duration of action than tubocurarine; however, in very large doses, its duration of action may be longer.

## Parenteral Dosage Forms

### GALLAMINE TRIETHIODIDE INJECTION USP

**Usual adult and adolescent dose**
Intravenous, initially 1 mg per kg of body weight, not to exceed 100 mg per dose; then 500 mcg (0.5 mg) to 1 mg per kg of body weight after an interval of thirty to forty minutes, if necessary, for prolonged procedures.

Note: A dose of 1 mg per kg of body weight produces a 50% reduction in respiratory minute volume; a dose of 1.5 mg per kg of body weight produces a 75% reduction in respiratory minute volume.

**Usual pediatric dose**
See *Usual adult and adolescent dose*.

Note: Caution in use is recommended, especially for patients weighing less than 5 kg.

**Strength(s) usually available**
U.S.—
 20 mg per mL (Rx) [*Flaxedil* (edetate disodium; sodium bisulfite)].
Canada—
 20 mg per mL (Rx) [*Flaxedil* (potassium metabisulfite; sodium sulfite)].

**Packaging and storage**
Store below 40 °C (104 °F), preferably between 15 and 30 °C (59 and 86 °F), unless otherwise specified by manufacturer. Protect from light. Protect from freezing.

## METOCURINE

## Summary of Differences

Pharmacology/pharmacokinetics:
 Mechanism of action/effect—
  A nondepolarizing neuromuscular blocking agent.
  Action is usually antagonized by anticholinesterase agents.
 Other actions/effects—
  May cause histamine release.
 Protein-binding—
  Moderate; primarily to beta and gamma globulins.
 Half-life—
  Distribution: 1.9 minutes.
  Elimination: 216 minutes.
 Onset of action—
  Initial effect within 1–4 minutes.
 Time to peak effect—
  1.5–10 (average 3–5) minutes.
 Duration of peak effect—
  35–60 minutes (maximum effect); average duration of relaxation 60 (range 25–90) minutes; increased by repeated dosing.
 Time to recovery—
  From time of injection:
  50% of twitch response achieved in >360 minutes.
 Elimination—
  Renal (50% within 48 hours as unchanged metocurine) and biliary (2% as unchanged metocurine).
Precautions:
 Cross-sensitivity and/or related problems—
  Cross-sensitivity may occur in patients sensitive to iodine or iodides.
 Drug interactions and/or related problems—
  May increase incidence and severity of bradycardia and hypotension when used together with opioid analgesics; also, histamine release may be additive to that induced by many opioids.
  Use with digitalis glycosides not reported to cause cardiac arrhythmias or other undesirable cardiac effects.
  Effects not prolonged by cholinesterase inhibitors or hexafluorenium.
  Serious side effects with concurrent use of methotrimeprazine have not been reported.
  Additive effects with physostigmine have not been reported.
 Medical considerations/contraindications—
  Caution required in patients with cardiovascular function impairment.
  Efficacy may be reduced by hepatic function impairment.
  Caution required in patients with pre-existing hypotension.
  Effects may be prolonged by renal function impairment or shock, but to a lesser extent than for gallamine.
Side/adverse effects:
 Moderate risk of side effects associated with histamine release.

## Additional Dosing Information

See also *General Dosing Information*.

Metocurine is approximately twice as potent as tubocurarine; 1 mg of metocurine may be expected to produce a therapeutic response comparable to that obtained with 1.8 mg of tubocurarine.

Rapid intravenous injection and/or large doses of metocurine may cause an increased release of histamine, resulting in hypotension and in decreased respiratory capacity due to bronchospasm combined with drug-induced paralysis of the respiratory muscles. Hypotension may also occur because of ganglionic blockade or as a complication of positive pressure respiration.

Intramuscular administration of metocurine iodide injection is not recommended.

## Parenteral Dosage Forms

### METOCURINE IODIDE INJECTION USP

**Usual adult and adolescent dose**
Intravenous, 150 to 400 mcg (0.15 to 0.4 mg) per kg of body weight, administered over thirty to sixty seconds, initially. Supplemental doses of 500 mcg (0.5 mg) to 1 mg may be administered every thirty to ninety minutes as required.

Enflurane or isoflurane anesthesia—A 33% to 50% reduction in dosage may be required. A reduction in dosage may also be required during halothane anesthesia.

In electroshock therapy—Intravenous, 2 to 3 mg (range, 1.75 to 5.5 mg).

**Usual pediatric dose**
Dosage has not been established.

**Strength(s) usually available**
U.S.—
   2 mg per mL (Rx) [*Metubine Iodide* (phenol); GENERIC].
Canada—
   2 mg per mL (Rx) [*Metubine Iodide* (phenol)].

**Packaging and storage**
Store below 40 °C (104 °F), preferably between 15 and 30 °C (59 and 86 °F), unless otherwise specified by manufacturer. Protect from freezing.

**Stability**
Metocurine iodide is unstable in alkaline solutions. When metocurine iodide injection is mixed with a barbiturate solution such as methohexital sodium or thiopental sodium, a precipitate may form because of the high pH of the barbiturate solution. Solutions containing barbiturates, meperidine, or morphine sulfate should not be administered from the same syringe as metocurine.

---

## PANCURONIUM

## Summary of Differences

Pharmacology/pharmacokinetics:
   Mechanism of action/effect—
      A nondepolarizing neuromuscular blocking agent.
      Action is usually antagonized by anticholinesterase agents.
   Other actions/effects—
      Has vagolytic activity.
      Less likely than most other neuromuscular blocking agents to cause histamine release.
   Protein-binding—
      Very low.
   Biotransformation—
      Hepatic, in small quantities.
   Half-life—
      Distribution: 10–13 minutes.
      Elimination: 114–116 minutes.
   Onset of action—
      Initial effect within 1 minute; intubation conditions in 2–3 minutes.
   Time to peak effect—
      3–4.5 minutes, depending on dose.
   Duration of peak effect—
      35–45 minutes; increased by repeated dosing.
   Time to recovery—
      From time of injection: 90% of twitch response achieved in <60 minutes.
   Elimination—
      Renal (about 80% as unchanged pancuronium); about 10% biliary (up to 10% as unchanged pancuronium).
Precautions:
   Cross-sensitivity and/or related problems—
      Cross-sensitivity may occur in patients sensitive to bromides.
   Drug interactions and/or related problems—
      Vagolytic activity may decrease risk of opioid analgesic–induced bradycardia and/or hypotension, but may increase risk of tachycardia and/or hypertension in some patients.
      Use with digitalis glycosides may cause cardiac arrhythmias or other undesirable cardiac effects.
      Effects may be enhanced or prolonged by beta-adrenergic blocking agents.
      Effects may be enhanced or prolonged in patients receiving chronic lithium therapy.
      Effects not prolonged by cholinesterase inhibitors or hexafluorenium.
      Serious side effects with concurrent use of methotrimeprazine have not been reported.
      Additive effects with physostigmine have not been reported.
      Effects may be decreased by hydrocortisone or prednisone.
   Medical considerations/Contraindications—
      More likely than most other neuromuscular blocking agents to cause problems in patients with cardiac conditions in which tachycardia would be undesirable.
      Caution required in patients for whom histamine release would be hazardous.
      Effects may be prolonged by hepatic function impairment.

Effects may be prolonged by renal function impairment, but to a lesser extent than for gallamine.
Side/adverse effects:
   Relatively low risk of side effects associated with histamine release.
   May cause itching of skin more frequently than other neuromuscular blocking agents.
   Excessive salivation has been reported.

## Additional Dosing Information

See also *General Dosing Information*.

Pancuronium is approximately 5 times as potent as tubocurarine.

## Parenteral Dosage Forms
### PANCURONIUM BROMIDE INJECTION

**Usual adult and adolescent dose**
Initial—
   Intravenous, 40 to 100 mcg (0.04 to 0.1 mg) per kg of body weight. Incremental doses starting at 10 mcg (0.01 mg) per kg of body weight may then be administered, generally every twenty to sixty minutes, the dosage being adjusted as needed.
   For administration after steady-state enflurane or isoflurane anesthesia has been established and/or after succinylcholine-assisted endotracheal intubation—
      Intravenous, 40 mcg (0.04 mg) per kg of body weight, initially, then adjusted according to patient response.
   For endotracheal intubation—
      Intravenous, 60 to 100 mcg (0.06 to 0.1 mg) per kg of body weight.

**Usual pediatric dose**
Neonates up to 1 month of age—
   Dosage must be individualized by the physician. Dosage may be based on the patient's response to a test dose of 20 mcg (0.02 mg) per kg of body weight.
Children 1 month of age and over—
   See *Usual adult and adolescent dose*.

**Strength(s) usually available**
U.S.—
   1 mg per mL (Rx) [*Pavulon* (benzyl alcohol); GENERIC].
   2 mg per mL (Rx) [*Pavulon* (benzyl alcohol); GENERIC].
Canada—
   1 mg per mL (Rx) [*Pavulon*].
   2 mg per mL (Rx) [*Pavulon*].

**Packaging and storage**
Store between 2 and 8 °C (36 and 46 °F), unless otherwise specified by manufacturer. Protect from freezing.

---

## SUCCINYLCHOLINE

## Summary of Differences

Pharmacology/pharmacokinetics:
   Mechanism of action/effect—
      A depolarizing neuromuscular blocking agent.
      Action not antagonized by anticholinesterase agents.
   Other actions/effects—
      May cause histamine release.
   Biotransformation—
      In plasma; rapidly hydrolyzed by pseudocholinesterase.
   Onset of action—
      Intravenous: Initial effect within 0.5–1 minute.
      Intramuscular: Initial effect within 3 minutes.
   Time to peak effect—
      Intravenous: 1–2 minutes.
   Duration of peak effect—
      Intravenous: 4–10 minutes.
      Intramuscular: 10–30 minutes.
   Elimination—
      Renal; about 10% as unchanged succinylcholine.
Precautions:
   Pediatrics—
      Pediatric patients may be especially susceptible to succinylcholine-induced myoglobinemia, myoglobinuria, and cardiac effects.
   Drug interactions and/or related problems—
      May increase incidence and severity of bradycardia and hypotension when used together with opioid analgesics; also, histamine release may be additive to that induced by many opioids.
      Potentiation of effect by hydrocarbon inhalation anesthetics less than for nondepolarizing neuromuscular blocking agents.

Effects not enhanced or prolonged by beta-adrenergic blocking agents.

Effects not reversed by calcium salts.

Effects prolonged by cholinesterase inhibitors or hexafluorenium.

Use with digitalis glycosides may cause cardiac arrhythmias or other undesirable cardiac effects.

Effects may be enhanced or prolonged in patients receiving chronic lithium therapy.

Serious side effects with concurrent use of methotrimeprazine have been reported.

Additive effects with physostigmine have been reported.

Effects may be enhanced by potassium-depleting medications.

Laboratory value alterations—

Serum potassium concentration may be increased.

Medical considerations/contraindications—

Caution required in patients with cardiovascular function impairment.

Effects may be prolonged in patients with renal function impairment, but to a lesser extent than for gallamine.

Caution also required in:

Conditions that may be adversely affected by increased potassium concentrations (severe burns, digitalis toxicity or recent digitalization, degenerative or dystrophic neuromuscular disease, paraplegia, pre-existing hyperkalemia, spinal cord injury, severe trauma).

Conditions that may lead to low plasma pseudocholinesterase activity (severe anemia, dehydration, exposure to neurotoxic insecticides or other cholinesterase inhibitors, severe hepatic disease or cirrhosis, malnutrition, pregnancy, recessive hereditary trait).

Conditions that may be adversely affected by increase in intraocular pressure (open eye injury, glaucoma, ocular surgery).

Fractures or muscle spasm.

Malignant hyperthermia, history of in patient or close relative.

Side/adverse effects:

Moderate risk of side effects associated with histamine release.

More likely than other neuromuscular blocking agents to cause bradycardia or cardiac arrhythmias.

Increased intraocular pressure, malignant hyperthermia, rhabdomyolysis leading to myoglobinemia and myoglobinuria, postoperative muscle pains and stiffness, and excessive salivation have been reported.

## Additional Dosing Information

See also *General Dosing Information*.

Succinylcholine is usually administered intravenously but may be administered intramuscularly if necessary.

When administered intramuscularly, the injection should be deep and high into the deltoid muscle.

An initial test dose of 10 mg may be administered to determine the sensitivity of the patient and recovery time.

Patients with low levels of pseudocholinesterase activity may require reduced doses, because they may be unusually sensitive to the effects of succinylcholine.

If low pseudocholinesterase activity is suspected, a test dose of 5 to 10 mg may be administered.

Premedication with atropine or scopolamine is recommended to prevent excessive salivation.

To reduce the severity of muscle fasciculations, a small dose of a nondepolarizing agent may be administered prior to administration of succinylcholine.

Following administration, succinylcholine may cause transient bradycardia accompanied by hypotension, cardiac arrhythmias, and possibly a short period of sinus arrest due to vagal stimulation, especially with repeated administration and in children. These effects may be inhibited by prior administration of atropine or thiopental sodium.

Succinylcholine may cause myoglobinemia and myoglobinuria, especially in children. Administration of small doses of tubocurarine prior to succinylcholine has been shown to decrease the incidence of myoglobinuria.

Repeated doses of succinylcholine may result in tachyphylaxis.

## Parenteral Dosage Forms

### SUCCINYLCHOLINE CHLORIDE INJECTION USP

**Usual adult and adolescent dose**

For short surgical procedures—

Intravenous, usually 600 mcg (0.6 mg) (range 300 mcg [0.3 mg] to 1.1 mg) per kg of body weight, initially. Repeated doses may be administered, if necessary, calculated on the basis of response to the first dose.

Intramuscular, 3 to 4 mg per kg of body weight, not to exceed a total dose of 150 mg.

For prolonged surgical procedures—

Intravenous, initially 600 mcg (0.6 mg) to 1.1 mg per kg of body weight; subsequent doses to be individualized for maintaining degree of relaxation required.

Note: Administration of repeated fractional doses is generally not recommended because of possible tachyphylaxis and prolonged apnea; continuous infusion is preferred for prolonged surgical procedures.

Intravenous infusion, as a 0.1 to 0.2% solution in 5% dextrose injection, sodium chloride injection, or other appropriate diluent, administered at a rate of 500 mcg (0.5 mg) to 10 mg per minute, depending on patient response and degree of relaxation required, for up to one hour.

Note: When succinylcholine is administered by infusion, careful monitoring of neuromuscular function with a peripheral nerve stimulator is recommended to avoid overdose and to detect development of a nondepolarizing block.

Electroshock therapy—

Intravenous, 10 to 30 mg administered approximately one minute before the shock, although dosage must be individualized according to the size and physical condition of the patient.

Intramuscular, up to 2.5 mg per kg of body weight, not to exceed a total dose of 150 mg.

**Usual pediatric dose**

Endotracheal intubation—

Intramuscular, up to 2.5 mg per kg of body weight, not to exceed a total dose of 150 mg.

Intravenous, 1 to 2 mg per kg of body weight. Repeated doses may be administered, if necessary, calculated on the basis of response to the first dose.

Note: Administration of succinylcholine by continuous intravenous infusion is considered to be unsafe in neonates and children because of the risk of malignant hyperpyrexia.

**Strength(s) usually available**

U.S.—

20 mg per mL (Rx) [*Anectine* (methylparaben); *Quelicin* (methylparaben; propylparaben); *Sucostrin* (methylparaben; propylparaben); GENERIC].

50 mg per mL (Rx) [*Quelicin*].

100 mg per mL (Rx) [*Sucostrin High Potency* (methylparaben; propylparaben)].

Canada—

20 mg per mL (Rx) [*Anectine* (methylparaben [multiple-dose vials only]); *Quelicin* (methylparaben; propylparaben); GENERIC].

100 mg per mL (Rx) [*Quelicin*].

**Packaging and storage**

Store between 2 and 8 °C (36 and 46 °F). Protect from freezing.

**Stability**

Do not use if the solution is not absolutely clear.

Only freshly prepared solutions of succinylcholine should be used.

The stability of diluted solutions may vary, depending on the specific product. See the manufacturer's prescribing information for product-specific information.

Succinylcholine is rapidly hydrolyzed, quickly loses potency, and may cause formation of a precipitate when mixed with alkaline solutions of other medications. Therefore, succinylcholine should not be mixed in the same syringe or administered simultaneously through the same needle with solutions of short-acting barbiturates such as thiopental sodium or other medications that have an alkaline pH. It should be injected separately.

### SUCCINYLCHOLINE CHLORIDE STERILE USP

**Usual adult and adolescent dose**

Intravenous infusion, as a 0.1 to 0.2% solution in 5% dextrose injection, sodium chloride injection, or other appropriate diluent, administered at a rate of 500 mcg (0.5 mg) to 10 mg per minute, depending on patient response and degree of relaxation required, for up to one hour.

Note: When succinylcholine is administered by infusion, careful monitoring of neuromuscular function with a peripheral nerve stimulator is recommended to avoid overdose and to detect development of a nondepolarizing block.

**Usual pediatric dose**

Use of succinylcholine by continuous intravenous infusion is not recommended, because of the risk of malignant hyperpyrexia.

**Size(s) usually available**

U.S.—

　500 mg (Rx) [*Anectine Flo-Pack*].

　1 gram (Rx) [*Anectine Flo-Pack*].

Canada—

　500 mg (Rx) [*Anectine Flo-Pack*].

　1 gram (Rx) [*Anectine Flo-Pack*].

**Packaging and storage**

Prior to reconstitution, store below 40 °C (104 °F), preferably between 15 and 30 °C (59 and 86 °F), unless otherwise specified by manufacturer.

**Preparation of dosage form**

For intravenous infusion, sterile succinylcholine chloride may be dissolved in 0.9% sodium chloride injection, 5% dextrose injection, or other appropriate infusion solution.

**Stability**

Only freshly prepared solutions of succinylcholine should be used. The reconstituted solution should be used within 24 hours.

Succinylcholine is rapidly hydrolyzed, quickly loses potency, and may cause formation of a precipitate when mixed with alkaline solutions of other medications. Therefore, succinylcholine should not be mixed in the same syringe or administered simultaneously through the same needle with solutions of short-acting barbiturates such as thiopental sodium or other medications that have an alkaline pH. It should be injected separately.

---

### TUBOCURARINE

## Summary of Differences

Indications:

　Also indicated as a diagnostic aid for myasthenia gravis.

Pharmacology/pharmacokinetics:

　Mechanism of action/effect—

　　A nondepolarizing neuromuscular blocking agent.

　　Action is usually antagonized by anticholinesterase agents.

　Other actions/effects—

　　Most likely of the neuromuscular blocking agents to cause histamine release.

　Protein-binding—

　　Moderate.

　Biotransformation—

　　Hepatic.

　Half-life—

　　Distribution: 4.8–6.4 minutes.

　　Elimination: 84–120 minutes.

　Onset of action—

　　Intravenous: Initial effect within 1 minute.

　　Intramuscular: Initial effect within 15–25 minutes.

　Time to peak effect—

　　Intravenous: 2–5 minutes.

　Duration of peak effect—

　　20–40 minutes; increased with repeated dosing.

　Time to recovery—

　　From time of injection: 50% of twitch response achieved in 50 minutes and 95% of twitch response achieved in 74–90 minutes.

　Elimination—

　　Renal (about 40% as unchanged tubocurarine) and biliary (about 12% as unchanged tubocurarine).

Precautions:

　Pregnancy—

　　May cause congenital fetal contractures if large and repeated doses are administered during the early months of pregnancy.

　　Also, diminished skeletal muscle activity of the newborn may occur if large and repeated doses are administered near delivery.

　Drug interactions and/or related problems—

　　May increase incidence and severity of bradycardia and hypotension when used together with opioid analgesics; also, histamine release may be additive to that induced by many opioids.

　　Use with digitalis glycosides not reported to cause cardiac arrhythmias or other undesirable cardiac effects.

Effects not prolonged by cholinesterase inhibitors or hexafluorenium.

Effects may be prolonged or enhanced by calcium salts.

Serious side effects with concurrent use of methotrimeprazine have not been reported.

Additive effects with physostigmine have not been reported.

Medical considerations/Contraindications—

　Caution required in patients with cardiovascular function impairment.

　Effects may be reduced by hepatic function impairment.

　Caution required in patients with pre-existing hypotension.

　Effects may be prolonged in patients with renal function impairment or shock, but to a lesser extent than for gallamine.

Side/adverse effects:

　Relatively high risk of side effects associated with histamine release. Decrease in blood pressure occurs more frequently than with other neuromuscular blocking agents.

## Additional Dosing Information

See also *General Dosing Information.*

Tubocurarine is usually administered intravenously as a sustained injection over a period of 1 to 1.5 minutes. It may also be administered intramuscularly, if necessary, but is slowly and irregularly absorbed.

Rapid intravenous injection and/or large doses of tubocurarine may cause an increased release of histamine, resulting in hypotension and in decreased respiratory capacity due to bronchospasm combined with drug-induced paralysis of the respiratory muscles. Hypotension may also occur because of ganglionic blockade or as a complication of positive pressure respiration.

## Parenteral Dosage Forms

### TUBOCURARINE CHLORIDE INJECTION USP

**Usual adult and adolescent dose**

Neuromuscular blocking agent—

　Adjunct to surgical anesthesia:

　　Intramuscular or intravenous, 6 to 9 mg initially, then 3 to 4.5 mg in three to five minutes if necessary. For prolonged procedures, supplemental doses of 3 mg may be administered.

　　Note: Dosage may generally be calculated on the basis of 165 mcg (0.165 mg) per kg of body weight.

　Aid to controlled respiration:

　　Intravenous, initially 16.5 mcg (0.0165 mg) per kg of body weight, the subsequent doses being adjusted as needed.

　Electroshock therapy:

　　Intravenous, 165 mcg (0.165 mg) per kg of body weight, administered over a period of thirty to ninety seconds.

　　Note: Initially, a dose of 3 mg less than the calculated total dose should be used.

Diagnostic aid (myasthenia gravis)—

　Intravenous, 4 to 33 mcg (0.004 to 0.033 mg) per kg of body weight.

　Note: It is recommended that the test be terminated within two to three minutes by intravenous injection of 1.5 mg of neostigmine, since the marked exaggeration of myasthenia gravis symptoms may result in prolonged respiratory paralysis.

**Usual pediatric dose**

Neuromuscular blocking agent—Adjunct to surgical anesthesia:

　Neonates up to 4 weeks of age—Intravenous, 250 to 500 mcg (0.25 to 0.5 mg) per kg of body weight initially; then subsequent doses in increments of one-fifth or one-sixth of the initial doses, if necessary.

　Infants and children—Intravenous, 500 mcg (0.5 mg) per kg of body weight.

**Strength(s) usually available**

U.S.—

　3 mg (20 Units) per mL (Rx) [GENERIC].

Canada—

　3 mg (20 Units) per mL (Rx) [*Tubarine;* GENERIC].

**Packaging and storage**

Store below 40 °C (104 °F), preferably between 15 and 30 °C (59 and 86 °F), unless otherwise specified by manufacturer. Protect from freezing.

**Stability**

When tubocurarine is mixed with a barbiturate solution such as methohexital sodium or thiopental sodium, a precipitate may form because of the high pH of the barbiturate solution. Each medication should be given in a separate syringe.

## VECURONIUM

## Summary of Differences

Pharmacology/pharmacokinetics:
  Mechanism of action/effect—
    A nondepolarizing neuromuscular blocking agent.
    Action is usually antagonized by anticholinesterase agents.
  Other actions/effects—
    Less likely than most other neuromuscular blocking agents to cause histamine release.
  Protein-binding—
    Moderate to high.
  Biotransformation—
    Hepatic; only 5–10% of a dose is metabolized. One metabolite has some neuromuscular blocking activity.
  Half-life—
    Distribution: 2–3.4 minutes.
    Elimination: 20 minutes.
  Onset of action—
    Initial effect within 1 minute; intubation conditions in 2.5–3 minutes.
  Time to peak effect—
    3–5 minutes.
  Duration of peak effect—
    25–30 minutes (balanced anesthesia); not changed by repeated dosing, provided that recovery from the prior dose begins before subsequent doses are given.
  Time to recovery—
    From time of injection (balanced anesthesia): 25% of twitch response achieved in 25–40 minutes and 95% of twitch response achieved in 45–65 minutes.
  Elimination—
    Biliary (25–50% of a dose) and renal (3–35% of a dose).
Precautions:
  Cross-sensitivity and/or related problems—
    Cross-sensitivity may occur in patients sensitive to bromides.
  Pregnancy/reproduction—
    Has been shown to cross the human placenta.
  Pediatrics—
    Patients 7 weeks to 1 year of age are more sensitive to the effects of vecuronium than are adults; recovery time may be 1½ times that of adults.
  Drug interactions and/or related problems—
    May increase incidence and severity of bradycardia and hypotension when used together with opioid analgesics.
    Use with digitalis glycosides not reported to cause cardiac arrhythmias or other undesirable cardiac effects.
    Effects not prolonged by cholinesterase inhibitors or hexafluorenium.
    Serious side effects with concurrent use of methotrimeprazine have not been reported.
    Additive effects with physostigmine have not been reported.
  Medical considerations/Contraindications—
    Caution required in patients with cardiovascular function impairment.
    Effects may be prolonged by hepatic function impairment.
Side/adverse effects:
  Relatively low risk of side effects caused by histamine release.

## Additional Dosing Information

See also *General Dosing Information.*
Vecuronium is to be administered by intravenous injection only.

## Parenteral Dosage Forms

### VECURONIUM BROMIDE FOR INJECTION

**Usual adult and adolescent dose**
Initial—
  For intubation:
    Intravenous, 80 to 100 mcg (0.08 to 0.1 mg) per kg of body weight.
  For administration after the patient has been anesthetized with enflurane or isoflurane (i.e., more than 5 minutes after anesthesia has been instituted or after steady state has been achieved):
    Intravenous, 60 to 85 mcg (0.06 to 0.085 mg) per kg of body weight, or approximately 15% less than the usual initial dose.
  For administration after succinylcholine-assisted endotracheal intubation:
    Intravenous, 40 to 60 mcg (0.04 to 0.06 mg) per kg of body weight under inhalation anesthesia, or 50 to 60 mcg (0.05 to 0.06 mg)

per kg of body weight under balanced anesthesia. The effects of succinylcholine, as determined with a peripheral nerve stimulator, should be permitted to subside prior to administration of vecuronium.
  Note: If larger initial doses are required by the individual patient, initial doses ranging from 150 to 280 mcg (0.15 to 0.28 mg) per kg of body weight have been administered during surgery with halothane anesthesia without adverse effects on the cardiovascular system occurring, provided that adequate ventilation was maintained.
Supplemental—
  Intravenous, 10 to 15 mcg (0.01 to 0.015 mg) per kg of body weight, administered twenty-five to forty minutes following the initial dose, then every twelve to fifteen minutes or as required by clinical conditions; or
  Intravenous infusion (initiated after recovery from the effects of an initial intravenous dose of 80 to 100 mcg per kg of body weight has begun): 1 mcg (0.001 mg) per kg of body weight per minute, initially, then adjusted according to clinical requirements and patient response. Average infusion rates may range from 0.8 to 1.2 mcg (0.0008 to 0.0012 mg) per kg of body weight per minute. After steady-state enflurane or isoflurane anesthesia has been established—
    The required rate of infusion may be reduced by 25 to 60%. This reduction may not be required for patients anesthetized with halothane.

**Usual pediatric dose**
Neonates—
  Dosage has not been established.
Patients 7 weeks to 1 year of age—
  Dosage must be individualized.
Patients 1 to 10 years of age—
  Dosage must be individualized. These patients may require a slightly higher initial dose and slightly more frequent supplemental doses than adults.
Patients 10 years of age and older—
  Initial:
    See *Usual adult and adolescent dose.*
  Supplemental:
    Intravenous—See *Usual adult and adolescent dose.*
    Intravenous infusion—Dosage has not been established.

**Size(s) usually available**
U.S.—
  10 mg (Rx) [*Norcuron;* GENERIC].
Canada—
  10 mg (Rx) [*Norcuron*].

**Packaging and storage**
Prior to reconstitution, store between 15 and 30 °C (59 and 86 °F), protected from light, unless otherwise specified by manufacturer.

**Preparation of dosage form**
Reconstitute using bacteriostatic water for injection (provided by the manufacturer in some packages of vecuronium bromide for injection) or another compatible intravenous solution, such as 5% dextrose injection, 0.9% sodium chloride injection, 5% dextrose in sodium chloride injection, or lactated Ringer's injection. For direct intravenous injection, the medication is generally reconstituted using 5 or 10 mL of diluent. For intravenous infusion, the medication is diluted to a convenient concentration, such as 10 or 20 mg per 100 mL of infusion solution.

**Stability**
After reconstitution with bacteriostatic water for injection, the solution may be stored at room temperature or in a refrigerator; it should be used within 5 days. After reconstitution with other compatible intravenous solutions, the solution should be stored in a refrigerator and used within 24 hours. Reconstituted solutions are intended to be used only once; unused portions should be discarded.

**Incompatibilities**
Alkaline solutions such as barbiturate injections should not be mixed in the same syringe, or administered simultaneously through the same intravenous needle, with vecuronium.

Revised: September 1990
Interim revision: 07/26/96

## Table 1. Pharmacology/Pharmacokinetics

| Drug | Protein Binding | Biotransformation | Half-life Distribution/ Elimination (min) | Elimination Primary (% excreted unchanged)/Secondary (% excreted unchanged) |
|---|---|---|---|---|
| **Depolarizing** | | | | |
| Succinylcholine | — | In plasma, by pseudocholinesterase* | — | Renal (about 10) |
| **Nondepolarizing** | | | | |
| Atracurium | High | In plasma† | 2–3.4/20 | Renal and biliary (<10) |
| Gallamine | — | Essentially none | 16/150 | Renal (almost 100) |
| Metocurine | Moderate‡ | — | 1.9/216 | Renal (about 50 within 48 hr)/ biliary (2) |
| Pancuronium | Very low | Hepatic (in small quantities) | 10–13/114–116 | Renal (about 80)/10% biliary (up to 10) |
| Tubocurarine | Moderate§ | Hepatic | 4.8–6.4/84–120 | Renal (about 40)/biliary (12) |
| Vecuronium | Moderate to high# | Hepatic** | 4/65–75†† | 25–50% Biliary within 42 hr/3–35% renal within 24 hr‡‡ |

*Hydrolyzed rapidly to succinylmonocholine (a weak nondepolarizing neuromuscular blocking agent that is one-twentieth as potent as succinylcholine), then more slowly to succinic acid and choline.

†Metabolized by ester hydrolysis catalyzed by nonspecific esterases and by Hofmann elimination, a nonenzymatic chemical process that occurs at plasma pH; is independent of hepatic or renal function or plasma pseudocholinesterase activity.

‡Bound primarily to beta and gamma globulins.

§With plasma concentrations of 5 to 50 mcg/mL.

#With doses of 40 to 100 mcg per kg of body weight.

**Only 5 to 10% of a dose is metabolized. However, one metabolite, 3-deacetyl vecuronium, has been shown in animal studies to have neuromuscular blocking activity that is 50% as potent as that of vecuronium.

††May be decreased to 35 to 40 minutes in late pregnancy and prolonged in patients with cirrhosis or cholestasis.

‡‡Up to 25% of a dose may be excreted in bile, and up to 10% of a dose may be excreted in urine, as 3-deacetyl vecuronium.

## Table 2. Pharmacology/Pharmacokinetics*

| Drug | Initial Dose (mg/kg) | Onset of Initial Action (Time to Intubation Conditions) (min) | Time to Peak Effect (min) | Duration of Peak Effect (min)/Effect of Repeated Dosing | Time to Recovery in min (% of twitch response attained) |
|---|---|---|---|---|---|
| **Depolarizing** | | | | | |
| Succinylcholine | | | | | |
| Intramuscular | 3–4 | Up to 3 | — | 10–30† | — |
| Intravenous | 0.3–1.0 | 0.5–1 | 1–2 | 4–10† | — |
| **Nondepolarizing** | | | | | |
| Atracurium | | | | | |
| Intravenous | 0.4–0.5 | Within 2 (2–2.5) | 3–5 (range 1.7–10) | 20–35 under balanced anesthesia/no change‡ | From time of injection— balanced anesthesia‡: 35–45 (25); 60–70 (95) From beginning of recovery§— balanced anesthesia: 30 (95) inhalation anesthesia: 40 (95) |
| Gallamine | | | | | |
| Intravenous | 1.0 | 1–2 | 3–5 | 15–30/increased# | — |

*Onset of initial action and of effective skeletal muscle relaxation (peak effect) are dose-dependent and decrease with increasing doses. Duration of effective skeletal muscle relaxation and time to recovery are also dose-dependent and increase with increasing doses. Other factors, especially administration of hydrocarbon inhalation anesthetics or other potentiating medications, also influence the duration of effective skeletal muscle relaxation and time to recovery.

†Duration of action and time to recovery with succinylcholine may be increased when plasma pseudocholinesterase activity is decreased.

‡The duration of peak effect and time to recovery with atracurium or vecuronium are not affected by repeated administration of recommended maintenance doses, provided that recovery from the effects of the previous dose begins prior to administration of a subsequent dose.

§Once recovery begins, the rate of recovery is independent of atracurium dosage; however, it is affected by the type of anesthesia administered.

#Following a single dose, the action of the medication is terminated by redistribution into inactive sites. However, following multiple doses, the inactive sites of uptake become saturated, and factors of degradation and/or elimination then directly influence the duration of action and time to recovery.

## Table 2. Pharmacology/Pharmacokinetics* *(continued)*

| Drug | Initial Dose (mg/kg) | Onset of Initial Action (Time to Intubation Conditions) (min) | Time to Peak Effect (min) | Duration of Peak Effect (min)/Effect of Repeated Dosing | Time to Recovery in min (% of twitch response attained) |
|---|---|---|---|---|---|
| Metocurine Intravenous | 0.2–0.4 | 1–4 | 1.5–10; usually 3–5 | 35–60 (maximum effect); average duration of relaxation 60 (range 25–90)/increased | From time of injection#: >360 (50); may be decreased with lower doses |
| Pancuronium Intravenous | 0.04 0.06 0.08 | Within 0.75 (2–3) 0.5 | 4.5 — Within 3 | —/increased# 35–45/increased# —/increased# | From time of injection#: <60 (90) — — |
| Tubocurarine Intramuscular Intravenous | 0.1–0.3 0.1–0.3 | 15–25 Within 1 | — 2–5 | — 20–40/ increased# | — From time of injection: 50 (50); 74–90 (95) |
| Vecuronium Intravenous | 0.08–0.1 | 1 (2.5–3) | 3–5 | 25–30 under balanced anesthesia/ no change‡ | From time of injection— balanced anesthesia‡: 25–40 (25); 45–65 (95) |

*Onset of initial action and of effective skeletal muscle relaxation (peak effect) are dose-dependent and decrease with increasing doses. Duration of effective skeletal muscle relaxation and time to recovery are also dose-dependent and increase with increasing doses. Other factors, especially administration of hydrocarbon inhalation anesthetics or other potentiating medications, also influence the duration of effective skeletal muscle relaxation and time to recovery.

†Duration of action and time to recovery with succinylcholine may be increased when plasma pseudocholinesterase activity is decreased.

‡The duration of peak effect and time to recovery with atracurium or vecuronium are not affected by repeated administration of recommended maintenance doses, provided that recovery from the effects of the previous dose begins prior to administration of a subsequent dose.

§Once recovery begins, the rate of recovery is independent of atracurium dosage; however, it is affected by the type of anesthesia administered.

#Following a single dose, the action of the medication is terminated by redistribution into inactive sites. However, following multiple doses, the inactive sites of uptake become saturated, and factors of degradation and/or elimination then directly influence the duration of action and time to recovery.

## Table 3. Drug Interactions and/or Related Problems

| The following drug interactions and/or related problems have been selected on the basis of their potential clinical significance (possible mechanism in parentheses where appropriate)—not necessarily inclusive (» = major clinical significance): Note: Combinations containing any of the following medications, depending on the amount present, may also interact with this medication. | Depolarizing | Nondepolarizing | | | | | |
|---|---|---|---|---|---|---|---|
| | Legend: I=Succinyl-choline | II=Atracurium III=Gallamine IV=Metocurine | | | V=Pancuronium VI=Tubocurarine VII=Vecuronium | | |
| | I | II | III | IV | V | VI | VII |
| » Aminoglycosides, possibly including oral neomycin (if significant quantities are absorbed in patients with renal function impairment), or » Anesthetics, parenteral-local (large doses leading to significant plasma concentrations) or » Capreomycin or » Citrate-anticoagulated blood (massive transfusions) or » Clindamycin or Lidocaine (intravenous doses > 5 mg per kg) or » Lincomycin or » Polymyxins or Procaine (intravenous) or Trimethaphan (large doses) (neuromuscular blocking activity of these medications may be additive to that of neuromuscular blocking agents)* | ✔ | ✔ | ✔ | ✔ | ✔ | ✔ | ✔ |

## Table 3. Drug Interactions and/or Related Problems (continued)

| | Depolarizing | Nondepolarizing | | | | | |
|---|---|---|---|---|---|---|---|
| | Legend:<br>I = Succinyl-<br>choline | II = Atracurium<br>III = Gallamine<br>IV = Metocurine | | | V = Pancuronium<br>VI = Tubocurarine<br>VII = Vecuronium | | |
| | I | II | III | IV | V | VI | VII |
| **Analgesics, opioid (narcotic), especially those commonly used as adjuncts to anesthesia** | | | | | | | |
| (central respiratory depressant effects of opioid analgesics may be additive to the respiratory depressant effects of neuromuscular blocking agents)* | ✓ | ✓ | ✓ | ✓ | ✓ | ✓ | ✓ |
| (high doses of sufentanil may reduce the initial dosage requirements for a nondepolarizing neuromuscular blocking agent; it is recommended that a peripheral nerve stimulator be used to determine dosage) | | ✓ | ✓ | ✓ | ✓ | ✓ | ✓ |
| (concurrent use of a neuromuscular blocking agent prevents or reverses muscle rigidity induced by sufficiently high doses of most opioid analgesics, especially alfentanil, fentanyl, or sufentanil) | ✓ | ✓ | ✓ | ✓ | ✓ | ✓ | ✓ |
| (gallamine and pancuronium, because of their vagolytic activity, may decrease the risk of opioid analgesic–induced bradycardia or hypotension [especially in patients receiving chronic therapy with beta-adrenergic blocking agents and/or vasodilators for treatment of coronary artery disease], but may also increase the risk of tachycardia or hypertension in some patients) | | | ✓ | | ✓ | | |
| (a nonvagolytic neuromuscular blocking agent will not decrease the risk of opioid analgesic–induced bradycardia or hypotension; in some patients [especially patients with compromised cardiac function and/or those receiving a beta-adrenergic blocking agent preoperatively], the incidence and/or severity of these effects may be increased) | ✓ | ✓ | | ✓ | | ✓ | ✓ |
| (histamine release induced by tubocurarine or, to a lesser extent, atracurium, metocurine, or succinylcholine, may be additive to that induced by many opioid analgesics [except alfentanil, fentanyl, and sufentanil, which do not cause histamine release], leading to increased risk of hypotension; administration of histamine [both H$_1$ and H$_2$] receptor–blocking agents may prevent or reduce this effect) | ✓ | ✓ | | ✓ | | ✓ | |
| **Anesthetics, hydrocarbon inhalation, such as:**<br>Chloroform<br>Cyclopropane<br>Enflurane<br>Ether<br>Halothane<br>Isoflurane<br>Methoxyflurane<br>Trichloroethylene | | | | | | | |
| (concurrent use with succinylcholine may increase the potential for malignant hyperthermia; also, repeated concurrent use may enhance the initial transient bradycardia produced by succinylcholine) | ✓ | | | | | | |
| (neuromuscular blocking activity of inhalation anesthetics, especially enflurane or isoflurane, may be additive to that of the nondepolarizing neuromuscular blocking agents; dosage of vecuronium should be reduced by 15%, and dosage of other neuromuscular blocking agents should be reduced by ⅓ to ½ of the usual dose or as determined with a peripheral nerve stimulator)* | | ✓ | ✓ | ✓ | ✓ | ✓ | ✓ |
| (halogenated hydrocarbon anesthetics may also potentiate succinylcholine-induced neuromuscular blockade, but to a lesser extent than they potentiate the effects of nondepolarizing neuromuscular blocking agents)* | ✓ | | | | | | |

*Increased or prolonged respiratory depression or paralysis (apnea) may occur but is of minor clinical significance while the patient is being mechanically ventilated. However, caution and careful monitoring of the patient are recommended during and following concurrent or sequential use, especially if there is a possibility of incomplete reversal of neuromuscular blockade postoperatively.

## Table 3. Drug Interactions and/or Related Problems (continued)

| | Depolarizing | Nondepolarizing | | | | | |
| --- | --- | --- | --- | --- | --- | --- | --- |
| | Legend:<br>I=Succinyl-<br>choline | II=Atracurium<br>III=Gallamine<br>IV=Metocurine | | | V=Pancuronium<br>VI=Tubocurarine<br>VII=Vecuronium | | |
| | I | II | III | IV | V | VI | VII |
| **Antimyasthenics or**<br>**Edrophonium**<br>(these agents may antagonize the effects of nondepolarizing neuromuscular blocking agents; parenteral neostigmine or pyridostigmine are indicated to reverse neuromuscular blockade following surgery; although the usefulness of edrophonium for this purpose has been considered to be limited because of its brief duration of action, recent studies indicate that edrophonium is equivalent to neostigmine in reversing the effects of tubocurarine) | | ✔ | ✔ | ✔ | ✔ | ✔ | ✔ |
| (these agents may prolong phase I block when used concurrently with succinylcholine*; however, if succinylcholine has been used for a prolonged period of time and the depolarization block has changed to a nondepolarization block, edrophonium, neostigmine, or pyridostigmine may reverse the nondepolarization block) | ✔ | | | | | | |
| (neuromuscular blocking agents may antagonize the effects of antimyasthenics on skeletal muscle; temporary dosage adjustment may be required to control symptoms of myasthenia gravis following surgery) | ✔ | ✔ | ✔ | ✔ | ✔ | ✔ | ✔ |
| **Beta-adrenergic blocking agents**<br>(concurrent use may enhance or prolong the blockade of the nondepolarizing neuromuscular blocking agents)* | | | ✔ | ✔ | ✔ | ✔ | |
| **Calcium salts**<br>(calcium salts usually reverse the effects of nondepolarizing neuromuscular blocking agents) | | ✔ | ✔ | ✔ | ✔ | ✔ | ✔ |
| (concurrent use has been reported to enhance or prolong the neuromuscular blocking action of tubocurarine)* | | | | | | ✔ | |
| » **Cholinesterase inhibitors, especially echothiophate, demecarium, and isoflurophate,**<br>or<br>**Cyclophosphamide or**<br>» **Insecticides, neurotoxic, exposure to, possibly including large quantities of topical malathion, or**<br>**Phenelzine or**<br>**Thiotepa**<br>(may decrease plasma concentrations or activity of pseudocholinesterase, the enzyme that metabolizes succinylcholine, thereby enhancing the neuromuscular blockade of succinylcholine; effects of echothiophate, demecarium, or isoflurophate may persist for weeks or months after the cholinesterase inhibitor has been discontinued)* | ✔ | | | | | | |
| » **Digitalis glycosides**<br>(cardiac effects may be increased when digitalis glycosides are used concurrently with succinylcholine and, to a lesser extent, with pancuronium, possibly resulting in cardiac arrhythmias) | ✔ | | | | ✔ | | |
| **Doxapram**<br>(the residual effects of neuromuscular blocking agents may be masked temporarily by doxapram when it is used post-anesthesia) | ✔ | ✔ | ✔ | ✔ | ✔ | ✔ | ✔ |
| **Hexafluorenium**<br>(concurrent use may prolong the action of succinylcholine and may minimize or prevent the muscle fasciculations and pain that may occur when succinylcholine is used alone; however, concurrent use may increase the potential for development of a dual block)* | ✔ | | | | | | |
| **Lithium (chronic therapy)**<br>(concurrent use may enhance or prolong the neuromuscular blockade of atracurium, succinylcholine, or pancuronium)* | ✔ | ✔ | | | ✔ | | |

Table 3. Drug Interactions and/or Related Problems *(continued)*

| | Depolarizing | Nondepolarizing | | | | | |
|---|---|---|---|---|---|---|---|
| | Legend:<br>**I**=Succinyl-<br>choline | **II**=Atracurium<br>**III**=Gallamine<br>**IV**=Metocurine | | | **V**=Pancuronium<br>**VI**=Tubocurarine<br>**VII**=Vecuronium | | |
| | **I** | **II** | **III** | **IV** | **V** | **VI** | **VII** |
| Magnesium salts, parenteral, or<br>»  Procainamide or<br>»  Quinidine<br>    (concurrent use may enhance the blockade of the neuromuscular blocking agents)* | ✔ | ✔ | ✔ | ✔ | ✔ | ✔ | ✔ |
| Methotrimeprazine<br>    (concurrent use with succinylcholine may cause tachycardia, a fall in blood pressure, CNS stimulation and delirium, and an aggravation of extrapyramidal effects) | ✔ | | | | | | |
| Neuromuscular blocking agents, depolarizing<br>    (prior administration may enhance the blockade of nondepolarizing neuromuscular blocking agents; if a depolarizing agent is used before a nondepolarizing agent, administration of the nondepolarizing agent should be delayed until the effects of the depolarizing agent have decreased) | | ✔ | ✔ | ✔ | ✔ | ✔ | ✔ |
| Neuromuscular blocking agents, nondepolarizing<br>    (concurrent use may enhance the blockade of depolarizing neuromuscular blocking agents if they have been administered over a prolonged period of time and the depolarized block has gradually changed to a nondepolarized block)<br>    (concurrent use of pancuronium and another nondepolarizing neuromuscular blocking agent may substantially reduce the required dose of both medications) | ✔ | <br><br><br>✔ | | <br><br><br>✔ | <br><br><br>✔ | <br><br><br>✔ | <br><br><br>✔ |
| »  Physostigmine<br>    (concurrent use with succinylcholine is not recommended since high doses of physostigmine may cause muscle fasciculation and ultimately, a depolarization block, which may be additive to that produced by succinylcholine) | ✔ | | | | | | |
| Potassium-depleting medications, such as:<br>  Amphotericin B<br>  Bumetanide<br>  Carbonic anhydrase inhibitors<br>  Corticosteroids, glucocorticoid, especially with significant mineralo-<br>    corticoid activity<br>  Corticosteroids, mineralocorticoid<br>  Corticotropin, chronic therapeutic use<br>  Ethacrynic acid<br>  Furosemide<br>  Indapamide<br>  Thiazide diuretics<br>    (hypokalemia induced by these medications may enhance the blockade of nondepolarizing neuromuscular blocking agents; serum potassium determinations and correction of serum potassium concentration may be necessary prior to administration of nondepolarizing neuromuscular blocking agents)*<br>    (hydrocortisone and prednisone have also been reported to decrease the efficacy of pancuronium by an unknown mechanism; increased dosage of pancuronium or use of an alternate neuromuscular blocking agent may be necessary) | | ✔ | ✔ | ✔ | ✔<br><br>✔ | ✔ | ✔ |

*Increased or prolonged respiratory depression or paralysis (apnea) may occur but is of minor clinical significance while the patient is being mechanically ventilated. However, caution and careful monitoring of the patient are recommended during and following concurrent or sequential use, especially if there is a possibility of incomplete reversal of neuromuscular blockade postoperatively.

## Table 4. Medical considerations/Contraindications

Note: A blank space usually signifies lack of information; it is not necessarily an indication that a given medical problem is of no concern. However, the pharmacologic similarity of the nondepolarizing neuromuscular blocking agents may suggest that if caution is required in particular medical problems for one agent, then it may be required for the others as well.

The medical considerations/contraindications included have been selected on the basis of their potential clinical significance (reasons given in parentheses where appropriate)—not necessarily inclusive (» = major clinical significance).

| Risk-benefit should be considered when the following medical problems exist: | Depolarizing Legend: I=Succinylcholine | Nondepolarizing II=Atracurium III=Gallamine IV=Metocurine | | | V=Pancuronium VI=Tubocurarine VII=Vecuronium | | |
|---|---|---|---|---|---|---|---|
| | I | II | III | IV | V | VI | VII |
| Allergic reaction to the neuromuscular blocker considered for use, history of | ✔ | ✔ | ✔ | ✔ | ✔ | ✔ | ✔ |
| Burns, severe, or Digitalis toxicity or in patients recently digitalized or Neuromuscular disease, degenerative or dystrophic, or Paraplegia or Spinal cord injury or Trauma, severe (serious cardiac arrhythmias or cardiac arrest may occur as a result of increased serum potassium concentrations) | ✔ | | | | | | |
| Carcinoma, bronchogenic (action of neuromuscular blocking agent may be enhanced) | ✔ | ✔ | ✔ | ✔ | ✔ | ✔ | ✔ |
| Cardiac conditions in which tachycardia would be undesirable (gallamine and pancuronium may cause tachycardia) | | | ✔ | | ✔ | | |
| Cardiovascular function impairment | | | | | | ✔ | ✔ |
| Conditions in which histamine release would be hazardous (these neuromuscular blocking agents may cause histamine release) | ✔ | ✔ | | ✔ | ✔ | ✔ | ✔ |
| Conditions in which low levels of plasma pseudocholinesterase activity may exist, such as: Anemia, severe Dehydration Exposure to neurotoxic insecticides or other cholinesterase inhibitors Hepatic disease, severe, or cirrhosis Malnutrition Pregnancy Recessive hereditary trait (prolonged respiratory depression or apnea may occur) | ✔ | | | | | | |
| Dehydration or Electrolyte or acid-base imbalance (action of neuromuscular blocking agent may be altered) | ✔ | ✔ | ✔ | ✔ | ✔ | ✔ | ✔ |
| Eye injury, open, or Glaucoma or Ocular surgery (succinylcholine may increase intraocular pressure) | ✔ | | | | | | |
| Fractures or muscle spasm (initial muscle fasciculations may cause additional trauma) | ✔ | | | | | | |
| Hepatic function impairment (patients may have decreased levels of pseudocholinesterase activity, possibly resulting in prolonged respiratory depression or apnea) | ✔ | | | | | | |
| (effect of metocurine, panuronium, or tubocurarine may be reduced) | | | | ✔ | ✔ | ✔ | |
| (effect of vecuronium may be prolonged) | | | | | | | ✔ |
| Hyperkalemia, preexisting (may be exacerbated by succinylcholine-induced increases in serum potassium concentration) | ✔ | | | | | | |
| Hypertension (gallamine may increase blood pressure) | | | ✔ | | | | |
| Hyperthermia (intensity and duration of action of depolarizing agents may be decreased and that of nondepolarizing agents may be increased) | ✔ | | ✔ | ✔ | ✔ | ✔ | |
| Hypotension (rapid IV administration and/or large doses of atracurium, metocurine, and tubocurarine may cause hypotension) | | ✔ | | ✔ | | ✔ | |

## Table 4. Medical considerations/Contraindications *(continued)*

| | Depolarizing | Nondepolarizing | | | | | |
|---|---|---|---|---|---|---|---|
| | Legend:<br>**I**=Succinyl-<br>choline | **II**=Atracurium<br>**III**=Gallamine<br>**IV**=Metocurine | | | **V**=Pancuronium<br>**VI**=Tubocurarine<br>**VII**=Vecuronium | | |
| | **I** | **II** | **III** | **IV** | **V** | **VI** | **VII** |
| Hypothermia<br>(intensity and/or duration of action of succinylcholine and atracurium may be increased and that of gallamine, metocurine, pancuronium, and tubocurarine may be decreased) | ✔ | ✔ | ✔ | ✔ | ✔ | ✔ | |
| » Malignant hyperthermia, history of in patient or close relative, or suspected predisposition to<br>(may be induced by succinylcholine) | ✔ | | | | | | |
| Myasthenia gravis, except when tubocurarine is used as a diagnostic agent | ✔ | ✔ | ✔ | ✔ | ✔ | ✔ | ✔ |
| Pulmonary function impairment or<br>Respiratory depression<br>(risk of additive respiratory depression) | ✔ | ✔ | ✔ | ✔ | ✔ | ✔ | ✔ |
| Renal function impairment<br>(eliminated by kidneys; prolonged neuromuscular blockade may occur) | ✔ | | | | ✔ | ✔ | ✔ |
| » Renal function impairment<br>(eliminated by kidneys primarily as unchanged drug; prolonged neuromuscular blockade may occur) | | | ✔ | | | | |
| » Shock<br>(action of gallamine may be prolonged) | | | ✔ | | | | |
| Shock<br>(action of metocurine and tubocurarine may be prolonged) | | | | | | ✔ | ✔ |

## Table 5. Side/Adverse Effects*

| | Depolarizing | Nondepolarizing | | | | | |
|---|---|---|---|---|---|---|---|
| | Legend:<br>**I**=Succinyl-<br>choline | **II**=Atracurium<br>**III**=Gallamine<br>**IV**=Metocurine | | | **V**=Pancuronium<br>**VI**=Tubocurarine<br>**VII**=Vecuronium | | |
| The following side/adverse effects have been selected on the basis of their potential clinical significance (possible signs and symptoms in parentheses where appropriate)—not necessarily inclusive: | **I** | **II** | **III** | **IV** | **V** | **VI** | **VII** |
| **Medical attention needed**<br>*Anaphylactic, anaphylactoid, or other hypersensitivity reaction* | R | R | R | R | R | R | R |
| *Bradycardia* | L† | R‡ | U | U | U | R | R‡ |
| *Bronchospasm* | R§ | R§ | U | R§ | R§ | R§ | R§ |
| *Cardiac arrhythmias* | L† | U | U | U | U | R | U |
| *Circulatory depression or collapse*—may occur in overdose | R§ | R§ | U | R§ | R§ | R§ | R§ |
| *Decreased blood pressure*—may reach hypotensive levels; with usual doses of metocurine or tubocurarine, or larger-than-recommended doses of atracurium, may be caused by ganglionic blockade; may also occur as a complication of high-dose positive pressure respiration | R†§ | L§ | U | L§ | R§ | M§ | R§ |
| *Edema* | R§ | R§ | U | R§ | R§ | R§ | R§ |
| *Erythema* | R§ | R§ | U | R§ | R§ | R§ | R§ |

*Differences in frequency of occurrence may reflect either lack of clinical-use data or actual pharmacologic distinctions among agents (although their pharmacologic similarity suggests that side effects occurring with one may occur with the others). M=more frequent; L=less frequent; R=rare; U=unknown.

†Succinylcholine may cause transient bradycardia accompanied by hypotension, cardiac arrhythmias, and possibly a short period of sinus arrest due to increased vagal stimulation, especially with repeated administration and in children. Following these effects, tachycardia and hypertension may occur due to asphyxial pressor response and mild sympathetic ganglion stimulation.

‡Atracurium and vecuronium have little or no direct effect on heart rate; bradycardia may occur because these medications do not counteract the bradycardia caused by other medications (e.g., anesthetics, opioid analgesics) or vagal stimulation.

§May be caused by histamine release, especially following rapid intravenous injection and/or large doses, or an overdose. The risk of clinically significant histamine release is highest with tubocurarine; moderate with atracurium, metocurine, or succinylcholine; relatively low with pancuronium or vecuronium; and least with gallamine.

## Table 5. Side/Adverse Effects* *(continued)*

|  | Depolarizing | Nondepolarizing | | | | | |
|---|---|---|---|---|---|---|---|
|  | Legend:<br>**I**=Succinyl-<br>choline | **II**=Atracurium<br>**III**=Gallamine<br>**IV**=Metocurine | | | **V**=Pancuronium<br>**VI**=Tubocurarine<br>**VII**=Vecuronium | | |
|  | **I** | **II** | **III** | **IV** | **V** | **VI** | **VII** |
| *Flushing of skin* | R§ | M§ | U | R§ | R§ | R§ | R§ |
| *Hives* | U | R | U | U | U | U | U |
| *Increased blood pressure*—may reach hypertensive levels; with gallamine or pancuronium, may be caused by vagolytic activity | R† | L | M | U | L | U | U |
| *Increased intraocular pressure*—possibly caused by contraction of extraocular muscle; occurs immediately after injection and during the fasciculation phase | M | U | U | U | U | U | U |
| *Laryngospasm* | U | R | U | U | U | U | U |
| *Malignant hyperthermic crisis* | R | U | U | U | U | U | U |
| *Myoglobinemia and myoglobinuria caused by rhabdomyolysis*—especially in children; may lead to myoglobinuric acute renal failure | R | U | U | U | U | U | U |
| *Tachycardia*—with gallamine, occurs after doses of 500 mcg (0.5 mg) per kg of body weight and reaches a maximum within 3 minutes, then declines gradually to the control level; with gallamine and pancuronium, may be due to vagolytic activity | L†§ | L§ | M | R§ | L§ | R§ | R§ |
| **Medical attention needed only if continuing or bothersome**<br>*Itching of skin* | R§ | R§ | U | R§ | L§ | R§ | R§ |
| *Muscle pain and stiffness, postoperative*—possibly caused by muscle fasciculations that occur immediately following injection; incidence may vary from 10% in patients maintained on bed rest for 1 day to 70% in ambulatory patients; symptoms usually appear 12 to 24 hours following administration and last for several hours to a few days | M | — | — | — | — | — | — |
| *Salivation, excessive* | L | U | U | U | L | U | U |
| *Skin rash* | R§ | R§ | U | R§ | L§ | R§ | R§ |

*Differences in frequency of occurrence may reflect either lack of clinical-use data or actual pharmacologic distinctions among agents (although their pharmacologic similarity suggests that side effects occurring with one may occur with the others). M=more frequent; L=less frequent; R=rare; U=unknown.

†Succinylcholine may cause transient bradycardia accompanied by hypotension, cardiac arrhythmias, and possibly a short period of sinus arrest due to increased vagal stimulation, especially with repeated administration and in children. Following these effects, tachycardia and hypertension may occur due to asphyxial pressor response and mild sympathetic ganglion stimulation.

‡Atracurium and vecuronium have little or no direct effect on heart rate; bradycardia may occur because these medications do not counteract the bradycardia caused by other medications (e.g., anesthetics, opioid analgesics) or vagal stimulation.

§May be caused by histamine release, especially following rapid intravenous injection and/or large doses, or an overdose. The risk of clinically significant histamine release is highest with tubocurarine; moderate with atracurium, metocurine, or succinylcholine; relatively low with pancuronium or vecuronium; and least with gallamine.

# NIACIN   Systemic

This monograph includes information on the following: Niacin; Niacinamide.

INN:

Niacin—Nicotinic acid
Niacinamide—Nicotinamide

VA CLASSIFICATION (Primary/Secondary): VT103/CV350

Other commonly used names are: Nicotinamide [Niacinamide], Nicotinic acid [Niacin], Vitamin B₃ [Niacin; Niacinamide].

Note: For a listing of dosage forms and brand names by country availability, see *Dosage Forms* section(s). For a listing of brand names for the articles in this monograph, refer to the General Index.

## Category

Note: Niacin and niacinamide (vitamin B₃) are water-soluble vitamins.

Nutritional supplement (vitamin)—Niacin; Niacinamide.
Antihyperlipidemic—Niacin.

## Indications

### Accepted

Niacin deficiency (prophylaxis and treatment)—Niacin and niacinamide are indicated for prevention and treatment of vitamin B₃ deficiency states. Vitamin B₃ deficiency may occur as a result of inadequate nutrition or intestinal malabsorption but does not occur in healthy individuals receiving an adequate balanced diet. Simple nutritional deficiency of individual B vitamins is rare since dietary inadequacy usually results in multiple deficiencies. For prophylaxis of niacin deficiency, dietary improvement, rather than supplementation, is advisable. For treatment of niacin deficiency, supplementation is preferred.

Deficiency of niacin may lead to pellagra.

Recommended intakes may be increased and/or supplementation may be necessary in the following persons or conditions (based on documented niacin deficiency):

Diabetes mellitus
Fever, chronic
Gastrectomy
Hartnup disease
Hepatic-biliary tract disease—cirrhosis
Hyperthyroidism

Infection, chronic

Intestinal diseases—celiac disease, persistent diarrhea, tropical sprue, regional enteritis

Malabsorption syndromes associated with pancreatic insufficiency

Malignancy

Oropharyngeal lesions

Stress, continuing

Some unusual diets (e.g., reducing diets that drastically restrict food selection) may not supply minimum daily requirements of niacin. Supplementation is necessary in patients receiving total parenteral nutrition (TPN) or undergoing rapid weight loss or in those with malnutrition, because of inadequate dietary intake.

Recommended intakes for all vitamins and most minerals are increased during pregnancy. Many physicians recommend that pregnant women receive multivitamin and mineral supplements, especially those pregnant women who do not consume an adequate diet and those in high-risk categories (i.e., women carrying more than one fetus, heavy cigarette smokers, and alcohol and drug abusers). However, taking excessive amounts of a multivitamin and mineral supplement may be harmful to the mother and/or fetus and should be avoided.

Recommended intakes for all vitamins and most minerals are increased during breast-feeding.

Hyperlipidemia (treatment)—Niacin (but not niacinamide) is also indicated in the treatment of hyperlipidemia. Niacin is recommended for use only in patients with primary hyperlipidemia (type IIa, IIb, III, IV, or V hyperlipoproteinemia) and a significant risk of coronary artery disease who have not responded to other measures alone. It is one of the drugs of first choice for initiating therapy to reduce low density lipoprotein (LDL)–cholesterol concentrations and triglycerides, and to increase high density lipoprotein (HDL)–cholesterol concentrations.

Studies have suggested that control of elevated cholesterol and triglycerides may not lessen the danger of cardiovascular disease and mortality, although incidence of nonfatal myocardial infarctions may be decreased.

For additional information on initial therapeutic guidelines related to the treatment of hyperlipidemia, see *Appendix III*.

**Unaccepted**

Niacin is not useful for treatment of schizophrenia and other mental disorders not related to niacin deficiency. Niacin also has not been proven effective for treatment of acne, alcohol dependence, drug-induced hallucinations, hyperkinesis, leprosy, livedoid vasculitis, peripheral vascular disease, motion sickness, or for prevention of heart attacks.

## Pharmacology/Pharmacokinetics

**Physicochemical characteristics**

Molecular weight—

Niacin: 123.11.

Niacinamide: 122.13.

pKa—

Niacin: 4.85.

Niacinamide: 0.5 and 3.35.

**Mechanism of action/Effect**

Nutritional supplement—Niacin, after conversion to niacinamide, is a component of two coenzymes, nicotinamide adenine dinucleotide (NAD) and nicotinamide adenine dinucleotide phosphate (NADP), which are necessary for tissue respiration; glycogenolysis; and lipid, amino acid, protein, and purine metabolism.

Antihyperlipidemic—Niacin lowers serum cholesterol and triglyceride concentrations by inhibiting the synthesis of very low density lipoproteins (VLDL), which are precursors to the formation of low-density lipoproteins, the principal carrier of blood cholesterol.

**Other actions/effects**

Niacin (but not niacinamide) causes direct peripheral vasodilation.

**Absorption**

The B vitamins, including niacin and niacinamide, are readily absorbed from the gastrointestinal tract, except in malabsorption syndromes.

**Biotransformation**

Hepatic. Dietary tryptophan is converted by intestinal bacteria to niacin and niacinamide (about 60 mg of tryptophan is equivalent to 1 mg of niacin). Niacin is also converted to niacinamide as needed.

**Half-life**

Elimination—Approximately 45 minutes.

**Onset of action**

Reduced cholesterol concentrations—Oral: Several days.

Reduced triglyceride concentrations—Oral: Several hours.

**Time to peak serum concentration**

Oral—45 minutes.

**Elimination**

Renal (almost entirely as metabolites). Excess beyond daily needs is excreted, largely unchanged, in urine.

## Precautions to Consider

**Pregnancy/Reproduction**

Problems in humans have not been documented with intake of normal daily recommended amounts. Studies have not been done in humans. Studies have not been done in animals.

**Breast-feeding**

Problems in humans have not been documented with intake of normal daily recommended amounts.

**Pediatrics**

Problems in pediatrics have not been documented with intake of normal daily recommended amounts. Appropriate studies of niacin as an antihyperlipidemic have not been performed in the pediatric population. However, use of niacin as an antihyperlipidemic in children under 2 years of age is not recommended since cholesterol is required for normal development.

**Geriatrics**

Problems in geriatrics have not been documented with intake of normal daily recommended amounts.

**Drug interactions and/or related problems**

The following drug interactions and/or related problems have been selected on the basis of their potential clinical significance (possible mechanism in parentheses where appropriate)—not necessarily inclusive (» = major clinical significance):

Chenodiol or
Ursodiol
(effect may be decreased when chenodiol or ursodiol is used concurrently with antihyperlipidemics, which tend to increase cholesterol saturation of bile)

HMG-CoA reductase inhibitors
(concurrent use with niacin may be associated with an increased risk of rhabdomyolysis and acute renal failure; combined therapy with lovastatin, pravastatin, or simvastatin should include careful monitoring for symptoms of myopathy or rhabdomyolysis)

**Laboratory value alterations**

The following have been selected on the basis of their potential clinical significance (possible effect in parentheses where appropriate)—not necessarily inclusive (» = major clinical significance):

Note: Usually occur only with large doses.

With diagnostic test results
Urinary catecholamine concentration, measurements by fluorimetric methods
(niacin may produce fluorescent substances and falsely elevated results)

Urine glucose determinations using cupric sulfate (Benedict's reagent)
(niacin may produce false-positive reactions)

With physiology/laboratory test values
Uric acid concentrations in blood
(may be increased by large doses of niacin)

**Medical considerations/Contraindications**

The medical considerations/contraindications included here have been selected on the basis of their potential clinical significance (reasons given in parentheses where appropriate)—not necessarily inclusive (» = major clinical significance).

*Risk-benefit should be considered when the following medical problems exist:*

» Arterial bleeding or hemorrhage or
Glaucoma
(these conditions may be exacerbated)

» Diabetes mellitus
(large doses of niacin may cause impaired glucose tolerance)

Gout
(large doses may cause hyperuricemia)

» Hepatic disease
(large doses may cause hepatic damage)

Hypotension
(may worsen due to vasodilating effects of niacin)

» Peptic ulcer
(large doses may activate peptic ulcer)

Sensitivity to niacin or niacinamide

**Patient monitoring**

The following may be especially important in patient monitoring (other tests may be warranted in some patients, depending on condition; » = major clinical significance):

Cholesterol concentrations, serum
(determinations recommended at periodic intervals during antihyperlipidemic therapy)

Glucose concentrations, blood and
Hepatic function determinations and
Uric acid concentrations
(determinations recommended at periodic intervals in patients receiving high doses of niacin or niacinamide for prolonged periods)

## Side/Adverse Effects

Note: Flushing and pruritus may be reduced with the extended-release dosage form of niacin.

The following side/adverse effects have been selected on the basis of their potential clinical significance (possible signs and symptoms in parentheses where appropriate)—not necessarily inclusive:

**Those indicating need for medical attention**
Incidence rare
*Allergic reaction, anaphylactic* (skin rash or itching; wheezing)—after intravenous administration

With long-term use of extended-release niacin
*Hepatotoxicity or cholestasis* (darkening of urine; light gray-colored stools; loss of appetite; severe stomach pain; yellow eyes or skin)

**Those indicating need for medical attention only if they continue or are bothersome**
Incidence less frequent—with niacin only
*Feeling of warmth; flushing or redness of skin, especially on face and neck; headache*
With high oral doses
*Cardiac arrhythmias* (unusually fast, slow, or irregular heartbeat); *diarrhea; dizziness or faintness; dryness of skin or eyes; hyperglycemia* (frequent urination or unusual thirst)—may occasionally be fatal; *hyperuricemia* (joint pain; side, lower back, or stomach pain; swelling of feet or lower legs); *myalgia* (fever; muscle aching or cramping; unusual tiredness or weakness); *nausea or vomiting; peptic ulcer, aggravation of* (stomach pain); *pruritus* (itching of skin)—may be severe
Note: Rarely, along with markedly elevated creatine kinase (CK) concentrations, fever, muscle aching or cramping, or unusual tiredness or weakness may be symptoms of myositis or rhabdomyolysis; incidence may be increased in patients treated concurrently with lovastatin, pravastatin, or simvastatin.

## Patient Consultation

As an aid to patient consultation, refer to *Advice for the Patient, Niacin (Vitamin B₃) (Systemic)* or *Niacin—For High Cholesterol (Systemic)*.

In providing consultation, consider emphasizing the following selected information (» = major clinical significance):

**Description of use**
Description should include function in the body, signs of deficiency, and unproven uses

**Importance of diet**
*For use as a vitamin supplement*
Importance of proper nutrition; supplement may be needed because of inadequate dietary intake
Food sources of niacin; effects of processing
Not using vitamins as substitute for balanced diet
Recommended daily intake for niacin

**Before using this medication**
*For use as a vitamin supplement*
See *Indications* for conditions and medications affecting requirements.
*For use as an antihyperlipidemic (niacin only)*
Diet as preferred therapy
» Conditions affecting use, especially:
Sensitivity to niacin or niacinamide
Use in children—Not recommended as antihyperlipidemic in children under 2 years of age since cholesterol is required for normal development
Other medical problems, especially arterial bleeding or hemorrhage, diabetes mellitus, hepatic disease, or peptic ulcer

**Proper use of this medication**
Possibility of stomach upset; taking with meals or milk; checking with physician if stomach upset continues

Proper administration of extended-release dosage forms: Swallowing whole without crushing, breaking, or chewing; contents of capsule may be mixed with jam or jelly and swallowed without chewing
» Proper storage
*For use as a vitamin supplement*
» Proper dosing
Missed dose: No cause for concern because of length of time necessary for depletion; remembering to take as directed
*For use as an antihyperlipidemic (niacin only)*
» Importance of not taking more or less medication than prescribed
Niacin does not cure the condition but instead helps control it
» Importance of following prescribed diet
Missed dose: Taking as soon as possible; not taking if almost time for next dose; not doubling doses

**Precautions while using this medication**
Caution if dizziness or faintness occurs
*For use as an antihyperlipidemic (niacin only)*
» Importance of close monitoring by physician to check progress
» Checking with physician before discontinuing medication; blood lipid concentrations may increase significantly

**Side/adverse effects**
Signs of potential side effects, especially anaphylactic reaction with injection only; hepatotoxicity or cholestasis with high doses of extended-release niacin

## General Dosing Information

Dosages of niacin and niacinamide as vitamin supplements are equal; some clinicians prefer niacinamide because of its lack of vasodilating effect.

Because of the infrequency of single B vitamin deficiencies, combinations are commonly administered. Many commercial combinations of B vitamins are available.

When used for treatment of pellagra, niacin or niacinamide is usually given in combination with 5 mg each of thiamine, riboflavin, and pyridoxine.

**For parenteral dosage forms only**
In most cases, parenteral administration is indicated only when oral administration is not acceptable (for example, in nausea, vomiting, and preoperative and postoperative conditions) or possible (for example, in malabsorption syndromes or following gastric resection).

When administered intravenously, niacin or niacinamide should be given at a rate not exceeding 2 mg per minute.

**Diet/Nutrition**
Niacin or niacinamide may be taken with meals or milk if nausea, vomiting, or diarrhea occurs. A physician should be consulted if stomach upset continues.

Recommended dietary intakes for niacin are defined differently worldwide.

For U.S.—
The Recommended Dietary Allowances (RDAs) for vitamins and minerals are determined by the Food and Nutrition Board of the National Research Council and are intended to provide adequate nutrition in most healthy persons under usual environmental stresses. In addition, a different designation may be used by the FDA for food and dietary supplement labeling purposes, as with Daily Value (DV). DVs replace the previous labeling terminology United States Recommended Daily Allowances (USRDAs).

For Canada—
Recommended Nutrient Intakes (RNIs) for vitamins, minerals, and protein are determined by Health and Welfare Canada and provide recommended amounts of a specific nutrient while minimizing the risk of chronic diseases.

Daily recommended intakes for niacin are generally defined as follows:

| Persons | U.S. (mg) | Canada (mg) |
|---|---|---|
| Infants and children | | |
| Birth to 3 years of age | 5–9 | 4–9 |
| 4 to 6 years of age | 12 | 13 |
| 7 to 10 years of age | 13 | 14–18 |
| Adolescent and adult males | 15–20 | 14–23 |
| Adolescent and adult females | 13–15 | 14–16 |
| Pregnant females | 17 | 14–16 |
| Breast-feeding females | 20 | 14–16 |

These are usually provided by adequate diets.

Best dietary sources of niacin include meats, eggs, and milk and dairy products; dietary tryptophan (from protein) is converted to niacin. There is little loss of niacin from foods with ordinary cooking.

**For treatment of adverse effects**

Tolerance to the vasodilating and gastrointestinal effects of niacin usually occurs within 2 weeks.

The severe flushing, pruritus, and gastrointestinal effects may be minimized by starting therapy with a low dose and increasing the dosage gradually, and by taking niacin with meals or milk.

Persistent flushing may sometimes be controlled with 300 mg of aspirin taken 30 minutes before each niacin dose.

---

## NIACIN

# Oral Dosage Forms

## NIACIN EXTENDED-RELEASE CAPSULES

Note: Dose-related hepatotoxicity may be more prevalent with high doses of the extended-release dosage form of niacin.

Flushing and pruritus may be reduced with the extended-release dosage form of niacin.

**Usual adult and adolescent dose**

Antihyperlipidemic—

Initial: Oral, 1 gram three times a day, the dosage being increased in increments of 500 mg a day every two to four weeks as needed.

Note: Some clinicians may begin with 500 mg per day and gradually increase the dosage to 4 grams a day.

Maintenance: Oral, 1 to 2 grams three times a day.

Deficiency (prophylaxis)—

Oral, amount based on normal daily recommended intakes:

| Persons | U.S. (mg) | Canada (mg) |
|---|---|---|
| Adolescent and adult males | 15–20 | 14–23 |
| Adolescent and adult females | 13–15 | 14–16 |
| Pregnant females | 17 | 14–16 |
| Breast-feeding females | 20 | 14–16 |

Deficiency (treatment)—

Treatment dose is individualized by prescriber based on severity of deficiency.

**Usual adult prescribing limits**

Oral, 6 grams a day.

**Usual pediatric dose**

Dosage form is not recommended for use in children.

**Strength(s) usually available**

U.S.—

125 mg [*Nicobid Tempules* (OTC); GENERIC (Rx/OTC)].

250 mg [*Nicobid Tempules* (OTC); GENERIC (Rx/OTC)].

300 mg (OTC) [*Niac*].

400 mg [*Nia-Bid* (OTC); *Niacels* (OTC); *Nico-400* (OTC); GENERIC (Rx/OTC)].

500 mg [*Nicobid Tempules* (OTC); GENERIC (Rx/OTC)].

Canada—

Not commercially available.

Note: For use as a dietary supplement, some strengths of these niacin preparations may exceed the dosage range recommended by USP DI Advisory Panels based on the amount necessary to meet normal nutritional needs.

**Packaging and storage**

Store below 40 °C (104 °F), preferably between 15 and 30 °C (59 and 86 °F), in a well-closed container, unless otherwise specified by manufacturer.

**Auxiliary labeling**

• Swallow capsules whole.

• Take with meals or milk.

**Note**

Contents of capsule may be mixed with jelly or jam and swallowed without chewing.

## NIACIN ORAL SOLUTION

**Usual adult and adolescent dose**

Antihyperlipidemic—

Initial: Oral, 1 gram three times a day, the dosage being increased in increments of 500 mg a day every two to four weeks as needed.

Maintenance: Oral, 1 to 2 grams three times a day.

Deficiency (prophylaxis or treatment)—

See *Niacin Extended-release Capsules*.

**Usual adult prescribing limits**

Oral, 6 grams a day.

**Usual pediatric dose**

Deficiency (prophylaxis)—

Oral, amount based on normal daily recommended intakes:

| Persons | U.S. (mg) | Canada (mg) |
|---|---|---|
| Infants and children | | |
| Birth to 3 years of age | 5–9 | 4–9 |
| 4 to 6 years of age | 12 | 13 |
| 7 to 10 years of age | 13 | 14–18 |

Deficiency (treatment)—

Treatment dose is individualized by prescriber based on severity of deficiency.

**Strength(s) usually available**

U.S.—

50 mg per 5 mL (OTC) [*Nicotinex Elixir* (alcohol 14%)].

Canada—

Not commercially available.

Note: For use as a dietary supplement, the strength of this niacin preparation may exceed the dosage range recommended by USP DI Advisory Panels based on the amount necessary to meet normal nutritional needs.

**Packaging and storage**

Store below 40 °C (104 °F), preferably between 15 and 30 °C (59 and 86 °F), in a tight container, unless otherwise specified by manufacturer. Protect from freezing.

**Auxiliary labeling**

• Take with meals or milk.

## NIACIN TABLETS USP

**Usual adult and adolescent dose**

Antihyperlipidemic—

Initial: Oral, 1 gram three times a day, the dosage being increased in increments of 500 mg a day every two to four weeks as needed.

Note: Some clinicians may begin with 100 mg per day and gradually increase the dosage to 4 grams per day.

Maintenance: Oral, 1 to 2 grams three times a day.

Deficiency (prophylaxis or treatment)—

See *Niacin Extended-release Capsules*.

**Usual adult prescribing limits**

Oral, 6 grams a day.

**Usual pediatric dose**

Deficiency (prophylaxis or treatment)—

See *Niacin Oral Solution*.

**Strength(s) usually available**

U.S.—

25 mg (OTC) [GENERIC].

50 mg (OTC) [GENERIC].

100 mg (OTC) [GENERIC].

125 mg (OTC) [GENERIC].

250 mg (OTC) [GENERIC].

400 mg (OTC) [GENERIC].

500 mg [*Niacor* (Rx) (scored); *Nicolar* (Rx) (scored; tartrazine); GENERIC (Rx/OTC)].

Canada—

50 mg (OTC) [*Novo-Niacin;* GENERIC].

100 mg (OTC) [GENERIC].

500 mg (OTC) [GENERIC].

Note: For use as a dietary supplement, some strengths of these niacin preparations may exceed the dosage range recommended by USP DI Advisory Panels based on the amount necessary to meet normal nutritional needs.

**Packaging and storage**

Store below 40 °C (104 °F), preferably between 15 and 30 °C (59 and 86 °F), unless otherwise specified by manufacturer. Store in a well-closed container.

**Auxiliary labeling**

• Take with meals or milk.

## NIACIN EXTENDED-RELEASE TABLETS

Note: Dose-related hepatotoxicity may be more prevalent with high doses of the extended-release dosage form.

Flushing and pruritus may be reduced with the extended-release dosage form of niacin.

### Usual adult and adolescent dose

Antihyperlipidemic—
  Initial: Oral, 1 gram three times a day, the dosage being increased in increments of 500 mg a day every two to four weeks as needed and tolerated.
  Note: Some clinicians may begin with 500 mg per day and gradually increase the dosage to 3 grams a day.
  Maintenance: Oral, 1 to 2 grams three times a day.
  Note: Some clinicians may use a maintenance dose of 500 mg to 1 gram two to three times a day.

Deficiency (prophylaxis and treatment)—
  See *Niacin Extended-release Capsules.*

### Usual adult prescribing limits

Oral, 6 grams a day.

### Usual pediatric dose

Dosage form is not recommended for use in children.

### Strength(s) usually available

U.S.—
  125 mg (Rx) [GENERIC].
  250 mg [*Endur-Acin* (OTC); *Slo-Niacin* (OTC) (scored); GENERIC (Rx/OTC)].
  400 mg (OTC) [GENERIC].
  500 mg [*Endur-Acin* (OTC); *Slo-Niacin* (OTC) (scored); GENERIC (Rx/OTC)].
  750 mg [*Slo-Niacin* (OTC) (scored); GENERIC (Rx/OTC)].
  1000 mg (OTC) [GENERIC].

Canada—
  500 mg (OTC) [GENERIC].

Note: For use as a dietary supplement, some strengths of these niacin preparations may exceed the dosage range recommended by USP DI Advisory Panels based on the amount necessary to meet normal nutritional needs.

### Packaging and storage

Store below 40 °C (104 °F), preferably between 15 and 30 °C (59 and 86 °F), in a well-closed container, unless otherwise specified by manufacturer.

### Auxiliary labeling

• Swallow tablets whole.
• Take with meals or milk.

### Note

If tablets are scored, they may be broken, but not crushed or chewed, before swallowing.

## Parenteral Dosage Forms

### NIACIN INJECTION USP

#### Usual adult and adolescent dose

Deficiency (prophylaxis)—
  Intravenous infusion, as part of total parenteral nutrition solutions, the specific amount determined by individual patient need.
Deficiency (treatment)—
  Intramuscular, 50 to 100 mg five or more times a day.
  Intravenous (slow), 25 to 100 mg two or more times a day.

#### Usual pediatric dose

Deficiency (prophylaxis)—
  Intravenous infusion, as part of total parenteral nutrition solutions, the specific amount determined by individual patient need.
Deficiency (treatment)—
  Intravenous (slow), up to 300 mg a day.

#### Strength(s) usually available

U.S.—
  100 mg per mL (Rx) [GENERIC].
Canada—
  Not commercially available.

#### Packaging and storage

Store below 40 °C (104 °F), preferably between 15 and 30 °C (59 and 86 °F), unless otherwise specified by manufacturer. Protect from freezing.

#### Preparation of dosage form

For administration by the intravenous route, niacin injection should be diluted to a strength of 2 mg per mL or added to 500 mL of sodium chloride injection and administered at a rate not exceeding 2 mg per minute.

---

### *NIACINAMIDE*

## Oral Dosage Forms

### NIACINAMIDE TABLETS USP

#### Usual adult and adolescent dose

Deficiency (prophylaxis)—
  Oral, amount based on normal daily recommended intakes:

| Persons | U.S. (mg) | Canada (mg) |
|---|---|---|
| Adolescent and adult males | 15–20 | 14–23 |
| Adolescent and adult females | 13–15 | 14–16 |
| Pregnant females | 17 | 14–16 |
| Breast-feeding females | 20 | 14–16 |

Deficiency (treatment)—
  Treatment dose is individualized by prescriber based on severity of deficiency.

#### Usual pediatric dose

Deficiency (prophylaxis)—
  Oral, amount based on normal daily recommended intakes:

| Persons | U.S. (mg) | Canada (mg) |
|---|---|---|
| Infants and children | | |
| Birth to 3 years of age | 5–9 | 4–9 |
| 4 to 6 years of age | 12 | 13 |
| 7 to 10 years of age | 13 | 14–18 |

Deficiency (treatment)—
  Treatment dose is individualized by prescriber based on severity of deficiency.

#### Strength(s) usually available

U.S.—
  50 mg (OTC) [GENERIC].
  100 mg (OTC) [GENERIC].
  125 mg (OTC) [GENERIC].
  250 mg (OTC) [GENERIC].
  500 mg (Rx/OTC) [GENERIC].
Canada—
  100 mg (OTC) [GENERIC].
  500 mg (OTC) [GENERIC].

Note: For use as a dietary supplement, some strengths of these niacinamide preparations may exceed the dosage range recommended by USP DI Advisory Panels based on the amount necessary to meet normal nutritional needs.

#### Packaging and storage

Store below 40 °C (104 °F), preferably between 15 and 30 °C (59 and 86 °F), unless otherwise specified by manufacturer. Store in a tight container.

## Parenteral Dosage Forms

### NIACINAMIDE INJECTION USP

#### Usual adult and adolescent dose

Deficiency (prophylaxis)—
  Intravenous infusion, as part of total parenteral nutrition solutions, the specific amount determined by individual patient need.
Deficiency (treatment)—
  Intramuscular, 50 to 100 mg five or more times a day.
  Intravenous (slow), 25 to 100 mg two or more times a day.

#### Usual pediatric dose

Deficiency (prophylaxis)—
  Intravenous infusion, as part of total parenteral nutrition solutions, the specific amount determined by individual patient need.
Deficiency (treatment)—
  Intravenous (slow), up to 300 mg a day.

#### Strength(s) usually available

U.S.—
  100 mg per mL (Rx) [GENERIC].
Canada—
  Not commercially available.

#### Packaging and storage

Store below 40 °C (104 °F), preferably between 15 and 30 °C (59 and 86 °F), unless otherwise specified by manufacturer. Protect from freezing.

---

Revised: 11/09/91
Interim revision: 08/10/94; 05/26/95; 07/11/95

**NIACINAMIDE**—See *Niacin (Systemic)*

**NICARDIPINE**—See *Calcium Channel Blocking Agents (Systemic)*

# NICLOSAMIDE    Oral-Local†

**VA CLASSIFICATION (Primary): AP200**

Note: For a listing of dosage forms and brand names by country availability, see *Dosage Forms* section(s). For a listing of brand names for the articles in this monograph, refer to the General Index.

†Not commercially available in Canada.

## Category

Anthelmintic (oral-local).

## Indications

Note: Bracketed information in the *Indications* section refers to uses that are not included in U.S. product labeling.

**Accepted**

Diphyllobothriasis (treatment)—Niclosamide is indicated in the treatment of diphyllobothriasis caused by *Diphyllobothrium latum* (broad or fish tapeworm).

Hymenolepiasis (treatment)—Niclosamide is indicated in the treatment of hymenolepiasis caused by *Hymenolepis nana* (dwarf tapeworm) and [*H. diminuta* (rat tapeworm)].

Taeniasis (treatment)—Niclosamide is indicated in the treatment of taeniasis caused by *Taenia saginata* (beef tapeworm) and [*T. solium* (pork tapeworm)].

[Dipylidiasis (treatment)]—Niclosamide is used in the treatment of dipylidiasis caused by *Dipylidium caninum* (dog and cat tapeworm).

Although niclosamide is effective in the treatment of cestode infections caused by *T. solium*, it causes disintegration of the proglottids with release of viable eggs into the intestinal lumen. Since this may theoretically result in cysticercosis, quinacrine, which expels *T. solium* intact, may be preferred by some medical experts even though it may be less convenient to administer and is more toxic. However, quinacrine commonly causes vomiting, which may predispose to egg activation in the gastrointestinal lumen.

Niclosamide is effective only in the treatment of intestinal cestodes.

Not all species or strains of a particular helminth may be susceptible to niclosamide.

**Unaccepted**

Niclosamide is not effective against cysticercosis.

## Pharmacology/Pharmacokinetics

**Physicochemical characteristics**

Molecular weight—327.12.

**Mechanism of action/Effect**

Inhibits oxidative phosphorylation in mitochondria of cestodes; anaerobic metabolism, on which many cestodes are dependent, may also be inhibited; scolex and proximal proglottids are rapidly killed on contact; scolex is loosened from intestinal wall and may be digested.

**Absorption**

Not significantly absorbed from the gastrointestinal tract.

**Elimination**

Fecal.

## Precautions to Consider

**Carcinogenicity**

Although carcinogenicity studies have not been done, long-term feeding of the ethanolamine salt of niclosamide to rats and mice has not shown that niclosamide is carcinogenic.

**Mutagenicity**

Studies have not been done.

**Pregnancy/Reproduction**

Fertility—Studies in rats and rabbits given 25 times the human therapeutic dose and studies in mice given 12 times the human therapeutic dose have not shown that niclosamide causes impaired fertility.

Pregnancy—Adequate and well-controlled studies in humans have not been done.

Studies in rats and rabbits given 25 times the human therapeutic dose and studies in mice given 12 times the human therapeutic dose have not shown that niclosamide causes adverse effects in the fetus.

FDA Pregnancy Category B.

**Breast-feeding**

It is not known whether niclosamide is distributed into breast milk. However, problems in humans have not been documented.

**Pediatrics**

Appropriate studies on the relationship of age to the effects of niclosamide have not been performed in children up to 2 years of age. However, no pediatrics-specific problems have been documented to date in children over the age of 2.

**Geriatrics**

No information is available on the relationship of age to the effects of niclosamide in geriatric patients.

**Medical considerations/Contraindications**

The medical considerations/contraindications included here have been selected on the basis of their potential clinical significance (reasons given in parentheses where appropriate)—not necessarily inclusive (» = major clinical significance).

*Risk-benefit should be considered when the following medical problem exists:*

Hypersensitivity to niclosamide

**Patient monitoring**

The following may be especially important in patient monitoring (other tests may be warranted in some patients, depending on condition; » = major clinical significance):

» Stool examinations

(may be required approximately 1 month and 3 months following treatment with niclosamide to determine efficacy or proof of cure; where expulsion of the tapeworm[s] is uncertain, stool examinations for the presence of ova or segments of the worm[s] may be required periodically; no patient should be considered cured unless stool examinations have been negative for 3 months)

## Side/Adverse Effects

The following side/adverse effects have been selected on the basis of their potential clinical significance (possible signs and symptoms in parentheses where appropriate)—not necessarily inclusive:

**Those indicating need for medical attention only if they continue or are bothersome**

Incidence less frequent (1 to 3%)

*Gastrointestinal disturbances* (abdominal or stomach cramps or pain; diarrhea; loss of appetite; nausea or vomiting)

Incidence rare

*Dizziness or lightheadedness; drowsiness; itching of the rectal area; skin rash; unpleasant taste*

## Overdose

For specific information on the agents used in the management of niclosamide overdose, see:

• *Laxatives (Local)* monograph.

For more information on the management of overdose or unintentional ingestion, **contact a Poison Control Center** (see *Poison Control Center Listing*).

**Treatment of overdose**

Recommended treatment consists of the following:

To decrease absorption—

Administering a fast-acting laxative and enema.

Not inducing vomiting.

Supportive care—

Patients in whom intentional overdose is confirmed or suspected should be referred for psychiatric consultation.

## Patient Consultation

As an aid to patient consultation, refer to *Advice for the Patient, Niclosamide (Oral)*.

In providing consultation, consider emphasizing the following selected information (» = major clinical significance):

**Before using this medication**
» Conditions affecting use, especially:
    Hypersensitivity to niclosamide

**Proper use of this medication**
    No special preparations or additional measures (e.g., dietary restrictions or fasting, concurrent medications, purging, or cleansing enemas) required before, during, or immediately after therapy
    Taking on an empty stomach or after a light meal (for example, breakfast)
    Chewing or crushing tablets; in young children, crushing tablets and mixing with small amount of water to form a paste
» Proper storage
*For beef, fish, and dwarf tapeworms*
» Compliance with full course of therapy; second course may be required
» Proper dosing
» Missed dose: Taking as soon as possible; not taking if almost time for next dose; do not double doses

**Precautions while using this medication**
*For beef, fish, and dwarf tapeworms*
    Regular visits to physician to check progress
    Checking with physician if no improvement within a few days

## General Dosing Information

No special preparations or additional measures (e.g., dietary restrictions or fasting, concurrent medications, purging, or cleansing enemas) are required before, during, or immediately after treatment with niclosamide.

Niclosamide should preferably be taken after a light meal (for example, breakfast). However, it may also be taken on an empty stomach (either 1 hour before or 2 hours after a meal).

In *Diphyllobothrium latum* (broad or fish tapeworm) and *Taenia saginata* (beef tapeworm) infections in which proglottids and/or ova persist for 7 days after treatment, a second course of niclosamide may be administered.

In *Hymenolepis nana* (dwarf tapeworm) infections, both mature cestodes and cysticerci (larvae) are found in the intestine. Cysticerci maturing in the intestinal wall are generally resistant to niclosamide. Therefore, therapy should be continued for 7 days to cover adequately all stages of maturation. A second course of niclosamide may be administered 7 to 14 days after initial treatment if necessary.

To prevent the development of cysticercosis in the treatment of *T. solium* (pork tapeworm) infections, a magnesium sulfate or other saline purge should be administered approximately 1 to 2 hours after niclosamide. This may also aid in the identification of the tapeworm by permitting the expulsion of an intact scolex.

## Oral Dosage Forms

Note: Bracketed uses in the *Dosage Forms* section refer to categories of use and/or indications that are not included in U.S. product labeling.

### NICLOSAMIDE CHEWABLE TABLETS

**Usual adult and adolescent dose**
*Diphyllobothrium latum*, [*Dipylidium caninum*], *Taenia saginata*, and [*T. solium*] infections—
    Oral, 2 grams as a single dose. May be repeated in seven days if required.
*Hymenolepis nana* and [*H. diminuta*] infections—
    Oral, 2 grams once a day for seven days. May be repeated in seven to fourteen days in *H. nana* infections if required.
    Note: Some medical experts recommend a dose of 2 grams as a single dose the first day, then 1 gram once a day for the next six days for *Hymenolepis nana* and [*H. diminuta*] infections.

**Usual pediatric dose**
*Diphyllobothrium latum*, [*Dipylidium caninum*], *Taenia saginata*, and [*T. solium*] infections—
    Children 11 to 34 kg of body weight: Oral, 1 gram as a single dose. May be repeated in seven days if required.
    Children over 34 kg of body weight: Oral, 1.5 grams as a single dose. May be repeated in seven days if required.
*Hymenolepis nana* and [*H. diminuta*] infections—
    Children 11 to 34 kg of body weight: Oral, 1 gram as a single dose the first day, then 500 mg once a day for the next six days. May be repeated in seven to fourteen days in *H. nana* infections if required.
    Children over 34 kg of body weight: Oral, 1.5 grams as a single dose the first day, then 1 gram once a day for the next six days. May be repeated in seven to fourteen days in *H. nana* infections if required.
Note: Children under 2 years of age—Dosage has not been established.

**Strength(s) usually available**
U.S.—
    500 mg (Rx) [*Niclocide* (sodium saccharin)].
Canada—
    Not commercially available.

**Packaging and storage**
Store below 30 °C (86 °F), in a well-closed container, unless otherwise specified by manufacturer.

**Auxiliary labeling**
• Chew or crush tablets before swallowing.
• Continue medication for full time of treatment (dwarf tapeworm infections).

Revised: 06/23/95

---

# NICOTINE   Systemic

VA CLASSIFICATION (Primary): AD900
Note: For a listing of dosage forms and brand names by country availability, see *Dosage Forms* section(s). For a listing of brand names for the articles in this monograph, refer to the General Index.

## Category
Smoking cessation adjunct.

## Indications

**Accepted**
Nicotine dependence (treatment adjunct)—Nicotine chewing gum and nicotine transdermal systems are indicated as temporary aids to the cigarette smoker who wants to give up smoking while participating in a behavior modification program. They provide an alternate source of nicotine for nicotine-dependent individuals acutely withdrawing from cigarette smoking.

Behavior modification encompasses supervised programs of education, counseling, and psychological support. The efficacy of these nicotine products without concomitant participation in such a program has not been established.

Generally, smokers who have a strong physical nicotine dependence are more likely to benefit from the use of these nicotine products.

Smoking withdrawal effects such as irritability, drowsiness, fatigue, headache, and nicotine craving are lessened with their use.

Nicotine chewing gum has not been shown to be beneficial for longer than 3 months. The use of nicotine transdermal systems for longer than 12 to 20 weeks, depending on the product, has not been evaluated and is not recommended.

**Unaccepted**
Nicotine chewing gum and transdermal systems are not recommended for use by nonsmokers because increase in heart rate and blood pressure and central nervous system (CNS)–mediated symptoms such as hiccups, nausea, and vomiting are associated with even small doses of nicotine from these products. Also, nicotine in these products may cause dependence in nonsmokers.

## Pharmacology/Pharmacokinetics

**Physicochemical characteristics**
Molecular weight—Nicotine: 162.2.

**Mechanism of action/Effect**
Nicotine acts as an agonist at the nicotinic receptors in the peripheral and central nervous systems, producing both stimulant and depressant phases of action on all autonomic ganglia.

When the gum is chewed, nicotine is displaced from polacrilex by alkaline saliva.

#### Other actions/effects

Has actions on the chemoreceptors of the aortic and carotid bodies, resulting in reflex vasoconstriction, tachycardia, elevated blood pressure, and stimulation of respiration.

Stimulates sympathetic ganglia and adrenal medulla, causing release of catecholamines, resulting in direct sympathomimetic effects on the heart and peripheral vasculature.

Has actions that tend to reduce blood pressure and heart rate. In low concentrations, stimulates certain chemoreceptors in the pulmonary and coronary circulation, leading to reflex bradycardia and hypotension.

Causes release of antidiuretic hormone (ADH) by stimulation of hypothalamus.

Stimulation of emetic chemoreceptor trigger zone of medulla oblongata and vagal reflex activation may result in vomiting.

Parasympathetic stimulation increases tone and motor activity of the gastrointestinal tract, leading to nausea, vomiting, and occasionally diarrhea.

Effects of nicotine on exocrine glands cause an initial stimulation followed by inhibition of salivary and bronchial secretions.

Action on CNS may result in respiratory failure due to both central paralysis and peripheral blockade of muscles of respiration.

#### Absorption

Chewing gum—
> Buccal mucosa: Absorption enhanced by buffering of gum to pH 8.5; rate of absorption is slower than from lungs during smoking.
> Stomach: Not absorbed in significant amounts when gum is swallowed because of poor release of nicotine from gum in acidic pH of stomach.

Transdermal systems—
> Skin: Well absorbed.

#### Distribution

Nicotine passes into breast milk.

#### Biotransformation

Primarily hepatic; smaller amounts are metabolized in the kidneys and lungs; metabolites include cotinine and nicotine-1'-N-oxide.

#### Half-life

Nicotine—1 to 2 hours.

Cotinine—15 to 20 hours.

#### Time to peak concentration

Chewing gum—
> 15 to 30 minutes after start of chewing.

Transdermal systems (at steady state)—
> *Habitrol:* 5 to 6 hours after application.
> *Nicoderm:* 4 hours after application.
> *ProStep:* 9 hours after application.

#### Peak serum concentration

Average steady-state—
> Chewing gum:
> 7.9 to 10.8 nanograms per mL.
> Transdermal systems:
> *Habitrol*—17 nanograms per mL following application of the 21 mg/day patch.
> *Nicoderm*—23 nanograms per mL following application of the 21 mg/day patch; 17 nanograms per mL following application of the 14 mg/day patch; 8 nanograms per mL following application of the 7 mg/day patch.
> *ProStep*—16 nanograms per mL following application of the 22 mg/day patch.

#### Elimination

Renal, 10 to 20% unchanged; up to 30% may be excreted in acidified urine (pH <5) and with high urine flow rate.

### Precautions to Consider

#### Carcinogenicity

Nicotine does not appear to be carcinogenic in laboratory animals. Inconclusive evidence suggests that cotinine, an oxidized metabolite, may be carcinogenic in rats.

#### Tumorigenicity

When given in combination with tumor initiators, nicotine and its metabolites increased the incidence of tumors in hamsters and rats.

#### Mutagenicity

Neither nicotine nor its metabolite, cotinine, was shown to be mutagenic in the Ames *Salmonella* test. Nicotine induced repairable DNA dam-

age in an *E. coli* test system. Nicotine was shown to be genotoxic in Chinese hamster ovary cells.

#### Pregnancy/Reproduction

Fertility—Impaired fertility has been demonstrated in mice. In addition, implantation was delayed or inhibited in rats and rabbits by reduction in DNA synthesis that appears to be caused by nicotine. Rats treated with nicotine during the time of gestation have produced decreased litter sizes.

Pregnancy—Nicotine replacement therapy is not recommended during pregnancy and should be used only if the likelihood of smoking cessation justifies the potential risk in pregnant patients who continue to smoke. Pregnant smokers should be encouraged to attempt smoking cessation using education and behavioral interventions before using pharmacological measures.

Cigarette smoking may cause low birth weight, increased risk of spontaneous abortion, and increased perinatal mortality. Spontaneous abortion during nicotine replacement therapy has been reported, and possibly may be due to the nicotine.

Studies in pregnant rhesus monkeys have shown that nicotine administered intravenously produces acidosis, hypoxia, and hypercarbia in the fetus. Teratogenicity has been demonstrated in offspring of mice given toxic doses of nicotine.

Nicotine chewing gum—FDA Pregnancy Category X.

Nicotine transdermal systems—FDA Pregnancy Category D.

#### Breast-feeding

Nicotine is distributed into breast milk. Problems in humans have not been documented; however, because of the potential for serious adverse effects, risk-benefit must be considered.

#### Pediatrics

Small amounts of nicotine can cause serious harm in children. Even used nicotine transdermal systems contain enough nicotine to cause potential problems in children.

#### Geriatrics

Appropriate studies on the relationship of age to the effects of nicotine have not been performed in the geriatric population. However, evidence to date from a limited number of geriatric patients has not indicated geriatrics-specific problems.

#### Dental

When used over an extended period of time, nicotine gum may cause severe occlusal stress because its viscosity is heavier than ordinary chewing gum. This can cause loosening of inlays or fillings, can stick to dentures, and can cause damage to oral mucosa and natural teeth. The use of hard sugarless candy between doses of gum is recommended to help alleviate mucosal discomfort and to provide oral stimulation required by some patients. Also, some temporomandibular joint dysfunction and pain have been associated with excessive chewing.

#### Drug interactions and/or related problems

The following drug interactions and/or related problems have been selected on the basis of their potential clinical significance (possible mechanism in parentheses where appropriate)—not necessarily inclusive (» = major clinical significance):

Note: Combinations containing any of the following medications, depending on the amount present, may also interact with this medication.

» Bronchodilators, xanthine-derivative, except dyphylline or
» Propoxyphene or
» Propranolol, and possibly other beta-adrenergic blocking agents
> (smoking cessation may increase therapeutic effects of these agents by decreasing metabolism, thereby increasing serum concentrations; dosage adjustments may be necessary)

» Insulin
> (smoking cessation and concurrent therapy with nicotine chewing gum, transdermal systems, or other smoking deterrents, such as lobeline sulfate and silver acetate, may increase the therapeutic effects of insulin by increasing absorption, thereby increasing serum concentrations; dosage reduction of insulin may be necessary when an insulin-dependent diabetic patient suddenly stops smoking)

#### Medical considerations/Contraindications

The medical considerations/contraindications included here have been selected on the basis of their potential clinical significance (reasons given in parentheses where appropriate)—not necessarily inclusive (» = major clinical significance).

*Except under special circumstances, this medication should not be used when the following medical problems exist:*

» Angina pectoris, severe or
» Cardiac arrhythmias, life-threatening or

» Post-myocardial infarction
(may be exacerbated by action on heart of catecholamines released from adrenal medulla; tolerance to this effect does not develop)

*Risk-benefit should be considered when the following medical problems exist:*
Angina pectoris or
Cardiac arrhythmias or
Diabetes mellitus, insulin-dependent or
Hypertension or
Hyperthyroidism or
Myocardial infarction, history of or
Pheochromocytoma or
Vasospastic diseases, such as Buerger's disease and Prinzmetal's (or variant) angina
(increases in blood pressure, heart rate, and plasma glucose concentrations may result from effects of nicotine-induced catecholamine release)
Peptic ulcer disease, history of
(may be exacerbated)
Sensitivity to nicotine

*For the chewing gum only (in addition to the above)*
Dental problems or
Temporomandibular joint (TMJ) disorder
(injury to teeth or aggravation of TMJ may result from mechanical effects of chewing gum)
Esophagitis, history of or
Inflammation of mouth or throat
(may be exacerbated)

*For the transdermal systems only (in addition to the above)*
Skin diseases
(may be exacerbated)

**Patient monitoring**
The following may be especially important in patient monitoring (other tests may be warranted in some patients, depending on condition; » = major clinical significance):
» Evaluation of progress of smoking cessation
(recommended periodically during therapy to assess therapeutic efficacy of nicotine replacement products and to re-evaluate their use)

## Side/Adverse Effects

Note: Side effects are dose-dependent; extremely high doses can produce toxic symptoms, even in nicotine-tolerant individuals.

The following side/adverse effects have been selected on the basis of their potential clinical significance (possible signs and symptoms in parentheses where appropriate)—not necessarily inclusive:

**Those indicating need for medical attention**
Incidence more frequent
*For chewing gum only*
*Injury to mouth, teeth, or dental work*
Note: Nicotine gum is stickier and of heavier viscosity than ordinary gum, making it harder to chew.

Incidence rare
*For all nicotine replacement products*
*Atrial fibrillation, reversible* (irregular heartbeat); *hypersensitivity reactions, local or generalized, including edema* (swelling); *erythema* (redness); *pruritus* (itching); *rash; or urticaria* (hives)

**Those indicating need for medical attention only if they continue or are bothersome**
Incidence more frequent
*For all nicotine replacement products*
*Fast heartbeat; headache, mild; increased appetite*
*For chewing gum only*
*Belching*—may be minimized by modifying chewing technique; *increased watering of mouth, mild; jaw muscle ache; sore mouth or throat*
*For transdermal systems only*
*Erythema, pruritus, and/or burning at site of application* (redness, itching, and/or burning)—usually subsides within an hour
Incidence less frequent or rare
*For all nicotine replacement products*
*Constipation; coughing, increased; diarrhea; dizziness or lightheadedness, mild; drowsiness; dryness of mouth; dysmenorrhea* (menstrual pain); *insomnia* (trouble in sleeping); *or abnormal dreams; loss of appetite; muscle or joint pain; stomach upset or*

*indigestion, mild; sweating, increased; unusual irritability or nervousness*
*For chewing gum only*
*Hiccups; hoarseness*

## Overdose

For specific information on the agents used in the management of nicotine overdose, see:
• Atropine in *Anticholinergics/Antispasmodics (Systemic)* monograph;
• *Barbiturates (Systemic)* monograph;
• *Charcoal, Activated (Oral-Local)* monograph;
• *Diazepam* in *Benzodiazepines (Systemic)* monograph; and/or
• *Ipecac (Oral-Local)* monograph.

For more information on the management of overdose or unintentional ingestion, **contact a Poison Control Center** (see *Poison Control Center Listing*).

**Clinical effects of overdose**
The following effects have been selected on the basis of their potential clinical significance (possible signs and symptoms in parentheses where appropriate)—not necessarily inclusive:
Early effects of overdose (in possible order of occurrence)
*Nausea and/or vomiting; increased watering of mouth, severe; abdominal pain, severe; diarrhea, severe; cold sweat; headache, severe; dizziness, severe; drooling; disturbed hearing and vision; confusion; weakness, severe*
Late effects of overdose (in possible order of occurrence)
*Fainting; hypotension; difficulty in breathing, severe; fast, weak, or irregular pulse; convulsions*
Note: *Overdose* may occur if many pieces of gum are chewed simultaneously or in rapid succession, or may occur after a single piece of gum in some patients; absorption may be reduced by the early nausea and vomiting known to occur with excessive nicotine intake; if gum is swallowed without chewing, little nicotine will be released or absorbed in significant amounts because of acid pH of stomach.

**Treatment of overdose**
For chewing gum only—
To decrease absorption—In a conscious patient, if emesis has not occurred, induction of vomiting with ipecac syrup. In an unconscious patient with a clear airway, gastric lavage followed by a suspension of activated charcoal left in the stomach.
To enhance elimination—A saline cathartic will hasten the gastrointestinal passage of the gum.
For transdermal systems only—
To decrease absorption—Remove patch and flush skin surface with water and dry. Do not use soap, because it may increase nicotine absorption. If patch has been ingested, administer activated charcoal. Repeated doses of charcoal should be administered as long as the patch remains in the gastrointestinal tract because it will continue to release nicotine.
To enhance elimination—A saline cathartic or sorbitol may be added to the first dose of activated charcoal to speed passage of the patch.
For all nicotine replacement products—
Supportive care—Respiratory support for respiratory failure. Intensive treatment of hypotension and cardiovascular collapse. Anticonvulsants such as diazepam or barbiturates for seizures. Administration of atropine for excessive bronchial secretions or diarrhea. Patients in whom intentional overdose is confirmed or suspected should be referred for psychiatric consultation.

## Patient Consultation

As an aid to patient consultation, refer to *Advice for the Patient, Nicotine (Systemic)*.

In providing consultation, consider emphasizing the following selected information (» = major clinical significance):

**Before using this medication**
» Conditions affecting use, especially:
Pregnancy—Not recommended during pregnancy; spontaneous abortions have been reported; use only if the likelihood of smoking cessation justifies the potential risk in pregnant patients who continue to smoke
Breast-feeding—Distributed into breast milk
Use in children—Small amounts of nicotine can cause serious harm in children
Dental—Chewing gum may cause severe occlusive stress resulting in damage to teeth, dentures, or dental work
Other medications, especially insulin, propoxyphene, propranolol, or xanthine-derivative bronchodilators (except dyphylline)

Other medical problems, especially severe angina pectoris, life-threatening cardiac arrhythmias, postmyocardial infarction state

**Proper use of this medication**

*Proper administration of the chewing gum*
» Reading patient instructions carefully before using
» Participating in a supervised stop-smoking program
» Using gum only when there is an urge to smoke
» Chewing gum slowly and intermittently for 30 minutes
» Not chewing too fast, not chewing more than one piece of gum at a time, and not chewing one piece too soon after another, to avoid adverse effects or overdose

*Compliance with chewing gum therapy*
» Reducing number of pieces chewed each day over a 2- to 3-month period
» Importance of carrying gum at all times during therapy
» Using hard sugarless candy between doses of gum to help alleviate mucosal discomfort

*Proper administration of the transdermal systems*
» Reading patient instructions carefully before using
» Participating in a supervised stop-smoking program
» Keeping patch in sealed pouch until ready to apply to skin
» Not trimming or cutting patch
» Applying to clean, dry skin area on upper arm or torso free of oil, hair, scars, cuts, burns, or irritation
» Pressing the patch firmly in place with palm for about 10 seconds; making sure there is good contact, especially around edges
» Keeping patch in place even during showering, bathing, or swimming; replacing systems that have fallen off
» Washing hands with plain water after handling patches; soap will enhance transdermal absorption of nicotine
» Alternating application sites
» Folding used patches in half with adhesive sides together, and replacing in protective pouch or aluminum foil; disposing of patch carefully, out of reach of children or pets
» Getting into the habit of changing patch at the same time each day to help increase compliance
» Proper dosing
» Proper storage

**Precautions while using this medication**
» Regular visits to physician to check progress in smoking cessation
» Not smoking during treatment with nicotine replacement products
» Not using nicotine replacement products during pregnancy
» Prevention of accidental ingestion of nicotine replacement products by children or pets to prevent poisoning

*For the chewing gum only*
» Not chewing more than 24 pieces of gum a day
» Not using gum for longer than 6 months to avoid physical dependence
» Discontinuing use and consulting physician or dentist if excessive sticking to dental work occurs; gum may damage dental work or dentures

*For the transdermal systems only*
» Calling physician and not applying new patch if evidence of allergic reaction; knowing that allergic reaction to nicotine patch could cause reaction to use of cigarettes or other products containing nicotine
» Not using patches for longer than 20 weeks

**Side/adverse effects**
Signs of potential side effects, especially injury to mouth, teeth, or dental work (with gum only); irregular heartbeat; or hypersensitivity reaction (with transdermal systems only)

## General Dosing Information

The necessity of immediate cessation of smoking upon initiation of therapy must be emphasized.

Overdose of nicotine can be fatal, especially in small children. Immediate treatment is necessary.

**For chewing gum only**

When there is an urge to smoke, one piece of gum is chewed very slowly and intermittently for about 30 minutes until most (90%) of the nicotine is released.

The amount of nicotine released depends on the rate of chewing and the amount of time the saliva is in contact with the resin.

The use of nicotine polacrilex for longer than 3 months may be an indication that this medication is being used as a substitute source of nicotine to maintain nicotine dependence. If gum consumption has not been spontaneously reduced within 6 months, a gradual withdrawal should be initiated.

**For transdermal systems only**

If a patient is unable to stop smoking by the 4th week of therapy, treatment should be discontinued, as the patient is unlikely to quit on that attempt.

The use of nicotine patches for longer than 12 to 20 weeks (depending on the product) in patients who have stopped smoking has not been evaluated and is not recommended because chronic use of nicotine can be harmful and addictive.

Most manufacturers supply supportive instructional materials and provide telephone information accessible by patients.

## Oral Dosage Forms

### NICOTINE POLACRILEX GUM USP

**Usual adult and adolescent dose**

Smoking cessation adjunct—
  Oral, 2 or 4 mg as a chewing gum, the dose being repeated as determined by individual's urge to smoke and rate of chewing.

Note: Most patients require approximately 20 mg a day during first month of treatment.

  Some clinicians maintain that patients initially need at least 12 pieces daily and recommend regular dosing, such as 1 piece per hour while awake, in addition to doses taken in response to an individual's urge to smoke.

**Usual adult prescribing limits**

96 mg a day.

**Usual pediatric dose**

Safety and efficacy have not been established.

**Strength(s) usually available**

U.S.—

  2 mg (OTC) [*Nicorette* (flavors; glycerin; gum base; sodium bicarbonate; sodium carbonate; sorbitol)].

  4 mg (OTC) [*Nicorette* (flavors; glycerin; gum base; sodium carbonate; sorbitol; D&C Yellow No. 10)].

Canada—

  2 mg (OTC) [*Nicorette* (gum; menthol; magnesium oxide; peppermint oil; sodium bicarbonate; sodium carbonate; xylitol)].

  4 mg (Rx) [*Nicorette Plus* (gum; magnesium oxide; menthol; peppermint oil; sodium carbonate; xylitol; D&C Yellow No. 10)].

**Packaging and storage**

Store below 40 °C (104 °F), preferably between 15 and 30 °C (59 and 86 °F), unless otherwise specified by manufacturer. Protect from light.

**Auxiliary labeling**
• Chew slowly.
• Do not chew more than 24 pieces in one day.

## Topical Dosage Forms

### NICOTINE TRANSDERMAL SYSTEM

**Usual adult dose**

Smoking cessation adjunct; depending on the product—
  Patients weighing more than 100 pounds, smoking more than 10 cigarettes a day, and without cardiovascular disease:
    16-hour system: Topical, to intact skin—
      *Nicotrol*: Initially one 15-mg system applied for sixteen hours per day for four to twelve weeks. Patients who have successfully abstained from smoking should have their dose reduced to one 10-mg system applied for sixteen hours per day for the next two to four weeks, and then to one 5-mg system applied for sixteen hours per day for the following two to four weeks.
    24-hour system: Topical, to intact skin—
      *Habitrol*: Initially one 21-mg system per day for four to eight weeks. Patients who have successfully abstained from smoking should have their dose reduced to one 14-mg system per day for the next two to four weeks. The dosage should be further reduced to one 7-mg system per day for the following two to four weeks.
      *Nicoderm*: Initially one 21-mg system per day for six weeks. Patients who have successfully abstained from smoking should have their dose reduced to one 14-mg system per day for two weeks. The dosage should be further reduced to one 7-mg system per day for two weeks.
      *ProStep*: Initially one 22-mg system per day for four to eight weeks. Patients who have successfully abstained from smoking should have their dose reduced to one 11-mg system per day for two to four weeks.

Patients weighing less than 100 pounds, smoking less than 10 cigarettes a day, or with cardiovascular disease:
24-hour system: Topical, to intact skin—
> *Habitrol*: Initially one 14-mg system per day for four to eight
> weeks. Patients who have successfully abstained from
> smoking should have their dose reduced to one 7-mg sys-
> tem per day for the next two to four weeks.
>
> *Nicoderm*: Initially one 14-mg system per day for six weeks.
> Patients who have successfully abstained from smoking
> should have their dose reduced to one 7-mg system per day
> for two to four weeks.
>
> *ProStep*: Initially one 11-mg system per day for four to eight
> weeks.

**Usual pediatric dose**
Safety and efficacy have not been established.

**Usual geriatric dose**
See *Usual adult dose.*

**Strength(s) usually available**
U.S.—
16-hour Systems
5 mg (Rx) [*Nicotrol*].
10 mg (Rx) [*Nicotrol*].
15 mg (Rx) [*Nicotrol*].
24-hour Systems
7 mg (Rx) [*Habitrol; Nicoderm*].
11 mg (Rx) [*ProStep*].
14 mg (Rx) [*Habitrol; Nicoderm*].

21 mg (Rx) [*Habitrol; Nicoderm*].
22 mg (Rx) [*ProStep*].
Canada—
16-hour Systems
5 mg (Rx) [*Nicotrol*].
10 mg (Rx) [*Nicotrol*].
15 mg (Rx) [*Nicotrol*].
24-hour Systems
7 mg (Rx) [*Habitrol; Nicoderm*].
11 mg (Rx) [*ProStep*].
14 mg (Rx) [*Habitrol; Nicoderm*].
21 mg (Rx) [*Habitrol; Nicoderm*].
22 mg (Rx) [*ProStep*].

Note: Nicotine transdermal systems are designed to release a constant,
controlled dose of nicotine over the period during which they are
applied to the skin. Systems are labeled by the dose actually absorbed by the patient, not by the total nicotine content.

**Packaging and storage**
Store below 30 °C (86 °F), in the intact pouch. Because nicotine is volatile,
the system may lose strength if removed from pouch prematurely.

**Auxiliary labeling**
• For external use only.
• Follow the manufacturer's directions carefully.

Revised: 09/08/92
Interim revision: 05/19/94; 07/11/96

# NICOTINYL ALCOHOL    Systemic*

VA CLASSIFICATION (Primary): CV500
Note: For a listing of dosage forms and brand names by country availability, see *Dosage Forms* section(s). For a listing of brand names
for the articles in this monograph, refer to the General Index.

*Not commercially available in the U.S.

## Category
Vasospastic therapy adjunct.

## Indications

**Accepted**
Vascular disease, peripheral (treatment)
Vascular spasm (treatment)
Ulcer, varicose (treatment)
Ulcer, decubital (treatment)
Frostbite (treatment)
Ear, inner, circulatory disturbances of (Menière's syndrome) (treatment)
or
Vertigo (treatment)—Nicotinyl alcohol may be effective for its labeled
indications, which include peripheral vascular disease, vascular spasm,
varicose ulcers, decubital ulcers, chilblains (frostbite), Menière's syn-
drome, and vertigo.

## Pharmacology/Pharmacokinetics

**Physicochemical characteristics**
Molecular weight—109.13.

**Mechanism of action/Effect**
Nicotinyl alcohol's action occurs as a result of its *in vivo* conversion to
niacin (nicotinic acid). Nicotinic acid produces weak peripheral vasodilation by a direct effect on vascular smooth muscle; however, in
usual doses it is probable that only cutaneous vessels are affected.

**Onset of action**
Vasodilator effect—Extended-release tablets: 30 minutes.

**Time to peak effect**
Clinical improvement may occur gradually over several weeks.

**Duration of action**
Vasodilator effect—Extended-release tablets: 6–12 hours.

## Precautions to Consider

**Pregnancy/Reproduction**
Pregnancy—Studies have not been done in humans.
Studies have not been done in animals.

**Breast-feeding**
It is not known whether nicotinyl alcohol is excreted in breast milk. However, problems in humans have not been documented.

**Geriatrics**
Appropriate studies on the relationship of age to the effects of nicotinyl
alcohol have not been performed in the geriatric population. However,
the risk of nicotinyl alcohol–induced hypothermia may be increased
in elderly patients.

**Drug interactions and/or related problems**
The following drug interactions and/or related problems have been selected on the basis of their potential clinical significance (possible
mechanism in parentheses where appropriate)—not necessarily inclusive (» = major clinical significance):
Smoking, tobacco
(heavy smoking may interfere with the therapeutic effect of nicotinyl alcohol because nicotine constricts blood vessels)

**Laboratory value alterations**
The following have been selected on the basis of their potential clinical
significance (possible effect in parentheses where appropriate)—not
necessarily inclusive (» = major clinical significance):
With physiology/laboratory test values
Alanine aminotransferase (ALT [SGPT]), serum and
Alkaline phosphatase, serum and
Aspartate aminotransferase (AST [SGOT]), serum and
Bilirubin, serum and
Lactate dehydrogenase (LDH), serum
(concentrations may be increased, indicating hepatotoxicity, with
long-term, high-dose administration)

Glucose, blood and urine
(concentrations may be increased in diabetic or pre-diabetic patients or when high doses are administered to patients with
hypercholesterolemia)

**Medical considerations/Contraindications**
The medical considerations/contraindications included here have been selected on the basis of their potential clinical significance (reasons given
in parentheses where appropriate)—not necessarily inclusive (» =
major clinical significance).

*Risk-benefit should be considered when the following medical problems exist:*

» Active peptic ulcer or gastritis
» Cerebrovascular disease, severe or
» Myocardial infarction, recent or
» Obliterative coronary artery disease, severe
      (a "steal effect" may occur, since nicotinyl alcohol has a greater effect on peripheral vessels than on cerebral and coronary vessels, leading to a further decrease in flow to ischemic areas)
    Diabetes mellitus
      (nicotinyl alcohol may increase fasting blood sugar concentrations)
    Glaucoma, predisposition to
    Hyperlipidemia
      (large doses necessary to treat this condition may cause impaired glucose tolerance)
    Sensitivity to nicotinyl alcohol

## Side/Adverse Effects

The following side/adverse effects have been selected on the basis of their potential clinical significance (possible signs and symptoms in parentheses where appropriate)—not necessarily inclusive:

**Those indicating need for medical attention**
Incidence rare—dose-related
    *Hepatotoxicity* (swelling of feet or lower legs; yellow eyes or skin)
    Note: *Hepatotoxicity* occurs only with very high doses.

**Those indicating need for medical attention only if they continue or are bothersome**
Incidence more frequent
    *Vasodilation, especially on face and neck* (flushing; warmth or tingling)
Incidence less frequent or rare
    *Allergic reaction* (skin rash); *diarrhea; hypotension* (dizziness or faintness); *increased hair loss; nausea and vomiting*

## Patient Consultation

As an aid to patient consultation, refer to *Advice for the Patient, Nicotinyl Alcohol (Systemic)*.

In providing consultation, consider emphasizing the following selected information (» = major clinical significance):

**Before using this medication**
» Conditions affecting use, especially:
    Sensitivity to nicotinyl alcohol
    Use in the elderly—Increased risk of hypothermia
    Other medical problems, especially peptic ulcer or gastritis (active), cerebrovascular disease, recent myocardial infarction, or obliterative coronary artery disease (severe)

**Proper use of this medication**
    Swallowing tablets whole; not breaking, crushing, or chewing prior to swallowing

» Proper dosing
    Missed dose: Taking as soon as possible; not taking if almost time for next dose; not doubling doses
» Proper storage

**Precautions while using this medication**
    Checking with physician before discontinuing medication
    Avoiding smoking (nicotine constricts blood vessels)

**Side/adverse effects**
    Signs of potential side effects, especially hepatotoxicity

## Oral Dosage Forms

Note: The dosage and strengths of the dosage form available are expressed in terms of nicotinyl alcohol.

### NICOTINYL ALCOHOL TARTRATE EXTENDED-RELEASE TABLETS

**Usual adult dose**
Vasospastic therapy adjunct—
    Oral, 150 to 300 mg (nicotinyl alcohol) two times a day, in the morning and evening.

**Strength(s) usually available**
U.S.—
    Not commercially available.
Canada—
    150 mg (nicotinyl alcohol) (OTC) [*Roniacol* (sucrose)].

**Packaging and storage**
Store below 40 °C (104 °F), preferably between 15 and 30 °C (59 and 86 °F), in a well-closed container, unless otherwise specified by manufacturer.

**Auxiliary labeling**
• Swallow tablets whole.

Revised: 04/06/93

---

**NIFEDIPINE**—See *Calcium Channel Blocking Agents (Systemic)*

---

**NIFURTIMOX**—Since Nifurtimox is not commercially available in the U.S. or Canada, the *Nifurtimox (Systemic)* monograph is not included in this published version of the USP DI database. Copies of the monograph are available on request from the USP Division of Information Development, 12601 Twinbrook Parkway, Rockville, MD 20852; telephone (301) 816-8351; telefax (301) 816-8374.

---

**NIMODIPINE**—See *Calcium Channel Blocking Agents (Systemic)*

---

# NITRATES   Systemic

This monograph includes information on the following: Erythrityl Tetranitrate; Isosorbide Dinitrate; Isosorbide Mononitrate†; Nitroglycerin; Pentaerythritol Tetranitrate.

INN:
    Erythrityl Tetranitrate—Eritrityl Tetranitrate
    Pentaerythritol Tetranitrate—Pentaerithrityl Tetranitrate
VA CLASSIFICATION (Primary/Secondary):
    Erythrityl tetranitrate—CV250/CV900
    Isosorbide dinitrate—CV250/CV900
    Isosorbide mononitrate—CV250
    Nitroglycerin—CV250/CV490; CV900
    Pentaerythritol tetranitrate—CV250/CV900

Other commonly used names are: Eritrityl tetranitrate [Erythrityl Tetranitrate], Erythritol tetranitrate [Erythrityl Tetranitrate], Glyceryl trinitrate [Nitroglycerin], Pentaerithrityl tetranitrate [Pentaerythritol Tetranitrate], P.E.T.N. [Pentaerythritol Tetranitrate]

Note: For a listing of dosage forms and brand names by country availability, see *Dosage Forms* section(s). For a listing of brand names for the articles in this monograph, refer to the General Index.

†Not commercially available in Canada.

## Category

Note: All of the nitrates have similar pharmacologic actions; however, clinical uses among specific agents may vary because of actual pharmacokinetic differences, availability of specific testing, and/or availability of clinical-use data.

Antianginal—Erythrityl Tetranitrate; Isosorbide Dinitrate; Isosorbide Mononitrate; Nitroglycerin; Pentaerythritol Tetranitrate.
Antihypertensive—Nitroglycerin Injection.
Vasodilator, congestive heart failure—Erythrityl Tetranitrate; Isosorbide Dinitrate; Nitroglycerin; Pentaerythritol Tetranitrate.

## Indications

Note: Bracketed information in the *Indications* section refers to uses that are not included in U.S. product labeling.

See *Table 1*, page 2151.

**Accepted**
Angina pectoris, acute (treatment)—The sublingual, lingual, and extended-release buccal[1] dosage forms of nitroglycerin and the sublingual[1] and chewable dosage forms of isosorbide dinitrate are indicated for the relief of pain of an acute episode of angina pectoris due to coronary

artery disease. Sublingual or lingual nitroglycerin is preferred; isosorbide dinitrate should be used in patients intolerant of or unresponsive to nitroglycerin. Sublingual isosorbide dinitrate[1] or sublingual or lingual nitroglycerin may be administered to relieve acute anginal attacks that may occur while the patient is on oral prophylactic therapy.

Angina pectoris, acute (prophylaxis)—The sublingual, lingual[1], and extended-release buccal dosage forms of nitroglycerin; the sublingual dosage form of erythrityl tetranitrate; and the sublingual or chewable dosage forms of isosorbide dinitrate are indicated for prophylaxis of acute angina attacks in situations (such as stress or exertion) likely to provoke such attacks.

Angina pectoris, chronic (treatment)—The oral/sublingual dosage form of erythrityl tetranitrate; the regular, chewable, sublingual, and extended-release oral dosage forms of isosorbide dinitrate; the regular and extended-release oral dosage forms of isosorbide mononitrate; and the extended-release oral and buccal dosage forms of nitroglycerin are indicated for the prophylaxis and long-term treatment of angina pectoris due to coronary artery disease, but not in the treatment of acute anginal attacks (except for chewable isosorbide dinitrate and buccal nitroglycerin). Rapid first-pass hepatic destruction of nitroglycerin may increase the dosage requirements of the oral extended-release capsules and tablets in the prophylaxis and treatment of angina.

FDA has classified the oral dosage forms of pentaerythritol tetranitrate as *possibly effective* in the prophylaxis of angina pectoris, but not in the treatment of acute attacks. This classification requires the submission of adequate and well-controlled studies in order to provide substantial evidence of effectiveness.

Nitroglycerin injection is indicated in the treatment of unstable angina pectoris in patients who have not responded to recommended doses of other organic nitrates and/or a beta-blocker.

Nitroglycerin ointment and nitroglycerin transdermal systems are indicated for the prophylaxis and long-term treatment of angina pectoris but are not indicated for the relief of an acute angina episode.

Hypertension (treatment) or
Hypotension, controlled—Nitroglycerin injection is indicated for blood pressure control during certain surgical procedures and for controlled hypotension during surgery to reduce bleeding into the surgical field.

Myocardial infarction (treatment adjunct) or
Congestive heart failure (treatment)—Nitroglycerin injection is indicated in the adjunctive therapy for congestive heart failure associated or not associated with acute myocardial infarction. (Treatment of congestive heart failure not associated with acute myocardial infarction is not included in Canadian product labeling.) [Sublingual][1], [lingual][1], and [topical][1] nitroglycerin; [regular oral and sublingual erythrityl tetranitrate][1]; [regular oral][1], [chewable], and [sublingual][1] isosorbide dinitrate; and [regular oral pentaerythritol tetranitrate][1] are also being used for treatment of congestive heart failure, whether or not it is associated with acute myocardial infarction. In general, the oral extended-release dosage forms are not recommended because the effects are difficult to terminate if excessive hypotension or tachycardia develops, although these dosage forms may be acceptable once the patient is stabilized.

---

[1]Not included in Canadian product labeling.

# Pharmacology/Pharmacokinetics

## Physicochemical characteristics
Molecular weight—
Erythrityl tetranitrate: 302.11.
Isosorbide dinitrate: 236.14.
Isosorbide mononitrate: 191.14.
Nitroglycerin: 227.09.
Pentaerythritol tetranitrate: 316.14.

## Mechanism of action/Effect
Antianginal or cardiac load–reducing agent—Not specifically known but thought to cause a reduction of myocardial oxygen demand. This is attributed to a reduction in left ventricular preload and afterload because of venous (predominantly) and arterial dilation with a more efficient redistribution of blood flow within the myocardium.
Antihypertensive—Peripheral vasodilation.

## Absorption
Erythrityl tetranitrate—Readily absorbed after oral or sublingual administration.
Isosorbide dinitrate—Bioavailability is 59% after sublingual administration and 22% after oral administration.
Isosorbide mononitrate—Nearly 100%.

## Protein binding
Nitroglycerin—Moderate (60%).
Isosorbide mononitrate—Very low (< 4%).

## Biotransformation
Hepatic (very rapid and nearly complete) and in blood (enzymatically). Oral dosage forms undergo extensive first-pass metabolism.

## Half-life
Isosorbide dinitrate—
Sublingual: 60 minutes.
Oral: 4 hours.
Isosorbide mononitrate—
5 hours.
Nitroglycerin—
1 to 4 minutes.

## Onset of action
Note: Although information is limited, pharmacokinetics of sublingual tablets administered buccally are probably similar to those after sublingual administration.
Erythrityl tetranitrate—
Oral tablets: 15 to 30 minutes.
Sublingual tablets: 5 minutes.
Isosorbide dinitrate—
Oral capsules and tablets: 15 to 40 minutes.
Chewable tablets: 2 to 5 minutes.
Extended-release capsules and tablets: 30 minutes.
Sublingual tablets: 2 to 5 minutes.
Isosorbide mononitrate—
Oral tablets: 1 hour.
Nitroglycerin—
Buccal tablets: 3 minutes.
Lingual aerosol: 2 to 4 minutes.
Intravenous infusion: Immediate.
Sublingual tablets: 1 to 3 minutes.
Ointment: Within 30 minutes.
Transdermal systems: Within 30 minutes.
Pentaerythritol tetranitrate—
Oral tablets: 30 minutes.
Extended-release capsules and tablets: Slow.

## Duration of action
Note: Although information is limited, pharmacokinetics of sublingual tablets administered buccally are probably similar to those after sublingual administration.
Erythrityl tetranitrate—
Oral tablets: Up to 6 hours.
Sublingual tablets: 2 to 3 hours.
Isosorbide dinitrate—
Oral capsules and tablets: 4 to 6 hours.
Chewable tablets: 1 to 2 hours.
Extended-release capsules and tablets: 12 hours.
Sublingual tablets: 1 to 2 hours.
Nitroglycerin—
Buccal extended-release tablets: Approximately 5 hours.
Extended-release capsules and tablets: 8 to 12 hours.
Intravenous infusion: Several minutes (dose-dependent).
Sublingual tablets: 30 to 60 minutes.
Ointment: 4 to 8 hours.
Transdermal systems: 8 to 24 hours.
Pentaerythritol tetranitrate—
Oral tablets: 4 to 5 hours.
Extended-release capsules and tablets: 12 hours.

## Elimination
Renal (after nearly total metabolism).

# Precautions to Consider

## Cross-sensitivity and/or related problems
Patients sensitive to one nitrate may be sensitive to other nitrates also, although the reaction is rare.
Patients sensitive to nitrites may be sensitive to nitrates also, although the reaction is rare.

## Carcinogenicity
Studies with erythrityl tetranitrate, isosorbide dinitrate, or nitroglycerin have not been done. Studies in mice given oral isosorbide mononitrate at doses of up to 900 mg per kg of body weight (mg/kg) per day (102 times the human exposure comparing body surface area) did not reveal evidence of carcinogenicity.

## Pregnancy/Reproduction
Fertility—
*Isosorbide dinitrate:* Studies in rats given isosorbide dinitrate at doses of 25 or 100 mg/kg per day found no impairment of fertility.
*Isosorbide mononitrate:* No adverse effect on fertility was observed in male and female rats given isosorbide mononitrate at doses of up to

500 mg/kg per day (125 times the human exposure comparing body surface area).

Pregnancy—Adequate and well-controlled studies in humans have not been done.

Studies in rabbits given isosorbide dinitrate in oral doses of 35 and 150 times the maximum daily recommended human dose have shown a dose-related increase in embryotoxicity. Administration of isosorbide mononitrate to rats at doses of 500 mg/kg per day (125 times the human exposure comparing body surface area) was associated with increased rates of prolonged gestation, prolonged parturition, stillbirths and neonatal death, and decreases in birth weight, live litter size, and pup survival. No evidence of developmental abnormalities, fetal abnormalities, or other effects on reproductive performance was observed in rats and rabbits given isosorbide mononitrate at doses of 250 mg/kg per day.

FDA Pregnancy Category C.

### Breast-feeding
It is not known whether nitrates are distributed into breast milk. However, problems in humans have not been documented.

### Pediatrics
Appropriate studies on the relationship of age to the effects of nitrates have not been performed in the pediatric population.

### Geriatrics
Appropriate studies on the relationship of age to the effects of nitrates have not been performed in the geriatric population. However, elderly patients may be more sensitive to the hypotensive effects of nitrates. In addition, elderly patients are more likely to have age-related renal function impairment, which may require caution in patients receiving nitrates.

### Drug interactions and/or related problems
The following drug interactions and/or related problems have been selected on the basis of their potential clinical significance (possible mechanism in parentheses where appropriate)—not necessarily inclusive (» = major clinical significance):

Note: Combinations containing any of the following medications, depending on the amount present, may also interact with this medication.

Acetylcholine or
Histamine or
Norepinephrine (levarterenol)
(effects of these medications may be decreased when they are used concurrently with nitrates)

» Alcohol, moderate or excessive amounts or
» Antihypertensives or
Hypotension-producing medications, other, (see *Appendix II*) or
Opioid (narcotic) analgesics or
» Vasodilators, other
(concurrent use may intensify the orthostatic hypotensive effects of nitrates; dosage adjustments may be necessary)

Heparin
(the anticoagulant effect of heparin may be decreased in patients receiving nitroglycerin via intravenous infusion; adjustment of heparin dosage may be required to maintain the desired degree of anticoagulation during and following administration of a nitroglycerin infusion)

Sympathomimetics
(concurrent use may reduce the antianginal effects of nitrates)
(nitrates may counteract the pressor effect of sympathomimetics, possibly resulting in hypotension)

### Laboratory value alterations
The following have been selected on the basis of their potential clinical significance (possible effect in parentheses where appropriate)—not necessarily inclusive (» = major clinical significance):

With diagnostic test results
Serum cholesterol determinations by the Zlatkis-Zak color reaction method
(may be falsely decreased)

With physiology/laboratory test values
Methemoglobin concentrations in blood
(may be increased by excessive doses of nitrates)

Urine catecholamine concentrations (epinephrine and norepinephrine) and
Urine vanillylmandelic acid (VMA) concentrations
(may be markedly increased by nitroglycerin)

### Medical considerations/Contraindications
The medical considerations/contraindications included here have been selected on the basis of their potential clinical significance (reasons given in parentheses where appropriate)—not necessarily inclusive (» = major clinical significance).

*Except under special circumstances, this medication should not be used when the following medical problems exist:*

*For nitroglycerin injection only*
» Cerebral hemorrhage or
» Head trauma, recent
(nitroglycerin may increase cerebrospinal fluid pressure)
» Pericardial tamponade
» Pericarditis, constrictive

*Risk-benefit should be considered when the following medical problems exist:*

*For all nitrates*
» Anemia, severe
» Cerebral hemorrhage or
» Head trauma, recent
(nitrates may increase cerebrospinal fluid pressure)
» Glaucoma
(nitrates may increase intraocular pressure)
Hepatic function impairment, severe
(increased risk of methemoglobinemia)
» Hyperthyroidism
Hypertrophic cardiomyopathy
(angina may be aggravated)
Hypotension, with low systolic pressure
(may be aggravated, accompanied by paradoxical bradycardia and increased angina pectoris)
» Myocardial infarction, recent
(risk of hypotension and tachycardia, which may aggravate ischemia)
Renal function impairment, severe
Sensitivity to the nitrate prescribed

*For oral dosage forms only (in addition to the above)*
Gastrointestinal hypermotility or
Malabsorption syndrome
(use of extended-release dosage forms should be avoided because they may not dissolve and may be excreted intact)

*For nitroglycerin injection only (in addition to the above)*
» Hypovolemia
(risk of producing severe hypotension and shock; should be corrected prior to use of nitroglycerin)
» Normal or low pulmonary capillary wedge pressure
(patients may be unusually sensitive to hypotensive effects)

### Patient monitoring
The following may be especially important in patient monitoring (other tests may be warranted in some patients, depending on condition; » = major clinical significance):

Blood pressure determinations and
Heart rate determinations
(recommended at periodic intervals in patients using nitrates regularly to aid in dosage adjustment)

## Side/Adverse Effects
The following side/adverse effects have been selected on the basis of their potential clinical significance (possible signs and symptoms in parentheses where appropriate)—not necessarily inclusive:

### Those indicating need for medical attention
Incidence rare
*Blurred vision; dryness of mouth; headache, severe or prolonged; skin rash*

### Those indicating need for medical attention only if they continue or are bothersome
Incidence more frequent—dose-related
*Flushing of face and neck; headache; nausea or vomiting; orthostatic hypotension* (dizziness or lightheadedness, especially when getting up from a lying or sitting position); *restlessness; tachycardia* (fast heartbeat)

Incidence less frequent
*Sore, reddened skin*—topical nitroglycerin dosage forms

# Overdose

For more information on the management of overdose or unintentional ingestion, **contact a Poison Control Center** (see *Poison Control Center Listing*).

## Clinical effects of overdose

The following effects have been selected on the basis of their potential clinical significance (possible signs and symptoms in parentheses where appropriate)—not necessarily inclusive:

Signs and symptoms of overdose (in order of occurrence)

*Bluish-colored lips, fingernails, or palms of hands; dizziness, extreme, or fainting; feeling of extreme pressure in head; shortness of breath; unusual tiredness or weakness; weak and fast heartbeat; fever; convulsions*

Note: Cyanosis may occur at blood methemoglobin concentrations of 1.5 grams per 100 mL. More pronounced signs of methemoglobinemia (pressure in head, tiredness or weakness, shortness of breath) occur at concentrations of 20 to 50 grams per 100 mL.

## Treatment of overdose

Any remaining nitroglycerin should be removed (e.g., ointment, transdermal system). Buccal or sublingual tablets should be removed and the gum wiped clean at the site of insertion.

If excessive hypotension occurs, elevate the legs to aid venous return.

The rapid metabolism of nitroglycerin usually makes additional measures unnecessary. However, if additional correction of severe hypotension is required, administration of an intravenous alpha-adrenergic agonist such as methoxamine or phenylephrine may be considered; epinephrine should be avoided since it aggravates the shock-like reaction.

Methemoglobin concentrations in blood should be monitored and methemoglobinemia treated with high-flow oxygen and intravenous methylene blue.

# Patient Consultation

See *Table 2*, page 2152.

# General Dosing Information

Dosage must be adjusted to the needs and tolerance of the individual patient. Dosage requirements may be increased by a worsening of the patient's condition or a loss of medication potency.

Tolerance to the pharmacologic and therapeutic effects of nitrate medications may occur. Nitrate tolerance manifests as a decrease in patient response to the nitrate or as a need for progressively higher doses to maintain therapeutic effect. The development of nitrate tolerance may occur with any nitrate dosage form that maintains continuous medication blood levels.Tolerance can be managed by adjustments in dosing strategy. Intermittent nitrate therapy appears to be effective. An optimal nitrate-free period of at least 8 to 12 hours appears to be effective in preventing attenuation of nitrate effect. Careful monitoring is recommended to make sure that the desired therapeutic effect is being maintained.

Nitrate therapy should be discontinued if blurred vision or dry mouth continues or is severe.

When this medication is to be discontinued following high-dose or long-term administration, dosage should be reduced gradually to prevent possible withdrawal rebound angina.

## For oral dosage forms only

There have been reports of patients finding intact or partially dissolved extended-release isosorbide dinitrate or pentaerythritol tetranitrate tablets in the stool. Some patients may benefit by a change from the extended-release tablet to the extended-release capsule or the regular oral tablet and an increase in dosage to an effective level for each individual patient.

## For buccal extended-release nitroglycerin tablets or sublingual tablets administered buccally only

The tablet should be placed between upper lip and gum (above the incisors) or between cheek and upper gum, and allowed to dissolve in place. Tablet placement sites may be alternated as patient desires.

The dissolution time of the buccal extended-release tablet may vary from 3 to 5 hours in most patients. The dissolution rate is increased when the tablet is touched with the tongue or the patient drinks hot liquids. The buccal extended-release tablet utilizes an inert polymer vehicle which enables a metered nitroglycerin release not affected by pH, food, or drink (placement is suggested behind the upper lip if food and drink are to be taken during dosing).

Use at bedtime is not recommended because of the risk of aspiration.

Sublingual erythrityl tetranitrate, isosorbide dinitrate, and nitroglycerin tablets may also be administered buccally. Although information is limited, onset and duration of action are probably similar to sublingual dosing.

## Diet/Nutrition

The regular oral dosage forms of this medication should preferably be taken with a glass of water on an empty stomach (either 1 hour before or 2 hours after meals) for faster absorption.

---

## ERYTHRITYL TETRANITRATE

# Summary of Differences

Indications: Although available in sublingual dosage form, is not useful for treatment of acute angina attacks.

# Oral Dosage Forms

## ERYTHRITYL TETRANITRATE TABLETS USP

### Usual adult dose

Antianginal—

Oral, sublingual, or buccal, 5 to 10 mg three or four times a day, the dosage being adjusted as needed and tolerated.

Note: The regular tablet of erythrityl tetranitrate currently marketed may be utilized for oral, sublingual, or buccal dosage.

### Usual adult prescribing limits

Up to 100 mg daily.

### Usual pediatric dose

Dosage has not been established.

### Strength(s) usually available

U.S.—

10 mg (Rx) [*Cardilate*].

Canada—

10 mg (Rx) [*Cardilate*].

### Packaging and storage

Store below 40 °C (104 °F), preferably between 15 and 30 °C (59 and 86 °F), unless otherwise specified by manufacturer. Store in a tight container.

### Stability

Loss of potency is accelerated by exposure to heat and moisture.

### Auxiliary labeling

• Caution with alcoholic beverages.
• Keep container tightly closed.
• Store in a cool, dry place.

---

## ISOSORBIDE DINITRATE

# Oral Dosage Forms

## ISOSORBIDE DINITRATE CAPSULES

### Usual adult dose

Antianginal—

Oral, 5 to 20 mg every six hours, the dosage being adjusted as needed and tolerated. The dosage range is 5 to 40 mg four times a day, with the usual dosage range being 20 to 40 mg four times a day.

### Usual pediatric dose

Dosage has not been established.

### Strength(s) usually available

U.S.—

40 mg (Rx) [GENERIC].

Canada—

Not commercially available.

### Packaging and storage

Store below 40 °C (104 °F), preferably between 15 and 30 °C (59 and 86 °F), in a well-closed container, unless otherwise specified by manufacturer.

### Stability

Loss of potency is accelerated by exposure to heat and moisture.

### Auxiliary labeling

• Caution with alcoholic beverages.
• Store in a cool, dry place.

# ISOSORBIDE DINITRATE EXTENDED-RELEASE CAPSULES USP

**Usual adult dose**
Antianginal—
   Oral, 40 to 80 mg every eight to twelve hours.

**Usual pediatric dose**
Dosage has not been established.

**Strength(s) usually available**
U.S.—
   40 mg (Rx) [*Dilatrate-SR; Iso-Bid; Isorbid; Isordil; Isotrate;* GENERIC].
Canada—
   Not commercially available.

**Packaging and storage**
Store below 40 °C (104 °F), preferably between 15 and 30 °C (59 and 86 °F), unless otherwise specified by manufacturer. Store in a well-closed container.

**Stability**
Loss of potency is accelerated by exposure to heat and moisture.

**Auxiliary labeling**
• Caution with alcoholic beverages.
• Swallow capsules whole.
• Store in a cool, dry place.

# ISOSORBIDE DINITRATE TABLETS USP

**Usual adult dose**
Antianginal—
   Oral, 5 to 20 mg every six hours, the dosage being adjusted as needed and tolerated. The dosage range is 5 to 40 mg four times a day, with the usual dosage range being 20 to 40 mg four times a day.

**Usual pediatric dose**
Dosage has not been established.

**Strength(s) usually available**
U.S.—
   2.5 mg (Rx) [GENERIC].
   5 mg (Rx) [*Isonate; Isorbid; Isordil; Sorbitrate;* GENERIC].
   10 mg (Rx) [*Isonate; Isorbid; Isordil; Sorbitrate;* GENERIC].
   20 mg (Rx) [*Isonate; Isorbid; Isordil; Sorbitrate;* GENERIC].
   30 mg (Rx) [*Isonate; Isorbid; Isordil; Sorbitrate;* GENERIC].
   40 mg (Rx) [*Isordil; Sorbitrate*].
Canada—
   10 mg (Rx) [*Apo-ISDN; Coronex; Isordil; Novosorbide*].
   30 mg (Rx) [*Apo-ISDN; Coronex; Isordil; Novosorbide*].

**Packaging and storage**
Store below 40 °C (104 °F), preferably between 15 and 30 °C (59 and 86 °F), unless otherwise specified by manufacturer. Store in a well-closed container.

**Stability**
Loss of potency is accelerated by exposure to heat and moisture.

**Auxiliary labeling**
• Caution with alcoholic beverages.
• Store in a cool, dry place.

# ISOSORBIDE DINITRATE CHEWABLE TABLETS USP

**Usual adult dose**
Antianginal—
   Oral, 5 mg chewed well every two to three hours, the dosage being adjusted as needed and tolerated.

Note: Chewed tablet is to be held in mouth for one or two minutes to allow time for absorption through buccal tissues.

**Usual pediatric dose**
Dosage has not been established.

**Strength(s) usually available**
U.S.—
   5 mg (Rx) [*Sorbitrate*].
   10 mg (Rx) [*Sorbitrate*].
Canada—
   Not commercially available.

**Packaging and storage**
Store below 40 °C (104 °F), preferably between 15 and 30 °C (59 and 86 °F), unless otherwise specified by manufacturer. Store in a glass container.

**Stability**
Loss of potency is accelerated by exposure to heat and moisture.

**Auxiliary labeling**
• Caution with alcoholic beverages.
• Chew well before swallowing.
• Store in a cool, dry place.

**Note**
Chewable tablets up to 10 mg each are exempt from child-resistant container regulations.

# ISOSORBIDE DINITRATE EXTENDED-RELEASE TABLETS USP

**Usual adult dose**
Antianginal—
   Oral, 20 to 80 mg every eight to twelve hours.

**Usual pediatric dose**
Dosage has not been established.

**Strength(s) usually available**
U.S.—
   40 mg (Rx) [*Isonate; Isorbid; Isordil; Sorbitrate SA;* GENERIC].
Canada—
   20 mg (Rx) [*Cedocard-SR*].

**Packaging and storage**
Store below 40 °C (104 °F), preferably between 15 and 30 °C (59 and 86 °F), unless otherwise specified by manufacturer. Store in a well-closed container.

**Stability**
Loss of potency is accelerated by exposure to heat and moisture.

**Auxiliary labeling**
• Caution with alcoholic beverages.
• Swallow tablets whole.
• Store in a cool, dry place.

# Sublingual Dosage Forms

## ISOSORBIDE DINITRATE SUBLINGUAL TABLETS USP

**Usual adult dose**
Antianginal—
   Sublingual or buccal, 2.5 to 5 mg every two to three hours as needed.

**Usual pediatric dose**
Dosage has not been established.

**Strength(s) usually available**
U.S.—
   2.5 mg (Rx) [*Isonate; Isorbid; Isordil; Sorbitrate;* GENERIC].
   5 mg (Rx) [*Isonate; Isorbid; Isordil; Sorbitrate;* GENERIC].
   10 mg (Rx) [*Isonate; Isorbid; Isordil; Sorbitrate;* GENERIC].
Canada—
   5 mg (Rx) [*Apo-ISDN; Coronex; Isordil*].

**Packaging and storage**
Store below 40 °C (104 °F), preferably between 15 and 30 °C (59 and 86 °F), unless otherwise specified by manufacturer. Store in a well-closed container.

**Stability**
Loss of potency is accelerated by exposure to heat and moisture.

**Auxiliary labeling**
• Caution with alcoholic beverages.
• Dissolve tablets under tongue.
• Store in a cool, dry place.

**Note**
Do not dispense sublingual tablets in child-resistant containers. Sublingual tablets up to 10 mg each are exempt from child-resistant container regulations.

---

## ISOSORBIDE MONONITRATE

# Summary of Differences

Pharmacology/pharmacokinetics:
   Protein binding—Very low.
   Half-life—5 hours.

# Oral Dosage Form

## ISOSORBIDE MONONITRATE TABLETS

**Usual adult dose**
Antianginal—
   Oral, 20 mg two times a day, with the two doses given seven hours apart.

Note: An initial dose of 5 mg may be appropriate for patients of particularly small stature; the dosage being increased to at least 10 mg by the second or third day of therapy.

**Usual pediatric dose**
Safety and efficacy have not been established.

**Strength(s) usually available**
U.S.—
    10 mg (Rx) [*Monoket* (scored)].
    20 mg (Rx) [*ISMO; Monoket* (scored)].
Canada—
    Not commercially available.

**Packaging and storage**
Store below 40 °C (104 °F), preferably between 15 and 30 °C (59 and 86 °F) in a tight container, unless otherwise specified by manufacturer.

**Stability**
Loss of potency is accelerated by exposure to heat and moisture.

**Auxiliary labeling**
• Caution with alcoholic beverages.
• Store in a cool, dry place.

## ISOSORBIDE MONONITRATE EXTENDED-RELEASE TABLETS

**Usual adult dose**
Antianginal—
    Oral, 30 or 60 mg once a day, the dosage being increased after several days to 120 mg once a day, as needed and tolerated. Rarely, 240 mg once a day may be needed.

**Usual pediatric dose**
Safety and efficacy have not been established.

**Strength(s) usually available**
U.S.—
    60 mg (Rx) [*IMDUR* (scored; ethanol, trace)].
Canada—
    Not commercially available.

**Packaging and storage**
Store between 2 and 30 °C (36 and 86 °F) in a tight container.

**Stability**
Loss of potency is accelerated by exposure to heat and moisture.

**Auxiliary labeling**
• Caution with alcoholic beverages.
• Store in a cool, dry place.
• Do not crush or chew.

---

### NITROGLYCERIN

## Summary of Differences

Category:
    Antihypertensive; cardiac load–reducing agent.
Indications:
    Hypertension (parenteral dosage form); hypotension, controlled (parenteral dosage form); acute myocardial infarction; congestive heart failure.
Pharmacology/pharmacokinetics:
    Half-life—1 to 4 minutes.
Precautions:
    Medical considerations/contraindications—Contraindicated in increased intracranial pressure, constrictive pericarditis (parenteral dosage form); caution needed in hypovolemia or severe hepatic or renal function impairment (parenteral dosage form).

## Additional Dosing Information

See also *General Dosing Information*.

**For sublingual tablets only**
Judging the ability of a sublingual tablet to relieve angina by the presence of a tingling or burning sensation after a tablet has been dissolved under the tongue, is not completely reliable since some patients may be unable to detect these effects. Newer, stabilized sublingual nitroglycerin tablets are making such potency testing less useful, since the stabilized tablets may be less likely to produce these detectable effects.
Nitroglycerin tablets should maintain their potency through the expiration date on the bottle, provided the cap is tightly replaced after each use and proper storage instructions are adhered to.
A supplementary stainless steel container has been developed and approved for temporary storage of small quantities of nitroglycerin tablets. The pendant-type container on a chain, which can be worn around

the patient's neck, is intended to provide a convenient source of nitroglycerin for emergency use.

**For intravenous infusion form only**
Special nitroglycerin infusion sets made of non-PVC plastic cause minimal absorption; therefore, nearly all the calculated dose will be delivered to the patient. When these sets are used, *dosage instructions should be followed with care,* as changing from a standard set (PVC) to a special set (non-PVC) may result in excessive nitroglycerin dosage unless allowances are made for the difference in the amount of nitroglycerin actually delivered to the patient.

**For ointment dosage form only**
The dose should be individualized starting with ¹/₂ to 1 inch of ointment as squeezed from the tube and then increasing the dose by ¹/₂ inch at each application until the desired clinical effect and the greatest asymptomatic decrease in resting blood pressure occur. The largest dose that does not cause symptomatic hypotension is used as the patient's individualized dose.
The ointment is applied with the dose-measuring application papers supplied with the medicine. The ointment is squeezed onto the measuring scale printed on the paper. The paper is then used to spread the ointment onto the skin in a thin, even layer, covering an area (at least 2 by 3 inches) of the same size at each dose without rubbing or massage.
The site of ointment application may be the non-hairy skin of the chest, stomach, front of the thighs, or any other accessible area of clean, dry skin. Application to the chest is commonly preferred since the patient also benefits psychologically from applying medication to the area where the pain is experienced.

**For transdermal dosage forms only**
Application should preferably be made at the same time each day (after removal of the previous system) to areas of clean, dry, hairless skin on the chest, inner side of the upper arm, or shoulders; application to extremities below the knee or elbow should be avoided. Skin areas with extensive scarring, calluses, or irritation should also be avoided. Application sites should be varied to avoid causing skin irritation.
All available transdermal systems provide therapeutic effects within 30 minutes and sustain the required plasma concentration of nitroglycerin for 8 to 24 hours.
The transdermal units *should not* be cut or trimmed in an attempt to adjust dosage.
A new dosage unit should be applied if the first becomes loosened or falls off.
Removal of the transdermal unit before defibrillation or cardioversion is recommended because of the potential for altered electrical conductivity and enhanced risk of arcing associated with use of defibrillators.

## Buccal Dosage Forms

### NITROGLYCERIN EXTENDED-RELEASE BUCCAL TABLETS

**Usual adult dose**
Antianginal—
    Buccal, 1 mg dissolved in place on the oral mucosa every five hours during waking hours, the dosage being increased by frequency and/or strength as required.

**Usual pediatric dose**
Dosage has not been established.

**Strength(s) usually available**
U.S.—
    1 mg (Rx) [*Nitrogard*].
    2 mg (Rx) [*Nitrogard*].
    3 mg (Rx) [*Nitrogard*].
Canada—
    1 mg (Rx) [*Nitrogard SR*].
    2 mg (Rx) [*Nitrogard SR*].
    3 mg (Rx) [*Nitrogard SR*].
    5 mg (Rx) [*Nitrogard SR*].

**Packaging and storage**
Store between 15 and 30 °C (59 and 86 °F), unless otherwise specified by manufacturer. Store in a glass container with a tight screw cap.

**Stability**
Loss of potency is accelerated by exposure to heat and moisture.

**Auxiliary labeling**
• Caution with alcoholic beverages.
• Dissolve tablet between lip or cheek and upper gum.
• Do not chew or swallow.
• Keep in original container, tightly closed.
• Store in a cool, dry place.

# Lingual Dosage Forms

## NITROGLYCERIN LINGUAL AEROSOL

### Usual adult dose
Antianginal—
 On or under the tongue, 1 or 2 metered doses (400 or 800 mcg [0.4 or 0.8 mg]) repeated at five-minute intervals as needed for relief of angina attack.

Note: If relief is not obtained after a total of 3 metered doses in a fifteen-minute period, the physician should be contacted or the patient taken to a hospital.

### Usual adult prescribing limits
Up to 1.2 mg per day.

### Usual pediatric dose
Dosage has not been established.

### Strength(s) usually available
U.S.—
 400 mcg (0.4 mg) per metered dose (Rx) [*Nitrolingual*].
Canada—
 400 mcg (0.4 mg) per metered dose (Rx) [*Nitrolingual*].

### Packaging and storage
Store below 40 °C (104 °F), preferably between 15 and 30 °C (59 and 86 °F), unless otherwise specified by manufacturer. Protect from freezing.

### Auxiliary labeling
• Do not shake.
• Caution with alcoholic beverages.
• Store in a cool place.

# Oral Dosage Forms

## NITROGLYCERIN EXTENDED-RELEASE CAPSULES

### Usual adult dose
Antianginal—
 Oral, 2.5, 6.5, or 9 mg every twelve hours, the dosage being increased to every eight hours if needed and tolerated.

### Usual pediatric dose
Dosage has not been established.

### Strength(s) usually available
U.S.—
 2.5 mg (Rx) [*Nitrocap T.D; Nitroglyn; Nitrolin; Nitrospan;* GENERIC].
 6.5 mg (Rx) [*Nitrocap; Nitroglyn; Nitrolin; Nitrospan;* GENERIC].
 9 mg (Rx) [*Nitroglyn; Nitrolin;* GENERIC].
Canada—
 Not commercially available.

### Packaging and storage
Store between 15 and 30 °C (59 and 86 °F), unless otherwise specified by manufacturer. Store in a container with a tight screw cap.

### Stability
Loss of potency is accelerated by exposure to heat and moisture.

### Auxiliary labeling
• Caution with alcoholic beverages.
• Swallow capsules whole.
• Keep container tightly closed.
• Store in a cool, dry place.

## NITROGLYCERIN EXTENDED-RELEASE TABLETS

### Usual adult dose
Antianginal—
 Oral, 1.3, 2.6, or 6.5 mg every twelve hours, the dosage being increased to every eight hours as needed and tolerated.

### Usual pediatric dose
Dosage has not been established.

### Strength(s) usually available
U.S.—
 2.6 mg (Rx) [*Klavikordal; Niong; Nitronet; Nitrong*].
 6.5 mg (Rx) [*Klavikordal; Niong; Nitronet; Nitrong*].
 9 mg (Rx) [*Nitrong*].
Canada—
 2.6 mg (Rx) [*Nitrong SR*].

### Packaging and storage
Store between 15 and 30 °C (59 and 86 °F), unless otherwise specified by manufacturer. Store in a glass container with a tight screw cap.

### Stability
Loss of potency is accelerated by exposure to heat and moisture.

### Auxiliary labeling
• Caution with alcoholic beverages.
• Swallow tablets whole.
• Keep container tightly closed.
• Store in a cool, dry place.

# Parenteral Dosage Forms

## NITROGLYCERIN INJECTION USP

### Usual adult dose
Antianginal or
Antihypertensive or
Cardiac load–reducing agent—
 Intravenous infusion, initially administered at a rate of 5 mcg (0.005 mg) per minute, the dosage being increased by increments of 5 mcg per minute at three- to five-minute intervals until an effect is obtained or until the rate is 20 mcg (0.02 mg) per minute. If no effect is obtained at 20 mcg per minute, the dosage may be increased further by increments of 10 mcg (0.01 mg) per minute at the same time intervals, and later increased by increments of 20 mcg (0.02 mg) per minute if necessary to obtain an effect. The dosage increments should be reduced and the time interval between dosage increases lengthened when a partial effect is observed, to attain the desired response cautiously.

Note: Close attention must be given to manufacturers' instructions for dilution, dosage, and administration because concentrations and/or volume per vial of nitroglycerin may differ among the several products available from different manufacturers.

 Stated dosage is based on use of special, non-polyvinylchloride (non-PVC) intravenous infusion sets. Dosage requirements may vary when standard infusion sets of polyvinyl chloride (PVC) are used. Continuous concurrent monitoring of blood pressure and heart rate in *all patients* must be performed to establish the correct effective dose.

 To achieve optimal control of dosage and effects, it is recommended that nitroglycerin be administered intravenously by means of an infusion pump, a micro-drip regulator, or a similar device to allow precise adjustment of the flow rate.

 Standard intravenous infusion sets made of PVC plastic may unpredictably absorb 40 to 80% of the nitroglycerin from a diluted solution for infusion.

 Some intravenous filters may also absorb nitroglycerin, but the effect is variable; since nitroglycerin dosage is titrated according to response, no precaution is necessary.

 Extra caution should be observed when non-PVC infusion sets are used to administer intravenous nitroglycerin. Some infusion pumps—
 • When turned off may not completely stop the flow of infusion solution with these non-PVC sets.
 • May not accurately deliver the infusion solution at low rates of flow.
 • Require extension sets and other connecting equipment made of PVC, thus partially negating the advantage of the non-PVC infusion set.
 Close monitoring of patient hemodynamic response is required. All infusion pumps should be tested with the infusion set being used to ensure accurate delivery of nitroglycerin at low flow rates and complete interruption of flow when the set is turned off.

### Usual adult prescribing limits
No fixed maximum dose established. Dosage is titrated to individual patient response beginning with small doses (to which hypersensitive patients may respond).

### Usual pediatric dose
Dosage has not been established.

### Strength(s) usually available
U.S.—
 500 mcg (0.5 mg) per mL (Rx) [*Tridil*].
 800 mcg (0.8 mg) per mL (Rx) [*Nitrol; Nitrostat*].
 1 mg per mL (Rx) [*Nitroject*].
 5 mg per mL (Rx) [*Nitro-Bid; Nitroject; Nitrol; Nitrostat; Tridil;* GENERIC].
 10 mg per mL (Rx) [*Nitro-Bid; Nitrostat*].
Canada—
 800 mcg (0.8 mg) per mL (Rx) [*Nitrostat*].
 1 mg per mL (Rx) [*Nitroject*].
 5 mg per mL (Rx) [*Nitro-Bid; Nitroject; Nitrostat; Tridil;* GENERIC].

### Packaging and storage
Store between 15 and 30 °C (59 and 86 °F), unless otherwise specified by manufacturer. Protect from light. Protect from freezing.

## Preparation of dosage form
• *Not for direct intravenous injection.*
• Must be diluted prior to infusion. Dilution may be in 5% dextrose injection or 0.9% sodium chloride injection, followed by thorough mixing. Dilution and storage of nitroglycerin injection should be made only in glass parenteral solution bottles, to avoid absorption of nitroglycerin into plastic containers.
• *Must not be admixed with other medications.*

## Stability
It is recommended that diluted solutions of nitroglycerin not be kept or used longer than 24 hours, unless otherwise specified by the manufacturer. Solution is *not* explosive either before or after dilution.

## Note
Manufacturer's package information must be checked for dilution, administration, and dosage because of product differences.

Some products contain substantial amounts of propylene glycol or ethanol.

# Sublingual Dosage Forms
## NITROGLYCERIN TABLETS (SUBLINGUAL) USP

### Usual adult dose
Antianginal—
   Sublingual or buccal, 150 to 600 mcg (0.15 to 0.6 mg) repeated at five-minute intervals as needed for relief of angina attack.

Note: If relief is not obtained after a total of 3 tablets used over a fifteen-minute period, the physician should be contacted or the patient taken to a hospital.

### Usual adult prescribing limits
Up to 10 mg per day.

### Usual pediatric dose
Dosage has not been established.

### Strength(s) usually available
U.S.—
   150 mcg (0.15 mg) (Rx) [*Nitrostat;* GENERIC].
   300 mcg (0.3 mg) (Rx) [*Nitrostat;* GENERIC].
   400 mcg (0.4 mg) (Rx) [*Nitrostat;* GENERIC].
   600 mcg (0.6 mg) (Rx) [*Nitrostat;* GENERIC].
Canada—
   300 mcg (0.3 mg) (Rx) [*Nitrostat;* GENERIC].
   600 mcg (0.6 mg) (Rx) [*Nitrostat;* GENERIC].

### Packaging and storage
Store between 15 and 30 °C (59 and 86 °F), unless otherwise specified by manufacturer. Store in original container with tight metal screw cap.

### Stability
Loss of potency through volatilization of nitroglycerin from tablets is accelerated by exposure to air, heat, and moisture. After the bottle is opened, stabilized tablets will maintain potency through the expiration date provided the bottle cap is replaced tightly after each use.

### Auxiliary labeling
• Caution with alcoholic beverages.
• Dissolve tablets under tongue.
• Keep in original container, tightly closed.
• Store in a cool, dry place.

### Note
Do not dispense sublingual nitroglycerin tablets in child-resistant containers.

Suggest to the patient that the cotton be removed from the container *before* the tablets are required for angina attack.

USP requires that sublingual forms of nitroglycerin be dispensed in the original unopened manufacturer's container.

Sublingual nitroglycerin tablets should not be placed in containers with other medications.

# Topical Dosage Forms
## NITROGLYCERIN OINTMENT USP

### Usual adult dose
Antianginal—
   Topical, to the skin, 15 to 30 mg of nitroglycerin (contained in 2.5 to 5 cm [1 to 2 inches] of ointment as squeezed from the tube) every eight hours during the day and at bedtime. If angina occurs between doses, frequency of application may be increased to every six hours.

Note: Ointment is applied in a thin, even layer covering an area of the same size (measuring at least 2 by 3 inches) at each use, but is not to be rubbed or massaged into the skin.

### Usual adult prescribing limits
Up to 75 mg of nitroglycerin (contained in 12.5 cm [5 inches] of ointment as squeezed from the tube) per application. Rarely, application as frequently as every four hours may be necessary.

### Usual pediatric dose
Dosage has not been established.

### Strength(s) usually available
U.S.—
   2% (Rx) [*Nitro-Bid; Nitrol; Nitrong; Nitrostat;* GENERIC].
Canada—
   2% (Rx) [*Nitro-Bid; Nitrol; Nitrong*].

### Packaging and storage
Store between 15 and 30 °C (59 and 86 °F), unless otherwise specified by manufacturer. Store in a tight container.

### Auxiliary labeling
• Caution with alcoholic beverages.
• For external use only.
• Store in a cool place.
• Keep tightly closed.

### Note
Dispense ointment in original manufacturer's tube together with patient instructions and dose-measuring papers.

## NITROGLYCERIN TRANSDERMAL SYSTEM

### Usual adult dose
Antianginal—
   Topical, to the intact skin, 1 transdermal dosage system, delivering the smallest available dose of nitroglycerin in its dosage series, every twenty-four hours. Dosage adjustments may be made by changing to the next larger dosage system in the series or to a combination of systems.

Note: To prevent tolerance, it is recommended that the patch be left on only 12 to 14 hours a day, with a patch-off period of 10 to 12 hours before the next daily patch is applied.

### Usual pediatric dose
Dosage has not been established.

### Strength(s) usually available
U.S.—
   Dose of nitroglycerin delivered per hour
   0.1 mg (Rx) [*Nitro-Dur II; Transderm-Nitro*].
   0.2 mg (Rx) [*Deponit; Nitrodisc; Nitro-Dur; Nitro-Dur II; NTS; Transderm-Nitro;* GENERIC].
   0.3 mg (Rx) [*Nitrodisc; Nitro-Dur II*].
   0.4 mg (Rx) [*Deponit; Nitrodisc; Nitro-Dur; Nitro-Dur II; Transderm-Nitro;* GENERIC].
   0.6 mg (Rx) [*Nitro-Dur II; NTS; Transderm-Nitro;* GENERIC].
Canada—
   Dose of nitroglycerin delivered per hour
   0.2 mg (Rx) [*Transderm-Nitro*].
   0.4 mg (Rx) [*Transderm-Nitro*].

### Packaging and storage
Store between 15 and 30 °C (59 and 86 °F), unless otherwise specified by manufacturer.

### Auxiliary labeling
• Caution with alcoholic beverages.
• For external use only.
• Store in a cool place.

### Note
Include patient instructions when dispensing.

Products should be prescribed and dispensed on the basis of the amount of nitroglycerin delivered in 24 hours; use of brand names alone may be confusing because numbers within the brand name may refer to the surface area of the patch, which is different from the dose of nitroglycerin delivered.

---

## *PENTAERYTHRITOL TETRANITRATE*

# Oral Dosage Forms
## PENTAERYTHRITOL TETRANITRATE EXTENDED-RELEASE CAPSULES

### Usual adult dose
Antianginal—
   Oral, 30 to 80 mg two times a day.

### Usual adult prescribing limits
Up to 160 mg daily.

**Usual pediatric dose**
Dosage has not been established.

**Strength(s) usually available**
U.S.—
30 mg (Rx) [*Duotrate*].
45 mg (Rx) [*Duotrate*].
80 mg (Rx) [GENERIC].
Canada—
Not commercially available.

**Packaging and storage**
Store below 40 °C (104 °F), preferably between 15 and 30 °C (59 and 86 °F), unless otherwise specified by manufacturer. Store in a tight container.

**Stability**
Loss of potency is accelerated by exposure to heat and moisture.

**Auxiliary labeling**
• Caution with alcoholic beverages.
• Swallow capsules whole.
• Keep container tightly closed.
• Store in a cool, dry place.

## PENTAERYTHRITOL TETRANITRATE TABLETS USP

**Usual adult dose**
Antianginal—
Oral, 10 to 20 mg four times a day, the dosage being adjusted as needed and tolerated.

**Usual adult prescribing limits**
Up to 160 mg daily.

**Usual pediatric dose**
Dosage has not been established.

**Strength(s) usually available**
U.S.—
10 mg (Rx) [*Pentylan;* GENERIC].
20 mg (Rx) [*Pentylan; Peritrate;* GENERIC].
80 mg (Rx) [GENERIC].
Canada—
10 mg (Rx) [*Peritrate*].
20 mg (Rx) [*Peritrate*].
80 mg (Rx) [*Peritrate Forte*].

**Packaging and storage**
Store below 40 °C (104 °F), preferably between 15 and 30 °C (59 and 86 °F), unless otherwise specified by manufacturer. Store in a tight container.

**Stability**
Loss of potency is accelerated by exposure to heat and moisture.

**Auxiliary labeling**
• Caution with alcoholic beverages.
• Keep container tightly closed.
• Store in a cool, dry place.

## PENTAERYTHRITOL TETRANITRATE EXTENDED-RELEASE TABLETS

**Usual adult dose**
Antianginal—
Oral, up to 80 mg two times a day.

**Usual adult prescribing limits**
Oral, up to 160 mg daily.

**Usual pediatric dose**
Dosage has not been established.

**Strength(s) usually available**
U.S.—
80 mg (Rx) [*Peritrate SA;* GENERIC].
Canada—
80 mg (Rx) [*Peritrate SA*].

**Packaging and storage**
Store below 40 °C (104 °F), preferably between 15 and 30 °C (59 and 86 °F), unless otherwise specified by manufacturer. Store in a tight container.

**Stability**
Loss of potency is accelerated by exposure to heat and moisture.

**Auxiliary labeling**
• Caution with alcoholic beverages.
• Swallow tablets whole.
• Keep container tightly closed.
• Store in a cool, dry place.

Revised: 10/06/93
Interim revision: 02/22/94; 06/06/95

## Table 1. Indications

Note: Bracketed information in the *Indications* section refers to uses that are not included in U.S. product labeling.

Legend:
I=Angina pectoris, acute (treatment)
II=Angina pectoris, acute (prophylaxis)
III=Angina pectoris, chronic (treatment)
IV=Hypertension (treatment); or Hypotension, controlled
V=Myocardial infarction (treatment adjunct)
VI=Congestive heart failure (treatment)

| | I | II | III | IV | V | VI |
|---|---|---|---|---|---|---|
| Erythrityl tetranitrate Oral/Sublingual | | ✔ | ✔ | [✔][1] | [✔][1] | |
| Isosorbide dinitrate Oral Capsules and tablets, regular | | | | ✔ | [✔][1] | [✔][1] |
| Extended-release capsules or tablets | | | | ✔ | | |
| Chewable tablets | ✔ | ✔ | ✔ | [✔] | [✔] | |
| Sublingual | ✔[1] | ✔ | ✔ | [✔][1] | [✔][1] | |
| Isosorbide mononitrate Oral Tablets, regular | | | ✔ | | | |

[1]Not included in Canadian product labeling.

## Table 1. Indications *(continued)*

| | Legend:<br>**I** = Angina pectoris, acute (treatment)<br>**II** = Angina pectoris, acute (prophylaxis)<br>**III** = Angina pectoris, chronic (treatment) | | | **IV** = Hypertension (treatment); or Hypotension, controlled<br>**V** = Myocardial infarction (treatment adjunct)<br>**VI** = Congestive heart failure (treatment) | | |
|---|---|---|---|---|---|---|
| | **I** | **II** | **III** | **IV** | **V** | **VI** |
| Nitroglycerin<br>  Buccal, extended-release | ✔[1] | ✔ | ✔ | | | |
| Lingual, aerosol | ✔ | ✔[1] | | | [✔][1] | [✔][1] |
| Oral, extended-release | | | ✔ | | | |
| Parenteral | | | ✔ | ✔ | ✔ | ✔ |
| Sublingual | ✔ | ✔ | | | [✔][1] | [✔][1] |
| Topical<br>  Ointment<br>  Transdermal systems | | | | ✔<br>✔ | [✔][1]<br>[✔] | [✔][1]<br>[✔] |
| Pentaerythritol tetranitrate<br>Oral<br>  Tablets, regular | | | | ✔ | [✔][1] | [✔][1] |
| Extended-release capsules and tablets | | | ✔ | | | |

[1]Not included in Canadian product labeling.

## Table 2. Patient Consultation

| | Buccal | Lingual | Oral | | | Sublingual | | | Topical | |
|---|---|---|---|---|---|---|---|---|---|---|
| As an aid to patient consultation, refer to *Advice for the Patient, Nitrates—Lingual Aerosol (Systemic), Nitrates—Oral (Systemic), Nitrates—Sublingual, Chewable, or Buccal (Systemic),* or *Nitrates—Topical (Systemic).*<br><br>Consider advising the patient on the following: | Legend:<br>**I** = Extended-release nitroglycerin | **II** = Aerosol nitroglycerin | **III** = Regular<br>**IV** = Chewable<br>**V** = Extended-release | | | **VI** = Erythrityl tetranitrate<br>**VII** = Isosorbide dinitrate<br>**VIII** = Nitroglycerin | | | **IX** = Nitroglycerin ointment<br>**X** = Transdermal nitroglycerin | |
| | **I** | **II** | **III** | **IV** | **V** | **VI** | **VII** | **VIII** | **IX** | **X** |
| **Before using this medication**<br>See *Precautions to Consider.* | ✔ | ✔ | ✔ | ✔ | ✔ | ✔ | ✔ | ✔ | ✔ | ✔ |
| **Proper use of this medication**<br>» Compliance with therapy | ✔ | ✔ | ✔ | ✔ | ✔ | ✔ | ✔ | ✔ | ✔ | ✔ |
| » Reading patient instructions carefully | | ✔ | | | | | | | ✔ | ✔ |
| Proper administration:<br>» Regular or extended-release capsule or tablet—Taking with full glass of water on empty stomach | | | ✔ | | ✔ | | | | | |
| » Buccal—<br>Under upper lip (above incisors) against gum or between cheek and upper gum; placing between upper lip (above incisors) and gum if food or drink to be taken within 3 to 5 hours; patients with dentures may place anywhere between cheek and gum | ✔ | | | | | ✔ | ✔ | ✔ | | |
| Touching with tongue or drinking hot liquids may increase rate of dissolution | ✔ | | | | | ✔ | ✔ | ✔ | | |
| Bedtime use not recommended because of risk of aspiration | ✔ | | | | | ✔ | ✔ | ✔ | | |
| Replacing tablet if inadvertently swallowed | ✔ | | | | | ✔ | ✔ | ✔ | | |
| Not using chewing tobacco while tablet in place | ✔ | | | | | | | | | |
| » Chewable tablet—Chewing well and holding in mouth for approximately 2 minutes | | | | ✔ | | | | | | |
| » Lingual aerosol—<br>Removing plastic cover; not shaking container | | ✔ | | | | | | | | |
| Holding container vertically and spraying onto or under tongue; not inhaling spray | | ✔ | | | | | | | | |

## Table 2. Patient Consultation (continued)

| | Buccal | Lingual | Oral | | | Sublingual | | | Topical | |
|---|---|---|---|---|---|---|---|---|---|---|
| Legend: | I=Extended-release nitroglycerin | II=Aerosol nitroglycerin | III=Regular IV=Chewable V=Extended-release | | | VI=Erythrityl tetranitrate VII=Isosorbide dinitrate VIII=Nitroglycerin | | | IX=Nitroglycerin ointment X=Transdermal nitroglycerin | |
| | **I** | **II** | **III** | **IV** | **V** | **VI** | **VII** | **VIII** | **IX** | **X** |
| Closing mouth after each spray; not swallowing immediately | | ✔ | | | | | | | | |
| » Sublingual tablet—Under the tongue; avoiding eating, drinking, smoking, or using chewing tobacco while tablet is dissolving | | | | | | ✔ | ✔ | ✔ | | |
| » Ointment—Cleansing skin before applying; measuring; using applicator; spreading evenly over same size of skin area in each application; not rubbing into skin; applying to skin free of hair, in different areas; proper application of occlusive dressing, if ordered | | | | | | | | | ✔ | |
| Transdermal—Not trimming or cutting patch; applying to clean, dry skin free of hair, scars, cuts, or irritation (after removal of previous system); replacing systems that have loosened or fallen off; alternating application sites | | | | | | | | | | ✔ |
| » Not chewing, crushing, or swallowing | ✔ | | | | | ✔ | ✔ | ✔ | | |
| » Not breaking, crushing, or chewing before swallowing | | | | | ✔ | | | | | |

*For use in treating acute angina attacks*

| | I | II | III | IV | V | VI | VII | VIII | IX | X |
|---|---|---|---|---|---|---|---|---|---|---|
| » Sitting down and using medication at first sign of angina attack; caution if dizziness or faintness occurs | ✔ | ✔ | | ✔ | | ✔ | ✔ | ✔ | | |
| Remaining calm until medicine has opportunity to work | ✔ | ✔ | | ✔ | | | ✔ | ✔ | | |
| » Relief usually occurs within 5 minutes— | ✔ | ✔ | | ✔ | | | ✔ | ✔ | | |
| Dose may be repeated if pain not relieved in 5 to 10 minutes; calling physician or going to emergency room if angina pain not relieved by 3 doses in 15 minutes | | ✔ | | ✔ | | | | ✔ | | |
| Not repeating dose; using sublingual nitroglycerin and calling physician or going to emergency room if angina pain not relieved in 15 minutes | ✔ | | | | | | | | | |

*For use in preventing angina*

| | I | II | III | IV | V | VI | VII | VIII | IX | X |
|---|---|---|---|---|---|---|---|---|---|---|
| » This dosage form does not relieve angina attacks but rather prevents them (exceptions are chewable and sublingual isosorbide dinitrate) | | | ✔ | ✔ | ✔ | ✔ | | | ✔ | ✔ |
| Using 5 to 10 minutes prior to anticipated stress to prevent attack | ✔ | ✔ | | | | ✔ | ✔ | | | |
| Missed dose: | | | | | | | | | | |
| Taking/using as soon as possible unless next scheduled dose is within: | | | | | | | | | | |
| —2 hours (exception is oral extended-release); | ✔ | | | ✔ | ✔ | | ✔ | ✔ | | ✔ |
| —6 hours (for oral extended-release); | | | | | ✔ | | | | | |
| Returning to regular dosing schedule; not doubling doses | ✔ | | | ✔ | | ✔ | ✔ | | | ✔ |
| » Proper storage | ✔ | ✔ | ✔ | ✔ | ✔ | ✔ | ✔ | ✔ | ✔ | ✔ |
| Protecting from freezing | | ✔ | | | | | | | | |
| Not puncturing, breaking, or burning aerosol container | | ✔ | | | | | | | | |
| Storing in cool place, tightly closed | | | | | | | | | ✔ | |
| Lack of reliability of flushing or headache as test of potency | | | | | | | | | | ✔ |
| » Keeping sublingual nitroglycerin in original glass, screw-cap bottle (unless using special nitroglycerin container) with cotton plug removed; avoiding handling tablets; capping quickly and tightly after each use; not storing in same container as other medications; not carrying close to body or in auto glove compartment; not storing in refrigerator or bathroom medicine cabinet | | | | | | | | ✔ | | |

**Precautions while using this medication**

| | I | II | III | IV | V | VI | VII | VIII | IX | X |
|---|---|---|---|---|---|---|---|---|---|---|
| » Checking with physician before discontinuing medication; gradual dosage reduction may be needed | ✔ | ✔ | ✔ | ✔ | ✔ | ✔ | ✔ | ✔ | ✔ | ✔ |
| » Caution when getting up suddenly from a lying or sitting position | ✔ | ✔ | ✔ | ✔ | ✔ | ✔ | ✔ | ✔ | ✔ | ✔ |

## Table 2. Patient Consultation (continued)

| | Buccal | Lingual | Oral | | | Sublingual | | | Topical | |
|---|---|---|---|---|---|---|---|---|---|---|
| | Legend:<br>I=Extended-release nitroglycerin | II=Aerosol nitroglycerin | III=Regular<br>IV=Chewable<br>V=Extended-release | | | VI=Erythrityl tetranitrate<br>VII=Isosorbide dinitrate<br>VIII=Nitroglycerin | | | IX=Nitroglycerin ointment<br>X=Transdermal nitroglycerin | |
| | I | II | III | IV | V | VI | VII | VIII | IX | X |
| » Caution in using alcohol, while standing for long periods or exercising, and during hot weather because of enhanced orthostatic hypotensive effects | ✔ | ✔ | ✔ | ✔ | ✔ | ✔ | ✔ | ✔ | ✔ | ✔ |
| » Headache as a common effect; should decrease with continuing therapy; checking with physician if continuing or severe | ✔ | ✔ | ✔ | ✔ | ✔ | ✔ | ✔ | ✔ | ✔ | ✔ |
| Notifying physician if undigested extended-release tablets are found in stools (for isosorbide dinitrate and pentaerythritol tetranitrate only) | | | | | | ✔ | | | | |
| **Side/adverse effects**<br>Signs of potential side effects, especially blurred vision, dryness of mouth, severe or prolonged headache, and skin rash | ✔ | ✔ | ✔ | ✔ | ✔ | ✔ | ✔ | ✔ | ✔ | ✔ |

**NITRAZEPAM**—See *Benzodiazepines (Systemic)*

# NITROFURANTOIN   Systemic

**VA CLASSIFICATION (Primary): AM600**

Note: For a listing of dosage forms and brand names by country availability, see *Dosage Forms* section(s). For a listing of brand names for the articles in this monograph, refer to the General Index.

## Category

Antibacterial (systemic).

## Indications

Note: Bracketed information in the *Indications* section refers to uses that are not included in U.S. product labeling.

### Accepted

Urinary tract infections, bacterial (treatment)—Nitrofurantoin is indicated in the treatment of urinary tract infections caused by susceptible strains of *Escherichia coli*, enterococci, *Staphylococcus aureus*, *S. saprophyticus*, *Klebsiella* species, *Enterobacter* species, and *Proteus* species.

[Urinary tract infections, bacterial (prophylaxis)][1]—Nitrofurantoin is used in the prophylaxis of urinary tract infections.

Not all species or strains of a particular organism may be susceptible to nitrofurantoin.

[1]Not included in Canadian product labeling.

## Pharmacology/Pharmacokinetics

### Physicochemical characteristics

Molecular weight—238.16.

### Mechanism of action/Effect

Nitrofurantoin, a synthetic, broad-spectrum, weakly acidic antibacterial, is generally bactericidal at therapeutic concentrations. Therapeutic concentrations are achieved only in the urine. The mechanism of antimicrobial action is unique among antibacterials. Nitrofurantoin is reduced by bacterial flavoproteins to reactive intermediates, which inactivate or alter bacterial ribosomal proteins and other macromolecules.

### Absorption

Microcrystalline—Rapidly and completely absorbed in the small intestine.

Macrocrystalline—More slowly absorbed and usually causes less gastrointestinal irritation.

The presence of food can increase the bioavailability of both forms of nitrofurantoin; this also increased the duration of therapeutic urinary concentrations.

### Distribution

High concentrations are achieved in urine and the kidneys; serum concentrations are very low; crosses the placenta and blood-brain barrier.

### Protein binding

Moderate (60%).

### Biotransformation

Approximately two-thirds of the drug is rapidly metabolized and inactivated in most body tissues, including the liver.

### Half-life

0.3 to 1 hour.

### Elimination

Renal—Primarily excreted by glomerular filtration with some tubular secretion and reabsorption; 30 to 40% rapidly excreted unchanged; the macrocrystalline form is excreted more slowly; active drug accumulates in patients with impaired renal function and may reach toxic concentrations.

Biliary—May also be excreted in the bile.

In dialysis—Nitrofurantoin is dialyzable.

## Precautions to Consider

### Cross-sensitivity and/or related problems

Patients hypersensitive to one nitrofuran may be hypersensitive to other nitrofurans also.

### Carcinogenicity

Nitrofurantoin, given as 0.3% of the diet to female Holtzman rats for up to 44.5 weeks or given as 0.1% to 0.187% of the diet to female Sprague-Dawley rats for 75 weeks, has not been shown to be carcinogenic. No evidence of carcinogenicity was found in 2 chronic rodent bioassays in male and female Sprague-Dawley rats and 2 chronic bioassays in Swiss mice and in BDF₁ mice. Increased incidences of tubular adenomas, benign mixed tumors, and granulosa cell tumors of the ovary were seen in female B6C3F₁ mice. There was an increased incidence of uncommon kidney tubular cell neoplasms, osteosarcomas, and neoplasms of the subcutaneous tissue in male F344/N rats. Lung papillary adenomas of unknown significance were observed in the F1 generation of pregnant mice given 75 mg per kg of body weight (mg/kg) of nitrofurantoin by subcutaneous injection.

### Mutagenicity

Nitrofurantoin has induced point mutations in certain strains of *Salmonella typhimurium* and forward mutations in L5178Y mouse lymphoma cells. It has also induced increased numbers of sister chromatid exchanges and chromosomal aberrations in Chinese hamster ovary cells but not in human cells in culture. Results of the sex-linked recessive lethal assay in *Dro-*

*sophila* were negative after oral or parenteral administration of nitrofurantoin. The medication did not induce heritable mutation in the rodent models examined.

### Pregnancy/Reproduction
Fertility—Nitrofurantoin, given in high doses in rats, has been shown to cause temporary spermatogenic arrest, which was reversible upon discontinuation of the medication. Nitrofurantoin, in doses of 10 mg/kg per day or greater, may produce slight to moderate spermatogenic arrest, with decreased sperm counts, in human males.

Pregnancy—Nitrofurantoin crosses the placenta. Use is contraindicated in pregnancy at term and during labor and delivery, or when the onset of labor is imminent, because of the possibility of hemolytic anemia due to immature enzyme systems in the fetus.

Reproduction studies have been performed in rabbits and rats given doses up to 6 times the human dose; these studies have revealed no evidence of impaired fertility or harm to the fetus due to nitrofurantoin. In a single study conducted in mice given 68 times the human dose (based on mg/kg administered to the dam), growth retardation and a low incidence of minor and common malformations were observed. However, fetal malformations were not observed at 25 times the human dose.

FDA Pregnancy Category B.

### Breast-feeding
Nitrofurantoin is excreted in breast milk in trace amounts. Hemolytic anemia may occur, especially in glucose-6-phosphate dehydrogenase (G6PD)–deficient infants.

### Pediatrics
Use of nitrofurantoin is contraindicated in infants up to 1 month of age because of the possibility of hemolytic anemia due to immature enzyme systems.

### Geriatrics
No information is available on the relationship of age to the effects of nitrofurantoin in geriatric patients. However, elderly patients are more likely to have an age-related decrease in renal function, which may require a decrease in dosage or change in medication. Side effects, such as acute pneumonitis and peripheral polyneuropathy, may also occur more frequently in elderly patients.

### Drug interactions and/or related problems
The following drug interactions and/or related problems have been selected on the basis of their potential clinical significance (possible mechanism in parentheses where appropriate)—not necessarily inclusive (» = major clinical significance):

Note: Combinations containing any of the following medications, depending on the amount present, may also interact with this medication.

» Hemolytics, other (See *Appendix II*)
   (concurrent use with nitrofurantoin may increase the potential for toxic side effects)

Hepatotoxic medications, other (See *Appendix II*)
   (concurrent use of nitrofurantoin with other hepatotoxic medications may increase the potential for hepatotoxicity)

Magnesium trisilicate
   (magnesium trisilicate reduces both the rate and extent of absorption of nitrofurantoin, probably by adsorption of nitrofurantoin to its surface)

Nalidixic acid
   (nitrofurantoin interferes with the therapeutic effects of nalidixic acid)

» Neurotoxic medications, other (See *Appendix II*)
   (concurrent use of nitrofurantoin with other neurotoxic medications may increase the potential for neurotoxicity)

» Probenecid or
» Sulfinpyrazone
   (these medications may inhibit renal tubular secretion of nitrofurantoin, resulting in increased serum concentrations and/or toxicity, prolonged elimination half-life, and reduced urinary concentrations and effectiveness; dosage adjustment of probenecid may be necessary)

### Laboratory value alterations
The following have been selected on the basis of their potential clinical significance (possible effect in parentheses where appropriate)—not necessarily inclusive (» = major clinical significance):

With diagnostic test results

Glucose, urine
   (nitrofurantoin may produce metabolites in the urine that may give false-positive results with copper sulfate reduction tests, such as *Benedict's* solution)

### Medical considerations/Contraindications
The medical considerations/contraindications included here have been selected on the basis of their potential clinical significance (reasons given in parentheses where appropriate)—not necessarily inclusive (» = major clinical significance).

*Risk-benefit should be considered when the following medical problems exist:*
» Glucose-6-phosphate dehydrogenase (G6PD) deficiency
   (hemolysis may occur in patients with G6PD deficiency who take nitrofurantoin)

   Hypersensitivity to nitrofurans
» Neuropathy, peripheral
   (nitrofurantoin may cause peripheral neuropathy)
» Pulmonary disease
   (nitrofurantoin may cause acute, subacute, and chronic pulmonary reactions, including pneumonitis)
» Renal function impairment
   (because nitrofurantoin is excreted through the kidneys, it is recommended that nitrofurantoin not be given to patients with a creatinine clearance of less than 40 to 60 mL per minute [0.67 to 1.00 mL per second]; nitrofurantoin loses its effectiveness in patients with renal function impairment, and toxic effects are increased)

### Patient monitoring
The following may be especially important in patient monitoring (other tests may be warranted in some patients, depending on condition; » = major clinical significance):

Hepatic function determinations
   (may be required periodically during long-term therapy to detect changes in hepatic function; if hepatitis occurs, nitrofurantoin should be discontinued immediately and appropriate measures taken)
» Pulmonary function determinations
   (may be required periodically during long-term therapy if pulmonary reactions [e.g., diffuse interstitial pneumonitis, pulmonary fibrosis] occur; if pulmonary reactions occur, nitrofurantoin should be discontinued and appropriate measures taken)

## Side/Adverse Effects
Note: Acute pneumonitis is more common in the elderly; symptoms usually occur within the first week of therapy. The pneumonitis is often reversible with discontinuation of the drug; corticosteroids may be beneficial in severe cases. Chronic pulmonary reactions, including diffuse interstitial pneumonitis and fibrosis, are insidious in onset and are more likely to occur in patients who have been on nitrofurantoin therapy for at least 6 months. Pulmonary function may be permanently impaired even after the drug has been stopped, especially if pulmonary reactions are not recognized early.

Peripheral polyneuropathy is an ascending sensorimotor neuropathy, which may be progressive if the drug is not discontinued immediately. Polyneuropathy occurs more frequently in patients with renal dysfunction and in the elderly; however, it also occurs in patients with normal renal function who have received nitrofurantoin for prolonged periods of time. Demyelination and degeneration of both sensory and motor nerves occur. Nitrofurantoin should be stopped at the first signs of neuritis.

The following side/adverse effects have been selected on the basis of their potential clinical significance (possible signs and symptoms in parentheses where appropriate)—not necessarily inclusive:

### Those indicating need for medical attention
Incidence more frequent
   *Pneumonitis* (chest pain; chills; cough; fever; troubled breathing)
Incidence less frequent
   *Hematologic reactions, specifically granulocytopenia* (sore throat and fever); *leukopenia* (sore throat and fever); *or megaloblastic anemia* (unusual tiredness or weakness); *neurotoxicity* (dizziness; drowsiness; headache; unusual tiredness or weakness); *polyneuropathy* (numbness, tingling, or burning of face or mouth; unusual muscle weakness)
Incidence rare
   *Hemolytic anemia* (pale skin; unusual tiredness or weakness); *hepatitis* (yellow eyes or skin); *hypersensitivity* (skin rash; itching; arthralgia; fever; chills)

### Those indicating need for medical attention only if they continue or are bothersome
Incidence more frequent
   *Gastrointestinal disturbances* (abdominal or stomach pain or upset; diarrhea; loss of appetite; nausea or vomiting)

### Those not indicating need for medical attention
   *Rust-yellow to brown discoloration of urine*

## Overdose

For more information on the management of overdose or unintentional ingestion, **contact a Poison Control Center** (see *Poison Control Center Listing*).

### Treatment of overdose

Recommended treatment consists of the following:

To decrease absorption—Induction of emesis if vomiting has not already occurred.

Specific treatment—Maintaining a high fluid intake to promote urinary excretion of nitrofurantoin.

Supportive care—Patients in whom intentional overdose is known or suspected should be referred for psychiatric consultation.

## Patient Consultation

As an aid to patient consultation, refer to *Advice for the Patient, Nitrofurantoin (Systemic)*.

In providing consultation, consider emphasizing the following selected information (» = major clinical significance):

### Before using this medication

» Conditions affecting use, especially:

  Hypersensitivity to nitrofurans

  Pregnancy—Nitrofurantoin is contraindicated at term and during labor and delivery because of the possibility of hemolytic anemia in the fetus

  Breast-feeding—Not recommended since hemolytic anemia may occur in G6PD-deficient infants

  Use in children—Nitrofurantoin is contraindicated in infants up to 1 month of age because of the possibility of hemolytic anemia

  Use in the elderly—Side effects, such as acute pneumonitis and peripheral polyneuropathy, may occur more frequently in elderly patients

  Other medications, especially other hemolytics, other neurotoxic medications, probenecid, or sulfinpyrazone

  Other medical problems, especially G6PD deficiency, peripheral neuropathy, pulmonary disease, or renal function impairment

### Proper use of this medication

» Not giving to infants up to 1 month of age

  Taking with food or milk

*Proper administration technique for oral liquid:*

  Shaking well before each dose

  Using a specially marked measuring spoon or other device

  May be mixed with water, milk, fruit juices, or infants' formulas

  Proper administration technique for extended-release tablets: Swallowing tablet whole; not breaking, crushing, or chewing before swallowing

» Compliance with full course of therapy

» Proper dosage

  Missed dose: Taking as soon as possible; not taking if almost time for next dose; not doubling doses

» Proper storage

### Precautions while using this medication

  Regular visits to physician to check progress if on long-term therapy

  Checking with physician if no improvement within a few days

» Diabetics: False-positive reactions with copper sulfate urine glucose tests may occur

### Side/adverse effects

  Rust-yellow to brown discoloration of urine may be alarming to patient although medically insignificant

  Signs of potential side effects, especially hemolytic anemia, jaundice, neurotoxicity, pneumonitis, and polyneuropathy

## General Dosing Information

Nitrofurantoin should preferably be taken with food or milk. This minimizes gastrointestinal irritation, delays and increases absorption of both the macrocrystalline and microcrystalline forms, increases the peak concentration of the macrocrystalline form, and prolongs the duration of therapeutic concentrations in the urine.

Patients on long-term suppressive therapy require a reduction in dose.

Patients with impaired renal function (creatinine clearance less than 40 to 60 mL per minute [0.67 to 1.00 mL per second]) should not receive nitrofurantoin since increased toxicity due to possible accumulation of toxic metabolites may occur. Also, nitrofurantoin is ineffective in patients whose creatinine clearance is less than 40 mL per minute.

## Oral Dosage Forms

Note: Bracketed uses in the *Dosage Forms* section refer to categories of use and/or indications that are not included in U.S. product labeling.

### NITROFURANTOIN CAPSULES USP

#### Usual adult and adolescent dose

Antibacterial—

  Oral, 50 to 100 mg every six hours.

Note: [Urinary tract infections, bacterial (prophylaxis)][1]—Oral, 50 to 100 mg once a day at bedtime.

  Most uncomplicated infections caused by susceptible bacteria are adequately treated with 50 mg three times a day.

#### Usual adult prescribing limits

Up to 600 mg daily; or up to 10 mg per kg of body weight daily.

#### Usual pediatric dose

Antibacterial—

  Infants up to 1 month of age: Use is contraindicated because of the possibility of hemolytic anemia due to immature enzyme systems.

  Infants and children 1 month of age and over: Oral, 0.75 to 1.75 mg per kg of body weight every six hours.

Note: [Urinary tract infections, bacterial (prophylaxis)][1]—Oral, 1 mg per kg of body weight once a day at bedtime.

  Therapeutic doses up to 10 mg per kg of body weight daily in four evenly divided doses have been used.

#### Strength(s) usually available

U.S.—

  25 mg (Rx) [*Macrodantin* (macrocrystalline)].

  50 mg (Rx) [*Macrodantin* (macrocrystalline); GENERIC (macrocrystalline and microcrystalline)].

  100 mg (Rx) [*Macrodantin* (macrocrystalline); GENERIC (macrocrystalline and microcrystalline)].

Canada—

  25 mg (Rx) [*Macrodantin* (macrocrystalline)].

  50 mg (Rx) [*Macrodantin* (macrocrystalline)].

  100 mg (Rx) [*Macrodantin* (macrocrystalline)].

#### Packaging and storage

Store below 40 °C (104 °F), preferably between 15 and 30 °C (59 and 86 °F), unless otherwise specified by manufacturer. Store in a tight, light-resistant container.

#### Auxiliary labeling

• Continue medicine for full time of treatment.

• Take with food or milk.

• May discolor urine.

### NITROFURANTOIN EXTENDED-RELEASE CAPSULES

#### Usual adult and adolescent dose

Antibacterial—

  Oral, 100 mg every twelve hours for seven days.

#### Usual pediatric dose

Antibacterial—

  Safety and efficacy have not been established in children up to 12 years of age.

#### Strength(s) usually available

U.S.—

  100 mg (Rx) [*Macrobid* (macrocrystalline 25 mg; monohydrate 75 mg)].

Canada—

  Not commercially available.

#### Packaging and storage

Store below 40 °C (104 °F), preferably between 15 and 30 °C (59 and 86 °F), unless otherwise specified by manufacturer. Store in a tight, light-resistant container.

#### Auxiliary labeling

• Continue medicine for full time of treatment.

• Take with food or milk.

• May discolor urine.

### NITROFURANTOIN ORAL SUSPENSION USP

#### Usual adult and adolescent dose

See *Nitrofurantoin Capsules USP*.

#### Usual adult prescribing limits

See *Nitrofurantoin Capsules USP*.

#### Usual pediatric dose

See *Nitrofurantoin Capsules USP*.

**Strength(s) usually available**
U.S.—
  25 mg per 5 mL (Rx) [*Furadantin* (methylparaben; propylparaben; saccharin; sorbitol)].
Canada—
  Not commercially available.

**Packaging and storage**
Store below 40 °C (104 °F), preferably between 15 and 30 °C (59 and 86 °F), unless otherwise specified by manufacturer. Store in a tight, light-resistant container. Protect from freezing.

**Incompatibilities**
Nitrofurantoin and its solutions are discolored by alkalis and by exposure to strong light and decompose upon contact with metals other than stainless steel or aluminum.

**Auxiliary labeling**
• Shake well.
• Continue medicine for full time of treatment.
• Take with food or milk.
• May discolor urine.

**Note**
Dispense in amber bottles.

When dispensing, include a calibrated liquid-measuring device.

**Additional information**
The oral suspension dosage form is readily miscible with water, milk, fruit juices, or infants' formulas.

## NITROFURANTOIN TABLETS USP

**Usual adult and adolescent dose**
See *Nitrofurantoin Capsules USP.*

**Usual adult prescribing limits**
See *Nitrofurantoin Capsules USP.*

**Usual pediatric dose**
See *Nitrofurantoin Capsules USP.*

**Strength(s) usually available**
U.S.—
  50 mg (Rx) [*Furalan; Furatoin; Nitrofuracot;* GENERIC].
  100 mg (Rx) [*Furalan;* GENERIC].
Canada—
  50 mg (Rx) [*Apo-Nitrofurantoin*].
  100 mg (Rx) [*Apo-Nitrofurantoin*].

**Packaging and storage**
Store below 40 °C (104 °F), preferably between 15 and 30 °C (59 and 86 °F), unless otherwise specified by manufacturer. Store in a tight, light-resistant container.

**Incompatibilities**
Nitrofurantoin and its solutions are discolored by alkalis and by exposure to strong light and decompose upon contact with metals other than stainless steel or aluminum.

**Auxiliary labeling**
• Continue medicine for full time of treatment.
• Take with food or milk.
• May discolor urine.

**Note**
Dispense in amber bottles.

[1]Not included in Canadian product labeling.

Revised: 01/19/93

## NITROGLYCERIN—See *Nitrates (Systemic)*

---

# NITROPRUSSIDE   Systemic

VA CLASSIFICATION (Primary/Secondary): CV490/CV500; CV900
Note: For a listing of dosage forms and brand names by country availability, see *Dosage Forms* section(s). For a listing of brand names for the articles in this monograph, refer to the General Index.

## Category

Antihypertensive; vasodilator, congestive heart failure; myocardial infarction therapy adjunct; antidote (to ergot alkaloid poisoning).

## Indications

Note: Bracketed information in the *Indications* section refers to uses that are not included in U.S. product labeling.

**Accepted**
Congestive heart failure (treatment)[1]—Nitroprusside is indicated for the management of acute congestive heart failure.

Hypertension (treatment)—Nitroprusside is indicated for the immediate reduction of blood pressure of patients in hypertensive crisis.

Hypotension, controlled—Nitroprusside is indicated for producing controlled hypotension during surgery to reduce bleeding into the surgical field.

[Hypertension, paroxysmal, in surgery for pheochromocytoma (treatment)][1]—Nitroprusside is used to control paroxysmal hypertension prior to and during surgery for pheochromocytoma.

[Myocardial infarction (treatment adjunct)][1]—Use of nitroprusside to reduce afterload is also recommended in patients with acute myocardial infarction who are hypertensive with persistent chest pain or left ventricular failure.

[Valvular regurgitation (treatment adjunct)][1]—Nitroprusside is also used as an adjunct to standard treatment of aortic or mitral regurgitation prior to surgical intervention.

[Toxicity, ergot alkaloid (treatment)][1]—Nitroprusside is also used for treatment of peripheral vasospasm caused by ergot alkaloid overdose.

**Unaccepted**
Nitroprusside should *not* be used in the treatment of compensatory hypertension (such as in arteriovenous shunt or coarctation of the aorta).

[1]Not included in Canadian product labeling.

## Pharmacology/Pharmacokinetics

**Physicochemical characteristics**
Molecular weight—297.95.

**Mechanism of action/Effect**
Antihypertensive—Hypertension or controlled hypotension: Causes vasodilation by a direct effect on arterial and venous smooth muscle, with no effect on uterine or duodenal smooth muscle or on myocardial contractility; regional distribution of blood flow is only marginally affected. Reduces peripheral resistance and has a variable effect on cardiac output. Is more active on veins than arteries (but less markedly so than nitroglycerin). Increases renin activity.

Vasodilator, congestive heart failure—Beneficial effects in congestive heart failure are due to decreased systemic resistance, preload and afterload reduction, and improved cardiac output.

Myocardial infarction therapy adjunct—The effect of nitroprusside on ischemic myocardial areas is not totally known. It dilates coronary arteries. The medication reportedly reduces myocardial oxygen consumption and relieves persistent chest pain but has also been found to aggravate ischemia by redistributing blood flow away from ischemic myocardium.

Valvular regurgitation therapy adjunct—In the treatment of valvular regurgitation, nitroprusside reduces aortic and left ventricular impedance.

Antidote (to ergot alkaloid poisoning)—Causes vasodilation.

**Other actions/effects**
Slightly increases heart rate. Decreases platelet aggregation.

**Biotransformation**
By intraerythrocytic reaction with hemoglobin to produce cyanmethemoglobin and cyanide ion. Exogenous cyanide is sequestered by erythrocyte methemoglobin as cyanmethemoglobin until intraerythrocytic methemoglobin is saturated. Some cyanide ion is eliminated from the body as expired hydrogen cyanide, but most is enzymatically converted to thiocyanate, which is eliminated in the urine; this reaction requires a hepatic mitochondrial enzyme, rhodanase (thiosulfate-cyanide sulfur transferase), and a sulfur donor, especially thiosulfate, cystine, and cysteine. Cyanide not removed by any of these methods binds to mitochondrial cytochromes and prevents oxidative metabolism; cells either are forced to provide for their energy needs via anaerobic pathways, generating lactic acid, or die hypoxic deaths.

Cyanide is normally found in serum and is derived from dietary substrates and tobacco smoke. Normal cyanide ion concentrations in packed erythrocytes are less than 1 micromole per liter (25 mg per liter); these concentrations are doubled in heavy smokers.

At healthy steady state, less than 1% of hemoglobin is in the form of methemoglobin. Nitroprusside metabolism leads to methemoglobin formation either through dissociation of cyanmethemoglobin formed in the original reaction of nitroprusside with hemoglobin or by direct oxidation of hemoglobin by the released nitroso group. A patient with normal red-cell mass and normal methemoglobin concentrations can buffer about 175 mcg of cyanide ion per kg of body weight (mcg/kg), corresponding to a little less than 500 mcg/kg of infused sodium nitroprusside.

Thiosulfate is a normal constituent of serum, produced by cysteine. Normal physiological concentrations of 0.1 millimole per liter (11 mg per liter) are approximately double in children and in adults who are not eating. When thiosulfate is being supplied only by normal physiologic mechanisms, conversion of cyanide ion to thiocyanate generally occurs at about 1 mcg/kg per minute. This rate of cyanide clearance corresponds to steady-state processing of a sodium nitroprusside infusion of slightly more than 2 mcg/kg per minute. Cyanide begins to accumulate when sodium nitroprusside infusions exceed this rate.

### Half-life
Nitroprusside—Circulatory: About 2 minutes.

Thiosulfate—After intravenous infusion: About 20 minutes.

Thiocyanate—About 3 days; may be doubled or tripled in renal failure.

### Onset of action
Hypotensive—Within 1 to 2 minutes after start of an adequate infusion.

### Time to peak effect
Hypotensive—Almost immediate.

### Duration of action
Hypotensive—1 to 10 minutes after infusion is stopped.

### Elimination
Thiocyanate and infused thiosulfate—Renal.

## Precautions to Consider

### Carcinogenicity/Mutagenicity
Studies have not been done in either animals or humans.

### Pregnancy/Reproduction
Pregnancy—Adequate and well-controlled studies in humans have not been done. Birth of a stillborn infant without any obvious anomalies was reported after one woman was given nitroprusside to control gestational hypertension; however, cyanide concentrations in the infant's liver were well below usual toxic levels and the mother demonstrated no cyanide toxicity.

Teratogenicity studies in laboratory animals have not been done. In three studies in pregnant ewes, nitroprusside was shown to cross the placenta; fetal cyanide levels were dose-related to maternal levels; fatal cyanide levels could be produced in fetuses by using high rates of nitroprusside administration to the pregnant ewes.

FDA Pregnancy Category C.

### Breast-feeding
It is not known whether nitroprusside is excreted in breast milk. Problems in humans have not been documented.

### Pediatrics
Appropriate studies on the relationship of age to the effects of nitroprusside have not been performed in the pediatric population. However, pediatrics-specific problems that would limit the usefulness of this medication in children are not expected.

### Geriatrics
Although appropriate studies on the relationship of age to the effects of nitroprusside have not been performed in the geriatric population, the elderly may be more sensitive to the hypotensive effects. In addition, elderly patients are more likely to have age-related renal function impairment, which may require caution in patients receiving nitroprusside.

### Drug interactions and/or related problems
The following drug interactions and/or related problems have been selected on the basis of their potential clinical significance (possible mechanism in parentheses where appropriate)—not necessarily inclusive (» = major clinical significance):

Note: Combinations containing any of the following medications, depending on the amount present, may also interact with this medication.

Dobutamine
(concurrent use with nitroprusside may result in a higher cardiac output and a lower pulmonary wedge pressure)

Estrogens or
Sympathomimetics
(hypotensive effects of nitroprusside may be reduced when it is used concurrently with estrogens or sympathomimetics; dosage adjustment based on careful blood pressure monitoring is recommended)

Hypotension-producing medications, other (see *Appendix II*)
(concurrent use may result in increased hypotensive effects which may be severe; dosage adjustment based on careful blood pressure monitoring is recommended)

### Laboratory value alterations
The following have been selected on the basis of their potential clinical significance (possible effect in parentheses where appropriate)—not necessarily inclusive (» = major clinical significance):

With physiology/laboratory test values
Bicarbonate concentrations, blood and
$PCO_2$ and
pH
(may be decreased, indicating metabolic acidosis, during cyanide toxicity; however, may not be present until an hour or more after toxic cyanide concentrations are reached)

Cyanide, serum
(concentrations increased with excessive rate of nitroprusside infusion; except at low nitroprusside infusion rates [less than 2 mcg per kg of body weight (mcg/kg) per minute] or with brief use, concentrations produced are significant, potentially reaching toxic or lethal levels; venous blood appears bright red because of hyperoxemia)

Lactate, arterial blood
(concentrations may be increased in overdose, indicating metabolic acidosis, during cyanide toxicity; however, may not be present until an hour or more after toxic cyanide concentrations are reached)

Methemoglobin, blood
(concentrations may rarely be increased if amount of nitroprusside administered exceeds rate at which back-conversion of methemoglobin to hemoglobin can occur; blood appears chocolate brown, without color change on exposure to air)

Oxygen, venous blood
(concentrations increased in cyanide toxicity; venous blood appears bright red)

Thiocyanate, serum
(concentrations increased as a result of cyanide enzymatic reaction with thiosulfate; with prolonged infusions, the steady-state concentration is increased with increased infusion rate)

### Medical considerations/Contraindications
The medical considerations/contraindications included here have been selected on the basis of their potential clinical significance (reasons given in parentheses where appropriate)—not necessarily inclusive (» = major clinical significance).

### *Risk-benefit should be considered when the following medical problems exist:*
Anemia—for use in producing controlled hypotension during anesthesia only; patient's capacity to compensate may be diminished; should be corrected prior to use of nitroprusside

» Cerebrovascular or coronary artery insufficiency
(reduced tolerance of hypotension)

» Encephalopathy or other conditions where intracranial pressure is elevated
(intracranial pressure may be further increased; nitroprusside should be used only with extreme caution)

» Hepatic function impairment
(hepatic enzyme is involved in metabolism of nitroprusside)

Hypothyroidism
(thiocyanate, one of the metabolic products of nitroprusside, inhibits both uptake and binding of iodine)

Hypovolemia—for use in producing controlled hypotension during anesthesia only; patient's capacity to compensate may be diminished; should be corrected prior to use of nitroprusside

» Leber's hereditary optic atrophy or
» Tobacco amblyopia
(deficiency or absence of enzyme [rhodanase] needed for metabolism of nitroprusside)

Pulmonary function impairment
(aggravation of hypoxemia)
» Renal function impairment
(reduced excretion of thiocyanate)
Sensitivity to nitroprusside
» Vitamin B₁₂ deficiency
(related to metabolism)

### Patient monitoring
The following may be especially important in patient monitoring (other tests may be warranted in some patients, depending on condition; » = major clinical significance):

Acid-base balance and
Oxygen concentrations, venous
(may indicate metabolic acidosis resulting from cyanide toxicity; however, because measurable effects may be delayed an hour or more after toxic cyanide concentrations are reached, these values should not be used to decide when to treat for cyanide toxicity)

» Blood pressure determinations
(should be made continuously, either with a continually reinflated sphygmomanometer or, preferably, an intra-arterial pressure sensor)
(pulmonary artery diastolic or wedge pressure determinations may be required in patients with acute myocardial infarction)

Cyanide concentrations, serum
(may be determined; however, not particularly useful because the cyanide assay is technically difficult and cyanide concentrations in body fluids other than packed red cells are difficult to interpret)

Methemoglobin concentrations, blood
(recommended in patients who have received more than 10 mg of nitroprusside per kg of body weight and who exhibit signs of impaired oxygen delivery despite adequate cardiac output and adequate arterial pO₂)

Thiocyanate concentrations, serum
(recommended at daily intervals in patients receiving prolonged nitroprusside infusions at a rate greater than 3 mcg per kg of body weight [mcg/kg] per minute [1 mcg/kg per minute in anuric patients]; should not exceed 1 millimole per liter)

*For congestive heart failure*
Invasive hemodynamic monitoring and
Urine output
(recommended to guide titration of infusion rate)

## Side/Adverse Effects

Note: A severe rebound hypertension has been reported after discontinuation of an infusion used to produce controlled hypotension during surgery.

The following side/adverse effects have been selected on the basis of their potential clinical significance (possible signs and symptoms in parentheses where appropriate)—not necessarily inclusive:

### Those indicating need for medical attention
Signs and/or symptoms of excessively rapid fall in blood pressure (appear to be related to rate of administration rather than total dose)
*Abdominal pain* (stomach pain); *dizziness; excessive sweating; headache; muscle twitching; nervousness or anxiety; restlessness; retching; tachycardia, reflex*

Note: Excessive *hypotension,* sometimes to levels low enough to compromise perfusion of vital organs, may be produced by small transient excesses in the infusion rate. Excessively rapid decreases in blood pressure can lead to irreversible ischemic injuries or death if patients are not properly monitored.

Signs and/or symptoms of thiocyanate toxicity
*Ataxia; blurred vision; delirium; dizziness; headache; loss of consciousness; nausea and vomiting; shortness of breath; tinnitus* (ringing in ears)

Note: Mild neurotoxicity (*tinnitus, miosis, hyperreflexia*) occurs at serum thiocyanate concentrations of 1 millimole per liter (60 mg per liter). Thiocyanate toxicity becomes life-threatening at serum concentrations of 200 mg per liter.

Signs and/or symptoms of cyanide toxicity
*Absence of reflexes; coma; distant heart sounds; hypotension; imperceptible pulse; metabolic acidosis; pink color; very shallow breathing; widely dilated pupils*

Note: Nitroprusside infusion rates greater than 2 mcg per kg of body weight (mcg/kg) per minute generate cyanide ion faster than the body can normally eliminate it (administration of thiosulfate greatly increases the body's capacity for cyanide elimination). The capacity of methemoglobin to buffer cyanide is exhausted from about 500 mcg/kg of nitroprusside (the amount administered in less than an hour at a rate of 10 mcg/kg per minute). Above this level, toxic effects of cyanide may be rapid, serious, and lethal.

Elevated cyanide concentrations, metabolic acidosis, and marked clinical deterioration have occasionally been reported in patients given infusions at recommended rates for only a few hours (in one case, for only 35 minutes).

Incidence less frequent or rare
*Flushing; hypothyroidism; ileus; increased intracranial pressure; methemoglobinemia*—concentrations greater than 10%; *pain or redness at site of injection; skin rash*

Note: *Hypothyroidism*—Thiocyanate interferes with iodine uptake by the thyroid.

*Methemoglobinemia* is usually rare, because the back-conversion process returning methemoglobin to hemoglobin is normally rapid. Even in patients congenitally incapable of back-converting methemoglobin, a cumulative dose of 10 mg of nitroprusside per kg of body weight (mg/kg) (e.g., given at a rate of 10 mcg/kg per minute for 16 hours) would be required to produce 10% methemoglobinemia.

## General Dosing Information

Nitroprusside should be administered *only* by intravenous infusion by means of an infusion pump, preferably a volumetric pump.

It is recommended that patients receiving nitroprusside be in a setting with available equipment and personnel to allow blood pressure to be monitored continuously.

Care should be taken to avoid extravasation because of possible irritation.

Larger than ordinary doses may be required for hypotensive anesthesia in young, vigorous males.

It is recommended that administration of nitroprusside be discontinued immediately if administration of 10 mcg (0.01 mg) (sodium nitroprusside dihydrate) per kg of body weight per minute for 10 minutes does not produce adequate reduction of blood pressure.

Concurrent administration of sodium thiosulfate (at 5 to 10 times the rate of sodium nitroprusside administration) may reduce the risk of cyanide toxicity by increasing the rate of cyanide conversion. However, it has not been extensively studied, and in one study appeared to potentiate nitroprusside's hypotensive effect. Caution is necessary to avoid prolonged or high doses of sodium nitroprusside with sodium thiosulfate, which could lead to thiocyanate toxicity and hypovolemia.

Apparent tolerance has occurred occasionally. Although a correlation between tachyphylaxis and concomitant cyanide toxicity has been proposed, no correlation has been demonstrated.

### For use in treatment of hypertension
It is recommended that oral antihypertensive therapy be instituted while the patient is receiving nitroprusside and that nitroprusside be withdrawn as soon as the patient has stabilized. Patients receiving concomitant antihypertensive medication require lower doses of nitroprusside.

### For use in treatment of congestive heart failure
Addition of a potent inotropic medication such as dopamine or dobutamine may be useful when doses of nitroprusside that are effective in restoring pump function in left ventricular congestive heart failure cause excessive hypotension.

### For treatment of adverse effects/overdose
For methemoglobinemia
• Intravenous administration of methylene blue in a dose of 1 to 2 mg per kg of body weight (mg/kg) given over several minutes. Extreme caution is necessary in patients likely to have substantial amounts of cyanide bound to methemoglobin as cyanmethemoglobin.

For excessive hypotension
- Slowing or discontinuation of infusion; symptoms disappear quickly (within 1 to 10 minutes). Placement of the patient in the Trendelenberg position to maximize venous return may be helpful.

For thiocyanate toxicity
- Hemodialysis; clearance rates during dialysis can approach the blood flow rate of the dialyzer.

For cyanide toxicity
- Discontinuation of nitroprusside administration. Because metabolic acidosis may not be evident until more than an hour after the appearance of dangerous cyanide concentrations, laboratory test results should not be awaited; treatment should be initiated with reasonable suspicion of cyanide toxicity.
- Intravenous administration of sodium nitrite (as a 3% solution), in a dose of 4 to 6 mg/kg over 2 to 4 minutes. Sodium nitrite provides a buffer for cyanide by converting as much hemoglobin into methemoglobin as the patient can safely tolerate; this dose can be expected to convert about 10% of the patient's hemoglobin, and this level of methemoglobinemia is not associated with any known hazards. Sodium nitrite infusion may cause transient vasodilation and hypotension, which should be managed as necessary. Amyl nitrite inhalations may be used in environments where intravenous administration of sodium nitrite may be delayed.
- Immediately following sodium nitrite infusion, intravenous infusion of sodium thiosulfate in a sufficient amount to convert the cyanide into thiocyanate. The recommended dose of sodium thiosulfate is 150 to 200 mg/kg; a typical adult dose is 50 mL of a 25% solution (sodium thiosulfate is also available as a 50% solution). Thiocyanate concentrations will be raised in acutely cyanide-toxic patients, but not to a dangerous level.
- Hemodialysis is not effective in removing cyanide.
- If necessary, the nitrite/thiosulfate regimen may be repeated, at half the original doses, after 2 hours.

## Parenteral Dosage Forms
### STERILE SODIUM NITROPRUSSIDE

**Usual adult and adolescent dose**
Antihypertensive—
Intravenous infusion, initially, 0.3 mcg (0.0003 mg) (sodium nitroprusside dihydrate) per kg of body weight per minute, adjusted every few minutes according to response; usual dose is 3 mcg (0.003 mg) per kg of body weight per minute.

Note: Geriatric patients may be more sensitive to the usual adult dose of nitroprusside.

**Usual adult prescribing limits**
Up to 10 mcg (0.01 mg) per kg of body weight per minute for a maximum period of 10 minutes, or a total dose of 3.5 mg per kg of body weight (500 mcg [0.5 mg] per kg of body weight during short-term infusions such as in controlled hypotension during surgery). To keep the steady-state thiocyanate concentration below 1 millimole per liter, the rate of a prolonged infusion should be no more than 3 mcg per kg of body weight per minute (1 mcg per kg of body weight per minute in anuric patients).

**Usual pediatric dose**
Antihypertensive—
See *Usual adult and adolescent dose.*

**Size(s) usually available**
U.S.—
50 mg (sodium nitroprusside dihydrate) (Rx) [*Nitropress;* GENERIC].
Canada—
50 mg (sodium nitroprusside dihydrate) (Rx) [*Nipride*].

**Packaging and storage**
Store below 40 °C (104 °F), preferably between 15 and 30 °C (59 and 86 °F), unless otherwise specified by manufacturer. Protect from light.

**Preparation of dosage form**
Nitroprusside is prepared for intravenous infusion by dissolving the contents of a 50-mg vial in 2.3 mL of 5% dextrose injection only and shaking gently to dissolve. The reconstituted solution must be diluted further in 250 to 1000 mL of 5% dextrose injection to achieve the desired concentration and the container is wrapped in a supplied opaque sleeve, aluminum foil, or other opaque material to protect it from light (it is not necessary to wrap the infusion drip chamber or the tubing).

**Stability**
Solutions of nitroprusside should be freshly prepared and any unused portion discarded. A freshly prepared solution has a slight brownish tint and should be discarded if the color is dark brown, orange, or blue.

It is recommended that solutions of nitroprusside not be kept or used longer than 24 hours, unless otherwise specified by the manufacturer.

No other medications should be added to infusion fluid containing nitroprusside.

Sodium nitroprusside solution is rapidly degraded by trace contaminants, often with resulting color changes. A change in color to blue, green, or bright red indicates reaction of nitroprusside ion with another substance, and the solution must be replaced and discarded.

Sodium nitroprusside solution is sensitive to certain wavelengths of light and therefore must be protected from light. After preparation of the medication, the container should be promptly wrapped in the supplied opaque sleeve, aluminum foil, or other opaque material (it is not necessary to wrap the infusion drip chamber or the tubing).

## Selected Bibliography
Kreye VAW. Sodium nitroprusside. In: Scriabine A, ed. Pharmacology of antihypertensive drugs. New York: Raven Press, 1980: 373-96.
Gaskins JD, Holt RJ, Kessler C. Comparative review of intravenous nitroglycerin and nitroprusside sodium. Hosp Form 1982 Jul; 928-34.

Revised: 08/07/92

---

**NITROPRUSSIDE URINE KETONE TEST**—See *Urine Glucose and Ketone Test Kits for Home Use*

---

**NITROUS OXIDE**—See *Anesthetics, Inhalation (Systemic)*

---

**NIZATIDINE**—See *Histamine $H_2$-receptor Antagonists (Systemic)*

---

**NONOXYNOL 9**—See *Spermicides (Vaginal)*

---

**NOREPINEPHRINE**—See *Sympathomimetic Agents—Cardiovascular Use (Parenteral-Systemic)*

---

**NOREPINEPHRINE-CONTAINING COMBINATIONS**—
Propoxycaine, Procaine, and Norepinephrine (Parenteral-Local)—See *Anesthetics (Parenteral-Local)*

---

**NORETHINDRONE**—See *Progestins (Systemic)*

---

**NORFLOXACIN**—See *Fluoroquinolones (Systemic); Norfloxacin (Ophthalmic)*

# NORFLOXACIN Ophthalmic

VA CLASSIFICATION (Primary): OP201

Note: For a listing of dosage forms and brand names by country availability, see *Dosage Forms* section(s). For a listing of brand names for the articles in this monograph, refer to the General Index.

## Category

Antibacterial (ophthalmic).

## Indications

### Accepted

Conjunctivitis, bacterial (treatment)—Ophthalmic norfloxacin is indicated for the treatment of conjunctivitis caused by susceptible strains of: *Acinetobacter calcoaceticus, Aeromonas hydrophila, Haemophilus influenzae, Proteus mirabilis, Pseudomonas aeruginosa, Serratia marcescens, Staphylococcus aureus, S. epidermidis, S. warnerii,* and *Streptococcus pneumoniae.*

Note: Not all species or strains of a particular organism may be susceptible to norfloxacin.

## Pharmacology/Pharmacokinetics

### Physicochemical characteristics

Chemical group—Norfloxacin, a fluoroquinolone, is a synthetic pyridone carboxylic acid analog of nalidixic acid. Norfloxacin differs from quinolones by having a fluorine atom at the 6 position and a piperazine moiety at the 7 position

Molecular weight—319.34.

pKa—Approximately 6.34 and 8.75 at 25 °C for $pKa_1$ and $pKa_2$, respectively.

pH—Approximately 5.2.

Osmolarity—Approximately 285 mOsmol per liter.

### Mechanism of action/Effect

Norfloxacin is bactericidal and acts by inhibiting bacterial deoxyribonucleic acid (DNA) synthesis. Norfloxacin is a broad-spectrum anti-infective, active against a wide range of aerobic gram-positive and gram-negative organisms. The fluorine atom at the 6 position increases potency against gram-negative organisms, and the piperazine moiety at the 7 position is responsible for anti-pseudomonal activity.

### Absorption

In animals, systemic absorption following ophthalmic administration was minimal.

### Distribution

There is no information on ophthalmic norfloxacin. However, systemic norfloxacin is widely distributed to most body fluids and tissues, such as the prostate, testicles, uterus, cervix, vagina, fallopian tubes, liver, seminal fluid, sputum, blister fluid, and serum. Substantial concentrations are reached in kidney tissue, urine, feces, and bile.

### Protein binding

Low, between 10 and 15%.

### Biotransformation

Norfloxacin has 6 active metabolites, which have less antibacterial potency than the drug itself. Norfloxacin is metabolized in the liver and kidney.

### Half-life

In serum and plasma—3 to 4 hours.

In the elderly, in serum and plasma—4 hours.

### Onset of action

One hour for ophthalmic norfloxacin.

### Peak serum concentration

A maximum of 10.2 nanograms per mL for a daily ophthalmic dose of 2.5 mg.

### Elimination

Biliary—

In the feces, 28% of a single oral dose is excreted in 24 to 36 hours. The rate of excretion following oral administration is 207 to 2716 mcg per gram at peak levels.

In the bile, the rate of excretion following oral administration is 7.4 mcg/mL at peak levels.

Renal—

Occurs by glomerular filtration and tubular secretion.

Renal clearance is approximately 275 mL per minute.

In the urine, 26 to 32% of a single oral dose is excreted in 24 hours.

## Precautions to Consider

### Cross-sensitivity and/or related problems

Patients sensitive to systemic norfloxacin or to other quinolones (e.g., cinoxacin, ciprofloxacin, enoxacin, lomefloxacin, nalidixic acid, ofloxacin), may be sensitive to ophthalmic norfloxacin also.

### Carcinogenicity

In a study lasting up to 96 weeks, no increase in neoplastic changes was observed in rats administered doses 8 to 9 times the usual human oral dose of norfloxacin.

### Mutagenicity

Norfloxacin had no mutagenic effect in the dominant lethal test in mice. In doses 30 to 60 times the usual human oral dose, norfloxacin did not cause chromosomal aberrations in hamsters or rats. Norfloxacin had no mutagenic activity in the Ames microbial mutagen test or in Chinese hamster fibroblasts. Although norfloxacin was weakly positive in the Rec-assay for DNA repair, it had no mutagenic activity in the more sensitive V-79 mammalian cell assay.

### Pregnancy/Reproduction

Fertility—In male and female mice, oral doses of norfloxacin up to 33 times the usual human oral dose did not adversely affect fertility.

Pregnancy—Since systemic norfloxacin has been shown to cause arthropathy in immature animals (see *Pediatrics*) and there is no information on ophthalmic norfloxacin, use of ophthalmic norfloxacin is not recommended during pregnancy.

Adequate and well controlled studies in humans have not been done. Systemic norfloxacin crosses the placenta. The umbilical cord serum concentration ranged from undetectable to 0.5 mg/mL and the amniotic fluid concentration ranged from undetectable to 0.92 mg/mL following the administration of a single 200 mg dose of norfloxacin.

At oral doses 6 to 50 times the human oral dose, there has been no evidence of a teratogenic effect in rats, rabbits, mice, or monkeys. However, in monkeys administered oral doses 10 times the maximum human oral dose (800 mg daily), norfloxacin has been shown to produce embryonic loss. Peak plasma levels reached 2 to 3 times those obtained in humans.

FDA Pregnancy Category C.

### Breast-feeding

It is not known whether ophthalmic norfloxacin is distributed into breast milk. Systemic norfloxacin has not been detected in breast milk when it was given in low (200-mg) doses to nursing mothers. However, other systemic quinolone derivatives are distributed into breast milk, and systemic norfloxacin causes arthropathy in immature animals (see *Pediatrics*). Therefore, use of ophthalmic norfloxacin is not recommended in nursing mothers.

### Pediatrics

Appropriate studies on the relationship of age to the effects of ophthalmic norfloxacin have not been performed in infants up to 1 year of age. Safety and efficacy have not been established.

Although there is no information on ophthalmic norfloxacin, other ophthalmic quinolones have not been shown to cause arthropathy in immature animals. In addition, there is no evidence that these ophthalmic quinolones have any effects on the weight-bearing joints.

### Geriatrics

Appropriate studies on the relationship of age to the effects of ophthalmic norfloxacin have not been performed in the geriatric population. However, no geriatrics-specific problems have been documented to date.

When systemic norfloxacin was administered to 6 patients, 67 to 74 years old, with normal renal function (creatinine clearance 91 mL/min/1.73 $m^2$), the plasma half-life was slightly prolonged (3.9 vs 3.2 hours) and there was a small increase in the plasma concentration (2.0 vs 1.5 hours). Alterations in dosage have not been recommended unless the patient has severe renal function impairment (creatinine clearance ≤ 30 mL/min/1.73 $m^2$).

### Laboratory value alterations

The following have been selected on the basis of their potential clinical significance (possible effect in parentheses where appropriate)—not necessarily inclusive (» = major clinical significance):

With physiology/laboratory test values
    Alanine aminotransferase (ALT [SGPT]), serum and
    Alkaline phosphatase, serum and
    Aspartate aminotransferase (AST [SGOT]), serum and
    Blood urea nitrogen (BUN) and
    Creatinine, serum and
    Lactate dehydrogenase (LDH) serum
       (although there is no information on ophthalmic norfloxacin, increased values have been observed with systemic norfloxacin)

### Medical considerations/Contraindications

The medical considerations/contraindications included here have been selected on the basis of their potential clinical significance (reasons given in parentheses where appropriate)—not necessarily inclusive (» = major clinical significance).

*Except under special circumstances, this medication should not be used when the following medical problem exists:*

» Hypersensitivity to norfloxacin or other quinolones

## Side/Adverse Effects

The following side/adverse effects have been selected on the basis of their potential clinical significance (possible signs and symptoms in parentheses where appropriate)—not necessarily inclusive:

### Those indicating need for medical attention
Incidence rare
    *Skin rash or other sign of hypersensitivity* (allergic reaction)

### Those indicating need for medical attention only if they continue or are bothersome
Incidence more frequent
    *Burning or other eye discomfort*

Incidence less frequent
    *Bitter taste following instillation; chemosis* (swelling of the membrane covering the white part of the eye); *hyperemia, conjunctival* (redness of the lining of the eyelids); *photophobia* (increased sensitivity of eye to light)

## Patient Consultation

As an aid to patient consultation, refer to *Advice for the Patient, Norfloxacin (Ophthalmic)*.

In providing consultation, consider emphasizing the following selected information (» = major clinical significance):

### Before using this medication
» Conditions affecting use, especially:
    Sensitivity to norfloxacin or other quinolone derivatives
    Pregnancy—Ophthalmic norfloxacin is not recommended during pregnancy, because it is not known whether it can cause arthropathy in immature animals as can systemic norfloxacin
    Breast-feeding—Ophthalmic norfloxacin is not recommended, because it is not known whether it can cause arthropathy in immature animals as can systemic norfloxacin
    Use in children—Ophthalmic norfloxacin is not recommended in infants, because it is not known whether it can cause arthropathy in immature animals as can systemic norfloxacin

### Proper use of this medication
Proper administration technique
» Proper dosage
» Compliance with full course of therapy
    Missed dose: Applying as soon as possible; not applying if almost time for next dose
» Proper storage

### Precautions while using this medication
Checking with physician if no improvement within a few days

Possible photophobic reactions; wearing sunglasses and avoiding prolonged exposure to bright light

### Side/adverse effects
Signs of potential side effects, especially skin rash or other sign of hypersensitivity

## General Dosing Information

### For treatment of adverse effects
Recommended treatment consists of the following:
- For mild hypersensitivity reaction—Administering antihistamines and, if necessary, glucocorticoids.
- For severe hypersensitivity or anaphylactic reaction—Administering epinephrine. Antihistamines and/or glucocorticoids may also be administered as required.

## Ophthalmic Dosage Forms

### NORFLOXACIN OPHTHALMIC SOLUTION

**Usual adult and adolescent dose**
Topical, to the conjunctiva, 1 drop four times a day for up to 7 days.

Note: For severe infections, the dosage may be increased to 1 drop every two hours while awake.

**Usual pediatric dose**
Infants up to 1 year of age—Safety and efficacy have not been established.
Children 1 year of age and over—See *Usual adult and adolescent dose*.

**Strength(s) usually available**
U.S.—
    0.3% (Rx) [*Chibroxin* (benzalkonium chloride 0.0025%)].
Canada—
    0.3% (Rx) [*Noroxin* (benzalkonium chloride 0.0025%)].

**Packaging and storage**
Store below 40 °C (104 °F), preferably between 15 and 30 °C (59 and 86 °F), unless otherwise specified by manufacturer. Protect from freezing and light.

**Stability**
Norfloxacin ophthalmic solution is a clear, colorless to light yellow solution. The solution should not be used if it is discolored or contains a precipitate.
The solution is stable for at least 2 years if stored at room temperature and protected from light.
Norfloxacin solution is stable at a pH of 5.0 to 5.4.

**Auxiliary labeling**
- For the eye.

## Selected Bibliography

Chibroxin Formulary Information monograph (MSD—US), Rev 1991, Rec 11/91.
Goldstein EJG, et al. Potential of topical norfloxacin therapy. Comparative in vitro activity against clinical ocular bacterial isolates. Arch Ophthalmol 1987 Jul; 105 (7): 991-4.
Shungu DL, et al. In vitro antibacterial activity of norfloxacin and other agents against ocular pathogens. Chemotherapy 1985; 31: 112-8.

Revised: 12/22/93

---

**NORGESTREL**—See *Progestins (Systemic)*

---

**NORTRIPTYLINE**—See *Antidepressants, Tricyclic (Systemic)*

# NYLIDRIN    Systemic*

VA CLASSIFICATION (Primary): CV500

Note: For a listing of dosage forms and brand names by country availability, see *Dosage Forms* section(s). For a listing of brand names for the articles in this monograph, refer to the General Index.

*Not commercially available in the U.S.

## Category
Vasospastic therapy adjunct.

## Indications

### Accepted
Vascular disease, peripheral (treatment)—Nylidrin is considered only "possibly" effective for its labeled indication, which includes peripheral vasospastic disorders such as arteriosclerosis obliterans; thromboangiitis obliterans; diabetic vascular disease; night leg cramps; Raynaud's phenomenon and disease; frostbite; acrocyanosis; acroparesthesia; thrombophlebitis; and cold feet, legs, and hands.

### Unaccepted
FDA has classified nylidrin as "lacking substantial evidence of effectiveness" in cerebral ischemia, cerebral arteriosclerosis, and other circulatory insufficiencies of the brain. Therefore, the FDA has withdrawn nylidrin from the U.S. market.

## Pharmacology/Pharmacokinetics

### Physicochemical characteristics
Molecular weight—335.87.

### Mechanism of action/Effect
Vasodilation of skeletal arteries and arterioles via beta-adrenergic receptor stimulation and possibly also a direct effect.

### Absorption
Readily absorbed from the gastrointestinal tract.

### Onset of action
10 minutes.

### Time to peak effect
30 minutes.

### Duration of action
2 hours.

## Precautions to Consider

### Pregnancy/Reproduction
Pregnancy—Studies have not been done in humans.
Studies have not been done in animals.

### Breast-feeding
Problems in humans have not been documented.

### Geriatrics
Appropriate studies on the relationship of age to the effects of nylidrin have not been performed in the geriatric population. However, the risk of nylidrin-induced hypothermia may be increased in elderly patients.

### Drug interactions and/or related problems
The following drug interactions and/or related problems have been selected on the basis of their potential clinical significance (possible mechanism in parentheses where appropriate)—not necessarily inclusive (» = major clinical significance):
Smoking, tobacco
  (heavy smoking may interfere with the therapeutic effect of nylidrin because nicotine constricts blood vessels)

### Medical considerations/Contraindications
The medical considerations/contraindications included here have been selected on the basis of their potential clinical significance (reasons given in parentheses where appropriate)—not necessarily inclusive (» = major clinical significance).

*Risk-benefit should be considered when the following medical problems exist:*
»  Angina pectoris, progressive, or
»  Myocardial infarction, recent
    (a "steal effect" may occur, since nylidrin has a greater effect on peripheral than on coronary vessels, leading to a further decrease in flow to ischemic areas)
   Cardiac disease or
   Congestive heart failure, uncompensated, or
»  Tachycardia, paroxysmal, or
»  Thyrotoxicosis
    (nylidrin may aggravate these conditions)
   Peptic ulcer
    (nylidrin increases gastric acid secretion and may aggravate this condition)
   Sensitivity to nylidrin

## Side/Adverse Effects
The following side/adverse effects have been selected on the basis of their potential clinical significance (possible signs and symptoms in parentheses where appropriate)—not necessarily inclusive:

### Those indicating need for medical attention
Incidence less frequent
  *Anemia* (continuing tiredness or weakness); *dizziness; fast or irregular heartbeat*

### Those indicating need for medical attention only if they continue or are bothersome
Incidence less frequent
  *Chilliness; flushing or redness of face; headache; nausea and vomiting; nervousness; trembling*

## Overdose
For more information on the management of overdose or unintentional ingestion, **contact a Poison Control Center** (see *Poison Control Center Listing*).

### Clinical effects of overdose
The following effects have been selected on the basis of their potential clinical significance (possible signs and symptoms in parentheses where appropriate)—not necessarily inclusive:
  *Blurred vision; chest pain; decrease in urination or inability to urinate; fever; metallic taste*

## Patient Consultation
As an aid to patient consultation, refer to *Advice for the Patient, Nylidrin (Systemic)*.

In providing consultation, consider emphasizing the following selected information (» = major clinical significance):

**Before using this medication**
»  Conditions affecting use, especially:
    Sensitivity to nylidrin
    Use in the elderly—Increased risk of hypothermia
    Other medical problems, especially angina pectoris, recent myocardial infarction, paroxysmal tachycardia, and thyrotoxicosis

**Proper use of this medication**
   Timing of doses to minimize interference with sleep due to palpitations; avoiding taking last dose at bedtime
»  Proper dosing
   Missed dose: Taking as soon as possible; not taking if almost time for next dose; not doubling doses
»  Proper storage

**Precautions while using this medication**
   Checking with physician before discontinuing medication
   Avoiding smoking (nicotine constricts blood vessels)

**Side/adverse effects**
   Signs of potential side effects, especially anemia, dizziness, and fast or irregular heartbeat

## Oral Dosage Forms

### NYLIDRIN HYDROCHLORIDE TABLETS USP

**Usual adult dose**
Vasospastic therapy adjunct—
    Oral, 3 to 12 mg three or four times a day.

**Strength(s) usually available**
U.S.—
    Not commercially available.

Canada—
    6 mg (Rx) [*Arlidin* (scored); *PMS Nylidrin* (scored)].
    12 mg (Rx) [*Arlidin Forte* (scored)].

**Packaging and storage**
Store below 40 °C (104 °F), preferably between 15 and 30 °C (59 and 86 °F), unless otherwise specified by manufacturer. Store in a tight container.

Revised: 05/14/93

---

# NYSTATIN    Oral-Local

**VA CLASSIFICATION (Primary): AM700**
Note: For a listing of dosage forms and brand names by country availability, see *Dosage Forms* section(s). For a listing of brand names for the articles in this monograph, refer to the General Index.

## Category
Antifungal (oral-local).

## Indications
Note: Bracketed information in the *Indications* section refers to uses that are not included in U.S. product labeling.

**Accepted**
Candidiasis, oropharyngeal (treatment)—Nystatin lozenges (pastilles), nystatin oral suspension, and nystatin for oral suspension are indicated in the local treatment of fungal infections of the oral cavity caused by *Candida albicans* and other *Candida* species.

[Candidiasis, oropharyngeal (prophylaxis)]—Nystatin oral suspension, lozenges (pastilles), and nystatin for oral suspension are used in the prophylaxis of oropharyngeal candidiasis.

Not all species or strains of a particular organism may be susceptible to nystatin.

**Unaccepted**
Nystatin is not indicated in the treatment of systemic fungal infections since it is not absorbed from the gastrointestinal tract.

USP medical experts do not recommend nystatin oral tablets for any indication.

## Pharmacology/Pharmacokinetics

**Mechanism of action/Effect**
Binds to sterols in the fungal cell membrane, resulting in the cell membrane's inability to function as a selective barrier, thus allowing loss of essential cellular constituents.

**Absorption**
Not absorbed from the gastrointestinal tract.

**Saliva concentrations**
Saliva concentrations of nystatin are maintained above those required *in vitro* to inhibit the growth of clinically significant *Candida* species for approximately 2 hours after the start of oral dissolution of 2 nystatin lozenges (400,000 units).

**Elimination**
Fecal. Orally administered nystatin is excreted almost entirely as unchanged drug.

## Precautions to Consider

**Carcinogenicity/Mutagenicity**
Studies have not been done to evaluate the carcinogenic or mutagenic potential of nystatin.

**Pregnancy/Reproduction**
Fertility—Studies have not been done to evaluate the effect of nystatin on fertility in either males or females.

Pregnancy—Studies in humans have not shown that nystatin causes adverse effects on the fetus.

**Breast-feeding**
It is not known whether oral nystatin is excreted in breast milk. However, problems in humans have not been documented.

**Pediatrics**
Use of nystatin lozenges is not recommended in infants and children up to 5 years of age since this age group may not be capable of using the lozenges or tablets safely. However, no pediatrics-specific problems have been documented to date with nystatin oral suspension.

**Geriatrics**
No information is available on the relationship of age to the effects of oral nystatin in geriatric patients.

**Dental**
Patients with full or partial dentures who have symptomatic oral candidiasis may need to soak their dentures nightly in reconstituted nystatin for oral suspension to eliminate *Candida* species from the dentures. In rare cases when this does not eliminate the fungus, it may be necessary to have new dentures made.

**Medical considerations/Contraindications**
The medical considerations/contraindications included here have been selected on the basis of their potential clinical significance (reasons given in parentheses where appropriate)—not necessarily inclusive (» = major clinical significance).

*Risk-benefit should be considered when the following medical problem exists:*
    Intolerance to nystatin

## Side/Adverse Effects
The following side/adverse effects have been selected on the basis of their potential clinical significance (possible signs and symptoms in parentheses where appropriate)—not necessarily inclusive:

**Those indicating need for medical attention only if they continue or are bothersome**
Incidence less frequent
    *Gastrointestinal disturbances* (diarrhea; nausea or vomiting; stomach pain)

## Patient Consultation
As an aid to patient consultation, refer to *Advice for the Patient, Nystatin (Oral)*.

In providing consultation, consider emphasizing the following selected information (» = major clinical significance):

**Before using this medication**
» Conditions affecting use, especially:
    Intolerance to nystatin
    Use in children—Nystatin lozenges or tablets are not recommended in infants and children up to 5 years of age since this age group may not be capable of using the lozenges or tablets safely

**Proper use of this medication**
    Proper administration technique for dry powder, lozenges, and oral suspension
» Compliance with full course of therapy
» Proper dosing
    Missed dose: Taking as soon as possible; not taking if almost time for next dose; not doubling doses
» Proper storage

**Side/adverse effects**
    Signs of potential side effects, especially gastrointestinal disturbance

## General Dosing Information
The oral suspension should be administered by placing 1/2 of the dose in each side of the mouth. The patient should hold the suspension in the mouth or swish it throughout the mouth for as long as possible, then gargle and swallow.

Lozenges (pastilles) should be allowed to dissolve slowly and completely in the mouth. They should not be chewed or swallowed whole.

To prevent relapse, therapy should be continued for 48 hours after symptoms have disappeared and the cultures have returned to normal.

## Oral Dosage Forms
### NYSTATIN LOZENGES (PASTILLES)
**Usual adult and adolescent dose**
Candidiasis—
Oral, as a lozenge dissolved slowly and completely in the mouth, 200,000 to 400,000 Units four or five times a day for up to fourteen days.

**Usual pediatric dose**
Candidiasis—
Infants and children up to 5 years of age: Use is not recommended since this age group may not be capable of using the lozenges safely.
Children 5 years of age and over: See *Usual adult and adolescent dose*.

**Strength(s) usually available**
U.S.—
200,000 Units (Rx) [*Mycostatin*].
Canada—
Not commercially available.

**Packaging and storage**
Store between 2 and 8 °C (36 and 46 °F), in a well-closed container, unless otherwise specified by manufacturer.

**Auxiliary labeling**
• Refrigerate.
• Dissolve slowly in mouth.
• Continue medicine for full time of treatment.

### NYSTATIN ORAL SUSPENSION USP
**Usual adult and adolescent dose**
Candidiasis—
Oral, 400,000 to 600,000 Units four times a day.

**Usual pediatric dose**
Candidiasis—
Premature and low-birth-weight infants: Oral, 100,000 Units four times a day.
Older infants: Oral, 200,000 Units four times a day.
Children: See *Usual adult and adolescent dose*.

**Strength(s) usually available**
U.S.—
100,000 Units per mL (Rx) [*Mycostatin; Nilstat; Nystex;* GENERIC].
Canada—
100,000 Units per mL (Rx) [*Mycostatin; Nadostine; Nilstat; PMS Nystatin*].

**Packaging and storage**
Store below 40 °C (104 °F), preferably between 15 and 30 °C (59 and 86 °F), unless otherwise specified by manufacturer. Store in a tight, light-resistant container. Protect from freezing.

**Auxiliary labeling**
• Shake well.
• Continue medicine for full time of treatment.

**Note**
When dispensing, include a calibrated liquid-measuring device.

### NYSTATIN FOR ORAL SUSPENSION USP
**Usual adult and adolescent dose**
See *Nystatin Oral Suspension USP*.

**Usual pediatric dose**
See *Nystatin Oral Suspension USP*.

**Size(s) usually available**
U.S.—
50,000,000 Units (Rx) [GENERIC].
150,000,000 Units (Rx) [GENERIC].
500,000,000 Units (Rx) [GENERIC].
1,000,000,000 Units (Rx) [*Nilstat;* GENERIC].
2,000,000,000 Units (Rx) [*Nilstat;* GENERIC].
5,000,000,000 Units (Rx) [GENERIC].
10,000,000,000 Units (Rx) [GENERIC].
Canada—
1,000,000,000 Units (Rx) [*Nilstat*].
2,000,000,000 Units (Rx) [*Nilstat*].
Note: One-eighth ($^1/_8$) teaspoonful of nystatin for oral suspension is approximately equal to 500,000 units.

**Packaging and storage**
Prior to reconstitution, store below 40 °C (104 °F), preferably between 15 and 30 °C (59 and 86 °F), unless otherwise specified by manufacturer. Store in a tight container.

**Preparation of dosage form**
Add $^1/_8$ teaspoonful (approximately 500,000 Units) of dry powder to approximately 120 mL of water. Stir well.

**Stability**
After mixing, suspension should be used immediately since nystatin for oral suspension contains no preservatives.

**Auxiliary labeling**
• Dissolve in water immediately before taking.
• Continue medicine for full time of treatment.

**Note**
Explain administration technique.

### NYSTATIN TABLETS USP
**Usual adult and adolescent dose**
Candidiasis—
Oral, 500,000 to 1,000,000 Units three times a day.

**Usual pediatric dose**
Candidiasis—
Infants and children up to 5 years of age: Use is not recommended since this age group may not be capable of using the tablet safely.
Children 5 years of age and over: Oral, 500,000 Units four times a day.

**Strength(s) usually available**
U.S.—
500,000 Units (Rx) [*Mycostatin* (film-coated); *Nilstat* (film-coated); GENERIC].
Canada—
500,000 Units (Rx) [*Mycostatin* (film-coated); *Nadostine* (film-coated); *Nilstat* (film-coated)].

**Packaging and storage**
Store below 40 °C (104 °F), preferably between 15 and 30 °C (59 and 86 °F), unless otherwise specified by manufacturer. Store in a tight, light-resistant container.

**Auxiliary labeling**
• Continue medicine for full time of treatment.

Revised: 01/19/93
Interim revision: 04/14/95

# NYSTATIN Topical

VA CLASSIFICATION (Primary): DE102
Note: For a listing of dosage forms and brand names by country availability, see *Dosage Forms* section(s). For a listing of brand names for the articles in this monograph, refer to the General Index.

## Category
Antifungal (topical).

## Indications
Note: Bracketed information in the *Indications* section refers to uses that are not included in U.S. product labeling.

**Accepted**
Candidiasis, cutaneous (treatment) or
Candidiasis, mucocutaneous, chronic (treatment)—Topical nystatin is indicated in the treatment of cutaneous and chronic mucocutaneous candidiasis caused by *Candida (Monilia) albicans* and other *Candida* species.

[Tinea barbae (treatment)] or

[Tinea capitis (treatment)]—Topical nystatin is used in the treatment of tinea barbae and tinea capitis.

Not all species or strains of a particular organism may be susceptible to nystatin.

## Pharmacology/Pharmacokinetics

### Mechanism of action/Effect
Topical nystatin binds to sterols in the fungal cell membrane, resulting in the cell membrane's inability to function as a selective barrier, allowing loss of essential cellular constituents.

### Absorption
Not absorbed following topical application to intact skin or mucous membranes.

## Precautions to Consider

### Pregnancy/Reproduction
Pregnancy—Problems in humans have not been documented.

### Breast-feeding
It is not known whether topically applied nystatin is distributed into breast milk. However, problems in humans have not been documented.

### Pediatrics
Appropriate studies on the relationship of age to the effects of topical nystatin have not been performed in the pediatric population. However, no pediatrics-specific problems have been documented to date. When this medication is used in the treatment of candidiasis, occlusive dressings (e.g., tight-fitting diaper, plastic pants) should be avoided since they provide conditions that favor growth of yeast and release of its irritating endotoxin.

### Geriatrics
No information is available on the relationship of age to the effects of topical nystatin in geriatric patients.

### Medical considerations/Contraindications
The medical considerations/contraindications included here have been selected on the basis of their potential clinical significance (reasons given in parentheses where appropriate)—not necessarily inclusive (» = major clinical significance).

*Risk-benefit should be considered when the following medical problem exists:*
   Hypersensitivity to nystatin

## Side/Adverse Effects
The following side/adverse effects have been selected on the basis of their potential clinical significance (possible signs and symptoms in parentheses where appropriate)—not necessarily inclusive:

**Those indicating need for medical attention**
   *Skin irritation not present before therapy*

## Patient Consultation
As an aid to patient consultation, refer to *Advice for the Patient, Nystatin (Topical)*.

In providing consultation, consider emphasizing the following selected information (» = major clinical significance):

**Before using this medication**
» Conditions affecting use, especially:
      Hypersensitivity to nystatin

**Proper use of this medication**
   Not for ophthalmic use
   Applying sufficient medication to cover affected area
   Proper administration technique for topical powder
» Not applying occlusive dressing over this medication unless directed to do so by physician; avoiding tight-fitting diapers and plastic pants on diaper area of children
» Compliance with full course of therapy
» Proper dosing
   Missed dose: Applying as soon as possible
» Proper storage

**Side/adverse effects**
   Signs of potential side effects, especially skin irritation not present before therapy

## General Dosing Information
The cream is usually preferred to the ointment for candidiasis involving intertriginous areas. However, very moist lesions involving intertriginous areas are usually best treated with the topical powder.

For fungal infection of the feet, the powder should be dusted freely on the feet as well as in the shoes and socks.

Symptomatic relief usually occurs within 24 to 72 hours following initiation of therapy.

Therapy for a period of 2 weeks is usually sufficient, but more prolonged treatment may be necessary.

When this medication is used in the treatment of candidiasis, occlusive dressings should be avoided since they provide conditions that favor growth of yeast and release of its irritating endotoxin. An oleaginous ointment, a thin film of polyethylene, a bandage, a tight-fitting diaper, plastic pants, or tape may constitute an occlusive dressing.

## Topical Dosage Forms

### NYSTATIN CREAM USP

**Usual adult and adolescent dose**
Candidiasis—
   Topical, to the skin, two or three times a day.

**Usual pediatric dose**
See *Usual adult and adolescent dose.*

**Strength(s) usually available**
U.S.—
   100,000 Units per gram (Rx) [*Mycostatin; Nilstat; Nystex;* GENERIC].
Canada—
   100,000 Units per gram (OTC) [*Mycostatin; Nadostine; Nilstat; Nyaderm*].

**Packaging and storage**
Store below 40 °C (104 °F), in a collapsible tube, or in other tight container. Protect from freezing.

**Auxiliary labeling**
• For external use only.
• Continue medication for full time of treatment.

### NYSTATIN OINTMENT USP

**Usual adult and adolescent dose**
See *Nystatin Cream USP.*

**Usual pediatric dose**
See *Nystatin Cream USP.*

**Strength(s) usually available**
U.S.—
   100,000 Units per gram (Rx) [*Mycostatin; Nilstat; Nystex;* GENERIC].
Canada—
   100,000 Units per gram (OTC) [*Mycostatin; Nadostine; Nilstat; Nyaderm*].

**Packaging and storage**
Store in a well-closed container, preferably between 15 and 30 °C (59 and 86 °F), unless otherwise specified by manufacturer. Protect from freezing.

**Auxiliary labeling**
• For external use only.
• Continue medication for full time of treatment.

### NYSTATIN TOPICAL POWDER USP

**Usual adult and adolescent dose**
See *Nystatin Cream USP.*

**Usual pediatric dose**
See *Nystatin Cream USP.*

**Strength(s) usually available**
U.S.—
   100,000 Units per gram (Rx) [*Mycostatin*].
Canada—
   100,000 Units per gram (OTC) [*Mycostatin*].

**Packaging and storage**
Store in a well-closed container below 40 °C (104 °F), preferably between 15 and 30 °C (59 and 86 °F), unless otherwise specified by manufacturer.

**Auxiliary labeling**
• For external use only.
• Keep container tightly closed.
• Continue medication for full time of treatment.

Revised: 07/25/94

# NYSTATIN   Vaginal

VA CLASSIFICATION (Primary): GU300

Note: For a listing of dosage forms and brand names by country availability, see *Dosage Forms* section(s). For a listing of brand names for the articles in this monograph, refer to the General Index.

## Category
Antifungal (vaginal).

## Indications

Note: Bracketed information in the *Indications* section refers to uses that are not included in U.S. product labeling.

### Accepted
Candidiasis, vulvovaginal (treatment)—Vaginal nystatin is indicated in the local treatment of vulvovaginal candidiasis caused by *Candida (Monilia) albicans* and other *Candida* species.

[Candidiasis, oropharyngeal (treatment)]—Nystatin vaginal tablets are used as lozenges to treat oropharyngeal candidiasis since their slow dissolution rate provides prolonged oral contact.

Not all species or strains of a particular organism may be susceptible to nystatin.

### Unaccepted
Nystatin is not effective against *Trichomonas vaginalis* or *Gardnerella vaginalis (Haemophilus vaginalis).*

## Pharmacology/Pharmacokinetics

### Physicochemical characteristics
Source—Derived from *Streptomyces noursei.*
Chemical group—Polyene antifungal.

### Mechanism of action/Effect
Binds to sterols in the fungal cell membrane, resulting in the cell membrane's inability to function as a selective barrier, which allows loss of essential cellular constituents.

## Precautions to Consider

### Carcinogenicity/Mutagenicity
Long-term studies in animals have not been done to evaluate the carcinogenic or mutagenic potential of nystatin.

### Pregnancy/Reproduction
Fertility—Long-term studies in animals have not been done to evaluate the effect of nystatin on fertility in females.

Pregnancy—Studies in animals have not been done. However, studies in humans have not shown that nystatin causes adverse effects on the fetus.

FDA Pregnancy Category A.

### Breast-feeding
It is not known whether vaginal nystatin is distributed into breast milk. However, problems in humans have not been documented.

### Pediatrics
No information is available on the relationship of age to the effects of vaginal nystatin in pediatric patients.

### Geriatrics
No information is available on the relationship of age to the effects of vaginal nystatin in geriatric patients.

### Medical considerations/Contraindications
The medical considerations/contraindications included here have been selected on the basis of their potential clinical significance (reasons given in parentheses where appropriate)—not necessarily inclusive (» = major clinical significance).

*Risk-benefit should be considered when the following medical problem exists:*
Sensitivity to nystatin

## Side/Adverse Effects

The following side/adverse effects have been selected on the basis of their potential clinical significance (possible signs and symptoms in parentheses where appropriate)—not necessarily inclusive:

### Those indicating need for medical attention
Incidence rare
*Vaginal irritation not present before therapy*

## Patient Consultation

As an aid to patient consultation, refer to *Advice for the Patient, Nystatin (Vaginal).*

In providing consultation, consider emphasizing the following selected information (» = major clinical significance):

### Before using this medication
» Conditions affecting use, especially:
Sensitivity to nystatin

### Proper use of this medication
Reading patient instructions before using medication
Proper administration technique
» Compliance with full course of therapy
» Proper dosing
Missed dose: Inserting as soon as possible; not inserting if almost time for next dose
» Proper storage

### Precautions while using this medication
» Using hygienic measures to control sources of infection or reinfection
Checking with physician about douching or intercourse during therapy
Protection of clothing because of possible vaginal drainage

### Side/adverse effects
Signs of potential side effects, especially vaginal irritation not present before therapy

## General Dosing Information

Therapy for a period of 2 weeks is usually sufficient, but more prolonged treatment may be necessary.

To prevent thrush in the newborn, it is suggested that nystatin vaginal tablets be administered to pregnant patients with candidal vaginitis in a dosage of 100,000 to 200,000 Units daily for 3 to 6 weeks prior to delivery.

## Vaginal Dosage Forms

### NYSTATIN VAGINAL CREAM

#### Usual adult and adolescent dose
Antifungal—
Intravaginal, 1 (100,000-Unit) applicatorful one or two times a day for two weeks; or 1 (500,000-Unit) applicatorful once daily.

Note: For severe infections, *Nilstat* vaginal cream may be repeated every 12 hours.

#### Usual pediatric dose
Dosage has not been established.

#### Strength(s) usually available
U.S.—
Not commercially available.
Canada—
25,000 Units per gram (100,000 Units per applicatorful) (Rx) [*Mycostatin; Nadostine; Nyaderm*].
100,000 Units per gram (500,000 Units per applicatorful) (Rx) [*Nilstat*].

#### Packaging and storage
Store below 40 °C (104 °F), preferably between 15 and 30 °C (59 and 86 °F), unless otherwise specified by manufacturer. Store in a tight, light-resistant container.

#### Auxiliary labeling
• Continue medicine for full time of treatment.
• For vaginal use only

#### Note
Include patient instructions when dispensing.
Explain administration technique.
Medication should be continued even during menstruation.

## NYSTATIN VAGINAL TABLETS USP

**Usual adult and adolescent dose**
Antifungal—
Intravaginal, 100,000 Units one or two times a day for two weeks.

**Usual pediatric dose**
Dosage has not been established.

**Strength(s) usually available**
U.S.—
100,000 Units (Rx) [*Mycostatin; Nilstat*; GENERIC].
Canada—
100,000 Units (Rx) [*Mycostatin; Nadostine; Nilstat*].

**Packaging and storage**
Store below 40 °C (104 °F), preferably between 15 and 30 °C (59 and 86 °F), unless otherwise specified by manufacturer. Store in a tight, light-resistant container.

Note: Some manufacturers recommend storage in a refrigerator.

**Auxiliary labeling**
• Continue medicine for full time of treatment.
• For vaginal use only

**Note**
Include patient instructions when dispensing.
Explain administration technique (for use as oral lozenge).
Medication should be continued even during menstruation.

Revised: 09/08/92
Interim revision: 06/30/94

---

## NYSTATIN-CONTAINING COMBINATIONS—
Nystatin and Triamcinolone (Topical)

---

# NYSTATIN AND TRIAMCINOLONE  Topical

VA CLASSIFICATION (Primary): DE250

**NOTE:** The *Nystatin and Triamcinolone (Topical)* monograph is maintained on the USP DI electronic data base. For a printed copy of the most recent revision of the complete monograph, contact the USP Division of Information Development, 12601 Twinbrook Parkway, Rockville, MD 20852.

For information on the specific components of this combination, see the *USP DI* monographs for *Corticosteroids (Topical)* and *Nystatin (Topical)*.

The information that follows is selectively abstracted from the complete monograph and is provided to facilitate drug use review and patient counseling.

Note: For a listing of dosage forms and brand names by country availability, see *Dosage Forms* section(s). For a listing of brand names for the articles in this monograph, refer to the General Index.

## Category
Antifungal-corticosteroid (topical).

## Indications
Note: Bracketed information in the *Indications* section refers to uses that are not included in U.S. product labeling.

**Accepted**
Candidiasis, cutaneous (treatment)—Nystatin and triamcinolone combination is indicated as a secondary agent in the topical treatment of cutaneous candidiasis, [accompanied by inflammation], caused by *Candida albicans (Monilia albicans)* and other *Candida* species.

The use of nystatin and triamcinolone combination has been shown to provide greater benefit than nystatin alone during the first few days of treatment [or for as long as inflammation persists. After this time, USP medical experts recommend the use of plain nystatin or other topical antifungal agents. Also, nystatin and triamcinolone combination is recommended only for short-term (less than 2 weeks) treatment of inflammatory candidiasis confined to limited areas of the skin].

Not all species or strains of a particular organism may be susceptible to nystatin.

**Unaccepted**
Nystatin and triamcinolone combination is not recommended in the treatment of mucocutaneous candidiasis. In addition, nystatin is not effective against bacteria, protozoa, trichomonads, or viruses.

## Patient Consultation
As an aid to patient consultation, refer to *Advice for the Patient, Nystatin and Triamcinolone (Topical)*.

In providing consultation, consider emphasizing the following selected information (» = major clinical significance):

**Before using this medication**
» Conditions affecting use, especially:
Sensitivity to nystatin or corticosteroids
Pregnancy—Topical corticosteroids may be systemically absorbed; potent corticosteroids have been shown to be teratogenic in animals following topical application

Breast-feeding—Systemic corticosteroids are distributed into breast-milk and may cause growth suppression in the infant; topical corticosteroids may be systemically absorbed
Use in children—Children may absorb a proportionately larger amount of topical corticosteroid than adults, making them more susceptible to HPA axis suppression and Cushing's syndrome
Other medical problems, especially Herpes simplex; tubercular infections of the skin; vaccinia, eczema vaccinatum, varicella, or other viral infections of the skin

**Proper use of this medication**
» Not for ophthalmic use
» Checking with physician before using medication on other skin problems
Applying a thin layer of medication to affected area and rubbing in gently and thoroughly
» Not applying occlusive dressing over this medication unless directed to do so by physician; wearing loose-fitting clothing when using on inguinal area; avoiding tight-fitting diapers and plastic pants on diaper area of children
» Compliance with full course of therapy; not using more often or longer than directed by physician; excessive use on thin skin areas may result in skin atrophy and stretch marks
» Proper dosing
Missed dose: Applying as soon as possible; not applying if almost time for next dose
» Proper storage

**Precautions while using this medication**
» Using hygienic measures to cure infection or prevent reinfection; keeping affected area as cool and dry as possible
Checking with physician if no improvement within 2 or 3 weeks
» May be more likely to cause systemic toxicity in children; chronic use may interfere with growth and development also; having children closely monitored by their physician
» Diabetics: May rarely cause hyperglycemia and glucosuria; checking with physician before changing diet or dosage of antidiabetic medication

**Side/adverse effects**
Side effects more likely to occur in children
Signs of potential side effects, especially hypersensitivity; acne or oily skin; increased hair growth especially on the face; increased loss of hair, especially on the scalp; reddish purple lines on arms, face, legs, trunk, or groins; skin atrophy

## Topical Dosage Forms

### NYSTATIN AND TRIAMCINOLONE ACETONIDE CREAM USP

**Usual adult and adolescent dose**
Antifungal—
Topical, to the skin, two times a day, morning and evening.

**Usual pediatric dose**
See *Usual adult and adolescent dose.*

**Strength(s) usually available**

U.S.—

    100,000 Units of nystatin and 1 mg of triamcinolone acetonide per gram [*Dermacomb; Myco II; Mycobiotic II; Mycogen II; Mycolog II; Myco-Triacet II; Mykacet II; Mytrex; Tristatin II;* GENERIC].

Canada—

    Not commercially available.

**Auxiliary labeling**

- For external use only.
- Continue medication for full time of treatment.
- Do not use in or around the eyes.

# NYSTATIN AND TRIAMCINOLONE ACETONIDE OINTMENT USP

**Usual adult and adolescent dose**

Antifungal—

    Topical, to the skin, two or three times a day.

**Usual pediatric dose**

See *Usual adult and adolescent dose.*

**Strength(s) usually available**

U.S.—

    100,000 Units of nystatin and 1 mg of triamcinolone acetonide per gram [*Myco II; Mycobiotic II; Mycogen II; Mycolog II; Myco-Triacet II; Mykacet; Mytrex; Tristatin II;* GENERIC].

Canada—

    Not commercially available.

**Auxiliary labeling**

- For external use only.
- Continue medication for full time of treatment.
- Do not use in or around the eyes.

Revised: 08/15/94

## OCTOCRYLENE-CONTAINING COMBINATIONS—

Avobenzone, Octocrylene, Octyl Salicylate, and Oxybenzone (Topical)—See *Sunscreen Agents (Topical)*

Homosalate, Octocrylene, Octyl Methoxycinnamate, and Oxybenzone (Topical)—See *Sunscreen Agents (Topical)*

Menthyl Anthranilate, Octocrylene, and Octyl Methoxycinnamate (Topical)—See *Sunscreen Agents (Topical)*

Menthyl Anthranilate, Octocrylene, Octyl Methoxycinnamate, and Oxybenzone (Topical)—See *Sunscreen Agents (Topical)*

Octocrylene and Octyl Methoxycinnamate (Topical)—See *Sunscreen Agents (Topical)*

Octocrylene, Octyl Methoxycinnamate, Octyl Salicylate, and Oxybenzone (Topical)—See *Sunscreen Agents (Topical)*

Octocrylene, Octyl Methoxycinnamate, Octyl Salicylate, Oxybenzone, and Titanium Dioxide (Topical)—See *Sunscreen Agents (Topical)*

Octocrylene, Octyl Methoxycinnamate, and Oxybenzone (Topical)—See *Sunscreen Agents (Topical)*

Octocrylene, Octyl Methoxycinnamate, Oxybenzone, and Titanium Dioxide (Topical)—See *Sunscreen Agents (Topical)*

Octocrylene, Octyl Methoxycinnamate, and Titanium Dioxide (Topical)—See *Sunscreen Agents (Topical)*

## OCTOXYNOL 9—See *Spermicides (Vaginal)*

# OCTREOTIDE    Systemic

VA CLASSIFICATION (Primary/Secondary): GA400/CV900; HS900

Note: For a listing of dosage forms and brand names by country availability, see *Dosage Forms* section(s). For a listing of brand names for the articles in this monograph, refer to the General Index.

## Category

Antidiarrheal (gastrointestinal tumor; acquired immune deficiency syndrome [AIDS]); antihypotensive (carcinoid crisis); growth hormone suppressant (acromegaly); antihypoglycemic (pancreatic tumor).

## Indications

Note: Bracketed information in the *Indications* section refers to uses that are not included in U.S. product labeling.

### Accepted

Tumors, gastrointestinal (treatment adjunct)—Octreotide is indicated for palliative management of gastrointestinal endocrine tumors, such as: Carcinoid tumors—To suppress or inhibit the associated severe diarrhea and facial flushing episodes.

Vasoactive intestinal peptide tumors (VIPomas)—For the treatment of the profuse watery diarrhea associated with vasoactive intestinal peptide (VIP)–secreting tumors.

[Hypotension (treatment)][1]—Octreotide is used to reverse life-threatening hypotension due to carcinoid crisis during induction of anesthesia.

Acromegaly (treatment)[1]—Octreotide is used to decrease secretion of growth hormone from pituitary tumors and decrease blood concentrations of insulin-like growth factor-I (IGF-I or somatomedin-C) in patients with acromegaly who have not optimally responded to or cannot be treated with surgical resection or pituitary irradiation, or have been unable to tolerate bromocriptine. Octreotide may be used as adjunctive therapy with irradiation treatment to help relieve symptoms of acromegaly and possibly suppress the rate of tumor growth.

[Tumors, pancreatic (treatment adjunct)][1]—Octreotide is used as palliative treatment of the symptoms resulting from hyperinsulinemia from severe refractory metastatic insulinoma.

[Diarrhea, AIDS-associated (treatment)][1]—Octreotide is used in AIDS patients with severe secretory diarrhea who have failed to respond to antimicrobial or antimotility agents.

[1]Not included in Canadian product labeling.

## Pharmacology/Pharmacokinetics

### Physicochemical characteristics
Molecular weight—1019.26.

### Mechanism of action/Effect
Action similar to naturally occurring somatostatin, but with a prolonged duration of action. Like the naturally occurring hormone, octreotide suppresses secretion of serotonin and the gastroenteropancreatic peptides. Stimulates fluid and electrolyte absorption from the gastrointestinal tract, and prolongs intestinal transit time. It blocks the carcinoid flush, decreases circulating levels of serotonin metabolite 5-hydroxyindoleacetic acid (5-HIAA), and controls other symptoms associated with the carcinoid syndrome.

### Other actions/effects
Suppresses growth hormone, insulin, and glucagon. Decreases splanchnic blood flow. Inhibits gallbladder contractions. Slows gastrointestinal transit time.

### Absorption
Absorbed rapidly and completely from injection site.

### Protein binding
High (65%, to lipoproteins and to a lesser extent to albumin).

### Half-life
Elimination—1.5 hours.

### Time to peak concentration
≤0.5 hours.

### Peak serum concentration
5.5 nanograms/mL (with 100-mcg dose).

### Duration of action
Up to 12 hours (depending on type of tumor).

### Elimination
Renal (32% of dose).

## Precautions to Consider

### Carcinogenicity/Mutagenicity
No long-term studies to assess carcinogenic potential of octreotide have been completed in animals or humans. Studies in animals have demonstrated no mutagenic potential.

### Pregnancy/Reproduction
Pregnancy—Appropriate studies in humans have not been performed.

Studies in rats and rabbits at doses up to 30 times the maximum human dose have not shown that octreotide causes adverse effects on the fetus.

FDA Pregnancy Category B.

### Breast-feeding
It is not known whether octreotide is distributed into breast milk. However, problems in humans have not been documented.

### Pediatrics
Appropriate studies with octreotide have not been performed in the pediatric population. However, doses of 1 to 10 mcg per kg of body weight, given to children as young as 1 month old, were well tolerated. One case in which an infant (a case of nesidioblastosis) suffered a seizure while undergoing octreotide therapy was thought to be unrelated to octreotide administration.

### Geriatrics
Studies performed to date in patients as old as 83 years of age have not demonstrated geriatrics-specific problems that would limit the usefulness of this medication in the elderly.

### Drug interactions and/or related problems
The following drug interactions and/or related problems have been selected on the basis of their potential clinical significance (possible mechanism in parentheses where appropriate)—not necessarily inclusive (» = major clinical significance):

Note: Combinations containing any of the following medications, depending on the amount present, may also interact with this medication.

»   Antidiabetic agents, sulfonlyurea or
»   Glucagon or
»   Growth hormone or
»   Insulin
       (use of these medications during octreotide therapy may result in hypo- or hyperglycemia; patient monitoring and dosage adjustment of these medications may be necessary)

Cyclosporine
(a single case of transplant rejection [renal/whole pancreas] in a patient who was receiving octreotide and who was immunosuppressed with cyclosporine has been reported; the use of octreotide to reduce exocrine secretion and close a fistula in this patient resulted in a decrease in the blood levels of cyclosporine, thus possibly contributing to the rejection episode)

### Laboratory value alterations
The following have been selected on the basis of their potential clinical significance (possible effect in parentheses where appropriate)—not necessarily inclusive (» = major clinical significance):

With physiology/laboratory test values
Thyroid hormones
(serum concentration of thyroxine [$T_4$] may be decreased; hypothyroidism occurred in 1 clinical trial patient after 19 months of receiving 1.5 mg of octreotide daily)

### Medical considerations/Contraindications
The medical considerations/contraindications included here have been selected on the basis of their potential clinical significance (reasons given in parentheses where appropriate)—not necessarily inclusive (» = major clinical significance).

*Risk-benefit should be considered when the following medical problems exist:*

Diabetes mellitus
(therapy used to control glycemic states may need to be adjusted)
» Gallbladder disease or gallstones, or history of
(increased risk of cholelithiasis possibly due to alteration of fat absorption and decrease in gallbladder motility caused by octreotide)
Renal function impairment, severe
(half-life of octreotide may be increased; dosage adjustment may be necessary)
Sensitivity to octreotide

### Patient monitoring
The following may be especially important in patient monitoring (other tests may be warranted in some patients, depending on condition; » = major clinical significance):

Carotene, serum concentrations and
Fat content, fecal
(octreotide therapy may alter absorption of dietary fats; periodic 72-hour fecal fat and serum carotene determinations are recommended to assess possible aggravation of fat malabsorption)
Glucose
(measurement of blood concentrations is recommended at beginning of octreotide therapy and at each change of dosage if clinical signs of increase or decrease occur)
Plasma vasoactive intestinal peptide (VIP)
(determinations recommended periodically during therapy of patients with VIPomas to assess patient response)
Thyroid function determinations
(baseline and periodic thyroid function tests using total and free serum thyroxine [$T_4$] are recommended during chronic therapy)
» Ultrasonograms
(therapy with octreotide, like the natural hormone somatostatin, may be associated with cholelithiasis presumably due to an alteration of fat absorption and possibly to a decrease in the motility of the gallbladder; baseline and periodic ultrasonograms may be required to assess the presence of gallstones)
» Urinary 5-hydroxyindoleacetic acid (5-HIAA) and
Plasma substance P
(determinations recommended periodically during therapy of patients with carcinoid tumors to assess patient response)

## Side/Adverse Effects
Note: Isolated reports of hepatic dysfunctions associated with octreotide administration include acute hepatitis without cholestasis, slow development of hyperbilirubinemia, and gallstone formation.

The risk of cholelithiasis increases with long-term therapy, as is usually required in the treatment of acromegaly.

The following side/adverse effects have been selected on the basis of their potential clinical significance (possible signs and symptoms in parentheses where appropriate)—not necessarily inclusive:

### Those indicating need for medical attention
Incidence less frequent or rare
*Hyperglycemia* (drowsiness; dry mouth; flushed, dry skin; fruit-like breath odor; increased urination; loss of appetite; rapid weight loss;

stomachache, nausea, or vomiting; trouble in breathing; unusual thirst; unusual tiredness); *hypoglycemia* (anxious feeling; chills; cool, pale skin; difficulty in concentrating; headache; hunger; nausea; nervousness; shakiness; sweating; unconsciousness; unusual tiredness; weakness)

Note: Octreotide therapy is occasionally associated with mild transient *hypo-* or *hyperglycemia* due to alteration in the balance between the counter regulatory hormones, insulin, glucagon, and growth hormone.

### Those indicating need for medical attention only if they continue or are bothersome
Incidence more frequent (3 to 10%)
*Gastrointestinal symptoms* (abdominal or stomach pain or discomfort; diarrhea; nausea and vomiting); *pain, stinging, tingling, or burning sensation at injection site, with redness and swelling*

Note: *Gastrointestinal symptoms* are usually self-limiting and usually are resolved after 2 to 3 weeks of therapy.

Incidence less frequent or rare (1 to 3%)
*Dizziness or lightheadedness; edema* (swelling of feet or lower legs); *fatigue; headache; redness or flushing of face; unusual weakness*

## Overdose
For more information on the management of overdose or unintentional ingestion, **contact a Poison Control Center** (see *Poison Control Center Listing*).

### Clinical effects of overdose
Although octreotide overdosage in humans has not been reported, based on the pharmacological properties of octreotide, acute overdosage may be expected to produce hyper- or hypoglycemia depending on the endocrine status of the patient and the type of tumor involved. Temporary withdrawal of octreotide and symptomatic treatment should alleviate this condition.

### Treatment of overdose
Supportive care—Recommended treatment consists of temporary withdrawal of octreotide and symptomatic treatment of hyper- or hypoglycemia.

## Patient Consultation
As an aid to patient consultation, refer to *Advice for the Patient, Octreotide (Systemic).*

In providing consultation, consider emphasizing the following selected information (» = major clinical significance):

### Before using this medication
» Conditions affecting use, especially:
Sensitivity to octreotide
Other medications, especially oral antidiabetics, glucagon, growth hormone, insulin
Other medical problems, especially diabetes, severe renal function impairment, or gallbladder disease or gallstones

### Proper use of this medication
» Using medication only as directed by physician; taking in evenly spaced doses as ordered
» Reading directions in starter kit before using
» Proper dosing
Missed dose: Using as soon as possible unless almost time for next dose, then going back to regular dosing schedule; not doubling doses
» Proper storage

### Precautions while using this medication
» Importance of close monitoring by physician
» Carefully selecting and rotating injection sites

### Side/adverse effects
Signs of potential side effects, especially hyperglycemia or hypoglycemia

## General Dosing Information
Preferred sites for subcutaneous injection of octreotide are the hip, thigh, or abdomen.

Multiple injections at the same injection site within short periods of time are not recommended. This is to avoid irritating the area.

To avoid the occurrence of gastrointestinal side effects, injections of octreotide should be scheduled between meals and at bedtime.

Local reactions at injection site may be reduced by allowing the solution to reach room temperature before injection and by administering slowly.

## Parenteral Dosage Forms

Note: Bracketed uses in the *Dosage Forms* section refer to categories of use and/or indications that are not included in U.S. product labeling.

### OCTREOTIDE ACETATE INJECTION

#### Usual adult and adolescent dose

Antidiarrheal (gastrointestinal tumor)—

Subcutaneous, 50 mcg (0.05 mg) initially, administered one or two times a day, the dose being increased gradually according to patient tolerance and response. The following dosages are recommended for specific tumors:

Carcinoid tumors—Subcutaneous, 100 to 600 mcg (0.1 to 0.6 mg) per day, administered in two to four divided doses, for the first two weeks of therapy.

Vasoactive intestinal peptide tumors (VIPomas)—Subcutaneous, 200 to 300 mcg (0.2 to 0.3 mg) per day, administered in two to four divided doses, for the first two weeks of therapy.

[Antidiarrheal (AIDS)][1]—

Subcutaneous, 100 to 1800 mcg (0.1 to 1.8 mg) per day.

Growth hormone suppressant (acromegaly)[1]—

Subcutaneous or intravenous, initially 50 mcg (0.05 mg) injected two or three times a day. Dosage is titrated every two weeks as needed, according to IGF-I blood concentrations, to reach a dose of 100 mcg (0.1 mg) three times a day; or, for rapid titration, dosage increase may be based on multiple serum growth hormone concentrations taken at one- to four-hour intervals over eight to twelve hours. Doses up to 500 mcg (0.5 mg) three times a day have been used rarely.

Note: Octreotide injection may be administered subcutaneously (the preferred route) or intravenously. To help prevent pain at the injection site, octreotide should be given in the smallest volume needed to achieve the proper dose. In emergencies, intravenous injections may be used cautiously.

[Antihypoglycemic (pancreatic tumor)][1]—

Subcutaneous, 50 to 150 mcg (0.05 to 0.15 mg) initially, administered two times a day thirty minutes before meals, the dose being increased gradually according to patient tolerance and response.

#### Usual adult prescribing limits

Up to 750 mcg (0.75 mg) daily.

#### Usual pediatric dose

Subcutaneous, 1 to 10 mcg (0.001 to 0.01 mg) per kg of body weight per day.

#### Usual geriatric dose

See *Usual adult and adolescent dose.*

#### Strength(s) usually available

U.S.—

0.05 mg per mL (Rx) [*Sandostatin*].
0.1 mg per mL (Rx) [*Sandostatin*].
0.2 mg per mL (Rx) [*Sandostatin*].
0.5 mg per mL (Rx) [*Sandostatin*].
1 mg per mL (Rx) [*Sandostatin*].

Note: 0.05 mg per mL, 0.1 mg per mL, and 0.5 mg per mL are packaged as single-use ampules; the remaining strengths are packaged as multiple-dose vials.

Canada—

0.05 mg per mL (Rx) [*Sandostatin*].
0.1 mg per mL (Rx) [*Sandostatin*].
0.5 mg per mL (Rx) [*Sandostatin*].

#### Packaging and storage

Store at 2 to 8 °C (36 to 46 °F), unless otherwise specified by manufacturer. Protect from freezing. Protect from light.

Note: Solution should be allowed to warm to room temperature before administration. Do not warm artificially before injection. Single-use ampules should be opened just prior to use and any unused portion discarded.

#### Preparation of dosage form

Octreotide is stable when diluted for intravenous use when diluted in 50 to 200 mL of either sterile 0.9% sodium chloride injection or 5% dextrose in sterile water for injection. The diluted solution can be infused intravenously and administered over a 15- to 30-minute period or administered via a direct intravenous injection over a 3-minute period. In emergencies, rapid intravenous injections may be used cautiously.

#### Stability

If protected from light, octreotide injection is stable at room temperature, preferably between 15 and 30 °C (59 and 86 °F), for 14 days. Octreotide should not be used if discolored or if particulate matter forms in solution.

#### Incompatibilities

Octreotide is not compatible with total parenteral nutrition (TPN) solutions; decreased efficacy may result if glycosyl octreotide conjugates form.

#### Auxiliary labeling

• Refrigerate.

#### Note

Subcutaneous injection sites should be rotated.

---

[1]Not included in Canadian product labeling.

### Selected Bibliography

Lamberts SW. A guide to the clinical use of the somatostatin analogue SMS 201-995 (Sandostatin). Acta Endocrinol Suppl 1987; 286: 54-66.

O'Donnell LJ, Farthing MJ. Therapeutic potential of a long-acting somatostatin analogue in gastrointestinal diseases. Gut 1989; 30 (9): 1165-72.

---

Revised: 12/15/92
Interim revision: 06/30/94; 08/08/95

---

## OCTYL METHOXYCINNAMATE—See *Sunscreen Agents (Topical)*

---

## OCTYL METHOXYCINNAMATE-CONTAINING COMBINATIONS—

Avobenzone and Octyl Methoxycinnamate (Topical)—See *Sunscreen Agents (Topical)*

Avobenzone, Octyl Methoxycinnamate, Octyl Salicylate, and Oxybenzone (Topical)—See *Sunscreen Agents (Topical)*

Avobenzone, Octyl Methoxycinnamate, and Oxybenzone (Topical)—See *Sunscreen Agents (Topical)*

Homosalate, Menthyl Anthranilate, and Octyl Methoxycinnamate (Topical)—See *Sunscreen Agents (Topical)*

Homosalate, Menthyl Anthranilate, Octyl Methoxycinnamate, Octyl Salicylate, and Oxybenzone (Topical)—See *Sunscreen Agents (Topical)*

Homosalate, Octocrylene, Octyl Methoxycinnamate, and Oxybenzone (Topical)—See *Sunscreen Agents (Topical)*

Homosalate, Octyl Methoxycinnamate, Octyl Salicylate, and Oxybenzone (Topical)—See *Sunscreen Agents (Topical)*

Homosalate, Octyl Methoxycinnamate, and Oxybenzone (Topical)—See *Sunscreen Agents (Topical)*

Menthyl Anthranilate, Octocrylene, and Octyl Methoxycinnamate (Topical)—See *Sunscreen Agents (Topical)*

Menthyl Anthranilate, Octocrylene, Octyl Methoxycinnamate, and Oxybenzone (Topical)—See *Sunscreen Agents (Topical)*

Menthyl Anthranilate and Octyl Methoxycinnamate (Topical)—See *Sunscreen Agents (Topical)*

Menthyl Anthranilate, Octyl Methoxycinnamate, and Octyl Salicylate (Topical)—See *Sunscreen Agents (Topical)*

Menthyl Anthranilate, Octyl Methoxycinnamate, Octyl Salicylate, and Oxybenzone (Topical)—See *Sunscreen Agents (Topical)*

Menthyl Anthranilate, Octyl Methoxycinnamate, and Oxybenzone (Topical)—See *Sunscreen Agents (Topical)*

Octocrylene and Octyl Methoxycinnamate (Topical)—See *Sunscreen Agents (Topical)*

Octocrylene, Octyl Methoxycinnamate, Octyl Salicylate, and Oxybenzone (Topical)—See *Sunscreen Agents (Topical)*

Octocrylene, Octyl Methoxycinnamate, Octyl Salicylate, Oxybenzone, and Titanium Dioxide (Topical)—See *Sunscreen Agents (Topical)*

Octocrylene, Octyl Methoxycinnamate, and Oxybenzone (Topical)—See *Sunscreen Agents (Topical)*

Octocrylene, Octyl Methoxycinnamate, Oxybenzone, and Titanium Dioxide (Topical)—See *Sunscreen Agents (Topical)*

Octocrylene, Octyl Methoxycinnamate, and Titanium Dioxide (Topical)—See *Sunscreen Agents (Topical)*

Octyl Methoxycinnamate and Octyl Salicylate (Topical)—See *Sunscreen Agents (Topical)*

Octyl Methoxycinnamate, Octyl Salicylate, and Oxybenzone (Topical)—See *Sunscreen Agents (Topical)*

Octyl Methoxycinnamate, Octyl Salicylate, Oxybenzone, and Padimate O (Topical)—See *Sunscreen Agents (Topical)*

Octyl Methoxycinnamate, Octyl Salicylate, Oxybenzone, Padimate O, and Titanium Dioxide (Topical)—See *Sunscreen Agents (Topical)*

Octyl Methoxycinnamate, Octyl Salicylate, Oxybenzone, Phenylbenzimidazole, and Titanium Dioxide (Topical)—See *Sunscreen Agents (Topical)*

Octyl Methoxycinnamate, Octyl Salicylate, Oxybenzone, and Titanium Dioxide (Topical)—See *Sunscreen Agents (Topical)*

Octyl Methoxycinnamate, Octyl Salicylate, Phenylbenzimidazole, and Titanium Dioxide (Topical)—See *Sunscreen Agents (Topical)*

Octyl Methoxycinnamate, Octyl Salicylate, and Titanium Dioxide (Topical)—See *Sunscreen Agents (Topical)*

Octyl Methoxycinnamate and Oxybenzone (Topical)—See *Sunscreen Agents (Topical)*

Octyl Methoxycinnamate, Oxybenzone, and Padimate O (Topical)—See *Sunscreen Agents (Topical)*

Octyl Methoxycinnamate, Oxybenzone, Padimate O, and Titanium Dioxide (Topical)—See *Sunscreen Agents (Topical)*

Octyl Methoxycinnamate, Oxybenzone, and Titanium Dioxide (Topical)—See *Sunscreen Agents (Topical)*

Octyl Methoxycinnamate and Padimate O (Topical)—See *Sunscreen Agents (Topical)*

Octyl Methoxycinnamate and Phenylbenzimidazole (Topical)—See *Sunscreen Agents (Topical)*

---

## OCTYL SALICYLATE—See *Sunscreen Agents (Topical)*

## OCTYL SALICYLATE-CONTAINING COMBINATIONS—

Avobenzone, Octocrylene, Octyl Salicylate, and Oxybenzone (Topical)—See *Sunscreen Agents (Topical)*

Avobenzone, Octyl Methoxycinnamate, Octyl Salicylate, and Oxybenzone (Topical)—See *Sunscreen Agents (Topical)*

Homosalate, Menthyl Anthranilate, Octyl Methoxycinnamate, Octyl Salicylate, and Oxybenzone (Topical)—See *Sunscreen Agents (Topical)*

Homosalate, Octyl Methoxycinnamate, Octyl Salicylate, and Oxybenzone (Topical)—See *Sunscreen Agents (Topical)*

Menthyl Anthranilate, Octyl Methoxycinnamate, and Octyl Salicylate (Topical)—See *Sunscreen Agents (Topical)*

Menthyl Anthranilate, Octyl Methoxycinnamate, Octyl Salicylate, and Oxybenzone (Topical)—See *Sunscreen Agents (Topical)*

Octocrylene, Octyl Methoxycinnamate, Octyl Salicylate, and Oxybenzone (Topical)—See *Sunscreen Agents (Topical)*

Octocrylene, Octyl Methoxycinnamate, Octyl Salicylate, Oxybenzone, and Titanium Dioxide (Topical)—See *Sunscreen Agents (Topical)*

Octyl Methoxycinnamate and Octyl Salicylate (Topical)—See *Sunscreen Agents (Topical)*

Octyl Methoxycinnamate, Octyl Salicylate, and Oxybenzone (Topical)—See *Sunscreen Agents (Topical)*

Octyl Methoxycinnamate, Octyl Salicylate, Oxybenzone, and Padimate O (Topical)—See *Sunscreen Agents (Topical)*

Octyl Methoxycinnamate, Octyl Salicylate, Oxybenzone, Padimate O, and Titanium Dioxide (Topical)—See *Sunscreen Agents (Topical)*

Octyl Methoxycinnamate, Octyl Salicylate, Oxybenzone, Phenylbenzimidazole, and Titanium Dioxide (Topical)—See *Sunscreen Agents (Topical)*

Octyl Methoxycinnamate, Octyl Salicylate, Oxybenzone, and Titanium Dioxide (Topical)—See *Sunscreen Agents (Topical)*

Octyl Methoxycinnamate, Octyl Salicylate, Phenylbenzimidazole, and Titanium Dioxide (Topical)—See *Sunscreen Agents (Topical)*

Octyl Methoxycinnamate, Octyl Salicylate, and Titanium Dioxide (Topical)—See *Sunscreen Agents (Topical)*

Octyl Salicylate and Padimate O (Topical)—See *Sunscreen Agents (Topical)*

---

## OFLOXACIN—See *Fluoroquinolones (Systemic)*; *Ofloxacin (Ophthalmic)*

---

# OFLOXACIN Ophthalmic†

VA CLASSIFICATION (Primary): OP201

Note: For a listing of dosage forms and brand names by country availability, see *Dosage Forms* section(s). For a listing of brand names for the articles in this monograph, refer to the General Index.

†Not commercially available in Canada.

## Category
Antibacterial (ophthalmic).

## Indications

### Accepted
Conjunctivitis, bacterial (treatment)—Ophthalmic ofloxacin is indicated in the treatment of conjunctivitis caused by susceptible strains of *Enterobacter cloacae, Haemophilus influenzae, Proteus mirabilis, Pseudomonas aeruginosa, Staphylococcus aureus, S. epidermidis,* and *Streptococcus pneumoniae.*

Not all species or strains of a particular organism may be susceptible to ofloxacin.

## Pharmacology/Pharmacokinetics

### Physicochemical characteristics
Chemical group—Fluoroquinolone.
Molecular weight—361.37.
pH—6.4 (range 6.0 to 6.8).
Osmolarity—300 mOsmol per kilogram.

### Mechanism of action/Effect
Ofloxacin's bactericidal action results from interference with the enzyme, DNA gyrase, which is needed for synthesis of bacterial DNA.

### Absorption
In one study in which ophthalmic ofloxacin was administered 4 times a day for 10½ days, the maximum plasma concentration was approximately 1.9 nanograms per mL.

### Elimination
Excreted in the urine, primarily as unchanged drug.

## Precautions to Consider

### Cross-sensitivity and/or related problems
Patients sensitive to fluoroquinolones or their derivatives, such as cinoxacin, ciprofloxacin, enoxacin, lomefloxacin, nalidixic acid, or norfloxacin, may be sensitive to ofloxacin also.

### Carcinogenicity
Studies to determine the carcinogenic potential of ofloxacin have not been done.

### Mutagenicity
Ofloxacin was mutagenic in the unscheduled DNA synthesis (UDS) test using rat hepatocytes and in the mouse lymphoma assay. However, ofloxacin was not mutagenic in the UDS assay using human fibroblasts, the Ames test, *in vitro* and *in vivo* cytogenic assay, sister chromatid exchange assay (Chinese hampster and human cell lines), dominant lethal assay, or mouse micronucleus assay.

### Pregnancy/Reproduction
Fertility—In studies in rats, ofloxacin did not affect male or female fertility when given orally in doses of up to 360 mg per kg of body weight (mg/kg) per day.

Pregnancy—Adequate and well-controlled studies have not been done in humans.

Studies using ophthalmic ofloxacin have not been done in animals. However, systemic doses below 810 mg/kg per day in rats and below 160 mg/kg per day in rabbits were not shown to be teratogenic. Doses of 810 mg/kg per day in rats resulted in decreased fetal body weight and minor fetal skeletal variations; rabbits given doses of 160 mg/kg per day showed an increase in fetal mortality.

In addition, although systemic ofloxacin has been shown to cause arthropathy in immature animals, ophthalmic ofloxacin has not caused arthropathy or had any other effect on weight bearing joints in immature animals.

FDA Pregnancy Category C.

Labor—Studies in rats given systemic doses of ofloxacin of up to 360 mg/kg per day during late gestation showed no adverse effect of the medication on labor.

Delivery—Studies in rats given systemic doses of ofloxacin of up to 360 mg/kg per day during late gestation showed no adverse effect of the medication on delivery.

**Breast-feeding**

It is not known whether ophthalmic ofloxacin is distributed into breast milk. An orally administered dose of 200 mg of ofloxacin in nursing women resulted in concentrations of ofloxacin in the milk that were similar to its concentrations in plasma. However, for ophthalmic ofloxacin, the dose is much smaller and the plasma concentration is much lower than those of oral ofloxacin.

**Pediatrics**

Appropriate studies on the relationship of age to the effects of ophthalmic ofloxacin have not been performed in children up to 1 year of age. Safety and efficacy have not been established.

Although ofloxacin and other quinolones cause arthropathy in immature animals after oral administration, ophthalmic ofloxacin administered to immature animals did not cause arthropathy. In addition, there is no evidence that the ophthalmic dosage form has any effect on the weight bearing joints.

**Geriatrics**

Appropriate studies on the relationship of age to the effects of ophthalmic ofloxacin have not been performed in the geriatric population. However, no geriatrics-specific problems have been documented to date.

**Medical considerations/Contraindications**

The medical considerations/contraindications included here have been selected on the basis of their potential clinical significance (reasons given in parentheses where appropriate)—not necessarily inclusive ( ≫ = major clinical significance).

*Except under special circumstances, this medication should not be used when the following medical problem exists:*
≫  Sensitivity to ofloxacin or other fluoroquinolones or their derivatives

## Side/Adverse Effects

The following side/adverse effects have been selected on the basis of their potential clinical significance (possible signs and symptoms in parentheses where appropriate)—not necessarily inclusive:

**Those indicating need for medical attention**

Incidence rare
 *Dizziness*

**Those indicating need for medical attention only if they continue or are bothersome**

Incidence more frequent
 *Burning of eye*

Incidence less frequent
 *Photophobia* (increased sensitivity of eye to light); *stinging, redness, itching, tearing, or dryness of eye*

## Patient Consultation

As an aid to patient consultation, refer to *Advice for the Patient, Ofloxacin (Ophthalmic)* .

In providing consultation, consider emphasizing the following selected information ( ≫ = major clinical significance):

**Before using this medication**
≫  Conditions affecting use, especially:
  Sensitivity to ofloxacin or other fluoroquinolones or their derivatives
  Pregnancy—Studies using ophthalmic ofloxacin have not been done; however, studies in animals given very high doses of systemic ofloxacin have shown fetotoxicity
  Breast-feeding—Oral ofloxacin is distributed into breast milk; it is not known whether ophthalmic ofloxacin is distributed into breast milk
  Use in children—Safety and efficacy have not been established in infants up to 1 year of age

**Proper use of this medication**

Proper administration technique
≫  Compliance with full course of therapy
≫  Proper dosing
  Missed dose: Applying as soon as possible; not applying if almost time for next dose
≫  Proper storage

**Precautions while using this medication**

Checking with physician if no improvement within 7 days
Possible photophobic reactions; wearing sunglasses and avoiding prolonged exposure to bright light

**Side/adverse effects**

Signs of potential side effects, especially dizziness

## General Dosing Information

Ofloxacin ophthalmic solution is not for injection into the eye.

Although some manufacturers recommend doses of 2 drops of ophthalmic solutions at appropriate intervals, the conjunctival sac usually holds less than 1 drop.

If hypersensitivity develops, therapy with ophthalmic ofloxacin should be discontinued.

**For treatment of adverse effects**

Recommended treatment consists of the following:
  • For mild hypersensitivity reaction—Administering antihistamines and, if necessary, glucocorticoids.
  • For severe hypersensitivity or anaphylactic reaction—Administering epinephrine. Antihistamines and/or glucocorticoids may also be administered as required.

## Ophthalmic Dosage Forms

### OFLOXACIN OPHTHALMIC SOLUTION

**Usual adult and adolescent dose**

Bacterial conjunctivitis—
  Topical, to the conjunctiva, 1 drop in each eye every two to four hours, while patient is awake, for two days; then, 1 drop four times a day for up to five more days.

**Usual pediatric dose**

Bacterial conjunctivitis—
  Infants up to 1 year of age: Safety and efficacy have not been established.
  Children 1 year of age and older: See *Usual adult and adolescent dose*.

**Strength(s) usually available**

U.S.—
  0.3% (Rx) [*Ocuflox* (benzalkonium chloride 0.005%)].

Canada—
  Not commercially available.

**Packaging and storage**

Store between 15 and 25 °C (59 and 77 °F), unless otherwise specified by manufacturer.

**Auxiliary labeling**
 • For the eye.

## Selected Bibliography

Gwon A. Topical ofloxacin compared with gentamicin in the treatment of external ocular infection. Ofloxacin Study Group. Br J Ophthalmol 1992 Dec; 76 (12): 714-8.

Gwon A. Ofloxacin vs tobramycin for the treatment of external ocular infection. Ofloxacin Study Group II. Arch Ophthalmol 1992 Sep; 110 (9): 1234-7.

Borrmann L, Tang-Liu DD, Kann J, Nista J, Lin ET, Frank J. Ofloxacin in human serum, urine, and tear film after topical application. Cornea 1992 May; 11 (3): 226-30.

Developed: 12/21/93

# OLSALAZINE    Oral-Local

VA CLASSIFICATION (Primary): GA900

Other commonly used names are azodisal sodium and sodium azodisalicylate.

Note: For a listing of dosage forms and brand names by country availability, see *Dosage Forms* section(s). For a listing of brand names for the articles in this monograph, refer to the General Index.

## Category

Bowel disease (inflammatory) suppressant.

## Indications

Note: Bracketed information in the *Indications* section refers to uses that are not included in U.S. product labeling.

### Accepted

Bowel disease, inflammatory (prophylaxis)—Olsalazine is indicated to maintain remission of ulcerative colitis in patients who are intolerant of sulfasalazine.

[Bowel disease, inflammatory (treatment)]—Olsalazine is indicated to treat acute ulcerative colitis of mild to moderate severity.

## Pharmacology/Pharmacokinetics

### Physicochemical characteristics
Molecular weight—346.21.

### Mechanism of action/Effect

Bowel disease (inflammatory) suppressant—

Uncertain. Unabsorbed olsalazine is cleaved in the colon by colonic bacteria to form 2 molecules of mesalamine (5-aminosalicylic acid; 5-ASA), the therapeutically active moiety in the management of ulcerative colitis. Mucosal production of arachidonic acid metabolites, both through the cyclooxygenase and lipoxygenase pathways, is increased in patients with inflammatory bowel disease. Mesalamine appears to diminish inflammation by inhibiting cyclooxygenase and lipoxygenase, thereby decreasing the production of prostaglandins, and leukotrienes and hydroxyeicosatetraenoic acids (HETEs), respectively.

It is also believed that mesalamine acts as a scavenger of oxygen-derived free radicals, which are produced in greater numbers in patients with inflammatory bowel disease.

### Absorption
Limited systemic bioavailability; approximately 2.4% of a single 1-gram dose of olsalazine is absorbed.

### Distribution
Approximately 99% of an oral dose (unabsorbed) of olsalazine reaches the colon.

### Protein binding
Olsalazine—Very high (>99%).
Olsalazine-O-sulfate (olsalazine-S)—Very high (>99%).
Mesalamine (5-ASA)—High (74%).
*N*-acetyl-5-ASA (Ac-5-ASA)—High (81%).

### Biotransformation
Absorbed—Approximately 0.1% of an oral dose of olsalazine is metabolized in the liver to olsalazine-S.

Unabsorbed—Each molecule of olsalazine that reaches the colon is rapidly converted into 2 molecules of mesalamine by colonic bacteria, and the low prevailing redox potential found in this environment. The liberated mesalamine is then absorbed slowly, resulting in very high local concentrations in the colon. The absorbed mesalamine is acetylated to Ac-5-ASA; however, it is not known whether acetylation takes place at colonic or systemic sites. Ac-5-ASA is further acetylated (deactivated) in at least 2 sites, the colonic epithelium and the liver.

### Half-life
Elimination—
Olsalazine: 0.9 hours.
Olsalazine-S: 7 days.

### Time to peak concentration
Olsalazine—Approximately 1 hour.
Mesalamine—4 to 8 hours.

### Peak serum concentration
Following a single 1-gram dose of olsalazine, peak serum concentrations were—
Olsalazine: 1.6 to 6.2 micromoles per L.

Mesalamine: 0 to 4.3 micromoles per L.
Ac-5-ASA: 1.7 to 8.7 micromoles per L.

### Elimination
Renal—
As olsalazine: <1% of administered dose.
As Ac-5-ASA (major metabolite): Approximately 20% of the total mesalamine.
Fecal—
Approximately 80% of the total mesalamine (partially acetylated).

## Precautions to Consider

### Cross-sensitivity and/or related problems
Because olsalazine is a sodium salt of a salicylate derivative, patients sensitive to salicylates may be sensitive to olsalazine also. In addition, patients sensitive to mesalamine or sulfasalazine may be sensitive to this medication.

### Carcinogenicity
In a 2-year study in male and female rats, olsalazine given orally in doses corresponding to 10 to 40 times the human dose caused an increase in the incidence of urinary bladder transitional cell carcinomas in males receiving the highest dose.

### Mutagenicity
No evidence of mutagenicity was observed in *in vitro* Ames tests, mouse lymphoma cell mutation assays, human lymphocyte chromosomal aberration tests, or an *in vivo* rat bone marrow cell chromosomal aberration test.

### Pregnancy/Reproduction
Fertility—Oligospermia and infertility in men, which have been reported in association with sulfasalazine, have not been seen with olsalazine.

Olsalazine was found to have no effect on the fertility of male and female rats when given orally at a dose corresponding to 5 to 20 times the human dose.

Pregnancy—Adequate and well-controlled studies in humans have not been done.

Fetotoxic effects, such as decreased fetal weight, retarded ossification, and immaturity of the fetal visceral organs, were seen in rats given doses corresponding to 5 to 20 times the human dose.

FDA Pregnancy Category C.

### Breast-feeding
It is not known whether olsalazine or its metabolites are distributed into breast milk. However, olsalazine administered to nursing rats at a dose corresponding to 5 to 20 times the human dose caused growth retardation in the pups.

### Pediatrics
Appropriate studies on the relationship of age to the effects of olsalazine have not been performed in the pediatric population. Safety and efficacy have not been established.

### Geriatrics
Appropriate studies on the relationship of age to the effects of olsalazine have not been performed in the geriatric population. However, geriatrics-specific problems that would limit the usefulness of this medication in the elderly are not expected.

### Drug interactions and/or related problems
The following drug interactions and/or related problems have been selected on the basis of their potential clinical significance (possible mechanism in parentheses where appropriate)—not necessarily inclusive (» = major clinical significance):

Note: Combinations containing any of the following medications, depending on the amount present, may also interact with this medication.

Anticoagulants, coumarin- or indandione-derivative
(olsalazine may prolong the prothrombin time, which is used for dosage adjustments of anticoagulants)

### Medical considerations/Contraindications
The medical considerations/contraindications included here have been selected on the basis of their potential clinical significance (reasons given in parentheses where appropriate)—not necessarily inclusive (» = major clinical significance).

*Risk-benefit should be considered when the following medical problems exist:*

Renal function impairment
(increased risk of renal tubular damage)

Sensitivity to olsalazine, mesalamine, sulfasalazine, or salicylates

### Patient monitoring

The following may be especially important in patient monitoring (other tests may be warranted in some patients, depending on condition; » = major clinical significance):

Blood urea nitrogen (BUN) and
Creatinine, serum and
Urinalysis
(determinations may be required in patients with renal function impairment)

Proctoscopy and
Sigmoidoscopy
(may be required periodically during treatment to determine patient response and dosage adjustments)

## Side/Adverse Effects

The following side/adverse effects have been selected on the basis of their potential clinical significance (possible signs and symptoms in parentheses where appropriate)—not necessarily inclusive:

### Those indicating need for medical attention
Incidence rare
*Exacerbation of ulcerative colitis* (bloody diarrhea; fever; skin rash); *hepatitis* (yellow eyes or skin); *pancreatitis* (back or stomach pain, severe; fast heartbeat; fever; nausea or vomiting; swelling of the stomach)

### Those indicating need for medical attention only if they continue or are bothersome
Incidence more frequent
*Gastrointestinal disturbances* (abdominal or stomach pain or upset; diarrhea; loss of appetite; nausea or vomiting)

Note: In controlled studies, *diarrhea* has been reported in approximately 11% of patients receiving olsalazine, resulting in treatment withdrawal in approximately 6% of patients. *Diarrhea* appeared to be dose-related and coincident with the start of olsalazine therapy; it was distinguishable from disease-related diarrhea by its watery appearance and absence of blood.

Incidence less frequent
*Aching joints and muscles; acne; anxiety or depression; dizziness or drowsiness; headache; insomnia* (trouble in sleeping)

## Patient Consultation

As an aid to patient consultation, refer to *Advice for the Patient, Olsalazine (Oral).*

In providing consultation, consider emphasizing the following selected information (» = major clinical significance):

### Before using this medication
» Conditions affecting use, especially:
Sensitivity to olsalazine, mesalamine, sulfasalazine, or salicylates

### Proper use of this medication
Taking with food to lessen gastrointestinal irritation

» Compliance with full course of therapy
» Proper dosing
Missed dose: Taking as soon as possible; not taking if almost time for next dose; not doubling doses
» Proper storage

### Precautions while using this medication
» Regular visits to physician to check progress in patients on long-term therapy

### Side/adverse effects
Signs of potential side effects, especially exacerbation of ulcerative colitis, hepatitis, and pancreatitis

## General Dosing Information

Olsalazine should be taken with food to decrease gastrointestinal irritation. The total daily dose should be taken in evenly divided doses.

## Oral Dosage Forms

Note: Bracketed uses in the *Dosage Forms* section refer to categories of use and/or indications that are not included in U.S. product labeling.

### OLSALAZINE SODIUM CAPSULES

#### Usual adult and adolescent dose
Bowel disease, inflammatory (prophylaxis)—
Oral, 500 mg two times a day.
[Bowel disease, inflammatory (treatment)]—
Oral, 500 mg four times a day.

#### Usual pediatric dose
Safety and efficacy have not been established.

#### Usual geriatric dose
See *Usual adult and adolescent dose.*

#### Strength(s) usually available
U.S.—
250 mg (Rx) [*Dipentum* (magnesium stearate)].
Canada—
250 mg (Rx) [*Dipentum*].

#### Packaging and storage
Store below 40 °C (104 °F), preferably between 15 and 30 °C (59 and 86 °F), unless otherwise specified by manufacturer. Store in a well-closed container.

#### Auxiliary labeling
• Continue medicine for full time of treatment.
• Take with food.

## Selected Bibliography
Wadworth AN, Fitton A. Olsalazine. A review of its pharmacodynamic and pharmacokinetic properties, and therapeutic potential in inflammatory bowel disease. Drugs 1991; 41: 647-64.
Segars LW, Gales BJ. Mesalamine and olsalazine: 5-aminosalicylic acid agents for the treatment of inflammatory bowel disease. Clin Pharm 1992; 11: 514-28.
Ruderman WB. Newer pharmacologic agents for the therapy of inflammatory bowel disease. Med Clin North Am 1990; 74: 133-53.

Revised: 03/15/95

# OMEPRAZOLE   Systemic

VA CLASSIFICATION (Primary/Secondary): GA900/GA309
Note: For a listing of dosage forms and brand names by country availability, see *Dosage Forms* section(s). For a listing of brand names for the articles in this monograph, refer to the General Index.

## Category
Gastric acid pump inhibitor; antiulcer agent.

## Indications

### Accepted
Reflux, gastroesophageal (prophylaxis and treatment)—Omeprazole is indicated for the short-term treatment of severe erosive esophagitis associated with gastroesophageal reflux disease and for symptomatic gastroesophageal reflux disease poorly responsive to customary medical treatment, including $H_2$-receptor antagonist therapy. Omeprazole also is indicated in the prevention of erosive esophagitis recurrence after initial healing has occurred.

Hypersecretory conditions, gastric (treatment)
Zollinger-Ellison syndrome (treatment)
Mastocytosis, systemic (treatment) or
Adenoma, multiple endocrine (treatment)—Omeprazole is indicated for the long-term treatment of pathologic gastric hypersecretion associated with Zollinger-Ellison syndrome (alone or as part of multiple endocrine neoplasia Type-1), systemic mastocytosis, and multiple endocrine adenoma.

Ulcer, duodenal (treatment)—Omeprazole is indicated in the short-term treatment of active duodenal ulcer.

Ulcer, gastric (treatment)—Omeprazole is indicated in the short-term treatment of active benign gastric ulcer.

# Pharmacology/Pharmacokinetics

## Physicochemical characteristics
Molecular weight—345.42.
pKa—4 and 8.8.

## Mechanism of action/Effect
Omeprazole is activated at an acidic pH to a sulphenamide derivative that binds irreversibly to H+, K+-ATPase, an enzyme system found at the secretory surface of parietal cells. It thereby inhibits the final transport of hydrogen ions (via exchange with potassium ions) into the gastric lumen. Since the H+, K+-ATPase enzyme system is regarded as the acid (proton) pump of the gastric mucosa, omeprazole is known as a gastric acid pump inhibitor. Omeprazole inhibits both basal and stimulated acid secretion irrespective of the stimulus.

## Other actions/effects
Inhibits hepatic cytochrome P-450 mixed function oxidase system.

## Absorption
Rapid.

## Distribution
Distributed in tissue, particularly gastric parietal cells.

## Protein binding
Very high, approximately 95% bound to albumin and alpha₁-acid glycoprotein.

## Biotransformation
Hepatic, extensive.

## Half-life
Plasma—
  Normal hepatic function—30 minutes to 1 hour.
  Chronic hepatic disease—3 hours.

## Onset of action
Within one hour.

## Time to peak concentration
Within 30 minutes to 3.5 hours.

## Time to peak effect
Within 2 hours.

## Duration of action
Up to 72 hours or more (96 hours required for full restoration of acid production).

## Elimination
Renal—72 to 80%.
Fecal—18 to 23%.
In dialysis—Not readily dialyzable, because of extensive protein binding.

# Precautions to Consider

## Carcinogenicity/Tumorigenicity/Mutagenicity
In two 2-year studies in rats, omeprazole, given in doses corresponding to 4 to 352 times the human dose, caused end-life gastric carcinoid tumors and enterochromaffin-like (ECL) cell hyperplasia in a dose-related manner in both male and female animals. These ECL cell changes have been shown to be caused by high levels of gastrin (or hypergastrinemia). Pronounced acid inhibition at extremely high doses of gastric acid pump inhibitors or H₂-receptor antagonists results in the same feedback elevation of gastrin and subsequent ECL cell changes of the stomach.

## Pregnancy/Reproduction
Fertility—In a rat fertility and general reproductive performance test, omeprazole, in a dose 35 to 345 times the human dose, was not toxic or deleterious to the reproductive performance of parental animals.

Pregnancy—Adequate and well-controlled studies in humans have not been done.

Studies in pregnant rats did not show omeprazole to have any teratogenic potential at doses 345 times the human dose. Omeprazole produced dose-related increases in embryo-lethality, fetal resorptions, and pregnancy disruptions in rabbits receiving 17 to 172 times the human dose. In rats, dose-related embryo/fetal toxicity and postnatal developmental toxicity were observed in offspring resulting from parents treated with 35 to 345 times the human dose.

FDA Pregnancy Category C.

## Breast-feeding
It is not known whether omeprazole is distributed into human milk. However, because omeprazole has been shown to cause tumorigenic and carcinogenic effects in animals, a decision should be made on whether nursing should be discontinued or the medication withdrawn, taking into account the importance of the omeprazole to the mother.

## Pediatrics
Appropriate studies on the relationship of age to the effects of omeprazole have not been performed in the pediatric population.

## Geriatrics
No information is available on the relationship of age to the effects of omeprazole in geriatric patients. However, a somewhat decreased rate of elimination and an increased bioavailability are more likely to occur in geriatric patients taking omeprazole.

## Pharmacogenetics
Pharmacokinetic studies in Asian subjects receiving single 20-mg doses of omeprazole showed an approximately fourfold increase in the area under the plasma concentration-time curve (AUC) as compared to Caucasian subjects. Dosage adjustments should be considered for Asian patients, especially for prophylaxis of recurrence of erosive esophagitis.

## Drug interactions and/or related problems
The following drug interactions and/or related problems have been selected on the basis of their potential clinical significance (possible mechanism in parentheses where appropriate)—not necessarily inclusive (» = major clinical significance):

Note: Only specific interactions between omeprazole and other medications have been identified in this monograph. However, omeprazole, by increasing gastric pH, has the potential to affect the bioavailability of any medication for which absorption is pH-dependent. Also, omeprazole may prevent the degradation of acid-labile drugs.

In addition, because of omeprazole's ability to inhibit hepatic microsomal drug metabolism, elimination of other medications that require hepatic metabolism via the cytochrome P-450 system or that are highly extracted by the liver may be decreased during concurrent use with omeprazole.

Combinations containing any of the following medications, depending on the amount present, may also interact with this medication.

Ampicillin esters

Iron salts or
Ketoconazole
  (omeprazole may increase gastrointestinal pH; concurrent use with omeprazole may result in a reduction in absorption of ampicillin esters, iron salts, or ketoconazole)

» Anticoagulants, coumarin- or indandione-derivative or
» Diazepam or
» Phenytoin
  (inhibition of the cytochrome P-450 enzyme system by omeprazole, especially in high doses, may cause a decrease in the hepatic metabolism of these medications, which may result in delayed elimination and increased blood concentrations, when these medications are used concurrently with omeprazole)

  (monitoring of blood concentrations, or prothrombin time for anticoagulants, is recommended as a guide to dosage since dosage adjustment of these medications may be necessary during and after omeprazole therapy to prevent bleeding due to anticoagulant potentiation)

Bone marrow depressants (See *Appendix II*)
  (concurrent use of omeprazole with these medications may increase the leukopenic and/or thrombocytopenic effects of both these medications; if concurrent use is required, close observation for toxic effects should be considered)

## Laboratory value alterations
The following have been selected on the basis of their potential clinical significance (possible effect in parentheses where appropriate)—not necessarily inclusive (» = major clinical significance):

With physiology/laboratory test values
  Alanine aminotransferase (ALT [SGPT]) and
  Alkaline phosphatase and
  Aspartate aminotransferase (AST [SGOT])
    (serum values may be increased)

  Gastrin, serum
    (concentrations will increase during the first 1 to 2 weeks of omeprazole therapy and return to normal after the medication is discontinued; this increase is probably due to the inhibition of acid secretion, which eliminates the negative feedback effect of acid on gastrin secretion; in addition to stimulating gastric acid secretion, gastrin promotes the growth and proliferation of endocrine or enterochromaffin-like [ECL] cells in the gastric mucosa)

**Medical considerations/Contraindications**

The medical considerations/contraindications included here have been selected on the basis of their potential clinical significance (reasons given in parentheses where appropriate)—not necessarily inclusive (» = major clinical significance).

*Risk-benefit should be considered when the following medical problems exist:*

» Hepatic disease, chronic, current or history of
      (dosage reduction may be required due to increased half-life in chronic hepatic disease)
   Sensitivity to omeprazole

## Side/Adverse Effects

Note: Gastric fundic gland polyps have occurred rarely in patients receiving omeprazole; these appear to be benign and reversible upon discontinuance of omeprazole.

   Gastroduodenal carcinoids have been reported in patients with Zollinger-Ellison syndrome who have received long-term omeprazole therapy. These carcinoids are believed to be a manifestation of the underlying syndrome, which is known to be associated with such tumors.

   Atrophic gastritis has been noted occasionally in gastric corpus biopsies from patient receiving long-term omeprazole therapy.

The following side/adverse effects have been selected on the basis of their potential clinical significance (possible signs and symptoms in parentheses where appropriate)—not necessarily inclusive:

**Those indicating need for medical attention**
Incidence rare
   *Hematologic abnormalities, specifically anemia* (unusual tiredness or weakness); *eosinopenia; leukocytosis* (sore throat and fever); *neutropenia* (continuing ulcers or sores in mouth); *pancytopenia or thrombocytopenia* (unusual bleeding or bruising); *hematuria* (bloody urine); *proteinuria* (cloudy urine); *urinary tract infection* (bloody or cloudy urine; difficult, burning, or painful urination; frequent urge to urinate)

**Those indicating need for medical attention only if they continue or are bothersome**
Incidence more frequent
   *Abdominal pain or colic*
Incidence less frequent
   *Asthenia* (muscle pain; unusual tiredness); *central nervous system (CNS) disturbances, specifically dizziness, headache, somnolence* (unusual drowsiness); *or unusual tiredness; chest pain; gastrointestinal disturbances, specifically acid regurgitation* (heartburn); *constipation; diarrhea or loose stools, flatulence* (gas), *or nausea and vomiting; skin rash or itching*)

## Overdose

For more information on the management of overdose or unintentional ingestion, **contact a Poison Control Center** (see *Poison Control Center Listing*).

**Clinical effects of overdose**
The following effects have been selected on the basis of their potential clinical significance (possible signs and symptoms in parentheses where appropriate)—not necessarily inclusive:

   *Blurred vision; confusion; diaphoresis* (increased sweating); *drowsiness; dryness of mouth; flushing; headache; nausea; tachycardia* (fast or irregular heartbeat)

**Treatment of overdose**
Since there is no specific antidote for overdose with omeprazole, treatment should be symptomatic and supportive. Due to extensive protein binding, omeprazole is not readily dialyzable. Patients in whom intentional overdose is confirmed or suspected should be referred for psychiatric consultation.

## Patient Consultation

As an aid to patient consultation, refer to *Advice for the Patient, Omeprazole (Systemic)*.

In providing consultation, consider emphasizing the following selected information (» = major clinical significance):

**Before using this medication**
» Conditions affecting use, especially:
      Sensitivity to omeprazole
      Breast-feeding—May be distributed into breast milk; may cause potentially serious adverse effects in nursing infants
      Other medications, especially anticoagulants, diazepam, or phenytoin

Other medical problems, especially chronic hepatic disease or history of

**Proper use of this medication**
   Taking the capsule form of this medication immediately before a meal, preferably the morning meal
   May take antacids for relief of pain, unless otherwise instructed by physician
   Swallowing capsule whole; not crushing, breaking, chewing, or opening the capsule
» Compliance with full course of therapy
» Proper dosing
   Missed dose: Taking as soon as possible; not taking if almost time for next dose; not doubling doses
» Proper storage

**Precautions while using this medication**
   Checking with physician if condition does not improve or worsens

**Side/adverse effects**
   Signs of potential side effects, especially hematologic abnormalities, hematuria, proteinuria, and urinary tract infection

## General Dosing Information

For therapy of gastrointestinal reflux disease, omeprazole usually is used for short-term (4- to 8-week) courses; however, additional 4- to 8-week courses of treatment may be considered if there is recurrence of severe or symptomatic gastroesophageal reflux poorly responsive to customary medical treatment. Controlled studies of omeprazole used as maintenance therapy to prevent erosive eophagitis recurrence have not been conducted beyond 12 months., although a limited number of patients have received continuous maintenance treatment for up to 6 years. Dosage adjustments should be considered for Asian patients, especially for prophylaxis of erosive esophagitis recurrence, since pharmacokinetic studies in Asian subjects receiving single 20-mg doses of omeprazole showed an approximately fourfold increase in the area under the plasma concentration-time curve (AUC) as compared to Caucasian subjects.

Although the symptoms of duodenal ulcers may subside within 1 or 2 weeks after initiation of therapy, unless healing has been documented by endoscopic examination or x-rays, therapy should be continued for at least 4 to 6 weeks.

Omeprazole may be taken with antacids, especially for the first few doses, to aid in the relief of pain.

Initial titration of doses and subsequent dosage adjustment of omeprazole is recommended in the long-term treatment of pathological hypersecretory conditions (e.g., Zollinger-Ellison syndrome, systemic mastocytosis, multiple endocrine adenomas). Doses of up to 120 mg three times a day have been administered. Patients may require at least one increase in dose per year. If the daily dose is greater than 80 mg, it should be administered in divided doses. Zollinger-Ellison syndrome has been treated continuously with omeprazole for more than 5 years.

**Diet/Nutrition**
Omeprazole capsules should be taken immediately before meals, preferably in the morning. Omeprazole tablets may be taken with food or on an empty stomach.

## Oral Dosage Forms

### OMEPRAZOLE DELAYED-RELEASE CAPSULES

**Usual adult dose**
Gastroesophageal reflux (treatment)—
   Oral, 20 mg once a day for four to eight weeks.
   Note: A dosage of 40 mg once a day has been used for esophagitis associated with gastroesophageal reflux disease refractory to other treatment regimens.
Erosive esophagitis (prophylaxis)—
   Oral, 20 mg once a day.
Gastric hypersecretory conditions (e.g., Zollinger-Ellison syndrome, systemic mastocytosis, multiple endocrine adenomas)—
   Oral, 60 mg once a day, the dosage being adjusted as needed, and therapy continued for as long as clinically indicated. Doses of up to 120 mg three times a day have been used. If the total daily dose is greater than 80 mg, it should be administered in divided doses.
Duodenal ulcer—
   Oral, 20 mg once a day.
   Note: The dosage can be increased to 40 mg once a day for duodenal ulcer refractory to other treatment regimens.
Gastric ulcer, active—
   Oral, 40 mg once a day for four to eight weeks.

Note: The dosage can be increased to 40 mg once a day for gastric ulcer refractory to other treatment regimens.

      If healing of gastric ulcer has not occurred within four weeks, an additional four weeks of treatment is recommended.

**Usual pediatric dose**
Dosage has not been established.

**Strength(s) usually available**
U.S.—

    10 mg (Rx) [*Prilosec*].

    20 mg (Rx) [*Prilosec*].

Canada—

    Not commercially available.

**Packaging and storage**
Store between 15 and 30 °C (59 and 86 °F), in a tight container, unless otherwise specified by manufacturer. Protect from light.

**Auxiliary labeling**
• Take before meals.
• Swallow capsules whole.

## OMEPRAZOLE DELAYED-RELEASE TABLETS

**Usual adult dose**
See *Omeprazole Delayed-release Capsules.*

**Usual pediatric dose**
See *Omeprazole Delayed-release Capsules.*

**Strength(s) usually available**
U.S.—

    Not commercially available.

Canada—

    20 mg (Rx) [*Losec*].

**Packaging and storage**
Store between 15 and 30 °C (59 and 86 °F), in a tight container, unless otherwise specified by manufacturer.

Revised: 08/05/96

# ONDANSETRON   Systemic

VA CLASSIFICATION (Primary/Secondary): GA700

Note: For a listing of dosage forms and brand names by country availability, see *Dosage Forms* section(s). For a listing of brand names for the articles in this monograph, refer to the General Index.

## Category
Antiemetic.

## Indications
Note: Bracketed information in the *Indications* section refers to uses that are not included in U.S. product labeling.

**Accepted**
Nausea and vomiting, cancer chemotherapy–induced (prophylaxis)—Ondansetron is indicated for the prevention of nausea and vomiting associated with initial and repeat courses of moderately or highly emetogenic cancer chemotherapy, including high-dose cisplatin.

    Studies done to date comparing ondansetron to high-dose metoclopramide have shown ondansetron to be more effective in preventing nausea and vomiting induced by emetogenic chemotherapy agents during the acute phase lasting 24 hours after the start of chemotherapy.

    The combination of ondansetron plus dexamethasone has been shown to provide better emetic control over cisplatin-induced emesis than ondansetron alone.

Nausea and vomiting, postoperative (prophylaxis)—Ondansetron is indicated for the prevention of postoperative nausea and vomiting. Patients at greatest risk of developing postoperative nausea and vomiting include patients who have previously experienced postoperative nausea, patients predisposed to motion sickness, and patients with high levels of preoperative anxiety. The incidence of postoperative nausea and vomiting is also higher in women and children than in men and adults, respectively. Routine prophylaxis is not recommended for patients in whom there is little expectation that postoperative nausea and vomiting will occur, except in cases in which the stress of vomiting may damage the operation site.

Nausea and vomiting, radiotherapy-induced (prophylaxis)—Ondansetron tablets are indicated for the prevention of nausea and vomiting associated with radiotherapy in patients receiving total body irradiation, single high-dose fraction, or daily fractions to the abdomen.

[Nausea and vomiting, postoperative (treatment)]—Ondansetron injection is indicated for the treatment of postoperative nausea and vomiting.

**Unaccepted**
Ondansetron is not effective in preventing motion-induced nausea and vomiting.

## Pharmacology/Pharmacokinetics

**Physicochemical characteristics**
Molecular weight—365.86.
pH—Injection: 3.3 to 4

**Mechanism of action/Effect**
Antiemetic—Ondansetron is a competitive, highly selective antagonist of 5-hydroxytryptamine (serotonin) subtype 3 (5-HT₃) receptors. 5-HT₃ receptors are present peripherally on vagal nerve terminals and centrally in the area postrema of the brain. It is not certain whether ondansetron's action is mediated peripherally, centrally, or both. Cytotoxic drugs and radiation appear to damage gastrointestinal mucosa, causing the release of serotonin from the enterochromaffin cells of the gastrointestinal tract. Stimulation of 5-HT₃ receptors causes transmission of sensory signals to the vomiting center via vagal afferent fibers to induce vomiting. By binding to 5-HT₃ receptors, ondansetron blocks vomiting mediated by serotonin release.
Ondansetron has no dopamine-receptor antagonist activity.

**Other actions/effects**
Multiple oral doses of ondansetron administered to healthy volunteers slowed colonic transit time. However, no effects have been demonstrated on esophageal motility, gastric motility lower esophageal sphincter pressure, small intestine transit time, or plasma prolactin concentrations.

**Absorption**
Ondansetron is well absorbed after oral administration and undergoes limited first-pass metabolism. The extent and rate of ondansetron's absorption following a single oral dose is greater in women than in men. However, it is not known if this difference is clinically significant.

**Distribution**
The volume of distribution (Vol_D) in healthy young males following administration of 8 mg of ondansetron as an intravenous infusion over 5 minutes was about 160 L. Patients 4 to 12 years of age reportedly have a Vol_D somewhat larger than do adults.
Thirty-six percent of circulating ondansetron is distributed into erythrocytes.

**Protein binding**
High (70 to 76%).

**Biotransformation**
Hepatic; extensive. Primarily hydroxylation, followed by glucuronide or sulfate conjugation.

**Half-life**
The mean elimination half-life in adult cancer patients is 4 hours. Elderly patients and patients with severe hepatic function impairment tend to have an increased elimination half-life, while most pediatric patients less than 15 years of age have shorter plasma half-lives (about 2.4 hours) than patients older than 15 years of age.

**Peak plasma concentration**
Following administration of a single intravenous dose of 0.15 mg of ondansetron per kg of body weight to healthy volunteers—

| Age group (years) | Peak plasma concentration (nanograms per mL) |
|---|---|
| 19–40 | 102 |
| 61–74 | 106 |
| 75–82 | 170 |

Following administration of a single oral dose of 8 mg of ondansetron to healthy volunteers—

| Age group (years) | Gender | Peak plasma concentration (nanograms per mL) |
|---|---|---|
| 19–40 | M | 26.2 |
| | F | 42.7 |
| 61–74 | M | 24.1 |
| | F | 52.4 |
| ≥75 | M | 37 |
| | F | 46.1 |

The higher plasma concentrations in females may be attributed to slower clearance, smaller apparent $Vol_D$ (adjusted for weight), and higher absolute bioavailability in females than in males.

### Elimination

Predominantly hepatic; less than 5% of an intravenous dose of ondansetron is recovered unchanged in the urine.

Following administration of a single intravenous dose of 0.15 mg of ondansetron per kg of body weight to healthy volunteers, plasma clearance values were:

| Age group (years) | Plasma clearance (L per hour per kg) |
|---|---|
| 19–40 | 0.381 |
| 61–74 | 0.319 |
| 75–82 | 0.262 |

Elderly patients tended to have lower clearance values than did younger adults, while most pediatric patients 4 to 12 years of age had greater clearance values than adults.

## Precautions to Consider

### Cross-sensitivity and/or related problems

Patients sensitive to granisetron may also be sensitive to ondansetron.

### Carcinogenicity

Carcinogenic effects were not seen in 2-year studies in rats and mice given ondansetron orally in doses up to 10 and 30 mg per kg of body weight (mg/kg) per day, respectively.

### Mutagenicity

Standard tests showed no mutagenic activity of ondansetron.

### Pregnancy/Reproduction

Fertility—Ondansetron had no effect on the fertility or reproductive performance of male and female rats when given in oral doses up to 15 mg/kg per day.

Pregnancy—Adequate and well-controlled studies in humans have not been done.

Studies in pregnant rats and rabbits given intravenous doses of up to 4 mg/kg per day, and oral doses of up to 15 and 30 mg/kg per day, respectively, have not shown that ondansetron causes adverse effects in the fetus.

FDA Pregnancy Category B.

### Breast-feeding

It is not known whether ondansetron is distributed into human breast milk. However, ondansetron is distributed into the milk of rats.

### Pediatrics

Studies performed to date that included cancer patients aged 4 to 18 years have not demonstrated pediatrics-specific problems that would limit the usefulness of ondansetron in children.

### Geriatrics

Studies performed to date that included cancer patients over 65 years of age have not demonstrated geriatrics-specific problems that would limit the usefulness of ondansetron in the elderly.

### Drug interactions and/or related problems

The following drug interactions and/or related problems have been selected on the basis of their potential clinical significance (possible mechanism in parentheses where appropriate)—not necessarily inclusive (» = major clinical significance):

Hepatic enzyme inducers (See *Appendix II*) or
Hepatic enzyme inhibitors (See *Appendix II*)
   (because ondansetron is metabolized by hepatic cytochrome P450 enzymes, inducers or inhibitors of these enzymes potentially may alter its clearance and half-life; ondansetron does not appear to induce or inhibit the cytochrome P450 enzyme system of the liver)

### Laboratory value alterations

The following have been selected on the basis of their potential clinical significance (possible effect in parentheses where appropriate)—not necessarily inclusive (» = major clinical significance):

With physiology/laboratory test values
   Alanine aminotransferase (ALT [SGPT]) and
   Aspartate aminotransferase (AST [SGOT])
      (values may be increased; increases reportedly are transient and unrelated to dose or duration of therapy)
   Bilirubin, serum
      (concentrations may be increased; increases reportedly are transient and unrelated to dose or duration of therapy)

### Medical considerations/Contraindications

The medical considerations/contraindications included here have been selected on the basis of their potential clinical significance (reasons given in parentheses where appropriate)—not necessarily inclusive (» = major clinical significance).

*Risk-benefit should be considered when the following medical problems exist:*

Hepatic function impairment
   (use of ondansetron may result in increases in hepatic enzymes)
Surgery, abdominal
   (use of ondansetron may mask a progressive ileus and/or gastric distension)
Sensitivity to ondansetron or granisetron

## Side/Adverse Effects

Note: Since ondansetron is used in conjunction with cancer chemotherapeutic agents, it is difficult to attribute some side effects, such as diarrhea and fever, to ondansetron alone.

   Signs and symptoms consistent with extrapyramidal effects have been reported in a very small number of patients receiving ondansetron; however, a causal relationship has not been established.

The following side/adverse effects have been selected on the basis of their potential clinical significance (possible signs and symptoms in parentheses where appropriate)—not necessarily inclusive:

**Those indicating need for medical attention**

Incidence rare
   *Anaphylaxis* (hypotension; skin rash, hives, and/or itching; troubled breathing); *bronchospasm* (shortness of breath, tightness in chest, troubled breathing, or wheezing); *chest pain*

**Those indicating need for medical attention only if they continue or are bothersome**

Incidence more frequent
   *Constipation; diarrhea; fever; headache*

Incidence less frequent or rare
   *Abdominal pain or stomach cramps; dizziness or lightheadedness; drowsiness; dryness of mouth; skin rash; unusual tiredness or weakness*

## Patient Consultation

As an aid to patient consultation, refer to *Advice for the Patient, Ondansetron (Systemic)*.

In providing consultation, consider emphasizing the following selected information (» = major clinical significance):

**Before using this medication**
» Conditions affecting use, especially:
      Sensitivity to ondansetron or granisetron

**Proper use of this medication**
   Taking additional dose if vomiting occurs within 30 minutes after a dose; checking with doctor if vomiting persists
» Proper dosing
      Missed dose: Taking missed dose as soon as possible if nausea or vomiting occurs
» Proper storage

**Side/adverse effects**
   Signs of potential side effects, especially anaphylaxis, bronchospasm, or chest pain

## Oral Dosage Forms

Note: The oral dosage form of ondansetron is indicated for prevention of nausea and vomiting induced by *moderately* emetogenic cancer chemotherapy. For prophylaxis against nausea and vomiting induced by *highly* emetogenic chemotherapeutic agents, the injection dosage form is recommended.

# ONDANSETRON HYDROCHLORIDE TABLETS

## Usual adult and adolescent dose
Nausea and vomiting, cancer chemotherapy–induced (prophylaxis)—
Initial: Oral, 8 mg thirty minutes prior to chemotherapy.
Post-chemotherapy: Oral, 8 mg eight hours after the initial dose, followed by 8 mg every twelve hours for one to two days.
Nausea and vomiting, postoperative (prophylaxis)—
Oral, 16 mg one hour prior to induction of anesthesia.
Nausea and vomiting, radiotherapy-induced (prophylaxis)—
Initial: Oral, 8 mg one to two hours prior to radiotherapy.
Post-radiotherapy: Oral, 8 mg every eight hours each day radiotherapy is given.
Note: In patients with hepatic function impairment, the maximum recommended dose of ondansetron is 8 mg a day.

## Usual pediatric dose
Nausea and vomiting, cancer chemotherapy–induced (prophylaxis)—
Children up to 4 years of age:
Dosage has not been established.
Children 4 to 12 years of age:
Initial—Oral, 4 mg thirty minutes prior to chemotherapy.
Post-chemotherapy—Oral, 4 mg four and eight hours after the initial dose, followed by 4 mg every eight hours for one to two days.
Children 12 years of age and older:
See *Usual adult and adolescent dose.*
Nausea and vomiting, postoperative (prophylaxis) or
Nausea and vomiting, radiotherapy-induced (prophylaxis)—
Dosage has not been established.

## Usual geriatric dose
See *Usual adult and adolescent dose.*

## Strength(s) usually available
U.S.—
4 mg (Rx) [*Zofran* (lactose; microcrystalline cellulose; pregelatinized starch; hydroxypropyl methylcellulose; magnesium stearate; titanium dioxide; sodium benzoate)].
8 mg (Rx) [*Zofran* (lactose; microcrystalline cellulose; pregelatinized starch; hydroxypropyl methylcellulose; magnesium stearate; titanium dioxide; iron oxide)].
Canada—
4 mg (Rx) [*Zofran*].
8 mg (Rx) [*Zofran*].

## Packaging and storage
Store between 2 and 30 °C (36 and 86 °F), unless otherwise specified by manufacturer. Protect from light.

## Preparation of dosage form
For patients who cannot take oral solids—Ondansetron oral suspension may be prepared by crushing twelve 8-mg tablets and grinding them to a very fine powder. Sixty mL of a suspending agent, e.g., *Ora Plus*, is added to the powder and the preparation mixed to a pasty consistency. A flavored syrup should then be added in 25-mL increments to make 120 mL. The final concentration is 4 mg per 5 mL. Ondansetron oral suspension may be stored at 4 °C (39 °F) for up to 6 weeks.

## Auxiliary labeling
For ondansetron oral suspension—
• Refrigerate.
• Shake well.

# Parenteral Dosage Forms

Note: Bracketed uses in the *Dosage Forms* section refer to categories of use and/or indications that are not included in U.S. product labeling.

## ONDANSETRON HYDROCHLORIDE INJECTION

### Usual adult dose
Nausea and vomiting, cancer chemotherapy–induced (prophylaxis)—
Intravenous, 32 mg administered over fifteen minutes beginning thirty minutes prior to chemotherapy. Alternatively, three doses of 150 mcg (0.15 mg) per kg of body weight, each administered over fifteen minutes, with the initial dose beginning thirty minutes prior to chemotherapy, and subsequent doses administered four and eight hours after the first dose. [Or, 8 mg administered over fifteen minutes beginning thirty minutes prior to chemotherapy, followed immediately by a continuous infusion of 1 mg per hour for up to twenty-four hours.]
Nausea and vomiting, postoperative (prophylaxis)—
Intravenous, 4 mg administered over not less than thirty seconds, and preferably over two to five minutes, beginning immediately prior to induction of anesthesia.
[Nausea and vomiting, postoperative (treatment)]—
Intravenous, 4 mg administered over not less than thirty seconds, and preferably over two to five minutes.
Note: In patients with hepatic function impairment, the maximum recommended dose of ondansetron is 8 mg a day.

## Usual pediatric dose
Nausea and vomiting, cancer chemotherapy–induced (prophylaxis)—
Children up to 4 years of age: Dosage has not been established.
Children 4 to 18 years of age: Intravenous, three doses of 150 mcg (0.15 mg) per kg of body weight, each administered over fifteen minutes, with the initial dose beginning thirty minutes prior to chemotherapy, and subsequent doses administered four and eight hours after the first dose. [Alternatively, 3 to 5 mg per square meter of body surface area administered over fifteen minutes beginning immediately prior to chemotherapy, followed after therapy by oral ondansetron 4 mg every eight hours for up to five days.]
Nausea and vomiting, postoperative—
Dosage has not been established.

## Usual geriatric dose
See *Usual adult dose.*

## Strength(s) usually available
U.S.—
2 mg per mL (Rx) [*Zofran* (sodium chloride; citric acid monohydrate 0.5 mg; sodium citrate dihydrate 0.25 mg; [may contain methylparaben 1.2 mg, propylparaben 0.15 mg])].
32 mg per 50 mL (premixed) (Rx) [*Zofran* (dextrose 2500 mg; citric acid 26 mg; sodium citrate 11.5 mg)].
Canada—
2 mg per mL (Rx) [*Zofran*].

## Packaging and storage
Store between 2 and 30 °C (36 and 86 °F), unless otherwise specified by manufacturer. Protect from light.

## Preparation of dosage form
For prevention of cancer chemotherapy–induced nausea and vomiting—The manufacturer recommends that the dose of ondansetron be diluted in 50 mL of 5% dextrose injection or 0.9% sodium chloride injection; however, ondansetron also has been shown to be stable in dextrose and sodium chloride injections, 3% sodium chloride injection, 10% mannitol injection, and Ringer's injection.
For prevention of postoperative nausea and vomiting—Dilution of ondansetron is not necessary.

## Stability
Intravenous infusions of ondansetron retain their potency for 48 hours at room temperature under normal lighting after dilution with 5% dextrose injection, dextrose and sodium chloride injections, 0.9% sodium chloride injection, and 3% sodium chloride injection.

## Incompatibilities
The following medications may be incompatible with ondansetron and should be avoided in admixtures: acyclovir, aminophylline, amphotericin B, ampicillin, ampicillin and sulbactam, amsacrine, cefoperazone, furosemide, ganciclovir, lorazepam, methylprednisolone, mezlocillin, piperacillin, and sargramostim. In addition, alkaline solutions and fluorouracil in concentrations greater than 0.8 mg per mL have been shown to be physically incompatible with ondansetron.

# Selected Bibliography

Markham A, Sorkin EM, Ondansetron. An update of its therapeutic use in chemotherapy-induced and postoperative nausea and vomiting. Drugs 1993; 45: 931-52.

Revised: 01/19/95
Interim revision: 08/15/95

# OPIOID (NARCOTIC) ANALGESICS Systemic

This monograph includes information on the following: Butorphanol†; Codeine; Hydrocodone‡; Hydromorphone; Levorphanol; Meperidine; Methadone; Morphine; Nalbuphine; Opium; Oxycodone; Oxymorphone; Pentazocine; Propoxyphene.

Note: See also individual *Buprenorphine (Systemic)* and *Dezocine (Systemic)* monographs.

See also *Fentanyl Derivatives (Systemic)* for information on alfentanil, fentanyl, and sufentanil.

INN:

Meperidine—Pethidine
Propoxyphene—Dextropropoxyphene

VA CLASSIFICATION (Primary/Secondary):
Butorphanol—CN101/CN205
Codeine—
  Oral: CN101/RE301; GA400
  Parenteral: CN101/GA400
Hydrocodone—CN101/RE301
Hydromorphone—
  Oral: CN101/RE301
  Parenteral: CN101/CN205; RE301
  Rectal: CN101
Levorphanol—
  Oral: CN101
  Parenteral: CN101/CN205
Meperidine—
  Oral: CN101
  Parenteral: CN101/CN205
Methadone—CN101/AD900; RE301
Morphine—
  Oral: CN101/RE301; GA400
  Parenteral: CN101/CN205; RE301; GA400
  Rectal: CN101/RE301
Nalbuphine—CN101/CN205
Opium—
  Oral: GA400/CN101
  Parenteral: CN101
Oxycodone—CN101
Oxymorphone—
  Parenteral: CN101/CN205
  Rectal: CN101
Pentazocine—
  Oral: CN101
  Parenteral: CN101/CN205
Propoxyphene—CN101

Note: Controlled substances in the U.S. and Canada as follows:

| Drug | U.S. | Canada |
|---|---|---|
| Butorphanol | ** | †† |
| Codeine | II | N |
| Hydrocodone | ‡‡ | N |
| Hydromorphone | II | N |
| Levorphanol | II | N |
| Meperidine | II | N |
| Methadone | II | N§§ |
| Morphine | II | N |
| Nalbuphine | ** | C |
| Opium | II | N |
| Oxycodone | II | N |
| Oxymorphone | II | N |
| Pentazocine | IV | N |
| Propoxyphene | IV | N |

**Not a controlled substance in the U.S.
††Not commercially available in Canada.
‡‡Commercially available in the U.S. only in combination with other active ingredients.
§§Available in Canada only through practitioners authorized to treat opioid addicts.

Other commonly used names are: Dextropropoxyphene [Propoxyphene], Dihydromorphinone [Hydromorphone], Laudanum [Opium Tincture], Levorphan [Levorphanol], Pethidine [Meperidine], Papaveretum [Opium (Parenteral)].

Note: For a listing of dosage forms and brand names by country availability, see *Dosage Forms* section(s). For a listing of brand names for the articles in this monograph, refer to the General Index.

†Not commercially available in Canada.

‡Commercially available in the U.S. only in combination with other active ingredients. See *Cough/Cold Combinations (Systemic)*, *Opioid (Narcotic) Analgesics and Acetaminophen (Systemic)*, and *Opioid (Narcotic) Analgesics and Aspirin (Systemic)*.

## Category

Note: All of the opioid analgesics have similar pharmacologic actions; however, clinical uses among specific agents may vary because of actual pharmacokinetic differences, differences in potential for causing adverse effects, lack of specific testing, and/or lack of clinical-use data.

Analgesic—Butorphanol; Codeine; Hydrocodone; Hydromorphone; Levorphanol; Meperidine; Methadone; Morphine; Nalbuphine; Opium; Oxycodone; Oxymorphone; Pentazocine; Propoxyphene.

Note: Butorphanol, nalbuphine, and pentazocine are opioid agonist/antagonist analgesics; the other agents in this group are opioid agonist analgesics.

Anesthesia adjunct (opioid analgesic)—Parenteral dosage forms only: Butorphanol; Hydromorphone; Levorphanol; Meperidine; Morphine; Nalbuphine; Oxymorphone; Pentazocine.

Note: For other opioids used primarily as anesthesia adjuncts, see *Fentanyl Derivatives (Systemic)*.

Antidiarrheal—Codeine; Morphine; Opium Tincture.

Note: For other opioids used only as antidiarrheals, see individual monograph listings for *Difenoxin and Atropine*, *Diphenoxylate and Atropine*, *Loperamide*, and *Paregoric*.

Antitussive—Codeine (oral dosage forms only); Hydrocodone; Hydromorphone; Methadone; Morphine.

Note: For use of hydromorphone as an antitussive, see *Cough-Cold Combinations (Systemic)—Hydromorphone and Guaifenesin*.

Suppressant (narcotic abstinence syndrome)—Methadone; Opium Tincture.

Pulmonary edema therapy adjunct—Morphine.

## Indications

Note: Bracketed information in the *Indications* section refers to uses that are not included in U.S. product labeling.

### Accepted

Pain (treatment)—Morphine, methadone, and parenteral opium are indicated for relief of severe pain; codeine and propoxyphene are indicated for relief of mild to moderate pain; and the other opioid analgesics are indicated for relief of moderate to severe pain.

Epidural or intrathecal administration of small doses of opioid analgesics may provide prolonged pain relief. Although administration via these routes may decrease the risk of some side/adverse effects, respiratory depression may occur. Solutions containing a preservative must *not* be used. Only morphine sulfate is currently commercially available in a dosage form that is FDA-approved for administration via these routes.

For relief of pain due to acute myocardial infarction, morphine is usually considered the drug of choice. Butorphanol and pentazocine are less desirable than other opioid analgesics for this purpose because they have cardiovascular effects that tend to increase cardiac work. Although nalbuphine has not been reported to adversely affect cardiovascular function in patients with acute myocardial infarction (and may be less likely than morphine to cause hypotension), its effects in patients with severely compromised cardiac function caused by acute myocardial infarction have not been fully determined. Therefore, these agents should be used with caution in such patients.

Parenterally administered opioid analgesics (except for methadone) are indicated to provide obstetrical analgesia.

Controlled clinical studies have shown that intrathecal, but not epidural, administration of opioid analgesics provides adequate relief of labor pain. Only a preservative-free solution should be used. Morphine sulfate is the only opioid analgesic currently commercially available in a dosage form that is FDA-approved for administration via these routes.

Anesthesia, general or local, adjunct—Parenteral dosage forms of butorphanol, [hydromorphone], levorphanol, meperidine, morphine, nalbuphine, oxymorphone, and pentazocine are indicated to supplement general, regional, or local anesthesia. During surgery, they are often used in conjunction with other agents, such as a combination of an ultrashort-acting barbiturate, a neuromuscular blocking agent, and an inhalation anesthetic (usually nitrous oxide), for the maintenance of "balanced" anesthesia.

Parenteral dosage forms of most opioid analgesics are indicated to provide analgesic, antianxiety, and sedative effects as presurgical medication. However, other medications, such as benzodiazepines, are more commonly used if the patient is not in pain.

Diarrhea (treatment)—[Codeine][1], [morphine], and opium tincture are indicated for treatment of diarrhea. In diarrhea caused by poisoning, these agents should not be used until the toxic material has been eliminated from the gastrointestinal tract.

Cough (treatment)—Although only codeine (oral dosage forms), hydrocodone, and hydromorphone are indicated as antitussives, all opioid analgesics depress the cough reflex. Meperidine, oxymorphone, and propoxyphene have relatively less antitussive activity than other opioid analgesics, especially in low or moderate doses.

[Methadone and morphine are sometimes used as antitussives when severe pain is present and coughing cannot be relieved by other means.]

Opioid (narcotic) abstinence syndrome (prophylaxis and treatment); or

Opioid (narcotic) drug use, illicit (treatment)—Methadone is indicated as a suppressant to permit detoxification. Oral methadone is also indicated as maintenance therapy to discourage addicts from returning to illicit use of other opioid drugs.

Edema, pulmonary, acute (treatment adjunct)—Morphine is indicated as adjunctive therapy in the treatment of acute pulmonary edema secondary to left ventricular failure.

Oxymorphone is also FDA-approved as an adjunct in the treatment of acute pulmonary edema. However, oxymorphone is rarely if ever used for this indication; morphine is the preferred medication.

[Opioid (narcotic) dependence, neonatal (treatment)]—Opium tincture is used in diluted form in the treatment of neonatal opioid dependence.

### Unaccepted

Methadone is not recommended for obstetrical analgesia because its long duration of action increases the risk of neonatal respiratory depression.

---

[1]Not included in Canadian product labeling.

## Pharmacology/Pharmacokinetics

See *Table 1*, page 2203.
See *Table 2*, page 2204.

### Physicochemical characteristics

Molecular weight—
  Butorphanol tartrate: 477.55.
  Codeine phosphate: 406.37 (hemihydrate); 397.36 (anhydrous).
  Codeine sulfate: 750.86 (trihydrate); 696.81 (anhydrous).
  Hydrocodone bitartrate: 494.50 (hydrate); 449.46 (anhydrous).
  Hydromorphone hydrochloride: 321.80.
  Levorphanol tartrate: 443.49 (dihydrate); 407.46 (anhydrous).
  Meperidine hydrochloride: 283.80.
  Methadone hydrochloride: 345.91.
  Morphine sulfate: 758.83 (pentahydrate); 668.76 (anhydrous).
  Nalbuphine hydrochloride: 393.91.
  Oxycodone hydrochloride: 351.83.
  Oxymorphone hydrochloride: 337.80.
  Pentazocine hydrochloride: 321.89.
  Pentazocine lactate: 375.51.
  Propoxyphene hydrochloride: 375.94.
  Propoxyphene napsylate: 565.72 (monohydrate); 547.71 (anhydrous).

### Mechanism of action/Effect

Opioid analgesics bind with stereospecific receptors at many sites within the central nervous system (CNS) to alter processes affecting both the perception of pain and the emotional response to pain. Although the precise sites and mechanisms of action have not been fully determined, alterations in release of various neurotransmitters from afferent nerves sensitive to painful stimuli may be partially responsible for the analgesic effects. When these medications are used as adjuncts to anesthesia, analgesic actions may provide dose-related protection against hemodynamic responses to surgical stress.

It has been proposed that there are multiple subtypes of opioid receptors, each mediating various therapeutic and/or side effects of opioid drugs. The actions of an opioid analgesic may therefore depend upon its binding affinity for each type of receptor and on whether it acts as a full agonist or a partial agonist or is inactive at each type of receptor.

At least two types of opioid receptors (mu and kappa) mediate analgesia. A third type of receptor (sigma) may not mediate analgesia; actions at this receptor may produce the subjective and psychotomimetic effects characteristic of pentazocine and, to a lesser extent, butorphanol and nalbuphine. Morphine and other opioid agonists exert their agonist

activity primarily at the mu receptor, whereas buprenorphine, nalbuphine, and pentazocine exert agonist activity at the kappa and sigma receptors. Mu receptors are widely distributed throughout the CNS, especially in the limbic system (frontal cortex, temporal cortex, amygdala, and hippocampus), thalamus, striatum, hypothalamus, and midbrain as well as laminae I, II, IV, and V of the dorsal horn in the spinal cord. Kappa receptors are localized primarily in the spinal cord and in the cerebral cortex.

Nalbuphine and pentazocine may displace opioids having only agonist activity from their receptor binding sites and competitively inhibit their actions. The medications may therefore precipitate withdrawal symptoms in patients who are physically dependent on such agonists. Butorphanol appears to have no significant antagonist activity at the mu receptor; in some studies, it failed to produce withdrawal symptoms in patients physically dependent on morphine. However, butorphanol does not substitute for mu-receptor agonists sufficiently to prevent or attenuate withdrawal symptoms caused by abrupt discontinuation of these agonists in physically dependent patients. Also, opioid agonist/antagonist drugs share several pharmacologic actions that differ from those of opioids having only agonist activity; i.e., different respiratory depressant, subjective, psychotomimetic, and hemodynamic effects; lower dependence liability; and reduced severity of withdrawal symptoms produced when they are discontinued after prolonged use.

Antidiarrheal—
  Act locally and possibly centrally to alter intestinal motility.

Antitussive—
  Suppress the cough reflex by a direct central action, probably in the medulla or pons.

Suppressant (narcotic abstinence syndrome)—
  Substitute for other opioid drugs when administered orally and prevent or attenuate withdrawal symptoms during detoxification. Withdrawal symptoms that may occur when the substituted opioid is discontinued are usually greatly reduced in severity. With continued administration, methadone may produce cross-tolerance to the euphoric effects of other opioid drugs, thereby reducing the patient's desire for such drugs.

### Biotransformation

Hepatic; also in intestinal mucosa.

## Precautions to Consider

### Pregnancy/Reproduction

Pregnancy—Risk-benefit must be considered because opioid analgesics cross the placenta. Regular use during pregnancy may cause physical dependence in the fetus, leading to withdrawal symptoms (convulsions, irritability, excessive crying, tremors, hyperactive reflexes, fever, vomiting, diarrhea, sneezing, and yawning) in the neonate. Use of methadone by pregnant women participating in methadone maintenance programs has also been associated with fetal distress in utero and low birth weight.

For butorphanol, nalbuphine, pentazocine, and propoxyphene: Although studies in humans have not been done, studies in animals have not shown that these agents cause adverse effects on fetal development (Pentazocine and naloxone tablets—FDA Pregnancy Category C).

For codeine, hydrocodone, hydromorphone, morphine, and opium: Although teratogenic effects in humans have not been documented, controlled studies have not been done. Studies in animals have shown codeine (single dose of 100 mg per kg) to cause delayed ossification in mice and (in doses of 120 mg per kg) increased resorptions in rats, and hydrocodone, hydromorphone, and morphine to be teratogenic in very high doses (FDA Pregnancy Category C).

For levorphanol, meperidine, methadone, oxycodone, and oxymorphone: Although teratogenic effects in humans have not been documented, controlled studies have not been done.

Labor and delivery—Opioid analgesics, including epidurally or intrathecally administered opioids, readily enter the fetal circulation when used during labor and may cause respiratory depression in the neonate, especially the premature neonate. These agents should be used with caution, if at all, during the delivery of a premature infant. Methadone is not recommended for obstetrical analgesia because its long duration of action increases the risk of neonatal respiratory depression. Also, morphine, hydromorphone, codeine, and possibly other opioids may prolong labor. Intrathecal administration of up to 1 mg of morphine sulfate has little effect on the first stage of labor but may prolong the second stage of labor.

### Breast-feeding

Problems in humans with most opioid analgesics have not been documented. Butorphanol, codeine, meperidine, methadone, morphine, and propoxyphene are distributed into breast milk. Information concerning the excretion of other opioid analgesics in breast milk is lacking. With usual analgesic doses, concentrations of those drugs known to be distributed into breast milk are generally low. However, risk-benefit must be considered when methadone is administered to a nursing mother in a methadone maintenance program because use of maintenance doses may cause physical dependence in the infant.

### Pediatrics
Children up to 2 years of age may be more susceptible to the effects, especially the respiratory depressant effects, of these medications.
Paradoxical excitation is especially likely to occur in pediatric patients receiving opioid analgesics.

### Geriatrics
Geriatric patients may be more susceptible to the effects, especially the respiratory depressant effects, of these medications. Also, geriatric patients are more likely to have prostatic hypertrophy or obstruction and age-related renal function impairment, and are therefore more likely to be adversely affected by opioid-induced urinary retention. In addition, geriatric patients may metabolize or eliminate these medications more slowly than younger adults. Lower doses or longer dosing intervals than those usually recommended for adults may be required, and are usually therapeutically effective, for these patients.

### Dental
Opioid analgesics may decrease or inhibit salivary flow, thus contributing to the development of caries, periodontal disease, oral candidiasis, and discomfort.

### Drug interactions and/or related problems
See *Table 3*, page 2206.

### Laboratory value alterations
The following have been selected on the basis of their potential clinical significance (possible effect in parentheses where appropriate)—not necessarily inclusive (» = major clinical significance):

With diagnostic test results
Gastric emptying studies
(opioid analgesics delay gastric emptying, thereby invalidating test results)
Hepatobiliary imaging using technetium Tc 99m disofenin
(delivery of technetium Tc 99m disofenin to the small bowel may be prevented because opioid analgesics [except for butorphanol] may cause constriction of the sphincter of Oddi and increased biliary tract pressure; these actions result in delayed visualization and thus resemble obstruction of the common bile duct)

With physiology/laboratory test values
Cerebrospinal fluid (CSF) pressure
(may be increased; effect is secondary to respiratory depression–induced carbon dioxide retention)
Plasma amylase activity and
Plasma lipase activity
(may be increased because opioid analgesics [except butorphanol] can cause contractions of the sphincter of Oddi and increased biliary tract pressure; the diagnostic utility of determinations of these enzymes may be compromised for up to 24 hours after the medication has been given)
Serum alanine aminotransferase (ALT [SGPT]) and
Serum alkaline phosphatase and
Serum aspartate aminotransferase (AST [SGOT]) and
Serum bilirubin and
Serum lactate dehydrogenase (LDH)
(activity may be increased in patients receiving propoxyphene)

### Medical considerations/Contraindications
The medical considerations/contraindications included here have been selected on the basis of their potential clinical significance (reasons given in parentheses where appropriate)—not necessarily inclusive (» = major clinical significance).

*Except under special circumstances, this medication should not be used when the following medical problems exist:*

*For all opioid analgesic usage*
» Diarrhea associated with pseudomembranous colitis caused by cephalosporins, lincomycins (possibly including topical clindamycin), or penicillins or
» Diarrhea caused by poisoning, until toxic material has been eliminated from gastrointestinal tract
(opioid analgesics may slow elimination of toxic material, thereby worsening and/or prolonging the diarrhea)
» Respiratory depression, acute
(may be exacerbated)

*For epidural or intrathecal administration*
» Any condition that precludes epidural or intrathecal administration, such as:
» Coagulation defects caused by anticoagulant therapy or hematologic disorders
(trauma to a blood vessel during administration may result in uncontrollable CNS or soft tissue hemorrhage)
» Infection at or near site of administration
(risk of spreading the infection into the CNS)

*Risk-benefit should be considered when the following medical problems exist:*

*For all opioid analgesics*
Abdominal conditions, acute
(diagnosis or clinical course may be obscured)
Allergic reaction to the opioid analgesic considered for use, history of
» Asthma, acute attack or
» Respiratory impairment or disease, chronic
(opioids may decrease respiratory drive and increase airway resistance in patients with these conditions)
Cardiac arrhythmias or
Convulsions, history of
(may be induced or exacerbated by opioids; meperidine and propoxyphene may be especially likely to induce or exacerbate convulsions; with meperidine, the proconvulsant activity of its metabolite normeperidine may be responsible)
Drug abuse or dependence, current or history of, including alcoholism, or
Emotional instability or
Suicidal ideation or attempts
(patient predisposition to drug abuse)
Gallbladder disease or gallstones
(opioids [except butorphanol] may cause biliary contraction)
Gastrointestinal tract surgery, recent
(opioids may alter gastrointestinal motility)
Head injury or
Increased intracranial pressure, pre-existing or
Intracranial lesions
(risk of respiratory depression and further elevation of cerebrospinal fluid pressure is increased; also, opioids may cause sedation and pupillary changes that may obscure clinical course of head injury)
Hepatic function impairment
(opioids metabolized in liver)
Hypothyroidism
(risk of respiratory depression and prolonged CNS depression is greatly increased)
» Inflammatory bowel disease, severe
(risk of toxic megacolon may be increased, especially with repeated dosing)
Prostatic hypertrophy or obstruction or
Urethral stricture or
Urinary tract surgery, recent
(opioids may cause urinary retention)
Renal function impairment
(increased risk of convulsions [with meperidine] or other adverse effects because opioids and/or their metabolites excreted primarily via kidneys; also, opioids may cause urinary retention)
Caution is also advised in administration to very young, elderly, or very ill or debilitated patients, who may be more sensitive to the effects, especially the respiratory depressant effects, of these medications.

*For butorphanol, nalbuphine, or pentazocine only (in addition to those medical problems listed above)*
Dependence on opioid agonist analgesics, current
(nalbuphine and pentazocine may precipitate, and butorphanol does not prevent occurrence of, withdrawal symptoms)
Hypertension
(butorphanol may increase blood pressure in these patients when used as presurgical medication)
» Myocardial infarction, acute
(pentazocine and butorphanol may increase cardiac work; effects of nalbuphine in patients with severely compromised cardiac function have not been fully evaluated)

*For epidural or intrathecal administration (in addition to those medical problems listed above as applying to all opioid analgesics)*

Dependence on opioid analgesics, current

(low doses of opioids administered via epidural or intrathecal injection will not prevent withdrawal symptoms from occurring in a physically dependent patient)

**Patient monitoring**

The following may be especially important in patient monitoring (other tests may be warranted in some patients, depending on condition; » = major clinical significance):

» Respiratory function

(monitoring recommended for at least 24 hours following epidural or intrathecal injection because delayed respiratory depression may occur up to 24 hours after administration via these routes)

## Side/Adverse Effects

See *Table 4*, page 2210.

Note: Physical dependence, with or without psychological dependence, may occur with chronic administration of opioid analgesics; an abstinence syndrome may occur when these drugs are discontinued. Specific withdrawal symptoms that may occur, and their severity, depend upon the specific drug used, the abruptness of withdrawal, and the degree to which dependence has developed. Butorphanol, nalbuphine, and pentazocine have lower dependence liability and potential for abuse than opioid agonists; codeine and propoxyphene have lower dependence liability and potential for abuse than other agonists because of their comparatively lower potency with usual doses.

Epidural or intrathecal administration does not eliminate the risk of severe side effects common to systemic opioid analgesics. Respiratory depression may occur shortly after administration because of direct venous redistribution to the respiratory centers in the CNS. Also, delayed respiratory depression may occur up to 24 hours after administration, possibly as the result of rostral spread of the medication. Intrathecal administration and/or injection into thoracic sites are more likely to cause respiratory depression than epidural administration and/or injection into lumbar sites.

Following epidural or intrathecal administration of morphine, urinary retention occurs very frequently (incidence about 90% in males and somewhat lower in females) and may persist for 10 to 20 hours following injection. Catheterization may be required. Also, dose-related generalized pruritus occurs frequently. Excessive sedation is uncommon, and loss of motor, sensory, or sympathetic function does not occur.

**Those indicating possible withdrawal and the need for medical attention if they occur after medication is discontinued**

*Body aches; diarrhea; fast heartbeat; fever, runny nose, or sneezing; gooseflesh; increased sweating; increased yawning; loss of appetite; nausea or vomiting; nervousness, restlessness, or irritability; shivering or trembling; stomach cramps; trouble in sleeping; unusually large pupils; weakness*

Note: *The signs and symptoms of withdrawal* listed above are characteristic of the abstinence syndrome produced by abrupt discontinuation of mu-receptor agonists such as morphine. The milder abstinence syndrome produced by abrupt discontinuation of opioids having mixed agonist/antagonist activity may also include some of these signs and symptoms.

It has been proposed that adverse effects (such as tachycardia, hypertension, hyperpnea, hyperalgesia, nausea, and vomiting) occurring (rarely) after naloxone is administered for postoperative reversal of opioid effects following a lengthy surgical procedure may be manifestations of an induced abstinence syndrome in acutely dependent individuals. However, other symptoms more commonly associated with an opioid withdrawal syndrome have not been reported.

## Overdose

For specifc information on the agents used in the management of opioid (narcotic) analgesics overdose, see:
• *Naloxone (Systemic)* monograph.

For more information on the management of overdose or unintentional ingestion, **contact a Poison Control Center** (see *Poison Control Center Listing*).

**Clinical effects of overdose**

The following effects have been selected on the basis of their potential clinical significance (possible signs and symptoms in parentheses where appropriate)—not necessarily inclusive:

Acute and chronic

*Cold, clammy skin; confusion; convulsions; dizziness, severe; drowsiness, severe; low blood pressure; nervousness or restlessness, severe; pinpoint pupils of eyes; slow heartbeat; slow or troubled breathing; unconsciousness; weakness, severe*

Note: *Convulsions* are more likely to occur with meperidine or propoxyphene than with other opioids.

**Treatment of overdose**

To decrease absorption—Emptying the stomach via induction of emesis or gastric lavage (if the opioid was taken orally). However, treatment of respiratory depression or other potentially life-threatening adverse effects must take precedence.

Specific treatment—Administering the opioid antagonist naloxone. However, larger doses of naloxone may be required for treatment of overdose with butorphanol, nalbuphine, pentazocine, or propoxyphene. Naloxone injections may be repeated at two- to three-minute intervals as needed. The fact that naloxone may also antagonize the analgesic actions of opioid analgesics and may precipitate withdrawal symptoms in physically dependent patients must be kept in mind. For reversal of postoperative opioid depression, dosage of naloxone must be carefully titrated to avoid interference with control of postoperative pain or causing other adverse effects; hypertension and tachycardia, sometimes resulting in left ventricular failure and pulmonary edema, have occurred following naloxone administration in these circumstances (especially in cardiac patients). See the package insert or *Naloxone (Systemic)* for specific dosing guidelines for use of this product.

Monitoring—Continuing to monitor the patient (mandatory because the duration of action of the opioid analgesic may exceed that of the antagonist) and administering additional naloxone as needed. Alternatively, initial treatment may be followed by continuous intravenous infusion of naloxone, with the rate of infusion being adjusted according to patient response.

Supportive care—Establishing adequate respiratory exchange through provision of a patent airway and institution of assisted or controlled respiration. Administering intravenous fluids and/or vasopressors and using other supportive measures as needed. Patients in whom intentional overdose is known or suspected should be referred for psychiatric consultation.

## Patient Consultation

As an aid to patient consultation, refer to *Advice for the Patient, Narcotic Analgesics—For Pain Relief (Systemic), Narcotic Analgesics—For Surgery and Obstetrics (Systemic),* and *Opium Preparations (Systemic).*

In providing consultation, consider emphasizing the following selected information (» = major clinical significance):

**Before using this medication**

» Conditions affecting use, especially:

Sensitivity to the opioid considered for use, history of

Pregnancy—Opioids cross the placenta; regular use by pregnant women may cause physical dependence in the fetus and withdrawal symptoms in the neonate

Breast-feeding—Butorphanol, codeine, meperidine, methadone, morphine, and propoxyphene are known to be distributed into breast milk; high-dose methadone may cause dependence in nursing infants

Use in children—Children up to 2 years of age are more susceptible to the effects of opioids, especially respiratory depression; also, children may be more likely to experience paradoxical CNS excitation during therapy

Use in the elderly—Geriatric patients are more susceptible to the effects of opioids, especially respiratory depression

Dental—May cause dryness of mouth, which can lead to caries, periodontal disease, oral candidiasis, and discomfort

Other medications, especially alcohol or other CNS depressants, monoamine oxidase inhibitors, naltrexone, rifampin, and zidovudine

Other medical problems, especially diarrhea caused by antibiotics or poisoning, asthma or other respiratory problems, and severe inflammatory bowel disease

**Proper use of this medication**

*Proper administration of*

» Injections (if dispensed to the patient for home use)

» Meperidine syrup—Mixing with ½ glass (4 ounces) of water to lessen numbing effect in mouth and throat

» Methadone oral concentrate—Diluting with water to at least 1 ounce before taking, unless premixed at a methadone treatment center

» Methadone dispersible tablets—Must be dissolved in water or fruit juice before taking

Morphine oral liquid—May be mixed with fruit juice to improve taste

» Morphine extended-release tablets—Swallowing tablets whole; not breaking, crushing, or chewing

Suppository dosage forms—proper administration technique

*Proper administration of opium tincture*
Medication may be diluted in water, which will cause it to turn milky
Taking with food or meals if gastrointestinal irritation occurs

» Importance of not taking more medication than the amount prescribed because of danger of overdose and habit-forming potential

» Not increasing dose if medication is less effective after a few weeks; checking with physician

» Missed dose (if on scheduled dosing): Taking as soon as possible; not taking if almost time for next dose; not doubling doses

» Proper storage

**Precautions while using this medication**
Regular visits to physician to check progress during long-term therapy

» Avoiding use of alcoholic beverages or other CNS depressants during therapy, unless prescribed or otherwise approved by physician

» Caution if dizziness, drowsiness, lightheadedness, or false sense of well-being occurs

» Caution when getting up suddenly from a lying or sitting position

Lying down if nausea or vomiting, or dizziness or lightheadedness occurs

Need to inform physician or dentist of use of medication if any kind of surgery (including dental surgery) or emergency treatment is required

Possible dryness of mouth; using sugarless gum or candy, ice, or saliva substitute for relief; checking with dentist if dry mouth continues for more than 2 weeks

» Checking with physician before discontinuing medication after prolonged use of high doses; gradual dosage reduction may be necessary to avoid withdrawal symptoms

» Suspected overdose: Getting emergency help at once

*For opium tincture when used as antidiarrheal only*

» Consulting physician if diarrhea continues and/or fever develops

**Side/adverse effects**
Signs of potential side effects, especially respiratory depression or impairment; allergic reactions; confusion, convulsions, hallucinations, mental depression, or other signs of CNS toxicity; hepatotoxicity; hypertension; and paradoxical CNS excitation, especially in children

## General Dosing Information

These medications may suppress respiration, especially in very young, elderly, very ill, or debilitated patients and those with respiratory problems. Lower doses may be required for these patients. However, elderly patients may also be more sensitive to the analgesic effects of these medications so that lower doses or an increased dosing interval may be sufficient to provide effective analgesia.

Dosage and dosing intervals should be individualized on the basis of the potency and duration of action of the specific drug used, the severity of pain, the condition of the patient, other medications given concurrently, and patient response.

Concurrent administration of a nonopioid analgesic (such as aspirin or other salicylates, other nonsteroidal anti-inflammatory analgesics, or acetaminophen) with opioid analgesics provides additive analgesia and may permit lower doses of the opioid analgesic to be utilized.

Some clinicians recommend that patients in severe chronic pain receive opioid analgesics on a fixed dosage schedule so that they remain free of pain rather than on an as needed basis after pain recurs. The medication should be given orally if possible.

Tolerance to many of the effects of these medications may develop with repeated administration. The first sign of tolerance is usually a decrease in the duration of adequate analgesia. Tolerance to the respiratory depressant effects of opioid analgesics develops concurrently with tolerance to their analgesic effects. Careful adjustment of dosage as required to provide adequate analgesia is not likely to increase the risk of respiratory depression. Patients who become tolerant to one of these agents may be partially cross-tolerant to the others. However, when an alternate opioid analgesic is substituted for one to which tolerance has developed, it is recommended that one-half of the equianalgesic dose of the new medication be used initially. Dosage of the new medication may then be adjusted as necessary.

Psychological and physical dependence may occur with chronic administration of opioid analgesics, including epidurally or intrathecally administered opioid analgesics; an abstinence syndrome may occur when these drugs are discontinued. Physical dependence in patients receiving prolonged therapy for severe chronic pain rarely leads to true addiction, i.e., a desire to continue taking the drug (for its euphoric effect) after it is no longer required for treatment. Fear of causing addiction should not result in failure to provide adequate pain relief, although caution is advised if patient predisposition toward drug abuse is known or strongly suspected. Gradual withdrawal may minimize the development of withdrawal symptoms following prolonged use.

**For parenteral dosage forms only**
Rapid intravenous injection of most opioid analgesics has caused anaphylactoid reactions, severe respiratory depression, hypotension, peripheral circulatory collapse, and cardiac arrest. It is recommended that when an opioid analgesic must be given intravenously, dosage should be reduced and a dilute solution should be injected slowly over a period of several minutes. An opioid antagonist and equipment for artificial ventilation should be available.

When an opioid analgesic is administered parenterally, the patient usually should be lying down and should remain recumbent for a period of time to minimize side effects such as hypotension, dizziness, lightheadedness, nausea, and vomiting. If these side effects occur in an ambulatory patient, they may be relieved if the patient lies down.

In patients with shock, impaired perfusion may prevent complete absorption following intramuscular or subcutaneous injection. Repeated administration may result in overdose due to an excessive amount suddenly being absorbed when circulation is restored.

Opioid analgesics may not provide sufficient analgesia to prevent or overcome hemodynamic responses to surgical stress when used as the sole intravenous supplement to nitrous oxide for the maintenance of balanced anesthesia. Concurrent use of other medications, such as a benzodiazepine, an ultrashort-acting barbiturate, or a potent hydrocarbon inhalation anesthetic, may be required.

Epidural or intrathecal administration of opioid analgesics should be performed only by physicians experienced in these techniques. Solutions containing a preservative must *not* be injected via these routes. *Resuscitative equipment and medications should be immediately available for management of respiratory depression or other complications that may arise from inadvertent intrathecal or intravascular administration. Also, facilities for adequate monitoring of the patient's respiratory status must be available.*

For epidural or intrathecal administration, injection into the lumbar area may be preferred because of the increased risk of respiratory depression with injection into the thoracic area. Also, the epidural route is preferred, whenever possible, because of the increased risk of respiratory depression with intrathecal administration.

Prior to epidural administration, proper placement of the needle or catheter in the epidural space must be verified. Aspiration to check for blood in the cerebrospinal fluid may be performed; however, the fact that intravascular administration is possible even when aspiration for blood is negative must be kept in mind. Alternatively, administration of 5 mL (3 mL for obstetrical patients) of preservative-free 1.5% lidocaine hydrochloride with epinephrine 1:200,000 injection may be used to verify placement in the epidural space. Tachycardia occurring after injection of the test medication indicates that the medication has entered the circulation; sudden onset of segmental anesthesia indicates that the medication has been administered intrathecally.

Following epidural or intrathecal injection of an opioid analgesic, administration of low doses of naloxone via continuous intravenous infusion for 24 hours may decrease the incidence of potential side effects without interfering with the analgesic effectiveness of the medication.

---

### *BUTORPHANOL*

## Summary of Differences

Indications:
Caution required when used as analgesic to relieve pain due to acute myocardial infarction because of cardiovascular effects that tend to increase cardiac work.

Pharmacology/pharmacokinetics:
Mechanism of action/effect—
An opioid agonist/antagonist analgesic.
Agonist: Has agonist activity at the kappa and sigma receptors.
Antagonist: Probably has no direct antagonist activity at the mu receptor; antagonist effects may result from failure to substitute for mu-receptor agonists sufficiently to prevent or attenuate withdrawal symptoms in physically dependent patients.

Equivalence—
  2 mg via intramuscular injection therapeutically equivalent to 10 mg of intramuscular morphine.
Protein binding—
  High.
Half-life—
  2.5–4 hours.
Onset of action—
  Intramuscular: 10–30 minutes.
  Intravenous: 2–3 minutes.
Time to peak concentration—
  0.5–1 hour.
Peak plasma concentration—
  2.2 nanograms/mL.
Time to peak effect—
  Intramuscular: 30–60 minutes.
  Intravenous: 30 minutes.
Duration of action (nontolerant patients only; decreases as tolerance develops during chronic therapy)—
  Intramuscular: 3–4 hours.
  Intravenous: 2–4 hours.
Elimination—
  72% Renal, <5% as unchanged buprenorphine; 15% biliary.
Precautions:
  Laboratory value alterations—
    Does not intefere with hepatobiliary imaging.
    Does not increase plasma amylase or lipase activity.
  Medical considerations/contraindications—
    Caution not required in gallbladder disease or gallstones.
    Also, should be used with caution in patients physically dependent on opioid agonists, in hypertensive patients (when used preoperatively), and in patients with acute myocardial infarction.
Side/adverse effects:
  Less likely to cause constipation than most other opioids.
  Biliary spasm has not been reported.
  Rarely, may cause subjective and psychotomimetic effects characteristic of sigma receptor agonists.
  Has lower dependence liability than opioid agonists.
  Withdrawal symptoms less severe than those produced by opioid agonist analgesics.

## Parenteral Dosage Forms

### BUTORPHANOL TARTRATE INJECTION USP

**Usual adult dose**
Analgesic—
  Intramuscular, 1 to 4 mg (usually 2 mg) every three to four hours as needed.
  Intravenous, 500 mcg (0.5 mg) to 2 mg (usually 1 mg) every three to four hours as needed.
Anesthesia adjunct—
  Preoperative:
    Intravenous, usually 2 mg sixty to ninety minutes prior to surgery, although dosage must be individualized.
  Balanced anesthesia:
    Intravenous, initially 1 to 4 mg, followed by supplemental doses of 500 mcg (0.5 mg) to 1 mg as needed.
    Note: Dosage must be individualized. Supplemental doses of up to 60 mcg (0.06 mg) per kg of body weight may be necessary in some patients.
      The total quantity of butorphanol required during surgery usually ranges between 60 and 180 mcg (0.06 and 0.18 mg) per kg of body weight.

**Usual pediatric dose**
Dosage in patients up to 18 years of age has not been established.

**Strength(s) usually available**
U.S.—
  With preservative (benzethonium chloride 0.1 mg/mL)
    2 mg per mL (Rx) [Stadol].
  Without preservative
    1 mg per mL (Rx) [Stadol].
    2 mg per mL (Rx) [Stadol].
Canada—
  Not commercially available.

**Packaging and storage**
Store between 15 and 30 °C (59 and 86 °F), unless otherwise specified by manufacturer. Protect from light. Protect from freezing.

**Auxiliary labeling**
• May cause drowsiness.
• Avoid alcoholic beverages.

**Note**
Not a controlled substance in the U.S.

***

### CODEINE

## Summary of Differences

Indications:
  Oral dosage forms also indicated as antitussive.
  Also, used as antidiarrheal.
Pharmacology/pharmacokinetics:
  Mechanism of action/effect—
    An opioid agonist analgesic; exerts agonist activity primarily at the mu receptor, but with usual doses is relatively weak.
  Equivalence—
    120 mg via intramuscular injection or 200 mg via oral administration therapeutically equivalent to 10 mg of intramuscular morphine.
  Protein binding—
    Very low.
  Half-life—
    2.5–4 hours
  Biotransformation—
    Hepatic; about 10% demethylated to morphine.
  Onset of action—
    Analgesic:
      Intramuscular—10–30 minutes.
      Subcutaneous—10–30 minutes.
      Oral—30–45 minutes.
  Time to peak effect—
    Analgesic:
      Intramuscular—30–60 minutes.
      Oral—1–2 hours.
  Duration of action—
    Analgesic (in nontolerant patients only; decreases as tolerance develops during chronic therapy): Intramuscular, subcutaneous, or oral—4 hours.
    Antitussive: Oral—4–6 hours.
  Elimination—
    Renal, 5–15% as unchanged codeine and 10% as unchanged or conjugated morphine.
Side/adverse effects:
  More likely than most other opioids to cause constipation, especially during chronic therapy.
  Has lower dependence liability than most other opioid agonists.
  Withdrawal symptoms less severe than those produced by stronger opioid agonist analgesics.

## Additional Dosing Information

See also *General Dosing Information.*

**For parenteral dosage forms only**
Local tissue irritation, pain, and induration may occur with repeated subcutaneous injection.

## Oral Dosage Forms

Note: Bracketed uses in the *Dosage Forms* section refer to categories of use and/or indications that are not included in U.S. product labeling.

### CODEINE PHOSPHATE ORAL SOLUTION

**Usual adult dose**
Analgesic—
  Oral, 15 to 60 mg (usually 30 mg) every three to six hours as needed.
[Antidiarrheal][1]—
  Oral, 30 mg up to four times a day.
Antitussive—
  Oral, 10 to 20 mg every four to six hours.

**Usual adult prescribing limits**
Antitussive—
  Up to 120 mg in twenty-four hours.

**Usual pediatric dose**
Analgesic—
  Premature infants: Use is not recommended.
  Newborn infants: Dosage has not been established.
  Infants and children: Oral, 500 mcg (0.5 mg) per kg of body weight or 15 mg per square meter of body surface every four to six hours as needed.
[Antidiarrheal][1]—
  Oral, 500 mcg (0.5 mg) per kg of body weight up to four times a day.

Antitussive—
  Children up to 2 years of age:
    Use is not recommended.
  Children 2 to 5 years of age:
    Oral, 1 mg per kg of body weight per day, administered in four
      equal divided doses, or for
    Children 2 years of age (average body weight 12 kg)—Oral, 3 mg
      every four to six hours, not to exceed 12 mg per day.
    Children 3 years of age (average body weight 14 kg)—Oral, 3.5
      mg every four to six hours, not to exceed 14 mg per day.
    Children 4 years of age (average body weight 16 kg)—Oral, 4 mg
      every four to six hours, not to exceed 16 mg per day.
    Children 5 years of age (average body weight 18 kg)—Oral, 4.5
      mg every four to six hours, not to exceed 18 mg per day.
  Children 6 to 12 years of age:
    Oral, 5 to 10 mg every four to six hours, not to exceed 60 mg per
      day.
Note: Use of a calibrated measure is recommended to prevent possible
  overdosage in children up to 6 years of age.

**Strength(s) usually available**
U.S.—
  15 mg per 5 mL (Rx) [GENERIC].
Canada—
  10 mg per mL (Rx) [*Paveral*].

**Packaging and storage**
Store below 40 °C (104 °F), preferably between 15 and 30 °C (59 and 86
  °F), in a tight, light-resistant container, unless otherwise specified by
  manufacturer. Protect from freezing.

**Auxiliary labeling**
• May cause drowsiness.
• Avoid alcoholic beverages.
• May be habit-forming.

**Note**
Controlled substance in both the U.S. and Canada.

**CODEINE PHOSPHATE TABLETS USP**

**Usual adult dose**
Analgesic—
  Oral, 15 to 60 mg (usually 30 mg) every three to six hours as needed.
[Antidiarrheal][1]—
  Oral, 30 mg up to four times a day.
Antitussive—
  Oral, 10 to 20 mg every four to six hours.

**Usual adult prescribing limits**
Antitussive—
  Up to 120 mg in twenty-four hours.

**Usual pediatric dose**
Analgesic—
  Premature infants: Use is not recommended.
  Newborn infants: Dosage has not been established.
  Infants and children: Oral, 500 mcg (0.5 mg) per kg of body weight
    or 15 mg per square meter of body surface every four to six hours
    as needed.
[Antidiarrheal][1]—
  Oral, 500 mcg (0.5 mg) per kg of body weight up to four times a day.
Antitussive—
  Children up to 2 years of age:
    Use is not recommended.
  Children 2 to 5 years of age:
    Oral, 1 mg per kg of body weight per day, administered in four
      equal divided doses, or for
    Children 2 years of age (average body weight 12 kg)—Oral, 3 mg
      every four to six hours, not to exceed 12 mg per day.
    Children 3 years of age (average body weight 14 kg)—Oral, 3.5
      mg every four to six hours, not to exceed 14 mg per day.
    Children 4 years of age (average body weight 16 kg)—Oral, 4 mg
      every four to six hours, not to exceed 16 mg per day.
    Children 5 years of age (average body weight 18 kg)—Oral, 4.5
      mg every four to six hours, not to exceed 18 mg per day.
  Children 6 to 12 years of age:
    Oral, 5 to 10 mg every four to six hours, not to exceed 60 mg per
      day.

**Strength(s) usually available**
U.S.—
  30 mg (Rx) [GENERIC].
  60 mg (Rx) [GENERIC].
Canada—
  15 mg (Rx) [GENERIC].
  30 mg (Rx) [GENERIC].

Note: Strengths of commercially available tablets do not correspond to
  recommended antitussive doses.

**Packaging and storage**
Store below 40 °C (104 °F), preferably between 15 and 30 °C (59 and 86
  °F). Store in a well-closed, light-resistant container.

**Auxiliary labeling**
• May cause drowsiness.
• Avoid alcoholic beverages.
• May be habit-forming.

**Note**
Controlled substance in both the U.S. and Canada.

**CODEINE SULFATE TABLETS USP**

**Usual adult dose**
Analgesic—
  Oral, 15 to 60 mg (usually 30 mg) every three to six hours as needed.
[Antidiarrheal]—
  Oral, 30 mg up to four times a day.
Antitussive—
  Oral, 10 to 20 mg every four to six hours.

**Usual pediatric dose**
Analgesic—
  Premature infants: Use is not recommended.
  Newborn infants: Dosage has not been established.
  Infants and children: Oral, 500 mcg (0.5 mg) per kg of body weight
    or 15 mg per square meter of body surface every four to six hours
    as needed.
[Antidiarrheal]—
  Oral, 500 mcg (0.5 mg) per kg of body weight up to four times a day.
Antitussive—
  Children up to 2 years of age:
    Use is not recommended.
  Children 2 to 5 years of age:
    Oral, 1 mg per kg of body weight per day, administered in four
      equal divided doses, or for
    Children 2 years of age (average body weight 12 kg)—Oral, 3 mg
      every four to six hours, not to exceed 12 mg per day.
    Children 3 years of age (average body weight 14 kg)—Oral, 3.5
      mg every four to six hours, not to exceed 14 mg per day.
    Children 4 years of age (average body weight 16 kg)—Oral, 4 mg
      every four to six hours, not to exceed 16 mg per day.
    Children 5 years of age (average body weight 18 kg)—Oral, 4.5
      mg every four to six hours, not to exceed 18 mg per day.
  Children 6 to 12 years of age:
    Oral, 5 to 10 mg every four to six hours, not to exceed 60 mg per
      day.

**Strength(s) usually available**
U.S.—
  15 mg (Rx) [GENERIC].
  30 mg (Rx) [GENERIC].
  60 mg (Rx) [GENERIC].
Canada—
  Not commercially available.

Note: Strengths of commercially available tablets do not correspond to
  recommended antitussive doses.

**Packaging and storage**
Store below 40 °C (104 °F), preferably between 15 and 30 °C (59 and 86
  °F). Store in a well-closed container.

**Auxiliary labeling**
• May cause drowsiness.
• Avoid alcoholic beverages.
• May be habit-forming.

# Parenteral Dosage Forms
**CODEINE PHOSPHATE INJECTION USP**

**Usual adult dose**
Analgesic—
  Intramuscular, intravenous, or subcutaneous, 15 to 60 mg (usually 30
    mg) every four to six hours as needed.

**Usual pediatric dose**
Analgesic—
  Premature infants: Use is not recommended.
  Newborn infants: Dosage has not been established.
  Infants and children: Intramuscular or subcutaneous, 500 mcg (0.5 mg)
    per kg of body weight or 15 mg per square meter of body surface
    every four to six hours as needed.

**Strength(s) usually available**

U.S.—

With preservative

30 mg per mL (Rx) [GENERIC].

60 mg per mL (Rx) [GENERIC].

Canada—

30 mg per mL (Rx) [GENERIC].

60 mg per mL (Rx) [GENERIC].

**Packaging and storage**

Store below 40 °C (104 °F), preferably between 15 and 30 °C (59 and 86 °F), unless otherwise specified by manufacturer. Protect from light. Protect from freezing.

**Auxiliary labeling**

• May cause drowsiness.

• Avoid alcoholic beverages.

• May be habit-forming.

**Note**

Controlled substance in both the U.S. and Canada.

## CODEINE PHOSPHATE SOLUBLE TABLETS

**Usual adult dose**

Analgesic—

Intramuscular or subcutaneous, 15 to 60 mg (usually 30 mg) every four to six hours as needed.

**Usual pediatric dose**

Analgesic—

Premature infants: Use is not recommended.

Newborn infants: Dosage has not been established.

Infants and children: Intramuscular or subcutaneous, 500 mcg (0.5 mg) per kg of body weight or 15 mg per square meter of body surface every four to six hours as needed.

**Strength(s) usually available**

U.S.—

30 mg (Rx) [GENERIC].

60 mg (Rx) [GENERIC].

Canada—

Not commercially available.

**Packaging and storage**

Store between 15 and 30 °C (59 and 86 °F), in a tight, light-resistant container, unless otherwise specified by manufacturer.

**Preparation of dosage form**

For parenteral administration—Dissolve the required number of tablets in a suitable volume of sterile water for injection, then filter through a 0.22–micron membrane filter.

**Auxiliary labeling**

• May cause drowsiness.

• Avoid alcoholic beverages.

• May be habit-forming.

**Note**

Controlled substance in the U.S.

## CODEINE SULFATE SOLUBLE TABLETS

**Usual adult dose**

Analgesic—

Intramuscular or subcutaneous, 15 to 60 mg (usually 30 mg) every four to six hours as needed.

**Usual pediatric dose**

Analgesic—

Premature infants: Use is not recommended.

Newborn infants: Dosage has not been established.

Infants and children: Intramuscular or subcutaneous, 500 mcg (0.5 mg) per kg of body weight or 15 mg per square meter of body surface every four to six hours as needed.

**Strength(s) usually available**

U.S.—

30 mg (Rx) [GENERIC].

60 mg (Rx) [GENERIC].

Canada—

Not commercially available.

**Packaging and storage**

Store between 15 and 30 °C (59 and 86 °F), in a tight, light-resistant container, unless otherwise specified by manufacturer.

**Preparation of dosage form**

For parenteral administration—Dissolve the required number of tablets in a suitable volume of sterile water for injection, then filter through a 0.22–micron membrane filter.

**Auxiliary labeling**

• May cause drowsiness.

• Avoid alcoholic beverages.

• May be habit-forming.

**Note**

Controlled substance in the U.S.

¹Not included in Canadian product labeling.

---

### *HYDROCODONE*

## Summary of Differences

Indications:

Also, indicated as an antitussive.

Pharmacology/pharmacokinetics—

Mechanism of action/effect—

An opioid agonist analgesic; exerts agonist activity primarily at the mu receptor.

Half-life—

3.8 hours.

Onset of action—

Analgesic: Oral 10–30 minutes.

Time to peak effect—

Analgesic: Oral 30–60 minutes

Duration of action—

Analgesic (nontolerant patients only; decreases as tolerance develops during chronic therapy): Oral—4–6 hours.

Antitussive: Oral—4–6 hours.

Elimination—

Renal.

Side/adverse effects:

More likely than most other opioids to cause side effects associated with histamine release.

## Oral Dosage Forms

### HYDROCODONE BITARTRATE SYRUP

**Usual adult dose**

Antitussive—

Oral, 5 mg every four to six hours as needed.

**Usual pediatric dose**

Dosage has not been established.

**Strength(s) usually available**

U.S.—

Not commercially available.

Canada—

5 mg per 5 mL (Rx) [*Hycodan* (sucrose); *Robidone* (alcohol 3.2%; sugar)].

Note: In Canada, *Hycodan* contains only hydrocodone bitartrate; in the U.S., *Hycodan* contains homatropine in addition to hydrocodone bitartrate.

**Packaging and storage**

Store below 40 °C (104 °F), preferably between 15 and 30 °C (59 and 86 °F), in a well-closed container, unless otherwise specified by manufacturer. Protect from freezing.

**Auxiliary labeling**

• May cause drowsiness.

• Avoid alcoholic beverages.

• May be habit-forming.

**Note**

Controlled substance in Canada.

### HYDROCODONE BITARTRATE TABLETS USP

**Usual adult dose**

Analgesic—

Oral, 5 to 10 mg every four to six hours as needed.

Antitussive—

Oral, 5 mg every four to six hours as needed.

**Usual pediatric dose**

Analgesic—

Oral, 150 mcg (0.15 mg) per kg of body weight every six hours as needed.

**Strength(s) usually available**

U.S.—

Not commercially available.

Canada—

5 mg (Rx) [*Hycodan* (scored; lactose)].

Note: In Canada, *Hycodan* contains only hydrocodone bitartrate; in the U.S., *Hycodan* contains homatropine in addition to hydrocodone bitartrate.

**Packaging and storage**
Store below 40 °C (104 °F), preferably between 15 and 30 °C (59 and 86 °F). Store in a tight, light-resistant container.

**Auxiliary labeling**
• May cause drowsiness.
• Avoid alcoholic beverages.
• May be habit-forming.

**Note**
Controlled substance in Canada.

---

### *HYDROMORPHONE*

## Summary of Differences

Indications:
    Also, indicated as an antitussive; see also *Cough/Cold Combinations (Systemic)—Hydromorphone and Guaifenesin.*
Pharmacology/pharmacokinetics:
    Mechanism of action/effect—
        An opioid agonist analgesic; exerts agonist activity primarily at the mu receptor.
    Equivalence—
        1.5 mg via intramuscular injection, 7.5 mg via oral administration, or 3 mg via rectal administration therapeutically equivalent to 10 mg of intramuscular morphine.
    Half-life—
        2.6–4 hours
    Onset of action—
        Intramuscular: 15 minutes.
        Intravenous: 10–15 minutes.
        Oral: 30 minutes.
        Subcutaneous: 15 minutes.
    Time to peak effect—
        Intramuscular: 30–60 minutes.
        Intravenous: 15–30 minutes.
        Oral: 90–120 minutes.
        Subcutaneous: 30–90 minutes.
    Duration of action (nontolerant patients only; decreases as tolerance develops during chronic therapy)—
        Intramuscular: 4–5 hours.
        Intravenous: 2–3 hours.
        Oral: 4 hours.
        Subcutaneous: 4 hours.
    Elimination—
        Renal.

## Oral Dosage Forms

### HYDROMORPHONE HYDROCHLORIDE ORAL SOLUTION

**Usual adult dose**
Oral, 2.5 to 10 mg every three to six hours, depending on the severity of pain and patient tolerance.

**Usual pediatric dose**
Dosage must be individualized by physician, depending on the severity of pain and the patient's age, size, and opioid tolerance.

**Strength(s) usually available**
U.S.—
    5 mg per 5 mL [*Dilaudid-5*].
Canada—
    5 mg per 5 mL [*Dilaudid* (sucrose); *PMS-Hydromorphone Syrup*].

### HYDROMORPHONE HYDROCHLORIDE TABLETS USP

**Usual adult dose**
Analgesic—
    Oral, 2 mg every three to six hours as needed.
Note: Dosage may be increased to 4 mg or more every four to six hours, depending on the severity of pain and patient tolerance.

**Usual pediatric dose**
Dosage must be individualized by physician, depending on the severity of pain and the patient's age, size, and opioid tolerance.

**Strength(s) usually available**
U.S.—
    1 mg (Rx) [*Hydrostat IR*].
    2 mg (Rx) [*Dilaudid* (lactose); *Hydrostat IR;* GENERIC].

    3 mg (Rx) [*Hydrostat IR*].
    4 mg (Rx) [*Dilaudid* (lactose); *Hydrostat IR;* GENERIC].
    8 mg (Rx) [*Dilaudid*].
Canada—
    1 mg (Rx) [*Dilaudid; PMS-Hydromorphone*].
    2 mg (Rx) [*Dilaudid; PMS-Hydromorphone;* GENERIC].
    4 mg (Rx) [*Dilaudid; PMS-Hydromorphone;* GENERIC].
    8 mg (Rx) [*Dilaudid; PMS-Hydromorphone*].

**Packaging and storage**
Store below 40 °C (104 °F), preferably between 15 and 30 °C (59 and 86 °F), unless otherwise specified by manufacturer. Store in a tight, light-resistant container.

**Auxiliary labeling**
• May cause drowsiness.
• Avoid alcoholic beverages.
• May be habit-forming.

**Note**
Controlled substance in both the U.S. and Canada.

## Parenteral Dosage Forms

### HYDROMORPHONE HYDROCHLORIDE INJECTION USP

**Usual adult dose**
Analgesic—
    Intramuscular or subcutaneous, 1 to 2 mg every three to six hours as needed; may be increased to 3 or 4 mg every four to six hours if pain is severe.
    Note: For opioid-tolerant patients requiring high-dose therapy, the 10-mg-per-mL concentration may be substituted for lower strengths of hydromorphone hydrochloride injection or for other opioid analgesics. Dosage must be individualized, depending on the severity of pain, opioid requirements at the time therapy with the high-potency injection is initiated, and patient response. Although patients who have become tolerant to another opioid may be at least partially cross-tolerant to hydromorphone also, it is recommended that one-half of the equianalgesic dose of hydromorphone be used initially, then adjusted as necessary.
    Intravenous, 500 mcg (0.5 mg) to 1 mg every three hours as needed; administered slowly.

**Usual pediatric dose**
Dosage must be individualized by physician on the basis of patient's age and size.

**Strength(s) usually available**
U.S.—
    With preservatives
        1 mg per mL (Rx) [GENERIC].
        2 mg per mL (Rx) [*Dilaudid* (methylparaben and propylparaben); GENERIC].
        3 mg per mL (Rx) [GENERIC].
        4 mg per mL (Rx) [GENERIC].
    Without preservative
        1 mg per mL (Rx) [*Dilaudid*].
        2 mg per mL (Rx) [*Dilaudid*].
        4 mg per mL (Rx) [*Dilaudid*].
        10 mg per mL (Rx) [*Dilaudid-HP*].
Canada—
    Without preservative
        2 mg per mL (Rx) [*Dilaudid*].
        10 mg per mL (Rx) [*Dilaudid-HP*].

**Packaging and storage**
Store below 40 °C (104 °F), preferably between 15 and 30 °C (59 and 86 °F), unless otherwise specified by manufacturer. Protect from light. Protect from freezing.

**Auxiliary labeling**
• May cause drowsiness.
• Avoid alcoholic beverages.
• May be habit-forming.

**Note**
Controlled substance in both the U.S. and Canada.

## Rectal Dosage Forms

### HYDROMORPHONE HYDROCHLORIDE SUPPOSITORIES

**Usual adult dose**
Analgesic—
    Rectal, 3 mg every four to eight hours as needed.

**Usual pediatric dose**
Dosage has not been established.

**Strength(s) usually available**
U.S.—
   3 mg (Rx) [*Dilaudid*].
Canada—
   3 mg (Rx) [*Dilaudid; PMS-Hydromorphone*].

**Packaging and storage**
Store between 2 and 8 °C (36 and 46 °F), in a well-closed container, unless otherwise specified by manufacturer. Protect from freezing.

**Auxiliary labeling**
• May cause drowsiness.
• Avoid alcoholic beverages.
• May be habit-forming.
• Store in refrigerator.

**Note**
Controlled substance in both the U.S. and Canada.

---

## *LEVORPHANOL*

## Summary of Differences
Pharmacology/pharmacokinetics:
   Mechanism of action/effect—
      An opioid agonist analgesic; exerts agonist activity primarily at the mu receptor.
   Equivalence—
      2 mg via intramuscular injection or 4 mg via oral administration therapeutically equivalent to 10 mg of intramuscular morphine.
   Protein binding—
      Moderate.
   Onset of action—
      Oral: 10–60 minutes.
   Time to peak effect—
      Intramuscular: 60 minutes.
      Intravenous: Within 20 minutes.
      Oral: 90–120 minutes.
      Subcutaneous: 60–90 minutes.
   Duration of action (nontolerant patients only; duration decreases as tolerance develops during chronic therapy)—
      Intramuscular, intravenous, oral, or subcutaneous: 4–5 hours.
   Elimination—
      Renal.

## Oral Dosage Forms
### LEVORPHANOL TARTRATE TABLETS USP

**Usual adult dose**
Analgesic—
   Oral, 2 mg; may be increased to 3 or 4 mg if pain is severe.

**Usual pediatric dose**
Dosage must be individualized by physician on the basis of patient's age and size.

**Strength(s) usually available**
U.S.—
   2 mg (Rx) [*Levo-Dromoran* (scored; lactose); GENERIC].
Canada—
   2 mg (Rx) [*Levo-Dromoran* (scored; lactose)].

**Packaging and storage**
Store between 15 and 30 °C (59 and 86 °F), in a light-resistant container, unless otherwise specified by manufacturer. Store in a well-closed container.

**Auxiliary labeling**
• May cause drowsiness.
• Avoid alcoholic beverages.
• May be habit-forming.

**Note**
Controlled substance in both the U.S. and Canada.

## Parenteral Dosage Forms
### LEVORPHANOL TARTRATE INJECTION USP

**Usual adult dose**
Analgesic—
   Subcutaneous, 2 mg; may be increased to 3 mg if pain is severe.

Note: The medication may also be given intravenously.
      For preoperative analgesia—Subcutaneous, 1 to 2 mg ninety minutes prior to surgery.

**Usual pediatric dose**
Dosage must be individualized by physician on the basis of patient's age and size.

**Strength(s) usually available**
U.S.—
   With preservatives
      2 mg per mL (Rx) [*Levo-Dromoran* (methylparaben and propylparaben [1-mL ampuls]; or 0.45% phenol [10-mL vials])].
Canada—
   With preservatives
      2 mg per mL (Rx) [*Levo-Dromoran* (0.45% phenol)].

**Packaging and storage**
Store below 40 °C (104 °F), preferably between 15 and 30 °C (59 and 86 °F), unless otherwise specified by manufacturer. Protect from freezing.

**Auxiliary labeling**
• May cause drowsiness.
• Avoid alcoholic beverages.
• May be habit-forming.

**Note**
Controlled substance in both the U.S. and Canada.

---

## *MEPERIDINE*

## Summary of Differences
Pharmacology/pharmacokinetics:
   Mechanism of action/effect—
      An opioid agonist analgesic; exerts agonist activity primarily at the mu receptor.
   Equivalence—
      75 mg via intramuscular injection or 300 mg via oral administration therapeutically equivalent to 10 mg of intramuscular morphine.
   Protein binding—
      High.
   Half-life—
      2.4–4 hours
   Biotransformation—
      Metabolized to normeperidine, which is active and toxic.
   Onset of action—
      Intramuscular: 10–15 minutes.
      Intravenous: 1 minute.
      Oral: 15 minutes.
      Subcutaneous: 10–15 minutes.
   Time to peak effect—
      Intramuscular: 30–50 minutes.
      Intravenous: 5–7 minutes.
      Oral: 60–90 minutes.
      Subcutaneous: 30–50 minutes.
   Duration of action (nontolerant patients only; decreases as tolerance develops during chronic therapy)—
      Intramuscular, intravenous, oral, or subcutaneous: 2–4 hours.
   Elimination—
      Renal, 5% as unchanged meperidine.
Precautions:
   Drug interactions and/or related problems—
      May increase effects of coumarin- or indandione-derivative anticoagulants.
      Contraindicated in patients who have received a monoamine oxidase (MAO) inhibitor within past 14–21 days; concurrent use has produced serious, sometimes fatal, reactions.
      Concurrent use with amphetamines, which have some MAO inhibiting activity, not recommended because of risk of serious reactions similar to those reported with other MAO inhibitors.
Side/adverse effects:
   More likely than most other opioids to cause side effects associated with histamine release, convulsions, or constipation.

## Additional Dosing Information
See also *General Dosing Information*.

**For oral dosage forms only**
The syrup may be diluted with ½ glass (120 mL) of water to prevent a slight topical anesthetic effect on the mucous membranes.

**For parenteral dosage forms only**
Intramuscular administration is preferred when repeated doses are required. Repeated subcutaneous administration causes local tissue irritation and induration.

Inadvertent injection around a nerve trunk may cause sensory-motor paralysis, which is usually, but not always, transitory.

## Oral Dosage Forms
### MEPERIDINE HYDROCHLORIDE SYRUP USP

**Usual adult dose**
Analgesic—
    Oral, 50 to 150 mg (usually 100 mg) every three to four hours as needed.

**Usual pediatric dose**
Analgesic—
    Oral, 1.1 to 1.76 mg per kg of body weight, not to exceed 100 mg, every three to four hours as needed. Use of a calibrated measure is recommended to prevent possible overdosage in children up to 6 years of age.

**Strength(s) usually available**
U.S.—
    50 mg per 5 mL (Rx) [*Demerol* (glucose; saccharin sodium); GENERIC].
Canada—
    Not commercially available.

**Packaging and storage**
Store below 40 °C (104 °F), preferably between 15 and 30 °C (59 and 86 °F). Store in a tight, light-resistant container. Protect from freezing.

**Auxiliary labeling**
• May cause drowsiness.
• Avoid alcoholic beverages.
• May be habit-forming.

**Note**
Controlled substance in the U.S.

### MEPERIDINE HYDROCHLORIDE TABLETS USP

**Usual adult dose**
Analgesic—
    Oral, 50 to 150 mg (usually 100 mg) every three to four hours as needed.

**Usual pediatric dose**
Analgesic—
    Oral, 1.1 to 1.76 mg per kg of body weight, not to exceed 100 mg, every three to four hours as needed.

**Strength(s) usually available**
U.S.—
    50 mg (Rx) [*Demerol;* GENERIC].
    100 mg (Rx) [*Demerol;* GENERIC].
Canada—
    50 mg (Rx) [*Demerol* (scored)].

**Packaging and storage**
Store below 40 °C (104 °F), preferably between 15 and 30 °C (59 and 86 °F). Store in a well-closed, light-resistant container.

**Auxiliary labeling**
• May cause drowsiness.
• Avoid alcoholic beverages.
• May be habit-forming.

**Note**
Controlled substance in both the U.S. and Canada.

## Parenteral Dosage Forms
### MEPERIDINE HYDROCHLORIDE INJECTION USP

**Usual adult dose**
Analgesic—
    Intramuscular (preferred) or subcutaneous, 50 to 150 mg (usually 100 mg) every three to four hours as needed.
    Intravenous infusion, 15 to 35 mg per hour as required, administered using an infusion pump.
    Note: Dosage must be adjusted according to the severity of pain and patient response.
    Obstetrical analgesia: Intramuscular (preferred) or subcutaneous, 50 to 100 mg administered when pains become regular. May be repeated at one- to three-hour intervals as needed.
Anesthesia adjunct—
    Preoperative: Intramuscular (preferred) or subcutaneous, 50 to 100 mg thirty to ninety minutes prior to anesthesia.
    Intravenous, by repeated slow injection of fractional doses of a solution diluted to 10 mg per mL.
    Intravenous infusion, as a solution diluted to 1 mg per mL.

Note: Dosage must be titrated to the needs of the patient, depending on the premedication given, the type of anesthesia, and the nature and duration of the surgical procedure.

**Usual pediatric dose**
Analgesic—
    Intramuscular (preferred) or subcutaneous, 1.1 to 1.76 mg per kg of body weight, not to exceed 100 mg, every three to four hours as needed.
Preoperative—
    Intramuscular (preferred) or subcutaneous, 1 to 2.2 mg per kg of body weight, not to exceed 100 mg, thirty to ninety minutes prior to anesthesia.

**Strength(s) usually available**
U.S.—
    With preservative
        25 mg per mL (Rx) [GENERIC].
        50 mg per mL (Rx) [*Demerol* (metacresol); GENERIC].
        75 mg per mL (Rx) [GENERIC].
        100 mg per mL (Rx) [*Demerol* (metacresol); GENERIC].
    Without preservative
        10 mg per mL (Rx) [GENERIC].
        25 mg per mL (Rx) [*Demerol;* GENERIC].
        50 mg per mL (Rx) [*Demerol;* GENERIC].
        75 mg per mL (Rx) [*Demerol;* GENERIC].
        100 mg per mL (Rx) [*Demerol;* GENERIC].
    Note: In addition to being available in single- or multiple-dose units containing the concentrations listed above, *Demerol* is available in single-dose ampuls that contain 0.5, 1.5, or 2 mL of the 50 mg per mL concentration (providing 25, 75, or 100 mg of meperidine hydrochloride, respectively).
Canada—
    With preservative
        50 mg per mL (Rx) [*Demerol* (metacresol)].
        100 mg per mL (Rx) [*Demerol* (metacresol)].
    Without preservative
        10 mg per mL (Rx) [GENERIC].
        25 mg per mL (Rx) [GENERIC].
        50 mg per mL (Rx) [*Demerol;* GENERIC].
        75 mg per mL (Rx) [*Demerol;* GENERIC].
        100 mg per mL (Rx) [*Demerol;* GENERIC].

**Packaging and storage**
Store below 40 °C (104 °F), preferably between 15 and 30 °C (59 and 86 °F), unless otherwise specified by manufacturer. Protect from light. Protect from freezing.

**Incompatibilities**
Solutions of meperidine are chemically incompatible with aminophylline, barbiturates, heparin, iodides, methicillin, phenytoin, sodium bicarbonate, sulfadiazine, and sulfisoxazole.

**Auxiliary labeling**
• May cause drowsiness.
• Avoid alcoholic beverages.
• May be habit-forming.

**Note**
Controlled substance in both the U.S. and Canada.

---

## METHADONE

## Summary of Differences

Note: In the U.S., methadone may be dispensed for treatment of opioid addiction only through treatment programs that have been approved by the Food and Drug Administration (FDA), Drug Enforcement Administration (DEA), and designated state authorities. Use of methadone in such programs is subject to treatment requirements stipulated in the Code of Federal Regulations.

In Canada, methadone is a controlled substance (Classification N). It is available only through physicians who have received special authorization to prescribe the medication for treatment of opioid addiction.

Indications:
    Also, indicated as narcotic abstinence syndrome suppressant.
    Also, used as antitussive.
    Not recommended for obstetrical analgesia.
Pharmacology/pharmacokinetics:
    Mechanism of action/effect—
        An opioid agonist analgesic; exerts agonist activity primarily at the mu receptor.

Equivalence—
   10 mg via intramuscular injection or 20 mg via oral administration
      therapeutically equivalent to 10 mg of intramuscular morphine.
Protein binding—
   High.
Half-life—
   15–25 hours; increases with repeated administration.
Onset of action—
   Intramuscular: 10–20 minutes.
   Oral: 30–60 minutes.
Time to peak effect—
   Intramuscular: 1–2 hours.
   Intravenous: 15–30 minutes.
   Oral: 1.5–2 hours.
Duration of action (in nontolerant patients, may increase considerably
   with chronic use because of accumulation of methadone or active
   metabolites; may then decrease as tolerance develops during
   chronic therapy)—
   Intramuscular: 4–5 hours.
   Intravenous: 3–4 hours.
   Oral: 4–6 hours.
Elimination—
   Primarily renal (rate increased in acidic urine); also some biliary
      elimination.
Precautions:
Drug interactions and/or related problems—
   Urinary acidifiers may increase methadone elimination, thereby re-
      ducing the plasma concentration; withdrawal symptoms may
      occur in some physically dependent patients.
   Phenytoin or rifampin may increase methadone metabolism and
      precipitate withdrawal symptoms in physically dependent
      patients.
Side/adverse effects:
   May be more likely than most other opioids to cause constipation.

## Additional Dosing Information

See also *General Dosing Information*.

U.S. Federal regulations permit methadone to be used in detoxification
   and maintenance treatment programs for opioid addiction. Short-term
   (up to 30 days) or long-term (up to 180 days) detoxification programs
   use methadone to alleviate adverse physiological or psychological consequences of withdrawal from illicit opioids, with dosage gradually
   being decreased until a drug-free state is achieved. After 180 days,
   patients who have not achieved a drug-free state are considered to be
   receiving maintenance treatment. Patients 18 years of age or older may
   also be enrolled directly into a maintenance program without first attempting detoxification. In maintenance treatment programs, relatively
   stable doses of opioid are given on a continuing basis as a substitute
   for illicit opioids.

Detoxification and comprehensive maintenance programs must include a
   full range of medical and rehabilitative services in addition to opioid
   administration. However, patients who are awaiting admission to a
   comprehensive maintenance program may receive up to 120 days of
   interim maintenance treatment, which consists only of opioid administration and needed medical services.

Oral administration is preferred for detoxification and mandatory for
   maintenance.

### For parenteral dosage forms only

Intramuscular administration is recommended when repeated doses are
   required. Repeated subcutaneous administration causes local tissue irritation and induration.

## Oral Dosage Forms

### METHADONE HYDROCHLORIDE ORAL CONCENTRATE USP

**Usual adult dose**
Analgesic—
   Oral, 5 to 20 mg every four to eight hours. Dosage may be increased
      or the interval between doses decreased if pain is very severe or
      if the patient becomes tolerant to the medication.
Suppressant (narcotic abstinence syndrome)—
   Detoxification: Oral, 15 to 40 mg once a day or as needed to control
      observed withdrawal symptoms; dosage to be reduced at one- or
      two-day intervals according to patient response.
   Maintenance: Dosage must be individualized.

**Usual adult prescribing limits**
Up to 120 mg per day.

**Usual pediatric dose**
Analgesic—
   Dosage must be individualized by physician on the basis of patient's
      age and size. Use of a calibrated measure is recommended to pre-
      vent possible overdosage in children up to 6 years of age.
Suppressant (narcotic abstinence syndrome)—
   Dosage must be individualized by physician according to the needs of
      the specific patient. Dosage must not exceed 120 mg per day.
   Note: Patients younger than 18 years of age may be admitted to meth-
      adone maintenance programs only after 2 documented attempts
      at short-term (up to 30 days) detoxification or drug-free treat-
      ment have failed. A one-week waiting period is required be-
      tween a detoxification attempt and admission to a methadone
      maintenance program. A parent, legal guardian, or other re-
      sponsible adult designated by the State authority must complete
      and sign a consent to treatment form for all such minors.

**Strength(s) usually available**
U.S.—
   10 mg per mL (Rx) [*Methadose;* GENERIC].

**Packaging and storage**
Store between 15 and 30 °C (59 and 86 °F). Store in a tight container.
   Protect from light. Protect from freezing.

**Preparation of dosage form**
Each dose must be diluted with water or another liquid before administration. For use in the treatment of chronic pain, each dose should be
   diluted to at least 30 mL. U.S. Federal regulations stipulate that the
   oral concentrate be diluted with water or other suitable liquid before
   being administered to a patient undergoing treatment for opioid addiction. It is recommended that each dose be diluted to 90 mL or more
   as a deterrent to misuse by injection. Treatment centers that dispense
   both methadone and levomethadyl (which must also be dispensed as
   a diluted liquid) should use liquids of different colors for preparing
   each medication, so that they can be readily distinguished from each
   other.

**Auxiliary labeling**
• May cause drowsiness.
• Avoid alcoholic beverages.
• May be habit-forming.

**Note**
Controlled substance in the U.S.

When preparing the label, indicate that the medication must be diluted
   with water or another liquid to 30 mL or more prior to administration.

If the concentrate is being taken home, make sure the patient understands
   the dilution requirements.

### METHADONE HYDROCHLORIDE ORAL SOLUTION USP

**Usual adult dose**
Analgesic—
   Oral, 5 to 20 mg every four to eight hours. Dosage may be increased
      or the interval between doses decreased if pain is very severe or
      if the patient becomes tolerant to the medication.

**Usual pediatric dose**
Analgesic—
   Dosage must be individualized by physician on the basis of patient's
      age and size. Use of a calibrated measure is recommended to pre-
      vent possible overdosage in children up to 6 years of age.

**Strength(s) usually available**
U.S.—
   5 mg per 5 mL (Rx) [GENERIC].
   10 mg per 5 mL (Rx) [GENERIC].
Canada—
   Not commercially available.

**Packaging and storage**
Store between 15 and 30 °C (59 and 86 °F). Store in a tight container.
   Protect from light. Protect from freezing.

**Auxiliary labeling**
• May cause drowsiness.
• Avoid alcoholic beverages.
• May be habit-forming.

**Note**
Controlled substance in the U.S.

## METHADONE HYDROCHLORIDE TABLETS USP

**Usual adult dose**
Analgesic—
    Oral, 2.5 to 10 mg every three to four hours as needed initially. For chronic use, dose and dosing interval to be adjusted according to patient response.

**Usual pediatric dose**
Analgesic—
    Dosage must be individualized by physician on the basis of patient's age and size.

**Strength(s) usually available**
U.S.—
    5 mg (Rx) [*Dolophine* (lactose; sucrose); *Methadose;* GENERIC].
    10 mg (Rx) [*Dolophine* (lactose; sucrose); *Methadose;* GENERIC].
Canada—
    Not commercially available.

**Packaging and storage**
Store below 40 °C (104 °F), preferably between 15 and 30 °C (59 and 86 °F). Store in a well-closed container.

**Auxiliary labeling**
• May cause drowsiness.
• Avoid alcoholic beverages.
• May be habit-forming.

**Note**
Controlled substance in the U.S.

## METHADONE HYDROCHLORIDE TABLETS (DISPERSIBLE) USP

**Usual adult dose**
Suppressant (narcotic abstinence syndrome)—
    Detoxification: Oral, 15 to 40 mg once a day or as needed to control observed withdrawal symptoms; dosage to be reduced at one- or two-day intervals according to patient response.
    Maintenance: Dosage must be individualized.

**Usual adult prescribing limits**
Up to 120 mg per day.

**Usual pediatric dose**
Suppressant (narcotic abstinence syndrome)—
    Dosage must be individualized by physician according to the needs of the specific patient. Dosage must not exceed 120 mg per day.

Note: Patients younger than 18 years of age may be admitted to methadone maintenance programs only after 2 documented attempts at short-term (up to 30 days) detoxification or drug-free treatment have failed. A 1-week waiting period is required between a detoxification attempt and admission to a methadone maintenance program. A parent, legal guardian, or other responsible adult designated by the State authority must complete and sign a consent to treatment form for all such minors.

**Strength(s) usually available**
U.S.—
    40 mg (Rx) [*Methadose;* GENERIC].

**Packaging and storage**
Store between 15 and 30 °C (59 and 86 °F). Store in a well-closed container.

**Preparation of dosage form**
U.S. Federal regulations stipulate that the tablets must be dispersed in water or other suitable liquid before being administered to the patient. Treatment centers that dispense both methadone and levomethadyl (which must also be dispensed as a diluted liquid) should use liquids of different colors for preparing each medication, so that they can be readily distinguished from each other. The dispersible tablets have been formulated with insoluble excipients as a deterrent to misuse of the medication by injection.

**Auxiliary labeling**
• May cause drowsiness.
• Avoid alcoholic beverages.
• May be habit-forming.

**Note**
Controlled substance in the U.S.

## Parenteral Dosage Forms
### METHADONE HYDROCHLORIDE INJECTION USP

**Usual adult dose**
Analgesic—
    Intramuscular or subcutaneous, 2.5 to 10 mg every three to four hours as needed.
Suppressant (narcotic abstinence syndrome)—
    For detoxification only: Intramuscular or subcutaneous, 15 to 40 mg once a day or as needed to control observed withdrawal symptoms; dosage to be reduced at one- or two-day intervals according to patient response.
    Note: Parenteral administration in a detoxification regimen is recommended only for patients unable to take medication orally.

**Usual pediatric dose**
Analgesic—
    Dosage must be individualized by physician on the basis of patient's age and size

**Strength(s) usually available**
U.S.—
    With preservative
        10 mg per mL (Rx) [*Dolophine* (chlorobutanol)].
    Without preservative
        10 mg per mL (Rx) [*Dolophine*].

**Packaging and storage**
Store below 40 °C (104 °F), preferably between 15 and 30 °C (59 and 86 °F), in a light-resistant container. Protect from freezing.

**Auxiliary labeling**
• May cause drowsiness.
• Avoid alcoholic beverages.
• May be habit-forming.

**Note**
Controlled substance in the U.S.

---

### MORPHINE

## Summary of Differences

Indications:
    Drug of choice to relieve pain due to acute myocardial infarction.
    Also, indicated as adjunctive therapy in the treatment of acute pulmonary edema secondary to left ventricular failure.
    Also, used as antitussive.
Pharmacology/pharmacokinetics:
    Mechanism of action/effect—
        An opioid agonist analgesic; exerts agonist activity primarily at the mu receptor.
    Equivalence—
        60 mg via oral administration therapeutically equivalent to 10 mg intramuscularly; however, with chronic use on a fixed schedule may decrease to 20–30 mg.
    Protein binding—
        Low.
    Half-life—
        2–3 hours
    Onset of action—
        Epidural: 15–60 minutes.
        Intramuscular: 10–30 minutes.
        Intrathecal: 15–60 minutes.
        Rectal: 20–60 minutes.
        Subcutaneous: 10–30 minutes.
    Time to peak effect—
        Intramuscular: 30–60 minutes.
        Intravenous: 20 minutes.
        Oral (immediate-release dosage forms): 1–2 hours.
        Subcutaneous: 50–90 minutes.
    Duration of action (nontolerant patients only; may decrease as tolerance develops during chronic therapy)—
        Epidural: Up to 24 hours.
        Intramuscular: 4–5 hours.
        Intrathecal: Up to 24 hours.
        Intravenous: 4–5 hours.
        Oral: 4–5 hours with immediate-release dosage forms; 8 or 12 hours (depending on specific product) with extended-release dosage forms.
        Subcutaneous: 4–5 hours.
    Elimination—
        85% Renal, 9–12% as unchanged morphine; 7–10% biliary.

Precautions:

Drug interactions and/or related problems—

Also may decrease clearance of zidovudine; toxicity of either or both medications may be potentiated.

Side/adverse effects:

More likely than most other opioids to cause constipation and to produce symptoms associated with histamine release.

## Additional Dosing Information

See also *General Dosing Information.*

### For oral dosage forms only

The oral dosage forms are recommended for administration via a fixed dosage schedule to patients with severe, chronic pain. However, low doses of an immediate-release oral dosage form may be used on an as-needed basis to relieve ''breakthrough'' pain that occurs during chronic treatment with an extended-release dosage form.

Periodic attempts should be made to reduce the dosage after an initial response has been achieved and maintained for at least 3 days.

The oral liquid may be diluted in a glass of fruit juice just prior to ingestion, if desired, to improve the taste.

The extended-release tablets are to be swallowed whole. They should not be broken, crushed, or chewed.

### For parenteral dosage forms only

Intramuscular administration is recommended when repeated doses are required. Repeated subcutaneous administration causes local tissue irritation, pain, and induration.

The 25- or 50-mg per mL concentration of morphine sulfate injection available in Canada may be administered undiluted to opioid-tolerant patients requiring high-dose therapy. The 25-mg-per-mL concentration of morphine sulfate injection available in the U.S. is intended only for the preparation of intravenous infusion solutions and is not to be administered via other parenteral routes.

### Bioequivalence information

Bioavailability or bioequivalence problems among different brands of Morphine Sulfate Tablets (immediate-release) and different brands of Morphine Sulfate Oral Solution have not been documented.

Morphine Sulfate Extended-release Capsules (available in Canada) should not be interchanged with other extended-release dosage forms containing morphine hydrochloride or morphine sulfate. Bioavailability or bioequivalence studies comparing the products have not been done.

## Oral Dosage Forms

### MORPHINE HYDROCHLORIDE SYRUP

**Usual adult dose**

Analgesic—

Chronic pain: Dosage and dosing interval must be individualized by the physician according to the severity of pain and patient response. Initial oral doses of 10 to 30 mg every four hours are recommended by most manufacturers of oral morphine products. However, some patients receiving the medication via the recommended fixed dosing schedule may respond to lower doses, while others have required 75 mg or more.

**Usual pediatric dose**

Analgesic—

Dosage must be individualized by the physician according to the severity of pain as well as on the basis of the patient's age and size. Use of calibrated measure is recommended to prevent possible overdosage in children up to 6 years of age.

**Strength(s) usually available**

U.S.—

Not commercially available.

Canada—

1 mg per mL (Rx) [*Morphitec* (alcohol 5%; tartrazine); *M.O.S*].

5 mg per mL (Rx) [*Morphitec* (alcohol 5%; tartrazine); *M.O.S*].

10 mg per mL (Rx) [*Morphitec* (alcohol 5%; tartrazine); *M.O.S*].

20 mg per mL (Rx) [*Morphitec* (alcohol 5%; tartrazine); *M.O.S*].

50 mg per mL (Rx) [*M.O.S*].

**Packaging and storage**

Store below 40 °C (104 °F), preferably between 15 and 30 °C (59 and 86 °F), in a well-closed container, unless otherwise specified by manufacturer. Protect from freezing.

**Auxiliary labeling**

• May cause drowsiness.

• Avoid alcoholic beverages.

• May be habit-forming.

**Note**

Controlled substance in Canada.

### MORPHINE HYDROCHLORIDE TABLETS

**Usual adult dose**

Analgesic—

Chronic pain: Dosage and dosing interval must be individualized by the physician according to the severity of pain and patient response. Initial oral doses of 10 to 30 mg every four hours are recommended by most manufacturers of oral morphine products. However, some patients receiving the medication via the recommended fixed dosing schedule may respond to lower doses, while others have required 75 mg or more.

**Usual pediatric dose**

Analgesic—

Dosage must be individualized by the physician according to the severity of pain as well as on the basis of the patient's age and size.

**Strength(s) usually available**

U.S.—

Not commercially available.

Canada—

10 mg (Rx) [*M.O.S*].

20 mg (Rx) [*M.O.S*].

40 mg (Rx) [*M.O.S*].

60 mg (Rx) [*M.O.S*].

**Packaging and storage**

Store below 40 °C (104 °F), preferably between 15 and 30 °C (59 and 86 °F), in a well-closed container, unless otherwise specified by manufacturer. Protect from freezing.

**Auxiliary labeling**

• May cause drowsiness.

• Avoid alcoholic beverages.

• May be habit-forming.

**Note**

Controlled substance in Canada.

### MORPHINE HYDROCHLORIDE EXTENDED-RELEASE TABLETS

**Usual adult dose**

Analgesic—

Chronic pain: Dosage must be individualized by the physician according to the severity of pain and patient response.

**Usual pediatric dose**

Dosage has not been established.

**Strength(s) usually available**

U.S.—

Not commercially available.

Canada—

30 mg (Rx) [*M.O.S.-S.R*].

60 mg (Rx) [*M.O.S.-S.R*].

**Packaging and storage**

Store below 40 °C (104 °F), preferably between 15 and 30 °C (59 and 86 °F), in a well-closed container, unless otherwise specified by manufacturer.

**Auxiliary labeling**

• Swallow tablets whole.

• May cause drowsiness.

• Avoid alcoholic beverages.

• May be habit-forming.

**Note**

Controlled substance in Canada.

### MORPHINE SULFATE CAPSULES

**Usual adult dose**

Analgesic—

Chronic pain: Dosage and dosing interval must be individualized by the physician according to the severity of pain and patient response. Initial oral doses of 10 to 30 mg every four hours are recommended by most manufacturers of oral morphine products. However, some patients receiving the medication via the recommended fixed dosing schedule may respond to lower doses, while others have required 75 mg or more.

**Usual pediatric dose**

Analgesic—

Dosage must be individualized by the physician according to the severity of pain as well as on the basis of the patient's age and size.

**Strength(s) usually available**
U.S.—
   15 mg (Rx) [*MSIR*].
   30 mg (Rx) [*MSIR*].
Canada—
   Not commercially available.

## MORPHINE SULFATE EXTENDED-RELEASE CAPSULES

Note: The extended-release capsule dosage form has not been evaluated for bioequivalence with other extended-release dosage forms containing morphine hydrochloride or morphine sulfate and should not be interchanged with them.

**Usual adult dose**
Analgesic—
   Chronic pain: Oral, 30 mg every twelve hours, initially, with dosage then being adjusted according to the requirements of the individual patient.

Note: Patients being transferred from other opioid analgesics or other morphine dosage forms to the morphine sulfate extended-release capsules should receive a total daily dose of oral morphine sulfate equivalent to the established total daily dose of previously administered medication, administered in divided doses at twelve-hour intervals. The manufacturers' prescribing information contains recommendations for calculating equivalent dosage.

**Usual pediatric dose**
Dosage has not been established.

**Strength(s) usually available**
U.S.—
   Not commercially available.
Canada—
   10 mg (Rx) [*M-Eslon*].
   30 mg (Rx) [*M-Eslon*].
   60 mg (Rx) [*M-Eslon*].
   100 mg (Rx) [*M-Eslon*].

**Packaging and storage**
Store between 15 and 30 °C (59 and 86 °F).

**Auxiliary labeling**
• May cause drowsiness.
• Avoid alcoholic beverages.
• May be habit-forming.

**Note**
Controlled substance in Canada.

## MORPHINE SULFATE ORAL SOLUTION

Note: Bioavailability or bioequivalence problems among different brands of Morphine Sulfate Oral Solution have not been documented.

**Usual adult dose**
Analgesic—
   Chronic pain: Dosage and dosing interval must be individualized by the physician according to the severity of pain and patient response. Initial oral doses of 10 to 30 mg every four hours are recommended by most manufacturers of oral morphine products. However, some patients receiving the medication via the recommended fixed dosing schedule may respond to lower doses, while others have required 75 mg or more.

**Usual pediatric dose**
Analgesic—
   Dosage must be individualized by the physician according to the severity of pain as well as on the basis of the patient's age and size. Use of calibrated measure is recommended to prevent possible overdosage in children up to 6 years of age.

**Strength(s) usually available**
U.S.—
   10 mg per 2.5 mL (unit dose) (Rx) [*Rescudose; Roxanol UD*].
   10 mg per 5 mL (Rx) [*MSIR* (sucrose); *MS/L;* GENERIC].
   20 mg per 5 mL (Rx) [*MSIR; Roxanol UD;* GENERIC].
   20 mg per mL (Rx) [*MSIR; MS/L Concentrate; OMS Concentrate; Roxanol*].
   30 mg per 1.5 mL (Rx) [*Roxanol UD*].
   100 mg per 5 mL (Rx) [*Roxanol 100*].
Canada—
   2 mg per mL (Rx) [GENERIC].
   4 mg per mL (Rx) [GENERIC].
   20 mg per mL (Rx) [*Statex Drops*].
   50 mg per mL (Rx) [*Statex Drops*].

**Packaging and storage**
Store between 15 and 30 °C (59 and 86 °F), in a tight, light-resistant container, unless otherwise specified by manufacturer. Protect from freezing.

**Auxiliary labeling**
• May cause drowsiness.
• Avoid alcoholic beverages.
• May be habit-forming.

**Note**
Controlled substance in both the U.S. and Canada.

## MORPHINE SULFATE SYRUP

**Usual adult dose**
Analgesic—
   Chronic pain: Dosage and dosing interval must be individualized by the physician according to the severity of pain and patient response. Initial oral doses of 10 to 30 mg every four hours are recommended by most manufacturers of oral morphine products. However, some patients receiving the medication via the recommended fixed dosing schedule may respond to lower doses, while others have required 75 mg or more.

**Usual pediatric dose**
Analgesic—
   Dosage must be individualized by the physician according to the severity of pain as well as on the basis of the patient's age and size.

**Strength(s) usually available**
U.S.—
   Not commercially available.
Canada—
   1 mg per mL (Rx) [*Statex*].
   5 mg per mL (Rx) [*Statex*].
   10 mg per mL (Rx) [*Statex*].

**Packaging and storage**
Store below 40 °C (104 °F), preferably between 15 and 30 °C (59 and 86 °F), in a well-closed container, unless otherwise specified by manufacturer. Protect from freezing.

**Auxiliary labeling**
• May cause drowsiness.
• Avoid alcoholic beverages.
• May be habit-forming.

**Note**
Controlled substance in Canada.

## MORPHINE SULFATE TABLETS

Note: Bioavailability or bioequivalence problems among different brands of Morphine Sulfate Tablets have not been documented.

**Usual adult dose**
Analgesic—
   Chronic pain: Dosage and dosing interval must be individualized by the physician according to the severity of pain and patient response. Initial oral doses of 10 to 30 mg every four hours are recommended by most manufacturers of oral morphine products. However, some patients receiving the medication via the recommended fixed dosing schedule may respond to lower doses, while others have required 75 mg or more.

**Usual pediatric dose**
Analgesic—
   Chronic pain: Dosage must be individualized by the physician according to the severity of pain as well as on the basis of the patient's age and size.

**Strength(s) usually available**
U.S.—
   15 mg (Rx) [*MSIR* (scored); GENERIC].
   30 mg (Rx) [*MSIR* (scored); GENERIC].
Canada—
   5 mg (Rx) [*MS•IR* (scored); *Statex* (scored)].
   10 mg (Rx) [*MS•IR* (scored); *Statex* (scored)].
   15 mg (Rx) [GENERIC].
   20 mg (Rx) [*MS•IR* (scored)].
   25 mg (Rx) [*Statex* (scored)].
   30 mg (Rx) [*MS•IR* (scored); GENERIC].
   50 mg (Rx) [*Statex* (scored)].

**Packaging and storage**
Store below 40 °C (104 °F), preferably between 15 and 30 °C (59 and 86 °F), in a well-closed container, unless otherwise specified by manufacturer.

**Auxiliary labeling**
- May cause drowsiness.
- Avoid alcoholic beverages.
- May be habit-forming.

**Note**
Controlled substance in both the U.S. and Canada.

## MORPHINE SULFATE EXTENDED-RELEASE TABLETS

**Usual adult dose**
Analgesic—
   Chronic pain: Oral, 30 mg every twelve hours, initially, with dosage and dosing interval then being adjusted according to the requirements of the individual patient.

Note: Patients being transferred from other opioid analgesics or other morphine dosage forms to the morphine sulfate extended-release tablets should receive a total daily dose of oral morphine sulfate equivalent to the established total daily dose of previously administered medication, administered in divided doses at twelve-hour intervals. The manufacturers' prescribing information contains recommendations for calculating equivalent dosage.

**Usual pediatric dose**
Dosage has not been established.

**Strength(s) usually available**
U.S.—
   15 mg (Rx) [*M S Contin;* GENERIC].
   30 mg (Rx) [*M S Contin; Oramorph SR;* GENERIC].
   60 mg (Rx) [*M S Contin; Oramorph SR;* GENERIC].
   100 mg (Rx) [*M S Contin; Oramorph SR;* GENERIC].
   200 mg (Rx) [*M S Contin*].
Canada—
   15 mg (Rx) [*M S Contin*].
   30 mg (Rx) [*M S Contin; Oramorph SR*].
   60 mg (Rx) [*M S Contin; Oramorph SR*].
   100 mg (Rx) [*M S Contin; Oramorph SR*].
   200 mg (Rx) [*M S Contin* (scored)].

**Packaging and storage**
Store below 40 °C (104 °F), preferably between 15 and 30 °C (59 and 86 °F), in a well-closed container, unless otherwise specified by manufacturer.

**Auxiliary labeling**
- Swallow tablets whole.
- May cause drowsiness.
- Avoid alcoholic beverages.
- May be habit-forming.

**Note**
Controlled substance in both the U.S. and Canada.

# Parenteral Dosage Forms
## MORPHINE SULFATE INJECTION USP

**Usual adult dose**
Analgesic—
   Intramuscular or subcutaneous, 5 to 20 mg (usually 10 mg, initially) every four hours as needed. For severe, chronic pain the medication may also be administered by subcutaneous infusion, using a portable pump, at a rate titrated to the requirements and response of the individual patient.

Note: The recommendation of an initial 10-mg dose is based on a 70-kg person.

   In Canada, the 25- or 50-mg-per-mL concentration may be substituted for lower strengths of morphine sulfate injection or for other opioid analgesics in opioid-tolerant patients requiring high-dose therapy. Dosage must be individualized, depending on the severity of pain, opioid requirements at the time therapy with the high-potency injection is initiated, and patient response. Although patients who have become tolerant to another opioid may be at least partially cross-tolerant to morphine also, it is recommended that one-half of the equianalgesic dose of morphine be used initially, then adjusted as necessary.

Intravenous, 4 to 10 mg diluted in 4 to 5 mL of sterile water for injection, administered slowly. For severe, chronic pain the medication may also be administered via intravenous infusion at a rate titrated to the requirements and response of the individual patient.
Epidural (in the lumbar region), 5 mg.

Note: If adequate pain relief is not achieved within one hour, incremental doses of 1 to 2 mg may be administered at intervals sufficient to assess effectiveness, up to a maximum of 10 mg per twenty-four hours.

Intrathecal, 200 mcg (0.2 mg) to 1 mg as a single dose.

Note: Clinical experience with repeated intrathecal injections is limited. Therefore, repeated administration via this route is not recommended. Alternate routes of administration should be considered for treating recurrent or chronic pain.

**Usual pediatric dose**
Analgesic—
   Subcutaneous, 100 to 200 mcg (0.1 to 0.2 mg) per kg of body weight every four hours as needed, not to exceed 15 mg per dose.
   Intravenous, 50 to 100 mcg (0.05 to 0.1 mg) per kg of body weight, administered very slowly.
Preoperative—
   Intramuscular, 50 to 100 mcg (0.05 to 0.1 mg) per kg of body weight, not to exceed 10 mg per dose.

**Strength(s) usually available**
U.S.—
   With preservative
      1 mg per mL (Rx) [GENERIC].
      2 mg per mL (Rx) [GENERIC].
      4 mg per mL (Rx) [GENERIC].
      5 mg per mL (Rx) [GENERIC].
      8 mg per mL (Rx) [GENERIC].
      10 mg per mL (Rx) [GENERIC].
      15 mg per mL (Rx) [GENERIC].
      25 mg per mL (Rx) [GENERIC].
      50 mg per mL (Rx) [GENERIC].
   Without preservative
      500 mcg (0.5 mg) per mL (Rx) [*Astramorph PF; Duramorph;* GENERIC].
      1 mg per mL (Rx) [*Astramorph PF; Duramorph;* GENERIC].
      50 mg per mL (Rx) [GENERIC].
Canada—
   With preservative
      1 mg per mL (Rx) [GENERIC].
      2 mg per mL (Rx) [GENERIC].
      5 mg per mL (Rx) [GENERIC].
      10 mg per mL (Rx) [GENERIC].
      15 mg per mL (Rx) [GENERIC].
      25 mg per mL (Rx) [*Morphine Forte*].
      50 mg per mL (Rx) [*Morphine Extra-Forte*].
   Without preservative
      500 mcg (0.5 mg) per mL (Rx) [*Epimorph;* GENERIC].
      1 mg per mL (Rx) [*Epimorph;* GENERIC].
      2 mg per mL (Rx) [GENERIC].
      25 mg per mL (Rx) [*Morphine H.P;* GENERIC].
      50 mg per mL (Rx) [*Morphine H.P;* GENERIC].

**Packaging and storage**
Store below 40 °C (104 °F), preferably between 15 and 30 °C (59 and 86 °F), unless otherwise specified by manufacturer. Protect from light. Protect from freezing.

**Stability**
Do not autoclave the preservative-free injection.
Unused portion of preservative-free injection must be discarded.

**Incompatibilities**
Morphine Sulfate Injection USP is incompatible with soluble barbiturates.

**Auxiliary labeling**
- May cause drowsiness.
- Avoid alcoholic beverages.
- May be habit-forming.

**Note**
Controlled substance in both the U.S. and Canada.

## MORPHINE SULFATE SOLUBLE TABLETS

**Usual adult dose**
Analgesic—
   Intramuscular or subcutaneous, 5 to 20 mg (usually 10 mg, initially) every four hours as needed.

Note: The recommendation of an initial 10-mg dose is based on a 70-kg person.

**Usual pediatric dose**
Analgesic—
   Subcutaneous, 100 to 200 mcg (0.1 to 0.2 mg) per kg of body weight every four hours as needed, not to exceed 15 mg per dose.

**Strength(s) usually available**
U.S.—
   10 mg (Rx) [GENERIC].
   15 mg (Rx) [GENERIC].
   30 mg (Rx) [GENERIC].

Canada—
    Not commercially available.

**Packaging and storage**
Store between 15 and 30 °C (59 and 86 °F), in a tight, light-resistant container, unless otherwise specified by manufacturer.

**Preparation of dosage form**
For parenteral administration—Dissolve the required number of tablets in a suitable volume of sterile water for injection, then filter through a 0.22–micron membrane filter.

**Auxiliary labeling**
• May cause drowsiness.
• Avoid alcoholic beverages.
• May be habit-forming.

**Note**
Controlled substance in the U.S.

# Rectal Dosage Forms
## MORPHINE HYDROCHLORIDE SUPPOSITORIES

**Usual adult dose**
Analgesic—
    Rectal, 20 to 30 mg every four to six hours.

**Usual pediatric dose**
Analgesic—
    Dosage must be individualized by the physician according to the severity of pain as well as on the basis of the patient's age and size.

**Strength(s) usually available**
U.S.—
    Not commercially available.
Canada—
    10 mg (Rx) [*M.O.S*].
    20 mg (Rx) [*M.O.S*].
    30 mg (Rx) [*M.O.S*].

**Packaging and storage**
Store below 40 °C (104 °F), preferably between 15 and 30 °C (59 and 86 °F), in a well-closed container, unless otherwise specified by manufacturer. Protect from freezing.

**Auxiliary labeling**
• May cause drowsiness.
• Avoid alcoholic beverages.
• May be habit-forming.

**Note**
Controlled substance in Canada.

## MORPHINE SULFATE SUPPOSITORIES

**Usual adult dose**
Analgesic—
    Rectal, 10 to 30 mg every four hours or as required.

    Note: Dosage must be individualized according to the severity of pain and the response of the patient.

**Usual pediatric dose**
Analgesic—
    Dosage must be individualized by physician on the basis of the patient's age and size.

**Strength(s) usually available**
U.S.—
    5 mg (Rx) [*MS/S; RMS Uniserts; Roxanol;* GENERIC].
    10 mg (Rx) [*MS/S; RMS Uniserts; Roxanol;* GENERIC].
    20 mg (Rx) [*MS/S; RMS Uniserts; Roxanol;* GENERIC].
    30 mg (Rx) [*MS/S; RMS Uniserts; Roxanol;* GENERIC].
Canada—
    5 mg (Rx) [*Statex*].
    10 mg (Rx) [*MS•IR; Statex*].
    20 mg (Rx) [*MS•IR; Statex*].
    30 mg (Rx) [*MS•IR; Statex*].

**Packaging and storage**
Store between 15 and 30 °C (59 and 86 °F), in a well-closed container, unless otherwise specified by manufacturer. Protect from freezing.

**Auxiliary labeling**
• May cause drowsiness.
• Avoid alcoholic beverages.
• May be habit-forming.

**Note**
Controlled substance in both the U.S. and Canada.

---

## NALBUPHINE

# Summary of Differences
Indications:
    Caution required when used as analgesic to relieve pain in patients with severely compromised cardiac function; cardiovascular effects in these patients have not been fully evaluated.
Pharmacology/pharmacokinetics:
    Mechanism of action/effect—
        An opioid agonist/antagonist analgesic.
        Agonist: Has agonist activity at the kappa and sigma receptors.
        Antagonist: Has antagonist activity at the mu receptor; may precipitate withdrawal symptoms in patients who are physically dependent on mu-receptor agonists.
    Equivalence—
        10 mg via intramuscular injection therapeutically equivalent to 10 mg of intramuscular morphine.
    Half-life—
        5 hours
    Onset of action—
        Intramuscular: Within 15 minutes.
        Intravenous: 2–3 minutes.
        Subcutaneous: Within 15 minutes.
    Time to peak concentration—
        Intramuscular: 0.5 hour.
    Peak plasma concentration—
        48 nanograms per mL.
    Time to peak effect—
        Intramuscular: 60 minutes.
        Intravenous: 30 minutes.
    Duration of action (nontolerant patients only; decreases as tolerance develops during chronic therapy)—
        Intramuscular: 3–6 hours.
        Intravenous: 3–4 hours.
        Subcutaneous: 3–6 hours.
    Elimination—
        Renal.
Precautions:
    Drug interactions and/or related problems—
        May antagonize effects of mu-receptor agonists.
    Medical considerations/contraindications—
        Also should be used with caution in patients who are physically dependent on opioid agonists.
Side/adverse effects:
    Rarely, may cause subjective and psychotomimetic effects characteristic of sigma receptor agonists.
    Respiratory depression subject to a "ceiling effect," after which the depth of respiratory depression does not increase with dose.
    More likely than most other opioid analgesics to produce symptoms associated with histamine release.
    Has lower dependence liability than opioid agonists.
    Withdrawal symptoms less severe than those produced by opioid agonist analgesics.

# Parenteral Dosage Forms
## NALBUPHINE HYDROCHLORIDE INJECTION

**Usual adult dose**
Analgesic—
    Intramuscular, intravenous, or subcutaneous, 10 mg every three to six hours as needed.

    Note: The usual adult dose is based on a 70-kg person.
Anesthesia adjunct (balanced anesthesia)—
    Initial: Intravenous, 300 mcg (0.3 mg) to 3 mg per kg of body weight, administered over a ten- to fifteen-minute period.
    Supplemental: Intravenous, 250 to 500 mcg (0.25 to 0.5 mg) per kg of body weight, as required.

**Usual adult prescribing limits**
For nontolerant patients—
Up to 20 mg as a single dose and up to 160 mg as a total daily dose.

**Usual pediatric dose**
Dosage has not been established.

**Strength(s) usually available**
U.S.—
    With preservatives
        10 mg per mL (Rx) [*Nubain* (methylparaben; propylparaben; sodium metabisulfite); GENERIC].
        20 mg per mL (Rx) [*Nubain* (methylparaben; propylparaben; sodium metabisulfite); GENERIC].

Without preservatives
10 mg per mL (Rx) [*Nubain*].
20 mg per mL (Rx) [*Nubain*].
Canada—
With preservatives
10 mg per mL (Rx) [*Nubain* (methylparaben; propylparaben; sodium metabisulfite)].
20 mg per mL (Rx) [*Nubain* (methylparaben; propylparaben; sodium metabisulfite)].

**Packaging and storage**
Store between 15 and 30 °C (59 and 86 °F), unless otherwise specified by manufacturer. Protect from light. Protect from freezing.

**Auxiliary labeling**
• May cause drowsiness.
• Avoid alcoholic beverages.

**Note**
Controlled substance in Canada.

---

## OPIUM

## Summary of Differences

Indications:
Oral dosage form—
Indicated as antidiarrheal.
Also, used as narcotic abstinence syndrome suppressant in neonates.
Pharmacology/pharmacokinetics:
Mechanism of action/effect—An opioid agonist analgesic; has agonist activity primarily at the mu receptor.
Equivalence—13.3 mg parenterally is therapeutically equivalent to 10 mg of intramuscular morphine.
Elimination—Renal and biliary.

## Additional Dosing Information

See also *General Dosing Information.*

The effects of opium preparations are due primarily to the morphine component.

**For oral dosage form only**
Alteration of intestinal motility in patients with traveler's diarrhea may result in prolonged fever by slowing expulsion of infectious organisms that penetrate intestinal mucosa (for example, *Shigella, Salmonella,* and certain strains of *Escherichia coli*).
Opium may produce fluid retention in the bowel, which may mask dehydration and electrolyte depletion caused by severe diarrhea, especially in young children. Patients with severe or prolonged diarrhea should be monitored for signs of dehydration or electrolyte imbalance, and corrective therapy administered as required.
To reduce the risk of toxic megacolon in patients with acute inflammatory bowel disease, treatment with opium tincture should be discontinued promptly if abdominal distention or other gastrointestinal symptoms occur.
Tolerance to the antidiarrheal effects of opium tincture may develop with prolonged use.
Following prolonged administration of high doses, opium tincture should be withdrawn gradually in order to reduce the possibility of withdrawal symptoms.
Many clinicians have recommended use of diluted opium tincture instead of paregoric in the treatment of neonatal narcotic dependence, because of the risks associated with two of the components of the paregoric formulation. Opium tincture is diluted to produce the same concentration of morphine as paregoric and may be administered every 3 hours, with gradual withdrawal over 2 to 4 weeks when symptoms are controlled.

**For parenteral dosage form only**
This formulation contains all of the alkaloids of opium as the hydrochlorides.

## Oral Dosage Forms

### OPIUM TINCTURE (Laudanum) USP

**Usual adult dose**
Antidiarrheal—
Oral, 0.3 to 1.0 mL (usually 0.6 mL) (the equivalent of morphine—3 to 10 mg) four times a day.

**Usual adult prescribing limits**
A single dose of 1 mL, or a total of 6 mL within twenty-four hours.

**Usual pediatric dose**
Dosage has not been established.

**Strength(s) usually available**
U.S.—
10% of opium (the equivalent of 900 mg to 1.10 grams of anhydrous morphine per 100 mL) (Rx) [GENERIC (alcohol 17–21%)].
Canada—
10% of opium (the equivalent of 900 mg to 1.10 grams of anhydrous morphine per 100 mL) (Rx) [GENERIC (alcohol 17–21%)].

**Packaging and storage**
Store below 40 °C (104 °F), preferably between 15 and 30 °C (59 and 86 °F), unless otherwise specified by manufacturer. Store in a tight, light-resistant container. Avoid exposure to direct sunlight and excessive heat. Protect from freezing.

**Auxiliary labeling**
• May cause drowsiness.
• Avoid alcoholic beverages.
• Do not take other medicines without your doctor's advice.
• Keep out of reach of children.
• May be habit-forming.

**Note**
Caution—Be careful not to confuse opium tincture with camphorated tincture of opium (paregoric).

Controlled substance in both the U.S. and Canada.

Refrigeration is not recommended because decreased solubility and precipitation of some of the ingredients may occur. If this occurs, the preparation must be discarded.

## Parenteral Dosage Forms

### OPIUM ALKALOIDS HYDROCHLORIDES INJECTION (Papaveretum)

**Usual adult dose**
Analgesic—
Intramuscular or subcutaneous, 5 to 20 mg every four to five hours as needed.

**Usual pediatric dose**
Dosage has not been established.

**Strength(s) usually available**
U.S.—
Not commercially available.
Canada—
With preservatives
20 mg, as hydrochlorides of opium alkaloids, per mL (Rx) [*Pantopon* (methylparaben; propylparaben)].
Note: Contains 10 mg of anhydrous morphine per mL.

**Packaging and storage**
Store between 15 and 30 °C (59 and 86 °F), unless otherwise specified by manufacturer. Protect from freezing.

**Auxiliary labeling**
• May cause drowsiness.
• Avoid alcoholic beverages.
• May be habit-forming.

**Note**
Controlled substance in Canada.

---

## OXYCODONE

## Summary of Differences

Pharmacology/pharmacokinetics:
Mechanism of action/effect—An opioid agonist analgesic; has agonist activity primarily at the mu receptor.
Equivalence—30 mg via oral administration therapeutically equivalent to 10 mg of intramuscular morphine.
Half-life—2–3 hours.
Time to peak effect—Oral: 1 hour.
Duration of action (nontolerant patients only; duration decreases as tolerance develops during chronic therapy)—Oral: 3–4 hours.
Elimination—Renal.

# Oral Dosage Forms

## OXYCODONE HYDROCHLORIDE ORAL SOLUTION USP

**Usual adult dose**
Analgesic—
  Oral, 5 mg every three to six hours as needed; may be increased if severe pain is present.

**Usual pediatric dose**
Dosage must be individualized by physician on the basis of patient's age and size. Use of calibrated measure is recommended to prevent possible overdosage in children up to 6 years of age.

**Strength(s) usually available**
U.S.—
  5 mg per 5 mL (Rx) [*Roxicodone* (alcohol 7–9%)].
  20 mg per mL (Rx) [*Roxicodone Intensol*].
Canada—
  Not commercially available.

**Packaging and storage**
Store between 15 and 30 °C (59 and 86 °F), unless otherwise specified by manufacturer. Store in a tight, light-resistant container. Protect from freezing.

**Auxiliary labeling**
• May cause drowsiness.
• Avoid alcoholic beverages.
• May be habit-forming.

**Note**
Controlled substance in the U.S.

## OXYCODONE HYDROCHLORIDE TABLETS USP

**Usual adult dose**
Analgesic—
  Oral, 5 mg every three to six hours or 10 mg three or four times a day as needed; may be increased if severe pain is present.

**Usual pediatric dose**
Dosage must be individualized by physician on the basis of patient's age and size.

**Strength(s) usually available**
U.S.—
  5 mg (Rx) [*Roxicodone* (scored)].
Canada—
  5 mg (Rx) [*Supeudol*].
  10 mg (Rx) [*Supeudol*].

**Packaging and storage**
Store below 40 °C (104 °F), preferably between 15 and 30 °C (59 and 86 °F). Store in a tight, light-resistant container.

**Auxiliary labeling**
• May cause drowsiness.
• Avoid alcoholic beverages.
• May be habit-forming.

**Note**
Controlled substance in both the U.S. and Canada.

# Rectal Dosage Forms

## OXYCODONE HYDROCHLORIDE SUPPOSITORIES

**Usual adult dose**
Analgesic—
  Rectal, 10 to 40 mg three or four times a day.

**Usual pediatric dose**
Dosage must be individualized by physician on the basis of patient's age and size.

**Strength(s) usually available**
U.S.—
  Not commercially available.
Canada—
  10 mg (Rx) [*Supeudol*].
  20 mg (Rx) [*Supeudol*].

**Packaging and storage**
Store between 2 and 8 °C (36 and 46 °F), in a well-closed container, unless otherwise specified by manufacturer. Protect from freezing.

**Auxiliary labeling**
• May cause drowsiness.
• Avoid alcoholic beverages.
• May be habit-forming.
• Store in refrigerator. Protect from freezing.

**Note**
Controlled substance in Canada.

---

## OXYMORPHONE

# Summary of Differences

Indications:
  Also, FDA-approved, but rarely if ever used, as adjunctive therapy in the treatment of acute pulmonary edema secondary to left ventricular failure.
Pharmacology/pharmacokinetics:
  Mechanism of action/effect—
    An opioid agonist analgesic; has agonist activity primarily at the mu receptor.
  Equivalence—
    1 mg via intramuscular injection or 10 mg rectally therapeutically equivalent to 10 mg of intramuscular morphine.
  Onset of action—
    Intramuscular: 10–15 minutes.
    Intravenous: 5–10 minutes.
    Subcutaneous: 10–20 minutes.
    Rectal: 15–30 minutes.
  Time to peak effect—
    Intramuscular: 30–90 minutes.
    Intravenous: 15–30 minutes.
    Rectal: 2 hours.
  Duration of action (nontolerant patients only; duration decreases as tolerance develops during chronic therapy)—
    Intramuscular: 3–6 hours.
    Intravenous: 3–4 hours.
    Subcutaneous: 3–6 hours.
    Rectal: 3–6 hours.
  Elimination—
    Renal.

# Parenteral Dosage Forms

## OXYMORPHONE HYDROCHLORIDE INJECTION USP

**Usual adult dose**
Analgesic—
  Intramuscular or subcutaneous, 1 to 1.5 mg every three to six hours as needed.
  Intravenous, 500 mcg (0.5 mg).
Note: Doses may be cautiously increased, if necessary, if pain is severe. For obstetrical analgesia—Intramuscular, 500 mcg (0.5 mg) to 1 mg.

**Usual pediatric dose**
Dosage has not been established.

**Strength(s) usually available**
U.S.—
  With preservatives
    1 mg per mL (Rx) [*Numorphan* (methylparaben; propylparaben)].
    1.5 mg per mL (Rx) [*Numorphan* (methylparaben; propylparaben)].
Canada—
  With preservatives
    1.5 mg per mL (Rx) [*Numorphan* (methylparaben; propylparaben)].

**Packaging and storage**
Store below 40 °C (104 °F), preferably between 15 and 30 °C (59 and 86 °F), unless otherwise specified by manufacturer. Protect from light. Protect from freezing.

**Auxiliary labeling**
• May cause drowsiness.
• Avoid alcoholic beverages.
• May be habit-forming.

**Note**
Controlled substance in both the U.S. and Canada.

# Rectal Dosage Forms

## OXYMORPHONE HYDROCHLORIDE SUPPOSITORIES USP

**Usual adult dose**
Analgesic—
  Rectal, 5 mg every four to six hours as needed.

**Usual pediatric dose**
Dosage has not been established.

**Strength(s) usually available**
U.S.—
    5 mg (Rx) [*Numorphan*].
Canada—
    5 mg (Rx) [*Numorphan*].

**Packaging and storage**
Store between 2 and 8 °C (36 and 46 °F), in a well-closed container. Protect from freezing.

**Auxiliary labeling**
• May cause drowsiness.
• Avoid alcoholic beverages.
• May be habit-forming.
• Store in refrigerator. Protect from freezing.

**Note**
Controlled substance in both the U.S. and Canada.

---

## PENTAZOCINE

## Summary of Differences

Indications:
    Less desirable than morphine or other opioid agonist analgesics for relief of pain due to acute myocardial infarction because of cardiovascular effects that tend to increase cardiac work.
Pharmacology/pharmacokinetics:
    Mechanism of action/effect—
        An opioid agonist/antagonist analgesic.
        Agonist: Has agonist activity at the kappa and sigma receptors.
        Antagonist: Has antagonist activity at the mu receptor; may precipitate withdrawal symptoms in patients who are physically dependent on mu-receptor agonists.
    Equivalence—
        60 mg via intramuscular injection or 180 mg via oral administration therapeutically equivalent to 10 mg of intramuscular morphine.
    Protein binding—
        Moderate.
    Half-life—
        2–3 hours.
    Onset of action—
        Intramuscular: 15–20 minutes.
        Intravenous: 2–3 minutes.
        Oral: 15–30 minutes.
        Subcutaneous: 15–20 minutes.
    Time to peak effect—
        Intramuscular: 30–60 minutes.
        Intravenous: 15–30 minutes.
        Oral: 60–90 minutes.
        Subcutaneous: 30–60 minutes.
    Duration of action (nontolerant patients only; decreases as tolerance develops during chronic therapy)—
        Intramuscular: 2–3 hours.
        Intravenous: 2–3 hours.
        Oral: 3 hours.
        Subcutaneous: 2–3 hours.
    Elimination—
        Renal, 5–23% as unchanged pentazocine, and biliary.
Precautions:
    Drug interactions and/or related problems—
        May antagonize the effects of mu-receptor agonists.
    Medical considerations/contraindications—
        Also must be used with caution in patients physically dependent on opioid agonists and in patients with acute myocardial infarction.
Side/adverse effects:
    Although occurs rarely, more likely than butorphanol or nalbuphine to cause subjective and psychotomimetic effects characteristic of sigma receptor agonists.
    Respiratory depression subject to a ''ceiling effect,'' after which the depth of respiratory depression does not increase with dose.
    Has lower dependence liability than opioid agonists.
    Withdrawal symptoms less severe than those produced by opioid agonist analgesics.

## Additional Dosing Information

See also *General Dosing Information*.

The naloxone present in the pentazocine and naloxone dosage formulation has no pharmacologic activity when administered orally. If the product is misused by injection, the naloxone antagonizes the effects of pentazocine. Also, injection of the medication will precipitate withdrawal symptoms if the patient is physically dependent on an opioid agonist.

For long-term administration, the oral form of the medication is preferred. If the parenteral form is used instead, dosage should be reduced gradually when the medication is to be discontinued to reduce the risk of withdrawal symptoms.

The extent to which pentazocine may produce withdrawal symptoms in patients who are physically dependent on opioid analgesics depends upon the dose of pentazocine, the specific opioid drug involved, and the degree to which physical dependence has developed.

**For parenteral dosage forms only**
Intravenous or intramuscular administration is recommended, especially when repeated doses are required. Subcutaneous administration may lead to severe tissue damage at the injection site. When the intramuscular route is used, rotation of injection sites is essential to prevent tissue damage.

## Oral Dosage Forms
### PENTAZOCINE HYDROCHLORIDE TABLETS USP

**Usual adult dose**
Analgesic—
    Oral, 50 mg of pentazocine (base) every three to four hours as needed. The dose may be increased to 100 mg (base) if necessary, but total daily dosage should not exceed 600 mg (base).

**Usual adult prescribing limits**
Analgesic—
    Up to 600 mg of pentazocine (base) per day

**Usual pediatric dose**
Dosage has not been established.

**Strength(s) usually available**
U.S.—
    Not commercially available.
Canada—
    50 mg (base) (Rx) [*Talwin* (scored; sulfites)].

**Packaging and storage**
Store below 40 °C (104 °F), preferably between 15 and 30 °C (59 and 86 °F), unless otherwise specified by manufacturer. Store in a tight, light-resistant container.

**Auxiliary labeling**
• May cause drowsiness.
• Avoid alcoholic beverages.
• May be habit-forming.

**Note**
Controlled substance in Canada.

### PENTAZOCINE AND NALOXONE HYDROCHLORIDES TABLETS USP

**Usual adult dose**
Analgesic—
    Oral, 50 mg of pentazocine (base) every three to four hours as needed. The dose may be increased to 100 mg (base) if necessary, but total daily dosage should not exceed 600 mg (base).

**Usual adult prescribing limits**
Analgesic—
    Up to 600 mg of pentazocine (base) per day.

**Usual pediatric dose**
Dosage has not been established.

**Strength(s) usually available**
U.S.—
    50 mg (base), with 500 mcg (0.5 mg) of naloxone hydrochloride (Rx) [*Talwin-Nx* (scored)].
Canada—
    Not commercially available.

**Packaging and storage**
Store below 40 °C (104 °F), preferably between 15 and 30 °C (59 and 86 °F), unless otherwise specified by manufacturer. Store in a tight, light-resistant container.

**Auxiliary labeling**
• May cause drowsiness.
• Avoid alcoholic beverages.
• May be habit-forming.

**Note**
Controlled substance in the U.S.

## Parenteral Dosage Forms
### PENTAZOCINE LACTATE INJECTION USP

**Usual adult dose**
Analgesic—
    Intramuscular, intravenous, or subcutaneous, 30 mg (base) every three to four hours as needed.
Obstetrical analgesia—
    Intramuscular, 30 mg (base) as a single dose; or
    Intravenous, 20 mg (base) administered when contractions become regular and repeated two or three times at two- to three-hour intervals as needed.

**Usual adult prescribing limits**
Up to 360 mg (base) daily.
As a single dose, up to 30 mg (base) intravenously or 60 mg (base) intramuscularly.

**Usual pediatric dose**
Dosage has not been established.

**Strength(s) usually available**
U.S.—
    With preservative
        30 mg (base) per mL (Rx) [*Talwin* (acetone sodium bisulfite; methylparaben)].
    Without preservative
        30 mg (base) per mL (Rx) [*Talwin* (may contain acetone sodium bisulfite)].
Canada—
    Without preservative
        30 mg (base) per mL (Rx) [*Talwin*].

**Packaging and storage**
Store below 40 °C (104 °F), preferably between 15 and 30 °C (59 and 86 °F), unless otherwise specified by manufacturer. Protect from freezing.

**Incompatibilities**
Precipitation will occur if a soluble barbiturate is mixed in the same syringe as pentazocine.

**Auxiliary labeling**
• May cause drowsiness.
• Avoid alcoholic beverages.
• May be habit-forming.

**Note**
Controlled substance in both the U.S. and Canada.

---

### *PROPOXYPHENE*

## Summary of Differences
Pharmacology/pharmacokinetics:
    Mechanism of action/effect—
        An opioid agonist analgesic; has agonist activity at the mu receptor.
    Equivalence—
        Dose therapeutically equivalent to 10 mg of intramuscular morphine too toxic to administer.
    Protein binding—
        High.
    Biotransformation—
        Metabolite norpropoxyphene is toxic.
    Half-life—
        Propoxyphene: 6–12 hours
        Norpropoxyphene: 30–36 hours
    Onset of action—
        Oral: 15–60 minutes.
    Time to peak concentration:
        Oral: 2–2.5 hours.
    Peak plasma concentration:
        0.05–0.1 mcg per mL.
    Time to peak effect:
        Oral: 2 hours.
    Duration of action (nontolerant patients only; decreases as tolerance develops during chronic therapy):
        Oral: 4–6 hours.

Elimination:
    Renal, <10% as unchanged propoxyphene; biliary.
Precautions:
    Drug interactions and/or related problems:
        Risk of convulsions if overdose of propoxyphene administered to amphetamine-treated patients.
        May increase effects of coumarin- or indandione-derivative anticoagulants.
        Concurrent use with carbamazepine not recommended because may decrease carbamazepine metabolism, leading to increased risk of toxicity.
        Effects may be decreased in patients who smoke because tobacco smoking increases propoxyphene metabolism.
    Laboratory value alterations:
        May elevate levels of enzymes in liver function tests.
Side/adverse effects—
    May be more likely than most opioid analgesics to cause convulsions.
    Hepatotoxicity has been reported.
    Has lower dependence liability than other opioid agonists.
    Withdrawal symptoms less severe than those produced by stronger opioid agonist analgesics.

## Additional Dosing Information
See also *General Dosing Information.*
100 mg of propoxyphene napsylate are equivalent to 65 mg of propoxyphene hydrochloride.

## Oral Dosage Forms
### PROPOXYPHENE HYDROCHLORIDE CAPSULES USP

**Usual adult dose**
Analgesic—
    Oral, 65 mg every four hours as needed.

**Usual adult prescribing limits**
Up to 390 mg daily.

**Usual pediatric dose**
Dosage has not been established.

**Strength(s) usually available**
U.S.—
    65 mg (Rx) [*Cotanal-65; Darvon; PP-Cap;* GENERIC].
Canada—
    Not commercially available.

**Packaging and storage**
Store below 40 °C (104 °F), preferably between 15 and 30 °C (59 and 86 °F). Store in a tight container.

**Auxiliary labeling**
• May cause drowsiness.
• Avoid alcoholic beverages.
• May be habit-forming.

**Note**
Controlled substance in both the U.S. and Canada.

### PROPOXYPHENE HYDROCHLORIDE TABLETS

**Usual adult dose**
Analgesic—
    Oral, 65 mg every four hours as needed.

**Usual adult prescribing limits**
Analgesic—
    Oral, up to 390 mg daily.

**Usual pediatric dose**
Dosage has not been established.

**Strength(s) usually available**
U.S.—
    Not commercially available.
Canada—
    65 mg (Rx) [*642* (scored)].

**Packaging and storage**
Store below 40 °C (104 °F), preferably between 15 and 30 °C (59 and 86 °F), in a well-closed container, unless otherwise specified by manufacturer.

**Auxiliary labeling**
• May cause drowsiness.
• Avoid alcoholic beverages.
• May be habit-forming.

**Note**
Controlled substance in Canada.

## PROPOXYPHENE NAPSYLATE CAPSULES

**Usual adult dose**
Analgesic—
Oral, 100 mg every four hours as needed.

**Usual adult prescribing limits**
Analgesic—
Up to 600 mg daily.

**Usual pediatric dose**
Dosage has not been established.

**Strength(s) usually available**
U.S.—
Not commercially available.
Canada—
100 mg (Rx) [*Darvon-N*].

**Packaging and storage**
Store below 40 °C (104 °F), preferably between 15 and 30 °C (59 and 86 °F), unless otherwise specified by manufacturer. Store in a tight container.

**Auxiliary labeling**
• May cause drowsiness.
• Avoid alcoholic beverages.
• May be habit-forming.

**Note**
Controlled substance in Canada.

## PROPOXYPHENE NAPSYLATE ORAL SUSPENSION USP

**Usual adult dose**
Analgesic—
Oral, 100 mg every four hours as needed.

**Usual adult prescribing limits**
Analgesic—
Up to 600 mg daily.

**Usual pediatric dose**
Dosage has not been established.

**Strength(s) usually available**
U.S.—
50 mg per 5 mL (Rx) [*Darvon-N* (butylparaben; methylparaben; propylparaben; saccharin; sucrose)].

Canada—
Not commercially available.

**Packaging and storage**
Store below 40 °C (104 °F), preferably between 15 and 30 °C (59 and 86 °F), unless otherwise specified by manufacturer. Store in a tight container. Protect from light. Protect from freezing.

**Auxiliary labeling**
• Shake well.
• May cause drowsiness.
• Avoid alcoholic beverages.
• May be habit-forming.

**Note**
Controlled substance in the U.S.

## PROPOXYPHENE NAPSYLATE TABLETS USP

**Usual adult dose**
Analgesic—
Oral, 100 mg every four hours as needed.

**Usual adult prescribing limits**
Analgesic—
Up to 600 mg daily.

**Usual pediatric dose**
Dosage has not been established.

**Strength(s) usually available**
U.S.—
100 mg (Rx) [*Darvon-N;* GENERIC].
Canada—
Not commercially available.

**Packaging and storage**
Store below 40 °C (104 °F), preferably between 15 and 30 °C (59 and 86 °F), unless otherwise specified by manufacturer. Store in a tight container.

**Auxiliary labeling**
• May cause drowsiness.
• Avoid alcoholic beverages.
• May be habit-forming.

**Note**
Controlled substance in the U.S.

Revised: July 1990
Interim revision: 06/28/95

## Table 1. Pharmacology/Pharmacokinetics

| Drug | Protein Binding | Half-life (hr)* | Elimination | |
|------|-----------------|-----------------|-------------|--|
| | | | Primary (% excreted unchanged)† | Secondary |
| Butorphanol | High | 2.5–4 | 72% Renal (<5) | 15% biliary |
| Codeine‡ | Very low | 2.5–4 | Renal (5–15); 10% as unchanged or conjugated morphine | |
| Hydrocodone | | 3.8 | Renal | |
| Hydromorphone | | 2.6–4 | Renal | |
| Levorphanol | Moderate | | Renal | |
| Meperidine§ | High | 2.4–4 | Renal (5) | |

*Half-life may be increased in geriatric patients because of decreased clearance rate. Also, significant increases have been reported in patients with hepatic cirrhosis for meperidine (6 to 7 hr), morphine, and pentazocine.

†All opioid analgesics are excreted primarily as metabolites.

‡About 10% of a dose is demethylated to morphine, which may contribute to the therapeutic actions.

§Metabolite normeperidine is active and toxic (having CNS excitatory [proconvulsant] activity) and accumulates in patients with renal function impairment.

#Some metabolites are active; drug and/or metabolites may accumulate with repeated administration.

**Metabolite norpropoxyphene may be toxic; it is not known whether this metabolite has analgesic activity.

## Table 1. Pharmacology/Pharmacokinetics *(continued)*

| Drug | Protein Binding | Half-life (hr)* | Elimination Primary (% excreted unchanged)† | Elimination Secondary |
|---|---|---|---|---|
| Methadone# | High | 15–25; increases with repeated administration | Renal; rate increased in acidic urine | Biliary |
| Morphine | Low | 2–3 | 85% Renal (9–12) | 7–10% Biliary |
| Nalbuphine | | 5 | Renal | |
| Opium | | | Renal | Biliary |
| Oxycodone | | 2–3 | Renal | |
| Oxymorphone | | | Renal | |
| Pentazocine | Moderate | 2–3 | Renal (5–23) | Biliary |
| Propoxyphene** | High | 6–12 (propoxyphene) 30–36 (norpropoxyphene) | Renal (<10) | Biliary |

\*Half-life may be increased in geriatric patients because of decreased clearance rate. Also, significant increases have been reported in patients with hepatic cirrhosis for meperidine (6 to 7 hr), morphine, and pentazocine.

†All opioid analgesics are excreted primarily as metabolites.

‡About 10% of a dose is demethylated to morphine, which may contribute to the therapeutic actions.

§Metabolite normeperidine is active and toxic (having CNS excitatory [proconvulsant] activity) and accumulates in patients with renal function impairment.

#Some metabolites are active; drug and/or metabolites may accumulate with repeated administration.

\*\*Metabolite norpropoxyphene may be toxic; it is not known whether this metabolite has analgesic activity.

## Table 2. Pharmacology/Pharmacokinetics

| Drug and Route* | Equivalence† | Time to Peak Concentration (hr) | Peak Plasma Concentration | Therapeutic Effects Onset of Analgesic Action (min) | Therapeutic Effects Peak Analgesic Effect (min) | Therapeutic Effects Duration of Action Analgesic (hr)‡/ Antitussive (hr) |
|---|---|---|---|---|---|---|
| **Butorphanol** | | | | | | |
| IM | 2 | 0.5–1 | 2.2 ng§/mL | 10–30 | 30–60 | 3–4 |
| IV | | | | 2–3 | 30 | 2–4 |
| **Codeine** | | | | | | |
| Oral | 200 | | | 30–45 | 60–120 | 4/4–6 |
| IM | 120 | | | 10–30 | 30–60 | 4 |
| SC | | | | 10–30 | | 4 |
| **Hydrocodone** | | | | | | |
| Oral | | | | 10–30 | 30–60 | 4–6/4–6 |
| **Hydromorphone** | | | | | | |
| Oral | 7.5 | | | 30 | 90–120 | 4 |
| IM | 1.5 | | | 15 | 30–60 | 4–5 |
| IV | | | | 10–15 | 15–30 | 2–3 |
| SC | | | | 15 | 30–90 | 4 |
| Rectal | 3 | | | | | |
| **Levorphanol** | | | | | | |
| Oral | 4 | | | 10–60 | 90–120 | 4–5 |
| IM | 2 | | | | 60 | 4–5 |
| IV | | | | | Within 20 | 4–5 |
| SC | | | | | 60–90 | 4–5 |
| **Meperidine** | | | | | | |
| Oral | 300 | | | 15 | 60–90 | 2–4 |
| IM | 75 | | | 10–15 | 30–50 | 2–4 |
| IV | | | | 1 | 5–7 | 2–4 |
| SC | | | | 10–15 | 30–50 | 2–4 |
| **Methadone** | | | | | | |
| Oral | 20 | | | 30–60 | 90–120 | 4–6# |
| IM | 10 | | | 10–20 | 60–120 | 4–5# |
| IV | | | | | 15–30 | 3–4# |

## Table 2. Pharmacology/Pharmacokinetics (continued)

| Drug and Route* | Equivalence† | Time to Peak Concentration (hr) | Peak Plasma Concentration | Therapeutic Effects | | |
| --- | --- | --- | --- | --- | --- | --- |
| | | | | Onset of Analgesic Action (min) | Peak Analgesic Effect (min) | Duration of Action Analgesic (hr)‡/ Antitussive (hr) |
| **Morphine** | | | | | | |
| Oral | 60** | | | | | |
|   Extended-release tablets | | | | | | 8–12 |
|   Other oral dosage forms | | | | Slower than IM | 60–120 | 4–5 |
| IM | 10 | | | 10–30 | 30–60 | 4–5 |
| IV | | | | | 20 | 4–5 |
| SC | | | | 10–30 | 50–90 | 4–5 |
| Epidural | | | | 15–60 | | Up to 24 |
| Intrathecal | | | | 15–60 | | Up to 24 |
| Rectal | | | | 20–60 | | |
| **Nalbuphine** | | | | | | |
| IM | 10 | 0.5 | 48 ng§/mL | Within 15 | 60 | 3–6 |
| IV | | | | 2–3 | 30 | 3–4 |
| SC | | | | Within 15 | | 3–6 |
| **Opium** | | | | | | |
| Parenteral | 13.3 | | | | | |
| **Oxycodone** | | | | | | |
| Oral | 30 | | | | 60 | 3–4 |
| **Oxymorphone** | | | | | | |
| IM | 1 | | | 10–15 | 30–90 | 3–6 |
| IV | | | | 5–10 | 15–30 | 3–4 |
| SC | | | | 10–20 | | 3–6 |
| Rectal | 10 | | | 15–30 | 120 | 3–6 |
| **Pentazocine** | | | | | | |
| Oral | 180 | | | 15–30 | 60–90 | 3 |
| IM | 60 | | | 15–20 | 30–60 | 2–3 |
| IV | | | | 2–3 | 15–30 | 2–3 |
| SC | | | | 15–20 | 30–60 | 2–3 |
| **Propoxyphene** | | | | | | |
| Oral | †† | 2–2.5 | 0.05–0.1 mcg/mL | 15–60 | 120 | 4–6 |

*IM=Intramuscular; IV=Intravenous; SC=Subcutaneous.

†Dose in mg therapeutically equivalent to a 10-mg intramuscular dose of morphine.

‡In nontolerant patients only. The first sign of tolerance is usually a decrease in the duration of adequate analgesia. Also, may be increased in geriatric patients because of decreased clearance rate.

§Nanograms.

#Increases with repeated dosing because of accumulation of drug and/or active metabolites.

**For single doses or occasional use only; with chronic dosing on a fixed schedule, may decrease to 20 or 30 mg.

††Dose equivalent to 10 mg of morphine would be too toxic to administer. Values reported under *time to peak concentration* and *peak plasma concentration* were determined following a 65-mg dose of propoxyphene hydrochloride or a 100-mg dose of propoxyphene napsylate.

## Table 3. Drug Interactions and/or Related Problems

The following drug interactions and/or related problems have been selected on the basis of their potential clinical significance (possible mechanism in parentheses where appropriate)—not necessarily inclusive (» = major clinical significance):

Note: Combinations containing any of the following medications, depending on the amount present, may also interact with this medication.

**Legend:**

Agonist
- I = Codeine
- II = Hydrocodone
- III = Hydromorphone
- IV = Levorphanol
- V = Meperidine
- VI = Methadone
- VII = Morphine
- VIII = Opium
- IX = Oxycodone
- X = Oxymorphone
- XI = Propoxyphene

Agonist/Antagonist
- XII = Butorphanol
- XIII = Nalbuphine
- XIV = Pentazocine

| Interaction | I | II | III | IV | V | VI | VII | VIII | IX | X | XI | XII | XIII | XIV |
|---|---|---|---|---|---|---|---|---|---|---|---|---|---|---|
| Acidifiers, urinary, such as: Ammonium chloride; Ascorbic acid; Potassium or sodium phosphate (acidification of the urine by these medications increases methadone excretion, resulting in decreased methadone plasma concentrations; high doses of urinary acidifiers, such as several grams daily of ammonium chloride, may cause withdrawal symptoms in patients who are dependent on methadone) | | | | | | ✓ | | | | | | | | |
| » Alcohol or » CNS depression–producing medications, other (See *Appendix II*) (concurrent use with opioid analgesics may result in increased CNS depressant, respiratory depressant, and hypotensive effects; caution is recommended and dosage of one or both agents should be reduced. In addition, some phenothiazines increase, while others decrease, the effects of opioid analgesics used as adjuncts to anesthesia) | | ✓ | ✓ | ✓ | ✓ | ✓ | ✓ | ✓ | ✓ | ✓ | | ✓ | ✓ | ✓ |
| (concurrent use with other CNS depressants having habituation potential may increase the risk of habituation) | | ✓ | ✓ | ✓ | ✓ | ✓ | ✓ | ✓ | ✓ | ✓ | | ✓ | ✓ | ✓ |
| Amphetamines (amphetamines may potentiate the analgesic effects of meperidine; however, concurrent use of the 2 medications is not recommended because the monoamine oxidase inhibiting effect of amphetamines may increase the risk of hypotension, severe respiratory depression, coma, convulsions, hyperpyrexia, vascular collapse, and death) | | | | | ✓ | | | | | | | | | |
| (an overdose of propoxyphene may potentiate the CNS stimulating effects of amphetamines; fatal convulsions can result) | | | | | | | | | | | ✓ | | | |
| Anticholinergics or other medications with anticholinergic activity (See *Appendix II*) (concurrent use with opioid analgesics may result in increased risk of severe constipation, which may lead to paralytic ileus, and/or urinary retention) | | ✓ | ✓ | | | ✓ | | ✓ | ✓ | | | ✓ | ✓ | ✓ |
| Anticoagulants, coumarin- or indandione-derivative (meperidine and propoxyphene have been reported to increase the effects of these anticoagulants; although clinical significance has not been established, the possibility should be considered that adjustment of anticoagulant dosage may be necessary during and following concurrent use) | | | | | ✓ | | | | | | ✓ | | | |
| Antidiarrheals, antiperistaltic, such as: Difenoxin and atropine; Diphenoxylate and atropine; Kaolin, pectin, belladonna alkaloids, and opium; Loperamide; Opium tincture; Paregoric (concurrent use with an opioid analgesic may increase the risk of severe constipation as well as central nervous system [CNS] depression) | ✓ | ✓ | | | | ✓ | | ✓ | ✓ | | | ✓ | ✓ | ✓ |

Table 3. Drug Interactions and/or Related Problems (continued)

Legend:
I = Codeine
II = Hydrocodone
III = Hydromorphone
IV = Levorphanol
V = Meperidine
VI = Methadone
VII = Morphine
VIII = Opium
IX = Oxycodone
X = Oxymorphone
XI = Propoxyphene
XII = Butorphanol
XIII = Nalbuphine
XIV = Pentazocine

Columns I–XI = Agonist; Columns XII–XIV = Agonist/Antagonist

| Drug Interactions and/or Related Problems | I | II | III | IV | V | VI | VII | VIII | IX | X | XI | XII | XIII | XIV |
|---|---|---|---|---|---|---|---|---|---|---|---|---|---|---|
| **Antihypertensives, especially ganglionic blockers such as guanadrel, guanethidine, and mecamylamine, or Diuretics or Hypotension-producing medications, other** (See Appendix II) (hypotensive effects of these medications may be potentiated when used concurrently with opioid analgesics, leading to increased risk of orthostatic hypotension; patients should be monitored during concurrent use) | ✓ | ✓ | ✓ | ✓ | ✓ | ✓ | ✓ | ✓ | ✓ | ✓ | ✓ | ✓ | ✓ | ✓ |
| » **Buprenorphine** (buprenorphine is a partial mu-receptor agonist with high affinity for, and a slow rate of dissociation from, the mu receptor; if administered prior to another opioid agonist, it may reduce the therapeutic effects of the other opioid; in one study in opioid addicts receiving chronic administration of 8 mg of buprenorphine per day, the effects of large doses [up to 120 mg] of morphine were blocked during buprenorphine therapy and for at least 30 hours following the last dose of buprenorphine) (buprenorphine may also have some antagonist activity at the kappa receptor; the possibility should be considered that it may also reduce the therapeutic effects of subsequently administered butorphanol, nalbuphine, or pentazocine) (buprenorphine antagonizes the respiratory depressant effects of large doses of previously administered mu-receptor agonists; however, additive respiratory depression may occur if buprenorphine is administered in conjunction with low doses of other mu-receptor agonists or with kappa-receptor agonists) (buprenorphine may precipitate withdrawal symptoms in physically dependent patients who are chronically receiving potent mu-receptor agonists; however, because of its partial agonist activity, buprenorphine may partially suppress spontaneous withdrawal symptoms caused by abrupt discontinuation of these agonists) | ✓ | ✓ | ✓ | ✓ | ✓ | ✓ | ✓ | ✓ | ✓ | ✓ | ✓ | ✓ | ✓ | ✓ |
| » **Carbamazepine** (concurrent use with propoxyphene may result in decreased carbamazepine metabolism and lead to increased carbamazepine blood concentration and toxicity; concurrent use is not recommended) | | | | | | | | | | | ✓ | | | |
| **Hydroxyzine** (concurrent use with opioid analgesics ; ay result in increased analgesia as well as increased CNS depressant and hypotensive effects) | ✓ | ✓ | ✓ | ✓ | ✓ | ✓ | ✓ | ✓ | ✓ | ✓ | ✓ | ✓ | ✓ | ✓ |
| **Metoclopramide** (opioid analgesics may antagonize the effects of metoclopramide on gastrointestinal motility) | ✓ | ✓ | ✓ | ✓ | ✓ | ✓ | ✓ | ✓ | ✓ | ✓ | ✓ | ✓ | ✓ | ✓ |

Table 3. Drug Interactions and/or Related Problems *(continued)*

Legend:
I = Codeine
II = Hydrocodone
III = Hydromorphone
IV = Levorphanol
V = Meperidine
VI = Methadone
VII = Morphine
VIII = Opium
IX = Oxycodone
X = Oxymorphone
XI = Propoxyphene
XII = Butorphanol
XIII = Nalbuphine
XIV = Pentazocine

| Drug Interactions and/or Related Problems | Agonist | | | | | | | | | | | Agonist/Antagonist | | |
|---|---|---|---|---|---|---|---|---|---|---|---|---|---|---|
| | I | II | III | IV | V | VI | VII | VIII | IX | X | XI | XII | XIII | XIV |
| » **Monoamine oxidase (MAO) inhibitors**, including furazolidone, pargyline, and procarbazine<br>(concurrent use with meperidine has resulted in unpredictable, severe, and sometimes fatal reactions, including immediate excitation, sweating, rigidity, and severe hypertension, or, in some patients, hypotension, severe respiratory depression, coma, seizures, hyperpyrexia, and cardiovascular collapse; meperidine is contraindicated in patients who have received an MAO inhibitor within 14 to 21 days)<br>(other opioid analgesics may be used cautiously and in reduced dosage in patients receiving MAO inhibitors; however, it is recommended that a small test dose [ of the usual dose] or several small incremental test doses over a period of several hours first be administered to permit observation of any interaction) | | | | | ✓ | | | | | | | | | |
| **Naloxone**<br>(antagonizes the analgesic, CNS, and respiratory depressant effects of opioid analgesics; however, larger doses may be required to reverse the effects of butorphanol, nalbuphine, pentazocine, or propoxyphene than are needed to reverse the effects of other opioids; also, because naloxone may precipitate withdrawal symptoms in physically dependent patients, dosage of naloxone should be carefully titrated when used to treat opioid overdosage in dependent patients) | ✓ | ✓ | ✓ | ✓ | ✓ | ✓ | ✓ | ✓ | ✓ | ✓ | ✓ | ✓ | ✓ | ✓ |
| » **Naltrexone**<br>(administration of naltrexone to a patient physically dependent on opioid drugs will precipitate withdrawal symptoms; symptoms may appear within 5 minutes of naltrexone administration, persist for up to 48 hours, and be difficult to reverse)<br>(naltrexone blocks the therapeutic effects of opioids [i.e., analgesic, antidiarrheal, and antitussive]; naltrexone therapy should not be initiated in patients receiving these agents for therapeutic purposes; also, patients receiving naltrexone should be advised to use alternative medications when necessary)<br>(administration of increased doses of opioids to override naltrexone blockade of opioid receptors may result in increased and prolonged respiratory depression and/or circulatory collapse)<br>(naltrexone should be discontinued several days prior to elective surgery if administration of an opioid prior to, during, or following surgery is unavoidable)<br>(the efficacy of naltrexone in antagonizing opioid effects not mediated via opioid receptors [i.e., those that may be caused by histamine release, such as facial swelling, itching, generalized erythema, hives, and, to some extent, hypotension] has not been fully determined; naltrexone may not antagonize these effects completely) | ✓ | ✓ | ✓ | ✓ | ✓ | ✓ | ✓ | ✓ | ✓ | ✓ | ✓ | ✓ | ✓ | ✓ |
| **Neuromuscular blocking** agents and possibly other medications having some neuromuscular blocking activity<br>(respiratory depressant effects of neuromuscular blockade may be additive to central respiratory depressant effects of opioid analgesics; increased or prolonged respiratory depression [apnea] or paralysis may occur but is of minor clinical significance if the patient is being mechanically ventilated; however, caution and careful monitoring of the patient are recommended during and following concurrent or sequential use, especially if there is a possibility of incomplete reversal of neuromuscular blockade postoperatively) | ✓ | ✓ | ✓ | ✓ | ✓ | ✓ | ✓ | ✓ | ✓ | ✓ | ✓ | ✓ | ✓ | ✓ |

## Table 3. Drug Interactions and/or Related Problems (continued)

Legend:
I = Codeine
II = Hydrocodone
III = Hydromorphone
IV = Levorphanol

Agonist:
V = Meperidine
VI = Methadone
VII = Morphine
VIII = Opium
IX = Oxycodone
X = Oxymorphone
XI = Propoxyphene

Agonist/Antagonist:
XII = Butorphanol
XIII = Nalbuphine
XIV = Pentazocine

| Drug Interaction and/or Related Problem | I | II | III | IV | V | VI | VII | VIII | IX | X | XI | XII | XIII | XIV |
|---|---|---|---|---|---|---|---|---|---|---|---|---|---|---|
| Nicotine chewing gum or Other smoking deterrents or Smoking, tobacco, or cessation of (tobacco smoking may increase the metabolism of propoxyphene leading to decreased therapeutic effects; also, smoking cessation by a patient receiving propoxyphene chronically may increase its effects) | | | | | | | | | | | ✓ | | | |
| Opioid agonist analgesics, including alfentanil, fentanyl, and sufentanil (additive CNS depressant, respiratory depressant, and hypotensive effects may occur if two or more opioid agonist analgesics are used concurrently) | ✓ | ✓ | ✓ | ✓ | ✓ | ✓ | ✓ | ✓ | ✓ | ✓ | ✓ | | | |
| (pentazocine and nalbuphine may partially antagonize the analgesic and CNS depressant effects of opioid agonists) | | | | | | | | | | | | | ✓ | ✓ |
| (in patients who are not physically dependent on opioid agonists, concurrent use of butorphanol, nalbuphine, or pentazocine may result in additive side effects) | | | | | | | | | | | | ✓ | ✓ | ✓ |
| (in patients who are physically dependent on opioid agonists, nalbuphine and pentazocine may precipitate, and butorphanol will not prevent or attenuate, withdrawal symptoms) | | | | | | | | | | | | ✓ | ✓ | ✓ |
| » Phenytoin, chronic use of, or » Rifampin (these medications may increase methadone metabolism, probably via induction of hepatic microsomal enzyme activity, and may precipitate withdrawal symptoms in patients being treated for opioid dependence; methadone dosage adjustments may be necessary when phenytoin or rifampin therapy is initiated or discontinued) | | | | | | ✓ | | | | | | | | |
| » Zidovudine (morphine may competitively inhibit the hepatic glucuronidation and decrease the clearance of zidovudine; concurrent use should be avoided because the toxicity of either or both of these medications may be potentiated) | | | | | | | ✓ | | | | | | | |

## Table 4. Side/Adverse Effects*

The following side/adverse effects have been selected on the basis of their potential clinical significance (possible signs and symptoms in parentheses where appropriate)—not necessarily inclusive:

Legend:
I=Butorphanol
II=Codeine
III=Hydrocodone
IV=Hydromorphone
V=Levorphanol
VI=Meperidine
VII=Methadone
VIII=Morphine
IX=Nalbuphine
X=Opium
XI=Oxycodone
XII=Oxymorphone
XIII=Pentazocine
XIV=Propoxyphene

| | I | II | III | IV | V | VI | VII | VIII | IX | X | XI | XII | XIII | XIV |
|---|---|---|---|---|---|---|---|---|---|---|---|---|---|---|
| **Medical attention needed** | | | | | | | | | | | | | | |
| *Allergic reaction* (skin rash, hives, and/or itching†; swelling of face) | R (<1%) | L | R | R | R | R | R | L | L | R | R | R | L | L |
| *Atelectasis; bronchospastic allergic reaction; laryngeal edema, allergic; laryngospasm, allergic; or respiratory depression‡* (shortness of breath, slow or irregular breathing, troubled breathing) | R (<1%) | L | L | L | L | L | L | L | R (<1%) | R | R | R | L | U |
| *CNS stimulation, paradoxical* (unusual excitement or restlessness)—especially in children | R | L | R | R | R | R | R | R | R | R | R | R | R | R |
| *Confusion§*—may include delusions and feelings of depersonalization or unreality | R (<1%) | L | L | L | L | L | L | L | R (<1%) | L | R | L | R | R |
| *Convulsions* | U | R | R | U | U | L | U | U | U | U | U | U | U | L |
| *Fast, slow, or pounding heartbeat* | R (<1%) | L | L | L | L | L | L | L | R (<1%) | R | U | L | L | U |
| *Hallucinations§* | R (<1%) | R | R | R | R | R | R | R | R (<1%) | R | R | R | R | U |
| *Hepatotoxicity* (dark urine, pale stools, yellow eyes or skin) | U | U | U | U | U | U | U | U | U | U | U | U | U | U |
| *Histamine release* (decreased blood pressure, fast heartbeat, increased sweating, redness or flushing of face, wheezing or troubled breathing) | L | L | M | L | R | M | M | M | M | L | L | L | L | L |
| *Increased blood pressure* | R (<1%) | U | R | U | U | U | U | U | R | U | U | U | L | R |
| *Mental depression* | R (<1%) | R | R | R | R | R | R | R | R (<1%) | R | R | R | R | R |
| *Muscle rigidity, especially in muscles of respiration*—with large doses | U | R | R | U | U | U | U | R | U | U | U | U | U | R |
| *Paralytic ileus or toxic megacolon* (severe constipation, bloating, nausea, stomach cramps or pain, vomiting)—in patients with inflammatory bowel disease | R | R | R | R | R | R | R | R | R | R | R | R | R | R |
| *Ringing or buzzing in the ears* | R | U | R | U | U | U | U | U | U | U | U | U | U | L |
| *Trembling or uncontrolled muscle movements* | U | R | R | L | U | L | U | L | U | L | U | U | R | L |
| **Medical attention needed only if continuing or bothersome** | | | | | | | | | | | | | | |
| *Antidiuretic effect* (decreased urination) | L | L | L | L | L | L | L | L | R (<1%) | L | L | L | L | L |
| *Biliary spasm* (stomach cramps or pain) | U | R | R | L | L | L | L (<1%) | L | R (<1%) | R | U | L | R | R |
| *Blurred or double vision or other changes in vision* | R (<1%) | L | L | L | L | L | L | L | R (<1%) | L | U | L | L | L |
| *Constipation* | R | M | L | L | L | M | M | M | U | R | L | L | L | L |
| *Dizziness, feeling faint, or lightheadedness*—especially in ambulatory patients. | L | L | M | M | M | M | M | M | L | M | M | M | L | M |

## Table 4. Side/Adverse Effects* *(continued)*

| | Legend:<br>**I**=Butorphanol<br>**II**=Codeine<br>**III**=Hydrocodone<br>**IV**=Hydromorphone | | | | **V**=Levorphanol<br>**VI**=Meperidine<br>**VII**=Methadone | | | **VIII**=Morphine<br>**IX**=Nalbuphine<br>**X**=Opium | | | **XI**=Oxycodone<br>**XII**=Oxymorphone<br>**XIII**=Pentazocine<br>**XIV**=Propoxyphene | | | |
|---|---|---|---|---|---|---|---|---|---|---|---|---|---|---|
| | **I** | **II** | **III** | **IV** | **V** | **VI** | **VII** | **VIII** | **IX** | **X** | **XI** | **XII** | **XIII** | **XIV** |
| *Drowsiness* | M (40%) | M | M | M | M | M | M | M | M (36%) | M | M | M | M | M |
| *Dry mouth* | R (<1%) | L | L | L | L | L | L | L | L (4%) | L | L | L | L | L |
| *False sense of well-being* | R (<1%) | L | L | L | U | L | L | L | R (<1%) | L | U | L | M | L |
| *Gastrointestinal irritation* (stomach cramps or pain) | R | R | R | L | L | L | L | L | R | R | U | L | R | R |
| *General feeling of discomfort or illness*§ | L | L | L | L | L | L | L | L | R (<1%) | L | L | L | L | L |
| *Headache* | L (3%) | L | L | L | L | L | L | L | L (3%) | L | L | L | L | L |
| *Hypotension* (dizziness, feeling faint, light-headedness, unusual tiredness or weakness)—although hypotension may occur in recumbent patients, orthostatic hypotension commonly occurs in ambulatory patients | L | L | M | M | M | M | M | M | L | M | M | M | L | M |
| *Loss of appetite* | L | L | L | M | L | L | L | L | L | R | U | R | R | R |
| *Nausea or vomiting*—occurs more frequently in ambulatory patients; are more frequent with initial doses, and are less likely to occur with subsequent doses | L (6%) | L | L | L | M | M | M | M | L (6%) | R | M | M | M | M |
| *Nervousness or restlessness*§ | R (<1%) | L | L | L | L | L | L | L | R (<1%) | L | L | L | L | L |
| *Nightmares or unusual dreams*§ | R (<1%) | R | R | U | U | L | U | U | R (<1%) | U | U | U | L | L |
| *Redness, swelling, pain, or burning at site of injection* | R | L | — | L | L | L | R | L | L | L | — | L | L | — |
| *Unusual tiredness or weakness* | L | L | M | M | M | M | M | M | L | M | M | M | L | M |
| *Ureteral spasm* (difficult or painful urination, frequent urge to urinate) | L | L | L | L | L | L | L | L | R (<1%) | L | L | L | L | L |
| *Trouble in sleeping* | R | R | R | R | R | R | R | R | R | R | R | R | R | R |

*Differences in frequency of occurrence may reflect either lack of clinical-use data or actual pharmacologic distinctions among agents (although their pharmacologic similarity suggests that side effects occurring with one may occur with the others). M = more frequent; L = less frequent; R = rare; U = unknown.

†*Generalized or facial pruritus* may represent an opioid-induced dysesthesia rather than an allergic reaction, especially following epidural or intrathecal administration, and requires medical attention only if bothersome to the patient.

‡*Respiratory depression* induced by butorphanol, nalbuphine, and pentazocine differs from that due to other opioid analgesics in that the depth of respiratory depression is not increased with higher doses (ceiling effect); however, with butorphanol the duration of respiratory depression is increased with higher doses.

§Although these effects may occur with large doses of any opioid analgesic, with butorphanol, nalbuphine, and pentazocine they may be part of a group of subjective and psychotomimetic effects characteristic of opioids having sigma-receptor activity. These effects include *confusion, delusions, feelings of depersonalization or unreality, hallucinations* (usually visual), *dysphoria, nightmares, and nervousness or anxiety*. These effects generally occur with large doses of these drugs; although they occur rarely with any of them, they may be most likely to occur with pentazocine.

# OPIOID (NARCOTIC) ANALGESICS AND ACETAMINOPHEN    Systemic

This monograph includes information on the following: Acetaminophen and Codeine; Dihydrocodeine and Acetaminophen; Hydrocodone and Acetaminophen; Oxycodone and Acetaminophen; Pentazocine and Acetaminophen; Propoxyphene and Acetaminophen.

PEN:

Acetaminophen and Codeine—Co-codAPAP
Hydrocodone and Acetaminophen—Co-hycodAPAP
Oxycodone and Acetaminophen—Co-oxycodAPAP
Propoxyphene napsylate and Acetaminophen—Co-proxAPAP

INN:

Acetaminophen—Paracetamol
Propoxyphene—Dextropropoxyphene

VA CLASSIFICATION (Primary): CN101

NOTE: The *Opioid (Narcotic) Analgesics and Acetaminophen (Systemic)* monograph is maintained on the USP DI electronic data base. For a printed copy of the most recent revision of the complete monograph, contact the USP Division of Information Development, 12601 Twinbrook Parkway, Rockville, MD 20852.

For information on the specific components of this combination, see the *USP DI* monographs for *Acetaminophen (Systemic)* and *Opioid (Narcotic) Analgesics (Systemic)*.

The information that follows is selectively abstracted from the complete monograph and is provided to facilitate drug use review and patient counseling.

Note: For a listing of dosage forms and brand names by country availability, see *Dosage Forms* section(s). For a listing of brand names for the articles in this monograph, refer to the General Index.

## Category

Analgesic.

Note: Opioid agonist analgesics—Codeine, Dihydrocodeine, Hydrocodone, Oxycodone, and Propoxyphene.

Opioid agonist/antagonist analgesic—Pentazocine.

## Indications

### Accepted

Pain (treatment)—Indicated for the symptomatic relief of:

Mild to moderate pain—Pentazocine and acetaminophen; propoxyphene and acetaminophen.

Mild to severe pain (depending on the dose of codeine)—Acetaminophen and codeine.

Moderate to moderately severe pain—Dihydrocodeine and acetaminophen; hydrocodone and acetaminophen; oxycodone and acetaminophen.

## Patient Consultation

As an aid to patient consultation, refer to *Advice for the Patient, Narcotic Analgesics and Acetaminophen (Systemic)*.

In providing consultation, consider emphasizing the following selected information (≫ = major clinical significance):

### Before using this medication

≫ Conditions affecting use, especially:

Sensitivity to acetaminophen or to opioid analgesic considered for use, history of

Pregnancy—Acetaminophen and opioid analgesics cross the placenta; regular use of opioids by pregnant women may cause physical dependence in the fetus and withdrawal symptoms in the neonate

Breast-feeding—Acetaminophen, codeine, and propoxyphene are distributed into breast milk

Use in children—Children up to 2 years of age are more susceptible to the effects of opioids, especially respiratory depression; also, children may be more likely to experience paradoxical CNS excitation during therapy

Use in the elderly—Geriatric patients are more susceptible to the effects of opioids, especially respiratory depression

Other medications, especially alcohol or other CNS depressants, monoamine oxidase inhibitors, tricyclic antidepressants, zidovudine, and naltrexone

Other medical problems, especially alcoholism (active or in remission), diarrhea caused by antibiotics or poisoning, asthma or other respiratory problems, hepatic disease, viral hepatitis, and severe inflammatory bowel disease

### Proper use of this medication

≫ Importance of not taking more medication than the amount prescribed because of danger of overdose and habit-forming potential of opioid analgesics; also, acetaminophen may cause liver damage with long-term or high-dose use

≫ Not increasing dose if medication is less effective after a few weeks; checking with physician

≫ Missed dose (if on scheduled dosing): Taking as soon as possible; not taking if almost time for next dose; not doubling doses

≫ Proper storage

### Precautions while using this medication

Regular visits to physician to check progress during long-term or high-dose therapy

≫ Caution if other medications containing opioid analgesics or acetaminophen are used

≫ Avoiding use of alcohol or other central nervous system (CNS) depressants during therapy unless prescribed or otherwise approved by physician

Possibility that drinking large amounts of alcohol may increase risk of liver damage with acetaminophen

Not regularly taking aspirin or other salicylates or other nonsteroidal anti-inflammatory drugs concurrently, unless directed by physician or dentist

≫ Caution if dizziness, drowsiness, lightheadedness, or false sense of well-being occurs

Caution when getting up suddenly from a lying or sitting position

Lying down if nausea or vomiting, or dizziness or lightheadedness occurs

Caution if any kind of surgery (including dental surgery) or emergency treatment is required

Possible dryness of mouth; using sugarless gum or candy, ice, or saliva substitute for relief; checking with dentist if dry mouth continues for more than 2 weeks

≫ Checking with physician before discontinuing medication after prolonged use of high doses; gradual dosage reduction may be necessary to avoid withdrawal symptoms

≫ Suspected overdose: Getting emergency help at once

### Side/adverse effects

Signs of potential side effects, especially respiratory depression or impairment; allergic reactions; confusion, convulsions, hallucinations, mental depression, or other signs of CNS toxicity; agranulocytosis; hepatotoxicity; hypertension; paradoxical CNS excitation, especially in children; renal function impairment; and thrombocytopenia

---

### *ACETAMINOPHEN AND CODEINE*

## Oral Dosage Forms

### ACETAMINOPHEN AND CODEINE PHOSPHATE CAPSULES USP

**Usual adult dose**

Analgesic—

Oral, 1 or 2 capsules containing 325 mg of acetaminophen and 30 mg of codeine phosphate every four hours as needed; or

Oral, 1 capsule containing 325 mg of acetaminophen and 60 mg of codeine phosphate every four hours as needed.

**Usual pediatric dose**

Dosage must be individualized by the physician.

**Strength(s) usually available**

U.S.—

325 mg of acetaminophen and 30 mg of codeine phosphate (Rx) [*Phenaphen with Codeine No.3* (D&C Yellow 10,; edible ink; FD&C Blue 1; FD&C Yellow 6; gelatin; magnesium stearate; sodium starch glycolate; stearic acid)].

325 mg of acetaminophen and 60 mg of codeine phosphate (Rx) [*Phenaphen with Codeine No.4* (lactose; cornstarch; D&C Yellow 10; edible ink; FD&C Green 3 or Blue 1; FD&C Yellow 6; gelatin; magnesium stearate; sodium starch glycolate; stearic acid)].

Canada—

Not commercially available.

Note: In Canada, *Phenaphen with Codeine* contains phenobarbital, aspirin, and codeine. See *Barbiturates and Analgesics (Systemic)*.

**Auxiliary labeling**
- May cause drowsiness.
- Avoid alcoholic beverages.
- May be habit-forming.

## ACETAMINOPHEN AND CODEINE PHOSPHATE ORAL SOLUTION USP

**Usual adult dose**
Analgesic—
    Oral, 15 mL every four hours, as needed.

**Usual pediatric dose**
Analgesic—
    Children up to 3 years of age: Dosage has not been established.
    Children 3 to 7 years of age: Oral, 5 mL three or four times a day, as needed.
    Children 7 to 12 years of age: Oral, 10 mL three or four times a day, as needed.

**Strength(s) usually available**
U.S.—
    120 mg of acetaminophen and 12 mg of codeine phosphate, per 5 mL (Rx) [*Tylenol with Codeine Elixir* (alcohol 7%); GENERIC].
Canada—
    160 mg of acetaminophen and 8 mg of codeine phosphate, per 5 mL (Rx) [*PMS-Acetaminophen with Codeine* (alcohol 7%); *Tylenol with Codeine Elixir* (alcohol 7%)].

**Auxiliary labeling**
- May cause drowsiness.
- Avoid alcoholic beverages.
- May be habit-forming.

## ACETAMINOPHEN AND CODEINE PHOSPHATE ORAL SUSPENSION USP

**Usual adult dose**
See *Acetaminophen and Codeine Phosphate Oral Solution USP.*

**Usual pediatric dose**
See *Acetaminophen and Codeine Phosphate Oral Solution USP.*

**Strength(s) usually available**
U.S.—
    120 mg of acetaminophen and 12 mg of codeine phosphate, per 5 mL (Rx) [*Capital with Codeine*].
Canada—
    Not commercially available.

**Auxiliary labeling**
- May cause drowsiness.
- Avoid alcoholic beverages.
- Shake well.
- May be habit-forming.

## ACETAMINOPHEN AND CODEINE PHOSPHATE TABLETS USP

**Usual adult dose**
Analgesic—
    Oral, 1 or 2 tablets containing 300 mg of acetaminophen and 15 or 30 mg of codeine phosphate every four hours as needed; or
    Oral, 1 tablet containing 300 mg of acetaminophen and 60 mg of codeine phosphate every four hours as needed; or
    Oral, 1 tablet containing 650 mg of acetaminophen and 30 mg of codeine phosphate every four hours as needed.

**Usual pediatric dose**
Dosage must be individualized by the physician.

**Strength(s) usually available**
U.S.—
    300 mg of acetaminophen and 15 mg of codeine phosphate (Rx) [*Tylenol with Codeine No.2* (sodium metabisulfite); GENERIC].
    300 mg of acetaminophen and 30 mg of codeine phosphate (Rx) [*Pyregesic-C; Tylenol with Codeine No.3* (sodium metabisulfite); GENERIC].
    300 mg of acetaminophen and 60 mg of codeine phosphate (Rx) [*Tylenol with Codeine No.4* (sodium metabisulfite); GENERIC].
    650 mg of acetaminophen and 30 mg of codeine phosphate (Rx) [*EZ III; Margesic #3*].
Canada—
    300 mg of acetaminophen and 30 mg of codeine phosphate (Rx) [*Acet Codeine 30* (scored); *Empracet-30* (scored); *Emtec-30; Triatec-30*].
    300 mg of acetaminophen and 60 mg of codeine phosphate (Rx) [*Acet Codeine 60* (scored); *Empracet-60; Lenoltec with Codeine No.4; Tylenol with Codeine No.4*].

**Auxiliary labeling**
- May cause drowsiness.
- Avoid alcoholic beverages.
- May be habit-forming.

## ACETAMINOPHEN, CODEINE PHOSPHATE, AND CAFFEINE TABLETS

**Usual adult dose**
Analgesic—
    Oral, 1 or 2 tablets every four hours as needed.

**Usual pediatric dose**
Dosage must be individualized by the physician.

**Strength(s) usually available**
U.S.—
    Not commercially available.
Canada—
    300 mg of acetaminophen, 8 mg of codeine phosphate, and 15 mg of caffeine (OTC) [*Lenoltec with Codeine No.1; Novo-Gesic C8; Tylenol with Codeine No.1;* GENERIC (may be scored)].
    300 mg of acetaminophen, 8 mg of codeine phosphate, and 30 mg of caffeine citrate (OTC) [*Exdol-8* (scored)].
    300 mg of acetaminophen, 15 mg of codeine phosphate, and 15 mg of caffeine (Rx) [*Acet-2* (scored); *Lenoltec with Codeine No.2; Novo-Gesic C15* (scored); *Tylenol with Codeine No.2*].
    300 mg of acetaminophen, 30 mg of codeine phosphate, and 15 mg of caffeine (Rx) [*Acet-3* (scored); *Lenoltec with Codeine No.3; Novo-Gesic C30* (scored); *Tylenol with Codeine No.3*].
    325 mg of acetaminophen, 8 mg of codeine phosphate, and 15 mg of caffeine (OTC) [*Cetaphen with Codeine*].
    325 mg of acetaminophen, 8 mg of codeine phosphate, and 30 mg of caffeine citrate (OTC) [*Atasol-8* (scored); *Cotabs; Triatec-8*].
    325 mg of acetaminophen, 15 mg of codeine phosphate, and 30 mg of caffeine citrate (Rx) [*Atasol-15* (scored)].
    325 mg of acetaminophen, 30 mg of codeine phosphate, and 30 mg of caffeine citrate (Rx) [*Atasol-30* (scored)].
    500 mg of acetaminophen, 8 mg of codeine phosphate, and 15 mg of caffeine (OTC) [*Cetaphen Extra Strength with Codeine; Tylenol with Codeine No.1 Forte;* GENERIC].
    500 mg of acetaminophen, 8 mg of codeine phosphate, and 30 mg of caffeine citrate (OTC) [*Triatec-8 Strong*].

**Auxiliary labeling**
- May cause drowsiness.
- Avoid alcoholic beverages.
- May be habit-forming.

---

### *DIHYDROCODEINE AND ACETAMINOPHEN*

## Oral Dosage Forms

### DIHYDROCODEINE BITARTRATE, ACETAMINOPHEN, AND CAFFEINE CAPSULES

**Usual adult dose**
Analgesic—
    Oral, 2 capsules every four hours.

**Usual pediatric dose**
Dosage has not been established.

**Strength(s) usually available**
U.S.—
    16 mg of dihydrocodeine bitartrate, 356.4 mg of acetaminophen, and 30 mg of caffeine (Rx) [*DHCplus* (croscarmellose sodium; FD&C Blue 1; FD&C Green 3; gelatin; silica gel,; silicon dioxide; sodium lauryl sulfate; cornstarch; titanium dioxide; zinc stearate)].
Canada—
    Not commercially available.

**Auxiliary labeling**
- May cause drowsiness.
- Avoid alcoholic beverages.
- May be habit-forming.

---

### *HYDROCODONE AND ACETAMINOPHEN*

## Oral Dosage Forms

### HYDROCODONE BITARTRATE AND ACETAMINOPHEN CAPSULES

**Usual adult dose**
Analgesic—
    Oral, one capsule every four to six hours, as needed. Dosage may be increased to two capsules every six hours if necessary.

**Usual adult prescribing limits**

Analgesic—
Up to eight capsules per 24 hours.

**Usual pediatric dose**

Dosage has not been established.

**Strength(s) usually available**

U.S.—
5 mg of hydrocodone bitartrate and 500 mg of acetaminophen (Rx)
[*Allay; Anolor DH 5; Bancap-HC; Dolacet; Dolagesic; Hycomed; Hyco-Pap; Hydrocet; Hydrogesic; Lorcet-HD; Margesic-H; Panlor; Polygesic; Stagesic; T-Gesic; Ugesic; Vendone; Zydone* (FD&C Yellow 6); GENERIC].

Canada—
Not commercially available.

**Auxiliary labeling**
• May cause drowsiness.
• Avoid alcoholic beverages.
• May be habit-forming.

## HYDROCODONE BITARTRATE AND ACETAMINOPHEN ORAL SOLUTION

**Usual adult dose**

Analgesic—
Oral, 5 to 15 mL every four to six hours as needed.

**Usual pediatric dose**

Dosage has not been established.

**Strength(s) usually available**

U.S.—
2.5 mg of hydrocodone bitartrate and 167 mg of acetaminophen per 5 mL (Rx) [*Lortab* (alcohol 7%; citric acid; ethyl maltol; glycerin, methylparaben; propylene glycol; propylparaben; saccharin sodium; sorbitol solution; sucrose; D&C Yellow #10; FD&C Yellow #6)].

Canada—
Not commercially available.

**Auxiliary labeling**
• May cause drowsiness.
• Avoid alcoholic beverages.
• May be habit-forming.

## HYDROCODONE BITARTRATE AND ACETAMINOPHEN TABLETS USP

**Usual adult dose**

Analgesic—
Oral, 1 or 2 tablets containing 2.5 mg of hydrocodone bitartrate and 500 mg of acetaminophen every four to six hours; or

Oral, 1 tablet containing 5 mg of hydrocodone bitartrate and 500 mg of acetaminophen every four to six hours as needed, with dosage being increased to 2 tablets every six hours if necessary; or

Oral, 1 tablet containing 7.5 mg of hydrocodone bitartrate and 650 mg of acetaminophen every four to six hours as needed, with dosage being increased to 2 tablets every six hours if necessary; or

Oral, 1 tablet containing 7.5 mg of hydrocodone bitartrate and 750 mg of acetaminophen every four to six hours as needed; or

Oral, 1 tablet containing 10 mg of hydrocodone bitartrate and 650 mg of acetaminophen every four to six hours as needed.

**Usual adult prescribing limits**

Up to 40 mg of hydrocodone bitartrate and 4 grams of acetaminophen in twenty-four hours.

**Usual pediatric dose**

Dosage has not been established.

**Strength(s) usually available**

U.S.—
2.5 mg of hydrocodone bitartrate and 500 mg of acetaminophen (Rx) [*Lortab2.5/500* (scored); GENERIC].

5 mg of hydrocodone bitartrate and 500 mg of acetaminophen (Rx) [*Anexsia 5/500* (scored); *Co-Gesic* (scored); *Duocet* (scored); *HY-PHEN* (scored); *Lortab 5/500* (scored); *Oncet; Panacet 5/500* (scored); *Vanacet; Vicodin* (scored); GENERIC].

7.5 mg of hydrocodone bitartrate and 500 mg of acetaminophen (Rx) [*Lortab 7.5/500* (scored); GENERIC].

7.5 mg of hydrocodone bitartrate and 650 mg of acetaminophen (Rx) [*Anexsia 7.5/650* (scored); *Lorcet Plus* (scored); GENERIC].

7.5 mg of hydrocodone bitartrate and 750 mg of acetaminophen (Rx) [*Vicodin ES* (scored); GENERIC].

10 mg of hydrocodone bitartrate and 650 mg of acetaminophen (Rx) [*Lorcet 10/650* (scored; colloidal silicon dioxide,; croscarmellose sodium; crospovidone; microcrystalline cellulose; povidone; pregelatinized starch; stearic acid; FD&C Blue #1 Lake)].

Canada—
Not commercially available.

**Auxiliary labeling**
• May cause drowsiness.
• Avoid alcoholic beverages.
• May be habit-forming.

---

### *OXYCODONE AND ACETAMINOPHEN*

## Oral Dosage Forms

### OXYCODONE AND ACETAMINOPHEN CAPSULES USP

**Usual adult dose**

Analgesic—
Oral, 1 capsule every four to six hours as needed.

**Usual pediatric dose**

Dosage has not been established.

**Strength(s) usually available**

U.S.—
5 mg of oxycodone hydrochloride and 500 mg of acetaminophen (Rx) [*Roxilox; Tylox* (sodium metabisulfite); GENERIC].

Canada—
Not commercially available.

**Auxiliary labeling**
• May cause drowsiness.
• Avoid alcoholic beverages.
• May be habit-forming.

### OXYCODONE AND ACETAMINOPHEN ORAL SOLUTION

**Usual adult dose**

Analgesic—
Oral, 5 mL every four to six hours as needed.

**Usual pediatric dose**

Dosage has not been established.

**Strength(s) usually available**

U.S.—
5 mg of oxycodone hydrochloride and 325 mg of acetaminophen per 5 mL (Rx) [*Roxicet* (alcohol 0.4%; edetic acid; saccharin)].

Canada—
Not commercially available.

**Auxiliary labeling**
• May cause drowsiness.
• Avoid alcoholic beverages.
• May be habit-forming.

### OXYCODONE AND ACETAMINOPHEN TABLETS USP

**Usual adult dose**

Oral, 1 tablet every four to six hours as needed.

**Usual pediatric dose**

Dosage has not been established.

**Strength(s) usually available**

U.S.—
5 mg of oxycodone hydrochloride and 325 mg of acetaminophen (Rx) [*Endocet; Percocet* (scored); *Roxicet* (scored); GENERIC].

5 mg of oxycodone hydrochloride and 500 mg of acetaminophen (Rx) [*Roxicet 5/500* (scored); GENERIC].

Canada—
2.5 mg of oxycodone hydrochloride and 325 mg of acetaminophen (Rx) [*Percocet-Demi* (double-scored)].

5 mg of oxycodone hydrochloride and 325 mg of acetaminophen (Rx) [*Endocet* (scored); *Oxycocet* (scored); *Percocet* (scored); *Roxicet* (scored)].

**Auxiliary labeling**
• May cause drowsiness.
• Avoid alcoholic beverages.
• May be habit-forming.

---

## PENTAZOCINE AND ACETAMINOPHEN

## Oral Dosage Forms

### PENTAZOCINE HYDROCHLORIDE AND ACETAMINOPHEN TABLETS

**Usual adult dose**
Analgesic—
   Oral, 1 tablet every four hours.

**Usual adult prescribing limits**
Up to 6 tablets daily.

**Usual pediatric dose**
Dosage has not been established.

**Strength(s) usually available**
U.S.—
   650 mg of acetaminophen and 25 mg of pentazocine base (Rx) [*Talacen* (scored; colloidal silicon dioxide; FD&C Blue #1; gelatin; microcrystalline cellulose; potassium sorbate; pregelatinized starch; sodium lauryl sulfate; sodium metabisulfite; sodium starch glycolate; stearic acid)].
Canada—
   Not commercially available.

**Auxiliary labeling**
• May cause drowsiness.
• Avoid alcoholic beverages.
• May be habit-forming.

---

## PROPOXYPHENE AND ACETAMINOPHEN

## Oral Dosage Forms

### PROPOXYPHENE HYDROCHLORIDE AND ACETAMINOPHEN TABLETS USP

**Usual adult dose**
Analgesic—
   Oral, 1 tablet every four hours, as needed.

**Usual pediatric dose**
Dosage has not been established.

**Strength(s) usually available**
U.S.—
   65 mg of propoxyphene hydrochloride and 650 mg of acetaminophen (Rx) [*E-Lor; Wygesic* (scored); GENERIC].
Canada—
   Not commercially available.

**Auxiliary labeling**
• May cause drowsiness.
• Avoid alcoholic beverages.
• May be habit-forming.

### PROPOXYPHENE NAPSYLATE AND ACETAMINOPHEN TABLETS USP

**Usual adult dose**
Analgesic—
   Oral, 2 tablets containing 50 mg of propoxyphene napsylate and 325 mg of acetaminophen every four hours, as needed; or
   Oral, 1 tablet containing 100 mg of propoxyphene napsylate and 650 mg of acetaminophen every four hours, as needed.

**Usual pediatric dose**
Dosage has not been established.

**Strength(s) usually available**
U.S.—
   50 mg of propoxyphene napsylate and 325 mg of acetaminophen (Rx) [*Darvocet-N 50*; GENERIC].
   100 mg of propoxyphene napsylate and 650 mg of acetaminophen (Rx) [*Darvocet-N 100* (cellulose; cornstarch; FD&C Yellow #6; magnesium stearate; stearic acid,; titanium dioxide); *Propacet 100*; GENERIC].
Canada—
   Not commercially available.

**Auxiliary labeling**
• May cause drowsiness.
• Avoid alcoholic beverages.
• May be habit-forming.

Revised: July 1990
Interim revision: 07/11/95

---

# OPIOID (NARCOTIC) ANALGESICS AND ASPIRIN   Systemic

This monograph includes information on the following: Aspirin and Codeine‡; Aspirin and Codeine, Buffered‡; Aspirin and Dihydrocodeine; Hydrocodone and Aspirin; Oxycodone and Aspirin‡; Pentazocine and Aspirin; Propoxyphene and Aspirin‡.

PEN:
   Aspirin and Codeine—Co-codaprin
INN:
   Propoxyphene—Dextropropoxyphene

VA CLASSIFICATION (Primary): CN101

**NOTE:** The *Opioid (Narcotic) Analgesics and Aspirin (Systemic)* monograph is maintained on the USP DI electronic data base. For a printed copy of the most recent revision of the complete monograph, contact the USP Division of Information Development, 12601 Twinbrook Parkway, Rockville, MD 20852.

For information on the specific components of this combination, see the *USP DI* monographs for *Opioid (Narcotic) Analgesics (Systemic)* and *Salicylates (Systemic)*.

The information that follows is selectively abstracted from the complete monograph and is provided to facilitate drug use review and patient counseling.

---

‡*Aspirin* is a brand name in Canada; acetylsalicylic acid is the generic name. ASA, a commonly used designation for aspirin (or acetylsalicylic acid) in both the U.S. and Canada, is the term used in Canadian product labeling.

Note: For a listing of dosage forms and brand names by country availability, see *Dosage Forms* section(s). For a listing of brand names for the articles in this monograph, refer to the General Index.

---

## Category

Analgesic.

Note: Opioid agonist analgesics—Codeine, dihydrocodeine, hydrocodone, oxycodone, and propoxyphene.

Opioid agonist/antagonist analgesic—Pentazocine.

## Indications

**Accepted**
Pain (treatment)—Indicated for symptomatic relief of:
   Mild to severe pain (depending on the dose of codeine)—Aspirin and codeine; buffered aspirin and codeine.
   Mild to moderate pain—Propoxyphene and aspirin.
   Moderate pain—Pentazocine and aspirin.
   Moderate to moderately severe pain—Aspirin and dihydrocodeine; oxycodone and aspirin.
   Moderate to severe pain—Hydrocodone and aspirin.

## Patient Consultation

As an aid to patient consultation, refer to *Advice for the Patient, Narcotic Analgesics and Aspirin (Systemic)*.

In providing consultation, consider emphasizing the following selected information (» = major clinical significance):

**Before using this medication**
» Conditions affecting use, especially:
   Sensitivity to the opioid considered for use, to aspirin, or to nonsteroidal anti-inflammatory drugs (NSAIDs), history of
   Pregnancy—Aspirin and opioid analgesics cross the placenta; high-dose chronic use or abuse of aspirin in the third trimester may be hazardous to the mother as well as the fetus and/or neonate, causing heart problems in fetus or neonate and/or bleeding in mother, fetus, or neonate; high-dose chronic use or abuse may also prolong and complicate labor and delivery; also, regular use of opioids by pregnant women may cause physical dependence in the fetus and withdrawal symptoms in the neonate; not taking aspirin during the third trimester unless prescribed by physician
   Breast-feeding—Aspirin, codeine, and propoxyphene are distributed into breast milk

Use in children and in teenagers—Checking with physician before giving to children or teenagers with symptoms of acute febrile illness, especially influenza or varicella, because of the risk of Reye's syndrome; also, increased susceptibility to aspirin toxicity in children, especially with fever and dehydration; also, children up to 2 years of age are more susceptible to the effects of opioids, especially respiratory depression; in addition, children may be more likely to experience opioid-induced paradoxical CNS excitation during therapy

Use in the elderly—Increased risk of aspirin toxicity and of opioid-induced adverse effects, especially respiratory depression

Other medications, especially alcohol or other CNS depressants, anticoagulants, antidiabetic agents (oral), those cephalosporins that may cause hypoprothrombinemia, methotrexate, monoamine oxidase inhibitors, naltrexone, nonsteroidal anti-inflammatory drugs (NSAIDs), platelet aggregation inhibitors, plicamycin, probenecid, sulfinpyrazone, urinary alkalizers, valproic acid, vancomycin, and zidovudine

Other medical problems, especially coagulation or platelet function disorders, diarrhea caused by antibiotics or poisoning, asthma or other respiratory problems, and gastrointestinal problems such as ulceration or erosive gastritis (especially a bleeding ulcer) or other severe inflammatory bowel disease

**Proper use of this medication**

» Taking with food or a full glass (240 mL) of water to minimize stomach irritation

» Not taking medication if it has a strong vinegar-like odor

» Importance of not taking more medication than the amount prescribed because of danger of overdose of aspirin or opioid analgesics and habit-forming potential of opioid analgesics

» Not increasing dose if medication seems less effective after a few weeks; checking with physician instead

» Proper dosing

» Missed dose (if on scheduled dosing): Taking as soon as possible; not taking if almost time for next dose; not doubling doses

» Proper storage

**Precautions while using this medication**

Regular visits to physician to check progress during long-term therapy

» Caution if other medications containing aspirin or other salicylates or opioid analgesics are used

» Avoiding use of alcohol or other central nervous system (CNS) depressants during therapy unless prescribed or otherwise approved by physician; also, alcohol consumption may increase risk of aspirin-induced stomach problems

Not taking acetaminophen or ibuprofen or other NSAIDs concurrently for more than a few days unless directed by physician or dentist

» Caution if dizziness, drowsiness, lightheadedness, or false sense of well-being occurs

Caution when getting up suddenly from a lying or sitting position

Lying down if nausea or vomiting, or dizziness or lightheadedness occurs

Need to inform physician or dentist of use of medication if any kind of surgery (including dental surgery) or emergency treatment is required

Caution if any kind of surgery is required; aspirin should be discontinued 5 days prior to surgery unless otherwise directed by physician or dentist

Checking with pharmacist before using the buffered formulation (available in Canada) with any other oral medication; antacids in the formulation may interfere with absorption of many oral medications

Diabetics: Aspirin may cause false urine sugar test results with prolonged use of 8 or more 325-mg (5-grain), or 4 or more 650-mg (10-grain), doses per day

Possible dryness of mouth; using sugarless gum or candy, ice, or saliva substitute for relief; checking with dentist if dry mouth continues for more than 2 weeks

» Checking with physician before discontinuing medication after prolonged use of high doses; gradual dosage reduction may be necessary to avoid withdrawal symptoms

» Suspected overdose: Getting emergency help at once

**Side/adverse effects**

Signs of potential side effects, especially respiratory depression or impairment; allergic reactions; confusion, convulsions, hallucinations, mental depression, or other signs of CNS toxicity; gastrointestinal toxicity; hepatotoxicity; hypertension, and paradoxical CNS excitation, especially in children

---

## ASPIRIN AND CODEINE

## Oral Dosage Forms

### ASPIRIN AND CODEINE PHOSPHATE TABLETS USP

**Usual adult dose**
Oral, 1 or 2 tablets every four hours as needed.

**Usual pediatric dose**
Dosage has not been established.

**Strength(s) usually available**
U.S.—
    325 mg of aspirin and 15 mg of codeine phosphate (Rx) [GENERIC].
    325 mg of aspirin and 30 mg of codeine phosphate (Rx) [*Empirin with Codeine No.3;* GENERIC].
    325 mg of aspirin and 60 mg of codeine phosphate (Rx) [*Empirin with Codeine No.4;* GENERIC].
Canada—
    Not commercially available.

**Auxiliary labeling**
• May cause drowsiness.
• Avoid alcoholic beverages.
• Take with food or with a full glass of water.
• May be habit-forming.

### ASPIRIN, CODEINE PHOSPHATE, AND CAFFEINE TABLETS USP

**Usual adult dose**
Analgesic—
    Oral, 1 or 2 tablets every four hours as needed.

**Usual pediatric dose**
Dosage has not been established.

**Strength(s) usually available**
U.S.—
    Not commercially available.
Canada—
    325 mg of ASA, 8 mg of codeine phosphate, and 15 mg of caffeine (OTC) [*C2 with Codeine;* GENERIC].
    325 mg of ASA, 8 mg of codeine phosphate, and 32 mg of caffeine (OTC) [*Anacin with Codeine*].
    375 mg of ASA, 8 mg of codeine phosphate, and 30 mg of caffeine (OTC) [GENERIC].
    375 mg of ASA, 8 mg of codeine phosphate, and 30 mg of caffeine citrate (OTC) [*222 (double-scored)*].
    375 mg of ASA, 15 mg of codeine phosphate, and 30 mg of caffeine citrate (Rx) [*282 (scored)*].
    375 mg of ASA, 30 mg of codeine phosphate, and 30 mg of caffeine citrate (Rx) [*292 (scored)*].
    400 mg of ASA, 8 mg of codeine phosphate, and 15 mg of caffeine (OTC) [*Novo-AC and C*].
    500 mg of ASA, 8 mg of codeine phosphate, and 15 mg of caffeine (OTC) [GENERIC].

    Note: 30 mg of caffeine citrate are equivalent to 15 mg of caffeine base.

**Auxiliary labeling**
• May cause drowsiness.
• Avoid alcoholic beverages.
• Take with food or with a full glass of water.
• May be habit-forming.

---

## ASPIRIN AND CODEINE, BUFFERED

## Oral Dosage Forms

### ASPIRIN, CODEINE PHOSPHATE, CAFFEINE, ALUMINA, AND MAGNESIA TABLETS

**Usual adult dose**
Analgesic—
    Oral, 1 or 2 tablets every four hours as needed.

**Usual pediatric dose**
Dosage has not been established.

**Strength(s) usually available**
U.S.—
    Not commercially available.

Canada—
    325 mg of ASA, 8 mg of codeine phosphate, and 15 mg of caffeine, with 35 mg of aluminum hydroxide and 70 mg of magnesium hydroxide (OTC) [*C2 Buffered with Codeine*].

### Auxiliary labeling
- May cause drowsiness.
- Avoid alcoholic beverages.
- Take with food or with a full glass of water.
- May be habit-forming.

---

## ASPIRIN AND DIHYDROCODEINE

# Oral Dosage Forms
## ASPIRIN, CAFFEINE, AND DIHYDROCODEINE BITARTRATE CAPSULES USP

### Usual adult dose
Analgesic—
    Oral, 2 capsules every four hours as needed.

### Usual pediatric dose
Dosage has not been established.

### Strength(s) usually available
U.S.—
    356.4 mg of aspirin, 30 mg of caffeine, and 16 mg of dihydrocodeine bitartrate (Rx) [*Synalgos-DC*].
Canada—
    Not commercially available.

### Auxiliary labeling
- May cause drowsiness.
- Avoid alcoholic beverages.
- Take with food or with a full glass of water.
- May be habit-forming.

---

## HYDROCODONE AND ASPIRIN

# Oral Dosage Forms
## HYDROCODONE BITARTRATE AND ASPIRIN TABLETS

### Usual adult dose
Analgesic—
    Oral, 1 or 2 tablets every four to six hours as needed.

### Usual pediatric dose
Dosage has not been established.

### Strength(s) usually available
U.S.—
    5 mg of hydrocodone bitartrate and 500 mg of aspirin (Rx) [*Azdone* (scored); *Damason-P; Lortab ASA; Panasal 5/500*].
Canada—
    Not commercially available.

### Auxiliary labeling
- May cause drowsiness.
- Avoid alcoholic beverages.
- Take with food or with a full glass of water.
- May be habit-forming.

---

## OXYCODONE AND ASPIRIN

# Oral Dosage Forms
## OXYCODONE AND ASPIRIN TABLETS USP

### Usual adult dose
Analgesic—
    Oral, 1 or 2 half-strength tablets or 1 full-strength tablet, every four to six hours as needed. Dosage may be increased if necessary for severe pain.

### Usual pediatric dose
Analgesic—
    Children up to 6 years of age—Use is not recommended.
    Children 6 to 12 years of age—Oral, ¼ half-strength tablet every six hours as needed.
    Children 12 years of age and over—Oral, ½ half-strength tablet every six hours as needed.

### Strength(s) usually available
U.S.—
    Half-strength: 2.25 mg of oxycodone hydrochloride and 190 mcg (0.19 mg) of oxycodone terephthalate, with 325 mg of aspirin (Rx) [*Percodan-Demi* (scored)].
    Full-strength: 4.5 mg of oxycodone hydrochloride and 380 mcg (0.38 mg) of oxycodone terephthalate, with 325 mg of aspirin (Rx) [*Endodan; Percodan* (scored); *Roxiprin;* GENERIC].
Canada—
    Half-strength: 2.5 mg of oxycodone hydrochloride and 325 mg of ASA (Rx) [*Percodan-Demi* (scored)].
    Full-strength: 5 mg of oxycodone hydrochloride and 325 mg of ASA (Rx) [*Endodan* (scored); *Oxycodan* (scored); *Percodan* (scored)].

### Auxiliary labeling
- May cause drowsiness.
- Avoid alcoholic beverages.
- Take with food or with a full glass of water.
- May be habit-forming.

---

## PENTAZOCINE AND ASPIRIN

# Oral Dosage Forms
## PENTAZOCINE HYDROCHLORIDE AND ASPIRIN TABLETS USP

### Usual adult dose
Analgesic—
    Oral, 2 tablets three or four times a day as needed.

### Usual pediatric dose
Dosage has not been established.

### Strength(s) usually available
U.S.—
    12.5 mg of pentazocine (base) and 325 mg of aspirin (Rx) [*Talwin Compound*].
Canada—
    Not commercially available.

### Auxiliary labeling
- May cause drowsiness.
- Avoid alcoholic beverages.
- Take with food or with a full glass of water.
- May be habit-forming.

---

## PROPOXYPHENE AND ASPIRIN

# Oral Dosage Forms
## PROPOXYPHENE HYDROCHLORIDE, ASPIRIN, AND CAFFEINE CAPSULES USP

### Usual adult dose
Oral, 1 capsule every four hours, as needed.

### Usual adult prescribing limits
Up to 390 mg of propoxyphene hydrochloride a day.

### Usual pediatric dose
Dosage has not been established.

### Strength(s) usually available
U.S.—
    65 mg of propoxyphene hydrochloride, 389 mg of aspirin, and 32.4 mg of caffeine (Rx) [*Darvon Compound-65; PC-Cap; Propoxyphene Compound-65;* GENERIC].
Canada—
    Not commercially available.

### Auxiliary labeling
- May cause drowsiness.
- Avoid alcoholic beverages.
- Take with food or with a full glass of water.
- May be habit-forming.

## PROPOXYPHENE HYDROCHLORIDE, ASPIRIN, AND CAFFEINE TABLETS

### Usual adult dose
Analgesic—
    Oral, 1 tablet every four hours, as needed.

### Usual adult prescribing limits
Up to 390 mg of propoxyphene hydrochloride a day.

**Usual pediatric dose**
Dosage has not been established.

**Strength(s) usually available**
U.S.—
    Not commercially available.
Canada—
    65 mg of propoxyphene hydrochloride, 375 mg of ASA, and 30 mg
        of caffeine (Rx) [*692* (scored)].

**Auxiliary labeling**
• May cause drowsiness.
• Avoid alcoholic beverages.
• Take with food or with a full glass of water.
• May be habit-forming.

## PROPOXYPHENE NAPSYLATE AND ASPIRIN CAPSULES

**Usual adult dose**
Analgesic—
    Oral, 1 capsule every four hours, as needed.

**Usual adult prescribing limits**
Up to 600 mg of propoxyphene napsylate a day.

**Usual pediatric dose**
Dosage has not been established.

**Strength(s) usually available**
U.S.—
    Not commercially available.
Canada—
    100 mg of propoxyphene napsylate and 325 mg of ASA (Rx) [*Darvon-
        N with A.S.A.*].

**Auxiliary labeling**
• May cause drowsiness.
• Avoid alcoholic beverages.
• Take with food or with a full glass of water.
• May be habit-forming.

## PROPOXYPHENE NAPSYLATE, ASPIRIN, AND CAFFEINE CAPSULES

**Usual adult dose**
Analgesic—
    Oral, 1 capsule every four hours, as needed.

**Usual adult prescribing limits**
Up to 600 mg of propoxyphene napsylate a day.

**Usual pediatric dose**
Dosage has not been established.

**Strength(s) usually available**
U.S.—
    Not commercially available.
Canada—
    100 mg of propoxyphene napsylate, 375 mg of ASA, and 30 mg of
        caffeine (Rx) [*Darvon-N Compound*].

**Auxiliary labeling**
• May cause drowsiness.
• Avoid alcoholic beverages.
• Take with food or with a full glass of water.
• May be habit-forming.

Revised: July 1990
Interim revision: 07/05/95

---

**OPIUM**—See *Opioid (Narcotic) Analgesics (Systemic)*

---

**ORAL REHYDRATION SALTS**—See *Carbohydrates and Electrolytes (Systemic)*

---

**ORPHENADRINE**—See *Skeletal Muscle Relaxants (Systemic)*

---

# ORPHENADRINE AND ASPIRIN   Systemic

VA CLASSIFICATION (Primary): MS200

**NOTE:** The *Orphenadrine and Aspirin (Systemic)* monograph is main-
    tained on the USP DI electronic data base. For a printed copy of
    the most recent revision of the complete monograph, contact the
    USP Division of Information Development, 12601 Twinbrook
    Parkway, Rockville, MD 20852.

    For information on the specific components of this combination,
    see the *USP DI* monographs for *Salicylates (Systemic)* and *Skel-
    etal Muscle Relaxants (Systemic)*.

    The information that follows is selectively abstracted from the
    complete monograph and is provided to facilitate drug use review
    and patient counseling.

Note: For a listing of dosage forms and brand names by country availa-
    bility, see *Dosage Forms* section(s). For a listing of brand names
    for the articles in this monograph, refer to the General Index.

## Category

Analgesic–skeletal muscle relaxant.

## Indications

**Accepted**

Spasm, skeletal muscle, accompanied by pain (treatment)—Indicated as
    an adjunct to other measures, such as rest and physical therapy, for
    relief of pain and muscle spasm associated with acute painful mus-
    culoskeletal conditions.

## Patient Consultation

As an aid to patient consultation, refer to *Advice for the Patient,
    Orphenadrine and Aspirin (Systemic)*.

In providing consultation, consider emphasizing the following selected
    information (» = major clinical significance):

**Before using this medication**
» Conditions affecting use, especially:
    Allergic reaction to orphenadrine, aspirin, or nonsteroidal anti-in-
        flammatory drugs (NSAIDs), history of
    Pregnancy—High-dose chronic use or abuse of aspirin in third tri-
        mester may be hazardous to the mother as well as the fetus
        and/or neonate, causing heart problems in fetus or neonate and/
        or bleeding in mother, fetus, or neonate; high-dose chronic use
        or abuse may also prolong and complicate labor and delivery;
        not taking aspirin in third trimester unless prescribed by
        physician
    Use in children and teenagers—Checking with physician before
        giving to children or teenagers with symptoms of acute febrile
        illness, especially influenza or varicella, because of the risk of
        Reye's syndrome; also, increased susceptibility to aspirin tox-
        icity in children, especially with fever and dehydration
    Use in the elderly—Increased risk of aspirin toxicity
    Other medications, especially anticoagulants, antidiabetic agents
        (oral), CNS depression–producing medications, those cepha-
        losporins that may cause hypoprothrombinemia, moxalactam,
        plicamycin, valproic acid, methotrexate, NSAIDs, platelet ag-
        gregation inhibitors, probenecid, sulfinpyrazone, urinary alkal-
        izers, vancomycin, and zidovudine
    Other medical problems, especially achalasia, bladder neck ob-
        struction, coagulation or platelet function disorders, gastroin-
        testinal problems such as ulceration or erosive gastritis (espe-
        cially a bleeding ulcer or a stenosing peptic ulcer), glaucoma
        (or predisposition to), myasthenia gravis, prostatic hypertrophy,
        and pyloric or duodenal obstruction

**Proper use of this medication**
» Taking with food or full glass (240 mL) of water to minimize stomach
    irritation
» Not taking medication if it has a strong vinegar-like odor
» Importance of not taking more medication than the amount prescribed
» Proper dosing

Missed dose: Taking if remembered within an hour; not taking if not remembered until later; not doubling doses

» Proper storage

**Precautions while using this medication**

Regular visits to physician to check progress during prolonged therapy

» Caution if other medications containing aspirin or other salicylates or orphenadrine are used

Not taking acetaminophen or ibuprofen or other nonsteroidal anti-inflammatory analgesics concurrently for more than a few days unless directed by physician

Diabetics: May cause false urine sugar test results

Caution if any kind of surgery is required; aspirin should be discontinued 5 days prior to surgery

» Avoiding use of alcohol or other central nervous system (CNS) depressants unless prescribed or otherwise approved by physician

Alcohol consumption may increase probability of stomach problems

» Caution if blurred vision, drowsiness, dizziness, lightheadedness, or faintness occurs

Possible dryness of mouth; using sugarless gum or candy, ice, or saliva substitute for relief; checking with dentist if dry mouth continues for more than 2 weeks

» Suspected overdose: Getting emergency help at once

**Side/adverse effects**

Signs and symptoms of possible side effects, especially allergic reactions (including anaphylaxis and angioedema), blood dyscrasias, fainting, fast or pounding heartbeat, gastrointestinal toxicity, and hallucinations

## Oral Dosage Forms

### ORPHENADRINE CITRATE, ASPIRIN, AND CAFFEINE TABLETS

**Usual adult and adolescent dose**

Oral, 1 or 2 tablets containing 25 mg of orphenadrine citrate three or four times a day; or

Oral, ½ or 1 tablet containing 50 mg of orphenadrine citrate three or four times a day.

**Usual pediatric dose**

Dosage has not been established.

**Strength(s) usually available**

U.S.—

25 mg of orphenadrine citrate, 385 mg of aspirin, and 30 mg of caffeine (Rx) [*Norgesic; Norphadrine; N3 Gesic; Orphenagesic*].

50 mg of orphenadrine citrate, 770 mg of aspirin, and 60 mg of caffeine (Rx) [*Norgesic Forte; Norphadrine Forte; N3 Gesic Forte; Orphenagesic Forte*].

Canada—

25 mg of orphenadrine citrate, 385 mg of ASA, and 30 mg of caffeine (OTC) [*Norgesic*].

50 mg of orphenadrine citrate, 770 mg of ASA, and 60 mg of caffeine (OTC) [*Norgesic Forte*].

Note: *Aspirin* is a brand name in Canada; acetylsalicylic acid is the generic name. ASA, a commonly used designation for aspirin (or acetylsalicylic acid) in both the U.S. and Canada, is the term used in Canadian product labeling.

**Auxiliary labeling**
• May cause drowsiness.
• Avoid alcoholic beverages.
• Take with food or with a full glass of water.

Revised: July 1990
Interim revision: 08/11/94

## ORPHENADRINE-CONTAINING COMBINATIONS—

Orphenadrine, Aspirin, and Caffeine (Systemic)—See *Orphenadrine and Aspirin (Systemic)*

# OVULATION PREDICTION TEST KITS FOR HOME USE

This monograph includes information on the following: Enzyme Immunoassay Ovulation Prediction Test Kits for Home Use.

VA CLASSIFICATION (Primary): DX900

Note: For a listing of product forms and brand names by country availability, see *Diagnostic Product Forms* section.

## Category

Diagnostic aid (ovulation).

## Indications

Note: Bracketed information in the *Indications* section refers to uses that are not included in U.S. product labeling.

**Accepted**

Infertility, female or male (treatment adjunct)—Ovulation prediction test kits are used to identify the fertile period in the menstrual cycle as a means of enhancing chances of conception. These products are intended primarily for use by couples having fertility problems or with particular concern for timing of conception.

[May be used to coordinate insemination of sperm, endometrial biopsy, other infertility evaluations, or oocyte retrieval for *in vitro* fertilization.]

**Unaccepted**

Not marketed as a means of contraception.

## Pharmacology/Pharmacokinetics

**Physicochemical characteristics**

Luteinizing hormone (LH), normally present in the plasma and urine in very small amounts, increases sharply 24 to 38 hours prior to ovulation in humans. This sharp increase (the LH surge) is an accurate predictor of ovulation. Conception is most likely if the woman has intercourse or is otherwise inseminated within 24 hours of the beginning of the surge.

The ovulation predictor kits are marketed in 6- and 9-test units. Testing of the urine is begun 2 to 3 days before the expected date of ovulation, based on menstrual cycle length, and continues daily or as directed by the physician. The normal low LH level will give a white to pale blue

result. The LH surge will result in a brighter blue color, predicting ovulation.

An enzyme immunoassay uses antibodies (monoclonal or polyclonal) specific to LH. The test kit supplies a test stick or solution containing the antibody. Urine to be tested for LH is added, and any LH present binds to the antibody. A second antibody form which is linked to an enzyme is then applied, and binds to the LH/antibody complex. After a washing step which removes any unlinked products, a chromogen is added, which will react with the enzyme in the bound complex. The intensity of the color on the test stick or in solution is directly proportional to the amount of LH in the urine sample.

## Precautions to Consider

**Laboratory value alterations**

The following have been selected on the basis of their potential clinical significance (possible effect in parentheses where appropriate)—not necessarily inclusive (» = major clinical significance):

With results of *this* test

*Due to medications*

Anticonvulsants or

Antiparkinsonism agents or

Antipsychotics

(luteinizing hormone levels are increased by some anticonvulsant, antiparkinsonism, and antipsychotic agents and may produce confusing results)

Clomiphene

(clomiphene elevates LH levels during administration, usually the fifth through ninth days of the cycle. LH levels should drop somewhat before the date on which testing is begun, and the LH surge is usually distinguishable. However, the couple should consult their fertility specialist about the appropriate use of the test kit)

Estrogens or

Estrogens and progestins or

Progestins

(oral contraceptives, other hormones, and steroids may cause false-positive results)

Menotropins
(administration of sufficient quantities of menotropins may interfere with the detection of the LH surge)

*Due to medical problems or conditions*
Dilute urine
(substantial intake of fluids such as water or ethanol may cause
dilution of urine, which will produce abnormal test results)
Endometriosis or
Hypothyroidism or
Menopause or
Ovarian cysts or
Ovarian failure or
Pregnancy
(because of the structural similarities between LH and thyroid-
stimulating hormone, human chorionic gonadotropin, and follicle-
stimulating hormone, these conditions may produce abnormal test
results)
Hematuria or
Proteinuria or
Urinary tract infection
(proteinuria or hematuria may interfere with test results)

*Due to test procedures*
Contamination
(traces of detergent may affect test results; patients should not reuse test materials except where specifically indicated)
Outdated test materials and improper storage
(chilled test materials or urine or outdated or heat-exposed test
materials may not react accurately

## Patient Consultation

As an aid to patient consultation, refer to *Advice for the Patient, Ovulation
Prediction Test Kits for Home Use.*

In providing consultation, consider emphasizing the following selected
information (» = major clinical significance):

**Before using this test**
Noting possible interference with other medications or conditions
Getting assistance in reading results if vision is impaired or if having
problems in reading or understanding written instructions
» Conditions affecting use, especially:

**Proper use of this test**
Checking package expiration date and not using outdated materials
Storing test kits as package directs
Keeping materials out of the reach of children
Reading and following instructions for the individual products
Beginning testing 2 to 3 days before expected date of ovulation or as
instructed
Working in well-lighted area with normal temperature and humidity
Storing urine sample for testing as package insert directs
Using timing devices as necessary to perform tests correctly
Avoiding touching test reaction areas
Observing for an increase in color intensity
Recording test results as kit instructs
Consulting a health care professional or calling the toll-free number
in the kit if questions on procedure remain
Discarding test materials in trash, with liquids poured down a drain

Noting that advice of the patient's fertility specialist may differ slightly
from package instructions, such as in frequency or timing of testing

**Follow-up**
Pregnancy is most likely to occur if patient has intercourse or is inseminated within 24 hours of the detection of the LH surge. Couples having difficulty achieving pregnancy should be encouraged
to consult a physician after 6 to 12 months (or sooner if desired)
of attempts
Asking physician, nurse, or pharmacist questions about results; also,
most kits provide a toll-free number

---

### *ENZYME IMMUNOASSAY*

## Diagnostic Product Forms
### ENZYME IMMUNOASSAY OVULATION PREDICTION TEST KITS FOR HOME USE

**Administration**
Products vary in steps and timing. A specified number of drops of urine
(usually not first morning void) are added to a test surface that is
coated with monoclonal antibodies (MCA) specific for luteinizing hormone. A second, enzyme-linked MCA is added in solution. After
washing, a color-development step generates a color reaction. A negative result is no or faint color, compared to a scale in the kit instructions. A positive result is a distinct change in color intensity. Some
kits include a control test and means of recording results.

**Product(s) usually available**
U.S.—
[*Answer Ovulation; Clearplan Easy; Color Ovulation Test; Conceive
Ovulation Predictor; First Response; Fortel; OvuGen; OvuKIT;
OvuQUICK; Q-test*].
Canada—
[*Clearplan Easy; First Response; Ovukit; OvuQuick*].
Note: Products are labeled as to number of tests per kit, with refills of
additional units available for some kits.

**Packaging and storage**
Store between 15 and 30 °C (59 and 86 °F), out of direct sunlight. Avoid
excess humidity and freezing.

## Selected Bibliography

Corson SL, Batzer FR, McCarthy JJ, et al. Ovulation prediction in the
treatment of infertility: a symposium. J Repro Med 1986; 311 (8)
suppl: 739-63.
Vermesh M, et al. Monitoring techniques to predict and detect ovulation.
Fertil Steril 1987; 47 (2): 259-64.
Batzer FR. Test kits for ovulation and pregnancy, Contemp Ob Gyn 1986;
27 (Technology 1987): 7-16.

Revised: 10/08/91
Interim revision: 07/05/94

---

## OXACILLIN—See *Penicillins (Systemic)*

---

# OXAMNIQUINE    Systemic†

VA CLASSIFICATION (Primary): AP200
Note: For a listing of dosage forms and brand names by country availability, see *Dosage Forms* section(s). For a listing of brand names
for the articles in this monograph, refer to the General Index.

†Not commercially available in Canada.

## Category
Anthelmintic (systemic).

## Indications

**Accepted**
Schistosomiasis (treatment)—Oxamniquine is indicated as alternative therapy in the treatment of all stages, including the acute phase and
chronic phase with hepatosplenic involvement, of schistosomiasis (bil-
harziasis) caused by *Schistosoma mansoni*. Praziquantel is considered

to be the drug of choice. Oxamniquine is also indicated in the treatment of decompensated hepatosplenic disease and in severe diffuse
colonic polyposis caused by *S. mansoni*.

**Unaccepted**
Oxamniquine is not effective against other *Schistosoma* species.

## Pharmacology/Pharmacokinetics

**Physicochemical characteristics**
Molecular weight—279.34.

**Mechanism of action/Effect**
Schistosomicidal against both immature and mature worms. Oxamniquine
causes the worms to shift from the mesenteric veins to the liver where
they are destroyed. Male schistosomes are more susceptible than females; however, after successful treatment with oxamniquine, the residual female schistosomes cease to lay eggs.

**Absorption**

Well absorbed orally; however, food significantly delays absorption.

**Biotransformation**

Probably hepatic; extensively metabolized to inactive acidic metabolites; primary metabolite is the 6-carboxy metabolite.

**Half-life**

1 to 2.5 hours.

**Time to peak serum concentration**

1 to 1.5 hours.

**Elimination**

Renal, 0.4 to 1.9% excreted unchanged in urine; approximately 40 to 70% excreted as 6-carboxy metabolite; primary metabolite largely excreted within first 12 hours.

Fecal, minimal (in animals).

## Precautions to Consider

### Pregnancy/Reproduction

Pregnancy—Oxamniquine crosses the placenta. Adequate and well-controlled studies in humans have not been done. However, there have been no reports of abnormalities in the pregnancies, births, or children of women who received oxamniquine during pregnancy.

Studies in animals have shown that oxamniquine is embryocidal in rabbits and mice when given in doses 10 times the usual human dose.

FDA Pregnancy Category C.

### Breast-feeding

It is not known whether oxamniquine is distributed into breast milk. However, problems in humans have not been documented.

### Pediatrics

Oxamniquine has been used in children, and no pediatrics-specific problems have been documented to date. Because strains of *S. mansoni* in South America and the Caribbean are more difficult to eradicate in children than adults, the total dosage for children in these areas is higher than for adults.

### Geriatrics

No information is available on the relationship of age to the effects of oxamniquine in geriatric patients.

### Medical considerations/Contraindications

The medical considerations/contraindications included here have been selected on the basis of their potential clinical significance (reasons given in parentheses where appropriate)—not necessarily inclusive (» = major clinical significance).

*Risk-benefit should be considered when the following medical problems exist:*

» Epilepsy or other seizure disorders, history of
(seizures may be more likely to occur in patients receiving oxamniquine who have a history of seizure disorders)

Hypersensitivity to oxamniquine

## Side/Adverse Effects

The following side/adverse effects have been selected on the basis of their potential clinical significance (possible signs and symptoms in parentheses where appropriate)—not necessarily inclusive:

### Those indicating need for medical attention

Incidence rare

*Fever*—seen primarily in Egyptian patients; *neuropsychiatric reactions* (auditory or visual hallucinations); *seizures*—more frequent in patients with history of seizure disorders; *skin rash or hives*

### Those indicating need for medical attention only if they continue or are bothersome

Incidence more frequent—about 33%

*Dizziness; drowsiness; headache*

Incidence less frequent

*Gastrointestinal disturbances* (abdominal or stomach pain; diarrhea; loss of appetite; nausea or vomiting)

### Those not indicating need for medical attention

*Reddish orange discoloration of urine*

## Patient Consultation

As an aid to patient consultation, refer to *Advice for the Patient, Oxamniquine (Systemic).*

In providing consultation, consider emphasizing the following selected information (» = major clinical significance):

### Before using this medication

» Conditions affecting use, especially:

Hypersensitivity to oxamniquine

Pregnancy—Oxamniquine crosses the placenta

Other medical problems, especially epilepsy or a history of seizure disorders

### Proper use of this medication

No special preparations (e.g., dietary restrictions or fasting, concurrent medications, purging, or cleansing enemas) required before, during, or immediately after therapy

» Taking after meals to minimize possibility of side effects (gastric irritation, drowsiness, or dizziness)

» Compliance with therapy

» Proper dosing

Missed dose: Taking as soon as possible; not taking if almost time for next dose; not doubling doses

» Proper storage

### Precautions while using this medication

Regular visits to physician to check progress

Checking with physician if no improvement after completing course of therapy

» Caution if dizziness or drowsiness occurs

### Side/adverse effects

Reddish orange discoloration of urine may be alarming to patient although medically insignificant

Signs of potential side effects, especially fever, hallucinations, seizures, and skin rash or hives

## General Dosing Information

No special preparations (e.g., dietary restrictions or fasting, concurrent medications, purging, or cleansing enemas) are required before, during, or immediately after treatment with oxamniquine.

Oxamniquine should be taken after meals to minimize possibility of side effects.

Oxamniquine has also been administered intramuscularly in doses of 7.5 mg per kg of body weight (mg/kg) as a single dose. However, because of severe local pain at the injection site, oxamniquine is recommended only for oral use.

## Oral Dosage Forms

### OXAMNIQUINE CAPSULES USP

**Usual adult and adolescent dose**

Schistosomiasis—

East African strains of *S. mansoni*:

Oral, 15 mg per kg of body weight two times a day for one day.

North and South African strains of *S. mansoni*:

Oral, 15 mg per kg of body weight two times a day for two days.

West African and Western Hemisphere strains of *S. mansoni*:

Oral, 15 mg per kg of body weight as a single dose.

**Usual pediatric dose**

Schistosomiasis—

East African strains of *S. mansoni*:

Oral, 15 mg per kg of body weight two times a day for one day.

North and South African strains of *S. mansoni*:

Oral, 15 mg per kg of body weight two times a day for two or three days.

West African and Western Hemisphere strains of *S. mansoni*:

Children weighing up to 30 kg: Oral, 10 mg per kg of body weight per dose for two doses given two to eight hours apart.

Children weighing 30 kg and over: See *Usual adult and adolescent dose.*

**Strength(s) usually available**

U.S.—

250 mg (Rx) [*Vansil*].

Canada—

Not commercially available.

**Packaging and storage**

Store below 40 °C (104 °F), preferably between 15 and 30 °C (59 and 86 °F), unless otherwise specified by manufacturer. Store in a tight container.

**Auxiliary labeling**
• May cause dizziness or drowsiness.
• Take after meals.
• Continue medication for full time of treatment.

Revised: 01/19/93
Interim revision: 07/21/94

---

**OXANDROLONE**—See *Anabolic Steroids (Systemic)*

---

**OXAPROZIN**—See *Anti-inflammatory Drugs, Nonsteroidal (Systemic)*

---

**OXAZEPAM**—See *Benzodiazepines (Systemic)*

---

# OXICONAZOLE    Topical†

VA CLASSIFICATION (Primary): DE102

Note: For a listing of dosage forms and brand names by country availability, see *Dosage Forms* section(s). For a listing of brand names for the articles in this monograph, refer to the General Index.

†Not commercially available in Canada.

## Category
Antifungal (topical).

## Indications
**Accepted**
Tinea corporis (treatment)
Tinea cruris (treatment) or
Tinea pedis (treatment)—Oxiconazole is indicated in the topical treatment of tinea corporis (ringworm of the body), tinea cruris (ringworm of the groin; jock itch), and tinea pedis (ringworm of the foot; athlete's foot) caused by *Trichophyton rubrum*, *T. mentagrophytes*, and *Epidermophyton floccosum*.

## Pharmacology/Pharmacokinetics

**Physicochemical characteristics**
Molecular weight—Oxiconazole nitrate: 492.15.

**Mechanism of action/Effect**
Inhibits ergosterol biosynthesis, which is necessary for fungal cellular membrane integrity.

**Absorption**
Low.

**Elimination**
Less than 0.3% of a topically applied dose of oxiconazole cream (2.5 mg per square cm of body surface area) was recovered in the urine.

## Precautions to Consider

**Carcinogenicity**
No studies have been done.

**Mutagenicity**
No evidence of mutagenic effect was found in 2 mutation assays (Ames test and Chinese hamster V79 *in vitro* cell mutation assay) and in 2 cytogenetic assays (human peripheral blood lymphocyte *in vitro* chromosome aberration assay and *in vivo* micronucleus assay in mice).

**Pregnancy/Reproduction**
Fertility—Fertility was not impaired in female rats given oral doses of 3 mg per kg of body weight (mg/kg) a day and in male rats given 15 mg/kg a day. However, rats given higher oral doses than those listed above exhibited reduced sperm counts, extended estrous cycles, and decreased mating frequency.
Pregnancy—Adequate and well-controlled studies in humans have not been done.
Teratogenic studies in rabbits, rats, and mice given oral doses of 100, 150, and 200 mg/kg a day, respectively, have not shown that oxiconazole causes adverse effects on the fetus.
FDA Pregnancy Category B.

**Breast-feeding**
Topical oxiconazole is distributed into breast milk.

**Pediatrics**
Appropriate studies on the relationship of age to the effects of topical oxiconazole have not been performed in the pediatric population.

However, no pediatrics-specific problems have been documented to date.

**Geriatrics**
Appropriate studies on the relationship of age to the effects of topical oxiconazole have not been performed in the geriatric population. However, no geriatrics-specific problems have been documented to date.

**Medical considerations/Contraindications**
The medical considerations/contraindications included here have been selected on the basis of their potential clinical significance (reasons given in parentheses where appropriate)—not necessarily inclusive (» = major clinical significance).

*Risk-benefit should be considered when the following medical problem exists:*
Sensitivity to oxiconazole

## Side/Adverse Effects
The following side/adverse effects have been selected on the basis of their potential clinical significance (possible signs and symptoms in parentheses where appropriate)—not necessarily inclusive:

**Those indicating need for medical attention**
Incidence rare
   *Hypersensitivity* (rash)

**Those indicating need for medical attention only if they continue or are bothersome**
Incidence less frequent
   *Local irritation* (burning, stinging, itching, redness, or other sign of irritation not present before use of this medicine)

## Patient Consultation
As an aid to patient consultation, refer to *Advice for the Patient, Oxiconazole (Topical)*.

In providing consultation, consider emphasizing the following selected information (» = major clinical significance):

**Before using this medication**
» Conditions affecting use, especially:
      Sensitivity to oxiconazole
      Breast-feeding—Distributed into breast milk

**Proper use of this medication**
Applying sufficient medication to cover affected and surrounding areas, and rubbing in gently
» Avoiding contact with the eyes; not using in vagina
» Compliance with full course of therapy; fungal infections may require prolonged therapy
» Proper dosing
      Missed dose: Applying as soon as possible; not applying if almost time for next dose
» Proper storage

**Precautions while using this medication**
Checking with physician if no improvement occurs within 2 to 4 weeks
» Using hygienic measures to cure infection and prevent reinfection:
*For tinea cruris*
      Avoiding underwear that is tight-fitting or made from synthetic materials; wearing loose-fitting cotton underwear instead
      Using a bland, absorbent powder or an antifungal powder on the skin; using the powder between administration times for oxiconazole

*For tinea pedis*
      Carefully drying feet, especially between toes, after bathing

Avoiding socks made from wool or synthetic materials; wearing clean, cotton socks and changing them each day or more often if feet perspire excessively

Wearing sandals or well-ventilated shoes

Using bland, absorbent powder or an antifungal powder between toes, on feet, and in socks and shoes 1 or 2 times a day; using the powder between administration times for oxiconazole

**Side/adverse effects**

Signs of potential side effects, especially hypersensitivity

## General Dosing Information

To reduce the possibility of recurrence, tinea corporis and tinea cruris should be treated for at least 2 weeks; tinea pedis should be treated for at least 4 weeks.

## Topical Dosage Forms

Note: The dosing and strength of the dosage forms available are expressed in terms of oxiconazole base.

### OXICONAZOLE NITRATE CREAM

**Usual adult and adolescent dose**
Topical antifungal—
Topical, to the skin and surrounding areas, one to two times a day.

**Usual pediatric dose**
See *Usual adult and adolescent dose.*

**Strength(s) usually available**
U.S.—
1% (base) (Rx) [*Oxistat*].
Canada—
Not commercially available.

**Packaging and storage**
Store below 40 °C (104 °F), preferably between 15 and 30 °C (59 and 86 °F), unless otherwise specified by manufacturer.

**Auxiliary labeling**
• For external use only.
• Continue medicine for full time of treatment.

### OXICONAZOLE NITRATE LOTION

**Usual adult and adolescent dose**
Topical antifungal—
Topical, to the skin and surrounding areas, one to two times a day.

**Usual pediatric dose**
See *Usual adult and adolescent dose.*

**Strength(s) usually available**
U.S.—
1% (base) (Rx) [*Oxistat*].
Canada—
Not commercially available.

**Packaging and storage**
Store below 40 °C (104 °F), preferably between 15 and 30 °C (59 and 86 °F), unless otherwise specified by manufacturer.

**Auxiliary labeling**
• For external use only.
• Continue medicine for full time of treatment.

## Selected Bibliography

Cleary JD, et al. Imidazoles and triazoles in antifungal therapy. DICP Ann Pharmacother (USA) 1990; 24 (2): 148-52.

Jegasothy BV, Pakes GE. Oxiconazole nitrate: pharmacology, efficacy, and safety of a new imidazole antifungal agent. Clin Ther 1991 Jan-Feb; 13 (1): 126-41.

Revised: 07/06/93

---

**OXPRENOLOL**—See *Beta-adrenergic Blocking Agents (Systemic)*

---

**OXTRIPHYLLINE**—See *Bronchodilators, Theophylline (Systemic)*

---

# OXTRIPHYLLINE AND GUAIFENESIN    Systemic

VA CLASSIFICATION (Primary): RE109

NOTE: The *Oxtriphylline and Guaifenesin (Systemic)* monograph is maintained on the USP DI electronic data base. For a printed copy of the most recent revision of the complete monograph, contact the USP Division of Information Development, 12601 Twinbrook Parkway, Rockville, MD 20852.

> For information on the specific components of this combination, see the *USP DI* monographs for *Bronchodilators, Theophylline (Systemic)* and *Guaifenesin (Systemic).*

> The information that follows is selectively abstracted from the complete monograph and is provided to facilitate drug use review and patient counseling.

Note: For a listing of dosage forms and brand names by country availability, see *Dosage Forms* section(s). For a listing of brand names for the articles in this monograph, refer to the General Index.

---

## Category

Asthma prophylactic; bronchodilator.

## Indications

### Accepted

Asthma (prophylaxis and treatment)—Oxtriphylline and guaifenesin combination is indicated in the management of asthma symptoms. Oxtriphylline may benefit those patients with an inadequate response to anti-inflammatory medications and beta-adrenergic bronchodilators; however, theophylline bronchodilators are not considered to be first-line therapy.

Bronchitis, chronic (treatment) or
Emphysema, pulmonary (treatment) or
Pulmonary disease, chronic obstructive, other (treatment)—Oxtriphylline and guaifenesin combination may be indicated in the management of bronchitis, pulmonary emphysema, or other chronic obstructive lung diseases.

## Patient Consultation

As an aid to patient consultation, refer to *Advice for the Patient, Oxtriphylline and Guaifenesin (Systemic).*

In providing consultation, consider emphasizing the following selected information (» = major clinical significance):

**Before using this medication**
» Conditions affecting use, especially:
Sensitivity to oxtriphylline, other theophylline bronchodilators, or guaifenesin
Pregnancy—Theophylline crosses the placenta; decreased elimination during third trimester may require more frequent serum concentration determinations; guaifenesin is associated with an increased incidence of inguinal hernias in the babies of one group of women taking guaifenesin during pregnancy; however, this did not occur in other groups
Breast-feeding—Theophylline distributes into breast milk; may result in irritability in infants
Use in children—Not recommended due to high alcohol content
Use in the elderly—Possible decreased theophylline clearance in patients 60 years of age or older may result in lower dosage requirements; severe signs or symptoms of toxicity are more common in these patients following chronic overdose that results in serum concentrations >30 mcg per mL (165 micromoles per L)
Other medications, especially beta-adrenergic blocking agents; cimetidine; ciprofloxacin; clarithromycin; enoxacin; erythromycin; fluvoxamine; mexiletine; moricizine; pentoxifylline; phenytoin; rifampin; tacrine; thiabendazole; ticlopidine; or troleandomycin
Other medical problems, especially congestive heart failure, convulsions (seizures), hepatic disease, or hypothyroidism

**Proper use of this medication**
» Taking on empty stomach with a glass of water for faster absorption or, if necessary, taking with meals or immediately after meals to lessen gastrointestinal irritation

» Importance of not taking more medication than the amount prescribed
» Compliance with therapy; not missing any doses
» Proper dosing
  Missed dose: Taking as soon as possible; not taking if almost time for next dose; not doubling doses
» Proper storage

**Precautions while using this medication**

Regular visits to physician to check progress during initial period of therapy, including blood levels

» Caution in eating or drinking large amounts of caffeine-containing foods or beverages during therapy with this medication
» Notifying physician of factors that may alter theophylline concentrations, such as:
  —fever (≥102 °F ≥24 hours or a lower temperature elevation for a longer period)
  —other medicines started or stopped
  —smoking started or stopped
  —an extended change in diet
» Notifying the physician before having myocardial perfusion studies; results may be affected by this medicine

**Side/adverse effects**

Signs of potential side effects, especially heartburn and/or vomiting

# Oral Dosage Forms

Note: The dose of oxtriphylline and guaifenesin combination should be determined on the basis of the anhydrous theophylline content of the oxtriphylline component.

## OXTRIPHYLLINE AND GUAIFENESIN ELIXIR

**Usual adult dose**

Bronchodilator—
  Loading dose:
    For patients *not* currently receiving theophylline preparations—Oral, the equivalent of 5 mg of anhydrous theophylline per kg of lean (ideal) body weight as a single dose to provide an average peak serum concentration of 10 mcg per mL (55 micromoles per L), range 5 to 15 mcg per mL (27.5 to 82.5 micromoles per L).
    For patients currently receiving theophylline preparations—Obtaining a serum theophylline concentration prior to administering a partial loading dose is recommended. Once the theophylline concentration is known, the loading dose for theophylline is based on the principle that each 0.5 mg of theophylline per kg of lean (ideal) body weight will result in a 1 mcg per mL (5.5 micromoles per L) increase in serum theophylline concentration.
  Maintenance:
    Oral, the equivalent of anhydrous theophylline, initially, 300 mg per day. After three days, the dosage may be increased, if tolerated, to 400 mg per day. After three more days, the dosage may be increased, if tolerated, to 600 mg per day without measurement of serum concentration.
    The total daily adult dose is administered in three or four divided doses given about six to eight hours apart. Patients with risk factors for impaired theophylline clearance may require a dosing interval of every twelve hours. Young adult smokers and patients with more rapid metabolism may require a dosing interval of every six hours.
    Note: **If the 600-mg-per-day dose is to be maintained or exceeded, monitoring of serum theophylline concentration and patient response is recommended to achieve the optimal therapeutic oxtriphylline dosage and minimize the risk of toxicity.**

**Usual pediatric dose**

Use is not recommended in children due to high alcohol content of elixir.

**Strength(s) usually available**

U.S.—
  100 mg of oxtriphylline (equivalent to 64 mg of anhydrous theophylline) and 50 mg of guaifenesin, per 5 mL (Rx) [*Brondelate* (alcohol); GENERIC (may contain alcohol)].

Canada—
  100 mg of oxtriphylline (equivalent to 64 mg of anhydrous theophylline) and 50 mg of guaifenesin, per 5 mL (Rx) [*Choledyl Expectorant* (alcohol 20%; sodium 10.4 mg; sucrose)].

**Auxiliary labeling**
• Keep container tightly closed.

Revised: 06/21/96

# OXTRIPHYLLINE-CONTAINING COMBINATIONS—

Oxtriphylline and Guaifenesin (Systemic)

# OXYBENZONE-CONTAINING COMBINATIONS—

Aminobenzoic Acid, Padimate O, and Oxybenzone (Topical)—See *Sunscreen Agents (Topical)*

Avobenzone, Octocrylene, Octyl Salicylate, and Oxybenzone—See *Sunscreen Agents (Topical)*

Avobenzone, Octyl Methoxycinnamate, Octyl Salicylate, and Oxybenzone (Topical)—See *Sunscreen Agents (Topical)*

Avobenzone, Octyl Methoxycinnamate, and Oxybenzone—See *Sunscreen Agents (Topical)*

Dioxybenzone, Oxybenzone, and Padimate O (Topical)—See *Sunscreen Agents (Topical)*

Homosalate, Menthyl Anthranilate, Octyl Methoxycinnamate, Octyl Salicylate, and Oxybenzone (Topical)—See *Sunscreen Agents (Topical)*

Homosalate, Octocrylene, Octyl Methoxycinnamate, and Oxybenzone (Topical)—See *Sunscreen Agents (Topical)*

Homosalate, Octyl Methoxycinnamate, Octyl Salicylate, and Oxybenzone (Topical)—See *Sunscreen Agents (Topical)*

Homosalate, Octyl Methoxycinnamate, and Oxybenzone (Topical)—See *Sunscreen Agents (Topical)*

Homosalate and Oxybenzone (Topical)—See *Sunscreen Agents (Topical)*

Lisadimate, Oxybenzone, and Padimate O (Topical)—See *Sunscreen Agents (Topical)*

Menthyl Anthranilate, Octocrylene, Octyl Methoxycinnamate, and Oxybenzone (Topical)—See *Sunscreen Agents (Topical)*

Menthyl Anthranilate, Octyl Methoxycinnamate, Octyl Salicylate, and Oxybenzone (Topical)—See *Sunscreen Agents (Topical)*

Menthyl Anthranilate, Octyl Methoxycinnamate, and Oxybenzone (Topical)—See *Sunscreen Agents (Topical)*

Octocrylene, Octyl Methoxycinnamate, Octyl Salicylate, and Oxybenzone (Topical)—See *Sunscreen Agents (Topical)*

Octocrylene, Octyl Methoxycinnamate, Octyl Salicylate, Oxybenzone, and Titanium Dioxide (Topical)—See *Sunscreen Agents (Topical)*

Octocrylene, Octyl Methoxycinnamate, and Oxybenzone (Topical)—See *Sunscreen Agents (Topical)*

Octocrylene, Octyl Methoxycinnamate, Oxybenzone, and Titanium Dioxide (Topical)—See *Sunscreen Agents (Topical)*

Octyl Methoxycinnamate, Octyl Salicylate, and Oxybenzone (Topical)—See *Sunscreen Agents (Topical)*

Octyl Methoxycinnamate, Octyl Salicylate, Oxybenzone, and Padimate O (Topical)—See *Sunscreen Agents (Topical)*

Octyl Methoxycinnamate, Octyl Salicylate, Oxybenzone, Padimate O, and Titanium Dioxide (Topical)—See *Sunscreen Agents (Topical)*

Octyl Methoxycinnamate, Octyl Salicylate, Oxybenzone, Phenylbenzimidazole, and Titanium Dioxide (Topical)—See *Sunscreen Agents (Topical)*

Octyl Methoxycinnamate, Octyl Salicylate, Oxybenzone, and Titanium Dioxide (Topical)—See *Sunscreen Agents (Topical)*

Octyl Methoxycinnamate and Oxybenzone (Topical)—See *Sunscreen Agents (Topical)*

Octyl Methoxycinnamate, Oxybenzone, and Padimate O (Topical)—See *Sunscreen Agents (Topical)*

Octyl Methoxycinnamate, Oxybenzone, Padimate O, and Titanium Dioxide (Topical)—See *Sunscreen Agents (Topical)*

Octyl Methoxycinnamate, Oxybenzone, and Titanium Dioxide (Topical)—See *Sunscreen Agents (Topical)*

Oxybenzone and Padimate O (Topical)—See *Sunscreen Agents (Topical)*

Oxybenzone and Roxadimate (Topical)—See *Sunscreen Agents (Topical)*

# OXYBUTYNIN   Systemic

VA CLASSIFICATION (Primary): GU201

Note: For a listing of dosage forms and brand names by country availability, see *Dosage Forms* section(s). For a listing of brand names for the articles in this monograph, refer to the General Index.

## Category

Antispasmodic (urinary tract).

## Indications

### Accepted

Urologic disorders, symptoms of (treatment) and

Irritative voiding, symptoms of (treatment)—Oxybutynin is indicated for the relief of symptoms associated with voiding, such as frequent urination, urgency, urge incontinence, nocturia, and incontinence in patients with uninhibited neurogenic bladder contractions and in those patients with reflex neurogenic bladder.

### Unaccepted

Oxybutynin has been used as an antispasmodic in the symptomatic treatment of gastrointestinal disorders; however, its effectiveness has not been established.

## Pharmacology/Pharmacokinetics

### Physicochemical characteristics

Molecular weight—393.95.
pKa—6.96.

### Mechanism of action/Effect

Exerts direct antispasmodic effect on smooth muscle and inhibits the action of acetylcholine at postganglionic cholinergic sites, thus increasing bladder capacity and delaying the initial desire to void by reducing the number of motor impulses reaching the detrusor muscle. It does not block acetylcholine effects at skeletal myoneural junctions or at autonomic ganglia; neither does it have effect on the smooth muscle of blood vessels.

### Other actions/effects

Oxybutynin has also shown (in animal studies) moderate antihistaminic, some local anesthetic, mild analgesic, and very low mydriatic and antisialagogue activity.

### Absorption

Rapidly absorbed from gastrointestinal tract.

### Biotransformation

Hepatic.

### Onset of action

30 minutes to 1 hour.

### Time to peak effect:

3 to 6 hours.

### Duration of action

6 to 10 hours (antispasmodic effect).

### Elimination

Primarily renal.

## Precautions to Consider

### Pregnancy/Reproduction

Fertility—Reproduction studies in the hamster, rabbit, rat, and mouse have not shown oxybutynin to impair fertility.

Pregnancy—Adequate and well-controlled studies in humans have not been done.

Reproduction studies in the hamster, rabbit, rat, and mouse have not shown oxybutynin to harm the fetus.

FDA Pregnancy Category B.

### Breast-feeding

Problems in humans have not been documented. However, oxybutynin may inhibit lactation.

### Pediatrics

Appropriate studies on the relationship of age to the effects of oxybutynin have not been performed in children up to 5 years of age.

### Geriatrics

Geriatric patients may be more sensitive than younger adults to the anticholinergic effects of oxybutynin.

Oxybutynin may also exacerbate underlying disease states in these patients.

### Dental

Prolonged use of oxybutynin may decrease or inhibit salivary flow, thus contributing to the development of caries, periodontal disease, oral candidiasis, and discomfort.

### Drug interactions and/or related problems

The following drug interactions and/or related problems have been selected on the basis of their potential clinical significance (possible mechanism in parentheses where appropriate)—not necessarily inclusive (» = major clinical significance):

Note: Combinations containing any of the following medications, depending on the amount present, may also interact with this medication.

» Anticholinergics or other medications with anticholinergic activity (See *Appendix II*)
(concurrent use may intensify the anticholinergic effects of oxybutynin)

Central nervous system (CNS) depression–producing medications, other (See *Appendix II*)
(concurrent use may increase the sedative effects of either these medications or oxybutynin)

### Medical considerations/Contraindications

The medical considerations/contraindications included here have been selected on the basis of their potential clinical significance (reasons given in parentheses where appropriate)—not necessarily inclusive (» = major clinical significance).

*Risk-benefit should be considered when the following medical problems exist:*

» Cardiac disease, especially mitral stenosis, cardiac arrhythmias, congestive heart failure, coronary heart disease or

» Hemorrhage, acute, with unstable cardiovascular status
(increase in heart rate may be undesirable)

» Gastrointestinal tract obstructive disease as in achalasia and pyloroduodenal stenosis
(decrease in motility and tone may occur, resulting in obstruction and gastric retention)

» Glaucoma, angle-closure, or predisposition to
(possible mydriatic effect of oxybutynin resulting in increased intraocular pressure may precipitate an acute attack of angle-closure glaucoma)

Hepatic function impairment
(decreased metabolism of oxybutynin)

» Hernia, hiatal, associated with reflux esophagitis or
Hypertension
(may be aggravated)

Hyperthyroidism
(characterized by tachycardia, which may be increased)

» Intestinal atony in the elderly or debilitated patient or

» Paralytic ileus
(use of oxybutynin may lead to obstruction)

» Myasthenia gravis
(oxybutynin may aggravate condition because of inhibition of acetylcholine action)

Neuropathy, autonomic
(urinary retention and cycloplegia may be aggravated)

» Prostatic hypertrophy, nonobstructive
(reduction in tone of urinary bladder may lead to complete urinary retention)

Renal function impairment
(decreased excretion may increase the risk of side effects)

Sensitivity to oxybutynin

» Tachycardia
(may be increased)

Toxemia of pregnancy
(hypertension may be aggravated)

» Ulcerative colitis, severe
(large doses may suppress intestinal motility and may cause paralytic ileus; also, use may precipitate or aggravate the serious complication of toxic megacolon)

» Urinary retention or
» Uropathy, obstructive, such as bladder neck obstruction due to prostatic hypertrophy
(urinary retention may be precipitated or aggravated)
Xerostomia
(prolonged use may further reduce limited salivary flow)
Caution in use is also recommended in patients over 40 years of age because of danger of precipitating undiagnosed glaucoma.
In patients with diarrhea the possibility of intestinal obstruction should be excluded before oxybutynin is administered.

### Patient monitoring
The following may be especially important in patient monitoring (other tests may be warranted in some patients, depending on condition; » = major clinical significance):
Cystometry
(recommended at periodic intervals to evaluate response to therapy)

## Side/Adverse Effects
Note: When oxybutynin is given to patients where the environmental temperature is high, there is risk of a rapid increase in body temperature because of suppression of sweat gland activity.

The following side/adverse effects have been selected on the basis of their potential clinical significance (possible signs and symptoms in parentheses where appropriate)—not necessarily inclusive:

### Those indicating need for medical attention
Incidence rare
*Allergic reaction* (skin rash or hives); *increased intraocular pressure* (eye pain)

### Those indicating need for medical attention only if they continue or are bothersome
Incidence more frequent
*Constipation; decreased sweating; drowsiness; dryness of mouth, nose, and throat*
Incidence less frequent or rare
*Decreased flow of breast milk; decreased saliva secretion* (difficulty in swallowing); *decreased sexual ability; difficult urination; difficulty in accommodation* (blurred vision); *headache; mydriatic effect* (increased sensitivity of eyes to light); *nausea or vomiting; trouble in sleeping; unusual tiredness or weakness*

## Overdose
For specific information on the agents used in the management of oxybutynin overdose, see:
• *Physostigmine (Systemic)* monograph
For more information on the management of overdose or unintentional ingestion, **contact a Poison Control Center** (see *Poison Control Center Listing*).

### Clinical effects of overdose
The following effects have been selected on the basis of their potential clinical significance (possible signs and symptoms in parentheses where appropriate)—not necessarily inclusive:
*Clumsiness or unsteadiness; confusion; dizziness; severe drowsiness; fast heartbeat; fever; flushing or redness of face; hallucinations; respiratory depression* (shortness of breath or troubled breathing); *unusual excitement, nervousness, restlessness, or irritability*

### Treatment of overdose
To decrease absorption—
Immediate gastric lavage.
Specific treatment—
*Slow* intravenous administration of 0.5 to 2 mg of physostigmine, repeated as needed up to a total of 5 mg.
Supportive care—
In the event of respiratory depression, starting and maintaining artificial respiration. Treating fever symptomatically with ice packs or alcohol sponging.

## Patient Consultation
As an aid to patient consultation, refer to *Advice for the Patient, Oxybutynin (Systemic)*.
In providing consultation, consider emphasizing the following selected information » = major clinical significance):

### Before using this medication
» Conditions affecting use, especially:
Sensitivity to oxybutynin
Use in the elderly—Increased sensitivity to anticholinergic effects

Dental—Possible development of dental problems because of decreased salivary flow
Other medications, especially other anticholinergics
Other medical problems, especially cardiac diseases, glaucoma, hemorrhage, hiatal hernia, intestinal atony, myasthenia gravis, paralytic ileus, prostatic hypertrophy, obstruction in gastrointestinal or urinary tract, tachycardia, ulcerative colitis, urinary retention

### Proper use of this medication
Taking medication on an empty stomach with water, or with food or milk to reduce gastric irritation
» Importance of not taking more medication than the amount prescribed
» Proper dosing
Missed dose: Taking as soon as possible; if almost time for next dose, not taking at all; not doubling doses
» Proper storage

### Precautions while using this medication
» Avoiding use of alcohol or other CNS depressants
Possible increased sensitivity of eyes to light
» Caution if drowsiness or blurred vision occurs
» Caution during exercise and hot weather; overheating may result in heat stroke
Possible dryness of mouth, nose, and throat; using sugarless gum or candy, ice, or saliva substitute for relief of dry mouth; checking with physician or dentist if dry mouth continues for more than 2 weeks

### Side/adverse effects
Signs of potential side effects, especially allergic reaction or increased intraocular pressure

## General Dosing Information
Oxybutynin may be taken on an empty stomach with water; however, if gastric irritation occurs it may be taken with food or milk.
Cystometry and other appropriate diagnostic procedures should precede treatment with oxybutynin.
If urinary tract infection is present, appropriate antibacterial therapy should be administered.

## Oral Dosage Forms
### OXYBUTYNIN CHLORIDE SYRUP USP

**Usual adult and adolescent dose**
Antispasmodic (urinary tract)—
Oral, 5 mg two or three times a day, the dosage being adjusted as needed and tolerated.

**Usual adult prescribing limits**
Antispasmodic (urinary tract)—
Oral, 5 mg four times a day or 20 mg daily.

**Usual pediatric dose**
Antispasmodic (urinary tract)—
Children up to 5 years of age: Dosage has not been established.
Children 5 years of age and over: Oral, 5 mg two or three times a day, not to exceed 15 mg per day.

**Usual geriatric dose**
See *Usual adult and adolescent dose.*
Note: Geriatric patients may be more sensitive to the effects of the usual adult dose.

**Strength(s) usually available**
U.S.—
5 mg per 5 mL (Rx) [*Ditropan* (methylparaben; sucrose)].
Canada—
5 mg per 5 mL (Rx) [*Ditropan* (methylparaben; sucrose)].

**Packaging and storage**
Store below 40 °C (104 °F), preferably between 15 and 30 °C (59 and 86 °F), unless otherwise specified by manufacturer. Store in a tight, light-resistant container. Protect from freezing.

**Auxiliary labeling**
• May cause drowsiness or blurred vision.

### OXYBUTYNIN CHLORIDE TABLETS USP

**Usual adult and adolescent dose**
See *Oxybutynin Chloride Syrup USP.*

**Usual adult prescribing limits**
See *Oxybutynin Chloride Syrup USP.*

**Usual pediatric dose**
See *Oxybutynin Chloride Syrup USP.*

**Usual geriatric dose**
See *Oxybutynin Chloride Syrup USP*.

Note: Geriatric patients may be more sensitive to the effects of the usual adult dose.

**Strength(s) usually available**
U.S.—
 5 mg (Rx) [*Ditropan* (scored); GENERIC].
Canada—
 5 mg (Rx) [*Ditropan* (scored)].

**Packaging and storage**
Store below 40 °C (104 °F), preferably between 15 and 30 °C (59 and 86 °F), unless otherwise specified by manufacturer. Store in a tight, light-resistant container.

**Auxiliary labeling**
• May cause drowsiness or blurred vision.

Revised: 06/16/93

## OXYCODONE—See *Opioid (Narcotic) Analgesics (Systemic)*

## OXYCODONE-CONTAINING COMBINATIONS—

Oxycodone and Acetaminophen (Systemic)—See *Opioid (Narcotic) Analgesics and Acetaminophen (Systemic)*
Oxycodone and Aspirin (Systemic)—See *Opioid (Narcotic) Analgesics and Aspirin (Systemic)*

# OXYMETAZOLINE   Nasal

VA CLASSIFICATION (Primary): NT100

Note: For a listing of dosage forms and brand names by country availability, see *Dosage Forms* section(s). For a listing of brand names for the articles in this monograph, refer to the General Index.

## Category
Decongestant (topical).

## Indications

Note: Bracketed information in the *Indications* section refers to uses that are not included in U.S. product labeling.

**Accepted**
Congestion, nasal (treatment)—Oxymetazoline is indicated for temporary relief of nasal congestion due to the common cold, sinusitis, hay fever, or other upper respiratory allergies.

[Congestion, sinus (treatment)]—Nasal oxymetazoline is used for the relief of sinus congestion.

## Pharmacology/Pharmacokinetics

**Physicochemical characteristics**
Molecular weight—296.84.
pH—Approximately 6.4.

**Mechanism of action/Effect**
Oxymetazoline is a direct-acting sympathomimetic amine. It acts on alpha-adrenergic receptors in the arterioles of the nasal mucosa to produce constriction, resulting in decreased blood flow and decreased nasal congestion.

## Precautions to Consider

**Cross-sensitivity and/or related problems**
Patients sensitive to other nasal decongestants may be sensitive to this medication also.

**Pregnancy/Reproduction**
Oxymetazoline may be systemically absorbed. However, problems in humans have not been documented.

**Breast-feeding**
Oxymetazoline may be systemically absorbed. However, problems in humans have not been documented.

**Pediatrics**
Children may be especially prone to systemic absorption of oxymetazoline with resulting side/adverse effects.

**Geriatrics**
Although appropriate studies on the relationship of age to the effects of oxymetazoline have not been performed in the geriatric population, no geriatrics-specific problems have been documented to date.

**Drug interactions and/or related problems**
The following drug interactions and/or related problems have been selected on the basis of their potential clinical significance (possible mechanism in parentheses where appropriate)—not necessarily inclusive (» = major clinical significance):

Note: Combinations containing any of the following medications, depending on the amount present, may also interact with this medication.

Antidepressants, tricyclic or
Maprotiline
 (if significant systemic absorption of nasal oxymetazoline occurs, concurrent use of maprotiline or tricyclic antidepressants may potentiate the pressor effect of oxymetazoline)

**Medical considerations/Contraindications**
The medical considerations/contraindications included here have been selected on the basis of their potential clinical significance (reasons given in parentheses where appropriate)—not necessarily inclusive (» = major clinical significance).

*Risk-benefit should be considered when the following medical problems exist:*
Coronary artery disease or
Heart disease, including angina or
Hypertension
 (condition may be exacerbated due to drug-induced cardiovascular effects)
Diabetes mellitus
Hyperthyroidism
Sensitivity to oxymetazoline or other nasal decongestants

## Side/Adverse Effects

The following side/adverse effects have been selected on the basis of their potential clinical significance (possible signs and symptoms in parentheses where appropriate)—not necessarily inclusive:

**Those indicating need for medical attention**
 *Rebound congestion* (increase in runny or stuffy nose)

**Symptoms of systemic absorption**
 *Fast, irregular, or pounding heartbeat; headache or lightheadedness; nervousness; trembling; trouble in sleeping*

**Those indicating need for medical attention only if they continue or are bothersome**
 *Burning, dryness, or stinging of nasal mucosa; sneezing*

## Patient Consultation

As an aid to patient consultation, refer to *Advice for the Patient, Oxymetazoline (Nasal)*.

In providing consultation, consider emphasizing the following selected information (» = major clinical significance):

**Before using this medication**
» Conditions affecting use, especially:
  Sensitivity to oxymetazoline or other nasal decongestants
  Use in children—Children may be especially sensitive to the effects of oxymetazoline

**Proper use of this medication**
 Proper administration technique
 Preventing contamination: Wiping tip of applicator with clean, damp tissue; replacing cap right after use
 Preventing spread of infection: Not using bottle for more than 1 person
» Importance of not using more medication than the amount recommended; not using medication for more than 3 days without checking with physician
» Proper dosing
 Missed dose: If on scheduled dosing regimen—Using right away if remembered within an hour or so; if not remembered until later,

skipping missed dose and returning to regular dosing schedule; not doubling doses

» Proper storage

**Side/adverse effects**

Signs of potential side effects, especially rebound congestion or systemic sympathomimetic effects

## General Dosing Information

Prolonged or excessive use of this medication will cause rebound congestion with chronic swelling of nasal mucosa.

## Nasal Dosage Forms

### OXYMETAZOLINE HYDROCHLORIDE NASAL SOLUTION USP

**Usual adult and adolescent dose**

Decongestant—

Intranasal, 2 or 3 drops or sprays of a 0.05% solution into each nostril two times a day, morning and evening.

Note: The nasal spray form of the medication is more effective and less likely to cause systemic absorption.

**Usual pediatric dose**

Decongestant—

Children up to 2 years of age: Dosage has not been established.

Children 2 to 6 years of age: Intranasal, 2 or 3 drops of a 0.025% solution into each nostril two times a day, morning and evening.

Children 6 years of age and older: See *Usual adult and adolescent dose.*

**Strength(s) usually available**

U.S.—

0.025% (nasal drops) (OTC) [*Afrin Children's Strength Nose Drops*].

0.05% (nasal drops) (OTC) [*Afrin Nose Drops; NTZ Long Acting Decongestant Nose Drops;* GENERIC].

0.05% (nasal spray) (OTC) [*Afrin Cherry Scented Nasal Spray; Afrin Extra Moisturizing Nasal Decongestant Spray; Afrin Menthol Nasal Spray; Afrin Nasal Spray; Afrin Sinus Spray* (benzyl alcohol); *Afrin Spray Pump; Allerest 12 Hour Nasal Spray; Cheracol Nasal Spray; Cheracol Nasal Spray Pump Cherry Scented; Dristan 12-Hr Nasal Spray; Duramist Plus Up To 12 Hours Decongestant Nasal Spray; Duration 12 Hour Nasal Spray; Duration 12 Hour Nasal Spray Pump; Nasal-12 Hour; Nasal Relief; Nasal Spray 12-Hour; Nasal Spray Long Acting; Neo-Synephrine 12 Hour Nasal Spray; Neo-Synephrine 12 Hour Nasal Spray Pump; Nostrilla Long-Acting Nasal Decongestant; NTZ Long Acting Decongestant Nasal Spray; Sinarest 12 Hour Nasal Spray; Vicks Sinex Long-Acting 12-Hour Formula Decongestant Nasal Spray; Vicks Sinex Long-Acting 12-Hour Formula Decongestant Ultra Fine Mist; 4-Way Long Lasting Nasal Spray;* GENERIC].

Canada—

0.05% (nasal spray) (OTC) [*Dristan; Dristan Mentholated* (alcohol); *Drixoral*].

**Packaging and storage**

Store below 40 °C (104 °F), preferably between 15 and 30 °C (59 and 86 °F), unless otherwise specified by manufacturer. Store in a tight container. Protect from freezing.

**Auxiliary labeling**

• For the nose.

Revised: 04/19/94
Interim revision: 03/28/95; 05/24/95

---

# OXYMETAZOLINE  Ophthalmic

VA CLASSIFICATION (Primary): OP800

Note: For a listing of dosage forms and brand names by country availability, see *Dosage Forms* section(s). For a listing of brand names for the articles in this monograph, refer to the General Index.

## Category

Decongestant (ophthalmic).

## Indications

**Accepted**

Ocular redness (treatment)—Oxymetazoline is indicated for the temporary relief of redness associated with minor irritations of the eye, such as those caused by pollen-related allergies, colds, dust, smog, wind, swimming, or wearing contact lenses.

## Pharmacology/Pharmacokinetics

**Physicochemical characteristics**

Molecular weight—260.37.

**Mechanism of action/Effect**

Oxymetazoline is a direct-acting sympathomimetic amine. It acts on alpha-adrenergic receptors in the arterioles of the conjunctiva to produce vasoconstriction, resulting in decreased conjunctival congestion.

**Onset of action**

Within 5 minutes.

**Duration of action**

Approximately 6 hours.

## Precautions to Consider

**Cross-sensitivity and/or related problems**

Patients sensitive to other ophthalmic sympathomimetics may be sensitive to this medication also.

**Pregnancy/Reproduction**

Pregnancy—Oxymetazoline may be systemically absorbed.

Studies have not been done in humans or animals.

**Breast-feeding**

Problems in humans have not been documented; however, oxymetazoline may be systemically absorbed.

**Pediatrics**

Check with physician before using oxymetazoline ophthalmic solution in children up to 6 years of age. Eye redness in children can occur with illnesses, such as allergies, fevers, colds, and measles, that may require medical attention.

**Geriatrics**

Appropriate studies on the relationship of age to the effects of oxymetazoline have not been performed in the geriatric population. However, no geriatrics-specific problems have been documented to date.

**Drug interactions and/or related problems**

The following drug interactions and/or related problems have been selected on the basis of their potential clinical significance (possible mechanism in parentheses where appropriate)—not necessarily inclusive (» = major clinical significance):

Antidepressants, tricyclic or

Maprotiline

(if significant systemic absorption of ophthalmic oxymetazoline occurs, concurrent use may potentiate the pressor effect of oxymetazoline)

**Medical considerations/Contraindications**

The medical considerations/contraindications included here have been selected on the basis of their potential clinical significance (reasons given in parentheses where appropriate)—not necessarily inclusive (» = major clinical significance).

*Risk-benefit should be considered when the following medical problems exist:*

Coronary artery disease or

Heart disease, including angina or

Hypertension

(if significant systemic absorption of ophthalmic oxymetazoline occurs, condition may be exacerbated due to drug-induced cardiovascular effects)

Eye disease, infection, or injury

(may mask symptoms and delay treatment)

Glaucoma, narrow-angle, or predisposition to

(may precipitate an attack by dilating pupil)

Hyperthyroidism
    (may exacerbate existing tachycardia or elevated blood pressure)
Sensitivity to oxymetazoline

## Side/Adverse Effects

Note: Excessive dosage and/or prolonged use may cause increased irritation of the conjunctiva. Prolonged use may also cause reactive hyperemia.

The following side/adverse effects have been selected on the basis of their potential clinical significance (possible signs and symptoms in parentheses where appropriate)—not necessarily inclusive:

**Those indicating need for medical attention**
With excessive dosage and/or prolonged use
    *Hyperemia, reactive* (increase in irritation or redness of eyes)
Symptoms of systemic absorption
    *Fast, irregular, or pounding heartbeat; headache or lightheadedness; nervousness; trembling; trouble in sleeping*

## Patient Consultation

As an aid to patient consultation, refer to *Advice for the Patient, Oxymetazoline (Ophthalmic).*

In providing consultation, consider emphasizing the following selected information (» = major clinical significance):

**Before using this medication**
» Conditions affecting use, especially:
        Sensitivity to oxymetazoline or any other eye decongestant
        Use in children—Checking with physician before using medication in children up to 6 years of age; eye redness in children can occur with illnesses, such as allergies, fevers, colds, and measles, that may require medical attention

**Proper use of this medication**
    Not using if solution becomes cloudy or changes color
    Proper administration technique
    Preventing contamination: Not touching applicator tip to any surface and keeping container tightly closed
» Importance of not using more medication than the amount recommended and not using for more than 72 hours, unless directed to do so by physician; overuse may increase eye irritation and the chance of side effects
» Proper dosing
» Proper storage

**Precautions while using this medication**
» Stopping medication and checking with physician if eye pain or change in vision occurs or if redness or irritation continues, gets worse, or lasts for more than 72 hours

**Side/adverse effects**
    Side effects usually are rare when medication is used for short periods of time at low doses
    Signs of potential side effects, especially reactive hyperemia or symptoms of systemic absorption

## General Dosing Information

Treatment should not be continued for more than 72 hours unless otherwise directed by physician.

Although the manufacturer recommends that patients remove soft contact lenses before using oxymetazoline ophthalmic solution, USP medical experts do not believe this precaution is necessary unless the patient has corneal epithelial problems. No significant problems have been documented with ophthalmic solutions containing 0.03% or less of benzalkonium chloride as a preservative when they are used as eye drops in patients with no significant corneal surface problem.

## Ophthalmic Dosage Forms

### OXYMETAZOLINE HYDROCHLORIDE OPHTHALMIC SOLUTION USP

**Usual adult and adolescent dose**
Topical, to the conjunctiva, 1 drop of a 0.025% solution every six hours as needed, or as directed by physician.

**Usual pediatric dose**
Children up to 6 years of age—Dosage must be individualized by physician.
Children 6 years of age and older—See *Usual adult and adolescent dose.*

**Strength(s) usually available**
U.S.—
    0.025% (OTC) [*OcuClear; Visine L.R.*].
Canada—
    0.025% (OTC) [*OcuClear*].

**Packaging and storage**
Store between 2 and 30 °C (36 and 86 °F), unless otherwise specified by manufacturer. Store in a tight container. Protect from freezing.

**Stability**
Do not use if solution contains a precipitate or changes color.

**Auxiliary labeling**
• For the eye.
• Keep container tightly closed.

Revised: 04/29/92
Interim revision: 02/17/94

---

**OXYMETHOLONE**—See *Anabolic Steroids (Systemic)*

---

**OXYMORPHONE**—See *Opioid (Narcotic) Analgesics (Systemic)*

---

**OXYTETRACYCLINE**—See *Tetracyclines (Systemic)*

---

# OXYTOCIN    Systemic

VA CLASSIFICATION (Primary/Secondary): GU600/DX900; HS900
Note: For a listing of dosage forms and brand names by country availability, see *Dosage Forms* section(s). For a listing of brand names for the articles in this monograph, refer to the General Index.

## Category

Oxytocic—Oxytocin.
Antihemorrhagic (postpartum and postabortal uterine bleeding)—Oxytocin Injection.
Lactation stimulant—Oxytocin Nasal Solution.
Diagnostic aid (utero-placental insufficiency; placental reserve)—Oxytocin Injection.

## Indications

Note: Bracketed information in the *Indications* section refers to uses that are not included in U.S. product labeling.

**Accepted**
Labor, medical induction of or
Labor, augmentation of or
Abortion, incomplete (treatment)—Parenterally administered oxytocin is indicated for induction and augmentation of labor. Parenteral oxytocin is also indicated for management of incomplete abortion. Oxytocin is sometimes used in combination with prostaglandins.
Abortion, therapeutic—Parenterally administered oxytocin is indicated for performance of therapeutic abortion. Oxytocin is sometimes used in combination with hypertonic sodium chloride, urea, or prostaglandins.
Hemorrhage, postabortion and postpartum (treatment)—Oxytocin is indicated in the management of postabortion and postpartum bleeding or hemorrhage.
Lactation deficiency (treatment)—Intranasally administered oxytocin is indicated for stimulation of impaired milk ejection (lack of let-down). Nasal oxytocin is recommended for short-term use, generally during the first week postpartum.

[Fetal distress (diagnosis)][1] or
[Utero-placental insufficiency (diagnosis)][1]—Oxytocin is administered parenterally to assess fetal-placental respiratory capabilities in high-risk pregnancies. This is also referred to as the oxytocin challenge test.

---

[1]Not included in Canadian product labeling.

## Pharmacology/Pharmacokinetics

### Physicochemical characteristics
Source—Synthetically produced pituitary hormone.
Molecular weight—1007.19.

### Mechanism of action/Effect
Uterine—
The uterine myometrium contains receptors specific to oxytocin. Oxytocin stimulates contraction of uterine smooth muscle by increasing intracellular calcium concentrations, thus mimicking contractions of normal, spontaneous labor and transiently impeding uterine blood flow. Amplitude and duration of uterine contractions are increased, leading to dilation and effacement of the cervix. The number of oxytocin receptors and, therefore, uterine response to oxytocin increases gradually throughout pregnancy, reaching its peak at term.

For diagnosis of fetal distress and utero-placental insufficiency: By comparing baseline and oxytocin-induced fetal heart rate patterns and uterine contraction patterns, the oxytocin challenge test may aid in determining if there is adequate placental reserve for continuation of a high-risk pregnancy. The occurrence of a fetal heart rate pattern exhibiting late decelerations with administration of oxytocin may indicate utero-placental insufficiency.

Lactation—
Stimulates smooth muscle to facilitate ejection of milk from breasts. Oxytocin does not increase milk production.

### Absorption
Rapidly absorbed through nasal mucous membranes; may be erratic.

### Protein binding
Low (30%).

### Biotransformation
Enzymatic hydrolysis, primarily by tissue oxytocinase. Oxytocinase is also found in placental tissue and plasma.

### Half-life
1 to 6 minutes (decreased in late pregnancy and lactation).

### Onset of action
Nasal—Within a few minutes.
Intramuscular—3 to 5 minutes.
Intravenous—Immediate.

### Duration of action
Nasal—20 minutes.
Intramuscular—2 to 3 hours.
Intravenous—Uterine activity generally subsides within one hour.

### Elimination
Only small amounts are excreted unchanged.

## Precautions to Consider

### Carcinogenicity/Mutagenicity
No animal or human studies have been conducted to evaluate the carcinogenic or mutagenic potential of oxytocin.

### Pregnancy/Reproduction
Pregnancy—
*For augmentation or stimulation of labor—*
Oxytocin is not indicated for use in the first trimester of pregnancy, other than for the treatment of incomplete abortion or therapeutic abortion.
Animal reproductive studies have not been conducted.
*For stimulation of lactation—*
Not recommended for use during pregnancy because its use may result in contractions and abortion.
FDA Pregnancy Category X.

Labor and delivery—Based on extensive clinical use and known pharmacologic properties of oxytocin, it is not expected to cause an increased risk of fetal abnormalities when used as indicated. Because of maternal and fetal risks, oxytocin must be administered with caution. It has been reported to cause fetal bradycardia, neonatal retinal hemorrhage, and neonatal jaundice, in addition to maternal effects.

Fetal deaths due to various causes have reportedly been associated with the parenteral use of oxytocics for induction or augmentation of labor.

Excessive dosage or administration of oxytocin to hypersensitive patients may cause uterine hypertonicity with spasm and tetanic contraction or uterine rupture. Abruptio placentae, impaired uterine blood flow, amniotic fluid embolism, and fetal trauma including cardiac arrhythmias, intracranial hemorrhage, and asphyxia may occur as a result.

Oxytocin may inhibit, rather than promote, expulsion of the placenta and increase the risk of hemorrhage and infection.

### Breast-feeding
For stimulation of milk ejection—Problems in humans have not been documented. Only minimal amounts pass into breast milk.

### Drug interactions and/or related problems
The following drug interactions and/or related problems have been selected on the basis of their potential clinical significance (possible mechanism in parentheses where appropriate)—not necessarily inclusive (» = major clinical significance):

Note: Combinations containing any of the following medications, depending on the amount present, may also interact with this medication.

Anesthetics, hydrocarbon inhalation, such as
  Cyclopropane
  Enflurane
  Halothane
  Isoflurane
  (cyclopropane anesthesia may lessen tachycardia but worsen hypotension caused by oxytocin; maternal sinus bradycardia and abnormal atrioventricular rhythms have been reported with concurrent use, although the correlation is controversial)
  (enflurane [concentrations > 1.5%], halothane [concentrations > 1%], and possibly isoflurane produce a dose-dependent decrease in the uterine response to oxytocics and may abolish the response if sufficient concentrations [> 3% of enflurane] are administered; uterine hemorrhage may result)

Caudal block anesthesia with a vasoconstrictor or
Vasopressors
  (concurrent use with oxytocin may potentiate the pressor effect of the sympathomimetic pressor amines with possible severe hypertension and rupture of cerebral blood vessels)
  (severe hypertension has been reported when oxytocin was given 3 to 4 hours after caudal block anesthesia with a vasoconstrictor)

» Sodium chloride, intra-amniotic for abortion or
» Urea, intra-amniotic for abortion or
» Oxytocics, other
  (concurrent use with oxytocin may result in uterine hypertonus, possibly causing uterine rupture or cervical laceration, especially in the absence of adequate cervical dilation; although combinations are sometimes used for therapeutic advantage, patient should be monitored closely during concurrent use; when used as an adjunct to abortifacients, it is recommended that oxytocin not be administered until the oxytocic effect of the abortifacient has subsided, to reduce the risk of uterine rupture and cervical laceration; water intoxication may also occur in patients given oxytocin following the use of intra-amniotic hypertonic saline for abortion)

### Laboratory value alterations
The following have been selected on the basis of their potential clinical significance (possible effect in parentheses where appropriate)—not necessarily inclusive (» = major clinical significance):

With physiology/laboratory test values
  Bilirubin, neonatal serum concentrations
    (neonatal jaundice has been reported, although it is not clear whether jaundice is due to oxytocin or labor process itself)
  Chloride and
  Sodium
    (antidiuretic effect of oxytocin may cause reduced maternal serum concentrations and water intoxication)

### Medical considerations/Contraindications
The medical considerations/contraindications included here have been selected on the basis of their potential clinical significance (reasons given in parentheses where appropriate)—not necessarily inclusive (» = major clinical significance).

*Except under special circumstances, this medication should not be used when the following medical problems exist:*

*For all indications*
» Allergy to oxytocin, history of

*For augmentation or induction of labor*
» Absolute contraindications to vaginal delivery
» Hypertonic uterine patterns

*Risk-benefit should be considered when the following medical problems exist:*

*For all indications, except for stimulation of lactation*
Cardiac disease, especially involving fixed cardiac output or
Hypertension or
Renal function impairment
(increased susceptibility to fluid overload, arrhythmia, or hypotension and reflex tachycardia; reduction in dosage is recommended)

Exaggerated response to oxytocin or other oxytocics, history of
(excessive dosage or administration of oxytocin to hypersensitive patients may cause uterine hypertonicity with spasm and tetanic contraction, which can lead to uterine rupture, cervical lacerations, abruptio placentae, impaired uterine blood flow, amniotic fluid embolism, and fetal trauma including cardiac arrhythmias, intracranial hemorrhage, and asphyxia)

*For augmentation or induction of labor only, in addition to those problems listed above*
» Relative contraindications to vaginal delivery
» Uterine inertia
(*prolonged use* of oxytocin is not recommended; in cases of uterine inertia, it is recommended that oxytocin be administered for no longer than 6 to 8 hours)

### Patient monitoring
The following may be especially important in patient monitoring (other tests may be warranted in some patients, depending on condition; » = major clinical significance):

Acid-base equilibrium determinations, fetal and
Contractions—frequency, duration, and force of and
Fetal heart rate monitoring, continuous and
Heart rate and blood pressure determinations, maternal and
Uterine tone, resting
(recommended at frequent intervals during labor and delivery)

Fluid intake and output determinations
(recommended to reduce the risk of water intoxication, especially during prolonged administration of oxytocin)

## Side/Adverse Effects
The following side/adverse effects have been selected on the basis of their potential clinical significance (possible signs and symptoms in parentheses where appropriate)—not necessarily inclusive:

**Those indicating need for medical attention**
Incidence rare
*With nasal use*
***Psychotic reaction***—one case reported; *seizures*—one case reported; *unexpected uterine bleeding or contractions*

*With parenteral use*
***Afibrinogenemia or pelvic hematoma or postpartum hemorrhage*** (increased or continuing vaginal bleeding); ***allergy or*** (skin rash or itching; hives); ***generalized anaphylaxis*** (difficulty in breathing; skin rash or itching; hives); ***cardiac arrhythmias or premature ventricular contractions*** (fast or irregular heartbeat); ***hypotension*** (weakness; dizziness); *followed by hypertension and* (continuing or severe headache); ***reflexive tachycardia*** (fast heartbeat); ***uterine rupture*** (increased or continuing vaginal bleeding; severe pelvic or abdominal pain); ***water intoxication*** (seizures; coma; confusion; continuing headache; rapid weight gain)

Note: Fatal *allergic reactions* have occurred with the use of oxytocin.
*Hypotension* may be caused by administration of large doses or rapid intravenous infusion.
Maternal death due to *uterine rupture* has been reported to be associated with the parenteral administration of oxytocics for the induction or augmentation of labor.
Because of its slight antidiuretic effect, prolonged intravenous administration of oxytocin (usually in doses of 40 to 50 milliunits or more per minute) with large volumes of fluid may produce severe *water intoxication*. Maternal deaths due to hypertensive episodes and subarachnoid hemorrhage have been reported.

**Those indicating need for medical attention only if they continue or are bothersome**
Incidence rare
*With parenteral use*
***Nausea; vomiting***

*With nasal use*
***Lacrimation*** (tearing of the eyes); ***nasal irritation; rhinorrhea*** (runny nose)

## Patient Consultation
As an aid to patient consultation, refer to *Advice for the Patient, Oxytocin (Systemic)*.

In providing consultation, consider emphasizing the following selected information (» = major clinical significance):

**Before using this medication**
» Conditions affecting use, especially:
Allergy to oxytocin

**Proper use of this medication**
*For intranasal use only*
Proper administration
» Proper dosing

**Precautions while using this medication**
Possible therapeutic failure of nasal spray when used as lactation stimulant

**Side/adverse effects**
Signs of potential side effects, especially:
For parenteral use—Water intoxication, afibrinogenemia, pelvic hematoma, postpartum hemorrhage, anaphylaxis, allergy, cardiac arrhythmias, premature ventricular contractions, hypotension, and uterine rupture
For nasal use—Unexpected uterine bleeding or contractions, psychotic reaction, and seizures

## General Dosing Information
Patients receiving oxytocin should be hospitalized and under the supervision of a physician experienced in its use.

Therapeutic failure frequently occurs with the administration of nasal spray for stimulation of lactation.

**For parenteral dosage forms only**
Oxytocin must be diluted and administered by intravenous infusion for induction or stimulation of labor. Intramuscular administration of oxytocin is not recommended for induction or stimulation of labor, since intramuscular administration is difficult to regulate and may lead to uterine hyperactivity and fetal distress.

It is recommended that oxytocin infusion be administered intravenously by means of an infusion pump, a microdrip regulator, or a similar device to allow precise adjustment of the flow rate.

Dosage must be adjusted to meet the individual requirements of each patient, on the basis of maternal and fetal response.

Oxytocin should not be used simultaneously by more than one route.

**For treatment of adverse effects**
Oxytocin infusion should be discontinued or the rate of infusion decreased at the first sign of uterine hyperactivity or fetal distress. Supportive care, including administration of oxygen to the mother, is also recommended.

## Nasal Dosage Forms
### OXYTOCIN NASAL SOLUTION USP

**Usual adult dose**
Lactation stimulant—
Intranasal, 1 spray into one or both nostrils two to three minutes before nursing or pumping of breasts.

**Strength(s) usually available**
U.S.—
40 Units per mL (Rx) [*Syntocinon*].
Canada—
40 Units per mL (Rx) [*Syntocinon*].

**Packaging and storage**
Store below 40 °C (104 °F), preferably between 15 and 30 °C (59 and 86 °F), unless otherwise specified by manufacturer.

## Parenteral Dosage Forms
Note: Bracketed uses in the *Dosage Forms* section refer to categories of use and/or indications that are not included in U.S. product labeling.

# OXYTOCIN INJECTION USP

## Usual adult dose

**Augmentation or**
**Induction of labor—**

Intravenous infusion, initially no more than 0.5 to 2 milliunits per minute, increased every fifteen to sixty minutes in increments of 1 to 2 milliunits per minute until adequate uterine activity is established, up to 20 milliunits per minute (usually 2 to 5 milliunits per minute). Occasionally, doses higher than 20 milliunits per minute may be required.

The infusion rate may be reduced by similar increments, once labor is established.

**Abortion, incomplete (treatment) or**
**Abortion, therapeutic—**

Intravenous infusion, 10 Units at a rate of 20 to 40 milliunits per minute.

**Hemorrhage, postpartum (treatment)—**

Intravenous infusion, 10 Units at a rate of 20 to 40 milliunits per minute following delivery of the infant(s) and preferably the placenta(s).

Intramuscular, 10 Units after delivery of the placenta(s).

**Hemorrhage, postabortion (treatment)—**

Intravenous infusion, 10 Units at a rate of 20 to 100 milliunits per minute.

**[Utero-placental insufficiency (diagnosis)][1]—**

Intravenous infusion, initially 0.5 milliunits per minute, doubled every twenty minutes as necessary to the effective dose (usually 5 to 6 milliunits per minute). When three moderate uterine contractions (duration of forty to sixty seconds) occur in one ten-minute interval, the infusion is discontinued and baseline and oxytocin-induced fetal heart rate and uterine contraction patterns are compared.

## Strength(s) usually available

U.S.—

10 Units per mL (Rx) [*Pitocin; Syntocinon;* GENERIC].

Canada—

5 Units per mL (Rx) [*Syntocinon*].

10 Units per mL (Rx) [*Syntocinon*].

## Packaging and storage

Store below 40 °C (104 °F), preferably between 15 and 30 °C (59 and 86 °F), unless otherwise specified by manufacturer. Protect from freezing.

## Preparation of dosage form

For augmentation or induction of labor—Using standard aseptic technique, add 10 units of Oxytocin Injection USP to 1000 mL of normal saline (0.9% sodium chloride injection), lactated Ringer's solution, or other nonhydrating diluent. Final solution concentration is 10 milliunits per mL.

For control of postabortion or postpartum uterine bleeding—Using standard aseptic technique, add 10 to 40 units of Oxytocin Injection USP to 1000 mL of a nonhydrating diluent. Final solution concentration is 10 to 40 milliunits per mL.

---

[1]Not included in Canadian product labeling.

Revised: 07/14/93
Interim revision: 06/30/94

# PACLITAXEL    Systemic

VA CLASSIFICATION (Primary): AN900

Note: For a listing of dosage forms and brand names by country availability, see *Dosage Forms* section(s). For a listing of brand names for the articles in this monograph, refer to the General Index.

## Category
Antineoplastic.

## Indications

Note: Bracketed information in the *Indications* section refers to uses that are not included in the U.S. product labeling.

**Accepted**

Carcinoma, ovarian (treatment)—Paclitaxel is indicated for treatment of metastatic ovarian carcinoma after failure of first-line or subsequent chemotherapy.

[Carcinoma, breast (treatment)][1]—Paclitaxel is accepted for treatment of metastatic breast carcinoma, based upon reports of objective tumor responses, most of which were partial.

[Carcinoma, lung, non–small cell (treatment)][1]—Paclitaxel is accepted for treatment of non–small cell lung carcinoma, based upon reports of objective tumor responses, almost all of which were partial, in two small studies.

---

[1]Not included in Canadian product labeling.

## Pharmacology/Pharmacokinetics

Note: Pharmacokinetic studies were conducted in adult cancer patients who received single doses of 15–135 mg per square meter of body surface given by 1-hour infusions (15 patients), 30–275 mg per square meter of body surface given by 6-hour infusions (36 patients), and 135–275 mg per square meter of body surface given by 24-hour infusions (54 patients).

**Physicochemical characteristics**

Source—Natural. Extracted from the bark of the Pacific yew (*Taxus brevifolia*) tree.

Chemical group—Paclitaxel is a diterpenoid taxane.

Molecular weight—853.9.

**Mechanism of action/Effect**

Paclitaxel belongs to the class of medications known as antimicrotubule agents. It promotes the assembly of microtubules from tubulin dimers and stabilizes microtubules by preventing depolymerization. This stability results in the inhibition of the normal dynamic reorganization of the microtubule network that is essential for vital interphase and mitotic cellular functions. In addition, paclitaxel induces abnormal arrays or "bundles" of microtubules throughout the cell cycle and multiple asters of microtubules during mitosis.

**Other actions/effects**

Paclitaxel enhances the cytotoxic effects of ionizing radiation *in vitro*.

**Protein binding**

Very high (89–98%).

**Biotransformation**

Probably hepatic.

**Half-life**

Terminal—Mean (standard deviation): Range 5.3 (4.6) to 17.4 (4.7) hours, following 1-hour and 6-hour infusions at doses of 15–275 mg per square meter of body surface.

**Elimination**

Not completely understood. Mean (standard deviation) values for urinary recovery of unchanged drug following 1-, 6-, and 24-hour infusions at doses of 15–275 mg per square meter of body surface ranged from 1.3% (0.5%) to 12.6% (16.2%) of the dose, indicating extensive non-renal clearance. High concentrations of paclitaxel and metabolites have been reported in the bile.

The decline in plasma concentrations is biphasic; the initial rapid decline represents distribution to the peripheral compartment and significant elimination. The later phase is due, in part, to a relatively slow efflux from the peripheral compartment.

The mean (standard deviation) steady state volume of distribution ranged from 42 (15) to 162 (133) liters per square meter of body surface, indicating extensive extravascular distribution and/or tissue binding.

Mean (standard deviation) values for total body clearance following 24-hour infusions at doses of 200–275 mg per square meter of body surface ranged from 14.2 (2.3) to 17.2 (2.8) liters per hour per square meter of body surface.

## Precautions to Consider

**Cross-sensitivity and/or related problems**

Patients sensitive to polyoxyethylated castor oil may be sensitive to paclitaxel also, since the injection contains a polyoxyethylated castor oil vehicle.

**Carcinogenicity**

Studies with paclitaxel have not been done.

Secondary malignancies are potential delayed effects of many antineoplastic agents, although it is not clear whether the effect is related to their mutagenic or immunosuppressive action. The effect of dose and duration of therapy is also unknown, although risk seems to increase with long-term use. Although information is limited, available data seem to indicate that the carcinogenic risk is greatest with the alkylating agents.

**Mutagenicity**

Paclitaxel is mutagenic *in vitro* (chromosome aberrations in human lymphocytes) and *in vivo* (micronucleus test in mice) mammalian test systems. However, it was not mutagenic in the Ames test or the CHO/HGPRT gene mutation assay.

**Pregnancy/Reproduction**

Fertility—Studies in rats at doses of 1 mg per kg of body weight (mg/kg; 6 mg per square meter of body surface) found that paclitaxel reduced fertility.

Pregnancy—Adequate and well-controlled studies in women have not been done.

First trimester: It is usually recommended that use of antineoplastics, especially combination chemotherapy, be avoided whenever possible, especially during the first trimester. Although information is limited because of the relatively few instances of antineoplastic administration during pregnancy, the mutagenic, teratogenic, and carcinogenic potential of these medications must be considered.

Other hazards to the fetus include adverse reactions seen in adults.

In general, use of contraception is recommended during cytotoxic drug therapy.

Paclitaxel was found to be maternal and embryo-fetal toxic in rabbits at intravenous doses of 3 mg/kg (33 mg per square meter of body surface) given during organogenesis. In rats and rabbits, paclitaxel was found to produce abortions, decreased corpora lutea, a decrease in implantations and live fetuses, and increased resorptions and embryo-fetal deaths. No gross external, soft tissue, or skeletal alterations occurred.

FDA Pregnancy Category D.

**Breast-feeding**

Although very little information is available regarding distribution of antineoplastic agents into breast milk, breast-feeding is not recommended during chemotherapy because of the potential risks to the infant (adverse effects, mutagenicity, carcinogenicity). It is not known whether paclitaxel is distributed into breast milk.

**Pediatrics**

No information is available on the relationship of age to the effects of paclitaxel in pediatric patients, although phase I studies in children have been reported. Safety and efficacy have not been established.

**Geriatrics**

One retrospective study on the relationship of age to the effects of paclitaxel found no difference in dose intensity achieved.

**Dental**

The bone marrow depressant effects of paclitaxel may result in an increased incidence of microbial infection, delayed healing, and gingival bleeding. Dental work, whenever possible should be completed prior to initiation of therapy or deferred until blood counts have returned to normal. Patients should be instructed in proper oral hygiene during treatment, including caution in use of regular toothbrushes, dental floss, and toothpicks.

Paclitaxel also may cause mucositis, which is usually mild but which at high doses may be associated with considerable discomfort.

**Drug interactions and/or related problems**

The following drug interactions and/or related problems have been selected on the basis of their potential clinical significance (possible mechanism in parentheses where appropriate)—not necessarily inclusive (» = major clinical significance):

Note: Combinations containing any of the following medications, depending on the amount present, may also interact with this medication.

Blood dyscrasia–causing medications (See *Appendix II*)
(leukopenic and/or thrombocytopenic effects of paclitaxel may be increased with concurrent or recent therapy if these medications cause the same effects; dosage adjustment of paclitaxel, if necessary, should be based on blood counts)

» Bone marrow depressants, other (See *Appendix II*) or
Radiation therapy
(additive bone marrow depression may occur; dosage reduction may be required when two or more bone marrow depressants, including radiation, are used concurrently or consecutively)

(severity of paclitaxel-induced neutropenia may be related to the extent of prior myelotoxic therapy)

(in one Phase I study, administration of cisplatin before paclitaxel, rather than after, was found to reduce paclitaxel clearance by approximately 25%)

Vaccines, killed virus
(because normal defense mechanisms may be suppressed by paclitaxel therapy, the patient's antibody response to the vaccine may be decreased. The interval between discontinuation of medications that cause immunosuppression and restoration of the patient's ability to respond to the vaccine depends on the intensity and type of immunosuppression-causing medication used, the underlying disease, and other factors; estimates vary from 3 months to 1 year)

» Vaccines, live virus
(because normal defense mechanisms may be suppressed by paclitaxel therapy, concurrent use with a live virus vaccine may potentiate the replication of the vaccine virus, may increase the side/adverse effects of the vaccine virus, and/or may decrease the patient's antibody response to the vaccine; immunization of these patients should be undertaken only with extreme caution after careful review of the patient's hematologic status and only with the knowledge and consent of the physician managing the paclitaxel therapy. The interval between discontinuation of medications that cause immunosuppression and restoration of the patient's ability to respond to the vaccine depends on the intensity and type of immunosuppression-causing medication used, the underlying disease, and other factors; estimates vary from 3 months to 1 year. In addition, immunization with oral poliovirus vaccine should be postponed in persons in close contact with the patient, especially family members)

**Laboratory value alterations**
The following have been selected on the basis of their potential clinical significance (possible effect in parentheses where appropriate)—not necessarily inclusive (» = major clinical significance):

With physiology/laboratory test values
Alkaline phosphatase and
Aspartate aminotransferase (AST [SGOT]) and
Bilirubin
(serum values may be increased transiently; elevations of alkaline phosphatase and bilirubin may be dose-related)
Triglycerides
(elevations in serum concentrations have been reported)

**Medical considerations/Contraindications**
The medical considerations/contraindications included here have been selected on the basis of their potential clinical significance (reasons given in parentheses where appropriate)—not necessarily inclusive (» = major clinical significance).

*Risk-benefit should be considered when the following medical problems exist:*

» Bone marrow depression
(will be increased; it is recommended that paclitaxel not be administered when baseline neutrophil counts are lower than 1500 cells per cubic millimeter, and that subsequent doses not be administered until neutrophil counts have returned to greater than 1500 cells per cubic millimeter and platelet counts to greater than 100,000 cells per cubic millimeter or to baseline values)

Cardiac function impairment, including:
Angina
» Cardiac conduction abnormalities
Congestive heart failure, history of
Myocardial infarction within the past 6 months
(the patient's ability to tolerate the cardiovascular side effects of paclitaxel may be reduced)

» Chickenpox, existing or recent (including recent exposure) or
» Herpes zoster
(risk of severe generalized disease)

» Infection
» Sensitivity to paclitaxel
» Caution should be used also in patients who have had previous cytotoxic drug therapy or radiation therapy.

**Patient monitoring**
The following may be especially important in patient monitoring (other tests may be warranted in some patients, depending on condition; » = major clinical significance):

» Hematocrit or hemoglobin and
» Leukocyte count, total and, if appropriate, differential and
» Platelet count
(determinations recommended prior to initiation of therapy and at periodic intervals during therapy; frequency varies according to clinical state, agent, dose, and other agents being used concurrently)

» Vital signs
(recommended frequently, especially during the first hour of paclitaxel infusions)

## Side/Adverse Effects

Note: Neutropenia is the major dose-limiting effect.

The following side/adverse effects have been selected on the basis of their potential clinical significance (possible signs and symptoms in parentheses where appropriate)—not necessarily inclusive:

**Those indicating need for medical attention**
Incidence more frequent
*Anemia* (usually asymptomatic); *hypersensitivity reaction* (flushing of face; skin rash or itching; shortness of breath; rarely [with proper premedication], severe shortness of breath; severe skin reaction); *leukopenia or neutropenia, with or without infection* (fever or chills; cough or hoarseness; lower back or side pain; painful or difficult urination); *thrombocytopenia* (usually asymptomatic; less frequently, unusual bleeding or bruising; black, tarry stools; blood in urine or stools; pinpoint red spots on skin)

Note: Incidence and severity of *anemia* seem to increase with increasing exposure to paclitaxel.

With proper premedication, *hypersensitivity reactions* are usually mild (flushing of face, skin rash, shortness of breath). However, severe reactions (hypotension requiring treatment, dyspnea requiring bronchodilators, angioedema or generalized urticaria, chest pain) can occur, even with premedication, and necessitate immediate discontinuation of paclitaxel and aggressive symptomatic therapy. Severe symptoms usually occur within the first 10 minutes of paclitaxel infusion, after the first or second dose of paclitaxel. A fatal reaction occurred in a patient who was not premedicated. In general, it is recommended that paclitaxel not be readministered to patients who have experienced a severe hypersensitivity reaction. However, in patients with objective tumor responses and without other options to paclitaxel therapy, retreatment may be attempted with extreme caution and aggressive premedication by experienced practitioners.

Severe *neutropenia* (neutrophil count below 500 cells per cubic millimeter) is common but only infrequently persists for more than 7 days. The nadir of the neutrophil counts usually occurs at approximately Day 11 of paclitaxel therapy; in general, neutropenia is rapidly reversible, with recovery by Day 15 to 21. Cumulative neutropenia does not occur. The most common infections associated with neutropenia are urinary tract infections, upper respiratory infections, and sepsis. Fatalities have occurred from neutropenia-related sepsis.

In *thrombocytopenia*, the nadir of the platelet counts usually occurs at approximately Day 8 or 9 of paclitaxel therapy. Platelet counts generally do not fall below 100,000 cells per cubic millimeter. Hemorrhagic episodes may also be disease-related.

Incidence less frequent
*Cardiovascular effects, including bradycardia; hypotension; or abnormal electrocardiogram (ECG)* (usually asymptomatic); *elevated serum hepatic enzymes* (asymptomatic)

Note: *Cardiovascular effects* have also included more severe atrioventricular (AV) blocks, occasionally resulting in third-degree block requiring cardiac pacing. Atypical chest pains and a fatal myocardial infarction have also occurred, as well as asymptomatic bundle branch block and transient ventricular tachycardia, although the exact relationship to paclitaxel is unknown.

Incidence rare

*Extravasation, with phlebitis or cellulitis* (pain or redness at site of injection); *mucositis* (sores in mouth and on lips)

Note: Oropharyngeal *mucositis* is dose-related; it is infrequent or mild at usual recommended doses and usually resolves 5 to 7 days following treatment. However, esophageal and intestinal epithelial necrosis and ulceration have been reported.

### Those indicating need for medical attention only if they continue or are bothersome

Incidence more frequent

*Arthralgias or myalgias* (pain in joints or muscles, especially in arms or legs); *diarrhea; nausea and vomiting; peripheral neuropathy, including mild paresthesia* (numbness, burning, or tingling in hands or feet)

Note: *Arthralgias or myalgias* usually begin 2 to 3 days after treatment and resolve within 5 days. Pain is usually relieved by analgesics, but occasionally may be severe enough to require narcotics.

*Nausea and vomiting* are usually mild or moderate.

Incidence and severity of *peripheral neuropathy* are dose-related; at usual doses, a sensory neuropathy in a glove-and-stocking distribution occurs. Only rarely is withdrawal of paclitaxel necessary. Symptoms usually appear after multiple doses and improve or resolve within several months after paclitaxel is discontinued. High doses (over 250 mg per square meter of body surface) may cause dose-limiting motor and autonomic dysfunction, especially in patients with pre-existing neuropathies, beginning as early as 24 to 72 hours after treatment.

### Those not indicating need for medical attention

Incidence more frequent

*Loss of hair*

Note: Complete *loss of hair* (including scalp hair, eyebrows, eyelashes, and pubic hair) occurs in almost all patients between Days 14 and 21, but is reversible after therapy has ended.

## Patient Consultation

As an aid to patient consultation, refer to *Advice for the Patient, Paclitaxel (Systemic)*.

In providing consultation, consider emphasizing the following selected information (» = major clinical significance):

### Before using this medication

» Conditions affecting use, especially:

Sensitivity to paclitaxel

Pregnancy—Use not recommended because of mutagenic, teratogenic, and carcinogenic potential; advisability of using contraception; telling physician immediately if pregnancy is suspected

Breast-feeding—Not recommended because of risk of serious side effects

Other medications, especially other bone marrow depressants, or other cytotoxic drugs or radiation therapy

Other medical problems, especially cardiac conduction abnormalities, chickenpox, herpes zoster, or infection

### Proper use of this medication

Frequency of nausea and vomiting; importance of continuing medication despite stomach upset

» Proper dosing

### Precautions while using this medication

» Importance of close monitoring by the physician

» Avoiding immunizations unless approved by physician; other persons in patient's household should avoid immunizations with oral poliovirus vaccine; avoiding other persons who have taken oral poliovirus vaccine or wearing a protective mask that covers nose and mouth

*Caution if bone marrow depression occurs:*

» Avoiding exposure to persons with bacterial infections, especially during periods of low blood counts; checking with physician immediately if fever or chills, cough or hoarseness, lower back or side pain, or painful or difficult urination occur

» Checking with physician immediately if unusual bleeding or bruising; black, tarry stools; blood in urine or stools; or pinpoint red spots on skin occur

Caution in use of regular toothbrush, dental floss, or toothpick; physician, dentist, or nurse may suggest alternatives; checking with physician before having dental work done

Not touching eyes or inside of nose unless hands washed immediately before

Using caution to avoid accidental cuts with use of sharp objects such as safety razor or fingernail or toenail cutters

Avoiding contact sports or other situations where bruising or injury could occur

### Side/adverse effects

May cause adverse effects such as blood problems; importance of discussing possible effects with physician

Signs of potential side effects, especially hypersensitivity reaction, leukopenia or neutropenia, thrombocytopenia, extravasation, and mucositis

Asymptomatic side effects, including anemia, leukopenia or neutropenia, thrombocytopenia, cardiovascular effects, and elevated hepatic enzymes

Physician or nurse can help in dealing with side effects

Possibility of hair loss; hair should return after treatment has ended

## General Dosing Information

Patients receiving paclitaxel should be under supervision of a physician experienced in cancer chemotherapy.

It is recommended that patients receiving paclitaxel be under continuous observation for at least the first 30 minutes of the infusion and at frequent intervals after that. Equipment and medications (including epinephrine and oxygen) necessary for treatment of a possible anaphylactic reaction should be immediately available during each administration of paclitaxel.

*Paclitaxel concentrate for injection must be diluted before administration by intravenous infusion.*

The needle should be carefully positioned in the vein to avoid extravasation and resulting phlebitis and cellulitis.

In order to prevent severe hypersensitivity reactions, it is recommended that all patients be premedicated with corticosteroids (such as dexamethasone), diphenhydramine, and histamine $H_2$-receptor antagonists (such as cimetidine or ranitidine) (see *Parenteral Dosage Forms* for specific dosing).

Mild hypersensitivity symptoms (flushing, skin reactions, dyspnea, hypotension, tachycardia) do not require interruption of paclitaxel therapy. However, severe reactions (hypotension requiring treatment, dyspnea requiring bronchodilators, angioedema or generalized urticaria) require immediate withdrawal of paclitaxel and aggressive symptomatic therapy. It is generally recommended that paclitaxel administration not be repeated in patients who have experienced severe hypersensitivity reactions to the medication. However, in patients with objective tumor responses and without other options to paclitaxel therapy, retreatment may be attempted with extreme caution and aggressive premedication by experienced practitioners.

If severe peripheral neuropathy occurs, it is recommended that subsequent dosage of paclitaxel be reduced by 20%.

If significant cardiac conduction abnormalities occur during administration of paclitaxel, appropriate therapy is recommended, along with continuous cardiac monitoring during subsequent paclitaxel administration.

If severe neutropenia (neutrophil counts of less than 500 cells per cubic millimeter for seven days or more) occurs during a course of paclitaxel, it is recommended that the paclitaxel dose for subsequent courses be reduced by 20%.

Patients who develop leukopenia should be observed carefully for signs of infection. Antibiotic support may be required. In neutropenic patients who develop fever, broad-spectrum antibiotic coverage should be initiated empirically, pending bacterial cultures and appropriate diagnostic tests.

Special precautions are recommended in patients who develop thrombocytopenia as a result of administration of paclitaxel. These may include extreme care in performing invasive procedures; regular inspection of intravenous sites, skin (including perirectal area), and mucous membrane surfaces for signs of bleeding or bruising; limiting frequency of venipuncture and avoiding intramuscular injections; testing urine, emesis, stool, and secretions for occult blood; care in use of regular toothbrushes, dental floss, toothpicks, safety razors, and fingernail and toenail cutters; avoiding constipation; and using caution to prevent falls and other injuries. Such patients should avoid alcohol and aspirin intake because of the risk of gastrointestinal bleeding. Platelet transfusions may be required.

### Safety considerations for handling this medication

There is limited but increasing evidence and concern that personnel involved in preparation and administration of parenteral antineoplastics may be at some risk because of the potential mutagenicity, teratogenicity, and/or carcinogenicity of these agents, although the actual risk is unknown. USP advisory panels recommend cautious handling both

in preparation and disposal of antineoplastic agents. Precautions that have been suggested include:
• Use of a biological containment cabinet during reconstitution and dilution of parenteral medications and wearing of disposable surgical gloves and masks.
• Use of proper technique to prevent contamination of the medication, work area, and operator during transfer between containers (including proper training of personnel in this technique).
• Cautious and proper disposal of needles, syringes, vials, ampuls, and unused medication.
A number of medical centers have developed detailed guidelines for handling of antineoplastic agents.

## Parenteral Dosage Forms

### PACLITAXEL CONCENTRATE FOR INJECTION

**Usual adult dose**
Ovarian carcinoma—
Intravenous (as a twenty-four–hour infusion), 135 mg per square meter of body surface, repeated every twenty-one days. (Canadian product labeling recommends a dose of 170 mg per square meter of body surface as a twenty-four-hour intravenous infusion, repeated every twenty-one days.)

Note: To prevent severe hypersensitivity reactions, all patients should be premedicated with corticosteroids (e.g., dexamethasone 20 mg orally or intravenously approximately twelve and six hours prior to paclitaxel); diphenhydramine (e.g., 50 mg intravenously thirty to sixty minutes prior to paclitaxel) or its equivalent; and cimetidine (e.g., 300 mg intravenously thirty to sixty minutes prior to paclitaxel), ranitidine (e.g., 50 mg intravenously thirty to sixty minutes prior to paclitaxel), or famotidine (e.g., 20 mg intravenously thirty to sixty minutes prior to paclitaxel).

Contact of paclitaxel with plasticized polyvinyl chloride (PVC) equipment or devices must be avoided because of the risk of patient exposure to the plasticizer DEHP (di-[2-ethylhexyl]phthalate), which may be leached from PVC infusion bags or sets. Paclitaxel solutions should be diluted and stored in glass or polypropylene bottles or in plastic bags (polypropylene, polyolefin) and administered through polyethylene-lined administrations sets.

Paclitaxel intravenous infusion should be administered through an in-line filter with a microporous membrane not greater than 0.22 microns. Use of filter devices that incorporate short inlet and outlet PVC-coated tubing has not resulted in significant leaching of DEHP. Frequent changing of filters (e.g., every twelve hours) may be necessary because of clogging during the infusion.

**Usual pediatric dose**
Safety and efficacy have not been established.

**Strength(s) usually available**
U.S.—
6 mg per mL (5-mL vials) (Rx) [*Taxol* (polyoxyethylated castor oil 527 mg per mL; dehydrated alcohol USP 49.7% v/v)].
Canada—
6 mg per mL (5-mL vials) (Rx) [*Taxol* (polyoxyethylated castor oil 527 mg per mL; dehydrated alcohol USP 49.7% v/v)].

**Packaging and storage**
Store between 2 and 8 °C (36 and 46 °F), unless otherwise specified by manufacturer. Not adversely affected by freezing.

**Preparation of dosage form**
*Paclitaxel concentrate for injection must be diluted before administration.* Paclitaxel concentrate for injection is prepared for administration by intravenous infusion by diluting it to a concentration of 0.3 to 1.2 per mL in 5% dextrose injection, 0.9% sodium chloride injection, or 5% dextrose in Ringer's injection.

Note: Diluted solutions of paclitaxel may show haziness, which is attributed to the formulation vehicle.

**Stability**
Diluted solutions of paclitaxel are physically and chemically stable for up to 27 hours at ambient room temperature (approximately 25 °C) and room lighting conditions.

**Auxiliary labeling**
• Must be diluted prior to administration.

**Note**
If paclitaxel solution contacts the skin, the skin should be washed immediately and thoroughly with soap and water. If paclitaxel contacts mucous membranes, thorough flushing with water is recommended.

## Selected Bibliography

Rowinsky EK, Onetto N, Canetta RM, et al. Taxol: the first of the taxanes, an important new class of antitumor agents. Semin Oncol 1992 Dec; 19 (6): 646-62.
Einzig AI, Wiernik PH, Schwartz EL. Taxol: a new agent active in melanoma and ovarian cancer. In: Muggia FM, editor. New drugs concepts and results in cancer chemotherapy. Boston: Kluwer Academic Publishers, 1992: 89-100.

Revised: 09/15/93
Interim revision: 07/05/94

---

## PADIMATE O—See *Sunscreen Agents (Topical)*

---

## PADIMATE O–CONTAINING COMBINATIONS—

Aminobenzoic Acid, Padimate O, and Oxybenzone (Topical)—See *Sunscreen Agents (Topical)*
Dioxybenzone, Oxybenzone, and Padimate O (Topical)—See *Sunscreen Agents (Topical)*
Lisadimate, Oxybenzone, and Padimate O (Topical)—See *Sunscreen Agents (Topical)*
Lisadimate and Padimate O (Topical)—See *Sunscreen Agents (Topical)*
Menthyl Anthranilate and Padimate O (Topical)—See *Sunscreen Agents (Topical)*
Octyl Methoxycinnamate, Octyl Salicylate, Oxybenzone, and Padimate O (Topical)—See *Sunscreen Agents (Topical)*
Octyl Methoxycinnamate, Octyl Salicylate, Oxybenzone, Padimate O, and Titanium Dioxide (Topical)—See *Sunscreen Agents (Topical)*
Octyl Methoxycinnamate, Oxybenzone, and Padimate O (Topical)—See *Sunscreen Agents (Topical)*
Octyl Methoxycinnamate, Oxybenzone, Padimate O, and Titanium Dioxide (Topical)—See *Sunscreen Agents (Topical)*
Octyl Methoxycinnamate and Padimate O (Topical)—See *Sunscreen Agents (Topical)*
Octyl Salicylate and Padimate O (Topical)—See *Sunscreen Agents (Topical)*
Oxybenzone and Padimate O (Topical)—See *Sunscreen Agents (Topical)*

---

# PAMIDRONATE   Systemic

VA CLASSIFICATION (Primary): HS900
Another commonly used name is APD.
Note: For a listing of dosage forms and brand names by country availability, see *Dosage Forms* section(s). For a listing of brand names for the articles in this monograph, refer to the General Index.

---

## Category
Bone resorption inhibitor; antihypercalcemic.

## Indications
Note: Bracketed information in the *Indications* section refers to uses that are not included in U.S. product labeling.

**Accepted**
Hypercalcemia, associated with neoplasms (treatment)—Pamidronate disodium is indicated for the treatment of hypercalcemia of malignancy, with or without bone metastases, that is inadequately managed by oral hydration alone. It is used with saline hydration and may be used with loop diuretics.

Paget's disease of bone (treatment)—Pamidronate is indicated in the treatment of symptomatic Paget's disease (osteitis deformans), characterized by abnormal and accelerated bone metabolism in one or more bones. Signs and symptoms may include bone pain, deformity, and/or fractures; increased concentrations of serum alkaline phosphatase and/or urinary hydroxyproline; neurologic disorders associated with skull lesions and spinal deformities; and elevated cardiac output and other vascular disorders associated with increased vascularity of bones.

Metastases, osteolytic (treatment adjunct)[1]—Pamidronate is used in the treatment of osteolytic bone metastases sometimes found with [breast cancer] and myeloma.

### Unaccepted

The safety and efficacy of pamidronate disodium in the treatment of hypercalcemia associated with hyperparathyroidism or other nontumor-related conditions have not been established.

---

[1]Not included in Canadian product labeling.

## Pharmacology/Pharmacokinetics

### Physicochemical characteristics
Molecular weight—369.11.

### Mechanism of action/Effect
Pamidronate inhibits bone resorption and is believed to accomplish this by several mechanisms. It adsorbs onto the surface of hydroxyapatite crystals in mineralized bone matrix, thus reducing the solubility of the mineralized matrix and rendering it more resistant to osteoclastic resorption. By impairing attachment of osteoclast precursors to mineralized matrix, pamidronate blocks their transformation into mature, functioning osteoclasts.

Hypercalcemia of malignancy—Bone resorption is increased in the presence of neoplastic tissue. Pamidronate inhibits abnormal bone resorption and reduces the flow of calcium from the resorbing bone into the blood, effectively decreasing total and ionized serum calcium. When kidney function is adequate for the fluid load, hydration with saline increases urine output and the use of loop diuretics increases the rate of calcium excretion.

Paget's disease—Pamidronate reduces the rate of bone turnover, by an initial blocking of bone resorption, resulting in decreases in serum alkaline phosphatase (reflecting decreased bone formation) and decreases in urinary hydroxyproline excretion (reflecting decreased bone resorption, i.e., breakdown of collagen).

Osteolytic metastases—Osteolytic metastases result from accelerated bone resorption induced by the tumor via an activation of osteoclasts. By inhibiting bone resorption, pamidronate may reduce morbidity of bone metastases from breast cancer and myeloma.

### Distribution
In cancer patients, 45 to 53% of an intravenous dose of 60 mg infused over 24 hours is adsorbed to bone preferentially in areas of high turnover.

### Half-life
Alpha—1.6 hours.
Beta—27.2 hours.

### Elimination
51% of drug excreted unchanged in urine within 24 hours after an intravenous dose of 60 mg infused over 4 to 24 hours.

## Precautions to Consider

### Cross-sensitivity and/or related problems
Patients sensitive to any bisphosphonate may also be sensitive to pamidronate.

### Carcinogenicity
A 104-week carcinogenicity study with daily oral pamidronate administration in rats found a positive dose-response relationship for benign adrenal pheochromocytoma in males. The condition was observed in females, but was not statistically significant. Another 80-week study in mice found that daily oral pamidronate administration was not carcinogenic.

### Mutagenicity
Pamidronate was nonmutagenic in the Ames test, nucleus-anomaly test, sister-chromatid-exchange study, and point-mutation test.

### Pregnancy/Reproduction
Fertility—In rats, decreased fertility occurred in first-generation offspring of parents who had received 150 mg of oral pamidronate per kg of body weight (mg/kg). This occurred only when animals were mated with members of the same dose group.

Pregnancy—Adequate and well-controlled studies have not been done in pregnant women.

Adequate and well-controlled studies with intravenous pamidronate have not been done in animals. However, oral doses of 60 and 150 mg/kg of body weight a day increased the length of gestation and parturition in rats and increased pup mortality. Oral doses of 25 to 150 mg/kg a

day during gestation failed to demonstrate any teratogenic, fetotoxic, or embryotoxic effects in rats or rabbits.

FDA Pregnancy Category C.

### Breast-feeding
It is not known if pamidronate is distributed into breast milk.

### Pediatrics
No information is available on the relationship of age to the effects of pamidronate in pediatric patients. Safety and efficacy have not been established.

### Geriatrics
Appropriate studies have not been performed in the geriatric population. However, elderly patients may be more prone to overhydration when treated with parenteral pamidronate in conjunction with hydration therapy. Careful monitoring of fluid and electrolyte status or infusing pamidronate in a smaller volume of fluid is recommended.

### Drug interactions and/or related problems
The following drug interactions and/or related problems have been selected on the basis of their potential clinical significance (possible mechanism in parentheses where appropriate)—not necessarily inclusive (» = major clinical significance):

Note: Combinations containing any of the following, depending on the amount present, may also interact with this medication.

» Calcium-containing preparations or
» Vitamin D, including calcifediol and calcitriol
    (concurrent use may antagonize the effects of pamidronate in the treatment of hypercalcemia)

### Medical considerations/Contraindications
The medical considerations/contraindications included here have been selected on the basis of their potential clinical significance (reasons given in parentheses where appropriate)—not necessarily inclusive (» = major clinical significance).

*Risk-benefit should be considered when the following medical problems exist:*

» Cardiac failure
    (overhydration should be avoided when pamidronate is used in patients with cardiac failure; infusing pamidronate in a smaller volume of fluid is recommended)

» Renal function impairment when serum creatinine is 5 mg per dL or greater
    (pamidronate is excreted via the kidneys; use of pamidronate in patients with renal function impairment may require a lower dose and slower rate of infusion)

### Patient monitoring
The following may be especially important in patient monitoring (other tests may be warranted in some patients, depending on condition; » = major clinical significance):

Alkaline phosphatase concentrations serum
    (determinations recommended periodically during therapy for Paget's disease as a marker for disease activity)

Calcium, serum and
Magnesium, serum and
Phosphate, serum and
Potassium, serum
    (determinations recommended periodically during therapy; some clinicians recommend monitoring serum magnesium and potassium concentrations only with concurrent diuretic use; serum ionized calcium concentrations are preferable to determine free and bound calcium, but may not be available from a reliable lab)

Complete blood count with differential and
Hematocrit and
Hemoglobin
    (determinations recommended periodically during therapy, especially for patients who develop fever during pamidronate use; patients with pre-existing anemia, leukopenia, or thrombocytopenia should be carefully monitored for the first 2 weeks of therapy)

Creatinine, serum and
Renal function
    (determinations recommended periodically during therapy; if serum creatinine exceeds 5 mg per dL, risk-benefit of continued treatment or reduction of dosage should be considered)

## Side/Adverse Effects

Note: Fluid overload, hypokalemia, hypomagnesemia, and hypophosphatemia may occur due to concurrent fluid and diuretic use.

The following side/adverse effects have been selected on the basis of their potential clinical significance (possible signs and symptoms in parentheses where appropriate)—not necessarily inclusive:

**Those indicating need for medical attention**
Incidence more frequent
*Hypocalcemia* (abdominal cramps; confusion; muscle spasms); *leukopenia or lymphopenia* (fever, chills, or sore throat)
Note: *Hypocalcemia* occurs less frequently when doses of 60 mg, rather than 90 mg, are used.

**Those indicating need for medical attention only if they continue or are bothersome**
Incidence more frequent—at higher doses
*Fever, transient; nausea; pain and swelling at injection site*
Incidence less frequent
*Muscle stiffness*

## Overdose

For specific information on the agents used in the management of pamidronate overdose, see:
• *Calcium Supplements (Systemic)* monograph.

For more information on the management of overdose or unintentional ingestion, **contact a Poison Control Center** (see *Poison Control Center Listing*).

**Specific treatment**
Hypocalcemia resulting from overdose should be treated with intravenous calcium.

## Patient Consultation

As an aid to patient consultation, refer to *Advice for the Patient, Pamidronate (Systemic)*.

In providing consultation, consider emphasizing the following selected information (» = major clinical significance):

**Before using this medication**
» Conditions affecting use, especially:
Sensitivity to etidronate or pamidronate
Use in the elderly—Elderly patients may be more prone to overhydration when treated with pamidronate in conjunction with hydration therapy
Other medications, especially calcium- and vitamin D–containing preparations
Other medical problems, especially cardiac failure and renal function impairment

**Proper use of this medication**
» Proper dosing

**Precautions while using this medication**
Importance of close monitoring by physician
*For patients with hypercalcemia*
Possible need for calcium and vitamin D restriction, including calcifediol and calcitriol

**Side/adverse effects**
Signs of potential adverse effects, especially hypocalcemia, leukopenia, and lymphopenia

## General Dosing Information

The U.S. product manufacturer recommends that the daily dose of pamidronate be reconstituted and diluted in 1000 mL of 0.45% or 0.9% sodium chloride or 5% dextrose injection. The Canadian products should be reconstituted and diluted in 0.9% sodium chloride or 5% dextrose injection to a maximum concentration of 30 mg of pamidronate per 250 mL of solution. The diluted dose should be administered over a period of 24 hours. However, some clinicians recommend that the daily dose be diluted in as little as 500 mL of fluid and administered over 4 to 24 hours.

Fluid overload, hypokalemia, hypomagnesemia, and hypophosphatemia may occur due to concurrent fluid and diuretic use.

## Parenteral Dosage Forms

Note: Bracketed information in the *Indications* section refers to uses that are not included in the U.S. product labeling.

### PAMIDRONATE DISODIUM FOR INJECTION

**Usual adult dose**
Hypercalcemia—
Intravenous infusion, 60 mg administered over a period of four to twenty-four hours.
Note: Patients with renal failure or mild hypercalcemia may receive 30 mg of pamidronate over a period of four to twenty-four hours.

Patients with more severe hypercalcemia (corrected serum calcium greater than 13.5 mg per dL) may receive 90 mg of pamidronate over a period of twenty-four hours. Retreatment with pamidronate may be considered if hypercalcemia recurs; however, seven days should elapse before retreatment.
Paget's disease of bone (treatment)—
Intravenous infusion, a total dose of 90 to 180 mg per treatment period, administered at a rate of 15 mg per hour. Dosage may be administered between the range of 30 mg per day on three consecutive days up to 30 mg once a week for six weeks. Alternatively, three doses of 60 mg may be administered every second week. The regimen may need to be repeated in some patients.
Note: Some clinicians have found that a single dose of 60 to 90 mg is effective in some cases.
Osteolytic metastases (treatment adjunct)—
In myeloma[1] or
In [breast cancer][1]—
Intravenous infusion, 90 mg over a period of two to four hours once a month

**Usual pediatric dose**
Safety and efficacy have not been established.

**Strength(s) usually available**
U.S.—
30 mg per vial (Rx) [*Aredia*].
60 mg per vial (Rx) [*Aredia*].
90 mg per vial (Rx) [*Aredia*].
Canada—
30 mg per vial (Rx) [*Aredia*].
60 mg per vial (Rx) [*Aredia*].
90 mg per vial (Rx) [*Aredia*].

**Packaging and storage**
Store below 40 °C (104 °F), preferably between 15 and 30 °C (59 and 86 °F), unless otherwise specified by manufacturer. Protect from freezing.

**Preparation of dosage form**
Each vial should be reconstituted with 10 mL of sterile water for injection. The daily dose should then be diluted in 1000 mL of 0.45% or 0.9% sodium chloride or 5% dextrose injection.

**Stability**
The diluted infusion solution is stable for 24 hours at room temperature.

**Incompatibilities**
Pamidronate should not be mixed with calcium-containing infusion solutions, such as Ringer's solution.

---

[1]Not included in Canadian product labeling.

## Selected Bibliography

Fitton A, McTavish D. Pamidronate: a review of its pharmacological properties and therapeutic efficacy in resorptive bone diseases. Drugs 1991; 41[2]: 289-318.

---

Developed: 06/02/93
Interim revision: 08/07/95; 06/07/96

# PANCRELIPASE Systemic

VA CLASSIFICATION (Primary): GA500

Another commonly used name is lipancreatin.

Note: For a listing of dosage forms and brand names by country availability, see *Dosage Forms* section(s). For a listing of brand names for the articles in this monograph, refer to the General Index.

## Category

Enzyme (pancreatic) replenisher; digestant; diagnostic aid (pancreatic function).

## Indications

Note: Bracketed information in the *Indications* section refers to uses that are not included in U.S. product labeling.

### Accepted

Pancreatic insufficiency (treatment)—Pancrelipase is indicated as a pancreatic enzyme supplement and replacement therapy in conditions where pancreatic enzymes are either absent or deficient, resulting in inadequate fat and carbohydrate digestion. Such conditions are usually due to chronic pancreatitis, pancreatectomy, cystic fibrosis, gastrointestinal bypass surgery (Billroth II and total), and ductal obstruction from neoplasm (of the pancreas or common bile duct).

Steatorrhea (treatment)—Indicated for treating steatorrhea associated with the postgastrectomy syndrome and bowel resection, and for decreasing malabsorption in these patients.

[Pancreatic insufficiency (diagnosis)][1]—Pancrelipase is used as a presumptive test for pancreatic function, especially in pancreatic insufficiency due to chronic pancreatitis.

### Unaccepted

Pancrelipase is not effective in the treatment of gastrointestinal disorders unrelated to pancreatic enzyme insufficiency.

---

[1]Not included in Canadian product labeling.

## Pharmacology/Pharmacokinetics

### Mechanism of action/Effect

Proteolytic, amylolytic, and lipolytic enzymes in pancrelipase enhance the digestion of proteins, starches, and fats in the gastrointestinal tract, primarily in the duodenum and upper jejunum. The activity of pancrelipase is greater in neutral or faintly alkaline media. Pancrelipase has about 12 times the lipolytic activity, 4 times the proteolytic activity, and 4 times the amylolytic activity of pancreatin.

The efficacy of pancrelipase activity is dependent on how much of the enzyme reaches the small intestine. This can be influenced by the enzyme dose, the prevention of release of pancrelipase in the stomach, the microsphere size of the delayed-release product, and the pH at which the microsphere dissolves and releases the enzyme, with activity being greater at a neutral or alkaline pH.

## Precautions to Consider

### Cross-sensitivity and/or related problems

Patients sensitive to pancreatin or pork protein may be sensitive to this medication also.

### Pregnancy/Reproduction

Pregnancy—Studies have not been done in humans.

Studies have not been done in animals.

FDA Pregnancy Category C.

### Breast-feeding

It is not known whether pancrelipase is distributed into breast milk. However, problems in humans have not been documented.

### Pediatrics

Appropriate studies on the relationship of age to the effects of pancrelipase have not been performed in children up to 6 months of age.

### Geriatrics

Appropriate studies on the relationship of age to the effects of pancrelipase have not been performed in the geriatric population. However, geriatrics-specific problems that would limit the usefulness of this medication in the elderly are not expected.

### Drug interactions and/or related problems

The following drug interactions and/or related problems have been selected on the basis of their potential clinical significance (possible mechanism in parentheses where appropriate)—not necessarily inclusive (» = major clinical significance):

Note: Combinations containing any of the following medications, depending on the amount present, may also interact with this medication.

Antacids, calcium carbonate– and/or magnesium hydroxide–containing (concurrent administration of antacids may be required to prevent inactivation of pancrelipase [except the enteric-coated dosage forms] by gastric pepsin and acid pH; however, calcium carbonate– and/or magnesium hydroxide–containing antacids are not recommended since they may decrease the effectiveness of pancrelipase)

Iron, supplements or preparations (iron absorption may be decreased when used concurrently with pancrelipase)

### Laboratory value alterations

The following have been selected on the basis of their potential clinical significance (possible effect in parentheses where appropriate)—not necessarily inclusive (» = major clinical significance):

With physiology/laboratory test values

Uric acid (blood and urine concentrations may be increased; ribonuclease present in pancreatic extracts catalyzes the formation of purine precursors of uric acid, thus increasing the risk of hyperuricosuria, especially with large doses of the purine-rich older formulations of pancrelipase)

### Medical considerations/Contraindications

The medical considerations/contraindications included here have been selected on the basis of their potential clinical significance (reasons given in parentheses where appropriate)—not necessarily inclusive (» = major clinical significance).

*Except under special circumstances, this medication should not be used if the following medical problems exist:*

» Pancreatitis, acute

» Sensitivity to pork protein, pancrelipase, or pancreatin

## Side/Adverse Effects

The following side/adverse effects have been selected on the basis of their potential clinical significance (possible signs and symptoms in parentheses where appropriate)—not necessarily inclusive:

### Those indicating need for medical attention

Incidence rare

*Allergic reaction* (skin rash or hives); *irritation of the mouth*—induced by enzymatic digestion of mucous membranes when tablet dosage form is retained in mouth; *sensitization* (shortness of breath; stuffy nose; troubled breathing; wheezing; tightness in chest)—induced by repeated inadvertent inhalation of powder dosage form or the powder from opened capsules

With high doses

*Gastrointestinal effects, specifically diarrhea; intestinal obstruction; nausea; stomach cramps or pain; hyperuricemia or hyperuricosuria* (blood in urine; joint pain; swelling of feet or lower legs)—more frequent with extremely high doses of the purine-rich older formulations of pancrelipase

Note: There have been reports of gastrointestinal stricture requiring surgery in cystic fibrosis patients receiving high potency pancrelipase for 12 months or longer. The pathogenesis is unknown at this time. The U. S. Food and Drug Administration has issued a voluntary recall of pancrelipase products that contain greater than 20,000 Units of lipase.

## Patient Consultation

As an aid to patient consultation, refer to *Advice for the Patient, Pancrelipase (Systemic)*.

In providing consultation, consider emphasizing the following selected information (» = major clinical significance):

### Before using this medication

» Conditions affecting use, especially:
   Sensitivity to pork protein, pancrelipase, or pancreatin
   Other medical problems, especially acute pancreatitis

### Proper use of this medication

Taking dose before or with meals for maximum effectiveness

» Importance of following diet ordered by physician

»   Not chewing tablets; swallowing them quickly with liquid to lessen potential for mouth irritation

     Not chewing or crushing capsules containing enteric-coated spheres

»   Proper dosing

     Missed dose: Not taking missed dose at all; not doubling doses

»   Proper storage

### Precautions while using this medication

     Possible concurrent use with antacids that contain calcium carbonate and/or magnesium hydroxide

     Not changing brands or dosage forms of pancrelipase without checking with physician

     Possible sensitization resulting from repeated inhalation of powder, either from opened capsules or from powder dosage form

### Side/adverse effects

     Signs of potential side effects, especially allergic reaction, hyperuricemia or hyperuricosuria (with extremely high doses); gastrointestinal effects; irritation of mucous membranes; and respiratory problems (with inhalation of powder)

## General Dosing Information

The destruction of pancrelipase's enzymes by gastric pepsin or their inactivation by acid pH may be prevented by the use of enteric-coated dosage forms, particularly the enteric-coated spheres. Or, if dosage forms of pancrelipase which are not enteric-coated are used, the gastric and duodenal pH may be raised instead by the concurrent administration of sodium bicarbonate, aluminum hydroxide, histamine $H_2$-receptor antagonists, misoprostol, or omeprazole (also, antacid, $H_2$-receptor antagonist, misoprostol, or omeprazole administration may be necessary in patients with deficient pancreatic bicarbonate secretion for the control of steatorrhea). An $H_2$-receptor antagonist administered with meals may be preferred instead of antacids, especially in patients with high rates of acid secretion.

Dosage should be individualized and determined by the degree of maldigestion and malabsorption, the fat content of the diet, and the enzyme activity of each preparation rather than by the weight of the extract. Ideally, a starting dose of 8,000 to 10,000 Units of lipase should be given with each meal.

To avoid irritation of the mouth, lips, and tongue, the tablets should not be chewed. Instead, the tablets should be swallowed quickly, preferably with some liquid, since proteolytic enzymes (trypsin and chymotrypsin) present in pancrelipase, when retained in the mouth may begin to digest the mucous membranes and cause ulcerations.

Retention of the tablet dosage form in the esophagus may occur in some patients with esophageal abnormalities or in patients taking the tablet in a recumbent position. To decrease the likelihood of mucous membrane digestion, 1 or 2 mouthfuls of solid food should be swallowed after each dose.

### Diet/Nutrition

Pancrelipase should preferably be taken before or with meals for maximum effectiveness.

In pancreatic insufficiency, a high-calorie diet which is high in protein and low in fat is recommended. In severe cases, higher doses of pancrelipase and dietary adjustment may be necessary. Some clinicians recommend that cystic fibrosis patients consume a liberal fat diet along with an increase in pancelipase dosage to ensure adequate energy intake.

Capsule dosage forms may be opened and sprinkled on food for administration to young children. However, capsules containing the enteric-coated spheres should be taken with liquids or small amounts of soft foods (e.g., applesauce, gelatin) that do not require chewing.

### Bioequivalence information

The microsphere size of the delayed-release product, among other factors, determines how much of the enzyme reaches the small intestine. It has been found that some delayed-release pancrelipase products provide higher levels of enzyme activity than labeled. Since substitution of one manufacturer's delayed-release product for another may sometimes be accompanied by therapeutic failure, caution should be exercised in substituting.

## Oral Dosage Forms

### PANCRELIPASE CAPSULES USP

#### Usual adult and adolescent dose

Enzyme (pancreatic) replenisher and

Digestant—

     Oral, 1 to 3 capsules before or with meals and snacks, the dosage being adjusted as needed and tolerated.

#### Usual pediatric dose

Enzyme (pancreatic) replenisher and

Digestant—

     Oral, contents of 1 to 3 capsules with meals, the dosage being adjusted as needed and tolerated.

#### Usual geriatric dose

See *Usual adult and adolescent dose.*

#### Strength(s) usually available

U.S.—

     8000 USP Units of lipase, 30,000 USP Units of protease, and 30,000 USP Units of amylase, per capsule (Rx) [*Cotazym* (calcium carbonate 25 mg); *Ku-Zyme HP*].

Canada—

     8000 USP Units of lipase, 30,000 USP Units of protease, and 30,000 USP Units of amylase, per capsule (Rx) [*Cotazym; Cotazym-65 B* (bile salts 65 mg; cellulase 2 mg)].

#### Packaging and storage

Store below 25 °C (77 °F), in a tight container, unless otherwise specified by manufacturer. Store with a desiccant.

#### Auxiliary labeling

• Take before or with meals.

• If capsules are opened, do not inhale powder.

### PANCRELIPASE DELAYED-RELEASE CAPSULES

Note: Substitution of one manufacturer's delayed-release product for another has resulted in therapeutic failure.

#### Usual adult and adolescent dose

Enzyme (pancreatic) replenisher and

Digestant—

     Oral, 1 or 2 capsules before or with meals and snacks, the dosage being adjusted as needed and tolerated.

#### Usual pediatric dose

Enzyme (pancreatic) replenisher and

Digestant—

     Oral, contents of 1 or 2 capsules with meals, the dosage being adjusted as needed and tolerated.

Note: Contents of capsules containing the enteric-coated spheres should be taken with liquids or a small amount of soft foods that do not require chewing.

#### Usual geriatric dose

See *Usual adult and adolescent dose.*

#### Strength(s) usually available

U.S.—

     4000 USP Units of lipase, 12,000 USP Units of protease, and 12,000 USP Units of amylase, per capsule (Rx) [*Pancrease MT 4*].

     4000 USP Units of lipase, 25,000 USP Units of protease, and 20,000 USP Units of amylase, per capsule (Rx) [*Pancoate; Pancrease; Protilase;* GENERIC].

     5000 USP Units of lipase, 20,000 USP Units of protease, and 20,000 USP Units of amylase, per capsule (Rx) [*Cotazym-S*].

     10,000 USP Units of lipase, 30,000 USP Units of protease, and 30,000 USP Units of amylase, per capsule (Rx) [*Pancrease MT 10*].

     12,000 USP Units of lipase, 24,000 USP Units of protease, and 24,000 USP Units of amylase, per capsule (Rx) [*Zymase*].

     12,000 USP Units of lipase; 39,000 USP Units of protease, and 39,000 USP Units of amylase, per capsule (Rx) [*Ultrase MT 12*].

     16,000 USP Units of lipase, 48,000 USP Units of protease, and 48,000 USP Units of amylase, per capsule (Rx) [*Enzymase-16; Pancrease MT 16;* GENERIC].

     20,000 USP Units of lipase, 44,000 USP Units of protease, and 56,000 USP Units of amylase, per capsule (Rx) [*Pancrease MT 20*].

     20,000 USP Units of lipase, 65,000 USP Units of protease, and 65,000 USP Units of amylase, per capsule (Rx) [*Ultrase MT 20*].

Canada—

     4000 USP Units of lipase, 12,000 USP Units of protease, and 12,000 USP Units of amylase, per capsule (Rx) [*Pancrease MT 4*].

     4000 USP Units of lipase, 25,000 USP Units of protease, and 20,000 USP Units of amylase, per capsule (Rx) [*Pancrease*].

     8000 USP Units of lipase, 30,000 USP Units of protease, and 30,000 USP Units of amylase, per capsule (Rx) [*Cotazym E.C.S. 8*].

     10,000 USP Units of lipase, 30,000 USP Units of protease, and 30,000 USP Units of amylase, per capsule (Rx) [*Pancrease MT 10*].

     16,000 USP Units of lipase, 48,000 USP Units of protease, and 48,000 USP Units of amylase, per capsule (Rx) [*Pancrease MT 16*].

     20,000 USP Units of lipase, 55,000 USP Units of protease, and 55,000 USP Units of amylase, per capsule (Rx) [*Cotazym E.C.S. 20*].

**Packaging and storage**
Store below 25 °C (77 °F), in a tight container, unless otherwise specified by manufacturer. Store with a desiccant.

**Auxiliary labeling**
• Take before or with meals.
• Do not chew or crush (for capsules containing the enteric-coated spheres only).

## PANCRELIPASE POWDER

**Usual adult and adolescent dose**
Enzyme (pancreatic) replenisher and
Digestant—
    Oral, 0.7 gram with meals and snacks, the dosage being adjusted as needed and tolerated.

**Usual pediatric dose**
Enzyme (pancreatic) replenisher and
Digestant—
    Oral, 0.7 gram with meals, the dosage being adjusted as needed and tolerated.

**Usual geriatric dose**
See *Usual adult and adolescent dose.*

**Strength(s) usually available**
U.S.—
    16,800 USP Units of lipase, 70,000 USP Units of protease, and 70,000 USP Units of amylase, per 0.7 gram (Rx) [*Viokase*].
Canada—
    Not commercially available.

**Packaging and storage**
Store below 25 °C (77 °F), unless otherwise specified by manufacturer.

**Auxiliary labeling**
• Take with meals.
• Do not inhale.

## PANCRELIPASE TABLETS USP

**Usual adult and adolescent dose**
Enzyme (pancreatic) replenisher and
Digestant—
    Oral, 1 to 3 tablets before or with meals and snacks, the dosage being adjusted as needed and tolerated.

**Usual pediatric dose**
Enzyme (pancreatic) replenisher and
Digestant—
    Oral, 1 or 2 tablets with meals.

**Usual geriatric dose**
See *Usual adult and adolescent dose.*

**Strength(s) usually available**
U.S.—
    8000 USP Units of lipase, 30,000 USP Units of protease, and 30,000 USP Units of amylase, per tablet (Rx) [*Panokase; Viokase*].
    11,000 USP Units of lipase, 30,000 USP Units of protease, and 30,000 USP Units of amylase, per tablet (Rx) [*Ilozyme*].
Canada—
    Not commercially available.

**Packaging and storage**
Store below 25 °C (77 °F), in a tight container, unless otherwise specified by manufacturer. Store with a desiccant.

**Auxiliary labeling**
• Take before or with meals.
• Do not chew.

Revised: 02/13/92
Interim revision: 08/01/94; 08/01/95

---

**PANCURONIUM**—See *Neuromuscular Blocking Agents (Systemic)*

---

# PANTOTHENIC ACID    Systemic†

VA CLASSIFICATION (Primary): VT107
Other commonly used names are vitamin B₅ and calcium pantothenate.
Note: For a listing of dosage forms and brand names by country availability, see *Dosage Forms* section(s). For a listing of brand names for the articles in this monograph, refer to the General Index.

    †Not commercially available in Canada.

## Category
Nutritional supplement (vitamin).
Note: Pantothenic acid (vitamin B₅) is a water-soluble vitamin.

## Indications
### Accepted
Pantothenic acid deficiency (prophylaxis and treatment)—The B vitamins are indicated for prevention and treatment of vitamin B deficiency. Vitamin B deficiency may occur as a result of inadequate nutrition or intestinal malabsorption but does not occur in healthy individuals receiving an adequate balanced diet. Simple nutritional deficiency of individual B vitamins is rare since dietary inadequacy usually results in multiple deficiencies. For prophylaxis of pantothenic acid deficiency, dietary improvement, rather than supplementation, is advisable. For treatment of pantothenic acid deficiency, supplementation is preferred.

There is no indication for pantothenic acid alone, since deficiency is virtually unknown except with administration of pantothenic acid antagonists, which may result in burning foot syndrome. Requirements may be increased in malabsorption syndromes such as tropical sprue, celiac disease, or regional enteritis.

### Unaccepted
Pantothenic acid has not been proven effective for treatment of diabetic neuropathy; preventing gray hair or restoring its color; improvement of mental processes; increasing gastrointestinal peristalsis; prevention of arthritis, Addison's disease, or allergies; prevention of birth defects and some respiratory disorders; relief of itching and healing of minor dermatoses (topical); or treatment of streptomycin and salicylate toxicities.

## Pharmacology/Pharmacokinetics

**Physicochemical characteristics**
Molecular weight—Calcium pantothenate: 476.54.

**Mechanism of action/Effect**
Pantothenic acid is a precursor of coenzyme A and is required for various metabolic functions, including metabolism of carbohydrates, proteins, and lipids. It is also used in the synthesis of steroids, porphyrins, acetylcholine, and other substances. Pantothenic acid may also be necessary for normal epithelial function.

**Absorption**
The B vitamins are readily absorbed from the gastrointestinal tract, except in malabsorption syndromes.

**Distribution**
Pantothenic acid is distributed into body tissues mainly as coenzyme A. Highest concentrations are found in the liver, adrenal glands, heart, and kidneys.

**Biotransformation**
Pantothenic acid is not metabolized.

**Elimination**
Renal, 70% (unchanged).
Fecal, 30%.

## Precautions to Consider

**Pregnancy/Reproduction**
Pregnancy—Problems in humans have not been documented with intake of normal daily recommended amounts.

**Breast-feeding**
Problems in humans have not been documented with intake of normal daily recommended amounts.

**Pediatrics**
Problems in pediatrics have not been documented with intake of normal daily recommended amounts.

**Geriatrics**
Problems in geriatrics have not been documented with intake of normal daily recommended amounts.

## Side/Adverse Effects

No side effects have been reported with pantothenic acid.

## Patient Consultation

As an aid to patient consultation, refer to *Advice for the Patient, Pantothenic Acid (Vitamin B₅) (Systemic)*.

In providing consultation, consider emphasizing the following selected information (» = major clinical significance):

**Description of use**
Description should include function in the body, signs of deficiency, and unproven uses

**Importance of diet**
Importance of proper nutrition; supplement may be needed because of inadequate dietary intake
Food sources of pantothenic acid; effects of processing
Not using vitamins as substitute for balanced diet
Recommended daily intake for pantothenic acid

**Proper use of this dietary supplement**
» Proper dosing
Missed dose: No cause for concern because of length of time necessary for depletion; remembering to take as directed
» Proper storage

## General Dosing Information

Because of the infrequency of single B vitamin deficiencies, combinations are commonly administered. Many commercial combinations of B vitamins are available.

Each 10 mg of calcium pantothenate is equivalent to 9.2 mg of pantothenic acid.

**Diet/Nutrition**
Recommended dietary intakes for pantothenic acid are defined differently worldwide.
For U.S.—
The Recommended Dietary Allowances (RDAs) for vitamins and minerals are determined by the Food and Nutrition Board of the National Research Council and are intended to provide adequate nutrition in most healthy persons under usual environmental stresses. In addition, a different designation may be used by the FDA for food and dietary supplement labeling purposes, as with Daily Value (DV). DVs replace the previous labeling terminology United States Recommended Daily Allowances (USRDAs).
For Canada—
Recommended Nutrient Intakes (RNIs) for vitamins, minerals, and protein are determined by Health and Welfare Canada and provide recommended amounts of a specific nutrient while minimizing the risk of chronic diseases.
There is no RDA or RNI established for pantothenic acid. The following daily intakes are considered adequate for all individuals—
Infants and children:
Birth to 3 years of age: 2–3 mg.
4 to 6 years of age: 3–4 mg.
7 to 10 years of age: 4–5 mg.
Adolescents and adults:
4–7 mg.
The best dietary sources of pantothenic acid include peas and beans (except green beans), lean meat, poultry, fish, and whole-grain cereals. There is little loss of pantothenic acid from foods with ordinary cooking.

## Oral Dosage Forms

### CALCIUM PANTOTHENATE TABLETS USP

Note: The dosing and strengths of the dosage forms available are expressed in terms of pantothenic acid (not the calcium salt).

**Usual adult and adolescent dose**
Deficiency (prophylaxis)—
Oral, amount based on normal daily recommended intakes of 4 to 7 mg (base).
Deficiency (treatment)—
Dose is individualized by prescriber based on severity of deficiency.

**Usual pediatric dose**
Deficiency (prophylaxis)—Oral, amount based on normal daily recommended intakes:—
Birth to 3 years of age—2–3 mg (base).
4 to 6 years of age—3–4 mg (base).
7 to 10 years of age—4–5 mg (base).
Deficiency (treatment)—
Dose is individualized by prescriber based on severity of deficiency.

**Strength(s) usually available**
U.S.—
10 mg (base) (OTC) [GENERIC].
25 mg (base) (OTC) [GENERIC].
50 mg (base) (OTC) [GENERIC].
100 mg (base) (OTC) [GENERIC].
218 mg (base) (OTC) [GENERIC].
250 mg (base) (OTC) [GENERIC].
500 mg (base) (OTC) [GENERIC].
545 mg (base) (OTC) [GENERIC].
Canada—
Not commercially available.
Note: Some strengths of these calcium pantothenate preparations may exceed the dosage range recommended by USP DI Advisory Panels based on the amount necessary to meet normal nutritional needs.

**Packaging and storage**
Store below 40 °C (104 °F), preferably between 15 and 30 °C (59 and 86 °F), unless otherwise specified by manufacturer. Store in a tight container.

**Additional information**
Each 10 mg of calcium pantothenate is equivalent to 9.2 mg of pantothenic acid.

### PANTOTHENIC ACID CAPSULES

**Usual adult and adolescent dose**
See *Calcium Pantothenate Tablets USP*.

**Usual pediatric dose**
See *Calcium Pantothenate Tablets USP*.

**Strength(s) usually available**
U.S.—
200 mg (OTC) [GENERIC].
250 mg (OTC) [GENERIC].
Canada—
Not commercially available.
Note: Some strengths of these pantothenic acid preparations may exceed the dosage range recommended by USP DI Advisory Panels based on the amount necessary to meet normal nutritional needs.

**Packaging and storage**
Store below 40 °C (104 °F), preferably between 15 and 30 °C (59 and 86 °F), unless otherwise specified by manufacturer. Store in a tight container.

### PANTOTHENIC ACID ORAL SOLUTION

**Usual adult and adolescent dose**
See *Calcium Pantothenate Tablets USP*.

**Usual pediatric dose**
See *Calcium Pantothenate Tablets USP*.

**Strength(s) usually available**
U.S.—
200 mg per 5 mL (OTC) [GENERIC].
Canada—
Not commercially available.
Note: The strength of this pantothenic acid preparation may exceed the dosage range recommended by USP DI Advisory Panels based on the amount necessary to meet normal nutritional needs.

**Packaging and storage**
Store below 40 °C (104 °F), preferably between 15 and 30 °C (59 and 86 °F), unless otherwise specified by manufacturer. Store in a tight container.

### PANTOTHENIC ACID TABLETS

**Usual adult and adolescent dose**
See *Calcium Pantothenate Tablets USP*.

**Usual pediatric dose**
See *Calcium Pantothenate Tablets USP*.

**Strength(s) usually available**
U.S.—
50 mg (OTC) [GENERIC].
100 mg (OTC) [GENERIC].
200 mg (OTC) [GENERIC].
250 mg (OTC) [GENERIC].
500 mg (OTC) [GENERIC].
1 gram (OTC) [GENERIC].
Canada—
Not commercially available.

Note: Some strengths of these pantothenic acid preparations may exceed the dosage range recommended by USP DI Advisory Panels based on the amount necessary to meet normal nutritional needs.

**Packaging and storage**
Store below 40 °C (104 °F), preferably between 15 and 30 °C (59 and 86 °F), unless otherwise specified by manufacturer. Store in a tight container.

## PANTOTHENIC ACID EXTENDED-RELEASE TABLETS

**Usual adult and adolescent dose**
*See Calcium Pantothenate Tablets USP.*

**Usual pediatric dose**
Dosage form not appropriate for pediatric patients.

**Strength(s) usually available**
U.S.—
500 mg (OTC) [GENERIC].
Canada—
Not commercially available.

Note: The strength of this pantothenic acid preparation may exceed the dosage range recommended by USP DI Advisory Panels based on the amount necessary to meet normal nutritional needs.

**Packaging and storage**
Store below 40 °C (104 °F), preferably between 15 and 30 °C (59 and 86 °F), in a well-closed container, unless otherwise specified by manufacturer.

Revised: 07/16/92
Interim revision: 08/15/94

---

# PAPAVERINE   Intracavernosal

VA CLASSIFICATION (Primary/Secondary): CV500/GU900
Note: For a listing of dosage forms and brand names by country availability, see *Dosage Forms* section(s). For a listing of brand names for the articles in this monograph, refer to the General Index.

## Category
Impotence therapy.

## Indications
Note: Bracketed information in the *Indications* section refers to uses that are not included in U.S. product labeling.
Note: For information pertaining to the use of papaverine for other indications, see *Papaverine (Systemic)*.

**Accepted**
[Impotence (treatment)][1]—Papaverine is used, sometimes in combination with an alpha-adrenergic blocking agent such as phentolamine, by intracavernosal injection to facilitate erections in men with impotence. In general, it is most useful in patients with organic impotence (neurogenic and, to a lesser extent, vascular). It is less useful in patients with impotence due to endocrine problems (hypogonadism, hyper- or hypothyroidism) or medications.

[Impotence (diagnosis)][1]—Papaverine is used, sometimes in combination with phentolamine, by intracavernosal injection as an aid in the evaluation of penile vasculature, alone or prior to angiography, corpus cavernosography, or cavernosometry.

**Unaccepted**
Use of papaverine to enhance erections in men who are not impotent is not recommended because of the risk of priapism and permanent damage to penile tissues.

---

[1]Not included in Canadian product labeling.

## Pharmacology/Pharmacokinetics

**Physicochemical characteristics**
Molecular weight—375.85.

**Mechanism of action/Effect**
Papaverine has a direct, nonspecific relaxant effect on smooth muscle. When administered by intracavernous injection, it is thought to cause relaxation of the trabecular cavernous smooth muscles and vasodilation of the penile arteries. This results in increased arterial blood flow into the corpus cavernosa, and swelling and elongation of the penis; the glans and corpus spongiosum swell very little, if at all. Venous outflow is also reduced, possibly as a result of increased venous resistance.

**Absorption**
Slowly released into venous circulation; minimal, if any, systemic effects.

**Time to peak effect**
Variable, but usually within 10 minutes.

**Duration of action**
1 to 6 hours; dose-related; prolonged by concurrent administration with phentolamine.

## Precautions to Consider

**Pregnancy/Reproduction**
Problems in humans have not been documented.

**Geriatrics**
No information is available on the relationship of age to the use of papaverine intracavernosally in geriatric patients. However, geriatrics-specific problems that would limit the usefulness of this medication in the elderly are not expected.

**Drug interactions and/or related problems**
The following drug interactions and/or related problems have been selected on the basis of their potential clinical significance (possible mechanism in parentheses where appropriate)—not necessarily inclusive (» = major clinical significance):
Sympathomimetics, alpha-adrenergic, especially metaraminol, epinephrine, and phenylephrine
(reverse the vasodilating effect of papaverine; may be used to treat priapism or overdose)

**Medical considerations/Contraindications**
The medical considerations/contraindications included here have been selected on the basis of their potential clinical significance (reasons given in parentheses where appropriate)—not necessarily inclusive (» = major clinical significance).

*Risk-benefit should be considered when the following medical problems exist:*
Allergy to papaverine
» Coagulation defects, severe
(risk of bleeding at injection site)
Hepatic function impairment
(papaverine may cause hepatotoxicity when used systemically, but is only slowly absorbed systemically after intracavernosal administration)
» Priapism, history of or
» Sickle cell disease
(increased risk of priapism)

**Patient monitoring**
The following may be especially important in patient monitoring (other tests may be warranted in some patients, depending on condition; » = major clinical significance):
Hepatic function tests
(recommended at periodic intervals because of potential hepatotoxicity)
Palpation of penis
(recommended at regular intervals by both the patient and the physician to check for developing fibrosis or curvature)

## Side/Adverse Effects

The following side/adverse effects have been selected on the basis of their potential clinical significance (possible signs and symptoms in parentheses where appropriate)—not necessarily inclusive:

**Those indicating need for medical attention**
Incidence rare
>*Dizziness; fibrosis* (lumps in penis); *priapism* (erection, continuing for more than 4 hours, or painful erection)

>Note: *Fibrosis* of the corpus cavernosum, resulting in blockage and inability to insert a penile prosthesis, has been reported.

>*Priapism* is usually due to excessive dosage. Prolonged erection may resolve spontaneously, but in most cases will require treatment.

**Those indicating need for medical attention only if they continue or are bothersome**
Incidence less frequent or rare
>*Burning, mild, along penis; difficulty in ejaculating; inadvertent subcutaneous administration* (bruising or bleeding at site of injection; swelling at site of injection); *superficial hematoma* (bruising or bleeding at site of injection)

>Note: *Burning* may be more severe with inadvertent subcutaneous administration.

**Those not indicating need for medical attention**
Incidence more frequent
>*Tingling at tip of penis*

## Patient Consultation

As an aid to patient consultation, refer to *Advice for the Patient, Papaverine (Intracavernosal)* or *Phentolamine and Papaverine (Intracavernosal)*.

In providing consultation, consider emphasizing the following selected information (» = major clinical significance):

**Before using this medication**
» Conditions affecting use, especially:
   Allergy to papaverine
   Other medical problems, especially severe coagulation defects, history of priapism, or sickle cell disease

**Proper use of this medication**
*Proper administration*
» Cleansing injection site with alcohol; injecting slowly and directly into corpus cavernosum at base of penis; avoiding subcutaneous administration; if inadvertently injected subcutaneously (as evidenced by pain at injection site), stopping, withdrawing, and repositioning needle
   Putting pressure on injection site for 1 to 2 minutes to prevent bruising; massaging penis, as directed by physician, to distribute medication
   Effect begins in about 10 minutes; attempting intercourse within 2 hours after administration
» Proper dosing
» Proper storage

**Precautions while using this medication**
» Compliance with therapy; importance of not exceeding prescribed dosage and frequency of use; risk of priapism, tissue ischemia, and permanent damage with overdose
» Telling physician immediately if erection persists longer than 4 hours or becomes painful
   If bleeding occurs at injection site, applying pressure; checking with physician if bleeding persists
   Examining penis regularly for signs of fibrosis at injection site or for curvature; checking with physician if either of these occurs

**Side/adverse effects**
   Signs of potential side effects, especially dizziness, priapism, and fibrosis
   Injection may cause tingling at tip of penis; no cause for concern

## General Dosing Information

Patients receiving intracavernosal papaverine should be under supervision of a physician experienced in its use and familiar with proper management of sustained erection and priapism.

Dosage adjustment should be made carefully, based on the degree and duration of tumescence achieved with the previous dose. In general, patients with neurogenic impotence may be more sensitive to the effects of intracavernosal vasodilators and may require lower doses.

Intracavernosal papaverine may be self-administered by the patient, but only after careful training in the technique to reduce the incidence of inadvertent subcutaneous administration, ecchymosis, and urethral injury.

For treatment of impotence, papaverine is injected slowly (over 1 to 2 minutes), directly into the corpus cavernosum at the base of the penis. A characteristic give should be noticed as the needle penetrates the tunica albuginea and enters the corpus cavernosum. Proper injection technique is necessary to avoid injury or injection of the urethra or vessels on the dorsal aspect of the penis.

After completion of the injection, pressure is applied to the injection site to prevent bleeding. Then the entire length of the corpus cavernosum should be squeezed firmly to distribute medication to the other side, followed by the same procedure on the other side. The penis should then be pinched transversely in several places to distribute medication to both ends of the corpus cavernosa.

If a sustained erection occurs, the next dose of papaverine should be reduced.

Intercourse should be attempted within 2 hours after administration.

If fibrosis occurs, discontinuation of papaverine therapy may be necessary, especially if a penile implant is planned in the future.

**For treatment of prolonged erection or priapism**
A sustained erection should be treated if it persists for longer than 4 hours; priapism should be treated promptly. If tumescence is not reversed, interruption of blood flow may result in penile tissue ischemia and permanent damage.

Depending on the severity, treatment may include:
• Aspiration of intracavernous blood.
• Irrigation of the corpus cavernosa with saline to remove clotted blood.
• Intracavernous administration of an alpha-adrenergic agonist, such as metaraminol, epinephrine, or phenylephrine.
• Surgery.

## Parenteral Dosage Forms

Note: Bracketed uses in the *Dosage Forms* section refer to categories of use and/or indications that are not included in U.S. product labeling.

### PAPAVERINE HYDROCHLORIDE INJECTION USP

**Usual adult dose**
[Impotence therapy][1]—
   Intracavernosal, a mixture of 30 mg Papaverine Hydrochloride Injection USP and 0.5 to 1.0 mg of reconstituted Phentolamine Mesylate for Injection USP (5 mg per mL), the dosage being adjusted according to response, or
   Intracavernosal, initially 30 mg of Papaverine Hydrochloride Injection USP alone, the dosage being adjusted, up to 60 mg, according to response.

Note: Patients with neurogenic impotence may require lower doses or use of papaverine alone.

**Usual adult prescribing limits**
Impotence therapy—
   Up to 60 mg of papaverine hydrochloride per dose. The injection should not be given more than three times weekly or two days in succession.

**Strength(s) usually available**
U.S.—
   30 mg per mL (Rx) [GENERIC].
Canada—
   32.5 mg per mL (Rx) [GENERIC].

**Packaging and storage**
Store below 40 °C (104 °F), preferably between 15 and 30 °C (59 and 86 °F), unless otherwise specified by manufacturer. Protect from freezing.

**Incompatibilities**
Papaverine Hydrochloride Injection USP is physically incompatible with lactated Ringer's injection (precipitate will form).

[1]Not included in Canadian product labeling.

## Selected Bibliography

Morley JE. Impotence. Am J Med 1986 May; 80 (5): 897-905.
Sidi AA, Lange PH. Recent advances in the diagnosis and management of impotence. Urol Clin North Am 1986 Aug; 13 (3): 489-500.
Lue TF, Tanagho EA. Physiology of erection and pharmacological management of impotence. J Urol 1987 May; 137 (5): 829-36.

Revised: 08/06/92
Interim revision: 06/07/94

# PAPAVERINE   Systemic

VA CLASSIFICATION (Primary): CV500

Note: For information pertaining to the use of papaverine for impotence, see *Papaverine (Intracavernosal)*.

Note: For a listing of dosage forms and brand names by country availability, see *Dosage Forms* section(s). For a listing of brand names for the articles in this monograph, refer to the General Index.

## Category
Vasodilator.

## Indications

### Unaccepted
Although papaverine has previously been classed as a "grandfather drug" and exempted from FDA's DESI classification, the Peripheral and Central Nervous System Drugs Advisory Committee of the FDA has concluded after studies and hearings that, in spite of its proven vasodilating effects, the medication has not been shown to be effective for its claimed indications. These include use as a smooth muscle relaxant in the treatment of cerebral and peripheral ischemia associated with arterial spasm and myocardial ischemia complicated by arrhythmias; and for visceral spasm as in ureteral colic, biliary colic, or gastrointestinal colic.

## Pharmacology/Pharmacokinetics

### Physicochemical characteristics
Molecular weight—375.85.

### Mechanism of action/Effect
Papaverine has a direct, nonspecific relaxant effect on vascular, cardiac, and other smooth muscle.

### Absorption
Variable; oral bioavailability is usually about 54%, but absorption from extended-release dosage forms is poor.

### Protein binding
Very high (approximately 90%).

### Biotransformation
Hepatic.

### Half-life
0.5 to 2 hours (variable; may be as long as 24 hours).

### Elimination
Renal (as metabolites).
In dialysis—Removable by hemodialysis.

## Precautions to Consider

### Pregnancy/Reproduction
Pregnancy—Studies have not been done in humans.
Studies have not been done in animals.

FDA Pregnancy Category C.

### Breast-feeding
It is not known whether papaverine is distributed into breast milk. However, problems in humans have not been documented.

### Pediatrics
Appropriate studies on the relationship of age to the effects of papaverine have not been performed in the pediatric population. However, pediatrics-specific problems that would limit the usefulness of this medication in children are not expected.

### Geriatrics
Appropriate studies on the relationship of age to the effects of papaverine have not been performed in the geriatric population. However, the risk of papaverine-induced hypothermia may be increased in elderly patients.

### Drug interactions and/or related problems
The following drug interactions and/or related problems have been selected on the basis of their potential clinical significance (possible mechanism in parentheses where appropriate)—not necessarily inclusive (» = major clinical significance):

Note: Combinations containing any of the following medications, depending on the amount present, may also interact with this medication.

Levodopa
(concurrent use may decrease the therapeutic effects of levodopa because of possible blockade of dopamine receptors by papaverine)

Smoking, tobacco
(heavy smoking may interfere with the therapeutic effect of papaverine because nicotine constricts blood vessels)

### Laboratory value alterations
The following have been selected on the basis of their potential clinical significance (possible effect in parentheses where appropriate)—not necessarily inclusive (» = major clinical significance):

With physiology/laboratory test values
Alanine aminotransferase (ALT [SGPT]) concentration, serum and
Alkaline phosphatase concentration, serum and
Aspartate aminotransferase (AST [SGOT]) concentration, serum and
Bilirubin concentration, serum and
Eosinophil count
(may be increased; signs of hepatic hypersensitivity)

### Medical considerations/Contraindications
The medical considerations/contraindications included here have been selected on the basis of their potential clinical significance (reasons given in parentheses where appropriate)—not necessarily inclusive (» = major clinical significance).

*Except under special circumstances, this medication should not be used intravenously when the following medical problem exists:*
» Atrioventricular (AV) heart block, complete
(large doses can depress AV and intraventricular conduction and produce serious arrhythmias)

*Risk-benefit should be considered when the following medical problems exist:*
Angina or
Myocardial infarction, recent or
Stroke, recent
(ischemia may be exacerbated by a possible "steal effect" since papaverine has a greater effect on peripheral than cerebral and coronary vessels, leading to a further decrease in flow to ischemic areas)

Glaucoma
» Myocardial depression
(large doses may cause further depression)
Sensitivity to papaverine

### Patient monitoring
The following may be especially important in patient monitoring (other tests may be warranted in some patients, depending on condition; » = major clinical significance):

Hepatic function tests
(may be indicated if patient develops gastrointestinal symptoms or jaundice suggesting hepatic hypersensitivity)

Intraocular pressure measurements
(recommended at periodic intervals in glaucoma patients who are receiving papaverine)

## Side/Adverse Effects
The following side/adverse effects have been selected on the basis of their potential clinical significance (possible signs and symptoms in parentheses where appropriate)—not necessarily inclusive:

### Those indicating need for medical attention
Incidence rare
*Hepatic hypersensitivity* (yellow eyes or skin)
With parenteral administration
*Thrombosis* (redness, swelling, or pain at injection site)

### Those indicating need for medical attention only if they continue or are bothersome
With rapid parenteral administration
*Deep breathing; fast heartbeat; flushing of face; hypotension* (dizziness)

## Overdose
For more information on the management of overdose or unintentional ingestion, **contact a Poison Control Center** (see *Poison Control Center Listing*).

**Clinical effects of overdose**

The following effects have been selected on the basis of their potential clinical significance (possible signs and symptoms in parentheses where appropriate)—not necessarily inclusive:

*Blurred or double vision; drowsiness; weakness*

**Treatment of overdose**

Treatment of acute poisoning consists of: Removal or delay of absorption of papaverine by administration of tap water, milk, or activated charcoal, and removal of stomach contents by gastric lavage or emesis, followed by catharsis; appropriate measures for treatment of coma or respiratory depression and maintenance of blood pressure; hemodialysis may be useful.

## Patient Consultation

As an aid to patient consultation, refer to *Advice for the Patient, Papaverine (Systemic).*

In providing consultation, consider emphasizing the following selected information (» = major clinical significance):

**Before using this medication**

» Conditions affecting use, especially:

     Sensitivity to papaverine

     Use in the elderly—Increased risk of hypothermia

     Other medical problems, especially complete atrioventricular heart block (for intravenous administration only) and myocardial depression

**Proper use of this medication**

Taking with or following meals, milk, or antacids, to reduce nausea

Proper administration of extended-release capsules: Swallowing whole without crushing, breaking, or chewing before swallowing or, if too large to swallow, mixing contents with jam or jelly and swallowing without chewing

» Proper dosing

Missed dose: Taking as soon as possible; not taking if almost time for next dose; not doubling doses

» Proper storage

**Precautions while using this medication**

Checking with physician before discontinuing medication

Avoiding smoking because nicotine constricts blood vessels

» Caution when getting up from a lying or sitting position or when climbing stairs

**Side/adverse effects**

Signs of potential side effects, especially hepatic hypersensitivity and (for parenteral administration only) thrombosis

## General Dosing Information

Dosage of papaverine should be reduced if drowsiness occurs.

If signs of hepatic hypersensitivity occur, it is recommended that papaverine therapy be withdrawn.

**For oral dosage forms only**

Oral papaverine may be administered with or following meals, milk, or antacids to reduce stomach upset.

**For parenteral dosage forms only**

The intra-arterial route should be used only by those experienced in the procedure.

Intravenous administration may be used when an immediate effect is desired, but should be done slowly over 1 or 2 minutes to avoid adverse effects (arrhythmias and fatal apnea).

## Oral Dosage Forms

### PAPAVERINE HYDROCHLORIDE EXTENDED-RELEASE CAPSULES

**Usual adult dose**

Vasospastic therapy adjunct—

     Oral, 150 mg every twelve hours, the dosage being increased to 150 mg every eight hours or 300 mg every twelve hours if necessary.

**Strength(s) usually available**

U.S.—

     150 mg (Rx) [*Cerespan; Genabid; Pavabid* (sucrose); *Pavacels; Pavacot; Pavagen; Pavarine; Pavased; Pavatine; Pavatym; Paverolan;* GENERIC].

Canada—

     Not commercially available.

**Packaging and storage**

Store below 40 °C (104 °F), preferably between 15 and 30 °C (59 and 86 °F), in a well-closed container, unless otherwise specified by manufacturer.

### PAPAVERINE HYDROCHLORIDE TABLETS USP

**Usual adult dose**

Vasospastic therapy adjunct—

     Oral, 100 to 300 mg three to five times a day.

**Strength(s) usually available**

U.S.—

     30 mg (Rx) [GENERIC].

     60 mg (Rx) [*Pavacot;* GENERIC].

     100 mg (Rx) [*Pavacot;* GENERIC].

     200 mg (Rx) [GENERIC].

     300 mg (Rx) [*Pavabid HP;* GENERIC].

Canada—

     100 mg (OTC) [GENERIC].

**Packaging and storage**

Store below 40 °C (104 °F), preferably between 15 and 30 °C (59 and 86 °F), unless otherwise specified by manufacturer. Store in a tight container.

## Parenteral Dosage Forms

### PAPAVERINE HYDROCHLORIDE INJECTION USP

**Usual adult dose**

Vasospastic therapy adjunct—

     Intra-arterial, 40 mg, administered slowly over a one- to two-minute period.

     Intramuscular or intravenous, 30 to 120 mg every three hours, administered slowly over a one- to two-minute period. In the treatment of cardiac asystole, two doses may be given ten minutes apart.

**Usual pediatric dose**

Intramuscular or intravenous, 1.5 mg per kg of body weight four times a day.

**Strength(s) usually available**

U.S.—

     30 mg per mL (Rx) [GENERIC].

Canada—

     32.5 mg per mL (OTC) [GENERIC].

**Packaging and storage**

Store below 40 °C (104 °F), preferably between 15 and 30 °C (59 and 86 °F), unless otherwise specified by manufacturer. Protect from freezing.

**Incompatibilities**

Papaverine hydrochloride injection is physically incompatible with lactated Ringer's injection (precipitate will form).

Revised: 04/13/93

# PARALDEHYDE   Systemic

VA CLASSIFICATION (Primary): CN400

Note: Controlled substance in the U.S.—Schedule IV.

Note: For a listing of dosage forms and brand names by country availability, see *Dosage Forms* section(s). For a listing of brand names for the articles in this monograph, refer to the General Index.

## Category

Anticonvulsant.

## Indications

### Accepted

Convulsions (treatment) or

Status epilepticus (treatment)—Parenteral paraldehyde may be indicated in the emergency treatment of status epilepticus and of convulsions induced by tetanus or eclampsia, when other agents are not effective. Oral paraldehyde may be used in the management of convulsions induced by tetanus when other agents are not effective.

### Unaccepted

Paraldehyde has been used as a sedative-hypnotic; however, it generally has been replaced by safer and/or more effective agents for the following indications:

Insomnia

Sedation

Delirium tremens and other psychiatric states characterized by excitement, to quiet the patient and produce sleep (generally replaced by benzodiazepines such as chlordiazepoxide and diazepam)

Convulsions caused by convulsant drug toxicity

Parenterally for intractable pain not responsive to other types of therapy (e.g., in an occasional patient with acute coronary thrombosis who fails to obtain relief from repeated injections of morphine sulfate)

Intramuscularly to induce artificial sleep and thereby to facilitate electroencephalographic study, especially in children

## Pharmacology/Pharmacokinetics

### Physicochemical characteristics

Molecular weight—132.16.

### Mechanism of action/Effect

The precise mechanism of action of paraldehyde is unknown. It may depress many levels of the central nervous system (CNS) including the ascending reticular activating system to produce imbalances between facilitatory and inhibitory mechanisms.

### Absorption

Rapidly absorbed from the gastrointestinal tract and from intramuscular injection sites.

### Biotransformation

Hepatic. Approximately 70 to 90% of a dose of paraldehyde is metabolized.

### Half-life

Biological—3.4 to 9.8 hours.

### Onset of action

Hypnotic—Within 15 minutes.

### Time to peak serum concentration

Oral—30 to 60 minutes.

Rectal—About 2.5 hours.

### Duration of action

Hypnotic—About 8 to 12 hours.

### Elimination

Unmetabolized paraldehyde (11 to 28%) is excreted via exhalation. Trace amounts are excreted in the urine.

## Precautions to Consider

### Pregnancy/Reproduction

Pregnancy—Paraldehyde crosses the placenta. Studies have not been done in humans.

Studies have not been done in animals.

FDA Pregnancy Category C.

Labor—Use of paraldehyde during labor may cause respiratory depression in the neonate.

### Breast-feeding

Problems in humans have not been documented.

### Pediatrics

Appropriate studies on the relationship of age to the effects of paraldehyde have not been performed in the pediatric population. However, no pediatrics-specific problems have been documented to date.

### Geriatrics

No information is available on the relationship of age to the effects of paraldehyde in geriatric patients.

### Drug interactions and/or related problems

The following drug interactions and/or related problems have been selected on the basis of their potential clinical significance (possible mechanism in parentheses where appropriate)—not necessarily inclusive (» = major clinical significance):

Note: Combinations containing any of the following medications, depending on the amount present, may also interact with this medication.

Addictive medications, other, especially central nervous system (CNS) depressants with habituating potential

(prolonged concurrent use may increase the risk of habituation; caution is recommended)

» Alcohol or

» CNS depression–producing medications, other (See *Appendix II*)

(concurrent use may increase the CNS depressant effects of either these medications or paraldehyde; caution is recommended and dosage of one or both agents should be reduced)

» Disulfiram

(concurrent use with paraldehyde is not recommended because disulfiram may decrease the metabolism of paraldehyde by inhibition of acetaldehyde dehydrogenase, resulting in increased blood concentrations of paraldehyde and acetaldehyde)

### Laboratory value alterations

The following have been selected on the basis of their potential clinical significance (possible effect in parentheses where appropriate)—not necessarily inclusive (» = major clinical significance):

With diagnostic test results

Metyrapone test

(paraldehyde may interfere with the assay for urine 17-ketosteroids or 17-ketogenic steroids)

Phentolamine test

(paraldehyde may cause false-positive phentolamine test; it is recommended that all medications be withdrawn at least 24 hours, preferably 48 to 72 hours, prior to a phentolamine test)

Urinary 17-hydroxycorticosteroid determinations

(may be interfered with when a modification of the Reddy, Jenkins, and Thorn procedure is used)

### Medical considerations/Contraindications

The medical considerations/contraindications included here have been selected on the basis of their potential clinical significance (reasons given in parentheses where appropriate)—not necessarily inclusive (» = major clinical significance).

*Risk-benefit should be considered when the following medical problems exist:*

Alcoholism, active or in remission or

Drug abuse or dependence, history of

(predisposition of patient to habituation and dependence)

» Bronchopulmonary disease

(paraldehyde excreted via lungs)

» Hepatic function impairment

(paraldehyde metabolized in liver; patients may be more susceptible to effects of paraldehyde)

Sensitivity to paraldehyde

*With oral use*

Gastroenteritis or

» Peptic ulcer

(condition may be exacerbated)

*With rectal use*

Colitis

(condition may be exacerbated)

## Side/Adverse Effects

The following side/adverse effects have been selected on the basis of their potential clinical significance (possible signs and symptoms in parentheses where appropriate)—not necessarily inclusive:

**Those indicating need for medical attention**
Incidence more frequent
   *Effects on pulmonary capillaries* (coughing)—with intravenous administration only; *skin rash*
Incidence less frequent
   *Thrombophlebitis* (redness, swelling, or pain at injection site)
With prolonged use
   *Hepatitis* (yellow eyes or skin)

**Those indicating need for medical attention only if they continue or are bothersome**
Incidence more frequent
   *Drowsiness; unpleasant breath odor; nausea or vomiting*—with oral use; *stomach pain*—with oral use
Incidence less frequent
   *Clumsiness or unsteadiness; dizziness; "hangover" effect*

**Those indicating possible withdrawal and the need for medical attention if they occur after medication is discontinued**
   *Convulsions; hallucinations; increased sweating; muscle cramps; nausea or vomiting; stomach cramps; trembling*

## Overdose

For specific information on the agents used in the management of paraldehyde overdose, see:
   • *Mineral Oil* in *Laxatives (Local)* monograph; and/or
   • *Sodium Bicarbonate (Systemic)* monograph.

For more information on the management of overdose or unintentional ingestion, **contact a Poison Control Center** (see *Poison Control Center Listing*).

**Clinical effects of overdose**
The following effects have been selected on the basis of their potential clinical significance (possible signs and symptoms in parentheses where appropriate)—not necessarily inclusive:
   *Cloudy urine; decreased urination; fast and deep breathing; metabolic acidosis* (confusion; muscle tremors; continuing or severe nausea or vomiting; nervousness; restlessness; irritability; severe stomach cramps); *shortness of breath or slow or troubled breathing; slow heartbeat; weakness, severe*

**Treatment of overdose**
Recommended treatment for paraldehyde overdose includes the following:
   To decrease absorption—
      For oral overdose, performing gastric lavage (provided an endotracheal tube with cuff inflated is in place to prevent aspiration of vomitus), followed by administering a demulcent (e.g., mineral oil) to relieve gastric irritation.
      For rectal overdose, performing rectal lavage.
   Specific treatment—
      Correcting metabolic acidosis, if necessary, by intravenous administration of sodium bicarbonate or sodium lactate.
   Supportive care—
      Re-establishing adequate respiratory exchange by maintaining an adequate airway, controlling respiration, and administering oxygen.
      Maintaining body temperature.
      Supporting circulation.
      Patients in whom intentional overdose is known or suspected should be referred for psychiatric consultation.

## Patient Consultation

As an aid to patient consultation, refer to *Advice for the Patient, Paraldehyde (Systemic)*.

In providing consultation, consider emphasizing the following selected information (» = major clinical significance):

**Before using this medication**
» Conditions affecting use, especially:
      Sensitivity to paraldehyde
      Pregnancy—Paraldehyde crosses placenta
      Labor—Use of paraldehyde during labor may cause respiratory depression in neonate
      Other medications, especially alcohol or other CNS depression–producing medications or disulfiram
      Other medical problems, especially bronchopulmonary disease, hepatic function impairment, or peptic ulcer (with oral use only)

**Proper use of this medication**
» Importance of not using more medication than the amount prescribed because of habit-forming potential
» Not using medication if it is brownish in color or has a strong vinegar-like odor
      Avoiding contact with eyes, skin, and clothing
      Keeping away from heat, open flame, and sparks
» Not using plastic containers for administration of this medication
» Proper dosing
      Missed dose: If on scheduled dosing regimen—Taking right away if remembered within an hour or so; not taking if remembered later; not doubling doses
» Proper storage
*For oral use*
» Taking liquid diluted in milk or iced fruit juice to mask odor and taste and to minimize gastric irritation

*For rectal use*
   Proper administration: Paraldehyde may need diluting before using

**Precautions while using this medication**
   Regular visits to physician to check progress during prolonged therapy
   Checking with physician before discontinuing medication after prolonged use; gradual dosage reduction may be necessary to avoid possibility of withdrawal symptoms
» Avoiding use of alcohol or other CNS depressants
   Caution if any laboratory tests required; possible interference with metyrapone or phentolamine test results
» Suspected overdose: Getting emergency help at once
» Caution if drowsiness occurs

**Side/adverse effects**
   Signs of potential side effects, especially effects on pulmonary capillaries (with intravenous use only), skin rash, thrombophlebitis (with injection only), and, with prolonged use, hepatitis
   Strong unpleasant breath odor may be alarming to patient although medically insignificant

## General Dosing Information

Do not use plastic containers or plastic syringes or tubing for administration since paraldehyde is incompatible with many plastics.

Prolonged use of larger than usual therapeutic doses may result in tolerance and psychic or physical dependence.

Following prolonged administration, paraldehyde should be withdrawn gradually in order to avoid the possibility of precipitating withdrawal symptoms.

**For oral use only**
When paraldehyde is administered orally, it should be well diluted in milk or iced fruit juice to mask the odor and taste and to minimize gastric irritation.

**For parenteral use only**
Intramuscular injection is the preferred route of administration. The paraldehyde injection should be administered deeply into the gluteus maximus muscle, care being taken to avoid nerve trunks because paraldehyde may cause nerve injury and paralysis. No more than 5 mL should be administered at each injection site.

Paraldehyde should not be administered subcutaneously because it is irritating to tissue.

Intravenous administration is not recommended except in emergencies, since it may produce circulatory collapse or pulmonary edema.

If administered intravenously, paraldehyde should be diluted with several volumes of 0.9% sodium chloride injection and injected slowly at a rate not to exceed 1 mL per minute.

**For rectal use only**
For rectal administration, paraldehyde should be diluted with 1 or 2 parts of olive oil, cottonseed oil, or 0.9% sodium chloride solution to prevent rectal irritation.

## Oral/Rectal Dosage Forms

### PARALDEHYDE USP

**Usual adult dose**
Anticonvulsant—
   Oral, up to 12 mL (diluted to a 10% solution) via gastric tube every four hours as needed.
   Rectal, 10 to 20 mL.

**Usual pediatric dose**
Anticonvulsant—
   Oral, 0.3 mL per kg of body weight or 12 mL per square meter of body surface.

Rectal, 0.3 mL per kg of body weight or 12 mL per square meter of body surface.

**Size(s) usually available**

U.S.—

   30 mL (Rx) [*Paral;* GENERIC].

Canada—

   Not commercially available.

   Note: In Canada, the sterile paraldehyde dosage form can be used whenever oral or rectal paraldehyde is prescribed.

**Packaging and storage**

Store below 25 °C (77 °F), in a tight, light-resistant container holding not more than 30 mL. Paraldehyde solidifies at approximately 12 °C (54 °F) and must be liquefied before use. Keep paraldehyde away from heat, open flame, or sparks. Store in glass containers since paraldehyde is incompatible with many plastics.

**Preparation of dosage form**

For rectal administration, dilute paraldehyde with 1 or 2 parts of olive oil, cottonseed oil, or 0.9% sodium chloride solution.

**Stability**

When exposed to light and air, paraldehyde decomposes to form acetaldehyde, which is oxidized to acetic acid. If liquid turns brownish in color and has a sharp penetrating odor of acetic acid, it should not be used. The unused contents of any container that has been opened for more than 24 hours should be discarded.

**Incompatibilities**

Paraldehyde is incompatible with most plastics; therefore, plastic containers should not be used for administration of the medication.

**Auxiliary labeling**

* Avoid alcoholic beverages.
* May cause drowsiness.
* Discard any unused liquid if container has been opened for more than 24 hours.

**Note**

Controlled substance in the U.S.

## Parenteral Dosage Forms

### PARALDEHYDE STERILE USP

**Usual adult dose**

Anticonvulsant—

   Intramuscular, 5 to 10 mL.

Intravenous infusion, 5 mL diluted with at least 100 mL of 0.9% sodium chloride injection and administered slowly at a rate not exceeding 1 mL per minute.

**Usual pediatric dose**

Anticonvulsant—

   Intramuscular, 0.15 mL per kg of body weight or 6 mL per square meter of body surface.

   Intravenous, 0.1 to 0.15 mL per kg of body weight diluted with 0.9% sodium chloride injection and administered slowly.

**Size(s) usually available**

U.S.—

   Not commercially available.

Canada—

   5 mL (Rx) [GENERIC].

**Packaging and storage**

Store below 25 °C (77 °F), in a light-resistant container. Paraldehyde solidifies at approximately 12 °C (54 °F) and must be liquefied before use. Keep paraldehyde away from heat, open flame, and sparks.

**Preparation of dosage form**

For intravenous administration, paraldehyde should be diluted with several volumes of 0.9% sodium chloride injection.

**Stability**

When exposed to light and air, paraldehyde decomposes to form acetaldehyde, which is oxidized to acetic acid. If injection turns brownish in color and has a sharp penetrating odor of acetic acid, it should not be used. Any unused portion of the injection should be discarded.

**Incompatibilities**

Paraldehyde is incompatible with most plastics; therefore, a glass syringe should be used for administration of the medication.

**Auxiliary labeling**

* For single dose only. Discard unused portion.

Revised: 03/19/93

---

**PARAMETHADIONE**—See *Anticonvulsants, Dione (Systemic)*

---

**PARAMETHASONE**—See *Corticosteroids—Glucocorticoid Effects (Systemic)*

---

# PAREGORIC   Systemic

VA CLASSIFICATION (Primary/Secondary): GA400/CN101

Note: Controlled substance classification—

   U.S.: III.

   Canada: N.

A commonly used name is camphorated opium tincture. In the U.S., however, camphor is no longer a required ingredient in the formulation.

Note: For a listing of dosage forms and brand names by country availability, see *Dosage Forms* section(s). For a listing of brand names for the articles in this monograph, refer to the General Index.

## Category

Antidiarrheal.

## Indications

**Unaccepted**

Paregoric has been replaced by equally or more effective, and safer, agents for treatment of diarrhea. However, the efficacy of any antidiarrheal medication for treatment of childhood diarrhea is questionable; preferred treatment consists of fluid and electrolyte replacement, nutritional therapy, and, if possible, elimination of the underlying cause of the diarrhea.

Paregoric is not recommended for ameliorating withdrawal symptoms in opioid-dependent neonates. Because paregoric contains ingredients that are potentially hazardous to infants (alcohol, benzoic acid, and, in most products, camphor), it has been replaced for this purpose by other opioid preparations having fewer or no hazardous additional ingredients, such as diluted tincture of opium or morphine sulfate oral solution, or by benzodiazepines, barbiturates, and/or clonidine.

Although paregoric was at one time applied to the gums of a teething infant (to provide local anesthesia and permit sleep), such use is not recommended.

## Pharmacology/Pharmacokinetics

**Mechanism of action/Effect**

Most of the effects of paregoric are due to the morphine component. Usefulness in the treatment of diarrhea is due to alteration of intestinal motility.

**Absorption**

Morphine—Well absorbed from the gastrointestinal tract but undergoes rapid metabolism so that the effect is less than after parenteral administration.

**Protein binding**

Morphine—Low.

**Biotransformation**

Hepatic.

**Half-life**

Morphine—2 to 3 hours.

**Elimination**

Renal and biliary.

## Precautions to Consider

**Cross-sensitivity and/or related problems**

Patients hypersensitive to other opium alkaloids may be hypersensitive to this medication also.

**Pregnancy/Reproduction**
Pregnancy—
*First trimester—*
Problems in humans have not been documented; however, opium alkaloids cross the placenta. Camphor, which may be present in some formulations, and alcohol also cross the placenta.

Morphine has been shown to be teratogenic in animals in very high doses.
*Third trimester—*
Regular use of an opiate by a pregnant woman late in pregnancy may cause physical dependence in the fetus, leading to withdrawal symptoms in the neonate. Also, administration of an opiate to a pregnant woman shortly before delivery may cause respiratory depression in the neonate, especially the premature neonate.

Camphor, which may be present in some formulations, may cause respiratory depression and death in the neonate if administered to a pregnant woman shortly before delivery.

**Breast-feeding**
Problems in humans have not been documented; however, opium alkaloids (particularly morphine) are distributed into breast milk.

**Pediatrics**
Children up to 2 years of age may be more susceptible to the effects, especially the respiratory depressant effects, of opiates. Preferred measures for treating childhood diarrhea consist of fluid and electrolyte replacement, nutritional therapy, and, if possible, eliminating the cause of the diarrhea; whether antidiarrheals are beneficial for this condition is questionable. It is recommended that paregoric not be used for treatment of diarrhea in infants and children up to 2 years of age. In older children, paregoric should be used with caution (if at all), for as short a time as possible, and only in addition to the preferred treatment measures.

Paregoric contains 45% alcohol, which is considered an undesirable ingredient in medications administered to pediatric patients.

Neonates may also be susceptible to serious toxicity induced by camphor, including convulsions and respiratory depression, and to benzoic acid–induced hyperbilirubinemia. Whenever possible, other medications (e.g., diluted tincture of opium, morphine sulfate oral solution, barbiturates, benzodiazepines, clonidine) should be used for ameliorating withdrawal symptoms in opioid-dependent neonates.

**Geriatrics**
Geriatric patients may be more susceptible to the effects, especially the respiratory depressant effects, of opiates. Also, geriatric patients are more likely to have prostatic hypertrophy or obstruction and age-related renal function impairment; opiate-induced urinary retention may be detrimental to these patients.

**Drug interactions and/or related problems**
The following drug interactions and/or related problems have been selected on the basis of their potential clinical significance (possible mechanism in parentheses where appropriate)—not necessarily inclusive (» = major clinical significance):

Note: Combinations containing any of the following medications, depending on the amount present, may also interact with this medication.

Addictive medications, other, especially central nervous system (CNS) depressants with habituating potential
(prolonged concurrent use may increase the risk of habituation; caution is recommended)

» Alcohol or
» Antidiarrheals, antiperistaltic, other, such as:
» Difenoxin and atropine
» Diphenoxylate and atropine
» Kaolin, pectin, belladonna alkaloids and opium
» Loperamide
» Opium tincture or
» CNS depression–producing medications, other (See *Appendix II*)
(concurrent use of these medications with paregoric may result in increased CNS depressant, respiratory depressant, and hypotensive effects; concurrent use should be undertaken with caution, and dosage of one or both agents should be reduced)

(concurrent use of any opioid-containing analgesic or antidiarrheal with paregoric may also increase the risk of severe constipation)

Anticholinergics or other medications with anticholinergic activity (See *Appendix II*)
(concurrent use with paregoric may result in increased risk of severe constipation, which may lead to paralytic ileus, and/or urinary retention)

Metoclopramide
(paregoric may antagonize the effects of metoclopramide on gastrointestinal motility)

Monoamine oxidase (MAO) inhibitors, including furazolidone, procarbazine, and selegiline
(caution is recommended when using any opioid in patients who have received an MAO inhibitor within 14 days because concurrent use of MAO inhibitors with meperidine has resulted in unpredictable, severe, and sometimes fatal reactions, including immediate excitation, sweating, rigidity, and severe hypertension, or, in some patients, hypotension, severe respiratory depression, coma, convulsions, hyperpyrexia, and vascular collapse)

» Naloxone
(naloxone reverses the effects of paregoric and may precipitate withdrawal symptoms in opioid-dependent patients)

» Naltrexone
(naltrexone blocks the therapeutic effects of paregoric and may precipitate withdrawal symptoms in opioid-dependent patients; naltrexone therapy should not be initiated in a patient receiving paregoric; patients receiving naltrexone should be treated with nonopioid medications when antidiarrheal treatment is required)

**Laboratory value alterations**
The following have been selected on the basis of their potential clinical significance (possible effect in parentheses where appropriate)—not necessarily inclusive (» = major clinical significance):

With diagnostic test results
Gastric emptying studies
(paregoric may delay gastric emptying, thereby invalidating test results)

Hepatobiliary imaging using technetium Tc 99m disofenin
(delivery of technetium Tc 99m disofenin to the small bowel may be prevented because paregoric may cause constriction of the sphincter of Oddi and increased biliary tract pressure; these actions result in delayed visualization and thus resemble obstruction of the common bile duct)

With physiology/laboratory test values
Amylase, plasma and
Lipase, plasma
(values may be increased because opiates can cause contractions of the sphincter of Oddi and increased biliary tract pressure; the diagnostic utility of determinations of these enzymes may be compromised for up to 24 hours after medication has been given)

**Medical considerations/Contraindications**
The medical considerations/contraindications included here have been selected on the basis of their potential clinical significance (reasons given in parentheses where appropriate)—not necessarily inclusive (» = major clinical significance).

*Except under special circumstances, this medication should not be used when the following medical problems exist:*

» Diarrhea associated with pseudomembranous colitis caused by cephalosporins; lincomycins, possibly including topical clindamycin; or penicillins or
» Diarrhea caused by poisoning, until after the toxic material has been eliminated from the gastrointestinal tract
(paregoric may delay removal of toxins from the colon, thereby prolonging and/or worsening the diarrhea)
» Diarrhea caused by infectious organisms, including:
» Dysentery, acute, characterized by bloody stools and elevated temperature
(paregoric may slow recovery by delaying removal of infectious organisms or toxins, prolonging contact between infectious organisms and the mucosa, and delaying other appropriate treatment; antimicrobial treatment may be necessary)

» Respiratory depression, acute
(may be exacerbated)

*Risk-benefit should be considered (if paregoric is to be used over prolonged periods) when the following medical problems exist:*

Alcohol abuse or history of or
Drug abuse or dependence, history of
(patient predisposition to drug abuse)
» Asthma, acute attack or
» Respiratory disease or impairment, especially chronic obstructive pulmonary disease
(paregoric may decrease respiratory drive and increase airway resistance in these patients)

Cardiac arrhythmias or
Convulsions, history of
>> (may be exacerbated)

>> Dehydration, especially in infants and children
(rehydration therapy is essential if signs of dehydration, such as
dry mouth, excessive thirst, wrinkled skin, decreased urination,
rapid or racing pulse, and dizziness or lightheadedness, are present
[especially when caused by diarrhea]; fluid loss may have serious
consequences, such as circulatory collapse and renal failure, especially in young children)

Gallbladder disease or gallstones
(paregoric may cause biliary contraction)

Head injury or
Increased intracranial pressure, pre-existing or
Intracranial lesions
(increased risk of respiratory depression and further increase in
cerebrospinal fluid pressure)

Hepatic function impairment

Hypersensitivity to paregoric or other opiates, history of

Hypothyroidism
(increased risk of respiratory depression and CNS depression)

>> Inflammatory bowel disease, severe
(risk of toxic megacolon may be increased, especially with repeated dosing, although antidiarrheals may be used in moderation
to provide symptomatic relief)

Prostatic hypertrophy or obstruction or
Urethral stricture
(paregoric may cause urinary retention)

Renal function impairment
(components of this formulation excreted primarily via kidneys;
also, paregoric may cause urinary retention)

Caution is also advised in administration to very young, elderly, or
very ill or debilitated patients, who may be more sensitive to the
effects, especially the respiratory depressant effects, of opiates.

## Side/Adverse Effects

Note: At high doses, paregoric exhibits effects of opiates.
Physical dependence with or without psychological dependence
may occur with chronic administration of high doses of paregoric;
an abstinence syndrome may occur when the medication is
discontinued.

Dizziness, feeling faint, or lightheadedness occurs more frequently
in ambulatory patients receiving opiates and may be a sign of orthostatic hypotension; however, these effects may also reflect the
CNS depressant effects of opiates and may occur independently of
hypotension.

The following side/adverse effects have been selected on the basis of their
potential clinical significance (possible signs and symptoms in parentheses where appropriate)—not necessarily inclusive:

### Those indicating need for medical attention
Incidence rare
*Allergic reaction* (skin rash, hives, itching); *histamine release* (decreased blood pressure; fast heartbeat; increased sweating; redness or
flushing of face; shortness of breath, wheezing, or troubled breathing);
*mental depression; toxic megacolon* (bloating; constipation; loss of
appetite; nausea or vomiting; stomach pain)

### Those indicating need for medical attention only if they continue or are bothersome
Incidence more frequent with large doses
*Antidiuretic effect* (decreased urination); *CNS effects* (dizziness; feeling faint; lightheadedness; unusual tiredness or weakness; drowsiness;
nervousness or restlessness); *hypotension, including orthostatic hypotension* (dizziness; feeling faint; lightheadedness; unusual tiredness
or weakness); *ureteral spasm* (difficult or painful urination; frequent
urge to urinate)

### Those indicating possible withdrawal and the need for medical attention if they occur after medication is discontinued
*Body aches; diarrhea; fast heartbeat; fever, runny nose, or sneezing;
gooseflesh; increased sweating; increased yawning; loss of appetite;
nausea or vomiting; nervousness, restlessness, or irritability; shivering or trembling; stomach cramps; trouble in sleeping; unusually
large pupils; weakness, severe*

## Overdose
For specific information on the agents use in the management of paregoric
overdose, see:
• *Naloxone (Systemic)* monograph.

For more information on the management of overdose or unintentional
ingestion, **contact a Poison Control Center** (see *Poison Control Center Listing*).

### Clinical effects of overdose
The following effects have been selected on the basis of their potential
clinical significance (possible signs and symptoms in parentheses
where appropriate)—not necessarily inclusive:
Acute and chronic
*Cold, clammy skin; confusion; convulsions; severe dizziness, drows-
iness, nervousness, restlessness, or weakness; low blood pressure;
pinpoint pupils; respiratory depression* (slow or irregular breathing);
*slow heartbeat; unconsciousness*

### Treatment of overdose
To decrease absorption—Emptying the stomach by induction of emesis
or gastric lavage. However, treatment of respiratory depression or
other potentially life-threatening adverse effects must take precedence.

Specific treatment—Use of the opioid antagonist naloxone. See the package insert or *Naloxone (Systemic)* for specific dosing guidelines for
use of this product.

Monitoring—Continuing to monitor the patient (mandatory because the
duration of action of the opioid may exceed that of naloxone) so that
additional antagonist may be administered as needed. Alternatively,
initial treatment may be followed by continuous intravenous infusion
of naloxone, with the rate of infusion being adjusted according to
patient response. The fact that naloxone may precipitate withdrawal
symptoms in physically dependent patients must be kept in mind.

Supportive care—Establishing adequate respiratory exchange through provision of a patent airway and institution of assisted or controlled respiration. Administration of intravenous fluids, vasopressors, and other
supportive measures as needed. Patients in whom intentional overdose
is known or suspected should be referred for psychiatric consultation.

## Patient Consultation
As an aid to patient consultation, refer to *Advice for the Patient, Opium
Preparations (Systemic)*.

In providing consultation, consider emphasizing the following selected
information (>> = major clinical significance):

### Before using this medication
>> Conditions affecting use, especially:
Hypersensitivity to paregoric or other opiates, history of
Pregnancy—Opiates and camphor cross the placenta; regular use
of opiates may cause physical dependence in the fetus, leading
to withdrawal symptoms in the neonate; camphor may cause
respiratory depression and other serious adverse effects in the
neonate
Breast-feeding—Opium alkaloids distributed into breast milk
Use in children—Increased sensitivity to respiratory depressant effects in children up to 2 years of age
Use in the elderly—Increased sensitivity to respiratory depressant
effects in geriatric patients
Other medications, especially alcohol or other CNS depressants,
other antiperistaltic antidiarrheals, and naltrexone
Other medical problems, especially asthma or other respiratory disease or impairment; and severe inflammatory bowel disease

### Proper use of this medication
Proper administration
Taking with food or meals if gastrointestinal irritation occurs
>> Importance of not taking more medication than the amount prescribed
because of danger of overdose and habit-forming potential
>> Proper dosing
>> Missed dose: Taking as soon as possible; not taking if almost time for
next dose; not doubling doses
>> Proper storage

### Precautions while using this medication
>> Consulting physician if diarrhea continues and/or fever develops
>> Avoiding use of alcoholic beverages or other CNS depressants during
therapy unless prescribed or otherwise approved by physician
>> Caution if drowsiness, dizziness, or lightheadedness occurs
Caution when getting up suddenly from a lying or sitting position
>> Checking with physician before discontinuing medication after pro-
longed use of high doses; gradual dosage reduction may be necessary to avoid possible withdrawal symptoms
>> Suspected overdose: Getting emergency help at once

**Side/adverse effects**

Signs of potential side effects, especially allergic reaction, histamine release, mental depression, and toxic megacolon

## General Dosing Information

Alteration of intestinal motility in patients with traveler's diarrhea may result in prolonged fever by slowing expulsion of infectious organisms that penetrate the intestinal mucosa (for example, *Shigella*, *Salmonella*, and certain strains of *Escherichia coli*).

Paregoric may produce fluid retention in the bowel, which may mask dehydration and electrolyte depletion caused by severe diarrhea, especially in infants and young children. Patients with severe or prolonged diarrhea should be monitored for signs of dehydration or electrolyte imbalances, and corrective therapy administered as required.

To reduce the risk of toxic megacolon in patients with acute inflammatory bowel disease, treatment with paregoric should be discontinued promptly if abdominal distention or other gastrointestinal symptoms occur.

Prolonged use of larger than usual therapeutic doses may result in physical and psychological dependence.

Tolerance to the antidiarrheal effects of paregoric may develop with prolonged use.

Following prolonged administration of high doses, paregoric should be withdrawn gradually in order to reduce the possibility of precipitating withdrawal symptoms.

This medication may suppress respiration, especially in very young, elderly, very ill, or debilitated patients, and patients with respiratory problems. Lower doses may be required for these patients.

A reduction in dosage is recommended for patients with impaired hepatic function who require prolonged treatment with this medication.

The effect of 4 mL of paregoric is similar to that of 2.5 mg of diphenoxylate.

## Oral Dosage Forms

### PAREGORIC USP

**Usual adult dose**
Antidiarrheal—
Oral, 5 to 10 mL (the equivalent of 2 to 4 mg of anhydrous morphine) one to four times a day until diarrhea is controlled.

**Usual adult prescribing limits**
Oral, 10 mL four times a day.

**Usual pediatric dose**
Antidiarrheal—
Children 2 years of age and older: Oral, 0.25 to 0.5 mL (the equivalent of 100 to 200 mcg [0.1 to 0.2 mg] of anhydrous morphine) per kg of body weight one to four times a day.

Note: For treatment of neonatal opioid withdrawal—Oral, 0.2 mL (the equivalent of 80 mcg [0.08 mg] of anhydrous morphine) every three hours. The dose may be increased, if necessary, by 0.05 mL (the equivalent of 20 mcg [0.02 mg] of anhydrous morphine) every three hours until symptoms are controlled, up to a maximum of 0.7 mL (the equivalent of 280 mcg [0.28 mg] of anhydrous morphine) per dose. After symptoms have remained stable for three to five days, dosage should be reduced gradually over a period of two to four weeks before treatment is discontinued.

It is recommended that a standard scoring system that provides objective assessment of symptom severity be used as a guide to the treatment of opioid-dependent neonates.

**Strength(s) usually available**
U.S.—
The equivalent of 2 mg of anhydrous morphine per 5 mL (Rx) [GENERIC].
Canada—
The equivalent of 2 mg of anhydrous morphine per 5 mL (Rx) [GENERIC].

Paregoric contains:

| | |
|---|---|
| Powdered opium | 4.3 grams |
| Suitable essential oil (s) | |
| Benzoic acid | 3.8 grams |
| Diluted alcohol | 900 mL |
| Glycerin | 38 mL |
| To make about | 950 mL |

Note: Paregoric may also be prepared with opium or opium tincture instead of powdered opium, the anhydrous morphine content being adjusted to 40 mg in each 100 mL and the alcohol content being adjusted to 45%.

Paregoric may also be prepared using 3.8 grams of camphor instead of the suitable essential oil (s).

**Packaging and storage**
Store below 40 °C (104 °F), preferably between 15 and 30 °C (59 and 86 °F), unless otherwise specified by manufacturer. Store in a tight, light-resistant container. Avoid exposure to direct sunlight and to excessive heat. Protect from freezing.

**Auxiliary labeling**
- May cause drowsiness.
- Avoid alcoholic beverages.
- Do not take other medicines without your doctor's advice.
- Keep out of reach of children.
- May be habit-forming.
- Shake well before using.

**Note**
Controlled substance in both the U.S. and Canada.

Caution: Be careful not to confuse paregoric (Camphorated opium tincture) with Opium tincture (Laudanum).

Refrigeration is not recommended because decreased solubility and precipitation of some of the ingredients may occur. If this occurs, filtration may be used to remove the sediment.

## Selected Bibliography

The rational use of drugs in the management of acute diarrhoea in children. Geneva: World Health Organization; 1990.
de L Costello AM, Bhutta TI. Antidiarrhoeal drugs for acute diarrhoea in children. None work, and many may be dangerous. Br Med J 1992; 304: 1-2.

Revised: 09/08/94
Interim revision: 07/05/95

## PAREGORIC-CONTAINING COMBINATIONS—

Kaolin, Pectin, and Paregoric (Systemic)

# PAROXETINE    Systemic

VA CLASSIFICATION (Primary): CN609

Note: For a listing of dosage forms and brand names by country availability, see *Dosage Forms* section(s). For a listing of brand names for the articles in this monograph, refer to the General Index.

## Category

Antidepressant.

## Indications

**Accepted**
Depression, mental (treatment)—Paroxetine is indicated for the treatment of major depressive disorder.

## Pharmacology/Pharmacokinetics

Note: A wide range of intersubject variability has been observed in the pharmacokinetic parameters of paroxetine.

**Physicochemical characteristics**
Chemically unrelated to other selective serotonin reuptake inhibitors (SSRIs), or to tricyclic, tetracyclic, or any other currently available antidepressants.
Chemical group—Phenylpiperidine.
Molecular weight—374.8.

**Mechanism of action/Effect**
Paroxetine is a potent and selective inhibitor of neuronal serotonin reuptake. Its antidepressant activity is presumed to be linked to potentiation of serotonergic activity in the central nervous system (CNS). Paroxe-

tine inhibits the active membrane transport mechanism for reuptake of serotonin, which increases concentration of the neurotransmitter at the synaptic cleft and prolongs its activity at the postsynaptic receptor sites. Inhibition of serotonin reuptake also enhances serotonergic neurotransmission by reducing turnover of the neurotransmitter via a negative feedback mechanism. Paroxetine inhibits serotonin reuptake more selectively and more potently than do fluoxetine, sertraline, fluvoxamine, zimeldine, or clomipramine. Paroxetine only very weakly inhibits reuptake of norepinephrine and dopamine.

Receptor binding studies have demonstrated that paroxetine does not interact directly with any of the central neurotransmitter receptor sites, including alpha$_1$-, alpha$_2$-, or beta- adrenoreceptors, and (D$_2$) dopamine, (5HT$_1$ or 5HT$_2$) serotonin, or (H$_1$) histamine receptors. Paroxetine has only very weak affinity for the muscarinic-cholinergic receptor, and does not inhibit monoamine oxidase.

### Other actions/effects

Selective serotonin reuptake inhibitors (SSRIs), including paroxetine, inhibit the P$_{450}$ IID$_6$ isoenzyme of the hepatic cytochrome P$_{450}$ system. At therapeutic doses, paroxetine does not significantly impair psychomotor function and exerts no significant effects on heart rate, blood pressure, or electrocardiogram (ECG) parameters. Also, paroxetine does not appear to induce epileptiform activity or to lower the seizure threshold.

### Absorption

Paroxetine is well absorbed, with bioavailability ranging from 50 to 100%. Bioavailability increases after multiple dosing due to partial saturation of first-pass metabolism. Absorption is not influenced by the presence of food, milk, or antacids.

### Distribution

Paroxetine is extensively distributed into tissues, with only 1% remaining in the systemic circulation. The volume of distribution (Vol$_D$) is large due to the lipophilic nature of paroxetine; values of 13 (range, 3 to 28) L per kilogram of body weight (L/kg) have been reported. Paroxetine is distributed into breast milk in concentrations similar to plasma concentrations.

### Protein binding
Very high (95%).

### Biotransformation

Paroxetine undergoes extensive first-pass metabolism in the liver. At least 85% of a paroxetine dose is oxidized to a catechol intermediate that undergoes subsequent methylation and conjugation to clinically inactive glucuronide and sulfate metabolites.

Metabolism is accomplished in part by cytochrome P$_{450}$ IID$_6$; partial saturation of this enzyme at clinical doses appears to account for the nonlinear kinetics observed with increasing dose and duration of paroxetine treatment. The elderly may be more susceptible to the saturation of hepatic metabolic capacity, leading to conversion to nonlinear kinetics, which results in increased plasma concentrations of paroxetine at lower than usual doses. Paroxetine inhibits cytochrome P$_{450}$ enzymes to a lesser degree than fluoxetine, but more than sertraline.

### Half-life

Elimination—
About 24 hours (range, 3 to 65 hours) in healthy adults. Due to partially saturable kinetics, the elimination half-life may be increased in the elderly. However, there is wide intersubject variability. Half-life is prolonged in patients with severe hepatic or renal function impairment.

### Onset of action

Within 1 to 4 weeks, with improvement in sleep parameters usually occurring in 1 to 2 weeks.

### Time to peak concentration
Range, 2 to 8 hours.

### Peak serum concentration

Following multiple dosing in volunteers, peak paroxetine plasma concentrations (C$_{max}$) ranged from 8.6 to 105 micrograms per L (mcg/L) (0.02 to 0.21 micromoles per L). Peak serum concentrations are subject to broad interpatient variability because of first-pass metabolism.

### Time to steady-state serum concentration

Usually achieved by 7 to 14 days in most patients, although it may take considerably longer in some patients.

### Steady-state serum concentration

In non-elderly depressed patients receiving chronic doses of 20 to 50 mg of paroxetine a day, mean steady-state serum concentrations ranged from 48.7 to 117 mcg/L (0.13 to 0.31 micromoles per L). There appears to be no correlation between paroxetine plasma concentrations and clinical efficacy or incidence of adverse effects. Linear kinetics were observed in patients with high initial plasma concentrations of

paroxetine, in contrast to nonlinear kinetics observed in patients with low initial plasma concentrations. Nonlinearity is thought to be the result of increased systemic availability, rather than a decrease in systemic clearance.

### Elimination

Renal—
In the 10-day period following administration of 30 mg of a paroxetine solution, approximately 64% of the dose was excreted in the urine, of which 2% or less was the parent compound.

Fecal—
In the 10-day period following administration of 30 mg of a paroxetine solution, about 36% of the dose was excreted in the feces, of which unchanged paroxetine comprised less than 1%.

## Precautions to Consider

### Carcinogenicity

In two-year carcinogenicity studies, a significantly greater number of male rats in the group receiving 20 times the maximum recommended human dose (MRHD) on a mg/kg basis exhibited reticulum cell sarcomas than did rats receiving lower doses. Also, there was a significantly increased linear trend across dose groups for occurrence of lymphoreticular tumors in male rats. Female rats were unaffected. In mice receiving 25 times the MRHD, there was a dose-related increase in the number of tumors in mice, but no drug-related increase in the number of mice with tumors. The relevance of these findings to humans is not known.

### Mutagenicity

Paroxetine demonstrated no genotoxic effects in a battery of 5 *in vitro* and 2 *in vivo* assays, including the bacterial mutation assay, mouse lymphoma mutation assay, unscheduled DNA synthesis assay, tests for cytogenetic aberrations *in vivo* in mouse bone marrow and *in vitro* in human lymphocytes, and a dominant lethal test in rats.

### Pregnancy/Reproduction

Fertility—Serotonin (5-hydroxytryptamine [5HT]) and compounds that modulate 5HT, are known to affect reproduction function in animals. Rats administered paroxetine at doses 15 or more times the highest recommended human dose had impaired reproductive function, including reduced pregnancy rates and increased pre- and post-implantation losses.

Pregnancy—Adequate and well-controlled studies in humans have not been done.

No teratogenic effects or selective toxicity to the fetus were demonstrated in studies in rats and rabbits receiving 50 and 6 times the maximum daily human mg/kg dose, respectively. However, decreased pup viability occurred in rats given doses 15 or more times the MRHD.

FDA Pregnancy Category B.

Labor and delivery—The effect of paroxetine on labor and delivery is not known.

### Breast-feeding

Paroxetine is distributed into breast milk in concentrations similar to those found in plasma.

### Pediatrics

No information is available on the relationship of age to the effects of paroxetine in pediatric patients. Safety and efficacy have not been established.

### Geriatrics

No geriatrics-related problems have been documented in studies done to date that included geriatric patients.

### Dental

Prolonged use of paroxetine may decrease or inhibit salivary flow, thus contributing to the development of caries, periodontal disease, oral candidiasis, and discomfort.

### Drug interactions and/or related problems

The following drug interactions and/or related problems have been selected on the basis of their potential clinical significance (possible mechanism in parentheses where appropriate)—not necessarily inclusive (» = major clinical significance):

Note: Possible interactions with hepatic enzyme inducers, hepatic enzyme inhibitors, and medications that are metabolized by the hepatic P$_{450}$ enzyme system (including tricyclic antidepressants, phenothiazines, and type IC antiarrhythmics), other than those listed below, have not been studied, but the possibility of a significant interaction should be considered. Lower initial doses and gradual dose titration may be necessary, and the patient should be carefully monitored during and following concurrent use. Paroxetine is not a general inducer or inhibitor of hepatic oxidation processes.

*In vitro* studies have shown little chance of paroxetine being displaced by other highly protein-bound agents; also, paroxetine is unlikely to displace other highly protein-bound medications. *In vivo*, however, the potential exists for displacement of one highly protein-bound medication by another; increased free concentrations of the displaced agent could result, increasing the likelihood of adverse effects.

A potentially lethal hyperserotonergic state known as the serotonin syndrome may occur if a serotonergic agent such as paroxetine is administered with MAO inhibitors or other agents that affect serotonergic mechanisms. The syndrome may be manifested by mental status changes, restlessness, myoclonus, hyperreflexia, diaphoresis, shivering, tremor, diarrhea, incoordination, and/or fever. If recognized early, the syndrome usually resolves quickly upon withdrawal of the offending agents.

Combinations containing any of the following medications, depending on the amount present, may also interact with this medication.

Alcohol
(although paroxetine has not been shown to alter alcohol metabolism and does not appear to potentiate cognitive and psychomotor effects of alcohol in normal subjects, concomitant use in depressed patients is not recommended)

Cimetidine
(in one study, steady-state plasma concentrations of paroxetine were increased by approximately 50% during concurrent administration of cimetidine; although the clinical significance of this interaction has not been definitively established, initial dosage reductions are not thought to be necessary, but subsequent dose titration should be based on clinical effects)

Digoxin
(mean digoxin area under the concentration-time curve [AUC] decreased 15% in the presence of paroxetine; since there is little clinical experience with this combination, concurrent administration should be undertaken with caution)

Lithium
(although no pharmacokinetic or pharmacodynamic interactions have been reported, there is little clinical experience with this combination; because lithium may activate serotonergic mechanisms, caution should be exercised during concomitant use to avoid adverse events such as the serotonin syndrome)

» Monoamine oxidase (MAO) inhibitors, including furazolidone, procarbazine, and selegiline
(concurrent use of MAO inhibitors with paroxetine may result in confusion, agitation, restlessness, and gastrointestinal symptoms, or possibly hyperpyretic episodes, severe convulsions, hypertensive crises, or the serotonin syndrome; at least 14 days should elapse between discontinuation of one medication and initiation of another)

Phenobarbital or
Primidone
(because primidone is partially metabolized to phenobarbital, which induces many cytochrome P$_{450}$ enzymes, administration of either of these agents concomitantly with paroxetine may reduce the systemic availability of paroxetine; no initial dosage adjustments are recommended, but subsequent titration should be based on clinical effects)

Phenytoin
(concomitant administration with paroxetine may decrease the systemic availability of either agent; also, both medications may exhibit nonlinear pharmacokinetic properties; no initial dosage adjustments are recommended, but subsequent titration should be based on clinical effects)

Procyclidine
(concurrent use may increase the systemic availability of procyclidine; if anticholinergic effects occur, the dosage of procyclidine should be reduced)

» Tryptophan
(because tryptophan can be metabolized to serotonin, the risk of serious serotonin-associated side effects, including the serotonin syndrome, is increased; concomitant use is not recommended)

» Warfarin
(although paroxetine does not alter *in vitro* protein binding of warfarin, a pharmacodynamic interaction may exist that causes an increased bleeding diathesis despite unaltered prothrombin time; since there is little clinical experience, caution is advised when using these agents concomitantly)

**Laboratory value alterations**
The following have been selected on the basis of their potential clinical significance (possible effect in parentheses where appropriate)—not necessarily inclusive (» = major clinical significance):

With physiology/laboratory test values
    Hematocrit or
    Hemoglobin or
    White blood cell counts
        (may be decreased)

**Medical considerations/Contraindications**
The medical considerations/contraindications included here have been selected on the basis of their potential clinical significance (reasons given in parentheses where appropriate)—not necessarily inclusive (» = major clinical significance).

*Risk-benefit should be considered when the following medical problems exist:*
Drug abuse or dependence, history of
    (patients with a history of drug abuse should be observed closely for signs of misuse or abuse of paroxetine, as with any new central nervous system [CNS] drug)
Hepatic function impairment, severe
    (metabolism of paroxetine may be altered; initial dosage should be reduced, starting at 10 mg once a day)
Mania, history of
    (activation of hypomania or mania has been reported in depressed patients treated with paroxetine)
Renal function impairment, severe
    (excretion of paroxetine may be altered; initial dosage should be reduced, starting at 10 mg once a day)
Seizures, history of
    (as with other antidepressants, paroxetine should be introduced with caution; if seizures develop, paroxetine should be discontinued)

**Patient monitoring**
The following may be especially important in patient monitoring (other tests may be warranted in some patients, depending on condition; » = major clinical significance):

Careful supervision of depressed patients with suicidal tendencies
    (recommended especially during early treatment phase before peak effectiveness of paroxetine is achieved; prescribing the smallest number of tablets necessary for good patient management is recommended to decrease risk of overdose)

# Side/Adverse Effects

Note: Side effects are usually mild and transient, with evidence of dose-dependency for some of the most common adverse effects. In addition, there is evidence of adaptation with continuing therapy (over 4 to 6 weeks) to some effects such as nausea and dizziness.

The following side/adverse effects have been selected on the basis of their potential clinical significance (possible signs and symptoms in parentheses where appropriate)—not necessarily inclusive:

**Those indicating need for medical attention**
Incidence less frequent
    *Agitation; myalgia, myasthenia, or myopathy* (muscle pain or weakness); *orthostatic hypotension* (lightheadedness or fainting); *skin rash*
Incidence rare
    *Extrapyramidal symptoms, including; akinesia or hypokinesia* (absence of or decrease in body movements); *dyskinesia* (unusual or incomplete body movements); *dystonia* (unusual or sudden body or facial movements; inability to move eyes); *and dysarthria* (difficulty in speaking); *hyponatremia* (drowsiness; dryness of mouth; increased thirst; lack of energy); *mania or hypomania* (talking, feeling, and acting with excitement and activity you cannot control); *serotonin syndrome* (diarrhea; fever; increased sweating; mood or behavior changes; overactive reflexes; racing heartbeat; restlessness; shivering or shaking)

Note: *Hyponatremia* has been reported mostly in elderly patients, some of whom were taking diuretics or were otherwise volume-depleted.

Activation of *mania/hypomania* occurred in about 1% of unipolar and in about 2% of a subset of bipolar patients during premarketing testing.

**Those indicating need for medical attention only if they continue or are bothersome**

Incidence more frequent

*Asthenia* (unusual tiredness or weakness); *constipation; diarrhea; dizziness; drowsiness; dryness of mouth; headache; increased sweating; insomnia* (trouble in sleeping); *nausea; sexual dysfunction, especially ejaculatory disturbances* (decreased sexual ability); *tremor; urinary frequency or retention* (problems in urinating); *vomiting*

Note: *Dryness of mouth* is probably due to a direct effect on the serotonin system rather than cholinergic blockade.

Incidence less frequent

*Anxiety or nervousness; blurred vision; decreased libido* (decreased sexual desire); *decreased or increased appetite; palpitation* (fast or irregular heartbeat); *paresthesia* (tingling, burning, or prickly sensations); *taste perversion* (change in your sense of taste); *weight loss or gain*

Note: Paroxetine may cause less *weight loss* than fluoxetine or sertraline; also, it may cause less *weight gain* than imipramine, especially in females. Long-term paroxetine treatment may cause *increased appetite* and *weight gain*.

**Those indicating the need for medical attention if they occur after medication is discontinued**

*Agitation, confusion, or restlessness; diarrhea; dizziness, vertigo, or lightheadedness; headache; insomnia; migraine-like visual disturbances* (vision changes); *myalgia; nausea or vomiting; rhinorrhea* (runny nose); *sweating; tremor; unusual tiredness or weakness*

Note: Withdrawal symptoms, if they occur, usually start 1 to 4 days after stopping paroxetine; however, some patients may experience effects immediately. Instances of withdrawal symptoms occurring in patients after paroxetine dosage was tapered over 7 to 10 days have been reported. Although most effects are generally mild and transient, some patients may experience more severe symptoms.

## Overdose

For specific information on the agents used in the management of paroxetine overdose, see:

• *Charcoal, Activated (Oral-Local)* monograph.

For more information on the management of overdose or unintentional ingestion, **contact a Poison Control Center** (see *Poison Control Center Listing*).

### Clinical effects of overdose

The following effects have been selected on the basis of their potential clinical significance (possible signs and symptoms in parentheses where appropriate)—not necessarily inclusive:

*Dilated pupils* (large pupils); *drowsiness, severe; dryness of mouth, severe; irritability; nausea, severe; sinus tachycardia* (racing heartbeat); *tremor, severe; vomiting, severe*

### Treatment of overdose

There is no specific antidote for paroxetine. Treatment is essentially symptomatic and supportive, possibly including:

To decrease absorption—

Decontaminating gastrointestinal tract by emesis, lavage, or both, followed by administering 20 to 30 grams of activated charcoal during the first 24 to 48 hours following ingestion.

Monitoring—

Monitoring cardiac function and vital signs.

Supportive care—

Establishing and monitoring airway. Patients in whom intentional overdose is known or suspected should be referred for psychiatric consultation.

Note: Due to the large volume of distribution of paroxetine, forced diuresis, hemodialysis, hemoperfusion, or exchange transfusions are not likely to be of benefit.

## Patient Consultation

As an aid to patient consultation, refer to *Advice for the Patient, Paroxetine (Systemic)*.

In providing consultation, consider emphasizing the following selected information (» = major clinical significance):

### Before using this medication

» Conditions affecting use, especially:

Sensitivity to paroxetine

Pregnancy—Studies in rats using higher than the maximum human mg/kg doses have shown increased pre-and post-implantation losses and decreased viability of pups; clinical significance is unknown

Breast-feeding—Distributed into breast milk

Dental—Decreased salivary flow may contribute to caries, periodontal disease, candidiasis, and discomfort

Other medications, especially monoamine oxidase (MAO) inhibitors, tryptophan, and warfarin

### Proper use of this medication

» Compliance with therapy; not taking more or less medicine than prescribed

» Up to 4 weeks or more of therapy may be required before antidepressant effects are achieved

» Proper dosing

Missed dose: Taking as soon as possible; continuing on regular schedule with next dose; not doubling doses

» Proper storage

### Precautions while using this medication

Regular visits to physician to check progress of therapy

Checking with physician before discontinuing medication

» Avoiding use of alcoholic beverages; not taking other CNS depressants unless prescribed by physician

» Possible blurred vision, drowsiness, impairment of judgment, thinking, or motor skills; caution when driving or doing jobs requiring alertness

» Possible dizziness or lightheadedness; caution when getting up suddenly from a lying or sitting position

» Possible dryness of mouth; using sugarless gum or candy, ice, or saliva substitute for relief; checking with physician or dentist if dry mouth continues for more than 2 weeks

### Side/adverse effects

Possibility of withdrawal symptoms

Signs of potential side effects, especially agitation; myalgia, myasthenia, or myopathy; orthostatic hypotension; rash; extrapyramidal symptoms; hyponatremia; mania or hypomania; serotonin syndrome

## General Dosing Information

Paroxetine may be administered once daily, usually in the morning, to diminish sleep disturbances and other adverse effects.

Abrupt discontinuation of paroxetine may result in symptoms of withdrawal, including agitation, confusion, or restlessness; diarrhea; dizziness, vertigo, or lightheadedness; headache; insomnia; migraine-like visual disturbances; myalgia; nausea or vomiting; rhinorrhea; sweating; tremor; or unusual tiredness or weakness

Potentially suicidal patients should not have access to large quantities of this medication since depressed patients, particularly those who may use alcohol excessively, may continue to exhibit suicidal tendencies until significant improvement occurs. Some clinicians recommend that the patient be supplied with the smallest quantity of medication necessary for satisfactory patient management.

Activation of hypomania or mania has been reported in depressed patients treated with paroxetine.

### Diet/Nutrition

Paroxetine may be taken with or without food. Some clinicians advise their patients to take this medication with food to lessen gastrointestinal side effects.

## Oral Dosage Forms

### PAROXETINE HYDROCHLORIDE TABLETS

**Usual adult dose**

Antidepressant—

Oral, initially 20 mg once a day, usually in the morning. The dose may be increased, as needed and tolerated, by 10 mg a day at intervals of at least 7 days, up to a maximum dose of 50 mg a day.

Note: For most patients, 20 mg a day is the optimal dose. Geriatric or debilitated patients, and patients with severe renal or hepatic function impairment should receive an initial dose of 10 mg a day, with upward titration as needed up to a maximum of 40 mg a day.

**Usual adult prescribing limits**

50 mg a day.

**Usual pediatric dose**

Safety and efficacy in children have not been established.

**Usual geriatric dose**

Antidepressant—
  Oral, initially 10 mg once a day, usually in the morning. Dose may
    be increased as needed and tolerated, up to a maximum dose of
    40 mg a day

**Strength(s) usually available**

U.S.—
  20 mg (Rx) [*Paxil*].
  30 mg (Rx) [*Paxil*].
Canada—
  20 mg (Rx) [*Paxil*].
  30 mg (Rx) [*Paxil*].

**Auxiliary labeling**

• Avoid alcoholic beverages.
• May cause drowsiness.

## Selected Bibliography

Dechant KL, Clissold SP. Paroxetine. A review of its pharmacodynamic
  and pharmacokinetic properties, and therapeutic potential in depressive
  illness. Drugs 1991 Feb; 41 (2): 225-53.
Caley CF, Weber SS. Paroxetine: A selective serotonin reuptake inhibiting
  antidepressant. Ann Pharmacother 1993 Oct; 27: 1212-22.
Nemeroff CB. The clinical pharmacology and use of paroxetine, a new
  selective serotonin reuptake inhibitor. Pharmacotherapy 1994; 14 (2):
  127-38.

Developed: 08/22/94

## PECTIN-CONTAINING COMBINATIONS—

Kaolin and Pectin (Oral-Local)
Kaolin, Pectin, Hyoscyamine, Atropine, and Scopolamine (Systemic)—
  See *Kaolin, Pectin, and Belladonna Alkaloids (Systemic)*
Kaolin, Pectin, and Paregoric (Systemic)

# PEGADEMASE    Systemic†

VA CLASSIFICATION (Primary): IM900

Some other commonly used names are PEG-ADA and PEG-adenosine
  deaminase.

Note: For a listing of dosage forms and brand names by country availability, see *Dosage Forms* section(s). For a listing of brand names
  for the articles in this monograph, refer to the General Index.

  †Not commercially available in Canada.

## Category

Enzyme, adenosine deaminase, replenisher.

## Indications

**Accepted**

Adenosine deaminase deficiency (treatment)—Pegademase bovine is indicated for enzyme replacement therapy for adenosine deaminase
  (ADA) deficiency in patients with severe combined immunodeficiency
  disease (SCID) who are not suitable candidates for, or who have failed,
  bone marrow transplantation.

**Unaccepted**

Pegademase bovine is not intended as a replacement for HLA identical
  bone marrow transplant therapy and there is no evidence supporting
  safety and efficacy as preparatory or support therapy for bone marrow
  transplantation.

## Pharmacology/Pharmacokinetics

**Physicochemical characteristics**

Source—Pegademase bovine is a conjugate of the enzyme adenosine deaminase (ADA) covalently attached to numerous strands of monomethoxypolyethylene glycol (which permits prolonged circulation of
  ADA in the blood). Adenosine deaminase used in the manufacture of
  pegademase bovine is derived from bovine intestine.
Molecular weight—Pegademase bovine: 90,000.
Monomethoxypolyethylene glycol (PEG): 5000.

**Mechanism of action/Effect**

In the absence of ADA, accumulation of the purine substrates adenosine
  and 2'-deoxyadenosine occurs; these substrates and their metabolites
  are toxic to lymphocytes. Replacement of the ADA results in correction of the metabolic abnormalities, which leads to improvement in
  immune function, reduced frequency of opportunistic infections, and
  fewer complications of infections. Pegademase bovine reduces elevated deoxyadenosine triphosphate (dATP) in erythrocytes and increases diminished levels of S-adenosylhomocysteine hydrolase
  (SAHase).

**Half-life**

ADA—3 to more than 6 days; variable, even for the same patient.

**Onset of action**

Between correction of the metabolic abnormality and improvement in immune function—2 to 6 months; improvement in clinical status is usually evident by the end of the first year of therapy.

**Time to peak plasma concentration**

For ADA activity—2 to 3 days.

Note: Average trough plasma ADA activity, with weekly injections of 15
  Units per kg of body weight is 20 to 25 micromoles per hour per
  mL.

## Precautions to Consider

**Carcinogenicity**

Studies have not been done.

**Mutagenicity**

Mutagenicity tests against *Salmonella typhimurium* strains in the Ames
  assay were negative.

**Pregnancy/Reproduction**

Pregnancy—Studies have not been done in either animals or humans.
FDA Pregnancy Category C.

**Breast-feeding**

It is not known whether pegademase bovine is excreted in breast milk.

**Pediatrics**

Pegademase bovine is used primarily in infants and children. No pediatrics-specific problems have been documented in studies in children
  age 6 weeks to 12 years.

**Geriatrics**

No published geriatrics-specific information is available.

**Drug interactions and/or related problems**

The following drug interactions and/or related problems have been selected on the basis of their potential clinical significance (possible
  mechanism in parentheses where appropriate)—not necessarily inclusive (» = major clinical significance):
  Vidarabine
    (because vidarabine is a substrate for adenosine deaminase [ADA],
    the activities of one or both medications could potentially be al-
    tered with concurrent use)

**Medical considerations/Contraindications**

The medical considerations/contraindications included here have been selected on the basis of their potential clinical significance (reasons given
  in parentheses where appropriate)—not necessarily inclusive (» =
  major clinical significance).

*Except under special circumstances, this medication should not be used
  when the following medical problem exists:*

» Thrombocytopenia, severe
    (risk of bleeding with intramuscular injection)

*Risk-benefit should be considered when the following medical problems
  exist:*

Sensitivity to pegademase

» Thrombocytopenia
    (risk of bleeding with intramuscular injection)

**Patient monitoring**

The following may be especially important in patient monitoring (other tests may be warranted in some patients, depending on condition; » = major clinical significance):

» Plasma adenosine (ADA) activity, trough (pre-injection)

(recommended prior to initiation of therapy and every 1 to 2 weeks during the first 8 to 12 weeks of therapy to establish an effective dose; a minimum trough level before maintenance injection of 15 to 35 micromoles per hour per mL [assayed at 37 °C] should be maintained to ensure that plasma ADA activity from dose to dose is maintained above the level of total erythrocyte ADA activity in the blood of normal individuals; between 3 and 9 months, should be determined twice a month, then monthly until after 18 to 24 months of therapy; after 2 years of therapy, should be determined every 2 to 4 months [more frequently if therapy is interrupted or if clearance rate of plasma ADA activity is increased])

» Red blood cell deoxyadenosine triphosphate (dATP) concentrations

(determinations recommended prior to initiation of therapy and after 2 months of treatment; concentrations should decrease to range of less than or equal to 0.005 to 0.015 micromoles per mL [normal value is 0.001 micromoles per mL] or less than or equal to 1% of the total erythrocyte adenine nucleotide [ATP plus dATP] content, with a normal ATP level, as measured in a pre-injection sample; once the concentration of dATP has fallen adequately, determinations are recommended 2 to 4 times during the remainder of the first year and 2 to 3 times a year thereafter [more frequently if therapy is interrupted or if clearance rate of plasma ADA activity is increased])

Immune function and
Clinical status

(monitoring at regular intervals is recommended)

Assay for antibody to ADA and pegademase bovine, by ELISA or enzyme inhibition

(recommended if a persistent fall in plasma ADA activity to less than 10 micromoles per hour per mL occurs, which has been determined not to be caused by improper storage of pegademase bovine injection or improper handling of plasma samples or by interruption of therapy)

## Side/Adverse Effects

Note: Increased clearance of plasma ADA activity in association with presence of an antibody that directly inhibited ADA and pegademase bovine has been reported. Temporarily increasing the dose of pegademase bovine restored ADA activity to effective levels, and after a few months reduction to the usual dose resulted in continued effective plasma activity.

Plasma levels of ADA activity more than twice the upper limit of 35 micromoles per hour per mL occurring for as long as several weeks have not resulted in adverse effects.

The following side/adverse effects have been selected on the basis of their potential clinical significance (possible signs and symptoms in parentheses where appropriate)—not necessarily inclusive:

**Those indicating need for medical attention only if they continue or are bothersome**
Incidence rare
*Headache; pain at site of injection*

## Patient Consultation

As an aid to patient consultation, refer to *Advice for the Patient, Pegademase (Systemic).*

In providing consultation, consider emphasizing the following selected information (» = major clinical significance):

**Before using this medication**
» Conditions affecting use, especially:
    Sensitivity to pegademase
    Other medical problems, especially thrombocytopenia

**Proper use of this medication**
» Proper dosing
    Missed dose: Resuming therapy as soon as possible

**Precautions while using this medication**
» Importance of lifelong treatment with pegademase bovine; impaired immunity and risk of serious infection if regular treatment not continued

## General Dosing Information

Pegademase bovine injection is for intramuscular use only.

One Unit of activity is defined as the amount of adenosine deaminase (ADA) that converts 1 micromole of adenosine to inosine per minute at 25 °C and pH 7.3.

Dosage of pegademase bovine injection should be individualized on the basis of plasma ADA activity and red blood cell deoxyadenosine nucleotide (dATP) concentrations.

Until an improvement in immune function has been confirmed, patients should receive appropriate care to protect against infection and other related illnesses.

Lifelong replacement therapy with pegademase bovine injection is necessary.

A decline in immune function may occur during therapy if adequate levels of ADA activity are not maintained, which may occur if an antibody to pegademase bovine injection develops, dosage is miscalculated, therapy is interrupted, or the injection is improperly stored. If a persistent decline in plasma ADA activity occurs, immune function and clinical status should be monitored closely and precautions taken to minimize the risk of infection.

If a persistent fall in plasma ADA activity is determined to be caused by development of an antibody to ADA or pegademase bovine, dosage adjustment is recommended.

Testing prior to distribution may not assure the initial and continuing potency of each new lot of pegademase bovine injection. If, after adequate ADA plasma activity has been achieved, a fall in activity below 10 micromoles per hour per mL occurs, which cannot be attributed to improper dosing or sample handling or to antibody development, the following is recommended:

• All patients receiving the same lot of the injection as the patient in whom the fall in ADA activity occurred (Patient 1) are required to have a blood sample for plasma ADA determinations taken prior to the next injection.

• The index patient (Patient 1) requires retesting for determination of plasma ADA activity prior to the next injection.

• If both values (the second value in Patient 1 and the value from one of the other patients who received the same lot of the injection as Patient 1) are less than 10 micromoles per hour per mL, the manufacturer will recall and replace the lot in question.

## Parenteral Dosage Forms
### PEGADEMASE BOVINE INJECTION

**Usual pediatric dose**

Initial—Intramuscular, 10 Units per kg of body weight, followed seven days later by 15 Units per kg of body weight, followed seven days later by 20 Units per kg of body weight.

Maintenance—Intramuscular, 20 Units per kg of body weight once a week.

Note: Further increases of 5 Units per kg of body weight per week may be necessary, but a maximum single dose of 30 Units per kg of body weight should not be exceeded.

Twice weekly dosing may be necessary if antibodies to ADA or pegademase bovine develop.

Pegademase bovine injection may be used in infants from birth or in children of any age.

**Strength(s) usually available**
U.S.—
    250 Units per mL (375 Units per 1.5-mL single-use vial) (Rx) [*Adagen*].
Canada—
    Not commercially available.

**Packaging and storage**
Store between 2 and 8 °C (36 and 46 °F), unless otherwise specified by manufacturer. Protect from freezing.

**Incompatibilities**
Should not be diluted or mixed with any other medication prior to administration.

**Auxiliary labeling**
• Do not freeze.

## Selected Bibliography

Hershfield MS, Buckley RH, Greenberg ML, et al. Treatment of adenosine deaminase deficiency with polyethylene glycol–modified adenosine deaminase. New Engl J Med 1987; 316: 589-96.

Levy Y, Hershfield MS, Fernandez-Mejia C, et al. Adenosine deaminase deficiency with late onset of recurrent infections: response to treatment with polyethylene glycol–modified adenosine deaminase. J Pediatr 1988; 113: 312-7.

Kredich NM, Hershfield MS. Immunodeficiency diseases caused by adenosine deaminase deficiency and purine nucleoside phosphorylase deficiency. In: Scriver CR, Beaudet AL, Sly WS, Valle D, eds. The metabolic basis of inherited disease, 6th ed. New York: McGraw-Hill, 1989: 1045-75.

Revised: 09/90
Interim revision: 07/11/94

# PEMOLINE   Systemic

VA CLASSIFICATION (Primary): CN809

Note: Controlled substance in the U.S.—Schedule IV.

Note: For a listing of dosage forms and brand names by country availability, see *Dosage Forms* section(s). For a listing of brand names for the articles in this monograph, refer to the General Index.

## Category

Central nervous system stimulant.

## Indications

### Accepted

Attention-deficit hyperactivity disorder (treatment)—Pemoline is indicated in attention-deficit hyperactivity disorder (ADHD) as an integral part of a total treatment program that includes other remedial measures (psychological, educational, and social) for a stabilizing effect in some children with ADHD. This complex behavioral syndrome has been known in the past as hyperkinetic child syndrome, minimal brain damage, minimal cerebral dysfunction, or minor cerebral dysfunction. The syndrome is characterized by moderate to severe distractibility, short attention span, hyperactivity, emotional lability, and impulsivity.

## Pharmacology/Pharmacokinetics

### Physicochemical characteristics

Molecular weight—176.17.

### Mechanism of action/Effect

Pemoline's mechanism and site of action have not been conclusively determined; however, animal studies suggest that pemoline may act through dopaminergic mechanisms. In children with attention deficit disorder, pemoline decreases hyperactivity and prolongs attention span. However, the mechanism by which pemoline produces mental and behavioral effects in children has not been established.

### Protein binding

Moderate (50%).

### Biotransformation

Hepatic; metabolites include pemoline conjugate, pemoline dione, mandelic acid, and unidentified polar compounds.

### Half-life

12 hours.

### Time to peak serum concentration

2 to 4 hours; steady state reached in 2 to 3 days.

### Time to peak effect

3 to 4 weeks.

### Elimination

Renal; about 75% of an oral dose of pemoline is excreted in the urine within 24 hours and about 50% is excreted unchanged.

## Precautions to Consider

### Carcinogenicity

There was no significant difference in the incidence of neoplasms between rats given doses as high as 150 mg per kg per day for 18 months and untreated rats.

### Mutagenicity

Data are not available concerning long-term effects on mutagenicity in humans or animals.

### Pregnancy/Reproduction

Pregnancy—Problems in humans have not been documented.

Animal studies have shown an increased incidence of stillbirths when pemoline was administered at a dose of 37.5 mg per kg of body weight (mg/kg) a day. Postnatal survival rate of offspring was reduced at doses of 18.75 and 37.5 mg/kg a day.

FDA Pregnancy Category B.

### Breast-feeding

It is not known if pemoline is excreted in breast milk; however, problems in humans have not been documented.

### Pediatrics

Monitoring of growth should be conducted in children during long-term treatment with pemoline since suppression of growth has been reported with the use of central nervous system (CNS) stimulants in children.

Some medical authorities recommend drug-free periods during treatment. Pemoline may exacerbate symptoms of behavior disturbance and thought disorder in psychotic children.

### Drug interactions and/or related problems

The following drug interactions and/or related problems have been selected on the basis of their potential clinical significance (possible mechanism in parentheses where appropriate)—not necessarily inclusive (» = major clinical significance):

Note: Combinations containing any of the following medications, depending on the amount present, may also interact with this medication.

Anticonvulsants
(pemoline may decrease the seizure threshold; therefore, dosage adjustments of the anticonvulsant may be necessary during concurrent use)

CNS stimulation–producing medications, other (See *Appendix II*)
(concurrent use of other CNS stimulation–producing medications with pemoline may result in additive CNS stimulation to excessive levels causing nervousness, irritability, insomnia, or possibly convulsions or cardiac arrhythmias; close observation is recommended)

### Laboratory value alterations

The following have been selected on the basis of their potential clinical significance (possible effect in parentheses where appropriate)—not necessarily inclusive (» = major clinical significance):

With physiology/laboratory test values
Alanine aminotransferase (ALT [SGPT]) and
Aspartate aminotransferase (AST [SGOT]) and
Lactate dehydrogenase (LDH)
(serum values may be increased; increases usually occur after several months of therapy; effects are possibly caused by a delayed hypersensitivity reaction and appear to be reversible upon withdrawal of pemoline)

### Medical considerations/Contraindications

The medical considerations/contraindications included here have been selected on the basis of their potential clinical significance (reasons given in parentheses where appropriate)—not necessarily inclusive (» = major clinical significance):

*Except under special circumstances, this medication should not be used if the following medical problem exists:*

» Hepatic function impairment
(may be exacerbated)

*Risk-benefit should be considered when the following medical problems exist:*

» Gilles de la Tourette's disorder or other tics
(attacks may be precipitated)

» Psychosis
(symptoms of behavior disturbance and thought disorder may be exacerbated in psychotic children)

» Renal function impairment
(excretion may be altered)

Sensitivity to pemoline

## Patient monitoring

The following may be especially important in patient monitoring (other tests may be warranted in some patients, depending on condition; » = major clinical significance):

Assessment of potential tolerance, dependence, or drug-seeking behavior
(recommended at periodic intervals during long-term therapy)

Hepatic function determinations
(recommended prior to and at periodic intervals during therapy)

Monitoring for motor or vocal tics
(recommended periodically during therapy)

Monitoring of growth, both height and weight gain, in children
(recommended during long-term therapy since suppression of growth has been reported with use of CNS stimulants in children)

Reassessment of need for therapy for attention-deficit hyperactivity disorder in children
(interruption of therapy at periodic intervals is recommended to determine if a recurrence of behavioral symptoms is sufficient to continue therapy)

## Side/Adverse Effects

The following side/adverse effects have been selected on the basis of their potential clinical significance (possible signs and symptoms in parentheses where appropriate)—not necessarily inclusive:

**Those indicating need for medical attention**
Incidence rare
*Jaundice* (yellow eyes or skin)

**Those indicating need for medical attention only if they continue or are bothersome**
Incidence more frequent
*Anorexia* (loss of appetite); *insomnia* (trouble in sleeping); *weight loss*
Incidence less frequent
*Dizziness; drowsiness; increased irritability; mental depression; nausea; skin rash; stomach ache*

**Those indicating possible withdrawal and the need for medical attention if they occur after medication is discontinued**
*Mental depression, severe; unusual behavior; unusual tiredness or weakness*

## Overdose

For specific information on the agents used in the management of pemoline overdose, see:
- *Chlorpromazine* in *Phenothiazines (Systemic)* monograph; and/or
- *Phentolamine (Systemic)* monograph.

For more information on the management of overdose or unintentional ingestion, **contact a Poison Control Center** (see *Poison Control Center Listing*).

### Clinical effects of overdose

The following effects have been selected on the basis of their potential clinical significance (possible signs and symptoms in parentheses where appropriate)—not necessarily inclusive:

*Agitation; confusion; convulsions; false sense of well-being; fast heartbeat; hallucinations; headache, severe; high fever with sweating; hypertension* (high blood pressure); *large pupils; muscle trembling or twitching; nervousness or restlessness; uncontrolled movements of the eyes or other parts of the body; vomiting*

### Treatment of overdose

Treatment is symptomatic and supportive, and is essentially the same as that for an overdosage of any CNS stimulant. Treatment may include the following:

To decrease absorption—Inducing emesis and/or using gastric lavage.

Specific treatment—Sometimes using chlorpromazine to control excessive CNS stimulation and sympathomimetic effects. Using intravenous phentolamine to control hypertension.

Monitoring—Monitoring cardiovascular and respiratory functioning.

Supportive care—Using intravenous fluids to control hypotension. Protecting patient from self-injury by use of restraints if necessary. Patients in whom intentional overdose is known or suspected should be referred for psychiatric consultation.

## Patient Consultation

As an aid to patient consultation, refer to *Advice for the Patient, Pemoline (Systemic)*.

In providing consultation, consider emphasizing the following selected information (» = major clinical significance):

**Before using this medication**
» Conditions affecting use, especially:
Sensitivity to pemoline
Pregnancy—Animal studies have shown an increase in stillbirths and reduced postnatal survival rate
Use in children—Inhibition of growth reported with CNS stimulants, but data inconclusive; drug-free periods recommended; symptoms of behavior disturbance and thought disorder exacerbated in psychotic children
Other medical problems, especially hepatic function impairment; Tourette's disorder; psychosis; or renal function impairment

**Proper use of this medication**
Proper administration of chewable tablet: Tablet must be chewed
» May require 3 to 4 weeks of therapy to obtain optimal effects
» Importance of not taking more medication than the amount prescribed because of possible habit-forming potential
» Proper dosing
Missed dose: Taking as soon as possible; if remembered the next day, skipping missed dose; continuing on schedule; not doubling doses
» Proper storage

**Precautions while using this medication**
Regular visits to physician to check progress during therapy
Checking with physician before discontinuing medication after long-term and high-dose therapy; gradual dosage reduction may be necessary to avoid possibility of withdrawal symptoms
» Caution if dizziness occurs
» Suspected physical or psychological dependence; checking with physician

**Side/adverse effects**
Signs of potential side effects, especially jaundice

## General Dosing Information

Significant beneficial effects of pemoline may not be evident until the third or fourth week of therapy since clinical improvement is gradual.

Prolonged use of pemoline may result in psychological or physical dependence.

When symptoms of attention-deficit hyperactivity disorder are controlled in children, dosage reduction or interruption in therapy may be possible during the summer months and at other times when the child is under less stress; medication may be given on each of the 5 school days during the week, with medication-free weekends and school holidays.

When the medication is to be discontinued following high-dose and long-term administration, the dosage should be reduced gradually since abrupt withdrawal may result in extreme fatigue, mental depression, and unusual behavior.

## Oral Dosage Forms

### PEMOLINE TABLETS

**Usual pediatric dose**
Attention-deficit hyperactivity disorder—
Children up to 6 years of age: Dosage has not been established.
Children 6 years of age and over: Oral, 37.5 mg as a single dose each morning, the dosage being increased by 18.75 mg a day at one-week intervals until the desired response is obtained, up to a maximum of 112.5 mg a day.

**Strength(s) usually available**
U.S.—
18.75 mg (Rx) [*Cylert* (scored; corn starch; gelatin; lactose; magnesium hydroxide; polyethylene glycol; talc)].
37.5 mg (Rx) [*Cylert* (scored; corn starch; FD&C Yellow No. 6; gelatin; lactose; magnesium hydroxide; polyethylene glycol; talc)].
75 mg (Rx) [*Cylert* (scored; corn starch; gelatin; iron oxide; lactose; magnesium hydroxide; polyethylene glycol; talc)].
Canada—
37.5 mg (Rx) [*Cylert* (scored)].
75 mg (Rx) [*Cylert* (scored)].

**Packaging and storage**
Store below 40 °C (104 °F), preferably between 15 and 30 °C (59 and 86 °F), in a well-closed container, unless otherwise specified by manufacturer.

**Note**
Controlled substance in the U.S.

## PEMOLINE CHEWABLE TABLETS

### Usual pediatric dose
See *Pemoline Tablets*.

### Strength(s) usually available
U.S.—
   37.5 mg (Rx) [*Cylert Chewable* (corn starch; FD&C Yellow No. 6; magnesium hydroxide; magnesium stearate; mannitol; polyethylene glycol; povidone; talc; artificial flavor)].
Canada—
   Not commercially available.

### Packaging and storage
Store below 40 °C (104 °F), preferably between 15 and 30 °C (59 and 86 °F), in a well-closed container, unless otherwise specified by manufacturer.

### Auxiliary labeling
• Must be chewed.

### Note
Controlled substance in the U.S.

Revised: 04/16/93

---

**PENBUTOLOL**—See *Beta-adrenergic Blocking Agents (Systemic)*

---

# PENICILLAMINE   Systemic

VA CLASSIFICATION (Primary/Secondary): MS104/GU900; AD300
Note: For a listing of dosage forms and brand names by country availability, see *Dosage Forms* section(s). For a listing of brand names for the articles in this monograph, refer to the General Index.

## Category
Chelating agent; antirheumatic (disease-modifying); antiurolithic (cystine calculi); antidote (to heavy metals).

## Indications
Note: Bracketed information in the *Indications* section refers to uses that are not included in U.S. product labeling.

### Accepted
Wilson's disease (treatment)—Penicillamine is indicated in the treatment of symptomatic patients (those with tissue damage due to deposition of excessive copper in various tissues) and as prophylaxis against the development of tissue damage in asymptomatic patients.

Arthritis, rheumatoid (treatment);
[Felty's syndrome (treatment)][1] or
[Vasculitis, rheumatoid (treatment)][1]—Penicillamine is indicated in the treatment of patients with severe, active rheumatoid arthritis [including Felty's syndrome or rheumatoid vasculitis] who have not responded to other therapy.

Cystinuria (treatment) or
Renal calculi, cystine, recurrence (prophylaxis)—Penicillamine is indicated in the treatment of patients with excessive urinary cystine concentration and/or recurrent cystine stone formation who have not responded to or will not comply with other prophylactic measures.

[Toxicity, heavy metal (treatment)]—Penicillamine is less effective than other chelating agents (edetate calcium disodium or dimercaprol) for the treatment of severe lead poisoning. It is used as adjunctive treatment following initial therapy with another chelating agent. It may also be used as sole therapy in the treatment of asymptomatic patients with moderately elevated blood concentrations of lead. Penicillamine is also used in the treatment of poisoning due to other heavy metals, including mercury.

### Unaccepted
Penicillamine is not effective in treating ankylosing spondylitis or psoriatic arthritis.

---

[1]Not included in Canadian product labeling.

## Pharmacology/Pharmacokinetics

### Physicochemical characteristics
Molecular weight—149.21.

### Mechanism of action/Effect
Chelating agent—
   Penicillamine chelates mercury, lead, copper, iron, and probably other heavy metals to form stable, soluble complexes that are readily excreted in the urine.
Antirheumatic—
   The mechanism of action of penicillamine in rheumatoid arthritis is not known, but may involve improvement of lymphocyte function. It markedly reduces IgM rheumatoid factor and immune complexes in serum and synovial fluid, but does not significantly lower absolute concentrations of serum immunoglobulins. *In vitro*, penicillamine depresses T-cell but not B-cell activity. However, the relationship of these effects to the activity of penicillamine in rheumatoid arthritis is not known.
Antiurolithic (cystine calculi)—
   Penicillamine combines chemically with cystine (cysteine–cysteine disulfide) to form penicillamine–cysteine disulfide, which is more soluble than cystine and is readily excreted. As a result, urinary cystine concentrations are lowered and the formation of cystine calculi is prevented. With prolonged treatment, existing cystine calculi may be gradually dissolved.
Antidote (to heavy metals)—
   See *Chelating agent* above.

### Biotransformation
Hepatic.

### Onset of action
Wilson's disease—1 to 3 months.
Rheumatoid arthritis—2 to 3 months.

### Elimination
Renal and fecal.

## Precautions to Consider

### Cross-sensitivity and/or related problems
Patients sensitive to penicillin may be sensitive to this medication also.

### Carcinogenicity
Long-term animal carcinogenicity studies with penicillamine have not been done. However, in one study in autoimmune disease–prone NZB Hybrid mice receiving 400 mg per kg of body weight (mg/kg) intraperitoneally 5 days a week for 6 months, 5 of 10 of the animals tested developed lymphocytic leukemia.

### Pregnancy/Reproduction
Pregnancy—Controlled studies have not been done in pregnant women. However, birth defects have occurred in infants born to women who received penicillamine for rheumatoid arthritis or cystinuria during pregnancy.
In rheumatoid arthritis: It is recommended that penicillamine not be used in pregnant women with rheumatoid arthritis.
In cystinuria: It is recommended that penicillamine be avoided if possible in pregnant patients with cystinuria.
In Wilson's disease: Although birth defects have not been reported in infants of women receiving penicillamine for Wilson's disease, it is recommended that the daily dose be limited to 1 gram. Also, if cesarean section is planned, it is recommended that the daily dose be limited to 250 mg during the last 6 weeks of pregnancy and following surgery until wound healing is complete.
Studies in animals have shown that penicillamine causes skeletal defects, cleft palates, and an increased number of resorptions when administered to rats in doses 6 times the maximum recommended human dose.

### Breast-feeding
It is not known whether penicillamine is distributed into breast milk.

### Pediatrics
Appropriate studies with penicillamine have not been performed in the pediatric population. Efficacy for treatment of juvenile arthritis has not been established. However, pediatrics-specific problems that would limit the usefulness of this medication for other indications in children are not expected.

## Geriatrics

Patients 65 years of age or older may be more likely to develop hematologic toxicity with penicillamine. Also, elderly patients are more likely to have age-related renal function impairment, which increases the risk of adverse renal effects in patients receiving penicillamine for the treatment of rheumatoid arthritis.

## Dental

The leukopenic and thrombocytopenic effects of penicillamine may result in an increased incidence of microbial infection, delayed healing, and gingival bleeding. If leukopenia or thrombocytopenia occurs, dental work should be delayed until blood counts have returned to normal, and patients should be instructed in proper oral hygiene, including caution in use of regular toothbrushes, dental floss, and toothpicks.

Penicillamine may cause oral ulcerations, which in some cases have the appearance of aphthous stomatitis, and, rarely, cheilosis, glossitis, or gingivostomatitis.

## Drug interactions and/or related problems

The following drug interactions and/or related problems have been selected on the basis of their potential clinical significance (possible mechanism in parentheses where appropriate)—not necessarily inclusive (» = major clinical significance):

Note: Combinations containing any of the following medications, depending on the amount present, may also interact with this medication.

4-Aminoquinolines or
Bone marrow depressants (See *Appendix II*) or
» Gold compounds or
Immunosuppressants, except glucocorticoids or
» Phenylbutazone
   (concurrent use with penicillamine may increase the potential for serious hematologic and/or renal adverse reactions; concurrent use with gold compounds or phenylbutazone is not recommended)
   (concurrent use with 4-aminoquinolines may also increase the risk of severe dermatologic reactions)

Iron supplements
   (concurrent use may decrease the effects of penicillamine; if necessary, iron may be administered in short courses, but a period of 2 hours should elapse between administration of penicillamine and iron)

Pyridoxine
   (penicillamine may cause anemia or peripheral neuritis by acting as a pyridoxine antagonist or increasing renal excretion of pyridoxine; requirements for pyridoxine may be increased during penicillamine therapy)

## Laboratory value alterations

The following have been selected on the basis of their potential clinical significance (possible effect in parentheses where appropriate)—not necessarily inclusive (» = major clinical significance):

With physiology/laboratory test values
Renal imaging using technetium Tc 99m gluceptate
   (penicillamine may cause transchelation of technetium Tc 99m gluceptate to a compound excreted through the hepatobiliary system, resulting in gallbladder visualization; gallbladder visualization may mimic abnormal kidney localization on posterior views of renal images)

## Medical considerations/Contraindications

The medical considerations/contraindications included here have been selected on the basis of their potential clinical significance (reasons given in parentheses where appropriate)—not necessarily inclusive (» = major clinical significance).

*Risk-benefit should be considered when the following medical problems exist:*

» Agranulocytosis or aplastic anemia, penicillamine-related, history of
   (risk of recurrence)

Sensitivity to penicillamine, history of

*In rheumatoid arthritis patients*
Renal function impairment, current or history of
   (increased risk of adverse renal effects)

## Patient monitoring

The following may be especially important in patient monitoring (other tests may be warranted in some patients, depending on condition; » = major clinical significance):

Blood cell counts, white and differential and
Hemoglobin determinations and
Platelet counts, direct and

Urinalyses, especially for protein and cells
   (recommended at least every 2 weeks during the first 6 months of therapy, then monthly thereafter during therapy; however, more frequent testing of blood cell count and urinalyses may be advisable during the first 6 weeks of therapy and for several weeks following an increase in maintenance dosage)

Hepatic function determinations
   (recommended every 6 months during the first 18 months of therapy because of possible intrahepatic cholestasis and toxic hepatitis)

*In cystinuria*
X-ray for renal calculi
   (recommended annually during therapy since cystine stones may form rapidly, sometimes within 6 months)

*In rheumatoid arthritis*
Urinary protein determinations, 24-hour
   (recommended at 1- to 2-week intervals for those patients who develop moderate degrees of proteinuria)

*In Wilson's disease*
Urinary copper analyses, 24-hour
   (recommended prior to and soon after initiation of therapy to determine optimal dosage; during continued therapy, recommended approximately every 3 months; urine specimens must be collected in copper-free glassware)

## Side/Adverse Effects

The following side/adverse effects have been selected on the basis of their potential clinical significance (possible signs and symptoms in parentheses where appropriate)—not necessarily inclusive:

### Those indicating need for medical attention
Incidence more frequent
   *Allergic reaction* (fever; joint pain; skin rash, hives, and/or itching; swelling of lymph glands); *stomatitis* (ulcers, sores, or white spots in mouth)
Incidence less frequent
   *Agranulocytosis* (sore throat and fever with or without chills; sores, ulcers, or white spots on lips or in mouth); *aplastic anemia* (shortness of breath, troubled breathing, tightness in chest, and/or wheezing; sores, ulcers, or white spots on lips or in mouth; swollen and/or painful glands; unusual bleeding or bruising; unusual tiredness or weakness); *glomerulopathy, possible impending* (bloody or cloudy urine; swelling of face, feet, or lower legs; weight gain)—glomerulopathy may progress to nephrotic syndrome; *hemolytic anemia* (troubled breathing, exertional; unusual tiredness or weakness); *leukopenia* (usually asymptomatic; fever or chills; cough or hoarseness; lower back or side pain; painful or difficult urination)—rarely; *thrombocytopenia* (usually asymptomatic; rarely, unusual bleeding or bruising; black, tarry stools; blood in urine or stools; pinpoint red spots on skin)
Incidence rare
   *Bronchiolitis, obstructive* (coughing, wheezing, or shortness of breath); *dermatitis, exfoliative* (fever with or without chills; red, thickened, or scaly skin; swollen and/or painful glands; unusual bruising); *Goodpasture's syndrome* (difficulty in breathing, spitting blood, unusual tiredness or weakness); *jaundice, cholestatic* (dark urine, itching, pale stools, yellow eyes or skin); *myasthenia gravis syndrome* (difficulty in breathing, chewing, talking, or swallowing; double vision; muscle weakness); *necrolysis, toxic epidermal* (redness, tenderness, itching, burning, or peeling of skin; sore throat; fever with or without chills; red or irritated eyes); *neuritis, optic* (eye pain, blurred vision, or any change in vision)—may be caused by pyridoxine deficiency; *pancreatitis or peptic ulcer reactivation;* (abdominal or stomach pain, severe); *ringing or buzzing in ears; systemic lupus erythematosus (SLE)–like syndrome* (skin rash, hives, and/or itching; blisters on skin; chest pain; general feeling of discomfort or illness; joint pain)

### Those indicating need for medical attention only if continuing or bothersome
Incidence more frequent
   *Diarrhea; lessening or loss of taste sense; loss of appetite; nausea or vomiting; stomach pain, mild*

## Patient Consultation

As an aid to patient consultation, refer to *Advice for the Patient, Penicillamine (Systemic)*.

In providing consultation, consider emphasizing the following selected information (» = major clinical significance):

### Before using this medication
» Conditions affecting use, especially:
   Sensitivity to penicillamine or penicillin, history of
   Pregnancy—Has been reported to cause birth defects in humans

Use in the elderly—Increased risk of hematologic toxicity
Other medications, especially gold compounds and phenylbutazone
Other medical problems, especially a history of penicillamine-in-
    duced agranulocytosis or aplastic anemia

### Proper use of this medication
*For patients with cystinuria*
Importance of high fluid intake, especially at night
Possible need for low-methionine diet

*For patients with rheumatoid arthritis*
Taking medication on an empty stomach
Improvement in condition may require 2 to 3 months of therapy

*For patients with Wilson's disease*
Taking medication on an empty stomach
Possible need for low-copper diet
Improvement in condition may require 1 to 3 months of therapy

*For patients with lead poisoning*
Taking medication on an empty stomach

*For all patients*
» Compliance with therapy; checking with physician before discontin-
    uing medication since interruption of therapy may cause sensitivity
    reactions when therapy is reinstituted
» Proper dosing
Missed dose: If dosing schedule is—
    Once a day: Taking as soon as possible; not taking if not remem-
        bered until next day; not doubling doses
    Two times a day: Taking as soon as possible; not taking if almost
        time for next dose; not doubling doses
    More than two times a day: Taking if remembered within an hour;
        not taking if not remembered until later; not doubling doses
» Proper storage

### Precautions while using this medication
Regular visits to physician to check progress during therapy
Caution if any kind of surgery (including dental surgery) is required
    because of the effects of penicillamine on collagen and elastin
Avoiding concurrent use of iron-containing medications

### Side/adverse effects
Signs of potential side effects, especially allergic reactions, stomatitis,
    blood dyscrasias, glomerulopathy, obstructive bronchiolitis, exfo-
    liative dermatitis, Goodpasture's syndrome, jaundice, myasthenia
    gravis syndrome, toxic epidermal necrolysis, optic neuritis, pan-
    creatitis, peptic ulcer reactivation, ringing or buzzing in ears, and
    SLE-like syndrome

## General Dosing Information

Penicillamine therapy should be continued on a daily basis because inter-
    ruptions for even a few days may cause sensitivity reactions following
    reinstitution of therapy.

If surgery is necessary during penicillamine therapy, the dosage should
    be reduced to 250 mg daily because of the effects on collagen and
    elastin. Reinstitution of full therapy should be delayed until wound
    healing is complete.

In the treatment of cystinuria or Wilson's disease, a daily dose of 250 mg
    may be administered with the dosage being increased gradually to the
    optimum dosage if the patient cannot tolerate the usual initial dose of
    penicillamine. This may also help to reduce the incidence of adverse
    reactions.

Patients with rheumatoid arthritis (whose nutrition is impaired), cystinuria,
    or Wilson's disease should be given 25 mg of pyridoxine daily during
    therapy because penicillamine increases the intake requirement for this
    vitamin.

Impairment of taste may occur with penicillamine therapy. Except for
    patients with Wilson's disease, normal taste acuity may be restored
    while therapy with penicillamine is continued by administering 5 to
    10 mg of copper daily (5 to 10 drops of a 4% cupric sulfate solution
    may be administered in fruit juice 2 times a day).

If therapy is interrupted for any reason, it should be reinstituted with a
    small dosage, which is gradually increased until full dosage is
    achieved.

### In cystinuria
The daily dosage of penicillamine may range from 1 to 4 grams.

The dosage of penicillamine should be based on measurements of urinary
    cystine excretion. Urinary cystine excretion should be maintained at
    less than 100 mg daily in patients with a history of renal calculi and/or
    pain, or at 100 to 200 mg daily in patients without a history of renal
    calculi.

If administration in 4 equally divided doses is not possible, the larger dose
    should be given at bedtime; or, if the occurrence of side effects re-

quires dosage reduction, the bedtime dose should be one of the doses
    retained.

To help prevent the formation of cystine stones, a high fluid intake is
    recommended. The patient should drink 500 mL of water at bedtime
    and another 500 mL once during the night when the urine is more
    concentrated and more acidic than during the day. Usually the greater
    the fluid intake, the lower the required dose of penicillamine.

A diet low in methionine may be necessary to minimize cystine produc-
    tion. This diet is not recommended in growing children or during preg-
    nancy because of its low protein content.

### In lead poisoning
Penicillamine should be administered on an empty stomach, 2 hours be-
    fore meals or at least 3 hours after meals.

### In rheumatoid arthritis
Penicillamine should be given on an empty stomach (at least 1 hour before
    meals or 2 hours after meals) and at least 1 hour apart from any other
    medication, food, or milk in order to achieve maximum absorption
    and to reduce the possibility of inactivation by metal binding.

Dosage up to 500 mg per day may be given as a single dose. Dosage
    above 500 mg per day should be administered in divided doses.

During initial therapy, if the dosage has been increased up to 1 to 1.5
    grams of penicillamine per day and after 3 to 4 months there is still
    no improvement in the patient's condition, the medication should be
    discontinued.

The maintenance dosage of penicillamine may need adjustment during the
    course of treatment. Changes in maintenance dosage levels may not
    be noticed clinically or in the erythrocytic sedimentation rate for 2 or
    3 months after each dosage adjustment.

For those patients who require an increase in the maintenance dosage to
    achieve maximal disease suppression after the first 6 to 9 months of
    therapy, the daily dosage may be increased by 125 or 250 mg per day
    at 3-month intervals up to 1.5 grams per day.

### In Wilson's disease
Dosage of penicillamine should be determined by measurements of uri-
    nary copper excretion to achieve and maintain a negative copper
    balance.

Penicillamine should be administered on an empty stomach (30 minutes
    to 1 hour before meals and at least 2 hours after the evening meal).

The dosage may be increased as indicated by urinary copper analyses, but
    dosage greater than 2 grams daily is usually not necessary.

In conjunction with penicillamine therapy, a low-copper diet of less than
    2 mg daily should be maintained. Such a diet should exclude, most
    importantly, chocolate, nuts, shellfish, mushrooms, liver, molasses,
    broccoli, and cereals enriched with copper. Distilled or demineralized
    water should be used if the patient's drinking water contains more
    than 100 mcg (0.1 mg) of copper per liter.

Sulfurated potash (10 to 40 mg) may be administered with meals to min-
    imize absorption of copper (capsules of sulfurated potash may be pre-
    pared by using light magnesium oxide as a diluent).

## Oral Dosage Forms

Note: Bracketed uses in the *Dosage Forms* section refer to categories of
    use and/or indications that are not included in U.S. product labeling.

### PENICILLAMINE CAPSULES USP

**Usual adult and adolescent dose**
Chelating agent—
    Oral, 250 mg four times a day.
Antirheumatic—
    Oral, initially 125 or 250 mg once a day as a single dose, the dosage
        being increased, if necessary and tolerated, by adding 125 or 250
        mg per day at two- to three-month intervals up to a maximum of
        1.5 grams per day.
    Note: Some clinicians recommend a maximum dose of 1 gram per
        day in rheumatoid arthritis.
Antiurolithic—
    Oral, 500 mg four times a day.
[Antidote (to heavy metals)]—
    Oral, 500 mg to 1.5 grams per day for one to two months.

**Usual pediatric dose**
Chelating agent—
    Infants over 6 months of age and young children: Oral, 250 mg as a
        single dose administered in fruit juice.
    Older children: See *Usual adult and adolescent dose.*
Antirheumatic—
    Efficacy and dosage have not been established.

Antiurolithic—
Oral, 7.5 mg per kg of body weight four times a day.
[Antidote (to heavy metals)]—
Oral, 30 to 40 mg per kg of body weight or 600 to 750 mg per square meter of body surface per day for one to six months.

### Usual geriatric dose
Oral, initially 125 mg per day. Dosage may be increased, if necessary and tolerated, by adding 125 mg per day at two- to three-month intervals, up to a maximum of 750 mg per day.

### Strength(s) usually available
U.S.—
125 mg (Rx) [*Cuprimine* (lactose)].
250 mg (Rx) [*Cuprimine* (lactose)].
Canada—
125 mg (Rx) [*Cuprimine* (lactose)].
250 mg (Rx) [*Cuprimine* (lactose)].

### Packaging and storage
Store below 40 °C (104 °F), preferably between 15 and 30 °C (59 and 86 °F), unless otherwise specified by manufacturer. Store in a tight container.

### Auxiliary labeling
• Take on an empty stomach.

## PENICILLAMINE TABLETS USP

### Usual adult and adolescent dose
Chelating agent—
Oral, 250 mg four times a day.
Antirheumatic—
Oral, initially 125 or 250 mg once a day as a single dose, the dosage being increased, if necessary and tolerated, by adding 125 or 250 mg per day at two- to three-month intervals up to a maximum of 1.5 grams per day.
Note: Some clinicians recommend a maximum dose of 1 gram per day in rheumatoid arthritis.
Antiurolithic—
Oral, 500 mg four times a day.

[Antidote (to heavy metals)]—
Oral, 500 mg to 1.5 grams per day for one to two months.

### Usual pediatric dose
Chelating agent—
Infants over 6 months of age and young children: Oral, 250 mg as a single dose administered in fruit juice.
Older children: See *Usual adult and adolescent dose.*
Antirheumatic—
Dosage has not been established.
Antiurolithic—
Oral, 7.5 mg per kg of body weight four times a day.
[Antidote (to heavy metals)]—
Oral, 30 to 40 mg per kg of body weight or 600 to 750 mg per square meter of body surface per day for one to six months.

### Usual geriatric dose
Oral, initially 125 mg per day. Dosage may be increased, if necessary and tolerated, by adding 125 mg per day at two- to three-month intervals, up to a maximum of 750 mg per day.

### Strength(s) usually available
U.S.—
250 mg (Rx) [*Depen* (scored; lactose)].
Canada—
250 mg (Rx) [*Depen* (scored; lactose)].

### Packaging and storage
Store below 40 °C (104 °F), preferably between 15 and 30 °C (59 and 86 °F), unless otherwise specified by manufacturer. Store in a tight container.

### Auxiliary labeling
• Take on an empty stomach.

Revised: July 1990
Interim revision: 09/01/94

## PENICILLIN G—See *Penicillins (Systemic)*

# PENICILLINS   Systemic

This monograph includes information on the following: Amoxicillin; Ampicillin; Bacampicillin; Carbenicillin; Cloxacillin; Dicloxacillin†; Flucloxacillin*; Methicillin†; Mezlocillin†; Nafcillin; Oxacillin†; Penicillin G; Penicillin V; Piperacillin; Pivampicillin*; Pivmecillinam*; Ticarcillin.

INN:
Amoxicillin—Amoxicilline
Carbenicillin indanyl sodium—Carindacillin
Methicillin—Meticillin
Penicillin G benzathine—Benzathine benzylpenicillin
Penicillin V—Phenoxymethylpenicillin
BAN:
Amoxicillin—Amoxycillin
Carbenicillin indanyl sodium—Carindacillin
Penicillin G benzathine—Benzathine penicillin
Penicillin G procaine—Procaine penicillin
Penicillin V—Phenoxymethylpenicillin
VA CLASSIFICATION (Primary):
Amoxicillin—AM052
Ampicillin—AM052
Bacampicillin—AM052
Carbenicillin—AM054
Cloxacillin—AM053
Dicloxacillin—AM053
Flucloxacillin—AM053
Methicillin—AM053
Mezlocillin—AM054
Nafcillin—AM053
Oxacillin—AM053
Penicillin G—AM051
Penicillin V—AM051
Piperacillin—AM054
Pivampicillin—AM052
Pivmecillinam—AM052
Ticarcillin—AM054

Note: For a listing of dosage forms and brand names by country availability, see *Dosage Forms* section(s). For a listing of brand names for the articles in this monograph, refer to the General Index.

*Not commercially available in the U.S.
†Not commercially available in Canada.

## Category
Antibacterial (systemic).

## Indications
Note: Bracketed information in the *Indications* section refers to uses that are not included in U.S. product labeling.

### General considerations
Penicillins can be classified into four broad categories, each covering a different spectrum of activity. The natural penicillins (penicillin G and penicillin V) have activity against many gram-positive organisms, gram-negative cocci, and some other gram-negative organisms. The aminopenicillins (ampicillin, amoxicillin, bacampicillin, and pivampicillin) have activity against penicillin-sensitive gram-positive bacteria, as well as *Escherichia coli, Proteus mirabilis, Salmonella* sp., *Shigella* sp., and *Haemophilus influenzae.* The antistaphylococcal penicillins (cloxacillin, dicloxacillin, flucloxacillin, methicillin, nafcillin, and oxacillin) are also active against beta-lactamase–producing staphylococci. The antipseudomonal penicillins (carbenicillin, mezlocillin, piperacillin, and ticarcillin) have less activity against gram-positive organisms than the natural penicillins or aminopenicillins; however, unlike the other penicillins, these penicillins are active against some gram-negative bacilli, including *Pseudomonas aeruginosa.*
Resistance to penicillins is thought to be due to 3 main mechanisms. The first is alteration of the antibiotic target sites' penicillin-binding proteins (PBPs); the second is inactivation of the penicillin by bacterially produced enzymes (beta-lactamases); and the third is decreased permeability of the cell wall to penicillins. Of these 3 mechanisms, production of beta-lactamase is the most common and the most important.

The spectrums of activity of penicillin G and penicillin V include *Staphylococcus* and *Streptococcus* species. However, most strains of *S. aureus* and *S. epidermidis* produce beta-lactamases, which destroy these penicillins. A small proportion of community-acquired strains (5 to 15%) of *S. aureus* remains susceptible to penicillin G. Penicillin G also has activity against the gram-negative cocci, *Neisseria meningitidis* and *N. gonorrhoeae*. However, resistance to penicillin G by beta-lactamase–producing *N. gonorrhoeae* has become a widespread problem in many parts of the world. Penicillin G is more active than penicillin V against *Haemophilus* and *Neisseria* species. Some other organisms for which penicillin G has good activity include *Actinomyces israelii*, *Bacillus anthracis*, oropharyngeal *Bacteroides* species, *Borrelia burgdorferi*, *Clostridium* sp., *Corynebacterium diphtheriae*, *Erysipelothrix rhusiopathiae*, *Listeria monocytogenes*, *Spirillium minor*, *Streptobacillus moniliformis*, and *Treponema pallidum*.

The aminopenicillins have activity against *H. influenzae*, *E. coli*, *P. mirabilis*, and *Salmonella* and some *Shigella* species, while also retaining activity against penicillin-sensitive gram-positive bacteria. However, many Enterobacteriaceae, *H. influenzae*, *Salmonella* and *Shigella* species are resistant to these penicillins because of beta-lactamase production by these organisms. Bacampicillin and pivampicillin are esters of ampicillin that are hydrolyzed during absorption to liberate ampicillin; this results in increased bioavailability and serum concentrations of ampicillin. Amoxicillin has the same *in vitro* activity as ampicillin, although amoxicillin has slightly better activity against *Enterococcus faecalis*, *E. coli*, and *Salmonella* sp.

The antistaphylococcal penicillins were developed to treat beta-lactamase–producing staphylococci. These penicillins are active against both penicillin-sensitive and penicillin-resistant staphylococci, as well as *S. pyogenes* and *S. pneumoniae*. However, they are less potent than penicillin G against penicillin-sensitive bacteria, and they have very little activity against *E. faecalis* and gram-negative organisms. Nafcillin has more intrinsic activity than methicillin against staphylococci and streptococci. The mechanism of methicillin-resistant *S. aureus* is not due to beta-lactamase production by the organism, but results from an alteration of penicillin binding proteins. Methicillin-resistant staphylococci are also resistant to the other penicillins in this category.

The antipseudomonal penicillins are active against a wide variety of gram-negative bacteria, including *Pseudomonas aeruginosa*, *Enterobacter*, *Morganella*, and *Providencia* species. These penicillins are less active than ampicillin against streptococci and enterococci; however, their activity against non-beta-lactamase–producing *Haemophilus*, *N. meningitidis*, and *N. gonorrhoeae* is similar to that of ampicillin. These agents are also destroyed by beta-lactamases produced by gram-positive and some gram-negative organisms. Ticarcillin is 2 to 4 times more active than carbenicillin against *P. aeruginosa*. Mezlocillin has a spectrum of activity similar to that of carbenicillin and ticarcillin; however, mezlocillin has better activity against non-beta-lactamase–producing strains of *Klebsiella*, *H. influenzae*, and *B. fragilis*. Piperacillin has excellent activity against streptococci, *Neisseria*, and *Haemophilus* species, and is the most active penicillin against *P. aeruginosa*.

Another penicillin, which does not neatly fit into any of these four categories, is pivmecillinam. Pivmecillinam is hydrolyzed during absorption to liberate the active agent, mecillinam. Mecillinam has poor activity against gram-positive organisms, *Haemophilus*, and *Neisseria* species; however, it has very good activity against many gram-negative bacteria, including *E. coli*, many *Klebsiella*, *Enterobacter*, and *Citrobacter* species. It has variable activity against *Proteus* sp. and does not inhibit *P. aeruginosa* or anaerobes, such as *B. fragilis* or *Clostridium* species.

## Accepted

Actinomycosis (treatment)—Penicillin G (parenteral) and [penicillin V][1] are indicated in the treatment of actinomycosis caused by *Actinomyces* sp.

Anthrax (treatment)—Penicillin G (parenteral), [penicillin V][1], and penicillin G procaine are indicated in the treatment of anthrax caused by *Bacillus anthracis*.

Arthritis, gonococcal (treatment)—Penicillin G (parenteral) is indicated in the treatment of infective arthritis caused by susceptible strains of *Neisseria gonorrhoeae*.

Bejel (treatment)—Penicillin G benzathine and penicillin G procaine are indicated in the treatment of bejel caused by *Treponema pallidum endemicum*.

Bone and joint infections (treatment)—Carbenicillin (parenteral), cloxacillin (parenteral), [methicillin][1], [nafcillin (parenteral)][1], [oxacillin (parenteral)][1], [penicillin G (parenteral)][1], and piperacillin are indicated in the treatment of bone and joint infections caused by susceptible organisms.

Bronchitis, bacterial exacerbations (treatment)—Amoxicillin, ampicillin, bacampicillin, cloxacillin (oral), dicloxacillin, penicillin V, and pivampicillin are indicated in the treatment of bronchitis caused by susceptible organisms.

Diphtheria (prophylaxis)—Penicillin G (parenteral), [penicillin G benzathine][1], penicillin G procaine, and penicillin V are indicated in the prophylaxis of diphtheria, caused by *Corynebacterium diphtheriae*, as an adjunct to antitoxin.

Endocarditis, bacterial (prophylaxis)—[Amoxicillin][1], [ampicillin][1], penicillin G (parenteral), and penicillin V are indicated in the prophylaxis of bacterial endocarditis caused by susceptible organisms.

Endocarditis, bacterial (treatment)—Ampicillin (parenteral), carbenicillin (parenteral), cloxacillin (parenteral), [methicillin][1], [nafcillin (parenteral)][1], [oxacillin (parenteral)], [penicillin G (parenteral)][1] and penicillin G procaine are indicated in the treatment of bacterial endocarditis caused by susceptible organisms.

Erysipelas (treatment)—Penicillin G (parenteral), penicillin V, and penicillin G procaine are indicated in the treatment of erysipelas caused by susceptible strains of group A streptococci.

Erysipeloid (treatment)—Penicillin G (parenteral), [penicillin V][1], [penicillin G benzathine][1], and [penicillin G procaine][1] are indicated in the treatment of erysipeloid, including endocarditis and septicemia, caused by *Erysipelothrix rhusiopathiae*.

Gingivitis, acute, necrotizing, ulcerative (treatment)—Penicillin G (oral and parenteral), penicillin V, and penicillin G procaine are indicated in the treatment of acute, necrotizing, ulcerative gingivitis, also called Vincent's angina or "trench mouth," a pharyngeal and tonsillar infection caused by anaerobes and spirochetes.

Gonorrhea, endocervical and urethral, uncomplicated (treatment)—Amoxicillin, in combination with probenecid, and [penicillin G (parenteral)][1] are indicated in the treatment of gonorrhea caused by susceptible strains of *Neisseria gonorrhoeae*. However, because of resistance to penicillin, other agents, such as ceftriaxone, cefixime, or ciprofloxacin, are considered to be first-line agents.

Intra-abdominal infections (treatment)—Carbenicillin (parenteral), mezlocillin, [penicillin G (parenteral)][1], piperacillin, and ticarcillin are indicated in the treatment of intra-abdominal infections caused by susceptible organisms.

Listeriosis (treatment)—[Ampicillin (parenteral)][1] and penicillin G (parenteral) are indicated in the treatment of listeriosis caused by *Listeria monocytogenes*.

Meningitis, bacterial (treatment)—Ampicillin (parenteral), carbenicillin (parenteral), [nafcillin (parenteral)][1], [oxacillin (parenteral)][1], penicillin G (parenteral), [piperacillin][1], and [ticarcillin][1] are indicated in the treatment of bacterial meningitis caused by susceptible organisms.

Otitis media, acute (treatment)—Amoxicillin, ampicillin, bacampicillin, penicillin G procaine, penicillin G (oral), penicillin V, and pivampicillin are indicated in the treatment of acute otitis media caused by susceptible organisms.

*Pasteurella multocida* infections (treatment)—[Ampicillin (parenteral)][1], penicillin G (parenteral), and [penicillin V][1] are indicated in the treatment of infections caused by *Pasteurella multocida*.

Pelvic infections, female (treatment)—[Carbenicillin (parenteral)][1], mezlocillin, piperacillin, and ticarcillin are indicated in the treatment of female pelvic infections caused by susceptible organisms.

Pericarditis, bacterial (treatment)—Penicillin G (parenteral), penicillin G procaine, and [nafcillin (parenteral)][1] are indicated in the treatment of bacterial pericarditis caused by susceptible organisms.

Pharyngitis, bacterial (treatment)—Amoxicillin, ampicillin, bacampicillin, cloxacillin (oral), dicloxacillin, flucloxacillin, penicillin G benzathine, penicillin G (oral), penicillin V, and pivampicillin are indicated in the treatment of bacterial pharyngitis caused by susceptible organisms.

Pinta (treatment)—Penicillin G benzathine and penicillin G procaine are indicated in the treatment of pinta caused by *Treponema carateum*.

Pneumonia, bacterial (treatment)—Amoxicillin, ampicillin, bacampicillin, carbenicillin (parenteral), cloxacillin, dicloxacillin, mezlocillin, penicillin G (parenteral), penicillin G procaine, piperacillin, and ticarcillin are indicated in the treatment of bacterial pneumonia caused by susceptible organisms.

Prostatitis (treatment)—Carbenicillin (oral) is indicated in the treatment of prostatitis caused by susceptible organisms.

Rat-bite fever (treatment)—Penicillin G (parenteral), penicillin G procaine, and [penicillin V][1] are indicated in the treatment of rat-bite fever caused by *Streptobacillus moniliformis* or *Spirillum minor*.

Rheumatic fever (prophylaxis)—Penicillin V, and penicillin G benzathine are indicated in the prophylaxis of rheumatic fever caused by group A streptococci.

Scarlet fever (treatment)—Penicillin V, penicillin G procaine, and [penicillin G (parenteral)][1] are indicated in the treatment of scarlet fever caused by group A streptococci.

Septicemia, bacterial (treatment)—Ampicillin (parenteral), carbenicillin (parenteral), cloxacillin (parenteral), methicillin, mezlocillin, nafcillin (parenteral), oxacillin (parenteral), penicillin G (parenteral), penicillin G procaine, piperacillin, and ticarcillin are indicated in the treatment of bacterial septicemia caused by susceptible organisms.

Sinusitis (treatment)—Amoxicillin, ampicillin, bacampicillin, cloxacillin, flucloxacillin, methicillin, nafcillin, oxacillin, and penicillin V are indicated in the treatment of sinusitis caused by susceptible organisms.

Skin and soft tissue infections (treatment)—Carbenicillin (parenteral), cloxacillin, dicloxacillin, flucloxacillin, methicillin, mezlocillin, nafcillin, oxacillin, penicillin G procaine, [penicillin G (parenteral)][1], penicillin V, piperacillin, pivampicillin, and ticarcillin are indicated in the treatment of skin and soft tissue infections caused by susceptible organisms.

Syphilis (treatment)—Penicillin G benzathine is indicated in the treatment of primary, secondary, and early and late latent syphilis. Penicillin G (parenteral) and penicillin G procaine, in combination with probenecid, are indicated in the treatment of tertiary syphilis. Penicillin G (parenteral) is indicated in the treatment of neurosyphilis. Penicillin G benzathine fails to achieve adequate concentrations in the cerebrospinal fluid.

Tetanus (treatment)—Penicillin G (parenteral) is indicated in the treatment of the infecting organism in tetanus, *Clostridium tetani*.

Urinary tract infections, bacterial (treatment)—Amoxicillin, ampicillin, bacampicillin, carbenicillin (oral and parenteral), mezlocillin, piperacillin, pivampicillin, pivmecillinam, and ticarcillin are indicated in the treatment of bacterial urinary tract infections caused by susceptible organisms.

Yaws (treatment)—Penicillin G benzathine, penicillin G procaine, and [penicillin G (parenteral)] are indicated in the treatment of yaws caused by *Treponema pallidum pertenue*.

[Chlamydial infections in pregnant women (treatment)][1]—Amoxicillin and ampicillin are used in the treatment of chlamydial infections in pregnant women who cannot tolerate erythromycin.

[Gas gangrene infections (treatment)][1]—Penicillin G (parenteral) is used in the treatment of gas gangrene caused by *Clostridium* sp.

[Gastritis, *Helicobacter pylori*-associated (treatment adjunct)][1] or
[Ulcer, peptic, *Helicobacter pylori*-associated (treatment adjunct)][1]—Amoxicillin is used, in combination with metronidazole and bismuth subsalicylate, in the treatment of gastritis and peptic ulcer disease caused by *H. pylori*.

[Leptospirosis (treatment)][1]—Ampicillin (parenteral) and penicillin G (parenteral) are used in the treatment of leptospirosis caused by *Leptospira* sp.

[Lyme disease (treatment)][1]—Amoxicillin and penicillin V are used in the treatment of early Lyme disease, caused by *Borrelia burgdorferi*. Amoxicillin, in combination with probenecid, and penicillin G (parenteral) are used to treat more advanced stages of Lyme disease, including mild neurological manifestations, cardiac manifestations, and arthritis.

[Typhoid fever (treatment)][1]—Amoxicillin and ampicillin are used in the treatment of typhoid fever caused by *Salmonella typhi*.

### Unaccepted

For carbenicillin (oral)—
Since effective serum concentrations are not achieved with oral carbenicillin, it is indicated only for urinary tract infections and prostatitis.

For nafcillin (oral)—
The oral absorption of nafcillin is erratic and the resulting serum concentrations are low; therefore, use of oral nafcillin is not recommended.

For penicillin G benzathine (parenteral)—
Parenteral penicillin G benzathine is not indicated for the treatment of meningitis or neurosyphilis because it fails to achieve adequate concentrations in the cerebrospinal fluid (CSF).

For penicillin G (oral)—
Because of the low serum concentrations achieved with oral penicillin G, it is not indicated for the treatment of severe infections.

---

[1]Not included in Canadian product labeling.

## Pharmacology/Pharmacokinetics

See also *Table 1*, page 2284, and *Table 2*, page 2285.

### Physicochemical characteristics

Chemical group—
Amoxicillin: Aminopenicillin
Ampicillin: Aminopenicillin
Bacampicillin: Aminopenicillin
Carbenicillin: Carboxypenicillin
Cloxacillin: Isoxazolyl penicillin
Dicloxacillin: Isoxazolyl penicillin
Flucloxacillin: Isoxazolyl penicillin
Mezlocillin: Acylureidopenicillin
Oxacillin: Isoxazolyl penicillin
Piperacillin: Acylureidopenicillin
Pivampicillin: Aminopenicillin
Ticarcillin: Carboxypenicillin

Molecular weight—
Amoxicillin: 419.45.
Ampicillin: 349.40.
Ampicillin sodium: 371.39.
Bacampicillin hydrochloride: 501.98.
Carbenicillin disodium: 422.36.
Carbenicillin indanyl sodium: 516.54.
Cloxacillin sodium: 475.88.
Dicloxacillin sodium: 510.32.
Flucloxacillin: 453.87.
Methicillin sodium: 420.41.
Mezlocillin sodium: 561.56.
Nafcillin sodium: 454.47.
Oxacillin sodium: 441.43.
Penicillin G benzathine: 981.19.
Penicillin G potassium: 372.48.
Penicillin G procaine: 588.72.
Penicillin G sodium: 356.37.
Penicillin V potassium: 388.48.
Piperacillin sodium: 539.54.
Pivampicillin hydrochloride: 500.01.
Pivmecillinam: 439.57.
Ticarcillin disodium: 428.38.

### Mechanism of action/Effect

Bactericidal; inhibit bacterial cell wall synthesis. Action is dependent on the ability of penicillins to reach and bind penicillin-binding proteins (PBPs) located on the inner membrane of the bacterial cell wall. PBPs (which include transpeptidases, carboxypeptidases, and endopeptidases) are enzymes that are involved in the terminal stages of assembling the bacterial cell wall and in reshaping the cell wall during growth and division. Penicillins bind to, and inactivate, PBPs, resulting in the weakening of the bacterial cell wall and lysis.

### Distribution

Penicillins are widely distributed to most tissues and body fluids, including peritoneal fluid, blister fluid, urine (high concentrations), pleural fluid, middle ear fluid, intestinal mucosa, bone, gallbladder, lung, female reproductive tissues, and bile. Distribution into the cerebrospinal fluid (CSF) is low in subjects with noninflamed meninges, as is penetration into purulent bronchial secretions.

Penicillins also cross the placenta and are distributed into breast milk.

### Biotransformation

Hepatic metabolism accounts for less than 30% of the biotransformation of most penicillins, with the exception of nafcillin and oxacillin.

Bacampicillin—A prodrug of ampicillin; bacampicillin is hydrolyzed by esterases in the intestinal wall during absorption to produce ampicillin. Bacampicillin provides earlier and higher peak concentrations of ampicillin than administration of ampicillin does.

Carbenicillin indanyl sodium—After absorption, carbenicillin indanyl sodium is rapidly converted to carbenicillin by hydrolysis of the ester linkage.

Penicillin G benzathine (intramuscular)—Slowly released from the intramuscular injection site and hydrolyzed to penicillin G, resulting in serum concentrations that are much lower but much more prolonged than other parenteral penicillins.

Penicillin G procaine—Dissolves slowly at the site of injection, giving a plateau-type blood level at 4 hours, which falls slowly over the next 15 to 20 hours.

Pivampicillin—A prodrug of ampicillin, which is converted during absorption to ampicillin, formaldehyde, and pivalic acid, by non-specific esterases in most body tissues. Pivampicillin provides earlier and higher peak concentrations of ampicillin than administration of ampicillin does.

Pivmecillinam—A prodrug of mecillinam, which is converted during absorption to mecillinam, formaldehyde, and pivalic acid, by non-specific esterases in most body tissues.

## Elimination

Primarily renal (glomerular filtration and tubular secretion).

Hepatic metabolism accounts for less than 30% of the elimination of most penicillins, with the exception of nafcillin and oxacillin.

Biliary—Some penicillins may be excreted in the bile in high concentrations, such as ampicillin, mezlocillin, nafcillin, penicillin G, piperacillin, and pivmecillinam. Approximately 10% of cloxacillin, dicloxacillin, flucloxacillin, and oxacillin is recovered in the bile.

# Precautions to Consider

## Cross-sensitivity and/or related problems

Patients allergic to one penicillin may be allergic to other penicillins also. Patients allergic to cephalosporins or cephamycins may be allergic to penicillins also. Patients allergic to procaine or other ester-type local anesthetics may also be allergic to sterile penicillin G procaine suspension, which is an equimolar compound of procaine and penicillin G.

## Carcinogenicity

*Amoxicillin, ampicillin, bacampicillin, cloxacillin, dicloxacillin, methicillin, nafcillin, oxacillin, penicillin G, penicillin V*—Long-term studies have not been performed in animals.

*Carbenicillin*—Long-term studies have not been performed in animals. Rats given 25 to 100 mg per kg of body weight (mg/kg) per day of carbenicillin for 18 months developed mild liver pathology (bile duct hyperplasia) at all dose levels, but there was no evidence of drug-related neoplasia.

## Mutagenicity

*Amoxicillin, ampicillin, bacampicillin, cloxacillin, dicloxacillin, methicillin, nafcillin, oxacillin, penicillin G, penicillin V*—Long-term studies have not been performed in animals.

## Pregnancy/Reproduction

Fertility—*Amoxicillin:* Studies in mice and rats at doses up to 10 times the human dose of amoxicillin revealed no evidence of impaired fertility.

*Bacampicillin:* Studies in mice and rats given doses of up to 750 mg/kg (more than 25 times the usual human dose) showed no evidence of impaired fertility. Also, bacampicillin had no effect on the reproductive organs of rats or dogs receiving daily oral doses of up to 800 and 650 mg, respectively, for 6 months.

*Carbenicillin:* Administration of carbenicillin at doses of up to 1000 mg/kg had no apparent effect on the fertility or reproductive performance of rats.

*Cloxacillin, dicloxacillin, methicillin, nafcillin, oxacillin, penicillin G, penicillin V:* Reproductive studies performed in the mouse, rat, and rabbit given these penicillins have revealed no evidence of impaired fertility.

*Mezlocillin:* Studies in mice and rats given doses up to twice the usual human dose have not shown that mezlocillin impairs fertility.

*Piperacillin:* Studies in mice and rats given doses up to 4 times the human dose of piperacillin have shown no evidence of impaired fertility.

*Ticarcillin:* Reproductive studies done in mice and rats given ticarcillin have revealed no evidence of impaired fertility.

Pregnancy—Penicillins cross the placenta. Adequate and well-controlled studies in humans have not been done to determine whether penicillins are teratogenic; however, penicillins are widely used in pregnant women and problems have not been documented.

*Amoxicillin:* Studies in mice and rats at doses up to 10 times the human dose of amoxicillin revealed no evidence of harm to the fetus.

FDA Pregnancy Category B.

*Ampicillin:* Studies in animals given doses several times the human dose have revealed no evidence of adverse effects in the fetus.

FDA Pregnancy Category B.

*Bacampicillin:* Studies in mice and rats given doses of up to 750 mg/kg (more than 25 times the usual human dose) have not shown that bacampicillin causes adverse effects in the fetus.

FDA Pregnancy Category B.

*Carbenicillin:* Reproductive studies using doses of 500 or 1000 mg/kg in rats, 200 mg/kg in mice, and 500 mg/kg in monkeys showed no harm to the fetus.

FDA Pregnancy Category B.

*Cloxacillin, dicloxacillin, methicillin, nafcillin, oxacillin, penicillin G, penicillin V:* Reproductive studies performed in the mouse, rat, and rabbit given these penicillins have revealed no evidence of impaired fertility or harm to the fetus.

FDA Pregnancy Category B.

*Flucloxacillin, pivampicillin, pivmecillinam:* Safety during pregnancy has not been established.

*Mezlocillin:* Studies in mice and rats given doses up to twice the usual human dose have not shown that mezlocillin causes adverse effects in the fetus.

FDA Pregnancy Category B.

*Piperacillin:* Studies in mice and rats given doses up to 4 times the usual human dose have not shown that piperacillin causes adverse effects in the fetus.

FDA Pregnancy Category B.

*Ticarcillin:* Reproductive studies done in mice and rats given ticarcillin have not shown that ticarcillin causes adverse effects in the fetus.

FDA Pregnancy Category B.

## Breast-feeding

Penicillins are distributed into breast milk, some in low concentrations. Although significant problems in humans have not been documented, the use of penicillins by nursing mothers may lead to sensitization, diarrhea, candidiasis, and skin rash in the infant.

## Pediatrics

Many penicillins have been used in pediatric patients and no pediatrics-specific problems have been documented to date. However, the incompletely developed renal function of neonates and young infants may delay the excretion of renally eliminated penicillins.

Because pivampicillin and pivmecillinam have been associated with a decrease in serum carnitine, it is recommended that these penicillins be avoided in children less than 3 months of age.

## Geriatrics

Penicillins have been used in geriatric patients and no geriatrics-specific problems have been documented to date. However, elderly patients are more likely to have age-related renal function impairment, which may require an adjustment in dosage in patients receiving penicillins.

## Dental

Prolonged use of penicillins may lead to the development of oral candidiasis.

## Drug interactions and/or related problems

The following drug interactions and/or related problems have been selected on the basis of their potential clinical significance (possible mechanism in parentheses where appropriate)—not necessarily inclusive (» = major clinical significance):

Note: Combinations containing any of the following medications, depending on the amount present, may also interact with this medication.

Allopurinol
(concurrent use with ampicillin or bacampicillin may significantly increase the possibility of skin rash, especially in hyperuricemic patients; however, it has not been established that allopurinol, rather than the presence of hyperuricemia, is responsible for this effect)

» Aminoglycosides
(mixing penicillins with aminoglycosides *in vitro* has resulted in substantial mutual inactivation; if these groups of antibacterials are to be administered concurrently, they should be administered at separate sites at least 1 hour apart)

» Angiotensin-converting enzyme (ACE) inhibitors or
» Diuretics, potassium-sparing or
» Potassium-containing medications, other or
» Potassium supplements
(concurrent administration of these medications with parenteral penicillin G potassium may promote serum potassium accumulation with possible resultant hyperkalemia, especially in patients with renal insufficiency; concurrent administration with ACE inhibitors may result in hyperkalemia since reduction of aldosterone production induced by ACE inhibitors may lead to elevation of serum potassium)

» Anticoagulants, coumarin- or indandione-derivative or
» Heparin or
» Thrombolytic agents
(concurrent use of these medications with high-dose parenteral carbenicillin, piperacillin, or ticarcillin may increase the risk of hemorrhage because these penicillins inhibit platelet aggregation; patients should be monitored carefully for signs of bleeding; concurrent use of these penicillins with thrombolytic agents may increase the risk of severe hemorrhage and is not recommended)

» Anti-inflammatory drugs, nonsteroidal (NSAIDs), especially aspirin or Diflunisal, very high doses or
Other salicylates or
» Platelet aggregation inhibitors, other (See *Appendix II*) or
» Sulfinpyrazone
(concurrent use of these medications with high-dose parenteral carbenicillin, piperacillin, or ticarcillin may increase the risk of hemorrhage because of additive inhibition of platelet function; in addition, hypoprothrombinemia induced by large doses of salicylates and the gastrointestinal ulcerative or hemorrhagic potential of

NSAIDs, salicylates, or sulfinpyrazone may also increase the risk of hemorrhage when these medications are used concurrently with these penicillins)

Chloramphenicol or
Erythromycins or
Sulfonamides or
Tetracyclines
(since bacteriostatic drugs may interfere with the bactericidal effect of penicillins in the treatment of meningitis or in other situations in which a rapid bactericidal effect is necessary, it is best to avoid concurrent therapy; however, chloramphenicol and ampicillin are sometimes administered concurrently to pediatric patients)

» Cholestyramine or
» Colestipol
(may impair absorption of oral penicillin G when used concurrently; patients should be advised to take oral penicillin G and these medications several hours apart)

» Contraceptives, estrogen-containing, oral
(there have been case reports of reduced oral contraceptive effectiveness in women taking ampicillin, amoxicillin, and penicillin V, resulting in unplanned pregnancy. This is thought to be due to a reduction in enterohepatic circulation of estrogens. Although the association is weak, patients should be advised of this information and given the option to use an alternate or additional method of contraception while taking any of these penicillins)

Disulfiram
(metabolism of the ester moiety of bacampicillin yields acetaldehyde and ethanol, which are later converted to acetaldehyde; furthermore, since disulfiram blocks the hepatic conversion of acetaldehyde to nontoxic compounds, concurrent use with bacampicillin may result in nausea, vomiting, confusion, and cardiovascular abnormalities)

Hepatotoxic medications, other (See *Appendix II*)
(concurrent use of other hepatotoxic medications with cloxacillin, dicloxacillin, flucloxacillin, mezlocillin, nafcillin, oxacillin, or piperacillin may increase the potential for hepatotoxicity)

» Methotrexate
(concurrent use with penicillins has resulted in decreased clearance of methotrexate and in methotrexate toxicity; this is thought to be due to competition for renal tubular secretion; patients should be closely monitored; leucovorin doses may need to be increased and administered for longer periods of time)

» Probenecid
(probenecid decreases renal tubular secretion of penicillins when used concurrently; this effect results in increased and prolonged serum concentrations, prolonged elimination half-life, and increased risk of toxicity. Penicillins and probenecid are often used concurrently to treat sexually transmitted diseases [STDs] or other infections in which high and/or prolonged antibiotic serum and tissue concentrations are required)

## Laboratory value alterations
The following have been selected on the basis of their potential clinical significance (possible effect in parentheses where appropriate)—not necessarily inclusive (» = major clinical significance):

With diagnostic test results
» Glucose, urine
(high urinary concentrations of a penicillin may produce false-positive or falsely elevated test results with copper sulfate tests [Benedict's, *Clinitest*, or Fehling's]; glucose enzymatic tests [*Clinistix* or *Testape*] are not affected)

Direct antiglobulin (Coombs') tests
(false-positive result may occur during therapy with any penicillin)

Protein, urine
(high urinary concentrations of mezlocillin or ticarcillin may produce false-positive protein reactions [pseudoproteinuria] with the sulfosalicylic acid and boiling test, the acetic acid test, the biuret reaction, and the nitric acid test; bromophenol blue reagent test strips [*Multi-stix*] are reportedly unaffected)

With physiology/laboratory test values
Alanine aminotransferase (ALT [SGPT]) and
Alkaline phosphatase and
Aspartate aminotransferase (AST [SGOT]) and
Lactate dehydrogenase (LDH), serum
(values may be increased)

Bilirubin, serum
(an increase has been associated with mezlocillin, piperacillin, and ticarcillin)

Blood urea nitrogen (BUN) and
Creatinine, serum
(an increase has been associated with flucloxacillin, mezlocillin, and piperacillin)

Estradiol or
Estriol, total conjugated or
Estriol-glucuronide or
Estrone, conjugated
(concentrations may be transiently decreased in pregnant women following administration of ampicillin and bacampicillin)

» Partial thromboplastin time (PTT) and
» Prothrombin time (PT)
(an increase has been associated with intravenous carbenicillin, piperacillin, and ticarcillin)

Potassium, serum
(hyperkalemia may occur following administration of large doses of parenteral penicillin G potassium because of high potassium content; hypokalemia may occur following administration of parenteral carbenicillin, mezlocillin, piperacillin, or ticarcillin, which may act as a nonreabsorbable anion in the distal renal tubules; this may cause an increase in pH and result in increased urinary potassium loss; the risk of hypokalemia increases with use of larger doses)

Sodium, serum
(hypernatremia may occur following administration of large doses of parenteral carbenicillin, mezlocillin, penicillin G sodium, or ticarcillin because of the high sodium content of these medications)

Uric acid, serum
(flucloxacillin may transiently decrease the serum uric acid concentration in some patients)

White blood cell count
(leukopenia or neutropenia is associated with the use of all penicillins; the effect is more likely to occur with prolonged therapy and severe hepatic function impairment)

## Medical considerations/Contraindications
The medical considerations/contraindications included here have been selected on the basis of their potential clinical significance (reasons given in parentheses where appropriate)—not necessarily inclusive (» = major clinical significance).

*Except under special circumstances, this medication should not be used when the following medical problem exists:*
» Allergy to penicillins

*Risk-benefit should be considered when the following medical problems exist:*
Allergy, general, history of sensitivity to multiple allergens
» Bleeding disorders, history of
(some penicillins, especially carbenicillin, piperacillin, and ticarcillin, may cause platelet dysfunction and hemorrhage)

Carnitine deficiency
(pivampicillin and pivmecillinam may reduce serum carnitine concentrations by increasing the urinary excretion of carnitine; use of these penicillins is not recommended in patients with carnitine deficiency or in infants up to 3 months of age)

» Congestive heart failure (CHF) or
Hypertension
(the sodium content of high doses of parenteral carbenicillin and ticarcillin should be considered in patients who require sodium restriction)

» Cystic fibrosis
(patients with cystic fibrosis may be at increased risk of fever and skin rash when given piperacillin)

» Gastrointestinal disease, history of, especially antibiotic-associated colitis
(penicillins may cause pseudomembranous colitis)

» Mononucleosis, infectious
(a morbilliform skin rash may occur in a high percentage [43 to 100%] of patients taking ampicillin, bacampicillin, or pivampicillin)

» Renal function impairment
(because most penicillins are excreted through the kidneys, a reduction in dosage, or increase in dosing interval, is recommended in patients with renal function impairment; also, the sodium content of high doses of parenteral carbenicillin and ticarcillin, and the potassium content of high doses of penicillin G potassium, should be considered in patients with severe renal function impairment)

**Patient monitoring**

The following may be especially important in patient monitoring (other tests may be warranted in some patients, depending on condition; » = major clinical significance):

*For carbenicillin (parenteral), piperacillin, ticarcillin*
» Partial thromboplastin time (PTT) and
» Prothrombin time (PT)
> (may be required prior to and during prolonged therapy in patients with renal function impairment who are receiving high doses since hemorrhagic manifestations may occur, although this effect is rare)

» Potassium, serum or
» Sodium, serum
> (determinations may be required periodically in patients with low potassium reserves and in patients receiving cytotoxic medications or diuretics who are also receiving high doses since hypokalemia may occur; also, because of the high sodium content of these medications, hypernatremia may occur)

*For methicillin*
» Renal function determinations
> (may be required during prolonged therapy since methicillin may cause interstitial nephritis in up to 33% of patients treated with methicillin for more than 10 days)

*For mezlocillin*
> Potassium, serum
> (may be required periodically during prolonged therapy in patients receiving high doses since hypokalemia may occur)

*For penicillin G (parenteral)*
> Potassium, serum or
» Sodium, serum
> (may be required periodically during therapy in patients receiving high doses of penicillin G potassium or penicillin G sodium since hyperkalemia or hypernatremia may occur; very high doses of penicillin G potassium may cause severe or fatal hyperkalemia; very high doses of penicillin G sodium may cause congestive heart failure)

*For all penicillins (if Clostridium difficile colitis occurs)*
» Stool cytotoxin assays
> (enzyme immunoassay of stool samples for the presence of *C. difficile* toxins may be required prior to treatment of patients with antibiotic-associated colitis to document the presence of *C. difficile* toxins; however, *C. difficile* and its toxins may persist following treatment with oral vancomycin, metronidazole, or cholestyramine, despite clinical improvement; follow-up cultures and toxin assays are not recommended if clinical improvement is complete)

## Side/Adverse Effects

The following side/adverse effects have been selected on the basis of their potential clinical significance (possible signs and symptoms in parentheses where appropriate)—not necessarily inclusive:

**Those indicating need for medical attention**

Incidence less frequent
> *Allergic reactions, specifically anaphylaxis* (fast or irregular breathing; puffiness or swelling around face; shortness of breath; sudden, severe decrease in blood pressure); *exfoliative dermatitis* (red, scaly skin); *serum sickness–like reactions* (skin rash; joint pain; fever); *skin rash, hives, or itching*

Incidence rare
> *Clostridium difficile colitis* (severe abdominal or stomach cramps and pain; abdominal tenderness; watery and severe diarrhea, which may also be bloody; fever); *hepatotoxicity* (fever; nausea and vomiting; yellow eyes or skin); *interstitial nephritis* (fever; possibly decreased urine output; skin rash); *leukopenia or neutropenia* (sore throat and fever); *mental disturbances* (anxiety; confusion; agitation or combativeness; depression; seizures; hallucinations; expressed fear of impending death); *pain at site of injection; platelet dysfunction or thrombocytopenia* (unusual bleeding or bruising); *seizures*

> Note: *Hepatotoxicity* has been associated with several penicillins, especially cloxacillin, dicloxacillin, flucloxacillin, and oxacillin; however, flucloxacillin appears to have a very high association with cholestatic jaundice, especially in older patients and those receiving flucloxacillin for more than 14 days. Also, one small study found HIV-infected patients to be more susceptible to oxacillin-hepatotoxicity (81%) than HIV-negative patients (4.5%).

> *Interstitial nephritis* is seen primarily with methicillin, and to a lesser degree with nafcillin and oxacillin, but may occur with any penicillin.

*Mental disturbances* are toxic reactions to the procaine content of penicillin G procaine; this reaction may be seen in patients who receive a large single dose of the medication, as in the treatment of gonorrhea.

*Platelet dysfunction* is primarily associated with carbenicillin, piperacillin, and ticarcillin; it may be more pronounced in patients with renal insufficiency due to the prolongation of the penicillin's half-life and uremic platelet dysfunction.

*Clostridium difficile colitis* may occur up to several weeks after discontinuation of these medications.

*Seizures* are more likely to occur in patients receiving high doses of a penicillin and/or patients with severe renal function impairment.

**Those indicating need for medical attention only if they continue or are bothersome**

Incidence more frequent
> *Gastrointestinal reactions* (mild diarrhea; nausea or vomiting); *headache; oral candidiasis* (sore mouth or tongue; white patches in mouth and/or on tongue); *vaginal candidiasis* (vaginal itching and discharge)

## Overdose

For more information on the management of overdose or unintentional ingestion, **contact a Poison Control Center** (see *Poison Control Center Listing*).

**Treatment of overdose**

Specific treatment—Hemodialysis may aid in the removal of penicillins from the blood.

Supportive care—Since there is no specific antidote, treatment of penicillin overdose should be symptomatic and supportive. Patients in whom intentional overdose is known or suspected should be referred for psychiatric consultation.

## Patient Consultation

As an aid to patient consultation, refer to *Advice for the Patient, Penicillins (Systemic)*.

In providing consultation, consider emphasizing the following selected information (» = major clinical significance):

**Before using this medication**
» Conditions affecting use, especially:
> Allergy to penicillins, cephalosporins, or cephamycins
> Pregnancy—Penicillins cross the placenta
> Breast-feeding—Penicillins are distributed into breast milk
> Use in children—Neonates and young infants may have reduced elimination of renally eliminated penicillins due to incompletely developed renal function
> Other medications, especially aminoglycosides; angiotensin-converting enzyme inhibitors; cholestyramine; colestipol; coumarin- or indandione-derivative anticoagulants; estrogen-containing oral contraceptives; heparin; methotrexate; nonsteroidal anti-inflammatory drugs (NSAIDs), especially aspirin; other platelet aggregation inhibitors; other potassium-containing medications; potassium-sparing diuretics; potassium supplements; probenecid; sulfinpyrazone; or thrombolytic agents
> Other medical problems, especially a history of bleeding disorders; congestive heart failure; cystic fibrosis; active or history of gastrointestinal disease, especially antibiotic-associated colitis; infectious mononucleosis; or renal function impairment

**Proper use of this medication**
> Taking on an empty stomach (for ampicillin, bacampicillin oral suspension, carbenicillin; cloxacillin, dicloxacillin, flucloxacillin, nafcillin, oxacillin, penicillin G)
> Taking on a full or empty stomach (for amoxicillin, bacampicillin tablets, penicillin V, pivampicillin, pivmecillinam)
> Taking amoxicillin suspension straight or mixed with formulas, milk, fruit juice, water, ginger ale, or other cold drinks; taking immediately after mixing; drinking full dose
> Not drinking acidic fruit juices or other acidic beverages within 1 hour of taking oral penicillin G
> Proper administration technique for oral liquids and/or pediatric drops
> Not using after expiration date
» Compliance with full course of therapy, especially in streptococcal infections
» Importance of not missing doses and taking at evenly spaced times
» Proper dosing
> Missed dose: Taking as soon as possible; not taking if almost time for next dose; not doubling doses
» Proper storage

### Precautions while using this medication
Checking with physician if no improvement within a few days
» For severe diarrhea, checking with physician before taking any anti-diarrheals; for mild diarrhea, kaolin- or attapulgite-containing antidiarrheals may be used, but antiperistaltic antidiarrheals should be avoided; checking with physician or pharmacist if mild diarrhea continues or worsens
» Possibly using an alternate or additional method of contraception if taking estrogen-containing oral contraceptives concurrently, especially with ampicillin, amoxicillin, or penicillin V
» Diabetics: False-positive reactions with copper sulfate urine glucose tests may occur
Possible interference with diagnostic tests

### Side/adverse effects
Signs of potential side effects, especially allergic reactions, *Clostridium difficile* colitis, hepatotoxicity, interstitial nephritis, leukopenia or neutropenia, mental disturbances, pain at site of injection, platelet dysfunction or thrombocytopenia, and seizures

## General Dosing Information

Therapy should be continued for at least 10 days in Group A beta-hemolytic streptococcal infections to help prevent the occurrence of acute rheumatic fever.

### For oral dosage forms only
Penicillins, except amoxicillin, bacampicillin hydrochloride tablets, penicillin V, pivampicillin, and pivmecillinam should preferably be taken with a full glass (240 mL) of water on an empty stomach (either 1 hour before or 2 hours after meals) to obtain optimum serum and/or urine concentrations. Amoxicillin, bacampicillin hydrochloride tablets, penicillin V, pivampicillin, and pivmecillinam may be taken on a full or empty stomach.

### For treatment of adverse effects
Serious anaphylactoid reactions require immediate emergency treatment, which consists of the following:
• Parenteral epinephrine.
• Oxygen.
• Intravenous corticosteroids.
• Airway management (including intubation).
For *Clostridium difficile* colitis—
• Some patients may develop *Clostridium difficile* colitis during or following administration of penicillins.
• *C. difficile* colitis may result in severe watery diarrhea, which may occur during therapy or up to several weeks after therapy is discontinued. If diarrhea occurs, administration of antiperistaltic antidiarrheals (e.g., opioids, diphenoxylate and atropine combination, loperamide, paregoric) is not recommended since they may delay the removal of toxins from the colon, thereby prolonging and/or worsening the condition.
• Mild cases may respond to discontinuation of the medication alone. Moderate to severe cases may require fluid, electrolyte, and protein replacement.
• In cases not responding to the above measures or in more severe cases, oral doses of vancomycin, metronidazole, or cholestyramine may be used. Oral vancomycin is effective in doses of 125 mg every 6 hours for 5 to 10 days. The dose of metronidazole is 250 to 500 mg every 8 hours and the dose of cholestyramine is 4 grams four times a day. Recurrences, which occur in approximately 25% of patients treated with vancomycin or metronidazole, may be treated with a second course of these medications.
• Cholestyramine resin has been shown to bind *C. difficile* toxin *in vitro*. If cholestyramine resin is administered in conjunction with oral vancomycin, the medications should be administered several hours apart since the resin has been shown to bind oral vancomycin also.

---

## *AMOXICILLIN*

## Summary of Differences

Category:
Aminopenicillin.
Pharmacology/pharmacokinetics:
High oral absorption (75 to 90%).
Precautions:
Drug interactions and/or related problems—May also interact with oral contraceptives.
Medical considerations/Contraindications—Caution also needed in infectious mononucleosis.

## Additional Dosing Information

Patients with impaired renal function do not generally require a reduction in dose unless the impairment is severe.

### For oral dosage forms only
Amoxicillin may be taken on a full or empty stomach.
Amoxicillin may be taken with formulas, milk, fruit juice, water, ginger ale, or other cold drinks.

## Oral Dosage Forms

Note: Bracketed uses in the *Dosage Forms* section refer to categories of use and/or indications that are not included in U.S. product labeling.

### AMOXICILLIN CAPSULES USP

#### Usual adult and adolescent dose
Antibacterial—
Oral, 250 to 500 mg every eight hours.
Endocarditis, bacterial (prophylaxis): Oral, 3 grams one hour before the procedure, then 1.5 grams six hours after the initial dose.
[Chlamydia, treatment in pregnant women][1]: Oral, 500 mg every eight hours for seven to ten days.
[Gastritis, *Helicobacter pylori*][1] or
[Ulcer, peptic, *Helicobacter pylori*][1]: Oral, 500 mg four times a day; or 750 mg three times a day.
[Lyme disease][1]: Oral, 250 to 500 mg three or four times a day for three to four weeks. Duration of therapy is based on clinical response. Treatment failures have occurred and retreatment may be necessary.

#### Usual adult prescribing limits
Up to 4.5 grams a day.

#### Usual pediatric dose
Antibacterial—
Gonorrhea, endocervical and urethral, uncomplicated: Oral, 50 mg per kg of body weight and 25 mg of probenecid per kg of body weight simultaneously as a single dose in prepubertal children. However, probenecid is not recommended in children under 2 years of age.
[Lyme disease][1]: Oral, 6.7 to 13.3 mg per kg of body weight every eight hours for ten to thirty days. Duration of therapy is based on clinical response. Treatment failures have occurred and retreatment may be necessary.
For all other indications: Infants and children up to 20 kg of body weight—A product of suitable strength is not available for infants and children up to 20 kg of body weight. See *Amoxicillin for Oral Suspension USP*.
Children 20 kg of body weight and over—See *Usual adult and adolescent dose*.

#### Strength(s) usually available
U.S.—
250 mg (Rx) [*Amoxil; Trimox; Wymox;* GENERIC].
500 mg (Rx) [*Amoxil; Trimox; Wymox;* GENERIC].
Canada—
250 mg (Rx) [*Amoxil; Apo-Amoxi; Novamoxin; Nu-Amoxi*].
500 mg (Rx) [*Amoxil; Apo-Amoxi; Novamoxin; Nu-Amoxi*].

#### Packaging and storage
Store between 15 and 30 °C (59 and 86 °F). Store in a tight container.

#### Auxiliary labeling
• Continue medication for full time of treatment.

### AMOXICILLIN FOR ORAL SUSPENSION USP

#### Usual adult and adolescent dose
See *Amoxicillin Capsules USP*.

#### Usual adult prescribing limits
See *Amoxicillin Capsules USP*.

#### Usual pediatric dose
Antibacterial—
Infants up to 6 kg of body weight: Oral, 25 to 50 mg every eight hours.
Infants 6 to 8 kg of body weight: Oral, 50 to 100 mg every eight hours.
Infants and children 8 to 20 kg of body weight: Oral, 6.7 to 13.3 mg per kg of body weight every eight hours.
Children 20 kg of body weight and over: See *Usual adult and adolescent dose*.

#### Strength(s) usually available
U.S.—
50 mg per mL (when reconstituted according to manufacturer's instructions) (Rx) [*Amoxil; Trimox; Polymox*].

125 mg per 5 mL (when reconstituted according to manufacturer's instructions) (Rx) [*Amoxil; Polymox; Trimox; Wymox;* GENERIC].
250 mg per 5 mL (when reconstituted according to manufacturer's instructions) (Rx) [*Amoxil; Polymox; Trimox; Wymox;* GENERIC].
Canada—
   50 mg per mL (when reconstituted according to manufacturer's instructions) (Rx) [*Amoxil*].
   125 mg per 5 mL (when reconstituted according to manufacturer's instructions) (Rx) [*Amoxil; Apo-Amoxi; Novamoxin; Nu-Amoxi*].
   250 mg per 5 mL (when reconstituted according to manufacturer's instructions) (Rx) [*Amoxil; Apo-Amoxi; Novamoxin; Nu-Amoxi*].

**Packaging and storage**
Prior to reconstitution, store between 15 and 30 °C (59 and 86 °F). Store in a tight container.

**Stability**
After reconstitution, suspensions retain their potency for up to 14 days at room temperature or for up to 14 days if refrigerated, depending on the manufacturer.
Note: Some manufacturers prefer refrigerated storage.

**Auxiliary labeling**
• Refrigerate.
• Shake well.
• Continue medication for full time of treatment.
• Beyond-use date.
• Take by mouth only (pediatric drops).

**Note**
Explain administration technique for pediatric drops (50 mg per mL).
When dispensing, include a calibrated liquid-measuring device.

## AMOXICILLIN TABLETS (CHEWABLE) USP

**Usual adult and adolescent dose**
See *Amoxicillin Capsules USP*.

**Usual adult prescribing limits**
See *Amoxicillin Capsules USP*.

**Usual pediatric dose**
See *Amoxicillin Capsules USP*.

**Strength(s) usually available**
U.S.—
   125 mg (Rx) [*Amoxil*].
   250 mg (Rx) [*Amoxil;* GENERIC].
Canada—
   125 mg (Rx) [*Amoxil*].
   250 mg (Rx) [*Amoxil*].

**Packaging and storage**
Store between 15 and 30 °C (59 and 86 °F). Store in a tight container.

**Auxiliary labeling**
• Should be chewed or crushed.
• Continue medication for full time of treatment.

---

[1]Not included in Canadian product labeling.

---

## *AMPICILLIN*

# Summary of Differences

Category:
   Aminopenicillin.
Precautions:
   Drug interactions and/or related problems—Also interacts with allopurinol and oral contraceptives.
   Medical considerations/contraindications—Caution also needed in infectious mononucleosis.

# Additional Dosing Information

Patients with impaired renal function do not generally require a reduction in dose unless the impairment is severe.

# Oral Dosage Forms

Note: Bracketed uses in the *Dosage Forms* section refer to categories of use and/or indications that are not included in U.S. product labeling.

## AMPICILLIN CAPSULES USP

**Usual adult and adolescent dose**
Antibacterial—
   Oral, 250 to 500 mg every six hours.
   [Typhoid fever][1]: Oral, 25 mg per kg of body weight every six hours.

**Usual adult prescribing limits**
Up to 4 grams a day.

**Usual pediatric dose**
Antibacterial—
   Infants and children up to 20 kg of body weight: A product of suitable strength is not available for infants and children up to 20 kg of body weight. See *Ampicillin for Oral Suspension USP*.
   Children 20 kg of body weight and over: See *Usual adult and adolescent dose*.

**Strength(s) usually available**
U.S.—
   250 mg (Rx) [*Omnipen; Principen; Totacillin;* GENERIC].
   500 mg (Rx) [*Omnipen; Principen; Totacillin;* GENERIC].
Canada—
   250 mg (Rx) [*Apo-Ampi; Novo-Ampicillin; Nu-Ampi; Penbritin*].
   500 mg (Rx) [*Apo-Ampi; Novo-Ampicillin; Nu-Ampi; Penbritin*].

**Packaging and storage**
Store below 40 °C (104 °F), preferably between 15 and 30 °C (59 and 86 °F), unless otherwise specified by manufacturer. Store in a tight container.

**Auxiliary labeling**
• Continue medication for full time of treatment.
• Take on empty stomach.

## AMPICILLIN FOR ORAL SUSPENSION USP

**Usual adult and adolescent dose**
See *Ampicillin Capsules USP*.

**Usual adult prescribing limits**
See *Ampicillin Capsules USP*.

**Usual pediatric dose**
Antibacterial—
   Infants and children up to 20 kg of body weight: Oral, 12.5 to 25 mg per kg of body weight every six hours; or 16.7 to 33.3 mg per kg of body weight every eight hours
   Children 20 kg of body weight and over: See *Usual adult and adolescent dose*.

**Strength(s) usually available**
U.S.—
   100 mg per mL (Rx) [*Polycillin*].
   125 mg per 5 mL (Rx) [*Omnipen; Polycillin; Principen; Totacillin;* GENERIC].
   250 mg per 5 mL (Rx) [*Omnipen; Polycillin; Principen; Totacillin;* GENERIC].
   500 mg per 5 mL (Rx) [*Polycillin*].
Canada—
   125 mg per 5 mL (Rx) [*Apo-Ampi; Novo-Ampicillin; Nu-Ampi*].
   250 mg per 5 mL (Rx) [*Apo-Ampi; Novo-Ampicillin; Nu-Ampi; Penbritin*].

**Packaging and storage**
Prior to reconstitution, store below 40 °C (104 °F), preferably between 15 and 30 °C (59 and 86 °F), unless otherwise specified by manufacturer. Store in a tight container.

**Stability**
After reconstitution, suspensions retain their potency for 7 days at room temperature or for 14 days if refrigerated, depending on manufacturer.

**Auxiliary labeling**
• Refrigerate.
• Shake well.
• Continue medication for full time of treatment.
• Beyond-use date.
• Take by mouth only (pediatric drops).
• Take on empty stomach.

**Note**
Explain administration technique for pediatric drops (100 mg per mL).
When dispensing, include a calibrated liquid-measuring device.

# Parenteral Dosage Forms

Note: Bracketed uses in the *Dosage Forms* section refer to categories of use and/or indications that are not included in U.S. product labeling.
   The dosing and strengths of the dosage forms available are expressed in terms of ampicillin base (not the sodium salt).

## AMPICILLIN SODIUM STERILE USP

**Usual adult and adolescent dose**
Antibacterial—
   Intramuscular or intravenous, 250 to 500 mg (base) every six hours.

Endocarditis, bacterial
Meningitis, bacterial or
Septicemia, bacterial: Intramuscular or intravenous, 1 to 2 grams
  (base) every three to four hours.
Listeriosis: Intramuscular or intravenous, 50 mg per kg of body weight
  every six hours.
[Leptospirosis][1]: Intramuscular or intravenous, 500 mg to 1 gram every
  six hours.
[Typhoid fever][1]: Intramuscular or intravenous, 25 mg per kg of body
  weight every six hours.

## Usual adult prescribing limits
Up to 14 grams a day.

## Usual pediatric dose
Antibacterial—
  Meningitis, bacterial:
    Neonates up to 2 kg of body weight—Intramuscular or intrave-
      nous, 25 to 50 mg per kg of body weight every twelve hours
      during the first week of life, then 50 mg per kg of body weight
      every eight hours thereafter.
    Neonates 2 kg of body weight and over—Intramuscular or intra-
      venous, 50 mg per kg of body weight every eight hours during
      the first week of life, then 50 mg per kg of body weight every
      six hours thereafter.
  For all other indications:
    Infants up to 20 kg of body weight—Intramuscular or intravenous,
      12.5 mg (base) per kg of body weight every six hours.
    Infants and children 20 kg of body weight and over—See *Usual
      adult and adolescent dose.*

## Size(s) usually available
U.S.—
  125 mg (base) (Rx) [*Omnipen-N; Polycillin-N;* GENERIC].
  250 mg (base) (Rx) [*Omnipen-N; Polycillin-N; Totacillin-N;*
    GENERIC].
  500 mg (base) (Rx) [*Omnipen-N; Polycillin-N; Totacillin-N;*
    GENERIC].
  1 gram (base) (Rx) [*Omnipen-N; Polycillin-N; Totacillin-N;* GENERIC].
  2 grams (base) (Rx) [*Omnipen-N; Polycillin-N; Totacillin-N;*
    GENERIC].
  10 grams (base) (Rx) [*Omnipen-N; Polycillin-N;* GENERIC].
Canada—
  125 mg (base) (Rx) [*Ampicin; Penbritin*].
  250 mg (base) (Rx) [*Ampicin; Penbritin*].
  500 mg (base) (Rx) [*Ampicin; Penbritin*].
  1 gram (base) (Rx) [*Ampicin; Penbritin*].
  2 grams (base) (Rx) [*Ampicin; Penbritin*].

## Packaging and storage
Prior to reconstitution, store below 40 °C (104 °F), preferably between 15
  and 30 °C (59 and 86 °F), unless otherwise specified by manufacturer.
  Protect the reconstituted solution from freezing.

## Preparation of dosage form
To prepare initial dilution for intramuscular use, depending on the manufacturer, add 0.9 to 1.2 mL of sterile water for injection or bacteriostatic water for injection to each 125-mg vial, 0.9 to 1.9 mL of diluent
  to each 250-mg vial, 1.2 to 1.8 mL of diluent to each 500-mg vial,
  2.4 to 7.4 mL of diluent to each 1-gram vial, and 6.8 mL of diluent
  to each 2-gram vial.
To prepare initial dilution for direct intermittent intravenous use, add 5
  mL of sterile water for injection or bacteriostatic water for injection
  to each 125-, 250-, or 500-mg vial or at least 7.4 to 10 mL of diluent
  to each 1- or 2-gram vial. The resulting solution should be administered slowly over a 3- to 5-minute period for each 125- to 500-mg
  dose or over a 10- to 15-minute period for each 1- to 2-gram dose.
  More rapid administration may result in convulsive seizures.
Intravenous infusions of sterile ampicillin sodium should be administered
  in a suitable diluent in a concentration not exceeding 30 mg per mL
  (see manufacturer's package insert).
For reconstitution of pharmacy bulk vials or piggyback infusion bottles,
  see manufacturer's labeling for instructions.

## Stability
After reconstitution for intramuscular or direct intravenous use, solutions
  retain their potency for 1 hour.
After reconstitution for intravenous infusion, solutions in concentrations
  up to 30 mg per mL retain at least 90% of their potency for 2 to 8
  hours at room temperature or for up to 72 hours if refrigerated in
  suitable diluents (see manufacturer's package insert).
Concentrated solutions (100 mg per mL) prepared from pharmacy bulk
  vials retain their potency for 2 hours at room temperature or for 4
  hours if refrigerated.

Diluted solutions (20 mg per mL or less) in 5% dextrose injection retain
  their potency for 2 hours at room temperature or for 3 hours if
  refrigerated.

## Incompatibilities
Extemporaneous admixtures of beta-lactam antibacterials (penicillins and
  cephalosporins) and aminoglycosides may result in substantial mutual
  inactivation. If these groups of antibacterials are administered concurrently, they should be administered in separate sites at least 1 hour
  apart. Do not mix them in the same intravenous bag, bottle, or tubing.
When aminoglycosides and penicillins are administered separately by different routes, a reduction in aminoglycoside serum concentration may
  occur. Usually this is clinically significant only in patients with severely impaired renal function when the excretion of both medications
  is delayed.

## Additional information
The sodium content is approximately 3.4 mEq (3.4 mmol) per gram of
  ampicillin, depending on the manufacturer. This must be considered
  in patients on a restricted sodium intake when calculating total daily
  sodium intake.

---

[1]Not included in Canadian product labeling.

---

## *BACAMPICILLIN*

# Summary of Differences
Category:
  Aminopenicillin.
Pharmacology/pharmacokinetics:
  Hydrolyzed to ampicillin during absorption.
Precautions:
  Drug interactions and/or related problems—Also interacts with allo-
    purinol and disulfiram.
  Medical considerations/contraindications—Caution also needed in in-
    fectious mononucleosis.

# Additional Dosing Information
Bacampicillin is stable in the presence of gastric acid. Also, food does
  not delay or reduce absorption of bacampicillin hydrochloride tablets.
  Therefore, the tablets may be taken on a full or empty stomach. However, bacampicillin hydrochloride oral suspension should preferably
  be taken with a full glass (240 mL) of water on an empty stomach
  (either 1 hour before or 2 hours after meals) to obtain optimum serum
  and/or urine concentrations.
Patients with impaired renal function do not generally require a reduction
  in dose unless the impairment is severe. The serum half-life increases
  when the creatinine clearance is below 30 mL per minute (0.50 mL
  per second).

# Oral Dosage Forms
Note: The dosing and strengths of the dosage forms available are expressed in terms of bacampicillin hydrochloride (not the base).

## BACAMPICILLIN HYDROCHLORIDE FOR ORAL SUSPENSION USP

### Usual adult and adolescent dose
Antibacterial—
  Oral, 400 to 800 mg every twelve hours.

### Usual adult prescribing limits
Up to 3.2 grams a day.

### Usual pediatric dose
Antibacterial—
  Oral, 12.5 to 25 mg per kg of body weight every twelve hours.

### Strength(s) usually available
U.S.—
  125 mg per 5 mL (Rx) [*Spectrobid*].
  Note: 125 mg of bacampicillin hydrochloride are equivalent to 87.5
    mg of ampicillin.
Canada—
  Not commercially available.

### Packaging and storage
Prior to reconstitution, store below 40 °C (104 °F), preferably between 15
  and 30 °C (59 and 86 °F), unless otherwise specified by manufacturer.
  Store in a tight container.

### Stability
After reconstitution, suspensions retain their potency for 10 days if
  refrigerated.

### Auxiliary labeling

- Refrigerate.
- Shake well.
- Continue medication for full time of treatment.
- Beyond-use date.
- Take on empty stomach.

### Note

When dispensing, include a calibrated liquid-measuring device.

## BACAMPICILLIN HYDROCHLORIDE TABLETS USP

### Usual adult and adolescent dose

See *Bacampicillin Hydrochloride for Oral Suspension USP*.

### Usual adult prescribing limits

See *Bacampicillin Hydrochloride for Oral Suspension USP*.

### Usual pediatric dose

Infants and children up to 25 kg of body weight—Use of the tablets is not recommended. See *Bacampicillin Hydrochloride for Oral Suspension USP*.

Children 25 kg of body weight and over—See *Usual adult and adolescent dose*.

### Strength(s) usually available

U.S.—
    400 mg (Rx) [*Spectrobid*].
Canada—
    400 mg (Rx) [*Penglobe* (scored)].
    800 mg (Rx) [*Penglobe* (scored)].

Note: 400 mg of bacampicillin hydrochloride are equivalent to 280 mg of ampicillin.

### Packaging and storage

Store below 40 °C (104 °F), preferably between 15 and 30 °C (59 and 86 °F), unless otherwise specified by manufacturer. Store in a tight container.

### Auxiliary labeling

- Continue medication for full time of treatment.

---

## CARBENICILLIN

## Summary of Differences

### Category:
Antipseudomonal penicillin.

### Pharmacology/pharmacokinetics:
Renal elimination of oral carbenicillin is approximately 36%, and 75 to 95% for intravenous carbenicillin.

### Precautions:
Drug interactions and/or related problems—Parenteral carbenicillin also interacts with anticoagulants and other medications that affect blood clotting.

Laboratory value alterations—May increase bleeding time; may also cause hypernatremia.

Medical considerations/contraindications—Caution in patients with a history of bleeding disorders, congestive heart failure, or hypertension.

Patient monitoring—Bleeding time and serum potassium and sodium determinations may be required (parenteral only).

## Additional Dosing Information

### For oral dosage forms only

Patients with severely impaired renal function (creatinine clearance less than 10 mL per minute) will not achieve therapeutic urine concentrations of carbenicillin.

### For parenteral dosage forms only

Intramuscular injections should not exceed 2 grams in each site.
Intermittent infusions may be administered over a 30- to 40-minute period.
Patients with impaired renal function may require a reduction in dose and should be observed for hemorrhagic complications.

## Oral Dosage Forms

Note: The dosing and strengths of the dosage forms available are expressed in terms of carbenicillin indanyl sodium (not the base).

## CARBENICILLIN INDANYL SODIUM TABLETS USP

### Usual adult and adolescent dose

Antibacterial—
    Oral, 500 mg to 1 gram every six hours.

### Usual pediatric dose

Dosage has not been established.

### Strength(s) usually available

U.S.—
    500 mg (Rx) [*Geocillin*].
Canada—
    500 mg (Rx) [*Geopen Oral*].

Note: 500 mg of carbenicillin indanyl sodium are equivalent to 382 mg of carbenicillin and 118 mg of indanyl sodium.

### Packaging and storage

Store below 40 °C (104 °F), preferably between 15 and 30 °C (59 and 86 °F), unless otherwise specified by manufacturer. Store in a tight container.

### Auxiliary labeling

- Continue medication for full time of treatment.

## Parenteral Dosage Forms

Note: The dosing and strengths of the dosage forms available are expressed in terms of carbenicillin disodium (not the base).

## STERILE CARBENICILLIN DISODIUM USP

### Usual adult and adolescent dose

Antibacterial—
    Intramuscular or intravenous, 50 to 83.3 mg per kg of body weight every four hours.
    Urinary tract infections: Intramuscular or intravenous, 1 to 2 grams every six hours; or up to 50 mg per kg of body weight every six hours.

### Usual adult prescribing limits

Up to 40 grams a day.

### Usual pediatric dose

Antibacterial—
    Neonates up to 2 kg of body weight: Intramuscular or intravenous, 75 mg per kg of body weight every twelve hours during the first week of life; followed by 75 mg per kg of body weight every eight hours thereafter.
    Neonates 2 kg of body weight and over: Intramuscular or intravenous, 75 mg per kg of body weight every eight hours during the first week of life; followed by 75 mg per kg of body weight every six hours thereafter.
    Older infants and children: Intramuscular or intravenous, 25 to 75 mg per kg of body weight every six hours; or 16.7 to 50 mg per kg of body weight every four hours.

### Size(s) usually available

U.S.—
    1 gram (Rx) [*Geopen*].
    2 grams (Rx) [*Geopen*].
    5 grams (Rx) [*Geopen*].
    10 grams (Rx) [*Geopen*].
    30 grams (Rx) [*Geopen*].
Canada—
    1 gram (Rx) [*Pyopen*].
    5 grams (Rx) [*Pyopen*].

### Packaging and storage

Prior to reconstitution, store below 40 °C (104 °F), preferably between 15 and 30 °C (59 and 86 °F), unless otherwise specified by manufacturer.

### Preparation of dosage form

To prepare initial dilution for intramuscular use, depending on the manufacturer, add 2 to 3.6 mL of sterile water for injection or bacteriostatic water for injection (preserved with 0.9% benzyl alcohol) to each 1-gram vial, 4 to 7.2 mL of diluent to each 2-gram vial, and 7 to 17 mL of diluent to each 5-gram vial. Lidocaine hydrochloride injection 0.5% (without epinephrine) may also be used as a diluent for intramuscular use.

To prepare initial dilution for direct intravenous use, reconstitute as directed above for intramuscular use. Each gram of carbenicillin should be further diluted with the addition of not less than 5 mL of diluent. The resulting solution should be administered as slowly as possible to avoid vein irritation.

For reconstitution of pharmacy bulk vials or piggyback infusion bottles, see manufacturer's labeling for instructions.

Caution: Use of diluents containing benzyl alcohol is not recommended for preparation of medications for use in neonates. A fatal toxic syndrome consisting of metabolic acidosis, CNS depression, respiratory problems, renal failure, hypotension, and possibly seizures and intracranial hemorrhages has been associated with this use.

### Stability

After reconstitution for intramuscular or direct intravenous use, solutions retain their potency for 24 hours at room temperature or for 72 hours if refrigerated.

Intravenous infusions in suitable diluents (see manufacturer's package insert), concentrated solutions (200 mg per mL), or diluted solutions (10 to 100 mg per mL) prepared from pharmacy bulk vials retain their potency for 24 hours at room temperature or for 72 hours if refrigerated.

### Incompatibilities

Extemporaneous admixtures of beta-lactam antibacterials (penicillins and cephalosporins) and aminoglycosides may result in substantial mutual inactivation. If these groups of antibacterials are administered concurrently, they should be administered in separate sites at least 1 hour apart. Do not mix them in the same intravenous bag, bottle, or tubing.

When aminoglycosides and penicillins are administered separately by different routes, a reduction in aminoglycoside serum concentration may occur. Usually this is clinically significant only in patients with severely impaired renal function when the excretion of both medications is delayed.

### Additional information

The sodium content is approximately 4.7 to 5.3 mEq (4.7 to 5.3 mmol), but may be as high as 6.5 mEq (6.5 mmol), per gram of carbenicillin. This must be considered in patients on a restricted sodium intake when calculating total daily sodium intake.

---

## CLOXACILLIN

## Summary of Differences

Category: Penicillinase-resistant penicillin.
Pharmacology/pharmacokinetics: Very high plasma protein binding (95%).
Precautions: Drug interactions and/or related problems—May interact with other hepatotoxic medications.
Side/adverse effects: May be an increased risk of hepatotoxicity.

## Additional Dosing Information

Patients with impaired renal function do not generally require a reduction in dose unless the impairment is severe.

Cloxacillin should be taken on an empty stomach, preferably, 1 hour before meals.

## Oral Dosage Forms

Note: The dosing and strengths of the dosage forms available are expressed in terms of cloxacillin base (not the sodium salt).

### CLOXACILLIN SODIUM CAPSULES USP

**Usual adult and adolescent dose**
Antibacterial—
Oral, 250 to 500 mg (base) every six hours.

**Usual adult prescribing limits**
Up to 6 grams (base) a day.

**Usual pediatric dose**
Antibacterial—
Infants and children up to 20 kg of body weight: Oral, 6.25 to 12.5 mg (base) per kg of body weight every six hours.
Children 20 kg of body weight and over: See *Usual adult and adolescent dose.*

**Strength(s) usually available**
U.S.—
250 mg (base) (Rx) [*Cloxapen;* GENERIC].
500 mg (base) (Rx) [*Cloxapen;* GENERIC].
Canada—
250 mg (base) (Rx) [*Apo-Cloxi; Novo-Cloxin; Nu-Cloxi; Orbenin*].
500 mg (base) (Rx) [*Apo-Cloxi; Novo-Cloxin; Nu-Cloxi; Orbenin*].

**Packaging and storage**
Store below 40 °C (104 °F), preferably between 15 and 30 °C (59 and 86 °F), unless otherwise specified by manufacturer. Store in a tight container.

**Auxiliary labeling**
• Continue medication for full time of treatment.
• Take on empty stomach.

### CLOXACILLIN SODIUM FOR ORAL SOLUTION USP

**Usual adult and adolescent dose**
See *Cloxacillin Sodium Capsules USP.*

**Usual adult prescribing limits**
See *Cloxacillin Sodium Capsules USP.*

**Usual pediatric dose**
See *Cloxacillin Sodium Capsules USP.*

**Strength(s) usually available**
U.S.—
125 mg per 5 mL (base) (Rx) [*Tegopen;* GENERIC].
Canada—
125 mg per 5 mL (base) (Rx) [*Apo-Cloxi; Novo-Cloxin; Nu-Cloxi; Orbenin*].

**Packaging and storage**
Prior to reconstitution, store below 40 °C (104 °F), preferably between 15 and 30 °C (59 and 86 °F), unless otherwise specified by manufacturer. Store in a tight container.

**Stability**
After reconstitution, solutions retain their potency for 14 days if refrigerated.

**Auxiliary labeling**
• Refrigerate.
• Continue medication for full time of treatment.
• Beyond-use date.
• Take on empty stomach.

**Note**
When dispensing, include a calibrated liquid-measuring device.

## Parenteral Dosage Forms

Note: The dosing and dosage forms available are expressed in terms of cloxacillin base (not the sodium salt).

### CLOXACILLIN SODIUM INJECTION

**Usual adult and adolescent dose**
Antibacterial—
Intravenous, 250 to 500 mg (base) every six hours.

**Usual adult prescribing limits**
Up to 6 grams (base) a day.

**Usual pediatric dose**
Antibacterial—
Infants and children up to 20 kg of body weight: Intravenous, 6.25 to 12.5 mg (base) per kg of body weight every six hours.
Children 20 kg of body weight and over: See *Usual adult and adolescent dose.*

Note: Cystic fibrosis patients: Intravenous, 25 mg (base) per kg of body weight every six hours.

**Strength(s) usually available**
U.S.—
Not commercially available.
Canada—
250 mg (base) (Rx) [*Orbenin; Tegopen*].
500 mg (base) (Rx) [*Orbenin; Tegopen*].
2 grams (base) (Rx) [*Orbenin; Tegopen*].

**Packaging and storage**
Prior to reconstitution, store between 15 and 30 °C (59 and 86 °F), unless otherwise specified by manufacturer.

**Preparation of dosage form**
To prepare for intramuscular injection, add 1.9 mL or 1.7 mL of sterile water for injection to each 250 mg or 500 mg vial, respectively, and shake to dissolve.
To prepare for intravenous injection, add 4.9 mL, 4.8 mL, or 6.8 mL of sterile water for injection to each 250 mg, 500 mg, or 2 gram vial, respectively, and shake to dissolve.
For direct intravenous use, the resulting solution should be administered slowly over a 2- to 4-minute period.
For intermittent intravenous use, the resulting solution should be further diluted with a suitable diluent (see manufacturer's package insert). It may be administered over a 30- to 40-minute period.

**Stability**
After reconstitution with suitable diluents (see manufacturer's package insert), solutions retain their potency for 24 hours at controlled room temperature (25 °C [77 °F]), or 72 hours if refrigerated.

**Incompatibilities**
Extemporaneous admixtures of beta-lactam antibacterials (penicillins and cephalosporins) and aminoglycosides may result in substantial mutual inactivation. If these groups of antibacterials are administered concurrently, they should be administered in separate sites at least 1 hour apart. Do not mix them in the same intravenous bag, bottle, or tubing.
When aminoglycosides and penicillins are administered separately by different routes, a reduction in aminoglycoside serum concentration may occur. Usually this is clinically significant only in patients with se-

verely impaired renal function when the excretion of both medications is delayed.

---

## DICLOXACILLIN

## Summary of Differences

Category: Penicillinase-resistant penicillin.
Pharmacology/pharmacokinetics: Very high plasma protein binding (95 to 98%).
Precautions: Drug interactions and/or related problems—May react with other hepatotoxic medications.
Side/adverse effects: May be an increased risk of hepatotoxicity.

## Additional Dosing Information

Patients with impaired renal function do not generally require a reduction in dose unless the impairment is severe.

Dicloxacillin should be taken on an empty stomach, preferably 1 hour before meals.

## Oral Dosage Forms

Note: The dosing and strengths of the dosage forms available are expressed in terms of dicloxacillin base (not the sodium salt).

### DICLOXACILLIN SODIUM CAPSULES USP

**Usual adult and adolescent dose**
Antibacterial—
Oral, 125 to 250 mg (base) every six hours.

**Usual adult prescribing limits**
Up to 6 grams (base) a day.

**Usual pediatric dose**
Antibacterial—
Infants and children up to 40 kg of body weight: Oral, 3.125 to 6.25 mg (base) per kg of body weight every six hours.
Children 40 kg of body weight and over: See *Usual adult and adolescent dose.*
Note: Cystic fibrosis patients: Oral, 12.5 to 25 mg (base) per kg of body weight every six hours.

**Strength(s) usually available**
U.S.—
125 mg (base) (Rx) [*Dynapen*].
250 mg (base) (Rx) [*Dycill; Dynapen; Pathocil;* GENERIC].
500 mg (base) (Rx) [*Dycill; Dynapen; Pathocil;* GENERIC].
Canada—
Not commercially available.

**Packaging and storage**
Store below 40 °C (104 °F), preferably between 15 and 30 °C (59 and 86 °F), unless otherwise specified by manufacturer. Store in a tight container.

**Auxiliary labeling**
• Continue medication for full time of treatment.
• Take on empty stomach.

### DICLOXACILLIN SODIUM FOR ORAL SUSPENSION USP

**Usual adult and adolescent dose**
See *Dicloxacillin Sodium Capsules USP.*

**Usual adult prescribing limits**
See *Dicloxacillin Sodium Capsules USP.*

**Usual pediatric dose**
See *Dicloxacillin Sodium Capsules USP.*

**Strength(s) usually available**
U.S.—
62.5 mg per 5 mL (base) (Rx) [*Dynapen; Pathocil*].
Canada—
Not commercially available.

**Packaging and storage**
Prior to reconstitution, store below 40 °C (104 °F), preferably between 15 and 30 °C (59 and 86 °F), unless otherwise specified by manufacturer. Store in a tight container.

**Stability**
After reconstitution, suspensions retain their potency for 7 days at room temperature or for 14 days if refrigerated.

---

**Auxiliary labeling**
• Refrigerate.
• Shake well.
• Continue medication for full time of treatment.
• Beyond-use date.
• Take on empty stomach.

**Note**
When dispensing, include a calibrated liquid-measuring device.

---

## FLUCLOXACILLIN

## Summary of Differences

Category:
Penicillinase-resistant penicillin.
Pharmacology/pharmacokinetics:
Very high plasma protein binding (94%).
Precautions:
Drug interactions and/or related problems—May react with other hepatotoxic medications.
Laboratory value alterations—May transiently decrease the serum uric acid concentration in some patients.
Side/adverse effects:
May be an increased risk of cholestatic jaundice.

## Additional Dosing Information

Patients with impaired renal function do not generally require a reduction in dose unless the impairment is severe.

Flucloxacillin should be taken on an empty stomach, preferably, 1 hour before meals.

## Oral Dosage Forms

Note: The dosing and strengths of the dosage forms available are expressed in terms of flucloxacillin sodium (not the base).

### FLUCLOXACILLIN SODIUM CAPSULES

**Usual adult and adolescent dose**
Antibacterial—
Oral, 250 to 500 mg every six hours.

**Usual pediatric dose**
Antibacterial—
Children less than 12 years of age and up to 40 kg of body weight: Oral, 125 to 250 mg every six hours; or 6.25 to 12.5 mg per kg of body weight every six hours
Infants up to 6 months of age: Oral, 6.25 mg per kg of body weight every six hours.

**Strength(s) usually available**
U.S.—
Not commercially available.
Canada—
250 mg (Rx) [*Fluclox*].
500 mg (Rx) [*Fluclox*].

**Packaging and storage**
Store between 15 and 30 °C (59 and 86 °F). Store in a tight container.

**Auxiliary labeling**
• Continue medication for full time of treatment.
• Take on empty stomach.

### FLUCLOXACILLIN FOR ORAL SUSPENSION USP

**Usual adult and adolescent dose**
See *Flucloxacillin Sodium Capsules.*

**Usual pediatric dose**
See *Flucloxacillin Sodium Capsules.*

**Strength(s) usually available**
U.S.—
Not commercially available.
Canada—
125 mg per 5 mL (Rx) [*Fluclox*].
250 mg per 5 mL (Rx) [*Fluclox*].

**Packaging and storage**
Prior to reconstitution, store between 15 and 30 °C (59 and 86 °F). Store in a tight container.

**Stability**
After reconstitution, the suspension retains its potency for 7 days when refrigerated.

**Auxiliary labeling**
- Refrigerate.
- Shake well.
- Continue medication for full time of treatment.
- Beyond-use date.
- Take on empty stomach.

**Note**
When dispensing, include a calibrated liquid-measuring device.

## METHICILLIN

## Summary of Differences

Category: Penicillinase-resistant penicillin.
Precautions: Patient monitoring—Renal function determinations may be required because of interstitial nephritis.
Side/adverse effects—May be increased risk of interstitial nephritis.

## Additional Dosing Information

Methicillin sodium for injection should be administered by deep intra-gluteal injection or by intravenous injection only.

Patients with impaired renal function require a reduction in dose.

## Parenteral Dosage Forms

Note: The dosing and strengths of the dosage forms available are expressed in terms of methicillin sodium (not the base).

### METHICILLIN SODIUM FOR INJECTION USP

**Usual adult and adolescent dose**
Antibacterial—
Intramuscular, 1 gram every four to six hours.
Intravenous, 1 gram every six hours.

**Usual adult prescribing limits**
Up to 24 grams a day.

**Usual pediatric dose**
Antibacterial—
Meningitis, bacterial:
Neonates up to 2 kg of body weight—Intramuscular or intravenous, 25 to 50 mg per kg of body weight every twelve hours during the first week of life, then 50 mg per kg of body weight every eight hours thereafter.
Neonates 2 kg of body weight and over—Intramuscular or intravenous, 50 mg per kg of body weight every eight hours during the first week of life, then 50 mg per kg of body weight every six hours thereafter.
For all other indications:
Infants and children up to 40 kg of body weight—Intramuscular or intravenous, 25 mg per kg of body weight every six hours.
Children 40 kg of body weight and over—See *Usual adult and adolescent dose.*

Note: Cystic fibrosis patients—Intramuscular or intravenous, 50 mg per kg of body weight every six hours.

**Size(s) usually available**
U.S.—
1 gram (Rx) [*Staphcillin*].
4 grams (Rx) [*Staphcillin*].
6 grams (Rx) [*Staphcillin*].
10 grams (Rx) [*Staphcillin*].
Canada—
Not commercially available.

**Packaging and storage**
Prior to reconstitution, store between 15 and 30 °C (59 and 86 °F).

**Preparation of dosage form**
To prepare initial dilution for intramuscular use, add 1.5 mL of sterile water for injection or 0.9% sodium chloride injection to each 1-gram vial, 5.7 mL of diluent to each 4-gram vial, and 8.6 mL of diluent to each 6-gram vial to provide a concentration of 500 mg per mL.
To prepare initial dilution for direct intravenous use, reconstitute as directed above for intramuscular use. Each mL (500 mg) of the resulting solution should be further diluted in 25 mL of 0.9% sodium chloride injection and administered at the rate of 10 mL per minute.
For reconstitution of pharmacy bulk vials or piggyback infusion bottles, see manufacturer's labeling for instructions.

**Stability**
After reconstitution for intramuscular use, solutions retain their potency for 24 hours at room temperature or for 4 days if refrigerated.

After reconstitution for intravenous use, solutions in concentrations of 2 to 20 mg per mL retain at least 90% of their potency for 8 hours at room temperature in suitable diluents (see manufacturer's package insert).

**Incompatibilities**
Extemporaneous admixtures of beta-lactam antibacterials (penicillins and cephalosporins) and aminoglycosides may result in substantial mutual inactivation. If these groups of antibacterials are administered concurrently, they should be administered in separate sites at least 1 hour apart. Do not mix them in the same intravenous bag, bottle, or tubing.
When aminoglycosides and penicillins are administered separately by different routes, a reduction in aminoglycoside serum concentration may occur. Usually this is clinically significant only in patients with severely impaired renal function when the excretion of both medications is delayed.
Extemporaneous admixtures of other drugs with methicillin sodium for injection are not recommended.

**Additional information**
The total sodium content is approximately 2.24 mEq (2.24 mmol) per gram of methicillin sodium. This must be considered in patients on a restricted sodium intake when calculating total daily sodium intake.

## MEZLOCILLIN

## Summary of Differences

Category:
Antipseudomonal penicillin.
Precautions:
Drug interactions and/or related problems—May also interact with other hepatotoxic medications.
Laboratory value alterations—May produce false-positive protein reactions with various urine protein tests.
Patient monitoring—Serum potassium determinations may be required.

## Additional Dosing Information

Intramuscular injections should not exceed 2 grams in each site.

Adults with impaired renal function may require a reduction in dose as follows:

| Creatinine Clearance (mL/min)/ (mL/sec) | Dose |
| --- | --- |
| >30/0.50 | See *Usual adult and adolescent dose* |
| 10–30/0.17–0.50 | 1.5 to 3 grams every 6 to 8 hours |
| <10/0.17 | 1.5 to 2 grams every 8 hours |
| Hemodialysis patients | 3 to 4 grams after each dialysis, then every 12 hours |
| Peritoneal dialysis patients | 3 grams every 12 hours |

## Parenteral Dosage Forms

Note: The dosing and strengths of the dosage forms available are expressed in terms of mezlocillin sodium (not the base).

### STERILE MEZLOCILLIN SODIUM USP

**Usual adult and adolescent dose**
Antibacterial—
Intramuscular or intravenous, 33.3 to 58.3 mg per kg of body weight every four hours; 50 to 87.5 mg per kg of body weight every six hours; or 3 to 4 grams every four to six hours.
Urinary tract infections, complicated: Intravenous, 37.5 to 50 mg per kg of body weight every six hours; or 3 grams every six hours.
Urinary tract infections, uncomplicated: Intramuscular or intravenous, 25 to 31.25 mg per kg of body weight every six hours; or 1.5 to 2 grams every six hours.

**Usual adult prescribing limits**
Up to 24 grams a day.

**Usual pediatric dose**
Antibacterial—
Neonates up to 2 kg of body weight: Intramuscular or intravenous, 50 to 75 mg per kg of body weight every twelve hours during the first week of life, then 50 mg per kg of body weight every eight hours thereafter.
Neonates 2 kg of body weight and over: Intramuscular or intravenous, 50 mg per kg of body weight every eight hours during the first week of life, then 50 mg per kg of body weight every six hours thereafter.

Infants over 1 month of age and children up to 12 years of age: Intramuscular or intravenous, 50 mg per kg of body weight every four hours.

**Size(s) usually available**
U.S.—
   1 gram (Rx) [*Mezlin*].
   2 grams (Rx) [*Mezlin*].
   3 grams (Rx) [*Mezlin*].
   4 grams (Rx) [*Mezlin*].
   20 grams (Rx) [*Mezlin*].
Canada—
   Not commercially available.

**Packaging and storage**
Prior to reconstitution, store below 30 °C (86 °F). After reconstitution, if precipitation occurs during refrigeration, the solution may be warmed to 37 °C (98.6 °F) for 20 minutes in a water bath, and shaken well.

**Preparation of dosage form**
To prepare initial dilution for intramuscular use, add 3 to 4 mL of sterile water for injection or 0.5 or 1% lidocaine hydrochloride injection (without epinephrine) to each 1-gram vial and shake vigorously. The resulting solution should be administered slowly over a 12- to 15-second period to minimize discomfort.

To prepare initial dilution for intravenous use, add at least 10 mL of sterile water for injection, 5% dextrose injection, or 0.9% sodium chloride injection to each 1-gram vial and shake vigorously. For direct intravenous use, the resulting solution should be administered slowly over a 3- to 5-minute period to minimize vein irritation. The concentration should not exceed 10% (100 mg per mL).

For intermittent intravenous use, the resulting solution should be further diluted in 50 to 100 mL of a suitable diluent (see manufacturer's package insert). It may be administered over a 30-minute period by direct infusion or by a Y-type hook-up.

For reconstitution of piggyback infusion bottles, see manufacturer's labeling for instructions. If the Y-type or piggyback method of administration is used, the primary infusion should be temporarily discontinued during infusion of mezlocillin.

**Stability**
After reconstitution with suitable diluents (see manufacturer's package insert), solutions at concentrations of 10 and 100 mg per mL retain at least 90% of their potency for 24 to 72 hours at controlled room temperature (15 to 30 °C [59 to 86 °F]) or for 1 to 7 days if refrigerated.

After reconstitution with sterile water for injection, 0.9% sodium chloride injection, or 5% dextrose injection, solutions at concentrations up to 100 mg per mL retain their potency for 4 weeks when frozen at −12 °C (10 °F).

After reconstitution with sterile water for injection, 0.9% sodium chloride injection, or 0.5 or 1% lidocaine hydrochloride injection (without epinephrine), solutions at concentrations up to 250 mg per mL retain their potency for 24 hours at room temperature.

Solutions range from clear and colorless to pale yellow in color. However, the powder and reconstituted solution may darken slightly during storage; this darkening does not affect their potency.

**Incompatibilities**
Extemporaneous admixtures of beta-lactam antibacterials (penicillins and cephalosporins) and aminoglycosides may result in substantial mutual inactivation. If these groups of antibacterials are administered concurrently, they should be administered in separate sites at least 1 hour apart. Do not mix them in the same intravenous bag, bottle, or tubing.

When aminoglycosides and penicillins are administered separately by different routes, a reduction in aminoglycoside serum concentration may occur. Usually this is clinically significant only in patients with severely impaired renal function when the excretion of both medications is delayed.

**Additional information**
The sodium content is approximately 1.9 mEq (43 mg) per gram of mezlocillin. This must be considered in patients on a restricted sodium intake when calculating total daily sodium intake.

---

## NAFCILLIN

## Summary of Differences

Category:
   Penicillinase-resistant penicillin.
Pharmacology/pharmacokinetics:
   Oral absorption—Erratic and poor.
   Protein binding—High (90%).
   Hepatic biotransformation—High (60–70%).

Precautions:
   Drug interactions and/or related problems—
      May also interact with other hepatotoxic medications.
Side/adverse effects:
   May be an increased risk of interstitial nephritis.

## Additional Dosing Information

Nafcillin sodium for injection should be administered by deep intragluteal injection or by intravenous injection only.

## Oral Dosage Forms

Note: The dosing and strengths of the dosage forms available are expressed in terms of nafcillin base (not the sodium salt).

### NAFCILLIN SODIUM CAPSULES USP

**Usual adult and adolescent dose**
Antibacterial—
   Oral, 250 mg to 1 gram (base) every four to six hours.

**Usual adult prescribing limits**
Up to 6 grams (base) daily.

**Usual pediatric dose**
Antibacterial—
   Pharyngitis, bacterial:
      Oral, 250 mg (base) every eight hours.
   For all other indications:
      Neonates—Oral, 10 mg (base) per kg of body weight every six to eight hours.
      Older infants and children—Oral, 6.25 to 12.5 mg (base) per kg of body weight every six hours.

**Strength(s) usually available**
U.S.—
   250 mg (base) (Rx) [*Unipen*].
Canada—
   Not commercially available.

**Packaging and storage**
Store below 40 °C (104 °F), preferably between 15 and 30 °C (59 and 86 °F), unless otherwise specified by manufacturer. Store in a tight container.

**Auxiliary labeling**
• Continue medication for full time of treatment.
• Take on empty stomach.

### NAFCILLIN SODIUM TABLETS USP

**Usual adult and adolescent dose**
See *Nafcillin Sodium Capsules USP*.

**Usual adult prescribing limits**
See *Nafcillin Sodium Capsules USP*.

**Usual pediatric dose**
See *Nafcillin Sodium Capsules USP*.

**Strength(s) usually available**
U.S.—
   500 mg (base) (Rx) [*Unipen*].
Canada—
   Not commercially available.

**Packaging and storage**
Store below 40 °C (104 °F), preferably between 15 and 30 °C (59 and 86 °F), unless otherwise specified by manufacturer. Store in a tight, light-resistant container.

**Auxiliary labeling**
• Continue medication for full time of treatment.
• Take on empty stomach.

## Parenteral Dosage Forms

Note: The dosing and strengths of the dosage forms available are expressed in terms of nafcillin base (not the sodium salt).

### NAFCILLIN SODIUM FOR INJECTION USP

**Usual adult and adolescent dose**
Antibacterial—
   Bone and joint infections
   Endocarditis, bacterial
   Meningitis, bacterial or
   Pericarditis, bacterial:
      Intravenous, 1.5 to 2 grams every four to six hours.

For all other indications:
>Intramuscular, 500 mg (base) every four to six hours.
>Intravenous, 500 mg to 1.5 grams (base) every four hours.

**Usual adult prescribing limits**
Intramuscular—Up to 12 grams (base) a day.
Intravenous—Up to 20 grams (base) a day.

**Usual pediatric dose**
Antibacterial—
>Meningitis, bacterial:
>>Neonates up to 2 kg of body weight—
>>>Intramuscular or intravenous, 25 to 50 mg per kg of body weight every twelve hours during the first week of life, then 50 mg per kg of body weight every eight hours thereafter.
>>Neonates 2 kg of body weight and over—
>>>Intramuscular or intravenous, 50 mg per kg of body weight every eight hours during the first week of life, then 50 mg per kg of body weight every six hours thereafter.
>For all other indications:
>>Neonates—
>>>Intramuscular, 10 mg (base) per kg of body weight every twelve hours.
>>>Intravenous, 10 to 20 mg (base) per kg of body weight every four hours; or 20 to 40 mg per kg of body weight every eight hours.
>>Older infants and children—
>>>Intramuscular, 25 mg (base) per kg of body weight every twelve hours.
>>>Intravenous, 10 to 20 mg (base) per kg of body weight every four hours; or 20 to 40 mg per kg of body weight every eight hours.

**Size(s) usually available**
U.S.—
>500 mg (base) (Rx) [*Nafcil; Nallpen;* GENERIC].
>1 gram (base) (Rx) [*Nafcil; Nallpen; Unipen;* GENERIC].
>2 grams (base) (Rx) [*Nafcil; Nallpen; Unipen;* GENERIC].
>10 grams (base) (Rx) [*Nafcil; Nallpen; Unipen;* GENERIC].
Canada—
>500 mg (base) (Rx) [*Unipen*].

**Packaging and storage**
Prior to reconstitution, store below 40 °C (104 °F), preferably between 15 and 30 °C (59 and 86 °F), unless otherwise specified by manufacturer.

**Preparation of dosage form**
To prepare initial dilution for intramuscular use, depending on the manufacturer, add 1.7 to 1.8 mL of sterile water for injection or bacteriostatic water for injection to each 500-mg vial, 3.4 mL of diluent to each 1-gram vial, or 6.6 to 6.8 mL of diluent to each 2-gram vial to provide 250 mg (base) per mL.

To prepare initial dilution for direct intravenous use, reconstitute as directed above for intramuscular use. The resulting solution should be further diluted in 15 to 30 mL of sterile water for injection or 0.9% sodium chloride injection and administered over a 5- to 10-minute period.

For reconstitution of pharmacy bulk vials or piggyback infusion bottles, see manufacturer's labeling for instructions.

Intravenous infusions of nafcillin sodium for injection should be administered in suitable diluents (see manufacturer's package insert) in a concentration of 2 to 40 mg per mL. Infusions should be administered over at least a 30- to 60-minute period to avoid vein irritation.

**Stability**
After reconstitution for intramuscular use, solutions retain their potency for 3 days at room temperature or for 7 days if refrigerated, depending on the manufacturer.

After reconstitution for intravenous use, solutions in concentrations of 2 to 40 mg per mL retain at least 90% of their potency for 24 hours at room temperature or for 96 hours if refrigerated (depending on the manufacturer) in suitable diluents (see manufacturer's package insert).

Concentrated solutions (100 mg per mL) prepared from pharmacy bulk vials retain their potency for 8 hours at room temperature or for 48 hours if refrigerated.

Concentrated solutions (250 mg per mL) retain their potency for 3 days at room temperature or for 7 days if refrigerated or frozen.

**Incompatibilities**
Extemporaneous admixtures of beta-lactam antibacterials (penicillins and cephalosporins) and aminoglycosides may result in substantial mutual inactivation. If these groups of antibacterials are administered concurrently, they should be administered in separate sites at least 1 hour apart. Do not mix them in the same intravenous bag, bottle, or tubing.

When aminoglycosides and penicillins are administered separately by different routes, a reduction in aminoglycoside serum concentration may

occur. Usually this is clinically significant only in patients with severely impaired renal function when the excretion of both medications is delayed.

**Additional information**
The total sodium content is approximately 2.9 mEq (2.9 mmol) per gram of nafcillin. This must be considered in patients on a restricted sodium intake when calculating total daily sodium intake.

---

## *OXACILLIN*

## Summary of Differences

Category: Penicillinase-resistant penicillin.
Pharmacology/pharmacokinetics: High plasma protein binding (90%).
Precautions: Drug interactions and/or related problems—May also interact with other hepatotoxic medications.
Side/adverse effects: May be an increased risk of hepatotoxicity and interstitial nephritis.

## Additional Dosing Information

Patients with impaired renal function do not generally require a reduction in dose.

## Oral Dosage Forms

Note: The dosing and strengths of the dosage forms available are expressed in terms of oxacillin base (not the sodium salt).

### OXACILLIN SODIUM CAPSULES USP

**Usual adult and adolescent dose**
Antibacterial—
>Oral, 500 mg to 1 gram (base) every four to six hours.

**Usual adult prescribing limits**
Up to 6 grams (base) a day.

**Usual pediatric dose**
Antibacterial—
>Children up to 40 kg of body weight: Oral, 12.5 to 25 mg (base) per kg of body weight every six hours.
>Children 40 kg of body weight and over: See *Usual adult and adolescent dose*.

**Strength(s) usually available**
U.S.—
>250 mg (base) (Rx) [*Bactocill; Prostaphlin;* GENERIC].
>500 mg (base) (Rx) [*Bactocill; Prostaphlin;* GENERIC].
Canada—
>Not commercially available.

**Packaging and storage**
Store between 15 and 30 °C (59 and 86 °F). Store in a tight container.

**Auxiliary labeling**
• Continue medication for full time of treatment.
• Take on empty stomach.

### OXACILLIN SODIUM FOR ORAL SOLUTION USP

**Usual adult and adolescent dose**
See *Oxacillin Sodium Capsules USP*.

**Usual adult prescribing limits**
See *Oxacillin Sodium Capsules USP*.

**Usual pediatric dose**
See *Oxacillin Sodium Capsules USP*.

**Strength(s) usually available**
U.S.—
>250 mg per 5 mL (base) (Rx) [*Prostaphlin;* GENERIC].
Canada—
>Not commercially available.

**Packaging and storage**
Prior to reconstitution, store between 15 and 30 °C (59 and 86 °F). Store in a tight container.

**Stability**
After reconstitution, solutions retain their potency for 7 days at room temperature or for 14 days if refrigerated.

**Auxiliary labeling**
• Refrigerate.
• Continue medication for full time of treatment.
• Beyond-use date.
• Take on empty stomach.

**Note**
When dispensing, include a calibrated liquid-measuring device.

# Parenteral Dosage Forms

## OXACILLIN SODIUM FOR INJECTION USP

### Usual adult and adolescent dose
Antibacterial—
>Intramuscular or intravenous, 250 mg to 1 gram (base) every four to six hours.
>Meningitis, bacterial: Intravenous, 1.5 to 2 grams every four hours.

### Usual pediatric dose
Antibacterial—
>Meningitis, bacterial:
>>Neonates up to 2 kg of body weight—Intramuscular or intravenous, 25 to 50 mg per kg of body weight every twelve hours during the first week of life, then 50 mg per kg of body weight every eight hours thereafter.
>>Neonates 2 kg of body weight and over—Intramuscular or intravenous, 50 mg per kg of body weight every eight hours during the first week of life, then 50 mg per kg of body weight every six hours thereafter.
>For all other indications:
>>Premature infants and neonates—Intramuscular or intravenous, 6.25 mg (base) every six hours.
>>Children up to 40 kg of body weight—Intramuscular or intravenous, 12.5 to 25 mg (base) per kg of body weight every six hours; or 16.7 mg per kg of body weight every four hours.
>>Children 40 kg of body weight and over—See *Usual adult and adolescent dose.*

### Size(s) usually available
U.S.—
>250 mg (base) (Rx) [*Prostaphlin*].
>500 mg (base) (Rx) [*Bactocill; Prostaphlin;* GENERIC].
>1 gram (base) (Rx) [*Bactocill; Prostaphlin;* GENERIC].
>2 grams (base) (Rx) [*Bactocill; Prostaphlin;* GENERIC].
>4 grams (base) (Rx) [*Bactocill; Prostaphlin*].
>10 grams (base) (Rx) [*Bactocill; Prostaphlin;* GENERIC].

Canada—
>Not commercially available.

### Packaging and storage
Prior to reconstitution, store between 15 and 30 °C (59 and 86 °F).

### Preparation of dosage form
To prepare initial dilution for intramuscular use, depending on the manufacturer, add 1.4 mL of sterile water for injection to each 250-mg vial, 2.7 to 2.8 mL of diluent to each 500-mg vial, 5.7 mL of diluent to each 1-gram vial, 11.4 to 11.5 mL of diluent to each 2-gram vial, and 21.8 to 23 mL of diluent to each 4-gram vial to provide a concentration of 250 mg per 1.5 mL.

To prepare initial dilution for direct intravenous use, add 5 mL of sterile water for injection or 0.9% sodium chloride injection to each 250- or 500-mg vial, 10 mL of diluent to each 1-gram vial, 20 mL of diluent to each 2-gram vial, and 40 mL of diluent to each 4-gram vial. The resulting solution should be administered slowly over a 10-minute period.

Intravenous infusions of oxacillin sodium for injection should be administered in a suitable diluent in a concentration of up to 40 mg per mL (see manufacturer's package insert).

For reconstitution of pharmacy bulk vials, piggyback infusion bottles, and dual-compartment vials, see manufacturer's labeling for instructions.

### Stability
After reconstitution for intramuscular use, solutions retain their potency for 4 days at room temperature or for 7 days if refrigerated.

Concentrated solutions (100 mg per mL) prepared from pharmacy bulk vials retain their potency for 48 hours at room temperature or for 7 days if refrigerated.

Diluted solutions (up to 40 mg per mL) retain their potency for 72 hours at room temperature, for 7 days if refrigerated, or for 30 days if frozen.

Solutions (10 to 50 mg per mL) prepared from piggyback infusion bottles retain their potency for 24 hours at room temperature.

### Incompatibilities
Extemporaneous admixtures of beta-lactam antibacterials (penicillins and cephalosporins) and aminoglycosides may result in substantial mutual inactivation. If these groups of antibacterials are administered concurrently, they should be administered in separate sites at least 1 hour apart. Do not mix them in the same intravenous bag, bottle, or tubing.

When aminoglycosides and penicillins are administered separately by different routes, a reduction in aminoglycoside serum concentration may occur. Usually this is clinically significant only in patients with severely impaired renal function when the excretion of both medications is delayed.

### Additional information
The total sodium content (derived from dibasic sodium phosphate buffer and oxacillin sodium) is approximately 2.8 to 3.1 mEq (64 to 71 mg) per gram of oxacillin. This must be considered in patients on a restricted sodium intake when calculating total daily sodium intake.

---

## PENICILLIN G

# Summary of Differences
Category:
>Natural penicillin.

Pharmacology/pharmacokinetics:
>Oral absorption low (15 to 30%).
>>Time to peak serum concentration—
>>>Benzathine salt: 24 hours.
>>>Procaine salt: 4 hours.

Precautions:
>Cross-sensitivity and/or related problems—
>>Cross-sensitivity with other ester-type local anesthetics may also occur with administration of penicillin G procaine.
>Drug interactions and/or related problems—
>>Use of angiotensin-converting enzyme (ACE) inhibitors, potassium-sparing diuretics, other potassium-containing medications, or potassium supplements with parenteral penicillin G potassium may promote hyperkalemia; also oral penicillin G may interact with cholestyramine and colestipol.
>Patient monitoring—
>>Serum potassium or sodium determinations may be required (parenteral only).

Side/adverse effects:
>May be an increased risk of mental disturbances with administration of penicillin G procaine.

# Additional Dosing Information
Patients with impaired renal function do not generally require a reduction in dose unless the impairment is severe.

### For oral dosage forms only
Oral administration of penicillin G commonly results in low serum concentrations. Therefore, severe infections should not be treated with oral penicillin during the acute stage.

Penicillin G is an acid-labile penicillin; therefore, concurrent administration with acidic fruit juices and other acidic beverages should be avoided.

# Oral Dosage Forms
Note: The dosing and strengths of the dosage forms available are expressed in terms of penicillin G benzathine (not the base).

## PENICILLIN G BENZATHINE SUSPENSION

### Usual adult and adolescent dose
Antibacterial—
>Oral, 200,000 to 500,000 Units (125 to 312 mg) every four to six hours.
>Continuous prophylaxis of streptococcal infections in patients with a history of rheumatic heart disease: Oral, 200,000 to 250,000 Units (125 to 156 mg) every twelve hours.

### Usual adult prescribing limits
Up to 2,000,000 Units a day.

### Usual pediatric dose
Antibacterial—
>Infants and children up to 12 years of age: Oral, 4167 to 15,000 Units per kg of body weight every four hours; 6250 to 22,500 Units per kg of body weight every six hours; or 8333 to 30,000 Units per kg of body weight every eight hours.
>Children 12 years of age and over: See *Usual adult and adolescent dose.*

### Strength(s) usually available
U.S.—
>Not commercially available.

Canada—
>250,000 Units (156 mg) per 5 mL (Rx) [*Megacillin*].
>500,000 Units (312 mg) per 5 mL (Rx) [*Megacillin*].

### Packaging and storage
Store between 15 and 30 °C (59 and 86 °F), unless otherwise specified by manufacturer.

**Stability**
The reconstituted suspension may be stored at room temperature until the labeled expiration date.

**Auxiliary labeling**
- Continue medication for full time of treatment.
- Take on empty stomach.
- Beyond-use date.

## PENICILLIN G POTASSIUM FOR ORAL SOLUTION USP

**Usual adult and adolescent dose**
See *Penicillin G Benzathine Suspension.*

**Usual adult prescribing limits**
See *Penicillin G Benzathine Suspension.*

**Usual pediatric dose**
See *Penicillin G Benzathine Suspension.*

**Strength(s) usually available**
U.S.—
   400,000 Units (250 mg) per 5 mL (Rx) [GENERIC].
Canada—
   Not commercially available.

**Packaging and storage**
Prior to reconstitution, store below 40 °C (104 °F), preferably between 15 and 30 °C (59 and 86 °F), unless otherwise specified by manufacturer. Store in a tight container.

**Stability**
After reconstitution, solutions retain their potency for 14 days if refrigerated.

**Auxiliary labeling**
- Refrigerate.
- Continue medication for full time of treatment.
- Beyond-use date.
- Take on empty stomach.

**Note**
When dispensing, include a calibrated liquid-measuring device.

## PENICILLIN G POTASSIUM TABLETS USP

**Usual adult and adolescent dose**
See *Penicillin G Benzathine for Oral Solution.*

**Usual adult prescribing limits**
See *Penicillin G Benzathine for Oral Solution.*

**Usual pediatric dose**
See *Penicillin G Benzathine for Oral Solution.*

**Strength(s) usually available**
U.S.—
   200,000 Units (125 mg) (Rx) [GENERIC].
   250,000 Units (156 mg) (Rx) [GENERIC].
   400,000 Units (250 mg) (Rx) [*Pentids;* GENERIC].
   800,000 Units (500 mg) (Rx) [GENERIC].
Canada—
   500,000 Units (312 mg) (Rx) [*Megacillin* (scored)].

**Packaging and storage**
Store below 40 °C (104 °F), preferably between 15 and 30 °C (59 and 86 °F), unless otherwise specified by manufacturer. Store in a tight container.

**Auxiliary labeling**
- Continue medication for full time of treatment.
- Take on empty stomach.

## Parenteral Dosage Forms

Note: Bracketed uses in the *Dosage Forms* section refer to categories of use and/or indications that are not included in U.S. product labeling.
    The dosing and strengths of the dosage forms available are expressed in terms of penicillin G salt (not the base).

## STERILE PENICILLIN G BENZATHINE SUSPENSION USP

**Usual adult and adolescent dose**
Antibacterial—
   Bejel
   Pinta or
   Yaws: Intramuscular, 1,200,000 Units as a single dose.
   Continuous prophylaxis of streptococcal infections in patients with a history of rheumatic heart disease: Intramuscular, 1,200,000 Units every three to four weeks.

   Pharyngitis, streptococcal: Intramuscular, 1,200,000 Units as a single dose.
   Syphilis (primary, secondary, and early latent): Intramuscular, 2,400,000 Units as a single dose.
   Syphilis (tertiary and late latent, excluding neurosyphilis): Intramuscular, 2,400,000 Units once a week for three weeks.

**Usual adult prescribing limits**
Up to 2,400,000 Units a day.

**Usual pediatric dose**
Antibacterial—
   Pharyngitis, group A streptococcal:
      Infants and children up to 27.3 kg of body weight—Intramuscular, 300,000 to 600,000 Units as a single dose.
      Children 27.3 kg of body weight and over—Intramuscular, 900,000 Units as a single dose.
   Rheumatic fever (prophylaxis):
      Intramuscular, 1,200,000 Units every two or three weeks.
   Syphilis (primary, secondary, and early latent):
      Intramuscular, 50,000 Units per kg of body weight, up to 2,400,000 Units, as a single dose.
   Syphilis (late latent or latent of unknown duration):
      Intramuscular, 50,000 Units per kg of body weight once a week for three weeks.

**Strength(s) usually available**
U.S.—
   600,000 Units in 1 mL (Rx) [*Bicillin L-A; Permapen*].
   1,200,000 Units in 2 mL (Rx) [*Bicillin L-A*].
   2,400,000 Units in 4 mL (Rx) [*Bicillin L-A*].
   3,000,000 Units in 10 mL (Rx) [*Bicillin L-A*].
Canada—
   1,200,000 Units in 2 mL (Rx) [*Bicillin L-A*].

**Packaging and storage**
Store between 2 and 8 °C (36 and 46 °F).

**Additional information**
For deep intramuscular use only. Do not administer intravenously, intra-arterially, subcutaneously, by fat-layer injection, or into or near a nerve. Intravenous injection may cause embolic or toxic reactions. Intra-arterial injection may cause extensive necrosis of the extremity or organ, especially in children. Subcutaneous and fat-layer injection may cause pain and induration. Injection into or near a nerve may result in permanent neurological damage.

Injection of penicillin G benzathine should be made at a slow, steady rate to prevent blockage of the needle because of the high concentration of suspended material.

Intramuscular administration of penicillin G benzathine results in much lower and more prolonged serum concentrations than those attained with other parenteral penicillins.

## PENICILLIN G POTASSIUM FOR INJECTION USP

**Usual adult and adolescent dose**
Antibacterial—
   Intramuscular or intravenous, 1,000,000 to 5,000,000 Units every four to six hours.
   Actinomycosis: Intramuscular or intravenous, 10,000,000 to 20,000,000 Units a day for two to six weeks.
   Anthrax: Intramuscular or intravenous, 2,000,000 Units every six hours.
   Clostridial infections: Intramuscular or intravenous, 20,000,000 Units a day.
   Erysipelas: Intramuscular or intravenous, 600,000 to 2,000,000 Units every six hours.
   Erysipeloid endocarditis: Intramuscular or intravenous, 12,000,000 to 20,000,000 Units a day.
   Listeriosis: Intramuscular or intravenous, 300,000 Units per kg of body weight a day.
   Meningitis, bacterial: Intramuscular or intravenous, 50,000 Units per kg of body weight every four hours; or 24,000,000 Units daily divided every two to four hours.
   Neurosyphilis: Intravenous, 2,000,000 to 4,000,000 Units every four hours for ten to fourteen days.
   *Pasteurella multocida* septicemia and meningitis: Intramuscular or intravenous, 4,000,000 to 6,000,000 Units a day.
   Pericarditis, bacterial: Intramuscular or intravenous, 20,000,000 to 30,000,000 Units a day for four to six weeks.
   Rat-bite fever: Intramuscular or intravenous, 20,000,000 Units a day.
   [Leptospirosis][1]: Intramuscular or intravenous, 1,500,000 Units every six hours.
   [Lyme disease][1]: Intravenous, 20,000,000 to 24,000,000 Units a day for two to three weeks. Duration of therapy is based on clinical

response. Treatment failures have occurred and retreatment may
be necessary.

**Usual adult prescribing limits**
Up to 80,000,000 Units a day.

**Usual pediatric dose**
Antibacterial—

Listeriosis in neonates:
500,000 to 1,000,000 Units daily.

Meningitis, bacterial:

Neonates up to 2 kg of body weight—Intramuscular or intravenous, 25,000 to 50,000 Units per kg of body weight every
twelve hours during the first week of life, then 50,000 Units
per kg of body weight every eight hours thereafter.

Neonates 2 kg of body weight and over—Intramuscular or intravenous, 50,000 Units per kg of body weight every eight hours
during the first week of life, then 50,000 Units per kg of body
weight every six hours thereafter.

Syphilis, congenital:

Intramuscular or intravenous, 50,000 Units per kg of body weight
every twelve hours for the first week of life, then 50,000 Units
per kg of body weight every eight hours for the next ten to
fourteen days.

[Lyme disease][1]:

Intravenous, 250,000 to 400,000 Units per kg of body weight daily
for two to three weeks. Duration of therapy is based on clinical
response. Treatment failures have occurred and retreatment
may be necessary.

For all other indications:

Premature and full-term neonates—Intramuscular or intravenous,
30,000 Units per kg of body weight every twelve hours.

Older infants and children—Intramuscular or intravenous, 8333 to
16,667 Units per kg of body weight every four hours; or 12,500
to 25,000 Units per kg of body weight every six hours.

**Size(s) usually available**
U.S.—

1,000,000 Units (Rx) [GENERIC].
5,000,000 Units (Rx) [*Pfizerpen;* GENERIC].
10,000,000 Units (Rx) [GENERIC].
20,000,000 Units (Rx) [*Pfizerpen;* GENERIC].

Canada—

1,000,000 Units (Rx) [GENERIC].
5,000,000 Units (Rx) [GENERIC].
10,000,000 Units (Rx) [GENERIC].

**Packaging and storage**
Prior to reconstitution, store below 40 °C (104 °F), preferably between 15
and 30 °C (59 and 86 °F), unless otherwise specified by manufacturer.

**Preparation of dosage form**
To prepare initial dilution for intramuscular or intravenous use, see manufacturer's labeling for instructions.

To prepare for further dilution for intravenous use, see manufacturer's
labeling for instructions.

**Stability**
After reconstitution, solutions retain their potency for 24 hours at room
temperature or for 7 days if refrigerated.

**Incompatibilities**
Penicillin G potassium is rapidly inactivated by oxidizing and reducing
agents, such as alcohols and glycols.

Extemporaneous admixtures of beta-lactam antibacterials (penicillins and
cephalosporins) and aminoglycosides may result in substantial mutual
inactivation. If these groups of antibacterials are administered concurrently, they should be administered in separate sites at least 1 hour
apart. Do not mix them in the same intravenous bag, bottle, or tubing.

When aminoglycosides and penicillins are administered separately by different routes, a reduction in aminoglycoside serum concentration may
occur. Usually this is clinically significant only in patients with severely impaired renal function when the excretion of both medications
is delayed.

**Additional information**
Daily doses of 10,000,000 Units or more should be administered by slow
intravenous infusion or by intermittent piggyback infusion because of
possible electrolyte imbalance.

The potassium content and sodium content (derived from sodium citrate
buffer) of penicillin G potassium for injection are approximately 1.7
mEq (66.3 mg) and 0.3 mEq (6.9 mg) per 1,000,000 Units of penicillin
G, respectively. The sodium content must be considered in patients on
a restricted sodium intake when calculating total daily sodium intake.

# STERILE PENICILLIN G PROCAINE SUSPENSION USP

**Usual adult and adolescent dose**
Antibacterial—

Intramuscular, 600,000 to 1,200,000 Units a day.

Diphtheria: Intramuscular, 300,000 to 600,000 Units a day as adjunctive therapy to diphtheria antitoxin.

Neurosyphilis: Intramuscular, 2,400,000 Units a day, and 500 mg of
probenecid orally four times a day, for ten to fourteen days.

Rat-bite fever: Intramuscular, 600,000 Units every twelve hours for
ten to fourteen days.

**Usual pediatric dose**
Antibacterial—

Syphilis, congenital: Intramuscular, 50,000 Units per kg of body
weight a day for ten to fourteen days.

**Strength(s) usually available**
U.S.—

600,000 Units in 1 mL (Rx) [*Wycillin*].
1,200,000 Units in 2 mL (Rx) [*Wycillin*].
2,400,000 Units in 4 mL (Rx) [*Wycillin*].
3,000,000 Units in 10 mL (Rx) [*Crysticillin 300 A.S; Pfizerpen-AS*].

Canada—

3,000,000 Units per 10 mL (Rx) [*Ayercillin* (propylparaben 0.013%)].
5,000,000 Units per 10 mL (base) (Rx) [*Wycillin*].

**Packaging and storage**
Store between 2 and 8 °C (36 and 46 °F).

**Additional information**
For deep intramuscular use only. Do not administer intravenously, intra-
arterially, or into or near a nerve. Intravenous injection may cause
embolic or toxic reactions. Intra-arterial injection may cause extensive
necrosis of the extremity or organ, especially in children.

Some patients may experience immediate toxic reactions to procaine, especially when administered in large single doses. These reactions, usually transient, may be characterized by anxiety, confusion, agitation or
combativeness, depression, seizures, hallucinations, or expressed fear
of impending death.

# PENICILLIN G SODIUM FOR INJECTION USP

**Usual adult and adolescent dose**
See *Penicillin G Potassium for Injection USP.*

**Usual adult prescribing limits**
See *Penicillin G Potassium for Injection USP.*

**Usual pediatric dose**
See *Penicillin G Potassium for Injection USP.*

**Size(s) usually available**
U.S.—

5,000,000 Units (Rx) [GENERIC].

Canada—

1,000,000 Units (Rx) [GENERIC].
5,000,000 Units (Rx) [GENERIC].
10,000,000 Units (Rx) [GENERIC].

**Packaging and storage**
Prior to reconstitution, store below 40 °C (104 °F), preferably between 15
and 30 °C (59 and 86 °F), unless otherwise specified by manufacturer.

**Preparation of dosage form**
To prepare initial dilution for intramuscular or intravenous use, see manufacturer's labeling for instructions.

**Stability**
After reconstitution, solutions retain their potency for 24 hours at room
temperature or for 7 days if refrigerated.

**Incompatibilities**
Penicillin G sodium is rapidly inactivated by acids, alkalies, and oxidizing
agents and in carbohydrate solutions at alkaline pH.

Extemporaneous admixtures of beta-lactam antibacterials (penicillins and
cephalosporins) and aminoglycosides may result in substantial mutual
inactivation. If these groups of antibacterials are administered concurrently, they should be administered in separate sites at least 1 hour
apart. Do not mix them in the same intravenous bag, bottle, or tubing.

When aminoglycosides and penicillins are administered separately by different routes, a reduction in aminoglycoside serum concentration may
occur. Usually this is clinically significant only in patients with severely impaired renal function when the excretion of both medications
is delayed.

**Additional information**
Daily doses of 10,000,000 Units or more should be administered by slow
intravenous infusion to avoid causing possible electrolyte imbalance.

The sodium content is approximately 2 mEq (2 mmol) per million Units of penicillin G. This must be considered in patients on a restricted sodium intake when calculating total daily sodium intake.

---

[1]Not included in Canadian product labeling.

---

## PENICILLIN V

## Summary of Differences

Category: Penicillin G-related natural penicillin.

Precautions: Drug interactions and/or related problems—Also interacts with oral contraceptives.

## Additional Dosing Information

Penicillin V may be taken on a full or empty stomach.

Patients with impaired renal function do not generally require a reduction in dose unless the impairment is severe.

## Oral Dosage Forms

Note: Bracketed uses in the *Dosage Forms* section refer to categories of use and/or indications that are not included in U.S. product labeling.

    The dosing and strengths of the dosage forms available are expressed in terms of penicillin V salt (not the base).

### PENICILLIN V BENZATHINE SUSPENSION

**Usual adult and adolescent dose**

Antibacterial—

Oral, 200,000 to 500,000 Units every six to eight hours.

Continuous prophylaxis of streptococcal infections in patients with a history of rheumatic heart disease: Oral, 200,000 Units every twelve hours.

**Usual pediatric dose**

Antibacterial—

Infants and children up 60 kg of body weight: Oral, 100,000 to 250,000 Units every six to eight hours.

Children 60 kg of body weight and over: See *Usual adult and adolescent dose.*

**Strength(s) usually available**

U.S.—

Not commercially available.

Canada—

250,000 Units (156 mg) per 5 mL (Rx) [*PVF*].

300,000 Units (180 mg) per 5 mL (Rx) [*Pen-Vee*].

500,000 Units (300 mg) per 5 mL (Rx) [*Pen-Vee; PVF*].

**Packaging and storage**

Prior to reconstitution, store below 40 °C (104 °F), preferably between 15 and 30 °C (59 and 86 °F), unless otherwise specified by manufacturer. Store in a tight container.

**Stability**

Store at room temperature.

**Auxiliary labeling**

• Continue medication for full time of treatment.

• Beyond-use date.

**Note**

When dispensing, include a calibrated liquid-measuring device.

### PENICILLIN V POTASSIUM FOR ORAL SOLUTION USP

**Usual adult and adolescent dose**

Antibacterial—

Oral, 125 to 500 mg (200,000 to 800,000 Units) every six to eight hours.

Continuous prophylaxis of streptococcal infections in patients with a history of rheumatic heart disease: Oral, 125 to 250 mg (200,000 to 400,000 Units) every twelve hours.

Erysipelas: Oral, 500 mg every six hours.

Erysipeloid, uncomplicated: Oral, 250 mg every six hours for five to ten days.

Gingivitis, acute, necrotizing, ulcerative: Oral, 500 mg every six hours.

*Pasteurella* infections: Oral, 500 mg every six hours for ten to fourteen days.

Rat-bite fever: Oral, 500 mg every six hours for fourteen days.

[Lyme disease][1]: Oral, 250 to 500 mg three or four times a day for three to four weeks. Duration of therapy is based on clinical response. Treatment failures have occurred and retreatment may be necessary.

**Usual adult prescribing limits**

Up to 7.2 grams (11,520,000 Units) a day.

**Usual pediatric dose**

Antibacterial—

[Lyme disease][1]:

Oral, 5 to 12.5 mg per kg of body weight four times a day for three to four weeks. Duration of therapy is based on clinical response. Treatment failures have occurred and retreatment may be necessary.

For all other indications:

Infants and children up to 12 years of age—Oral, 2.5 to 8.3 mg (4167 to 13,280 Units) per kg of body weight every four hours; 3.75 to 12.5 mg (6250 to 20,000 Units) per kg of body weight every six hours; or 5 to 16.7 mg (8333 to 26,720 Units) per kg of body weight every eight hours.

Children 12 years of age and over—See *Usual adult and adolescent dose.*

**Strength(s) usually available**

U.S.—

125 mg (200,000 Units) per 5 mL (Rx) [*Beepen-VK; Betapen-VK; Ledercillin VK; Pen Vee K; Veetids;* GENERIC].

250 mg (400,000 Units) per 5 mL (Rx) [*Beepen-VK; Betapen-VK; Ledercillin VK; Pen Vee K; V-Cillin K; Veetids;* GENERIC].

Canada—

125 mg (200,000 Units) per 5 mL (Rx) [*Apo-Pen VK; Nadopen-V 200; V-Cillin K*].

250 mg (400,000 Units) per 5 mL (Rx) [*Nadopen-V 400; V-Cillin K*].

300 mg (500,000 Units) per 5 mL (Rx) [*Apo-Pen VK; Novo-Pen-VK*].

**Packaging and storage**

Prior to reconstitution, store below 40 °C (104 °F), preferably between 15 and 30 °C (59 and 86 °F), unless otherwise specified by manufacturer. Store in a tight container.

**Stability**

After reconstitution, solutions retain their potency for 14 days if refrigerated.

**Auxiliary labeling**

• Refrigerate.

• Continue medication for full time of treatment.

• Beyond-use date.

• Shake well.

**Note**

When dispensing, include a calibrated liquid-measuring device.

### PENICILLIN V POTASSIUM TABLETS USP

**Usual adult and adolescent dose**

See *Penicillin V Potassium for Oral Solution USP.*

**Usual adult prescribing limits**

See *Penicillin V Potassium for Oral Solution USP.*

**Usual pediatric dose**

See *Penicillin V Potassium for Oral Solution USP.*

**Strength(s) usually available**

U.S.—

250 mg (400,000 Units) (Rx) [*Beepen-VK; Ledercillin VK; Pen Vee K; V-Cillin K; Veetids;* GENERIC].

500 mg (800,000 Units) (Rx) [*Beepen-VK; Ledercillin VK; Pen Vee K; V-Cillin K; Veetids;* GENERIC].

Canada—

250 mg (400,000 Units) (Rx) [*Ledercillin VK* (scored); *V-Cillin K*].

300 mg (500,000 Units) (Rx) [*Apo-Pen VK; Nadopen-V* (scored); *Novo-Pen-VK; Nu-Pen-VK; Pen Vee* (scored); *PVF K* (scored)].

500 mg (800,000 Units) (Rx) [*Ledercillin VK*].

**Packaging and storage**

Store below 40 °C (104 °F), preferably between 15 and 30 °C (59 and 86 °F), unless otherwise specified by manufacturer. Store in a tight container.

**Auxiliary labeling**

• Continue medication for full time of treatment.

---

[1]Not included in Canadian product labeling.

---

## PIPERACILLIN

## Summary of Differences

Category:

Antipseudomonal penicillin.

**Precautions:**

Drug interactions and/or related problems—Also interacts with anti-coagulants and other medications that affect blood clotting, and other hepatotoxic medications.

Laboratory value alterations—May increase bleeding time.

Medical considerations/contraindications—Caution in patients with a history of bleeding disorders and cystic fibrosis.

Patient monitoring—Serum potassium and sodium determinations may be required.

## Additional Dosing Information

Intramuscular injections should not exceed 2 grams in each site.

Adults with impaired renal function may require a reduction in dose as follows:

| Creatinine Clearance (mL/min)/(mL/sec) | Dose (base) |
|---|---|
| >40/0.67 | See *Usual adult and adolescent dose* |
| 20–40/0.33–0.67 | 3 to 4 grams every 8 hours |
| <20/0.33 | 3 to 4 grams every 12 hours |
| Hemodialysis patients | 1 gram after each dialysis, then 2 grams every 8 hours |

## Parenteral Dosage Forms

Note: The dosing and strengths of the dosage forms available are expressed in terms of piperacillin base (not the sodium salt).

### PIPERACILLIN SODIUM STERILE USP

**Usual adult and adolescent dose**

Antibacterial—

Intramuscular or intravenous, 3 to 4 grams (base) every four to six hours.

Meningitis, bacterial: Intravenous, 4 grams every four hours; or 75 mg per kg of body weight every six hours.

Urinary tract infections, complicated: Intravenous, 3 to 4 grams (base) every six to eight hours.

Urinary tract infections, uncomplicated: Intramuscular or intravenous, 1.5 to 2 grams (base) every six hours or 3 to 4 grams every twelve hours.

**Usual adult prescribing limits**

Up to 24 grams (base) a day.

**Usual pediatric dose**

Antibacterial—

Meningitis, bacterial:

Neonates up to 2 kg of body weight—Intramuscular or intra-venous, 50 mg per kg of body weight every twelve hours during the first week of life, then 50 mg per kg of body weight every eight hours thereafter.

Neonates 2 kg of body weight and over—Intramuscular or intra-venous, 50 mg per kg of body weight every eight hours during the first week of life, then 50 mg per kg of body weight every six hours thereafter.

For all other indications:

Infants and children under 12 years of age—Dosage has not been established.

Children 12 years of age and over—See *Usual adult and adolescent dose.*

Note: Cystic fibrosis patients—Intravenous, 350 to 450 mg per kg of body weight daily.

**Size(s) usually available**

U.S.—

2 grams (base) (Rx) [*Pipracil*].

3 grams (base) (Rx) [*Pipracil*].

4 grams (base) (Rx) [*Pipracil*].

40 grams (base) (Rx) [*Pipracil*].

Canada—

2 grams (base) (Rx) [*Pipracil*].

3 grams (base) (Rx) [*Pipracil*].

4 grams (base) (Rx) [*Pipracil*].

**Packaging and storage**

Prior to reconstitution, store below 40 °C (104 °F), preferably between 15 and 30 °C (59 and 86 °F), unless otherwise specified by manufacturer.

**Preparation of dosage form**

To prepare initial dilution for intramuscular use, add 4 mL of sterile water for injection or 0.5 or 1% lidocaine hydrochloride injection (without epinephrine) to each 2-gram vial, 6 mL of diluent to each 3-gram vial, and 7.8 mL of diluent to each 4-gram vial to provide a concentration of 1 gram (base) per 2.5 mL.

To prepare initial dilution for intravenous use, add at least 5 mL of a suitable diluent (see manufacturer's package insert) for each gram of piperacillin and shake well until dissolved. For direct intravenous use, the resulting solution should be administered slowly over a 3- to 5-minute period. For intermittent intravenous use, the resulting solution should be further diluted with a suitable diluent (see manufacturer's package insert) to at least 50 mL. It should be administered over approximately a 20- to 30-minute period.

For reconstitution of pharmacy bulk vials or piggyback infusion bottles, see manufacturer's labeling for instructions.

**Stability**

After reconstitution with suitable diluents (see manufacturer's package insert), solutions retain their potency for 24 hours at controlled room temperature, 7 days if refrigerated, or 1 month if frozen at −15 °C (5 °F).

**Incompatibilities**

Because of chemical instability, piperacillin should not be used for intra-venous admixtures with solutions containing *only* sodium bicarbonate.

Extemporaneous admixtures of beta-lactam antibacterials (penicillins and cephalosporins) and aminoglycosides may result in substantial mutual inactivation. If these groups of antibacterials are administered concurrently, they should be administered in separate sites at least 1 hour apart. Do not mix them in the same intravenous bag, bottle, or tubing.

When aminoglycosides and penicillins are administered separately by different routes, a reduction in aminoglycoside serum concentration may occur. Usually this is clinically significant only in patients with severely impaired renal function when the excretion of both medications is delayed.

**Additional information**

The sodium content is approximately 1.98 mEq (45.5 mg) per gram of piperacillin. This must be considered in patients on a restricted sodium intake when calculating total daily sodium intake.

---

## PIVAMPICILLIN

## Summary of Differences

Category: Aminopenicillin.

Pharmacology/pharmacokinetics: Converted to ampicillin during absorption.

Pediatrics: Should be avoided in children up to 3 months of age since pivampicillin decreases serum carnitine concentrations.

Precautions: Medical considerations/contraindications—Caution in patients with carnitine deficiency.

## Additional Dosing Information

Patients with impaired renal function do not generally require a reduction in dose unless the impairment is severe.

Pivampicillin may be taken on a full or empty stomach.

## Oral Dosage Forms

Note: The dosing and strengths of the dosage forms available are expressed in terms of pivampicillin (not the ampicillin base).

### PIVAMPICILLIN FOR ORAL SUSPENSION USP

**Usual adult and adolescent dose**

Antibacterial—

Oral, 525 to 1050 mg two times a day.

**Usual pediatric dose**

Antibacterial—

Infants 3 to 12 months of age: Oral, 20 to 30 mg per kg of body weight two times a day.

Children 1 to 3 years of age: Oral, 175 mg two times a day.

Children 4 to 6 years of age: Oral, 262.5 mg two times a day.

Children 7 to 10 years of age: Oral, 350 mg two times a day.

Children 10 years of age and older: See *Usual adult and adolescent dose.*

**Strength(s) usually available**

U.S.—

Not commercially available.

Canada—

35 mg per mL (Rx) [*Pondocillin*].

Note: 35 mg of pivampicillin are equivalent to 26.4 mg of ampicillin.

**Packaging and storage**

Prior to reconstitution, store between 15 and 30 °C (59 and 86 °F). Store in a tight container.

**Auxiliary labeling**
• Shake well.
• Continue medication for full time of treatment.
• Beyond-use date.

**Note**
When dispensing, include a calibrated liquid-measuring device.

## PIVAMPICILLIN TABLETS

**Usual adult and adolescent dose**
Antibacterial—
  Oral, 500 mg to 1 gram two times a day.

**Usual pediatric dose**
Antibacterial—
  Children 10 years of age and over: See *Usual adult and adolescent dose.*
  Children up to 10 years of age: A product of suitable strength is not available for infants and children up to 10 years of age. See *Pivampicillin for Oral Suspension USP.*

**Strength(s) usually available**
U.S.—
  Not commercially available.
Canada—
  500 mg (Rx) [*Pondocillin*].

Note: 500 mg of pivampicillin are equivalent to 377 mg of ampicillin.

**Packaging and storage**
Store between 15 and 30 °C (59 and 86 °F). Store in a tight container.

**Auxiliary labeling**
• Continue medication for full time of treatment.

---

### PIVMECILLINAM

## Summary of Differences

Category: Aminopenicillin.
Pharmacology/pharmacokinetics: Converted to mecillinam during absorption.
Pediatrics: Should be avoided in children up to 3 months of age since pivmecillinam decreases serum carnitine concentrations.
Precautions: Medical considerations/contraindications—Caution in patients with carnitine deficiency.

## Additional Dosing Information

Patients with impaired renal function do not generally require a reduction in dose unless the impairment is severe.

Pivmecillinam may be taken on a full or empty stomach.

## Oral Dosage Forms

Note: The dosing and strengths of the dosage forms available are expressed in terms of pivmecillinam hydrochloride (not the mecillin base).

## PIVMECILLINAM HYDROCHLORIDE TABLETS

**Usual adult and adolescent dose**
Antibacterial—
  Oral, 200 mg two to four times a day for three days.

**Usual pediatric dose**
Antibacterial—
  Children up to 40 kg of body weight: Dosage has not been established.
  Children 40 kg of body weight and over: See *Usual adult and adolescent dose.*

**Strength(s) usually available**
U.S.—
  Not commercially available.
Canada—
  200 mg (Rx) [*Selexid*].

Note: 200 mg of pivmecillinam hydrochloride is equivalent to 137 mg of mecillinam.

**Packaging and storage**
Store between 15 and 30 °C (59 and 86 °F). Store in a tight container.

**Auxiliary labeling**
• Continue medication for full time of treatment.

---

## Summary of Differences

Category:
  Antipseudomonal penicillin.
Precautions:
  Drug interactions and/or related problems—Also interacts with anticoagulants and other medications that affect blood clotting.
  Laboratory value alterations—May increase bleeding time and may cause false-positive protein reaction for various urine protein tests.
  Medical considerations/contraindications—Caution in patients with a history of bleeding disorders, and congestive heart failure or hypertension.
  Patient monitoring—Bleeding time and serum potassium and sodium determinations may be required.

## Additional Dosing Information

Intramuscular injections should not exceed 2 grams in each site.

Patients with impaired renal function should be observed for hemorrhagic complications.

Note: After an initial intravenous loading dose of 3 grams (base), adults with impaired renal function may require a reduction in dose as follows:

| Creatinine Clearance (mL/min)/ (mL/sec) | Dose (base) |
| --- | --- |
| >60/1.00 | 3 grams every 4 hours |
| 30–60/0.50–1.00 | 2 grams every 4 hours |
| 10–30/0.17–0.50 | 2 grams every 8 hours |
| <10/0.17 | 2 grams every 12 hours |
| <10 with impaired hepatic function | 2 grams every 24 hours |
| Hemodialysis | 2 grams every 12 hours plus 3 grams after dialysis |
| Peritoneal dialysis | 3 grams every 12 hours |

## Parenteral Dosage Forms

Note: The dosing and strengths of the dosage forms available are expressed in terms of ticarcillin base (not the sodium salt).

## TICARCILLIN DISODIUM STERILE USP

**Usual adult and adolescent dose**
Antibacterial—
  Intravenous infusion, 3 grams (base) every four hours; or 4 grams every six hours.
  Meningitis, bacterial: Intravenous infusion, 75 mg per kg of body weight every six hours.
  Urinary tract infections, complicated: Intravenous infusion, 3 grams (base) every six hours.
  Urinary tract infections, uncomplicated: Intramuscular or intravenous, 1 gram (base) every six hours.

**Usual adult prescribing limits**
Up to 24 grams a day.

**Usual pediatric dose**
Antibacterial—
  Neonates up to 2 kg of body weight:
    Intramuscular or intravenous, 75 mg per kg of body weight every twelve hours during the first week of life; followed by 75 mg per kg of body weight every eight hours thereafter.
  Neonates 2 kg of body weight and over:
    Intramuscular or intravenous, 75 mg per kg of body weight every eight hours during the first week of life; followed by 75 mg per kg of body weight every six hours thereafter.
  Children up to 40 kg of body weight:
    Intravenous infusion, 33.3 to 50 mg (base) per kg of body weight every four hours; or 50 to 75 mg per kg of body weight every six hours.
    Urinary tract infections, bacterial (complicated)—Intravenous infusion, 25 to 33.3 mg (base) per kg of body weight every four hours; or 37.5 to 50 mg per kg of body weight every six hours.
    Urinary tract infections, bacterial (uncomplicated)—Intramuscular or intravenous, 12.5 to 25 mg (base) per kg of body weight every six hours; or 16.7 to 33.3 mg per kg of body weight every eight hours.
  Children 40 kg of body weight and over:
    See *Usual adult and adolescent dose.*

## Size(s) usually available
U.S.—
- 1 gram (base) (Rx) [*Ticar*].
- 3 grams (base) (Rx) [*Ticar*].
- 6 grams (base) (Rx) [*Ticar*].
- 20 grams (base) (Rx) [*Ticar*].
- 30 grams (base) (Rx) [*Ticar*].

Canada—
- 1 gram (base) (Rx) [*Ticar*].
- 3 grams (base) (Rx) [*Ticar*].
- 6 grams (base) (Rx) [*Ticar*].
- 20 grams (base) (Rx) [*Ticar*].

## Packaging and storage
Prior to reconstitution, store below 40 °C (104 °F), preferably between 15 and 30 °C (59 and 86 °F), unless otherwise specified by manufacturer.

## Preparation of dosage form
To prepare initial dilution for intramuscular use, add 2 mL of sterile water for injection, 1% lidocaine hydrochloride injection (without epinephrine), or sodium chloride injection to each 1-gram vial to provide a concentration of 1 gram per 2.6 mL.

To prepare initial dilution for direct intravenous use, add at least 4 mL of 5% dextrose, 0.9% sodium chloride, or lactated Ringer's injection to each 1-gram vial. Each gram of ticarcillin may be further diluted if desired. The resulting solution should be administered as slowly as possible to avoid vein irritation.

Intermittent infusions may be administered over a 30-minute to 2-hour period in adults. In neonates, intermittent infusions may be administered over a 10- to 20-minute period.

For reconstitution of pharmacy bulk vials or piggyback infusion bottles, see manufacturer's labeling for instructions.

## Stability
After reconstitution for intramuscular use, solutions retain their potency for 12 hours at room temperature or for 24 hours if refrigerated.

After reconstitution for intravenous use, solutions in concentrations of 10 to 50 mg per mL retain at least 90% of their potency for 48 to 72 hours at room temperature or for 14 days if refrigerated in suitable diluents (see manufacturer's package insert).

If frozen after reconstitution with sterile water for injection, 0.9% sodium chloride injection, 5% dextrose injection, Ringer's injection, or lactated Ringer's injection, solutions in concentrations up to 100 mg per mL retain their potency up to 30 days at −18 °C (0 °F). Once thawed, solutions must be used within 24 hours.

## Incompatibilities
Extemporaneous admixtures of beta-lactam antibacterials (penicillins and cephalosporins) and aminoglycosides may result in substantial mutual inactivation. If these groups of antibacterials are administered concurrently, they should be administered in separate sites at least 1 hour apart. Do not mix them in the same intravenous bag, bottle, or tubing.

When aminoglycosides and penicillins are administered separately by different routes, a reduction in aminoglycoside serum concentration may occur. Usually this is clinically significant only in patients with severely impaired renal function when the excretion of both medications is delayed.

## Additional information
The sodium content is approximately 5.2 mEq (5.2 mmol), but may be as high as 6.5 mEq (6.5 mmol), per gram of ticarcillin. This must be considered in patients on a restricted sodium intake when calculating total daily sodium intake.

Revised: 08/25/94
Interim revision: 04/26/95

## Table 1. Pharmacology/Pharmacokinetics

| Drug | Oral Absorption (%) | Time to Peak Serum Concentration (hr) | Peak Serum Concentration Dose | Peak Serum Concentration mcg/mL | Half-life (hr) Creatinine Clearance > 50 mL/min (0.83 mL/sec) | Half-life (hr) Creatinine Clearance 10–30 mL/min (0.17–0.83 mL/sec) | Half-life (hr) Creatinine Clearance < 10 mL/min (0.17 mL/sec) |
|---|---|---|---|---|---|---|---|
| Amoxicillin | 75–90 | 1–2 (oral) | 250 mg (oral) | 3.5–5 | 1 | 4.5 | 12.6 |
| Ampicillin | 35–50 | 1.5–2 (oral) 1 (IM)* | 500 mg (oral) 500 mg (IM) 500 mg (IV)* | 3–6 7–14 12–29 | 1–1.5 | 3.4 | 19 |
| Bacampicillin | 35–50† | 0.5–1† (oral) | 400 mg (oral) | 7.9† | 1† | 4.5† | 12.6† |
| Carbenicillin | 30 | 0.5–1 (oral and IM) | 500 mg (oral) 1 gram (IM) 2 grams (IV) | 6.5 20 241 | 1–1.5 | 9.6 | 18.2 |
| Cloxacillin | 50 | 1–2 (oral) | 500 mg (oral) 500 mg (IM) | 8 16 | 0.5–1 | | 2.5 |
| Dicloxacillin | 37–50 | 0.5–1 (oral) | 125 mg (oral) | 4.7 | 0.5–1 | | 1.8 |
| Flucloxacillin | 30–50 | 1 (oral) | 250 mg (oral) | 6–10 | 0.7–1.3 | | |
| Methicillin | | 0.5–1 (IM) | 1 gram (IM) 1 gram (IV) | 12 60 | 0.3–1 | | 4 |
| Mezlocillin | | 0.5–1 (IM) | 1 gram (IM) 4 grams (IV) | 35–45 254 | 0.8–1.1 | 2 | 2.6 |
| Nafcillin | Erratic; poor | 1–2 (oral) 0.5–1 (IM) | 1 gram (IM) | 7.6 | 0.5–1.5 | 1.9 | 2.1 |
| Oxacillin | 30–35 | 0.5–1 (oral and IM) | 500 mg (oral) 500 mg (IM) | 5–7 15 | 0.4–0.7 | | 0.8 |
| Penicillin G Oral IV Benzathine (IM) Procaine (IM) | 15–30 | 1–2 24 4 | 3,200,000 units (IV) 300,000 units (IM) | 2.2–17 0.03–0.05 | 0.5–0.7 | | 4.1 |
| Penicillin V | 60–73 | 0.5–1 (oral) | 250 mg (oral) | 2–3 | 0.5–1 | | 4.1 |

## Table 1. Pharmacology/Pharmacokinetics *(continued)*

| Drug | Oral Absorption (%) | Time to Peak Serum Concentration (hr) | Peak Serum Concentration | | Half-life (hr) | | |
| | | | Dose | mcg/mL | Creatinine Clearance > 50 mL/min (0.83 mL/sec) | Creatinine Clearance 10–30 mL/min (0.17–0.83 mL/sec) | Creatinine Clearance < 10 mL/min (0.17 mL/sec) |
|---|---|---|---|---|---|---|---|
| Piperacillin | | 0.5 (IM) | 4 grams (IV) | 412 | 0.6–1.2 | 2 | 2.8 |
| Pivampicillin | 35–50† | 1† (oral) | 500 mg (oral) | 13† | 1† | | |
| Pivmecillinam | Poor‡ | 0.5–1.5‡ (oral) | 200 mg (oral) | 3.3‡ | 1‡ | | |
| Ticarcillin | | 0.5–1 (IM) | 3 grams (IV) | 190 | 1–1.2 | 5.2 | 8.9 |

*IV=intravenous; IM=intramuscular.
†As ampicillin.
‡As mecillinam.

## Table 2. Pharmacology/Pharmacokinetics

| Drug | Protein Binding (%) | Hepatic Biotransformation (%) | Renal Elimination (% unchanged) | Vol$_D$ (L/kg) | Removal by Hemodialysis |
|---|---|---|---|---|---|
| Amoxicillin | Low (20) | 10 | 60–75 | 0.36 | Yes |
| Ampicillin | Low (20) | 10 | 75–90 | 0.29 | Yes |
| Bacampicillin | Low (18–20)* | 10* | 70–75* | 0.29* | Yes |
| Carbenicillin | Moderate (50) | 0–2 | 36 (oral) 75–95 (intravenous) | 0.12 | Yes |
| Cloxacillin | Very high (95) | 20 | 30–60 | 0.11 | No |
| Dicloxacillin | Very high (95–98) | 10 | 50–70 | 0.08 | No |
| Flucloxacillin | Very high (94) | | 50–65 | | No |
| Methicillin | Low to moderate (40) | 10 | 60–80 | 0.36 | No |
| Mezlocillin | Low to moderate (16–42) | 20–30 | 55–60 | 0.23 | Yes |
| Nafcillin | High (90) | 60–70 | 11–30 | 1.1 | No |
| Oxacillin | High (90–94) | 45 | 55–60 | 0.4 | No |
| Penicillin G Oral Parenteral Benzathine IM Procaine | Moderate (60) | 20 | 20 60–90 | 0.5–0.7 | Yes |
| Penicillin V | High (80) | 55 | 20–40 | 0.5 | Yes |
| Piperacillin | Low (16) | 20–30 | 60–80 | 0.23 | Yes† |
| Pivampicillin | Low (20)* | 10* | 25–30* | | Yes |
| Pivmecillinam | Low (5–10)‡ | | 60–80‡ | | Yes§ |
| Ticarcillin | Moderate (45–60) | 15 | 60–80 | 0.16 | Yes |

*As ampicillin.
†Hemodialysis removes 30–50% of piperacillin in 4 hours.
‡As mecillinam.
§Hemodialysis removes 50–70% of pivmecillinam in 4 hours.

# PENICILLINS AND BETA-LACTAMASE INHIBITORS   Systemic

This monograph includes information on the following: Amoxicillin and Clavulanate; Ampicillin and Sulbactam†; Piperacillin and Tazobactam; Ticarcillin and Clavulanate.

INN:
Amoxicillin—Amoxicilline

BAN:
Amoxicillin—Amoxycillin

VA CLASSIFICATION (Primary):
Amoxicillin and Clavulanate—AM052
Ampicillin and Sulbactam—AM052
Piperacillin and Tazobactam—AM054
Ticarcillin and Clavulanate—AM054

Note: For a listing of dosage forms and brand names by country availability, see *Dosage Forms* section(s). For a listing of brand names for the articles in this monograph, refer to the General Index.

†Not commercially available in Canada.

## Category

Antibacterial (systemic).

## Indications

Note: Bracketed information in the *Indications* section refers to uses that are not included in U.S. product labeling.

### General considerations

Ampicillin and amoxicillin have activity against *Haemophilus influenzae*, *Escherichia coli*, and *Salmonella* and *Shigella* species, and also retain activity against penicillin-sensitive gram-positive bacteria. However, many Enterobacteriaceae and *H. influenzae* are resistant as a result of beta-lactamase production. Amoxicillin has the same spectrum of activity as ampicillin, although amoxicillin has slightly better activity against *Enterococcus faecalis*, *E. coli*, and *Salmonella* sp., and slightly less activity against *Shigella* sp.

Ticarcillin combines the gram-negative spectrum of ampicillin with activity against most species of *Enterobacter*, *Providencia*, and *Morganella* sp. It also has some activity against *Pseudomonas aeruginosa* and some indole-positive *Proteus* sp.

Piperacillin is more active than ticarcillin against *P. aeruginosa* and *Klebsiella* sp., but has activity similar to that of ticarcillin against most other gram-negative bacteria. Piperacillin also inhibits *P. cepacia*, *P. maltophilia*, and *P. fluorescens*.

Resistance to penicillins is thought to be due to 3 main mechanisms. The first is alteration of the antibiotic target sites' penicillin-binding proteins (PBPs); the second is inactivation of the penicillin by bacterially produced enzymes (beta-lactamases); and the third is decreased permeability of the cell wall to penicillins. Of these 3 mechanisms, production of beta-lactamase is the most common and the most important.

When combined with a penicillin, beta-lactamase inhibitors, which include clavulanic acid (clavulanate), sulbactam, and tazobactam, have effectively extended the penicillin's spectrum of activity. Like penicillins, the beta-lactamase inhibitors are beta-lactam compounds; however, they have minimal intrinsic antibacterial activity. Instead of being hydrolyzed by beta-lactamases, they irreversibly bind to these enzymes, thereby protecting the penicillin from hydrolysis ('suicide' inhibition). Beta-lactamase inhibitors only work when a beta-lactamase enzyme is present. They will not alter the susceptibility of organisms inherently resistant to the penicillin; nor will they alter resistance patterns due to other causes, e.g., alteration of the penicillin-binding proteins (PBPs) (the mechanism of resistance for methicillin-resistant staphylococci).

Clavulanate, sulbactam, and tazobactam are irreversible inhibitors of a wide variety of plasmid-mediated and some chromosomally mediated bacterial beta-lactamases. Clavulanate and tazobactam are highly active, and sulbactam is moderately active, against transferable plasmid-mediated beta-lactamases. The inhibitory effect on chromosomally mediated type I enzymes is variable. Any beta-lactam agent, including beta-lactamase inhibitors and penicillins, may induce beta-lactamase production. Therefore, organisms such as *Enterobacter*, *Serratia*, *Morganella*, and *Pseudomonas* species may produce more beta-lactamase enzyme when they are exposed to a penicillin or a beta-lactamase inhibitor. Clavulanate is a moderate inducer of the chromosomal enzymes in these organisms; sulbactam and tazobactam are weaker inducers. Also, if the complex with the beta-lactamase inhibitor is not stable, regeneration of the beta-lactamase may occur. If so, the enzyme must be repeatedly inactivated for inhibition to be maintained. It is also easier to protect a beta-lactam antibiotic against organisms that

produce a small amount of enzyme than it is to protect against organisms producing a large amount.

All 3 beta-lactamase inhibitors inactivate staphylococcal penicillinase. Beta-lactamase inhibitors inactivate the chromosomally mediated beta-lactamases of *Proteus vulgaris* and *Bacteroides* sp., and the class IV beta-lactamases present in some *Klebsiella* sp. Resistance in *H. influenzae* and *Neisseria gonorrhoeae* that produce TEM beta-lactamases is rare since these organisms produce only a small quantity of enzyme and are very permeable to the inhibitor.

Clavulanate is a potent inhibitor of plasmid-mediated enzymes, most commonly found in Enterobacteriaceae. However, all beta-lactamases are not equally susceptible. The class I beta-lactamases of the Richmond-Sykes classification are often resistant, including beta-lactamases typically produced by *Enterobacter*, *Citrobacter*, and *Serratia* species, and *P. aeruginosa*. Clavulanic acid is available as a combined product with both amoxicillin and ticarcillin, resulting in products with broad-spectrum antibacterial activity against beta-lactamase–producing strains of *E. coli*, *H. influenzae*, *Moraxella (Branhamella) catarrhalis*, many *Klebsiella* sp., most *Bacteroides* sp., *S. aureus*, and *S. epidermidis*, except methicillin-resistant staphylococcal strains. Combining ticarcillin with clavulanic acid increases the activity of ticarcillin to include 60 to 80% of ticarcillin-resistant strains of Enterobacteriaceae and all beta-lactamase–producing strains of *Staphylococcus aureus*, *H. influenzae*, and *Bacteroides* sp. No increase in activity is provided against *P. aeruginosa*.

Sulbactam also inhibits many beta-lactamases, including those produced by *Bacteroides*, *Haemophilus*, and *Klebsiella* sp., and *N. gonorrhoeae*, but it appears to be less potent than clavulanic acid against several beta-lactamases, including staphylococcal beta-lactamases, TEM-type enzymes, especially strains of *E. coli* and other pathogens producing TEM-1 and TEM-2 beta-lactamases, and the beta-lactamases typically present in *B. fragilis*.

Tazobactam also has a broad spectrum of activity, and appears to be at least as effective as clavulanic acid against a wide variety of beta-lactamases. Tazobactam may have greater activity than clavulanate against some Enterobacteriaceae class I chromosomally mediated beta-lactamases, such as those of *Morganella morganii*, *E. coli*, *K. pneumoniae*, *Citrobacter diversus*, *P. mirabilis*, *Providencia stuartii*, and *Pseudomonas aeruginosa*. Both tazobactam and clavulanate have greater activity against these organisms than sulbactam has. The piperacillin and tazobactam combination also has good activity against staphylococci, streptococci, *H. influenzae*, *Moraxella catarrhalis*, *Enterococcus faecalis*, and *Listeria monocytogenes*. Greater resistance was seen with *E. faecium*, *Enterobacter* sp., *Citrobacter freundii*, *Serratia* sp., and *Xanthomonas maltophilia*.

### Accepted

Bone and joint infections (treatment)—Ticarcillin and clavulanate combination and [ampicillin and sulbactam combination][1] are indicated in the treatment of bone and joint infections caused by susceptible organisms.

Intra-abdominal infections (treatment)—Ampicillin and sulbactam combination, piperacillin and tazobactam combination, and ticarcillin and clavulanate combination are indicated in the treatment of intra-abdominal infections caused by susceptible organisms.

Otitis media, acute (treatment)—Amoxicillin and clavulanate combination is indicated in the treatment of acute otitis media caused by susceptible organisms.

Pelvic infections, female (treatment)—Ampicillin and sulbactam combination, piperacillin and tazobactam combination, and ticarcillin and clavulanate combination are indicated in the treatment of female pelvic infections caused by susceptible organisms.

Pneumonia, bacterial (treatment)—Amoxicillin and clavulanate combination, piperacillin and tazobactam combination, and ticarcillin and clavulanate combination are indicated in the treatment of bacterial pneumonia caused by susceptible organisms.

Septicemia, bacterial (treatment)—Ticarcillin and clavulanate combination and [piperacillin and tazobactam combination][1] are indicated in the treatment of bacterial septicemia caused by susceptible organisms.

Sinusitis (treatment)—Amoxicillin and clavulanate combination is indicated in the treatment of sinusitis caused by susceptible organisms.

Skin and soft tissue infections (treatment)—Amoxicillin and clavulanate combination, ampicillin and sulbactam combination, piperacillin and tazobactam combination, and ticarcillin and clavulanate combination are indicated in the treatment of skin and soft tissue infections caused by susceptible organisms.

Urinary tract infections, bacterial (treatment)—Amoxicillin and clavulanate combination and ticarcillin and clavulanate combination are indicated in the treatment of bacterial urinary tract infections caused by susceptible organisms.

[Bronchitis (treatment)][1]—Amoxicillin and clavulanate combination is used in the treatment of bronchitis caused by susceptible organisms.

[Chancroid (treatment)][1]—Amoxicillin and clavulanate combination is used in the treatment of chancroid caused by *Haemophilus ducreyi*.

[Gonorrhea, endocervical and urethral (treatment)][1]—Ampicillin and sulbactam combination is used in the treatment of uncomplicated endocervical and urethral gonorrhea caused by *Neisseria gonorrhoeae*.

[Perioperative infection prophylaxis for colorectal surgery, abdominal hysterectomy, and high-risk cesarean section]—Ticarcillin and clavulanate combination is used prophylactically to help prevent perioperative infections that may result from colorectal surgery, abdominal hysterectomy, and high-risk cesarean section; however, other agents (i.e., cefazolin for hysterectomy and high-risk cesarean section, and neomycin plus erythromycin base for colorectal surgery) are preferred for use as perioperative prophylaxis in these procedures.

### Unaccepted
Piperacillin and tazobactam combination should not be used for the treatment of complicated urinary tract infections because of inadequate efficacy at the usual dose (3.375 grams every six hours).

---

[1]Not included in Canadian product labeling.

## Pharmacology/Pharmacokinetics

### Physicochemical characteristics
Source—
  Clavulanate: Naturally occurring compound produced by *Streptomyces clavuligerus*
  Sulbactam: Synthetic penicillanic acid sulfone
  Tazobactam: Analog of sulbactam
Chemical group—
  Amoxicillin: Aminopenicillin
  Ampicillin: Aminopenicillin
  Piperacillin: Acylureidopenicillin
  Ticarcillin: Carboxypenicillin
Molecular weight—
  Amoxicillin: 419.45.
  Ampicillin sodium: 371.39.
  Clavulanate potassium: 237.25.
  Piperacillin sodium: 539.54.
  Sulbactam sodium: 255.22.
  Tazobactam sodium: 322.27.
  Ticarcillin disodium: 428.39.

### Mechanism of action/Effect
Penicillins—Bactericidal; inhibit bacterial cell wall synthesis. Action is dependent on the ability of penicillins to reach and bind penicillin-binding proteins (PBPs) located on the inner membrane of the bacterial cell wall. PBPs (which include transpeptidases, carboxypeptidases, and endopeptidases) are enzymes that are involved in the terminal stages of assembling the bacterial cell wall and in reshaping the cell wall during growth and division. Penicillins bind to, and inactivate, PBPs, resulting in the weakening of the bacterial cell wall and lysis.
Beta-lactamase inhibitors—Act by irreversibly binding to the beta-lactamase enzyme, preventing hydrolysis of the beta-lactam ring of the penicillin. The inhibitor first forms a noncovalent complex, which is fully reversible, with a beta-lactam agent. Beta-lactamase inhibitors then act by recognizing the serine residue at the active site of the beta-lactamase enzyme. The structure of the inhibitor is opened and a covalent acyl-enzyme complex is formed with the serine residue. This prevents the beta-lactamase enzyme from hydrolyzing the penicillin and the liberation of the beta-lactamase enzyme.

### Absorption
Amoxicillin and clavulanate are both well absorbed after oral administration and are stable in the presence of gastric acid. Food does not affect absorption, and this combination product may be given without regard to meals. Oral bioavailability of amoxicillin and clavulanic acid is approximately 90% and 75%, respectively. Orally administered sulbactam is poorly absorbed.

### Distribution
The penicillins and beta-lactamase inhibitors are widely distributed to most tissues and body fluids, including peritoneal fluid, blister fluid, urine (high concentrations), pleural fluid, middle ear fluid, intestinal mucosa, bone, gallbladder, lung, female reproductive tissues, and bile. Distribution into the cerebrospinal fluid (CSF) is low in subjects with noninflamed meninges, as is penetration into purulent bronchial secretions.

Penicillins also cross the placenta and are distributed into breast milk.
  Volume of distribution (Vol_D)—
    Amoxicillin: 0.36 L/kg.
    Ampicillin: 0.29 L/kg.
    Piperacillin: 0.23 L/kg.
    Ticarcillin: 0.16 L/kg.

### Protein binding
Amoxicillin—Low (17 to 20%).
Ampicillin—Low (20 to 28%).
Clavulanic acid—Low (22 to 30%).
Piperacillin—Low (Approximately 16 to 30%).
Sulbactam—Moderate (38%).
Tazobactam—Low (Approximately 30%).
Ticarcillin—Moderate (45 to 60%).

### Biotransformation
Hepatic—
  Amoxicillin: Approximately 10% of a dose is metabolized.
  Ampicillin: Approximately 10% of a dose is metabolized to inactive penicilloic acid.
  Clavulanic acid: Less than 50% of a dose is metabolized.
  Piperacillin: Metabolized to the desethyl metabolite, which has minor activity.
  Sulbactam: Less than 25% of a dose is metabolized.
  Tazobactam: Metabolized to a single, inactive metabolite.
  Ticarcillin: Less than 15% of a dose is metabolized.

### Half-life
Normal renal function—
  Amoxicillin: Approximately 1.3 hours.
  Ampicillin: Approximately 1 hour.
  Clavulanic acid: Approximately 1 hour.
  Piperacillin: 0.7 to 1.2 hours.
  Sulbactam: Approximately 1 hour.
  Tazobactam: 0.7 to 1.2 hours.
  Ticarcillin: 1 to 1.2 hours.
Impaired renal function (severe)—
  Amoxicillin: Approximately 12 hours.
  Ampicillin: 9 to 19 hours.
  Clavulanate: Approximately 3 hours.
  Piperacillin: 1.4 to 2.8 hours.
  Sulbactam: Approximately 9 hours.
  Tazobactam: 2.8 to 4.8 hours.
  Ticarcillin: Approximately 9 hours.

### Time to peak serum concentration
Amoxicillin and clavulanic acid combination—1 to 2 hours.
Ampicillin and sulbactam combination—End of infusion.
Piperacillin and tazobactam combination—End of infusion.
Ticarcillin and clavulanate combination—End of infusion.

### Peak serum concentration
Amoxicillin and clavulanic acid combination—
  Chewable tablets and oral suspension: Approximately 6.9 mcg per mL (mcg/mL) amoxicillin and 1.6 mcg/mL clavulanic acid after an oral dose of 250 mg amoxicillin and 62.5 mg clavulanic acid.
  Tablets (film-coated): Approximately 4.4 to 4.7 mcg/mL amoxicillin and 2.3 to 2.5 mcg/mL clavulanic acid after an oral dose of 250 mg amoxicillin and 125 mg clavulanic acid.
Ampicillin and sulbactam combination—
  Intramuscular: Approximately 8 to 35 mcg/mL ampicillin and 6 to 25 mcg/mL sulbactam following an intramuscular dose of 1.5 grams (1 gram of ampicillin and 500 mg of sulbactam).
  Intravenous: Approximately 40 to 70 mcg/mL ampicillin and 20 to 40 mcg/mL sulbactam following an intravenous dose of 1.5 grams (1 gram of ampicillin and 500 mg of sulbactam).
Piperacillin and tazobactam combination—
  Approximately 242 mcg/mL piperacillin and 24 mcg/mL tazobactam following an intravenous dose of 3.375 grams (3 grams of piperacillin and 0.375 gram of sulbactam).
Ticarcillin and clavulanic acid combination—
  Approximately 330 mcg/mL ticarcillin and 8 mcg/mL clavulanic acid following an intravenous dose of 3.1 grams (3 grams of ticarcillin and 0.1 gram of clavulanic acid).

### Elimination
Primarily renal (glomerular filtration and tubular secretion)—
  Amoxicillin and clavulanic acid combination:
    50 to 78%, and 25 to 40% of an administered dose of amoxicillin and clavulanic acid, respectively, are excreted unchanged in the urine within first 6 hours after administration.

Ampicillin and sulbactam combination:
    75 to 85% of an administered dose of both ampicillin and sulbactam is excreted unchanged in the urine within first 8 hours after administration.
Piperacillin and tazobactam combination:
    Approximately 68% and 80% of an administered dose of piperacillin and tazobactam, respectively, are excreted unchanged in the urine.
Ticarcillin and clavulanic acid combination:
    60 to 70%, and 35 to 45% of an administered dose of ticarcillin and clavulanic acid, respectively, are excreted unchanged in the urine within first 6 hours after administration.
Biliary—
    Ampicillin and sulbactam:
        Less than 1%.
    Piperacillin and tazobactam combination:
        Less than 2%.
In dialysis—
    Hemodialysis:
        Hemodialysis removes amoxicillin, ampicillin, clavulanate, piperacillin, sulbactam, tazobactam, and ticarcillin from the blood.
        Piperacillin and tazobactam combination—30 to 40% of an administered dose is removed, plus an additional 5% of the tazobactam dose as the metabolite.
    Peritoneal dialysis:
        Piperacillin and tazobactam combination—6 to 21% of an administered dose is removed, plus an additional 16% of the tazobactam dose as the metabolite.

## Precautions to Consider

### Cross-sensitivity and/or related problems
Patients allergic to one penicillin may be allergic to other penicillins also.
Patients allergic to cephalosporins, cephamycins, or beta-lactamase inhibitors may be allergic to penicillin and beta-lactamase inhibitor combinations also.

### Carcinogenicity
Long-term carcinogenicity studies in animals have not been done on any of the penicillin and beta-lactamase inhibitor combinations.

### Mutagenicity
*Amoxicillin and clavulanic acid combination*—Long-term studies in animals have not been done to evaluate the mutagenic potential of this combination.
*Ampicillin and sulbactam combination*—Long-term studies in animals have not been done to evaluate the mutagenic potential of this combination.
*Piperacillin and tazobactam combination*—Microbial mutagenicity studies with piperacillin and tazobactam combination at concentrations of up to 14.84 and 1.86 mcg, respectively, per plate were negative. Negative results were also found in the unscheduled DNA synthesis (UDS) test at concentrations of up to 5689 and 711 mcg per mL (mcg/mL), respectively, in the mammalian point mutation (Chinese hamster ovary cell HPRT) assay at concentrations of up to 8000 and 1000 mcg/mL, respectively, and in the mammalian cell (BALB/c-3T3) transformation assay at concentrations of up to 8 and 1 mcg/mL, respectively. *In vivo*, piperacillin and tazobactam combination did not induce chromosomal aberrations in rats administered intravenous doses of 1500 and 187.5 mg per kg of body weight (mg/kg), respectively; this dose is similar to the maximum recommended human daily dose based on mg per square meter of body surface area (mg/m²).
*Ticarcillin and clavulanic acid combination*—Studies performed *in vitro* and *in vivo* did not indicate a potential for mutagenicity.

### Pregnancy/Reproduction
Fertility—*Amoxicillin and clavulanic acid combination:* Studies in rats and mice given doses up to 10 times the usual human dose have not shown that amoxicillin and clavulanate combination impairs fertility.
*Ampicillin and sulbactam combination:* Studies in mice, rats, and rabbits given doses up to 10 times the human dose have not shown that ampicillin and sulbactam combination causes adverse effects on fertility.
*Piperacillin and tazobactam combination:* Reproduction studies in rats revealed no evidence of impaired fertility when piperacillin and tazobactam combination was administered at doses similar to the maximum recommended human daily dose based on body surface area (mg/m²). There was also no evidence of impaired fertility when tazobactam was administered at doses up to 3 times the maximum recommended human daily dose based on body surface area (mg/m²).
*Ticarcillin and clavulanic acid combination:* Studies in rats given daily doses of up to 1050 mg/kg have not shown that ticarcillin and clavulanate combination impairs fertility.

Pregnancy—Penicillins cross the placenta. Clavulanic acid also crosses the placenta. Adequate and well-controlled studies in humans have not been done; however, problems in humans have not been documented.
*Amoxicillin and clavulanate combination:* Studies in rats and mice given doses up to 10 times the usual human dose have not shown that amoxicillin and clavulanate combination causes adverse effects in the fetus.
FDA Pregnancy Category B.
*Ampicillin and sulbactam combination:* Studies in mice, rats, and rabbits given doses up to 10 times the human dose have not shown that ampicillin and sulbactam combination causes adverse effects in the fetus.
FDA Pregnancy Category B.
*Piperacillin and tazobactam combination:* Teratology studies performed in mice and rats given piperacillin and tazobactam combination at doses 1 to 2 times, respectively, the human dose based on body surface area (mg/m²) revealed no evidence of harm to the fetus. In addition, no evidence of harm to the fetus was found when tazobactam was administered to mice and rats at doses up to 6 and 14 times the human dose, respectively, based on body surface area (mg/m²). Tazobactam crosses the placenta in mice; concentrations in the fetus are 10% or less those found in maternal plasma.
FDA Pregnancy Category B.
*Ticarcillin and clavulanate combination:* Studies in rats given daily doses of up to 1050 mg/kg have not shown that ticarcillin and clavulanate combination causes adverse effects in the fetus.
FDA Pregnancy Category B.

### Breast-feeding
Penicillins and sulbactam are distributed into breast milk in low concentrations; it is not known whether clavulanic acid and tazobactam are distributed into breast milk. Although significant problems in humans have not been documented, the use of penicillins by nursing mothers may lead to sensitization, diarrhea, candidiasis, and skin rash in the infant.

### Pediatrics
Many penicillins have been used in pediatric patients, and no pediatrics-specific problems have been documented to date. However, the incompletely developed renal function of neonates and young infants may delay the excretion of renally eliminated penicillins.
*Piperacillin and tazobactam combination:* Although safety and efficacy have not been established in pediatric patients, the results of one study found the clearance and elimination half-life to be increased in infants < 6 months of age. Piperacillin and tazobactam combination had no effect on bilirubin-albumin binding *in vitro*.

### Geriatrics
Penicillins have been used in geriatric patients and no geriatrics-specific problems have been documented to date. However, elderly patients are more likely to have an age-related decrease in renal function, which may require an adjustment in dosage in patients receiving penicillins.

### Dental
Prolonged use of penicillins may lead to the development of oral candidiasis.

### Drug interactions and/or related problems
The following drug interactions and/or related problems have been selected on the basis of their potential clinical significance (possible mechanism in parentheses where appropriate)—not necessarily inclusive (» = major clinical significance):

Note: Combinations containing any of the following medications, depending on the amount present, may also interact with this medication.

Allopurinol
    (concurrent use with ampicillin may significantly increase the possibility of skin rash, especially in hyperuricemic patients; however, it has not been established that allopurinol, rather than the presence of hyperuricemia, is responsible for this effect)
» Aminoglycosides
    (mixing penicillins with aminoglycosides *in vitro* has resulted in substantial mutual inactivation; concurrent administration of piperacillin and tazobactam combination with tobramycin decreased the urinary recovery of tobramycin by 38%; concurrent administration of tobramycin and ticarcillin resulted in a decrease in serum tobramycin concentration by 11%; if these groups of antibacterials are to be administered concurrently, they should be administered at separate sites at least 1 hour apart)
» Anticoagulants, coumarin- or indandione-derivative or
» Heparin or
» Thrombolytic agents
    (concurrent use of these medications with high-dose piperacillin or ticarcillin may increase the risk of hemorrhage because these penicillins inhibit platelet aggregation; patients should be monitored

carefully for signs of bleeding; concurrent use of piperacillin or ticarcillin with thrombolytic agents may increase the risk of severe hemorrhage and is not recommended)

» Anti-inflammatory drugs, nonsteroidal (NSAIDs), especially aspirin or Diflunisal, very high doses or
Other salicylates or

» Platelet aggregation inhibitors, other, (See *Appendix II*) or

» Sulfinpyrazone
(concurrent use of these medications with high-dose piperacillin or ticarcillin may increase the risk of hemorrhage because of additive inhibition of platelet function; in addition, hypoprothrombinemia induced by large doses of salicylates and the gastrointestinal ulcerative or hemorrhagic potential of NSAIDs, salicylates, or sulfinpyrazone may also increase the risk of hemorrhage when these medicines are used concurrently with piperacillin or ticarcillin)

Chloramphenicol or
Erythromycins or
Sulfonamides or
Tetracyclines
(since bacteriostatic drugs may interfere with the bactericidal effect of penicillins in the treatment of meningitis or in other situations in which a rapid bactericidal effect is necessary, it is best to avoid concurrent therapy; however, chloramphenicol and ampicillin are sometimes administered concurrently in pediatric patients)

» Probenecid
(probenecid decreases renal tubular secretion of penicillins, sulbactam, and tazobactam [but not clavulanic acid, which is cleared primarily by glomerular filtration] when used concurrently; this effect results in increased and more prolonged serum concentrations, prolonged elimination half-life [half-life of piperacillin increased by 21%, that of tazobactam by 71%, and that of sulbactam by 40%], and increased risk of toxicity. Penicillins and probenecid are often used concurrently to treat sexually transmitted diseases [STDs] or other infections in which high and/or prolonged antibiotic serum and tissue concentrations are required)

## Laboratory value alterations

The following have been selected on the basis of their potential clinical significance (possible effect in parentheses where appropriate)—not necessarily inclusive (» = major clinical significance):

With diagnostic test results

» Glucose, urine
(high urinary concentrations of a penicillin may produce false-positive or falsely elevated test results with copper-reduction tests [Benedict's, *Clinitest*, or Fehling's]; glucose enzymatic tests [*Clinistix* or *Testape*] are not affected)

Direct antiglobulin (Coombs') tests
(false-positive result may occur during therapy with any penicillin)

Protein, urine
(high urinary concentrations of piperacillin or ticarcillin may produce false-positive protein reactions [pseudoproteinuria] with the sulfosalicylic acid and boiling test, the acetic acid test, the biuret reaction, and the nitric acid test; bromophenol blue reagent test strips [*Multi-stix*] are reportedly unaffected)

With physiology/laboratory test values

Alanine aminotransferase (ALT [SGPT]) and
Alkaline phosphatase and
Aspartate aminotransferase (AST [SGOT]) and
Bilirubin, serum
Lactate dehydrogenase (LDH), serum
(values may be increased)

Blood urea nitrogen (BUN) and
Creatinine, serum
(increased concentrations have been associated with ampicillin and sulbactam, piperacillin, and ticarcillin)

Estradiol or
Estriol, total conjugated or
Estriol-glucuronide or
Estrone, conjugated
(concentrations may be transiently decreased in pregnant women following administration of amoxicillin and ampicillin)

» Partial thromboplastin time (PTT) and

» Prothrombin time (PT)
(an increase has been associated with piperacillin and ticarcillin)

Potassium, serum
(hypokalemia may occur following administration of piperacillin or ticarcillin, either of which may act as a nonreabsorbable anion

in the distal renal tubules; this may cause an increase in pH and result in increased urinary potassium loss; the risk of hypokalemia increases with use of larger doses)

Sodium, serum
(hypernatremia may occur following administration of large doses of ticarcillin because of the medication's high sodium content)

Uric acid, serum
(ticarcillin may transiently decrease the serum concentration in some patients)

White blood count
(leukopenia or neutropenia is associated with the use of all penicillins; the effect is more likely to occur with prolonged therapy and severe hepatic function impairment)

## Medical considerations/Contraindications

The medical considerations/contraindications included here have been selected on the basis of their potential clinical significance (reasons given in parentheses where appropriate)—not necessarily inclusive (» = major clinical significance).

*Except under special circumstances, this medication should not be used when the following medical problem exists:*

» Allergy to penicillins or beta-lactamase inhibitors

*Risk-benefit should be considered when the following medical problems exist:*

Allergy, general, history of, such as asthma, eczema, hay fever, hives

» Bleeding disorders, history of
(some penicillins, especially piperacillin and ticarcillin, may cause platelet dysfunction and hemorrhage)

» Congestive heart failure (CHF) or
Hypertension
(the sodium content of high doses of ticarcillin should be considered in patients who require sodium restriction)

» Cystic fibrosis
(patients with cystic fibrosis may be at increased risk of fever and skin rash when given piperacillin)

» Gastrointestinal disease, active or a history of, especially antibiotic-associated colitis
(penicillins may cause pseudomembranous colitis)

» Mononucleosis, infectious
(a morbilliform skin rash may occur in a high percentage of patients taking ampicillin)

» Renal function impairment
(because most penicillins are excreted through the kidneys, a reduction in dosage, or an increase in dosing interval, is recommended in patients with renal function impairment; also, the sodium content of high doses of ticarcillin should be considered in patients with severe renal function impairment)

## Patient monitoring

The following may be especially important in patient monitoring (other tests may be warranted in some patients, depending on condition; » = major clinical significance):

*For piperacillin and tazobactam combination and ticarcillin and clavulanate combination*

» Partial thromboplastin time (PTT) and

» Prothrombin time (PT)
(may be required prior to and during prolonged therapy in patients with renal function impairment who are receiving high doses, since hemorrhagic manifestations may occur, although the effect is rare)

*For piperacillin and ticarcillin*

Potassium, serum
(determinations may be required periodically during therapy in patients with low potassium reserves and in patients receiving cytotoxic medications or diuretics, since hypokalemia may occur)

*For all penicillin and beta-lactamase inhibitor combinations (if C. difficile colitis occurs)*

» Stool toxin assays
(enzyme immunoassay of stool samples for the presence of *Clostridium difficile* toxins may be required prior to treatment of patients with antibiotic-associated colitis to document the presence of *C. difficile* toxins; however, *C. difficile* and its toxins may persist following treatment with oral vancomycin, metronidazole, or cholestyramine, despite clinical improvement; follow-up cultures and toxin assays are not recommended if clinical improvement is complete)

## Side/Adverse Effects

The following side/adverse effects have been selected on the basis of their potential clinical significance (possible signs and symptoms in parentheses where appropriate)—not necessarily inclusive:

### Those indicating need for medical attention
Incidence less frequent
*Allergic reactions, specifically anaphylaxis* (fast or irregular breathing; puffiness or swelling around face; shortness of breath; sudden, severe decrease in blood pressure); *serum sickness–like reactions* (skin rash; joint pain; fever); *skin rash, hives, or itching*

Incidence rare
*Leukopenia or neutropenia* (sore throat and fever); *pain at site of injection; platelet dysfunction* (unusual bleeding or bruising); *Clotridium difficile colitis* (severe abdominal or stomach cramps and pain; abdominal tenderness; watery and severe diarrhea, which may also be bloody; fever); *seizures*

Note: *Platelet dysfunction* is primarily associated with piperacillin and ticarcillin.

     *Clotridium difficile colitis* may occur up to several weeks after discontinuation of these medications.

     *Seizures* are more likely to occur in patients receiving high doses of a penicillin and/or patients with severe renal function impairment.

### Those indicating need for medical attention only if they continue or are bothersome
Incidence more frequent
*Gastrointestinal reactions* (mild diarrhea; nausea or vomiting; stomach pain); *headache; oral candidiasis* (sore mouth or tongue; white patches in mouth and/or on tongue); *vaginal candidiasis* (vaginal itching and discharge)

## Overdose

For more information on the management of overdose or unintentional ingestion, **contact a Poison Control Center** (see *Poison Control Center Listing*).

### Treatment of overdose
Since there is no specific antidote, treatment of penicillin overdose should be symptomatic and supportive.

Specific treatment—Hemodialysis may aid in the removal of penicillins from the blood.

Supportive care—Patients in whom intentional overdose is known or suspected should be referred for psychiatric consultation.

## Patient Consultation

As an aid to patient consultation, refer to *Advice for the Patient, Penicillins and Beta-lactamase Inhibitors (Systemic)*.

In providing consultation, consider emphasizing the following selected information (» = major clinical significance):

### Before using this medication
» Conditions affecting use, especially:
     Allergy to penicillins, cephalosporins, cephamycins, or beta-lactamase inhibitors
     Pregnancy—Penicillins cross the placenta
     Breast-feeding—Penicillins and sulbactam are distributed into breast milk
     Use in children—Neonates and young infants may have reduced elimination of renally eliminated penicillins due to incompletely developed renal function
     Other medications, especially aminoglycosides; coumarin- or indandione-derivative anticoagulants; heparin; nonsteroidal antiinflammatory drugs (NSAIDs), especially aspirin; other platelet aggregation inhibitors; probenecid; sulfinpyrazone; or thrombolytic agents
     Other medical problems, especially a history of bleeding disorders; congestive heart failure; cystic fibrosis; active or history of gastrointestinal disease, especially antibiotic-associated colitis; infectious mononucleosis; or renal function impairment

### Proper use of this medication
     Taking amoxicillin and clavulanate combination on a full or empty stomach; administration with food may decrease the incidence of gastrointestinal side effects (diarrhea, nausea and vomiting)
     Proper administration technique for oral liquids
     Not using after expiration date
» Importance of taking at evenly spaced times and not missing doses
» Proper dosing
     Missed dose: Taking as soon as possible; not taking if almost time for next dose; not doubling doses

» Proper storage

### Precautions while using this medication
     Checking with physician if no improvement within a few days
» For severe diarrhea, checking with physician before taking any antidiarrheals; for mild diarrhea, kaolin- or attapulgite-containing, but not other, antidiarrheals may be tried; checking with physician or pharmacist if mild diarrhea continues or worsens
» Diabetics: False-positive reactions with copper sulfate urine glucose tests may occur, especially with amoxicillin and clavulanate, ampicillin and sulbactam, and piperacillin and tazobactam combinations
     Possible interference with diagnostic tests

### Side/adverse effects
     Signs of potential side effects, especially allergic reactions, leukopenia or neutropenia, pain at site of injection, platelet dysfunction, pseudomembranous colitis, and seizures

## General Dosing Information

### For oral dosage forms only
Amoxicillin and clavulanate combination may be taken on a full or empty stomach. Administration with food may decrease the incidence of gastrointestinal side effects (diarrhea, nausea and vomiting).

### For treatment of adverse effects
Serious anaphylactoid reactions require immediate emergency treatment, which consists of the following:
  • Parenteral epinephrine.
  • Oxygen.
  • Intravenous corticosteroids.
  • Airway management (including intubation).

For *Clostridium difficile* colitis—
  • Some patients may develop *C. difficile* colitis during or following administration of penicillins.
  • *C. difficile* colitis may result in severe watery diarrhea, which may occur during therapy or up to several weeks after therapy is discontinued. If diarrhea occurs, administration of antiperistaltic antidiarrheals (e.g., opioids, diphenoxylate and atropine combination, loperamide, paregoric) is not recommended since they may delay the removal of toxins from the colon, thereby prolonging and/or worsening the condition.
  • Mild cases may respond to discontinuation of the medication alone. Moderate to severe cases may require fluid, electrolyte, and protein replacement.
  • In cases not responding to the above measures or in more severe cases, oral doses of vancomycin, metronidazole, or cholestyramine may be used. Oral vancomycin is effective in doses of 125 mg every 6 hours for 5 to 10 days. The dose of metronidazole is 250 to 500 mg every 8 hours, and the dose of cholestyramine is 4 grams four times a day. Recurrences, which occur in approximately 25% of patients treated with vancomycin or metronidazole, may be treated with a second course of these medications.
  • Cholestyramine resin has been shown to bind *C. difficile* toxin *in vitro*. If cholestyramine resin is administered in conjunction with oral vancomycin, the medications should be administered several hours apart since the resin has been shown to bind oral vancomycin also.

---

### AMOXICILLIN AND CLAVULANATE

## Summary of Differences

Precautions:
     Drug interactions and/or related problems—Clavulanic acid does not interact with probenecid.
     Laboratory value alterations—Amoxicillin may decrease total conjugated estriol, estriol-glucuronide, conjugated estrone, and estradiol concentrations in pregnant women.

## Additional Dosing Information

Absorption of amoxicillin and clavulanate combination is not affected by food. The medication may be taken on a full or empty stomach. Administration with food may decrease the incidence of gastrointestinal side effects (diarrhea, nausea and vomiting).

Amoxicillin and clavulanate 250-mg tablets and 250-mg chewable tablets do not contain the same amount of clavulanate. The 250-mg tablets contain 125 mg of clavulanate, and the 250-mg chewable tablets contain 62.5 mg of clavulanate. Therefore, these products should not be substituted for each other or used interchangeably. This is important to ensure that there is a sufficient concentration of clavulanate at the site of infection to inhibit the beta-lactamase that is present.

The 250-mg tablet should not be used in children who weigh less than 40 kg.

Since the 250-mg and the 500-mg strengths of amoxicillin and clavulanate combination tablets contain the same amount of clavulanate (125 mg), two 250-mg tablets are not equivalent to one 500-mg tablet.

Adults and adolescents with impaired renal function may receive the usual dose with the dosing interval increased as follows:

| Creatinine Clearance (mL/min)/ (mL/sec) | Dosing interval (hours) |
|---|---|
| >30/0.50 | 8 |
| 10–30/0.17–0.50 | 12 |
| 2–10/0.03–0.17 | 24 |

## Oral Dosage Forms

Note: Bracketed uses in the *Dosage Forms* section refer to categories of use and/or indications that are not included in U.S. product labeling.

### AMOXICILLIN AND CLAVULANATE POTASSIUM FOR ORAL SUSPENSION USP

**Usual adult and adolescent dose**
Antibacterial—
Pneumonia and other severe infections:
Oral, 500 mg of amoxicillin and 125 mg of clavulanic acid every eight hours for seven to ten days.
Other infections:
Oral, 250 mg of amoxicillin and 62.5 mg of clavulanic acid every eight hours for seven to ten days.

**Usual pediatric dose**
Antibacterial—
Infants and children up to 40 kg of body weight:
Otitis media, acute
Pneumonia
Sinusitis
Other severe infections—Oral, 13.3 mg of amoxicillin and 3.3 mg of clavulanic acid per kg of body weight every eight hours for seven to ten days.
Other infections—Oral, 6.7 mg of amoxicillin and 1.7 mg of clavulanic acid per kg of body weight every eight hours for seven to ten days.
Children 40 kg of body weight and over:
See *Usual adult and adolescent dose.*

**Strength(s) usually available**
U.S.—
125 mg of amoxicillin and 31.25 mg of clavulanic acid per 5 mL (when reconstituted according to manufacturer's instructions) (Rx) [*Augmentin*].
250 mg of amoxicillin and 62.5 mg of clavulanic acid per 5 mL (when reconstituted according to manufacturer's instructions) (Rx) [*Augmentin*].
Canada—
125 mg of amoxicillin and 31.25 mg of clavulanic acid per 5 mL (when reconstituted according to manufacturer's instructions) (Rx) [*Clavulin-125F*].
250 mg of amoxicillin and 62.5 mg of clavulanic acid per 5 mL (when reconstituted according to manufacturer's instructions) (Rx) [*Clavulin-250F*].

**Packaging and storage**
Prior to reconstitution, store between 15 and 30 °C (59 and 86 °F). Store in a tight container.

**Stability**
After reconstitution, suspensions retain their potency for 10 days if refrigerated.

**Auxiliary labeling**
• Refrigerate.
• Shake well.
• Continue medication for full time of treatment.
• Beyond-use date.

**Note**
When dispensing, include a calibrated liquid-measuring device.

### AMOXICILLIN AND CLAVULANATE POTASSIUM TABLETS USP

**Usual adult and adolescent dose**
Antibacterial—
Pneumonia and other severe infections:
Oral, 500 mg of amoxicillin and 125 mg of clavulanic acid every eight hours for seven to ten days.

Other infections:
Oral, 250 mg of amoxicillin and 125 mg of clavulanic acid every eight hours for seven to ten days.
[Chancroid][1]:
Oral, 500 mg of amoxicillin and 125 mg of clavulanic acid, or 500 mg of amoxicillin and 250 mg of clavulanic acid every eight hours for three to seven days.

**Usual pediatric dose**
Antibacterial—
Infants and children up to 40 kg of body weight:
Otitis media, acute
Pneumonia
Sinusitis
Other severe infections—Oral, 13.3 mg of amoxicillin and 3.3 mg of clavulanic acid per kg of body weight every eight hours for seven to ten days.
Other infections—Oral, 6.7 mg of amoxicillin and 1.7 mg of clavulanic acid per kg of body weight every eight hours for seven to ten days.
Children 40 kg of body weight and over:
See *Usual adult and adolescent dose.*

**Strength(s) usually available**
U.S.—
250 mg of amoxicillin and 125 mg of clavulanic acid (Rx) [*Augmentin*].
500 mg of amoxicillin and 125 mg of clavulanic acid (Rx) [*Augmentin*].
Canada—
250 mg of amoxicillin and 125 mg of clavulanic acid (Rx) [*Clavulin-250*].
500 mg of amoxicillin and 125 mg of clavulanic acid (Rx) [*Clavulin-500F*].

Note: Two 250-mg tablets are not equivalent to one 500-mg tablet since both strengths contain equal amounts of clavulanate potassium.

**Packaging and storage**
Store below 40 °C (104 °F), preferably between 15 and 30 °C (59 and 86 °F), unless otherwise specified by manufacturer. Store in a tight container.

**Auxiliary labeling**
• Continue medication for full time of treatment.

### AMOXICILLIN AND CLAVULANATE POTASSIUM TABLETS (CHEWABLE) USP

**Usual adult and adolescent dose**
See *Amoxicillin and Clavulanate Potassium for Oral Suspension.*

**Usual pediatric dose**
See *Amoxicillin and Clavulanate Potassium for Oral Suspension.*

**Strength(s) usually available**
U.S.—
125 mg of amoxicillin and 31.25 mg of clavulanic acid (Rx) [*Augmentin*].
250 mg of amoxicillin and 62.5 mg of clavulanic acid (Rx) [*Augmentin*].
Canada—
Not commercially available.

**Packaging and storage**
Store below 40 °C (104 °F), preferably between 15 and 30 °C (59 and 86 °F), unless otherwise specified by manufacturer. Store in a tight container.

**Auxiliary labeling**
• Should be chewed or crushed.
• Continue medication for full time of treatment.

[1]Not included in Canadian product labeling.

---

### *AMPICILLIN AND SULBACTAM*

## Summary of Differences

Precautions:
Drug interactions and/or related problems—Concurrent use with allopurinol may increase the risk of skin rash.
Laboratory value alterations—Ampicillin may decrease total conjugated estriol, estriol-glucuronide, conjugated estrone, and estradiol concentrations in pregnant women.
Medical considerations/contraindications—Use in patients with infectious mononucleosis may increase the risk of skin rash.

## Additional Dosing Information

Ampicillin and sulbactam combination should be administered by deep intramuscular injection or by direct, slow intravenous injection over at least a 10- to 15-minute period. It may also be administered by intravenous infusion in 50 to 100 mL of a suitable diluent over a 15- to 30-minute period.

Adults with impaired renal function may require an increase in the dosing interval as follows:

| Creatinine Clearance (mL/min)/ (mL/sec) | Dosing interval (hours) |
|---|---|
| ≥30/0.50 | 6 to 8 |
| 15–29/0.25–0.48 | 12 |
| 5–14/0.08–0.23 | 24 |
| <5/0.08 | 48 |

## Parenteral Dosage Forms

Note: Bracketed uses in the *Dosage Forms* section refer to categories of use and/or indications that are not included in U.S. product labeling.

### STERILE AMPICILLIN SODIUM AND SULBACTAM SODIUM USP

**Usual adult and adolescent dose**
Antibacterial—
Intramuscular or intravenous, 1.5 to 3 grams (1 to 2 grams of ampicillin and 500 mg to 1 gram of sulbactam) every six hours.
[Gonorrhea][1]—
Intramuscular, 1.5 grams (1 gram of ampicillin and 500 mg of sulbactam) as a single dose with 1 gram of oral probenecid.

**Usual adult prescribing limits**
Up to 4 grams of sulbactam daily.

**Usual pediatric dose**
Antibacterial—
Children up to 12 years of age: Dosage has not been established. However, doses of 200 to 400 mg per kg of body weight of ampicillin and 100 to 200 mg per kg of body weight of sulbactam per day, administered in divided doses, have been used.

**Size(s) usually available**
U.S.—
1.5 grams (1 gram of ampicillin and 500 mg of sulbactam) (Rx) [*Unasyn* (sodium 5 mEq [5 mmol])].
3 grams (2 grams of ampicillin and 1 gram of sulbactam) (Rx) [*Unasyn* (sodium 10 mEq [10 mmol])].
Canada—
Not commercially available.

**Packaging and storage**
Prior to reconstitution, store below 30 °C (86 °F), unless otherwise specified by manufacturer.

**Preparation of dosage form**
To prepare initial dilution for intramuscular use, add 3.2 mL of sterile water for injection or of 0.5 or 2% lidocaine hydrochloride injection (without epinephrine) to each 1.5-gram vial and 6.4 mL of diluent to each 3-gram vial to provide an ampicillin concentration of 250 mg per mL and a sulbactam concentration of 125 mg per mL.
To prepare initial dilution for direct intermittent intravenous use, add 3.2 mL of sterile water for injection to each 1.5-gram vial and 6.4 mL of diluent to each 3-gram vial to provide an ampicillin concentration of 250 mg per mL and a sulbactam concentration of 125 mg per mL. The resulting solution should be immediately diluted with a suitable diluent (see manufacturer's package insert) to a final ampicillin concentration of 2 to 30 mg per mL and a final sulbactam concentration of 1 to 15 mg per mL.
Solutions should be allowed to stand following dissolution to allow any foaming to dissipate.
For reconstitution of piggyback infusion bottles, consult manufacturer's labeling.

**Stability**
After reconstitution for intramuscular use, solutions retain their potency for 1 hour.
After reconstitution for intravenous infusion, solutions containing 30 mg of ampicillin and 15 mg of sulbactam per mL retain their potency for 8 hours at 25 °C (77 °F) or for 48 hours at 4 °C (39 °F) in sterile water for injection or 0.9% sodium chloride injection. Solutions containing 20 mg of ampicillin and 10 mg of sulbactam per mL retain their potency for 72 hours at 4 °C (39 °F) in sterile water for injection or 0.9% sodium chloride injection. Solutions containing 20 mg of ampicillin and 10 mg of sulbactam per mL retain their potency for 2 hours at 25 °C (77 °F) or for 4 hours at 4 °C (39 °F) in 5% dextrose

injection. Solutions containing 2 mg of ampicillin and 1 mg of sulbactam per mL retain their potency for 4 hours at 25 °C (77 °F) in 5% dextrose injection. For stability in other diluents, consult manufacturer's package insert.
Solutions (250 mg of ampicillin and 125 mg of sulbactam per mL) may vary in color from pale yellow to yellow. Dilute solutions (up to 30 mg of ampicillin and 15 mg of sulbactam per mL) may vary in color from colorless to pale yellow.

**Incompatibilities**
Extemporaneous admixtures of beta-lactam antibacterials (penicillins) and aminoglycosides may result in substantial mutual inactivation. If these groups of antibacterials are administered concurrently, they should be administered at separate sites at least 1 hour apart. Do not mix them in the same intravenous bag, bottle, or tubing.
When aminoglycosides and penicillins are administered separately by different routes, a reduction in aminoglycoside serum concentration may occur. Usually this is clinically significant only in patients with severely impaired renal function in whom the excretion of both medications is delayed.

**Additional information**
The sodium content (derived from ampicillin sodium and sulbactam sodium) is approximately 5 mEq (5 mmol) per 1.5 grams (1 gram of ampicillin and 500 mg of sulbactam). This must be considered in patients on a restricted sodium intake when calculating total daily sodium intake.

[1]Not included in Canadian product labeling.

---

## PIPERACILLIN AND TAZOBACTAM

## Summary of Differences

Precautions:
Drug interactions and/or related problems—Piperacillin also interacts with anticoagulants and other medications that affect blood clotting.
Laboratory value alterations—May cause false-positive protein reaction in various urine protein tests; may decrease serum potassium concentrations; may increase prothrombin time and partial thromboplastin time.
Medical considerations/contraindications—Caution required in patients with history of bleeding problems; patients with cystic fibrosis may be at increased risk of fever and skin rash.
Side/adverse effects:
Increased risk of platelet dysfunction.

## Additional Dosing Information

Piperacillin and tazobactam combination should be administered by intravenous infusion over a 30-minute period.
The half-life of piperacillin and tazobactam is increased by 25% and 18%, respectively, in patients with hepatic cirrhosis. However, this difference does not warrant an adjustment in dose.
Patients with impaired renal function may require a reduction in dose and should be observed for hemorrhagic complications. Reductions in dose for adults and adolescents with impaired renal function are as follows:

| Creatinine Clearance (mL/min)/ (mL/sec) | Dose/Dosing interval (piperacillin and tazobactam) |
|---|---|
| >40/0.67 | 3.375 grams every 6 hours |
| 20–40/0.33–0.67 | 2.25 grams every 6 hours |
| <20/0.33 | 2.25 grams every 8 hours |
| Hemodialysis patients | 2.25 grams every 8 hours and 0.75 grams after each dialysis |

## Parenteral Dosage Forms

### STERILE PIPERACILLIN SODIUM AND TAZOBACTAM SODIUM

**Usual adult and adolescent dose**
Antibacterial—
Intravenous infusion, 3.375 grams to 4.5 grams (3 to 4 grams of piperacillin and 0.375 to 0.5 grams of tazobactam) every six to eight hours for seven to ten days.

**Usual pediatric dose**
Antibacterial—
Infants and children up to 12 years of age: Dosage has not been established.

Children 12 years of age and older: See *Usual adult and adolescent dose.*

### Size(s) usually available
U.S.—
2.25 grams (2 grams of piperacillin and 0.25 grams of tazobactam) (Rx) [*Zosyn* (sodium 4.7 mEq [4.7 mmol])].
3.375 grams (3 grams of piperacillin and 0.375 grams of tazobactam) (Rx) [*Zosyn* (sodium 7.1 mEq [7.1 mmol])].
4.5 grams (4 grams of piperacillin and 0.5 grams of tazobactam) (Rx) [*Zosyn* (sodium 9.4 mEq [9.4 mmol])].
Canada—
2.25 grams (2 grams of piperacillin and 0.25 grams of tazobactam) (Rx) [*Tazocin*].
3.375 grams (3 grams of piperacillin and 0.375 grams of tazobactam) (Rx) [*Tazocin*].
4.5 grams (4 grams of piperacillin and 0.5 grams of tazobactam) (Rx) [*Tazocin*].

### Packaging and storage
Prior to reconstitution, store below 40 °C (104 °F), preferably between 15 and 30 °C (59 and 86 °F), unless otherwise specified by manufacturer.

### Preparation of dosage form
To prepare initial dilution for intravenous use, add 5 mL of sterile water for injection, 5% dextrose injection, or sodium chloride injection to each vial and shake well until dissolved. This solution may be further diluted to the desired final volume with compatible intravenous diluents. Lactated Ringer's injection is *not* compatible as an initial diluent with piperacillin and tazobactam combination.

### Stability
After reconstitution for intravenous use, solutions retain their potency for 24 hours at room temperature (21 to 24 °C [70 to 75 °F]) or for up to 7 days if refrigerated at 4 °C (39 °F). Lactated Ringer's injection is compatible with piperacillin and tazobactam combination for up to 2 hours when used as a diluent after initial reconstitution with 5% dextrose injection or sodium chloride injection.

### Incompatibilities
Lactated Ringer's injection is *not* compatible as an initial diluent with piperacillin and tazobactam combination.
Extemporaneous admixtures of beta-lactam antibacterials (penicillins) and aminoglycosides may result in substantial mutual inactivation. If these groups of antibacterials are administered concurrently, they should be administered in separate sites at least 1 hour apart. Do not mix them in the same intravenous bag, bottle, or tubing.
When aminoglycosides and penicillins are administered separately by different routes, a reduction in aminoglycoside serum concentration may occur. Usually this is clinically significant only in patients with severely impaired renal function in whom the excretion of both medications is delayed.

### Additional information
The sodium content is approximately 2.35 mEq (2.35 mmol) per gram of piperacillin. This must be considered in patients on a restricted sodium intake when calculating total daily sodium intake.

---

## *TICARCILLIN AND CLAVULANATE*

## Summary of Differences
Precautions:
Drug interactions and/or related problems—Ticarcillin interacts with anticoagulants and other medications that affect blood clotting; clavulanic acid does not interact with probenecid.
Laboratory value alterations—May cause false-positive protein reaction for various urine protein tests; may decrease serum potassium concentrations; may increase prothrombin time and partial thromboplastin time; may increase serum sodium concentrations; may decrease uric acid.
Medical considerations/contraindications—Caution required in patients with history of bleeding problems; caution also required in patients with congestive heart failure, hypertension, or renal function impairment because of sodium content.
Side/adverse effects:
Increased risk of platelet dysfunction.

## Additional Dosing Information
Sterile ticarcillin disodium and clavulanate potassium and ticarcillin disodium and clavulanate potassium injection should be administered by intravenous infusion over a 30-minute period.

Patients with impaired renal function may require a reduction in dose and should be observed for hemorrhagic complications. After an initial loading dose of 3 grams of ticarcillin and 100 mg of clavulanic acid, adults with impaired renal function may require a reduction in dose as follows:

| Creatinine Clearance (mL/min)/ (mL/sec) | Dose/Dosing interval (based on ticarcillin content) |
|---|---|
| >60/1.0 | 3 grams every 4 hours |
| 30–60/0.50–1.0 | 2 grams every 4 hours |
| 10–30/0.17–0.50 | 2 grams every 8 hours |
| <10/0.17 | 2 grams every 12 hours |
| <10 with hepatic dysfunction | 2 grams every 24 hours |
| Peritoneal dialysis patients | 3 grams every 12 hours |
| Hemodialysis patients | 2 grams every 12 hours; and 3 grams after each dialysis |

## Parenteral Dosage Forms
Note: Bracketed uses in the *Dosage Forms* section refer to categories of use and/or indications that are not included in U.S. product labeling.

### STERILE TICARCILLIN DISODIUM AND CLAVULANATE POTASSIUM USP

### Usual adult and adolescent dose
Antibacterial—
Treatment:
Adults and adolescents up to 60 kg of body weight—Intravenous infusion, 33.3 to 50 mg of ticarcillin and 1.1 to 1.7 mg of clavulanic acid per kg of body weight every four hours; or 50 to 75 mg of ticarcillin and 1.7 to 2.5 mg of clavulanic acid per kg of body weight every six hours.
Adults and adolescents 60 kg of body weight and over—Intravenous infusion, 3 grams of ticarcillin and 100 mg of clavulanic acid every four to six hours.
[Surgical prophylaxis]:
Intravenous infusion, 3 grams of ticarcillin and 100 mg of clavulanic acid one-half to one hour prior to the start of surgery, or (for cesarean section) as soon as the umbilical cord is clamped, then 3.1 grams at four-hour intervals for a total of three doses.

### Usual pediatric dose
Antibacterial—
Infants less than 1 month of age:
Dosage has not been established.
Infants and children 1 month to 12 years of age:
Intravenous infusion, 50 mg of ticarcillin and 1.7 mg of clavulanic acid per kg of body weight every four to six hours.
Note: Children with cystic fibrosis—Intravenous infusion, 350 to 450 mg of ticarcillin and 11.7 to 17 mg of clavulanic acid per kg of body weight a day in divided doses.
Children 12 years of age and older:
See *Usual adult and adolescent dose (Adults and adolescents up to 60 kg of body weight).*

### Size(s) usually available
U.S.—
3.1 grams (3 grams of ticarcillin and 100 mg of clavulanic acid) (Rx) [*Timentin* (sodium 4.75 mEq [4.75 mmol] per gram)].
31 grams (30 grams of ticarcillin and 1 gram of clavulanic acid) (Rx) [*Timentin*].
Note: Although listed in the U.S. package insert, the 3.2-gram vial is not currently available, according to the manufacturer.
Canada—
3.1 grams (3 grams of ticarcillin and 100 mg of clavulanic acid) (Rx) [*Timentin* (sodium 4.75 mEq [4.75 mmol] per gram)].

### Packaging and storage
Prior to reconstitution, store below 40 °C (104 °F), preferably between 15 and 30 °C (59 and 86 °F), unless otherwise specified by manufacturer.

### Preparation of dosage form
To prepare initial dilution for direct intravenous use, add 13 mL of sterile water for injection or sodium chloride injection to each 3.1-gram vial to provide a ticarcillin concentration of approximately 200 mg per mL and a clavulanic acid concentration of approximately 6.7 mg per mL. The resulting solution should be further diluted to desired volume in sodium chloride injection, 5% dextrose injection, or lactated Ringer's injection and administered over a 30-minute period.
For reconstitution of piggyback infusion bottles or pharmacy bulk vials, see manufacturer's labeling for instructions. If the Y-type method of administration is used, the primary infusion should be temporarily discontinued during infusion of ticarcillin and clavulanate combination.

**Stability**

After reconstitution for intravenous use, solutions containing 200 mg of ticarcillin per mL retain their potency for 6 hours at room temperature (21 to 24 °C [70 to 75 °F]) or for up to 72 hours if refrigerated at 4 °C (39 °F). Solutions containing 10 to 100 mg of ticarcillin per mL in sodium chloride injection or lactated Ringer's injection retain their potency for 24 hours at room temperature (21 to 24 °C [70 to 75 °F]) or for 7 days if refrigerated at 4 °C (39 °F). Solutions containing 10 to 100 mg of ticarcillin per mL in 5% dextrose injection retain their potency for 24 hours at room temperature or for 3 days if refrigerated.

After reconstitution, solutions containing 100 mg of ticarcillin or less per mL in sodium chloride injection or lactated Ringer's injection may be frozen and stored for up to 30 days. Solutions in 5% dextrose injection may be frozen for 7 days. Thawed solutions should be used within 8 hours.

Solutions may vary in color from colorless to pale yellow.

**Incompatibilities**

Extemporaneous admixtures of beta-lactam antibacterials (penicillins) and aminoglycosides may result in substantial mutual inactivation. If these groups of antibacterials are administered concurrently, they should be administered in separate sites at least 1 hour apart. Do not mix them in the same intravenous bag, bottle, or tubing.

When aminoglycosides and penicillins are administered separately by different routes, a reduction in aminoglycoside serum concentration may occur. Usually this is clinically significant only in patients with severely impaired renal function in whom the excretion of both medications is delayed.

Sterile ticarcillin disodium and clavulanate potassium combination is incompatible with sodium bicarbonate.

**Additional information**

The sodium content is approximately 4.75 mEq (4.75 mmol) per gram of ticarcillin. This must be considered in patients on a restricted sodium intake when calculating total daily sodium intake.

The potassium content is approximately 0.15 mEq (6 mg) per 100 mg of clavulanic acid.

## TICARCILLIN DISODIUM AND CLAVULANATE POTASSIUM INJECTION

**Usual adult and adolescent dose**

See *Sterile Ticarcillin Disodium and Clavulanate Potassium USP.*

**Usual pediatric dose**

See *Sterile Ticarcillin Disodium and Clavulanate Potassium USP.*

**Strength(s) usually available**

U.S.—

3.1 grams (3 grams of ticarcillin and 100 mg of clavulanic acid) in 50 mL (Rx) [*Timentin* (sodium 4.75 mEq [4.75 mmol] per gram)].

3.1 grams (3 grams of ticarcillin and 100 mg of clavulanic acid) in 100 mL (Rx) [*Timentin* (sodium 4.75 mEq [4.75 mmol] per gram)].

Canada—

Not commercially available.

**Packaging and storage**

Do not store above −10 °C (14 °F), unless otherwise specified by manufacturer.

**Preparation of dosage form**

Thaw container at room temperature before administration, making sure that all ice crystals have melted.

Minibags should not be used in series connections. Doing so may result in air embolism because of residual air being drawn from the primary container before administration of intravenous solution from the secondary container is complete.

**Stability**

Thawed solutions should be used within 8 hours. Once thawed, solutions should not be refrozen.

**Incompatibilities**

Extemporaneous admixtures of beta-lactam antibacterials (penicillins) and aminoglycosides may result in substantial mutual inactivation. If these groups of antibacterials are administered concurrently, they should be administered in separate sites at least 1 hour apart. Do not mix them in the same intravenous bag, bottle, or tubing.

When aminoglycosides and penicillins are administered separately by different routes, a reduction in aminoglycoside serum concentration may occur. Usually this is clinically significant only in patients with severely impaired renal function in whom the excretion of both medications is delayed.

**Additional information**

The sodium content is approximately 4.75 mEq (4.75 mmol) per gram of ticarcillin. This must be considered in patients on a restricted sodium intake when calculating total daily sodium intake.

The potassium content is approximately 0.15 mEq (6 mg) per 100 mg of clavulanic acid.

---

Developed: 07/29/94
Revised: 04/19/95

---

## PENICILLIN V—See *Penicillins (Systemic)*

---

## PENTAERYTHRITOL TETRANITRATE—See *Nitrates (Systemic)*

---

# PENTAGASTRIN    Systemic

VA CLASSIFICATION (Primary): DX900

Note: For a listing of dosage forms and brand names by country availability, see *Dosage Forms* section(s). For a listing of brand names for the articles in this monograph, refer to the General Index.

## Category

Diagnostic aid (gastric function).

## Indications

**Accepted**

Anacidity (diagnosis)—Pentagastrin is indicated as a diagnostic aid for evaluation of gastric acid secretory function. It is effective in testing for anacidity (achlorhydria) in patients with suspected pernicious anemia, atrophic gastritis, or gastric carcinoma. It is also effective in determining the reduction in acid output after operations for peptic ulcer, such as vagotomy or gastric resection.

Hypersecretory conditions, gastric (diagnosis)—Pentagastrin is indicated as a diagnostic aid in testing for gastric hypersecretion in patients with suspected duodenal ulcer or postoperative stomal ulcer, and for the diagnosis of Zollinger-Ellison tumor.

## Pharmacology/Pharmacokinetics

**Mechanism of action/Effect**

The exact mechanism by which pentagastrin stimulates gastric acid, pepsin, and intrinsic factor secretion is unknown; however, since pentagastrin is an analogue of natural gastrin, it is believed that it excites the oxyntic cells of the stomach to secrete to their maximum capacity.

Pentagastrin stimulates pancreatic secretion, especially when administered in large intramuscular doses. Pentagastrin also increases gastrointestinal motility by a direct effect on the intestinal smooth muscle. However, it delays gastric emptying time probably by stimulation of terminal antral contractions, which enhance retropulsion.

**Other actions/effects**

Pentagastrin increases blood flow in the gastric mucosa, inhibits absorption of water and electrolytes from the ileum, and promotes sodium and chloride diuresis. It causes contraction of the smooth muscle of the lower esophageal sphincter when administered intravenously. Pentagastrin produces an increase in the motor activity of the colon and rectum.

**Absorption**

Rapidly absorbed after parenteral administration.

**Biotransformation**

Primarily hepatic.

**Half-life**

10 minutes or less.

**Onset of action**

10 minutes.

**Time to peak effect**

20 to 30 minutes.

**Duration of action**

60 to 80 minutes.

**Elimination**

Renal.

# Precautions to Consider

## Pregnancy/Reproduction
Pregnancy—Studies have not been done in humans.
Studies have not been done in animals.
FDA Pregnancy Category C.

## Breast-feeding
It is not known whether pentagastrin is distributed into breast milk. However, problems in humans have not been documented.

## Pediatrics
Appropriate studies on the relationship of age to the effects of pentagastrin have not been performed in the pediatric population. Safety and efficacy have not been established.

## Geriatrics
No information is available on the relationship of age to the effects of pentagastrin in geriatric patients.

## Drug interactions and/or related problems
The following drug interactions and/or related problems have been selected on the basis of their potential clinical significance (possible mechanism in parentheses where appropriate)—not necessarily inclusive (» = major clinical significance):

See *Diagnostic interference.*

## Diagnostic interference
The following have been selected on the basis of their potential clinical significance (possible effect in parentheses where appropriate)—not necessarily inclusive (» = major clinical significance):

With results of *this test*
~*Due to other medications*
» Antacids
(administration on the morning of the test may decrease the total effects of pentagastrin and thus is not recommended)
» Anticholinergics, or other medications with anticholinergic activity (see *Appendix II*) or
» Histamine H$_2$-receptor antagonists, such as, cimetidine, famotidine, nizatidine, and ranitidine
(concurrent use may antagonize the effect of pentagastrin; administration of these medications is not recommended during the 24 hours preceding the test)
» Omeprazole
(concurrent use may antagonize the effect of pentagastrin on gastric acid secretion; administration of omeprazole is not recommended during the 96 hours preceding the test)

With physiology/laboratory test values
Bicarbonate secretion and
Biliary flow and
Pancreatic enzyme secretion
(may be increased)

## Medical considerations/Contraindications
The medical considerations/contraindications included here have been selected on the basis of their potential clinical significance (reasons given in parentheses where appropriate)—not necessarily inclusive (» = major clinical significance).

*Except under special circumstances, this medication should not be used when the following medical problem exists:*
» Peptic ulcer, acute, obstructing, penetrating, or bleeding
(condition may be exacerbated)

*Risk-benefit should be considered when the following medical problems exist:*
Biliary disease or
Hepatic function impairment or
Pancreatitis, acute
(stimulation of secretion of pancreatic enzymes and bicarbonate, and increased flow of bile may be undesirable in these conditions)
Sensitivity to pentagastrin

# Side/Adverse Effects
The following side/adverse effects have been selected on the basis of their potential clinical significance (possible signs and symptoms in parentheses where appropriate)—not necessarily inclusive:

## Those indicating need for medical attention
Incidence rare
*Allergic reaction* (skin rash or hives)

## Those indicating need for medical attention only if they continue or are bothersome
Incidence more frequent
*Gas; gastrointestinal effects* (nausea or vomiting; stomach pain; urge to have bowel movement)—usually disappear within 15 minutes after subcutaneous administration

Incidence less frequent or rare
*Blurred vision; cardiovascular effects* (fast heartbeat; unusual warmth or flushing of skin)—usually transient; *chills; dizziness, faintness, or lightheadedness; drowsiness; feeling of heaviness of arms and legs; headache; increased sweating; numbness, tingling, pain, or weakness in hands or feet; shortness of breath; unusual tiredness*

# Patient Consultation
As an aid to patient consultation, refer to *Advice for the Patient, Pentagastrin (Diagnostic).*

In providing consultation, consider emphasizing the following selected information (» = major clinical significance):

## Description of use
Procedure for pentagastrin test: Dose of pentagastrin based on body weight and must be determined by doctor; pentagastrin is injected subcutaneously; 10 or 15 minutes after injection, stomach contents emptied and tested for volume and acidity; procedure may be repeated 4 or 6 times

## Before having this test
» Conditions affecting use, especially:
Sensitivity to pentagastrin
Other medications, especially antacids, anticholinergics, histamine H$_2$-receptor antagonists, or omeprazole
Other medical problems, especially acute, obstructing, penetrating, or bleeding peptic ulcer

## Preparation for this test
Not eating prior to the test beginning the night before or drinking for at least 4 hours before test is administered
» Not taking antacids on morning of test
» Not taking anticholinergics, cimetidine, famotidine, nizatidine, ranitidine, or other medications that inhibit gastric secretion within 24 hours before test; not taking omeprazole within 96 hours before test

## Side/adverse effects
Signs of potential side effects, especially allergic reaction

# General Dosing Information
Not eating prior to the test beginning the night before the test and abstaining from liquids at least 4 hours before the test are usually recommended since the presence of food or liquid in the stomach may interfere with the interpretation of test results.

After the injection of pentagastrin, four aspirates at 15-minute intervals or six aspirates at 10-minute intervals are collected and examined to determine the stimulated acid output.

Use of doses larger than the recommended dose may cause inhibition of gastric acid secretion.

Pentagastrin has also been administered intramuscularly, intravenously, and as a powder by nasal inhalation. The intramuscular dose used has been the same as the subcutaneous dose. The intravenous infusion dose has ranged from 0.1 to 12 mcg (0.0001 to 0.012 mg) per kg of body weight per hour administered in a 0.9% sodium chloride injection. By nasal inhalation, 1 mg of the powder has been administered every 10 minutes for 1 hour.

# Parenteral Dosage Forms

## PENTAGASTRIN INJECTION

### Usual adult and adolescent dose
Gastric function diagnosis—
Subcutaneous, 6 mcg (0.006 mg) per kg of body weight.

### Usual pediatric dose
Dosage has not been established.

### Usual geriatric dose
See *Usual adult and adolescent dose.*

### Strength(s) usually available
U.S.—
250 mcg (0.25 mg) per mL (Rx) [*Peptavlon*].
Canada—
250 mcg (0.25 mg) per mL (Rx) [*Peptavlon*].

### Packaging and storage
Store between 2 and 8 °C (36 to 46 °F), unless otherwise specified by manufacturer. Protect from freezing.

Revised: 07/14/93
Interim revision: 07/01/94

# PENTAMIDINE    Inhalation

VA CLASSIFICATION (Primary): AP109
Note: For a listing of dosage forms and brand names by country availability, see *Dosage Forms* section(s). For a listing of brand names for the articles in this monograph, refer to the General Index.

## Category
Antiprotozoal.

## Indications
Note: Bracketed information in the *Indications* section refers to uses that are not included in U.S. product labeling.

**Accepted**

Pneumonia, *Pneumocystis carinii* (PCP) (prophylaxis)—Aerosolized pentamidine is indicated in both secondary prophylaxis (patients who have already had at least one episode of *Pneumocystis carinii* pneumonia), and primary prophylaxis (HIV-infected patients with a CD4 lymphocyte count less than or equal to 200 cells per cubic millimeter) of *Pneumocystis carinii* pneumonia.

[Pneumonia, *Pneumocystis carinii* (PCP) (treatment)][1]—Aerosolized pentamidine is used in the treatment of mild (A-a gradient < 30 mm Hg) *Pneumocystis carinii* pneumonia. However, preliminary studies have suggested that aerosolized pentamidine may be less effective than conventional systemic therapies; patients receiving this regimen should be followed closely for evidence of progressive disease.

---

[1]Not included in Canadian product labeling.

## Pharmacology/Pharmacokinetics

**Physicochemical characteristics**

Molecular weight—340.42.

**Mechanism of action/Effect**

Not clearly defined; pentamidine may interfere with incorporation of nucleotides into RNA and DNA and may inhibit oxidative phosphorylation, resulting in inhibition of DNA, RNA, phospholipid, and protein biosynthesis; may also interfere with folate transformation.

**Absorption**

Systemic absorption of inhaled pentamidine is minimal, with serum pentamidine concentrations less than 20 nanograms per mL after a nebulized dose of 4 mg per kg in most cases (versus 612 nanograms per mL after a single intravenous dose of 4 mg per kg). Peak systemic absorption occurs at, or near, completion of inhalation therapy.

**Distribution**

Aerosolized pentamidine produces concentrations approximately 10 to 100 times higher in the lungs than would a comparable dose of intravenous pentamidine.

**Elimination**

Unknown; in one study, cumulative percentage of total dose renally excreted was 0.4% over a 72-hour period.

## Precautions to Consider

**Carcinogenicity/Mutagenicity**

Pentamidine has not been shown to be mutagenic in Ames studies. Carcinogenicity studies have not been done.

**Pregnancy/Reproduction**

Fertility—Studies have not been done.

Pregnancy—Studies with aerosolized pentamidine have not been done in humans.

Studies with aerosolized pentamidine have not been done in animals. However, studies in rabbits have shown that systemic pentamidine was associated with an increased incidence of post-implantation losses and delayed fetal ossification.

FDA Pregnancy Category C.

**Breast-feeding**

It is not known whether pentamidine is distributed into breast milk.

**Pediatrics**

No information is available on the relationship of age to the effects of aerosolized pentamidine in pediatric patients. Safety and efficacy have not been established. However, if sulfamethoxazole and trimethoprim combination is not tolerated, aerosolized pentamidine is recommended for children 5 years of age and older.

**Geriatrics**

No information is available on the relationship of age to the effects of pentamidine in geriatric patients.

**Dental**

Pentamidine may cause a bitter or metallic taste, gingivitis, hypersalivation, or dry mouth.

**Drug interactions and/or related problems**

At this time, no clinically significant drug interactions and/or related problems have been documented in patients receiving prophylactic aerosolized pentamidine.

**Medical considerations/Contraindications**

The medical considerations/contraindications included here have been selected on the basis of their potential clinical significance (reasons given in parentheses where appropriate)—not necessarily inclusive (» = major clinical significance).

***Except under special circumstances, this medication should not be used when the following medical problem exists:***

» Allergy to pentamidine

(aerosolized pentamidine is contraindicated in patients with a history of an anaphylactic reaction to inhaled or systemic pentamidine)

***Risk-benefit should be considered when the following medical problem exists:***

Asthma

(aerosolized pentamidine may induce acute bronchospasm, usually in patients with a history of asthma; this may be reduced by pretreatment with a bronchodilator)

**Patient monitoring**

The following may be especially important in patient monitoring (other tests may be warranted in some patients, depending on condition; » = major clinical significance):

At this time, there are no particular laboratory tests or monitoring parameters recommended routinely for patients receiving prophylactic aerosolized pentamidine. However, baseline parameters, including pulmonary function tests, serum amylase and lipase, may be obtained for the first treatment, and then followed as needed.

## Side/Adverse Effects

Note: The prophylactic use of aerosolized pentamidine has a very low incidence of severe side effects. Many adverse reactions will be due to other medications, other concurrent infections, or the HIV disease itself, and may be difficult to differentiate.

Coughing and bronchospasm occur primarily in patients who are cigarette smokers and continue to smoke, or have an underlying pulmonary disease, such as asthma.

A number of cases of extrapulmonary pneumocystosis and pneumothorax have been reported in patients receiving aerosolized pentamidine. These are thought to be infectious complications due to subclinical, peripheral infection and poor systemic distribution of aerosolized pentamidine. Although the incidence is not known at this time, one study found that extrapulmonary pneumocystosis appears to occur more frequently in, but is not limited to, patients who have been diagnosed with AIDS for longer than 12 months. These patients usually have had prior episodes of *Pneumocystis carinii* pneumonia (PCP), often do not have concurrent pneumonia, are receiving concurrent zidovudine, and have had prolonged treatment with aerosolized pentamidine. It is suggested that use of zidovudine and prophylactic aerosolized pentamidine may allow for the emergence of extrapulmonary pneumocystosis.

The following side/adverse effects have been selected on the basis of their potential clinical significance (possible signs and symptoms in parentheses where appropriate)—not necessarily inclusive:

**Those indicating need for medical attention**

Incidence more frequent

*Chest pain or congestion; coughing; dyspnea* (difficulty in breathing); *pharyngitis* (burning pain, dryness, or sensation of lump in throat; difficulty in swallowing); *skin rash; wheezing*

Incidence rare

*Extrapulmonary pneumocystosis*—most frequent sites include the spleen, liver, lymph nodes, and eyes; *pancreatitis* (nausea; pain in upper abdomen, possibly radiating to the back; vomiting)—may occur more frequently with prolonged use; *pneumothorax* (sudden onset of severe breathing difficulty; severe pain in chest)

Incidence rare—with daily treatment doses only

*Hypoglycemia, mild* (anxiety; chills; cold sweats; cool, pale skin; headache; increased hunger; nausea; nervousness; shakiness); *renal insufficiency* (decreased urination; loss of appetite; nausea; unusual tiredness)

**Those not indicating need for medical attention**
Incidence less frequent
*Bitter or metallic taste*

## Patient Consultation

As an aid to patient consultation, refer to *Advice for the Patient, Pentamidine (Inhalation)*.

In providing consultation, consider emphasizing the following selected information (» = major clinical significance):

**Before using this medication**
» Conditions affecting use, especially:
   Allergy to pentamidine

**Proper use of this medication**
Importance of receiving medication for full course of therapy and on regular schedule
» Proper dosing
Missed dose: Receiving therapy as soon as possible

**Precautions while using this medication**
If also using a bronchodilator inhaler, using about 5 to 10 minutes prior to aerosolized pentamidine
Possible bitter or metallic taste; dissolving a hard candy in mouth after administration of medication
Cigarette smokers who continue to smoke are more likely to experience coughing and bronchospasm during aerosolized pentamidine therapy

**Side/adverse effects**
Signs of potential side effects, especially chest pain or congestion, coughing, dyspnea, pharyngitis, skin rash, wheezing, extrapulmonary pneumocystosis, pancreatitis, pneumothorax, hypoglycemia, and renal insufficiency
A bitter or metallic taste may occur; however, it is medically insignificant

## General Dosing Information

Coughing and bronchospasm occur primarily in cigarette smokers who continue to smoke, or patients with an underlying pulmonary disease, such as asthma. A higher incidence of coughing and bronchospasm may be related to larger particle sizes; however, these symptoms appear to occur most frequently due to an increased particle load with larger doses. Pretreatment with a bronchodilator, e.g., albuterol, metaproterenol, or terbutaline, helps to alleviate this problem and may improve pentamidine distribution in the lung.

It is important that as much medication as possible reach the upper lobes of the lungs, since upper lobe *P. carinii* pneumonia relapses have occurred in patients while they were receiving aerosolized pentamidine. There appears to be a more uniform distribution of aerosolized pentamidine in the lungs when it is administered to patients in a supine or recumbent position.

Before aerosolized pentamidine treatment is started, a tuberculin skin test, chest x-ray, and sputum culture, if possible, should be performed to rule out tuberculosis due to *Mycobacterium tuberculosis*. A tuberculin skin test alone may not be useful because false negative readings often occur in AIDS patients. The risk of active disease or reactivation of latent tuberculosis infection is more prevalent in HIV-infected people. Also, the risk of transmission of tuberculosis to health care workers or others in the vicinity may exist.

Health care workers are advised to administer aerosolized pentamidine in a well-ventilated room if possible. Although one study found the environmental levels of pentamidine in a treatment room to be low, long-term occupational studies have not been done and the risk has not been established. Of primary concern is the previously mentioned risk of transmission of tuberculosis or other respiratory pathogens via aerosols, as well as anecdotal reports of a reversible decrease in pulmonary function testing parameters and chemical conjunctivitis due to ocular exposure to aerosolized pentamidine.

Two types of nebulizers have been shown to be effective in decreasing the incidence of *P. carinii* pneumonia. Respirgard II is a jet nebulizer and is used with NebuPent and Pentacarinat; Fisoneb is an ultrasonic nebulizer and is used with Pneumopent. Jet nebulizers use a high-flow gas to shear liquid strands from a thin layer of solution. The liquid strands hit a baffle, creating a wide variety of particle sizes. Larger particles generally fall by gravity and get reincorporated into the solution. Ultrasonic nebulizers generate an ultrahigh frequency sound, creating a geyser from which particles are expelled. When the flow through the nebulizer is interrupted, as with tidal breathing, the smaller particles coalesce into larger particles. Because of this, measurements of output and particle size will vary with different operating conditions.

Particle size produced by the nebulizer is an important factor in the location of aerosol deposition. The optimal size for deposition in the alveoli, where *Pneumocystis carinii* pneumonia (PCP) causes damage, is 1 to 2 microns; the optimal size for tracheobronchial deposition is 4 to 7 microns. Many factors can affect and limit aerosol deposition into the alveoli, including inspiratory flowrates, frequency of respiration, breath-holding, tidal volumes, and airway narrowing from bronchospasm, emphysema, mucus, and PCP.

Because of the differences in nebulizers and the efficacy with which they deliver aerosolized pentamidine, the nebulizers should not be utilized interchangeably with the different dosing regimens. The two regimens shown to be effective are described below.

## Inhalation Dosage Forms

Note: Bracketed uses in the *Dosage Forms* section refer to categories of use and/or indications that are not included in U.S. product labeling.

### PENTAMIDINE ISETHIONATE FOR INHALATION SOLUTION

**Usual adult and adolescent dose**
Pneumonia, *Pneumocystis carinii*—
For *NebuPent* and *Pentacarinat* using the Respirgard II jet nebulizer:
Prophylaxis—
Oral inhalation, 300 mg every four weeks, administered via the Respirgard II nebulizer. The aerosol treatment should be continued over a period of approximately thirty to forty-five minutes, until the nebulizer chamber is empty.
Note: A prophylactic dose of 150 mg every two weeks, administered via the Respirgard II nebulizer, has also been used if the patient cannot tolerate a single monthly dose. One study found that although patients who received 300 mg monthly had a lower rate of PCP than those receiving 150 mg every two weeks, the difference was not significant.
[Treatment][1]—
Oral inhalation, 600 mg a day, administered via the Respirgard II nebulizer for twenty-one days. Continue the aerosol treatment over a period of approximately twenty-five to thirty minutes.
Note: The flow rate for the nebulizer should be 5 to 7 liters per minute from a 40- to 50-pounds-per-square-inch (PSI) air or oxygen source.
Low pressure compressors (<20 PSI) should not be used.
For *Pneumopent* using the Fisoneb ultrasonic nebulizer:
Loading dose (prophylaxis)—
Oral inhalation, 60 mg, administered via the Fisoneb ultrasonic nebulizer, every twenty-four to seventy-two hours for a total of 5 doses over a two week period. The aerosol treatment should be continued over a period of approximately fifteen minutes, until the nebulizer chamber is empty.
Maintenance dose (prophylaxis)—
Oral inhalation, 60 mg, administered via the Fisoneb ultrasonic nebulizer, every two weeks.
Note: The flow rate of the nebulizer should be set at the mid-flow mark.

**Usual pediatric dose**
Pneumonia, *Pneumocystis carinii*—
Prophylaxis: Dosage has not been established. However, 300 mg every four weeks has been used in children 5 years of age and older who cannot tolerate sulfamethoxazole and trimethoprim combination.

**Size(s) usually available**
U.S.—
300 mg (Rx) [*NebuPent* (Respirgard II nebulizer)].
Canada—
60 mg (Rx) [*Pneumopent* (Fisoneb nebulizer)].
300 mg (Rx) [*Pentacarinat* (Respirgard II nebulizer)].

**Packaging and storage**
Prior to reconstitution, store between 15 and 30 °C (59 and 86 °F), unless otherwise specified by manufacturer.

**Preparation of dosage form**

For *NebuPent* and *Pentacarinat*—

To prepare pentamidine for oral inhalation *prophylaxis*, add 6 mL of sterile water for injection to each 300-mg vial of sterile pentamidine isethionate.

To prepare pentamidine for oral inhalation *treatment*, add 6 mL of sterile water for injection to 600 mg of sterile pentamidine isethionate.

For administration, place the entire reconstituted contents into the reservoir chamber of the Respirgard II nebulizer.

For *Pneumopent*—

To prepare for oral inhalation, remove the rubber stopper and put it aside, upside down, on a clean surface for later use. Add 3 to 5 mL of sterile water for inhalation or sterile water for injection to the vial. Do not use tap water and do not use normal saline. Replace the rubber stopper. The powder should dissolve immediately; if it does not, gently shake the vial to mix it. It should form a clear, colorless solution; if the solution is cloudy, do not use it.

For administration, place the entire reconstituted contents into the chamber of the Fisoneb ultrasonic nebulizer.

**Stability**

For *NebuPent*—

After reconstitution, solutions in concentrations of 93 mg per mL retain at least 90% of their potency for up to 4 months when frozen in plastic syringes at-20 °C. Do not defrost and refreeze.

For *Pentacarinat*—

Store unopened vials at room temperature; protect from light.

After reconstitution, solutions in concentrations of approximately 2 mg per mL are stable for up to 24 hours at room temperature.

For *Pneumopent*—

Store unopened vials at room temperature.

After reconstitution, solution may be stored for up to 24 hours at room temperature or up to 48 hours in a refrigerator. Do not freeze.

**Incompatibilities**

Reconstitution of pentamidine with saline solutions may cause pentamidine to precipitate out of solution.

**Additional information**

Pentamidine inhalation solution should not be mixed with any other medications.

Do not use the Respirgard II nebulizer to administer a bronchodilator.

---

[1]Not included in Canadian product labeling.

## Selected Bibliography

Monk JP, Benfield P. Inhaled pentamidine. An overview of its pharmacological properties and a review of its therapeutic use in Pneumocystis carinii pneumonia. Drugs 1990; 39 (5): 741-56.

Revised: 03/03/92
Interim revision: 03/28/94

---

# PENTAMIDINE   Systemic

VA CLASSIFICATION (Primary): AP109

Note: For a listing of dosage forms and brand names by country availability, see *Dosage Forms* section(s). For a listing of brand names for the articles in this monograph, refer to the General Index.

---

## Category

Antiprotozoal.

## Indications

Note: Bracketed information in the *Indications* section refers to uses that are not included in U.S. product labeling.

**Accepted**

Pneumonia, *Pneumocystis carinii* (treatment)—Pentamidine is indicated in the treatment of *Pneumocystis carinii* pneumonia (PCP) in immunocompromised patients, including patients with acquired immunodeficiency syndrome (AIDS). Sulfamethoxazole and trimethoprim combination is considered to be the primary agent for PCP in patients who can tolerate it.

[Leishmaniasis, visceral (treatment)][1]—Pentamidine is used as a secondary agent in the treatment of visceral leishmaniasis (kala-azar) caused by *Leishmania donovani*. Stibogluconate sodium, a pentavalent antimony derivative, is considered to be the primary agent for visceral leishmaniasis.

[Leishmaniasis, cutaneous (treatment)][1]—Pentamidine is used as a secondary agent in the treatment of cutaneous leishmaniasis caused by *Leishmania tropica, L. major, L. mexicana, L. aethiopica, L. peruviana, L. guyanensis,* and *L. braziliensis*. Stibogluconate sodium, a pentavalent antimony derivative, is considered to be the primary agent for cutaneous leishmaniasis.

[Trypanosomiasis, African (treatment)][1]—Pentamidine is used as a secondary agent in the treatment of African trypanosomiasis (trypanosome fever; African sleeping sickness) caused by *Trypanosoma brucei gambiense* and *T. b. rhodesiense* in patients with early or hemolymphatic disease without central nervous system (CNS) involvement. Suramin is considered to be the primary agent for African trypanosomiasis in these patients.

In patients with late or chronic trypanosomiasis involving the CNS, melarsoprol, an arsenical complexed with dimercaprol, is considered the primary agent.

Not all species or strains of a particular organism may be susceptible to pentamidine.

**Unaccepted**

Since pentamidine does not cross the blood-brain barrier, it is not useful in patients with late or chronic trypanosomiasis involving the CNS.

---

[1]Not included in Canadian product labeling.

## Pharmacology/Pharmacokinetics

**Physicochemical characteristics**

Molecular weight—Pentamidine: 340.42.

**Mechanism of action/Effect**

Not clearly defined; pentamidine may interfere with incorporation of nucleotides into RNA and DNA and inhibit oxidative phosphorylation and biosynthesis of DNA, RNA, protein, and phospholipid; may also interfere with folate transformation.

**Other actions/effects**

May also have antifungal activity.

**Absorption**

Poorly absorbed from the gastrointestinal tract; must be given parenterally.

**Distribution**

Rapidly distributed after administration; distribution half-life of 5 to 15 minutes after intravenous administration, 0.9 hours after intramuscular administration. In humans, highest concentrations of pentamidine were found in the liver, kidneys, adrenal glands, and spleen; lung concentrations were lower than concentrations in these organs, and accumulated over a 4 to 5 day period. There were indications of very slow uptake into the CNS, with pentamidine being detected in brain tissue approximately 30 days after the start of daily therapy.

Apparent Vol$_D$ at steady state—3 to 32 liters per kg (L/kg).

**Protein binding**

High (69%). Rapidly bound to tissues following administration.

**Storage**

In humans, appears to be stored in the body to some extent, and slowly excreted; in mice, may be stored for months in the kidneys and liver.

**Biotransformation**

In rats, metabolized to as many as 6 primary metabolic forms; human metabolism is unknown.

**Half-life**

Intramuscular—9.1 to 13.2 hours.

Intravenous—Approximately 6.5 hours.

Terminal half-life—2 to 4 weeks.

Renal function impairment—Pentamidine half-life may be prolonged in patients with renal dysfunction; however, no correlation between renal function and plasma clearance of pentamidine has been found.

**Time to peak serum concentration**
Intramuscular—0.5 to 1 hour.
Intravenous—End of infusion (1 to 2 hours).

**Peak serum concentration**
Intramuscular—0.2 to 1.4 mcg per mL (mcg/mL) after 4 mg per kg of body weight (mg/kg).
Intravenous—0.5 to 3.4 mcg/mL after 4 mg/kg infused over 1 to 2 hours.
Multiple dosing results in progressive drug accumulation; this may occur even in patients with normal renal function who receive a reduced daily dose of intravenous pentamidine.

**Elimination**
Renal—4 to 17% of intramuscular dose excreted in urine over 24 hours; approximately 2.5% of intravenous dose excreted in urine over 24 hours. Patients may continue to excrete decreasing amounts in urine for up to 8 weeks following discontinuation of therapy.
Fecal—In humans, no information available; in mice, excreted in feces in an amount approximately ¼ that in urine.
In dialysis—Neither peritoneal dialysis nor hemodialysis appears to significantly reduce plasma pentamidine concentrations.

## Precautions to Consider

### Carcinogenicity/Mutagenicity
No studies have been conducted to evaluate the potential of pentamidine as a carcinogen or mutagen.

### Pregnancy/Reproduction
Fertility—Studies have not been done.

Pregnancy—Adequate and well-controlled studies in humans have not been done.

Pentamidine has been found to cross the placenta in rats given high doses late in pregnancy. Studies in rabbits have also shown pentamidine to be mildly embryotoxic, with an increase in post-implantation losses and delayed fetal ossification at doses of 1, 3, and 8 mg per kg of body weight (mg/kg)

FDA Pregnancy Category C.

### Breast-feeding
It is not known whether pentamidine is distributed into breast milk. However, because of the potential risks to the newborn, breast-feeding is not recommended during pentamidine therapy.

### Pediatrics
Limited clinical and pharmacokinetic data are available in children; however, the mg/kg dose used in children is the same as that used in adults, and side effects seen in children are similar to those seen in adults. No pediatrics-specific problems have been documented to date.

### Geriatrics
No information is available on the relationship of age to the effects of pentamidine in geriatric patients.

### Dental
Systemic pentamidine may rarely cause an unpleasant metallic taste.
Pentamidine may cause leukopenia and thrombocytopenia, resulting in an increased incidence of certain microbial infections, delayed healing, and gingival bleeding. Dental work, whenever possible, should be completed prior to initiation of therapy or deferred until blood counts have returned to normal. Patients should be instructed in proper oral hygiene during treatment, including caution in use of regular toothbrushes, dental floss, and toothpicks.

### Drug interactions and/or related problems
The following drug interactions and/or related problems have been selected on the basis of their potential clinical significance (possible mechanism in parentheses where appropriate)—not necessarily inclusive (» = major clinical significance):

Note: Combinations containing any of the following medications, depending on the amount present, may also interact with this medication.

Blood dyscrasia–causing medications (See *Appendix II*) or
» Bone marrow depressants, other (See *Appendix II*) or
» Radiation therapy
(concurrent use with pentamidine may increase the abnormal hematologic effects of these medications and radiation therapy; dosage reduction may be required)
» Didanosine
(concurrent use with pentamidine may increase the potential for development of pancreatitis)
Erythromycin
(concurrent use of intravenous erythromycin with pentamidine may increase the potential for development of torsades de pointes)

» Foscarnet
(concurrent use with pentamidine may result in severe, but reversible, hypocalcemia, hypomagnesemia, and nephrotoxicity)
» Nephrotoxic medications, other (See *Appendix II*)
(concurrent use of other nephrotoxic medications with pentamidine may increase the potential for nephrotoxicity; renal function determinations, dosage reductions, and/or dosage interval adjustments may be required)

### Laboratory value alterations
The following have been selected on the basis of their potential clinical significance (possible effect in parentheses where appropriate)—not necessarily inclusive (» = major clinical significance):

With physiology/laboratory test values
Alanine aminotransferase (ALT [SGPT]) and
Alkaline phosphatase, serum, and
Aspartate aminotransferase (AST [SGOT]) and
Bilirubin, serum
(values may be increased)
» Blood urea nitrogen (BUN) and
» Creatinine, serum
(concentrations may be increased)
Calcium, serum and
Magnesium, serum
(concentrations may be decreased)
» Glucose, blood
(concentrations may be increased or decreased since both hypoglycemia and hyperglycemia have occurred)
Potassium, serum
(concentrations may be increased)

### Medical considerations/Contraindications
The medical considerations/contraindications included here have been selected on the basis of their potential clinical significance (reasons given in parentheses where appropriate)—not necessarily inclusive (» = major clinical significance).

*Except under special circumstances, this medication should not be used when the following medical problem exists:*
» Previous allergic reaction to pentamidine
(pentamidine is contraindicated in patients with a history of an anaphylactic reaction to inhaled or systemic pentamidine)

*Risk-benefit should be considered when the following medical problems exist:*
Anemia or
» Bleeding disorders, history of, or
» Bone marrow depression
(pentamidine may cause hematologic abnormalities, resulting in anemia, leukopenia, and thrombocytopenia)
» Cardiac disease or arrhythmias
(pentamidine may cause fatal cardiac arrhythmias, tachycardia, torsades de pointes, or other cardiotoxicity)
» Dehydration or
» Renal function impairment
(pentamidine may cause azotemia or acute renal insufficiency; dehydration may contribute to renal toxicity)
» Diabetes mellitus or
» Hypoglycemia
(pentamidine may cause hypoglycemia or hyperglycemia and may aggravate diabetes mellitus)
Hepatic function impairment
(pentamidine may cause an increase in AST [SGOT], ALT [SGPT], bilirubin, and alkaline phosphatase)
» Hypotension
(pentamidine may cause sudden severe hypotension; this is seen most frequently after intramuscular injections and rapid intravenous infusions)
» Risk-benefit should also be considered in patients who have had previous cytotoxic drug therapy or radiation therapy.

### Patient monitoring
The following may be especially important in patient monitoring (other tests may be warranted in some patients, depending on condition; » = major clinical significance):
» Blood pressure determinations
(since sudden, severe hypotension may occur, even after a single intramuscular or intravenous dose of pentamidine, patients should be lying down and their blood pressure should be closely monitored during administration and several times thereafter until blood pressure is stable)

» Blood urea nitrogen (BUN) and
» Creatinine, serum
    (concentrations may be required prior to and daily during therapy
    since pentamidine may be nephrotoxic; serum creatinine concen-
    trations up to 6 mg per dL, as well as acute renal failure with even
    higher serum creatinine concentrations, have been reported; pa-
    tients with severely impaired renal function may require a reduc-
    tion in dose)
  Calcium, serum and
  Magnesium, serum
    (concentrations may be required prior to and every 3 days during
    therapy since hypocalcemia and hypomagnesemia due to pentam-
    idine-induced tubular injury may occur)
» Complete blood counts (CBCs) or
» Platelet counts
    (may be required prior to and every 3 days during therapy since
    pentamidine may cause severe leukopenia, thrombocytopenia, and,
    occasionally, anemia)
» Electrocardiograms (ECGs)
    (may be required at regular intervals during therapy since fatalities
    due to cardiac arrhythmias, tachycardia, torsades de pointes, or
    other cardiotoxicity have been reported; potassium and magnesium
    concentrations should also be monitored; patients who develop
    monomorphic and polymorphic ventricular tachycardia may benefit
    from rapid intravenous injection of magnesium sulfate)
» Glucose concentrations, blood
    (pentamidine may cause hypoglycemia, which may be associated
    with pancreatic islet cell necrosis and inappropriately high plasma
    insulin concentrations; blood glucose concentrations below 20 mg
    per dL have been reported; hyperglycemia and permanent diabetes
    mellitus, with or without preceding hypoglycemia, have also oc-
    curred, sometimes up to several months after therapy is discontin-
    ued; therefore, blood glucose determinations may be required prior
    to therapy, daily during therapy, and up to several months follow-
    ing therapy)
  Liver function tests
    (hepatic function determinations, including bilirubin, alkaline
    phosphatase, AST [SGOT], and ALT [SGPT], may be required
    prior to and every 3 days during therapy since elevated hepatic
    function test results have been reported)

## Side/Adverse Effects

Note: Rapid intravenous infusion may result in a precipitous drop in blood
    pressure. The risk of hypotension is decreased if pentamidine is
    administered by slow intravenous infusion, over at least 60 minutes,
    and preferably over 2 hours.

    Pentamidine can produce prolonged, severe hypoglycemia lasting
    from 1 day to several weeks. This hypoglycemia has been associ-
    ated with a direct cytolytic effect on pancreatic beta islet cells,
    leading to insulin release. It usually occurs after 5 to 7 days of
    therapy; however, it may not occur until after pentamidine has been
    discontinued. One study found the risk of hypoglycemia to be in-
    creased with higher doses, longer duration of therapy, and retreat-
    ment within 3 months.

    Hyperglycemia and diabetes mellitus may occur up to several
    months after pentamidine therapy has been discontinued.

The following side/adverse effects have been selected on the basis of their
potential clinical significance (possible signs and symptoms in parentheses where appropriate)—not necessarily inclusive:

### Those indicating need for medical attention
Incidence more frequent
    *Diabetes mellitus or hyperglycemia* (drowsiness; flushed, dry skin;
    fruit-like breath odor; increased thirst; increased urination; loss of ap-
    petite); *elevated liver function tests; hypoglycemia* (anxiety; chills;
    cold sweats; cool, pale skin; headache; increased hunger; nausea; nerv-
    ousness; shakiness); *hypotension* (blurred vision; confusion; dizziness;
    fainting; lightheadedness; unusual tiredness or weakness); *leukopenia
    or neutropenia* (sore throat and fever); *nephrotoxicity* (decreased fre-
    quency of urination; loss of appetite; weakness); *thrombocytopenia*
    (unusual bleeding or bruising)
Incidence less frequent
    *Anemia* (unusual tiredness or weakness); *cardiac arrhythmias* (rapid
    or irregular pulse; ECG abnormalities; torsades de pointes)—primarily
    ventricular tachycardia; *hypersensitivity* (skin rash, redness, or itching;
    fever); *pancreatitis* (pain in upper abdomen; nausea and vomiting);
    *phlebitis* (pain at site of injection)—with intravenous injection; *sterile*

*abscess* (pain, redness, and hardness at site of injection)—with intramuscular injection

### Those indicating need for medical attention only if they continue or are bothersome
Incidence more frequent
    *Gastrointestinal disturbances* (nausea and vomiting; loss of appetite;
    diarrhea)

### Those not indicating need for medical attention
Incidence less frequent
    *Unpleasant metallic taste*

### Those indicating possible hyperglycemia or hypoglycemia and the need for medical attention if they occur after medication is discontinued
Signs of hyperglycemia
    *Drowsiness; flushed, dry skin; fruit-like breath odor; increased
    thirst; increased urination; loss of appetite*
Signs of hypoglycemia
    *Anxiety; chills and cold sweats; cool, pale skin; headache; increased
    hunger; nausea; nervousness; shakiness*

## Patient Consultation

As an aid to patient consultation, refer to *Advice for the Patient,
Pentamidine (Systemic)*.

In providing consultation, consider emphasizing the following selected
information (» = major clinical significance):

### Before using this medication
» Conditions affecting use, especially:
    Allergy to pentamidine
    Pregnancy—Pentamidine crosses the placenta in animals; studies
      have found it to be mildly embryotoxic in rabbits
    Use in children—There are limited data available on the use of
      pentamidine in children; however, the dose used in children is
      the same as that used in adults and the side effects seen appear
      to be similar to those seen in adults
    Other medications, especially bone marrow depressants, didano-
      sine, foscarnet, other nephrotoxic medications, or radiation
      therapy
    Other medical problems, especially a history of bleeding disorders,
      bone marrow depression, cardiac disease, dehydration, diabetes
      mellitus, hypoglycemia, hypotension, or renal function
      impairment

### Proper use of this medication
» Importance of receiving medication for full course of therapy and on
    regular schedule
» Proper dosing

### Precautions while using this medication
» Severe hypotension may occur; patient should be lying down during
    administration; physician may need to monitor blood pressure dur-
    ing administration and several times thereafter until blood pressure
    stabilizes
*To reduce the risk of bleeding during periods of low blood counts:*
» Checking with physician immediately if unusual bleeding or bruising
    occurs
    Using caution in use of regular toothbrushes, dental floss, and tooth-
      picks; physician, dentist, or nurse may suggest alternative methods
      for cleaning teeth and gums; checking with physician before hav-
      ing dental work done
    Avoiding use of safety razor; using electric shaver instead; using cau-
      tion in use of fingernail or toenail cutters

*For visceral leishmaniasis or African trypanosomiasis*
*Measures for sandfly and tsetse fly control:*
    Sleeping under fine-mesh netting
    Wearing long-sleeved shirts or blouses and long trousers; wearing
      clothing of moderately heavy material to protect from tsetse fly
      bites
    Applying insect repellant to uncovered areas of skin

### Side/adverse effects
    Unpleasant metallic taste may occur, although medically insignificant
    Signs of potential side effects, especially diabetes mellitus, hypergly-
      cemia, hypoglycemia, hypotension, leukopenia, neutropenia, ne-
      phrotoxicity, thrombocytopenia, anemia, cardiac arrhythmias, hy-
      persensitivity, pancreatitis, phlebitis, and sterile abscess

## General Dosing Information

Slow intravenous infusion, over 1 to 2 hours, is the preferred route of
    administration. Intramuscular administration can cause a sterile ab-

scess at the site of injection. If pentamidine must be given intramuscularly, it should be reserved for patients with adequate muscle mass, and the daily dose of pentamidine should be administered by deep injection only.

Pentamidine may cause sudden, severe hypotension, even after a single dose. Therefore, patients should be lying down and their blood pressure should be closely monitored during administration and several times thereafter until blood pressure is stable.

No adjustment of the pentamidine dose is needed in patients with renal impairment. Because less than 3% of a dose of pentamidine is excreted through the kidneys, no correlation has been seen between renal function and plasma drug clearance. Also, the renal excretion increased only marginally with repeated pentamidine dosing.

## Parenteral Dosage Forms

Note: Bracketed uses in the *Dosage Forms* section refer to categories of use and/or indications that are not included in U.S. product labeling.

### STERILE PENTAMIDINE ISETHIONATE

**Usual adult and adolescent dose**
Pneumonia, *Pneumocystis carinii*—
Intravenous infusion, 4 mg per kg of body weight, administered over one to two hours, once a day for fourteen to twenty-one days, depending on clinical response.

Note: In preliminary studies, a reduced intravenous dose of 3 mg per kg of body weight once a day was used successfully in the treatment of mild to moderate *P. carinii* pneumonia.

[Leishmaniasis, visceral][1]—
Intravenous infusion, 2 to 4 mg per kg of body weight, administered over one to two hours, once a day for up to fifteen days. Administration may be repeated in one to two weeks if required.

[Leishmaniasis, cutaneous][1]—
Intravenous infusion, 2 to 4 mg per kg of body weight, administered over one to two hours, once or twice a week until the lesions heal.

[Trypanosomiasis, African (without CNS involvement)][1]—
Treatment: Intravenous infusion, 4 mg per kg of body weight, administered over one to two hours, once a day for ten days.

Note: The dose of pentamidine isethionate is based on the total weight of the salt, whereas the dose of pentamidine mesylate (methanesulfonate) is based on the weight of pentamidine base. Since both preparations are available in some countries, clinicians should calculate the dose for pentamidine preparations on the basis that 2.4 mg of pentamidine mesylate is equivalent to 4 mg of pentamidine isethionate.

**Usual adult prescribing limits**
Trypanosomiasis, African—
3 to 5 mg per kg of body weight a day.

**Usual pediatric dose**
See *Usual adult and adolescent dose.*

**Size(s) usually available**
U.S.—
300 mg (Rx) [*Pentam 300;* GENERIC].

Canada—
200 mg (Rx) [*Pentacarinat*].
300 mg (Rx) [*Pentacarinat;* GENERIC].

**Packaging and storage**
Prior to reconstitution, store between 2 and 8 °C (36 and 46 °F), unless otherwise specified by manufacturer. Protect dry powder and reconstituted solution from light.

**Preparation of dosage form**
To prepare initial dilution for intramuscular use, add 3 mL of sterile water for injection to each 300-mg vial.
To prepare initial dilution for intermittent intravenous use, add 2.1 mL of sterile water for injection to each 200-mg vial, or add 3 to 5 mL of sterile water for injection or 5% dextrose injection to each 300-mg vial. The solution may be further diluted in 50 to 250 mL of 5% dextrose injection and administered over a period of *at least 1 hour, and preferably up to 2 hours.*

**Stability**
After reconstitution in 5% dextrose injection, pentamidine solutions with concentrations of 1 and 2.5 mg per mL retain their potency for up to 24 hours at room temperature. Discard any unused portion. Reconstituted pentamidine should not be mixed with any solutions other than 5% dextrose.

---

[1]Not included in Canadian product labeling.

---

Revised: 05/27/94
Interim revision: 04/24/95

---

## PENTAZOCINE—See *Opioid (Narcotic) Analgesics (Systemic)*

---

## PENTAZOCINE-CONTAINING COMBINATIONS—

Pentazocine and Acetaminophen (Systemic)—See *Opioid (Narcotic) Analgesics and Acetaminophen (Systemic)*
Pentazocine and Aspirin (Systemic)—See *Opioid (Narcotic) Analgesics and Aspirin (Systemic)*
Pentazocine and Naloxone (Systemic)—See *Opioid (Narcotic) Analgesics (Systemic)*

---

## PENTOBARBITAL—See *Barbiturates (Systemic)*

---

## PENTOBARBITAL-CONTAINING COMBINATIONS—

Ergotamine, Caffeine, Belladonna Alkaloids, and Pentobarbital (Systemic)—See *Vascular Headache Suppressants, Ergot Derivative–containing (Systemic)*

---

# PENTOSTATIN  Systemic

---

VA CLASSIFICATION (Primary): AN900
Other commonly used names are 2'-deoxycoformycin and 2'DCF.

Note: For a listing of dosage forms and brand names by country availability, see *Dosage Forms* section(s). For a listing of brand names for the articles in this monograph, refer to the General Index.

## Category
Antineoplastic.

## Indications
Note: Bracketed information in the *Indications* section refers to uses that are not included in U.S. product labeling.

**Accepted**
Leukemia, hairy cell (treatment)—Pentostatin is indicated as a single agent for treatment of adult patients with hairy cell leukemia who have not responded after a minimum of 6 months of alpha interferon treatment or have progressed after a minimum of 3 months' treatment with alpha interferon.

[There is also some evidence that pentostatin is useful for treatment of hairy cell leukemia not refractory to interferon treatment.]

## Pharmacology/Pharmacokinetics

**Physicochemical characteristics**
Source—Isolated from fermentation cultures of *Streptomyces antibioticus*
Chemical group—Pentostatin is a purine (deoxyinosine) analog.
Molecular weight—268.21.

**Mechanism of action/Effect**
Pentostatin is an antimetabolite. Its exact mechanism of action in hairy cell leukemia is unknown. Pentostatin is a potent transition state inhibitor of adenosine deaminase (ADA), the greatest activity of which is found in cells of the lymphoid system. T-cells have higher ADA activity than B-cells, and T-cell malignancies have higher activity than B-cell malignancies. The cytotoxicity that results from prevention of catabolism of adenosine or deoxyadenosine is thought to be due to elevated intracellular levels of dATP, which can block DNA synthesis through inhibition of ribonucleotide reductase. Inhibition of RNA synthesis may also contribute to the cytotoxic effect. Although pentostatin arrests cells in the $G_1$ or S phase of cell division, it is also reported

to have cell cycle–phase nonspecific actions (including increased DNA strand breaks).

### Other actions/effects
Pentostatin appears to have immunosuppressant activity; significant reductions in T- and B-cells occur during treatment and T4 reductions persist, sometimes for months or years, after treatment.

### Distribution
Pentostatin crosses the blood-brain barrier; cerebrospinal fluid concentrations achieved are 10 to 12.5% of serum concentrations within 24 hours after a single dose.

### Protein binding
Low (4%).

### Biotransformation
Hepatic; however, only small amounts are metabolized.

### Half-life
Distribution—
11 minutes (following a single dose of 4 mg per square meter of body surface infused over 5 minutes). A range of 17 to 85 minutes has also been reported.
Terminal—
Normal: 5.7 hours (following a single dose of 4 mg per square meter of body surface infused over 5 minutes). A range of 2.6 to 15 hours has been reported.
Renal function impairment (creatinine clearance less than 50 mL per minute): 18 hours.

### Onset of action
Time to achieve response—Median 4.7 months (range 2.9 to 24.1 months).

### Duration of action
Pharmacologic—Inhibition of ADA: More than 1 week after a single dose.

### Elimination
Renal, 90%, as unchanged drug and metabolites as measured by adenosine deaminase inhibitory activity. In two small studies, 32 to 73% was recovered unchanged.

## Precautions to Consider

### Carcinogenicity
Secondary malignancies are potential delayed effects of many antineoplastic agents, although it is not clear whether the effect is related to their mutagenic or immunosuppressive action. The effect of dose and duration of therapy is also unknown, although risk seems to increase with long-term use. Although information is limited, available data seem to indicate that the carcinogenic risk is greatest with the alkylating agents.
Antimetabolites have been shown to be carcinogenic in animals and may be associated with an increased risk of development of secondary carcinomas in humans, although the risk appears to be less than with alkylating agents.
Lymphoid neoplasms have been reported in humans.
Studies with pentostatin in animals have not been done.

### Mutagenicity
Pentostatin was not found to be mutagenic in several strains of *Salmonella typhimurium*, including TA-98, TA-1535, TA-1537, and TA-1538. When tested with strain TA-100, a repeatable statistically significant response trend was observed with and without metabolic activation. The response was 2.1 to 2.2 fold higher than the background at 10 mg/plate, the maximum possible drug concentration. Formulated pentostatin was clastogenic in the *in vivo* mouse bone marrow micronucleus assay at 20, 120, and 240 mg per kg of body weight (mg/kg). Pentostatin was non-mutagenic to V79 Chinese hamster lung cells at the hypoxanthine-guanine-phosphororibosyltransferase (HGPRT) locus exposed for 3 hours to concentrations of 1 to 3 mg per mL, with or without metabolic activation. Pentostatin did not significantly increase chromosomal aberrations in V79 Chinese hamster lung cells exposed for 3 hours to 1 to 3 mg per mL in the presence or absence of metabolic activation.

### Pregnancy/Reproduction
Fertility—Gonadal suppression, resulting in amenorrhea or azoospermia, may occur in patients taking antineoplastic therapy, especially with the alkylating agents. In general, these effects appear to be related to dose and length of therapy and may be irreversible. Prediction of the degree of testicular or ovarian function impairment is complicated by the common use of combinations of several antineoplastics, which makes it difficult to assess the effects of individual agents. Fertility studies with pentostatin have not been done in animals; however, mild seminiferous tubular degeneration was observed in a 5-day intravenous toxicity study at doses of 1 and 4 mg/kg in dogs.

Pregnancy—Adequate and well-controlled studies in women have not been done.
First trimester: It is usually recommended that use of antineoplastics, especially combination chemotherapy, be avoided whenever possible, especially during the first trimester. Although information is limited because of the relatively few instances of antineoplastic administration during pregnancy, the mutagenic, teratogenic, and carcinogenic potential of these medications must be considered.
Other hazards to the fetus include adverse reactions seen in adults.
In general, use of contraception is recommended during cytotoxic drug therapy.
Studies in rats at intravenous doses of 0, 0.01, 0.1, or 0.75 mg/kg (0, 0.06, 0.6, or 4.5 mg per square meter of body surface, respectively) per day on days 6 through 15 of gestation found drug-related maternal toxicity at doses of 0.1 and 0.75 mg/kg per day (0.6 and 4.5 mg per square meter of body surface, respectively). Teratogenic effects (increased incidence of various skeletal malformations) were observed at doses of 0.75 mg/kg (4.5 mg per square meter of body surface per day). In a dose range–finding study in rats at intravenous doses of 0, 0.05, 0.1, 0.5, 0.75, or 1 mg/kg (0, 0.3, 0.6, 3, 4.5, or 6 mg per square meter of body surface, respectively, per day) on days 6 through 15 of gestation, fetal malformations were observed, including an omphalocele at 0.05 mg/kg (0.3 mg per square meter of body surface), gastroschisis at 0.75 mg/kg and 1 mg/kg (4.5 and 6 mg per square meter of body surface, respectively), and a flexure defect of the hindlimbs at 0.75 mg/kg (4.5 mg per square meter of body surface). Pentostatin was also teratogenic in mice in single intraperitoneal doses of 2 mg/kg (6 mg per square meter of body surface) on day 7 of gestation. Pentostatin was not teratogenic in rabbits at intravenous doses of 0, 0.005, 0.01, or 0.02 mg/kg per day (0, 0.015, 0.03, or 0.06 mg per square meter of body surface per day, respectively); however, maternal toxicity, abortions, early deliveries, and deaths occurred in all drug-treated groups.

FDA Pregnancy Category D.

### Breast-feeding
Although very little information is available regarding excretion of antineoplastic agents in breast milk, breast-feeding is not recommended during chemotherapy because of the potential risks to the infant (adverse effects, mutagenicity, carcinogenicity). It is not known whether pentostatin is excreted in breast milk.

### Pediatrics
No information is available on the relationship of age to the effects of pentostatin in pediatric patients. Safety and efficacy have not been established.

### Geriatrics
Although appropriate studies on the relationship of age to the effects of pentostatin have not been performed in the geriatric population, clinical trials have included elderly patients and geriatrics-specific problems that would limit the usefulness of this medication in the elderly are not expected. However, elderly patients are more likely to have age-related renal function impairment, which may require caution in patients receiving pentostatin.

### Dental
The bone marrow depressant effects of pentostatin may result in an increased incidence of microbial infection, delayed healing, and gingival bleeding. Dental work, whenever possible should be completed prior to initiation of therapy or deferred until blood counts have returned to normal. Patients should be instructed in proper oral hygiene during treatment, including caution in use of regular toothbrushes, dental floss, and toothpicks.
Pentostatin also sometimes causes stomatitis associated with considerable discomfort.

### Drug interactions and/or related problems
The following drug interactions and/or related problems have been selected on the basis of their potential clinical significance (possible mechanism in parentheses where appropriate)—not necessarily inclusive (» = major clinical significance):

Note: Combinations containing any of the following medications, depending on the amount present, may also interact with this medication.

Allopurinol or
Colchicine or
» Probenecid or
» Sulfinpyrazone
(pentostatin may raise the concentration of blood uric acid; dosage adjustment of antigout agents may be necessary to control hyperuricemia and gout; allopurinol may be preferred to prevent or reverse pentostatin-induced hyperuricemia because of risk of uric acid nephropathy with uricosuric antigout agents)

(one case has been reported in which a patient receiving both allopurinol and pentostatin developed a fatal hypersensitivity vasculitis, although a definite connection with the combination has not been established)

Blood dyscrasia–causing medications (See *Appendix II*)
(leukopenic and/or thrombocytopenic effects of pentostatin may be increased with concurrent or recent therapy if these medications cause the same effects; dosage adjustment of pentostatin, if necessary, should be based on blood counts)

» Bone marrow depressants, other (See *Appendix II*) or
Radiation therapy
(additive bone marrow depression may occur; dosage reduction may be required when two or more bone marrow depressants, including radiation, are used concurrently or consecutively)

Fludarabine
(concurrent use with pentostatin is not recommended because of a possible increased risk of fatal pulmonary toxicity)

Vaccines, killed virus
(because normal defense mechanisms may be suppressed by pentostatin therapy, the patient's antibody response to the vaccine may be decreased. The interval between discontinuation of medications that cause immunosuppression and restoration of the patient's ability to respond to the vaccine depends on the intensity and type of immunosuppression-causing medication used, the underlying disease, and other factors; estimates vary from 3 months to 1 year)

» Vaccines, live virus
(because normal defense mechanisms may be suppressed by pentostatin therapy, concurrent use with a live virus vaccine may potentiate the replication of the vaccine virus, may increase the side/adverse effects of the vaccine virus, and/or may decrease the patient's antibody response to the vaccine; immunization of these patients should be undertaken only with extreme caution after careful review of the patient's hematologic status and only with the knowledge and consent of the physician managing the pentostatin therapy. The interval between discontinuation of medications that cause immunosuppression and restoration of the patient's ability to respond to the vaccine depends on the intensity and type of immunosuppression-causing medication used, the underlying disease, and other factors; estimates vary from 3 months to 1 year. Patients with leukemia in remission should not receive live virus vaccine until at least 3 months after their last chemotherapy. In addition, immunization with oral poliovirus vaccine should be postponed in persons in close contact with the patient, especially family members)

Vidarabine
(biochemical studies have shown an enhancement of vidarabine's effects by pentostatin, which could result in an increase in adverse effects of each)

**Laboratory value alterations**
The following have been selected on the basis of their potential clinical significance (possible effect in parentheses where appropriate)—not necessarily inclusive (» = major clinical significance):

With physiology/laboratory test values
Alanine aminotransferase (ALT [SGPT]) and
Alkaline phosphatase and
Aspartate aminotransferase (AST [SGOT]) and
Lactate dehydrogenase (LDH)
(serum values are transiently increased in most patients)

Creatinine
(dose-related increases in serum concentrations may occur, indicating renal toxicity, but increases are usually minor and transient at recommended doses in patients with normal baseline renal function)

Uric acid concentrations in blood and urine
(may be increased)

**Medical considerations/Contraindications**
The medical considerations/contraindications included here have been selected on the basis of their potential clinical significance (reasons given in parentheses where appropriate)—not necessarily inclusive (» = major clinical significance).

***Risk-benefit should be considered when the following medical problems exist:***

» Bone marrow depression
Cardiovascular function impairment, including coronary artery disease, congestive heart failure, hypertension
(cardiac effects of pentostatin may be more likely)

» Chickenpox, existing or recent (including recent exposure) or
» Herpes zoster
(risk of severe generalized disease)

Gout, history of or
Urate renal stones, history of
(risk of hyperuricemia)

» Infection
(pentostatin should be withheld until active infection is controlled)

» Renal function impairment
(reduced elimination; in patients with increased serum creatinine concentrations, pentostatin should be withheld and creatinine clearance determined)

» Sensitivity to pentostatin

» Caution should be used also in patients who have had previous cytotoxic drug therapy or radiation therapy.

**Patient monitoring**
The following are especially important in patient monitoring (other tests may be warranted in some patients, depending on condition; » = major clinical significance):

» Creatinine clearance and/or
Creatinine concentrations, serum
(creatinine clearance and/or serum creatinine concentration determinations are recommended prior to initiation of therapy; serum creatinine concentration determinations are recommended before each dose and at other appropriate intervals during therapy)

» Hematocrit or hemoglobin and
» Leukocyte count, total and, if appropriate, differential and
» Platelet count
(determinations recommended prior to initiation of therapy and at periodic intervals during therapy, especially during early courses; frequency varies according to clinical state, agent, dose, and other agents being used concurrently)

Uric acid concentrations, serum
(determinations recommended prior to initiation of therapy and at periodic intervals during therapy; frequency varies according to clinical state, agent, dose, and other agents being used concurrently)

# Side/Adverse Effects

Note: In patients with progressive hairy cell leukemia, neutropenia may worsen during the initial courses of pentostatin therapy.

Most side/adverse effects decrease in severity with continued treatment.

The following side/adverse effects have been selected on the basis of their potential clinical significance (possible signs and symptoms in parentheses where appropriate)—not necessarily inclusive:

**Those indicating need for medical attention**
Incidence more frequent
*Allergic reaction* (sudden skin rash or itching)—11%; *anemia* (usually asymptomatic)—35%; *CNS (central nervous system) toxicity* (unusual tiredness; less frequently, anxiety or nervousness; confusion; mental depression; numbness or tingling of hands or feet; sleepiness; trouble in sleeping); *hepatic function impairment* (usually asymptomatic)—19%; *leukopenia or infection* (fever or chills; cough or hoarseness; lower back or side pain; painful or difficult urination)—60% or 36%, respectively; *pain; thrombocytopenia* (usually asymptomatic; less frequently [less than 10%], unusual bleeding or bruising; black, tarry stools; blood in urine or stools; pinpoint red spots on skin)—32%

Note: *Unusual tiredness* has been reported to increase with repeated weekly dosing and has been reduced by limiting pentostatin to three weekly doses or giving it every other week.

With high doses, *CNS toxicity* may lead to seizures, coma, and death.

Although hepatic enzyme elevations are usually transient, severe *hepatotoxicity* requiring withdrawal of pentostatin has been reported.

Severe *neutropenia* has occurred during early courses of treatment with pentostatin.

*Infections* may be bacterial, viral, or fungal, may occur even in the absence of leukopenia, and may be life-threatening.

Incidence less frequent—less than 10%
*Cardiac effects, including angina and myocardial infarction, congestive heart failure, and acute arrhythmias* (chest pain; swelling of feet or lower legs); *changes in vision; keratoconjunctivitis* (sore, red eyes); *pulmonary toxicity, including bronchitis, dyspnea, epistaxis, lung edema, pneumonia, pharyngitis, rhinitis, or sinusitis* (cough;

nosebleed; shortness of breath); *renal toxicity* (asymptomatic; seen as increases in serum creatinine); *stomatitis* (sores in mouth or on lips); *stomach pain; thrombophlebitis* (cramps in lower legs)

Note: *Cardiac effects* tend to occur in patients with pre-existing cardiovascular conditions. Fatalities have occurred.

*Keratoconjunctivitis* is transient but may recur with subsequent doses.

**Those indicating need for medical attention only if they continue or are bothersome**
Incidence more frequent
*Diarrhea*—15%; *headache*—13%; *loss of appetite*—16%; *muscle pain*—11%; *nausea and vomiting*—53%; *skin rash*—26%

Note: Maculopapular *skin rashes* are occasionally severe and may worsen with continued treatment, necessitating withdrawal of pentostatin. *Herpes simplex* and *herpes zoster* infections may also occur. Inflammation of multiple actinic (solar) keratoses has been reported.

Incidence less frequent—less than 10%
*Back pain; constipation; dry skin; flatulence* (bloating or gas); *flu-like syndrome* (general feeling of discomfort or illness); *itching; joint pain; weakness; weight loss*

## Overdose

For more information on the management of overdose or unintentional ingestion, **contact a Poison Control Center** (see *Poison Control Center Listing*).

**Treatment of overdose**
Treatment consists of withdrawal of pentostatin and supportive therapy.

## Patient Consultation

As an aid to patient consultation, refer to *Advice for the Patient, Pentostatin (Systemic)*.

In providing consultation, consider emphasizing the following selected information (» = major clinical significance):

**Before using this medication**
» Conditions affecting use, especially:
　Sensitivity to pentostatin
　Pregnancy—Use not recommended because of mutagenic, teratogenic, and carcinogenic potential; advisability of using contraception; telling physician immediately if pregnancy is suspected
　Breast-feeding—Not recommended because of risk of serious side effects
　Other medications, especially probenecid, sulfinpyrazone, other bone marrow depressants, or other cytotoxic drug or radiation therapy
　Other medical problems, especially chickenpox, herpes zoster, renal function impairment, or infection

**Proper use of this medication**
　Frequency of nausea and vomiting; importance of continuing medication despite stomach upset
» Proper dosing

**Precautions while using this medication**
» Importance of close monitoring by the physician
» Avoiding immunizations unless approved by physician; other persons in patient's household should avoid immunizations with oral poliovirus vaccine; avoiding other persons who have taken oral poliovirus vaccine or wearing a protective mask that covers nose and mouth
*Caution if bone marrow depression occurs:*
» Avoiding exposure to persons with bacterial infections, especially during periods of low blood counts; checking with physician immediately if fever or chills, cough or hoarseness, lower back or side pain, or painful or difficult urination occur
» Checking with physician immediately if unusual bleeding or bruising; black, tarry stools; blood in urine or stools; or pinpoint red spots on skin occur
　Caution in use of regular toothbrush, dental floss, or toothpick; physician, dentist, or nurse may suggest alternatives; checking with physician before having dental work done
　Not touching eyes or inside of nose unless hands washed immediately before
　Using caution to avoid accidental cuts with use of sharp objects such as safety razor or fingernail or toenail cutters
　Avoiding contact sports or other situations where bruising or injury could occur

**Side/adverse effects**
　May cause adverse effects such as blood problems; importance of discussing possible effects with physician
　Signs of potential side effects, especially allergic reaction, CNS toxicity, leukopenia or infection, pain, thrombocytopenia, cardiac effects, changes in vision, keratoconjunctivitis, pulmonary toxicity, stomatitis, stomach pain, and thrombophlebitis
　Asymptomatic side effects, including anemia, hepatic function impairment, thrombocytopenia, and renal function impairment
　Physician or nurse can help in dealing with side effects

## General Dosing Information

Patients receiving pentostatin should be under supervision of a physician experienced in cancer chemotherapy.

It is recommended that antiemetics be prescribed for 48 to 74 hours after pentostatin administration.

If CNS toxicity occurs, it is recommended that pentostatin be withheld or discontinued.

If severe skin rash occurs, it is recommended that pentostatin be withheld.

If elevated serum creatinine occurs, it is recommended that pentostatin be withheld and creatinine clearance determined. No recommendations are available for dosage adjustment in renal function impairment (creatinine clearance less than 60 mL per minute).

Development of uric acid nephropathy in patients with leukemia or lymphoma may be prevented by adequate oral hydration and, in some cases, administration of allopurinol. Alkalinization of urine may be necessary if serum uric acid concentrations are elevated.

Special precautions are recommended in patients who develop thrombocytopenia as a result of administration of pentostatin. These may include extreme care in performing invasive procedures; regular inspection of intravenous sites, skin (including perirectal area), and mucous membrane surfaces for signs of bleeding or bruising; limiting frequency of venipuncture and avoiding intramuscular injections; testing urine, emesis, stool, and secretions for occult blood; care in use of regular toothbrushes, dental floss, toothpicks, safety razors, and fingernail and toenail cutters; avoiding constipation; and using caution to prevent falls and other injuries. Such patients should avoid alcohol and aspirin intake because of the risk of gastrointestinal bleeding. Platelet transfusions may be required.

It is recommended that pentostatin be temporarily withheld if the absolute neutrophil count (ANC) falls below 200 per cubic millimeter in patients who had an initial count of greater than 500 per cubic millimeter. Treatment with pentostatin may be resumed when the ANC returns to pretreatment levels.

Patients who develop leukopenia should be observed carefully for signs of infection. Antibiotic support may be required. In neutropenic patients who develop fever, broad-spectrum antibiotic coverage should be initiated empirically, pending bacterial cultures and appropriate diagnostic tests.

If active infection occurs during pentostatin treatment, it is recommended that pentostatin be withheld until the infection is controlled.

**Safety considerations for handling this medication**
There is limited but increasing evidence and concern that personnel involved in preparation and administration of parenteral antineoplastics may be at some risk because of the potential mutagenicity, teratogenicity, and/or carcinogenicity of these agents, although the actual risk is unknown. USP advisory panels recommend cautious handling both in preparation and disposal of antineoplastic agents. Precautions that have been suggested include:
• Use of a biological containment cabinet during reconstitution and dilution of parenteral medications and wearing of disposable surgical gloves and masks.
• Use of proper technique to prevent contamination of the medication, work area, and operator during transfer between containers (including proper training of personnel in this technique).
• Cautious and proper disposal of needles, syringes, vials, ampuls, and unused medication.
A number of medical centers have developed detailed guidelines for handling of antineoplastic agents.

## Parenteral Dosage Forms
### PENTOSTATIN FOR INJECTION

**Usual adult dose**
Hairy cell leukemia—
　Intravenous (by rapid injection or diluted in a larger volume and given over twenty to thirty minutes), 4 mg per square meter of body surface every other week.

Note: Hydration with 500 to 1000 mL of 5% dextrose in 0.45% sodium chloride injection or the equivalent before administration and 500 mL after administration is recommended.

Higher doses are not recommended because of the risk of renal, hepatic, pulmonary, and CNS toxicity.

It is recommended that pentostatin treatment be continued until two doses after a complete response is achieved. If the best response achieved is a partial response, it is recommended that pentostatin be discontinued after twelve months of treatment. If a complete or partial response is not achieved after six months of treatment, it is recommended that pentostatin be discontinued.

### Usual pediatric dose
Safety and efficacy have not been established.

### Size(s) usually available
U.S.—

10 mg (Rx) [*Nipent* (mannitol 50 mg; sodium hydroxide or hydrochloric acid)].

Canada—

10 mg (Rx) [*Nipent* (mannitol 50 mg; sodium hydroxide or hydrochloric acid)].

### Packaging and storage
Store between 2 and 8 °C (36 and 46 °F), unless otherwise specified by manufacturer.

### Preparation of dosage form
Pentostatin for injection is prepared for intravenous use by aseptically adding 5 mL of sterile water for injection to the 10-mg vial, producing a solution containing 2 mg of pentostatin per mL.

Pentostatin solutions may be given intravenously by rapid injection or further diluted in 25 to 50 mL of 5% dextrose injection or 0.9% sodium chloride injection (producing a solution containing 0.33 mg per mL or 0.18 mg per mL, respectively) for administration by intravenous infusion.

### Stability
Reconstituted solutions contain no preservative and should be used within 8 hours of reconstitution.

### Note
The manufacturer recommends that spills and wastes be treated with 5% sodium hypochlorite solution prior to disposal.

## Selected Bibliography

Kane BJ, Kuhn JG, Roush MK. Pentostatin: an adenosine deaminase inhibitor for the treatment of hairy cell leukemia. Ann Pharmacother 1992 Jul/Aug; 26: 939-47.

O'Dwyer PJ, Wagner B, Leyland-Jones B, et al. 2'-Deoxycoformycin (pentostatin) for lymphoid malignancies. Rational development of an active new drug. Ann Intern Med 1988 May; 108: 733-43.

Revised: 05/06/93
Interim revision: 06/30/94

---

# PENTOXIFYLLINE    Systemic

VA CLASSIFICATION (Primary): CV900
Another commonly used name is oxypentifylline.

Note: For a listing of dosage forms and brand names by country availability, see *Dosage Forms* section(s). For a listing of brand names for the articles in this monograph, refer to the General Index.

## Category
Blood viscosity–reducing agent.

## Indications
Note: Bracketed information in the *Indications* section refers to uses that are not included in U.S. product labeling.

### Accepted
Vascular disease, peripheral (treatment)—Pentoxifylline is indicated to provide symptomatic relief of intermittent claudication [and other signs and symptoms, including trophic ulcers] associated with chronic occlusive arterial disorders of the limbs. Although pentoxifylline may improve function as well as provide symptomatic relief, it is not intended as a replacement for more definitive therapy that may be needed, such as surgical bypass procedures or removal of arterial obstructions.

### Unaccepted
Pentoxifylline is used, in conjunction with other forms of treatment, to promote healing of stasis ulcers associated with venous insufficiency. However, further study is needed to determine the efficacy of the medication for this purpose.

## Pharmacology/Pharmacokinetics

### Physicochemical characteristics
Chemical group—A dimethylxanthine derivative.
Molecular weight—278.31.

### Mechanism of action/Effect
Pentoxifylline reduces blood viscosity and improves erythrocyte flexibility, microcirculatory flow, and tissue oxygen concentrations. Improvement in erythrocyte flexibility appears to be due to inhibition of phosphodiesterase and a resultant increase in cyclic AMP in red blood cells. Reduction of blood viscosity may be the result of decreased plasma fibrinogen concentrations and inhibition of red blood cell and platelet aggregation.

### Absorption
Almost completely absorbed; absorption is slowed but not reduced by food. Some first-pass metabolism occurs.

### Protein binding
Bound to erythrocyte membrane.

### Biotransformation
First by erythrocytes and then hepatic. Some metabolites are active.

### Half-life
Unchanged drug—0.4 to 0.8 hours.
Metabolites—1 to 1.6 hours.

### Onset of action
Multiple doses—2 to 4 weeks.

### Time to peak concentration
Within 2 to 4 hours.

### Elimination
Renal (as metabolites).
Fecal—Less than 4%.

## Precautions to Consider

### Cross-sensitivity and/or related problems
Patients sensitive to methylxanthines such as caffeine, theophylline, or theobromine may be sensitive to pentoxifylline also.

### Carcinogenicity
Studies in mice given pentoxifylline at doses up to 24 times the maximum recommended human dose for 18 months found no evidence of carcinogenicity.

### Tumorigenicity
Studies in rats given pentoxifylline at doses up to 24 times the maximum recommended human dose for 18 months, with a 6-month drug-free period, showed an increase in benign mammary fibroadenomas in females at the highest dose.

### Mutagenicity
Pentoxifylline was not found to be mutagenic in Ames tests in the presence and absence of metabolic activation.

### Pregnancy/Reproduction
Pregnancy—Adequate and well-controlled studies have not been done in humans.

Studies in rabbits and rats given up to about 10 and 25 times the maximum recommended human dose, respectively, have found an increased incidence of fetal resorptions in rats when pentoxifylline was given at the highest dose. No fetal malformations were observed.

FDA Pregnancy Category C.

### Breast-feeding
Pentoxifylline and its metabolites are distributed into breast milk. Although problems in humans have not been documented, breast-feeding during treatment is not recommended because pentoxifylline may be

tumorigenic (as demonstrated by the occurrence of benign mammary fibroadenomas in animal studies).

### Pediatrics

No information is available on the relationship of age to the effects of pentoxifylline in pediatric patients. Safety and efficacy have not been established.

### Geriatrics

Bioavailability of pentoxifylline may be increased and excretion decreased in the elderly, with resulting increased potential for toxicity. In addition, elderly patients are more likely to have age-related renal function impairment, which may require caution in patients receiving pentoxifylline.

### Drug interactions and/or related problems

The following drug interactions and/or related problems have been selected on the basis of their potential clinical significance (possible mechanism in parentheses where appropriate)—not necessarily inclusive (» = major clinical significance):

Note: Combinations containing any of the following medications, depending on the amount present, may also interact with this medication.

Anticoagulants, coumarin- or indandione-derivative, or
Heparin or
Other medications that may interfere with blood clotting by interfering with platelet function and/or by causing hypoprothrombinemia, such as:
  Cefamandole
  Cefoperazone
  Cefotetan
  Plicamycin
  Valproic acid, ór
Platelet aggregation inhibitors, other (See *Appendix II*), or
Thrombolytic agents
  (pentoxifylline inhibits platelet aggregation and has also caused prolongation of prothrombin time and bleeding; concurrent use with any of these medications may increase the risk of bleeding because of additive interferences with blood clotting; caution, increased monitoring of the patient for any indication of bleeding, and, when applicable, more frequent monitoring of the prothrombin time are recommended)

Antihypertensives
  (antihypertensive effects may be potentiated when these medications are used concurrently with pentoxifylline; dosage adjustments of both pentoxifylline and the antihypertensive may be necessary)

Cimetidine
  (cimetidine significantly increases the steady-state plasma concentration of pentoxifylline, which may increase the chance of side effects during concurrent use)

Smoking, tobacco
  (although pentoxifylline is not a peripheral vasodilator, smoking may interfere with the therapeutic effect because nicotine constricts blood vessels, which may worsen the condition for which pentoxifylline is being used; avoidance of smoking is recommended)

Sympathomimetic agents or
Xanthines, other
  (concurrent use with pentoxifylline may lead to excessive central nervous system [CNS] stimulation)

### Medical considerations/Contraindications

The medical considerations/contraindications included here have been selected on the basis of their potential clinical significance (reasons given in parentheses where appropriate)—not necessarily inclusive (» = major clinical significance).

*Risk-benefit should be considered when the following medical problems exist:*

» Any condition in which there is a risk of bleeding, especially recent cerebral or retinal hemorrhage, or
Bleeding, active
  (pentoxifylline may cause or exacerbate bleeding; careful patient selection and monitoring of at risk patients via hematocrit and/or hemoglobin determinations are recommended)

Cerebrovascular disease or
Coronary artery disease
  (angina, arrhythmia, and/or hypotension have occurred in some patients with these medical problems during treatment with pentoxifylline)

» Hepatic function impairment or
» Renal function impairment
  (medication may accumulate; lower doses may be required; therapy may be inadvisable in patients with severe impairment; patients with mild to moderate impairment should be closely monitored)
Sensitivity to pentoxifylline or other methylxanthines

## Side/Adverse Effects

The following side/adverse effects have been selected on the basis of their potential clinical significance (possible signs and symptoms in parentheses where appropriate)—not necessarily inclusive:

### Those indicating need for medical attention

Incidence rare
  *Arrhythmias* (irregular heartbeat); *chest pain*

### Those indicating need for medical attention only if they continue or are bothersome

Incidence less frequent—dose-related
  *Dizziness; headache; nausea or vomiting; stomach discomfort*

## Overdose

For more information on the management of overdose or unintentional ingestion, **contact a Poison Control Center** (see *Poison Control Center Listing*).

### Clinical effects of overdose

The following effects have been selected on the basis of their potential clinical significance (possible signs and symptoms in parentheses where appropriate)—not necessarily inclusive:

Acute effects—in order of occurrence
  *Drowsiness; flushing; faintness; unusual excitement; convulsions*

### Treatment of overdose

To decrease absorption—Immediate evacuation of the stomach.

Supportive care—Symptomatic and supportive treatment, including respiratory support, maintenance of blood pressure, and control of convulsions.

## Patient Consultation

As an aid to patient consultation, refer to *Advice for the Patient, Pentoxifylline (Systemic)*.

In providing consultation, consider emphasizing the following selected information (» = major clinical significance):

### Before using this medication

» Conditions affecting use, especially:
  Sensitivity to pentoxifylline or other methylxanthines
  Breast-feeding—Passes into breast milk; breast-feeding may be inadvisable on the basis of tumorigenic effects in animal studies
  Use in the elderly—Increased risk of side effects because of decreased clearance
  Other medical problems, especially hepatic or renal function impairment or any condition in which there is a risk of bleeding

### Proper use of this medication

  Swallowing whole without crushing, breaking, or chewing
» Taking with meals and/or antacids to reduce gastrointestinal irritation
» Proper dosing
  Missed dose: Taking as soon as possible; not taking if almost time for next dose; not doubling doses
» Proper storage

### Precautions while using this medication

  Checking with physician before discontinuing medication; pentoxifylline may take several weeks to work
  Avoiding smoking (nicotine constricts blood vessels)

### Side/adverse effects

  Signs of potential side effects, especially arrhythmias and chest pain

## General Dosing Information

Pentoxifylline should be administered with meals and/or with antacids to reduce gastrointestinal irritation.

It is recommended that dosage be reduced if gastrointestinal or central nervous system (CNS) side effects develop. If symptoms persist, pentoxifylline therapy should be withdrawn.

## Oral Dosage Forms

### PENTOXIFYLLINE EXTENDED-RELEASE TABLETS

**Usual adult dose**
Peripheral vascular disease—
    Oral, 400 mg three times a day with meals.

Note: Dosage should be reduced to 400 mg two times a day if gastrointestinal or CNS side effects occur.

    Geriatric patients may be more sensitive to the effects of the usual adult dose.

**Usual pediatric dose**
Safety and efficacy have not been established.

**Strength(s) usually available**
U.S.—
    400 mg (Rx) [*Trental*].

Canada—
    400 mg (Rx) [*Trental*].

**Packaging and storage**
Store below 40 °C (104 °F), preferably between 15 and 30 °C (59 and 86 °F), in a well-closed container, unless otherwise specified by manufacturer. Protect from light.

**Auxiliary labeling**
• Take with meals or food.
• Swallow tablets whole.

## Selected Bibliography

Ward A, Clissold SP. Pentoxifylline. A review of its pharmacodynamic and pharmacokinetic properties, and its therapeutic efficacy. Drugs 1987; 34: 50-97.

Revised: 07/13/93

---

# PERFLUBRON   Oral-Local†

VA CLASSIFICATION (Primary): DX900
Another commonly used name is perfluorooctylbromide.

Note: For a listing of dosage forms and brand names by country availability, see *Dosage Forms* section(s). For a listing of brand names for the articles in this monograph, refer to the General Index.

†Not commercially available in Canada.

## Category

Diagnostic aid, radiopaque (gastrointestinal disorders).

## Indications

**Accepted**

Gastrointestinal imaging, magnetic resonance—Perflubron is indicated to enhance delineation of the bowel during magnetic resonance imaging (MRI) in order to differentiate it from adjacent structures and from pathologic masses.

## Pharmacology/Pharmacokinetics

**Physicochemical characteristics**
Molecular weight—498.96.

**Mechanism of action/Effect**
Perflubron acts as a negative bowel contrast agent. It generates no signal during proton MRI. Bowel loops filled with perflubron appear black with all pulse sequences because the contrast agent lacks mobile protons (hydrogen has been replaced with halogen atoms). Due to its insolubility in water it does not mix with intestinal secretions; thus bowel lumina appear homogeneously black on MR images when perflubron replaces bowel contents.

**Absorption**
Minimal absorption (less than 0.001% of the administered dose) has occurred in persons with normal gastrointestinal tracts.

**Distribution**
Rapid transit through the gastrointestinal tract; reaches rectum within 30 to 40 minutes in most patients.

**Elimination**
Through rectum within 30 minutes of ingestion; usually completely eliminated within 24 to 48 hours.

## Precautions to Consider

**Carcinogenicity**
Long-term animal studies to evaluate carcinogenic potential of perflubron have not been performed.

**Mutagenicity**
In the Ames test, in a chromosome aberration study conducted in cultured human lymphocytes, and in a mouse micronucleus assay *in vivo*, perflubron was not shown to cause mutagenesis.

**Pregnancy/Reproduction**
Pregnancy—Adequate and well-controlled studies in humans have not been done. However, although there is no evidence that the magnetic and electric fields associated with MRI have an effect on human development, *in vitro* studies and theoretical predictions raise concern regarding the risk of the developing embryo's or fetus's exposure to MR. More studies are needed to establish the safety of MRI in pregnant patients.

Studies in animals have not been done.

FDA Pregnancy Category C.

**Breast-feeding**
It is not known whether perflubron is distributed into breast milk.

**Pediatrics**
Appropriate studies on the relationship of age to the effects of perflubron have not been performed in the pediatric population. However, clinical trials, which included children, were conducted and pediatrics-specific problems that would limit the usefulness of this agent were not reported.

**Geriatrics**
Appropriate studies on the relationship of age to the effects of perflubron have not been performed in the geriatric population. However, clinical trials, which included older patients, were conducted and geriatrics-specific problems that would limit the usefulness of this medication in the elderly were not reported.

**Laboratory value alterations**
The following have been selected on the basis of their potential clinical significance (possible effect in parentheses where appropriate)—not necessarily inclusive (» = major clinical significance):

With physiology/laboratory test values
    Aspartate aminotransferase (AST [SGOT])
        (although rare, serum values may be increased)
    Bilirubin, serum
        (although rare, concentrations may be decreased)
    Leukocyte count
        (may be increased rarely)

**Diagnostic interference**
The following have been selected on the basis of their potential clinical significance (possible effect in parentheses where appropriate)—not necessarily inclusive (» = major clinical significance):

With *other* diagnostic test results
    Computed tomography studies and
    Radiographic images
        (perflubron may interfere with image interpretation if these studies are done prior to elimination of perflubron)

**Medical considerations/Contraindications**
The medical considerations/contraindications included here have been selected on the basis of their potential clinical significance (reasons given in parentheses where appropriate)—not necessarily inclusive (» = major clinical significance).

*Risk-benefit should be considered when the following medical problems exist:*
    Bowel perforation, known or suspected or
    Bowel obstruction, complete
        (increased risk of absorption)
» Sensitivity to perflubron

## Side/Adverse Effects

The following side/adverse effects have been selected on the basis of their potential clinical significance (possible signs and symptoms in parentheses where appropriate)—not necessarily inclusive:

**Those indicating need for medical attention only if they continue or are bothersome**
Incidence more frequent
  *Abdominal fullness*—incidence 5.1%; *diarrhea*—incidence 14.3%; *nausea and vomiting*—incidence 15.8%; *oily taste in mouth*—incidence 30%; *rectal incontinence*

  Note: The incidence of *nausea and vomiting* may be associated with the concurrent administration of glucagon; *diarrhea* may be dose-related.

Incidence less frequent (1–3%)
  *Abdominal pain*—incidence 2.2%; *rectal flatulence*—incidence 2.2%; *rectal leakage of solution*

Incidence rare (<1%)
  *Chills; dizziness; headache; numb mouth; tremors; vasodilation* (flushing or redness of skin)

## Patient Consultation

As an aid to patient consultation, refer to *Advice for the Patient, Perflubron (Diagnostic).*

In providing consultation, consider emphasizing the following selected information (» = major clinical significance):

**Description of use**
  Action in the body: Passage through gastrointestinal tract allows bowel delineation and improved visualization with MR imaging instruments

**Before having this test**
» Conditions affecting use, especially:
    Sensitivity to perflubron
    Pregnancy—Safety concerns with use of magnetic and electric fields associated with MRI
    Other medical problems, especially bowel perforation or complete obstruction

**Preparation for this test**
  Special preparatory instructions may apply; patient should inquire in advance
  Fasting for at least 4 hours prior to test is recommended to facilitate ingestion of large volume of contrast agent

**Precautions after this test**
  Leakage of solution from rectum, for the first 3 hours, may require protection of clothing

## General Dosing Information

Imaging of the upper abdominal region should begin within 15 minutes of ingestion of perflubron. Imaging of the pelvic region should begin 15 to 60 minutes after ingestion.

Glucagon may be administered after ingestion of perflubron to reduce bowel motion and promote uniform gastrointestinal distribution of the contrast agent. This results in a greater degree of bowel darkening and, thus, increased clarity of bowel wall visualization.

## Oral Dosage Forms

### PERFLUBRON ORAL SOLUTION

**Usual adult and adolescent dose**
Gastrointestinal imaging, magnetic resonance—
  Oral, 9 mL per kg of body weight (usual range, 600 to 1000 mL total dose).

**Usual adult prescribing limits**
Up to a total dose of 1000 mL.

**Usual pediatric dose**
Dosage has not been established.

**Usual geriatric dose**
See *Usual adult and adolescent dose.*

**Size(s) usually available**
U.S.—
  200 mL (Rx) [*Imagent GI*].
Canada—
  Not commercially available.

**Packaging and storage**
Store between 15 and 30 °C (59 and 86 °F), in a light-resistant container, unless otherwise specified by manufacturer. Protect from light.

## Selected Bibliography

Brown JJ, Duncan JR, Heiken JP, et al. Perfluorooctylbromide as a gastrointestinal contrast agent for MR imaging: use with and without glucagon. Radiology 1991; 181: 455-60.

Developed: 01/25/94

---

# PERFLUOROCHEMICAL EMULSION    Systemic†

VA CLASSIFICATION (Primary): CV900
Note: For a listing of dosage forms and brand names by country availability, see *Dosage Forms* section(s). For a listing of brand names for the articles in this monograph, refer to the General Index.

  †Not commercially available in Canada.

## Category
Myocardial ischemia prophylactic.

## Indications

**Accepted**
Ischemia, myocardial (prophylaxis and treatment)—Perfluorochemical emulsion is indicated to prevent or diminish myocardial ischemia, as manifested by decreased ventricular wall motion and global ejection fraction, occurring during percutaneous transluminal coronary angioplasty (PTCA) in patients at high risk of ischemic complications of angioplasty (e.g., those with low baseline ejection fraction [less than 45%], large areas of myocardium at risk, recent myocardial infarction, or unstable angina or refractory angina requiring hospitalization).

## Pharmacology/Pharmacokinetics

**Physicochemical characteristics**
Formulation—Stable emulsion of synthetic perfluorochemicals (perfluorodecalin, perfluorotri-n-propylamine) in Water for Injection. Also contains Poloxamer 188, glycerin, egg yolk phospholipids, dextrose, and the potassium salt of oleic acid, plus electrolytes in physiologic concentrations.
Osmolarity—Approximately 410 mOsmol per liter.

Mean particle diameter—Less than 270 nanometers as determined by laser light scattering spectrophotometry. The content of particles greater than 400 nanometers is less than 10%.
pH—After preparation for administration: 7.3.
Solubility of oxygen—At 37 °C and at partial pressure of oxygen ($pO_2$) of 760 mm Hg:7 volume %. Increases with decreasing temperature; at 10 °C and $pO_2$ of 760 mm Hg, is 9 volume %.
Solubility of carbon dioxide—At 37 °C and at partial pressure of carbon dioxide ($pCO_2$) of 760 mm Hg: 66 volume %.
Viscosity—Less viscous than whole blood at 37 °C and physiological shear rates.

**Mechanism of action/Effect**
The perfluorochemical phase of the emulsion dissolves oxygen and carbon dioxide. When prepared for use during PTCA, the emulsion carries oxygen preferentially dissolved in the perfluorochemical emulsion particles. Oxygenation of the emulsion and transluminal injection through a coronary angioplasty balloon catheter delivers oxygen to the myocardium distal to the point of balloon inflation. This results in preservation of ventricular wall motion and global left ventricular ejection fraction, reduced ST segment deviation at the end of balloon inflation, and reduced incidence of severe angina and delayed onset of angina, as compared with routine, unprotected PTCA.
Poloxamer 188 contained in the emulsion is a nonionic surfactant. Phospholipids are the hydrophobic components of membranes and provide electrically insulated layers; they are involved in the formation of membrane structures. Choline prevents deposition of fat in the liver. Glycerol is used in the synthesis of body fats. Free fatty acids such as oleic acid are oxidized or converted in the liver to very low density lipoproteins (VLDL) that re-enter the bloodstream. Glucose is metabolized as an energy source.

## Distribution

Perfluorodecalin and perfluorotri-n-propylamine—

Taken up by the reticuloendothelial system, primarily in the liver, spleen, and bone marrow; none detected in the brain. Following a single dose of 10 mL per kg of body weight, trace amounts of perfluorochemicals will be present in the liver and spleen for up to 80 days, and in fat, bone marrow, adrenal, kidneys, lungs, and other organs for lesser periods, although presence in tissues for longer periods has been reported.

In breast milk: One day after peripheral intravenous infusion of perfluorochemical emulsion 20 mL per kg of body weight when the fluorocrit was 0.5%, the concentration of perfluorodecalin in the breast milk was 0.58 mg per mL; no perfluorotri-n-propylamine was detected.

## Biotransformation

Perfluorochemicals—None.

Poloxamer 188—None.

Glycerol—Metabolized to carbon dioxide and glycogen or used in the synthesis of body fats.

Oleic acid—Either enters the tissues where it may be oxidized or synthesized into triglycerides, or circulates in the plasma, bound to albumin.

Glucose—Metabolized as an energy source.

## Half-life

Perfluorochemicals—8 hours at doses of 10 mL per kg of body weight; dose-dependent.

## Elimination

Perfluorochemicals—Pulmonary, in expiratory gases, unchanged.

Poloxamer 188—Renal.

## Precautions to Consider

### Mutagenicity

Mutagenicity studies were negative.

### Pregnancy/Reproduction

Fertility—Administration to male and female rats prior to mating produced no evidence of impaired fertility.

Pregnancy—Adequate and well-controlled studies in humans have not been done.

Studies in rats at approximately 3 times the human dose found no adverse effects on the fetus.

FDA Pregnancy Category B.

### Breast-feeding

Perfluorochemicals are distributed into breast milk. One day after peripheral intravenous infusion of perfluorochemical emulsion 20 mL per kg of body weight when the fluorocrit was 0.5%, the concentration of perfluorodecalin in the breast milk was 0.58 mg per mL; no perfluorotri-n-propylamine was detected. Although perfluorochemicals will not be absorbed orally, breast-feeding is not recommended after administration of perfluorochemical emulsion.

### Pediatrics

No information is available on the relationship of age to the effects of perfluorochemical emulsion in pediatric patients. Safety and efficacy have not been established.

### Geriatrics

No information is available on the relationship of age to the effects of perfluorochemical emulsion in geriatric patients.

### Drug interactions and/or related problems

The following drug interactions and/or related problems have been selected on the basis of their potential clinical significance (possible mechanism in parentheses where appropriate)—not necessarily inclusive (» = major clinical significance):

Anesthetics, lipid soluble
(action may be prolonged by perfluorochemical emulsion)

### Laboratory value alterations

The following have been selected on the basis of their potential clinical significance (possible effect in parentheses where appropriate)—not necessarily inclusive (» = major clinical significance):

With diagnostic test results

Radioimmunoassays
(at concentrations in blood well above those expected in angioplasty perfusion, perfluorochemical emulsion may cause an upward displacement of the standard curve in some radioimmunoassays)

Spectrophotometric tests
(at high concentrations in the blood, perfluorochemical emulsion may interfere with some tests because of turbidity)

With physiology/laboratory test values

Electrocardiographic change, specifically:

ST segment elevation
(a characteristic pattern, reaching a plateau at 30 to 45 seconds of balloon inflation with an amplitude of 1–2 mm, has been observed in many patients; in contrast, in patients not treated with perfluorochemical emulsion, the ST segment elevation continues to rise after balloon inflation)

Fluorocrit
(centrifuged samples of blood containing perfluorochemical emulsion may contain a packed layer of perfluorochemicals at the bottom of the tube; packed red blood cells will be above the layer of perfluorochemicals and plasma will be at the top; the volume % of perfluorochemicals in the sample is referred to as the fluorocrit)

### Medical considerations/Contraindications

The medical considerations/contraindications included here have been selected on the basis of their potential clinical significance (reasons given in parentheses where appropriate)—not necessarily inclusive (» = major clinical significance).

*Except under special circumstances, this medication should not be used when the following medical problem exists:*

» Stenosis, functionally critical secondary, in the dilated and perfused vessel distal to the treated lesion

*Risk-benefit should be considered when the following medical problems exist:*

Asplenia
(half-life of perfluorochemical particles in circulation may be increased and accumulation in liver and other tissues may be greater)

» Sensitivity to any component of the emulsion

### Patient monitoring

The following may be especially important in patient monitoring (other tests may be warranted in some patients, depending on condition; » = major clinical significance):

» Electrocardiogram (ECG)
(recommended throughout the procedure)

» Monitoring for signs of ischemia
(recommended throughout the procedure)

## Side/Adverse Effects

Note: Side/adverse reactions to perfluorochemical emulsion perfusion may be difficult to distinguish from complications associated with the procedure itself.

The following side/adverse effects have been selected on the basis of their potential clinical significance (possible signs and symptoms in parentheses where appropriate)—not necessarily inclusive:

### Those indicating need for medical attention

Incidence less frequent

*Bradycardia; dyspnea or increased respiratory rate; hypotension; pulmonary wedge pressure elevation, transient; ventricular tachycardia and/or ventricular fibrillation*

Note: *Elevation of pulmonary wedge pressure* has been observed with multiple balloon inflations with perfluorochemical emulsion perfusion. Wedge pressure returned to near baseline levels within 3 to 5 minutes after the procedure.

Intracoronary infusion of perfluorochemical emulsion at ambient room temperature rather than at the recommended temperature of 37 °C has been associated with *ventricular fibrillation* requiring cardioversion.

Incidence rare

*Ischemia* (ST segment elevation; angina); *reaction to test dose* (mild generalized pruritus; mild chills; nausea; vomiting; urticaria; mild back pain)

Note: If the position of the catheter is such that it occludes side branches that will not receive perfusion from perfluorochemical emulsion, *ischemic ST changes, angina,* and *creatine kinase* elevation may result.

### Those indicating need for medical attention only if they continue or are bothersome

Incidence less frequent

*Cough; pruritus, mild*

## General Dosing Information

It is recommended that supportive personnel and procedures be immediately available during perfusion because of the potential risk of coronary arterial dissection with occlusion, coronary artery spasm and vasospastic angina, myocardial infarction, distal intraluminal thrombus, arrhythmia, tachycardia, bradycardia, and ventricular fibrillation requiring cardioversion, which may occur during any coronary angioplasty. Institutional policy should be followed regarding surgical standby for emergency coronary artery bypass graft surgery.

Oxygenated perfluorochemical emulsion must be warmed to approximately 37 °C prior to administration. Intracoronary infusion at ambient room temperature has been associated with ventricular fibrillation requiring cardioversion.

An intravenous test dose, with or without prior oxygenation of perfluorochemical emulsion, is recommended 10 minutes before the intracoronary perfusion is begun. If an adverse reaction to the test dose occurs, perfluorochemical emulsion perfusion should not be administered; instead, the patient should be treated by an alternative procedure, such as angioplasty without distal perfusion or coronary artery bypass graft surgery. Intravenous diphenhydramine and/or methylprednisolone may be given to treat such reactions.

Oxygenated perfluorochemical emulsion should be administered only via intracoronary perfusion during balloon angioplasty by means of an angiographic power injector, kept warm by means of a warming jacket on the injector.

Perfusion with oxygenated perfluorochemical emulsion should be performed only with lumened catheters and guidewire systems that permit pressure monitoring and/or contrast agent delivery with the guidewire in place.

Prior to initiating oxygenated perfluorochemical emulsion perfusion, the operator must verify proper positioning of the balloon catheter.

## Parenteral Dosage Forms

### PERFLUOROCHEMICAL EMULSION FOR INJECTION

**Usual adult dose**

Test dose—Intravenous (into a peripheral vein), 0.5 mL (withdrawn from the container prepared for administration). The patient is observed for ten minutes after administration and if an adverse reaction does not occur, the perfusion may proceed.

Intracoronary perfusion (by means of an angiographic power injector through the central lumen of the angioplasty balloon catheter without removing the guidewire), 60 to 90 mL (depending on the size of the distal vessel bed) per minute at approximately 37 °C during the period of balloon inflation.

Note: It may be helpful to initiate oxygenated perfluorochemical emulsion perfusion shortly before balloon inflation and to continue momentarily after balloon deflation. Balloon inflation time should be limited by the patient's tolerance and by the physician's judgment of clinical status and desired therapeutic result. An angiographic power injector reservoir, filled with 260 mL of oxygenated perfluorochemical emulsion will allow more than four minutes of perfusion time at a flow rate of 60 mL per minute (1 mL per second). Perfusion rates above 120 mL per minute and total intracoronary perfusion volumes above 500 mL have not been studied.

A minimum lumen diameter of 0.004 inch for the angioplasty balloon catheter with the guidewire in place is adequate to allow perfusion at the recommended rate.

Filters should not be used when perfluorochemical emulsion is administered as this may disturb the emulsion.

If any evidence of emulsion instability is found during the preparation procedure or during the infusion, administration should be discontinued and the emulsion discarded.

**Usual adult prescribing limits**

Should not be used more than one time in six months.

**Usual pediatric dose**

Safety and efficacy have not been established.

**Strength(s) usually available**

U.S.—

20% (when prepared for administration, contains 14 grams of perfluorodecalin and 6 grams of perfluorotri-n-propylamine per 100 mL) (Rx) [*Fluosol*].

Canada—

Not commercially available.

Note: *Fluosol* comes as a kit containing perfluorochemical emulsion, two additive solutions (Solution 1 and 2; to adjust pH, ionic strength, and osmotic pressure in the final preparation), a continuous oxygenation kit, and directions for use. The content of each constituent is:

Perfluorochemical emulsion—
Perfluorodecalin: 17.5 grams per 100 mL
Perfluorotri-n-propylamine: 7.5 grams per 100 mL
Poloxamer 188: 3.4 grams per 100 mL

Glycerin USP: 1.0 gram per 100 mL
Egg yolk phospholipids: 0.5 gram per 100 mL
Potassium oleate: 0.04 gram per 100 mL
Water for Injection USP: qs

Solution 1—
Sodium Bicarbonate USP: 3.5% w/v (1.05 grams per 30 mL)
Potassium Chloride USP: 0.56% w/v (0.168 gram per 30 mL)
Water for Injection USP: qs
pH adjusted with carbon dioxide gas

Solution 2—
Sodium Chloride USP: 4.29% w/v (3.004 grams per 70 mL)
Dextrose USP, Anhydrous: 1.29% w/v (0.901 gram per 70 mL)
Magnesium Chloride • 6H$_2$O USP: 0.305% w/v (0.214 gram per 70 mL)
Calcium Chloride • 2H$_2$O USP: 0.254/5 w/v (0.178 gram per 70 mL)
Water for Injection USP: qs

The composition of perfluorochemical emulsion when prepared for administration is:

Perfluorodecalin—14 grams per 100 mL
Perfluorotri-n-propylamine—6 grams per 100 mL
Poloxamer 188—2.72 grams per 100 mL
Glycerin USP—0.8 gram per 100 mL
Sodium Chloride USP—0.6 gram per 100 mL
Egg yolk phospholipids—0.4 gram per 100 mL
Sodium Bicarbonate USP—0.21 gram per 100 mL
Dextrose USP, Anhydrous—0.18 gram per 100 mL
Magnesium Chloride • 6H$_2$O USP—0.043 gram per 100 mL
Calcium Chloride • 2H$_2$O USP—0.036 gram per 100 mL
Potassium Chloride USP—0.034 gram per 100 mL
Potassium oleate—0.032 gram per 100 mL
Water for Injection USP—qs

**Packaging and storage**

Store perfluorochemical emulsion between −30 and −5 °C (−20 and +23 °F), unless otherwise specified by manufacturer. Once thawed, the emulsion should not be refrozen. Solutions 1 and 2 should be stored at a temperature not exceeding 30 °C (86 °F) and protected from freezing.

**Preparation of dosage form**

Perfluorochemical emulsion must be thawed in a water bath or warming cabinet at 37 °C (takes about 30 minutes) and mixed with Solutions 1 and 2 prior to administration. It should not be thawed in a microwave oven because that could cause uneven warming and localized overheating. The thawed and reconstituted emulsion must be oxygenated to greater than 600 mm Hg partial pressure of oxygen prior to use. *Perfluorochemical emulsion must be reconstituted and oxygenated according to the manufacturer's directions provided with the kit, using materials included in the kit.*

Note: Additives other than Solution 1, Solution 2, and Carbogen (95% O$_2$ /5% CO$_2$) gas must not be made to the container of *Fluosol* emulsion. Oxygen 100% should not be used for the oxygenation procedure because it may adversely affect the pH of the emulsion.

Aseptic technique should be used in thawing, addition and mixing of additive solutions, oxygenation, and filling the power injector.

Solutions 1 and 2 must be added separately and sequentially to perfluorochemical emulsion prior to administration.

**Stability**

Must be used within 8 hours of thawing. Contents of any container in which there appears to be a separation of the emulsion or which may have thawed during storage should not be administered. Any unused contents of a container should be discarded.

**Auxiliary labeling**

Perfluorochemical emulsion
• Must be kept frozen prior to use.

## Selected Bibliography

Zalewski A, Savage M, Goldberg S. Protection of the ischemic myocardium during percutaneous transluminal coronary angioplasty. Am J Cardiol 1988; 61: 54G-60G.

Cleman J, Jaffe CC, Wohlgelernter D. Prevention of ischemia during percutaneous transluminal coronary angioplasty by transcatheter infusion of oxygenated Fluosol-DA 10%. Circulation 1986; 74: 555-62.

Jaffe CC, Wohlgelernter D, Cabin H, et al. Preservation of left ventricular ejection fraction during percutaneous transluminal angioplasty by distal transcatheter coronary perfusion of oxygenated Fluosol DA 20%. Am Heart J 1988; 115: 1156-64.

Revised: 09/30/92

# PERGOLIDE  Systemic

VA CLASSIFICATION (Primary): CN500

Note: For a listing of dosage forms and brand names by country availability, see *Dosage Forms* section(s). For a listing of brand names for the articles in this monograph, refer to the General Index.

## Category

Antidyskinetic (dopamine agonist).

## Indications

### Accepted

Parkinsonism (treatment adjunct)—Pergolide is indicated, as an adjunct to levodopa or levodopa/carbidopa therapy, for treatment of the signs and symptoms of idiopathic or postencephalitic Parkinson's disease to allow achievement of symptomatic relief with lower doses of levodopa or levodopa/carbidopa.

## Pharmacology/Pharmacokinetics

### Physicochemical characteristics

Source—Pergolide is a semisynthetic ergot alkaloid derivative
Molecular weight—410.59.

### Mechanism of action/Effect

Stimulation of post-synaptic dopamine receptors (at both $D_1$ and $D_2$ receptor sites) in the nigrostriatal system. Unlike bromocriptine, but similar to apomorphine and lysuride, postsynaptic dopamine agonist properties are independent of presynaptic dopamine synthesis or stores.

### Other actions/effects

Inhibits secretion of prolactin; causes transient rise in serum concentration of growth hormone in normal patients while in patients with acromegaly it causes a decrease; causes decrease in serum concentrations of luteinizing hormone (LH).

### Absorption

Significant amount may be absorbed (at present, data on systemic bioavailability is insufficient).

### Protein binding

Very high (approximately 90%).

### Elimination

Primarily renal.

## Precautions to Consider

### Cross-sensitivity and/or related problems

Patients sensitive to other ergot derivatives may be sensitive to this medication also.

### Carcinogenicity

Uterine neoplasms in rats and mice, and endometrial adenomas and carcinomas in rats, occurred with doses as high as 340 and 12 times (in mice and rats, respectively) the maximum human oral dose. It is believed that this was due to the high estrogen/progesterone ratio that may occur in rodents as a result of inhibition of prolactin secretion. Human data are not available.

### Pregnancy/Reproduction

Pregnancy—Adequate and well-controlled studies in humans have not been done.

Reproduction studies in mice and rabbits with doses as high as 375 and 133 times, respectively, the maximum human dose administered in clinical trials (6 mg/day) have not shown that pergolide causes adverse effects on the fetus.

FDA Pregnancy Category B.

### Breast-feeding

This medication should not be administered to mothers who intend to breast-feed, since pergolide may inhibit lactation.

### Pediatrics

No published pediatrics-specific information is available. Safety and efficacy have not been established.

### Geriatrics

Studies performed to date have not demonstrated geriatrics-specific problems that would limit the usefulness of pergolide in the elderly.

### Dental

Pergolide may decrease or inhibit salivary flow, thus contributing to the development of caries, periodontal disease, oral candidiasis, and discomfort.

### Drug interactions and/or related problems

The following drug interactions and/or related problems have been selected on the basis of their potential clinical significance (possible mechanism in parentheses where appropriate)—not necessarily inclusive (» = major clinical significance):

Note: Combinations containing any of the following medications, depending on the amount present, may also interact with this medication.

Droperidol or
Haloperidol or
Loxapine or
Methyldopa or
Metoclopramide or
Molindone or
Papaverine or
Phenothiazines or
Reserpine or
Thioxanthenes
  (dopamine antagonists may decrease the effectiveness of pergolide)

Hypotension-producing medications, other (See *Appendix II*)
  (concurrent use may result in additive hypotensive effects)

### Laboratory value alterations

The following have been selected on the basis of their potential clinical significance (possible effect in parentheses where appropriate)—not necessarily inclusive (» = major clinical significance):

With physiology/laboratory test values
Plasma growth hormone concentrations
  (may be transiently increased in individuals with normal concentrations; paradoxically reduced in patients with acromegaly)

### Medical considerations/Contraindications

The medical considerations/contraindications included here have been selected on the basis of their potential clinical significance (reasons given in parentheses where appropriate)—not necessarily inclusive (» = major clinical significance):

*Except under special circumstances, this medication should not be used when the following medical problem exists:*

» Sensitivity to pergolide or other ergot alkaloids

*Risk-benefit should be considered when the following medical problems exist:*

Cardiac dysrhythmias
  (increased risk of atrial premature contractions and sinus tachycardia)

Psychiatric disorders
  (pre-existing states of confusion and hallucinations may be exacerbated)

### Patient monitoring

The following may be especially important in patient monitoring (other tests may be warranted in some patients, depending on condition; » = major clinical significance):

» Blood pressure measurements
  (pergolide commonly decreases or less frequently increases blood pressure)

## Side/Adverse Effects

The following side/adverse effects have been selected on the basis of their potential clinical significance (possible signs and symptoms in parentheses where appropriate)—not necessarily inclusive:

### Those indicating need for medical attention

Incidence more frequent
  *CNS effects* (confusion; dyskinesias [uncontrolled movements of the body, such as the face, tongue, arms, hands, head, and upper body]; hallucinations); *urinary tract infections* (pain or burning while urinating)

Incidence less frequent
  *Hypertension*

Incidence rare
> *Cerebrovascular hemorrhage* (severe or continuing headache; seizures; vision changes, such as blurred vision or temporary blindness; sudden weakness); *myocardial infarction* (severe chest pain; fainting; fast heartbeat; increased sweating; continuing or severe nausea and vomiting; nervousness; unexplained shortness of breath; weakness)

### Those indicating need for medical attention only if they continue or are bothersome
Incidence more frequent
> *Abdominal or stomach pain; constipation; dizziness or drowsiness; flu-like symptoms; hypotension* (dizziness or lightheadedness, especially when getting up from a lying or sitting position); *lower back pain; nausea; rhinitis* (runny nose); *weakness*

> Note: Approximately 10% of patients experience *orthostatic hypotension* during initial treatment. Tolerance usually develops with gradual dosage titration.

Incidence less frequent
> *Chills; diarrhea; dryness of mouth; facial edema* (swelling of the face); *loss of appetite; vomiting*

## Overdose
For specific information on the agents used in the management of pergolide overdose, see:
- *Charcoal, Activated (Oral-Local)* monograph; and/or
- *Phenothiazines (Systemic)* monograph.

For more information on the management of overdose or unintentional ingestion, **contact a Poison Control Center** (see *Poison Control Center Listing*).

### Treatment of overdose
Treatment is symptomatic and supportive, with possible utilization of the following:

To decrease absorption—Administration of activated charcoal instead of or in addition to gastric emptying.

Specific treatment—Antiarrhythmic medication, if necessary. Phenothiazine or other neuroleptic agent, to treat CNS stimulation.

Monitoring—Monitoring of cardiac function.

Supportive care—Maintenance of arterial blood pressure. Patients in whom intentional overdose is confirmed or suspected should be referred for psychiatric consultation.

## Patient Consultation
As an aid to patient consultation, refer to *Advice for the Patient, Pergolide (Systemic).*

In providing consultation, consider emphasizing the following selected information (» = major clinical significance):

### Before using this medication
» Conditions affecting use, especially:
>> Sensitivity to pergolide or other ergot alkaloids
>> Breast-feeding—May prevent lactation in mothers who intend to breast-feed
>> Dental—Reduced salivary flow may contribute to dental problems

### Proper use of this medication
> Taking with meals to reduce gastric effects
» Proper dosing
> Missed dose: Taking as soon as possible; not taking if almost time for next dose; not doubling doses
» Proper storage

### Precautions while using this medication
> Regular visits to physician to check progress
» Caution when driving or doing jobs requiring alertness, because of possible drowsiness or dizziness
> Dizziness may be more likely to occur after initial doses; taking first dose at bedtime or while lying down; getting up slowly from sitting or lying position
> Possible dryness of mouth; using sugarless gum or candy, ice, or saliva substitute for relief; checking with physician or dentist if dry mouth continues for more than 2 weeks
> Checking with physician before reducing dosage or discontinuing medication

### Side/adverse effects
> Signs of potential side effects, especially CNS effects, urinary tract infection, hypertension, cerebrovascular hemorrhage, and myocardial infarction

## General Dosing Information
Titrated dosage is necessary to achieve the individual therapeutic blood concentration requirements and to minimize the risk of side effects.

Nausea and dizziness associated with initiation of pergolide therapy usually resolve with continued therapy; however, incidence and severity of these side effects may be reduced with a decrease in pergolide dose. Dizziness and nausea may be better tolerated by administering the initial dose at bedtime or while lying down. Also, administration of pergolide with food may alleviate the nausea.

## Oral Dosage Forms
Note: The dosing and strengths of the dosage forms available are expressed in terms of pergolide base, not the mesylate salt.

### PERGOLIDE MESYLATE TABLETS
#### Usual adult and adolescent dose
Parkinsonism—
> Oral, 50 mcg (0.05 mg) (base) a day for the first two days; the dosage being increased gradually by 100 or 150 mcg (0.1 or 0.15 mg) (base) every third day over the next twelve days of therapy. Afterwards, the dose may be increased by 250 mcg (0.25 mg) (base) every third day until optimum therapeutic effect is achieved.

Note: Usually administered in divided doses three times a day.
> During dosage titration of pergolide the concurrent dose of levodopa or levodopa/carbidopa may be decreased with caution according to clinical response.

#### Usual adult prescribing limits
Up to 5 mg daily.

#### Usual pediatric dose
Safety and efficacy have not been established.

#### Usual geriatric dose
See *Usual adult and adolescent dose.*

#### Strength(s) usually available
U.S.—
> 50 mcg (0.05 mg) (base) (Rx) [*Permax* (scored; carboxymethylcellulose sodium; iron oxide; lactose; magnesium stearate; povidone)].
> 250 mcg (0.25 mg) (base) (Rx) [*Permax* (scored; carboxymethylcellulose sodium; iron oxide; lactose; magnesium stearate; povidone; FD&C Blue No. 1)].
> 1 mg (base) (Rx) [*Permax* (scored; carboxymethylcellulose sodium; iron oxide; lactose; magnesium stearate; povidone)].

Canada—
> 50 mcg (0.05 mg) (base) (Rx) [*Permax* (scored; croscarmellose sodium; iron oxide yellow; lactose; magnesium stearate; povidine; FD &C Blue No. 2 Aluminum Lake)].
> 250 mcg (0.25 mg) (base) (Rx) [*Permax* (scored; croscarmellose sodium; iron oxide yellow; lactose; l-methionine; magnesium stearate; povidine)].
> 1 mg (base) (Rx) [*Permax* (scored; croscarmellose sodium; iron oxide red pure; lactose; magnesium stearate; povidine)].

#### Packaging and storage
Store between 15 and 30 °C (59 and 86 °F), unless otherwise specified by manufacturer.

#### Auxiliary labeling
- May cause drowsiness.

## Selected Bibliography
Lieberman AN, Goldstein M, Gopinathan G, et al. D$_1$ and D$_2$ agonists in Parkinson's disease. Can J Neurol Sci 1987 Aug; 14 (3 Suppl): 466-73.

Lieberman AN, Gopinathan G, Neophytides A, et al. Management of levodopa failures: the use of dopamine agonists. Clin Neuropharmacol 1986; 9 (Suppl 2): S9-21.

Factor SA, Sanchez-Ramos JR, Weiner WJ. Parkinson's disease: An open label trial of pergolide in patients failing bromocriptine therapy. J Neurol Neurosurg Psychiatry 1988 Apr; 51 (4): 529-33.

Revised: 03/19/93

---

**PERICYAZINE**—See *Phenothiazines (Systemic)*

# PERMETHRIN  Topical

VA CLASSIFICATION (Primary): AP300

Note: For a listing of dosage forms and brand names by country availability, see *Dosage Forms* section(s). For a listing of brand names for the articles in this monograph, refer to the General Index.

## Category
Pediculicide.

## Indications

### Accepted
Pediculosis capitis (treatment)—Permethrin is indicated for the treatment of infestation caused by *Pediculus humanus* var. *capitis* (head louse) and its ova.

## Pharmacology/Pharmacokinetics

### Physicochemical characteristics
Source—Permethrin is a mixture of the *cis* and *trans* isomers of a synthetic pyrethroid. Permethrin is the first pyrethroid formulated for human use.
Molecular weight—391.29.

### Mechanism of action/Effect
Permethrin acts on the nerve cell membrane of the louse to disrupt the sodium channel current that regulates the polarization of the membrane. This leads to delayed repolarization and subsequent paralysis of the louse.

### Other actions/effects
Pharmacologically active against lice, ticks, mites, and fleas.

### Absorption
Not determined precisely; however, preliminary data suggest that less than 2% of the amount applied is absorbed systemically.
Permethrin is detectable in residual amounts on the hair for at least 10 days following a treatment.

### Biotransformation
Rapidly metabolized by ester hydrolysis to inactive metabolites.

### Duration of action
14 days.

### Elimination
Primarily in the urine.

## Precautions to Consider

### Cross-sensitivity and/or related problems
Patients sensitive to veterinary insecticides containing permethrin will be sensitive to permethrin lotion. In addition, patients sensitive to other synthetic pyrethroids, such as those found in household insecticides, or sensitive to pyrethrins or chrysanthemums may be sensitive to this medication also.

### Carcinogenicity/Tumorigenicity
Carcinogenicity bioassays with permethrin were evaluated using 3 rat studies and 3 mice studies. In the 3 mice studies, there were increases in pulmonary adenomas. In addition, in the females in one of the mice studies, there was increased incidence of pulmonary alveolar-cell carcinomas and benign liver adenomas when the mice were given permethrin at 5000 ppm in their food. No tumorigenicity was evident in the rat studies.

### Mutagenicity
Permethrin showed no evidence of mutagenic potential in a battery of *in vitro* and *in vivo* genetic toxicity studies in rodents.

### Pregnancy/Reproduction
Fertility—In a 3-generation rat study, permethrin did not have any adverse effect on reproductive function at an oral dose of 180 mg per kg of body weight (mg/kg) per day. In addition, reproductive studies performed in mice, rats, and rabbits given oral doses of 200 to 400 mg of permethrin per kg of body weight per day revealed no evidence of impaired fertility.

Pregnancy—There are no adequate and well-controlled studies in pregnant women.
Reproductive studies performed in mice, rats, and rabbits given oral doses of 200 to 400 mg of permethrin per kg of body weight per day revealed no evidence of harm to the fetus.

FDA Pregnancy Category B.

### Breast-feeding
Problems in humans have not been documented. Although it is not known whether permethrin is distributed into human milk, permethrin has been shown to have tumorigenic potential in some animal studies.

### Pediatrics
Appropriate studies on the relationship of age to the effects of permethrin have not been performed in the pediatric population. However, no pediatrics-specific problems have been documented to date.

### Geriatrics
Appropriate studies on the relationship of age to the effects of permethrin have not been performed in the geriatric population. However, no geriatrics-specific problems have been documented to date.

### Medical considerations/Contraindications
The medical considerations/contraindications included here have been selected on the basis of their potential clinical significance (reasons given in parentheses where appropriate)—not necessarily inclusive (» = major clinical significance):

*Risk-benefit should be considered when the following medical problems exist:*
Inflammation of the scalp, acute
   (condition may be exacerbated)
Sensitivity to permethrin

## Side/Adverse Effects
The following side/adverse effects have been selected on the basis of their potential clinical significance (possible signs and symptoms in parentheses where appropriate)—not necessarily inclusive:

**Those indicating need for medical attention only if they continue or are bothersome**
Incidence less frequent or rare
   *Burning, itching, numbness, rash, redness, stinging, swelling, or tingling of the scalp*
   Note: *Itching, redness,* and *swelling* often accompany lice infestations; the use of permethrin may temporarily increase this discomfort.

## Patient Consultation
As an aid to patient consultation, refer to *Advice for the Patient, Permethrin (Topical).*

In providing consultation, consider emphasizing the following selected information (» = major clinical significance):

### Before using this medication
» Conditions affecting use, especially:
      Sensitivity to permethrin; to other synthetic pyrethroids, such as those found in household insecticides; to pyrethrins or chrysanthemums; or to veterinary insecticides containing permethrin
      Breast-feeding—Animal studies have shown that permethrin can cause tumors

### Proper use of this medication
» Avoiding contact with the eyes; flushing eyes thoroughly with water if medication accidentally gets in eyes
   Container usually holds one treatment; using as much as needed and disposing of the remainder
*Proper administration*
   Shampooing the hair and scalp first using regular shampoo
   Thoroughly rinsing and towel drying hair and scalp
   Shaking lotion well before applying
   Thoroughly wetting hair and scalp with lotion; covering the areas behind the ears and on the nape of the neck also; allowing lotion to remain in place for 10 minutes
   Rinsing hair and scalp thoroughly and drying with clean towel
   If desired, using fine-toothed comb to remove dead lice and eggs
» Importance of having household members examined for infestation and treated if infested
» Proper dosing
» Proper storage

### Precautions while using this medication
   Using hygienic measures to control reinfestation or spread of infestation:
      Machine washing all clothing (including hats, scarves, and coats), bedding, towels, and washcloths in very hot water and drying them by using hot cycle of dryer for at least 20 minutes; for clothing or bedding that are not washable, dry cleaning or sealing in an airtight plastic bag for 2 weeks
      Shampooing all wigs and hairpieces
      Washing hairbrushes and combs in very hot soapy water (at least 130 °F) for 5 to 10 minutes; not sharing them with other people
      Cleaning house or room by thoroughly vacuuming upholstered furniture, rugs, and floors

Washing all toys in very hot soapy water (at least 130 °F) for 5 to 10 minutes or sealing in an airtight plastic bag for 2 weeks; especially important for stuffed toys used on the bed.

## General Dosing Information

Permethrin is used as a single-application treatment. Less than 1% of patients will require an additional treatment. If live lice are observed after 7 or more days following initial treatment, a second treatment may be administered.

Shampoo, rinse, and dry hair and scalp before application of permethrin.

The lotion should be worked into dry hair until the hair and scalp are thoroughly wet. The lotion should be allowed to remain in place for 10 minutes. Then the hair and scalp should be rinsed thoroughly and dried with a clean towel.

Although not necessary for the success of the treatment, when the hair is dry after the treatment, the patient may use a fine-toothed comb to remove any remaining nits or nit shells.

After treatment, a residual amount of permethrin remains on the hair providing protection against reinfestation for approximately 2 weeks. This protection is unaffected by regular shampooing.

## Topical Dosage Forms

### PERMETHRIN LOTION

**Usual adult and adolescent dose**
Pediculosis capitis—
Topical, to the hair and scalp, for one application.

**Usual pediatric dose**
Pediculosis capitis—
Children up to 2 years of age: Dosage has not been established.
Children 2 years of age and older: See *Usual adult and adolescent dose.*

**Strength(s) usually available**
U.S.—
1% (OTC) [*Nix Cream Rinse* (isopropyl alcohol 20%)].
Canada—
1% (OTC) [*Nix Cream Rinse* (isopropyl alcohol 20%)].

**Packaging and storage**
Store between 15 and 25 °C (59 and 77 °F), unless otherwise specified by manufacturer. Protect from freezing.

**Auxiliary labeling**
• Shake well.
• For external use only.

Revised: 07/25/94

**PERPHENAZINE**—See *Phenothiazines (Systemic)*

---

# PERPHENAZINE AND AMITRIPTYLINE    Systemic

**VA CLASSIFICATION (Primary): CN900**

**NOTE:**   The *Perphenazine and Amitriptyline (Systemic)* monograph is maintained on the USP DI electronic data base. For a printed copy of the most recent revision of the complete monograph, contact the USP Division of Information Development, 12601 Twinbrook Parkway, Rockville, MD 20852.

For information on the specific components of this combination, see the *USP DI* monographs for *Antidepressants, Tricyclic (Systemic)* and *Phenothiazines (Systemic).*

The information that follows is selectively abstracted from the complete monograph and is provided to facilitate drug use review and patient counseling.

Note: For a listing of dosage forms and brand names by country availability, see *Dosage Forms* section(s). For a listing of brand names for the articles in this monograph, refer to the General Index.

## Category

Antipsychotic-antidepressant.

## Indications

**Accepted**
Anxiety associated with mental depression (treatment)—Perphenazine and amitriptyline combination is indicated in the treatment of patients with moderate to severe anxiety and/or agitation and depression, anxiety and depression associated with chronic physical disease, anxiety and depression that cannot be differentiated, and symptoms of depression in schizophrenia.

## Patient Consultation

As an aid to patient consultation, refer to *Advice for the Patient, Perphenazine and Amitriptyline (Systemic).*

In providing consultation, consider emphasizing the following selected information (» = major clinical significance):

**Before using this medication**
» Conditions affecting use, especially:
    Sensitivity to phenothiazines, tricyclic antidepressants, or possibly maprotiline or trazodone
    Pregnancy—
       Amitriptyline: Animal studies have shown teratogenic effects when amitriptyline was given in doses many times larger than the human dose; reports of cardiac problems, muscle spasms, respiratory distress, or urinary retention in neonates of mothers taking amitriptyline just prior to delivery
       Perphenazine: Phenothiazines have been found to depress spermatogenesis in animals; not recommended for use during

pregnancy, because of reports of prolonged jaundice, hypo- or hyperreflexia, and extrapyramidal effects in neonates
    Breast-feeding—Distributed into breast milk, possibly causing drowsiness, dystonias, and tardive dyskinesia in the baby; increased prolactin secretion in mother
    Use in children—Adolescents more sensitive to effects, requiring lower doses; children more prone to develop extrapyramidal reactions
    Use in the elderly—Elderly more likely to develop extrapyramidal, anticholinergic, hypotensive, and sedative effects; lower doses and more gradual increases required
    Dental—Decreased salivary flow contributes to caries, periodontal disease, candidiasis, and discomfort; blood dyscrasias may cause increased infections, delayed healing, and gingival bleeding; increased extrapyramidal motor activity of head, face, and neck may cause difficulty with occlusal and other procedures
    Other medications, especially alcohol and other CNS depressants, antithyroid agents, epinephrine, levodopa, lithium, cimetidine, other EPS-causing medications, MAO inhibitors, metrizamide, or sympathomimetics
    Other medical problems, especially alcoholism (active), bipolar disorder, blood disorders, cardiovascular disorders, gastrointestinal disorders, glaucoma, hepatic function impairment, renal function impairment, hyperthyroidism, prostatic hypertrophy, latent psychosis, Reye's syndrome, severe CNS depression, seizures, or urinary retention

**Proper use of this medication**
    Taking after meals or with food to reduce gastrointestinal irritation
» Compliance with therapy; not taking more or less medication than the amount prescribed
» Several weeks of therapy may be required to produce optimal therapeutic effects
» Proper dosing
    Missed dose: Taking as soon as possible; not taking at all if less than 2 hours to next dose; not doubling doses
» Proper storage

**Precautions while using this medication**
    Regular visits to physician to check progress of therapy
» Checking with physician before discontinuing medication; gradual dosage reduction may be needed
    Avoiding use of antacids or antidiarrheals within 2 hours of taking this medication
» Avoiding use of alcoholic beverages or other CNS depressants during therapy
» Caution if any kind of surgery, dental treatment, or emergency treatment is required
» Possible drowsiness or blurred vision; caution when driving, using machines or doing jobs requiring alertness or accurate vision

» Possible dizziness or lightheadedness; caution when getting up suddenly from a lying or sitting position
» Possible heat stroke: caution during exercise, hot weather, or hot baths or saunas
　Possible dryness of mouth; using sugarless gum or candy, ice, or saliva substitute for relief; checking with physician or dentist if dry mouth continues for more than 2 weeks
　Possible skin photosensitivity; avoiding unprotected exposure to sun; using protective clothing; using a sun block product that includes protection against both UVA-caused photosensitivity reactions and UVB-caused sunburn reactions; avoiding use of sunlamp, tanning bed, or tanning booth
　Observing precautions for 3 to 7 days after stopping medication

### Side/adverse effects

» Stopping medication and getting emergency treatment if symptoms of neuroleptic malignant syndrome (NMS) appear
» Notifying physician as soon as possible if early symptoms of tardive dyskinesia appear
　Possibility of withdrawal symptoms
　Signs of potential side effects, especially anticholinergic effects; hypotension; dystonias; fast, slow, or irregular heartbeat; tardive dyskinesia or Parkinsonian syndrome; akathisia; shakiness or tremors; NMS; heat stroke; testicular swelling; allergic reactions; alopecia; blood dyscrasias; cholestatic jaundice; photosensitivity; ophthalmologic effects; melanosis; priapism; seizures; SIADH; or tinnitus

## Oral Dosage Forms

### PERPHENAZINE AND AMITRIPTYLINE HYDROCHLORIDE TABLETS USP

#### Usual adult dose
Oral, 2 mg of perphenazine and 25 mg of amitriptyline hydrochloride to 4 mg of perphenazine and 25 mg of amitriptyline hydrochloride three or four times a day initially, the daily dosage being adjusted as needed and tolerated.

Note: Debilitated patients usually require a lower initial dose, which is then gradually increased as needed and tolerated.

#### Usual adult prescribing limits
Up to a total of 32 mg of perphenazine and 200 mg of amitriptyline hydrochloride daily.

#### Usual pediatric dose
Children up to 12 years of age—Safety and efficacy have not been established.

Children over 12 years of age—Adolescent patients usually require a lower initial dose, which is then gradually increased as needed and tolerated. Dosage must be individualized by physician.

#### Usual geriatric dose
Oral, 4 mg of perphenazine and 10 mg of amitriptyline hydrochloride three or four times a day initially, the dosage being adjusted as needed and tolerated.

#### Strength(s) usually available
U.S.—

　2 mg of perphenazine and 10 mg of amitriptyline hydrochloride (Rx)
　　[*Etrafon; Triavil;* GENERIC].
　2 mg of perphenazine and 25 mg of amitriptyline hydrochloride (Rx)
　　[*Etrafon; Triavil;* GENERIC].
　4 mg of perphenazine and 10 mg of amitriptyline hydrochloride (Rx)
　　[*Etrafon-A; Triavil;* GENERIC].
　4 mg of perphenazine and 25 mg of amitriptyline hydrochloride (Rx)
　　[*Etrafon-Forte; Triavil;* GENERIC].
　4 mg of perphenazine and 50 mg of amitriptyline hydrochloride (Rx)
　　[*Triavil;* GENERIC].

Canada—

　2 mg of perphenazine and 10 mg of amitriptyline hydrochloride (Rx)
　　[*Etrafon*].
　2 mg of perphenazine and 25 mg of amitriptyline hydrochloride (Rx)
　　[*Elavil Plus; Etrafon-D; PMS Levazine*].
　3 mg of perphenazine and 15 mg of amitriptyline hydrochloride (Rx)
　　[*Triavil*].
　4 mg of perphenazine and 10 mg of amitriptyline hydrochloride (Rx)
　　[*Etrafon-A*].
　4 mg of perphenazine and 25 mg of amitriptyline hydrochloride (Rx)
　　[*Etrafon-F; PMS Levazine*].

#### Auxiliary labeling
• May cause drowsiness.
• Avoid alcoholic beverages.

Revised: 01/27/92
Interim revision: 08/09/94

## PERPHENAZINE-CONTAINING COMBINATIONS—
Perphenazine and Amitriptyline (Systemic)

# PHENACEMIDE　Systemic†

VA CLASSIFICATION (Primary): CN400
Another commonly used name is phenacetylcarbamide.

Note: For a listing of dosage forms and brand names by country availability, see *Dosage Forms* section(s). For a listing of brand names for the articles in this monograph, refer to the General Index.

†Not commercially available in Canada.

## Category
Anticonvulsant.

## Indications

#### Accepted
Epilepsy, complex partial seizure pattern (treatment)—Phenacemide is indicated for control of severe epilepsy, particularly mixed forms of complex partial (psychomotor or temporal lobe) seizures, refractory to other anticonvulsants. Phenacemide should not be used unless other less toxic anticonvulsants have been ineffective in controlling seizures.

## Pharmacology/Pharmacokinetics

#### Physicochemical characteristics
Molecular weight—178.19.

#### Mechanism of action/Effect
The mechanism of action in humans has not been established. However, in animals, at doses well below those causing neurological signs, phenacemide elevates the threshold for minimal electroshock convulsions and abolishes the tonic phase of maximal electroshock seizures. It also prevents or modifies seizures induced by pentylenetetrazol or other convulsants.

#### Absorption
Almost completely absorbed.

#### Biotransformation
Metabolized in the liver by hepatic microsomal enzymes, where it is inactivated by *p*-hydroxylation.

#### Half-life
In one study using 1 control subject and 3 epileptic patients, the half-life of phenacemide was demonstrated to be 22 to 25 hours.

## Precautions to Consider

#### Carcinogenicity
Studies have not been done to determine the carcinogenic potential of phenacemide.

#### Pregnancy/Reproduction
Pregnancy—Phenacemide may cause fetal damage when used during pregnancy. Also, teratogenic effects have been associated with other anticonvulsant medications. Risk-benefit must be carefully considered when this medication is required in life-threatening situations or in serious diseases for which other medications cannot be used or are ineffective.

FDA Pregnancy Category D.

Delivery—Exposure to phenacemide prior to delivery may lead to an increased risk of life-threatening hemorrhage in the neonate, usually within 24 hours of birth. Phenacemide may also produce a deficiency of vitamin K in the mother, causing increased maternal bleeding during delivery. Risk of maternal and infant bleeding may be reduced by administering water-soluble vitamin K prophylactically to the mother 1 month prior to and during delivery and to the neonate, intramuscularly or subcutaneously, immediately after birth.

**Breast-feeding**

It is not known whether phenacemide is excreted in breast milk.

**Pediatrics**

Appropriate studies on the relationship of age to the effects of phenacemide have not been performed in the pediatric population. However, no pediatrics-specific problems have been documented to date.

**Geriatrics**

No information is available on the relationship of age to the effects of phenacemide in geriatric patients.

**Drug interactions and/or related problems**

The following drug interactions and/or related problems have been selected on the basis of their potential clinical significance (possible mechanism in parentheses where appropriate)—not necessarily inclusive (» = major clinical significance):

Note: Combinations containing any of the following medications, depending on the amount present, may also interact with this medication.

Alcohol and
Central nervous system (CNS) depression–producing medications, other
    (See *Appendix II*)
    (CNS depression may be enhanced)

» Anticonvulsants, other, especially ethotoin
    (risk of additive toxicity when these medications are used concurrently with phenacemide; concurrent use of ethotoin with phenacemide has been reported to cause paranoid symptoms; extreme caution is recommended during concurrent use of phenacemide with other anticonvulsants)

**Medical considerations/Contraindications**

The medical considerations/contraindications included here have been selected on the basis of their potential clinical significance (reasons given in parentheses where appropriate)—not necessarily inclusive (» = major clinical significance).

*Risk-benefit should be considered when the following medical problems exist:*

» Blood dyscrasias, history of
    (deaths due to phenacemide-induced aplastic anemia have occurred)

» Hepatic function impairment, history of
    (deaths due to phenacemide-induced liver damage have occurred)

» Personality disorders, history of
    (personality changes including attempts at suicide and psychoses requiring hospitalization have occurred; patient hospitalization during the first week of treatment may be advisable)

» Renal function impairment, history of
    (condition may be aggravated)

» Sensitivity to phenacemide or history of allergy to other anticonvulsants

**Patient monitoring**

The following may be especially important in patient monitoring (other tests may be warranted in some patients, depending on condition; » = major clinical significance):

» Blood cell counts, including platelets
    (recommended before and at monthly intervals after initiation of therapy; if no abnormalities are detected after 12 months, the testing intervals may be extended. The total number of each cellular element per cubic millimeter is a better index of possible blood dyscrasias than the percentage of cells)

» Hepatic function determinations and
Renal function determinations and
Urinalyses
    (recommended before and during therapy)

    Note: If severe depression of the blood count or abnormal urinary findings occur, the medication should be withdrawn.

## Side/Adverse Effects

The following side/adverse effects have been selected on the basis of their potential clinical significance (possible signs and symptoms in parentheses where appropriate)—not necessarily inclusive:

**Those indicating need for medical attention**

Incidence more frequent
    *Behavior or mood changes*

Incidence rare
    *Allergic reactions* (skin rash); *blood dyscrasias, such as aplastic anemia* (shortness of breath; troubled breathing, wheezing, or tightness in chest; sores, ulcers, or white spots on lips or in mouth; swollen or painful glands; unusual bleeding or bruising); *leukopenia* (fever, chills, or sore throat); *or neutropenia* (fever, chills, or continuing ulcers or sores in mouth or throat); *hepatitis* (dark-colored urine; flu-like symptoms; fever with or without chills; headache; body ache; yellow eyes or skin); *nephritis* (difficulty in breathing; drowsiness or unusual tiredness or weakness; nausea or vomiting; blood in urine; unusual weight gain; or swelling of face, feet, or lower legs)

    Note: If *hepatitis* or *jaundice* occurs, the medication should be discontinued.

**Those indicating need for medical attention only if they continue or are bothersome**

Incidence more frequent
    *Anorexia* (loss of appetite); *drowsiness; headache*

Incidence less frequent or rare
    *Dizziness; fever; insomnia* (trouble in sleeping); *muscle pain; palpitation* (pounding heartbeat); *paresthesias* (tingling, burning, or prickly sensations); *unusual tiredness or weakness; weight loss*

## Overdose

For more information on the management of overdose or unintentional ingestion, **contact a Poison Control Center** (see *Poison Control Center Listing*).

**Clinical effects of overdose**

The following effects have been selected on the basis of their potential clinical significance (possible signs and symptoms in parentheses where appropriate)–not necessarily inclusive:

Symptoms of overdose (in order of occurrence)
    *Excitement or mania* (unusual nervousness or irritability); *ataxia* (clumsiness or unsteadiness); *drowsiness, severe*

**Treatment of overdose**

There is no specific antidote for phenacemide overdose. Recommended treatment consists of the following:

To decrease absorption—Evacuation of stomach by induction of emesis or lavage.

Supportive care—Patients in whom intentional overdose is confirmed or suspected should be referred for psychiatric consultation.

Following recovery, evaluation of hepatic and renal function, mental state, and blood-forming organs should be performed.

## Patient Consultation

As an aid to patient consultation, refer to *Advice for the Patient, Phenacemide (Systemic)*.

In providing consultation, consider emphasizing the following selected information (» = major clinical significance):

**Before using this medication**

» Conditions affecting use, especially:
    Sensitivity to phenacemide or history of allergy to other anticonvulsants
    Pregnancy—Increased risk of fetal damage
    Delivery—Possibility of life-threatening hemorrhage in the neonate
    Other medications, especially other anticonvulsants
    Other medical problems, especially a history of personality disorders, blood dyscrasias, or hepatic or renal function impairment

**Proper use of this medication**

» Compliance with therapy; taking every day as directed by physician
» Proper dosing
    Missed dose: Taking as soon as possible; not taking if almost time for next scheduled dose; not doubling doses
» Proper storage

**Precautions while using this medication**

» Regular visits to physician to check progress of therapy
» Checking with physician before discontinuing this medication; gradual dosage reduction may be necessary
» Reporting sore throat, fever, and any unusual bleeding or bruising to physician as soon as possible
» Reporting behavioral changes such as decreased interest in surroundings, depression, or aggressiveness to physician as soon as possible
» Avoiding the use of alcoholic beverages; not taking other medication unless prescribed by physician
» Possibility of drowsiness; caution if driving or doing things requiring alertness

**Side/adverse effects**

» Potential side effects, especially behavior changes, allergic reaction, or symptoms of blood dyscrasias, hepatitis, and nephritis

## General Dosing Information

Because of the potential for serious toxic effects, the dosage of phenacemide should be maintained at the minimum amount necessary to achieve seizure control.

Withdrawal of phenacemide or transition to or from other anticonvulsants should be made gradually to maintain seizure control.

## Oral Dosage Forms

### PHENACEMIDE TABLETS USP

**Usual adult and adolescent dose**
Anticonvulsant—
    Oral, initially 500 mg three times a day; after 1 week, an additional 500 mg may be taken upon arising; in the third week, if necessary, the dose may be increased by adding 500 mg at bedtime.

**Usual adult prescribing limits**
Up to 5 grams daily.

**Usual pediatric dose**
Anticonvulsant—
    Children up to 5 years of age: Dosage has not been established.

Children 5 years of age and over—Oral, initially 250 mg three times a day, the dosage being increased by 250 mg at one week intervals until seizure control is obtained or a total dose of 1.5 grams per day is reached.

**Strength(s) usually available**
U.S.—
    500 mg (Rx) [*Phenurone* (lactose)].
Canada—
    Not commercially available.

**Packaging and storage**
Store below 40 °C (104 °F), preferably between 15 and 30 °C (59 and 86 °F), unless otherwise specified by manufacturer. Store in a well-closed container.

Revised: 03/09/93

---

# PHENAZOPYRIDINE   Systemic

VA CLASSIFICATION (Primary): GU100
Note: For a listing of dosage forms and brand names by country availability, see *Dosage Forms* section(s). For a listing of brand names for the articles in this monograph, refer to the General Index.

## Category
Analgesic (urinary).

## Indications

**Accepted**
Urinary tract irritation (treatment)—Phenazopyridine is indicated for short-term use to relieve symptoms such as pain, burning, and urinary urgency and/or frequency caused by irritation of the lower urinary tract mucosa. The underlying cause of the irritation must be determined and treated (for example, antibacterial therapy for infection).

## Pharmacology/Pharmacokinetics

**Physicochemical characteristics**
Chemical group—Azo dye.
Molecular weight—249.70.

**Mechanism of action/Effect**
Exerts a topical analgesic or local anesthetic action on the urinary tract mucosa. The exact mechanism of action is unknown.

**Biotransformation**
Probably hepatic; also in other tissues. One of the metabolites is acetaminophen.

**Elimination**
Renal. Up to 90% of a dose is excreted within 24 hours, as unchanged drug and metabolites. About 18% of a dose is eliminated as acetaminophen. Up to 65% of a dose may be excreted unchanged.

## Precautions to Consider

**Carcinogenicity**
Long-term administration of phenazopyridine has caused neoplasia of the large intestine in rats and neoplasia of the liver in mice. No association between use of the medication in humans and development of neoplasia has been reported; however, studies in humans have not been done.

**Pregnancy/Reproduction**
Fertility—Studies in rats with doses up to 50 mg per kg of body weight (mg/kg) per day have not shown evidence of impaired fertility.

Pregnancy—Adequate and well-controlled studies have not been done in humans.
Studies in rats with doses up to 50 mg/kg per day have not shown evidence of harm to the fetus.

FDA Pregnancy Category B.

**Breast-feeding**
It is not known whether phenazopyridine or any of its metabolites are distributed into breast milk. However, problems in humans have not been documented.

**Pediatrics**
Appropriate studies with phenazopyridine have not been performed in the pediatric population. However, no pediatrics-specific problems have been documented to date.

**Geriatrics**
Although appropriate studies with phenazopyridine have not been performed in the geriatric population, no geriatrics-specific problems have been documented to date. However, elderly patients are more likely to have age-related renal function impairment, which may increase the risk of accumulation and toxicity in patients receiving phenazopyridine.

**Laboratory value alterations**
The following have been selected on the basis of their potential clinical significance (possible effect in parentheses where appropriate)—not necessarily inclusive (» = major clinical significance):

With physiology/laboratory test values
    Urinalyses based on color reaction or spectroscopy, for example:
      Bilirubin, urine, determined via foam test, talc-disk–Fouchetspot test, or Franklin's tablet-Fouchet test methods
      Glucose, urine, determined using glucose oxidase
      17-Hydroxycorticosteroids, urine, determined via Glenn-Nelson method
      Ketones, urine, determined using sodium nitroprusside or Gerhardt ferric chloride test
      17-Ketosteroids, urine, determined via Haltorff Koch modification of Zimmerman reaction
      Kidney function tested via phenolsulfonphthalein (PSP) excretion
      Protein, urine, determined using bromophenol blue test reagent strips or nitric acid ring test
      Urobilinogen, urine, determined using Ehrlich's reagent
      (phenazopyridine may interfere with test results by causing discoloration of the urine)

**Medical considerations/Contraindications**
The medical considerations/contraindications included here have been selected on the basis of their potential clinical significance (reasons given in parentheses where appropriate)—not necessarily inclusive (» = major clinical significance).

*Risk-benefit should be considered when the following medical problems exist:*
    Allergic reaction to phenazopyridine, history of
» Glucose-6-phosphate dehydrogenase (G6PD) deficiency
    (increased risk of severe hemolytic anemia)
    Hepatitis
    (increased risk of adverse effects)
    Renal function impairment
    (increased risk of accumulation and toxicity)

## Side/Adverse Effects

Note: In addition to the side effects reported below, an anaphylactoid-like reaction has been reported.

The following side/adverse effects have been selected on the basis of their potential clinical significance (possible signs and symptoms in parentheses where appropriate)—not necessarily inclusive:

**Those indicating need for medical attention**
Incidence rare
    *Anemia, hemolytic* (troubled breathing, exertional; unusual tiredness or weakness); *aseptic meningitis* (fever; confusion)—reported in 1 patient; causal relationship verified via rechallenge; *dermatitis, allergic* (skin rash); *hepatotoxicity* (yellow eyes or skin); *methemoglobinemia* (blue or blue-purple discoloration of skin; shortness of breath); *renal function impairment or failure* (increased blood pressure; shortness of breath; troubled breathing; tightness in chest,

and/or wheezing; sudden decrease in amount of urine; swelling of face, fingers, feet, and/or lower legs; thirst, continuing; unusual tiredness or weakness; weight gain)

Note: *Hemolytic anemia* or *methemoglobinemia* may be more likely with an overdose or if the medication is administered to patients with renal function impairment, but have also been reported with therapeutic doses in patients with normal renal function. Also, *hemolytic anemia* is especially likely to occur in patients with glucose-6-phosphate dehydrogenase deficiency.

*Hepatotoxicity* has been reported in conjunction with impaired renal excretion of the medication; however, yellowish discoloration of eyes or skin may also occur independently of hepatotoxicity, indicating accumulation. Permanent staining of soft contact lenses has also been reported.

**Those indicating need for medical attention only if they continue or are bothersome**
Incidence less frequent or rare
*Dizziness; headache; indigestion; stomach cramps or pain*

## Patient Consultation

As an aid to patient consultation, refer to *Advice for the Patient, Phenazopyridine (Systemic).*

In providing consultation, consider emphasizing the following selected information (» = major clinical significance):

**Before using this medication**
» Conditions affecting use, especially:
Allergic reaction to phenazopyridine, history of
Other medical problems, especially glucose-6-phosphate dehydrogenase (G6PD) deficiency

**Proper use of this medication**
Taking with or following food (a meal or a snack) to reduce gastric upset
» Not using any saved portion of medication in the future unless authorized by physician
» Proper dosing
Missed dose: Taking as soon as possible; not taking if almost time for next dose; not doubling doses
» Proper storage

**Precautions while using this medication**
» Informing physician if symptoms worsen
» Medication causes urine to turn reddish orange and may stain clothing
Not wearing soft contact lenses during therapy because of possible permanent staining
Diabetics: May cause false urine sugar and urine ketone test results
Possible interference with laboratory test results; notifying person in charge that medication is being used

**Side/adverse effects**
Signs of potential side effects, especially allergic dermatitis, aseptic meningitis, hemolytic anemia, hepatotoxicity, methemoglobinemia, and renal impairment or failure

## General Dosing Information

This medication should be taken with or following food to lessen gastric irritation.

When phenazopyridine is used concurrently with an antibacterial agent in the treatment of a urinary tract infection, the duration of phenazopyridine therapy should not exceed 2 days. Adequate evidence that more prolonged phenazopyridine therapy provides greater therapeutic benefit than is achieved with the antibacterial agent alone is not available.

**For treatment of adverse effects**
Recommended treatment consists of the following:
• For methemoglobinemia—Administering methylene blue (1 to 2 mg per kg of body weight (mg/kg), intravenously) or ascorbic acid (100 to 200 mg orally).

## Oral Dosage Forms

### PHENAZOPYRIDINE HYDROCHLORIDE TABLETS USP

**Usual adult and adolescent dose**
Analgesic (urinary)—
Oral, 200 mg three times a day, with or following food.

**Usual pediatric dose**
Analgesic (urinary)—
Oral, 4 mg per kg of body weight three times a day, with food.

**Strength(s) usually available**
U.S.—
100 mg (Rx) [*Azo-Standard; Baridium; Eridium; Geridium; Phenazodine; Pyridiate; Pyridium; Urodine; Urogesic;* GENERIC].
200 mg (Rx) [*Geridium; Phenazodine; Pyridiate; Pyridium; Urodine; Viridium;* GENERIC].
Canada—
100 mg (OTC) [*Phenazo; Pyridium*].
200 mg (OTC) [*Phenazo; Pyridium*].

**Packaging and storage**
Store below 40 °C (104 °F), preferably between 15 and 30 °C (59 and 86 °F), unless otherwise specified by manufacturer. Store in a tight container.

**Auxiliary labeling**
• May discolor urine.
• Take with food.

**Note**
Stains on clothing may be removed with a 0.25% solution of sodium dithionate or sodium hydrosulfite.

Revised: 06/08/92
Interim revision: 08/24/94

## PHENAZOPYRIDINE-CONTAINING COMBINATIONS—

Sulfamethoxazole and Phenazopyridine (Systemic)—See *Sulfonamides and Phenazopyridine (Systemic)*
Sulfisoxazole and Phenazopyridine (Systemic)—See *Sulfonamides and Phenazopyridine (Systemic)*

## PHENDIMETRAZINE—See *Appetite Suppressants (Systemic)*

## PHENELZINE—See *Antidepressants, Monoamine Oxidase (MAO) Inhibitor (Systemic)*

## PHENINDAMINE—See *Antihistamines (Systemic)*

## PHENINDAMINE-CONTAINING COMBINATIONS—

Chlorpheniramine, Phenindamine, Phenylephrine, Dextromethorphan, Acetaminophen, Salicylamide, Caffeine, and Ascorbic Acid (Systemic)—See *Cough/Cold Combinations (Systemic)*
Chlorpheniramine, Phenindamine, and Phenylpropanolamine (Systemic)—See *Antihistamines and Decongestants (Systemic)*

## PHENIRAMINE-CONTAINING COMBINATIONS—

Chlorpheniramine, Pheniramine, Pyrilamine, Phenylephrine, Hydrocodone, Salicylamide, Caffeine, and Ascorbic Acid (Systemic)—See *Cough/Cold Combinations (Systemic)*
Pheniramine, Codeine, and Guaifenesin (Systemic)—See *Cough/Cold Combinations (Systemic)*
Pheniramine and Phenylephrine (Systemic)—See *Antihistamines and Decongestants (Systemic)*
Pheniramine, Phenylephrine, and Acetaminophen (Systemic)—See *Antihistamines, Decongestants, and Analgesics (Systemic)*
Pheniramine, Phenylephrine, Codeine, Sodium Citrate, Sodium Salicylate, and Caffeine (Systemic)—See *Cough/Cold Combinations (Systemic)*
Pheniramine, Phenylephrine, and Dextromethorphan (Systemic)—See *Cough/Cold Combinations (Systemic)*
Pheniramine, Phenylephrine, Phenylpropanolamine, Hydrocodone, and Guaifenesin (Systemic)—See *Cough/Cold Combinations (Systemic)*
Pheniramine, Phenylephrine, Sodium Salicylate, and Caffeine (Systemic)—See *Antihistamines, Decongestants, and Analgesics (Systemic)*
Pheniramine, Phenyltoloxamine, Pyrilamine, and Phenylpropanolamine (Systemic)—See *Antihistamines and Decongestants (Systemic)*
Pheniramine, Pyrilamine, Hydrocodone, Potassium Citrate, and Ascorbic Acid (Systemic)—See *Cough/Cold Combinations (Systemic)*
Pheniramine, Pyrilamine, Phenylephrine, Phenylpropanolamine, and Hydrocodone (Systemic)—See *Cough/Cold Combinations (Systemic)*
Pheniramine, Pyrilamine, and Phenylpropanolamine (Systemic)—See *Antihistamines and Decongestants (Systemic)*
Pheniramine, Pyrilamine, Phenylpropanolamine, and Codeine (Systemic)—See *Cough/Cold Combinations (Systemic)*

Pheniramine, Pyrilamine, Phenylpropanolamine, Codeine, Acetaminophen, and Caffeine (Systemic)—See *Cough/Cold Combinations (Systemic)*

Pheniramine, Pyrilamine, Phenylpropanolamine, and Dextromethorphan (Systemic)—See *Cough/Cold Combinations (Systemic)*

Pheniramine, Pyrilamine, Phenylpropanolamine, Dextromethorphan, and Ammonium Chloride (Systemic)—See *Cough/Cold Combinations (Systemic)*

Pheniramine, Pyrilamine, Phenylpropanolamine, Dextromethorphan, and Guaifenesin (Systemic)—See *Cough/Cold Combinations (Systemic)*

Pheniramine, Pyrilamine, Phenylpropanolamine, and Guaifenesin (Systemic)—See *Cough/Cold Combinations (Systemic)*

Pheniramine, Pyrilamine, Phenylpropanolamine, and Hydrocodone (Systemic)—See *Cough/Cold Combinations (Systemic)*

Pheniramine, Pyrilamine, Phenylpropanolamine, Hydrocodone, and Guaifenesin (Systemic)—See *Cough/Cold Combinations (Systemic)*

---

## PHENOBARBITAL—See *Barbiturates (Systemic)*

---

## PHENOBARBITAL-CONTAINING COMBINATIONS—

Atropine, Hyoscyamine, Scopolamine, and Phenobarbital (Systemic)—See *Belladonna Alkaloids and Barbiturates (Systemic)*

Atropine and Phenobarbital (Systemic)—See *Belladonna Alkaloids and Barbiturates (Systemic)*

Belladonna and Phenobarbital (Systemic)—See *Belladonna Alkaloids and Barbiturates (Systemic)*

Ergotamine, Belladonna Alkaloids, and Phenobarbital (Systemic)

Hyoscyamine and Phenobarbital (Systemic)—See *Belladonna Alkaloids and Barbiturates (Systemic)*

Phenobarbital, ASA, and Codeine (Systemic)—See *Barbiturates and Analgesics (Systemic)*

Theophylline, Ephedrine, Guaifenesin, and Phenobarbital (Systemic)

Theophylline, Ephedrine, and Phenobarbital (Systemic)

---

## PHENOLPHTHALEIN—See *Laxatives (Local)*

---

## PHENOLPHTHALEIN-CONTAINING COMBINATIONS—

Cascara Sagrada and Phenolphthalein (Oral-Local)—See *Laxatives (Local)*

Dehydrocholic Acid, Docusate, and Phenolphthalein (Oral-Local)—See *Laxatives (Local)*

Docusate and Phenolphthalein (Oral-Local)—See *Laxatives (Local)*

Mineral Oil, Glycerin, and Phenolphthalein (Oral-Local)—See *Laxatives (Local)*

Mineral Oil and Phenolphthalein (Oral-Local)—See *Laxatives (Local)*

Phenolphthalein and Senna (Oral-Local)—See *Laxatives (Local)*

---

# PHENOLSULFONPHTHALEIN   Systemic

VA CLASSIFICATION (Primary): DX900

Some other commonly used names are phenol red and PSP.

Note: For a listing of dosage forms and brand names by country availability, see *Dosage Forms* section(s). For a listing of brand names for the articles in this monograph, refer to the General Index.

## Category

Diagnostic aid (renal function; residual bladder urine).

Note: Phenolsulfonphthalein is a pH indicator dye.

## Indications

### Accepted

Renal function studies—PSP is indicated for evaluation of renal blood flow to aid in determination of renal function. Because the maximum plasma concentrations of PSP produced by the usual dose do not approach the maximum concentrations that the renal tubules can handle, the PSP excretion test is more a test of renal perfusion than of tubular function.

In general, the PSP excretion test has been replaced by more accurate tests of renal function, such as creatinine clearance.

Bladder urine, residual, determinations—PSP is indicated as a qualitative test for residual bladder urine.

## Pharmacology/Pharmacokinetics

### Physicochemical characteristics

Molecular weight—354.38.

pKa—7.9.

### Mechanism of action/Effect

PSP's usefulness as a diagnostic agent is based on its rapid excretion from the body. It is not reabsorbed by the renal tubules but is secreted predominantly by a single tubular transport path. The excretory rate of PSP is directly related to renal blood flow.

PSP excretion correlates well with the glomerular filtration rate (GFR), although PSP clearance is greater than GFR. Therefore, a normal PSP excretion indicates a normal GFR; a 15% PSP excretion at 15 minutes, for example, indicates a GFR of about 45% of normal.

### Protein binding

High (75 to 80%) *in vitro* (reportedly much lower *in vivo*).

### Biotransformation

Not metabolized, although about 20% of an injected dose is removed by the liver.

### Elimination

Renal, up to 85% (4 to 6% by glomerular filtration, with the remainder secreted by the proximal tubules).

In normal renal function, approximately 25 to 45% of an intravenous dose is excreted in 15 minutes, 50 to 65% in 30 minutes, 65 to 80% in 60 minutes, and up to 85% in 120 minutes.

Excretion is delayed after intramuscular administration (40 to 50% after 1 hour, 60 to 75% after 2 hours).

Biliary.

## Precautions to Consider

### Pregnancy/Reproduction

Pregnancy—Studies have not been done in humans.

It is believed that the PSP excretion test is invalid during pregnancy because of back-diffusion that occurs in dilated ureters (normal part of pregnancy).

Studies have not been done in animals.

FDA Pregnancy Category C.

### Breast-feeding

It is not known if PSP is distributed into breast milk. Problems in humans have not been documented.

### Pediatrics

Appropriate studies on the relationship of age to the effects of PSP have not been performed in the pediatric population. However, pediatrics-specific problems that would limit the use of PSP in children are not expected.

### Geriatrics

Although appropriate studies on the relationship of age to the effects of PSP have not been performed in the geriatric population, geriatrics-specific problems that would limit the usefulness of this medication in the elderly are not expected. However, elderly patients are more likely to have age-related renal function impairment, which in severe cases is a contraindication to use of PSP.

### Drug interactions and/or related problems

See *Laboratory value alterations*.

### Laboratory value alterations

The following have been selected on the basis of their potential clinical significance (possible effect in parentheses where appropriate)—not necessarily inclusive (» = major clinical significance):

With results of *this* test

  *Due to other medications*

    Acidic medications

      (competitive inhibition of transport may result in decreased urinary excretion of PSP)

»  Aminohippurate sodium or

»  Atropine or

»  Diatrizoates or

»  Diuretics, thiazide or

»  Penicillins or

» Salicylates or
» Sulfonamides or
» Uricosurics (such as probenecid and sulfinpyrazone)
  (utilize the same tubular mechanism of secretion as PSP, resulting in decreased urinary excretion of PSP; PSP excretion test is not recommended in patients receiving these medications)

Methylene blue
  (methylene blue may cause a false positive PSP excretion test result)

Substances that discolor the urine (such as sulfobromophthalein, formaldehyde-forming medications, nitrofurantoin, phenazopyridine, and danthron and other anthraquinone-containing medications such as cascara)
  (it is recommended that these medications be avoided for 24 hours prior to the PSP excretion test)

*Due to medical problems or conditions*
Cardiac failure or
Renal diseases, primary or
Vascular diseases, primary
  (impaired renal function may reduce excretion of PSP)

Gout
  (urinary excretion of PSP may be decreased by competitive inhibition of transport)

Hepatic function impairment or
Hypoalbuminemia or
Multiple myeloma
  (may increase the excretion rate of PSP)

Pregnancy
  (back-diffusion that occurs in dilated ureters may make PSP excretion test invalid)

With *other* diagnostic test results
Colorimetric measurements of serum sulfobromophthalein (BSP); serum and urinary creatinine; and urinary creatine, acetone, color, ketones, and vanillylmandelic acid
  (PSP may discolor the urine, resulting in false elevations; PSP causes a pink or red color in alkaline urine)

**Medical considerations/Contraindications**
The medical considerations/contraindications included here have been selected on the basis of their potential clinical significance (reasons given in parentheses where appropriate)—not necessarily inclusive (» = major clinical significance).
See also *Laboratory value alterations.*

*Except under special circumstances, this medication should not be used when the following medical problems exist:*
» Cardiac failure, severe or
» Renal insufficiency, severe
  (rapid hydration necessary for the PSP excretion test may be dangerous)

*Risk-benefit should be considered when the following medical problem exists:*
  Sensitivity to PSP

**Patient monitoring**
The following may be especially important in patient monitoring (other tests may be warranted in some patients, depending on condition; » = major clinical significance):

*For PSP excretion test*
Urinary PSP determinations by colorimetric methods, after alkalinization of the sample
  (recommended on urinary samples collected exactly 15, 30, 60, and 120 minutes after intravenous administration or 1 and 2 hours after intramuscular administration of PSP; the 15-minute value is used most commonly after intravenous administration and is the most useful)

## Side/Adverse Effects

The following side/adverse effects have been selected on the basis of their potential clinical significance (possible signs and symptoms in parentheses where appropriate)—not necessarily inclusive:

**Those indicating need for medical attention**
Incidence rare
  *Idiosyncratic reaction* (skin rash or itching; wheezing)

## Patient Consultation

As an aid to patient consultation, refer to *Advice for the Patient, Phenolsulfonphthalein (Diagnostic).*

In providing consultation, consider emphasizing the following selected information (» = major clinical significance):

**Description of use**
Test procedure: Empty bladder; receive injection; empty bladder again
Proper dosing
» Importance of emptying the bladder completely when asked to do so; otherwise test results may be affected

**Before having this test**
» Conditions affecting use, especially:
    Sensitivity to PSP
    Other medications, especially atropine, thiazide diuretics, penicillins, salicylates, probenecid, sulfinpyrazone, or sulfonamides

**Preparation for this test**
» Importance of fluid intake prior to test; following physician's instructions carefully

**Side/adverse effects**
Signs of potential side effects, especially idiosyncratic reaction

## General Dosing Information

PSP may be administered intravenously or intramuscularly.

**For PSP excretion test**
Results of the PSP excretion test should be interpreted by someone familiar with renal physiology and the clinical status of the patient.

It is recommended that the patient ingest 500 to 1000 mL of water 30 to 90 minutes prior to administration of PSP to ensure adequate hydration and excretion. If necessary, additional fluids may be administered during the test.

Urine collections (emptying of the bladder) are made 15, 30, 60, and 120 minutes after PSP is administered intravenously (1 and 2 hours after intramuscular administration) and analyzed immediately for PSP concentration. If the amount of urine collected is less than 40 mL, results may be distorted.

If PSP excretion is increased at later times over the 15-minute value, there may have been residual urine present in the bladder due to obstructive uropathy or incomplete bladder emptying.

Results of the PSP excretion test may also be distorted by abnormal drainage sites (such as fistulas) or the presence of interfering substances (such as in hematuria).

**For residual bladder urine test**
After emptying the bladder, the patient ingests 600 mL of water, after which no further fluids are administered for the duration of the test.

PSP is administered 30 minutes after ingestion of the water.

A urine collection (emptying of the bladder) is made 2 hours after PSP is administered and that collection and the next voiding are analyzed immediately for PSP concentration. If the patient is not retaining urine and has good kidney function, the second collection should contain no PSP; if it does contain PSP, the two concentrations can be used to calculate the volume of retained urine.

**For treatment of adverse effects**
Adverse effects or idiosyncratic reactions respond to antihistamines or epinephrine.

## Parenteral Dosage Forms

### PHENOLSULFONPHTHALEIN INJECTION

**Usual adult and adolescent dose**
Renal function studies and
Residual bladder urine determinations—
  Intravenous (rapid) or intramuscular, 6 mg.

**Usual pediatric dose**
Renal function studies and
Residual bladder urine determinations—
  See *Usual adult and adolescent dose.*

**Usual geriatric dose**
See *Usual adult and adolescent dose.*

**Strength(s) usually available**
U.S.—
  6 mg per mL (Rx) [GENERIC].

**Packaging and storage**
Store below 40 °C (104 °F), preferably between 15 and 30 °C (59 and 86 °F), unless otherwise specified by manufacturer. Protect from freezing.

Revised: 10/07/91
Interim revision: 08/11/92

# PHENOTHIAZINES  Systemic

This monograph includes information on the following: Acetophenazine†; Chlorpromazine; Fluphenazine; Mesoridazine; Methotrimeprazine; Pericyazine\*; Perphenazine; Pipotiazine\*; Prochlorperazine; Promazine; Thiopropazate\*; Thioproperazine\*; Thioridazine; Trifluoperazine; Triflupromazine†.

INN:
Methotrimeprazine—Levomepromazine
Pericyazine—Periciazine

VA CLASSIFICATION (Primary/Secondary):
Acetophenazine—CN701
Chlorpromazine—CN701/GA700; AU350
Fluphenazine—CN701/CN103
Mesoridazine—CN701
Methotrimeprazine—CN701/CN103; CN309
Pericyazine—CN701
Perphenazine—CN701/GA700
Pipotiazine—CN701
Prochlorperazine—CN701/GA700
Promazine—CN701
Thiopropazate—CN701
Thioproperazine—CN701
Thioridazine—CN701/AU350
Trifluoperazine—CN701
Triflupromazine—CN701/GA700

Note: For a listing of dosage forms and brand names by country availability, see *Dosage Forms* section(s). For a listing of brand names for the articles in this monograph, refer to the General Index.

\*Not commercially available in the U.S.
†Not commercially available in Canada.

## Category

Antipsychotic—Acetophenazine; Chlorpromazine; Fluphenazine; Mesoridazine; Methotrimeprazine; Pericyazine; Perphenazine; Pipotiazine; Prochlorperazine; Promazine; Thiopropazate; Thioproperazine; Thioridazine; Trifluoperazine; Triflupromazine.
Antiemetic—Chlorpromazine; Perphenazine; Prochlorperazine; Triflupromazine.
Analgesic—Methotrimeprazine.
Sedative (preoperative)—Methotrimeprazine.
Antidyskinetic (Huntington's disease)—Chlorpromazine; Thioridazine.
Antineuralgia adjunct—Fluphenazine.

## Indications

Note: Bracketed information in the *Indications* section refers to uses that are not included in U.S. product labeling.

**Accepted**
Psychotic disorders (treatment)—Acetophenazine, chlorpromazine, fluphenazine, mesoridazine, [methotrimeprazine], pericyazine, perphenazine, pipotiazine, prochlorperazine, promazine, thiopropazate, thioproperazine, thioridazine, trifluoperazine, and triflupromazine are indicated in the management of psychotic conditions. They are clearly effective in schizophrenia, and for production of a quieting effect in hyperactive or excited psychotic patients.

Chlorpromazine, mesoridazine, and thioridazine are used for the treatment of children or adults with severe behavior problems associated with psychotic disorders or neurologic disease, who show combativeness and/or explosive, hyperexcitable behavior that is out of proportion to the immediate provocation. These agents are also used in the short-term treatment of hyperactive children who show excessive motor activity with accompanying conduct disorders such as impulsivity, mood lability, aggressiveness, short attention span, and poor frustration tolerance. Pericyazine is a more sedative phenothiazine with weak antipsychotic properties. It is indicated as an adjunctive medication in some psychotic patients for the control of residual prevailing hostility, impulsiveness, and aggressiveness.

Long-acting parenteral forms, fluphenazine decanoate and enanthate and pipotiazine palmitate, are indicated for the maintenance treatment of chronic, non-agitated schizophrenic patients stabilized with shorter-acting neuroleptics, who may benefit from a transfer to the longer-acting drug.

Thioridazine is indicated for the short-term treatment of adult patients with moderate to severe mental depression with varying degrees of anxiety and geriatric patients with multiple symptoms such as anxiety, agitation, depressed mood, tension, sleep disturbances, and fears.

Chlorpromazine is used for anxiety, apprehension, and restlessness before surgery.

Nausea and vomiting (treatment)—Prochlorperazine, chlorpromazine, perphenazine, and triflupromazine are indicated in the control of severe nausea and vomiting in selected patients, with prochlorperazine being superior to other phenothiazines.

Pain (treatment)—Methotrimeprazine is indicated for the relief of moderate to severe pain in nonambulatory patients, and to produce obstetrical analgesia when respiratory depression should be avoided.

Sedation—Methotrimeprazine is indicated as a presurgical or obstetrical medication to produce sedation and somnolence.

[Anesthesia, general, adjunct]—Intravenous administration of methotrimeprazine is indicated as an adjunct to anesthesia, to increase the effects of anesthetics. The dose of a barbiturate or narcotic should be reduced by half when used with methotrimeprazine during surgery or labor.

Tetanus (treatment adjunct)—Chlorpromazine is indicated, usually in conjunction with a barbiturate, for the treatment of tetanus.

Porphyria, acute, intermittent (treatment)—Chlorpromazine is indicated in the treatment of acute intermittent porphyria.

Hiccups, intractable (treatment)—Chlorpromazine is indicated in the control of intractable hiccups.

[Pain, neurogenic (treatment adjunct)][1]—Fluphenazine has been used as an adjunct to tricyclic antidepressant therapy for some chronic pain states, as in patients trying to withdraw from narcotics, and in treatment of symptoms of diabetic neuropathy.

[Huntington's disease, choreiform movement of (treatment)][1]—Chlorpromazine and thioridazine are effective in reducing choreiform movement in Huntington's disease, and have been used as alternatives to haloperidol.

[1]Not included in Canadian product labeling.

## Pharmacology/Pharmacokinetics

**Physicochemical characteristics**
Chemical group—
Aliphatic: Chlorpromazine; methotrimeprazine; promazine; triflupromazine
Piperazine: Acetophenazine; fluphenazine; perphenazine; prochlorperazine; thiopropazate; thioproperazine; trifluoperazine
Piperidine: Mesoridazine; pericyazine; pipotiazine; thioridazine
Molecular weight—
Acetophenazine maleate: 643.71.
Chlorpromazine: 318.86.
Chlorpromazine hydrochloride: 355.32.
Fluphenazine decanoate: 591.8.
Fluphenazine enanthate: 549.69.
Fluphenazine hydrochloride: 510.44.
Mesoridazine besylate: 544.74.
Methotrimeprazine: 328.47.
Pericyazine: 365.19.
Perphenazine: 403.97.
Pipotiazine palmitate: 714.08.
Prochlorperazine: 373.94.
Prochlorperazine edisylate: 564.13.
Prochlorperazine maleate: 606.09.
Prochlorperazine mesylate: 566.1.
Promazine hydrochloride: 320.88.
Thiopropazate hydrochloride: 518.94.
Thioproperazine mesylate: 638.8.
Thioridazine: 370.57.
Thioridazine hydrochloride: 407.03.
Trifluoperazine hydrochloride: 480.42.
Triflupromazine: 352.42.
Triflupromazine hydrochloride: 388.88.

**Mechanism of action/Effect**
Antipsychotic—Thought to improve psychotic conditions by blocking postsynaptic mesolimbic dopaminergic receptors in the brain. Phenothiazines also produce an alpha-adrenergic blocking effect and depress the release of hypothalamic and hypophyseal hormones. However, blockade of dopamine receptors increases prolactin release by the pituitary.
Antiemetic—Phenothiazines act centrally to inhibit or block the dopamine ($D_2$) receptors in the medullary chemoreceptor trigger zone (CTZ) and peripherally by blocking the vagus nerve in the gastrointestinal tract.

The antiemetic effects of phenothiazines may be augmented by their anticholinergic, sedative, and antihistaminic effects.

Antianxiety—Thought to cause indirect reduction in arousal and increased filtering of internal stimuli to the brainstem reticular system.

Analgesic; sedative—Methotrimeprazine raises pain threshold and produces amnesia by suppression of sensory impulses. The alpha-adrenergic blocking effects of phenothiazines may produce sedation and tranquilization.

| Drug | Action* | | | | |
|------|---------|---|---|---|---|
| | Legend:<br>**I**=Antiemetic<br>**II**=Anticholinergic<br>**III**=Extrapyramidal<br>**IV**=Hypotensive<br>**V**=Sedative | | | | |
| | **I** | **II** | **III** | **IV** | **V** |
| **Aliphatic** | | | | | |
| Chlorpromazine | S | M–S | W–M | S | S |
| Methotrimeprazine | W | M | W–M | S | S |
| Promazine | M | S | W | S | S |
| Triflupromazine | S | S | M–S | M | M–S |
| **Piperazine** | | | | | |
| Acetophenazine | W | W | M | W | M |
| Fluphenazine | W | W | S | W | W |
| Perphenazine | S | W–M | S | W | W–M |
| Prochlorperazine | S | W | S | W | W |
| Thiopropazate | W | W | S | W | W |
| Thioproperazine | W | W | S | W | W |
| Trifluoperazine | S | W | S | W | W |
| **Piperidine** | | | | | |
| Mesoridazine | W | M | W | M–S | S |
| Pericyazine | S | S | M | M | S |
| Pipotiazine | W | W | S | W | W |
| Thioridazine | W | M | W | M–S | M |

*S=strong; M=moderate; W=weak

**Protein binding**
Very high (90% or more).

**Biotransformation**
Hepatic.

**Onset of action**
Antipsychotic effect—
Gradual (up to several weeks) and variable between patients.
Long-acting parenteral dosage forms—
Fluphenazine decanoate injection—Antipsychotic effects usually begin between 24 and 72 hours after administration and become significant within 48 to 96 hours.
Pipotiazine palmitate injection—Antipsychotic effects usually begin within the first 48 to 72 hours after administration and become significant within 1 week.

**Time to peak effect**
Antipsychotic effect—Approximately 4 to 7 days to achieve steady-state plasma concentrations; peak therapeutic effects may take from 6 weeks to 6 months.
Analgesic effect (methotrimeprazine)—Within 20 to 40 minutes after intramuscular injection, maintained for about 4 hours.

**Elimination**
Primarily renal; biliary.
In dialysis—Phenothiazines are not successfully dialyzed because of their high protein binding.

## Precautions to Consider

### Cross-sensitivity and/or related problems
Patients sensitive to one phenothiazine may be sensitive to other phenothiazines also.

### Tumorigenicity
Antipsychotic medications produce an elevation in prolactin concentrations, which persists during chronic administration. Tissue culture experiments indicate that approximately one-third of human breast cancers are prolactin-dependent *in vitro*, a factor of potential importance if the prescription of these medications is contemplated in a patient with a previously detected breast cancer. Although disturbances such as galactorrhea, amenorrhea, gynecomastia, and impotence have been reported, the clinical significance of elevated serum prolactin concentrations is unknown for most patients. An increase in mammary neoplasms has been found in rodents after chronic administration of an-

tipsychotic medications. However, neither clinical studies nor epidemiologic studies conducted to date have shown an association between chronic administration of these medications and mammary tumorigenesis; the available evidence is considered too limited to be conclusive at this time.

### Pregnancy/Reproduction
Fertility—Phenothiazines have been found to depress spermatogenesis in animals at doses greatly exceeding the human dose.

Pregnancy—Although adequate and well-controlled studies in humans have not been done, there have been reports of prolonged jaundice, hypo- or hyperreflexia, and extrapyramidal effects in the neonates of mothers who received phenothiazines near term. Phenothiazines are not recommended for use during pregnancy.

For chlorpromazine: Chlorpromazine crosses the placenta. Reproductive studies in rodents have shown a potential for embryotoxicity, increased neonatal mortality and decreased performance. The possibility of permanent neurological damage in offspring of rodent mothers cannot be excluded.

For methotrimeprazine: Reproductive studies in animals and clinical experience have failed to show a teratogenic effect. However, a possible antifertility effect has been suggested since successive generations of animals administered methotrimeprazine have shown smaller litter sizes than those of controls.

For thioridazine: Reproductive studies in animals and clinical experience have failed to show a teratogenic effect.

For trifluoperazine: Reproductive studies in rats given 600 times the human dose showed an increased incidence of malformations and reduced weight and litter size linked to maternal toxicity.

### Breast-feeding
Phenothiazines are distributed into breast milk, possibly causing drowsiness and an increased risk of dystonias and tardive dyskinesia in the baby. Most phenothiazines increase prolactin secretion in the mother.

### Pediatrics
Children appear to be prone to develop neuromuscular or extrapyramidal reactions, especially dystonias, and should be closely monitored while receiving therapeutic doses of phenothiazines. Children with acute illnesses, such as chickenpox, CNS infections, measles, gastroenteritis, or dehydration, are especially at risk.

### Geriatrics
Geriatric patients tend to develop higher plasma concentrations of phenothiazines because of changes in distribution due to decreases in lean body mass, total body water, and albumin, and often an increase in total body fat composition. Therefore, these patients usually require lower initial dosage and a more gradual titration of dose.

Elderly patients appear to be more prone to orthostatic hypotension and exhibit an increased sensitivity to the anticholinergic and sedative effects of phenothiazines. In addition, they are more prone to develop extrapyramidal side effects, such as tardive dyskinesia and parkinsonism. The symptoms of tardive dyskinesia are persistent, difficult to control, and, in some patients, appear to be irreversible. There is no known effective treatment. Careful observation during treatment for early signs of tardive dyskinesia and reduction of dosage or discontinuation of medication may prevent a more severe manifestation of the syndrome.

It has been suggested that elderly patients receive half the usual adult dose. Patients with organic brain syndrome or acute confusional states, should initially receive one-third to one-half the usual adult dose, with the dose being increased no more frequently than every 2 or 3 days, preferably at intervals of 7 to 10 days, if possible. After clinical improvement occurs, periodic attempts should be made to discontinue medication.

### Dental
The peripheral anticholinergic effects of phenothiazines may decrease or inhibit salivary flow, especially in middle-aged or elderly patients, thus contributing to the development of caries, periodontal disease, oral candidiasis, and discomfort.

Extrapyramidal reactions induced by phenothiazines will result in increased motor activity of the head, face, and neck. Occlusal adjustments, bite registrations, and treatment for bruxism may be made less reliable.

The leukopenic and thrombocytopenic effects of phenothiazines may result in an increased incidence of microbial infection, delayed healing, and gingival bleeding. If leukopenia or thrombocytopenia occurs, dental work should be deferred until blood counts have returned to normal, and patients should be instructed in proper oral hygiene, including caution in use of regular toothbrushes, dental floss, and toothpicks.

### Drug interactions and/or related problems
The following drug interactions and/or related problems have been selected on the basis of their potential clinical significance (possible

mechanism in parentheses where appropriate)—not necessarily inclusive (» = major clinical significance):

Note: Combinations containing any of the following medications, depending on the amount present, may also interact with this medication.

» Alcohol or
» CNS depression–producing medications, other (See *Appendix II*)
   (concurrent use with phenothiazines may result in increased CNS and respiratory depression and increased hypotensive effects; dosage reductions of either drug may be necessary during concurrent use or when sequence of use enhances CNS effects)

   (alcohol may increase the risk of heat stroke when taken concurrently with phenothiazines)

   (in addition, barbiturates increase the metabolism of chlorpromazine by induction of hepatic microsomal enzymes, thus decreasing plasma concentrations, and possibly the therapeutic effect, of chlorpromazine; conversely, thioridazine may reduce serum phenobarbital concentrations)

Amantadine or
Antidyskinetics or
Antihistamines or
Anticholinergics or other medications with anticholinergic action (See *Appendix II*)
   (concurrent use with phenothiazines may intensify anticholinergic side effects, especially confusion, hallucinations, and nightmares, because of the phenothiazines' secondary anticholinergic effects; medications with anticholinergic effects may potentiate the hyperpyretic effect of phenothiazines, especially when environmental temperatures are high, by preventing sweating as a cooling mechanism; this effect could lead to heat stroke; also, patients should be advised to report occurrence of gastrointestinal problems since paralytic ileus may occur with concurrent therapy)

   (trihexyphenidyl may decrease plasma phenothiazine concentrations by decreasing gastrointestinal motility and increasing metabolism of the phenothiazine; since the antipsychotic effectiveness may be reduced, dosage adjustment of the phenothiazine may be required)

   (parenteral methotrimeprazine, used as preanesthetic medication, may be administered concurrently, but with caution, with lowered doses of atropine or scopolamine; tachycardia and a fall in blood pressure may occur, and CNS reactions, such as stimulation, delirium, and extrapyramidal reactions, may be aggravated)

Amphetamines
   (stimulant effects may be decreased when amphetamines are used concurrently with phenothiazines since phenothiazines produce alpha-adrenergic blockade; also, the antipsychotic effectiveness of phenothiazines may be reduced)

Antacids, aluminum- or magnesium-containing or
Antidiarrheals, adsorbent
   (concurrent use of these medications with phenothiazines may inhibit the absorption of orally administered phenothiazines, especially chlorpromazine; simultaneous use should be avoided)

Anticonvulsants, including barbiturates
   (phenothiazines may lower the seizure threshold; dosage adjustment of anticonvulsant medications may be necessary)

   (phenothiazines may inhibit phenytoin metabolism, leading to phenytoin toxicity)

» Antidepressants, tricyclic or
Maprotiline or
Monoamine oxidase (MAO) inhibitors, including furazolidone, procarbazine, and selegiline
   (concurrent use may prolong and intensify the sedative and anticholinergic effects of either these medications or phenothiazines; phenothiazines may increase plasma concentrations of cyclic antidepressants by inhibiting metabolism; conversely, cyclic antidepressants may inhibit phenothiazine metabolism; also, the risk of neuroleptic malignant syndrome [NMS] may be increased)

» Antithyroid agents
   (concurrent use with phenothiazines may increase the risk of agranulocytosis)

Apomorphine
   (prior ingestion of phenothiazine antiemetics may decrease the emetic response to apomorphine; also, the CNS depressant effects of phenothiazine antiemetics are additive to those of apomorphine and may induce dangerous respiratory depression, circulatory system effects, or prolonged sleep)

Appetite suppressants
   (concurrent use with phenothiazines may antagonize the anorectic effect of appetite suppressants, with the exception of fenfluramine and phenmetrazine)

Beta-adrenergic blocking agents
   (concurrent use of beta-blockers, possibly including ophthalmics, with phenothiazines may result in an increased plasma concentration of each medication because of inhibition of metabolism; this may result in additive hypotensive effects, irreversible retinopathy, cardiac arrhythmias, and tardive dyskinesia)

Bromocriptine
   (concurrent use may increase serum prolactin concentrations and interfere with effects of bromocriptine; dosage adjustments may be necessary)

Cimetidine
   (concurrent use may decrease steady-state chlorpromazine concentrations by impairing its gastrointestinal absorption)

Diuretics, thiazide
   (concurrent use may potentiate hyponatremia and water intoxication; alternate methods of hypertension control should be considered)

Dopamine
   (concurrent use may antagonize the peripheral vasoconstriction produced by high doses of dopamine, because of the alpha-adrenergic blocking action of phenothiazines)

Ephedrine
   (concurrent use with phenothiazines may decrease the pressor response to ephedrine)

» Epinephrine
   (the use of epinephrine to treat phenothiazine-induced hypotension should be avoided because the alpha-adrenergic effects of epinephrine may be blocked, resulting in beta stimulation only and causing severe hypotension and tachycardia)

» Extrapyramidal reaction–causing medications, other (See *Appendix II*)
   (concurrent use with phenothiazines may increase the severity and frequency of extrapyramidal effects)

Hepatotoxic medications, other (See *Appendix II*)
   (concurrent use of phenothiazines with medications known to alter hepatic microsomal enzyme activity may result in an increased incidence of hepatotoxicity; patients, especially those on prolonged administration or with a history of liver disease, should be carefully monitored)

» Hypotension–producing medications, other (See *Appendix II*)
   (concurrent use with phenothiazines may produce severe hypotension with postural syncope)

» Levodopa
   (antiparkinsonian effects of levodopa may be inhibited when it is used concurrently with phenothiazines, because of blockade of dopamine receptors in brain; levodopa has not been shown to be effective in the treatment of phenothiazine-induced parkinsonism)

» Lithium
   (concurrent use with chlorpromazine and possibly other phenothiazines may reduce gastrointestinal absorption of the phenothiazine, thereby decreasing its serum concentrations by as much as 40%; concurrent use may increase rate of renal excretion of lithium; extrapyramidal symptoms may be increased; also, nausea and vomiting, early indications of lithium toxicity, may be masked by the antiemetic effect of some phenothiazines)

Metaraminol
   (concurrent use with phenothiazines usually decreases, but does not reverse or completely block, the pressor effect of metaraminol because of the alpha-adrenergic blocking action of phenothiazines)

Mephentermine
   (concurrent use with phenothiazines, especially chlorpromazine, may antagonize the antipsychotic effect of the phenothiazine or the pressor effect of mephentermine by exerting opposing effects on monoaminergic functions in the central and peripheral nervous systems)

Methoxamine
   (prior administration of phenothiazines may decrease the pressor effect and shorten the duration of action of methoxamine, because of the alpha-adrenergic blocking action of phenothiazines)

» Metrizamide
   (concurrent use with phenothiazines may lower the seizure threshold; phenothiazines should be discontinued at least 48 hours before, and not resumed for at least 24 hours following, myelography)

Ototoxic medications, especially ototoxic antibiotics (See *Appendix II*)
(concurrent use with phenothiazines may mask some symptoms of ototoxicity such as tinnitus, dizziness, or vertigo)

Opioid (narcotic) analgesics
(in addition to increased CNS and respiratory depression, concurrent use with phenothiazines increases orthostatic hypotension and increases the risk of severe constipation, which may lead to paralytic ileus, and/or urinary retention)

Phenylephrine
(prior administration of phenothiazines may decrease the pressor effect and shorten the duration of action of phenylephrine)

Photosensitizing medications, other
(concurrent use with phenothiazines may cause additive photosensitizing effects)

(in addition, concurrent use of systemic methoxsalen, trioxsalen, or tetracyclines with phenothiazines may potentiate intraocular photochemical damage to the choroid, retina, or lens)

Probucol
(additive QT interval prolongation may increase the risk of ventricular tachycardia)

Succinylcholine
(concurrent use with methotrimeprazine may cause tachycardia and a fall in blood pressure, CNS stimulation and delirium, and an aggravation of extrapyramidal effects)

## Laboratory value alterations
The following have been selected on the basis of their potential clinical significance (possible effect in parentheses where appropriate)—not necessarily inclusive (» = major clinical significance):

With diagnostic test results
Bilirubin tests, urine
(phenothiazine use may produce false-positive results)

Electrocardiogram (ECG) readings
(may cause Q- and T-wave changes, such as increased QT intervals, ST depression, and changes in AV conduction; these are usually reversible)

Gonadorelin test
(phenothiazines may blunt the response to gonadorelin by increasing serum prolactin concentrations)

Pregnancy tests, immunologic urine
(phenothiazines may produce false-positive or false-negative results, depending on the test used)

Metyrapone tests
(adrenocorticotropic hormone [ACTH] secretion may be reduced)

## Medical considerations/Contraindications
The medical considerations/contraindications included here have been selected on the basis of their potential clinical significance (reasons given in parentheses where appropriate)—not necessarily inclusive (» = major clinical significance).

*Except under special circumstances, this medicine should not be used when the following medical problems exist:*

» Cardiovascular disease, severe or
» CNS depression, severe or
» Comatose states
(may be exacerbated)

*Risk-benefit should be considered when the following medical problems exist:*

» Alcoholism, active
(CNS depression may be potentiated; risk of heat stroke may be increased; chronic alcohol abusers may be predisposed to hepatotoxic reactions during phenothiazine therapy)

Angina pectoris
(pain may be increased with use of trifluoperazine)

» Blood dyscrasias
(may be exacerbated; treatment may have to be discontinued)

Breast cancer
(potentially higher risk of disease progression and possible increased resistance to endocrine and cytotoxic treatment, due to phenothiazine-induced prolactin secretion)

Cardiovascular disease
(increased risk of hypotension; myocardial depression, cardiomegaly, congestive heart failure [CHF], and arrhythmias may be induced)

Glaucoma, or predisposition to
(may be potentiated)

» Hepatic function impairment
(metabolism may be decreased; higher serum phenothiazine concentrations may increase sensitivity to CNS effects)

Parkinson's disease
(potentiation of extrapyramidal effects)

Peptic ulcer or
Urinary retention
(may be exacerbated)

Prostatic hypertrophy, symptomatic
(increased risk of urinary retention)

Respiratory disorders, chronic, especially in children
(may be potentiated)

» Reye's syndrome
(increased risk of hepatotoxicity in children and adolescents whose signs and symptoms suggest Reye's syndrome)

Seizure disorders
(seizures may be precipitated)

Sensitivity to any phenothiazine
(may be potentiated upon re-exposure to any phenothiazine in patients with a history of phenothiazine-induced blood dyscrasias, jaundice, or skin reactions)

Vomiting
(antiemetic action of phenothiazines may mask vomiting caused by overdose of other medications)

Caution should also be used in geriatric, emaciated, and debilitated patients, who usually require a lower initial dose.

## Patient monitoring
The following may be especially important in patient monitoring (other tests may be warranted in some patients, depending on condition; » = major clinical significance):

Abnormal-movement determinations
(recommended every 2 months during therapy for institutionalized patients, using the abnormal involuntary movement scale [AIMS], and again at 8 to 12 weeks after therapy has been discontinued)

Blood cell counts and differential in patients with sore throat and fever or infections
(may be required during high-dose or prolonged therapy when symptoms of infection develop; agranulocytosis is more likely to occur between the 4th and 10th weeks of therapy; if significant cellular depression occurs, medication should be discontinued and appropriate therapy initiated; rechallenge in recovered patients will usually cause a recurrence of agranulocytosis; use of alternate neuroleptics such as haloperidol or thioxanthenes is recommended)

Blood pressure measurements
(recommended periodically to detect hypotension)

Careful observation for early signs of tardive dyskinesia
(recommended at periodic intervals, especially in the elderly and other patients on high or extended maintenance dosage; since there is no known effective treatment if syndrome should develop, the phenothiazine should be discontinued at earliest signs, usually fine, worm-like movements of the tongue, to stop further development)

Hepatic function determinations and
Urine tests for bilirubin and bile
(may be required at periodic intervals during prolonged therapy, or if jaundice or grippe-like symptoms occur, to detect liver function impairment; these side effects are more likely to occur between the 2nd and 4th weeks of therapy; phenothiazine should be discontinued if bilirubinemia, bilirubinuria, or icterus occurs)

Ophthalmologic examinations
(recommended, if possible, prior to initiation of phenothiazine therapy as a baseline; initial screening should include measurement of visual acuity with and without refraction, a color vision test to detect possible central defects, and, if feasible, a slit-lamp microscopy study of the fundus and examination of the visual fields. Tests may be required at periodic intervals [usually every 6 to 12 months] during high-dose or prolonged therapy, since deposition of particulate matter in the lens and cornea has occurred with some phenothiazines; therapy should be discontinued if corneal, retinal, or lens changes are noticed; blurred vision, defective color vision, and night blindness are early symptoms of pigmentary retinopathy and may be reversible if detected and the phenothiazine discontinued in the early stages)

Phenothiazine concentrations, serum
(determinations recommended when toxicity or poor response occurs, or when noncompliance is suspected)

# Side/Adverse Effects

The following side/adverse effects have been selected on the basis of their potential clinical significance (possible signs and symptoms in parentheses where appropriate)—not necessarily inclusive:

**Those indicating need for medical attention**
Incidence more frequent
*Akathisia* (restlessness or need to keep moving); *blurred vision associated with anticholinergic effect; deposition of opaque material in lens, cornea, and retina* (blurred vision); *dystonic extrapyramidal effects* (muscle spasms of face, neck, and back; tic-like or twitching movements, twisting movements of body; inability to move eyes; weakness of arms and legs); *parkinsonian extrapyramidal effects* (difficulty in speaking or swallowing; loss of balance control; mask-like face; shuffling walk; stiffness of arms or legs; trembling and shaking of hands and fingers); *hypotension* (fainting)—less common with the piperazine phenothiazines; *pigmentary retinopathy* (blurred vision; defective color vision; difficulty seeing at night)—more frequent with high doses of thioridazine; *tardive dyskinesia* (lip smacking or puckering; puffing of cheeks; rapid or worm-like movements of tongue; uncontrolled chewing movements; uncontrolled movements of arms and legs)—more frequent in elderly patients, women, and patients with brain damage

Note: *Parkinsonian* effects are more frequent in the elderly, whereas *dystonias* occur more often in younger patients. Symptoms may be seen in the first few days of treatment or after prolonged treatment, and can recur after even a single dose. The effects are more common with the piperazine phenothiazines.

Incidence less frequent
*Difficulty in urinating; increased sensitivity of skin to sun* (rash; severe sunburn); *skin rash*—associated with contact dermatitis (with liquid products), or other allergic reaction, or cholestatic jaundice

Incidence rare
*Agranulocytosis* (sore throat; fever; unusual bleeding or bruising; unusual tiredness or weakness)—more frequent with aliphatic phenothiazines; *cholestatic jaundice* (abdominal or stomach pains; aching muscles and joints; fever and chills; severe skin itching; yellow eyes or skin; fatigue; nausea, vomiting, or diarrhea); *heat stroke* (hot dry skin; inability to sweat; muscle weakness; confusion); *neuroleptic malignant syndrome (NMS)* (convulsions; difficult or fast breathing; fast heartbeat or irregular pulse; fever; high or low [irregular] blood pressure; increased sweating; loss of bladder control; severe muscle stiffness; unusually pale skin; unusual tiredness or weakness); *priapism* (prolonged, painful, inappropriate penile erection); *melanosis* (tanning or blue-gray discoloration of skin)—more common with long-term, high-dose, low-potency chlorpromazine and thioridazine

Note: *Agranulocytosis* can develop within the first 3 months of treatment, with recovery within 1 to 2 weeks after medication is discontinued; may recur upon rechallenge in recovered patients.

Liver function tests may be abnormal without overt jaundice. *Jaundice* may appear about 2 weeks after severe pruritus and may progress to chronic active hepatitis. Discontinuing medication may be necessary.

*Heat stroke,* caused by phenothiazine-induced suppression of central and peripheral temperature regulation in the hypothalamus, may occur in environmental conditions of high heat and high humidity. The effectiveness of sweating as a cooling mechanism may be reduced by humid conditions and by the *anticholinergic effects* of phenothiazines or their combination with other anticholinergic medications such as nonprescription cold medications or antihistamines. Adequate interior temperature control (air-conditioning) must be maintained for institutionalized patients during hot weather because of the increased risk of *heat stroke* and *neuroleptic malignant syndrome (NMS)*. Patients should be advised to avoid exertion, stay in cool areas, and avoid dehydration and other anticholinergic medications. Phenothiazines may also cause hypothermia in cold weather, since the disruption of the thermoregulatory mechanisms results in a poikilothermic state.

*NMS* may occur at any time during neuroleptic therapy and is potentially fatal. It is more commonly seen soon after start of therapy or after patient has switched from one neuroleptic to another, during combined therapy with another psychotropic medication, or after a dosage increase. Along with the overt signs of skeletal muscle rigidity, hyperthermia, autonomic dysfunction, and altered consciousness, differential diagnosis may reveal leukocytosis (9500 to 26,000 cells per cubic millimeter), elevated liver enzyme tests, and elevated creatine phosphokinase (CPK).

**Those indicating need for medical attention only if they continue or are bothersome**
Incidence more frequent
*Anticholinergic effects* (constipation; decreased sweating; dizziness [orthostatic hypotension]; drowsiness; dry mouth)—less frequent with piperazine phenothiazines; *nasal congestion*

Incidence less frequent
*Changes in menstrual period; decreased sexual ability; secretion of milk, unusual; swelling or pain in breasts; weight gain, unusual*

**Those indicating need for medical attention if they occur after the medication is discontinued**
Incidence more frequent
*Tardive dyskinesia, persistent* (lip smacking or puckering; puffing of cheeks; rapid or worm-like movements of tongue; uncontrolled chewing movements; uncontrolled movements of arms and legs)—more frequent in elderly patients, women, and patients with brain damage

Incidence less frequent
*Dizziness; nausea and vomiting; stomach pain; trembling of fingers and hands*

# Overdose

For specific information on the agents used in the management of phenothiazine overdose, see:
*Benztropine* in *Antidyskinetics (Systemic)* monograph;
*Charcoal, Activated (Oral-Local)* monograph;
*Diazepam* in *Benzodiazepines (Systemic)* monograph;
*Digitalis Glycosides (Systemic)* monograph;
*Diphenhydramine* in *Antihistamines (Systemic)* monograph;
*Norepinephrine* and/or *Phenylephrine* in *Sympathomimetic Agents—Cardiovascular Use (Parenteral-Systemic)* monograph; and/or
*Phenytoin* in *Anticonvulsants, Hydantoin (Systemic)* monograph.

For more information on the management of overdose or unintentional ingestion, **contact a Poison Control Center** (see *Poison Control Center Listing*).

**Treatment of overdose**
Treatment is essentially symptomatic and supportive. The following may be considered:
To decrease absorption—
  Attempting early gastric lavage; avoiding induction of vomiting because potential phenothiazine-induced dystonic reactions of the head and neck may result in aspiration of vomitus.
  Administering activated charcoal slurry.
  Administering saline cathartic.
Specific treatment—
  Controlling cardiac arrhythmias with intravenous phenytoin, 9 to 11 mg per kg of body weight (mg/kg).
  Digitalizing for cardiac failure.
  Administering vasopressor such as norepinephrine or phenylephrine for hypotension (not using epinephrine, because it may cause paradoxical hypotension).
  Controlling convulsions with diazepam followed by phenytoin, 15 mg/kg, while monitoring ECG.
  Administering benztropine or diphenhydramine to manage acute, parkinson-like symptoms that may occur.
Monitoring—
  Monitoring cardiovascular function for not less than 5 days.
Supportive care—
  Maintaining respiratory function.
  Maintaining body temperature.
  Patients in whom intentional overdose is known or suspected should be referred for psychiatric consultation.

Note: Dialysis of phenothiazines has not been successful.

# Patient Consultation

As an aid to patient consultation, refer to *Advice for the Patient, Phenothiazines (Systemic)*.

In providing consultation, consider emphasizing the following selected information (» = major clinical significance):

**Before using this medication**
» Conditions affecting use, especially:
  Sensitivity to any phenothiazine
  Pregnancy—Not recommended for use during pregnancy because of reports of jaundice, hypo- or hyperreflexia, and extrapyramidal symptoms in neonates
  Breast-feeding—Distributed into breast milk; may cause drowsiness, dystonias, and tardive dyskinesia in the baby
  Use in children—Children, especially those with acute illnesses, are more prone to extrapyramidal symptoms

Use in the elderly—Elderly patients are more likely to develop extrapyramidal, anticholinergic, hypotensive, and sedative effects; reduced dosage recommended

Dental—Phenothiazine-induced blood dyscrasias may result in infections, delayed healing, and bleeding; dry mouth may cause caries and candidiasis; increased motor activity of face, head, and neck may interfere with some dental procedures

Other medications, especially alcohol, other CNS depression-producing medications, tricyclic antidepressants, antithyroid agents, epinephrine, other hypotension-producing medications, other extrapyramidal-producing medications, levodopa, lithium, or metrizamide

Other medical problems, especially cardiovascular disease, severe CNS depression, active alcoholism, blood dyscrasias, liver disease, or Reye's syndrome

## Proper use of this medication

Proper administration of this medication
*For oral dosage forms*
 Taking with food, milk, or water to reduce stomach irritation
» Diluting medication that comes in dropper bottle with recommended beverages prior to use
 Swallowing the extended-release dosage form whole
*For rectal dosage forms*
 Chilling suppository if too soft to insert
 How to insert suppository
» Compliance with therapy; not taking more or less medication than prescribed
» Several weeks of therapy may be required to produce desired effects in treatment of nervous, mental, or emotional conditions
» Proper dosing
 Missed dose: When dosing schedule is—
  One dose a day: Taking as soon as possible unless almost time for next dose, then going back to regular dosing schedule; not doubling doses
  More than one dose a day: Taking as soon as possible if within an hour or so of missed dose; skipping missed dose if not remembered until later; going back to regular dosing schedule; not doubling doses
» Proper storage

## Precautions while using this medication

Regular visits to physician to check progress of therapy
» Checking with physician before discontinuing medication; gradual dosage reduction may be needed
 Avoiding use of antacids or antidiarrheal medication within 2 hours of taking phenothiazine
» Avoiding use of alcoholic beverages or other CNS depressants during therapy
 Avoiding the use of over-the-counter medications for colds or allergies, to prevent increased anticholinergic effects and risk of heat stroke
 Caution if any laboratory tests required; possible interference with ECG readings, and with gonadorelin, immunologic urine pregnancy, metyrapone, and urine bilirubin test results
» Caution if any kind of surgery, dental treatment, or emergency treatment is required; telling physician or dentist in charge about phenothiazine because of possible drug interactions or blood dyscrasias
» Possible drowsiness or blurred vision; caution when driving, using machines, or doing other things requiring alertness or accurate vision
» Possible dizziness or lightheadedness (orthostatic hypotension); caution when getting up suddenly from a lying or sitting position
» Possible heat stroke: Caution during exercise, hot weather, or when taking hot baths
 Possible hypothermia: Caution during prolonged exposure to cold
» Possible dryness of mouth; using sugarless gum or candy, ice, or saliva substitute for relief; checking with physician or dentist if dry mouth continues for more than 2 weeks
» Possible skin photosensitivity; avoiding unprotected exposure to sun; using protective clothing; using a sun block product that includes protection against both UVA-caused photosensitivity reactions and UVB-caused sunburn reactions; avoiding use of sunlamp, tanning bed, or tanning booth
» Possible eye photosensitivity; wearing sunglasses that block ultraviolet light
» Avoiding spilling liquid dosage form on skin or clothing; may cause skin irritation
» Observing precautions for up to 12 weeks with long-acting parenteral forms

## Side/adverse effects

Side effects more likely to occur in the elderly
Signs of potential side effects, especially tardive dyskinesia, dystonias, parkinsonian effects, anticholinergic effects, blurred vision, possible pigmentary retinopathy, allergic skin reactions, photosensitivity, agranulocytosis, cholestatic jaundice, heat stroke, neuroleptic malignant syndrome, priapism, melanosis, dryness of mouth, orthostatic hypotension, or akathisia
» Stopping medication and notifying physician immediately if symptoms of neuroleptic malignant syndrome (NMS) appear, especially muscle rigidity, fever, difficult or fast breathing, seizures, fast heartbeat, increased sweating, loss of bladder control, unusually pale skin, unusual tiredness or weakness
» Notifying physician immediately if early symptoms of tardive dyskinesia appear, such as fine worm-like movements of the tongue or other uncontrolled movements of the mouth, tongue, jaw, or arms and legs; dosage adjustment or discontinuation may be needed to prevent irreversibility
Possibility of withdrawal symptoms

# General Dosing Information

Dosage must be individualized by titration from the lower dose range. After a favorable psychiatric response is noted (within several days to several months), that dosage should be continued for about 2 weeks, then gradually decreased to the lowest level that will maintain an adequate clinical response.

When extended therapy is discontinued, a gradual reduction in phenothiazine dosage over several weeks is recommended, since abrupt withdrawal may cause some patients on high or long-term dosage to experience transient dyskinetic signs, nausea, vomiting, gastritis, trembling, and dizziness.

The antiemetic effect of some phenothiazines may mask signs of drug toxicity or obscure diagnosis of conditions whose primary symptom is nausea. Phenothiazines have no antiemetic effect when nausea is a result of vestibular stimulation or local gastrointestinal irritation.

Antidyskinetic agents such as trihexyphenidyl or benztropine may be used concurrently to control phenothiazine-induced extrapyramidal symptoms. They should be used only when required (not prophylactically), and, generally, are only needed for a few weeks to two or three months.

Avoid skin contact with liquid forms of phenothiazine medication; contact dermatitis has resulted.

## For parenteral dosage forms only

Because hypotension is a possible side effect of phenothiazines, parenteral administration should be used only in patients who are bedfast or for appropriate acute therapy in ambulatory patients who can be closely monitored. A possible exception may be those patients who are dose-stabilized on the extended-action injectable forms.

Intramuscular injections should be administered slowly and deeply into the upper outer quadrant of the buttock. Patient should remain lying down for at least $^{1}/_{2}$ hour after injection to avoid possible hypotensive effects.

To prevent irritation or sterile abscesses at the site of intramuscular injection, rotation of the injection sites, dilution of the phenothiazine injection with sodium chloride injection, and/or addition of 2% procaine are recommended.

Effects of the extended-action injectable forms may last for up to 12 weeks in some patients. The side effects information and precautions apply during this period of time.

The dose of the extended-action injectable forms should *not* be increased to prolong the dosing interval. Each patient must be carefully supervised to determine the optimal dosing interval and lowest effective dose, depending on patient's response, age, physical condition, symptoms, severity of illness, and drug history.

Geriatric and pediatric patients, especially those acutely ill or dehydrated, should be monitored very carefully during parenteral therapy because of a higher incidence of hypotensive and extrapyramidal reactions in these age groups.

## Diet/Nutrition

The oral dosage forms of this medication may be taken with food or a full glass (240 mL) of water or milk, if necessary, to lessen stomach irritation.

Requirements for riboflavin may be increased in patients receiving phenothiazines.

## For treatment of adverse effects

Neuroleptic malignant syndrome (NMS)—
 Treatment is essentially symptomatic and supportive and may include the following

• *Discontinuing phenothiazine immediately.*
• Hyperthermia—Administering antipyretics (aspirin or acetaminophen); using cooling blanket.
• Dehydration—Restoring fluids and electrolytes.
• Cardiovascular instability—Monitoring blood pressure and cardiac rhythm closely. Use of sodium nitroprusside may allow vasodilation with subsequent heat loss from the skin in patients with less dominant muscle rigidity.
• Hypoxia—Administering oxygen; considering airway insertion and assisted ventilation.
• Muscle rigidity—Administering dantrolene sodium (100 to 300 mg per day in divided doses or 1.25 to 1.5 mg/kg, intravenously) for muscle relaxation; or administering amantadine (100 mg twice daily) or bromocriptine (5 mg three times a day) to restore central balance of dopamine and acetylcholine at the receptor site.
• If neuroleptics must be continued because of severe psychosis, rechallenge should consist of:
—at least five days of neuroleptic abstinence before rechallenge.
—a low-potency neuroleptic.
—a neuroleptic of a different class from the one causing NMS.
—a low dose.
—using a neuroleptic only for controlling the psychosis.
—avoiding parenteral and extended-action dosage forms.
Parkinsonism—
Treatment may include:
• Reducing the antipsychotic dosage, if possible, for treatment of milder effects.
• Administering oral antiparkinsonian agents (of the anticholinergic type) such as trihexyphenidyl, 2 mg three times per day, or benztropine for treatment of more severe parkinsonism and acute motor restlessness; using sparingly, only when side effects appear, and then usually for no longer than 3 months. Observing caution to prevent hyperpyrexia with concomitant use of phenothiazines and other medications with anticholinergic action.
• In the elderly patient, using amantadine, 100 to 200 mg at bedtime, to minimize severe anticholinergic effects that may occur with other antidyskinetics.
• Levodopa is *not* useful in the treatment of phenothiazine-induced parkinsonism because the dopamine receptors are blocked by the phenothiazine.
Restlessness (akathisia)—
May respond to antiparkinsonian drugs or propranolol, 30 to 80 mg per day; nadolol, 40 mg per day; or diazepam, 2 mg two or three times a day, but often requires dosage reduction of the phenothiazine or substitution of a less potent neuroleptic.
Dystonia—
Acute dystonic postures or oculogyric crisis may be relieved by parenteral administration of benztropine, 2 mg intramuscularly or intravenously; diphenhydramine, 50 mg intramuscularly; or diazepam, 5 to 7.5 mg intravenously, to be followed by oral antidyskinetic medication for one or two days to prevent recurrent dystonic episodes. Dosage adjustments of the phenothiazine may control these effects, and discontinuation of the phenothiazine may reverse severe symptoms.
Tardive dyskinesia—
No known effective treatment. Dosage of phenothiazine should be lowered or medication discontinued at earliest signs of tardive dyskinesia to prevent irreversible effects.
Pruritus associated with cholestasis—
• Topical treatment may include:
—Topical adrenocorticoids combined with cool-water compresses, aluminum acetate solution, or calamine lotion.
—For widespread itching, baths containing colloidal oatmeal or baking soda (2 cups per tubful).
—For severe itching, topical anesthetics containing 20% benzocaine or 5% lidocaine; however, itching may be relieved for only 30 to 60 minutes.
• Oral treatment may include:
—Initially, diphenhydramine, cyproheptadine, or hydroxyzine.
—Bile acid sequestrants or cholestyramine, but only when topical and oral antipruritic agents fail to control symptoms.
—Supplementation with fat-soluble vitamins (A, D, E, K) for patients with protracted jaundice.
—Resuming therapy with a nonphenothiazine neuroleptic, such as loxapine, thioxanthenes, and molindone.

---

## ACETOPHENAZINE

## Summary of Differences
Pharmacology/pharmacokinetics:
    Chemical Group—
        Piperazine
    Actions—
        Antiemetic: Weak
        Anticholinergic: Weak
        Extrapyramidal: Moderate
        Hypotensive: Weak
        Sedative: Moderate

## Oral Dosage Forms
### ACETOPHENAZINE MALEATE TABLETS USP

**Usual adult and adolescent dose**
Psychotic disorders—
    Oral, 20 mg three times a day, the dosage being adjusted as needed and tolerated.
Note: Geriatric, emaciated, or debilitated patients usually require a lower initial dose, the dosage being gradually increased as needed and tolerated.

**Usual adult prescribing limits**
Up to 120 mg a day.

**Usual pediatric dose**
Psychotic disorders—
    Children up to 12 years of age: Dosage has not been established.
    Children 12 years of age and over: See *Usual adult and adolescent dose.*

**Strength(s) usually available**
U.S.—
    20 mg (Rx) [*Tindal*].
Canada—
    Not commercially available.

**Packaging and storage**
Store below 40 °C (104 °F), preferably between 15 and 30 °C (59 and 86 °F), unless otherwise specified by manufacturer. Store in a tight, light-resistant container.

**Auxiliary labeling**
• May cause drowsiness.
• Avoid alcoholic beverages.

---

## CHLORPROMAZINE

## Summary of Differences
Category:
    Includes antiemetic and antidyskinetic (Huntington's disease) uses.
Pharmacology/pharmacokinetics:
    Chemical group—
        Aliphatic
    Actions—
        Antiemetic: Strong
        Anticholinergic: Moderate to strong
        Extrapyramidal: Weak to moderate
        Hypotensive: Strong
        Sedative: Strong

## Additional Dosing Information
See also *General Dosing Information.*

For intractable hiccups, chlorpromazine is initially administered orally. If symptoms persist for 2 or 3 days, intramuscular administration is indicated, followed by slow intravenous infusion if hiccups continue.

*For parenteral use*
Chlorpromazine injection must not be administered subcutaneously, because it causes severe tissue necrosis.
For intramuscular injection, diluting chlorpromazine injection with sodium chloride injection and/or adding 2% procaine may prevent irritation at the injection site.
The intravenous route of administration is used only for severe hiccups, surgery, and tetanus.
Before intravenous injection, chlorpromazine hydrochloride injection should be diluted with sodium chloride injection.
Close monitoring of blood pressure for hypotension is necessary during parenteral administration.

## Oral Dosage Forms

Note: The dosing and strengths of the dosage forms available are expressed in terms of chlorpromazine base (not the hydrochloride salt).

### CHLORPROMAZINE HYDROCHLORIDE EXTENDED-RELEASE CAPSULES

#### Usual adult and adolescent dose
Psychotic disorders—
Oral, 30 to 300 mg (base) one to three times a day, the dosage being adjusted as needed and tolerated.

Note: Geriatric, emaciated, or debilitated patients usually require a lower initial dose, the dosage being gradually increased as needed and tolerated.

The 300-mg extended-release capsules are used only in severe neuropsychiatric conditions.

#### Usual adult prescribing limits
Up to 1 gram (base) a day.

Note: Although doses are sometimes gradually increased to 2 grams a day or more for short periods, 1 gram or less is usually sufficient for extended therapy.

#### Usual pediatric dose
The extended-release dosage form is not recommended for use in children.

#### Strength(s) usually available
U.S.—
30 mg (base) (Rx) [*Thorazine Spansule* (benzyl alcohol; calcium sulfate; cetylpyridinium chloride; FD&C Yellow No. 6; gelatin; glyceryl distearate; glyceryl monostearate; iron oxide; povidone; silicon dioxide; sodium lauryl sulfate; starch; sucrose; titanium dioxide; wax)].

75 mg (base) (Rx) [*Thorazine Spansule* (benzyl alcohol; calcium sulfate; cetylpyridinium chloride; FD&C Yellow No. 6; gelatin; glyceryl distearate; glyceryl monostearate; iron oxide; povidone; silicon dioxide; sodium lauryl sulfate; starch; sucrose; titanium dioxide; wax)].

150 mg (base) (Rx) [*Thorazine Spansule* (benzyl alcohol; calcium sulfate; cetylpyridinium chloride; FD&C Yellow No. 6; gelatin; glyceryl distearate; glyceryl monostearate; iron oxide; povidone; silicon dioxide; sodium lauryl sulfate; starch; sucrose; titanium dioxide; wax)].

200 mg (base) (Rx) [*Thorazine Spansule* (benzyl alcohol; calcium sulfate; cetylpyridinium chloride; FD&C Yellow No. 6; gelatin; glyceryl distearate; glyceryl monostearate; iron oxide; povidone; silicon dioxide; sodium lauryl sulfate; starch; sucrose; titanium dioxide; wax)].

300 mg (base) (Rx) [*Thorazine Spansule* (benzyl alcohol; calcium sulfate; cetylpyridinium chloride; FD&C Yellow No. 6; gelatin; glyceryl distearate; glyceryl monostearate; iron oxide; povidone; silicon dioxide; sodium lauryl sulfate; starch; sucrose; titanium dioxide; wax)].

Canada—
Not commercially available.

#### Packaging and storage
Store below 40 °C (104 °F), preferably between 15 and 30 °C (59 and 86 °F), in a tight, light-resistant container, unless otherwise specified by manufacturer.

#### Auxiliary labeling
• May cause drowsiness.
• Avoid alcoholic beverages.

### CHLORPROMAZINE HYDROCHLORIDE ORAL CONCENTRATE USP

#### Usual adult and adolescent dose
Psychotic disorders—
Oral, 10 to 25 mg (base) two to four times a day, the dosage being increased by 20 to 50 mg a day every three or four days as needed and tolerated.
Nausea and vomiting—
Oral, 10 to 25 mg (base) every four hours, the dosage being increased as needed and tolerated.
Anxiety, presurgical—
Oral, 25 to 50 mg (base) two to three hours before surgery.
Hiccups or
Porphyria—
Oral, 25 to 50 mg (base) three or four times a day.

Note: Geriatric, emaciated, or debilitated patients usually require a lower initial dose, the dosage being gradually increased as needed and tolerated.

#### Usual adult prescribing limits
Up to 1 gram (base) a day.

Note: Although doses are sometimes gradually increased to 2 grams a day or more for short periods, 1 gram or less is usually sufficient for extended therapy.

#### Usual pediatric dose
Psychotic disorders or
Nausea and vomiting—
Children up to 6 months of age: Dosage has not been established.
Children 6 months of age and older: Oral, 550 mcg (0.55 mg) (base) per kg of body weight or 15 mg per square meter of body surface every four to six hours, the dosage being adjusted as needed and tolerated.
Anxiety, presurgical—
Oral, 550 mcg (0.55 mg) (base) per kg of body weight or 15 mg per square meter of body surface two or three hours before surgery.

#### Strength(s) usually available
U.S.—
30 mg (base) per mL (Rx) [*Thorazine Concentrate;* GENERIC].
100 mg (base) per mL (Rx) [*Thorazine Concentrate; Thor-Prom;* GENERIC].
Canada—
40 mg (base) per mL (Rx) [*Chlorpromanyl-40; Largactil Oral Drops* (alcohol 17.5%)].

#### Packaging and storage
Store below 40 °C (104 °F), preferably between 15 and 30 °C (59 and 86 °F), in a tight container, unless otherwise specified by manufacturer. Protect from light. Protect from freezing.

#### Stability
A slight yellowing will not alter potency; however, do not use if markedly discolored or if a precipitate is present.

#### Auxiliary labeling
• May cause drowsiness.
• Avoid alcoholic beverages.
• Do not spill on skin or clothing.
• Must be diluted before use.

#### Note
Avoid skin contact with liquid forms of this medication; contact dermatitis has resulted.

Each dose must be diluted just before administration in a half glass (120 mL) of coffee, tea, milk, tomato or fruit juice, water, soup, or carbonated beverage.

Explain dilution and dosage measurement to patient if self-administered.

### CHLORPROMAZINE HYDROCHLORIDE SYRUP USP

#### Usual adult and adolescent dose
Psychotic disorders—
Oral, 10 to 25 mg (base) two to four times a day, the dosage being increased by 20 to 50 mg a day every three or four days as needed and tolerated.
Nausea and vomiting—
Oral, 10 to 25 mg (base) every four hours, the dosage being increased as needed and tolerated.
Anxiety, presurgical—
Oral, 25 to 50 mg (base) two to three hours before surgery.
Hiccups or
Porphyria—
Oral, 25 to 50 mg (base) three or four times a day.

Note: Geriatric, emaciated, or debilitated patients usually require a lower initial dose, the dosage being gradually increased as needed and tolerated.

#### Usual adult prescribing limits
Up to 1 gram (base) a day.

Note: Although doses are sometimes gradually increased to 2 grams a day or more for short periods, 1 gram or less is usually sufficient for extended therapy.

#### Usual pediatric dose
Psychotic disorders or
Nausea and vomiting—
Children up to 6 months of age: Dosage has not been established.
Children 6 months of age and older: Oral, 550 mcg (0.55 mg) (base) per kg of body weight or 15 mg per square meter of body surface every four to six hours, the dosage being adjusted as needed and tolerated.
Anxiety, presurgical—
Oral, 550 mcg (0.55 mg) (base) per kg of body weight or 15 mg per square meter of body surface two or three hours before surgery.

## Strength(s) usually available

U.S.—

    10 mg (base) per 5 mL (Rx) [*Thorazine;* GENERIC].

Canada—

    25 mg (base) per 5 mL (Rx) [*Chlorpromanyl-5; Largactil Liquid* (alcohol 0.5%; sucrose)].

    100 mg (base) per 5 mL (Rx) [*Chlorpromanyl-20; Largactil Liquid* (alcohol 0.5%; sucrose)].

### Packaging and storage

Store below 40 °C (104 °F), preferably between 15 and 30 °C (59 and 86 °F), unless otherwise specified by manufacturer. Store in a tight, light-resistant container. Protect from freezing.

### Stability

A slight yellowing will not alter potency; however, do not use if markedly discolored or if a precipitate is present.

### Auxiliary labeling

• May cause drowsiness.

• Avoid alcoholic beverages.

• Do not spill on skin or clothing.

### Note

Avoid skin contact with liquid forms of this medication; contact dermatitis has resulted.

## CHLORPROMAZINE HYDROCHLORIDE TABLETS USP

### Usual adult and adolescent dose

Psychotic disorders—

    Oral, 10 to 25 mg (base) two to four times a day, the dosage being increased by 20 to 50 mg a day every three to four days as needed and tolerated.

Nausea and vomiting—

    Oral, 10 to 25 mg (base) every four hours, the dosage being increased as needed and tolerated.

Anxiety, presurgical—

    Oral, 25 to 50 mg (base) two to three hours before surgery.

Hiccups or

Porphyria—

    Oral, 25 to 50 mg (base) three or four times a day.

Note: Geriatric, emaciated, or debilitated patients usually require a lower initial dose, the dosage being gradually increased as needed and tolerated.

       The 100- and 200-mg tablets are for use in severe neuropsychiatric conditions.

### Usual adult prescribing limits

Up to 1 gram (base) a day.

Note: Although doses are sometimes gradually increased to 2 grams a day or more for short periods, 1 gram or less is usually sufficient for extended therapy.

### Usual pediatric dose

Psychotic disorders or

Nausea and vomiting—

    Children up to 6 months of age: Dosage has not been established.

    Children 6 months of age and older: Oral, 550 mcg (0.55 mg) (base) per kg of body weight or 15 mg per square meter of body surface every four to six hours, the dosage being adjusted as needed and tolerated.

Anxiety, presurgical—

    Oral, 550 mcg (0.55 mg) (base) per kg of body weight or 15 mg per square meter of body surface two or three hours before surgery.

Note: Since tablets are not suitable for many pediatric patients' requirements, the oral solution or syrup dosage forms are usually preferred.

### Strength(s) usually available

U.S.—

    10 mg (base) (Rx) [*Thorazine; Thor-Prom;* GENERIC].

    25 mg (base) (Rx) [*Thorazine; Thor-Prom;* GENERIC].

    50 mg (base) (Rx) [*Thorazine; Thor-Prom;* GENERIC].

    100 mg (base) (Rx) [*Thorazine; Thor-Prom;* GENERIC].

    200 mg (base) (Rx) [*Thorazine; Thor-Prom;* GENERIC].

Canada—

    10 mg (base) (Rx) [*Largactil; Novo-Chlorpromazine*].

    25 mg (base) (Rx) [*Largactil; Novo-Chlorpromazine;* GENERIC].

    50 mg (base) (Rx) [*Largactil; Novo-Chlorpromazine;* GENERIC].

    100 mg (base) (Rx) [*Largactil; Novo-Chlorpromazine;* GENERIC].

    200 mg (base) (Rx) [*Largactil; Novo-Chlorpromazine*].

### Packaging and storage

Store below 40 °C (104 °F), preferably between 15 and 30 °C (59 and 86 °F), unless otherwise specified by manufacturer. Store in a well-closed, light-resistant container.

### Auxiliary labeling

• May cause drowsiness.

• Avoid alcoholic beverages.

# Parenteral Dosage Forms

Note: The dosing and strengths of the dosage forms available are expressed in terms of chlorpromazine base (not the hydrochloride salt).

## CHLORPROMAZINE HYDROCHLORIDE INJECTION USP

### Usual adult dose

Psychotic disorders (severe)—

    Intramuscular, 25 to 50 mg (base), the dose being repeated in one hour if needed, and every three to twelve hours thereafter as needed and tolerated. The dosage may be gradually increased over several days as needed and tolerated.

Nausea and vomiting—

    Intramuscular, 25 mg (base) in a single dose, the dosage being increased to 25 to 50 mg every three to four hours as needed and tolerated until vomiting stops.

Nausea and vomiting during surgery—

    Intramuscular: 12.5 mg (base) in a single dose, the dose being repeated in thirty minutes as needed and tolerated.

    Intravenous infusion: Up to 25 mg (base), diluted to a concentration of at least 1 mg per mL of 0.9% sodium chloride injection, administered at a rate of no more than 2 mg every 2 minutes.

Anxiety, presurgical—

    Intramuscular, 12.5 to 25 mg (base) one or two hours before surgery.

Hiccups—

    Intramuscular: 25 to 50 mg (base) three or four times a day.

    Intravenous infusion: 25 to 50 mg (base), diluted in 500 to 1000 mL sodium chloride injection, administered slowly at a rate of 1 mg per minute.

Porphyria—

    Intramuscular, 25 mg (base) every six or eight hours until patient can take oral therapy.

Tetanus—

    Intramuscular: 25 to 50 mg (base) three or four times a day, the dosage being increased gradually as needed and tolerated.

    Intravenous infusion: 25 to 50 mg (base), diluted to a concentration of at least 1 mg per mL with sodium chloride injection, administered at a rate of 1 mg per minute.

Note: Geriatric, emaciated, or debilitated patients usually require a lower initial dose, the dosage being gradually increased as needed and tolerated.

### Usual adult prescribing limits

Up to 1 gram (base) a day.

Note: Although antipsychotic doses are sometimes gradually increased to 2 grams a day or more for short periods, 1 gram or less is usually sufficient for extended therapy.

### Usual pediatric dose

Psychotic disorders or

Nausea and vomiting—

    Children up to 6 months of age: Dosage has not been established.

    Children 6 months of age and over: Intramuscular, 550 mcg (0.55 mg) (base) per kg of body weight or 15 mg per square meter of body surface every six to eight hours as needed.

Nausea and vomiting during surgery—

    Intramuscular: 275 mcg (0.275 mg) (base) per kg of body weight, the dosage being repeated in thirty minutes as needed and tolerated.

    Intravenous infusion: 275 mcg (0.275 mg) (base) per kg of body weight, diluted to a concentration of at least 1 mg per mL with 0.9% sodium chloride injection, administered at a rate of no more than 1 mg every 2 minutes.

Anxiety, presurgical—

    Intramuscular, 550 mcg (0.55 mg) (base) per kg of body weight one to two hours before surgery.

Tetanus—

    Intramuscular: 550 mcg (0.55 mg) (base) per kg of body weight every six to eight hours.

    Intravenous infusion: 550 mcg (0.55 mg) (base) per kg of body weight, diluted to a concentration of at least 1 mg per mL with 0.9% sodium chloride injection, administered at a rate of 1 mg per 2 minutes.

Note: Children 6 months to 5 years of age (up to 23 kg) should receive no more than 40 mg a day.

       Children 5 to 12 years of age (23 to 46 kg) should receive no more than 75 mg a day, except in unmanageable cases.

## Strength(s) usually available

U.S.—

25 mg (base) per mL (Rx) [*Ormazine; Thorazine* (sulfite; vials, benzyl alcohol 2%); GENERIC].

Canada—

25 mg (base) per mL (Rx) [*Largactil* (sodium sulfite; potassium metabisulfite); GENERIC].

## Packaging and storage

Store below 40 °C (104 °F), preferably between 15 and 30 °C (59 and 86 °F), unless otherwise specified by manufacturer. Protect from light. Protect from freezing.

## Stability

A slight yellowing will not alter potency; however, do not use if markedly discolored or if a precipitate is present.

## Incompatibilities

A precipitate will form if chlorpromazine hydrochloride injection is mixed with thiopental, atropine, or solutions not having a pH of 4 to 5. Mixing chlorpromazine hydrochloride injection with other agents in the syringe is not recommended.

## Note

Avoid skin contact with liquid forms of this medication; contact dermatitis has resulted.

# Rectal Dosage Forms

## CHLORPROMAZINE SUPPOSITORIES USP

### Usual adult and adolescent dose

Nausea and vomiting—

Rectal, 50 to 100 mg every six to eight hours as needed.

Note: Geriatric, emaciated, or debilitated patients usually require a lower initial dose, the dosage being gradually increased as needed and tolerated.

### Usual adult prescribing limits

Up to 400 mg a day.

### Usual pediatric dose

Nausea and vomiting—

Children up to 6 months of age: Dosage has not been established.

Children 6 months of age and over: Rectal, 1 mg per kg of body weight every six to eight hours as needed.

Note: The 100-mg suppository dosage form is not recommended for pediatric use.

### Strength(s) usually available

U.S.—

25 mg (Rx) [*Thorazine* (glycerin; glyceryl monopalmitate; glyceryl monostearate; hydrogenated coconut oil fatty acids; hydrogenated palm kernel oil fatty acids)].

100 mg (Rx) [*Thorazine* (glycerin; glyceryl monopalmitate; glyceryl monostearate; hydrogenated coconut oil fatty acids; hydrogenated palm kernel oil fatty acids)].

Canada—

100 mg (Rx) [*Largactil*].

### Packaging and storage

Store between 15 and 30 °C (59 and 86 °F). Store in a well-closed, light-resistant container.

### Auxiliary labeling

• May cause drowsiness.
• Avoid alcoholic beverages.
• For rectal use only.

### Note

Explain administration technique.

---

## *FLUPHENAZINE*

---

# Summary of Differences

Category:

Includes use as antineuralgia adjunct in patients with chronic pain.

Pharmacology/pharmacokinetics:

Chemical group—

Piperazine

Actions—

Antiemetic: Weak

Anticholinergic: Weak

Extrapyramidal: Strong

Hypotensive: Weak

Sedative: Weak

# Additional Dosing Information

See also *General Dosing Information.*

## For long-acting parenteral dosage forms

A dry syringe and needle (at least 21 gauge) should be used, since use of a wet needle may cause the solution to become cloudy.

After the initial dose of the decanoate or enanthate extended-action injection, dosages and dosing intervals are determined by the patient's response.

# Oral Dosage Forms

## FLUPHENAZINE HYDROCHLORIDE ELIXIR USP

### Usual adult and adolescent dose

Psychotic disorders—

Initial: Oral, 2.5 to 10 mg a day in divided doses every six to eight hours, the dosage being increased gradually as needed and tolerated.

Maintenance: Oral, 1 to 5 mg a day as a single dose or in divided doses.

Note: Emaciated or debilitated patients usually require a lower initial dosage (1 to 2.5 mg daily), the dosage being gradually increased as needed and tolerated.

### Usual adult prescribing limits

Up to 20 mg a day.

### Usual pediatric dose

Psychotic disorders—

Oral, 250 to 750 mcg (0.25 to 0.75 mg) one to four times a day.

### Usual geriatric dose

Psychotic disorders—

Oral, 1 to 2.5 mg a day, the dosage being gradually increased as needed and tolerated.

### Strength(s) usually available

U.S.—

2.5 mg per 5 mL (0.5 mg per mL) (Rx) [*Prolixin* (alcohol 14%; FD&C Yellow No. 6; flavors; glycerin; polysorbate 40; purified water; sodium benzoate; sucrose)].

Canada—

2.5 mg per 5 mL (0.5 mg per mL) (Rx) [*Moditen HCl* (alcohol 14%)].

### Packaging and storage

Store below 40 °C (104 °F), preferably between 15 and 30 °C (59 and 86 °F), unless otherwise specified by manufacturer. Store in a tight container. Protect from light. Protect from freezing.

### Auxiliary labeling

• May cause drowsiness.
• Avoid alcoholic beverages.
• Do not spill on skin or clothing.
• Keep container tightly closed.

### Note

Avoid skin contact with liquid forms of this medication; contact dermatitis has resulted.

## FLUPHENAZINE HYDROCHLORIDE ORAL SOLUTION USP

### Usual adult and adolescent dose

Psychotic disorders—

Initial: Oral, 2.5 to 10 mg a day in divided doses every six to eight hours, the dosage being increased gradually as needed and tolerated.

Maintenance: Oral, 1 to 5 mg a day as a single dose or in divided doses.

Note: Emaciated or debilitated patients usually require a lower initial dosage (1 to 2.5 mg daily), the dosage being gradually increased as needed and tolerated.

### Usual adult prescribing limits

Up to 20 mg a day.

### Usual pediatric dose

Psychotic disorders—

Oral, 250 to 750 mcg (0.25 to 0.75 mg) one to four times a day.

### Usual geriatric dose

Psychotic disorders—

Oral, 1 to 2.5 mg a day, the dosage being gradually increased as needed and tolerated.

### Strength(s) usually available

U.S.—

5 mg per mL (Rx) [*Permitil Concentrate* (alcohol 1%); *Prolixin Concentrate* (alcohol 14%; sodium benzoate); GENERIC].

**Canada—**
   Not commercially available.

**Packaging and storage**
Store below 40 °C (104 °F), preferably between 15 and 30 °C (59 and 86 °F), unless otherwise specified by manufacturer. Store in a tight container. Protect from light. Protect from freezing.

**Auxiliary labeling**
- May cause drowsiness.
- Avoid alcoholic beverages.
- Do not spill on skin or clothing.
- Must be diluted before use.

**Note**
Avoid skin contact with liquid forms of this medication; contact dermatitis has resulted.

Each dose must be diluted just before administration in a half (120 mL) to a full (240 mL) glass of milk, tomato or fruit juice, water, soup, or carbonated beverage.

Explain dilution and dosage measurement to patient if self-administered.

## FLUPHENAZINE HYDROCHLORIDE TABLETS USP

**Usual adult and adolescent dose**
Psychotic disorders—
   Initial: Oral, 2.5 to 10 mg a day in divided doses every six to eight hours, the dosage being increased gradually as needed and tolerated.
   Maintenance: Oral, 1 to 5 mg a day as a single dose or in divided doses.
   Note: Emaciated or debilitated patients usually require a lower initial dosage (1 to 2.5 mg daily), the dosage being gradually increased as needed and tolerated.

**Usual adult prescribing limits**
Up to 20 mg a day.

**Usual pediatric dose**
Psychotic disorders—
   Oral, 250 to 750 mcg (0.25 to 0.75 mg) one to four times a day.

**Usual geriatric dose**
Psychotic disorders—
   Oral, 1 to 2.5 mg a day, the dosage being gradually increased as needed and tolerated.

**Strength(s) usually available**
U.S.—
   1 mg (Rx) [*Prolixin;* GENERIC].
   2.5 mg (Rx) [*Permitil; Prolixin* (tartrazine); GENERIC].
   5 mg (Rx) [*Permitil; Prolixin* (tartrazine); GENERIC].
   10 mg (Rx) [*Permitil; Prolixin* (tartrazine); GENERIC].
Canada—
   1 mg (Rx) [*Apo-Fluphenazine; Moditen HCl; Permitil*].
   2 mg (Rx) [*Apo-Fluphenazine; Moditen HCl* (tartrazine)].
   5 mg (Rx) [*Apo-Fluphenazine; Moditen HCl; Permitil*].
   10 mg (Rx) [*Moditen HCl*].

**Packaging and storage**
Store below 40 °C (104 °F), preferably between 15 and 30 °C (59 and 86 °F), unless otherwise specified by manufacturer. Store in a tight, light-resistant container.

**Auxiliary labeling**
- May cause drowsiness.
- Avoid alcoholic beverages.

# Parenteral Dosage Forms

## FLUPHENAZINE DECANOATE INJECTION

**Usual adult dose**
Psychotic disorders—
   Initial: Intramuscular or subcutaneous, 12.5 to 25 mg, the dose being repeated or increased every one to three weeks as needed and tolerated.
   Maintenance: Intramuscular or subcutaneous, usually up to 50 mg every one to four weeks, as needed and tolerated.
   Note: For doses greater than 50 mg, increases should be made cautiously in increments of 12.5 mg.

**Usual adult prescribing limits**
Up to 100 mg per dose.

**Usual pediatric dose**
Psychotic disorders—
   Children 5 to 12 years of age: Intramuscular or subcutaneous, 3.125 to 12.5 mg, the dosage being repeated every one to three weeks as needed and tolerated.
   Children 12 years of age and over: Intramuscular or subcutaneous, initially 6.25 to 18.75 mg a week, the dosage being increased to 12.5 to 25 mg and administered every one to three weeks as needed and tolerated.

**Strength(s) usually available**
U.S.—
   25 mg per mL (Rx) [*Prolixin Decanoate* (sesame oil; benzyl alcohol 1.2% w/v); GENERIC].
Canada—
   25 mg per mL (Rx) [*Modecate* (sesame oil; benzyl alcohol 1.2% w/v)].
   100 mg per mL (Rx) [*Modecate Concentrate* (sesame oil; benzyl alcohol 1.5% w/v)].

**Packaging and storage**
Store below 40 °C (104 °F), preferably between 15 and 30 °C (59 and 86 °F), unless otherwise specified by manufacturer. Protect from light. Protect from freezing.

**Note**
Avoid skin contact with liquid forms of this medication; contact dermatitis has resulted.

**Additional information**
The onset of action of the initial dose is generally between 24 and 72 hours after administration, and antipsychotic effects become significant within 48 to 96 hours.

The effects of a single injection of the extended-action injectable forms may last for up to 6 weeks in some patients. The side effects information and precautions apply during this period of time.

The time to steady-state from a dosage change requires 6 to 12 weeks or longer.

## FLUPHENAZINE ENANTHATE INJECTION USP

**Usual adult and adolescent dose**
Psychotic disorders—
   Intramuscular or subcutaneous, 25 mg, the dosage being repeated or increased every one to three weeks as needed and tolerated.
   Note: For doses greater than 50 mg, increases should be made cautiously in increments of 12.5 mg.

**Usual adult prescribing limits**
Up to 100 mg per dose.

**Usual pediatric dose**
Psychotic disorders—
   Children up to 12 years of age: Dosage has not been established.
   Children 12 years of age and over: See *Usual adult and adolescent dose.*

**Strength(s) usually available**
U.S.—
   25 mg per mL (Rx) [*Prolixin Enanthate* (sesame oil; benzyl alcohol 1.5% w/v)].
Canada—
   25 mg per mL (Rx) [*Moditen Enanthate* (sesame oil; benzyl alcohol 1.5% w/v)].

**Packaging and storage**
Store below 40 °C (104 °F), preferably between 15 and 30 °C (59 and 86 °F), unless otherwise specified by manufacturer. Protect from light. Protect from freezing.

**Note**
Avoid skin contact with liquid forms of this medication; contact dermatitis has resulted.

**Additional information**
The effects of a single dose of the extended-action injectable forms may last for up to 6 weeks in some patients. The side effects information and precautions apply during this period of time.

## FLUPHENAZINE HYDROCHLORIDE INJECTION USP

**Usual adult and adolescent dose**
Psychotic disorders—
   Intramuscular, 1.25 to 2.5 mg every six to eight hours as needed and tolerated.
   Note: Emaciated or debilitated patients usually require a lower initial dose (1 to 2.5 mg daily), the dosage being increased gradually as needed and tolerated.

**Usual adult prescribing limits**
Up to 10 mg a day.

**Usual pediatric dose**
Psychotic disorders—
  Children up to 12 years of age: Dosage has not been established.
  Children 12 years of age and over: See *Usual adult and adolescent dose.*

**Usual geriatric dose**
Psychotic disorders—
  Intramuscular, 1 to 2.5 mg a day, the dosage being increased gradually as needed and tolerated.

**Strength(s) usually available**
U.S.—
  2.5 mg per mL (Rx) [*Prolixin* (methylparaben 0.1%; propylparaben 0.01%); GENERIC].
Canada—
  10 mg per mL (Rx) [*Moditen HCl-H.P.* (benzyl alcohol 1.5%)].

**Packaging and storage**
Store below 40 °C (104 °F), preferably between 15 and 30 °C (59 and 86 °F), unless otherwise specified by manufacturer. Protect from light. Protect from freezing.

**Stability**
A slight yellowing to a light amber color will not alter potency; however, do not use if markedly discolored or if a precipitate is present.

**Note**
Avoid skin contact with liquid forms of this medication; contact dermatitis has resulted.

---

## MESORIDAZINE

## Summary of Differences

Pharmacology/pharmacokinetics:
  Chemical group—
    Piperidine
  Actions—
    Antiemetic: Weak
    Anticholinergic: Moderate
    Extrapyramidal: Weak
    Hypotensive: Strong
    Sedative: Strong

## Oral Dosage Forms

Note: The dosing and strengths of the dosage forms available are expressed in terms of mesoridazine base (not the besylate salt).

### MESORIDAZINE BESYLATE ORAL SOLUTION USP

**Usual adult and adolescent dose**
Psychotic disorders—
  Oral, 30 to 150 mg (base) a day in two or three divided doses, the dosage being adjusted as needed and tolerated.
Note: Geriatric, emaciated, or debilitated patients usually require a lower initial dose, the dosage being increased gradually as needed and tolerated.

**Usual pediatric dose**
Psychotic disorders—
  Children up to 12 years of age: Dosage has not been established.
  Children 12 years of age and over: See *Usual adult and adolescent dose.*

**Strength(s) usually available**
U.S.—
  25 mg (base) per mL (Rx) [*Serentil Concentrate* (alcohol 0.6% v/v)].
Canada—
  Not commercially available.

**Packaging and storage**
Store below 25 °C (77 °F). Store in a tight, light-resistant container. Protect from freezing.

**Auxiliary labeling**
• May cause drowsiness.
• Avoid alcoholic beverages.
• Do not spill on skin or clothing.
• Must be diluted before use.

**Note**
Avoid skin contact with liquid forms of this medication; contact dermatitis has resulted.

Each dose must be diluted just before administration in distilled water, acidified tap water, orange juice, or grapefruit juice. The recommended dilution is 25 mg in 2 teaspoonfuls of diluent. Higher doses require more diluent. Preparation and storage of bulk dilution is not recommended.

Explain dilution and dosage measurement to patient if self-administered.

### MESORIDAZINE BESYLATE TABLETS USP

**Usual adult and adolescent dose**
Psychotic disorders—
  Oral, 30 to 150 mg (base) a day in two or three divided doses, the dosage being adjusted as needed and tolerated.
Note: Geriatric, emaciated, or debilitated patients usually require a lower initial dose, the dosage being increased gradually as needed and tolerated.

**Usual pediatric dose**
Psychotic disorders—
  Children up to 12 years of age: Dosage has not been established.
  Children 12 years of age and older: See *Usual adult and adolescent dose.*

**Strength(s) usually available**
U.S.—
  10 mg (base) (Rx) [*Serentil* (acacia; carnauba wax; colloidal silicon dioxide; FD&C Red No. 40 aluminum lake; microcrystalline cellulose; povidone; sodium benzoate; stearic acid; sucrose; lactose; talc; titanium dioxide; starch)].
  25 mg (base) (Rx) [*Serentil* (acacia; carnauba wax; colloidal silicon dioxide; FD&C Red No. 40 aluminum lake; microcrystalline cellulose; povidone; sodium benzoate; stearic acid; sucrose; lactose; talc; titanium dioxide)].
  50 mg (base) (Rx) [*Serentil* (acacia; carnauba wax; colloidal silicon dioxide; FD&C Red No. 40 aluminum lake; microcrystalline cellulose; povidone; sodium benzoate; stearic acid; sucrose; lactose; talc; titanium dioxide; starch; gelatin)].
  100 mg (base) (Rx) [*Serentil* (acacia; carnauba wax; colloidal silicon dioxide; FD&C Red No. 40 aluminum lake; microcrystalline cellulose; povidone; sodium benzoate; stearic acid; sucrose; lactose; talc; titanium dioxide; starch; gelatin)].
Canada—
  10 mg (base) (Rx) [*Serentil* (cornstarch; lactose)].
  25 mg (base) (Rx) [*Serentil* (cornstarch; lactose)].
  50 mg (base) (Rx) [*Serentil* (cornstarch; lactose)].

**Packaging and storage**
Store below 30 °C (86 °F), unless otherwise specified by manufacturer. Store in a well-closed, light-resistant container.

**Auxiliary labeling**
• May cause drowsiness.
• Avoid alcoholic beverages.

## Parenteral Dosage Forms

Note: The dosing and strengths of the dosage forms available are expressed in terms of mesoridazine base (not the besylate salt).

### MESORIDAZINE BESYLATE INJECTION USP

**Usual adult and adolescent dose**
Psychotic disorders—
  Intramuscular, 25 mg (base), the dose being repeated in one-half to one hour as needed and tolerated.
Note: Geriatric, emaciated, or debilitated patients usually require a lower initial dose, the dosage being gradually increased as needed and tolerated.

**Usual pediatric dose**
Psychotic disorders—
  Children up to 12 years of age: Dosage has not been established.
  Children 12 years of age and older: See *Usual adult and adolescent dose.*

**Strength(s) usually available**
U.S.—
  25 mg (base) per mL (Rx) [*Serentil* (edetate sodium)].
Canada—
  Not commercially available.

**Packaging and storage**
Store below 30 °C (86 °F), unless otherwise specified by manufacturer. Protect from light. Protect from freezing.

**Stability**
A slight yellowing will not alter potency; however, do not use if markedly discolored or if a precipitate is present.

**Note**

Avoid skin contact with liquid forms of this medication; contact dermatitis has resulted.

---

## METHOTRIMEPRAZINE

## Summary of Differences

Category:

In addition to being used as an antipsychotic, methotrimeprazine is used as an analgesic, antianxiety agent, and sedative.

Indications:

Also indicated for relief of moderate to severe pain in nonambulatory patients, and for obstetrical pain and sedation when respiratory depression should be avoided; anxiety, apprehension, restlessness, and sedation before surgery; adjunctive therapy in general anesthesia to increase effects of anesthetics.

Pharmacology/pharmacokinetics:

Chemical group—

Aliphatic

Actions—

Antiemetic: Weak

Anticholinergic: Moderate

Extrapyramidal: Weak to moderate

Hypotensive: Strong

Sedative: Strong

## Oral Dosage Forms

Note: The dosing and strengths of the dosage forms available are expressed in terms of methotrimeprazine base (not the hydrochloride or maleate salts).

### METHOTRIMEPRAZINE HYDROCHLORIDE ORAL SOLUTION

**Usual adult and adolescent dose**

Psychotic disorders or

Pain—

Oral, initially, 6 to 25 mg (base) a day in three divided doses with meals (mild to moderate pain or psychosis), or 50 to 75 mg a day in two or three divided doses with meals (severe pain or psychosis), the dosage being gradually increased as needed and tolerated.

Note: If doses of 100 to 200 mg a day are required, the patient should be confined to bed for the first few days to prevent orthostatic hypotension.

Sedation, presurgical—

Oral, initially, 6 to 25 mg (base) a day in three divided doses with meals, the dosage being increased gradually as needed and tolerated.

**Usual pediatric dose**

Psychotic disorders or

Pain or

Sedation, presurgical—

Oral, initially, 250 mcg (0.25 mg) per kg (base) of body weight a day in two or three divided doses with meals, the dosage being increased gradually as needed and tolerated.

Note: Dosage must not exceed 40 mg a day in children under twelve years of age.

**Strength(s) usually available**

U.S.—

Not commercially available.

Canada—

40 mg (base) per mL (Rx) [*Nozinan Oral Drops* (alcohol 16.5%; sucrose)].

**Packaging and storage**

Store below 40 °C (104 °F), preferably between 15 and 30 °C (59 and 86 °F), protected from light, unless otherwise specified by manufacturer. Protect from freezing.

**Auxiliary labeling**

• May cause drowsiness.

• Avoid alcoholic beverages.

• Do not spill on skin or clothing.

**Note**

Avoid skin contact with liquid forms of this medication; contact dermatitis may result.

**Additional information**

Only enclosed calibrated dropper should be used for measuring dose.

### METHOTRIMEPRAZINE HYDROCHLORIDE SYRUP

**Usual adult and adolescent dose**

Psychotic disorders or

Pain—

Oral, initially, 6 to 25 mg (base) a day in three divided doses with meals (mild to moderate pain or psychosis), or 50 to 75 mg a day in two or three divided doses with meals (severe pain or psychosis), the dosage being increased gradually as needed and tolerated.

Note: If doses of 100 to 200 mg a day are required, the patient should be confined to bed for the first few days to prevent orthostatic hypotension.

Sedation, presurgical—

Oral, initially, 6 to 25 mg (base) a day in three divided doses with meals, the dosage being increased gradually as needed and tolerated.

**Usual pediatric dose**

Psychotic disorders or

Pain or

Sedation—

Oral, initially, 250 mcg (0.25 mg) (base) per kg of body weight a day in two or three divided doses with meals, the dosage being increased gradually as needed and tolerated.

Note: Dosage must not exceed 40 mg a day in children under twelve years of age.

**Strength(s) usually available**

U.S.—

Not commercially available.

Canada—

25 mg (base) per 5 mL (Rx) [*Nozinan Liquid* (alcohol 2%; sucrose)].

**Packaging and storage**

Store below 40 °C (104 °F), preferably between 15 and 30 °C (59 and 86 °F), protected from light, unless otherwise specified by manufacturer. Protect from freezing.

**Auxiliary labeling**

• May cause drowsiness.

• Avoid alcoholic beverages.

• Do not spill on skin or clothing.

**Note**

Avoid skin contact with liquid forms of this medication; contact dermatitis may result.

### METHOTRIMEPRAZINE MALEATE TABLETS

**Usual adult and adolescent dose**

Psychotic disorders or

Pain—

Oral, initially, 6 to 25 mg (base) a day in three divided doses with meals (mild to moderate pain or psychosis), or 50 to 75 mg a day in two or three divided doses with meals (severe pain or psychosis), the dosage being increased gradually as needed and tolerated.

Note: If doses of 100 to 200 mg a day are required, the patient should be confined to bed for the first few days to prevent orthostatic hypotension.

Sedation, presurgical—

Oral, initially, 6 to 25 mg (base) a day in three divided doses with meals, the dosage being gradually increased as needed and tolerated.

**Usual pediatric dose**

Psychotic disorders or

Pain or

Sedation—

Oral, initially, 250 mcg (0.25 mg) (base) per kg of body weight a day in two or three divided doses with meals, the dosage being increased gradually as needed and tolerated.

Note: Doses must not exceed 40 mg a day in children under twelve years of age.

**Strength(s) usually available**

U.S.—

Not commercially available.

Canada—

2 mg (base) (Rx) [*Nozinan*].

5 mg (base) (Rx) [*Nozinan*].

25 mg (base) (Rx) [*Nozinan*].

50 mg (base) (Rx) [*Nozinan*].

**Packaging and storage**

Store below 40 °C (104 °F), preferably between 15 and 30 °C (59 and 86 °F), protected from light, unless otherwise specified by manufacturer.

**Auxiliary labeling**
• May cause drowsiness.
• Avoid alcoholic beverages.

## Parenteral Dosage Forms

Note: Bracketed uses in the *Dosage Forms* section refer to categories of use and/or indications that are not included in U.S. product labeling.

### METHOTRIMEPRAZINE INJECTION USP

**Usual adult and adolescent dose**
[Psychotic disorders, severe or]
Pain, acute or intractable—
    Intramuscular, initially, 10 to 20 mg at four- to six-hour intervals, the dosage being increased as needed for pain and sedation.
Pain, obstetrical—
    Intramuscular, initially 15 to 20 mg, the dose being adjusted and repeated as needed.
Pain, postoperative—
    Intramuscular, 2.5 to 7.5 mg immediately after surgery, the dosage being adjusted and repeated every three to four hours as needed.
    Note: After initial dose, the patient should be confined to bed or carefully supervised for at least 6 hours following administration, to prevent orthostatic hypotension, dizziness, or fainting.
    Residual effects of anesthetic agents may be additive to the effects of methotrimeprazine.
Sedation, preanesthetic—
    Intramuscular, 2 to 20 mg administered forty-five minutes to three hours before surgery.
[Anesthesia adjunct during surgery or labor]—
    Intravenous infusion, 10 to 25 mg in 500 mL of 5% dextrose injection administered at a rate of 20 to 40 drops a minute.

**Usual pediatric dose**
Pain—
    Intramuscular, 62.5 to 125 mcg (0.062 to 0.125 mg) per kg of body weight a day in single or divided doses.
[Anesthesia adjunct during surgery]—
    Intravenous infusion, 62.5 to 125 mcg (0.062 to 0.125 mg) per kg of body weight a day in 250 mL of 5% dextrose injection, administered at a rate of 20 to 40 drops a minute.

**Usual geriatric dose**
Pain—
    Intramuscular, initially, 5 to 10 mg every four to six hours, the dosage being increased gradually as needed and tolerated.

**Strength(s) usually available**
U.S.—
    20 mg per mL (Rx) [*Levoprome* (benzyl alcohol 0.9% w/v; disodium edetate; sodium metabisulfite)].
Canada—
    25 mg per mL (Rx) [*Nozinan* (sodium sulfite)].

**Packaging and storage**
Store below 40 °C (104 °F), preferably between 15 and 30 °C (59 and 86 °F), unless otherwise specified by manufacturer. Protect from light. Protect from freezing.

**Incompatibilities**
Methotrimeprazine should not be mixed in the same syringe with any drug except atropine sulfate or scopolamine hydrobromide.

**Note**
Avoid skin contact with liquid forms of this medication; contact dermatitis may result.

---

### PERICYAZINE

## Summary of Differences

Indications:
    Indicated in some psychotic patients for the control of residual prevailing hostility, impulsivity, and aggressiveness.
Pharmacology/pharmacokinetics:
    Chemical group—
        Piperidine
    Actions—
        Antiemetic: Strong
        Anticholinergic: Strong
        Extrapyramidal: Moderate
        Hypotensive: Moderate
        Sedative: Strong

## Oral Dosage Forms

### PERICYAZINE CAPSULES

**Usual adult dose**
Psychotic disorders—
    Initial: Oral, 5 to 20 mg in the morning and 10 to 40 mg in the evening as needed and tolerated.
    Maintenance: Oral, 2.5 to 15 mg in the morning and 5 to 30 mg in the evening.

**Usual pediatric dose**
Psychotic disorders—
    Children 5 years of age to adolescence: Oral, 2.5 to 10 mg in the morning and 5 to 30 mg in the evening as needed and tolerated.

**Usual geriatric dose**
Psychotic disorders—
    Oral, initially, 5 mg a day, the dosage being increased gradually as needed and tolerated, up to about 30 mg a day.

**Strength(s) usually available**
U.S.—
    Not commercially available.
Canada—
    5 mg (Rx) [*Neuleptil*].
    10 mg (Rx) [*Neuleptil*].
    20 mg (Rx) [*Neuleptil*].

**Packaging and storage**
Store below 40 °C (104 °F), preferably between 15 and 30 °C (59 and 86 °F), protected from light, unless otherwise specified by manufacturer.

**Auxiliary labeling**
• May cause drowsiness.
• Avoid alcoholic beverages.

### PERICYAZINE ORAL SOLUTION

**Usual adult dose**
Psychotic disorders—
    Initial: Oral, 5 to 20 mg in the morning and 10 to 40 mg in the evening as needed and tolerated.
    Maintenance: Oral, 2.5 to 15 mg in the morning and 5 to 30 mg in the evening.

**Usual pediatric dose**
Psychotic disorders—
    Children 5 years of age to adolescence: Oral, 2.5 to 10 mg in the morning and 5 to 30 mg in the evening as needed and tolerated.

**Usual geriatric dose**
Psychotic disorders—
    Oral, initially, 5 mg a day, the dosage being increased gradually as needed and tolerated up to about 30 mg a day.

**Strength(s) usually available**
U.S.—
    Not commercially available.
Canada—
    10 mg per mL (Rx) [*Neuleptil*].

**Packaging and storage**
Store below 40 °C (104 °F), preferably between 15 and 30 °C (59 and 86 °F), protected from light, unless otherwise specified by manufacturer.

**Auxiliary labeling**
• May cause drowsiness.
• Avoid alcoholic beverages.
• Do not spill on skin or clothing.

**Note**
Avoid skin contact with liquid forms of this medication; contact dermatitis may result.

**Additional information**
Only enclosed calibrated dropper should be used for measuring dose.

---

### PERPHENAZINE

## Summary of Differences

Category:
    Includes antiemetic use.
Pharmacology/pharmacokinetics:
    Chemical group—
        Piperazine
    Actions—
        Antiemetic: Strong
        Anticholinergic: Weak to moderate

Extrapyramidal: Strong
Hypotensive: Weak
Sedative: Weak to moderate

# Oral Dosage Forms

Note: Bracketed uses in the *Dosage Forms* section refer to categories of use and/or indications that are not included in U.S. product labeling.

## PERPHENAZINE ORAL SOLUTION USP

### Usual adult and adolescent dose
Psychotic disorders (hospitalized patients)—
Oral, 8 to 16 mg two to four times a day, up to 64 mg a day, the dosage being adjusted as needed and tolerated.

Note: Geriatric, emaciated, or debilitated patients usually require a lower initial dose, the dosage being gradually increased as needed and tolerated.

Adolescents usually require the lowest limit of the adult dose range.

### Usual pediatric dose
Psychotic disorders—
Children up to 12 years of age: Dosage has not been established.
Children 12 years of age and over: See *Usual adult and adolescent dose.*

### Strength(s) usually available
U.S.—
16 mg per 5 mL (Rx) [*Trilafon Concentrate*].
Canada—
16 mg per 5 mL (Rx) [*PMS Perphenazine; Trilafon Concentrate*].

### Packaging and storage
Store below 40 °C (104 °F), preferably between 15 and 30 °C (59 and 86 °F), unless otherwise specified by manufacturer. Store in a well-closed, light-resistant container. Protect from freezing.

### Auxiliary labeling
• May cause drowsiness.
• Avoid alcoholic beverages.
• Do not spill on skin or clothing.
• Must be diluted before use.

### Note
The oral solution is intended primarily for institutional usage.
Avoid skin contact with liquid forms of this medication; contact dermatitis has resulted.
Each dose must be measured with accompanying dropper and diluted before administration in water, salt solution, milk, tomato or fruit juice (except apple juice), soup, or carbonated beverage. The oral solution should not be mixed with beverages containing caffeine or tannins (colas, coffee, or tea). The recommended dilution is 2 fluid ounces (60 mL) of diluent for each teaspoonful (5 mL) of perphenazine oral solution.
Explain dilution and dosage measurement to patient if self-administered.

## PERPHENAZINE SYRUP USP

### Usual adult and adolescent dose
Psychotic disorders—
Oral, 2 to 16 mg two to four times a day, the dosage being adjusted gradually as needed and tolerated.
Nausea and vomiting—
Oral, 2 to 4 mg two to four times a day, the dosage being adjusted gradually as needed and tolerated.

Note: Geriatric, emaciated, or debilitated patients usually require a lower initial dose, the dosage being gradually increased as needed and tolerated.

Adolescents usually require the lowest limit of the adult dose range.

### Usual pediatric dose
Psychotic disorders or
Nausea and vomiting—
Children up to 12 years of age: Dosage has not been established.
Children 12 years of age and over: See *Usual adult and adolescent dose.*

### Strength(s) usually available
U.S.—
Not commercially available.
Canada—
2 mg per 5 mL (Rx) [*Trilafon* (methylparaben; propylparaben; sorbitol; sucrose)].

### Packaging and storage
Store below 40 °C (104 °F), preferably between 15 and 30 °C (59 and 86 °F), unless otherwise specified by manufacturer. Store in a well-closed, light-resistant container. Protect from freezing.

### Auxiliary labeling
• May cause drowsiness.
• Avoid alcoholic beverages.
• Do not spill on skin or clothing.

### Note
Avoid skin contact with liquid forms of this medication; contact dermatitis has resulted.

## PERPHENAZINE TABLETS USP

### Usual adult and adolescent dose
Psychotic disorders—
Oral, 4 to 16 mg two to four times a day, the dosage being adjusted gradually as needed and tolerated.
Nausea and vomiting—
Oral, 8 to 16 mg a day in divided doses, the dosage being decreased as early as possible.

Note: Geriatric, emaciated, or debilitated patients usually require a lower initial dose, the dosage being increased gradually as needed and tolerated.

Adolescents usually require the lowest limit of the adult dose range.

### Usual adult prescribing limits
Psychotic disorders—
Up to 64 mg a day.
Nausea and vomiting—
Up to 24 mg a day.

### Usual pediatric dose
Psychotic disorders or
Nausea and vomiting—
Children up to 12 years of age: Dosage has not been established.
Children 12 years of age and over: See *Usual adult and adolescent dose.*

### Strength(s) usually available
U.S.—
2 mg (Rx) [*Trilafon;* GENERIC].
4 mg (Rx) [*Trilafon;* GENERIC].
8 mg (Rx) [*Trilafon;* GENERIC].
16 mg (Rx) [*Trilafon;* GENERIC].
Canada—
2 mg (Rx) [*Apo-Perphenazine; PMS Perphenazine; Trilafon;* GENERIC].
4 mg (Rx) [*Apo-Perphenazine; PMS Perphenazine; Trilafon;* GENERIC].
8 mg (Rx) [*Apo-Perphenazine; PMS Perphenazine; Trilafon;* GENERIC].
16 mg (Rx) [*Apo-Perphenazine; PMS Perphenazine; Trilafon;* GENERIC].

### Packaging and storage
Store below 40 °C (104 °F), preferably between 15 and 30 °C (59 and 86 °F), unless otherwise specified by manufacturer. Store in a tight, light-resistant container.

### Auxiliary labeling
• May cause drowsiness.
• Avoid alcoholic beverages.

# Parenteral Dosage Forms

## PERPHENAZINE INJECTION USP

### Usual adult and adolescent dose
Psychotic disorders—
Intramuscular, 5 to 10 mg every six hours, the dosage being adjusted as needed and tolerated.
Nausea and vomiting—
Intramuscular, 5 mg, the dose being increased to 10 mg as needed and tolerated for rapid control of severe vomiting.
Intravenous, up to 5 mg diluted to 0.5 mg per mL with 0.9% sodium chloride injection, in divided doses, not more than 1 mg administered not less than every one to two minutes; or administered as an infusion at a rate not to exceed 1 mg per minute.

Note: Geriatric, emaciated, or debilitated patients usually require a lower initial dose, the dosage being gradually increased as needed and tolerated.

Adolescents usually require the lowest limit of the adult dose range.

In psychotic conditions, most patients are controlled and amenable to oral therapy within a maximum of 24 to 48 hours.

### Usual adult prescribing limits
Ambulatory patients: Up to 15 mg daily.
Institutionalized patients: Up to 30 mg daily.
Intravenous administration: Up to 5 mg.

**Usual pediatric dose**
Psychotic disorders—
    Children up to 12 years of age: Dosage has not been established.
    Children 12 years of age and over: See *Usual adult and adolescent dose.*

**Strength(s) usually available**
U.S.—
    5 mg per mL (Rx) [*Trilafon* (sodium bisulfite)].
Canada—
    5 mg per mL (Rx) [*Trilafon* (sodium bisulfite)].

**Packaging and storage**
Store below 40 °C (104 °F), preferably between 15 and 30 °C (59 and 86 °F), unless otherwise specified by manufacturer. Protect from light. Protect from freezing.

**Stability**
A slight yellowing will not alter potency; however, do not use if markedly discolored or if a precipitate is present.

**Note**
Avoid skin contact with liquid forms of this medication; contact dermatitis has resulted.

---

## PIPOTIAZINE

## Summary of Differences
Indications:
    For the maintenance treatment of chronic, non-agitated schizophrenic patients stabilized on shorter-acting neuroleptics.
Pharmacology/pharmacokinetics:
    Chemical group—
        Piperidine
    Actions—
        Antiemetic: Weak
        Anticholinergic: Weak
        Extrapyramidal: Strong
        Hypotensive: Weak
        Sedative: Weak

## Additional Dosing Information
See also *General Dosing Information*.

A dry syringe and needle (at least 21-gauge) should be used, since use of a wet needle or syringe may cause the solution to become cloudy.

After the initial dose of pipotiazine palmitate extended-action injection, dosages and dosing intervals are determined by the patient's response.

## Parenteral Dosage Forms
### PIPOTIAZINE PALMITATE INJECTION
**Usual adult and adolescent dose**
Psychotic disorders—
    Intramuscular, initially, 50 to 100 mg, the dosage being increased in increments of 25 mg every two to three weeks, as needed and tolerated, usually up to a maintenance dose of 75 to 150 mg every four weeks.
Note: Geriatric patients usually require lower initial doses and, after initial titration, dosage should be reduced to the lowest effective maintenance dosage as soon as possible.

**Usual pediatric dose**
Dosage has not been established.

**Strength(s) usually available**
U.S.—
    Not commercially available.
Canada—
    25 mg per mL (Rx) [*Piportil L₄* (sesame oil)].
    50 mg per mL (Rx) [*Piportil L₄* (sesame oil)].

**Packaging and storage**
Store below 40 °C (104 °F), preferably between 15 and 30 °C (59 and 86 °F), protected from light, unless otherwise specified by manufacturer. Protect from freezing.

**Note**
Avoid skin contact with liquid forms of this medication; contact dermatitis may result.

**Additional information**
The onset of action is usually within the first 2 or 3 days after injection, and antipsychotic effects become significant within 1 week.

The effects of a single injection may last from 3 to 6 weeks, but adequate symptom control may be maintained with one injection every 4 weeks.

---

## PROCHLORPERAZINE

## Summary of Differences
Category:
    Includes antiemetic use.
Pharmacology/pharmacokinetics:
    Chemical group—
        Piperazine
    Actions—
        Antiemetic: Strong
        Anticholinergic: Weak
        Extrapyramidal: Strong
        Hypotensive: Weak
        Sedative: Moderate

## Additional Dosing Information
See also *General Dosing Information*.
For parenteral dosage forms only
    • Must be injected deep into upper outer quadrant of the buttock.
    • Subcutaneous administration is not recommended because of irritation at injection site and a potential for sterile abscesses.

## Oral Dosage Forms
Note: The dosing and strengths of the dosage forms available are expressed in terms of prochlorperazine base (not the edisylate, maleate, or mesylate salts).

### PROCHLORPERAZINE EDISYLATE SYRUP USP
**Usual adult and adolescent dose**
Psychotic disorders—
    Oral, 5 to 10 mg (base) three or four times a day, the dosage being gradually increased every two to three days as needed and tolerated.
Anxiety—
    Oral, 5 mg (base) three or four times a day, up to 20 mg a day, for no longer than twelve weeks.
Nausea and vomiting—
    Oral, 5 to 10 mg (base) three or four times a day, up to 40 mg a day.
Note: Geriatric, emaciated, or debilitated patients usually require a lower initial dose, the dosage being gradually increased as needed and tolerated.

**Usual adult prescribing limits**
Up to 150 mg (base) a day.

**Usual pediatric dose**
Psychotic disorders—
    Children up to 2 years of age or 9 kg of body weight: Dosage has not been established.
    Children 2 to 12 years of age: Oral, 2.5 mg (base) two or three times a day.
    Children 12 years of age and over: See *Usual adult and adolescent dose.*
Nausea and vomiting—
    Children 9 to 13 kg of body weight: Oral, 2.5 mg (base) one or two times a day, not to exceed 7.5 mg per day.
    Children 14 to 17 kg of body weight: Oral, 2.5 mg (base) two or three times a day, not to exceed 10 mg per day.
    Children 18 to 39 kg of body weight: Oral, 2.5 mg (base) three times a day or 5 mg two times a day, not to exceed 15 mg per day.
Note: The total daily dose for any child should not exceed 10 mg the first day. On subsequent days the total daily dose should not exceed 20 mg for children 2 to 5 years of age or 25 mg for children 6 to 12 years of age.

**Strength(s) usually available**
U.S.—
    5 mg (base) per 5 mL (Rx) [*Compazine* (FD&C Yellow No. 6; flavors; polyoxyethylene polyoxypropylene glycol; sodium benzoate; sodium citrate; sucrose; water)].
Canada—
    Not commercially available.

**Packaging and storage**
Store below 40 °C (104 °F), preferably between 15 and 30 °C (59 and 86 °F), unless otherwise specified by manufacturer. Store in a tight, light-resistant container. Protect from freezing.

## Stability

A slight yellowing will not affect potency; however, do not use if markedly discolored or if a precipitate is present.

### Auxiliary labeling

- May cause drowsiness.
- Avoid alcoholic beverages.
- Do not spill on skin or clothing.

### Note

Avoid skin contact with liquid forms of this medication; contact dermatitis has resulted.

## PROCHLORPERAZINE MALEATE EXTENDED-RELEASE CAPSULES

### Usual adult and adolescent dose

Psychotic disorders—
  Oral, 5 to 10 mg (base) every three or four hours, the dosage being increased gradually every two or three days as needed and tolerated, up to 100 to 150 mg a day.

Anxiety—
  Oral, 15 mg (base) in the morning; or 10 mg every twelve hours, up to 20 mg a day for no longer than 12 weeks.

Nausea and vomiting—
  Oral, 15 to 30 mg (base) once a day in the morning; or 10 mg every twelve hours, up to 40 mg a day as needed and tolerated.

  Note: Daily dosages above 40 mg should be used only in resistant cases.

Note: Geriatric, emaciated, or debilitated patients usually require a lower initial dose, the dosage being gradually increased as needed and tolerated.

### Usual adult prescribing limits

Psychotic disorders—
  Up to 150 mg (base) daily.

### Usual pediatric dose

The extended-release dosage form is not recommended for use in children.

### Strength(s) usually available

U.S.—
  10 mg (base) (Rx) [*Compazine Spansule* (benzyl alcohol; cetylpyridinium chloride; D&C Green No. 5; D&C Yellow No. 10; FD&C Blue No. 1; FD&C Red No. 40; FD&C Yellow No. 6; gelatin; glyceryl monostearate; sodium lauryl sulfate; starch; sucrose; wax)].
  15 mg (base) (Rx) [*Compazine Spansule* (benzyl alcohol; cetylpyridinium chloride; D&C Green No. 5; D&C Yellow No. 10; FD&C Blue No. 1; FD&C Red No. 40; FD&C Yellow No. 6; gelatin; glyceryl monostearate; sodium lauryl sulfate; starch; sucrose; wax)].
  30 mg (base) (Rx) [*Compazine Spansule* (benzyl alcohol; cetylpyridinium chloride; D&C Green No. 5; D&C Yellow No. 10; FD&C Blue No. 1; FD&C Red No. 40; FD&C Yellow No. 6; gelatin; glyceryl monostearate; sodium lauryl sulfate; starch; sucrose; wax)].

Canada—
  Not commercially available.

### Packaging and storage

Store below 40 °C (104 °F), preferably between 15 and 30 °C (59 and 86 °F), in a well-closed container, unless otherwise specified by manufacturer. Protect from light.

### Auxiliary labeling

- May cause drowsiness.
- Avoid alcoholic beverages.
- Swallow capsule whole.

## PROCHLORPERAZINE MALEATE TABLETS USP

### Usual adult and adolescent dose

Psychotic disorders—
  Oral, 5 to 10 mg (base) three or four times a day, the dosage being gradually increased every two or three days as needed and tolerated.

Anxiety—
  Oral, 5 mg (base) three or four times a day, up to 20 mg a day, for no longer than twelve weeks.

Nausea and vomiting—
  Oral, 5 to 10 mg (base) three or four times a day, up to 40 mg a day.

  Note: Daily dosages above 40 mg should be used only in resistant cases.

Note: Geriatric, emaciated, or debilitated patients usually require a lower initial dose, the dosage being gradually increased as needed and tolerated.

### Usual adult prescribing limits

Psychotic disorders—
  Up to 150 mg (base) a day.

### Usual pediatric dose

Since tablets are not suitable for many pediatric patients' requirements, the oral syrup dosage form is usually preferred.

### Strength(s) usually available

U.S.—
  5 mg (base) (Rx) [*Compazine;* GENERIC].
  10 mg (base) (Rx) [*Compazine;* GENERIC].
  25 mg (base) (Rx) [*Compazine;* GENERIC].

Canada—
  5 mg (base) (Rx) [*PMS Prochlorperazine; Prorazin; Stemetil*].
  10 mg (base) (Rx) [*PMS Prochlorperazine; Prorazin; Stemetil*].

### Packaging and storage

Store below 40 °C (104 °F), preferably between 15 and 30 °C (59 and 86 °F), unless otherwise specified by manufacturer. Store in a well-closed container. Protect from light.

### Auxiliary labeling

- May cause drowsiness.
- Avoid alcoholic beverages.

## PROCHLORPERAZINE MESYLATE SYRUP

### Usual adult and adolescent dose

Psychotic disorders—
  Oral, 5 to 10 mg (base) three or four times a day, the dosage being gradually increased every two to three days as needed and tolerated.

Anxiety—
  Oral, 5 mg (base) three or four times a day, up to 20 mg a day, for no longer than twelve weeks.

Nausea and vomiting—
  Oral, 5 to 10 mg (base) three or four times a day, up to 40 mg a day.

Note: Geriatric, emaciated, or debilitated patients usually require a lower initial dose, the dosage being gradually increased as needed and tolerated.

### Usual pediatric dose

Psychotic disorders—
  Children up to 2 years of age or 9 kg of body weight: Dosage has not been established.
  Children 2 to 12 years of age: Oral, 2.5 mg (base) two or three times a day.
  Children 12 years of age and older: See *Usual adult and adolescent dose.*

Nausea and vomiting—
  Children 9 to 13 kg of body weight: Oral, 2.5 mg (base) one or two times a day, not to exceed 7.5 mg a day.
  Children 14 to 17 kg of body weight: Oral, 2.5 mg (base) two or three times a day, not to exceed 10 mg a day.
  Children 18 to 39 kg of body weight: Oral, 2.5 mg (base) three times a day or 5 mg two times a day, not to exceed 15 mg a day.

Note: The total daily dose for any child should not exceed 10 mg the first day. On subsequent days the total daily dose should not exceed 20 mg for children 2 to 5 years of age or 25 mg for children 6 to 12 years of age.

### Strength(s) usually available

U.S.—
  Not commercially available.

Canada—
  5 mg (base) per 5 mL (Rx) [*Stemetil Liquid* (sucrose)].

### Packaging and storage

Store below 40 °C (104 °F), preferably between 15 and 30 °C (59 and 86 °F), in a tight container, protected from light, unless otherwise specified by manufacturer. Protect from freezing.

### Auxiliary labeling

- May cause drowsiness.
- Avoid alcoholic beverages.
- Do not spill on skin or clothing.

### Note

Avoid skin contact with liquid forms of this medication; contact dermatitis has resulted.

## Parenteral Dosage Forms

Note: The dosing and strengths of the dosage forms available are expressed in terms of prochlorperazine base (not the edisylate or mesylate salts).

## PROCHLORPERAZINE EDISYLATE INJECTION USP

**Usual adult and adolescent dose**

Nausea and vomiting—
Intramuscular, 5 to 10 mg (base), the dosage to be repeated every three to four hours as needed.
Intravenous, 2.5 to 10 mg as a slow injection or infusion, at a rate not exceeding 5 mg per minute, up to 40 mg a day.
Note: May be administered undiluted or diluted in isotonic solution.
Single dose should not exceed 10 mg.

Nausea and vomiting in surgery—
Intramuscular, 5 to 10 mg (base) one to two hours before induction of anesthesia, or to control acute symptoms during or after surgery, the dose being repeated once in thirty minutes if needed.
Intravenous, 5 to 10 mg (base), administered as a slow injection or infusion fifteen to thirty minutes before induction of anesthesia, or to control acute symptoms during or after surgery, at a rate not exceeding 5 mg per mL per minute, the dose being repeated once if needed.
Note: May be administered undiluted or diluted in isotonic solution.
Single dose should not exceed 10 mg.

Psychotic disorders—
Initial (for immediate control of severely disturbed patients): Intramuscular, 10 to 20 mg (base), the dose being repeated every two to four hours as needed, usually up to three or four doses.
Maintenance: Intramuscular, 10 to 20 mg (base) every four to six hours.

Anxiety—
Intramuscular, 5 to 10 mg (base), the dosage to be repeated every three to four hours as needed.
Intravenous, 2.5 to 10 mg as a slow injection or infusion, at a rate not exceeding 5 mg per minute, up to 40 mg a day.
Note: May be administered undiluted or diluted in isotonic solution.
Single dose should not exceed 10 mg.

Note: Geriatric, emaciated, or debilitated patients usually require a lower dose, the dosage being increased gradually as needed and tolerated.

**Usual adult prescribing limits**

Nausea and vomiting or anxiety—
Up to 40 mg (base) a day.
Psychotic disorders—
Up to 200 mg (base) a day.

**Usual pediatric dose**

Nausea and vomiting or
Psychotic disorders or anxiety—
Children up to 2 years of age or 9 kg of body weight: Dosage has not been established.
Children 2 to 12 years of age: Intramuscular, 132 mcg (0.132 mg) (base) per kg of body weight.
Children 12 years of age and older: See *Usual adult and adolescent dose.*
Note: Usual pediatric prescribing limits are 20 mg a day for children 2 to 5 years of age, and 25 mg a day for children 6 to 12 years old.
Control is usually obtained after one dose, after which patient may be switched to an oral dosage form at the same dosage level or higher.
Not recommended in pediatric surgery.

**Strength(s) usually available**

U.S.—
5 mg (base) per mL (Rx) [*Compa-Z; Compazine* (ampuls: sulfite; vials: benzyl alcohol 0.75%); *Cotranzine; Ultrazine-10;* GENERIC].
Canada—
Not commercially available.

**Packaging and storage**

Store below 40 °C (104 °F), preferably between 15 and 30 °C (59 and 86 °F), unless otherwise specified by manufacturer. Protect from light. Protect from freezing.

**Stability**

A slight yellowing will not alter potency; however, do not use if markedly discolored or if a precipitate is present.

**Incompatibilities**

A white milky precipitate may form when prochlorperazine edisylate injection is mixed in the same syringe with morphine sulfate injection produced by certain manufacturers.

**Note**

Avoid skin contact with liquid forms of this medication; contact dermatitis has resulted.

## PROCHLORPERAZINE MESYLATE INJECTION

**Usual adult and adolescent dose**

Nausea and vomiting—
Intramuscular, 5 to 10 mg (base), the dose being repeated every three to four hours if needed.

Nausea and vomiting in surgery—
Intramuscular, 5 to 10 mg (base) one to two hours before induction of anesthesia, or to control acute symptoms during or after surgery, the dose being repeated once in thirty minutes if needed.
Intravenous, 5 to 10 mg (base), administered fifteen to thirty minutes before induction of anesthesia, or to control acute symptoms during or after surgery, at a rate not to exceed 5 mg per mL per minute, the dose being repeated once if needed.
Intravenous infusion, 20 mg (base) in no less than 1 liter of isotonic solution, administered fifteen to thirty minutes before induction of anesthesia.

Psychotic disorders—
Initial (for immediate control of severely disturbed patients): Intramuscular, 10 to 20 mg (base), the dose being repeated every two to four hours as needed, usually up to three or four doses.
Maintenance: Intramuscular, 10 to 20 mg (base) every four to six hours.

Anxiety—
Intramuscular, 5 to 10 mg (base), the dose being repeated every three to four hours if needed.

Note: Geriatric, emaciated, or debilitated patients usually require a lower dose, the dosage being increased gradually as needed and tolerated.

**Usual adult prescribing limits**

Nausea and vomiting—
Up to 40 mg (base) a day.
Psychotic disorders—
Up to 200 mg (base) a day.

**Usual pediatric dose**

Nausea and vomiting or
Psychotic disorders or anxiety—
Children up to 2 years of age or 9 kg of body weight: Dosage has not been established.
Children 2 to 12 years of age: Intramuscular, 132 mcg (0.132 mg) (base) per kg of body weight, not exceeding 10 mg the first day, the dosage being increased, thereafter, as needed and tolerated.
Children 12 years of age and over: See *Usual adult or adolescent dose.*
Note: Usual pediatric prescribing limits are 20 mg a day for children 2 to 5 years of age, and 25 mg a day for children 6 to 12 years old.
Not recommended in pediatric surgery.

**Strength(s) usually available**

U.S.—
Not commercially available.
Canada—
5 mg (base) per mL (Rx) [*PMS Prochlorperazine; Stemetil* (sulfite); GENERIC].

**Packaging and storage**

Store below 40 °C (104 °F), preferably between 15 and 30 °C (59 and 86 °F), protected from light, unless otherwise specified by manufacturer. Protect from freezing.

**Stability**

A slight yellowing will not alter potency; however, do not use if markedly discolored or if a precipitate is present.

**Note**

Avoid skin contact with liquid forms of this medication; contact dermatitis has resulted.

# Rectal Dosage Forms

## PROCHLORPERAZINE SUPPOSITORIES USP

**Usual adult and adolescent dose**

Nausea and vomiting—
Rectal, 25 mg two times a day.
Psychotic disorders—
Rectal, 10 mg three or four times a day, the dosage being increased gradually by 5 to 10 mg every two to three days as needed and tolerated.
Note: Geriatric, emaciated, or debilitated patients usually require a lower initial dose, the dosage being gradually increased as needed and tolerated.

**Usual pediatric dose**

Nausea and vomiting—

Children up to 2 years of age or 9 kg of body weight: Dosage has not been established.

Children 9 to 13 kg of body weight: Rectal, 2.5 mg one or two times a day, not to exceed 7.5 mg per day.

Children 14 to 17 kg of body weight: Rectal, 2.5 mg two or three times a day, not to exceed 10 mg per day.

Children 18 to 39 kg of body weight: Rectal, 2.5 mg three times a day or 5 mg two times a day, not to exceed 15 mg per day.

Note: The total daily dose for any child should not exceed 10 mg the first day. On subsequent days, the total daily dose should not exceed 20 mg for children 2 to 5 years of age or 25 mg for children 6 to 12 years of age.

The 25-mg suppository is not recommended for use in children.

**Strength(s) usually available**

U.S.—

2.5 mg (Rx) [Compazine].

5 mg (Rx) [Compazine].

25 mg (Rx) [Compazine; GENERIC].

Canada—

10 mg (Rx) [PMS Prochlorperazine; Prorazin; Stemetil; GENERIC].

**Packaging and storage**

Store below 37 °C (98 °F). Store in a tight container. Protect from light.

**Auxiliary labeling**

• May cause drowsiness.

• Avoid alcoholic beverages.

• For rectal use only.

**Note**

Explain administration technique.

---

## PROMAZINE

## Summary of Differences

Pharmacology/pharmacokinetics:

Chemical group—

Aliphatic

Actions—

Antiemetic: Moderate

Anticholinergic: Strong

Extrapyramidal: Weak

Hypotensive: Strong

Sedative: Strong

## Oral Dosage Forms

### PROMAZINE HYDROCHLORIDE TABLETS USP

**Usual adult dose**

Psychotic disorders—

Oral, 10 to 200 mg every four to six hours, the dosage being adjusted gradually as needed and tolerated.

Note: Geriatric, emaciated, or debilitated patients usually require a lower initial dose, the dosage being gradually increased as needed and tolerated.

**Usual adult prescribing limits**

Up to 1 gram a day.

**Usual pediatric dose**

Psychotic disorders—

Children up to 12 years of age: Dosage has not been established.

Children 12 years of age and over: Oral, 10 to 25 mg every four to six hours, the dosage being adjusted as needed and tolerated.

**Strength(s) usually available**

U.S.—

25 mg (Rx) [Sparine (tartrazine; sucrose)].

50 mg (Rx) [Sparine (sucrose)].

100 mg (Rx) [Sparine (sucrose)].

Canada—

Not commercially available.

**Packaging and storage**

Store below 40 °C (104 °F), preferably between 15 and 30 °C (59 and 86 °F), unless otherwise specified by manufacturer. Store in a tight, light-resistant container.

**Auxiliary labeling**

• May cause drowsiness.

• Avoid alcoholic beverages.

## Parenteral Dosage Forms

### PROMAZINE HYDROCHLORIDE INJECTION USP

**Usual adult dose**

Psychotic disorders—

Intramuscular:

Initial—50 to 150 mg, the dosage being increased, if necessary, after thirty minutes.

Maintenance—10 to 200 mg, the dose being repeated at four- to six-hour intervals as needed and tolerated.

Intravenous:

Administered slowly after being diluted to 25 mg or less per mL with 0.9% sodium chloride injection.

Note: Geriatric, emaciated, or debilitated patients usually require a lower initial dose, the dosage being gradually increased as needed and tolerated.

Intravenous injection should be reserved for severely agitated hospitalized patients.

In acutely inebriated patients, the initial dose should not exceed 50 mg.

**Usual adult prescribing limits**

Up to 1 gram a day.

Note: Although doses are sometimes gradually increased to 2 grams a day or more for short periods, extended therapy with 1 gram or less is usually sufficient.

**Usual pediatric dose**

Psychotic disorders—

Children up to 12 years of age: Dosage has not been established.

Children 12 years of age and over: Intramuscular, 10 to 25 mg every four to six hours, up to 1 gram a day.

**Strength(s) usually available**

U.S.—

50 mg per mL (Rx) [Primazine; Prozine-50; Sparine; GENERIC (syringe units; sulfite)].

Canada—

50 mg per mL (Rx) [GENERIC].

**Packaging and storage**

Store below 40 °C (104 °F), preferably between 15 and 30 °C (59 and 86 °F), unless otherwise specified by manufacturer. Protect from light. Protect from freezing.

**Stability**

A slight yellowing will not alter potency; however, do not use if markedly discolored or if a precipitate is present.

**Note**

Avoid skin contact with liquid forms of this medication; contact dermatitis has resulted.

---

## THIOPROPAZATE

## Summary of Differences

Pharmacology/pharmacokinetics:

Chemical group—

Piperazine

Actions—

Antiemetic: Weak

Anticholinergic: Weak

Extrapyramidal: Strong

Hypotensive: Weak

Sedative: Weak

## Oral Dosage Forms

### THIOPROPAZATE HYDROCHLORIDE TABLETS

**Usual adult and adolescent dose**

Psychotic disorders—

Initial: Oral, 10 mg three times a day, the dosage being adjusted gradually by 10 mg every three or four days as needed and tolerated.

Maintenance: Oral, 10 to 20 mg two to four times a day.

Note: Geriatric, emaciated, or debilitated patients usually require a lower initial dose, the dosage being increased gradually as needed and tolerated, and decreased to the lowest effective dose as soon as possible.

**Usual adult prescribing limits**

Up to 100 mg a day.

**Usual pediatric dose**
Dosage has not been established.

**Strength(s) usually available**
U.S.—
Not commercially available.
Canada—
5 mg (Rx) [*Dartal* (acacia; activated charcoal; cornstarch; lactose; light liquid parafin; magnesium stearate; sodium sulfate; talc; tapioca starch; sodium 3.5 mmol [80 mg])].

**Packaging and storage**
Store below 40 °C (104 °F), in a well-closed, light-resistant container, unless otherwise specified by manufacturer.

**Auxiliary labeling**
• May cause drowsiness.
• Avoid alcoholic beverages.

---

## THIOPROPERAZINE

## Summary of Differences

Pharmacology/pharmacokinetics:
Chemical group—
Piperazine
Actions—
Antiemetic: Weak
Anticholinergic: Weak
Extrapyramidal: Strong
Hypotensive: Weak
Sedative: Weak

## Oral Dosage Forms

Note: The dosing and strengths of the dosage forms available are expressed in terms of thioproperazine base (not the mesylate salt).

### THIOPROPERAZINE MESYLATE TABLETS

**Usual adult and adolescent dose**
Psychotic disorders—
Oral, initially, 5 mg (base) a day, the dosage being adjusted gradually by 5 mg every two or three days as needed and tolerated.
Note: The usual effective dose is about 30 to 40 mg a day. In some patients, 90 mg or more a day may be necessary to control symptoms. Once symptoms are controlled, dosage should be reduced gradually to the lowest effective maintenance dose.

**Usual pediatric dose**
Dosage has not been established.

**Strength(s) usually available**
U.S.—
Not commercially available.
Canada—
10 mg (base) (Rx) [*Majeptil*].

**Packaging and storage**
Store below 40 °C (104 °F), in a well-closed, light-resistant container, unless otherwise specified by manufacturer.

**Auxiliary labeling**
• May cause drowsiness.
• Avoid alcoholic beverages.

---

## THIORIDAZINE

## Summary of Differences

Pharmacology/pharmacokinetics:
Chemical group—
Piperidine
Actions—
Antiemetic: Weak
Anticholinergic: Moderate
Extrapyramidal: Weak
Hypotensive: Moderate to strong
Sedative: Moderate
Side/adverse effects:
In high doses, more likely to cause pigmentary retinopathy than other phenothiazines.

## Oral Dosage Forms

### THIORIDAZINE ORAL SUSPENSION USP

**Usual adult and adolescent dose**
Psychotic disorders—
Initial: Oral, 25 to 100 mg (hydrochloride) three times a day, the dosage being adjusted gradually as needed and tolerated.
Maintenance: Oral, 10 to 200 mg (hydrochloride) two to four times a day.
Note: Geriatric, emaciated, or debilitated patients usually require a lower initial dose, the dosage being gradually increased as needed and tolerated.

**Usual adult prescribing limits**
Up to 800 mg (hydrochloride) a day.

**Usual pediatric dose**
Psychotic disorders—
Children up to 2 years of age: Dosage has not been established.
Children 2 to 12 years of age: Oral, 250 mcg (0.25 mg) to 3 mg (hydrochloride) per kg of body weight or 7.5 mg per square meter of body surface four times a day; or 10 to 25 mg two or three times a day.
Children 12 years of age and over: See *Usual adult and adolescent dose.*

**Strength(s) usually available**
U.S.—
25 mg (hydrochloride) per 5 mL (Rx) [*Mellaril-S* (carbomer 934; flavor; polysorbate 80; purified water; sodium hydroxide; sucrose)].
100 mg (hydrochloride) per 5 mL (Rx) [*Mellaril-S* (carbomer 934; flavor; polysorbate 80; purified water; sodium hydroxide; sucrose; D&C Yellow No. 10; FD&C Yellow No. 6)].
Canada—
10 mg (hydrochloride) per 5 mL (Rx) [*Mellaril* (alcohol; parabens)].

**Packaging and storage**
Store below 30 °C (86 °F). Store in a tight, light-resistant container. Protect from freezing.

**Auxiliary labeling**
• Shake well before using.
• May cause drowsiness.
• Avoid alcoholic beverages.
• Do not spill on skin or clothing.

**Note**
Avoid skin contact with liquid forms of this medication; contact dermatitis has resulted.

### THIORIDAZINE HYDROCHLORIDE ORAL SOLUTION USP

**Usual adult and adolescent dose**
Psychotic disorders—
Initial: Oral, 25 to 100 mg three times a day, the dosage being adjusted gradually as needed and tolerated.
Maintenance: Oral, 10 to 200 mg two to four times a day.
Note: Geriatric, emaciated, or debilitated patients usually require a lower initial dose, the dosage being gradually increased as needed and tolerated.

**Usual adult prescribing limits**
Up to 800 mg a day.

**Usual pediatric dose**
Psychotic disorders—
Children up to 2 years of age: Dosage has not been established.
Children 2 to 12 years of age: Oral, 250 mcg (0.25 mg) to 3 mg per kg of body weight or 7.5 mg per square meter of body surface four times a day; or 10 to 25 mg two or three times a day.
Children 12 years of age and over: See *Usual adult and adolescent dose.*

**Strength(s) usually available**
U.S.—
30 mg per mL (Rx) [*Mellaril Concentrate* (alcohol 3%); GENERIC].
100 mg per mL (Rx) [*Mellaril Concentrate* (alcohol 4.2%); GENERIC].
Canada—
30 mg per mL (Rx) [*Mellaril* (alcohol 3%; parabens)].

**Packaging and storage**
Store between 15 and 30 °C (59 and 86 °F), unless otherwise specified by manufacturer. Store in a tight, light-resistant container. Protect from freezing.

**Auxiliary labeling**
• May cause drowsiness.
• Avoid alcoholic beverages.

• Do not spill on skin or clothing.
• Must be diluted before use.

**Note**

Avoid skin contact with liquid forms of this medication; contact dermatitis has resulted.

Each dose must be diluted just before administration in a half glass (120 mL) of distilled water, acidified tap water, orange juice, or grapefruit juice.

Explain dilution and dosage measurement to patient if self-administered.

## THIORIDAZINE HYDROCHLORIDE TABLETS USP

**Usual adult and adolescent dose**

Psychotic disorders—
Initial: Oral, 25 to 100 mg three times a day, the dosage being adjusted gradually as needed and tolerated.
Maintenance: Oral, 10 to 200 mg two to four times a day.

Note: Geriatric, emaciated, or debilitated patients usually require a lower initial dose, the dosage being gradually increased as needed and tolerated.

**Usual adult prescribing limits**

Up to 800 mg a day.

**Usual pediatric dose**

Psychotic disorders—
Children up to 2 years of age: Dosage has not been established.
Children 2 to 12 years of age: Oral, 250 mcg (0.25 mg) to 3 mg per kg of body weight or 7.5 mg per square meter of body surface four times a day; or 10 to 25 mg two or three times a day.
Children 12 years of age and over: See *Usual adult and adolescent dose.*

Note: Since tablets are not suitable for many pediatric patients' requirements, the oral solution may be preferred.

**Strength(s) usually available**

U.S.—
10 mg (Rx) [*Mellaril;* GENERIC].
15 mg (Rx) [*Mellaril;* GENERIC].
25 mg (Rx) [*Mellaril;* GENERIC].
50 mg (Rx) [*Mellaril;* GENERIC].
100 mg (Rx) [*Mellaril;* GENERIC].
150 mg (Rx) [*Mellaril;* GENERIC].
200 mg (Rx) [*Mellaril;* GENERIC].
Canada—
10 mg (Rx) [*Apo-Thioridazine; Mellaril; Novo-Ridazine; PMS Thioridazine*].
25 mg (Rx) [*Apo-Thioridazine; Mellaril; Novo-Ridazine; PMS Thioridazine*].
50 mg (Rx) [*Apo-Thioridazine; Mellaril; Novo-Ridazine; PMS Thioridazine*].
100 mg (Rx) [*Apo-Thioridazine; Mellaril; Novo-Ridazine; PMS Thioridazine*].
200 mg (Rx) [*Mellaril; Novo-Ridazine*].

**Packaging and storage**

Store below 40 °C (104 °F), preferably between 15 and 30 °C (59 and 86 °F), unless otherwise specified by manufacturer. Store in a tight, light-resistant container.

**Auxiliary labeling**

• May cause drowsiness.
• Avoid alcoholic beverages.

---

### *TRIFLUOPERAZINE*

---

## Summary of Differences

Pharmacology/pharmacokinetics:
Chemical group—
Piperazine
Actions—
Antiemetic: Strong
Anticholinergic: Weak
Extrapyramidal: Strong
Hypotensive: Weak
Sedative: Weak

## Oral Dosage Forms

Note: The dosing and strengths of the dosage forms available are expressed in terms of trifluoperazine base (not the hydrochloride salt).

## TRIFLUOPERAZINE HYDROCHLORIDE ORAL SOLUTION

**Usual adult and adolescent dose**

Psychotic disorders—
Oral, 2 to 5 mg (base) two times a day initially, the dosage being gradually increased as needed and tolerated.
Anxiety—
1 to 2 mg (base) a day, up to a total of 6 mg a day, for no longer than twelve weeks.

Note: Geriatric, emaciated, or debilitated patients usually require a lower initial dose, the dosage being gradually increased as needed and tolerated.

**Usual adult prescribing limits**

Up to 40 mg (base) a day.

**Usual pediatric dose**

Psychotic disorders—
Children up to 6 years of age: Dosage has not been established.
Children 6 years of age and over: Oral, 1 mg (base) one or two times a day, the dosage being adjusted gradually as needed and tolerated.

**Strength(s) usually available**

U.S.—
10 mg (base) per mL (Rx) [*Stelazine Concentrate* (sulfite); GENERIC].
Canada—
10 mg (base) per mL (Rx) [*Stelazine Concentrate* (sulfite); *Terfluzine Concentrate*].

**Packaging and storage**

Store below 40 °C (104 °F), preferably between 15 and 30 °C (59 and 86 °F), in a tight, light-resistant container, unless otherwise specified by manufacturer. Protect from freezing.

**Stability**

A slight yellowing will not alter potency; however, do not use if markedly discolored or if a precipitate is present.

**Auxiliary labeling**

• May cause drowsiness.
• Avoid alcoholic beverages.
• Do not spill on skin or clothing.
• Must be diluted before use.

**Note**

The oral solution is intended primarily for institutional usage.

Avoid skin contact with liquid forms of this medication; contact dermatitis has resulted.

Each dose must be diluted just before administration in a half glass (120 mL) of milk, tomato or fruit juice, water, or soup.

Explain dilution and dosage measurement to patient if self-administered.

## TRIFLUOPERAZINE HYDROCHLORIDE SYRUP USP

**Usual adult and adolescent dose**

Psychotic disorders—
Oral, 2 to 5 mg (base) two times a day initially, the dosage being gradually increased as needed and tolerated.
Anxiety—
1 to 2 mg (base) a day, up to a total of 6 mg a day, for no longer than twelve weeks.

Note: Geriatric, emaciated, or debilitated patients usually require a lower initial dose, the dosage being gradually increased as needed and tolerated.

**Usual adult prescribing limits**

Up to 40 mg (base) a day.

**Usual pediatric dose**

Psychotic disorders—
Children up to 6 years of age: Dosage has not been established.
Children 6 years of age and over: Oral, 1 mg (base) one or two times a day, the dosage being adjusted gradually as needed and tolerated.

**Strength(s) usually available**

U.S.—
Not commercially available.
Canada—
1 mg (base) per mL (Rx) [*PMS Trifluoperazine*].
10 mg (base) per mL (Rx) [*PMS Trifluoperazine; Terfluzine*].

**Packaging and storage**

Store below 40 °C (104 °F), preferably between 15 and 30 °C (59 and 86 °F), in a tight, light-resistant container, unless otherwise specified by manufacturer. Protect from freezing.

**Auxiliary labeling**
• May cause drowsiness.
• Avoid alcoholic beverages.

## TRIFLUOPERAZINE HYDROCHLORIDE TABLETS USP

**Usual adult and adolescent dose**
Psychotic disorders—
    Oral, 2 to 5 mg (base) two times a day initially, the dosage being gradually increased as needed and tolerated.
Anxiety—
    1 to 2 mg (base) a day, up to a total of 6 mg a day, for not longer than twelve weeks.
Note: Geriatric, emaciated, or debilitated patients usually require a lower initial dose, the dosage being gradually increased as needed and tolerated.

**Usual adult prescribing limits**
Up to 40 mg (base) a day.

**Usual pediatric dose**
Psychotic disorders—
    Children up to 6 years of age: Dosage has not been established.
    Children 6 years of age and over: Oral, 1 mg (base) one or two times a day, the dosage being adjusted gradually as needed and tolerated.

**Strength(s) usually available**
U.S.—
    1 mg (base) (Rx) [*Stelazine;* GENERIC].
    2 mg (base) (Rx) [*Stelazine;* GENERIC].
    5 mg (base) (Rx) [*Stelazine;* GENERIC].
    10 mg (base) (Rx) [*Stelazine;* GENERIC].
Canada—
    1 mg (base) (Rx) [*Apo-Trifluoperazine; Novo-Flurazine; PMS Trifluoperazine; Stelazine; Terfluzine*].
    2 mg (base) (Rx) [*Apo-Trifluoperazine; Novo-Flurazine; PMS Trifluoperazine; Solazine; Stelazine; Terfluzine*].
    5 mg (base) (Rx) [*Apo-Trifluoperazine; Novo-Flurazine; PMS Trifluoperazine; Solazine; Stelazine; Terfluzine*].
    10 mg (base) (Rx) [*Apo-Trifluoperazine; Novo-Flurazine; PMS Trifluoperazine; Solazine* (tartrazine); *Stelazine; Terfluzine*].
    20 mg (base) (Rx) [*Apo-Trifluoperazine; Novo-Flurazine; PMS Trifluoperazine*].

**Packaging and storage**
Store below 40 °C (104 °F), preferably between 15 and 30 °C (59 and 86 °F), unless otherwise specified by manufacturer. Store in a well-closed, light-resistant container.

**Auxiliary labeling**
• May cause drowsiness.
• Avoid alcoholic beverages.

## Parenteral Dosage Forms

Note: The dosing and strengths of the dosage forms available are expressed in terms of trifluoperazine base (not the hydrochloride salt).

## TRIFLUOPERAZINE HYDROCHLORIDE INJECTION USP

**Usual adult and adolescent dose**
Psychotic disorders—
    Intramuscular, 1 to 2 mg (base) every four to six hours as needed.
Note: Geriatric, emaciated, or debilitated patients usually require a lower initial dose, the dosage being increased gradually as needed and tolerated.

**Usual adult prescribing limits**
Up to 10 mg (base) a day.

**Usual pediatric dose**
Psychotic disorders—
    Children up to 6 years of age: Dosage has not been established.
    Children 6 years of age and over: Intramuscular, 1 mg (base) one or two times a day.

**Strength(s) usually available**
U.S.—
    2 mg (base) per mL (Rx) [*Stelazine* (benzyl alcohol 0.75%; sodium tartrate; sodium biphosphate; sodium saccharin); GENERIC].
Canada—
    1 mg (base) per mL (Rx) [*Stelazine* (sulfite; benzyl alcohol 0.75%)].

**Packaging and storage**
Store below 40 °C (104 °F), preferably between 15 and 30 °C (59 and 86 °F), unless otherwise specified by manufacturer. Protect from light. Protect from freezing.

**Stability**
A slight yellowing will not alter potency; however, do not use if markedly discolored or if a precipitate is present.

**Note**
Avoid skin contact with liquid forms of this medication; contact dermatitis has resulted.

---

## *TRIFLUPROMAZINE*

## Summary of Differences

Category:
    Includes antiemetic use.
Pharmacology/pharmacokinetics:
    Chemical group—
        Aliphatic
    Actions—
        Antiemetic: Strong
        Anticholinergic: Strong
        Extrapyramidal: Moderate to strong
        Hypotensive: Moderate
        Sedative: Moderate to strong

## Parenteral Dosage Forms

## TRIFLUPROMAZINE HYDROCHLORIDE INJECTION USP

**Usual adult and adolescent dose**
Psychotic disorders—
    Intramuscular, 60 mg as needed.
Nausea and vomiting—
    Intramuscular, 5 to 15 mg every four hours.
    Intravenous, 1 mg as needed.
Note: Geriatric, emaciated, or debilitated patients usually require a lower initial dose, the dosage being increased as needed and tolerated.

**Usual adult prescribing limits**
Psychotic disorders—
    Intramuscular, up to 150 mg a day.
Nausea and vomiting—
    Intramuscular, up to 60 mg a day.
    Intravenous, up to 3 mg a day.

**Usual pediatric dose**
Psychotic disorders or
Nausea and vomiting—
    Children up to 2½ years of age: Dosage has not been established.
    Children 2½ years of age and over: Intramuscular, 200 to 250 mcg (0.2 to 0.25 mg) per kg of body weight, not to exceed 10 mg per day.
Note: Intravenous administration is not recommended in children because of hypotension and rapid onset of severe extrapyramidal reactions.

**Strength(s) usually available**
U.S.—
    10 mg per mL (Rx) [*Vesprin* (benzyl alcohol 1.5%)].
    20 mg per mL (Rx) [*Vesprin* (benzyl alcohol 1.5%)].
Canada—
    Not commercially available.

**Packaging and storage**
Store between 15 and 30 °C (59 and 86 °F), unless otherwise specified by manufacturer. Protect from light. Protect from freezing.

**Stability**
A slight yellowing to a light amber color will not alter potency; however, do not use if markedly discolored or if a precipitate is present.

**Note**
Avoid skin contact with liquid forms of this medication; contact dermatitis has resulted.

---

Revised: 03/16/92
Interim revision: 08/23/94

# PHENOXYBENZAMINE Systemic

VA CLASSIFICATION (Primary/Secondary): AU200/CV490; GU900

Note: For a listing of dosage forms and brand names by country availability, see *Dosage Forms* section(s). For a listing of brand names for the articles in this monograph, refer to the General Index.

## Category

Antihypertensive (pheochromocytoma); benign prostatic hypertrophy therapy.

## Indications

Note: Bracketed information in the *Indications* section refers to uses that are not included in U.S. product labeling.

### Accepted

Pheochromocytoma (treatment)—Phenoxybenzamine is indicated to control episodes of hypertension and sweating in the treatment of pheochromocytoma as preoperative preparation for surgery, in management of patients when surgery is contraindicated, and in chronic management of patients with malignant pheochromocytoma.

[Benign prostatic hypertrophy (treatment)]—Phenoxybenzamine is used for the treatment of urinary symptoms associated with benign prostatic hypertrophy (BPH).

### Unaccepted

Phenoxybenzamine is not useful in the treatment of essential hypertension because of its side effects, particularly reflex tachycardia.

## Pharmacology/Pharmacokinetics

### Physicochemical characteristics
Molecular weight—340.29.
pKa—4.4.

### Mechanism of action/Effect
Nonselective alpha-adrenergic blockade; phenoxybenzamine combines irreversibly with postganglionic alpha-adrenergic receptor sites, preventing or reversing effects of endogenous or exogenous catecholamines; no effect on beta-adrenergic receptors.

### Absorption
Variable following oral administration. Approximately 20 to 30% absorbed in the active form.

### Biotransformation
Hepatic.

### Half-life
Approximately 24 hours.

### Onset of action
Alpha-adrenergic blockade—Several hours.

Note: Alpha-adrenergic blocking effects are cumulative over approximately 7 days with daily dosing.

### Duration of action
Alpha-adrenergic blockade—3 to 4 days after a single dose.

### Elimination
Renal/biliary.

## Precautions to Consider

### Carcinogenicity
Repeated intraperitoneal administration of phenoxybenzamine to rats and mice caused peritoneal sarcomas, and chronic oral dosing in rats caused malignant tumors of the gastrointestinal tract (primarily in the nonglandular stomach). Chronic oral studies in rats found probable drug-related development of ulcerative and/or erosive gastritis of the glandular stomach.

### Mutagenicity
Phenoxybenzamine has been found to be mutagenic *in vitro* in the Ames test and in the mouse lymphoma assay. However, it has not shown mutagenic activity in the micronucleus test in mice.

### Pregnancy/Reproduction
Pregnancy—Studies have not been done in humans.
Studies have not been done in animals.
FDA Pregnancy Category C.

### Breast-feeding
It is not known whether phenoxybenzamine is distributed into breast milk. However, problems in humans have not been documented.

### Pediatrics
Appropriate studies on the relationship of age to the effects of phenoxybenzamine have not been performed in the pediatric population. However, pediatrics-specific problems that would limit the usefulness of this medication in children are not expected.

### Geriatrics
Although appropriate studies on the relationship of age to the effects of phenoxybenzamine have not been performed in the geriatric population, no geriatrics-specific problems have been documented to date. However, the elderly may be more sensitive to the hypotensive effects and the risk of phenoxybenzamine-induced hypothermia may be increased in elderly patients. Furthermore, elderly patients are also more likely to have age-related renal function impairment, which may require caution in patients receiving phenoxybenzamine.

### Dental
Use of phenoxybenzamine may decrease or inhibit salivary flow, thus contributing to the development of caries, periodontal disease, oral candidiasis, and discomfort.

### Drug interactions and/or related problems
The following drug interactions and/or related problems have been selected on the basis of their potential clinical significance (possible mechanism in parentheses where appropriate)—not necessarily inclusive (» = major clinical significance):

Note: Combinations containing any of the following medications, depending on the amount present, may also interact with this medication.

Diazoxide
(concurrent use with phenoxybenzamine antagonizes the inhibition of insulin release by diazoxide)

Guanadrel or
Guanethidine
(concurrent use with phenoxybenzamine may cause an increased incidence of orthostatic hypotension or bradycardia)

Sympathomimetics, such as:
Dopamine
Ephedrine
» Epinephrine
» Metaraminol
» Methoxamine
» Phenylephrine
(concurrent use of dopamine with phenoxybenzamine antagonizes the peripheral vasoconstriction produced by high doses of dopamine)
(concurrent use of ephedrine with phenoxybenzamine may decrease the pressor response to ephedrine)
(concurrent use of epinephrine with phenoxybenzamine may block the alpha-adrenergic effects of epinephrine, possibly resulting in severe hypotension and tachycardia)
(alpha-adrenergic blocking agents such as phenoxybenzamine usually decrease, but do not reverse, pressor response to metaraminol)
(prior administration of phenoxybenzamine may block the pressor response to methoxamine, possibly resulting in severe hypotension)
(prior administration of phenoxybenzamine may decrease the pressor response to phenylephrine)

### Medical considerations/Contraindications
The medical considerations/contraindications included here have been selected on the basis of their potential clinical significance (reasons given in parentheses where appropriate)—not necessarily inclusive (» = major clinical significance).

*Risk-benefit should be considered when the following medical problems exist:*

Cerebrovascular insufficiency
(reduced blood pressure may aggravate ischemia)

Congestive heart failure, compensated or
Coronary artery disease
(reflex tachycardia may precipitate frank congestive heart failure and angina)

Renal function impairment

Respiratory infection
(symptoms such as nasal congestion may be aggravated)

Sensitivity to phenoxybenzamine

**Patient monitoring**

The following may be especially important in patient monitoring (other tests may be warranted in some patients, depending on condition; » = major clinical significance):

» Blood pressure measurements and

» Urinary catecholamine measurements
  (recommended at periodic intervals during initial therapy to determine maximal dose)

## Side/Adverse Effects

The following side/adverse effects have been selected on the basis of their potential clinical significance (possible signs and symptoms in parentheses where appropriate)—not necessarily inclusive:

**Those indicating need for medical attention only if they continue or are bothersome**

Incidence more frequent—resulting from alpha-adrenergic blockade
*Miosis* (pinpoint pupils); *nasal congestion* (stuffy nose); *postural hypotension* (dizziness or lightheadedness, especially when getting up from a lying or sitting position); *tachycardia, reflex* (fast heartbeat)

Incidence less frequent
*Confusion; drowsiness; dryness of mouth; headache; inability to ejaculate; lack of energy; unusual tiredness or weakness*

Note: *Inability to ejaculate* is caused by alpha-adrenergic blockade.

## Overdose

For more information on the management of overdose or unintentional ingestion, **contact a Poison Control Center** (see *Poison Control Center Listing*).

**Treatment of overdose**

Treatment of circulatory failure, either by placing the patient in the recumbent position with legs elevated or additional measures if shock is present.

The usual pressor agents are not effective; epinephrine should not be used because of the risk of further hypotension.

Intravenous administration of levarterenol bitartrate may be useful.

## Patient Consultation

As an aid to patient consultation, refer to *Advice for the Patient, Phenoxybenzamine (Systemic)*.

In providing consultation, consider emphasizing the following selected information (»= major clinical significance):

**Before using this medication**

» Conditions affecting use, especially:
  Sensitivity to phenoxybenzamine
  Use in the elderly—Elderly patients may be more sensitive to the hypotensive effects; risk of phenoxybenzamine-induced hypothermia may be increased
  Dental—May decrease or inhibit salivary flow

**Proper use of this medication**

Getting into the habit of taking at same times each day to help increase compliance

» Proper dosing
  Missed dose: Taking as soon as possible; not taking if almost time for next dose; not doubling doses

» Proper storage

**Precautions while using this medication**

Regular visits to physician to check progress during therapy

» Not taking other medications, especially nonprescription sympathomimetics, unless discussed with physician

» Caution when driving or doing things requiring alertness because of possible dizziness or drowsiness

» Caution when getting up suddenly from a lying or sitting position

» Caution in using alcohol, while standing for long periods or exercising, and during hot weather because of enhanced orthostatic hypotensive effects

» Caution if any kind of surgery (including dental surgery) or emergency treatment is required
  Possible dryness of mouth; using sugarless candy or gum, ice, or saliva substitute for relief; checking with physician or dentist if dry mouth continues for more than 2 weeks

## General Dosing Information

Dosage must be adjusted to meet the individual requirements of each patient, on the basis of clinical response and urinary catecholamine determinations.

Incidence and severity of side effects may be reduced by initiating therapy at a low dose and increasing gradually to the minimum effective dose.

It is recommended that dosage increments be made no more frequently than every 4 days.

Concurrent administration of a beta-adrenergic blocker may be necessary if reflex tachycardia is severe.

If gastrointestinal irritation occurs, phenoxybenzamine may be administered with meals or milk; dosage reduction may be necessary.

## Oral Dosage Forms

**PHENOXYBENZAMINE HYDROCHLORIDE CAPSULES USP**

**Usual adult dose**

Antihypertensive (pheochromocytoma)—
  Initial: Oral, 10 mg twice a day, increased by increments of 10 mg every other day until an adequate response is achieved.
  Maintenance: Oral, 20 to 40 mg two or three times a day.
[Benign prostatic hypertrophy therapy]—
  10 to 20 mg per day.

Note: Geriatric patients may be more sensitive to the effects of the usual adult dose.

**Usual pediatric dose**

Antihypertensive (pheochromocytoma)—
  Initial: Oral, 200 mcg (0.2 mg) per kg of body weight or 6 mg per square meter of body surface, up to a maximum dose of 10 mg, once a day. Dosage is increased gradually at four-day intervals, until an adequate response is achieved.
  Maintenance: Oral, 400 mcg (0.4 mg) to 1.2 mg per kg of body weight or 12 to 36 mg per square meter of body surface a day in three or four divided doses.

**Strength(s) usually available**

U.S.—
  10 mg (Rx) [*Dibenzyline* (lactose)].

**Packaging and storage**

Store below 40 °C (104 °F), preferably between 15 and 30 °C (59 and 86 °F), unless otherwise specified by manufacturer. Store in a well-closed container.

---

Revised: 09/20/92
Interim revision: 07/20/94

---

**PHENSUXIMIDE**—See *Anticonvulsants, Succinimide (Systemic)*

---

**PHENTERMINE**—See *Appetite Suppressants (Systemic)*

---

# PHENTOLAMINE   Intracavernosal

VA CLASSIFICATION (Primary/Secondary): AU200/GU900

Note: For a listing of dosage forms and brand names by country availability, see *Dosage Forms* section(s). For a listing of brand names for the articles in this monograph, refer to the General Index.

## Category

Impotence therapy adjunct.

## Indications

Note: Bracketed information in the *Indications* section refers to uses that are not included in U.S. product labeling.

Information pertaining to the use of phentolamine for other indications, see *Phentolamine (Systemic)*.

**Accepted**

[Impotence (treatment adjunct)][1]—Phentolamine is used in combination with papaverine, by intracavernosal injection, to facilitate erections in men with impotence. In general, the combination is most useful in patients with organic impotence (neurogenic and, to a lesser extent, vascular). It is less useful in patients with impotence due to endocrine problems (hypogonadism, hyper- or hypothyroidism) or medications.

[Impotence (diagnosis)][1]—Phentolamine is used with papaverine, by intracavernosal injection, as an aid in the evaluation of penile vasculature, alone or prior to angiography, corpus cavernosography, or cavernosometry.

## Unaccepted
Use of phentolamine and papaverine to enhance erections in men who are not impotent is not recommended because of the risk of priapism and permanent damage to penile tissues.

---

[1]Not included in Canadian product labeling.

## Pharmacology/Pharmacokinetics

### Physicochemical characteristics
Molecular weight—377.46.

### Mechanism of action/Effect
Alpha-adrenergic blockade (alpha$_1$ and alpha$_2$ receptors) and antagonism of effects of circulating epinephrine and norepinephrine to cause vasodilation and reduction in peripheral resistance. When administered by intracavernous injection, it is thought to cause relaxation of the trabecular cavernous smooth muscles and vasodilation of the penile arteries. This results in increased arterial blood flow into the corpus cavernosa, and swelling and elongation of the penis; the glans and corpus spongiosum swell very little, if at all. Venous outflow is also reduced by papaverine, possibly as a result of increased venous resistance.

### Absorption
Slowly released into venous circulation; minimal, if any, systemic effects.

### Time to peak effect
In combination with papaverine—Variable, but usually within 10 minutes.

### Duration of action
In combination with papaverine—1 to 6 hours; dose-related.

## Precautions to Consider

### Pregnancy/Reproduction
Problems in humans have not been documented.

### Geriatrics
No information is available on the relationship of age to the effects of phentolamine for impotence in geriatric patients. However, geriatrics-specific problems that would limit the usefulness of this medication in the elderly are not expected.

### Drug interactions and/or related problems
The following drug interactions and/or related problems have been selected on the basis of their potential clinical significance (possible mechanism in parentheses where appropriate)—not necessarily inclusive (» = major clinical significance):
Sympathomimetics, alpha-adrenergic, especially metaraminol, epinephrine, and phenylephrine
(reverse the vasodilating effect of phentolamine; may be used to treat priapism or overdose)

### Medical considerations/Contraindications
The medical considerations/contraindications included here have been selected on the basis of their potential clinical significance (reasons given in parentheses where appropriate)—not necessarily inclusive (» = major clinical significance).

*Risk-benefit should be considered when the following medical problems exist:*
Allergy to phentolamine
» Coagulation defects, severe
(risk of bleeding at injection site)
» Priapism, history of
» Sickle cell disease
(increased risk of priapism)

### Patient monitoring
The following may be especially important in patient monitoring (other tests may be warranted in some patients, depending on condition; » = major clinical significance):
Palpation of penis
(recommended at regular intervals by both the patient and the physician to check for developing fibrosis or curvature)

## Side/Adverse Effects
The following side/adverse effects have been selected on the basis of their potential clinical significance (possible signs and symptoms in parentheses where appropriate)—not necessarily inclusive:

### Those indicating need for medical attention
Incidence rare
*Dizziness; fibrosis* (lumps in penis); *priapism* (erection, continuing for more than 4 hours, or painful erection)
Note: *Fibrosis* of the corpus cavernosum, resulting in blockage and inability to insert a penile prosthesis, has been reported in a patient using papaverine injection.
*Priapism* is usually due to excessive dosage. Prolonged erection may resolve spontaneously, but in most cases will require treatment.

### Those indicating need for medical attention only if they continue or are bothersome
Incidence less frequent or rare
*Burning, mild, along penis; difficulty in ejaculating; inadvertent subcutaneous administration* (bruising or bleeding at site of injection, swelling at site of injection); *superficial hematoma* (bruising or bleeding at site of injection)
Note: *Burning* may be more severe with inadvertent subcutaneous administration.

### Those not indicating need for medical attention
Incidence more frequent
*Tingling at tip of penis*

## Patient Consultation
As an aid to patient consultation, refer to *Advice for the Patient, Phentolamine and Papaverine (Intracavernosal)*.

In providing consultation, consider emphasizing the following selected information (» = major clinical significance):

### Before using this medication
» Conditions affecting use, especially:
Allergy to phentolamine
Other medical problems, especially severe coagulation defects, history of priapism, or sickle cell disease

### Proper use of this medication
*Proper administration*
» Cleansing injection site with alcohol; injecting slowly and directly into corpus cavernosum at base of penis; avoiding subcutaneous administration; if inadvertently injected subcutaneously (as evidenced by pain at injection site), stopping, withdrawing, and repositioning needle
Putting pressure on injection site for 1 to 2 minutes to prevent bruising; massaging penis, as directed by physician, to distribute medication
Effect begins in about 10 minutes; attempting intercourse within 2 hours after administration
» Proper dosing
» Proper storage

### Precautions while using this medication
» Compliance with therapy; importance of not exceeding prescribed dosage and frequency of use; risk of priapism, tissue ischemia, and permanent damage with overdose
» Telling physician immediately if erection persists longer than 4 hours or becomes painful
If bleeding occurs at injection site, applying pressure; checking with physician if bleeding persists
Examining penis regularly for signs of fibrosis at injection site or for curvature; checking with physician if either of these occurs

### Side/adverse effects
Signs of potential side effects, especially dizziness, fibrosis, priapism
Injection may cause tingling at tip of penis; no cause for concern

## General Dosing Information
Patients receiving intracavernosal phentolamine and papaverine should be under supervision of a physician experienced in their use and familiar with proper management of sustained erection and priapism.

Dosage adjustment should be made carefully, based on the degree and duration of tumescence achieved with the previous dose. In general, patients with neurogenic impotence may be more sensitive to the effects of intracavernosal vasodilators and may require lower doses.

Intracavernosal phentolamine and papaverine may be self-administered by the patient, but only after careful training in the technique to reduce the incidence of inadvertent subcutaneous administration, ecchymosis, and urethral injury.

For treatment of impotence, phentolamine and papaverine are injected slowly (over 1 to 2 minutes), directly into the corpus cavernosum at the base of the penis. A characteristic give should be noticed as the needle penetrates the tunica albuginea and enters the corpus cavernosum. Proper injection technique is necessary to avoid injury or injection of the urethra or vessels on the dorsal aspect of the penis.

After completion of the injection, pressure is applied to the injection site to prevent bleeding. Then the entire length of the corpus cavernosum should be squeezed firmly to distribute medication to the other side, followed by the same procedure on the other side. The penis should then be pinched transversely in several places to distribute medication to both ends of the corpus cavernosa.

If a sustained erection occurs, the next dose of phentolamine and papaverine should be reduced.

Intercourse should be attempted within 2 hours after administration.

If fibrosis occurs, discontinuation of phentolamine and papaverine therapy may be necessary, especially if a penile implant is planned in the future.

### For treatment of prolonged erection or priapism

A sustained erection should be treated if it persists for longer than 4 hours; priapism should be treated promptly. If tumescence is not reversed, interruption of blood flow may result in penile tissue ischemia and permanent damage.

Depending on the severity, treatment may include
- Aspiration of intracavernous blood.
- Irrigation of the corpus cavernosa with saline to remove clotted blood.
- Intracavernous administration of an alpha-adrenergic agonist, such as metaraminol, epinephrine, or phenylephrine.
- Surgery.

## Parenteral Dosage Forms

Note: Bracketed uses in the *Dosage Forms* section refer to categories of use and/or indications that are not included in U.S. product labeling.

### PHENTOLAMINE MESYLATE FOR INJECTION USP

**Usual adult dose**
[Impotence therapy][1]—
Intracavernosal, a mixture of 30 mg Papaverine Hydrochloride Injection USP and 0.5 to 1.0 mg of reconstituted Phentolamine Mesylate

for Injection USP, the dosage being adjusted according to response.

Note: Patients with neurogenic impotence may require lower doses or use of papaverine alone.

**Usual adult prescribing limits**
Impotence therapy—
Up to 60 mg of papaverine hydrochloride per dose. The injection should not be given more than three times weekly or two days in succession.

**Size(s) usually available**
U.S.—
5 mg (Rx) [*Regitine*].
Canada—
5 mg (Rx) [*Rogitine*].

**Packaging and storage**
Store below 40 °C (104 °F), preferably between 15 and 30 °C (59 and 86 °F), unless otherwise specified by manufacturer.

**Preparation of dosage form**
Phentolamine Mesylate for Injection USP is reconstituted for parenteral use by adding 1 mL of sterile water for injection to the vial, producing a solution containing 5 mg of phentolamine mesylate per mL.

**Stability**
Any unused portion should be discarded. There are no data available on stability of admixtures of phentolamine injection and Papaverine Hydrochloride Injection USP.

[1]Not included in Canadian product labeling.

## Selected Bibliography

Morley JE. Impotence. Am J Med 1986 May; 80 (5): 897-905.
Sidi AA, Lange PH. Recent advances in the diagnosis and management of impotence. Urol Clin North Am 1986 Aug; 13 (3): 489-500.
Lue TF, Tanagho EA. Physiology of erection and pharmacological management of impotence. J Urol 1987 May; 137 (5): 829-36.

Revised: 09/20/92
Interim revision: 06/07/94

---

# PHENTOLAMINE    Systemic

VA CLASSIFICATION (Primary/Secondary): AU200/CV150; CV900

Note: For information pertaining to use of phentolamine for impotence, see *Phentolamine (Intracavernosal)*.

Note: For a listing of dosage forms and brand names by country availability, see *Dosage Forms* section(s). For a listing of brand names for the articles in this monograph, refer to the General Index.

## Category

Antiadrenergic; vasodilator, congestive heart failure.

## Indications

Note: Bracketed information in the *Indications* section refers to uses that are not included in U.S. product labeling.

### Accepted

Hypertension, paroxysmal, in surgery for pheochromocytoma (prophylaxis and treatment)—Phentolamine is indicated to prevent or control paroxysmal hypertension prior to and during surgery for pheochromocytoma.

Necrosis, dermal (prophylaxis)—Parenteral phentolamine is indicated to prevent dermal necrosis and sloughing following intravenous administration or extravasation of norepinephrine.

[Congestive heart failure (treatment)][1]—Phentolamine has been used in treating left ventricular failure, reduced cardiac output, and increased pulmonary pressure that occur in various conditions (for example, myocardial infarction, acute and chronic congestive heart failure, mitral or aortic insufficiency) and following open-heart surgery.

### Unaccepted

Although phentolamine is indicated as an aid in the diagnosis of pheochromocytoma, determinations of blood and urine catecholamine concentrations are considered safer and more reliable.

[1]Not included in Canadian product labeling.

## Pharmacology/Pharmacokinetics

**Physicochemical characteristics**
Molecular weight—377.46.

**Mechanism of action/Effect**
Hypertension—Alpha-adrenergic blockade (alpha $_1$ and alpha $_2$ receptors) and antagonism of effects of circulating epinephrine and norepinephrine to cause vasodilation and reduction in peripheral resistance. Phentolamine has little effect on the blood pressure of healthy individuals or patients with essential hypertension.

Vasodilator, congestive heart failure—Reduction in afterload and pulmonary arterial pressure; increased cardiac output; positive inotropic effect.

**Half-life**
Intravenous—Approximately 19 minutes.

**Elimination**
Not completely known; however, approximately 13% of a single intravenous dose is excreted in urine as unmetabolized drug.

## Precautions to Consider

**Carcinogenicity/Mutagenicity**
Studies have not been done.

## Pregnancy/Reproduction

Pregnancy—Adequate and well-controlled studies in humans have not been done. However, one death has been reported with use of the phentolamine test for pheochromocytoma during pregnancy.

Studies in rats and mice at oral doses of 24 to 30 times the usual daily human dose (based on a 60-kg woman) found that phentolamine causes slightly decreased growth and slight skeletal immaturity (increased incidence of incomplete or unossified calcanei and phalangeal nuclei of the hind limb and of incompletely ossified sternebrae) of the fetuses. Studies in rats at oral doses of 60 times the usual daily human dose found a slightly lower implantation rate. Embryonic or fetal development was not affected in rabbits at oral doses of 20 times the usual daily human dose. No teratogenicity or embryotoxicity was found in the rat, mouse, or rabbit studies.

FDA Pregnancy Category C.

## Breast-feeding

It is not known whether phentolamine is distributed into breast milk. However, problems in humans have not been documented.

## Pediatrics

Appropriate studies on the relationship of age to the effects of phentolamine have not been performed in the pediatric population. However, pediatrics-specific problems that would limit the usefulness of this medication in children are not expected.

## Geriatrics

No information is available on the relationship of age to the effects of phentolamine in geriatric patients. However, the risk of phentolamine-induced hypothermia may be increased in elderly patients.

## Drug interactions and/or related problems

The following drug interactions and/or related problems have been selected on the basis of their potential clinical significance (possible mechanism in parentheses where appropriate)—not necessarily inclusive (» = major clinical significance):

Note: Combinations containing any of the following medications, depending on the amount present, may also interact with this medication.

Diazoxide
(concurrent use with phentolamine antagonizes the inhibition of insulin release by diazoxide)

Guanadrel or
Guanethidine
(concurrent use of phentolamine with guanadrel or guanethidine may cause an increased incidence of orthostatic hypotension or bradycardia)

Sympathomimetics, such as:
Dopamine
Ephedrine
» Epinephrine
» Metaraminol
» Methoxamine
» Phenylephrine
(concurrent use of dopamine with phentolamine antagonizes the peripheral vasoconstriction produced by high doses of dopamine)
(concurrent use of ephedrine with phentolamine may decrease the pressor response to ephedrine)
(concurrent use of epinephrine with phentolamine may block the alpha-adrenergic effects of epinephrine, possibly resulting in severe hypotension and tachycardia)
(alpha-adrenergic blocking agents such as phentolamine usually decrease, but do not reverse, pressor response to metaraminol)
(prior administration of phentolamine may block the pressor response to methoxamine, possibly resulting in severe hypotension)
(prior administration of phentolamine may decrease the pressor response to phenylephrine)

## Medical considerations/Contraindications

The medical considerations/contraindications included here have been selected on the basis of their potential clinical significance (reasons given in parentheses where appropriate)—not necessarily inclusive (» = major clinical significance).

*Risk-benefit should be considered when the following medical problems exist:*
» Angina or
» Coronary artery insufficiency or
» Myocardial infarction, or history of
(reflex tachycardia may precipitate frank congestive heart failure and angina; use of phentolamine is not recommended by the man-

ufacturer, but it has been used investigationally in patients with cardiac failure)
Gastritis or
Peptic ulcer
(may be exacerbated)
Sensitivity to phentolamine

## Side/Adverse Effects

Note: Parenteral administration of phentolamine has been associated with acute and prolonged hypotension, tachycardia, cardiac arrhythmias, myocardial infarction, and cerebrovascular spasm or occlusion; deaths have been reported.

The following side/adverse effects have been selected on the basis of their potential clinical significance (possible signs and symptoms in parentheses where appropriate)—not necessarily inclusive:

### Those indicating need for medical attention
Incidence more frequent
*Reflex tachycardia* (fast or irregular heartbeat)

Incidence less frequent
*Fainting; weakness*

Incidence rare—most frequent after parenteral administration
*Cerebrovascular spasm or occlusion* (confusion, severe or sudden headache, sudden loss of coordination, sudden slurring of speech); *myocardial infarction* (chest pain, sudden shortness of breath)

### Those indicating need for medical attention only if they continue or are bothersome
Incidence more frequent
*Diarrhea; nausea or vomiting; orthostatic hypotension* (dizziness or lightheadedness, especially when getting up from a lying or sitting position); *abdominal pain*
Incidence less frequent
*Flushing or redness of face; nasal stuffiness*

## Overdose

### Treatment of overdose
Treatment of acute hypotension includes: supportive measures, elevation of patient's legs and administration of a plasma expander, and intravenous infusion of norepinephrine. Epinephrine is not recommended since it may cause a further paradoxical decrease in blood pressure.

## Parenteral Dosage Forms

Note: Bracketed uses in the *Dosage Forms* section refer to categories of use and/or indications that are not included in U.S. product labeling.

### PHENTOLAMINE MESYLATE FOR INJECTION USP

**Usual adult dose**
Prevention of dermal necrosis and sloughing—
During intravenous administration of norepinephrine: 10 mg added to each liter of intravenous fluid containing norepinephrine.
Following extravasation of intravenous fluids containing norepinephrine: Infiltration, 5 to 10 mg in 10 mL of sodium chloride injection; effective only if given within twelve hours after extravasation.
Antiadrenergic—
Preoperative: Intravenous, 5 mg one to two hours before surgery, repeated if necessary.
During surgery (to prevent or control symptoms of excessive epinephrine release due to manipulation of the tumor): Intravenous, 5 mg; or intravenous infusion, 500 mcg (0.5 mg) to 1 mg per minute, adjusted according to response.
[Vasodilator, congestive heart failure][1]—
Intravenous infusion, 170 to 400 mcg (0.17 to 0.4 mg) per minute.

**Usual pediatric dose**
Antiadrenergic—
Preoperative: Intramuscular or intravenous, 1 mg; or 100 mcg (0.1 mg) per kg of body weight or 3 mg per square meter of body surface, one to two hours before surgery; may be repeated if necessary.
During surgery (to prevent symptoms of excessive epinephrine release due to manipulation of the tumor): Intravenous, 1 mg; or 100 mcg (0.1 mg) per kg of body weight or 3 mg per square meter of body surface.

**Size(s) usually available**
U.S.—
5 mg (Rx) [*Regitine*].
Canada—
5 mg (Rx) [*Rogitine*].

**Packaging and storage**

Store below 40 °C (104 °F), preferably between 15 and 30 °C (59 and 86 °F), unless otherwise specified by manufacturer.

**Preparation of dosage form**

Phentolamine Mesylate for Injection USP is reconstituted for parenteral use by adding 1 mL of sterile water for injection to the vial, producing a solution containing 5 mg of phentolamine mesylate per mL.

Phentolamine Mesylate for Injection USP is prepared for administration by intravenous infusion by adding 5 to 10 mg to 500 mL of 5% dextrose injection.

**Stability**

It is recommended that any unused portion be discarded.

---

¹Not included in Canadian product labeling.

---

Revised: 08/06/92

---

**PHENYLBENZIMIDAZOLE**—See *Sunscreen Agents (Topical)*

---

**PHENYLBENZIMIDAZOLE-CONTAINING COMBINATIONS—**

Octyl Methoxycinnamate, Octyl Salicylate, Oxybenzone, Phenylbenzimidazole, and Titanium Dioxide (Topical)—See *Sunscreen Agents (Topical)*

Octyl Methoxycinnamate, Octyl Salicylate, Phenylbenzimidazole, and Titanium Dioxide (Topical)—See *Sunscreen Agents (Topical)*

Octyl Methoxycinnamate and Phenylbenzimidazole (Topical)—See *Sunscreen Agents (Topical)*

Phenylbenzimidazole and Sulisobenzone (Topical)—See *Sunscreen Agents (Topical)*

---

**PHENYLBUTAZONE**—See *Anti-inflammatory Drugs, Nonsteroidal (Systemic)*

---

**PHENYLEPHRINE**—See *Phenylephrine (Nasal); Sympathomimetic Agents—Cardiovascular Use (Parenteral-Systemic)*

---

# PHENYLEPHRINE   Nasal

VA CLASSIFICATION (Primary): NT100

Note: For a listing of dosage forms and brand names by country availability, see *Dosage Forms* section(s). For a listing of brand names for the articles in this monograph, refer to the General Index.

## Category

Decongestant (topical).

## Indications

Note: Bracketed information in the *Indications* section refers to uses that are not included in U.S. product labeling.

**Accepted**

Congestion, nasal (treatment)—Nasal phenylephrine is indicated for the symptomatic relief of nasal congestion due to the common cold or hay fever, sinusitis, or other upper respiratory allergies.

[Congestion, sinus (treatment)]—Nasal phenylephrine is used for relief of sinus congestion.

Congestion, eustachian tube (treatment)—Nasal phenylephrine may be useful in the adjunctive therapy of middle ear infections by decreasing congestion around the eustachian ostia.

## Pharmacology/Pharmacokinetics

**Physicochemical characteristics**

Molecular weight—203.67.

**Mechanism of action/Effect**

Phenylephrine is primarily a direct-acting sympathomimetic amine. It acts on alpha-adrenergic receptors in the arterioles of the nasal mucosa to produce constriction, resulting in decreased nasal congestion.

**Duration of action**

30 minutes to 4 hours.

## Precautions to Consider

**Cross-sensitivity and/or related problems**

Patients sensitive to other nasal decongestants may be sensitive to this medication also.

**Pregnancy/Reproduction**

Pregnancy—Problems in humans have not been documented; however, nasal phenylephrine may be systemically absorbed.

**Breast-feeding**

Problems in humans have not been documented; however, nasal phenylephrine may be systemically absorbed.

**Pediatrics**

Children may be especially prone to systemic absorption of nasal phenylephrine and resulting side/adverse effects.

**Geriatrics**

Appropriate studies on the relationship of age to the effects of phenylephrine have not been performed in the geriatric population. However, no geriatrics-specific problems have been documented to date.

**Drug interactions and/or related problems**

The following drug interactions and/or related problems have been selected on the basis of their potential clinical significance (possible mechanism in parentheses where appropriate)—not necessarily inclusive (» = major clinical significance):

Note: Combinations containing any of the following medications, depending on the amount present, may also interact with this medication.

Antidepressants, tricyclic or
Maprotiline or
Monoamine oxidase (MAO) inhibitors, including furazolidone, procarbazine, and selegiline
(if significant systemic absorption of nasal phenylephrine occurs, concurrent use of these medications may potentiate the pressor effect of phenylephrine; nasal phenylephrine should not be administered within 14 days following the administration of MAO inhibitors)

Guanadrel or
Guanethidine
(if significant systemic absorption of nasal phenylephrine occurs, concurrent use of guanadrel or guanethidine may potentiate the pressor effect of phenylephrine, possibly resulting in hypertension and/or cardiac arrhythmias)

**Medical considerations/Contraindications**

The medical considerations/contraindications included here have been selected on the basis of their potential clinical significance (reasons given in parentheses where appropriate)—not necessarily inclusive (» = major clinical significance).

*Risk-benefit should be considered when the following medical problems exist:*

Coronary artery disease or
Heart disease, including angina or
Hypertension
(condition may be exacerbated because of drug-induced cardiovascular effects)

Diabetes mellitus

Hyperthyroidism

Sensitivity to phenylephrine or other nasal decongestants

## Side/Adverse Effects

The following side/adverse effects have been selected on the basis of their potential clinical significance (possible signs and symptoms in parentheses where appropriate)—not necessarily inclusive:

**Those indicating need for medical attention**
*Rebound congestion* (increase in runny or stuffy nose)

**Symptoms of systemic absorption**
*Fast, irregular, or pounding heartbeat; headache or dizziness; increased sweating; nervousness; paleness; trembling; trouble in sleeping*

**Those indicating need for medical attention only if they continue or are bothersome**
*Burning, dryness, or stinging of nasal mucosa*

## Patient Consultation

As an aid to patient consultation, refer to *Advice for the Patient, Phenylephrine (Nasal).*

In providing consultation, consider emphasizing the following selected information (» = major clinical significance):

**Before using this medication**
» Conditions affecting use, especially:
    Sensitivity to phenylephrine or other nasal decongestants
    Use in children—Children may be especially prone to systemic absorption of nasal phenylephrine and resulting side/adverse effects

**Proper use of this medication**
Proper administration technique
*Preventing contamination:*
    Replacing cap right after use
*For nasal drops*
    After using—Rinsing dropper with hot water and drying with clean tissue
*For nasal spray*
    After using—Rinsing tip of spray bottle with hot water, taking care not to suck water into bottle, and drying with clean tissue
*For nasal jelly*
    After using—Wiping tip of tube with clean, damp tissue

    Preventing spread of infection: Not using container for more than one person
» Importance of not using more medication than the amount recommended
» Proper dosing
    Missed dose: If on scheduled dosing regimen—Using right away if remembered within an hour or so; not using if remembered later; not doubling doses
» Proper storage

**Side/adverse effects**
Signs of potential side effects, especially rebound congestion and sympathomimetic systemic effects

## General Dosing Information

Prolonged or excessive use of this medication will cause rebound congestion with chronic swelling of nasal mucosa.

To reduce the chance of rebound congestion and systemic side effects, the weakest strength that is effective should be used.

## Nasal Dosage Forms

### PHENYLEPHRINE HYDROCHLORIDE NASAL JELLY USP

**Usual adult and adolescent dose**
Decongestant, topical—
    Intranasal, a small quantity of a 0.5% jelly placed into each nostril and sniffed well back into the nasal passages every three or four hours as needed.

**Usual pediatric dose**
Pediatric strength not available.

**Strength(s) usually available**
U.S.—
    0.5% (OTC) [*Neo-Synephrine Nasal Jelly*].

Canada—
    Not commercially available.

**Packaging and storage**
Store below 40 °C (104 °F), preferably between 15 and 30 °C (59 and 86 °F), unless otherwise specified by manufacturer. Store in a tight container. Protect from light. Protect from freezing.

**Stability**
Prolonged exposure to air, strong light, or heat results in oxidation and some loss of potency. Do not use if jelly is brown.

**Incompatibilities**
Medication is incompatible with butacaine, alkalies, ferric salts, oxidizing agents, and metals.

**Auxiliary labeling**
• For the nose.

### PHENYLEPHRINE HYDROCHLORIDE NASAL SOLUTION USP

**Usual adult and adolescent dose**
Decongestant, topical—
    Intranasal, 2 or 3 drops or sprays of a 0.25 to 0.5% solution into each nostril every four hours as needed

Note: The nasal spray form of this medication is more effective and less likely to cause systemic absorption than is the drop form.

    In cases of extreme nasal congestion, the 1% solution may be used initially.

**Usual pediatric dose**
Decongestant, topical—
    Infants and children up to 2 years of age: Dosage must be individualized by physician.
    Children 2 to 6 years of age: Intranasal, 2 or 3 drops of a 0.125 or 0.16% solution into each nostril every four hours as needed.
    Children 6 to 12 years of age: Intranasal, 2 or 3 drops or sprays of a 0.25% solution into each nostril every four hours as needed.
    Children 12 years of age and over: See *Usual adult and adolescent dose.*

**Strength(s) usually available**
U.S.—
    0.125% (drops) (OTC) [*Neo-Synephrine Pediatric Nasal Drops*].
    0.16% (drops) (OTC) [*Alconefrin Nasal Drops 12*].
    0.2% (drops) (OTC) [*Rhinall-10 Children's Flavored Nose Drops*].
    0.25% (drops) (OTC) [*Alconefrin Nasal Drops 25; Doktors; Neo-Synephrine Nasal Drops; Rhinall;* GENERIC].
    0.25% (spray) (OTC) [*Alconefrin Nasal Spray 25; Doktors; Neo-Synephrine Nasal Spray; Nostril Spray Pump Mild; Rhinall*].
    0.5% (drops) (OTC) [*Alconefrin Nasal Drops 50; Neo-Synephrine Nasal Drops*].
    0.5% (spray) (OTC) [*Duration; Neo-Synephrine Nasal Spray; Nostril Spray Pump; Vicks Sinex;* GENERIC].
    1% (drops) (OTC) [*Neo-Synephrine Nasal Drops*].
    1% (spray) (OTC) [*Neo-Synephrine Nasal Spray;* GENERIC].
Canada—
    0.25% (drops) (OTC) [*Neo-Synephrine Nasal Drops*].
    0.25% (spray) (OTC) [*Neo-Synephrine Nasal Spray*].
    0.5% (drops) (OTC) [*Neo-Synephrine Nasal Drops*].
    0.5% (spray) (OTC) [*Neo-Synephrine Nasal Spray*].
    1% (drops) (OTC) [*Neo-Synephrine Nasal Drops*].

**Packaging and storage**
Store below 40 °C (104 °F), preferably between 15 and 30 °C (59 and 86 °F), unless otherwise specified by manufacturer. Store in a tight, light-resistant container. Protect from freezing.

**Stability**
Prolonged exposure to air, strong light, or heat results in oxidation and some loss of potency. Do not use if solution is brown or contains a precipitate.

**Incompatibilities**
Medication is incompatible with butacaine, alkalies, ferric salts, oxidizing agents, and metals.

**Auxiliary labeling**
• For the nose.

Revised: 05/16/94

# PHENYLEPHRINE    Ophthalmic

VA CLASSIFICATION (Primary/Secondary): OP600/OP800; DX900

Note: For a listing of dosage forms and brand names by country availability, see *Dosage Forms* section(s). For a listing of brand names for the articles in this monograph, refer to the General Index.

## Category

Mydriatic; decongestant (ophthalmic); diagnostic aid (mydriatic).

## Indications

### Accepted

Note: The 2.5 and 10% phenylephrine ophthalmic solutions are indicated when rapid dilation of the pupil and reduction of congestion in the capillary bed are desired.

Uveitis with posterior synechiae (treatment) or

Synechiae, posterior (prophylaxis)—The 2.5 and 10% phenylephrine ophthalmic solutions are indicated in patients with uveitis when synechiae are present or may develop. The formation of synechiae may be prevented by concurrent use of either of these concentrations with atropine to produce wide dilation of the pupil; however, the vasoconstrictor effect of phenylephrine may be antagonistic to the increase of local blood flow in uveal inflammation.

Mydriasis, preoperative—The 2.5 and 10% phenylephrine ophthalmic solutions are indicated to produce dilation of the pupil prior to intraocular surgery.

Mydriasis, in diagnostic procedures—Refraction: Prior to determination of refractive errors, the 2.5% phenylephrine ophthalmic solution may be used effectively with homatropine, atropine, cyclopentolate, or tropicamide.

Ophthalmoscopy: The 2.5% phenylephrine ophthalmic solution is indicated to produce mydriasis for ophthalmoscopic examination.

Retinoscopy (shadow test): The 2.5% phenylephrine ophthalmic solution may be used alone when dilation of the pupil without cycloplegic action is desired for retinoscopy (shadow test).

Blanching test: The 2.5% phenylephrine ophthalmic solution is indicated for the blanching test. If blanching occurs, the congestion is superficial and probably does not indicate iritis.

Ocular redness (treatment)—The 0.12% phenylephrine ophthalmic solution is indicated to provide temporary relief of redness associated with minor eye irritations, such as those caused by hay fever, colds, dust, wind, swimming, sun, smog, smoke, or wearing contact lenses.

## Pharmacology/Pharmacokinetics

### Physicochemical characteristics
Molecular weight—203.67.

### Mechanism of action/Effect
Phenylephrine is primarily a direct-acting sympathomimetic amine, which stimulates alpha-adrenergic receptors.
Mydriatic—
Phenylephrine acts on alpha-adrenergic receptors in the dilator muscle of the pupil, producing contraction.
Decongestant (ophthalmic)—
Phenylephrine acts on alpha-adrenergic receptors in the arterioles of the conjunctiva, producing constriction.

### Time to peak effect
Mydriasis—
2.5% solution: 15 to 60 minutes.
10% solution: 10 to 90 minutes.

### Duration of action
Mydriasis recovery time—
2.5% solution: 1 to 3 hours.
10% solution: 3 to 7 hours.

## Precautions to Consider

### Carcinogenicity
Long-term studies have not been done.

### Pregnancy/Reproduction
Pregnancy—Studies have not been done in humans; however, ophthalmic phenylephrine may be systemically absorbed.
Studies have not been done in animals.
FDA Pregnancy Category C.

### Breast-feeding
It is not known whether phenylephrine is distributed into breast milk and problems in humans have not been documented; however, ophthalmic phenylephrine may be systemically absorbed.

### Pediatrics
The recommended dose should not be exceeded in pediatric patients, especially for the 2.5 and 10% solutions, since high doses of phenylephrine can increase blood pressure and cause irregular heartbeat. In addition, repeated use of 2.5 or 10% phenylephrine may result in rebound miosis and a reduced mydriatic effect. Moreover, the 10% phenylephrine solution is not recommended for use in infants, since a pronounced increase in blood pressure may occur. Also, the 2.5 and 10% concentrations are not recommended for use in low birth weight infants.

### Geriatrics
Cardiovascular reactions, such as marked increase in blood pressure, syncope, myocardial infarction, tachycardia, arrhythmia, and fatal subarachnoid hemorrhage, have occurred primarily in elderly patients. In addition, repeated use of 2.5 or 10% phenylephrine, especially in older patients, may result in rebound miosis and a reduced mydriatic effect. Also, older patients may develop transient pigment floaters in the aqueous humor 40 to 45 minutes following administration of the 2.5 or 10% concentrations, the appearance of which may be similar to anterior uveitis or to a microscopic hyphema.

### Drug interactions and/or related problems
The following drug interactions and/or related problems have been selected on the basis of their potential clinical significance (possible mechanism in parentheses where appropriate)—not necessarily inclusive (» = major clinical significance):

Note: Combinations containing any of the following medications, depending on the amount present, may also interact with this medication.

*For 2.5 or 10% strengths only*
Antidepressants, tricyclic or
Maprotiline or
Monoamine oxidase (MAO) inhibitors, including furazolidone, procarbazine, and selegiline
(if significant systemic absorption of ophthalmic phenylephrine occurs, concurrent use of these medications may potentiate the pressor effect of phenylephrine; in addition, if ophthalmic phenylephrine is administered during or within 21 days following the administration of MAO inhibitors, careful supervision with possible adjustment of dosage is recommended, since exaggerated adrenergic response may occur)

Guanadrel or
Guanethidine
(if significant systemic absorption of ophthalmic phenylephrine occurs, concurrent use of guanadrel or guanethidine may increase the mydriatic effect of phenylephrine; also, concurrent use may potentiate the pressor effect of phenylephrine, possibly resulting in hypertension and cardiac arrhythmias)

### Medical considerations/Contraindications
The medical considerations/contraindications included here have been selected on the basis of their potential clinical significance (reasons given in parentheses where appropriate)—not necessarily inclusive (» = major clinical significance).

*Risk-benefit should be considered when the following medical problems exist:*

*For 2.5 or 10% strengths only*
Arteriosclerotic changes, advanced
Cardiac disease
Diabetes mellitus
» Glaucoma, angle-closure, predisposition to
Hypertension
Idiopathic orthostatic hypotension
(a marked increase in blood pressure may occur)
Sensitivity to phenylephrine or sulfites

## Side/Adverse Effects

The following side/adverse effects have been selected on the basis of their potential clinical significance (possible signs and symptoms in parentheses where appropriate)—not necessarily inclusive:

**Those indicating need for medical attention**
Incidence less frequent with 10% solution; incidence rare with 2.5% or weaker solution
*Signs and symptoms of systemic absorption*
    *Dizziness; fast, irregular, or pounding heartbeat; increase in blood pressure; increase in sweating; paleness; trembling*

**Those indicating need for medical attention only if they continue or are bothersome**
Incidence more frequent with 2.5 or 10% solution
    *Burning or stinging of eyes; headache; browache; sensitivity of eyes to light; watering of eyes*
Incidence less frequent
    *Eye irritation not present before therapy*

## Overdose

For specific information on the agents used in the management of phenylephrine ophthalmic overdose, see:
• *Phentolamine (Systemic)* monograph.

For more information on the management of overdose or unintentional ingestion, **contact a Poison Control Center** (see *Poison Control Center Listing*).

**Treatment of overdose**
Specific treatment—The hypertensive effects of phenylephrine may be treated with an alpha-adrenergic blocker, such as phentolamine 5 to 10 mg intravenously, repeated as necessary.

## Patient Consultation

As an aid to patient consultation, refer to *Advice for the Patient, Phenylephrine (Ophthalmic).*

In providing consultation, consider emphasizing the following selected information (» = major clinical significance):

**Before using this medication**
» Conditions affecting use, especially:
    Sensitivity to phenylephrine or to sulfites
    Use in children—May be especially sensitive to the effects of phenylephrine; also, the 10% strength is not recommended for use in infants, and the 2.5 and 10% strengths are not recommended for use in low birth weight infants
    Use in the elderly—Repeated use of 2.5 or 10% phenylephrine may increase the chance of side/adverse effects; also, cardiovascular reactions have occurred more often in elderly patients
    Other medical problems, especially, predisposition to angle-closure glaucoma

**Proper use of this medication**
Not using if solution turns brown or contains a precipitate
Proper administration technique
Preventing contamination: Not touching applicator tip to any surface; keeping container tightly closed
» Proper dosing
» Proper storage
*For the 2.5 and 10% solutions*
» Importance of not using more medication than the amount prescribed
    Missed dose: Applying as soon as possible; not applying if almost time for next dose; applying next dose at regularly scheduled time

**Precautions while using this medication**
» Stopping medication and checking with physician if eye pain or change in vision occurs or if redness or irritation continues, gets worse, or lasts for more than 72 hours
*For the 2.5 and 10% solutions*
» Medication may cause increased sensitivity of eyes to light; wearing sunglasses that block ultraviolet light to protect eyes from sunlight and other bright lights; checking with physician if this effect continues longer than 12 hours after discontinuation of medication

**Side/adverse effects**
Signs of potential side effects, especially systemic absorption

## General Dosing Information

Although some manufacturers recommend a dose of 2 drops of an ophthalmic solution at appropriate intervals, the conjunctival sac will usually hold only 1 drop.

To avoid excessive systemic absorption, patient should apply digital pressure to the lacrimal sac during and for 2 or 3 minutes following instillation of medication.

Although some manufacturers recommend that patients not wear soft contact lenses during treatment with phenylephrine ophthalmic solution, USP medical experts do not believe this precaution is necessary unless the patient has corneal epithelial problems and the medication is to be used more often than once every 1 to 2 hours. No significant problems have been documented with ophthalmic solutions containing 0.03% or less of benzalkonium chloride as a preservative that are used in patients with no significant corneal surface problems.

**For the 2.5 and 10% solutions**
To prevent pain and subsequent lacrimation on administration, a suitable topical anesthetic may be applied a few minutes before use of phenylephrine solution.

The recommended dose should not be exceeded, especially in children and in individuals with high blood pressure or heart disease, since high doses of phenylephrine can increase blood pressure and cause irregular heartbeat.

Repeated use of phenylephrine, especially in older patients, may result in rebound miosis and a reduced mydriatic effect.

## Ophthalmic Dosage Forms

### PHENYLEPHRINE HYDROCHLORIDE OPHTHALMIC SOLUTION USP

**Usual adult and adolescent dose**
Mydriasis and vasoconstriction—
    Topical, to the conjunctiva, 1 drop of a 2.5 or 10% solution, repeated in one hour if necessary.
Chronic mydriasis—
    Topical, to the conjunctiva, 1 drop of a 2.5 or 10% solution two or three times a day.
Uveitis with posterior synechiae (treatment) or
Synechiae, posterior (prophylaxis)—
    Topical, to the conjunctiva, 1 drop of a 2.5 or 10% solution, repeated in one hour if necessary, not to exceed three times a day. Treatment may be continued the following day, if necessary.
    Note: Atropine sulfate and the application of hot compresses should also be used if indicated.
Mydriasis, preoperative—
    Topical, to the conjunctiva, 1 drop of a 2.5 or 10% solution thirty to sixty minutes prior to surgery.
Mydriasis, in diagnostic procedures—
    Refraction:
        Topical, to the conjunctiva, 1 drop of a cycloplegic followed in five minutes by 1 drop of a 2.5% solution of phenylephrine. The need for additional drops of the cycloplegic, and the waiting period before adequate cycloplegia occurs, depend on the cycloplegic used.
        Note: For a "one application method," the 2.5% solution may be used in combination with a cycloplegic for synergistic action.
    Ophthalmoscopy:
        Topical, to the conjunctiva, 1 drop of a 2.5% solution fifteen to thirty minutes prior to examination.
    Retinoscopy (shadow test):
        Topical, to the conjunctiva, as a 2.5% solution.
    Blanching test:
        Topical, to the infected eye, 1 drop of a 2.5% solution.
        Note: Eye should be examined for perilimbal blanching 5 minutes after application of phenylephrine.
Ocular redness (treatment)—
    Topical, to the conjunctiva, 1 drop of a 0.12% solution every three or four hours as needed.

**Usual pediatric dose**
Mydriasis and vasoconstriction—
    Topical, to the conjunctiva, 1 drop of a 2.5% solution, repeated in one hour if necessary.
Chronic mydriasis—
    Topical, to the conjunctiva, 1 drop of a 2.5% solution two or three times a day.
Uveitis with posterior synechiae (treatment)—
    Topical, to the conjunctiva, 1 drop of a 2.5% solution, repeated in one hour if necessary. Treatment may be continued the following day, if necessary.
    Note: Atropine sulfate and application of hot compresses should also be used if indicated.

Mydriasis, preoperative—
Topical, to the conjunctiva, 1 drop of a 2.5% solution thirty to sixty minutes prior to surgery.

Mydriasis, in diagnostic procedures—
Refraction:
Topical, to the conjunctiva, 1 drop of a 1% solution of atropine, followed in ten to fifteen minutes by 1 drop of a 2.5% solution of phenylephrine and in five to ten minutes by a second drop of a 1% solution of atropine. In one to two hours, the eyes are ready for refraction.

Note: For a ''one application method,'' the 2.5% solution of phenylephrine may be used in combination with a cycloplegic for synergistic action.

Ophthalmoscopy:
See *Usual adult and adolescent dose.*
Retinoscopy (shadow test):
See *Usual adult and adolescent dose.*
Blanching test:
See *Usual adult and adolescent dose.*

Ocular redness (treatment)—
See *Usual adult and adolescent dose.*

Note: The 10% phenylephrine solution is not recommended for use in infants, since a pronounced increase in blood pressure may occur following instillation. Also, the 2.5 and 10% concentrations are not recommended for use in low birth weight infants.

**Strength(s) usually available**
U.S.—
0.12% (OTC) [*Ak-Nefrin; Isopto Frin; Ocu-Phrin Sterile Eye Drops; Prefrin Liquifilm* (polyvinyl alcohol 1.4%); *Relief Eye Drops for Red Eyes* (polyvinyl alcohol 1.4%); GENERIC].
2.5% (Rx) [*Ak-Dilate* (sodium bisulfite; benzalkonium chloride 0.01%); *Dilatair; I-Phrine; Mydfrin* (sodium bisulfite; benzalkonium chloride 0.01%; boric acid; edetate disodium; sodium hydroxide or hydrochloric acid); *Neo-Synephrine; Ocugestrin; Ocu-Phrin Sterile Ophthalmic Solution; Phenoptic;* GENERIC].
10% (Rx) [*Ak-Dilate* (sodium bisulfite; benzalkonium chloride 0.01%); *I-Phrine; Neo-Synephrine; Ocu-Phrin Sterile Ophthalmic Solution;* GENERIC].

Canada—
0.12% (OTC) [*Prefrin Liquifilm* (sodium bisulfite; polyvinyl alcohol 1.4%)].
2.5% (OTC) [*Ak-Dilate* (sodium bisulfite); *Mydfrin; Spersaphrine*].
10% (OTC) [*Minims Phenylephrine*].

**Packaging and storage**
Store below 40 °C (104 °F), preferably between 15 and 30 °C (59 and 86 °F), unless otherwise specified by manufacturer. Store in a tight, light-resistant container of not more than 15-mL size. Protect from freezing.

**Stability**
Prolonged exposure to air or strong light may cause oxidation and discoloration. Do not use if solution is brown or contains a precipitate.

**Incompatibilities**
Phenylephrine is chemically incompatible with the local anesthetic butacaine.

**Auxiliary labeling**
• For the eye.
• Keep container tightly closed.

Revised: 07/14/95

# PHENYLEPHRINE-CONTAINING COMBINATIONS—

Brompheniramine and Phenylephrine (Systemic)—See *Antihistamines and Decongestants (Systemic)*
Brompheniramine, Phenylephrine, and Phenylpropanolamine (Systemic)—See *Antihistamines and Decongestants (Systemic)*
Brompheniramine, Phenylephrine, Phenylpropanolamine, and Codeine (Systemic)—See *Cough/Cold Combinations (Systemic)*
Brompheniramine, Phenylephrine, Phenylpropanolamine, Codeine, and Guaifenesin (Systemic)—See *Cough/Cold Combinations (Systemic)*
Brompheniramine, Phenylephrine, Phenylpropanolamine, and Dextromethorphan (Systemic)—See *Cough/Cold Combinations (Systemic)*
Brompheniramine, Phenylephrine, Phenylpropanolamine, and Guaifenesin (Systemic)—See *Cough/Cold Combinations (Systemic)*
Brompheniramine, Phenylephrine, Phenylpropanolamine, Hydrocodone, and Guaifenesin (Systemic)—See *Cough/Cold Combinations (Systemic)*

Chlorpheniramine, Ephedrine, Phenylephrine, and Carbetapentane (Systemic)—See *Cough/Cold Combinations (Systemic)*
Chlorpheniramine, Ephedrine, Phenylephrine, Dextromethorphan, Ammonium Chloride, and Ipecac (Systemic)—See *Cough/Cold Combinations (Systemic)*
Chlorpheniramine, Phenindamine, Phenylephrine, Dextromethorphan, Acetaminophen, Salicylamide, Caffeine, and Ascorbic Acid (Systemic)—See *Cough/Cold Combinations (Systemic)*
Chlorpheniramine, Pheniramine, Pyrilamine, Phenylephrine, Hydrocodone, Salicylamide, Caffeine, and Ascorbic Acid (Systemic)—See *Cough/Cold Combinations (Systemic)*
Chlorpheniramine and Phenylephrine (Systemic)—See *Antihistamines and Decongestants (Systemic)*
Chlorpheniramine, Phenylephrine, and Acetaminophen (Systemic)—See *Antihistamines, Decongestants, and Analgesics (Systemic)*
Chlorpheniramine, Phenylephrine, Acetaminophen, and Salicylamide (Systemic)—See *Antihistamines, Decongestants, and Analgesics (Systemic)*
Chlorpheniramine, Phenylephrine, Acetaminophen, Salicylamide, and Caffeine (Systemic)—See *Antihistamines, Decongestants, and Analgesics (Systemic)*
Chlorpheniramine, Phenylephrine, Codeine, and Ammonium Chloride (Systemic)—See *Cough/Cold Combinations (Systemic)*
Chlorpheniramine, Phenylephrine, Codeine, and Potassium Iodide (Systemic)—See *Cough/Cold Combinations (Systemic)*
Chlorpheniramine, Phenylephrine, and Dextromethorphan (Systemic)—See *Cough/Cold Combinations (Systemic)*
Chlorpheniramine, Phenylephrine, Dextromethorphan, Acetaminophen, and Salicylamide (Systemic)—See *Cough/Cold Combinations (Systemic)*
Chlorpheniramine, Phenylephrine, Dextromethorphan, and Guaifenesin (Systemic)—See *Cough/Cold Combinations (Systemic)*
Chlorpheniramine, Phenylephrine, Dextromethorphan, Guaifenesin, and Ammonium Chloride (Systemic)—See *Cough/Cold Combinations (Systemic)*
Chlorpheniramine, Phenylephrine, and Guaifenesin (Systemic)—See *Cough/Cold Combinations (Systemic)*
Chlorpheniramine, Phenylephrine, and Hydrocodone (Systemic)—See *Cough/Cold Combinations (Systemic)*
Chlorpheniramine, Phenylephrine, Hydrocodone, Acetaminophen, and Caffeine (Systemic)—See *Cough/Cold Combinations (Systemic)*
Chlorpheniramine, Phenylephrine, and Methscopolamine (Systemic)—See *Antihistamines, Decongestants, and Anticholinergics (Systemic)*
Chlorpheniramine, Phenylephrine, and Phenylpropanolamine (Systemic)—See *Antihistamines and Decongestants (Systemic)*
Chlorpheniramine, Phenylephrine, Phenylpropanolamine, Atropine, Hyoscyamine, and Scopolamine (Systemic)—See *Antihistamines, Decongestants, and Anticholinergics (Systemic)*
Chlorpheniramine, Phenylephrine, Phenylpropanolamine, Carbetapentane, and Potassium Guaiacolsulfonate (Systemic)—See *Cough/Cold Combinations (Systemic)*
Chlorpheniramine, Phenylephrine, Phenylpropanolamine, and Codeine (Systemic)—See *Cough/Cold Combinations (Systemic)*
Chlorpheniramine, Phenylephrine, Phenylpropanolamine, and Dextromethorphan (Systemic)—See *Cough/Cold Combinations (Systemic)*
Chlorpheniramine, Phenylephrine, Phenylpropanolamine, Dextromethorphan, Guaifenesin, and Acetaminophen (Systemic)—See *Cough/Cold Combinations (Systemic)*
Chlorpheniramine, Phenylephrine, Phenylpropanolamine, and Dihydrocodeine (Systemic)—See *Cough/Cold Combinations (Systemic)*
Chlorpheniramine, Phenyltoloxamine, and Phenylephrine (Systemic)—See *Antihistamines and Decongestants (Systemic)*
Chlorpheniramine, Phenyltoloxamine, Phenylephrine, and Phenylpropanolamine (Systemic)—See *Antihistamines and Decongestants (Systemic)*
Chlorpheniramine, Pyrilamine, and Phenylephrine (Systemic)—See *Antihistamines and Decongestants (Systemic)*
Chlorpheniramine, Pyrilamine, Phenylephrine, and Acetaminophen (Systemic)—See *Antihistamines, Decongestants, and Analgesics (Systemic)*
Chlorpheniramine, Pyrilamine, Phenylephrine, and Phenylpropanolamine (Systemic)—See *Antihistamines and Decongestants (Systemic)*
Chlorpheniramine, Pyrilamine, Phenylephrine, Phenylpropanolamine, and Acetaminophen (Systemic)—See *Antihistamines, Decongestants, and Analgesics (Systemic)*
Isoproterenol and Phenylephrine (Systemic)
Pheniramine and Phenylephrine (Systemic)—See *Antihistamines and Decongestants (Systemic)*
Pheniramine, Phenylephrine, and Acetaminophen (Systemic)—See *Antihistamines, Decongestants, and Analgesics (Systemic)*
Pheniramine, Phenylephrine, Codeine, Sodium Citrate, Sodium Salicylate, and Caffeine (Systemic)—See *Cough/Cold Combinations (Systemic)*

Pheniramine, Phenylephrine, and Dextromethorphan (Systemic)—See *Cough/Cold Combinations (Systemic)*

Pheniramine, Phenylephrine, Phenylpropanolamine, Hydrocodone, and Guaifenesin (Systemic)—See *Cough/Cold Combinations (Systemic)*

Pheniramine, Phenylephrine, Sodium Salicylate, and Caffeine (Systemic)—See *Antihistamines, Decongestants, and Analgesics (Systemic)*

Pheniramine, Pyrilamine, Phenylephrine, Phenylpropanolamine, and Hydrocodone (Systemic)—See *Cough/Cold Combinations (Systemic)*

Phenylephrine and Acetaminophen (Systemic)—See *Decongestants and Analgesics (Systemic)*

Phenylephrine and Codeine (Systemic)—See *Cough/Cold Combinations (Systemic)*

Phenylephrine, Dextromethorphan, and Guaifenesin (Systemic)—See *Cough/Cold Combinations (Systemic)*

Phenylephrine and Guaifenesin (Systemic)—See *Cough/Cold Combinations (Systemic)*

Phenylephrine, Guaifenesin, Acetaminophen, Salicylamide, and Caffeine (Systemic)—See *Cough/Cold Combinations (Systemic)*

Phenylephrine and Hydrocodone (Systemic)—See *Cough/Cold Combinations (Systemic)*

Phenylephrine, Hydrocodone, and Guaifenesin (Systemic)—See *Cough/Cold Combinations (Systemic)*

Phenylephrine, Phenylpropanolamine, Carbetapentane, and Potassium Guaiacolsulfonate (Systemic)—See *Cough/Cold Combinations (Systemic)*

Phenylephrine, Phenylpropanolamine, and Guaifenesin (Systemic)—See *Cough/Cold Combinations (Systemic)*

Promethazine and Phenylephrine (Systemic)—See *Antihistamines and Decongestants (Systemic)*

Promethazine, Phenylephrine, and Codeine (Systemic)—See *Cough/Cold Combinations (Systemic)*

Promethazine, Phenylephrine, Codeine, and Potassium Guaiacolsulfonate (Systemic)—See *Cough/Cold Combinations (Systemic)*

Promethazine, Phenylephrine, and Potassium Guaiacolsulfonate (Systemic)—See *Cough/Cold Combinations (Systemic)*

Pyrilamine, Phenylephrine, Aspirin, and Caffeine (Systemic)—See *Antihistamines, Decongestants, and Analgesics (Systemic)*

Pyrilamine, Phenylephrine, and Codeine (Systemic)—See *Cough/Cold Combinations (Systemic)*

Pyrilamine, Phenylephrine, and Dextromethorphan (Systemic)—See *Cough/Cold Combinations (Systemic)*

Pyrilamine, Phenylephrine, and Hydrocodone (Systemic)—See *Cough/Cold Combinations (Systemic)*

Pyrilamine, Phenylephrine, Hydrocodone, and Ammonium Chloride (Systemic)—See *Cough/Cold Combinations (Systemic)*

# PHENYLPROPANOLAMINE Systemic†

VA CLASSIFICATION (Primary/Secondary): AU100/GA751; RE200

Another commonly used name is PPA.

Note: For a listing of dosage forms and brand names by country availability, see *Dosage Forms* section(s). For a listing of brand names for the articles in this monograph, refer to the General Index.

†Not commercially available in Canada.

## Category

Sympathomimetic (adrenergic) agent; appetite suppressant; decongestant, nasal (systemic).

## Indications

Note: Bracketed information in the *Indications* section refers to uses that are not included in U.S. product labeling.

### Accepted

Obesity, exogenous (treatment)—Phenylpropanolamine (PPA) is indicated in the management of exogenous obesity for short-term use (6 to 12 weeks) in conjunction with a regimen of weight reduction based on caloric restriction, exercise, and behavior modification.

Nasal congestion (treatment)—Administered orally, phenylpropanolamine is indicated in the temporary, symptomatic relief of local swelling and congestion of nasal mucous membranes.

[Urinary incontinence (treatment)]—Phenylpropanolamine is used in the treatment of mild to moderate stress incontinence; it may be effective in up to 75% of patients with mild to moderate conditions. In females, phenylpropanolamine may be used in combination with estrogen therapy for a synergistic clinical effect.

## Pharmacology/Pharmacokinetics

### Physicochemical characteristics

Molecular weight—187.67.

pKa—9.

Other characteristics—Similar in structure and action to ephedrine and amphetamine but with less central nervous system (CNS) stimulation

### Mechanism of action/Effect

Appetite suppression—A mixed-acting sympathomimetic amine with predominantly alpha-adrenergic activity, phenylpropanolamine is believed to suppress the appetite control center in the hypothalamus. Other CNS actions and/or metabolic effects may also be involved. PPA acts as an agonist at central norepinephrine receptors and may also have dopamine agonist properties.

Decongestion, nasal—Phenylpropanolamine acts on alpha-adrenergic receptors in the mucosa of the respiratory tract to produce vasoconstriction, which temporarily reduces the swelling associated with inflammation of the mucous membranes lining the nasal passages.

Urinary incontinence—Phenylpropanolamine produces contraction of the bladder neck and of the smooth muscle of the urethra, possibly due to stimulation of alpha-adrenergic receptors.

### Other actions/effects

Increases heart rate, force of contraction, and cardiac output and excitability, possibly by stimulating beta-adrenergic receptors in the heart.

Causes CNS stimulation by releasing norepinephrine from storage sites.

Produces mydriasis.

### Absorption

Readily absorbed.

### Biotransformation

Hepatic, to an active hydroxylated metabolite.

### Onset of action

Nasal decongestion—15 to 30 minutes.

### Duration of action

Capsules and tablets—3 hours.

Extended-release—12 to 16 hours.

### Elimination

Renal; about 80 to 90% excreted unchanged within 24 hours.

## Precautions to Consider

### Cross-sensitivity and/or related problems

Patients sensitive to other sympathomimetics (for example, amphetamines, ephedrine, epinephrine, isoproterenol, metaproterenol, norepinephrine, phenylephrine, pseudoephedrine, terbutaline) may be sensitive to this medication also.

### Pregnancy/Reproduction

Pregnancy—Problems with teratogenicity in humans have not been documented.

Postpartum—Evidence shows that postpartum women may be at greater risk than the rest of the population of developing psychiatric disorders with the use of phenylpropanolamine at recommended doses and with overdose.

### Breast-feeding

Problems in humans have not been documented.

### Pediatrics

Appropriate studies have not been performed in children up to 12 years of age. However, recent evidence shows that children under 6 years of age may be at greater risk than the rest of the population of developing psychiatric disorders with the use of phenylpropanolamine at recommended doses and with overdose.

Phenylpropanolamine is not recommended as an appetite suppressant in children up to 12 years of age. In children between 12 and 18 years of age, the use of phenylpropanolamine as an appetite suppressant must be carefully supervised by a physician.

### Geriatrics

No information is available on the relationship of age to the effects of phenylpropanolamine in geriatric patients.

### Drug interactions and/or related problems

The following drug interactions and/or related problems have been selected on the basis of their potential clinical significance (possible

mechanism in parentheses where appropriate)—not necessarily inclusive (» = major clinical significance):

Note: Combinations containing any of the following medications, depending on the amount present, may also interact with this medication.

» Anesthetics, hydrocarbon inhalation
(chronic use of phenylpropanolamine prior to anesthesia with these agents may increase the risk of cardiac arrhythmias, since these medications may sensitize the myocardium to the effects of phenylpropanolamine; arrhythmias may respond to a beta-adrenergic blocking agent such as propranolol)

Antidepressants, tricyclic
(tricyclic antidepressants may potentiate the response to sympathomimetic amines such as PPA by blocking the reuptake of biogenic amines by nerve terminals)

Antihypertensives or
Diuretics used as antihypertensives
(hypotensive effects of these medications may be reduced during concurrent use with phenylpropanolamine; the patient should be carefully monitored to confirm that the desired effect is being obtained)

» Beta-adrenergic blocking agents
(concurrent use with phenylpropanolamine may result in significant hypertension and excessive bradycardia with possible heart block; concurrent use requires careful monitoring)

» CNS stimulation–producing medications (see *Appendix II*) or
» Sympathomimetics, other
(concurrent use with phenylpropanolamine may result in additive CNS stimulation to excessive levels, causing nervousness, irritability, insomnia, or possibly seizures or cardiac arrhythmias; close monitoring is recommended)
(also, concurrent use of other sympathomimetics with phenylpropanolamine may increase pressor or cardiovascular effects of either medication)

» Digitalis glycosides
(concurrent use may result in cardiac arrhythmias)

» Monoamine oxidase (MAO) inhibitors, including furazolidone, procarbazine, and selegiline
(concurrent use may potentiate the pressor effect of phenylpropanolamine with resultant hypertensive crisis by releasing catecholamines, which accumulate during therapy with MAO inhibitors, from intraneuronal storage sites; phenylpropanolamine should not be administered during or within 14 days following administration of MAO inhibitors)

» Rauwolfia alkaloids
(concurrent use may inhibit the indirect-acting sympathomimetic action of phenylpropanolamine by depleting catecholamine stores)

**Medical considerations/Contraindications**
The medical considerations/contraindications included here have been selected on the basis of their potential clinical significance (reasons given in parentheses where appropriate)—not necessarily inclusive (» = major clinical significance).

*Except under special circumstances, this medication should not be used when the following medical problems exist:*

» Coronary artery disease, severe
(phenylpropanolamine may increase heart rate and force of contraction, with resultant decreased cardiac efficiency)

» Hypertension, severe
(pressor effect of phenylpropanolamine may result in hypertensive crisis)

*Risk-benefit should be considered when the following medical problems exist:*

» Cardiovascular disorders
(phenylpropanolamine may cause cardiac excitation leading to arrhythmias)

Diabetes mellitus
(adrenergic properties of phenylpropanolamine may lead to increased blood glucose concentrations)

Glaucoma, angle-closure
(condition may be aggravated)

» Hypertension, mild
(vasoconstrictive properties of phenylpropanolamine may exacerbate condition)

Hyperthyroidism
(symptoms may be exacerbated by cardiac stimulant properties of phenylpropanolamine)

Prostatic hypertrophy
(urinary retention may be precipitated)

Psychosis or other psychiatric disorders, history of
(phenylpropanolamine may precipitate psychiatric disorders)

Sensitivity to phenylpropanolamine or other sympathomimetics

## Side/Adverse Effects

Note: The safety profile of phenylpropanolamine is controversial. Most controlled studies have demonstrated minimal side effects from PPA. Serious adverse reactions including hypertensive crises, stroke, arrhythmias, acute renal failure, rhabdomyolysis, psychotic disturbances, hallucinations, and seizures have been reported following consumption of PPA; however, case studies in many of these patients have revealed confounding factors such as pre-existing conditions and/or consumption of medications in addition to PPA.

Some investigators have suggested that serious cardiovascular side effects may be more likely to occur in patients prone to hypertension (such as obese patients, patients under stress, elderly patients, or female patients receiving oral contraceptives); in patients with eating disorders, such as anorexia nervosa or bulimia (these patients may tend to abuse weight control medications); and in females and children who, because of their smaller size, receive a greater dose per unit of body weight.

Similarly, serious CNS side effects may occur more frequently in patients with a history of pre-existing neurological or psychiatric conditions. In addition, one study noted that organic symptoms (such as dizziness, loss of motor coordination, confusion, and photophobia) that have occurred in many patients are comparable to CNS dysfunction due to increased blood pressure.

Increases in blood pressure and CNS toxicity may represent idiosyncratic reactions in some patients.

The following side/adverse effects have been selected on the basis of their potential clinical significance (possible signs and symptoms in parentheses where appropriate)—not necessarily inclusive:

### Those indicating need for medical attention
Incidence rare
*Headache, severe*—may be prodromal of severe side effects related to elevated blood pressure; *increased blood pressure; painful or difficult urination; tightness in chest*

### Those indicating need for medical attention only if they continue or are bothersome
Incidence less frequent—more frequent with high doses
*Dizziness; dryness of nose or mouth; false sense of well-being; headache, mild; insomnia* (trouble in sleeping); *nausea, mild; nervousness, mild; restlessness, mild*

## Overdose

For more information on the management of overdose or unintentional ingestion, **contact a Poison Control Center** (see *Poison Control Center Listing*).

### Clinical effects of overdose
The following have been selected on the basis of their potential clinical significance (possible signs and symptoms in parentheses where appropriate)—not necessarily inclusive:

Early symptoms of overdose
*Abdominal or stomach pain; fast, pounding, or irregular heartbeat; headache, severe; increased sweating not associated with exercise; nausea and vomiting, severe; nervousness or restlessness, severe*

Late symptoms of overdose
*Confusion; convulsions; fast breathing; fast and irregular pulse; hallucinations; hostile behavior; muscle trembling*

### Treatment of overdose
Since there is no specific antidote for overdosage with phenylpropanolamine, treatment is symptomatic and supportive with possible use of the following—
Induction of emesis and/or use of gastric lavage is primary.
Barbiturate sedatives are sometimes used to control excessive CNS stimulation.
Cardiovascular and respiratory monitoring.
Intravenous fluids to control hypotension.
Intravenous phentolamine or nitrates to control hypertension.
Acidification of urine and forced diuresis.
Protecting patient from self-injury by use of restraints if necessary.

# Patient Consultation

As an aid to patient consultation, refer to *Advice for the Patient, Phenylpropanolamine (Systemic)*.

In providing consultation, consider emphasizing the following selected information (» = major clinical significance):

## Before using this medication
» Conditions affecting use, especially:

Sensitivity to phenylpropanolamine or other sympathomimetics

Pregnancy—Psychiatric side effects more likely in postpartum women

Use in children—Psychiatric side effects more likely in children up to 6 years of age; not recommended for use as appetite suppressant in children up to 12 years of age; in adolescents between 12 and 18 years of age, use for appetite suppression recommended only with doctor's supervision

Other medications, especially beta-adrenergic blocking agents, CNS stimulation–producing medications, other sympathomimetics, digitalis glycosides, monoamine oxidase (MAO) inhibitors, or rauwolfia alkaloids

Other medical problems, especially severe coronary artery disease, other cardiovascular disorders, or hypertension

## Proper use of this medication

Proper administration of extended-release dosage forms: swallowing whole; not breaking, crushing, or chewing; taking with a full glass of water; taking around 10 am if taking only one dose of medication a day

» Importance of not taking more medication than the amount recommended or for a longer period of time than directed

Taking the last dose of medication a few hours before bedtime to minimize the possibility of insomnia

» Proper dosing

» Proper storage

*For decongestant use only*

Missed dose: Taking as soon as possible; not taking within 2 hours (12 hours for extended-release dosage forms) of next scheduled dose; not doubling doses

*For appetite suppressant use only*

Not taking for longer than a few weeks without physician's permission

## Precautions while using this medication

Not drinking large amounts of caffeine-containing coffee, tea, or colas

» Caution if dizziness occurs; not driving, using machines, or doing anything else that requires alertness while taking medication

*For decongestant use only*

» Checking with physician if cold symptoms do not improve within 7 days or if fever is present

## Side/adverse effects

Signs of potential side effects, especially severe headache, increased blood pressure, painful or difficult urination, or tightness in chest

# General Dosing Information

To minimize the possibility of insomnia, the last dose of phenylpropanolamine for each day should be administered a few hours before bedtime.

With prolonged use or too frequent administration, tolerance to the therapeutic effects of phenylpropanolamine may develop. Phenylpropanolamine is effective as an appetite suppressant only for a few weeks.

# Oral Dosage Forms

Note: Bracketed uses in the *Dosage Forms* section refer to categories of use and/or indications not included in U.S. product labeling.

## PHENYLPROPANOLAMINE HYDROCHLORIDE CAPSULES

### Usual adult dose

Appetite suppressant—

Oral, 25 mg three times a day, not to exceed 75 mg in twenty-four hours.

Decongestant—

Oral, 25 mg every four hours as needed, not to exceed 150 mg in twenty-four hours.

[Urinary incontinence]—

Oral, 50 to 150 mg a day, in divided doses.

### Usual pediatric dose

Appetite suppressant—

Children up to 12 years of age: Use is not recommended.

Children 12 to 18 years of age: Dosage must be individualized by physician.

Decongestant—

Children up to 2 years of age: Dosage must be individualized by physician.

Children 2 to 6 years of age: Oral, 6.25 mg every four hours as needed, not to exceed 37.5 mg in twenty-four hours.

Children 6 to 12 years of age: Oral, 12.5 mg every four hours as needed, not to exceed 75 mg in twenty-four hours.

Children 12 to 18 years of age: See *Usual adult dose.*

### Strength(s) usually available

U.S.—

25 mg (OTC) [*Efed II Yellow*].

37.5 mg (OTC) [*Prolamine*].

Canada—

Not commercially available.

### Packaging and storage

Store below 40 °C (104 °F), preferably between 15 and 30 °C (59 and 86 °F), in a tight container, unless otherwise specified by manufacturer. Protect from light.

## PHENYLPROPANOLAMINE HYDROCHLORIDE EXTENDED-RELEASE CAPSULES USP

### Usual adult dose

Appetite suppressant—

Oral, 75 mg once a day at mid-morning (10 a.m.) with a full glass of water.

Decongestant—

Oral, 75 mg every twelve hours.

[Urinary incontinence]—

Oral, 50 to 150 mg a day, in divided doses.

### Usual pediatric dose

Appetite suppressant—

Children up to 12 years of age: Use is not recommended.

Children 12 to 18 years of age: Dosage must be individualized by physician.

Decongestant—

Dosage has not been established.

### Strength(s) usually available

U.S.—

75 mg (OTC) [*Control* (OTC); *Dexatrim Maximum Strength Capsules* (OTC); *Diet-Aid Maximum Strength* (OTC); GENERIC (OTC)].

Canada—

Not commercially available.

### Packaging and storage

Store below 40 °C (104 °F), preferably between 15 and 30 °C (59 and 86 °F), unless otherwise specified by manufacturer. Store in a tight, light-resistant container.

### Auxiliary labeling

• Swallow capsules whole.

## PHENYLPROPANOLAMINE HYDROCHLORIDE TABLETS

### Usual adult dose

See *Phenylpropanolamine Hydrochloride Capsules.*

### Usual pediatric dose

See *Phenylpropanolamine Hydrochloride Capsules.*

### Strength(s) usually available

U.S.—

25 mg (OTC) [*Propagest;* GENERIC].

50 mg (OTC) [GENERIC].

Canada—

Not commercially available.

### Packaging and storage

Store below 40 °C (104 °F), preferably between 15 and 30 °C (59 and 86 °F), in a tight container, unless otherwise specified by manufacturer. Protect from light.

## PHENYLPROPANOLAMINE HYDROCHLORIDE EXTENDED-RELEASE TABLETS

### Usual adult dose

See *Phenylpropanolamine Hydrochloride Extended-release Capsules USP.*

### Usual pediatric dose

See *Phenylpropanolamine Hydrochloride Extended-release Capsules USP.*

**Strength(s) usually available**
U.S.—
 75 mg (OTC) [*Acutrim 16 Hour; Acutrim Late Day* (isopropyl alcohol); *Acutrim II Maximum Strength; Dexatrim Maximum Strength Caplets; Dexatrim Maximum Strength Tablets; Phenyldrine*].
Canada—
 Not commercially available.

**Packaging and storage**
Store below 40 °C (104 °F), preferably between 15 and 30 °C (59 and 86 °F), in a tight container, unless otherwise specified by manufacturer. Protect from light.

**Auxiliary labeling**
• Swallow tablets whole.

Revised: 06/21/94

# PHENYLPROPANOLAMINE-CONTAINING COMBINATIONS—

Brompheniramine, Phenylephrine, and Phenylpropanolamine (Systemic)—See *Antihistamines and Decongestants (Systemic)*

Brompheniramine, Phenylephrine, Phenylpropanolamine, and Codeine (Systemic)—See *Cough/Cold Combinations (Systemic)*

Brompheniramine, Phenylephrine, Phenylpropanolamine, Codeine, and Guaifenesin (Systemic)—See *Cough/Cold Combinations (Systemic)*

Brompheniramine, Phenylephrine, Phenylpropanolamine, and Dextromethorphan (Systemic)—See *Cough/Cold Combinations (Systemic)*

Brompheniramine, Phenylephrine, Phenylpropanolamine, and Guaifenesin (Systemic)—See *Cough/Cold Combinations (Systemic)*

Brompheniramine, Phenylephrine, Phenylpropanolamine, Hydrocodone, and Guaifenesin (Systemic)—See *Cough/Cold Combinations (Systemic)*

Brompheniramine and Phenylpropanolamine (Systemic)—See *Antihistamines and Decongestants (Systemic)*

Brompheniramine, Phenylpropanolamine, and Acetaminophen (Systemic)—See *Antihistamines, Decongestants, and Analgesics (Systemic)*

Brompheniramine, Phenylpropanolamine, and Codeine (Systemic)—See *Cough/Cold Combinations (Systemic)*

Brompheniramine, Phenylpropanolamine, and Dextromethorphan (Systemic)—See *Cough/Cold Combinations (Systemic)*

Chlorpheniramine, Phenindamine, and Phenylpropanolamine (Systemic)—See *Antihistamines and Decongestants (Systemic)*

Chlorpheniramine, Phenylephrine, and Phenylpropanolamine (Systemic)—See *Antihistamines and Decongestants (Systemic)*

Chlorpheniramine, Phenylephrine, Phenylpropanolamine, Atropine, Hyoscyamine, and Scopolamine (Systemic)—See *Antihistamines, Decongestants, and Anticholinergics (Systemic)*

Chlorpheniramine, Phenylephrine, Phenylpropanolamine, Carbetapentane, and Potassium Guaiacolsulfonate (Systemic)—See *Cough/Cold Combinations (Systemic)*

Chlorpheniramine, Phenylephrine, Phenylpropanolamine, and Codeine (Systemic)—See *Cough/Cold Combinations (Systemic)*

Chlorpheniramine, Phenylephrine, Phenylpropanolamine, and Dextromethorphan (Systemic)—See *Cough/Cold Combinations (Systemic)*

Chlorpheniramine, Phenylephrine, Phenylpropanolamine, Dextromethorphan, Guaifenesin, and Acetaminophen (Systemic)—See *Cough/Cold Combinations (Systemic)*

Chlorpheniramine, Phenylephrine, Phenylpropanolamine, and Dihydrocodeine (Systemic)—See *Cough/Cold Combinations (Systemic)*

Chlorpheniramine and Phenylpropanolamine (Systemic)—See *Antihistamines and Decongestants (Systemic)*

Chlorpheniramine, Phenylpropanolamine, and Acetaminophen (Systemic)—See *Antihistamines, Decongestants, and Analgesics (Systemic)*

Chlorpheniramine, Phenylpropanolamine, Acetaminophen, and Caffeine (Systemic)—See *Antihistamines, Decongestants, and Analgesics (Systemic)*

Chlorpheniramine, Phenylpropanolamine, and Aspirin (Systemic)—See *Antihistamines, Decongestants, and Analgesics (Systemic)*

Chlorpheniramine, Phenylpropanolamine, Aspirin, and Caffeine (Systemic)—See *Antihistamines, Decongestants, and Analgesics (Systemic)*

Chlorpheniramine, Phenylpropanolamine, and Caramiphen (Systemic)—See *Cough/Cold Combinations (Systemic)*

Chlorpheniramine, Phenylpropanolamine, Codeine, Guaifenesin, and Acetaminophen (Systemic)—See *Cough/Cold Combinations (Systemic)*

Chlorpheniramine, Phenylpropanolamine, and Dextromethorphan (Systemic)—See *Cough/Cold Combinations (Systemic)*

Chlorpheniramine, Phenylpropanolamine, Dextromethorphan, and Acetaminophen (Systemic)—See *Cough/Cold Combinations (Systemic)*

Chlorpheniramine, Phenylpropanolamine, Dextromethorphan, and Ammonium Chloride (Systemic)—See *Cough/Cold Combinations (Systemic)*

Chlorpheniramine, Phenylpropanolamine, Dextromethorphan, and Aspirin (Systemic)—See *Cough/Cold Combinations (Systemic)*

Chlorpheniramine, Phenylpropanolamine, and Guaifenesin (Systemic)—See *Cough/Cold Combinations (Systemic)*

Chlorpheniramine, Phenylpropanolamine, Guaifenesin, Sodium Citrate, and Citric Acid (Systemic)—See *Cough/Cold Combinations (Systemic)*

Chlorpheniramine, Phenylpropanolamine, and Methscopolamine (Systemic)—See *Antihistamines, Decongestants, and Anticholinergics (Systemic)*

Chlorpheniramine, Phenyltoloxamine, Phenylephrine, and Phenylpropanolamine (Systemic)—See *Antihistamines and Decongestants (Systemic)*

Chlorpheniramine, Phenyltoloxamine, Phenylpropanolamine, and Acetaminophen (Systemic)—See *Antihistamines, Decongestants, and Analgesics (Systemic)*

Chlorpheniramine, Pyrilamine, Phenylephrine, and Phenylpropanolamine (Systemic)—See *Antihistamines and Decongestants (Systemic)*

Chlorpheniramine, Pyrilamine, Phenylephrine, Phenylpropanolamine, and Acetaminophen (Systemic)—See *Antihistamines, Decongestants, and Analgesics (Systemic)*

Clemastine and Phenylpropanolamine (Systemic)—See *Antihistamines and Decongestants (Systemic)*

Diphenhydramine, Phenylpropanolamine, and Aspirin (Systemic)—See *Antihistamines, Decongestants, and Analgesics (Systemic)*

Diphenylpyraline, Phenylpropanolamine, Acetaminophen, and Caffeine (Systemic)—See *Antihistamines, Decongestants, and Analgesics (Systemic)*

Doxylamine, Phenylpropanolamine, Dextromethorphan, and Aspirin (Systemic)—See *Cough/Cold Combinations (Systemic)*

Pheniramine, Phenylephrine, Phenylpropanolamine, Hydrocodone, and Guaifenesin (Systemic)—See *Cough/Cold Combinations (Systemic)*

Pheniramine, Phenyltoloxamine, Pyrilamine, and Phenylpropanolamine (Systemic)—See *Antihistamines and Decongestants (Systemic)*

Pheniramine, Pyrilamine, Phenylephrine, Phenylpropanolamine, and Hydrocodone (Systemic)—See *Cough/Cold Combinations (Systemic)*

Pheniramine, Pyrilamine, and Phenylpropanolamine (Systemic)—See *Antihistamines and Decongestants (Systemic)*

Pheniramine, Pyrilamine, Phenylpropanolamine, and Codeine (Systemic)—See *Cough/Cold Combinations (Systemic)*

Pheniramine, Pyrilamine, Phenylpropanolamine, Codeine, Acetaminophen, and Caffeine (Systemic)—See *Cough/Cold Combinations (Systemic)*

Pheniramine, Pyrilamine, Phenylpropanolamine, and Dextromethorphan (Systemic)—See *Cough/Cold Combinations (Systemic)*

Pheniramine, Pyrilamine, Phenylpropanolamine, Dextromethorphan, and Ammonium Chloride (Systemic)—See *Cough/Cold Combinations (Systemic)*

Pheniramine, Pyrilamine, Phenylpropanolamine, Dextromethorphan, and Guaifenesin (Systemic)—See *Cough/Cold Combinations (Systemic)*

Pheniramine, Pyrilamine, Phenylpropanolamine, and Guaifenesin (Systemic)—See *Cough/Cold Combinations (Systemic)*

Pheniramine, Pyrilamine, Phenylpropanolamine, and Hydrocodone (Systemic)—See *Cough/Cold Combinations (Systemic)*

Pheniramine, Pyrilamine, Phenylpropanolamine, Hydrocodone, and Guaifenesin (Systemic)—See *Cough/Cold Combinations (Systemic)*

Phenylephrine, Phenylpropanolamine, Carbetapentane, and Potassium Guaiacolsulfonate (Systemic)—See *Cough/Cold Combinations (Systemic)*

Phenylephrine, Phenylpropanolamine, and Guaifenesin (Systemic)—See *Cough/Cold Combinations (Systemic)*

Phenylpropanolamine and Acetaminophen (Systemic)—See *Decongestants and Analgesics (Systemic)*

Phenylpropanolamine, Acetaminophen, and Aspirin (Systemic)—See *Decongestants and Analgesics (Systemic)*

Phenylpropanolamine, Acetaminophen, and Caffeine (Systemic)—See *Decongestants and Analgesics (Systemic)*

Phenylpropanolamine, Acetaminophen, Salicylamide, and Caffeine (Systemic)—See *Decongestants and Analgesics (Systemic)*

Phenylpropanolamine and Aspirin (Systemic)—See *Decongestants and Analgesics (Systemic)*

Phenylpropanolamine and Caramiphen (Systemic)—See *Cough/Cold Combinations (Systemic)*

Phenylpropanolamine, Codeine, and Guaifenesin (Systemic)—See *Cough/Cold Combinations (Systemic)*

Phenylpropanolamine and Dextromethorphan (Systemic)—See *Cough/Cold Combinations (Systemic)*

Phenylpropanolamine, Dextromethorphan, and Acetaminophen (Systemic)—See *Cough/Cold Combinations (Systemic)*

Phenylpropanolamine, Dextromethorphan, and Guaifenesin (Systemic)—See *Cough/Cold Combinations (Systemic)*

Phenylpropanolamine and Guaifenesin (Systemic)—See *Cough/Cold Combinations (Systemic)*

Phenylpropanolamine and Hydrocodone (Systemic)—See *Cough/Cold Combinations (Systemic)*

Phenylpropanolamine, Hydrocodone, Guaifenesin, and Salicylamide (Systemic)—See *Cough/Cold Combinations (Systemic)*

Phenyltoloxamine, Phenylpropanolamine, and Acetaminophen (Systemic)—See *Antihistamines, Decongestants, and Analgesics (Systemic)*

Pyrilamine, Phenylpropanolamine, Acetaminophen, and Caffeine (Systemic)—See *Antihistamines, Decongestants, and Analgesics (Systemic)*

Pyrilamine, Phenylpropanolamine, Dextromethorphan, Guaifenesin, Potassium Citrate, and Citric Acid (Systemic)—See *Cough/Cold Combinations (Systemic)*

Pyrilamine, Phenylpropanolamine, Dextromethorphan, and Sodium Salicylate (Systemic)—See *Cough/Cold Combinations (Systemic)*

## PHENYL SALICYLATE–CONTAINING COMBINATIONS—

Atropine, Hyoscyamine, Methenamine, Methylene Blue, Phenyl Salicylate, and Benzoic Acid (Systemic)

## PHENYLTOLOXAMINE-CONTAINING COMBINATIONS—

Chlorpheniramine, Phenyltoloxamine, Ephedrine, Codeine, and Guaiacol Carbonate (Systemic)—See *Cough/Cold Combinations (Systemic)*

Chlorpheniramine, Phenyltoloxamine, and Phenylephrine (Systemic)—See *Antihistamines and Decongestants (Systemic)*

Chlorpheniramine, Phenyltoloxamine, Phenylephrine, and Phenylpropanolamine (Systemic)—See *Antihistamines and Decongestants (Systemic)*

Chlorpheniramine, Phenyltoloxamine, Phenylpropanolamine, and Acetaminophen (Systemic)—See *Antihistamines, Decongestants, and Analgesics (Systemic)*

Pheniramine, Phenyltoloxamine, Pyrilamine, and Phenylpropanolamine (Systemic)—See *Antihistamines and Decongestants (Systemic)*

Phenyltoloxamine and Hydrocodone (Systemic)—See *Cough/Cold Combinations (Systemic)*

Phenyltoloxamine, Phenylpropanolamine, and Acetaminophen (Systemic)—See *Antihistamines, Decongestants, and Analgesics (Systemic)*

## PHENYTOIN—See *Anticonvulsants, Hydantoin (Systemic)*

# PHOSPHATES    Systemic

This monograph includes information on the following: Potassium Phosphates; Potassium and Sodium Phosphates; Sodium Phosphates†.

VA CLASSIFICATION (Primary/Secondary): TN408/GU900

Note: For a listing of dosage forms and brand names by country availability, see *Dosage Forms* section(s). For a listing of brand names for the articles in this monograph, refer to the General Index.

†Not commercially available in Canada.

## Category

Acidifier (urinary)—Monobasic Potassium Phosphate; Potassium and Sodium Phosphates.

Antiurolithic (calcium calculi)—Monobasic Potassium Phosphate; Potassium and Sodium Phosphates.

Electrolyte replenisher—Potassium Phosphates; Potassium and Sodium Phosphates; Sodium Phosphates.

## Indications

### Accepted

Hypophosphatemia (prophylaxis and treatment)—Phosphates, both oral and parenteral, provide supplemental ionic phosphorus for correction of hypophosphatemia in patients with low or restricted oral intake or conditions with increased requirements for phosphorus, such as premature infants fed human milk, or patients who have inadequately controlled diabetes mellitus, hyperparathyroidism, hyperthyroidism, chronic alcoholism, renal tubular defects leading to increased urinary phosphate loss, respiratory alkalosis, gastrectomy, vitamin D deficiency, total parenteral nutrition (TPN) therapy, or patients who use thiazide diuretics, intravenous dextrose solutions, or those who chronically use aluminum- or magnesium-containing antacids. For prophylaxis of phosphorus deficiency, dietary improvement, rather than supplementation, is advisable. For treatment of phosphorus deficiency, supplementation is preferred.

Requirements for all vitamins and most minerals are increased during pregnancy. Many physicians recommend that pregnant women receive multivitamin and mineral supplements, especially those pregnant women who do not consume an adequate diet and those in high-risk categories (i.e., women carrying more than one fetus, heavy cigarette smokers, and alcohol and drug abusers). Taking excessive amounts of a multivitamin and mineral supplement may be harmful to the mother and/or fetus and should be avoided.

Recommended intakes for all vitamins and most minerals are increased during breast-feeding.

Urinary tract infections (treatment adjunct)—Urinary acidification by potassium and sodium phosphates combination and monobasic potassium phosphate augments the efficacy of methenamine mandelate and methenamine hippurate, which are dependent upon an acid medium for antibacterial activity. Phosphates eliminate the odor, rash, and turbidity present with ammoniacal urine associated with urinary tract infections. However, use of phosphates for urea splitting urinary tract infections may predispose to struvite stones that form in alkaline urine.

Renal calculi, calcium (prophylaxis)—Potassium and sodium phosphates combination and monobasic potassium phosphate have been used to reduce urinary calcium concentration and help prevent precipitation of calcium deposits in the urinary tract.

### Unaccepted

Although sodium and/or potassium phosphates have been used in the treatment of hypercalcemia, USP medical advisory panels do not recommend this use since these medications have been replaced by safer and more effective agents.

## Pharmacology/Pharmacokinetics

### Physicochemical characteristics

Molecular weight—
Dibasic potassium phosphate: 174.18.
Dibasic sodium phosphate (heptahydrate): 268.07.
Monobasic potassium phosphate: 136.09.
Monobasic sodium phosphate (anhydrous): 119.98.

### Mechanism of action/Effect

Urinary acidification—At the renal distal tubule, the secretion of hydrogen by the tubular cell in exchange for sodium in the tubular urine converts dibasic phosphate salts to monobasic phosphate salts. Therefore, large amounts of acid can be excreted without lowering the pH of the urine to a degree that would block hydrogen transport by a high concentration gradient between the tubular cell and luminal fluid.

Antiurolithic—Phosphates inhibit spontaneous nucleation of calcium oxalate, thus reducing the possibility of calcium urolithiasis.

Electrolyte replenisher—Phosphorus modifies the steady state of calcium concentrations, has a buffering effect on acid-base equilibrium, and influences the renal excretion of hydrogen ion.

### Absorption

Ingested phosphates are absorbed from the gastrointestinal tract. However, the presence of large amounts of calcium or aluminum may lead to formation of insoluble phosphate and reduce the net absorption. Vitamin D stimulates phosphate absorption.

### Elimination

Renal (90%) and fecal (10%).

## Precautions to Consider

### Pregnancy/Reproduction

Pregnancy—Adequate and well-controlled studies have not been done in humans. However, problems in humans have not been documented with intakes of normal daily recommended amounts.

Studies have not been done in animals.

FDA Pregnancy Category C.

**Breast-feeding**

It is not known if phosphates are distributed into breast milk. However, problems in nursing infants have not been documented with intake of normal daily recommended amounts.

**Pediatrics**

Problems in pediatrics have not been documented with intake of normal daily recommended amounts. However, there have been several case reports of phosphate toxicity in pediatric patients from use of phosphate-containing enemas..

**Geriatrics**

Problems in geriatrics have not been documented with intakes of normal daily recommended amounts.

**Drug interactions and/or related problems**

The following drug interactions and/or related problems have been selected on the basis of their potential clinical significance (possible mechanism in parentheses where appropriate)—not necessarily inclusive (» = major clinical significance):

Note: Combinations containing any of the following, depending on the amount present, may also interact with this medication.

Anabolic steroids or
Androgens or
Estrogens
> (concurrent use with sodium phosphates may increase the risk of edema, due to the sodium content)

» Angiotensin-converting enzyme (ACE) inhibitors or
» Anti-inflammatory drugs, nonsteroidal (NSAIDs) or
» Cyclosporine or
» Diuretics, potassium-sparing or
» Heparin, chronic use of or
» Low-salt milk or
» Potassium-containing medications, other or
» Salt substitutes
> (concurrent use with potassium phosphate may result in hyperkalemia, especially in patients with renal impairment; patient should have serum potassium concentration determinations at periodic intervals)

» Antacids, aluminum- or magnesium-containing or
Oxalates, found in large quantities in rhubarb and spinach or
Phytates, in bran and whole-grain cereals
> (concurrent use with phosphates may bind the phosphate and prevent its absorption)

» Calcium-containing medications, including dietary supplements and antacids
> (concurrent use with phosphates may increase risk of deposition of calcium in soft tissues, if serum ionized calcium is high; also, phosphate absorption may be reduced because of formation of large amounts of insoluble phosphate)

» Corticosteroids, glucocorticoid, especially with significant mineralocorticoid activity or
» Corticosteroids, mineralocorticoid or
» Corticotropin (ACTH)
> (concurrent use with sodium phosphates may result in edema, due to the sodium content)

» Digitalis glycosides
> (use of potassium phosphates injection in digitalized patients with severe or complete heart block is not recommended because of possible hyperkalemia)

Iron supplements
> (concurrent use with foods or medicines containing phosphates will decrease iron absorption because of the formation of less soluble or insoluble complexes; iron supplements should not be taken within 1 hour before or 2 hours after ingestion of phosphates)

» Phosphate-containing medication, other
> (concurrent use with other phosphate containing medications may increase the risk of hyperphosphatemia, especially in patients with renal disease)

Salicylates
> (concurrent use with potassium and sodium phosphates combination or monobasic potassium phosphate may increase plasma concentrations of salicylates since salicylate excretion is decreased in acidified urine; addition of these phosphates to patients stabilized on a salicylate may lead to toxic salicylate concentrations)

» Sodium-containing medications
> (concurrent use with sodium phosphates may increase the risk of edema, especially in patients with renal disease)

Vitamin D, including calcifediol and calcitriol
> (concurrent use with phosphorus-containing medications in high doses may increase the potential for hyperphosphatemia because of vitamin D enhancement of phosphate absorption)

Zinc supplements
> (concurrent use of phosphorus-containing medications with zinc supplements may reduce zinc absorption by formation of nonabsorbable complexes; phosphorus-containing medications should be taken 2 hours after zinc supplements)

**Laboratory value alterations**

The following have been selected on the basis of their potential clinical significance (possible effect in parentheses where appropriate)—not necessarily inclusive (» = major clinical significance):

With diagnostic tests results
Skeletal imaging
> (saturation of bone binding sites by phosphorus ions in phosphates may cause decreased bone uptake of technetium Tc 99m–labeled diagnostic aids during bone imaging)

**Medical considerations/Contraindications**

The medical considerations/contraindications included here have been selected on the basis of their potential clinical significance (reasons given in parentheses where appropriate)—not necessarily inclusive (» = major clinical significance).

*Except under special circumstances, this medication should not be used when the following medical problems exist:*

» Hyperphosphatemia
> (phosphates may further increase serum phosphate concentrations, especially in patients with renal disease)

» Renal function impairment, severe—less than 30% of normal
> (use may result in increased serum phosphate concentrations)

Urinary tract infections caused by urea splitting organisms
> (use of phosphates may predispose to struvite stone formation)

» Urolithiasis, magnesium ammonium phosphate, infected
> (condition may be exacerbated)

*Risk-benefit should be considered when the following medical problems exist:*

*For all phosphates*
» Conditions in which high phosphate concentrations may be encountered, such as:
Hypoparathyroidism
Renal disease, chronic
Rhabdomyolysis
> (administration of phosphates may further increase serum phosphate concentrations)

» Conditions in which low calcium concentrations may be encountered, such as:
Hypoparathyroidism
Osteomalacia
Pancreatitis, acute
Renal disease, chronic
Rhabdomyolysis
Rickets
> (administration of phosphates may further decrease serum calcium concentrations)

Sensitivity to potassium, sodium, or phosphates

*For potassium-containing phosphates only*
Cardiac disease, particularly in digitalized patients
> (condition may be exacerbated)

» Conditions in which high potassium concentrations may be encountered, such as:
Adrenal insufficiency, severe—Addison's disease
Dehydration, acute
Pancreatitis
Physical exercise, strenuous, in unconditioned persons
Renal insufficiency, severe
Rhabdomyolysis
Tissue breakdown, extensive, such as severe burns
> (increased serum potassium concentrations leading to cardiac arrest may occur; exercise-induced hyperkalemia is transient and is a problem only in patients with renal insufficiency or those taking medications that increase serum potassium)

Myotonia congenita
> (condition may be exacerbated)

*For sodium-containing phosphates only*
Cardiac failure or
Cirrhosis of liver or severe hepatic disease or
Edema, peripheral and pulmonary or

» Hypernatremia or
Hypertension or
Renal function impairment or
Toxemia of pregnancy
(sodium salts should be used cautiously in patients with these conditions to prevent exacerbation; also, patients on sodium restricted
diets should not use sodium phosphates)

**Patient monitoring**
The following may be especially important in patient monitoring (other
tests may be warranted in some patients, depending on condition;
» = major clinical significance):

*For all phosphates*
Calcium concentrations, serum and
Phosphorus concentrations, serum and
Potassium concentrations, serum and
Renal function and
Sodium concentrations, serum
(determinations may be required at frequent intervals during ther-
apy, especially during intravenous therapy; high serum phosphate
concentrations increase the incidence of extraskeletal calcification)

*For potassium phosphates injection only*
Electrocardiogram (ECG)
(may be required at frequent intervals during intravenous therapy)

## Side/Adverse Effects

The following side/adverse effects have been selected on the basis of their
potential clinical significance (possible signs and symptoms in parentheses where appropriate)—not necessarily inclusive:

**Those indicating need for medical attention**
Incidence less frequent or rare
*Fluid retention* (swelling of feet or lower legs; weight gain); *hyperkalemia* (confusion; tiredness or weakness; irregular or slow heartbeat;
numbness or tingling around lips, hands, or feet; unexplained anxiety;
weakness or heaviness of legs; shortness of breath or troubled
breathing); *hypernatremia* (confusion; tiredness or weakness;
convulsions; decrease in amount of urine or in frequency of urination;
fast heartbeat; headache or dizziness; increased thirst);
*hyperphosphatemia or hypocalcemic tetany* (convulsions, muscle
cramps, numbness, tingling, pain, or weakness in hands or feet; shortness of breath, tremor or troubled breathing); *metastatic calcification*

**Those indicating need for medical attention only if they continue
or are bothersome**
Incidence less frequent—for oral dosage forms only
*Laxative effect or diarrhea; nausea or vomiting; stomach pain*

## Patient Consultation

As an aid to patient consultation, refer to *Advice for the Patient,
Phosphates (Systemic)*.

In providing consultation, consider emphasizing the following selected
information (» = major clinical significance):

**Importance of diet**
Importance of proper nutrition; supplement under physician's care may
be needed because of inadequate dietary intake or increased
requirements
Food sources of phosphorus
Recommended daily intake for phosphorus

**Before using this medication**
» Conditions affecting use, especially:
Sensitivity to potassium, sodium, or phosphates
Other medications, especially angiotensin-converting (ACE) inhibitors, antacids, calcium-containing medications, corticosteroids,
corticotropin (ACTH), cyclosporine, digitalis glycosides,
chronic use of heparin, low-salt milk, nonsteroidal anti-inflammatory drugs, potassium-containing medications, potassium-
sparing diuretics, salt substitutes, or sodium-containing
medicines
Other medical problems, especially acute dehydration, acute pancreatitis, Addison's disease, edema, hypernatremia, hyperphosphatemia, hypoparathyroidism, infected urolithiasis, osteomalacia, rickets, severe dehydration, severe kidney disease

**Proper use of this medication**
Taking dissolved in water
» Taking after meals or with food to minimize possible stomach upset
or laxative action
» Importance of high fluid intake (8-ounce glass of water every hour)
to prevent kidney stones

» Importance of not taking more medication than the amount
recommended
» For patients taking sodium-containing phosphates: Importance of low-
sodium diet
» Proper dosing
Missed dose: Taking as soon as possible; not taking if within 1 or 2
hours of next dose; not doubling doses
» Proper storage

**Precautions while using this medication**
Regular visits to physician to check progress during therapy
Not taking iron supplements within 1 to 2 hours of phosphates
Checking with physician before beginning exercise program if on po-
tassium-containing phosphate
Possible need for potassium or sodium restriction

**Side/adverse effects**
Signs of potential side effects, especially hyperkalemia, hypernatremia,
hyperphosphatemia, hypocalcemic tetany, or fluid retention

## General Dosing Information

The normal concentration of serum inorganic phosphate is 3 to 4.5 mg
(0.1 to 0.15 mmol) per 100 mL in adults and 4 to 7 mg (0.13 to 0.2
mmol) per 100 mL in children.

**For oral dosage forms**
Before this medication is taken, it must be thoroughly dissolved in water.

**For parenteral dosage forms**
Before administration, the concentrated phosphates injection (3 mmol of
phosphorus per mL) must be diluted and thoroughly mixed with a
larger volume of fluid.

The dose and rate of administration must be individualized.

When used as an electrolyte replenisher, a dose of the equivalent of 10
to 15 mmol (310 mg to 465 mg) of phosphorus a day is usually sufficient to maintain normal serum phosphate, although larger amounts
may be required in hypermetabolic states.

The solution should be infused slowly to avoid phosphate intoxication.

Intravenous infusion of phosphates in high concentrations may cause
hypocalcemia.

**Diet/Nutrition**
This medication should be taken immediately after a meal or with food
to minimize possible stomach upset or laxative action.

Recommended dietary intakes for phosphorus are defined differently
worldwide.
For U.S.—

The Recommended Dietary Allowances (RDAs) for vitamins and
minerals are determined by the Food and Nutrition Board of
the National Research Council and are intended to provide adequate nutrition in most healthy persons under usual environmental stresses. In addition, a different designation may be
used by the FDA for food and dietary supplement labeling
purposes, as with Daily Value (DV). DVs replace the previous
labeling terminology United States Recommended Daily Allowances (USRDAs).

For Canada—

Recommended Nutrient Intakes (RNIs) for vitamins, minerals, and
protein are determined by Health and Welfare Canada and provide
recommended amounts of a specific nutrient while minimizing the
risk of chronic diseases.

Daily recommended intakes for phosphorus are generally defined as
follows:

| Persons | U.S. (mg) | Canada (mg) |
| --- | --- | --- |
| Infants and children | | |
| Birth to 3 years of age | 300–800 | 150–350 |
| 4 to 6 years of age | 800 | 400 |
| 7 to 10 years of age | 800 | 500–800 |
| Adolescent and adult males | 800–1200 | 700–1000 |
| Adolescent and adult females | 800–1200 | 800–850 |
| Pregnant females | 1200 | 1050 |
| Breast-feeding females | 1200 | 1050 |

The best dietary sources of phosphorus include dairy products, meat, poultry, fish, and cereal products.

**For treatment of adverse effects**
Recommended treatment consists of the following:
• Withholding administration of phosphates.
• Correcting deficient serum electrolyte concentrations (such as that
of calcium).

## POTASSIUM PHOSPHATES

# Oral Dosage Forms

## MONOBASIC POTASSIUM PHOSPHATE TABLETS FOR ORAL SOLUTION

**Usual adult and adolescent dose**
Acidifier (urinary) or
Antiurolithic or
Electrolyte replenisher—
  Oral, 1 gram (228 mg or 7.4 mmol of phosphorus) in 180 to 240 mL of water four times a day, with meals and at bedtime.

**Usual pediatric dose**
Electrolyte replenisher—
  Children up to 4 years of age: Oral, the equivalent of 200 mg (6.4 mmol) of phosphorus in 60 mL of water four times a day, after meals and at bedtime.
  Children 4 years of age and over: See *Usual adult and adolescent dose.*

**Strength(s) usually available**
U.S.—
  500 mg (114 mg [3.7 mmol] of phosphorus) (Rx) [*K-Phos Original* (scored)].
Canada—
  Not commercially available.

**Packaging and storage**
Store below 40 °C (104 °F), preferably between 15 and 30 °C (59 and 86 °F), in a well-closed container, unless otherwise specified by manufacturer.

**Preparation of dosage form**
Soak the tablets in 60 or 75 mL of water for 2 to 5 minutes. Stir well to dissolve completely before swallowing.

**Auxiliary labeling**
• Do not swallow tablet.
• Dissolve tablet in a full glass (8 ounces) of water.

**Additional information**
Each 500-mg tablet supplies 114 mg (3.7 mmol) of phosphorus and 3.7 mEq (144 mg) of potassium.

## POTASSIUM PHOSPHATES CAPSULES FOR ORAL SOLUTION

**Usual adult and adolescent dose**
Electrolyte replenisher—
  Oral, 1.45 grams (250 mg or 8 mmol of phosphorus) in 75 mL of water or juice four times a day, after meals and at bedtime.

**Usual pediatric dose**
Electrolyte replenisher—
  Children up to 4 years of age: Oral, the equivalent of 200 mg (6.4 mmol) of phosphorus in 60 mL of water or juice four times a day, after meals and at bedtime.
  Children 4 years of age and over: See *Usual adult and adolescent dose.*

**Strength(s) usually available**
U.S.—
  1.45 grams (250 mg [8 mmol] of phosphorus) (OTC) [*Neutra-Phos-K*].
Canada—
  Not commercially available.

**Packaging and storage**
Store below 40 °C (104 °F), preferably between 15 and 30 °C (59 and 86 °F), in a well-closed container, unless otherwise specified by manufacturer.

**Preparation of dosage form**
Empty contents of capsule into 60 or 75 mL of water or juice and stir well.

**Auxiliary labeling**
• Do not swallow filled capsule.
• Mix contents of each capsule with one-third glass of water or juice.

**Additional information**
Each 1.45-gram capsule supplies 250 mg (8 mmol) of phosphorus and 14.25 mEq (556 mg) of potassium, as monobasic and dibasic potassium phosphates per 75 mL of water or juice, or 200 mg (6.4 mmol) per 60 mL of water or juice, when reconstituted according to manufacturer's instructions.

## POTASSIUM PHOSPHATES FOR ORAL SOLUTION

**Usual adult and adolescent dose**
Electrolyte replenisher—
  Oral, the equivalent of 250 mg (8 mmol) of phosphorus four times a day, after meals and at bedtime.

**Usual pediatric dose**
Electrolyte replenisher—
  Children up to 4 years of age: Oral, the equivalent of 200 mg (6.4 mmol) of phosphorus four times a day, after meals and at bedtime.
  Children 4 years of age and over: See *Usual adult and adolescent dose.*

**Size(s) usually available**
U.S.—
  1.45 grams (250 mg [8mmol] of phosphorus) (OTC) [*Neutra-Phos-K*].
  71 grams (250 mg [8 mmol] of phosphorus) (OTC) [*Neutra-Phos-K*].
Canada—
  Not commercially available.

**Packaging and storage**
Store below 40 °C (104 °F), preferably between 15 and 30 °C (59 and 86 °F), in a well-closed container, unless otherwise specified by manufacturer.

**Preparation of dosage form**
To prepare solution, add the contents of one bottle (71 grams) of powder concentrate, supplied by the manufacturer, to a sufficient amount of water to make 1 gallon (3.785 liters) of solution or the contents of one packet of powder concentrate to a sufficient amount of water to make 1/3 of a glass (approximately 2.5 ounces) of water. Shake the container for 2 or 3 minutes or until all the powder is dissolved. Solution should not be diluted.

**Stability**
Solution can be stored for 60 days.

**Additional information**
Each 75 mL of solution or the solution prepared from one packet, when constituted according to manufacturer's instructions, supplies 250 mg (8 mmol) of phosphorus and 14.25 mEq (556 mg) of potassium, as monobasic and dibasic potassium phosphates.

# Parenteral Dosage Forms

## POTASSIUM PHOSPHATES INJECTION USP

Note: **Potassium phosphates injection must be diluted prior to intravenous administration.**

**Usual adult and adolescent dose**
Electrolyte replenisher—
  Intravenous infusion, the equivalent of 10 mmol (310 mg) of phosphorus a day.

**Usual pediatric dose**
Electrolyte replenisher—
  Intravenous infusion, the equivalent of 1.5 to 2 mmol (46.5 to 62 mg) of phosphorus a day.

**Strength(s) usually available**
U.S.—
  224 mg of monobasic potassium phosphate and 236 mg of dibasic potassium phosphate (3 mmol [93 mg] of phosphorus) per mL (Rx) [GENERIC].
Canada—
  224 mg of monobasic potassium phosphate and 236 mg of dibasic potassium phosphate (3 mmol [93 mg] of phosphorus) per mL (Rx) [GENERIC].

**Packaging and storage**
Store between 15 and 30 °C (59 and 86 °F), unless otherwise specified by manufacturer.

**Incompatibilities**
Precipitate may form when phosphates are added to solution containing calcium or magnesium.

**Additional information**
Each mL of potassium phosphates injection supplies 283.5 mg of phosphate (approximately 3 mmol [93 mg] of phosphorus) and 4.4 mEq (170.2 mg) of potassium.

## POTASSIUM AND SODIUM PHOSPHATES

# Oral Dosage Forms

## MONOBASIC POTASSIUM AND SODIUM PHOSPHATES TABLETS FOR ORAL SOLUTION

### Usual adult and adolescent dose
Acidifier (urinary) or
Antiurolithic or
Electrolyte replenisher—
    Oral, 250 mg (8 mmol) of phosphorus with a full glass (240 mL) of water four times a day, after meals and at bedtime.

Note: When the urine is difficult to acidify, a dose of the equivalent of 250 mg (8 mmol) of phosphorus may be administered every two hours, not to exceed 2 grams of phosphorus in a twenty-four–hour period.

### Usual pediatric dose
Electrolyte replenisher—
    Children up to 4 years of age: Oral, 200 mg (6.4 mmol) of phosphorus in 60 mL of water four times a day, after meals and at bedtime.
    Children 4 years of age and over: See *Usual adult and adolescent dose.*

### Strength(s) usually available
U.S.—
    155 mg of monobasic potassium phosphate and 350 mg of anhydrous monobasic sodium phosphate (125.6 mg [4 mmol] of phosphorus) (Rx) [*K-Phos M. F* (scored)].
    155 mg of monobasic potassium phosphate, 130 mg of hydrous monobasic sodium phosphate, and 852 mg of anhydrous dibasic sodium phosphate (250 mg [8 mmol] of phosphorus) (Rx) [*K-Phos Neutral*].
    305 mg of monobasic potassium phosphate and 700 mg of anhydrous monobasic sodium phosphate (250 mg [8 mmol] of phosphorus) (Rx) [*K-Phos No. 2*].
Canada—
    Not commercially available.

### Packaging and storage
Store between 15 and 30 °C (59 and 86 °F), in a well-closed container, unless otherwise specified by manufacturer.

### Auxiliary labeling
- Do not swallow tablet.
- Dissolve tablet in a full glass (8 ounces) of water.

### Additional information
A dose of 155 mg of monobasic potassium phosphate and 350 mg of anhydrous monobasic sodium phosphate supplies 125.6 mg (4 mmol) of phosphorus, 1.14 mEq (44.5 mg) of potassium, and 2.9 mEq (67 mg) of sodium.

A dose of 305 mg of monobasic potassium phosphate and 700 mg of anhydrous monobasic sodium phosphate supplies 250 mg (8 mmol) of phosphorus, 2.3 mEq (88 mg) of potassium, and 5.8 mEq (134 mg) of sodium.

A dose of 155 mg of monobasic potassium phosphate, 130 mg of hydrous monobasic sodium phosphate, and 852 mg of anhydrous dibasic sodium phosphate supplies 250 mg (8 mmol) of phosphorus, 1.15 mEq (45 mg) of potassium, and 12.9 mEq (298 mg) of sodium.

## POTASSIUM AND SODIUM PHOSPHATES CAPSULES FOR ORAL SOLUTION

### Usual adult and adolescent dose
Electrolyte replenisher—
    Oral, 1.25 grams (250 mg or 8 mmol of phosphorus) in 75 mL of water or juice four times a day, after meals and at bedtime.

### Usual pediatric dose
Electrolyte replenisher—
    Children up to 4 years of age: Oral, the equivalent of 200 mg (6.4 mmol) of phosphorus in 60 mL of water or juice four times a day, after meals and at bedtime.
    Children 4 years of age and over: See *Usual adult and adolescent dose.*

### Strength(s) usually available
U.S.—
    1.25 grams (250 mg [8 mmol] of phosphorus) (OTC) [*Neutra-Phos*].
Canada—
    Not commercially available.

### Packaging and storage
Store below 40 °C (104 °F), preferably between 15 and 30 °C (59 and 86 °F), in a well-closed container, unless otherwise specified by manufacturer.

### Preparation of dosage form
Empty contents of capsule into 75 mL of water or juice and stir well.

### Auxiliary labeling
- Do not swallow filled capsule.
- Mix contents of each capsule with one-third glass of water or juice.

### Additional information
Each 1.25-gram capsule supplies 250 mg (8 mmol) of phosphorus, 278 mg (7.125 mEq) of potassium, and 164 mg (7.125 mEq) of sodium.

## POTASSIUM AND SODIUM PHOSPHATES FOR ORAL SOLUTION

### Usual adult and adolescent dose
Electrolyte replenisher—
    Oral, 250 mg (8 mmol) of phosphorus four times a day, after meals and at bedtime.

### Usual pediatric dose
Electrolyte replenisher—
    Children up to 4 years of age: Oral, 200 mg (6.4 mmol) four times a day after meals and at bedtime.
    Children 4 years of age and over: See *Usual adult and adolescent dose.*

### Size(s) usually available
64 grams (250 mg or 8 mmol of phosphorus per 75 mL, when reconstituted according to manufacturer's instruction).
U.S.—
    1.25 grams (250 mg [8mmol] of phosphorus) (OTC) [*NeutraPhos*].
    64 grams (250 mg [8 mmol] of phosphorus) (OTC) [*Neutra-Phos*].
Canada—
    Not commercially available.

### Packaging and storage
Store between 15 and 30 °C (59 and 86 °F), in a well-closed container, unless otherwise specified by manufacturer.

### Preparation of dosage form
To prepare solution, add the contents of one bottle (64 grams) of dibasic potassium and sodium phosphates and monobasic potassium sodium phosphates powder concentrate, supplied by the manufacturer, to a sufficient amount of water to make 1 gallon (3.785 liters) of solution or the contents of one packet, supplied by the manufacturer, to a sufficient amount of water to make 1/3 glass of water (approximately 2.5 ounces) of solution. Shake for 2 or 3 minutes or until all the powder is dissolved. Solution should not be diluted.

### Stability
Solution can be stored for 60 days.

### Additional information
Each 75 mL of solution or solution prepared from one packet supplies 250 mg (8 mmol) of phosphorus, 7.125 mEq (278 mg) of potassium, and 7.125 mEq (164 mg) of sodium.

## POTASSIUM AND SODIUM PHOSPHATES TABLETS FOR ORAL SOLUTION

### Usual adult and adolescent dose
Electrolyte replenisher—
    Oral, the equivalent of 250 mg (8 mmol) of phosphorus with a full glass (240 mL) of water four times a day.

### Usual pediatric dose
Electrolyte replenisher—
    Children up to 4 years of age: Oral, 200 mg (6.4 mmol) of phosphorus in 60 mL of water four times a day, after meals and at bedtime.
    Children 4 years of age and over: See *Usual adult and adolescent dose.*

### Strength(s) usually available
U.S.—
    250 mg (8 mmol) of phosphorus (Rx) [*Uro-KP-Neutral*].
Canada—
    250 mg (8 mmol) of phosphorus (Rx) [*Uro-KP-Neutral*].

### Packaging and storage
Store below 40 °C (104 °F), preferably between 15 and 30 °C (59 and 86 °F), in a well-closed container, unless otherwise specified by manufacturer.

### Auxiliary labeling
- Do not swallow tablet.
- Dissolve tablet in a full glass (8 ounces) of water.

**Additional information**
Each tablet supplies 250 mg (8 mmol) of phosphorus, 1.28 mEq (50 mg)
of potassium, and 10.8 mEq (250 mg) of sodium, as anhydrous dibasic
sodium phosphate, anhydrous dibasic potassium phosphate, and anhydrous monobasic sodium phosphate.

## SODIUM PHOSPHATES

## Parenteral Dosage Forms

Note: **Sodium phosphates injection must be diluted prior to intravenous administration.**

### SODIUM PHOSPHATES INJECTION USP

**Usual adult and adolescent dose**
Electrolyte replenisher—
    Intravenous infusion, 10 to 15 mmol (310 to 465 mg) of phosphorus
    a day.

**Usual pediatric dose**
Electrolyte replenisher—
    Intravenous infusion, 1.5 to 2 mmol of phosphorus per kg of body
    weight a day.

**Strength(s) usually available**
U.S.—
    276 mg of hydrous monobasic sodium phosphate and 142 mg of an-
    hydrous dibasic sodium phosphate (3 mmol [93 mg] of phospho-
    rus) per mL (Rx) [GENERIC].
Canada—
    Not commercially available.

**Packaging and storage**
Store below 40 °C (104 °F), preferably between 15 and 30 °C (59 and 86
°F), unless otherwise specified by manufacturer. Protect from freezing.

**Incompatibilities**
Precipitate may form when sodium phosphates injection is added to solution containing calcium or magnesium.

**Additional information**
Each mL of sodium phosphates injection supplies 285 mg of phosphate
(approximately 3 mmol [93 mg] of phosphorus) and 4 mEq (92 mg)
of sodium.

Revised: 04/16/92
Interim revision: 08/30/94; 07/18/95

---

# PHYSOSTIGMINE    Ophthalmic†

VA CLASSIFICATION (Primary): OP102

Note: For a listing of dosage forms and brand names by country availa-
    bility, see *Dosage Forms* section(s). For a listing of brand names
    for the articles in this monograph, refer to the General Index.

    †Not commercially available in Canada.

## Category

Antiglaucoma agent (ophthalmic); miotic.

## Indications

Note: Bracketed information in the *Indications* section refers to uses that
    are not included in U.S. product labeling.

**Accepted**
Glaucoma, open-angle (treatment)—Indicated for reduction of intraocular
    pressure in open-angle glaucoma. Physostigmine may be used in con-
    junction with beta-adrenergic blockers, carbonic anhydrase inhibitors,
    or hyperosmotic agents.
[Glaucoma, angle-closure, *during* or *after* iridectomy (treatment)]—Phy-
    sostigmine is used in the treatment of angle-closure glaucoma during
    or after iridectomy.
[Glaucoma, secondary (treatment)]—Physostigmine is used in the treat-
    ment of secondary glaucoma if there is no active intraocular inflam-
    mation present.

## Pharmacology/Pharmacokinetics

**Physicochemical characteristics**
Molecular weight—Physostigmine salicylate: 413.47.
Physostigmine sulfate: 648.77.

**Mechanism of action/Effect**
Physostigmine is an indirect-acting parasympathomimetic drug that pro-
    motes accumulation and potentiation of the actions of endogenous ace-
    tylcholine via a temporary inactivation of cholinesterase. It produces
    contraction of the iris sphincter muscle, resulting in pupillary constric-
    tion (miosis); constriction of the ciliary muscle, resulting in increased
    accommodation; and a reduction in intraocular pressure associated
    with decreased resistance to aqueous humor outflow.
In chronic open-angle glaucoma, the exact mechanism by which miotics
    lower intraocular pressure is not precisely known; however, contrac-
    tion of the ciliary muscle apparently opens the intertrabecular spaces
    and facilitates aqueous humor outflow.

**Onset of action**
Miosis—Within 10 to 30 minutes.

**Duration of action**
Miosis—12 to 48 hours.

## Precautions to Consider

**Pregnancy/Reproduction**
Pregnancy—Studies have not been done in humans; however, ophthalmic
    physostigmine may be systemically absorbed.
Studies have not been done in animals.
FDA Pregnancy Category C.

**Breast-feeding**
Problems in humans have not been documented; however, ophthalmic
    physostigmine may be systemically absorbed.

**Pediatrics**
Appropriate studies on the relationship of age to the effects of physostig-
    mine have not been performed in the pediatric population. However,
    no pediatrics-specific problems have been documented to date.

**Geriatrics**
Appropriate studies on the relationship of age to the effects of physostig-
    mine have not been performed in the geriatric population. However,
    no geriatrics-specific problems have been documented to date.

**Drug interactions and/or related problems**
The following drug interactions and/or related problems have been se-
    lected on the basis of their potential clinical significance (possible
    mechanism in parentheses where appropriate)—not necessarily inclu-
    sive (» = major clinical significance):
Note: Combinations containing any of the following medications, de-
    pending on the amount present, may also interact with this
    medication.

    Belladonna alkaloids, ophthalmic
        (concurrent use may antagonize the antiglaucoma and miotic ac-
        tions of physostigmine)

    Echothiophate or
    Isoflurophate
        (duration of action may be shortened by prior use of
        physostigmine)

**Medical considerations/Contraindications**
The medical considerations/contraindications included here have been se-
    lected on the basis of their potential clinical significance (reasons given
    in parentheses where appropriate)—not necessarily inclusive (» =
    major clinical significance).

*Risk-benefit should be considered when the following medical problems
exist:*
    Corneal injury
    Sensitivity to physostigmine
» Uveitis, active

**Patient monitoring**
The following may be especially important in patient monitoring (other tests may be warranted in some patients, depending on condition; » = major clinical significance):

Intraocular pressure determinations
(recommended at periodic intervals during therapy)

## Side/Adverse Effects

The following side/adverse effects have been selected on the basis of their potential clinical significance (possible signs and symptoms in parentheses where appropriate)—not necessarily inclusive:

**Those indicating need for medical attention**
Symptoms of systemic absorption
*Increased sweating; loss of bladder control; muscle weakness; nausea, vomiting, diarrhea, or stomach cramps or pain; shortness of breath, tightness in chest, or wheezing; slow or irregular heartbeat; unusual tiredness or weakness; watering of mouth*

**Those indicating need for medical attention only if they continue or are bothersome**
Incidence more frequent
*Blurred vision or change in near or distant vision; eye pain*
Incidence less frequent
*Burning, redness, stinging, or other eye irritation; headache or browache; twitching of eyelids; watering of eyes*

## Patient Consultation

As an aid to patient consultation, refer to *Advice for the Patient, Physostigmine (Ophthalmic).*

In providing consultation, consider emphasizing the following selected information (» = major clinical significance):

**Before using this medication**
» Conditions affecting use, especially:
Sensitivity to physostigmine
Other medical problems, especially active uveitis

**Proper use of this medication**
Not using solution if it becomes discolored
Proper administration technique
Washing hands immediately after application to remove any medication that may be on them
» Importance of not using more medication than the amount prescribed
» Proper dosing
Missed dose: If dosing schedule is—
One dose a day: Applying as soon as possible; not applying if not remembered until next day; applying next regularly scheduled dose
More than one dose a day: Applying as soon as possible; not applying if almost time for next dose; applying next dose at regularly scheduled time
*Preventing contamination*
For solution dosage form—Not touching applicator tip to any surface; keeping container tightly closed
For ointment dosage form—Not touching applicator tip to any surface; wiping tip of ointment tube with clean tissue; keeping tube tightly closed
» Proper storage

**Precautions while using this medication**
Regular visits to physician to check eye pressure during therapy
» Caution if blurred vision or change in near or distant vision occurs, especially at night

**Side/adverse effects**
Signs of potential side effects, especially systemic absorption

## General Dosing Information

Although some manufacturers recommend a dose of 2 drops of an ophthalmic solution at appropriate intervals, the conjunctival sac will usually hold only 1 drop.
More frequent instillation or use of a stronger concentration may be required to produce adequate miosis and reduction in intraocular pressure in eyes with brown or hazel irides than in eyes with blue or light-colored irides.

Tolerance to physostigmine may develop with prolonged use. Effectiveness may be restored by changing to another miotic for a short time and then resuming the original medication.

**For the ointment dosage form only**
At night, the ophthalmic ointment may be used to provide prolonged contact with the medication.

**For the solution dosage form only**
To avoid excessive systemic absorption, patient should press finger to the lacrimal sac during and for 1 or 2 minutes following instillation of the ophthalmic solution.

## Ophthalmic Dosage Forms
### PHYSOSTIGMINE SALICYLATE OPHTHALMIC SOLUTION USP

**Usual adult and adolescent dose**
Open-angle glaucoma—
Topical, to the conjunctiva, 1 drop of a 0.25 or 0.5% solution up to four times a day.

**Usual pediatric dose**
See *Usual adult and adolescent dose.*

**Usual geriatric dose**
See *Usual adult and adolescent dose.*

**Strength(s) usually available**
U.S.—
0.25% (Rx) [*Isopto Eserine*].
0.5% (Rx) [*Eserine Salicylate* (sodium bisulfite); *Isopto Eserine*].
Canada—
Not commercially available.

**Packaging and storage**
Store below 40 °C (104 °F), preferably between 15 and 30 °C (59 and 86 °F), unless otherwise specified by manufacturer. Store in a tight, light-resistant container. Protect from freezing.

**Stability**
Physostigmine solutions are sensitive to heat and light and should not be used if they become cloudy or dark brown.

**Auxiliary labeling**
• For the eye.
• Keep container tightly closed.

### PHYSOSTIGMINE SULFATE OPHTHALMIC OINTMENT USP

**Usual adult and adolescent dose**
Open-angle glaucoma—
Topical, to the conjunctiva, 1 cm of a 0.25% ointment one to three times a day.

**Usual pediatric dose**
See *Usual adult and adolescent dose.*

**Usual geriatric dose**
See *Usual adult and adolescent dose.*

**Strength(s) usually available**
U.S.—
0.25% (Rx) [*Eserine Sulfate;* GENERIC].
Canada—
Not commercially available.

**Packaging and storage**
Store below 40 °C (104 °F), preferably between 15 and 30 °C (59 and 86 °F), unless otherwise specified by manufacturer. Store in a tight container. Protect from freezing.

**Auxiliary labeling**
• For the eye.
• Keep container tightly closed.

Revised: 07/01/93

# PHYSOSTIGMINE   Systemic

VA CLASSIFICATION (Primary): AU300
Another commonly used name is eserine.

Note: For a listing of dosage forms and brand names by country availability, see *Dosage Forms* section(s). For a listing of brand names for the articles in this monograph, refer to the General Index.

## Category

Cholinergic (cholinesterase inhibitor); antidote (to anticholinergics).

## Indications

Note: Bracketed information in the *Indications* section refers to uses that are not included in U.S. product labeling.

**Accepted**

Toxicity, anticholinergic agent (treatment)—Physostigmine is indicated to reverse toxic effects on the central nervous system (CNS) caused by drugs and plants capable of producing anticholinergic poisoning in clinical or toxic dosages. Physostigmine is not recommended for treatment of routine anticholinergic poisoning or those not responding to less toxic alternatives because of potential complications such as bradycardia, seizures, and asystole.

[Ataxias, hereditary (treatment)][1]—FDA has granted physostigmine an orphan drug designation for use in Friedreich's and other inherited ataxias.

**Unaccepted**

Physostigmine has been reported to antagonize the CNS depressant effects of benzodiazepines; however, physostigmine should not be used in benzodiazepine overdosage because of its nonspecific action and potential toxicity.

---

[1]Not included in Canadian product labeling.

## Pharmacology/Pharmacokinetics

**Mechanism of action/Effect**

Antidote (to anticholinergics)—
 Antagonizes action of anticholinergics, which block the postsynaptic receptor sites of acetylcholine, by reversibly inhibiting the destruction of acetylcholine by acetylcholinesterase, thereby increasing the concentration of acetylcholine at sites of cholinergic transmission.
 Since physostigmine is a lipid-soluble tertiary amine, which (unlike the quaternary amines neostigmine and pyridostigmine) can cross the blood-brain barrier, it acts against both central and peripheral anticholinergic effects.

**Distribution**

Easily penetrates the blood-brain barrier.

**Biotransformation**

Rapidly hydrolyzed by cholinesterases.

**Time to peak effect**

Intramuscular—20 to 30 minutes.
Intravenous—Within 5 minutes.

**Duration of action**

Intramuscular and intravenous—30 to 60 minutes.

**Elimination**

Very small amounts eliminated in urine; largely destroyed in body by hydrolysis.

## Precautions to Consider

**Pregnancy/Reproduction**

Pregnancy—Studies in humans have not been done. Physostigmine crosses the blood-brain barrier and would be expected to cross the placenta.

**Breast-feeding**

It is not known whether physostigmine is excreted in breast milk.

**Pediatrics**

No information is available on the relationship of age to the effects of physostigmine in pediatric patients. However, physostigmine should be used in children only in life-threatening situations.

Physostigmine injection that contains benzyl alcohol as a preservative should not be used in newborn and immature infants. The use of benzyl alcohol in neonates has been associated with a fatal toxic syndrome consisting of metabolic acidosis and CNS, respiratory, circulatory, and renal function impairment.

**Geriatrics**

No information is available on the relationship of age to the effects of physostigmine in geriatric patients.

**Drug interactions and/or related problems**

The following drug interactions and/or related problems have been selected on the basis of their potential clinical significance (possible mechanism in parentheses where appropriate)—not necessarily inclusive (» = major clinical significance):

Note: Combinations containing any of the following medications, depending on the amount present, may also interact with this medication.

» Choline esters (acetylcholine, bethanechol, carbachol, methacholine)
  (effects of acetylcholine and methacholine are markedly enhanced by prior administration of physostigmine, since these medications are hydrolyzed by acetylcholinesterase; physostigmine produces only additive effects when used concurrently with carbachol or bethanechol)

» Succinylcholine
  (concurrent use with physostigmine is not recommended since high doses of physostigmine may cause muscle fasciculation and ultimately, a depolarization block, which may be additive to that produced by the depolarizing neuromuscular blocking agents)

**Medical considerations/Contraindications**

The medical considerations/contraindications included here have been selected on the basis of their potential clinical significance (reasons given in parentheses where appropriate)—not necessarily inclusive (» = major clinical significance).

*Risk-benefit should be considered when the following medical problems exist:*

» Asthma
  (increase in bronchial secretions and other respiratory effects of physostigmine may aggravate condition)

» Cardiovascular disease or
» Gangrene or
» Intestinal or urogenital tract obstruction, mechanical, or any vagotonic state
  (these conditions may be exacerbated by physostigmine)

 Parkinsonism
  (akinesia, rigidity, and tremor may be increased)

» Organophosphate poisoning
  (physostigmine may potentiate anticholinesterase activity)

 Sensitivity to physostigmine

**Patient monitoring**

The following may be especially important in patient monitoring (other tests may be warranted in some patients, depending on condition; » = major clinical significance):

 Blood pressure and
 Heart rate and rhythm
  (monitoring is recommended because physostigmine has been reported to cause bradycardia and hypotension)

## Side/Adverse Effects

The following side/adverse effects have been selected on the basis of their potential clinical significance (possible signs and symptoms in parentheses where appropriate)—not necessarily inclusive:

**Those indicating need for medical attention**

Incidence less frequent or rare
 *Irregular heartbeat; muscle twitching; shortness of breath, troubled breathing, wheezing, or tightness in chest; unusual tiredness or weakness*

With too rapid intravenous administration
 *Convulsions; difficulty in breathing; slow heartbeat*

**Those indicating need for medical attention only if they continue or are bothersome**

Incidence more frequent
 *Diarrhea; increased sweating; increased watering of mouth; nausea or vomiting; stomach cramps or pain*

Incidence less frequent
*Frequent urge to urinate; increase in bronchial secretions; nervousness or restlessness; unusually small pupils; unusual watering of eyes*

## Overdose

For specific information on the agents used in the management of physostigmine overdose, see:
• *Atropine* in *Anticholinergics/Antispasmodics (Systemic)* monograph.

For more specific information on the management of overdose or unintentional ingestion, **contact a Poison Control Center** (see *Poison Control Center Listing*).

**Treatment of overdose**
Specific treatment—

Use of the antagonist atropine sulfate injection. See the package insert or *Atropine* in *Anticholinergic/Antispasmodics (Systemic)* for specific dosing guidelines for use of this product.

Use of intravenous administration of pralidoxime chloride to counteract ganglionic and skeletal muscle effects. See the package insert for specific dosing guidelines for use of this product.

Treatment of convulsions or shock as appropriate.

Monitoring— May include monitoring of cardiac function.

Supportive care—Maintenance of open airway (possible suction of bronchial secretions); use of assisted respiration.

## General Dosing Information

The dosage of physostigmine should be reduced if excessive sweating or nausea occurs.

Physostigmine should be discontinued if excessive symptoms of salivation, vomiting, urination, or diarrhea occur.

Rapid intravenous administration may cause bradycardia, hypersalivation resulting in breathing difficulties, and possibly convulsions.

## Parenteral Dosage Forms

### PHYSOSTIGMINE SALICYLATE INJECTION USP

**Usual adult and adolescent dose**
Antidote—
Intramuscular or intravenous, 500 mcg (0.5 mg) to 2 mg, administered at a rate of not more than 1 mg per minute; doses of 1 to 4 mg may be repeated, if necessary, at intervals of 20 to 30 minutes as life-threatening signs recur.

**Usual pediatric dose**
Antidote—
Intravenous, initially no more than 20 mcg (0.02 mg) per kilogram of body weight administered over a period of at least one minute; if toxic effects persist and there is no sign of cholinergic effects, dose may be repeated at five- to ten-minute intervals, if necessary, up to a maximum dose of 2 mg.

Note: Use should be reserved for life-threatening situations only.

Physostigmine injection that contains benzyl alcohol as a preservative should not be used in newborn and immature infants. The use of benzyl alcohol in neonates has been associated with a fatal toxic syndrome consisting of metabolic acidosis and CNS, respiratory, circulatory, and renal function impairment.

**Strength(s) usually available**
U.S.—
1 mg per mL (Rx) [*Antilirium* (benzyl alcohol 2%); GENERIC].
Canada—
1 mg per mL (Rx) [*Antilirium* (benzyl alcohol 2%)].

**Packaging and storage**
Store below 40 °C (104 °F), preferably between 15 and 30 °C (59 and 86 °F), unless otherwise specified by manufacturer. Protect from light. Protect from freezing.

Revised: 08/21/92

---

**PHYTONADIONE**—See *Vitamin K (Systemic)*

---

# PILOCARPINE    Ophthalmic

VA CLASSIFICATION (Primary): OP102
Note: For a listing of dosage forms and brand names by country availability, see *Dosage Forms* section(s). For a listing of brand names for the articles in this monograph, refer to the General Index.

## Category

Antiglaucoma agent (ophthalmic); miotic.

## Indications

**Accepted**

Glaucoma, open-angle (treatment)—Pilocarpine is indicated primarily for the treatment of open-angle (chronic simple) glaucoma. It may be used in conjunction with a carbonic anhydrase inhibitor, epinephrine, timolol, fluorescein, or anesthetic, antibiotic, or anti-inflammatory steroid ophthalmic solutions.

Glaucoma, angle-closure (treatment)—Pilocarpine (hydrochloride or nitrate) ophthalmic solution is indicated for use alone or in combination with carbonic anhydrase inhibitors or hyperosmotic agents to lower intraocular pressure in the emergency treatment of acute angle-closure glaucoma prior to surgery or laser iridotomy. In addition, pilocarpine may be indicated for the treatment of chronic angle-closure glaucoma.

Glaucoma, angle-closure, *during* or *after* iridectomy (treatment)—Pilocarpine (hydrochloride or nitrate) ophthalmic solution may be indicated for the treatment of angle-closure glaucoma *during* or *after* iridectomy.

Glaucoma, secondary (treatment)—Pilocarpine may be indicated for the treatment of nonuveitic secondary glaucoma.

Miosis induction, postoperative or
Miosis induction, following ophthalmoscopy—Pilocarpine (hydrochloride or nitrate) ophthalmic solution is indicated to produce miosis in order to counteract the effects of cycloplegics and mydriatics following surgery or ophthalmoscopic examination.

## Pharmacology/Pharmacokinetics

**Physicochemical characteristics**
Molecular weight—Pilocarpine: 208.26.
Pilocarpine hydrochloride: 244.72.
Pilocarpine nitrate: 271.27.

**Mechanism of action/Effect**
Pilocarpine is a parasympathomimetic that directly stimulates cholinergic receptors. It produces contraction of the iris sphincter muscle, resulting in pupillary constriction (miosis); constriction of the ciliary muscle, resulting in increased accommodation; and reduction in intraocular pressure associated with an increase in the outflow and a decrease in the inflow of aqueous humor.

In chronic open-angle glaucoma, the exact mechanism by which miotics lower intraocular pressure is not precisely known; however, contraction of the ciliary muscle apparently opens the intertrabecular spaces and facilitates aqueous humor outflow. There is also a decrease in the rate of inflow of aqueous humor.

In angle-closure glaucoma, constriction of the pupil apparently pulls the iris away from the trabeculum, thereby relieving blockage of the trabecular meshwork.

**Onset of action**
Miosis—Solution (1%): Within 10 to 30 minutes.

**Time to peak effect**
Reduction in intraocular pressure—
Ocular system: 1.5 to 2 hours.
Solution: Within 75 minutes, depending on strength used.

**Duration of action**
Miosis—
Solution: About 4 to 8 hours.
Reduction in intraocular pressure—
Ocular system: 7 days.
Solution: 4 to 14 hours, depending on strength used.

## Precautions to Consider

### Carcinogenicity
No long-term studies have been done.

### Pregnancy/Reproduction
Pregnancy—Studies have not been done in humans; however, ophthalmic pilocarpine may be systemically absorbed.

Studies have not been done in animals.

FDA Pregnancy Category C.

### Breast-feeding
It is not known whether pilocarpine is distributed into breast milk and problems in humans have not been documented. However, ophthalmic pilocarpine may be systemically absorbed.

### Pediatrics
Appropriate studies on the relationship of age to the effects of pilocarpine have not been performed in the pediatric population. However, no pediatrics-specific problems have been documented to date.

### Geriatrics
Appropriate studies on the relationship of age to the effects of pilocarpine have not been performed in the geriatric population. However, no geriatrics-specific problems have been documented to date.

### Drug interactions and/or related problems
The following drug interactions and/or related problems have been selected on the basis of their potential clinical significance (possible mechanism in parentheses where appropriate)—not necessarily inclusive (» = major clinical significance):

Belladonna alkaloids, ophthalmic or
Cyclopentolate
   (concurrent use may interfere with the antiglaucoma action of pilocarpine; also, concurrent use with pilocarpine counteracts the mydriatic effects of these medications; this anti-mydriatic effect may be used to therapeutic advantage)

### Medical considerations/Contraindications
The medical considerations/contraindications included here have been selected on the basis of their potential clinical significance (reasons given in parentheses where appropriate)—not necessarily inclusive (» = major clinical significance):

*Risk-benefit should be considered when the following medical problems exist:*

Asthma, bronchial

Infectious conjunctivitis or keratitis, acute—for ocular system dosage form only

» Iritis, acute, or other conditions in which pupillary constriction is undesirable

Retinal detachment, history of or predisposition to

Sensitivity to pilocarpine

### Patient monitoring
The following may be especially important in patient monitoring (other tests may be warranted in some patients, depending on condition; » = major clinical significance):

Intraocular pressure determinations
   (recommended at periodic intervals during therapy)

## Side/Adverse Effects
The following side/adverse effects have been selected on the basis of their potential clinical significance (possible signs and symptoms in parentheses where appropriate)—not necessarily inclusive:

### Those indicating need for medical attention
Symptoms of systemic absorption
   *Increased sweating; muscle tremors; nausea, vomiting, or diarrhea; troubled breathing or wheezing; watering of mouth*

Incidence less frequent or rare
   *Eye pain*

### Those indicating need for medical attention only if they continue or are bothersome
Incidence more frequent
   *Blurred vision or change in near or far vision; decrease in night vision*

Incidence less frequent
   *Eye irritation; headache or browache*

## Overdose
For specific piiformation on the agents used in the management of ophthalmic pilocarpine overdose, see:
   • *Atropine* in *Anticholinergics/Antispasmodics (Systemic)* monograph.

For more information on the management of overdose or unintentional ingestion, **contact a Poison Control Center** (see *Poison Control Center Listing*).

### Treatment of overdose
If accidental overdosage occurs in the eye, flushing the eye with water or normal saline.

If medication is accidentally ingested, inducing emesis or performing gastric lavage. Patients should be observed for signs of pilocarpine toxicity (i.e., unusual watering of mouth, unusual sweating, nausea, vomiting, and diarrhea); if these occur, therapy with anticholinergics, such as atropine, may be necessary.

## Patient Consultation
As an aid to patient consultation, refer to *Advice for the Patient, Pilocarpine (Ophthalmic)*.

In providing consultation, consider emphasizing the following selected information (» = major clinical significance):

### Before using this medication
» Conditions affecting use, especially:
      Sensitivity to pilocarpine
      Other medical problems, especially acute iritis or other conditions in which pupillary constriction is undesirable

### Proper use of this medication
   Proper administration technique
   Washing hands immediately after application to remove any medication that may be on them
» Importance of not using more medication than the amount prescribed
» Proper dosing
   Missed dose:
      For solution dosage form—Using as soon as possible; not using if almost time for next dose; using next dose at regularly scheduled time
      For gel dosage form—Using as soon as possible; not using if not remembered until next day; using next dose at regularly scheduled time
      For eye system dosage form—Replacing as soon as possible; inserting next eye system at regularly scheduled time
» Proper storage
*For gel or solution dosage forms*
   Preventing contamination: Not touching applicator tip to any surface; keeping container tightly closed
*For ocular system dosage form*
   Reading patient instructions carefully before using
   Not using if damaged
   Removing and replacing with new unit if too much medicine is being released

### Precautions while using this medication
   Regular visits to physician to check eye pressure during therapy
» Caution if blurred vision or change in near or far vision occurs, especially at night

### Side/adverse effects
   Signs of potential side effects, especially symptoms of systemic absorption or eye pain

## General Dosing Information
Tolerance to pilocarpine may develop with prolonged use. Effectiveness may be restored by changing to another miotic for a short time and then resuming the original medication.

### For the ocular system dosage form
The system should be placed in the eye at bedtime so that the pilocarpine-induced myopia may reach a stable level by morning.

Damaged or deformed systems should not be placed or retained in the eye. If a system is believed to be associated with an unexpected increase in action of the medication, it should be removed and replaced with a new system.

### For the solution dosage forms
Although some manufacturers recommend a dose of 2 drops of an ophthalmic solution at appropriate intervals, the conjunctival sac will usually hold only 1 drop.

To avoid excessive systemic absorption, patient should press finger to the lacrimal sac during and for 1 or 2 minutes following instillation of the solution.

Although some manufacturers recommend that patients not wear soft contact lenses during treatment with pilocarpine ophthalmic solution, USP medical experts do not believe this precaution is necessary unless the patient has corneal epithelial problems and the medication is to be used more often than once every 1 to 2 hours. No significant problems have been documented with ophthalmic solutions containing 0.03% or less of benzalkonium chloride as a preservative that are used in patients with no significant corneal surface problems.

# Ophthalmic Dosage Forms

## PILOCARPINE OCULAR SYSTEM USP

### Usual adult and adolescent dose
Antiglaucoma agent (ophthalmic)—
    Topical, to the conjunctiva, 1 ocular system delivering 20 or 40 mcg (0.02 or 0.04 mg) per hour, once every seven days.

### Usual pediatric dose
Antiglaucoma agent (ophthalmic)—
    Infants: Safety and efficacy have not been established.
    Children: See *Usual adult and adolescent dose.*

### Usual geriatric dose
See *Usual adult and adolescent dose.*

### Strength(s) usually available
U.S.—
    20 mcg (0.02 mg) per hour for seven days (Rx) [*Ocusert Pilo-20*].
    40 mcg (0.04 mg) per hour for seven days (Rx) [*Ocusert Pilo-40*].
Canada—
    20 mcg (0.02 mg) per hour for seven days (Rx) [*Ocusert Pilo-20*].
    40 mcg (0.04 mg) per hour for seven days (Rx) [*Ocusert Pilo-40*].

### Packaging and storage
Store between 2 and 8 °C (36 and 46 °F).

### Auxiliary labeling
• For the eye.
• Refrigerate.

### Note
Include patient instructions when dispensing.

## PILOCARPINE HYDROCHLORIDE OPHTHALMIC GEL

### Usual adult and adolescent dose
Antiglaucoma agent (ophthalmic)—
    Topical, to the conjunctiva, approximately 1.5 cm (1/2-inch strip) of a 4% gel once a day at bedtime.

### Usual pediatric dose
Antiglaucoma agent (ophthalmic)—
    Safety and efficacy have not been established.

### Usual geriatric dose
See *Usual adult and adolescent dose.*

### Strength(s) usually available
U.S.—
    4% (Rx) [*Pilopine HS*].
Canada—
    4% (Rx) [*Pilopine HS*].

### Packaging and storage
Store between 2 and 8 °C (36 and 46 °F), in a tight container, unless otherwise specified by manufacturer. Protect from freezing.

### Stability
The 5-gram size requires refrigeration; the 3.5-gram size can be stored at room temperature.

### Auxiliary labeling
• For the eye.
• Keep container tightly closed.

## PILOCARPINE HYDROCHLORIDE OPHTHALMIC SOLUTION USP

### Usual adult and adolescent dose
Antiglaucoma agent (ophthalmic)—
    Chronic glaucoma:
        Topical, to the conjunctiva, 1 drop of a 0.5 to 4% solution up to four times a day.
    Acute angle-closure glaucoma:
        Topical, to the conjunctiva, 1 drop of a 1 or 2% solution every five to ten minutes for three to six doses, then 1 drop every one to three hours until intraocular pressure is reduced.
    Note: To possibly avoid a bilateral attack of angle-closure glaucoma, 1 drop of a 1 or 2% solution may be instilled in the unaffected eye every six to eight hours. However, more intensive treatment may precipitate an attack in the unaffected eye and should be avoided.
Miotic—
    To counteract mydriatic effects of sympathomimetics:
        Topical, to the conjunctiva, 1 drop of a 1% solution.

Prior to surgery for congenital glaucoma (goniotomy):
    Topical, to the conjunctiva, 1 drop of a 2% solution every four to six hours (usually for one or two doses) before surgery.
Prior to iridectomy:
    Topical, to the conjunctiva, 1 drop of a 2% solution for four doses immediately before surgery.

### Usual pediatric dose
See *Usual adult and adolescent dose.*
Note: For infants, the administration of solutions with strengths greater than 1% is not recommended.

### Usual geriatric dose
See *Usual adult and adolescent dose.*

### Strength(s) usually available
U.S.—
    0.25% (Rx) [*Isopto Carpine;* GENERIC].
    0.5% (Rx) [*Isopto Carpine; Ocu-Carpine; Pilocar; Piloptic-1/2; Pilostat;* GENERIC].
    1% (Rx) [*Adsorbocarpine; Akarpine; Isopto Carpine; Ocu-Carpine; Pilocar; Piloptic-1; Pilostat;* GENERIC].
    2% (Rx) [*Adsorbocarpine; Akarpine; Isopto Carpine; Ocu-Carpine; Pilocar; Piloptic-2; Pilostat;* GENERIC].
    3% (Rx) [*Isopto Carpine; Ocu-Carpine; Pilocar; Piloptic-3; Pilostat;* GENERIC].
    4% (Rx) [*Adsorbocarpine; Akarpine; Isopto Carpine; Ocu-Carpine; Pilocar; Piloptic-4; Pilostat;* GENERIC].
    5% (Rx) [*Isopto Carpine; Ocu-Carpine;* GENERIC].
    6% (Rx) [*Isopto Carpine; Ocu-Carpine; Pilocar; Piloptic-6; Pilostat;* GENERIC].
    8% (Rx) [*Isopto Carpine;* GENERIC].
    10% (Rx) [*Isopto Carpine*].
Canada—
    0.5% (Rx) [*Isopto Carpine*].
    1% (Rx) [*Isopto Carpine; Miocarpine; Pilostat; Spersacarpine*].
    2% (Rx) [*Isopto Carpine; Miocarpine; Pilostat; Spersacarpine*].
    4% (Rx) [*Isopto Carpine; Miocarpine; Pilostat; Spersacarpine*].
    6% (Rx) [*Isopto Carpine; Miocarpine*].

### Packaging and storage
Store below 40 °C (104 °F), preferably between 15 and 30 °C (59 and 86 °F), unless otherwise specified by manufacturer. Store in a tight container. Protect from freezing.

### Auxiliary labeling
• For the eye.
• Keep container tightly closed.

## PILOCARPINE NITRATE OPHTHALMIC SOLUTION USP

### Usual adult and adolescent dose
Antiglaucoma agent (ophthalmic)—
    Chronic glaucoma:
        Topical, to the conjunctiva, 1 drop of a 1 to 4% solution two to four times a day.
    Acute angle-closure glaucoma:
        Topical, to the conjunctiva, 1 drop of a 1 or 2% solution every five to ten minutes for three to six doses, then 1 drop every one to three hours until intraocular pressure is reduced.
    Note: To possibly avoid a bilateral attack of angle-closure glaucoma, 1 drop of a 1 or 2% solution may be instilled in the unaffected eye every six to eight hours. However, more intensive treatment may precipitate an attack in the unaffected eye and should be avoided.
Miotic—
    To counteract mydriatic effects of sympathomimetics:
        Topical, to the conjunctiva, 1 drop of a 1% solution.
    Prior to surgery for congenital glaucoma (goniotomy):
        Topical, to the conjunctiva, 1 drop of a 2% solution every four to six hours (usually for one or two doses) before surgery.
    Prior to iridectomy:
        Topical, to the conjunctiva, 1 drop of a 2% solution for four doses immediately before surgery.

### Usual pediatric dose
See *Usual adult and adolescent dose.*
Note: For infants, the administration of solutions with strengths greater than 1% is not recommended.

### Usual geriatric dose
See *Usual adult and adolescent dose.*

**Strength(s) usually available**

U.S.—

1% (Rx) [*Pilagan*].

2% (Rx) [*Pilagan*].

4% (Rx) [*Pilagan*].

Canada—

1% (Rx) [*P.V. Carpine Liquifilm*].

2% (Rx) [*Minims Pilocarpine; P.V. Carpine Liquifilm*].

4% (Rx) [*Minims Pilocarpine; P.V. Carpine Liquifilm*].

**Packaging and storage**

Store below 40 °C (104 °F), preferably between 15 and 30 °C (59 and 86 °F), unless otherwise specified by manufacturer. Store in a tight, light-resistant container. Protect from freezing.

**Auxiliary labeling**

• For the eye.

• Keep container tightly closed.

• Shake well.

Revised: 06/21/95

---

# PILOCARPINE    Systemic†

VA CLASSIFICATION (Primary): XX000

Note: For a listing of dosage forms and brand names by country availability, see *Dosage Forms* section(s). For a listing of brand names for the articles in this monograph, refer to the General Index.

†Not commercially available in Canada.

## Category

Cholinergic.

## Indications

**Accepted**

Xerostomia (treatment)—Pilocarpine is indicated for the treatment of xerostomia from salivary gland hypofunction caused by radiotherapy for cancer of the head and neck.

## Pharmacology/Pharmacokinetics

**Physicochemical characteristics**

Molecular weight—Pilocarpine hydrochloride: 244.72.

pKa—7.15.

**Mechanism of action/Effect**

Pilocarpine is a cholinergic parasympathomimetic agent that exerts a broad spectrum of pharmacologic effects with predominantly muscarinic action, including stimulation of exocrine function. This stimulation results in increased secretion by the exocrine glands, including the salivary glands.

**Other actions/effects**

Other exocrine glands, such as the sweat, lacrimal, gastric, pancreatic, and intestinal glands, may be stimulated.

Pulmonary effects may include stimulation of the mucous cells of the respiratory tract, increased airway resistance, and increased bronchial smooth muscle tone and secretions.

Cardiovascular effects may include changes in hemodynamics and cardiac rhythm. However, pilocarpine may have paradoxical effects. Instead of the expected muscarinic effect of vasodepression occurring, pilocarpine may produce short-lived hypotension followed by hypertension. In addition, both bradycardia and tachycardia have been reported.

Gastrointestinal effects include smooth muscle stimulation of the intestinal tract that may result in increased tone and motility, spasm, and tenesmus. The tone and motility of the urinary tract, gallbladder, and biliary duct smooth muscle may be enhanced.

**Biotransformation**

Not fully understood; inactivation of pilocarpine is thought to occur at the neuronal synapses and in the plasma.

**Half-life**

Elimination—0.76 hours after 2 days of 5 mg of pilocarpine administered orally 3 times daily; 1.35 hours after 2 days of 10 mg of pilocarpine administered orally 3 times daily.

**Onset of action**

20 minutes.

**Time to peak concentration**

1.25 or 0.85 hours, after 2 days of 5 or 10 mg, respectively, of pilocarpine administered orally 3 times daily.

**Peak serum concentration**

15 or 41 nanograms per mL (72 or 196.8 nanomoles per L), after 2 days of 5 or 10 mg, respectively, of pilocarpine administered orally 3 times daily.

Pharmacokinetic studies were done in young men and men and women over 65 years of age after administration of 5 or 10 mg oral pilocarpine 3 times daily for 2 days. The pharmacokinetics were comparable in men under and over 65 years. However, all 5 of the women over 65 years of age in the study had mean maximum concentrations ($C_{max}$) that were approximately twice as high as the men's values. The men's $C_{max}$ values were 15 and 41 nanograms per mL (72 and 196.8 nanomoles per L) after the 5 and 10 mg dosage, respectively. No pharmacokinetic values are available for younger women.

**Time to peak effect**

1 hour.

**Duration of action**

3 to 5 hours.

**Elimination**

Not fully understood; in the urine, as unchanged pilocarpine and its minimally active or inactive degradation products, such as pilocarpic acid.

In dialysis—It is not known if pilocarpine is dialyzable.

## Precautions to Consider

**Cross-sensitivity and/or related problems**

Patients sensitive to ophthalmic pilocarpine may be sensitive to oral pilocarpine also.

**Carcinogenicity**

Studies have not been done.

**Mutagenicity**

Pilocarpine did not cause genetic toxicity in bacterial assays (*Salmonella* and *E. coli*) for reverse gene mutations, *in vitro* chromosome aberration assay (micronucleus test) in mice, and primary DNA damage assay (unscheduled DNA synthesis) in rat hepatocyte primary cultures.

**Pregnancy/Reproduction**

Fertility—Studies have not been done in humans.

Male rats given 39 mg per kg of body weight (mg/kg) per day of pilocarpine (approximately 10 times the usual human dose) exhibited morphologic evidence of reduced spermatogenesis.

Pregnancy—Studies have not been done in humans.

Fetuses of pregnant rats given 90 mg/kg per day of pilocarpine (approximately 26 times the maximum recommended human dose) had reduced mean body weight and an increased incidence of skeletal variations. However, these effects may have been secondary to maternal toxicity.

FDA Pregnancy Category C.

**Breast-feeding**

It is not known whether pilocarpine is distributed into breast milk. However, problems in humans have not been documented.

**Pediatrics**

Appropriate studies on the relationship of age to the effects of oral pilocarpine have not been performed in the pediatric population. Safety and efficacy have not been established.

**Geriatrics**

Appropriate studies performed to date have not demonstrated geriatric-specific problems that would limit the usefulness of oral pilocarpine in the elderly.

Clinical trials were conducted in both men and women under and over 65 years of age. The adverse events reported by these 4 groups were comparable. In addition, pharmacokinetic studies were done in young men and men and women over 65 years of age after administration of 5 or 10 mg oral pilocarpine 3 times daily for 2 days. The pharmacokinetics were comparable in men under and over 65 years. However, all 5 of the women over 65 years of age in the study had mean maximum concentrations ($C_{max}$) and trapezoidal values of the areas under the curve (AUC) that were approximately twice as high as the men's values. The men's $C_{max}$ values were 15 and 41 nanograms per mL (72 and 196.8 nanomoles per L) after the 5 and 10 mg dosage, respectively. The men's AUC trapezoidal values were 33 and 108 h (nanograms per mL) after the 5 and 10 mg dosage, respectively.

**Drug interactions and/or related problems**
The following drug interactions and/or related problems have been selected on the basis of their potential clinical significance (possible mechanism in parentheses where appropriate)—not necessarily inclusive (» = major clinical significance):

Note: Combinations containing any of the following medications, depending on the amount present, may also interact with this medication.

» Anticholinergics or other medications with anticholinergic activity
(See *Appendix II*)
(concurrent use may cause an antagonism of pilocarpine's therapeutic cholinergic effect)

(concurrent use may cause an antagonism of the anticholinergic drug's anticholinergic effects; this may be important not only when the drug is being used therapeutically for its anticholinergic effects, but also when the drug has other therapeutic effects and its anticholinergic side effects are being used as indicators of impending adverse effects)

» Antiglaucoma agents, cholinergic, long acting, ophthalmic or
» Antiglaucoma agents, cholinergic, short acting, ophthalmic or
» Bethanechol or
» Cholinergics, other, or other medications with cholinergic activity, such as antimyasthenics
(concurrent use with pilocarpine may result in additive cholinergic effects)

» Beta-adrenergic blocking agents, systemic and ophthalmic
(concurrent use with pilocarpine may increase the possibility of conduction disturbances)

**Medical considerations/Contraindications**
The medical considerations/contraindications included here have been selected on the basis of their potential clinical significance (reasons given in parentheses where appropriate)—not necessarily inclusive (» = major clinical significance).

*Except under special circumstances, this medication should not be used when the following medical problems exist:*

» Asthma, uncontrolled
(pilocarpine may stimulate the mucous cells of the respiratory tract and may increase airway resistance and bronchial smooth muscle tone)

» Glaucoma, angle closure or
» Iritis, acute
(pilocarpine may cause miosis)

» Sensitivity to pilocarpine

*Risk-benefit should be considered when the following medical problems exist:*

» Asthma, controlled or
» Bronchitis, chronic or
» Chronic obstructive pulmonary disease
(pilocarpine may stimulate the mucous cells of the respiratory tract and may increase airway resistance and bronchial smooth muscle tone)

» Biliary tract disease or
» Cholelithiasis, known or suspected
(pilocarpine may cause contractions of the gallbladder or biliary smooth muscle and cholecystitis, cholangitis, or biliary obstruction may occur)

» Cardiovascular disease
(patients with significant cardiovascular disease may be unable to compensate for the transient changes in hemodynamics or heart rhythm that are induced by pilocarpine; pulmonary edema has occurred as a complication of pilocarpine toxicity from high ophthalmic doses and may occur with oral pilocarpine also)

» Cognitive disturbances or
» Psychiatric disturbances
(pilocarpine may have central nervous system effects, which may exacerbate these conditions)

Nephrolithiasis
(pilocarpine may increase ureteral smooth muscle tone and may theoretically precipitate renal colic, especially in patients with nephrolithiasis)

» Retinal detachment, predisposition to or
» Retinal disease
(an association between use of ophthalmic pilocarpine and retinal detachment has been reported in patients with pre-existing retinal disease; it is not known whether this association may occur with oral pilocarpine)

**Patient monitoring**
The following may be especially important in patient monitoring (other tests may be warranted in some patients, depending on condition; » = major clinical significance):

Fundus examination
(should be performed periodically in patients with pre-existing retinal disease, since an association between use of ophthalmic pilocarpine and retinal detachment has been reported in patients with pre-existing retinal disease; it is not known whether this association may occur with oral pilocarpine)

# Side/Adverse Effects

Note: Pilocarpine toxicity is characterized by an exaggeration of its parasympathomimetic effects.

The following side/adverse effects have occurred in less than 1% of patients treated with pilocarpine; however, the causal relationship is unknown: anorexia, anxiety, deafness, depression, dysuria, electrocardiogram abnormality, esophagitis, eye pain, glaucoma, hyperkinesia, hypoesthesia, hypothermia, leukopenia, lymphadenopathy, metrorrhagia, paresthesias, seborrhea, speech disorder, stridor, syncope, and urinary impairment. In addition, 1 patient experienced a myocardial infarction and 1 patient had an episode of syncope; both patients had underlying cardiovascular disease.

The following side/adverse effects have occurred rarely in patients treated with ophthalmic pilocarpine: agitation, atrioventricular block, ciliary congestion, confusion, delusion, depression, dermatitis, iris cysts, macular hole, malignant glaucoma, middle ear disturbance, shock, and visual hallucination.

The following side/adverse effects have been selected on the basis of their potential clinical significance (possible signs and symptoms in parentheses where appropriate)—not necessarily inclusive:

**Those indicating need for medical attention only if they continue or are bothersome**
Incidence more frequent
*Sweating*
Incidence less frequent or rare
*Amblyopia* (trouble seeing); *asthenia* (unusual weak feeling); *chills; diarrhea; dizziness; dyspepsia* (indigestion); *dysphagia* (trouble swallowing); *edema* (holding more body water; swelling of face, fingers, ankles, or feet); *epistaxis* (nosebleeds); *flushing* (redness of face or feeling of warmth); *headache; hypertension; nausea; rhinitis* (runny nose); *tachycardia* (fast heartbeat); *tremors* (trembling or shaking); *urinary frequency* (passing urine more often); *voice change; vomiting*

# Overdose

For specific information on the agents used in the management of systemic pilocarpine overdose, see:
• *Atropine* in *Anticholinergics/Antispasmodics (Systemic)* monograph; and/or
• *Epinephrine* in *Bronchodilators, Adrenergic (Systemic)* monograph.

For more information on the management of overdose or unintentional ingestion, **contact a Poison Control Center** (see *Poison Control Center Listing*).

Pilocarpine toxicity is characterized by an exaggeration of its parasympathomimetic effects. One hundred mg of pilocarpine is considered to be potentially fatal.

**Clinical effects of overdose**
The following effects have been selected on the basis of their potential clinical significance (possible signs and symptoms in parentheses where appropriate)—not necessarily inclusive:

Acute and chronic
*Arrhythmia* (irregular heartbeat, continuing or severe); *atrioventricular block* (chest pain or fainting); *bradycardia* (slow heartbeat, con-

tinuing or severe); *confusion; diarrhea, continuing or severe; gastrointestinal spasm* (stomach cramps or pain); *headache, continuing or severe; hypertension; hypotension* (tiredness or weakness, continuing or severe); *nausea, continuing or severe; respiratory distress* (shortness of breath or troubled breathing); *shock* (fainting or tiredness or weakness, continuing or severe); *tachycardia* (fast heartbeat, continuing or severe); *tremors* (trembling or shaking, continuing or severe); *visual disturbance, continuing or severe* (trouble seeing, continuing or severe); *vomiting, continuing or severe*

### Treatment of overdose

0.5 to 1 mg of atropine should be administered subcutaneously or intravenously.

Supportive measures to maintain respiration and circulation should be used.

For severe cardiovascular depression or bronchoconstriction, 0.3 to 1 mg of epinephrine should be administered subcutaneously or intramuscularly.

## Patient Consultation

As an aid to patient consultation, refer to *Advice for the Patient, Pilocarpine (Systemic)*.

In providing consultation, consider emphasizing the following selected information (» = major clinical significance):

### Before using this medication
» Conditions affecting use, especially:
  Sensitivity to ophthalmic or oral pilocarpine
  Use in children—Safety and efficacy have not been established
  Other medications, especially anticholinergics or other medications with anticholinergic activity; antiglaucoma agents, cholinergic, long acting, ophthalmic; antiglaucoma agents, cholinergic, short acting, ophthalmic; beta-adrenergic blocking agents, systemic and ophthalmic; bethanechol; or cholinergics, other, or other medications with cholinergic activity
  Other medical problems, especially asthma, controlled; asthma, uncontrolled; biliary tract disease; bronchitis, chronic; cardiovascular disease; cholelithiasis, known or suspected; chronic obstructive pulmonary disease; cognitive disturbances; glaucoma, angle closure; iritis, acute; psychiatric disturbances; retinal detachment, predisposition to; or retinal disease

### Proper use of this medication
» Taking medication only as directed; not taking it more often and not taking larger dose than directed; doing so may increase chance of side/adverse effects
  Importance of seeing dentist regularly to prevent dental and other mouth problems, which are more likely to occur in patients with xerostomia
» Proper dosing
  Missed dose: Taking as soon as possible; skipping missed dose if it is almost time for next dose; not doubling doses
» Proper storage

### Precautions while using this medication
» Caution if difficulty in reading or other vision problems occur; caution if dizziness or lightheadedness occurs; not driving, using machines, or doing anything else that could be dangerous if not alert or able to see well; checking with physician if reactions are especially bothersome
» Importance of drinking enough liquids to offset the sweating that medication may cause

### Side/adverse effects
Signs of potential side effects, especially signs of overdose

## General Dosing Information

The lowest dosage that is effective should be used, since the incidence of side/adverse effects is dose dependent.

## Oral Dosage Forms

### PILOCARPINE HYDROCHLORIDE TABLETS

#### Usual adult and adolescent dose
Xerostomia (treatment)——
  Oral, 5 mg three times a day. Dosage may be increased up to 10 mg three times a day for patients who do not respond to lower doses; however, increasing the dose also increases the incidence of side/adverse effects. The lowest dose that is tolerated and effective should be used for maintenance.

#### Usual pediatric dose
Safety and efficacy have not been established.

#### Strength(s) usually available
U.S.—
  5 mg (Rx) [*Salagen*].
Canada—
  Not commercially available.

#### Packaging and storage
Store at controlled room temperature between 15 and 30 °C (59 and 86 °F).

## Selected Bibliography

LeVeque FG, Montgomery M, Potter D, et al. A multicenter, randomized, double-blind, placebo-controlled, dose-titration study of oral pilocarpine for treatment of radiation-induced xerostomia in head and neck cancer patients. J Clin Oncol 1993 Jun; 11 (6): 1124-31.

Johnson JT, Ferretti GA, Nethery WJ, et al. Oral pilocarpine for post-irradiation xerostomia in patients with head and neck cancer. N Engl J Med 1993 Aug 5; 329 (6): 390-5.

Wolff A, Atkinson JC, Macynski AA, et al. Oral complications of cancer therapies. Pretherapy interventions to modify salivary dysfunction. NCI Monogr 1990; (9): 87-90.

Developed: 01/17/95
Interim revision: 03/15/95

---

# PIMOZIDE    Systemic

VA CLASSIFICATION (Primary/Secondary): CN900/CN709

Note: For a listing of dosage forms and brand names by country availability, see *Dosage Forms* section(s). For a listing of brand names for the articles in this monograph, refer to the General Index.

## Category

Antidyskinetic (Gilles de la Tourette's syndrome); antipsychotic.

## Indications

Note: Bracketed information in the *Indications* section refers to uses that are not included in U.S. product labeling.

### Accepted

Gilles de la Tourette's syndrome (treatment)[1]—Pimozide is indicated for the suppression of motor and vocal tics in patients with Tourette's disorder whose symptoms are severe and who cannot tolerate or have failed to respond satisfactorily to haloperidol.

[Psychotic disorders (treatment)]—Pimozide is used for maintenance therapy in the management of *chronic* schizophrenic patients *without* symptoms of excitement, agitation, or hyperactivity.

### Unaccepted
Pimozide must not be used for simple tics or tics that are not associated with Tourette's disorder because of the high risk of cardiovascular and extrapyramidal effects.

Pimozide is ineffective and should not be used for the management of patients with mania or acute schizophrenia.

---

[1]Not included in Canadian product labeling.

## Pharmacology/Pharmacokinetics

### Physicochemical characteristics
Chemical group—A diphenylbutylpiperidine analog of butyrophenone and a derivative of the meperidine-like analgesics.
Molecular weight—461.55.

### Mechanism of action/Effect
Pimozide's exact mechanism of action in Tourette's disorder has not been established; however, pimozide is thought to block dopamine nonselectively at both the pre- and postsynaptic receptors on neurons in the central nervous system (CNS).

Secondary changes in central dopamine function and metabolism, such as altered dopamine release and increased brain turnover of dopamine (but not of norepinephrine), may also contribute to both therapeutic and adverse effects. There are also various effects, not fully characterized, on other CNS receptor systems.

In psychotic disorders, pimozide is thought to have more specific dopamine receptor blocking activity, less potential for inducing sedation, and fewer autonomic effects than other neuroleptic agents.

### Absorption
Poor; 50% absorbed after oral administration.

### Biotransformation
Significant first-pass metabolism, primarily by N-dealkylation in the liver; two major metabolites of undetermined neuroleptic activity.

### Half-life
Plasma—
    Average: 29 hours.
    Range: 19 to 39 hours.
Elimination—
    55 hours in schizophrenic patients, with significant interindividual variation.

### Time to peak concentration
6 to 8 hours (range, 4 to 12 hours).

### Elimination
Within 1 week—
    Renal—50%.
    Fecal—20%.

## Precautions to Consider

### Cross-sensitivity and/or related problems
Patients sensitive to neuroleptic agents such as haloperidol, loxapine, molindone, phenothiazines, or thioxanthenes may also be sensitive to pimozide.

### Carcinogenicity
In a 24-month carcinogenicity study of rats receiving up to 50 times the maximum recommended human dose (MRHD), no increased incidence of overall tumors or tumors at any site was observed in either sex. The meaning of these results is unclear because of the limited number of animals that survived the study.

### Tumorigenicity
Studies in mice have shown that pimozide causes a dose-related increase in benign pituitary and mammary gland tumors. The mechanism for induction is unknown.

Pituitary gland tumors, in female mice only, developed as hyperplasia at doses approximating the human dose, and as adenoma at doses about 15 times the MRHD, on a mg-per-kg basis.

Mammary gland tumors increased in female mice treated with pimozide, which elevates serum prolactin concentrations. Prolactin concentrations increase in humans, also, with chronic administration of antipsychotic agents. Tissue culture experiments indicate that after chronic administration of antipsychotic agents, approximately $^1/_3$ of human breast cancers are prolactin-dependent *in vitro,* a factor of potential importance if the prescription of these drugs is contemplated in a patient with previously detected breast cancer or if the patient is young and chronic use of the medication is anticipated.

### Mutagenicity
Pimozide did not have mutagenic activity in the Ames test with four bacterial test strains, in the mouse dominant lethal test, or in the micronucleus test in rats.

### Pregnancy/Reproduction
Fertility—Studies in rats have shown prolonged estrus cycles and fewer pregnancies. These effects are thought to be due to an inhibition of or delay in implantation, which has also been observed in rodents administered other antipsychotic agents.

Pregnancy—Adequate and well-controlled studies in humans have not been done.

Studies in rats given doses 8 times the maximum human dose showed retarded fetal development. In rabbits, maternal toxicity, mortality, decreased weight gain, and embryotoxicity, including increased resorptions, were dose-related.

FDA Pregnancy Category C.

### Breast-feeding
It is not known whether pimozide is excreted in breast milk. Problems in humans have not been documented, although there is potential for maternal mammary gland tumor formation and unknown cardiovascular effects in the infant.

### Pediatrics
Because its use and safety have not been evaluated in other childhood disorders, pimozide is not recommended for use in children with any condition other than Tourette's disorder.

In Tourette's disorder, a gradual initiation of pimozide therapy in patients up to 12 years of age is recommended since information on safety and efficacy is very limited. Children may be especially sensitive to the effects of pimozide.

### Geriatrics
Geriatric patients tend to develop higher plasma concentrations because of changes in distribution due to decreases in lean body mass, total body water, and albumin, and often an increase in total body fat composition. These patients usually require lower initial dosage and a more gradual titration of dose. Also, elderly patients are more prone to develop transient hypotension and exhibit an increased sensitivity to the anticholinergic and sedative effects of pimozide.

In addition, older patients tend to develop extrapyramidal side effects more frequently, especially persistent tardive dyskinesia and parkinsonism. Tardive dyskinesia may be difficult to control and, in some patients, appears to be irreversible. The symptoms of tardive dyskinesia may be masked during therapy but may appear after reduction of dose or withdrawal of pimozide. There is no known effective treatment. Careful observation during pimozide therapy for early signs of tardive dyskinesia and reduction of dosage or discontinuation of medication may prevent a more severe manifestation of the syndrome.

### Dental
The peripheral anticholinergic effects of pimozide may decrease or inhibit salivary flow, especially in middle-aged or elderly patients, thus contributing to the development of caries, periodontal disease, oral candidiasis, and discomfort.

Extrapyramidal reactions induced by pimozide will result in increased motor activity of the head, face, and neck. Occlusal adjustments, bite registrations, and treatment for bruxism may be made less reliable.

The blood dyscrasia–causing effects of pimozide may result in an increased incidence of microbial infection, delayed healing, and gingival bleeding. If leukopenia or thrombocytopenia occurs, dental work should be deferred until blood counts have returned to normal. Patients should be instructed in proper oral hygiene, including caution in use of regular toothbrushes, dental floss, and toothpicks.

### Drug interactions and/or related problems
The following drug interactions and/or related problems have been selected on the basis of their potential clinical significance (possible mechanism in parentheses where appropriate)—not necessarily inclusive (» = major clinical significance):

Note: Combinations containing any of the following medications, depending on the amount present, may also interact with this medication.

» Alcohol or
» CNS depression–producing medications, other (See *Appendix II*)
    (concurrent use with pimozide may potentiate the CNS depressant effects of these medications)

» Amphetamines or
» Methylphenidate or
» Pemoline
    (concurrent use with pimozide may mask the cause of tics since these medications themselves may provoke tics; before therapy with pimozide is initiated, these medications should be withdrawn)

» Anticholinergics or other medications with anticholinergic activity (See *Appendix II*)
    (concurrent use with pimozide may intensify anticholinergic effects, especially those of dry mouth, constipation, and unusual excitability, because of secondary anticholinergic effects of pimozide)

Anticonvulsants
    (although there has been no primary documentation for a drug interaction with pimozide and anticonvulsants, the potential exists for a lowering of the convulsive threshold with concurrent use; dosage adjustment of anticonvulsant may be necessary when pimozide treatment is initiated or discontinued or when the dose is reduced)

» Antidepressants, tricyclic or
» Disopyramide or
» Maprotiline or
» Phenothiazines or
» Procainamide or
» Quinidine
    (concurrent use of these agents with pimozide may potentiate cardiac arrhythmias, which are seen on electrocardiogram [ECG] as prolongation of the QT interval)

    (in addition, concurrent use of phenothiazines with pimozide may potentiate the anticholinergic, CNS depressant, and extrapyramidal effects of both medications)

» Extrapyramidal reaction–causing medications, other (See *Appendix II*) (concurrent use of these agents with pimozide may increase the anticholinergic, CNS depressant, and extrapyramidal effects of both medications)

**Laboratory value alterations**
The following have been selected on the basis of their potential clinical significance (possible effect in parentheses where appropriate)—not necessarily inclusive (» = major clinical significance):

With diagnostic test results
» Electrocardiogram [ECG]
(may result in prolongation of QT interval; flattening, notching, and inversion of the T-wave; and the appearance of U-waves)
Pregnancy tests, immunologic urine
(pimozide may produce false-positive results)

**Medical considerations/Contraindications**
The medical considerations/contraindications included here have been selected on the basis of their potential clinical significance (reasons given in parentheses where appropriate)—not necessarily inclusive (» = major clinical significance).

*Except under special circumstances, this medication should not be used when the following medical problems exist:*
» Cardiac arrhythmias, history of or
» Long QT syndrome, congenital
(may be aggravated by use of pimozide, predisposing patients to ventricular arrhythmias)
» CNS depression, severe or
» Comatose states
(may be potentiated)
» Tics, motor or vocal, other than those caused by Tourette's disorder
(risk of cardiovascular and extrapyramidal effects)

*Risk-benefit should be considered when the following medical problems exist:*
» Breast cancer, history of
(may be aggravated by increased serum prolactin concentrations)
Hepatic function impairment or
Renal function impairment
(metabolism and excretion of pimozide may be altered)
» Hypokalemia
(potassium deficiency, especially from diarrhea or use of diuretics, should be corrected before initiation of pimozide therapy because of risk of ventricular arrhythmias)
Sensitivity to pimozide or other neuroleptics, such as haloperidol, loxapine, molindone, phenothiazines, or thioxanthenes

**Patient monitoring**
The following may be especially important in patient monitoring (other tests may be warranted in some patients, depending on condition; » = major clinical significance):
» Electrocardiogram [ECG]
(recommended at initiation of therapy, as baseline, and periodically thereafter, especially during dosage adjustment; any indications of prolongation of the QT interval beyond an absolute limit of 0.47 seconds in children, 0.52 seconds in adults, or more than 25% of the patient's original baseline, should be considered a basis for stopping increase of dosage or reducing dose)
Careful observation for early signs of tardive dyskinesia, especially in the elderly or patients on high or extended maintenance dosage
(recommended at periodic intervals, especially in the elderly and patients on high or extended maintenance dosage; since there is no known effective treatment if syndrome should develop, pimozide should be discontinued, if clinically feasible, at earliest signs, usually fine, worm-like movements of the tongue, to stop further development)
Careful observation for early symptoms of tardive dystonia
(recommended at periodic intervals; since there is no known effective treatment if syndrome should develop, pimozide should be discontinued, if clinically feasible, at the earliest signs)

## Side/Adverse Effects

The following side/adverse effects have been selected on the basis of their potential clinical significance (possible signs and symptoms in parentheses)—not necessarily inclusive:

**Those indicating need for medical attention**
Incidence more frequent
*Akathisia* (restlessness or need to keep moving); *arrhythmias, ventricular* (fast or irregular heartbeat)—seen on ECG as prolonged QT interval; *extrapyramidal effects, parkinsonian* (difficulty in speaking; loss of balance control; mask-like face; shuffling walk; slowed movements; stiffness of arms and legs; trembling and shaking of fingers and hands); *mood or behavior changes*
Note: *Parkinsonian extrapyramidal effects* often occur during first few days of treatment, even at relatively low doses, and are usually mild to moderately severe.

Incidence less frequent
*Extrapyramidal reactions, dystonic* (difficulty in swallowing; inability to move eyes; muscle spasms, especially of the face, neck, or back; twisting movements of the body); *tardive dyskinesia, persistent* (lip smacking or puckering; puffing of cheeks; rapid or worm-like movements of tongue; uncontrolled chewing movements; uncontrolled movements of arms and legs)
Note: *Tardive dyskinesia* is initially dose related, but may increase with long-term treatment and total cumulative dose; may persist after discontinuation of pimozide.

Incidence rare
*Blood dyscrasias* (sore throat and fever; unusual bleeding or bruising); *jaundice, obstructive* (yellow eyes or skin); *neuroleptic malignant syndrome (NMS)* (convulsions; difficult or unusually fast breathing; high fever; high or low [irregular] blood pressure; increased sweating; loss of bladder control; severe muscle stiffness); *tardive dystonia* (increased blinking or spasms of eyelid; unusual facial expressions or body positions; uncontrolled twisting movements of neck, trunk, arms, or legs); *tiredness or weakness; unusually pale skin*
Note: Additional signs of *NMS* may include fast heartbeat, elevated creatine phosphokinase (CPK), myoglobinuria [rhabdomyolysis], and acute renal failure. NMS may occur at any time during neuroleptic therapy, but is more commonly seen soon after start of therapy, or after patient has switched from one neuroleptic to another, during combined therapy with another psychotropic medication, or after a dosage increase.

**Those indicating need for medical attention only if they continue or are bothersome**
Incidence more frequent
*Blurred vision or other vision problems; constipation; drowsiness; dryness of mouth; hypotension, orthostatic* (dizziness, lightheadedness, or fainting, especially when getting up from a lying or sitting position); *skin rash, itching, or discoloration; swelling or soreness of breasts; unusual secretion of milk*
Incidence less frequent
*Decreased sexual ability; diarrhea; headache; loss of appetite and weight; mental depression; nausea and vomiting; swelling of the face*

**Those indicating the need for medical attention if they occur after the medication is discontinued**
*Dyskinesia, withdrawal emergent* (lip smacking or puckering; puffing of cheeks; rapid or worm-like movements of tongue; uncontrolled chewing movements; uncontrolled movements of arms and legs)

## Overdose

For specific information on the agents used in the management of pimozide overdose, see:
• *Albumin Human (Systemic)* monograph;
• *Benztropine* in *Antidyskinetics (Systemic)* monograph;
• *Diphenhydramine* in *Antihistamines (Systemic)* monograph; and/or
• *Norepinephrine* in *Sympathomimetic Agents–Cardiovascular Use (Parenteral-Systemic)* monograph.

For more information on the management of overdose or unintentional ingestion, **contact a Poison Control Center** (see *Poison Control Center Listing*).

**Clinical effects of overdose**
The following effects have been selected on the basis of their potential clinical significance (possible signs and symptoms in parentheses where appropriate)—not necessarily inclusive:
*Drowsiness or dizziness, severe, or comatose state; muscle trembling, jerking, stiffness, or uncontrolled movements, severe; troubled breathing, severe; unusual tiredness or weakness, severe*

**Treatment of overdose**
Treatment is essentially symptomatic and supportive and may include:
To decrease absorption—
Inducing emesis or initiating gastric lavage.
Specific treatment—
Counteracting hypotension and circulatory collapse with use of intravenous fluids, plasma, or concentrated albumin, and vasopressor agents such as norepinephrine. Epinephrine should *not* be used since it may cause paradoxical hypotension.

Administering benztropine or diphenhydramine to manage severe extrapyramidal reactions.

Monitoring—

Immediately monitoring ECG and continuing until parameters are
within normal range.

Observing patients for at least 4 days because of long half-life of
pimozide.

Supportive care—

Establishing a patent airway.

Mechanically assisting respiration, if necessary.

Patients in whom intentional overdose is known or suspected should
be referred for psychiatric consultation.

## Patient Consultation

As an aid to patient consultation, refer to *Advice for the Patient, Pimozide
(Systemic)*.

In providing consultation, consider emphasizing the following selected
information (» = major clinical significance):

**Before using this medication**

» Conditions affecting use, especially:

Sensitivity to pimozide or other neuroleptic agents

Pregnancy—Animal studies have shown fewer pregnancies; retarded fetal development; maternal toxicity; mortality; decreased weight gain; embryotoxicity; increased resorptions

Use in children—Not recommended for any condition other than
Tourette's syndrome; therapy should be initiated gradually in
patients up to 12 years of age; children are more sensitive to
effects of pimozide

Use in the elderly—Elderly patients are more likely to develop
extrapyramidal, anticholinergic, hypotensive, and sedative effects; reduced dosage recommended

Dental—Pimozide-induced blood dyscrasias may result in infections, delayed healing, and bleeding; dry mouth may cause caries, candidiasis, periodontal disease, and discomfort; increased
motor activity of face, head, and neck may interfere with some
dental procedures

Other medications, especially alcohol, other CNS depression–producing medications, amphetamines, methylphenidate, pemoline, tricyclic antidepressants, disopyramide, maprotiline, phenothiazines, other extrapyramidal reaction–producing
medications, procainamide, quinidine, or anticholinergics

Other medical problems, especially cardiac arrhythmias, tics other
than those caused by Tourette's disorder, severe CNS depression, history of breast cancer, or hypokalemia

**Proper use of this medication**

» Importance of not taking more medication than the amount prescribed

» Proper dosing

Missed dose: Taking as soon as possible; taking any remaining doses
for that day at regularly spaced intervals; not doubling doses

» Proper storage

**Precautions while using this medication**

Regular visits to physician to check progress of therapy

» Checking with physician before discontinuing medication; gradual
dosage reduction may be needed

» Avoiding use of alcoholic beverages or other CNS depressants during
therapy

» Possible drowsiness, blurred vision, or muscle stiffness; caution when
driving, using machinery, or doing other things requiring alertness,
clear vision, and good muscle control

Possible dizziness or lightheadedness; avoiding getting up suddenly
from a sitting or lying position

» Caution if any kind of surgery, dental treatment, or emergency surgery
is required

Possible dryness of mouth; using sugarless gum or candy, ice, or saliva
substitute for relief; checking with physician or dentist if dry
mouth continues for more than 2 weeks

**Side/adverse effects**

Side effects more likely in children and elderly or debilitated patients

» Stopping medication and notifying physician immediately if symptoms
of neuroleptic malignant syndrome (NMS) appear

» Notifying physician as soon as possible if early symptoms of tardive
dyskinesia appear

Possibility of withdrawal symptoms

Signs of potential side effects, especially akathisia, ventricular arrhythmias, parkinsonism, mood or behavior changes, dystonic reactions,
tardive dyskinesia or dystonia, blood dyscrasias, obstructive jaundice, or NMS

## General Dosing Information

Periodic attempts should be made to reduce the dosage of pimozide gradually to see whether tics persist at the level and extent first identified.
In doing so, consideration should be given to the possibility that any
increases in tic intensity and frequency may represent a transient with-
drawal-related phenomenon rather than a return of disease symptoms.
Two to three weeks should elapse before a final conclusion is reached
that an increase in tic manifestations is a function of the underlying
disease syndrome rather than a response to pimozide withdrawal. Also,
spontaneous remission and fluctuating symptoms may occur in many
patients, since pimozide's poor absorption and presystemic metabolism
profile may result in a highly variable absorption from day to day.

**For treatment of adverse reactions**

Neuroleptic malignant syndrome (NMS)—

Treatment is essentially symptomatic and supportive and may include the following:

• *Discontinuing pimozide immediately*.

• Hyperthermia—Administering antipyretics (aspirin or acetaminophen); using cooling blanket.

• Dehydration—Restoring fluids and electrolytes.

• Cardiovascular instability—Monitoring blood pressure and
cardiac rhythm closely.

• Hypoxia—Administering oxygen; consider airway insertion
and assisted ventilation.

• Muscle rigidity—Dantrolene sodium may be administered
(100 to 300 mg per day in divided doses; 1.25 to 1.5 mg per
kg of body weight [mg/kg], intravenously). Bromocriptine (5
to 7.5 mg every eight hours) has been used to reverse hyperpyrexia and muscle rigidity.

Parkinsonism—

Many medical authorities advise that the only appropriate treatment
of extrapyramidal symptoms is reduction of the antipsychotic dosage, if possible, to the lowest effective dose. Oral antidyskinetic
agents, such as trihexyphenidyl (2 mg three times a day) or benztropine, may be effective in treating more severe parkinsonism and
acute motor restlessness but are used sparingly, and then usually
for no longer than 3 months. Extrapyramidal symptoms may reappear if both pimozide and the antidyskinetic agent are discontinued
simultaneously. The antidyskinetic agent may have to be continued
after pimozide is discontinued because of different excretion rates.
Milder effects may be treated by adjusting dosage.

Akathisia—

Restlessness may be treated with antiparkinsonian medications, or with
propranolol (30 to 120 mg a day), nadolol (40 mg a day), pindolol
(5 to 60 mg a day), lorazepam (1 or 2 mg two or three times a
day), or diazepam (2 mg two or three times a day).

Dystonia—

Acute dystonic postures or oculogyric crisis may be relieved by parenteral administration of benztropine (2 mg intramuscularly); diphenhydramine (50 mg intramuscularly); or diazepam (5 to 7.5 mg
intravenously), to be followed by oral antidyskinetic medication
for one or two days to prevent recurrent dystonic episodes. Dosage
adjustments of pimozide may control these effects.

Tardive dyskinesia or tardive dystonia—

No known effective treatment. Dosage of pimozide should be lowered
or medication discontinued, if clinically feasible, at earliest signs
of tardive dyskinesia or tardive dystonia, to prevent irreversible
effects.

## Oral Dosage Forms

Note: Bracketed uses in the *Dosage Forms* section refer to categories of
use and/or indications that are not included in U.S. product labeling.

### PIMOZIDE TABLETS USP

**Usual adult and adolescent dose**

Tourette's disorder[1]—

Oral, initially, 1 to 2 mg a day in divided doses, the dosage being
increased gradually every other day as needed and tolerated.

Note: Most patients are maintained at daily doses of up to 200 mcg
(0.2 mg) per kg of body weight, or 10 mg a day, whichever is
less.

[Psychotic disorders]—

Oral, 2 to 4 mg once a day, the dosage being increased at weekly
intervals by 2 to 4 mg a day.

Note: The average maintenance dose is 6 mg a day, with a usual range
of 2 to 12 mg a day. Daily doses above 30 mg are seldom
required.

**Usual adult prescribing limits**
Up to 300 mcg (0.3 mg) per kg of body weight a day or 20 mg a day in
divided doses.

**Usual pediatric dose**
Tourette's disorder[1] or
[Psychotic disorders]—
Children up to 12 years of age: Dosage has not been established.
Children 12 years of age and over: See *Usual adult and adolescent
dose.*

**Strength(s) usually available**
U.S.—
2 mg (Rx) [*Orap* (scored; calcium stearate; cellulose; lactose; corn
starch)].
Canada—
2 mg (Rx) [*Orap* (scored; tartrazine; lactose)].
4 mg (Rx) [*Orap* (scored; tartrazine; lactose)].
10 mg (Rx) [*Orap* (scored; tartrazine; lactose)].

**Packaging and storage**
Store below 40 °C (104 °F), preferably between 15 and 30 °C (59 and 86
°F), unless otherwise specified by manufacturer. Store in a tight, light-
resistant container.

**Auxiliary labeling**
• May cause drowsiness.
• Avoid alcoholic beverages.

[1]Not included in Canadian product labeling.

Revised: 04/16/93

---

**PINDOLOL**—See *Beta-adrenergic Blocking Agents (Systemic)*

---

# PINDOLOL-CONTAINING COMBINATIONS—
Pindolol and Hydrochlorothiazide (Systemic)—See *Beta-adrenergic
Blocking Agents and Thiazide Diuretics (Systemic)*

---

# PIPECURONIUM   Systemic†

VA CLASSIFICATION (Primary): MS300
Note: For a listing of dosage forms and brand names by country availability, see *Dosage Forms* section(s). For a listing of brand names
for the articles in this monograph, refer to the General Index.

†Not commercially available in Canada.

## Category
Neuromuscular blocking agent.

## Indications
**Accepted**
Muscle (skeletal) relaxation, for surgery—Pipecuronium is indicated as an
adjunct to anesthesia to induce skeletal muscle relaxation and to facilitate the management of patients undergoing mechanical ventilation.
Pipecuronium has a long duration of action and is recommended only
for surgical procedures expected to last 90 minutes or longer.

**Unaccepted**
Pipecuronium has not been adequately studied, and is not presently recommended, for facilitating prolonged mechanical ventilation in intensive care patients, for administration prior to or following use of other
nondepolarizing neuromuscular blocking agents, or for obstetrical use
(Cesarean section).

## Pharmacology/Pharmacokinetics
Note: Pharmacokinetic studies on the volume of distribution, distribution
and elimination half-lives, and clearance of pipecuronium have
been done in a limited number of patients; data presented below
must be considered preliminary and subject to interpatient
variability.

**Physicochemical characteristics**
Molecular weight—798.74.

**Mechanism of action/Effect**
Pipecuronium is a nondepolarizing neuromuscular blocking agent. Neuromuscular blocking agents produce skeletal muscle paralysis by
blocking neural transmission at the myoneural junction. The paralysis
is selective initially and usually appears in the following muscles consecutively: levator muscles of eyelids, muscles of mastication, limb
muscles, abdominal muscles, muscles of the glottis, and finally, the
intercostal muscles and the diaphragm. Neuromuscular blocking agents
have no clinically significant effect on consciousness or the pain
threshold.
Nondepolarizing neuromuscular blocking agents inhibit neuromuscular
transmission by competing with acetylcholine for the cholinergic receptors of the motor end plate, thereby reducing the response of the
end plate to acetylcholine. This type of neuromuscular block is usually
antagonized by anticholinesterase agents.

**Distribution**
Volume of distribution (steady-state)—
Normal renal function: 0.25 (range, 0.12–0.37) L per kg of body
weight.
Renal function impairment: 0.37 (range, 0.28–0.51) L per kg of body
weight.

**Half-life**
Distribution—
Normal renal function: 6.22 (range, 1.34–10.66) minutes.
Renal function impairment: 4.33 (range, 1.69–6.17) minutes.
Elimination—
Normal renal function: 1.7 (range, 0.9–2.7) hours. The elimination
half-life is not altered by hypothermia and bypass.
Renal function impairment: 4 (range, 2.0–8.2) hours.

**Onset of action**
Intubating conditions are achieved in 2.5 to 3 minutes with doses of 70
to 100 mcg per kg of body weight (mcg/kg). The time to achieve
intubating conditions may be somewhat longer when lower doses are
administered.

**Time to peak effect**
In adults, maximum (95%) suppression of the twitch response to peripheral nerve stimulation is achieved in about 5.5 to 6 minutes following
a dose of 50 mcg/kg and in about 3 to 5 minutes after single doses of
70 to 85 mcg/kg. The peak effect time is not significantly affected by
the type of anesthesia administered.

**Duration of action**
Initial dose—
Adults:
Long-acting; dependent on dose and on type of anesthesia. With
neurolept (nitrous oxide/fentanyl/droperidol) anesthesia, the expected duration of clinical effect (time until the twitch response
returns to 25% of the control value as determined using a peripheral nerve stimulator) is about 30 minutes following a dose
of 50 mcg/kg. With "balanced" anesthesia (in which a neuromuscular blocking agent may be used together with other
medications, such as an induction agent [e.g., an ultrashort-
acting barbiturate or propofol], an opioid analgesic, and an inhalation anesthetic [usually nitrous oxide]), doses of 70 to 85
mcg/kg usually provide about 1 to 2 hours of clinical relaxation. Values ranging from 30 to 175 minutes have been reported with 70 mcg/kg and values ranging from 40 to 211
minutes have been reported with 80 to 85 mcg/kg. After the
twitch response has recovered to 25% of control, spontaneous
recovery to 50% of the control value takes about 24 minutes
(range, 8 to 131 minutes) and spontaneous recovery to 75% of
the control value takes about 33 minutes.
When pipecuronium is administered following recovery from succinylcholine-assisted endotracheal intubation, a dose of 50
mcg/kg provides about 45 minutes of clinical relaxation, and a
dose of 70 to 85 mcg/kg provides the same clinical duration
as without prior administration of succinylcholine.

Infants and children:

Intermediate- to long-acting and age-dependent; the expected duration of clinical effect (time until the twitch response returns to 25% of the control value as determined using a peripheral nerve stimulator) provided by an effective dose is about 13 minutes in infants < 3 months of age, 10 to 44 minutes in infants 3 months to 1 year of age, and 18 to 52 minutes in children 1 to 14 years of age. After the twitch response has recovered to 25% of control, spontaneous recovery to 75% of the control value takes about 25 to 30 minutes.

Maintenance doses—

Adults:

The expected clinical duration of additional doses of 10 to 15 mcg/kg, administered when the twitch response has returned to 25% of the control value, is about 50 (range, 17 to 175) minutes.

Note: The clinical duration of initial and maintenance doses is increased by use of enflurane or isoflurane, and possibly by other potentiating medications, but is not significantly prolonged by halothane.

In patients with renal function impairment, the duration of action is more variable than in patients with normal renal function; accumulation of pipecuronium may lead to a significant prolongation of neuromuscular blockade.

No significant correlation was found between the duration of pipecuronium-induced neuromuscular blockade and the pharmacokinetic variables studied (volume of distribution, distribution and elimination half-lives, and plasma clearance) in a study in patients with normal renal function.

## Elimination

Renal—In one study in patients undergoing coronary artery bypass surgery who received 200 mcg/kg (double the currently recommended maximum adult dose), 56% of the administered dose was excreted in the urine within 24 hours, 41% of the dose as unchanged pipecuronium and 15% as the active 3-decacetyl metabolite. In animals, this metabolite has about 40 to 50% of the activity of the parent compound.

Clearance—0.12 to 0.15 L per kg of body weight per hour (L/kg/hr) in patients with normal renal function and 0.08 L/kg/hr in patients with renal function impairment.

# Precautions to Consider

## Cross-sensitivity and/or related problems

Patients sensitive to bromides may be sensitive to pipecuronium bromide also.

## Mutagenicity

No evidence of mutagenicity was found in the Ames test or the Sister Chromatid Exchange test.

## Pregnancy/Reproduction

Fertility—Animal studies have not been done.

Pregnancy—Adequate and well-controlled studies have not been done in pregnant women.

Pipecuronium did not cause teratogenicity in rats receiving up to 50 mcg per kg of body weight intravenously. However, the highest dose caused embryotoxicity (increase in early fetal resorptions) secondary to maternal toxicity.

FDA Pregnancy Category C.

Labor and delivery—Pipecuronium is not recommended for use in obstetrics (Cesarean section) because of insufficient information on placental transfer and possible consequent effects on the neonate. Also, pipecuronium's duration of action exceeds the expected duration of Cesarean section.

## Breast-feeding

It is not known whether pipecuronium is distributed into breast milk. However, problems in nursing babies have not been reported.

## Pediatrics

Children 1 to 14 years of age are less sensitive to the effects of pipecuronium than are adults or infants < 1 year of age. The duration of clinical effect (time to recovery of the twitch response to 25% of the control value) is shorter in infants and children than in adults.

## Geriatrics

One study in patients 66 to 79 years of age has shown that response and dosage requirements for pipecuronium are not significantly different in geriatric patients than in younger adults. However, whether the results reported in the relatively few elderly patients studied to date can be applied to the geriatric population in general has not been determined. Also, elderly patients are more likely to have age-related renal function impairment, which requires caution and possibly dosage reduction and/or longer intervals between doses in patients receiving pipecuronium.

## Drug interactions and/or related problems

The following drug interactions and/or related problems have been selected on the basis of their potential clinical significance (possible mechanism in parentheses where appropriate)—not necessarily inclusive (» = major clinical significance):

Note: Combinations containing any of the following medications, depending on the amount present, may also interact with this medication.

Some of the following interactions have not been documented with pipecuronium. However, because they have been reported to occur with other nondepolarizing neuromuscular blocking agents, the possibility of a significant interaction with pipecuronium must be considered.

» Aminoglycosides, possibly including oral neomycin (if significant quantities are absorbed in patients with renal function impairment) or

» Anesthetics, parenteral-local (large doses leading to significant plasma concentrations) or

Bacitracin or

» Capreomycin or

» Citrate-anticoagulated blood (massive transfusions) or

» Clindamycin or

Colistin or

Colistimethate sodium or

Lidocaine (intravenous doses > 5 mg/kg) or

» Lincomycin or

» Polymyxins or

Procaine (intravenous) or

Tetracyclines or

Trimethaphan (large doses)

(neuromuscular blocking activity of these medications may be additive to that of neuromuscular blocking agents; increased or prolonged respiratory depression or paralysis [apnea] may occur, but is of minor clinical significance while the patient is being mechanically ventilated; however, caution and careful monitoring of the patient are recommended during and following concurrent or sequential use, especially if there is a possibility of incomplete reversal of neuromuscular blockade postoperatively)

Analgesics, opioid (narcotic), especially those commonly used as adjuncts to anesthesia

(central respiratory depressant effects of opioid analgesics may be additive to the respiratory depressant effects of neuromuscular blocking agents; increased or prolonged respiratory depression or paralysis [apnea] may occur, but is of minor clinical significance while the patient is being mechanically ventilated; however, caution and careful monitoring of the patient are recommended during and following concurrent or sequential use, especially if there is a possibility of incomplete reversal of neuromuscular blockade postoperatively)

(although specific information for pipecuronium is not available, high doses of sufentanil reduce initial dosage requirements for other nondepolarizing neuromuscular blocking agents; it is recommended that a peripheral nerve stimulator be used to determine dosage)

(concurrent use of a neuromuscular blocking agent prevents or reverses muscle rigidity induced by sufficiently high doses of most opioid analgesics, especially alfentanil, fentanyl, or sufentanil)

(pipecuronium has no vagolytic activity and will therefore not decrease the risk of opioid analgesic–induced bradycardia or hypotension; in some patients [especially patients with compromised cardiac function and/or those receiving a beta-adrenergic blocking agent preoperatively], the incidence and/or severity of these effects may be increased)

Anesthetics, hydrocarbon inhalation, such as:

Chloroform

Cyclopropane

Enflurane

Ether

Halothane

Isoflurane

Methoxyflurane

Trichloroethylene

(neuromuscular blocking activity of inhalation hydrocarbon anesthetics, especially enflurane or isoflurane, may be additive to that of nondepolarizing neuromuscular blocking agents; enflurane and isoflurane have been shown to increase pipecuronium's duration of action by about 50% and 12%, respectively, but halothane has not been shown to prolong pipecuronium's effects significantly)

Antimyasthenics or
Edrophonium
  (these agents antagonize the effects of nondepolarizing neuromuscular blocking agents; parenteral neostigmine or pyridostigmine are indicated to reverse neuromuscular blockade following surgery; edrophonium in a dose of 0.5 mg per kg of body weight [mg/kg] is not recommended for reversal of pipecuronium because it has been reported to be less effective than neostigmine [dose of 40 mcg (0.04 mg)/kg]; use of higher doses of edrophonium or of pyridostigmine for reversal of pipecuronium has not been studied)
  (neuromuscular blocking agents may antagonize the effects of antimyasthenics on skeletal muscle; temporary dosage adjustment may be required to control symptoms of myasthenia gravis following surgery)

Calcium salts
  (calcium salts may reverse the effects of nondepolarizing neuromuscular blocking agents)

Doxapram
  (the residual effects of neuromuscular blocking agents may be masked temporarily by doxapram when it is used post-anesthesia)

Magnesium salts, parenteral or
» Procainamide or
» Quinidine
  (these medications may enhance the blockade of the neuromuscular blocking agents; increased or prolonged respiratory depression or paralysis [apnea] may occur but is of minor clinical significance while the patient is being mechanically ventilated; however, caution and careful monitoring of the patient are recommended during and following concurrent or sequential use, especially if there is a possibility of incomplete reversal of neuromuscular blockade postoperatively)

Neuromuscular blocking agents, other
  (pipecuronium may be administered following recovery from succinylcholine when the latter has been administered to facilitate endotracheal intubation; administration of pipecuronium prior to succinylcholine, to prevent or attenuate succinylcholine-induced side effects, has not been studied)
  (administration of pipecuronium in conjunction with other nondepolarizing neuromuscular blocking agents has not been studied)

Potassium-depleting medications, such as:
Adrenocorticoids, glucocorticoid, especially with significant mineralocorticoid activity
Adrenocorticoids, mineralocorticoid
Amphotericin B
Bumetanide
Carbonic anhydrase inhibitors
Corticotropin, chronic therapeutic use of
Ethacrynic acid
Furosemide
Indapamide
Thiazide diuretics
  (serum potassium determinations and correction of serum potassium concentration may be necessary prior to administration of pipecuronium because hypokalemia induced by these medications may enhance the blockade of nondepolarizing neuromuscular blocking agents; increased or prolonged respiratory depression or paralysis [apnea] may occur but is of minor clinical significance while the patient is being mechanically ventilated; however, caution and careful monitoring of the patient are recommended during and following concurrent or sequential use, especially if there is a possibility of incomplete reversal of neuromuscular blockade postoperatively)

**Laboratory value alterations**
The following have been selected on the basis of their potential clinical significance (possible effect in parentheses where appropriate)—not necessarily inclusive (» = major clinical significance):

With physiology/laboratory test values
Creatinine concentration and
Potassium concentration
  (may be increased—incidence of each < 1%)

Glucose concentration, in blood
  (may be increased—incidence < 1%)

**Medical considerations/Contraindications**
The medical considerations/contraindications included here have been selected on the basis of their potential clinical significance (reasons given in parentheses where appropriate)—not necessarily inclusive (» = major clinical significance).

*Risk-benefit should be considered when the following medical problems exist:*
Biliary obstruction or
Hepatic function impairment
  (time to onset and maximum effect, pharmacokinetics, and dosage requirements of pipecuronium have not been studied in patients with moderate or severe hepatic function impairment or biliary obstruction)

Carcinoma, bronchogenic
  (duration of action of neuromuscular blocking agents may be prolonged)

Cardiovascular disease leading to slower circulation time or
Edema or
Other conditions associated with increased distribution volume
  (time to onset of action and maximum effect of pipecuronium may be prolonged; a delay in readiness for intubation or surgery should be anticipated and allowed; administration of higher doses of pipecuronium to compensate for a delayed response is not recommended)

Dehydration or
Electrolyte or acid-base imbalance
  (action of neuromuscular blocking agents may be altered; neuromuscular blockade is usually counteracted by alkalosis and enhanced by acidosis, but mixed imbalances may be present, leading to unpredictable responses)

Hypothermia
  (intensity and duration of action of nondepolarizing neuromuscular blocking agents may be increased)

Myasthenia gravis or
Myasthenic syndrome (Eaton-Lambert syndrome)
  (risk of severe and prolonged muscle paralysis or weakness; a neuromuscular blocking agent with a shorter duration of action may be preferable [although caution is required even with shorter-acting agents])

Pulmonary function impairment or
Respiratory depression
  (risk of additive respiratory depression or impairment)

Renal function impairment, mild or moderate or
» Renal function impairment, severe
  (duration of action of pipecuronium may be prolonged or unpredictable; a reduction in dosage may be necessary, but use of a neuromuscular blocking agent with a more predictable duration of action in patients with renal function impairment [e.g., atracurium or vecuronium] may be preferable)

Sensitivity to pipecuronium or to bromides

## Side/Adverse Effects

Note: Unlike gallamine and pancuronium, pipecuronium has no vagolytic activity. Also, unlike several other neuromuscular blocking agents [especially tubocurarine, and, to a somewhat lesser extent, atracurium, metocurine, or succinylcholine], pipecuronium has not been reported to cause histamine release. It therefore causes minimal hemodynamic disturbance, although bradycardia and/or hypotension may occur because pipecuronium does not counteract the bradycardia and/or hypotension induced by other medications (e.g., anesthetics, opioid analgesics) or vagal stimulation.

The following side/adverse effects have been selected on the basis of their potential clinical significance (possible signs and symptoms in parentheses where appropriate)—not necessarily inclusive:

**Those indicating need for medical attention**
Incidence less frequent (1% or higher)
  *Bradycardia, clinically significant*—incidence 1.4%; *hypotension, clinically significant*—incidence 2.5%
Incidence rare (< 1%)
  *Anuria; atelectasis; atrial fibrillation; cerebrovascular accident; CNS depression; dyspnea; hypertension; hypesthesia; laryngismus; muscle atrophy; myocardial ischemia; respiratory depression; skin rash; thrombosis; urticaria; ventricular extrasystole*

## Overdose

For specific information on the agents used in the management of pipecuronium overdose, see:
  • *Atropine (Systemic)* in *Anticholinergics/Antispasmodics (Systemic)* monograph; and/or
  • *Neostigmine* in *Antimyasthenics (Systemic)* monograph.

For more information on the management of overdose, **contact a Poison Control Center** (see *Poison Control Center Listing*).

**Treatment of overdose**
Specific treatment—
  Administering anticholinesterase agents, such as neostigmine, to antagonize the action of pipecuronium. Edrophonium (0.5 mg/kg) does not sufficiently antagonize the effects of the medication, i.e., it does not increase the twitch response to peripheral nerve stimulation to 70% of the control value or higher, especially when potent hydrocarbon inhalation anesthetics (enflurane or isoflurane) have been administered. Use of higher doses of edrophonium or of pyridostigmine for antagonism of pipecuronium has not been studied. It is recommended that atropine or another suitable anticholinergic agent be administered prior to or concurrently with the antagonist to counteract its muscarinic side effects. However, use of an antagonist is merely an adjunct to, and not to be substituted for, the institution of measures to ensure adequate ventilation. Ventilatory assistance must be continued until the patient can maintain an adequate ventilatory exchange unassisted.
Monitoring—
  Determining the nature and degree of the neuromuscular blockade, using a peripheral nerve stimulator.
  Monitoring of vital organ function for the period of paralysis and for an extended period post-recovery.
  Monitoring the patient following successful antagonism, because the duration of action of pipecuronium may exceed that of the antagonist.
Supportive care for apnea or prolonged paralysis—
  Maintaining an adequate airway and assisting or controlling ventilation. Artificial respiration should be continued until adequate spontaneous ventilation can be maintained.

# General Dosing Information

Neuromuscular blocking agents have no clinically significant effect on consciousness or the pain threshold; therefore, when used as an adjunct to surgery, the neuromuscular blocking agent should always be used with adequate anesthesia.

Since neuromuscular blocking agents may cause respiratory depression, they should be used only by those individuals experienced in the techniques of tracheal intubation, artificial respiration, and the administration of oxygen under positive pressure; facilities for these procedures should be immediately available.

Pipecuronium is intended for intravenous administration only.

The stated doses are intended as a guideline. Actual dosage must be individualized. It is recommended that a peripheral nerve stimulator be used to monitor response, need for additional doses, and reversal.

The $ED_{95}$ (dose of pipecuronium that will produce a 95% suppression of the twitch response to peripheral nerve stimulation) during balanced anesthesia in adults (geriatric patients as well as younger adults) may range from 21 to 77 (average, 41) mcg per kg of body weight. In infants < 1 year of age, the $ED_{95}$ is within the same range as for adults (generally about 33 to 48 mcg/kg). In children 1 to 14 years of age, the $ED_{95}$ may range from 47 to 80 mcg/kg. In patients of all ages, the $ED_{95}$ is significantly reduced with enflurane or isoflurane, but not halothane, anesthesia (as compared with balanced or neurolept anesthesia).

For obese patients (> 30% above ideal body weight for height), dosage of pipecuronium should be calculated on the basis of ideal body weight. Administration of pipecuronium to obese patients in doses based on actual body weight significantly prolongs the medication's effects.

When nondepolarizing neuromuscular blocking agents are administered concurrently with potent general anesthetics such as enflurane, ether, isoflurane, methoxyflurane, or cyclopropane, a reduction in dosage, as determined using a peripheral nerve stimulator, may be required. However, halothane has not been shown to potentiate significantly the effect of pipecuronium.

It is recommended that reversal of pipecuronium-induced neuromuscular blockade with an antagonist (e.g., neostigmine) be attempted only after some spontaneous recovery, as demonstrated using a peripheral nerve stimulator, has first taken place. Recovery will not occur as rapidly if the antagonist is administered earlier.

# Parenteral Dosage Forms

## PIPECURONIUM BROMIDE FOR INJECTION

**Usual adult dose**
Initial:
  For intubation: Intravenous, 70 to 85 mcg (0.07 to 0.085 mg) per kg of actual body weight (normal weight patients) or ideal body weight (obese patients). The lowest dose recommended to provide adequate intubation conditions is 50 mcg per kg of body weight, but the onset of action may be delayed with this dose.
  For administration following recovery from succinylcholine-facilitated endotracheal intubation: Intravenous, 50 mcg (0.05 mg) per kg of actual body weight (normal weight patients) or ideal body weight (obese patients) to provide about 45 minutes of relaxation, or 70 to 85 mcg (0.07 to 0.085 mg) per kg of body weight to provide about 1 to 2 hours of muscle paralysis.
Maintenance:
  Intravenous, after recovery of the twitch response to peripheral nerve stimulation to 25% of control, 10 to 15 mcg (0.01 to 0.015 mg) per kg of body weight. Lower doses may be sufficient for patients receiving inhalation anesthesia.
Note: For patients with renal function impairment, dosage should be based on creatinine clearance as well as body weight. The following initial doses are recommended:

| Creatinine Clearance (mL/min) | Dose (mcg/kg ideal body weight) |
|---|---|
| <40 | 50 |
| 60 | 55 |
| 80 | 70 |
| 100 | 85 |
| >100 | Up to 100 |

**Usual adult prescribing limits**
Intravenous, 100 mcg (0.1 mg) per kg of actual body weight (normal weight patients) or ideal body weight (obese patients).

**Usual pediatric and adolescent dose**
Initial—
  Infants up to 3 months of age: Dosage has not been established.
  Infants 3 to 12 months of age: Intravenous, 40 mcg (0.04 mg) per kg of body weight (provides about 10 to 44 minutes of clinical relaxation).
  Children 1 to 14 years of age: Intravenous, 57 mcg (0.057 mg) per kg of body weight (provides 18 to 52 minutes of clinical relaxation).
  Adolescents over 14 years of age: See *Usual adult dose*.
Maintenance—
  Dosage has not been established.

**Usual geriatric dose**
See *Usual adult dose*.

**Size(s) usually available**
U.S.—
  10 mg (Rx) [*Arduan* (mannitol 380 mg)].
Canada—
  Not commercially available.

**Packaging and storage**
Before reconstitution—
  Store between 2 and 30 °C (36 and 86 °F), protected from light, unless otherwise specified by manufacturer.
After reconstitution—
  Bacteriostatic water for injection as diluent: Store at room temperature (15 to 30 °C [59 to 86 °F]) or in a refrigerator (2 to 8 °C [36 to 46 °F]).
  Other injections as diluent: Store in a refrigerator.

**Preparation of dosage form**
Pipecuronium bromide for injection may be reconstituted with 0.9% sodium chloride injection, 5% dextrose in sodium chloride injection, 5% dextrose in water injection, lactated Ringer's injection, sterile water for injection, or bacteriostatic water for injection. Reconstitution using 10 mL of diluent provides a solution containing 10 mg per mL of pipecuronium bromide.
Caution: Use of diluents containing benzyl alcohol (e.g., bacteriostatic water for injection) is not recommended for preparation of medications for use in neonates. A fatal toxic syndrome consisting of metabolic acidosis, CNS depression, respiratory problems, renal failure, hypotension, and possibly seizures and intracranial hemorrhages has been associated with this use.

**Stability**
The vial of pipecuronium bromide is intended for single-dose use only; unused portions of the reconstituted solution should be discarded.
After reconstitution with bacteriostatic water for injection, pipecuronium should be administered within 5 days.
After reconstitution with injections other than bacteriostatic water for injection, pipecuronium should be administered within 24 hours.

## Selected Bibliography

Larijani GE, Bartkowski RR, Azad SS et al. Clinical pharmacology of pipecuronium bromide. Anesth Analg 1989; 68: 734-9.

Foldes FF, Nagashima H, Nguyen HD, Duncalf D, Goldiner PL. Neuromuscular and cardiovascular effects of pipecuronium. Can J Anaesth 1990 Jul; 37: 549-55.

Pittet JF, Tassonyi E, Morel DR et al. Pipecuronium-induced neuromuscular blockade during nitrous oxide–fentanyl, isoflurane, and halothane anesthesia in adults and children. Anesthesiology 1989 71; 210-3.

Revised: 08/13/91

---

**PIPERACILLIN**—See *Penicillins (Systemic)*

---

## PIPERACILLIN-CONTAINING COMBINATIONS—

Piperacillin and Tazobactam (Systemic)—See *Penicillins and Beta-lactamase Inhibitors (Systemic)*

---

# PIPERAZINE    Systemic

VA CLASSIFICATION (Primary): AP200

Note: For a listing of dosage forms and brand names by country availability, see *Dosage Forms* section(s). For a listing of brand names for the articles in this monograph, refer to the General Index.

## Category

Anthelmintic (systemic).

## Indications

### Accepted

Ascariasis (treatment); or

Enterobiasis (treatment)—Piperazine is indicated as alternative treatment for ascariasis caused by *Ascaris lumbricoides* (roundworm) and enterobiasis (oxyuriasis) caused by *Enterobius vermicularis* (pinworm). Piperazine is especially useful in the treatment of partial intestinal obstruction caused by *Ascaris* worms, which is a condition primarily seen in children. The use of albendazole, flubendazole, mebendazole, or pyrantel pamoate is generally preferred in the treatment of ascariasis and enterobiasis because they are effective in single doses.

## Pharmacology/Pharmacokinetics

### Physicochemical characteristics

Molecular weight—Piperazine adipate: 232.3.
Piperazine citrate: 642.66.

### Mechanism of action/Effect

Piperazine blocks the response of the worm muscle (best studied in *Ascaris*), causing flaccid paralysis of the worm. While the worm is paralyzed, it is dislodged from the intestinal lumen and expelled live from the body by normal intestinal peristalsis.

### Absorption

Rapidly absorbed from the gastrointestinal tract.

### Biotransformation

Approximately 25% is metabolized in the liver. Piperazine is nitrosated to form N-mononitrosopiperazine (MNPz) in gastric juice and further metabolized to N-nitroso-3-hydroxypyrrolidine (NHPYR).

### Half-life

Plasma half-life is highly variable.

### Time to peak plasma concentration:

2 to 4 hours.

### Elimination

Renal—Approximately 20% is excreted unchanged in the urine within 24 hours.

## Precautions to Consider

### Cross-sensitivity and/or related problems

There has been a report of cross-reactivity between piperazine and ethylenediamine, a substance used as a stabilizer in topical creams. Piperazine can cause a contact allergy that could be life-threatening in a person who has been sensitized to ethylenediamine either by topical application or by occupational exposure. Although rare, adverse dermatologic problems also may occur due to the cross-sensitivity of these two medications.

### Carcinogenicity

A potentially carcinogenic nitrosamine derivative, N-mononitrosopiperazine (MNPz), has been found in gastric juice and urine of volunteers given therapeutic doses of piperazine. However, the significance of this finding is unknown.

### Tumorigenicity/Mutagenicity

Studies have not been done to determine the tumorigenicity or mutagenicity of piperazine.

### Pregnancy/Reproduction

Pregnancy—Adequate and well-controlled studies in humans have not been done. Piperazine has been used without apparent adverse effects during pregnancy. In three cases of first-trimester exposures to piperazine by pregnant women, no malformations were seen in the fetuses. However, because a study showed that orally administered piperazine undergoes partial conversion to a potentially carcinogenic nitrosamine derivative, it is recommended that piperazine be given to pregnant women only if clearly indicated and then only if alternative drugs are not available.

Studies in animals (rats and pigs) have failed to demonstrate any teratogenic effects of piperazine on the fetus.

### Breast-feeding

Piperazine is thought to be distributed into breast milk but no definitive information is available. However, problems in humans have not been documented.

### Pediatrics

Appropriate studies on the relationship of age to the effects of piperazine have not been performed in the pediatric population. No pediatrics-specific problems have been documented to date. However, because of piperazine's potential neurotoxicity, it should be used with caution in children. Prolonged or repeated treatment with piperazine in children should be avoided.

### Geriatrics

No information is available on the relationship of age to the effects of piperazine in geriatric patients.

### Drug interactions and/or related problems

The following drug interactions and/or related problems have been selected on the basis of their potential clinical significance (possible mechanism in parentheses where appropriate)—not necessarily inclusive (» = major clinical significance):

Note: Combinations containing any of the following medications, depending on the amount present, may also interact with this medication.

» Phenothiazines, such as chlorpromazine
   (high doses of piperazine may enhance the effects of chlorpromazine and increase the risk of seizures; concurrent use is not recommended)

» Pyrantel
   (pyrantel may antagonize the anthelmintic effects of piperazine; concurrent use is not recommended)

### Medical considerations/Contraindications

The medical considerations/contraindications included here have been selected on the basis of their potential clinical significance (reasons given in parentheses where appropriate)—not necessarily inclusive (» = major clinical significance).

### *Risk-benefit should be considered when the following medical problems exist:*

» Hepatic function impairment
   (because piperazine is partially metabolized in the liver, accumulation of piperazine may occur, with an increased incidence of side effects)

Hypersensitivity reactions to piperazine and its salts, history of

» Renal function impairment
(urinary excretion is the primary route of elimination of piperazine; therefore, high concentrations of piperazine may accumulate in patients with renal dysfunction, resulting in neurotoxicity)

» Seizure disorders, especially a history of epilepsy
(seizures may be exacerbated)

**Patient monitoring**

The following may be especially important in patient monitoring (other tests may be warranted in some patients, depending on condition; » = major clinical significance):

*For pinworms*

» Perianal examinations
(cellophane tape swabbing of the perianal area to detect the presence of eggs may be required prior to treatment to confirm the diagnosis of pinworms; swabbing is done again one week following treatment with piperazine, especially in patients with persisting symptoms; swabbing should be done every morning prior to defecation and bathing for at least 3 days to determine efficacy or proof of cure; perianal examinations may also be required to detect the presence of adult worms in the perianal area; no patient should be considered cured unless perianal swabbings have been negative for 7 consecutive days)

*For roundworms*

» Stool examinations
(may be required prior to treatment and approximately 2 to 6 weeks following treatment with piperazine to determine efficacy or proof of cure)

## Side/Adverse Effects

The following side/adverse effects have been selected on the basis of their potential clinical significance (possible signs and symptoms in parentheses where appropriate)—not necessarily inclusive:

**Those indicating need for medical attention**

Incidence rare
*Hypersensitivity* (fever; joint pain; skin rash or itching)

**Those indicating need for medical attention only if they continue or are bothersome**

Incidence less frequent
*CNS effects* (dizziness; drowsiness; headache; muscle weakness; tremors); *gastrointestinal disturbances* (abdominal cramps or pain; diarrhea; nausea; vomiting)

## Overdose

For more information on the management of overdose or unintentional ingestion, **contact a Poison Control Center** (see *Poison Control Center Listing*).

**Clinical effects of overdose**

The following effects have been selected on the basis of their potential clinical significance (possible signs and symptoms in parentheses where appropriate)—not necessarily inclusive:

Acute
*Muscle weakness of the extremities, transient; respiratory depression* (difficulty in breathing); *seizures*

**Treatment of overdose**

Recommended treatment consists of the following:

To decrease absorption—
Emesis or gastric lavage may be performed within a few hours of ingestion.

Specific treatment—
Symptomatic treatment may be given.

Supportive care—
Supportive measures such as maintaining an open airway, respiration, and circulation may be administered. Patients in whom intentional overdose is known or suspected should be referred for psychiatric consultation.

## Patient Consultation

As an aid to patient consultation, refer to *Advice for the Patient, Piperazine (Systemic)*.

In providing consultation, consider emphasizing the following selected information (» = major clinical significance):

**Before using this medication**

» Conditions affecting use, especially:
Hypersensitivity to piperazine or its salt, or ethylenediamine
Pregnancy—Piperazine partially converts to a potentially carcinogenic nitrosamine derivative; therefore its use in pregnant

women is recommended only if clearly indicated and then only if alternative drugs are not available

Use in children—Cautious and short-term use is recommended because of potential neurotoxic effects

Other medications, especially pyrantel and phenothiazines, such as chlorpromazine

Other medical problems, especially hepatic or renal function impairment and seizure disorders, such as epilepsy

**Proper use of this medication**

No special preparation (e.g., dietary restrictions or fasting, concurrent medications, purging, or cleansing enemas) is required before, during, or immediately after therapy

Taking on full or empty stomach as directed by physician

*Proper administration for granules for oral solution dosage form*

Dissolving contents of 1 packet of granules in 57 mL (about 2 ounces) of water, milk, or fruit juice

Drinking all of liquid to get the full dose of the medication

» Importance of not taking more medication than the amount recommended

» Compliance with full course of therapy

» Treatment program may be repeated in 1 to 2 weeks for heavy infection or reinfestation

» Proper dosing
Missed dose: Taking as soon as possible; not taking if almost time for next dose; not doubling doses

» Proper storage

*For pinworms*

Treating all household members simultaneously

**Precautions while using this medication**

Regular visits to physician to check progress

Checking with physician if no improvement after the full course of treatment or if symptoms persist

*For pinworms*

Washing (not shaking) all bedding and nightclothes after treatment to prevent reinfection

**Side/adverse effects**

Signs of potential side effects, especially hypersensitivity

## General Dosing Information

Patients who are heavily infected with helminths may require a second treatment.

**For pinworms**

Because of the high probability of transfer of pinworms, it is often recommended that all members of the household be treated concurrently. Retreatment is recommended 1 to 2 weeks following initial treatment.

## Oral Dosage Forms

### PIPERAZINE ADIPATE GRANULES FOR ORAL SOLUTION

**Usual adult and adolescent dose**

Ascariasis or
Enterobiasis—
Patients weighing 41 kg of body weight and over: Oral, 2 grams three times a day for one day. Treatment may be repeated in two weeks.

**Usual pediatric dose**

Ascariasis or
Enterobiasis—
Children 2 to 8 years of age (13.5 to 27.5 kg of body weight): Oral, 2 grams once a day for one day. Treatment may be repeated in two weeks.

Children 8 to 14 years of age (27.5 to 41 kg of body weight): Oral, 2 grams two times a day for one day. Treatment may be repeated in two weeks.

Children 14 years of age and over (41 kg of body weight and over): See *Usual adult and adolescent dose.*

**Strength(s) usually available**

U.S.—
Not commercially available.

Canada—
2 grams per packet (Rx) [*Entacyl* (sodium <19.2 mg)].

**Packaging and storage**

Store below 40 °C (104 °F), preferably between 15 and 30 °C (59 and 86 °F), in a well-closed container, unless otherwise specified by manufacturer.

## PIPERAZINE ADIPATE ORAL SUSPENSION

**Usual adult and adolescent dose**
Ascariasis or
Enterobiasis—
Oral, 1.8 grams every four hours three times a day for one day. Treatment may be repeated in two weeks.

**Usual pediatric dose**
Ascariasis or
Enterobiasis—
Children up to 2 years of age: Oral, 600 mg (0.6 gram) every four hours three times a day for one day. Treatment may be repeated in two weeks.
Children 2 to 8 years of age: Oral, 1.2 grams every six hours two times a day for one day. Treatment may be repeated in two weeks.
Children 8 to 14 years of age: Oral, 1.2 grams every four hours three times a day for one day. Treatment may be repeated in two weeks.
Children 14 years of age and over: See *Usual adult and adolescent dose.*

**Strength(s) usually available**
U.S.—
Not commercially available.
Canada—
600 mg per 5 ml (Rx) [*Entacyl* (sodium <0.8 mg)].

**Packaging and storage**
Store below 40 °C (104 °F), preferably between 15 and 30 °C (59 and 86 °F), in a well-closed container, unless otherwise specified by manufacturer. Protect from freezing.

**Auxiliary labeling**
• Shake well.

## PIPERAZINE CITRATE TABLETS USP

Note: The dosing and strength of the dosage form available are expressed in terms of piperazine hexahydrate.

**Usual adult and adolescent dose**
Ascariasis—
Oral, 3.5 grams (hexahydrate) per day for two consecutive days. Treatment may be repeated after one week for heavy infection.
Enterobiasis—
Oral, 65 mg (hexahydrate) per kg of body weight per day for seven consecutive days. Treatment may be repeated after one week for heavy infection.

**Usual adult prescribing limits**
Ascariasis—Up to 3.5 grams (hexahydrate) per day.
Enterobiasis—Up to 2.5 grams (hexahydrate) per day.

**Usual pediatric dose**
Ascariasis—
Oral, 75 mg (hexahydrate) per kg of body weight per day for two consecutive days. Treatment may be repeated after one week for heavy infection.

Enterobiasis—
See *Usual adult and adolescent dose.*

**Usual pediatric prescribing limits**
Ascariasis—Up to 3.5 grams (hexahydrate) per day.
Enterobiasis—Up to 2.5 grams (hexahydrate) per day.

**Strength(s) usually available**
U.S.—
250 mg (hexahydrate) (275.75 mg piperazine citrate anhydrous) (Rx) [GENERIC].
Canada—
Not commercially available.

**Packaging and storage**
Store below 40 °C (104 °F), preferably between 15 and 30 °C (59 and 86 °F) in a well-closed container, unless otherwise specified by manufacturer.

## Selected Bibliography
Nanivadekar AS, Gadgil SD, Apte VV. Efficacy of levamisole, mebendazole, piperazine and pyrantel in roundworm infection: by national anthelmintic study group. J Postgrad Med 1984 Jul; 30 (3): 144-52.
Tricker AR, Kumar R, Siddiqi M, Khuroo MS, Preussmann R. Endogenous formation of N-nitrosamines from piperazine and their urinary excretion following anthelmintic treatment with piperazine citrate. Carcinogenesis 1991; 12 (9): 1595-9.

Revised: 08/02/93

---

**PIPOTIAZINE**—See *Phenothiazines (Systemic)*

---

**PIRBUTEROL**—See *Bronchodilators, Adrenergic (Systemic)*

---

**PIRENZEPINE**—See *Anticholinergics/Antispasmodics (Systemic)*

---

**PIROXICAM**—See *Anti-inflammatory Drugs, Nonsteroidal (Systemic)*

---

**PIVAMPICILLIN**—See *Penicillins (Systemic)*

---

**PIVMECILLINAM**—See *Penicillins (Systemic)*

---

# PLAGUE VACCINE    Systemic†

VA CLASSIFICATION (Primary): IM100

Note: For a listing of dosage forms and brand names by country availability, see *Dosage Forms* section(s). For a listing of brand names for the articles in this monograph, refer to the General Index.

†Not commercially available in Canada.

## Category
Immunizing agent (active).

## Indications

**General considerations**
In the U.S., the important reservoirs of *Yersinia pestis* are the ground squirrel, rock squirrel, prairie dog, and pack rat. Worldwide, rats, camels, goats, sheep, coyotes, deer, dogs, and cats may become carriers of *Y. pestis* by feeding on infected carcasses or being bitten by infected fleas.
Travel to countries where plague occurs presents low risk of acquiring the disease under normal circumstances. To further reduce risks, travelers should be told to avoid known plague outbreak areas and follow the preventive measures described below:
• Travelers should avoid exposure to fleas from diseased rats. The risk of being bitten by infected fleas is especially high after large numbers of plague-infected rats have died. In these instances, infected, starving fleas aggressively seek new hosts. Places having large numbers of rats, and where large numbers of rats have reportedly died, should be avoided. If travel to such areas is essential, insect repellent containing *N,N*-diethylmethyltoluamide (DEET) should be applied to exposed parts of the body, such as legs and ankles. Also, DEET or other repellents and insecticides should be applied to clothes and outer bedding according to manufacturers' directions. Preventive antibiotics should be taken if risk of exposure is high.
• Travelers should avoid close contact with infected animals. Sick or dead animals should not be handled. In addition to rats and other rodents, cats can acquire plague and directly transmit the disease to humans. Plague in cats is characterized by fever; sores of the head, neck, and mouth; and sometimes cough.
• Travelers should avoid close contact with pneumonic plague patients. All suspected pneumonic plague patients should be hospitalized, be placed in isolation, have specimens obtained for plague diagnosis, and immediately be given antibiotic therapy. Persons in close contact with the patient should receive preventive antibiotic therapy. Close

contact is defined as face-to-face contact, or being within the same closed space, such as a room or vehicle. Household contacts of persons with bubonic plague are also advised to receive preventive antibiotic treatment.

The most common form of human plague is the bubonic form, transmitted by the bites of infected fleas. However, pneumonic plague can also be acquired by handling infected animals or by exposure to respiratory droplets from persons or animals with pneumonic plague. Untreated patients with cough or other signs of pneumonia, whether or not vaccinated, may transmit the plague bacillus to other persons through airborne droplets. The degree of protection afforded against the pneumonic form by plague vaccine is unknown and vaccinated persons exposed to the pneumonic form should be treated with suitable antibiotics.

### Accepted

Plague (prophylaxis)—Plague vaccine is indicated for active immunization of adults and children against bubonic plague caused by *Yersinia pestis*. However, safety and immunogenicity data supporting the use of plague vaccine in persons younger than 18 and older than 61 years of age are not available.

    Routine plague vaccination is not recommended in the U.S. However, selective vaccination is indicated for the following groups
• Laboratory personnel regularly working with *Y. pestis* or *Y. pestis*–infected rodents, particularly those personnel engaged in *Y. pestis* aerosol experiments or working with *Y. pestis* organisms resistant to antimicrobials.
• Persons engaged in field operations or workers who reside in rural areas with enzootic or epidemic plague where avoidance of rodents and fleas is impossible.
• Persons whose vocation brings them into regular contact with wild rodents or infected animals in areas with enzootic plague.
Plague vaccine may be considered for persons traveling to, or residing in, endemic and epizootic areas following natural disasters, and when regular sanitary practices are interrupted such that plague can extend from its usual areas of endemicity into urban centers.

## Pharmacology/Pharmacokinetics

### Physicochemical characteristics

Plague vaccine contains *Yersinia pestis* (formerly *Pasteurella pestis*), Indian isolate 195/P strain that is grown on E-broth agar overlay production medium containing beef heart infusion, soytone (or phytone), casamino acids, sodium sulfite, L-cysteine hydrochloride, and yeast extract at pH 7.3 ± 0.2.

### Mechanism of action/Effect

The induction of anti-F1 antibodies following immunization with whole cell *Y. pestis* vaccine is thought to be a major element contributing to protection conferred by plague vaccine.

### Protective effect

Vaccination of humans with plague vaccine promotes immunity against systemic (bubonic) infection by *Y. pestis*. The degree of protection afforded against primary pneumonic infection is not known. Field experience indicates that vaccination with plague vaccine reduces the incidence and severity of disease resulting from the bite of infected rodent fleas. The factors influencing protection are not well understood. Various plasmid and chromosomally encoded functions have been associated with virulence in *Y. pestis*. Among these virulence-associated factors in *Y. pestis* are antigenic components, including capsular fraction 1 (F1) antigen, V and W antigens, murine exotoxins A and B, yersiniae outer membrane proteins (Yops), and endotoxin (lipopolysaccharide). The induction of anti-F1 antibodies following immunization with whole cell *Y. pestis* vaccine is thought to be a major element contributing to protection conferred by plague vaccine. In one study, 29 human subjects were immunized with 1 mL, and then 0.2 mL at three months, and 0.2 mL six months later. Thirty days after the initial dose of vaccine, 86% of the vaccinees had detectable passive hemagglutination (PHA) antibody titers against *Y. pestis* F1 antigen on sensitized sheep red blood cells. After the second and third doses, 90 and 93%, respectively, of the subjects had detectable PHA titers. Two individuals (7%) did not develop detectable antibodies after three doses. Subsequent booster doses of vaccine stimulated increased titers of PHA anti-F1 antibodies.

Time to protective effect—
    The protective titer of antibody to F1 antigen is generally reached following administration of the first two doses (1 mL and 0.2 mL, respectively). The titer increases following administration of the third dose of 0.2 mL of the vaccine.

### Duration of protective effect

The duration of protection against plague infection following the primary series of immunizations with plague vaccine is approximately 6 to 12

months. Therefore, under conditions of repeated exposure (for individuals remaining in a known plague area), a single booster dose should be given every 6 months.

## Precautions to Consider

### Carcinogenicity/Mutagenicity

No animal or human studies have been conducted to evaluate the carcinogenic or mutagenic potential of plague vaccine.

### Pregnancy/Reproduction

Fertility—Studies of effects of plague vaccine on fertility have not been done.

Pregnancy—Studies have not been done in humans.
Studies have not been done in animals.

FDA Pregnancy Category C.

### Breast-feeding

It is not known whether plague vaccine is distributed into breast milk. However, problems in humans have not been documented.

### Pediatrics

Safety and immunogenicity data supporting the use of plague vaccine in persons younger than 18 years of age are not available. However, the U.S. Public Health Service Advisory Committee on Immunization Practices (ACIP) recommends immunization of children who are at risk of plague infection.

### Geriatrics

Appropriate studies on the relationship of age to the effects of plague vaccine have not been performed in geriatric populations older than 61 years of age. However, vaccination may be considered if there is a risk of plague infection.

### Drug interactions and/or related problems

The following drug interactions and/or related problems have been selected on the basis of their potential clinical significance (possible mechanism in parentheses where appropriate)—not necessarily inclusive (» = major clinical significance):

Cholera vaccine or
Typhoid vaccine
    (concurrent use of plague vaccine may increase the risk of local and systemic adverse effects)

### Medical considerations/Contraindications

The medical considerations/contraindications included here have been selected on the basis of their potential clinical significance (reasons given in parentheses where appropriate)—not necessarily inclusive (» = major clinical significance).

*Except under special circumstances, this medication should not be used when the following medical problems exist:*

»  Febrile illness, acute
    (administration of plague vaccine should be postponed to avoid confusing manifestations of acute febrile illness with possible side/adverse effects of the vaccine; minor illnesses, such as upper respiratory infections, with or without low grade fever or mild diarrhea, do not preclude administration of vaccine)

»  Previous sensitivity reaction to plague vaccine
    (plague vaccine is contraindicated in patients with a history of a severe systemic or allergic reaction to a previous administration of plague vaccine)

## Side/Adverse Effects

The following side/adverse effects have been selected on the basis of their potential clinical significance (possible signs and symptoms in parentheses where appropriate)—not necessarily inclusive:

### Those indicating need for medical attention

Incidence rare
    *Anaphylactic reaction* (difficulty in breathing or swallowing; hives; itching, especially of soles or palms; reddening of skin, especially around ears; swelling of eyes, face, or inside of nose; unusual tiredness or weakness, sudden and severe)

### Those indicating need for medical attention only if they continue or are bothersome

Incidence more frequent
    *Arthralgia* (joint pain); *fever; headache; lymphadenopathy* (swollen glands); *malaise* (general feeling of discomfort or illness); *myalgia* (muscle pain); *nausea and/or vomiting; pain, redness, or swelling at injection site*

## Patient Consultation

As an aid to patient consultation, refer to *Advice for the Patient, Plague Vaccine (Systemic)*.

In providing consultation, consider emphasizing the following selected information (» = major clinical significance):

**Before receiving this vaccine**
» Conditions affecting use, especially:
   Sensitivity to plague vaccine
   Other medical problems, especially acute febrile illness and previous sensitivity reaction to plague vaccine

**Proper use of this vaccine**
» Proper dosing

**Side/adverse effects**
   Signs of potential side effects, especially anaphylactic reaction

## General Dosing Information

Even after immunization with plague vaccine, not all recipients of the vaccine will be fully protected against plague. Travelers to endemic and epidemic plague areas should be advised to take all necessary precautions to avoid contact with wild rodents or their fleas or other infected domestic and wild animals.

For immediate protection in outbreak situations, plague vaccines are of unproven effectiveness and are not recommended.

Appropriate precautions should be taken prior to plague vaccine administration to prevent allergic or other unwanted reactions. These precautions should include review of the patient's history regarding possible sensitivity to plague vaccine or similar vaccines and the ready availability of epinephrine 1:1000 and other appropriate agents used for control of immediate allergic reactions.

Primary immunization with plague vaccine consists of three doses. Patients should be informed of the importance of completing the immunization schedule.

Under conditions of continued or repeated exposure (for individuals remaining in a known plague area), a single booster dose should be given every 6 months. It is not necessary to repeat the primary immunization series. Booster doses at intervals of 1 to 2 years may be appropriate for persons who have received three or more booster doses at 6-month intervals. Where available, the determination of hemagglutination titers may be helpful in determining the need for a booster immunization.

Plague vaccine is administered by intramuscular injection, preferably into the deltoid muscle, and should not be administered by intravenous injection.

## Parenteral Dosage Forms

### PLAGUE VACCINE USP

**Usual adult and adolescent dose**
Immunizing agent (active)—
   Primary immunization:
      First dose—Intramuscular, 1 mL at initial visit.
      Second dose—Intramuscular, 0.2 mL one to three months after the first dose.
      Third dose—Intramuscular, 0.2 mL five or six months after the second dose.

Booster dose:
   Intramuscular, 0.1 to 0.2 mL every six months.

**Usual pediatric dose**
Immunizing agent (active)—
   Primary immunization:
      First dose—
         Infants and children up to 1 year of age: Intramuscular, 0.2 mL at initial visit.
         Children 1 to 5 years of age: Intramuscular, 0.4 mL at initial visit.
         Children 5 to 10 years of age: Intramuscular, 0.6 mL at initial visit.
         Children 10 years of age and over: See *Usual adult and adolescent dose.*
      Second dose—
         Infants and children up to 1 year of age: Intramuscular, 0.04 mL one to three months after the first dose.
         Children 1 to 5 years of age: Intramuscular, 0.08 mL one to three months after the first dose.
         Children 5 to 10 years of age: Intramuscular, 0.12 mL one to three months after the first dose.
         Children 10 years of age and over: See *Usual adult and adolescent dose.*
      Third dose—
         Infants and children up to 1 year of age: Intramuscular, 0.04 mL five or six months after the second dose.
         Children 1 to 5 years of age: Intramuscular, 0.08 mL five or six months after the second dose.
         Children 5 to 10 years of age: Intramuscular, 0.12 mL five or six months after the second dose.
         Children 10 years of age and over: See *Usual adult and adolescent dose.*
   Booster doses:
      Infants and children up to 1 year of age—
         Intramuscular, 0.02 to 0.04 mL every six months.
      Children 1 to 5 years of age—
         Intramuscular, 0.04 to 0.08 mL every six months.
      Children 5 to 10 years of age—
         Intramuscular, 0.06 to 0.12 mL every six months.
      Children 10 years of age and over—
         See *Usual adult and adolescent dose.*

**Strength(s) usually available**
U.S.—
   1.8–2.2 × 10⁹ formaldehyde-killed whole bacilli (*Yersinia pestis*) per mL (Rx) [GENERIC].
Canada—
   Not commercially available.

**Packaging and storage**
Store between 2 and 8 °C (36 and 46 °F). Protect from freezing.

**Auxiliary labeling**
• Do not freeze.
• Shake well.

Developed: 02/23/96

---

# PLICAMYCIN    Systemic†

VA CLASSIFICATION (Primary/Secondary): AN200/HS900
Another commonly used name in the U.S. is mithramycin.
Note: For a listing of dosage forms and brand names by country availability, see *Dosage Forms* section(s). For a listing of brand names for the articles in this monograph, refer to the General Index.

†Not commercially available in Canada.

## Category

Antineoplastic; antihypercalcemic; antihypercalciuric; bone resorption inhibitor.

## Indications

Note: Bracketed information in the *Indications* section refers to uses that are not included in U.S. product labeling.

**Accepted**
Carcinoma, testicular (treatment)—Plicamycin is indicated for treatment of testicular carcinoma, although use has been replaced by that of more effective agents.

Hypercalcemia, associated with neoplasms (treatment) and
Hypercalciuria, associated with neoplasms (treatment)—Plicamycin is indicated in the treatment of hypercalcemia and hypercalciuria associated with neoplasms, although use has generally been replaced by other agents. Some clinicians have found that a single dose of plicamycin is effective and eliminates the possibility of toxicity.

[Paget's disease of bone (treatment)]—Plicamycin is used in the treatment of Paget's disease; however, its use should be reserved for those patients refractory to other agents.

## Pharmacology/Pharmacokinetics

**Physicochemical characteristics**
Molecular weight—1085.16.

## Mechanism of action/Effect

Antineoplastic—The exact mechanism of action is unknown. However, it has been shown that plicamycin forms a complex with DNA in the presence of magnesium or other divalent cations, thereby inhibiting DNA-dependent or DNA-directed RNA synthesis.

Antihypercalcemic or

Paget's disease—Plicamycin is believed to lower serum calcium concentrations, but the exact mechanism is unknown. It may act by blocking hypercalcemic action of vitamin D or by inhibiting the effect of parathyroid hormone on osteoclasts. Plicamycin's inhibition of DNA-dependent RNA synthesis appears to render osteoclasts unable to fully respond to parathyroid hormone with the biosynthesis necessary for osteolysis.

## Distribution

Plicamycin is concentrated in the Kupffer cells of the liver, in renal tubular cells, and along formed bone surfaces. It may localize in areas of active bone resorption. Plicamycin also crosses the blood-brain barrier and enters the cerebrospinal fluid (CSF).

## Onset of action

When used for hypercalcemia, a reduction in plasma calcium usually occurs within 24 to 48 hours following administration.

## Time to peak effect

72 hours with a single dose.

## Duration of action

7 to 10 days with a single dose.

## Elimination

Renal.

# Precautions to Consider

Note: Although lower doses are used in the treatment of hypercalcemia than in antitumor treatment, the same precautions and contraindications apply.

## Pregnancy/Reproduction

Fertility—Studies in male rats receiving doses of 0.6 mg and above per kg of body weight per day showed histologic evidence of inhibition of spermatogenesis.

Pregnancy—Plicamycin is not recommended for use during pregnancy. Although studies have not been done and problems have not been documented in humans, risk-benefit must be considered since the use of plicamycin during pregnancy may be toxic to the fetus.

FDA Pregnancy Category X.

## Breast-feeding

It is not known whether plicamycin is excreted in breast milk.

## Pediatrics

No information is available on the relationship of age to the effects of plicamycin in pediatric patients.

## Geriatrics

No information is available on the relationship of age to the effects of plicamycin in geriatric patients.

## Dental

The leukopenic and thrombocytopenic effects of plicamycin may result in an increased incidence of microbial infection, delayed healing, and gingival bleeding. Dental work, whenever possible, should be completed prior to initiation of therapy or deferred until blood counts have returned to normal. Patients should be instructed in proper oral hygiene during treatment, including caution in use of regular toothbrushes, dental floss, and toothpicks. Plicamycin may also cause stomatitis associated with considerable discomfort.

## Drug interactions and/or related problems

The following drug interactions and/or related problems have been selected on the basis of their potential clinical significance (possible mechanism in parentheses where appropriate)—not necessarily inclusive ($\gg$ = major clinical significance):

Note: Combinations containing any of the following medications, depending on the amount present, may also interact with this medication.

In addition to the interactions listed below, the possibility should be considered that additive or multiple effects leading to impaired blood clotting and/or increased risk of bleeding may occur if plicamycin is used concurrently with any other medication having a significant potential for inhibiting platelet aggregation or causing hypoprothrombinemia, thrombocytopenia, or gastrointestinal ulceration or hemorrhage.

$\gg$ Anticoagulants, coumarin- or indandione-derivative or
$\gg$ Heparin or

$\gg$ Thrombolytic agents
(plicamycin-induced hypoprothrombinemia may increase the activity of coumarin- and indandione-derivative anticoagulants and may increase the risk of bleeding in patients receiving heparin or thrombolytic agents; concurrent use is not recommended)

(also, inhibition of platelet aggregation may increase the risk of hemorrhage in patients receiving anticoagulant or thrombolytic therapy)

$\gg$ Anti-inflammatory drugs, nonsteroidal (NSAIDs) or
$\gg$ Aspirin or
$\gg$ Dextran or
$\gg$ Dipyridamole or
$\gg$ Sulfinpyrazone or
$\gg$ Valproic acid
(concurrent use with plicamycin may increase the risk of hemorrhage because of additive or multiple actions, which may decrease the blood-clotting ability, i.e., inhibition of platelet aggregation, by these medications and/or plicamycin combined with induction of hypoprothrombinemia by plicamycin and large doses of aspirin; in addition, the gastrointestinal ulcerative or hemorrhagic potential of aspirin, the NSAIDs, or sulfinpyrazone may increase the risk of hemorrhage in plicamycin-treated patients)

$\gg$ Bone marrow depressants, other (See *Appendix II* ) or
$\gg$ Hepatotoxic medications (See *Appendix II* ) or
$\gg$ Nephrotoxic medications (See *Appendix II* )
(concurrent use with plicamycin may increase the potential for toxicity)

$\gg$ Calcium-containing preparations or
$\gg$ Vitamin D, including calcifediol and calcitriol
(concurrent use may antagonize the effect of plicamycin when used as a calcium antagonist)

$\gg$ Vaccines, live virus
(because normal defense mechanisms are suppressed by plicamycin therapy, the replication of the vaccine virus may be potentiated, the side/adverse effects of the vaccine virus may be increased, and/or the patient's response to the vaccine may be decreased; immunization of these patients should be undertaken only with extreme caution after careful review of the patient's hematologic status and only with the knowledge and consent of the physician managing the plicamycin therapy; immunization is also contraindicated in persons in close contact with the patient, especially family members)

## Medical considerations/Contraindications

The medical considerations/contraindications included here have been selected on the basis of their potential clinical significance (reasons given in parentheses where appropriate)—not necessarily inclusive ($\gg$ = major clinical significance).

*Except under special circumstances, this medication should not be used when the following medical problems exist:*

$\gg$ Blood dyscrasias, including thrombocytopathy and thrombocytopenia (condition may be exacerbated)

$\gg$ Chickenpox, existing or recent, including recent exposure or
$\gg$ Herpes zoster
(risk of severe generalized disease)

$\gg$ Coagulation disorders or increased susceptibility to bleeding due to other causes, including ingestion of aspirin or other potent platelet-aggregation inhibitors within the week prior to plicamycin therapy (increased risk of hemorrhage)

*Risk-benefit should be considered when the following medical problems exist:*

Electrolyte imbalance, especially hypocalcemia, hypokalemia, or hypophosphatemia or
$\gg$ Hepatic function impairment, severe or
$\gg$ Renal function impairment, severe
(condition may be exacerbated)

Sensitivity to plicamycin

$\gg$ Caution should be used also in patients who have had previous cytotoxic drug therapy and radiation therapy, and in cases of general debility.

## Patient monitoring

The following may be especially important in patient monitoring (other tests may be warranted in some patients, depending on condition; $\gg$ = major clinical significance):

Bleeding time determinations and
Complete blood count and differential and

Platelet count determinations and
Prothrombin time determinations
  (recommended before therapy and then at intervals during therapy
  that depend on frequency of dose and patient status; a significant
  increase in prothrombin or bleeding times, which may be early
  signs of impending hemorrhage, or a significant decrease in the
  platelet count are indications for discontinuing the medication)

Calcium concentrations, serum and
Phosphorus concentrations, serum and
Potassium concentrations, serum
  (any electrolyte imbalance should be corrected before initiation of
  therapy and at intervals during therapy with plicamycin depending
  on frequency of dose and patient status)

Hepatic function determinations and
Renal function determinations
  (recommended before therapy and then at intervals during therapy
  that depend on frequency of dose and patient status)

## Side/Adverse Effects

The following side/adverse effects have been selected on the basis of their
potential clinical significance (possible signs and symptoms in parentheses where appropriate)—not necessarily inclusive:

**Those indicating need for medical attention**
Incidence less frequent
  *Hypocalcemia* (muscle and abdominal cramps)

**Those indicating need for medical attention only if they continue
or are bothersome**
Incidence more frequent
  *Anorexia* (loss of appetite); *diarrhea; irritation or soreness of mouth;
  nausea or vomiting*—may occur 1 to 2 hours after initiation of therapy
  and continue for 12 to 24 hours
  Note: Incidence and severity of *gastrointestinal side effects* may in-
    crease with too rapid a rate of administration.

Incidence less frequent
  *Drowsiness; fever; headache; mental depression; pain, redness, sore-
  ness, or swelling at injection site; unusual tiredness or weakness*

**Those indicating possible hematologic abnormalities and the need
for medical attention if they occur after medication is
discontinued**
  *Bloody or black, tarry stools; nosebleed; sore throat and fever; un-
  usual bleeding or bruising; vomiting of blood*

## Overdose

For information on the management of overdose, **contact a Poison Control Center** (see *Poison Control Center Listing* ).

**Clinical effects of overdose**
The following effects have been selected on the basis of their potential
clinical significance (possible signs and symptoms in parentheses
where appropriate)–not necessarily inclusive:
  *Gastrointestinal bleeding* (bloody or black, tarry stools; vomiting of
  blood); *hepatotoxicity* (yellow eyes or skin); *nosebleed or other bleeding; leukopenia* (sore throat and fever)—incidence about 6%; *petechial bleeding* (small red spots on skin); *thrombocytopenia* (unusual
  bleeding or bruising); *toxic epidermal necrolysis* (flushing or redness
  or swelling of face; skin rash)—possible early symptoms
  Note: *Hemorrhagic diathesis*—Incidence more frequent with doses of
    more than 30 mcg (0.03 mg) per kg of body weight a day and/
    or for more than 10 doses.

## Patient Consultation

As an aid to patient consultation, refer to *Advice for the Patient,
Plicamycin (Systemic)*.

In providing consultation, consider emphasizing the following selected
information (» = major clinical significance):

**Before receiving this medication**
» Conditions affecting use, especially:
    Sensitivity to plicamycin
    Pregnancy—Use not recommended during pregnancy; possible
      toxicity to the fetus
    Dental—Blood dyscrasias may result in increased incidence of gin-
      gival bleeding, delayed healing, and microbial infection
    Other medications, especially anticoagulants, aspirin, bone marrow
      depressants, calcium- or vitamin D–containing preparations,
      dextran, dipyridamole, hepatotoxic medications, nephrotoxic
      medications, nonsteroidal anti-inflammatory drugs, sulfinpyra-
      zone, thrombolytics, or valproic acid

Other medical problems, especially blood disorders, chickenpox,
  herpes zoster, severe hepatic function impairment, or severe
  renal function impairment

**Proper use of this medication**
Frequency of nausea and vomiting; importance of continuing treatment
» Proper dosing

**Precautions after receiving this medication**
Importance of close monitoring by the physician
» Avoiding salicylate-containing products, which may increase risk of
  hemorrhage
Possible need to avoid calcium- and vitamin D–containing products
» Avoiding immunizations unless approved by physician; other persons
  in patient's household should avoid immunizations with oral poliovirus vaccine; avoiding other persons who have taken oral poliovirus vaccine or wearing a protective mask that covers nose and
  mouth
Caution if bone marrow depression occurs:
» Avoiding exposure to persons with bacterial infections, especially during periods of low blood counts; checking with physician immediately if fever or chills, cough or hoarseness, lower back or side
  pain, or painful or difficult urination occurs
» Checking with physician immediately if unusual bleeding or bruising;
  black, tarry stools; blood in urine or stools; or pinpoint red spots
  on skin occur
Caution in use of regular toothbrush, dental floss, or toothpick; physician, dentist, or nurse may suggest alternatives; checking with
  physician before having dental work done
Not touching eyes or inside of nose unless hands washed immediately
  before
Using caution to avoid accidental cuts with use of sharp objects such
  as safety razor or fingernail or toenail cutters
Avoiding contact sports or other situations where bruising or injury
  could occur

## General Dosing Information

It is recommended that plicamycin be administered by intravenous infusion only to hospitalized patients by or under the supervision of a
physician experienced in the use of cancer chemotherapeutic agents
because of the possibility of severe reactions.

Before plicamycin therapy is initiated, dehydration or volume depletion
should be corrected.

Rapid direct intravenous injection of plicamycin should be avoided since
it may be associated with a higher incidence and greater severity of
gastrointestinal side effects.

Special precautions are recommended in patients who develop thrombocytopenia as a result of administration of plicamycin. These may include extreme care in performing invasive procedures; regular inspection of intravenous sites, skin (including perirectal area), and mucous
membrane surfaces for signs of bleeding or bruising; limiting frequency of venipuncture and avoiding intramuscular injections; testing
urine, emesis, stool and secretions for occult blood; care in use of
regular toothbrushes, dental floss, toothpicks, safety razors, and fingernail and toenail cutters; avoiding constipation; and using caution to
prevent falls and other injuries. Such patients should avoid alcohol and
any aspirin intake because of the risk of gastrointestinal bleeding.
Platelet transfusions may be required.

Patients who develop leukopenia should be observed carefully for signs
of infection. Antibiotic support may be required. In neutropenic patients who develop fever, broad-spectrum antibiotic coverage should
be initiated empirically, pending bacterial cultures and appropriate diagnostic tests.

**Safety considerations for handling this medication**
There is limited but increasing evidence and concern that personnel involved in preparation and administration of parenteral antineoplastics
may be at some risk because of the potential mutagenicity, teratogenicity, and/or carcinogenicity of these agents, although the actual risk
is unknown. USP advisory panels recommend cautious handling both
in preparation and disposal of antineoplastic agents. Precautions that
have been suggested include:
• Use of a biological containment cabinet during reconstitution and
  dilution of parenteral medications and wearing of disposable surgical
  gloves and masks.
• Use of proper technique to prevent contamination of the medication,
  work area, and operator during transfer between containers (including
  proper training of personnel in this technique).
• Cautious and proper disposal of needles, syringes, vials, ampuls, and
  unused medication.
A number of medical centers have developed detailed guidelines for
handling of antineoplastic agents.

### For treatment of adverse effects

Nausea and vomiting—The use of antiemetics prior to and during treatment with plicamycin may help relieve nausea and vomiting, which may begin 1 to 2 hours after initiation of therapy and persist for 12 to 24 hours.

Extravasation—If local irritation or cellulitis occurs at the injection site, immediate application of a cold pack to the site may prevent pain and swelling. If swelling develops, application of moderate heat may help disperse the medication and reduce the discomfort. If cellulitis occurs, the infusion should be discontinued and then reinstituted at another site.

## Parenteral Dosage Forms

### PLICAMYCIN FOR INJECTION USP

**Usual adult dose**

Antineoplastic—

Intravenous infusion, 25 to 30 mcg (0.025 to 0.03 mg) per kg of body weight a day, administered over a period of four to six hours, for eight to ten days unless significant side effects or toxicity symptoms occur; or 25 to 50 mcg (0.025 to 0.05 mg) per kg of body weight once a day every other day for up to eight doses or until toxicity requires discontinuation of medication. Additional courses of therapy may be administered at one-month intervals.

Note: The same dose may be given by intravenous push over 20 to 30 minutes to reduce the risk of extravasation.

Doses of more than 30 mcg (0.03 mg) per kg of body weight a day and/or a duration of therapy longer than ten days increases the potential of a hemorrhagic diathesis.

The alternate-day dosage schedule has been shown to decrease the toxicity potential.

Delayed toxicity may occur for as long as seventy-two hours after medication has been discontinued following daily administration, but does not occur when the alternate-day dosage schedule is used.

Antihypercalcemic and
Antihypercalciuric—

Intravenous infusion, initially 15 to 25 mcg (0.015 to 0.025 mg) per kg of body weight a day, to be administered over a period of four to six hours, for three to four days, the dose to be repeated at one-week or more intervals, if necessary, until the desired response is obtained.

Note: The same dose may be given by intravenous push over 20 to 30 minutes to reduce the risk of extravasation.

Alternatively, normal calcium balance may be maintained by administering one to three doses a week, depending upon the patient's response. Some clinicians recommend a single dose of plicamycin with one repeat dose at 48 hours if normalization of calcium levels has not been achieved.

**Usual pediatric dose**

Dosage has not been established.

**Strength(s) usually available**

U.S.—

2500 mcg (2.5 mg) (Rx) [*Mithracin*].

Canada—

Not commercially available.

**Packaging and storage**

Prior to reconstitution, store between 2 and 8 °C (36 and 46 °F). Store in a light-resistant container.

**Preparation of dosage form**

To prepare initial dilution of 500 mcg (0.5 mg) of plicamycin per mL, add 4.9 mL of sterile water for injection to the 2500-mcg vial and shake to dissolve. After the appropriate dose has been withdrawn from the vial, discard the unused portion.

For intravenous infusion, the daily dose should be further diluted in 1000 mL of 5% dextrose injection or 0.9% sodium chloride injection and administered by infusion over a period of 4 to 6 hours.

**Stability**

Reconstituted solution (500 mcg per mL) should be freshly prepared for each dose and used immediately. Infusion solution is stable for 4 to 6 hours at room temperature. Discard any unused portion of either solution.

Revised: 09/14/92
Interim revision: 08/02/94

---

# PNEUMOCOCCAL VACCINE POLYVALENT    Systemic

VA CLASSIFICATION (Primary): IM100

Note: This monograph refers to the 23-valent vaccine licensed in the U.S. in 1983. This vaccine replaces the 14-valent vaccine licensed in the U.S. in 1977.

Note: For a listing of dosage forms and brand names by country availability, see *Dosage Forms* section(s). For a listing of brand names for the articles in this monograph, refer to the General Index.

## Category

Immunizing agent (active).

## Indications

### Accepted

Pneumococcal disease (prophylaxis)—Pneumococcal vaccine polyvalent is a vaccine consisting of purified bacterial capsular polysaccharides and containing no viable components. It is indicated for immunization against pneumococcal disease caused by any of the 23 pneumococcal types included in the vaccine. These 23 types are responsible for approximately 90% of serious pneumococcal disease. The main objective of pneumococcal immunization is to prevent the severe effects, such as pneumonia, meningitis, bacteremia, and death, that may occur from a pneumococcal infection.

Pneumococcal vaccine polyvalent is recommended for adults and children 2 years of age or older, who are considered to be at increased risk of pneumococcal infection or its complications, particularly:

• Older adults, especially those 50 years of age and older.

• Adults of any age with chronic illnesses, such as cardiovascular disease, pulmonary disease, Hodgkin's disease, multiple myeloma, cirrhosis, alcoholism, renal failure, cerebrospinal fluid leaks, and conditions associated with immunosuppression.

• Adults and children 2 years of age and older with asymptomatic or symptomatic human immunodeficiency virus (HIV) infection.

• Children 2 years of age or older with chronic illnesses, such as nephrotic syndrome, cerebrospinal fluid leaks, and conditions associated with immunosuppression.

• Persons without a spleen or with splenic dysfunction because of sickle cell disease or other causes. Persons scheduled for elective splenectomy should have the vaccine administered at least 2 weeks prior to surgery to receive the full immunizing effect of the vaccine.

• Persons who are to undergo therapy with medications that cause immunosuppression, including candidates for organ transplants and persons with Hodgkin's disease. When possible, the vaccine should be administered at least 10 days, preferably more than 14 days, prior to the immunosuppression-causing medication to achieve the full immunizing effect of the vaccine. Patients with Hodgkin's disease should not receive the vaccine less than 10 days prior to, or during, immunosuppressive therapy, since some patients so immunized have exhibited post-immunization antibody levels below their preimmunization levels. Since response to vaccination is inadequate for the first 6 months following an organ transplant, if the vaccine is not administered before the organ transplant, administration of the vaccine should wait until 6 months following the transplant to elicit a better antibody response. If the vaccine is not administered to persons with Hodgkin's disease before treatment starts, it should be administered 3 months after treatment ends. However, patients with Hodgkin's disease who have received extensive chemotherapy and/or nodal irradiation should not receive the vaccine at all, since immunization of some intensively treated patients has caused depression of pre-existing levels of antibody to some pneumococcal types.

• Persons in residence institutions, such as orphanages and nursing homes.

• Persons at increased risk of pneumococcal infection who will be traveling outside the U.S., since pneumococcal pneumonia is very common in many developing countries and good medical care may not always be readily available.

• Bedridden persons, since persons with limited mobility tend to pool pulmonary secretions and, therefore, are at increased risk for pulmonary infection.

• Selected persons who have been discharged from a hospital within the past 5 years. Studies have shown that approximately two-thirds of all patients with pneumococcal bacteremia have been discharged from a hospital within the past 5 years. Previous hospital care appears to be a dynamic expression of the impact of age and/or medical condition on a person's risk status.

In general, repeat doses of pneumococcal vaccine are not recommended. Increased frequency and severity of side/adverse effects, including Arthus and systemic reactions, are thought to be caused by pre-existing high antibody levels in persons who have previously received a pneumococcal vaccine of any valence. However, when there is doubt or no information on whether an individual at high risk has previously received a pneumococcal vaccine, the vaccine should be administered. In addition, repeat doses of pneumococcal vaccine may be desirable in patients at high risk of severe illness or death from pneumococcal disease, such as children without a spleen or with sickle cell disease, or persons with chronic renal failure whose antibody levels are likely to decline more rapidly than normally, despite the risk of increased side/adverse effects. The optimum interval between revaccinations is not known. However, for adults at highest risk, reimmunization should be considered 6 or more years after the initial dose. For children with nephrotic syndrome, asplenia, or sickle cell anemia, reimmunization should be considered 3 to 5 years after the initial dose, as long as the child will be 10 years of age or less at the time of reimmunization.

### Unaccepted

Pneumococcal vaccine is not indicated for recurrent otitis media, because the vaccine has not shown significant benefit in preventing otitis media in children.

## Pharmacology/Pharmacokinetics

### Physicochemical characteristics

Source—The currently available vaccines in the U.S. (*Pneumovax 23*, MSD, and *Pnu-Imune 23*, Lederle) contain a mixture of purified capsular polysaccharides from the 23 most prevalent pneumococcal types responsible for approximately 90% of serious pneumococcal disease. Each of the pneumococcal polysaccharide types is produced separately. The resultant 23 polysaccharides are separated from the cells, purified, and combined to give 25 mcg of each type per 0.5-mL dose of the final vaccine

*Pneumovax 23*, MSD (Canada) brand of pneumococcal vaccine polyvalent also contains 23 polysaccharides

Other characteristics—The U.S. nomenclature for these 23 types is: 1, 2, 3, 4, 5, 26, 51, 8, 9, 68, 34, 43, 12, 14, 54, 17, 56, 57, 19, 20, 22, 23, 70

The Danish nomenclature for these 23 types is: 1, 2, 3, 4, 5, 6B, 7F, 8, 9N, 9V, 10A, 11A, 12F, 14, 15B, 17F, 18C, 19A, 19F, 20, 22F, 23F, 33F

### Mechanism of action/Effect

Pneumococcal bacteria are surrounded by polysaccharide capsules, which make the bacteria resistant to attack by white blood cells. However, human blood serum contains antibodies, which render the bacteria vulnerable to attack. The vaccine, which is composed of the purified polysaccharides from bacterial cells, stimulates production of these antibodies and provides active immunity to the 23 types of pneumococcal bacteria represented in the vaccine.

### Protective effect

The vaccine is about 60 to 80% effective in preventing infection to all 23 types of pneumococcal bacteria represented in the vaccine in persons with normal immune systems, including the elderly. Since the vaccine contains 23 types of antigens, the overall efficacy of the vaccine will be less than the efficacy of each individual type of antigen. In addition, efficacy may be reduced or nonexistent in persons with certain disease states, especially those who are immunocompromised.

Although the 23-valent vaccine contains only 25 mcg of each antigen per dose as compared to the 14-valent vaccine, which contained 50 mcg of antigen per dose, there appear to be comparable levels of antigenicity.

### Time to protective effect

Approximately 2 to 3 weeks.

### Duration of protective effect

Antibody levels for most antigen types in healthy adults remain elevated for at least 5 years. In some persons, the levels fall to prevaccination levels within 10 years. A more rapid reduction in antibody levels may occur in children. In addition, in children without spleens, with sickle cell disease, or with nephrotic syndrome, there may be a decline of antibody levels for some antigen types to prevaccination levels within 3 to 5 years.

## Precautions to Consider

### Cross-sensitivity and/or related problems

Patients allergic to thimerosal may be allergic to the pneumococcal vaccine available in the U.S. because it may contain a small amount of thimerosal.

### Pregnancy/Reproduction

Pregnancy—Studies have not been done in humans. However, if the vaccine is administered during pregnancy, it should be given after the first trimester and only to women at high risk of pneumococcal disease. Studies have not been done in animals.

FDA Pregnancy Category C.

### Breast-feeding

It is not known whether pneumococcal vaccine is distributed into breast milk. However, problems in humans have not been documented.

### Pediatrics

Infants and children younger than 2 years of age—Immunization is not recommended for infants and children younger than 2 years of age, since this age group may not show adequate response to many of the antigens, and antibody levels stimulated by the vaccine may not persist.

Children 2 years of age and older—Response to one of the important pediatric pneumococcal types, type 14, is decreased in children who are less than 5 years of age. Other pediatrics-specific problems that would limit the usefulness of this vaccine in children 2 years of age and older are not expected.

### Geriatrics

Appropriate studies on the relationship of age to the effects of pneumococcal vaccine have not been performed in the geriatric population. However, geriatrics-specific problems that would limit the usefulness of this vaccine in the elderly are not expected.

### Drug interactions and/or related problems

The following drug interactions and/or related problems have been selected on the basis of their potential clinical significance (possible mechanism in parentheses where appropriate)—not necessarily inclusive (» = major clinical significance):

Note: Combinations containing any of the following medications, depending on the amount present, may also interact with this medication.

Immunosuppressive agents or
Radiation therapy
(because normal defense mechanisms are suppressed, the patient's antibody response to the pneumococcal vaccine may be decreased. If possible, persons who are to undergo therapy with medications that cause immunosuppression, including candidates for organ transplants, should receive the vaccine at least 10 days, and preferably more than 14 days, prior to receiving the immunosuppression-causing medication to receive the full immunizing effect of the vaccine. The precaution does not apply to corticosteroids used as replacement therapy, for short-term [less than 2 weeks] systemic therapy, or by other routes of administration that do not cause immunosuppression)
(patients with Hodgkin's disease should not receive the vaccine less than 10 days prior to, or during, immunosuppressive therapy, since some patients so immunized have exhibited post-immunization antibody levels below their preimmunization levels. In addition, patients with Hodgkin's disease who have received extensive chemotherapy and/or nodal irradiation should not receive the vaccine at all, since immunization of some intensively treated patients caused depression of pre-existing levels of antibody to some pneumococcal types)

» Pneumococcal vaccine polyvalent, other
(persons previously immunized with pneumococcal vaccine of any valence generally should not be revaccinated with pneumococcal vaccine polyvalent 23, because of increased frequency and severity of side/adverse effects, including Arthus and systemic reactions. However, it may be desirable to administer subsequent doses of vaccine to patients at high risk of severe illness or death from pneumococcal disease [See *Indications*.])

### Medical considerations/Contraindications

The medical considerations/contraindications included here have been selected on the basis of their potential clinical significance (reasons given in parentheses where appropriate)—not necessarily inclusive (» = major clinical significance).

*Risk-benefit should be considered when the following medical problems exist:*

Febrile illness, severe
(to avoid confusing manifestations of illness with possible side/adverse effects of vaccine; minor illnesses, such as upper respiratory infection, do not preclude administration of vaccine)

Sensitivity to pneumococcal vaccine

Thrombocytopenic purpura, idiopathic
(in one report, two stabilized patients experienced a relapse 2 to 14 days after vaccination; this relapse lasted up to 2 weeks)

## Side/Adverse Effects

Note: Neurological disorders, such as paresthesias and acute radiculoneuropathy, including Guillain-Barré syndrome (GBS), have been reported rarely in temporal association with pneumococcal vaccine administration; however, no causal relationship has been established, and the incidence of GBS in vaccinated persons appears to be no greater than the incidence in the general population.

Some persons previously vaccinated with a pneumococcal vaccine of any valence and subsequently revaccinated with the same or a different polyvalent pneumococcal vaccine have experienced increased frequency and severity of side/adverse effects, including Arthus and systemic reactions.

It is recommended that persons who experience neurological symptoms or signs following administration of pneumococcal vaccine should not be reimmunized.

The following side/adverse effects have been selected on the basis of their potential clinical significance (possible signs and symptoms in parentheses where appropriate)—not necessarily inclusive:

**Those indicating need for medical attention**
Incidence rare
*Anaphylactic reaction* (difficulty in breathing or swallowing; hives; itching, especially of soles or palms; reddening of skin, especially around ears; swelling of eyes, face, or inside of nose; unusual tiredness or weakness, sudden and severe); *fever over 39 °C (102 °F)*

**Those indicating need for medical attention only if they continue or are bothersome**
Incidence more frequent
*Redness, soreness, hard lump, swelling, or pain at injection site*
Incidence less frequent or rare
*Adenitis* (swollen glands); *arthralgia or myalgia* (aches or pain in joints or muscles); *asthenia* (unusual tiredness or weakness); *fever of 38.3 °C (101 °F) or less; malaise* (vague feeling of bodily discomfort); *skin rash*

## Patient Consultation

As an aid to patient consultation, refer to *Advice for the Patient, Pneumococcal Vaccine Polyvalent (Systemic).*

In providing consultation, consider emphasizing the following selected information (» = major clinical significance):

**Before receiving this vaccine**
» Conditions affecting use, especially:
Sensitivity to pneumococcal vaccine or thimerosal
Pregnancy—If needed, administer vaccine following the first trimester and only to women at high risk of pneumococcal disease
Use in children—Not recommended for infants and children younger than 2 years of age
Other medications, especially previous use of any pneumococcal vaccine

**Proper use of this vaccine**
» Proper dosing

**Precautions after receiving this vaccine**
» Notifying all patient's physicians that patient has received pneumococcal vaccine polyvalent 23 so that the information can be included in patient's medical records; the vaccine is usually administered only once

**Side/adverse effects**
Signs of potential side effects, especially anaphylactic reaction or fever over 39 °C (102 °F)

## General Dosing Information

The dosage of pneumococcal vaccine polyvalent is the same for all persons: children and adults.

When sterilizing syringes before vaccination, care should be taken to avoid preservatives, antiseptics, detergents, and disinfectants, since the vaccine is easily inactivated by these substances.

Pneumococcal vaccine polyvalent is administered by subcutaneous or intramuscular injection. It is not recommended for intradermal injection, because it may cause severe local reactions. Also, intravenous administration is not recommended.

Pneumococcal vaccine polyvalent, a polysaccharide vaccine, can be administered concurrently with the following, using separate body sites, separate syringes, and the precautions that apply to each immunizing agent:
• Polysaccharide vaccines, other, such as haemophilus b polysaccharide vaccine, haemophilus b conjugate vaccine, or meningococcal polysaccharide vaccine.
• Influenza vaccine, whole or split virus.
• Diphtheria toxoid, tetanus toxoid, and/or pertussis vaccine.
• Live virus vaccines, such as measles, mumps, and/or rubella vaccines.
• Poliovirus vaccines (oral [OPV], inactivated [IPV], or enhanced-potency inactivated [enhanced-potency IPV]).
• Immune globulin and disease-specific immune globulins.
• Hepatitis B recombinant or plasma-derived vaccine, or other inactivated vaccines, except cholera, typhoid, and plague. It is recommended that cholera, typhoid, and plague vaccines be administered on separate occasions because of these vaccines' propensity to cause side/adverse effects.

Patients who require antibiotic prophylaxis against pneumococcal infection should continue to receive antibiotic therapy after vaccination with pneumococcal vaccine.

**For treatment of adverse effects**
Recommended treatment includes
• For mild hypersensitivity reaction—Administering antihistamines, and, if necessary, corticosteroids.
• For severe hypersensitivity or anaphylactic reaction—Administering epinephrine. Antihistamines or corticosteroids may also be administered as required.

## Parenteral Dosage Forms

### PNEUMOCOCCAL VACCINE POLYVALENT INJECTION

**Usual adult and adolescent dose**
Immunizing agent (active)—
Intramuscular or subcutaneous, 0.5 mL, preferably into the outer aspect of the upper arm or into the lateral mid-thigh.

**Usual pediatric dose**
Immunizing agent (active)—
Infants and children up to 2 years of age: Use is not recommended, since this age group may not show adequate response to many of the antigens, and antibody levels stimulated by the vaccine may not persist.
Children 2 years of age and older: See *Usual adult and adolescent dose.*

**Strength(s) usually available**
U.S.—
25 mcg of polysaccharide from each of the 23 capsular types of pneumococci represented in the vaccine in each 0.5 mL dose (Rx) [*Pneumovax 23* (phenol 0.25%); *Pnu-Imune 23* (thimerosal 0.01%)].
Canada—
25 mcg of polysaccharide from each of the 23 capsular types of pneumococci represented in the vaccine in each 0.5 mL dose (Rx) [*Pneumovax 23* (phenol 0.25%)].

**Packaging and storage**
Store manufacturer-supplied filled syringes, unopened vials, and partially used vials of the vaccine between 2 and 8 °C (36 and 46 °F), unless otherwise specified by manufacturer. Protect from freezing.

**Stability**
The vaccine is a clear, colorless solution. It should not be used if it is discolored or contains a precipitate.

**Incompatibilities**
A sterile syringe free of preservatives, antiseptics, disinfectants, and detergents should be used for each injection because these substances may inactivate the vaccine.

**Auxiliary labeling**
• Store in refrigerator.

Revised: 07/12/94

# PODOPHYLLUM    Topical†

VA CLASSIFICATION (Primary): DE500

Note: For a listing of dosage forms and brand names by country availability, see *Dosage Forms* section(s). For a listing of brand names for the articles in this monograph, refer to the General Index.

†Not commercially available in Canada.

## Category
Cytotoxic (topical).

## Indications

### Accepted
Condylomata acuminata (treatment)—Podophyllum is indicated for the treatment of condylomata acuminata (venereal warts).

Epitheliomatosis, multiple superficial (treatment) or
Keratosis, pre-epitheliomatosis (treatment) or
Papilloma, of the larynx, juvenile (treatment)—Podophyllum is used in the treatment of multiple superficial epitheliomatosis, such as multiple superficial or infiltrating basal cell epithelioma, squamous cell epithelioma (prickle cell epithelioma), and basal-squamous cell epithelioma (mixed or transitional cell epithelioma); seborrheic, actinic, and roentgen ray keratoses; and juvenile papilloma of the larynx.

### Unaccepted
Podophyllum has been used in the treatment of general types of verrucae, such as vulgaris (common warts), filiformis (filiform warts), plana (flat warts), and plantaris (plantar warts); however, it is much less effective in these types of warts than in venereal warts. Also, podophyllum therapy is less effective than other types of treatment for these warts.

## Pharmacology/Pharmacokinetics

### Physicochemical characteristics
Source—Dried resin from the roots and rhizomes of *Podophyllum peltatum* (mandrake or May apple plant), the North American variety; active constituents are lignans including podophyllotoxin (20%), alpha-peltatin (10%), and beta-peltatin (5%).

### Mechanism of action/Effect
Podophyllum resin's major active constituent, podophyllotoxin, is a lipid-soluble compound that easily crosses cell membranes. Podophyllotoxin and its derivatives are potent cytotoxic agents that inhibit cell mitosis and deoxyribonucleic acid (DNA) synthesis in a manner similar to that of colchicine. Cell division is arrested, and other cellular processes are impaired, gradually resulting in the disruption of cells and erosion of the tissue.

### Absorption
Topical podophyllum is systemically absorbed; absorption may be increased if podophyllum is applied to friable, bleeding, or recently biopsied warts.

## Precautions to Consider

### Cross-sensitivity and/or related problems
Patients sensitive to benzoin may be sensitive to this medication also because some preparations may contain tincture of benzoin.

### Pregnancy/Reproduction
Pregnancy—Topical podophyllum is absorbed systemically and can cross the placenta. It should not be used during any phase of pregnancy, because of its teratogenic potential. Following oral administration during pregnancy, podophyllum has been reported to cause fetal abnormalities, such as skin tags on the ears and cheeks, limb malformations, and septal heart defects, as well as polyneuritis. Intrauterine death has occurred following topical application to vulval warts during the 32nd week of pregnancy. In one patient, minor fetal anomalies, including preauricular skin tags and a simian crease on the left hand, occurred following topical application during the 23rd, 24th, 25th, 28th, and 29th weeks of pregnancy.

Warts of the vaginal, perianal, or anal areas requiring treatment during pregnancy should be treated by alternative methods, such as electro-desiccation, diathermy, curettage, surgical excision, or cryosurgery with liquid nitrogen or dry ice.

### Breast-feeding
Topical podophyllum is systemically absorbed. However, it is not known whether topical podophyllum is distributed into breast milk. Problems in humans have not been documented.

### Pediatrics
Appropriate studies on the relationship of age to the effects of topical podophyllum have not been performed in the pediatric population. However, no pediatrics-specific problems have been documented to date.

### Geriatrics
Appropriate studies on the relationship of age to the effects of topical podophyllum have not been performed in the geriatric population. However, no geriatrics-specific problems have been documented to date.

### Laboratory value alterations
The following have been selected on the basis of their potential clinical significance (possible effect in parentheses where appropriate)—not necessarily inclusive ($\gg$ = major clinical significance):

With physiology/laboratory test values
Alkaline phosphatase and
Aspartate aminotransferase (AST [SGOT]) and
Lactate dehydrogenase (LDH)
(serum values may be increased in association with renal failure and hepatotoxicity)

### Medical considerations/Contraindications
The medical considerations/contraindications included here have been selected on the basis of their potential clinical significance (reasons given in parentheses where appropriate)—not necessarily inclusive ($\gg$ = major clinical significance).

*Risk-benefit should be considered when the following medical problems exist:*
$\gg$  Friable, bleeding, or recently biopsied warts
(risk of systemic toxicity may be increased)
Sensitivity to podophyllum

## Side/Adverse Effects

Note: Podophyllum resin topical solution is highly irritating to the eye and to mucous membranes in general.

Podophyllum can cause severe systemic toxicity, which may result from either topical application or ingestion. The toxic effects are usually reversible but have been fatal. Death can occur with ingestion of podophyllum in amounts as small as 300 mg.

Serious systemic toxicity has occurred following topical application of podophyllum to large areas or in excessive amounts, or when the medication was allowed to remain in contact with the skin or mucous membranes for a prolonged period of time.

The risk of systemic toxicity may be increased when podophyllum is applied to friable, bleeding, or recently biopsied warts, or when the medication is inadvertently applied to normal skin or mucous membranes surrounding the affected area(s).

Renal failure and hepatotoxicity have occurred following topical application of podophyllum.

Adverse effects on the nervous system may occur following topical application of podophyllum; these are usually delayed in onset and prolonged in duration.

Cerebral toxicity (manifested by altered sensorium ranging from mild confusion to coma) may occur following topical application of podophyllum and continue for 7 to 10 days during which the electroencephalogram (EEG) may show generalized slowing.

The following side/adverse effects have been selected on the basis of their potential clinical significance (possible signs and symptoms in parentheses where appropriate)—not necessarily inclusive:

### Those indicating need for medical attention
*Burning, redness, or other irritation of affected area; skin rash or itching*—allergic reaction to benzoin, which may be present in some preparations

## Overdose
For specific information on the agents used in the management of podophyllum overdose, see:
• *Charcoal, Activated (Oral-Local)* monograph.

For more information on the management of overdose or unintentional ingestion, **contact a Poison Control Center** (see *Poison Control Center Listing*).

**Clinical effects of overdose**

The following effects have been selected on the basis of their potential clinical significance (possible signs and symptoms in parentheses where appropriate)—not necessarily inclusive:

Initial symptoms of systemic toxicity

*Abdominal or stomach pain; clumsiness or unsteadiness; confusion; decreased or loss of reflexes; diarrhea*—sometimes severe and prolonged; *excitement, irritability, or nervousness; hallucinations; leukopenia* (sore throat and fever); *muscle weakness; nausea or vomiting; thrombocytopenia* (unusual bleeding or bruising)

Delayed symptoms of systemic toxicity

*Autonomic neuropathy* (difficult or painful urination; dizziness or lightheadedness, especially when getting up from a lying or sitting position; fast heartbeat); *difficulty in breathing; drowsiness; paralytic ileus* (constipation; nausea and vomiting; pain in upper abdomen or stomach, mild, dull, and continuing); *peripheral neuropathy* (numbness, tingling, pain, or weakness in hands or feet); *seizures*

Note: If *peripheral neuropathy* occurs, it usually appears about 2 weeks after podophyllum application, may worsen progressively for up to 3 months, and may persist for up to 9 months or longer.

**Treatment of overdose**

Treatment of systemic toxicity or accidental ingestion is essentially supportive and may included the following:

To decrease absorption—If podophyllum is accidentally ingested and the patient is conscious, emesis should be immediately induced. If the patient is unconscious, gastric lavage should be performed. Activated charcoal may also be administered.

To enhance elimination—Charcoal hemoperfusion may be beneficial in life-threatening or deteriorating conditions.

Monitoring—Electrolytes, serum calcium, and hemoglobin concentrations should be closely monitored.

Supportive care—Intravenous therapy and respiratory support should be administered if necessary. Patients in whom intentional overdose is known or suspected should be referred for psychiatric consultation.

## Patient Consultation

As an aid to patient consultation, refer to *Advice for the Patient, Podophyllum (Topical)*.

In providing consultation, consider emphasizing the following selected information (» = major clinical significance):

**Before using this medication**

» Conditions affecting use, especially:
   Sensitivity to podophyllum or benzoin
   Pregnancy—Podophyllum should not be used during pregnancy, because it is absorbed through the mother's skin
   Breast-feeding—Podophyllum is absorbed through the mother's skin
   Other medical problems, especially friable, bleeding, or recently biopsied warts, because of increased risk of systemic toxicity

**Proper use of this medication**

» Importance of keeping away from mouth; medication is poisonous
» Avoiding contact with the eyes and mucous membranes; if contact occurs, immediately flushing eyes with water for 15 minutes, and thoroughly washing skin with soap and water or (if preparation contains tincture of benzoin) swabbing it with rubbing alcohol
» Not using near heat, open flame, or while smoking
» Importance of not using more medication than the amount prescribed
» Not using on moles or birthmarks
» Not using on friable, bleeding, or recently biopsied warts
*Proper administration*
» Preventing dissemination of podophyllum to uninvolved skin—Applying petrolatum around affected areas before applying podophyllum and/or applying talcum powder to treated area immediately after applying podophyllum
   Using a toothpick or a cotton-tipped or glass applicator to apply medication
   Applying one drop at a time, allowing time between drops for drying, until affected area is covered
   Following application of podophyllum, allowing medication to remain on affected area for 1 to 6 hours as directed by physician; removing medication by thoroughly washing affected area with soap and water or, if preparation contains tincture of benzoin, swabbing it with rubbing alcohol
   Washing hands immediately after using medication
» Proper dosing
   Missed dose: Applying as soon as possible
» Proper storage

**Side/adverse effects**

Signs of potential side effects, especially burning, redness, or other irritation of affected area; skin rash or itching; or initial or delayed symptoms of systemic toxicity

## General Dosing Information

Some clinicians recommend that podophyllum be used only under medical supervision because of its potentially serious adverse effects.

Old, discolored, dried, or gritty preparations of podophyllum should not be used.

Podophyllum should not be applied to friable, bleeding, or recently biopsied warts, because systemic absorption of the medication may be increased.

Podophyllum should not be used on moles or birthmarks, since acute inflammation or ulceration may occur.

Podophyllum is most frequently used in a concentration of 25%; however, concentrations of 5 to 10% have been recommended for very large lesions (>10 to 20 cm²) in order to minimize the risk of toxicity.

Also, to minimize the risk of toxicity, application of podophyllum should be limited to small areas of intact skin.

If podophyllum is to be self-administered, patients should be instructed to use the medication with great caution. It should be applied only to the affected areas, avoiding contact with normal tissue. This medication can cause severe erosive damage to normal skin.

If podophyllum accidentally comes in contact with normal tissue, it should be removed, preferably by thoroughly washing with soap and water, or, if the podophyllum preparation contains tincture of benzoin, swabbing with rubbing alcohol.

Great care should be taken to avoid contact with the eyes because podophyllum can cause corneal damage. If contact does occur, the eyes should be immediately and thoroughly flushed with water for 15 minutes.

To prevent dissemination of the medication to uninvolved skin, petrolatum may be applied to normal skin surrounding the affected areas prior to application of podophyllum and/or talcum powder may be applied to the treated area immediately following application of podophyllum.

A toothpick or a cotton-tipped or glass applicator should be used to apply the topical solution one drop at a time, until the affected area is covered. Sufficient time should be allowed between drops for drying.

**For condylomata acuminata**

Following application of podophyllum, the medication should be allowed to remain on the affected area for a period of 1 to 6 hours as prescribed by the physician.

At the end of the treatment period, the medication should be removed, preferably by thoroughly washing with soap and water. Some clinicians recommend removing podophyllum preparations that contain tincture of benzoin by swabbing with rubbing alcohol; however, this may be more irritating than washing with soap and water.

A minimum of 7 days should elapse between treatments because of the risk of systemic toxicity. Treatment may be repeated at weekly intervals for up to 4 weeks; however, if a beneficial effect does not occur within 4 weeks, alternative therapy should be considered.

**For multiple superficial epitheliomatosis or pre-epitheliomatosis keratoses**

Before each subsequent application of the medication, the necrotic tissue should be removed by curettage or wiped away with gauze.

In response to treatment, the lesion usually sloughs off leaving a superficial ulcer and a moderate degree of dermatitis of the immediate surrounding tissue. When treatment is discontinued, the lesion may be dressed with a mild antiseptic ointment; healing usually occurs in a few days, except in very large lesions, which may take longer to heal.

## Topical Dosage Forms

### PODOPHYLLUM RESIN TOPICAL SOLUTION USP

**Usual adult and adolescent dose**

Condylomata acuminata—
   Topical, to the skin, as a 10 to 25% solution for a period of one to six hours; treatment may be repeated at one-week intervals for up to four weeks.

Multiple superficial epitheliomatosis or
Pre-epitheliomatosis keratoses—
   Topical, to the skin, as a 25% solution once a day; treatment should be continued for several days following the initial slough.

Juvenile papilloma of the larynx—
   Topical, to the lesion, as a 12.5% solution once a day. The intervals of treatment can be gradually increased as the lesions become

smaller; however, applications at short intervals give the best results.

**Usual pediatric dose**
See *Usual adult and adolescent dose.*

**Strength(s) usually available**
U.S.—
25% (Rx) [*Podocon-25; Podofin*].
Note: Other strengths are currently not commercially available; compounding required for prescriptions.
Canada—
Podophyllum resin of the North American variety is not commercially available.

**Packaging and storage**
Store below 40 °C (104 °F), preferably between 15 and 30 °C (59 and 86 °F), unless otherwise specified by manufacturer. Store in a tight, light-resistant container. Protect from freezing.

**Preparation of dosage form**
For treatment of juvenile papilloma of the larynx, the 25% solution should be diluted with an equal volume of 95% alcohol to yield the 12.5% solution.
A 25% Podophyllum Resin Topical Solution USP may be prepared extemporaneously by mixing 25 grams of the alcohol-soluble extractive

of podophyllum resin in alcohol and 10 grams of the alcohol-soluble extractive of benzoin in alcohol, and diluting with alcohol to make 100 mL.
The solution should be prepared with native North American podophyllum resin, rather than a mixture of North American and Indian resins, because the Indian resin is stronger and more irritating than the North American variety. Also, the resin should be free of guaiacium gum, which may be a sensitizer.
Other vehicles that may be used for preparation of podophyllum resin topical solution include mineral oil or collodion.

**Stability**
Exposure to light, air, and warmth may cause precipitation and darkening of the solution because of evaporation and decomposition; such solutions should be discarded.

**Auxiliary labeling**
• Poison.
• For external use only.
• Shake well.
• Keep container tightly closed.

Revised: 08/15/94

# POLIOVIRUS VACCINE    Systemic

This monograph includes information on the following: Poliovirus Vaccine Inactivated; Poliovirus Vaccine Inactivated Enhanced Potency; Poliovirus Vaccine Live Oral.

VA CLASSIFICATION (Primary): IM100

Other commonly used names are: Enhanced-potency IPV [Poliovirus Vaccine Inactivated Enhanced Potency], IPV [Poliovirus Vaccine Inactivated], N-IPV [Poliovirus Vaccine Inactivated Enhanced Potency], OPV [Poliovirus Vaccine Live Oral], Sabin vaccine [Poliovirus Vaccine Live Oral], Salk vaccine [Poliovirus Vaccine Inactivated], TOPV [Poliovirus Vaccine Live Oral]

Note: For a listing of dosage forms and brand names by country availability, see *Dosage Forms* section(s). For a listing of brand names for the articles in this monograph, refer to the General Index.

## Category

Immunizing agent (active).

## Indications

**Accepted**
Poliomyelitis (prophylaxis)—IPV, enhanced-potency IPV, and OPV are indicated for immunization against poliomyelitis caused by poliovirus types 1, 2, and 3 according to the following recommendations.

Unless otherwise contraindicated, all infants from age 6 to 12 weeks, all children, all adolescents up to 18 years of age, and adults at greater risk of exposure to polioviruses than the general population who do not have time to receive IPV immunization should be immunized against poliomyelitis with OPV.

OPV is the vaccine of choice for infants and children up to 18 years of age because the vaccine induces intestinal immunity that provides resistance to reinfection with polioviruses, is easy to administer, is well accepted by parents, results in immunization of some contacts of the vaccinated children, and has a record of having essentially eliminated poliomyelitis associated with wild poliovirus in the U.S.

Immunization with IPV or enhanced-potency IPV is recommended for adults who are at greater risk of exposure to polioviruses than the general population. However, since enhanced-potency IPV is more consistently immunogenic than IPV, it is generally preferred to IPV. IPV or enhanced-potency IPV is the vaccine of choice over OPV, with certain exceptions, for adults 18 years of age and older, especially those with no history of poliovirus vaccination, because the risk of vaccine-associated paralysis following OPV is slightly higher for adults than for children. However, routine primary poliovirus vaccination with IPV or enhanced-potency IPV of adults (18 years of age or older) residing in the U.S. and Canada who have not had a primary series as children is not necessary. Most adults are already immune and also have a very small risk of exposure to polioviruses in the U.S. and Canada.

In addition, the following persons should be immunized against poliomyelitis:
• Persons traveling to countries with endemic or epidemic poliomyelitis, whether or not they have been previously immunized.
• Unimmunized adults at increased risk of exposure to polioviruses.
• Incompletely immunized adults at increased risk of exposure to polioviruses.
• Previously vaccinated adults at increased risk of exposure to polioviruses.
• Personnel in day-care centers and custodial institutions for children.
• Medical personnel and employees in medical facilities should be immunized with IPV or enhanced-potency IPV instead of OPV because virus may be shed after receipt of OPV and inadvertent contact with susceptible immunocompromised patients may occur.
• Persons at risk during a poliomyelitis epidemic. OPV should be administered to all persons within the epidemic area who are over 6 weeks of age and have not been completely immunized or whose immunization status is unknown, with the exception of persons with immunodeficiency considerations. Infants can receive OPV at birth, but because successful immunization is less likely in newborn infants, a complete series of OPV beginning when the infants are 6 weeks of age should also be administered.
• Members of communities or specific population groups with disease caused by wild polioviruses.
• Newborn infants living in tropical endemic areas where the incidence of poliomyelitis is increasing should receive OPV at birth. However, because successful immunization is less likely in newborn infants, a complete series of OPV beginning when the infants are 6 weeks of age should also be administered. There should be a minimum interval of 4 weeks between the neonatal dose and the first dose of the primary series of OPV; in addition, subsequent doses of the primary series should be administered at 4-week intervals. Optimally, the neonate should be immunized with OPV 3 days after birth, and breast-feeding should be withheld for 2 or 3 hours before and after immunization to allow for the establishment of the vaccine viruses in the infant's gut.
• Laboratory workers handling specimens that may contain polioviruses.
• Immunodeficient patients and their household contacts, whether or not the immunodeficient patient had at some earlier time received a poliovirus immunization when his/her immune status was normal. This is because some immunodeficiencies impair the immune response to antigens against which the immune system was previously primed. IPV or enhanced-potency IPV is the poliovirus vaccine of choice. Although patients with immune deficiency diseases may not develop a protective immune response, immunization with IPV or enhanced-potency IPV should be attempted anyway. OPV should not be given to persons residing in the household of an immunocompromised or immunosuppressed person, because live poliovirus is excreted by the recipient of OPV and may be communicable to the immunocompromised or immunosuppressed person. If protection against poliomyelitis is required, IPV or enhanced-potency IPV should be used for immu-

nizing household contacts of immunocompromised or immunosuppressed persons.
- Members of a household in which there is a family history of acquired or hereditary immunodeficiency. IPV or enhanced-potency IPV is the poliovirus vaccine of choice. OPV should not be given to a member of a household in which there is a family history of acquired or hereditary immunodeficiency unless or until the immune status of the family members as well as the patient is known.

Adults who have not been immunized or who are inadequately immunized with either OPV, IPV, or enhanced-potency IPV are at a very small risk (approximately 1 case in 5 million doses of OPV distributed) of developing OPV-associated paralytic poliomyelitis when children in the household are given OPV. These adults should receive IPV or enhanced-potency IPV. However, because of the overriding importance of ensuring timely immunization of children and the extreme rarity of OPV-associated disease in contacts, children should be immunized on schedule with OPV regardless of the poliovirus-vaccine status of adult household contacts. Only if the child's immunization will not be jeopardized or unduly delayed should the adult be immunized before administering OPV to the child. Adults who want to be immunized should receive at least 2 doses of IPV or enhanced-potency IPV a month apart before the children are immunized, and preferably, the full primary series. The children may receive their first dose of OPV at the same time that the adults receive their third dose of IPV or their second dose of enhanced-potency IPV. Adult household contacts who are not adequately immunized prior to the child's receiving OPV should be informed of the small risk involved and of the precautions to be taken, such as hand washing after changing the immunized infant's diaper.

Poliovirus vaccines are not effective in modifying cases of existing poliomyelitis or preventing cases of incubating poliomyelitis.

## Pharmacology/Pharmacokinetics

### Physicochemical characteristics
Source—
Produced from a mixture of 3 types of attenuated polioviruses that have been propagated in monkey kidney cell culture
Poliovirus vaccine inactivated (IPV) and Poliovirus vaccine inactivated enhanced potency (enhanced-potency IPV): The polioviruses are inactivated with formaldehyde
Poliovirus vaccine live oral (OPV): Contains the live, attenuated polioviruses

### Mechanism of action/Effect
Administration of poliovirus vaccine inactivated (IPV), poliovirus vaccine inactivated enhanced potency (enhanced-potency IPV), or poliovirus vaccine live oral (OPV) simulates natural infection by inducing systemic immunity. In addition, OPV induces active mucosal immunity because the live viruses multiply in the intestinal tract. These live viruses persist in the intestinal tract for at least 4 to 6 weeks. The antibodies formed by the administration of a primary series of IPV, enhanced-potency IPV, or OPV protect the person against clinical poliomyelitis infection by any of the 3 types of poliovirus.

### Other actions/effects
Live poliovirus is excreted by persons recently immunized with OPV, especially following the first dose. The vaccine viruses are excreted in the immunized person's feces for at least 6 to 8 weeks and also from the nose or throat for 7 to 10 days.

OPV induces intestinal immunity that provides resistance to reinfection with polioviruses, including the simultaneous infection by wild polioviruses. This is of special value in epidemic-control campaigns. Persons immunized with IPV or enhanced-potency IPV are more likely to be subclinically infected with and excrete in the feces either wild strains or attenuated vaccine virus strains. Immunization with IPV, enhanced-potency IPV, or especially OPV has greatly reduced the circulation of wild polioviruses, and inapparent infection with wild strains no longer contributes significantly to establishing or maintaining immunity; this makes universal vaccination of infants and children even more important.

### Protective effect
A primary vaccination series with 3 doses of OPV, 3 doses of enhanced-potency IPV, or 4 doses of IPV produces immunity to all three poliovirus types in more than 95% of recipients. When OPV is used, many persons are protected after a single dose and most are protected after 2 doses. When enhanced-potency IPV is used, most persons are protected after the second dose. An antibody response to OPV usually occurs within 7 to 10 days after administration and peaks approximately 21 days later.

### Duration of protective effect
With IPV, although vaccine-induced antibodies have persisted for 12 years in some persons, the duration of immunity following primary immunization with the currently available IPV has not been established.
Although conclusive studies are not yet available with enhanced-potency IPV, unpublished studies of an enhanced-potency IPV with a lower antigen content than the U.S. product have shown 100% seropositivity 5 years after the third dose.
With OPV, 95% of children studied 5 years after full immunization had protective antibodies to all 3 types of poliovirus, and some studies show persistence of local intestinal immunity in some persons for more than 6 years; however, the duration of humoral and intestinal immunity following primary immunization with OPV has not been established.

## Precautions to Consider

### Cross-sensitivity and/or related problems
Persons sensitive to one poliovirus vaccine may be sensitive to the other poliovirus vaccines also.
In addition, in the U.S., patients allergic to the following may be allergic to poliovirus vaccines also:
- Neomycin, which may be contained in IPV, enhanced-potency IPV, and OPV.
- Polymyxin B, which may be contained in enhanced-potency IPV.
- Streptomycin, which may be contained in IPV, enhanced-potency IPV, and OPV.
In Canada, patients allergic to the following may be allergic to poliovirus vaccines also:
- Neomycin, which may be contained in IPV, enhanced-potency IPV, and OPV.
- Penicillin, which may be contained in OPV.
- Polymyxin B, which may be contained in OPV.
- Streptomycin, which may be contained in IPV, enhanced-potency IPV, and OPV.
A history of hypersensitivity reactions other than anaphylaxis, such as delayed-type allergic reaction (contact dermatitis), generally does not preclude immunization.

### Carcinogenicity/Mutagenicity
Studies have not been done.

### Pregnancy/Reproduction
Fertility—Studies have not been done.

Pregnancy—Studies have not been done in humans, and problems in humans have not been documented. Although routine immunization of pregnant women is not recommended, if the risk of exposure is or will be high during pregnancy, it is recommended that OPV be administered. However, if time is available before the risk of exposure occurs, some experts recommend that IPV be administered. Enhanced-potency IPV is not recommended for use in pregnant women, because of the lack of data on possible adverse effects.
Although live poliovirus is shed by persons recently immunized with OPV, especially following the first dose, OPV can be administered to children of pregnant women without special risk to the pregnant woman or the fetus.
Studies have not been done in animals.
FDA Pregnancy Category C.

### Breast-feeding
IPV—Problems in humans have not been documented.
Enhanced-potency IPV—Problems in humans have not been documented.
OPV—Although poliovirus antibodies may be distributed into breast milk, mothers who breast-feed can receive OPV without any interruption in the feeding schedule. In addition, breast-feeding does not interfere with the usual immunization of infants with OPV. However, when a neonate is immunized at birth, as may occur in tropical endemic areas or during a poliomyelitis epidemic, breast-feeding should be withheld for 2 or 3 hours before and after immunization with OPV because the colostrum may interfere with the establishment of the vaccine viruses in the neonate's gut.

### Pediatrics
Infants up to 6 weeks of age—Use is not recommended.
Infants and children 6 weeks of age and older—Pediatrics-specific problems that would limit the usefulness of this vaccine in children in this age group are not expected.

### Geriatrics
Appropriate studies on the relationship of age to the effects of poliovirus vaccine have not been performed in the geriatric population. However, geriatrics-specific problems that would limit the usefulness of this vaccine in the elderly are not expected.

## Drug interactions and/or related problems

The following drug interactions and/or related problems have been selected on the basis of their potential clinical significance (possible mechanism in parentheses where appropriate)—not necessarily inclusive (» = major clinical significance):

Note: Combinations containing any of the following medications, depending on the amount present, may also interact with this vaccine.

Blood products, antibody-containing or
Immune globulin (IG)
  (do not appear to interfere with the immune response to OPV; OPV may be administered concurrently with immune globulins if necessary. Since IPV and enhanced-potency IPV are inactivated products, there is no reason to suspect interference, and IPV or enhanced-potency IPV can be administered without regard to immune globulins)

» Immunosuppressants or
» Radiation therapy
  (because normal defense mechanisms are suppressed, the patient's antibody response to any of the poliovirus vaccines may be decreased; in addition, the use of a live virus vaccine, such as OPV, may potentiate the replication of the vaccine virus, possibly causing poliomyelitis infection secondary to the vaccine; therefore, OPV should not be administered to these patients; IPV or enhanced-potency IPV should be administered instead. The precaution does not apply to corticosteroids used as replacement therapy, for short-term [less than 2 weeks] systemic therapy, or by other routes of administration that do not cause immunosuppression)

  (where there is a family history of congenital or hereditary immune deficiency conditions, the patient should not be vaccinated with OPV until his/her immune competence is demonstrated; IPV or enhanced-potency IPV should be administered instead)

Live virus vaccines, other
  (although data are lacking on impairment of antibody responses to rubella, measles, mumps, or OPV when these vaccines are administered on different days within 1 month of each other, the chance exists that the immune responses may be impaired when live virus vaccines are administered in this manner; therefore, when feasible, live virus vaccines not administered on the same day should be given at least 1 month apart)

## Medical considerations/Contraindications

The medical considerations/contraindications included here have been selected on the basis of their potential clinical significance (reasons given in parentheses where appropriate)—not necessarily inclusive (» = major clinical significance).

Note: A past history of clinical poliomyelitis in otherwise healthy persons does not preclude the administration of IPV, enhanced-potency IPV, or OPV if such administration is otherwise indicated.

  Persons who are immunized with OPV should avoid close contact for at least 6 to 8 weeks with persons with altered immune status.

*Except under special circumstances, this vaccine should not be used when the following medical problems exist:*

» Debilitated condition, advanced or
» Illness, moderate or severe, with or without fever
  (administration of IPV, enhanced-potency IPV, or OPV should be postponed or avoided; minor illnesses, such as mild upper respiratory infections, do not preclude administration of vaccine)

» Diarrhea, persistent or
» Viral infection or
» Vomiting, persistent
  (the presence of other viruses, including poliovirus and other enteroviruses, in the intestinal tract may interfere with the replication of OPV and therefore with final immunity. Alternatives in the presence of the above illnesses include administration of IPV or, in the case of persistent diarrhea, the administration of OPV without it counting as part of the primary series)

» Immune deficiency conditions, congenital or hereditary, family history of or
» Immune deficiency conditions, primary or acquired
  (because of reduced or suppressed defense mechanisms, patients who are immunocompromised or immunosuppressed should not receive live virus vaccines, such as OPV; IPV or enhanced-potency IPV should be administered instead)

  (persons with leukemia in remission may receive live virus vaccines, such as OPV, if at least 3 months have passed since their last chemotherapy treatment)

  (persons with asymptomatic or symptomatic human immunodeficiency virus [HIV] infection may receive IPV or enhanced-potency IPV, but not OPV)

(when there is a family history of congenital or hereditary immune deficiency conditions, the patient should not be vaccinated with OPV until his/her immune competence is demonstrated; IPV or enhanced-potency IPV should be administered instead)

Sensitivity to poliovirus vaccine

## Side/Adverse Effects

Note: The risk of developing OPV-associated paralytic poliomyelitis is as follows in unimmunized persons:
  • Approximately 1 case in 5 million doses of OPV distributed, in adults living in the same household as children who are given OPV.
  • Approximately 1 case in 3.2 million doses of OPV distributed, in all normal vaccine recipients or their close contacts.
  • Approximately 1 case in 2.6 million doses of OPV distributed, in all cases (normal as well as immune-deficient recipients and all close contacts).

No paralytic poliomyelitis reactions to poliovirus vaccine inactivated (IPV) have occurred since the 1955 incident in which the vaccine contained live viruses that had escaped inactivation. Although Guillain-Barré syndrome (GBS) has occurred following IPV, no causal relationship has been established. In addition, no other serious side effects of IPV have been documented.

Since there is no evidence that IPV causes serious side effects, poliovirus vaccine inactivated enhanced potency (enhanced-potency IPV) is not expected to cause serious side effects either.

A history of hypersensitivity reactions other than anaphylaxis, such as delayed-type allergic reaction (contact dermatitis), generally does not preclude immunization.

The following side/adverse effects have been selected on the basis of their potential clinical significance (possible signs and symptoms in parentheses where appropriate)—not necessarily inclusive:

### Those indicating need for medical attention
Incidence rare
  *Anaphylactic reaction* (difficulty in breathing or swallowing; hives; itching, especially of soles or palms; reddening of skin, especially around ears; swelling of eyes, face, or inside of nose; unusual tiredness or weakness, sudden and severe)

### Those indicating need for medical attention only if they continue or are bothersome
Incidence less frequent
  *Delayed-type allergic reaction, cell-mediated* (itching or skin rash)—with injection; *fever over 38.5 °C (101.3 °F)*—incidence 5% with injection; *redness, soreness, hard lump, tenderness, or pain at injection site*—with injection

## Patient Consultation

As an aid to patient consultation, refer to *Advice for the Patient, Poliovirus Vaccine (Systemic).*

In providing consultation, consider emphasizing the following selected information (» = major clinical significance):

### Before using this vaccine
» Conditions affecting use, especially:
  Sensitivity to poliovirus vaccine or allergy to neomycin, penicillin, polymyxin B, or streptomycin
  Use in children—Not recommended in infants up to 6 weeks of age
  Other medications, especially immunosuppressants or radiation therapy
  Other medical problems, especially advanced debilitated condition; moderate or severe illness, with or without fever; persistent diarrhea or vomiting; viral infection; family history of congenital or hereditary immune deficiency conditions; or primary or acquired immune deficiency conditions
  Diet—Patients on low-sugar diets should be cautioned that the oral solution form of poliovirus vaccine may be administered on a sugar cube

### Proper use of this vaccine
» Proper dosing

### Precautions after receiving this vaccine
  Checking with physician before receiving any other live virus vaccines within 1 month of this vaccine

### Side/adverse effects
  In rare instances (approximately 1 case in 3.2 million doses of distributed vaccine), healthy persons who have taken the live oral polio vaccine (OPV) and healthy persons who are close contacts

of adults or children who have taken OPV have been infected by the poliovirus and become paralyzed

No paralysis caused by polio infection has occurred with the injected inactivated polio vaccine (IPV) since 1955 when the vaccine contained live viruses that accidentally had not been inactivated

Signs of potential side effects, especially anaphylactic reaction

# General Dosing Information

Poliovirus vaccine inactivated (IPV) and poliovirus vaccine inactivated enhanced potency (enhanced-potency IPV) are administered subcutaneously. The vaccines should not be administered intravenously.

Poliovirus vaccine live oral (OPV) is administered orally. The vaccine should not be administered parenterally.

A primary series of IPV is 4 doses; a primary series of enhanced-potency IPV or of OPV is 3 doses. If a combination of IPV and OPV or a combination of IPV and enhanced-potency IPV is used, a total of 4 doses constitutes a primary series. If a combination of enhanced-potency IPV and OPV is used, a total of 3 doses constitutes a primary series.

The multiple doses of IPV, enhanced-potency IPV, or OPV in the primary series are not administered as boosters, but to ensure that immunity to all three types of poliovirus has been achieved.

For IPV, enhanced-potency IPV, or OPV, time intervals between doses that are longer than those recommended for routine primary immunization do not require additional doses of vaccine.

Although the fourth dose of diphtheria-tetanus-pertussis (DTP) vaccine and the third dose of OPV have traditionally been administered to children 18 months of age, and measles-mumps-rubella (MMR) vaccine has traditionally been administered to children 15 months of age, it is now recommended that DTP, OPV, and MMR be administered concurrently to children 15 months of age. MMR should not be postponed in order to administer these vaccines concurrently at 18 months of age. In addition, the traditional method is still an acceptable alternative.

OPV, a live virus vaccine, can be administered concurrently with the following, using separate body sites, separate syringes, and the precautions that apply to each immunizing agent:
- Polysaccharide vaccines, such as haemophilus b polysaccharide vaccine, haemophilus b conjugate vaccine, meningococcal polysaccharide vaccine, or pneumococcal polyvalent vaccine.
- Influenza vaccine, whole or split virus.
- Diphtheria toxoid, tetanus toxoid, and/or pertussis vaccine.
- Live virus vaccines, other, such as measles, mumps, and/or rubella vaccines, but only if the vaccines are administered on the same day; otherwise they should be administered at least 1 month apart.
- Immune globulin and disease-specific immune globulins.
- Hepatitis B recombinant or plasma-derived vaccine.
- Inactivated vaccines, except cholera, parenteral typhoid, and plague. It is recommended that cholera, parenteral typhoid, and plague vaccines be administered on separate occasions because of these vaccines' propensity to cause side/adverse effects.
- Typhoid vaccine, live, oral. May be administered concurrently with, or at any interval before or after, OPV.

IPV or enhanced-potency IPV, an inactivated vaccine, can be administered concurrently with the following, using separate body sites, separate syringes, and the precautions that apply to each immunizing agent:
- Polysaccharide vaccines, such as haemophilus b polysaccharide vaccine, haemophilus b conjugate vaccine, meningococcal polysaccharide vaccine, or pneumococcal polyvalent vaccine.
- Influenza vaccine, whole or split virus.
- Diphtheria toxoid, tetanus toxoid, and/or pertussis vaccine.
- Live virus vaccines, such as measles, mumps, and/or rubella vaccines.
- Immune globulin and disease-specific immune globulins.
- Hepatitis B recombinant or plasma-derived vaccine.
- Inactivated vaccines, other, except cholera, parenteral typhoid, and plague. It is recommended that cholera, parenteral typhoid, and plague vaccines be administered on separate occasions because of these vaccines' propensity to cause side/adverse effects.

Persons traveling to countries with endemic or epidemic poliomyelitis:
- At a minimum, all travelers should receive a complete primary series of OPV, IPV, or enhanced-potency IPV, depending on age. In addition, travelers, regardless of age, who have previously completed the primary series of OPV, IPV, or enhanced-potency IPV should receive an additional dose of OPV or enhanced-potency IPV.
- If at least 4 weeks remain before departure, inadequately vaccinated adults 18 years of age and older should receive, at intervals of not less

than 4 weeks, additional doses of IPV or enhanced-potency IPV up to the total number of doses recommended to complete the primary series.
- Regardless of age, travelers who have not had a primary series and who have less than 4 weeks before beginning their travels should receive one dose of either OPV or enhanced-potency IPV. Such travelers who are under 18 years of age should then complete the primary series of OPV, at the recommended intervals, whether they remain in the foreign country or return to the U.S. or Canada; such travelers 18 years of age and older should complete the primary series of OPV, IPV, or enhanced-potency IPV only if they remain in the foreign country or plan to travel again to a country with endemic or epidemic poliomyelitis.
- If time permits, infants and children under 2 years of age should receive at least 3 doses of OPV before travel. Intervals between doses may be reduced to 4 weeks to maximize immunization status before departure. If the infant is under 6 weeks of age, a dose of OPV should be given before travel, but the dose should not be counted as part of the 3-dose primary series of OPV. Thereafter, if the infant remains in the foreign country or if there are plans to travel again before the primary series is completed, doses of the primary 3-dose series of OPV should be scheduled at 4-week intervals, otherwise the regular immunization schedule may be used.

Unimmunized adults at increased risk of exposure to polioviruses:
- Primary immunization with IPV or enhanced-potency IPV is recommended whenever possible. If time allows and IPV is being administered, 3 doses should be given at intervals of 1 to 2 months with a fourth dose given 6 to 12 months after the third dose. If time allows and enhanced-potency IPV is being administered, 2 doses should be given at intervals of 1 to 2 months with a third dose given 6 to 12 months after the second dose.
- If at least 8 weeks are available before protection is required, 3 doses of enhanced-potency IPV should be given at least 4 weeks apart.
- If less than 8, but at least 4 weeks are available before protection is required, 2 doses of IPV or enhanced-potency IPV should be given at least 4 weeks apart.
- If less than 4 weeks are available before protection is required, a single dose of either OPV or enhanced-potency IPV should be given.
- Generally, if the person remains at increased risk, the remaining doses of IPV, enhanced-potency IPV, or OPV should be given at the usual intervals.

Incompletely immunized adults who are at increased risk of exposure to polioviruses and who have previously received only 1 dose of OPV, fewer than 3 doses of IPV, or a combination of OPV and IPV totaling fewer than 3 doses should receive at least 1 dose of either OPV or enhanced-potency IPV. If time permits, the remaining required doses of OPV, IPV, or enhanced-potency IPV should be administered regardless of the interval since the previously administered dose (s) or the type of vaccine previously received.

Adults who have previously completed a primary course of OPV, IPV, or enhanced-potency IPV and who are at increased risk of exposure to polioviruses should receive an additional dose of OPV, IPV, or enhanced-potency IPV, regardless of which vaccine was previously used. For OPV, IPV, and enhanced-potency IPV, the need for further supplementary doses has not been established. However, if OPV has been used exclusively, further supplementary doses are probably not necessary. If IPV has been used exclusively, further supplementary doses may be given every 5 years (U.S.) or 10 years (Canada).

Pregnant women at increased risk of poliomyelitis:
- Although routine immunization of pregnant women is not recommended, if the risk of exposure is or will be high during pregnancy, it is recommended that OPV be administered. However, if time is available before the risk of exposure occurs, some experts recommend that IPV be administered instead.
- Enhanced-potency IPV is not recommended for use in pregnant women, because of the lack of data on possible adverse effects.
- If OPV is used, 2 doses should be administered at a 6- to 8-week interval with a third dose given at least 6 weeks later (customarily 8 to 12 months later).
- If IPV is used, 3 doses should be administered at intervals of 1 to 2 months with a fourth dose given 6 to 12 months later.
- If there is not time for either of the above schedules and at least 4 weeks are available, 2 doses of IPV should be given 4 weeks apart. If less than 4 weeks are available, a single dose of OPV should be given.
- The remaining required doses of either IPV or OPV should be given at the appropriate intervals only if the woman remains at increased risk.

**For treatment of adverse effects**
Recommended treatment includes:
- For mild hypersensitivity reaction—Administering antihistamines and, if necessary, corticosteroids.
- For severe hypersensitivity or anaphylactic reaction—Administering epinephrine. Antihistamines or corticosteroids may also be administered as required.

---

## *POLIOVIRUS VACCINE INACTIVATED*

# Parenteral Dosage Forms

## POLIOVIRUS VACCINE INACTIVATED (Injection) USP

**Usual adult dose**
Immunizing agent (active)—
Subcutaneously, 1 mL:
First dose:
At initial visit.
Second dose:
Four to eight weeks after the first dose.
Third dose:
Four to eight weeks after the second dose.
Fourth dose:
Six to twelve months after the third dose.
Note: If a booster is required following the primary series, either IPV or OPV may be administered.

If immediate protection is needed against poliomyelitis, OPV or enhanced-potency IPV should be administered.

**Usual pediatric dose**
Immunizing agent (active)—
Subcutaneously, 1 mL:
First dose:
At initial visit, preferably at 6 to 12 weeks of age, commonly with the first DTP inoculation at 2 months of age.
Second dose:
Four to eight weeks after the first dose, commonly with the second DTP inoculation at 4 months of age.
Third dose:
Four to eight weeks after the second dose, commonly with the third DTP inoculation at 6 months of age.
Fourth dose:
Six to twelve months after the third dose, commonly with the MMR and fourth DTP inoculations at 15 months of age.
First booster dose:
Children who have completed the primary series of 4 doses of IPV should receive a booster dose of IPV or enhanced-potency IPV or 1 dose of OPV upon entering school, usually between 4 to 6 years of age. However, this booster dose of IPV or enhanced-potency IPV or the OPV dose is not required in children who receive the fourth dose of the primary series of IPV on or after their fourth birthday.
Additional booster doses:
In the U.S.: Every five years after the last dose of the primary series or after the first booster dose, whichever occurs last, up until 18 years of age unless a complete primary series of OPV has been administered.
In Canada: Every ten years after the last dose of the primary series or after the first booster dose, whichever occurs last.
Note: In the U.S. and Canada, OPV is the poliovirus vaccine of choice for infants and children up to 18 years of age.

**Strength(s) usually available**
U.S.—
The vaccine meets the requirements of the specific monkey potency test by virus-neutralizing antibody production, based on the U.S. Reference Poliovirus Antiserum, such that the ratio of the geometric mean titer of the group of monkey serums representing the vaccine to the mean titer value of the reference serum is not less than 1.29 for Type 1 (Mahoney), 1.13 for Type 2 (M.E.F.1), and 0.72 for Type 3 (Saukett) (Rx) [GENERIC].
Canada—
The vaccine contains three types of poliovirus: Type 1 (Mahoney), Type 2 (M.E.F.1), and Type 3 (Saukett), grown in monkey kidney cell cultures (Rx) [GENERIC].

**Packaging and storage**
Store between 2 and 8 °C (36 and 46 °F). Do not freeze.

**Auxiliary labeling**
- Shake well.
- Do not freeze.

---

## *POLIOVIRUS VACCINE INACTIVATED ENHANCED POTENCY*

# Parenteral Dosage Forms

## POLIOVIRUS VACCINE INACTIVATED ENHANCED POTENCY (Injection)

**Usual adult dose**
Immunizing agent (active)—
Subcutaneously, 0.5 mL:
First dose:
At initial visit.
Second dose:
Four to eight weeks (preferably eight weeks) after the first dose.
Third dose:
Six to twelve months (preferably closer to twelve months) after the second dose.
Note: If a booster is required following the primary series, either enhanced-potency IPV or OPV may be administered.

If immediate protection is needed against poliomyelitis, OPV or enhanced-potency IPV should be administered.

**Usual pediatric dose**
Immunizing agent (active)—
Subcutaneously, 0.5 mL:
First dose:
At 6 to 8 weeks of age (preferably at 8 weeks of age), commonly with the first DTP inoculation at 2 months of age.
Second dose:
Four to eight weeks (preferably eight weeks) after the first dose, commonly with the second DTP inoculation at 4 months of age.
Third dose:
Six to twelve months (preferably closer to twelve months) after the second dose, commonly with the MMR and fourth DTP inoculations at 15 months of age.
First booster dose:
Children who have completed the primary series of 3 doses of enhanced-potency IPV should receive a booster dose of enhanced-potency IPV or 1 dose of OPV upon entering school, usually between 4 to 6 years of age. However, this booster dose of enhanced-potency IPV or the OPV dose is not required in children who receive the third dose of the primary series of enhanced-potency IPV on or after their fourth birthday.
Additional booster doses:
The need for routinely administered booster doses of enhanced-potency IPV is not known at this time.
Note: In the U.S. and Canada, OPV is the poliovirus vaccine of choice for infants and children up to 18 years of age.

**Strength(s) usually available**
U.S.—
40, 8, and 32 D-Antigen units of types 1, 2, and 3, respectively, determined by comparison to a reference preparation, per 0.5 mL (Rx) [*Ipol;* GENERIC].
Canada—
40, 8, and 32 D-Antigen units of types 1, 2, and 3, respectively, determined by comparison to a reference preparation, per 0.5 mL (Rx) [GENERIC].

**Packaging and storage**
Store between 2 and 8 °C (36 and 46 °F). Do not freeze.

**Auxiliary labeling**
- Shake well.
- Do not freeze.

---

## *POLIOVIRUS VACCINE LIVE ORAL*

# Oral Dosage Forms

## POLIOVIRUS VACCINE LIVE ORAL (Oral Solution) USP

**Usual adult dose**
Immunizing agent (active)—
Oral, 0.5 mL (U.S.) or 0.5 mL or 3 drops (Canada—specific dose depends on manufacturer)

U.S.:

2 doses administered not less than six and preferably eight weeks apart, with the third dose administered six to twelve months following the second dose.

Canada:

2 or 3 doses administered six to twelve weeks apart.

Note: Except in certain circumstances as specified in *General Dosing Information* and *Indications*, in the U.S. and Canada, OPV is not indicated for adults; IPV or enhanced-potency IPV is the poliovirus vaccine of choice in the U.S. and Canada when immunization is indicated for adults. Where OPV *is* indicated for adults, the frequency and number of doses may be different from the *Usual adult dose* above according to the specific circumstances (see *General Dosing Information*).

## Usual pediatric dose

Immunizing agent (active)—

Oral, 0.5 mL (U.S.) or 0.5 mL or 3 drops (Canada—specific dose depends on manufacturer).

Infants:

First dose—

U.S.—At 6 to 12 weeks of age, commonly with the first DTP inoculation at 2 months of age.

Canada—Not earlier than 2 months of age.

Second dose—

U.S.—Not less than six and preferably eight weeks after the first dose, commonly with the second DTP inoculation at 4 months of age.

Canada—Six to twelve weeks after the first dose.

Third dose—

U.S.—Eight to twelve months after the second dose, commonly with the MMR and fourth DTP inoculations at 15 months of age, but may be administered at any time between 12 and 24 months of age.

Canada—Six to twelve weeks after the second dose.

Booster doses—

U.S.—Upon entering school, usually between 4 to 6 years of age. However, this booster dose is not required in children who receive the third dose of the primary series on or after their fourth birthday.

Canada—Eight to fifteen months after the third dose; during the first school year; and around 15 years of age.

Note: U.S.—An optional additional dose may be administered at 6 months of age (along with the third DTP inoculation) in areas with a high risk of poliovirus exposure.

Children up to age 18 who did not follow the above schedule:

U.S.: The first two doses should be administered not less than six and preferably eight weeks apart, and the third dose should be administered six to twelve months following the second dose.

Canada: 2 doses six to twelve weeks apart, followed by the booster doses above.

Note: When there are time constraints with regard to immunization, the vaccination schedule may be accelerated for infants and children up to 18 years of age so that the first dose may be given at or after 6 weeks of age, the second dose given 6 to 8 weeks later, and the third dose given 6 weeks to 12 months later. Moreover, the second and third doses may be given as close as 4 weeks apart if necessary.

## Strength(s) usually available

U.S.—

The equivalent of $10^{5.4}$ to $10^{6.4}$ for Type 1, $10^{4.5}$ to $10^{5.5}$ for Type 2, and $10^{5.2}$ to $10^{6.2}$ for Type 3 of the TCID$_{50}$ (quantity of virus

estimated to infect 50% of inoculated cultures) of the U.S. Reference Poliovirus, Live, Attenuated, per 0.5 mL (Rx) [*Orimune*].

Canada—

Approximately 1,000,000 infectious particles of Type 1, approximately 100,000 infectious particles of Type 2, and approximately 300,000 infectious particles of Type 3, per 0.5 mL (Rx) [GENERIC (I.A.F.)].

Approximately 1,000,000 infectious particles of Type 1, approximately 100,000 infectious particles of Type 2, and approximately 300,000 infectious particles of Type 3, per 3-drop dose (Rx) [GENERIC (Connaught)].

## Packaging and storage

Preserve at a temperature that will maintain ice continuously in a solid state. Because of its sorbitol content, this vaccine may remain fluid at temperatures above −14 °C (+7 °F). If frozen, the vaccine must be completely thawed prior to use. Preserve thawed vaccine at a temperature between 2 and 8 °C (36 and 46 °F). Vaccine that has been thawed may be carried through a maximum of 10 freeze-thaw cycles, provided the temperature does not exceed 8 °C (46 °F) during the periods of thaw and provided the total cumulative duration of thaw does not exceed 24 hours. If the 24-hour period is exceeded, the vaccine must be used within 30 days, during which time it must be stored at a temperature between 2 and 8 °C (36 and 46 °F).

## Preparation of dosage form

The vaccine must be completely thawed prior to use.

The vaccine may be administered directly or mixed with distilled water, chlorine-free tap water, Syrup NF, or milk. Alternatively, it may be adsorbed on foods, such as bread, cake, or cube sugar.

## Stability

The vaccine contains phenol red as a pH indicator. The usual color of the vaccine is pink, although some containers of vaccine may exhibit a yellow coloration. The color of the vaccine prior to use (red-pink-yellow) has no effect on the virus or efficacy of the vaccine.

## Auxiliary labeling

• For oral use only.

Revised: 07/12/94

---

**POLIOVIRUS VACCINE INACTIVATED**—See *Poliovirus Vaccine (Systemic)*

---

**POLIOVIRUS VACCINE INACTIVATED ENHANCED POTENCY**—See *Poliovirus Vaccine (Systemic)*

---

**POLIOVIRUS VACCINE LIVE ORAL**—See *Poliovirus Vaccine (Systemic)*

---

**POLOXAMER 188**—See *Laxatives (Local)*

---

**POLYCARBOPHIL**—See *Laxatives (Local)*

---

# POLYETHYLENE GLYCOL AND ELECTROLYTES   Local

VA CLASSIFICATION (Primary): GA209

Note: For a listing of dosage forms and brand names by country availability, see *Dosage Forms* section(s). For a listing of brand names for the articles in this monograph, refer to the General Index.

## Category

Evacuant (bowel).

## Indications

### Accepted

Bowel evacuation, preoperative, and

Bowel evacuation, pre-radiography—Polyethylene glycol (PEG) 3350 and electrolytes oral solution is indicated for bowel cleansing prior to gastrointestinal examination (e.g., colonoscopy, barium enema, intravenous pyelography) and colon surgery.

For double contrast barium enema, administration of the PEG-electrolyte solution alone has not been found to be an adequate method of bowel cleansing. PEG-electrolyte solution followed by oral administration of bisacodyl has been reported to achieve better removal of feces and correct degraded mucosal coating.

# Pharmacology/Pharmacokinetics

**Physicochemical characteristics**
Molecular weight—Potassium chloride: 74.55.
Sodium bicarbonate: 84.01.
Sodium chloride: 58.44.
Sodium sulfate: 322.20.
Osmolality—280 mOsmol per kg of water.

**Mechanism of action/Effect**
Evacuant (bowel)—Cleansing of the bowel is achieved by fluid overload with the osmotically balanced PEG-electrolyte solution, which induces a liquid stool within a short period of time. The concentration of electrolytes in the solution causes no net absorption or secretion of ions; thus no significant changes in water or electrolyte balance occur.

**Absorption**
Negligible absorption from gastrointestinal tract.

**Onset of action**
30 to 60 minutes.

**Elimination**
Negligible renal excretion (<0.1%).

# Precautions to Consider

**Carcinogenicity/Mutagenicity**
Studies to evaluate carcinogenic or mutagenic potential have not been performed.

**Pregnancy/Reproduction**
Pregnancy—Studies have not been done in humans.
Studies have not been done in animals.
FDA Pregnancy Category C.

**Breast-feeding**
It is not known whether PEG-electrolyte solution is distributed into breast milk. However, problems in humans have not been documented.

**Pediatrics**
Studies performed in children ranging in age from 6 months to 18 years have not demonstrated pediatrics-specific problems that would limit the usefulness of PEG-electrolyte solution in children.

**Geriatrics**
Appropriate studies performed to date have not demonstrated geriatrics-specific problems that would limit the usefulness of PEG-electrolyte solution in the elderly.

**Drug interactions and/or related problems**
The following drug interactions and/or related problems have been selected on the basis of their potential clinical significance (possible mechanism in parentheses where appropriate)—not necessarily inclusive (» = major clinical significance):
» Oral medications, other
(other oral medications administered within 1 hour of administration of PEG-electrolyte solution may be flushed from the gastrointestinal tract and not absorbed)

**Laboratory value alterations**
The following have been selected on the basis of their potential clinical significance (possible effect in parentheses where appropriate)—not necessarily inclusive (» = major clinical significance):

With diagnostic test results
Barium sulfate, rectal
(administration of PEG-electrolyte solution on the same day as a barium enema [either single or double contrast] may result in retained fluid and thus barium dilution and may prevent barium coating of the intestinal wall)

**Medical considerations/Contraindications**
The medical considerations/contraindications included here have been selected on the basis of their potential clinical significance (reasons given in parentheses where appropriate)—not necessarily inclusive (» = major clinical significance).

*Except under special circumstances, this medication should not be used when the following medical problems exist:*

» Intestinal obstruction or
» Paralytic ileus or
» Perforated bowel or
» Toxic colitis or
» Toxic megacolon
(condition may be aggravated; colonic perforation may occur in patients with intestinal obstruction or toxic colitis)

*Risk-benefit should be considered when the following medical problems exist:*
Aspiration, predisposition to or
Impaired gag reflex or
Regurgitation, predisposition to or
Unconscious or semiconscious state
(administration via nasogastric tube may increase risk of complications)
Ulcerative colitis, severe
(condition may be aggravated)

# Side/Adverse Effects

Note: Hypothermia was reported in one patient after ingestion of 5 liters of chilled PEG-electrolyte solution.

One patient experienced cardiac asystole after a large bowel movement following administration of PEG-electrolyte solution. Further studies are needed to establish a causal relationship.

The following side/adverse effects have been selected on the basis of their potential clinical significance (possible signs and symptoms in parentheses where appropriate)—not necessarily inclusive:

**Those indicating need for medical attention**
Incidence rare
*Allergic reaction* (skin rash)

**Those indicating need for medical attention only if they continue or are bothersome**
Incidence more frequent
*Bloating; nausea*
Incidence less frequent
*Abdominal or stomach cramps; anal irritation; vomiting*

# Patient Consultation

As an aid to patient consultation, refer to *Advice for the Patient, Polyethylene Glycol and Electrolytes (Local).*

In providing consultation, consider emphasizing the following selected information (» = major clinical significance):

**Before using this medication**
» Conditions affecting use, especially:
Other oral medicines administered within 1 hour of solution
Other medical problems, especially intestinal obstruction, paralytic ileus, perforated bowel, toxic colitis, or toxic megacolon

**Proper use of this medication**
Special preparatory instructions may be given; patient should inquire in advance
» Taking solution exactly as directed for best test results
» Drinking all the solution for best results, unless otherwise directed by physician
» Fasting for at least 3 hours prior to ingestion of solution; clear liquids are allowed after ingestion of solution
Directions for the preparation of the powder dosage form
» Proper dosing
» Proper storage

**Side/adverse effects**
Signs of potential side effects, especially allergic reaction

# General Dosing Information

**Diet/Nutrition**
Fasting is recommended for at least 3 hours prior to administration of the PEG-electrolyte solution.

The PEG-electrolyte solution may be administered on the morning of the examination, as long as enough time is allowed for the patient to drink the solution (3 hours) and for complete bowel evacuation (1 additional hour). If the patient is having a barium enema examination, the PEG-electrolyte solution should be administered early (e.g., 6 pm) the evening before the examination to permit proper mucosal coating by barium. No foods except clear liquids are allowed after administration of the solution.

Rapid drinking of each portion of the the PEG-electrolyte solution is recommended rather than drinking small amounts continuously.

## Oral Dosage Forms

### POLYETHYLENE GLYCOL 3350 AND ELECTROLYTES ORAL SOLUTION

**Usual adult and adolescent dose**
Bowel evacuant—
Oral, 240 mL every ten minutes, up to 4 L, or until the fecal discharge is clear and free of solid matter.

Note: May also be given via nasogastric tube at a rate of 20 to 30 mL per minute (1.2 to 1.8 L per hour).

**Usual pediatric dose**
Bowel evacuant—Oral or by continuous nasogastric drip, 25 to 40 mL per kg of body weight per hour until the fecal discharge is clear and free of solid matter.

**Usual geriatric dose**
See *Usual adult and adolescent dose.*

**Strength(s) usually available**
U.S.—

|  | Content (mg/100 mL) | | | | |
| Product | PEG 3350 | NaCl | NaHCO$_3$ | Na$_2$SO$_4$ | KCl |
|---|---|---|---|---|---|
| U.S.— | | | | | |
| OCL (Rx) | 6000 | 146 | 168 | 569 | 75 |
| Canada— | | | | | |
| Peglyte (OTC) | 5960 | 150 | 170 | 570 | 80 |

**Packaging and storage**
Store between 15 and 30 °C (59 and 86 °F). Store in a tight container.

**Incompatibilities**
The addition of flavoring agents, such as sugar, nutritional supplements, or other sweeteners, is *not* recommended. Such additives may change the osmolality of the solution; sucrose or glucose may cause fluid and electrolyte absorption. Additives may also predispose to colonic bacterial fermentation and formation of combustible gases.

### POLYETHYLENE GLYCOL 3350 AND ELECTROLYTES FOR ORAL SOLUTION USP

**Usual adult and adolescent dose**
See *Polyethylene Glycol 3350 and Electrolytes Oral Solution.*

**Usual pediatric dose**
See *Polyethylene Glycol 3350 and Electrolytes Oral Solution.*

**Usual geriatric dose**
See *Polyethylene Glycol 3350 and Electrolytes Oral Solution.*

**Size(s) usually available**
U.S.—

|  | Content (mg/100 mL) | | | | |
| Product | PEG 3350 | NaCl | NaHCO$_3$ | Na$_2$SO$_4$ | KCl |
|---|---|---|---|---|---|
| U.S.— | 6000 | 146 | 168 | 568 | 74.5 |
| Co-Lav (Rx) | | | | | |
| Colovage (Rx) | | | | | |
| Colyte (Rx) | | | | | |
| Colyte-flavored (Rx) | | | | | |
| Go-Evac (Rx) | | | | | |
| GoLYTELY (Rx) | | | | | |
| NuLYTELY (Rx) | 10500 | 280 | 143 | — | 37 |
| NuLYTELY, Cherry Flavor (Rx) | | | | | |
| Canada— | 6000 | 146 | 168 | 568 | 75 |
| Colyte (OTC) | | | | | |
| GoLYTELY (OTC) | | | | | |
| Klean-Prep (OTC) | | | | | |
| Peglyte (OTC) | 6000 | 150 | 170 | 570 | 80 |

**Packaging and storage**
Store below 40 °C (104 °F), preferably between 15 and 30 °C (59 and 86 °F), unless otherwise specified by manufacturer. Store in a tight container.

Note: After reconstitution, solution should be refrigerated to improve palatability.

**Preparation of dosage form**
See manufacturer's package label for complete instructions on reconstitution.
Tap water must be used for reconstitution.
To assure that all ingredients have dissolved, solution must be shaken vigorously.

**Stability**
Reconstituted solution should be used within 48 hours. Unused portion should be discarded.

**Incompatibilities**
The addition of flavoring agents, such as sugar, nutritional supplements, or other sweeteners, is *not* recommended. Such additives may change the osmolality of the solution; sucrose or glucose may cause fluid and electrolyte absorption. Additives may also predispose to colonic bacterial fermentation and formation of combustible gases.

Revised: 08/15/95

### POLYMERIC ENTERAL NUTRITION FORMULAS—
See *Enteral Nutrition Formulas (Systemic)*

### POLYMYXIN B–CONTAINING COMBINATIONS—
Neomycin and Polymyxin B (Topical)
Neomycin, Polymyxin B, and Bacitracin (Ophthalmic)
Neomycin, Polymyxin B, and Bacitracin (Topical)
Neomycin, Polymyxin B, and Gramicidin (Ophthalmic)
Neomycin, Polymyxin B, and Hydrocortisone (Ophthalmic)
Neomycin, Polymyxin B, and Hydrocortisone (Otic)

### POLYTHIAZIDE—See *Diuretics, Thiazide (Systemic)*

### POLYTHIAZIDE-CONTAINING COMBINATIONS—
Prazosin and Polythiazide (Systemic)
Reserpine and Polythiazide (Systemic)—See *Rauwolfia Alkaloids and Thiazide Diuretics (Systemic)*

### POTASSIUM ACETATE—See *Potassium Supplements (Systemic)*

### POTASSIUM BICARBONATE—See *Potassium Supplements (Systemic)*

### POTASSIUM BICARBONATE AND POTASSIUM CHLORIDE—See *Potassium Supplements (Systemic)*

### POTASSIUM BICARBONATE AND POTASSIUM CITRATE—See *Potassium Supplements (Systemic)*

### POTASSIUM BITARTRATE AND SODIUM BICARBONATE—See *Laxatives (Local)*

### POTASSIUM CHLORIDE—See *Potassium Supplements (Systemic)*

### POTASSIUM CITRATE—See *Citrates (Systemic)*

### POTASSIUM CITRATE AND CITRIC ACID—See *Citrates (Systemic)*

## POTASSIUM CITRATE AND SODIUM CITRATE—
See *Citrates (Systemic)*

## POTASSIUM GLUCONATE—See *Potassium Supplements (Systemic)*

## POTASSIUM GLUCONATE AND POTASSIUM CHLORIDE—See *Potassium Supplements (Systemic)*

## POTASSIUM GLUCONATE AND POTASSIUM CITRATE—See *Potassium Supplements (Systemic)*

## POTASSIUM GUAIACOLSULFONATE-CONTAINING COMBINATIONS—
Bromodiphenhydramine, Diphenhydramine, Codeine, Ammonium Chloride, and Potassium Guaiacolsulfonate (Systemic)—See *Cough/Cold Combinations (Systemic)*

Chlorpheniramine, Phenylephrine, Phenylpropanolamine, Carbetapentane, and Potassium Guaiacolsulfonate (Systemic)—See *Cough/Cold Combinations (Systemic)*

Hydrocodone and Potassium Guaiacolsulfonate (Systemic)—See *Cough/Cold Combinations (Systemic)*

Phenylephrine, Phenylpropanolamine, Carbetapentane, and Potassium Guaiacolsulfonate (Systemic)—See *Cough/Cold Combinations (Systemic)*

Promethazine, Codeine, and Potassium Guaiacolsulfonate (Systemic)—See *Cough/Cold Combinations (Systemic)*

Promethazine, Phenylephrine, Codeine, and Potassium Guaiacolsulfonate (Systemic)—See *Cough/Cold Combinations (Systemic)*

Promethazine, Phenylephrine, and Potassium Guaiacolsulfonate (Systemic)—See *Cough/Cold Combinations (Systemic)*

# POTASSIUM IODIDE    Systemic

VA CLASSIFICATION (Primary/Secondary): HS852/AD900; AM700; TN499

Other commonly used names are KI and SSKI.

Note: For a listing of dosage forms and brand names by country availability, see *Dosage Forms* section(s). For a listing of brand names for the articles in this monograph, refer to the General Index.

## Category

Antihyperthyroid agent; radiation protectant (thyroid gland); thyroid inhibitor; antifungal (systemic); iodine replenisher.

## Indications

Note: Bracketed information in the *Indications* section refers to uses that are not included in U.S. product labeling.

**Accepted**

Hyperthyroidism (treatment)[1]—Potassium iodide is indicated in the treatment of hyperthyroidism.

Radiation protection, thyroid gland—Potassium iodide is indicated as a radiation protectant (thyroid gland) prior to and following oral administration or inhalation of radioactive isotopes of iodine or in radiation emergencies.

[Erythema nodosum (treatment)][1]—Potassium iodide is used in the treatment of erythema nodosum.

[Iodine deficiency (treatment)][1]—Potassium iodide is used in the treatment of iodine deficiency.

[Sporotrichosis, cutaneous lymphatic (treatment)][1]—Potassium iodide is used in the treatment of cutaneous lymphatic sporotrichosis.

[Thyroid involution, preoperative][1]—Potassium iodide is used concurrently with an antithyroid agent to induce thyroid involution prior to thyroidectomy.

**Unaccepted**

Potassium iodide has not been shown to have a clinically significant expectorant action.

[1]Not included in Canadian product labeling.

## Pharmacology/Pharmacokinetics

**Physicochemical characteristics**

Molecular weight—166.00.

**Mechanism of action/Effect**

Antihyperthyroid agent—

In hyperthyroid patients, potassium iodide produces rapid remission of symptoms by inhibiting the release of thyroid hormone into the circulation. The effects of potassium iodide on the thyroid gland include reduction of vascularity, a firming of the glandular tissue, shrinkage of the size of individual cells, reaccumulation of colloid in the follicles, and increases in bound iodine. These actions may facilitate thyroidectomy when the medication is given prior to surgery.

Radiation protectant—

When administered prior to and following administration of radioactive isotopes and in radiation emergencies involving the release of radioactive iodine, potassium iodide protects the thyroid gland by blocking the thyroidal uptake of radioactive isotopes of iodine.

When potassium iodide is administered simultaneously with radiation exposure, the protectant effect is approximately 97%. Potassium iodide given 12 and 24 hours before exposure yields a 90% and 70% protectant effect, respectively. However, potassium iodide administered 1 and 3 hours after exposure results in an 85% and 50% protectant effect, respectively. Potassium iodide administered more than 6 hours after exposure is thought to have a negligible protectant effect.

## Precautions to Consider

**Pregnancy/Reproduction**

Potassium iodide crosses the placenta; use during pregnancy may result in abnormal thyroid function and/or goiter in the infant.

**Breast-feeding**

Potassium iodide is distributed into breast milk; use by nursing mothers may cause skin rash and thyroid suppression in the infant.

**Pediatrics**

Potassium iodide may cause skin rash and thyroid suppression in infants. Appropriate studies have not been performed for use as a systemic antifungal.

**Geriatrics**

Appropriate studies on the relationship of age to the effects of potassium iodide have not been performed in the geriatric population. However, geriatrics-specific problems that would limit the usefulness of this medication in the elderly are not expected.

**Dental**

Potassium iodide may cause salivary gland swelling or tenderness, burning of mouth or throat, metallic taste, soreness of teeth and gums, and unusual increase in salivation.

**Drug interactions and/or related problems**

The following drug interactions and/or related problems have been selected on the basis of their potential clinical significance (possible mechanism in parentheses where appropriate)—not necessarily inclusive (» = major clinical significance):

Note: Combinations containing any of the following medications, depending on the amount present, may also interact with this medication.

» Antithyroid agents
(concurrent use of these medications with potassium iodide may potentiate the hypothyroid and goitrogenic effects of antithyroid agents or potassium iodide; baseline thyroid status should be determined at periodic intervals to detect changes in the thyroid-pituitary response)

Captopril or
Enalapril or
Lisinopril
(concurrent use of captopril, enalapril, or lisinopril with potassium iodide may result in hyperkalemia; serum potassium concentrations should be monitored)

» Diuretics, potassium-sparing
(concurrent use with potassium iodide may increase the effects of potassium, possibly resulting in hyperkalemia and cardiac arrhythmias or cardiac arrest; serum potassium concentrations should be monitored)

» Lithium
(concurrent use with potassium iodide may potentiate the hypothyroid and goitrogenic effects of either medication; baseline thyroid status should be determined at periodic intervals to detect changes in the thyroid-pituitary response)

Sodium iodide I 131, therapeutic
(potassium iodide may decrease thyroidal uptake of I 131)

### Laboratory value alterations
The following have been selected on the basis of their potential clinical significance (possible effect in parentheses where appropriate)—not necessarily inclusive (» = major clinical significance):

With diagnostic test results
Thyroid function studies
Thyroid imaging, radionuclide and
Thyroid uptake tests
(potassium iodide may decrease thyroidal uptake of I 131, I 123, and sodium pertechnetate Tc 99m)

### Medical considerations/Contraindications
The medical considerations/contraindications included here have been selected on the basis of their potential clinical significance (reasons given in parentheses where appropriate)—not necessarily inclusive (» = major clinical significance).

*Risk-benefit should be considered when the following medical problems exist:*

» Hyperkalemia
(condition may be exacerbated)

Hyperthyroidism (for use other than thyroid inhibitor)
(prolonged use of iodine may cause thyroid gland hyperplasia, thyroid adenoma, goiter, or hypothyroidism)

Myotonia congenita
(condition may be exacerbated by potassium)

» Renal function impairment
(may cause excessive serum potassium concentrations)

Sensitivity to potassium iodide

Tuberculosis
(may cause irritation and increase secretions)

### Patient monitoring
The following may be especially important in patient monitoring (other tests may be warranted in some patients, depending on condition; » = major clinical significance):

Serum potassium concentrations
(recommended at periodic intervals during therapy in patients with renal function impairment)

## Side/Adverse Effects
The following side/adverse effects have been selected on the basis of their potential clinical significance (possible signs and symptoms in parentheses where appropriate)—not necessarily inclusive:

### Those indicating need for medical attention
Incidence less frequent
*Allergic reactions, specifically angioedema* (swelling of the arms, face, legs, lips, tongue, and/or throat); *arthralgia* (joint pain); *eosinophilia; swelling of lymph nodes; urticaria* (hives)

With prolonged use
*Iodism* (burning of mouth or throat; gastric irritation; increased watering of mouth; metallic taste; severe headache; skin lesions; soreness of teeth and gums; symptoms of head cold); *potassium toxicity* (confusion; irregular heartbeat; numbness, tingling, pain, or weakness in hands or feet; unusual tiredness; weakness or heaviness of legs)

### Those indicating need for medical attention only if they continue or are bothersome
Incidence less frequent
*Diarrhea; nausea or vomiting; stomach pain*

## Patient Consultation
As an aid to patient consultation, refer to *Advice for the Patient, Potassium Iodide (Systemic).*

In providing consultation, consider emphasizing the following selected information (» = major clinical significance):

### Before using this medication
» Conditions affecting use, especially:
Sensitivity to iodine or potassium iodide
Pregnancy—May cause thyroid problems or goiter in the newborn infant
Breast-feeding—May cause skin rash and thyroid problems in nursing babies
Use in children—May cause skin rash and thyroid problems in nursing infants
Dental—May cause swelling of salivary glands, burning of mouth or throat, metallic taste, soreness of teeth and gums, or increase in salivation
Other medications, especially antithyroid agents, diuretics (potassium sparing), or lithium
Other medical problems, especially hyperkalemia or renal function impairment

### Proper use of this medication
» Taking after meals or with food or milk to minimize gastrointestinal irritation
*Proper administration technique for oral liquids:*
Taking medication by mouth even if dispensed in a dropper bottle
Not using if solution turns brownish yellow
Taking medication in a full glass (240 mL) of water or in fruit juice, milk, or broth to improve taste and lessen gastric upset; drinking full dose
If crystals form in solution, warming closed container in warm water and gently shaking container
*Proper administration technique for uncoated tablets:*
Dissolving each tablet in ½ glass (120 mL) of water or milk before taking; drinking full dose
» Compliance with full course of therapy (fungal infections)
» Proper dosing
Missed dose: Taking as soon as possible; not taking if almost time for next dose; not doubling doses
» Proper storage
*For use as a radiation protectant (thyroid gland)*
Taking medication only upon instructions from state or local health authorities
» Taking medication daily for 10 days, unless otherwise instructed; not taking more medication or more often than instructed

### Precautions while using this medication
Regular visits to physician to check progress during therapy
» Caution in patients on potassium-restricted diet

### Side/adverse effects
Signs of potential side effects, especially allergic reactions, iodism, or potassium toxicity

## General Dosing Information
The potassium content is 6 mEq (234 mg) per gram of potassium iodide.

To minimize stomach upset, the medication may be administered after meals and at bedtime with food or milk.

To protect against possible gastrointestinal injury, which has been associated with the oral ingestion of concentrated potassium salt preparations, it is recommended that the oral solution be administered in a full glass (240 mL) of water, or in fruit juice, milk, or broth. It is also recommended that each regular tablet be dissolved in ½ glass (120 mL) of water or milk before ingestion.

Prolonged use may result in hypothyroidism, parotitis, iodism, and, particularly in postpubescent patients, acneiform skin lesions.

## Oral Dosage Forms
Note: Bracketed uses in the *Dosage Forms* section refer to categories of use and/or indications that are not included in U.S. product labeling.

### POTASSIUM IODIDE ORAL SOLUTION USP

**Usual adult and adolescent dose**
Antihyperthyroid agent[1]—
Oral, 250 mg three times a day.
Radiation protectant (thyroid gland)—
Oral, 100 to 150 mg twenty-four hours prior to and once a day for three to ten days following administration of, or exposure to, radioactive isotopes of iodine.

[Antifungal (systemic)][1]—
  Oral, 600 mg three times a day, the dosage being increased by 60 mg at each dose until the maximum tolerated dose is reached.

[Iodine replenisher][1]—
  Oral, 5 to 10 mg per day.

[Thyroid inhibitor—Thyroid involution, preoperative][1]: Prior to thyroidectomy—
  Oral, 5 drops of a 1-gram-per-mL solution (approximately 250 mg) three times a day for ten days before surgery, usually administered concurrently with an antithyroid agent.

## Usual adult prescribing limits
Up to 12 grams daily.

## Usual pediatric dose
Radiation protectant (thyroid gland)—
  Infants up to 1 year of age: Oral, 65 mg once a day for ten days following administration of, or exposure to, radioactive isotopes of iodine.
  Infants and children 1 year of age and older: Oral, 130 mg once a day for ten days following administration of, or exposure to, radioactive isotopes of iodine.

[Antifungal (systemic)][1]—
  Dosage has not been established.

[Iodine replenisher][1]—
  Oral, 1 mg per day.

[Thyroid inhibitor—Thyroid involution, preoperative][1]—
  See *Usual adult and adolescent dose.*

## Strength(s) usually available
U.S.—
  1 gram per mL (Rx) [GENERIC].

## Packaging and storage
Store below 40 °C (104 °F), preferably between 15 and 30 °C (59 and 86 °F), unless otherwise specified by manufacturer. Store in a tight, light-resistant container. Protect from freezing.

## Stability
Crystallization may occur under normal conditions of storage, especially if refrigerated; however, on warming and shaking, the crystals will redissolve.

Free iodine may be liberated by oxidation of the potassium iodide, causing the solution to turn brownish yellow in color. If this occurs, the solution should be discarded.

## Auxiliary labeling
• For oral use only.
• Do not refrigerate.
• Continue medicine for full time of treatment (antifungal).

## POTASSIUM IODIDE SYRUP

### Usual adult and adolescent dose
Radiation protectant (thyroid gland)—
  Oral, 100 to 150 mg twenty-four hours prior to and once a day for three to ten days following administration of, or exposure to, radioactive isotopes of iodine.

[Antifungal (systemic)][1]—
  Oral, 600 mg three times a day, the dosage being increased by 60 mg at each dose until the maximum tolerated dose is reached.

[Iodine replenisher][1]—
  Oral, 5 to 10 mg per day.

[Thyroid inhibitor—Thyroid involution, preoperative][1]: Prior to thyroidectomy—
  Oral, 4 mL (approximately 260 mg) three times a day for ten days before surgery, usually administered concurrently with an antithyroid agent.

### Usual adult prescribing limits
Up to 12 grams daily.

### Usual pediatric dose
Radiation protectant (thyroid gland)—
  Infants up to 1 year of age: Oral, 65 mg once a day for ten days following administration of, or exposure to, radioactive isotopes of iodine.
  Infants and children 1 year of age and older: Oral, 130 mg once a day for ten days following administration of, or exposure to, radioactive isotopes of iodine.

[Antifungal (systemic)][1]—
  Dosage has not been established.

[Iodine replenisher][1]—
  Oral, 1 mg per day.

[Thyroid inhibitor—Thyroid involution, preoperative][1]—
  See *Usual adult and adolescent dose.*

## Strength(s) usually available
U.S.—
  325 mg per 5 mL (Rx) [*Pima*].

## Packaging and storage
Store below 40 °C (104 °F), preferably between 15 and 30 °C (59 and 86 °F), in a well-closed container, unless otherwise specified by manufacturer. Protect from freezing.

## Auxiliary labeling
• For oral use only.
• Continue medicine for full time of treatment (for 3-day uncinariasis treatment).

Note: When dispensing, include a calibrated liquid-measuring device.

## POTASSIUM IODIDE TABLETS USP

### Usual adult and adolescent dose
Radiation protectant (thyroid gland)—
  Oral, 100 to 150 mg twenty-four hours prior to and once a day for three to ten days following administration of, or exposure to, radioactive isotopes of iodine.

[Antifungal (systemic)][1]—
  Oral, 600 mg three times a day, the dosage being increased by 60 mg at each dose until the maximum tolerated dose is reached.

[Iodine replenisher][1]—
  Oral, 5 to 10 mg per day.

[Thyroid inhibitor—Thyroid involution, preoperative][1]: Prior to thyroidectomy—
  Oral, Dissolve 2 tablets (approximately 260 mg) in 1 glassful of water, three times a day for ten days before surgery, usually administered concurrently with an antithyroid agent.

### Usual adult prescribing limits
Up to 12 grams daily.

### Usual pediatric dose
Radiation protectant (thyroid gland)—
  Infants up to 1 year of age: Oral, 65 mg once a day for ten days following administration of, or exposure to, radioactive isotopes of iodine.
  Infants and children 1 year of age and older: Oral, 130 mg once a day for ten days following administration of, or exposure to, radioactive isotopes of iodine.

[Antifungal (systemic)][1]—
  Dosage has not been established.

[Iodine replenisher][1]—
  Oral, 1 mg per day.

[Thyroid inhibitor—Thyroid involution, preoperative][1]—
  See *Usual adult and adolescent dose.*

### Strength(s) usually available
U.S.—
  Not commercially available; however, potassium iodide tablets are available to government and public health organizations for use in radiation emergencies.
Canada—
  130 mg (Rx) [*Thyro-Block*].

### Packaging and storage
Store below 40 °C (104 °F), preferably between 15 and 30 °C (59 and 86 °F), unless otherwise specified by manufacturer. Store in a tight container.

### Auxiliary labeling
• Dissolve in liquid before taking.
• Continue medicine for full time of treatment (for 3-day uncinariasis treatment).

## POTASSIUM IODIDE TABLETS (ENTERIC-COATED) USP

Note: Enteric-coated potassium iodide tablets are not recommended since the administration of this dosage form has been associated with small bowel lesions, which can cause obstruction, hemorrhage, perforation, and possibly death.

### Strength(s) usually available
U.S.—
  300 mg (Rx) [GENERIC].

---

[1]Not included in Canadian product labeling.

---

Revised: 04/14/92
Interim revision: 08/26/94

## POTASSIUM AND SODIUM PHOSPHATES—See *Phosphates (Systemic)*

## POTASSIUM PHOSPHATES—See *Phosphates (Systemic)*

# POTASSIUM SUPPLEMENTS    Systemic

This monograph includes information on the following: Potassium Acetate†; Potassium Bicarbonate; Potassium Bicarbonate and Potassium Chloride; Potassium Bicarbonate and Potassium Citrate†; Potassium Chloride; Potassium Gluconate; Potassium Gluconate and Potassium Chloride†; Potassium Gluconate and Potassium Citrate†; Trikates†.

VA CLASSIFICATION (Primary): TN403

Another commonly used name in the U.S. for trikates is potassium triplex.

Note: For a listing of dosage forms and brand names by country availability, see *Dosage Forms* section(s). For a listing of brand names for the articles in this monograph, refer to the General Index.

†Not commercially available in Canada.

## Category

Antihypokalemic; electrolyte replenisher.

## Indications

### Accepted

Hypokalemia (treatment)—Potassium supplements are indicated in patients with hypokalemia, with or without metabolic alkalosis; in chronic digitalis intoxication; and in patients with hypokalemic familial periodic paralysis. Potassium supplementation is indicated in severe hypokalemia in patients receiving potassium-wasting diuretics for uncomplicated essential hypertension, when dosage adjustment of the diuretic is ineffective or unwarranted. Potassium supplementation may be needed in patients receiving antibiotics that cause potassium depletion, either by drug-induced nephrotoxicity (e.g., amphotericin B, polymyxin B, or gentamicin) or by a nonreabsorbable anion effect (e.g., azlocillin, carbenicillin, mezlocillin, penicillin, piperacillin, or ticarcillin). Potassium chloride is usually the salt of choice in the treatment of hypokalemia, since it is better absorbed from the gastrointestinal tract than the nonchloride potassium salts, and the chloride ion may be required to correct hypochloremia, which often occurs with hypokalemia. In rare circumstances (e.g., patients with renal tubular acidosis), potassium depletion may be associated with metabolic acidosis and hyperchloremia. In such patients, potassium replacement should be accomplished with potassium salts other than chloride, such as potassium acetate, potassium bicarbonate, potassium citrate, or potassium gluconate.

Hypokalemia (prophylaxis)—Potassium supplements are indicated to prevent hypokalemia in patients who would be at particular risk if hypokalemia were to develop (e.g., digitalized patients with significant cardiac arrhythmias). Potassium depletion will occur when the rate of loss through renal excretion and/or loss from the gastrointestinal tract exceeds the rate of potassium intake. Potassium supplements may also be indicated in patients who suffer from hepatic cirrhosis with ascites; states of aldosterone excess with normal renal function; certain diarrheal states, including those induced by chronic laxative use; prolonged vomiting; Bartter's syndrome; potassium-losing nephropathy; and in patients, including children, on long-term corticosteroid therapy.

Deficiency of potassium may lead to muscle weakness, irregular heartbeat, mood or mental changes, or nausea or vomiting.

### Acceptance not established

There are insufficient data to show that potassium supplementation lowers *blood pressure* in hypertensive patients.

### Unaccepted

Enteric-coated tablets of potassium chloride are no longer recommended for use because of the high incidence of severe injury to adjacent gastrointestinal tissues during tablet dissolution.

## Pharmacology/Pharmacokinetics

### Physicochemical characteristics

Molecular weight—
    Potassium acetate: 98.14.
    Potassium bicarbonate: 100.12.
    Potassium chloride: 74.55.
    Potassium citrate: 324.41.
    Potassium gluconate: 234.25.

### Mechanism of action/Effect

Potassium is the predominant cation (approximately 150 to 160 mEq per liter) within cells. Intracellular sodium content is relatively low. In extracellular fluid, sodium predominates and the potassium content is low (3.5 to 5 mEq per liter). A membrane-bound enzyme, sodium-potassium–activated adenosinetriphosphatase ($Na^+K^+$ ATPase), actively transports or pumps sodium out and potassium into cells to maintain these concentration gradients. The intracellular to extracellular potassium gradients are necessary for the conduction of nerve impulses in such specialized tissues as the heart, brain, and skeletal muscle, and for the maintenance of normal renal function and acid-base balance. High intracellular potassium concentrations are necessary for numerous cellular metabolic processes.

### Elimination

Renal—90%.
Fecal—10%.

## Precautions to Consider

### Carcinogenicity

No data are available on long-term potential for carcinogenicity in animals or humans. Potassium is a normal dietary constituent.

### Pregnancy/Reproduction

Pregnancy—Studies have not been done in humans.
Studies have not been done in animals.

FDA Pregnancy Category C.

### Breast-feeding

Problems in humans have not been documented.

### Pediatrics

Appropriate studies on the relationship of age to the effects of potassium supplements have not been performed in the pediatric population. However, no pediatrics-specific problems have been documented to date.

### Geriatrics

Although appropriate studies on the relationship of age to the effects of potassium supplements have not been performed in the geriatric population, no geriatrics-specific problems have been sufficiently documented to date. However, elderly patients are at greater risk of developing hyperkalemia due to age-related changes in the ability of the kidneys to excrete potassium.

### Drug interactions and/or related problems

The following drug interactions and/or related problems have been selected on the basis of their potential clinical significance (possible mechanism in parentheses where appropriate)—not necessarily inclusive (» = major clinical significance):

Note: Combinations containing any of the following, depending on the amount present, may also interact with this medication.

Amphotericin B or
Corticosteroids, glucocorticoid, especially with significant mineralocorticoid activity or
Corticosteroids, mineralocorticoid or
Corticotropin (ACTH) or
Gentamicin or
Penicillins (including azlocillin, carbenicillin, mezlocillin, piperacillin, ticarcillin) or
Polymyxin B
    (potassium requirements may be increased in patients receiving these medications, due to renal potassium wasting; close monitoring of serum potassium is recommended)
» Angiotensin-converting enzyme (ACE) inhibitors or
» Anti-inflammatory drugs, nonsteroidal (NSAIDs) or
» Beta-adrenergic blocking agents or
Blood from blood bank (may contain up to 30 mEq of potassium per liter of plasma or up to 65 mEq per liter of whole blood when stored for more than 10 days) or
Cyclosporine or
» Diuretics, potassium-sparing or

» Heparin or
» Low-salt milk or
   Potassium-containing medications, other or
   Salt substitutes
      (concurrent use with potassium supplements may increase serum
      potassium concentrations, which may cause severe hyperkalemia
      and lead to cardiac arrest, especially in renal insufficiency; low-
      salt milk may contain up to 60 mEq of potassium per liter and
      most salt substitutes contain substantial amounts of potassium; in
      addition, use of NSAIDs in combination with potassium supple-
      ments may increase the risk of gastrointestinal side effects)

» Anticholinergics or other medications with anticholinergic activity
   (See *Appendix II*)
      (concurrent use with potassium chloride oral supplements, espe-
      cially solid dosage forms, may increase severity of gastrointestinal
      lesions produced by potassium chloride alone; if symptoms de-
      velop, patients should be carefully monitored endoscopically for
      evidence of lesions)

   Calcium salts, parenteral
      (potassium supplements should be used cautiously in patients re-
      ceiving parenteral calcium salts because of the danger of precipi-
      tating cardiac arrhythmias)

» Digitalis glycosides, in the presence of heart block
      (potassium supplements are not recommended for concurrent use
      in digitalized patients with severe or complete heart block; how-
      ever, if potassium supplements must be used to prevent or correct
      hypokalemia in digitalized patients, careful monitoring of serum
      potassium concentrations is extremely important)

» Diuretics, thiazide
      (increased risk of hyperkalemia when a potassium-wasting diuretic
      is discontinued after concurrent use with a potassium supplement)

   Exchange resins, sodium cycle, such as sodium polystyrene sulfonate
      (whether these medications are administered orally or rectally, se-
      rum potassium concentrations are reduced by sodium replacement
      of the potassium; fluid retention may occur in some patients be-
      cause of the increased sodium intake)

   Insulin or
   Sodium bicarbonate
      (concurrent use of these medications decreases serum potassium
      concentration by promoting a shift of potassium ion into the cells)

   Laxatives
      (chronic use or overuse of laxatives may reduce serum potassium
      concentrations by promoting excessive potassium loss from the
      intestinal tract)

### Medical considerations/Contraindications

The medical considerations/contraindications included here have been selected on the basis of their potential clinical significance (reasons given
   in parentheses where appropriate)—not necessarily inclusive (» =
   major clinical significance).

**Except under special circumstances, this medication should not be
used when hyperkalemia exists, because further increases in serum
potassium may cause cardiac arrest.**

*Risk-benefit should be considered when the following medical problems
exist:*

*For potassium acetate only*
   Alkalosis, metabolic or respiratory
      (acetate is a precursor to bicarbonate, which may exacerbate the
      condition)

*For all potassium supplements*
» Diarrhea, prolonged or severe, resulting in severe dehydration
      (the loss of fluid in combination with use of potassium supplements
      may cause renal toxicity, which may increase the risk of hyper-
      kalemia; if potassium supplements are given in the presence of
      diarrhea, serum potassium should be monitored)

» Esophageal compression or
» Gastric emptying, delayed or
» Intestinal obstruction or stricture or
» Peptic ulcer
      (delayed passage of potassium supplements through the gastro-
      intestinal tract may cause or worsen gastrointestinal irritation, es-
      pecially with solid dosage forms)

» Familial periodic paralysis or
   Myotonia congenita
      (potassium supplements may aggravate these conditions, although
      some patients with familial periodic paralysis may require potas-
      sium supplementation)

» Heart block, severe or complete
      (increased risk of hyperkalemia, especially in digitalized patients;
      careful monitoring of serum potassium concentrations is
      recommended)

» Hyperkalemia, or conditions predisposing to hyperkalemia, such as:
   Acidosis, metabolic, acute
   Adrenal insufficiency
   Dehydration, acute
   Diabetes mellitus, uncontrolled
   Physical exercise, strenuous, in unconditioned persons
   Renal failure, chronic
   Tissue breakdown, extensive
      (increased serum potassium concentrations possibly leading to car-
      diac arrest may occur; exercise-induced hyperkalemia is transient
      and is a problem only in patients with renal insufficiency from
      dehydration or those taking medications that increase serum
      potassium)

   Sensitivity to potassium

### Patient monitoring

The following may be especially important in patient monitoring (other
   tests may be warranted in some patients, depending on condition;
   » = major clinical significance):

   Electrocardiograms (ECG) and
   Potassium concentrations, serum and
   Renal function determinations, especially serum creatinine and urine
   output
      (monitoring recommended at periodic intervals during oral ther-
      apy; recommended concurrently during parenteral therapy)

   Magnesium concentrations, serum
      (determinations recommended in patients with refractory hypoka-
      lemia; coexisting magnesium depletion may need correction to re-
      plenish serum potassium and/or cell potassium concentrations)

   pH determinations, serum
      (used to help determine existence of acidosis or alkalosis and thus
      allow improved interpretation of serum potassium measurements;
      utilized more often during parenteral therapy)

## Side/Adverse Effects

The following side/adverse effects have been selected on the basis of their
   potential clinical significance (possible signs and symptoms in parentheses where appropriate)—not necessarily inclusive:

### Those indicating need for medical attention

Incidence less frequent
   *Hyperkalemia* (confusion; irregular or slow heartbeat; numbness or
   tingling in hands, feet, or lips; shortness of breath or difficult
   breathing; unexplained anxiety; unusual tiredness or weakness; weakness or heaviness of legs)

   Note: *Hyperkalemia* side effects are considered rare when oral dosage
      forms of potassium are administered to patients having normal
      renal function. When hyperkalemia is present, severe muscle
      weakness and a slow, irregular heartbeat are the most common
      symptoms. When the medication is administered parenterally,
      the incidence of irregular heartbeat (arrhythmias) may become
      more frequent.

      Irregular heartbeat is usually the earliest clinical indication of
      hyperkalemia and is readily detected by ECG.

Incidence rare
   *Irritation, contact, of the alimentary tract* (continuing abdominal or
   stomach pain, cramping, or soreness; chest or throat pain, especially
   when swallowing; stools containing fresh or digested blood)

   Note: *Irritation of the alimentary tract* may occur when potassium is
      in contact with ulcerous areas, or when there is a high concen-
      tration of potassium in one area; the latter has resulted from
      improper release from oral dosage form, or from delayed pas-
      sage of the dosage form through the alimentary tract.

### Those indicating need for medical attention only if they continue or are bothersome

Incidence more frequent
   *For oral dosage forms*
      *Diarrhea; nausea; stomach pain, discomfort, or gas, mild;
      vomiting*

      Note: These side effects occur more frequently when the medi-
      cation is not taken with food or is not diluted properly.

# Patient Consultation

As an aid to patient consultation, refer to *Advice for the Patient, Potassium Supplements (Systemic).*

In providing consultation, consider emphasizing the following selected information (» = major clinical significance):

**Description of use**
Description should include function in the body; signs of deficiency

**Importance of diet**
Importance of proper nutrition
Potassium content of selected foods
Recommended daily intake for potassium
Not exceeding recommended amounts of potassium

**Before using this medication**
» Conditions affecting use, especially:
Sensitivity to potassium
Use in the elderly—Risk of developing hyperkalemia due to age-related changes in ability of kidneys to excrete potassium
Other medications, especially beta adrenergic blocking agents, nonsteroidal anti-inflammatory drugs, anticholinergics, potassium-sparing and thiazide diuretics, low-salt milk, other potassium-containing medications, ACE inhibitors, digitalis glycosides, or heparin
Other medical problems, especially delayed gastric emptying, esophageal compression, or intestinal obstruction or stricture, peptic ulcer; heart block; hyperkalemia or conditions predisposing to hyperkalemia for all potassium supplements; metabolic or respiratory acidosis for potassium acetate

**Proper use of this medication**
*Proper administration technique*
Necessary dilution of liquid dosage forms
Taking tablets and capsules with adequate liquids
Complete dissolution of effervescent dosage forms prior to taking
Not using tomato juice for dilution if on a sodium-restricted diet
Not crushing or chewing extended-release dosage forms, unless otherwise directed
Sprinkling contents of some extended-release capsules and some tablets over soft food such as applesauce or mixing with fruit juice, if unable to swallow whole, but only when directed to do so
» Taking each dose immediately after a meal or with food
» Compliance with therapy, especially when taking diuretics and digitalis
» Proper dosing
Missed dose: Taking as soon as possible if remembered within 2 hours; going back to regular dosage schedule; not doubling doses
» Proper storage

**Precautions while using this medication**
Regular visits to physician to check progress of therapy; serum potassium monitoring may be necessary
» Not taking salt substitutes or low-salt milk or food unless approved by physician; importance of carefully reading labels of all low-salt foods to prevent excess intake of potassium
Checking with physician before beginning strenuous physical exercise if out of condition, to prevent possible hyperkalemia
» Checking with physician at once if signs of gastrointestinal bleeding are observed

**Side/adverse effects**
Expended wax matrix from some potassium chloride extended-release tablets may be seen in stool and be alarming to patient, although not necessarily an indication of improper dissolution of tablet or lack of bioavailability of potassium chloride
Signs of potential side effects, especially hyperkalemia or contact irritation of the alimentary tract

# General Dosing Information

Caution must be observed in the attempt to correct hypokalemia in order to avoid overcompensation and a resultant hyperkalemia with accompanying cardiac arrhythmias.

The normal adult concentration of serum potassium is 3.5 to 5.0 millimoles or mEq per liter with 4.5 millimoles or mEq often being used for a reference point. Potassium concentrations exceeding 5.5 mEq per liter are dangerous because of possible initiation of cardiac arrhythmias. Normal potassium concentrations tend to be higher in neonates (7.7 mEq per liter) than in adults.

Serum potassium concentrations do not necessarily indicate the true body potassium content. A rise in plasma pH (alkalosis) and chronic acidosis may decrease plasma potassium concentration by promoting potassium excretion and increase the intracellular potassium concentra-

tion. Conversely, a decrease in blood pH (acute acidosis) can cause an increase in serum potassium by inhibiting potassium excretion. However, it is necessary to attempt to restore serum potassium to normal in familial periodic paralysis, even though there is no total body potassium depletion.

Adequate renal function is essential for therapy with potassium supplements, since the kidneys maintain normal potassium balance. A gradual increase in the amount of potassium ingested leads to an increased ability of the kidneys to excrete potassium, thus preventing lethal hyperkalemia. The risk-benefit of potassium supplements should be considered in any patient with a higher-than-normal serum creatinine concentration.

Abrupt discontinuation of supplemental potassium to a patient suffering concurrent potassium losses, and also receiving digitalis preparations, may result in digitalis toxicity.

One gram of potassium acetate provides 10.26 mEq of potassium.
One gram of potassium bicarbonate provides 10 mEq of potassium.
One gram of potassium chloride provides 13.41 mEq of potassium.
One gram of potassium citrate provides 9.26 mEq of potassium.
One gram of potassium gluconate provides 4.27 mEq of potassium.

**For oral dosage forms only**
*Because of their ulcerogenic tendency and the incidence of local tissue destruction produced from their dissolution, use of compressed tablets or enteric-coated tablets is not recommended.*

Solid tablet dosage forms should not be used in patients with delayed gastric emptying, esophageal compression, or intestinal obstruction or stricture. The use of potassium tablets in such conditions increases the possibility of tissue destruction by high, local concentrations of potassium released by the tablet.

**For parenteral dosage forms only**
Infusion of insulin- or glucose-containing or sodium bicarbonate solutions may decrease serum potassium concentrations because of a shift of potassium into the cells.

Before commencing intravenous administration of potassium chloride for large-dose replacement therapy:
• Serum potassium concentrations should be determined.
• Renal function should be determined. Adequate urine output should be ensured.
• Concentrated potassium chloride injection must be diluted and thoroughly mixed with a larger volume (1000 mL) of fluid suitable for intravenous administration, preferably to a concentration of 40 mEq of potassium per liter, not to exceed 80 mEq per liter.
• When mixing in soft or bag-type containers of large-volume parenteral fluids, extra care must be used to ensure complete mixing and absence of pools of concentrated material.
• In dehydrated patients, a liter of potassium-free hydrating solution such as 0.2 or 0.45% sodium chloride injection is sometimes rapidly infused to ensure hydration and adequate renal function in select patients whose condition will tolerate bolus fluids. In such patients, serum potassium should be measured, and potassium added to the solution if serum potassium levels fall.

During intravenous potassium chloride administration:
• To avoid hyperkalemia, the infusion rate must not be rapid; a rate of 10 mEq of potassium per hour is usually considered to be safe as long as urine output is adequate. As a general rule, the rate should never exceed 1 mEq per minute for adults, or 0.02 mEq per kg of body weight per minute for children.
• Close patient monitoring by clinical observation, frequent electrocardiograms (especially during administration at the higher rates), and serum potassium determinations may be desirable as indicated by the situation.
• If renal dysfunction, especially acute renal failure as evidenced by oliguria and/or rising serum creatinine, should occur during infusion of potassium chloride, the infusion should be stopped at once. Subsequent infusion, if needed, should be administered very cautiously and with close monitoring.

**Diet/Nutrition**
Oral potassium supplements should be taken with or immediately after a meal to minimize possible stomach upset or laxative action. Most oral tablets or capsules should be swallowed whole, never crushed or chewed. However, some commercial extended-release products, because of microencapsulation, may be crushed, chewed, or sprinkled on a spoonful of soft food if the patient is unable to swallow the solid dosage form whole. The oral solution, soluble tablet, and powder forms should be completely dissolved in at least one-half glass (120 mL) of cold water or juice, then sipped slowly over a 5- to 10-minute period.

Recommended dietary intakes for potassium are defined differently worldwide.

For U.S.—

The Recommended Dietary Allowances (RDAs) for vitamins and minerals are determined by the Food and Nutrition Board of the National Research Council and are intended to provide adequate nutrition in most healthy persons under usual environmental stresses. In addition, a different designation may be used by the FDA for food and dietary supplement labeling purposes, as with Daily Value (DV). DVs replace the previous labeling terminology United States Recommended Daily Allowances (USRDAs).

For Canada—

Recommended Nutrient Intakes (RNIs) for vitamins, minerals, and protein are determined by Health and Welfare Canada and provide recommended amounts of a specific nutrient while minimizing the risk of chronic diseases.

There is no RDA or RNI established for potassium; 1600 to 2000 mg (40 to 50 mEq) per day is considered adequate for adults.

Low-salt milk and salt substitutes may contain substantial amounts of potassium. These and other low-salt foods, especially breads and canned foods, should be avoided during treatment with potassium supplements, unless otherwise specified by the health care professional. Serum potassium may increase with resulting hyperkalemia, especially in patients with renal insufficiency.

The following table indicates the potassium content of selected foods:

| Food (amount) | Milligrams of potassium | Milliequivalents of potassium |
| --- | --- | --- |
| Acorn squash, cooked (1 cup) | 896 | 23 |
| Potato with skin, baked (1 long) | 844 | 22 |
| Spinach, cooked (1 cup) | 838 | 21 |
| Lentils, cooked (1 cup) | 731 | 19 |
| Kidney beans, cooked (1 cup) | 713 | 18 |
| Split peas, cooked (1 cup) | 710 | 18 |
| White navy beans, cooked (1 cup) | 669 | 17 |
| Butternut squash, cooked (1 cup) | 583 | 15 |
| Watermelon (1/16) | 560 | 14 |
| Raisins (1/2 cup) | 553 | 14 |
| Yogurt, low-fat, plain (1 cup) | 531 | 14 |
| Orange juice, frozen (1 cup) | 503 | 13 |
| Brussel sprouts, cooked (1 cup) | 494 | 13 |
| Zucchini, cooked, sliced (1 cup) | 456 | 12 |
| Banana (medium) | 451 | 12 |
| Collards, frozen, cooked (1 cup) | 427 | 11 |
| Cantaloupe (1/4) | 412 | 11 |
| Milk, low-fat 1% (1 cup) | 348 | 9 |
| Broccoli, frozen, cooked (1 cup) | 332 | 9 |

**For treatment of adverse effects**

Treatment of hyperkalemia includes:

• If appropriate, discontinuing blood products, foods and medication that contain potassium, as well as ACE inhibitors, beta blocking agents, nonsteroidal anti-inflammatory drugs (NSAIDs), heparin, cyclosporine, and potassium-sparing diuretics.

• Administering 10% dextrose containing 10 to 20 units of insulin per liter at a rate of 300 to 500 mL of solution per hour. This will facilitate a shift of potassium into the cells.

• Correcting any existing acidosis with 50 mEq intravenous sodium bicarbonate over 5 minutes. The dose may be repeated in 10 to 15 minutes if needed. This will facilitate a shift of potassium into the cells.

• Administering a calcium salt (calcium gluconate, 0.5 to 1 gram, over a 2-minute period) to antagonize the cardiotoxic effects in patients whose electrocardiograms (ECGs) show absent P waves, or a broad QRS complex, and who are not receiving digitalis glycosides. Doses may be repeated after 2-minute intervals.

• Utilizing exchange resins to remove excess potassium from the body by adsorption and/or exchange of potassium. The oral dose of sodium polystyrene sulfonate is 20 to 50 grams of the resin dissolved in 100 to 200 mL of 20% sorbitol. The dose may by given every 4 hours up to four or five daily doses until potassium levels return to normal. It may also be given as a retention enema by mixing 8 grams of sodium polystyrene sulfonate and 50 grams of sorbitol in 200 mL of water. The retention enema exchanges potassium faster than the oral sodium polystyrene sulfonate.

• Utilizing hemodialysis or peritoneal dialysis to reduce serum potassium concentrations. May be necessary in patients with renal function impairment.

• Ascertaining adequate urine output and, if not contraindicated by the clinical condition of the patient, maintaining a high urine output with normal saline solutions and loop diuretics.

Caution must be observed when treating hyperkalemia in digitalized patients, since rapid reduction of serum potassium concentrations may induce digitalis toxicity.

---

## POTASSIUM ACETATE

# Parenteral Dosage Forms

Note: **Injectable potassium products must be diluted prior to intravenous administration. Direct patient injection of potassium concentrate may be instantaneously fatal.**

### POTASSIUM ACETATE INJECTION USP

**Usual adult and adolescent dose**

Electrolyte replenisher or

Hypokalemia (treatment)—

Intravenous infusion, the dose and rate of infusion to be determined by the individual requirements of each patient, up to 400 mEq of potassium a day (usually not more than 3 mEq per kg of body weight). The response of the patient, as determined by the measurement of serum potassium concentration and the electrocardiogram following the initial 40 to 60 mEq infused, should indicate the subsequent infusion rate required.

Serum potassium *greater* than 2.5 mEq per liter: Intravenous infusion, up to 200 mEq of potassium a day in a concentration less than 30 mEq per liter and at a rate not exceeding 10 mEq per hour.

Serum potassium *less* than 2.0 mEq per liter with ECG changes or paralysis (urgent treatment): Intravenous infusion, up to 400 mEq of potassium a day in a suitable concentration and at a rate up to, but usually not exceeding, 20 mEq per hour.

Note: Some urgent situations may require a dosage and/or rate of administration that temporarily exceeds those stated above.

Hypokalemia (prophylaxis)—

Intravenous infusion, as part of total parenteral nutrition solutions, the specific amount determined by individual patient need.

**Usual pediatric dose**

Electrolyte replenisher or

Hypokalemia (treatment)—

Intravenous infusion, up to 3 mEq of potassium per kg of body weight or 40 mEq per square meter of body surface a day. Volume of administered fluids must be adjusted to body size.

Hypokalemia (prophylaxis)—

Intravenous infusion, as part of total parenteral nutrition solutions, the specific amount determined by individual patient need.

**Strength(s) usually available**

U.S.—

2 mEq of potassium per mL (Rx) [GENERIC].

4 mEq of potassium per mL (Rx) [GENERIC].

Canada—

Not commercially available.

**Packaging and storage**

Store below 40 °C (104 °F), preferably between 15 and 30 °C (59 and 86 °F), unless otherwise specified by manufacturer. Protect from freezing.

---

## POTASSIUM BICARBONATE

# Oral Dosage Forms

### POTASSIUM BICARBONATE EFFERVESCENT TABLETS FOR ORAL SOLUTION USP

**Usual adult and adolescent dose**

Hypokalemia (prophylaxis or treatment)—

Oral, 25 to 50 mEq of potassium dissolved in one-half to one glass (120 to 240 mL) of cold water one or two times a day, the dosage being adjusted as needed and tolerated.

**Usual adult prescribing limits**

Up to 100 mEq of potassium a day.

**Usual pediatric dose**

Dosage has not been established.

**Strength(s) usually available**

U.S.—

6.5 mEq of potassium (650 mg) (Rx) [GENERIC].

20 mEq of potassium (Rx) [*K+ Care ET*].

25 mEq of potassium (Rx) [*K+ Care ET; K-Electrolyte; K-Ide; Klor-Con/EF; K-Lyte; K-Vescent;* GENERIC].

Canada—
25 mEq of potassium (Rx) [*K-Lyte*].

### Packaging and storage
Store below 40 °C (104 °F), preferably between 15 and 30 °C (59 and 86 °F), unless otherwise specified by manufacturer. Store in a tight container or original foil packaging.

### Auxiliary labeling
• Take dissolved in cold water.
• Take with or immediately after food.

### Note
Dispense in original foil packaging to help maintain moisture-free condition until use.

---

## POTASSIUM BICARBONATE AND POTASSIUM CHLORIDE

# Oral Dosage Forms

## POTASSIUM BICARBONATE AND POTASSIUM CHLORIDE FOR EFFERVESCENT ORAL SOLUTION USP

### Usual adult and adolescent dose
Hypokalemia (prophylaxis or treatment)—
Oral, 20 mEq of potassium dissolved in one-half to one glass (120 to 240 mL) of cold water one or two times a day, the dosage being adjusted as needed and tolerated.

### Usual adult prescribing limits
Up to 100 mEq of potassium a day.

### Usual pediatric dose
Dosage has not been established.

### Strength(s) usually available
U.S.—
20 mEq of potassium per 2.8-gram packet (Rx) [*Klorvess Effervescent Granules*].

Canada—
20 mEq of potassium per 2.8-gram packet (Rx) [*Neo-K*].

### Packaging and storage
Store below 40 °C (104 °F), preferably between 15 and 30 °C (59 and 86 °F), unless otherwise specified by manufacturer. Store in a tight container or original foil packaging.

### Auxiliary labeling
• Take dissolved in cold water.
• Take with or immediately after food.

### Note
Dispense in original foil packaging to help maintain moisture-free condition until use.

## POTASSIUM BICARBONATE AND POTASSIUM CHLORIDE EFFERVESCENT TABLETS FOR ORAL SOLUTION USP

### Usual adult and adolescent dose
Hypokalemia (prophylaxis or treatment)—
Oral, 20, 25, or 50 mEq of potassium dissolved in one-half to one glass (120 to 240 mL) of cold water one or two times a day, the dosage being adjusted as needed and tolerated.

### Usual adult prescribing limits
Up to 100 mEq of potassium a day.

### Usual pediatric dose
Dosage has not been established.

### Strength(s) usually available
U.S.—
20 mEq of potassium (Rx) [*Klorvess*].
25 mEq of potassium (Rx) [*K-Lyte/Cl*].
50 mEq of potassium (Rx) [*K-Lyte/Cl 50*].

Canada—
12 mEq of potassium (Rx) [*Potassium-Sandoz*].

### Packaging and storage
Store below 40 °C (104 °F), preferably between 15 and 30 °C (59 and 86 °F), unless otherwise specified by manufacturer. Store in a tight container or original foil packaging.

### Auxiliary labeling
• Take dissolved in cold water.
• Take with or immediately after food.

### Note
Dispense in original foil packaging to help maintain moisture-free condition until use.

---

## POTASSIUM BICARBONATE AND POTASSIUM CITRATE

# Oral Dosage Forms

## POTASSIUM BICARBONATE AND POTASSIUM CITRATE EFFERVESCENT TABLETS FOR ORAL SOLUTION

### Usual adult and adolescent dose
Hypokalemia (prophylaxis or treatment)—
Oral, 25 or 50 mEq of potassium dissolved in one-half to one glass (120 to 240 mL) of cold water one or two times a day, the dosage being adjusted as needed and tolerated.

### Usual adult prescribing limits
Up to 100 mEq of potassium a day.

### Usual pediatric dose
Dosage has not been established.

### Strength(s) usually available
U.S.—
25 mEq of potassium (Rx) [*Effer-K*].
50 mEq of potassium (Rx) [*K-Lyte DS*].

Canada—
Not commercially available.

### Packaging and storage
Store below 40 °C (104 °F), preferably between 15 and 30 °C (59 and 86 °F), unless otherwise specified by manufacturer. Store in original foil packaging.

### Auxiliary labeling
• Take dissolved in cold water.
• Take with or immediately after food.

### Note
Dispense in original foil packaging to help maintain moisture-free condition until use.

---

## POTASSIUM CHLORIDE

# Oral Dosage Forms

## POTASSIUM CHLORIDE EXTENDED-RELEASE CAPSULES USP

### Usual adult and adolescent dose
Hypokalemia (prophylaxis)—
Oral, the equivalent of 16 to 24 mEq of potassium a day, divided into two or three doses, the dosage being adjusted as needed and tolerated.
Hypokalemia (treatment)—
Oral, 40 to 100 mEq of potassium a day, divided into two or three doses, the dosage being adjusted as needed and tolerated.

### Usual adult prescribing limits
Up to 100 mEq of potassium a day.

### Usual pediatric dose
Dosage has not been established.

### Strength(s) usually available
U.S.—
8 mEq (600 mg) of potassium (Rx) [*Micro-K;* GENERIC].
10 mEq (750 mg) of potassium (Rx) [*K-Lease; K-Norm; Micro-K 10;* GENERIC].

Canada—
8 mEq (600 mg) of potassium (Rx) [*Micro-K*].
10 mEq (750 mg) of potassium (Rx) [*Micro-K 10*].

### Packaging and storage
Store below 30 °C (86 °F). Store in a tight container.

### Auxiliary labeling
• Swallow capsules whole with a full glass of water.
• Do not chew or crush.
• Take with or immediately after food.

**Note**

Extended release over an 8- to 10-hour period. Polymeric particle coating of one product allows contents of the capsule to be sprinkled over soft food or mixed with juice.

## POTASSIUM CHLORIDE ORAL SOLUTION USP

**Usual adult and adolescent dose**

Hypokalemia (prophylaxis or treatment)—
   Oral, 20 mEq of potassium diluted in one-half glass (120 mL) of cold water or juice one to four times a day, the dosage being adjusted as needed and tolerated.

**Usual adult prescribing limits**

Up to 100 mEq of potassium a day.

**Usual pediatric dose**

Hypokalemia (prophylaxis or treatment)—
   Oral, 15 to 40 mEq of potassium per square meter of body surface or 1 to 3 mEq of potassium per kg of body weight a day administered in divided doses and well diluted in water or juice.

**Strength(s) usually available**

U.S.—
   10 mEq (750 mg) of potassium per 15 mL (Rx) [GENERIC (alcohol 5%)].
   20 mEq (1.5 grams) of potassium per 15 mL (Rx) [*Cena-K; Kaochlor 10%* (alcohol 5%; tartrazine); *Kaochlor S-F 10%* (alcohol 5%); *Kay Ciel* (alcohol 4%); *Klorvess 10% Liquid* (alcohol 0.75%); *Potasalan* (alcohol 4%); GENERIC].
   30 mEq (2.25 grams) of potassium per 15 mL (Rx) [*Rum-K*].
   40 mEq (3 grams) of potassium per 15 mL (Rx) [*Cena-K; Kaon-Cl 20% Liquid* (alcohol 5%); GENERIC].

Canada—
   10 mEq (750 mg) of potassium per 15 mL (Rx) [*KCL 5%*].
   20 mEq (1.5 grams) of potassium per 15 mL (Rx) [*K-10; Kaochlor-10; Roychlor-10%*].
   40 mEq (3 grams) of potassium per 15 mL (Rx) [*Kaochlor-20*].

**Packaging and storage**

Store below 40 °C (104 °F), preferably between 15 and 30 °C (59 and 86 °F), unless otherwise specified by manufacturer. Store in a tight container. Protect from freezing.

**Stability**

Some commercial preparations contain coloring agents that fade when exposed to light. Active ingredients are not affected by light.

**Auxiliary labeling**

• Take mixed in cold water or juice.
• Take with or immediately after food.

## POTASSIUM CHLORIDE FOR ORAL SOLUTION USP

**Usual adult and adolescent dose**

Hypokalemia (prophylaxis or treatment)—
   Oral, 15 to 25 mEq of potassium diluted in four to six ounces (180 mL) of cold water two to four times a day, the dosage being adjusted as needed and tolerated.

**Usual adult prescribing limits**

Up to 100 mEq of potassium a day.

**Usual pediatric dose**

Hypokalemia (prophylaxis or treatment)—
   Oral, 15 to 25 mEq of potassium per square meter of body surface, or 1 to 3 mEq of potassium per kg of body weight a day administered in divided doses and well diluted in water or juice.

**Strength(s) usually available**

U.S.—
   10 mEq (745 mg) of potassium per packet (Rx) [GENERIC].
   15 mEq (1.12 grams) of potassium per packet (Rx) [*K+ Care; K-Lor*].
   20 mEq (1.5 grams) of potassium per packet (Rx) [*Gen-K; Kato; Kay Ciel; K+ Care; K-Ide; K-Lor; Klor-Con Powder; K-Sol*; GENERIC].
   25 mEq (1.8 grams) of potassium per packet or dose (Rx) [*Gen-K; K+ Care; Klor-Con/25 Powder; K-Lyte/Cl Powder* (bulk or packet); GENERIC].

Canada—
   20 mEq (1.5 grams) of potassium per packet (Rx) [*K-Lor*].
   25 mEq (1.8 grams) of potassium per packet (Rx) [*K-Lyte/Cl*].

**Packaging and storage**

Store below 40 °C (104 °F), preferably between 15 and 30 °C (59 and 86 °F), unless otherwise specified by manufacturer. Store in a tight container.

**Auxiliary labeling**

• Take dissolved in cold water or juice.
• Take with or immediately after food.

## POTASSIUM CHLORIDE FOR ORAL SUSPENSION

**Usual adult and adolescent dose**

Hypokalemia (prophylaxis or treatment)—
   Oral, 20 mEq of potassium mixed in two to six ounces (180 mL) of cold water one to five times a day, the dosage being adjusted as needed and tolerated.

**Usual adult prescribing limits**

Up to 100 mEq of potassium a day.

**Usual pediatric dose**

Dosage has not been established.

**Strength(s) usually available**

U.S.—
   20 mEq (1.5 grams) of potassium per packet (Rx) [*Micro-K LS*].

Canada—
   Not commercially available.

**Packaging and storage**

Store below 40 °C (104 °F), preferably between 15 and 30 °C (59 and 86 °F), in a tight container, unless otherwise specified by manufacturer.

**Preparation of dosage form**

Add granules to 2 to 6 ounces of water or juice, and stir for 1 minute before swallowing. The granules may also be added to 2 ounces of orange juice, tomato juice, apple juice, or milk.

**Auxiliary labeling**

• Take dissolved in cold water or juice.
• Take with or immediately after food.

Note: May be sprinkled on food.

## POTASSIUM CHLORIDE EXTENDED-RELEASE TABLETS USP

**Usual adult and adolescent dose**

Hypokalemia (prophylaxis or treatment)—
   Oral, 6.7 to 20 mEq of potassium (approximately 500 to 1.5 grams of potassium chloride, respectively) three times a day.

**Usual adult prescribing limits**

Up to 100 mEq of potassium a day.

**Usual pediatric dose**

Dosage has not been established.

**Strength(s) usually available**

U.S.—
   6.7 mEq (500 mg) of potassium (Rx) [*Kaon-Cl* (tartrazine)].
   8 mEq (600 mg) of potassium (Rx) [*K-8; Klor-Con 8; Slow-K*; GENERIC].
   10 mEq (750 mg) of potassium (Rx) [*K+ 10; Kaon-Cl-10* (tartrazine); *K-Dur; Klor-Con 10; Klotrix; K-Tab; Ten-K* (scored); GENERIC].
   20 mEq (1.5 grams) of potassium (Rx) [*K-Dur* (scored)].

Canada—
   6.7 mEq (500 mg) of potassium (Rx) [*K-Long*].
   8 mEq (600 mg) of potassium (Rx) [*Apo-K; Slow-K*].
   10 mEq (750 mg) of potassium (Rx) [*Kalium Durules*].
   12 mEq (900 mg) of potassium (Rx) [*K-Med 900*].
   20 mEq (1500 mg) of potassium (Rx) [*K-Dur* (scored)].

**Packaging and storage**

Store below 30 °C (86 °F). Store in a tight container.

**Auxiliary labeling**

• Swallow tablets whole with a full glass of water.
• Do not chew or crush unless otherwise directed.
• Take with or immediately after food.

**Additional information**

Most extended-release tablets utilize an inert wax matrix from which the drug is slowly leached out as it passes through the gastrointestinal tract. The expended wax matrix may appear intact in the stool.

The extended-release tablets without a wax matrix may be swallowed whole or broken or crushed and sprinkled on food.

# Parenteral Dosage Forms

## POTASSIUM CHLORIDE FOR INJECTION CONCENTRATE USP

Note: **Injectable potassium chloride products in strengths of 1.5 mEq and 2 mEq per mL must be diluted prior to intravenous administration. Direct patient injection of potassium concentrate may be instantaneously fatal. However, injectable potassium** chloride products in strengths of 0.1, 0.2, 0.3, and 0.4 mEq per mL are intended for use with a calibrated infusion device and do not require dilution.

**Usual adult and adolescent dose**
Electrolyte replenisher or
Hypokalemia (treatment)—

Intravenous infusion, the dose and rate of infusion to be determined by the individual requirements of each patient, up to 400 mEq of potassium a day (usually not more than 3 mEq per kg of body weight). The response of the patient, as determined by the measurement of serum potassium concentration and the electrocardiogram following the initial 40 to 60 mEq infused, should indicate the subsequent infusion rate required.

Serum potassium *greater* than 2.5 mEq per liter: Intravenous infusion, up to 200 mEq of potassium a day in a concentration less than 30 mEq per liter and at a rate not exceeding 10 mEq per hour.

Serum potassium *less* than 2.0 mEq per liter with ECG changes or paralysis (urgent treatment): Intravenous infusion, up to 400 mEq of potassium a day in a suitable concentration and at a rate up to, but usually not exceeding, 20 mEq per hour.

Note: Some urgent situations may require a dosage and/or rate of administration that temporarily exceeds those stated above.

Hypokalemia (prophylaxis)—

Intravenous infusion, as part of total parenteral nutrition solutions, the specific amount determined by individual patient need.

**Usual pediatric dose**
Electrolyte replenisher or
Hypokalemia (treatment)—

Intravenous infusion, up to 3 mEq of potassium per kg of body weight or 40 mEq per square meter of body surface a day. Volume of administered fluids must be adjusted to body size.

Hypokalemia (prophylaxis)—

Intravenous infusion, as part of total parenteral nutrition solutions, the specific amount determined by individual patient need.

**Strength(s) usually available**
U.S.—

0.1 mEq of potassium per mL (Rx) [GENERIC].
0.2 mEq of potassium per mL (Rx) [GENERIC].
0.3 mEq of potassium per mL (Rx) [GENERIC].
0.4 mEq of potassium per mL (Rx) [GENERIC].
1.5 mEq of potassium per mL (Rx) [GENERIC].
2 mEq of potassium per mL (Rx) [GENERIC].
3 mEq of potassium per mL (Rx) [GENERIC].
10 mEq of potassium per mL (Rx) [GENERIC].

Note: To alert the practitioner to the potential danger of administering potassium chloride not intended for use in a calibration device (e.g., 1.5 or 2 mEq per mL) undiluted, USP requires that Potassium Chloride for Injection Concentrate products in vials be identified with black caps and ferrules. Ampuls must have a black band above the constriction. In addition, the words "Must Be Diluted" must appear on the cap and overseal of the cap, and the product label must bear the boxed warning "Concentrate Must Be Diluted Before Use."

Potassium chloride products in strengths of 0.1, 0.2, 0.3, and 0.4 mEq per mL are intended for use with a calibrated infusion device and do not require dilution.

Canada—
2 mEq of potassium per mL (Rx) [GENERIC].

**Packaging and storage**
Store below 40 °C (104 °F), preferably between 15 and 30 °C (59 and 86 °F), unless otherwise specified by manufacturer. Protect from freezing.

**Incompatibilities**
Potassium chloride should not be added to mannitol, blood or blood products, or amino acid or lipid-containing solutions because it may precipitate these substances from solution or cause lysis of infused red blood cells.

---

## *POTASSIUM GLUCONATE*

# Oral Dosage Forms
## POTASSIUM GLUCONATE ELIXIR USP

**Usual adult and adolescent dose**
Hypokalemia (prophylaxis or treatment)—

Oral, 20 mEq of potassium diluted in one-half glass (120 mL) of cold water or juice two to four times a day, the dosage being adjusted as needed and tolerated.

**Usual adult prescribing limits**
Up to 100 mEq of potassium daily.

**Usual pediatric dose**
Antihypokalemic—

Oral, 20 to 40 mEq of potassium per square meter of body surface, or 2 to 3 mEq per kg of body weight a day, administered in divided doses and well diluted in water or juice.

**Strength(s) usually available**
U.S.—

20 mEq of potassium (4.68 grams of potassium gluconate) per 15 mL (Rx) [*Kaon* (alcohol 5%); *Kaylixir* (alcohol 5%); *K-G Elixir* (alcohol 5%); GENERIC].

Canada—

20 mEq of potassium (4.68 grams of potassium gluconate) per 15 mL (Rx) [*Kaon; Potassium-Rougier*].

**Packaging and storage**
Store below 40 °C (104 °F), preferably between 15 and 30 °C (59 and 86 °F), unless otherwise specified by manufacturer. Store in a tight, light-resistant container. Protect from freezing.

**Stability**
Some commercial preparations contain coloring agents that fade when exposed to light. Active ingredients are not affected by light.

**Auxiliary labeling**
• Take mixed in cold water or juice.
• Take with or immediately after food.
• Keep container tightly closed.

## POTASSIUM GLUCONATE TABLETS USP

Note: Certain strengths of potassium gluconate may be available over-the-counter in some stores. Unless directed by the physician, use of these products should be discouraged.

**Usual adult and adolescent dose**
Hypokalemia (prophylaxis or treatment)—

Oral, 5 to 10 mEq of potassium two to four times a day.

**Usual adult prescribing limits**
Up to 100 mEq of potassium a day.

**Usual pediatric dose**
Dosage has not been established.

**Strength(s) usually available**
U.S.—

2 mEq of potassium (500 mg of potassium gluconate) [*Glu-K* (Rx); GENERIC (Rx/OTC)].
2.3 mEq of potassium (550 mg of potassium gluconate) (Rx/OTC) [GENERIC].
2.5 mEq of potassium (595 mg of potassium gluconate) (Rx/OTC) [GENERIC].

Canada—
Not commercially available.

**Packaging and storage**
Store below 40 °C (104 °F), preferably between 15 and 30 °C (59 and 86 °F), unless otherwise specified by manufacturer. Store in a tight container.

**Auxiliary labeling**
• Take with or immediately after food.
• Swallow tablet whole with a full glass of water.
• Do not chew or crush.

---

## *POTASSIUM GLUCONATE AND POTASSIUM CHLORIDE*

# Oral Dosage Forms
## POTASSIUM GLUCONATE AND POTASSIUM CHLORIDE ORAL SOLUTION USP

**Usual adult and adolescent dose**
Hypokalemia (prophylaxis or treatment)—

Oral, 20 mEq of potassium diluted in 30 mL or more of cold water or juice two to four times a day, the dosage being adjusted as needed and tolerated.

**Usual adult prescribing limits**
Up to 100 mEq of potassium a day.

**Usual pediatric dose**
Hypokalemia (prophylaxis or treatment)—

Oral, 20 to 40 mEq of potassium per square meter of body surface or 2 to 3 mEq per kg of body weight a day, administered in divided doses and well diluted in water or juice.

**Strength(s) usually available**

U.S.—

20 mEq of potassium per 15 mL (Rx) [*Kolyum*].

Canada—

Not commercially available.

**Packaging and storage**

Store below 40 °C (104 °F), preferably between 15 and 30 °C (59 and 86 °F), unless otherwise specified by manufacturer. Store in a tight container. Protect from freezing.

**Stability**

Some commercial preparations contain coloring agents that fade when exposed to light. Active ingredients are not affected by light.

**Auxiliary labeling**

• Take mixed in cold water or juice.
• Take with or immediately after food.
• Keep container tightly closed.

## POTASSIUM GLUCONATE AND POTASSIUM CHLORIDE FOR ORAL SOLUTION USP

**Usual adult and adolescent dose**

Hypokalemia (prophylaxis or treatment)—

Oral, 20 mEq of potassium diluted in 30 mL or more of cold water or juice two to four times a day, the dosage being adjusted as needed and tolerated.

**Usual adult prescribing limits**

Up to 100 mEq of potassium a day.

**Usual pediatric dose**

Hypokalemia (prophylaxis or treatment)—

Oral, 20 to 40 mEq of potassium per square meter of body surface or 2 to 3 mEq per kg of body weight a day, administered in divided doses and well diluted in water or juice.

**Strength(s) usually available**

U.S.—

20 mEq of potassium per 5-gram packet (Rx) [*Kolyum*].

Canada—

Not commercially available.

**Packaging and storage**

Store below 40 °C (104 °F), preferably between 15 and 30 °C (59 and 86 °F), unless otherwise specified by manufacturer. Store in a tight container or original package.

**Auxiliary labeling**

• Take mixed in cold water or juice.
• Take with or immediately after food.

**Note**

Dispense in original packet to help maintain moisture-free condition until use.

## *POTASSIUM GLUCONATE AND POTASSIUM CITRATE*

## Oral Dosage Forms

### POTASSIUM GLUCONATE AND POTASSIUM CITRATE ORAL SOLUTION USP

**Usual adult and adolescent dose**

Hypokalemia (prophylaxis or treatment)—

Oral, 20 mEq of potassium diluted in one-half glass (120 mL) of cold water or juice two to four times a day, the dosage being adjusted as needed and tolerated.

**Usual adult prescribing limits**

Up to 100 mEq of potassium a day.

**Usual pediatric dose**

Hypokalemia (prophylaxis or treatment)—

Oral, 20 to 40 mEq of potassium per square meter of body surface or 2 to 3 mEq per kg of body weight a day, administered in divided doses and well diluted in water or juice.

**Strength(s) usually available**

U.S.—

20 mEq of potassium per 15 mL (Rx) [*Twin-K*].

Canada—

Not commercially available.

**Packaging and storage**

Store below 40 °C (104 °F), preferably between 15 and 30 °C (59 and 86 °F), unless otherwise specified by manufacturer. Store in a tight container. Protect from freezing.

**Stability**

Some commercial preparations contain coloring agents that fade when exposed to light. Active ingredients are not affected by light.

**Auxiliary labeling**

• Take mixed in cold water or juice.
• Take with or immediately after food.
• Keep container tightly closed.

## *TRIKATES*

Note: Trikates consists of potassium acetate, potassium bicarbonate, and potassium citrate.

## Oral Dosage Forms

### TRIKATES ORAL SOLUTION USP

**Usual adult and adolescent dose**

Hypokalemia (prophylaxis or treatment)—

Oral, 15 mEq of potassium three or four times a day diluted in one-half glass (120 mL) of cold water or juice, the dosage being adjusted as needed and tolerated.

**Usual adult prescribing limits**

Up to 100 mEq of potassium a day.

**Usual pediatric dose**

Hypokalemia (prophylaxis or treatment)—

Oral, 15 to 30 mEq of potassium per square meter of body surface or 2 to 3 mEq per kg of body weight a day, administered in divided doses and well diluted in water or juice.

**Strength(s) usually available**

U.S.—

15 mEq of potassium per 5 mL (Rx) [*Tri-K*].

Canada—

Not commercially available.

**Packaging and storage**

Store below 40 °C (104 °F), preferably between 15 and 30 °C (59 and 86 °F), unless otherwise specified by manufacturer. Store in a tight, light-resistant container. Protect from freezing.

**Auxiliary labeling**

• Take mixed in cold water or juice.
• Take with or immediately after food.

Revised: 07/16/92
Interim revision: 07/11/95

# PRALIDOXIME   Systemic

VA CLASSIFICATION (Primary): AD900

Other commonly used names are: 2-PAM and 2-PAM chloride.

Note: For a listing of dosage forms and brand names by country availability, see *Dosage Forms* section(s). For a listing of brand names for the articles in this monograph, refer to the General Index.

## Category

Antidote (to organophosphate pesticides); antidote (to organophosphate chemicals); antidote (to cholinesterase inhibitors).

## Indications

**Accepted**

Toxicity, organophosphate pesticide (treatment adjunct)

Toxicity, organophosphate chemical (treatment adjunct) or

Toxicity, cholinesterase inhibitor (treatment adjunct)—Pralidoxime is indicated as an adjunct in the treatment of moderate and severe poisoning caused by organophosphate pesticides that have anticholinesterase activity or by chemicals with anticholinesterase activity such as some chemicals used as nerve agents during chemical warfare. Pralidoxime is also indicated as an adjunct in the management of overdose of cholinesterase inhibitors, such as ambenonium, neostigmine, and pyridostigmine, used in the treatment of myasthenia gravis.

Pralidoxime, used in conjunction with atropine, reverses nicotinic effects, such as muscle weakness and fasciculation, respiratory depression, and central nervous system (CNS) effects, associated with toxic exposure to organophosphate anticholinesterase pesticides and chemicals and with cholinesterase inhibitor overdose. Atropine, by antagonizing the action of cholinesterase inhibitors at muscarinic receptor sites, reverses muscarinic effects, such as tracheobronchial and salivary secretion, bronchoconstriction, bradycardia, and, to a moderate extent, CNS effects. Atropine does not reverse nicotinic effects.

Pralidoxime should also be used in poisonings in which the patient presents with symptoms typical of acetylcholinesterase inhibition, although the source of the poisoning is not known, or in which the patient suffers from mixed organophosphate-carbamate pesticide poisoning.

### Acceptance not established
Use of pralidoxime in the treatment of carbamate pesticide poisoning is controversial (except in carbaryl poisoning, in which the use of pralidoxime is not recommended). In a manner similar to that of organophosphates, carbamates inhibit acetylcholinesterase; but unlike the bond formed between organophosphates and cholinesterase, the carbamate-cholinesterase bond is reversible and readily dissociates. The effects of the poisoning are short-lived and usually can be resolved with atropine and supportive care. Pralidoxime has been used in a small number of patients to treat the nicotinic effects of carbamate poisoning. However, more experience is needed to determine that resolution of nicotinic effects of carbamate poisoning is actually potentiated by administration of pralidoxime, and not merely due to spontaneous recovery of acetylcholinesterase activity.

### Unaccepted
Pralidoxime should not be used in the treatment of poisoning caused by the carbamate pesticide, carbaryl. Pralidoxime has been shown in animal studies to enhance the severity of the poisoning.

Pralidoxime is not effective in the treatment of poisoning caused by phosphorus, inorganic phosphates, or organophosphates not having anticholinesterase activity.

## Pharmacology/Pharmacokinetics

### Physicochemical characteristics
Molecular weight—172.61.
pH—Auto-injection: 2 to 3.
Reconstituted solution: 3.5 to 4.5.

### Mechanism of action/Effect
Antidote to organophosphate pesticides and chemicals and to cholinesterase inhibitors—Organophosphates bind to the esteratic site of acetylcholinesterase, resulting initially in reversible inactivation of the enzyme. If given within 24 hours, and possibly up to 48 hours, after organophosphate exposure, pralidoxime reactivates the enzyme by cleaving the phosphate-ester bond formed between the organophosphate and acetylcholinesterase. After 24 to 48 hours, the bond "ages" and acetylcholinesterase cannot be reactivated by pralidoxime. Pralidoxime also slows the process of aging of phosphorylated acetylcholinesterase to a nonreactivatable form and detoxifies certain organophosphates by direct chemical action.

Note: In high doses, pralidoxime may inhibit acetylcholinesterase and cause neuromuscular blockade.

### Distribution
Distributed throughout the extracellular water.

### Protein binding
Not bound to plasma proteins.

### Biotransformation
Metabolized largely by the liver.

### Half-life
Elimination—Approximately 1.2 hours.

### Onset of action
Within 10 to 40 minutes.

### Minimum therapeutic concentration:
4 mcg per mL (23.17 micromoles per L).

### Elimination
Rapidly excreted in the urine, partly unchanged, and partly as a metabolite produced by the liver.

## Precautions to Consider

### Carcinogenicity/Mutagenicity
Studies have not been done to evaluate the carcinogenic or mutagenic potential of pralidoxime.

### Pregnancy/Reproduction
Pregnancy—Studies have not been done in humans.
Studies have not been done in animals.

FDA Pregnancy Category C.

### Breast-feeding
It is not known whether pralidoxime is distributed into breast milk.

### Pediatrics
Appropriate studies on the relationship of age to the effects of pralidoxime have not been performed in the pediatric population. However, pediatrics-specific problems that would limit the usefulness of this medication in children are not expected.

### Geriatrics
Appropriate studies on the relationship of age to the effects of pralidoxime have not been performed in the geriatric population. However, no geriatrics-specific problems have been documented to date.

### Drug interactions and/or related problems
The following drug interactions and/or related problems have been selected on the basis of their potential clinical significance (possible mechanism in parentheses where appropriate)—not necessarily inclusive (» = major clinical significance):

Note: Combinations containing any of the following medications, depending on the amount present, may also interact with this medication.

　Barbiturates
　　(poisoning with organophosphates sensitizes the medullary centers to depression by barbiturates)

　CNS depression–producing medications (See *Appendix II*) or Xanthines, such as:
» 　Aminophylline
» 　Caffeine
» 　Theophylline
　　(use of these medications may exacerbate the effects of organophosphate poisoning)

» 　Succinylcholine
　　(succinylcholine is metabolized by plasma cholinesterases, which are inhibited in organophosphate poisoning or cholinesterase inhibitor overdose; therefore, prolonged respiratory paralysis could occur)

　Thiamine
　　(concurrent administration of intravenous thiamine may delay initial excretion of pralidoxime, probably by competing at a common renal excretory site)

### Laboratory value alterations
The following have been selected on the basis of their potential clinical significance (possible effect in parentheses where appropriate)—not necessarily inclusive (» = major clinical significance):

With physiology/laboratory test values
　Alanine aminotransferase (ALT [SGPT]) and
　Aspartate aminotransferase (AST [SGOT]) and
　Creatine kinase (CK)
　　(transient increases in values have been seen in healthy volunteers; values returned to normal within approximately 2 weeks)

### Medical considerations/Contraindications
The medical considerations/contraindications included here have been selected on the basis of their potential clinical significance (reasons given in parentheses where appropriate)—not necessarily inclusive (» = major clinical significance).

*Risk-benefit should be considered when the following medical problems exist:*
» 　Myasthenia gravis
　　(pralidoxime should be used with caution to avoid precipitating a myasthenic crisis)

» 　Renal function impairment
　　(pralidoxime is excreted via the kidneys; reduction in dose is recommended)

　Sensitivity to pralidoxime

**Patient monitoring**

The following may be especially important in patient monitoring (other tests may be warranted in some patients, depending on condition; » = major clinical significance:

Note: Initiation of therapy must **not** be delayed until the results of the tests recommended below are available. However, blood should be drawn prior to initiation of pralidoxime therapy to establish baseline red blood cell acetylcholinesterase and pseudocholinesterase concentrations. Pralidoxime causes these concentrations to lose their diagnostic significance.

Acetylcholinesterase, red blood cell (RBC)

(a measure of true cholinesterase activity that correlates with the concentration of acetylcholine present at receptor sites; recommended prior to administration of pralidoxime to confirm diagnosis of organophosphate poisoning; a history of exposure to organophosphates and a reduction in acetylcholinesterase concentration below 50% of normal laboratory or pre-exposure values are consistent with poisoning)

Electrocardiogram (ECG)

(recommended to detect arrhythmias, especially in patients with pulmonary edema or patients who are severely poisoned or unconscious)

Paranitrophenol, urinary

(recommended to confirm diagnosis and monitor clinical progress of parathion toxicity)

Pseudocholinesterase, serum

(a measure of cholinesterase found in the liver and serum; recommended to assess the degree of exposure to organophosphate pesticides or chemicals and to monitor clinical progress; pseudocholinesterase concentrations may be decreased in patients with liver disease, malnutrition, acute infections, anemias, myocardial infarction, dermatomyositis, and a genetically determined enzyme deficiency, as well as in patients with organophosphate poisoning; low concentrations may also be seen in patients taking estrogens or oral contraceptives)

## Side/Adverse Effects

Note: Many of the following side/adverse effects have been reported only in normal volunteers given pralidoxime, not in patients given pralidoxime after exposure to organophosphate pesticides or chemicals.

In patients treated for poisoning it is difficult to differentiate the side/adverse effects produced by atropine or the organophosphate pesticides or chemicals from those produced by pralidoxime.

The following side/adverse effects have been selected on the basis of their potential clinical significance (possible signs and symptoms in parentheses where appropriate)—not necessarily inclusive:

**Those indicating need for medical attention**

Incidence more frequent

*Blurred or double vision; dizziness; hyperventilation* (rapid breathing); *impaired accommodation* (difficulty in focusing eyes); *increased blood pressure; laryngospasm* (difficulty in speaking or breathing); *muscle rigidity or weakness; pain at injection site—* following intramuscular administration; *tachycardia* (fast heartbeat)

Note: *Increased blood pressure, laryngospasm, muscle rigidity,* and *tachycardia* may be caused by a too-rapid rate of intravenous administration. These effects may be avoided by keeping the rate of injection at less than 500 mg per minute.

**Those indicating need for medical attention only if they continue or are bothersome**

Incidence more frequent

*Drowsiness; headache; nausea*

## Patient Consultation

As an aid to patient consultation, refer to *Advice for the Patient, Pralidoxime (Systemic)*.

In providing consultation, consider emphasizing the following selected information (» = major clinical significance):

**Before using this medication**

» Conditions affecting use, especially:

Sensitivity to pralidoxime

Other medications, especially xanthines, such as aminophylline, caffeine, and theophylline

Other medical problems, especially myasthenia gravis or renal function impairment

**Proper use of this medication**

*For auto-injector dosage form*

Receiving training and reading patient instructions carefully before need to use medication

Importance of not removing safety cap before ready to use

Procedures for using auto-injector

Removing gray safety cap

Placing black tip of device on thigh with injector pointed at thigh

Pressing hard into thigh until auto-injector functions; holding in place several seconds; removing and discarding as directed

Massaging injected area for 10 seconds

» Importance of not using more medication than the amount recommended

*For all dosage forms*

» Proper dosing

» Proper storage

**Precautions while using this medication**

Avoiding use of CNS depressants

**Side/adverse effects**

Signs of potential side effects, especially blurred or double vision, dizziness, hyperventilation, impaired accommodation, increased blood pressure, laryngospasm, muscle rigidity or weakness, pain at injection site, and tachycardia

## General Dosing Information

For more information on the management of organophosphate pesticide or chemical toxicity, or cholinesterase inhibitor overdose, **contact a poison control center** (see *Poison Control Center Listing*).

**For treatment of organophosphate pesticide or chemical toxicity**

Initial treatment of organophosphate pesticide or chemical toxicity should be directed toward decontamination and maintenance or restoration of adequate ventilation. Removing nasopharyngeal secretions and administering oxygen or otherwise assisting respiration are essential. Provision of an artificial airway may also be necessary. It is important that those attending to the patient protect themselves from contamination. If the patient has had dermal exposure, the clothing should be removed and the hair, skin, and fingernails washed thoroughly, first with sodium bicarbonate, then with alcohol. Soap and water may be used if sodium bicarbonate and alcohol are not available. If there has been ocular involvement, the eyes should be flushed with a gentle stream of water for at least 15 minutes.

If the organophosphate has been inhaled, exposure should be terminated by removing the patient from the environment and, if the air remains contaminated, administering oxygen.

Ingested organophosphates should be removed by gastric lavage with protection of the airway, if necessary. Gastric lavage is most effective when instituted within 30 minutes after ingestion because organophosphates are rapidly absorbed from the gastrointestinal tract. Activated charcoal should be administered to reduce further absorption. Induced emesis with ipecac syrup should be avoided because unconsciousness may develop before emesis occurs.

Once adequate ventilation has been established, atropine should be administered intravenously. For adults, the dose is 2 to 4 mg, repeated every 5 to 10 minutes; for children, the dose is 0.05 to 0.1 mg per kg of body weight administered on a similar schedule. In severe poisoning, a more aggressive escalation of the dose may be needed. Administration of atropine should be continued until signs of atropine toxicity (delirium; dilated pupils; dry mouth; muscle twitching; tachycardia—if bradycardia was an earlier sign; warm, dry, and flushed skin) appear or until secretions are inhibited. Atropine should not be given in the presence of hypoxia because of the risk of inducing ventricular fibrillation. Some degree of atropinization should be maintained for at least 48 hours.

Pralidoxime should be administered after the effects of atropine become apparent. However, pralidoxime becomes ineffective as an antidote when administered more than 24 to 48 hours postexposure as a result of aging of the phosphate-ester bond. The preferred route of administration of pralidoxime is intravenous. However, pralidoxime may be administered intramuscularly or subcutaneously if intravenous administration is not possible. Treatment with atropine and pralidoxime should continue until there is symptomatic improvement and restoration of acetylcholinesterase activity, as determined by measurement of red blood cell acetylcholinesterase. The patient should be monitored closely for 48 to 72 hours.

Many of the alkyl phosphates are extremely lipid soluble, and if extensive partitioning into body fat has occurred, the onset of symptoms may be delayed and may recur after initial treatment. In some cases it has been necessary to continue treatment with atropine and pralidoxime for several weeks.

Diazepam may be given to relieve anxiety or to control seizures not responsive to atropine.

### For treatment of cholinesterase inhibitor toxicity

Cholinesterase inhibitor toxicity, or cholinergic crisis, must be distinguished from myasthenic crisis, either on the basis of presenting signs and symptoms or through the use of edrophonium.

To control the increased gastrointestinal stimulation and muscarinic effects associated with cholinergic crisis, atropine may be administered intravenously at an initial dose of 2 to 4 mg followed by 2 mg every 5 to 10 minutes until muscarinic effects disappear or signs of atropine toxicity appear. Pralidoxime may then be administered to treat the nicotinic effects.

## Parenteral Dosage Forms

### PRALIDOXIME CHLORIDE USP

Note: The pralidoxime chloride auto-injector is specifically designed for use by military personnel or qualified civilian emergency responders.

#### Usual adult dose

Toxicity, organophosphate chemical—
Intramuscular, 600 mg. The dose may be repeated two times at fifteen-minute intervals, if necessary.

#### Usual pediatric dose

Dosage has not been established.

#### Usual geriatric dose

See *Usual adult dose*.

#### Strength(s) usually available

U.S.—
600 mg per 2 mL (Rx) [GENERIC (benzyl alcohol 20 mg per mL; aminoacetic acid 11.26 mg per mL; water for injection)].

Note: Pralidoxime auto-injectors are available through the Directorate of Medical Material of the Defense Personnel Support Center or other analogous local, state, or federal agencies.

Canada—
Not commercially available.

#### Packaging and storage

Store below 40 °C (104 °F), preferably between 15 and 30 °C (59 and 86 °F), unless otherwise specified by manufacturer. Protect from freezing.

### PRALIDOXIME CHLORIDE STERILE USP

#### Usual adult and adolescent dose

Toxicity, organophosphate pesticide—
Intravenous: 1 to 2 grams injected at a rate not to exceed 500 mg per minute or infused over fifteen to thirty minutes. The dose may be repeated after one hour, and then at eight- to twelve-hour intervals if muscle weakness persists.
Toxicity, cholinesterase inhibitor—
Intravenous, initially, 1 to 2 grams followed by 250 mg every five minutes.

Note: Reduction in dose is recommended in the presence of renal function impairment.

#### Usual adult prescribing limits

Twelve grams within twenty-four hours.

#### Usual pediatric dose

Toxicity, organophosphate pesticide—
Intravenous infusion: 25 to 50 mg per kg of body weight over fifteen to thirty minutes. The dose may be repeated after one hour, and then at eight- to twelve-hour intervals if muscle weakness persists.
Toxicity, cholinesterase inhibitor—
Dosage has not been established.

#### Usual geriatric dose

See *Usual adult and adolescent dose*.

#### Size(s) usually available

U.S.—
1 gram (Rx) [*Protopam Chloride*].
Canada—
1 gram (Rx) [*Protopam Chloride*].

#### Packaging and storage

Store below 40 °C (104 °F), preferably between 15 and 30 °C (59 and 86 °F), unless otherwise specified by manufacturer.

#### Preparation of dosage form

For intravenous injection, 20 mL of sterile water for injection should be added to each 1-gram vial.
For intravenous infusion, the solution should be prepared as described for preparation of injection. This solution may be further diluted with 0.9% sodium chloride injection to a final concentration of 1 to 2%.

#### Stability

Pralidoxime should be used promptly after reconstitution and any remaining solution discarded.

## Selected Bibliography

Haddad LM. Organophosphates and other insecticides. In: Haddad LM, Winchester JF. Clinical management of poisoning and drug overdose. 2nd ed. Philadelphia: W.B. Saunders Company, 1990: 1076-87.
Minton NA, Murray VSG. A review of organophosphate poisoning. Med Toxicol 1988; 3: 350-75.

Developed: 04/01/96

---

**PRAMOXINE**—See *Anesthetics (Mucosal-Local)*; *Anesthetics (Topical)*

---

**PRAMOXINE AND MENTHOL**—See *Anesthetics (Topical)*

---

**PRAVASTATIN**—See *HMG-CoA Reductase Inhibitors (Systemic)*

---

**PRAZEPAM**—See *Benzodiazepines (Systemic)*

---

# PRAZIQUANTEL   Systemic†

VA CLASSIFICATION (Primary): AP200

Note: For a listing of dosage forms and brand names by country availability, see *Dosage Forms* section(s). For a listing of brand names for the articles in this monograph, refer to the General Index.

†Not commercially available in Canada.

## Category

Anthelmintic (systemic).

Note: Praziquantel is an unusually broad-spectrum anthelmintic.

## Indications

Note: Bracketed information in the *Indications* section refers to uses that are not included in U.S. product labeling.

### Accepted

Clonorchiasis (treatment)—Praziquantel is indicated in the treatment of clonorchiasis caused by *Clonorchis sinensis* (Chinese or Oriental liver fluke).

Opisthorchiasis (treatment)—Praziquantel is indicated in the treatment of opisthorchiasis caused by *Opisthorchis viverrini* and *O. felineus* (liver flukes).

Schistosomiasis (treatment)—Praziquantel is indicated in the treatment of schistosomiasis caused by *Schistosoma mekongi*, *S. japonicum*, *S. mansoni*, and *S. hematobium*.

[Cysticercosis (treatment)] or
[Neurocysticercosis (treatment)]—Praziquantel is used in the treatment of all types of cysticercosis (except ocular cysticercosis). Concurrent use of corticosteroids may also be necessary in the treatment of neurocysticercosis to control edema and/or other reactions to death of the cysticerci.

[Diphyllobothriasis (treatment)]—Praziquantel is used in the treatment of diphyllobothriasis.

[Dipylidiasis (treatment)]—Praziquantel is used in the treatment of dipylidiasis.

[Hymenolepiasis (treatment)]—Praziquantel is used in the treatment of hymenolepiasis caused by *Hymenolepis nana* (dwarf tapeworm).

[Metagonimiasis (treatment)]—Praziquantel is used in the treatment of metagonimiasis caused by *Metagonimus yokogawai* (intestinal fluke).

[Paragonimiasis (treatment)]—Praziquantel is used in the treatment of paragonimiasis caused by *Paragonimus westermani* (Oriental lung fluke) and other *Paragonimus* species.

[Taeniasis (treatment)]—Praziquantel is used in the treatment of taeniasis caused by *Taenia solium* (pork tapeworm) and *T. saginata* (beef tapeworm).

Not all species or strains of a particular helminth may be susceptible to praziquantel.

### Unaccepted

Praziquantel is not indicated in the treatment of ocular cysticercosis since destruction of the parasite in the eye may result in irreparable lesions.

Praziquantel is not likely to be effective in the treatment of human echinococcosis caused by *Echinococcus* species or fascioliasis caused by *Fasciola hepatica* (sheep liver fluke).

## Pharmacology/Pharmacokinetics

### Physicochemical characteristics
Molecular weight—312.41.

### Mechanism of action/Effect
Vermicidal; precise mechanism of action unknown, but may involve synergy between praziquantel and the host's humoral immune response in *S. mansoni*; praziquantel is rapidly taken up by helminths and also appears to increase permeability of helminth's cell membrane, leading to a loss of intracellular calcium; massive contraction and paralysis of the helminth's musculature rapidly result; after exposure to praziquantel, tegument in neck region of adult helminths develops blebs, which appear to burst and disintegrate; praziquantel also produces intense vacuolization at several sites in tegument of adult schistosomes; in *S. mansoni*, this is followed by phagocytic attachment to parasite and, ultimately, death.

### Absorption
Helminth—Rapidly taken up by schistosomes, other flukes, and adult tapeworms.

Human—Rapidly absorbed following oral administration, even when taken with meals; however, praziquantel undergoes extensive first-pass metabolism with only a small amount of active drug likely to reach the systemic circulation.

### Distribution
Helminth—Appears evenly distributed throughout.

Human—Distributed to serum and cerebrospinal fluid (CSF); concentrations in CSF are approximately 15 to 20% of the total amount of free and bound praziquantel in serum. Praziquantel levels in the bile, feces, and breast milk range from less than 10% to 20% of plasma concentrations.

### Protein binding
High (80 to 85%).

### Biotransformation
Helminth—Does not appear to be metabolized by cestodes or schistosomes.

Human—Pronounced first-pass effect; rapidly and completely metabolized to inactive mono- and polyhydroxylated derivatives.

### Half-life
Praziquantel—0.8 to 1.5 hours.

Metabolites—4 to 6 hours.

### Time to peak serum concentration
1 to 3 hours.

### Peak serum concentration
Normal liver function—0.2 to 2.0 mcg per mL after therapeutic doses.

Moderate to severe liver function impairment—Plasma concentrations significantly elevated (2 to 4 times) in one study.

### Elimination
Renal, rapid; metabolites excreted primarily in urine; 72% excreted within 24 hours; approximately 80% excreted within 4 days; small amounts also excreted in feces.

## Precautions to Consider

### Carcinogenicity
Long-term carcinogenicity studies in rats and golden hamsters have not shown any carcinogenic effects.

### Mutagenicity
Mutagenicity studies have not shown mutagenic activity in tissue-, host-, and urine-mediated assays with *Salmonella typhimurium;* in dominant lethal and micronucleus tests in mice; and in spermatogonial tests in Chinese hamsters. Also, studies using other species of organisms (e.g., *Schizosaccharomyces, Saccharomyces, Drosophila*) have not shown mutagenic activity. Although mutagenic effects in *Salmonella* tests have been reported by one laboratory, they were not confirmed in the same strain by other laboratories.

### Pregnancy/Reproduction
Pregnancy—Adequate and well-controlled studies in humans have not been done.

Studies in rats and rabbits given up to 40 times the usual human dose have not shown that praziquantel impairs fertility or is teratogenic. However, praziquantel has been shown to cause an increase in the abortion rate in rats given 3 times the single human dose.

FDA Pregnancy Category B.

### Breast-feeding
Praziquantel is excreted in breast milk; concentrations are approximately 25% of those found in the maternal serum. Nursing mothers should stop breast-feeding when beginning treatment with praziquantel. Breast-feeding should not be resumed until 72 hours after treatment is completed. During this time, the breast milk should be expressed and discarded.

### Pediatrics
Appropriate studies on the relationship of age to the effects of praziquantel have not been performed in children up to 4 years of age. However, no pediatrics-specific problems have been documented to date in children 4 years of age and older.

### Geriatrics
No information is available on the relationship of age to the effects of praziquantel in geriatric patients.

### Drug interactions and/or related problems
The following drug interactions and/or related problems have been selected on the basis of their potential clinical significance (possible mechanism in parentheses where appropriate)—not necessarily inclusive (» = major clinical significance):

Note: Combinations containing any of the following medications, depending on the amount present, may also interact with this medication.

Carbamazepine or
Phenytoin
(one small, single-dose, controlled study found that epileptic patients taking carbamazepine or phenytoin had significantly lower plasma concentrations of praziquantel [7.9% and 24% of the control group, respectively]; this effect is thought to be due to induction of the cytochrome P-450 microsomal enzyme system by carbamazepine and phenytoin; patients on carbamazepine or phenytoin may require a larger dose of praziquantel)

Dexamethasone
(one study found that concurrent administration of dexamethasone with praziquantel reduced praziquantel plasma concentrations by approximately 50%)

### Medical considerations/Contraindications
The medical considerations/contraindications included here have been selected on the basis of their potential clinical significance (reasons given in parentheses where appropriate)—not necessarily inclusive (» = major clinical significance).

*Except under special circumstances, this medication should not be used when the following medical problem exists:*

» Ocular cysticercosis
(destruction of parasites in the eye may result in irreparable ocular lesions)

*Risk-benefit should be considered when the following medical problems exist:*

Hypersensitivity to praziquantel

Liver disease, moderate to severe
(peak plasma concentrations were found to be significantly higher in patients with moderate to severe liver disease; higher concentrations were associated with an increased incidence of side effects; the increased bioavailability in patients with hepatosplenic schis-

tosomiasis is presumed to be a result of decreased first-pass metabolism; however, the elimination half-life was not found to be significantly different between patients with and patients without liver disease)

**Patient monitoring**

The following may be especially important in patient monitoring (other tests may be warranted in some patients, depending on condition; » = major clinical significance):

*For Schistosoma hematobium*
» Urine examinations

(examinations for eggs may be required approximately 1, 3, and 6 months following treatment with praziquantel to determine efficacy or provide proof of cure; no patient should be considered cured unless urine examinations have been negative for several months)

*For tapeworms, flukes, and other Schisotosoma species*
» Stool examinations

(may be required approximately 1, 3, and 12 months following treatment with praziquantel to determine efficacy or provide proof of cure; where expulsion of the tapeworm[s] is uncertain, stool examinations for the presence of eggs or segments of the worm[s] may be required periodically; no patient should be considered cured unless stool examinations have been negative for 3 months)

## Side/Adverse Effects

The following side/adverse effects have been selected on the basis of their potential clinical significance (possible signs and symptoms in parentheses where appropriate)—not necessarily inclusive:

**Those indicating need for medical attention only if they continue or are bothersome**
Incidence more frequent
*Central nervous system effects* (dizziness; drowsiness; headache; malaise); *fever; gastrointestinal effects* (abdominal cramps or pain; loss of appetite; nausea or vomiting; bloody diarrhea); *increased sweating*
Incidence less frequent
*Skin rash, hives, or itching*

## Patient Consultation

As an aid to patient consultation, refer to *Advice for the Patient, Praziquantel (Systemic)*.

In providing consultation, consider emphasizing the following selected information (» = major clinical significance):

**Before using this medication**
» Conditions affecting use, especially:
Hypersensitivity to praziquantel
Breast-feeding—Praziquantel is excreted in breast milk
Other medical problems, especially ocular cysticercosis

**Proper use of this medication**
No special preparations (e.g., dietary restrictions or fasting, concurrent medications, purging, or cleansing enemas) required before, during, or immediately after therapy
» Not chewing tablets; swallowing tablets whole with small amount of liquid during meals to avoid bitter taste, which may cause gagging and vomiting
» Compliance with therapy
» Proper dosing
Missed dose: Taking as soon as possible; not taking if almost time for next dose; not doubling doses
» Proper storage

**Precautions while using this medication**
Importance of physician checking progress after treatment
Checking with physician if no improvement after completing course of therapy
» Caution if dizziness or drowsiness occurs; not driving, using machines, or doing other jobs that require alertness while taking praziquantel and for 24 hours after discontinuing it

## General Dosing Information

No special preparations (e.g., dietary restrictions or fasting, concurrent medications, purging, or cleansing enemas) are required before, during, or immediately after treatment with praziquantel.

A bitter taste develops if praziquantel tablets are held in the mouth or chewed; this may result in gagging or vomiting. Therefore, praziquantel tablets, either whole or partial, should be swallowed unchewed with a small amount of liquid during meals.

Patients with severely impaired hepatic function may require a reduction in dose because elevated plasma concentrations have been associated with an increased incidence of side effects.

In the treatment of neurocysticercosis, praziquantel may be most effective in symptomatic patients with viable cysts within the cerebral parenchyma and in the rapidly progressive form of cysticercosis. Patients with intraventricular cysts, meningeal cysts, and old, dead, calcified cysts will probably not benefit from treatment with praziquantel. Also, a single ring-enhancing lesion with surrounding edema likely represents a dying cyst for which praziquantel will not be useful.

## Oral Dosage Forms

Note: Bracketed uses in the *Dosage Forms* section refer to categories of use and/or indications that are not included in U.S. product labeling.

### PRAZIQUANTEL TABLETS USP

**Usual adult and adolescent dose**
Clonorchiasis—
Oral, 25 mg per kg of body weight three times a day for one day. May be repeated if required.
Schistosomiasis—
*S. haematobium* and
*S. mansoni:* Oral, 20 mg per kg of body weight two times a day for one day.
*S. japonicum* and
*S. mekongi:* Oral, 20 mg per kg of body weight three times a day for one day.
Note: Doses should be spaced not less than four and not more than six hours apart.
40 to 60 mg per kg of body weight as a single dose may also be given.
[Diphyllobothriasis]—
*D. latum:* Oral, 10 to 20 mg per kg of body weight as a single dose.
*D. pacificum:* Oral, 10 to 20 mg per kg of body weight as a single dose.
[Dipylidiasis]—
Oral, 10 to 20 mg per kg of body weight as a single dose.
[Hymenolepiasis]—
Oral, 25 mg per kg of body weight as a single dose. Heavy infection may require repeated therapy after ten days.
[Metagonimiasis]—
Oral, 25 mg per kg of body weight three times a day for one day.
[Neurocysticercosis]—
Oral, 16.7 to 33 mg per kg of body weight three times a day for fourteen to thirty days. May be repeated in two to six months if required.
Opisthorchiasis—
Oral, 25 mg per kg of body weight three times a day for one day. May be repeated if required.
[Paragonimiasis]—
Oral, 25 mg per kg of body weight three times a day for two days.
[Taeniasis—*Taenia solium* infections]:
Oral, 10 mg per kg of body weight as a single dose.

**Usual adult prescribing limits**
Doses up to 75 mg per kg of body weight daily have been tolerated without serious adverse effects.

**Usual pediatric dose**
Children up to 4 years of age—Dosage has not been established.
Children 4 years of age and over—See *Usual adult and adolescent dose.*

**Strength(s) usually available**
U.S.—
600 mg (Rx) [*Biltricide*].
Canada—
Not commercially available.
Note: Tablets are triple-scored for dosage adjustment (e.g., pediatric use).

**Packaging and storage**
Store below 30 °C (86 °F), unless otherwise specified by manufacturer.

**Auxiliary labeling**
• May cause dizziness or drowsiness.
• Swallow tablets whole.
• Take with liquid during meals.
• Continue medicine for full time of treatment.

Revised: 03/23/93

# PRAZOSIN  Systemic

VA CLASSIFICATION (Primary/Secondary): CV150/CV490; CV900; AD900; GU900

Note: For a listing of dosage forms and brand names by country availability, see *Dosage Forms* section(s). For a listing of brand names for the articles in this monograph, refer to the General Index.

## Category

Antihypertensive; vasodilator, congestive heart failure; antidote (to ergot alkaloid poisoning); vasospastic therapy adjunct; benign prostatic hyperplasia therapy agent.

## Indications

Note: Bracketed information in the *Indications* section refers to uses that are not included in U.S. product labeling.

### Accepted

Hypertension (treatment)—Prazosin is indicated in the treatment of hypertension.

For additional information on initial therapeutic guidelines related to the treatment of hypertension, see *Appendix III.*

[Congestive heart failure (treatment)][1]—Prazosin may be used as an adjunct to digoxin and diuretics for the treatment of congestive heart failure. However, prazosin has not been shown to improve survival in these patients.

[Toxicity, ergot alkaloid (treatment)][1]—Prazosin is used for treatment of peripheral vasospasm caused by ergot alkaloid overdose.

[Pheochromocytoma (treatment)][1]—Prazosin is used for the management of hypertension associated with pheochromocytoma.

[Raynaud's phenomenon (treatment)][1]—Prazosin is used for treatment of Raynaud's phenomenon.

[Benign prostatic hyperplasia (BPH) (treatment)][1]—Prazosin is used for the treatment of urinary symptoms associated with benign prostatic hyperplasia. Prazosin has been shown to improve urinary flow and symptoms of BPH. However, the long-term effects of prazosin on the incidence of acute urinary obstruction or other complications of BPH or on the need for surgery have not yet been determined.

---

[1]Not included in Canadian product labeling.

## Pharmacology/Pharmacokinetics

### Physicochemical characteristics

Molecular weight—419.87.
pKa—6.5.

### Mechanism of action/Effect

Prazosin is a selective alpha$_1$-adrenergic blocking agent. The alpha$_1$-adrenergic blocking action is thought to account primarily for its effects.

Hypertension—
Prazosin produces vasodilation and reduces peripheral resistance but generally has little effect on cardiac output. Antihypertensive effect is usually not accompanied by reflex tachycardia. There is little or no effect on renal blood flow or glomerular filtration rate.

Congestive heart failure—
Beneficial vasodilator effects are due to decreased systemic resistance, preload and afterload reduction, and resulting improved cardiac output.

Raynaud's phenomenon—
Therapeutic effect for vasospasm is due to inhibition of vasoconstriction by blocking of postsynaptic alpha$_1$ receptors.

Benign prostatic hyperplasia—
Relaxation of smooth muscle in the bladder neck, prostate, and prostate capsule produced by alpha$_1$-adrenergic blockade results in a reduction in urethral resistance and pressure, bladder outlet resistance, and urinary symptoms.

### Other actions/effects

Prazosin may affect serum lipids. The most consistent changes observed are a decrease in levels of serum total cholesterol and low density lipoprotein (LDL) cholesterol. However, the implications of these changes are unclear.

### Absorption

Well-absorbed from gastrointestinal tract; bioavailability is variable (50 to 85%).

### Protein binding

Very high (97%; 20% to red blood cells).

### Biotransformation

Primarily hepatic. Several metabolites have been identified in humans and animals (6-O-demethyl, 7-O-demethyl, 2-[1-piperazinyl]-4-amino-6, 7-dimethoxyquinazoline, 2,4-diamino-6,7-dimethoxyquinazoline); in dog studies, three of the metabolites were shown to be responsible for approximately 10 to 25% of prazosin's hypotensive activity.

### Half-life

2 to 3 hours; unchanged in renal function impairment, but may increase to more than double (6 to 8 hours) in congestive heart failure.

### Onset of action

Hypertension—Within 30 to 90 minutes after a single dose.
Congestive heart failure—Rapid.

### Time to peak concentration

1 to 3 hours.

### Time to peak effect

Hypertension—
Single dose: 2 to 4 hours.
Multiple doses: Up to 3 to 4 weeks of therapy may be required for maximal therapeutic effect.
Congestive heart failure—
1 hour.

### Duration of action

Hypertension—Single dose: 7 to 10 hours.
Congestive heart failure—6 hours.

### Elimination

Primarily in bile and feces; 6 to 10% in urine. Excreted as unchanged drug (5 to 11%) and metabolites. Elimination of prazosin may be slower in patients with congestive heart failure than in normal subjects.
In dialysis—Not dialyzable.

## Precautions to Consider

### Cross-sensitivity and/or related problems

Patients sensitive to other quinazolines (doxazosin, terazosin) may also be sensitive to prazosin.

### Carcinogenicity

An 18-month study in rats given prazosin at doses of more than 225 times the usual maximum recommended human dose of 20 mg per day did not demonstrate carcinogenic potential.

### Mutagenicity

Prazosin was not mutagenic in *in vitro* genetic toxicology studies.

### Pregnancy/Reproduction

Fertility—A study in male rats given subcutaneous injections of prazosin (1.4 mg per kg of body weight [mg/kg]) revealed reduced fertility manifested by a suppression of the fertilizing potential of spermatozoa.
A fertility and general reproductive performance study in male and female rats given prazosin at a dose of 75 mg/kg (225 times the usual maximum recommended human dose) demonstrated decreased fertility. However, when rats were given 25 mg/kg (75 times the usual maximum recommended human dose) decreased fertility was not seen.

Pregnancy—Adequate and well-controlled studies in humans have not been done. However, limited uncontrolled use of prazosin and a beta-blocking agent for the control of severe hypertension in 44 pregnant women revealed no drug-related fetal abnormalities or adverse effects. Also, use of prazosin during the last trimester in 8 pregnant women with hypertension produced no prolonged clinical problems. All infants were developing normally 6 to 30 months following delivery.
In rats given doses more than 225 times the usual maximum recommended human dose, prazosin has been shown to be associated with decreased litter weight at birth and at 1, 4, and 21 days of age. There was no evidence, however, of drug-related external, visceral, or skeletal abnormalities.
In pregnant rabbits and pregnant monkeys given doses of more than 225 times and 12 times the usual maximum recommended human dose, respectively, no drug-related external, visceral, or skeletal abnormalities were observed in the fetuses.

FDA Pregnancy Category C.

### Breast-feeding

Prazosin is distributed into breast milk in small amounts.

### Pediatrics

Appropriate studies on the relationship of age to the effects of prazosin have not been performed in the pediatric population. However, no pediatrics-specific problems have been documented to date.

### Geriatrics

Although appropriate studies on the relationship of age to the effects of prazosin have not been performed in the geriatric population, geriatrics-specific problems are not expected to limit the usefulness of prazosin in the elderly. However, elderly patients may be more sensitive to the hypotensive effects and are more likely to have age-related renal function impairment, which may require lower prazosin doses. In addition, the risk of prazosin-induced hypothermia may be increased in elderly patients.

### Drug interactions and/or related problems

The following drug interactions and/or related problems have been selected on the basis of their potential clinical significance (possible mechanism in parentheses where appropriate)—not necessarily inclusive (» = major clinical significance):

Note: Combinations containing any of the following medications, depending on the amount present, may also interact with this medication.

Anti-inflammatory drugs, nonsteroidal (NSAIDs), especially indomethacin
(antihypertensive effects of prazosin may be reduced when it is used concurrently with these agents; indomethacin, and possibly other NSAIDs, may antagonize the antihypertensive effect by inhibiting renal prostaglandin synthesis and/or by causing sodium and fluid retention; the patient should be carefully monitored to confirm that the desired effect is being obtained)

Estrogens
(estrogen-induced fluid retention tends to increase blood pressure)

Hypotension-producing medications, other (see *Appendix II*)
(antihypertensive effects may be potentiated when these medications are used concurrently with prazosin; although some antihypertensive and/or diuretic combinations are frequently used to therapeutic advantage, dosage adjustments are necessary when these medications are used concurrently)

Sympathomimetics
(antihypertensive effects of prazosin may be reduced when it is used concurrently with these agents; the patient should be carefully monitored to confirm that the desired effect is being obtained)

(concurrent use of prazosin antagonizes the peripheral vasoconstriction produced by high doses of dopamine)

(concurrent use of prazosin may decrease the pressor response to ephedrine)

(concurrent use of prazosin may block the alpha-adrenergic effects of epinephrine, possibly resulting in severe hypotension and tachycardia)

(concurrent use of prazosin usually decreases, but does not reverse or completely block, the pressor effect of metaraminol)

(prior administration of prazosin may decrease the pressor effect and shorten the duration of action of methoxamine and phenylephrine)

### Laboratory value alterations

The following have been selected on the basis of their potential clinical significance (possible effect in parentheses where appropriate)—not necessarily inclusive (» = major clinical significance):

With diagnostic test results
Vanillylmandelic acid (VMA), urinary
(concentrations may be increased; false positive results may occur in screening tests for pheochromocytoma)

### Medical considerations/Contraindications

The medical considerations/contraindications included here have been selected on the basis of their potential clinical significance (reasons given in parentheses where appropriate)—not necessarily inclusive (» = major clinical significance).

*Risk-benefit should be considered when the following medical problems exist:*

Angina pectoris
(may induce angina or aggravate pre-existing angina)

» Cardiac disease, severe
(prazosin is usually not used alone, although it may improve cardiac performance in some patients with severe refractory congestive heart failure)

Narcolepsy
(may exacerbate cataplexy; however, a clear cause-effect relationship has not been established)

Renal function impairment
(increased sensitivity to prazosin's effects; lower doses may be required)

Sensitivity to prazosin

### Patient monitoring

The following may be especially important in patient monitoring (other tests may be warranted in some patients, depending on condition; » = major clinical significance):

» Blood pressure measurements
(recommended at periodic intervals in patients being treated for hypertension; selected patients may be trained to perform blood pressure measurements at home and report the results at regular physician visits)

## Side/Adverse Effects

Note: A "first-dose orthostatic hypotensive reaction" sometimes occurs, most frequently 30 to 90 minutes after the initial dose of prazosin, and may be severe. Syncope or other postural symptoms, such as dizziness, may occur. Subsequent occurrence with dosage increases is also possible. Incidence appears to be dose-related; thus, it is important that therapy be initiated with the lowest possible dose. Patients who are volume-depleted or sodium-restricted may be more sensitive to the orthostatic hypotensive effects of prazosin, and the effect may be exaggerated after exercise.

Hypotensive side effects may be more likely to occur in geriatric patients.

The following side/adverse effects have been selected on the basis of their potential clinical significance (possible signs and symptoms in parentheses where appropriate)—not necessarily inclusive:

### Those indicating need for medical attention

Incidence more frequent
*Dizziness; orthostatic hypotension* (dizziness or lightheadedness when getting up from a lying or sitting position; sudden fainting)

Incidence less frequent
*Edema* (swelling of feet or lower legs); *palpitations* (pounding heartbeat); *urinary incontinence* (loss of bladder control)

Incidence rare
*Angina* (chest pain); *dyspnea* (shortness of breath); *priapism* (painful, inappropriate erection of the penis, continuing)

### Those indicating need for medical attention only if they continue or are bothersome

Incidence more frequent
*Drowsiness; headache; malaise* (lack of energy)

Incidence less frequent
*Dryness of mouth; fatigue* (unusual tiredness or weakness); *nervousness*

Incidence rare
*Nausea; urinary frequency* (frequent urge to urinate)

## Overdose

For more information on the management of overdose or unintentional ingestion, **contact a Poison Control Center** (see *Poison Control Center Listing*).

### Treatment of overdose

Recommended treatment for prazosin overdose includes: Treatment of circulatory failure, either by placing the patient in the supine position and elevating the legs or by using additional measures if shock is present, is most important; volume expanders may be used to treat shock, followed, if necessary, by administration of a vasopressor; symptomatic, supportive treatment and monitoring of fluid and electrolyte status.

## Patient Consultation

As an aid to patient consultation, refer to *Advice for the Patient, Prazosin (Systemic)*.

In providing consultation, consider emphasizing the following selected information (» = major clinical significance):

### Before using this medication

» Conditions affecting use, especially:
Sensitivity to quinazolines
Breast-feeding—Distributed into breast milk in small amounts
Use in the elderly—Increased sensitivity to hypotensive effects and increased risk of prazosin-induced hypothermia
Other medical problems, especially severe cardiac disease

## Proper use of this medication

Getting into the habit of taking at same times each day to help increase compliance

» Proper dosing

Missed dose: Taking as soon as possible; not taking if almost time for next dose; not doubling doses

» Proper storage

*For use as an antihypertensive*

Possible need for control of weight and diet, especially sodium intake

» Patient may not experience symptoms of hypertension; importance of taking medication even if feeling well

» Does not cure, but helps control hypertension; possible need for life-long therapy; serious consequences of untreated hypertension

*For use in benign prostatic hyperplasia (BPH)*

Relieves symptoms of BPH but does not change the size of the prostate; may not prevent the need for surgery in the future

## Precautions while using this medication

Regular visits to physician to check progress

» Caution if dizziness, lightheadedness, or sudden fainting occurs, especially after initial dose; taking first dose at bedtime

» Caution when getting up suddenly from a lying or sitting position

» Caution in using alcohol, while standing for long periods or exercising, and during hot weather because of enhanced orthostatic hypotensive effects

» Possibility of drowsiness

» Caution when driving or doing anything else requiring alertness because of possible drowsiness, dizziness, or lightheadedness

» Not taking other medications, especially nonprescription sympathomimetics, unless discussed with physician

## Side/adverse effects

Signs of potential side effects, especially dizziness, orthostatic hypotension, edema, palpitations, urinary incontinence, angina, dyspnea, and priapism

# General Dosing Information

Dosage of prazosin should be adjusted to meet the individual requirements of each patient, on the basis of blood pressure response.

Prazosin may be used alone or in combination with a thiazide diuretic or beta-adrenergic blocker, both of which reduce the tendency for sodium and water retention, although they also produce additive hypotension. If combination therapy is indicated, individual titration is required to ensure the lowest possible therapeutic dose of each drug.

In order to minimize the "first-dose orthostatic hypotensive reaction," an initial dose of 1 mg is recommended, with gradual increments as needed. Administration of the initial dose at bedtime is recommended, as well as the initial dose of each increment.

When a diuretic or other antihypertensive agent is added to prazosin therapy, the dose of prazosin should be reduced to 1 or 2 mg three times a day, followed by titration of dosage of the combination. When prazosin is added to existing diuretic or antihypertensive therapy, the dose of the other agent should be reduced and prazosin started at a dose of 0.5 or 1 mg two or three times a day.

Tolerance to the effects of prazosin may occur during treatment of congestive heart failure but usually not during treatment of hypertension. An early, transient (usually within the first few doses) blunting of hemodynamic effect may occur due to reflex activation of the sympathetic nervous system. The hemodynamic effect may spontaneously restore with uninterrupted therapy or the blunted effect may be overcome by temporarily interrupting prazosin therapy. A later apparent tolerance may result from fluid retention, requiring increased doses of diuretics; this effect may be minimized by increasing the dose of prazosin, temporarily interrupting prazosin therapy, or substituting another vasodilator.

# Oral Dosage Forms

Note: Bracketed uses in the *Dosage Forms* section refer to categories of use and/or indications that are not included in U.S. product labeling.

## PRAZOSIN HYDROCHLORIDE CAPSULES USP

Note: The dosing and strengths of the dosage forms available are expressed in terms of prazosin base (not the hydrochloride salt).

### Usual adult dose

Antihypertensive—

Initial: Oral, 1 mg (base) two or three times a day.

Maintenance: Oral, adjusted gradually to meet individual requirements, most commonly 6 to 15 mg (base) a day in two or three divided doses.

[Toxicity, ergot alkaloid]—

Oral, 1 mg three times a day.

[Vasospastic therapy adjunct—Raynaud's phenomenon]—

Oral, 1 mg three times a day.

[Benign prostatic hyperplasia]—

Initial: Oral, 1 mg (base) two times a day.

Maintenance: Oral, 1 to 5 mg (base) two times a day.

Note: Geriatric patients may be more sensitive to the effects of the usual adult dose.

### Usual adult prescribing limits

Daily doses higher than 20 mg (base) usually do not have increased efficacy, although some patients respond to up to 40 mg a day.

### Usual pediatric dose

Antihypertensive—

Oral, 50 to 400 mcg (0.05 to 0.4 mg) (base) per kg of body weight per day in two or three divided doses. Single doses should not exceed 7 mg, and the total daily dose should not exceed 15 mg per day.

### Strength(s) usually available

U.S.—

1 mg (base) (Rx) [*Minipress* (sucrose); GENERIC (sucrose)].

2 mg (base) (Rx) [*Minipress* (sucrose); GENERIC (sucrose)].

5 mg (base) (Rx) [*Minipress* (sucrose); GENERIC (sucrose)].

Canada—

Not commercially available.

### Packaging and storage

Store below 40 °C (104 °F), preferably between 15 and 30 °C (59 and 86 °F), unless otherwise specified by manufacturer. Store in a well-closed, light-resistant container.

### Auxiliary labeling

• Do not take other medicines without your doctor's advice.

• May cause dizziness.

### Note

Check refill frequency to determine compliance in hypertensive patients.

## PRAZOSIN HYDROCHLORIDE TABLETS

Note: The dosing and strengths of the dosage forms available are expressed in terms of prazosin base (not the hydrochloride salt).

### Usual adult dose

Antihypertensive—

Initial: Oral, 500 mcg (0.5 mg) two or three times a day for at least 3 days. If tolerated, increase to 1 mg (base) two or three times a day for a further 3 days.

Maintenance: Oral, adjusted gradually to meet individual requirements, most commonly 6 to 15 mg (base) a day in two or three divided daily doses.

Toxicity, ergot alkaloid[1]—

Oral, 1 mg three times a day.

Vasospastic therapy adjunct—Raynaud's phenomenon[1]—

Oral, 1 mg three times a day.

Benign prostatic hyperplasia[1]—

Initial: Oral, 1 mg (base) two times a day.

Maintenance: Oral, 1 to 5 mg (base) two times a day.

Note: Geriatric patients may be more sensitive to the effects of the usual adult dose.

### Usual adult prescribing limits

Daily doses higher than 20 mg (base) usually do not have increased efficacy, although some patients respond to up to 40 mg a day.

### Usual pediatric dose

Antihypertensive—

See *Prazosin Hydrochloride Capsules USP.*

### Strength(s) usually available

U.S.—

Not commercially available.

Canada—

1 mg (base) (Rx) [*Minipress* (scored); GENERIC].

2 mg (base) (Rx) [*Minipress* (scored); GENERIC].

5 mg (base) (Rx) [*Minipress* (scored); GENERIC].

### Packaging and storage

Store below 40 °C (104 °F), preferably between 15 and 30 °C (59 and 86 °F), unless otherwise specified by manufacturer. Store in a well-closed, light-resistant container.

### Auxiliary labeling

• Do not take other medicines without your doctor's advice.

• May cause dizziness.

**Note**
Check refill frequency to determine compliance in hypertensive patients.

¹Not included in Canadian product labeling.

## Selected Bibliography
The fifth report of the Joint National Committee on Detection, Evaluation, and Treatment of High Blood Pressure. Arch Intern Med 1993; 153: 154-83.

Revised: 08/02/94

---

**PRAZOSIN-CONTAINING COMBINATIONS—**
Prazosin and Polythiazide (Systemic)

---

# PRAZOSIN AND POLYTHIAZIDE  Systemic

VA CLASSIFICATION (Primary): CV400

**NOTE:** The *Prazosin and Polythiazide (Systemic)* monograph is maintained on the USP DI electronic data base. For a printed copy of the most recent revision of the complete monograph, contact the USP Division of Information Development, 12601 Twinbrook Parkway, Rockville, MD 20852.

For information on the specific components of this combination, see the *USP DI* monographs for *Diuretics, Thiazide (Systemic)* and *Prazosin (Systemic)*.

The information that follows is selectively abstracted from the complete monograph and is provided to facilitate drug use review and patient counseling.

Note: For a listing of dosage forms and brand names by country availability, see *Dosage Forms* section(s). For a listing of brand names for the articles in this monograph, refer to the General Index.

## Category
Antihypertensive.

## Indications

### Accepted
Hypertension (treatment)—Prazosin and polythiazide combination is indicated in the treatment of hypertension.

Fixed-dosage combinations are generally not recommended for initial therapy and are useful for subsequent therapy only when the proportion of the component agents corresponds to the dose of the individual agents, as determined by titration.

For additional information on initial therapeutic guidelines related to the treatment of hypertension, see *Appendix III*.

## Patient Consultation

As an aid to patient consultation, refer to *Advice for the Patient, Prazosin and Polythiazide (Systemic)*.

In providing consultation, consider emphasizing the following selected information (» = major clinical significance):

**Before using this medication**
» Conditions affecting use, especially:
  Sensitivity to quinazolines, thiazide diuretics, other sulfonamide-type medications, bumetanide, furosemide, or carbonic anhydrase inhibitors
  Pregnancy—Not recommended for routine use; thiazide diuretics may cause jaundice, thrombocytopenia, hypokalemia in infant
  Breast-feeding—Distributed into breast milk; recommended that nursing mothers avoid thiazides diuretics during first month of breast-feeding because of reports of suppression of lactation
  Use in children—Caution if giving to infants with jaundice
  Use in the elderly—Elderly patients may be more sensitive to hypotensive effects; potential for increased risk of prazosin-induced hypothermia and electrolyte effects of polythiazide
  Other medications, especially cholestyramine, colestipol, digitalis glycosides, or lithium
  Other medical problems, especially anuria, severe cardiac disease, severe renal function impairment, or infants with jaundice

**Proper use of this medication**
  Possible need for control of weight and diet, especially sodium intake
» Patient may not experience symptoms of hypertension; importance of taking medication even if feeling well
» Does not cure, but helps control hypertension; possible need for lifelong therapy; serious consequences of untreated hypertension
  Diuretic effects of the medication and timing of doses to minimize inconvenience of diuresis
  Getting into the habit of taking at same time each day to help increase compliance

» Proper dosing
  Missed dose: Taking as soon as possible; not taking if almost time for next dose; not doubling doses
» Proper storage

**Precautions while using this medication**
  Regular visits to physician to check progress
» Not taking other medications, especially nonprescription sympathomimetics, unless discussed with physician
  Possibility of hypokalemia; possible need for additional potassium in diet; not changing diet without first checking with physician
  To prevent dehydration, checking with physician if severe nausea, vomiting, or diarrhea occurs and continues
  May increase blood sugar levels in diabetics
  Possible photosensitivity; avoiding unprotected exposure to sun; using protective clothing and sun block product; avoiding use of sunlamp, tanning bed, or tanning booth
» Caution if dizziness, lightheadedness, or sudden fainting occurs, especially after initial dose; taking first dose at bedtime
» Caution when getting up suddenly from a lying or sitting position
» Caution in using alcohol, while standing for long periods or exercising, and during hot weather because of enhanced orthostatic hypotensive effects
» Possibility of drowsiness
» Caution when driving or doing anything else requiring alertness because of possible drowsiness, dizziness, or lightheadedness

**Side/adverse effects**
  Signs of potential side effects, especially dizziness, edema, urinary incontinence, priapism, electrolyte imbalance, orthostatic hypotension, agranulocytosis, allergic reaction, angina, cholecystitis, pancreatitis, hepatic function impairment, palpitations, shortness of breath, hyperuricemia, gout, and thrombocytopenia

## Oral Dosage Forms

### PRAZOSIN HYDROCHLORIDE AND POLYTHIAZIDE CAPSULES

**Usual adult dose**
Antihypertensive—
Oral, 1 capsule two or three times a day, as determined by individual titration with the component agents.

Note: Geriatric patients may be more sensitive to the effects of the usual adult dose and may require a lower dose in order to prevent syncope.

**Usual pediatric dose**
Antihypertensive—
As determined by individual titration with the component agents.

**Strength(s) usually available**
U.S.—
  1 mg of prazosin (base) and 500 mcg (0.5 mg) of polythiazide (Rx) [*Minizide* (sucrose)].
  2 mg of prazosin (base) and 500 mcg (0.5 mg) of polythiazide (Rx) [*Minizide* (sucrose)].
  5 mg of prazosin (base) and 500 mcg (0.5 mg) of polythiazide (Rx) [*Minizide* (sucrose)].
Canada—
  Not commercially available.

**Auxiliary labeling**
• Do not take other medicines without your doctor's advice.

Revised: 07/21/92
Interim revision: 07/20/94

**PREDNISOLONE**—See *Corticosteroids (Ophthalmic); Corticosteroids—Glucocorticoid Effects (Systemic)*

**PREDNISONE**—See *Corticosteroids—Glucocorticoid Effects (Systemic)*

---

# PREGNANCY TEST KITS FOR HOME USE

This monograph includes information on the following: Colloidal Gold Particle Pregnancy Immunoassay Test Kits; Enzyme Immunoassay Pregnancy Test Kits; Hemagglutination Inhibition Pregnancy Test Kits.

VA CLASSIFICATION (Primary): DX900

Note: For a listing of product forms and brand names by country availability, see *Diagnostic Product Forms* section.

---

## Category

Diagnostic aid (pregnancy).

## Indications

Note: Bracketed information in the *Indications* section refers to uses that are not included in U.S. product labeling.

**Accepted**

Pregnancy (diagnosis)—Pregnancy test kits are intended for patient use in early detection of pregnancy, as an adjunct to health care professional confirmation by examination for intrauterine pregnancy and dating. Early detection of pregnancy at home may encourage the patient to make earlier decisions concerning prenatal care and lifestyle changes to limit fetal exposure to drugs, alcohol, tobacco, and radiation.

[Pregnancy test kits for home use are also used for decision-making in continuation of drugs for the treatment of infertility or contraceptive drug therapy.]

## Pharmacology/Pharmacokinetics

**Physicochemical characteristics**

Human chorionic gonadotropin (HCG) is a hormone produced by the outer cells (trophoblast) of the fertilized ovum. Once the ovum implants in the endometrium, HCG is secreted into maternal fluids. HCG helps to maintain the corpus luteum's production of progesterone and estrogen, which sustain the endometrium and thus maintain the pregnancy until placental development is adequate. It is therefore considered a diagnostic marker for pregnancy. HCG is detectable in maternal urine and serum within 1 to 2 weeks of implantation, increases for 8 to 12 weeks, and then drops. It disappears from the blood within weeks after the termination of pregnancy.

HCG or subunits of it are also produced by trophoblastic tumors such as hydatidiform mole and choriocarcinoma, and some types of cancer (ovarian, bronchogenic, and others). HCG is a glycoprotein composed of two dissimilar subunits, termed alpha and beta. The alpha subunit is common to the structurally similar hormones luteinizing hormone (LH), follicle-stimulating hormone (FSH), and thyroid-stimulating hormone (TSH). The beta subunit is unique to each. Therefore, there can be false-positive results with less specific tests for HCG when levels of any of these hormones are elevated. However, newer tests with monoclonal antibodies specific to the beta subunit are quite sensitive and specific to HCG.

Most kits on the market utilize monoclonal or polyclonal antibodies in an enzyme immunoassay. Some kits use a hemagglutination inhibition process on erythrocytes coated with antibodies.

*Colloidal gold particle immunoassay and enzyme immunoassay (EIA, ELISA)*—Antibodies (monoclonal or polyclonal) against HCG are bound to a solid phase (stick, bead, diaphragm) or in solution. Drops of the urine sample are added. HCG in the urine will complex with the antibodies. In ELISA kits, a second bound antibody (usually specific for beta-HCG) is covalently bonded to an enzyme such as alkaline phosphatase that is added in solution. The colloidal gold particle immunoassay utilizes a colloidal gold particle covalently bonded to the second antibody, rather than an enzyme. This sandwiches the HCG between the solid phase and enzyme, or in solution. A washing or filtering step removes unbound compounds, and an agent that will produce a color on reaction with the enzyme is added. The color is produced in proportion to the amount of antibody-HCG complex present. Some kits provide a control reaction area to verify that the test reaction took place.

*Hemagglutination inhibition (HAI)*—A urine sample is added to a suspension of red blood cells coated with antibodies to HCG. HCG in the urine binds with the antibodies. An antiserum to the antibodies is added to the test tube. The antiserum will bind with the antibodies if HCG is not present, and the cells will form a mat in the bottom of the test tube. If HCG is present, bonding between the antibodies and antiserum will not take place, and the cells will settle in a ring or donut pattern at the bottom of the tube.

## Precautions to Consider

**Laboratory value alterations**

The following have been selected on the basis of their potential clinical significance (possible effect in parentheses where appropriate)—not necessarily inclusive (» = major clinical significance):

With results of *this* test

*Due to medications*

Anticonvulsants or
Antiparkinsonism agents or
Antipsychotics
    (luteinizing hormone levels are increased by some anticonvulsant, antiparkinsonism, and antipsychotic agents; applies only to HAI tests, which are less specific to HCG)

*Due to medical problems or conditions*

Abortion, incomplete or
Blighted ovum or
Tubal pregnancy
    (false-negative results may be encountered in tubal pregnancy, missed abortion, or blighted ovum cases)

Abortion, spontaneous or induced or
Delivery, normal or
Tubal pregnancy, removal of
    (HCG levels may be detectable for several weeks after spontaneous or induced abortion and after removal of a tubal pregnancy as well as after normal delivery)

Amenorrhea or
Pregnancy, symptoms of, other
    (negative results in the presence of amenorrhea and other symptoms of pregnancy should be reported to a physician, to rule out tubal pregnancy, incomplete abortion, or a possible endocrine disorder)

Cancer
    (elevated HCG levels may be a sign of some types of cancer)

Endometriosis or
Menopause or
Ovarian disorders
    (luteinizing hormone levels are increased in some ovarian disorders, during menopause, and with endometriosis)

Hematuria or
Proteinuria or
Urinary tract infection
    (proteinuria or hematuria may confound test results)

Hypothyroidism
    (thyroid-stimulating hormone may be elevated in hypothyroidism)

*Due to test procedures*

Improper storage or
Outdated test materials
    (chilled test materials or urine may not react accurately)

    (outdated or heat-exposed test materials may not react appropriately; direct, intense sunlight should also be avoided)

Timing
    (testing too early or late in pregnancy may produce false-negative results)

Vibration
    (hemagglutination tests may be disturbed by vibration, including vibration from household appliance motors, or movement of the tube, giving false results)

## Patient Consultation

As an aid to patient consultation, refer to *Advice for the Patient, Pregnancy Test Kits for Home Use.*

In providing consultation, consider emphasizing the following selected information (» = major clinical significance):

**Before using this test**

Getting assistance in reading results if vision is impaired, if color-blind, or if having problems in reading or understanding written instructions

Noting possible interference with test results caused by other medications or conditions

» Conditions affecting use, especially:

**Proper use of this test**

Checking the expiration date and not using outdated materials

Reading and following kit instructions

*Proper test procedures*

Using first morning urine, collected in container that is free of detergent or traces of chemicals

Working on a clean, dry surface in normal humidity and temperature, near a source of cold water

Avoiding touching test reaction areas; skin oils or perspiration may affect test results

Carefully timing steps, using a stopwatch or timer, according to kit instructions

Observing for increase in color intensity

Recording and dating test results for discussion with health care professional

» Proper storage

**Follow-up**

Importance of contacting physician, regardless of test results

If test is positive, importance of seeking prenatal care, including examination for confirmation and dating of pregnancy

If test is negative, importance of repeating test in 7 days and reporting continued amenorrhea or other signs of pregnancy to health care professional

Consulting physician, nurse, or pharmacist, or calling the toll-free phone number accompanying the kit with questions concerning how to perform test or about results

---

### COLLOIDAL GOLD PARTICLE PREGNANCY IMMUNOASSAY TEST KITS

## Diagnostic Product Forms

### COLLOIDAL GOLD PARTICLE PREGNANCY IMMUNOASSAY TEST KITS

**Administration**

Most kits will produce a response the first day or one day after menstrual period is missed. A specified quantity of urine is added to test material. Steps and timing vary among kits. Results are read in approximately three to ten minutes, depending upon kit, and are in the form of a color change.

**Product(s) usually available**

U.S.—

[*Answer Quick & Simple; e.p.t. Quick Stick; First Response; Fortel Midstream; Fortel Plus*].

**Packaging and storage**

Store between 15 and 30 °C (59 and 86 °F), out of direct sunlight. Avoid excess humidity.

---

### ENZYME IMMUNOASSAY PREGNANCY TEST KITS

## Diagnostic Product Forms

### ENZYME IMMUNOASSAY PREGNANCY TEST KITS

**Administration**

Most kits will produce response one day after period is missed. A specified number of drops of first morning voided urine are added to test material. Steps and timing vary among kits. Results are read in one to thirty minutes, depending on kit, and may be in the form of color change or plus/minus sign.

**Product(s) usually available**

U.S.—

[*Advance; Answer Plus; Answer Plus II; Clearblue Easy; Daisy 2; Fact Plus; Q-test; SureCell hCG-Urine Test*].

Canada—

[*Clearblue Easy*].

Note: Products are labeled to indicate whether they contain 1 or 2 tests; several are packaged with enough materials to repeat test in seven days if the first one is negative.

**Packaging and storage**

Store between 15 and 30 °C (59 and 86 °F), out of direct sunlight. Avoid excess humidity.

---

### HEMAGGLUTINATION INHIBITION PREGNANCY TEST KITS

## Diagnostic Product Forms

### HEMAGGLUTINATION INHIBITION PREGNANCY TEST KITS

**Administration**

Usual test instructions state test will give response three to seven days after missed period. Steps and timing vary among products. Specified number of drops of first morning voided urine are added to test solution in tube and allowed to stand. A second solution is added, and the tube is set aside to allow for undisturbed settling. Results are read as a ring or button (positive) or mat formation (negative) in bottom of test tube.

**Product(s) usually available**

U.S.—

[*Answer*].

Note: Products are labeled to indicate whether they contain 1 or 2 tests; some are packaged with enough materials to repeat test in seven days if the first one is negative.

**Packaging and storage**

Store between 15 and 30 °C (59 and 86 °F), out of direct sunlight. Avoid excess humidity.

---

Revised: 07/20/93
Interim revision: 06/30/94

---

## PRILOCAINE—See *Anesthetics (Parenteral-Local)*

## PRILOCAINE-CONTAINING COMBINATIONS—

Lidocaine and Prilocaine (Topical)
Prilocaine and Epinephrine (Parenteral-Local)—See *Anesthetics (Parenteral-Local)*

---

# PRIMAQUINE Systemic

VA CLASSIFICATION (Primary): AP101

Note: For a listing of dosage forms and brand names by country availability, see *Dosage Forms* section(s). For a listing of brand names for the articles in this monograph, refer to the General Index.

## Category

Antiprotozoal.

## Indications

Note: Bracketed information in the *Indications* section refers to uses that are not included in U.S. product labeling.

**Accepted**

Malaria (treatment)—Primaquine is indicated for the prevention of relapses (radical cure) of malaria caused by *Plasmodium vivax* [and *P. ovale*]. Primaquine is also effective against the gametocytes of *P. falciparum*.

[Pneumonia, *Pneumocystis carinii* (treatment)][1]—Primaquine is used in combination with clindamycin in the treatment of *Pneumocystis carinii* pneumonia (PCP) in patients unresponsive or intolerant to standard therapy.

---

[1]Not included in Canadian product labeling.

## Pharmacology/Pharmacokinetics

### Physicochemical characteristics
Chemical group—8-aminoquinoline.
Molecular weight—455.34.

### Mechanism of action/Effect
The precise mechanism of action has not been determined, but may be based on primaquine's ability to bind to and alter the properties of DNA. Primaquine is highly active against the exoerythrocytic stages of *P. vivax* and *P. ovale* and against the primary exoerythrocytic stages of *P. falciparum*. It is also highly active against the sexual forms (gametocytes) of plasmodia, especially *P. falciparum*, disrupting transmission of the disease by eliminating the reservoir from which the mosquito carrier is infected.

### Absorption
Rapidly absorbed; bioavailability is approximately 96%.

### Distribution
Extensively distributed; unlike the 4-aminoquinoline antimalarials, there is no evidence of accumulation of primaquine or carboxyprimaquine in blood cells; the whole blood to plasma distribution ratio was 0.93 in one study of patients being treated with 15 mg (base) daily for 14 days.
Apparent $Vol_D$ = mean 248 L (range, 149 to 303 L).

### Biotransformation
Rapidly converted to carboxyprimaquine, the principal plasma metabolite. It is not known whether this metabolite has antimalarial activity.

### Half-life
Primaquine—Mean, 5.8 hours (range, 3.7 to 7.4 hours).
Carboxyprimaquine—22 to 30 hours.

### Time to peak concentration
Primaquine—Approximately 2 to 3 hours.
Carboxyprimaquine—Approximately 7 hours (range, 2.6 to 8).

### Peak serum concentration
Primaquine (steady state)—
    15 mg (base): 50 to 66 nanograms per mL.
    30 mg (base): Approximately 104 nanograms per mL.
Carboxyprimaquine—
    15 mg (base) single dose: 291 to 736 nanograms per mL.
    15 mg (base) daily, on day 14: 432 to 1240 nanograms per mL.

### Elimination
Less than 2% of oral primaquine dose excreted in urine within 24 hours.

## Precautions to Consider

### Cross-sensitivity and/or related problems
Patients hypersensitive to iodoquinol, a chemically related 8-aminoquinoline, may be hypersensitive to this medication also.

### Pregnancy/Reproduction
Pregnancy—Primaquine is not recommended during pregnancy because it may cross the placenta and may cause hemolytic anemia in utero in G6PD-deficient fetuses.

### Breast-feeding
It is not known whether primaquine is excreted in breast milk. However, problems in humans have not been documented.

### Pediatrics
Appropriate studies on the relationship of age to the effects of primaquine have not been performed in the pediatric population. However, no pediatrics-specific problems have been documented to date.

### Geriatrics
No information is available on the relationship of age to the effects of primaquine in geriatric patients.

### Drug interactions and/or related problems
The following drug interactions and/or related problems have been selected on the basis of their potential clinical significance (possible mechanism in parentheses where appropriate)—not necessarily inclusive (» = major clinical significance):

Note: Combinations containing any of the following medications, depending on the amount present, may also interact with this medication.

Bone marrow depressants (See *Appendix II*) or
» Hemolytics, other (See *Appendix II*)
    (concurrent use of primaquine with bone marrow depressants may increase the leukopenic effects; if concurrent use is required, close observation for myelotoxic effects should be considered)
    (concurrent use of primaquine with other hemolytics may increase the potential for toxic side effects)
» Quinacrine
    (concurrent use is not recommended since it may increase the toxic effects of primaquine)

### Medical considerations/Contraindications
The medical considerations/contraindications included here have been selected on the basis of their potential clinical significance (reasons given in parentheses where appropriate)—not necessarily inclusive (» = major clinical significance).

*Risk-benefit should be considered when the following medical problems exist:*

Favism or acute hemolytic anemia, history of (family or personal) or
» Glucose-6-phosphate dehydrogenase (G6PD) deficiency
    (primaquine may cause hemolytic anemia, especially in G6PD-deficient patients)
Hypersensitivity to primaquine
Nicotinamide adenine dinucleotide (NADH) methemoglobin reductase deficiency
    (primaquine may cause methemoglobinemia, especially in patients with NADH methemoglobin reductase deficiency)

### Patient monitoring
The following may be especially important in patient monitoring (other tests may be warranted in some patients, depending on condition; » = major clinical significance):
Blood cell counts and
Hemoglobin determinations
    (recommended at weekly intervals during therapy in patients with G6PD deficiency since anemia, methemoglobinemia, and leukopenia have been reported following administration of large doses of primaquine; a mild leukocytosis has also been observed; primaquine should be discontinued immediately if a sudden decrease in hemoglobin concentration, erythrocyte count, or leukocyte count occurs)
» Glucose-6-phosphate dehydrogenase (G6PD) determinations
    (required prior to treatment, especially in Caucasians of Mediterranean origin, Blacks, Asians, and Orientals; if a deficiency is found, primaquine should be given with caution since hemolytic effects may be exaggerated)

## Side/Adverse Effects
The following side/adverse effects have been selected on the basis of their potential clinical significance (possible signs and symptoms in parentheses where appropriate)—not necessarily inclusive:

### Those indicating need for medical attention
Incidence more frequent
    *Hemolytic anemia* (dark urine; back, leg, or stomach pains; loss of appetite; pale skin; unusual tiredness or weakness; fever)—severity of hemolysis in patients with G6PD deficiency is directly related to the degree of deficiency and the dose of primaquine administered
Incidence less frequent
    *Methemoglobinemia* (cyanosis—bluish fingernails, lips, or skin; dizziness or lightheadedness; difficulty breathing; unusual tiredness or weakness)—especially with high doses or in patients with NADH methemoglobin reductase deficiency
Incidence rare
    *Leukopenia* (sore throat and fever)

### Those indicating need for medical attention only if they continue or are bothersome
Incidence more frequent
    *Gastrointestinal effects* (abdominal pain or cramps, nausea or vomiting)

## Patient Consultation
As an aid to patient consultation, refer to *Advice for the Patient, Primaquine (Systemic).*

In providing consultation, consider emphasizing the following selected information (» = major clinical significance):

### Before using this medication
» Conditions affecting use, especially:
    Hypersensitivity to primaquine

Pregnancy—Use is not recommended
Other medications, especially other hemolytics and quinacrine
Other medical problems, especially G6PD deficiency

### Proper use of this medication
» Taking with meals or antacids to minimize gastric irritation
» Compliance with full course of therapy
» Proper dosing
Missed dose: Taking as soon as possible; not taking if almost time for next dose; not doubling doses
» Proper storage

### Precautions while using this medication
Regular visits to physician to check progress during therapy

### Side/adverse effects
Signs of potential side effects, especially hemolytic anemia, leukopenia, and methemoglobinemia.

## General Dosing Information

Primaquine may be taken with meals or antacids to minimize gastric irritation.

When used to prevent relapses, primaquine may be administered concurrently or consecutively with chloroquine or hydroxychloroquine.

## Oral Dosage Forms

Note: Bracketed uses in the *Dosage Forms* section refer to categories of use and/or indications that are not included in U.S. product labeling.

### PRIMAQUINE PHOSPHATE TABLETS USP

#### Usual adult and adolescent dose
Malaria—
Oral, 26.3 mg (15 mg base) once a day for fourteen days.

Note: For some strains of *Plasmodium vivax* (particularly those from Southeast Asia), a dose of 39.4 to 52.6 mg (22.5 to 30 mg base) daily for fourteen days may be required for radical cure of malaria.
To eliminate gametocytes of *P. falciparum*, a single dose of 78.9 mg (45 mg base) may be administered.
[*Pneumocystis carinii* pneumonia][1]—
Oral, 26.3 mg to 52.6 mg (15 to 30 mg base) once a day for twenty-one days.

#### Usual pediatric dose
Malaria—
Oral, 680 mcg (390 mcg base) (0.68 mg [0.39 mg base]) per kg of body weight once a day for fourteen days.

#### Strength(s) usually available
U.S.—
26.3 mg (15 mg base) (Rx) [GENERIC].
Canada—
26.3 mg (15 mg base) (Rx) [GENERIC].

#### Packaging and storage
Store below 40 °C (104 °F), preferably between 15 and 30 °C (59 and 86 °F), unless otherwise specified by manufacturer. Store in a well-closed, light-resistant container.

#### Auxiliary labeling
• Continue medicine for full time of treatment.

[1]Not included in Canadian product labeling.

Revised: 01/19/93

---

# PRIMIDONE Systemic

VA CLASSIFICATION (Primary): CN400
Note: For a listing of dosage forms and brand names by country availability, see *Dosage Forms* section(s). For a listing of brand names for the articles in this monograph, refer to the General Index.

## Category
Anticonvulsant.

## Indications
Note: Bracketed information in the *Indications* section refers to uses that are not included in U.S. product labeling.

### Accepted
Epilepsy (treatment)—Primidone, either alone or used concomitantly with other anticonvulsants, is indicated in the control of generalized tonic-clonic (grand mal), nocturnal myoclonic, complex partial (psychomotor), and simple partial (cortical focal) epileptic seizures.

[Essential tremor (treatment)][1]—Primidone is used in the treatment of essential (familial) tremor. Although propranolol is considered to be the treatment of choice for essential tremor, primidone provides effective treatment for some patients.

[1]Not included in Canadian product labeling.

## Pharmacology/Pharmacokinetics

### Physicochemical characteristics
Molecular weight—218.25.

### Mechanism of action/Effect
Unknown, but anticonvulsant effects are thought to be due to the parent compound, primidone, as well as its two active metabolites, phenobarbital and phenylethylmalonamide (PEMA), whose actions may be synergistic.

### Absorption
Rapid, usually complete with wide individual variation. Bioavailability—90 to 100% (indirect estimates).

### Distribution
Primidone has a volume of distribution ($V_D$) of 0.64 to 0.86 liters per kg. Primidone and its metabolites pass into breast milk, reaching a mean concentration of 75% of maternal steady-state serum levels.

### Half-life
Primidone—3 to 23 hours.
Phenobarbital metabolite—75 to 126 hours.
PEMA metabolite—10 to 25 hours.

### Time to peak concentration
Average 3 to 4 hours.

### Therapeutic serum concentration
5 to 12 mcg of primidone per mL (mcg/mL) (23 to 55 mmol/L), which produces phenobarbital serum concentrations of 20 to 40 mcg/mL (86 to 172 mmol/L). Some clinicians have suggested that the optimal mean plasma primidone concentration is 12 mcg/mL with an associated mean derived phenobarbital concentration of 15 mcg/mL resulting in a primidone-to-phenobarbital ratio of 0.8; however, much variation occurs among patients.

| | Protein Binding (%) | Biotransformation | Elimination (% unchanged) |
|---|---|---|---|
| Primidone | 0–20 | Hepatic; 2 active metabolites: phenobarbital (15–25%) and PEMA. PEMA is the major metabolite and less active than phenobarbital | Renal (64) |
| PEMA (metabolite) | Negligible | No further metabolism | Renal (6.6) |
| Phenobarbital (metabolite) | 50 | Hepatic (therapeutic doses of primidone produce therapeutic blood concentrations of phenobarbital) | Renal (5.1) |

## Precautions to Consider

### Cross-sensitivity and/or related problems
Patients sensitive to barbiturates may be sensitive to this medication also.

### Pregnancy/Reproduction
Pregnancy—Adequate and well-controlled studies in humans have not been done. However, reports have suggested an association between

the use of other anticonvulsant drugs and an increased incidence of birth defects (fetal hydantoin syndrome) in newborns. Symptoms similar to fetal hydantoin syndrome, i.e., growth retardation, craniofacial and heart abnormalities, and hypoplasia of the fingernails and distal phalanges, have been shown to occur with primidone also.

Neonatal hemorrhage, with a coagulation defect resembling vitamin K deficiency, has been described in newborns whose mothers were taking primidone and other anticonvulsants. Risk may be reduced by administering water-soluble vitamin K prophylactically to the mother 1 month prior to and during delivery and also to the neonate, intramuscularly or subcutaneously, immediately after birth.

**Breast-feeding**
Primidone is distributed into breast milk in substantial amounts, and the use of primidone by nursing mothers may cause unusual drowsiness in the neonate.

**Pediatrics**
Some children may react to primidone with paradoxical excitement and restlessness.

**Geriatrics**
Unusual restlessness and excitement may sometimes occur as a paradoxical reaction in the elderly.

**Drug interactions and/or related problems**
The following drug interactions and/or related problems have been selected on the basis of their potential clinical significance (possible mechanism in parentheses where appropriate)—not necessarily inclusive (» = major clinical significance):

Note: Combinations containing any of the following medications, depending on the amount present, may also interact with this medication.

Although not all of the following interactions have been documented to pertain specifically to primidone, a potential exists for their occurrence because of the barbiturate metabolite of primidone.

Acetaminophen
(when acetaminophen in therapeutic doses is used concurrently in patients receiving chronic primidone therapy, its effects may be decreased because of increased metabolism resulting from induction of hepatic microsomal enzymes by the phenobarbital metabolite; also, risk of hepatotoxicity with single toxic doses or prolonged use of acetaminophen may be increased in chronic alcoholics or in patients regularly using hepatic-enzyme inducing agents)

» Adrenocorticoids, glucocorticoid and mineralocorticoid or
» Anticoagulants, coumarin- or indandione-derivative or
Antidepressants, tricyclic or
Chloramphenicol or
» Contraceptives, oral, estrogen-containing or
» Corticotropin (ACTH) or
Cyclosporine or
Dacarbazine or
Digitalis glycosides, with possible exception of digoxin or
Disopyramide or
Doxycycline or
Levothyroxine or
Metronidazole or
Mexiletine or
Quinidine
(concurrent use with primidone may decrease the effects of these medications because of increased metabolism resulting from induction of hepatic microsomal enzymes by the barbiturate metabolite; dosage increases may be necessary during and after primidone therapy)

(use of a nonhormonal method of birth control or a progestin-only oral contraceptive may be necessary during primidone therapy)

(also, concurrent use of tricyclic antidepressants with primidone may enhance central nervous system [CNS] depression, lower convulsive threshold, and decrease the effects of primidone; dosage adjustments may be necessary to control seizures)

» Alcohol or
» CNS depression–producing medications, other (See *Appendix II*)
(concurrent use may potentiate the CNS and respiratory depressant effects of either these medications or primidone; dosage adjustment of primidone may be necessary)

Amphetamines
(concurrent use may cause a delay in the intestinal absorption of the phenobarbital metabolite)

» Anticonvulsants, other
(concurrent use may cause a change in the pattern of epileptiform seizures because of altered medication metabolism; monitoring of

plasma concentrations of both medications is recommended; dosage adjustments may be necessary)

(carbamazepine induces metabolism and decreases effects of primidone; monitoring of plasma concentrations is recommended as a guide to dosage if either medication is added or withdrawn from an existing regimen)

(concurrent use of valproic acid with primidone may cause higher serum concentrations of primidone leading to increased CNS depression and neurological toxicity because of protein binding displacement and reduced metabolism; half-life of valproic acid may be decreased; in addition, primidone may enhance valproic acid hepatotoxicity, presumably through the formation of hepatotoxic valproate metabolites; dosage adjustment of primidone may be necessary)

Carbonic anhydrase inhibitors
(osteopenia induced by primidone may be enhanced; it is recommended that patients receiving concurrent therapy be monitored for early signs of osteopenia and that the carbonic acid anhydrase inhibitor be discontinued and appropriate treatment initiated if necessary)

Cyclophosphamide
(concurrent use with primidone may induce microsomal metabolism to increase the formation of alkylating metabolites of cyclophosphamide, thereby reducing the half-life and increasing the leukopenic activity of cyclophosphamide)

Enflurane or
Halothane or
Methoxyflurane
(chronic use of primidone prior to anesthesia may increase anesthetic metabolism, leading to increased risk of hepatotoxicity)

(also, chronic use of primidone prior to anesthesia with methoxyflurane may increase formation of nephrotoxic metabolites, leading to increased risk of nephrotoxicity)

Fenoprofen
(concurrent use with primidone may decrease the elimination half-life of fenoprofen, possibly because of increased metabolism resulting from induction of hepatic microsomal enzyme activity; fenoprofen dosage adjustment may be required)

Folic acid
(requirements for folic acid may be increased in patients receiving anticonvulsant therapy)

Griseofulvin
(antifungal effects may be decreased when griseofulvin is used concurrently with primidone because of impaired absorption resulting in decreased serum concentrations; although the effect of decreased serum concentrations on therapeutic response has not been established, concurrent use preferably should be avoided)

Guanadrel or
Guanethidine
(concurrent use with primidone may aggravate orthostatic hypotension)

Haloperidol or
Loxapine or
Maprotiline or
Molindone or
Phenothiazines or
Thioxanthenes
(concurrent use may lower the seizure threshold because of altered metabolism; CNS depression may be increased; decreases in primidone dosage may be necessary)

(serum concentrations of neuroleptics may be significantly reduced when these medications are used concurrently with primidone because of increased metabolism)

Leucovorin
(large doses may counteract the anticonvulsant effects of primidone)

Methylphenidate
(concurrent use may increase serum concentrations of primidone because of metabolism inhibition, possibly resulting in toxicity; dosage adjustments may be necessary)

» Monoamine oxidase (MAO) inhibitors, including furazolidone, procarbazine, or selegiline
(concurrent use may prolong the effects of primidone because metabolism of the barbiturate metabolite may be inhibited; changes in the pattern of epileptiform seizures may occur; dosage adjustments of primidone may be necessary)

Phenobarbital
(although concurrent use with primidone is rarely indicated, since primidone is metabolized to phenobarbital, it may cause a change in the pattern of epileptiform seizures because of altered medication metabolism and also increase the sedative effect of either primidone or the barbiturate anticonvulsant; decreases in primidone dosage may be necessary)

Phenylbutazone
(concurrent use may decrease the efficacy of the phenobarbital metabolite of primidone by inducing hepatic microsomal enzymes and increasing its metabolism; also, hepatic enzyme inducers such as barbiturates may increase phenylbutazone metabolism and decrease its half-life)

Posterior pituitary
(concurrent use with primidone may increase the risk of cardiac arrhythmias and coronary insufficiency)

Rifampin
(concurrent use of rifampin with barbiturates may enhance the metabolism of hexobarbital by induction of hepatic microsomal enzymes, resulting in lower serum concentrations; there is conflicting data on rifampin's effect on phenobarbital blood levels; dosage adjustment may be required)

Vitamin D
(effects may be reduced by primidone, because of accelerated metabolism by hepatic microsomal enzyme induction; vitamin D supplementation may be required in patients on long-term primidone therapy to prevent osteomalacia, although rickets is rare)

Xanthines, such as:
Aminophylline
Caffeine
Oxtriphylline
Theophylline
(concurrent use with primidone, because of the barbiturate metabolite, may increase metabolism of the xanthines [except dyphylline] by induction of hepatic microsomal enzymes, resulting in increased theophylline clearance)

## Laboratory value alterations
The following have been selected on the basis of their potential clinical significance (possible effect in parentheses where appropriate)—not necessarily inclusive (» = major clinical significance):

With diagnostic test results
Cyanocobalamin Co 57
(absorption of radioactive cyanocobalamin may be impaired by concurrent use of primidone)

Metyrapone test
(increased metabolism of metyrapone by an hepatic enzyme inducer such as primidone may decrease the response to metyrapone)

Phentolamine test
(primidone may cause a false-positive phentolamine test; it is recommended that all medications be withdrawn at least 24 hours, preferably 48 to 72 hours, prior to a phentolamine test)

With physiology/laboratory test values
Bilirubin concentrations, serum
(may be decreased in patients with congenital nonhemolytic unconjugated hyperbilirubinemia and in epileptics; this effect is presumably due to induction of glucuronyl transferase, the enzyme responsible for the conjugation of bilirubin)

## Medical considerations/Contraindications
The medical considerations/contraindications included here have been selected on the basis of their potential clinical significance (reasons given in parentheses where appropriate)—not necessarily inclusive (» = major clinical significance).

*This medication should not be used when the following medical problem exists:*
» Porphyria, acute intermittent or variegate, or history of
(barbiturate metabolite of primidone may aggravate symptoms of porphyria by inducing enzymes responsible for porphyrin synthesis)

*Risk-benefit should be considered when the following medical problems exist:*
Hepatic function impairment
(possible systemic accumulation of barbiturate metabolite)

Hyperkinesia
(may be precipitated or aggravated by primidone)

Renal function impairment
(possible systemic accumulation of barbiturate metabolite)

» Respiratory diseases such as asthma, emphysema, or those involving dyspnea or obstruction
(serious ventilatory depression may occur)

Sensitivity to primidone or barbiturates

## Patient monitoring
The following may be especially important in patient monitoring (other tests may be warranted in some patients, depending on condition; » = major clinical significance):

Blood cell counts, complete and
Blood chemistry profiles
(manufacturer recommends that these tests be completed every 6 months)

Folate concentrations, serum
(determinations recommended periodically because of increased folate requirements of patients on long-term anticonvulsant therapy)

Phenobarbital concentrations, serum, and
Primidone concentrations, serum
(since phenobarbital is a major metabolite of primidone, serum concentrations of both may be required in some patients at periodic intervals to maintain maximum therapeutic efficacy)

# Side/Adverse Effects
The following side/adverse effects have been selected on the basis of their potential clinical significance (possible signs and symptoms in parentheses where appropriate)—not necessarily inclusive:

**Those indicating need for medical attention**
Incidence less frequent
*Paradoxical reaction* (unusual excitement or restlessness)—especially in children and the elderly

Incidence rare
*Anemia, megaloblastic* (unusual tiredness or weakness); *skin rash*

Note: *Megaloblastic anemia* may respond to folic acid without discontinuation of anticonvulsant therapy.

Signs of intolerance or overdose
*Confusion; diplopia* (double vision); *nystagmus* (continuous, uncontrolled back-and-forth and/or rolling eye movements); *shortness of breath or troubled breathing*

**Those indicating need for medical attention only if they continue or are bothersome**
Incidence more frequent
*Ataxia* (clumsiness or unsteadiness); *dizziness*

Incidence less frequent
*Anorexia* (loss of appetite); *drowsiness; impotence* (decreased sexual ability); *mood or mental changes; nausea or vomiting*—usually decreases or disappears with continued use of medication

# Patient Consultation
As an aid to patient consultation, refer to *Advice for the Patient, Primidone (Systemic)*.

In providing consultation, consider emphasizing the following selected information (» = major clinical significance):

**Before using this medication**
» Conditions affecting use, especially:
Sensitivity to primidone or barbiturates
Pregnancy—Abnormalities similar to fetal hydantoin syndrome may occur; neonatal hemorrhaging may occur at delivery
Breast-feeding—Distributed into breast milk, causing drowsiness in the baby
Use in children—Paradoxical excitement and restlessness may occur
Use in the elderly—Paradoxical excitement and restlessness may occur
Other medications, especially adrenocorticoids, anticoagulants, estrogens, estrogen-containing contraceptives, CNS depression–producing medications, other anticonvulsants, or monoamine oxidase inhibitors
Other medical problems, especially acute intermittent porphyria, or respiratory diseases

**Proper use of this medication**
» Compliance with therapy; taking every day in doses spaced as directed
» Proper dosing
   Missed dose: Taking as soon as possible, unless within an hour of next scheduled dose; not doubling doses
» Proper storage

**Precautions while using this medication**
   Regular visits to physician to check progress of therapy
   Checking with physician before discontinuing medication; gradual dosage reduction may be needed
   Caution if any kind of surgery, dental treatment, or emergency treatment is required
» Avoiding use of alcoholic beverages; not taking other CNS depressants unless prescribed by physician
» Possible drowsiness; caution when driving or doing other things requiring alertness
» Possible dizziness or lightheadedness; caution when getting up suddenly from a lying or sitting position
   Caution if any laboratory tests required; possible interference with results of cyanocobalamin Co 57, metyrapone, or phentolamine tests.

**Side/adverse effects**
   Signs of potential side effects, especially excitement or restlessness, allergic reaction, or megaloblastic anemia

## General Dosing Information

Because primidone serum concentrations vary greatly among patients after oral administration, it is very important that the dosage be individualized. One of primidone's metabolites, phenobarbital, greatly influences its serum concentration, side effects, and interactions, as well as its therapeutic effect.

When primidone is to be discontinued, dosage should be reduced gradually. Abrupt withdrawal may precipitate status epilepticus.

When used with or to replace other anticonvulsant therapy, the dosage of primidone should be increased gradually while that of the other medication is maintained or decreased gradually in order to maintain seizure control. When therapy with primidone alone is the objective, the transition should not be completed in less than 2 weeks.

Many of the common side effects such as nausea, dizziness, and drowsiness diminish in frequency and intensity with continued use of the medication or reduction of dosage.

### Diet/Nutrition
Patients on long-term anticonvulsant therapy have increased folate requirements. In addition, patients on long-term therapy may require vitamin D supplementation to prevent osteomalacia.

## Oral Dosage Forms

Note: Bracketed uses in the *Dosage Forms* section refer to categories of use and/or indications that are not included in U.S. product labeling.

### PRIMIDONE ORAL SUSPENSION USP

**Usual adult and adolescent dose**
Anticonvulsant—
   Initial:
      Oral, 100 or 125 mg once a day at bedtime for the first three days, the daily dose being increased to 100 or 125 mg two times a day for the fourth, fifth, and sixth days, and then increased to 100 or 125 mg three times a day for the seventh, eighth, and ninth days. On the tenth day a maintenance dosage of 250 mg three times a day may be established and then adjusted according to patient needs and tolerance but not to exceed 2 grams a day.
      Note: Initial doses as low as 25 mg twice a day have been used in patients experiencing troublesome nausea and vomiting.
   Maintenance:
      Oral, 250 mg three or four times a day.
   [Tremorlytic][1]—
      Oral, initially 50 to 62.5 mg a day, the dosage being increased as needed and tolerated up to a maximum of 750 mg a day.

**Usual pediatric dose**
Anticonvulsant—
   Children up to 8 years of age:
      Initial—Oral, 50 mg at bedtime for the first three days, the daily dose being increased to 50 mg two times a day for the fourth,

fifth, and sixth days and then increased to 100 mg two times a day for the seventh, eighth, and ninth days.
      Maintenance—Oral, on the tenth day, 125 to 250 mg three times a day (or 10 to 25 mg per kg of body weight a day given in divided doses), the dosage being adjusted according to patient needs and tolerance.
   Children 8 years of age and over:
      See *Usual adult and adolescent dose*.

**Strength(s) usually available**
U.S.—
   250 mg per 5 mL (Rx) [*Mysoline* (ammonia solution [diluted]; citric acid; D&C Yellow No. 10; FD&C Yellow No. 6; magnesium aluminum silicate; methylparaben; propylparaben; saccharin sodium; sodium alginate; sodium citrate; sodium hypochlorite solution; sorbic acid; sorbitan monolaurate; purified water; flavors)].
Canada—
   Not commercially available.

**Packaging and storage**
Store below 40 °C (104 °F), preferably between 15 and 30 °C (59 and 86 °F), unless otherwise specified by manufacturer. Store in a tight, light-resistant container. Protect from freezing.

**Auxiliary labeling**
• Shake well.
• May cause drowsiness.
• Avoid alcoholic beverages.
• Do not freeze.

### PRIMIDONE TABLETS USP

**Usual adult and adolescent dose**
See *Primidone Oral Suspension USP*.

**Usual pediatric dose**
See *Primidone Oral Suspension USP*.

**Strength(s) usually available**
U.S.—
   50 mg (Rx) [*Mysoline* (lactose)].
   250 mg (Rx) [*Myidone; Mysoline;* GENERIC].
Canada—
   125 mg (Rx) [*Apo-Primidone; PMS Primidone; Sertan*].
   250 mg (Rx) [*Apo-Primidone; Mysoline* (lactose); *PMS Primidone; Sertan;* GENERIC].

**Packaging and storage**
Store below 40 °C (104 °F), preferably between 15 and 30 °C (59 and 86 °F), unless otherwise specified by manufacturer. Store in a well-closed container.

**Auxiliary labeling**
• May cause drowsiness.
• Avoid alcoholic beverages.

### PRIMIDONE CHEWABLE TABLETS

**Usual adult and adolescent dose**
See *Primidone Oral Suspension USP*.

**Usual pediatric dose**
See *Primidone Oral Suspension USP*.

**Strength(s) usually available**
U.S.—
   Not commercially available.
Canada—
   125 mg (Rx) [*Mysoline* (lactose)].

**Packaging and storage**
Store below 40 °C (104 °F), preferably between 15 and 30 °C (59 and 86 °F), in a well-closed container unless otherwise specified by manufacturer.

**Auxiliary labeling**
• Chew tablets before swallowing
• May cause drowsiness.
• Avoid alcoholic beverages.

---

[1]Not included in Canadian product labeling.

---

Revised: 01/27/92
Interim revision: 08/16/94

# PROBENECID  Systemic

VA CLASSIFICATION (Primary): MS400

Note: For a listing of dosage forms and brand names by country availability, see *Dosage Forms* section(s). For a listing of brand names for the articles in this monograph, refer to the General Index.

## Category

Antigout agent; antibiotic therapy adjunct; antihyperuricemic.

## Indications

Note: Bracketed information in the *Indications* section refers to uses that are not included in U.S. product labeling.

### Accepted

Gouty arthritis, chronic (treatment) or

Hyperuricemia (treatment)—Probenecid is indicated for the long-term management of hyperuricemia associated with chronic gout. It is recommended only for patients whose 24-hour renal excretion of urate is 800 mg (4.8 mmol) or lower (i.e., patients who are hyperuricemic as a result of underexcretion, rather than overproduction, of urate). The aim of probenecid therapy is to reduce the number of acute gout attacks.

Probenecid is not effective in the treatment of acute gout attacks and does not eliminate the need to use colchicine or a nonsteroidal anti-inflammatory drug (NSAID) to relieve an attack. Also, probenecid therapy should not be initiated during an attack, because it may induce fluctuations in urate concentration that may result in prolongation of the attack or initiation of a new attack.

[Probenecid is sometimes used in the treatment of hyperuricemia not associated with gout. However, treatment of asymptomatic hyperuricemia is often unnecessary; the need for such therapy should be determined on an individual basis][1].

Antibiotic therapy, adjunct—Probenecid is indicated as an adjunct to therapy with penicillins [and some of the cephalosporin antibiotics][1]. It is used primarily when high antibiotic plasma and tissue concentrations are required. Adjunctive use of probenecid is included in some of the U.S. Centers for Disease Control (CDC) guidelines for the treatment of sexually transmitted diseases such as gonorrhea, acute pelvic inflammatory disease (outpatient treatment), and neurosyphilis.

### Unaccepted

Probenecid is not recommended in circumstances in which there is an especially high risk of adverse effects associated with crystallization and deposition of urate in renal tissues, such as formation of renal calculi and uric acid nephropathy. It therefore should not be used for treatment of gout in patients whose 24-hour urate excretion exceeds 800 mg (4.8 mmol) or who have extensive tophi, or for treatment of hyperuricemia associated with neoplastic disease or its treatment (chemotherapy with rapidly cytolytic antineoplastic agents or radiation therapy). Allopurinol, which decreases the quantity of urate that reaches the kidneys in addition to decreasing the concentration of urate in the blood, is recommended in these circumstances.

[1]Not included in Canadian product labeling.

## Pharmacology/Pharmacokinetics

### Physicochemical characteristics

Molecular weight—285.36.

pKa—3.4.

### Mechanism of action/Effect

Antigout agent; antihyperuricemic—Probenecid is a uricosuric agent. By competitively inhibiting the active reabsorption of urate at the proximal renal tubule, it increases the urinary excretion of uric acid and lowers serum urate concentrations. By lowering serum concentrations of uric acid below its solubility limits, probenecid may decrease or prevent urate deposition, tophi formation, and chronic joint changes; promote resolution of existing urate deposits; and, after several months of therapy, reduce the frequency of acute attacks of gout. Probenecid has no anti-inflammatory or analgesic activity.

Antibiotic therapy adjunct—Probenecid is a competitive inhibitor of the secretion of weak organic acids, including penicillins and some of the cephalosporin antibiotics, at the proximal and distal renal tubules. It thereby increases blood concentrations of these antibiotics (penicillin concentrations may increase 2- to 4-fold), increases their elimination half-life, and prolongs their duration of action.

### Other actions/effects

Probenecid also inhibits the renal and/or biliary transport, as well as transport into or out of the cerebrospinal fluid (CSF), of many other endogenous compounds and medications.

### Absorption

Rapid and complete.

### Protein binding

High to very high (75 to 95%); primarily to albumin.

### Biotransformation

Hepatic; rapid and extensive. Metabolites include probenecid monoacyl glucuronide, a carboxylated metabolite, and hydroxylated compounds that have uricosuric activity.

### Half-life

Dose-dependent; 3 to 8 hours following administration of a 500-mg dose; 6 to 12 hours following administration of larger doses.

### Time to peak concentration

Adults—2 to 4 hours following a single 1-gram dose; 4 hours following a single 2-gram dose.

### Peak serum concentration

> 30 mcg per mL (mcg/mL) (105 micromoles/L) following a single 1-gram dose; 150 to 200 mcg/mL (525 to 700 micromoles/L) following a single 2-gram dose.

### Therapeutic plasma concentration

Uricosuric effect—100 to 200 mcg/mL (350 to 700 micromoles/L).

Suppression of penicillin excretion—40 to 60 mcg/mL (140 to 210 micromoles/L).

### Time to peak effect

Uricosuric—30 minutes.

Suppression of penicillin excretion—2 hours.

### Duration of action

The effect on penicillin plasma concentration persists for about 8 hours following a single dose.

### Elimination

Primarily via hepatic metabolism, followed by renal excretion of metabolites. About 5 to 10% of a dose is excreted unchanged within 24 to 48 hours. Probenecid excretion is dependent upon urinary pH and is increased in alkaline urine; however, the uricosuric activity is not altered.

## Precautions to Consider

### Pregnancy/Reproduction

Pregnancy—Probenecid crosses the placenta and appears in cord blood. However, the medication has been administered to pregnant women without known adverse effects occurring.

### Breast-feeding

It is not known whether probenecid is excreted in breast milk. However, problems in humans have not been documented.

### Pediatrics

Antibiotic therapy adjunct—Studies performed to date have not demonstrated pediatrics-specific problems that would limit the usefulness of probenecid in children 2 to 14 years of age. Use in children younger than 2 years of age is not recommended.

Antigout agent or

Antihyperuricemic—No information is available on the relationship of age to the effects of probenecid as an antigout or antihyperuricemic agent in pediatric patients.

### Geriatrics

No information is available on the relationship of age to the effects of probenecid in geriatric patients. However, elderly patients are more likely to have age-related renal function impairment, which requires caution in patients receiving probenecid.

### Drug interactions and/or related problems

The following drug interactions and/or related problems have been selected on the basis of their potential clinical significance (possible mechanism in parentheses where appropriate)—not necessarily inclusive (» = major clinical significance):

See also *Laboratory value alterations*.

Note: Combinations containing any of the following medications, depending on the amount present, may also interact with this medication.

Acyclovir, systemic
(probenecid may decrease renal tubular secretion of acyclovir, resulting in increased and prolonged acyclovir serum and cerebrospinal fluid [CSF] concentrations, prolonged elimination half-life in serum and CSF, and, potentially, increased toxicity)

Alcohol or
Diazoxide or
Mecamylamine or
Pyrazinamide
(these medications may increase serum uric acid concentrations; pyrazinamide may also more directly antagonize probenecid's uricosuric activity; dosage adjustment of probenecid may be necessary to control hyperuricemia and gout)

Allopurinol
(probenecid increases urinary excretion of oxipurinol, the active metabolite of allopurinol; however, the antihyperuricemic effects of the two medications are additive and increased therapeutic benefit has been reported with concurrent use)

Aminosalicylate sodium
(probenecid may decrease renal tubular secretion of aminosalicylate sodium, resulting in increased and prolonged serum concentrations and/or toxicity; however, probenecid is not currently recommended as an adjunct to therapy with this medication; patients should be monitored and dosage adjustments made as necessary during and after concurrent therapy)

Anti-inflammatory drugs, nonsteroidal (NSAIDs), especially:
» Indomethacin and
» Ketoprofen
(probenecid decreases the renal clearance of ketoprofen by approximately 66%, ketoprofen protein binding by 28%, and formation and renal clearance of ketoprofen conjugates, leading to greatly increased ketoprofen plasma concentration and risk of toxicity; concurrent use is not recommended)

(probenecid may decrease renal excretion and biliary clearance of indomethacin, leading to increased plasma concentration, elimination half-life [in one study, the elimination half-life was increased from 10.1 to 17.6 hours], and toxicity, and possibly resulting in increased effectiveness; if concurrent use is required, it is recommended that indomethacin be administered in reduced dosage and that increases in dosage be made slowly and in small increments)

(probenecid has also been shown to increase the plasma concentration of naproxen [by 50%], and meclofenamate, and may also increase the plasma concentration of other NSAIDs, possibly enhancing effectiveness and/or increasing the potential for toxicity; a reduction of NSAID dosage may be required if adverse effects occur)

(probenecid may increase the plasma concentrations of sulindac and its sulfone metabolite and slightly decrease the plasma concentrations of the active sulfide metabolite)

» Antineoplastic agents, rapidly cytolytic
(concurrent use with probenecid is not recommended because of the risk of uric acid nephropathy; allopurinol is the antihyperuricemic agent of choice for reducing risks [gout and/or urate nephropathy] associated with chemotherapy-induced hyperuricemia; also, rapidly cytolytic antineoplastic agents may increase serum uric acid concentrations and interfere with control of pre-existing hyperuricemia and gout)

» Aspirin or other salicylates, including bismuth subsalicylate
(chronic administration of a salicylate with probenecid may interfere with probenecid's uricosuric effect [but not its effect on penicillin excretion]; also, probenecid inhibits the uricosuria induced by high doses of salicylates and may inhibit salicylate excretion, possibly leading to increased salicylate concentrations and toxicity; chronic use of a salicylate, especially in large [antirheumatic] doses, together with probenecid is not recommended)

(occasional use of a salicylate in low to moderate analgesic doses, or chronic administration of 80 mg per day of aspirin as an antithrombotic, is not likely to interfere with probenecid's uricosuric effect)

» Cephalosporins or
» Penicillins
(probenecid decreases renal tubular secretion of penicillins and those cephalosporins excreted by this mechanism, resulting in increased and prolonged antibiotic serum concentrations, prolonged elimination half-life, and increased risk of toxicity; adjunctive use

of probenecid provides therapeutic benefit when high and/or prolonged plasma and tissue concentrations of these antibiotics are required; however, probenecid has no effect on the secretion of cefoperazone, ceforanide, ceftazidime, ceftriaxone, or moxalactam)

(probenecid also decreases renal tubular secretion of sulbactam, resulting in increased sulbactam plasma concentrations, but has no effect on renal tubular secretion of clavulanic acid [agents used in combination with some of the beta-lactam antibiotics to protect the antibiotics from enzymatic degradation])

Chlorpropamide and possibly other sulfonylurea antidiabetic agents
(probenecid decreases chlorpropamide elimination, leading to increased plasma concentration and elimination half-life and possibly to an enhanced or prolonged hypoglycemic effect; although an effect of probenecid on the elimination of other sulfonylurea antidiabetic agents has not been determined, the possibility of similar effects should be considered)

Ciprofloxacin or
Norfloxacin
(probenecid decreases renal tubular secretion of ciprofloxacin [by about 50%] and norfloxacin, leading to increased and more prolonged serum concentrations, prolonged elimination half-life, and increased risk of toxicity of the antibacterials)

Clofibrate
(probenecid may decrease renal and metabolic clearances and alter the protein binding of clofibrate, thereby increasing clofibrate's therapeutic and toxic effects)

Dapsone
(concurrent administration with probenecid results in dapsone plasma concentrations being increased by 50% 4 hours after administration and by 25% 8 hours after administration; the patient should be observed for signs of dapsone toxicity and dosage decreased if necessary)

Dyphylline
(probenecid may increase the half-life of dyphylline, possibly permitting less frequent dyphylline dosing)

Furosemide
(probenecid may inhibit renal tubular secretion of furosemide, leading to increased furosemide serum concentrations)

Ganciclovir
(probenecid may decrease the renal clearance of ganciclovir)

» Heparin
(probenecid may increase and prolong the anticoagulant effects of heparin)

Imipenem (available only as imipenem and cilastatin combination)
(since concurrent use with probenecid results in only minimal increase in the serum concentration and half-life of imipenem, such concurrent use to increase imipenem blood concentration is not recommended)

Lorazepam or
Oxazepam or
Temazepam
(probenecid may impair glucuronide conjugation of these benzodiazepines, resulting in increased effects and possibly excessive sedation)

» Methotrexate
(when methotrexate is used as an antineoplastic agent, concurrent use of probenecid is not recommended because of the risk of uric acid nephropathy; allopurinol is the antihyperuricemic agent of choice in this situation)

(probenecid may inhibit renal excretion of methotrexate, possibly leading to toxic plasma concentrations even with the relatively low doses of methotrexate used for noncancerous indications; if used concurrently with probenecid, methotrexate dosage should be decreased, the patient observed for signs of toxicity, and/or methotrexate plasma concentration monitored)

» Nitrofurantoin
(probenecid may inhibit renal tubular secretion of nitrofurantoin, resulting in increased serum concentrations and/or toxicity and reduced urinary concentrations and effectiveness as a urinary antiseptic; a reduction of probenecid dosage may be necessary to ensure effectiveness against urinary tract infection)

Riboflavin (vitamin $B_2$)
(probenecid decreases gastrointestinal absorption of riboflavin; requirements for riboflavin may be increased in patients receiving probenecid)

Rifampin
(probenecid may compete with rifampin for hepatic uptake when the two medications are used concurrently, resulting in increased and prolonged rifampin blood concentrations and/or toxicity; however, the effect on rifampin blood concentrations is inconsistent and concurrent use of probenecid to increase rifampin blood concentrations is not recommended)

Sodium benzoate and sodium phenylacetate
(probenecid may interfere with renal elimination of the conjugated products of these agents)

Sulfinpyrazone
(probenecid inhibits the renal secretion of sulfinpyrazone and its active metabolite; however, the uricosuric effects of the medications are additive, and increased therapeutic benefit has been reported with concurrent use)

Sulfonamides
(probenecid decreases renal excretion of sulfonamides, resulting in increased total serum concentrations of these medications, which may increase the risk of toxicity, but concurrent use provides no therapeutic advantage because free serum concentrations of antibacterial sulfonamides are not increased; sulfonamide serum concentrations should be determined at periodic intervals when these medications are used concurrently with probenecid for a prolonged period of time)

Thiopental
(administration of probenecid 3 hours prior to induction of anesthesia with thiopental significantly reduced the required dose of thiopental and prolonged its effects)

» Zidovudine
(probenecid inhibits hepatic glucuronidation and renal tubular secretion of zidovudine, resulting in increased serum concentrations and prolonged elimination half-life; this may increase the risk of toxicity, or possibly permit a reduction in daily zidovudine dosage; however, in 1 small trial, a very high incidence of skin rash occurred in patients receiving the medications concurrently)

## Laboratory value alterations
The following have been selected on the basis of their potential clinical significance (possible effect in parentheses where appropriate)—not necessarily inclusive (» = major clinical significance):

With diagnostic test results
Aminohippuric acid (PAH) clearance studies and
Phenolsulfonphthalein (PSP) clearance studies
(probenecid decreases renal clearance of PAH and PSP, leading to reduced urine concentrations and misleading test results)

Glucose, urine, determinations
(a reducing substance present in the urine of patients receiving probenecid may cause false-positive test results with copper sulfate urine sugar tests, but not with glucose enzymatic urine sugar tests)

Renal function studies using iodohippurate sodium I 123, iodohippurate sodium I 131, or technetium Tc 99m gluceptate
(probenecid may decrease kidney uptake of these diagnostic aids because of probenecid's inhibitory action on the enzyme transport system in the proximal tubule)

With physiology/laboratory test values
Homovanillic acid (HVA) and
5-Hydroxyindoleacetic acid (5-HIAA)
(probenecid inhibits transport of these substances from the cerebrospinal fluid [CSF] into the blood, resulting in increased CSF concentrations and reduced urine concentrations; however, the changes in HVA and 5-HIAA concentrations are not as great in patients with parkinsonian syndrome and mental depression, respectively, as in healthy individuals)

17-Ketosteroid concentrations, urine
(may be decreased)

Phosphorus
(reabsorption may be increased in hypoparathyroid, but not euparathyroid, individuals)

## Medical considerations/Contraindications
The medical considerations/contraindications included here have been selected on the basis of their potential clinical significance (reasons given in parentheses where appropriate)—not necessarily inclusive (» = major clinical significance).

*Except under special circumstances, this medication should not be used when the following medical conditions exist:*
» Any condition in which there is an increased risk of uric acid renal

calculus formation or urate nephropathy, such as:
» Cancer chemotherapy with rapidly cytolytic antineoplastic agents
» Radiation therapy for malignancy
» Renal calculi or history of, especially uric acid calculi
» Urate excretion higher than 800 mg (4.8 mmol) in 24 hours
» Urate nephropathy or history of
(probenecid is likely to induce, or to exacerbate pre-existing, renal calculi and/or urate nephropathy; allopurinol is recommended instead)

» Renal function impairment, moderate to severe
(probenecid's efficacy decreases with increasing degrees of renal function impairment; the medication is completely ineffective when the patient's creatinine clearance is lower than 30 mL per minute)

*Risk-benefit should be considered when the following medical problems exist:*
Allergic reaction to probenecid, history of
» Blood dyscrasias
(may be exacerbated)
Peptic ulcer, history of
(increased risk of gastrointestinal side effects)
» Renal function impairment, mild
(probenecid's efficacy begins to decrease when the creatinine clearance is 80 mL per minute; although higher doses may be effective in patients with gout who have mild renal function impairment, use of probenecid to increase penicillin concentrations is not recommended for these patients)

## Patient monitoring
The following may be especially important in patient monitoring (other tests may be warranted in some patients, depending on condition; » = major clinical significance):

Acid-base balance determinations
(recommended at periodic intervals if urinary alkalizers are used concurrently with probenecid in uricosuric therapy)
» Serum uric acid concentrations and/or
» Urine uric acid (24-hour) determinations
(monitoring may be required for proper dosing when probenecid is used as an antihyperuricemic; the effect of probenecid may be measured by a reduction of serum uric acid concentration [the upper limit of normal is about 7 mg per 100 mL (420 micromoles/L) for men and postmenopausal women and about 6 mg per 100 mL (360 micromoles/L) for premenopausal women but may vary, depending on the patient and laboratory methodology] or, more directly, by a significant increase in 24-hour uric acid excretion)

# Side/Adverse Effects
The following side/adverse effects have been selected on the basis of their potential clinical significance (possible signs and symptoms in parentheses where appropriate)—not necessarily inclusive:

## Those indicating need for medical attention
Incidence less frequent
*Renal calculi, urate* (lower back and/or side pain; painful urination, with or without blood in urine); *dermatitis, allergic* (skin rash, hives, and/or itching)

Incidence rare
*Anaphylaxis* (changes in facial skin color; skin rash, hives, and/or itching; fast or irregular breathing; puffiness or swelling of the eyelids or around the eyes; shortness of breath, troubled breathing, tightness in chest, and/or wheezing); *anemia* (unusual tiredness and/or weakness if severe)—often asymptomatic; *aplastic anemia* (shortness of breath, troubled breathing, tightness in chest, and/or wheezing; sores, ulcers, or white spots on lips or in mouth; swollen and/or painful glands; unusual bleeding or bruising; unusual tiredness or weakness); *hemolytic anemia* (troubled breathing, exertional; unusual tiredness or weakness)—may be associated with glucose-6-phosphate dehydrogenase (G6PD) deficiency; *fever, allergic; hepatic necrosis* (yellow eyes or skin); *leukopenia* (rarely, fever or chills; cough or hoarseness; lower back or side pain; painful or difficult urination)—usually asymptomatic; *nephrotic syndrome* (cloudy urine; swelling of face); *pain in back and/or ribs; renal colic* (pain, severe and/or sharp, in lower back and/or side); *urate nephropathy* (symptoms of renal impairment, e.g., increased blood pressure; shortness of breath, troubled breathing, tightness in chest, and/or wheezing; sudden decrease in amount of urine; swelling of face, fingers, feet, and/or lower legs; unusual tiredness or weakness; weight gain)

**Those indicating need for medical attention only if they continue or are bothersome**
Incidence more frequent
    *Gouty arthritis, acute attack* (joint pain; redness; swelling); *headache; loss of appetite; nausea or vomiting, mild*
    Note: An increase in the frequency of *acute attacks of gout* during the first few months of therapy may be anticipated, unless adequate prophylaxis with colchicine (or, if the patient is unable to take colchicine, a nonsteroidal anti-inflammatory drug [NSAID]) is given concurrently with the probenecid. Up to 20% of patients started on treatment with probenecid alone may experience acute attacks within the first few days of treatment.

Incidence less frequent
    *Dizziness; flushing or redness of face; frequent urge to urinate; sore gums*

## Overdose

For specific information on the agents in the management of probenecid overdose, see:
    • *Acetazolamide* in *Carbonic Anhydrase Inhibitors (Systemic)* monograph;
    • *Allopurinol (Systemic)* monograph;
    • *Diazepam* in *Benzodiazepines (Systemic)* monograph; and/or
    • *Potassium Citrate* in *Citrates (Systemic)* monograph.

For more information on the management of overdose or unintentional ingestion, **contact a Poison Control Center** (see *Poison Control Center Listing*).

**Clinical effects of overdose**
The following effects have been selected on the basis of their potential clinical significance (possible signs and symptoms in parentheses where appropriate)—not necessarily inclusive:

Acute
    Note: One case of overdose has been reported, in which an extremely high dose (> 45 grams) produced central nervous system (CNS) stimulation, clonic-tonic seizures, severe vomiting, and respiratory failure.

**Treatment of overdose**
Specific treatment—
For uric acid calculi or urate nephropathy:
Recommended measures include administration of large quantities of fluids and of allopurinol to increase urine flow and reduce uric acid formation, respectively. A urinary pH of 6 to 6.5 should be achieved and maintained by administration of alkali such as potassium citrate. If necessary to maintain the desired urinary pH through the night acetazolamide may also be given at bedtime. Other interventions designed to facilitate removal of renal calculi may also be needed. See the package inserts or *Acetazolamide* in *Carbonic Anhydrase Inhibitors (Systemic)*, *Allopurinol (Systemic)*, or *Potassium Citrate* in *Citrates (Systemic)* for specific dosing guidelines for use of these products.

For convulsions:
Administering appropriate anticonvulsive therapy such as intravenous diazepam. See the package insert or *Diazepam* in *Benzodiazepines (Systemic)* for specific dosing guidelines for use of this product.

Supportive care—General measures, such as monitoring the patient and instituting supportive treatment as needed. Patients in whom intentional overdose is known or suspected should be referred for psychiatric consultation.

## Patient Consultation

As an aid to patient consultation, refer to *Advice for the Patient, Probenecid (Systemic)*.

In providing consultation, consider emphasizing the following selected information (»= major clinical significance):

**Before using this medication**
»   Conditions affecting use, especially:
    Allergic reaction to probenecid, history of
    Pregnancy—Probenecid crosses the placenta
    Other medications, especially antibiotics, antivirals, indomethacin, ketoprofen, antineoplastic agents, aspirin or other salicylates, including bismuth subsalicylate (when probenecid used as antihyperuricemic or antigout agent), heparin, methotrexate, nitrofurantoin, or zidovudine
    Other medical problems, especially cancer being treated by cytolytic medication or radiation (x-ray) therapy; kidney stones or other kidney problems, especially if caused by uric acid, or history of; renal function impairment; and blood dyscrasias

**Proper use of this medication**
    Taking with food or an antacid to minimize gastric irritation
    Missed dose: Taking as soon as possible; not taking if almost time for next dose; not doubling doses
»   Proper dosing
»   Proper storage
*For use as antigout agent*
    Several months of continuous therapy may be required for maximum effectiveness
»   Medication does not relieve acute attacks but rather helps to prevent them; need to continue taking probenecid with medication prescribed for gout attacks
*For use as antihyperuricemic (including gout therapy)*
    Importance of high fluid intake and compliance with therapy for alkalinization of urine, if prescribed

**Precautions while using this medication**
    Regular visits to physician to check progress during long-term therapy
    Caution if any laboratory tests required; possible interference with test results
    Diabetics: May cause false results with copper sulfate urine sugar tests, but not with glucose enzymatic urine sugar tests
*For use as antihyperuricemic (including gout therapy)*
»   Aspirin or other salicylates may decrease uricosuric effects of probenecid; checking with physician regarding concurrent use, since effect is dependent on salicylate dose and duration of use
»   Possibility that alcohol taken in large amounts may increase blood uric acid concentration and reduce effectiveness of medication

**Side/adverse effects**
    Signs and symptoms of potential side effects, especially renal calculi, allergic dermatitis, anaphylaxis, anemia, aplastic anemia, hemolytic anemia, fever, hepatic necrosis, leukopenia, nephrotic syndrome, pain in back and/or ribs, renal colic, and urate nephropathy

## General Dosing Information

Probenecid therapy for gouty arthritis should not be initiated until 2 to 3 weeks after an acute attack has subsided. However, if an acute attack occurs in a patient already receiving probenecid, the medication should be continued at the same dose while full therapeutic doses of colchicine or a nonsteroidal anti-inflammatory drug (NSAID) are given to relieve the attack.

Probenecid may be administered with food or an antacid to minimize gastric irritation. A reduction in the dose may reduce gastrointestinal intolerance.

Determination of serum or 24-hour urine uric acid concentrations may be necessary for proper dosing in uricosuric therapy.

To reduce the risk of urate stone formation in patients with hyperuricemia, a high fluid intake (no less than 2.5 to 3 liters daily) and maintenance of an alkaline urine by administration of sodium bicarbonate (3 to 7.5 grams daily), potassium citrate (7.5 grams daily), or acetazolamide (250 mg daily) are recommended. The risk of urate stone formation is highest during the first few weeks of therapy, when urate excretion is high; after hyperuricemia has been controlled, and urinary excretion of uric acid decreases, the need for these measures is reduced.

Since probenecid may increase the frequency of acute attacks of gout during the early months of therapy, prophylactic doses of colchicine (or, if the patient cannot take colchicine, an NSAID) should be administered concurrently during the first 3 to 6 months of probenecid therapy. However, even with colchicine prophylactic therapy, acute attacks of gout requiring treatment with full therapeutic doses of colchicine or an NSAID may occur.

In gouty arthritis, higher doses may be required for patients with mild renal function impairment. However, it is recommended that dosage be reduced in geriatric patients with possible renal function impairment.

Probenecid is included as an adjunct to antibiotic therapy in some of the U.S. Centers for Disease Control (CDC) recommendations for the treatment of sexually transmitted diseases. The current CDC recommendations may be consulted for a complete description of all of the recommended treatment regimens.

## Oral Dosage Forms

### PROBENECID TABLETS USP

**Usual adult and adolescent dose**
Antigout agent or
Antihyperuricemic—
    Initial: Oral, 250 mg two times a day for one week.

Maintenance: Oral, 500 mg two times a day. In nongeriatric patients, if this dose does not control symptoms, or if the 24-hour uric acid excretion is not above 700 mg, the daily dose may be increased by 500 mg per day at 4-week intervals, if necessary, up to a maximum of 3 grams per day.

Note: The initial dose may be eliminated, and treatment started with the usual maintenance dose, when patients previously controlled with other uricosuric therapy are transferred to probenecid.

When acute attacks of gout have not occurred for at least 6 months, and the serum uric acid concentrations remain within normal limits, the daily dose of probenecid may be reduced by 500 mg every 6 months until the lowest effective maintenace dose is reached.

Antibiotic therapy adjunct—

Penicillin or cephalosporin therapy (general): Oral, 500 mg four times a day. If the antibiotic is being administered parenterally, the probenecid should be administered at least thirty minutes prior to the antibiotic.

Treatment of sexually transmitted diseases: Oral, 1 gram as a single dose, administered simultaneously or concurrently with appropriate antibiotic therapy.

Note: For treatment of neurosyphilis—Oral, 500 mg four times a day, concurrently with one dose of 2.4 million units of penicillin G procaine per day, for ten to fourteen days.

### Usual adult prescribing limits

Antigout agent or
antihyperuricemic agent—
Oral, 3 grams per day.

### Usual pediatric dose

Antihyperuricemic—
Dosage has not been established.

Antibiotic therapy adjunct—

Penicillin or cephalosporin therapy (general):
Children up to 2 years of age—Use is not recommended.
Children 2 to 14 years of age or
Children weighing up to 50 kg—Oral, initially 25 mg per kg of body weight or 700 mg per square meter of body surface area, then 10 mg per kg of body weight or 300 mg per square meter of body surface area, four times a day.
Children weighing over 50 kg—See *Usual adult and adolescent dose*.

Note: If the antibiotic is being administered parenterally, the probenecid should be administered at least thirty minutes prior to the antibiotic.

Treatment of gonorrhea:
Postpubertal children and/or children weighing over 45 kg—Oral, 1 gram as a single dose, administered simultaneously or concurrently with appropriate antibiotic therapy.

### Strength(s) usually available

U.S.—
500 mg (Rx) [*Benemid* (scored); *Probalan;* GENERIC].
Canada—
500 mg (OTC) [*Benemid* (scored); *Benuryl*].

### Packaging and storage

Store below 40 °C (104 °F), preferably between 15 and 30 °C (59 and 86 °F), unless otherwise specified by manufacturer. Store in a well-closed container.

Revised: 09/01/92

---

# PROBENECID AND COLCHICINE   Systemic

VA CLASSIFICATION (Primary): MS400

NOTE: The *Probenecid and Colchicine (Systemic)* monograph is maintained on the USP DI electronic data base. For a printed copy of the most recent revision of the complete monograph, contact the USP Division of Information Development, 12601 Twinbrook Parkway, Rockville, MD 20852.

For information on the specific components of this combination, see the *USP DI* monographs for *Colchicine (Systemic)* and *Probenecid (Systemic)*.

The information that follows is selectively abstracted from the complete monograph and is provided to facilitate drug use review and patient counseling.

Note: For a listing of dosage forms and brand names by country availability, see *Dosage Forms* section(s). For a listing of brand names for the articles in this monograph, refer to the General Index.

## Category

Antigout agent.

## Indications

### Accepted

Gouty arthritis, chronic (treatment)—Probenecid and colchicine combination is indicated for the treatment of chronic gouty arthritis in patients having frequent, recurrent acute attacks.

Probenecid is used to control hyperuricemia. Therapy with this uricosuric agent is recommended only for patients whose 24-hour renal excretion of urate is 800 mg (4.8 mmol) or lower (i.e., patients who are hyperuricemic as a result of underexcretion, rather than overproduction, of urate). The aim of probenecid therapy is to reduce the number of acute gout attacks. Probenecid therapy should not be initiated during an acute attack because it may produce fluctuations in urate concentration that may result in prolongation of the attack or initiation of a new attack. Even when probenecid therapy is started several weeks after an acute attack, the frequency of acute attacks may be increased during the early months of therapy. Therefore, prophylactic doses of the colchicine in this combination medication are usually administered for the first 3 to 6 months of probenecid therapy.

### Unaccepted

Probenecid is not recommended in circumstances in which there is an especially high risk of adverse effects associated with crystallization and deposition of urate in renal tissues, such as formation of renal calculi and uric acid nephropathy. It therefore should not be used for treatment of gout in patients whose 24-hour urate excretion exceeds 800 mg (4.8 mmol) or who have extensive tophi. Allopurinol, which decreases the quantity of urate that reaches the kidneys in addition to decreasing the concentration of urate in the blood, is recommended in these circumstances.

## Patient Consultation

As an aid to patient consultation, refer to *Advice for the Patient, Probenecid and Colchicine (Systemic)*.

In providing consultation, consider emphasizing the following selected information (» = major clinical significance):

### Before using this medication

» Conditions affecting use, especially:
Allergic reaction to probenecid or sensitivity to colchicine, history of
Pregnancy—Probenecid crosses the placenta; colchicine reported to be teratogenic in humans
Use in the elderly—Increased susceptibility to cumulative colchicine toxicity
Other medications, especially antibiotics, antivirals, bone marrow depressants or blood dyscrasia–causing medications, indomethacin, ketoprofen, antineoplastic agents, aspirin or other salicylates, including bismuth subsalicylate, heparin, methotrexate, nitrofurantoin, or zidovudine
Other medical problems, especially alcohol abuse, severe cardiac or gastrointestinal disorders; cancer being treated by cytolytic medication or radiation (x-ray) therapy; kidney stones or other kidney problems, especially if caused by uric acid, or history of; renal function impairment; hepatic function impairment; stomach ulcer or other stomach problems, and blood dyscrasias

### Proper use of this medication

Taking with food or an antacid to minimize gastric irritation
Importance of not taking more medication than the amount prescribed
Several months of continuous therapy may be required for maximum effectiveness

» Medication does not relieve acute attacks of gout but rather helps to prevent them; need to continue taking probenecid and colchicine with medication prescribed for gout attacks

Importance of high fluid intake and compliance with therapy for alkalinization of urine, if prescribed

» Proper dosing

Missed dose: Taking as soon as possible; not taking if almost time for next dose; not doubling doses

» Proper storage

**Precautions while using this medication**

Regular visits to physician to check progress during therapy

Caution if any laboratory tests required; possible interference with test results

Diabetics: May cause false results with copper sulfate urine sugar tests, but not with glucose enzymatic urine sugar tests

» Aspirin or other salicylates may decrease uricosuric effects of probenecid; checking with physician regarding concurrent use, since effect is dependent on salicylate dose and duration of use

» Possibility that alcohol taken in large amounts may increase the risk of colchicine-induced gastrointestinal toxicity; also, may increase uric acid concentrations and thereby reduce effectiveness of medication

» For patients taking high doses (4 tablets a day): Discontinuing at once and notifying physician as soon as possible if symptoms of gastrointestinal toxicity occur

**Side/adverse effects**

Signs and symptoms of potential side effects, especially renal calculi, allergic dermatitis, anaphylaxis, anemia, aplastic anemia, hemolytic anemia, fever, hepatic necrosis, leukopenia, nephrotic syndrome, pain in back and/or ribs, renal colic, urate nephropathy, colchicine-induced gastrointestinal toxicity, and peripheral neuritis

## Oral Dosage Forms

### PROBENECID AND COLCHICINE TABLETS USP

**Usual adult dose**

Antigout agent—

Initial: Oral, 1 tablet a day for one week.

Maintenance: Oral, 1 tablet two times a day. In nongeriatric patients, if this dose does not control symptoms or if the 24-hour uric acid excretion is not above 700 mg, the daily dosage may be increased by 1 tablet every four weeks as tolerated (usually not above 4 tablets per day). If the increase in colchicine dosage is not desired or tolerated, administration of additional probenecid alone may be required.

Note: The initial dose may be eliminated, and treatment started with the usual maintenance dose, when patients previously controlled with other uricosuric therapy are transferred to probenecid.

When acute attacks of gout have not occurred for at least six months, and the serum uric acid concentrations remain within normal limits, the daily dose may be reduced by 1 tablet every six months until the lowest effective maintenance dose is reached. Alternatively, prophylactic use of colchicine may be discontinued and the patient treated with maintenance doses of probenecid alone.

**Usual pediatric dose**

Dosage has not been established.

**Strength(s) usually available**

U.S.—

500 mg of probenecid and 500 mcg (0.5 mg) of colchicine (Rx) [ColBenemid; Col-Probenecid; Proben-C; GENERIC].

Revised: 09/09/92
Interim revision: 08/27/94

---

## PROBENECID-CONTAINING COMBINATIONS—

Probenecid and Colchicine (Systemic)

---

# PROBUCOL   Systemic

VA CLASSIFICATION (Primary): CV350

Note: For a listing of dosage forms and brand names by country availability, see Dosage Forms section(s). For a listing of brand names for the articles in this monograph, refer to the General Index.

## Category

Antihyperlipidemic.

## Indications

**Accepted**

Hyperlipidemia (treatment)—Probucol is recommended for use as an adjunct to dietary measures in patients with primary hypercholesterolemia (type IIa hyperlipoproteinemia) and a significant risk of coronary artery disease, who have not responded to diet or other measures alone. Probucol reduces plasma cholesterol concentrations, but has a variable effect on serum triglyceride concentrations, and so is not useful in patients with elevated triglyceride concentrations alone. Its use is limited in other types of hyperlipidemia (including type IIb) because it may cause further elevation of triglycerides. Its main advantage over the anion exchange resins is its ease of administration and better acceptance and tolerance by the patient.

For additional information on initial therapeutic guidelines related to the treatment of hyperlipidemia, see Appendix III.

## Pharmacology/Pharmacokinetics

**Physicochemical characteristics**

Molecular weight—516.84.

**Mechanism of action/Effect**

Lorelco lowers serum cholesterol by increasing the fractional rate of low-density lipoprotein (LDL) catabolism in the final metabolic pathway for cholesterol elimination from the body. Additionally, probucol may inhibit early stages of cholesterol biosynthesis and slightly inhibit dietary cholesterol absorption. Recent information suggests that probucol

may inhibit the oxidation and tissue deposition of LDL cholesterol, thereby inhibiting atherogenesis.

**Absorption**

Absorption from the gastrointestinal tract is limited and variable (about 7%).

**Distribution**

Accumulates in fat tissue with prolonged treatment.

**Half-life**

Ranges from 12 hours to more than 500 hours, the longest half-life probably being in adipose tissue.

**Time to peak plasma concentration**

Plasma concentrations increase slowly and reach steady state after 3 to 4 months; they also decline slowly after withdrawal, by 60% after 6 weeks and by 80% after 6 months.

**Time to peak effect**

Maximal reduction in plasma cholesterol concentrations usually occurs within 20 to 50 days after initiation of probucol therapy, although a further decrease may occur gradually over several months. A clinical response usually occurs within 1 to 3 months.

**Elimination**

Biliary (slowly in the feces).

Renal, very little (mainly as unchanged drug).

## Precautions to Consider

**Carcinogenicity**

Two-year studies in rats did not reveal carcinogenicity.

**Mutagenicity**

Mutagenic studies were negative.

**Pregnancy/Reproduction**

Fertility—Studies in rats and rabbits did not reveal adverse effects on fertility.

Pregnancy—Studies in humans have not been done.

Studies in rats and rabbits at doses up to 50 times the human dose have not shown that probucol causes adverse effects on the fetus.

FDA Pregnancy Category B.

### Breast-feeding

It is not known whether probucol is distributed into human breast milk. However, it is distributed into the milk of animals. Use of probucol while breast-feeding is not recommended, because of potentially serious adverse effects on nursing infants.

### Pediatrics

Appropriate studies on the relationship of age to the effects of probucol have not been performed in the pediatric population. However, use in children under 2 years of age is not recommended since cholesterol is required for normal development.

### Geriatrics

No information is available on the relationship of age to the effects of probucol in geriatric patients.

### Drug interactions and/or related problems

The following drug interactions and/or related problems have been selected on the basis of their potential clinical significance (possible mechanism in parentheses where appropriate)—not necessarily inclusive (» = major clinical significance):

Note: Combinations containing any of the following medications, depending on the amount present, may also interact with this medication.

Antiarrhythmics with QT interval prolongation, such as:
Amiodarone
Bretylium
Disopyramide
Encainide
Flecainide
Lidocaine
Mexiletine
Moricizine
Procainamide
Propafenone
Quinidine
Sotalol
Tocainide or
Antidepressants, tricyclic or
Phenothiazines
(additive QT interval prolongation may increase risk of ventricular tachycardia)

Beta-adrenergic blocking agents or
Digoxin
(the effect of beta-adrenergic blocking agents on the atrial rate and the effect of digoxin on AV block can cause bradycardia; when these medications are given in conjunction with a medication that prolongs the QT interval [i.e. probucol], the risk of ventricular tachycardia may be increased)

Chenodiol or
Ursodiol
(effect may be decreased when chenodiol or ursodiol is used concurrently with antihyperlipidemics since they tend to increase cholesterol saturation of bile)

### Laboratory value alterations

The following have been selected on the basis of their potential clinical significance (possible effect in parentheses where appropriate)—not necessarily inclusive (» = major clinical significance):

With physiology/laboratory test values
Alanine aminotransferase (ALT [SGPT]), serum and
Alkaline phosphatase, serum and
Aspartate aminotransferase (AST [SGOT]), serum and
Bilirubin and
Blood urea nitrogen (BUN) and
Creatine phosphokinase (CPK) and
Glucose, blood, and
Uric acid, serum
(concentrations may be slightly increased)
Electrocardiogram (ECG)
(QT interval prolongation may occur)
Eosinophil concentrations in blood and
Hematocrit and
Hemoglobin concentrations
(may be decreased)

### Medical considerations/Contraindications

The medical considerations/contraindications included here have been selected on the basis of their potential clinical significance (reasons given in parentheses where appropriate)—not necessarily inclusive (» = major clinical significance).

***Except under special circumstances, this medication should not be used when the following medical problems exist:***

» Primary biliary cirrhosis
(may further raise the cholesterol concentration)

» QT interval prolongation
(probucol may prolong QT interval)

***Risk-benefit should be considered when the following medical problems exist:***

Bradycardia, intrinsic, severe or
Hypokalemia or
Hypomagnesemia
(the risk of ventricular tachycardia may be increased because probucol prolongs the QT interval)

» Cardiac arrhythmias or evidence of recent or progressive myocardial damage
(condition may be exacerbated; probucol should be used only with periodic electrocardiogram [ECG] monitoring)

» Congestive heart failure, unresponsive or
Gallstones
(conditions may be exacerbated)

Hepatic function impairment
(higher blood levels of probucol may result)

Sensitivity to probucol

### Patient monitoring

The following may be especially important in patient monitoring (other tests may be warranted in some patients, depending on condition; » = major clinical significance):

» Cholesterol, serum and
» Triglycerides, serum
(determinations recommended prior to initiation of therapy and every 3 to 4 months during therapy to confirm efficacy; if an increase in serum triglyceride concentrations occurs, adjustment of the diet is recommended; if the increase persists, it is recommended that probucol therapy be withdrawn)

ECG
(recommended at periodic intervals in patients with a history of cardiac arrhythmias; probucol therapy should be withdrawn if cardiac arrhythmias or a prolonged QT interval occurs)

## Side/Adverse Effects

Note: Prolongation of QT interval associated with serious arrhythmias has been reported in patients treated with probucol.

The following side/adverse effects have been selected on the basis of their potential clinical significance (possible signs and symptoms in parentheses where appropriate)—not necessarily inclusive:

### Those indicating need for medical attention

Incidence more frequent
***Eosinophilia; QT interval prolongation and ventricular arrhythmias*** (dizziness or fainting; pounding heartbeat; fast or irregular heartbeat)

Incidence rare
***Anemia*** (unusual tiredness or weakness); ***angioneurotic edema*** (swellings on face, hands, or feet, or in mouth); ***thrombocytopenia*** (unusual bleeding or bruising)

### Those indicating need for medical attention only if they continue or are bothersome

Incidence more frequent
***Gastrointestinal irritation*** (bloating; diarrhea; nausea and vomiting; stomach pain)

Note: *Gastrointestinal irritation* is usually transient and mild.

Incidence less frequent
***Dizziness; headache; paresthesia*** (numbness or tingling of fingers, toes, or face)

## Patient Consultation

As an aid to patient consultation, refer to *Advice for the Patient, Probucol (Systemic).*

In providing consultation, consider emphasizing the following selected information (» = major clinical significance):

### Before using this medication

Diet as preferred therapy; importance of following prescribed diet
» Conditions affecting use, especially:
Sensitivity to probucol

Breast-feeding—Use not recommended because of potentially serious adverse effects on nursing infants

Use in children—Not recommended in children under 2 years of age since cholesterol is required for normal development

Other medical problems, especially primary biliary cirrhosis, and cardiac abnormalities including congestive heart failure and QT interval prolongation

### Proper use of this medication
» Importance of not taking more or less medication than the amount prescribed

This medication does not cure the condition but rather helps control it
» Compliance with prescribed diet

Taking with meals, since medication is more effective with food
» Proper dosing

Missed dose: Taking as soon as possible; not taking if almost time for next dose; not doubling doses
» Proper storage

### Precautions while using this medication
» Importance of close monitoring by the physician
» Checking with physician before discontinuing medication; blood lipid concentrations may increase significantly

### Side/adverse effects
Signs of potential side effects, especially angioneurotic edema, blood dyscrasias, QT interval prolongation, and tachycardia

## General Dosing Information

See also *Patient Monitoring*.

If unexplained or cardiovascular-related syncope occurs, probucol therapy should be withdrawn and ECG monitored.

If response is inadequate after 4 months of treatment, probucol therapy should be re-evaluated and possibly withdrawn, except in the case of xanthoma tuberosum, which may require up to 1 year of treatment as long as reduction in size and/or number of xanthomata occurs.

When probucol is discontinued, an appropriate hypolipidemic diet and monitoring of serum lipids are recommended until the patient stabilizes, since a rise in serum cholesterol concentrations to or above the original base may occur.

### Diet/Nutrition
It is recommended that probucol be taken with food to maximize absorption.

## Oral Dosage Forms
### PROBUCOL TABLETS
**Usual adult dose**
Antihyperlipidemic—
Oral, 500 mg two times a day with the morning and evening meals.

**Usual pediatric dose**
Dosage has not been established.

**Strength(s) usually available**
U.S.—
250 mg (Rx) [*Lorelco* (lactose; polysorbate 80)].
500 mg (Rx) [*Lorelco* (lactose; polysorbate 80)].
Canada—
250 mg (Rx) [*Lorelco*].

**Packaging and storage**
Store below 40 °C (104 °F), preferably between 15 and 30 °C (59 and 86 °F), in a well-closed, light-resistant container, unless otherwise specified by manufacturer.

**Auxiliary labeling**
• Take with meals.

## Selected Bibliography
Howard P. Probucol in hypercholesterolemia. Ann Pharmacother 1989; 23: 880-1.

National Cholesterol Education Program. Second Report of the Expert Panel on Detection, Evaluation, and Treatment of High Blood Cholesterol in Adults (Adult Treatment Panel II). Circulation 1994; 89 (3): 1329-445.

Knodel LC, Talbert RL. Adverse effects of hypolipidaemic drugs. Med Toxicol 1987; 2: 10-32.

Revised: 04/13/93
Interim revision: 06/28/95

---

# PROCAINAMIDE   Systemic

VA CLASSIFICATION (Primary): CV300
Note: For a listing of dosage forms and brand names by country availability, see *Dosage Forms* section(s). For a listing of brand names for the articles in this monograph, refer to the General Index.

## Category
Antiarrhythmic.

## Indications
Note: Bracketed information in the *Indications* section refers to uses that are not included in U.S. product labeling.

### Accepted
Arrhythmias, ventricular (treatment)—Procainamide is indicated in the treatment of life-threatening ventricular arrhythmias, such as sustained ventricular tachycardia. Parenteral procainamide also is indicated for treatment of ventricular extrasystoles and cardiac arrhythmias associated with anesthesia and surgery.

[Arrhythmias, supraventricular (treatment)]—Procainamide is used for the conversion and management of atrial fibrillation and paroxysmal atrial tachycardia.

## Pharmacology/Pharmacokinetics

### Physicochemical characteristics
Molecular weight—271.79.
pKa—9.23.

### Mechanism of action/Effect
Direct cardiac effect—Decreases excitability, conduction velocity, automaticity, and membrane responsiveness with prolonged refractory period. No effect on contractility or cardiac output unless myocardial damage present. Larger doses may induce atrioventricular (AV) block.

In the Vaughan Williams classification of antiarrhythmics, procainamide is considered to be a Class I antiarrhythmic.

### Other actions/effects
Relatively weak anticholinergic action diminishes vagal transmission, resulting in increased heart rate, usually with higher dosages. Alpha-adrenergic blockade does not occur. Also causes peripheral vasodilation.

### Absorption
Oral—Rapid; 75 to 95% complete but may vary.
Intramuscular—Rapid.
Intravenous—Immediate.

### Protein binding
Low (15 to 20%).

### Biotransformation
Hepatic; approximately 25% of dose is converted to the active metabolite *N*-acetylprocainamide (NAPA); up to 40% conversion occurs in patients who are rapid acetylators or those with renal function impairment.

### Half-life
Procainamide—About 2.5 to 4.5 hours (11 to 20 hours in renal function impairment).

*N*-acetylprocainamide—About 6 hours.

### Therapeutic serum concentration
Procainamide—4 to 10 mg per L; higher levels may be needed in some patients such as those with sustained ventricular tachycardia.
NAPA—10 to 30 mg per L.

### Time to peak effect
Oral—60 to 90 minutes.
Intravenous—Immediately.
Intramuscular—15 to 60 minutes.

**Elimination**

Renal, 50 to 60% unchanged. The cardioactive metabolite, NAPA, has a slower excretion rate than the parent compound. In cases of renal function impairment or congestive heart failure, this metabolite tends to accumulate rapidly in the serum to toxic concentrations, while the serum concentration of procainamide appears to be within acceptable limits.

In dialysis—Procainamide and NAPA are removable by hemodialysis but not by peritoneal dialysis.

# Precautions to Consider

**Cross-sensitivity and/or related problems**

Patients sensitive to procaine or other related agents may be sensitive to procainamide also.

**Carcinogenicity/Mutagenicity**

Long-term studies in animals have not been done.

**Pregnancy/Reproduction**

Pregnancy—Procainamide crosses the placenta. Adequate and well-controlled studies have not been done in humans. Some reports of procainamide use in pregnant women seem to indicate that although procainamide and N-acetylprocainamide (NAPA) appear in fetal serum, no adverse effects on the fetus or neonate have been noted. However, there is a potential risk of drug accumulation and maternal hypotension leading to uteroplacental insufficiency and ventricular arrhythmias.

FDA Pregnancy Category C.

**Breast-feeding**

Procainamide and NAPA are distributed into breast milk.

**Pediatrics**

Appropriate studies on the relationship of age to the effects of procainamide have not been performed in the pediatric population. Occasional use in pediatric patients has not demonstrated pediatrics-specific problems that would limit the usefulness of procainamide in these patients. However, dosage requirements to achieve and maintain effective therapeutic concentrations may be higher in some pediatric patients than in adults.

**Geriatrics**

Appropriate studies on the relationship of age to the effects of procainamide have not been performed in the geriatric population. However, elderly patients may be more prone to hypotension, especially with parenteral use or when very high doses are given. In addition, elderly patients are more likely to have age-related renal function impairment, which may require lower doses in patients receiving procainamide.

**Dental**

The leukopenic and thrombocytopenic effects of procainamide may result in an increased incidence of microbial infection, delayed healing, and gingival bleeding. If leukopenia or thrombocytopenia occurs, dental work should be deferred until blood counts have returned to normal, and patients should be instructed in proper oral hygiene, including caution in use of regular toothbrushes, dental floss, and toothpicks.

The secondary anticholinergic effects of procainamide may decrease or inhibit salivary flow, especially in middle-aged or elderly patients, thus contributing to the development of caries, periodontal disease, oral candidiasis, and discomfort.

**Drug interactions and/or related problems**

The following drug interactions and/or related problems have been selected on the basis of their potential clinical significance (possible mechanism in parentheses where appropriate)—not necessarily inclusive (» = major clinical significance):

Note: Combinations containing any of the following medications, depending on the amount present, may also interact with this medication.

» Antiarrhythmics, other
(concurrent use with procainamide may produce additive cardiac effects)

Anticholinergics, especially atropine or related compounds (see *Appendix II* ), or
Antidyskinetics or
Antihistamines
(concurrent use with procainamide may intensify atropine-like side effects because of the secondary anticholinergic activities of procainamide; patients should be advised to report occurrence of gastrointestinal problems promptly since paralytic ileus may occur with concurrent therapy)

» Antihypertensives
(concurrent use with procainamide, especially intravenous procainamide, may produce additive hypotensive effects)

» Antimyasthenics
(neuromuscular blocking action and/or secondary anticholinergic activity of procainamide may antagonize the effect of antimyasthenics on skeletal muscle; dosage adjustments of antimyasthenics may be necessary to control symptoms of myasthenia gravis)

Bethanechol
(concurrent use with procainamide may antagonize the cholinergic effects of bethanechol)

Bone marrow depressants (see *Appendix II* )
(concurrent use of procainamide with these medications may increase the leukopenic and/or thrombocytopenic effects; if concurrent use is required, close observation for toxic effects should be considered)

Bretylium
(concurrent administration may counteract inotropic effect of bretylium and potentiate hypotension)

» Neuromuscular blocking agents
(effects of these medications may be prolonged or enhanced when they are used concurrently with procainamide; careful postoperative monitoring of the patient may be necessary following concurrent or sequential use, especially if there is a possibility of incomplete reversal of neuromuscular blockade)

» Pimozide
(concurrent use with procainamide may potentiate cardiac arrhythmias, which are seen on electrocardiogram [ECG] as prolongation of QT interval)

**Laboratory value alterations**

The following have been selected on the basis of their potential clinical significance (possible effect in parentheses where appropriate)—not necessarily inclusive (» = major clinical significance):

With diagnostic test results

Bentiromide
(administration of procainamide during a bentiromide test period will invalidate test results since procainamide is also metabolized to arylamines and will thus increase the percent of para-aminobenzoic acid [PABA] recovered; discontinuation of procainamide at least 3 days prior to the administration of bentiromide is recommended)

Edrophonium tests
(may be altered)

With physiology/laboratory test values

Alanine aminotransferase (ALT [SGPT]), serum and
Alkaline phosphatase, serum and
Aspartate aminotransferase (AST [SGOT]), serum and
Bilirubin, serum and
Lactate dehydrogenase (LDH), serum
(concentrations may be increased)

Antinuclear antibody (ANA) titers
(occur in 60 to 70% of patients after 1 to 2 months of procainamide therapy; may increase with continued therapy)

Direct antiglobulin (Coombs') tests
(may produce positive results)

ECG changes such as:
QRS widening, and less frequently
PR and QT prolongation and
Reduced voltage of QRS and T waves
(may occur with large doses)

Leukocyte counts, including neutrophils and
Platelet counts
(may rarely be decreased)

**Medical considerations/Contraindications**

The medical considerations/contraindications included here have been selected on the basis of their potential clinical significance (reasons given in parentheses where appropriate)—not necessarily inclusive (» = major clinical significance).

*Except under special circumstances, this medication should not be used when the following medical problems exist:*

» Atrioventricular (AV) block, complete, and also 2nd and 3rd degree AV block unless controlled by electrical pacemaker
(risk of additive cardiac depression)

» Torsades de pointes
(procainamide may aggravate this arrhythmia)

*Risk-benefit should be considered when the following medical problems exist:*

» AV block or
» Bundle branch block or

>> Digitalis intoxication, severe
    (risk of additive cardiac depression and ventricular asystole or fibrillation)
  Bronchial asthma
    (possible hypersensitivity)
>> Congestive heart failure or
  Hepatic function impairment or
>> Renal function impairment
    (possible accumulation leading to toxicity; lower doses may be required in patients with congestive heart failure or renal function impairment)
>> Lupus erythematosus, history of
    (procainamide may precipitate active lupus)
>> Myasthenia gravis
    (procainamide may increase muscle weakness)
  Sensitivity to procainamide
>> Ventricular tachycardia during an occlusive coronary episode

### Patient monitoring

The following may be especially important in patient monitoring (other tests may be warranted in some patients, depending on condition; » = major clinical significance):

Antinuclear antibody (ANA) titers
    (recommended at periodic intervals during prolonged use of procainamide or if symptoms of a lupus-like reaction occur; procainamide should be withdrawn if a steady increase in ANA titer occurs)

Blood pressure determinations and
>> Cardiac function monitoring, including ECG
    (recommended at periodic intervals with oral therapy and concurrently with parenteral administration; procainamide should be withdrawn if an excessive blood pressure reduction or QRS widening occurs, and immediately if signs of impending heart block occur)

Complete blood cell counts (especially leukocyte counts)
    (recommended every 2 weeks during the first 3 months of therapy, then at longer intervals throughout maintenance, especially in patients taking the extended-release dosage form or after cardiovascular surgery; procainamide should be withdrawn if leukocyte counts fall)

Plasma procainamide and *N*-acetylprocainamide (NAPA) concentrations
    (recommended at periodic intervals to aid in dosage adjustment, especially in patients with congestive heart failure or hepatic or renal function impairment, and when switching from regular oral to extended-release dosage form; risk of toxicity may be increased when the summed concentration of procainamide and NAPA exceeds 25 to 30 mg/L)

## Side/Adverse Effects

Note: Agranulocytosis, bone marrow depression, neutropenia, hypoplastic anemia, and thrombocytopenia have been reported with an incidence of about 0.5% in patients receiving procainamide. Fatalities have been reported, especially in cases of agranulocytosis (20 to 25% mortality in reported cases). Most cases have been noted in the first 12 weeks of therapy.

In the National Heart, Lung, and Blood Institute's Cardiac Arrhythmias Suppression Trial (CAST), treatment with encainide or flecainide was found to be associated with excessive mortality or increased nonfatal cardiac arrest rate, as compared with placebo, in patients with asymptomatic, non–life-threatening arrhythmias who had a recent myocardial infarction. The implications of these results for other patient populations or other antiarrhythmic agents are uncertain.

Tachycardia may occur at high plasma procainamide concentrations as a reflex sympathetic response to the hypotensive effect, due to the anticholinergic effect on the atrioventricular (AV) node, or in response to slowing of the atrial rate in treatment of atrial fibrillation. Tachycardia is especially hazardous in patients with myocardial damage, because of the risk of emboli. Adequate digitalization reduces, but does not abolish, the risk.

Intravenous administration may cause a transient but sometimes severe reduction in blood pressure, especially in conscious patients. Hypotension is less frequent with intramuscular administration and rare with oral use (except with excessive doses).

Ventricular asystole or fibrillation may occur, especially with too-rapid intravenous administration or excessive doses; death has occurred rarely.

The following side/adverse effects have been selected on the basis of their potential clinical significance (possible signs and symptoms in parentheses where appropriate)—not necessarily inclusive:

### Those indicating need for medical attention

Incidence less frequent
  *Allergic reaction or systemic lupus erythematosus (SLE)–like syndrome* (fever and chills; joint pain or swelling; pains with breathing; skin rash or itching)
  Note: After extended maintenance therapy nearly 80% of patients treated show an increased titer of antinuclear antibodies (an early sign of developing SLE), often within 1 to 12 months of commencing therapy. Nearly 30% of these patients develop clinical symptoms that resemble SLE. This *SLE-like condition* is usually reversible with discontinuation of procainamide therapy.

Incidence rare
  *Central nervous system (CNS) effects* (confusion; hallucinations; mental depression); *Coombs' positive hemolytic anemia* (unusual tiredness or weakness); *leukopenia (neutropenia) and possible agranulocytosis, which may be fatal* (fever, chills, or sore mouth, gums, or throat); *thrombocytopenia* (unusual bleeding or bruising)
  Note: *Coombs' positive hemolytic anemia* may be related to the SLE-like syndrome.
    *Leukopenia* may be more likely to occur with use of the extended-release dosage form, especially after cardiovascular surgery. Leukopenia usually occurs within the first 3 months of therapy, and counts recover within a few weeks after procainamide is withdrawn. Leukopenia also may occur in association with the SLE-like syndrome.
    *Thrombocytopenia* may be related to the SLE-like syndrome.

### Those indicating need for medical attention only if they continue or are bothersome

Incidence more frequent, especially with daily doses > 4 grams
  *Diarrhea; loss of appetite*
Incidence less frequent
  *Dizziness or lightheadedness*

## Overdose

For more information on the management of overdose or unintentional ingestion, **contact a Poison Control Center** (see *Poison Control Center Listing*).

### Clinical effects of overdose

The following effects have been selected on the basis of their potential clinical significance (possible signs and symptoms in parentheses where appropriate)—not necessarily inclusive:

  *Confusion; decrease in urination; dizziness, severe, or fainting; drowsiness; fast or irregular heartbeat; nausea and vomiting*

### Treatment of overdose

Treatment is primarily symptomatic and supportive. Gastric lavage, emesis, hemodialysis, pressor medication, and maintenance of airway are of possible benefit, according to the patient's condition.

## Patient Consultation

As an aid to patient consultation, refer to *Advice for the Patient, Procainamide (Systemic)*.

In providing consultation, consider emphasizing the following selected information (» = major clinical significance):

### Before using this medication

>> Conditions affecting use, especially:
    Sensitivity to procaine or other related agents
    Pregnancy—Procainamide crosses the placenta
    Breast-feeding—Procainamide and NAPA are distributed into breast milk
    Use in children—Higher doses may be needed to maintain adequate therapeutic concentrations in some patients
    Use in the elderly—May be more susceptible to hypotension
    Dental—May be more susceptible to microbial infection, delayed healing, and gingival bleeding because of risk of leukopenia and thrombocytopenia; may cause dryness of mouth
    Other medications, especially other antiarrhythmics, antihypertensives, antimyasthenics, neuromuscular blocking agents, and pimozide
    Other medical problems, especially atrioventricular block, torsades de pointes, severe digitalis intoxication, congestive heart failure, renal function impairment, lupus erythematosus, myasthenia gravis, or ventricular tachycardia during an occlusive coronary episode

## Proper use of this medication

» Taking exactly as directed even if feeling well

Taking on empty stomach for faster absorption, or with food or milk to reduce stomach irritation

Proper administration of extended-release tablets: Swallowing tablets whole, without breaking, crushing, or chewing

» Importance of not missing doses and of taking at evenly spaced intervals

» Proper dosing

Missed dose: Taking as soon as possible if remembered within 2 hours (4 hours for extended-release tablets); not taking if remembered later; not doubling doses

» Proper storage

## Precautions while using this medication

Regular visits to physician to check progress

» Checking with physician before discontinuing medication; gradual dosage reduction may be necessary to avoid worsening of condition

» Caution if any kind of surgery (including dental surgery) or emergency treatment is required

Carrying medical identification card or bracelet

» Possibility of dizziness with high dosage, especially in elderly; caution when driving or doing things requiring alertness

Caution if any laboratory tests required; possible interference with test results

## Side/adverse effects

Signs of potential side effects, especially allergic reaction, SLE-like syndrome, CNS effects, Coombs' positive hemolytic anemia, leukopenia, and thrombocytopenia

Extended-release tablet matrix may be seen in stool and is to be expected

# General Dosing Information

Dosage must be adjusted to meet the individual requirements of each patient, on the basis of clinical response.

Procainamide therapy should be withdrawn if signs or symptoms of systemic lupus erythematosus (SLE)–like syndrome, leukopenia, or hemolytic anemia occur.

## For treatment of atrial fibrillation

Patients should be digitalized prior to administration of procainamide to reduce the risk of enhancing atrioventricular (AV) conduction, which may result in ventricular rate acceleration.

## For oral dosage forms only

A period of 3 to 4 hours should elapse after the last intravenous dose before administration of the first oral dose.

## For parenteral dosage forms only

Procainamide Hydrochloride Injection USP is always diluted before intravenous administration.

Intravenous administration should be limited to hospitals where monitoring facilities are available.

Intramuscular injection usually is used only when the oral or intravenous routes are not feasible.

Procainamide intravenous injection should be administered at a rate not exceeding 50 mg per minute.

Because hypotension may develop rapidly during intravenous administration, it is highly recommended that blood pressure be monitored continuously, with the patient in a supine position. Phenylephrine and norepinephrine injections should be available to counteract severe hypotension.

## Diet/Nutrition

Oral procainamide should preferably be taken with a glass of water on an empty stomach (either 1 hour before or 2 hours after meals) for faster absorption; however, it may be taken with meals or immediately after meals to lessen gastrointestinal irritation.

# Oral Dosage Forms

Note: Bracketed information in the *Indications* section refers to uses that are not included in U.S. product labeling.

## PROCAINAMIDE HYDROCHLORIDE CAPSULES USP

### Usual adult dose

[Atrial arrhythmias]—

Initial: Oral, 1.25 grams, followed in one to two hours by 750 mg if necessary; then 500 mg to 1 gram every two or three hours as needed and tolerated.

Maintenance: Oral, 500 mg to 1 gram every four to six hours, the dosage being adjusted as needed and tolerated.

Ventricular arrhythmias—

Oral, 50 mg per kg of body weight per day in eight divided doses (every three hours), the dosage being adjusted as needed and tolerated.

Note: Geriatric patients may be more sensitive to the hypotensive effects of the usual adult dose.

Geriatric patients or patients with renal, hepatic, or cardiac insufficiency may require lower doses or longer dosing intervals.

### Usual adult prescribing limits

Maintenance—Up to 6 grams daily.

### Usual pediatric dose

Antiarrhythmic—

Oral, 12.5 mg per kg of body weight or 375 mg per square meter of body surface four times a day.

### Strength(s) usually available

U.S.—

250 mg (Rx) [*Promine; Pronestyl* (lactose); GENERIC].

375 mg (Rx) [*Promine; Pronestyl* (lactose); GENERIC].

500 mg (Rx) [*Promine; Pronestyl;* GENERIC].

Canada—

250 mg (Rx) [*Pronestyl*].

375 mg (Rx) [*Pronestyl*].

500 mg (Rx) [*Pronestyl;* GENERIC].

### Packaging and storage

Store below 40 °C (104 °F), preferably between 15 and 30 °C (59 and 86 °F), unless otherwise specified by manufacturer. Store in a tight container.

### Stability

Procainamide is hygroscopic.

### Auxiliary labeling

• Keep container tightly closed.

• Do not take other medicines without your doctor's advice.

## PROCAINAMIDE HYDROCHLORIDE TABLETS USP

### Usual adult dose

See *Procainamide Hydrochloride Capsules USP.*

### Usual pediatric dose

See *Procainamide Hydrochloride Capsules USP.*

### Strength(s) usually available

U.S.—

250 mg (Rx) [*Pronestyl* (tartrazine); GENERIC].

375 mg (Rx) [*Pronestyl* (tartrazine)].

500 mg (Rx) [*Pronestyl* (tartrazine)].

Canada—

Not commercially available.

### Packaging and storage

Store below 40 °C (104 °F), preferably between 15 and 30 °C (59 and 86 °F), unless otherwise specified by manufacturer. Store in a tight container.

### Stability

Procainamide is hygroscopic.

### Auxiliary labeling

• Keep container tightly closed.

• Do not take other medicines without your doctor's advice.

## PROCAINAMIDE HYDROCHLORIDE EXTENDED-RELEASE TABLETS USP

### Usual adult dose

[Atrial arrhythmias]—

Maintenance: Oral, 1 gram every six hours, the dosage being adjusted as needed and tolerated.

Ventricular arrhythmias—

Maintenance: Oral, 50 mg per kg of body weight per day in four divided doses (every six hours), the dosage being adjusted as needed and tolerated.

Note: The extended-release dosage form is intended for maintenance dosage, and not for initial dosage.

Geriatric patients may be more sensitive to the hypotensive effects of the usual adult dose.

### Usual adult prescribing limits

Maintenance—Up to 6 grams daily.

### Usual pediatric dose

Not generally used in children. See instead *Procainamide Hydrochloride Capsules USP.*

## Strength(s) usually available
U.S.—
   250 mg (Rx) [*Procan SR* (lactose; methylparaben; propylparaben); GENERIC].
   500 mg (Rx) [*Procan SR* (scored; lactose; methylparaben; propylparaben); *Pronestyl-SR;* GENERIC].
   750 mg (Rx) [*Procan SR;* GENERIC].
   1 gram (Rx) [*Procan SR*].
Canada—
   250 mg (Rx) [*Procan SR* (lactose; parabens)].
   500 mg (Rx) [*Procan SR* (parabens); *Pronestyl-SR*].
   750 mg (Rx) [*Procan SR* (scored)].
   1 gram (Rx) [*Procan SR* (scored)].

## Packaging and storage
Store below 30 °C (86 °F), unless otherwise specified by manufacturer. Store in a tight container.

## Stability
Procainamide is hygroscopic.

## Auxiliary labeling
• Keep container tightly closed.
• Do not take other medicines without your doctor's advice.
• Swallow tablets whole.

## Note
Extended-release tablets utilize a wax matrix, which may be detected in the stool.

# Parenteral Dosage Forms

## PROCAINAMIDE HYDROCHLORIDE INJECTION USP

### Usual adult dose
Antiarrhythmic—
   Intramuscular:
      50 mg per kg of body weight per day in divided doses given every three to six hours.
   Intravenous:
      Initial—
         Intravenous (direct), 100 mg (diluted in an appropriate volume of 5% dextrose injection to facilitate control of dosage rate) administered slowly (not exceeding 50 mg per minute) and repeated every five minutes until arrhythmia is controlled or up to a maximum total dose of 1 gram, or

Intravenous infusion, 500 to 600 mg diluted and administered at a constant rate over a period of twenty-five to thirty minutes.
   Maintenance—
      Intravenous infusion, diluted and administered at a rate of 2 to 6 mg per minute to maintain control of arrhythmia.

### Usual pediatric dose
Dosage has not been established.

### Strength(s) usually available
U.S.—
   100 mg per mL (Rx) [*Pronestyl* (benzyl alcohol; sodium bisulfite); GENERIC].
   500 mg per mL (Rx) [*Pronestyl* (sodium bisulfite; methylparaben); GENERIC].
Canada—
   100 mg per mL (Rx) [*Pronestyl* (benzyl alcohol; sodium bisulfite)].
   500 mg per mL (Rx) [*Pronestyl* (sodium bisulfite; methylparaben)].

### Packaging and storage
Store between 15 and 30 °C (59 and 86 °F), unless otherwise specified by manufacturer. Protect from freezing. Protect from light.

### Preparation of dosage form
For administration by intravenous infusion, dilute 200 mg to 1 gram of Procainamide Hydrochloride Injection USP to a concentration of 2 or 4 mg per mL using a suitable volume of 5% dextrose injection.

### Stability
A slight yellowing will not alter potency; however, do not use if markedly discolored (darker than light amber) or if a precipitate is present.

Revised: 08/04/93

---

**PROCAINE**—See *Anesthetics (Parenteral-Local)*

---

## PROCAINE-CONTAINING COMBINATIONS—

Propoxycaine, Procaine, and Levonordefrin (Parenteral-Local)—See *Anesthetics (Parenteral-Local)*
Propoxycaine, Procaine, and Norepinephrine (Parenteral-Local)—See *Anesthetics (Parenteral-Local)*

---

# PROCARBAZINE   Systemic

VA CLASSIFICATION (Primary): AN900
Note: For a listing of dosage forms and brand names by country availability, see *Dosage Forms* section(s). For a listing of brand names for the articles in this monograph, refer to the General Index.

## Category
Antineoplastic.

## Indications
Note: Bracketed information in the *Indications* section refers to uses that are not included in U.S. product labeling.

### Accepted
Lymphomas, Hodgkin's (treatment) or
[Lymphomas, non-Hodgkin's (treatment)][1]—Procarbazine is indicated, in combination with other agents, for treatment of Hodgkin's disease (Stage III and IV) and some non-Hodgkin's lymphomas.

[Tumors, brain, primary (treatment)][1] or
[Carcinoma, lung (treatment)][1]—Procarbazine is used for treatment of brain tumors and bronchogenic carcinoma.

[Malignant melanoma (treatment)][1]—Procarbazine is used for treatment of malignant melanoma.

[Multiple myeloma (treatment)][1]—Procarbazine is used for treatment of multiple myeloma.

[Polycythemia vera (treatment)][1]—Procarbazine is used for treatment of polycythemia vera.

---
[1]Not included in Canadian product labeling.

## Pharmacology/Pharmacokinetics

### Physicochemical characteristics
Molecular weight—257.76.

### Mechanism of action/Effect
Procarbazine is an alkylating agent and a monoamine oxidase (MAO) inhibitor. Procarbazine causes weak inhibition of monoamine oxidase (MAO). The exact mechanism of antineoplastic action is unknown but is thought to resemble that of the alkylating agents; procarbazine is cell cycle–specific for the S phase of cell division. Procarbazine is thought to inhibit DNA, RNA, and protein synthesis.

### Other actions/effects
MAO inhibitors prevent the inactivation of tyramine by hepatic and gastrointestinal monoamine oxidase. Tyramine in the bloodstream releases norepinephrine from the sympathetic nerve terminals and produces a sudden increase in blood pressure.

### Absorption
Almost completely absorbed from the gastrointestinal tract.

### Distribution
Crosses the blood-brain barrier.

### Biotransformation
Hepatic (to active metabolite).

### Half-life
Approximately 10 minutes.

### Elimination
Renal—70% (less than 5% unchanged).
Respiratory (as methane and carbon dioxide).

# Precautions to Consider

## Carcinogenicity/Mutagenicity

Secondary malignancies are potential delayed effects of many antineoplastic agents, although it is not clear whether the effect is related to their mutagenic or immunosuppressive action. The effect of dose and duration of therapy is also unknown, although risk seems to increase with long-term use. Although information is limited, available data seem to indicate that the carcinogenic risk is greatest with the alkylating agents.

Procarbazine is a potent carcinogen in animals and, because it is an alkylating agent, is also likely to be carcinogenic in humans.

## Pregnancy/Reproduction

Fertility—Gonadal suppression, resulting in amenorrhea or azoospermia, may occur in patients taking antineoplastic therapy, especially with the alkylating agents. In general, these effects appear to be related to dose and length of therapy and may be irreversible. Prediction of the degree of testicular or ovarian function impairment is complicated by the common use of combinations of several antineoplastics, which makes it difficult to assess the effects of individual agents. Procarbazine affects spermatogenesis in humans.

Pregnancy—Procarbazine is frequently teratogenic in animals and there have been reports of minor malformations or premature births when it is given later in pregnancy in humans.

First trimester: It is usually recommended that use of antineoplastics, especially combination chemotherapy, be avoided whenever possible, especially during the first trimester. Although information is limited because of the relatively few instances of antineoplastic administration during pregnancy, the mutagenic, teratogenic, and carcinogenic potential of these medications must be considered.

Other hazards to the fetus include adverse reactions seen in adults.

In general, use of a contraceptive is recommended during cytotoxic drug therapy.

## Breast-feeding

Although very little information is available regarding excretion of antineoplastic agents in breast milk, breast-feeding is not recommended while procarbazine is being administered because of the risks to the infant (adverse effects, mutagenicity, carcinogenicity).

## Pediatrics

Appropriate studies with procarbazine have not been performed in the pediatric population. However, pediatrics-specific problems that would limit the usefulness of this medication in children are not expected.

## Geriatrics

Although appropriate studies with procarbazine have not been performed in the geriatric population, the potential for increased vascular accidents (especially in the event of sudden hypertensive episodes), increased sensitivity to hypotensive effects, and reduced metabolic capacity discourages the first-time use of MAO inhibitors in patients over 60 years of age. When an MAO inhibitor is prescribed for an elderly patient, the patient's history of depression, ability to comply with prescribing instructions, and any potential drug interactions must also be considered. In addition, elderly patients are more likely to have age-related renal function impairment, which may require a lower dosage or, in severe cases, avoidance of use of procarbazine.

## Dental

The bone marrow depressant effects of procarbazine may result in an increased incidence of microbial infection, delayed healing, and gingival bleeding. Dental work, whenever possible, should be completed prior to initiation of therapy or deferred until blood counts have returned to normal. Patients should be instructed in proper oral hygiene during treatment, including caution in use of regular toothbrushes, dental floss, and toothpicks.

Procarbazine may also cause stomatitis associated with considerable discomfort.

The secondary anticholinergic effects of procarbazine may decrease or inhibit salivary flow, especially in middle-aged or elderly patients, thus contributing to the development of caries, periodontal disease, oral candidiasis, and discomfort.

## Drug interactions and/or related problems

The following drug interactions and/or related problems have been selected on the basis of their potential clinical significance (possible mechanism in parentheses where appropriate)—not necessarily inclusive (» = major clinical significance):

Note: Combinations containing any of the following medications, depending on the amount present, may also interact with this medication.

Most drug interactions are due to procarbazine's monoamine oxidase–inhibiting activity.

» Alcohol
(concurrent use with procarbazine may result in a disulfiram-like reaction and additive central nervous system (CNS) depression and postural hypotension; also, possible tyramine content in alcoholic beverages, especially beer, wine, or ale, may induce hypertensive reactions)

» Anesthetics, local, with epinephrine or levonordefrin or
» Cocaine
(concurrent use with procarbazine may cause severe hypertension due to sympathomimetic effects)
(cocaine should not be administered during or within 14 days following administration of an MAO inhibitor)

» Anesthetics, spinal
(hypotensive effects may be potentiated when spinal anesthetics are used concurrently with procarbazine; discontinuation of procarbazine at least 10 days before elective surgery if spinal anesthesia is planned may be advisable)

» Anticholinergics or other medications with anticholinergic activity (See *Appendix II*) or
Antidyskinetic agents or
» Antihistamines
(concurrent use with procarbazine may intensify anticholinergic effects because of the secondary anticholinergic activities of MAO inhibitors; also, MAO inhibitors may block detoxification of anticholinergics, thus potentiating their action; patients should be advised to report occurrence of gastrointestinal problems promptly since paralytic ileus may occur with concurrent therapy)
(concurrent use with MAO inhibitors may also prolong and intensify CNS depressant and anticholinergic effects of antihistamines; concurrent use is not recommended)

Anticoagulants, coumarin- and indandione-derivative
(concurrent use may increase anticoagulant activity; although the mechanism of action and clinical significance are unknown, caution is recommended)

Anticonvulsants
(concurrent use of anticonvulsants with procarbazine may lead to increased CNS depressant effects as well as a change in the pattern of epileptiform seizures; dosage adjustment of anticonvulsant may be necessary)

» Antidepressants, tricyclic
(in addition to increased anticholinergic effects, concurrent use with procarbazine may result in hyperpyretic crises, severe convulsions, and death; however, recent studies have shown that some tricyclic antidepressants can be used concurrently with MAO inhibitors with no adverse effects if both medications are initiated simultaneously at lower than usual doses and the doses raised gradually, or if the MAO inhibitor is gradually added to the tricyclic also at low doses; tricyclics should not be added to an established MAO inhibitor regimen; careful monitoring for side effects of either medication is necessary)

» Antidiabetic agents, oral or
» Insulin
(procarbazine may enhance hypoglycemic effects; dosage reduction of hypoglycemic medication may be necessary during and after such combined therapy)

Antihypertensives or
Diuretics or
Hypotension-producing medications, other (See *Appendix II*)
(concurrent use with procarbazine may result in an enhanced hypotensive effect; dosage adjustment may be necessary)
(antihypertensives with CNS depressant effects, such as clonidine, guanabenz, methyldopa, or metyrosine, may increase CNS depression)

Beta-adrenergic blocking agents, including ophthalmic beta-blockers absorbed systemically
(possible significant hypertension may theoretically occur up to 14 days following discontinuation of procarbazine; however, sufficient clinical reports are lacking)

Blood dyscrasia–causing medications (See *Appendix II*)
(leukopenic and/or thrombocytopenic effects of procarbazine may be increased with concurrent or recent therapy if these medications cause the same effects; dosage adjustment of procarbazine, if necessary, should be based on blood counts)

» Bone marrow depressants, other (See *Appendix II*) or
Radiation therapy
(additive bone marrow depression may occur; dosage reduction may be required when two or more bone marrow depressants, including radiation, are used concurrently or consecutively)

Bromocriptine
(concurrent use may increase serum prolactin concentrations and interfere with effects of bromocriptine; dosage adjustment of bromocriptine may be necessary)

» Buspirone
(concurrent use with MAO inhibitors is not recommended because elevation of blood pressure may occur)

» Caffeine-containing preparations
(concurrent use of excessive amounts of caffeine, consumed in chocolate, coffee, cola, tea, or "stay awake" products, with procarbazine may produce dangerous cardiac arrhythmias or severe hypertension because of sympathomimetic effects of caffeine)

» Carbamazepine or
» Cyclobenzaprine or
» Maprotiline or
» Monoamine oxidase (MAO) inhibitors, other, including furazolidone and pargyline
(concurrent use with procarbazine is not recommended on an outpatient basis, as hyperpyretic crises, severe seizures, and death could result; prior to initiation of procarbazine therapy, 14 days should elapse after discontinuance of one of these medications)

» CNS depression–producing medications, other (See *Appendix II*)
(CNS depression and postural hypotension may be enhanced; concurrent use with antihistamines is not recommended)

» Dextromethorphan
(concurrent use with procarbazine may cause excitation, hypertension, and hyperpyrexia)

» Doxapram
(concurrent use may increase the pressor effects of either doxapram or procarbazine)

» Fluoxetine
(concurrent use may result in confusion, agitation, restlessness, and gastrointestinal symptoms, or possibly hyperpyretic episodes, severe convulsions, and hypertensive crises. Based on experience with tricyclic antidepressants, at least 14 days should elapse between discontinuation of an MAO inhibitor and initiation of fluoxetine. However, because of the long half-lives of fluoxetine and its active metabolite, at least 5 weeks [approximately 5 half-lives of norfluoxetine] should elapse between discontinuation of fluoxetine and initiation of therapy with an MAO inhibitor. Administration of an MAO inhibitor within 5 weeks of discontinuation of fluoxetine may increase the risk of serious events. While a causal relationship to fluoxetine has not been established, death has been reported following the initiation of an MAO inhibitor shortly after fluoxetine administration was stopped)

» Guanadrel or
» Guanethidine or
» Rauwolfia alkaloids
(administration to patients receiving procarbazine may result in sudden release of accumulated catecholamines and a hypertensive reaction; parenteral administration is not recommended during and for 1 week following procarbazine therapy)

(when an MAO inhibitor is added to existing therapy with a rauwolfia alkaloid, serious potentiation of CNS depressant effects may result; however, if a rauwolfia alkaloid is added to an MAO inhibitor regimen, CNS excitation and hypertension may result from release of excessive amounts of accumulated norepinephrine and serotonin)

Haloperidol or
Loxapine or
Molindone or
Phenothiazines or
Pimozide or
Thioxanthenes
(concurrent use may prolong and intensify the sedative, hypotensive, and anticholinergic effects of either these medications or procarbazine)

» Levodopa
(concurrent use with MAO inhibitors is not recommended, as the combination may result in sudden moderate to severe hypertensive crisis; a period of 2 to 4 weeks is recommended after withdrawal of MAO inhibitors before levodopa is administered)

» Meperidine and possibly other opioid (narcotic) analgesics
(concurrent use with procarbazine may produce immediate excitation, sweating, rigidity, and severe hypertension; in some patients, hypotension, severe respiratory depression, coma, convulsions, hyperpyrexia, vascular collapse, and death may occur; reactions may be due to accumulation of serotonin resulting from MAO inhibition; avoidance of meperidine use within 2 to 3 weeks

following procarbazine is recommended; other opioid analgesics, such as morphine, are not likely to cause such severe reactions and may be used cautiously in reduced dosage in patients receiving MAO inhibitors; however, it is recommended that a small test dose [one-quarter of the usual dose] or several small incremental test doses over a period of several hours should first be administered to permit observation of any adverse effects)

(caution is also recommended in the use of alfentanil, fentanyl, or sufentanil as an adjunct to anesthesia if the patient has received procarbazine within 14 days; although the risk of a significant interaction has been questioned, the use of a small test dose is advised to detect any possible interaction)

» Methyldopa
(concurrent use with procarbazine may cause hyperexcitability; also headache, severe hypertension, and hallucinations have been reported)

» Methylphenidate
(concurrent use with procarbazine may potentiate the CNS stimulant effects of methylphenidate, possibly resulting in a hypertensive crisis; should not be administered during or within 14 days following the administration of procarbazine)

Metrizamide
(concurrent use with procarbazine may lower the seizure threshold; procarbazine should be discontinued at least 48 hours before myelography and should not be resumed for at least 24 hours after procedure)

Phenylephrine, nasal or ophthalmic
(if significant systemic absorption of nasal or ophthalmic phenylephrine occurs, concurrent use with procarbazine may potentiate pressor effects; these medications should not be administered during or within 14 days following the administration of procarbazine)

» Sympathomimetics
(concurrent use with procarbazine may prolong and intensify cardiac stimulant and vasopressor effects [including headache, cardiac arrhythmias, vomiting, sudden and severe hypertensive and hyperpyretic crises] of these medications because of release of catecholamines which accumulate in intraneuronal storage sites during MAO inhibitor therapy; these medications should not be administered during or within 14 days following the administration of procarbazine)

» Tryptophan
(concurrent use with MAO inhibitors may cause hyperreflexia, shivering, hyperventilation, hyperthermia, mania or hypomania, and disorientation or confusion; when tryptophan is added to an MAOI regimen, it should be started in low dosages and the dose titrated upwards gradually with close monitoring of mental status and blood pressure)

» Tyramine- or other high pressor amine–containing foods and beverages, such as aged cheese; beer; reduced-alcohol and alcohol-free beer and wine; red and white wines; sherry; liqueurs; yeast/protein extracts; fava or broad bean pods; smoked or pickled meats, poultry, or fish; fermented sausage (bologna, pepperoni, salami, summer sausage) or other fermented meat; and any overripe fruit
(concurrent use with procarbazine may cause sudden and severe hypertensive reactions; reactions are usually limited to a few hours and easily treated with phentolamine; severity depends on amount of tyramine ingested, rate of gastric emptying, and length of interval between dose of procarbazine and ingestion of tyramine; when procarbazine is discontinued, dietary restrictions must continue for at least 2 weeks; other tyramine- or high pressor amine–containing foods, such as yogurt, sour cream, cream cheese, cottage cheese, chocolate, and soy sauce, if eaten when fresh and in moderation, are considered unlikely to cause serious problems)

Vaccines, killed virus
(because normal defense mechanisms may be suppressed by procarbazine therapy, the patient's antibody response to the vaccine may be decreased. The interval between discontinuation of medications that cause immunosuppression and restoration of the patient's ability to respond to the vaccine depends on the intensity and type of immunosuppression-causing medication used, the underlying disease, and other factors; estimates vary from 3 months to 1 year)

» Vaccines, live virus
(because normal defense mechanisms may be suppressed by procarbazine therapy, concurrent use with a live virus vaccine may potentiate the replication of the vaccine virus, may increase the side/adverse effects of the vaccine virus, and/or may decrease the patient's antibody response to the vaccine; immunization of these patients should be undertaken only with extreme caution after care-

ful review of the patient's hematologic status and only with the knowledge and consent of the physician managing the procarbazine therapy. The interval between discontinuation of medications that cause immunosuppression and restoration of the patient's ability to respond to the vaccine depends on the intensity and type of immunosuppression-causing medication used, the underlying disease, and other factors; estimates vary from 3 months to 1 year. Patients with leukemia in remission should not receive live virus vaccine until at least 3 months after their last chemotherapy. Immunization with oral poliovirus vaccine should also be postponed in persons in close contact with the patient, especially family members)

## Medical considerations/Contraindications

The medical considerations/contraindications included here have been selected on the basis of their potential clinical significance (reasons given in parentheses where appropriate)—not necessarily inclusive (» = major clinical significance):

*Except under special circumstances, this medication should not be used when the following medical problems exist:*

»  Alcoholism, active

»  Congestive heart failure

»  Hepatic function impairment, severe
    (procarbazine may precipitate hepatic precoma in patients with cirrhosis, who are extremely sensitive to effects)

»  Pheochromocytoma
    (pressor substances secreted by such tumors may alter blood pressure during therapy with MAO inhibitors)

»  Renal function impairment, severe
    (cumulative effects of procarbazine may occur because of reduced renal excretion)

*Risk-benefit should be considered when the following medical problems exist:*

»  Bone marrow depression

»  Cardiac arrhythmias

»  Cardiovascular disease or coronary insufficiency
    (ischemia may be aggravated as a result of reduced blood pressure)

Cerebrovascular disease
    (cerebral ischemia may be aggravated as a result of reduced blood pressure)

»  Chickenpox, existing or recent (including recent exposure) or

»  Herpes zoster
    (risk of severe generalized disease)

Diabetes mellitus
    (procarbazine may alter insulin or oral hypoglycemic requirements)

Epilepsy
    (pattern of epileptiform seizures may be changed)

»  Headaches, severe or frequent
    (headache as a first sign of hypertensive reaction during therapy may be masked)

»  Hepatic function impairment
    (procarbazine may precipitate hepatic precoma in patients with cirrhosis, who are extremely sensitive to effects; lower dosage is recommended; use not recommended in severe function impairment)

Hyperthyroidism
    (sensitivity to pressor amines may be increased)

»  Infection

»  Paranoid schizophrenia or other hyperexcitable personality states
    (MAO inhibitors may cause excessive stimulation in schizophrenic patients; in manic-depressive states, may effect a swing from depressive to manic phase)

Parkinsonism
    (may be aggravated)

»  Renal function impairment
    (cumulative effects may occur; lower dosage is recommended; use not recommended in severe function impairment)

Sensitivity to procarbazine

»  Caution should be used also in patients who have had previous cytotoxic drug therapy or radiation therapy.

»  In addition, caution should be used in patients who have undergone sympathectomy, who may be more sensitive to the hypotensive effects of MAO inhibitors.

## Patient monitoring

The following procedures are especially important in patient monitoring (other tests may be warranted in some patients, depending on condition; » = major clinical significance):

Blood urea nitrogen (BUN) concentrations and

Serum creatinine concentrations
    (recommended prior to initiation of therapy and at periodic intervals during therapy; frequency varies according to clinical state, agent, dose, and other agents being used concurrently)

»  Bone marrow aspiration studies
    (recommended prior to initiation of procarbazine therapy and at time of maximum hematologic response to ensure adequate bone marrow reserve)

»  Hematocrit or hemoglobin and

»  Platelet count and

»  Total and, if appropriate, differential leukocyte count
    (determinations recommended prior to initiation of therapy and at periodic intervals during therapy; frequency varies according to clinical state, agent, dose, and other agents being used concurrently)

»  Serum alanine aminotransferase (ALT [SGPT]) concentrations and

»  Serum aspartate aminotransferase (AST [SGOT]) concentrations and

»  Serum bilirubin concentrations and

»  Serum lactate dehydrogenase (LDH) concentrations
    (recommended prior to initiation of therapy and at periodic intervals during therapy; frequency varies according to clinical state, agent, dose, and other agents being used concurrently)

## Side/Adverse Effects

Note: Many "side effects" of antineoplastic therapy are unavoidable and represent the medication's pharmacologic action. Some of these (for example, leukopenia and thrombocytopenia) are actually used as parameters to aid in individual dosage titration.

Except for hematologic, pulmonary, and gastrointestinal toxicity, adverse effects of procarbazine resemble those of the MAO inhibitors used in treating psychiatric disorders.

Toxicity is increased in patients with renal or hepatic function impairment or bone marrow depression.

The following side/adverse effects have been selected on the basis of their potential clinical significance (possible signs and symptoms in parentheses where appropriate)—not necessarily inclusive:

### Those indicating need for medical attention

Incidence more frequent
    *Anemia; CNS stimulation, excessive* (confusion; convulsions; hallucinations); *immunosuppression, infection, or leukopenia* (usually asymptomatic; less frequently, fever or chills; cough or hoarseness; lower back or side pain; painful or difficult urination); *thrombocytopenia* (usually asymptomatic; less frequently, unusual bleeding or bruising; black, tarry stools; blood in urine or stools; pinpoint red spots on skin); *hemolytic anemia* (continuing tiredness or weakness); *missing menstrual periods; pneumonitis* (cough; shortness of breath; thickening of bronchial secretions)

    Note: With *leukopenia* and *thrombocytopenia*, the nadir of the platelet count occurs after about 4 weeks, followed by the leukocyte count, with recovery complete in about 6 weeks.
        *Missing menstrual periods* occur with high doses.

Incidence less frequent
    *Gastrointestinal toxicity* (diarrhea); *hepatotoxicity* (yellow eyes or skin); *peripheral neuropathy* (tingling or numbness of fingers or toes; unsteadiness or awkwardness); *stomatitis* (sores in mouth and on lips)

Incidence rare
    *Allergic reaction* (skin rash, hives or itching; wheezing); *hypertensive crisis* (severe chest pain; enlarged pupils; fast or slow heartbeat; severe headache; increased sensitivity of eyes to light; increased sweating, possibly with fever or cold, clammy skin; stiff or sore neck); *orthostatic hypotension* (fainting)

### Those indicating need for medical attention only if they continue or are bothersome

Incidence more frequent
    *CNS stimulation, excessive* (drowsiness; muscle or joint pain; muscle twitching; nervousness; nightmares; trouble in sleeping); *nausea and vomiting; unusual tiredness or weakness*

Incidence less frequent
    *Constipation; darkening of skin; difficulty in swallowing; dry mouth; feeling of warmth and redness in face; headache; loss of appetite;*

*mental depression; orthostatic hypotension* (dizziness or lightheadedness when getting up from a lying or sitting position)

**Those not indicating need for medical attention**
Incidence less frequent
*Loss of hair*

## Overdose

For more information on the management of overdose or unintentional intestion, **contact a Poison Control Center** (see *Poison Control Center listing*).

**Treatment of overdose**

Note: Symptoms resulting from overdosage may be absent or minimal for nearly 12 hours following ingestion, and develop slowly thereafter, reaching a maximum in 24 to 48 hours. Immediate hospitalization and close monitoring of patient are essential during this period.

Treatment may include the following:
- Induction of vomiting or gastric lavage with protected airway followed by instillation of charcoal slurry in early overdose.
- Treatment of signs and symptoms of CNS stimulation with diazepam, administered intravenously and slowly.
- Treatment of hypotension and vascular collapse with intravenous fluids and a dilute pressor agent.
- Support of respiration by management of the airway, and mechanical ventilation with the use of supplemental oxygen, as required.
- Close monitoring of body temperature and vigorous treatment of hyperpyrexia with antipyretics and a cooling blanket. Maintenance of fluid and electrolyte balance is essential.
- Reduction of symptoms of hypermetabolic state (coma, respiratory failure, hyperpyrexia, tachycardia, muscular rigidity, tremor, and hyperreflexia) with intravenous dantrolene sodium at 2.5 mg per kg of body weight (mg/kg) a day in divided doses, with careful monitoring for signs of hepatotoxicity and pleural or pericardial effusions.
- Hemodialysis may be beneficial but is of unproven value.
- Pathophysiologic effects of massive overdose may persist for several days; recovery from mild overdose may take 3 to 4 days.

## Patient Consultation

As an aid to patient consultation, refer to *Advice for the Patient, Procarbazine (Systemic)*.

Consider advising the patient on the following (» = major clinical significance):

**Before using this medication**
» Conditions affecting use, especially:
  Pregnancy—Advisability of using contraception; telling physician immediately if pregnancy is suspected
  See also *Precautions to Consider*.

**Proper use of this medication**
» Importance of not taking more or less medication than the amount prescribed
  Caution in taking combination chemotherapy; taking each medication at the right time
» Frequency of nausea and vomiting; importance of continuing medication despite stomach upset
  Checking with physician if vomiting occurs shortly after dose is taken
» Proper dosing
  Missed dose: Taking as soon as remembered if within a few hours; not taking if several hours have passed or if almost time for next dose; not doubling doses
» Proper storage

**Precautions while using this medication**
» Importance of close monitoring by the physician
» Checking with hospital emergency room or physician if symptoms of hypertensive crisis develop
» Avoiding use of tyramine-containing foods, alcoholic beverages and large quantities of caffeine-containing beverages, over-the-counter cold and cough medicines, and other medication unless prescribed; having list of such for reference
» Obeying rules of caution during 14 days after discontinuing medication
» Caution in taking alcohol or other CNS depressants
» Caution if drowsiness occurs, especially when driving or doing things requiring alertness
» Avoiding immunizations unless approved by physician; other persons in patient's household should avoid immunizations with oral poliovirus vaccine; avoiding other persons who have taken oral poliovirus vaccine or wearing a protective mask that covers nose and mouth

*Caution if bone marrow depression occurs:*
» Avoiding exposure to persons with bacterial infections, especially during periods of low blood counts; checking with physician immediately if fever or chills, cough or hoarseness, lower back or side pain, or painful or difficult urination occur
» Checking with physician immediately if unusual bleeding or bruising; black, tarry stools; blood in urine or stools; or pinpoint red spots on skin occur
  Caution in use of regular toothbrush, dental floss, or toothpick; physician, dentist, or nurse may suggest alternatives; checking with physician before having dental work done
  Not touching eyes or inside of nose unless hands washed immediately before
  Using caution to avoid accidental cuts with use of sharp objects such as safety razor or fingernail or toenail cutters
  Avoiding contact sports or other situations where bruising or injury could occur

  Diabetics: Checking urine or blood sugar levels
» Caution if any kind of surgery (including dental surgery) or emergency treatment is required
  Carrying medical identification card

**Side/adverse effects**
  May cause adverse effects such as blood problems, loss of hair, hypertensive crisis, and cancer; importance of discussing possible effects with physician
  Signs of potential side effects, especially anemia, excessive CNS stimulation, immunosuppression, infection, leukopenia, thrombocytopenia, hemolytic anemia, missing menstrual periods, pneumonitis, gastrointestinal toxicity, hepatotoxicity, peripheral neuropathy, stomatitis, allergic reaction, hypertensive crisis, and orthostatic hypotension
  Physician or nurse can help in dealing with side effects

## General Dosing Information

Patients receiving procarbazine should be under supervision of a physician experienced in cancer chemotherapy.

A variety of dosage schedules and regimens of procarbazine, alone or in combination with other antitumor agents, are used. The prescriber may consult medical literature as well as the manufacturer's literature in choosing a specific dosage.

Dosage must be adjusted to meet the individual requirements of each patient, based on clinical response and appearance or severity of toxicity.

Although dosages are based on the patient's actual weight, use of estimated lean body mass (dry weight) is recommended in obese patients or those with weight gain due to edema, ascites, or other abnormal fluid retention.

It is recommended that procarbazine therapy be discontinued promptly if any of the following occur:
Allergic reaction
Diarrhea
Hemorrhage or bleeding tendencies
Leukopenia (particularly granulocytopenia), marked
Stomatitis
Thrombocytopenia, marked
Therapy may be resumed at a lower dosage when the clinical and laboratory examinations are satisfactory.

Because of the risk of enhanced bone marrow toxicity, an interval of at least 1 month (based on bone marrow studies) is recommended before starting procarbazine therapy after a patient has received radiation or chemotherapy with medications that depress bone marrow function.

After dosage is stopped, monoamine oxidase (MAO) inhibitor effects of this medication may persist for up to 2 weeks after withdrawal (time required for regeneration of enzyme). During this period, food and drug contraindications must be observed.

Special precautions are recommended in patients who develop thrombocytopenia as a result of administration of procarbazine. These may include extreme care in performing invasive procedures; regular inspection of intravenous sites, skin (including perirectal area), and mucous membrane surfaces for signs of bleeding or bruising; limiting frequency of venipuncture and avoiding intramuscular injections; testing urine, emesis, stool, and secretions for occult blood; care in use of regular toothbrushes, dental floss, toothpicks, safety razors, and fingernail and toenail cutters; avoiding constipation; and using caution to prevent falls and other injuries. Such patients should avoid alcohol and any aspirin intake because of the risk of gastrointestinal bleeding. Platelet transfusions may be required.

Patients who develop leukopenia should be observed carefully for signs of infection. Antibiotic support may be required. In neutropenic patients who develop fever, broad-spectrum antibiotic coverage should be initiated empirically, pending bacterial cultures and appropriate diagnostic tests.

### Diet/Nutrition

Foods and beverages containing tyramine or other high pressor amines, such as aged cheese; beer; reduced-alcohol and alcohol-free beer and wine; red and white wines; sherry; liqueurs; yeast/protein extracts; fava or broad bean pods; smoked or pickled meats, poultry, or fish; fermented sausage (bologna, pepperoni, salami, summer sausage) or other fermented meat; and any overripe fruit, when used concurrently with MAO inhibitors, may cause sudden and severe hypertensive reactions. The reactions are usually limited to a few hours and are easily treated with phentolamine. The severity depends on the amount of tyramine ingested, rate of gastric emptying, and length of the interval between the dose of MAO inhibitor and ingestion of tyramine. When MAO inhibitors are discontinued, dietary restrictions must continue for at least 2 weeks. Other foods, such as yogurt, sour cream, cream cheese, cottage cheese, chocolate, and soy sauce, if eaten when fresh and in moderation, are considered unlikely to cause serious problems.

### For treatment of hypertensive crisis

Recommended treatment includes:
- Discontinuing MAO inhibitor.
- Lowering blood pressure immediately with intravenous administration of 5 mg of phentolamine, with care being taken to inject slowly, to prevent excessive hypotensive effect.
- Reducing fever by external cooling.

### Combination chemotherapy

Procarbazine may be used in combination with other agents in various regimens. As a result, incidence and/or severity of side effects may be altered and different dosages (usually reduced) may be used. For example, procarbazine is part of the following chemotherapeutic combinations (some commonly used acronyms are in parentheses):
—doxorubicin, cyclophosphamide, vincristine, procarbazine, and prednisone (A-COPP).
—carmustine, cyclophosphamide, vinblastine, procarbazine, and prednisone (BCVPP).
—cyclophosphamide, doxorubicin, methotrexate, and procarbazine (CAMP).
—cyclophosphamide, vincristine, procarbazine, and prednisone (COPP or "C"MOPP).
—mechlorethamine, vincristine, procarbazine, and prednisone (MOPP).
—mechlorethamine, vincristine, procarbazine, prednisone, and bleomycin (MOPP-LO BLEO).
—procarbazine, vincristine, cyclophosphamide, and lomustine (POCC).

For specific dosages and schedules, consult the literature. For information regarding each agent, consult the individual monographs.

## Oral Dosage Forms

### PROCARBAZINE HYDROCHLORIDE CAPSULES USP

#### Usual adult dose

Lymphomas, Hodgkin's—
Initial: Oral, 2 to 4 mg (base) per kg of body weight (to the nearest 50 mg) a day in single or divided doses for the first week, followed by 4 to 6 mg per kg of body weight a day until leukopenia, thrombocytopenia, or maximum response occurs.
Note: If hematologic toxicity occurs, the medication is withdrawn until the toxicity is resolved, then treatment may be resumed with 1 to 2 mg (base) per kg of body weight a day.
Maintenance: Oral, 1 to 2 mg (base) per kg of body weight a day.

#### Usual pediatric dose

Lymphomas, Hodgkin's—
Initial:
Oral, 50 mg (base) a day for the first week, followed by 100 mg per square meter of body surface (to the nearest 50 mg) a day until leukopenia, thrombocytopenia, or maximum response occurs.
Note: If hematologic toxicity occurs, the medication is withdrawn until the toxicity is resolved, then treatment may be resumed with 50 mg (base) a day.
Maintenance:
Oral, 50 mg (base) a day.
Note: This dosage schedule is a guideline only. Undue toxicity in the form of tremors, coma, and seizures has occurred; therefore, dosage must be individualized based on clinical response and appearance of toxicity.

#### Strength(s) usually available

U.S.—
50 mg (base) (Rx) [Matulane].
Canada—
50 mg (base) (Rx) [Natulan].

#### Packaging and storage

Store below 40 °C (104 °F), preferably between 15 and 30 °C (59 and 86 °F), unless otherwise specified by manufacturer. Store in a tight, light-resistant container.

#### Auxiliary labeling

- Avoid alcoholic beverages.
- May cause drowsiness.
- Do not take other medicines without your doctor's advice.
- Avoid certain foods as directed.

Revised: 08/90
Interim revision: 08/05/93; 06/30/94

---

**PROCATEROL**—See *Bronchodilators, Adrenergic (Systemic)*

---

**PROCHLORPERAZINE**—See *Phenothiazines (Systemic)*

---

**PROCYCLIDINE**—See *Antidyskinetics (Systemic)*

---

**PROGESTERONE**—See *Progestins (Systemic)*

---

# PROGESTERONE INTRAUTERINE DEVICE (IUD)†

VA CLASSIFICATION (Primary): GU900
Note: For a listing of dosage forms and brand names by country availability, see *Dosage Forms* section(s). For a listing of brand names for the articles in this monograph, refer to the General Index.

†Not commercially available in Canada.

## Category

Contraceptive (intrauterine-local).

## Indications

### Accepted

Pregnancy (prophylaxis)—Progesterone intrauterine devices are recommended as a contraceptive method, primarily for parous women who are in a mutually monogamous relationship and have no history of pelvic inflammatory disease (PID).

An IUD may **not** be an appropriate choice for nulliparous or low parity women whose lifestyle (involvement in multiple relationships or in a nonmonogamous relationship) may expose them to sexually transmitted diseases (STDs) or for women at risk of developing PID because PID, if it develops, potentially may be more severe for these women. The IUD is **not** generally recommended for women whose uterine cavity measures less than 6.5 centimeters (cm).

IUDs do not protect against sexually transmitted diseases including human immunodeficiency virus (HIV) infection or acquired immunodeficiency syndrome (AIDS).

The following table presents the results of studies examining contraceptive failure rates calculated using the life-table method. The first column lists the contraceptive method used. The second column indicates the percentage of women experiencing an accidental pregnancy in the first year of use of a contraceptive method while using the method perfectly under clinical conditions. The range of failure rates in the clinical trials may be explained by interstudy variations in study design or patient population characteristics, such as motivation, fecundity, or socioeconomic factors (including education). The third column indicates contraceptive failure rates in the first year of contraceptive use under clinical conditions for typical couples who start using a method (not necessarily for the first time). Failure rates among adolescents may be higher due to poorer compliance than in other age groups.

| Method used | Failure rate range (over 12 months) in clinical studies (%) | Typical first year failure rate (%) |
|---|---|---|
| None | 78–94 | 85 |
| Spermicides[1] | 0.3–37 | 21 |
| Periodic abstinence[2] | 13–35 | 20 |
| Withdrawal | 7–22 | 19 |
| Cervical cap with spermicide | 6–27 | 18 |
| Diaphragm with spermicide | 2–23 | 18 |
| Condom without spermicide | 2–14 | 12 |
| IUD | | |
|   Progesterone-releasing | 1.9–2.0 | 2 |
|   Copper-T 200 | 3.0–3.6 | |
|   Copper-T 200Ag[3] | 0–1.2 | |
|   Copper-T 220C[4] | 0.9–1.8 | |
|   Copper-T 380A | 0.5–0.8 | 0.8 |
|   Copper-T 380S | 0.9 | |
| Oral contraceptive | 3 | |
|   Estrogen and progestin | 0–6 | |
|   Progestin only | 1–10 | |
| Medroxyprogesterone injection (90-day) | 0–0.3 | 0.3 |
| Levonorgestrel (implants) | | |
|   Six capsules | 0–0.09 | 0.09 |
|   Two rods | 0–0.2 | 0.3 |
| Sterilization | | |
|   Female[5] | 0–8 | 0.4 |
|   Male | 0–0.5 | 0.15 |

[1]Spermicides studied include creams, foams, gels, jellies, and suppositories.

[2]Methods studied include calendar, ovulation method, and symptothermal (cervical mucus method supplemented by basal body temperature in post-ovulatory phases, post-ovulation phases, post-ovulation).

[3]Life-table method rate is unavailable for Copper-T 200Ag and the Pearl method rate at 12 months was reported; these methods at 12 months are considered comparable.

[4]Copper-T 220C is manufactured with copper sleeves instead of copper wire; often used as a control in clinical studies.

[5]Methods studied include culdotomy, laparoscopy, minilaparotomy, electrocoagulation, laparotomy, tubal diathermy and/or use of rings or clips.

## Pharmacology/Pharmacokinetics

### Physical description—Physicochemical characteristics
The ethylene/vinyl coacetate polymer (EVA) T-shaped body has a 36 millimeter tubular vertical stem that contains a reservoir of 38 mg of microcrystallized progesterone (initially) and radiopaque barium sulfate (to monitor location) dispersed in silicone fluid; the horizontal arms measure 32 millimeters. In addition, the T-shaped body contains two blue-black monofilament threads (to monitor placement and aid in IUD removal).

### Mechanism of action/Effect
Contraceptive, intrauterine-local—

The progesterone intrauterine device prevents pregnancy in 98% of users in the first year of use. The precise mechanism of action has not been fully elucidated; a number of mechanisms may contribute to the contraceptive effect.

Progesterone is thought to enhance an unfavorable uterine environment for implantation by suppressing endometrial proliferation and to inhibit sperm penetration by causing cervical mucus to become thick and scanty. Progesterone also may directly inhibit metabolism, capacitation, and swimming speed of the sperm. Other normal cyclic reproductive function, including ovulation, continues as it does with other IUDs.

In general, IUDs produce cellular reactions that can lead to local superficial ulceration in adjacent uterine cells. This causes a foreign-

body inflammatory response leading to biochemical and morphological changes in the endometrial tissue and uterine fluid, including increased infiltration of leukocytes, especially macrophages. This action adds to progesterone's ability to interfere with sperm migration, fertilization and, to a lesser extent, with implantation.

### Other actions/effects
Progesterone may decrease the endometrial content of prostaglandins and decrease the concentration of blood vessels in the endometrium which may result in fewer complaints of dysmenorrhea and a lower total volume of menstrual blood loss in women using a progesterone IUD.

### Absorption
Readily absorbed into uterine epithelium; systemic progesterone absorption is low and not considered to be clinically significant. Progesterone IUDs release progesterone continuously into the uterus at an average rate of 65 mcg per day by membrane controlled diffusion from the reservoir. This membrane barrier allows delivery of progesterone but prevents diffusion of silicone fluid and barium sulfate from the reservoir.

### Distribution
Local, uterine.

### Biotransformation
Rapid metabolism by endometrium.

### Half-life
Several minutes.

### Onset of action
Local contraceptive action begins immediately after insertion.

### Duration of action
The manufacturer recommends progesterone IUD replacement within 12 months. Local contraceptive action terminates quickly on removal.

## Precautions to Consider

### Carcinogenicity/Tumorigenicity/Mutagenicity
Studies have not been done in either animals or humans.

### Pregnancy/Reproduction
Fertility—In most women, fertility resumes on removal of the IUD. Up to 76% of women desiring pregnancy conceive successfully within 12 months after IUD removal, and 49% of women conceive within the first 3 months.

Monogamous women with monogamous partners have little risk of primary tubal infertility attributable to progesterone IUDs unless there are other risk factors, such as endometriosis or past history of surgery on the female reproductive system. IUDs increase the risk of tubal infertility caused by obstruction in or damage to the fallopian tubes, which are problems associated with pelvic inflammatory disease (PID) or an infection in the uterus or fallopian tubes. This risk from the insertion procedure is highest within the first few months after IUD insertion.

Pregnancy—Use of a progesterone IUD is not recommended during pregnancy although there is no clear evidence of adverse effects for infants conceived with an IUD in situ. Long-term effects on the offspring if conceived with a progesterone IUD present are not known. A congenital anomaly, bilateral inguinal hernia, has occurred, but causal relationship was not established.

An IUD in utero during pregnancy has resulted in maternal sepsis (usually, but not exclusively, in the second trimester, secondary to a septic abortion or chorioamnionitis) and, rarely, death. If pregnancy occurs with an IUD in situ, risk-benefit of leaving the IUD in situ versus IUD removal must be carefully considered. If an IUD remains in utero, possible complications include a 50% risk of spontaneous abortion and an increased risk of premature rupture of membranes, labor, and delivery.

If a pregnancy occurs with a progesterone IUD in place, the IUD should be removed if the string is visible and the removal is easy. However, manipulation of the IUD may stimulate spontaneous abortion. If the string is not visible, removal of the IUD may be attempted under ultrasound guidance, and/or the termination of the pregnancy should be considered.

When a pregnancy occurs with a progesterone IUD in situ, the possibility of an ectopic pregnancy should be considered as the IUD protects against intrauterine pregnancy more than it protects against extrauterine pregnancy. Studies indicate that about 1 ectopic pregnancy per 200 users per year occurs with a progesterone IUD in situ, a rate similar to that of noncontracepting sexually active women but approximately 6 times higher than that of women using nonmedicated IUDs. Clinical trials also show that the risk of ectopic pregnancy occurring in nulliparous women is twice that of parous women, 1 ectopic pregnancy of

3.6 pregnancies versus 1 ectopic pregnancy in 6.2 pregnancies, respectively.

Diagnosis of ectopic pregnancy may be difficult because early symptoms (enlarged and tender breasts, dizziness, faintness, nausea, unusual tiredness or weakness, lower abdominal pain, cramping or tenderness [possibly severe], vaginal bleeding [possibly heavy and/or unexpected], or absent or delayed menstrual cycle) are nonspecific and variable. Also, 83% of patients continue to have menses, and 53% do not suspect pregnancy.

Delivery—If an intrauterine pregnancy continues with an IUD *in situ*, the risk for premature delivery is increased along with the usual complications of premature infants.

Postpartum—It is recommended that postpartum IUD insertion be performed 8 weeks or more after delivery (interval insertion) or after complete involution of the uterus has occurred, although individual needs and desires should be taken into consideration by the physician. The risk of an IUD expulsion or uterine perforation caused by an IUD is lower for interval insertions than for postplacental insertions (insertions performed within 10 minutes after delivery). Immediate postpartum insertions (insertions performed within 48 hours after delivery) or immediate postabortion insertions may involve a risk of uterine perforation by the IUD similar to that for interval insertions, but the expulsion rate is higher. Higher expulsion rates in postpartum women may be due to the difficulty in placing the IUD sufficiently high in the fundus.

### Breast-feeding

Problems in humans have not been documented. IUDs are recommended by the World Health Organization (WHO) for use as a contraceptive method because IUDs do not interfere with lactation.

### Adolescents

Sexually active adolescents may be better served with a contraceptive method that also protects against sexually transmitted diseases (STDs). In general, young age and nulliparity in women appear to be associated with a higher expulsion rate, possibly due to a more reactive myometrium and irregular and heavy menses.

### Drug interactions and/or related problems

The following drug interactions and/or related problems have been selected on the basis of their potential clinical significance (possible mechanism in parentheses where appropriate)—not necessarily inclusive (» = major clinical significance):

Note: Combinations containing the following medication, depending on the amount present, may also interact with this device.

Anticoagulants
(use of anticoagulants may initially potentiate the risk of abnormal uterine bleeding around the time of the progesterone IUD insertion; risk lessens with use but spotting may persist)

### Laboratory value alterations

The following have been selected on the basis of their potential clinical significance (possible effect in parentheses where appropriate)—not necessarily inclusive (» = major clinical significance):

With physiology/laboratory test values

Glucose, plasma
(glucose measurements induced by glucose tolerance tests were slightly elevated at 3 hours according to studies in women using progesterone IUDs at 6 and 12 months; fasting and 0.5 hour glucose measurements were unchanged)

Insulin concentration, serum
(measurements induced by glucose tolerance tests in women using progesterone IUDs for 12 months have shown that insulin concentrations taken at fasting, 0.5 hour, and 3 hours increased from 10.3, 69, and 40.5 microunits/mL to 18.1, 118.4, and 68.5 microunits/mL, respectively; insulin concentrations at 1 and 2 hours were not significantly changed)

Triglyceride, plasma, fasting
(although no change was shown at 6 months, a study showed that triglyceride concentrations decreased at 12 months from 76.3 to 61.8 mg/dL for women using progesterone IUDs for 12 months)

### Medical considerations/Contraindications

The medical considerations/contraindications included here have been selected on the basis of their potential clinical significance (reasons given in parentheses where appropriate)—not necessarily inclusive (» = major clinical significance).

*Except under special circumstances, this device should not be used when the following medical problems exist:*

» Acquired immunodeficiency syndrome (AIDS) or
» Autoimmune diseases or
» Malignancy treated with antineoplastic agents and/or radiation or
» Malignancy, uterine or cervical, known or suspected or
» Any other condition associated with or resulting in decreased immunity and/or increased susceptibility to infection
(possible increased risk of infection with an IUD when a patient lacks an intact immune system)

» Bleeding, genital, of unknown etiology
(insertion of a progesterone IUD may initially exacerbate uterine bleeding, then, with continued use, decrease uterine bleeding; this could mask other serious underlying conditions and delay the diagnosis of the condition)

» Ectopic pregnancy, history of
(may increase risk of ectopic pregnancy with contraceptive failure, especially in nulliparous women)

» Infection or inflammation in female reproductive tract, including
Abortion, recent septic
Cervicitis
Endometritis
Genital actinomyces-like infection
PID, acute or history of
Sexually transmitted diseases during last 12 months
Vaginitis, excluding candidiasis but including bacterial vaginosis, until controlled
(use of an IUD, when any of the above conditions is present, may predispose the patient to upper genital tract infections that may range in severity from mild to life-threatening; risk is highest within the first 30 days after IUD insertion)
(women with a history of PID may be at increased risk of developing PID; nulliparous women may be at greater risk than parous women)
(significant risk of infection progressing to PID may be related to acquisition of or exposure to PID-associated sexually transmitted diseases)

» Surgery involving the uterus or fallopian tubes
(women currently using an IUD may have an increased risk of surgical complications; also, in cases of contraception failure, women having had surgery involving the uterus or fallopian tubes may have additional risk for developing an ectopic pregnancy)

» Uterine abnormalities or cavity distortion
(possibility of decreased contraceptive effectiveness; increased risk of IUD expulsion or IUD perforation of the uterus)

*Risk-benefit should be considered when the following medical problems exist:*

Bradycardia, neurovascular, history of or
Syncope, neurovascular, history of
(short-term syncope or bradycardia may occur with IUD insertion; increased risk if these conditions are present)

Cervical stenosis
(may prevent ease of insertion of IUD; excessive force to overcome this resistance is not advised)

» Coagulopathy
(use of a progesterone IUD when increased vascularity and permeability and decreased hemostatic response exists may increase risk of of an IUD expulsion)

Diabetes, insulin-dependent
(IUDs may be a good choice for diabetics; however, complications from infection, if infection occurs, are potentially more likely)

Heart defect, valvular or congenital
(insertion of an IUD may represent a potential source of septic emboli, since these patients are prone to develop subacute bacterial endocarditis)

### Patient monitoring

The following may be especially important in patient monitoring (other tests may be warranted in some patients, depending on condition; » = major clinical significance):

Papanicolaou (Pap) test
(recommended annually; examination for actinomycosis-like organisms and, if appropriate, gonococcal and chlamydial tests should be performed)

Physical examination
(recommended once during the first 3 months and at 12 months after insertion for removal; special attention should be given to reports of delayed menses and/or pelvic pain because of the possibility of ectopic pregnancies with failed IUD contraception)

## Side/Adverse Effects

Note: Cervical laceration, cervical or uterine perforations, and/or abdominal displacement of the IUD may progress to peritonitis, sepsis, pelvic inflammatory disease (PID), abdominal adhesions, intestinal penetration, intestinal obstruction, cystic masses in the pelvis, and local inflammatory reaction with abscess formation, including tubo-ovarian abscess. Certain of these adverse effects of IUDs, although very rare, can lead to a loss of fertility, require partial or total removal of reproductive organs, and, in extremely rare circumstances, cause death. An IUD must be surgically removed as soon as feasible after IUD displacement has been diagnosed.

Because many of the side effects listed below present with uterine bleeding and pain, these symptoms should always be evaluated even though they may not signify a serious problem. Persistent or recurring abnormal uterine bleeding and/or abdominal pain may lessen with continued progesterone IUD use. Other problems such as cervical or uterine perforation, IUD displacement, ectopic pregnancy, PID, and IUD embedment should be ruled out.

The following side/adverse effects have been selected on the basis of their potential clinical significance (possible signs and symptoms in parentheses where appropriate)—not necessarily inclusive:

### Those indicating need for medical attention
Incidence more frequent
*Abdominal pain or cramping on insertion, continuing; intermenstrual spotting or uterine bleeding* (uterine bleeding between menstrual periods); *uterine bleeding on insertion, continuing*

Note: *Abdominal pain* or *uterine bleeding* should be investigated if it continues beyond several days after IUD insertion. *Intermenstrual spotting* can be expected for up to 6 months after insertion and *intermenstrual uterine bleeding* may stop within 3 months. The amount of menstrual blood loss usually is less than preinsertion levels.

Incidence rare
*Cervical perforation or laceration; embedment of IUD or perforation of the uterus* (severe abdominal pain or cramping; unexpected, heavy vaginal bleeding, sharp pain on insertion); *fragmentation of device; neurovascular episodes* (dizziness; faintness)—at time of insertion; *PID* (dull or aching abdominal pain, continuing; fever; odorous vaginal discharge; unusual tiredness or weakness; unusual uterine bleeding)—2 to 3.1%

Note: Increased risk of *PID* occurs within the first 3 months of IUD insertion; ectopic pregnancy should be ruled out before treatment of PID because of similar presenting symptoms. Also, PID and actinomycosis-like infection may be asymptomatic.

## Patient Consultation

As an aid to patient consultation, refer to *Advice for the Patient, Progesterone Intrauterine Device (IUD).*

In providing consultation, consider emphasizing the following selected information (» = major clinical significance):

### Before using this device
Note: In the U.S., the health care professional is required by U.S. federal regulation to provide a patient information brochure to the patient regarding the use of IUDs for contraception, discussing it and other methods of contraception.
» Conditions affecting use, especially:
Pregnancy—IUD use is not recommended for women during pregnancy, those planning to become pregnant shortly, or women who have had an ectopic pregnancy. If contraception fails with a progesterone IUD, complications to the mother or infant are possible whether the pregnancy continues with the IUD *in situ* or the device is removed; also, the risk of uterine perforation and expulsion of the IUD may be increased when an IUD is inserted before 8 weeks postpartum
Use in adolescents—Sexually active adolescents may be better served with a contraceptive method that also protects against sexually transmitted diseases (STDs); IUD use in adolescents

of young age and nulliparous women appears to be associated with a higher expulsion rate
Other medical problems, especially acquired immunodeficiency syndrome (AIDS), autoimmune diseases, immunosuppressive therapy, malignancy of the cervix or uterus, or any other conditions of decreased immunity or increased risk of infection; coagulopathy; genital bleeding of unknown etiology; history of ectopic pregnancy; infection or inflammation in female reproductive tract; surgery involving the uterus or fallopian tubes; or uterine abnormalities or cavity distortion

### Proper use of this device
» Reading a copy of the patient information brochure provided by the health care professional helps explain possible side effects, risks, and warning signs of trouble with the IUD
Spermicides are not needed with a properly placed IUD
» Checking for changes in the IUD thread length after the monthly menses, if not more often, as instructed by physician
» Proper dosing, including IUD removal or replacement times

### Precautions while using this device
» Visiting physician regularly to check progress, especially within the first 3 months, preferably the first month, and at 12 months for removal
» Alerting medical personnel before having diagnostic or therapeutic procedures such as surgery involving the uterus or fallopian tubes
» Notifying physician immediately if a partial or complete expulsion is suspected; using another form of nonhormonal contraception until evaluated by a physician; patient should not try to remove the IUD or re-insert it
» Reporting missed or scanty menses to physician immediately and using other nonhormonal contraceptive methods
» Reporting symptoms of possible pregnancy, including ectopic pregnancy, to physician in the rare case when IUD contraceptive effects fail
» Notifying physician and using other nonhormonal contraceptive methods if any of the following occur:
—Abnormal vaginal bleeding
—Exposure to sexually transmitted diseases
—Feeling the tip of the IUD at the cervix or pain during sexual intercourse
—Change in length of IUD threads or disappearance of IUD threads on periodic observation after menses
—Lifestyle change from a mutually monogamous relationship
—Pelvic/lower abdominal pain or cramping, unusual or severe, possibly with fever
—Vaginal discharge or signs of genital lesions or sores
Progesterone IUDs should not interfere with the proper use of other vaginal products such as tampons or condoms

### Side/adverse effects
Signs of potential side effects, especially abdominal pain or cramping on insertion (continuing), intermenstrual spotting or uterine bleeding, uterine bleeding on insertion (continuing), cervical perforation or laceration, embedment of IUD, fragmentation of device, perforation of the uterus, neurovascular episodes on insertion, pelvic inflammatory disease (PID)

## General Dosing Information

In the U.S., the health care professional is required by U.S. Federal Regulations (21 CFR 310.502) to give the patient a copy of the Patient Information for an Informed Decision to ensure complete understanding of the risks and benefits, safety, and efficacy of the progesterone IUD.

It is generally believed that perforations occur at the time of insertion, although they may not be detected until later. Adequate training of those health care professionals inserting the device may help prevent cervical or uterine perforation. A number of supervised insertions may be necessary before a solo attempt. The degree of training needed depends on the health care professional's skill and experience with IUD aseptic insertion techniques and uterus manipulation.

The manufacturer's product information should be consulted for specific directions.

The IUD may be inserted at any time during the menstrual cycle. Many physicians prefer insertion at the end of or within 2 days after a menstrual period to reduce the possibility of inserting an IUD in the presence of an undiagnosed pregnancy. However, the optimal time for insertion appears to be the periovulatory period. Caution should be used to avoid inserting a second IUD, as patients may forget about a previously inserted IUD or may assume it to be expelled.

Using aseptic technique and removing the IUD from the sterile packaging no more than 5 minutes before the insertion procedure are recommended. Prophylactic treatment with antibiotics theoretically may reduce the risk of infection, which is 6 times higher within the first 20 days after insertion. Regimens include doxycycline 200 mg orally one hour before insertion, or erythromycin 500 mg orally one hour before insertion and 500 mg orally six hours after insertion. This may be of limited benefit and unnecessary for women at low risk of sexually transmitted disease (STDs).

It is recommended that an IUD be removed for the following medical reasons: pelvic infection, genital actinomycosis, dyspareunia, pregnancy (when able to remove the IUD), endometrial or cervical malignancy, uterine or cervical perforation, or partial expulsion.

If the retrieval threads cannot be seen, they may have retracted into the uterus or have been broken, or the IUD may have been expelled. Pregnancy, both uterine and ectopic, should be considered before attempting to locate the IUD. Although ultrasound is the preferred method of locating a malpositioned IUD, high- or intermediate-strength magnetic resonance imaging (MRI), uterine probe, or x-rays may also be used.

Removing an intraperitoneal progesterone IUD as soon as medically feasible after the diagnosis is recommended because of the possibility of abdominal adhesion formation, intestinal penetration, and local inflammatory reaction with abscess formation and erosion of adjacent viscera, maternal sepsis, or, rarely, death.

The manufacturer's information should be consulted for the recommended removal procedure. If an IUD is difficult to remove, the procedure may need to be done in a hospital or operating room. Another type of contraception should begin immediately after IUD removal if contraception is desired.

**For treatment of adverse effects**
Recommended treatment consists of the following:
- For pain—Treating with mild analgesics for several hours after IUD insertion.
- For pelvic inflammatory disease (PID)—Removing the progesterone IUD and treating the patient with appropriate broad-spectrum antibi-

otics; the patient's partner may require treatment with broad-spectrum antibiotics as well.

Note: HIV-infected women with PID who are immunocompromised may be at increased risk of a complicated clinical course and should be hospitalized for intravenous therapy.

## Intrauterine Dosage Form
### PROGESTERONE INTRAUTERINE CONTRACEPTIVE SYSTEM USP

**Usual adult and adolescent dose**
Contraceptive—
Intrauterine, one device; the maximum duration of use is 12 months.

**Strength(s) usually available**
U.S.—
38 mg progesterone (Rx) [*Progestasert*].
Canada—
Not commercially available.

**Packaging and storage**
Store below 40 °C (104 °F), preferably between 15 and 30 °C (59 and 86 °F), unless otherwise specified by manufacturer. Preserve in sealed, single-unit containers.

**Note**
Provide patient with patient package insert (PPI).

## Selected Bibliography
Farley TM, Rosenberg MJ, Rowe PJ, et al. Intrauterine devices and pelvic inflammatory disease: an international perspective. Lancet 1992 Mar 28; 339: 785-8.
Liskin L, Fox G. IUDs: an appropriate contraceptive for many women. Popul Rep B; Intrauterine Devices, (4), Washington, DC, 1982.
Trussell J, Hatcher RA, Cates W Jr, et al. Contraceptive failure in the United States: an update. Stud Fam Plann 1990; 21 (1): 51-4.

Developed: 12/04/95

---

# PROGESTINS　Systemic

This monograph includes information on the following: Hydroxyprogesterone†; Levonorgestrel; Medrogestone*; Medroxyprogesterone; Megestrol; Norethindrone; Norgestrel†; Progesterone.

INN:
　Hydroxyprogesterone caproate—Hydroxyprogesterone
　Medroxyprogesterone acetate—Medroxyprogesterone
　Megestrol acetate—Megestrol
　Norethindrone—Norethisterone

BAN:
　Hydroxyprogesterone caproate—Hydroxyprogesterone
　Medroxyprogesterone acetate—Medroxyprogesterone
　Megestrol acetate—Megestrol
　Norethindrone—Norethisterone

VA CLASSIFICATION (Primary/Secondary):
　Hydroxyprogesterone—HS800
　Levonorgestrel—HS800/HS200
　Medrogestone—HS800
　Medroxyprogesterone—HS800/AN500; HS200
　Megestrol—HS800/AN500
　Norethindrone—HS800/HS200
　Norgestrel—HS800/HS200
　Progesterone—HS800

Another commonly used name for norethindrone is norethisterone.

Note: For a listing of dosage forms and brand names by country availability, see *Dosage Forms* section(s). For a listing of brand names for the articles in this monograph, refer to the General Index.

---

*Not commercially available in the U.S.
†Not commercially available in Canada.

---

## Category
Progestational agent—Hydroxyprogesterone; Medrogestone; Medroxyprogesterone (oral); Norethindrone; Norgestrel; Progesterone.
Antianoretic—Megestrol.
Anticachectic—Megestrol.
Antineoplastic—Medroxyprogesterone (parenteral); Megestrol.

Contraceptive (systemic)—Levonorgestrel; Medroxyprogesterone (parenteral); Norethindrone (base); Norgestrel.
Diagnostic aid (estrogen production)—Hydroxyprogesterone; Medroxyprogesterone (oral); Progesterone.

## Indications
Note: Bracketed information in the *Indications* section refers to uses that are not included in U.S. product labeling.

**Accepted**
Amenorrhea, secondary or
Dysfunctional uterine bleeding (DUB) or
Menses, induction of (treatment)—Hydroxyprogesterone, medrogestone, oral medroxyprogesterone, norethindrone acetate, and progesterone are indicated in the treatment of menstrual disorders, including secondary amenorrhea and dysfunctional uterine bleeding (DUB) caused by hormonal imbalance in the absence of organic pathology. Hydroxyprogesterone is also indicated for the production of a secretory endometrium and desquamation. The uterus must be sufficiently primed with endogenous or exogenous estrogen for the progestins to produce a secretory-like endometrium and endometrial shedding after progestin use ends. Withdrawal bleeding usually occurs 3 to 7 days after discontinuation of the progestin for women with an intact uterus.

Anorexia (treatment) or
Cachexia (treatment) or
Weight loss, significant, AIDS-associated (treatment)—Megestrol is indicated in the treatment of unexplained significant weight loss (loss of 10% or more of base-line body weight).

Endometriosis (treatment)—Norethindrone acetate and [medroxyprogesterone][1] are indicated in the treatment of endometriosis.

Estrogen production, endogenous (diagnosis)—Hydroxyprogesterone, [oral medroxyprogesterone], and [parenteral progesterone] are indicated as a test for endogenous estrogen production and can be used to determine whether low levels of estrogen are present if withdrawal bleeding does not occur after a progestin challenge in menopausal women before estrogen-progestin replacement therapy is considered. However, determination that serum gonadotropins are elevated is the standard way to confirm menopause.

Carcinoma (treatment)—[Oral] or parenteral medroxyprogesterone, and megestrol are indicated for the treatment of endometrial carcinoma.

Parenteral medroxyprogesterone is also indicated in the treatment of metastatic renal carcinoma.

Megestrol and [oral and parenteral medroxyprogesterone] are indicated in the treatment of breast carcinoma; [medroxyprogesterone] is indicated for use in postmenopausal women only.

[Megestrol] is indicated in the treatment of hormonally dependent and advanced prostate carcinoma.

Note: Progestins are recommended only for adjunctive and/or palliative therapy when used in the treatment of advanced (inoperable, recurrent, or metastatic) hormonally dependent carcinoma.

Hormone replacement, female, menopause (treatment)—[Oral medroxyprogesterone], [norethindrone][1], and medrogestone can be used for hormonal replacement therapy to oppose the effects of estrogen on the endometrium in estrogen-treated menopausal women. All menopausal patients receiving progestins do not have recognized endometrial shedding; there is frequently amenorrhea after several months treatment with estrogen-progestin regimens. Optimal or recommended length of replacement after menopause has not been established. Studies have shown that administration of a progestin for a minimum of 10 to 14 days of an estrogen cycle in women with an intact uterus is required for major reduction of endometrial hyperplasia and endometrial carcinoma compared with an estrogen-only cycle. Other dosing regimens for estrogens and progestins, including low continuous daily dosing, are also used. Progestins without estrogens may be used for debilitating menopausal symptoms in patients who have breast cancer and are candidates for progestin therapy but cannot take estrogens.

Pregnancy (prophylaxis)—Levonorgestrel, parenteral medroxyprogesterone[1], norethindrone (base), and norgestrel are indicated for the prevention of pregnancy.

The following table presents the results of studies examining contraceptive failure rates calculated using the life-table method. The first column lists the contraceptive method used. The second column indicates the percentage of women experiencing an accidental pregnancy in the first year of use of a contraceptive method while using the method perfectly under clinical conditions. The range of failure rates in the clinical trials may be explained by interstudy variations in study design or patient population characteristics, such as motivation, fecundity, or socioeconomic factors (including education). The third column indicates contraceptive failure rates in the first year of contraceptive use under clinical conditions for typical couples who start using a method (not necessarily for the first time). Failure rates among adolescents may be higher due to poorer compliance than in other age groups.

| Method used | Failure rate range (over 12 months) in clinical studies (%) | Typical first year failure rate (%) |
|---|---|---|
| None | 78–94 | 85 |
| Spermicides[1] | 0.3–37 | 21 |
| Periodic abstinence[2] | 13–35 | 20 |
| Withdrawal | 7–22 | 19 |
| Cervical cap with spermicide | 6–27 | 18 |
| Diaphragm with spermicide | 2–23 | 18 |
| Condom without spermicide | 2–14 | 12 |
| IUD | | |
|   Progesterone-releasing | 1.9–2 | 2 |
|   Copper-T 200 | 3–3.6 | |
|   Copper-T 200Ag[3] | 0–1.2 | |
|   Copper-T 220C[4] | 0.9–1.8 | |
|   Copper-T 380A | 0.5–0.8 | 0.8 |
|   Copper-T 380S | 0.9 | |
| Oral contraceptive | | 3 |
|   Estrogen and progestin | 0–6 | |
|   Progestin only | 1–10 | |
| Progestin injection | | |
|   Medroxyprogesterone (90-day) | 0–0.3 | 0.3 |
| Levonorgestrel (subdermal) | | |
|   Six capsules | 0–0.09 | 0.09 |
|   Two rods | 0–0.2 | 0.3 |
| Sterilization | | |
|   Female[5] | 0–8 | 0.4 |
|   Male | 0–0.5 | 0.15 |

[1]Spermicides studied include creams, foams, gels, jellies, and suppositories.

[2]Methods studied include calendar, ovulation method, symptothermal (cervical mucus method supplemented by basal body temperature post-ovulation).

[3]Life table method rate is unavailable for Copper-T 200Ag and the Pearl method rate at 12 months was reported; these methods at 12 months are considered comparable.

[4]Copper-T 220C is manufactured with copper sleeves instead of copper wire; often used as a control in clinical studies.

[5]Methods studied include culdotomy laparoscopy, minilaparotomy, electrocoagulation, laparotomy, tubal diathermy and/or use of rings or clips.

[Corpus luteum insufficiency (treatment)][1]—Progesterone is used to treat corpus luteum dysfunction.

[Hyperplasia, endometrial (treatment)][1]—Megestrol and oral medroxyprogesterone have been used to treat endometrial hyperplasia without atypia, which is usually not a precursor of carcinoma. Complex atypical hyperplasia (previously called adenomatous hyperplasia) is usually best treated surgically, but in some high risk patients or when future pregnancy is desired, high continuous doses of progestins have been used.

[Polycystic ovary syndrome (treatment)][1]—Medroxyprogesterone is used in the treatment of endometrial hyperplasia and its consequences in syndromes, such as polycystic ovary syndrome.

[Puberty, precocious (treatment)][1]—Parenteral medroxyprogesterone is accepted therapy for use in the treatment of precocious puberty but has been replaced by other treatment modalities.

**Unaccepted**

There is no evidence that progesterone is effective in the treatment of premenstrual syndrome.

Progestins are no longer recommended for use as pregnancy tests because of possible teratogenic effects with synthetic progestins; also, other tests available are quicker and easier to perform.

With the exception of progesterone in patients who are progesterone deficient, progestins have no proven value in the treatment of threatened abortion and are no longer recommended for such use.

Unlike oral medroxyprogesterone, parenteral medroxyprogesterone is not recommended by the manufacturer for treatment of secondary amenorrhea or dysfunctional uterine bleeding.

Megestrol is not recommended for prophylactic use to avoid weight loss.

[1]Not included in Canadian product labeling.

# Pharmacology/Pharmacokinetics

See also *Table 1*, page 2456.

**Physicochemical characteristics**

Molecular weight—
  Hydroxyprogesterone caproate: 428.62.
  Levonorgestrel: 312.45.
  Medrogestone: 340.51.
  Medroxyprogesterone acetate: 386.53.
  Megestrol acetate: 384.52.
  Norethindrone: 298.43.
  Norethindrone acetate: 340.47.
  Norgestrel: 312.45.
  Progesterone: 314.47.

**Mechanism of action/Effect**

Progestins enter target cells by passive diffusion and bind to cytosolic (soluble) receptors that are loosely bound in the nucleus. The steroid receptor complex initiates transcription, resulting in an increase in protein synthesis.

Progestins are capable of affecting serum concentrations of other hormones, particularly estrogen. Estrogenic effects are modified by the progestins, either by reducing the availability or stability of the hormone receptor complex or by turning off specific hormone-responsive genes by direct interaction with the progestin receptor in the nucleus. In addition, estrogen priming is necessary to increase progestin effects by upregulating the number of progestin receptors and/or increasing progesterone production, causing a negative feedback mechanism that inhibits estrogen receptors.

Depending on the progestin and its dose, progestin may demonstrate varying degrees of progestational effects. Also, other hormonal effects, such as estrogenic-, anabolic-, androgenic-, or glucocorticoid-inducing or suppressing effects are demonstrated to different degrees and depend on the progestin type and dose. For example, an androgenic effect may be expressed by 19-nor derivatives of testosterone but not by other progestins. The androgenic effects of norethindrone are minor to moderate; norethindrone acetate is twice as potent as norethindrone. Norgestrel and levonorgestrel have androgenic effects at high doses if unopposed by estrogens. While the progestational effects dominate, the other effects can become important when choosing the appropriate progestin or monitoring side effects. Progestins are not used exclusively for other than their progestational effects, as the other effects are highly variable and unreliable.

Progestational agents—Progestins produce histologic changes in the vaginal epithelium and induce secretory-like changes in the endometrium in the second half of the menstrual cycle. As progestin levels fall after estrogen priming, uterine bleeding occurs.

Antianoretic

    Anticachectic—The mechanism that produces weight gain has not been fully elucidated; however, megestrol appears to have appetite-stimulant and metabolic effects that result in weight gain while causing minimal fluid retention. The underlying cause of wasting should be treated concurrently to optimize management of catabolism.

Antineoplastic—The mechanism has not been fully elucidated; however, several mechanisms may be involved that are dependent on the type and dose of progestin. In certain doses, progestins can produce a diminished response to endogenous hormones in tumor cells by decreasing the number of steroid hormone receptors (estrogen, progesterone, androgen, and glucocorticoid); the degree of variation of response is tissue- and progestin-dependent. The suppression of the growth of hormone-sensitive cells may be due to a direct cytotoxic effect or anti-proliferative effects on cell cycle growth and an increased terminal cell differentiation. At higher doses, some progestins compete for the glucocorticoid receptor, resulting in suppressed adrenal production of estradiol and androstenedione. Still-higher progestin doses are able to completely suppress the hypothalamic-pituitary-adrenal axis (HPA-axis), an effect that is important in the treatment of estrogen- or testosterone-sensitive tumors.

Contraceptive (systemic)—Inhibition of the secretion of gonadotropins from the anterior pituitary prevents ovulation and follicular maturation and is one of the contraceptive actions of levonorgestrel, parenteral medroxyprogesterone, norethindrone, and norgestrel. These effects do not occur with low-dose oral medroxyprogesterone, which is not used for contraception. In some patients using low-dose progestin-only contraceptives, particularly norethindrone (base) and levonorgestrel subdermal capsules, ovulation is not suppressed consistently from cycle to cycle. The contraceptive effect is achieved through other mechanisms that result in interference with implantation and fertilization, such as thickening of the cervical mucus and changes in the endometrium. In males, medroxyprogesterone suppresses the Leydig cell function.

### Other actions/effects

Progestins increase body temperature, stimulate the respiratory center, and, in some cases, may provide pain relief. The mechanism by which progesterone and medroxyprogesterone mediate thermogenic effects is not clear. It has been suggested that progesterone influences neurotransmitters and neuropeptides in the brain, notably endogenous opioids, interleukin-1, and serotonin, that raise body temperature. Also, medroxyprogesterone may reduce hypercapnia in certain patients by stimulating the respiratory center. Pain relief from high-dose progestins may be due in part to an anti-inflammatory action.

Locally the progestins relax the uterine smooth muscle, sustain pregnancy, decrease the immune response, and, acting with estrogen, stimulate breast tissue growth.

Some progestins cause sodium and water retention. Progesterone doses of 50 to 100 mg may produce a moderate catabolic effect and transient increase in sodium chloride excretion. In addition, use of some progestins may result in dose-related adverse effects on carbohydrate and lipid metabolism.

Progestins influence bone density. When progestins have been used without estrogen, a positive effect has been shown in postmenopausal women and a possible negative effect in premenopausal women; the latter may depend on the degree to which a progestin can reduce ovarian estrogen production, a dose-dependent effect. When progestins have been used sequentially with continuously administered estrogen, a synergistic protective effect on bone density has been shown. Specifically, placebo-controlled studies of postmenopausal women showed that medroxyprogesterone decreased the rate of cortical bone loss but did not protect trabecular areas of the skeleton, such as the spine, equally from bone loss in all studies. A low-dose combination of continuously administered estrogen and sequentially administered progestin therapy showed protective effects against bone loss that were similar to those of higher doses of estrogen therapy alone. This effect may be due to an increase of progestin receptors caused by estrogen, to an antagonistic effect of progestin binding to glucocorticoid receptors, or to a stimulatory effect of progestin acting on progestin receptors within osteoblasts. Additional studies are needed to confirm and fully characterize these results.

Other health benefits of progestational hormone therapy may include less painful menstruation, less menstrual blood loss and anemia, fewer pelvic infections, and lower incidence of uterine cancers.

### Absorption

Progestins—Well absorbed, except for oral progesterone, which is not easily absorbed even when micronized.

Levonorgestrel subdermal capsules and parenteral medroxyprogesterone acetate—Well-absorbed during controlled release with wide intra- and intersubject variability; initial release rate for a set of implanted levonorgestrel subdermal capsules is approximately 80 micrograms of levonorgestrel per 24 hours, declining over the first 6 to 18 months to an approximately constant release rate of 30 micrograms of levonorgestrel per 24 hours over the remainder of the 5 years.

## Precautions to Consider

### Carcinogenicity

The benefit of lowering the incidence of endometrial hyperplasia and endometrial cancer by adding progestin to an estrogen replacement modality to counter estrogen's effect on the uterus has been established.

*Medroxyprogesterone—*

    Long-term studies in humans using parenteral medroxyprogesterone for contraception have found no increase in the overall risk of ovarian, liver, breast, or cervical cancer and have found a prolonged, protective effect of reducing the risk of endometrial cancer for at least 8 years. The possible protective effect may be lessened with concomitant use of estrogen; however, the lifetime risk for developing endometrial cancer is not increased in women with a uterus who take estrogen plus a progestin for 10 to 20 years. In the short-term, the initial risk of breast cancer with parenteral medroxyprogesterone exposure may be increased in the first 4 years after initial exposure in women under 35 years of age. The risk lessens with duration of use and results in no overall increase of risk for developing breast cancer.

    Studies of monkeys administered doses of 3, 30, and 150 mg per kg (mg/kg) of body weight every 90 days for 10 years produced undifferentiated carcinoma of the uterus in a few monkeys dosed at 150 mg/kg. No uterine malignancies were reported in monkeys taking other doses or in the control monkeys; no uterine abnormalities were produced in similar studies of rats after 2 years. The relevance of these findings to humans is not known.

### Tumorigenicity/Mutagenicity

*Hydroxyprogesterone, levonorgestrel, medrogestone, norgestrel, norethindrone, and progesterone—*

    Studies have not been done.

*Medroxyprogesterone—*

    Studies in humans have not been done.

    Mammary nodules, some of which were malignant in the high-dose group, developed in a number of beagles given doses of 3 or 75 mg/kg of medroxyprogesterone every 90 days for 7 years. In studies of monkeys, doses of 3, 30, or 150 mg/kg of medroxyprogesterone given every 90 days for 10 years produced transient mammary nodules in the 3 and 30 mg/kg groups, with none reported in the 150 mg/kg group during the study; hyperplastic nodules had developed in 3 monkeys that had been administered 30 mg/kg of medroxyprogesterone; no breast abnormalities were produced in rats after 2 years. Caution is warranted in applying these results of animal studies of progestins to their use in humans because of the hormonal differences between species. Also, humans and beagles metabolize medroxyprogesterone differently, and beagles are particularly susceptible to this type of breast tumor and develop these tumors spontaneously without progestin use.

There was no mutagenic response in the Ames and micronucleus tests.

*Megestrol—*

    Studies in humans have not been done.

    Studies of female dogs given megestrol for up to 7 years showed an increased incidence of both benign and malignant tumors; 2-year studies of female rats demonstrated an increased incidence of pituitary tumors. These effects were not found in monkey studies.

### Pregnancy/Reproduction

Fertility—Progestins cause a decrease in quantity and/or change the quality of cervical mucus and may interfere with sperm function, fertilization, and subsequently, the occurrence of pregnancy. This effect depends on the dose and type of the progestin. High-dose or long-term use of progestins may cause a delayed return to fertility.

*Levonorgestrel subdermal capsules—*

    After removal, 40% of those women wanting to conceive did so by 3 months; 76% conceived within 1 year.

*Medroxyprogesterone—*

It has been reported that of the women who discontinued parenteral medroxyprogesterone to become pregnant, 68% conceived within 12 months, 83% conceived within 15 months, and 93% conceived within 18 months after discontinuation (range, 4 to 31 months; median 10 months). The return of fertility is a function of the uptake and metabolism of parenteral medroxyprogesterone; follicular activity has been reported to return 3 to 37 days after parenteral medroxyprogesterone is nondetectable in serum, whereas luteal function is delayed by 14 to 102 days.

Animal studies with medroxyprogesterone have reported no impairment of fertility in first or second generation studies.

*Megestrol—*

Studies in humans have not been done.

Studies of rats given megestrol in doses of 0.05 to 12.5 mg per kg of body weight (mg/kg), which are lower than the human dose of 13.3 mg/kg, resulted in impaired reproductive capability of male offspring produced from megestrol-treated females; similar results were found in studies of dogs.

*Progesterone—*

Progesterone has been used successfully with assisted reproductive technologies.

Pregnancy—Progestins, in general, should be withheld during pregnancy. Progestins cross the placenta. Although many studies fail to demonstrate an increase in teratogenicity when progestins are given in the first trimester, the possibility that genital abnormalities may appear in male and female fetuses exposed to progestins during that period has been suggested by some studies. The low number of abnormalities reported include an increased risk of hypospadias in male fetuses exposed to intrauterine progesterone and virilization of the female fetus' external genitalia when exposed to ethisterone and norethindrone. There is some controversy about the reliability of these reports. The significant concentration of endogenous natural progesterone produced during pregnancy is devoid of teratogenic effects.

Ectopic pregnancy is possible with contraception failure because some progestin-only contraceptives protect mainly against intrauterine pregnancy. For progestin-only oral contraceptives, the ectopic pregnancy rate reported is 4.1 per 100 pregnancies. The rate of ectopic pregnancy for the first year of use of a set of levonorgestrel subdermal capsules is 1.3 per 1000 woman-years. This is lower than those for women not using any contraceptive method (2.7 to 3 ectopic pregnancies per 1000 woman-years). However, the risk may increase with longer duration of use of levonorgestrel subdermal capsules and increased weight of the user; risk does not increase in women of normal weight.

*Hydroxyprogesterone and progesterone—*

Use is generally not recommended during pregnancy. Hydroxyprogesterone and progesterone have been used to prevent habitual or threatened abortion within the first few months of pregnancy. Progesterone may be used for corpus luteum deficiency in early pregnancy. There are no adequate and well-controlled studies in humans to document that such use is effective during the first 4 months of pregnancy in preventing miscarriage; use is generally limited to certain cases of hormonal imbalance. When there is a hormone imbalance, including a progesterone deficiency, use of these hormones appears to be beneficial. It does not appear to be efficacious when a hormone imbalance does not exist. In addition, the progesterone's effects on the uterus may delay the spontaneous miscarriage of a defective ovum.

FDA Pregnancy Category D.

*Levonorgestrel, norethindrone, and norgestrel—*

Use is not recommended during pregnancy. Virilization of the female fetus has been reported with norethindrone in a few cases, but a causal relationship has not been conclusively proven.

FDA Pregnancy Category X.

*Medroxyprogesterone—*

Use is not recommended in pregnancy. Studies in humans have shown that medroxyprogesterone may decrease intrauterine growth. Polysyndactyly in the offspring of women who had used parenteral medroxyprogesterone during pregnancy was reported in a few case-reports; this effect has not been seen in major studies. Furthermore, there has been no evidence of problems associated with growth and development in children exposed *in utero* to medroxyprogesterone and followed to adolescence.

In studies of pregnant beagles given doses of 1, 10, and 30 mg/kg of body weight per day for 6 months, clitoral hypertrophy appeared in the female pups of the high-dose group; no abnormalities were reported in the male pups. No abnormalities were detected in the treated female pups' offspring. Caution is war-

ranted in transferring this information to humans because beagle dogs metabolize medroxyprogesterone differently than do humans.

Medroxyprogesterone, parenteral—FDA Pregnancy Category X.

Note: An FDA category has not been assigned for medroxyprogesterone tablets.

*Megestrol—*

Use is not recommended during pregnancy. Risk-benefit must be carefully considered.

Studies in pregnant rats given high doses of megestrol decreased fetal birth weight, produced fewer live births, and resulted in reversible feminization of some male fetuses.

Megestrol suspension—FDA Pregnancy Category X.

Megestrol tablets—FDA Pregnancy Category D.

## Breast-feeding

Progestins are distributed into breast milk in variable amounts and, depending on the progestin and dose, may increase or decrease quantity or quality or have no effect on breast milk. No adverse effects on breast milk's quantity or quality have been seen with progestin-only contraceptives, or specifically, when norethindrone or levonorgestrel was used for contraception within 5 days postpartum or after the establishment of lactation. Progestin-only contraceptives are recommended in breast-feeding women when oral contraception is desired. The manufacturers of levonorgestrel subdermal capsules and parenteral medroxyprogesterone for contraception recommend that their initial use for contraception begin at 6 weeks postpartum for exclusively breast-feeding mothers. Additionally, no adverse effects have been reported in a study of nursing infants exposed to parenteral medroxyprogesterone and followed through puberty or in another study of 80 nursing infants exposed to levonorgestrel subdermal capsules 6 weeks after delivery and followed for 3 years.

Progestins used in very high doses are not recommended for use by nursing mothers.

## Pediatrics

No information is available on the relationship of age to the effects of progestins in pediatric patients. Safety and efficacy have not been established. Serious adverse effects have not been reported in small children who ingested large doses of oral contraceptives.

## Adolescents

Special counseling for drug dosing compliance and prevention of sexually transmitted diseases (STDs) is needed. Studies have shown that adolescents tend to have a higher failure rate with the use of any type of contraceptive that requires strict compliance, such as oral progestins for contraception and its use is not generally recommended in this age group. Although parenteral medroxyprogesterone and levonorgestrel subdermal capsules do not require daily compliance, readministration of their doses after 3 months (13 weeks) and after 5 years, respectively, is important. Furthermore, none of the progestin contraceptives protect against STDs, which are significant risk-factors for this age group.

## Geriatrics

No information is available on the relationship of age to the effects of progestins in geriatric patients.

## Dental

Increased concentrations of progestins increase the normal oral flora growth rate, leading to an increase in inflammation of the gingival tissues and increased bleeding. A strictly enforced program of teeth cleaning by a professional, combined with plaque control by the patient, will minimize severity.

## Drug interactions and/or related problems

The following drug interactions and/or related problems have been selected on the basis of their potential clinical significance (possible mechanism in parentheses where appropriate)—not necessarily inclusive (» = major clinical significance):

Note: Combinations containing any of the following medications, depending on the amount present, may also interact with this medication.

» Aminoglutethimide

(may significantly lower the serum concentrations of oral and parenteral medroxyprogesterone by an undetermined mechanism; it has been suggested that aminoglutethimide may decrease the intestinal absorption of oral medroxyprogesterone)

» Hepatic enzyme inducing medications, such as
Carbamazepine or
Phenobarbital or
Phenytoin or

Rifabutin or
Rifampin
 (decreased efficacy of some progestins, including levonorgestrel subdermal capsules, has been suggested to be caused by enhanced metabolism of the progestins by these drugs)

 (phenytoin and rifampin increase the serum concentrations of sex-hormone binding globulin [SHBG]; this significantly decreases the serum concentration of free drug for some progestins)

 (drug interaction data are not available for rifabutin, but because its structure is similar to that of rifampin, similar precautions with its use with progestins may be warranted)

## Laboratory value alterations

The following have been selected on the basis of their potential clinical significance (possible effect in parentheses where appropriate)—not necessarily inclusive (» = major clinical significance):

With diagnostic test results
 Biopsy
  (pathologist should be notified of relevant specimens)

 Glucose tolerance test
  (may be decreased)

 Metapyrone
  (lower response than normally expected)

With laboratory test values
 Apolipoprotein A and
 High-density lipoproteins (HDL) and
 Total cholesterol and
 Triglycerides
  (serum concentrations may be increased or decreased and may differ depending on type of progestin, dose, dosing, and duration of therapy. In general, all progestins will lower triglyceride and total cholesterol concentrations. Parenteral medroxyprogesterone, in low doses, produces no significant decrease in HDL cholesterol concentrations; oral doses may blunt an estrogen-induced increase of HDL. In contrast, 19-nor-testosterone derived progestins significantly lower HDL cholesterol as well as total cholesterol)

 Apolipoprotein B and
 Low-density lipoproteins (LDL)
  (serum concentrations may be increased and may differ depending on type of progestin, dose, dosing, and duration of therapy)

  (LDL concentrations increased initially in some studies and then returned to normal or below normal baseline levels when progestins were given for a year. Additionally, serum estrogen concentrations seemed to influence the cyclicality and degree to which LDL concentration increased; progestins affected the values to a lesser extent when estrogen levels were normal)

 Clotting factors II, VII, VIII, IX, and X and
 Prothrombin
  (serum concentrations may be increased although studies have not shown consistent results; no change in clotting factors has been reported with parenteral medroxyprogesterone for contraception)

 Gonadotropin and
 Sex-hormone binding globulin (SHBG)
  (serum concentration may be decreased)

 Liver function tests and
 Sulfobromophthalein
  (values may be increased; if abnormal with parenteral medroxyprogesterone use, liver tests may be repeated 4 to 6 months after its discontinuation)

 Steroid, serum and
 Steroid, urinary
  (urinary and serum concentrations of pregnanediol, testosterone, cortisol, estradiol, and progesterone may be decreased)

 $T_3$-uptake
  (values may be decreased because of increase in thyroid-binding globulin [TBG]; free $T_4$ concentration is unaltered)

 $T_4$, total
  (unaffected by most progestins but concentrations are slightly decreased with levonorgestrel; free $T_4$ concentration is unaltered)

## Medical considerations/Contraindications

The medical considerations/contraindications included here have been selected on the basis of their potential clinical significance (reasons given in parentheses where appropriate)—not necessarily inclusive (» = major clinical significance).

*Except under special circumstances, these medications should not be used when the following medical problems exist:*

» Breast malignancies or tumors, known or suspected
  (may worsen conditions in some nonresponsive patients; however, some progestins are used for palliative treatment in select patients)

» Hepatic disease, acute, including benign or malignant liver tumors
  (metabolism of 19-nor derivatives of testosterone-type progestins may be impaired; also, progestins may worsen the condition)

» Pregnancy, known or suspected
  (use of synthetic progestins during pregnancy may result in virilization of a female fetus and, in a small number of cases, increase risk of hypospadia in a male fetus)

  (use for pregnancy diagnosis is contraindicated)

» Sensitivity to progestins

» Thrombophlebitis or thromboembolic disease, active
  (the large doses of progestins used to treat breast and prostate cancer have been associated with a slight risk of thrombogenic conditions; mechanism is unclear and may be due to underlying condition. Problems have not been associated with low doses used for contraception, including parenteral medroxyprogesterone, progestin-only oral contraceptives, and levonorgestrel subdermal capsules)

 Urinary tract bleeding, undiagnosed or
 Uterine or genital bleeding, undiagnosed
  (use of a progestin may delay diagnosis by masking underlying conditions, including cancer)

*Risk-benefit should be considered when the following medical problems exist:*

 Asthma or
 Cardiac insufficiency, significant or
 Epilepsy or
 Hypertension or
 Migraine headaches or
 Renal dysfunction, significant
  (fluid retention may be caused by some progestins, especially in high doses, and may aggravate these conditions)

 CNS disorders, such as depression or convulsions, history of
  (progestins, such as levonorgestrel, medroxyprogesterone, or norethindrone, may make these conditions worse; cases of convulsions have been reported with use of parenteral medroxyprogesterone; however, a clear association has not been established)

 Diabetes mellitus
  (high doses of progestins may alter carbohydrate metabolism by an unknown mechanism, producing a mild decrease in glucose tolerance in some patients; progestin-only contraception does not usually affect carbohydrate metabolism. Time to start and maximal effects may differ between progestins and their doses with intraindividual variability; no clinical significance on fasting blood glucose is seen in nondiabetics receiving low doses)

  (levonorgestrel's effects on carbohydrate metabolism appear to be minimal for nondiabetics but are considered inconclusive for prediabetics and diabetics)

  (parenteral medroxyprogesterone may be used with caution for contraception in diabetics)

 Hepatic disease or dysfunction, history of
  (metabolism of progestins, specifically androgenic progestins, may be impaired and contribute to the hepatic condition)

 Hyperlipidemia
  (some progestins, specifically androgenic progestins, might increase LDL and lower HDL levels and aggravate problems in controlling hyperlipidemia)

 Significant risk factors for low bone mineral content
  (the overall effect on bone density for progestins has yet to be established and may depend on type of progestin, dose, and gender and age of patient. A retrospective cross-sectional study has reported that women using parenteral medroxyprogesterone for contraception had bone density measurements lower than the control group of premenopausal women but higher than the control group of postmenopausal women. Specifically, medroxyprogesterone may temporarily increase the loss of trabecular bone and additionally increase the risk of osteoporosis. The greatest bone loss is evident in the early years of use and is usually reversible and possibly reflects other factors, such as hypoestrogenism, when progestin is used alone. A prospective study has reported that the use of oral medroxyprogesterone alone for hormone replacement in postmenopausal women showed a protective effect; other studies,

particularly those in which a progestin was combined with estrogen, have also shown a protective effect)

» Thromboembolic disorders, including cerebrovascular disease, pulmonary embolism, retinal thrombosis, history of or
Thrombophlebitis, history of
(the large doses of progestins used to treat breast and prostate cancer have been associated with a slight risk of thrombogenic conditions; mechanism is unclear and may be due to the underlying condition. Problems have not been associated with low doses used for contraception, including parenteral medroxyprogesterone, progestin-only oral contraceptives, or levonorgestrel subdermal capsules for patients with a history of thromboembolic disorders or thrombophlebitis)

**Patient monitoring**
The following may be especially important in patient monitoring (other tests may be warranted in some patients, depending on condition; » = major clinical significance):

Breast examinations
(should be performed routinely, especially with prolonged progestin use)
Papanicolaou (Pap) test and
Physical examination
(as determined by physician, with special attention being given to abdomen, breast and pelvic organs; pre- and post-inspection of site of insertion and removal of implanted levonorgestrel subdermal capsules with annual inspection of implantation site during use)

## Side/Adverse Effects

The following side/adverse effects have been selected on the basis of their potential clinical significance (possible signs and symptoms in parentheses where appropriate)—not necessarily inclusive:

**Those indicating need for medical attention**
Incidence more frequent
*Amenorrhea* (stopping of menstrual periods); *breakthrough uterine bleeding or metromenorrhagia* (medium to heavy uterine bleeding between regular monthly periods); *hyperglycemia* (dry mouth; frequent urination; loss of appetite; unusual thirst)—16% with high doses of megestrol; *menorrhagia* (increased amount of menstrual bleeding occurring at regular monthly periods); *spotting* (light uterine bleeding between regular monthly periods)—17% for levonorgestrel subdermal capsules or oral progestins for contraception

Note: *For all progestins,* if *abnormal uterine bleeding* is persistent (longer than 10 days at a time) or recurring (heavier than normal menses occurring longer than 10 months after beginning therapy or more often than monthly), malignancy should be considered as a cause of the bleeding.

*For progestins used for cycle control or as part of hormone replacement therapy: Breakthrough uterine bleeding* is not as prevalent as it is with progestin-only contraceptives; therefore, any uterine bleeding that persists for 3 to 6 months should be investigated.

*For oral progestins for contraception: Breakthrough uterine bleeding* or *spotting* is common.

*For parenteral medroxyprogesterone: Amenorrhea* increases with duration of use (12 months—55% and 24 months—68%). *Breakthrough bleeding* occurs in 90% of users.

*For levonorgestrel subdermal capsules:* After 1 year of use of levonorgestrel subdermal capsules, total uterine blood loss decreases from baseline levels of 31 mL per month to 24 mL per month. *Amenorrhea* occurs in 9.4 to 15% of users of the subdermal capsules and *breakthrough bleeding* occurs in 28% of users, persisting throughout treatment.

Incidence less frequent
*Galactorrhea* (unexpected or increased flow of breast milk); *mental depression; skin rash*
Incidence rare
*Thromboembolism or thrombus formation* (headache or migraine; loss of or change in speech, coordination, or vision; pain or numbness in chest, arm, or leg; shortness of breath, unexplained)—severe and sudden, with high doses of progestins for noncontraceptive uses

Note: It is not clear if the *thromboembolism or thrombus formation* associated with use of progestins in high doses is due to the treatment or to the underlying condition that is being treated, such as cancer.

**Those indicating need for medical attention only if they continue or are bothersome**
Incidence more frequent
*Abdominal pain or cramping; bloating or swelling of face, ankles, or feet*—including, Cushing-like "moon face" with high doses of medroxyprogesterone; *headache, mild*—up to 24% with levonorgestrel subdermal capsules; *mood changes*—up to 16% for levonorgestrel subdermal capsules; *nervousness; ovarian enlargement or ovarian cyst formation* (abdominal pain)—10% for levonorgestrel subdermal capsules; *pain, redness, or skin irritation at the site of injection or implantation*—including, local skin color change and residual lump; *unusual tiredness or weakness; weight gain*

Note: For parenteral medroxyprogesterone for contraception: Average *weight gain* is 2.5 to 7.5 kilograms (kg) after 1 to 6 years of use.

*Ovarian enlargement or ovarian cyst formation* occurring with levonorgestrel subdermal capsules is almost always transient and rarely requires surgery.

Incidence less frequent
*Acne; breast pain or tenderness; hot flashes; insomnia* (trouble in sleeping); *libido decrease* (loss of sexual desire); *loss or gain of body, facial, or scalp hair; melasma* (brown spots on exposed skin, which may persist after treatment stops); *nausea*—subsides in 3 months for low dose progestins for contraception

**Those indicating need for medical attention if they occur after medication is discontinued**
*Delayed return to fertility*

## Patient Consultation

As an aid to patient consultation, refer to *Advice for the Patient, Progestins—For Noncontraceptive Use (Systemic)* or *Progestins—For Contraceptive Use (Systemic).*

In providing consultation, consider emphasizing the following selected information (» = major clinical significance):

**Before using this medication**
» Conditions affecting use, especially:
Allergy to progestins
Carcinogenicity—Studies are ongoing and have not been done with all progestins. Use of progestins with hormone replacement therapy lowers the incidences of endometrial hyperplasia and endometrial cancer. Significantly, a prolonged (8-year) study in women using injectable medroxyprogesterone for contraception has found a protective effect against endometrial cancer. Long-term studies of parenteral medroxyprogesterone have found no increase in overall risk of breast, ovarian, liver, or cervical cancer. Women 35 years of age or younger may have an increased risk of breast cancer during the first four years following initial use
Pregnancy—With the exception of hydroxyprogesterone and progesterone, use is not recommended during pregnancy. When progestins are used in doses for contraception, ectopic pregnancy is possible, although rare. Alternative methods of contraception should be used by fertile and sexually active females when high dose progestins are used for noncontraceptive purposes, such as in treatment of cancer; physician should be told immediately if pregnancy is suspected
Breast-feeding—Progestins are distributed into breast milk in variable amounts; high doses may increase or decrease the quantity or quality of breast milk while low doses have no effect on breast milk and are recommended for use in breast-feeding women needing contraception; adverse effects in the nursing infant have not been reported
Dental—May predispose patient to increased bleeding and inflammation of the gingival tissues; teeth cleaning and plaque control should minimize severity
Other medications, especially aminoglutethimide and hepatic enzyme inducers, such as carbamazepine, phenobarbital, phenytoin, rifabutin, or rifampin
Other medical problems, especially active thrombophlebitis or thromboembolic disease; acute hepatic disease, including benign or malignant tumors; history of thromboembolic disease; known or suspected breast malignancy or tumor; known or suspected pregnancy

**Proper use of this medication**
Reading patient directions
» Importance of not taking more or less medication than the amount prescribed
» Proper dosing
Missed dose

» Proper storage

*For contraception use*

Caution that progestins do not protect against sexually transmitted diseases, including human immunodeficiency virus (HIV) infection or acquired immunodeficiency syndrome (AIDS)

*For levonorgestrel subdermal capsules*

Insertion procedure by a health care professional takes 15 minutes under local anesthesia

» Caring for insertion site requires removing pressure dressing in 24 hours, leaving steristrips (sterile tape) on incisions for 3 days, keeping covered and dry, taking care not to bump site or to lift heavy objects for 24 hours, and expecting some swelling and bruising at site of insertion

» Full contraceptive protection begins within 24 hours when insertion is done within 7 days of the beginning of the menstrual period; otherwise, another birth control method must be used during the rest of the first menstrual cycle; protection ends immediately after removal

» Removal procedure may be done at any time by a health care professional. After 5 years of use the subdermal capsules should be removed and, if desired, a new set of subdermal capsules can be inserted at this time; the removal procedure takes 20 minutes or longer under local anesthesia; rarely, some difficult cases may require skin healing between unsuccessful attempts

*For medroxyprogesterone for contraception*

» Importance of receiving an injection by a health care professional every 3 months (13 weeks)

Stopping use by simply not receiving the injection

Full contraceptive protection begins immediately after initial injection without need for additional birth control methods if given within the first 5 days of a normal menstrual period, within the first 5 days postpartum if not breast-feeding, and, if exclusively breast-feeding, at the sixth postpartum week. Protection continues when an injection is given every 3 months (13 weeks)

*For oral progestins for contraception*

» Compliance with therapy, taking medication at the same time each day at 24-hour intervals

*For noncontraception use*

Caution in taking combination therapy; taking each medication at the right time

## Precautions while using this medication

» Regular visits to health care professional

Checking with doctor immediately if uterine bleeding continues or if menstruation is delayed by 45 days

» Contacting doctor immediately if pregnancy is suspected

If scheduled for laboratory tests, tell physician if taking progestins; certain blood tests may be affected

Possibility of dental problems, such as tenderness, swelling, or bleeding of gums; checking with dentist if there are questions about care of teeth or gums or if tenderness, swelling, or bleeding of gums occurs; patient should follow good cleaning procedures, such as regular brushing and flossing teeth, massaging gums, and having dentist clean teeth regularly

*For contraceptive use*

» Using a second method of birth control when taking medications that reduce effectiveness of progestins

*For noncontraceptive use*

» Advisability of using contraceptive methods while taking progestins for noncontraceptive uses if fertile and sexually active

## Side/adverse effects

Signs of potential side effects, especially amenorrhea; breakthrough bleeding; hyperglycemia; menorrhagia; spotting; galactorrhea; mental depression; skin rash; thromboembolism or thrombus formation

# General Dosing Information

## For all progestins

The cyclical administration of progestins is based on an assumed menstrual cycle of 28 days.

Onset of the female menopause may be masked by the use of progestins.

Follicular atresia may be delayed, allowing the growth and development of follicles that clinically may appear to be ovarian cysts, especially with levonorgestrel subdermal capsules. In most cases, enlarged follicles disappear spontaneously, but, rarely, they may rupture, causing abdominal pain and requiring surgical intervention.

Discontinue medication pending eye examination if there is sudden partial or complete loss of vision or sudden onset of proptosis (exophthalmos or abnormal protusion of the eyeball), diplopia (seeing double), or migraine. Also, discontinue medication if examination reveals papilledema or if thrombotic disorder occurs or is suspected.

The patient package insert is mandatory for progestational drugs to convey information regarding birth defects to premenopausal women unless childbearing is impossible. However, it is recommended that the patient package insert also be given to patients taking or using progestins for noncontraceptive purposes.

## For noncontraceptive uses

For those women using progestins for other reasons besides contraception, concurrent contraceptive methods should be used if fertile and sexually active.

Response rates are about 15 to 16% in patients using progestins for treating endometrial carcinoma with high-grade resistant tumors and may be significantly better with low-grade malignancy; response rate decreases for tumors of increasing grade and in those tumors negative for both estrogen and progesterone receptors; median survival is approximately 9 to 10 months.

Response rates are approximately 5% and of short duration in patients using progestins for treating renal carcinoma; routine receptor assay is not helpful in predicting appropriate patients.

Response rates of up to about 40% have been reported when high-dose oral medroxyprogesterone has been used to treat breast cancer.

Decisions to treat menopausal symptoms with hormones for a limited time (1 to 5 years) or to use hormones to prevent diseases in postmenopausal women for a longer period of time (10 to 20 years), or a lifetime, should be separate decisions. Counseling asymptomatic postmenopausal women about the benefits and risks of long-term estrogen and progestin hormone replacement therapy to prevent disease and prolong life is complex. It is dependent on an individual's risk of breast cancer, osteoporosis, and coronary heart disease and whether a uterus is present (progestins are not needed when the uterus is absent). Adding a progestin to estrogen therapy may benefit postmenopausal women at risk for osteoporosis, slightly reduce estrogen's protective effect against coronary heart disease (women at more risk are provided the greatest benefit), and slightly increase the risk of breast cancer over that of non-users. Women should understand that the benefits and risks of preventive hormone therapy depend on their risk status.

## For progesterone

Rapid transformation renders oral administration ineffective, although there has been some success with micronized progesterone capsules. The parenteral dose is absorbed and metabolized so rapidly after injection that frequent doses are needed to be effective. Synthetic progestins are generally used for oral administration and are more potent than natural progesterone; i.e., 20 to 25 mg progesterone (intramuscular) has an effect equivalent to 100 mg progesterone (vaginal suppository) or 5 to 10 mg medroxyprogesterone (oral).

## For medroxyprogesterone

Re-establishment of menstrual cycle may be delayed (up to 18 months or longer) and is difficult to predict following the intramuscular administration of medroxyprogesterone. Because of the prolonged action and the resulting difficulty in predicting the time of withdrawal bleeding following injection, parenteral medroxyprogesterone is not recommended for treatment of secondary amenorrhea or dysfunctional uterine bleeding; oral medroxyprogesterone is the preferred mode of therapy.

## For megestrol

The magnitude and rate of weight gain are highly dependent on megestrol dose and are significantly greater with higher doses. The greatest effect can be maintained at a lower dose of 400 mg a day in the second to fourth months when 800 mg a day is taken in the first month, although some studies have reported further benefit when the dose is not lowered.

Adrenal suppression may occur with normal dosing range; effects on HIV viral replication have not been determined.

## For contraception use

When used as oral contraceptives, progestins are administered daily without interruption, regardless of menstrual cycle. Although some progestin products protect against pregnancy, none protects against HIV infection or AIDS.

Another contraceptive method should be used and pregnancy should be ruled out before resuming use of hormonal contraceptives if two tablets or an injection is missed.

## For levonorgestrel subdermal capsules

Insertion (usually a 15-minute procedure using local anesthesia) should be performed within the first 7 days of a normal menstrual period or immediately postabortion. Furthermore, insertion is not recommended by the manufacturer in the first 6-weeks postpartum for breast-feeding women.

All 6 subdermal capsules are inserted subdermally in a fanlike pattern about 15 degrees apart (totaling 75 degrees) in the midportion of the upper arm (8 to 10 centimeters above the crease in the elbow).

Knowledge of proper insertion technique for insertion or removal of subdermal capsules reduces the incidence of hard-to-remove subdermal capsules, expulsions, and improper placement of subdermal capsules. Bruising and some scarring may occur with insertion or removal procedures. Insertion site complications at one year follow-up include 0.8% skin infection, 0.4% expulsion, and 4.7% local skin reaction; in 40.9% of women with a skin infection, an expulsion of an implanted capsule resulted.

When an implanted capsule is expelled, a new subdermal capsule may be inserted in the same incision, although any infection or unusual wound or incision site problems should heal before a new sterile subdermal capsule is inserted. Other contraceptive methods should be used concurrently when fewer than 6 subdermal capsules are in place. Also, if removal of all subdermal capsules is not successful with the first attempt, the skin should be allowed to heal completely before a second attempt of removal.

Removal of the levonorgestrel implanted capsules (usually a 20-minute procedure) may occur on request at any time or at the end of the fifth year of use, and should be considered if prolonged immobilization is anticipated or if persistent infection develops at the implantation site. Used subdermal capsules should be disposed of by using the Centers for Disease Control guidelines for biohazardous waste.

### For parenteral medroxyprogesterone

The formulation of parenteral medroxyprogesterone for noncontraceptive use (400 mg/mL) should not be used for contraceptive uses, even if the proper dose (150 mg) is considered. Efficacy issues arose and resulted in discontinuation of a clinical trial conducted by the manufacturer using a lower volume dose than that used in the formulation of medroxyprogesterone for contraception. Dose adjustment is not necessary for body weight but it is reported that plasma concentration and duration decreased by a mean of 3.3 picograms/mL per kg increase of body weight because of its accumulation in fat cells; therefore, return to fertility may be especially prolonged in obese women.

Injecting into the deltoid muscle as opposed to the gluteal muscle is recommended by some clinicians to lessen absorption problems that may occur because of rubbing the injection site while sitting.

---

## *HYDROXYPROGESTERONE*

## Summary of Differences

Category:
  Progestational agent; diagnostic aid.
Indications:
  Amenorrhea, dysfunctional uterine bleeding, induction of menses, and test for endogenous estrogen production.
Pharmacology/pharmacokinetics:
  More potent than progesterone with longer duration of action.
  Synthetic 17-hydroxy derivative of progesterone with progestogenic, androgenic, and glucocorticoid effects.

## Parenteral Dosage Forms

### HYDROXYPROGESTERONE CAPROATE INJECTION USP

#### Usual adult and adolescent dose

Amenorrhea or
Dysfunctional uterine bleeding—
  Intramuscular, 375 mg.
Menses, induction of or
Test for endogenous estrogen production—
  Intramuscular, 125 to 250 mg given on day ten of menstrual cycle, repeated every seven days until suppression is no longer desired.
  Note: Withdrawal bleeding usually occurs within three to seven days after discontinuing therapy.

#### Strength(s) usually available

U.S.—
  125 mg per mL (Rx) [GENERIC].
  250 mg per mL (Rx) [*Gesterol LA 250; Hy/Gestrone; Hylutin; Prodrox; Pro-Span;* GENERIC].
Canada—
  Not commercially available.

### Packaging and storage

Store below 40 °C (104 °F), preferably between 15 and 30 °C (59 and 86 °F), unless otherwise specified by manufacturer. Protect from freezing.

### Note

Castor or sesame oils are commonly used as the vehicle for intramuscular injection.

Include mandatory patient package insert (PPI) when dispensing to premenopausal patient unless reproduction is impossible.

---

## *LEVONORGESTREL*

## Summary of Differences

Category:
  Contraceptive.
Indications:
  Pregnancy prophylaxis.
Pharmacology/pharmacokinetics:
  19-nor derivative of testosterone; has progestational and androgenic effects.
Precautions:
  Breast-feeding—Generally recommended for use 6 weeks postpartum in breast-feeding women but has been used 5 days postpartum after establishment of lactation.
  Laboratory value alterations—Serum $T_3$ concentrations may be slightly elevated and $T_4$ concentrations may be decreased; total serum $T_4$ concentrations are unaffected.
  Medical considerations/contraindications—Levonorgestrel subdermal capsules have not caused thrombogenic disorders, but caution may be necessary with use in patients with a history of thrombosis. Caution is necessary in patients with a history of CNS disorders, such as depression or history of convulsions.
Side effects:
  Breakthrough bleeding or spotting, reduced amount of menstrual bleeding, and amenorrhea are predominant side effects. These bleeding irregularities may persist but are less problematic with time. Other side effects include ovarian enlargement or cysts—usually reversible with continued use, acne, headaches, and mood changes.

## Additional Dosing Information

See also *General Dosing Information.*

Special training for insertion, removal, and disposal of levonorgestrel subdermal capsules includes knowledge and familiarity of procedures by physician and patient.

## Subdermal Dosage Form

### LEVONORGESTREL IMPLANT CAPSULES

#### Usual adult and adolescent dose

Contraception—
  Subdermally, one set of six Silastic closed-capsules implanted every five years.

#### Strength(s) usually available

U.S.—
  216 mg (Rx) [*NORPLANT*].
Canada—
  216 mg (Rx) [*NORPLANT*].

### Packaging and storage

Store below 40 °C (104 °F), preferably between 15 and 30 °C (59 and 86 °F), unless otherwise specified by manufacturer. Store away from excess heat or moisture.

### Note

Include mandatory patient package insert (PPI) when dispensing progestins to premenopausal patient unless reproduction is impossible.

---

## *MEDROGESTONE*

## Summary of Differences

Category:
  Progestational agent.
Indications:
  Secondary amenorrhea, dysfunctional uterine bleeding, induction of menses, and, in conjunction with estrogens, for endometrial shedding in menopausal women.

Pharmacology/pharmacokinetics:
17-hydroxy derivative of progesterone; highly progestational, devoid of estrogenic, androgenic, glucocorticoid, or anti-androgenic effects.

# Oral Dosage Forms
## MEDROGESTONE TABLETS
### Usual adult and adolescent dose
Amenorrhea, secondary or
Dysfunctional uterine bleeding or
Hormone replacement, female menopause or
Menses, induction of—
Oral, 5 to 10 mg a day on days fifteen through twenty-five of monthly cycle.

Note: Withdrawal bleeding usually occurs within three to seven days after discontinuing therapy.

An optimum secretory transformation of an endometrium that has been adequately primed with either endogenous or exogenous estrogens (days five to twenty-five of menstrual cycle) may be reestablished with three or more cycles.

### Strength(s) usually available
U.S.—
Not commercially available.
Canada—
5 mg (Rx) [*Colprone* (scored)].

### Packaging and storage
Store below 40 °C (104 °F), preferably between 15 and 30 °C (59 and 86 °F), unless otherwise specified by manufacturer. Store in a well-closed container.

---

## *MEDROXYPROGESTERONE*

# Summary of Differences
Category:
Oral medroxyprogesterone used as a progestational agent, antineoplastic agent, and diagnostic aid (test for endogenous estrogen production). Parenteral medroxyprogesterone used as adjunct in antineoplastic therapy and indicated as contraceptive agent in a special parenteral formulation.
Indications:
Oral and parenteral medroxyprogesterone indicated to treat breast carcinoma in postmenopausal women and endometrial hyperplasia in conditions such as polycystic ovary syndrome; however, only parenteral medroxyprogesterone is indicated for adjunct treatment of metastatic renal or endometrial carcinoma and endometriosis. Parenteral medroxyprogesterone is accepted therapy for precocious puberty, but has been replaced by other modalities. Unlike parenteral medroxyprogesterone, oral medroxyprogesterone is indicated for secondary amenorrhea, dysfunctional uterine bleeding, induction of menses, carcinoma, female hormone replacement in menopause, and testing for endogenous estrogen production.
Unlike oral medroxyprogesterone, parenteral medroxyprogesterone is not recommended for treatment of secondary amenorrhea or dysfunctional uterine bleeding.
Pharmacology/pharmacokinetics:
17-hydroxy derivative of progesterone with progestogenic, androgenic, and glucocorticoid effects.
Precautions:
Fertility—Luteal function may be delayed after cessation of parenteral medroxyprogesterone treatment for contraception, especially in obese females of reproductive age.
Pregnancy—Use in pregnancy has produced problems in the fetus and is not recommended. Doses used for contraception have not appeared to produce problems for nursing infants after lactation is established.
Drug interactions—Use of aminoglutethimide may lower serum concentrations of medroxyprogesterone and interfere with intestinal absorption of oral dose.
Medical considerations/contraindications—Low dose parenteral medroxyprogesterone can be used with caution for contraception in women with diabetes mellitus. High doses (but not low doses) have rarely been associated with thromboembolic disorders or thrombophlebitis.
Side/adverse effects:
Bloating or swelling of face, ankles, or feet more likely with higher doses.

# Additional Dosing Information
See also *General Dosing Information*.
Re-establishment of menstrual cycle can be delayed and difficult to predict following the parenteral dose. Also, only the 150 mg/mL formulation and a 150-mg dose should be used for contraception; a special dose adjustment for the obese patient is not needed; however, contraceptive efficacy in patients over 90 kg has not been evaluated.

# Oral Dosage Forms
Note: Bracketed uses in the *Dosage Forms* section refer to categories of use or indications that are not included in U.S. product labeling.

## MEDROXYPROGESTERONE ACETATE TABLETS USP
### Usual adult or adolescent dose
Amenorrhea, secondary—
Oral, 5 to 10 mg a day for five to ten days, started any time during cycle.
Dysfunctional uterine bleeding—
Oral, 5 to 10 mg a day for five to ten days, commencing on the calculated day sixteen or day twenty-one of the menstrual cycle.
Menses, induction of—
Oral, 10 mg daily for ten days starting on day sixteen of the menstrual cycle. If bleeding is controlled satisfactorily, two or more subsequent cycles of the treatment should be given.
[Hormonal replacement therapy, female, menopause]—

There are several recommended dosing schedules:
Oral, 5 to 10 mg medroxyprogesterone a day for ten or fourteen days beginning on days twelve or sixteen through day twenty-five, estrogen is taken on day one through twenty-five, and neither estrogen or medroxyprogesterone is taken on the twenty-fifth day through the end of the month.
Oral, 5 to 10 mg medroxyprogesterone a day taken on the first ten to fourteen days along with continuous estrogen dosing.
Oral, 2.5 mg medroxyprogesterone a day taken continuously with continuous estrogen dosing.
Note: Other regimens may differ but also may be appropriate. Withdrawal bleeding usually occurs within three to seven days after discontinuing therapy.
[Carcinoma, breast, postmenopausal women]—
Oral, 400 mg a day in divided doses.
[Carcinoma, endometrial]—
Initial: Oral, 200 to 400 mg a day for two to three months.
Maintenance: Oral, 200 mg a day.
Note: Improvement may not be evident until eight to ten weeks following initiation of therapy for breast or endometrial carcinoma. However, treatment should be discontinued when there is rapid progression of the disease at any time during therapy.
[Endometriosis]¹—
Oral, 10 to 40 mg a day for six to nine months.
[Estrogen production, endogenous]—
Oral, 10 mg a day for five to ten days. Withdrawal bleeding will occur three to seven days following therapy if the uterus has been sufficiently primed with endogenous estrogen.
[Hyperplasia, endometrial]¹—

There are several recommended dosing schedules:
Oral, 10 mg a day for three to six months.
Oral, 10 mg a day for twenty-one days each month for three months. Then the dose is reduced to 10 mg a day for ten to fourteen days a month.
Oral, 20 mg a day for thirty days every six months.
Note: Other regimens may differ but also may be appropriate.

### Strength(s) usually available
U.S.—
2.5 mg (Rx) [*Cycrin* (scored); *Provera* (scored); GENERIC].
5 mg (Rx) [*Cycrin* (scored); *Provera* (scored); GENERIC].
10 mg (Rx) [*Amen* (scored); *Curretab* (scored); *Cycrin* (scored); *Provera* (scored); GENERIC].
Canada—
2.5 mg (Rx) [*Provera*].
5 mg (Rx) [*Provera* (scored)].
10 mg (Rx) [*Provera* (scored)].
100 mg (Rx) [*Provera* (scored)].

### Packaging and storage
Store below 40 °C (104 °F), preferably between 15 and 30 °C (59 and 86 °F), unless otherwise specified by manufacturer.

**Note**
Include mandatory patient package insert (PPI) when dispensing progestins to premenopausal patient unless reproduction is impossible.

## Parenteral Dosage Forms

Note: Bracketed uses in the *Dosage Forms* section refer to categories of use or indications that are not included in U.S. product labeling.

### STERILE MEDROXYPROGESTERONE ACETATE SUSPENSION USP

**Usual adult or adolescent dose**
Carcinoma, endometrial or
Carcinoma, renal—
    Initial: Intramuscular, 400 mg to 1 gram once a week until improvement and stabilization occur.
    Maintenance: Intramuscular, 400 mg or more once a month.
[Carcinoma, breast]—
    Initial: Intramuscular, 500 mg a day for twenty-eight days.
    Maintenance: Intramuscular, 500 mg two times a week.

Note: Improvement may not be evident for eight to ten weeks of therapy for breast or endometrial carcinoma. However, treatment should be discontinued with rapid progression of the disease at any time during therapy.
Contraceptive[1]—
    Intramuscular, 150 mg every three months.

Note: Dosage does not need to be adjusted for body weight in patients weighing less than 90 kg, but this has not been studied in patients weighing more than 90 kg. It is recommended that the first injection be given during the first five days after onset of a normal menstrual period; within five days postpartum if not breast-feeding, and if exclusively breast-feeding, at six weeks postpartum. A physician should determine that a patient is not pregnant if more than thirteen weeks will elapse between injections.
[Endometriosis]—

There are several dosage schedules:
    Intramuscular, 50 mg once a week for at least six months.
    Intramuscular, 100 mg every two weeks for at least six months.
    Intramuscular, 150 mg every 3 months for at least six months.

**Strength(s) usually available**
U.S.—
    150 mg per mL (Rx) [*Depo-Provera Contraceptive Injection*].
    400 mg per mL (Rx) [*Depo-Provera*].
Canada—
    50 mg per mL (Rx) [*Depo-Provera*].
    100 mg per mL (Rx) [*Depo-Provera*].

**Packaging and storage**
Store below 40 °C (104 °F), preferably between 15 and 30 °C (59 and 86 °F), unless otherwise specified by manufacturer. Protect from freezing.

**Preparation of dosage form**
Should be shaken vigorously before administration.

**Auxiliary labeling**
• Shake well.

**Note**
Include mandatory patient package insert (PPI) when dispensing progestins to premenopausal patient unless reproduction is impossible.

[1]Not included in Canadian product labeling.

---

### MEGESTROL

## Summary of Differences

Category:
    Antianoretic, anticachectic, antineoplastic.
Indications:
    Endometrial or breast carcinoma, anorexia, cachexia and significant weight loss; used for advanced prostate carcinoma. Not recommended for prophylactic avoidance of weight loss.
Pharmacology/pharmacokinetics:
    17-hydroxy derivative of progesterone; progestogenic, glucocorticoid, and anti-estrogenic effects.
Precautions:
    Fertility—Impaired fertility shown in male offspring of megestrol-treated females in studies in rats and dogs.
    Pregnancy—Use is not recommended.

## Additional Dosing Information

See also *General Dosing Information*.

Magnitude and rate of weight gain are dose-related; lower doses of 400 mg are recommended after the first month, although some results have shown weight gain continuing with 800 mg given continuously for 4 months.

## Oral Dosage Forms

Note: Bracketed uses in the *Dosage Forms* section refer to categories of use or indications that are not included in U.S. product labeling.

### MEGESTROL ACETATE SUSPENSION

**Usual adult dose**
Anorexia, AIDS-associated or
Cachexia, AIDS-associated or
Weight-loss, significant, AIDS-associated—
    Oral, 800 mg a day the first month, then 400 or 800 mg a day for three more months.

**Strength(s) usually available**
U.S.—
    40 mg per milliliter (mL) (Rx) [*Megace* (alcohol 0.06%)].
Canada—
    Not commercially available.

**Packaging and storage**
Store at or below 25 °C (77 °F). Protect from heat. Store in a well-closed container.

**Auxiliary labeling**
• Shake well.

**Note**
Include patient package insert (PPI) when dispensing.

### MEGESTROL ACETATE TABLETS USP

**Usual adult and adolescent dose**
Carcinoma, breast—
    Oral, 160 mg a day as a single dose or in divided doses.
Carcinoma, endometrial—
    Oral, 40 to 320 mg a day in divided doses.
[Carcinoma, prostate, advanced]—
    Oral, 120 mg once a day with 0.1 mg diethylstilbesterol a day.

Note: At least two months of continuous treatment is considered an adequate period for determining the efficacy of megestrol.
[Hyperplasia, endometrial][1]—
    Oral, 20 to 40 mg a day for 14 days or longer every month.

**Strength(s) usually available**
U.S.—
    20 mg (Rx) [*Megace* (scored); GENERIC].
    40 mg (Rx) [*Megace* (scored); GENERIC].
Canada—
    40 mg (Rx) [*Megace* (scored)].
    160 mg (Rx) [*Megace*].

**Packaging and storage**
Store below 40 °C (104 °F), preferably between 15 and 30 °C (59 and 86 °F), unless otherwise specified by manufacturer. Store in a well-closed container.

**Note**
Include patient package insert (PPI) when dispensing.

[1]Not included in Canadian product labeling.

---

### NORETHINDRONE

## Summary of Differences

Category:
    Indicated as a progestational agent (norethindrone base and acetate) and contraceptive agent (norethindrone base).
Indication:
    Norethindrone acetate indicated for secondary amenorrhea, dysfunctional uterine bleeding, induction of menses, and endometriosis. Norethindrone base is indicated for contraception while the acetate form is not.

## Oral Dosage Forms
### NORETHINDRONE TABLETS USP

**Usual adult and adolescent dose**
Contraceptive—
 Oral, 350 mcg (0.35 mg) a day, starting on day one of menstrual cycle and continuing uninterrupted at the same time every day of the year, whether or not menstrual bleeding occurs.

**Strength(s) usually available**
U.S.—
 350 mcg (0.35 mg) (Rx) [*Micronor; Nor-QD*].
Canada—
 350 mcg (0.35 mg) (Rx) [*Micronor*].

**Packaging and storage**
Store below 40 °C (104 °F), preferably between 15 and 30 °C (59 and 86 °F), unless otherwise specified by manufacturer. Store in a well-closed container.

**Note**
Include mandatory patient package insert (PPI) when dispensing progestins to premenopausal patient unless reproduction is impossible.

### NORETHINDRONE ACETATE TABLETS USP

**Usual adult and adolescent dose**
Amenorrhea, secondary or
Dysfunctional uterine bleeding—
 Oral, 2.5 to 10 mg a day on day five through day twenty-five of the menstrual cycle or for five to ten days during the last half of menstrual cycle.
 Note: Withdrawal bleeding occurs within three to seven days after progestin treatment ends.
Endometriosis—
 Initial: Oral, 5 mg a day for two weeks, increasing by 2.5 mg a day at two-week intervals to reach a total dose of 15 mg a day.
 Maintenance: Oral, 15 mg a day for six to nine months, unless temporarily discontinued because of breakthrough bleeding.

**Strength(s) usually available**
U.S.—
 5 mg (Rx) [*Aygestin* (scored)].
Canada—
 5 mg (Rx) [*Norlutate*].

**Packaging and storage**
Store below 40 °C (104 °F), preferably between 15 and 30 °C (59 and 86 °F), unless otherwise specified by manufacturer. Store in a well-closed container.

**Note**
Include mandatory patient package insert (PPI) when dispensing progestins to premenopausal patients unless reproduction is impossible.

---
### NORGESTREL
---

## Summary of Differences
Category:
 Contraceptive agent.
Indication:
 Pregnancy prophylaxis.
Pharmacology/pharmacokinetics:
 19-nor derivative of testosterone; has progestogenic, estrogenic, androgenic, and anti-estrogenic effects.

## Oral Dosage Forms
### NORGESTREL TABLETS USP

**Usual adult and adolescent dose**
Contraceptive—
 Oral, 75 mcg (0.075 mg) a day, starting on day one of menstrual cycle and continuing uninterrupted at the same time every day of the year whether or not menstrual bleeding occurs.

**Strength(s) usually available**
U.S.—
 75 mcg (0.075 mg) (Rx) [*Ovrette*].
Canada—
 Not commercially available.

**Packaging and storage**
Store below 40 °C (104 °F), preferably between 15 and 30 °C (59 and 86 °F), unless otherwise specified by manufacturer. Store in a well-closed container.

**Note**
Include mandatory patient package insert (PPI) when dispensing progestins to premenopausal patients unless reproduction is impossible.

---
### PROGESTERONE
---

## Summary of Differences
Category:
 Progestational agent.
Indications:
 Indicated for secondary amenorrhea and dysfunctional uterine bleeding but is also used for corpus luteum insufficiency.
Pharmacology/pharmacokinetics:
 Natural hormone with progestational, androgenic, and anti-estrogenic effects.
Precautions:
 Pregnancy—Although not proven effective, progesterone has been used during first few months of pregnancy to prevent habitual or threatened abortion due to hormonal imbalance but may also delay expulsion of a defective ovum.

## Additional Dosing Information
See also *General Dosing Information*.

Twenty to 25 mg progesterone (intramuscular) produces an equivalent progestogenic effect compared to 100 mg progesterone (vaginal suppository).

## Parenteral Dosage Forms
Note: Bracketed uses in the *Dosage Forms* section refer to categories of use or indications that are not included in U.S. product labeling.

### PROGESTERONE INJECTION USP

**Usual adult dose**
Amenorrhea, secondary—
 Intramuscular, 5 to 10 mg a day for six to ten consecutive days or 100 to 150 mg injected intramuscularly as a single dose.
 Note: If there has been sufficient ovarian activity to produce a proliferative endometrium or two weeks of prior estrogen therapy, withdrawal bleeding will occur forty-eight to seventy-two hours after the last injection. The patient should discontinue therapy if menstrual cycle occurs. This may be followed by spontaneous normal cycles. Progesterone should be discontinued if menses occurs during the series of injections.
Dysfunctional uterine bleeding—
 Intramuscular, 5 to 10 mg a day for six consecutive days.
 Note: Bleeding should cease within six days. When estrogen is being given, the administration of progesterone should begin after two weeks of estrogen therapy. Progesterone should be discontinued if menses occurs during the series of injections.
[Corpus luteum insufficiency][1]—
 Intramuscular, 12.5 mg or more a day initiated within several days of ovulation. Treatment duration is usually two weeks, but it may be continued, if necessary, up to eleventh week of gestation.
[Estrogen production, endogenous, diagnosis][1]—
 Intramuscular, 100 mg as a single dose.

**Usual adult prescribing limits**
Up to 50 mg daily.

**Strength(s) usually available**
U.S.—
 50 mg per mL (Rx) [*Gesterol 50* (in sesame seed oil; benzyl alcohol 10%); GENERIC (in sesame seed or peanut oil)].
Canada—
 50 mg per mL (Rx) [*PMS-Progesterone* (in sesame seed oil; benzyl alcohol 10%)].

**Packaging and storage**
Store below 40 °C (104 °F), preferably between 15 and 30 °C (59 and 86 °F), unless otherwise specified by manufacturer. Protect from freezing.

**Note**
Include mandatory patient package insert (PPI) when dispensing progestins to premenopausal patients unless reproduction is impossible.

## Vaginal Dosage Forms
Note: Bracketed uses in the *Dosage Forms* section refer to categories of use or indications that are not included in U.S. product labeling.

## PROGESTERONE SUPPOSITORIES

### Usual adult and adolescent dose

[Corpus luteum insufficiency][1]—

Vaginal, 25 to 100 mg one to two times a day initiated within several days of ovulation. Treatment duration is usually continued if the patient is pregnant up to about the eleventh week of gestation.

Note: Vaginal suppositories are better tolerated than other dosage forms of progesterone and are therefore more frequently prescribed for this indication.

### Strength(s) usually available

U.S.—

Not commercially available. Compounding required for prescription.

Canada—

Not commercially available. Compounding required for prescription.

### Packaging and storage

Store below 40 °C (104 °F), preferably between 15 and 30 °C (59 and 86 °F), in a tight container, unless otherwise specified by manufacturer.

### Preparation of dosage form

A formulation that has been used for the extemporaneous compounding of progesterone suppositories is as follows:

• 710 mg (0.71 grams) progesterone powder

• 33.7 grams polyethylene glycol 400
• 22.3 grams polyethylene glycol 6000

Makes 28 suppositories, 25 mg progesterone per suppository.

### Auxiliary labeling

• For vaginal use only.

[1]Not included in Canadian product labeling.

## Selected Bibliography

Grady D, Rubin SM, Petitti DB, et al. Hormone therapy to prevent disease and prolong life in postmenopausal women. Ann Intern Med 1992 Dec; 117 (12): 1016-37.

American College of Physicians. Clinical Guideline. Guidelines for counseling postmenopausal women about preventive hormone therapy. Ann Intern Med 1992 Dec; 117 (12): 1038-41.

Revised: 08/08/95
Interim revision: 06/26/96

## Table 1. Pharmacokinetics

| Drug | Protein* binding (%) | Biotransformation | Elimination half-life (hrs) | Time to peak concentration (hrs) | Peak serum concentration ng/ml | Peak serum concentration Dose (mg) | Renal elimination (%) | Fecal elimination (%) |
|---|---|---|---|---|---|---|---|---|
| Natural: Progesterone | Very high† (90% or more) | Hepatic | Several minutes | | | | 50–60 | 10 |
| Synthetic 17-hydroxy derivatives: Hydroxyprogesterone caproate | Very high (90% or more) | Hepatic | | | | | | |
| Medroxyprogesterone acetate | Very high (90% or more) | Hepatic | | | | | 15–22 | 45–80 |
| Oral | | | 30 | within 2–4 | 19–35 | 10 | | |
| IM | | No first-pass hepatic effect | 50 days | 3 weeks | 1–7 | 150‡ | | |
| Medrogestone | | | 4 | 1 | | | | |
| Megestrol acetate | Very high (90% or more) | Hepatic | 38 (13–104) | | | | 66 | 20 |
| Oral | | | | 2–3 | 200 | 160 | | |
| Oral | | | | 2–3 | 753 | 600 | | |
| Synthetic 19-nor derivatives: Levonorgestrel subdermal capsules | Very high§ (90% or more) | No first-pass hepatic effect | 16 (8–30) | 24 | 1.6 | 216 | 45 | 32 |
| 3 months | | | | | 0.4 | | | |
| 12 months | | | | | 0.32 | | | |
| 60 months | | | | | 0.26 | | | |
| Norgestrel | Very high (90% or more) | | 20 | | | | | |
| Norethindrone | Very high# (90% or more) | Hepatic first pass effect | 8 (6–12) | 2 | | | 50 | 20–40 |
| Norethindrone acetate | Very high (90% or more) | Hepatic first pass effect | 8 | | | | | |

* Sex hormone binding globulin (SHBG) synthesis is stimulated by estrogens and inhibited by androgens; levels are twice as high in women as in men.

† Progesterone binds strongly to cortisol binding globulin (CBG) 17.7%, SHBG 0.6%, and weakly to albumin 79.3%.

‡ Pertains to parenteral medroxyprogesterone for contraception injection formulation (150mg/mL) only.

§ Levonorgestrel: Free, 1.1–1.7%; SHBG 92–62%; albumin 37.56%, but suppresses SHBG by 33%.

# Norethindrone: Free 3.5%; SHBG 35.5%; albumin 61%.

# PROGUANIL    Systemic*

VA CLASSIFICATION (Primary): AP101

Note: For a listing of dosage forms and brand names by country availability, see *Dosage Forms* section(s). For a listing of brand names for the articles in this monograph, refer to the General Index.

*Not commercially available in the U.S.

## Category

Antimalarial.

## Indications

Note: Because proguanil is not commercially available in the U.S., the bracketed information in this monograph reflects the lack of labeled (approved) indications for this medication in this country.

### Accepted

[Malaria (prophylaxis)]—Proguanil is indicated for the causal prevention and suppression of malaria caused by susceptible strains of *Plasmodium falciparum* and other species of *Plasmodium* found in some geographic areas of the world. This medication acts against the pre-erythrocytic intrahepatic forms of the parasite. The efficacy of proguanil when used alone as a chemoprophylactic agent for malaria is uncertain because of the widespread resistance documented globally due to the extensive use of the medication.

Proguanil is recommended for use daily in combination with weekly chloroquine in multi-drug resistant areas as an alternative regimen for long or short-term prophylaxis against malaria for persons who cannot tolerate mefloquine or doxycycline. However, limited data suggest that this combination regimen is more effective than using chloroquine alone in sub-Saharan Africa but not in Thailand or Papua New Guinea.

## Pharmacology/Pharmacokinetics

### Physicochemical characteristics

Source—Synthetic biguanide derivative of pyrimidine.
Molecular weight—Proguanil: 253.7.
Proguanil hydrochloride: 290.2.

### Mechanism of action/Effect

Proguanil is a slow-acting blood schizonticidal (suppresses intraerythrocytic schizogony). Proguanil acts through its active metabolite, cycloguanil. The mechanism of action is probably due to interference of cycloguanil with the folic-folinic system of the parasite through inhibition of the plasmodial enzyme, dihydrofolate reductase. This inhibition results in the depletion of folate, an essential cofactor in the biosynthesis of nucleic acids, thus resulting in interference with the synthesis of protozoal nucleic acids and protein production.

Proguanil may also have some sporonticidal activity, rendering the gametocyte non-infective to the mosquito vector.

### Absorption

Rapidly and well absorbed in humans following oral doses ranging from 50 to 500 mg.

### Protein binding

High (approximately 75%).

### Biotransformation

Variably metabolized in the liver by cytochrome P450 isoenzymes to the active triazine metabolite, cycloguanil. This variable metabolism of proguanil may have profound clinical importance in poor metabolizers such as the Asian and African populations at risk of malaria infection. Prophylaxis with proguanil may not be effective in these persons because they may not achieve adequate therapeutic levels of the active compound, cycloguanil, even after multiple doses.

### Half-life

Approximately 20 hours.

### Time to peak concentration

Following an oral 200-mg dose——
Proguanil: Approximately 3 to 4 hours.
Cycloguanil: Approximately 1 hour.

### Peak plasma concentration

Following an oral 200-mg dose——
Proguanil: Approximately 140 nanograms per mL.
Cycloguanil: Approximately 75 nanograms per mL.

### Elimination

Renal—40 to 60% of the proguanil is excreted in the urine, of which 60% is unchanged drug and 30% is the active metabolite cycloguanil.
Fecal—About 10%.

## Precautions to Consider

### Pregnancy/Reproduction

Pregnancy—Problems in humans have not been documented. Proguanil has been widely used for more than 30 years and has been shown to be safe for use in pregnancy. Folate supplements, however, are recommended with use of proguanil during pregnancy because proguanil, as a folate antagonist, tends to deplete folate and may cause or accentuate anemia in pregnancy.

### Breast-feeding

Proguanil is distributed into breast milk. However, problems in humans have not been documented. The amount of proguanil distributed is insufficient to provide any prophylactic benefit to the infant against malaria. Therefore, a separate chemoprophylaxis may be required for the nursing infant.

### Pediatrics

Appropriate studies on the relationship of age to the effects of proguanil have not been performed in the pediatric population. However, no pediatrics-specific problems have been documented to date.

### Geriatrics

Appropriate studies on the relationship of age to the effects of proguanil have not been performed in the geriatric population. However, no geriatrics-specific problems have been documented to date.

### Medical considerations/Contraindications

The medical considerations/contraindications included here have been selected on the basis of their potential clinical significance (reasons given in parentheses where appropriate)—not necessarily inclusive (» = major clinical significance).

*Risk-benefit should be considered when the following medical problems exist:*
Hypersensitivity to proguanil
» Renal failure, severe
(impaired elimination may result in accumulation of proguanil and an increased incidence of side effects; use when renal failure is present has been associated with blood dyscrasias such as pancytopenia and megaloblastic anemia)

## Side/Adverse Effects

The following side/adverse effects have been selected on the basis of their potential clinical significance (possible signs and symptoms in parentheses where appropriate)—not necessarily inclusive:

**Those indicating need for medical attention**
Incidence rare
*Skin rash or itching*

**Those indicating need for medical attention only if they continue or are bothersome**
Incidence more frequent
*Anorexia* (lack of appetite); *gastric intolerance, mild* (diarrhea; nausea; vomiting)—usually subsides as treatment continues; *headache; stomatitis* (mouth sores or ulcers)

**Those not indicating need for medical attention**
Incidence less frequent or rare
*Alopecia, reversible* (temporary hair loss)

## Overdose

For more information on the management of overdose or unintentional ingestion, **contact a Poison Control Center** (see *Poison Control Center Listing*).

### Clinical effects of overdose

The following effects have been selected on the basis of their potential clinical significance (possible signs and symptoms in parentheses where appropriate)—not necessarily inclusive:

Acute
*Epigastric discomfort* (abdominal or stomach pain); *renal irritation with hematuria* (blood in urine)

**Treatment of overdose**
Because there is no specific antidote for proguanil overdose, treatment should include the following:
Specific treatment—
   Symptomatic treatment may be given.
Supportive care—
   Supportive measures necessary for maintaining the vital functions of the patient may be administered. Patients in whom intentional overdose is known or suspected should be referred for psychiatric consultation.

## Patient Consultation

As an aid to patient consultation, refer to *Advice for the Patient, Proguanil (Systemic)*.

In providing consultation, consider emphasizing the following selected information (» = major clinical significance):

**Before using this medication**
» Conditions affecting use, especially:
   Hypersensitivity to proguanil
   Pregnancy—Folate supplements should be taken by pregnant women receiving proguanil
   Breast-feeding—Proguanil is distributed into breast milk
   Other medical problems, especially severe renal failure

**Proper use of this medication**
   Taking medication with water after meals to minimize adverse effects
   Crushing the tablet and mixing it with milk, honey, or jam when giving to young children
» Compliance with full course of therapy
» Taking the medication at least 24 hours before arrival in a malarious area, then daily while staying in the malarious area; continuing to take medication daily for 4 weeks after leaving the malarious area
» Proper dosing
   Missed dose
» Proper storage

**Precautions while using this medication**
*Personal protection measures to prevent malaria such as*
   Avoiding exposure to mosquitoes, especially at peak feeding times (between dusk and dawn)
   Wearing suitable clothing (long-sleeved shirt and long trousers) to protect arms and legs when mosquitoes are out
   Applying insect repellant (containing diethylmetatoluamide [DEET]) sparingly to exposed skin
   Sleeping in screened or air-conditioned room
   Using bed netting impregnated with insecticides
   Using mosquito coils or sprays
» Checking with physician if fever or "flu-like" symptoms develop during travel or within a year (particularly within the first 2 months) after leaving the malarious area

## General Dosing Information

Proguanil should be taken with water after meals, at the same time each day. For young children, proguanil tablets should be given by crushing the tablet and mixing with milk, honey, or jam.

Generally, antimalarial medications for prophylaxis are taken at least a week prior to travel to a malarious area in order to ensure an adequate blood concentration of the medication. This regimen also allows evaluation of any potential adverse effects so that if the need arises, an alternative medication may be prescribed. Proguanil may be taken at least 24 hours prior to arrival in a malarious area, and taken daily throughout the stay in the malarious area. Proguanil should be continuously taken daily for 4 weeks after departure from a malarious area to ensure that the medication will be in the blood circulation to kill any malaria parasites that may be released from the liver into the blood.

Proguanil is usually taken daily in combination with weekly chloroquine. Although widely practiced, the safety of this therapeutic regimen has not been formally established.

For prevention of malaria after departure from areas where the other species (*P. vivax* and *P. ovale*) are endemic, which includes almost all areas where malaria is found (except Haiti), some medical experts prescribe, in addition, primaquine phosphate 15 mg base (26.3 mg) per day for adults or 0.3 mg base per kg (0.5 mg per kg) of body weight per day for children during the last two weeks of prophylaxis. However, other medical experts prefer to avoid the toxicity of primaquine and rely on surveillance to detect cases when they occur, especially when exposure has been limited or is doubtful.

## Oral Dosage Forms

Note: Because proguanil is not commercially available in the U.S., the bracketed information in the *Dosage Forms* section reflects the lack of labeled (approved) indications for this product in this country.

### PROGUANIL HYDROCHLORIDE TABLETS

**Usual adult and adolescent dose**
[Malaria (prophylaxis)]—
   Oral, 200 mg a day, taken after meals, starting at least twenty-four hours before arrival in a malarious region, and continuing every day during stay in the malarious region, and for four weeks after departure from the endemic area.

**Usual pediatric dose**
[Malaria (prophylaxis)]—
   Infants and children up to 1 year of age: Oral, 25 mg a day, taken after meals, starting at least twenty-four hours before arrival in a malarious region, and continuing every day during stay in the malarious region, and for four weeks after departure from the endemic area.
   Children 1 to 4 years of age: Oral, 50 mg a day, taken after meals, starting at least twenty-four hours before arrival in a malarious region, and continuing every day during stay in the malarious region, and for four weeks after departure from the endemic area.
   Children 5 to 8 years of age: Oral, 75 to 100 mg a day, taken after meals, starting at least twenty-four hours before arrival in a malarious region, and continuing every day during stay in the malarious region, and for four weeks after departure from the endemic area.
   Children 9 to 12 years of age: Oral, 100 to 150 mg a day, taken after meals, starting at least twenty-four hours before arrival in a malarious region, and continuing every day during stay in the malarious region, and for four weeks after departure from the endemic area.
   Children 12 years of age and over: See *Usual adult and adolescent dose*.

**Strength(s) usually available**
U.S.—
   Not commercially available.
Canada—
   100 mg (Rx) [*Paludrine*].
Other (United Kingdom)—
   100 mg (Rx) [*Paludrine*].

**Packaging and storage**
Store below 40 °C (104 °F), preferably between 15 and 30 °C (59 and 86 °F), in a well-closed container, unless otherwise specified by manufacturer. Protect from light.

**Auxiliary labeling**
• Take with food.
• Continue medication for full time of treatment.

## Selected Bibliography

Fogh S, Schapira A, Bygbjerg IC, Jepsen S, Mordhorst CH, Kuijlen K, et al. Malaria chemoprophylaxis in travellers to east Africa: a comparative prospective study of chloroquine plus proguanil with chloroquine plus sulfadoxine-pyrimethamine. Br Med J 1988; 296: 820-2.
Steffen R, Fuchs E, Schildknecht J, Naef U, Funk M, Schlagenhauf P, et al. Mefloquine compared with other malaria chemoprophylactic regimens in tourists visiting East Africa. Lancet 1993; 341: 1299-303.

Developed: 04/18/94

**PROMAZINE**—See *Phenothiazines (Systemic)*

**PROMETHAZINE**—See *Antihistamines, Phenothiazine-derivative (Systemic)*

## PROMETHAZINE-CONTAINING COMBINATIONS—

Promethazine and Codeine (Systemic)—See *Cough/Cold Combinations (Systemic)*
Promethazine, Codeine, and Potassium Guaiacolsulfonate (Systemic)—See *Cough/Cold Combinations (Systemic)*
Promethazine and Dextromethorphan (Systemic)—See *Cough/Cold Combinations (Systemic)*

Promethazine and Phenylephrine (Systemic)—See *Antihistamines and Decongestants (Systemic)*

Promethazine, Phenylephrine, and Codeine (Systemic)—See *Cough/Cold Combinations (Systemic)*

Promethazine, Phenylephrine, Codeine, and Potassium Guaiacolsulfonate (Systemic)—See *Cough/Cold Combinations (Systemic)*

Promethazine, Phenylephrine, and Potassium Guaiacolsulfonate (Systemic)—See *Cough/Cold Combinations (Systemic)*

# PROPAFENONE   Systemic

VA CLASSIFICATION (Primary): CV300

Note: For a listing of dosage forms and brand names by country availability, see *Dosage Forms* section(s). For a listing of brand names for the articles in this monograph, refer to the General Index.

## Category
Antiarrhythmic.

## Indications

Note: Bracketed information in the *Indications* section refers to uses that are not included in U.S. product labeling.

### Accepted

Arrhythmias, ventricular (treatment)—Propafenone is indicated for suppression of documented life-threatening ventricular arrhythmias, including sustained ventricular tachycardia.

[Arrhythmias, supraventricular (treatment)][1]—Propafenone may be used for the treatment of supraventricular arrhythmias such as, intranodal and extranodal (e.g., Wolff-Parkinson-White Syndrome) reentrant tachycardias. Data for use of propafenone in the treatment of atrial fibrillation/flutter are less convincing, although it may help some patients. Caution is warranted when administering propafenone to patients in atrial fibrillation/flutter and structural heart disease because of the possibility of serious proarrhythmia, including ventricular tachycardia.

### Unaccepted

Use of propafenone is not recommended in the U.S. for treatment of less severe arrhythmias such as nonsustained ventricular tachycardias or frequent premature ventricular contractions, even if patients are symptomatic, because of results of a study in patients following a myocardial infarction that found increased mortality in patients with non–life-threatening ventricular arrhythmias who were treated with encainide and flecainide.

---

[1]Not included in Canadian product labeling.

## Pharmacology/Pharmacokinetics

### Physicochemical characteristics
Molecular weight—377.91.
pKa—9.

### Mechanism of action/Effect
Reduces the inward sodium current in Purkinje and myocardial cells. Decreases excitability, conduction velocity, and automaticity in atrioventricular (AV) nodal, His-Purkinje, and intraventricular tissue, and causes a slight but significant prolongation of refractory periods in AV nodal tissue. The greatest effect is on the His-Purkinje system. Decreases the rate of rise of the action potential without markedly affecting its duration. Also, prolongs conduction velocity and effective refractory periods in accessory pathways in both directions. Electrophysiologic effects are greater in ischemic than in normal myocardial tissue. In the Vaughan Williams classification of antiarrhythmics, propafenone is considered to be a class IC agent.

### Other actions/effects
Negative inotropic effect. Has approximately one-fortieth the beta-adrenergic blocking activity of propranolol, which may become clinically significant in some patients. Has weak calcium channel blocking properties. Has local anesthetic activity approximately equal to that of procaine.

### Absorption
Rapid and nearly complete, with more than 90% of an oral dose absorbed. Systemic bioavailability ranges from 5 to 50%, reflecting significant first-pass metabolism. Such a wide range in systemic bioavailability is related to two factors. The presence of food increases bioavailability for extensive metabolizers (more than 90% of patients). In addition, bioavailability increases as dosage increases. Absolute bioavailability is 3.4% for a 150-mg tablet compared to 10.6% for a 300-mg tablet.

### Protein binding
Very high (97%).

### Biotransformation
Hepatic; significant first-pass effect. In over 90% of patients, rapidly and extensively metabolized to 2 active metabolites, 5-hydroxypropafenone and N-depropylpropafenone, which have antiarrhythmic activity comparable to propafenone but which are present in concentrations less than 20% of propafenone concentrations. In less than 10% of patients and in patients also receiving quinidine, more slowly metabolized (these patients also have a diminished ability to metabolize debrisoquin, encainide, metoprolol, and dextromethorphan); little, if any, 5-hydroxypropafenone is present in plasma.

### Half-life
In extensive metabolizers (more than 90% of patients)—2 to 10 hours.
In poor metabolizers (less than 10% of patients)—10 to 32 hours.

### Time to peak plasma concentration
1 to 3.5 hours.

### Time to steady-state plasma concentration
Multiple doses—4 to 5 days.

### Steady-state plasma concentrations
Wide interindividual variability. In extensive metabolizers, pharmacokinetics are nonlinear; because of saturable first-pass metabolism, a 3-fold increase in dose may result in a 10-fold increase in steady-state plasma concentrations; however, in poor metabolizers, pharmacokinetics are linear.

### Peak plasma concentration
In poor metabolizers, concentrations are 1.5 to 2 times those of extensive metabolizers at doses of 675 to 900 mg per day.

### Elimination
Renal—38% as metabolites; less than 1% as unchanged drug.
Fecal—53% as metabolites.

## Precautions to Consider

### Carcinogenicity
Studies in rats and mice at oral doses of up to 270 mg per kg of body weight (mg/kg) per day and 360 mg/kg per day, respectively, revealed no evidence of carcinogenicity.

### Mutagenicity
The mouse dominant lethal test, rat bone marrow chromosome analysis, Chinese hamster bone marrow and spermatogonia chromosome analysis, Chinese hamster micronucleus test, and Ames bacterial test were negative.

### Pregnancy/Reproduction
Fertility—A reversible reduction in sperm count (within normal range) occurred after short-term administration in humans, but chronic administration did not have this effect.

Reversible impairment of spermatogenesis occurs in monkeys, dogs, and rabbits after high intravenous doses.

Pregnancy—Adequate and well-controlled studies in humans have not been done.

Studies in rats and rabbits at doses of up to 40 and 10 times the maximum recommended human dose, respectively, have not shown that propafenone causes teratogenicity in the fetus; however, a perinatal and postnatal study in rats at doses of 6 times the maximum recommended human dose or greater found a dose-related increase in maternal and neonatal mortality, decreased maternal and pup body weight gain, and reduced neonatal physiological development.

FDA Pregnancy Category C.

### Breast-feeding
Propafenone and 5-OH-propafenone are excreted in breast milk at concentrations lower than those found in maternal plasma. However, problems in humans have not been documented.

### Pediatrics
Safety and efficacy have not been established. However, limited use of propafenone in neonates, infants, and children seems to indicate that

the incidence of side effects in pediatric patients is similar to that reported in adults. Proarrhythmic effects have been reported in the pediatric population, as in the adult population, including an incident of sudden death which may or may not have been related to propafenone. Therefore, propafenone should be used with caution in pediatric patients.

## Geriatrics

Although appropriate studies on the relationship of age to the effects of propafenone have not been performed in the geriatric population, no geriatrics-specific problems have been documented to date. However, elderly patients are more likely to have age-related hepatic and renal function impairment, which may require dosage reduction in patients receiving propafenone.

## Drug interactions and/or related problems

The following drug interactions and/or related problems have been selected on the basis of their potential clinical significance (possible mechanism in parentheses where appropriate)—not necessarily inclusive (» = major clinical significance):

Anesthetics, local
(concurrent use with propafenone may increase the risk of central nervous system [CNS] side effects)

Antiarrhythmics, other
(although some antiarrhythmic agents may be used in combination for therapeutic advantage, combined use may sometimes potentiate risk of adverse cardiac effects)

Beta-adrenergic blocking agents
(concurrent use with propafenone results in significant increases in plasma concentrations and half-life of propranolol and metoprolol, without affecting plasma propafenone concentrations; dosage reduction of the beta-blocker may be necessary)

Cimetidine
(concurrent use of cimetidine produces a 20% [approximate] increase in plasma concentrations of propafenone; however, because of wide interindividual variability in plasma concentrations and, therefore, lack of direct correlation with clinical effect, effects of propafenone on electrocardiogram parameters are unchanged)

» Digoxin
(concurrent use with propafenone results in an increase in serum digoxin concentrations ranging from 35 to 85%, which appears to be unrelated to digoxin renal clearance but which may be related to a decrease in volume of distribution and nonrenal clearance; careful monitoring of digoxin concentrations and dosage reduction of digoxin are recommended when propafenone is initiated; subsequent dosage adjustments should be based on plasma digoxin concentrations)

Quinidine
(small doses completely inhibit hydroxylation of propafenone, effectively making patients poor metabolizers of propafenone; however, dosage adjustment of propafenone is usually not necessary)

» Warfarin
(concurrent use with propafenone results in a significant increase [approximately 40%] in mean steady-state warfarin plasma concentrations, with a corresponding increase in prothrombin time of approximately 25%; monitoring of prothrombin time and appropriate adjustment of warfarin dosage are recommended during concurrent use)

## Laboratory value alterations

The following have been selected on the basis of their potential clinical significance (possible effect in parentheses where appropriate)—not necessarily inclusive (» = major clinical significance):

With physiology/laboratory test values
Electrocardiogram (ECG) changes such as:
QRS widening and
PR prolongation
(occur in most patients; dose-related)
Note: ECG changes produced by propafenone do not necessarily indicate efficacy, toxicity, or overdose.

Antinuclear antibody (ANA) titers, positive
(may occur rarely; reversible after withdrawal and sometimes during continued propafenone treatment; usually not symptomatic, but one case of lupus erythematosus, which reversed on withdrawal, has been reported)

## Medical considerations/Contraindications

The medical considerations/contraindications included here have been selected on the basis of their potential clinical significance (reasons given in parentheses where appropriate)—not necessarily inclusive (» = major clinical significance).

*Except under special circumstances, this medication should not be used when the following medical problems exist:*

» Atrioventricular (AV) block, pre-existing second or third degree without pacemaker, or

» Right bundle branch block associated with a left hemiblock (bifascicular block) without pacemaker
(risk of complete heart block)

*Risk-benefit should be considered when the following medical problems exist:*

Asthma or
Bronchospasm, nonallergenic (e.g., chronic bronchitis, emphysema)
(because of its beta-adrenergic blocking effect, propafenone may promote bronchospasm)

» Cardiogenic shock or

» Sinus bradycardia
(risk of further myocardial depression)

Cardiomyopathy

» Congestive heart failure
(negative inotropic effect of propafenone; also, risk of further depression of myocardial contractility because of beta-adrenergic blocking activity of propafenone)

Hepatic function impairment
(reduced first-pass effect results in increased bioavailability, to approximately 70%; increased half-life; dosage of propafenone should be reduced to approximately 20 to 30% of the usual dose, with careful monitoring)

Hypokalemia or hyperkalemia
(effects of propafenone may be altered; any electrolyte imbalance should be corrected prior to beginning therapy with propafenone)

Hypotension, marked
(may be aggravated)

Myocardial infarction, history of, especially with associated left ventricular function impairment

Renal function impairment
(reduced elimination; dosage reduction may be necessary)

Sensitivity to propafenone

» Sick sinus syndrome
(sinus node recovery time prolonged; sinus bradycardia, sinus pause, or sinus arrest may occur)

Caution is recommended in patients with permanent pacemakers or temporary pacing electrodes; propafenone may increase endocardial pacing thresholds and may suppress ventricular escape rhythms; use is not recommended in patients with existing poor thresholds or nonprogrammable pacemakers unless suitable pacing rescue is available.

## Patient monitoring

The following may be especially important in patient monitoring (other tests may be warranted in some patients, depending on condition; » = major clinical significance):

» Electrocardiogram (ECG)
(recommended prior to initiation of therapy and at periodic intervals during therapy to help assess efficacy and detect possible proarrhythmic effects)

# Side/Adverse Effects

Note: In the National Heart, Lung and Blood Institute's Cardiac Arrhythmia Suppression Trial (CAST), encainide and flecainide treatment were found to be associated with excessive mortality or increased nonfatal cardiac arrest rate as compared with placebo in patients with asymptomatic, non–life-threatening arrhythmias who had a recent myocardial infarction. The implications of these results for other patient populations or other antiarrhythmic agents are uncertain.

Adverse cardiac effects reported with propafenone administration include new or exacerbated ventricular arrhythmias in about 4.7% of patients; new or exacerbated congestive heart failure in 1% or less of patients; first, second, or third degree atrioventricular (AV) block in 2.5%, 0.6%, and 0.2% of patients, respectively; sinus bradycardia in 1.5% of patients; and rarely, sinus pause or sinus arrest.

Incidence of cardiac and other effects is at least partially dose-related.

Signs of overdose, usually most severe within 3 hours of ingestion, include hypotension, somnolence, bradycardia, AV dissociation, and intra-arterial and intraventricular conduction disturbances; asystole may develop. Convulsions and high grade ventricular arrhythmias have been reported rarely.

The following side/adverse effects have been selected on the basis of their potential clinical significance (possible signs and symptoms in parentheses where appropriate)—not necessarily inclusive:

**Those indicating need for medical attention**
Incidence more frequent
*Ventricular tachyarrhythmias* (fast or irregular heartbeat)
Note: Like other antiarrhythmic agents, propafenone may induce new arrhythmias and/or worsen an existing arrhythmia. *Ventricular tachyarrhythmias* are dose-related and potentially fatal; incidence increased in patients with sustained ventricular tachycardia, coronary artery disease, or history of myocardial infarction. Proarrhythmic effects usually occur during the first week of therapy, although effects are also seen later.

Incidence less frequent
*Angina* (chest pain); *bradycardia* (slow heartbeat); *congestive heart failure* (shortness of breath, swelling of feet or lower legs)

Incidence rare
*Agranulocytosis* (fever or chills); *conduction abnormalities, including atrioventricular block, bundle branch block; hypotension* (low blood pressure); *joint pain; supraventricular tachyarrhythmias, including atrial flutter, atrial fibrillation; trembling or shaking*

**Those indicating need for medical attention only if they continue or are bothersome**
Incidence more frequent
*Dizziness; taste disturbance* (change in taste; bitter or metallic taste)
Incidence less frequent
*Blurred vision; constipation or diarrhea; dryness of mouth; headache; nausea and/or vomiting; skin rash; unusual tiredness or weakness*

## Overdose

For more information on the management of overdose or unintentional ingestion, **contact a Poison Control Center** (see *Poison Control Center Listing*).

### Treatment of overdose

Treatment is primarily supportive and symptomatic and may include: Defibrillation and infusion of dopamine and isoproterenol to control rhythm and blood pressure; intravenous diazepam for convulsions; mechanical respiratory assistance and external cardiac massage.

## Patient Consultation

As an aid to patient consultation, refer to *Advice for the Patient, Propafenone (Systemic).*

In providing consultation, consider emphasizing the following selected information (» = major clinical significance):

**Before using this medication**
» Conditions affecting use, especially:
    Sensitivity to propafenone
    Pregnancy—Reduces fertility in monkeys, dogs, and rabbits; in rats, causes increased maternal and neonatal mortality, decreased maternal and infant weight gain, and reduced neonatal development
    Other medications, especially digoxin or warfarin
    Other medical problems, especially second or third degree atrioventricular (AV) block, right bundle branch block associated with a left hemiblock, cardiogenic shock, congestive heart failure, sick sinus syndrome, or sinus bradycardia

**Proper use of this medication**
» Compliance with therapy; taking as directed even if feeling well
» Importance of not missing doses and taking at evenly spaced intervals
    Missed dose: Taking as soon as possible if remembered within 4 hours; not taking if remembered later; not doubling doses
» Proper storage

**Precautions while using this medication**
    Regular visits to physician to check progress
    Carrying medical identification card or bracelet
» Caution if any kind of surgery (including dental surgery) or emergency treatment is required

Caution when driving or doing things requiring alertness because of possible dizziness
**Side/adverse effects**
    Signs of potential side effects, especially ventricular tachyarrhythmias, angina, congestive heart failure, agranulocytosis, bradycardia, conduction abnormalities, hypotension, joint pain, and trembling or shaking

## General Dosing Information

Because of wide interindividual variability in plasma concentrations, careful titration of dosage is recommended. However, because steady-state concentrations are achieved after the same amount of time in both extensive and poor metabolizers, and because the difference in peak plasma concentrations decreases at high doses and the active 5-hydroxy metabolite is absent in poor metabolizers, the recommended dosage regimen is the same for both groups of patients.

Dosage increments should be made no more frequently than every 3 to 4 days.

It is recommended that treatment be initiated in the hospital because of the increased risk of proarrhythmic effects associated with propafenone administration.

In general, it is recommended that previous antiarrhythmic therapy be withdrawn 2 to 5 half-lives before initiation of propafenone therapy.

In patients with pacemakers, pacing threshold should be monitored and programmed at periodic intervals during propafenone therapy.

## Oral Dosage Forms

### PROPAFENONE HYDROCHLORIDE TABLETS

**Usual adult dose**
Antiarrhythmic—Ventricular or
[Antiarrhythmic—Supraventricular][1]—
    Oral, initially 150 mg every eight hours, increased, if necessary, after three to four days to 225 mg every eight hours (U.S. labeling) or 300 mg every twelve hours (Canadian labeling); may be further increased after an additional three to four days, if necessary, to 300 mg every eight hours.

**Usual pediatric dose**
Safety and efficacy have not been established.

**Strength(s) usually available**
U.S.—
    150 mg (Rx) [*Rythmol* (scored)].
    225 mg (Rx) [*Rythmol* (scored)].
    300 mg (Rx) [*Rythmol* (scored)].
Canada—
    150 mg (Rx) [*Rythmol*].
    300 mg (Rx) [*Rythmol* (scored)].

**Packaging and storage**
Store between 15 and 30 °C (59 and 86 °F), in a tight, light-resistant container, unless otherwise specified by manufacturer.

---

[1]Not included in Canadian product labeling.

## Selected Bibliography

Chow MS, Lebsack C, Hilleman D. Propafenone: A new antiarrhythmic agent. Clin Pharm 1988; 7: 869-77.
Harron DW, Brogden RN. Propafenone. A review of its pharmacodynamic and pharmacokinetic properties, and therapeutic use in the treatment of arrhythmias. Drugs 1987; 34: 617-47.
Funck-Brentano C, Kroemer HK, Lee JT, Roden DM. Propafenone. N Engl J Med 1990; 322 (8): 518-25.

---

Revised: 10/07/92
Interim revision: 08/02/93

---

**PROPANTHELINE**—See *Anticholinergics/Antispasmodics (Systemic)*

---

**PROPARACAINE**—See *Anesthetics (Ophthalmic)*

# PROPIOMAZINE   Systemic†

VA CLASSIFICATION (Primary): CN309

Note: For a listing of dosage forms and brand names by country availability, see *Dosage Forms* section(s). For a listing of brand names for the articles in this monograph, refer to the General Index.

†Not commercially available in Canada.

## Category
Sedative-hypnotic.

## Indications

### Accepted
Anesthesia, adjunct—Propiomazine is indicated for the relief of restlessness and apprehension, preoperatively or during surgery.

Analgesia adjunct, during labor—Propiomazine is indicated as an adjunct to analgesics for the relief of restlessness and apprehension during labor.

## Pharmacology/Pharmacokinetics

### Physicochemical characteristics
Molecular weight—376.94.

### Mechanism of action/Effect
Unknown. Propiomazine is a phenothiazine compound with sedative action.

### Other actions/effects
Propiomazine also has antiemetic and antihistaminic properties.

### Biotransformation
Unknown, but probably hepatic as with other phenothiazines.

### Time to peak serum concentration
1 to 3 hours following intramuscular administration.

### Time to peak effect
Intramuscular—Within 40 to 60 minutes.
Intravenous—Within 15 to 30 minutes.

### Duration of action
About 3 to 6 hours.

### Elimination
Unknown, but probably renal and biliary as with other phenothiazines.

## Precautions to Consider

### Cross-sensitivity and/or related problems
Patients sensitive to other phenothiazines may be sensitive to this medication also.

### Pregnancy/Reproduction
Problems in humans have not been documented.

### Breast-feeding
Problems in humans have not been documented.

### Pediatrics
Appropriate studies on the relationship of age to the effects of propiomazine have not been performed in the pediatric population. However, no pediatrics-specific problems have been documented to date.

### Geriatrics
No information is available on the relationship of age to the effects of propiomazine in geriatric patients.

### Drug interactions and/or related problems
The following drug interactions and/or related problems have been selected on the basis of their potential clinical significance (possible mechanism in parentheses where appropriate)—not necessarily inclusive (» = major clinical significance):

Note: Combinations containing any of the following medications, depending on the amount present, may also interact with this medication.

» Alcohol or
» Central nervous system (CNS) depression–producing medications, other (See *Appendix II*)
     (concurrent use may increase the CNS depressant effects of either these medications or propiomazine; caution is recommended and dosage of one or both agents should be reduced; dosage adjustments of barbiturates to approximately one-half of the usual dose

and narcotic analgesics to approximately one-fourth to one-half of the usual dose are recommended)

Epinephrine
     (concurrent use with propiomazine may block the alpha-adrenergic effects of epinephrine, allowing beta-adrenergic effects to predominate, thus possibly resulting in severe hypotension)

Hypotension-producing medications, other (See *Appendix II*)
     (concurrent use may potentiate the hypotensive effect of propiomazine; dosage adjustments may be necessary)

     (concurrent use of mecamylamine or trimethaphan with propiomazine may potentiate the hypotensive response, with increased risk of severe hypotension, shock, and cardiovascular collapse during surgery)

     (caution is advised during titration of calcium channel blocker dosage for those patients taking medication, such as propiomazine, known to promote hypotension, since the combination may result in excessive hypotension)

Ketamine
     (concurrent use of ketamine, especially in high doses or when rapidly administered, with propiomazine may increase the risk of hypotension and/or respiratory depression)

### Laboratory value alterations
The following have been selected on the basis of their potential clinical significance (possible effect in parentheses where appropriate)—not necessarily inclusive (» = major clinical significance):

With diagnostic test results
Phentolamine
     (propiomazine may cause false-positive phentolamine test; it is recommended that all medications be withdrawn at least 24 hours, preferably 48 to 72 hours, prior to a phentolamine test)

### Medical considerations/Contraindications
The medical considerations/contraindications included here have been selected on the basis of their potential clinical significance (reasons given in parentheses where appropriate)—not necessarily inclusive (» = major clinical significance).

*Risk-benefit should be considered when the following medical problem exists:*

Sensitivity to propiomazine or other phenothiazines

## Side/Adverse Effects
The following side/adverse effects have been selected on the basis of their potential clinical significance (possible signs and symptoms in parentheses where appropriate)—not necessarily inclusive:

### Those indicating need for medical attention
*Thrombophlebitis* (redness, swelling, or pain at injection site)

Incidence rare
*Neuroleptic malignant syndrome (NMS)* (difficult or unusually fast breathing; fast or irregular heartbeat or pulse; high fever; high or low [irregular] blood pressure; loss of bladder control; mental changes; severe muscle stiffness; seizures; unusual increase in sweating; unusually pale skin; unusual tiredness or weakness)

Note: *NMS* has been reported in association with antipsychotic medications; occurrence of NMS does not appear to be related to the dose or the duration of therapy; propiomazine should be discontinued immediately because of possible fatal results

### Those indicating need for medical attention only if they continue or are bothersome

Incidence more frequent
*Dizziness; drowsiness, prolonged; dryness of mouth*

Incidence less frequent
*Confusion; diarrhea; fast heartbeat; nausea or vomiting; restlessness; shortness of breath or troubled breathing; skin rash; stomach pain*

## Patient Consultation
As an aid to patient consultation, refer to *Advice for the Patient, Propiomazine (Systemic).*

In providing consultation, consider emphasizing the following selected information (» = major clinical significance):

**Before receiving this medication**
» Conditions affecting use, especially:
  Sensitivity to propiomazine or other phenothiazines
  Other medications, especially alcohol or other CNS depression–producing medications

**Proper use of this medication**
» Proper dosing

**Precautions after receiving this medication**
» Possibility of psychomotor impairment following use of propiomazine; using caution in driving or performing other tasks requiring alertness and coordination until the effects of propiomazine have subsided or until the day after receiving propiomazine, whichever is longer
» Avoiding use of alcohol or other CNS depressants within 24 hours after receiving propiomazine except as directed by physician or dentist

**Side/adverse effects**
  Signs of potential side effects, especially thrombophlebitis and neuroleptic malignant syndrome (NMS)

## General Dosing Information

Intra-arterial injection is not recommended because of chemical irritation, which may be severe enough to cause arteriospasm, possibly resulting in local impairment of circulation.

Intravenous injections should be made only into undamaged veins since propiomazine may cause irritation, possibly resulting in thrombophlebitis.

Intravenous injections should be administered slowly, as too rapid administration may produce a transient fall in blood pressure.

Care should be used to avoid perivascular extravasation since chemical irritation may be severe.

**For treatment of adverse effects**
  Neuroleptic malignant syndrome (NMS)—
    Treatment is essentially symptomatic and supportive and may include the following
    • *Discontinuing propiomazine immediately.*
    • Hyperthermia—Administering antipyretics (aspirin or acetaminophen); using cooling blanket.
    • Dehydration—Restoring fluids and electrolytes.
    • Cardiovascular instability—Monitoring blood pressure and cardiac rhythm closely. Use of sodium nitroprusside may allow vasodilation with subsequent heat loss from the skin in patients with less dominant muscle rigidity.

• Hypoxia—Administering oxygen; intubation and mechanical ventilation may be necessary.
• Muscle rigidity—Administering dantrolene sodium (100 to 300 mg per day in divided doses; 1.25 to 1.5 mg per kg of body weight [mg/kg], intravenously); or administering amantadine 100 mg twice daily, or bromocriptine, 5 mg three times a day, to restore central balance of dopamine and acetylcholine at the receptor site.

## Parenteral Dosage Forms

### PROPIOMAZINE HYDROCHLORIDE INJECTION USP

**Usual adult dose**
Preoperative—
  Intramuscular or intravenous, 20 to 40 mg administered in conjunction with 50 mg of meperidine.
Sedation during surgery with local, nerve block, or spinal anesthesia—
  Intramuscular or intravenous, 10 to 20 mg.
Analgesia adjunct, during labor—
  Intramuscular or intravenous, 20 to 40 mg in the early stages of labor, then 20 to 40 mg of propiomazine administered in conjunction with 25 to 75 mg of meperidine when labor is definitely established. Doses may be repeated every three hours, if necessary.

**Usual pediatric dose**
Sedation prior to surgery; preanesthetic; or postoperative—
  Children up to 27 kg: Intramuscular or intravenous, 550 mcg (0.55 mg) to 1.1 mg per kg of body weight; or for
  Children 2 to 4 years of age: Intramuscular or intravenous, 10 mg.
  Children 4 to 6 years of age: Intramuscular or intravenous, 15 mg.
  Children 6 to 12 years of age: Intramuscular or intravenous, 25 mg.

**Strength(s) usually available**
U.S.—
  20 mg per mL (Rx) [*Largon* (sodium acetate; sodium formaldehyde sulfoxylate not more than 1 mg)].
Canada—
  Not commercially available.

**Packaging and storage**
Store between 15 and 30 °C (59 and 86 °F). Protect from light.

**Stability**
Do not use the injection if it is cloudy or contains a precipitate.

**Incompatibilities**
Aqueous solutions of propiomazine are incompatible with barbiturate salts and other alkaline substances.

Revised: 04/16/93
Interim revision: 07/26/94

# PROPOFOL Systemic

VA CLASSIFICATION (Primary/Secondary): CN203/CN205; CN309
Another commonly used name is disoprofol.
Note: For a listing of dosage forms and brand names by country availability, see *Dosage Forms* section(s). For a listing of brand names for the articles in this monograph, refer to the General Index.

## Category

Anesthetic, general; anesthesia adjunct; sedative-hypnotic.

## Indications

Note: Bracketed information in the *Indications* section refers to uses that are not included in U.S. product labeling.

**Accepted**
Anesthesia, general or
Anesthesia, general, adjunct—Propofol is indicated for the induction of general anesthesia. It is also indicated for maintenance of anesthesia utilizing balanced techniques with other appropriate agents such as opioids and inhalation anesthetics.

[Sedation][1]—Propofol is used to produce sedation or amnesia as a supplement to regional anesthetics. Propofol is also used in procedures not requiring analgesia, such as endoscopy.

Propofol may be useful for sedation in critically ill patients confined to intensive care units. Although cardiovascular, respiratory, and sedative effects must be carefully monitored, propofol reportedly provides

good control of depth of sedation, and the rapid return of spontaneous ventilation following discontinuation of propofol infusion allows early extubation. Tachyphylaxis, delayed awakening, or cumulative effects have not been reported after prolonged administration of propofol as they have with prolonged infusion of thiopental, diazepam, or midazolam. In addition, propofol does not suppress adrenocortical function as does etomidate.

[1]Not included in Canadian product labeling.

## Pharmacology/Pharmacokinetics

**Physicochemical characteristics**
Molecular weight—178.27.
pH—Propofol emulsion: 7 to 8.5

**Mechanism of action/Effect**
Propofol is a short-acting hypnotic. Its mechanism of action has not been well defined.

**Other actions/effects**
Hemodynamic effects—
  Propofol's hemodynamic effects are generally more pronounced than those of other intravenous anesthetic agents. Arterial hypotension, with readings decreased by as much as 30% or more, has been reported. Hypotensive effects are generally proportional to dose and rate of administration of propofol, and may be potentiated by opioid analgesics. Endotracheal intubation and surgical stimulation may increase arterial pressure; increases in heart rate and/or blood

pressure to greater than baseline values, which occur frequently with other agents, are not as significant with propofol, possibly due to central sympatholytic and/or vagotonic effects. Propofol may also decrease systemic vascular resistance and myocardial oxygen blood flow and consumption. The mechanism for these effects may involve direct vasodilation and negative inotropy. Effects such as decreased stroke volume and cardiac output have been demonstrated in some studies.

Respiratory effects—
Propofol is a respiratory depressant, frequently producing apnea that may persist for longer than 60 seconds, depending on factors such as premedication, rate of administration, dose administered, and presence of hyperventilation or hyperoxia. In addition, propofol may produce significant decreases in respiratory rate, minute volume, tidal volume, mean inspiratory flow rate, and functional residual capacity. These respiratory depressant effects may be the result of depression of the central inspiratory drive as opposed to a change in central timing. The ventilatory depressant effects of propofol may be counteracted by painful surgical stimulation.

Cerebral effects—
Propofol decreases cerebral blood flow, cerebral metabolic oxygen consumption, and intracranial pressure, and increases cerebrovascular resistance. It does not appear to affect cerebrovascular reactivity to changes in arterial carbon dioxide tension.

Other effects—
Preliminary findings suggest that in patients with normal intraocular pressure, propofol decreases intraocular pressure by as much as 30 to 50%. This decrease may be associated with a concomitant decrease in systemic vascular resistance.

Clinical studies have shown that propofol does not cause significant signs of histamine release or significant increases in plasma immunoglobulin or complement $C_3$ levels.

Although propofol has the potential for affecting adrenal steroidogenesis, it does not appear to block cortisol and aldosterone secretion in response to surgical stress or adrenocorticotropic hormone (ACTH) in clinical practice. Although transient decreases in plasma cortisol concentrations have occurred, these reductions have not been sustained.

Propofol appears to have no analgesic activity. In addition, animal studies have demonstrated no significant effect on coagulation profiles.

Limited experience with propofol in susceptible patients and animal studies has not demonstrated a propensity to induce malignant hyperthermia.

Some investigators have attributed antiemetic properties to propofol, which reportedly causes less nausea and vomiting than do thiopental or methohexital.

**Distribution**
Propofol is rapidly and extensively distributed in the body. It crosses the blood-brain barrier quickly, and its short duration of action is due to rapid redistribution from the CNS to other tissues, high metabolic clearance, and high lipophilicity.
Volumes of distribution—
Initial apparent ($vol_D$)—Relatively large, 13 to 76 liters.
Steady-state ($V_{DSS}$)—171 to 349 liters.
Elimination ($vol_D$)—209 to 1008 liters.
Propofol crosses the placenta; although maternal concentrations of drug significantly exceed cord concentrations, there is no apparent barrier.

**Protein binding**
Very high (95-99%).

**Biotransformation**
Hepatic; rapidly undergoes glucuronide conjugation to inactive metabolites. An unidentified route of extrahepatic metabolism may also exist, suggested by the fact that propofol clearance exceeds estimated hepatic blood flow.

**Half-life**
Distribution—
Two distribution phases:
Rapid—2 to 4 minutes.
Slower—30 to 64 minutes.
Elimination—
Terminal elimination half-life is 3 to 12 hours; prolonged administration of propofol may result in a longer duration.
Note: The long terminal elimination half-life of propofol does not reflect elimination, as more than 70% is eliminated during the first 2 phases. Some investigators believe that the second exponential phase half-life (30–64 minutes) best explains the properties of propofol in clinical practice.
Other—
Blood-brain equilibration half-life: 2.9 minutes.

**Onset of action**
Loss of consciousness occurs rapidly and smoothly, usually within 40 seconds (one arm-brain circulation time) from the start of intravenous injection of propofol. Loss of consciousness is dependent on the dose administered, the rate of administration, and the extent of premedication.

**Plasma concentrations**
Propofol concentrations of 1.5 to 6 mcg per mL will maintain hypnosis, although needs vary with type of surgery and use of other anesthetic agents.

**Duration of action**
Mean duration following a single bolus dose of 2 to 2.5 mg per kg of body weight is 3 to 5 minutes.

**Time to recovery**
Recovery from anesthesia with propofol is rapid, with minimal psychomotor impairment. Emergence following induction (with 2 to 2.5 mg of propofol per kg) and maintenance (with 0.1 to 0.2 mg of propofol per kg per minute) for up to 2 hours occurs in most patients within 8 minutes. If an opioid has been used, recovery may take up to 19 minutes.

Recovery reportedly occurs faster than that following the use of thiopental, etomidate, methohexital, or midazolam. When anesthesia has included use of an opioid with propofol, recovery has occurred more quickly than with similar use of etomidate, midazolam, or thiopental.

Many investigators have noted clearheadedness in patients emerging from propofol anesthesia, and less residual impairment of performance than in patients who received methohexital has been reported.

**Elimination**
Renal; approximately 70% of a dose excreted in the urine within 24 hours after administration, and 90% excreted within 5 days. Clearance of propofol ranges from 1.6 to 3.4 liters per minute in healthy 70 kg patients. As the age of the patient increases, total body clearance of propofol may decrease. Clearance rates ranging from 1.4 to 2.2 liters per minute in patients 18 to 35 years of age have been reported, in contrast to clearance rates of 1.0 to 1.8 liters per minute in patients 65 to 80 years of age.

Note: Pharmacokinetic parameters of propofol appear to be unaffected by gender, obesity, chronic hepatic cirrhosis, and possibly chronic renal failure.

## Precautions to Consider

**Carcinogenicity**
Studies have not been done.

**Mutagenicity**
The Ames mutation test using *Salmonella* species, gene mutation/gene conversion using *Saccharomyces cerevisiae*, cytogenetic studies in Chinese hamsters, and a mouse micronucleus test have failed to demonstrate mutagenic potential by propofol.

**Pregnancy/Reproduction**
Fertility—Studies in rats given doses up to 6 times the human dose for varying lengths of time have shown no evidence of impaired fertility.

Pregnancy—Propofol crosses the placenta. Adequate and well-controlled studies in humans have not been done.

Studies in animals have shown propofol to cause increased maternal deaths in rats and rabbits and decreased pup survival during the lactating period when the dams received 6 times the recommended human dose

FDA Pregnancy Category B.

Labor and delivery—The manufacturer states that use of propofol is not recommended since data are insufficient to support its use in obstetrics, including cesarean section deliveries.

**Breast-feeding**
Propofol is reportedly distributed into breast milk. However, the effects of oral administration of small amounts of propofol are not known.

**Pediatrics**
Appropriate studies with propofol have not been performed in the pediatric population.

**Geriatrics**
Propofol should be used with caution in the elderly, as these patients may be more sensitive to its effects than are younger adults. Lower induction doses and a slower maintenance infusion rate should be used in geriatric patients, due to reduced total body clearance and volume of distribution in these patients.

**Drug interactions and/or related problems**
The following drug interactions and/or related problems have been selected on the basis of their potential clinical significance (possible mechanism in parentheses where appropriate)—not necessarily inclusive (» = major clinical significance):

Note: Combinations containing any of the following medications, depending on the amount present, may also interact with this medication.

» Alcohol or
» CNS depression–producing medications, other, including those commonly used for preanesthetic medication or induction or supplementation of anesthesia (See *Appendix II*)
(concurrent administration may increase the CNS depressant, respiratory depressant, or hypotensive effects of propofol as well as decreasing anesthetic requirements and prolonging recovery from anesthesia; dosage adjustments may be required)

### Medical considerations/Contraindications

The medical considerations/contraindications included here have been selected on the basis of their potential clinical significance (reasons given in parentheses where appropriate)—not necessarily inclusive (» = major clinical significance).

*Risk-benefit should be considered when the following medical problems exist:*

Circulatory disorders or
Compromised cardiovascular function
(may be aggravated by cardiovascular-depressant and hypotensive effects)

Disorders of lipid metabolism, such as primary hyperlipoproteinemia, diabetic hyperlipemia, or pancreatitis
(may be aggravated by emulsion vehicle of propofol)

Increased intracranial pressure or
Impaired cerebral circulation
(substantial decreases in mean arterial pressure and cerebral perfusion may occur)

Sensitivity to propofol or its emulsion vehicle

Caution is also recommended in geriatric, debilitated, and/or hypovolemic patients, because they may require lower induction and maintenance doses.

## Side/Adverse Effects

Note: Postoperative infections and subsequent deaths have been reported following the use of propofol that was not administered using strict aseptic technique.

Rarely, a clinical syndrome including bronchospasm, erythema, and hypotension has occurred shortly after administration of propofol, and sequelae including anoxic brain damage and death have been reported; concurrent use of other agents makes a causal relationship unclear.

The following side/adverse effects have been selected on the basis of their potential clinical significance (possible signs and symptoms in parentheses where appropriate)—not necessarily inclusive:

**Those indicating need for medical attention**
Incidence more frequent
*Apnea; bradycardia; hypotension*

Incidence less frequent or rare
*Hypertension; perioperative myoclonia, rarely including opisthotonus*

**Those indicating need for medical attention only if they continue or are bothersome**
Incidence more frequent
*Involuntary muscle movements, temporary; nausea and/or vomiting; pain, burning, or stinging at injection site*

Note: *Excitatory movements* reportedly occur more often than with thiopental but less often than with etomidate or methohexital.

*Pain* is usually mild and short-lived, and may be decreased by using the larger veins of the forearm or anticubital fossa or a dedicated intravenous catheter. Pain may be decreased by prior intravenous injection of 10 to 20 mg of lidocaine. Post-injection thrombosis or phlebitis is rare.

Incidence less frequent or rare
*Abdominal cramping; cough; dizziness; fever; flushing; headache; hiccups; tingling, numbness, or coldness at injection site*

## Overdose

For specific information on the management of a propofol overdose, see:
• *Atropine* in *Anticholinergics/Antispasmodics* monograph; and/or
• *Sympathomimetic Agents—Cardiovascular Use (Parenteral-Systemic)* monograph.

For more information on the management of overdose, **contact a Poison Control Center** (see *Poison Control Center Listing*).

### Clinical effects of overdose
The following effects have been selected on the basis of their potential clinical significance (possible signs and symptoms in parentheses where appropriate)—not necessarily inclusive:
Acute
*Cardiovascular depression; respiratory depression*

### Treatment of overdose
Specific treatment—
Discontinuation of propofol.
For respiratory depression—artificial ventilation with oxygen.
For cardiovascular depression—elevation of legs, increasing flow rate of intravenous fluids, and administration of pressor agents and/or anticholinergic agents.
Monitoring—
Patients should be continuously monitored for signs of significant hypotension and/or bradycardia.

## Patient Consultation

As an aid to patient consultation, refer to *Advice for the Patient, Anesthetics, General (Systemic)*.

In providing consultation, consider emphasizing the following selected information (» = major clinical significance):

**Before using this medication**
» Conditions affecting use, especially:
Sensitivity to propofol or its emulsion vehicle
Pregnancy—Propofol crosses the placenta
Labor and delivery—Use of propofol is not recommended since data are insufficient to support its use in obstetrics
Use in the elderly—Lower induction and maintenance doses are recommended
Other medications, especially other CNS depressants

**Proper use of this medication**
Proper dosing

**Precautions after receiving this medication**
Possibility of psychomotor impairment following use of anesthetics; for about 24 hours following anesthesia, using added caution in driving or performing other tasks requiring alertness and coordination
Avoiding use of alcohol or other CNS depressants within 24 hours following anesthesia except as directed by physician or dentist

**Side/adverse effects**
Signs of potential side effects, especially apnea, bradycardia, hypotension, hypertension, and perioperative myoclonia

## General Dosing Information

**Propofol should be administered only by individuals qualified in the use of general anesthetics. Appropriate resuscitative and endotracheal intubation equipment, oxygen, and medications for prevention and treatment of anesthetic emergencies must be immediately available. Airway patency must be maintained at all times.**

Propofol emulsion is for intravenous administration only. Although clinical experience and animal studies have shown that inadvertent intra-arterial injection of propofol usually produces minimal tissue reaction, intra-arterial injection of propofol is not recommended.

Dosage of propofol must be individualized for each patient, with the dose titrated to achieve the desired clinical effect. Lower doses are usually required for elderly, debilitated, or higher risk surgical patients, or those with circulatory disorders. The dosage of intravenously administered propofol should be adjusted according to the type and amount of premedication used.

When propofol is administered by infusion, it is recommended that drop counters, syringe pumps, or volumetric pumps be utilized to control infusion rates.

When nitrous oxide, oxygen, and propofol are used for maintenance of general anesthesia, supplemental analgesic agents are generally required; neuromuscular blocking agents may also be required. Concurrent use of propofol with neuromuscular blocking agents does not significantly alter the onset, intensity, or duration of action of these agents.

**For treatment of adverse effects**
Patients should be continuously monitored for early signs of significant hypotension and/or bradycardia.
Recommended treatment may include
• Increasing the rate of intravenous fluid administration.
• Elevation of the lower extremities.

- Use of pressor agents.
- Administration of atropine.

# Parenteral Dosage Forms

Note: Bracketed uses in the *Dosage Forms* section refer to categories of use and/or indications that are not included in U.S. product labeling.

## PROPOFOL INJECTION

### Usual adult and adolescent dose

Dosage must be individualized and titrated to the desired clinical effect; however, as a general guideline—

Anesthesia, general (induction):

    Adults up to 55 years of age and/or ASA I or II patients—
      Intravenous, 2.0 to 2.5 mg per kg of body weight (approximately 40 mg every ten seconds until onset of induction).

    Elderly, debilitated, hypovolemic, and/or ASA III or IV patients—
      Intravenous, 1.0 to 1.5 mg per kg of body weight (approximately 20 mg every ten seconds until onset of induction).

    Note: Slow injection of the induction dose of propofol may result in longer induction times and a lower percentage of successful inductions, probably due to rapid redistribution from the CNS; however, some investigators believe slower injection of larger doses is preferable, in order to diminish some of the cardiovascular effects.

Anesthesia, general, adjunct (maintenance):

    Intravenous (infusion)—

      Adults up to 55 years of age and/or ASA I or II patients:
        100 to 200 mcg (0.1 to 0.2 mg) per kg of body weight per minute (6 to 12 mg per kg of body weight per hour).

      Note: During the initial ten to fifteen minutes following induction, higher infusion rates of 150 to 200 mcg (0.15 to 0.2 mg) per kg of body weight per minute are generally required. Infusion rates should subsequently be decreased by 30 to 50% during the first half-hour of maintenance.

      Infusion rates should always be titrated downward in the absence of light anesthesia to avoid administration of propofol at rates higher than clinically necessary. In general, rates of 50 to 100 mcg (0.05 to 0.1 mg) per kg of body weight per minute should be achieved during maintenance to optimize recovery times.

      Elderly, debilitated, hypovolemic, and/or ASA III or IV patients:
        50 to 100 mcg (0.05 to 0.1 mg) per kg of body weight per minute (3 to 6 mg per kg of body weight per hour).

    Intravenous (intermittent)—
      25 to 50 mg increments, administered as needed. Alternatively, some clinicians recommend increments of 500 mcg (0.5 mg) per kg of body weight.

[Sedation][1]:
    Intravenous infusion, 1 to 6 mg per kg of body weight per hour.

### Usual pediatric dose
Dosage has not been established.

### Strength(s) usually available
U.S.—
    10 mg per mL (Rx) [*Diprivan* (soybean oil 10% w/v; glycerol 2.25% w/v; purified egg phosphatide (lecithin) 1.2% w/v)].
Canada—
    10 mg per mL (Rx) [*Diprivan* (soybean oil 10% w/v; glycerol 2.25% w/v; purified egg phosphatide (lecithin) 1.2% w/v)].

### Packaging and storage
Store between 4 and 22 °C (40 and 72 °F). Refrigeration is not recommended. Protect from light.

### Preparation of dosage form
Propofol is compatible with 5% dextrose in water, lactated Ringer's solution, and combinations of 5% dextrose with 0.45% or 0.2% sodium chloride.

If propofol is diluted prior to administration, only 5% Dextrose Injection USP should be used as a diluent, and the final concentration should not be less than 2 mg per mL to preserve the emulsion base. The dilution appears to be more stable in glass than in plastic.

### Stability
Propofol injection contains no antimicrobial preservatives, and the vehicle is capable of supporting the rapid growth of microorganisms; particulate or bacterial contamination may be difficult to detect because propofol injection is opaque. Therefore, strict aseptic technique must be maintained. Propofol injection should be drawn into sterile syringes or connected to a volumetric infusion device immediately after the

container is opened, and administered promptly. Unused portions of the injection as well as reservoirs, IV lines, or solutions containing propofol injection, must be discarded at the end of the procedure or within 6 hours, whichever occurs sooner.

Propofol should not be used if there is evidence of separation of the emulsion phases.

### Incompatibilities
The manufacturer states that propofol emulsion should not be mixed with other therapeutic agents prior to administration. In addition, propofol should not be coadministered through the same IV catheter with blood or plasma; although the clinical significance is not known, *in vitro* studies have shown that the globular component of the emulsion vehicle has formed aggregates when in contact with human and animal blood, plasma, and serum.

### Auxiliary labeling
- Shake well before use.
- Protect from light.

[1]Not included in Canadian product labeling.

## Selected Bibliography

G E Larijani et al. Clinical pharmacology of propofol: an intravenous anesthetic agent. DICP, Ann Pharmacother (Oct) 1989; 23: 743-9.

L Kiser. Correction: propofol dosage. (letter) and G E Larijani. (response). DICP, Ann Pharmacother (Jan) 1990; 24: 102.

P S Sebel and J D Lowdon. Propofol: A new intravenous anesthetic. Anesthesiology 1989; 71: 260-77.

M S Langley and R C Heel. Propofol. A review of its pharmacodynamic and pharmacokinetic properties and use as an intravenous anaesthetic. Drugs 1988; 35: 334-72.

White PF. Propofol: pharmacokinetics and pharmacodynamics. Seminars in Anesthesia (Mar) 1988; 7 (1) (suppl 1): 4–20.

Revised: 02/12/91
Interim revision: 07/03/91

# PROPOXYCAINE-CONTAINING COMBINATIONS—

Propoxycaine, Procaine, and Levonordefrin (Parenteral-Local)—See *Anesthetics (Parenteral-Local)*

Propoxycaine, Procaine, and Norepinephrine (Parenteral-Local)—See *Anesthetics (Parenteral-Local)*

# PROPOXYPHENE—See *Opioid (Narcotic) Analgesics (Systemic)*

# PROPOXYPHENE-CONTAINING COMBINATIONS—

Propoxyphene and Acetaminophen (Systemic)—See *Opioid (Narcotic) Analgesics and Acetaminophen (Systemic)*

Propoxyphene and Aspirin (Systemic)—See *Opioid (Narcotic) Analgesics and Aspirin (Systemic)*

Propoxyphene, Aspirin, and Caffeine (Systemic)—See *Opioid (Narcotic) Analgesics and Aspirin (Systemic)*

# PROPRANOLOL—See *Beta-adrenergic Blocking Agents (Systemic)*

# PROPRANOLOL-CONTAINING COMBINATIONS—

Propranolol and Hydrochlorothiazide (Systemic)—See *Beta-adrenergic Blocking Agents and Thiazide Diuretics (Systemic)*

# PROPYLTHIOURACIL—See *Antithyroid Agents (Systemic)*

# PROTAMINE    Systemic

BAN: Protamine sulphate

VA CLASSIFICATION (Primary): BL200

Note: For a listing of dosage forms and brand names by country availability, see *Dosage Forms* section(s). For a listing of brand names for the articles in this monograph, refer to the General Index.

## Category

Antidote (to heparin).

## Indications

Note: Bracketed information in the *Indications* section refers to uses that are not included in U.S. product labeling.

### Accepted

Toxicity, heparin (treatment) or

[Toxicity, enoxaparin (treatment)][1]—Protamine is indicated in the treatment of severe heparin overdose resulting in hemorrhage; it is also used to neutralize the hemorrhagic effects following overdose of the low molecular weight heparin, enoxaparin. Transfusion of whole blood or fresh frozen plasma may also be required to replace lost volume if hemorrhaging has been severe; this may dilute, but will not neutralize the effects of, heparin.

Protamine is also indicated for administration following cardiac or arterial surgery or dialysis procedures when required to neutralize the effects of heparin administered during extracorporeal circulation.

### Unaccepted

Protamine is not used in treating minor heparin overdose that may respond to withdrawal of heparin, or in treating hemorrhage not caused by heparin.

---

[1] Not included in Canadian product labeling.

## Pharmacology/Pharmacokinetics

### Mechanism of action/Effect

Protamine is a strongly basic substance that combines with the strongly acidic heparin to form a stable complex. Heparin produces its effects indirectly, apparently by forming a complex with and producing a conformational change in the antithrombin III (heparin cofactor) molecule, resulting in potentiation of antithrombin III activity. One study has indicated that by combining with heparin, protamine causes a dissociation of the heparin-antithrombin III complex, resulting in loss of anticoagulant activity.

### Other actions/effects

Protamine has some anticoagulant activity of its own when administered in the absence of heparin or in doses larger than those required to neutralize heparin, but it is not used as an anticoagulant. This anticoagulant effect may be caused by protamine's antithromboplastin activity, which results in inhibition of thrombin generation.

### Onset of action

30 seconds to 1 minute.

### Duration of action

2 hours; dependent on body temperature.

## Precautions to Consider

### Pregnancy/Reproduction

Pregnancy—Studies have not been done in humans.
Studies have not been done in animals.

FDA Pregnancy Category C.

### Breast-feeding

It is not known whether protamine is distributed into breast milk. However, problems in humans have not been documented.

### Pediatrics

Appropriate studies performed to date have not demonstrated pediatrics-specific problems that would limit the usefulness of protamine in children.

### Geriatrics

Appropriate studies on the relationship of age to the effects of protamine have not been performed in the geriatric population. However, geriatrics-specific problems that would limit the usefulness of this medication in the elderly are not expected.

### Medical considerations/Contraindications

The medical considerations/contraindications included here have been selected on the basis of their potential clinical significance (reasons given in parentheses where appropriate)—not necessarily inclusive (» = major clinical significance).

*Risk-benefit should be considered when the following medical problems exist:*

» Allergic reaction to protamine, history of

  Antibodies to protamine in the sera of infertile or vasectomized men or

  Prior exposure to protamine or other protamine-containing medications, e.g., protamine insulin
  (increased risk of allergic reaction)

### Patient monitoring

The following may be especially important in patient monitoring (other tests may be warranted in some patients, depending on condition; » = major clinical significance):

Blood coagulation tests
  (recommended as a guide to protamine efficacy and dosage; in the operating room, activated clotting time [ACT], either manual or automated, is most often used to monitor neutralization of large doses of heparin)

Blood titration tests with protamine
  (may be necessary as a guide to protamine dosage, especially when large doses of heparin have been administered)

## Side/Adverse Effects

The following side/adverse effects have been selected on the basis of their potential clinical significance (possible signs and symptoms in parentheses where appropriate)—not necessarily inclusive:

### Those indicating need for medical attention

Incidence more frequent—usually caused by too-rapid administration of medication
  *Bradycardia; cardiovascular collapse or shock*—may be caused by a direct myocardial effect and/or peripheral vasodilatation; *decrease in blood pressure, sudden*—may reach hypotensive levels; *dyspnea*

Incidence less frequent
  *Anaphylactic or anaphylactoid reaction; bleeding*—may be caused by protamine overdose or by a rebound of heparin activity; *hypertension, pulmonary and/or systemic; noncardiogenic pulmonary edema*—reported in patients on cardiopulmonary bypass undergoing cardiovascular surgery

  Note: *Anaphylactic or anaphylactoid reactions* may be more likely to occur in patients with a history of allergy to fish (because protamine is prepared from the sperm or mature testes of fish [salmon or related species]), patients who have been previously exposed to protamine, and patients with protamine antibodies; however, a definite relationship between allergy to fish and allergic reactions to protamine sulfate has not been established. In addition, a reaction similar to anaphylaxis may occur when protamine is administered too rapidly.

### Those indicating need for medical attention only if they continue or are bothersome

Incidence less frequent or rare
  *Back pain*—reported rarely in conscious patients undergoing procedures such as cardiac catheterization; *feeling of warmth; feeling of weakness; flushing; nausea or vomiting*

## General Dosing Information

Protamine sulfate is administered by intravenous injection only. A concentration of 10 mg of protamine sulfate per mL is usually used.

Facilities for treating shock and other symptoms of anaphylaxis should be available whenever protamine sulfate is administered.

Prior to administration of protamine, it is recommended that care be taken to assure that the patient's blood volume is adequate. Hypovolemia may increase the risk of peripheral vasodilatation, which may lead to cardiovascular collapse, especially following too-rapid administration of protamine.

The stated doses are intended as a guideline only. It is strongly recommended that blood coagulation tests be used to determine optimum dosage of protamine, especially when neutralizing large doses of heparin given during cardiac or arterial surgery.

Tests used to monitor protamine therapy include activated clotting time (ACT), activated partial thromboplastin time (APTT), thrombin time (TT), and/or direct titration of a sample of the patient's blood with protamine. The tests should be performed at least 5 to 15 minutes following initial administration of protamine and repeated as necessary. Neutralization of heparin used during extracorporeal circulation may be monitored using sequential ACT testing with a dose/response curve that correlates the test results with the quantity of heparin remaining to be neutralized. However, hypothermia may decrease the accuracy of these tests.

APTT and TT may not be useful in monitoring protamine therapy after administration of enoxaparin because enoxaparin, in therapeutic doses, does not alter the value of these tests.

Bleeding may recur if too much protamine, which has anticoagulant activity of its own, is administered or if the effects of heparin persist longer than the effects of protamine. The half-life of heparin is 60 to 360 minutes with an average of 90 minutes. The half-life is dose dependent (the larger the dose, the longer the half-life) and subject to intra- and interpatient variation. It has been proposed that the rebound of heparin effect may be caused by metabolism of protamine with resultant dissociation of the heparin-protamine complex and/or by release of heparin from storage or binding sites. Heparin rebound is especially likely to occur following administration of large doses of heparin, such as those used during cardiopulmonary bypass procedures, and has been reported to occur as late as 18 hours following initial complete neutralization of heparin. Prolonged monitoring of the patient is necessary so that additional doses of protamine may be administered if coagulation test results indicate that they are required.

As time elapses following intravenous administration of heparin, less protamine is required because of rapidly decreasing heparin blood concentrations. For example, 30 minutes after the intravenous administration of heparin, approximately one-half the amount of protamine sulfate is sufficient for neutralization. However, absorption of heparin may be prolonged following subcutaneous administration. For neutralizing heparin given subcutaneously, an initial loading dose of 25 to 50 mg of protamine sulfate, followed by administration of the remainder of the calculated protamine sulfate dose as an intravenous infusion over a period of 8 to 16 hours, has been recommended.

## Parenteral Dosage Forms

Note: Bracketed uses in the *Dosage Forms* section refer to categories of use and/or indications that are not included in U.S. product labeling.

### PROTAMINE SULFATE INJECTION USP

#### Usual adult and adolescent dose
Heparin toxicity—
    Intravenous, 1 mg of protamine sulfate for approximately every 100 USP units of heparin to be neutralized, or as determined by blood coagulation test results.
[Enoxaparin toxicity][1]—
    Intravenous, 1 mg of protamine sulfate for approximately every 1 mg of enoxaparin to be neutralized.

Note: Protamine sulfate should be administered at a rate of 5 mg per minute, not to exceed 50 mg in any ten-minute period.

    Additional doses may be required as indicated by blood coagulation studies.

    Since protamine has anticoagulant activity of its own, it is not advisable to administer more than 100 mg of protamine sulfate over a 2-hour period of time (the duration of action of protamine), unless blood coagulation tests indicate a larger requirement.

#### Usual pediatric dose
See *Usual adult and adolescent dose.*

#### Strength(s) usually available
U.S.—
    10 mg per mL (Rx) [GENERIC].
Canada—
    10 mg per mL (Rx) [GENERIC].

#### Packaging and storage
Store between 2 and 8 °C (36 and 46 °F), or between 15 and 30 °C (59 and 86 °F), as directed by the manufacturer. Protect from freezing.

#### Preparation of dosage form
Protamine sulfate injection is intended for use without further dilution; however, if further dilution is desired, 5% dextrose injection or 0.9% sodium chloride injection may be used.

#### Stability
Contains no preservatives; discard unused portion of opened container. Diluted solutions should not be stored because they contain no preservative.

#### Incompatibilities
Protamine sulfate solutions are incompatible with certain antibiotics, including several of the cephalosporins and penicillins. It is recommended that no other medications be mixed with protamine sulfate unless they are known to be compatible.

### PROTAMINE SULFATE FOR INJECTION USP

#### Usual adult and adolescent dose
See *Protamine Sulfate Injection USP.*

#### Usual pediatric dose
See *Protamine Sulfate Injection USP.*

#### Size(s) usually available
U.S.—
    Not commercially available.
Canada—
    Not commercially available.

#### Packaging and storage
Store below 40 °C (104 °F), preferably between 15 and 30 °C (59 and 86 °F), unless otherwise specified by manufacturer.

#### Preparation of dosage form
Five mL of bacteriostatic water for injection containing 0.9% benzyl alcohol should be added to the vial containing 50 mg of protamine sulfate and shaken vigorously to dissolve. Each mL of the resultant solution will contain 10 mg of protamine sulfate.

#### Stability
Reconstituted solutions should be refrigerated and used within 24 hours.

#### Incompatibilities
Protamine sulfate solutions are incompatible with certain antibiotics, including several of the cephalosporins and penicillins. It is recommended that no other medications be mixed with protamine sulfate unless they are known to be compatible.

---

[1]Not included in Canadian product labeling.

---

Revised: 03/24/94

---

# PROTIRELIN    Systemic

VA CLASSIFICATION (Primary): DX900
Note: For a listing of dosage forms and brand names by country availability, see *Dosage Forms* section(s). For a listing of brand names for the articles in this monograph, refer to the General Index.

---

## Category
Diagnostic aid (hypothalamic-pituitary-thyroid axis function).

## Indications
Note: Bracketed information in the *Indications* section refers to uses that are not included in U.S. product labeling.

**Accepted**
Thyroid function studies and
Pituitary function studies—Protirelin is indicated as an adjunct in the diagnostic assessment of thyroid function in patients with pituitary or hypothalamic function impairment and to help evaluate the effectiveness or adjust the dosage of thyroid hormone in patients with nodular or diffuse goiter or primary hypothyroidism.

    As an adjunct to other diagnostic procedures, protirelin serves to evaluate pituitary function when hypothalamic or pituitary lesions are suspected.

    [Protirelin is also used to detect inhibition of thyroid-stimulating hormone (TSH) secretion that occurs in hyperthyroidism.][1]

---

[1]Not included in Canadian product labeling.

# Pharmacology/Pharmacokinetics

## Physicochemical characteristics
Molecular weight—362.39.

## Mechanism of action/Effect
Diagnostic aid (thyroid function)—Like naturally occurring thyrotropin-releasing hormone (TRH), protirelin stimulates release of thyroid-stimulating hormone (TSH) from the anterior pituitary. As a result, protirelin can be used to detect an increase in or blunting of TSH response due to a variety of medical conditions or to confirm adequate suppression of TSH response by administration of thyroid hormones.

## Other actions/effects
Protirelin appears to increase plasma growth hormone concentrations in some acromegalic patients. It also increases serum prolactin concentrations.

## Half-life
5 minutes.

## Time to peak TSH concentration
Normal—20 to 30 minutes.

## Duration of action
Approximately 3 hours for TSH concentrations to return to baseline.

## Elimination
Renal.

# Precautions to Consider

## Pregnancy/Reproduction
Pregnancy—Studies in humans have not been done.
Studies in rabbits have shown that protirelin at doses $1\frac{1}{2}$ and 6 times the human dose caused an increase in the number of resorption sites in the pregnant rabbit.

## Breast-feeding
Problems in humans have not been documented; however, breast enlargement and leaking of milk have occurred in lactating women, persisting for up to 2 to 3 days after administration of protirelin.

## Pediatrics
Diagnostic studies performed to date have not demonstrated pediatrics-specific problems that would limit the usefulness of protirelin in children.

## Geriatrics
Caution in interpreting thyroid-stimulating hormone (TSH) response is recommended in elderly males because of a natural decrease in responsiveness to thyrotropin-releasing hormone (TRH).

## Drug interactions and/or related problems
See *Laboratory value alterations.*

## Laboratory value alterations
The following have been selected on the basis of their potential clinical significance (possible effect in parentheses where appropriate)—not necessarily inclusive (» = major clinical significance):

With results of *this* test
 *Due to other medications*
  Adrenocorticoids, glucocorticoid with mineralocorticoid activity
   (physiologic doses have no effect but pharmacologic doses may reduce the thyroid-stimulating hormone [TSH] response to protirelin; in general, however, withdrawal of adrenocorticoids in patients with known hypopituitarism is not recommended)

  Aspirin
   (doses of 2 to 3.6 grams per day may inhibit the TSH response to protirelin; peak TSH concentrations occur at the same time after administration but are reduced)

  Levodopa, or other dopaminergic medications
   (chronic use may inhibit the TSH response to protirelin)

  Thyroid hormones
   (concurrent use decreases the TSH response to protirelin administration; withdrawal of liothyronine 7 days [or of levothyroxine, liotrix, thyroglobulin, or thyroid extract at least 14 days and preferably 4 to 6 weeks] prior to testing is recommended *except* in patients being evaluated for effectiveness of levothyroxine for nodular or diffuse goiter or when dosage of thyroid hormone for primary hypothyroidism is being adjusted)

 *Due to medical problems or conditions*
  Renal function impairment
   (may produce unreliable test results)

With physiology/laboratory test values
 Growth hormone
  (plasma concentrations may be increased in patients with acromegaly; however, protirelin may also inhibit release of growth hormone caused by levodopa)

 Prolactin
  (serum concentrations may be increased in euthyroid and also to a lesser extent in hyperthyroid individuals)

## Medical considerations/Contraindications
The medical considerations/contraindications included here have been selected on the basis of their potential clinical significance (reasons given in parentheses where appropriate)—not necessarily inclusive (» = major clinical significance).
See also *Laboratory value alterations.*

*Risk-benefit should be considered when the following medical problems exist:*
» Conditions in which sudden changes in blood pressure would be dangerous, such as:
  Cerebrovascular disease
  Coronary insufficiency
  Hypertension
  Occlusive vascular disease
 Sensitivity to protirelin

## Patient monitoring
The following may be especially important in patient monitoring (other tests may be warranted in some patients, depending on condition; » = major clinical significance):

 Blood pressure measurements
  (recommended prior to and at frequent intervals during the first 15 minutes following administration of protirelin; if a clinically significant change occurs, monitoring should be continued until blood pressure returns to baseline levels)
» Thyroid-stimulating hormone (TSH), serum concentrations
  (blood samples should be drawn immediately prior to and at specific intervals [30 and 60 minutes; or 20, 40, and 60 minutes] following protirelin administration; because of possible variation, the physician should be familiar with the assay method used and the normal range for the particular laboratory being utilized)

# Side/Adverse Effects

Note: Hypotension or hypertension, which rarely may be severe (including possible syncope), occurs frequently immediately after injection, usually persisting for no more than 15 minutes following administration.
   Most side effects persist for only a few minutes following administration.

The following side/adverse effects have been selected on the basis of their potential clinical significance (possible signs and symptoms in parentheses where appropriate)—not necessarily inclusive:

**Those indicating need for medical attention**
Incidence rare
  *Amaurosis, in patients with pituitary tumors* (temporary loss of vision); *hypotension, severe* (fainting)

**Those indicating need for medical attention only if they continue or are bothersome**
Incidence more frequent
  *Flushing or redness of skin; frequent urge to urinate; headache, sometimes severe; lightheadedness; nausea; stomach pain; unpleasant taste in mouth or dryness of mouth*
Incidence less frequent
  *Anxiety; drowsiness; pressure in the chest or tightness in throat; sweating; tingling*

# Patient Consultation

As an aid to patient consultation, refer to *Advice for the Patient, Protirelin (Diagnostic).*

In providing consultation, consider emphasizing the following selected information (» = major clinical significance):

## Description of use
  Test procedure: Blood sample taken; injection given; one or more blood samples taken again; lying down before, during, and for at least 15 minutes after administration to avoid dizziness or lightheadedness

## Before having this test
» Conditions affecting use, especially:
  Sensitivity to protirelin

Breast-feeding—Breast enlargement and leaking of milk possible; may persist for 2 to 3 days after administration

Use in the elderly—Decreased response in males to thyrotropin-releasing hormone; caution in interpreting test results

Other medical problems, especially cerebrovascular disease, coronary insufficiency, hypertension, occlusive vascular disease

### Preparation for this test
» Physician may recommend fasting or a low-fat meal prior to the test; following instructions carefully

### Side/adverse effects
Signs of potential side effects, especially amaurosis and severe hypotension

## General Dosing Information

Results of the protirelin test should be interpreted by someone familiar with thyroid-pituitary-hypothalamic physiology and the clinical status of the patient. The physician should also be familiar with the thyroid-stimulating hormone (TSH) assay method used and the normal range for the laboratory performing the assay.

Fasting for 6 hours prior to the test or a low-fat meal prior to the test is recommended for patients (except those with hypopituitarism) to prevent interference with the TSH test by elevated serum lipids.

It is recommended that the patient be supine before, during, and for at least 15 minutes following administration of protirelin to reduce the risk or severity of hypotension.

Protirelin is administered as an intravenous injection over 15 to 30 seconds.

Because repeated administration of protirelin leads to a reduced TSH response, an interval of at least 7 days is recommended between tests with protirelin.

## Parenteral Dosage Forms

### PROTIRELIN INJECTION

**Usual adult dose**
Diagnostic aid (thyroid function)—
   Intravenous, 500 mcg (0.5 mg).

**Usual pediatric dose**
Diagnostic aid (thyroid function)—
   Children up to 6 years of age: Experience is limited with the use of protirelin in this age group; however, doses of 7 mcg (0.007 mg) per kg of body weight administered intravenously have been used.
   Children 6 to 16 years of age: Intravenous, 7 mcg (0.007 mg) per kg of body weight, up to 500 mcg (0.5 mg).

**Strength(s) usually available**
U.S.—
   500 mcg (0.5 mg) per mL (Rx) [*Relefact TRH*].
Canada—
   200 mcg (0.2 mg) per mL (Rx) [*Relefact TRH*].

**Packaging and storage**
Store below 40 °C (104 °F), preferably between 15 and 30 °C (59 and 86 °F), unless otherwise specified by manufacturer. Protect from freezing.

Revised: 09/19/91
Interim revision: 07/05/94

---

## PROTRIPTYLINE—See *Antidepressants, Tricyclic (Systemic)*

---

## PRUSSIAN BLUE—Since Prussian Blue is not commercially available in the U.S. or Canada, the *Prussian Blue (Oral-Local)* monograph is not included in this published version of the USP DI database. Copies of the monograph are available on request from the USP Division of Information Development, 12601 Twinbrook Parkway, Rockville, MD 20852; telephone (301) 816-8351; telefax (301) 816-8374.

---

# PSEUDOEPHEDRINE   Systemic

VA CLASSIFICATION (Primary): RE200

Note: For a listing of dosage forms and brand names by country availability, see *Dosage Forms* section(s). For a listing of brand names for the articles in this monograph, refer to the General Index.

## Category
Decongestant, nasal (systemic).

## Indications

**Accepted**
Congestion, nasal (treatment)
Congestion, sinus (treatment) or
Congestion, eustachian tube (treatment)—Pseudoephedrine is indicated for temporary relief of congestion associated with acute coryza, acute eustachian salpingitis, serous otitis media with eustachian tube congestion, vasomotor rhinitis, and aerotitis (barotitis) media. Pseudoephedrine also may be indicated as an adjunct to analgesics, antihistamines, antibiotics, antitussives, or expectorants for optimum results in allergic rhinitis, croup, acute and subacute sinusitis, acute otitis media, and acute tracheobronchitis.

## Pharmacology/Pharmacokinetics

**Physicochemical characteristics**
Molecular weight—Pseudoephedrine hydrochloride: 201.70.
Pseudoephedrine sulfate: 428.54.

**Mechanism of action/Effect**
Pseudoephedrine acts on alpha-adrenergic receptors in the mucosa of the respiratory tract, producing vasoconstriction. The medication shrinks swollen nasal mucous membranes; reduces tissue hyperemia, edema, and nasal congestion; and increases nasal airway patency. Also, drainage of sinus secretions may be increased and obstructed eustachian ostia may be opened.

**Biotransformation**
Pseudoephedrine is incompletely metabolized in the liver.

**Onset of action**
15 to 30 minutes.

**Time to peak effect**
Within 30 to 60 minutes.

**Duration of action**
Tablets, oral solution, and syrup–3 to 4 hours.
Extended-release capsules and tablets–8 to 12 hours.

**Elimination**
Renal. About 55 to 75% of a dose is excreted unchanged. The rate of excretion is accelerated in acidic urine.

## Precautions to Consider

**Cross-sensitivity and/or related problems**
Patients sensitive to other sympathomimetics (for example, albuterol, amphetamines, ephedrine, epinephrine, isoproterenol, metaproterenol, norepinephrine, phenylephrine, phenylpropanolamine, terbutaline) may be sensitive to this medication also.

**Pregnancy/Reproduction**
Pregnancy—Studies in humans have not been done.
Studies in animals have not shown that pseudoephedrine causes teratogenic effects in the fetus. However, pseudoephedrine reduced average weight, length, and rate of skeletal ossification in the animal fetus.

FDA Pregnancy Category B.

**Breast-feeding**
Pseudoephedrine is distributed into breast milk; use by nursing mothers is not recommended, because of the higher than usual risk to infants, especially newborn and premature infants, of side effects from sympathomimetic amines.

**Pediatrics**

Pseudoephedrine should be used with caution in infants, especially newborn and premature infants, because of the higher than usual risk of side/adverse effects.

**Geriatrics**

No information is available on the relationship of age to the effects of pseudoephedrine in geriatric patients. However, elderly patients are more likely to have age-related prostatic hypertrophy, which may require adjustment of dosage in patients receiving pseudoephedrine.

**Drug interactions and/or related problems**

The following drug interactions and/or related problems have been selected on the basis of their potential clinical significance (possible mechanism in parentheses where appropriate)—not necessarily inclusive (» = major clinical significance):

Note: Combinations containing any of the following medications, depending on the amount present, may also interact with this medication.

Anesthetics, hydrocarbon inhalation, such as:

  Chloroform

  Cyclopropane

  Enflurane

  Halothane

  Isoflurane

  Methoxyflurane

  Trichloroethylene

    (administration of pseudoephedrine prior to or shortly after anesthesia with chloroform, cyclopropane, halothane, or trichloroethylene may increase the risk of severe ventricular arrhythmias, especially in patients with pre-existing heart disease, because these anesthetics greatly sensitize the myocardium to the effects of sympathomimetics)

    (enflurane, isoflurane, or methoxyflurane may also cause some sensitization of the myocardium to the effects of sympathomimetics; caution is recommended in patients taking pseudoephedrine)

Antihypertensives or

Diuretics used as antihypertensives

    (antihypertensive effects may be reduced when these medications are used concurrently with pseudoephedrine; the patient should be carefully monitored to confirm that the desired effect is being obtained)

» Beta-adrenergic blocking agents

    (concurrent use with pseudoephedrine may inhibit the therapeutic effect of these medications; beta-blockade may result in unopposed alpha-adrenergic activity of pseudoephedrine with a risk of hypertension and excessive bradycardia and possible heart block)

Central nervous system (CNS) stimulation–producing medications, other (see *Appendix II*)

    (concurrent use with pseudoephedrine may result in additive CNS stimulation to excessive levels, which may cause unwanted effects such as nervousness, irritability, insomnia, or possibly convulsions or cardiac arrhythmias; close observation is recommended)

Citrates

    (concurrent use may inhibit urinary excretion and prolong the duration of action of pseudoephedrine)

» Cocaine, mucosal-local

    (in addition to increasing CNS stimulation, concurrent use with pseudoephedrine may increase the cardiovascular effects of either or both medications and the risk of adverse effects)

Digitalis glycosides

    (concurrent use with pseudoephedrine may increase the risk of cardiac arrhythmias; caution and electrocardiographic monitoring are very important if concurrent use is necessary)

Levodopa

    (concurrent use with pseudoephedrine may increase the possibility of cardiac arrhythmias; dosage reduction of the sympathomimetic is recommended)

» Monoamine oxidase (MAO) inhibitors, including furazolidone, procarbazine, and selegiline

    (concurrent use may prolong and intensify the cardiac stimulant and vasopressor effects of pseudoephedrine because of release of catecholamines, which accumulate in intraneuronal storage sites during MAO inhibitor therapy, resulting in headache, cardiac arrhythmias, vomiting, or sudden and severe hypertensive and/or hyperpyretic crises; pseudoephedrine should not be administered during or within 14 days following administration of MAO inhibitors)

Nitrates

    (concurrent use with pseudoephedrine may reduce the antianginal effects of these medications)

Rauwolfia alkaloids

    (concurrent use may inhibit the action of pseudoephedrine by depleting catecholamine stores)

Sympathomimetics, other

    (in addition to possibly increasing CNS stimulation, concurrent use may increase the cardiovascular effects of either the other sympathomimetics or pseudoephedrine and the potential for side effects)

Thyroid hormones

    (concurrent use may increase the effects of either these medications or pseudoephedrine; thyroid hormones enhance risk of coronary insufficiency when sympathomimetic agents are administered to patients with coronary artery disease; dosage adjustment is recommended, although problem is reduced in euthyroid patients)

**Medical considerations/Contraindications**

The medical considerations/contraindications included here have been selected on the basis of their potential clinical significance (reasons given in parentheses where appropriate)—not necessarily inclusive (» = major clinical significance).

*Risk-benefit should be considered when the following medical problems exist:*

  Cardiovascular disease, including ischemic heart disease, or

» Coronary artery disease, severe or

  Hypertension, mild to moderate or

» Hypertension, severe

    (condition may be exacerbated due to drug-induced cardiovascular effects)

  Diabetes mellitus

  Glaucoma, predisposition to

  Hyperthyroidism

  Prostatic hypertrophy

  Sensitivity to pseudoephedrine or other sympathomimetics

# Side/Adverse Effects

The following side/adverse effects have been selected on the basis of their potential clinical significance (possible signs and symptoms in parentheses where appropriate)—not necessarily inclusive:

**Those indicating need for medical attention**

Incidence rare—more frequent with high doses

    *Convulsions; hallucinations; irregular or slow heartbeat; shortness of breath or troubled breathing*

**Those indicating need for medical attention only if they continue or are bothersome**

Incidence more frequent

    *Nervousness; restlessness; trouble in sleeping*

Incidence less frequent

    *Difficult or painful urination; dizziness or lightheadedness; fast or pounding heartbeat; headache; increased sweating; nausea or vomiting; trembling; troubled breathing; unusual paleness; weakness*

# Overdose

For more information on the management of overdose or unintentional ingestion, **contact a Poison Control Center** (see *Poison Control Center Listing*).

**Clinical effects of overdose**

The following effects have been selected on the basis of their potential clinical significance (possible signs and symptoms in parenthesis where appropriate)–not necessarily inclusive:

Acute and chronic effects

    *Convulsions; fast breathing; hallucinations; increase in blood pressure; irregular heartbeat, continuing; shortness of breath or troubled breathing, severe or continuing; slow or fast heartbeat, severe or continuing; unusual nervousness, restlessness, or excitement*

**Treatment of overdose**

To decrease absorption—

    Because pseudoephedrine is rapidly absorbed from the gut, emetics and gastric lavage should be instituted within 4 hours of overdosage in order to be effective. Charcoal is useful only if administered within 1 hour. However, if an extended-release preparation was taken, there will be more time for benefit from these measures.

To enhance elimination—

    Forced diuresis will increase elimination of pseudoephedrine provided renal function is adequate; however, diuresis is not recommended for severe overdosage.

Specific treatment—
> For delirium or convulsions, intravenous diazepam may be administered.
> The cardiac state should be monitored and serum electrolytes measured. If there are signs of cardiac toxicity, intravenous propranolol may be indicated.
> Hypokalemia may be treated, if necessary, with a slow infusion of a dilute potassium chloride solution; serum potassium concentration should be monitored during and for several hours after administration of potassium chloride.

## Patient Consultation

As an aid to patient consultation, refer to *Advice for the Patient, Pseudoephedrine (Systemic).*

In providing consultation, consider emphasizing the following selected information (» = major clinical significance):

**Before using this medication**
» Conditions affecting use, especially:
     Sensitivity to pseudoephedrine or other sympathomimetics
     Pregnancy—In animal studies, pseudoephedrine caused reduced average weight, length, and rate of skeletal ossification in animal fetus
     Breast-feeding—Pseudoephedrine distributed into breast milk; use by nursing mothers not recommended because of higher than usual risk of side effects for infants, especially newborn and premature infants
     Use in children—Caution should be used in infants, especially newborn and premature infants, because of higher than usual risk of side/adverse effects
     Other medications, especially beta-adrenergic blocking agents, mucosal-local cocaine, or monoamine oxidase (MAO) inhibitors
     Other medical problems, especially severe coronary artery disease or severe hypertension

**Proper use of this medication**
*Proper administration of extended-release dosage forms*
     Swallowing capsules or tablets whole; if capsule too large to swallow, mixing contents with jam or jelly and swallowing without chewing
     Not crushing or chewing capsules; not crushing, breaking, or chewing tablets
» Taking the medication a few hours before bedtime to minimize the possibility of insomnia
» Importance of not taking more medication than the amount recommended
» Proper dosing
     Missed dose: Taking right away if remembered within an hour or so; not taking if remembered later; not doubling doses
» Proper storage

**Precautions while using this medication**
» Checking with physician if symptoms do not improve within 7 days or if fever is present

**Side/adverse effects**
     Signs of potential side effects, especially convulsions, hallucinations, irregular or slow heartbeat, and shortness of breath or troubled breathing

## General Dosing Information

To minimize the possibility of insomnia, the last dose of pseudoephedrine for each day should be administered a few hours before bedtime.

For patients who have difficulty in swallowing the extended-release capsule, the contents of the capsule may be mixed with jam or jelly and taken without chewing.

## Oral Dosage Forms

### PSEUDOEPHEDRINE HYDROCHLORIDE CAPSULES

**Usual adult and adolescent dose**
Decongestant, nasal—
     Oral, 60 mg every four to six hours.

**Usual adult prescribing limits**
240 mg in twenty-four hours.

**Usual pediatric dose**
Decongestant, nasal—
     Children up to 12 years of age: Use is not recommended.
     Children 12 years of age and over: See *Usual adult and adolescent dose.*

**Strength(s) usually available**
U.S.—
     Not commercially available.
Canada—
     60 mg (OTC) [*Benylin Decongestant*].

**Packaging and storage**
Store below 40 °C (104 °F), preferably between 15 and 30 °C (59 and 86 °F), in a well-closed container, unless otherwise specified by manufacturer.

### PSEUDOEPHEDRINE HYDROCHLORIDE EXTENDED-RELEASE CAPSULES

**Usual adult and adolescent dose**
Decongestant, nasal—
     Oral, 120 mg every twelve hours, or 240 mg every twenty-four hours.

**Usual adult prescribing limits**
240 mg in twenty-four hours.

**Usual pediatric dose**
Decongestant, nasal—
     Children up to 12 years of age: Use is not recommended.
     Children 12 years of age and over: See *Usual adult and adolescent dose.*

**Strength(s) usually available**
U.S.—
     120 mg (Rx) [*Novafed*].
Canada—
     120 mg (OTC) [*Eltor 120;* GENERIC].

**Packaging and storage**
Store below 40 °C (104 °F), preferably between 15 and 30 °C (59 and 86 °F), in a tight container, unless otherwise specified by manufacturer. Protect from light.

**Auxiliary labeling**
• Swallow capsules whole.

### PSEUDOEPHEDRINE HYDROCHLORIDE ORAL SOLUTION

**Usual adult and adolescent dose**
Decongestant, nasal—
     See *Pseudoephedrine Hydrochloride Capsules.*

**Usual adult prescribing limits**
See *Pseudoephedrine Hydrochloride Capsules.*

**Usual pediatric dose**
Decongestant, nasal—
     Oral, 4 mg per kg of body weight or 125 mg per square meter of body surface per day, administered in four divided doses; or for
     Children up to 2 years of age: Dosage must be individualized.
     Children 2 to 6 years of age: Oral, 15 mg every four to six hours, not to exceed 60 mg in twenty-four hours.
     Children 6 to 12 years of age: Oral, 30 mg every four to six hours, not to exceed 120 mg in twenty-four hours.
     Children 12 years of age and over: See *Pseudoephedrine Hydrochloride Capsules.*

**Strength(s) usually available**
U.S.—
     7.5 mg per 0.8 mL (OTC) [*PediaCare Infants' Oral Decongestant Drops*].
     15 mg per 5 mL (OTC) [*Dorcol Children's Decongestant Liquid*].
     30 mg per 5 mL (OTC) [*Myfedrine; Sudafed Liquid, Children's*].
Canada—
     Not commercially available.

**Packaging and storage**
Store below 40 °C (104 °F), preferably between 15 and 30 °C (59 and 86 °F), in a well-closed container, unless otherwise specified by manufacturer. Protect from freezing. Protect from light.

### PSEUDOEPHEDRINE HYDROCHLORIDE SYRUP USP

**Usual adult and adolescent dose**
Decongestant, nasal—
     See *Pseudoephedrine Hydrochloride Capsules.*

**Usual adult prescribing limits**
See *Pseudoephedrine Hydrochloride Capsules.*

**Usual pediatric dose**
Decongestant, nasal—
     Children up to 12 years of age: See *Pseudoephedrine Hydrochloride Oral Solution.*
     Children 12 years of age and over: See *Pseudoephedrine Hydrochloride Capsules.*

**Strength(s) usually available**

U.S.—

    30 mg per 5 mL (OTC) [*Cenafed; Decofed; Pseudogest; Sufedrin;* GENERIC].

Canada—

    30 mg per 5 mL (OTC) [*Balminil Decongestant Syrup* (alcohol, parabens); *Robidrine* (alcohol 1.4%, sugar); *Sudafed* (methylparaben, sucrose)].

**Packaging and storage**

Store below 40 °C (104 °F), preferably between 15 and 30 °C (59 and 86 °F), unless otherwise specified by manufacturer. Store in a tight, light-resistant container. Protect from freezing.

## PSEUDOEPHEDRINE HYDROCHLORIDE TABLETS USP

**Usual adult and adolescent dose**

Decongestant, nasal—

    See *Pseudoephedrine Hydrochloride Capsules.*

**Usual adult prescribing limits**

See *Pseudoephedrine Hydrochloride Capsules.*

**Usual pediatric dose**

Decongestant, nasal—

    Children up to 12 years of age: See *Pseudoephedrine Hydrochloride Oral Solution.*

    Children 12 years of age and over: See *Pseudoephedrine Hydrochloride Capsules.*

**Strength(s) usually available**

U.S.—

    30 mg (OTC) [*Decofed; Genaphed; Halofed; Pseudo; Pseudogest; Sudafed* (povidone, sodium benzoate); GENERIC].

    60 mg (OTC) [*Cenafed; Decofed; Halofed Adult Strength; Pseudo; Pseudogest; Sudafed* (sodium starch glycolate, sucrose); *Sufedrin;* GENERIC].

Canada—

    60 mg (OTC) [*Robidrine* (scored, lactose); *Sudafed* (scored)].

**Packaging and storage**

Store below 40 °C (104 °F), preferably between 15 and 30 °C (59 and 86 °F), unless otherwise specified by manufacturer. Store in a tight container.

## PSEUDOEPHEDRINE HYDROCHLORIDE EXTENDED-RELEASE TABLETS

**Usual adult and adolescent dose**

Decongestant, nasal—

    See *Pseudoephedrine Hydrochloride Extended-Release Capsules.*

**Usual adult prescribing limits**

See *Pseudoephedrine Hydrochloride Extended-Release Capsules.*

**Usual pediatric dose**

Decongestant, nasal—

    Children up to 12 years of age: Use is not recommended.

    Children 12 years of age and over: See *Pseudoephedrine Hydrochloride Extended-Release Capsules.*

**Strength(s) usually available**

U.S.—

    120 mg (OTC) [*Sudafed 12 Hour*].

    240 mg (OTC) [*Efidac/24*].

Canada—

    120 mg (OTC) [*Maxenal; Sudafed 12 Hour*].

**Packaging and storage**

Store below 40 °C (104 °F), preferably between 15 and 30 °C (59 and 86 °F), in a tight container, unless otherwise specified by manufacturer. Protect from light.

**Auxiliary labeling**

• Swallow tablets whole.

## PSEUDOEPHEDRINE SULFATE TABLETS

**Usual adult and adolescent dose**

Decongestant, nasal—

    See *Pseudoephedrine Hydrochloride Capsules.*

**Usual adult prescribing limits**

See *Pseudoephedrine Hydrochloride Capsules.*

**Usual pediatric dose**

Decongestant, nasal—

    Children up to 12 years of age: See *Pseudoephedrine Hydrochloride Oral Solution.*

    Children 12 years of age and over: See *Pseudoephedrine Hydrochloride Capsules.*

**Strength(s) usually available**

U.S.—

    60 mg (OTC) [*Chlor-Trimeton Non-Drowsy Decongestant 4 Hour* (scored, lactose, povidone)].

Canada—

    Not commercially available.

**Packaging and storage**

Store between 2 and 30 °C (36 and 86 °F), in a well-closed container, unless otherwise specified by manufacturer. Protect from light.

## PSEUDOEPHEDRINE SULFATE EXTENDED-RELEASE TABLETS

**Usual adult and adolescent dose**

Decongestant, nasal—

    See *Pseudoephedrine Hydrochloride Extended-Release Capsules.*

**Usual adult prescribing limits**

See *Pseudoephedrine Hydrochloride Extended-Release Capsules.*

**Usual pediatric dose**

Decongestant, nasal—

    Children up to 12 years of age: Use is not recommended.

    Children 12 years of age and over: See *Pseudoephedrine Hydrochloride Extended-Release Capsules.*

**Strength(s) usually available**

U.S.—

    120 mg (OTC) [*Drixoral Non-Drowsy Formula* (butylparaben, lactose, povidone, sugar)].

Canada—

    Not commercially available.

**Packaging and storage**

Store between 2 and 30 °C (36 and 86 °F), in a well-closed container, unless otherwise specified by manufacturer. Protect from light.

**Auxiliary labeling**

• Swallow tablets whole.

Revised: 04/19/94

## PSEUDOEPHEDRINE-CONTAINING COMBINATIONS—

Acrivastine and Pseudoephedrine (Systemic)—See *Antihistamines and Decongestants (Systemic)*

Azatadine and Pseudoephedrine (Systemic)—See *Antihistamines and Decongestants (Systemic)*

Brompheniramine and Pseudoephedrine (Systemic)—See *Antihistamines and Decongestants (Systemic)*

Brompheniramine, Pseudoephedrine, and Acetaminophen (Systemic)—See *Antihistamines, Decongestants, and Analgesics (Systemic)*

Brompheniramine, Pseudoephedrine, and Dextromethorphan (Systemic)—See *Cough/Cold Combinations (Systemic)*

Carbinoxamine and Pseudoephedrine (Systemic)—See *Antihistamines and Decongestants (Systemic)*

Carbinoxamine, Pseudoephedrine, and Dextromethorphan (Systemic)—See *Cough/Cold Combinations (Systemic)*

Chlorpheniramine and Pseudoephedrine (Systemic)—See *Antihistamines and Decongestants (Systemic)*

Chlorpheniramine, Pseudoephedrine, and Acetaminophen (Systemic)—See *Antihistamines, Decongestants, and Analgesics (Systemic)*

Chlorpheniramine, Pseudoephedrine, and Codeine (Systemic)—See *Cough/Cold Combinations (Systemic)*

Chlorpheniramine, Pseudoephedrine, and Dextromethorphan (Systemic)—See *Cough/Cold Combinations (Systemic)*

Chlorpheniramine, Pseudoephedrine, Dextromethorphan, and Acetaminophen (Systemic)—See *Cough/Cold Combinations (Systemic)*

Chlorpheniramine, Pseudoephedrine, Dextromethorphan, Acetaminophen, and Caffeine (Systemic)—See *Cough/Cold Combinations (Systemic)*

Chlorpheniramine, Pseudoephedrine, and Guaifenesin (Systemic)—See *Cough/Cold Combinations (Systemic)*

Chlorpheniramine, Pseudoephedrine, and Hydrocodone (Systemic)—See *Cough/Cold Combinations (Systemic)*

Dexbrompheniramine and Pseudoephedrine (Systemic)—See *Antihistamines and Decongestants (Systemic)*

Dexbrompheniramine, Pseudoephedrine, and Acetaminophen (Systemic)—See *Antihistamines, Decongestants, and Analgesics (Systemic)*

Dexchlorpheniramine, Pseudoephedrine, and Guaifenesin (Systemic)—See *Cough/Cold Combinations (Systemic)*

Diphenhydramine and Pseudoephedrine (Systemic)—See *Antihistamines and Decongestants (Systemic)*

Diphenhydramine, Pseudoephedrine, and Acetaminophen (Systemic)—See *Antihistamines, Decongestants, and Analgesics (Systemic)*

Diphenhydramine, Pseudoephedrine, Dextromethorphan, and Acetaminophen (Systemic)—See *Cough/Cold Combinations (Systemic)*

Doxylamine, Pseudoephedrine, Dextromethorphan, and Acetaminophen (Systemic)—See *Cough/Cold Combinations (Systemic)*

Loratadine and Pseudoephedrine (Systemic)—See *Antihistamines and Decongestants (Systemic)*

Pseudoephedrine and Acetaminophen (Systemic)—See *Decongestants and Analgesics (Systemic)*

Pseudoephedrine and Aspirin (Systemic)—See *Decongestants and Analgesics (Systemic)*

Pseudoephedrine and Codeine (Systemic)—See *Cough/Cold Combinations (Systemic)*

Pseudoephedrine, Codeine, and Guaifenesin (Systemic)—See *Cough/Cold Combinations (Systemic)*

Pseudoephedrine and Dextromethorphan (Systemic)—See *Cough/Cold Combinations (Systemic)*

Pseudoephedrine, Dextromethorphan, and Acetaminophen (Systemic)—See *Cough/Cold Combinations (Systemic)*

Pseudoephedrine, Dextromethorphan, and Guaifenesin (Systemic)—See *Cough/Cold Combinations (Systemic)*

Pseudoephedrine, Dextromethorphan, Guaifenesin, and Acetaminophen (Systemic)—See *Cough/Cold Combinations (Systemic)*

Pseudoephedrine and Guaifenesin (Systemic)—See *Cough/Cold Combinations (Systemic)*

Pseudoephedrine and Hydrocodone (Systemic)—See *Cough/Cold Combinations (Systemic)*

Pseudoephedrine, Hydrocodone and Guaiacolsulfonate (Systemic)—See *Cough/Cold Combinations (Systemic)*

Pseudoephedrine, Hydrocodone and Guaifenesin (Systemic)—See *Cough/Cold Combinations (Systemic)*

Pseudoephedrine and Ibuprofen (Systemic)—See *Decongestants and Analgesics (Systemic)*

Pyrilamine, Pseudoephedrine, Dextromethorphan, and Acetaminophen (Systemic)—See *Cough/Cold Combinations (Systemic)*

Terfenadine and Pseudoephedrine (Systemic)—See *Antihistamines and Decongestants (Systemic)*

Triprolidine and Pseudoephedrine (Systemic)—See *Antihistamines and Decongestants (Systemic)*

Triprolidine, Pseudoephedrine, and Acetaminophen (Systemic)—See *Antihistamines, Decongestants, and Analgesics (Systemic)*

Triprolidine, Pseudoephedrine, and Codeine (Systemic)—See *Cough/Cold Combinations (Systemic)*

Triprolidine, Pseudoephedrine, Codeine, and Guaifenesin (Systemic)—See *Cough/Cold Combinations (Systemic)*

Triprolidine, Pseudoephedrine, and Dextromethorphan (Systemic)—See *Cough/Cold Combinations (Systemic)*

---

**PSYLLIUM**—See *Laxatives (Local)*

---

## PSYLLIUM-CONTAINING COMBINATIONS—

Malt Soup Extract and Psyllium (Oral-Local)—See *Laxatives (Local)*

Psyllium Hydrophilic Mucilloid and Carboxymethylcellulose (Oral-Local)—See *Laxatives (Local)*

Psyllium Hydrophilic Mucilloid and Senna (Oral-Local)—See *Laxatives (Local)*

Psyllium Hydrophilic Mucilloid and Sennosides (Oral-Local)—See *Laxatives (Local)*

Psyllium and Senna (Oral-Local)—See *Laxatives (Local)*

---

**PSYLLIUM HYDROPHILIC MUCILLOID**—See *Laxatives (Local)*

---

# PYRANTEL    Oral-Local

VA CLASSIFICATION (Primary): AP200

Note: For a listing of dosage forms and brand names by country availability, see *Dosage Forms* section(s). For a listing of brand names for the articles in this monograph, refer to the General Index.

## Category
Anthelmintic (oral-local).

## Indications
Note: Bracketed information in the *Indications* section refers to uses that are not included in U.S. product labeling.

**Accepted**

Ascariasis (treatment)—Pyrantel is indicated in the treatment of ascariasis caused by *Ascaris lumbricoides* (common roundworm).

Enterobiasis (treatment)—Pyrantel is indicated in the treatment of enterobiasis (oxyuriasis) caused by *Enterobius vermicularis (Oxyuris vermicularis)* (pinworm).

Helminth infections, multiple (treatment)—Pyrantel is indicated in the treatment of multiple helminth infections.

[Hookworm infection (treatment)]—Pyrantel is used in the treatment of hookworm infection (uncinariasis) caused by *Ancylostoma duodenale* (common hookworm; Old World hookworm) and *Necator americanus* (American hookworm; New World hookworm).

[Trichostrongyliasis (treatment)][1]—Pyrantel is used in the treatment of trichostrongyliasis caused by *Trichostrongylus* species.

Not all species or strains of a particular helminth may be susceptible to pyrantel.

---

[1]Not included in Canadian product labeling.

## Pharmacology/Pharmacokinetics

**Physicochemical characteristics**
Molecular weight—594.68.

**Mechanism of action/Effect**
Not vermicidal or ovicidal; acts as a depolarizing neuromuscular blocking agent, thereby causing sudden contraction, followed by paralysis, of the helminths; also acts as a cholinesterase inhibitor and ganglionic stimulant; helminths are rendered unable to maintain their position in the intestinal lumen and are expelled from the body in the fecal stream by peristalsis.

**Absorption**
Poorly and incompletely absorbed from gastrointestinal tract.

**Time to peak serum concentration**
1 to 3 hours.

**Peak serum concentration:**
0.05 to 0.13 mcg/mL.

**Elimination**
Fecal (unchanged)—>50%.
Renal—<15% excreted in urine as unchanged drug and metabolites.

## Precautions to Consider

**Pregnancy/Reproduction**

*Pregnancy*—Adequate and well-controlled studies in humans have not been done.

Studies in animals have not shown that pyrantel causes adverse effects in the fetus.

**Breast-feeding**
Pyrantel is poorly and incompletely absorbed from the gastrointestinal tract and resulting maternal serum concentrations are low (0.05 to 0.13 mcg/mL). Therefore, it is unlikely that significant amounts of pyrantel would be excreted in breast milk. Problems in humans have not been documented.

**Pediatrics**
Appropriate studies on the relationship of age to the effects of pyrantel have not been performed in children up to the age of 2. However, no pediatrics-specific problems have been documented to date.

**Geriatrics**
No information is available on the relationship of age to the effects of pyrantel in geriatric patients.

**Drug interactions and/or related problems**
The following drug interactions and/or related problems have been selected on the basis of their potential clinical significance (possible

mechanism in parentheses where appropriate)—not necessarily inclusive (» = major clinical significance):

Note: Combinations containing any of the following medications, depending on the amount present, may also interact with this medication.

» Piperazine
(may antagonize the anthelmintic effects of pyrantel; concurrent use is not recommended)

## Medical considerations/Contraindications

The medical considerations/contraindications included here have been selected on the basis of their potential clinical significance (reasons given in parentheses where appropriate)—not necessarily inclusive (» = major clinical significance).

*Risk-benefit should be considered when the following medical problem exists:*

Hypersensitivity to pyrantel

## Patient monitoring

The following may be especially important in patient monitoring (other tests may be warranted in some patients, depending on condition; » = major clinical significance):

*For pinworms*
» Perianal examinations
(cellophane tape swabs of the perianal area to detect the presence of ova may be required prior to and starting 1 week following treatment with pyrantel, especially in patients with persisting symptoms; swabs should be taken every morning prior to defecation and bathing for at least 3 days to determine efficacy or provide proof of cure; perianal examinations may also be required to detect the presence of adult worms in the perianal area; no patient should be considered cured unless perianal swabs have been negative for 7 consecutive days)

*For roundworms*
» Stool examinations
(may be required prior to and approximately 2 weeks following treatment with pyrantel to determine efficacy or provide proof of cure; because of colonic mixing, ova may persist in the stool for up to 1 week following cure)

## Side/Adverse Effects

Note: Side/adverse effects are generally infrequent at usual doses (11 mg [base] per kg of body weight [mg/kg]). However, they may be considerably more frequent at higher doses without any significant increase in efficacy of the medication.

The following side/adverse effects have been selected on the basis of their potential clinical significance (possible signs and symptoms in parentheses where appropriate)—not necessarily inclusive:

**Those indicating need for medical attention**
Incidence rare
*Hypersensitivity* (skin rash)

**Those indicating need for medical attention only if they continue or are bothersome**
Incidence less frequent
*CNS effects* (dizziness; drowsiness; headache; trouble in sleeping); *gastrointestinal disturbances* (abdominal or stomach cramps or pain; diarrhea; loss of appetite; nausea or vomiting)

## Patient Consultation

As an aid to patient consultation, refer to *Advice for the Patient, Pyrantel (Oral).*

In providing consultation, consider emphasizing the following selected information (» = major clinical significance):

**Before using this medication**
» Conditions affecting use, especially:
Hypersensitivity to pyrantel
Other medications, especially piperazine

**Proper use of this medication**
No special preparations (e.g., dietary restrictions or fasting, concurrent medications, purging, or cleansing enemas) required before, during, or immediately after therapy
Proper administration technique for oral liquids
» Second dose may be required in some infections
*For pinworms*
Treating all household members concurrently; treating again in 2 to 3 weeks

» Proper dosing
» Proper storage

**Precautions while using this medication**
Checking with physician if no improvement within a few days
» Caution if dizziness or drowsiness occurs
*For pinworms*
Washing (not shaking) all bedding and nightclothes after treatment to prevent reinfection
Other measures may be recommended by some physicians
*For hookworms*
Importance of taking iron supplements daily during treatment and for up to 6 months following treatment if anemia was present prior to treatment

**Side/adverse effects**
Signs of potential side effects, especially hypersensitivity

## General Dosing Information

No special preparations (e.g., dietary restrictions or fasting, concurrent medications, purging, or cleansing enemas) are required before, during, or immediately after treatment with pyrantel.

**For hookworms**
In the treatment of hookworms, especially in patients who are heavily infected or have inadequate dietary intake of iron, concurrent iron therapy may be required if anemia occurs. Iron therapy may need to be continued for up to 6 months to replenish iron stores.

**For pinworms**
Because of the high probability of transfer of pinworms, it is usually recommended that all members of the household be treated concurrently. Retreatment of entire household is recommended 2 to 3 weeks following initial treatment.

## Oral Dosage Forms

Note: Bracketed uses in the *Dosage Forms* section refer to categories of use and/or indications that are not included in U.S. product labeling.

The dosing and strengths of the dosage forms available are expressed in terms of pyrantel base (not the pamoate salt).

## PYRANTEL PAMOATE ORAL SUSPENSION USP

**Usual adult and adolescent dose**
Ascariasis—
Oral, 11 mg (base) per kg of body weight as a single dose. May be repeated in two to three weeks if required.
Enterobiasis—
Oral, 11 mg (base) per kg of body weight as a single dose. Repeat in two to three weeks.
[Hookworm infection]—
Oral, 11 mg (base) per kg of body weight once a day for three days.
[Trichostrongyliasis][1]—
Oral, 11 mg (base) per kg of body weight as a single dose.

**Usual adult prescribing limits**
Up to 1 gram per day.

**Usual pediatric dose**
Infants and children up to 2 years of age—Dosage has not been established.
Children 2 years of age and over—See *Usual adult and adolescent dose.*
Note: The following amounts have also been given—
Infants and children weighing:
12 to 23 kg—125 to 250 mg (base).
24 to 45 kg—250 to 500 mg (base).
6 to 68 kg—500 to 750 mg (base).
Over 68 kg—1 gram (base).
In the treatment of ascariasis, enterobiasis, or uncinariasis (hookworm infection), pyrantel may be given in the above amounts as a single dose. Alternatively, in the treatment of uncinariasis, pyrantel may be given in the above amounts once a day for three days.

**Strength(s) usually available**
U.S.—
250 mg (base) per 5 mL (OTC) [*Antiminth; Reese's Pinworm Medicine;* GENERIC].
Canada—
250 mg (base) per 5 mL (OTC) [*Combantrin*].

**Packaging and storage**
Store below 40 °C (104 °F), preferably between 15 and 30 °C (59 and 86 °F), unless otherwise specified by manufacturer. Store in a tight, light-resistant container. Protect from freezing.

**Auxiliary labeling**
* Shake well.
* May cause dizziness or drowsiness.
* Continue medicine for full time of treatment (for 3-day uncinariasis treatment).

**Note**
When dispensing, include a calibrated liquid-measuring device.

## PYRANTEL PAMOATE TABLETS

**Usual adult and adolescent dose**
See *Pyrantel Pamoate Oral Suspension USP* .

**Usual adult prescribing limits**
See *Pyrantel Pamoate Oral Suspension USP*.

**Usual pediatric dose**
See *Pyrantel Pamoate Oral Suspension USP*.

**Strength(s) usually available**
U.S.—
  Not commercially available.
Canada—
  125 mg (base) (OTC) [*Combantrin* (scored)].

**Packaging and storage**
Store below 40 °C (104 °F), preferably between 15 and 30 °C (59 and 86 °F), unless otherwise specified by manufacturer. Store in a tight, light-resistant container.

**Auxiliary labeling**
* May cause dizziness or drowsiness.
* Continue medicine for full time of treatment (for 3-day uncinariasis treatment).

---

[1]Not included in Canadian product labeling.

Revised: 01/19/93

---

# PYRAZINAMIDE   Systemic

VA CLASSIFICATION (Primary): AM500
Note: For a listing of dosage forms and brand names by country availability, see *Dosage Forms* section(s). For a listing of brand names for the articles in this monograph, refer to the General Index.

## Category
Antibacterial (antimycobacterial).

## Indications

**Accepted**
Tuberculosis (treatment)—Pyrazinamide is indicated, in combination with other antimycobacterial drugs, in the treatment of tuberculosis. Pyrazinamide is effective only against mycobacteria.

Not all species or strains of a particular organism may be susceptible to pyrazinamide.

## Pharmacology/Pharmacokinetics

**Physicochemical characteristics**
Molecular weight—123.11.

**Mechanism of action/Effect**
Unknown; pyrazinamide may be bacteriostatic or bactericidal, depending on its concentration and the susceptibility of the organism. It is active *in vitro* at an acidic pH of 5.6 or less, similar to that found in early, active tubercular inflammatory lesions.

**Absorption**
Rapidly and almost completely absorbed from the gastrointestinal tract.

**Distribution**
Wide, to most fluids and tissues, including liver, lungs, kidneys, and bile. Pyrazinamide has excellent penetration into the cerebrospinal fluid (CSF), ranging from 87 to 105% of the corresponding serum concentration.
$Vol_D$ =0.57 to 0.74 L per kg.

**Protein binding**
Pyrazinamide—Low (10 to 20%).
Pyrazinoic acid—Low (approximately 31%).

**Biotransformation**
Hepatic; hydrolyzed by a microsomal deamidase to pyrazinoic acid, an active metabolite, and then hydroxylated by xanthine oxidase to 5-hydroxypyrazinoic acid.

**Half-life**
Distribution—
  Approximately 1.6 hours.
Elimination—
  Pyrazinamide:
    Normal renal function—Approximately 9.5 hours.
    Chronic renal failure—Approximately 26 hours.
  Pyrazinoic acid:
    Normal renal function—Approximately 12 hours.
    Chronic renal failure—Approximately 22 hours.

**Time to peak serum concentration**
Pyrazinamide—1 to 2 hours.
Pyrazinoic acid—4 to 5 hours.

**Peak serum concentration**
Pyrazinamide—
  Approximately 19 mcg/mL after a single dose of 14 mg per kg of body weight (mg/kg).
  Approximately 39 mcg/mL after a single dose of 27 mg/kg.
Pyrazinoic acid—
  Approximately 3 mcg/mL after a single dose of 14 mg/kg.
  Approximately 4.5 mcg/mL after a single dose of 27 mg/kg.

**Elimination**
Renal; approximately 3% of unchanged pyrazinamide, 33% of pyrazinoic acid, and 36% of remaining identifiable metabolites excreted in urine within 72 hours.
In dialysis—A single 3 to 4 hour hemodialysis session reduced serum pyrazinamide concentrations by approximately 55% and pyrazinoic acid concentrations by 50 to 60%.

## Precautions to Consider

**Cross-sensitivity and/or related problems**
Patients hypersensitive to ethionamide, isoniazid, niacin (nicotinic acid), or other chemically related medications may be hypersensitive to this medication also.

**Carcinogenicity**
Pyrazinamide was administered in the diet of rats and mice. The estimated daily dose was 2 grams per kg (grams/kg), or 40 times the maximum human dose, for the mouse, and 0.5 gram/kg, or 10 times the maximum human dose, for the rat. Pyrazinamide was not carcinogenic in rats or male mice. No conclusion was possible for female mice due to insufficient numbers of surviving control mice.

**Mutagenicity**
Pyrazinamide was not mutagenic in the Ames bacterial test, but it did induce chromosomal aberrations in human lymphocyte cell cultures.

**Pregnancy/Reproduction**
Pregnancy—Adequate and well-controlled studies in humans have not been done; the risk for teratogenicity has not been determined. If the organism is drug-susceptible, pregnant women can be safely treated with isoniazid, rifampin, and ethambutol for 9 months. If resistance to any of these medications is probable and susceptibility to pyrazinamide is likely, its use should be considered.
Animal reproduction studies have not been conducted with pyrazinamide.
FDA Pregnancy Category C.

**Breast-feeding**
Pyrazinamide is distributed into breast milk in small amounts.

**Pediatrics**
Appropriate studies on the relationship of age to the effects of pyrazinamide have not been performed in the pediatric population. However, no pediatrics-specific problems have been documented to date.

**Geriatrics**
Appropriate studies on the relationship of age to the effects of pyrazinamide have not been performed in the geriatric population. However, no geriatrics-specific problems have been documented to date.

### Drug interactions and/or related problems

The following drug interactions and/or related problems have been selected on the basis of their potential clinical significance (possible mechanism in parentheses where appropriate)—not necessarily inclusive (» = major clinical significance):

Note: Combinations containing any of the following medications, depending on the amount present, may also interact with this medication.

Allopurinol or
Colchicine or
Probenecid or
Sulfinpyrazone
    (pyrazinamide may increase serum uric acid concentrations and decrease the efficacy of gout therapy; dosage adjustments of these medications may be necessary to control hyperuricemia and gout when antigout medications are used concurrently with pyrazinamide)

Cyclosporine
    (concurrent use with pyrazinamide may decrease the serum concentrations of cyclosporine, possibly leading to inadequate immunosuppression; cyclosporine serum concentrations should be monitored)

### Laboratory value alterations

The following have been selected on the basis of their potential clinical significance (possible effect in parentheses where appropriate)—not necessarily inclusive (» = major clinical significance):

With diagnostic test results
    Ketone determinations, urine
        (may react with sodium nitroprusside tests, such as *Acetest* or *Chemstrip K*; both pyrazinamide and pyrazinoic acid produce an interfering pink-brown color reaction with nitroprusside)

With physiology/laboratory test values
    Alanine aminotransferase (ALT [SGPT]) and
    Aspartate aminotransferase (AST [SGOT])
        (values may be increased)

    Uric acid, serum
        (concentration may be increased)

### Medical considerations/Contraindications

The medical considerations/contraindications included here have been selected on the basis of their potential clinical significance (reasons given in parentheses where appropriate)—not necessarily inclusive (» = major clinical significance).

*Risk-benefit should be considered when the following medical problems exist:*

Gout, history of
    (pyrazinamide can increase serum uric acid concentrations and precipitate an acute attack of gout)

» Hepatic function impairment, severe
    (pyrazinamide is metabolized in the liver and, in high doses, can be hepatotoxic)

» Hypersensitivity to pyrazinamide, ethionamide, isoniazid, niacin (nicotinic acid), or other chemically related medications

### Patient monitoring

The following may be especially important in patient monitoring (other tests may be warranted in some patients, depending on condition; » = major clinical significance):

Hepatic function determinations
    (AST [SGOT] and ALT [SGPT] determinations may be required prior to and every 2 to 4 weeks during treatment; however, elevated serum enzyme values may not be predictive of clinical hepatitis and values may return to normal despite continued treatment; patients with impaired hepatic function should not receive pyrazinamide unless crucial to therapy)

Uric acid concentrations, serum
    (may be required during treatment since elevated serum uric acid concentrations frequently occur, possibly resulting in precipitation of acute gout)

## Side/Adverse Effects

The following side/adverse effects have been selected on the basis of their potential clinical significance (possible signs and symptoms in parentheses where appropriate)—not necessarily inclusive:

**Those indicating need for medical attention**
Incidence more frequent
    *Arthralgia* (pain in the large and small joints)—related to hyperuricemia; usually mild and self-limiting

Incidence rare
    *Gouty arthritis* (pain and swelling of joints, especially big toe, ankle, and knee; tense, hot skin over affected joints); *hepatotoxicity* (loss of appetite; unusual tiredness or weakness; yellow eyes or skin)—related to large doses, i.e., 40–50 mg per kg of body weight per day for prolonged periods of time

**Those indicating need for medical attention only if they continue or are bothersome**
Incidence rare
    *Itching; skin rash*

## Patient Consultation

As an aid to patient consultation, refer to *Advice for the Patient, Pyrazinamide (Systemic)*.

In providing consultation, consider emphasizing the following selected information (» = major clinical significance):

**Before using this medication**
» Conditions affecting use, especially:
    Hypersensitivity to pyrazinamide, ethionamide, isoniazid, niacin (nicotinic acid), or other chemically related medications
    Breast-feeding—Pyrazinamide is distributed into breast milk
    Other medical problems, especially severe hepatic function impairment

**Proper use of this medication**
» Compliance with full course of therapy, which may take months
» Proper dosing
    Missed dose: Taking as soon as possible; not taking if almost time for next dose; not doubling doses
» Proper storage

**Precautions while using this medication**
    Regular visits to physician to check progress
    Checking with physician if no improvement within 2 to 3 weeks
» Diabetics: May interfere with urine ketone determinations

**Side/adverse effects**
    Signs of side effects, especially arthralgia, gouty arthritis, and hepatotoxicity

## General Dosing Information

Since bacterial resistance may develop rapidly when pyrazinamide is administered alone in the treatment of tuberculosis, it should only be administered concurrently with other antituberculars.

Tuberculosis therapy must be continued for 6 months to 2 years, depending on the treatment regimen and local resistance patterns. Uncomplicated pulmonary tuberculosis is often successfully treated within 6 to 12 months. There are 3 treatment regimen options available for non–HIV-infected patients:

• An initial 4-drug regimen of isoniazid, rifampin, pyrazinamide, and streptomycin or ethambutol, taken under direct observation, in geographic areas where the isoniazid resistance rate is not documented to be <4%. This regimen should be administered for 8 weeks. After that time, isoniazid and rifampin are administered daily, or 2 or 3 times a week, under direct observation, for 16 weeks. When results of susceptibility tests for these medications become available, the regimen should be altered as appropriate.

• Isoniazid, rifampin, pyrazinamide, and streptomycin or ethambutol taken daily under direct observation for 2 weeks, followed by twice-weekly administration of all 4 medications for 6 weeks, under direct observation. This is then followed by twice-weekly administration, directly observed, of isoniazid and rifampin for 16 weeks.

• Isoniazid, rifampin, pyrazinamide, and streptomycin or ethambutol taken 3 times a week under direct observation for 6 months.

HIV-infected patients may use any of the above 3 options; however, treatment regimens should continue for a total of 9 months and at least 6 months beyond culture conversion.

Healthcare or correctional institutions experiencing outbreaks of tuberculosis that are resistant to isoniazid and rifampin, or that are resuming therapy for a patient with a prior history of antitubercular therapy, may need to begin 5- or 6-drug regimens as initial therapy. These regimens should include the 4-drug regimen and at least 3 medications to which the suspected multi-drug-resistant strain may be susceptible.

The regimen for treating pulmonary tuberculosis should be effective in treating extrapulmonary tuberculosis. Some experts recommend extending the duration of therapy to 9 months in patients with disseminated disease, miliary tuberculosis, disease involving bones or joints, or tuberculosis lymphadenitis. Adjunctive therapies, such as surgery and corticosteroids, may be beneficial.

Patients with concomitant human immunodeficiency virus (HIV) infection may require a longer course of treatment.

Patients with impaired renal function do not require a reduction in dose; however, patients on hemodialysis should receive the usual dose at the end of each dialysis session.

## Oral Dosage Forms
### PYRAZINAMIDE TABLETS USP

**Usual adult and adolescent dose**
Tuberculosis—
> In combination with other antitubercular drugs: Oral, 15 to 30 mg per kg of body weight once a day; or 50 to 70 mg per kg of body weight two or three times a week, depending on the treatment regimen.

> Note: The usual dose of pyrazinamide for persons infected with human immunodeficiency virus (HIV) is 20 to 30 mg per kg of body weight per day for the first two months of therapy.

**Usual adult prescribing limits**
Up to a maximum of 2 grams when taken daily, 3 grams per dose for the three times a week regimen, 4 grams per dose for the two times a week regimen.

**Usual pediatric dose**
See *Usual adult and adolescent dose.*

> Note: The usual maximum dose in children is 2 grams when taken daily, 3 grams per dose for the three times a week regimen, 4 grams per dose for the two times a week regimen.

**Strength(s) usually available**
U.S.—
> 500 mg (Rx) [GENERIC].

Canada—
> 500 mg (Rx) [*pms-Pyrazinamide; Tebrazid*].

**Packaging and storage**
Store below 40 °C (104 °F), preferably between 15 and 30 °C (59 and 86 °F), unless otherwise specified by manufacturer. Store in a well-closed container.

**Auxiliary labeling**
• Continue medicine for full time of treatment.

## Selected Bibliography
Initial therapy for tuberculosis in the era of multidrug resistance: recommendations of the advisory council for the elimination of tuberculosis. MMWR 1993; 42 (RR-7): 1-8.

Revised: 05/02/94

## PYRAZINAMIDE-CONTAINING COMBINATIONS—
Rifampin, Isoniazid, and Pyrazinamide (Systemic)

---

# PYRETHRINS AND PIPERONYL BUTOXIDE     Topical

VA CLASSIFICATION (Primary): AP300
> Note: For a listing of dosage forms and brand names by country availability, see *Dosage Forms* section(s). For a listing of brand names for the articles in this monograph, refer to the General Index.

## Category
Pediculicide.

## Indications
**Accepted**
Pediculosis corporis (treatment)
Pediculosis capitis (treatment) or
Pediculosis pubis (treatment)—Pyrethrins and piperonyl butoxide combination is indicated for the treatment of pediculosis (lice) infestations caused by *Pediculus humanus* var. *corporis* (body louse), *P. humanus* var. *capitis* (head louse), and *Phthirus pubis* (pubic or crab louse).

## Pharmacology/Pharmacokinetics

**Physicochemical characteristics**
Source—Pyrethrins: Obtained from flowers of the pyrethrum plant, *Chrysanthemum cincerariaefolium*, which is related to the ragweed plant; esters formed by the combination of chrysanthemic and pyrethric acids and pyrethrolone, cinerolone, and jasmolone alcohols.
Piperonyl butoxide: A synthetic piperic acid derivative.

**Mechanism of action/Effect**
Pyrethrins—Are absorbed through the chitinous exoskeleton of arthropods and stimulate the nervous system, probably by competitively interfering with cationic conductances in the lipid layer of nerve cells, thereby blocking nerve impulse transmissions, which results in paralysis and death.
Piperonyl butoxide—Has little or no insecticidal activity but potentiates that of pyrethrins by inhibiting the hydrolytic enzymes responsible for metabolism of pyrethrins in arthropods, thereby increasing the insecticidal activity of pyrethrins by 2 to 12 times.

**Absorption**
Pyrethrins and piperonyl butoxide are poorly absorbed through intact skin when applied topically; if pyrethrins are absorbed, they are rapidly metabolized in mammals.

## Precautions to Consider

**Cross-sensitivity and/or related problems**
Patients allergic to the ragweed or chrysanthemum plant may be allergic to the pyrethrins in this medication also.

Patients sensitive to kerosene may also be sensitive to the pyrethrins and piperonyl butoxide combination preparations that contain kerosene.

**Pregnancy/Reproduction**
Pregnancy—Problems in humans have not been documented; however, pyrethrins and piperonyl butoxide may be absorbed systemically in small amounts through intact skin.

**Breast-feeding**
Problems in humans have not been documented; however, pyrethrins and piperonyl butoxide may be absorbed systemically in small amounts through intact skin.

**Pediatrics**
Appropriate studies on the relationship of age to the effects of pyrethrins and piperonyl butoxide have not been performed in the pediatric population. However, no pediatrics-specific problems have been documented to date.

**Geriatrics**
Appropriate studies on the relationship of age to the effects of pyrethrins and piperonyl butoxide have not been performed in the geriatric population. However, no geriatrics-specific problems have been documented to date.

**Medical considerations/Contraindications**
The medical considerations/contraindications included here have been selected on the basis of their potential clinical significance (reasons given in parentheses where appropriate)—not necessarily inclusive (» = major clinical significance).

*Risk-benefit should be considered when the following medical problems exist:*
> Inflammation of skin, acute
> (condition may be exacerbated)
> Sensitivity to pyrethrins or piperonyl butoxide

## Side/Adverse Effects
> Note: Pyrethrins and piperonyl butoxide combination applied topically in recommended dosage appears to be relatively free of the risk of causing systemic toxicity.

> When pyrethrins are injected or inhaled, they can cause nausea, vomiting, muscle paralysis, and even death; however, severe poisoning from pyrethrins is rare.

> Piperonyl butoxide has been reported to cause nausea, vomiting, diarrhea, central nervous system (CNS) depression, and hemorrhagic enteritis when large amounts are ingested orally.

The following side/adverse effects have been selected on the basis of their potential clinical significance (possible signs and symptoms in parentheses where appropriate)—not necessarily inclusive:

**Those indicating need for medical attention**
Incidence less frequent or rare
>    *Allergic reaction* (skin rash; sudden attacks of sneezing; stuffy or runny nose; wheezing or difficulty in breathing); *skin infection; skin irritation not present before therapy*

## Patient Consultation

As an aid to patient consultation, refer to *Advice for the Patient, Pyrethrins and Piperonyl Butoxide (Topical)*.

In providing consultation, consider emphasizing the following selected information (» = major clinical significance):

**Before using this medication**
» Conditions affecting use, especially:
     Allergy to ragweed or chrysanthemum plants or sensitivity to pyrethrins, piperonyl butoxide, or kerosene or other petroleum products

**Proper use of this medication**
» Importance of not using more medication than the amount recommended
» Importance of keeping away from mouth and not inhaling; harmful if swallowed or inhaled
» Applying in a well-ventilated room to minimize possibility of inhalation
» Avoiding contact with the eyes and mucous membranes, such as the inside of the nose, mouth, or vagina; flushing eyes thoroughly with water if medication accidentally gets in eyes
» Not using on eyelashes or eyebrows; checking with physician if they become infested
*Proper administration*
     Reading patient directions carefully before using
     Applying sufficient amount to thoroughly wet the dry hair and scalp or skin of affected areas
     Allowing to remain on affected areas for exactly 10 minutes
     Then—
         For gel and solution dosage forms: Thoroughly washing affected areas with warm water and soap or regular shampoo
         For shampoo dosage form: Using small amount of water and working shampoo into the hair and scalp or skin until a lather forms
     Rinsing thoroughly; drying with clean towel
     Using nit removal comb to remove dead lice and eggs from hair
     Washing hands immediately after using medication
     Repeating treatment once in 7 to 10 days to kill any newly hatched lice
» Importance of all members of household being examined for infestation, and treated if infested
     Importance of concurrent treatment of sexual partner in pediculosis pubis
» Proper dosing
» Proper storage

**Precautions while using this medication**
*Using hygienic measures to control reinfestation or spread of infestation*
*For head lice*
     Machine washing all clothing (including hats, scarves, and coats), bedding, towels, and washcloths in very hot water and drying them by using hot cycle of dryer for at least 20 minutes; for clothing or bedding not washable, dry-cleaning or sealing in a plastic bag for 2 weeks
     Shampooing all wigs and hairpieces
     Washing hairbrushes and combs in very hot soapy water (at least 130 °F) for 5 to 10 minutes; not sharing them with other people
     Cleaning house or room by thoroughly vacuuming upholstered furniture, rugs, and floors
*For body lice*
     Machine washing all clothing, bedding, towels, and washcloths in very hot water and drying them by using hot cycle of dryer for at least 20 minutes; for clothing or bedding not washable, dry-cleaning or sealing in a plastic bag for 2 weeks
     Cleaning house or room by thoroughly vacuuming upholstered furniture, rugs, and floors
*For pubic lice*
     Machine washing all clothing (especially underwear), bedding, towels, and washcloths in very hot water and drying them by using hot

cycle of dryer for at least 20 minutes; for clothing or bedding not washable, dry-cleaning or sealing in a plastic bag for 2 weeks
     Scrubbing toilet seats frequently

**Side/adverse effects**
     Signs of potential side effects, especially allergic reaction, skin infection, or skin irritation not present before therapy

## General Dosing Information

Following the initial treatment, a second treatment should be made in 7 to 10 days to kill any newly hatched lice.

When used in the treatment of pediculosis pubis (pubic or crab lice), the sexual partner should receive concurrent therapy, since the infestation may spread to persons in close contact.

**For treatment of systemic toxicity**
• For accidental ingestion—Primarily supportive treatment; induction of vomiting if patient is conscious; gastric lavage if patient is unconscious. Saline cathartics may be administered to minimize absorption of pyrethrins and piperonyl butoxide.
• For accidental inhalation—Artificial respiration, if necessary.

## Topical Dosage Forms
### PYRETHRINS AND PIPERONYL BUTOXIDE GEL

**Usual adult and adolescent dose**
Pediculicide—
     Topical, to the hair and scalp or skin, for one application, repeated once in seven to ten days.

**Usual adult prescribing limits**
No more than two applications within twenty-four hours.

**Usual pediatric dose**
See *Usual adult and adolescent dose*.

**Strength(s) usually available**
U.S.—
     0.18% pyrethrins, 2.2% piperonyl butoxide technical (equivalent to 1.76% [butylcarbityl] [6-propylpiperonyl] ether and 0.44% related compounds), and 4.80% petroleum distillate (OTC) [*Barc*].
     0.3% pyrethrins, 3% piperonyl butoxide technical (equivalent to 2.4% [butylcarbityl] [6-propylpiperonyl] ether and 0.6% related compounds), and 1.2% petroleum distillate (OTC) [*Blue; Tisit Blue*].
     0.33% pyrethrins, 4% piperonyl butoxide technical (equivalent to 3.2% [butylcarbityl] [6-propylpiperonyl] ether and 0.8% related compounds) (OTC) [*A-200 Gel Concentrate* (benzyl alcohol)].
Canada—
     Not commercially available.

**Packaging and storage**
Store below 40 °C (104 °F), preferably between 15 and 30 °C (59 and 86 °F), in a well-closed container, unless otherwise specified by manufacturer. Protect from freezing.

**Auxiliary labeling**
• For external use only.
• Harmful if swallowed or inhaled.

**Note**
When dispensing, include patient instructions.

### PYRETHRINS AND PIPERONYL BUTOXIDE SOLUTION SHAMPOO

**Usual adult and adolescent dose**
See *Pyrethrins and Piperonyl Butoxide Gel*.

**Usual adult prescribing limits**
See *Pyrethrins and Piperonyl Butoxide Gel*.

**Usual pediatric dose**
See *Usual adult and adolescent dose*.

**Strength(s) usually available**
U.S.—
     0.3% pyrethrins, 3% piperonyl butoxide technical (equivalent to 2.4% [butylcarbityl] [6-propylpiperonyl] ether and 0.6% related compounds), and 1.2% petroleum distillate (OTC) [*R & C*].
     0.3% pyrethrins, 3% piperonyl butoxide technical (equivalent to 2.4% [butylcarbityl] [6-propylpiperonyl] ether and 0.6% related compounds), 1.2% petroleum distillate, and 2.4% benzyl alcohol (OTC) [*Triple X*].
     0.33% pyrethrins, 4% piperonyl butoxide technical (equivalent to 3.2% [butylcarbityl] [6-propylpiperonyl] ether and 0.8% related compounds) (OTC) [*A-200 Shampoo Concentrate* (benzyl alcohol); *Pronto Lice Killing Shampoo Kit*].

Canada—
  0.3% pyrethrins, 3% piperonyl butoxide technical (equivalent to 2.4% [butylcarbityl] [6-propylpiperonyl] ether and 0.6% related compounds), and 1.2% petroleum distillate (OTC) [*R & C*].

**Packaging and storage**
Store below 40 °C (104 °F), preferably between 15 and 30 °C (59 and 86 °F), in a well-closed container, unless otherwise specified by manufacturer. Protect from freezing.

**Auxiliary labeling**
• For external use only.
• Harmful if swallowed or inhaled.

**Note**
When dispensing, include patient instructions.

## PYRETHRINS AND PIPERONYL BUTOXIDE TOPICAL SOLUTION

**Usual adult and adolescent dose**
See *Pyrethrins and Piperonyl Butoxide Gel.*

**Usual adult prescribing limits**
See *Pyrethrins and Piperonyl Butoxide Gel.*

**Usual pediatric dose**
See *Usual adult and adolescent dose.*

**Strength(s) usually available**
U.S.—
  0.18% pyrethrins, 2.2% piperonyl butoxide (equivalent to 1.76% [butylcarbityl] [6-propylpiperonyl] ether and 0.44% related compounds), and 5.52% petroleum distillate (OTC) [*Barc*].

---

0.2% pyrethrins, 2% piperonyl butoxide technical (equivalent to 1.6% [butylcarbityl] [6-propylpiperonyl] ether and 0.4% related compounds), and 0.8% deodorized kerosene or petroleum distillate (OTC) [*Licetrol; Pyrinyl*].
0.3% pyrethrins and 2% piperonyl butoxide technical (equivalent to 1.6% [butylcarbityl] [6-propylpiperonyl] ether and 0.4% related compounds) (OTC) [*Tisit*].
0.3% pyrethrins, 3% piperonyl butoxide technical (equivalent to 2.4% [butylcarbityl] [6-propylpiperonyl] ether and 0.6% related compounds), 1.2% petroleum distillate, and 2.4% benzyl alcohol (OTC) [*Rid; Tisit Shampoo*].

Canada—
  Not commercially available.

**Packaging and storage**
Store below 40 °C (104 °F), preferably between 15 and 30 °C (59 and 86 °F), in a well-closed container, unless otherwise specified by manufacturer. Protect from freezing.

**Auxiliary labeling**
• For external use only.
• Harmful if swallowed or inhaled.

**Note**
When dispensing, include patient instructions.

---

Revised: 07/26/93
Interim revision: 02/18/94

---

## PYRIDOSTIGMINE—See *Antimyasthenics (Systemic)*

# PYRIDOXINE    Systemic

VA CLASSIFICATION (Primary): VT104
Another commonly used name is vitamin B₆.
Note: For a listing of dosage forms and brand names by country availability, see *Dosage Forms* section(s). For a listing of brand names for the articles in this monograph, refer to the General Index.

## Category

Nutritional supplement (vitamin); antidote (to cycloserine poisoning; to isoniazid poisoning).

Note: Pyridoxine is a water-soluble vitamin.

## Indications

Note: Bracketed information in the *Indications* section refers to uses that are not included in U.S. product labeling.

**Accepted**

Pyridoxine deficiency (prophylaxis and treatment)—Pyridoxine is indicated for prevention and treatment of pyridoxine deficiency states. Pyridoxine deficiency may occur as a result of inadequate nutrition or intestinal malabsorption but does not occur in healthy individuals receiving an adequate balanced diet. Simple nutritional deficiency of individual B vitamins is rare since dietary inadequacy usually results in multiple deficiencies. For prophylaxis of pyridoxine deficiency, dietary improvement, rather than supplementation, is advisable. For treatment of pyridoxine deficiency, supplementation is preferred.

Deficiency of pyridoxine may lead to xanthurenic aciduria, sideroblastic anemia, neurologic problems, seborrheic dermatitis, and cheilosis.

Recommended intakes may be increased and/or supplementation may be necessary in the following conditions or persons (based on documented pyridoxine deficiency):
Alcoholism
Burns
Congenital metabolic dysfunction—cystathioninuria, homocystinuria, hyperoxaluria, xanthurenic aciduria
Congestive heart failure
Fever, chronic
Gastrectomy
Hemodialysis
Hyperthyroidism
Infants receiving unfortified formulas such as evaporated milk
Infection
Intestinal diseases—celiac, diarrhea, regional enteritis, sprue

Malabsorption syndromes associated with hepatic-biliary tract disease such as alcoholism with cirrhosis
Stress, prolonged

Recommended intakes for pyridoxine are related to protein intake.

Some unusual diets (e.g., reducing diets that drastically restrict food selection) may not supply minimum daily requirements of pyridoxine. Supplementation is necessary in patients receiving total parenteral nutrition (TPN) or undergoing rapid weight loss or in those with malnutrition, because of inadequate dietary intake.

Recommended intakes for all vitamins and most minerals are increased during pregnancy. Many physicians recommend that pregnant women receive multivitamin and mineral supplements, especially those pregnant women who do not consume an adequate diet and those in high-risk categories (i.e., women carrying more than one fetus, heavy cigarette smokers, and alcohol and drug abusers). Taking excessive amounts of a multivitamin and mineral supplement may be harmful to the mother and/or fetus and should be avoided.

Recommended intakes for all vitamins and most minerals are increased during breast-feeding.

Recommended intakes may be increased by the following medications: Cycloserine, ethionamide, hydralazine, immunosuppressants, isoniazid, penicillamine, and estrogen-containing oral contraceptives.

Some neonates exhibit a hereditary pyridoxine dependency syndrome and require pyridoxine in the first week of life to prevent anemia and mental retardation; the cause is unknown but signs are hyperirritability and epileptiform seizures.
[Cycloserine toxicity (treatment)] or
[Isoniazid toxicity (treatment)]—Pyridoxine is also used as an antidote in cycloserine poisoning and to terminate seizures and prevent neuropathy associated with isoniazid poisoning.

**Unaccepted**

Pyridoxine has not been proven effective for treatment of acne and other dermatoses, alcohol intoxication, asthma, hemorrhoids, kidney stones, mental disorders, migraine headaches, morning sickness or radiation sickness, premenstrual tension, or for stimulation of lactation or appetite.

## Pharmacology/Pharmacokinetics

**Physicochemical characteristics**
Molecular weight—205.64.

### Mechanism of action/Effect

Nutritional supplement—Pyridoxine is converted in erythrocytes to pyridoxal phosphate and to a lesser extent pyridoxamine phosphate, which act as coenzymes for various metabolic functions affecting protein, carbohydrate, and lipid utilization. Pyridoxine is involved in conversion of tryptophan to niacin or serotonin, breakdown of glycogen to glucose-1-phosphate, conversion of oxalate to glycine, synthesis of gamma aminobutyric acid (GABA) within the CNS, and synthesis of heme.

Antidote—Pyridoxine increases the excretion of certain drugs (e.g., cycloserine and isoniazid) that act as pyridoxine antagonists.

### Absorption

The B vitamins are readily absorbed from the gastrointestinal tract, except in malabsorption syndromes. Pyridoxine is absorbed mainly in the jejunum.

### Protein binding

Pyridoxal phosphate—Totally bound to plasma proteins.
Pyridoxine—Not bound to plasma proteins.

### Storage:

Pyridoxine is stored mainly in the liver, with lesser amounts stored in muscle and brain.

### Biotransformation

Hepatic.

### Half-life

15 to 20 days.

### Elimination

Renal (almost entirely as metabolites). Excess beyond daily needs is excreted, largely unchanged, in urine.

In dialysis—Removed by hemodialysis; dialysis patients should receive increased amounts (100 to 300% of USRDA).

## Precautions to Consider

### Pregnancy/Reproduction

Pregnancy—Problems in humans have not been documented with intake of normal daily recommended amounts. However, exposure to large doses of pyridoxine *in utero* may result in a pyridoxine dependency syndrome in the neonate.

FDA Pregnancy Category A (parenteral pyridoxine).

### Breast-feeding

Problems in humans have not been documented with intake of normal daily recommended amounts.

### Pediatrics

Problems in pediatrics have not been documented with intake of normal daily recommended amounts.

### Geriatrics

Problems in geriatrics have not been documented with intake of normal daily recommended amounts.

### Drug interactions and/or related problems

The following drug interactions and/or related problems have been selected on the basis of their potential clinical significance (possible mechanism in parentheses where appropriate)—not necessarily inclusive (» = major clinical significance):

Note: Combinations containing any of the following medications, depending on the amount present, may also interact with pyridoxine.

Cycloserine or
Ethionamide or
Hydralazine or
Immunosuppressants, such as:
  Azathioprine
  Chlorambucil
  Corticosteroids
  Corticotropin (ACTH)
  Cyclophosphamide
  Cyclosporine
  Mercaptopurine, or
Isoniazid or
Penicillamine
  (may cause anemia or peripheral neuritis by acting as pyridoxine antagonists or increasing renal excretion of pyridoxine; recommended intakes for pyridoxine may be increased in patients receiving these medications)

Estrogens or
Contraceptives, estrogen-containing, oral
  (may increase recommended intakes for pyridoxine)

» Levodopa
  (concurrent use with pyridoxine is not recommended since levodopa's antiparkinsonian effects are reversed by as little as 5 mg of pyridoxine orally; this problem does not occur with the carbidopa-levodopa combination)

### Laboratory value alterations

The following have been selected on the basis of their potential clinical significance (possible effect in parentheses where appropriate)—not necessarily inclusive (» = major clinical significance):

With diagnostic test results
  Urobilinogen determinations using Ehrlich's reagent
    (pyridoxine may produce false-positive results)

### Medical considerations/Contraindications

The medical considerations/contraindications included here have been selected on the basis of their potential clinical significance (reasons given in parentheses where appropriate)—not necessarily inclusive (» = major clinical significance).

*Risk-benefit should be considered when the following medical problem exists:*

Sensitivity to pyridoxine

## Side/Adverse Effects

Doses of 200 mg per day for over 30 days have been reported to produce a pyridoxine dependency syndrome.

High doses of pyridoxine (2 to 6 grams per day) taken for several months have caused a severe sensory neuropathy, progressing from unstable gait and numb feet to numbness and clumsiness of hands. This condition seems to be reversible on withdrawal of pyridoxine, although some residual weakness has been observed.

## Patient Consultation

As an aid to patient consultation, refer to *Advice for the Patient, Pyridoxine (Vitamin B₆) (Systemic)*.

In providing consultation, consider emphasizing the following selected information (» = major clinical significance):

### Description of use

Description should include function in the body, signs of deficiency, and unproven uses

### Importance of diet

Importance of proper nutrition; supplement may be needed because of inadequate dietary intake
Food sources of pyridoxine; effects of processing
Not using vitamins as substitute for balanced diet
Recommended daily intakes for pyridoxine

### Before using this dietary supplement

» Conditions affecting use, especially:
  Sensitivity to pyridoxine
  Pregnancy—Use of large doses in pregnancy may cause pyridoxine dependency syndrome in the neonate
  Other medications, especially levodopa

### Proper use of this dietary supplement

» Proper dosing
  Proper administration of extended-release capsule dosage forms: Swallowing whole without crushing, breaking, or chewing; contents of capsule may be mixed with jam or jelly and swallowed without chewing
  Proper administration of extended-release tablet dosage forms: Swallowing whole without crushing, breaking, or chewing
  Missed dose: No cause for concern because of length of time necessary for depletion; remembering to take as directed

» Proper storage

### Side/adverse effects

Signs of potential side effects, especially sensory neuropathy

## General Dosing Information

Because of the infrequency of single B vitamin deficiencies, combinations are commonly administered. Many commercial combinations of B vitamins are available.

### For parenteral dosage forms only

In most cases, parenteral administration is indicated only when oral administration is not acceptable (for example, in nausea, vomiting, preoperative and postoperative conditions) or possible (for example, in malabsorption syndromes or following gastric resection).

### Diet/Nutrition

Recommended dietary intakes for pyridoxine are defined differently worldwide.

**For U.S.—**

The Recommended Dietary Allowances (RDAs) for vitamins and minerals are determined by the Food and Nutrition Board of the National Research Council and are intended to provide adequate nutrition in most healthy persons under usual environmental stresses. In addition, a different designation may be used by the FDA for food and dietary supplement labeling purposes, as with Daily Value (DV). DVs replace the previous labeling terminology United States Recommended Daily Allowances (USRDAs).

**For Canada—**

Recommended Nutrient Intakes (RNIs) for vitamins, minerals, and protein are determined by Health and Welfare Canada and provide recommended amounts of a specific nutrient while minimizing the risk of chronic diseases.

Daily recommended intakes for pyridoxine are generally defined as follows:—

Infants and children:
Birth to 3 years of age: 0.3 to 1 mg.
4 to 6 years of age: 1.1 mg.
7 to 10 years of age: 1.4 mg.
Adolescent and adult males:
1.7 to 2 mg.
Adolescent and adult females:
1.4 to 1.6 mg.
Pregnant females:
2.2 mg.
Breast-feeding females:
2.1 mg.

The best dietary sources of pyridoxine include meats, bananas, lima beans, egg yolks, peanuts, and whole-grain cereals. Substantial loss of pyridoxal and pyridoxamine (but not pyridoxine) occurs during cooking.

# Oral Dosage Forms

## PYRIDOXINE HYDROCHLORIDE EXTENDED-RELEASE CAPSULES

**Usual adult and adolescent dose**
Deficiency (prophylaxis)—Oral, amount based on normal daily recommended intakes—
Adolescent and adult males—1.7 to 2 mg.
Adolescent and adult females—1.4 to 1.6 mg.
Pregnant females—2.2 mg.
Breast-feeding females—2.1 mg.
Deficiency (treatment)—
Treatment dose is individualized by prescriber based on severity of deficiency.

**Usual pediatric dose**
Dosage form not appropriate for pediatric patients.

**Strength(s) usually available**
U.S.—
150 mg (OTC) [*Rodex*].
Canada—
Not commercially available.
Note: The strength of this pyridoxine preparation may exceed the dosage range recommended by USP DI Advisory Panels based on the amount necessary to meet normal nutritional needs.

**Packaging and storage**
Store below 40 °C (104 °F), preferably between 15 and 30 °C (59 and 86 °F), in a well-closed container, unless otherwise specified by manufacturer. Protect from light.

**Auxiliary labeling**
• Swallow capsules whole.

## PYRIDOXINE HYDROCHLORIDE TABLETS USP

**Usual adult and adolescent dose**
See *Pyridoxine Hydrochloride Extended-release Capsules.*

**Usual pediatric dose**
Deficiency (prophylaxis)—Oral, amount based on normal daily recommended intakes—
Birth to 3 years of age—0.3 to 1 mg.
4 to 6 years of age—1.1 mg.
7 to 10 years of age—1.4 mg.
Deficiency (treatment)—
Treatment dose is individualized by prescriber based on severity of deficiency.

**Strength(s) usually available**
U.S.—
10 mg (OTC) [GENERIC].
25 mg (OTC) [*Nestrex;* GENERIC].

50 mg (OTC) [GENERIC].
100 mg (OTC) [GENERIC].
200 mg (OTC) [GENERIC].
250 mg (OTC) [GENERIC].
500 mg (OTC) [GENERIC].
Canada—
25 mg (OTC) [GENERIC].
50 mg (OTC) [GENERIC].
100 mg (OTC) [GENERIC].
250 mg (OTC) [GENERIC].
Note: Some strengths of these pyridoxine preparations may exceed the dosage range recommended by USP DI Advisory Panels based on the amount necessary to meet normal nutritional needs.

**Packaging and storage**
Store below 40 °C (104 °F), preferably between 15 and 30 °C (59 and 86 °F), unless otherwise specified by manufacturer. Store in a well-closed container. Protect from light.

## PYRIDOXINE HYDROCHLORIDE EXTENDED-RELEASE TABLETS

**Usual adult and adolescent dose**
See *Pyridoxine Hydrochloride Extended-release Capsules.*

**Usual pediatric dose**
Dosage form not appropriate for pediatric patients.

**Strength(s) usually available**
U.S.—
100 mg (OTC) [GENERIC].
200 mg (OTC) [GENERIC].
500 mg (OTC) [GENERIC].
Canada—
Not commercially available.
Note: Some strengths of these pyridoxine preparations may exceed the dosage range recommended by USP DI Advisory Panels based on the amount necessary to meet normal nutritional needs.

# Parenteral Dosage Forms

Note: Bracketed uses in the *Dosage Forms* section refer to categories of use and/or indications that are not included in U.S. product labeling.

## PYRIDOXINE HYDROCHLORIDE INJECTION USP

**Usual adult and adolescent dose**
Deficiency (prophylaxis)—
Intravenous infusion, as part of total parenteral nutrition solutions, the specific amount determined by individual patient need.
Deficiency (treatment)—
In patients receiving total parenteral nutrition: The specific amount determined by individual patient need.
Pyridoxine dependency syndrome: Initial—Intramuscular or intravenous, 30 to 600 mg per day.
Drug-induced deficiency: Intramuscular or intravenous, 50 to 200 mg per day for three weeks, followed by 25 to 100 mg per day as needed.
[Cycloserine poisoning]—
Intramuscular or intravenous, 300 mg or more per day.
[Isoniazid poisoning (10 grams or more)]—
An amount of pyridoxine equal to amount of isoniazid ingested—Intravenous, 4 grams followed by 1 gram intramuscular every 30 minutes.

**Usual pediatric dose**
Deficiency (prophylaxis)—
Intravenous infusion, as part of total parenteral nutrition solutions, the specific amount determined by individual patient need.
Deficiency (treatment)—
In patients receiving total parenteral nutrition: The specific amount determined by individual patient need.
Pyridoxine dependency syndrome in infants (with seizures): Initial—Intramuscular or intravenous, 10 to 100 mg.

**Strength(s) usually available**
U.S.—
100 mg per mL (Rx) [*Beesix* (1.5% benzyl alcohol); *Doxine; Pyri; Rodex; Vitabee 6;* GENERIC].
Canada—
100 mg per mL (Rx) [GENERIC].

**Packaging and storage**
Store below 40 °C (104 °F), preferably between 15 and 30 °C (59 and 86 °F), unless otherwise specified by manufacturer. Protect from light. Protect from freezing.

Revised: 09/21/92
Interim revision: 08/22/94; 05/01/95

---

**PYRILAMINE**—See *Antihistamines (Systemic)*

---

## PYRILAMINE-CONTAINING COMBINATIONS—

Chlorpheniramine, Pheniramine, Pyrilamine, Phenylephrine, Hydrocodone, Salicylamide, Caffeine, and Ascorbic Acid (Systemic)—See *Cough/Cold Combinations (Systemic)*

Chlorpheniramine, Pyrilamine, and Phenylephrine (Systemic)—See *Antihistamines and Decongestants (Systemic)*

Chlorpheniramine, Pyrilamine, Phenylephrine, and Acetaminophen (Systemic)—See *Antihistamines, Decongestants, and Analgesics (Systemic)*

Chlorpheniramine, Pyrilamine, Phenylephrine, and Phenylpropanolamine (Systemic)—See *Antihistamines and Decongestants (Systemic)*

Chlorpheniramine, Pyrilamine, Phenylephrine, Phenylpropanolamine, and Acetaminophen (Systemic)—See *Antihistamines, Decongestants, and Analgesics (Systemic)*

Pheniramine, Phenyltoloxamine, Pyrilamine, and Phenylpropanolamine (Systemic)—See *Antihistamines and Decongestants (Systemic)*

Pheniramine, Pyrilamine, Hydrocodone, Potassium Citrate, and Ascorbic Acid (Systemic)—See *Cough/Cold Combinations (Systemic)*

Pheniramine, Pyrilamine, Phenylephrine, Phenylpropanolamine, and Hydrocodone (Systemic)—See *Cough/Cold Combinations (Systemic)*

Pheniramine, Pyrilamine, and Phenylpropanolamine (Systemic)—See *Antihistamines and Decongestants (Systemic)*

Pheniramine, Pyrilamine, Phenylpropanolamine, and Codeine (Systemic)—See *Cough/Cold Combinations (Systemic)*

Pheniramine, Pyrilamine, Phenylpropanolamine, Codeine, Acetaminophen, and Caffeine (Systemic)—See *Cough/Cold Combinations (Systemic)*

Pheniramine, Pyrilamine, Phenylpropanolamine, and Dextromethorphan (Systemic)—See *Cough/Cold Combinations (Systemic)*

Pheniramine, Pyrilamine, Phenylpropanolamine, Dextromethorphan, and Ammonium Chloride (Systemic)—See *Cough/Cold Combinations (Systemic)*

Pheniramine, Pyrilamine, Phenylpropanolamine, Dextromethorphan, and Guaifenesin (Systemic)—See *Cough/Cold Combinations (Systemic)*

Pheniramine, Pyrilamine, Phenylpropanolamine, and Guaifenesin (Systemic)—See *Cough/Cold Combinations (Systemic)*

Pheniramine, Pyrilamine, Phenylpropanolamine, and Hydrocodone (Systemic)—See *Cough/Cold Combinations (Systemic)*

Pheniramine, Pyrilamine, Phenylpropanolamine, Hydrocodone, and Guaifenesin (Systemic)—See *Cough/Cold Combinations (Systemic)*

Pyrilamine and Codeine (Systemic)—See *Cough/Cold Combinations (Systemic)*

Pyrilamine, Phenylephrine, Aspirin, and Caffeine (Systemic)—See *Antihistamines, Decongestants, and Analgesics (Systemic)*

Pyrilamine, Phenylephrine, and Codeine (Systemic)—See *Cough/Cold Combinations (Systemic)*

Pyrilamine, Phenylephrine, and Dextromethorphan (Systemic)—See *Cough/Cold Combinations (Systemic)*

Pyrilamine, Phenylephrine, and Hydrocodone (Systemic)—See *Cough/Cold Combinations (Systemic)*

Pyrilamine, Phenylephrine, Hydrocodone, and Ammonium Chloride (Systemic)—See *Cough/Cold Combinations (Systemic)*

Pyrilamine, Phenylpropanolamine, Acetaminophen, and Caffeine (Systemic)—See *Antihistamines, Decongestants, and Analgesics (Systemic)*

Pyrilamine, Phenylpropanolamine, Dextromethorphan, Guaifenesin, Potassium Citrate, and Citric Acid (Systemic)—See *Cough/Cold Combinations (Systemic)*

Pyrilamine, Phenylpropanolamine, Dextromethorphan, and Sodium Salicylate (Systemic)—See *Cough/Cold Combinations (Systemic)*

Pyrilamine, Pseudoephedrine, Dextromethorphan,and Acetaminophen (Systemic)—See *Cough/Cold Combinations (Systemic)*

---

# PYRIMETHAMINE   Systemic

**VA CLASSIFICATION (Primary/Secondary): AP101/AP109**
Note: For a listing of dosage forms and brand names by country availability, see *Dosage Forms* section(s). For a listing of brand names for the articles in this monograph, refer to the General Index.

## Category
Antiprotozoal.

## Indications
Note: Bracketed information in the *Indications* section refers to uses that are not included in U.S. product labeling.

**Accepted**
Malaria (treatment)—Pyrimethamine is indicated in combination with sulfadoxine and quinine in the treatment of chloroquine-resistant *Plasmodium falciparum* malaria. It is also indicated in combination with mefloquine and sulfadoxine, or quinine and sulfadoxine in the treatment of chloroquine-resistant *P. falciparum* malaria acquired in Southeast Asia, Bangladesh, East Africa, or the Amazon basin. Pyrimethamine is indicated in combination with sulfadoxine in the presumptive treatment of chloroquine-resistant *P. falciparum* malaria for self-treatment of febrile illness when medical care is not immediately available.

Toxoplasmosis (treatment)—Pyrimethamine is indicated in combination with a sulfapyrimidine-type sulfonamide in the treatment of toxoplasmosis caused by *Toxoplasma gondii*.[Pyrimethamine is also used with clindamycin in the treatment of toxoplasmosis in patients who are unresponsive to or intolerant of standard therapy.][1]

[Isosporiasis (prophylaxis and treatment)][1]—Pyrimethamine is used with sulfadoxine in the prophylaxis and treatment of isosporiasis caused by *Isospora belli*. It has also been used alone in a limited number of patients in the prophylaxis and treatment of isosporiasis.

[Pneumonia, *Pneumocystis carinii* (treatment)][1]—Pyrimethamine is used in combination with sulfadiazine, sulfadoxine, or dapsone, in the treatment of mild to moderate pneumonia caused by *Pneumocystis carinii* in patients who are unresponsive to or intolerant of standard therapy.

Not all species or strains of a particular organism may be susceptible to pyrimethamine. Resistance to pyrimethamine has been reported in *P. falciparum* and *P. vivax* malaria and may be widespread in certain areas.

**Unaccepted**
Pyrimethamine is not indicated alone in the treatment of acute attacks of malaria in nonimmune patients. Fast-acting schizonticides (e.g., 4-aminoquinolines, quinine) are preferred for these patients.

[1]Not included in Canadian product labeling.

## Pharmacology/Pharmacokinetics

**Physicochemical characteristics**
Molecular weight—248.71.

**Mechanism of action/Effect**
Binds to and reversibly inhibits the protozoal enzyme dihydrofolate reductase, selectively blocking conversion of dihydrofolic acid to its functional form, tetrahydrofolic acid. This depletes folate, an essential cofactor in the biosynthesis of nucleic acids, resulting in interference with protozoal nucleic acid and protein production. Protozoal dihydrofolate reductase is many times more tightly bound by pyrimethamine than the corresponding mammalian enzyme.

Exerts its effect in the folate biosynthesis at a step immediately subsequent to the one at which sulfonamides exert their effect. When administered concurrently with sulfonamides, synergism occurs, which is attributed to inhibition of tetrahydrofolate production at 2 sequential steps in its biosynthesis.

Active against asexual erythrocytic forms and, to a lesser degree, tissue forms of *P. falciparum* malaria. Does not destroy gametocytes, but arrests sporogony in the mosquito. Used alone, pyrimethamine does not produce radical cure in vivax or ovale malaria since it does not kill the latent hepatic stages of these parasites.

**Absorption**
Well absorbed following oral administration.

**Distribution**

Widely distributed; mainly concentrated in blood cells, kidneys, lungs, liver, and spleen. Crosses into the cerebrospinal fluid (CSF), with concentrations ranging from 13 to 26% of the corresponding serum concentrations. The mean whole blood to plasma concentration ratio was 0.87 in 1 study. Also crosses the placenta and is excreted in breast milk.

Vol$_D$ ranges from 2.3 to 3.1 liters per kg.

**Protein binding**

High (87%).

**Biotransformation**

Hepatic.

**Half-life**

Adults—Range, 80 to 123 hours. However, the half-life of pyrimethamine has been found to be as short as 23 hours in studies in patients with acquired immunodeficiency syndrome (AIDS), suggesting the possibility of a genetic variation in the metabolism of pyrimethamine or altered hepatic function secondary to HIV infection.

Infants (approximately 1 year old)—Approximately 64 hours (range, 52 to 87 hours).

**Time to peak plasma concentration**

Approximately 3 hours (range, 2 to 6 hours).

**Peak plasma concentration**

Adults—0.13 to 0.31 mcg/mL after a 25 mg dose.

Infants (approximately 1 year old)—1.3 mcg/mL after a dose of 1 mg per kg of body weight (mg/kg) per day; 0.7 mcg/mL 4 hours after a dose when administered at 1 mg/kg every Monday, Wednesday, and Friday.

**Elimination**

Renal—Primary route; 20 to 30% excreted unchanged in urine. Urinary excretion may persist for 30 days or longer.

In dialysis—The serum concentration of pyrimethamine fell by approximately 47% after peritoneal dialysis in one patient.

# Precautions to Consider

**Carcinogenicity**

Pyrimethamine has been reported to be associated with 2 cases of cancer in humans. Chronic granulocytic leukemia and reticulum cell sarcoma developed in patients receiving long-term pyrimethamine therapy for toxoplasmosis. Pyrimethamine also produced a significant increase in the number of lung tumors in mice given high-dose intraperitoneal pyrimethamine.

**Mutagenicity**

An increase in the number of structural and numerical aberrations was found in the chromosomes analyzed from the bone marrow of rats dosed with pyrimethamine. Structural chromosome aberrations were induced by pyrimethamine in human blood lymphoctyes cultured *in vitro*. Pyrimethamine was positive in the L5178Y/TK +/− mouse lymphoma assay without metabolic activation. However, it was found to be nonmutagenic in the Ames point mutation assay, the Rec assay, and the *E. coli* WP2 assay.

**Pregnancy/Reproduction**

Fertility—The fertility index of rats treated with pyrimethamine was lowered when high doses were used, suggesting possible toxic effects on the whole organism and/or conceptuses.

Pregnancy—Pyrimethamine crosses the placenta. Studies in humans have not shown that pyrimethamine causes teratogenic effects. Also, use in pregnant women to date has not shown pyrimethamine to be teratogenic. However, use is not generally recommended during the first 14 to 16 weeks of pregnancy since studies in animals have shown that pyrimethamine may cause birth defects in the fetus and may interfere with folic acid metabolism, especially when given in large doses such as those required in the treatment of toxoplasmosis. If pyrimethamine is necessary in the treatment of toxoplasmosis during pregnancy, it is recommended that leucovorin (folinic acid) be given concurrently.

FDA Pregnancy Category C.

**Breast-feeding**

Pyrimethamine is excreted in breast milk. It is estimated that a nursing infant would ingest approximately 3 to 4 mg over 48 hours after the ingestion of a single 75 mg dose by the mother. Problems in humans have not been documented. However, pyrimethamine may interfere with folic acid metabolism in nursing infants, especially when given to nursing women in large doses such as those required in the treatment of toxoplasmosis.

**Pediatrics**

Pyrimethamine has been used in children, and no pediatrics-specific problems have been documented to date.

**Geriatrics**

No information is available on the relationship of age to the effects of pyrimethamine in geriatric patients.

**Dental**

High doses of pyrimethamine not supplemented by leucovorin (folinic acid) may cause a folic acid deficiency, which may be characterized by a change in or loss of taste, or pain, burning, or inflammation of the tongue.

The leukopenic and thrombocytopenic effects of high doses of pyrimethamine may result in an increased incidence of certain microbial infections, delayed healing, and gingival bleeding. If leukopenia or thrombocytopenia occurs, dental work should be deferred until blood counts have returned to normal. Patients should be instructed in proper oral hygiene, including caution in use of regular toothbrushes, dental floss, and toothpicks.

**Drug interactions and/or related problems**

The following drug interactions and/or related problems have been selected on the basis of their potential clinical significance (possible mechanism in parentheses where appropriate)—not necessarily inclusive (» = major clinical significance):

Note: Combinations containing any of the following medications, depending on the amount present, may also interact with this medication.

» Bone marrow depressants (See *Appendix II*)
   (concurrent use of pyrimethamine with bone marrow depressants may increase the leukopenic and/or thrombocytopenic effects; if concurrent use is required, the possibility of increased myelotoxic effects should be considered, especially when pyrimethamine is used in large doses such as those required in the treatment of toxoplasmosis)

Folate antagonists, other, (See *Appendix II*)
   (concurrent use of other folate antagonists with pyrimethamine or use of pyrimethamine between courses of other folate antagonists is not recommended because of the possible development of megaloblastic anemia)

**Medical considerations/Contraindications**

The medical considerations/contraindications included here have been selected on the basis of their potential clinical significance (reasons given in parentheses where appropriate)—not necessarily inclusive (» = major clinical significance).

*Risk-benefit should be considered when the following medical problems exist:*

» Anemia or
» Bone marrow depression
   (pyrimethamine may cause folic acid deficiency, resulting in megaloblastic anemia, and blood dyscrasias, including agranulocytosis and thrombocytopenia)

Hepatic function impairment
   (pyrimethamine is metabolized in the liver)

Hypersensitivity to pyrimethamine

» Seizure disorders, history of
   (pyrimethamine may cause central nervous system [CNS] toxicity when used in high doses, as in the treatment of toxoplasmosis)

**Patient monitoring**

The following may be especially important in patient monitoring (other tests may be warranted in some patients, depending on condition; » = major clinical significance):

» Complete blood counts (CBCs) and
» Platelet counts
   (may be required weekly during therapy in patients receiving high dosage, as in the treatment of toxoplasmosis)

# Side/Adverse Effects

Note: When pyrimethamine is used for malaria in usual recommended dosage, side/adverse effects usually are rare; however, with large doses, as for toxoplasmosis, side effects may occur more frequently unless pyrimethamine is given concurrently with folinic acid.

The following side/adverse effects have been selected on the basis of their potential clinical significance (possible signs and symptoms in parentheses where appropriate)—not necessarily inclusive:

**Those indicating need for medical attention**

Incidence more frequent with high doses

*Atrophic glossitis* (pain, burning, or inflammation of the tongue; change in or loss of taste)—due to folic acid deficiency; *blood dyscrasias, specifically agranulocytosis* (fever and sore throat); *megalo-*

*blastic anemia* (unusual tiredness or weakness); *or thrombocytopenia* (unusual bleeding or bruising)

Incidence rare
  *Hypersensitivity* (skin rash)

**Those indicating need for medical attention only if they continue or are bothersome**
Incidence more frequent with high doses
  *Gastrointestinal disturbances* (anorexia; diarrhea; nausea and vomiting)

## Overdose

For specific information on the agents used in the management of pyrimethamine overdose, see:
  • *Barbiturates (Systemic)* monograph;
  • *Benzodiazepines (Systemic)* monograph; and/or
  • *Leucovorin (Systemic)* monograph.

For more information on the management of overdose or unintentional ingestion, **contact a Poison Control Center** (see *Poison Control Center Listing*).

**Clinical effects of overdose**
The following effects have been selected on the basis of their potential clinical significance (possible signs and symptoms in parentheses where appropriate)—not necessarily inclusive:

Acute
  In order of occurrence:
  *Gastrointestinal toxicity* (abdominal pain; severe and repeated vomiting); *neurotoxicity* (hyperexcitability; seizures)—usually occurs within 30 minutes to 2 hours of ingestion; *respiratory depression; circulatory collapse*

**Treatment of overdose**
Recommended treatment for pyrimethamine overdose includes:
To decrease absorption—
  Gastric emptying by aspiration and lavage.
Specific treatment—
  Control of CNS stimulation, including seizures, by parenteral administration of benzodiazepines or short-acting barbiturates. Administration of leucovorin, 5 to 15 mg (up to 50 mg in cerebral toxoplasmosis) intramuscularly daily for 3 days or longer, to counteract the effects of folic acid antagonism (e.g., reduced white blood cell counts) induced by pyrimethamine.
Monitoring—
  Monitoring of hematopoietic status for at least 1 month following overdose.
Supportive care—
  Mechanical assistance of respiration, if necessary. Patients in whom intentional overdose is confirmed or suspected should be referred for psychiatric consultation.

## Patient Consultation

As an aid to patient consultation, refer to *Advice for the Patient, Pyrimethamine (Systemic)*.

In providing consultation, consider emphasizing the following selected information (» = major clinical significance):

**Before using this medication**
»  Conditions affecting use, especially:
    Hypersensitivity to pyrimethamine
    Pregnancy—Pyrimethamine crosses the placenta
    Breast-feeding—Pyrimethamine is excreted in breast milk
    Dental—High doses may cause atrophic glossitis, leukopenia, or thrombocytopenia
    Other medications, especially bone marrow depressants
    Other medical problems, especially anemia, bone marrow depression, or a history of seizure disorders

**Proper use of this medication**
»  Keeping medication out of reach of children; overdose is very dangerous
    Taking with meals or a snack if gastric irritation occurs
»  Compliance with full course of therapy
»  Importance of not missing doses and taking medication on a regular schedule
»  Proper dosing
    Missed dose: Taking as soon as possible; not taking if almost time for next dose; not doubling doses
»  Proper storage

**Precautions while using this medication**
»  Regular visits to physician to check blood counts, especially during high-dose therapy for toxoplasmosis

Checking with physician if no improvement within a few days
Importance of taking leucovorin concurrently if anemia occurs
Using caution in use of regular toothbrushes, dental floss, and toothpicks; deferring dental work until blood counts have returned to normal; checking with physician or dentist concerning proper oral hygiene

**Side/adverse effects**
Signs of potential side effects, especially blood dyscrasias, hypersensitivity, and symptoms of folic acid deficiency

## General Dosing Information

Pyrimethamine may cause gastric irritation, sometimes resulting in vomiting, when given in high doses. To minimize this, pyrimethamine may be taken with meals or a snack or the dosage may be reduced.

Therapy should be discontinued if symptoms of folic acid deficiency occur. However, to prevent folic acid deficiency, leucovorin (folinic acid) may be administered concurrently to restore normal hematopoiesis. Leucovorin does not interfere with the antiprotozoal activity of pyrimethamine. Since malarial parasites are unable to utilize preformed folic acid, the antimalarial effect of pyrimethamine should not be affected. However, folic acid may interfere with the action of pyrimethamine on *T. gondii*, and concurrent use in toxoplasmosis is not recommended. In adults, 5 to 15 mg of leucovorin may be given orally, intramuscularly, or intravenously once a day for 3 days or as required. Alternatively, adults may be given 9 mg of leucovorin 2 or 3 times a week. Doses of up to 50 mg per day of leucovorin have been used with pyrimethamine in AIDS patients. Infants may be given 1 mg of leucovorin once a day.

Patients with impaired renal function receiving pyrimethamine prophylactically do not generally require a reduction in dose. However, patients receiving pyrimethamine more frequently should be monitored closely for signs of toxicity.

**For toxoplasmosis**
The dose of pyrimethamine that is required in the treatment of toxoplasmosis is 10 to 20 times greater than the antimalarial dose. Concurrent prophylactic administration of leucovorin in doses up to 50 mg daily with pyrimethamine is recommended to avoid folic acid deficiency.

In patients with seizure disorders, small initial doses of pyrimethamine are recommended in the treatment of toxoplasmosis to avoid potential CNS toxicity.

In patients who also have AIDS, treatment with pyrimethamine and sulfonamides may be required indefinitely. Clindamycin has been used with pyrimethamine in doses of 900 mg to 2.4 grams daily in patients who experienced adverse reactions to sulfonamides.

## Oral Dosage Forms

Note: Bracketed uses in the *Dosage Forms* section refer to categories of use and/or indications that are not included in U.S. product labeling.

**PYRIMETHAMINE TABLETS USP**

**Usual adult and adolescent dose**
Malaria—
  Treatment:
    Chloroquine-resistant *P. falciparum* malaria—Oral, 75 mg of pyrimethamine in combination with 1.5 grams of sulfadoxine as a single dose on day three of quinine therapy.
    Chloroquine-resistant *P. falciparum* malaria acquired in Southeast Asia, Bangladesh, East Africa, or the Amazon basin—Oral, 75 mg of pyrimethamine in combination with 750 mg of mefloquine and 1.5 grams of sulfadoxine as a single dose.
  Presumptive treatment:
    Oral, 75 mg of pyrimethamine in combination with 1.5 grams of sulfadoxine as a single dose for self-treatment of febrile illness when medical care is not immediately available.
Toxoplasmosis—
  AIDS patients:
    Loading dose—Oral, 100 to 200 mg of pyrimethamine per day in combination with 500 mg to 1.5 grams of a sulfadiazine every six hours, or 600 mg of clindamycin every six hours, for one to two days.
    Treatment—Oral, 50 to 100 mg of pyrimethamine per day in combination with 500 mg to 1.5 grams of a sulfadiazine every six hours, or 600 mg of clindamycin every six hours, for three to six weeks.
    Maintenance—Oral, 25 to 50 mg of pyrimethamine per day in combination with 250 mg to 1 gram of a sulfadiazine every six hours, or 600 mg of clindamycin every six hours, as lifelong therapy.

Other patients:
Loading dose—Oral, 50 to 200 mg per day in combination with 250 mg to 1 gram of a sulfapyrimidine-type sulfonamide every six hours, for one to two days.
Treatment—Oral, 25 to 50 mg per day in combination with 125 to 500 mg of a sulfapyrimidine-type sulfonamide every six hours, for two to four weeks if patient is immunocompetent, and four to six weeks if patient is immunocompromised.

[Isosporiasis][1]—
Treatment: Oral, 50 to 75 mg of pyrimethamine per day for three to four weeks.
Prophylaxis: Oral, 25 mg of pyrimethamine in combination with 500 mg of sulfadoxine once a week; or 25 mg of pyrimethamine alone once a day.
Note: These doses are based on very limited data.

**Usual pediatric dose**
Malaria—
Treatment:
Chloroquine-resistant *P. falciparum* malaria—Oral, 1.25 mg per kg of body weight of pyrimethamine in combination with 25 mg per kg of body weight of sulfadoxine as a single dose on day three of quinine therapy.
Chloroquine-resistant *P. falciparum* malaria acquired in Southeast Asia, Bangladesh, East Africa, or the Amazon basin—Oral, 1 mg per kg of body weight of pyrimethamine in combination with 10 mg per kg of body weight of mefloquine and 20 mg per kg of body weight of sulfadoxine as a single dose.
Presumptive treatment, for self-treatment of febrile illness when medical care is not immediately available:
Children 5 to 10 kg of body weight—Oral, 12.5 mg of pyrimethamine and 250 mg of sulfadoxine combination ($^1/_2$ tablet) as a single dose.
Children 11 to 20 kg of body weight—Oral, 25 mg of pyrimethamine and 500 mg of sulfadoxine combination (1 tablet) as a single dose.
Children 21 to 30 kg of body weight—Oral, 37.5 mg of pyrimethamine and 750 mg of sulfadoxine combination ($1^1/_2$ tablets) as a single dose.
Children 31 to 45 kg of body weight—Oral, 50 mg of pyrimethamine and 1 gram of sulfadoxine combination (2 tablets) as a single dose.
Children greater than 45 kg of body weight—Oral, 75 mg of pyrimethamine and 1.5 grams of sulfadoxine combination (3 tablets) as a single dose.

Toxoplasmosis—
In combination with the usual pediatric dose of a sulfapyrimidine-type sulfonamide: Oral, 1 mg of pyrimethamine per kg of body weight once a day for one to three days; then 0.5 mg of pyrimethamine per kg of body weight once a day for four to six weeks.
Note: In infants with confirmed congenital toxoplasmosis, treatment should be continued for a minimum of six months if there are no signs of infection, and for one year if there are signs of significant infection.

**Strength(s) usually available**
U.S.—
25 mg (Rx) [*Daraprim* (scored)].
Canada—
25 mg (Rx) [*Daraprim* (scored)].

**Packaging and storage**
Store below 40 °C (104 °F), preferably between 15 and 30 °C (59 and 86 °F), unless otherwise specified by manufacturer. Store in a tight, light-resistant container.

**Preparation of dosage form**
For patients who cannot take oral solids—According to the manufacturer, the tablets may be crushed to prepare a 1% solution in normal saline. The solution is stable for 24 hours at room temperature. Cherry Syrup NF or sucrose-containing solutions may also be used as vehicles. However, pyrimethamine prepared in these vehicles should be used immediately after preparation.

**Auxiliary labeling**
• Continue medicine for full time of treatment.
• Keep out of reach of children.

**Note**
Explain potential danger of accidental overdose.
Consider dispensing in unit-dose packaging in child-resistant containers (''double-barrier'' packaging).

[1]Not included in Canadian product labeling.

Revised: 01/19/93

## PYRIMETHAMINE-CONTAINING COMBINATIONS—

Sulfadoxine and Pyrimethamine (Systemic)

# PYRITHIONE   Topical

VA CLASSIFICATION (Primary): DE400
Note: For a listing of dosage forms and brand names by country availability, see *Dosage Forms* section(s). For a listing of brand names for the articles in this monograph, refer to the General Index.

## Category
Antiseborrheic.

## Indications
**Accepted**
Dandruff (treatment) or
Dermatitis, seborrheic (treatment)—Indicated to help control dandruff and seborrheic dermatitis of the scalp.

## Pharmacology/Pharmacokinetics

**Physicochemical characteristics**
Molecular weight—317.69.

**Mechanism of action/Effect**
Pyrithione may act by an antimitotic action, resulting in a reduction in the turnover of epidermal cells. It also has bacteriostatic and fungistatic activity, but it is not known if this action contributes to the antiseborrheic effects of the drug.

## Precautions to Consider

**Pregnancy/Reproduction**
Problems in humans have not been documented.

**Breast-feeding**
Problems in humans have not been documented.

**Pediatrics**
Appropriate studies on the relationship of age to the effects of pyrithione have not been performed in the pediatric population. However, no pediatrics-specific problems have been documented to date.

**Geriatrics**
Appropriate studies on the relationship of age to the effects of pyrithione have not been performed in the geriatric population. However, no geriatrics-specific problems have been documented to date.

**Medical considerations/Contraindications**
The medical considerations/contraindications included here have been selected on the basis of their potential clinical significance (reasons given in parentheses where appropriate)—not necessarily inclusive (» = major clinical significance).

*Risk-benefit should be considered when the following medical problem exists:*
Sensitivity to pyrithione

## Side/Adverse Effects
The following side/adverse effects have been selected on the basis of their potential clinical significance (possible signs and symptoms in parentheses where appropriate)—not necessarily inclusive:

**Those indicating need for medical attention**
Incidence more frequent
*Irritation of skin*

## Overdose

For more information on the management of overdose or unintentional ingestion, **contact a Poison Control Center** (see *Poison Control Center Listing*).

**Treatment of overdose**

To decrease absorption—Emesis and gastric lavage for accidental ingestion.

Supportive care—Administration of fluids. Patients in whom intentional overdose is known or suspected should be referred for psychiatric consultation.

## Patient Consultation

As an aid to patient consultation, refer to *Advice for the Patient, Pyrithione (Topical)*.

In providing consultation, consider emphasizing the following selected information (» = major clinical significance):

**Before using this medication**
» Conditions affecting use, especially:
    Sensitivity to pyrithione

**Proper use of this medication**
For best results, using medication at least 2 times a week or as directed by physician
*Proper administration*
    Before applying—Wetting hair and scalp with lukewarm water
    Applying enough shampoo to work up lather; rubbing in well; rinsing
    Applying shampoo again and rinsing thoroughly
» Avoiding contact with the eyes; flushing thoroughly with water if medication accidentally gets in eyes
» Proper dosing
    Missed dose: Using as soon as possible; not using if almost time for next dose
» Proper storage

**Precautions while using this medication**
Checking with physician if condition does not get better after regular use, or if it gets worse

**Side/adverse effects**
Signs of potential side effects, especially skin irritation

## General Dosing Information

The scalp and hair should be wet with lukewarm water and enough shampoo massaged into the scalp to work up a lather; then the scalp and hair should be rinsed. Application should be repeated, then the scalp and hair rinsed thoroughly.

## Topical Dosage Forms

### PYRITHIONE ZINC BAR SHAMPOO

**Usual adult and adolescent dose**
Antiseborrheic—
    Topical, to the scalp, two times a week.

**Usual pediatric dose**
See *Usual adult and adolescent dose*.

**Strength(s) usually available**
U.S.—
    2% (OTC) [*ZNP Bar Shampoo*].

Canada—
    Not commercially available.

**Packaging and storage**
Store below 40 °C (104 °F), preferably between 15 and 30 °C (59 and 86 °F), in a well-closed container, unless otherwise specified by manufacturer.

**Auxiliary labeling**
• For external use only.

### PYRITHIONE ZINC CREAM SHAMPOO

**Usual adult and adolescent dose**
See *Pyrithione Zinc Bar Shampoo*.

**Usual pediatric dose**
See *Usual adult and adolescent dose*.

**Strength(s) usually available**
U.S.—
    1% (OTC) [*Head & Shoulders Antidandruff Cream Shampoo Normal to Dry Formula; Head & Shoulders Antidandruff Cream Shampoo Normal to Oily Formula*].
Canada—
    Not commercially available.

**Packaging and storage**
Store below 40 °C (104 °F), preferably between 15 and 30 °C (59 and 86 °F), in a well-closed container, unless otherwise specified by manufacturer. Protect from freezing.

**Auxiliary labeling**
• For external use only.

### PYRITHIONE ZINC LOTION SHAMPOO

**Usual adult and adolescent dose**
See *Pyrithione Zinc Bar Shampoo*.

**Usual pediatric dose**
See *Usual adult and adolescent dose*.

**Strength(s) usually available**
U.S.—
    1% (OTC) [*Danex; Head & Shoulders Antidandruff Lotion Shampoo Normal to Dry Formula; Head & Shoulders Antidandruff Lotion Shampoo Normal to Oily Formula; Head & Shoulders Antidandruff Lotion Shampoo 2 in 1 (Complete Dandruff Shampoo plus Conditioner in One) Formula; Head & Shoulders Dry Scalp Conditioning Formula Lotion Shampoo; Head & Shoulders Dry Scalp Regular Formula Lotion Shampoo; Head & Shoulders Dry Scalp 2 in 1 (Dry Scalp Shampoo Plus Conditioner in One) Formula Lotion Shampoo; Zincon Dandruff Lotion Shampoo; ZNP Shampoo*].
    2% (OTC) [*DHS Zinc Dandruff Shampoo; Sebex; Sebulon*].
Canada—
    2% (OTC) [*Dan-Gard; Sebulon*].

**Packaging and storage**
Store below 40 °C (104 °F), preferably between 15 and 30 °C (59 and 86 °F), in a well-closed container, unless otherwise specified by manufacturer. Protect from freezing.

**Auxiliary labeling**
• Shake well.
• For external use only.

Revised: 07/26/93

---

# PYRVINIUM    Oral-Local*

VA CLASSIFICATION (Primary): AP200
Another commonly used name is viprynium.

Note: For a listing of dosage forms and brand names by country availability, see *Dosage Forms* section(s). For a listing of brand names for the articles in this monograph, refer to the General Index.

*Not commercially available in the U.S.

## Category

Anthelmintic (oral-local).

## Indications

**Accepted**

Enterobiasis (treatment)—Pyrvinium is used in the treatment of enterobiasis caused by *Enterobius vermicularis* (pinworm). However, pyrvinium has generally been replaced by other anthelmintics (e.g., mebendazole or pyrantel).

## Pharmacology/Pharmacokinetics

**Physicochemical characteristics**
Molecular weight—1151.41.

**Mechanism of action/Effect**
Appears to prevent the parasite from utilizing exogenous carbohydrates.

**Absorption**
Not appreciably absorbed from gastrointestinal tract.

**Elimination**
Fecal (unchanged).

## Precautions to Consider

### Pregnancy/Reproduction
Pregnancy—Studies in humans have not been done. Problems in humans have not been documented. Since pyrvinium is not absorbed, it is the preferred medication for the treatment of pinworm infections in pregnant women.

Studies in animals have not been done.

### Breast-feeding
It is not known whether pyrvinium is excreted in breast milk. However, problems in humans have not been documented.

### Pediatrics
Gastrointestinal upset occurs more frequently in older children who have received large doses.

Because of limited experience, caution is recommended in the treatment of children weighing less than 10 kg.

### Geriatrics
No information is available on the relationship of age to the effects of pyrvinium in geriatric patients.

### Medical considerations/Contraindications
The medical considerations/contraindications included here have been selected on the basis of their potential clinical significance (reasons given in parentheses where appropriate)—not necessarily inclusive (» = major clinical significance).

*Risk-benefit should be considered when the following medical problems exist:*
Hypersensitivity to pyrvinium
Inflammatory bowel disease
(may increase absorption)

### Patient monitoring
The following may be especially important in patient monitoring (other tests may be warranted in some patients, depending on condition; » = major clinical significance):

» Perianal examinations
(cellophane tape swabs of the perianal area to detect the presence of ova may be required prior to and starting 1 week following treatment with pyrvinium, especially in patients with persisting symptoms; swabs should be taken every morning, for at least 3 days, prior to defecation and bathing, to determine efficacy or provide proof of cure; perianal examinations may also be required to ascertain the absence of adult worms in the perianal area; no patient should be considered cured unless perianal swabs have been negative for 7 consecutive days)

## Side/Adverse Effects
The following side/adverse effects have been selected on the basis of their potential clinical significance (possible signs and symptoms in parentheses where appropriate)—not necessarily inclusive:

**Those indicating need for medical attention**
Incidence rare
*Hypersensitivity* (skin rash)

**Those indicating need for medical attention only if they continue or are bothersome**
Incidence rare
*Gastrointestinal disturbances* (diarrhea; nausea and vomiting; stomach cramps); *photosensitivity* (increased sensitivity of skin to sunlight)

**Those not indicating need for medical attention**
*Bright red discoloration of stools and vomit*

## Patient Consultation
As an aid to patient consultation, refer to *Advice for the Patient, Pyrvinium (Oral).*

In providing consultation, consider emphasizing the following selected information (» = major clinical significance):

**Before using this medication**
» Conditions affecting use, especially:
Hypersensitivity to pyrvinium

**Proper use of this medication**
No special preparations (e.g., dietary restrictions or fasting, concurrent medications, purging, or cleansing enemas) required before, during, or immediately after therapy
Proper administration technique
Treating all household members concurrently; treating again in 2 to 3 weeks
» Compliance with therapy; second course may be required
» Proper dosing
» Proper storage

**Precautions while using this medication**
Checking with physician if no improvement within a few days
» Possible skin photosensitivity; avoiding unprotected exposure to sun; using protective clothing; using a sun block product that includes protection against both UVA-caused photosensitivity reactions and UVB-caused sunburn reaction; avoiding use of sunlamp, tanning bed, or tanning booth
Washing (not shaking) all bedding and nightclothes after treatment to prevent reinfection; other measures may be recommended by some physicians

**Side/adverse effects**
For 24 to 48 hours or longer, produces bright red stools, which may stain clothing
Signs of side effects, especially hypersensitivity

## General Dosing Information

No special preparations (e.g., dietary restrictions or fasting, concurrent medications, purging, or cleansing enemas) are required before, during, or immediately after treatment with pyrvinium.

Because of the high probability of transfer of pinworms, it is usually recommended that all members of the household be treated concurrently. Retreatment is recommended 2 to 3 weeks following initial treatment.

Gastrointestinal upset occurs more frequently in older children and adults who have received large doses.

## Oral Dosage Forms

Note: The dosing and strengths of the dosage forms are expressed in terms of pyrvinium base (not the pamoate salt).

### PYRVINIUM PAMOATE ORAL SUSPENSION USP

**Usual adult and adolescent dose**
Enterobiasis—
Oral, 5 mg (base) per kg of body weight as a single dose. Repeat in two to three weeks.

**Usual adult prescribing limits**
Enterobiasis—Up to a maximum of 350 mg (base), regardless of body weight.

**Usual pediatric dose**
Enterobiasis—
See *Usual adult and adolescent dose;* or
Oral, 150 mg (base) per square meter of body surface as a single dose, repeated in two or three weeks.

Note: Caution is recommended in children weighing less than 10 kg.

**Strength(s) usually available**
U.S.—
Not commercially available.
Canada—
10 mg per mL (Rx) [*Vanquin*].

**Packaging and storage**
Store below 40 °C (104 °F), preferably between 15 and 30 °C (59 and 86 °F), unless otherwise specified by manufacturer. Store in a tight, light-resistant container. Protect from freezing.

**Auxiliary labeling**
• Avoid too much sun or use of sunlamp.
• May discolor stools.
• Shake well.

**Note**
Attach label supplied by manufacturer to bottle.
When dispensing, include a calibrated liquid-measuring device.
Make sure that dose for each member of family is clearly understood.

Revised: 01/19/93

**QUAZEPAM**—See *Benzodiazepines (Systemic)*

# QUINACRINE   Systemic

INN: Mepacrine

VA CLASSIFICATION (Primary): AP109

Note: For a listing of dosage forms and brand names by country availability, see *Dosage Forms* section(s). For a listing of brand names for the articles in this monograph, refer to the General Index.

## Category

Antiprotozoal.

## Indications

Note: Bracketed information in the *Indications* section refers to uses that are not included in U.S. product labeling.

### Accepted

Giardiasis (treatment)—Quinacrine is indicated as a primary agent in the treatment of giardiasis caused by *Giardia lamblia*.

[Pneumothorax (prophylaxis)][1]—Quinacrine powder is used as an intrapleural sclerosing agent to prevent recurrence of pneumothorax in patients at high risk of recurrence, e.g., cystic fibrosis patients.

[Lupus erythematosus, discoid (treatment)][1]—Quinacrine is used in the treatment of mild to moderate discoid lupus erythematosus.

[Sterilization, female][1]—Quinacrine is used transcervically as a female sterilizing agent.

### Unaccepted

Although quinacrine has been used for the treatment of diphyllobothriasis, hymenolepiasis, malaria, and taeniasis, it has been superseded by safer and/or more effective agents (e.g., niclosamide, praziquantel, chloroquine, hydroxychloroquine).

[1]Not included in Canadian product labeling.

## Pharmacology/Pharmacokinetics

### Physicochemical characteristics

Molecular weight—508.91.

### Mechanism of action/Effect

Exact mechanism of antiparasitic action is unknown; however, quinacrine binds to deoxyribonucleic acid (DNA) by intercalation between adjacent base pairs, inhibiting transcription and translation to ribonucleic acid (RNA). It also inhibits succinate oxidation and interferes with electron transport. In addition, it binds to nucleoproteins, which can suppress the lupus erythematous (LE) cell factor, and acts as a strong inhibitor of cholinesterase.

### Absorption

Rapidly absorbed from the gastrointestinal tract following oral administration. Also rapidly absorbed after intrapleural administration.

### Distribution

Widely distributed; concentrates in the liver, spleen, lungs, and adrenal glands. Concentration in the liver may be 20,000 times that in the plasma. Also deposited in skin, fingernails, and hair. Cerebrospinal fluid (CSF) concentrations are 1 to 5% of corresponding plasma level. Lowest concentrations are found in the brain, heart, skeletal muscles, and breast milk.

### Protein binding

High (80 to 90%).

### Half-life

5 to 14 days.

### Time to peak plasma concentration

8 to 12 hours.

### Elimination

Renal; fecal—Less than 11% eliminated in the urine daily; acidification of urine increases urinary excretion of quinacrine by up to 14%; excreted slowly, significant amounts being excreted in the urine for 2 months or more after discontinuation of quinacrine.

Small amounts also excreted in bile, sweat, and saliva.

## Precautions to Consider

### Pregnancy/Reproduction

Pregnancy—Quinacrine crosses the placenta and reaches the fetal circulation. There is one case of possible renal agenesis and hydrocephalus in an infant, although normal pregnancies have been reported after quinacrine ingestion during the first 4 weeks of gestation. If possible, quinacrine treatment for giardiasis in asymptomatic pregnant women should be postponed until after delivery.

One study in rats showed an increased incidence of fetal death with high doses of quinacrine.

### Breast-feeding

A small amount of quinacrine is excreted in breast milk. However, problems in humans have not been documented.

### Pediatrics

Quinacrine may cause vomiting in children due to its bitter taste. The tablets may be crushed and mixed with jam, honey, or chocolate syrup or put in empty gelatin capsules to mask the taste.

Children also tolerate quinacrine less well than do adults.

### Geriatrics

Appropriate studies on the relationship of age to the effects of quinacrine have not been performed in the geriatric population. However, no geriatrics-specific problems have been documented to date.

### Drug interactions and/or related problems

The following drug interactions and/or related problems have been selected on the basis of their potential clinical significance (possible mechanism in parentheses where appropriate)—not necessarily inclusive (» = major clinical significance):

Note: Combinations containing any of the following medications, depending on the amount present, may also interact with this medication.

» Primaquine

(concurrent use with quinacrine may inhibit the metabolism of primaquine or may displace it from tissue-binding sites, thereby increasing serum concentrations and potential toxicity of primaquine)

### Medical considerations/Contraindications

The medical considerations/contraindications included here have been selected on the basis of their potential clinical significance (reasons given in parentheses where appropriate)—not necessarily inclusive (» = major clinical significance).

*Risk-benefit should be considered when the following medical problems exist:*

Hypersensitivity to quinacrine

Porphyria

(quinacrine may exacerbate porphyria)

» Psoriasis

(quinacrine may precipitate a severe attack of psoriasis)

» Psychosis, history of

(quinacrine may cause transitory psychosis)

### Patient monitoring

The following may be especially important in patient monitoring (other tests may be warranted in some patients, depending on condition; » = major clinical significance):

*For giardiasis*

» Stool examinations

(3 stool examinations, taken several days apart, beginning 3 to 4 weeks following treatment, are recommended if symptoms persist; however, in some successfully treated patients, the lactose intolerance brought on by the infection may persist for a period of some weeks or months, mimicking the symptoms of giardiasis; in cases of treatment failure, alternative medications may be used)

# Side/Adverse Effects

Note: Hepatitis, aplastic anemia, corneal edema, and retinopathy may occur with prolonged and/or high-dose therapy with quinacrine. However, these side/adverse effects occur rarely, if at all, with short-term therapy such as that used in giardiasis.

The following side/adverse effects have been selected on the basis of their potential clinical significance (possible signs and symptoms in parentheses where appropriate)—not necessarily inclusive:

**Those indicating need for medical attention**
Incidence less frequent
*Central nervous system (CNS) stimulation* (hallucinations; irritability; mood or other mental changes; nervousness; nightmares; psychosis); *skin rash, redness, itching, or peeling*

**Those indicating need for medical attention only if they continue or are bothersome**
Incidence more frequent
*Dizziness; gastrointestinal disturbances* (abdominal or stomach cramps; diarrhea; loss of appetite; nausea or vomiting); *headache*

**Those not indicating need for medical attention**
Incidence more frequent
*Yellow discoloration of skin and urine*—due to acridine dye characteristics

# Overdose

For specific information on the agents used in the management of quinacrine overdose, see:
- *Barbiturates (Systemic)* monograph;
- *Benzodiazepines (Systemic)* monograph; and/or
- *Vasopressors* in *Sympathomimetic Agents—Cardiovascular Use (Parenteral-Systemic)* monograph.

For more information on the management of overdose or unintentional ingestion, **contact a Poison Control Center** (see *Poison Control Center Listing*).

**Clinical effects of overdose**
The following effects have been selected on the basis of their potential clinical significance (possible signs and symptoms in parentheses where appropriate)—not necessarily inclusive:

Acute
In order of occurrence—
*Seizures; hypotension; cardiac arrhythmias; cardiovascular collapse*

**Treatment of overdose**
Recommended treatment consists of the following:
To decrease absorption—
Evacuating the stomach by gastric lavage or induction of emesis.
Specific treatment—
Controlling seizures with benzodiazepines or ultrashort-acting barbiturates.
Treating shock by administration of fluids and vasopressors.
Administering ammonium chloride, 8 grams daily in divided doses for adults, to acidify the urine and promote excretion of quinacrine by up to 14%.
Supportive care—
Administering supportive measures such as maintaining an open airway, breathing, and circulation. Closely observing for at least 6 hours those patients who have survived the acute phase and are asymptomatic. Patients in whom intentional overdose is known or suspected should be referred for psychiatric consultation.

# Patient Consultation

As an aid to patient consultation, refer to *Advice for the Patient, Quinacrine (Systemic)*.

In providing consultation, consider emphasizing the following selected information (» = major clinical significance):

**Before using this medication**
» Conditions affecting use, especially:
    Hypersensitivity to quinacrine
    Pregnancy—Quinacrine crosses the placenta
    Breast-feeding—Quinacrine is excreted in breast milk
    Use in children—Children tolerate quinacrine less well than do adults
    Other medicine, especially primaquine
    Other medical problems, especially psoriasis and a history of psychosis

**Proper use of this medication**
Taking after meals with a full glass (240 mL) of water, tea, or fruit juice
Crushing tablets and mixing with jam, honey, or chocolate syrup or placing in empty gelatin capsules to disguise bitter taste for patients unable to swallow tablets or unable to tolerate bitter taste
» Compliance with full course of therapy
» Proper dosing
Missed dose: Taking as soon as possible; not taking if almost time for next dose; not doubling doses
» Proper storage

**Precautions while using this medication**
Periodic visits to physician to check progress after treatment
Checking with physician if no improvement within a few days
» Caution if dizziness occurs

**Side/adverse effects**
Signs of potential side effects, especially central nervous system (CNS) stimulation and skin rash, redness, itching, or peeling
Yellow discoloration of skin and urine, due to dye-like characteristics of quinacrine, may be alarming to patient although medically insignificant

# General Dosing Information

Quinacrine should preferably be taken after meals with a full glass (240 mL) of water, tea, or fruit juice.

For patients unable to swallow tablets or unable to tolerate bitter taste, quinacrine tablets may be crushed and mixed with jam, honey, or chocolate syrup or placed in empty gelatin capsules to disguise the bitter taste. Quinacrine is not stable in solution for any length of time; it is converted to an insoluble precipitate.

# Oral Dosage Forms

## QUINACRINE HYDROCHLORIDE TABLETS USP

**Usual adult and adolescent dose**
Giardiasis—
Oral, 100 mg three times a day for five to seven days.

**Usual pediatric dose**
Giardiasis—
Oral, 2 mg per kg of body weight three times a day for five to seven days.

Note: The maximum dose in children is 300 mg daily.

**Strength(s) usually available**
U.S.—
100 mg (Rx) [*Atabrine*].
Canada—
100 mg (Rx) [*Atabrine* (scored)].

**Packaging and storage**
Store below 40 °C (104 °F), preferably between 15 and 30 °C (59 and 86 °F) in a light-resistant container, unless otherwise specified by manufacturer. Store in a tight container.

**Preparation of dosage form**
*For patients who cannot take oral solids*—Tablets may be crushed and mixed with jam, honey, or chocolate syrup or placed in empty gelatin capsules to disguise the bitter taste. Quinacrine is not stable in solution for any length of time; it is converted to an insoluble precipitate.

**Auxiliary labeling**
- Take after meals with liquids.
- May cause dizziness.
- Continue medicine for full time of treatment.

Revised: 02/01/93

---

**QUINAPRIL**—See *Angiotensin-converting Enzyme (ACE) Inhibitors (Systemic)*

---

**QUINESTROL**—See *Estrogens (Systemic)*

---

**QUINETHAZONE**—See *Diuretics, Thiazide (Systemic)*

# QUINIDINE    Systemic

VA CLASSIFICATION (Primary/Secondary): CV300/AP101

Note: For a listing of dosage forms and brand names by country availability, see *Dosage Forms* section(s). For a listing of brand names for the articles in this monograph, refer to the General Index.

## Category

Antiarrhythmic; antimalarial.

## Indications

### Accepted

Cardiac arrhythmias (prophylaxis and treatment)—Treatment and control of:

Atrial fibrillation, established
Atrial flutter
Paroxysmal atrial fibrillation
Paroxysmal atrial tachycardia
Paroxysmal atrioventricular (AV) junctional rhythm
Paroxysmal ventricular tachycardia not associated with complete heart block
Premature contractions, atrial and ventricular

Malaria (treatment)[1]—Intravenous quinidine is indicated in the treatment of life-threatening *Plasmodium falciparum* malaria.

---

[1]Not included in Canadian product labeling.

## Pharmacology/Pharmacokinetics

### Physicochemical characteristics

Molecular weight—Quinidine gluconate: 520.58.
Quinidine sulfate: 782.95.

### Mechanism of action/Effect

Quinidine has both direct and indirect (anticholinergic) effects on cardiac tissue. Automaticity, conduction velocity, and membrane responsiveness are decreased, possibly because quinidine inhibits movement of potassium ions across membranes. The effective refractory period is prolonged. The anticholinergic action reduces vagal tone. An alpha-adrenergic blocking action often produces increased beta-adrenergic effects such as peripheral vasodilation. In the Vaughan Williams classification of antiarrhythmics, quinidine is considered to be a Class I antiarrhythmic.

### Protein binding

High (70 to 80%).

### Biotransformation

Hepatic; some cardioactive metabolites.

### Half-life

About 6 hours.

### Time to peak concentration

Oral—
Quinidine gluconate: 3 to 4 hours.
Quinidine sulfate: 1 to 1.5 hours.
Intramuscular—
1 hour.

### Therapeutic serum concentration

Usually 3 to 6 mcg per mL; toxic effects commonly occur at concentrations above 8 mcg per mL.

### Duration of action

Oral—
Regular tablets or capsules: 6 to 8 hours.
Extended-release tablets: About 12 hours.

### Elimination

Renal, about 10 to 50% unchanged. Excretion is increased in acidic urine and decreased in alkaline urine.
In dialysis—Small amounts removed by hemodialysis, none by peritoneal dialysis.

## Precautions to Consider

### Cross-sensitivity and/or related problems

Patients sensitive to quinine may be sensitive to this medication also.

### Carcinogenicity/Mutagenicity

Studies have not been done in either animals or humans.

### Pregnancy/Reproduction

Pregnancy—Studies have not been done in humans. However, quinine, a closely related medication, has produced congenital abnormalities of the central nervous system (CNS) and extremities, has caused ototoxicity in the neonate, and has an oxytocic effect.

Studies have not been done in animals.

FDA Pregnancy Category C.

### Breast-feeding

Quinidine is distributed into breast milk. However, problems have not been documented.

### Pediatrics

Appropriate studies on the relationship of age to the effects of quinidine have not been performed in the pediatric population. Use of extended-release dosage forms is not recommended.

### Geriatrics

Although appropriate studies on the relationship of age to the effects of quinidine have not been performed in the geriatric population, geriatrics-specific problems that would limit the usefulness of this medication in the elderly are not expected. However, elderly patients are more likely to have age-related renal function impairment, which may require dosage adjustment in patients receiving quinidine.

### Dental

The secondary anticholinergic effects of quinidine may decrease or inhibit salivary flow, especially in middle-aged or elderly patients, thus contributing to the development of caries, periodontal disease, oral candidiasis, and discomfort.

### Drug interactions and/or related problems

The following drug interactions and/or related problems have been selected on the basis of their potential clinical significance (possible mechanism in parentheses where appropriate)—not necessarily inclusive (» = major clinical significance):

Note: Combinations containing any of the following medications, depending on the amount present, may also interact with this medication.

» Alkalizers, urinary, such as:
    Antacids, calcium- and/or magnesium-containing
    Carbonic anhydrase inhibitors
    Citrates
    Sodium bicarbonate
    (concurrent use may increase the potential for toxic effects of quinidine; serum quinidine concentration is increased by enhanced renal absorption, which is promoted by the higher urinary pH; dosage adjustments may be needed when urinary alkalizer therapy is initiated or discontinued or if the dosage is changed)

» Antiarrhythmics, other or
Phenothiazines or
Rauwolfia alkaloids
    (concurrent use with quinidine may result in additive cardiac effects)

Anticholinergics (see *Appendix II* )
    (concurrent use with quinidine may intensify atropine-like side effects because of the secondary anticholinergic activities of quinidine)

» Anticoagulants, coumarin- or indandione-derivative
    (concurrent use with quinidine may cause additive hypoprothrombinemia as a result of alteration of procoagulant factor synthesis or catabolism and increased receptor affinity for the anticoagulant; dosage adjustments of anticoagulant may be necessary during and after quinidine therapy)

Antimyasthenics
    (neuromuscular blocking and/or secondary anticholinergic actions of quinidine may antagonize the effect of antimyasthenics on skeletal muscle; dosage adjustments of antimyasthenics may be necessary to control symptoms of myasthenia gravis)

Bethanechol
    (concurrent use with quinidine may antagonize the cholinergic effects of bethanechol)

Bretylium
    (concurrent administration with quinidine may counteract inotropic effect of bretylium and potentiate hypotension)

Cimetidine
    (as a result of inhibition of hepatic microsomal enzymes, cimetidine reduces total body clearance and prolongs the half-life of quinidine; dosage adjustment may be necessary)

Digitalis glycosides
(concurrent use is reported to have increased serum concentrations of digoxin; studies also indicate possible increased serum concentrations of digitoxin when used concurrently with quinidine. Serum concentrations of the glycoside should be monitored and dosage adjusted as indicated)

Hepatic enzyme inducers (see *Appendix II* )
(concurrent use with quinidine may decrease serum quinidine concentrations because of enhanced hepatic metabolism; adjustments of quinidine dosage may be necessary)

» Neuromuscular blocking agents
(effects may be potentiated when these medications are used concurrently with quinidine; careful postoperative monitoring of the patient may be necessary following concurrent or sequential use, especially if there is a possibility of incomplete reversal of neuromuscular blockade)

» Pimozide
(concurrent use with quinidine may potentiate cardiac arrhythmias, which are seen on electrocardiogram [ECG] as prolongation of QT interval)

Potassium-containing medications
(concurrent use usually enhances quinidine's effects)

Quinine
(concurrent use with quinidine may increase the possibility of cinchonism)

### Medical considerations/Contraindications
The medical considerations/contraindications included here have been selected on the basis of their potential clinical significance (reasons given in parentheses where appropriate)—not necessarily inclusive (» = major clinical significance).

*Except under special circumstances, this medication should not be used when the following medical problems exist:*
» Atrioventricular (AV) block, complete or
» Digitalis toxicity with AV conduction disorder or
» Intraventricular conduction defects, severe
(additive cardiac depression)

*Risk-benefit should be considered when the following medical problems exist:*
Asthma or emphysema
(possible hypersensitivity)
» AV block, incomplete
(quinidine may produce complete block)
» Digitalis intoxication
(additive cardiac depression and intracardial conduction inhibition)
» Hepatic function impairment or
» Renal function impairment
(possible quinidine accumulation; dosage adjustment may be required)
Hyperthyroidism
Hypokalemia
(possible reduced effect of quinidine)
Infections, acute
» Myasthenia gravis
(quinidine may increase muscle weakness)
Psoriasis
Sensitivity to quinidine
» Thrombocytopenia, or history of

### Patient monitoring
The following may be especially important in patient monitoring (other tests may be warranted in some patients, depending on condition; » = major clinical significance):
Blood cell counts and
Hepatic function determinations and
Renal function determinations
(may be required during long-term therapy)
Blood pressure determinations
(recommended frequently during intravenous therapy)
ECG monitoring, continuous and
Potassium concentrations, serum and
Quinidine concentrations, serum
(recommended especially when daily oral dose exceeds 2 grams or during parenteral administration; widening of QRS complex by 50% is evidence of possible quinidine cardiotoxicity)

## Side/Adverse Effects
Note: Quinidine is potentially cardiotoxic, especially at dosages exceeding 2.4 grams per day. Possible cardiovascular effects include QRS widening, cardiac asystole, ventricular ectopic beats, idioventricular rhythms (including ventricular tachycardia and fibrillation), paradoxical tachycardia, and arterial embolism.

The following side/adverse effects have been selected on the basis of their potential clinical significance (possible signs and symptoms in parentheses where appropriate)—not necessarily inclusive:

### Those indicating need for medical attention
Incidence less frequent
*Allergic reaction* (fever; skin rash, hives, or itching; wheezing, shortness of breath, or troubled breathing); *cinchonism* (blurred vision or any change in vision; dizziness or lightheadedness, severe; headache; ringing or buzzing in ears or any loss of hearing); *hypotension or extreme CNS effects* (fainting)
Note: In sensitive patients, *cinchonism* may occur after a single dose.

Incidence rare
*Anemia* (unusual tiredness or weakness); *tachycardia, paradoxical* (fast heartbeat); *thrombocytopenia* (unusual bleeding or bruising)

### Those indicating need for medical attention only if they continue or are bothersome
Incidence more frequent
*Bitter taste; diarrhea; flushing of skin with itching; loss of appetite; nausea or vomiting; stomach pain or cramping*

Incidence less frequent
*Confusion*

## Overdose
For more information on the management of overdose or unintentional ingestion, **contact a Poison Control Center** (see *Poison Control Center Listing* ).

### Treatment of overdose
Treatment is primarily supportive and symptomatic.

Recent oral ingestion may benefit from emesis and/or gastric lavage.

Oxygen, mechanical respiratory assistance, electronic cardiac pacing, hypertensives, urine acidifiers, and intravenous fluids may be indicated.

Hemodialysis is rarely necessary, although reported to be slightly effective in reducing plasma quinidine concentrations.

## Patient Consultation
As an aid to patient consultation, refer to *Advice for the Patient, Quinidine (Systemic)*.

In providing consultation, consider emphasizing the following selected information (» = major clinical significance):

### Before using this medication
» Conditions affecting use, especially:
Sensitivity to quinine
Breast-feeding—Distributed into breast milk
Use in children—Use of extended-release dosage form not recommended
Dental—May decrease or inhibit salivary flow
Other medications, especially antiarrhythmics, anticoagulants, neuromuscular blocking agents, pimozide, and urinary alkalizers
Other medical problems, especially complete or incomplete atrioventricular block, digitalis toxicity, severe intraventricular conduction defects, hepatic or renal function impairment, myasthenia gravis, or thrombocytopenia

### Proper use of this medication
Taking medication with water at least 1 hour before or 2 hours after meals for better absorption; may be taken with food or milk to lessen gastrointestinal irritation
Proper administration of extended-release tablets: Swallowing tablet whole; not breaking, crushing, or chewing before swallowing
» Compliance with therapy; taking as directed even if feeling well
» Proper dosing
Missed dose: Taking as soon as possible if remembered within 2 hours; if remembered later, not taking at all; not doubling doses
» Proper storage

### Precautions while using this medication
Regular visits to physician to check progress
» Checking with physician before discontinuing medication
» Caution if any kind of surgery (including dental surgery) or emergency treatment is required

Carrying medical identification card

» Checking with physician if symptoms of quinidine intolerance occur

**Side/adverse effects**

Signs of potential side effects, especially allergic reaction, cinchonism, hypotension or extreme CNS effects, anemia, paradoxical tachycardia, and thrombocytopenia

# General Dosing Information

Dosage must be adjusted to meet the individual requirements of each patient, on the basis of clinical response.

A test dose of one regular oral tablet may be administered prior to quinidine therapy to check for intolerance.

Higher serum quinidine concentrations are usually required to correct atrial arrhythmias than to correct ventricular arrhythmias.

There is a risk that quinidine may enhance atrioventricular (AV) conduction resulting in ventricular rate acceleration during treatment of atrial fibrillation or flutter. Digitalization prior to quinidine administration may reduce this risk.

**Diet/Nutrition**

This medication is preferably taken with a full glass (240 mL) of water on an empty stomach 1 hour before or 2 hours after meals for better absorption; however, it may be taken with food or milk when necessary to lessen gastrointestinal irritation.

# Oral Dosage Forms

## QUINIDINE GLUCONATE TABLETS

**Usual adult dose**
Antiarrhythmic—
Oral, 325 to 650 mg every six hours as needed and tolerated.

**Usual pediatric dose**
Dosage has not been established.

**Strength(s) usually available**
U.S.—
Not commercially available.
Canada—
325 mg (Rx) [*Quinate*].

**Packaging and storage**
Store below 40 °C (104 °F), preferably between 15 and 30 °C (59 and 86 °F), in a well-closed container, unless otherwise specified by manufacturer. Protect from light.

**Auxiliary labeling**
• Do not take other medicines without advice from your doctor.

## QUINIDINE GLUCONATE EXTENDED-RELEASE TABLETS

**Usual adult dose**
Antiarrhythmic—
Oral, 324 to 660 mg every six to twelve hours as needed and tolerated.

**Usual pediatric dose**
Use is not recommended.

**Strength(s) usually available**
U.S.—
324 mg (equivalent to 243 mg of quinidine sulfate) (Rx) [*Quinaglute Dura-tabs; Quinalan;* GENERIC].
330 mg (equivalent to 248 mg of quinidine sulfate) (Rx) [*Duraquin*].
Canada—
324 mg (Rx) [*Quinaglute Dura-tabs*].

**Packaging and storage**
Store below 40 °C (104 °F), preferably between 15 and 30 °C (59 and 86 °F), in a well-closed container, unless otherwise specified by manufacturer. Protect from light.

**Auxiliary labeling**
• Swallow tablet whole. Do not break or chew.
• Do not take other medicines without advice from your doctor.

## QUINIDINE POLYGALACTURONATE TABLETS

**Usual adult dose**
Antiarrhythmic—
Initial—Oral, 275 to 825 mg every three to four hours for three or four doses with subsequent doses being increased by 137.5 to 275 mg every third or fourth dose until rhythm is restored or toxic effects occur.
Maintenance—Oral, 275 mg two or three times a day as needed and tolerated.

**Usual pediatric dose**
Antiarrhythmic—
Oral, 8.25 mg per kg of body weight or 247.5 mg per square meter of body surface five times a day.

**Strength(s) usually available**
U.S.—
275 mg (equivalent to 200 mg of quinidine sulfate) (Rx) [*Cardioquin*].
Canada—
275 mg (equivalent to 200 mg of quinidine sulfate) (Rx) [*Cardioquin*].

**Packaging and storage**
Store below 40 °C (104 °F), preferably between 15 and 30 °C (59 and 86 °F), in a well-closed container, unless otherwise specified by manufacturer.

**Auxiliary labeling**
• Do not take other medicines without advice from your doctor.

## QUINIDINE SULFATE CAPSULES USP

**Usual adult dose**
Antiarrhythmic—
Initial:
Premature atrial and ventricular contractions—Oral, 200 to 300 mg three or four times per day.
Paroxysmal supraventricular tachycardias—Oral, 400 to 600 mg every two or three hours until the paroxysm is terminated.
Atrial flutter—Oral, by individual titration following digitalization.
Conversion of atrial fibrillation—Oral, 200 mg every two or three hours for five to eight doses, with subsequent daily increases as needed and tolerated.
Maintenance:
Oral, 200 to 300 mg three or four times a day as needed and tolerated.

**Usual adult prescribing limits**
Up to 4 grams daily.

**Usual pediatric dose**
Antiarrhythmic—
Oral, 6 mg per kg of body weight or 180 mg per square meter of body surface five times a day.

**Strength(s) usually available**
U.S.—
200 mg (Rx) [*Cin-Quin;* GENERIC].
300 mg (Rx) [*Cin-Quin*].
Canada—
Not commercially available.

**Packaging and storage**
Store below 40 °C (104 °F), preferably between 15 and 30 °C (59 and 86 °F), unless otherwise specified by manufacturer. Store in a tight, light-resistant container.

**Auxiliary labeling**
• Do not take other medicines without advice from your doctor.

## QUINIDINE SULFATE TABLETS USP

**Usual adult dose**
Antiarrhythmic—See *Quinidine Sulfate Capsules USP.*

**Usual adult prescribing limits**
Up to 4 grams daily.

**Usual pediatric dose**
Antiarrhythmic—See *Quinidine Sulfate Capsules USP.*

**Strength(s) usually available**
U.S.—
100 mg (Rx) [*Cin-Quin*].
200 mg (Rx) [*Cin-Quin; Quinora;* GENERIC].
300 mg (Rx) [*Cin Quin; Quinora*].
Canada—
200 mg (Rx) [*Apo-Quinidine; Novoquinidin;* GENERIC].

**Packaging and storage**
Store below 40 °C (104 °F), preferably between 15 and 30 °C (59 and 86 °F), unless otherwise specified by manufacturer. Store in a well-closed, light-resistant container.

**Auxiliary labeling**
• Do not take other medicines without advice from your doctor.

## QUINIDINE SULFATE EXTENDED-RELEASE TABLETS USP

**Usual adult dose**
Antiarrhythmic—
Oral, 300 or 600 mg every eight to twelve hours as needed and tolerated.

**Usual pediatric dose**
Use is not recommended.

**Strength(s) usually available**
U.S.—
    300 mg (Rx) [*Quinidex Extentabs*].
Canada—
    300 mg (Rx) [*Quinidex Extentabs*].

**Packaging and storage**
Store between 15 and 30 °C (59 and 86 °F), unless otherwise specified by manufacturer. Store in a well-closed, light-resistant container.

**Auxiliary labeling**
• Swallow tablets whole. Do not break or chew.
• Do not take other medicines without advice from your doctor.

## Parenteral Dosage Forms

### QUINIDINE GLUCONATE INJECTION USP

Note: The dosing and strengths of the dosage form are expressed in terms of the gluconate salt.

**Usual adult dose**
Antiarrhythmic—
    Intramuscular, 600 mg (salt) initially; then 400 mg (salt) repeated as often as every two hours if necessary.
    Intravenous infusion, 800 mg (salt) in 40 mL of 5% Dextrose Injection USP administered at a rate of 1 mL per minute with electrocardiogram (ECG) and blood pressure monitoring.
Antimalarial[1]—
    Intravenous infusion, continuous, initially, 10 mg (salt) per kg of body weight in an appropriate volume of 5% dextrose or 0.9% sodium chloride infused over one to two hours; followed immediately by 20 mcg (0.02 mg) (salt) per kg of body weight per minute until parasitemia decreases to less than one percent or oral therapy can be instituted.
    Intravenous infusion, intermittent, initially, 24 mg (salt) per kg of body weight in a volume of 250 mL 5% dextrose or 0.9% sodium chloride infused over four hours; then, eight hours after the beginning of the initial dose, 12 mg (salt) per kg of body weight infused over four hours; this is administered every eight hours until parasitemia decreases to less than one percent or until oral therapy can be instituted.

Note: The intermittent intravenous infusion provides a larger dose of quinidine and may be potentially more toxic than the continuous intravenous infusion.

    Standard oral antiplasmodial therapy should be instituted as soon as it is practical. Usually this occurs within 24 to 48 hours of starting quinidine therapy. When the parasite density is < 1% or the patient can tolerate oral therapy, oral quinine may be substituted for intravenous quinidine. The standard duration of combined quinidine/quinine therapy is seventy-two hours when treatment with a

second drug (e.g., tetracycline or sulfadoxine/pyrimethamine) is given. However, *Plasmodium falciparum* acquired in Thailand requires seven days of quinidine and/or quinine and seven days of tetracycline.

    Continuous ECG and blood pressure monitoring are recommended. Quinidine infusion should be temporarily slowed or discontinued if prolongation of QT interval greater than 0.6 seconds, a QRS interval increase of more than 25% over baseline, or hypotension unresponsive to moderate fluid challenge occurs.

**Usual adult prescribing limits**
Up to 5 grams daily.

**Usual pediatric dose**
Dosage has not been established.

**Strength(s) usually available**
U.S.—
    80 mg per mL (Rx) [GENERIC].
Canada—
    Not commercially available.

**Packaging and storage**
Store below 40 °C (104 °F), preferably between 15 and 30 °C (59 and 86 °F), unless otherwise specified by manufacturer. Protect from freezing. Protect from light.

### QUINIDINE SULFATE INJECTION

**Usual adult dose**
Antiarrhythmic—
    Intramuscular, 190 to 380 mg every two to four hours, up to a total dose of 3 grams a day.
Note: An initial test dose of 95 mg given intramuscularly is recommended.

**Usual adult prescribing limits**
3 grams daily.

**Usual pediatric dose**
Dosage has not been established.

**Strength(s) usually available**
U.S.—
    Not commercially available.
Canada—
    190 mg per mL (Rx) [GENERIC (propylene glycol)].

**Packaging and storage**
Store below 40 °C (104 °F), preferably between 15 and 30 °C (59 and 86 °F), unless otherwise specified by manufacturer. Protect from freezing. Protect from light.

---

[1]Not included in Canadian product labeling.

---

Revised: 03/24/94

---

# QUININE   Systemic

VA CLASSIFICATION (Primary/Secondary): AP101/MS900
Note: For a listing of dosage forms and brand names by country availability, see *Dosage Forms* section(s). For a listing of brand names for the articles in this monograph, refer to the General Index.

## Category

Antiprotozoal; antimyotonic.

## Indications

Note: Bracketed information in the *Indications* section refers to uses that are not included in U.S. product labeling.

**Accepted**
Malaria (treatment)—Quinine is indicated concurrently with tetracycline, doxycycline, clindamycin, pyrimethamine plus sulfadiazine, or pyrimethamine plus sulfadoxine in the treatment of chloroquine-resistant malaria caused by *Plasmodium falciparum*.

[Leg cramps (prophylaxis and treatment)]—Quinine is indicated in the prophylaxis and treatment of nocturnal recumbency leg muscle cramps, including those associated with arthritis, diabetes, varicose veins, thrombophlebitis, arteriosclerosis, and static foot deformities.

[Babesiosis (treatment)][1]—Quinine is used concurrently with clindamycin in the treatment of severe babesiosis caused by *Babesia microti*.

---

[1]Not included in Canadian product labeling.

## Pharmacology/Pharmacokinetics

**Physicochemical characteristics**
Molecular weight—782.95.

**Mechanism of action/Effect**
Antiprotozoal—The precise mechanism of action of quinine in malaria has not been determined but may be based on its ability to concentrate in parasitic acid vesicles, causing an elevation of pH in intracellular organelles. This is thought to disrupt the intracellular transport of membrane components and macromolecules, and phospholipase activity. Quinine has a schizonticidal action. Its ability to concentrate in parasitized erythrocytes may account for its selective toxicity against the erythrocytic stages of the 4 malarial parasites, including *P. falciparum* strains resistant to chloroquine. The drug is also gametocidal against *P. vivax* and *P. malariae*.

Antimyotonic—Quinine increases the refractory period of skeletal muscle by direct action on the muscle fiber, and the distribution of calcium within the muscle fiber, thereby diminishing the response to tetanic stimulation. It also decreases the excitability of the motor end-plate region, reducing the responses to repetitive nerve stimulation and to acetylcholine.

### Absorption
Rapidly and almost completely absorbed. Bioavailability is approximately 80% in healthy subjects.

### Distribution
Distribution of quinine may vary depending on the degree of illness; the volume of distribution is smaller in patients with cerebral malaria and increases with recovery. Children and pregnant women have a smaller volume of distribution than do nonpregnant adults. Plasma and red blood cell (RBC) concentrations appear to be similar before infection; however, during a malaria attack, plasma concentrations are considerably higher than RBC concentrations. Quinine does not freely cross the blood-brain barrier; the cerebrospinal fluid to plasma ratio is approximately 7%. Quinine crosses the placenta and is distributed into breast milk; peak concentrations are reached in breast milk approximately 90 minutes after oral administration.

$Vol_D$—
  Adults:
    Cerebral malaria—Approximately 1.2 liters per kg.
    Uncomplicated malaria—Approximately 1.7 liters per kg.
  Children:
    Uncomplicated malaria—
      Approximately 0.8 liters per kg.

### Protein binding
Higher (>90%) in patients with cerebral malaria, pregnant women, and children; approximately 85 to 90% in patients with uncomplicated malaria; and approximately 70% in healthy adults.

### Biotransformation
Hepatic; >80% metabolized by the liver. Metabolites have less activity than the parent drug.

### Half-life
Adults—
  Cerebral malaria: Approximately 18 hours.
  Uncomplicated malaria: Approximately 16 hours.
  Healthy persons: Approximately 11 hours.
Children—
  Uncomplicated malaria: Approximately 12 hours.
Acute overdose—
  Approximately 26 hours.

### Time to peak serum concentration
Acute malaria—Approximately 5.9 hours.
Convalescence—Approximately 3.2 hours.

### Mean serum concentration:
Approximately 7 mcg per mL, following chronic administration of total daily doses of 1 gram. Plasma concentrations are higher in patients with cerebral malaria due to reduced clearance and volume of distribution; concentrations decrease as patient recovers.

### Elimination
Primarily renal, with about 20% excreted as unchanged drug. Excretion of quinine is increased in acidic urine.
Dialysis—Exchange transfusion, hemodialysis, peritoneal dialysis, and hemofiltration have little effect on plasma quinine concentrations.

## Precautions to Consider

### Cross-sensitivity and/or related problems
Patients hypersensitive to quinidine may be hypersensitive to this medication also.

### Carcinogenicity
A study in rats, given quinine sulfate in drinking water at a concentration of 0.1% for up to 20 months, has not shown that quinine is carcinogenic.

### Mutagenicity
Micronucleus tests in male and female mice, given 2 intraperitoneal injections of quinine dihydrochloride 24 hours apart in doses of 0.5 millimole per kg of body weight, have not shown that quinine is mutagenic. Direct *Salmonella typhimurium* tests were also negative. However, when mammalian liver homogenate was added, positive results were obtained.
Sister chromatid exchange (SCE) tests, micronucleus tests, and chromosome aberration tests in Chinese hamsters, given quinine hydrochloride orally in doses of 100 mg per kg of body weight (mg/kg), have not shown that quinine is mutagenic.
Micronucleus tests and chromosome aberration tests in mice, given quinine hydrochloride orally in doses of 100 mg/kg, have not shown that quinine is mutagenic. However, the SCE test showed an increase in SCEs per cell. Tests were repeated in 2 inbred strains of mice, using

oral doses of 55, 75, and 110 mg of quinine hydrochloride per kg of body weight. The effects were more pronounced in these mice and the increase in SCEs per cell demonstrated a linear dose relationship. One of the inbred strains of mice showed positive micronucleus test results. The chromosome aberration tests also showed an increase in chromatid breaks. In addition, the Ames test was negative for point mutation.

### Pregnancy/Reproduction
Fertility—No information is available on the effect of quinine on fertility in animals or humans.

Pregnancy—Quinine crosses the placenta; one study found the cord plasma concentration to be approximately one-third the concentration of quinine in maternal plasma. Quinine has been used to treat patients with *P. falciparum* malaria in the third trimester of pregnancy. However, the risk of quinine to the fetus must be balanced against the danger of *P. falciparum* malaria, which is potentially life-threatening, especially during pregnancy. Studies in humans have shown that quinine causes congenital malformations, especially when given in large doses (e.g., up to 30 grams for attempted abortion). These malformations include deafness related to auditory nerve hypoplasia, limb anomalies, visceral defects, and visual changes. In addition, quinine may have an oxytoxic action on the uterus and has been shown to cause abortion when taken in toxic amounts. Stillbirths have also been reported in mothers taking quinine during pregnancy.
Studies in rabbits and guinea pigs have shown that quinine is teratogenic. However, no teratogenic effects were seen in mice, rats, dogs, or monkeys.

FDA Pregnancy Category X.

### Breast-feeding
Quinine is distributed into breast milk in small amounts. One study suggests that a breast-fed infant will receive approximately 1.5 to 3.0 mg per day of quinine base from maternal therapy. Problems in humans have not been documented.

### Pediatrics
Appropriate studies on the relationship of age to the effects of quinine for use as an antimyotonic have not been performed in the pediatric population. Antimalarial studies performed to date have shown that children have a decreased elimination half-life and volume of distribution; however, pediatrics-specific problems that would limit the usefulness of quinine in children have not been documented.

### Geriatrics
No information is available on the relationship of age to the effects of quinine in geriatric patients.

### Drug interactions and/or related problems
The following drug interactions and/or related problems have been selected on the basis of their potential clinical significance (possible mechanism in parentheses where appropriate)—not necessarily inclusive (» = major clinical significance):
Note: Combinations containing any of the following medications, depending on the amount present, may also interact with this medication.

Antacids, aluminum-containing
  (concurrent use of aluminum-containing antacids with quinine may decrease or delay the absorption of quinine)

Anticoagulants, coumarin- or indandione-derivative
  (hypoprothrombinemic effects may be increased when these agents are used concurrently with quinine because of decreased hepatic synthesis of procoagulant factors; hypoprothrombinemia can be prevented by coadministration of vitamin K; dosage adjustments may be necessary during and after quinine therapy)

Antimyasthenics
  (concurrent use of medications with neuromuscular blocking action may antagonize the effect of antimyasthenics on skeletal muscle; temporary dosage adjustments of antimyasthenics may be necessary to control symptoms of myasthenia gravis during and following concurrent use)

Cimetidine
  (concurrent use of cimetidine with quinine may reduce the clearance of quinine)

Digitoxin or
Digoxin
  (concurrent use of digoxin with quinine may result in increased digoxin serum concentrations and increased digoxin effect by decreasing the nonrenal clearance of digoxin; concurrent use of quinidine with digitoxin has been reported to result in increased digitoxin serum concentrations and increased digitoxin effect as well; because of the similarities of the digitalis glycosides and the similarities of quinine and quinidine, serum digoxin and digitoxin con-

centrations should be monitored periodically during concurrent therapy with quinine, and dosage adjustments made as indicated)

Hemolytics, other (See *Appendix II* ) or
Neurotoxic medications, other (See *Appendix II* ) or
Ototoxic medications, other, (See *Appendix II* )
(concurrent use of these medications with quinine may increase the potential for toxicity)

» Mefloquine
(concurrent use with quinine may result in an increased incidence of seizures and of electrocardiogram abnormalities, predisposing the patient to arrhythmias; it is recommended that mefloquine be administered at least 12 hours after the last dose of quinine)

(patients taking weekly mefloquine prophylaxis may be found to have mefloquine-resistant malaria that requires treatment with quinine; because mefloquine has a very long half-life [approximately 20 days], it will remain in the body long after the drug has been discontinued. Although there is insufficient information available, it is recommended that if quinine must be given that the patient be hospitalized, if possible, and monitored for QT prolongation and possible rhythm disturbances. Seizure activity may also be potentiated in these patients. In patients considered to be at high risk for a seizure, additional precautions and interventions may be indicated)

Neuromuscular blocking agents
(neuromuscular blockade may be potentiated when these agents are used concurrently with quinine)

Quinidine
(concurrent use with quinine may increase the possibility of QT prolongation or cinchonism)

## Laboratory value alterations
The following have been selected on the basis of their potential clinical significance (possible effect in parentheses where appropriate)—not necessarily inclusive (» = major clinical significance):

With diagnostic test results
17-ketogenic steroid, urinary
(quinine may cause increased values for urinary 17-ketogenic steroids when the metyrapone or Zimmerman method is used)

## Medical considerations/Contraindications
The medical considerations/contraindications included here have been selected on the basis of their potential clinical significance (reasons given in parentheses where appropriate)—not necessarily inclusive (» = major clinical significance).

*Risk-benefit should be considered when the following medical problems exist:*

» Blackwater fever, history of
(interrupted or recurrent quinine therapy in patients with *P. falciparum* infections may predispose them to the complications of blackwater fever, including anemia and hemolysis with renal failure)

Cardiac arrhythmias, history of, or QT prolongation
(a prolonged QT interval has been noted in patients being treated for cerebral malaria, without correlation with plasma quinine concentration; patients with a history of cardiac arrhythmias or QT prolongation may be at risk for arrhythmias while taking quinine)

Glucose-6-phosphate dehydrogenase (G6PD) deficiency
(hemolysis or hemolytic anemia may occur in G6PD-deficient patients; however, quinine has been safely given in therapeutic doses to patients with G6PD deficiency)

» Hypersensitivity to quinine or quinidine

» Hypoglycemia
(quinine stimulates release of insulin from the pancreas; hypoglycemia may also be a complication of severe *P. falciparum* malaria, especially in children and during pregnancy)

» Myasthenia gravis
(quinine may exacerbate muscle weakness in myasthenia gravis due to its neuromuscular blocking effects)

» Purpura, thrombocytopenic, or history of
(quinine may cause thrombocytopenic purpura, especially in highly sensitive patients or in patients with a previous history of this reaction to quinine)

## Side/Adverse Effects
The following side/adverse effects have been selected on the basis of their potential clinical significance (possible signs and symptoms in parentheses where appropriate)—not necessarily inclusive:

**Those indicating need for medical attention**
Incidence rare
*Hematologic effects, specifically agranulocytosis* (sore throat and fever); *Coombs' positive hemolytic anemia* (back, leg, or stomach pains; loss of appetite; pale skin; unusual tiredness or weakness; fever); *hypoprothrombinemia* (unusual bleeding or bruising); *or thrombocytopenia* (unusual bleeding or bruising); *hypoglycemia* (anxiety; chills; cold sweats; cool, pale skin; headache; increased hunger; nausea; nervousness; shakiness); *hypersensitivity, specifically fever; hemolytic uremic syndrome* (often presents with abdominal pain, nausea and vomiting, muscle aches, bruising, fever and chills, sweating); *hepatotoxicity* (abdominal pain; nausea; pale stools; yellow skin and eyes); *skin rash; redness; hives; itching; wheezing; shortness of breath; or difficult breathing*

Note: *Hemolytic uremic syndrome* (HUS) is a multi-system disorder that is characterized by hemolytic anemia, thrombocytopenia, disseminated intravascular coagulation (DIC), and acute renal failure. This reaction may occur within hours of a single ingestion of quinine. Several case reports have been published describing patients who have had an acute hypersensitivity reaction to quinine that resulted in adult HUS.

*Hypoprothrombinemia* may be reversed with vitamin K administration.

**Those indicating need for medical attention only if they continue or are bothersome**
Incidence more frequent
*Cinchonism* (blurred vision or change in color vision; headache, severe; nausea or vomiting; ringing or buzzing in ears or transient loss of hearing)—usually develops when plasma concentrations exceed 7 to 10 mcg per mL, but may occur at lower levels; *gastrointestinal disturbances* (abdominal or stomach cramps or pain; diarrhea; nausea or vomiting)

## Overdose
For specific information on the agents used in the management of quinine overdose, see:
• *Charcoal, Activated (Oral-Local)* monograph; and/or
• *Ipecac (Oral-Local)* monograph.

For more information on the management of overdose or unintentional ingestion, **contact a Poison Control Center** (see *Poison Control Center Listing*).

**Clinical effects of overdose**
The following effects have been selected on the basis of their potential clinical significance (possible signs and symptoms in parentheses where appropriate)—not necessarily inclusive:

Acute and chronic
*Cardiovascular toxicity* (cardiac arrest; electromechanical dissociation; hypotension; left bundle branch block; myocardial depression; ventricular arrhythmias); *central nervous system toxicity* (coma; confusion; delirium; respiratory arrest; restlessness; seizures; somnolence); *ocular toxicity* (visual deficits, including peripheral field defects, scotoma, blindness)—some sight is usually recovered

**Treatment of overdose**
Recommended treatment consists of the following:
To decrease absorption—
Using gastric lavage or inducing emesis with ipecac syrup to remove residual quinine from the stomach. Repeated dosing of activated charcoal every 4 hours may be beneficial in shortening the half-life of quinine in an overdose.

To enhance elimination—
Although excretion of quinine is increased in acidic urine, administration of forced acid diuresis has had little impact on quinine elimination by the kidney, which accounts for only 20% of the total body clearance. Peritoneal dialysis, hemodialysis, exchange transfusion, charcoal hemoperfusion, resin hemoperfusion, and plasmapheresis have not been found to be effective in the management of quinine overdose.

Specific treatment—
Stellate ganglionic block has not been shown to be of value in treating quinine-induced blindness and may cause an increase in complications. Caution should be used in administration of antiarrhythmics since quinine has class 1 antiarrhythmic properties that can be potentiated.

Supportive care—
Supportive measures such as maintaining an open airway, respiration, and circulation may be administered. Patients in whom intentional overdose is confirmed or suspected should be referred for psychiatric consultation.

## Patient Consultation

As an aid to patient consultation, refer to *Advice for the Patient, Quinine (Systemic).*

In providing consultation, consider emphasizing the following selected information (» = major clinical significance):

**Before using this medication**
» Conditions affecting use, especially:
Hypersensitivity to quinine
Pregnancy—Quinine has been found to be teratogenic; it has also caused stillbirths and abortions in pregnant women
Breast-feeding—Quinine is distributed into breast milk
Other medications, especially mefloquine
Other medical problems, especially a history of blackwater fever, hypoglycemia, myasthenia gravis, and a history of thrombocytopenic purpura

**Proper use of this medication**
» Importance of not taking more medication than the amount recommended
» Taking medication with or after meals to minimize possible gastrointestinal irritation
» Compliance with full course of therapy in malaria
» Proper dosing
Missed dose: Taking as soon as possible; not taking if almost time for next dose; not doubling doses
» Proper storage

**Precautions while using this medication**
» Caution if blurred vision or change in color vision occurs

**Side/adverse effects**
Signs of side effects, especially hematologic effects, specifically agranulocytosis, Coombs' positive hemolytic anemia, hypoprothrombinemia, or thrombocytopenia; hypoglycemia; and hypersensitivity, specifically fever, hemolytic uremic syndrome, hepatotoxicity, skin rash, redness, hives, itching, wheezing, shortness of breath, or difficult breathing

## General Dosing Information

This medication should be taken with or after meals to minimize gastrointestinal irritation.

In the treatment of chloroquine-resistant *P. falciparum* malaria, quinine is given concurrently with tetracycline, clindamycin, or pyrimethamine in combination with sulfadiazine or sulfadoxine.

In the treatment of nocturnal recumbency leg cramps, quinine may be discontinued if leg cramps do not occur after several consecutive nights of therapy, to determine if continued therapy is needed.

Plasma concentrations above 10 mg per 100 mL may cause severe symptoms of cinchonism.

**Bioequivalence information**
Bioavailability of quinine is extensive and rapid in healthy subjects. Studies using various salts of quinine have indicated no marked difference in the rate and extent of absorption of quinine in the capsule and plain tablet dosage forms.

## Oral Dosage Forms

Note: Bracketed uses in the *Dosage Forms* section refer to categories of use and/or indications that are not included in U.S. product labeling. The dosing and dosage forms available are expressed in terms of quinine sulfate (salt). Bioavailability studies have indicated no marked difference in the rate and extent of absorption of quinine in the capsule and plain tablet dosage forms.

### QUININE SULFATE CAPSULES USP

**Usual adult and adolescent dose**
Malaria: For chloroquine-resistant *Plasmodium falciparum* malaria—
Oral, 600 to 650 mg every eight hours for at least three days in most areas of the world (seven days in Southeast Asia) with concurrent administration of 250 mg of tetracycline every six hours for seven days; or concurrent administration of 100 mg of doxycycline every twelve hours for seven days; or concurrent administration of 1.5 grams of sulfadoxine and 75 mg of pyrimethamine combination as a single dose; or concurrent administration of 900 mg of clindamycin three times a day for three days.

[Antimyotonic]—
Nocturnal recumbency leg cramps: Oral, 200 to 300 mg at bedtime; if an additional dose of 200 to 300 mg is needed, it may be taken following the evening meal.

[Babesiosis][1]—
Oral, 650 mg three or four times a day with concurrent intravenous administration of 300 to 600 mg clindamycin four times a day for seven to ten days.

**Usual pediatric dose**
Malaria: For chloroquine-resistant *Plasmodium falciparum* malaria—
Oral, 8.3 mg per kg of body weight every eight hours for at least three days in most areas of the world (seven days in Southeast Asia) with concurrent administration of 5 mg per kg of body weight of tetracycline every six hours for seven days in children over 8 years of age; or concurrent administration of 6.7 to 13.3 mg per kg of body weight of clindamycin three times a day for three days; or concurrent administration of 1.25 mg per kg of body weight of pyrimethamine in combination with 25 mg per kg of body weight of sulfadoxine as a single dose.

[Antimyotonic]—
Dosage has not been established.

[Babesiosis][1]—
Dosage has not been established; however, based on one case report in an infant, the suggested dose is: Oral, 25 mg per kg of body weight per day with concurrent intravenous or intramuscular administration of 20 mg per kg of body weight per day of clindamycin for seven to ten days.

**Strength(s) usually available**
U.S.—
200 mg (Rx) [GENERIC].
300 mg (Rx) [GENERIC].
325 mg (Rx) [GENERIC].
Canada—
200 mg (Rx) [GENERIC].
300 mg (Rx) [GENERIC].

**Packaging and storage**
Store below 40 °C (104 °F), preferably between 15 and 30 °C (59 and 86 °F), unless otherwise specified by manufacturer. Store in a well-closed container.

**Auxiliary labeling**
• May cause vision problems.
• Continue medication for full time of treatment.

### QUININE SULFATE TABLETS USP

**Usual adult and adolescent dose**
See *Quinine Sulfate Capsules USP.*

**Usual pediatric dose**
See *Quinine Sulfate Capsules USP.*

**Strength(s) usually available**
U.S.—
260 mg (Rx) [GENERIC].
325 mg (Rx) [GENERIC].
Canada—
Not commercially available.

**Packaging and storage**
Store below 40 °C (104 °F), preferably between 15 and 30 °C (59 and 86 °F), unless otherwise specified by manufacturer. Store in a well-closed container.

**Auxiliary labeling**
• May cause vision problems.
• Continue medication for full time of treatment.

[1]Not included in Canadian product labeling.

Revised: 02/23/93
Interim revision: 06/23/95

# RABIES IMMUNE GLOBULIN   Systemic

VA CLASSIFICATION (Primary): IM500

Other commonly used names are HRIG and RIG.

Note: For a listing of dosage forms and brand names by country availability, see *Dosage Forms* section(s). For a listing of brand names for the articles in this monograph, refer to the General Index.

## Category

Immunizing agent (passive).

## Indications

### Accepted

Rabies (prophylaxis)—Rabies immune globulin is indicated for post-exposure immunization against rabies infection in persons who have not been previously immunized against rabies with rabies vaccine. Rabies immune globulin is used in conjunction with rabies vaccine.

### Unaccepted

Post-exposure prophylaxis is not recommended for persons inadvertently exposed to modified live rabies virus (MLV) vaccines intended for animals. Although vaccine-induced rabies has occurred in animals administered these vaccines, there have been no reported rabies cases among humans resulting from exposure to needle sticks or sprays with licensed MLV vaccines.

## Pharmacology/Pharmacokinetics

### Physicochemical characteristics

Source—Rabies immune globulin is an antirabies gamma globulin obtained from the plasma of hyperimmunized human donors. It is concentrated by cold ethanol fractionation. The rabies neutralizing antibody content is usually standardized to contain 150 International Units (IU) per mL. One Canadian product is standardized to contain 300 International Units (IU) per mL. The International Unit of potency is equivalent to the U.S. unit of potency

### Mechanism of action/Effect

Following intramuscular administration, rabies immune globulin provides immediate passive antibodies for a short period of time. This protects the patient until the patient can produce active antibodies from the rabies vaccine.

### Protective effect

When the post-exposure prophylaxis regimen has included local wound treatment, passive immunization, and active immunization, 100% effectiveness has been shown. However, rabies has occasionally developed in persons when key elements of the rabies post-exposure prophylaxis regimen were omitted or incorrectly administered. This has occurred outside the United States in cases in which patients' wounds were not cleansed with soap and water or other antiviral agents, rabies vaccine was not administered in the deltoid area but rather in the gluteal area, and passive immunization was not administered around the wound site.

### Time to protective effect

An adequate titer of passive antibody is present 24 hours after injection.

### Duration of protective effect

Short; rabies immune globulin has a half-life of approximately 21 days.

## Precautions to Consider

### Cross-sensitivity and/or related problems

Patients sensitive to other human immune globulin products may be sensitive to rabies immune globulin (RIG) also.

### Pregnancy/Reproduction

Pregnancy—Studies have not been done in humans. Because of the potential consequences of rabies virus infection, and because there is no indication that fetal abnormalities have been associated with use of RIG in pregnant women, pregnancy is not considered to be a contraindication to use.

Studies have not been done in animals.

FDA Pregnancy Category C.

### Breast-feeding

Problems in humans have not been documented.

### Pediatrics

Appropriate studies on the relationship of age to the effects of RIG have not been performed in the pediatric population. However, pediatrics-specific problems that would limit the usefulness of this medicine in children are not expected.

### Geriatrics

No information is available on the relationship of age to the effects of RIG in geriatric patients.

### Drug interactions and/or related problems

The following drug interactions and/or related problems have been selected on the basis of their potential clinical significance (possible mechanism in parentheses where appropriate)—not necessarily inclusive (» = major clinical significance):

Note: Combinations containing any of the following medications, depending on the amount present, may also interact with this medication.

Live virus vaccines
(antibodies contained in RIG may interfere with the body's immune response to certain live virus vaccines; live virus vaccines, such as measles, mumps, and rubella, should be administered at least 14 days prior to, or at least 3 months after, administration of RIG)

### Medical considerations/Contraindications

The medical considerations/contraindications included here have been selected on the basis of their potential clinical significance (reasons given in parentheses where appropriate)—not necessarily inclusive (» = major clinical significance).

***Risk-benefit should be considered when the following medical problems exist:***

» Immunoglobulin A (IgA) deficiencies, in patients who have known antibody to IgA
(small amounts of IgA may be present in RIG and may cause a severe allergic reaction in patients with antibody to IgA)

Sensitivity to RIG

Sensitivity to thimerosal
(the RIG available in the U.S. and Canada contains thimerosal)

## Side/Adverse Effects

Note: Severe systemic adverse effects to rabies immune globulin (RIG) are rare.

Although not reported with RIG, anaphylaxis, angioneurotic edema, and nephrotic syndrome have been reported rarely with other immune globulin products.

If necessary, physicians should consult with the state public health department, the Centers for Disease Control (CDC), Canadian National Advisory Committee on Immunization (NACI), and/or the World Health Organization (WHO) regarding the management of serious adverse reactions.

There is no evidence that hepatitis B virus (HBV), human immunodeficiency virus (HIV), or other viruses have been transmitted by commercially available RIG in the U.S.

Since RIG is given in conjunction with rabies vaccine, adverse effects generally associated with rabies vaccine have also been temporally associated with RIG.

The following side/adverse effects have been selected on the basis of their potential clinical significance (possible signs and symptoms in parentheses where appropriate)—not necessarily inclusive:

### Those indicating need for medical attention only if they continue or are bothersome

Incidence less frequent
*Fever; pain, soreness, tenderness, or stiffness of the muscles at the place(s) of injection*—may persist for several hours following injection

## Patient Consultation

As an aid to patient consultation, refer to *Advice for the Patient, Rabies Immune Globulin (Systemic)*.

In providing consultation, consider emphasizing the following selected information (» = major clinical significance):

### Before using this medication

» Conditions affecting use, especially:
Sensitivity to rabies immune globulin, other human immune globulins, or thimerosal
Other medical problems, especially immunoglobulin A (IgA) deficiencies

**Proper use of this medication**

» Proper dosing

# General Dosing Information

The recommended dose of rabies immune globulin (RIG) is 20 International Units (IU) per kg of body weight. Since RIG may partially suppress active production of rabies antibody, it is recommended that no more than the recommended dose be administered.

If anatomically feasible, up to one-half of the dose of RIG should be thoroughly infiltrated into the area(s) around the wound(s) and the rest should be administered intramuscularly in the gluteal area.

Care should be taken to avoid injection of RIG into or near blood vessels or nerves.

All post-exposure therapy should begin with immediate and thorough cleansing of all the patient's wounds with soap and water. Studies have shown that wound cleansing greatly reduces the likelihood of rabies.

Appropriate management of persons who may have been exposed to rabies depends on the assessment of the risk of infection. The incubation period for rabies infection varies with respect to the location and severity of the bite. The incubation period is usually 2 to 6 weeks, but can be longer. For bites to the face or extensive bites elsewhere on the body, the incubation period may be as short as 10 to 17 days. Decisions about management should be made promptly. Persons who have been bitten by animals suspected of being, or proven, rabid should begin therapy within 24 hours. If necessary, physicians should consult with the local or state public health department, the Centers for Disease Control (CDC), the Canadian National Advisory Committee on Immunization (NACI), and/or the World Health Organization (WHO) regarding the need for rabies prophylaxis.

The essential components of the rabies post-exposure prophylaxis regimen are local wound treatment, passive immunization with RIG (unless the patient has been previously immunized against rabies), and active immunization with rabies vaccine. Rabies has occasionally developed in persons when key elements of this regimen were omitted or incorrectly performed. In addition, tetanus prophylaxis and antibacterial medications may be administered as required. Both passive immunization with RIG (except for patients who have been previously immunized against rabies) and active immunization with rabies vaccine are required regardless of the interval between exposure and initiation of therapy. However, RIG should not be administered in the same syringe or into the same body site as the rabies vaccine.

Persons are considered to have been previously immunized against rabies (and as such should not receive RIG as part of the post-exposure therapy) if they have previously received complete regimens of pre- or post-exposure rabies prophylaxis with human diploid cell rabies vaccine (HDCV) or rabies vaccine adsorbed (RVA) or if they have been documented to have had an adequate antibody response to another rabies vaccine, such as duck embryo rabies vaccine. Regardless of the antibody titer that is present before post-exposure therapy occurs, an anamnestic antibody response should occur following the administration of the next dose of rabies vaccine.

RIG, when indicated, is administered only once, usually at the beginning of the post-exposure therapy regimen. RIG provides immediate passive antibodies until the patient can produce active antibodies from the rabies vaccine. If not given on the first day, RIG may be given any time up through the 7th day of the therapy regimen. Beyond the 7th day, RIG is not indicated, since an active antibody response to the rabies vaccine is presumed to have begun, and passive antibody may interfere with the body's active response.

If post-exposure prophylaxis is administered outside the U.S., additional prophylaxis may be desirable when the patient returns to the U.S.

Physicians should contact the state public health department or the CDC for specific advice. This is important, since treatment regimens and products vary from country to country.

# Parenteral Dosage Forms

## RABIES IMMUNE GLOBULIN (HUMAN) (RIG) USP

**Usual adult and adolescent dose**

Immunizing agent (passive)—

Intramuscular: 20 International Units (IU) per kg of body weight. If anatomically feasible, up to one-half of the dose should be thoroughly infiltrated into the area(s) around the wound(s) and the rest should be administered intramuscularly in the gluteal area.

Note: Rabies immune globulin (RIG) is used in conjunction with rabies vaccine and should be administered at the time of the first rabies vaccine dose or no later than the 7th day of rabies vaccine therapy.

**Usual pediatric dose**

See *Usual adult and adolescent dose.*

**Strength(s) usually available**

U.S.—

150 International Units (IU) per mL (Rx) [*Imogam* (thimerosal); *Hyperab* (thimerosal)].

Canada—

150 International Units (IU) per mL (Rx) [*Imogam* (thimerosal); *Hyperab* (thimerosal)].

300 International Units (IU) per mL (Rx) [GENERIC (may contain thimerosal)].

Note: The International Unit of potency is equivalent to the U.S. unit of potency.

**Packaging and storage**

Store between 2 and 8 °C (35 and 46 °F), unless otherwise specified by manufacturer. Do not freeze.

**Stability**

The solution should be discarded if it has been frozen.

The solution should not be used if it is discolored or contains particulate matter.

Rabies immune globulin (RIG) should not be heated. It may be warmed slightly by holding the vial in one's hands, but it should not be placed in warm water or an incubator.

**Incompatibilities**

RIG should not be administered in the same syringe or into the same body site as the rabies vaccine.

**Auxiliary labeling**
• Store in refrigerator.
• Do not freeze.
• Discard if vaccine has been frozen.

## Selected Bibliography

Chabala S, Williams M, Amenta R, et al. Confirmed rabies exposure during pregnancy: treatment with human rabies immune globulin and human diploid cell vaccine. Am J Med 1991 Oct; 91: 423-4.

Centers for Disease Control and Prevention. Rabies prevention-United States, 1991: recommendations of the Immunization Practices Advisory Committee (ACIP). MMWR 1991 Mar 22; 40 (RR-3): 1-19.

Frenia ML, Lafin SM, Barone JA. Features and treatment of rabies. Clin Pharm 1992 Jan; 11 (1): 37-47.

Developed: 08/31/94

---

# RABIES VACCINE  Systemic

This monograph includes information on the following: Rabies Vaccine Adsorbed†; Rabies Vaccine, Human Diploid Cell.

VA CLASSIFICATION (Primary): IM100

Other commonly used names are: HDCV [Rabies Vaccine, Human Diploid Cell], RVA [Rabies Vaccine Adsorbed].

Note: For a listing of dosage forms and brand names by country availability, see *Dosage Forms* section(s). For a listing of brand names for the articles in this monograph, refer to the General Index.

---

†Not commercially available in Canada.

## Category

Immunizing agent (active).

## Indications

**Accepted**

Rabies (prophylaxis)—Rabies vaccine is indicated for post-exposure immunization against rabies infection. Rabies vaccine is also indicated for pre-exposure immunization of persons with a high risk of rabies infection, such as veterinarians, animal handlers, certain laboratory workers, persons spending more than 1 month in areas of foreign countries where rabies (usually canine) is endemic, and other persons whose activities bring them into frequent contact with rabies virus or potentially rabid animals, such as dogs, cats, skunks, raccoons, and bats. Pre-exposure immunization is also recommended for persons who frequently handle or administer modified live rabies virus (MLV) vaccines intended for animals because of the possibility of exposure via needle sticks or sprays. Pre-exposure immunization is indicated for several reasons. It may protect persons whose post-exposure therapy may be delayed and it simplifies post-exposure therapy, both of which may be important for persons in areas where immunizing products may not be available or where available products may carry a high risk of adverse reactions. In addition, pre-exposure immunization may protect persons with inapparent exposure to rabies.

### Unaccepted

Post-exposure prophylaxis is not recommended for persons inadvertently exposed to modified live rabies virus (MLV) vaccines intended for animals. Although vaccine-induced rabies has occurred in animals administered these vaccines, there have been no reported rabies cases among humans resulting from exposure to needle sticks or sprays with licensed MLV vaccines.

Rabies vaccine is not intended for use in persons who exhibit clinical manifestation of rabies infection.

## Pharmacology/Pharmacokinetics

### Physicochemical characteristics

Source—
Human diploid cell vaccine (HDCV): Most HDCV products are prepared from Wistar's Pitman-Moore strain of rabies virus grown in MRC-5 human diploid cell culture. The vaccine virus is concentrated and then inactivated by betapropiolactone. One Canadian product is prepared from the CL-77 strain of rabies virus grown in MRC-5 human diploid cell culture. This vaccine undergoes a unique purification process. It is also inactivated by betapropiolactone.
Rabies vaccine adsorbed (RVA): RVA is prepared from the CVS Kissling/MDPH strain of rabies virus grown in a diploid cell line derived from fetal rhesus monkey lung cells. The vaccine virus is inactivated by betapropiolactone and concentrated by adsorption to aluminum phosphate.

Description—
HDCV: Solid, having a creamy white to orange color, and having the characteristic appearance of substances dried from the frozen state. The reconstituted suspension is a pinkish-yellow to red color because of the presence of phenol red.
RVA: Suspension, having a pink color because of the presence of phenol red.

### Mechanism of action/Effect

Following intradermal or intramuscular administration, rabies vaccine induces the formation of protective antibodies to rabies virus, thereby providing active immunity to rabies virus.

### Protective effect

HDCV and RVA are considered equally effective and safe. When the post-exposure prophylaxis regimen has included local wound treatment, passive immunization, and active immunization, 100% effectiveness has been shown. However, rabies has occasionally developed in persons when key elements of the rabies post-exposure prophylaxis regimen were omitted or incorrectly administered. This has occurred outside the United States in cases in which patients' wounds were not cleansed with soap and water or other antiviral agents, rabies vaccine was not administered in the deltoid area, but rather in the gluteal area, and passive immunization was not administered around the wound site.
The presence of acceptable antibody titers following pre-exposure or post-exposure prophylaxis is demonstrated by complete neutralization of the challenge virus at a 1:25 serum dilution (from serum collected 2 to 4 weeks after therapy) by the rapid fluorescent focus inhibition test (RFFIT). This dilution is approximately equivalent to the minimum titer of 0.5 International Units (IU) recommended by the World Health Organization (WHO).
When considering the administration of booster doses of rabies vaccine, the minimum acceptable antibody titer is demonstrated by complete neutralization of the challenge virus at a 1:5 serum dilution by the RFFIT test.

### Time to protective effect

Induction of active antibody production begins within 7 to 10 days.

### Duration of protective effect

Two or more years. Studies have shown that 2 years after the 3-dose pre-exposure prophylaxis regimen with rabies vaccine, a 1:5 serum dilution failed to neutralize the challenge virus completely by the RFFIT test in 2 to 7% of persons who received the vaccine intramuscularly and 5 to 17% of persons who received the vaccine intradermally.

## Precautions to Consider

### Pregnancy/Reproduction

Pregnancy—Studies have not been done in humans. Because of the potential consequences of rabies virus infection, and because there is no indication that fetal abnormalities have been associated with use of rabies vaccine in pregnant women, pregnancy is not considered to be a contraindication to post-exposure prophylaxis. In addition, if there is a substantial risk of exposure to rabies, pre-exposure prophylaxis may also be administered during pregnancy.
Studies have not been done in animals.
FDA Pregnancy Category C.

### Breast-feeding

Problems in humans have not been documented.

### Pediatrics

*HDCV (intradermal)*—Appropriate studies on the relationship of age to the effects of rabies vaccine have not been performed in the pediatric population. However, pediatrics-specific problems that would limit the usefulness of this vaccine in children are not expected.
*HDCV (intramuscular)*—Appropriate studies performed to date have not demonstrated pediatrics-specific problems that would limit the usefulness of rabies vaccine in children.
*RVA*—Appropriate studies on the relationship of age to the effects of rabies vaccine have not been performed in children up to 6 years of age. However, pediatrics-specific problems that would limit the usefulness of this vaccine in children are not expected.

### Geriatrics

No information is available on the relationship of age to the effects of rabies vaccine in geriatric patients.

### Drug interactions and/or related problems

The following drug interactions and/or related problems have been selected on the basis of their potential clinical significance (possible mechanism in parentheses where appropriate)—not necessarily inclusive (» = major clinical significance):

Note: Combinations containing any of the following medications, depending on the amount present, may also interact with this medication.

» Chloroquine and possibly other related antimalarials, such as mefloquine
   (chloroquine, and possibly other related antimalarials, interferes with the antibody response to rabies vaccine. If the intradermal route is used for pre-exposure rabies immunization, rabies prophylaxis should be initiated at least one month prior to travel [i.e., at least 2 weeks before initiation of antimalarial therapy] to allow for the formation of adequate rabies antibodies; if rabies prophylaxis cannot be initiated at least one month prior to travel, the intramuscular route should be used for pre-exposure rabies prophylaxis, since the intramuscular route is considered to have an adequate margin of safety when given within 2 weeks of antimalarial therapy. If post-exposure therapy is required during concurrent use of chloroquine, it is prudent to test for an adequate response to the rabies vaccine)

» Corticosteroids or
» Immunosuppressive agents or
» Radiation therapy
   (because normal defense mechanisms are suppressed, concurrent use with rabies vaccine may decrease the patient's antibody response to rabies vaccine. During post-exposure prophylaxis against possible rabies infection, these agents should not be administered unless they are essential for the treatment of other conditions. If these agents must be used concurrently, it is important to test for an adequate response to the rabies vaccine. Pre-exposure prophylaxis for rabies should be postponed if possible. If persons are at risk of rabies exposure and must have pre-exposure prophylaxis, the intramuscular, not the intradermal, agent should be administered and the patient should be tested for an adequate response to the rabies vaccine)

### Medical considerations/Contraindications

The medical considerations/contraindications included here have been selected on the basis of their potential clinical significance (reasons given in parentheses where appropriate)—not necessarily inclusive (» = major clinical significance).

*Risk-benefit should be considered when the following medical problems exist:*

» Febrile illness, severe
   (to avoid confusing manifestations of illness with possible side/adverse effects of vaccine; minor illnesses, such as upper respiratory infection, do not preclude administration of vaccine. Al-

though pre-exposure prophylaxis may be postponed during severe
febrile illness, post-exposure prophylaxis should be initiated on
schedule)

» Immune complex–like hypersensitivity reaction to rabies vaccine, history of

(persons who have experienced an immune complex–like hypersensitivity reaction following immunization with either human diploid cell vaccine [HDCV] or rabies vaccine adsorbed [RVA]
should not receive further doses of the same type of rabies vaccine;
although it is not known whether cross-sensitivity exists between
the two types of rabies vaccine, it may be helpful to administer
the other type of rabies vaccine if additional treatment is necessary;
in addition, one specially purified Canadian HDCV vaccine [Ra-
bies Vaccine Inactivated, Diploid Cell Origin, Dried—Connaught]
has not been associated with this reaction [see *Side/Adverse Effects*
]; additional doses of the same type of rabies vaccine should be
administered only if the other types of rabies vaccine are not available and prophylaxis is essential [e.g., patient requires post-exposure prophylaxis or patient requires pre-exposure prophylaxis because of a high risk of rabies exposure and inadequate antibody
titers])

» Immune deficiency conditions, congenital or hereditary, family history
of, or

» Immune deficiency conditions, primary or acquired

(because normal defense mechanisms are suppressed or reduced,
there may be a decrease in the patient's antibody response to rabies
vaccine. Following post-exposure prophylaxis, it is essential to test
for an adequate response to the rabies vaccine. Pre-exposure prophylaxis should use the intramuscular, not the intradermal, route
of administration and the patient should be tested for an adequate
response to the rabies vaccine)

Sensitivity to bovine serum, human albumin, kanamycin, monkey proteins, neomycin, polymyxin B, or thimerosal

(the rabies vaccines available in the U.S. and Canada contain one
or more of these ingredients; it may be possible to select a product
not having the agent causing sensitivity)

Sensitivity to rabies vaccine

**Patient monitoring**

The following may be especially important in patient monitoring (other
tests may be warranted in some patients, depending on condition;
» = major clinical significance):

Rabies antibody titer, serum

(may be determined when there is doubt as to whether an adequate
antibody response has occurred following pre-exposure or post-
exposure prophylaxis; the acceptable antibody titer is demonstrated
by complete neutralization of the challenge virus at a 1:25 serum
dilution [from serum collected 2 to 4 weeks after therapy] by the
rapid fluorescent focus inhibition test [RFFIT]. This dilution is approximately equivalent to the minimum titer of 0.5 International
Units [IU] recommended by the World Health Organization
(WHO). Determination of the need for a booster dose of rabies
vaccine is based on the minimum acceptable antibody titer, which
is demonstrated by complete neutralization of the challenge virus
at a 1:5 serum dilution by the RFFIT test)

## Side/Adverse Effects

Note: All available methods of systemic prophylaxis against rabies are
complicated by occasional adverse effects; however, these adverse
effects are rarely severe.

If necessary, physicians should consult with the state public health
department, the Centers for Disease Control (CDC), Canadian National Advisory Committee on Immunization (NACI), and/or the
World Health Organization (WHO) regarding the management of
serious adverse reactions.

In approximately 6% of persons receiving a booster dose of human
diploid cell vaccine (HDCV), a non–life-threatening immune complex–like reaction occurs 2 to 21 days later. Patients develop a
generalized urticaria or rash, which is sometimes accompanied by
arthralgia, arthritis, angioedema, nausea, vomiting, fever, or malaise. The reaction occurs much less frequently among persons receiving a primary immunization series, and rarely, if at all, after
the first dose of a primary series. The reaction is thought to be
caused by human serum albumin present in the product that has
become allergenic by interaction with betapropiolactone. A similar
reaction occurs after 7 to 14 days in less than 1% of persons receiving a booster, but not a primary, dose of rabies virus adsorbed
(RVA), even though human serum albumin is not used in the production of RVA. However, RVA also is inactivated by betapropiolactone. It is not known whether a person hypersensitive to HDCV

is hypersensitive to RVA also, or vice versa. Administration of
booster doses of a specially purified HDCV vaccine, currently
available in Canada (Rabies Vaccine Inactivated, Diploid Cell Origin, Dried—Connaught), has not been associated with this
reaction.

Three cases of neurologic illness resembling Guillain-Barré syndrome that resolved without sequelae in 12 weeks have been reported following administration of rabies vaccine. In addition, a few
other subacute central and peripheral nervous system disorders have
been temporally associated with the vaccine, but a causal relationship has not been established.

The following side/adverse effects have been selected on the basis of their
potential clinical significance (possible signs and symptoms in parentheses where appropriate)—not necessarily inclusive:

**Those indicating need for medical attention**
Incidence rare
*Immune complex–like reaction* (hives or skin rash)—less frequent
with booster doses

**Those indicating need for medical attention only if they continue
or are bothersome**
Incidence more frequent
*Abdominal pain* (stomach or abdomen pain); *chills; dizziness; fatigue*
(tiredness or weakness); *fever; headache; itching, pain, redness, or
swelling at the place of injection; malaise* (general feeling of discomfort or illness); *muscle or joint aches; nausea*

## Patient Consultation

As an aid to patient consultation, refer to *Advice for the Patient, Rabies
Vaccine (Systemic)*.

In providing consultation, consider emphasizing the following selected
information (» = major clinical significance):

**Before using this medication**
» Conditions affecting use, especially:
Sensitivity to rabies vaccine or to bovine serum, human albumin,
kanamycin, monkey proteins, neomycin, polymyxin B, or thimerosal, which may also be present in the vaccine
Other medications, especially chloroquine and possibly other related antimalarials, such as mefloquine; corticosteroids; immunosuppressive agents; or radiation therapy
Other medical problems, especially febrile illness, severe; immune
complex–like hypersensitivity reaction to rabies vaccine, history of; immune deficiency conditions, congenital or hereditary, family history of; or immune deficiency conditions, primary or acquired

**Proper use of this medication**
» Importance of not missing doses; keeping appointments with physician
» Proper dosing
» Missed dose: Contacting physician as soon as possible

**Precautions while using this medication**
» Caution if dizziness occurs; not driving, using machines, or doing anything else that requires alertness while receiving rabies vaccine

**Side/adverse effects**
Signs of potential side effects, especially immune complex–like
reaction

## General Dosing Information

The dosage is the same for all persons, children and adults.

Rabies vaccine is administered either intramuscularly or intradermally,
depending on the product and the indication. The products are not
interchangable with respect to the route of administration. Care should
be taken to avoid injection of the vaccine into or near blood vessels
or nerves.

Rabies vaccine should not be administered into the gluteal area (buttocks),
since administration into this area of the body results in lower antibody
titers.

It is not considered necessary to document seroconversion by testing serum samples from patients completing pre- or post-exposure prophylaxis except under unusual instances, such as when the person is
known to be immunosuppressed. Studies at the Centers for Disease
Control (CDC) have shown that persons tested 2 to 4 weeks after
completion of pre- or post-exposure rabies prophylaxis, administered
according to Immunization Practices Advisory Committee (ACIP)
guidelines, developed adequate antibody response to rabies. If documentation of seroconversion is required, serum collected 2 to 4 weeks
after pre-exposure or post-exposure prophylaxis, and diluted 1:25,
should completely neutralize the challenge virus by the rapid fluorescent focus inhibition test (RFFIT). This dilution is approximately

equivalent to the minimum titer of 0.5 International Units (IU) recommended by the World Health Organization (WHO).

### For pre-exposure immunization only

For pre-exposure immunization, either the intradermal or intramuscular product may be used. If the intradermal vaccine is used and is inadvertently injected subcutaneously, another dose of intradermal vaccine should be administered at a different site.

Pre-exposure immunization does not eliminate the need for prompt post-exposure prophylaxis following an exposure. However, pre-exposure immunization eliminates the need for administration of rabies immune globulin and reduces the number of injections of rabies vaccine needed for post-exposure prophylaxis.

Pre-exposure booster immunization is administered to persons who have received the pre-exposure immunization series, who remain at risk of rabies exposure by reasons of occupation or avocation, and whose 1:5 diluted serum does not completely neutralize the challenge virus by the RFFIT test. Depending on the person's degree of risk of rabies exposure, serum testing should be performed every 6 months to 2 years. As an alternative to serum testing for those persons who, based on their degree of risk, would require serum testing every 2 years, a booster can be administered every 2 years.

### For post-exposure immunization only

All post-exposure therapy should begin with immediate and thorough cleansing of all the patient's wounds with soap and water. Studies have shown that wound cleansing greatly reduces the likelihood of rabies.

For post-exposure immunization, the intramuscular vaccine, not the intradermal vaccine, should be used.

Appropriate management of persons who may have been exposed to rabies depends on the assessment of the risk of infection. The incubation period for rabies infection varies with respect to the location and severity of the bite. For bites to the face or extensive bites elsewhere on the body, the incubation period may be as short as 17 days. Decisions about management should be made promptly. Persons who have been bitten by animals suspected of being, or proven, rabid should begin therapy within 24 hours. If necessary, physicians should consult with the local or state public health department, CDC, the Canadian National Advisory Commitee on Immunization (NACI), and/or WHO regarding the need for rabies prophylaxis.

The essential components of the rabies post-exposure prophylaxis regimen are local wound treatment, passive immunization with rabies immune globulin (RIG) (unless the patient has been previously immunized against rabies), and active immunization with rabies vaccine. Rabies has occasionally developed in persons when key elements of this regimen were omitted or incorrectly performed. In addition, tetanus prophylaxis and antibacterial medications may be administered as required. Both passive immunization with RIG (except for patients who have been previously immunized against rabies) and active immunization with rabies vaccine are required regardless of the interval between exposure and initiation of therapy.

Persons are considered to have been previously immunized against rabies (and as such should not receive RIG as part of the post-exposure therapy) if they have previously received complete regimens of pre- or post-exposure rabies prophylaxis with human diploid cell rabies vaccine (HDCV) or rabies vaccine adsorbed (RVA) or if they have been documented to have had an adequate antibody response to another rabies vaccine, such as duck embryo rabies vaccine. Regardless of the antibody titer that is present before post-exposure therapy occurs, an anamnestic antibody response should occur following the administration of the next dose of rabies vaccine.

RIG, when indicated, is administered only once, usually at the beginning of the post-exposure therapy regimen. RIG provides immediate passive antibodies until the patient can produce active antibodies from the rabies vaccine. If not given on the first day, RIG may be given any time up through the 7th day of the therapy regimen. Beyond the 7th day, RIG is not indicated, since an active antibody response to the rabies vaccine is presumed to have begun. RIG should not be administered in the same syringe or into the same body site as the rabies vaccine. In addition, since RIG may partially suppress active production of rabies antibody, it is recommended that no more than the recommended dose be administered.

WHO recommends a 6-dose series (administered on Days 0, 3, 7, 14, 30, and 90) of HDCV, and probably RVA, for persons not previously immunized with rabies vaccine. The WHO regimen is considered safe and effective. However, studies conducted at CDC have shown that a 5-dose regimen of HDCV or RVA was also safe and effective and induced an adequate antibody response in all recipients tested.

If post-exposure prophylaxis is administered outside the U.S., additional prophylaxis may be desirable when the patient returns to the U.S. Physicians should contact the state public health department or the CDC for specific advice. This is important, since treatment regimens and products vary from country to country.

### For treatment of adverse effects

Recommended treatment consists of the following:
- Antihistamines may be administered for mild hypersensitivity reactions.
- Anti-inflammatory and antipyretic agents (e.g., aspirin) may be administered for local or mild systemic adverse reactions.
- Epinephrine may be administered to treat severe hypersensitivity or anaphylactic reaction.
- If possible, corticosteroids should not be administered, because when given in immunosuppressive doses, they may reduce the production of rabies antibodies. If corticosteroids are administered, it is important to test for an adequate response to the rabies vaccine, especially during post-exposure prophylaxis.

---

## *RABIES VACCINE ADSORBED*

# Parenteral Dosage Forms

## RABIES VACCINE ADSORBED SUSPENSION (RVA) USP

### Usual adult and adolescent dose

Immunizing agent (active)—

    Intramuscular, into the deltoid muscle:

      Pre-exposure immunization:

        1 mL on Days 0, 7, and 21 or 28, for a total of three doses.

      Pre-exposure booster immunization, if required:

        1 mL as a single dose.

      Note: See *General Dosing Information* for the parameters for administering booster doses.

      Post-exposure immunization of persons who have been previously immunized against rabies:

        1 mL on Days 0 and 3, for a total of two doses.

      Post-exposure immunization of persons who have not been previously immunized against rabies:

        1 mL on Days 0, 3, 7, 14, and 28, for a total of five doses.

      Note: For persons who have not been previously immunized against rabies, rabies immune globulin (RIG) should be administered on Day 0 along with the first dose of the vaccine. See *General Dosing Information*.

### Usual pediatric dose

See *Usual adult and adolescent dose*.

Note: The vaccine may be administered into the anterolateral aspect of the thigh if the child does not have sufficient deltoid muscle mass.

### Strength(s) usually available

U.S.—

    Greater than or equal to 2.5 International Units (IU) of rabies antigen per mL (Rx) [GENERIC (no more than 2 mg aluminum phosphate per mL; 0.01% thimerosal)].

Canada—

    Not commercially available.

### Packaging and storage

Store between 2 and 8 °C (35 and 46 °F), unless otherwise specified by manufacturer. Do not freeze.

### Preparation of dosage form

The vial should be shaken gently to ensure complete suspension of the aluminum phosphate adjuvant before withdrawing the dose into a syringe.

### Stability

The suspension should be discarded if it has been frozen.

The suspension should not be used if it is discolored or contains particulate matter.

### Auxiliary labeling

- Do not freeze.
- Discard if vaccine has been frozen.
- Store in refrigerator

### Note

The suspension is a light pink color because of the presence of phenol red indicator.

---

### RABIES VACCINE, HUMAN DIPLOID CELL

## Parenteral Dosage Forms
### RABIES VACCINE, HUMAN DIPLOID CELL (FOR INTRADERMAL INJECTION) (HDCV)

#### Usual adult and adolescent dose
Immunizing agent (active)—
Intradermal, on the deltoid muscle:
Pre-exposure immunization:
0.1 mL on Days 0, 7, and 21 or 28, for a total of three doses.
Pre-exposure booster immunization, if required:
0.1 mL as a single dose.
Note: See *General Dosing Information* for the parameters for administering booster doses.

#### Usual pediatric dose
See *Usual adult and adolescent dose.*

#### Strength(s) usually available
U.S.—
Greater than or equal to 2.5 International Units (IU) of rabies antigen per mL of reconstituted suspension (Rx) [*Imovax I.D* (contains no preservatives or stabilizers)].
Canada—
Not commercially available.

#### Packaging and storage
Store between 2 and 8 °C (35 and 46 °F), unless otherwise specified by manufacturer. Do not freeze.

#### Preparation of dosage form
The freeze-dried vaccine is contained in the single-dose syringe. The plunger of the syringe should be pushed so that the leading edge of the black stopper is even with the broken blue line on the side of the syringe. The needle should be inserted into the diluent bottle in such a way that both syringe and bottle remain upright. The needle should be in the diluent at all times during withdrawal in order to prevent air bubbles. The diluent should be drawn into the syringe until the end of the syringe's black stopper is at the solid blue line on the side of the syringe. The protective rubber cap should be replaced on the needle, and the freeze-dried vaccine should be allowed to completely dissolve. The syringe may be shaken if necessary. The reconstituted vaccine should be used immediately.

#### Stability
The vaccine should be administered immediately following reconstitution, or reconstituted vaccine should be discarded.
The reconstituted vaccine should not be used if it is discolored or contains particulate matter.

#### Auxiliary labeling
• Use reconstituted vaccine immediately.

### RABIES VACCINE, HUMAN DIPLOID CELL (FOR INTRAMUSCULAR INJECTION) (HDCV) USP

#### Usual adult and adolescent dose
Immunizing agent (active)—
Intramuscular, into the deltoid muscle:
Pre-exposure immunization:
1 mL on Days 0, 7, and 21 or 28, for a total of three doses.
Pre-exposure booster immunization, if required:
1 mL as a single dose.
Note: See *General Dosing Information* for the parameters for administering booster doses.
Post-exposure immunization of persons who have been previously immunized against rabies:
1 mL on Days 0 and 3, for a total of two doses.

Post-exposure immunization of persons who have not been previously immunized against rabies:
1 mL on Days 0, 3, 7, 14, and 28, for a total of five doses.
Note: For persons who have not been previously immunized against rabies, rabies immune globulin (RIG) should be administered on Day 0 along with the first dose of the vaccine. See *General Dosing Information.*

#### Usual pediatric dose
See *Usual adult and adolescent dose.*
Note: The intramuscular vaccine may be administered into the anterolateral aspect of the thigh if the child does not have sufficient deltoid muscle mass.

#### Strength(s) usually available
U.S.—
Greater than or equal to 2.5 International Units (IU) of rabies antigen per mL of reconstituted suspension (Rx) [*Imovax* (contains no preservatives or stabilizers)].
Canada—
Greater than or equal to 2.5 International Units (IU) of rabies antigen per mL of reconstituted suspension (Rx) [GENERIC (diluent may contain 0.01% thimerosal)].

#### Packaging and storage
Store between 2 and 8 °C (35 and 46 °F), unless otherwise specified by manufacturer. Do not freeze.

#### Preparation of dosage form
The freeze-dried vaccine should be reconstituted in its vial by using the 1 mL of diluent supplied in the disposable syringe. The longer of the two needles should be used to introduce the diluent into the vaccine vial. The contents of the vial should be gently swirled until they are completely dissolved. The total amount of dissolved vaccine in the vial should be drawn into the syringe. In order to do this, the vial should be set in an upright position on a table. The needle used for reconstitution should be removed and replaced with the smaller needle that will be used for administration. The reconstituted vaccine should be used immediately.

#### Stability
The vaccine should be administered immediately following reconstitution, or the reconstituted vaccine should be discarded.
The reconstituted vaccine should not be used if it is discolored or contains particulate matter.

#### Auxiliary labeling
• Use reconstituted vaccine immediately.

## Selected Bibliography
Centers for Disease Control and Prevention. Rabies prevention-United States, 1991: recommendations of the Immunization Practices Advisory Committee (ACIP). MMWR 1991 Mar 22; 40 (RR-3): 1-19.
Centers for Disease Control and Prevention. Systemic allergic reactions following immunization with human diploid cell rabies vaccine. MMWR 1984 Apr 13; 33 (14): 185-7.
Frenia ML, Lafin SM, Barone JA. Features and treatment of rabies. Clin Pharm 1992 Jan; 11 (1): 37-47.

---

Developed: 08/31/94

---

## RABIES VACCINE ADSORBED—See *Rabies Vaccine (Systemic)*

---

## RABIES VACCINE, HUMAN DIPLOID CELL—See *Rabies Vaccine (Systemic)*

# RACEMETHIONINE Systemic†

INN: Methionine
JAN: DL-Methionine
VA CLASSIFICATION (Primary/Secondary): GU900/AD900
Note: For a listing of dosage forms and brand names by country availability, see *Dosage Forms* section(s). For a listing of brand names for the articles in this monograph, refer to the General Index.

†Not commercially available in Canada.

## Category

Acidifier (urinary); antidote (to acetaminophen overdose).

## Indications

Note: Bracketed information in the *Indications* section refers to uses that are not included in U.S. product labeling.

**Accepted**
Dermatitis, contact (treatment) and
Urine odor—Racemethionine is indicated for the treatment of dermatitis and ulcerations, and for the control of urine odor, caused by ammoniacal urine in incontinent adults. Racemethionine is also indicated in infants for the treatment of diaper rash.

[Toxicity, acetaminophen (treatment)]—Racemethionine may be used in the treatment of acetaminophen overdose to protect against hepatotoxicity. However, oral *N*-acetylcysteine is considered the treatment of choice for acetaminophe overdose. (See *Acetylcysteine [Systemic]* monograph.) Use of racemethionine should be limited to emergency situations in which *N*-acetylcysteine is not available.

## Pharmacology/Pharmacokinetics

**Physicochemical characteristics**
Molecular weight—149.21.

**Mechanism of action/Effect**
Acidifier, urinary—Racemethionine produces ammonia-free urine by lowering the urinary pH.
Antidote, to acetaminophen overdose—Racemethionine may protect against acetaminophen overdose–induced hepatotoxicity by maintaining or restoring hepatic concentrations of glutathione. Glutathione is required to inactivate an intermediate metabolite of acetaminophen, which is hepatotoxic. In acetaminophen overdose, excessive quantities of this metabolite are formed because the primary metabolic pathways (glucuronide and sulfate conjugation) become saturated. The excess metabolite binds irreversibly to essential hepatic proteins and enzymes, causing cell damage and death. Racemethionine serves as a precursor for the synthesis of glutathione and sulfate.

## Precautions to Consider

**Pregnancy/Reproduction**
Pregnancy—Problems in humans have not been documented.

**Breast-feeding**
It is not known whether racemethionine is distributed into breast milk.

**Pediatrics**
Appropriate studies performed to date have not demonstrated pediatrics-specific problems that would limit the usefulness of racemethionine in children.

**Geriatrics**
Appropriate studies on the relationship of age to the effects of racemethionine have not been performed in the geriatric population. However, geriatrics-specific problems that would limit the usefulness of this medication in the elderly are not expected.

**Drug interactions and/or related problems**
The following drug interactions and/or related problems have been selected on the basis of their potential clinical significance (possible mechanism in parentheses where appropriate)—not necessarily inclusive (» = major clinical significance):

Note: Combinations containing any of the following medications, depending on the amount present, may also interact with this medication.

Levodopa
    (concurrent use with racemethionine may decrease the therapeutic effects of levodopa)

**Laboratory value alterations**
The following have been selected on the basis of their potential clinical significance (possible effect in parentheses where appropriate)—not necessarily inclusive (» = major clinical significance):
With diagnostic test results
    Acetone, urine
        (test may show false positive results)

**Medical considerations/Contraindications**
The medical considerations/contraindications included here have been selected on the basis of their potential clinical significance (reasons given in parentheses where appropriate)—not necessarily inclusive (» = major clinical significance).

*Risk-benefit should be considered when the following medical problems exist:*
    Acidosis, metabolic
        (may be exacerbated)
    Hepatic function impairment, history of or
    Hepatic function impairment, severe
        (use of racemethionine for other than emergency uses may worsen hepatic toxemia)

**Patient monitoring**
The following may be especially important in patient monitoring (other tests may be warranted in some patients, depending on condition; » = major clinical significance):
*For treatment of acetaminophen toxicity*
» Acetaminophen concentration, plasma
        (should be determined not less than 4 hours following ingestion of acetaminophen overdose to determine the need for antidotal therapy)
    Alanine aminotransferase (ALT [SGPT]) and
    Aspartate aminotransferase (AST [SGOT]) and
    Bilirubin and
    Prothrombin time
        (serum determinations should be assessed daily for 3 or 4 consecutive days if plasma acetaminophen concentrations indicate potential hepatotoxicity)
    Blood urea nitrogen (BUN) and
    Creatinine, serum
        (recommended because of the potential for development of renal failure; however, BUN may not be elevated if the liver is unable to produce urea by-products)
    Complete blood counts
        (recommended daily for 3 or 4 days to detect thrombocytopenia)
    Glucose, blood
        (recommended daily for 3 or 4 days to detect hypoglycemia)
    Toxicology screen, urine
        (acetaminophen is commercially available in combination with other drugs; therefore, ingestion of other potentially toxic medications should be ruled out in overdose situations)

## Side/Adverse Effects

The following side/adverse effects have been selected on the basis of their potential clinical significance (possible signs and symptoms in parentheses where appropriate)—not necessarily inclusive:

**Those indicating need for medical attention only if they continue or are bothersome**
Incidence more frequent
    *Drowsiness; nausea and vomiting*

## Patient Consultation

As an aid to patient consultation, refer to *Advice for the Patient, Racemethionine (Systemic)*.

In providing consultation, consider emphasizing the following selected information (» = major clinical significance):

**Before using this medication**
» Conditions affecting use, especially:
        Other medical problems, especially history of, or severe hepatic function impairment, or metabolic acidosis

**Proper use of this medication**
*For treatment of contact dermatitis*
» Importance of not taking more medication than the amount prescribed, and getting enough protein in the diet in order to avoid abnormally low weight gain in infants

Taking medicine with, or just after meals

Adding contents of capsule to juice, water, or warm milk or infant formula, if necessary

Proper administration technique for oral solution

*For all uses*
» Proper dosing
» Proper storage

**Precautions while using this medication**
Checking with physician if no improvement after 10 days

# General Dosing Information

## For treatment of contact dermatitis
If there is no improvement after 10 days of therapy, it is recommended that racemethionine be discontinued because the probable cause of the rash is something other than ammoniacal urine.

## For treatment of acetaminophen toxicity
Oral *N*-acetylcysteine is considered the treatment of choice for acetaminophen overdose. (See *Acetylcysteine [Systemic]* monograph). *Use of racemethionine should be limited to emergency situations in which N-acetylcysteine is not available.*

Patients with suspected acetaminophen overdose should receive supportive therapy. This may include establishing and maintaining adequate airway, respiratory, and circulatory function; maintaining fluid and electrolyte balance; correcting hypoglycemia; and administering vitamin $K_1$ (if prothrombin time ratio exceeds 1.5) and fresh frozen plasma or prothrombin complex concentrate (if prothrombin time ratio exceeds 3).

Gastric decontamination, by means of lavage or ipecac-induced emesis may be beneficial if carried out within 4 hours after ingestion of potentially toxic doses of acetaminophen.

Administration of activated charcoal following acetaminophen overdose is controversial. Activated charcoal effectively adsorbs acetaminophen, but also adsorbs racemethionine, thereby diminishing the antidotal effectiveness of both agents.

Additional therapy to treat mixed overdose with other agents (i.e., naloxone for an opioid analgesic) may be needed, especially if symptoms of central nervous system (CNS) depression occur within a few hours after ingestion of potentially toxic doses of acetaminophen.

Racemethionine therapy must be instituted within 8 to 12 hours after acetaminophen ingestion. If given more than 15 hours postingestion, racemethionine may precipitate hepatic encephalopathy. *It is recommended that racemethionine be administered as soon as possible after ingestion of an overdose is suspected,* without waiting for the results of plasma acetaminophen concentrations or other laboratory tests.

Plasma acetaminophen concentration should be determined not less than 4 hours following ingestion of the overdose. Concentrations determined prior to this time are not reliable for assessing potential hepatotoxicity. The following chart, derived from the Rumack-Matthew nomogram, may be used to predict which patients may develop hepatotoxicity when the time of ingestion is known:

| Acetaminophen plasma concentration (mcg/mL) | Time after ingestion (hours) |
|---|---|
| > 150 | 4 |
| >100 | 6 |
| > 70 | 8 |
| > 50 | 10 |
| > 20 | 16 |
| > 8 | 20 |
| > 4 | 24 |

If the initial determination indicates a plasma concentration below those listed at the times indicated, cessation of antidotal therapy can be considered.

## Diet/Nutrition
For treatment of contact dermatitis—

It is essential that adequate protein intake be maintained during therapy with racemethionine and that the recommended dosage of medication not be exceeded. Excessive dosages of racemethionine added alone to the diet over an extended period of time may result in lower than normal weight gain in infants, when protein intake is insufficient.

# Oral Dosage Forms
Note: Bracketed uses in the *Dosage Forms* section refer to categories of use and/or indications that are not included in U.S. product labeling.

## RACEMETHIONINE CAPSULES USP

### Usual adult and adolescent dose
Acidifier, urinary—
Oral, 200 mg three or four times a day. Each dose should be taken with a meal.
[Antidote, to acetaminophen overdose]—
Oral, 2.5 grams every four hours, up to a total dose of 10 grams. The first dose must be given within eight to twelve hours after the toxic ingestion.

### Usual pediatric dose
Acidifier, urinary—
Oral, contents of 1 capsule (200 mg) added to the evening bottle, preferably while it is still warm, or added to a glass of juice or water.
[Antidote, to acetaminophen overdose]—
Children 12 years of age or older: See *Usual adult and adolescent dose.*
Children 3 to 11 years of age: Oral, 1 gram every four hours, up to a total dose of 4 grams. The first dose must be given within eight to twelve hours after the toxic ingestion.
Children up to 3 years of age: Dosage has not been established.

### Usual geriatric dose
See *Usual adult and adolescent dose.*

### Strength(s) usually available
U.S.—
200 mg (Rx) [*M-Caps; Pedameth; Uracid*].
Canada—
Not commercially available.

### Packaging and storage
Store below 40 °C (104 °F), preferably between 15 and 30 °C (59 and 86 °F), unless otherwise specified by manufacturer. Store in a well-closed, light-resistant container.

### Preparation of dosage form
For patients who cannot take oral solids—Contents of capsules may be added to juice, water, or warm milk or infant formula.

## RACEMETHIONINE ORAL SOLUTION

### Usual adult and adolescent dose
See *Racemethionine Capsules USP.*

### Usual pediatric dose
Acidifier, urinary—
Children over 14 months of age: See *Usual adult and adolescent dose.*
Children 6 to 14 months of age: Oral, 75 mg four times a day for three to five days.
Children 2 to 6 months of age: Oral, 75 mg three times a day for three to five days.
Children up to 2 months of age—Dosage has not been established.
Note: In severe cases, or when the infant is older than 1 year of age, the dosage may be doubled for the first two days of treatment.
[Antidote, to acetaminophen overdose]—
See *Racemethionine Capsules USP.*

### Usual geriatric dose
See *Racemethionine Capsules USP.*

### Strength(s) usually available
U.S.—
75 mg per 5 mL (Rx) [*Pedameth*].
Canada—
Not commercially available.

### Packaging and storage
Store below 40 °C (104 °F), preferably between 15 and 30 °C (59 and 86 °F), unless otherwise specified by manufacturer. Store in a well-closed, light-resistant container.

## RACEMETHIONINE TABLETS USP

### Usual adult and adolescent dose
Acidifier, urinary—
Oral, 500 mg three or four times a day. Each dose should be taken with a meal.
[Antidote, to acetaminophen overdose]—
See *Racemethionine Capsules USP.*

### Usual pediatric dose
The capsule or oral solution dosage form is recommended in pediatric patients.

**Usual geriatric dose**
See *Usual adult and adolescent dose.*

**Strength(s) usually available**
U.S.—
 500 mg (Rx) [GENERIC].

Canada—
 Not commercially available.

**Packaging and storage**
Store below 40 °C (104 °F), preferably between 15 and 30 °C (59 and 86 °F), unless otherwise specified by manufacturer. Store in a well-closed, light-resistant container.

**Selected Bibliography**
Lewis RK, Paloucek FP. Assessment and treatment of acetaminophen overdose. Clin Pharm 1991; 10: 765-74.

Developed: 12/05/94

---

# RADIOIODINATED ALBUMIN Systemic

VA CLASSIFICATION (Primary): DX202
Note: For a listing of dosage forms and brand names by country availability, see *Dosage Forms* section(s). For a listing of brand names for the articles in this monograph, refer to the General Index.

## Category
Diagnostic aid, radioactive (fluid and blood loss).

## Indications

### Accepted
Blood and plasma volumes determinations—Iodinated I 125 and I 131 albumin are indicated for use in determinations of total blood and plasma volumes.

### Unaccepted
Radioiodinated albumin has been used in determinations of cardiac and pulmonary blood volumes and circulation times and of cardiac output; in protein turnover studies to help determine gastrointestinal loss of protein. Iodinated I 131 albumin has been used for the delineation of the heart and great vessels; in placenta localization for the detection of placenta previa; and in brain scanning for the localization of cerebral neoplasms. However, these agents generally have been replaced by more effective and/or safer agents for these indications.

## Physical Properties

### Nuclear data

| Radionu-clide (half-life) | Decay constant | Mode of decay | Principal emissions (keV) | Mean number of emissions/ disintegration |
|---|---|---|---|---|
| I 125 (60.14 days) | 0.00048 h⁻¹ | Gamma and x-ray emissions | Gamma (35.0) | 0.067 |
| | | | x-ray (28.0) | 1.40 |
| I 131 (8.08 days) | 0.00358 h⁻¹ | Beta and gamma emissions | Beta (191.6) | 0.90 |
| | | | Gamma (364.4) | 0.81 |

## Pharmacology/Pharmacokinetics

### Mechanism of action/Effect
Human serum albumin occurs naturally as the major protein component of blood. When labeled with iodine I 125 or I 131 and given intravenously, it is distributed throughout the body similarly to the patient's serum albumin, and serves as a suitable tracer with which to determine plasma or blood volume. The radioconcentration can be quantitated in blood samples withdrawn at periodic intervals, after injection of the radioiodinated albumin. Although the gamma emissions of I 131 are suitable for external imaging, the biodistribution of iodinated I 131 albumin is seldom evaluated by *in vivo* imaging.

### Distribution
Radioiodinated serum albumin—Within 10 minutes throughout intravascular pool; more slowly into extravascular space. Can also be detected in the lymph and in certain body tissues within 10 minutes after injection; maximum distribution throughout the extravascular space does not occur until 2 to 4 days following injection.

Radioiodine—Small amount of released iodine I 125 or iodine I 131 (resulting from degradation of radioiodinated albumin) is selectively con-

centrated in thyroid gland; also concentrated in choroid plexus, gastric mucosa, salivary glands, stomach, and lactating breast.

### Radiation dosimetry

**I 125**
Estimated absorbed radiation dose*

| Organ | mGy/MBq | rad/mCi |
|---|---|---|
| Heart | 0.69 | 2.56 |
| Spleen | 0.59 | 2.19 |
| Lungs | 0.57 | 2.11 |
| Red marrow | 0.37 | 1.37 |
| Kidneys | 0.33 | 1.22 |
| Bone surfaces | 0.32 | 1.19 |
| Adrenals | 0.30 | 1.11 |
| Liver | 0.30 | 1.11 |
| Thyroid | 0.26 | 0.96 |
| Pancreas | 0.23 | 0.85 |
| Stomach wall | 0.21 | 0.78 |
| Small intestine | 0.21 | 0.78 |
| Large intestine (upper) | 0.21 | 0.78 |
| Large intestine (lower) | 0.20 | 0.74 |
| Bladder wall | 0.20 | 0.74 |
| Breast | 0.20 | 0.74 |
| Ovaries | 0.20 | 0.74 |
| Uterus | 0.20 | 0.74 |
| Testes | 0.16 | 0.59 |
| Other tissue | 0.19 | 0.70 |

Effective dose: 0.34 mSv/MBq (1.26 rem/mCi)

*For adults; intravenous injection

**I 131**
Estimated absorbed radiation dose*

| Organ | mGy/MBq | rad/mCi |
|---|---|---|
| Heart | 1.9 | 7.03 |
| Lungs | 1.5 | 5.55 |
| Spleen | 1.5 | 5.55 |
| Bone surfaces | 0.97 | 3.59 |
| Adrenals | 0.94 | 3.59 |
| Kidneys | 0.88 | 3.26 |
| Liver | 0.72 | 2.66 |
| Thyroid | 0.70 | 2.59 |
| Red marrow | 0.66 | 2.44 |
| Breast | 0.55 | 2.04 |
| Stomach wall | 0.53 | 1.96 |
| Small intestine | 0.52 | 1.92 |
| Large intestine (upper) | 0.52 | 1.92 |
| Uterus | 0.51 | 1.89 |
| Large intestine (lower) | 0.50 | 1.85 |
| Ovaries | 0.49 | 1.81 |
| Bladder wall | 0.49 | 1.81 |
| Testes | 0.46 | 1.70 |
| Other tissue | 0.47 | 1.74 |

Effective dose: 0.86 mSv/MBq (3.18 rem/mCi)

*For adults; intravenous injection

### Half-time:
Normal human serum albumin—Approximately 14 days (range, 10 to 20 days); dependent on initial rate of excretion, which is determined by the quality of the labeled albumin.

### Elimination
Primarily renal; about 2% eliminated in feces.

# Precautions to Consider

## Cross-sensitivity and/or related problems

Patients sensitive to human serum albumin–containing products may be sensitive to these products also.

## Pregnancy/Reproduction

Pregnancy—Iodine I 125 and I 131 cross the placenta and may cause severe and irreversible hypothyroidism in the fetus; the fetal thyroid begins to concentrate iodine during approximately the 12th week of gestation. Radioiodinated albumin is usually not recommended for use during pregnancy; however, if used, prior administration of potassium iodide (e.g., Lugol's solution or SSKI) may reduce the risk of fetal thyroid irradiation.

The possibility of pregnancy should be assessed in women of child-bearing potential. Clinical situations exist where the benefit to the patient and fetus, based on information derived from radiopharmaceutical use, outweighs the risks from fetal exposure to radiation. In these situations, the physician should use discretion and reduce the radiopharmaceutical dose to the lowest possible amount.

*Radioiodinated albumin—*
> Studies have not been done in humans with either iodinated I 131 albumin or iodinated I 125 albumin.
> Studies have not been done in animals.

FDA Pregnancy Category C.

## Breast-feeding

Iodine I 125 and I 131 are distributed into breast milk. Because of the potential risk to the infant from radiation exposure, temporary discontinuation of nursing is recommended for a length of time that may be assessed by measuring the activity of breast milk and estimating the radiation exposure to the infant.

## Pediatrics

Although radioiodinated albumin is used in children, there have been no specific studies evaluating its safety and efficacy in children. When this radiopharmaceutical is used in children, the diagnostic benefit should be judged to outweigh the potential risk of radiation.

## Geriatrics

Appropriate studies on the relationship of age to the effects of radioiodinated albumin have not been performed in the geriatric population. However, no geriatrics-specific problems have been documented to date.

## Diagnostic interference

The following have been selected on the basis of their potential clinical significance (possible effect in parentheses where appropriate)—not necessarily inclusive (» = major clinical significance):

With *other* diagnostic test results
  Thyroid function determinations and
  Thyroid imaging
    (potassium iodide [e.g., Lugol's solution] used prior to the administration of radioiodinated albumin may cause a decrease in radioactive iodine or pertechnetate ion uptake for several weeks)

## Medical considerations/Contraindications

The medical considerations/contraindications included here have been selected on the basis of their potential clinical significance (reasons given in parentheses where appropriate)—not necessarily inclusive (» = major clinical significance).

*Risk-benefit should be considered when the following medical problem exists:*
> Sensitivity to human serum albumin-containing products

# Side/Adverse Effects

Presently, there are no known side/adverse effects associated with the use of iodinated I 125 or I 131 albumin as a diagnostic aid. However, as with any protein-containing preparation, allergic reactions are possible.

# Patient Consultation

As an aid to patient consultation, refer to *Advice for the Patient, Radiopharmaceuticals (Diagnostic).*

In providing consultation, consider emphasizing the following selected information (» = major clinical significance):

## Description of use

Action in the body: Radioactive albumin's distribution in body same as normal albumin

Dilution of radioactivity in blood pool permits calculation of its volume
Small amounts of radioactivity used in diagnosis; radiation received is low and considered safe

## Before having this test

> Conditions affecting use, especially:
> Sensitivity to human serum albumin
> Pregnancy—Risk to fetus from radiation exposure as opposed to benefit derived from use should be considered; possibility of hypothyroidism in fetus
> Breast-feeding—Iodine I 125 and I 131 are distributed into breast milk; temporary discontinuation of nursing recommended because of risk to infant from radiation exposure
> Use in children—Risk from radiation exposure as opposed to benefit derived from use should be considered

## Preparation for this test

Special preparatory instructions may be given; patient should inquire in advance

## Precautions after having this test

Possible interference with future thyroid tests

## Side/adverse effects

No side/adverse effects reported; allergic reactions are possible

# General Dosing Information

Radiopharmaceuticals are to be administered only by or under the supervision of physicians who have had extensive training in the safe use and handling of radioactive materials and who are authorized by the Nuclear Regulatory Commission (NRC) or the appropriate Federal or Agreement State agency, if required or, outside the U.S., the appropriate authority.

Epinephrine, antihistamines, and corticosteroid agents should be available during the administration of radioiodinated albumin because of the possibility of allergic reactions.

To minimize the uptake of radioactive iodine by the thyroid, potassium iodide (e.g., Lugol's solution or SSKI) may be used one to three times daily, beginning at least 24 hours before and continuing for one or two weeks after administration of radioiodinated albumin.

## Safety considerations for handling this radiopharmaceutical

Improper handling of this radiopharmaceutical may cause radioactive contamination. Guidelines for handling radioactive material have been prepared by scientific, professional, state, federal, and international bodies and are available to the specially qualified and authorized users who have access to radiopharmaceuticals.

# Parenteral Dosage Forms

## IODINATED I 125 ALBUMIN INJECTION USP

### Usual adult and adolescent administered activity

Total blood and plasma volume determinations—
  Intravenous, 0.185 to 1.85 megabecquerels (5 to 50 microcuries).

> Note: For repeat blood volume determinations, the total dosage per week should not exceed 7.4 megabecquerels (200 microcuries).
>
> See manufacturer's package instructions for preparation of the reference solution and for formula used in the calculation of blood and plasma volumes.

### Usual pediatric administered activity

Dosage must be individualized by physician.

### Usual geriatric administered activity

See *Usual adult and adolescent administered activity.*

### Size(s) usually available

U.S.—
  At time of calibration: Per single-dose syringe
    0.37 megabecquerel (10 microcuries) per 1.5 mL (Rx) [*IHSA I 125*].
  At time of calibration: Per multiple-dose vial
    37 megabecquerels (1 millicurie) (Rx) [*Jeanatope*].
Canada—
  Content information not available at present (Rx) [GENERIC].

### Packaging and storage

Store between 2 and 8 °C (36 and 46 °F). Protect from freezing.

### Note

Caution—Radioactive material.

**IODINATED I 131 ALBUMIN INJECTION USP**

**Usual adult and adolescent administered activity**
Total blood and plasma volume determinations—
   Intravenous, 0.185 to 1.85 megabecquerels (5 to 50 microcuries).

   Note: For repeat blood volume determinations, the total dosage per
      week should not exceed 7.4 megabecquerels (200 microcuries).

      See manufacturer's package instructions for preparation of the
      reference solution and for formula used in the calculation of
      blood and plasma volumes.

**Usual pediatric administered activity**
Dosage must be individualized by physician.

**Usual geriatric administered activity**
See *Usual adult and adolescent administered activity.*

**Size(s) usually available**
U.S.—
   At time of calibration: Per multiple-dose vial
      37 megabecquerels (1 millicurie) per mL (Rx) [*Megatope*].
Canada—
   At time of calibration: Per multiple-dose vial

0.185 to 0.555 megabecquerels (5 to 15 microcuries) per mL (Rx)
   [GENERIC].
3.7 to 37 megabecquerels (0.1 to 1 millicurie) per mL (Rx)
   [GENERIC].

**Packaging and storage**
Store between 2 and 8 °C (36 and 46 °F). Protect from freezing.

**Note**
Caution—Radioactive material.

Revised: 07/20/93
Interim revision: 08/02/94

---

**RAMIPRIL**—See *Angiotensin-converting Enzyme (ACE) Inhibitors
   (Systemic)*

---

**RANITIDINE**—See *Histamine H₂-receptor Antagonists (Systemic)*

---

# RAUWOLFIA ALKALOIDS   Systemic

This monograph includes information on the following: Deserpidine†;
Rauwolfia Serpentina†; Reserpine.

VA CLASSIFICATION (Primary): CV490

Note: For a listing of dosage forms and brand names by country availability, see *Dosage Forms* section(s). For a listing of brand names
   for the articles in this monograph, refer to the General Index.

   †Not commercially available in Canada.

## Category

Antihypertensive; vasospastic therapy adjunct.

## Indications

Note: Bracketed information in the *Indications* section refers to uses that
   are not included in U.S. product labeling.

**Accepted**
Hypertension (treatment)—Rauwolfia alkaloids are indicated in the treatment of hypertension.

   For additional information on initial therapeutic guidelines related to
   the treatment of hypertension, see *Appendix III.*

[Raynaud's phenomenon (treatment)]¹—Reserpine has also been used to
   treat Raynaud's phenomenon.

**Unaccepted**
Rauwolfia alkaloids have been used for relief of symptoms in agitated
   psychotic states such as schizophrenia; however, use as antipsychotics
   and sedatives has been superseded by use of more effective, safer
   agents.

   ¹Not included in Canadian product labeling.

## Pharmacology/Pharmacokinetics

Note: Information (except physicochemical characteristics) available only
   for reserpine.

**Physicochemical characteristics**
Molecular weight—
   Reserpine: 608.69.
pKa—
   Deserpidine: 5.67.
   Reserpine: 6.6.

**Mechanism of action/Effect**
Acts at postganglionic sympathetic nerve endings; depletes tissue and central nervous system (CNS) stores of catecholamines and serotonin;
   antihypertensive activity thought to be due to reduced cardiac output
   and possibly some decrease in peripheral resistance.

**Absorption**
Reserpine is readily absorbed after oral administration.

**Protein binding**
None (bound to sites involved with storage of biogenic amines; may persist in body for several days).

**Biotransformation**
Hepatic.

**Half-life**
Normal—
   Initial: 4.5 hours.
   Terminal: 45 to 168 hours.
Anuric—
   Terminal: 87 to 323 hours.

**Onset of action**
Antihypertensive—Oral: Several days to 3 weeks (multiple doses).
Catecholamine depletion—Within 1 hour (single dose).

**Time to peak effect**
Antihypertensive—Oral: 3 to 6 weeks (multiple doses).
Catecholamine depletion—Within 24 hours (single dose).

**Duration of action**
Antihypertensive—Oral: 1 to 6 weeks.

**Elimination**
Fecal—More than 60%, mainly unchanged, in 4 days.
Renal—8%, less than 1% unchanged, in 4 days.

## Precautions to Consider

**Cross-sensitivity and/or related problems**
Patients sensitive to one rauwolfia alkaloid may be sensitive to other rauwolfia alkaloids also.

**Carcinogenicity/Tumorigenicity**
The suggestion that long-term use of reserpine (and also, presumably,
   other rauwolfia alkaloids) may increase the risk of breast cancer in
   postmenopausal women has been controversial. A few epidemiologic
   studies have suggested a slightly increased risk of breast cancer in
   women who have used reserpine. However, other studies have not
   confirmed this finding.
Studies in rats and mice at 100 to 300 times the usual human dose found
   an increased incidence of mammary fibroadenomas in females, and
   malignant tumors of the seminal vesicles and malignant adrenal medullary tumors in males.

**Pregnancy/Reproduction**
Fertility—Long-term animal studies have not been done with the rauwolfia
   alkaloids to determine their effect on fertility in males or females.

Pregnancy—Rauwolfia alkaloids cross the placenta. Adequate and well-
   controlled studies have not been done in humans. However, possible
   adverse effects in infants of mothers who received rauwolfia alkaloids
   include increased respiratory secretions, nasal congestion, cyanosis
   and anorexia.

Reserpine was found to be teratogenic in rats given parenteral doses of up to 2 mg per kg of body weight (mg/kg) and was embryocidal in guinea pigs given parenteral doses of 0.5 mg per day.

FDA Pregnancy Category C.

### Breast-feeding

Problems in humans have not been documented. However, rauwolfia alkaloids are distributed into breast milk. Possible adverse effects in infants of mothers who received rauwolfia alkaloids include increased respiratory secretions, nasal congestion, cyanosis, and anorexia.

### Pediatrics

Appropriate studies on the relationship of age to the effects of the rauwolfia alkaloids have not been performed in the pediatric population. However, pediatrics-specific problems that would limit the usefulness of these medications in children are not expected.

### Geriatrics

Although appropriate studies on the relationship of age to the effects of the rauwolfia alkaloids have not been performed in the geriatric population, the elderly may be more sensitive to the CNS depressant and hypotensive effects. In addition, elderly patients are more likely to have age-related renal function impairment, which may require caution in patients receiving rauwolfia alkaloids. A lower dose is recommended in the elderly.

### Dental

Use of rauwolfia alkaloids may decrease or inhibit salivary flow, thus contributing to the development of caries, periodontal disease, oral candidiasis, and discomfort.

### Drug interactions and/or related problems

The following drug interactions and/or related problems have been selected on the basis of their potential clinical significance (possible mechanism in parentheses where appropriate)—not necessarily inclusive (» = major clinical significance):

Note: Combinations containing any of the following medications, depending on the amount present, may also interact with this medication.

Alcohol or

CNS depression–producing medications (See *Appendix II*)
(concurrent use may enhance the CNS depressant effects of either these medications or rauwolfia alkaloids)

Anti-inflammatory drugs, nonsteroidal (NSAIDs), especially indomethacin
(antihypertensive effects of rauwolfia alkaloids may be reduced when used concurrently with these agents; indomethacin, and possibly other NSAIDs, may antagonize the antihypertensive effect by inhibiting renal prostaglandin synthesis and/or by causing sodium and fluid retention; the patient should be carefully monitored to confirm that the desired effect is being obtained)

Anticholinergics or other medications with anticholinergic action (See *Appendix II*)
(concurrent use of rauwolfia alkaloids may antagonize the inhibitory action of these medications on gastric acid secretion)

Beta-adrenergic blocking agents, including ophthalmic beta-blockers absorbed systemically
(concurrent administration with beta-blockers may result in additive and possibly excessive beta-adrenergic blockade; although this effect is largely theoretical, close observation is recommended since bradycardia and hypotension may occur)

Bromocriptine
(reserpine may increase serum prolactin concentrations, and interfere with effects of bromocriptine; dosage adjustment of bromocriptine may be necessary)

Digitalis glycosides or
Quinidine
(concurrent use may result in cardiac arrhythmias; although this interaction is controversial and does not appear to be significant with usual doses, caution is recommended, especially when large doses of rauwolfia alkaloids are used in digitalized patients)

Estrogens
(concurrent use may decrease the antihypertensive effect of rauwolfia alkaloids because estrogen-induced fluid retention may lead to increased blood pressure)

Extrapyramidal reaction–causing medications, other (See *Appendix II*)
(concurrent use with rauwolfia alkaloids may potentiate the extrapyramidal effects)

Hypotension-producing medications, other, except MAO inhibitors (See *Appendix II*)
(antihypertensive effects may be potentiated when these medications are used concurrently with rauwolfia alkaloids; although

some combinations are frequently used for therapeutic advantage, when used concurrently dosage adjustments may be necessary)
(concurrent use of guanadrel or guanethidine with rauwolfia alkaloids may cause an increased incidence of orthostatic hypotension or bradycardia)

Levodopa
(rauwolfia alkaloids may cause dopamine depletion and parkinsonian effects, decreasing the therapeutic effects of levodopa; dosage adjustments of either or both medications may be necessary)

» Monoamine oxidase (MAO) inhibitors, including furazolidone, procarbazine, and selegiline
(when an MAO inhibitor is added to existing therapy with rauwolfia alkaloids, serious potentiation of CNS depressant effect may result; however, if a rauwolfia alkaloid is added to an MAO inhibitor regimen, excessive stimulation of receptors caused by the sudden release of accumulated norepinephrine and serotonin may result in moderate to sudden and severe hypertension and hyperpyrexia, which can reach crisis levels; administration of rauwolfia alkaloids is not recommended during and for 1 week following MAO inhibitor therapy)

*Sympathomimetics*
(antihypertensive effects of rauwolfia alkaloids may be reduced when used concurrently with these agents; the patient should be carefully monitored to confirm that the desired effect is being obtained)
Indirect-acting amines, such as amphetamines, phenylpropanolamine, pseudoephedrine, and tyramine, or
Direct- and indirect-acting (primarily indirect-acting) amines, such as ephedrine and mephentermine
(rauwolfia alkaloids inhibit the action of indirect-acting sympathomimetics by depleting catecholamine stores)

Direct-acting amines such as epinephrine or norepinephrine (levarterenol) or
Direct- and indirect-acting (primarily direct-acting) amines such as appetite suppressants (except fenfluramine), dobutamine, dopamine, metaraminol, methoxamine, and phenylephrine
(rauwolfia alkaloids may theoretically prolong the action of direct-acting sympathomimetics by preventing uptake into storage granules; a "denervation supersensitivity" response is also possible; although concurrent use with rauwolfia alkaloids is not known to produce severe adverse effects, a significant increase in blood pressure has been documented when phenylephrine ophthalmic drops have been administered to patients taking reserpine, and caution and close observation are recommended; on the other hand, concurrent use with fenfluramine may increase the hypotensive effects of rauwolfia alkaloids)

### Laboratory value alterations

The following have been selected on the basis of their potential clinical significance (possible effect in parentheses where appropriate)—not necessarily inclusive (» = major clinical significance):

With diagnostic test results
Urinary steroid colorimetric determinations by modified Glenn-Nelson technique or Holtorff Koch modification of Zimmerman reaction
(falsely low because rauwolfia alkaloids slightly decrease absorbance)

With physiology/laboratory test values
Catecholamine excretion, urinary
(an overall decrease is usually noted with chronic administration of rauwolfia alkaloids)

Prolactin concentrations, serum
(may be increased)

Vanillylmandelic acid (VMA), urinary excretion
(chronic administration of rauwolfia alkaloids results in an overall decrease)

### Medical considerations/Contraindications

The medical considerations/contraindications included here have been selected on the basis of their potential clinical significance (reasons given in parentheses where appropriate)—not necessarily inclusive (» = major clinical significance).

*Risk-benefit should be considered when the following medical problems exist:*

Cardiac arrhythmias

Cardiac depression

Epilepsy

» Gallstones or
» Peptic ulcer or
» Ulcerative colitis
    (rauwolfia alkaloids increase gastrointestinal motility and secretion; may precipitate biliary colic)
» Mental depression, or history of
Parkinsonism
Pheochromocytoma
Renal function impairment
    (patients with renal insufficiency may adjust poorly to reduced blood pressure levels. However, dosage reduction is not necessary in these patients)
Respiratory problems
Sensitivity to the rauwolfia alkaloid prescribed
» Caution is required also in patients receiving electroconvulsive therapy, as well as in the severely debilitated.

**Patient monitoring**

The following may be especially important in patient monitoring (other tests may be warranted in some patients, depending on condition; » = major clinical significance):

» Blood pressure measurements
    (recommended at periodic intervals in patients being treated for hypertension; selected patients may be trained to perform blood pressure measurements at home and report the results at regular physician visits)

## Side/Adverse Effects

Note: Side effects occur more frequently with high-dose administration.

The following side/adverse effects have been selected on the basis of their potential clinical significance (possible cause in parentheses where appropriate)—not necessarily inclusive:

**Those indicating need for medical attention**
Incidence more frequent
    *Dizziness*
Incidence less frequent
    *Arrhythmias* (irregular heartbeat); *black, tarry stools; bloody vomit, stomach cramps or pain; bradycardia* (slow heartbeat); *chest pain; drowsiness or faintness; headache; impotence or decreased sexual interest; lack of energy or weakness; mental depression or inability to concentrate; nervousness or anxiety; shortness of breath; vivid dreams or nightmares or early-morning sleeplessness*
    Note: *CNS* effects are dose-related, occurring more frequently with doses exceeding 500 mcg (0.5 mg) per day.
Incidence rare
    *Painful or difficult urination; skin rash or itching; stiffness or trembling and shaking of hands and fingers; thrombocytopenia* (unusual bleeding or bruising)

**Those indicating need for medical attention only if they continue or are bothersome**
Incidence more frequent
    *Anorexia* (loss of appetite); *diarrhea; dryness of mouth; nasal congestion* (stuffy nose); *nausea and vomiting*
Incidence less frequent
    *Edema, peripheral* (swelling of feet and lower legs)

**Those indicating the need for medical attention if they occur after medication is discontinued**
    *Arrhythmias* (irregular heartbeat); *bradycardia* (slow heartbeat); *drowsiness or faintness; impotence or decreased sexual interest; lack of energy or weakness; mental depression or inability to concentrate; nervousness or anxiety; vivid dreams or nightmares or early-morning sleeplessness*
    Note: *Mental depression* may have an insidious onset, may be severe enough to cause suicide, and may persist for several months following withdrawal of this medication.

## Overdose

For more information on the management of overdose or unintentional ingestion, **contact a Poison Control Center** (see *Poison Control Center Listing*).

**Clinical effects of overdose**
The following effects have been selected on the basis of their potential clinical significance (possible signs and symptoms in parentheses where appropriate)—not necessarily inclusive:

    *Dizziness or drowsiness, severe; flushing of skin; pinpoint pupils of eyes; slow pulse*

**Treatment of overdose**
Immediate evacuation of the stomach and instillation of an activated charcoal slurry.

Supportive, symptomatic treatment.

If treatment with a vasopressor is necessary, one with a direct action on smooth muscle (phenylephrine, norepinephrine, metaraminol) should be used.

The patient should be observed for at least 72 hours.

## Patient Consultation

As an aid to patient consultation, refer to *Advice for the Patient, Rauwolfia Alkaloids (Systemic)*.

In providing consultation, consider emphasizing the following selected information (» = major clinical significance):

**Before using this medication**
» Conditions affecting use, especially:
    Sensitivity to any of the rauwolfia alkaloids
    Pregnancy—Teratogenic in animals
    Breast-feeding—Distributed into breast milk
    Use in the elderly—May be more sensitive to the CNS depressant and hypotensive effects
    Dental—May decrease or inhibit salivary flow
    Other medications, especially monoamine oxidase (MAO) inhibitors
    Other medical problems, especially gallstones, peptic ulcer, ulcerative colitis, or mental depression

**Proper use of this medication**
    Possible need for control of weight and diet, especially sodium intake
» Patient may not experience symptoms of hypertension; importance of taking medication even if feeling well
» Does not cure but helps control hypertension; possible need for life-long therapy; serious consequences of untreated hypertension
    Getting into the habit of taking at same time each day to help increase compliance
    Caution in taking combination therapy; taking each medication at the right time
    Taking with meals or milk to reduce gastrointestinal irritation
» Proper dosing
    Missed dose: Not taking missed dose at all and not doubling doses
» Proper storage

**Precautions while using this medication**
    Regular visits to physician to check progress
» Not taking other medications, especially nonprescription sympathomimetics, unless discussed with physician
» Caution if any kind of surgery (including dental surgery) or emergency treatment is required
» Caution if depression or changes in sleep pattern occur
» Caution in taking alcohol or other CNS depressants
» Caution when driving or doing things requiring alertness because of possible drowsiness or dizziness
    Possible dryness of mouth; using sugarless candy or gum, ice, or saliva substitute for relief; checking with physician or dentist if dry mouth continues for more than 2 weeks
    Nasal stuffiness may occur; nasal decongestants or other OTC preparations containing sympathomimetics should not be used without first consulting physician or pharmacist

**Side/adverse effects**
    Dizziness, arrhythmias, bradycardia, black, tarry stools, bloody vomit, chest pain, drowsiness or faintness, headache, impotence or decreased sexual interest, lack of energy or weakness, mental depression or inability to concentrate, nervousness or anxiety, vivid dreams or nightmares or early-morning sleeplessness, shortness of breath

## General Dosing Information

Dosage must be adjusted to meet the individual requirements of each patient, on the basis of clinical response, with the lowest effective dosage being utilized in order to minimize problems with mental depression, orthostatic hypotension, and other side effects.

Rauwolfia alkaloids are usually used in combination with a diuretic to prevent sodium and water retention.

A lower dose is recommended in the elderly or severely debilitated.

Doses higher than the recommended dose should be used with caution because of the risk of severe mental depression.

Antihypertensive effects of rauwolfia alkaloids may not be observed for a few days to several weeks after oral administration and may persist for 1 to 6 weeks after withdrawal of the medication. It is recommended that adjustments in dosage be made every 7 to 14 days to allow the full effects of the preceding dose to occur.

It is recommended that this medication be withdrawn at the first sign of despondency, early-morning insomnia, loss of appetite, impotence, or self-deprecation.

It is recommended that rauwolfia alkaloids be withdrawn 2 weeks before electroconvulsive therapy is employed.

Recent evidence suggests that withdrawal of catecholamine-depleting antihypertensive therapy prior to surgery is not necessary, but that the anesthesiologist must be aware of such therapy. Administration of atropine prior to induction may prevent excessive bradycardia. If a hypotensive episode occurs, use of a weak direct-acting sympathomimetic agent is recommended.

**Diet/Nutrition**

It is recommended that these medications be taken with food or milk to minimize gastrointestinal upset.

## DESERPIDINE

## Oral Dosage Forms

**DESERPIDINE TABLETS**

**Usual adult dose**

Antihypertensive—
Oral, 250 to 500 mcg (0.25 to 0.5 mg) a day as a single dose or in two divided daily doses.

Note: Geriatric patients may be more sensitive to the effects of the usual adult dose.

**Usual pediatric dose**

Dosage has not been established.

**Strength(s) usually available**

U.S.—
250 mcg (0.25 mg) (Rx) [*Harmonyl*].

Canada—
Not commercially available.

**Packaging and storage**

Store below 40 °C (104 °F), preferably between 15 and 30 °C (59 and 86 °F). Store in a tight container. Protect from light.

**Auxiliary labeling**

• Take with meals or milk.
• Do not take other medicines without your doctor's advice.

**Note**

Check refill frequency to determine compliance in hypertensive patients.

## RAUWOLFIA SERPENTINA

## Oral Dosage Forms

**RAUWOLFIA SERPENTINA TABLETS USP**

**Usual adult dose**

Antihypertensive—
Oral, 50 to 200 mg a day as a single dose or in two divided daily doses.

Note: Geriatric patients may be more sensitive to the effects of the usual adult dose.

**Usual pediatric dose**

Dosage has not been established.

**Strength(s) usually available**

U.S.—
50 mg (Rx) [*Raudixin; Rauval; Rauverid;* GENERIC].
100 mg (Rx) [*Raudixin; Rauval; Wolfina;* GENERIC].

Canada—
Not commercially available.

**Packaging and storage**

Store below 40 °C (104 °F), preferably between 15 and 30 °C (59 and 86 °F). Store in a tight, light-resistant container.

**Auxiliary labeling**

• Take with meals or milk.
• Do not take other medicines without your doctor's advice.

**Note**

Check refill frequency to determine compliance in hypertensive patients.

## RESERPINE

## Oral Dosage Forms

Note: Bracketed uses in the *Dosage Forms* section refer to categories of use and/or indications that are not included in U.S. product labeling.

**RESERPINE TABLETS USP**

**Usual adult dose**

Antihypertensive or
[Vasospastic therapy adjunct—Raynaud's phenomenon][1]—
Oral, 100 to 250 mcg (0.1 to 0.25 mg) a day.

Note: Geriatric patients may be more sensitive to the effects of the usual adult dose.

**Usual pediatric dose**

Antihypertensive—
Oral, 5 to 20 mcg (0.005 to 0.02 mg) per kg of body weight or 150 to 600 mcg (0.15 to 0.6 mg) per square meter of body surface a day in one or two divided daily doses.

**Strength(s) usually available**

U.S.—
100 mcg (0.1 mg) (Rx) [*Serpalan;* GENERIC].
250 mcg (0.25 mg) (Rx) [*Serpalan;* GENERIC].
1 mg (Rx) [GENERIC].

Canada—
250 mcg (0.25 mg) (Rx) [*Novoreserpine; Reserfia; Serpasil;* GENERIC].

**Packaging and storage**

Store below 40 °C (104 °F), preferably between 15 and 30 °C (59 and 86 °F). Store in a tight, light-resistant container.

**Auxiliary labeling**

• Take with meals or milk.
• Do not take other medicines without your doctor's advice.

**Note**

Check refill frequency to determine compliance in hypertensive patients.

[1]Not included in Canadian product labeling.

## Selected Bibliography

The fifth report of the Joint National Committee on Detection, Evaluation, and Treatment of High Blood Pressure (JNC V). Arch Intern Med 1993; 153 (2): 154-83.

Revised: 07/28/92
Interim revision: 07/20/94

# RAUWOLFIA ALKALOIDS AND THIAZIDE DIURETICS   Systemic

This monograph includes information on the following: Deserpidine and Hydrochlorothiazide; Deserpidine and Methyclothiazide; Rauwolfia Serpentina and Bendroflumethiazide; Reserpine and Chlorothiazide; Reserpine and Chlorthalidone; Reserpine and Hydrochlorothiazide; Reserpine and Hydroflumethiazide; Reserpine and Methyclothiazide; Reserpine and Polythiazide; Reserpine and Trichlormethiazide.

VA CLASSIFICATION (Primary): CV400

NOTE: The *Rauwolfia Alkaloids and Thiazide Diuretics (Systemic)* monograph is maintained on the USP DI electronic data base. For a printed copy of the most recent revision of the complete monograph, contact the USP Division of Information Development, 12601 Twinbrook Parkway, Rockville, MD 20852.

For information on the specific components of this combination, see the *USP DI* monographs for *Diuretics, Thiazide (Systemic)* and *Rauwolfia Alkaloids (Systemic)*.

The information that follows is selectively abstracted from the complete monograph and is provided to facilitate drug use review and patient counseling.

Note: For a listing of dosage forms and brand names by country availability, see *Dosage Forms* section(s). For a listing of brand names for the articles in this monograph, refer to the General Index.

# Category

Antihypertensive.

# Indications

## Accepted

Hypertension (treatment)—This combination is indicated for treatment of hypertension.

Fixed-dosage combinations are generally not recommended for initial therapy and are useful for subsequent therapy only when the proportion of the component agents corresponds to the dose of the individual agents, as determined by titration.

For additional information on initial therapeutic guidelines related to the treatment of hypertension, see *Appendix III*.

# Patient Consultation

As an aid to patient consultation, refer to *Advice for the Patient, Rauwolfia Alkaloids and Thiazide Diuretics (Systemic)*.

In providing consultation, consider emphasizing the following selected information (» = major clinical significance):

### Before using this medication
» Conditions affecting use, especially:
  Sensitivity to rauwolfia alkaloids, thiazide diuretics, other sulfonamide-type medications, bumetanide, furosemide, or carbonic anhydrase inhibitors
  Pregnancy—Reserpine is teratogenic in animals; thiazide diuretics are not recommended for routine use and may cause jaundice, thrombocytopenia, hypokalemia in infant
  Breast-feeding—Reserpine and thiazide diuretics are distributed into breast milk; recommended that nursing mothers avoid thiazide diuretics during first month of breast-feeding because of reports of suppression of lactation
  Use in the elderly—May be more sensitive to the hypotensive and electrolyte effects
  Other medications, especially monoamine oxidase (MAO) inhibitors, cholestyramine, colestipol, digitalis glycosides, or lithium
  Other medical problems, especially gallstones, peptic ulcer, ulcerative colitis, mental depression, or anuria or severe renal function impairment

### Proper use of this medication
  Possible need for control of weight and diet, especially sodium intake
» Patient may not experience symptoms of hypertension; importance of taking medication even if feeling well
» Does not cure, but helps control hypertension; possible need for lifelong therapy; serious consequences of untreated hypertension
  Diuretic effects of medications and timing of doses to minimize inconvenience of diuresis
  Getting into habit of taking at same time each day to help increase compliance
  Taking with meals or milk to reduce gastrointestinal irritation
» Proper dosing
  Missed dose: Taking as soon as possible; not taking if almost time for next dose; not doubling doses
» Proper storage

### Precautions while using this medication
  Regular visits to physician to check progress
» Not taking other medications, especially nonprescription sympathomimetics, unless discussed with physician
» Caution if any kind of surgery (including dental surgery) or emergency treatment is required
  Possibility of hypokalemia; possible need for additional potassium in diet; not changing diet without first checking with physician
  To prevent dehydration, checking with physician if severe nausea, vomiting, or diarrhea occurs and continues
» Caution when driving or doing things requiring alertness because of possible drowsiness or dizziness
» Caution if orthostatic hypotension occurs
» Caution if depression or changes in sleep pattern occur
» Caution in taking alcohol or other central nervous system (CNS) depressants
  Diabetics: May increase blood sugar levels
  Possible photosensitivity; avoiding unprotected exposure to sun; using protective clothing and sun block product; avoiding use of sunlamp, tanning bed, or tanning booth

Nasal stuffiness may occur; nasal decongestants or other OTC preparations containing sympathomimetics should not be used without first consulting physician or pharmacist
Possible dryness of mouth; using sugarless candy or gum, ice, or saliva substitute for relief; checking with physician or dentist if dry mouth continues for more than 2 weeks

### Side/adverse effects
  Signs and symptoms of potential side effects, especially electrolyte imbalance, agranulocytosis, allergic reaction, cholecystitis, pancreatitis, hepatic function impairment, hyperuricemia, gout, thrombocytopenia, dizziness, arrhythmias, bradycardia, black tarry stools, bloody vomit, chest pain, drowsiness or faintness, headache, impotence or decreased sexual interest, lack of energy or weakness, mental depression or inability to concentrate, nervousness or anxiety, vivid dreams or nightmares or early-morning sleeplessness, and shortness of breath

---

## DESERPIDINE AND HYDROCHLOROTHIAZIDE

# Oral Dosage Forms

## DESERPIDINE AND HYDROCHLOROTHIAZIDE TABLETS

### Usual adult dose
Antihypertensive—
  Oral, 1 tablet two times a day as determined by individual titration with the component agents.

Note: Geriatric patients may be more sensitive to the effects of the usual adult dose.

### Usual pediatric dose
Dosage has not been established.

### Strength(s) usually available
U.S.—
  125 mcg (0.125 mg) of deserpidine and 25 mg of hydrochlorothiazide (Rx) [*Oreticyl*].
  125 mcg (0.125 mg) of deserpidine and 50 mg of hydrochlorothiazide (Rx) [*Oreticyl*].
  250 mcg (0.25 mg) of deserpidine and 25 mg of hydrochlorothiazide (Rx) [*Oreticyl Forte*].
Canada—
  Not commercially available.

### Auxiliary labeling
· Take with meals or milk.
· Do not take other medicines without your doctor's advice.

---

## DESERPIDINE AND METHYCLOTHIAZIDE

# Oral Dosage Forms

## DESERPIDINE AND METHYCLOTHIAZIDE TABLETS

### Usual adult dose
Antihypertensive—
  Oral, ¹/₂ to 1 tablet a day as determined by individual titration with the component agents.

Note: Geriatric patients may be more sensitive to the effects of the usual adult dose.

### Usual pediatric dose
Dosage has not been established.

### Strength(s) usually available
U.S.—
  250 mcg (0.25 mg) of deserpidine and 5 mg of methyclothiazide (Rx) [*Enduronyl*].
  500 mcg (0.5 mg) of deserpidine and 5 mg of methyclothiazide (Rx) [*Enduronyl Forte;* GENERIC].
Canada—
  250 mcg (0.25 mg) of deserpidine and 5 mg of methyclothiazide (Rx) [*Dureticyl*].

### Auxiliary labeling
· Take with meals or milk.
· Do not take other medicines without your doctor's advice.

## *RAUWOLFIA SERPENTINA AND BENDROFLUMETHIAZIDE*

# Oral Dosage Forms

## RAUWOLFIA SERPENTINA AND BENDROFLUMETHIAZIDE TABLETS

### Usual adult dose
Antihypertensive—
> Oral, 1 to 4 tablets a day as determined by individual titration with the component agents.

Note: Geriatric patients may be more sensitive to the effects of the usual adult dose.

### Usual pediatric dose
Dosage has not been established.

### Strength(s) usually available
U.S.—
> 50 mg of rauwolfia serpentina and 4 mg of bendroflumethiazide (Rx) [*Rauzide*].

Canada—
> Not commercially available.

### Auxiliary labeling
* Take with meals or milk.
* Do not take other medicines without your doctor's advice.

## *RESERPINE AND CHLOROTHIAZIDE*

# Oral Dosage Forms

## RESERPINE AND CHLOROTHIAZIDE TABLETS USP

### Usual adult dose
Antihypertensive—
> Oral, 1 or 2 tablets one or two times a day as determined by individual titration with the component agents.

Note: Geriatric patients may be more sensitive to the effects of the usual adult dose.

### Usual pediatric dose
Dosage has not been established.

### Strength(s) usually available
U.S.—
> 125 mcg (0.125 mg) of reserpine and 250 mg of chlorothiazide (Rx) [*Diupres; Diurigen with Reserpine;* GENERIC].
> 125 mcg (0.125 mg) of reserpine and 500 mg of chlorothiazide (Rx) [*Diupres;* GENERIC].

Canada—
> Not commercially available.

### Auxiliary labeling
* Take with meals or milk.
* Do not take other medicines without your doctor's advice.

## *RESERPINE AND CHLORTHALIDONE*

# Oral Dosage Forms

## RESERPINE AND CHLORTHALIDONE TABLETS

### Usual adult dose
Antihypertensive—
> Oral, 1 or 2 tablets once a day as determined by individual titration with the component agents.

Note: Geriatric patients may be more sensitive to the effects of the usual adult dose.

### Usual pediatric dose
Dosage has not been established.

### Strength(s) usually available
U.S.—
> 125 mcg (0.125 mg) of reserpine and 25 mg of chlorthalidone (Rx) [*Demi-Regroton*].
> 250 mcg (0.25 mg) of reserpine and 50 mg of chlorthalidone (Rx) [*Regroton*].

Canada—
> Not commercially available.

### Auxiliary labeling
* Take with meals or milk.
* Do not take other medicines without your doctor's advice.

## *RESERPINE AND HYDROCHLOROTHIAZIDE*

# Oral Dosage Forms

## RESERPINE AND HYDROCHLOROTHIAZIDE TABLETS USP

### Usual adult dose
Antihypertensive—
> Oral, 1 tablet one to four times a day as determined by individual titration with the component agents.

Note: Geriatric patients may be more sensitive to the effects of the usual adult dose.

### Usual pediatric dose
Dosage has not been established.

### Strength(s) usually available
U.S.—
> 125 mcg (0.125 mg) of reserpine and 25 mg of hydrochlorothiazide (Rx) [*Hydropres; Hydrosine; Mallopres;* GENERIC].
> 125 mcg (0.125 mg) of reserpine and 50 mg of hydrochlorothiazide (Rx) [*Hydropres; Hydrosine; Hydrotensin;* GENERIC].

Canada—
> 125 mcg (0.125 mg) of reserpine and 25 mg of hydrochlorothiazide (Rx) [*Hydropres*].
> 125 mcg (0.125 mg) of reserpine and 50 mg of hydrochlorothiazide (Rx) [*Hydropres*].

### Auxiliary labeling
* Take with meals or milk.
* Do not take other medicines without your doctor's advice.

## *RESERPINE AND HYDROFLUMETHIAZIDE*

# Oral Dosage Forms

## RESERPINE AND HYDROFLUMETHIAZIDE TABLETS

Note: In Canada, *Salutensin* also contains 200 mcg (0.2 mg) of protoveratrine A.

### Usual adult dose
Antihypertensive—
> Oral, 1 tablet one or two times a day as determined by individual titration with the component agents.

Note: Geriatric patients may be more sensitive to the effects of the usual adult dose.

### Usual pediatric dose
Dosage has not been established.

### Strength(s) usually available
U.S.—
> 125 mcg (0.125 mg) of reserpine and 25 mg of hydroflumethiazide (Rx) [*Hydropine; Salutensin-Demi;* GENERIC].
> 125 mcg (0.125 mg) of reserpine and 50 mg of hydroflumethiazide (Rx) [*Hydropine H.P.; Salazide; Salutensin;* GENERIC].

Canada—
> 125 mcg (0.125 mg) of reserpine, 50 mg of hydroflumethiazide, and 200 mcg (0.2 mg) of protoveratrine A (Rx) [*Salutensin*].

### Auxiliary labeling
* Take with meals or milk.
* Do not take other medicines without your doctor's advice.

## *RESERPINE AND METHYCLOTHIAZIDE*

# Oral Dosage Forms

## RESERPINE AND METHYCLOTHIAZIDE TABLETS

### Usual adult dose
Antihypertensive—
> Oral, 1 to 4 tablets a day as determined by individual titration with the component agents.

Note: Geriatric patients may be more sensitive to the effects of the usual adult dose.

### Usual pediatric dose
Dosage has not been established.

### Strength(s) usually available
U.S.—
> 100 mcg (0.1 mg) of reserpine and 2.5 mg of methyclothiazide (Rx) [*Diutensen-R*].

Canada—
Not commercially available.

**Auxiliary labeling**
• Take with meals or milk.
• Do not take other medicines without your doctor's advice.

---

### RESERPINE AND POLYTHIAZIDE

## Oral Dosage Forms

### RESERPINE AND POLYTHIAZIDE TABLETS

**Usual adult dose**
Antihypertensive—
Oral, ¹/₂ to 2 tablets a day as determined by individual titration with the component agents.

Note: Geriatric patients may be more sensitive to the effects of the usual adult dose.

**Usual pediatric dose**
Dosage has not been established.

**Strength(s) usually available**
U.S.—
250 mcg (0.25 mg) of reserpine and 2 mg of polythiazide (Rx) [Renese-R].
Canada—
Not commercially available.

**Auxiliary labeling**
• Take with meals or milk.
• Do not take other medicines without your doctor's advice.

---

### RESERPINE AND TRICHLORMETHIAZIDE

## Oral Dosage Forms

### RESERPINE AND TRICHLORMETHIAZIDE TABLETS

**Usual adult dose**
Antihypertensive—
Oral, 1 or 2 tablets a day as a single dose or in divided daily doses as determined by individual titration with the component agents.

Note: Geriatric patients may be more sensitive to the effects of the usual adult dose.

**Usual pediatric dose**
Dosage has not been established.

**Strength(s) usually available**
U.S.—
100 mcg (0.1 mg) of reserpine and 2 mg of trichlormethiazide (Rx) [Metatensin].

100 mcg (0.1 mg) of reserpine and 4 mg of trichlormethiazide (Rx) [*Diurese-R; Metatensin; Naquival;* GENERIC].
Canada—
Not commercially available.

**Auxiliary labeling**
• Take with meals or milk.
• Do not take other medicines without your doctor's advice.

---

Revised: 09/22/92
Interim revision: 07/20/94

---

## RAUWOLFIA SERPENTINA—See *Rauwolfia Alkaloids (Systemic)*

---

## RAUWOLFIA SERPENTINA–CONTAINING COMBINATIONS—

Rauwolfia Serpentina and Bendroflumethiazide (Systemic)—See *Rauwolfia Alkaloids and Thiazide Diuretics (Systemic)*

---

## RESERPINE—See *Rauwolfia Alkaloids (Systemic)*

---

## RESERPINE-CONTAINING COMBINATIONS—

Reserpine and Chlorothiazide (Systemic)—See *Rauwolfia Alkaloids and Thiazide Diuretics (Systemic)*
Reserpine and Chlorthalidone (Systemic)—See *Rauwolfia Alkaloids and Thiazide Diuretics (Systemic)*
Reserpine, Hydralazine, and Hydrochlorothiazide (Systemic)
Reserpine and Hydrochlorothiazide (Systemic)—See *Rauwolfia Alkaloids and Thiazide Diuretics (Systemic)*
Reserpine and Hydroflumethiazide (Systemic)—See *Rauwolfia Alkaloids and Thiazide Diuretics (Systemic)*
Reserpine and Methyclothiazide (Systemic)—See *Rauwolfia Alkaloids and Thiazide Diuretics (Systemic)*
Reserpine and Polythiazide (Systemic)—See *Rauwolfia Alkaloids and Thiazide Diuretics (Systemic)*
Reserpine and Trichlormethiazide (Systemic)—See *Rauwolfia Alkaloids and Thiazide Diuretics (Systemic)*

---

# RESERPINE, HYDRALAZINE, AND HYDROCHLOROTHIAZIDE   Systemic

VA CLASSIFICATION (Primary): CV400
**NOTE:** The *Reserpine, Hydralazine, and Hydrochlorothiazide (Systemic)* monograph is maintained on the USP DI electronic data base. For a printed copy of the most recent revision of the complete monograph, contact the USP Division of Information Development, 12601 Twinbrook Parkway, Rockville, MD 20852.

For information on the specific components of this combination, see the *USP DI* monographs for *Diuretics, Thiazide (Systemic)*, *Hydralazine (Systemic)*, and *Rauwolfia Alkaloids (Systemic)*.

The information that follows is selectively abstracted from the complete monograph and is provided to facilitate drug use review and patient counseling.

Note: For a listing of dosage forms and brand names by country availability, see *Dosage Forms* section(s). For a listing of brand names for the articles in this monograph, refer to the General Index.

## Category
Antihypertensive.

## Indications

**Accepted**
Hypertension (treatment)—This combination is indicated for treatment of hypertension.

Fixed-dosage combinations are generally not recommended for initial therapy and are useful for subsequent therapy only when the proportion of the component agents corresponds to the dose of the individual agents, as determined by titration.

For additional information on initial therapeutic guidelines related to the treatment of hypertension, see *Appendix III*.

# Patient Consultation

As an aid to patient consultation, refer to *Advice for the Patient, Reserpine, Hydralazine, and Hydrochlorothiazide (Systemic)*.

In providing consultation, consider emphasizing the following selected information (» = major clinical significance):

## Before using this medication

» Conditions affecting use, especially:

Sensitivity to any of the rauwolfia alkaloids, hydralazine, thiazide diuretics, other sulfonamide-type medications, bumetanide, furosemide, or carbonic anhydrase inhibitors

Pregnancy—Reserpine teratogenic in animals; hydralazine reported to cause blood problems in infants of mothers who took hydralazine and causes birth defects in animals; hydrochlorothiazide not recommended for routine use and may cause jaundice, thrombocytopenia, hypokalemia in infant

Breast-feeding—Reserpine and hydrochlorothiazide distributed into breast milk; recommended that nursing mothers avoid hydrochlorothiazide during first month of breast-feeding because of reports of suppression of lactation

Use in the elderly—May be more sensitive to the CNS depressant, hypotensive, and electrolyte effects

Dental—May decrease or inhibit salivary flow

Other medications, especially monoamine oxidase (MAO) inhibitors, diazoxide, cholestyramine, colestipol, digitalis glycosides, or lithium

Other medical problems, especially gallstones, peptic ulcer, ulcerative colitis, mental depression, coronary artery disease, rheumatic heart disease, or anuria or severe renal function impairment

## Proper use of this medication

Possible need for control of weight and diet, especially sodium intake

» Patient may not experience symptoms of hypertension; importance of taking medication even if feeling well

» Does not cure, but helps control hypertension; possible need for lifelong therapy; serious consequences of untreated hypertension

Diuretic effects of medication and timing of doses to minimize inconvenience of diuresis

Getting into habit of taking at same time each day to help increase compliance

Taking with meals or milk to reduce gastrointestinal irritation

» Proper dosing

Missed dose: Taking as soon as possible; not taking if almost time for next dose; not doubling doses

» Proper storage

## Precautions while using this medication

Regular visits to physician to check progress

» Not taking other medications, especially nonprescription sympathomimetics, unless discussed with physician

» Caution if any kind of surgery (including dental surgery) or emergency treatment is required

» Caution when driving or doing things requiring alertness because of possible headache, drowsiness, or dizziness

Caution if orthostatic hypotension occurs

» Caution if depression or changes in sleep pattern occur

» Caution in taking alcohol or other central nervous system (CNS) depressants

Possibility of hypokalemia; possible need for additional potassium in diet; not changing diet without first checking with physician

To prevent dehydration, checking with physician if severe nausea, vomiting, or diarrhea occurs and continues

Diabetics: May increase blood sugar levels

Possible photosensitivity; avoiding unprotected exposure to sun; using protective clothing and sun block product; avoiding use of sunlamp, tanning bed, or tanning booth

Nasal stuffiness may occur; nasal decongestants or other OTC preparations containing sympathomimetics should not be used without first consulting physician or pharmacist

Possible dryness of mouth; using sugarless candy or gum, ice, or saliva substitute for relief; checking with physician or dentist if dry mouth continues for more than 2 weeks

## Side/adverse effects

Signs and symptoms of potential side effects, especially electrolyte imbalance, agranulocytosis, allergic reaction, angina pectoris, cutaneous vasculitis, lymphadenopathy, peripheral neuritis, SLE-like syndrome, cholecystitis, pancreatitis, hepatic function impairment, hyperuricemia, gout, thrombocytopenia, dizziness, arrhythmias, bradycardia, black tarry stools, bloody vomit, drowsiness or faintness, headache, impotence or decreased sexual interest, lack of energy or weakness, mental depression or inability to concentrate, nervousness or anxiety, vivid dreams or nightmares or early-morning sleeplessness, and shortness of breath

# Oral Dosage Forms

## RESERPINE, HYDRALAZINE HYDROCHLORIDE, AND HYDROCHLOROTHIAZIDE TABLETS USP

### Usual adult dose

Antihypertensive—

Oral, 1 or 2 tablets three times a day as determined by individual titration with the component agents.

Note: Geriatric patients may be more sensitive to the effects of the usual adult dose.

### Usual pediatric dose

Safety and efficacy have not been established.

### Strength(s) usually available

U.S.—

100 mcg (0.1 mg) of reserpine, 25 mg of hydralazine hydrochloride, and 15 mg of hydrochlorothiazide (Rx) [*Cam-Ap-Es; Cherapas; Ser-A-Gen; Seralazide; Ser-Ap-Es; Serpazide; Tri-Hydroserpine; Unipres;* GENERIC].

Canada—

100 mcg (0.1 mg) of reserpine, 25 mg of hydralazine hydrochloride, and 15 mg of hydrochlorothiazide (Rx) [*Ser-Ap-Es*].

### Auxiliary labeling

• Avoid alcoholic beverages.

• Take with meals or milk.

• Do not take other medicines without your doctor's advice.

Revised: 09/22/92
Interim revision: 07/20/94

# RESORCINOL Topical

VA CLASSIFICATION (Primary/Secondary): DE752/DE500

Note: For a listing of dosage forms and brand names by country availability, see *Dosage Forms* section(s). For a listing of brand names for the articles in this monograph, refer to the General Index.

## Category

Keratolytic (topical).

## Indications

### Accepted

Acne vulgaris (treatment)
Dermatitis, seborrheic (treatment)
Eczema (treatment)
Psoriasis (treatment)
Urticaria (treatment) or
Skin disorders, inflammatory (treatment)—Resorcinol may be used in the treatment of acne vulgaris, seborrheic dermatitis, eczema, psoriasis, urticaria, and other inflammatory disorders of the skin.

Calluses (treatment)
Corns (treatment) or
Verruca vulgaris (treatment)—Resorcinol may also be used in preparations for the removal of corns, warts, or calluses.

## Pharmacology/Pharmacokinetics

### Physicochemical characteristics

Molecular weight—110.11.

### Mechanism of action/Effect

The effectiveness of resorcinol in treating various dermatological conditions is probably related to its antibacterial, antifungal, local irritant, and keratolytic actions. Its antibacterial and antifungal actions may be the result of protein precipitation; however, its keratolytic action may contribute to the antifungal effect because removal of the stratum corneum suppresses fungal growth.

### Absorption

Resorcinol may be absorbed through the skin or from ulcerated surfaces.

## Precautions to Consider

### Pregnancy/Reproduction

Problems in humans have not been documented; however, resorcinol may be systemically absorbed.

### Breast-feeding

Problems in humans have not been documented; however, resorcinol may be systemically absorbed.

### Pediatrics

Appropriate studies on the relationship of age to the effects of this medicine have not been performed in the pediatric population. However, resorcinol may be absorbed through the skin and should not be used on large areas of the bodies of infants and children. In addition, application to wounds may cause methemoglobinemia.

### Geriatrics

Appropriate studies on the relationship of age to the effects of resorcinol have not been performed in the geriatric population. However, no geriatrics-specific problems have been documented to date.

### Drug interactions and/or related problems

The following drug interactions and/or related problems have been selected on the basis of their potential clinical significance (possible mechanism in parentheses where appropriate)—not necessarily inclusive (» = major clinical significance):

Note: Combinations containing any of the following medications, depending on the amount present, may also interact with this medication.

Abrasive or medicated soaps or cleansers or
Acne preparations or preparations containing a peeling agent such as
  Benzoyl peroxide
  Salicylic acid
  Sulfur
  Tretinoin or
Acne preparations, topical, other or
Alcohol-containing preparations, topical such as
  After-shave lotions
  Astringents

Perfumed toiletries
  Shaving creams or lotions or
Cosmetics or soaps with a strong drying effect or
Isotretinoin or
Medicated cosmetics or "cover-ups"
  (concurrent use with resorcinol may cause a cumulative irritant or drying effect, especially with the application of peeling, desquamating, or abrasive agents, resulting in excessive irritation of the skin)

### Medical considerations/Contraindications

The medical considerations/contraindications included here have been selected on the basis of their potential clinical significance (reasons given in parentheses where appropriate)—not necessarily inclusive (» = major clinical significance).

*Risk-benefit should be considered when the following medical problem exists:*

Sensitivity to resorcinol

## Side/Adverse Effects

The following side/adverse effects have been selected on the basis of their potential clinical significance (possible signs and symptoms in parentheses where appropriate)—not necessarily inclusive:

### Those indicating need for medical attention

Incidence less frequent or rare
  *Skin irritation not present before therapy*

Symptoms of systemic toxicity
  *Diarrhea, nausea, stomach pain, or vomiting; drowsiness; methemoglobinemia* (dizziness; severe or continuing headache; troubled breathing; unusual tiredness or weakness)—especially in children; *nervousness or restlessness; slow heartbeat, shortness of breath, or troubled breathing; sweating*

### Those indicating need for medical attention only if they continue or are bothersome

Incidence more frequent
  *Redness and peeling of skin*—may occur after a few days

## Patient Consultation

As an aid to patient consultation, refer to *Advice for the Patient, Resorcinol (Topical).*

In providing consultation, consider emphasizing the following selected information (» = major clinical significance):

### Before using this medication

» Conditions affecting use, especially:
    Sensitivity to resorcinol
    Use in children—Resorcinol may be absorbed through the skin and should not be used on large areas of the bodies of infants and children; resorcinol should not be used on wounds, since it may cause methemoglobinemia

### Proper use of this medication

» Importance of not using more medication than the amount prescribed
  Proper administration: Applying enough to cover affected areas; rubbing in gently
  Washing hands immediately after application to remove any medication that may be on them
» Avoiding contact with the eyes
» Proper dosing
  Missed dose: Applying as soon as possible; not applying if almost time for next dose
» Proper storage

### Precautions while using this medication

» Avoiding simultaneous use with other topical acne preparations or preparations containing peeling agents, alcohol-containing preparations, abrasive soaps or cleansers, cosmetics or soaps with drying effect, medicated cosmetics, or other topical skin medication, unless otherwise directed by physician
» Medication may darken light-colored hair

### Side/adverse effects

Signs of potential side effects, especially skin irritation not present before therapy or symptoms of resorcinol poisoning

## General Dosing Information

This medication is not recommended for application over large areas of the body, especially when used in high concentrations or in infants and children.

Prolonged use may lead to myxedema because of the antithyroid action of resorcinol, particularly when used on ulcerated surfaces.

Resorcinol is not recommended for use in blacks, since it may cause hyperpigmentation.

This medication may darken light-colored hair.

## Topical Dosage Forms

### RESORCINOL LOTION

**Usual adult and adolescent dose**
Keratolytic—
    Topical, to the skin.

**Usual pediatric dose**
See *Usual adult and adolescent dose.*

Note: Since resorcinol may be absorbed through the skin, application to wounds may cause methemoglobinemia in children.

**Strength(s) usually available**
U.S.—
    3% (OTC) [*RA* (alcohol 43%)].
Canada—
    Not commercially available.

**Packaging and storage**
Store below 40 °C (104 °F), preferably between 15 and 30 °C (59 and 86 °F), in a well-closed container. Protect from freezing. Protect from light.

**Auxiliary labeling**
• Shake well.
• For external use only.

### RESORCINOL OINTMENT

**Usual adult and adolescent dose**
Keratolytic—
    Topical, to the skin, as a 2 to 20% ointment.

**Usual pediatric dose**
See *Usual adult and adolescent dose.*

Note: Since resorcinol may be absorbed through the skin, application to wounds may cause methemoglobinemia in children.

**Strength(s) usually available**
U.S.—
    Dosage form not commercially available. Compounding required for prescriptions.
Canada—
    Dosage form not commercially available. Compounding required for prescriptions.

**Packaging and storage**
Store below 40 °C (104 °F), preferably between 15 and 30 °C (59 and 86 °F), in a well-closed container. Protect from freezing. Protect from light.

**Auxiliary labeling**
• For external use only.

Revised: 07/26/93

---

## RESORCINOL-CONTAINING COMBINATIONS—
Resorcinol and Sulfur (Topical)

---

# RESORCINOL AND SULFUR Topical

VA CLASSIFICATION (Primary/Secondary): DE752/DE500
**NOTE:** The *Resorcinol and Sulfur (Topical)* monograph is maintained on the USP DI electronic data base. For a printed copy of the most recent revision of the complete monograph, contact the USP Division of Information Development, 12601 Twinbrook Parkway, Rockville, MD 20852.

    For information on the specific components of this combination, see the *USP DI* monographs for *Resorcinol (Topical)* and *Sulfur (Topical).*

    The information that follows is selectively abstracted from the complete monograph and is provided to facilitate drug use review and patient counseling.

Note: For a listing of dosage forms and brand names by country availability, see *Dosage Forms* section(s). For a listing of brand names for the articles in this monograph, refer to the General Index.

## Category

Antiacne agent (topical); keratolytic (topical).

## Indications

### Accepted

Acne vulgaris (treatment) or
Skin conditions related to acne (treatment)—Resorcinol and sulfur combination is indicated as an aid in the drying and peeling of blemishes in acne and related skin conditions.

## Patient Consultation

As an aid to patient consultation, refer to *Advice for the Patient, Resorcinol and Sulfur (Topical).*

In providing consultation, consider emphasizing the following selected information (» = major clinical significance):

### Before using this medication
» Conditions affecting use, especially:
    Sensitivity to resorcinol or sulfur
    Use in children—Resorcinol may be absorbed through the skin and should not be used on large areas of the bodies of infants and

children; resorcinol should not be used on wounds, since it may cause methemoglobinemia

### Proper use of this medication
» Importance of not using more medication than the amount recommended
*Proper administration*
    Before using—Washing affected areas thoroughly; gently patting dry
    Applying small amount to affected areas; spreading on gently; not rubbing in
    Washing hands immediately after application to remove any medication that may be on them
    Avoiding contact with the eyes
» Proper dosing
    Missed dose: Applying as soon as possible; not applying if almost time for next dose
» Proper storage

### Precautions while using this medication
» Avoiding simultaneous use with other topical acne preparations or preparations containing peeling agents, alcohol-containing preparations, abrasive soaps or cleansers, cosmetics or soaps with drying effect, medicated cosmetics, or other topical skin medication, unless otherwise directed by physician
» Avoiding concurrent use with topical mercury-containing preparations
    Resorcinol may darken light-colored hair

### Side/adverse effects
Signs of potential side effects, especially skin irritation not present before therapy or symptoms of resorcinol poisoning

## Topical Dosage Forms

### RESORCINOL AND SULFUR CAKE

**Usual adult and adolescent dose**
Antiacne agent or
Keratolytic—
    Topical, to the skin, two or three times a day.

**Usual pediatric dose**
See *Usual adult and adolescent dose.*

**Strength(s) usually available**
U.S.—
Not commercially available.
Canada—
1% resorcinol and 4% sulfur (OTC) [*Acnomel Cake*].

**Auxiliary labeling**
• For external use only.

## RESORCINOL AND SULFUR CREAM

**Usual adult and adolescent dose**
Antiacne agent or
Keratolytic—
Topical, to the skin, one to three times a day.

**Usual pediatric dose**
See *Usual adult and adolescent dose.*

**Strength(s) usually available**
U.S.—
2% resorcinol and 8% sulfur (OTC) [*Acnomel Acne Cream* (alcohol 11%); *Bensulfoid Cream* (alcohol 10%); *Clearasil Adult Care Medicated Blemish Cream* (alcohol 10%)].
Canada—
2% resorcinol and 8% sulfur (OTC) [*Acnomel Cream* (isopropyl alcohol 11%); *Acnomel Vanishing Cream*].

**Auxiliary labeling**
• For external use only.

## RESORCINOL AND SULFUR GEL

**Usual adult and adolescent dose**
Antiacne agent or
Keratolytic—
Topical, to the skin.

**Usual pediatric dose**
See *Usual adult and adolescent dose.*

**Strength(s) usually available**
U.S.—
Not commercially available.
Canada—
1.25% resorcinol and 2.5% sulfur (OTC) [*Acne-Aid Gel*].

**Auxiliary labeling**
• For external use only.

## RESORCINOL AND SULFUR LOTION USP

**Usual adult and adolescent dose**
Antiacne agent or
Keratolytic—
Topical, to the skin, one or two times a day, preferably in the morning and at bedtime.

**Usual pediatric dose**
See *Usual adult and adolescent dose.*

**Strength(s) usually available**
U.S.—
2% resorcinol and 5% colloidal sulfur (OTC) [*Sulforcin* (alcohol 11.65%)].
2% resorcinol and 5% sulfur (OTC) [*Rezamid Acne Treatment* (alcohol 28.5%)].
2% resorcinol and 8% sulfur (OTC) [*Night Cast Special Formula Mask-lotion* (alcohol 31%)].
Canada—
2% resorcinol and 5% colloidal sulfur (OTC) [*Rezamid Lotion* (alcohol 19.4%; butylparaben; methylparaben; sodium bisulfite)].

**Auxiliary labeling**
• Shake well.
• For external use only.

## RESORCINOL AND SULFUR STICK

**Usual adult and adolescent dose**
Antiacne agent or
Keratolytic—
Topical, to the skin.

**Usual pediatric dose**
See *Usual adult and adolescent dose.*

**Strength(s) usually available**
U.S.—
1% resorcinol and 8% sulfur (OTC) [*Clearasil Adult Care Medicated Blemish Stick*].
Canada—
Not commercially available.

**Auxiliary labeling**
• For external use only.

Revised: 07/26/93

---

# RH$_O$(D) IMMUNE GLOBULIN    Systemic

VA CLASSIFICATION (Primary): IM 500

Other commonly used names are anti-D gammaglobulin; anti-D (Rh$_o$) immunoglobulin; anti-Rh immunoglobulin; anti-Rh$_o$(D); D (Rh$_o$) immune globulin; RhD immune globulin; Rh immune globulin; Rh-IG; and Rh$_o$(D) immune human globulin.

Note: For a listing of dosage forms and brand names by country availability, see *Dosage Forms* section(s). For a listing of brand names for the articles in this monograph, refer to the General Index.

## Category

Immunizing agent (passive).

## Indications

**Accepted**

Sensitization of Rh$_o$(D)–negative females to Rh$_o$(D)–positive blood (prophylaxis) or

Rh hemolytic disease of the newborn (prophylaxis)—Rh$_o$(D) immune globulin is indicated in Rh$_o$(D)–negative females of child-bearing age or younger who have not been previously sensitized to the Rh$_o$(D) erythrocyte factor and who may be exposed to the factor during one or more of the following events: the birth of an Rh$_o$(D)–positive infant; incomplete pregnancy terminating in the delivery of an Rh$_o$(D)–positive fetus (e.g., spontaneous or induced abortion or ruptured tubal pregnancy); amniocentesis, abdominal trauma during pregnancy, or transplacental hemorrhage, while carrying an Rh$_o$(D)–positive fetus; or transfusion involving mismatched Rh$_o$(D)–positive blood. Treating these females prophylactically prevents sensitization to the Rh$_o$(D) erythrocyte factor, which in turn prevents Rh hemolytic disease (erythroblastosis fetalis) in Rh$_o$(D)–positive neonates. See *Mechanism of action/Effect.*

## Pharmacology/Pharmacokinetics

**Physicochemical characteristics**
Source—A sterile, nonpyrogenic solution of immune globulin that contains antibody to the erythrocyte factor Rh$_o$(D). The solution is prepared from large pools of human blood plasma

**Mechanism of action/Effect**
By providing passive Rh$_o$(D) antibody, Rh$_o$(D) immune globulin suppresses the immune response to Rh$_o$(D)–positive blood in nonsensitized Rh$_o$(D)–negative females. This prevents sensitization to the Rh$_o$(D) erythrocyte factor and the subsequent formation of active Rh$_o$(D) antibody. This in turn prevents the occurrence of Rh hemolytic disease (erythroblastosis fetalis) in Rh$_o$(D)–positive neonates, which results from *in utero* exposure to maternal Rh$_o$(D) antibody.

**Protective effect**
Administration of Rh$_o$(D) immune globulin (full dose) within 72 hours of a delivery of a full-term Rh$_o$(D)–positive infant by an Rh$_o$(D)–negative mother reduces the incidence of Rh immunization from the usual 12 or 13% to 1 or 2%. The 1 or 2% treatment failures are thought to be due to immunization that occurred during the latter part of pregnancy. Studies have shown that 2 doses, the first given at 28 weeks gestation and the second given following delivery, can reduce treatment failures to 0.1%.

Studies have shown that administration of Rh$_o$(D) immune globulin (minidose) within 3 hours following termination of pregnancy prior to 13 weeks of gestation in Rh$_o$(D)–negative females who have not been previously sensitized to the Rh$_o$(D) factor was 100% effective in preventing Rh immunization.

**Duration of protective effect**
The half-life of Rh$_o$(D) immune globulin is 23 to 26 days.

# Precautions to Consider

### Cross-sensitivity and/or related problems
Patients sensitive to other human immune globulin products may be sensitive to Rh$_o$(D) immune globulin also.

### Pregnancy/Reproduction
Pregnancy—Adequate and well-controlled studies have not been done in pregnant women. However, use of Rh$_o$(D) immune globulin (full dose) during the third trimester has not produced evidence of hemolysis in the infant.

Studies have not been done in animals.

FDA Pregnancy Category C.

### Breast-feeding
Problems in humans have not been documented.

### Pediatrics
No information is available on the relationship of age to the effects of Rh$_o$(D) immune globulin in pediatric patients. Safety and efficacy have not been established.

### Drug interactions and/or related problems
The following drug interactions and/or related problems have been selected on the basis of their potential clinical significance (possible mechanism in parentheses where appropriate)—not necessarily inclusive (» = major clinical significance):

Note: Combinations containing any of the following medications, depending on the amount present, may also interact with this medication.

     Live virus vaccines
         (antibodies contained in Rh$_o$(D) immune globulin may interfere with the body's immune response to certain live virus vaccines; live virus vaccines, such as measles, mumps, and rubella, should be administered at least 3 months after administration of Rh$_o$(D) immune globulin)

### Laboratory value alterations
The following have been selected on the basis of their potential clinical significance (possible effect in parentheses where appropriate)—not necessarily inclusive (» = major clinical significance):

With diagnostic test results
     Antibody screening test, maternal
         (passively acquired anti-Rh$_o$(D) may be detected in maternal serum if antibody screening tests are performed subsequent to administration of Rh$_o$(D) immune globulin antepartum or postpartum)

     Direct antiglobulin test, neonate
         (infants born to women administered Rh$_o$(D) immune globulin antepartum may have a weakly positive direct antiglobulin test result at birth)

With physiology/laboratory test values
     Bilirubin, serum
         (concentrations may be elevated in persons receiving multiple doses of Rh$_o$(D) immune globulin, e.g., following a mismatched transfusion involving Rh$_o$(D)–positive blood. The elevation is believed to be due to a relatively rapid rate of foreign red cell destruction)

### Medical considerations/Contraindications
The medical considerations/contraindications included here have been selected on the basis of their potential clinical significance (reasons given in parentheses where appropriate)—not necessarily inclusive (» = major clinical significance).

*Risk-benefit should be considered when the following medical problems exist:*

»   Immunoglobulin A (IgA) deficiencies, selective, in patients who have known antibody to IgA
     (small amounts of IgA may be present in Rh$_o$(D) immune globulin and may cause a severe allergic reaction in patients with antibody to IgA)

     Sensitivity to Rh$_o$(D) immune globulin

     Sensitivity to thimerosal
     (the Rh$_o$(D) immune globulin available in the U.S. and Canada may contain thimerosal)

# Side/Adverse Effects

Note: Severe systemic adverse effects to Rh$_o$(D) immune globulin are rare.

The following side/adverse effects have been selected on the basis of their potential clinical significance (possible signs and symptoms in parentheses where appropriate)—not necessarily inclusive:

**Those indicating need for medical attention only if they continue or are bothersome**
Incidence less frequent
     *Fever; soreness at the place of injection*

# Patient Consultation
As an aid to patient consultation, refer to *Advice for the Patient, Rh$_o$(D) Immune Globulin (Systemic)*.

In providing consultation, consider emphasizing the following selected information (» = major clinical significance):

**Before using this medication**
»   Conditions affecting use, especially:
         Sensitivity to Rh$_o$(D) immune globulin, other human immune globulins, or thimerosal
         Other medical problems, especially immunoglobulin A (IgA) deficiencies

**Proper use of this medication**
»   Proper dosing

# General Dosing Information
Rh$_o$(D) immune globulin is *not* for use in neonates.

Rh$_o$(D) immune globulin should be administered only to Rh$_o$(D)–negative females. However, if there is doubt about the mother's Rh type, she should be given Rh$_o$(D) immune globulin. Doubt may arise when a large fetomaternal hemorrhage occurring late in pregnancy or during delivery infuses enough fetal red blood cells into the maternal circulation to cause a weak mixed field positive D$^u$ test result.

Although Rh$_o$(D) immune globulin is not effective in Rh$_o$(D)–negative females who have been already sensitized to the Rh$_o$(D) erythrocyte factor, administration to these females does not increase the risk of adverse effects.

When Rh typing of the fetus or newborn infant is not possible, the fetus or newborn infant should be assumed to be Rh$_o$(D)–positive, unless the father can be determined to be Rh$_o$(D)–negative.

Since 1 full dose of Rh$_o$(D) immune globulin available in the U.S. contains Rh$_o$(D) antibody sufficient to suppress the immunizing potential of approximately 15 mL of Rh$_o$(D)–positive packed red blood cells or 30 mL of Rh$_o$(D)–positive whole blood, the amount of Rh$_o$(D)–positive blood present in the mother's circulation should be carefully determined, since more than 1 dose of Rh$_o$(D) immune globulin may be required. A fetal red blood cell count can be performed on the maternal blood to determine the dosage of Rh$_o$(D) immune globulin required.

For all except one indication, at least 1 full dose of Rh$_o$(D) immune globulin is indicated. If a pregnancy is terminated prior to 13 weeks of gestation, the patient may be administered a mini-dose (approximately 1/6 of the full dose) of Rh$_o$(D) immune globulin instead of a full dose, since it is estimated that the total volume of red blood cells in a fetus at 12 weeks of gestation is less than 2.5 mL. For a pregnancy that is terminated at or beyond 13 weeks of gestation, the patient should receive at least 1 full dose of Rh$_o$(D) immune globulin.

Rh$_o$(D) immune globulin should be administered to the Rh$_o$(D)–negative female within 72 hours after the incompatible event involving Rh$_o$(D)–positive blood. If the event is a mismatched transfusion involving Rh$_o$(D)–positive blood, Rh$_o$(D) immune globulin should be administered within 72 hours, but preferably as soon as possible. If the event is a pregnancy terminated prior to 13 weeks of gestation, and the mini-dose of Rh$_o$(D) immune globulin will be given, the mini-dose should be administered within 72 hours, but preferably within 3 hours.

To maintain protection throughout pregnancy once Rh$_o$(D) immune globulin is administered, the level of passively acquired anti-Rh$_o$(D) should not be allowed to fall below the level required to prevent an immune response to Rh$_o$(D)–positive blood. Additional doses of Rh$_o$(D) immune globulin should be administered during pregnancy at approximately 12-week intervals following the first dose. In all cases, the postpartum dose of Rh$_o$(D) immune globulin should be administered, unless the previous dose was within 3 weeks of delivery and any fetomaternal hemorrhage that occurs during delivery produces less than 15 mL of red blood cells. For example, if an incompatible event involving Rh$_o$(D)–positive blood requires administration of Rh$_o$(D) immune globulin at 13 to 18 weeks of gestation, an additional dose should be administered at 26 to 28 weeks of gestation, followed by the postpartum dose within 72 hours of delivery. If the first dose is administered at 26 to 28 weeks of gestation, the postpartum dose is still required.

Rh$_o$(D) immune globulin should be administered by intramuscular injection. The U.S. products should not be administered intravenously. One Canadian product is indicated for either intravenous or intramuscular use.

## Parenteral Dosage Forms

### RH$_o$ (D) IMMUNE GLOBULIN (HUMAN) (FOR INJECTION)

**Usual adult and adolescent dose**
Immunizing agent (passive)—
  Intramuscular, into the deltoid muscle or the anterolateral aspect of the thigh, or intravenous: a sufficient amount of Rh$_o$(D) antibody to suppress the immunizing potential of the amount of Rh$_o$(D)–positive blood calculated or estimated to be present in the female's circulation because of pregnancy or transfusion.

**Usual pediatric dose**
Immunizing agent (passive)—
  Intramuscular, into the deltoid muscle or the anterolateral aspect of the thigh, or intravenous: a sufficient amount of Rh$_o$(D) antibody to suppress the immunizing potential of the amount of Rh$_o$(D)–positive blood calculated or estimated to be present in the female's circulation because of transfusion.

Note: See *General Dosing Information* for the parameters for administering Rh$_o$(D) immune globulin.

  If the patient requires administration of more than 1 vial/syringe of Rh$_o$(D) immune globulin, the contents of the vials/syringes may be administered at different sites at the same time or at intervals over time, provided that the entire dose is administered with 72 hours of the event.

**Strength(s) usually available**
U.S.—
  Not commercially available.
Canada—
  Sufficient Rh$_o$(D) antibody to suppress the immunizing potential of approximately 6 mL of Rh$_o$(D)–positive packed red blood cells or 12 mL of Rh$_o$(D)–positive whole blood (Rx) [*WinRho SD* (contains no preservatives)].
  Full dose: Sufficient Rh$_o$(D) antibody to suppress the immunizing potential of approximately 15 mL of Rh$_o$(D)–positive packed red blood cells or 30 mL of Rh$_o$(D)–positive whole blood (Rx) [*WinRho SD* (contains no preservatives)].

Note: Each full dose of Rh$_o$(D) immune globulin contains at least as much anti-Rh$_o$(D) as is contained in 1 mL of the U.S. Reference Rh$_o$(D) immune globulin. A full dose of Rh$_o$(D) immune globulin has traditionally been referred to as a "300 mcg" dose; however, this is *not* the actual anti-Rh$_o$(D) content of the product. Studies have shown that the U.S. Reference contains 820 International Units (IU) of anti-Rh$_o$(D) per mL, which is thought to be equivalent to 164 mcg per mL.

**Packaging and storage**
Store between 2 and 8 °C (36 and 46 °F), unless otherwise specified by manufacturer. Protect from freezing.

**Preparation of dosage form**
A suitable syringe and needle should be used to withdraw the diluent. 1.25 mL of diluent should be used for an intramuscular injection or 2.5 mL of diluent should be used for an intravenous injection. The diluent should be injected slowly into the vial containing the freeze-dried pellet so that the liquid is directed onto the inside glass wall of the vial. The pellet should be wet by gently tilting and inverting the vial. Frothing should be avoided. While the vial is held upright, it should be gently swirled until the pellet is dissolved. This should take less than 10 minutes.

**Stability**
The reconstituted solution may be stored at room temperature for up to 4 hours. It should be discarded if it is not used within 4 hours.
The solution should not be used if it is discolored or contains particulate matter.

**Auxiliary labeling**
• Do not freeze the powder, diluent, or the reconstituted solution.
• Use the reconstituted solution within 4 hours.

### RH$_o$ (D) IMMUNE GLOBULIN ( HUMAN) INJECTION USP

**Usual adult and adolescent dose**
Immunizing agent (passive)—
  Intramuscular, into the deltoid muscle or the anterolateral aspect of the thigh: a sufficient amount of Rh$_o$(D) antibody to suppress the immunizing potential of the amount of Rh$_o$(D)–positive blood calculated or estimated to be present in the female's circulation because of pregnancy or transfusion.

**Usual pediatric dose**
Immunizing agent (passive)—
  Intramuscular, into the deltoid muscle or the anterolateral aspect of the thigh: a sufficient amount of Rh$_o$(D) antibody to suppress the immunizing potential of the amount of Rh$_o$(D)–positive blood calculated or estimated to be present in the female's circulation because of transfusion.

Note: See *General Dosing Information* for the parameters for administering Rh$_o$(D) immune globulin.

  If the patient requires administration of more than 1 vial/syringe of Rh$_o$(D) immune globulin, the contents of the vials/syringes may be administered at different sites at the same time or at intervals over time, provided that the entire dose is administered with 72 hours of the event.

**Strength(s) usually available**
U.S.—
  Mini-dose: Sufficient Rh$_o$(D) antibody to suppress the immunizing potential of approximately 2.5 mL of Rh$_o$(D)–positive packed red blood cells or 5 mL of Rh$_o$(D)–positive whole blood (Rx) [*HypRho-D Mini-Dose* (thimerosal); *MICRhoGAM* (thimerosal); *Mini-Gamulin Rh* (thimerosal)].
  Full dose: Sufficient Rh$_o$(D) antibody to suppress the immunizing potential of approximately 15 mL of Rh$_o$(D)–positive packed red blood cells or 30 mL of Rh$_o$(D)–positive whole blood (Rx) [*Gamulin Rh* (thimerosal); *HypRho-D Full Dose* (thimerosal); *RhoGAM* (thimerosal)].
Canada—
  Full dose: Sufficient Rh$_o$(D) antibody to suppress the immunizing potential of approximately 15 mL of Rh$_o$(D)–positive packed red blood cells or 30 mL of Rh$_o$(D)–positive whole blood (Rx) [*HypRho-D Full Dose* (thimerosal)].

Note: Each full dose of Rh$_o$(D) immune globulin contains at least as much anti-Rh$_o$(D) as contained in 1 mL of the U.S. Reference Rh$_o$(D) immune globulin. A full dose of Rh$_o$(D) immune globulin has traditionally been referred to as a "300 mcg" dose; however, this is *not* the actual anti-Rh$_o$(D) content of the product. Studies have shown that the U.S. Reference contains 820 International Units (IU) of anti-Rh$_o$(D) per mL, which is thought to be equivalent to 164 mcg per mL.

  Each mini-dose of Rh$_o$(D) immune globulin contains not less than one-sixth of the amount of anti-Rh$_o$(D) that is contained in 1 mL of the U.S. Reference Rh$_o$(D) immune globulin.

**Packaging and storage**
Store between 2 and 8 °C (36 and 46 °F), unless otherwise specified by manufacturer. Protect from freezing.

**Stability**
The solution should be discarded if it has been frozen. The solution should not be used if it is discolored or contains particulate matter.

**Auxiliary labeling**
• Store in refrigerator.
• Do not freeze.
• Discard if solution has been frozen.

## Selected Bibliography

Bayliss KM, Kueck BD, Johnson ST, et al. Detecting fetomaternal hemorrhage: a comparison of five methods. Transfusion 1991 May; 31 (4): 303-7.
Duerbeck NB, Seeds JW. Rhesus immunization in pregnancy: a review. Obstet Gynecol Surv 1993 Dec; 48 (12): 801-10.

Developed: 08/31/94
Interim revision: 06/02/95

# RIBAVIRIN   Systemic

VA CLASSIFICATION (Primary): AM800

Another commonly used name is tribavirin.

Note: For a listing of dosage forms and brand names by country availability, see *Dosage Forms* section(s). For a listing of brand names for the articles in this monograph, refer to the General Index.

## Category

Antiviral (systemic)

Note: Ribavirin is a broad-spectrum antiviral active *in vitro* against a wide variety of DNA and RNA viruses.

## Indications

Note: Bracketed information in the *Indications* section refers to uses that are not included in U.S. product labeling.

### Accepted

Respiratory syncytial virus (RSV) infection, lower respiratory tract (treatment)—Ribavirin inhalation solution is indicated as a primary agent in the treatment of lower respiratory tract disease (including bronchiolitis and pneumonia) caused by respiratory syncytial virus (RSV) in hospitalized infants and young children who are at high risk for severe or complicated RSV infection; this category includes premature infants and infants with structural or physiologic cardiopulmonary disorders, bronchopulmonary dysplasia, immunodeficiency, or imminent respiratory failure. Ribavirin is indicated in the treatment of RSV infections in infants requiring mechanical ventilator assistance.

[Influenza A (treatment)][1] or
[Influenza B (treatment)][1]—Ribavirin inhalation solution is used as a secondary agent in the treatment of influenza A and B in young adults when treatment is started early (e.g., within 24 hours of initial symptoms) in the course of the disease.

[Lassa fever (prophylaxis and treatment)][1] or
[Viral hemorrhagic fever (prophylaxis and treatment)][1]—Oral and intravenous ribavirin are used in the treatment of Lassa fever and as post-exposure prophylaxis in contacts at high risk. It may be similarly effective with other viral hemorrhagic fevers, including hemorrhagic fever with renal syndrome, Crimean-Congo hemorrhagic fever, and Rift Valley fever.

### Unaccepted

Ribavirin is not indicated in children with mild RSV lower respiratory tract involvement who require a shorter hospitalization than that required for completion of a full course of ribavirin treatment (i.e., 3 to 7 days).

[1]Not included in Canadian product labeling.

## Pharmacology/Pharmacokinetics

### Physicochemical characteristics

Molecular weight—244.21.

### Mechanism of action/Effect

Virustatic; mechanism not completely understood, but does not alter viral attachment, penetration, or uncoating and does not induce cellular production of interferon; however, reversal of its antiviral action by guanosine and xanthosine suggests that ribavirin may act as a competitive inhibitor of cellular enzymes that act on these metabolites. Ribavirin is rapidly transported into cells and acts within virus-infected cells. Ribavirin is readily phosphorylated intracellularly by adenosine kinase to ribavirin mono-, di-, and triphosphate metabolites. Ribavirin triphosphate (RTP) is a potent competitive inhibitor of inosine monophosphate (IMP) dehydrogenase, influenza virus RNA polymerase, and messenger RNA (mRNA) guanylyltransferase, the latter resulting in inhibition of the capping of mRNA. These diverse effects result in a marked reduction of intracellular guanosine triphosphate (GTP) pools and inhibition of viral RNA and protein synthesis. Ultimately, viral replication and spreading to other cells are prevented or greatly inhibited.

### Other actions/effects

May have immunologic effects; decreases in neutralizing antibody responses to respiratory syncytial virus (RSV) infection have been reported in ribavirin-treated patients. The clinical significance of this effect is unknown. Ribavirin has also been shown to significantly reduce viral shedding in RSV-infected patients.

### Absorption

Inhalation—A small amount is systemically absorbed following inhalation.

Oral—Rapidly absorbed from the gastrointestinal tract following oral administration; bioavailability is approximately 45%.

### Distribution

Distributed to plasma, respiratory tract secretions, and erythrocytes (RBCs). Large amounts of ribavirin triphosphate are sequestered in RBCs, reaching a plateau in approximately 4 days and remaining sequestered for weeks after administration. Significant concentrations (greater than 67%) may be found in the cerebrospinal fluid after prolonged administration.

$Vol_D$ =Approximately 647 to 802 liters.

### Protein binding

No significant plasma protein binding.

### Biotransformation

Hepatic (probable); phosphorylated intracellularly to mono-, di-, and triphosphate metabolites, the latter being active; metabolized also to 1,2,4-triazole carboxamide metabolite; secondary metabolic pathway involves amide hydrolysis to tricarboxylic acid, deribosylation, and breakdown of the triazole ring.

### Half-life

Distribution—
    Intravenous:
        Approximately 0.2 hours.
Elimination—
    Inhalation: 9.5 hours.
    Intravenous and oral (single dose): 0.5 to 2 hours.
    In erythrocytes: 40 days.
Terminal—
    Intravenous and oral:
        Single dose—27 to 36 hours.
        Steady state—Approximately 151 hours.

### Time to peak plasma concentration

Intravenous—End of infusion.
Oral—1 to 1.5 hours.

### Therapeutic plasma concentration

Therapeutically effective concentrations depend primarily on the duration of exposure and patient minute volume. Concentrations in respiratory tract secretions are much higher than corresponding plasma concentrations.

### Mean peak plasma concentration

Inhalation—
    Approximately 0.2 mcg per mL (0.8 micromoles) in pediatric patients receiving ribavirin aerosol by face mask 2.5 hours per day for 3 days.
    Approximately 1.7 mcg per mL (6.8 micromoles) in pediatric patients receiving ribavirin aerosol by face mask or mist tent 20 hours per day for 5 days.
Intravenous—
    Approximately 43 micromoles per liter after a single 600 mg dose.
    Approximately 72 micromoles per liter after a single 1200 mg dose.
Oral—
    Approximately 5 micromoles per liter at the end of the first week of administration of 200 mg every 8 hours.
    Approximately 11 micromoles per liter at the end of the first week of administration of 400 mg every 8 hours.

### Elimination

Inhalation—
    Renal: Approximately 30 to 55% excreted as the 1,2,4-triazole carboxamide metabolite in urine within 72 to 80 hours.
    Fecal: Approximately 15% excreted in feces within 72 hours.
Intravenous—
    Approximately 19% excreted unchanged in 24 hours; approximately 24% excreted unchanged in 48 hours.
Oral—
    Approximately 7% excreted unchanged in 24 hours; approximately 10% excreted unchanged in 48 hours.
In dialysis—
    Significant amounts of ribavirin are not removed by hemodialysis.

# Precautions to Consider

## Carcinogenicity/Tumorigenicity
Studies have shown that ribavirin induces cell transformation in a mammalian system (Balb/C 3T3 cell line). Although carcinogenicity studies are incomplete and inconclusive, results thus far suggest that chronic feeding of ribavirin to rats in doses of 16 to 60 mg per kg of body weight (mg/kg) can induce benign mammary, pancreatic, pituitary, and adrenal gland tumors.

## Mutagenicity
Studies have shown that ribavirin is mutagenic to mammalian cells (L5178Y) in culture. However, microbial mutagenicity assays and dominant lethal assays in mice have not shown that ribavirin is mutagenic.

## Pregnancy/Reproduction
Fertility—Although the effects of lower doses have not been studied, studies have shown that ribavirin causes testicular lesions (tubular atrophy) in adult rats given oral doses as low as 16 mg/kg daily. However, the fertility of ribavirin-treated animals (male or female) has not been adequately investigated.

Pregnancy—Ribavirin is contraindicated during pregnancy. Studies in humans have not been done. Although ribavirin is not indicated for use in adults in the U.S., healthcare workers and visitors who spend time at the patient's bedside may become environmentally exposed to ribavirin. Female healthcare workers and visitors who are pregnant, or may become pregnant, should be advised of the potential risks of exposure.

Studies in primates (e.g., baboons) have not shown that ribavirin causes adverse effects on the fetus; however, ribavirin crosses the placenta and studies in other animals have shown that it is teratogenic and/or embryocidal in nearly all species tested; studies in hamsters given daily oral doses of 2.5 mg/kg and studies in rats given daily oral doses of 10 mg/kg have shown teratogenicity. Malformations of the skull, palate, eye, jaw, skeleton, and gastrointestinal tract have been observed in animal studies, and survival of fetuses and offspring was reduced. Studies in rabbits given daily oral doses as low as 1 mg/kg have shown that ribavirin is embryocidal.

FDA Pregnancy Category X.

## Breast-feeding
It is not known whether ribavirin is excreted in human breast milk. However, ribavirin is excreted in the breast milk of animals and has been shown to be toxic to lactating animals and their offspring. Ribavirin aerosol is not indicated in the treatment of nursing mothers since respiratory syncytial virus (RSV) infection is self-limited in this population.

## Pediatrics
Ribavirin inhalation solution is indicated in the treatment of RSV infection only in children.

## Geriatrics
Ribavirin inhalation solution is not indicated for use in geriatric patients.

## Drug interactions and/or related problems
The following drug interactions and/or related problems have been selected on the basis of their potential clinical significance (possible mechanism in parentheses where appropriate)—not necessarily inclusive (» = major clinical significance):

Note: Combinations containing any of the following medications, depending on the amount present, may also interact with this medication.

Zidovudine
(*in vitro* studies have shown that when combined, ribavirin and zidovudine are reproducibly antagonistic and should not be used concurrently; ribavirin inhibits the phosphorylation of zidovudine to its active triphosphate form)

## Medical considerations/Contraindications
The medical considerations/contraindications included here have been selected on the basis of their potential clinical significance (reasons given in parentheses where appropriate)—not necessarily inclusive (» = major clinical significance).

*Risk-benefit should be considered when the following medical problems exist:*

Anemia, severe
(intravenous and oral ribavirin may cause anemia that is reversible when the drug is discontinued)

Hypersensitivity to ribavirin

## Patient monitoring
The following may be especially important in patient monitoring (other tests may be warranted in some patients, depending on condition; » = major clinical significance):

Hematocrit
(hematocrit should be monitored periodically since intravenous and oral ribavirin may cause anemia)

# Side/Adverse Effects

Note: Although the manufacturer's literature includes a number of side effects, most studies indicate that ribavirin inhalation solution causes little or no systemic toxicity.

The following side/adverse effects have been selected on the basis of their potential clinical significance (possible signs and symptoms in parentheses where appropriate)—not necessarily inclusive:

## Those indicating need for medical attention
Incidence more frequent—intravenous and oral only
*Anemia* (unusual tiredness or weakness)
Note: Anemia is reversible with discontinuation of ribavirin.

## Those indicating need for medical attention only if they continue or are bothersome
Incidence less frequent—intravenous and oral only
*CNS effects* (fatigue; headache; insomnia)—usually with higher doses;
*gastrointestinal effects* (anorexia; nausea)
Incidence rare—inhalation only
*In patients*
**Skin irritation due to prolonged drug contact; skin rash**
*In healthcare worker*
**Headache; itching, redness, or swelling of eye**

# Patient Consultation
As an aid to patient consultation, refer to *Advice for the Patient, Ribavirin (Systemic)*.

In providing consultation, consider emphasizing the following selected information (» = major clinical significance):

## Before using this medication
» Conditions affecting use, especially:
Pregnancy—Ribavirin is contraindicated during pregnancy. Female healthcare workers and visitors who are pregnant or may become pregnant may become environmentally exposed to ribavirin and should be advised of the potential risks of exposure

## Proper use of this medication
» Importance of receiving medication for full course of therapy and on regular or continuous schedule
» Proper dosing

# General Dosing Information
Before using, become thoroughly familiar with the Viratek Small Particle Aerosol Generator (SPAG) Model SPAG-2 Operator's Manual for operating instructions.

According to the manufacturer, ribavirin inhalation solution should be administered using the Viratek SPAG Model SPAG-2 only. It should not be administered using any other aerosol-generating device. Ribavirin inhalation solution is usually administered using an infant oxygen hood attached to the SPAG-2 aerosol generator. However, administration by face mask may be necessary if an oxygen hood cannot be utilized (see SPAG-2 manual). With use of the recommended concentration (20 mg per mL) of ribavirin in the SPAG reservoir, the average ribavirin inhalation solution concentration over a 12-hour period is approximately 190 micrograms per liter of air.

Use of ribavirin inhalation solution in infants requiring mechanical ventilation should be undertaken only by health care workers familiar with this mode of administration and the specific ventilator being used. The dose for infants requiring mechanical ventilation is the same as for those who do not. Precipitation of ribavirin within the ventilator apparatus, including endotracheal tubes, may cause obstruction, resulting in increased positive end expiratory pressure and increased positive inspiratory pressure. Accumulation of fluid in the tubing ("rain out") has also been observed. To try to avoid this, instructions must be followed carefully. Either a pressure or volume cycle ventilator may be used in conjunction with the SPAG-2. Patients should have their endotracheal tubes suctioned every 1 to 2 hours, and their pulmonary pressures monitored frequently (every 2 to 4 hours). For both pressure and volume ventilators, heated wire connective tubing and bacteria filters in series in the expiratory limb of the system must be used to minimize the risk of ribavirin precipitation in the system and the subsequent risk of ventilator dysfunction. Bacteria filters must be changed frequently, i.e., every 4 hours. Water column pressure release valves should be used in the ventilator circuit for pressure cycled ventilators, and may be utilized with volume cycled ventilators. Refer to the SPAG-2 manual for detailed instructions.

Ribavirin aerosolization, using a small particle aerosol generator, produces particles of 1.2 to 1.6 microns (mass mean diameter) in size. Ribavirin inhalation solution has been administered by this method at the rate of 12.5 liters per minute via an infant oxygen hood or mask, tent, or tubing of a respirator. Using a ribavirin concentration of 20 mg per mL, this method delivers approximately 1.8 mg per kg of body weight (mg/kg) per hour in infants and children up to 6 years of age.

Although ribavirin inhalation solution has been administered using a tent, the volume of distribution and the condensation area are larger and the efficacy of this method has been evaluated in only a small number of patients.

Although ribavirin treatment may be initiated before the results of diagnostic tests are received, treatment should not be continued without laboratory confirmation of respiratory syncytial virus (RSV) infection.

Ribavirin inhalation solution treatment is generally effective when initiated within the first 3 days of RSV pneumonia. Early treatment may be necessary to achieve efficacy and to avoid further damage to the patient's lungs.

# Inhalation Dosage Forms

## RIBAVIRIN FOR INHALATION SOLUTION USP

### Usual adult and adolescent dose
Respiratory syncytial virus (RSV) infection, lower respiratory tract—
Dosage has not been established.

### Usual pediatric dose
Respiratory syncytial virus (RSV) infection, lower respiratory tract—
Oral inhalation, via a Viratek Small Particle Aerosol Generator (SPAG) Model SPAG-2 utilizing a 20-mg-per-mL ribavirin concentration in the reservoir, over a twelve- to eighteen-hour period per day for at least three to a maximum of seven days.

Note: Various ribavirin dosage regimens have been utilized in RSV pneumonia and other infections, including virtually continuous aerosolization for three to six days and aerosolization over a four-hour period three times a day for three days.

### Size(s) usually available
U.S.—
6 grams (Rx) [Virazole].
Canada—
6 grams (Rx) [Virazole].

### Packaging and storage
Prior to reconstitution, store between 15 and 25 °C (59 and 78 °F), in a dry place.

### Preparation of dosage form
To prepare initial dilution for oral inhalation, add a measured quantity of sterile water for injection (without antimicrobial agents or other added substances) or sterile water for inhalation, sufficient for dissolution, to each 6-gram vial. Transfer the resulting solution to a clean, sterilized 500-mL wide-mouth Erlenmeyer flask (SPAG-2 reservoir). Further dilute the solution to a final volume of 300 mL with sterile water for injection or sterile water for inhalation to provide a final concentration of 20 mg per mL.
Prior to administration, visually inspect the final solution for particulate matter and discoloration.
When the solution level in the SPAG-2 reservoir is low, discard the remaining solution before adding freshly reconstituted solution to the reservoir.

### Stability
The stability of ribavirin for inhalation solution (lyophilized powder) is unaffected by temperature, light, and moisture.
After reconstitution, solutions retain their potency at room temperature (20 to 30 °C [68 to 86 °F]) for 24 hours.
Ribavirin solutions are colorless.

### Incompatibilities
Ribavirin for inhalation solution should not be administered concurrently with other medications administered by aerosolization.

# Oral Dosage Forms

Note: Bracketed uses in the *Dosage Forms* section refer to categories of use and/or indications that are not included in U.S. product labeling.

## RIBAVIRIN FOR ORAL SOLUTION

Note: Ribavirin for Inhalation Solution USP is the dosage form being used because an oral solution is not commercially available.

### Usual adult and adolescent dose
[Lassa fever (prophylaxis)][1]—
Oral, 500 mg every six hours for seven to ten days.

### Usual pediatric dose
Children 10 years of age and older—See *Usual adult and adolescent dose*.
Children 6 to 9 years of age—Oral, 400 mg every six hours for seven to ten days.
Children less than 6 years of age—Dosage has not been established.

### Strength(s) usually available
U.S.—
Dosage form not commercially available. Compounding required for prescription.
Canada—
Dosage form not commercially available. Compounding required for prescription.

### Packaging and storage
Prior to reconstitution, store between 15 and 25 °C (59 and 78 °F), in a dry place.

### Preparation of dosage form
To prepare initial dilution for oral solution, add a measured quantity of sterile water for injection (without antimicrobial agents or other added substances) or sterile water for inhalation, sufficient for dissolution, to each 6-gram vial. Add dissolved solution to 0.9% sodium chloride or 5% dextrose in water.

### Stability
The stability of ribavirin for inhalation solution (lyophilized powder) is unaffected by temperature, light, and moisture.
After reconstitution, solutions retain their potency at room temperature (20 to 30 °C [68 to 86 °F]) for 24 hours.
Ribavirin solutions are colorless.

# Parenteral Dosage Forms

Note: Bracketed uses in the *Dosage Forms* section refer to categories of use and/or indications that are not included in U.S. product labeling.

## RIBAVIRIN FOR INJECTION

Note: Ribavirin for Inhalation Solution USP is the dosage form being used because a parenteral solution is not commercially available.

### Usual adult and adolescent dose
[Lassa fever (treatment)][1]—
Intravenous infusion, 30 mg per kg of body weight loading dose, then 16 mg per kg of body weight every six hours for four days, then 8 mg per kg of body weight every eight hours for six more days. Infuse over 15 to 20 minutes.

### Usual pediatric dose
Dosage has not been established.

### Strength(s) usually available
U.S.—
Dosage form not commercially available. Compounding required for prescription.
Canada—
Dosage form not commercially available. Compounding required for prescription.

### Packaging and storage
Prior to reconstitution, store between 15 and 25 °C (59 and 78 °F), in a dry place.

### Preparation of dosage form
To prepare initial dilution for parenteral use, add a measured quantity of sterile water for injection (without antimicrobial agents or other added substances) or sterile water for inhalation, sufficient for dissolution, to each 6-gram vial. Add to 0.9% sodium chloride or 5% dextrose in water and infuse over 15 to 20 minutes.

### Stability
The stability of ribavirin for inhalation solution (lyophilized powder) is unaffected by temperature, light, and moisture.
After reconstitution, solutions retain their potency at room temperature (20 to 30 °C [68 to 86 °F]) for 24 hours.
Ribavirin solutions are colorless.

---

[1]Not included in Canadian product labeling.

## Selected Bibliography

Demers RR, Parker J, Frankel LR, et al. Administration of ribavirin to neonatal and pediatric patients during mechanical ventilation. Respir Care 1986; 31: 1188-96.

Frankel LR, Wilson CW, Demers RR, et al. A technique for the administration of ribavirin to mechanically ventilated infants with severe respiratory syncytial virus infection. Crit Care Med 1987; 15: 1051-4.

McCormick JB, et al. Lassa fever-effective therapy with ribavirin. New Engl J Med 1986; 314 (1): 20-6.

Outwater KM, Meissner HC, Peterson MB. Ribavirin administration to infants receiving mechanical ventilation. Am J Dis Child 1988; 142: 512-5.

Revised: 02/23/93
Interim revision: 06/08/94

# RIBOFLAVIN   Systemic

VA CLASSIFICATION (Primary): VT106

A commonly used name is vitamin $B_2$.

Note: For a listing of dosage forms and brand names by country availability, see *Dosage Forms* section(s). For a listing of brand names for the articles in this monograph, refer to the General Index.

## Category

Nutritional supplement (vitamin)

Note: Riboflavin (vitamin $B_2$) is a water-soluble vitamin.

## Indications

### Accepted

Riboflavin deficiency (prophylaxis and treatment)—Riboflavin is indicated for prevention and treatment of riboflavin deficiency states. Riboflavin deficiency may occur as a result of inadequate nutrition or intestinal malabsorption but does not occur in healthy individuals receiving an adequate balanced diet. Simple nutritional deficiency of individual B vitamins is rare since dietary inadequacy usually results in multiple deficiencies. For prophylaxis of riboflavin deficiency, dietary improvement, rather than supplementation, is advisable. For treatment of riboflavin deficiency, supplementation is preferred.

Deficiency of riboflavin (ariboflavinosis) may lead to angular stomatitis, cheilosis, corneal vascularization, and dermatoses. Severe deficiency may cause normocytic, normochromic anemia and neuropathy.

Requirements for riboflavin may be increased and/or supplementation may be necessary in the following persons or conditions (although clinical deficiencies are usually rare):

Burns
Fever, chronic
Gastrectomy
Hepatic-biliary tract disease—alcoholism with cirrhosis, obstructive jaundice
Hyperbilirubinemia in neonates as phototherapy due to photo-decomposition of riboflavin by blue light
Hyperthyroidism
Infection, prolonged
Intestinal disease—celiac, tropical sprue, regional enteritis, persistent diarrhea
Malignancy
Stress, prolonged

Recommended intakes for riboflavin are related to caloric intake.

Some unusual diets (e.g., reducing diets that drastically restrict food selection) may not supply minimum daily requirements of riboflavin. Supplementation is necessary in patients receiving total parenteral nutrition (TPN) or undergoing rapid weight loss or in those with malnutrition, because of inadequate dietary intake.

Recommended intakes for all vitamins and most minerals are increased during pregnancy. Many physicians recommend that pregnant women receive multivitamin and mineral supplements, especially those pregnant women who do not consume an adequate diet and those in high-risk categories (i.e., women carrying more than one fetus, heavy cigarette smokers, and alcohol and drug abusers). Taking excessive amounts of a multivitamin and mineral supplement may be harmful to the mother and/or fetus and should be avoided.

Recommended intakes for all vitamins and most minerals are increased during breast-feeding.

Recommended intakes may be increased by the following medications: Phenothiazines, tricyclic antidepressants, and probenecid.

### Unaccepted

Riboflavin has not been proven effective for treatment of acne, burning foot syndrome, congenital methemoglobinemia, migraine headaches, or muscle cramps.

## Pharmacology/Pharmacokinetics

### Physicochemical characteristics

Molecular weight—376.37.

pKa—10.2.

### Mechanism of action/Effect

Riboflavin is converted to 2 coenzymes, flavin mononucleotide (FMN) and flavin adenine dinucleotide (FAD), which are necessary for normal tissue respiration. Riboflavin is also required for activation of pyridoxine, conversion of tryptophan to niacin, and may be involved in maintaining erythrocyte integrity.

### Absorption

The B vitamins are readily absorbed from the gastrointestinal tract, except in malabsorption syndromes. Riboflavin is absorbed mainly in the duodenum. Alcohol inhibits intestinal absorption of riboflavin.

### Protein binding

Metabolites (FAD and FMN)—Moderate (60%).

### Storage

Riboflavin and metabolites are distributed into all body tissues and breast milk. A small amount is stored in the liver, spleen, kidneys, and heart.

### Biotransformation

Hepatic.

### Half-life

Oral or intramuscular administration—66 to 84 minutes.

### Elimination

Renal (almost entirely as metabolites). Excess beyond daily needs is excreted, largely unchanged, in urine. Riboflavin is present in the feces.

In dialysis—Hemodialysis removes riboflavin, but more slowly than normal renal excretion.

## Precautions to Consider

### Pregnancy/Reproduction

Problems in humans have not been documented with intake of normal daily recommended amounts.

### Breast-feeding

Problems in humans have not been documented with intake of normal daily recommended amounts.

### Pediatrics

Problems in pediatrics have not been documented with intake of normal daily recommended amounts.

### Geriatrics

Problems in geriatrics have not been documented with intake of normal daily recommended amounts.

### Drug interactions and/or related problems

The following drug interactions and/or related problems have been selected on the basis of their potential clinical significance (possible mechanism in parentheses where appropriate)—not necessarily inclusive (» = major clinical significance):

Note: Combinations containing any of the following medications, depending on the amount present, may also interact with this medication.

Alcohol
   (impairs intestinal absorption of riboflavin)

Antidepressants, tricyclic or
Phenothiazines
(requirements for riboflavin may be increased in patients receiving
these medications)
Probenecid
(concurrent use decreases gastrointestinal absorption of riboflavin;
requirements for riboflavin may be increased in patients receiving
probenecid)

### Laboratory value alterations

The following have been selected on the basis of their potential clinical
significance (possible effect in parentheses where appropriate)—not
necessarily inclusive (» = major clinical significance):

Note: Usually occurs only with large doses.

With diagnostic test results
Urinary catecholamine concentration measurements by fluorimetric
methods
(riboflavin may produce fluorescent substances and falsely elevated
results)

Urobilinogen determinations using Ehrlich's reagent
(riboflavin may produce false-positive results)

## Side/Adverse Effects

While toxicity with high doses of riboflavin has not been reported, high
doses of other water-soluble vitamins have been known to cause
problems.

Large doses of riboflavin may cause yellow discoloration of urine.

## Patient Consultation

As an aid to patient consultation, refer to *Advice for the Patient, Riboflavin
(Vitamin B₂) (Systemic)*.

In providing consultation, consider emphasizing the following selected
information (» = major clinical significance):

### Description of use
Description should include function in the body, signs of deficiency,
and unproven uses

### Importance of diet
Importance of proper nutrition; supplement may be needed because of
inadequate dietary intake
Food sources of riboflavin; effects of processing
Not using vitamins as substitute for balanced diet
Recommended daily intake for riboflavin

### Proper use of this dietary supplement
» Proper dosing
Missed dose: No cause for concern because of length of time necessary
for depletion; remembering to take as directed
» Proper storage

### Side/adverse effects
Possible yellow discoloration of urine with large doses; no cause for
concern

## General Dosing Information

Because of the infrequency of single B vitamin deficiencies, combinations
are commonly administered. Many commercial combinations of B vitamins are available.

### Diet/Nutrition

Recommended dietary intakes for riboflavin are defined differently
worldwide.

For U.S.—

The Recommended Dietary Allowances (RDAs) for vitamins and minerals are determined by the Food and Nutrition Board of the National Research Council and are intended to provide adequate nutrition in most healthy persons under usual environmental stresses.
In addition, a different designation may be used by the FDA for
food and dietary supplement labeling purposes, as with Daily
Value (DV). DVs replace the previous labeling terminology United
States Recommended Daily Allowances (USRDAs).

For Canada—

Recommended Nutrient Intakes (RNIs) for vitamins, minerals, and
protein are determined by Health and Welfare in Canada and provide recommended amounts of a specific nutrient while minimizing
the risk of chronic diseases.

Daily recommended intakes for riboflavin are generally defined as follows:

| Persons | U.S. (mg) | Canada (mg) |
|---|---|---|
| Infants and children | | |
| Birth to 3 years of age | 0.4–0.8 | 0.3–0.7 |
| 4 to 6 years of age | 1.1 | 0.9 |
| 7 to 10 years of age | 1.2 | 1–1.3 |
| Adolescent and adult males | 1.4–1.8 | 1–1.6 |
| Adolescent and adult females | 1.2–1.3 | 1–1.1 |
| Pregnant females | 1.6 | 1.1–1.4 |
| Breast-feeding females | 1.7–1.8 | 1.4–1.5 |

These are ususally provided by adequate diets.

The best dietary sources of riboflavin include milk and dairy products,
fish, meats, green leafy vegetables, and whole grain and enriched cereals and bread. There is little loss of riboflavin from foods with ordinary cooking.

## Oral Dosage Forms

### RIBOFLAVIN TABLETS USP

#### Usual adult and adolescent dose
Deficiency (prophylaxis)—
Oral, amount based on normal daily recommended intakes:

| Persons | U.S. (mg) | Canada (mg) |
|---|---|---|
| Adolescent and adult males | 1.4–1.8 | 1–1.6 |
| Adolescent and adult females | 1.2–1.3 | 1–1.1 |
| Pregnant females | 1.6 | 1.1–1.4 |
| Breast-feeding females | 1.7–1.8 | 1.4–1.5 |

Deficiency (treatment)—
Treatment dose is individualized by prescriber based on severity of
deficiency.

#### Usual pediatric dose
Deficiency (prophylaxis)—
Oral, amount based on intake of normal daily recommended intakes:

| Persons | U.S. (mg) | Canada (mg) |
|---|---|---|
| Infants and children | | |
| Birth to 3 years of age | 0.4–0.8 | 0.3–0.7 |
| 4 to 6 years of age | 1.1 | 0.9 |
| 7 to 10 years of age | 1.2 | 1–1.3 |

Deficiency (treatment)—
Treatment dose is individualized by prescriber based on severity of
deficiency.

#### Strength(s) usually available
U.S.—
10 mg (OTC) [GENERIC].
25 mg (OTC) [GENERIC].
50 mg (OTC) [GENERIC].
100 mg (OTC) [GENERIC].
250 mg (OTC) [GENERIC].
Canada—
5 mg (OTC) [GENERIC].
100 mg (OTC) [GENERIC].
Note: Some strengths of these riboflavin preparations may exceed the
dosage range recommended by USP DI Advisory Panels based
on the amount necessary to meet normal nutritional needs.

#### Packaging and storage
Store below 40 °C (104 °F), preferably between 15 and 30 °C (59 and 86
°F), unless otherwise specified by manufacturer. Store in a tight, light-
resistant container.

Revised: 08/22/92
Interim revision: 07/29/94; 05/01/95

## RICE SYRUP SOLIDS AND ELECTROLYTES—See
*Carbohydrates and Electrolytes (Systemic)*

# RIFABUTIN    Systemic

VA CLASSIFICATION (Primary): AM900

Note: For a listing of dosage forms and brand names by country availability, see *Dosage Forms* section(s). For a listing of brand names for the articles in this monograph, refer to the General Index.

## Category

Antibacterial (antimycobacterial).

## Indications

### Accepted

*Mycobacterium avium* complex (MAC) disease (prophylaxis)—Rifabutin is indicated for the prevention of disseminated MAC disease in patients with advanced human immunodeficiency virus (HIV) infection.

Rifabutin also has *in vitro* activity against many strains of *Mycobacterium tuberculosis*. However, there is no evidence that rifabutin is effective as a prophylactic agent for tuberculosis. Isoniazid and rifabutin may be given concurrently for the prophylaxis of tuberculosis and MAC, respectively. Cross-resistance between rifampin and rifabutin is commonly observed with *M. tuberculosis* and *M. avium* complex isolates that are highly resistant to rifampin.

## Pharmacology/Pharmacokinetics

### Physicochemical characteristics
Molecular weight—847.02.

### Mechanism of action/Effect
Rifabutin inhibits DNA-dependent RNA polymerase in susceptible strains of *Escherichia coli* and *Bacillus subtilis*, but not in mammalian cells. Rifabutin does not inhibit this enzyme in resistant strains of *E. coli*. It is not known whether rifabutin inhibits DNA-dependent RNA polymerase in *Mycobacterium avium* or in *M. intracellulare*, which constitute *M. avium* complex (MAC).

### Absorption
Readily absorbed from the gastrointestinal tract. High-fat meals slow the rate, but not the extent, of absorption. Bioavailability is approximately 20%.

### Distribution
Highly lipophilic; widely distributed with extensive intracellular tissue uptake. Rifabutin crosses the blood-brain barrier; cerebrospinal fluid (CSF) concentrations are approximately 50% of the corresponding serum concentration.
Vol$_D$ =Approximately 9 liters per kg.

### Protein binding
High (approximately 85%).

### Biotransformation
Hepatic; 5 metabolites have been identified.

### Half-life
Mean terminal—45 hours (range, 16 to 69 hours).

### Time to peak concentration
2 to 4 hours.

### Peak serum concentration
375 nanograms per mL after a single oral dose of 300 mg in healthy volunteers.

### Elimination
30% fecal; 5% unchanged in the urine; 5% unchanged in the bile; 53% in urine as metabolites.
In dialysis—Hemodialysis is not expected to enhance elimination.

## Precautions to Consider

### Cross-sensitivity and/or related problems
Patients sensitive to other rifamycins (e.g., rifampin) may also be sensitive to rifabutin.

### Carcinogenicity
Long-term carcinogenicity studies found that rifabutin was not carcinogenic in mice at doses of up to 180 mg per kg of body weight (mg/kg) per day, or approximately 36 times the recommended human daily dose. Rifabutin was not carcinogenic in rats at doses of up to 60 mg/kg per day, or 12 times the recommended human dose.

### Mutagenicity
Rifabutin was not mutagenic in the Ames test using both rifabutin-susceptible and -resistant strains or in *Schizosaccharomyces pombe* $P_1$ and

was not genotoxic in V-79 Chinese hamster cells, human lymphocytes *in vitro*, or mouse bone marrow cells *in vivo*.

### Pregnancy/Reproduction
Fertility—Fertility was impaired in male rats given 160 mg/kg of rifabutin, or 32 times the recommended human daily dose.

Pregnancy—Adequate and well-controlled studies have not been done in humans.

No teratogenicity was seen in rats and rabbits given rifabutin at doses of up to 200 mg/kg (40 times the recommended human daily dose). There was a decrease in fetal viability in rats given 200 mg/kg per day. At 40 mg/kg per day, rifabutin caused an increase in rat fetal skeletal variants. In rabbits, rifabutin was maternotoxic and there was an increase in fetal skeletal anomalies at 80 mg/kg per day.

FDA Pregnancy Category B.

### Breast-feeding
It is not known whether rifabutin is distributed into human breast milk.

### Pediatrics
The safety and efficacy of rifabutin in the prophylaxis of *Mycobacterium avium* complex (MAC) in children have not been established. Limited data are available about the use of rifabutin in children; it was used, along with 2 other antimycobacterials, to treat MAC in 22 HIV-positive children. The mean doses used were 18.5 mg/kg in infants one year of age, 8.6 mg/kg in children 2 to 10 years of age, and 4 mg/kg in adolescents 14 to 16 years of age. Side effects seen in children were similar to those seen in adults.

### Geriatrics
No information is available on the relationship of age to the effects of rifabutin in geriatric patients.

### Drug interactions and/or related problems
The following drug interactions and/or related problems have been selected on the basis of their potential clinical significance (possible mechanism in parentheses where appropriate)—not necessarily inclusive (» = major clinical significance):

Note: Didanosine (ddI) and rifabutin coadministration has been studied in AIDS patients; rifabutin does not appear to affect the pharmacokinetics of didanosine and no dosage modifications are necessary.

   Combinations containing any of the following medications, depending on the amount present, may also interact with this medication.

Aminophylline or
Anticoagulants, coumarin- or indandione-derivative or
Antidiabetic agents, oral or
Barbiturates or
Beta-adrenergic blocking agents, systemic or
Chloramphenicol or
Clofibrate or
Contraceptives, estrogen-containing, oral or
Corticosteroids, glucocorticoid and mineralocorticoid or
Cyclosporine or
Dapsone or
Diazepam or
Digitalis glycosides or
Disopyramide or
Estramustine or
Estrogens or
Ketoconazole or
Mexiletine or
Oxtriphylline or
Phenytoin or
Quinidine or
Theophylline or
Tocainide or
Verapamil, oral
   (rifampin is structurally related to rifabutin; rifampin is known to reduce the activity of many drugs [including those listed above] due to its hepatic enzyme–inducing properties; rifabutin appears to be a less potent enzyme inducer of the hepatic cytochrome P-450 system than rifampin. Drug interaction data are unavailable for rifabutin itself; therefore, it is recommended that patients taking rifabutin concurrently with these medications be monitored since the significance of possible drug interactions is not known)

Fluconazole
   (pharmacokinetic studies with fluconazole and rifabutin show that fluconazole appears to increase the serum concentration of rifabutin; however, this is not thought to have clinical significance and

rifabutin dosing does not need to be modified in patients receiving fluconazole; in addition, the pharmacokinetics of fluconazole were unchanged)

Methadone
(concurrent administration with rifabutin has no significant effect on the pharmacokinetics of methadone; however, a few patients may require methadone dosage modification if symptoms of narcotic withdrawal occur)

» Zidovudine
(steady-state plasma concentrations and the area under the plasma concentration-time curve [AUC] of zidovudine were decreased after repeated rifabutin dosing in healthy volunteers and HIV-positive patients in phase I trials; the mean decreases in peak plasma concentration and AUC were 48% and 32%, respectively. However, a population pharmacokinetic analysis of zidovudine concentration versus time data from two phase III studies showed a nonsignificant trend for rifabutin to increase the apparent clearance of zidovudine. *In vitro* studies have demonstrated that rifabutin does not affect the inhibition of HIV by zidovudine)

### Laboratory value alterations
The following have been selected on the basis of their potential clinical significance (possible effect in parentheses where appropriate)—not necessarily inclusive (» = major clinical significance):

With physiology/laboratory test values
Neutrophil count
(rifabutin may cause neutropenia)

Platelet count
(rifabutin may, in rare cases, cause thrombocytopenia)

### Medical considerations/Contraindications
The medical considerations/contraindications included here have been selected on the basis of their potential clinical significance (reasons given in parentheses where appropriate)—not necessarily inclusive (» = major clinical significance).

*Except under special circumstances, this medication should not be used when the following medical problems exist:*

» Hypersensitivity to rifabutin or rifampin
» Tuberculosis, active
(patients with active tuberculosis must be treated with an effective combination of antitubercular agents; administration of single-agent rifabutin for prophylaxis of MAC to patients with active tuberculosis is likely to lead to the development of tuberculosis that is resistant to both rifabutin and rifampin)

### Patient monitoring
The following may be especially important in patient monitoring (other tests may be warranted in some patients, depending on condition; » = major clinical significance):

Platelet count

White blood cell count
(recommended periodically since rifabutin may cause neutropenia and, rarely, thrombocytopenia)

## Side/Adverse Effects
The following side/adverse effects have been selected on the basis of their potential clinical significance (possible signs and symptoms in parentheses where appropriate)—not necessarily inclusive:

### Those indicating need for medical attention
Incidence more frequent
*Skin rash*
Incidence rare
*Arthralgia* (joint pain); *dysgeusia* (change in taste); *myalgia* (muscle pain); *neutropenia* (fever and sore throat); *pseudojaundice* (yellow skin); *uveitis* (eye pain; loss of vision)
Note: Uveitis is usually associated with doses larger than 1050 mg per day.

### Those indicating need for medical attention only if they continue or are bothersome
Incidence more frequent
*Nausea; vomiting*

### Those not indicating need for medical attention
Incidence more frequent
*Reddish orange to reddish brown discoloration of urine, feces, saliva, skin, sputum, sweat, and tears*
Note: Tears discolored by rifabutin may also discolor soft contact lenses.

## Patient Consultation
As an aid to patient consultation, refer to *Advice for the Patient, Rifabutin (Systemic)*.

In providing consultation, consider emphasizing the following selected information (» = major clinical significance):

### Before using this medication
» Conditions affecting use, especially:
Hypersensitivity to rifabutin or rifampin
Other medications, especially zidovudine
Other medical problems, especially active tuberculosis

### Proper use of this medication
Taking on an empty stomach, or with food if gastrointestinal irritation occurs
» Compliance with full course of therapy, which may take months
» Proper dosing
» Missed dose: Taking as soon as possible; not taking if almost time for next dose; not doubling doses
» Proper storage

### Precautions while using this medication
» Regular visits to physician to check progress
» Medication causes tears to turn reddish orange to reddish brown and may also permanently discolor soft contact lenses; avoiding the use of soft contact lenses during treatment

### Side/adverse effects
Signs of potential side effects, especially skin rash, arthralgia, dysgeusia, myalgia, neutropenia, pseudojaundice, and uveitis
Reddish orange to reddish brown discoloration of urine, stools, saliva, skin, sputum, sweat, and tears may be alarming to patient, although medically insignificant

## General Dosing Information
Rifabutin is absorbed more rapidly if taken on an empty stomach. However, if gastrointestinal irritation occurs, administering rifabutin at doses of 150 mg two times a day with food may help reduce stomach upset.

Contents of rifabutin capsules may be mixed with applesauce for patients who are unable to swallow the capsules.

## Oral Dosage Forms
### RIFABUTIN CAPSULES

#### Usual adult and adolescent dose
*Mycobacterium avium* complex (MAC) disease (prophylaxis)—
Oral, 300 mg once a day, or 150 mg two times a day.

#### Usual pediatric dose
Dosage has not been established; however, MAC prophylaxis should follow recommendations similar to those for adults and adolescents. Limited data are available about the use of rifabutin in children; it has been used in the treatment of MAC in HIV-positive children. The mean doses used were 18.5 mg per kg of body weight in infants one year of age, 8.6 mg per kg of body weight in children 2 to 10 years of age, and 4 mg per kg of body weight in adolescents 14 to 16 years of age. Side effects seen in children were similar to those seen in adults.

#### Strength(s) usually available
U.S.—
150 mg (Rx) [*Mycobutin*].
Canada—
150 mg (Rx) [*Mycobutin*].

#### Packaging and storage
Store between 15 and 30 °C (59 and 86 °F). Store in a tightly closed container.

#### Auxiliary labeling
• Continue medicine for full time of treatment.
• May discolor body fluids.

Revised: 06/22/94

# RIFAMPIN    Systemic

INN: Rifampicin
VA CLASSIFICATION (Primary): AM500/AM900
Note: For a listing of dosage forms and brand names by country availability, see *Dosage Forms* section(s). For a listing of brand names for the articles in this monograph, refer to the General Index.

## Category

Antibacterial (antimycobacterial; antileprosy agent).

## Indications

Note: Bracketed information in the *Indications* section refers to uses that are not included in U.S. product labeling.

### Accepted

Tuberculosis (treatment)—Rifampin is indicated in combination with other antituberculosis medications in the treatment of all forms of tuberculosis, including tuberculous meningitis.

Meningococcal infections (prophylaxis)—Rifampin is indicated in the treatment of close contacts of patients with proved or suspected infection caused by *Neisseria meningitidis*. These contacts include other household members, children in nurseries, persons in day care centers, and closed populations, such as military recruits. Health care providers who have intimate exposure (e.g., mouth-to-mouth resuscitation) with index cases also should receive prophylactic therapy.

[*Haemophilus influenzae* type b infection (prophylaxis)][1]—Rifampin is used in the treatment of close contacts of patients with proved or suspected infections caused by *H. influenzae* type b if at least one of the contacts is 4 years of age or younger. A close contact is defined as one who has spent 4 or more hours per day for five of the seven most recent days with the index case.

[Leprosy (treatment)][1]—Rifampin is used in combination with other agents in the treatment of leprosy (Hansen's disease).

[Mycobacterial infections, atypical (treatment)][1]—Rifampin is used in combination with other agents in the treatment of certain atypical (nontuberculous) mycobacterial infections, such as those caused by *Mycobacterium avium* complex (MAC).

[Rifampin, administered concurrently with other antistaphylococcal agents, also may be used in the treatment of serious infections caused by *Staphylococcus* species (including methicillin- and multiresistant strains).][1]

### Unaccepted

Rifampin is not indicated as a sole agent in the treatment of meningococcal infections because of the possibility of the rapid emergence of resistant organisms.

---

[1]Not included in Canadian product labeling.

## Pharmacology/Pharmacokinetics

### Physicochemical characteristics

Molecular weight—822.95.

### Mechanism of action/Effect

Rifampin, a semisynthetic broad-spectrum bactericidal antibiotic, inhibits bacterial RNA synthesis by binding strongly to the beta subunit of DNA-dependent RNA polymerase, preventing attachment of the enzyme to DNA and thus blocking initiation of RNA transcription.

### Absorption

Well absorbed from the gastrointestinal tract.

### Distribution

Diffuses well to most body tissues and fluids, including the cerebrospinal fluid (CSF), where concentrations are increased if the meninges are inflamed; concentrations in the liver, gallbladder, bile, and urine are higher than those found in the blood; therapeutic concentrations are achieved in the saliva, reaching 20% of serum concentrations; crosses the placenta, with fetal serum concentrations at birth found to be approximately 33% of the maternal serum concentration; penetrates into aqueous humor; and is distributed into breast milk. Being lipid-soluble, rifampin may reach and kill susceptible intracellular, as well as extracellular, bacteria and *Mycobacteria* species.

$Vol_D = 1.6$ L per kg.

### Protein binding

High to very high (89%).

### Biotransformation

Hepatic; rapidly deacetylated by auto-induced microsomal oxidative enzymes to active metabolite (25-O-desacetylrifampin). Other identified metabolites include, rifampin quinone, desacetyl rifampin quinone, and 3-formylrifampin.

### Half-life

Absorption half-life—
    Approximately 0.6 hour.
Elimination half-life—
    Initially, 3 to 5 hours; with repeated administration, half-life decreases to 2 to 3 hours.

### Time to peak plasma concentration

1.5 to 4 hours after oral administration; peak concentration may be decreased and delayed following administration with food.

### Peak plasma concentration

Oral—
    Adults: 7 to 9 mcg/mL after 600 mg.
    Children (6 to 58 months old): Approximately 11 mcg/mL after a dose of 10 mg per kg of body weight (mg/kg) mixed in applesauce or simple syrup.
Intravenous—
    Adults: Approximately 17.5 mcg/mL after a 30 minute infusion of 600 mg.
    Children (3 months to 12 years old): Approximately 26 mcg/mL after a 30 minute infusion of 300 mg per m$^2$.

### Elimination

Biliary/fecal; enterohepatic recirculation of rifampin, but not of its deacetylated active metabolite; 60 to 65% of dose appears in feces.
Renal; 6 to 15% excreted as unchanged drug, and 15% excreted as active metabolite in urine; 7% excreted as inactive 3-formyl derivative.
Rifampin does not accumulate in patients with impaired renal function; its rate of excretion is increased during the first 6 to 10 days of therapy, probably because of auto-induction of hepatic microsomal oxidative enzymes; after high doses, excretion may be slower because of saturation of its biliary excretory mechanism.
In dialysis—
    Rifampin is not removed from the blood by either hemodialysis or peritoneal dialysis.

## Precautions to Consider

### Tumorigenicity

Studies in female mice of a strain known to be particularly susceptible to the spontaneous development of hepatomas have shown that rifampin, given in doses of 2 to 10 times the maximum human dose for 1 year, causes a significant increase in the development of hepatomas. However, studies in male mice of the same strain, in other strains of male or female mice, or in rats have not shown that rifampin is tumorigenic.

### Pregnancy/Reproduction

Pregnancy—Rifampin crosses the placenta. It is recommended that pregnant women with tuberculosis be treated for a minimum of 9 months with multi-drug therapy, including rifampin. It has rarely caused postnatal hemorrhages in the mother and infant when administered during the last few weeks of pregnancy; vitamin K may be indicated. Neonates should be carefully observed for evidence of adverse effects.
Imperfect osteogenesis and embryotoxicity were reported in rabbits given up to 20 times the usual daily human dose. Studies in rodents have shown that rifampin given in doses of 150 to 250 mg per kg of body weight (mg/kg) daily causes congenital malformations, primarily cleft palate and spina bifida.

FDA Pregnancy Category C.

### Breast-feeding

Rifampin is distributed into breast milk. Problems in humans have not been documented.

### Pediatrics

Appropriate studies performed to date have not demonstrated pediatrics-specific problems that would limit the usefulness of rifampin in children.

### Geriatrics

Appropriate studies on the relationship of age to the effects of rifampin have not been performed in the geriatric population. However, no geriatrics-specific problems have been documented to date.

### Dental

The leukopenic and thrombocytopenic effects of rifampin may result in an increased incidence of certain microbial infections, delayed healing, and gingival bleeding. If leukopenia or thrombocytopenia occurs, dental work should be deferred until blood counts have returned to normal. Patients should be instructed in proper oral hygiene, including caution in use of regular toothbrushes, dental floss, and toothpicks.

Rifampin may cause a hypersensitivity reaction of sore mouth or tongue.

## Drug interactions and/or related problems

The following drug interactions and/or related problems have been selected on the basis of their potential clinical significance (possible mechanism in parentheses where appropriate)—not necessarily inclusive (» = major clinical significance):

Note: Combinations containing any of the following medications, depending on the amount present, may also interact with this medication.

» Alcohol
(concurrent daily use of alcohol may result in increased incidence of rifampin-induced hepatotoxicity and increased metabolism of rifampin; dosage adjustments of rifampin may be necessary, and patients should be monitored closely for signs of hepatotoxicity)

» Aminophylline or
» Oxtriphylline or
» Theophylline
(rifampin may increase metabolism of theophylline, oxtriphylline, and aminophylline by induction of hepatic microsomal enzymes, resulting in increased theophylline clearance)

Anesthetics, hydrocarbon inhalation, except isoflurane
(chronic use of hepatic enzyme–inducing agents prior to anesthesia, except isoflurane, may increase anesthetic metabolism, leading to increased risk of hepatotoxicity)

» Anticoagulants, coumarin- or indandione-derivative
(concurrent use with rifampin may enhance the metabolism of these anticoagulants by induction of hepatic microsomal enzymes, resulting in a considerable decrease in the activity and effectiveness of the anticoagulants; prothrombin time determinations may be required as frequently as daily; dosage adjustments of anticoagulants may be required before and after rifampin therapy)

» Antidiabetic agents, oral
(concurrent use with rifampin may enhance the metabolism of tolbutamide, chlorpropamide, and glyburide by induction of hepatic microsomal enzymes, resulting in lower serum sulfonylurea concentrations; although not documented, other oral antidiabetic agents may also interact with rifampin; dosage adjustment may be required)

» Azole antifungals
(concurrent use may increase the metabolism of the azole antifungals, lowering their plasma concentrations; depending on the clinical situation, the dose of an azole antifungal may need to be increased during concurrent use with rifampin)

Barbiturates
(concurrent use with rifampin may enhance the metabolism of hexobarbital by induction of hepatic microsomal enzymes, resulting in lower serum concentrations; there are conflicting data on rifampin's effect on phenobarbital; dosage adjustment may be required)

Beta-adrenergic blocking agents, systemic
(concurrent use of metoprolol or propranolol with rifampin has resulted in reduced plasma concentrations of these 2 beta-adrenergic blocking agents due to enhanced metabolism of hepatic microsomal enzymes by rifampin; although not documented, other beta-adrenergic blocking agents may also interact with rifampin)

Bone marrow depressants (See *Appendix II*)
(concurrent use of bone marrow depressants with rifampin may increase the leukopenic and/or thrombocytopenic effects; if concurrent use is required, close observation for myelotoxic effects should be considered)

» Chloramphenicol
(concurrent use with rifampin may enhance the metabolism of chloramphenicol by induction of hepatic microsomal enzymes, resulting in significantly lower serum chloramphenicol concentrations; dosage adjustment may be necessary)

Clofazimine
(concurrent use with rifampin has resulted in reduced absorption of rifampin, delaying its time to peak concentration, and increasing its half-life)

Clofibrate
(concurrent use with rifampin may enhance the metabolism of clofibrate by induction of hepatic microsomal enzymes, resulting in significantly lower serum clofibrate concentrations)

» Contraceptives, estrogen-containing, oral
(concurrent use with rifampin may decrease the effectiveness of estrogen-containing oral contraceptives because of stimulation of estrogen metabolism or reduction in enterohepatic circulation of estrogens, resulting in menstrual irregularities, intermenstrual bleeding, and unplanned pregnancies; patients should be advised to use an additional method of contraception throughout the whole cycle while taking rifampin and estrogen-containing oral contraceptives concurrently)

» Corticosteroids, glucocorticoid and mineralocorticoid
(concurrent use with rifampin may enhance the metabolism of corticosteroids by induction of hepatic microsomal enzymes, resulting in a considerable decrease in corticosteroid plasma concentrations; dosage adjustment may be required; rifampin has also counteracted endogenous cortisol and produced acute adrenal insufficiency in patients with Addison's disease)

Cyclosporine
(rifampin may enhance metabolism of cyclosporine by induction of hepatic microsomal enzymes and intestinal cytochrome P-450 enzymes; dosage adjustment may be required)

Dapsone
(concurrent use with rifampin may decrease the effect of dapsone because of increased metabolism resulting from stimulation of hepatic microsomal enzyme activity; dapsone concentrations may be decreased by half; dapsone dosage adjustments are not required during concurrent therapy with rifampin for leprosy)

Diazepam
(concurrent use with rifampin may enhance the elimination of diazepam, resulting in decreased plasma concentrations; whether this effect applies to other benzodiazepines has not been determined; dosage adjustment may be necessary)

» Digitalis glycosides
(concurrent use with rifampin may enhance the metabolism of digoxin or digitoxin by induction of hepatic microsomal enzymes, resulting in significantly lower serum digoxin or digitoxin concentrations; dosage adjustment may be necessary)

» Disopyramide or
» Mexiletine or
Propafenone or
» Quinidine or
» Tocainide
(concurrent use with rifampin may enhance the metabolism of these antiarrhythmics by induction of hepatic microsomal enzymes, resulting in significantly lower serum antiarrhythmic concentrations; serum antiarrhythmic concentrations should be monitored and dosage adjustment may be necessary)

» Estramustine or
» Estrogens
(concurrent use of estramustine or estrogens with rifampin may result in significantly reduced estrogenic effect because of stimulation of estrogen metabolism or reduction in enterohepatic circulation of estrogens)

» Hepatotoxic medications, other (See *Appendix II*)
(concurrent use of rifampin and other hepatotoxic medications may increase the potential for hepatotoxicity; patients should be monitored closely for signs of hepatotoxicity)

» Isoniazid
(concurrent use of isoniazid with rifampin may increase the risk of hepatotoxicity, especially in patients with pre-existing hepatic function impairment and/or in fast acetylators of isoniazid; patients should be monitored closely for signs of hepatotoxicity during the first 3 months of therapy)

» Methadone
(concurrent use with rifampin may decrease the effects of methadone because of stimulation of hepatic microsomal enzyme activity and/or impaired absorption, resulting in symptoms of methadone withdrawal if the patient is dependent on methadone; dosage adjustments may be necessary during and after rifampin therapy)

» Phenytoin
(concurrent use with rifampin may stimulate the hepatic metabolism of phenytoin, increasing its elimination and thus counteracting its anticonvulsant effects; careful monitoring of serum hydantoin concentrations and dosage adjustments may be necessary before and after rifampin therapy)

Probenecid
(may compete with rifampin for hepatic uptake when used concurrently, resulting in increased and more prolonged rifampin serum concentrations and/or toxicity; however, the effect on rifampin serum concentrations is inconsistent, and concurrent use of pro-

benecid to increase rifampin serum concentrations is not recommended)

Trimethoprim
(concurrent use with rifampin may significantly increase the elimination and shorten the elimination half-life of trimethoprim)

» Verapamil, oral
(rifampin has been found to accelerate the metabolism of oral verapamil, resulting in a significant decrease in serum verapamil concentration and reversing its cardiovascular effects; concurrent use of intravenous verapamil with rifampin was found to have only minor effects on verapamil's clearance and no significant effect on cardiovascular effects)

## Laboratory value alterations

The following have been selected on the basis of their potential clinical significance (possible effect in parentheses where appropriate)—not necessarily inclusive (» = major clinical significance):

With diagnostic test results

Coombs' (antiglobulin) tests, direct
(may become positive rarely during rifampin therapy)

Dexamethasone suppression test
(rifampin may prevent the inhibitory action of a standard dexamethasone dose administered for the overnight suppression test, rendering the test abnormal; it is recommended that rifampin therapy be discontinued 15 days before administering the dexamethasone suppression test)

Folate determinations, serum and
Vitamin B$_{12}$ determinations, serum
(therapeutic concentrations of rifampin may interfere with standard microbiological assays for serum folate and vitamin B$_{12}$; alternate methods must be considered when determining serum folate and vitamin B$_{12}$ concentrations in patients taking rifampin)

Sulfobromophthalein (BSP) uptake and excretion
(hepatic uptake and excretion of BSP in liver function tests may be delayed by rifampin, resulting in BSP retention; the BSP test should be performed prior to the daily dose of rifampin to avoid false-positive test results)

Urinalyses based on spectrometry or color reaction
(rifampin may interfere with urinalyses that are based on spectrometry or color reaction due to rifampin's reddish orange to reddish brown discoloration of urine)

With physiology/laboratory test values

Alanine aminotransferase (ALT [SGPT]) and
Alkaline phosphatase and
Aspartate aminotransferase (AST [SGOT]) and
Bilirubin, serum concentrations and
Blood urea nitrogen (BUN) and
Uric acid, serum concentrations
(values may be increased)

## Medical considerations/Contraindications

The medical considerations/contraindications included here have been selected on the basis of their potential clinical significance (reasons given in parentheses where appropriate)—not necessarily inclusive (» = major clinical significance).

*Risk-benefit should be considered when the following medical problems exist:*

» Alcoholism, active or in remission or
» Hepatic function impairment
(rifampin is metabolized in the liver and may also be hepatotoxic)

Hypersensitivity to rifampin

## Patient monitoring

The following may be especially important in patient monitoring (other tests may be warranted in some patients, depending on condition; » = major clinical significance):

» Hepatic function determinations
(ALT [SGPT], AST [SGOT], alkaline phosphatase, and serum bilirubin determinations may be indicated prior to and monthly or more frequently during treatment; however, elevated serum enzyme values may not be predictive of clinical hepatitis and may return to normal despite continued treatment)

## Side/Adverse Effects

Note: Intermittent use of rifampin may increase the chance of a patient developing the "flu-like" syndrome, as well as acute hemolysis or renal failure. These reactions are thought to be immunologically mediated and intermittent use should be limited to those conditions, such as leprosy, where its safety and efficacy have been established.

The following side/adverse effects have been selected on the basis of their potential clinical significance (possible signs and symptoms in parentheses where appropriate)—not necessarily inclusive:

**Those indicating need for medical attention**

Incidence less frequent
*"Flu-like" syndrome* (chills; difficult breathing; dizziness; fever; headache; muscle and bone pain; shivering); *hypersensitivity* (itching; redness; skin rash)

Incidence rare
*Blood dyscrasias* (sore throat; unusual bleeding or bruising); *hepatitis* (yellow eyes or skin); *hepatitis prodromal symptoms* (loss of appetite; nausea or vomiting; unusual tiredness or weakness); *interstitial nephritis* (bloody or cloudy urine, greatly decreased frequency of urination or amount of urine)

**Those indicating need for medical attention only if they continue or are bothersome**

Incidence more frequent
*Gastrointestinal disturbances* (diarrhea; stomach cramps)

Incidence less frequent
*Fungal overgrowth* (sore mouth or tongue)

**Those not indicating need for medical attention**

Incidence more frequent
*Reddish orange to reddish brown discoloration of urine, feces, saliva, sputum, sweat, and tears*

Note: Tears discolored by rifampin may also discolor soft contact lenses.

## Overdose

The information below applies to the clinical effects and treatment of rifampin overdose.

### Clinical effects of rifampin overdose

The following effects have been selected on the basis of their potential clinical significance (possible signs and symptoms in parentheses where appropriate)—not necessarily inclusive

Acute and chronic effects
*Mental obtundation* (mental changes); *periorbital or facial edema* (swelling around the eyes or the whole face); *pruritus, generalized* (itching over the whole body); *Redman syndrome* (red-orange discoloration of skin, mucous membranes, and sclera)

Note: Fatalities are more likely to occur if there is underlying hepatic disease, frequent use or abuse of alcohol, or concurrent intake of other hepatotoxic medications.

### Treatment of rifampin overdose

To decrease absorption—
Evacuating stomach contents using ipecac syrup or gastric lavage.
Administering an activated charcoal slurry to help adsorb residual rifampin in the gastrointestinal tract.

Supportive care—
Supportive therapy.

## Patient Consultation

As an aid to patient consultation, refer to *Advice for the Patient, Rifampin (Systemic)*.

In providing consultation, consider emphasizing the following selected information (» = major clinical significance):

### Before using this medication

» Conditions affecting use, especially:
Hypersensitivity to rifampin
Pregnancy—Rifampin crosses the placenta and has rarely caused post-natal hemorrhages in the mother and infant when administered during the last few weeks of pregnancy
Breast-feeding—Rifampin is distributed into breast milk
Dental—Patients who develop blood dyscrasias may be at increased risk of microbial infections, delayed healing, and gingival bleeding
Other medications, especially azole antifungals, corticosteroids, coumarin- or indandione-derivative anticoagulants, oral antidiabetic agents, chloramphenicol, estrogen-containing oral contraceptives, digitalis glycosides, disopyramide, estramustine, estrogens, hepatotoxic medications, isoniazid, methadone, mexiletine, tocainide, phenytoin, quinidine, aminophylline, oxtriphylline, theophylline, or oral verapamil
Other medical problems, especially alcoholism, active or in remission, or impairment of hepatic function

## Proper use of this medication

Taking with a full glass (240 mL) of water on an empty stomach, 1 hour before or 2 hours after a meal, or with food if gastrointestinal irritation occurs

Proper administration technique for patients unable to swallow capsules

» Compliance with full course of therapy, which may take months or years

» Proper dosing

» Missed dose: Taking as soon as possible; not taking if almost time for next dose; not doubling doses; intermittent dosing may result in more frequent and/or severe side effects

» Proper storage

## Precautions while using this medication

» Regular visits to physician to check progress

Checking with physician if no improvement within 2 to 3 weeks

» Using an additional method of contraception if taking estrogen-containing oral contraceptives concurrently

» Avoiding alcoholic beverages concurrently with this medication

» Need to report prodromal signs of hepatotoxicity to physician

» Medication causes urine, feces, saliva, sputum, sweat, and tears to turn reddish orange to reddish brown and may also permanently discolor soft contact lenses; avoiding the wearing of soft contact lenses

Using caution in use of regular toothbrushes, dental floss, and toothpicks; deferring dental work until blood counts have returned to normal; checking with physician or dentist concerning proper oral hygiene

Possible interference with laboratory values

## Side/adverse effects

Reddish orange to reddish brown discoloration of urine, stools, saliva, sputum, sweat, and tears may be alarming to patient, although medically insignificant; however, tears discolored by rifampin may also discolor soft contact lenses

Signs of potential side effects, especially "flu-like" syndrome, hypersensitivity, blood dyscrasias, hepatitis, hepatitis prodromal symptoms, and interstitial nephritis

# General Dosing Information

Rifampin should preferably be taken with a full glass (240 mL) of water on an empty stomach (either 1 hour before or 2 hours after a meal) to obtain optimum absorption. However, it may be taken with food if gastrointestinal irritation occurs.

Contents of rifampin capsules may be mixed with applesauce or jelly for patients who are unable to swallow the capsules.

Since bacterial resistance may develop rapidly when rifampin is administered alone in the treatment of tuberculosis, it should be administered only concurrently with other antituberculosis medications.

Tuberculosis therapy must be continued for 6 months to 2 years, depending on the treatment regimen. Uncomplicated pulmonary tuberculosis is often successfully treated within 6 to 12 months. Several different treatment regimens are currently recommended.

- The Infectious Diseases Society of America recommends standard triple-drug therapy for patients born in the United States who have never been treated, do not reside in communities with a known high prevalence of drug-resistant *Mycobacterium* strains, and have no risk factors for drug-resistant tuberculosis.

—Isoniazid, rifampin, and, usually, pyrazinamide are given together daily for the first 2 months, then isoniazid and rifampin are continued daily or twice a week for the remainder of the treatment period. Directly observed therapy is recommended for patients suspected of being noncompliant. If a patient is at risk of being infected with drug-resistant organisms, 4-drug therapy, consisting of isoniazid, rifampin, pyrazinamide, and ethambutol, is recommended.

- The Centers for Disease Control recommend 3 other treatment regimen options available for non–HIV-infected patients:

—In geographic areas where the isoniazid resistance rate is documented to be ≥ 4%, an initial 4-drug regimen of isoniazid, rifampin, pyrazinamide, and streptomycin or ethambutol, taken under direct observation, is recommended. This should be administered for 8 weeks. After that time and provided that the organism is found to be susceptible, isoniazid and rifampin are administered daily, or 2 or 3 times a week, under direct observation, for 16 weeks. When results of susceptibility tests for these medications become available, the regimen should be altered as appropriate.

—Isoniazid, rifampin, pyrazinamide, and streptomycin or ethambutol taken daily under direct observation for 2 weeks, followed

by twice-weekly administration of all 4 medications for 6 weeks, under direct observation. This is then followed by twice-weekly administration, directly observed, of isoniazid and rifampin for 16 weeks.

—Isoniazid, rifampin, pyrazinamide, and streptomycin or ethambutol taken 3 times a week under direct observation for 6 months.

HIV-infected patients may use any of the 3 options recommended by the CDC; however, treatment regimens should continue for a total of 9 months and at least 6 months beyond culture conversion.

Healthcare or correctional institutions experiencing outbreaks of tuberculosis that are resistant to isoniazid and rifampin, or that are resuming therapy for a patient with a prior history of antitubercular therapy, may need to begin 5- or 6-drug regimens as initial therapy. These regimens should include the 4-drug regimen and at least 3 medications to which the suspected multi-drug-resistant strain may be susceptible.

The regimen for treating pulmonary tuberculosis should be effective in treating extrapulmonary tuberculosis. Some experts recommend extending the duration of therapy to 9 months in patients with disseminated disease, miliary tuberculosis, disease involving bones or joints, or tuberculosis lymphadenitis. Adjunctive therapies, such as surgery and corticosteroids, may be beneficial.

Side effects may be more frequent and/or severe with intermittent administration (600 mg once or twice weekly).

Patients with severe hepatic function impairment usually require a 50% reduction in dose of rifampin.

Patients with renal function impairment do not require a reduction in dose. In addition, rifampin plasma concentrations are not significantly altered in patients with decreased glomerular filtration rates (GFR) or in anuric patients.

# Oral Dosage Forms

Note: Bracketed uses in the *Dosage Forms* section refer to categories of use and/or indications that are not included in U.S. product labeling.

## RIFAMPIN CAPSULES USP

### Usual adult and adolescent dose

Tuberculosis—

In combination with other antituberculosis medications: Oral, 600 mg once a day for the entire treatment period; or 10 mg per kg of body weight, up to 600 mg, two or three times a week, depending on the treatment regimen.

Meningococcal infection (prophylaxis)—

Oral, 600 mg two times a day for two days.

[*Haemophilus influenzae* infection (prophylaxis)][1]—

Oral, 600 mg once a day for four days.

[Leprosy][1]—

In combination with other antileprosy agents:

For multibacillary leprosy—Oral, 600 mg once a month for a minimum of two years or until smear is negative, whichever is longer.

For paucilbacillary leprosy—Oral, 600 mg once a month for a minimum of six months.

Note: Debilitated patients—Oral, 10 mg per kg of body weight once a day.

### Usual adult prescribing limits

Up to 600 mg daily.

### Usual pediatric dose

Infants up to 1 month of age—

Tuberculosis: In combination with other antituberculosis medications—Oral, 10 to 20 mg per kg of body weight once a day; or 10 to 20 mg per kg of body weight, two or three times a week, depending on the treatment regimen.

Meningococcal infection (prophylaxis)—

Oral, 5 mg per kg of body weight every twelve hours for two days.

[*Haemophilus influenzae* infection (prophylaxis)][1]—

Oral, 10 mg per kg of body weight once a day for four days.

Children 1 month of age and over—

Tuberculosis: In combination with other antituberculosis medications—Oral, 10 to 20 mg per kg of body weight, up to 600 mg, once a day; or 10 to 20 mg per kg of body weight, up to 600 mg, two or three times a week, depending on the treatment regimen.

Meningococcal infection (prophylaxis): Oral, 10 mg per kg of body weight every twelve hours for two days.

[*Haemophilus influenzae* infection (prophylaxis)][1]—

Oral, 20 mg per kg of body weight once a day for four days.

Note: The maximum daily dose should not exceed 600 mg.

### Usual geriatric dose

Tuberculosis—

Oral, 10 mg per kg of body weight once a day.

**Strength(s) usually available**
U.S.—
   150 mg (Rx) [*Rifadin*].
   300 mg (Rx) [*Rifadin; Rimactane*].
Canada—
   150 mg (Rx) [*Rifadin; Rimactane; Rofact*].
   300 mg (Rx) [*Rifadin; Rimactane; Rofact*].

**Packaging and storage**
Store below 40 °C (104 °F). Store in a tight, light-resistant container.

**Preparation of dosage form**
For patients who cannot take oral solids—
If a liquid dosage form is preferred, a 1% (10-mg-per-mL) oral sus-
pension may be compounded as follows
   • Empty the contents of 4 capsules (300 mg each) or 8 capsules
    (150 mg each) onto a piece of glassine weighing paper.
   • If necessary, gently crush the contents of the capsules with a
    spatula to produce a fine powder.
   • Transfer the contents of the capsules to a 120-mL amber glass
    prescription bottle.
   • If necessary, rinse the glassine weighing paper and spatula with
    a 20-mL aliquot of simple syrup (Syrup NF), Wild Cherry Syrup,
    or other recommended syrup (see manufacturer's labeling). Add
    the rinse to the bottle. Shake vigorously.
   • Add sufficient syrup to the bottle so that the final volume meas-
    ures 120 mL. Shake vigorously.
The 1% suspension in syrup retains its potency for 4 weeks when
stored at room temperature (22 to 28 °C [72 to 83 °F]) or when re-
frigerated at 2 to 8 °C (36 to 46 °F). Dispense with a shake well label.

**Auxiliary labeling**
• Continue medicine for full time of treatment.
• Avoid alcoholic beverages.
• May discolor body fluids.

**Note**
Contents of the capsules may also be mixed with applesauce or jelly.

## Parenteral Dosage Forms

Note: Bracketed uses in the *Dosage Forms* section refer to categories of
   use and/or indications that are not included in U.S. product labeling.

### RIFAMPIN FOR INJECTION USP

**Usual adult and adolescent dose**
Tuberculosis—
   In combination with other antituberculosis medications: Intravenous,
   600 mg once a day for the entire treatment period; or 10 mg per
   kg of body weight, up to 600 mg, two or three times a week,
   depending on the treatment regimen.
   Meningococcal infection (prophylaxis)—Intravenous, 600 mg two
   times a day for two days.
   [Leprosy]—In combination with other antileprosy agents: Intravenous,
   600 mg once a month for a minimum of two years or until smear
   is negative, whichever is longer.
Note: Debilitated patients—Intravenous, 10 mg per kg of body weight
   once a day.

**Usual adult prescribing limits**
Up to 600 mg daily.

**Usual pediatric dose**
Infants up to 1 month of age—
   Tuberculosis: In combination with other antituberculosis medications—
    Intravenous, 10 to 20 mg per kg of body weight once a day; or
    10 to 20 mg per kg of body weight two or three times a week,
    depending on the treatment regimen.
   Meningococcal infection (prophylaxis): Intravenous, 5 mg per kg of
    body weight every twelve hours for two days.
Children 1 month of age and over—
   Tuberculosis: In combination with other antituberculosis medications—
    Intravenous, 10 to 20 mg per kg of body weight, up to 600 mg,
    once a day; or 10 to 20 mg per kg of body weight, up to 600 mg,
    two or three times a week, depending on the treatment regimen.
   Meningococcal infection (prophylaxis): Intravenous, 10 mg per kg of
    body weight every twelve hours for two days.
Note: The maximum daily dose should not exceed 600 mg.

**Usual geriatric dose**
Tuberculosis: Intravenous, 10 mg per kg of body weight once a day.

**Strength(s) usually available**
U.S.—
   600 mg (Rx) [*Rifadin IV*].
Canada—
   Not commercially available.

**Packaging and storage**
Store below 40 °C (104 °F). Store in a tight, light-resistant container.

**Preparation of dosage form**
To prepare for initial dilution for intravenous use, add 10 mL of sterile
   water for injection to each 600-mg vial. Gently swirl vial to completely
   dissolve the rifampin.
For intermittent infusion, add the calculated amount of reconstituted rifampin to be administered to 500 mL of 5% dextrose in water and
   infuse over 3 hours. In some cases, the calculated amount of rifampin
   may be added to 100 mL of 5% dextrose in water and infused over
   30 minutes.

**Stability**
5% dextrose in water is the recommended infusion medium. Sterile saline
   may be used; however, the stability of rifampin is slightly reduced.
   Other solutions are not recommended.
After reconstitution, the solution of 60 mg per mL is stable at room temperature for 24 hours. After dilution in 100 or 500 mL, solutions are
   also stable at room temperature for 24 hours.

---

¹Not included in Canadian product labeling.

## Selected Bibliography

Centers for Disease Control. Initial therapy for tuberculosis in the era of
   multidrug resistance: recommendations of the advisory council for the
   elimination of tuberculosis. MMWR 1993; 42 (RR-7): 1-8.

Revised: 06/22/94

---

## RIFAMPIN-CONTAINING COMBINATIONS—

Rifampin and Isoniazid (Systemic)
Rifampin, Isoniazid, and Pyrazinamide (Systemic)

---

# RIFAMPIN AND ISONIAZID    Systemic

INN: Rifampin—Rifampicin
VA CLASSIFICATION (Primary): AM500
**NOTE:** The *Rifampin and Isoniazid (Systemic)* monograph is maintained
   on the USP DI electronic data base. For a printed copy of the
   most recent revision of the complete monograph, contact the USP
   Division of Information Development, 12601 Twinbrook Parkway, Rockville, MD 20852.

   For information on the specific components of this combination,
   see the *USP DI* monographs for *Isoniazid (Systemic)* and *Rifampin (Systemic)*.

   The information that follows is selectively abstracted from the
   complete monograph and is provided to facilitate drug use review
   and patient counseling.

Note: For a listing of dosage forms and brand names by country availability, see *Dosage Forms* section(s). For a listing of brand names
   for the articles in this monograph, refer to the General Index.

## Category
Antibacterial (antimycobacterial).

## Indications

**Accepted**
Tuberculosis (treatment)—Rifampin and isoniazid combination is indicated in the treatment of pulmonary tuberculosis when the patient has
   been titrated on the individual components and the efficacy of the
   combination has been established.

## Unaccepted

Rifampin and isoniazid combination is not indicated for initial treatment or prophylaxis of pulmonary tuberculosis, for meningococcal infections, or in the treatment of asymptomatic meningococcal carriers to eliminate *Neisseria meningitidis* from the nasopharynx.

## Patient Consultation

As an aid to patient consultation, refer to *Advice for the Patient, Rifampin and Isoniazid (Systemic)*.

In providing consultation, consider emphasizing the following selected information (» = major clinical significance):

### Before using this medication

» Conditions affecting use, especially:

Hypersensitivity to rifampin, isoniazid, ethionamide, pyrazinamide, niacin (nicotinic acid), or other chemically related medications

Pregnancy—Isoniazid and rifampin cross the placenta. It is recommended that isoniazid and rifampin be used to treat pregnant women with tuberculosis; however, rifampin has rarely caused postnatal hemorrhage in the mother and infant when administered during the last few weeks of pregnancy

Breast-feeding—Isoniazid and rifampin are distributed into breast milk

Use in children—Use of the fixed-dose combination is not recommended in pediatric patients

Use in the elderly—Patients over the age of 50 have the highest incidence of hepatitis

Dental—Patients who develop blood dyscrasias may be at increased risk of microbial infections, delayed healing, and gingival bleeding

Other medicines, especially daily alcohol use, alfentanil, aminophylline, coumarin- or indandione-derivative anticoagulants, oral antidiabetic agents, azole antifungals, carbamazepine, chloramphenicol, corticosteroids, digitalis glycosides, disopyramide, disulfiram, estramustine, estrogens, fluconazole, other hepatotoxic medications, methadone, mexiletine, oral contraceptives, oxtriphylline, phenytoin, quinidine, theophylline, tocainide, or verapamil

Other medical problems, especially alcoholism, active or in remission, or hepatic function impairment

### Proper use of this medication

Taking this medication with food or antacids, but not within 1 hour of aluminum-containing antacids, if gastrointestinal irritation occurs

» Compliance with full course of therapy, which may take months or years

» Taking pyridoxine concurrently to prevent or minimize symptoms of peripheral neuritis

» Proper dosing

» Missed dose: Taking as soon as possible; not taking if almost time for next dose; not doubling doses; intermittent dosing may result in more frequent and/or severe side effects

» Proper storage

### Precautions while using this medication

» Regular visits to physician to check progress, as well as ophthalmologic examinations if signs of optic neuritis occur

Checking with physician if no improvement within 2 to 3 weeks

» Using an alternate method of contraception if taking estrogen-containing oral contraceptives concurrently

» Avoiding alcoholic beverages concurrently with this medication

Checking with physician if vascular reactions occur following concurrent ingestion of cheese or fish with isoniazid-containing medications

» Medication causes urine, feces, saliva, sputum, sweat, and tears to turn reddish-orange to reddish-brown and may also permanently discolor soft contact lenses; avoiding the wearing of soft contact lenses

» Need to report to physician promptly prodromal signs of hepatitis or peripheral neuritis

Using caution in use of regular toothbrushes, dental floss, and toothpicks; deferring dental work until blood counts have returned to normal; checking with physician or dentist concerning proper oral hygiene

Possible interference with diagnostic tests

### Side/adverse effects

Signs of potential side effects, especially blood dyscrasias, hepatitis, hepatitis prodromal symptoms, hypersensitivity, neurotoxicity, optic neuritis, peripheral neuritis, "flu-like" syndrome, and interstitial nephritis

Hepatitis may be more likely to occur in patients over 50 years of age

Reddish-orange to reddish-brown discoloration of urine, stools, saliva, sputum, sweat, and tears may be alarming to patient, although medically insignificant; however, tears discolored by rifampin may also discolor soft contact lenses

## Oral Dosage Forms

### RIFAMPIN AND ISONIAZID CAPSULES USP

**Usual adult and adolescent dose**
Tuberculosis—
Oral, 600 mg of rifampin and 300 mg of isoniazid once a day for the entire treatment period.

**Usual pediatric dose**
Use of the fixed-dose combination is not recommended in pediatric patients.

Note: See individual components for dosage recommendations.

**Strength(s) usually available**
U.S.—
300 mg of rifampin and 150 mg of isoniazid (Rx) [*Rifamate*].
Canada—
Not commercially available.

**Auxiliary labeling**
• Continue medicine for full time of treatment.
• Avoid alcoholic beverages.
• May discolor body fluids.

Revised: 07/17/96

---

# RIFAMPIN, ISONIAZID, AND PYRAZINAMIDE    Systemic

**VA CLASSIFICATION (Primary): AM500**

**NOTE:** The *Rifampin, Isoniazid, and Pyrazinamide (Systemic)* monograph is maintained on the USP DI electronic data base. For a printed copy of the most recent revision of the complete monograph, contact the USP Division of Information Development, 12601 Twinbrook Parkway, Rockville, MD 20852.

For information on the specific components of this combination, see the *USP DI* monographs for *Isoniazid (Systemic)*, *Pyrazinamide (Systemic)*, and *Rifampin (Systemic)*.

The information that follows is selectively abstracted from the complete monograph and is provided to facilitate drug use review and patient counseling.

Note: For a listing of dosage forms and brand names by country availability, see *Dosage Forms* section(s). For a listing of brand names for the articles in this monograph, refer to the General Index.

## Category

Antibacterial (antimycobacterial).

## Indications

### Accepted

Tuberculosis (treatment)—Rifampin, isoniazid, and pyrazinamide combination is indicated in the initial phase of the short-course treatment of all forms of tuberculosis. During this phase, which should last 2 months, rifampin, isoniazid, and pyrazinamide combination should be administered on a daily, continuous basis. Additional medications are indicated if multidrug-resistant tuberculosis is suspected.

## Patient Consultation

As an aid to patient consultation, refer to *Advice for the Patient, Rifampin, Isoniazid, and Pyrazinamide (Systemic)*.

In providing consultation, consider emphasizing the following selected information (» = major clinical significance):

### Before using this medication
» Conditions affecting use, especially:

Hypersensitivity to rifampin, isoniazid, pyrazinamide, ethionamide, niacin (nicotinic acid), rifabutin, or other chemically related medications

Pregnancy—Isoniazid and rifampin cross the placenta

Breast-feeding—Isoniazid, pyrazinamide, and rifampin are distributed into breast milk

Use in children—Use of the fixed-dose combination is not recommended in pediatric patients under the age of 15

Use in the elderly—Patients over the age of 50 have the highest incidence of hepatitis with use of isoniazid

Other medications, especially daily alcohol use, alfentanil, aminophylline, coumarin- or indandione-derivative anticoagulants, oral antidiabetic agents, azole antifungals, carbamazepine, chloramphenicol, oral contraceptives, corticosteroids, digitalis glycosides, disopyramide, disulfiram, estramustine, estrogens, other hepatotoxic medications, methadone, mexiletine, oxtriphylline, phenytoin, quinidine, theophylline, tocainide, or oral verapamil

Other medical problems, especially alcoholism, active or in remission, or hepatic function impairment

### Proper use of this medication
Taking this medication with food or antacids, but not within 1 hour of aluminum-containing antacids, if gastrointestinal irritation occurs

» Compliance with full course of therapy, which may take months or years

» Taking pyridoxine concurrently to prevent or minimize symptoms of peripheral neuritis

» Proper dosing

» Missed dose: Taking as soon as possible; not taking if almost time for next dose; not doubling doses; intermittent dosing may result in more frequent and/or severe side effects

» Proper storage

### Precautions while using this medication
» Regular visits to physician to check progress, as well as ophthalmologic examinations if signs of optic neuritis occur

Checking with physician if no improvement within 2 to 3 weeks

» Using an alternate method of contraception if taking estrogen-containing oral contraceptives concurrently

» Avoiding alcoholic beverages concurrently with this medication

» Checking with physician if vascular reactions occur following concurrent ingestion of cheese or fish with isoniazid-containing medication

» Medication causes urine, feces, saliva, sputum, sweat, and tears to turn reddish orange to reddish brown and may also permanently discolor soft contact lenses; avoiding the wearing of soft contact lenses

» Need to report to physician promptly prodromal signs of hepatitis or peripheral neuritis

Using caution in use of regular toothbrushes, dental floss, and toothpicks; deferring dental work until blood counts have returned to normal; checking with physician or dentist concerning proper oral hygiene

Possible interference with diagnostic tests

» Diabetics: May interfere with urine ketone determinations

### Side/adverse effects
Hepatitis caused by isoniazid may be more likely to occur in patients over 50 years of age

Reddish orange to reddish brown discoloration of urine, stools, saliva, sputum, sweat, and tears may be alarming to patient, although medically insignificant; however, tears discolored by rifampin may also discolor soft contact lenses

Signs of potential side effects, especially arthralgia, hepatitis, hepatitis prodromal symptoms, peripheral neuritis, "flu-like" syndrome, hypersensitivity, blood dyscrasias, interstitial nephritis, neurotoxicity, and optic neuritis

## Oral Dosage Forms

### RIFAMPIN, ISONIAZID AND PYRAZINAMIDE TABLETS

**Usual adult dose**
Tuberculosis—
Patients weighing 44 kg or less: Oral, 4 tablets once a day.
Patients weighing between 45 and 54 kg: Oral, 5 tablets once a day.
Patients weighing 55 kg or more: Oral, 6 tablets once a day.

**Usual pediatric dose**
Tuberculosis—
Children and adolescents up to 15 years of age: Use of the fixed-dose combination is not recommended.
Adolescents 15 years of age and older: See *Usual adult dose.*

Note: See individual components for dosage recommendations.

**Strength(s) usually available**
U.S.—
120 mg rifampin, 50 mg isoniazid, and 300 mg pyrazinamide (Rx) [*Rifater*].
Canada—
Not commercially available.

**Auxiliary labeling**
• Continue medicine for full time of treatment.
• Avoid alcoholic beverages.
• May discolor body fluids.

Developed: 01/04/96

---

# RILUZOLE    Systemic†

VA CLASSIFICATION (Primary): CN900
Note: For a listing of dosage forms and brand names by country availability, see *Dosage Forms* section(s). For a listing of brand names for the articles in this monograph, refer to the General Index.

†Not commercially available in Canada.

## Category
Amyotrophic lateral sclerosis (ALS) therapy agent.

## Indications
**Accepted**
Amyotrophic lateral sclerosis (ALS) (treatment)—Riluzole is indicated in the treatment of ALS; it may slow the progression of ALS by extending the survival and/or time to tracheostomy.

In two placebo-controlled studies, riluzole was shown to improve survival early in the trials; however, muscle strength and neurological functioning were not improved. Also, no statistically significant difference in mortality was seen at the conclusion of these studies.

## Pharmacology/Pharmacokinetics

**Physicochemical characteristics**
Chemical group—Benzothiazole
Molecular weight—234.20.

**Mechanism of action/Effect**
Riluzole presynaptically inhibits glutamate release in the central nervous system (CNS) and postsynaptically interferes with the effects of excitatory amino acids. Although the etiology of ALS is unknown, current hypotheses suggest that glutamic acid may play a secondary role in mediating the neurodegenerative processes in the disease. Another pharmacological property of riluzole that may be related to its effect is inactivation of voltage-dependent sodium channels.

**Other actions/effects**
In animal models, riluzole has demonstrated anticonvulsant effects at doses twice the recommended human daily dose, and myorelaxant and sedative properties at doses twenty times the recommended human daily dose. Anti-ischemic properties have also been reported.

**Absorption**
Riluzole is well absorbed (approximately 90%), and has an absolute bioavailability of about 60%. Administration with a high fat meal decreases absorption, decreasing the area under the plasma concentra-

tion–time curve (AUC) by about 20% and decreasing peak blood levels by about 45%.

**Distribution**
Riluzole penetrates the brain very readily.

**Protein binding**
Very high (96%); bound mainly to albumin and lipoproteins.

**Biotransformation**
Riluzole is extensively metabolized to six major and a number of minor metabolites, which have not all been identified to date. Metabolism is mostly hepatic, consisting of cytochrome P450–dependent hydroxylation and glucuronidation. P450 1A2 is the primary isozyme involved in N-hydroxylation; CYP 2D6, CYP 2C19, CYP 3A4, and CYP 2E1 are considered unlikely to contribute significantly to riluzole metabolism in humans.

**Half-life**
Elimination—Approximately 12 hours after multiple dosing.

**Time to steady-state concentration**
Steady-state is reached in less than 5 days. The pharmacokinetics of riluzole are linear over the dose range of 25 to 100 mg administered every 12 hours.

**Elimination**
There is marked interindividual variability in the clearance of riluzole, most likely due to variability of activity of the CYP 1A2 isoenzyme involved in the N-hydroxylation of the parent compound.
Renal: 90% of a single 150-mg radiolabeled dose administered to healthy males was recovered in the urine over 7 days, of which only 2% was unchanged riluzole. More than 85% of the metabolites recovered in the urine were glucuronide metabolites.
Fecal: 5% of a single 150-mg radiolabeled dose administered to healthy males was recovered in the feces over 7 days.

## Precautions to Consider

**Carcinogenicity**
Long-term studies to determine the carcinogenic potential of riluzole have not been completed to date.

**Mutagenicity**
There was no evidence of mutagenic or clastogenic potential in the Ames test, the mouse lymphoma assay, or the *in vivo* assays in the mouse and rat. There was an equivocal clastogenic response in the *in vitro* lymphocyte chromosomal aberration assay.

**Pregnancy/Reproduction**
Fertility—Riluzole impaired fertility when administered to male and female rats prior to and during mating at a dose of 15 mg per kg of body weight (mg/kg) or 1.5 times the maximum daily dose on a mg per square meter of body surface area basis.
Pregnancy—Adequate and well-controlled studies in humans have not been done.
Embryotoxicity and maternal toxicity were observed when riluzole was administered to pregnant rats and rabbits during the period of organogenesis at doses of 27 mg/kg and 60 mg/kg, respectively (2.6 and 11.5 times the maximum human recommended dose [MHRD], respectively). Administration of riluzole to rats during gestation and lactation at doses of 15 mg/kg (or 1.5 times the MHRD) produced adverse effects such as a decrease in implantations and an increase in intrauterine deaths. Viability and growth of the offspring also were adversely affected.
FDA Pregnancy Category C.

**Breast-feeding**
It is not known whether riluzole is distributed into human milk. However, it is distributed into maternal milk in rats. Because of the potential for serious adverse effects, it is recommended that women receiving riluzole not breast-feed.

**Pediatrics**
No information is available on the relationship of age to the effects of riluzole in pediatric patients. Safety and efficacy have not been established.

**Geriatrics**
Although appropriate studies on the relationship of age to the effects of riluzole have not been performed in the geriatric population, no geriatrics-specific problems have been documented to date. However, elderly patients are more likely to have age-related renal function impairment, which may cause decreased clearance of riluzole. About 30% of the patients included in controlled clinical trials were over 65 years of age; no differences in adverse effects between the younger and older patients were observed.

**Pharmacogenetics**
Riluzole clearance in Japanese subjects native to Japan has been shown to be 50% lower than riluzole clearance in Caucasians after adjusting for body weight. Although it is not clear if this effect is due to genetic or environmental factors, alcohol intake, coffee intake, other dietary preferences, or smoking, Japanese subjects may possess a lower capacity (oxidative and/or conjugative) for metabolizing riluzole.
Female subjects may possess lower metabolic capacity to eliminate riluzole as compared to males, due to lower activity of the CYP 1A2 isozyme. This gender effect may result in increased blood concentration of riluzole and its metabolites. However, in controlled trials, no gender effect on favorable or adverse effects of riluzole was noted.

**Drug interactions and/or related problems**
The following drug interactions and/or related problems have been selected on the basis of their potential clinical significance (possible mechanism in parentheses where appropriate)—not necessarily inclusive (» = major clinical significance):

Note: Clinical studies designed to evaluate the interaction of riluzole with other drugs have not been conducted.

Combinations containing any of the following medications, depending on the amount present, may also interact with this medication.

Alcohol
(it is not known if alcohol increases the risk of serious hepatotoxicity with riluzole; patients should be discouraged from drinking excessive amounts of alcohol)

Allopurinol or
Hepatotoxic agents or
Methyldopa or
Sulfasalazine
(because of the potential for additive hepatotoxic effects, caution should be exercised in prescribing these medications to a patient receiving riluzole)

Amitriptyline or
Caffeine or
Phenacetin or
Quinolones or
Tacrine or
Theophylline or
Other agents that potentially inhibit CYP 1A2
(inhibitors of CYP 1A2 may decrease the rate of elimination of riluzole)
(potential interactions may occur when riluzole is administered concomitantly with other agents that are also metabolized by CYP 1A2)

Charbroiled food or
Cigarette smoke or
Omeprazole or
Rifampicin
(inducers of CYP 1A2 may increase the rate of elimination of riluzole)

**Laboratory value alterations**
The following have been selected on the basis of their potential clinical significance (possible effect in parentheses where appropriate)—not necessarily inclusive (» = major clinical significance):

With diagnostic test results
Coombs' (antiglobulin) test, direct
(positive results may occur)

With physiology/laboratory test values
Alkaline phosphatase or
Gamma glutamyl transferase (GGT) or
Lactic dehydrogenase
(values may be increased)

» Aminotransferases, serum
(elevated values occur in many patients, even those with no prior history of liver disease; experience in nearly 800 ALS patients predicts that about 50% of riluzole-treated patients will experience at least one alanine aminotransferase [ALT (SGPT)] level above the upper limit of normal (ULN), about 8% will have elevations > 3 times the ULN, and about 2% will have elevations > 5 times the ULN)
(in clinical trials, maximum increases in serum ALT usually occurred within 3 months after initiation of therapy with riluzole; patients were continued on riluzole if ALT values were < 5 times the ULN, and levels usually decreased to < 2 times the ULN within 2 to 6 months; if ALT values exceeded 5 times the ULN, riluzole was discontinued, so there is no clinical experience to date

with continuing riluzole treatment in ALS patients with ALT values > 5 times the ULN)

Erythrocyte counts or
Hematocrit values or
Hemoglobin values
(levels may fall below the lower limit of normal; in clinical trials the changes were mostly mild and transient, and appeared to show a dose-response relationship)

Gamma globulins
(values may be increased)

### Medical considerations/Contraindications

The medical considerations/contraindications included here have been selected on the basis of their potential clinical significance (reasons given in parentheses where appropriate)—not necessarily inclusive (» = major clinical significance).

*Except under special circumstances, this medication should not be used when the following medical problem exists:*

» Severe hepatic function impairment
(increased risk of liver toxicity)

*Risk-benefit should be considered when the following medical problems exist:*

Hepatic function impairment
(metabolism of riluzole and its metabolites may be decreased, leading to higher plasma levels)

Renal function impairment
(excretion of riluzole and its metabolites may be decreased, leading to higher plasma levels)

Sensitivity to riluzole

### Patient monitoring

The following may be especially important in patient monitoring (other tests may be warranted in some patients, depending on condition; » = major clinical significance):

Hepatic function tests including:
Alanine aminotransferase (ALT [SGPT]) and
Aspartate aminotransferase (AST [SGOT]) and
Bilirubin and
Gamma glutamyl transferase (GGT)
(serum values of aminotransferases should be measured prior to and during riluzole treatment; serum ALT values should be monitored every month for the first 3 months of treatment, every 3 months during the remainder of the first year, and periodically thereafter)
(if riluzole therapy is continued in patients with ALT values > 5 times the upper limit of normal [ULN], frequent [at least weekly] monitoring of complete liver function is recommended; treatment should be discontinued if ALT values exceed 10 times the ULN or if clinical jaundice develops)

White blood cell counts
(because of the occurrence of rare but marked neutropenia [absolute neutrophil count less than 500 per cubic millimeter], patients reporting febrile illness should have white cell counts checked)

## Side/Adverse Effects

Note: Adverse effects can worsen the quality of life of ALS patients receiving riluzole; however, in one study, adverse reactions to the drug reportedly did not outweigh its therapeutic effect on survival.

The following side/adverse effects have been selected on the basis of their potential clinical significance (possible signs and symptoms in parentheses where appropriate)—not necessarily inclusive:

### Those indicating need for medical attention

Incidence more frequent
*Aggravation reaction* (worsening of symptoms of ALS); *including worsening of asthenia* (unusual tiredness or weakness); *and spasticity; diarrhea; nausea; vomiting*

Note: *Diarrhea, nausea,* and *worsening of asthenia* may be dose-related.

Incidence less frequent
*Respiratory disorders, including decreased lung function* (difficulty in breathing); *increased cough, and pneumonia*

Incidence rare
*Angioedema* (swelling of the eyelids, mouth, lips, tongue, and/or throat); *dysphagia* (trouble in swallowing); *exfoliative dermatitis* (redness, scaling, or peeling of the skin); *facial edema* (swelling of face); *hypertension, mild to moderate* (high blood pressure); *hypokalemia* (increased thirst; irregular heartbeat; mood or mental changes; muscle

cramps, pain, or weakness); *hyponatremia* (lack of energy); *incoordination* (lack of coordination); *jaundice* (yellow eyes or skin); *mental depression; neutropenia* (fever; chills; continuing sores in mouth); *phlebitis* (pain, tenderness, bluish color, or swelling of foot or leg); *seizures; tachycardia* (fast or pounding heartbeat); *urinary tract problems, including infections* (bloody or cloudy urine; frequent urge to urinate); *and dysuria* (painful or difficult urination)

### Those indicating need for medical attention only if they continue or are bothersome

Incidence more frequent
*Abdominal pain or gas; anorexia* (loss of appetite); *circumoral paresthesia* (numbness or tingling around the mouth); *dizziness; somnolence* (drowsiness); *vertigo*

Note: *Anorexia, circumoral paresthesia, dizziness, somnolence,* and *vertigo* may be dose-related. *Dizziness* may occur more commonly in females than in males.

Incidence less frequent
*Back or muscle pain or stiffness; constipation; dermatological problems, including alopecia* (hair loss); *eczema* (skin rash); *and pruritis* (itching); *headache; insomnia* (trouble in sleeping); *malaise* (general feeling of discomfort or illness); *peripheral edema* (swelling of feet or legs); *rhinitis* (runny nose); *stomatitis* (irritation or soreness of mouth)

## Overdose

For more information on the management of overdose or unintentional ingestion, **contact a Poison Control Center** (see *Poison Control Center Listing*).

### Clinical effects of overdose
No cases of overdose with riluzole have been reported to date.

### Treatment of overdose
No specific antidote or information on treatment is available.

If an overdose occurs, riluzole should be discontinued immediately.

Supportive care—Treatment should be directed toward alleviating symptoms of overdose. Patients in whom intentional overdose is confirmed or suspected should be referred for psychiatric consultation.

## Patient Consultation

As an aid to patient consultation, refer to *Advice for the Patient, Riluzole (Systemic).*

In providing consultation, consider emphasizing the following selected information (» = major clinical significance):

### Before using this medication
» Conditions affecting use, especially:
Sensitivity to riluzole
Pregnancy—Studies have shown adverse effects in animals receiving doses greater than recommended maximum human daily doses
Breast-feeding—Not recommended because of risk of serious side effects
Other medical problems, especially severe hepatic function impairment

### Proper use of this medication
Taking on a regular basis and at the same time of the day (e.g., morning and evening)
Taking on an empty stomach
Missed dose: skipping missed dose; starting again with next scheduled dose
» Proper storage

### Precautions while using this medication
Reporting any febrile illnesses promptly to physician
» Caution when driving or doing jobs requiring alertness, because of the potential for drowsiness, dizziness, or vertigo
Avoiding excessive alcohol intake

### Side/adverse effects
Aggravation reaction; asthenia; spasticity; diarrhea; nausea; vomiting; respiratory disorders, including decreased lung function, increased cough, and pneumonia; angioedema; dysphagia; exfoliative dermatitis; facial edema; hypertension; hypokalemia; hyponatremia; incoordination; jaundice; mental depression; neutropenia; phlebitis; seizures; tachycardia; and urinary tract problems including infections and dysuria

## General Dosing Information

Riluzole should be taken on a regular basis and at the same time of day (e.g., morning and evening). To avoid food-related decreases in bioavailability, riluzole should be given on an empty stomach, one hour before or two hours after meals.

## Oral Dosage Forms

### RILUZOLE TABLETS

**Usual adult dose**
Amyotrophic lateral sclerosis—Oral, 50 mg every twelve hours, taken on an empty stomach.

Note: Higher daily doses result in no increased benefit, but increased incidence of adverse effects.

**Usual adult prescribing limits**
100 mg a day.

**Usual pediatric dose**
Safety and efficacy have not been established.

**Usual geriatric dose**
See *Usual adult dose.*

**Strength(s) usually available**
U.S.—
    50 mg (Rx) [*Rilutek*].
Canada—
    Not commercially available.

**Packaging and storage**
Store between 20 and 25 °C (68 and 77 °F). Protect from bright light.

**Auxiliary labeling**
• May cause drowsiness.
• Take on an empty stomach.
• Avoid alcoholic beverages.

Developed: 07/30/96

# RIMANTADINE    Systemic†

VA CLASSIFICATION (Primary): AM800

Note: For a listing of dosage forms and brand names by country availability, see *Dosage Forms* section(s). For a listing of brand names for the articles in this monograph, refer to the General Index.

    †Not commercially available in Canada.

## Category
Antiviral (systemic).

## Indications

**Accepted**
Influenza A (prophylaxis and treatment)—Rimantadine is indicated for the prophylaxis of respiratory tract infections caused by influenza A virus in adults and children, and the treatment of respiratory tract infections caused by influenza A virus in adults.

Influenza A virus strains that are resistant to amantadine or rimantadine are cross-resistant to the other medication.

Although rimantadine is structurally similar to amantadine, differing only in the 10-carbon ring side chain, rimantadine, unlike amantadine, is not effective in the control of Parkinson's disease.

## Pharmacology/Pharmacokinetics

**Physicochemical characteristics**
Molecular weight—215.77.

**Mechanism of action/Effect**
Rimantadine is thought to exert its inhibitory effect early in the viral replicative cycle, possibly by blocking or greatly reducing the uncoating of viral RNA within host cells. Genetic studies suggest that a single amino acid change on the transmembrane portion of the M2 protein can completely eliminate influenza A virus' susceptibility to rimantadine.

**Absorption**
Well absorbed; tablets and syrup are absorbed equally well after oral administration.

**Distribution**
Vol$_D$—
    Adults: 17 to 25 L/kg.
    Children: Mean of 289 L.
Concentrations in the nasal mucus average 50% higher than those in plasma.

**Protein binding**
Moderate (approximately 40%).

**Biotransformation**
Extensively metabolized in the liver; glucuronidation and hydroxylation are the major metabolic pathways.

**Half-life**
Young adults (22 to 44 years old)—25 to 30 hours.

Older adults (71 to 79 years old) and patients with chronic liver disease—Approximately 32 hours.

Children (4 to 8 years old)—13 to 38 hours.

**Time to peak concentration**
1 to 4 hours.

**Peak serum concentration**
Steady state—
    100 mg once a day: Approximately 181 nanograms per mL.
    100 mg twice a day: Approximately 416 nanograms per mL.
Rimantadine concentrations in elderly nursing home patients were found to be nearly 3 times those of younger adults.

**Elimination**
Renal; > 90% recovered in the urine within 72 hours, mostly as metabolites. Less than 25% excreted in urine as unchanged drug.
In dialysis—Hemodialysis has a negligible effect on the clearance of rimantadine.

## Precautions to Consider

**Cross-sensitivity and/or related problems**
Patients who are hypersensitive to amantadine may also be hypersensitive to rimantadine.

**Carcinogenicity**
Carcinogenicity studies in animals have not been performed.

**Mutagenicity**
No mutagenic effects were seen when rimantadine was evaluated in several standard mutagenicity assays.

**Pregnancy/Reproduction**
Fertility—A study in male and female rats given doses of up to 60 mg per kg of body weight (mg/kg) per day (3 times the maximum human dose based on body surface area comparisons) showed no impairment of fertility.

Pregnancy—Adequate and well-controlled studies in humans have not been done.

Rimantadine crosses the placenta in mice. It has been shown to be embryotoxic in rats when given at a dose of 200 mg/kg per day (11 times the maximum human dose based on body surface area comparisons), and has caused fetal resorption. Maternal toxicity included ataxia, tremors, seizures, and significantly reduced weight gain. Rimantadine was not embryotoxic when given to rabbits in doses of up to 50 mg/kg per day (5 times the maximum human dose based on body surface area comparisons). However, there was evidence of a change in the ratio of fetuses with 12 ribs to fetuses with 13 ribs; normally the ratio is 50:50 in a litter, but the ratio was 80:20 after rimantadine treatment.

FDA Pregnancy Category C.

**Breast-feeding**
It is not known whether rimantadine is distributed into breast milk. However, it is distributed into the milk of rats. Rimantadine concentrations in the milk of rats were twice those found in serum 2 to 3 hours after administration.

**Pediatrics**
Appropriate studies on the relationship of age to the effects of rimantadine have not been performed in neonates and infants up to one year of age. However, use of rimantadine in children older than 1 year of age has not been shown to cause any pediatrics-specific problems that would limit its usefulness in children.

**Geriatrics**

Elderly patients, particularly those in chronic care facilities, are more likely than younger adults or children to experience adverse effects associated with rimantadine, primarily central nervous system (CNS) and gastrointestinal side effects.

**Drug interactions and/or related problems**

The following drug interactions and/or related problems have been selected on the basis of their potential clinical significance (possible mechanism in parentheses where appropriate)—not necessarily inclusive (» = major clinical significance):

Note: Combinations containing any of the following medications, depending on the amount present, may also interact with this medication.

Acetaminophen or
Aspirin
(concurrent use of acetaminophen or aspirin with rimantadine reduces the peak serum concentration of rimantadine by approximately 11%; the clinical significance is thought to be minimal at this time)

Cimetidine
(concurrent use of a single dose of rimantadine with cimetidine reduces rimantadine clearance by 18% in healthy adults; the clinical significance is thought to be minimal at this time)

**Medical considerations/Contraindications**

The medical considerations/contraindications included here have been selected on the basis of their potential clinical significance (reasons given in parentheses where appropriate)—not necessarily inclusive (» = major clinical significance).

*Risk-benefit should be considered when the following medical problems exist:*

» Epilepsy, history of, or other seizure disorders
(amantadine increases the risk of seizures; seizures have also been reported with rimantadine in 2 patients with a history of seizures who had previously been withdrawn from their anticonvulsants)

» Hepatic function impairment
(a single-dose study done in patients with severe liver dysfunction showed a reduction in rimantadine clearance by 50% compared to healthy subjects)

Hypersensitivity to amantadine or rimantadine

» Renal function impairment, severe
(a single-dose study done in patients with end-stage renal failure showed a reduction in rimantadine clearance by 40%, and an increase in elimination half-life by 60%, compared to healthy subjects; a dosage reduction is recommended in patients with a creatinine clearance of ≤ 10 mL/min [0.17 mL/second])

## Side/Adverse Effects

Note: Rimantadine has fewer CNS side effects than does amantadine. Elderly patients have a higher incidence of side effects, primarily CNS and gastrointestinal side effects, than do younger patients at conventional doses.

The following side/adverse effects have been selected on the basis of their potential clinical significance (possible signs and symptoms in parentheses where appropriate)—not necessarily inclusive:

**Those indicating need for medical attention only if they continue or are bothersome**

Incidence less frequent
*CNS effects* (difficulty in concentrating; difficulty in sleeping; dizziness; headache; nervousness; unusual tiredness); *gastrointestinal disturbances* (dryness of mouth; loss of appetite; nausea; stomach pain; vomiting)

## Patient Consultation

As an aid to patient consultation, refer to *Advice for the Patient, Rimantadine (Systemic).*

In providing consultation, consider emphasizing the following selected information (» = major clinical significance):

**Before using this medication**

» Conditions affecting use, especially:
Hypersensitivity to amantadine or rimantadine
Pregnancy—High doses were embryotoxic and maternotoxic in rats
Other medical problems, especially epilepsy or a history of seizures, liver function impairment and renal function impairment

**Proper use of this medication**

» Receiving a flu shot if recommended by your doctor

» Taking before exposure or as soon as possible after exposure
» Compliance with full course of therapy
» Importance of not missing doses and taking at evenly spaced times
Proper administration technique for oral liquid
» Proper dosing
Missed dose: Taking as soon as possible; not taking if almost time for next dose; not doubling doses
» Proper storage

**Precautions while using this medication**

Caution if dizziness occurs
Checking with physician if no improvement within a few days

## General Dosing Information

Chemoprophylactic administration should be started in anticipation of contact with, or as soon as possible after exposure to, persons having influenza A virus infections. Administration should be continued for at least 10 days following exposure. During an influenza epidemic, rimantadine should be given daily, usually for 6 to 8 weeks in most communities or until active immunity can be expected from administration of inactivated influenza A virus vaccine. Rimantadine has been reported to be effective for post-exposure prophylaxis of household contacts, but appeared to be less effective when used prophylactically in members of households in which index cases were being treated concurrently for influenza A. Failure was apparently due to transmission of drug-resistant strains of the virus.

If administered concurrently with inactivated influenza A virus vaccine until protective antibodies develop, rimantadine should be continued chemoprophylactically for 2 to 3 weeks after the vaccine has been administered. However, since the vaccine is only 70 to 80% effective, continued administration of rimantadine may be beneficial in elderly or high-risk patients. If the vaccine is unavailable or contraindicated, rimantadine should be administered for up to 90 days in cases of possible repeated or unknown exposure.

Treatment of influenza A virus infection with rimantadine should be started within 24 to 48 hours after the onset of symptoms and should be continued for 5 to 7 days. Optimal duration of therapy has not been established.

## Oral Dosage Forms

### RIMANTADINE HYDROCHLORIDE SYRUP

**Usual adult and adolescent dose**

Antiviral—
Prophylaxis: Oral, 100 mg two times a day.
Treatment: Oral, 100 mg two times a day for approximately five to seven days from the inital onset of symptoms.

Note: In adults with impaired renal function (creatinine clearance ≤ 10 mL/minute [0.17 mL/second]) or severe hepatic dysfunction, and in elderly nursing home patients, a dose of 100 mg once a day is recommended.

Although the manufacturer recommends twice-a-day dosing, once-a-day dosing has been well-tolerated and as effective because of the long elimination half-life of rimantadine.

**Usual pediatric dose**

Antiviral—Prophylaxis:—
Children up to 10 years of age: Oral, 5 mg per kg of body weight once a day. Maximum daily dose should not exceed 150 mg.
Children 10 years of age and over: See *Usual adult and adolescent dose.*

**Strength(s) usually available**

U.S.—
50 mg per 5 mL (Rx) [*Flumadine* (methylparaben; propylparaben; sodium saccharin)].

Canada—
Not commercially available.

**Packaging and storage**

Store below 40 °C (104 °F), preferably between 15 and 30 °C (59 and 86 °F), unless otherwise specified by manufacturer.

**Auxiliary labeling**

• Continue medicine for full time of treatment.

### RIMANTADINE HYDROCHLORIDE TABLETS

**Usual adult and adolescent dose**

See *Rimantadine Hydrochloride Syrup.*

**Usual pediatric dose**

See *Rimantadine Hydrochloride Syrup.*

**Strength(s) usually available**

U.S.—

100 mg (Rx) [*Flumadine*].

Canada—

Not commercially available.

**Packaging and storage**

Store below 40 °C (104 °F), preferably between 15 and 30 °C (59 and 86 °F), unless otherwise specified by manufacturer.

**Auxiliary labeling**

• Continue medicine for full time of treatment.

Developed: 03/29/94

---

# RISPERIDONE    Systemic

VA CLASSIFICATION (Primary): CN709

Note: For a listing of dosage forms and brand names by country availability, see *Dosage Forms* section(s). For a listing of brand names for the articles in this monograph, refer to the General Index.

## Category

Antipsychotic.

Note: Risperidone is considered by some experts to be an atypical antipsychotic. Universal acceptance of the exact parameters that define an antipsychotic as an atypical agent has not been established. Differences in binding affinities and activity at various receptor sites may explain the differing profiles of the newer antipsychotics.

## Indications

### Accepted

Psychotic disorders (treatment)—Risperidone is used to treat the manifestations of psychotic disorders. It appears to produce a significant improvement in both the positive and negative symptoms of schizophrenia.

## Pharmacology/Pharmacokinetics

### Physicochemical characteristics

Chemical group—A benzisoxazole derivative

Molecular weight—410.49.

$pKa_1$—8.24

$pKa_2$—3.11

### Mechanism of action/Effect

The mechanism by which risperidone exerts its antipsychotic effect is unknown. Risperidone is a selective monoaminergic antagonist with a strong affinity for serotonin type 2 ($5-HT_2$) receptors and a slightly weaker affinity for dopamine type 2 ($D_2$) receptors. The antipsychotic activity of risperidone may be mediated through antagonism at a combination of these receptor sites, particularly through blockade of cortical serotonin receptors and limbic dopamine systems.

Risperidone also has moderate affinity for the alpha-1 and alpha-2 adrenergic and $H_1$ histaminergic receptors. The affinity of risperidone for the serotonin $5HT_{1A}$, $5HT_{1C}$, and $5HT_{1D}$ receptors is low to moderate, while its affinity for dopamine $D_1$ receptors and the haloperidol-sensitive sigma site is weak.

Risperidone has negligible affinity for cholinergic-muscarinic, beta-adrenergic, and serotonin $5HT_{1B}$ and $5HT_3$ receptors.

### Other actions/effects

Cardiovascular effects reflect the vascular alpha-adrenergic antagonistic activity of risperidone, as evidenced by such dose-related effects as hypotension and reflex tachycardia. The potential for proarrhythmic effects exists, due to risperidone's ability to prolong the QT interval in some patients.

Risperidone changes sleep architecture by promoting deep slow-wave sleep, thereby improving sleep patterns. This effect is most likely due to risperidone's blockade of serotonin receptors.

Substantial and sustained elevations in serum prolactin levels are induced by risperidone. It appears that tolerance to hyperprolactinemia does not occur, but the condition is reversible upon withdrawal of risperidone. Increases in prolactin concentrations are likely due to risperidone's blockade of dopamine receptors.

Preliminary reports suggest that risperidone may suppress pre-existing dyskinesias and may exhibit a low propensity for inducing extrapyramidal symptoms or tardive dyskinesia. However, some clinicians believe that risperidone is likely to cause tardive movement disorders because of its relatively potent blockade of $D_2$ receptors. Additional data from long-term studies are needed to resolve these issues.

Risperidone exerts an antiemetic effect in animals that may also occur in humans, potentially masking signs and symptoms of other medical problems.

Although not yet documented with risperidone, disturbances of body temperature regulation have been reported with other antipsychotics.

### Absorption

Rapid and extensive. Food does not significantly affect the extent of absorption; therefore, risperidone may be given without respect to meals.

The relative bioavailability of risperidone from a tablet is 94% when compared with a solution. The absolute oral bioavailability of risperidone is 70%; the absolute bioavailability of the active moiety (risperidone plus 9-hydroxy-risperidone) approaches 100%, irrespective of the route of administration or the metabolic phenotype status of the patient.

### Distribution

Rapid and extensive. The volume of distribution ($Vol_D$) at steady state is about 1.1 L per kg. In animals, risperidone and 9-hydroxy-risperidone are distributed into breast milk, reaching concentrations comparable to plasma concentrations.

### Protein binding

Risperidone—Very high (90%).

9-hydroxy-risperidone—High (77%).

Note: In plasma, risperidone is predominantly bound to albumin and alpha$_1$-acid glycoprotein (AGP). Although the pharmacokinetics of risperidone in patients with hepatic function impairment are similar to those in healthy young controls, the mean free fraction of risperidone in plasma is increased by about 35% due to decreased concentrations of albumin and AGP.

### Biotransformation

Risperidone is extensively metabolized in the liver by the cytochrome $P_{450}$ $IID_6$ (CYP2D6) enzyme, which is under genetic control. The main metabolic pathway, hydroxylation, yields the major active metabolite 9-hydroxy-risperidone. The pharmacological activity, potency, and safety of this metabolite are comparable to those of its parent compound.

Hydroxylation of risperidone is subject to genetic polymorphism. Patients who are extensive metabolizers exhibit lower plasma concentrations of risperidone and higher concentrations of 9-hydroxy-risperidone than do patients who are poor metabolizers. Although blood levels of risperidone and 9-hydroxy-risperidone can differ by up to 7-fold, there is no difference in the area under the plasma concentration-time curve (AUC) for the combination, and clinical data do not indicate that the ratio of risperidone to 9-hydroxy-risperidone affects either therapeutics or incidence of adverse effects. Overall, the pharmacokinetic parameters of the active moiety (risperidone plus 9-hydroxy-risperidone) are similar in all metabolizers. Therefore, the metabolic phenotype status of patients is not considered to be clinically significant.

### Half-life

Elimination—

Overall mean elimination half-life of the active moiety (risperidone plus 9-hydroxy-risperidone) ranges from 20 to 24 hours.

In patients with renal function impairment, increased elimination half-lives have been reported. Dosage reductions for patients with renal function impairment are recommended.

### Time to peak concentration

Mean peak risperidone plasma concentrations occur within 1 to 2 hours following oral administration.

### Time to steady-state plasma concentrations

Steady-state concentrations of the active moiety (risperidone plus 9-hydroxy-risperidone) are achieved within 5 to 6 days.

### Peak plasma concentration

In one study in healthy volunteers, peak plasma concentrations of the active moiety (risperidone plus 9-hydroxy-risperidone) ranging from 9 to 16 nanograms/mL were reported following oral administration of 1 mg of risperidone. However, no correlation between plasma concentrations and therapeutic effect has been definitively established.

### Plasma concentrations
Although interindividual plasma concentrations vary considerably, plasma concentrations of risperidone, 9-hydroxy-risperidone, and the active moiety (risperidone plus 9-hydroxy-risperidone) are dose-proportional and linear over the therapeutic dosing range.

### Elimination
Renal—
    In patients with normal renal function: Approximately 70%.
    In patients with moderate to severe renal function impairment: Renal clearance of the active moiety (risperidone plus 9-hydroxy-risperidone) may be decreased by 60 to 80%.
Fecal—
    Approximately 15%.

## Precautions to Consider

### Carcinogenicity/Tumorigenicity
Significant increases in the incidence of mammary gland adenocarcinomas and pituitary adenomas occurred in female Swiss albino mice that received risperidone for 18 months at doses of 2.4 and 9.4 times, respectively, the maximum recommended human dose (MRHD) on a mg per kg of body weight (mg/kg) basis. Male Wistar rats that received risperidone for 25 months exhibited increased incidences of endocrine pancreas adenomas and mammary gland neoplasms after risperidone doses of 9.4 times the MRHD (on a mg/kg basis); mammary gland adenocarcinomas in females after risperidone doses of 2.4 times the MRHD (on a mg/kg basis) and in males after doses of 37.5 times the MRHD (on a mg/kg basis) were also reported.

Risperidone, like other agents that antagonize dopamine $D_2$ receptors, elevates prolactin concentrations; the elevation persists during chronic administration. Tissue culture experiments indicate that approximately one-third of human breast cancers are prolactin dependent *in vitro,* a factor of potential importance if use of this medication is contemplated in a patient with a previously detected breast cancer. Although disturbances such as galactorrhea, amenorrhea, gynecomastia, and impotence have been reported, the clinical significance of elevated serum prolactin concentrations is unknown for most patients. An increase in pituitary gland, mammary gland, and pancreatic islet cell hyperplasia and/or neoplasia has been found in rodents after chronic administration of medications (including risperidone) that increase prolactin release. However, neither clinical studies nor epidemiologic studies conducted to date have shown an association between chronic administration of these medications and tumorigenesis; the available evidence is considered too limited to be conclusive at this time.

### Mutagenicity
Risperidone demonstrated no mutagenic potential in the following tests: Ames reverse mutation test, mouse lymphoma assay, *in vitro* rat hepatocyte DNA-repair assay, *in vivo* micronucleus test in mice, the sex-linked recessive lethal test in Drosophila, and the chromosomal aberration test in human lymphocytes or Chinese hamster cells.

### Pregnancy/Reproduction
Fertility—In 3 reproductive studies, risperidone was shown to impair mating but not fertility in Wistar rats that received 0.1 to 3 times the MRHD (on a mg per square meter of body surface area [mg/m²] basis); this effect apparently occurred only in female rats. In a study in beagle dogs, sperm motility and concentration were decreased at risperidone doses of 0.6 to 10 times the MRHD (on a mg/m² basis). Dose-related decreases in serum testosterone were also noted. Serum testosterone and sperm parameters partially recovered but remained decreased after discontinuation of risperidone.

Pregnancy—Adequate and well-controlled studies in humans have not been done.

Agenesis of the corpus callosum in an infant exposed to risperidone in utero has been reported. However, a causal relationship to risperidone therapy has not been established.

In 3 teratogenicity studies conducted in rats and rabbits that received 0.4 to 6 times the MRHD of risperidone (on a mg/m² basis), the incidence of malformations was not increased as compared with controls. In 3 reproductive studies in rats, there was an increase in pup deaths during the first 4 days of lactation at doses of 0.1 to 3 times the MRHD (on a mg/m² basis); it is not known whether these deaths were due to a direct effect on the fetuses or pups, or to effects on the dams. In another study in rats receiving risperidone doses of 1.5 times the MRHD (on a mg/m² basis), there was an increase in the number of stillborn pups.

FDA Pregnancy Category C.

Labor and delivery—The effect of risperidone on labor and delivery is not known.

### Breast-feeding
Risperidone and 9-hydroxy-risperidone are distributed into animal milk in concentrations greater than or equal to plasma concentrations. It is not known if these substances are distributed into human milk.

### Pediatrics
No information is available on the relationship of age to the effects of risperidone in pediatric patients. Safety and efficacy in children up to 18 years of age have not been established.

### Geriatrics
There is limited experience in the use of risperidone in the elderly. In healthy elderly patients, decreases in renal clearance and increases in the elimination half-life of the active moiety (risperidone plus 9-hydroxy-risperidone) have been reported. Also, geriatric patients generally have decreased renal function, decreased hepatic function, decreased cardiac function, and an increased tendency to postural hypotension. Therefore, reduced risperidone doses are recommended.

### Pharmacogenetics
Hydroxylation of risperidone via the cytochrome $P_{450}$ $IID_6$ (CYP2D6) enzyme is subject to genetic polymorphism. About 6 to 8% of Caucasians and a low percentage of Asians have little or no enzyme activity and are considered poor metabolizers. Patients taking risperidone who are extensive metabolizers have lower plasma concentrations of risperidone and higher concentrations of 9-hydroxy-risperidone than do patients who are poor metabolizers. Although blood levels of risperidone and 9-hydroxy-risperidone can differ by up to 7-fold, there is no difference in the area under the plasma concentration-time curve (AUC) for the combination, and clinical data do not indicate that the ratio affects either therapeutics or incidence of adverse effects. Overall, the pharmacokinetic parameters of the active moiety (risperidone plus 9-hydroxy-risperidone) are similar in all metabolizers. Therefore, the metabolic phenotype status of patients is not considered to be clinically significant.

### Dental
Prolonged use of risperidone may decrease or inhibit salivary flow, thus contributing to the development of caries, periodontal disease, oral candidiasis, and discomfort. Conversely, some patients may experience an increase in salivation.

### Drug interactions and/or related problems
The following drug interactions and/or related problems have been selected on the basis of their potential clinical significance (possible mechanism in parentheses where appropriate)—not necessarily inclusive (» = major clinical significance):

Note: Medications that inhibit the cytochrome $P_{450}$ $IID_6$ (CYP2D6) isozyme potentially could inhibit the metabolism of risperidone. However, since only the relative amounts of risperidone and 9-hydroxy-risperidone and not the total concentration of active moiety (risperidone plus 9-hydroxy-risperidone) would be affected, no marked changes in activity should occur. Medications metabolized by other $P_{450}$ isozymes (including CYP1A1, CYP1A2, CYP2C9, CYP2C19, and CYP3A4) are only weak inhibitors of risperidone metabolism.

Similarly, risperidone potentially could interfere with the metabolism of other medications metabolized via $P_{450}$ $IID_6$ (CYP2D6); however, risperidone is bound relatively weakly to the enzyme, so these effects seem unlikely to be clinically significant.

*In vitro* studies have shown no significant interactions caused by other highly protein-bound agents displacing or being displaced by risperidone.

Combinations containing any of the following medications, depending on the amount present, may also interact with this medication.

» Alcohol or
» CNS depression–producing medications, other (See *Appendix II*)
    (additive CNS depressant effects may occur)

» Antihypertensive medications
    (potential hypotensive effects of these medications can enhance hypotensive effects of risperidone)

» Bromocriptine or
» Levodopa or
» Pergolide
    (risperidone may antagonize the effects of levodopa and dopamine agonists)

» Carbamazepine
    (chronic administration of carbamazepine may increase the clearance of risperidone)

» Clozapine
(chronic administration of clozapine may decrease the clearance of risperidone)

### Laboratory value alterations
The following have been selected on the basis of their potential clinical significance (possible effect in parentheses where appropriate)—not necessarily inclusive (» = major clinical significance):

With physiology/laboratory test values
Electrocardiogram
(prolongation of the QT interval may occur)

Prolactin concentrations, serum
(sustained elevations occur during therapy with risperidone)

### Medical considerations/Contraindications
The medical considerations/contraindications included here have been selected on the basis of their potential clinical significance (reasons given in parentheses where appropriate)—not necessarily inclusive (» = major clinical significance).

*Risk-benefit should be considered when the following medical problems exist:*

Brain tumor or
Intestinal obstruction or
Medication overdose or
Reye's syndrome
(risperidone's antiemetic effect may mask signs and symptoms of these conditions)

» Breast cancer
(prolactin-dependent cancer may be exacerbated)

» Cardiovascular disease, including heart failure, conduction abnormalities, or history of myocardial infarction or

» Cerebrovascular disease
(condition may be exacerbated)

» Dehydration or

» Hypovolemia
(risperidone-induced hypotension may exacerbate condition)

Drug abuse or dependence, history of
(patients with a history of drug abuse receiving risperidone should be observed closely, as with any new central nervous system [CNS] medication)

» Hepatic function impairment, severe
(metabolism of risperidone may be altered)

» Parkinson's disease
(may be exacerbated)

» Renal function impairment, severe
(excretion of risperidone may be altered)

» Risk factors for torsades de pointes, including bradycardia, electrolyte imbalance, or concomitant intake of other medications that prolong the QT interval
(risk of torsades de pointes may be increased)

» Seizures, history of
(seizure threshold may be lowered)

Sensitivity to risperidone

### Patient monitoring
The following may be especially important in patient monitoring (other tests may be warranted in some patients, depending on condition; » = major clinical significance):

Abnormal-movement determinations
(recommended at periodic intervals to detect extrapyramidal symptoms)

Careful observation for early signs of tardive dyskinesia
(recommended at periodic intervals; since there is no known effective treatment if the syndrome develops, risperidone should be discontinued, if clinically feasible, at the earliest signs, usually fine, worm-like movements of the tongue, to stop further development)

## Side/Adverse Effects

Note: Disturbances of body temperature regulation have been associated with use of other antipsychotic agents. Although this effect has not been reported to date with risperidone, caution is advised in administering this medication to patients who will be exposed to extreme heat.

The following side/adverse effects have been selected on the basis of their potential clinical significance (possible signs and symptoms in parentheses where appropriate)—not necessarily inclusive:

### Those indicating need for medical attention
Incidence more frequent
*Akathisia* (restlessness or need to keep moving); *anxiety or nervousness; changes in vision, including disturbances of accommodation and blurred vision; sexual dysfunction or decreased libido* (decreased sexual performance or desire); *dizziness; dysmenorrhea or menorrhagia* (menstrual changes); *extrapyramidal effects, dystonic* (muscle spasms of face, neck and back; tic-like or twitching movements; twisting movements of body; inability to move eyes; weakness of arms and legs); *extrapyramidal effects, parkinsonian* (difficulty in speaking or swallowing; loss of balance control; mask-like face; shuffling walk; stiffness of arms or legs; trembling and shaking of hands and fingers); *insomnia* (trouble in sleeping); *micturition disturbances or polyuria* (problems in urination or increase in amount of urine); *mood or mental changes, including aggressive behavior, agitation, difficulty in concentration, and memory problems; skin rash or itching*

Note: *Extrapyramidal symptoms* are dose-related; *sexual dysfunction* and *decreased libido,* or *vision changes* may be dose-related.

*Menorrhagia* may be associated with increased prolactin concentrations.

Incidence less frequent
*Amenorrhea* (menstrual changes); *back pain; cardiovascular effects, including orthostatic hypotension* (dizziness or lightheadedness); *orthostatic dizziness; hypotension; palpitations* (pounding heartbeat); *chest pain, and reflex tachycardia or tachycardia* (fast or racing heartbeat); *dyspnea* (trouble in breathing); *galactorrhea* (unusual secretion of milk); *seborrhea* (skin condition caused by excess release of oil—may be accompanied by dandruff and oily skin)

Note: *Amenorrhea* and *galactorrhea* are associated with increased prolactin concentrations. *Orthostatic dizziness, palpitations,* and *tachycardia* may be dose-related.

Incidence rare
*Anorexia* (loss of appetite); *mania or hypomania* (talking, feeling, and acting with excitement and activity you cannot control); *neuroleptic malignant syndrome (NMS)* (difficult or unusually fast breathing; fast heartbeat or irregular pulse; high fever; high or low [irregular] blood pressure; increased sweating; loss of bladder control; severe muscle stiffness; seizures; unusually pale skin; unusual tiredness or weakness); *polydipsia* (extreme thirst); *priapism* (prolonged, painful, inappropriate erection of the penis); *seizures* (convulsions); *tardive dyskinesia* (lip smacking or puckering; puffing of cheeks; rapid or worm-like movements of tongue; uncontrolled chewing movements; uncontrolled movements of arms and legs); *tardive dystonia* (increased blinking or spasms of eyelid; unusual facial expressions or body positions; uncontrolled twisting movements of neck, trunk, arms, or legs); *thrombocytopenic purpura* (unusual bleeding or bruising)

### Those indicating need for medical attention only if they continue or are bothersome
Incidence more frequent
*Asthenia, fatigue, or lassitude* (unusual tiredness or weakness); *constipation; cough; decreased salivation or dryness of mouth; diarrhea; drowsiness; dyspepsia* (heartburn); *headache; increased dream activity; increased duration of sleep; nausea; pharyngitis* (sore throat); *rhinitis* (runny nose); *weight gain*

Note: *Asthenia, lassitude, or fatigue, drowsiness, increased duration of sleep,* and *weight gain* may be dose-related. *Rhinitis* is most likely due to alpha-adrenoceptor-mediated nasal congestion.

Incidence less frequent
*Abdominal pain; arthralgia* (joint pain); *dry skin; increased pigmentation* (darkening of skin color); *increased salivation* (increased watering of mouth); *increased sweating; photosensitivity* (increased sensitivity of the skin to sun); *vomiting; weight loss*

Note: *Increased pigmentation* may be dose-related.

### Those indicating the need for medical attention if they occur after the medication is discontinued
*Withdrawal emergent dyskinesia* (lip smacking or puckering; puffing of cheeks; rapid or worm-like movements of tongue; uncontrolled chewing movements; uncontrolled movements of arms and legs)

## Overdose

For specific information on the agents used in the management of risperidone overdose, see:
• *Charcoal, Activated (Oral-Local)* monograph.

For more information on the management of overdose or unintentional ingestion, **contact a Poison Control Center** (see *Poison Control Center Listing*).

**Clinical effects of overdose**

The following effects have been selected on the basis of their potential clinical significance (possible signs and symptoms in parentheses where appropriate)—not necessarily inclusive:

Acute and chronic effects

*Drowsiness; extrapyramidal symptoms; electrocardiogram (ECG) abnormalities, especially prolonged QT interval; electrolyte disturbances; hypotension; seizures; tachycardia*

**Treatment of overdose**

There is no specific antidote for risperidone. Treatment is essentially symptomatic and supportive with possible utilization of the following:

To decrease absorption—
  Gastric lavage should be considered. Activated charcoal may be administered, and may be followed by administration of a laxative. The risk of aspiration with induced emesis is increased if the patient is obtunded, seizing, or experiencing dystonic movements of the head and neck.

Specific treatment—
  For treatment of severe extrapyramidal symptoms: Administration of anticholinergic agents may be indicated.
  For treatment of arrhythmias caused by risperidone toxicity: Selection of an appropriate antiarrhythmic agent—Use of disopyramide, procainamide, or quinidine may add to risperidone toxicity by prolonging the QT interval. Also, the alpha-adrenergic-blocking properties of bretylium may add to risperidone's effects, producing problematic hypotension.
  For treatment of hypotension or circulatory collapse: Selection of an appropriate sympathomimetic—Beta-adrenergic stimulation properties of epinephrine or dopamine may worsen the hypotension induced by risperidone's alpha-adrenergic blockade.

Monitoring—
  Cardiovascular monitoring should be initiated immediately to detect arrhythmias. Serum electrolytes should also be monitored.

Supportive care—
  Supportive measures such as establishing intravenous lines, hydration, correction of electrolyte imbalance, oxygenation, and support of ventilatory function are essential for maintaining the vital functions of the patient. Patients in whom intentional overdose is known or suspected should be referred for psychiatric consultation.

## Patient Consultation

As an aid to patient consultation, refer to *Advice for the Patient, Risperidone (Systemic)*.

In providing consultation, consider emphasizing the following selected information (» = major clinical significance):

**Before using this medication**
» Conditions affecting use, especially:
    Sensitivity to risperidone
    Pregnancy—Agenesis of the corpus callosum reported in 1 infant, but causal relationship not established
    Breast-feeding—Risperidone appears in animal milk at levels approximating plasma concentrations
    Use in the elderly—Older patients may be at increased risk for adverse effects
    Other medications, especially antihypertensives, bromocriptine, carbamazepine, clozapine, CNS depressants, levodopa, or pergolide
    Other medical problems, especially cardiovascular disease, cerebrovascular disease, hepatic function impairment, history of seizures, Parkinson's disease, renal function impairment, or risk factors for torsades de pointes

**Proper use of this medication**
» Compliance with therapy; not taking more or less medicine than prescribed
» Proper dosing
    Missed dose: Taking as soon as possible; if almost time for next dose, skipping missed dose; not doubling doses
» Proper storage

**Precautions while using this medication**
» Regular visits to physician to check progress of therapy
» Checking with physician before discontinuing medication; gradual dosage reduction may be needed
» Avoiding use of alcoholic beverages; not taking other CNS depressants unless prescribed by physician

» Caution if any kind of surgery, dental treatment, or emergency treatment is required; telling physician or dentist in charge about treatment with risperidone because of possible drug interactions or adverse effects
» Possible blurred vision, dizziness, or drowsiness; caution when driving or doing jobs requiring alertness or clear vision
» Possible dizziness or lightheadedness; caution when getting up suddenly from a lying or sitting position
» Possible skin photosensitivity; avoiding unprotected exposure to sun; wearing protective clothing; using a sun block product that includes protection against both UVA-caused photosensitivity reactions and UVB-caused sunburn reactions; avoiding use of sunlamp, tanning bed, or tanning booth
  Possible dryness of mouth; using sugarless gum or candy, ice, or saliva substitute for relief; checking with physician or dentist if dry mouth continues for more than 2 weeks
  Possible heatstroke; caution during exercise, hot baths, or hot weather

**Side/adverse effects**
  Akasthisia; anxiety or nervousness; changes in vision; sexual dysfunction or decreased libido; dizziness; dysmenorrhea or menorrhagia; extrapyramidal effects; insomnia; micturition disturbances or polyuria; mood or mental changes; skin rash or itching; amenorrhea; back pain; cardiovascular effects; dyspnea; galactorrhea; seborrhea; anorexia; mania or hypomania; neuroleptic malignant syndrome; polydipsia; priapism; seizures; tardive dyskinesia; tardive dystonia; thrombocytopenic purpura

## General Dosing Information

Risperidone dosage must be individualized by cautious titration from the lower dosage range, to avoid orthostatic hypotension. The need for risperidone should be reassessed periodically, and the patient maintained at the lowest possible dosage level.

Since the possiblity of suicide is inherent in schizophrenia, patients should not have access to large quantities of this medication. To reduce the risk of overdose, some clinicians recommend that the patient be supplied with the smallest quantity of medication necessary for satisfactory patient management.

There is a significant curvilinear dose-response relationship over the range of 1 to 16 mg of risperidone a day. This represents an "optimal dose" curve, along which maximum activity of risperidone occurs at doses of 4 to 8 mg a day. In general, daily doses greater than 6 mg of risperidone have not proven to be more efficacious than lower risperidone doses and were associated with increased adverse effects.

**Diet/Nutrition**
Risperidone may be given without regard to food.

**For treatment of adverse effects**
  Neuroleptic malignant syndrome (NMS)—Treatment is essentially symptomatic and supportive and may include the following
    • *Discontinuing risperidone immediately.*
    • Hyperthermia—Administering antipyretics (aspirin or acetaminophen); using cooling blanket.
    • Dehydration—Restoring fluids and electrolytes.
    • Cardiovascular instability—Monitoring blood pressure and cardiac rhythm closely; use of sodium nitroprusside may allow vasodilation with subsequent heat loss from the skin in patients with less dominant muscle rigidity.
    • Hypoxia—Administering oxygen; considering airway insertion and assisted ventilation.
    • Muscle rigidity—Administering dantrolene sodium (100 to 300 mg per day in divided doses, or 1.25 to 1.5 mg per kg of body weight, intravenously) for muscle relaxation; or amantadine (100 mg twice a day) or bromocriptine (5 mg three times a day) to restore central balance of dopamine and acetylcholine at the receptor site.
    • If neuroleptics must be continued because of severe psychosis, initial treatment may consist of
        —At least 5 days of neuroleptic abstinence before rechallenge.
        —Use of a neuroleptic of a different class from the one causing NMS.
        —Use of a low dose.
        —Using the neuroleptic only for controlling the psychosis.

  Tardive dyskinesia or tardive dystonia—No known effective treatment. Dosage of risperidone should be lowered or medication discontinued, if clinically feasible, at earliest signs of tardive dyskinesia or tardive dystonia, to prevent possible irreversible effects.

## Oral Dosage Forms
### RISPERIDONE TABLETS
**Usual adult dose**
Antipsychotic—
Oral, 1 mg two times a day on the first day; the dose may be increased to 2 mg two times a day on the second day, and further increased to 3 mg two times a day on the third day. Slower titration may be necessary in some patients. Further dosage adjustments should be made as needed and tolerated in small increments or decrements of 1 mg two times a day at intervals of no less than one week, thus enabling steady-state plasma concentrations to be reached before instituting further dosage changes.

Note: Dosing regimens for risperidone are somewhat controversial. The above recommendations represent those utilized in several premarketing clinical trials; many patients reportedly are unable to tolerate such rapid titrations, and alternative regimens are being utilized. For example, some clinicians advocate an initial dosing schedule of 0.5 to 1 mg two times a day, with the dose being increased as needed and tolerated at intervals of 3 to 5 days, until a total daily dose of 4 to 8 mg is reached; that dosage level is usually maintained for 1 to 2 weeks prior to any further changes in dose.

Debilitated patients, as well as those who have severe hepatic or renal function impairment, and those who are predisposed to hypotension or for whom hypotension would pose a risk should receive reduced doses, following the regimen described in the *Usual geriatric dose* section.

If risperidone treatment is to be reinitiated in a patient who was previously receiving risperidone therapy, the initial titration schedule should be followed.

When switching from other antipsychotics to risperidone, immediate discontinuation of the previous treatment may be acceptable for some patients, while more gradual discontinuation may be most appropriate for other patients. In all cases, the period of overlapping antipsychotic administration should be minimized. When switching patients from depot antipsychotics, risperdone may be instituted in place of the next scheduled depot injection, if medically appropriate. The need for continuing administration of medication to control extrapyramidal symptoms should be periodically reevaluated.

**Usual adult prescribing limits**
16 mg a day.

Note: In adults with severe hepatic function impairment, the usual prescribing limit is 4 mg a day.

**Usual pediatric dose**
Safety and efficacy in children up to 18 years of age have not been established.

**Usual geriatric dose**
Antipsychotic—
Oral, initially 0.5 mg two times a day. The dose may be increased as needed and tolerated in increments of 0.5 mg two times a day. Dosage increases exceeding 1.5 mg two times a day generally should occur only at intervals of at least one week.

Note: There is potential for accumulation of risperidone in the elderly.

**Usual geriatric prescribing limits**
3 mg a day.

**Strength(s) usually available**
U.S.—
1 mg (Rx) [*Risperdal* (scored; lactose)].
2 mg (Rx) [*Risperdal* (lactose)].
3 mg (Rx) [*Risperdal* (lactose)].
4 mg (Rx) [*Risperdal* (lactose)].
Canada—
1 mg (Rx) [*Risperdal* (scored; lactose)].
2 mg (Rx) [*Risperdal* (scored; lactose)].
3 mg (Rx) [*Risperdal* (scored; lactose)].
4 mg (Rx) [*Risperdal* (scored; lactose)].

**Packaging and storage**
Store below 40 °C (104 °F), preferably between 15 and 30 °C (59 and 86 °F), unless otherwise specified by manufacturer. Protect from light.

**Auxiliary labeling**
• Avoid alcoholic beverages.
• May cause drowsiness.

## Selected Bibliography
Grant S, Fitton A. Risperidone. A review of its pharmacology and therapeutic potential in the treatment of schizophrenia. Drugs 1994; 48 (2): 253-73.
Cohen LJ. Risperidone. Pharmacotherapy 1994; 14 (3): 253-65.
Ereshefsky L, Lacombe S. Pharmacological profile of risperidone. Can J Psychiatry 1993 Sept; 38 (Suppl 3): S80-S88.

Developed: 09/12/95

# RITODRINE   Systemic

VA CLASSIFICATION (Primary/Secondary): AU100/GU900
Note: For a listing of dosage forms and brand names by country availability, see *Dosage Forms* section(s). For a listing of brand names for the articles in this monograph, refer to the General Index.

## Category
Tocolytic.

## Indications
**Accepted**
Premature labor (prophylaxis and treatment)—Intravenous ritodrine is indicated in the treatment of preterm labor in patients with a pregnancy of 20 or more weeks' gestation. Preterm labor is defined as rhythmic uterine contractions less than 10 minutes apart accompanied by progressive cervical effacement and/or dilation before the end of the 37th week of gestation. By prolonging gestation, ritodrine may reduce the incidence of neonatal mortality and respiratory distress syndrome by allowing time for the fetus to age and the fetal lung to mature or time for corticosteroids to be administered to the mother to enhance lung maturity in the fetus. Suitable patients must have intact amniotic membranes, cervical dilation usually but not always less than 4 centimeters (cm), and cervical effacement less than 80%. Use is not recommended prior to the 20th week of pregnancy.

For intravenous ritodrine to be most effective, it is recommended that therapy begin as soon as the diagnosis of preterm labor is confirmed. Due to the potential risks for the patient and fetus, a physician experienced in the use of intravenous ritodrine should be present to intervene in case of an emergency.

Intravenous ritodrine is less likely to inhibit labor when labor is advanced (cervical dilation more than 4 cm or effacement more than 80%) or when patient is close to term; its use, according to one study, may be best in pregnancies of less than 28 weeks. Risk-benefit should be cautiously assessed for those women in advanced labor or whose amniotic membranes have ruptured as safety and efficacy have not been established for these patients; use of ritodrine is not recommended. Risk of intrauterine infection when amniotic membranes are ruptured must be considered.

Although oral ritodrine is indicated in the treatment of preterm labor in Canada, it is the opinion of the USP Obstetrics and Gynecology Advisory Panel that oral ritodrine cannot be recommended because its efficacy has not been established to be more effective than a placebo and alternative therapies may be more beneficial. Bed rest at home and early admission may be better alternatives than using oral ritodrine in treatment of preterm labor, including retreatment of recurrent preterm labor.

## Pharmacology/Pharmacokinetics

**Physicochemical characteristics**
Molecular weight—323.82.

**Mechanism of action/Effect**
Ritodrine, a beta-2–adrenergic agonist, relaxes the uterus by stimulating the beta-2–adrenergic receptors of the uterine muscle, which causes a decrease in the intensity and frequency of uterine contractions. Specifically, ritodrine decreases uterine myometrial contractility by increasing cellular cyclic adenosine monophosphate (cAMP) and increasing cell membrane cytokines that increase and sequester intracellular calcium. Without intracellular calcium, the activation of

contractile protein of smooth muscle is prevented and the uterus relaxes.

**Other actions/effects**

In addition to stimulating the beta-2–adrenergic receptors of the uterine smooth muscle, ritodrine stimulates beta-adrenergic receptors of bronchial and vascular smooth muscles. The cardiostimulatory effects, including increased cardiac output, increased maternal and fetal heart rates, and widening of the maternal pulse pressure, are probably due to relaxation of vascular smooth muscle. Relaxation of vascular smooth muscle stimulates the beta-1–adrenergic receptors and the reflex response to blood pressure. Also, during intravenous administration, ritodrine transiently increases maternal and fetal blood glucose and maternal plasma insulin concentrations. Other metabolic changes include increased cAMP, lactic acid, and free fatty acids, and decreased serum potassium concentration.

**Distribution**

Ritodrine and its conjugates transfer via placenta into the fetal circulation; fetal and maternal concencentrations may be equal.

**Protein binding**

Low (almost exclusively to albumin).

**Biotransformation**

Hepatic (inactive metabolites); metabolized to conjugates by both the mother and the fetus.

**Half-life**

Intravenous—Nonpregnant females—
Distribution: 6 to 9 minutes.
Elimination: 1.7 to 2.6 hours.

**Onset of action**

Intravenous—5 minutes (at effective dose).

**Peak serum concentration**

Intravenous—32 to 52 nanograms per mL after infusion of 9 mg over 60 minutes in nonpregnant females.

**Elimination**

Renal (71 to 93%; conjugated metabolites; with 90% of dose eliminated within 24 hours).
In dialysis—Removable by dialysis.

## Precautions to Consider

**Cross-sensitivity and/or related problems**

Patients sensitive to sulfites may be sensitive to intravenous ritodrine because of the sulfite preservative present.

**Carcinogenicity/Tumorigenicity**

Studies in rats receiving ritodrine orally found no increased risk of carcinogenicity or tumorigenicity.

**Pregnancy/Reproduction**

Pregnancy—Adequate and well-controlled studies in humans have not been done in women with a pregnancy of less than 20 weeks' gestation. A small number of children 7 to 9 years of age who had been exposed to ritodrine prenatally were studied for up to 2 years and did not show increased risk of abnormalities. Risk-benefit to the fetus must be considered since ritodrine crosses the placenta. Neonatal hypoglycemia, tachycardia, and ileus have been reported; ketoacidosis has resulted in fetal death. Neonatal hypocalcemia and hypotension have occurred with other beta-adrenergic stimulants, although they have not been reported with ritodrine.

Studies in animals have not shown that ritodrine causes adverse effects on the fetus.

FDA Pregnancy Category B.

**Drug interactions and/or related problems**

The following drug interactions and/or related problems have been selected on the basis of their potential clinical significance (possible mechanism in parentheses where appropriate)—not necessarily inclusive (» = major clinical significance):

Note: Combinations containing any of the following medications, depending on the amount present, may also interact with this medication.

Anesthetics, potent, general or
Diazoxide, parenteral or
Magnesium sulfate or
Meperidine
  (may potentiate cardiovascular effects of intravenous ritodrine, especially cardiac arrhythmias or hypotension)

» Beta-adrenergic agonists, other or
Parasympatholytic agents, such as atropine or

Sympathomimetics
  (concurrent use may cause an additive sympathomimetic effect and greatly increase the likelihood of developing side effects, including hypertension from a parasympatholytic agent or cardiac problems from another tocolytic agent. A sufficient time interval should elapse prior to administering another sympathomimetic agent [90% of an intravenous dose is eliminated within 24 hours])

» Beta-adrenergic blocking agents
  (these agents antagonize the effects of ritodrine, and although agents with greater beta-1–adrenergic selectivity may be less antagonistic, concurrent use is not recommended)

» Corticosteroids, long-acting
  (corticosteroids are often used concurrently to enhance fetal lung maturity; however, intravenous ritodrine and, to a lesser extent, corticosteroids each expand plasma volume by causing sodium retention. Intravenous ritodrine further increases plasma volume and may cause overhydration. One possible result of overhydration is maternal pulmonary edema, which has occurred with or without corticosteroid administration. Restricting and monitoring fluids helps prevent maternal pulmonary edema; however, on occurrence, discontinuance of ritodrine should be considered. Maternal ketoacidosis has also been reported with concurrent use of high doses of corticosteroids)

**Laboratory value alterations**

The following have been selected on the basis of their potential clinical significance (possible effect in parentheses where appropriate)—not necessarily inclusive (» = major clinical significance):

With physiology/laboratory test values

Alanine aminotransferase (ALT [SGPT]) or
Aspartate aminotransferase (AST [SGOT])
  (increased serum concentrations have been reported in less than 1% of patients receiving ritodrine and other beta-adrenergic agonists)

Blood pressure, maternal and
Cardiac output, maternal and
Heart rate, fetal and maternal
  (increased maternal heart rate, increased maternal systolic blood pressure, and decreased maternal diastolic blood pressure occur in 80 to 100% of patients treated with intravenous ritodrine; oral ritodrine frequently causes small increases in maternal heart rate but usually does not affect fetal heart rate or maternal blood pressure)

Free fatty acid, serum and
Glucose, blood and
Insulin, serum
  (concentrations may be transiently increased during intravenous infusion but usually return to pretreatment concentrations within 48 to 72 hours, even with continued infusion)

Potassium
  (serum concentration may be decreased during intravenous infusion; related to changes in glucose and insulin; maximum effect occurs within 2 hours after infusion is started and concentrations return to normal 30 minutes to 48 hours after withdrawal)

**Medical considerations/Contraindications**

The medical considerations/contraindications included here have been selected on the basis of their potential clinical significance (reasons given in parentheses where appropriate)—not necessarily inclusive (» = major clinical significance).

*Except under special circumstances, this medication should not be used when the following medical problems exist:*

» Cardiovascular diseases, maternal, especially those associated with arrhythmias or
» Hyperthyroidism, uncontrolled or
» Hypovolemia or
» Pheochromocytoma
  (ritodrine may precipitate arrhythmias or heart failure; occult cardiac disease may be unmasked)

» Chorioamnionitis or
» Intrauterine fetal death or
» Nonreassuring fetal status
  (premature labor should not be suppressed for these problems or conditions)

» Eclampsia and severe preeclampsia or
» Hypertension, uncontrolled or
» Pulmonary hypertension
  (ritodrine may aggravate these conditions and, if these conditions cannot be controlled, preterm labor should not be suppressed)

***Risk-benefit should be considered when the following medical problems exist:***

» Abruptio placentae or
» Hemorrhage, maternal or
» Placenta previa or
» Preeclampsia, mild to moderate
    (ritodrine may aggravate these conditions and, if they cannot be controlled, premature labor should not be suppressed)

Allergy or sensitivity to ritodrine or sulfites

» Diabetes mellitus
    (may be aggravated; maternal ketoacidosis has also been reported, especially in patients with poorly controlled diabetes; insulin dose may need to be increased; neonatal glucose should be checked after delivery)

Hypertension or
Migraine headaches, or history of
    (these conditions may be aggravated; also, transient cerebral ischemia has been reported with the use of other beta-adrenergic agonist therapy in patients who had migraines during ritodrine administration)

## Patient monitoring

The following may be especially important in patient monitoring (other tests may be warranted in some patients, depending on condition; » = major clinical significance):

Assessment of gestational age and fetal maturity
    (to diagnose preterm labor)

» Blood count determinations
    (patients using ritodrine long-term, especially intravenous use for 2 or 3 weeks, should be monitored for development of leukopenia or agranulocytosis)

» Blood glucose, maternal and neonatal and
» Fluid and electrolyte status, maternal and neonatal
    (should be monitored carefully during prolonged intravenous administration, especially in diabetic patients or those receiving corticosteroids, potassium-depleting diuretics, or digitalis glycosides; neonatal blood glucose should be determined promptly after delivery)

Cardiac function monitoring, maternal, such as electrocardiogram (ECG) and/or
Pulmonary function monitoring, maternal
    (baseline ECG should be done to rule out occult maternal cardiac disease; pulmonary function monitoring and an ECG should also be done immediately in patients complaining of chest pain or tightness during ritodrine therapy and ritodrine should be temporarily discontinued until ECG is assessed; a persistent high tachycardia [over 140 beats per minute] may be related to impending pulmonary edema)

Heart rate, fetal and
Heart rate and blood pressure, maternal and
Uterine activity
    (should be monitored frequently during intravenous administration)

## Side/Adverse Effects

Note: Most adverse effects of ritodrine are related to its beta-adrenergic stimulating activity and are usually dose-related.

    Maternal ketoacidosis has been reported, especially in patients also receiving high doses of corticosteroids or in patients with poorly controlled diabetes mellitus.

The following side/adverse effects have been selected on the basis of their potential clinical significance (possible signs and symptoms in parentheses where appropriate)—not necessarily inclusive:

**Those indicating need for medical attention**
Incidence more frequent
    ***Angina or cardiac disease, previously undiagnosed*** (chest pain or tightness)—15% with intravenous use; ***diastolic blood pressure reduction, maternal*** (lightheadedness or dizziness)—80 to 100% with intravenous use; ***hyperglycemia, maternal*** (blurred vision; drowsiness; dry mouth; flushed, dry skin; fruit-like breath odor; increased frequency and volume of urination; ketones in urine; loss of appetite; somnolence; stomachache, nausea, or vomiting; tiredness; troubled breathing, rapid and deep; unconsciousness; unusual thirst)—80 to 100% with intravenous use, transient for 48 to 72 hours; ***pulmonary edema*** (shortness of breath)—15% with intravenous use; ***tachycardia or other cardiac arrhythmias, maternal and fetal*** (fast or irregular heartbeat)—1% with oral use and 80 to 100% with intravenous use

    Note: Increased cardiac output resulting from the use of beta-adrenergic agonists may result in *cardiac arrhythmias* or *angina*

(with or without ECG changes) that has usually been associated with unrecognized cardiopulmonary disease, which may lead to myocardial ischemia, myocardial infarction, and possibly death.

At the recommended intravenous infusion rate in one study, the *maternal and fetal heartbeat* averaged 130 (range, 60 to 180) and 164 (range, 130 to 200) beats per minute, respectively. The maternal systolic and diastolic blood pressure measurements averaged 128 mm Hg (range, 96 to 162 mm Hg) and 48 mm Hg (range, 0 to 76 mm Hg), respectively. Only 1% of patients with persistent *tachycardia* or *severely decreased diastolic blood pressure* required withdrawal from the medication; these severe effects were managed successfully by dose reduction. Oral administration was associated with only a small increase in maternal heart rate and little or no effect on maternal blood pressure or fetal heart rate.

*Maternal hyperglycemia* may cause fetal or neonatal hypoglycemia.

Serious maternal *pulmonary edema* has occurred during intravenous administration of ritodrine or other beta-adrenergic agonists for premature labor or after delivery. Although the exact cause is unknown, it appears to be related to circulatory fluid overload with subsequent pulmonary edema, and has occurred more frequently with concurrent corticosteroid administration; maternal death has been reported with or without concomitantly administered corticosteroids. Other contributing factors may include hypokalemia, twin gestations, sustained tachycardia (> 140 beats per minute), undiagnosed cardiopulmonary disease, and catecholamine-induced cardiac injury. If pulmonary edema develops during administration, ritodrine should be discontinued.

Incidence rare
    ***Agranulocytosis or leukopenia*** (sore throat or fever)—with intravenous use for 2 to 3 weeks, reversible on discontinuation; ***hepatic function impairment or hepatitis*** (yellow eyes or skin)—reported in less than 1% of patients using ritodrine and other beta-adrenergic agonists

**Those indicating need for medical attention only if they continue or are bothersome**
Incidence more frequent
    ***Erythema*** (reddened skin)—10 to 50% with intravenous use; ***headache***—10 to 50% with intravenous use; ***nausea***—5 to 8% with oral use and 10 to 50% with intravenous use; ***palpitations*** (pounding or racing heartbeat)—10 to 15% with oral use and 33% with intravenous use; ***trembling***—10 to 15% with oral use and 10 to 50% with intravenous use; ***vomiting***—5 to 8% with oral use and 10 to 50% with intravenous use

Incidence less frequent or rare
    ***Psychological symptoms*** (anxiety, emotional upset, jitteriness, nervousness, restlessness)—5 to 8% with oral or intravenous use; ***skin rash***—3 to 4% with oral use and rare with intravenous use

**Those indicating possible maternal pulmonary edema and need for medical attention if they occur after medication is discontinued**
    ***Shortness of breath***

## Overdose

For specific information on the agents used in the management of ritodrine overdose, see:
    • *Beta-adrenergic Blocking Agents (Systemic)* monograph;
    • *Charcoal, Activated (Oral-Local)* monograph; and/or
    • *Furosemide (Systemic)* in the *Diuretics, Loop* monograph.

For more information on the management of overdose or unintentional ingestion, **contact a Poison Control Center** (see *Poison Control Center Listing*).

### Clinical effects of overdose

The following effects have been selected on the basis of their potential clinical significance (possible signs and symptoms in parentheses where appropriate)—not necessarily inclusive:
    ***Nausea or vomiting, severe; nervousness or trembling, severe; pulmonary edema*** (shortness of breath, severe); ***tachycardia*** (fast or irregular heartbeat, severe)
    Note: The dose required to produce overdose symptoms varies by individual.

### Treatment of overdose

Discontinuation of ritodrine is often all that is required if symptoms are not severe.

To enhance elimination—Renal dialysis for all dosage forms, if needed. Overdose of oral ritodrine may require induction of emesis, followed by administration of activated charcoal.

Specific treatment—Beta-adrenergic blocking agents are used to antagonize the actions of ritodrine and to treat arrhythmias. Loop diuretics are indicated as adjuncts to treat maternal pulmonary edema.

Supportive care—Supportive measures such as establishing intravenous lines, correction of hydration or electrolyte balance, especially potassium or calcium, oxygenation, and support of ventilatory function are essential for maintaining the vital functions of the patient.

## Patient Consultation

As an aid to patient consultation, refer to *Advice for the Patient, Ritodrine (Systemic)*.

In providing consultation, consider emphasizing the following selected information (» = major clinical significance):

### Before using this medication
» Conditions affecting use, especially:
   Sensitivity to ritodrine or sulfite preservative
   Other medications, especially beta-adrenergic agonists (other), beta-adrenergic blocking agents, or long-acting corticosteroids
   Other medical problems, especially abruptio placentae, cardiovascular disease (maternal), chorioamnionitis, diabetes mellitus, eclampsia, hemorrhage (maternal), hypertension (uncontrolled), hyperthyroidism (uncontrolled), hypovolemia, intrauterine fetal death, nonreassuring fetal status, pheochromocytoma, placenta previa, preeclampsia, or pulmonary hypertension

### Proper use of this medication
» Proper dosing
   Missed dose: Taking if remembered within an hour or so; not taking if remembered later; not doubling doses
» Proper storage

### Precautions while using this medication
» Checking with physician immediately if contractions begin again or in case of ruptured membranes
» Not taking other medications, especially OTC sympathomimetics, unless discussed with physician

### Side/adverse effects
   Signs of potential side effects, especially angina or cardiac disease (previously undiagnosed) (maternal), diastolic blood pressure reduction (maternal), hyperglycemia (maternal), tachycardia or other cardiac arrhythmias (maternal or fetal), agranulocytosis or leukopenia, hepatic function impairment or hepatitis, or pulmonary edema

## General Dosing Information

Side effects, including tachycardia (maternal heart rate of greater than 120 or fetal heart rate of greater than 170 to 180), may be reduced without reducing ritodrine's effectiveness by slowing the rate of infusion or decreasing the dose.

If labor persists despite administration of the maximum dose, it is recommended that ritodrine therapy be withdrawn; however, in cases of recurrence of unwanted preterm labor, ritodrine treatment may be repeated.

Ritodrine should be discontinued as soon as labor is irreversible in order to allow for metabolic recovery (reversal of maternal hyperglycemia or fetal hypoglycemia or hypocalcemia) before delivery.

### For parenteral dosage forms only
For better dose titration, it is recommended that ritodrine intravenous infusion be administered by means of a controlled infusion device, such as electronic volumetric controller, volumetric intravenous infusion pump, or intravenous microdrip chamber able to measure 60 drops per mL. The patient should be placed in the left lateral position to minimize hypotension. Fluids should be closely monitored to prevent circulatory fluid overload.

Concurrent administration of excessive intravenous fluids or saline intravenous solutions with ritodrine therapy may cause circulatory fluid overload and maternal pulmonary edema. Use of saline solutions, such as Sodium Chloride Injection USP, Ringer's Injection USP, or Hartmann's solution, should be avoided.

Ambulation may be resumed gradually after 36 to 48 hours if contractions do not recur and patient is clinically stable.

## Oral Dosage Forms

### RITODRINE HYDROCHLORIDE EXTENDED-RELEASE CAPSULES

**Usual adult dose**
Tocolytic—
   Initial: Oral, 40 mg thirty minutes before the intravenous infusion is discontinued, then 40 mg every eight hours for twenty-four hours.
   Maintenance: Oral, 40 mg every eight to twelve hours until term (or until the 37th week of gestation) or as medical judgment dictates.

**Usual adult prescribing limits**
Up to 120 mg a day.

**Strength(s) usually available**
U.S.—
   Not commercially available.
Canada—
   40 mg (Rx) [*Yutopar S.R*].

**Packaging and storage**
Store between 15 and 40 °C (59 and 104 °F), preferably below 30 °C (86 °F), unless otherwise specified by manufacturer. Store in a tight container.

### RITODRINE HYDROCHLORIDE TABLETS USP

**Usual adult dose**
Tocolytic—
   Initial: Oral, 10 mg thirty minutes before the intravenous infusion is discontinued, then 10 mg every two hours for twenty-four hours.
   Maintenance: Oral, 10 to 20 mg every four to six hours until term (or until the 37th week of gestation) or as medical judgment dictates.

**Usual adult prescribing limits**
Up to 120 mg a day.

**Strength(s) usually available**
U.S.—
   Not commercially available.
Canada—
   10 mg (Rx) [*Yutopar*].

**Packaging and storage**
Store between 15 and 40 °C (59 and 104 °F), preferably below 30 °C (86 °F). Store in a tight container.

## Parenteral Dosage Forms

### RITODRINE HYDROCHLORIDE INJECTION USP

**Usual adult dose**
Tocolytic—
   Initial: Intravenous, 50 to 100 mcg (0.05 to 0.1 mg) per minute, increased every ten minutes as necessary in increments of 50 mcg (0.05 mg) to the effective dose that balances uterine response and unwanted effects (increased maternal heart rate and decreased blood pressure and increased fetal heart rate), or until the maternal heart rate reaches 130 beats per minute.
   Maintenance: Intravenous, 150 to 350 mcg (0.15 to 0.35 mg) per minute at the lowest dose that maintains a relaxed uterus; however, as soon as labor is irreversible or the maximum dose of 350 mcg (0.35 mg) per minute is reached, ritodrine should be discontinued.
Note: Injection must be diluted before use unless premixed solution is used. Intravenous infusion should be continued for twelve to forty-eight hours after uterine contractions stop. Ritodrine should be administered in a separate intravenous line. Other medications of any type should not be administered via the same tubing.

**Usual adult prescribing limits**
Intravenous, up to 350 mcg (0.35 mg) per minute.

**Strength(s) usually available**
U.S.—
   10 mg per mL (Rx) [*Yutopar;* GENERIC].
   15 mg per mL (Rx) [*Yutopar;* GENERIC].
Canada—
   10 mg per mL (Rx) [*Yutopar*].

**Packaging and storage**
Store between 15 and 40°C (59 and 104 °F), preferably below 30 °C (86 °F).

**Preparation of dosage form**
Ritodrine Hydrochloride Injection USP may be prepared for intravenous infusion by dilution of 150 mg in 500 mL of 5% Dextrose Injection USP to produce a solution containing 300 mcg (0.3 mg) of ritodrine hydrochloride per mL. More concentrated solutions may be prepared in cases where fluid restriction is necessary. In general, use of saline

diluents, such as Sodium Chloride Injection USP, Ringer's Injection USP, or Hartmann's solution as the infusion solution should be avoided because of the risk of pulmonary edema.

### Stability
Ritodrine hydrochloride is stable for up to 48 hours following preparation of intravenous infusion containing 300 mcg (0.3 mg) per mL. Ritodrine Hydrochloride Injection USP should not be used if the solution is discolored or contains particulate matter.

## RITODRINE HYDROCHLORIDE IN 5% DEXTROSE INJECTION

### Usual adult dose
Tocolytic—See *Ritodrine Hydrochloride Injection USP.*

Note: Intravenous infusion should be continued for twelve to forty-eight hours after uterine contractions stop. Ritodrine should be administered in a separate intravenous line. Other medications of any type should not be administered via the same tubing.

### Usual adult prescribing limits
See *Ritodrine Hydrochloride Injection USP.*

### Strength(s) usually available
U.S.—
    150 mg per 500 mL of 5% Dextrose Injection USP (premix) (Rx) [GENERIC].
Canada—
    Not commercially available.

### Packaging and storage
Store below 40 °C (104 °F), preferably between 15 and 30 °C (59 and 86 °F), unless otherwise specified by manufacturer. Protect from freezing.

Note: If more concentrated solutions are needed when fluid restriction is necessary, ritodrine hydrochloride injection should be used to prepare the solution.

### Stability
Ritodrine Hydrochloride in 5% Dextrose Injection USP should not be used if the solution is discolored or contains particulate matter.

### Selected Bibliography
Wischnik A. Risk-benefit assessment of tocolytic drugs. Drug Safety 1991 6 (5): 371-80.

Revised: 06/28/96

---

# ROCURONIUM  Systemic

VA CLASSIFICATION (Primary): MS300

Note: For a listing of dosage forms and brand names by country availability, see *Dosage Forms* section(s). For a listing of brand names for the articles in this monograph, refer to the General Index.

## Category
Neuromuscular blocking agent.

## Indications

### Accepted
Muscle (skeletal) relaxation, for surgery—Rocuronium is indicated as an adjunct to general anesthesia to facilitate rapid-sequence or routine tracheal intubation and to induce skeletal muscle relaxation during surgery or mechanical ventilation.

### Acceptance not established
Rocuronium has not been studied for long-term use in the intensive care unit (ICU). Prolonged paralysis and/or skeletal muscle weakness may occur with chronic use in the ICU.

## Pharmacology/Pharmacokinetics

### Physicochemical characteristics
Chemical group—Aminosteroid compound
Molecular weight—609.69.

### Mechanism of action/Effect
Rocuronium is a nondepolarizing neuromuscular blocking agent with a rapid to intermediate onset of action depending on dose and with an intermediate duration of action. Rocuronium produces neuromuscular blockade by competing with acetylcholine for cholinergic receptors at the motor end plate.

### Other actions/effects
Rocuronium causes increases in heart rate of over 30% of baseline in some patients. While the etiology of the tachycardia is believed to be multifactorial, vagal blockade may contribute to tachycardia. Rocuronium is more likely than vecuronium but less likely than pancuronium to cause tachycardia.

Rocuronium may cause histamine release. In a study of histamine release, 1 of 88 (1.1%) patients receiving rocuronium had clinically significant concentrations of histamine. In pre-marketing clinical trials, rocuronium administration was accompanied by clinical signs of histamine release (e.g., flushing, rash, or bronchospasm) in 9 of 1137 (0.8%) patients. No clinical evidence of histamine release was observed in one study of 45 patients designed to provoke histamine release by the rapid injection of rocuronium.

### Distribution
Approximately 80% of the initial rocuronium dose is redistributed. As administration of rocuronium continues, tissue compartments fill. Within 4 to 8 hours, less rocuronium is redistributed away from the site of action, and the dosage requirement to maintain neuromuscular blockade via continuous infusion falls to about 20% of the initial infusion rate.

Volume of distribution—
    Adults with normal hepatic and renal function: 0.26 L per kg of body weight (L/kg).
    Adults with hepatic function impairment: 0.53 L/kg.
    Renal transplant patients (adults): 0.34 L/kg.
    Geriatric patients (>65 years of age): 0.22 L/kg.
    Infants 3 to 12 months of age: 0.3 L/kg.
    Children 1 to 3 years of age: 0.26 L/kg.
    Children 3 to 8 years of age: 0.21 L/kg.

### Protein binding
Low (30%).

### Biotransformation
Deacetylated in the liver to 17-desacetyl-rocuronium, a metabolite believed to have little neuromuscular blocking activity.

### Half-life
Distribution—
    Rocuronium has a biphasic distribution. The rapid distribution half-life is 1 to 2 minutes, and the slower distribution half-life is 14 to 18 minutes.
Elimination—
    Adult and geriatric patients with normal hepatic function: 1.4 to 2.4 hours.
    Adult and geriatric patients with hepatic function impairment: 4.3 hours.
    Renal transplant patients (adults): 2.4 hours.
    Infants 3 to 12 months of age: 1.3 hours.
    Children 1 to 3 years of age: 1.1 hours.
    Children 3 to 8 years of age: 0.8 hour.

### Onset of action
With doses of 0.6 mg rocuronium per kg of body weight administered over 5 seconds, effective intubating conditions are achieved within 60 to 70 seconds.

Note: Onset of action of rocuronium may be delayed in patients with conditions, such as cardiovascular disease and advanced age, associated with slowed circulation.

### Time to peak effect
The time to peak effect is dependent on dosage, the age of the patient, and the anesthetic administered concurrently. The median times to maximum block are given below.
Adults 18 to 64 years of age under opioid/nitrous oxide/oxygen anesthesia—
    0.45 mg per kg of body weight (mg/kg): 3 (range, 1.3–8.2) minutes.
    0.6 mg/kg: 1.8 (range, 0.6–13) minutes.
    0.9 mg/kg: 1.4 (range, 0.8–6.2) minutes.
    1.2 mg/kg: 1 (range, 0.6–4.7) minute.
Geriatric patients 65 years of age and older under opioid/nitrous oxide/oxygen anesthesia—
    0.6 mg/kg: 3.7 (range, 1.3–11.3) minutes.

0.9 mg/kg: 2.5 (range, 1.2–5) minutes.
1.2 mg/kg: 1.3 (range, 1.2–4.7) minutes.
Infants 3 months to 1 year of age under halothane anesthesia—
0.6 mg/kg: 0.8 (range, 0.3–3) minute.
0.8 mg/kg: 0.7 (range, 0.5–0.8) minute.
Children 1 to 12 years of age under halothane anesthesia—
0.6 mg/kg: 1 (range, 0.5–3.3) minute.
0.8 mg/kg: 0.5 (range, 0.3–1) minute.

### Duration of action
Duration of clinical effect (the time until spontaneous return of the twitch response to 25% of control value as determined using a peripheral nerve stimulator) is dependent on dosage—
Adults 18 to 64 years of age:
0.45 mg/kg—22 (range, 12–31) minutes.
0.6 mg/kg—31 (range, 15–85) minutes.
0.9 mg/kg—58 (range, 27–111) minutes.
1.2 mg/kg—67 (range, 38–160) minutes.
Geriatric patients 65 years of age and older:
0.6 mg/kg—46 (range, 22–73) minutes.
0.9 mg/kg—62 (range, 49–75) minutes.
1.2 mg/kg—94 (range, 64–138) minutes.
Infants 3 months to 1 year of age:
0.6 mg/kg—41 (range, 24–68) minutes.
0.8 mg/kg—40 (range, 27–70) minutes.
Children 1 to 12 years of age:
0.6 mg/kg—26 (range, 17–39) minutes.
0.8 mg/kg—30 (range, 17–56) minutes.
Median time to spontaneous recovery from 25 to 75% of the control value is 13 minutes in adults.

### Elimination
Biliary and renal.

## Precautions to Consider

### Carcinogenicity/Tumorigenicity
Studies have not been done to evaluate the carcinogenic or tumorigenic potential of rocuronium.

### Mutagenicity
No mutagenic effect was observed with the Ames test. No chromosomal abnormalities were induced in cultured mammalian cells. The micronucleus test did not suggest mutagenic potential.

### Pregnancy/Reproduction
Fertility—Studies have not been done.

Pregnancy—Rocuronium crosses the placenta. Adequate and well-controlled studies in humans have not been done.

No teratogenic effects were seen in a teratogenicity study in rats at dosages of 0.3 mg per kg of body weight (mg/kg).

FDA Pregnancy Category B.

Delivery—Rocuronium was administered in doses of 0.6 mg/kg to 55 patients for rapid-sequence induction of anesthesia for cesarean section. Patients were also given thiopental at doses of 4 to 6 mg/kg. Anesthesia was maintained with isoflurane, and nitrous oxide in oxygen. No neonate had an Apgar score below seven at 5 minutes after birth. Neonatal blood (umbilical venous) concentrations of rocuronium were 18% of maternal levels. Intubating conditions were poor or inadequate at 1 minute in four patients receiving 4 mg/kg of thiopental. Increasing the thiopental dose to 6 mg/kg improved intubating conditions; however, increasing the thiopental dose to improve intubating conditions is controversial and is not recommended due to an increased chance of central nervous system (CNS) depression in the neonate. Rocuronium is not recommended for rapid-sequence induction in cesarean section patients.

### Breast-feeding
It is not known if rocuronium is distributed into breast milk. However, problems in humans have not been documented.

### Pediatrics
Appropriate studies on the relationship of age to the effects of rocuronium have not been performed in infants less than 3 months of age. Rocuronium was studied in 228 pediatric patients 3 months to 12 years of age in pre-approval clinical trials. When halothane anesthesia was used without atropine pretreatment, a high incidence of tachycardia (exceeding 30% over baseline) was observed in patients given 0.6 to 0.8 mg/kg of rocuronium. A smaller, transient increase in heart rate was observed in another study of pediatric patients.

As compared to adults, children have increased clearance of rocuronium. As compared to children, infants have a longer duration of paralysis after an intubating dose of rocuronium.

Some pediatric patients have experienced tachycardia, increased blood pressure, and resistance to neuromuscular blockade when phenylephrine nose drops were administered after rocuronium.

### Geriatrics
Appropriate studies performed to date have not demonstrated geriatrics-specific problems that would limit the usefulness of rocuronium in the elderly. However, geriatric patients may have a delayed onset of effect as compared to other adult patients.

Geriatric patients have a slightly prolonged duration of clinical effect as compared to other adult patients, perhaps due to age-related changes in renal and hepatic perfusion. The rate of spontaneous recovery (25 to 75%) in geriatric patients is not different from that in other adults.

### Drug interactions and/or related problems
The following drug interactions and/or related problems have been selected on the basis of their potential clinical significance (possible mechanism in parentheses where appropriate)—not necessarily inclusive (» = major clinical significance):

Note: Combinations containing any of the following medications, depending on the amount present, may also interact with this medication.

» Aminoglycosides or
» Bacitracin or
» Colistin or
» Polymyxins or
» Sodium colistimethate or
  Tetracyclines or
» Vancomycin
    (neuromuscular blocking activity of these medications may be additive to that of rocuronium; prolongation of neuromuscular blocking activity is possible when these medications and rocuronium are used concurrently)

  Aminophylline or
  Theophylline
    (resistance to neuromuscular blockade may occur; higher doses of rocuronium may be needed)

» Anesthetics, inhalation, especially enflurane and isoflurane
    (the neuromuscular blocking activity of inhalation anesthetics may be additive to that of rocuronium; median spontaneous recovery time is prolonged by enflurane and isoflurane, but not by halothane; the infusion rate of rocuronium should be reduced by 40% when it is used concurrently with enflurane or isoflurane; the use of rocuronium with other inhalation anesthetics has not been fully studied)

  Atropine or
  Hyoscyamine
    (vagolytic activity of atropine and hyoscyamine may be additive or synergistic with the vagolytic activity of rocuronium; tachycardia has been observed when atropine or hyoscyamine was administered to patients with rocuronium-induced neuromuscular blockade; increased tachycardia also may occur with other anticholinergic drugs)

» Magnesium salts
    (magnesium in large doses [e.g., for management of toxemia of pregnancy] may cause enhancement of blockade)

  Neuromuscular blocking agents, nondepolarizing, other
    (the use of rocuronium with other nondepolarizing neuromuscular blocking agents has not been fully studied; interactions have been reported when other nondepolarizing neuromuscular blocking agents were used in succession)

    (the use of rocuronium with mivacurium results in synergistic activity)

    (the use of rocuronium before succinylcholine to reduce side effects of succinylcholine has not been studied; if rocuronium is used following use of succinylcholine, it should not be given until recovery from succinylcholine has been observed)

  Phenylephrine
    (resistance to neuromuscular blockade may occur, perhaps due to changes in perfusion of the muscle tissue; some pediatric patients receiving phenylephrine nose drops in conjunction with rocuronium experienced tachycardia)

  Phenytoin
    (resistance to neuromuscular blockade may occur with chronic phenytoin therapy, perhaps due to receptor up-regulation; diminished magnitude of blockade and shortened duration of blockade may occur)

» Quinidine
   (injection of quinidine during recovery from other neuromuscular blocking agents can cause recurrent paralysis; the same interaction is possible with rocuronium)

### Medical considerations/Contraindications

The medical considerations/contraindications included here have been selected on the basis of their potential clinical significance (reasons given in parentheses where appropriate)—not necessarily inclusive (» = major clinical significance).

*Except under special circumstances, this medication should not be used when the following medical problem exists:*

» Hypersensitivity to rocuronium bromide

*Risk-benefit should be considered when the following medical problems exist:*

Acid-base or electrolyte imbalance
   (action of rocuronium may be altered; resistance or enhanced effects may occur)

Burns
   (resistance to neuromuscular blocking agents may occur)

» Cachexia or debilitation
   (profound neuromuscular block may occur)

Cardiovascular disease
   (onset of action of rocuronium may be delayed in patients with conditions, such as cardiovascular disease, in which circulation is slowed)

Hepatic function impairment
   (duration of action may be prolonged as compared to patients with normal hepatic function; greater interpatient variability may be observed in patients with hepatic function impairment, necessitating close monitoring of twitch response)

» Neuromuscular diseases, such as myasthenia gravis or myasthenic syndrome
   (profound effects may occur with small doses of rocuronium)

Pulmonary hypertension or valvular heart disease
   (rocuronium may be associated with increased pulmonary vascular resistance)

Renal function impairment
   (duration of action may be prolonged as compared to patients with normal renal function; greater interpatient variability is observed in patients with renal function impairment, necessitating close monitoring of twitch response)

### Patient monitoring

The following may be especially important in patient monitoring (other tests may be warranted in some patients, depending on condition; » = major clinical significance):

Degree of neuromuscular blockade
   (a peripheral nerve stimulator may be used to determine the adequacy of spontaneous recovery or antagonism; recovery from neuromuscular blockade also should be evaluated clinically by assessment of 5-second head lift, phonation, ventilation, and ability to protect upper airway)

## Side/Adverse Effects

Note: It is not known whether rocuronium can precipitate malignant hyperthermia in susceptible humans, although it is believed to be unlikely. Malignant hyperthermia has not been reported with administration of rocuronium, nor did rocuronium precipitate malignant hyperthermia when tested in susceptible swine. However, clinicians using rocuronium should be familiar with the signs, symptoms, and treatment of malignant hyperthermia.

The following side/adverse effects have been selected on the basis of their potential clinical significance—not necessarily inclusive:

### Those indicating need for medical attention

Incidence less frequent
   *Hypertension; hypotension*

Incidence rare
   *Arrhythmia; bronchospasm; pruritus; rhonchi; skin rash; swelling at injection site; tachycardia; wheezing*

### Those indicating need for medical attention only if they continue or are bothersome

Incidence more frequent
   *Pain on injection*

Incidence rare
   *Hiccups; nausea; vomiting*

## Overdose

Note: No cases of overdose with rocuronium have been reported. Management of rocuronium overdose is the same as management of overdose of the other neuromuscular blocking agents.
   For specific information on the agents used in the management of rocuronium overdose, see:
   • *Atropine* in *Anticholinergics/Antispasmodics (Systemic)* monograph;
   • *Edrophonium (Systemic)* monograph;
   • *Glycopyrrolate* in *Anticholinergics/Antispasmodics (Systemic)* monograph;
   • *Neostigmine* in *Antimyasthenics (Systemic)* monograph; and/or
   • *Pyridostigmine* in *Antimyasthenics (Systemic)* monograph.

For more information on the management of overdose, **contact a Poison Control Center** (see *Poison Control Center Listing*).

### Clinical effects of overdose

The following effects have been selected on the basis of their potential clinical significance—not necessarily inclusive:

Acute effects
   *Apnea; prolonged paralysis*

### Treatment of overdose

The primary treatment consists of maintenance of a patent airway and controlled ventilation until recovery of neuromuscular function. After evidence of spontaneous recovery, further recovery may be facilitated by administration of an anticholinesterase agent (e.g., edrophonium, neostigmine, pyridostigmine) and an anticholinergic agent (e.g., atropine or glycopyrrolate). Use of a peripheral nerve stimulator to monitor recovery from paralysis is recommended.

## General Dosing Information

Rocuronium should be administered under the direct supervision of an experienced clinician familiar with the actions and potential complications of neuromuscular blocking agents. Equipment and materials for endotracheal intubation, assisted or controlled ventilation, and oxygen therapy, and an agent for reversal should be immediately available.

Rocuronium has no effect on consciousness or pain threshold. Therefore, when rocuronium is used, adequate analgesia and sedation should also be administered.

Doses must be individualized. The stated doses are to be used as a guideline. The degree of neuromuscular blockade should be monitored clinically and with a peripheral nerve stimulator. While the use of a peripheral nerve stimulator can help monitor neuromuscular function, studies comparing the action of rocuronium at the vocal cords and at the adductor pollicis show that onset is quicker at the vocal cords, but maximum block achieved with a given dose is less intense at the vocal cords as compared to the adductor pollicis. The diaphragm is more resistant to rocuronium than is the adductor pollicis. Differences in the action of rocuronium at these locations should be considered when using a peripheral nerve stimulator to monitor drug effect. Relaxation of the vocal cords and diaphragm is more likely to determine intubating conditions than is the degree of block achieved at the adductor pollicis, the site measured with a peripheral nerve stimulator.

Onset of action of rocuronium may be delayed in patients with conditions, such as cardiovascular disease and advanced age, associated with slowed circulation. More time should be allowed for onset of effect in these patients. Higher doses to facilitate more rapid onset should not be used since such doses will result in longer duration of action.

In most clinical trials, the dose for obese patients was determined using actual body weight (ABW). In one study in which the dose for obese patients was determined by ideal body weight (IBW), the patients experienced longer time to maximum block, shorter clinical duration, and unsatisfactory intubating conditions. In obese patients, it is recommended that the dose be determined according to ABW.

Extravasation of rocuronium may result in local irritation. If extravasation occurs, the injection or infusion should be terminated immediately and restarted in another vein.

Injection of rocuronium prior to loss of consciousness is associated with severe, burning pain at the site of injection when administered through a peripheral vein. Although some healthcare practitioners administer lidocaine prior to intravenous injection of rocuronium to attenuate this effect, this technique has not been tested by a controlled trial. Generally, rocuronium should not be administered until loss of consciousness.

Rocuronium is recommended for intravenous administration only.

Reversal of rocuronium blockade should not be attempted until demonstration of some spontaneous recovery from neuromuscular blockade.

Reversal of rocuronium can be accomplished more rapidly with edrophonium as compared to neostigmine at a return to 25% of control. At a return to 10% of control, reversal of neuromuscular blockade is accomplished more completely and rapidly with neostigmine as compared to edrophonium.

## Parenteral Dosage Forms

### ROCURONIUM BROMIDE FOR INJECTION

**Usual adult dose**
Neuromuscular blocking agent—
   Initial:
      For rapid sequence intubation—
         Intravenous, 0.6–1.2 mg per kg of body weight.
      For tracheal intubation—
         Intravenous, 0.6 mg per kg of body weight.

      Note: This dose results in blockade sufficient for intubation in one (range, 0.4–6) minute, allows intubation to be completed within two minutes, and achieves maximum blockade within three minutes. A lower dose of 0.45 mg per kg of body weight may be used with a small prolongation of time to blockade sufficient for intubation (1.3 minutes) and of time to achievement of maximum blockade (within 4 minutes). With a dose of 0.45 mg per kg of body weight, intubation can still be accomplished in most patients within two minutes. Doses of 0.9 and 1.2 mg per kg of body weight have been administered during surgery under opioid/nitrous oxide/oxygen anesthesia without adverse cardiovascular effects.

        The use of a priming dose (i.e., administration of 10% of the dose of rocuronium, followed three minutes later by the remaining 90% of the intubating dose) significantly shortened the onset time in one study. However, the peripheral intravenous injection of priming doses into patients who are conscious can be expected to be associated with burning pain on injection. Patients may experience sensations of weakness and difficulty breathing after receiving a priming dose.

   Maintenance:
      Intravenous—
         Doses of 0.1, 0.15, and 0.2 mg per kg of body weight given when twitch response returns to 25% of the control value provide a median of twelve (range, 2–31), seventeen (range, 6–50), and twenty-four (range, 7–69) minutes, respectively, of clinical relaxation under opioid/nitrous oxide/oxygen anesthesia. Additional maintenance doses should be guided by recovery of neuromuscular function following the initial dose and should not be administered until recovery of neuromuscular function is evident.
      Intravenous infusion—
         0.01 to 0.012 mg per kg of body weight per minute after evidence of recovery from the intubating dose. Additional doses may be needed until steady-state has been achieved. The rate of the maintenance infusion must be individualized for each patient and should be guided by the patient's twitch response to peripheral stimulation. In clinical trials, satisfactory blockade was obtained with maintenance infusion rates of 0.004 to 0.016 mg/kg per minute.

**Usual pediatric dose**
Neuromuscular blocking agent—
   Initial:
      Infants up to 3 months of age—Dosage has not been established.

Infants and children 3 months to 12 years of age—Intubation: Intravenous, 0.6 mg per kg of body weight.

Note: The median time to maximum blockade in pediatric patients is one (range, 0.5–3.3) minute. The intubating dose provides a median time of clinical relaxation of forty-one (range, 24–68) minutes in infants 3 months to 1 year of age and twenty-seven (range, 17–41) minutes in children 1 to 12 years of age.

   Maintenance:
      Intravenous—Doses of 0.075 to 0.125 mg per kg of body weight administered when twitch response returns to 25% of the control value to provide an additional seven to ten minutes of clinical relaxation.
      Intravenous infusion—0.012 mg per kg per minute administered when twitch response returns to 10% of the control value. The rate should be adjusted based on twitch response to peripheral nerve stimulation.

**Usual geriatric dose**
*See Usual adult dose.*

Note: Onset of action may be delayed in some geriatric patients. Geriatric patients exhibit a slightly prolonged duration of clinical effect.

**Strength(s) usually available**
U.S.—
   10 mg/mL (Rx) [*Zemuron*].
Canada—
   10 mg/mL (Rx) [*Zemuron*].

**Packaging and storage**
Store between 2 and 8 °C (36 and 46 °F). Protect from freezing.

**Preparation of dosage form**
Rocuronium may be prepared with 0.9% sodium chloride injection, 5% dextrose in sodium chloride injection, 5% dextrose in water injection, lactated Ringers injection, or sterile water for injection.

**Stability**
After reconstitution with one of the diluents listed above, rocuronium should be used within 24 hours. The prepared solution should be inspected for particulate matter and clarity before being administered to the patient, and should be discarded if particulate matter is present. Prior to reconstitution, rocuronium should be used within 30 days after removal from refrigeration.

**Incompatibilities**
Rocuronium is incompatible with alkaline solutions (e.g., barbiturate solutions). The immediate formation of a precipitate after sequential injection of thiopental and rocuronium through the same intravenous line has been reported, even with flushing of the line between injections.

## Selected Bibliography

Magorian T, Flannery KB, Miller RD. Comparison of rocuronium, succinylcholine, and vecuronium for rapid-sequence induction of anesthesia in adult patients. Anesthesiology 1993; 79: 913-8.

Bevan DR, Fiset P, Balendran P, et al. Pharmacodynamic behaviour of rocuronium in the elderly. Can J Anaesth 1993; 40: 127-32.

Hunter JM. New neuromuscular blocking drugs. N Engl J Med 1995; 332: 1691-9.

Developed: 06/28/96

## ROXADIMATE-CONTAINING COMBINATIONS—

Oxybenzone and Roxadimate (Topical)—See *Sunscreen Agents (Topical)*

# RUBELLA VIRUS VACCINE LIVE    Systemic

VA CLASSIFICATION (Primary): IM100

Note: This monograph is specific for the RA 27/3 strain of rubella virus vaccine live.

Note: For a listing of dosage forms and brand names by country availability, see *Dosage Forms* section(s). For a listing of brand names for the articles in this monograph, refer to the General Index.

## Category

Immunizing agent (active).

## Indications

### Accepted

Rubella (prophylaxis)—Rubella virus vaccine live is indicated for immunization against rubella (German measles). The main objective of rubella immunization is to prevent intrauterine infection of the fetus, which can result in miscarriage, abortion, or stillbirth, or in congenital rubella syndrome in the neonate.

   Unless otherwise contraindicated, all susceptible persons should be immunized against rubella, including
   • Females of child-bearing age, if they are not pregnant and if they are counseled not to become pregnant for 3 months following vac-

cination. Since there is an increased risk of acquiring rubella while traveling outside the U.S., females of child-bearing age should be immunized before leaving the country.

• Postpartum women who do not plan to breast-feed, preferably before discharge from the hospital. Although problems in humans have not been documented, postpartum women who plan to breast-feed should consult with their physician to consider risk-benefit before receiving immunization with rubella vaccine.

• Household contacts of susceptible pregnant women or other persons with medical contraindications to rubella vaccine, to reduce the risk to persons unable to receive rubella vaccine. Vaccinated persons do not transmit rubella vaccine virus.

• Persons traveling outside the U.S. Prior to international travel, persons should receive rubella vaccine, preferably as the measles, mumps, and rubella combination vaccine (MMR). MMR may be used regardless of the person's immune status to measles or mumps.

• Patients who in the past have abstained from immunization against rubella because of concern over hypersensitivity to vaccines grown in chicken or duck cultures. The current rubella vaccine, strain RA 27/3, available in the U.S. since 1979, is made using human diploid cell culture.

• Individuals who have been exposed to rubella, since a single exposure may not cause infection and post-exposure vaccination provides future protection. There is no evidence that vaccinating an individual incubating rubella is harmful, but neither will it prevent illness.

• Medical personnel and employees in medical facilities.

• Individuals in educational and training institutions (e.g., colleges, military bases).

• Children 12 months of age and older, including school-age children.

Persons should be considered immune to rubella only if they have documentation of immunization with rubella vaccine on or after their first birthday or if they have laboratory evidence of rubella immunity. Since the clinical diagnosis of rubella infection is unreliable, it should not be considered in assessing immune status.

Although serologic tests may be conducted to determine the susceptibility of persons of unknown immunity, studies have indicated there are no adverse effects from vaccinating persons already immune to rubella.

The measles, mumps, and rubella combination vaccine (MMR) should be used for vaccinating individuals who are likely to be susceptible to more than one of these viruses, unless otherwise contraindicated. Vaccines containing measles antigen should be administered to persons 15 months of age or older under routine conditions. Most individuals born before 1957 can generally be considered immune to measles and mumps because of probable previous infection, even though, in the case of mumps, the individuals may not have had clinically recognizable disease.

## Pharmacology/Pharmacokinetics

### Physicochemical characteristics
Source—The vaccine currently available in the U.S. contains a sterile, lyophilized preparation of live, attenuated Wistar Institute RA 27/3 strain of rubella virus. The virus is propagated in human diploid (WI-38) cell culture
The vaccines currently available in Canada also contain the RA 27/3 strain of rubella virus
Description—Solid, having the characteristic appearance of substances dried from the frozen state. Undergoes loss of potency on exposure to sunlight. The vaccine is to be constituted with a suitable diluent just prior to use

### Mechanism of action/Effect
Following subcutaneous injection, rubella vaccine induces the formation of protective antibodies in susceptible individuals. This produces a modified, non-communicable rubella infection and provides active immunity to rubella.

### Other actions/effects
The RA 27/3 strain, currently available in the U.S., produces a broader range of antibody responses than do the HPV-77 and Cendehill strains, which were available in the U.S. prior to 1979.
The RA 27/3 strain induces local secretory antibody in the oropharynx.

### Protective effect
Immunity to rubella occurs in approximately 95% of susceptible vaccinated individuals.

### Time to protective effect
Effective immunity occurs within 2 to 6 weeks.

### Duration of protective effect
At least 15 years and probably lifetime immunity.

## Precautions to Consider

### Cross-sensitivity and/or related problems
Patients allergic to systemic or topical neomycin may be allergic to the rubella virus vaccine available in the U.S. because it may contain a small amount of neomycin. Patients allergic to systemic or topical neomycin or to polymyxin B may be allergic to the rubella virus vaccine available in Canada because it may contain a small amount of neomycin and/or polymyxin B. The antibiotics are used in the production of the vaccine to prevent bacterial overgrowth in the viral culture. A history of hypersensitivity reactions other than anaphylaxis, such as delayed-type allergic reaction (contact dermatitis), generally does not preclude immunization.

### Pregnancy/Reproduction
Pregnancy—Although studies have not been done in humans, use in pregnant women is not recommended, because rubella vaccine virus crosses the placenta and has been recovered from the products of conception of some aborted women who received the vaccine just prior to or during pregnancy. In addition, it is recommended that pregnancy be avoided for 3 months following vaccination.
However, from 1971 through 1988 the Centers for Disease Control (CDC) monitored 210 susceptible pregnant women who had received the RA 27/3 strain of rubella virus vaccine within 3 months before or after conception and carried their pregnancies to term. Although some neonates had serological evidence of rubella virus infection, none had malformations associated with congenital rubella syndrome. Therefore, vaccination of a pregnant woman should not in itself indicate abortion, although the final decision rests with the woman and her physician.
The maximum estimated theoretical risk of serious malformations attributable to rubella vaccine is 1.7%. To date, the observed risk is zero. The risk of congenital rubella syndrome associated with maternal infection with the wild virus during the first trimester of pregnancy is at least 20%. Since the risk of teratogenicity is not fully known, and although the risk appears to be minimal, there is still a theoretical risk of fetal abnormality caused by the vaccine virus.
Studies have not been done in animals.
FDA Pregnancy Category C.

### Breast-feeding
Although rubella vaccine may be distributed into breast milk and infants may subsequently show serological evidence of rubella infection or mild clinical illness typical of acquired rubella, studies have not shown that these effects cause problems.

### Pediatrics
Immunization is not recommended for infants younger than 12 months of age, since maternal rubella-neutralizing antibodies may interfere with the immune response.
Children who were vaccinated when younger than 12 months of age should be revaccinated.
When rubella vaccine is part of a combination vaccination that includes measles vaccine, the minimum age for vaccination is 15 months in order to maximize measles seroconversion.

### Drug interactions and/or related problems
The following drug interactions and/or related problems have been selected on the basis of their potential clinical significance (possible mechanism in parentheses where appropriate)—not necessarily inclusive (» = major clinical significance):
Note: Combinations containing any of the following medications, depending on the amount present, may also interact with this medication.

Blood products or
Immune globulins
(concurrent administration with rubella vaccine may interfere with the patient's immune response to the virus because of the possibility of antibodies to rubella virus in these products. Rubella vaccine should be administered at least 14 days before, or more than 3 months after, administration of immune globulin; otherwise, seroconversion should be confirmed 6 to 8 weeks following vaccination. Studies suggest that rubella vaccine may be given with Rh₀(D) immune globulin or blood products without interfering with the vaccine's effectiveness; however, seroconversion should be confirmed 6 to 8 weeks following vaccination)

» Immunosuppressive agents or
» Radiation therapy
(because normal defense mechanisms are suppressed, concurrent use with rubella vaccine may potentiate the replication of the vaccine virus, may increase the side/adverse effects of the vaccine

virus, and/or may decrease the patient's antibody response to rubella vaccine. The interval between discontinuation of medications
that cause immunosuppression and restoration of the patient's ability to respond to rubella vaccine depends on the intensity and type
of immunosuppressive medication used, the underlying disease,
and other factors; estimates vary from 3 months to 1 year. Patients
with leukemia in remission should not receive rubella vaccine until
at least 3 months after their last chemotherapy. The precaution
does not apply to corticosteroids used as replacement therapy, for
short-term [less than 2 weeks] systemic therapy, or by other routes
of administration that do not cause immunosuppression)

Live virus vaccines, other
(although data are lacking on impairment of antibody responses to
rubella, measles, mumps, or oral polio vaccine when these vaccines
are administered on different days within 1 month of each other,
the chance exists that the immune responses may be impaired when
live virus vaccines are administered in this manner; therefore,
when feasible, live virus vaccines not administered on the same
day should be given at least 1 month apart)

### Laboratory value alterations
The following have been selected on the basis of their potential clinical
significance (possible effect in parentheses where appropriate)—not
necessarily inclusive (» = major clinical significance):

With diagnostic test results
Tuberculin skin test
(short-term suppression of 4 to 8 weeks may occur and may result
in false-negative tests; if required, tuberculin skin tests should be
done before, simultaneously with, or at least 8 weeks after administration of rubella vaccine)

With physiology/laboratory test values
Blood platelets
(counts may be decreased)

### Medical considerations/Contraindications
The medical considerations/contraindications included here have been selected on the basis of their potential clinical significance (reasons given
in parentheses where appropriate)—not necessarily inclusive (» =
major clinical significance):

*Except under special circumstances, this vaccine should not be used
when the following medical problems exist:*

» Febrile illness, severe
(to avoid confusing manifestations of illness with possible side/
adverse effects of vaccine; minor illnesses, such as upper respiratory infection, do not preclude administration of vaccine)

» Immune deficiency conditions, congenital or hereditary, family history
of, or

» Immune deficiency conditions, primary or acquired
(because of reduced or suppressed defense mechanisms, the use of
live virus vaccines, including rubella vaccine, may potentiate the
replication of the vaccine virus, may increase the side/adverse effects of the vaccine virus, and/or may decrease the patient's antibody response to rubella vaccine)

(persons with leukemia in remission may receive live virus vaccines if at least 3 months have passed since their last chemotherapy
treatment)

(persons infected with human immunodeficiency virus (HIV) may
receive this vaccine if they are asymptomatic; in addition, immunization with this vaccine should be considered for persons with
symptomatic HIV infection)

(when there is a family history of congenital or hereditary immune
deficiency conditions, the patient should not be vaccinated until
his/her immune competence is demonstrated)

*Risk-benefit should be considered when the following medical problems
exist:*

Sensitivity to rubella vaccine

» Tuberculosis, active, untreated
(since rubella vaccine suppresses the tuberculin skin test for 4 to
8 weeks, patients thought to have tuberculosis or at risk for tuberculosis should be tested before, or simultaneously with, administration of rubella vaccine [See also *Laboratory value alterations*.])

### Patient monitoring
The following may be especially important in patient monitoring (other
tests may be warranted in some patients, depending on condition;
» = major clinical significance):

Seroconversion test
(may be performed 6 to 8 weeks following vaccination in patients
in whom immunity is considered crucial [e.g., women in high risk

areas who intend to become pregnant], since vaccination with rubella vaccine may not result in seroconversion in all susceptible
patients)

## Side/Adverse Effects
Note: The incidence of side/adverse effects increases with age and is generally higher in females.

A history of hypersensitivity reactions other than anaphylaxis, such
as delayed-type allergic reaction (contact dermatitis), generally does
not preclude immunization.

Excretion of rubella virus from the nose or throat of the majority
of susceptible individuals has occurred 7 to 28 days after their vaccination; however, studies have documented the lack of commu-
nicability of the vaccine virus.

Patients who are immune to the rubella virus because of past vaccination or infection usually do not experience side/adverse effects
from the vaccine.

Isolated incidents of Guillain-Barré syndrome (GBS) have been reported after immunization with rubella vaccine.

The following side/adverse effects have been selected on the basis of their
potential clinical significance (possible signs and symptoms in parentheses where appropriate)—not necessarily inclusive:

### Those indicating need for medical attention
Incidence less frequent
*Optic neuritis* (pain or tenderness of eyes)—may occur from 1 to 4
weeks after immunization, lasting less than 1 week
Incidence rare
*Anaphylactic reaction* (difficulty in breathing or swallowing; hives;
itching, especially of soles or palms; reddening of skin, especially
around ears; swelling of eyes, face, or inside of nose; sudden and
severe unusual tiredness or weakness); *encephalitis or meningoencephalitis* (confusion, convulsions, severe or continuing headache, stiff
neck, unusual irritability, or vomiting); *peripheral neuropathy, polyneuritis, or polyneuropathy* (pain, numbness, or tingling of hands,
arms, legs, or feet)—may occur from 1 to 4 weeks after immunization,
lasting less than 1 week; *thrombocytopenic purpura* (bruising or purple spots on skin)

### Those indicating need for medical attention only if they continue
or are bothersome
Incidence more frequent
*Lymphadenopathy or parotitis*—incidence rare for parotitis (swelling
of glands in neck)—may occur from 1 to 4 weeks after immunization,
lasting less than 1 week; *reaction due to acid pH of vaccine* (burning
or stinging at injection site); *skin rash*
Incidence less frequent
*Arthralgia or arthritis* (aches or pain in joints)—may occur from 1 to
10 weeks after immunization, lasting less than 1 week; *delayed-type,
cell-mediated, allergic reaction* (itching, swelling, redness, tenderness,
or hard lump at injection site); *malaise* (vague feeling of bodily discomfort)—may occur from 1 to 4 weeks after immunization, lasting
less than 1 week; *mild headache, sore throat, runny nose, or fever*—
may occur from 1 to 4 weeks after immunization, lasting less than 1
week; *nausea*

Note: The incidence of *arthralgia and/or arthritis* is greatly increased
in females of child-bearing age. Generally, the older the female,
the greater the incidence, severity, and duration. However, even
in older females, the symptoms are generally well tolerated and
rarely interfere with normal activities. No joint destruction has
been reported.

## Patient Consultation
As an aid to patient consultation, refer to *Advice for the Patient, Rubella
Virus Vaccine Live (Systemic)*.

In providing consultation, consider emphasizing the following selected
information (» = major clinical significance):

### Before using this vaccine
» Conditions affecting use, especially:
Sensitivity to rubella vaccine or allergy to neomycin or polymyxin
B
Pregnancy—Rubella vaccine virus crosses the placenta; even
though the vaccine virus has not been reported to cause birth
defects, the vaccine is not recommended for pregnant women
Use in children—Not recommended for infants younger than 12
months of age, since maternal antibodies may interfere with
the infant's immune response
Other medications, especially immunosuppressive agents or radiation therapy

Other medical problems, especially severe febrile illness, family history of congenital or hereditary immune deficiency conditions, primary or acquired immune deficiency conditions, or active untreated tuberculosis

**Proper use of this vaccine**

» Proper dosing

*Precautions after receiving this vaccine*

» Not becoming pregnant for 3 months without first checking with physician, because of theoretical risk of birth defects

Checking with physician before receiving:

Tuberculin skin test within 8 weeks of this vaccine, since the results of the test may be affected by rubella vaccine

Any other live virus vaccines within 1 month of this vaccine

Blood transfusions or other blood products within 2 weeks of this vaccine

Gamma globulin or other globulins within 2 weeks of this vaccine

**Side/adverse effects**

The incidence of side/adverse effects, especially arthralgia and arthritis, increases with age and is generally higher in females

Some side/adverse effects, such as headache, sore throat, runny nose, or fever; peripheral neuropathy, polyneuritis, or polyneuropathy; optic neuritis; lymphadenopathy or parotitis; and malaise may occur from 1 to 4 weeks after immunization (arthralgia or arthritis may occur from 1 to 10 weeks after immunization) and usually last less than 1 week

Signs of potential side effects, especially anaphylactic reaction, encephalitis, meningoencephalitis, optic neuritis, peripheral neuropathy, polyneuritis, polyneuropathy, and thrombocytopenic purpura

# General Dosing Information

The dosage of rubella vaccine is the same for all persons: children and adults.

When sterilizing syringes and skin before vaccination, care should be taken to avoid preservatives, antiseptics, detergents, and disinfectants, since the vaccine virus is easily inactivated by these substances.

To prevent inactivation of the vaccine, it is recommended that only the diluent provided by the manufacturer be used.

A 25-gauge, 5/8th-inch needle is recommended for administration of the vaccine.

Rubella vaccine is administered subcutaneously. It should not be injected intravenously.

Although measles, mumps, and rubella vaccines are commercially available as a combination vaccine (MMR) and, as such, are administered as a single injection, the commercially available individual vaccines should not be mixed in the same syringe or administered at the same body site.

Although the fourth dose of diphtheria-tetanus-pertussis (DTP) and the third dose of oral poliovirus vaccine (OPV) have traditionally been administered to children 18 months of age and MMR has traditionally been administered to children 15 months of age, it is now recommended that DTP, OPV, and MMR be administered concurrently to children 15 months of age. MMR should not be postponed in order to administer these vaccines concurrently at 18 months of age. In addition, the traditional method is still an acceptable alternative.

Rubella vaccine, a live virus vaccine, can be administered concurrently with the following, using separate body sites, separate syringes, and the precautions that apply to each immunizing agent:

• Polysaccharide vaccines, such as haemophilus b polysaccharide vaccine, haemophilus b conjugate vaccine, meningococcal polysaccharide vaccine, or pneumococcal polyvalent vaccine.

• Influenza vaccine, whole or split virus.

• Diphtheria toxoid, tetanus toxoid, and/or pertussis vaccine.

• Live virus vaccines, other, such as measles, mumps, or oral polio vaccine (OPV), but only if the vaccines are administered on the same day; otherwise they should be administered at least 1 month apart.

• Inactivated poliovirus vaccine (IPV) or enhanced-potency inactivated vaccine (enhanced-potency IPV).

• Hepatitis B recombinant or plasma-derived vaccine.

• Inactivated vaccines, other, except cholera, typhoid, and plague.

It is recommended that cholera, typhoid, and plague vaccines be administered on separate occasions because of these vaccines' propensity to cause side/adverse effects.

Additional doses of rubella vaccine are not required for persons known to have been adequately vaccinated at 12 months of age or older because, even though some patients' antibody levels may appear to be low or nondetectable by some serologic procedures, any subsequent infection is asymptomatic and is not transmitted. However, if there is

doubt that the original vaccination was effective, the patient should be revaccinated, since studies have indicated that there are no adverse effects to vaccinating persons already immune to rubella.

**For treatment of adverse effects**

Recommended treatment includes:

• For mild hypersensitivity reaction—Administering antihistamines and, if necessary, corticosteroids.

• For severe hypersensitivity or anaphylactic reaction—Administering epinephrine. Antihistamines or corticosteroids may also be administered as required.

# Parenteral Dosage Forms

## RUBELLA VIRUS VACCINE LIVE (FOR INJECTION) USP

**Usual adult and adolescent dose**

Immunizing agent (active)—

Subcutaneous, 0.5 mL, preferably into the outer aspect of the upper arm.

**Usual pediatric dose**

Infants up to 12 months of age—

Use is not recommended, since maternal rubella-neutralizing antibodies may interfere with the immune response.

Infants and children 12 months of age and older—See *Usual adult and adolescent dose.*

**Strength(s) usually available**

U.S.—

Not less than the equivalent of 1000 $TCID_{50}$ (quantity of virus estimated to infect 50% of inoculated cultures times 1000) of the U.S. Reference Rubella Virus Live in each 0.5 mL dose (Rx) [*Meruvax II*].

Canada—

Not less than the equivalent of 1000 $TCID_{50}$ (quantity of virus estimated to infect 50% of inoculated cultures times 1000) of a reference rubella virus live in each 0.5 mL dose (Rx) [*Meruvax II;* GENERIC].

**Packaging and storage**

Store the lyophilized form of the vaccine, the diluent, and the reconstituted form of the vaccine between 2 and 8 °C (36 and 46 °F), unless otherwise specified by manufacturer.

Alternatively, the diluent for the single-dose vials only may be stored between 15 and 30 °C (59 and 86 °F).

Protect both the lyophilized form and the reconstituted form of the vaccine from light.

**Preparation of dosage form**

To reconstitute, use only the diluent provided by the manufacturer, since it is free of preservatives or other substances that might inactivate the vaccine.

Single-dose vial—Withdraw the entire volume of diluent (approximately 0.5 mL) into the syringe. Inject all the diluent in the syringe into the vial of lyophilized vaccine and agitate to mix thoroughly. Withdraw the entire contents into the syringe and inject the total volume of restored vaccine subcutaneously.

10-dose vial (in U.S., available only to government agencies/institutions)—Withdraw the entire contents (7 mL) of the diluent vial into the syringe to be used for reconstitution. Inject all of the diluent in the syringe into the 10-dose vial of lyophilized vaccine and agitate to mix thoroughly. The 10-dose container can be used with either syringes or jet injector. Since the vaccine and diluent do not contain preservatives, special care should be taken to prevent contamination of the multiple-dose vial of vaccine. In addition, the vial should be stored properly until the reconstituted vaccine is used. Discard unused vaccine after 8 hours.

50-dose vial (in U.S., available only to government agencies/institutions)—Withdraw the entire contents (30 mL) of the diluent vial into the syringe to be used for reconstitution. Inject all of the diluent in the syringe into the 50-dose vial of lyophilized vaccine and agitate to mix thoroughly. The 50-dose container is designed to be used only with a jet injector. Since the vaccine and diluent do not contain preservatives, special care should be taken to prevent contamination of the multiple-dose vial of vaccine. In addition, the vial should be stored properly until the reconstituted vaccine is used. Discard unused vaccine after 8 hours.

**Stability**

Both the lyophilized and reconstituted vaccine should be protected from light, which may inactivate the virus.

Use the reconstituted vaccine as soon as possible. Unused reconstituted vaccine should be discarded after 8 hours.

The reconstituted vaccine is clear yellow. It should not be used if it is discolored.

### Incompatibilities
Preservatives or other substances may inactivate the vaccine; therefore, only the diluent supplied by the manufacturer should be used for reconstitution.

Also, a sterile syringe free of preservatives, antiseptics, disinfectants, and detergents should be used for each injection and/or reconstitution of the vaccine because these substances may inactivate the live virus vaccine.

### Auxiliary labeling
• Protect from light.
• Store in refrigerator.
• Discard reconstituted vaccine if not used within 8 hours.

### Note
The date and time of reconstitution should be indicated on the vial if the reconstituted vaccine is not used at once.

Revised: 07/12/94

# RUBIDIUM RB 82   Systemic†

VA CLASSIFICATION (Primary): DX201

Note: For a listing of dosage forms and brand names by country availability, see *Dosage Forms* section(s). For a listing of brand names for the articles in this monograph, refer to the General Index.

†Not commercially available in Canada.

## Category
Diagnostic aid, radioactive (cardiac disease).

## Indications
Note: Bracketed information in the *Indications* section refers to uses that are not included in U.S. product labeling.

**Accepted**
Cardiac imaging, positron emission tomographic
Myocardial perfusion imaging, positron emission tomographic or
Myocardial infarction (diagnosis)—Positron emission tomography using rubidium Rb 82 ($^{82}$Rb-PET) is used to distinguish normal from abnormal regions of myocardial perfusion (blood flow) in patients with suspected myocardial infarction.

[Ischemia, myocardial (diagnosis)]—$^{82}$Rb-PET is used in studies of myocardial perfusion under resting conditions and after pharmacologic coronary vasodilation with dipyridamole or adenosine to detect myocardium with abnormal perfusion reserve secondary to coronary artery disease.

[Coronary artery disease (diagnosis)]—$^{82}$Rb-PET is used in studies of myocardial perfusion before and after physiologic or pharmacologic stress (either exercise or dipyridamole or adenosine infusion) to detect coronary artery disease and characterize its extent and severity.

## Physical Properties

**Nuclear data:**

| Radionuclide (half-life) | Mode of decay | Principal photon emissions (keV) | Mean number of emissions/ disintegration |
|---|---|---|---|
| Rb 82 (75 sec) | Positron decay | Gamma (511 each)* | 1.91 |

*Following positron emission, at the moment of annihilation two gamma rays are released, which are used for imaging purposes. Detection device used is a positron emission tomography (PET) unit.

## Pharmacology/Pharmacokinetics

**Mechanism of action/Effect**
Rubidium Rb 82 appears to accumulate, as a function of blood flow, in cells of myocardium and other tissues in a manner analogous to potassium. Compared with normal myocardium, areas of ischemia or infarction exhibit low Rb 82 uptake because of diminished blood flow and/or viability. Imaging equipment can record regional differences in rubidium Rb 82 uptake.

**Distribution**
Rapidly cleared from blood after intravenous administration. Myocardial activity noted within the first minute after injection. Also taken up to a variable degree by all other organs and tissues (with little uptake by normal brain because Rb 82 has limited ability to cross an intact blood-brain barrier).

**Time to radioactivity visualization**
2 to 7 minutes after injection.

## Radiation dosimetry

| Organ | Estimated absorbed radiation dose* | |
|---|---|---|
| | mGy/MBq | rad/mCi |
| Thyroid | 0.038 | 0.14 |
| Adrenals | 0.020 | 0.074 |
| Kidneys | 0.018 | 0.067 |
| Spleen | 0.0050 | 0.018 |
| Pancreas | 0.0045 | 0.017 |
| Small intestine | 0.0039 | 0.014 |
| Large intestine wall (upper) | 0.0039 | 0.014 |
| Large intestine wall (lower) | 0.0039 | 0.014 |
| Stomach wall | 0.0038 | 0.014 |
| Heart | 0.0033 | 0.012 |
| Lungs | 0.0024 | 0.0089 |
| Red marrow | 0.00099 | 0.0037 |
| Liver | 0.00097 | 0.0036 |
| Bone surfaces | 0.00067 | 0.0025 |
| Ovaries | 0.00024 | 0.00089 |
| Uterus | 0.00021 | 0.00078 |
| Breast | 0.00019 | 0.00070 |
| Other tissue | 0.00023 | 0.00085 |

Effective dose: 0.0048 mSv/MBq (0.018 rem/mCi)

*For adults; intravenous injection. Data based on the International Commission on Radiological Protection (ICRP) Publication 53—Radiation dose to patients from radiopharmaceuticals.

**Elimination**
Renal.

## Precautions to Consider

**Carcinogenicity/Mutagenicity**
Long-term animal studies to evaluate carcinogenic or mutagenic potential of rubidium Rb 82 have not been performed.

**Pregnancy/Reproduction**
Pregnancy—Adequate and well-controlled studies have not been done in humans. The possibility of pregnancy should be assessed in women of child-bearing potential. Clinical situations exist where the benefit to the patient and fetus, based on information derived from radiopharmaceutical use, outweighs the risks from fetal exposure to radiation. In this situation, the physician should use discretion and reduce the radiopharmaceutical dose to the lowest possible amount. However, exposure of the embryo or fetus to radiation with the use of rubidium Rb 82 is very low due to the rapid clearance of rubidium Rb 82 from the blood and its short physical half-life.
Studies have not been done in animals.

FDA Pregnancy Category C.

**Breast-feeding**
It is not known whether rubidium Rb 82 is distributed into breast milk; however, due to rubidium Rb 82's short physical half-life, excretion of the agent during lactation is unlikely to result in significant radiation exposure to the breast-feeding infant.
It is not known whether Sr 82 and Sr 85 contaminants are distributed into breast milk; however, due to the small amounts of these contaminants present, excretion during lactation is unlikely to result in significant exposure to the breast-feeding infant to radiation.

**Pediatrics**
No information is available on the relationship of age to the effects of rubidium Rb 82 in pediatric patients. When rubidium Rb 82 is used in children, the diagnostic benefit should be judged to outweigh the potential risk of radiation.

**Geriatrics**

Diagnostic studies performed to date using rubidium Rb 82 have not demonstrated geriatrics-specific problems that would limit its usefulness in the elderly.

**Drug interactions and/or related problems**

There are no known drug interactions and/or related problems associated with the use of rubidium Rb 82.

**Diagnostic interference**

The following have been selected on the basis of their potential clinical significance (possible effect in parentheses where appropriate)—not necessarily inclusive (» = major clinical significance):

With results of this test

*Due to medical problems or conditions*

Diabetes mellitus

(marked alterations in blood glucose, insulin, or pH may affect transport of rubidium Rb 82, possibly affecting quality of images)

**Medical considerations/Contraindications**

The medical considerations/contraindications included here have been selected on the basis of their potential clinical significance (reasons given in parentheses where appropriate)—not necessarily inclusive (» = major clinical significance).

See also *Diagnostic interference.*

*Risk-benefit should be considered when the following medical problem exists:*

Congestive heart failure

(hemodynamic disturbances may occur due to transitory increase in circulatory volume load)

## Side/Adverse Effects

There are no known side/adverse effects associated with the use of rubidium Rb 82.

## Patient Consultation

As an aid to patient consultation, refer to *Advice for the Patient, Radiopharmaceuticals (Diagnostic).*

In providing consultation, consider emphasizing the following selected information (» = major clinical significance):

**Description of use**

Action in the body: Concentration of radioactivity in heart allows images to be obtained

Small amounts of radioactivity used in diagnosis; radiation exposure is low and considered safe

**Before having this test**

» Conditions affecting use, especially:

Pregnancy—Risk to fetus from radiation exposure as opposed to benefit derived from use should be considered

Use in children—Risk of radiation exposure as opposed to benefit derived from use should be considered

**Preparation for this test**

Special preparatory instructions may be given; patient should inquire in advance

## General Dosing Information

Radiopharmaceuticals are to be administered only by or under the supervision of physicians who have had extensive training in the safe use and handling of radioactive materials and who are authorized by the appropriate Federal or state regulatory agency, if required, or, outside the U.S., the appropriate authority.

**Safety considerations for handling this radiopharmaceutical**

Improper handling of this radiopharmaceutical may cause radioactive contamination. Guidelines for handling radioactive material have been prepared by scientific, professional, state, federal, and international bodies and are available to the specially qualified and authorized users who have access to radiopharmaceuticals.

## Parenteral Dosage Forms

### RUBIDIUM CHLORIDE Rb 82 INJECTION

**Usual adult and adolescent administered activity**

Cardiac imaging—

Intravenous, 1480 megabecquerels (40 millicuries) (range, 1110 to 2220 megabecquerels [30 to 60 millicuries]), administered at a rate of 50 mL per minute not to exceed a cumulative volume of 200 mL.

**Usual adult prescribing limits**

Up to 2220 megabecquerels (60 millicuries), as a single dose. Limit for multiple injection series is 4440 megabecquerels (120 millicuries).

**Usual pediatric administered activity**

Dosage must be individualized by physician.

**Usual geriatric administered activity**

See *Usual adult and adolescent administered activity.*

**Strength(s) usually available**

U.S.—

The activity in megabecquerels (millicuries) of rubidium Rb 82 obtained in each elution depends on potency of generator (Rx) [*CardioGen-82*].

Note: Rubidium Rb 82 generator is supplied in the form of strontium Sr 82 adsorbed on a hydrous stannic oxide column with an activity of 3330 to 5550 megabecquerels (90 to 150 millicuries) of Sr 82 at calibration time.

Canada—

Not commercially available.

**Packaging and storage**

Store below 40 °C (104 °F), preferably between 15 and 30 °C (59 and 86 °F). Protect from freezing.

**Preparation of dosage form**

At least 10 minutes should be allowed between elutions for regeneration of Rb 82.

Additive-free sodium chloride injection must be used as the diluent.

The first 50 mL eluate should be discarded each day the generator is eluted.

For full preparation instructions, the rubidium Rb 82 generator package insert and the Rb 82 infusion system operator's manual should be consulted.

**Stability**

Almost all of the radioactivity in the eluate decays within 15 minutes after the end of elution.

**Note**

Caution—Radioactive material.

## Selected Bibliography

Williams KA, Ryan JW, Resnekov L, et al. Planar positron imaging of rubidium-82 for myocardial infarction: a comparison with thallium-201 and regional wall motion. Am Heart J 1989; 118 (3): 601-10.

Schwaiger M, Muzik O. Assessment of myocardial perfusion by positron emission tomography. Am J Cardiol 1991; 67: 35D-43D.

Gould KL. Clinical cardiac PET using generator-produced Rb 82: a review. Cardiovasc Intervent Radiol 1989; 12 (5): 245-51.

Revised: 06/14/93
Interim revision: 08/02/94

# SALICYLAMIDE-CONTAINING COMBINATIONS—

Acetaminophen, Aspirin, and Salicylamide, Buffered (Systemic)—See *Acetaminophen and Salicylates (Systemic)*

Acetaminophen, Aspirin, Salicylamide, and Caffeine (Systemic)—See *Acetaminophen and Salicylates (Systemic)*

Acetaminophen and Salicylamide (Systemic)—See *Acetaminophen and Salicylates (Systemic)*

Acetaminophen, Salicylamide, and Caffeine (Systemic)—See *Acetaminophen and Salicylates (Systemic)*

Chlorpheniramine, Phenindamine, Phenylephrine, Dextromethorphan, Acetaminophen, Salicylamide, Caffeine, and Ascorbic Acid (Systemic)—See *Cough/Cold Combinations (Systemic)*

Chlorpheniramine, Pheniramine, Pyrilamine, Phenylephrine, Hydrocodone, Salicylamide, Caffeine, and Ascorbic Acid (Systemic)—See *Cough/Cold Combinations (Systemic)*

Chlorpheniramine, Phenylephrine, Acetaminophen, and Salicylamide (Systemic)—See *Antihistamines, Decongestants, and Analgesics (Systemic)*

Chlorpheniramine, Phenylephrine, Acetaminophen, Salicylamide, and Caffeine (Systemic)—See *Antihistamines, Decongestants, and Analgesics (Systemic)*

Chlorpheniramine, Phenylephrine, Dextromethorphan, Acetaminophen, and Salicylamide (Systemic)—See *Cough/Cold Combinations (Systemic)*

Phenylephrine, Guaifenesin, Acetaminophen, Salicylamide, and Caffeine (Systemic)—See *Cough/Cold Combinations (Systemic)*

Phenylpropanolamine, Acetaminophen, Salicylamide, and Caffeine (Systemic)—See *Decongestants and Analgesics (Systemic)*

Phenylpropanolamine, Hydrocodone, Guaifenesin, and Salicylamide (Systemic)—See *Cough/Cold Combinations (Systemic)*

# SALICYLATES    Systemic

This monograph includes information on the following: Aspirin‡; Aspirin, Buffered‡; Choline Salicylate†; Choline and Magnesium Salicylates; Magnesium Salicylate; Salsalate; Sodium Salicylate.

VA CLASSIFICATION (Primary/Secondary):

Aspirin
> Tablets—CN103/CN104; CN850; MS101; BL700
> Chewable Tablets—CN103/CN104; CN850; MS101; BL700
> Chewing Gum Tablets—CN103
> Delayed-release Tablets—CN103/CN104; CN850; MS101; BL700
> Extended-release Tablets—CN103/CN104; CN850; MS101
> Suppositories—CN103/CN104; CN850; MS101

Aspirin and Caffeine—CN103/CN104; CN850; MS101

Aspirin, Buffered—CN103/CN104; CN850; MS101; BL700

Aspirin and Caffeine, Buffered—CN103/CN104; CN850; MS101; BL700

Choline Salicylate—CN103/CN104; CN850; MS101

Choline and Magnesium Salicylates—CN103/CN104; CN850; MS101

Magnesium Salicylate—CN103/CN104; CN850; MS101

Salsalate—MS101/CN103; CN104; CN850

Sodium Salicylate—CN103/CN104; CN850; MS101

Note: For information on a buffered aspirin product that is used for its antacid as well as its analgesic and antithrombotic effects, see *Aspirin, Sodium Bicarbonate, and Citric Acid (Systemic)*.

Other commonly used names are Acetylsalicylic Acid [Aspirin‡], ASA [Aspirin‡], Choline Magnesium Trisalicylate [Choline and Magnesium Salicylates], Salicylsalicylic Acid [Salsalate].

Note: For a listing of dosage forms and brand names by country availability, see *Dosage Forms* section(s). For a listing of brand names for the articles in this monograph, refer to the General Index.

---

†Not commercially available in Canada.

‡*Aspirin* is a brand name in Canada; acetylsalicylic acid is the generic name. ASA, a commonly used designation for aspirin (or acetylsalicylic acid) in both the U.S. and Canada, is the term used in Canadian product labeling. ·

---

# Category

Note: All of the salicylates have analgesic, anti-inflammatory, and antipyretic actions; however, clinical uses among specific agents or dosage formulations may vary because of actual pharmacokinetic differences, lack of specific testing, and/or lack of clinical-use data.

Analgesic—Aspirin; Aspirin, Buffered; Choline Salicylate; Choline and Magnesium Salicylates; Magnesium Salicylate; [Salsalate]; Sodium Salicylate.

Anti-inflammatory (nonsteroidal)—Aspirin; Aspirin, Buffered; Choline Salicylate; Choline and Magnesium Salicylates; Magnesium Salicylate; [Salsalate]; Sodium Salicylate.

Antipyretic—Aspirin; Aspirin, Buffered; Choline Salicylate; Choline and Magnesium Salicylates; [Magnesium Salicylate]; [Salsalate]; Sodium Salicylate.

Antirheumatic (nonsteroidal anti-inflammatory)—Aspirin; Aspirin, Buffered; Choline Salicylate; Choline and Magnesium Salicylates; Magnesium Salicylate; Salsalate; Sodium Salicylate.

Platelet aggregation inhibitor—Aspirin Tablets; Aspirin Tablets (Chewable); Aspirin Delayed-release Tablets; Aspirin, Buffered.

Antithrombotic—Aspirin Tablets; Aspirin Tablets (Chewable); Aspirin Delayed-release Tablets; Aspirin, Buffered.

Myocardial infarction prophylactic—Aspirin Tablets; Aspirin Tablets (Chewable); Aspirin Delayed-release Tablets; Aspirin, Buffered.

Myocardial reinfarction prophylactic—Aspirin Tablets; Aspirin Tablets (Chewable); Aspirin Delayed-release Tablets; Aspirin, Buffered.

# Indications

Note: Bracketed information in the *Indications* section refers to uses that are not included in U.S. product labeling.

**Accepted**

Pain (treatment) or

Fever (treatment)—Salicylates are indicated to relieve mild to moderate pain such as headache, toothache, and menstrual cramps and to reduce fever. These medications provide only symptomatic relief; additional therapy to treat the cause of the pain or fever should be instituted when necessary. However, the presence of an illness that may predispose toward Reye's syndrome (i.e., an acute febrile illness, especially influenza or varicella) should be ruled out before salicylate therapy is initiated in a pediatric or adolescent patient.

Salicylates are recommended for relief of mild to moderate bone pain caused by metastatic neoplastic disease. However, careful patient selection is necessary, especially in patients receiving chemotherapy, because of the platelet aggregation–inhibiting effect of aspirin and because salicylates may cause hypoprothrombinemia or gastrointestinal or renal toxicity.

Delayed-release formulations containing aspirin or sodium salicylate may not be as useful as immediate-release formulations for single-dose administration for analgesia or antipyresis because the delayed absorption prolongs the onset of action.

Note: The FDA has proposed that caffeine (present as an analgesic adjuvant in some aspirin products) be classified as a Category III ingredient (i.e., lacking documentation of efficacy) in OTC analgesic/antipyretic medications.

Inflammation, nonrheumatic (treatment)—Salicylates are indicated to relieve myalgia, musculoskeletal pain, and other symptoms of nonrheumatic inflammatory conditions such as athletic injuries, bursitis, capsulitis, tendinitis, and nonspecific acute tenosynovitis.

Arthritis, rheumatoid (treatment) or

Arthritis, juvenile (treatment) or

Osteoarthritis (treatment)—Salicylates are indicated for the symptomatic relief of acute and chronic rheumatoid arthritis, juvenile arthritis, osteoarthritis, and related rheumatic diseases. Aspirin is usually the first agent to be used and may be the drug of choice in patients able to tolerate prolonged therapy with high doses. These agents do not affect the progressive course of rheumatoid arthritis.

Concurrent treatment with a glucocorticoid or a disease-modifying antirheumatic agent may be needed, depending on the condition being treated and patient response.·

[Salicylates are also used to reduce arthritic complications associated with systemic lupus erythematosus.]

Rheumatic fever (treatment)—Salicylates are indicated to reduce fever and inflammation in rheumatic fever. However, they do not prevent cardiac or other complications associated with this condition. Sodium salicylate should be avoided in rheumatic fever if congestive cardiac complications are present because of its sodium content. Also, large doses of any salicylate should be avoided in rheumatic fever if severe carditis is present because of possible adverse cardiovascular effects.

Platelet aggregation (prophylaxis)—Aspirin (tablets, chewable tablets, delayed-release capsules or tablets, and buffered formulations) is indicated as a platelet aggregation inhibitor in the following:

Ischemic attacks, transient, in males (prophylaxis)

Thromboembolism, cerebral (prophylaxis) or

[Thromboembolism, cerebral, recurrence (prophylaxis)][1]—Aspirin is indicated in the treatment of men who have had transient brain ischemia due to fibrin platelet emboli to reduce the recurrence of transient ischemic attacks (TIAs) and the risk of stroke and death.

[Aspirin is also used in the treatment of women with transient brain ischemia due to fibrin platelet emboli. However, its efficacy in preventing stroke and death in female patients has not been established.][1]

[Aspirin is also indicated in the treatment of patients with documented, unexplained TIAs associated with mitral valve prolapse. However, if TIAs continue to occur after an adequate trial of aspirin therapy, aspirin should be discontinued and an oral anticoagulant administered instead.][1]

[Aspirin is also indicated to prevent initial or recurrent cerebrovascular embolism, TIAs, and stroke following carotid endarterectomy.]

[Aspirin is indicated in the treatment of patients who have had a completed thrombotic stroke, to prevent a recurrence.][1]

Myocardial infarction (prophylaxis) or

Myocardial reinfarction (prophylaxis)—Aspirin is indicated to prevent myocardial infarction in patients with unstable angina pectoris and to prevent recurrence of myocardial infarction in patients with a history of myocardial infarction.

In one study, aspirin significantly reduced the rate of reocclusion, reinfarction, stroke, and death when a single dose was administered within a few hours after the onset of symptoms of acute myocardial infarction and daily thereafter. The benefit of early treatment with aspirin was additive to that of streptokinase. Therefore, it is recommended that aspirin therapy be initiated as soon as possible after the onset of symptoms, even if the patient is receiving thrombolytic therapy.

[One study has shown that aspirin may also prevent myocardial infarction in individuals 50 years of age and older who have no history of unstable angina pectoris or myocardial infarction. However, the incidence of hemorrhagic stroke (but not the total number of hemorrhagic plus thrombotic strokes) was slightly increased in subjects receiving aspirin. Also, the incidence of myocardial infarction, although higher in the placebo group than in the aspirin group, was low in both groups. Therefore, aspirin's benefit in apparently healthy individuals has not been established. However, aspirin may be indicated for prevention of an initial myocardial infarction in selected patients, especially those who may be at risk because of the presence of chronic stable coronary artery disease (as shown by exertional or episodic angina pectoris, abnormal coronary arteriogram, or positive stress test) and/or other risk factors.][1]

[Thromboembolism (prophylaxis)]—Aspirin is used in low doses to decrease the risk of thromboembolism following orthopedic (hip) surgery (especially total hip replacement) and in patients with arteriovenous shunts.

Platelet aggregation inhibitors, although not as consistently effective as an anticoagulant or an anticoagulant plus dipyridamole, may provide some protection against the development of thromboembolic complications in patients with mechanical prosthetic heart valves. Therefore, administration of aspirin, alone or in combination with dipyridamole, may be considered if anticoagulant therapy is contraindicated for these patients. Patients with bioprosthetic cardiac valves who are in normal sinus rhythm generally do not require prolonged antithrombotic therapy, but long-term aspirin administration may be considered on an individual basis.[1]

Aspirin is also indicated, alone[1] or in combination with dipyridamole, to reduce the risk of thrombosis and/or reocclusion of saphenous vein aortocoronary bypass grafts following coronary bypass surgery.

Aspirin is also indicated, alone or in combination with dipyridamole, to reduce the risk of thrombosis and/or reocclusion of prosthetic or saphenous vein femoral popliteal bypass grafts.[1]

Because the patient may be at risk for thromboembolic complications, including myocardial infarction and stroke, long-term aspirin therapy may also be indicated for maintaining patency following coronary or peripheral vascular angioplasty and for treating patients with peripheral vascular insufficiency caused by arteriosclerosis.[1]

Prolonged antithrombotic therapy is generally not needed to maintain vessel patency following vascular reconstruction procedures in high-flow, low-resistance arteries larger than 6 mm in diameter. However, long-term aspirin therapy may be indicated, because patients requiring such procedures may be at risk for other thrombotic complications.[1]

[Kawasaki disease (treatment)][1]—Aspirin is indicated for its anti-inflammatory, antipyretic, and antithrombotic effects in the treatment of Kawasaki disease (Kawasaki syndrome, mucocutaneous lymph node syndrome) in children. It reduces fever, relieves inflammation (e.g., lymphadenitis, mucositis, conjunctivitis, serositis), and may reduce the occurrence of cardiovascular complications. However, the combination of high-dose intravenous gamma globulin and aspirin has been shown to be more effective than aspirin alone in reducing the formation of coronary artery abnormalities.

---

[1]Not included in Canadian product labeling.

## Pharmacology/Pharmacokinetics

### Physicochemical characteristics

Note: Aspirin is an acetylated salicylate; the other salicylates are nonacetylated.

Molecular weight—
Aspirin: 180.16.
Choline salicylate: 241.29.
Magnesium salicylate: 370.60 (tetrahydrate); 298.53 (anhydrous).
Salsalate: 258.23.
Sodium salicylate: 160.11.

pKa—
Aspirin: 3.5.
Note: The other salicylates are also acidic.

### Mechanism of action/Effect

The analgesic, antipyretic, and anti-inflammatory effects of aspirin are due to actions by both the acetyl and the salicylate portions of the intact molecule as well as by the active salicylate metabolite. The actions of other salicylates are due only to the salicylate portion of the molecule. Aspirin directly inhibits the activity of the enzyme cyclo-oxygenase to decrease the formation of precursors of prostaglandins and thromboxanes from arachidonic acid. Salicylate may competitively inhibit prostaglandin formation. Although many of the therapeutic and adverse effects of these medications may result from inhibition of prostaglandin synthesis (and consequent reduction of prostaglandin activity) in various tissues, other actions may also contribute significantly to the therapeutic effects.

Analgesic—
Salicylates: Produce analgesia through a peripheral action by blocking pain impulse generation and via a central action, possibly in the hypothalamus. The peripheral action may predominate and probably involves inhibition of the synthesis of prostaglandins, and possibly inhibition of the synthesis and/or actions of other substances, which sensitize pain receptors to mechanical or chemical stimulation.

Caffeine: A mild central nervous system (CNS) stimulant. Caffeine-induced constriction of cerebral blood vessels, which leads to a decrease in cerebral blood flow and in the oxygen tension of the brain, may contribute to relief of some types of headache. It has been suggested that the addition of caffeine to aspirin may provide a more rapid onset of action and/or enhanced pain relief with lower doses of analgesic. However, the FDA has determined that studies performed to date have not demonstrated that caffeine is an effective analgesic adjuvant or that it does not interfere with aspirin's efficacy as an antipyretic.

Anti-inflammatory (nonsteroidal)—
Exact mechanisms have not been determined. Salicylates may act peripherally in inflamed tissue, probably by inhibiting the synthesis of prostaglandins and possibly by inhibiting the synthesis and/or actions of other mediators of the inflammatory response. Inhibition of leukocyte migration, inhibition of the release and/or actions of lysosomal enzymes, and actions on other cellular and immunological processes in mesenchymal and connective tissues may be involved.

Antipyretic—
May produce antipyresis by acting centrally on the hypothalamic heat-regulating center to produce peripheral vasodilation resulting in increased cutaneous blood flow, sweating, and heat loss. The central action may involve inhibition of prostaglandin synthesis in the hypothalamus; however, there is some evidence that fevers caused by endogenous pyrogens that do not act via a prostaglandin mechanism may also respond to salicylate therapy.

Antirheumatic (nonsteroidal anti-inflammatory)—
Act via analgesic and anti-inflammatory mechanisms; the therapeutic effects are not due to pituitary-adrenal stimulation.

**Platelet aggregation inhibitor—**

The platelet aggregation–inhibiting effect of aspirin specifically involves the compound's ability to act as an acetyl donor to the platelet membrane; the nonacetylated salicylates have no clinically significant effect on platelet aggregation. Aspirin affects platelet function by inhibiting the enzyme prostaglandin cyclooxygenase in platelets, thereby preventing the formation of the aggregating agent thromboxane $A_2$. This action is irreversible; the effects persist for the life of the platelets exposed. Aspirin may also inhibit formation of the platelet aggregation inhibitor prostacyclin (prostaglandin $I_2$) in blood vessels; however, this action is reversible. These actions may be dose-dependent. Although there is some evidence that doses lower than 100 mg per day may not inhibit prostacyclin synthesis, optimum dosage that will suppress thromboxane $A_2$ formation without suppressing prostacyclin generation has not been determined.

**Other actions/effects**

It is proposed that the gastrointestinal toxicity of salicylates, especially aspirin, may be caused primarily by reduction of the activity of prostaglandins (which exert a protective effect on the gastrointestinal mucosa) because upper gastrointestinal toxicity has been reported following rectal or parenteral administration of nonsteroidal anti-inflammatory drugs. However, when administered orally, these acidic medications (unless administered in an enteric-coated formulation) probably also exert a direct irritant or erosive effect on the mucosa.

**Absorption**

Salicylates—

Absorption is generally rapid and complete following oral administration but may vary according to specific salicylate used, dosage form, and other factors such as tablet dissolution rate and gastric or intraluminal pH.

Food decreases the rate, but not the extent, of absorption.

Absorption from enteric-coated formulations is generally delayed.

Absorption of aspirin from the chewing gum tablet is incomplete as compared with absorption from the oral tablet.

Following rectal administration of aspirin, absorption is delayed and incomplete as compared with absorption following oral administration of equal doses.

Absorption of aspirin is impaired during the early febrile stage of Kawasaki disease, then increases toward normal in the convalescent stage.

Caffeine—

Well absorbed from the gastrointestinal tract.

**Distribution**

In breast milk—

Aspirin: Peak salicylate concentrations of 173 to 483 mcg per mL have been measured 5 to 8 hours after maternal ingestion of a single 650-mg dose.

Sodium salicylate: A total of 3 to 4 mg of salicylate is excreted following maternal ingestion of a single dose of 20 mg per kg of body weight (mg/kg).

**Protein binding**

Salicylate—High (to albumin); decreases as plasma salicylate concentration increases, with reduced plasma albumin concentration or renal dysfunction, and during pregnancy.

Caffeine—Low.

**Biotransformation**

Salicylate compounds are largely hydrolyzed in the gastrointestinal tract, liver, and blood to salicylate, which is further metabolized primarily in the liver.

Caffeine—Hepatic.

**Half-life**

Aspirin—

15 to 20 minutes (for intact molecule); rapidly hydrolyzed to salicylate.

In breast milk (as salicylate)—3.8 to 12.5 hours (average 7.1 hours) following a single 650-mg dose of aspirin.

Salicylate—

Dependent on dose and on urinary pH; about 2 to 3 hours with low or single doses and 20 hours or longer with very high doses; with repeated dosing using antirheumatic doses, may range from 5 to 18 hours.

Caffeine—

3 to 4 hours.

**Time to peak plasma concentration**

Generally 1 to 2 hours with single doses; may be more rapid with liquid dosage forms; may be delayed with salsalate (as compared with aspirin) or with delayed-release tablet or capsule formulations.

**Time to steady-state plasma concentration**

Increases as daily dosage and plasma concentrations are increased; with large (antirheumatic) doses of aspirin, may require up to 7 days.

**Therapeutic plasma concentration**

Salicylate—

Analgesic and antipyretic: 25 to 50 mcg per mL (2.5 to 5 mg per 100 mL); these concentrations are generally reached with single analgesic/antipyretic doses.

Anti-inflammatory/antirheumatic: 150 to 300 mcg per mL (15 to 30 mg per 100 mL). Steady-state plasma concentrations within this range are usually reached with therapeutic antirheumatic doses. However, because of interindividual differences in salicylate kinetics, wide variations in steady-state plasma concentrations may be produced in different patients by the same dose. Also, with large or repeated doses, major metabolic pathways become saturated; small changes in dosage may result in large changes in plasma concentration.

**Time to peak effect**

Antirheumatic—May require 2 to 3 weeks or more of continuous therapy.

**Elimination**

Aspirin and salicylate salts—

Renal; primarily as free salicylic acid and conjugated metabolites.

Salsalate—

About 13% of a dose excreted as conjugated salsalate; small amounts also excreted unchanged. The remainder of the dose is excreted as free or conjugated salicylate.

Note: Total salicylate excretion does not increase proportionately with dose, but excretion of unmetabolized salicylic acid is increased with higher doses; also, there are large interindividual differences in elimination kinetics. In addition, the rate of excretion of total salicylate and the quantity of free salicylic acid eliminated are increased in alkaline urine and decreased in acidic urine.

In dialysis—Salicylate—

Hemodialysis—Clearances of 35 to 100 mL per minute have been reported.

Peritoneal dialysis—Removed more slowly than with hemodialysis; clearances of 45 to 90 mL per hour have been reported in infants.

Caffeine—Renal; primarily as metabolites. About 1 to 2% of a dose is excreted unchanged.

# Precautions to Consider

**Cross-sensitivity and/or related problems**

Patients sensitive to one salicylate, including methyl salicylate (oil of wintergreen), or to other nonsteroidal anti-inflammatory drugs (NSAIDs) may be sensitive to other salicylates also.

Patients sensitive to aspirin may not necessarily be sensitive to nonacetylated salicylates.

Patients sensitive to tartrazine dye may be sensitive to aspirin also, and vice versa.

Cross-sensitivity between aspirin and other NSAIDs that results in bronchospastic or cutaneous reactions may be eliminated if the patient undergoes a desensitization procedure (See *General Dosing Information*).

Patients sensitive to other xanthines (aminophylline, dyphylline, oxtriphylline, theobromine, theophylline) may be sensitive to caffeine also.

**Pregnancy/Reproduction**

Fertility—Salicylates have caused increased numbers of fetal resorptions in animal studies.

Pregnancy—

*First trimester—*

For salicylates—Salicylates readily cross the placenta. Although it has been reported that salicylate use during pregnancy may increase the risk of birth defects in humans, controlled studies using aspirin have not shown proof of teratogenicity. Studies in humans with other salicylates have not been done. Studies in animals have shown that salicylates cause birth defects including fissure of the spine and skull; facial clefts; eye defects; and malformations of the CNS, viscera, and skeleton (especially the vertebrae and ribs). (Aspirin extended-release tablets: FDA Pregnancy Category D; Magnesium salicylate and salsalate: FDA Pregnancy Category C.)

For caffeine—Caffeine crosses the placenta and achieves blood and tissue concentrations similar to maternal concentrations. Studies in humans have not shown that caffeine causes birth defects. However, studies in animals have shown that caffeine causes skeletal abnormalities in the digits and phalanges (when given in doses equivalent to the caffeine content of 12 to 24 cups of coffee daily throughout pregnancy or when given in very large single doses, i.e., 50 to 100 mg per kg of body weight [mg/kg]) and retarded skeletal development (when given in lower doses).

*Third trimester—*

Chronic, high-dose salicylate therapy may result in prolonged gestation, increased risk of postmaturity syndrome (fetal damage or death due to decreased placental function if pregnancy is greatly prolonged), and increased risk of maternal antenatal hemorrhage. Also, ingestion of salicylates, especially aspirin, during the last 2 weeks of pregnancy may increase the risk of fetal or neonatal hemorrhage. The possibility that regular use late in pregnancy may result in constriction or premature closure of the fetal ductus arteriosus, possibly leading to persistent pulmonary hypertension and heart failure in the neonate, must also be considered. Overuse or abuse of aspirin late in pregnancy has been reported to increase the risk of stillbirth or neonatal death, possibly because of antenatal hemorrhage or premature ductus arteriosus closure, and to decrease birthweight; however, studies using therapeutic doses of aspirin have not shown these adverse effects. Pregnant women should be advised not to take aspirin during the last trimester of pregnancy unless such therapy is prescribed and monitored by a physician.

Labor and delivery—Chronic, high-dose salicylate therapy late in pregnancy may result in prolonged labor, complicated deliveries, and increased risk of maternal or fetal hemorrhage.

## Breast-feeding

*For salicylates—*

Problems in humans with usual analgesic doses have not been documented. However, salicylate is distributed into breast milk; with chronic, high-dose use, intake by the infant may be high enough to cause adverse effects.

In one study, peak salicylate concentrations of 173 to 483 mcg per mL were measured in breast milk 5 to 8 hours after maternal ingestion of a single dose of 650 mg of aspirin. The half-life in breast milk was 3.8 to 12.5 hours (average 7.1 hours).

Following maternal ingestion of 20 mg/kg of sodium salicylate, a total of 3 to 4 mg of salicylate is distributed into breast milk.

*For caffeine—*

Caffeine is distributed into breast milk in very small amounts; at recommended dosages, concentration in the infant is considered to be insignificant.

## Pediatrics

*For salicylates—*

Aspirin use may be associated with the development of Reye's syndrome in children and teenagers with acute febrile illnesses, especially influenza and varicella. It is recommended that salicylate therapy not be initiated in febrile pediatric or adolescent patients until after the presence of such an illness has been ruled out. Also, it is recommended that chronic salicylate therapy in these patients be discontinued if a fever occurs, and not resumed until it has been determined that an illness that may predispose to Reye's syndrome is not present or has run its course. Other forms of salicylate toxicity may also be more prevalent in pediatric patients, especially children who have a fever or are dehydrated.

Especially careful monitoring of the serum salicylate concentration is recommended in pediatric patients with Kawasaki disease. Absorption of aspirin is impaired during the early febrile stage of the disease; therapeutic anti-inflammatory plasma salicylate concentrations may be extremely difficult to achieve. Also, as the febrile stage passes, absorption is improved; salicylate toxicity may occur if dosage is not readjusted.

*For caffeine—*

Pediatric patients are especially susceptible to overdose of caffeine and its adverse CNS effects.

## Geriatrics

Geriatric patients may be more susceptible to the toxic effects of salicylates, possibly because of decreased renal function. Lower doses than those usually recommended for adults, especially for long-term use or for use of long-acting salicylates (such as choline and magnesium salicylates and salsalate), may be required.

## Drug interactions and/or related problems

The following drug interactions and/or related problems have been selected on the basis of their potential clinical significance (possible mechanism in parentheses where appropriate)—not necessarily inclusive (» = major clinical significance):

Note: Combinations containing any of the following medications, depending on the amount present, may also interact with this medication.

In addition to the interactions listed below, the possibility should be considered that additive or multiple effects leading to impaired blood clotting and/or increased risk of bleeding may occur if a salicylate, especially aspirin, is used concurrently with any medication having a significant potential for causing hypoprothrombinemia, thrombocytopenia, or gastrointestinal ulceration or hemorrhage.

*For all salicylates*

Acetaminophen

(prolonged concurrent use of acetaminophen with a salicylate is not recommended because chronic, high-dose administration of the combined analgesics [1.35 grams daily, or cumulative ingestion of 1 kg annually, for 3 years or longer] significantly increases the risk of analgesic nephropathy, renal papillary necrosis, end-stage renal disease, and cancer of the kidney or urinary bladder; also, it is recommended that for short-term use the combined dose of acetaminophen plus a salicylate not exceed that recommended for acetaminophen or a salicylate given individually)

Acidifiers, urinary, such as:

Ammonium chloride

Ascorbic acid (Vitamin C)

Potassium or sodium phosphates

(acidification of the urine by these medications decreases salicylate excretion, leading to increased salicylate plasma concentrations; initiation of therapy with these medications in patients stabilized on a salicylate may lead to toxic salicylate concentrations)

(aspirin may increase urinary excretion of ascorbic acid; clinical significance is unclear, but some clinicians recommend ascorbic acid supplementation in patients receiving prolonged high-dose aspirin therapy)

Alcohol or

» Nonsteroidal anti-inflammatory drugs (NSAIDs), other

(concurrent use of these medications with a salicylate may increase the risk of gastrointestinal side effects, including ulceration and gastrointestinal blood loss; also, concurrent use of a salicylate with an NSAID may increase the risk of severe gastrointestinal side effects without providing additional symptomatic relief and is therefore not recommended)

(aspirin may decrease the bioavailability of many NSAIDs, including diflunisal, fenoprofen, indomethacin, meclofenamate, piroxicam [to 80% of the usual plasma concentration], and the active sulfide metabolite of sulindac; aspirin has also been shown to decrease the protein binding and increase the plasma clearance of ketoprofen, and to decrease the formation and excretion of ketoprofen conjugates)

(concurrent use of other NSAIDs with aspirin may also increase the risk of bleeding at sites other than the gastrointestinal tract because of additive inhibition of platelet aggregation)

» Alkalizers, urinary, such as:

Carbonic anhydrase inhibitors

Citrates

Sodium bicarbonate or

Antacids, chronic high-dose use, especially calcium- and/or magnesium-containing

(alkalinization of the urine by these medications increases salicylate excretion, leading to decreased salicylate plasma concentrations, reduced effectiveness, and shortened duration of action; also, withdrawal of a urinary alkalizer from a patient stabilized on a salicylate may increase the plasma salicylate concentration to a toxic level; however, the antacids present in buffered aspirin formulations may not be present in sufficient quantity to alkalinize the urine)

(metabolic acidosis induced by carbonic anhydrase inhibitors may increase penetration of salicylate into the brain and increase the risk of salicylate toxicity in patients taking large [antirheumatic] doses of salicylate; if acetazolamide is used to produce forced alkaline diuresis in the treatment of salicylate poisoning, the increased risk of severe metabolic acidosis and increased salicylate toxicity must be considered and an alkaline intravenous solution given concurrently)

» Anticoagulants, coumarin- or indandione-derivative or

» Heparin or

» Thrombolytic agents, such as:

Alteplase

Anistreplase

Streptokinase

Urokinase

(salicylates may displace a coumarin- or indandione-derivative anticoagulant from its protein-binding sites, and, in high doses, may cause hypoprothrombinemia, leading to increased anticoagulation and risk of bleeding)

(the potential occurrence of gastrointestinal ulceration or hemorrhage during salicylate, especially aspirin, therapy may cause increased risk to patients receiving anticoagulant or thrombolytic therapy)

(because aspirin-induced inhibition of platelet function may lead to prolonged bleeding time and increased risk of hemorrhage, concurrent use of aspirin with an anticoagulant or a thrombolytic agent is recommended only within a carefully monitored antithrombotic regimen; although a recent study has shown that initiation of therapy with 160 mg of aspirin a day concurrently with short-term [1-hour] intravenous infusion of streptokinase in patients with acute coronary arterial occlusion significantly decreases the risk of reocclusion, reinfarction, stroke, and death without increasing the risk of adverse effects [as compared with streptokinase alone], other studies using higher doses of aspirin and/or more prolonged administration of a thrombolytic agent have demonstrated an increased risk of bleeding)

Anticonvulsants, hydantoin
(salicylates may decrease hydantoin metabolism, leading to increases in hydantoin plasma concentrations, efficacy, and/or toxicity; adjustment of hydantoin dosage may be required when chronic salicylate therapy is initiated or discontinued)

» Antidiabetic agents, oral or
Insulin
(effects of these medications may be increased by large doses of salicylates; dosage adjustments may be necessary; potentiation of oral antidiabetic agents may be caused partially by displacement from serum proteins; glipizide and glyburide, because of their nonionic binding characteristics, may not be affected as much as the other oral agents; however, caution in concurrent use is recommended)

Antiemetics, including antihistamines and phenothiazines
(antiemetics may mask the symptoms of salicylate-induced ototoxicity, such as dizziness, vertigo, and tinnitus)

Bismuth subsalicylate
(ingestion of large repeated doses as for traveler's diarrhea may produce substantial plasma salicylate concentrations; concurrent use with large doses of analgesic salicylates may increase the risk of salicylate toxicity)

» Cefamandole or
» Cefoperazone or
» Cefotetan or
» Plicamycin or
» Valproic acid
(these medications may cause hypoprothrombinemia; in addition, plicamycin or valproic acid may inhibit platelet aggregation; concurrent use with aspirin may increase the risk of bleeding because of additive interferences with blood clotting)

(hypoprothrombinemia induced by large doses of salicylates, and the potential occurrence of gastrointestinal ulceration or hemorrhage during salicylate, especially aspirin, therapy, may increase the risk of bleeding complications in patients receiving these medications)

(concurrent use of aspirin with valproic acid has also been reported to increase the plasma concentration of valproic acid and induce valproic acid toxicity)

Corticosteroids or
Corticotropin (ACTH), chronic therapeutic use of
(corticosteroids or corticotropin may increase salicylate excretion, resulting in lower plasma concentrations and increased salicylate dosage requirements; salicylism may result when corticosteroids or corticotropin dosage is subsequently decreased or discontinued, especially in patients receiving large [antirheumatic] doses of salicylate; also, the risk of gastrointestinal side effects, including ulceration and gastrointestinal blood loss, may be increased; however, concurrent use in the treatment of arthritis may provide additive therapeutic benefit and permit reduction of corticosteroid or corticotropin dosage)

(because corticosteroids and corticotropin may cause sodium and fluid retention, caution in concurrent use with large doses of sodium salicylate is recommended)

Furosemide
(in addition to increasing the risk of ototoxicity, concurrent use of furosemide with high doses of salicylate may lead to salicylate toxicity because of competition for renal excretory sites)

Laxatives, cellulose-containing
(concurrent use may reduce the salicylate effect because of physical binding or other absorptive hindrance; medications should be administered 2 hours apart)

» Methotrexate
(salicylates may displace methotrexate from its binding sites and decrease its renal clearance, leading to toxic methotrexate plasma concentrations; if they are used concurrently, methotrexate dosage should be decreased, the patient observed for signs of toxicity, and/or methotrexate plasma concentration monitored; also, it is recommended that salicylate therapy be discontinued 24 to 48 hours prior to administration of a high-dose methotrexate infusion, and not resumed until the plasma methotrexate concentration has decreased to a nontoxic level [usually at least 12 hours postinfusion])

Ototoxic medications, other (See *Appendix II* ), especially
» Vancomycin
(concurrent or sequential administration of these medications with a salicylate should be avoided because the potential for ototoxicity may be increased; hearing loss may occur and may progress to deafness even after discontinuation of the medication; these effects may be reversible, but usually are permanent)

» Platelet aggregation inhibitors (See *Appendix II* )
(concurrent use with aspirin is not recommended, except in a monitored antithrombotic regimen, because the risk of bleeding may be increased)

(the potential occurrence of gastrointestinal ulceration or hemorrhage during salicylate therapy, and the hypoprothrombinemic effect of large doses of salicylate, may cause increased risk to patients receiving a platelet aggregation inhibitor)

» Probenecid or
» Sulfinpyrazone
(concurrent use of a salicylate is not recommended when these medications are used to treat hyperuricemia or gout, because the uricosuric effect of these medications may be decreased by doses of salicylates that produce serum salicylate concentrations above 5 mg per 100 mL; also, these medications may inhibit the uricosuric effect achieved when serum salicylate concentrations are above 10 to 15 mg per 100 mL)

(probenecid may decrease renal clearance and increase plasma concentrations and toxicity of salicylates)

(sulfinpyrazone may decrease salicylate excretion and/or displace salicylate from its protein binding sites, possibly leading to increased salicylate concentrations and toxicity)

(although low doses of sulfinpyrazone and aspirin have been used concurrently to provide additive inhibition of platelet aggregation, the efficacy of the combination has not been established and the increased risk of bleeding must be considered; also, concurrent use of sulfinpyrazone with aspirin may increase the risk of gastrointestinal ulceration or hemorrhage)

Salicylic acid or other salicylates, topical
(concurrent use with systemic salicylates may increase the risk of salicylate toxicity if significant quantities are absorbed)

Vitamin K
(requirements for this vitamin may be increased in patients receiving high doses of salicylate)

Zidovudine
(in theory, aspirin may competitively inhibit the hepatic glucuronidation and decrease the clearance of zidovudine, leading to potentiation of zidovudine toxicity; the possibility must be considered that aspirin toxicity may also be increased)

*For buffered aspirin formulations, choline and magnesium salicylates, and magnesium salicylate (in addition to those interactions listed above as applying to all salicylates)*
» Ciprofloxacin or
» Enoxacin or
» Itraconazole or
» Ketoconazole or
» Lomefloxacin or
» Norfloxacin or
» Ofloxacin or
» Tetracyclines, oral
(antacids present in buffered aspirin formulations, and the magnesium in choline and magnesium salicylates or magnesium salicylate, interfere with absorption of these medications; if used concurrently, the interacting salicylate should be taken at least 6 hours before or 2 hours after ciprofloxacin or lomefloxacin, 8 hours before or 2 hours after enoxacin, 2 hours after itraconazole, 3 hours before or after ketoconazole, 2 hours before or after norfloxacin or ofloxacin, and 3 to 4 hours before or after a tetracycline)

*For enteric-coated formulations (in addition to those interactions listed above as applying to all salicylates)*

Antacids or

Histamine H$_2$-receptor antagonists

(concurrent administration of these medications, which increase intragastric pH, with an enteric-coated medication may cause premature dissolution, and loss of the protective effect, of the enteric coating)

*For formulations containing caffeine (in addition to those interactions listed above as applying to all salicylates)*

CNS stimulation–producing medications, other (See *Appendix II* )

(concurrent use with caffeine may result in excessive CNS stimulation, which may cause unwanted effects such as nervousness, irritability, insomnia, or possibly convulsions or cardiac arrhythmias; close observation is recommended)

Lithium

(caffeine increases urinary excretion of lithium, thereby possibly reducing its therapeutic effect)

Monoamine oxidase (MAO) inhibitors, including furazolidone, pargyline, and procarbazine

(concurrent use of large amounts of caffeine with MAO inhibitors may produce dangerous cardiac arrhythmias or severe hypertension because of the sympathomimetic side effects of caffeine)

**Laboratory value alterations**

The following have been selected on the basis of their potential clinical significance (possible effect in parentheses where appropriate)—not necessarily inclusive (» = major clinical significance):

With diagnostic test results

*For all salicylates*

Copper sulfate urine sugar tests

(false-positive test results may occur with chronic use of salicylates in doses equivalent in salicylate content to 2.4 grams or more of aspirin a day, i.e., 3.2 grams of choline salicylate, 2.4 grams of choline and magnesium salicylates, 2 grams of magnesium salicylate, 1.8 grams of salsalate, or 2.4 grams of sodium salicylate a day)

Gerhardt test for urine aceto-acetic acid

(interference may occur because reaction with ferric chloride produces a reddish color that persists after boiling)

Glucose enzymatic urine sugar tests

(false-negative test results may occur with chronic use of salicylates in doses equivalent in salicylate content to 2.4 grams or more of aspirin a day, i.e., 3.2 grams of choline salicylate, 2.4 grams of choline and magnesium salicylates, 2 grams of magnesium salicylate, 1.8 grams of salsalate, or 2.4 grams of sodium salicylate a day)

Renal function test using phenolsulfonphthalein (PSP)

(salicylate may competitively inhibit renal tubular secretion of PSP, thereby decreasing urinary PSP concentration and invalidating test results)

Serum uric acid determinations

(falsely increased values may occur with colorimetric assay methods when plasma salicylate concentrations exceed 13 mg per 100 mL; the uricase assay method is not affected)

Thyroid imaging, radionuclide

(chronic salicylate administration may depress thyroid function; salicylate therapy should be discontinued at least 1 week prior to administration of the radiopharmaceutical; however, a rebound effect may occur following discontinuation of salicylate therapy, resulting in a period of 3 to 10 days of increased thyroidal uptake)

Urine vanillylmandelic acid (VMA) determinations

(values may be falsely increased or decreased, depending on method used)

*For aspirin only (in addition to those interferences listed above for all salicylates)*

Protirelin-induced thyroid-stimulating hormone (TSH) release determinations

(TSH response to protirelin may be decreased by 2 to 3.6 grams of aspirin daily; peak TSH concentrations occur at the same time after administration, but are reduced)

Urine 5-hydroxyindoleacetic acid (5-HIAA) determinations

(aspirin may alter results when fluorescent method is used)

*For caffeine-containing formulations (in addition to the diagnostic interferences listed above)*

Myocardial perfusion imaging, radionuclide, when adenosine or dipyridamole is used as an adjunct to the radiopharmaceutical

(caffeine may reverse the effects of adenosine or dipyridamole on myocardial blood flow, thereby interfering with test results; patients should be advised to avoid caffeine for at least 8 to 12 hours prior to the test)

With physiology/laboratory test values

*For all salicylates*

Liver function tests, including:

Serum alanine aminotransferase (ALT [SGPT]) and

Serum alkaline phosphatase and

Serum aspartate aminotransferase (AST [SGOT])

(abnormalities may occur, especially in patients with juvenile rheumatoid arthritis, systemic lupus erythematosus, or pre-existing history of liver disease, or when plasma salicylate concentrations exceed 25 mg per 100 mL; liver function test values may return to normal despite continued use or when dosage is decreased; however, if severe abnormalities occur, or if there is evidence of active liver disease, the medication should be discontinued and used with caution in the future)

Prothrombin time

(may be prolonged with large doses of salicylates, especially if plasma concentrations exceed 30 mg per 100 mL)

Serum cholesterol concentrations

(may be decreased by chronic use of salicylates in doses equivalent in salicylate content to 5 grams or more of aspirin per day, i.e., 6.7 grams of choline salicylate, 5 grams of choline and magnesium salicylates, 4.1 grams of magnesium salicylate, 3.8 grams of salsalate, or 5 grams of sodium salicylate a day)

Serum potassium concentrations

(may be decreased because of increased potassium excretion caused by direct effect on renal tubules)

Serum thyroxine (T$_4$) concentrations and

Serum triiodothyronine (T$_3$) concentrations

(may be decreased when determined by radioimmunoassay—with large doses of salicylates)

Serum uric acid concentrations

(may be increased or decreased, depending on salicylate dosage; plasma salicylate concentrations below 10 to 15 mg per 100 mL increase serum uric acid concentrations and higher plasma salicylate concentrations decrease uric acid concentrations)

T$_3$ resin uptake

(may be increased with large doses of salicylates)

*For aspirin only (in addition to the interferences listed above)*

Bleeding time

(may be prolonged by aspirin for 4 to 7 days because of suppressed platelet aggregation; as little as 40 mg of aspirin affects platelet function for at least 96 hours following administration; however, clinical bleeding problems have not been reported with small doses [150 mg or less])

**Medical considerations/Contraindications**

The medical considerations/contraindications included here have been selected on the basis of their potential clinical significance (reasons given in parentheses where appropriate)—not necessarily inclusive (» = major clinical significance).

*Except under special circumstances, this medication should not be used when the following medical problems exist:*

*For all salicylates*

» Bleeding ulcers or

» Hemorrhagic states, other active

(may be exacerbated, especially by aspirin)

» Hemophilia or other bleeding problems, including coagulation or platelet function disorders

(increased risk of hemorrhage, especially with aspirin)

*For aspirin only (in addition to the contraindications listed above for all salicylates)*

» Angioedema, anaphylaxis, or other severe sensitivity reaction induced by aspirin or other NSAIDs, history of or

» Nasal polyps associated with asthma, induced or exacerbated by aspirin

(high risk of severe sensitivity reaction to aspirin)

» Thrombocytopenia

(increased risk of bleeding because aspirin inhibits platelet aggregation)

*For choline and magnesium salicylates and for magnesium salicylate only (in addition to the contraindications listed above for all salicylates)*
» Renal insufficiency, chronic advanced
     (risk of hypermagnesemic toxicity)

***Risk-benefit should be considered when the following medical problems exist:***

*For all salicylates*
Anemia
     (may be exacerbated by gastrointestinal blood loss during salicylate, especially aspirin, therapy; also, salicylate-induced peripheral vasodilation may lead to pseudoanemia)

Conditions predisposing to fluid retention, such as:
Compromised cardiac function or
Hypertension
     (in patients with carditis, high doses of salicylates may precipitate congestive heart failure or pulmonary edema)
     (patients with congestive heart disease may be more susceptible to adverse renal effects)
     (sodium content of sodium salicylate may be detrimental to these patients when large doses are administered chronically)

» Gastritis, erosive or
» Peptic ulcer
     (may be exacerbated because of ulcerogenic effects, especially with aspirin; risk of gastrointestinal bleeding is increased)

Gout
     (salicylates may increase serum uric acid concentrations and may interfere with efficacy of uricosuric agents)

Hepatic function impairment
     (salicylates metabolized hepatically; also, patients with decompensated hepatic cirrhosis may be more susceptible to adverse renal effects)
     (in severe hepatic impairment, inhibition of platelet function by aspirin may increase the risk of hemorrhage)

Hypoprothrombinemia or
Vitamin K deficiency
     (increased risk of bleeding because of antiplatelet action of aspirin and the hypoprothrombinemic effect of high doses of salicylates)

Renal function impairment
     (salicylate elimination may be reduced; also, the risk of renal adverse effects may be increased)
     (choline and magnesium salicylates or magnesium salicylate should be used with caution in patients with mild or moderate renal impairment because of the risk of hypermagnesemic toxicity; however, as stated above, these medications should *not* be used if chronic advanced renal insufficiency is present)

Sensitivity reaction, mild, to aspirin or other NSAIDs, history of
     (risk of sensitivity reaction, especially with aspirin)

Symptoms of nasal polyps associated with bronchospasm, or angioedema, anaphylaxis, or other severe allergic reactions induced by aspirin or other NSAIDs
     (although cross-sensitivity leading to severe reactions occurs very rarely with the nonacetylated salicylates, caution is recommended; however, as indicated above, aspirin should *not* be used)

Thyrotoxicosis
     (may be exacerbated by large doses)

*For aspirin only (in addition to those listed above for all salicylates)*
» Asthma
     (increased risk of bronchospastic sensitivity reaction)

Glucose-6-phosphate dehydrogenase (G6PD) deficiency
     (rarely, aspirin has caused hemolytic anemia in these patients)

*For formulations containing caffeine*
Cardiac disease, severe
     (high doses of caffeine may increase risk of tachycardia or extrasystoles, which may lead to heart failure)

Sensitivity to caffeine, history of
     (risk of allergic reaction)

**Patient monitoring**
The following may be especially important in patient monitoring (other tests may be warranted in some patients, depending on condition; » = major clinical significance):

*For all salicylates*
Hematocrit determinations
     (may be required at periodic intervals during prolonged high-dose therapy because of the possibility of gastrointestinal blood loss, especially with aspirin)

Hepatic function determinations
     (may be required prior to initiation of antirheumatic therapy and if symptoms of hepatotoxicity occur during therapy; salicylate-induced hepatotoxicity may be especially likely to occur in patients, especially children, with rheumatic fever, systemic lupus erythematosus, juvenile arthritis, or pre-existing hepatic disease)

Serum salicylate concentrations
     (monitoring required at periodic intervals during prolonged high-dose therapy as a guide to dosage, safety, and efficacy, especially in children; because aspirin absorption in children with Kawasaki disease is erratic and varies at different stages of the disease, monitoring of plasma salicylate concentration in these patients is critical)

*For choline and magnesium salicyltes and magnesium salicylate only (in addition to those listed above for all salicylates)*
Serum magnesium concentration
     (monitoring recommended during therapy with large doses in patients with renal insufficiency because of the possibility of hypermagnesemic toxicity)

## Side/Adverse Effects

Note:   Salicylates may decrease renal function, especially when serum salicylate concentrations reach 250 mcg per mL (25 mg per 100 mL). However, the risk of complications due to this action appears minimal in patients with normal renal function.

Aspirin-induced bronchospasm is most likely to occur in patients with the triad of asthma, allergies, and nasal polyps induced by aspirin. Nonacetylated salicylates may rarely cause bronchospastic reactions in susceptible people when very large doses are given.

Angioedema or urticaria may be more likely to occur in patients with a history of recurrent idiopathic angioedema or urticaria.

Gastrointestinal side effects are more likely to occur with aspirin than with other salicylates; also, they may be more likely to occur with chronic, high-dose administration than with occasional use. Use of enteric-coated formulations may reduce the potential for gastrointestinal side effects.

Adverse effects are more likely to occur at serum salicylate concentrations of 300 mcg per mL (30 mg per 100 mL) or above; however, they may also occur at lower serum concentrations, especially in patients 60 years of age or older. Serum concentrations at which adverse or toxic effects have been reported during chronic therapy include:

| Salicylate Concentration (mcg per mL/ mg per 100 mL) | Effect |
|---|---|
| 195–210/ 19.5–21 | Mild toxicity (tinnitus, decreased hearing) |
| 250/25 | Hepatotoxicity (abnormal liver function tests) |
| 250/25 | Decreased renal function |
| 300/30 | Decreased prothrombin time |
| 310/31 | Deafness |
| 350/35 | Hyperventilation |
| > 400/40 | Metabolic acidosis, other signs of severe toxicity |

The following side/adverse effects have been selected on the basis of their potential clinical significance (possible signs and symptoms in parentheses where appropriate)—not necessarily inclusive:

**Those indicating need for medical attention**
Incidence less frequent or rare
     ***Anaphylactoid reaction*** (bluish discoloration or flushing or redness of skin; coughing; difficulty in swallowing; dizziness or feeling faint, severe; skin rash, hives [may include giant urticaria], and/or itching; stuffy nose; swelling of eyelids, face, or lips; tightness in chest, troubled breathing, and/or wheezing, especially in asthmatic patients); ***anemia*** (unusual tiredness or weakness)—for aspirin or buffered aspirin only; may occur secondary to gastrointestinal microbleeding; ***anemia, hemolytic*** (troubled breathing, exertional; unusual tiredness or weakness)—reported with aspirin only, almost always in patients with glucose-6-phosphate (G6PD) deficiency; ***bronchospastic allergic reaction*** (shortness of breath, troubled breathing, tightness in chest, and/or wheezing); ***dermatitis, allergic*** (skin rash, hives, or itching); ***gastrointestinal ulceration, possibly with bleeding*** (bloody or black, tarry

stools; stomach pain, severe; vomiting of blood or material that looks
like coffee grounds)

Incidence unknown

*Rectal irritation*—for aspirin suppository dosage form

**Those indicating need for medical attention only if they continue
or are bothersome**

Incidence more frequent with aspirin; less frequent with enteric-coated or
buffered formulations and with other salicylates

*Gastrointestinal irritation* (mild stomach pain; heartburn or indigestion; nausea with or without vomiting)

Incidence less frequent

*For caffeine-containing formulations*

*CNS stimulation* (trouble in sleeping, nervousness, or jitters)

## Overdose

For specific information on the agents used in the management of salicylate overdose, see:

• Vitamin K₁—Phytonadione in *Vitamin K (Systemic)* monograph.

For more information on the management of overdose or unintentional
ingestion, **contact a Poison Control Center** (see *Poison Control Center Listing* ).

### Clinical effects of overdose

The following effects have been selected on the basis of their potential
clinical significance (possible signs and symptoms in parentheses
where appropriate)—not necessarily inclusive:

Acute and chronic

Mild overdose

*Salicylism* (Continuing ringing or buzzing in ears or hearing loss; confusion; severe or continuing diarrhea, stomach pain, and or headache;
dizziness or lightheadedness; severe drowsiness; fast or deep
breathing; continuing nausea and/or vomiting; uncontrollable flapping
movements of the hands, especially in elderly patients; increased thirst;
vision problems)—tinnitus and/or headache may be the earliest symptoms of salicylism

Severe overdose

*Bloody urine; convulsions; hallucinations; severe nervousness, ex-
citement, or confusion; shortness of breath or troubled breathing;
unexplained fever*

Note: In young children, the only signs of an overdose may be
changes in behavior, severe drowsiness or tiredness, and/or fast
or deep breathing.

Laboratory findings in overdose may indicate encephalographic
abnormalities, alterations in acid-base balance (especially respiratory alkalosis and metabolic acidosis), hyperglycemia or hypoglycemia (especially in children), ketonuria, hyponatremia,
hypokalemia, and proteinuria.

### Treatment of overdose

To decrease absorption—Emptying the stomach via induction of emesis
(taking care to guard against aspiration) or gastric lavage.

Administering activated charcoal.

To enhance elimination—Inducing forced alkaline diuresis to increase salicylate excretion. However, bicarbonate should not be administered
orally for this purpose because salicylate absorption may be increased.
Also, if acetazolamide is used, the increased risk of severe metabolic
acidosis and salicylate toxicity (caused by increased penetration of
salicylate into the brain because of metabolic acidosis) must be considered. Some emergency care practitioners recommend that acetazolamide not be used at all in the treatment of salicylate overdose. Others
state that acetazolamide may be used, provided that precautions are
taken to prevent systemic metabolic acidosis, such as concurrent administration of an alkaline intravenous solution, e.g., one that contains
sodium bicarbonate or sodium lactate.

Institution of exchange transfusion, hemodialysis, peritoneal dialysis, or
hemoperfusion as needed in severe overdose.

Specific treatment—Administering blood or vitamin K₁ if necessary to
treat hemorrhaging.

Monitoring—Monitoring for pulmonary edema and convulsions and instituting appropriate therapy if required.

Monitoring serum salicylate concentration until it is apparent that the concentration is decreasing to the nontoxic range. When a large single
dose of an immediate-release formulation has been ingested, salicylate
concentrations of 500 mcg per mL (50 mg per 100 mL; 3.62 mmol/
L) 2 hours after ingestion indicate serious toxicity; salicylate concentrations above 800 mcg per mL (80 mg per 100 mL; 5.79 mmol/L) 2
hours after ingestion indicate possible fatality. In addition, prolonged
monitoring may be necessary in massive overdosage because absorption may be delayed; if a determination performed prior to 6 hours

after ingestion fails to show a toxic salicylate concentration, the determination should be repeated. Although the following values are not
reliable for predicting the severity of toxicity after chronic or repeated
ingestions, or after ingestion of a large single dose of a delayed-release
(enteric-coated) or extended-release formulation, salicylate concentrations considered indicative of varying degrees of toxicity are as
follows:

| Time After Ingestion | Salicylate Concentration | | |
|---|---|---|---|
| | mcg/mL | mg/100 mL | mmol/L |
| Mild toxicity | | | |
| 6 hr | 450–650 | 45–65 | 3.26–4.71 |
| 12 hr | 350–550 | 35–55 | 2.53–3.98 |
| Moderate toxicity | | | |
| 6 hr | 650–900 | 65–90 | 4.71–6.52 |
| 12 hr | 550–750 | 55–75 | 3.98–5.43 |
| Severe toxicity | | | |
| 6 hr | > 900 | > 90 | > 6.52 |
| 12 hr | > 750 | > 75 | > 5.43 |

Supportive care—Monitoring and supporting vital functions. Correcting
hyperthermia; fluid, electrolyte, and acid-base imbalances; ketosis; and
plasma glucose concentration as needed. Patients in whom intentional
overdose is known or suspected should be referrred for psychiatric
consultation.

## Patient Consultation

As an aid to patient consultation, refer to *Advice for the Patient,
Salicylates (Systemic)*.

In providing consultation, consider emphasizing the following selected
information (» = major clinical significance):

**Before using this medication**

» Conditions affecting use, especially:

Sensitivity to any of the salicylates, including methyl salicylate, or
nonsteroidal anti-inflammatory drugs (NSAIDs), history of

Pregnancy—Salicylates and caffeine (present in some formulations) cross the placenta; high-dose chronic use or abuse of
aspirin in the third trimester may be hazardous to the mother
as well as the fetus and/or neonate, causing heart problems in
fetus or neonate and/or bleeding in mother, fetus, or neonate;
high-dose chronic use or abuse of any salicylate late in pregnancy may also prolong and complicate labor and delivery; not
taking aspirin during the third trimester unless prescribed by
physician

Breast-feeding—Salicylates and caffeine (present in some formulations) are excreted in breast milk

Use in children and teenagers—Checking with physician before
giving to children or teenagers with symptoms of acute febrile
illness, especially influenza or varicella, because of the risk of
Reye's syndrome; determining ahead of time what physician
wants done if a child receiving chronic therapy develops fever
or other symptoms of acute illness that may predispose to
Reye's syndrome; also, increased susceptibility to salicylate
toxicity in children, especially with fever and dehydration

Use in the elderly—Increased susceptibility to salicylate toxicity

Other medications, especially anticoagulants, antidiabetic agents
(oral), those cephalosporins that may cause hypoprothrombinemia, plicamycin, valproic acid, methotrexate, NSAIDs, platelet aggregation inhibitors, probenecid, sulfinpyrazone, urinary
alkalizers, and vancomycin; also, for buffered aspirin, choline
and magnesium salicylates, and magnesium salicylate: fluoroquinolone antibiotics, itraconazole, ketoconazole, and oral
tetracyclines

Other medical problems, especially coagulation or platelet function
disorders, gastrointestinal problems such as ulceration or erosive gastritis (especially a bleeding ulcer), thyrotoxicosis, and
(for choline and magnesium salicylates and for magnesium salicylate) chronic advanced renal insufficiency

Diet—Sodium content of sodium salicylate must be considered for
patients on a sodium-restricted diet, especially with chronic use
of antirheumatic doses

**Proper use of this medication**

» Taking nonenteric-coated oral dosage forms after meals or with food
to minimize stomach irritation

» Taking all tablet or capsule dosage forms with a full glass of water
and not lying down for 15 to 30 minutes after taking

» Not taking aspirin or buffered aspirin if it has a strong vinegar-like
odor

Not chewing aspirin or buffered aspirin dosage forms within 7 days
after tonsillectomy, tooth extraction, or other oral surgery

Not placing aspirin or buffered aspirin tablet directly on tooth or gum surface, to prevent tissue damage

*Proper administration of*

*Aspirin*

Chewable tablets—May be chewed, dissolved in liquid, crushed, or swallowed whole

Delayed-release tablets—Must be swallowed whole

Extended-release tablets—May be broken or crumbled (but not ground up) if necessary, unless specified by manufacturer to be swallowed whole; see manufacturer's prescribing information

Suppository—Proper administration technique

*Choline and magnesium salicylates oral solution*

Liquid may be mixed with fruit juice just prior to taking, if desired

*Sodium salicylate delayed-release tablets*

Tablets must be swallowed whole

Importance of not taking more medication than prescribed by physician or dentist or recommended on package label

Unless otherwise directed by physician, children not taking more often than 5 times daily

Compliance with therapy (for arthritis); may take 2 to 3 weeks or longer for maximum effectiveness

» Proper dosing

Missed dose: If on scheduled dosing regimen—taking as soon as possible; not taking if almost time for next dose; not doubling doses

» Proper storage

**Precautions while using this medication**

» Possibility of overdose if other medications containing aspirin or other salicylates (possibly including topical products) are used

» Regular visits to physician to check progress if long-term or high-dose therapy is prescribed

*Checking with physician if*

Taking for pain or fever, and pain persists for longer than 10 days for adults or 5 days for children, fever persists for longer than 3 days, condition becomes worse, new symptoms occur, or redness or swelling is present

Taking for sore throat, and sore throat is severe, persists for longer than 2 days, or occurs together with or is followed by fever, headache, rash, nausea, or vomiting

Symptoms of ringing or buzzing in ears or headache occur during long-term therapy

*Patients taking aspirin as a platelet aggregation inhibitor*

» Taking only the amount of aspirin prescribed; checking with prescribing physician about proper medication to use for relief of pain, fever, or arthritis

» Not discontinuing treatment for any reason without first consulting prescribing physician

» Not taking acetaminophen, ibuprofen, or other NSAIDs concurrently with salicylates for longer than a few days, unless specifically prescribed by physician or dentist, especially if using salicylates on a long-term and/or high-dose basis

*Diabetics: Possibility of false urine sugar test results with prolonged use (per day) of*—

8 or more 325-mg (5-grain), 4 or more 500-mg or 650-mg (10-grain), 3 or more 800-mg or 975-mg (15-grain) doses of aspirin

8 or more 325-mg (5-grain) or 4 or more 500-mg or 650-mg (10-grain) doses of buffered aspirin or sodium salicylate

4 or more 870-mg doses of choline salicylate

5 or more 500-mg, 4 or more 750-mg, or 2 or more 1000-mg, doses of choline and magnesium salicylates

7 or more regular strength, or 4 or more extra-strength, tablets of magnesium salicylate

4 or more 500-mg, or 3 or more 750-mg, doses of salsalate

Checking with physician, nurse, or pharmacist if unsure of daily dose being taken, if changes in urine sugar test results occur, or if any other questions, especially if diabetes not well-controlled

Caution if any kind of surgery is required; not taking aspirin for 5 days prior to surgery unless otherwise directed by physician or dentist because of risk of bleeding

Checking with health care professional before using buffered aspirin, choline and magnesium salicylates, or magnesium salicylate concurrently with a fluoroquinolone antibiotic, itraconazole, ketoconazole, or an oral tetracycline; these salicylate formulations may interfere with absorption of the anti-infective agent

Not taking a cellulose-containing laxative within 2 hours of a salicylate

Alcohol consumption may increase probability of stomach problems (for oral dosage forms only)

Checking with physician if rectal irritation occurs with aspirin suppositories

Caution if any laboratory tests required; possible interference with some test results by salicylates; possible interference with dipyridamole-assisted myocardial imaging by formulations containing caffeine

» Suspected overdose: Getting emergency help immediately

**Side/adverse effects**

Signs of potential side effects, especially allergic reactions, anemia, and gastrointestinal toxicity and, with aspirin suppositories, rectal irritation

# General Dosing Information

A reduction in initial dosage is recommended for geriatric patients, especially those receiving long-acting salicylates (e.g., choline and magnesium salicylates, salsalate) or prolonged therapy. These patients may be more susceptible to salicylate toxicity, especially if accumulation occurs because of impaired renal function. If the reduced dosage is not effective, dosage may gradually be increased as tolerated.

For treatment of arthritis, dosage is usually increased gradually until symptoms are relieved, therapeutic plasma concentrations are achieved, or signs of toxicity, such as tinnitus or headache, occur. If these signs should appear, dosage should be reduced. However, tinnitus is not a reliable index of maximum salicylate tolerance, especially in very young or geriatric patients or those with impaired hearing.

For treatment of arthritis, dosage adjustments should not be made more frequently than once weekly, unless a reduction in dosage is required because of side effects, because up to 7 days may be required to achieve steady-state plasma concentrations.

The risk of Reye's syndrome must be considered when salicylates are administered to children and teenagers. It is recommended that salicylates be withheld from pediatric and adolescent patients with a fever or other symptoms of an illness that may predispose to Reye's syndrome until it has been determined that such an illness is not present or has run its course.

Dosage should be reduced if fever or illness causes fluid depletion, especially in children.

In general, it is recommended that aspirin therapy be discontinued 5 days before surgery to prevent possible occurrence of bleeding problems.

Patients who experience bronchospastic or cutaneous allergic reactions to aspirin may be desensitized to these effects by administration of initially small and gradually increasing doses of aspirin. *Desensitization must be carried out only by clinicians who are familiar with the technique, and only in a facility having trained personnel, medications, and equipment immediately available for treating any adverse reaction to the medication (especially anaphylaxis or severe bronchospasm).* This procedure also desensitizes the patient to other nonsteroidal antiinflammatory drugs (NSAIDs). However, unless aspirin or another NSAID is then administered on a daily basis, sensitivity to these medications redevelops within a few days.

**For oral dosage forms only**

These medications (except enteric-coated formulations) should be administered after meals or with food to lessen gastric irritation.

It is recommended that tablet and capsule dosage forms of these medications always be administered with a full glass (240 mL) of water and that the patient remain in an upright position for 15 to 30 minutes after administration. These measures may reduce the risk of the medication becoming lodged in the esophagus, which has been reported to cause prolonged esophageal irritation and difficulty in swallowing in some patients receiving NSAIDs.

It is recommended that aspirin or buffered aspirin products not be chewed before swallowing for at least 7 days following tonsillectomy or oral surgery because of possible injury to oral tissues from prolonged contact with aspirin.

Aspirin or buffered aspirin tablets should not be placed directly on a tooth or gum surface because of possible injury to tissues.

Concurrent use of an antacid and/or a histamine ($H_2$)-receptor antagonist (cimetidine, famotidine, or ranitidine) may protect against salicylate-induced gastric irritation or ulceration. However, the fact that chronic, high-dose antacid use may alkalinize the urine and increase salicylate excretion must be considered. Also, because these medications may cause premature dissolution, and loss of the protective effect, of enteric coatings, they will not provide additive protection against gastric irritation when administered concurrently with enteric-coated dosage forms.

---

### ASPIRIN

## Summary of Differences

Category/indications:
Aspirin (tablets, chewable tablets, and delayed-release tablets) also indicated as a platelet aggregation inhibitor.

Pharmacology/pharmacokinetics:
Aspirin irreversibly inhibits platelet aggregation.

Precautions:
Cross-sensitivity and/or related problems—
Risk of cross-sensitivity with other nonsteroidal anti-inflammatory drugs (NSAIDs) significantly greater than with other salicylates.

Drug interactions and/or related problems—
May increase ascorbic acid requirement (prolonged high-dose use).
Theoretically, may decrease zidovudine clearance.
Higher risk of bleeding (compared with other salicylates) when used concurrently with other medications that may inhibit blood clotting or cause gastrointestinal ulceration or bleeding.

Laboratory value alterations—
Interferes with urine 5-hydroxyindoleacetic acid determinations.
Interferes with protirelin-induced thyroid-stimulating hormone release determinations.
Prolongs bleeding time.

Medical considerations/contraindications—
Should not be used in patients with a history of severe sensitivity reactions to aspirin, other NSAIDs, nasal polyps and asthma, or thrombocytopenia
Should be used with caution in patients with asthma or glucose-6-phosphate dehydrogenase (G6PD) deficiency.

Side/adverse effects:
More ulcerogenic than other salicylates.
Rarely, causes hemolytic anemia (in patients with G6PD deficiency).
Suppository dosage form may cause rectal bleeding.

## Additional Dosing Information

See also *General Dosing Information.*

Salicylate toxicity requiring treatment generally occurs with doses of 200 mg per kg of body weight (mg/kg), especially in children.

The general doses for aspirin products other than aspirin chewing gum tablets are based on the FDA's dosing recommendations for aspirin. The dosage unit of 80 mg (1.23 grains) is used for pediatric doses; the dosage unit of 325 mg (5 grains) is used for adult doses. The conversion factor of 1 grain equal to 65 mg is used. Strengths of specific products may vary, depending on the manufacturer.

The extended-release tablet, the suppository, and the chewing gum tablet dosage forms may give incomplete or unreliable absorption.

Chewable aspirin tablets may be chewed, dissolved in liquid, or swallowed whole.

The delayed-release tablets must be swallowed whole.

Some extended-release tablets may be broken or crumbled but must not be ground up before swallowing. Others must be swallowed whole. Consult manufacturers' prescribing information for individual products.

## Oral Dosage Forms

Note: Bracketed uses in the *Dosage Forms* section refer to categories of use and/or indications that are not included in U.S. product labeling.

### ASPIRIN TABLETS USP

**Usual adult and adolescent dose**

Analgesic/antipyretic—
Oral, 325 to 500 mg every three hours, 325 to 650 mg every four hours, or 650 mg to 1000 mg every six hours as needed, while symptoms persist.

Note: For patient self-medication, it is recommended that the total daily dose not exceed 4 grams, and that a physician be consulted if pain is not relieved within ten days, fever within three days, or sore throat within two days.

Antirheumatic (nonsteroidal anti-inflammatory)—
Oral, 3.6 to 5.4 grams a day in divided doses.

Note: In acute rheumatic fever, up to 7.8 grams a day in divided doses may be given.

Platelet aggregation inhibitor—
Oral, 80 to 325 mg a day, with the following exceptions
Ischemic attacks, transient, in males or

[Thromboembolism, cerebral, recurrence][1]—
Oral, 1 gram a day. Dosage may be reduced to 325 mg a day if the patient is unable to tolerate the higher dose.

[Ischemic attacks, transient, occurring in association with mitral valve prolapse][1]—
Oral, 325 mg to 1 gram a day.

[Prevention of thrombosis or occlusion of coronary bypass graft]—
Oral, 325 mg seven hours postoperatively (via a nasogastric tube), then 325 mg three times daily, concurrently with 75 mg of dipyridamole. Dipyridamole may be discontinued one week postoperatively, but aspirin should be continued indefinitely.

Platelet aggregation inhibitor therapy is most effective when it is initiated two days prior to scheduled surgery. However, preoperative administration of aspirin has been shown to increase perisurgical bleeding and is not recommended. Therapy is therefore initiated with dipyridamole (recommended dosage 100 mg four times a day for two days prior to surgery and 100 mg one hour postoperatively [via a nasogastric tube]). Dipyridamole therapy is continued postoperatively (recommended dosage 75 mg seven hours postoperatively, via a nasogastric tube, then 75 mg three times a day, concurrently with aspirin) for at least one week.

Note: Although the doses recommended above for use of aspirin as a platelet aggregation inhibitor have been found effective in clinical studies, optimum dosage has not been established. For indications other than prevention of transient ischemic attacks or recurrence of cerebral thromboembolism, lower doses are often used. A few studies have shown that 160 mg of aspirin every twenty-four hours, or 325 mg every forty-eight hours, may effectively inhibit platelet aggregation while minimizing the risk of aspirin-induced side effects. Other studies have shown that single doses of 40 to 80 mg also inhibit platelet aggregation.

**Usual pediatric dose**

Analgesic/antipyretic—
Oral, 1.5 grams per square meter of body surface a day in four to six divided doses; or for

Children up to 2 years of age: Dosage must be individualized by physician.

Children 2 to 4 years of age: Oral, 160 mg every four hours as needed, while symptoms persist.

Children 4 to 6 years of age: Oral, 240 mg every four hours as needed, while symptoms persist.

Children 6 to 9 years of age: Oral, 320 to 325 mg every four hours as needed, while symptoms persist.

Children 9 to 11 years of age: Oral, 320 to 400 mg every four hours as needed, while symptoms persist.

Children 11 to 12 years of age: Oral, 320 to 480 mg every four hours as needed, while symptoms persist.

Note: It is recommended that children up to 12 years of age receive no more than five doses in each twenty-four-hour period, unless otherwise directed by a physician, and that a physician be consulted if pain is not relieved within five days, fever within three days, or sore throat within two days.

Antirheumatic (nonsteroidal anti-inflammatory)—
Oral, 80 to 100 mg per kg of body weight a day in divided doses.

Note: If an adequate response is not achieved within one or two weeks, dosage adjustment should be based on measurement of plasma salicylate concentration. Up to 130 mg per kg of body weight per day may be required in some patients.

[Kawasaki disease][1]—
During the early febrile stage: Oral, 80 to 120 mg (average 100 mg) per kg of body weight a day in four divided doses for fourteen days or until inflammation has subsided. However, absorption may be impaired or erratic during this stage of the illness, and considerably higher doses may be required. It is recommended that dosage be adjusted to achieve and maintain a plasma salicylate concentration of 20 to 30 mg per 100 mL.

During the convalescent stage: Oral, 3 to 5 mg per kg of body weight a day as a single dose. If no coronary artery abnormalities occur, treatment is usually continued for a minimum of eight weeks. If coronary artery abnormalities occur, it is recommended that treatment be continued for at least one year, even if the abnormalities regress, and longer if abnormalities persist.

**Strength(s) usually available**

U.S.—
81 mg (OTC) [*Aspir-Low; Healthprin Adult Low Strength* (scored); GENERIC].

162.5 mg (OTC) [*Healthprin Half-Dose* (scored)].

325 mg (OTC) [*Aspirtab; Empirin; Genuine Bayer Aspirin Caplets; Genuine Bayer Aspirin Tablets; Healthprin Full Strength* (scored); *Norwich Aspirin;* GENERIC].

500 mg (OTC) [*Aspirtab-Max; Extra Strength Bayer Aspirin Caplets; Extra Strength Bayer Aspirin Tablets; Norwich Aspirin;* GENERIC].
650 mg (OTC) [GENERIC].

Canada—
300 mg of ASA (OTC) [*Headache Tablet*].
325 mg of ASA (OTC) [*Apo-ASA; Aspirin Caplets; Aspirin Tablets; PMS-ASA;* GENERIC].
500 mg of ASA (OTC) [*Aspirin Caplets; Aspirin Tablets*].

Note: Strengths of specific products labeled in grains may vary, depending on the manufacturer.

**Packaging and storage**
Store below 40 °C (104 °F), preferably between 15 and 30 °C (59 and 86 °F), unless otherwise specified by manufacturer. Store in a tight container.

**Auxiliary labeling**
• Take with food and a full glass of water.

## ASPIRIN TABLETS (CHEWABLE) USP

**Usual adult and adolescent dose**
See *Aspirin Tablets USP.*

**Usual pediatric dose**
See *Aspirin Tablets USP.*

**Strength(s) usually available**
U.S.—
81 mg (OTC) [*Bayer Children's Aspirin; St. Joseph Adult Chewable Aspirin;* GENERIC].

Canada—
80 mg of ASA (OTC) [*Aspirin Children's Tablets*].

**Packaging and storage**
Store below 40 °C (104 °F), preferably between 15 and 30 °C (59 and 86 °F), unless otherwise specified by manufacturer. Store in a tight container.

**Auxiliary labeling**
• May be chewed.
• Take with food and a full glass of water.

## ASPIRIN CHEWING GUM TABLETS

**Usual adult and adolescent dose**
Analgesic—
Oral, 454 to 650 mg. May be repeated every four hours as needed.

Note: For patient self-medication, it is recommended that a physician be consulted if pain is not relieved within ten days or sore throat within two days.

**Usual pediatric dose**
Analgesic—
Children up to 3 years of age: Dosage must be individualized by physician.
Children 3 to 6 years of age: Oral, 227 mg. May be repeated up to three times a day.
Children 6 to 12 years of age: Oral, 227 to 454 mg. May be repeated up to four times a day.

Note: It is recommended that children up to 12 years of age receive no more than five doses in each twenty-four-hour period, unless otherwise directed by a physician, and that a physician be consulted if pain is not relieved within five days or sore throat within two days.

**Strength(s) usually available**
U.S.—
227 mg (OTC) [*Aspergum*].
Canada—
325 mg of ASA (OTC) [*Aspergum*].

**Packaging and storage**
Store below 40 °C (104 °F), preferably between 15 and 30 °C (59 and 86 °F), unless otherwise specified by manufacturer.

**Auxiliary labeling**
• To be chewed.
• Take with food.
• Drink a full glass of water after chewing.

## ASPIRIN DELAYED-RELEASE TABLETS USP

**Usual adult and adolescent dose**
See *Aspirin Tablets USP.*

**Usual pediatric dose**
See *Aspirin Tablets USP.*

**Strength(s) usually available**
U.S.—
81 mg (OTC) [*Acuprin 81; Aspirin Regimen Bayer Adult Low Dose; Ecotrin Caplets; Ecotrin Tablets; Halfprin;* GENERIC].
162 mg (OTC) [*Halfprin*].
325 mg (OTC) [*Aspirin Regimen Bayer Regular Strength Caplets; Ecotrin Caplets; Ecotrin Tablets; Norwich Aspirin;* GENERIC].
500 mg (OTC) [*Ecotrin Caplets; Ecotrin Tablets; Extra Strength Bayer Arthritis Pain Formula Caplets; Maximum Strength Arthritis Foundation Safety Coated Aspirin; Norwich Aspirin;* GENERIC].
650 mg (OTC) [GENERIC].
975 mg (Rx) [*Easprin;* GENERIC].

Canada—
325 mg of ASA (OTC) [*Apo-ASEN; Aspirin, Coated; Astrin; Coryphen; Entrophen Caplets; Entrophen Tablets; Novasen; Novasen Sp.C;* GENERIC].
500 mg of ASA (OTC) [*Aspirin, Coated; Entrophen Extra Strength*].
650 mg of ASA (OTC) [*Apo-ASEN; Coryphen; Entrophen 10 Super Strength Caplets; Novasen; Novasen Sp.C;* GENERIC].
975 mg of ASA (OTC) [*Entrophen 15 Maximum Strength Tablets;* GENERIC].

**Packaging and storage**
Store below 40 °C (104 °F), preferably between 15 and 30 °C (59 and 86 °F), unless otherwise specified by manufacturer. Store in a tight container.

**Auxiliary labeling**
• Swallow tablets whole.
• Take with a full glass of water.

## ASPIRIN EXTENDED-RELEASE TABLETS USP

**Usual adult and adolescent dose**
Analgesic—
Oral, 650 mg to 1.3 grams as 650-mg tablets every eight hours, or 1.6 grams as 800-mg tablets twice a day.

Note: The extended-release tablets have not been recommended by FDA for use as a platelet aggregation inhibitor.
For treatment of arthritis, the recommended analgesic dose may be administered initially, then adjusted according to patient requirements and response.

**Usual pediatric dose**
Pediatric strength not available.

**Strength(s) usually available**
U.S.—
650 mg (OTC) [*Extended-release Bayer 8-Hour* (scored)].
800 mg (Rx) [*Sloprin; ZORprin;* GENERIC].
975 mg (Rx) [GENERIC].
Canada—
325 mg of ASA (OTC) [*Arthrisin*].
650 mg of ASA (OTC) [*Arthrisin; Artria S.R*].

**Packaging and storage**
Store below 40 °C (104 °F), preferably between 15 and 30 °C (59 and 86 °F), unless otherwise specified by manufacturer. Store in a tight container.

**Auxiliary labeling**
• Take with food and a full glass of water.
• Swallow tablets whole (if specified by manufacturer).

## ASPIRIN AND CAFFEINE CAPSULES

**Usual adult and adolescent dose**
See *Aspirin Tablets USP.* Dosage is based only on the aspirin component.

**Usual pediatric dose**
Analgesic/Antipyretic—
Children up to 6 years of age: Product of suitable strength not available.
Children 6 years of age and older: Oral, 325 mg every four hours as needed, while symptoms persist.

Note: It is recommended that children up to 12 years of age receive no more than five doses in each twenty-four-hour period, unless otherwise directed by a physician, and that a physician be consulted if pain is not relieved within five days, fever within three days, or sore throat within two days.

Antirheumatic (nonsteroidal anti-inflammatory)—
Oral, 80 to 100 mg per kg of body weight a day in divided doses.

Note: If an adequate response is not achieved within one or two weeks, dosage adjustment should be based on measurement of plasma salicylate concentration. Up to 130 mg per kg of body weight per day may be required in some patients.

### Strength(s) usually available

U.S.—

Not commercially available.

Canada—

325 mg of ASA and 55 mg of caffeine (OTC) [*Astone*].

### Packaging and storage

Store below 40 °C (104 °F), preferably between 15 and 30 °C (59 and 86 °F), in a well-closed container, unless otherwise specified by manufacturer.

### Auxiliary labeling

• Take with food and a full glass of water.

## ASPIRIN AND CAFFEINE TABLETS

### Usual adult and adolescent dose

See *Aspirin Tablets USP*. Dosage is based only on the aspirin component.

### Usual pediatric dose

Analgesic/Antipyretic—

Children up to 9 years of age: Product of suitable strength not available.

Children 9 years of age and older: Oral, 325 to 400 mg every four hours as needed, while symptoms persist.

Note: It is recommended that children up to 12 years of age receive no more than five doses in each twenty-four-hour period, unless otherwise directed by a physician, and that a physician be consulted if pain is not relieved within five days, fever within three days, or sore throat within two days.

Antirheumatic (nonsteroidal anti-inflammatory)—

Oral, 80 to 100 mg per kg of body weight a day in divided doses.

Note: If an adequate response is not achieved within one or two weeks, dosage adjustment should be based on measurement of plasma salicylate concentration. Up to 130 mg per kg of body weight per day may be required in some patients.

### Strength(s) usually available

U.S.—

400 mg of aspirin and 32 mg of caffeine (OTC) [*Anacin Caplets; Anacin Tablets; Gensan; P-A-C Revised Formula*].

500 mg of aspirin and 32 mg of caffeine (OTC) [*Anacin Maximum Strength*].

Canada—

325 mg of ASA and 4 mg of caffeine [*Kalmex*].

325 mg of ASA and 15 mg of caffeine (OTC) [*C2* (double-scored)].

325 mg of ASA and 30 mg of caffeine citrate equivalent to 15 mg of caffeine base (OTC) [*Herbopyrine; 217* (scored)].

325 mg of ASA and 30 mg of caffeine (OTC) [*Nervine*].

325 mg of ASA and 32 mg of caffeine (OTC) [*Anacin*].

325 mg of ASA and 32.4 mg of caffeine (OTC) [*Antidol*].

325 mg of ASA and 33 mg of caffeine (OTC) [*Calmine; Dolomine*].

325 mg of ASA and 65 mg of caffeine (OTC) [*Instantine*].

375 mg of ASA and 30 mg of caffeine citrate equivalent to 15 mg of caffeine base [*Arco Pain Tablet*].

500 mg of ASA and 30 mg of caffeine citrate equivalent to 15 mg of caffeine base (OTC) [*217 Strong*].

500 mg of ASA and 32 mg of caffeine (OTC) [*Anacin Extra Strength; Pain Aid*].

### Packaging and storage

Store below 40 °C (104 °F), preferably between 15 and 30 °C (59 and 86 °F), in a well-closed container, unless otherwise specified by manufacturer.

### Auxiliary labeling

• Take with food and a full glass of water.

# Rectal Dosage Forms

Note: Bracketed uses in the *Dosage Forms* section refer to categories of use and/or indications that are not included in U.S. product labeling.

## ASPIRIN SUPPOSITORIES USP

### Usual adult and adolescent dose

Analgesic/antipyretic—

Rectal, 325 to 650 mg every four hours as needed, while symptoms persist.

Note: For patient self-medication, it is recommended that the total daily dose not exceed 4 grams, and that a physician be consulted if pain is not relieved within ten days, fever within three days, or sore throat within two days.

Antirheumatic (nonsteroidal anti-inflammatory)—

Rectal, 3.6 to 5.4 grams a day in divided doses.

Note: In acute rheumatic fever, up to 7.8 grams a day in divided doses may be given.

Platelet aggregation inhibitor—

The suppositories have not been recommended by FDA for use as a platelet aggregation inhibitor.

### Usual pediatric dose

Analgesic/antipyretic—

Rectal, 1.5 grams per square meter of body surface a day in four to six divided doses; or for

Children up to 2 years of age—Dosage must be individualized by physician.

Children 2 to 4 years of age—Rectal, 160 mg every four hours as needed, while symptoms persist.

Children 4 to 6 years of age—Rectal, 240 mg every four hours as needed, while symptoms persist.

Children 6 to 9 years of age—Rectal, 325 mg every four hours as needed, while symptoms persist.

Children 9 to 11 years of age—Rectal, 325 to 400 mg every four hours as needed, while symptoms persist.

Children 11 to 12 years of age—Rectal, 325 to 480 mg every four hours as needed, while symptoms persist.

Note: Do not exceed 2.5 grams per square meter of body surface per day. It is recommended that children up to 12 years of age receive no more than five doses in each twenty-four-hour period, unless otherwise directed by a physician, and that a physician be consulted if pain is not relieved within five days, fever within three days, or sore throat within two days.

Antirheumatic (nonsteroidal anti-inflammatory)—

Rectal, 80 to 100 mg per kg of body weight a day in divided doses.

Note: If an adequate response is not achieved within one or two weeks, dosage adjustment should be based on measurement of plasma salicylate concentration. Up to 130 mg per kg of body weight per day may be required in some patients.

[Kawasaki disease][1]—

During the early febrile stage: Rectal, 80 to 120 mg (average 100 mg) per kg of body weight a day in four divided doses for fourteen days or until inflammation has subsided. However, absorption may be impaired or erratic during this stage of the illness, and considerably higher doses may be required. It is recommended that dosage be adjusted to achieve and maintain a plasma salicylate concentration of 20 to 30 mg per 100 mL.

During the convalescent stage: Rectal, 3 to 5 mg per kg of body weight a day as a single dose. If no coronary artery abnormalities occur, treatment is usually continued for a minimum of eight weeks. If coronary artery abnormalities occur, it is recommended that treatment be continued for at least one year, even if the abnormalities regress, and longer if abnormalities persist.

### Strength(s) usually available

U.S.—

60 mg (OTC) [GENERIC].

120 mg (OTC) [GENERIC].

125 mg (OTC) [GENERIC].

200 mg (OTC) [GENERIC].

300 mg (OTC) [GENERIC].

325 mg (OTC) [GENERIC].

600 mg (OTC) [GENERIC].

650 mg (OTC) [GENERIC].

1.2 grams (OTC) [GENERIC].

Canada—

150 mg of ASA (OTC) [*PMS-ASA;* GENERIC].

650 mg of ASA (OTC) [*PMS-ASA;* GENERIC].

Note: The strengths of the specific products may not conform to the recommended pediatric doses. Also, the strengths of some products labeled in grains may vary, depending on the manufacturer.

### Packaging and storage

Store between 8 and 15 °C (46 and 59 °F), unless otherwise specified by manufacturer. Store in a well-closed container, in a cool place.

### Auxiliary labeling

• Store in a cool place. May be refrigerated.

• For rectal use only.

---

[1]Not included in Canadian product labeling.

---

### *ASPIRIN, BUFFERED*

## Summary of Differences

Category/indications:

Aspirin, buffered, also indicated as a platelet aggregation inhibitor.

Pharmacology/pharmacokinetics:

Aspirin irreversibly inhibits platelet aggregation.

Precautions:
Cross-sensitivity and/or related problems—
Risk of cross-sensitivity with other nonsteroidal anti-inflammatory drugs (NSAIDs) significantly greater with aspirin than with other salicylates.
Drug interactions and/or related problems—
Aspirin may increase ascorbic acid requirement (prolonged high-dose use).
Theoretically, aspirin may decrease zidovudine clearance.
Higher risk of bleeding (compared with other salicylates) when aspirin is used concurrently with other medications that may inhibit blood clotting or cause gastrointestinal ulceration or bleeding.
Antacids present as buffering agents may decrease absorption of fluoroquinolone antibiotics, itraconazole, ketoconazole, and oral tetracyclines.
Laboratory value alterations—
Aspirin interferes with urine 5-hydroxyindoleacetic acid determinations.
Aspirin interferes with protirelin-induced thyroid stimulating hormone release determinations.
Aspirin prolongs bleeding time.
Medical considerations/contraindications—
Aspirin should not be used in patients with a history of severe sensitivity reactions to aspirin, other NSAIDs, nasal polyps and asthma, or thrombocytopenia.
Aspirin should be used with caution in patients with asthma or glucose-6-phosphate dehydrogenase (G6PD) deficiency.
Side/adverse effects:
Aspirin is more ulcerogenic than other salicylates.
Rarely, aspirin causes hemolytic anemia (in patients with G6PD deficiency).

## Additional Dosing Information

See also *General Dosing Information*.

The doses for buffered aspirin formulations are based on the FDA's dosing recommendations for aspirin. The dosage unit of 325 mg (5 grains) is used. The conversion factor of 1 grain equal to 65 mg is used. Strengths of specific products may vary, depending on the manufacturer.

The amount and type of buffering may vary among products.

## Oral Dosage Forms

Note: Bracketed uses in the *Dosage Forms* section refer to categories of use and/or indications that are not included in U.S. product labeling.

### ASPIRIN, ALUMINA, AND MAGNESIA TABLETS USP

**Usual adult and adolescent dose**
Analgesic/antipyretic—
Oral, 500 mg every three or four hours or 1000 mg every six hours as needed, while symptoms persist.
Note: For patient self-medication, it is recommended that the total daily dose not exceed 4 grams, and that a physician be consulted if pain is not relieved within ten days, fever within three days, or sore throat within two days.
Antirheumatic (nonsteroidal anti-inflammatory)—
Oral, 3.6 to 5.4 grams a day in divided doses.
Note: In acute rheumatic fever, up to 7.8 grams a day in divided doses may be given.
Platelet aggregation inhibitor—
Oral, 325 mg a day, with the following exceptions:
Ischemic attacks, transient, in males or—
[Thromboembolism, cerebral, recurrence][1]—
Oral, 1 gram a day. Dosage may be reduced to 325 mg a day if the patient is unable to tolerate the higher dose.
[Ischemic attacks, transient, occurring in association with mitral valve prolapse][1]—
Oral, 325 mg to 1 gram a day.
[Prevention of thrombosis or occlusion of coronary bypass graft]—
Oral, 325 mg seven hours postoperatively (via a nasogastric tube), then 325 mg three times daily, concurrently with 75 mg of dipyridamole. Dipyridamole may be discontinued one week postoperatively, but aspirin should be continued indefinitely.
Platelet aggregation inhibitor therapy is most effective when it is initiated two days prior to scheduled surgery. However, preoperative administration of aspirin has been shown to increase perisurgical bleeding and is not recommended. Therapy is therefore initiated with dipyridamole (recommended dosage 100 mg four times a day for two days prior to surgery and 100 mg one hour postoperatively [via a nasogastric tube]). Dipyridamole therapy is continued post-

operatively (recommended dosage 75 mg seven hours postoperatively, via a nasogastric tube, then 75 mg three times a day, concurrently with aspirin) for at least one week.
Note: Although the doses recommended above for use of aspirin as a platelet aggregation inhibitor have been found effective in clinical studies, optimum dosage has not been established. For indications other than prevention of transient ischemic attacks or recurrence of cerebral thromboembolism, lower doses are often used. A few studies have shown that 160 mg of aspirin every twenty-four hours, or 325 mg every forty-eight hours, may effectively inhibit platelet aggregation while minimizing the risk of aspirin-induced side effects.

For most antithrombotic indications, lower doses than can be achieved with the aspirin, alumina, and magnesia formulation are used. However, this formulation may be used when 500-mg or 1-gram doses are appropriate.

**Usual pediatric dose**
Analgesic/antipyretic—
Product of suitable strength not available.
Antirheumatic (nonsteroidal anti-inflammatory)—
Oral, 80 to 100 mg per kg of body weight a day in divided doses.
Note: If an adequate response is not achieved within one or two weeks, dosage adjustment should be based on measurement of plasma salicylate concentration. Up to 130 mg per kg of body weight per day may be required in some patients.
[Kawasaki disease][1]—
During the early febrile stage: Oral, 80 to 120 mg (average 100 mg) per kg of body weight a day in four divided doses for fourteen days or until inflammation has subsided. However, absorption may be impaired or erratic during this stage of the illness, and considerably higher doses may be required. It is recommended that dosage be adjusted to achieve and maintain a plasma salicylate concentration of 20 to 30 mg per 100 mL.
During the convalescent stage: Oral, 3 to 5 mg per kg of body weight a day as a single dose. If no coronary artery abnormalities occur, treatment is usually continued for a minimum of eight weeks. If coronary artery abnormalities occur, it is recommended that treatment be continued for at least one year, even if the abnormalities regress, and longer if abnormalities persist.

**Strength(s) usually available**
U.S.—
500 mg of aspirin, with 27 mg of aluminum hydroxide and 100 mg of magnesium hydroxide (OTC) [*Arthritis Pain Formula*].
Canada—
Not commercially available.

**Packaging and storage**
Store below 40 °C (104 °F), preferably between 15 and 30 °C (59 and 86 °F), unless otherwise specified by manufacturer. Store in a tight container.

**Auxiliary labeling**
• Take with food and a full glass of water.

### ASPIRIN, ALUMINA, AND MAGNESIUM OXIDE TABLETS USP

**Usual adult and adolescent dose**
Analgesic/antipyretic or
Antirheumatic (nonsteroidal anti-inflammatory)—
See *Aspirin, Alumina, and Magnesia Tablets USP*. Dosage is based only on the aspirin component.
Platelet aggregation inhibitor—
See *Aspirin, Alumina, and Magnesia Tablets USP*. Dosage is based only on the aspirin component. For most antithrombotic indications, lower doses than can be achieved with the aspirin, alumina, and magnesium oxide formulation are used. However, this formulation may be used when 500-mg or 1-gram doses are appropriate.

**Usual pediatric dose**
See *Aspirin, Alumina, and Magnesia Tablets USP*. Dosage is based only on the aspirin component.

**Strength(s) usually available**
U.S.—
500 mg of aspirin, with dried aluminum hydroxide gel equivalent to 125 mg of aluminum hydroxide and 150 mg of magnesium oxide (OTC) [*Cama Arthritis Pain Reliever*].
Canada—
Not commercially available.

**Packaging and storage**

Store below 40 °C (104 °F), preferably between 15 and 30 °C (59 and 86 °F), unless otherwise specified by manufacturer. Store in a tight container.

**Auxiliary labeling**
* Take with food and a full glass of water.

## BUFFERED ASPIRIN TABLETS USP

### Usual adult and adolescent dose
Analgesic/antipyretic—

Oral, 325 to 500 mg every three hours, 325 to 650 mg every four hours, or 650 mg to 1000 mg every six hours as needed, while symptoms persist.

Note: For patient self-medication, it is recommended that the total daily dose not exceed 4 grams, and that a physician be consulted if pain is not relieved within ten days, fever within three days, or sore throat within two days.

Platelet aggregation inhibitor—
See *Aspirin, Alumina, and Magnesia Tablets USP*.

### Usual pediatric dose
Analgesic/antipyretic—

Oral, 1.5 grams of aspirin per square meter of body surface a day in four to six divided doses; or for

Children up to 2 years of age: Dosage must be individualized by physician.

Children 2 to 4 years of age: Oral, ¹/₂ of a 325-mg tablet every four hours as needed, while symptoms persist.

Children 4 to 6 years of age: Oral, ³/₄ of a 325-mg tablet every four hours as needed, while symptoms persist.

Children 6 to 9 years of age: Oral, 1 tablet (325 mg) every four hours as needed, while symptoms persist.

Children 9 to 11 years of age: Oral, 1 to 1¹/₄ tablets (325 mg each) every four hours as needed, while symptoms persist.

Children 11 to 12 years of age: Oral, 1 to 1¹/₂ tablets (325 mg each) every four hours as needed, while symptoms persist.

Note: It is recommended that children up to 12 years of age receive no more than five doses in each twenty-four-hour period, unless otherwise directed by a physician, and that a physician be consulted if pain is not relieved within five days, fever within three days, or sore throat within two days.

Antirheumatic (nonsteroidal anti-inflammatory)—

Oral, 80 to 100 mg of aspirin per kg of body weight a day in divided doses.

Note: If an adequate response is not achieved within one or two weeks, dosage adjustment should be based on measurement of plasma salicylate concentration. Up to 130 mg per kg of body weight of aspirin per day may be required in some patients.

[Kawasaki disease][1]—

During the early febrile stage: Oral, 80 to 120 mg (average 100 mg) per kg of body weight a day in four divided doses for fourteen days or until inflammation has subsided. However, absorption may be impaired or erratic during this stage of the illness, and considerably higher doses may be required. It is recommended that dosage be adjusted to achieve and maintain a plasma salicylate concentration of 20 to 30 mg per 100 mL.

During the convalescent stage: Oral, 3 to 5 mg per kg of body weight a day as a single dose. If no coronary artery abnormalities occur, treatment is usually continued for a minimum of eight weeks. If coronary artery abnormalities occur, it is recommended that treatment be continued for at least one year, even if the abnormalities regress, and longer if abnormalities persist.

### Strength(s) usually available
U.S.—

325 mg of aspirin (OTC) [*Arthritis Pain Ascriptin; Bufferin Caplets; Bufferin Tablets; Buffex; Buffinol; Magnaprin; Regular Strength Ascriptin;* GENERIC].

500 mg of aspirin (OTC) [*Arthritis Strength Bufferin; Buffinol Extra; Extra Strength Bayer Plus Caplets; Maximum Strength Ascriptin*].

Canada—

325 mg of ASA (OTC) [*Aspirin Plus Stomach Guard Regular Strength; Bufferin Caplets; Tri-Buffered ASA;* GENERIC].

500 mg of ASA (OTC) [*Aspirin Plus Stomach Guard Extra Strength; Bufferin Extra Strength Caplets;* GENERIC].

Note: See individual product label for buffering agent (s).

The strengths of the specific products may not conform to the recommended pediatric doses.

---

**Packaging and storage**

Store below 40 °C (104 °F), preferably between 15 and 30 °C (59 and 86 °F), unless otherwise specified by manufacturer. Store in a tight container.

**Auxiliary labeling**
* Take with food and a full glass of water.

## BUFFERED ASPIRIN AND CAFFEINE TABLETS

### Usual adult and adolescent dose
See *Buffered Aspirin Tablets USP*. Dosage is based only on the aspirin component.

### Usual pediatric dose
Analgesic/antipyretic—

Oral, 1.5 grams of aspirin per square meter of body surface a day in four to six divided doses; or for

Children up to 2 years of age: Dosage must be individualized by physician.

Children 2 to 4 years of age: Oral, ¹/₂ of a 325-mg tablet every four hours as needed, while symptoms persist.

Children 4 to 6 years of age: Oral, ³/₄ of a 325-mg tablet every four hours as needed, while symptoms persist.

Children 6 to 9 years of age: Oral, 1 tablet (325 mg) every four hours as needed, while symptoms persist.

Children 9 to 11 years of age: Oral, 1 to 1¹/₄ tablets (325 mg each) every four hours as needed, while symptoms persist.

Children 11 to 12 years of age: Oral, 1 to 1¹/₂ tablets (325 mg each) or 1 tablet (421 mg) every four hours as needed, while symptoms persist.

Note: It is recommended that children up to 12 years of age receive no more than five doses in each twenty-four-hour period, unless otherwise directed by a physician, and that a physician be consulted if pain is not relieved within five days, fever within three days, or sore throat within two days.

Antirheumatic (nonsteroidal anti-inflammatory)—

Oral, 80 to 100 mg of aspirin per kg of body weight a day in divided doses.

Note: If an adequate response is not achieved within one or two weeks, dosage adjustment should be based on measurement of plasma salicylate concentration. Up to 130 mg per kg of body weight of aspirin per day may be required in some patients.

### Strength(s) usually available
U.S.—

421 mg of aspirin and 32 mg of caffeine (OTC) [*Cope*].

Canada—

325 mg of ASA and 15 mg of caffeine (OTC) [*C2 Buffered* (scored)].

Note: See individual product label for buffering agent(s).

The strengths of the specific products may not conform to the recommended pediatric doses.

### Packaging and storage
Store below 40 °C (104 °F), preferably between 15 and 30 °C (59 and 86 °F), unless otherwise specified by manufacturer. Store in a tight container.

### Auxiliary labeling
* Take with food and a full glass of water.

---

[1]Not included in Canadian product labeling.

---

## CHOLINE SALICYLATE

# Summary of Differences

Pharmacology/pharmacokinetics:

Choline salicylate does not have a clinically significant effect on platelet aggregation.

Precautions:

Cross-sensitivity and/or related problems—Lower risk than with aspirin of cross-sensitivity to nonsteroidal anti-inflammatory drugs (NSAIDs).

Drug interactions and/or related problems—Lower risk of bleeding (compared with aspirin) when used concurrently with other medications that may inhibit blood clotting or cause gastrointestinal ulceration or bleeding.

Medical considerations/contraindications—May be used in patients with a history of severe sensitivity reactions to aspirin or other NSAIDs, although caution is advised.

Side/adverse effects:

Less ulcerogenic than aspirin.

## Additional Dosing Information

See also *General Dosing Information*.

The nonarthritic doses are based on the FDA's dosing recommendations for aspirin.

A 435-mg dose of choline salicylate is equivalent in salicylate content to 325 mg of aspirin.

## Oral Dosage Forms

### CHOLINE SALICYLATE ORAL SOLUTION

**Usual adult and adolescent dose**
Analgesic/antipyretic—
Oral, 435 to 669 mg (equivalent in salicylate content to 325 to 500 mg of aspirin) every three hours, 435 to 870 mg (equivalent in salicylate content to 325 to 650 mg of aspirin) every four hours, or 870 to 1338 mg (equivalent in salicylate content to 650 to 1000 mg of aspirin) every six hours as needed, while symptoms persist.

Note: For patient self-medication, it is recommended that the total daily dose not exceed 5352 mg, and that a physician be consulted if pain is not relieved within ten days, fever within three days, or sore throat within two days.

Antirheumatic (nonsteroidal anti-inflammatory)—
Oral, 4.8 to 7.2 grams (equivalent in salicylate content to 3.6 to 5.4 grams of aspirin) a day in divided doses.

**Usual pediatric dose**
Analgesic/antipyretic—
Oral, 2 grams (equivalent in salicylate content to 1.5 grams of aspirin) per square meter of body surface a day in four to six divided doses; or for

Children up to 2 years of age: Dosage must be individualized by physician.

Children 2 to 4 years of age: Oral, 217.5 mg (equivalent in salicylate content to 162.5 mg of aspirin) every four hours as needed, while symptoms persist.

Children 4 to 6 years of age: Oral, 326.5 mg (equivalent in salicylate content to 243.8 mg of aspirin) every four hours as needed, while symptoms persist.

Children 6 to 9 years of age: Oral, 435 mg (equivalent in salicylate content to 325 mg of aspirin) every four hours as needed, while symptoms persist.

Children 9 to 11 years of age: Oral, 435 to 543.8 mg (equivalent in salicylate content to 325 to 406.3 mg of aspirin) every four hours as needed, while symptoms persist.

Children 11 to 12 years of age: Oral, 435 to 652.5 mg (equivalent in salicylate content to 325 to 487.5 mg of aspirin) every four hours as needed, while symptoms persist.

Note: It is recommended that children up to 12 years of age receive no more than five doses in each twenty-four-hour period, unless otherwise directed by a physician, and that a physician be consulted if pain is not relieved within five days, fever within three days, or sore throat within two days.

Antirheumatic (nonsteroidal anti-inflammatory)—
Oral, 107 to 133 mg (equivalent in salicylate content to 80 to 100 mg of aspirin) per kg of body weight a day in divided doses.

Note: If an adequate response is not achieved within one or two weeks, dosage adjustment should be based on measurement of plasma salicylate concentration. Up to 174 mg (equivalent in salicylate content to 130 mg of aspirin) per kg of body weight per day may be required in some patients.

**Strength(s) usually available**
U.S.—
870 mg (equivalent in salicylate content to 650 mg of aspirin) per 5 mL (OTC) [*Arthropan*].

Canada—
Not commercially available.

**Packaging and storage**
Store below 40 °C (104 °F), preferably between 15 and 30 °C (59 and 86 °F), in a well-closed container, unless otherwise specified by manufacturer. Protect from freezing.

**Auxiliary labeling**
• Take with food or a full glass of water.

---

## CHOLINE AND MAGNESIUM SALICYLATES

## Summary of Differences

Pharmacology/pharmacokinetics:
This medication does not have a clinically significant effect on platelet aggregation.

Precautions:
Cross-sensitivity and/or related problems—
Lower risk than with aspirin of cross-sensitivity to nonsteroidal anti-inflammatory drugs (NSAIDs).

Drug interactions and/or related problems—
Lower risk of bleeding (compared with aspirin) when used concurrently with other medications that may inhibit blood clotting or cause gastrointestinal ulceration or bleeding.

Magnesium may decrease absorption of fluoroquinolone antibiotics, itraconazole, ketoconazole, and oral tetracyclines.

Medical considerations/contraindications—
Should not be used in patients with chronic advanced renal impairment because of risk of hypermagnesemic toxicity.

May be used in patients with a history of severe sensitivity reactions to aspirin or other NSAIDs, although caution is advised.

Patient monitoring—
Monitoring of serum magnesium concentration recommended if large doses administered to patients with renal insufficiency.

Side/adverse effects:
Less ulcerogenic than aspirin.

## Additional Dosing Information

See also *General Dosing Information*.

Choline and magnesium salicylates oral solution may be mixed with fruit juices just prior to administration.

## Oral Dosage Forms

### CHOLINE AND MAGNESIUM SALICYLATES ORAL SOLUTION

**Usual adult and adolescent dose**
Analgesic or
Antipyretic—
Oral, 2 to 3 grams of salicylate a day in two or three divided doses.

Anti-inflammatory (nonsteroidal) or
Antirheumatic—
Oral, 3 grams of salicylate a day in a single dose at bedtime, or in two or three divided doses, initially. Dosage must then be adjusted according to the requirements and response of the individual patient.

**Usual pediatric dose**
Analgesic
Antipyretic or
Anti-inflammatory (nonsteroidal)—
Children weighing up to 37 kg: Oral, 50 mg of salicylate per kg of body weight per day in two divided doses.
Children weighing more than 37 kg: Oral, 2.2 grams of salicylate a day in two divided doses.

**Strength(s) usually available**
U.S.—
500 mg of salicylate (contains 293 mg of choline salicylate and 362 mg of magnesium salicylate) per 5 mL (Rx) [*Trilisate*].

Note: Each 5-mL dose of this medication is equivalent in salicylate content to 650 mg of aspirin.

Canada—
Not commercially available.

**Packaging and storage**
Store below 40 °C (104 °F), preferably between 15 and 30 °C (59 and 86 °F), unless otherwise specified by manufacturer. Protect from freezing.

**Auxiliary labeling**
• Take with food or a full glass of water.

### CHOLINE AND MAGNESIUM SALICYLATES TABLETS

**Usual adult and adolescent dose**
See *Choline and Magnesium Salicylates Oral Solution*.

**Usual pediatric dose**
See *Choline and Magnesium Salicylates Oral Solution*.

**Strength(s) usually available**
U.S.—

500 mg of salicylate (contains 293 mg of choline salicylate and 362 mg of magnesium salicylate) (Rx) [*CMT; Tricosal; Trilisate* (scored); GENERIC].

750 mg of salicylate (contains 440 mg of choline salicylate and 544 mg of magnesium salicylate) (Rx) [*CMT; Tricosal; Trilisate* (scored); GENERIC].

1000 mg of salicylate (contains 587 mg of choline salicylate and 725 mg of magnesium salicylate) (Rx) [*CMT; Tricosal; Trilisate* (scored); GENERIC].

Canada—

500 mg of salicylate (contains 293 mg of choline salicylate and 362 mg of magnesium salicylate) (Rx) [*Trilisate* (scored)].

Note: Each 500-mg tablet is equivalent in salicylate content to 650 mg of aspirin. Each 750-mg tablet is equivalent in salicylate content to 975 mg of aspirin. Each 1000-mg tablet is equivalent in salicylate content to 1.3 grams of aspirin.

**Packaging and storage**
Store below 40 °C (104 °F), preferably between 15 and 30 °C (59 and 86 °F), in a well-closed container, unless otherwise specified by manufacturer.

**Auxiliary labeling**
• Take with food and a full glass of water.

## MAGNESIUM SALICYLATE

## Summary of Differences

Pharmacology/pharmacokinetics:
Magnesium salicylate does not have a clinically significant effect on platelet aggregation.
Precautions:
Cross-sensitivity and/or related problems—
Lower risk than with aspirin of cross-sensitivity to nonsteroidal anti-inflammatory drugs (NSAIDs).
Drug interactions and/or related problems—
Lower risk of bleeding (compared with aspirin) when used concurrently with other medications that may inhibit blood clotting or cause gastrointestinal ulceration or bleeding.
Magnesium may decrease absorption of fluoroquinolone antibiotics, itraconazole, ketoconazole, and oral tetracyclines.
Medical considerations/contraindications—
Should not be used in patients with chronic advanced renal impairment.
May be used in patients with a history of severe sensitivity reactions to aspirin or other NSAIDs, although caution is advised.
Patient monitoring—
Monitoring of serum magnesium concentration recommended if large doses are administered to patients with renal insufficiency.
Side/adverse effects:
Less ulcerogenic than aspirin.

## Additional Dosing Information

See also *General Dosing Information*.

A 545-mg dose of magnesium salicylate is equivalent in salicylate content to 650 mg of aspirin.

## Oral Dosage Forms

### MAGNESIUM SALICYLATE TABLETS USP

**Usual adult and adolescent dose**
Analgesic/antipyretic
Antirheumatic (nonsteroidal anti-inflammatory)—
Oral, 2 regular-strength tablets (containing the equivalent of 303.7 mg of anhydrous magnesium salicylate per tablet) every four hours as needed, up to a maximum of 12 tablets a day, or
Oral, 2 extra-strength tablets (containing the equivalent of 467 mg of anhydrous magnesium salicylate, or more, per tablet) every six hours as needed, up to a maximum of 8 tablets a day.

Note: For patient self-medication, it is recommended that a physician be consulted if pain is not relieved within ten days, fever within three days, or sore throat within two days.

**Usual pediatric dose**
Dosage has not been established.

**Strength(s) usually available**
U.S.—

377 mg of magnesium salicylate tetrahydrate equivalent to 303.7 mg of anhydrous magnesium salicylate (OTC) [*Doan's Regular Strength Tablets*].

545 mg (Rx) [*Magan*].

580 mg of magnesium salicylate tetrahydrate equivalent to 467 mg of anhydrous magnesium salicylate (OTC) [*Backache Caplets; Bayer Select Maximum Strength Backache Pain Relief Formula; Maximum Strength Doan's Analgesic Caplets*].

600 mg (Rx) [*Mobidin* (scored)].

Canada—

325 mg (OTC) [*Doan's Backache Pills*].

650 mg (OTC) [*Sero-Gesic*].

**Packaging and storage**
Store below 40 °C (104 °F), preferably between 15 and 30 °C (59 and 86 °F), unless otherwise specified by manufacturer. Store in a tight container.

**Auxiliary labeling**
• Take with food and a full glass of water.

## SALSALATE

## Summary of Differences

Pharmacology/pharmacokinetics:
Salsalate does not have a clinically significant effect on platelet aggregation.
Precautions:
Cross-sensitivity and/or related problems—Lower risk than with aspirin of cross-sensitivity to nonsteroidal anti-inflammatory drugs (NSAIDs).
Drug interactions and/or related problems—Lower risk of bleeding (compared with aspirin) when used concurrently with other medications that may inhibit blood clotting or cause gastrointestinal ulceration or bleeding.
Medical considerations/contraindications—May be used in patients with a history of severe sensitivity reactions to aspirin or other NSAIDs, although caution is advised.
Side/adverse effects:
Less ulcerogenic than aspirin.

## Additional Dosing Information

**Bioequivalence information**
Bioavailability or bioequivalence problems among different brands of Salsalate Tablets USP have not been documented.

## Oral Dosage Forms

### SALSALATE CAPSULES USP

**Usual adult and adolescent dose**
Antirheumatic—
Oral, 1 gram three times a day initially. Dosage may then be titrated according to patient response.

**Usual pediatric dose**
Dosage has not been established.

**Strength(s) usually available**
U.S.—

500 mg (Rx) [*Disalcid;* GENERIC].

750 mg (Rx) [GENERIC].

Canada—

Not commercially available.

**Packaging and storage**
Store between 15 and 30 °C (59 and 86 °F), in a light-resistant container, unless otherwise specified by manufacturer. Store in a tight container.

**Auxiliary labeling**
• Take with food and a full glass of water.

### SALSALATE TABLETS USP

Note: Bioavailability or bioequivalence problems among different brands of Salsalate Tablets USP have not been documented.

**Usual adult and adolescent dose**
Analgesic/antipyretic or
Antirheumatic—
Oral, 500 mg to 1 gram two or three times a day initially. Dosage may then be titrated according to patient response.

**Usual pediatric dose**
Dosage has not been established.

**Strength(s) usually available**
U.S.—

500 mg (Rx) [*Amigesic; Disalcid* (scored); *Mono-Gesic; Salflex; Salsitab;* GENERIC].

750 mg (Rx) [*Amigesic* (scored); *Anaflex 750; Disalcid* (scored); *Marthritic; Mono-Gesic* (scored); *Salflex* (scored); *Salsitab* (scored); GENERIC].

Canada—

500 mg (Rx) [*Disalcid* (scored)].

750 mg (Rx) [*Disalcid* (scored)].

**Packaging and storage**
Store between 15 and 30 °C (59 and 86 °F), in a light-resistant container, unless otherwise specified by manufacturer. Store in a tight container.

**Auxiliary labeling**
• Take with food and a full glass of water.

---

## SODIUM SALICYLATE

## Summary of Differences

Pharmacology/pharmacokinetics:
Sodium salicylate does not have a clinically significant effect on platelet aggregation.
Precautions:
Cross-sensitivity and/or related problems—
Lower risk than with aspirin of cross-sensitivity to nonsteroidal anti-inflammatory drugs (NSAIDs).
Drug interactions and/or related problems—
Caution required when large doses administered concurrently with sodium-retaining medications.
Lower risk of bleeding (compared with aspirin) when used concurrently with other medications that may inhibit blood clotting or cause gastrointestinal ulceration or bleeding.
Medical considerations/contraindications—
Caution required in hypertensive patients or those on a sodium-restricted diet because of sodium content.
May be used in patients with a history of severe sensitivity reactions to aspirin or other NSAIDs, although caution is advised.
Side/adverse effects:
Less ulcerogenic than aspirin.

## Additional Dosing Information

See also *General Dosing Information.*

The nonarthritic doses are based on the FDA's dosing recommendations for sodium salicylate. The dosage unit of 325 mg (5 grains) is used for adult doses. The conversion factor of 65 mg equal to 1 grain is used. Strengths of specific products may vary, depending on the manufacturer.

The uncoated tablet form of sodium salicylate should be administered with food or a full glass (240 mL) of water to lessen gastric irritation.

Each 325-mg tablet of sodium salicylate contains 2 mEq (46 mg) of sodium.

## Oral Dosage Forms

### SODIUM SALICYLATE TABLETS USP

**Usual adult and adolescent dose**
Analgesic/antipyretic—
Oral, 325 to 650 mg every four hours as needed, while symptoms persist.
Note: For patient self-medication, it is recommended that the total daily dose not exceed 4 grams, and that a physician be consulted

if pain is not relieved within ten days, fever within three days, or sore throat within two days.
Antirheumatic (nonsteroidal anti-inflammatory)—
Oral, 3.6 to 5.4 grams a day in divided doses.

**Usual pediatric dose**
Analgesic/antipyretic—
Oral, 1.5 grams per square meter of body surface a day in four to six divided doses; or for
Children up to 6 years of age: Product of suitable strength not available.
Children 6 years of age and older: Oral, 325 mg every four hours as needed, while symptoms persist.
Note: It is recommended that children up to 12 years of age receive no more than five doses in each twenty-four-hour period, unless otherwise directed by a physician, and that a physician be consulted if pain is not relieved within five days, fever within three days, or sore throat within two days.
Antirheumatic (nonsteroidal anti-inflammatory)—
Oral, 80 to 100 mg per kg of body weight a day in divided doses.
Note: If an adequate response is not achieved within one or two weeks, dosage adjustment should be based on measurement of plasma salicylate concentration. Up to 130 mg per kg of body weight per day may be required in some patients.

**Strength(s) usually available**
U.S.—

Not commercially available.

Canada—

325 mg (OTC) [*Dodd's Pills; Gin Pain Pills*].

500 mg [*Dodd's Extra Strength*].

Note: The strengths of the specific products may not conform to the recommended pediatric dose. Also, the strengths of individual products labeled in grains may vary, depending on the manufacturer.

**Packaging and storage**
Store below 40 °C (104 °F), preferably between 15 and 30 °C (59 and 86 °F), unless otherwise specified by manufacturer. Store in a well-closed container.

**Auxiliary labeling**
• Take with food and a full glass of water.

### SODIUM SALICYLATE DELAYED-RELEASE TABLETS

**Usual adult and adolescent dose**
See *Sodium Salicylate Tablets USP.*

**Usual pediatric dose**
See *Sodium Salicylate Tablets USP.*

**Strength(s) usually available**
U.S.—

325 mg (OTC) [GENERIC].

650 mg (OTC) [GENERIC].

Canada—

Not commercially available.

Note: Strengths of individual products labeled in grains may vary, depending on the manufacturer.

**Packaging and storage**
Store between 15 and 30 °C (59 and 86 °F), in a well-closed container, unless otherwise specified by manufacturer.

**Auxiliary labeling**
• Swallow tablets whole.
• Take with a full glass of water.

---

Revised: August 1990
Interim revision: 07/25/95

# SALICYLIC ACID   Topical

VA CLASSIFICATION (Primary/Secondary):
   Salicylic Acid
     Cream—DE500
     Gel—DE500/DE752; DE802
     Lotion—DE500/DE752; DE900
     Ointment—DE500/DE752; DE802; DE900
     Pads—DE500/DE752
     Plaster—DE500
     Shampoo—DE500/DE900
     Soap—DE500/DE752
     Topical Solution—DE500/DE752

Note: For a listing of dosage forms and brand names by country availability, see *Dosage Forms* section(s). For a listing of brand names for the articles in this monograph, refer to the General Index.

## Category

Keratolytic (topical)—Salicylic Acid Cream; Salicylic Acid Gel USP; Salicylic Acid Lotion; Salicylic Acid Ointment; Salicylic Acid Pads; Salicylic Acid Plaster USP; Salicylic Acid Shampoo; Salicylic Acid Soap; Salicylic Acid Topical Solution.

Antiacne agent (topical)—Salicylic Acid Gel USP; Salicylic Acid Lotion; Salicylic Acid Ointment; Salicylic Acid Pads; Salicylic Acid Soap; Salicylic Acid Topical Solution.

Antiseborrheic—Salicylic Acid Lotion; Salicylic Acid Ointment; Salicylic Acid Shampoo.

Antipsoriatic (topical)—Salicylic Acid Gel USP; Salicylic Acid Ointment.

Caustic—Salicylic Acid Cream; Salicylic Acid Ointment; Salicylic Acid Plaster USP; Salicylic Acid Topical Solution.

## Indications

### Accepted

Acne vulgaris (treatment)—Salicylic acid gel, lotion, ointment, pads, soap, and topical solution are indicated as peeling and drying agents in the treatment of acne vulgaris.

Dandruff (treatment)

Dermatitis, seborrheic (treatment) or

Dermatitis, seborrheic, of scalp (treatment)—Salicylic acid lotion and shampoo are indicated to help control scaling of the scalp associated with dandruff and seborrheic dermatitis. Salicylic acid ointment is indicated in the treatment of seborrheic dermatitis.

Psoriasis (treatment)—Salicylic acid gel and ointment are indicated as adjuncts in the treatment of psoriasis.

Hyperkeratotic skin disorders (treatment)—Salicylic acid is indicated as a topical aid in the removal of excessive keratin in hyperkeratotic skin disorders, including verrucae and the various ichthyoses (vulgaris, sex-linked, and lamellar); keratosis palmaris and plantaris; keratosis pilaris; and pityriasis rubra pilaris. It is also indicated as a topical aid in the removal of excessive keratin on dorsal and plantar hyperkeratotic lesions. Salicylic acid cream, plaster, and topical solution are indicated to treat corns and calluses. Salicylic acid gel, ointment, plaster, and topical solution are indicated to treat common warts; the gel, plaster, and topical solution are indicated to treat plantar warts.

## Pharmacology/Pharmacokinetics

### Physicochemical characteristics
Molecular weight—138.12.

### Mechanism of action/Effect
Salicylic acid facilitates desquamation by solubilizing the intercellular cement that binds scales in the stratum corneum, thereby loosening the keratin. This keratolytic effect may provide an antifungal action because removal of the stratum corneum suppresses fungal growth; it also aids in the penetration of other antifungal agents. Salicylic acid also has a mild antiseptic action.

## Precautions to Consider

### Pregnancy/Reproduction
Pregnancy—Studies in humans have not been done; however, salicylic acid may be systemically absorbed. There is concern regarding the possibility of the premature closure of the ductus arteriosis.

Studies in rats and monkeys have shown that salicylic acid causes teratogenic effects. The oral dose given to monkeys may represent 6 times the maximum daily human dose of salicylic acid (as supplied in 28 grams of 6% salicylic acid gel) when applied topically over a large body surface.

FDA Pregnancy Category C.

### Breast-feeding
Problems in humans have not been documented; however, salicylic acid may be systemically absorbed.

### Pediatrics
Appropriate studies on the relationship of age to the effects of this medicine have not been performed in the pediatric population. However, young children may be at increased risk of toxicity because of increased absorption of salicylic acid through the skin and the increased ratio of total body surface area to treated area. In addition, young children may have a lower threshold for skin irritation from salicylic acid. Salicylic acid should not be applied to large areas of the body, for prolonged periods of time, or under occlusion to substantial areas.

### Geriatrics
Appropriate studies on the relationship of age to the effects of salicylic acid have not been performed in the geriatric population. However, elderly patients are more likely to have age-related peripheral vascular disease and, therefore, may be more prone to acute inflammation or ulceration of the extremities when they are treated with the 25 or 60% cream, 12 to 17% gel, 25 to 60% ointment, 12 to 50% plaster, and 5 to 27% topical solution.

### Drug interactions and/or related problems
The following drug interactions and/or related problems have been selected on the basis of their potential clinical significance (possible mechanism in parentheses where appropriate)—not necessarily inclusive (» = major clinical significance):

Note: Combinations containing any of the following medications, depending on the amount present, may also interact with this medication.

   Abrasive or medicated soaps or cleansers or
   Acne preparations or preparations containing a peeling agent such as
     Benzoyl peroxide
     Resorcinol
     Sulfur
     Tretinoin or
   Acne preparations, topical, other or
   Alcohol-containing preparations, topical such as
     After-shave lotions
     Astringents
     Perfumed toiletries
     Shaving creams or lotions or
   Cosmetics or soaps with a strong drying effect or
   Isotretinoin or
   Medicated cosmetics or "cover-ups"
     (concurrent use with salicylic acid may cause a cumulative irritant or drying effect, especially with the application of peeling, desquamating, or abrasive agents, resulting in excessive irritation of the skin)

### Medical considerations/Contraindications
The medical considerations/contraindications included here have been selected on the basis of their potential clinical significance (reasons given in parentheses where appropriate)—not necessarily inclusive (» = major clinical significance).

*Risk-benefit should be considered when the following medical problems exist:*

   Sensitivity to salicylic acid

*For 25 and 60% cream, 25 to 60% ointment, 12 to 50% plaster, 12 to 26% gel, and 5 to 27% topical solution*

   Diabetes mellitus or
   Peripheral vascular disease
     (acute inflammation or ulceration may occur, especially on the extremities)

   Inflammation, irritation, or infection of skin

## Side/Adverse Effects

Note: The treatment of warts using high concentrations of salicylic acid may cause skin erosion. This erosion may facilitate the spread of the warts.

The following side/adverse effects have been selected on the basis of their potential clinical significance (possible signs and symptoms in parentheses where appropriate)—not necessarily inclusive:

**Those indicating need for medical attention**
Incidence less frequent or rare
  *Skin irritation, moderate to severe, not present before therapy; skin ulceration or erosion*—especially when using medication with a high percentage of salicylic acid

**Those indicating need for medical attention only if they continue or are bothersome**
Incidence more frequent
  *Skin irritation, mild, not present before therapy; stinging*

## Overdose

For more information on the management of overdose or unintentional ingestion, **contact a Poison Control Center** (see *Poison Control Center Listing*).

**Clinical effects of overdose or salicylism**
The following effects have been selected on the basis of their potential clinical significance (possible signs and symptoms in parentheses where appropriate)—not necessarily inclusive:
  *Confusion; dizziness; headache, severe or continuing; rapid breathing; ringing or buzzing in ears, continuing*

## Patient Consultation

As an aid to patient consultation, refer to *Advice for the Patient, Salicylic Acid (Topical)*.

In providing consultation, consider emphasizing the following selected information (» = major clinical significance):

**Before using this medication**
» Conditions affecting use, especially:
    Sensitivity to salicylic acid
    Pregnancy—Medication may be absorbed through the skin; studies in animals have shown that salicylic acid causes birth defects when given orally in doses about 6 times the maximum daily human dose applied topically over a large body surface
    Use in children—Young children may be at increased risk of toxicity because of increased absorption of salicylic acid through the skin. Salicylic acid should not be applied to large areas of the body, for long periods of time, or under occlusion to substantial areas

**Proper use of this medication**
» Importance of using medication only as directed
    Proper use of occlusive dressing, if prescribed: Understanding exactly how to apply; using only as directed
» Avoiding contact with the eyes and other mucous membranes; if contact occurs, immediately flushing with water for 15 minutes
    Washing hands immediately after applying medication, unless hands are being treated
*Proper administration*
*For cream, lotion, or ointment dosage form*
    Applying enough to cover affected area; rubbing in gently
*For gel dosage form*
    Before using—Applying wet packs to affected area for at least 5 minutes
    Applying enough to cover affected area; rubbing in gently
*For pad dosage form*
    Wiping pad over affected area; not rinsing off medication after treatment
*For plaster dosage form*
    Reading patient instructions carefully before using medication
» Not using on irritated, inflamed, or infected skin, or if diabetic or have impaired blood circulation
» Not using on facial, genital, nasal, or oral warts; warts with hair growing from them; moles; or birthmarks
    Washing affected area and drying thoroughly; if treating warts, soaking warts in warm water for 5 minutes before drying
    Cutting plaster to fit wart, corn, or callus
    If treating corns or calluses, repeating application every 48 hours for up to 14 days; soaking corns or calluses in warm water for 5 minutes to assist in removal
    If treating warts, depending on product, either applying plaster and repeating every 48 hours or applying plaster at bedtime, leaving in place for at least 8 hours, removing in the morning, and repeating application every 24 hours; repeating application for up to 12 weeks
    Checking with doctor if discomfort increases during treatment or persists after treatment

*For shampoo dosage form*
    Before applying—Wetting hair and scalp with lukewarm water
    Applying enough to work up lather; rubbing well into scalp for 2 or 3 minutes; rinsing
    Applying again; rinsing thoroughly
*For soap dosage form*
    Working up lather with soap, using hot water
    Scrubbing entire affected area with a washcloth or facial sponge or mitt
    Using in a foot bath—Working up rich suds in hot water; soaking feet for 10 to 15 minutes; patting dry without rinsing
*For topical solution dosage form used for acne*
    Applying medication to cotton ball or pad; wiping over affected area; not rinsing off medication after treatment
*For topical solution dosage form used for corns, calluses, or warts*
    Reading patient instructions carefully before using medication
» Not using near heat or open flame or while smoking
» Not using on irritated, inflamed, or infected skin, or if diabetic or have impaired blood circulation
» Not using on facial, genital, nasal, or oral warts; warts with hair growing from them; moles; or birthmarks
    Avoiding inhalation of vapors
    Washing affected area and drying thoroughly; if treating warts, warts may be soaked in warm water for 5 minutes before drying
    Applying medication one drop at a time to sufficiently cover each wart, corn, or callus; letting dry
    If treating warts, repeating procedure once or twice daily for up to 12 weeks
    If treating corns or calluses, repeating procedure once or twice daily for up to 14 days
    Soaking corns and calluses in warm water for 5 minutes to assist in removal
    Checking with doctor if discomfort increases during treatment or persists after treatment
» Proper dosing
    Missed dose: Applying as soon as possible; not applying if almost time for next dose
» Proper storage

**Precautions while using this medication**
» Avoiding simultaneous use (at same site) with other topical acne preparations or preparations containing peeling agents, alcohol-containing preparations, abrasive soaps or cleansers, cosmetics or soaps with drying effect, medicated cosmetics, or other topical skin medication, unless otherwise directed by physician

**Side/adverse effects**
    Signs of potential side effects, especially skin irritation not present before therapy or symptoms of salicylism

## General Dosing Information

In young children, use is not recommended on large areas of the body, for prolonged periods of time, or under occlusion to sizable areas of the body.

**For the stronger strengths of salicylic acid, such as the 25 and 60% cream, 25 and 60% ointment, 12 to 50% plaster, 12 to 26% gel, and 5 to 27% topical solution**
These products are not recommended for use on irritated, inflamed, or infected skin; facial, genital, nasal, or oral warts; warts with hair growing from them; moles; or birthmarks. In addition, these products are not recommended for use on patients with diabetes mellitus or impaired blood circulation.

**For the gel dosage form**
Before application of the gel, wet packs should be applied to the affected areas for at least 5 minutes in order to enhance its effect.

The method of use usually preferred is application of the gel to the affected area with an occlusive dressing at night.

**For the 25 to 60% creams and ointments**
Application of these creams or ointments should be made only by a physician.

Caution should be used to avoid getting these creams or ointments on skin surrounding the area being treated.

Following application of these creams or ointments, an occlusive dressing is applied.

**For the 12 to 50% plaster dosage form**
The affected area should be washed and dried. Warts may be soaked in warm water for 5 minutes before drying.

The plaster should be cut to fit the wart, corn, or callus.

For corns and calluses: Application should be repeated every 48 hours as needed for up to 14 days until corn or callus is removed. The corn or callus may be soaked in warm water for 5 minutes to aid in removal.

For warts: Depending on the product, the plaster should either be applied every 48 hours or applied at bedtime, left in place for at least 8 hours, removed in the morning, and the application repeated every 24 hours. In either case, application should be repeated for up to 12 weeks until wart is removed.

### For the 5 to 27% topical solution dosage form for treatment of warts, corns, or calluses

The affected areas should be washed and dried. Warts may be soaked in warm water for 5 minutes before drying.

Medication should be applied one drop at a time to completely cover wart, corn, or callus.

Procedure should be repeated once or twice daily for up to 14 days for corns or calluses or up to 12 weeks for warts, until wart, corn, or callus is removed.

Corns and calluses may be soaked in water for 5 minutes to aid in removal.

## Topical Dosage Forms

### SALICYLIC ACID CREAM

**Usual adult and adolescent dose**
Keratolytic (topical)—
    Topical, to the skin, as a 2 to 10% cream.
Caustic—
    Topical, to the skin, as a 25 to 60% cream once every three to five days, under occlusion.

**Usual pediatric dose**
See *Usual adult and adolescent dose.*

**Strength(s) usually available**
U.S.—
    2% (OTC) [*Propa pH Medicated Acne Cream Maximum Strength*].
    3% (OTC) [*Antinea* (benzoic acid 6%)].
    10% (OTC) [*Calicylic Creme*].
    25% (Rx) [GENERIC].
    60% (Rx) [GENERIC].
Canada—
    Not commercially available.

**Packaging and storage**
Store below 40 °C (104 °F), preferably between 15 and 30 °C (59 and 86 °F), in a well-closed container, unless otherwise specified by manufacturer. Protect from freezing.

**Auxiliary labeling**
• For external use only.

### SALICYLIC ACID GEL USP

**Usual adult and adolescent dose**
Antiacne agent (topical)—
    Topical, to the skin, as a 0.5 to 5% gel once a day.
Antipsoriatic (topical)—
    Topical, to the skin, as a 5% gel once a day.
Keratolytic (topical)—
    Topical, to the skin, as a 5 to 26% gel once a day, preferably under occlusion.

**Usual pediatric dose**
See *Usual adult and adolescent dose.*

**Strength(s) usually available**
U.S.—
    0.5% (OTC) [*Noxzema Anti-Acne Gel*].
    5% (OTC) [*Saligel* (alcohol 14%)].
    6% [*Hydrisalic* (OTC); *Keralyt* (OTC) (alcohol 19.4%); *Keratex Gel* (Rx)].
    12% (Rx) [*Viranol* (alcohol)].
    17% (OTC) [*Compound W Gel*].
    26% (Rx) [*Viranol Ultra* (alcohol)].
Canada—
    10% (OTC) [*Cuplex Gel*].
    17% (OTC) [*Compound W Gel*].

**Packaging and storage**
Store below 40 °C (104 °F), preferably between 15 and 30 °C (59 and 86 °F), unless otherwise specified by manufacturer. Store in a tight container. Protect from freezing.

**Auxiliary labeling**
• For external use only.

### SALICYLIC ACID LOTION

**Usual adult and adolescent dose**
Antiacne agent (topical)—
    Topical, to the skin, as a 1 to 2% lotion one to three times a day.
Antiseborrheic or
Keratolytic (topical)—
    Topical, to the scalp, as a 1.8 to 2% lotion one or two times a day.

**Usual pediatric dose**
See *Usual adult and adolescent dose.*

**Strength(s) usually available**
U.S.—
    1% (OTC) [*Oxy Night Watch Sensitive Skin Lotion* (cetyl alcohol; stearyl alcohol)].
    1.8% (OTC) [*Sebucare*].
    2% (OTC) [*Listerex Golden Scrub Lotion; Listerex Herbal Scrub Lotion; Oxy Night Watch Maximum Strength Lotion* (cetyl alcohol; stearyl alcohol)].
Canada—
    1% (OTC) [*Oxy Night Watch Night Time Acne Medication Regular Strength Lotion*].
    2% (OTC) [*Oxy Night Watch Night Time Acne Medication Extra Strength Lotion; Oxy Sensitive Skin Vanishing Formula Lotion*].

**Packaging and storage**
Store below 40 °C (104 °F), preferably between 15 and 30 °C (59 and 86 °F), in a tight container, unless otherwise specified by manufacturer. Protect from freezing.

**Auxiliary labeling**
• For external use only.
• Keep container tightly closed.

### SALICYLIC ACID OINTMENT

**Usual adult and adolescent dose**
Antiacne agent (topical)—
    Topical, to the skin, as a 3 to 6% ointment.
Antipsoriatic (topical) or
Antiseborrheic or
Keratolytic (topical)—
    Topical, to the skin, as a 3 to 10% ointment.
Caustic—
    Topical, to the skin, as a 25 to 60% ointment once every three to five days, under occlusion.

**Usual pediatric dose**
See *Usual adult and adolescent dose.*

**Strength(s) usually available**
U.S.—
    25% (Rx) [*Salacid*].
    40% (Rx) [*Salonil*].
    60% (Rx) [*Salacid*].
    Note: Other strengths are currently not commercially available; compounding required for prescriptions.
Canada—
    Not commercially available. Compounding required for prescriptions.

**Packaging and storage**
Store below 40 °C (104 °F), preferably between 15 and 30 °C (59 and 86 °F), in a well-closed container, unless otherwise specified by manufacturer. Protect from freezing.

**Auxiliary labeling**
• For external use only.

### SALICYLIC ACID PADS

**Usual adult and adolescent dose**
Antiacne agent (topical)—
    Topical, to the skin, as a 0.5 to 2% pad one to three times a day.

**Usual pediatric dose**
See *Usual adult and adolescent dose.*

**Strength(s) usually available**
U.S.—
    0.5% (OTC) [*Noxzema Anti-Acne Pads Regular Strength; Oxy Clean Medicated Pads Regular Strength* (alcohol 40%); *Oxy Clean Medicated Pads Sensitive Skin* (alcohol 22%); *Propa pH Medicated Cleansing Pads Sensitive Skin* (alcohol 25%); *Stri-Dex Dual Textured Pads Regular Strength* (alcohol 28%); *Stri-Dex Dual Textured Pads Sensitive Skin* (alcohol 25%); *Stri-Dex Regular Strength Pads* (alcohol 28%)].
    1% (OTC) [*Clear by Design Medicated Cleansing Pads* (alcohol 29%)].

1.25% (OTC) [*Clearasil Double Textured Pads Regular Strength* (alcohol 40%)].

2% (OTC) [*Clearasil Double Textured Pads Maximum Strength* (alcohol 40%); *Noxzema Anti-Acne Pads Maximum Strength; Oxy Clean Medicated Pads Maximum Strength* (alcohol 50%); *Propa pH Medicated Cleansing Pads Maximum Strength* (alcohol 40%); *Stri-Dex Dual Textured Pads Maximum Strength* (alcohol 44%); *Stri-Dex Maximum Strength Pads* (alcohol 44%); *Stri-Dex Super Scrub Pads* (alcohol 50%)].

Canada—

0.5% (OTC) [*Oxy Clean Regular Strength Medicated Pads* (alcohol 40%); *Oxy Clean Sensitive Skin Pads* (alcohol 22%)].

2% (OTC) [*Oxy Clean Extra Strength Medicated Pads* (alcohol 50%)].

### Packaging and storage

Store below 40 °C (104 °F), preferably between 15 and 30 °C (59 and 86 °F), in a well-closed container, unless otherwise specified by manufacturer. Protect from freezing.

### Auxiliary labeling
• For external use only.

## SALICYLIC ACID PLASTER USP

### Usual adult and adolescent dose
Caustic or

Keratolytic (topical)—

Topical, to the skin, as a 12 to 50% plaster every other day or every day.

### Usual pediatric dose
See *Usual adult and adolescent dose.*

### Strength(s) usually available
U.S.—

15% (Rx) [*Trans-Ver-Sal*].

21% (Rx) [*Trans-Plantar*].

40% (OTC) [*Clear Away; Mediplast*].

50% (Rx) [*Sal-Acid Plaster*].

Canada—

15% (OTC) [*Trans-Ver-Sal*].

Note: Other strengths are currently not commercially available.

### Packaging and storage

Store below 40 °C (104 °F), preferably between 15 and 30 °C (59 and 86 °F), in a well-closed container, unless otherwise specified by manufacturer.

### Auxiliary labeling
• For external use only.

## SALICYLIC ACID SHAMPOO

### Usual adult and adolescent dose
Antiseborrheic or

Keratolytic (topical)—

Topical, to the scalp, as a 2 to 4% shampoo one or two times a week.

### Usual pediatric dose
See *Usual adult and adolescent dose.*

### Strength(s) usually available
U.S.—

2% (OTC) [*Ionil Plus Shampoo; Ionil Shampoo* (alcohol 12%; benzalkonium chloride); *P&S; Sal-Clens Plus Shampoo*].

4% (OTC) [*Sal-Clens Shampoo; X-Seb*].

Canada—

Not commercially available.

### Packaging and storage

Store below 40 °C (104 °F), preferably between 15 and 30 °C (59 and 86 °F), in a well-closed container, unless otherwise specified by manufacturer. Protect from freezing.

### Auxiliary labeling
• Shake well.
• For external use only.

## SALICYLIC ACID SOAP

### Usual adult and adolescent dose
Antiacne agent (topical) or

Keratolytic (topical)—

Topical, to the skin, as a 2 to 3.5% soap.

### Usual pediatric dose
See *Usual adult and adolescent dose.*

### Strength(s) usually available
U.S.—

2% (OTC) [*Buf-Puf Acne Cleansing Bar with Vitamin E; Salac*].

3.5% (OTC) [GENERIC].

Canada—

2% (OTC) [*Salac; Tersac Cleansing Gel*].

3.5% (OTC) [*Oxy Clean Medicated Soap*].

### Packaging and storage

Store below 40 °C (104 °F), preferably between 15 and 30 °C (59 and 86 °F), unless otherwise specified by manufacturer. Protect from freezing.

### Auxiliary labeling
• For external use only.

## SALICYLIC ACID TOPICAL SOLUTION

### Usual adult and adolescent dose
Antiacne agent (topical)—

Topical to the skin, as a 0.5 to 2% solution up to three times a day.

Keratolytic (topical)—

For warts: Topical, to the skin, as a 5 to 27% solution one or two times a day.

For corns and calluses: Topical, to the skin, as a 12 to 27% solution one or two times a day.

### Usual pediatric dose
See *Usual adult and adolescent dose.*

### Strength(s) usually available
U.S.—

0.5% (OTC) [*Clearasil Medicated Deep Cleanser Topical Solution* (alcohol 43%); *Oxy Clean Medicated Cleanser* (alcohol 40%); *Propa pH Perfectly Clear Skin Cleanser Topical Solution Normal/ Combination Skin* (alcohol 25%); *Propa pH Perfectly Clear Skin Cleanser Topical Solution Sensitive Skin Formula* (alcohol 25%)].

0.6% (OTC) [*Propa pH Perfectly Clear Skin Cleanser Topical Solution Oily Skin* (alcohol 51.21%)].

1.25% (OTC) [*Clearasil Clearstick Regular Strength Topical Solution* (alcohol 40%)].

1.4% (OTC) [*Ionax Astringent Skin Cleanser Topical Solution* (isopropyl alcohol; acetone)].

2% (OTC) [*Clearasil Clearstick Maximum Strength Topical Solution*].

13.6% (OTC) [*Freezone* (alcohol 20.5%)].

16.7% (Rx) [*Duofilm; Gordofilm; Lactisol* (lactic acid 16.7%); *Salactic Film Topical Solution; Viranol*].

17% [*Compound W Liquid* (OTC); *Occlusal Topical Solution* (OTC) (alcohol 20%); *Off-Ezy Topical Solution Corn & Callus Remover Kit* (OTC) (alcohol 21%); *Off-Ezy Topical Solution Wart Removal Kit* (OTC) (alcohol 21%); *Paplex* (Rx); *Verukan Topical Solution* (Rx) (lactic acid 17%; flexible collodion); *Wart-Off Topical Solution* (OTC) (alcohol 26.35%)].

26% (Rx) [*Occlusal-HP Topical Solution; Paplex Ultra; Verukan-HP Topical Solution* (flexible collodion)].

27% (Rx) [*Duoplant Topical Solution* (alcohol 50%); *Sal-Plant Gel Topical Solution* (alcohol; lactic acid; flexible collodion)].

Canada—

0.5% (OTC) [*Oxy Clean Regular Strength Medicated Cleanser Topical Solution* (alcohol 40%); *Oxy Clean Sensitive Skin Cleanser Topical Solution* (alcohol 22%)].

2% (OTC) [*Oxy Clean Extra Strength Skin Cleanser Topical Solution* (alcohol 50%)].

17% (OTC) [*Compound W Liquid; Occlusal Topical Solution*].

26% (Rx) [*Occlusal-HP Topical Solution*].

Note: Other strengths are currently not commercially available.

### Packaging and storage

Store between 15 and 30 °C (59 and 86 °F), in a tight container, unless otherwise specified by manufacturer.

### Auxiliary labeling
• Flammable.
• For external use only.

Revised: 07/26/93

---

# SALICYLIC ACID–CONTAINING COMBINATIONS—

Salicylic Acid and Sulfur (Topical)

Salicylic Acid, Sulfur, and Coal Tar (Topical)

# SALICYLIC ACID AND SULFUR   Topical

VA CLASSIFICATION (Primary/Secondary):
Cleansing Cream—DE500/DE752
Lotion—DE500/DE752
Cleansing Lotion—DE500/DE752
Cream Shampoo—DE500/DE900
Lotion Shampoo—DE500/DE900
Suspension Shampoo—DE500/DE900
Bar Soap—DE500/DE752
Cleansing Suspension—DE500/DE752
Topical Suspension—DE500/DE752

**NOTE:** The *Salicylic Acid and Sulfur (Topical)* monograph is maintained on the USP DI electronic data base. For a printed copy of the most recent revision of the complete monograph, contact the USP Division of Information Development, 12601 Twinbrook Parkway, Rockville, MD 20852.

For information on the specific components of this combination, see the *USP DI* monographs for *Salicylic Acid (Topical)* and *Sulfur (Topical)*.

The information that follows is selectively abstracted from the complete monograph and is provided to facilitate drug use review and patient counseling.

Note: For a listing of dosage forms and brand names by country availability, see *Dosage Forms* section(s). For a listing of brand names for the articles in this monograph, refer to the General Index.

## Category

Keratolytic (topical)—Salicylic Acid and Sulfur.
Antiacne agent (topical)—Salicylic Acid and Sulfur Cleansing Cream; Salicylic Acid and Sulfur Lotion; Salicylic Acid and Sulfur Cleansing Lotion; Salicylic Acid and Sulfur Bar Soap; Salicylic Acid and Sulfur Cleansing Suspension; Salicylic Acid and Sulfur Topical Suspension.
Antiseborrheic—Salicylic Acid and Sulfur Cream Shampoo; Salicylic Acid and Sulfur Lotion Shampoo; Salicylic Acid and Sulfur Suspension Shampoo.

## Indications

**Accepted**

Acne vulgaris (treatment) or
Oily skin (treatment)—Salicylic acid and sulfur combination (cleansing cream, lotion, cleansing lotion, bar soap, cleansing suspension, and topical suspension) is indicated for the treatment of acne and oily skin.

Dandruff (treatment) or
Dermatitis, seborrheic, of scalp (treatment)—Salicylic acid and sulfur shampoo is indicated for the temporary control of scaling and itching associated with dandruff and seborrheic dermatitis of the scalp.

## Patient Consultation

As an aid to patient consultation, refer to *Advice for the Patient, Salicylic Acid and Sulfur (Topical).*

In providing consultation, consider emphasizing the following selected information (» = major clinical significance):

**Before using this medication**
» Conditions affecting use, especially:
    Sensitivity to salicylic acid or sulfur
    Use in children—Young children may be at increased risk of toxicity because of increased absorption of salicylic acid through the skin

**Proper use of this medication**
» Importance of not using more medication than the amount recommended
    Washing hands immediately after application to remove any medication that may be on them
» Avoiding contact with the eyes
*Proper administration*
*For cleanser dosage forms*
    After wetting skin—Applying medication with fingertips or a wet sponge; rubbing in gently to work up lather; rinsing thoroughly and patting dry
*For lotion and topical suspension dosage form*
    Applying small amount to affected area; rubbing in gently
*For shampoo dosage form*
    Wetting hair and scalp with lukewarm water

Applying enough to work up lather; rubbing into scalp
Continuing to rub lather into scalp for several minutes or allowing to remain on scalp for about 5 minutes, depending on product
Applying medication again; rinsing thoroughly
*For bar soap dosage form*
    After wetting skin—Using to wash face and other affected areas; rinsing thoroughly; patting dry

» Proper dosing
    Missed dose: Using as soon as possible; not using if almost time for next dose
» Proper storage

**Precautions while using this medication**
» Avoiding simultaneous use with other topical acne preparations or preparations containing peeling agents, alcohol-containing preparations, abrasive soaps or cleansers, cosmetics or soaps with drying effect, medicated cosmetics, or other topical skin medication, unless otherwise directed by physician
» Avoiding concurrent use with topical mercury-containing preparations
    Caution if medications containing aspirin or other salicylates are used

**Side/adverse effects**
Signs of potential side effects, especially skin irritation not present before therapy

## Topical Dosage Forms

### SALICYLIC ACID AND SULFUR CLEANSING CREAM

**Usual adult and adolescent dose**
Antiacne agent (topical)—
    Topical, to the skin two or three times a day.

**Usual pediatric dose**
See *Usual adult and adolescent dose.*

**Strength(s) usually available**
U.S.—
    2% salicylic acid and 2% sulfur (OTC) [*Fostex Regular Strength Medicated Cleansing Cream*].
Canada—
    2% salicylic acid and 2% sulfur (OTC) [*Fostex Medicated Cleansing Cream*].
Note: *Fostex Regular Strength Medicated Cleansing Cream* and *Fostex Medicated Cleansing Cream* are used to treat face and scalp.

**Auxiliary labeling**
• For external use only.

### SALICYLIC ACID AND SULFUR LOTION

**Usual adult and adolescent dose**
Antiacne agent (topical)—
    Topical, to the skin, one or two times a day.

**Usual pediatric dose**
See *Usual adult and adolescent dose.*

**Strength(s) usually available**
U.S.—
    1.5% salicylic acid and 4% sulfur (OTC) [*Night Cast Regular Formula Mask-lotion* (alcohol 33%)].
    2% salicylic acid and 2% colloidal sulfur (OTC) [*Sebasorb Liquid*].
    2% salicylic acid and 3% sulfur (OTC) [*Acno*].
    25% salicylic acid and 8% sulfur (OTC) [*Acnotex* (isopropyl alcohol 22%; acetone; methylbenzethonium chloride)].
Canada—
    1.5% salicylic acid and 4% sulfur (OTC) [*Night Cast R*].

**Auxiliary labeling**
• Shake well.
• For external use only.

### SALICYLIC ACID AND SULFUR CLEANSING LOTION

**Usual adult and adolescent dose**
Antiacne agent (topical)—
    Topical, to the skin, one to three times a day.

**Usual pediatric dose**
See *Usual adult and adolescent dose.*

**Strength(s) usually available**
U.S.—
   1.5% salicylic acid and 2% sulfur (OTC) [*Pernox Lemon Medicated Scrub Cleanser; Pernox Regular Medicated Scrub Cleanser*].
   1.6% salicylic acid and 1.6% sulfur (OTC) [*Sastid (AL) Scrub* (aluminum oxide 20%); *Sastid Plain Shampoo and Acne Wash*].
Canada—
   1.5% salicylic acid and 2% sulfur (OTC) [*Pernox Lemon Medicated Scrub Cleanser; Pernox Regular Medicated Scrub Cleanser*].

**Auxiliary labeling**
• Shake well.
• For external use only.

## SALICYLIC ACID AND SULFUR CREAM SHAMPOO

**Usual adult and adolescent dose**
Antiseborrheic—
   Topical, to the scalp, one or two times a week or as needed.

**Usual pediatric dose**
See *Usual adult and adolescent dose.*

**Strength(s) usually available**
U.S.—
   1% salicylic acid and 2% sulfur (OTC) [*Vanseb Cream Dandruff Shampoo*].
   2% salicylic acid and 2% sulfur (OTC) [*Creamy SS Shampoo; Fostex Regular Strength Medicated Cleansing Cream; Sebulex Cream Medicated Shampoo*].
Canada—
   2% salicylic acid and 2% sulfur (OTC) [*Fostex Medicated Cleansing Cream*].
Note: *Fostex Regular Strength Medicated Cleansing Cream* and *Fostex Medicated Cleansing Cream* are used to treat face and scalp.

**Auxiliary labeling**
• For external use only.

## SALICYLIC ACID AND SULFUR LOTION SHAMPOO

**Usual adult and adolescent dose**
See *Salicylic Acid and Sulfur Cream Shampoo.*

**Usual pediatric dose**
See *Usual adult and adolescent dose.*

**Strength(s) usually available**
U.S.—
   1% salicylic acid and 2% sulfur (OTC) [*Vanseb Lotion Dandruff Shampoo*].
   1.6% salicylic acid and 1.6% sulfur (OTC) [*Sastid Plain Shampoo and Acne Wash*].
Canada—
   2% salicylic acid and 2% sulfur (OTC) [*Sebulex Lotion Shampoo*].

**Auxiliary labeling**
• Shake well.
• For external use only.

## SALICYLIC ACID AND SULFUR SUSPENSION SHAMPOO

**Usual adult and adolescent dose**
See *Salicylic Acid and Sulfur Cream Shampoo.*

**Usual pediatric dose**
See *Usual adult and adolescent dose.*

**Strength(s) usually available**
U.S.—
   2% salicylic acid and 2% colloidal sulfur (OTC) [*Sebex*].
   2% salicylic acid and 2% sulfur (OTC) [*Sebulex Antiseborrheic Treatment and Conditioning Shampoo; Sebulex Antiseborrheic Treatment Shampoo; Sebulex Medicated Dandruff Shampoo with Conditioners; Sebulex Regular Medicated Dandruff Shampoo*].
   3% salicylic acid and 5% sulfur (OTC) [*Meted Maximum Strength Anti-Dandruff Shampoo with Conditioners*].

Canada—
   2% salicylic acid and 2% sulfur (OTC) [*Sebulex Conditioning Suspension Shampoo; Sebulex Medicated Shampoo*].
   3% salicylic acid and 5% sulfur (OTC) [*Meted Maximum Strength Anti-Dandruff Shampoo with Conditioners*].

**Auxiliary labeling**
• Shake well.
• For external use only.

## SALICYLIC ACID AND SULFUR BAR SOAP

**Usual adult and adolescent dose**
Antiacne agent (topical)—
   Topical, to the skin, two or three times a day.

**Usual pediatric dose**
See *Usual adult and adolescent dose.*

**Strength(s) usually available**
U.S.—
   2% salicylic acid and 2% sulfur (OTC) [*Aveeno Cleansing Bar* (colloidal oatmeal 50%); *Fostex Regular Strength Medicated Cleansing Bar*].
   3% salicylic acid and 10% precipitated sulfur (OTC) [*Sastid Soap*; GENERIC].
Canada—
   2% salicylic acid and 2% sulfur (OTC) [*Aveeno Acne Bar* (colloidal oatmeal); *Fostex Medicated Cleansing Bar*].
   3% salicylic acid and 5% colloidal sulfur (OTC) [*Sulsal Soap*].
   3% salicylic acid and 10% precipitated sulfur (OTC) [*Sastid Soap*].

**Auxiliary labeling**
• For external use only.

## SALICYLIC ACID AND SULFUR CLEANSING SUSPENSION

**Usual adult and adolescent dose**
See *Salicylic Acid and Sulfur Lotion.*

**Usual pediatric dose**
See *Usual adult and adolescent dose.*

**Strength(s) usually available**
U.S.—
   1.5% salicylic acid and 2% sulfur (OTC) [*Pernox Lotion Lathering Abradant Scrub Cleanser*].
   2% salicylic acid and 2% sulfur (OTC) [*Pernox Lotion Lathering Scrub Cleanser*].
Canada—
   2% salicylic acid and 2% sulfur (OTC) [*Fostex Medicated Cleansing Liquid*].

**Auxiliary labeling**
• Shake well.
• For external use only.

## SALICYLIC ACID AND SULFUR TOPICAL SUSPENSION

**Usual adult and adolescent dose**
See *Salicylic Acid and Sulfur Lotion.*

**Usual pediatric dose**
See *Usual adult and adolescent dose.*

**Strength(s) usually available**
U.S.—
   2.35% salicylic acid and 4% sulfur (OTC) [*Therac Lotion*].
Canada—
   Not commercially available.

**Auxiliary labeling**
• Shake well.
• For external use only.

Revised: 07/26/93

# SALICYLIC ACID, SULFUR, AND COAL TAR    Topical

**VA CLASSIFICATION (Primary/Secondary): DE500/DE900; DE802**
**NOTE:** The *Salicylic Acid, Sulfur, and Coal Tar (Topical)* monograph is maintained on the USP DI electronic data base. For a printed copy of the most recent revision of the complete monograph, contact the USP Division of Information Development, 12601 Twinbrook Parkway, Rockville, MD 20852.

For information on the specific components of this combination, see the *USP DI* monographs for *Coal Tar (Topical)*, *Salicylic Acid (Topical)*, and *Sulfur (Topical)*.

The information that follows is selectively abstracted from the complete monograph and is provided to facilitate drug use review and patient counseling.

Note: For a listing of dosage forms and brand names by country availability, see *Dosage Forms* section(s). For a listing of brand names for the articles in this monograph, refer to the General Index.

## Category
Keratolytic (topical); antiseborrheic; antipsoriatic (topical).

## Indications

### Accepted
Dandruff (treatment) or

Dermatitis, seborrheic, of scalp (treatment)—Salicylic acid, sulfur, and coal tar cream shampoo and lotion shampoo are indicated as adjuncts in the treatment of dandruff and seborrheic dermatitis to relieve itching and scaling of the scalp.

Psoriasis, of scalp (treatment)—Salicylic acid, sulfur, and coal tar cream shampoo and lotion shampoo are indicated in the treatment of psoriasis to relieve itching and scaling of the scalp.

## Patient Consultation
As an aid to patient consultation, refer to *Advice for the Patient, Salicylic Acid, Sulfur, and Coal Tar (Topical)*.

In providing consultation, consider emphasizing the following selected information (» = major clinical significance):

### Before using this medication
» Conditions affecting use, especially:

Sensitivity to salicylic acid, sulfur, or coal tar

Use in children—Children may be at increased risk of toxicity because of increased absorption of salicylic acid through the skin

### Proper use of this medication
» Importance of not using more medication than the amount recommended

» Avoiding contact with the eyes

Washing hands immediately after application to remove any medication that may be on them

*Proper administration*

Before using—Wetting hair and scalp with lukewarm water

Applying a generous amount to scalp; working up a rich lather

Rubbing lather into scalp for 5 minutes; rinsing

Applying medication again; rinsing thoroughly

» Proper dosing

Missed dose: Using as soon as possible; not using if almost time for next dose

» Proper storage

### Precautions while using this medication
» Avoiding concurrent use with topical mercury-containing preparations

Medication may temporarily discolor blond, bleached, or tinted hair

### Side/adverse effects
Signs of potential side effects, especially skin irritation not present before therapy

## Topical Dosage Forms

### SALICYLIC ACID, SULFUR, AND COAL TAR CREAM SHAMPOO

#### Usual adult and adolescent dose
Dandruff

Psoriasis of scalp

Seborrheic dermatitis of scalp—

Topical, to the scalp, one or two times a week or as needed.

#### Usual pediatric dose
See *Usual adult and adolescent dose.*

#### Strength(s) usually available
U.S.—

1% salicylic acid, 2% sulfur, and 5% coal tar solution (OTC) [*Vanseb-T*].

2% salicylic acid, 2% sulfur, and 0.5% coal tar (OTC) [*Sebutone*].

Canada—

Not commercially available.

#### Auxiliary labeling
• For external use only.

### SALICYLIC ACID, SULFUR, AND COAL TAR LOTION SHAMPOO

#### Usual adult and adolescent dose
See *Salicylic Acid, Sulfur, and Coal Tar Cream Shampoo.*

#### Usual pediatric dose
See *Usual adult and adolescent dose.*

#### Strength(s) usually available
U.S.—

1% salicylic acid, 2% sulfur, and 5% coal tar solution (OTC) [*Vanseb-T*].

2% salicylic acid, 2% sulfur, and 0.5% coal tar (OTC) [*Sebutone*].

2% salicylic acid, 2% colloidal sulfur, and 5% coal tar solution (OTC) [*Sebex-T Tar Shampoo*].

Canada—

2% salicylic acid, 2% sulfur, and 0.5% coal tar (OTC) [*Sebutone*].

#### Auxiliary labeling
• Shake well.

• For external use only.

Revised: 07/26/93

# SALMETEROL　Inhalation-Local

VA CLASSIFICATION (Primary): RE102

Note: For a listing of dosage forms and brand names by country availability, see *Dosage Forms* section(s). For a listing of brand names for the articles in this monograph, refer to the General Index.

## Category
Bronchodilator.

## Indications

### Accepted
Asthma, bronchial, chronic (treatment)—Salmeterol is indicated to prevent bronchospasm and reduce the frequency of acute asthma attacks in patients with chronic asthma, including those patients with symptoms of nocturnal asthma, who are receiving optimal treatment with anti-inflammatory medication and still require regular treatment with an inhaled short-acting beta-adrenergic bronchodilator.

Bronchospasm, exercise-induced (prophylaxis)[1]—Salmeterol is indicated for prevention of exercise-induced bronchospasm.

### Unaccepted
*Salmeterol is not indicated for the treatment of acute or breakthrough asthma symptoms when rapid bronchodilation is needed* because of its slower onset of action compared to shorter-acting beta-adrenergic bronchodilators.

Salmeterol therapy *should not be initiated* in patients with significantly worsening or acutely deteriorating asthma.

[1]Not included in Canadian product labeling.

## Pharmacology/Pharmacokinetics

### Physicochemical characteristics
Molecular weight—603.8.

### Mechanism of action/Effect
Salmeterol produces its bronchodilating effect by stimulating beta-2-adrenergic receptors in the lungs to relax bronchial smooth muscle, thereby relieving bronchospasm, increasing vital capacity, decreasing residual volume, and reducing airway resistance. This action is believed to result from increased production of cyclic adenosine 3, 5-monophosphate (cyclic 3, 5-AMP; c-AMP) caused by activation of the enzyme that catalyzes the conversion of adenosine triphosphate (ATP) to c-AMP. In addition to relaxing bronchial smooth muscle, c-AMP inhibits release of mediators of immediate hypersensitivity from cells, especially mast cells.

### Other actions/effects
*In vitro* tests using human lung fragments and *in vivo* studies conducted in guinea pigs demonstrate that salmeterol has long-lasting inhibitory

effects on several inflammatory response mediators. Any potential anti-inflammatory effect of salmeterol in asthmatics is inferred from a small number of patients in allergen challenge studies. The exact mechanism of this effect and its clinical relevance are not clear.

### Absorption
Salmeterol acts locally in the lungs following inhalation. The resulting plasma concentrations are low or undetectable and are not predictive of therapeutic effect. The medication does not accumulate with repeated doses.

### Onset of action
Approximately 15 to 20 minutes; median time of onset reported in clinical trials varied from 10 to 25 minutes.

### Time to peak effect
3 to 4 hours; however, approximately 80% of the maximal increase in forced expiratory volume in 1 second (FEV$_1$) occurs within 1 hour after administration.

### Duration of action
Approximately 12 hours

Note: It is believed that the sustained pharmacological action of salmeterol is due to its lipophilicity and long $N$-substituted side chain. The side chain is thought to bind to the exo-site, an area in the beta-2-receptor adjacent to the active site. The phenylethanolamine portion of the salmeterol molecule is then in position to associate with and dissociate from the receptor's active site. This theory is supported by the fact that the pharmacologic effect of salmeterol *in vitro* is rapidly and completely reversed by beta-receptor antagonism and resumes once the antagonist is removed.

## Precautions to Consider

### Carcinogenicity/Tumorigenicity
An 18-month study in mice showed that salmeterol, administered orally in doses that provided 9 and 63 times the human exposure (based on comparison of area under the concentration-time curves [AUCs]), caused a dose-related increase in the incidences of smooth muscle hyperplasia, cystic glandular hyperplasia, leiomyomas of the uterus, and ovarian cysts.

A 24-month study in rats given salmeterol orally and by inhalation in doses approximately 55 and 215 times, respectively, the recommended human clinical dose based on mg per square meter of body surface area (mg/m²) showed dose-related increases in the incidences of mesovarian leiomyomas and ovarian cysts. Similar results have been reported with other beta-adrenergic bronchodilators. The relevance of these results to human use is unknown.

Salmeterol produced no significant carcinogenic effects in mice receiving doses that provided 1.3 times the human exposure based on AUC comparison, or in rats given 15 times the recommended human clinical dose based on mg/m².

### Mutagenicity
Salmeterol was not mutagenic in *in vitro* tests in microbial or mammalian genes or in human lymphocytes or in an *in vivo* rat micronucleus test.

### Pregnancy/Reproduction
Fertility—Reproduction studies in rats given oral salmeterol at doses up to approximately 160 times the recommended human clinical dose based on mg/m² showed no effects on fertility.

Pregnancy—Adequate and well-controlled studies have not been done in humans.

In rats, maternal exposure to salmeterol at doses up to approximately 160 times the recommended human clinical dose based on mg/m² produced no significant effects. However, Dutch rabbit fetuses exposed to high concentrations of salmeterol *in utero* developed effects considered to be characteristic of beta-adrenergic stimulation (i.e., precocious eyelid openings, cleft palate, sternebral fusion, limb and paw flexures, and delayed ossification of the frontal cranial bones). No significant effects occurred at 12 times the recommended human clinical dose based on AUC comparisons. In New Zealand rabbits, exposure to oral doses approximately 1600 times the recommended human clinical dose based on mg/m² produced only delayed ossification of frontal bones. There is no evidence that these beta-agonist effects in animals are relevant to human use.

FDA Pregnancy Category C.

Labor—No well-controlled studies have investigated the effects of salmeterol on preterm or term labor in humans; however, other beta-adrenergic agonists have been shown to decrease uterine contractions when administered systemically.

### Breast-feeding
It is not known whether salmeterol is distributed into the breast milk of humans; however, salmeterol is distributed into the milk of lactating rats in concentrations similar to those in plasma.

### Pediatrics
A limited number of children 4 to 12 years of age have been safely treated with salmeterol in clinical trials; however, the safety and efficacy of salmeterol in children younger than 12 years of age have not been established.

### Geriatrics
Clinical studies have been conducted in 241 patients 65 years of age and older. No apparent differences in the efficacy and safety of salmeterol were observed in these patients compared with younger patients.

### Drug interactions and/or related problems
The following drug interactions and/or related problems have been selected on the basis of their potential clinical significance (possible mechanism in parentheses where appropriate)—not necessarily inclusive (» = major clinical significance):

Note: Combinations containing any of the following medications, depending on the amount present, may also interact with this medication.

Because salmeterol is selective for beta-2-adrenoceptors and produces low systemic concentrations following inhalation, drug interactions known to occur with sympathomimetics as a class, especially with those possessing alpha-adrenoceptor activity, are unlikely to occur with use of salmeterol at recommended doses.

» Beta-adrenergic blocking agents, including ophthalmic agents
  (concurrent use with salmeterol may result in mutual inhibition of therapeutic effects; beta-blockade may antagonize the bronchodilating effect of salmeterol; although agents with beta-1-selectivity may be less antagonistic, extreme caution is recommended if these agents are used in patients with bronchospasm)

### Laboratory value alterations
The following have been selected on the basis of their potential clinical significance (possible effect in parentheses where appropriate)—not necessarily inclusive (» = major clinical significance):

With physiology/laboratory test values
  Electrocardiogram
    (minor or non-specific T-wave changes and prolongation of QT$_c$ interval reported rarely, at salmeterol doses about 8 times the recommended dose)

  Glucose, blood
    (concentrations may be increased, possibly due to glycogenolysis; clinically significant changes occurred rarely with recommended doses of salmeterol but may be more pronounced with frequent use of higher doses or an overdose)

  Potassium, serum
    (concentrations may be decreased, possibly through intracellular shunting; the decrease is dose-related, is usually transient, and may not require supplementation; clinically significant decreases occurred rarely with recommended doses of salmeterol in long-term clinical trials; effects may be more pronounced with frequent use of higher doses or an overdose)

### Medical considerations/Contraindications
The medical considerations/contraindications included here have been selected on the basis of their potential clinical significance (reasons given in parentheses where appropriate)—not necessarily inclusive (» = major clinical significance).

*Risk-benefit should be considered when the following medical problems exist:*

» Cardiac arrhythmias or
» Coronary insufficiency or
  Hyperthyroidism, not optimally controlled or
  Pheochromocytoma, diagnosed or suspected
    (signs or symptoms of excessive beta-adrenergic stimulation more likely to occur)
» Sensitivity to salmeterol or any aerosol component

### Patient monitoring
The following may be especially important in patient monitoring (other tests may be warranted in some patients, depending on condition; » = major clinical significance):

  Pulmonary function monitoring
    (recommended at periodic intervals as a guide to patient management)

## Side/Adverse Effects

Note: Fatalities have been reported in association with excessive use of inhaled sympathomimetics. The exact cause of death is unknown; however, cardiac arrest following development of a severe acute asthmatic crisis and subsequent hypoxia is suspected. Whether the fatalities are associated with disease severity, substandard quality of care, and/or patient noncompliance has not been established.

The following side/adverse effects have been selected on the basis of their potential clinical significance (possible signs and symptoms in parentheses where appropriate)—not necessarily inclusive:

**Those indicating need for medical attention**
Incidence rare
>*Bronchospasm, paradoxical or hypersensitivity-induced* (shortness of breath; troubled breathing; tightness in chest; wheezing); *dermatitis, hypersensitivity-induced* (angioedema [swelling of face, lips, or eyelids]); *skin rash; urticaria* (hives)

**Those indicating need for medical attention only if they continue or are bothersome**
Incidence more frequent (>3%)
>*Headache*

Incidence less frequent (1 to 3%)
>*Abdominal pain; cough; diarrhea; muscle cramps or soreness; nausea; nervousness; palpitations* (pounding heartbeat); *tachycardia* (fast heartbeat); *trembling*

## Overdose

For more information on the management of overdose or unintentional ingestion, **contact a Poison Control Center** (see *Poison Control Center Listing* ).

**Clinical effects of overdose**
The following have been selected on the basis of their potential clinical significance (possible signs and symptoms in parenthesis where appropriate)—not necessarily inclusive:

Symptoms of overdose of beta-adrenergic bronchodilators
>Note: Overdosage with salmeterol may be expected to result in symptoms of excessive beta-adrenergic stimulation.
>
>*Agitation, continuing* (nervousness or restlessness, continuing); *chest discomfort or pain; decreased blood pressure* (dizziness or lightheadedness); *hyperglycemia; hypokalemia; seizures; tachyarrhythmias* (fast and irregular heartbeat); *tachycardia, continuing* (fast heartbeat, continuing); *trembling, continuing; vomiting*

**Treatment of overdose**
Therapy with salmeterol and any other beta-adrenergic agonist should be stopped.

Monitoring the patient, especially cardiovascular status, and providing supportive treatment of observed symptoms.

Administering a cardioselective beta-adrenergic blocking agent, if necessary; however, caution is needed because beta-adrenergic blocking agents can induce bronchospasm.

## Patient Consultation

As an aid to patient consultation, refer to *Advice for the Patient, Salmeterol (Inhalation)*.

In providing consultation, consider emphasizing the following selected information (»=major clinical significance):

**Before using this medication**
» Conditions affecting use, especially:
> Other medications, especially beta-adrenergic blocking agents
> Other medical problems, especially cardiovascular disease

**Proper use of this medication**
» Importance of not using this medication to treat acute symptoms
» Having a rapid-acting inhaled beta-adrenergic bronchodilator available for symptomatic relief of acute asthma attacks
» Reading patient instructions carefully before using
» Importance of not using more medication than prescribed
> Saving inhaler; refill canister may be available
» Proper dosing
» Missed dose: If used regularly, using as soon as possible; resuming regular schedule; not doubling doses; using rapid-acting inhaled bronchodilator if symptoms occur before next dose is due
» Proper storage
*For salmeterol inhalation aerosol dosage form*
> Avoiding contact with the eyes
> Testing or priming inhaler before using first time
> Proper administration technique
> Proper cleaning procedure for inhaler

*For salmeterol powder for inhalation dosage form*
> Proper loading technique
> Proper administration technique
> Proper cleaning procedure for inhaler

**Precautions while using this medication**
> Regular visits to physician to check progress during therapy
» Checking with physician immediately if difficulty in breathing persists after use of this medication or if condition becomes worse
» Checking with physician immediately if more inhalations than usual of a rapid-acting beta-adrenergic bronchodilator are needed to relieve an acute attack
» Checking with physician if using 4 or more inhalations per day of a rapid-acting beta-adrenergic bronchodilator for 2 or more consecutive days or more than one canister (200 inhalations per canister) in an 8-week period
» For patients also using anti-inflammatory medication, checking with physician before stopping or reducing anti-inflammatory therapy

**Side/adverse effects**
> Signs of potential side effects, especially paradoxical bronchospasm or hypersensitivity

## General Dosing Information

It is not clear whether clinically significant tachyphylaxis, or tolerance to the bronchodilator effect of salmeterol develops with repeated use. In clinical trials, reduction of bronchodilator response was only reported in one 8-week study in which the effects of salmeterol on bronchodilation and on airway hyperresponsiveness to methacholine were studied in a small number of asthmatics. In another study duration of salmeterol's protective effect against exercise-induced bronchospasm, another potential marker of tolerance, decreased over a 4-week period in some patients.

The use of a spacer device with salmeterol has not been studied; however, with salmeterol, as with other inhaled medications, use of a spacer device may be beneficial, especially for young children and older adults. By reducing the need for proper coordination of timing of inhalation with activation of the inhaler and reducing the velocity and mean diameter of the aerosol particles, a spacer reduces the amount of medication deposited in the upper airways and increases the amount deposited in the lower respiratory tract.

## Inhalation Dosage Forms

Note: The doses and strengths of the available dosage forms are expressed in terms of salmeterol base (not the xinafoate salt).

### SALMETEROL XINAFOATE INHALATION AEROSOL

**Usual adult and adolescent dose**
Asthma, bronchial, chronic—
> Oral inhalation, 42 or 50 mcg (base) (two inhalations) two times a day, morning and evening, approximately twelve hours apart.
Bronchospasm, exercise-induced[1]—
> Oral inhalation, 42 mcg (base) (two inhalations) at least thirty to sixty minutes before exercise.

Note: Patients receiving chronic therapy should not use additional salmeterol for prevention of exercise-induced bronchospasm. Patients using salmeterol for exercise-induced bronchospasm should not use additional doses for twelve hours after each prophylactic administration.

**Usual pediatric dose**
Children up to 12 years of age—Safety and efficacy have not been established.

**Strength(s) usually available**
U.S.—
> 21 mcg (base) per metered spray (Rx) [Serevent].
Canada—
> 25 mcg (base) per metered spray (Rx) [Serevent].

Note: In Canada, metered dose inhalers are labeled according to the amount of salmeterol delivered at the valve; in the U.S., metered dose inhalers are labeled according to the amount of salmeterol delivered at the mouthpiece or actuator. Therefore, 25 mcg (base) of salmeterol delivered at the valve is equivalent to 21 mcg delivered at the actuator.

Note: The 13-gram canister provides 120 metered sprays; the 6.5-gram canister provides 60 metered sprays.

**Packaging and storage**
Store between 2 and 30 °C (36 and 86 °F). Protect from freezing.

**Auxiliary labeling**
• For oral inhalation only.
• Shake well before using.

## SALMETEROL XINAFOATE POWDER FOR INHALATION

**Usual adult and adolescent dose**
Asthma, bronchial (treatment)—
     Oral inhalation, 50 mcg (base) (the contents of one blister) two times a day.

**Usual pediatric dose**
Children up to 12 years of age—Safety and efficacy have not been established.

**Strength(s) usually available**
U.S.—
     Not commercially available.
Canada—
     50 mcg (base) per blister (Rx) [Serevent].

**Packaging and storage**
Store between 2 and 25 °C (36 and 77 °F). Protect from moisture.

**Auxiliary labeling**
• For oral inhalation only.

     [1]Not included in Canadian product labeling.

## Selected Bibliography

Meyer JM, Wenzel CL, Kradjan WA. Salmeterol: a novel, long-acting beta-2-agonist. Ann Pharmacother 1993; 27: 1478-87.

Brogden RN, Faulds D. Salmeterol xinafoate—a review of its pharmacological properties and therapeutic potential in reversible obstructive airways disease. Drugs 1991; 42: 895-912.

Kamada AK, Spahn JD, Blake KV. Salmeterol: its place in asthma management. Ann Pharmacother 1994; 28: 1100-2.

Developed: 04/28/95

---

**SALSALATE**—See *Salicylates (Systemic)*

---

**SARGRAMOSTIM**—See *Colony Stimulating Factors (Systemic)*

---

**SCOPOLAMINE**—See  *Anticholinergics/Antispasmodics (Systemic)*; *Scopolamine (Ophthalmic)*

---

# SCOPOLAMINE    Ophthalmic†

**VA CLASSIFICATION (Primary): OP600**
Another commonly used name is hyoscine.
Note: For a listing of dosage forms and brand names by country availability, see *Dosage Forms* section(s). For a listing of brand names for the articles in this monograph, refer to the General Index.

     †Not commercially available in Canada.

## Category

Cycloplegic; mydriatic.

## Indications

Note: Bracketed information in the *Indications* section refers to uses that are not included in U.S. product labeling.

**Accepted**
Refraction, cycloplegic—Scopolamine is indicated for measurement of refractive errors. Scopolamine is not useful for refraction in adults, because of its long duration of action.

Uveitis (treatment)—Scopolamine is indicated for pupil dilation and ciliary muscle relaxation, which are desirable in acute and sub-acute inflammatory conditions of the iris and uveal tract.

[Synechiae, posterior (prophylaxis)] or
Synechiae, posterior (treatment)—Scopolamine may be indicated for pupil dilation to break posterior synechiae. In addition, scopolamine is used in the prophylaxis of posterior synechiae.

Mydriasis, postoperative—Scopolamine may be indicated for postoperative mydriasis.

Iridocyclitis, postoperative (treatment) or
Iridocyclitis, preoperative (treatment)—Scopolamine is indicated in certain preoperative and postoperative conditions when a medication having mydriatic and cycloplegic properties is required in the treatment of iridocyclitis.

[Iridocyclitis (treatment)]—Scopolamine is also used in the treatment of iridocyclitis at times other than postoperative or preoperative conditions.

Mydriasis, in diagnostic procedures—Scopolamine is indicated in diagnostic procedures to produce mydriasis.

Note: Scopolamine may be useful in patients who are allergic to atropine.

## Pharmacology/Pharmacokinetics

**Mechanism of action/Effect**
Scopolamine (a belladonna alkaloid) is an anticholinergic agent that blocks the responses of the sphincter muscle of the iris and the accommodative muscle of the ciliary body to stimulation by acetylcholine. Dilation of the pupil (mydriasis) and paralysis of accommodation (cycloplegia) result.

**Duration of action**
Has shorter duration of action than atropine.
Residual cycloplegia and mydriasis may persist for approximately 3 to 7 days following instillation of medication.

## Precautions to Consider

**Cross-sensitivity and/or related problems**
Patients sensitive to any of the other belladonna alkaloids may be sensitive to scopolamine also.

**Pregnancy/Reproduction**
Pregnancy—Problems in humans have not been documented; however, ophthalmic scopolamine may be systemically absorbed.

**Breast-feeding**
Problems in humans have not been documented; however, ophthalmic scopolamine may be systemically absorbed.

**Pediatrics**
An increased susceptibility to scopolamine and similar drugs (such as atropine) has been reported in infants and young children and in children with blond hair, blue eyes, Down's syndrome, spastic paralysis, or brain damage; therefore, scopolamine should be used with great caution in these patients.

**Geriatrics**
Geriatric patients are more susceptible to the effects of scopolamine and similar drugs (such as atropine), thus increasing the potential for systemic side effects.

**Drug interactions and/or related problems**
The following drug interactions and/or related problems have been selected on the basis of their potential clinical significance (possible mechanism in parentheses where appropriate)—not necessarily inclusive (» = major clinical significance):

Note: Combinations containing any of the following medications, depending on the amount present, may also interact with this medication.

Anticholinergics or medications with anticholinergic activity, other (See *Appendix II* )
     (if significant systemic absorption of ophthalmic scopolamine occurs, concurrent use of other anticholinergics or medications with anticholinergic activity may result in potentiated anticholinergic effects)

Antiglaucoma agents, cholinergic, long-acting, ophthalmic
     (concurrent use with scopolamine may antagonize the antiglaucoma and miotic actions of ophthalmic long-acting cholinergic antiglaucoma agents, such as demecarium, echothiophate, and isoflurophate; concurrent use with scopolamine may also antagonize the

antiaccommodative convergence effects of these medications when they are used for the treatment of strabismus)

Antimyasthenics or
Potassium citrate or
Potassium supplements

    (if significant systemic absorption of ophthalmic scopolamine occurs, concurrent use may increase the chance of toxicity and/or side effects of these systemic medications because of the anticholinergic-induced slowing of gastrointestinal motility)

Carbachol or
Physostigmine or
Pilocarpine

    (concurrent use with scopolamine may interfere with the antiglaucoma action of carbachol, physostigmine, or pilocarpine. Also, concurrent use may counteract the mydriatic effect of scopolamine; this counteraction may be used to therapeutic advantage)

CNS depression–producing medications (See *Appendix II* )

    (if significant systemic absorption of ophthalmic scopolamine occurs, concurrent use of medications having CNS effects, such as antiemetic agents, phenothiazines, or barbiturates, may result in opisthotonos, convulsions, coma, and extrapyramidal symptoms)

**Medical considerations/Contraindications**

The medical considerations/contraindications included here have been selected on the basis of their potential clinical significance (reasons given in parentheses where appropriate)—not necessarily inclusive (» = major clinical significance).

*Risk-benefit should be considered when the following medical problems exist:*

Brain damage, in children

Down's syndrome (mongolism), in children and adults

» Glaucoma, primary, or predisposition to angle closure
Keratoconus

    (scopolamine may produce fixed dilated pupil)

Sensitivity to scopolamine

Spastic paralysis, in children

Synechiae between the iris and lens

## Side/Adverse Effects

Note:  An increased susceptibility to scopolamine and similar drugs (such as atropine) has been reported in infants, young children, children with blond hair or blue eyes, adults and children with Down's syndrome, children with brain damage or spastic paralysis, and the elderly. This susceptibility increases the potential for systemic side effects.

    Prolonged use of scopolamine may produce local irritation, resulting in follicular conjunctivitis, vascular congestion, edema, exudate, contact dermatitis, or an eczematoid dermatitis.

The following side/adverse effects have been selected on the basis of their potential clinical significance (possible signs and symptoms in parentheses where appropriate)—not necessarily inclusive:

**Those indicating need for medical attention**

Symptoms of systemic absorption

    *Clumsiness or unsteadiness; confusion or unusual behavior; dryness of skin; fever; flushing or redness of face; hallucinations; skin rash; slurred speech; swollen stomach in infants; tachycardia* (fast or irregular heartbeat); *unusual drowsiness; tiredness or weakness; xerostomia* (thirst or dryness of mouth)

**Those indicating need for medical attention only if they continue or are bothersome**

    *Blurred vision; eye irritation not present before therapy; increased sensitivity of eyes to light; swelling of the eyelids*

## Overdose

For specific information on the agents used in the management of ophthalmic scopolamine overdose, see:

- *Atropine* in *Anticholinergics/Antispasmodics (Systemic)* monograph;
- *Diazepam* in *Benzodiazepines (Systemic)* monograph;
- *Physostigmine (Systemic)* monograph.

For more information on the management of overdose or unintentional ingestion, **contact a Poison Control Center** (see *Poison Control Center Listing*).

**Treatment of overdose**

For accidental ingestion, emesis or gastric lavage with 4% tannic acid solution is recommended.

For systemic effects, 0.2 to 1 mg (0.2 mg in children) physostigmine should be administered intravenously as a dilution containing 1 mg in 5 mL of normal saline. The solution should be injected over a period of not less than 2 minutes. Dosage may be repeated every 5 minutes up to a total dose of 2 mg in children and 6 mg in adults in each 30-minute period.

Physostigmine is contraindicated in hypotensive reactions.

ECG monitoring is recommended during physostigmine administration.

Excitement may be controlled by diazepam or a short-acting barbiturate.

It is recommended that 1 mg of atropine be available for immediate injection if the physostigmine causes bradycardia, convulsion, or bronchoconstriction.

Supportive therapy may require oxygen and assisted respiration; cool water baths for fever, especially in children; and catheterization for urinary retention. In infants and small children, the body surface should be kept moist.

## Patient Consultation

As an aid to patient consultation, refer to *Advice for the Patient, Atropine/Homatropine/Scopolamine (Ophthalmic)*.

In providing consultation, consider emphasizing the following selected information (» = major clinical significance):

**Before using this medication**

» Conditions affecting use, especially:
    Sensitivity to atropine, homatropine, or scopolamine
    Use in children—Infants and young children and children with blond hair or blue eyes may be especially sensitive to the effects of scopolamine; this may increase the chance of side effects during treatment
    Use in the elderly—Geriatric patients are more susceptible to the effects of scopolamine and similar drugs (such as atropine), thus increasing the potential for systemic side effects
    Other medical problems, especially primary glaucoma or predisposition to angle closure

**Proper use of this medication**

Proper administration technique
    Washing hands immediately after application to remove any medication that may be on them; if applying medication to infants or children, washing their hands immediately afterwards also, and not letting any medication get into their mouths; wiping off any medication that may have accidentally gotten on the infant or child, including his or her face and eyelids
    Preventing contamination: Not touching applicator tip to any surface; keeping container tightly closed

» Importance of not using more medication than the amount prescribed
» Proper dosing
    Missed dose: If dosing schedule is—
        Once a day: Applying as soon as possible if remembered same day; if remembered later, skipping missed dose and going back to regular dosing schedule; not doubling doses
        More than once a day: Applying as soon as possible; if almost time for next dose, skipping missed dose and going back to regular dosing schedule; not doubling doses

» Proper storage

**Precautions while using this medication**

» Medication causes blurred vision and increased sensitivity of the eyes to light; checking with physician if these effects continue longer than 7 days after discontinuation of scopolamine

**Side/adverse effects**

    Signs of potential side effects, especially symptoms of systemic absorption

## General Dosing Information

Scopolamine has a cycloplegic effect comparable to that of atropine.

Although some manufacturers recommend a dose of 2 drops of an ophthalmic solution at appropriate intervals, the conjunctival sac will usually hold only 1 drop.

More frequent instillation or use of a stronger concentration may be required to produce adequate cycloplegia in eyes with brown or hazel irides than in eyes with blue irides.

To avoid excessive systemic absorption, patient should press finger to the lacrimal sac during, and for 2 or 3 minutes following, instillation of the solution.

## Ophthalmic Dosage Forms

Note:  Bracketed uses in the *Dosage Forms* section refer to categories of use and/or indications that are not included in U.S. product labeling.

## SCOPOLAMINE HYDROBROMIDE OPHTHALMIC SOLUTION USP

**Usual adult and adolescent dose**
Cycloplegic refraction—
Topical, to the conjunctiva, 1 drop of a 0.25% solution one hour prior to refraction.
Uveitis—
Topical, to the conjunctiva, 1 drop of a 0.25% solution up to four times a day, depending on the severity of the condition.
Posterior synechiae (treatment)—
Topical, to the conjunctiva, 1 drop of a 0.25% solution every ten minutes for three applications.

Note: To enhance the mydriatic effect of scopolamine, 1 drop of a 2.5 or 10% phenylephrine solution may be instilled every ten minutes for three applications. Extreme caution should be used if 10% phenylephrine is administered.

[Posterior synechiae (prophylaxis)]—
Topical, to the conjunctiva, 1 drop of a 0.25% solution one or two times a day as needed to maintain mydriasis.
Postoperative mydriasis—
Topical, to the conjunctiva, 1 drop of a 0.25% solution once a day. Administration two or three times a day may be necessary for patients with dark brown irides.
[Iridocyclitis (other than preoperative or postoperative)] or
Postoperative iridocyclitis or
Preoperative iridocyclitis—
Topical, to the conjunctiva, 1 drop of a 0.25% solution one to four times a day as needed to maintain mydriasis, the dose being decreased as the severity of the inflammation decreases.
Mydriasis in diagnostic procedures—
Topical, to the conjunctiva, 1 drop of a 0.25% solution as needed to maintain mydriasis.

**Usual pediatric dose**
Cycloplegic refraction—
Topical, to the conjunctiva, 1 drop of a 0.25% solution two times a day for two days prior to refraction.
Uveitis—
Topical, to the conjunctiva, 1 drop of a 0.25% solution up to four times a day, depending on the severity of the condition and the size and weight of the child.
[Posterior synechiae (prophylaxis)]—
See *Usual adult and adolescent dose.*
[Iridocyclitis (other than preoperative or postoperative)] or

Postoperative iridocyclitis or
Preoperative iridocyclitis—
See *Usual adult and adolescent dose.*

Note: The pediatric dose should be individualized based on the age and weight of the child as well as the severity of the inflammation.
Mydriasis in diagnostic procedures—
See *Usual adult and adolescent dose.*

**Strength(s) usually available**
U.S.—
0.25% (Rx) [*Isopto Hyoscine* (benzalkonium chloride 0.01%)].
Canada—
Not commercially available.

**Packaging and storage**
Store below 40 °C (104 °F), preferably between 15 and 30 °C (59 and 86 °F), unless otherwise specified by manufacturer. Store in a tight container. Protect from freezing. Protect from light.

**Auxiliary labeling**
• For the eye.
• Keep container tightly closed.

Revised: 06/21/94

## SCOPOLAMINE-CONTAINING COMBINATIONS—

Atropine, Hyoscyamine, Scopolamine, and Phenobarbital (Systemic)—See *Belladonna Alkaloids and Barbiturates (Systemic)*
Chlorpheniramine, Phenylephrine, Phenylpropanolamine, Atropine, Hyoscyamine, and Scopolamine (Systemic)—See *Antihistamines, Decongestants, and Anticholinergics (Systemic)*
Kaolin, Pectin, Hyoscyamine, Atropine, and Scopolamine (Systemic)—See *Kaolin, Pectin, and Belladonna Alkaloids (Systemic)*

## SECOBARBITAL—See *Barbiturates (Systemic)*

## SECOBARBITAL-CONTAINING COMBINATIONS—

Secobarbital and Amobarbital (Systemic)—See *Barbiturates (Systemic)*

# SELEGILINE    Systemic

VA CLASSIFICATION (Primary): CN500

Other commonly used names are deprenil and deprenyl.

Note: For a listing of dosage forms and brand names by country availability, see *Dosage Forms* section(s). For a listing of brand names for the articles in this monograph, refer to the General Index.

## Category
Antidyskinetic.

## Indications

Note: Bracketed information in the *Indications* section refers to uses that are not included in U.S. product labeling.

**Accepted**
Parkinsonism (treatment adjunct)—Selegiline is indicated for use with levodopa or levodopa and carbidopa combination in the treatment of idiopathic Parkinson's disease (paralysis agitans).

[Some studies have suggested that the initial use of selegiline may delay the need for addition of levodopa to the treatment regimen; in addition, these studies have shown that selegiline alone or in combination with levodopa may slow the progression of Parkinson's disease, possibly by preventing selective destruction of dopaminergic neurons in the substantia nigra. One retrospective study showed selegiline to possibly prolong the lifespan of patients with idiopathic Parkinson's disease.]

[The addition of selegiline to levodopa in patients experiencing fluctuating responses ("wearing off" effect or "on-off" phenomenon) may be of moderate benefit. However, the initial response to selegiline may not be sustained, with the degree of improvement declining over

6 months to 4 years. Selegiline is ineffective in advanced disease with extreme fluctuations. Motor control fluctuations may be due to factors other than the central pharmacokinetics of dopamine; hence prolongation of dopamine effects may fail in some cases to improve this problem.]

Note: Preliminary studies have demonstrated that selegiline may be useful as an antidepressant, usually when given in doses greater than those used for its antidyskinetic effect. However, there are *insufficient data* to definitively establish effectiveness of selegiline and criteria for its use in mental depression.

## Pharmacology/Pharmacokinetics

**Physicochemical characteristics**
Molecular weight—223.75.

**Mechanism of action/Effect**
The action of selegiline is thought to be related to its irreversible inhibition of monoamine oxidase type B (MAO B), the major form of the enzyme in the human brain. MAO B, which is involved in the oxidative deamination of dopamine in the brain, is inhibited when selegiline binds covalently and stoichiometrically to the isoalloxazine flavin adenine dinucleotide (FAD) at its active center. Administration of 10 mg of selegiline a day produces almost complete inhibition of MAO B in the brain. Selegiline becomes a non-selective inhibitor of all monoamine oxidase (MAO) at higher doses, possibly at 20 to 40 mg a day. At these doses, tyramine-mediated hypertensive reactions from MAO A blockade ("cheese reactions") may occur.
Selegiline (or its metabolites) may also act through other mechanisms to increase dopaminergic activity, including interfering with dopamine re-uptake at the synapse.

**Absorption**
Rapidly absorbed from the gastrointestinal tract.

**Distribution**
Crosses the blood-brain barrier.

**Biotransformation**
Rapidly and completely metabolized to *N*-desmethyldeprenyl, l-metham-phetamine, and l-amphetamine.

**Half-life**
The mean half-lives of the 3 active metabolites that were found in serum and urine following a single dose of selegiline are as follows—
N-desmethyldeprenyl: 2 hours.
l-amphetamine: 17.7 hours.
l-methamphetamine: 20.5 hours.
Elimination—
Selegiline: 39 (range, 16 to 69) hours.

**Time to peak plasma concentration**
0.5 to 2 hours.

**Duration of action**
Duration of clinical action depends on the regeneration time of MAO B.

**Elimination**
Renal; slow. 45% of a 10 mg dose appears in the urine as metabolites (*N*-desmethyldeprenyl, l-amphetamine, and l-methamphetamine) within 48 hours of ingestion.

# Precautions to Consider

**Carcinogenicity**
Long-term animal studies have revealed no evidence of carcinogenic effects.

**Pregnancy/Reproduction**
Pregnancy—Studies in humans have not been done.
Studies in animals have not shown that selegiline causes adverse effects on the fetus. Reproduction studies in rats and rabbits given approximately 250 and 350 times the comparable human dose, respectively, have revealed no evidence of teratogenic effects.
FDA Pregnancy Category C.

**Breast-feeding**
It is not known whether selegiline is excreted in breast milk.

**Pediatrics**
No published pediatrics-specific information is available. Safety and efficacy have not been established.

**Geriatrics**
No geriatrics-related problems have been documented in studies done to date that included elderly patients.

**Dental**
Selegiline may decrease or inhibit salivary flow, thus contributing to the development of caries, periodontal disease, oral candidiasis, and discomfort.

**Drug interactions and/or related problems**
The following drug interactions and/or related problems have been selected on the basis of their potential clinical significance (possible mechanism in parentheses where appropriate)—not necessarily inclusive (» = major clinical significance):
Note: Combinations containing any of the following medications, depending on the amount present, may also interact with this medication.

*For all doses of selegiline*
» Antidepressants, tricyclic
(asystole, diaphoresis, hypertension, syncope, changes in behavior and mental status, impaired consciousness, hyperpyrexia, seizures, muscular rigidity, and tremors have occurred with concurrent use of selegiline and tricyclic antidepressants. Concurrent use is not recommended; at least 14 days should elapse between discontinuation of selegiline and initiation of a tricyclic antidepressant)

» Fluoxetine or
» Fluvoxamine or
» Nefazodone or
» Paroxetine or
» Sertraline or
» Venlafaxine
(a reaction resembling the serotonin syndrome has been reported rarely following concurrent use of selegiline with selective sero-tonin re-uptake inhibitors (SSRIs). [The serotonin syndrome may occur as the result of combining a serotonergic agent with an MAO inhibitor. The syndrome may be manifest by mental status changes (confusion, hypomania), restlessness, myoclonus, hyperreflexia, di-aphoresis, shivering, tremor, diarrhea, incoordination, and/or fever. If recognized early, the syndrome usually resolves quickly upon withdrawal of the offending agents.] Concurrent use of selegiline with SSRIs is not recommended because of the potential for autonomic instability, muscular rigidity, severe agitation, or delirium. At least 14 days should elapse between discontinuation of an MAO inhibitor and initiation of an SSRI. However, because of the long half-lives of fluoxetine and its active metabolite, at least 5 weeks [approximately 5 half-lives] should elapse between discontinuation of fluoxetine and initiation of therapy with an MAO inhibitor. Also, based on the half life of venlafaxine, at least 7 days should elapse between discontinuation of venlafaxine and initiation of therapy with an MAO inhibitor)

Levodopa
(although selegiline is used in conjunction with levodopa, it may enhance levodopa-induced dyskinesias, nausea, orthostatic hypotension, confusion, and hallucinations; reduction of levodopa dosage may be necessary within 2 to 3 days after the initiation of selegiline therapy)

» Meperidine, and possibly other opioid (narcotic) analgesics
(at least one interaction of meperidine with selegiline has been reported; concurrent use of meperidine with non-selective mono-amine oxidase inhibitors [MAOIs] may produce immediate excitation, sweating, rigidity, and severe hypertension; in some patients, hypotension, severe respiratory depression, coma, convulsions, hyperpyrexia, vascular collapse, and death may occur; avoidance of meperidine use within 2 to 3 weeks following MAO inhibition is recommended; other opioid analgesics such as morphine are not likely to cause such severe reactions and may be used cautiously in reduced dosage in patients receiving MAOIs; however, it is recommended that a small test dose [¼ of the usual dose] or several small incremental test doses over a period of several hours should first be administered to permit observation of any adverse effects; caution is also recommended in the use of alfentanil, fentanyl, or sufentanil as an adjunct to anesthesia if the patient has received an MAOI within 14 days; because the risk of a significant interaction has been questioned, the use of a small test dose is advised to detect any possible interaction)

*For doses of 20 mg or more of selegiline per day*
» Tyramine- or other high pressor amine–containing foods and beverages, such as aged cheese; fava or broad bean pods; yeast/protein extracts; smoked or pickled meats, poultry, or fish; fermented sausage (bologna, pepperoni, salami, summer sausage) or other fermented meat; sauerkraut; any overripe fruit; beer; reduced-alcohol and alcohol-free beer and wine; red and white wines; sherry; and liqueurs
(concurrent use with MAOIs, including selegiline in doses of 20 mg a day or greater, may cause sudden and severe hypertensive reactions; reactions are usually limited to a few hours and are easily treated with rapidly acting hypotensive agents [such as labetalol, nifedipine, or, if necessary in severe cases refractory to other agents, phentolamine]; severity of reaction depends on amount of tyramine ingested, rate of gastric emptying, and length of interval between dose of MAOI and ingestion of tyramine; when MAOIs are discontinued, dietary restrictions must continue for at least 2 weeks; other tyramine- or high pressor amine–containing foods, such as yogurt, sour cream, cream cheese, cottage cheese, chocolate, and soy sauce, if eaten when fresh and in moderation, are considered unlikely to cause serious problems)

**Medical considerations/Contraindications**
The medical considerations/contraindications included here have been selected on the basis of their potential clinical significance (reasons given in parentheses where appropriate)—not necessarily inclusive (» = major clinical significance).

*Risk-benefit should be considered when the following medical problems exist:*
Dementia, profound or
Psychosis, severe or
Tardive dyskinesia or
Tremor, excessive
(condition may be exacerbated)

» Peptic ulcer disease, history of
(activation of pre-existing ulcers may occur, probably due to stimulation of the H₂ receptors in the stomach or inhibition of MAO-mediated gastric histamine catabolism)

Sensitivity to selegiline

## Side/Adverse Effects

Note: Selegiline enhances the dose-related side effects of levodopa, but few side effects are attributable to selegiline itself. When selegiline is used as an adjunct to levodopa or levodopa and carbidopa combination, adverse effects can usually be ameliorated by reducing the dose of levodopa or levodopa and carbidopa.

In addition, selegiline may cause elevation of liver enzymes.

The following side/adverse effects have been selected on the basis of their potential clinical significance (possible signs and symptoms in parentheses where appropriate)—not necessarily inclusive:

**Those indicating need for medical attention**
Incidence more frequent
*Dyskinesias* (increase in unusual movements of body); *mood or other mental changes*
Incidence less frequent or rare
*Angina pectoris, new or increased* (chest pain); *arrhythmias* (irregular heartbeat); *asthma* (wheezing, difficulty in breathing, or tightness in chest); *bradycardia, sinus* (slow heartbeat); *edema, peripheral* (swelling of feet or lower legs); *motor/coordination/extrapyramidal effects* (difficulty in speaking; loss of balance control; uncontrolled movements, especially of face, neck, and back; restlessness or desire to keep moving; twisting movements of body); *gastrointestinal bleeding* (bloody or black, tarry stools; severe stomach pain; vomiting of blood or material that looks like coffee grounds); *hallucinations; headache, severe; hypertension, severe; orthostatic hypotension* (dizziness or lightheadedness, especially when getting up from a lying or sitting position); *prostatic hypertrophy* (difficult or frequent urination); *tardive dyskinesia* (lip smacking or puckering; puffing of cheeks; rapid or worm-like movements of tongue; uncontrolled chewing movements; uncontrolled movements of arms and legs)
Symptoms of hypertensive crisis
*Chest pain, severe; enlarged pupils; fast or slow heartbeat; headache, severe; increased sensitivity of eyes to light; increased sweating, possibly with fever or cold, clammy skin; nausea or vomiting, severe; stiff or sore neck*

**Those indicating need for medical attention only if they continue or are bothersome**
Incidence more frequent
*Abdominal or stomach pain; dizziness or feeling faint; dryness of mouth; insomnia* (trouble in sleeping); *nausea or vomiting*
Incidence less frequent or rare
*Anxiety, nervousness, or restlessness; apraxia, increased* (inability to move); *blepharospasm* (sudden closing of eyelids); *blurred or double vision; body ache or back or leg pain; bradykinesia, increased* (slowed movements); *chills; constipation or diarrhea; diaphoresis* (increased sweating); *drowsiness; headache; heartburn; hypertension or hypotension* (high or low blood pressure); *impaired memory—* more frequent with doses greater than 10 mg a day; *slow or difficult urination; frequent urge to urinate; irritability, temporary; loss of appetite or weight loss; muscle cramps or numbness of fingers or toes; palpitations or tachycardia* (pounding or fast heartbeat); *paresthesias, circumoral* (burning of lips or mouth); *or burning of throat; photosensitivity* (increased sensitivity of skin and eyes to sunlight); *skin rash; tinnitus* (ringing or buzzing in ears); *taste changes; unusual feeling of well-being; unusual tiredness or weakness*
With doses greater than 10 mg a day
*Bruxism* (clenching, gnashing, or grinding teeth); *muscle twitches or myoclonic jerks* (sudden jerky movements of body)
Note: *Bruxism* and *myoclonic jerks* may be considered to be adverse effects only if not previously present and beginning shortly after the start of therapy with selegiline.

## Overdose

For specific information in the agents used in the management of selegiline overdose, see:
• *Charcoal, Activated (Oral-Local)* monograph.

For more information on the management of overdose of unintentional ingestion, **contact a Poison Control Center** (see *Poison Control Center Listing*).

**Clinical effects of overdose**
No specific information is available regarding overdoses with selegiline. Since overdose is likely to cause significant inhibition of both MAO type A and type B, symptoms of overdose may resemble those of non-selective MAO inhibitors.

Symptoms of MAOI overdose
*Agitation or irritability; chest pain; convulsions; cool, clammy skin; diaphoresis* (increased sweating); *dizziness, severe, or fainting; fast or irregular pulse, continuing; high or low blood pressure; hyperpyrexia* (high fever); *opisthotonus* (severe spasm where the head and heels are bent backward and the body arched forward); *respiratory depression* (troubled breathing); *trismus* (difficulty opening the mouth; lockjaw)

Note: Symptoms resulting from overdose may be absent or minimal for nearly 12 hours after ingestion, and develop slowly thereafter, reaching a maximum in 24 to 48 hours. Death has resulted. Immediate hospitalization and close monitoring of patient is essential during this period.

**Treatment of overdose**
Treatment may include the following:
To decrease absorption—
Induction of emesis or gastric lavage with protected airway followed by instillation of charcoal slurry in early overdose.
Specific treatment—
Treatment of signs and symptoms of central nervous system (CNS) stimulation with diazepam, administered intravenously and slowly. Phenothiazine derivatives should be avoided.
Treatment of hypotension and vascular collapse with intravenous fluids and, if necessary, a dilute pressor agent. Adrenergic agents may produce a markedly increased pressor response.
Vigorous treatment of hyperpyrexia with antipyretics and a cooling blanket.
Monitoring—
Close monitoring of body temperature.
Supportive care—
Maintenance of fluid and electrolyte balance is essential.
Support of respiration by management of the airway, and mechanical ventilation with the use of supplemental oxygen, as required.
Patients in whom intentional overdose is confirmed or suspected should be referred for psychiatric consultation.

## Patient Consultation

As an aid to patient consultation, refer to *Advice for the Patient, Selegiline (Systemic)*.

In providing consultation, consider emphasizing the following selected information (» = major clinical significance):

**Before using this medication**
» Conditions affecting use, especially:
Sensitivity to selegiline
Other medications, especially fluoxetine, fluvoxamine, meperidine and possibly other narcotic (opioid) analgesics, nefazodone, paroxetine, sertraline, tricyclic antidepressants, or venlafaxine
Other medical problems, especially a history of peptic ulcer disease

**Proper use of this medication**
» Importance of not taking more medication than the amount prescribed; to do so may increase the risk of side effects
Missed dose: Taking as soon as possible; not taking in the late afternoon or evening; not taking if almost time for next dose; not doubling doses.
» Proper storage

**Precautions while using this medication**
» If taking 20 mg or more of selegiline a day, avoiding tyramine-containing foods, alcoholic beverages, and large quantities of caffeine-containing beverages, over-the-counter cold and cough medicines, and other medications, unless prescribed
» Checking with hospital emergency room or physician if symptoms of hypertensive crisis develop
» Possibility of orthostatic hypotension; caution when getting up suddenly from a lying or sitting position
Possible dryness of mouth; using sugarless candy or gum, ice, or saliva substitute for relief; checking with physician or dentist if dryness of mouth continues for more than 2 weeks

**Side/adverse effects**
Signs of potential side effects, especially dyskinesias, mood or mental changes, angina pectoris, arrhythmias, asthma, bradycardia, peripheral edema, extrapyramidal effects, hallucinations, severe headache, severe hypertension, gastrointestinal bleeding, orthostatic hypotension, prostatic hypertrophy, and tardive dyskinesia

## General Dosing Information

Selegiline should not be used in the treatment of Parkinson's disease at doses exceeding 10 mg a day because of the risks associated with non-selective inhibition of monoamine oxidase (MAO). A tyramine-mediated hypertensive reaction has been reported when selegiline was administered at a dose of 20 mg a day. In addition, selegiline in doses greater than 10 mg a day has not demonstrated increased effectiveness in the treatment of Parkinson's disease.

When selegiline is used as an adjunct to levodopa or levodopa and carbidopa combination, adverse effects such as involuntary movements or hallucinations may result, and doses of levodopa may need to be reduced. If necessary, doses of levodopa should be reduced after 2 to 3 days by 10 to 30%, and possibly by as much as 50% with continued therapy.

Because selegiline may produce insomnia, it should not be administered in the late afternoon or evening.

### Diet/Nutrition

Selegiline should be administered with breakfast and lunch to minimize possible nausea and insomnia.

When monoamine oxidase inhibitors, including selegiline at doses of 20 mg a day or greater, are used concurrently with foods and beverages containing tyramine or other high pressor amines, sudden and severe hypertensive reactions may result. These reactions are usually limited to a few hours and are easily treated with rapidly acting hypotensive agents (such as labetalol, nifedipine, or, if necessary in severe cases refractory to other agents, phentolamine). The severity of the reaction depends on the amount of tyramine ingested, the rate of gastric emptying, and the length of the interval between the dose of MAO inhibitor and ingestion of tyramine. When MAO inhibitors are discontinued, dietary restrictions must continue for at least 2 weeks. Foods and beverages containing tyramine or other high pressor amines include aged cheese; fava or broad bean pods; yeast/protein extracts; smoked or pickled meats, poultry, or fish; fermented sausage (bologna, pepperoni, salami, summer sausage) or other fermented meat; sauerkraut; any overripe fruit; beer; reduced-alcohol and alcohol-free beer and wine; red and white wines; sherry; and liqueurs. Other foods, such as yogurt, sour cream, cream cheese, cottage cheese, chocolate, and soy sauce, if eaten when fresh and in moderation, are considered unlikely to cause serious problems.

## Oral Dosage Forms

### SELEGILINE HYDROCHLORIDE CAPSULES

**Usual adult dose**
Parkinsonism—
     Oral, 5 mg two times a day, at breakfast and lunch.

Note: In some cases, some clinicians recommend that the total daily dose be divided (2.5 mg four times a day) to decrease the side effects induced by concomitant administration of levodopa.

**Usual pediatric dose**
Safety and efficacy have not been established.

---

# SELENIUM SULFIDE    Topical

VA CLASSIFICATION (Primary): DE400

Note: For a listing of dosage forms and brand names by country availability, see *Dosage Forms* section(s). For a listing of brand names for the articles in this monograph, refer to the General Index.

---

## Category
Antiseborrheic.

## Indications

**Accepted**
Dandruff (treatment) or
Dermatitis, seborrheic, of scalp (treatment)—Selenium sulfide is indicated for the treatment of dandruff or seborrheic dermatitis of the scalp.

Tinea versicolor (treatment)—Selenium sulfide is indicated for the treatment of tinea versicolor.

## Pharmacology/Pharmacokinetics

**Physicochemical characteristics**
Molecular weight—143.08.

**Mechanism of action/Effect**
Selenium sulfide may act by an antimitotic action, resulting in a reduction in the turnover of epidermal cells. It also has local irritant, antibacterial, and mild antifungal activity, which may contribute to its effectiveness.

---

**Usual geriatric dose**
See *Usual adult dose.*

**Strength(s) usually available**
U.S.—
     5 mg (Rx) [*Eldepryl*].
Canada—
     Not commercially available.

**Packaging and storage**
Store below 40 °C (104 °F), preferably between 15 and 30 °C (59 and 86 °F), in a well-closed container, unless otherwise specified by manufacturer.

## SELEGILINE HYDROCHLORIDE TABLETS

**Usual adult dose**
See *Selegiline Hydrochloride Capsules.*

**Usual pediatric dose**
See *Selegiline Hydrochloride Capsules.*

**Usual geriatric dose**
See *Selegiline Hydrochloride Capsules.*

**Strength(s) usually available**
U.S.—
     5 mg (Rx) [GENERIC].
Canada—
     5 mg (Rx) [*Eldepryl; Novo-selegiline; SD Deprenyl*].

**Packaging and storage**
Store below 40 °C (104 °F), preferably between 15 and 30 °C (59 and 86 °F), in a well-closed container, unless otherwise specified by manufacturer.

## Selected Bibliography

Yahr MD. R- (—)-Deprenyl and parkinsonism. J Neural Transm 1987; 25 (Suppl): 5-12.
Golbe LI. Deprenyl as symptomatic therapy in Parkinson's disease. Clin Neuropharmacol 1988 Oct; 11 (5): 387-400.

---

Revised: 09/30/92
Interim revision: 08/20/96

---

## SELENIOUS ACID—See *Selenium Supplements (Systemic)*

---

## SELENIUM—See *Selenium Supplements (Systemic)*

---

## Precautions to Consider

**Carcinogenicity**
No carcinogenic effects were found after dermal applications of 0.625 and 1.25% selenium sulfide solutions were used on mice over an 88-week period.

**Pregnancy/Reproduction**
Pregnancy—Studies have not been done in humans. However, problems in humans have not been documented when selenium sulfide is used on the scalp.

It is recommended that selenium sulfide not be used for the treatment of tinea versicolor in pregnant women.

Studies have not been done in animals.

FDA Pregnancy Category C (for tinea versicolor).

**Breast-feeding**
Problems in humans have not been documented.

**Pediatrics**
Infants—Appropriate studies on the relationship of age to the effects of selenium sulfide have not been performed in infants. Safety and efficacy have not been established.

Children—Appropriate studies on the relationship of age to the effects of selenium sulfide have not been performed in children. However, pediatrics-specific problems that would limit the usefulness of this medication are not expected.

**Geriatrics**

Appropriate studies on the relationship of age to the effects of selenium sulfide have not been performed in the geriatric population. However, geriatrics-specific problems that would limit the usefulness of this medication in the elderly are not expected.

**Medical considerations/Contraindications**

The medical considerations/contraindications included here have been selected on the basis of their potential clinical significance (reasons given in parentheses where appropriate)—not necessarily inclusive (» = major clinical significance).

*Risk-benefit should be considered when the following medical problems exist:*

Inflammation or exudation of skin, acute (an increase in absorption may occur)

Sensitivity to selenium sulfide

## Side/Adverse Effects

The following side/adverse effects have been selected on the basis of their potential clinical significance (possible signs and symptoms in parentheses where appropriate)—not necessarily inclusive:

**Those indicating need for medical attention**

Incidence less frequent or rare

*Skin irritation*

**Those indicating need for medical attention only if they continue or are bothersome**

Incidence more frequent

*Unusual dryness or oiliness of hair or scalp*

Incidence less frequent

*Increase in normal hair loss*

## Overdose

For more information on the management of overdose or unintentional ingestion, **contact a Poison Control Center** (see *Poison Control Center Listing*).

**Treatment of overdose**

To decrease absorption—Institute emesis and gastric lavage if accidently ingested.

Supportive care—Patients in whom intentional overdose is known or suspected should be referred for psychiatric consultation.

## Patient Consultation

As an aid to patient consultation, refer to *Advice for the Patient, Selenium Sulfide (Topical).*

In providing consultation, consider emphasizing the following selected information (» = major clinical significance):

**Before using this medication**

» Conditions affecting use, especially:

Sensitivity to selenium sulfide

Pregnancy—Not using medication for the treatment of tinea versicolor

**Proper use of this medication**

» Importance of not using more of the 2.5% strength medication than the amount recommended

For best results, using the 1% strength medication at least 2 times a week or as directed by your doctor

*Proper administration of the medication for dandruff or seborrheic dermatitis*

Before using—Wetting hair and scalp with lukewarm water

Applying enough to scalp (approximately 1 or 2 teaspoonfuls) to work up lather

Allowing lather to remain on scalp for 2 to 3 minutes, then rinsing

Applying medication again and rinsing thoroughly

If using on light or blond, gray, or chemically treated (bleached, tinted, permanent-waved) hair, rinsing hair well for at least 5 minutes after using medication to lessen chance of hair discoloration

After treatment, washing your hands thoroughly

*Proper administration of the medication for tinea versicolor*

Applying medication to affected areas of body, except face and genitals

Working up lather using a small amount of water

Allowing medication to remain on skin for 10 minutes

Rinsing body well to remove all medication

» Not using medication if blistered, raw, or oozing areas are present on scalp or body

» Avoiding contact with the eyes; flushing thoroughly with water if medication accidentally gets in eyes

» Proper dosing

Missed dose: Using as soon as possible; not using if almost time for next dose

» Proper storage

**Precautions while using this medication**

Checking with physician if condition does not get better after regular use, or if it gets worse

**Side/adverse effects**

Signs of potential side effects, especially skin irritation

## General Dosing Information

Selenium sulfide should not be used when acute inflammation or exudate is present, because an increase in absorption may occur.

Discoloration of the hair may occur following use of selenium sulfide, especially if used on hair that is light, blond, or gray or on hair that has been chemically treated (i.e., bleached, tinted, or permanent-waved). The discoloration may be minimized or avoided by thoroughly rinsing the hair for at least 5 minutes after treatment.

## Topical Dosage Forms

### SELENIUM SULFIDE LOTION USP

**Usual adult and adolescent dose**

Dandruff or

Seborrheic dermatitis—

Topical, to the scalp as a 1% lotion, two times a week; or topical, to the scalp as a 2.5% lotion, two times a week for two weeks and then at less frequent intervals of once a week or once every two or more weeks.

Note: The medication should not be used more frequently than required to maintain control.

Tinea versicolor—

Topical, to the body as a 2.5% lotion, once a day for seven days.

Note: The lotion should be applied to all affected areas, except for the face and genitals, and left on for 10 minutes. Then the medication should be thoroughly rinsed off.

**Usual pediatric dose**

Dandruff or

Seborrheic dermatitis or

Tinea versicolor—

Infants: Safety and efficacy have not been established.

Children: See *Usual adult and adolescent dose.*

**Strength(s) usually available**

U.S.—

1% (OTC) [*Head & Shoulders Intensive Treatment Conditioning Formula Dandruff Lotion Shampoo; Head & Shoulders Intensive Treatment Regular Formula Dandruff Lotion Shampoo; Head & Shoulders Intensive Treatment 2 in 1 (Persistent Dandruff Shampoo plus Conditioner in One) Formula Dandruff Lotion Shampoo; Selsun Blue Dry Formula; Selsun Blue Extra Conditioning Formula; Selsun Blue Extra Medicated Formula; Selsun Blue Oily Formula; Selsun Blue Regular Formula;* GENERIC].

2.5% (Rx) [*Exsel Lotion Shampoo; Glo-Sel; Selsun;* GENERIC].

Canada—

1% (OTC) [*Selsun Blue; Selsun Blue Extra Conditioning Formula*].

2.5% (OTC) [*Selsun; Versel Lotion*].

**Packaging and storage**

Store below 40 °C (104 °F), preferably between 15 and 30 °C (59 and 86 °F), unless otherwise specified by manufacturer. Store in a tight container. Protect from freezing.

**Auxiliary labeling**

• Shake well.

• For external use only.

Revised: 07/26/93

# SELENIUM SUPPLEMENTS   Systemic

This monograph includes information on the following: Selenious Acid†; Selenium.

VA CLASSIFICATION (Primary): TN499

Note: For a listing of dosage forms and brand names by country availability, see *Dosage Forms* section(s). For a listing of brand names for the articles in this monograph, refer to the General Index.

---

†Not commercially available in Canada.

---

## Category

Nutritional supplement (mineral).

## Indications

### Accepted

Selenium deficiency (prophylaxis and treatment)—Selenium supplements are indicated in the prevention and treatment of selenium deficiency, which may result from inadequate nutrition or intestinal malabsorption, but does not occur in healthy individuals receiving an adequate balanced diet. For prophylaxis of selenium deficiency, dietary improvement, rather than supplementation, is advisable. For treatment of selenium deficiency, supplementation is preferred.

Deficiency of selenium may lead to lightening in color of the fingernail beds, muscle discomfort or weakness, and cardiomyopathy.

Clinical deficiencies of selenium in the U.S. are rare. Selenium supplements may be necessary in Keshan disease, a form of selenium deficiency that has been reported in areas of the world in which the soil is poor in selenium.

Some unusual diets (e.g., reducing diets that drastically restrict food selection) may not supply minimum daily requirements of selenium. Supplementation may be necessary in patients receiving total parenteral nutrition (TPN) or undergoing rapid weight loss or in those with malnutrition, because of inadequate dietary intake.

Recommended intakes for all vitamins and most minerals are increased during pregnancy. Many physicians recommend that pregnant women receive multivitamin and mineral supplements, especially those pregnant women who do not consume an adequate diet and those in high-risk categories (i.e., women carrying more than one fetus, heavy cigarette smokers, and alcohol and drug abusers). However, taking excessive amounts of multivitamin and mineral supplements may be harmful to the mother and/or fetus and should be avoided.

Recommended intakes for most vitamins and minerals are increased during breast-feeding.

### Acceptance not established

There are insufficient data to show that selenium may reduce the occurrence of certain types of *cancer*.

## Pharmacology/Pharmacokinetics

### Physicochemical characteristics

Molecular weight—
Elemental selenium: 78.96.
Selenious acid: 128.97.

### Mechanism of action/Effect

Selenium is necessary for the enzyme glutathione perioxidase, which facilitates the lowering of tissue peroxide levels in the body by destroying hydrogen peroxide. There is an overlap in action of selenium and vitamin E in that both are responsible for lowering tissue peroxide levels.

### Absorption

Readily absorbed.

### Storage

Selenium is stored primarily in red cells, liver, spleen, heart, nails, and tooth enamel, but also in testes and sperm.

### Elimination

Primarily in urine; to a lesser extent in the feces.

## Precautions to Consider

### Pregnancy/Reproduction

Pregnancy—Adequate and well controlled studies in humans have not been done and problems in humans have not been documented with intake of normal daily recommended amounts.

High doses of selenium (15 to 30 micrograms per egg) have been found to cause adverse embryological effects in chickens.

FDA Pregnancy Category C (parenteral selenium).

### Breast-feeding

Problems in humans have not been documented with intake of normal daily recommended amounts.

### Pediatrics

Problems in pediatrics have not been documented with intake of normal daily recommended amounts.

Selenium injection that contains benzyl alcohol as a preservative should not be used in newborn and immature infants. The use of benzyl alcohol in neonates has been associated with a fatal toxic syndrome consisting of metabolic acidosis and central nervous system (CNS), respiratory, circulatory, and renal function impairment.

### Geriatrics

Problems in geriatrics have not been documented with intake of normal daily recommended amounts.

### Medical considerations/Contraindications

The medical considerations/contraindications included here have been selected on the basis of their potential clinical significance (reasons given in parentheses where appropriate)—not necessarily inclusive (» = major clinical significance).

*Risk-benefit should be considered when the following medical problems exist:*
Gastrointestinal disease and
Renal function impairment
(may cause high levels of selenium; reduction of dosage may be necessary)

### Patient monitoring

The following may be especially important in patient monitoring (other tests may be warranted in some patients, depending on condition; » = major clinical significance):

Selenium, plasma
(weekly plasma selenium monitoring may be recommended by some clinicians for patients receiving short-term total parenteral nutrition [TPN]; monthly monitoring may be recommended with long-term use)

## Overdose

For more information on the management of overdose or unintentional ingestion, **contact a Poison Control Center** (see *Poison Control Center Listing* ).

Symptoms of overdose
*Dermatitis* (itching of skin); *diarrhea; fingernail weakening; garlic odor of breath and sweat; hair loss; irritability; metallic taste; nausea and vomiting; unusual tiredness and weakness*

## Patient Consultation

As an aid to patient consultation, refer to *Advice for the Patient, Selenium Supplements (Systemic).*

In providing consultation, consider emphasizing the following selected information (» = major clinical significance):

### Description of use

Description of use should include function in the body, signs of deficiency, conditions that may cause deficiency of selenium

### Importance of diet

Importance of proper nutrition; supplement may be needed because of inadequate dietary intake
Food sources of selenium
Recommended daily intake for selenium

### Proper use of this dietary supplement

»   Proper dosing
Missed dose: No cause for concern because of length of time necessary for depletion; remembering to take as directed
»   Proper storage

## General Dosing Information

Because of the infrequency of selenium deficiency alone, combinations of selenium with several vitamins and/or minerals are commonly administered. Many commercial vitamin-mineral complexes are available.

**For parenteral dosage forms only**
In most cases, parenteral administration is indicated only when oral administration is not acceptable (for example, in nausea, vomiting, preoperative and postoperative conditions) or possible (for example, in malabsorption syndromes or following gastric resection).

**Diet/Nutrition**
Recommended dietary intakes for selenium are defined differently worldwide.

For U.S.—

The Recommended Dietary Allowances (RDAs) for vitamins and minerals are determined by the Food and Nutrition Board of the National Research Council and are intended to provide adequate nutrition in most healthy persons under usual environmental stresses. In addition, a different designation may be used by the FDA for food and dietary supplement labeling purposes, as with Daily Value (DV). DV replaces the previous labeling terminology United States Recommended Daily Allowances (USRDAs).

For Canada—

Recommended Nutrient Intakes (RNIs) for vitamins, minerals, and protein are determined by Health and Welfare Canada and provide recommended amounts of a specific nutrient while minimizing the risk of chronic diseases.

Daily recommended intakes for selenium are generally defined as follows:

Infants and children—

Birth to 3 years: 10 to 20 mcg.

4 to 6 years: 20 mcg.

7 to 10 years: 30 mcg.

Adolescent and adult males—

40 to 70 mcg.

Adolescent and adult females—

45 to 55 mcg.

Pregnant females—

65 mcg.

Lactating females—

75 mcg.

The best sources of selenium include grains (depending on selenium content of soil), seafood, liver, and lean red meat.

---

## *SELENIOUS ACID*

## Parenteral Dosage Forms

### SELENIOUS ACID INJECTION USP

**Usual adult and adolescent dose**
Deficiency (treatment)—
Intravenous, 100 mcg a day of elemental selenium for 24 to 31 days, added to total parenteral nutrition (TPN).
Deficiency (prophylaxis)—
Intravenous, 20 to 40 mcg of elemental selenium a day, added to total parenteral nutrition (TPN).

**Usual pediatric dose**
Deficiency (prophylaxis and treatment)—
Intravenous, 3 mcg of elemental selenium per kilogram of body weight a day, added to total parenteral nutrition (TPN).

Note: Selenium injection that contains benzyl alcohol as a preservative should not be used in newborn and immature infants. The use of benzyl alcohol in neonates has been associated with a fatal toxic syndrome consisting of metabolic acidosis and CNS, respiratory, circulatory, and renal function impairment.

**Strength(s) usually available**
U.S.—
40 mcg elemental selenium per mL (Rx) [*Sele-Pak* (0.9% benzyl alcohol); *Selepen* (0.9% benzyl alcohol); GENERIC].
Canada—
Not commercially available.

**Packaging and storage**
Store below 40 °C (104 °F), preferably between 15 and 30 °C (59 and 86 °F), unless otherwise specified by manufacturer.

**Preparation of dosage form**
Selenious acid is compatible with amino acids, dextrose, electrolytes, and other trace elements usually used for total parenteral nutrition (TPN).

---

## *SELENIUM*

## Oral Dosage Forms

### SELENIUM TABLETS

**Usual adult and adolescent dose**
Deficiency (prophylaxis)—Oral, amount based on normal daily recommended intakes—
Adolescent and adult males—40 to 70 mcg.
Adolescent and adult females—45 to 55 mcg.
Pregnant females—65 mcg.
Lactating females—75 mcg.
Deficiency (treatment)—
Treatment dose is individualized by prescriber based on severity of deficiency.

**Usual pediatric dose**
Deficiency (prophylaxis)—Oral, amount based on normal daily recommended intakes—
Birth to 3 years of age—10 to 20 mcg.
4 to 6 years of age—20 mcg.
7 to 10 years of age—30 mcg.
Deficiency (treatment)—
Treatment dose is individualized by prescriber based on severity of deficiency.

**Strength(s) usually available**
U.S.—
50 mcg elemental selenium (OTC) [GENERIC (yeast)].
100 mcg elemental selenium (OTC) [GENERIC].
200 mcg elemental selenium (OTC) [GENERIC].
Canada—
50 mcg elemental selenium (OTC) [GENERIC (yeast)].
100 mcg elemental selenium (OTC) [GENERIC (yeast)].

Note: Some strengths of these selenium preparations may exceed the dosage range recommended by USP DI Advisory Panels based on the amount necessary to meet normal nutritional needs.

**Packaging and storage**
Store below 40 °C (104 °F), preferably between 15 and 30 °C (59 and 86 °F), unless otherwise specified by manufacturer.

Revised: 04/16/92
Interim revision: 06/06/92; 08/15/94; 05/01/95

---

**SENNA**—See *Laxatives (Local)*

---

**SENNA-CONTAINING COMBINATIONS**—

Phenolphthalein and Senna (Oral-Local)—See *Laxatives (Local)*
Psyllium Hydrophilic Mucilloid and Senna (Oral-Local)—See *Laxatives (Local)*
Psyllium and Senna (Oral-Local)—See *Laxatives (Local)*

---

**SENNOSIDES**—See *Laxatives (Local)*

---

**SENNOSIDES-CONTAINING COMBINATIONS**—

Psyllium Hydrophilic Mucilloid and Sennosides (Oral-Local)—See *Laxatives (Local)*
Sennosides and Docusate (Oral-Local)—See *Laxatives (Local)*

# SERTRALINE Systemic

VA CLASSIFICATION (Primary): CN609

Note: For a listing of dosage forms and brand names by country availability, see *Dosage Forms* section(s). For a listing of brand names for the articles in this monograph, refer to the General Index.

## Category
Antidepressant.

## Indications

**Accepted**

Depression, mental (treatment)—Sertraline is indicated for the treatment of major depressive disorder.

## Pharmacology/Pharmacokinetics

**Physicochemical characteristics**

Chemical group—Naphthylamine derivative antidepressant. Chemically unrelated to tricyclic, tetracyclic, or other available antidepressants. Molecular weight—342.7.

**Mechanism of action/Effect**

Sertraline is a potent and selective inhibitor of neuronal serotonin (5-HT) uptake. It has only weak effects on neuronal uptake of norepinephrine and dopamine. Chronic administration of sertraline in animals has resulted in downregulation of postsynaptic beta-adrenergic receptors. Sertraline's inhibition of serotonin reuptake enhances serotonergic transmission, which results in subsequent inhibition of adrenergic activity in the locus ceruleus. Specifically, sertraline depresses the firing of the raphe serotonin neurons; this, in turn, increases the activity of the locus ceruleus, with consequent desensitization of the postsynaptic beta-receptors and presynaptic alpha$_2$-receptors.

Sertraline has no specific affinity for adrenergic (alpha$_1$, alpha$_2$, or beta) receptors, muscarinic-cholinergic receptors, gamma aminobutyric acid (GABA) receptors, dopaminergic receptors, histaminergic receptors, serotonergic (5HT$_{1A}$, 5HT$_{1B}$, 5HT$_2$) receptors, or benzodiazepine receptors. Sertraline does not inhibit monoamine oxidase.

**Other actions/effects**

Sertraline has anorectic and anti-obsessional effects.

**Absorption**

Slow but consistent. Bioavailability is increased if sertraline is taken with food, possibly due to first-pass metabolism.

**Distribution**

Both sertraline and its metabolites are extensively distributed into tissues. In animal studies, the volume of distribution (Vol$_D$) exceeded 20 Liters/kilogram (L/kg).

**Protein binding**

Very high (98%).

**Biotransformation**

Undergoes extensive first-pass metabolism in liver. The primary initial pathway is N-demethylation to form N-desmethylsertraline, which is substantially less active than the parent compound, exhibiting only about 1/8 of its activity. Animal testing has shown that N-desmethylsertraline does not contribute to the antidepressant activity or toxicity of the parent compound. Both sertraline and N-desmethylsertraline undergo oxidative deamination and subsequent reduction, hydroxylation, and glucuronide conjugation.

**Half-life**

Elimination—

Sertraline: 24 to 26 hours.

N-desmethylsertraline: 62 to 104 hours.

**Onset of action**

Within 2 to 4 weeks.

**Time to peak concentration**

Time to reach mean peak plasma concentration (T$_{max}$) following administration of 50 to 200 mg of sertraline once daily for 14 days ranged from 4.5 to 8.4 hours. When sertraline was administered with food, T$_{max}$ fell from 8 hours to 5.5 hours post-dosing.

**Peak plasma concentration**

Mean peak plasma concentration (C$_{max}$) and area under the plasma concentration time curve (AUC) were proportional to dose over the range of 50 to 200 mg of sertraline, demonstrating linear pharmacokinetics. When sertraline was administered with food, C$_{max}$ increased by 25% and AUC increased slightly. After once-daily dosing of sertraline,

steady-state plasma concentrations were reached in about 7 days in adult subjects, and after 2 to 3 weeks in older patients.

**Elimination**

Renal—

About 40 to 45% of an administered radioactive dose was recovered in the urine within 9 days, with less than 0.2% recovered unchanged.

Fecal—

About 40 to 45% of an administered radioactive dose was recovered in feces within 9 days, including 12 to 14% unchanged sertraline.

In dialysis—

Due to large volume of distribution, dialysis is not believed to be effective.

Note: In one study, clearance of sertraline in 16 elderly patients was about 40% lower than that in a similar group of younger patients. Clearance of desmethylsertraline was also decreased in older men but not older women. Similarly, the half-life of desmethylsertraline in older men was 109 hours compared to 68 hours in older women. However, the significance of this difference is unknown since desmethylsertraline is less active than its parent compound.

## Precautions to Consider

**Carcinogenicity**

In lifetime carcinogenicity studies, there was a dose-related increase in the incidence of liver adenomas in male CD-1 mice receiving sertraline at doses of 10 to 40 mg per kg of body weight (mg/kg) (up to 10 times the maximum human recommended dose on a mg/kg or milligram per square meter of body surface [mg/m$^2$] basis). However, liver adenomas have a variable rate of spontaneous occurrence in the CD-1 mouse, and the significance of this finding to use in humans is unknown. No increase in liver adenomas or hepatocellular carcinomas was seen in Long-Evans rats or in female CD-1 mice receiving doses of up to 40 mg/kg. Female rats receiving 40 mg/kg had an increase in follicular adenomas of the thyroid, unaccompanied by thyroid hyperplasia. Rats receiving 10 to 40 mg/kg showed an increase in uterine adenocarcinomas compared with placebo controls, but this effect was not clearly drug related.

**Mutagenicity**

Sertraline had no genotoxic effects, with or without metabolic activation, based on the bacterial mutation assay, mouse lymphoma mutation assay, or tests for cytogenic aberrations *in vivo* in mouse bone marrow and *in vitro* in human lymphocytes.

**Pregnancy/Reproduction**

Fertility—A decrease in fertility was seen in 1 of 2 studies in rats that received 80 mg of sertraline per kg of body weight (20 times the maximum human dose on a mg/kg basis and 4 times the maximum human dose on a mg/m$^2$ basis).

Pregnancy—Adequate and well-controlled studies in humans have not been done.

No teratogenic effects were demonstrated in studies in rats and rabbits receiving 20 and 10 times the maximum daily human mg/kg dose, respectively. However, in fetuses of dams receiving doses approximately 2.5 to 10 times the maximum daily human mg/kg dose, sertraline was associated with delayed ossification, probably secondary to effects on the dams. At maternal doses as low as approximately 5 times the maximum human mg/kg dose, there was decreased neonatal survival. Decrease in pup survival was probably due to *in utero* exposure to sertraline, but the clinical significance of these effects is unknown.

FDA Pregnancy Category B.

Labor and delivery—The effect of sertraline on labor and delivery is not known.

**Breast-feeding**

It is not known whether sertraline is excreted in breast milk.

**Pediatrics**

No information is available on the relationship of age to the effects of sertraline in pediatric patients. Safety and efficacy have not been established.

**Geriatrics**

No geriatrics-related problems have been documented in studies done to date that included elderly patients.

**Dental**
Prolonged use of sertraline may decrease or inhibit salivary flow, thus contributing to the development of caries, periodontal disease, oral candidiasis, and discomfort.

**Drug interactions and/or related problems**
The following drug interactions and/or related problems have been selected on the basis of their potential clinical significance (possible mechanism in parentheses where appropriate)—not necessarily inclusive (» = major clinical significance):

Note: Combinations containing any of the following medications, depending on the amount present, may also interact with this medication.

Alcohol
(although sertraline has not been shown to alter alcohol metabolism and does not appear to potentiate cognitive and psychomotor effects of alcohol in normal subjects, concomitant use in depressed patients is not recommended)

Diazepam
(concurrent use of intravenous diazepam with sertraline may reduce the clearance and prolong the half-life of diazepam in some patients; however, the clinical significance of this interaction is unknown)

» Highly protein-bound medications, especially:
Digitoxin
Warfarin
(caution in concurrent use with sertraline is recommended because of possible displacement of either medication from protein-binding sites, leading to increased plasma concentrations of the free [unbound] medications and increased risk of adverse effects)
(prothrombin time should be carefully monitored when sertraline therapy is initiated or stopped in patients taking warfarin)

Lithium
(although the potential for an interaction of sertraline with lithium exists, a placebo-controlled clinical trial in normal volunteers demonstrated no alteration in steady-state lithium levels or renal clearance of lithium; however, close monitoring of lithium concentrations is recommended; also, concurrent use may lead to a high incidence of serotonin-associated side effects)

» Monoamine oxidase (MAO) inhibitors, including furazolidone, procarbazine, and selegiline
(a potentially lethal hyperserotonergic state known as the serotonin syndrome may occur if a serotonergic agent such as sertraline is administered with MAO inhibitors. The syndrome may be manifested by mental status changes [confusion, hypomania], restlessness, myoclonus, hyperreflexia, diaphoresis, shivering, tremor, diarrhea, incoordination, and/or fever. If recognized early, the syndrome usually resolves quickly upon withdrawal of the offending agents)
(concurrent use of MAO inhibitors with sertraline may also result in hyperpyretic episodes, severe convulsions, and hypertensive crises; fatalities have occurred. Concomitant use of MAO inhibitors with sertraline is contraindicated. A wash-out period of at least 14 days should elapse between discontinuation of one medication and initiation of the other)

Tolbutamide
(concomitant use may result in decreased clearance of tolbutamide, although the clinical significance of this interaction is unknown; blood glucose should be monitored, and the dosage of tolbutamide reduced if hypoglycemia occurs)

**Laboratory value alterations**
The following have been selected on the basis of their potential clinical significance (possible effect in parentheses where appropriate)—not necessarily inclusive (» = major clinical significance):

With physiology/laboratory test values
Alanine aminotransferase (ALT [SGPT]) or
Aspartate aminotransferase (AST [SGOT])
(increased values have been reported infrequently; increases usually occur within 1 to 9 weeks of initiation of therapy, with values generally normalizing after sertraline is discontinued)

Total cholesterol or
Triglycerides
(small mean increases have been reported)

Uric acid, serum
(mean decreases of approximately 7% have been reported)

**Medical considerations/Contraindications**
The medical considerations/contraindications included here have been selected on the basis of their potential clinical significance (reasons given in parentheses where appropriate)—not necessarily inclusive (» = major clinical significance).

*Risk-benefit should be considered when the following medical problems exist:*
Drug abuse or dependence, history of
(patients with a history of drug abuse should be observed closely for signs of misuse or abuse of sertraline, as with any new central nervous system [CNS] drug)

Hepatic function impairment
(metabolism of sertraline may be altered)

Renal function impairment
(excretion of sertraline may be altered; however, results of an open-label study showed no difference in pharmacokinetic parameters of sertraline in patients with renal impairment ranging from mild to severe [but not requiring regular hemodialysis] with those of a matched healthy group with no renal impairment)

Seizure disorders
(as with other antidepressants, sertraline should be introduced with care)

Sensitivity to sertraline

Weight loss
(significant weight loss, although only rarely reported, may be undesirable in some patients)

**Patient monitoring**
The following may be especially important in patient monitoring (other tests may be warranted in some patients, depending on condition; » = major clinical significance):

Careful supervision of depressed patients with suicidal tendencies
(recommended especially during early treatment phase before peak effectiveness of sertraline is achieved; prescribing the smallest number of tablets necessary for good patient management is recommended to decrease risk of overdose)

## Side/Adverse Effects

Note: Side effects may be dose-related and time-related. Severity of side effects appears to lessen with decreased doses or after administration for longer than 2 weeks.

The following side/adverse effects have been selected on the basis of their potential clinical significance (possible signs and symptoms in parentheses where appropriate)—not necessarily inclusive:

**Those indicating need for medical attention**
Incidence less frequent or rare
*Fever; mania or hypomania; skin rash, hives, or itching*

**Those indicating need for medical attention only if they continue or are bothersome**
Incidence more frequent
*Decreased appetite or weight loss; decreased sexual drive or ability; diarrhea; dizziness; drowsiness; dryness of mouth; headache; increased sweating; insomnia* (trouble in sleeping); *nausea; stomach or abdominal cramps, gas, or pain; tiredness or weakness; tremor*

Incidence less frequent
*Anxiety, agitation, nervousness, or restlessness; changes in vision, including blurred vision; constipation; flushing or redness of skin, with feeling of warmth or heat; increased appetite; palpitations* (fast or irregular heartbeat); *vomiting*

## Overdose

For specific information on the agents used in the management of sertraline overdose, see:
• *Charcoal, Activated (Oral-Local)* monograph.

For more information on the management of overdose or unintentional ingestion, **contact a Poison Control Center** (see *Poison Control Center Listing*).

**Treatment of overdose**
There is no specific antidote for sertraline. Treatment is essentially symptomatic and supportive, possibly including:
To decrease absorption—
Administering activated charcoal, which may be used with sorbitol, may be as or more effective than emesis or gastric lavage.
To enhance elimination—
Dialysis, forced diuresis, hemoperfusion, and exchange transfusions are unlikely to be of benefit due to sertraline's large volume of distribution and high degree of protein binding.
Monitoring—
Monitoring cardiac function and vital signs.

Supportive care—
   Establishing and monitoring airway. Patients in whom intentional overdose is known or suspected should be referred for psychiatric consultation.

## Patient Consultation

As an aid to patient consultation, refer to *Advice for the Patient, Sertraline (Systemic).*

In providing consultation, consider emphasizing the following selected information (» = major clinical significance):

**Before using this medication**
» Conditions affecting use, especially:
   Sensitivity to sertraline
   Pregnancy—Animal studies using higher than maximum human mg/kg doses have shown delayed ossification in fetuses and decreased pup survival, probably due to *in utero* exposure to sertraline; clinical significance is unknown
   Dental—Decreased salivary flow may contribute to caries, periodontal disease, candidiasis, and discomfort
   Other medications, especially digitoxin, warfarin, and MAO inhibitors
   Other medical problems, especially hepatic or renal dysfunction or history of drug dependence

**Proper use of this medication**
» Compliance with therapy; not taking more or less medicine than prescribed
» Up to 4 weeks or more of therapy may be required before antidepressant effects are achieved
» Proper dosing
   Missed dose: Discussing with doctor what to do about any missed doses
» Proper storage

**Precautions while using this medication**
   Regular visits to physician to check progress of therapy
» Avoiding use of alcoholic beverages; not taking other CNS depressants unless prescribed by physician
» Possible drowsiness, impairment of judgment, thinking, or motor skills; caution when driving or doing jobs requiring alertness
» Possible dryness of mouth; using sugarless gum or candy, ice, or saliva substitute for relief; checking with physician or dentist if dry mouth continues for more than 2 weeks

**Side/adverse effects**
   Fever; mania or hypomania; or skin rash, hives, or itching

## General Dosing Information

Potentially suicidal patients should not have access to large quantities of this medication since depressed patients, particularly those who may use alcohol excessively, may continue to exhibit suicidal tendencies until significant improvement occurs. Some clinicians recommend that the patient be supplied with the least amount of medication necessary for satisfactory patient management.

Activation of hypomania or mania has been reported in depressed patients treated with sertraline.

**Diet/Nutrition**
Sertraline may be taken with or without food. Some clinicians advise their patients to take this medication with food to lessen gastrointestinal side effects. However, sertraline should always be taken at the same time in relation to food intake in order to ensure consistent absorption.

## Oral Dosage Forms

Note: The dosing and strengths of the dosage forms available are expressed in terms of sertraline base.

## SERTRALINE HYDROCHLORIDE CAPSULES

**Usual adult dose**
Depression—
   Oral, initially 50 mg (base) a day as a single morning or evening dose. The dose may be increased after several weeks in increments of 50 mg, with increases made at intervals of at least 1 week, as needed and tolerated.

**Usual adult prescribing limits**
200 mg (base) a day.

**Usual pediatric dose**
Safety and efficacy have not been established.

**Strength(s) usually available**
U.S.—
   Not commercially available.
Canada—
   50 mg (base) (Rx) [*Zoloft*].
   100 mg (base) (Rx) [*Zoloft*].

**Packaging and storage**
Store below 40 °C (104 °F), preferably between 15 and 30 °C (59 and 86 °F), unless otherwise specified by manufacturer.

**Auxiliary labeling**
• Avoid alcoholic beverages.

## SERTRALINE HYDROCHLORIDE TABLETS

**Usual adult dose**
Depression—
   Oral, initially 50 mg (base) a day as a single morning or evening dose. The dose may be increased after several weeks in increments of 50 mg, with increases made at intervals of at least 1 week, as needed and tolerated.

Note: Some clinicians recommend an initial dose of 25 mg a day for 1 to 2 days.

**Usual adult prescribing limits**
200 mg (base) a day.

**Usual pediatric dose**
Safety and efficacy have not been established.

**Usual geriatric dose**
Initially 12.5 to 25 mg (base) a day, as a single morning or evening dose; dose may be increased gradually as needed and tolerated.

**Strength(s) usually available**
U.S.—
   50 mg (base) (Rx) [*Zoloft* (scored)].
   100 mg (base) (Rx) [*Zoloft* (scored)].
Canada—
   Not commercially available.

**Packaging and storage**
Store below 40 °C (104 °F), preferably between 15 and 30 °C (59 and 86 °F), unless otherwise specified by manufacturer.

**Auxiliary labeling**
• Avoid alcoholic beverages.

## Selected Bibliography

Guthrie SK. Sertraline: A new specific serotonin reuptake blocker. DICP Ann Pharmacother 1991 Sep; 25: 952-61.

Grimsley SR, Jann MW. Paroxetine, sertraline, and fluvoxamine: New selective serotonin reuptake inhibitors. Clin Pharm 1992 Nov; 11: 930-57.

Murdoch D, McTavish D. Sertraline. A review of its pharmacodynamic and pharmacokinetic properties, and therapeutic potential in depression and obsessive-compulsive disorder. Drugs 1992; 44 (4): 604-24.

Revised: 03/19/93
Interim revision: 08/14/95

# SEVOFLURANE  Inhalation-Systemic

VA CLASSIFICATION (Primary): CN201

Note: For a listing of dosage forms and brand names by country availability, see *Dosage Forms* section(s). For a listing of brand names for the articles in this monograph, refer to the General Index.

## Category
Anesthetic (general).

## Indications

### Accepted
Anesthesia, general—Sevoflurane is indicated for the induction and maintenance of general anesthesia in adult and pediatric patients during inpatient or outpatient surgery. Often, sevoflurane is used with other medications to induce or supplement anesthesia.

### Unaccepted
Sevoflurane does not have analgesic activity at subanesthetic concentrations and is not recommended as an analgesic.

## Pharmacology/Pharmacokinetics

Note: Concentration-response relationships for inhalation anesthetics are described in terms of the minimum alveolar concentration (MAC), which is defined as the alveolar concentration that prevents movement in 50% of patients after surgical skin incision. The MAC decreases with pregnancy, hypothermia, hypotension, increasing age, and concurrent use of other central nervous system (CNS) depressants, including other inhalation anesthetics. Average MAC values for sevoflurane (vaporized in oxygen) are 3%, 2.6%, and 1.7% for patients 1 to 6 months, 25 years, and 60 years of age, respectively. While MAC is commonly used to compare the concentration-response relationships for inhalation anesthetics, the $AD_{95}$ (the dose preventing 95% of patients from moving in response to skin incision) is more clinically relevant in dosing patients with inhalation anesthetics, if the inhalation anesthetic is used alone. Often, inhalation anesthetics are used in combination with other agents to supplement anesthesia.

### Physicochemical characteristics
Chemical group—A halogenated hydrocarbon (methyl ethyl ether) anesthetic.
Molecular weight—200.06.
Other characteristics—MAC in oxygen for adults 40 years of age: 2.1%.
Blood-to-gas partition coefficient (37 °C [98.6 °F]): 0.63 to 0.69.
Brain-to-gas partition coefficient (37 °C [98.6 °F]): 1.15.
Oil-to-gas partition coefficient (37 °C [98.6 °F]): 47 to 54.

### Mechanism of action/Effect
The precise mechanism by which inhalation anesthetics produce loss of perception of sensations and unconsciousness is not known. Inhaled anesthetics act at many areas in the CNS. The Meyer-Overton theory suggests that the site of action of inhalation anesthetics may be the lipid matrix of neuronal membranes or other lipophilic sites. Anesthetics may cause changes in membrane thickness, which in turn affect the gating properties of ion channels in neurons. Interference with the hydrophobic portion of neuronal ion channel membrane proteins may be an important mechanism.

### Other actions/effects
Cardiovascular system effects—
Sevoflurane has several effects that serve to lower blood pressure. It depresses cardiac function, decreases cardiac contractility, and decreases peripheral vascular resistance in a manner similar to that of isoflurane. These effects are dose-related; increasing the concentration of sevoflurane during maintenance of anesthesia results in a dose-dependent decrease in blood pressure. The effect of sevoflurane on the coronary arteries and the potential for "coronary steal" has been investigated in dogs. Sevoflurane administration to chronically instrumented dogs resulted in a reduced ratio of occluded/normal and stenotic/normal coronary artery flows. However, the ratios returned to normal when the arterial blood pressure and heart rate were restored to conscious values.
Sevoflurane has little effect on heart rate or rhythm. At clinically useful doses, sevoflurane does not increase heart rate or myocardial oxygen consumption. At higher concentrations, sevoflurane may increase heart rate. A study on the effects of sevoflurane on the arrhythmic response to epinephrine suggests that sevoflurane does not greatly sensitize the myocardium to the arrhythmogenic effect of catecholamines.

CNS—
Electroencephalogram (EEG): Sevoflurane causes a dose-dependent decrease in EEG activity. In dogs and rabbits, EEG burst suppression occurs at doses of 1 MAC or higher. Although sevoflurane is not believed to be epileptogenic, case reports describe clonic and tonic seizure-like movements and clinically silent electrical seizures during induction of anesthesia.
Effect on intracranial pressure: Sevoflurane did not impair cerebral autoregulation of blood flow when studied in patients with ischemic cerebrovascular disease. However, sevoflurane has the potential to increase intracranial pressure.
Neuromuscular effects—
Sevoflurane impairs neuromuscular conduction and decreases muscle contractility. Sevoflurane may produce sufficient muscle relaxation to allow some types of surgery to be performed without a neuromuscular blocker.
Respiratory system effects—
Respiration: Sevoflurane depresses ventilation in a dose-dependent manner, with apnea occurring between 1.5 and 2 MAC. Surgical stimulation changes the threshold at which apnea occurs. Sevoflurane increases carbon dioxide tension and decreases ventilatory response to increased carbon dioxide concentrations.
Effects on the airway: Sevoflurane results in a low incidence of respiratory irritation as evidenced by a low incidence of breath-holding, coughing, increased salivation, and laryngospasm during induction.

### Absorption
Sevoflurane is rapidly absorbed into the circulation via the lungs. Its solubility in the blood is low; for a given concentration of sevoflurane in the gas phase, only a small amount dissolved in the blood is necessary to achieve equilibrium between the alveolar partial pressure and the arterial partial pressure.

### Biotransformation
Approximately 5% of the sevoflurane dose is metabolized, primarily by cytochrome P450 2E1, with release of inorganic fluoride and carbon dioxide. The plasma inorganic fluoride concentration is increased to > 95 mcg per dL (mcg/dL) (50 micromoles per L [micromoles/L]) following surgery of long duration.

### Time to peak concentration
The alveolar concentration of sevoflurane increases rapidly toward the inspired concentration. The ratio of alveolar concentration to inspired concentration increases more rapidly with nitrous oxide and desflurane than with sevoflurane but more rapidly with sevoflurane than with isoflurane and halothane.

### Time to peak effect
Onset of anesthesia—Sevoflurane has a favorable rate of increase of the ratio of alveolar concentration to inspired concentration. When sevoflurane is used alone and is administered by conventional technique, induction is accomplished in 2 minutes. This time can be reduced by the addition of nitrous oxide or the use of a vital capacity breath technique. With the use of a vital capacity breath technique, induction can be accomplished in about 1 minute.

### Duration of action
Time to recovery—Recovery after discontinuation is rapid, but is subject to interpatient variability. Recovery time is affected by the administered concentration and other CNS depressants used concurrently. Emergence from sevoflurane is more rapid than emergence from isoflurane, but less rapid than from desflurane. Spontaneous eye opening, response to simple commands, extubation, and orientation are more quickly achieved with sevoflurane than with isoflurane. However, time to later recovery events (walking, tolerating oral fluids, voiding, and home readiness) does not differ between isoflurane and sevoflurane or desflurane and sevoflurane.

### Elimination
Rapidly eliminated via exhalation. The metabolite is conjugated with glucuronic acid and eliminated via the urine. Up to 3.5% of the sevoflurane dose appears in the urine as inorganic fluoride. Up to 50% of fluoride is taken up into the bone. As compared to the half-life in healthy individuals, the fluoride ion half-life is prolonged in patients with renal function impairment (33 hours versus 21 hours), and slightly prolonged in patients with hepatic function impairment.

# Precautions to Consider

## Cross-sensitivity and/or related problems
Patients sensitive to other halogenated ether hydrocarbons may be sensitive to sevoflurane also.

## Carcinogenicity
Studies have not been done.

## Mutagenicity
No mutagenic effect was observed in the Ames test. No chromosomal aberrations were induced in cultured mammalian cells. Problems in humans have not been documented.

## Pregnancy/Reproduction
Fertility—Reproduction studies performed in rats and rabbits at doses up to 1 minimum alveolar concentration (MAC) revealed no evidence of impaired fertility.

Pregnancy—Sevoflurane crosses the placenta. Adequate and well controlled studies have not been done in humans.

Studies in pregnant rabbits and rats at doses of 0.3 MAC, the highest nontoxic dose, revealed no fetal damage.

FDA Pregnancy Category B.

Labor and delivery—The safety of sevoflurane in labor and vaginal delivery has not been established. Sevoflurane was used as part of general anesthesia in 61 women undergoing elective cesarean section. There was no harmful effect in any mother or neonate. There was no difference between sevoflurane and isoflurane in recovery characteristics, Apgar score, or Neurological and Adaptive Capacity Score. In one study two of sixteen patients had poor spontaneous uterine contractions after receiving sevoflurane.

## Breast-feeding
It is not known if sevoflurane is distributed into breast milk. However, because of rapid washout, sevoflurane concentrations in milk are predicted to be below those found with other anesthetics. The concentrations of sevoflurane in milk are thought to be of no clinical importance 24 hours after anesthesia.

## Pediatrics
Due to its lack of pungency, sevoflurane is widely used in Japan for induction of anesthesia in pediatric patients. As compared to halothane, sevoflurane for induction is associated with a higher incidence of excitation. In one study, this led to a longer time to intubation with sevoflurane. The longer time to intubation was not seen in two other studies, perhaps due to differences in the speed with which maximum concentrations of anesthetic were reached.

Pediatric patients require a higher concentration of sevoflurane for maintenance of general anesthesia than that required by adults.

Sevoflurane is associated with a higher incidence of emergence excitation in children than is halothane, perhaps due to earlier emergence and the resultant earlier experience of pain in children receiving sevoflurane.

## Geriatrics
MAC decreases with increasing age. The average concentration of sevoflurane to achieve MAC in a patient 80 years of age is approximately 50% of that required in a patient 20 years of age.

Older adults may be slower than younger adults in achieving full cognitive recovery from general anesthesia with sevoflurane.

## Drug interactions and/or related problems
The following drug interactions and/or related problems have been selected on the basis of their potential clinical significance (possible mechanism in parentheses where appropriate)—not necessarily inclusive (» = major clinical significance):

Note: Combinations containing any of the following medications, depending on the amount present, may also interact with this medication.

Many of the following interactions have not been reported with sevoflurane. However, because they have been reported with other halogenated hydrocarbon anesthetics, the possibility of a significant interaction with sevoflurane must be considered.

Alcohol, chronic use
(anesthetic requirement may be increased; induction of cytochrome P450 2E1 hepatic enzymes increases the extent of metabolism of sevoflurane, increasing the production of inorganic fluoride)

» Aminoglycosides, systemic or
Anesthetics, parenteral-local or
Bacitracin or
» Capreomycin or
» Citrate-anticoagulated blood, massive transfusions of or
» Clindamycin or
Colistimethate sodium or

Colistin or
Lidocaine, systemic use or
» Lincomycin, systemic or
» Neuromuscular blocking agents or
» Polymyxins, systemic or
Procaine, systemic or
Tetracyclines or
Trimethaphan (large doses)
(neuromuscular blocking activities of these medications may be additive to that of sevoflurane, with the degree of potentiation increasing as the concentration of sevoflurane is increased)

Amiodarone
(concurrent use with inhalation anesthetics may potentiate hypotension and increase the risk of atropine-resistant bradycardia)

Antimyasthenics
(antimyasthenics may decrease the neuromuscular blocking activity of halogenated hydrocarbon anesthetics; also, the neuromuscular blocking activity of the anesthetic may interfere with the efficacy of antimyasthenics; neuromuscular blockade with vecuronium during sevoflurane anesthesia may be more difficult to reverse with neostigmine than when similar blockade is produced during isoflurane anesthesia)

Beta-adrenergic blocking agents, including ophthalmics
(severe hypotension may result because beta-blockade reduces the ability of the heart to respond to beta-adrenergically mediated sympathetic reflex stimuli)

Catecholamines, such as dopamine, epinephrine, or norepinephrine
(sevoflurane may cause some sensitization of the myocardium to the effects of catecholamines, increasing the risk of arrhythmias; this is similar to isoflurane's effect on the myocardium; sevoflurane sensitizes the myocardium much less than does halothane)

CNS depression–producing medications, other, including those commonly used for pre-anesthetic medications, or induction or supplementation of anesthesia (See Appendix II)
(may cause increased CNS depression, respiratory depression, and/or hypotension, decrease the anesthetic requirement, and prolong the recovery from anesthesia)

Hypotension-producing medications (See Appendix II)
(hypotensive effects may be potentiated when these medications are used concurrently with an inhalation anesthetic)

Isoniazid and other cytochrome P450 2E1 hepatic enzyme inducers
(enzyme induction increases the extent of metabolism of sevoflurane, increasing the production of inorganic fluoride; increased plasma fluoride concentrations have been associated with renal function impairment with other volatile inhalation anesthetics)

## Laboratory value alterations
The following have been selected on the basis of their potential clinical significance (possible effect in parentheses where appropriate)—not necessarily inclusive (» = major clinical significance):

With physiology/laboratory test values
Alanine aminotransferase (ALT [SGPT]), serum and
Aspartate aminotransferase (AST [SGOT]), serum and
Bilirubin, serum, indirect and
Lactate dehydrogenase, serum
(values may be transiently increased; the increases are dose-related)

Blood urea nitrogen (BUN) and
Creatinine, serum and
Fluoride, serum
(concentrations may be increased)

Glucose, serum
(concentration may be increased)

Leukocytes
(counts may be increased)

## Medical considerations/Contraindications
The medical considerations/contraindications included here have been selected on the basis of their potential clinical significance (reasons given in parentheses where appropriate)—not necessarily inclusive (» = major clinical significance).

*Except under special circumstances, this medication should not be used when the following medical problems exist:*
» Malignant hyperthermia, history of
(possible increased risk of malignant hyperthermia with sevoflurane; malignant hyperthermia has been associated with the use of sevoflurane in both children and adults)

» Sensitivity to halogenated ether anesthetic agents
  (possible increased risk of sensitivity to sevoflurane; although not yet reported with sevoflurane, cases of immune-mediated hepatitis have been reported with similar inhalation anesthetics)

*Risk-benefit should be considered when the following medical problems exist:*

Familial periodic paralysis or
Muscular dystrophy or
Myasthenia gravis or
Myasthenic syndrome or
Other neuromuscular disease leading to muscle weakness
  (the neuromuscular blocking activity of sevoflurane may increase the risk of severe muscle weakness in patients with these conditions; although use of an inhalation anesthetic with substantial neuromuscular blocking activity may be safer than [and eliminate the need for] a neuromuscular blocking agent in these patients, caution is recommended)

Head injury or
Increased intracranial pressure or
Intracranial lesions, space-occupying
  (sevoflurane may increase intracranial pressure to the same extent that isoflurane may; in a study on ten patients with ischemic cerebrovascular disease, carbon dioxide response and cerebral autoregulation were maintained under 0.88 MAC anesthesia)

Hepatic function impairment
  (in patients with mild to moderate hepatic function impairment, administration of sevoflurane resulted in prolonged terminal disposition of fluoride, as evidenced by longer inorganic fluoride half-life than that observed in patients with normal hepatic function; there is no published clinical experience with use of sevoflurane in patients with severe hepatic function impairment)

Pulsed dye laser therapy for portwine stain
  (sevoflurane anesthesia is associated with portwine stain fading and subsequent early termination of pulsed dye laser treatment, resulting in inadequate treatment of the stain; the incidence of portwine stain fade with sevoflurane is significantly higher than the incidence of fade with halothane, enflurane, or isoflurane)

Renal function impairment
  (extended anesthesia with sevoflurane is associated with hyperfluorinemia; with methoxyflurane, hyperfluorinemia in excess of 95 mcg per dL [mcg/dL] [50 micromoles per L (micromoles/L)] has been associated with renal function impairment; a tendency toward decreased urine concentrating ability and increased urinary excretion of N-acetyl-beta-glucosaminidase (NAG) has been associated with the use of sevoflurane; frank renal failure has not been observed, even when serum fluoride concentrations in excess of 95 mcg/dL [50 micromoles/L] are achieved; reaction of sevoflurane with carbon dioxide [$CO_2$] absorbents is associated with the formation of compound A, a nephrotoxin in rats; the toxicity of compound A has not been established in humans; caution is recommended in patients with renal function impairment because of limited studies in this patient population)

**Patient monitoring**

The following may be especially important in patient monitoring (other tests may be warranted in some patients, depending on condition; » = major clinical significance):

Note: Various organizations, including medical specialty societies, and institutions have established standards for the pre-, intra-, and postprocedural care, evaluation, and monitoring of patients receiving various forms of anesthesia. The following recommendations represent the minimum standards established by the American Society of Anesthesiologists for monitoring the status of patients receiving general anesthesia. Individual patients may require additional monitoring.

» Blood pressure and
» Body temperature and
» Cardiac/pulse rate and
» Cardiac rhythm and
» Pulse oximetry and
» Respiratory and ventilatory status
  (continuous monitoring is advisable during anesthetic administration; respiratory depression and excessive decreases in blood pressure may be related to the depth of anesthesia and may be corrected by decreasing the inspired concentration of sevoflurane)

## Side/Adverse Effects

The following side/adverse effects have been selected on the basis of their potential clinical significance (possible signs and symptoms in parentheses where appropriate)—not necessarily inclusive:

**Those indicating need for medical attention**

Incidence more frequent (greater than 3%)
  *During induction by mask (adult patients)*
    **Airway obstruction; bradycardia; breath-holding; cough, increased; hypotension; laryngospasm**

  *During induction by mask (pediatric patients)*
    **Breath-holding; cough, increased; hypotension; tachycardia**

  *During induction by mask (adult and pediatric patients)*
    **Agitation**

  *During maintenance and recovery (adult and pediatric patients)*
    **Bradycardia; excitement; hypotension**

Incidence less frequent (1 to 3%)
  *During induction by mask (adult patients)*
    **Tachycardia**

  *During induction by mask (pediatric patients)*
    **Apnea; laryngospasm**

  *During maintenance and recovery (adult and pediatric patients)*
    **Breath-holding; fever; hypertension; hypothermia; laryngospasm; tachycardia**

Incidence rare (less than 1%)
  **Acidosis; arrhythmias; bronchospasm; hypoxia; malignant hyperthermia; seizures; syncope; wheezing**

**Those indicating need for medical attention only if they continue or are bothersome**

Incidence more frequent (greater than 3%)
  *During maintenance and recovery (adult and pediatric patients)*
    **Cough, increased; dizziness; drowsiness, prolonged; nausea; salivation, increased; shivering; vomiting**

Incidence less frequent (1 to 3%)
  *During maintenance and recovery (adult and pediatric patients)*
    **Headache**

## Overdose

For more information on the management of overdose or unintentional ingestion, **contact a Poison Control Center** (see *Poison Control Center Listing*).

**Clinical effects of overdose**

The clinical effects of an overdose of sevoflurane represent an extension of its therapeutic effects. Some respiratory effects of increased depth of anesthesia (for example, respiratory depression and apnea) are not problematic if assisted or controlled ventilation is being used during the procedure. The following effects have been selected on the basis of their potential clinical significance (possible signs and symptoms in parentheses where appropriate)—not necessarily inclusive:

Acute effects
  **Apnea** (cessation of breathing); **bradycardia** (slowed heart rate); **cardiac arrest** (cessation of heartbeat); **circulatory collapse; circulatory depression** (bluish fingernails); **decreased cardiac contractility; decreased peripheral vascular resistance; EEG burst suppression; hypotension; respiratory depression** (slowed breathing)

**Treatment of overdose**

Discontinuing sevoflurane, maintaining a patent airway, initiating assisted or controlled ventilation with oxygen, and maintaining adequate cardiovascular function with general measures of circulatory support.

## Patient Consultation

As an aid to patient consultation, refer to *Advice for the Patient, Sevoflurane (Inhalation-Systemic)*.

In providing consultation, consider emphasizing the following selected information (» = major clinical significance):

**Before using this medication**

» Conditions affecting use, especially:
    Sensitivity to sevoflurane or other halogenated ether anesthetics
    Pregnancy—Sevoflurane crosses the placenta
    Other medications, especially aminoglycosides (systemic), capreomycin, citrate-anticoagulated blood (massive transfusions of), clindamycin, lincomycin, neuromuscular blocking agents, or polymyxins (systemic)
    Other medical problems, especially a history of or genetic susceptibility to malignant hyperthermia or renal function impairment

**Proper use of this medication**

» Proper dosing

**Precautions after receiving this medication**

» Possibility of psychomotor impairment following anesthesia; for 24 hours following anesthesia, avoiding driving or performing other tasks requiring alertness and coordination

» Avoiding use of alcohol or other CNS depressants within 24 hours following anesthesia, unless specifically prescribed or otherwise authorized by physician or dentist

**Side/adverse effects**

Signs of potential side effects, especially airway obstruction, bradycardia, breath-holding, increased cough, hypotension, laryngospasm, tachycardia, agitation, apnea, fever, hypertension, hypothermia, acidosis, arrhythmias, bronchospasm, hypoxia, malignant hyperthermia, seizures, syncope, and wheezing

Notifying physician if cough, drowsiness, nausea, or vomiting occurs or persists after discharge

# General Dosing Information

Sevoflurane is to be administered only by trained anesthesiologists or nurse anesthetists. Equipment and personnel for support of ventilation must be immediately available.

The dosage of sevoflurane must be individualized according to surgical requirements; concurrent use of adjuvant medications and/or nitrous oxide; and patient variables, especially age. Anesthetic requirements are increased in young children and decreased in geriatric patients.

The dosage requirement for neuromuscular blockers may change with sevoflurane anesthesia. The dose of neuromuscular blocker administered for endotracheal intubation should not be decreased, because delayed intubation may result. During maintenance of anesthesia with sevoflurane, the dose of neuromuscular blocker is likely to be lower than that required during anesthesia maintained with nitrous oxide and opioid agents. Neuromuscular blockade with vecuronium during sevoflurane anesthesia may be more difficult to reverse with neostigmine than when similar blockade is produced during isoflurane anesthesia.

Sevoflurane has a nonpungent odor and is associated with a low incidence of respiratory irritability, making it suitable for mask induction.

Sevoflurane may be vaporized in a flow of oxygen or a nitrous oxide–oxygen mixture. The concentration of sevoflurane being delivered from a vaporizer during anesthesia should be known. This may be accomplished by using a vaporizer calibrated specifically for sevoflurane. Fresh gas flow rates below 2 L per minute (L/min) are not recommended. A concern in low-flow systems is accumulation of compound A, a substance produced when sevoflurane interacts with carbon dioxide absorbents (e.g., soda lime or barium hydroxide). Compound A has been found to be a dose-dependent nephrotoxin in rats. The toxicity of compound A in humans has not been established.

During the maintenance of anesthesia, increasing the concentration of sevoflurane produces dose-dependent decreases in blood pressure. These hemodynamic changes may occur rapidly with sevoflurane due to its relative insolubility in blood. Excessive respiratory depression or decreases in blood pressure may be related to the depth of anesthesia and may be corrected by decreasing the inspired concentration of sevoflurane.

No specific premedication is indicated or contraindicated with the use of sevoflurane. The decisions regarding premedication should be based on the judgment of the health care professional.

**Safety considerations for handling this medication**

Acute overexposure of operating room personnel to sevoflurane may cause headache, dizziness, and, in extreme cases, unconsciousness.

The results of some epidemiological studies suggest a link between chronic exposure of operating room personnel to low concentrations of inhalation anesthetics (waste anesthetic gases [WAGs]) and increased health problems, including reproductive problems (increases in spontaneous abortions, stillbirths, and possibly birth defects). Although a causal relationship has not been established, measures to minimize exposure are recommended. Such measures include maintaining adequate general ventilation in the operating room, using a well-designed and well-maintained scavenging system, and, by employment of careful work procedures and routine equipment maintenance, minimizing leaks and spills while the anesthetic is in use.

Although no specific work exposure limit has been established for sevoflurane, the National Institute for Occupational Safety and Health Administration has recommended an 8-hour, time-weighted average limit of 2 parts per million (ppm) for halogenated anesthetic agents in general. The limit for halogenated anesthetics coupled with nitrous oxide is 0.5 ppm.

**For treatment of adverse effects**

Recommended treatment consists of the following:

• For malignant hyperthermic crisis—Discontinuation of possible triggering agents (such as inhalation anesthetics or succinylcholine), managing increased oxygen requirement, cooling the patient, and correcting fluid and electrolyte imbalances and metabolic acidosis. Dantrolene can be administered by rapid intravenous injection (See *Dantrolene [Systemic]* monograph).

# Inhalation Dosage Forms

## SEVOFLURANE

**Usual adult dose**

Anesthetic (general)—

Inhalation, vaporized in a flow of oxygen or nitrous oxide and oxygen:

Induction—Dosage must be individualized according to patient response.

Maintenance—Dosage must be individualized according to patient response. Surgical levels of anesthesia usually can be achieved with concentrations of 0.5 to 3% sevoflurane with or without concomitant use of nitrous oxide

Note: Anesthetic requirements decrease with increasing age. Minimum alveolar concentration (MAC) values for sevoflurane in oxygen are 2.6% for patients 25 years of age, 2.1% for patients 40 years of age, 1.7% for patients 60 years of age, and 1.4% for patients 80 years of age. Geriatric patients require lower doses of sevoflurane for induction and maintenance of anesthesia.

**Usual pediatric dose**

Anesthetic (general)—

Inhalation, vaporized in a flow of oxygen or nitrous oxide and oxygen:

Induction—Dosage must be individualized according to patient response.

Maintenance—Dosage must be individualized according to patient response. Surgical levels of anesthesia usually can be achieved with 0.5 to 3% sevoflurane with or without concomitant use of nitrous oxide.

Note: Anesthetic requirements decrease with increasing age. MAC values for sevoflurane in oxygen are 3.3% for neonates, 3% for infants less than 6 months of age, 2.8% for infants and children 6 months to 3 years of age, and 2.5% for children 3 to 12 years of age. MAC in premature neonates has not been determined.

MAC in adolescents has not been determined. The adolescent dose for other inhalation anesthetics is slightly higher than the dose for adult patients

**Usual geriatric dose**

Anesthetic (general)—

Geriatric patients require lower doses of sevoflurane for induction and maintenance of anesthesia. See *Usual adult dose.*

**Product(s) usually available**

U.S.—

(Rx) [*Ultane*].

Canada—

(Rx) [*Sevorane*].

**Packaging and storage**

Store below 40 °C (104 °F), preferably between 15 and 30 °C (59 and 86 °F), unless otherwise specified by manufacturer.

**Stability**

Stable at room temperature. No discernible degradation occurs in the presence of acid or heat. The only known degradation reaction in the clinical setting is through direct contact with carbon dioxide absorbents such as soda lime. This reaction produces pentafluoroisopropenyl fluoromethyl ether, also known as compound A, and trace amounts of pentafluoromethoxy isopropyl fluoromethyl ether, also known as compound B. The concentration of the degradants is inversely correlated with fresh gas flow rate.

With sevoflurane, unlike with desflurane, enflurane, and isoflurane, degradation of the anesthetic during use does not result in significant production of carbon monoxide.

# Selected Bibliography

Sarner JB, Levine M, Davis P, et al. Clinical characteristics of sevoflurane in children. A comparison with halothane. Anesthesiology 1995; 82 (1): 38-46.

Eger EI. New inhaled anesthetics. Anesthesiology 1994; 80: 906-22.

Frink EJ. Toxicologic potential of desflurane and sevoflurane. Acta Anaesthesiol Scand 1995; 39 (suppl 105): 120-2.

Developed: 06/28/96

# SILICONE OIL 5000 CENTISTOKES   Parenteral-Local†

VA CLASSIFICATION (Primary): OP900

Another commonly used name is polydimethylsiloxane.

Note: For a listing of dosage forms and brand names by country availability, see *Dosage Forms* section(s). For a listing of brand names for the articles in this monograph, refer to the General Index.

---

†Not commercially available in Canada.

## Category

Surgical aid (ophthalmic).

## Indications

### Accepted

Retinal detachment (treatment)—Silicone oil is indicated for use as a prolonged retinal tamponade in selected cases of complicated retinal detachments when other interventions are not appropriate for patient management. Complicated retinal detachments or recurrent retinal detachments occur most commonly following perforating injuries or in eyes with proliferative vitreoretinopathy (PVR), proliferative diabetic retinopathy (PDR), cytomegalovirus (CMV) retinitis, or giant tears.

Silicone oil is also indicated in the treatment of retinal detachments due to acquired immunodeficiency syndrome (AIDS)-related CMV retinitis and other viral infections.

## Pharmacology/Pharmacokinetics

### Physicochemical characteristics

Source—Silicone oil is a sterile, highly purified long chain polydimethylsiloxane. It is a clear colorless liquid at room temperature with a viscosity of 5000 to 5400 centistokes (nominal 5000 centistokes). It has a specific gravity of between 0.96 and 0.98 grams per cubic centimeter at 25° C. It has a refractive index of between 1.403 and 1.405 at 25° C.

### Mechanism of action/Effect

Provides a physical retinal tamponade.

### Onset of action

Immediately upon placement of product.

### Duration of action

Until product is physically removed.

## Precautions to Consider

### Pregnancy/Reproduction

Problems in humans have not been documented.

### Breast-feeding

Problems in humans have not been documented.

### Pediatrics

Appropriate studies performed to date have not demonstrated pediatrics-specific problems that would limit the usefulness of silicone oil in children.

### Geriatrics

Appropriate studies performed to date have not demonstrated geriatrics-specific problems that would limit the usefulness of silicone oil in the elderly.

### Medical considerations/Contraindications

The medical considerations/contraindications included here have been selected on the basis of their potential clinical significance (reasons given in parentheses where appropriate)—not necessarily inclusive (» = major clinical significance).

*Except under special circumstances, this product should not be used when the following medical problem exists:*
» Pseudophakia with silicone intraocular lenses (IOLs)
    (silicone oil can chemically interact with and opacify silicone elastomers; use of silicone oil is contraindicated in patients with pseudophakia who have IOLs)

*Risk-benefit should be considered when the following medical problem exists:*
    Sensitivity to silicone oil

## Patient monitoring

The following may be especially important in patient monitoring (other tests may be warranted in some patients, depending on condition; » = major clinical significance):
» Ophthalmologic examinations
    (patients should be scheduled for follow-up examinations at regular intervals; patients should be monitored for signs of glaucoma, cataracts, and keratopathy complications; in addition, since there is a possible correlation between the migration of silicone oil into the anterior chamber and the appearance of corneal changes, such as edema, hazing or opacification, Descemet folds, or decompensation, patients' corneal status should be regularly monitored and early corrective action should be taken, if necessary, including extraction of the oil from the anterior chamber; large bubbles or droplets of oil found in the anterior chamber can be removed manually by syringe)

## Side/Adverse Effects

Note: There is a possible correlation between the migration of silicone oil into the anterior chamber and the appearance of corneal changes, such as edema, hazing or opacification, Descemet folds, or decompensation.

Temporary increases in pressure that occur more than 3 weeks after silicone oil placement result from the silicone oil causing a mechanical blockage of the pupil, causing a mechanical blockage of a previously executed inferior iridectomy, or forcing its way anteriorly, thereby resulting in chamber angle closure. These conditions may normalize spontaneously or can be corrected by surgical treatment. If surgical treatment is needed, some of the oil may be withdrawn to relieve the mechanical force of the oil interface. Presence of silicone oil droplets in the anterior chamber may also cause a chronic outflow obstruction of the trabecular meshwork. In the majority of patients with outflow obstruction, elevated intraocular pressure can be managed with antiglaucoma medication.

The following side/adverse effects have been selected on the basis of their potential clinical significance (possible signs and symptoms in parentheses where appropriate)—not necessarily inclusive:

### Those indicating need for medical attention

Incidence more frequent
    *Anterior chamber oil migration* (blurred vision or other change in vision not present before treatment, or returning or getting worse after treatment; eye pain; eye redness; headache; tearing)—incidence 17 to 20%; *cataract* (blurred vision or other change in vision not present before treatment, or returning or getting worse after treatment)—incidence 50 to 70%; *glaucoma* (abdominal pain; eye pain; eye redness; headache; nausea or vomiting; tearing)—incidence approximately 20%; *keratopathy* (blurred vision or other change in vision not present before treatment, or returning or getting worse after treatment; eye pain; eye redness; swelling of eye; tearing)—incidence 8 to 20%

Incidence less frequent—incidence greater than 2%
    *Angle blockade* (abdominal pain; eye pain; eye redness; headache; nausea or vomiting; tearing); *macular pucker; optic nerve atrophy; traction detachment* (blurred vision or other change in vision not present before treatment, or returning or getting worse after treatment); *phthisis* (blurred vision or other change in vision not present before treatment, or returning or getting worse after treatment; eye pain; eye redness; tearing); *redetachment of retina; vitreous hemorrhage* (blurred vision or other change in vision not present before treatment, or returning or getting worse after treatment; seeing floaters or light flashes); *rubeosis iridis* (eye pain; eye redness; headache); *temporary intraocular pressure (IOP) increase* (abdominal pain; eye pain; eye redness; headache; nausea or vomiting; tearing)

Incidence rare—incidence less than 2%
    *Aniridia* (sensitivity to light); *choroidal detachment; cystoid macular edema; proliferative vitreoretinopathy (PVR) reproliferation; subretinal silicone oil* (blurred vision or other change in vision not present before treatment, or returning or getting worse after treatment); *endophthalmitis* (blurred vision or other change in vision not present before treatment, or returning or getting worse after treatment; eye pain; eye redness; headache; tearing); *retinal tear* (seeing floaters or light flashes)

## Patient Consultation

As an aid to patient consultation, refer to *Advice for the Patient, Silicone Oil 5000 Centistokes (Parenteral-Local)*.

In providing consultation, consider emphasizing the following selected information (» = major clinical significance):

**Before using this product**
» Conditions affecting use, especially:
    Sensitivity to silicone oil
    Other medical problems, especially pseudophakia with silicone intraocular lenses (IOLs)

**Proper use of this product**
» Proper dosing

**Precautions before receiving this product**
» Discussing with physician the possible serious or long-term side effects that may be caused by product
*Precautions after receiving this product*
» Importance of having progress checked regularly by physician

**Side/adverse effects**
Signs of potential side effects, especially anterior chamber oil migration, cataract, glaucoma, keratopathy, angle blockade, macular pucker, optic nerve atrophy, traction detachment, phthisis, redetachment of retina, vitreous hemorrhage, rubeosis iridis, temporary intraocular pressure (IOP) increase, aniridia, choroidal detachment, cystoid macular edema, proliferative vitreoretinopathy (PVR) reproliferation, subretinal silicone oil, endophthalmitis, or retinal tear

## General Dosing Information

Silicone oil can be used in conjunction with, or following, standard retinal surgical procedures, including scleral buckle surgery, vitrectomy, membrane peeling, and retinotomy or relaxing retinectomy.

The safety and effectiveness of long-term use of silicone oil have not been established. It is recommended that silicone oil be removed within 1 year following instillation if the retina is stable, attached, and without significant remnants of proliferation. There is insufficient clinical evidence to support justification for longer term tamponade. However, in patients at high risk for subsequent detachment or upon the development of phthisis and shrinkage due to hypotony, the physician should determine whether or not the oil should be removed. In addition, in order to minimize the number of invasive traumatic experiences, it may be desirable to avoid the removal of silicone oil in patients with acquired immunodeficiency syndrome (AIDS)-related cytomegalovirus (CMV) retinitis who are at high risk for subsequent detachment and who have a shortened expected lifespan.

Silicone oil can be removed from the posterior chamber by withdrawal with a normal 10 mL syringe and a wide bore 1 mm cannula. By repeated oil-fluid exchange, most of the remaining small silicone oil droplets can be mobilized and removed from the eye. Alternatively, oil can be passively removed by infusion of an appropriate aqueous solution under the oil bubble while the oil is allowed to effuse out of a sclerotomy incision or a limbal incision (in aphakic patients).

In clinical studies, successful reattachment of the retina occurred in 64 to 75% of the patients who were treated with silicone oil. This rate varied depending on the specific etiology of the disease and the severity of the condition. In AIDS-related CMV retinitis patients who received silicone oil as a primary means for reattaching the retina, attachment rates were as high as 90% within an average 6-month follow-up period.

In clinical studies, 45 to 70% of patients who received silicone oil showed improvement in visual acuity at 6 months after treatment. In 15 to 26% of patients, visual acuity did not change. In 15 to 30% of patients, worsening of visual acuity occurred. Deterioration of visual acuity in treated patients appeared to be related to subsequent detachment of the retina, further progression of retinal disease, or keratopathy and cataract complications. In AIDS-related CMV retinitis patients, improvement or maintenance of visual acuity occurred in 57% of the patients within an average 6-month follow-up period. In 33% of AIDS-related CMV retinitis patients, further decline in visual acuity occurred within 4 or 5 months of oil instillation and was due to the continuing progression of retinal and optic nerve disease or the development of oil-related cataracts.

## Parenteral Dosage Forms

### SILICONE OIL 5000 CENTISTOKES FOR INJECTION

**Usual adult and adolescent dose**
Surgical aid (ophthalmic)—
    Intracavitary, a sufficient quantity injected into the vitreous to achieve a retinal tamponade. Eighty percent to 100% of the vitreous space may be filled with the oil while existing fluid or air is exchanged at the same time. Care should be taken to prevent high intraocular pressure from developing during the exchange. Because the silicone oil is less dense than is the aqueous fluid in the eye, a basal iridectomy at the 6 o'clock meridian (Ando iridectomy) is recommended to minimize oil-induced pupillary block and early angle-closure glaucoma. It may be desirable to have the patient assume a face-down posture during the first 24 hours following surgery.

**Usual pediatric dose**
See *Usual adult and adolescent dose*.

**Usual geriatric dose**
See *Usual adult and adolescent dose*.

**Size(s) usually available**
U.S.—
    10 mL single-use vial (Rx) [*AdatoSil 5000*].
    Note: The product contains no additional ingredients.
Canada—
    Not commercially available.

**Packaging and storage**
Store between 8 and 24 °C (46 and 75 °F), unless otherwise specified by manufacturer. Protect from freezing.

**Preparation of dosage form**
The sterile vial of silicone oil should be aseptically removed from the peel-back pouch and deposited onto the sterile tray. The oil should be loaded into a sterile Luer-Lok screw syringe or Luer-Lok syringe adaptable to an automated pump system. Introduction of air bubbles into the oil should be avoided by careful withdrawal of the oil into the syringe. The oil may be injected into the vitreous from the syringe via a syringe needle or a single-use cannulated infusion line. Subretinal fluid may be drained with a flute needle concurrently with the silicone oil infusion.

**Stability**
Silicone oil should not be resterilized.
Silicone oil is stable for 2 years. See packaging for expiration date.

**Incompatibilities**
Silicone oil should not be mixed with any other substance prior to injection.

**Auxiliary labeling**
• For the eye.

## Selected Bibliography

Hutton WL, Azen SP, Blumenkranz MS, et al. The effects of silicone oil removal. Silicone Study Report 6. Arch Ophthalmol (Paris) 1994 Jun; 112 (6): 778-85.

Borislav D. Cataract after silicone oil implantation. Doc Ophthalmol 1993; 83 (1): 79-82.

Barr CC, Lai MY, Lean JS, et al. Postoperative intraocular pressure abnormalities in the Silicone Study. Silicone Study Report 4. Ophthalmology 1993 Nov; 100 (11): 1629-35.

Developed: 02/27/96

# SILVER SULFADIAZINE   Topical

VA CLASSIFICATION (Primary/Secondary): DE101/DE102

Note: For a listing of dosage forms and brand names by country availability, see *Dosage Forms* section(s). For a listing of brand names for the articles in this monograph, refer to the General Index.

## Category

Antibacterial (topical); antifungal (topical).

Note: Silver sulfadiazine is a broad-spectrum antibacterial agent having an antibacterial spectrum similar to that of mafenide.

## Indications

Note: Bracketed information in the *Indications* section refers to uses that are not included in U.S. product labeling.

**Accepted**

Burn wound infections (prophylaxis and treatment)—Silver sulfadiazine is indicated [as a primary agent] in the topical prophylaxis and treatment of burn wound infections caused by *Candida albicans (Monilia albicans), Citrobacter* species, *Enterobacter* species (including *E. cloacae*), enterococci, *Escherichia coli, Klebsiella* species, *Mima-Herellea* species, *Morganella morganii (Proteus morganii), P. mirabilis, P. vulgaris, Providencia rettgeri (Proteus rettgeri), Pseudomonas aeruginosa, Ps. maltophilia, Serratia* species, *Staphylococcus aureus, S. epidermidis*, and beta-hemolytic streptococci in patients with second- and third-degree burns.

[Skin infections, bacterial, minor (treatment)] or
[Ulcer, dermal (treatment)]—Silver sulfadiazine is used in the topical treatment of minor bacterial skin infections such as those involving skin grafts, incisions and other clean lesions, abrasions, minor cuts and wounds; and dermal ulcer such as leg ulcer.

Not all species or strains of a particular organism may be susceptible to silver sulfadiazine.

## Pharmacology/Pharmacokinetics

**Physicochemical characteristics**

Molecular weight—357.13.

Other characteristics—Sulfonamides have certain chemical similarities to some goitrogens, diuretics (acetazolamide and thiazides), and oral antidiabetic agents

**Mechanism of action/Effect**

Bactericidal for many gram-positive and gram-negative organisms. Mechanism of action differs from that of silver nitrate or sodium sulfadiazine. Acts only on the cell membrane and cell wall.

**Other actions/effects**

Also active against yeasts and *Candida albicans (M. albicans)*.

**Absorption**

Varies, depending on the percentage of body surface area to which silver sulfadiazine is applied and extent of tissue damage.

**Peak serum concentration**

Serum sulfadiazine concentrations may approach therapeutic concentrations (up to 8 to 12 mg per 100 mL) when used in burns over extensive areas of the body.

## Precautions to Consider

**Cross-sensitivity and/or related problems**

Patients sensitive to other sulfonamides, furosemide, thiazide diuretics, sulfonylureas, or carbonic anhydrase inhibitors may be sensitive to this medication also.

**Carcinogenicity**

Long-term dermal toxicity studies in rats (24 months) and mice (18 months), using 3 to 10% silver sulfadiazine, have shown no evidence of carcinogenicity.

**Pregnancy/Reproduction**

Pregnancy—Adequate and well-controlled studies in humans have not been done. However, absorbed sulfonamides may displace bilirubin from protein-binding sites in the fetal plasma, thus increasing the possibility of kernicterus in the neonate.

Studies in rabbits, treated with 3 to 10% silver sulfadiazine cream, have not shown that silver sulfadiazine causes adverse effects on the fetus.

FDA Pregnancy Category B.

**Breast-feeding**

It is not known whether silver sulfadiazine, applied topically, is distributed into breast milk. However, silver sulfadiazine may be absorbed systemically in variable amounts following topical application. Caution is recommended in nursing women since systemically administered sulfonamides are distributed into breast milk and may cause kernicterus in nursing infants. Also, sulfonamides may cause hemolytic anemia in glucose-6-phosphate dehydrogenase (G6PD)–deficient infants.

**Pediatrics**

Use is not recommended in premature or newborn infants up to 1 month of age since sulfonamides may cause kernicterus in these neonates. Appropriate studies on the relationship of age to the effects of silver sulfadiazine have not been performed in the pediatric population. However, pediatrics-specific problems that would limit the usefulness of this medication in older infants and children are not expected.

**Geriatrics**

No information is available on the relationship of age to the effects of silver sulfadiazine in geriatric patients.

**Drug interactions and/or related problems**

The following drug interactions and/or related problems have been selected on the basis of their potential clinical significance (possible mechanism in parentheses where appropriate)—not necessarily inclusive ($\gg$ = major clinical significance):

Note: Combinations containing any of the following medications, depending on the amount present, may also interact with this medication.

$\gg$  Collagenase or
$\gg$  Papain or
$\gg$  Sutilains
     (concurrent use of proteolytic enzymes with silver sulfadiazine is not recommended since heavy metal salts may inactivate the enzymes)

**Medical considerations/Contraindications**

The medical considerations/contraindications included here have been selected on the basis of their potential clinical significance (reasons given in parentheses where appropriate)—not necessarily inclusive ($\gg$ = major clinical significance).

*Risk-benefit should be considered when the following medical problems exist:*

Blood dyscrasias
     (sulfonamides may cause blood dyscrasias)

Glucose-6-phosphate dehydrogenase (G6PD) deficiency
     (sulfonamides may cause hemolytic anemia in G6PD-deficient patients)

Hepatic function impairment
     (sulfonamides are metabolized in the liver and may cause hepatitis; if hepatic function impairment occurs, discontinuation of therapy should be considered)

Porphyria
     (sulfonamides may precipitate an acute attack of porphyria)

Renal function impairment
     (if renal function impairment with decreased elimination occurs, discontinuation of therapy should be considered)

Sensitivity to silver sulfadiazine

**Patient monitoring**

The following may be especially important in patient monitoring (other tests may be warranted in some patients, depending on condition; $\gg$ = major clinical significance):

$\gg$  Complete blood counts (CBCs)
     (may be required prior to and weekly during treatment to detect blood dyscrasias in patients with extensive burns; therapy should be discontinued if a significant decrease in the count of any formed blood elements occurs)

Serum sulfadiazine concentrations
     (may be required periodically during treatment in patients with extensive burns since serum sulfadiazine concentrations may approach adult therapeutic concentrations)

Urinalyses
     (may be required prior to and periodically during treatment to detect crystalluria and/or urinary calculi formation in patients on long-term or high-dose therapy and in patients with impaired renal function)

## Side/Adverse Effects

Note: Hyperosmolality, due to the propylene glycol–containing vehicle, has been reported very rarely in infants during therapy with silver sulfadiazine cream.

    If significant absorption occurs, side/adverse effects (e.g., Stevens-Johnson syndrome, Lyell's syndrome, blood dyscrasias, crystalluria) usually seen with systemic sulfonamides may occur with silver sulfadiazine therapy, although few have been reported.

    If allergic reactions or hepatic or renal function impairment with decreased elimination occurs, discontinuation of therapy with silver sulfadiazine should be considered.

The following side/adverse effects have been selected on the basis of their potential clinical significance (possible signs and symptoms in parentheses where appropriate)—not necessarily inclusive:

**Those indicating need for medical attention**
Incidence rare
    *Increased sensitivity of skin to sunlight*—especially in patients with burns on large areas

**Those indicating need for medical attention only if they continue or are bothersome**
Incidence more frequent
    *Burning feeling on treated area(s)*

Incidence less frequent or rare
    *Brownish-gray skin discoloration; itching or skin rash*

## Patient Consultation

As an aid to patient consultation, refer to *Advice for the Patient, Silver Sulfadiazine (Topical)*.

In providing consultation, consider emphasizing the following selected information (» = major clinical significance):

**Before using this medication**
» Conditions affecting use, especially:
    Sensitivity to other sulfonamides, furosemide, thiazide diuretics, sulfonylureas, or carbonic anhydrase inhibitors
    Pregnancy—Absorbed sulfonamides may increase the possibility of kernicterus in the neonate
    Breast-feeding—May cause kernicterus in nursing infants; may cause hemolytic anemia in G6PD-deficient infants
    Use in children—Not recommended in premature or newborn infants up to 1 month of age; may cause kernicterus
    Other medications, especially collagenase, papain, or sutilains

**Proper use of this medication**
» Not using on premature or newborn infants up to 1 month of age; may cause kernicterus
*To use*
    Before applying, cleansing affected area(s); removing necrotic or burned skin and other debris
    Wearing a sterile glove to apply the medication; applying a thin layer (approximately 1.5 mm) to affected area(s); keeping affected area(s) covered with the medication at all times
    Reapplying silver sulfadiazine that has been removed by patient activity or washed off by bathing, showering, or use of a whirlpool bath
    After applying, covering treated area(s) with a dressing or leaving treated area(s) uncovered as desired
» Compliance with full course of therapy; continuing medication until burn has healed or is ready for skin grafting
» Proper dosing
    Missed dose: Applying as soon as possible; not applying if almost time for next dose
» Proper storage

**Precautions while using this medication**
    Regular visits to physician to check progress
    Checking with physician if no improvement within a few days or weeks (for more serious burns or burns over more extensive areas)
    May rarely stain skin brownish gray

**Side/adverse effects**
    Signs of potential side effects, especially photosensitivity reactions

## General Dosing Information

Before application, burn wounds should be cleansed and debrided following control of shock and pain. A sterile glove should be worn to apply the medication. A thin layer (approximately 1.5 mm) of silver sulfadiazine should then be applied to the affected area(s). The burn area(s) should be kept covered with silver sulfadiazine at all times. When necessary, silver sulfadiazine should be reapplied to any area(s) from which it has been removed by patient activity or washed off by bathing, showering, or use of a whirlpool bath.

Dressings, although not required, may be applied if necessary.

Treatment with silver sulfadiazine should be continued until satisfactory healing has occurred or until the burn site is ready for skin grafting. Therapy should not be discontinued while the possibility of infection exists, unless significant toxicity occurs.

Burn patients should be bathed daily, if feasible, to aid in debridement of the burned area(s). Whirlpool baths are particularly helpful, although burn patients may be bathed in bed or in a shower. Following this, silver sulfadiazine should be reapplied.

## Topical Dosage Forms

Note: Bracketed information in the *Indications* section refers to uses that are not included in U.S. product labeling.

### SILVER SULFADIAZINE CREAM USP

**Usual adult and adolescent dose**
Burn wound infections or
[Skin infections, bacterial, minor] or
[Ulcer, dermal]—
    Topical, to the affected area(s), one or two times a day, applied in a thin layer approximately 1.5 mm thick.
    Note: In some other countries, silver sulfadiazine is customarily applied less frequently (e.g., three times a week), in a 3- to 5-mm layer. However, USP medical experts prefer application one or two times a day in a 1.5-mm layer.

**Usual pediatric dose**
Burn wound infections or
[Skin infections, bacterial, minor] or
[Ulcer, dermal]—
    Premature and newborn infants up to 1 month of age—Use is not recommended, since sulfonamides may cause kernicterus in these neonates.
    Infants and children 1 month of age and over—See *Usual adult and adolescent dose*.

**Strength(s) usually available**
U.S.—
    1% (Rx) [*Flint SSD* (propylene glycol; methylparaben 0.3%); *Sildimac; Silvadene* (propylene glycol; methylparaben 0.3%); *SSD* (cetyl alcohol; propylene glycol; methylparaben 0.3%); *SSD AF* (propylene glycol; methylparaben 0.3%); *Thermazene* (propylene glycol; methylparaben 0.3%)].
Canada—
    1% (Rx) [*Flamazine*].

**Packaging and storage**
Store between 15 and 30 °C (59 and 86 °F), in a well-closed container, unless otherwise specified by manufacturer. Protect from freezing.

**Auxiliary labeling**
• For external use only.
• May discolor skin.
• Continue medicine for full time of treatment.

**Additional information**
Silver sulfadiazine cream is available in a water-miscible base containing silver sulfadiazine in micronized form.

Revised: 07/26/93

# SIMETHICONE   Oral-Local

VA CLASSIFICATION (Primary/Secondary): GA900/DX900

Note: For a listing of dosage forms and brand names by country availability, see *Dosage Forms* section(s). For a listing of brand names for the articles in this monograph, refer to the General Index.

## Category

Antiflatulent; diagnostic aid (gastroscopy; radiography of the bowel).

## Indications

Note: Bracketed information in the *Indications* section refers to uses that are not included in U.S. product labeling.

**Accepted**

Gas, gastrointestinal (treatment)—Simethicone's clinical use is based on its antifoam properties demonstrated *in vitro*. It is indicated in the treatment of functional conditions in which the retention of gas may be a problem.

[Gastroscopy adjunct][1] and
[Radiography, bowel, adjunct][1]—Simethicone is used as an antifoaming agent during gastroscopy to enhance visualization and prior to radiography of the bowel to reduce gas shadows.

**Unaccepted**

The clinical effectiveness of simethicone in such conditions as aerophagia, functional dyspepsia, peptic ulcer, spastic or irritable colon, or diverticulitis, beyond that of placebo, has not been established.

Simethicone is not recommended for use in infant colic.

[1]Not included in Canadian product labeling.

## Pharmacology/Pharmacokinetics

**Mechanism of action/Effect**

Acts *in vitro* to lower the surface tension of gas bubbles. Its relevance to action *in vivo* is not clearly established.

**Elimination**

Fecal, as unchanged drug.

## Precautions to Consider

**Pregnancy/Reproduction**

Pregnancy—Problems in humans have not been documented.

**Breast-feeding**

Problems in humans have not been documented.

**Pediatrics**

Appropriate studies performed to date have not demonstrated pediatrics-specific problems that would limit the usefulness of simethicone in children.

**Geriatrics**

No information is available on the relationship of age to the effects of simethicone in geriatric patients.

**Medical considerations/Contraindications**

The medical considerations/contraindications included here have been selected on the basis of their potential clinical significance (reasons given in parentheses where appropriate)—not necessarily inclusive (» = major clinical significance).

*Risk-benefit should be considered when the following medical problem exists:*
Sensitivity to simethicone

## Patient Consultation

As an aid to patient consultation, refer to *Advice for the Patient, Simethicone (Oral)*.

In providing consultation, consider emphasizing the following selected information (» = major clinical significance):

**Before using this medication**
» Conditions affecting use, especially:
  Sensitivity to simethicone
  —Importance of proper diet and exercise to prevent gas problem

**Proper use of this medication**
  Following physician's or manufacturer's instructions
» Taking after meals and at bedtime for best results
*For chewable tablet dosage form*
  Chewing tablets thoroughly for faster and more complete results

*For oral suspension dosage form*
  Proper use of dropper bottle or measuring spoon
» Proper dosing
  Missed dose: If on regular dosing schedule—Taking as soon as possible; not taking if almost time for next dose; not doubling doses
» Proper storage

## General Dosing Information

Dosage or frequency of administration may be doubled with the advice of a physician.

Pediatric dosage should be based on the severity of the condition and the surface area of the patient rather than on body weight.

## Oral Dosage Forms

Note: Bracketed uses in the *Dosage Forms* section refer to categories of uses and/or indications that are not included in the U.S. product labeling.

### SIMETHICONE CAPSULES USP

**Usual adult and adolescent dose**
Antiflatulent—
  Oral, 95 or 125 mg four times a day, after meals and at bedtime, or as needed.
Note: For OTC use, it is recommended that no more than 500 mg be taken in each twenty-four-hour period.

**Usual pediatric dose**
Dosage must be individualized by physician.

**Usual geriatric dose**
See *Usual adult and adolescent dose*.

**Strength(s) usually available**
U.S.—
  125 mg (OTC) [*Maximum Strength Phazyme*].
Canada—
  95 mg (OTC) [*Phazyme-95*].
  125 mg (OTC) [*Phazyme-125*].

**Packaging and storage**
Store between 15 and 30 °C (59 and 86 °F), unless otherwise specified by manufacturer. Store in a well-closed container.

### SIMETHICONE ORAL SUSPENSION USP

**Usual adult and adolescent dose**
Antiflatulent—
  Oral, 40 to 95 mg four times a day, after meals and at bedtime, or as needed.
[Diagnostic aid (gastroscopy; radiography of the bowel)][1]—
  Oral, 67 mg in 2.5 mL of water, as a single dose.
Note: For OTC use, it is recommended that no more than 500 mg be taken in each twenty-four-hour period.

**Usual pediatric dose**
Dosage must be individualized by physician.

**Usual geriatric dose**
See *Usual adult and adolescent dose*.

**Strength(s) usually available**
U.S.—
  40 mg per 0.6 mL (OTC) [*Flatulex; Gas Relief; My Baby Gas Relief Drops; Mylicon Drops; Phazyme;* GENERIC].
Canada—
  40 mg per 0.6 mL (OTC) [*Phazyme Drops*].
  40 mg per mL (OTC) [*Ovol*].
  95 mg per 1.425 mL (OTC) [*Phazyme-95*].

**Packaging and storage**
Store below 40 °C (104 °F), preferably between 15 and 30 °C (59 and 86 °F), unless otherwise specified by manufacturer. Store in a tight, light-resistant container. Protect from freezing.

**Auxiliary labeling**
• Shake well.

**Note**
Dispense in dropper bottle or with measuring spoon.

## SIMETHICONE TABLETS USP

**Usual adult and adolescent dose**
Antiflatulent—
   Oral, 60 to 95 mg four times a day, after meals and at bedtime, or as needed.

Note: For OTC use, it is recommended that no more than 500 mg be taken in each twenty-four-hour period.

**Usual pediatric dose**
Dosage must be individualized by physician.

**Usual geriatric dose**
See *Usual adult and adolescent dose.*

**Strength(s) usually available**
U.S.—
   60 mg (OTC) [*Phazyme* (sugar-coated)].
   80 mg (OTC) [*Flatulex; Genasyme* (scored); GENERIC].
   95 mg (OTC) [*Phazyme-95*].
Canada—
   Not commercially available.

**Packaging and storage**
Store below 40 °C (104 °F), preferably between 15 and 30 °C (59 and 86 °F), unless otherwise specified by manufacturer. Store in a well-closed container.

## SIMETHICONE TABLETS (CHEWABLE) USP

**Usual adult and adolescent dose**
Antiflatulent—
   Oral, 40 to 125 mg four times a day, after meals and at bedtime, or as needed; or, 150 mg three times a day, after meals, or as needed.

Note: For OTC use, it is recommended that no more than 500 mg be taken in each twenty-four-hour period.

**Usual pediatric dose**
Dosage must be individualized by physician.

**Usual geriatric dose**
See *Usual adult and adolescent dose.*

**Strength(s) usually available**
U.S.—
   40 mg (OTC) [*Mylanta Gas*].

   80 mg (OTC) [*Gas Relief; Gas-X* (scored); *Maalox Anti-Gas; Mylanta Gas Relief;* GENERIC].
   125 mg (OTC) [*Extra Strength Gas-X* (scored); *Maximum Strength Gas Relief; Maximum Strength Mylanta Gas Relief; Maximum Strength Phazyme*].
   150 mg (OTC) [*Extra Strength Maalox Anti-Gas*].
Canada—
   40 mg (OTC) [*Ovol-40* (scored)].
   80 mg (OTC) [*Maalox GRF Gas Relief Formula; Ovol-80* (scored)].
   150 mg (OTC) [*Extra Strength Maalox GRF Gas Relief Formula*].

**Packaging and storage**
Store below 40 °C (104 °F), preferably between 15 and 30 °C (59 and 86 °F), unless otherwise specified by manufacturer. Store in a well-closed container.

**Auxiliary labeling**
• Chew tablets well before swallowing.

[1]Not included in Canadian product labeling.

Revised: 06/16/93
Interim revision: 06/21/95

## SIMETHICONE-CONTAINING COMBINATIONS—

Alumina, Magnesia, Calcium Carbonate,, and Simethicone (Oral-Local)—See *Antacids (Oral-Local)*
Alumina, Magnesia, and Simethicone (Oral-Local)—See *Antacids (Oral-Local)*
Calcium Carbonate, Magnesia, and Simethicone (Oral-Local)—See *Antacids (Oral-Local)*
Calcium Carbonate and Simethicone (Oral-Local)—See *Antacids (Oral-Local)*
Magaldrate and Simethicone (Oral-Local)—See *Antacids (Oral-Local)*
Simethicone, Alumina, Magnesium Carbonate, and Magnesia (Oral-Local)—See *Antacids (Oral-Local)*

## SIMVASTATIN—See *HMG-CoA Reductase Inhibitors (Systemic)*

# SINCALIDE  Systemic

VA CLASSIFICATION (Primary/Secondary): HS900/DX900
Note: For a listing of dosage forms and brand names by country availability, see *Dosage Forms* section(s). For a listing of brand names for the articles in this monograph, refer to the General Index.

## Category
Cholecystokinetic; Diagnostic aid (gallbladder function; pancreatic function).

## Indications
Note: Bracketed information in the *Indications* section refers to uses that are not included in U.S. product labeling.

**Accepted**
Gallbladder disorders (diagnosis) or
Pancreas disorders (diagnosis)—Sincalide is indicated as a diagnostic aid for evaluation of gallbladder and pancreatic disorders. It is used to stimulate gallbladder contraction and emptying prior to or during cholecystography with contrast media or hepatobiliary scintigraphy (e.g., using technetium Tc 99m–labeled iminodiacetic acid derivatives) to aid in visualization of the cystic duct and gallbladder. Also, gallbladder contraction provides a sample of bile that may be aspirated from the duodenum for analysis of its composition (for example, to determine the degree of cholesterol saturation).

In conjuction with secretin, sincalide is used to stimulate pancreatic secretion for analysis of its composition and cytological examination, such as in suspected cancer of the pancreas.

Sincalide is used to accelerate small bowel transit time of contrast media, such as barium sulfate, thus decreasing the time and extent of radiation associated with fluoroscopy and x-ray examination of the intestinal tract.

[Ileus, postoperative (treatment)]—Sincalide is used to restore normal bowel activity in patients with postoperative ileus uncomplicated by

inflammatory processes such as pancreatitis and peritonitis, or by the presence of tumors or other obstructions in the lower digestive tract.

## Pharmacology/Pharmacokinetics

**Mechanism of action/Effect**
Sincalide, a synthetically-prepared C-terminal octapeptide of the natural hormone cholecystokinin, induces contraction of the gallbladder muscle, resulting in reduction of gallbladder size and evacuation of bile. Also, sincalide, like cholecystokinin, stimulates secretion of pancreatic enzymes.

**Other actions**
Sincalide decreases intestinal transit time; delays gastric emptying; decreases esophageal sphincter tone; inhibits gastric secretions; and stimulates intestinal muscle.

**Time to peak effect:**
Maximum contraction ($\geq$ 40% reduction in size) of gallbladder occurs 5 to 15 minutes after injection.

**Duration of action**
Gallbladder returns to basal size within 1 hour.

## Precautions to Consider

**Pregnancy/Reproduction**
Fertility—Although adequate studies in humans have not been done, studies in animals have not shown that sincalide causes impairment of fertility.
Pregnancy—Adequate and well-controlled studies in humans have not been done.
Studies in rats given doses up to 12.5 times the maximum recommended human dose have not shown that sincalide causes adverse effects in the fetus.
FDA Pregnancy Category B.

Labor—Although adequate studies in humans have not been done, sincalide should not be administered to pregnant women near term since sincalide, a smooth muscle stimulant, may induce spontaneous abortion or premature labor.

### Breast-feeding
It is not known whether sincalide is distributed into breast milk. However, problems in humans have not been documented.

### Pediatrics
Appropriate studies on the relationship of age to the effects of sincalide have not been performed in the pediatric population. Safety and efficacy have not been established.

### Geriatrics
No information is available on the relationship of age to the effects of sincalide in geriatric patients.

### Medical considerations/Contraindications
The medical considerations/contraindications included here have been selected on the basis of their potential clinical significance (reasons given in parentheses where appropriate)—not necessarily inclusive (» = major clinical significance).

*Except under special circumstances, this medication should not be used when the following medical problem exists:*
» Intestinal obstruction
   (condition may be aggravated)

*Risk-benefit should be considered when the following medical problems exist:*
Gallbladder stones
   (stimulation of gallbladder contraction in patients with small gallbladder stones may lead to the evacuation of the stones from the gallbladder resulting in their lodging in the cystic duct or in the common bile duct; however, this is unlikely with usual doses of sincalide since complete contraction of the gallbladder is not induced)
Sensitivity to sincalide

## Side/Adverse Effects
The following side/adverse effects have been selected on the basis of their potential clinical significance (possible signs and symptoms in parentheses where appropriate)—not necessarily inclusive:

**Those indicating need for medical attention**
Incidence less frequent or rare
   *Allergic reaction* (shortness of breath, skin rash); *hypotension* (dizziness, lightheadedness, or fainting); *increase in blood pressure*

**Those indicating need for medical attention only if they continue or are bothersome**
Incidence more frequent
   *Gastrointestinal effects* (nausea, abdominal or stomach pain, cramps, or discomfort)—20%
Incidence less frequent
   *Diarrhea; dizziness; flushing or redness of skin; headache; increased sweating; numbness; sneezing; urge to have bowel movement; vomiting*
   Note: The less frequent side effects listed occur in less than 1% of patients, except for *diarrhea*, which occurs in about 2% of patients.
       The above side effects are generally mild and of short duration; they are usually lessened by a slower injection rate.

## Patient Consultation
As an aid to patient consultation, refer to *Advice for the Patient, Sincalide (Diagnostic)*.

In providing consultation, consider emphasizing the following selected information (»= major clinical significance):

**Description of use**
Procedure for sincalide test: Dose of sincalide is based on body weight and must be determined by doctor; sincalide is injected intravenously

**Before having this test**
» Conditions affecting use, especially:
   Sensitivity to sincalide
   Other medical problems, especially gallbladder stones and intestinal obstruction

**Preparation for this test**
Special preparatory instructions may be given; patient should inquire in advance

### Side/adverse effects
Signs of potential side effects, especially allergic reaction, hypertension, and hypotension

## General Dosing Information

### For use in hepatobiliary imaging
During hepatobiliary imaging with technetium Tc 99m–labeled iminodiacetic acid (IDA) derivatives, prolonged fasting (e.g., more than 24 hours) may result in a false-positive hepatobiliary scan (i.e., nonvisualization of the gallbladder despite a patent cystic duct) due to the development of increased intraluminal gallbladder pressure (biliary stasis or sludge), which reduces radiotracer flow to the gallbladder. To avoid this, prior administration of sincalide (0.02 to 0.04 mcg per kg of body weight [mcg/kg]), to induce contraction of the gallbladder, is recommended for pre-emptying the gallbladder before the injection of the radiotracer. Whenever there is doubt about the dietary history of the patient, especially in emergency situations, a cholecystokinetic agent should be administered.

In patients receiving parenteral alimentation, the relative inactivity of the gallbladder results in bile stasis and the formation of thick viscous bile (sludge), which reduces the flow of the radiotracer into the gallbladder. Pretreatment with intravenous sincalide (0.02 to 0.04 mcg/kg administered slowly over a thirty- to sixty-second interval) may be useful to empty stored bile from the gallbladder, and thus may prevent a false-positive hepatobiliary scan.

In patients demonstrating radiotracer localization in the gallbladder, intravenous sincalide (0.02 to 0.04 mcg/kg) may be useful to stimulate gallbladder contraction, and thereby, evaluate the contractile function of the gallbladder. Quantitation of gallbladder emptying yields the ejection fraction (≥ 35% is usually considered normal).

## Parenteral Dosage Forms
Note: Bracketed uses in the *Dosage Forms* section refer to categories of use and/or indications that are not included in U.S. product labeling.

### SINCALIDE FOR INJECTION

**Usual adult and adolescent dose**
Gallbladder function diagnosis—
   For prompt contraction of gallbladder:
       Intravenous, 0.02 mcg per kg of body weight, administered over a thirty- to sixty-second period.
       Note: If satisfactory gallbladder contraction does not occur in fifteen minutes, a second dose of 0.04 mcg per kg of body weight may be administered.
           When used in cholecystography, radiographs are usually taken at five-minute intervals after the injection. However, for visualization of the cystic duct, it is recommended that radiographs be taken at one-minute intervals during the first five minutes after the injection.
           For reduction of side effects, an intravenous infusion of sincalide (0.12 mcg per kg of body weight diluted with 0.9% Sodium Chloride Injection USP to approximately 100 mL) may be administered at a rate of 2 mL per minute; alternatively, 0.1 mcg per kg of body weight may be used intramuscularly.
Pancreatic function diagnosis—
   Intravenous infusion, 0.02 mcg per kg of body weight, administered over a thirty-minute period.
   Note: Sincalide is administered, as a separate intravenous infusion, thirty minutes after the patient has started receiving secretin (0.25 units per kg of body weight) by intravenous infusion over a sixty-minute period.
To accelerate small bowel transit time of barium sulfate—
   Intravenous, 0.04 mcg per kg of body weight, administered over a thirty- to sixty-second period after the barium meal is beyond the proximal jejunum.
[Treatment of postoperative ileus]—
   Intravenous, 0.04 mcg per kg of body weight, administered over a thirty- to sixty-second period.
   Note: Dose may be repeated or increased to 0.08 mcg per kg of body weight at 4-hour intervals, up to a maximum of five doses of sincalide.

**Usual pediatric dose**
Safety and efficacy have not been established.

**Usual geriatric dose**
See *Usual adult and adolescent dose*.

**Strength(s) usually available**

U.S.—

5 mcg (0.005 mg) (Rx) [*Kinevac*].

Canada—

5 mcg (0.005 mg) (Rx) [*Kinevac*].

**Packaging and storage**

Store between 15 and 30 °C (59 to 86 °F), unless otherwise specified by manufacturer.

**Preparation of dosage form**

To prepare injection, 5 mL of Sterile Water for Injection USP is added to the vial containing sincalide. Additional dilutions should be made with 0.9% Sodium Chloride Injection USP.

**Stability**

Following reconstitution of—

U.S. product: Sincalide injection is stable for 24 hours at room temperature.

Canadian product: Sincalide injection may be stored under refrigeration for up to 24 hours.

## Selected Bibliography

Pickleman J, Peiss RL, Henkin R, et al. The role of sincalide cholescintigraphy in the evaluation of patients with acalculous gallbladder disease. Arch Surg 1985; 120: 693-7.

Developed: 02/27/95

---

# SKELETAL MUSCLE RELAXANTS Systemic

This monograph includes information on the following: Carisoprodol; Chlorphenesin; Chlorzoxazone†; Metaxalone†; Methocarbamol; Orphenadrine.

VA CLASSIFICATION (Primary/Secondary):

Carisoprodol—MS200

Chlorphenesin—MS200

Chlorzoxazone—MS200

Metaxalone—MS200

Methocarbamol—MS200

Orphenadrine Citrate—MS200

Orphenadrine Hydrochloride—AU350

Note: For a listing of dosage forms and brand names by country availability, see *Dosage Forms* section(s). For a listing of brand names for the articles in this monograph, refer to the General Index.

†Not commercially available in Canada.

## Category

Skeletal muscle relaxant—Carisoprodol; Chlorphenesin; Chlorzoxazone; Metaxalone; Methocarbamol; Orphenadrine Citrate.

Parkinsonism therapy adjunct—Orphenadrine Hydrochloride.

## Indications

### Accepted

Spasm, skeletal muscle (treatment)—Skeletal muscle relaxants are indicated as adjuncts to other measures, such as rest and physical therapy, for the relief of muscle spasm associated with acute, painful musculoskeletal conditions.

Parkinsonism (treatment adjunct)—Orphenadrine hydrochloride is indicated (but is rarely used) as an adjunct to physical therapy and other medications in the treatment of postencephalic, arteriosclerotic, or idiopathic parkinsonism. It produces symptomatic relief of tremor. The medication may be used concurrently with reduced dosages of more potent medications in treating patients who cannot tolerate effective doses of the other medications.

### Unaccepted

Methocarbamol is also FDA-approved for control of the neuromuscular manifestations of tetanus. However, it has largely been replaced in the treatment of tetanus by diazepam, or, in severe cases, a neuromuscular blocking agent such as pancuronium. Such therapy is used as an adjunct to other measures, such as debridement, tetanus antitoxin, penicillin, tracheotomy, fluid and electrolyte replacement, and supportive treatment.

## Pharmacology/Pharmacokinetics

See *Table 1*, page 2610, and *Table 2*, page 2610.

### Physicochemical characteristics

Molecular weight—

Carisoprodol: 260.34.

Chlorphenesin carbamate: 245.66.

Chlorzoxazone: 169.57.

Metaxalone: 221.26.

Methocarbamol: 241.25.

Orphenadrine citrate: 461.51.

Orphenadrine hydrochloride: 305.85.

### Mechanism of action/Effect

Skeletal muscle relaxant—Precise mechanism of action has not been determined. These agents act in the central nervous system (CNS) rather than directly on skeletal muscle. Several of these medications have been shown to depress polysynaptic reflexes preferentially. The muscle relaxant effects of most of these agents may be related to their CNS depressant (sedative) effects. Carisoprodol blocks interneuronal activity in the descending reticular formation and in the spinal cord. Chlorzoxazone acts primarily at the spinal cord level and at subcortical areas of the brain. Orphenadrine has analgesic activity, which may contribute to its skeletal muscle relaxant properties.

Parkinsonism therapy adjunct—Orphenadrine has mild anticholinergic actions, which produce its beneficial effect in parkinsonism.

### Other actions/effects

Orphenadrine also has anticholinergic properties.

## Precautions to Consider

### Cross-sensitivity and/or related problems

Patients sensitive to other carbamate derivatives (for example, carbromal, meprobamate, mebutamate, or tybamate) may be sensitive to carisoprodol also.

### Pregnancy/Reproduction

Pregnancy—

*Carisoprodol, chlorzoxazone, and methocarbamol—*

Problems in humans have not been documented.

*Chlorphenesin—*

Studies have not been done in either animals or humans.

*Metaxalone—*

Although studies in humans have not been done, studies in rats have not shown that metaxalone causes adverse effects in the fetus.

*Orphenadrine—*

Problems in humans have not been documented.

Studies in animals have not been done.

Orphenadrine citrate—FDA Pregnancy Category C.

### Breast-feeding

*Carisoprodol—*

Carisoprodol is distributed into breast milk in concentrations that may reach 2 to 4 times the maternal plasma concentrations; use by nursing mothers may cause sedation and gastrointestinal upset in the infant.

*Chlorphenesin, chlorzoxazone, metaxalone, methocarbamol, and orphenadrine—*

It is not known whether these medications are distributed into breast milk. However, problems in humans have not been documented.

### Pediatrics

*Carisoprodol—*

Although appropriate studies with carisoprodol have not been performed in the pediatric population, the medication has been used in children. Pediatrics-specific problems that would limit the use of carisoprodol in these patients have not been documented.

*Chlorphenesin, metaxalone, methocarbamol, and orphenadrine—*

No information is available on the relationship of age to the effects of these medications in pediatric patients. Safety and efficacy have not been established.

*Chlorzoxazone—*

This medication has been used in children. Pediatrics-specific problems that would limit use of chlorzoxazone in these patients have not been documented.

### Geriatrics

No information is available on the relationship of age to the effects of skeletal muscle relaxants in geriatric patients. However, elderly males are more likely to have age-related prostatic hypertrophy and may therefore be adversely affected by orphenadrine's anticholinergic activity. Also, elderly patients are more likely to have age-related renal function impairment, which may require that parenteral methocarbamol not be used at all and that other skeletal muscle relaxants be used with caution.

### Dental
*Orphenadrine—*
The peripheral anticholinergic effects of orphenadrine may decrease or inhibit salivary flow, thus contributing to the development of caries, periodontal disease, oral candidiasis, and discomfort.

### Drug interactions and/or related problems
The following drug interactions and/or related problems have been selected on the basis of their potential clinical significance (possible mechanism in parentheses where appropriate)—not necessarily inclusive (» = major clinical significance):

Note: Combinations containing any of the following medications, depending on the amount present, may also interact with this medication.

*For all skeletal muscle relaxants*
» Alcohol or
» CNS depression–producing medications, other (See *Appendix II* )
(concurrent use with a skeletal muscle relaxant may result in additive CNS depressant effects; caution is recommended and dosage of one or both agents should be reduced)

*For orphenadrine (in addition to the interaction listed above)*
Anticholinergics or other medications with anticholinergic action (See *Appendix II* )
(anticholinergic effects may be intensified when these medications are used concurrently with orphenadrine because of orphenadrine's secondary anticholinergic activity)

### Laboratory value alterations
The following have been selected on the basis of their potential clinical significance (possible effect in parentheses where appropriate)—not necessarily inclusive (» = major clinical significance):
With diagnostic test results
*For metaxalone*
Copper sulfate urine sugar tests
(false-positive test results may occur, possibly because of the presence of an unknown reducing substance; results of tests using glucose oxidase are not affected)

*For methocarbamol*
5-Hydroxyindoleacetic acid (5-HIAA), in urine, determinations
(values may be falsely increased when the nitrosonaphthol reagent is used)

Vanillylmandelic acid (VMA), in urine, determinations
(values may be falsely increased when the Gitlow screening method is used; no error occurs when the quantitative procedure of Sunderman is used)

With physiology/laboratory test values
*For metaxalone*
Cephalin flocculation tests
(elevations may occur without concurrent changes in other liver function tests)

### Medical considerations/Contraindications
See *Table 3*, page 2611.

### Patient monitoring
The following may be especially important in patient monitoring (other tests may be warranted in some patients, depending on condition; » = major clinical significance):

*For metaxalone*
Liver function tests
(recommended periodically during prolonged metaxalone therapy, especially if the patient has pre-existing hepatic function impairment or disease)

*For methocarbamol*
Renal function determinations
(recommended if parenteral therapy lasts 3 days or more because the polyethylene glycol 300 vehicle may be nephrotoxic)

*For orphenadrine*
Blood count and
Liver function tests and
Renal function tests
(recommended during prolonged therapy since the safety of continuous long-term use has not been established)

## Side/Adverse Effects
See *Table 4*, page 2612.

Note: Rarely, an idiosyncratic reaction to carisoprodol may occur within minutes or hours following the first dose of the medication. Reported symptoms include agitation, ataxia, confusion, disorientation, dizziness, euphoria, extreme weakness, speech disturbances, temporary loss of vision or other vision disturbances, and transient quadriplegia. Symptoms usually subside within several hours, but in some cases, supportive and symptomatic therapy, including hospitalization, may be necessary.

Psychological dependence and abuse have occurred very rarely with carisoprodol. Signs of abstinence have not been reported with clinical usage; however, in one study abrupt withdrawal of 100 mg per kg of body weight (mg/kg) per day of carisoprodol (5 times the recommended daily dose) produced withdrawal symptoms including abdominal cramps, insomnia, chills, headache, and nausea.

## Overdose
For more information on the management of overdose or unintentional ingestion, **contact a Poison Control Center** (see *Poison Control Center Listing*).

**Carisoprodol**
To decrease absorption—Emptying the stomach via induction of emesis or gastric lavage.
Specific treatment—Administering respiratory assistance, CNS stimulants, and pressor agents cautiously, if necessary.
To enhance elimination—Removing carisoprodol from the body via induction of diuresis, osmotic (mannitol) diuresis, peritoneal dialysis, or hemodialysis.
Monitoring—Monitoring urinary output.
Taking care to prevent overhydration.
Monitoring the patient for relapse due to incomplete gastric emptying and delayed absorption, and administering additional treatment as required.
Supportive care—Administering supportive treatment of observed symptoms.
Chlorphenesin—
To decrease absorption—Emptying the stomach via institution of saline catharsis or gastric lavage.
Supportive care—Administering supportive therapy of observed symptoms.
Chlorzoxazone—
To decrease absorption—Emptying the stomach via induction of emesis or gastric lavage.
Specific treatment—Administering oxygen and artificial respiration for respiratory depression and plasma volume expanders or vasopressors for hypotension.
Supportive care—Administering supportive treatment of observed symptoms.
Note: Cholinergic medications and analeptic medications are of no value in chlorzoxazone overdose and should not be used.
Metaxalone—
Experience with overdose causing major toxicity is extremely limited.
To decrease absorption—Emptying the stomach via induction of emesis or gastric lavage.
Supportive care—Administering supportive treatment of observed symptoms.
Methocarbamol—
To decrease absorption—Emptying the stomach via induction of emesis or gastric lavage (if administered orally).
To enhance elimination—The usefulness of forced diuresis or hemodialysis in treating overdose has not been determined.
Supportive care—Administering supportive treatment of observed symptoms.
Orphenadrine—
To decrease absorption—Emptying the stomach via induction of emesis or gastric lavage (if administered orally).
To enhance elimination—Maintaining a high-volume urinary output.
Institution of hemodialysis or peritoneal dialysis may be of some benefit if the serum concentration exceeds 4 mcg per mL.
Supportive care—Administering intravenous fluids and circulatory support as required. Administering supportive treatment of observed symptoms.

Note: Patients in whom intentional overdose is known or suspected should be referred for psychiatric consultation.

## Patient Consultation

See *Table 5*, page 2613.

---

### CARISOPRODOL

## Summary of Differences

Pharmacology/pharmacokinetics:
Physicochemical characteristics—Molecular weight: 260.34.
Biotransformation—Hepatic; one metabolite is meprobamate.
Half-life—8 hours
Onset of action—0.5 hour.
Time to peak concentration—4 hours (350-mg single dose).
Peak serum concentration—4–7 mcg per mL.
Duration of action—4–6 hours.
Elimination—Renal, <1% as unchanged carisoprodol. Carisoprodol is dialyzable.
Precautions:
Cross-sensitivity and/or related problems—May occur with other carbamate derivatives.
Breast-feeding—Distributed into breast milk in significant quantities; may cause sedation and gastrointestinal upset in the nursing infant.
Medical considerations/contraindications—
Should not be used in patients with known or suspected acute intermittent porphyria.
Caution also recommended in patients with a history of drug abuse or dependence.
Side/adverse effects:
Idiosyncratic reactions may occur shortly after first dose.
Psychological dependence and abuse reported very rarely.
Also may cause orthostatic hypotension, fast heartbeat, mental depression, clumsiness or unsteadiness, fever (allergic), stinging or burning of eyes, angioedema, bronchospastic allergic reaction, blurred vision, and flushing.

## Oral Dosage Forms

### CARISOPRODOL TABLETS USP

**Usual adult and adolescent dose**
Skeletal muscle relaxant—
Oral, 350 mg four times a day.

**Usual pediatric dose**
Skeletal muscle relaxant—
Children up to 5 years of age: Dosage has not been established.
Children 5 to 12 years of age: Oral, 6.25 mg per kg of body weight four times a day.

**Strength(s) usually available**
U.S.—
350 mg (Rx) [*Soma; Vanadom;* GENERIC].
Canada—
350 mg (Rx) [*Soma*].

**Packaging and storage**
Store below 40 °C (104 °F), preferably between 15 and 30 °C (59 and 86 °F), unless otherwise specified by manufacturer. Store in a well-closed container.

**Auxiliary labeling**
• May cause drowsiness.
• Avoid alcoholic beverages.

---

### CHLORPHENESIN

## Summary of Differences

Pharmacology/pharmacokinetics:
Physicochemical characteristics—Molecular weight: 245.66.
Absorption—Rapid; complete.
Biotransformation—Hepatic; at least partially metabolized.
Half-life—2.3–5 hours
Time to peak concentration—1–3 hours.
Peak serum concentration—3.8–17 mcg per mL (800-mg single dose).
Elimination—Renal; 85% of a dose excreted within 24 hours as the glucuronide metabolite.
Side/adverse effects:
Gastrointestinal bleeding reported, but causal relationship not established.

---

Also may cause fever (allergic), agranulocytosis, leukopenia, or thrombocytopenia.

## Additional Dosing Information

The safety of administering chlorphenesin for longer than 8 weeks has not been established.

## Oral Dosage Forms

### CHLORPHENESIN CARBAMATE TABLETS

**Usual adult and adolescent dose**
Skeletal muscle relaxant—
Oral, 800 mg three times a day initially; may be decreased to 400 mg four times a day or less, as required to maintain the desired response.

**Usual pediatric dose**
Safety and efficacy have not been established.

**Strength(s) usually available**
U.S.—
400 mg (Rx) [*Maolate*].
Canada—
Not commercially available.

**Packaging and storage**
Store below 40 °C (104 °F), preferably between 15 and 30 °C (59 and 86 °F), in a well-closed container, unless otherwise specified by manufacturer.

**Auxiliary labeling**
• May cause drowsiness.
• Avoid alcoholic beverages.

---

### CHLORZOXAZONE

## Summary of Differences

Pharmacology/pharmacokinetics:
Physicochemical characteristics—Molecular weight: 169.57.
Absorption—Rapid; complete.
Biotransformation—Hepatic.
Half-life—1.1 hours.
Onset of action—Within 1 hour.
Time to peak concentration—1–2 hours.
Peak serum concentration—10–30 mcg per mL (750-mg single dose).
Duration of action—3–4 hours.
Elimination—Renal; <1% as unchanged chlorzoxazone.
Precautions:
Medical considerations/contraindications: Also should be used with caution in patients with allergies (or history of).
Side/adverse effects:
Also may cause agranulocytosis, gastrointesinal bleeding, angioedema, anemia, diarrhea, heartburn, and constipation.
Hepatotoxicity reported, but causal association not established.

## Additional Dosing Information

Discontinuation of chlorzoxazone therapy is recommended if symptoms of hepatotoxicity or sensitivity (e.g., skin rash, hives, or itching) occur.

## Oral Dosage Forms

### CHLORZOXAZONE TABLETS USP

**Usual adult and adolescent dose**
Skeletal muscle relaxant—
Oral, 250 to 750 mg three or four times a day; usually 500 mg three or four times a day initially and increased or decreased as determined by patient response.

**Usual pediatric dose**
Skeletal muscle relaxant—
Oral, 20 mg per kg of body weight or 600 mg per square meter of body surface, in three or four divided doses; or 125 to 500 mg three or four times a day, according to the child's age and weight.

**Strength(s) usually available**
U.S.—
250 mg (Rx) [*Paraflex; Remular-S;* GENERIC].
500 mg (Rx) [*EZE-DS; Parafon Forte DSC* (scored); *Relaxazone; Remular; Strifon Forte DSC;* GENERIC].
Canada—
Not commercially available.

**Packaging and storage**
Store between 15 and 30 °C (59 and 86 °F), unless otherwise specified by manufacturer. Store in a tight container.

**Preparation of dosage form**
*Single dose*— Tablets may be crushed and mixed with food or liquid for ease of administration.

**Auxiliary labeling**
• May cause drowsiness.
• Avoid alcoholic beverages.

---

## METAXALONE

## Summary of Differences

Pharmacology/pharmacokinetics:
   Physicochemical characteristics—Molecular weight 221.26.
   Biotransformation—Hepatic.
   Half-life—2–3 hours
   Onset of action—1 hour.
   Time to peak concentration—2 hours (800-mg single dose).
   Peak serum concentration—295 mcg per mL (800-mg single dose).
   Elimination—Renal.
Precautions:
   Laboratory value alterations—
   May interfere with copper sulfate urine sugar test results.
   May cause liver function test abnormalities.
   Medical considerations/contraindications—Also should not be used in patients with hemolytic anemia or a history of hemolytic anemia, especially if drug-induced.
   Patient monitoring—Liver function tests recommended during prolonged therapy.
Side/adverse effects:
   Also may cause hemolytic anemia and hepatotoxicity.

## Additional Dosing Information

Discontinuation of metaxalone therapy is recommended if signs of hepatotoxicity occur.

## Oral Dosage Forms

### METAXALONE TABLETS

**Usual adult and adolescent dose**
Skeletal muscle relaxant—
   Oral, 800 mg three or four times a day.

**Usual pediatric dose**
Safety and efficacy have not been established.

**Strength(s) usually available**
U.S.—
   400 mg (Rx) [*Skelaxin* (scored)].
Canada—
   Not commercially available.

**Packaging and storage**
Store below 40 °C (104 °F), preferably between 15 and 30 °C (59 and 86 °F), in a well-closed container, unless otherwise specified by manufacturer.

**Auxiliary labeling**
• May cause drowsiness.
• Avoid alcoholic beverages.

---

## METHOCARBAMOL

## Summary of Differences

Pharmacology/pharmacokinetics:
   Physicochemical characteristics—Molecular weight: 241.25.
   Absorption—Rapid.
   Biotransformation—Probably hepatic.
   Half-life (elimination)—0.9–2.2 hours.
      Onset of action—
         Oral: Within 0.5 hour.
         Intravenous: Immediate.
      Time to peak concentration—
         Oral: 2 hours (2-gram single dose).
         Intravenous: Almost immediate.
      Peak serum concentration—
         Oral: 16 mcg per mL (2-gram single dose).
         Intravenous: 19 mcg per mL (1-gram single dose).

Elimination—
   Renal and fecal.
Precautions:
   Laboratory value alterations—Urinary 5-Hydroxyindoleacetic acid (5-HIAA) values may be falsely increased (with nitrosonaphthol reagent).
   Urinary vanillylmandelic acid (VMA) values may be falsely increased (with the Gitlow screening method).
   Medical considerations/contraindications—
   Parenteral dosage form should not be used in patients with renal function impairment or disease because the polyethylene glycol 300 vehicle is nephrotoxic.
   Parenteral dosage form also should be used with caution in patients with epilepsy.
   Patient monitoring—Renal function determinations recommended if parenteral therapy lasts 3 days or more.
Side/adverse effects:
   Parenteral dosage form also reported to cause convulsions, fainting, slow heartbeat, muscle weakness, nystagmus, and facial flushing, especially when given too rapidly.
   Parenteral dosage form may also cause pain or peeling of skin at injection site and thrombophlebitis.
   Also may cause fever (allergic), conjunctivitis and nasal congestion, and leukopenia.
   May be more likely than other muscle relaxants to cause blurred or double vision.

## Additional Dosing Information

**For parenteral dosage forms only**
The injection may be given intravenously or intramuscularly. Subcutaneous administration is not recommended.
The polyethylene glycol 300 vehicle in the parenteral dosage form may be nephrotoxic.
The medication may be administered intravenously undiluted at a rate not to exceed 3 mL (300 mg) per minute. It may also be given as an intravenous infusion in sodium chloride injection or 5% dextrose injection.
The patient should lie down during and for at least 10 to 15 minutes following intravenous administration.
Extravasation should be avoided, since the injection is hypertonic and may cause thrombophlebitis.
The manufacturer's labeling should be consulted for special directions for use in tetanus.
Not more than 5 mL (500 mg) should be given intramuscularly into each gluteal region at one time. The injections may be repeated at 8-hour intervals, if necessary.

## Oral Dosage Forms

### METHOCARBAMOL TABLETS USP

**Usual adult and adolescent dose**
Skeletal muscle relaxant—
   Initial: Oral, 1.5 grams four times a day for the first forty-eight to seventy-two hours of therapy. For severe conditions, 8 grams a day may be administered initially.
   Maintenance: Oral, 750 mg every four hours; 1 gram four times a day; or 1.5 grams three times a day.
Note: If used as adjunctive therapy in the treatment of tetanus—Via nasogastric tube, up to 24 grams a day depending on patient response.

**Usual pediatric dose**
Safety and efficacy have not been established.

**Strength(s) usually available**
U.S.—
   500 mg (Rx) [*Carbacot; Robaxin;* GENERIC].
   750 mg (Rx) [*Carbacot; Robaxin-750;* GENERIC].
Canada—
   500 mg (OTC) [*Robaxin* (scored)].
   750 mg (OTC) [*Robaxin-750* (scored)].

**Packaging and storage**
Store below 40 °C (104 °F), preferably between 15 and 30 °C (59 and 86 °F), unless otherwise specified by manufacturer. Store in a tight container.

**Preparation of dosage form**
For administration via nasogastric tube—Crush tablets and suspend in water or saline solution.

**Auxiliary labeling**
• May cause drowsiness.
• Avoid alcoholic beverages.

# Parenteral Dosage Forms

## METHOCARBAMOL INJECTION USP

### Usual adult and adolescent dose

Skeletal muscle relaxant—
  Intramuscular or intravenous, 1 to 3 grams a day for three days. Following a drug-free interval of forty-eight hours, the course may be repeated if necessary.

Note: If used as adjunctive therapy in the treatment of tetanus—Intravenous, 1 or 2 grams by direct intravenous injection. An additional 1 or 2 grams may be administered by intravenous infusion, so that a total initial dose of up to 3 grams is administered. This regimen should be repeated every six hours until therapy via a nasogastric tube can be instituted.

### Usual adult prescribing limits

Total adult dosage should not exceed 3 grams per day. Also, the medication should not be administered for more than three consecutive days except in the treatment of tetanus.

### Usual pediatric dose

Skeletal muscle relaxant—
  Safety and efficacy in children up to 12 years of age have not been established for conditions other than tetanus.

Note: If used as adjunctive therapy in the treatment of tetanus—Intravenous, 15 mg per kg of body weight every six hours.

### Strength(s) usually available

U.S.—
  100 mg per mL (1 gram per 10-mL single-dose ampul or vial) (Rx) [*Carbacot; Robaxin; Skelex;* GENERIC].

Canada—
  100 mg per mL (1 gram per 10-mL single-dose vial) (OTC) [*Robaxin*].

### Packaging and storage

Store below 40 °C (104 °F), preferably between 15 and 30 °C (59 and 86 °F), unless otherwise specified by manufacturer. Protect from freezing.

### Preparation of dosage form

For intravenous infusion—Dilute with sodium chloride injection or 5% dextrose injection; 10 mL (1 gram) of medication should be diluted to not more than 250 mL of infusion. After dilution, the injection should not be refrigerated.

---

## *ORPHENADRINE*

---

# Summary of Differences

Category:
  Hydrochloride salt indicated to relieve tremor in parkinsonism.
Pharmacology/pharmacokinetics—
  Physicochemical characteristics—Molecular weight—
    Orphenadrine citrate—461.51.
    Orphenadrine hydrochloride—305.85.
  Mechanism of action (parkinsonism therapy adjunct)—
    Has anticholinergic activity.
  Protein binding—
    Low.
  Biotransformation—
    Hepatic.
  Half-life—
    14 hours (parent compound; half-life of metabolites may range from 2 to 25 hours).
  Onset of action—
    Orphenadrine citrate:
      Oral (extended-release tablets)—Within 1 hour.
      Intramuscular—5 minutes.
      Intravenous—Immediate.
    Orphenadrine hydrochloride:
      Oral—Within 1 hour.
  Time to peak concentration:
    Orphenadrine citrate—
      Oral (extended-release tablets)—6–8 hours (100-mg single dose).
      Intramuscular—0.5 hour (60-mg single dose).
      Intravenous—Immediate.
    Orphenadrine hydrochloride—
      Oral—3 hours (50-mg single dose).
  Peak serum concentration—
    Orphenadrine citrate:
      Oral (extended-release tablets)—60–120 nanograms per mL (100-mg single dose).

Orphenadrine hydrochloride: Oral—110–210 nanograms per mL (100-mg single dose).
  Elimination:
    Renal and fecal.
Precautions:
  Dental—May cause dryness of mouth.
  Medical considerations/contraindications—
    Also should not be used in patients with medical conditions in which anticholinergic actions are detrimental.
    Also should be used with caution in patients with cardiac disease or arrhythmias, especially tachycardia.
  Patient monitoring—Blood count and hepatic and renal function tests recommended during prolonged therapy.
Side/adverse effects:
  Also may cause side effects typical of anticholinergics and aplastic anemia.
  Also may cause hallucinations, syncope, confusion (especially in the elderly), and blurred or double vision; anticholinergic as well as CNS actions may contribute to these effects.

## Additional Dosing Information

The safety of continuous long-term administration of orphenadrine has not been established.

## Oral Dosage Forms

### ORPHENADRINE CITRATE EXTENDED-RELEASE TABLETS

#### Usual adult and adolescent dose

Skeletal muscle relaxant—
  Oral, 100 mg two times a day, in the morning and evening.

#### Usual pediatric dose

Safety and efficacy have not been established.

#### Strength(s) usually available

U.S.—
  100 mg (Rx) [*Norflex;* GENERIC].

Canada—
  100 mg (OTC) [*Norflex*].

#### Packaging and storage

Store below 40 °C (104 °F), preferably between 15 and 30 °C (59 and 86 °F), in a tight, light-resistant container, unless otherwise specified by manufacturer.

#### Auxiliary labeling

• May cause drowsiness.
• Avoid alcoholic beverages.

### ORPHENADRINE HYDROCHLORIDE TABLETS

#### Usual adult and adolescent dose

Skeletal muscle relaxant
and Parkinsonism therapy adjunct—
  Oral, 50 mg three times a day.

Note: Smaller doses may suffice if other antiparkinson medications are being administered concurrently.

#### Usual adult prescribing limits

Up to 250 mg a day.

#### Usual pediatric dose

Dosage has not been established.

#### Strength(s) usually available

U.S.—
  Not commercially available.

Canada—
  50 mg (OTC) [*Disipal*].

#### Packaging and storage

Store below 40 °C (104 °F), preferably between 15 and 30 °C (59 and 86 °F), in a tight container, unless otherwise specified by manufacturer.

#### Auxiliary labeling

• May cause drowsiness.
• Avoid alcoholic beverages.

## Parenteral Dosage Forms

### ORPHENADRINE CITRATE INJECTION USP

#### Usual adult and adolescent dose

Skeletal muscle relaxant—
  Intramuscular or intravenous, 60 mg every twelve hours as needed.

#### Usual pediatric dose

Safety and efficacy have not been established.

**Strength(s) usually available**

U.S.—

    30 mg per mL (Rx) [*Antiflex; Banflex; Flexoject; Mio-Rel; Myolin; Myotrol; Norflex; Orfro; Orphenate;* GENERIC].

Canada—

    30 mg per mL (OTC) [*Norflex* (sodium bisulfite)].

**Packaging and storage**

Store below 40 °C (104 °F), preferably between 15 and 30 °C (59 and 86 °F), unless otherwise specified by manufacturer. Protect from light. Protect from freezing.

## Selected Bibliography

Elenbaas JK. Central acting oral skeletal muscle relaxants. Am J Hosp Pharm 1980; 37: 1313-23.

Waldman HJ. Centrally acting skeletal muscle relaxants and associated drugs. J Pain Symptom Manage 1994; 9: 434-41.

Revised: 08/11/95

## Table 1. Pharmacology/Pharmacokinetics

| Drug | Absorption | Protein Binding (%) | Biotransformation | Half-life (hr) | Elimination Primary (% Excreted Unchanged)/ Secondary |
|------|-----------|---------------------|-------------------|----------------|------------------------------------------------------|
| Carisoprodol | | | Hepatic* | 8 | Renal (<1)† |
| Chlorphenesin | Rapid; complete | | Hepatic‡ | 2.3–5 | Renal§ |
| Chlorzoxazone | Rapid; complete | | Hepatic | 1.1 | Renal (<1) |
| Metaxalone | | | Hepatic | 2–3 | Renal |
| Methocarbamol | Rapid | | Probably hepatic | 0.9–2.2 | Renal/fecal |
| Orphenadrine | | Low | Hepatic | 14# | Renal/fecal |

\*One of the metabolites is meprobamate.

†Distributed into breast milk; concentration may reach 2 to 4 times the maternal plasma concentration. Also, may be removed from the circulation via hemodialysis and peritoneal dialysis.

‡At least partially metabolized.

§85% of a dose excreted within 24 hours as the glucuronide metabolite.

#For the parent compound; half-life of metabolites may range from 2 to 25 hours.

## Table 2. Pharmacology/Pharmacokinetics

| Drug | Onset of Action | Time to Peak Concentration (hr) (single dose) | Peak Serum Concentration (single dose) | Duration of Action (hr) |
|------|-----------------|-----------------------------------------------|----------------------------------------|-------------------------|
| Carisoprodol | 0.5 hr | 4 (350 mg) | 4–7 mcg/mL | 4–6 |
| Chlorphenesin | | 1–3 | 3.8–17 mcg/mL (800 mg) | |
| Chlorzoxazone | Within 1 hr | 1–2 | 10–30 mcg/mL (750 mg) | 3–4 |
| Metaxalone | 1 hr | 2 (800 mg) | 295 mcg/mL (800 mg) | |
| Methocarbamol | | | | |
|   Oral | Within 0.5 hr | 2 (2 grams) | 16 mcg/mL (2 grams) | |
|   IV (300 mg/min) | Immediate | Almost immediate | 19 mcg/mL (1 gram) | |
| Orphenadrine citrate* | | | | |
|   Oral (extended-release tablets) | Within 1 hr | 6 to 8 (100 mg) | 60–120 nanograms/mL (100 mg) | 12 |
|   IM | 5 min | 0.5 (60 mg) | | |
|   IV | Immediate | Immediate | | |
| Orphenadrine hydrochloride† | Within 1 hr | 3 (50 mg) | 110–210 nanograms/mL (100 mg) | 8 |

\*Relief of muscle spasm.

†In parkinsonism.

## Table 3. Medical considerations/Contraindications

The medical considerations/contraindications included have been selected on the basis of their potential clinical significance (reasons given in parentheses where appropriate)—not necessarily inclusive (» = major clinical significance).

Legend:
I = Carisoprodol
II = Chlorphenesin
III = Chlorzoxazone
IV = Metaxalone
V = Methocarbamol
VI = Orphenadrine

| | I | II | III | IV | V | VI |
|---|---|---|---|---|---|---|
| ***Except under special circumstances, these medications should not be used when the following medical problems exist:*** | | | | | | |
| » Achalasia or | | | | | | ✔ |
| » Bladder neck obstruction or | | | | | | ✔ |
| » Glaucoma, or predisposition to, or | | | | | | ✔ |
| » Myasthenia gravis or | | | | | | ✔ |
| » Peptic ulcer, stenosing, or | | | | | | ✔ |
| » Prostatic hypertrophy or | | | | | | ✔ |
| » Pyloric or duodenal obstruction (anticholinergic actions detrimental in these conditions) | | | | | | ✔ |
| » Hemolytic anemia, or history of, especially if drug-induced (may be induced by metaxalone) | | | | ✔ | | |
| » Porphyria, acute intermittent, known or suspected | ✔ | | | | | |
| » Renal function impairment or disease (for parenteral dosage form only—polyethylene glycol 300 vehicle is nephrotoxic and may cause increased urea retention and acidosis in these patients) | | | | | ✔ | |
| ***Risk-benefit should be considered when the following medical problems exist:*** | | | | | | |
| Allergic reaction to the medication considered for use, history of | ✔ | ✔ | ✔ | ✔ | ✔ | ✔ |
| Allergies or history of | | | ✔ | | | |
| Cardiac disease or arrhythmias or Tachycardia (orphenadrine may cause tachycardia) | | | | | | ✔ |
| CNS depression (may be exacerbated) | ✔ | ✔ | ✔ | ✔ | ✔ | ✔ |
| Drug abuse or dependence, history of (psychological dependence and abuse reported rarely) | ✔ | | | | | |
| Epilepsy (for parenteral dosage form only—may increase risk of seizures) | | | | | ✔ | |
| Hepatic function impairment (metabolized in liver) | ✔ | ✔ | | | ✔ | ✔ |
| » Hepatic function impairment or disease (metabolized in liver; also, potentially hepatotoxic) | | | ✔ | ✔ | | |
| Renal function impairment (excreted via kidneys) | | | ✔ | | ✔ | ✔ |
| » Renal function impairment, severe (excreted via kidneys) | | | | ✔ | | |

Table 4. Side/Adverse Effects*

| The following side/adverse effects have been selected on the basis of their potential clinical significance (possible signs and symptoms in parentheses where appropriate)—not necessarily inclusive: | Legend:<br>I=Carisoprodol<br>II=Chlorphenesin<br>III=Chlorzoxazone | | | IV=Metaxalone<br>V=Methocarbamol<br>VI=Orphenadrine | | |
|---|---|---|---|---|---|---|
| | I | II | III | IV | V | VI |
| **Medical attention needed** | | | | | | |
| *Anticholinergic effects, specifically:* | | | | | | |
|   *Decreased urination* | — | — | — | — | — | L |
|   *Increased intraocular pressure* (eye pain) | — | — | — | — | — | L |
| *Cardiovascular effects, specifically:* | | | | | | |
|   *Fast heartbeat*—with orphenadrine, anticholinergic activity may contribute to this effect | L | U | U | U | U | L |
|   *Pounding heartbeat* | U | U | U | U | U | L |
|   *Slow heartbeat*—with parenteral dosage form only | — | — | — | — | L‡ | U |
|   *Thrombophlebitis* (local pain, tenderness, heat, redness, swelling at site of affected vein)—with parenteral administration only | — | | | | R | U |
| *Central nervous system effects, specifically:* | | | | | | |
|   *Convulsions* | U | U | U | U | R‡ | U |
|   *Fainting*—with carisoprodol, may also be caused by orthostatic hypotension | L | U | U | U | R‡ | L |
|   *Hallucinations*—orphenadrine's anticholinergic activity may contribute to this effect | U | U | U | U | U | R |
|   *Mental depression* | L | U | U | U | U | U |
| *Gastrointestinal bleeding* (bloody or black, tarry stools; vomiting of blood or material that looks like coffee grounds) | U | R† | R | U | U | U |
| *Hematologic effects, specifically:* | | | | | | |
|   *Agranulocytosis* (fever with or without chills; sores, ulcers, or white spots on lips or in mouth; sore throat) | U | R | R | U | U | U |
|   *Anemia* (unusual tiredness or weakness) | U | U | R | U | U | U |
|   *Anemia, aplastic [pancytopenia]* (shortness of breath, troubled breathing, tightness in chest, and/or wheezing; sores, ulcers, or white spots on lips or in mouth; swollen and/or painful glands; unusual bleeding or bruising; unusual tiredness or weakness) | R† | U | U | U | U | R |
|   *Anemia, hemolytic* (troubled breathing, exertional; unusual tiredness or weakness) | U | U | U | R | U | U |
|   *Leukopenia* (usually asymptomatic; rarely, fever or chills, cough or hoarseness, lower back or side pain, painful or difficult urination) | R† | R | U | R | R | U |
|   *Thrombocytopenia* (usually asymptomatic; rarely, unusual bleeding or bruising; black, tarry stools; blood in urine or stools; pinpoint red spots on skin) | U | R | U | U | U | U |
| *Hepatotoxicity* (yellow eyes or skin) | U | U | R† | R | U | U |
| *Hypersensitivity reactions, specifically:* | | | | | | |
|   *Anaphylactic or anaphylactoid reaction* (changes in facial skin color; skin rash, hives, and/or itching; fast or irregular breathing; puffiness or swelling of the eyelids or around the eyes; shortness of breath, troubled breathing, tightness in chest, and/or wheezing)—with carisoprodol, anaphylactic shock with sudden, severe decrease in blood pressure and collapse has also occurred | R | R | R | R | U | U |
|   *Angioedema* (hive-like swellings, large, on face, eyelids, mouth, lips, and/or tongue) | L | U | R | U | U | U |
|   *Bronchospastic allergic reaction* (shortness of breath, troubled breathing, tightness in chest, and/or wheezing) | L | U | U | U | U | U |
|   *Conjunctivitis and nasal congestion* (stuffy nose and red or bloodshot eyes) | U | U | U | U | L | U |
|   *Dermatitis, allergic* (skin rash, hives, itching, and/or redness)—with carisoprodol, fixed drug eruptions with cross-sensitivity to meprobamate have also been reported; with chlorzoxazone, petechial rashes and ecchymoses have also been reported | L | R | R | R | L | U |
|   *Eosinophilia* | R | U | U | U | U | U |
|   *Erythema multiforme* (fever with or without chills; muscle cramps or pain; skin rash; sores, ulcers, or white spots on lips or in mouth) | R | U | U | U | U | U |
|   *Fever, allergic* | L | R | U | U | L | U |
|   *Stinging or burning of eyes* | L | U | U | U | U | U |
| **Medical attention needed only if continuing or bothersome** | | | | | | |
| *Anticholinergic effects* (dryness of mouth [more frequent], confusion, difficult urination, constipation, unusually large pupils, blurred or double vision, weakness) | — | — | — | — | — | L |

## Table 4. Side/Adverse Effects* *(continued)*

| | Legend:<br>I = Carisoprodol<br>II = Chlorphenesin<br>III = Chlorzoxazone | | | IV = Metaxalone<br>V = Methocarbamol<br>VI = Orphenadrine | | |
|---|:---:|:---:|:---:|:---:|:---:|:---:|
| | **I** | **II** | **III** | **IV** | **V** | **VI** |
| ***Central nervous system effects, specifically:*** | | | | | | |
|   ***Blurred or double vision or any change in vision***—with orphenadrine, anticholinergic activity may also contribute to this effect | R | U | U | U | M | L |
|   ***Clumsiness or unsteadiness*** | R | U | U | U | U | U |
|   ***Confusion***—with orphenadrine, anticholinergic activity may also contribute to this effect, especially in elderly patients | U | L | U | U | U | L |
|   ***Dizziness or lightheadedness***—with carisoprodol, orthostatic hypotension may also contribute to this effect | L | L | M | M | M | L |
|   ***Drowsiness*** | M | L | M | M | M | L |
|   ***Headache*** | L | R | L | M | L | L |
|   ***Muscle weakness*** | U | R | U | U | L‡ | R |
|   ***Nystagmus*** (uncontrolled movements of eyes) | U | U | U | U | L‡ | U |
|   ***Stimulation, paradoxical*** (excitement, nervousness, restlessness, irritability, trouble in sleeping) | L | R | L | M | U | L |
|   ***Trembling*** | L | U | U | U | U | L |
| ***Flushing or redness of face*** | L | U | U | U | L‡ | U |
| ***Gastrointestinal irritation, specifically:***<br>  ***Abdominal or stomach cramps or pain*** | L | R | L | M | U | L |
|   ***Constipation***—with orphenadrine, anticholinergic activity may contribute to this effect | U | U | L | U | U | L |
|   ***Diarrhea*** | U | U | L | U | U | U |
|   ***Heartburn*** | U | U | L | U | U | U |
|   ***Hiccups*** | L | U | U | U | U | U |
|   ***Nausea or vomiting*** | L | R | L | M | L | L |
| ***Pain or peeling at place of injection*** | — | — | — | — | L‡ | U |

  *Differences in frequency of occurrence may reflect either lack of clinical-use data or actual pharmacologic distinctions among agents (although their pharmacologic similarity suggests that side effects occurring with one may occur with the others, except for those caused by anticholinergic activity, which is specific for orphenadrine). M = more frequent; L = less frequent; R = rare; U = unknown.

  †A causal association has not been established.

  ‡Usually reported with too-rapid intravenous administration.

## Table 5. Patient Consultation

| As an aid to patient consultation, refer to *Advice for the Patient, Skeletal Muscle Relaxants (Systemic)* or *Orphenadrine (Systemic)*.<br><br>In providing consultation, consider emphasizing the following selected information (» = major clinical significance): | Legend:<br>I = Carisoprodol<br>II = Chlorphenesin<br>III = Chlorzoxazone | | | IV = Metaxalone<br>V = Methocarbamol<br>VI = Orphenadrine | | |
|---|:---:|:---:|:---:|:---:|:---:|:---:|
| | **I** | **II** | **III** | **IV** | **V** | **VI** |
| **Before using this medication**<br>»  Conditions affecting use, especially: | | | | | | |
|     Sensitivity to the muscle relaxant considered for use, history of, and, for carisoprodol, sensitivity to other carbamate derivatives | ✔ | ✔ | ✔ | ✔ | ✔ | ✔ |
|     Breast-feeding—Carisoprodol distributed into breast milk and may cause sedation and gastrointestinal upset in the infant; problems in nursing infants have not been reported with other skeletal muscle relaxants | ✔ | | | | | |
|     Other medications, especially other CNS depression–producing medications | ✔ | ✔ | ✔ | ✔ | ✔ | ✔ |
|     Other medical problems, especially: | | | | | | |
|       Acute intermittent porphyria (known or suspected) | ✔ | | | | | |
|       Conditions that may be adversely affected by anticholinergic activity | | | | | | ✔ |
|       Hemolytic anemia, or history of | | | | ✔ | | |
|       Hepatic function impairment or disease | ✔ | ✔ | ✔ | ✔ | ✔ | ✔ |
|       Renal function impairment or disease | ✔ | ✔ | ✔ | ✔ | ✔ | ✔ |
| **Proper use of this medication**<br>  Tablets may be crushed and mixed with food or liquid for ease of administration | | | ✔ | ✔ | ✔ | |
| »  Proper dosing | ✔ | ✔ | ✔ | ✔ | ✔ | ✔ |

## Table 5. Patient Consultation *(continued)*

| | Legend:<br>**I**=Carisoprodol<br>**II**=Chlorphenesin<br>**III**=Chlorzoxazone | | | **IV**=Metaxalone<br>**V**=Methocarbamol<br>**VI**=Orphenadrine | | |
|---|---|---|---|---|---|---|
| | **I** | **II** | **III** | **IV** | **V** | **VI** |
| Missed dose: Taking if remembered within an hour or so; not taking if remembered later; not doubling doses | ✔ | ✔ | ✔ | ✔ | ✔ | ✔ |
| » Proper storage | ✔ | ✔ | ✔ | ✔ | ✔ | ✔ |
| **Precautions while using this medication** | | | | | | |
| Regular visits to physician to check progress during prolonged therapy | ✔ | ✔ | ✔ | ✔ | ✔ | ✔ |
| » Avoiding use of alcohol or other CNS depressants during therapy unless prescribed or otherwise approved by physician | ✔ | ✔ | ✔ | ✔ | ✔ | ✔ |
| » Caution if any of the following occur: | | | | | | |
|    Blurred vision or other vision problems | ✔ | | | | ✔ | ✔ |
|    Clumsiness or unsteadiness | ✔ | | | | ✔ | |
|    Dizziness or lightheadedness | ✔ | ✔ | ✔ | ✔ | ✔ | ✔ |
|    Drowsiness | ✔ | ✔ | ✔ | ✔ | ✔ | ✔ |
|    Faintness | ✔ | | | | ✔ | ✔ |
|    Muscle weakness | | | | | | ✔ |
| Possible dryness of mouth; using sugarless gum or candy, ice, or saliva substitute for relief; checking with dentist if dry mouth continues for more than 2 weeks | | | | | | ✔ |
| Diabetics: May cause false-positive urine sugar tests | | | | ✔ | | |
| **Side/adverse effects** | | | | | | |
| Signs and symptoms of potential side effects, especially: | | | | | | |
|    Allergic reactions | ✔ | ✔ | ✔ | ✔ | ✔ | ✔ |
|    Anticholinergic effects | | | | | | ✔ |
|    Blood dyscrasias | | ✔ | ✔ | ✔ | ✔ | |
|    Convulsions | | | | | ✔* | |
|    Fainting | ✔ | | | | ✔* | ✔ |
|    Fast heartbeat | ✔ | | | | | ✔ |
|    Gastrointestinal bleeding | | | | ✔ | | |
|    Hallucinations | | | | | | ✔ |
|    Hepatotoxicity | | | | ✔ | | |
|    Mental depression | ✔ | | | | | ✔ |
|    Pounding heartbeat | | | | | | ✔ |
|    Slow heartbeat | | | | | ✔* | |
| Medication may color urine orange or reddish purple | | | | ✔ | | |
| Medication may color urine black, brown, or green, especially if allowed to stand | | | | | ✔ | |

*For parenteral administration only.

---

**SODIUM ASCORBATE**—See *Ascorbic Acid (Systemic)*

---

# SODIUM BENZOATE AND SODIUM PHENYLACETATE   Systemic†

VA CLASSIFICATION (Primary): AD900

Note: For a listing of dosage forms and brand names by country availability, see *Dosage Forms* section(s). For a listing of brand names for the articles in this monograph, refer to the General Index.

†Not commercially available in Canada.

## Category

Antihyperammonemic.

## Indications

### Accepted

Hyperammonemia (prophylaxis and treatment)—Sodium benzoate and sodium phenylacetate combination is indicated as adjunctive therapy in the prevention and treatment of hyperammonemia in patients with urea cycle enzymopathy (UCE) due to carbamylphosphate synthetase, ornithine transcarbamylase, or arginosuccinate synthetase deficiency. Sodium benzoate and sodium phenylacetate combination is used in conjunction with a low protein diet and amino acid supplementation.

Beneficial use of sodium benzoate and sodium phenylacetate combi-nation in treating neonatal hyperammonemic coma has not been established. Treatment of choice for neonatal hyperammonemic coma is hemodialysis.

## Pharmacology/Pharmacokinetics

### Mechanism of action/Effect

Sodium benzoate and sodium phenylacetate combination decreases ammonia formation by conjugation reactions involving acylation of amino acids. Benzoate and phenylacetate activate conjugation pathways, which then substitute for or supplement the defective ureagenic pathway in patients with urea cycle enzymopathies. Benzoate conjugates with glycine to form hippurate, and phenylacetate conjugates with glutamine to form phenylacetylglutamine.

### Biotransformation

Hepatic and renal.

### Time to peak concentration

Within 1 hour in normal adults.

**Elimination**
Primarily renal; approximately 80 to 100% as the respective conjugation product, hippurate or phenylacetylglutamine, within 24 hours in normal adults.

## Precautions to Consider

### Carcinogenicity/Mutagenicity
Sodium benzoate has been tested as a food preservative and results indicate that it is not carcinogenic or mutagenic. Carcinogenic or mutagenic studies of sodium phenylacetate have not been conducted.

### Pregnancy/Reproduction
Fertility—Sodium benzoate has not been found to impair fertility. Fertility studies of sodium phenylacetate have not been conducted.

Pregnancy—Studies have not been done in humans.
Studies have not been done in animals.

FDA Pregnancy Category C.

### Breast-feeding
It is not known whether sodium benzoate or sodium phenylacetate combination is distributed into breast milk.

### Pediatrics
It is theorized that low birthweight infants with immature livers may not be capable of metabolizing benzoate and hippurate. Sodium benzoate and sodium phenylacetate combination should not be administered to low birthweight infants unless the benefits of treatment outweigh the risks.

### Geriatrics
No information is available on the relationship of age to the effects of sodium benzoate and sodium phenylacetate combination in geriatric patients. However, elderly patients are more likely to have age-related renal function impairment, which may require careful monitoring in patients receiving sodium benzoate and sodium phenylacetate combination.

### Drug interactions and/or related problems
The following drug interactions and/or related problems have been selected on the basis of their potential clinical significance (possible mechanism in parentheses where appropriate)—not necessarily inclusive (» = major clinical significance):

Note: Combinations containing any of the following medications, depending on the amount present, may also interact with this medication.

» Penicillins
(concurrent use with sodium benzoate and sodium phenylacetate combination is not recommended because penicillins may compete with the conjugated products of sodium benzoate and sodium phenylacetate for active secretion by renal tubules)

Probenecid
(probenecid inhibits the renal transport of many organic compounds, including aminohippuric acid, and may affect renal excretion of the conjugated products of sodium benzoate and sodium phenylacetate)

Valproic acid
(hyperammonemia, reported to be induced by valproic acid, may exacerbate urea cycle enzymopathy deficiency and antagonize the efficacy of sodium benzoate and sodium phenylacetate combination)

### Medical considerations/Contraindications
The medical considerations/contraindications included here have been selected on the basis of their potential clinical significance (reasons given in parentheses where appropriate)—not necessarily inclusive (» = major clinical significance).

*Risk-benefit should be considered when the following medical problems exist:*

Edematous sodium-retaining conditions, such as:
» Congestive heart failure or
» Renal function impairment or
» Toxemia of pregnancy
(fluid retention may be increased due to the sodium content of sodium benzoate and sodium phenylacetate)

Hyperbilirubinemia, neonatal
(benzoate may compete for bilirubin binding sites on albumin)

Peptic ulcer
(the condition may be exacerbated by sodium benzoate and sodium phenylacetate combination because of structural similarities between benzoate and salicylates)

Sensitivity to sodium benzoate or sodium phenylacetate combination, or either component

**Patient monitoring**
The following may be especially important in patient monitoring (other tests may be warranted in some patients, depending on condition; » = major clinical significance):

Ammonia concentrations, plasma
(determinations recommended at frequent intervals during therapy to confirm efficacy of sodium benzoate and sodium phenylacetate combination; excessive ammonia concentrations may lead to hyperammonemic coma)

## Side/Adverse Effects

Note: Because of structural similarities between benzoate and salicylates, sodium benzoate and sodium phenylacetate combination may have the potential to cause side effects associated with salicylates, such as exacerbation of peptic ulcers, mild hyperventilation, and mild respiratory alkalosis.

The following side/adverse effects have been selected on the basis of their potential clinical significance (possible signs and symptoms in parentheses where appropriate)—not necessarily inclusive:

**Those indicating need for medical attention only if they continue or are bothersome**
Incidence more frequent
*Nausea or vomiting*

## Overdose
For information on the management of overdose or unintentional ingestion, **contact a Poison Control Center** (see *Poison Control Center Listing* ).

**Clinical effects of overdose**
The following effects have been selected on the basis of their potential clinical significance (possible signs and symptoms in parentheses where appropriate)—not necessarily inclusive:

*Circulatory collapse* (feeling of faintness; rapid fall in blood pressure); *lethargy* (unusual drowsiness); *metabolic acidosis* (shortness of breath or troubled breathing); *respiratory alkalosis; unusual irritability; vomiting, persistent*

Note: *Circulatory collapse, lethargy,* and *metabolic acidosis* were reported after overdoses with intravenous sodium benzoate and sodium phenylacetate combination.

All side/adverse effects of sodium benzoate and sodium phenylacetate combination may also be symptoms of the disease state; however, they may be increased if overdose occurs.

**Treatment of overdose**
The medication should be discontinued. There is no known specific antidote for sodium benzoate and sodium phenylacetate combination overdose. Recommended treatment consists of the following
• Supportive care—Supportive therapy for metabolic acidosis and circulatory collapse. Hemodialysis or peritoneal dialysis.

## Patient Consultation
As an aid to patient consultation, refer to *Advice for the Patient, Sodium Benzoate and Sodium Phenylacetate (Systemic)*.

In providing consultation, consider emphasizing the following selected information (» = major clinical significance):

**Before using this medication**
» Conditions affecting use, especially:
Sensitivity to sodium benzoate and sodium phenylacetate combination, or either component
Use in children—Caution in low birthweight infants with immature livers
Other medicines, especially penicillins
Other medical problems, especially congestive heart failure, edema, renal function impairment, or toxemia of pregnancy

**Proper use of this medication**
Diluting medication in formula or milk before taking
Taking medication with meals
Importance of low protein diet
» Proper dosing
Missed dose: Taking as soon as possible; not taking if almost time for next dose; not doubling doses
» Proper storage

**Precautions while using this medication**
Regular visits to physician to check progress during therapy

## General Dosing Information

Sodium benzoate and sodium phenylacetate combination is a concentrated solution for oral use only. Each dose should be diluted in infant formula or milk before administration. If other beverages are used, particularly acidic beverages, precipitation of the medication may occur, depending on the pH and the final concentration. The mixture should be inspected for compatibility before administration.

Since sodium benzoate and sodium phenylacetate combination is a concentrated solution, care should be taken in calculating the dose to avoid the possibility of an overdose.

Since sodium phenylacetate has a lingering odor, caution should be used in mixing or administering the medication to minimize contact with skin and clothing.

### Diet/Nutrition

Sodium benzoate and sodium phenylacetate combination should be administered with meals.

Sodium benzoate and sodium phenylacetate combination should be combined with a low protein diet to reduce nitrogen intake and in some patients amino acid supplementation to provide a better tolerated type of dietary nitrogen.

Each dose of sodium benzoate and sodium phenylacetate combination must be diluted in 4 to 8 ounces of infant formula or milk before administration.

## Oral Dosage Forms

### SODIUM BENZOATE AND SODIUM PHENYLACETATE ORAL SOLUTION

#### Usual adult and adolescent dose
Antihyperammonemic—
    Oral, 250 mg of sodium benzoate and 250 mg of sodium phenylacetate (2.5 mL) per kg of body weight a day, in three to six equally divided doses, not to exceed 100 mL (10 grams each of sodium benzoate and sodium phenylacetate) a day.

#### Usual pediatric dose
See *Usual adult and adolescent dose.*

Note: Use in neonates with hyperammonemic coma has not been established.

#### Strength(s) usually available
U.S.—
    100 mg sodium benzoate and 100 mg sodium phenylacetate per mL (Rx) [*Ucephan*].

Canada—
    Not commercially available.

Note: The concentrated sodium benzoate and sodium phenylacetate solution, before dilution, contains 130 mEq (262 milliosmoles) of sodium per 100 mL.

#### Packaging and storage
Store below 40 °C (104 °F), preferably between 15 and 30 °C (59 and 86 °F), in a well-closed container, unless otherwise specified by manufacturer. Protect from freezing.

#### Preparation of dosage form
Each dose of sodium benzoate and sodium phenylacetate combination must be diluted in 4 to 8 ounces of infant formula or milk before administration.

#### Incompatibilities
Mixing with acidic beverages or medications may cause precipitation of sodium benzoate and sodium phenylacetate, depending on the pH and final concentration of the diluted solution.

#### Auxiliary labeling
• For oral use only.
• Take mixed in infant formula or milk.

Revised: 07/15/93

---

# SODIUM BICARBONATE    Systemic

VA CLASSIFICATION (Primary/Secondary): GA110/TN409

Note: For a listing of dosage forms and brand names by country availability, see *Dosage Forms* section(s). For a listing of brand names for the articles in this monograph, refer to the General Index.

## Category

Alkalizer (systemic; urinary)—Sodium Bicarbonate Injection USP; Sodium Bicarbonate Oral Powder USP; Sodium Bicarbonate Tablets USP.

Antacid—Effervescent Sodium Bicarbonate; Sodium Bicarbonate Oral Powder USP; Sodium Bicarbonate Tablets USP.

Electrolyte replenisher—Sodium Bicarbonate Injection USP.

## Indications

Note: Bracketed information in the *Indications* section refers to uses that are not included in U.S. product labeling.

### Accepted
Metabolic acidosis (treatment)—
Acute mild to moderate
In renal tubular disorders
In severe renal disease (renal tubular acidosis)
In circulatory insufficiency, due to shock or severe dehydration
In cardiac arrest
In extracorporeal circulation of blood and
In primary lactic acidosis, severe—Oral sodium bicarbonate is indicated in the treatment of metabolic acidosis. It is preferred over parenteral therapy in acute mild to moderate acidosis. Oral sodium bicarbonate is also indicated to correct acidosis in renal tubular disorders. Parenteral sodium bicarbonate is indicated to minimize risks of metabolic acidosis in severe renal disease, circulatory insufficiency due to shock or severe dehydration, extracorporeal circulation of blood, cardiac arrest, and severe primary lactic acidosis.

Intravenous sodium bicarbonate has been used to minimize the risks of metabolic acidosis in uncontrolled diabetes; however, it generally has been replaced by low-dose insulin therapy and saline, potassium, and fluid replacement. With low-dose insulin therapy there is less risk of developing serious hypoglycemia and/or hypokalemia.

Renal calculi, uric acid (prophylaxis)—Oral sodium bicarbonate is indicated to reduce uric acid crystallization as an adjuvant to uricosuric medication in gout.

Hyperacidity (treatment)—Also indicated orally to provide symptomatic relief of upset stomach associated with hyperacidity. It may also be used in the treatment of the symptoms of peptic ulcer disease.

Diarrhea (treatment adjunct)—Parenteral sodium bicarbonate is indicated in severe diarrhea in which the loss of bicarbonate is significant.

Toxicity, nonspecific (treatment)—Parenteral sodium bicarbonate is indicated in the treatment of certain drug intoxications, including barbiturates, and in poisoning by salicylates or methyl alcohol.

Sodium bicarbonate is not recommended for use as an antidote following the ingestion of strong mineral acids, since the formation of carbon dioxide may distend the weakened stomach and lead to gastric rupture.

Sodium bicarbonate has been used as a urinary alkalizer to increase sulfonamide solubility and prevent crystallization that may lead to renal calculi or nephrotoxicity; however, poorly soluble sulfonamides are rarely used now.

[Sodium bicarbonate has been used in the treatment of sickle cell anemia; however, it generally has been replaced by more effective agents.]

## Pharmacology/Pharmacokinetics

### Physicochemical characteristics
Molecular weight—84.01.

### Mechanism of action/Effect
Alkalizer, systemic—Increases the plasma bicarbonate, buffers excess hydrogen ion concentration, and raises blood pH, thereby reversing the clinical manifestations of acidosis.

Alkalizer, urinary—Increases the excretion of free bicarbonate ions in the urine, thus effectively raising the urinary pH. By maintaining an alkaline urine, the actual dissolution of uric acid stones may be accomplished.

Antacid—Reacts chemically to neutralize or buffer existing quantities of stomach acid but has no direct effect on its output. This action results in increased pH value of stomach contents, thus providing relief of hyperacidity symptoms.

## Elimination
Renal; $CO_2$ formed is eliminated via lungs.

# Precautions to Consider

## Pregnancy/Reproduction
Pregnancy—Problems in humans have not been documented; however, risk-benefit must be considered, since sodium bicarbonate is absorbed systemically. Chronic use may lead to systemic alkalosis. The sodium load that is absorbed can also cause edema and weight gain.

For parenteral dosage form: Studies have not been done in humans. Studies have not been done in animals.

FDA Pregnancy Category C.

## Breast-feeding
It is not known whether sodium bicarbonate is distributed into breast milk. However, problems in humans have not been documented.

## Pediatrics
Antacids should not be given to young children (up to 6 years of age) unless prescribed by a physician. Since children are not usually able to describe their symptoms precisely, proper diagnosis should precede the use of an antacid. This will avoid the complication of an existing condition (e.g., appendicitis) or the appearance of more severe adverse effects.

## Geriatrics
No information is available on the relationship of age to the effects of sodium bicarbonate in geriatric patients. However, elderly patients are more likely to have age-related renal function impairment, which may require caution in patients receiving sodium bicarbonate.

## Drug interactions and/or related problems
The following drug interactions and/or related problems have been selected on the basis of their potential clinical significance (possible mechanism in parentheses where appropriate)—not necessarily inclusive (» = major clinical significance):

Note: Not all interactions between sodium bicarbonate and other oral medications have been identified in this monograph. Because concurrent use may increase or reduce the rate and/or extent of absorption of other oral medications, patients should be advised not to take any other oral medications within 1 to 2 hours of sodium bicarbonate.

Combinations containing any of the following medications, depending on the amount present, may also interact with this medication.

Acidifiers, urinary, such as:
 Ammonium chloride
 Ascorbic acid
 Potassium or sodium phosphates
   (antacids may alkalinize the urine and counteract the effect of urinary acidifiers; frequent use of antacids, especially in high doses, is best avoided by patients receiving therapy to acidify the urine)

Amphetamines or
Quinidine
   (urinary excretion may be inhibited when these medications are used concurrently with sodium bicarbonate, possibly resulting in toxicity; dosage adjustment may be needed when sodium bicarbonate therapy is initiated or discontinued or if dosage is changed)

Anticholinergics or other medications with anticholinergic action (See *Appendix II*)
   (concurrent use with sodium bicarbonate may decrease absorption, reducing the effectiveness of the anticholinergic; doses of these medications should be spaced 1 hour apart from doses of sodium bicarbonate; also, urinary excretion may be delayed by alkalinization of the urine, thus potentiating the side effects of the anticholinergic)

Calcium-containing preparations or
Milk or milk products
   (concurrent and prolonged use with sodium bicarbonate may result in the milk-alkali syndrome)

Ciprofloxacin or
Norfloxacin or
Ofloxacin
   (alkalinization of the urine may reduce the solubility of ciprofloxacin, norfloxacin, or ofloxacin in the urine; patients should be observed for signs of crystalluria and nephrotoxicity)

Citrates
   (concurrent use with antacids containing sodium bicarbonate may result in systemic alkalosis)
   (concurrent use with sodium bicarbonate may promote the development of calcium stones in patients with uric acid stones, due to

sodium ion opposition to the hypocalciuric effect of the alkaline load; may also cause hypernatremia)

Enteric-coated medications, such as bisacodyl
   (concurrent administration of antacids with enteric-coated tablets may cause the enteric coating to dissolve too rapidly, resulting in gastric or duodenal irritation)

Ephedrine
   (urine alkalinization induced by sodium bicarbonate may increase the half-life of ephedrine and prolong its duration of action, especially if the urine remains alkaline for several days or longer; dosage adjustment of ephedrine may be necessary)

Histamine $H_2$-receptor antagonists, such as
 Cimetidine
 Famotidine
 Nizatidine
 Ranitidine
   (concurrent use with sodium bicarbonate may be indicated in the treatment of peptic ulcer to relieve pain; however, simultaneous administration of antacids of medium to high potency [80 mmol to 150 mmol HCl] is not recommended since absorption of these medications may be decreased; patients should be advised not to take any antacids within one-half to 1 hour of histamine $H_2$-receptor antagonists)

Iron supplements or preparations, oral
   (absorption may be decreased when these preparations are used concurrently with antacids containing carbonate; because of the formation of less soluble complexes, iron supplements should not be taken within 1 hour before or 2 hours after sodium bicarbonate)

» Ketoconazole
   (sodium bicarbonate may cause increased gastrointestinal pH; concurrent administration with sodium bicarbonate may result in a marked reduction in absorption of ketoconazole; patients should take sodium bicarbonate at least 2 hours after ketoconazole)

Lithium
   (sodium bicarbonate enhances lithium excretion, possibly resulting in decreased efficacy; this may be partly due to the sodium content)

» Mecamylamine
   (alkalinization of the urine caused by sodium bicarbonate slows excretion and prolongs the effects of mecamylamine; concurrent use is not recommended)

» Methenamine
   (alkalinization of the urine caused by sodium bicarbonate may reduce the effectiveness of methenamine by inhibiting its conversion to formaldehyde; concurrent use is not recommended)

Mexiletine
   (marked alkalinization of the urine caused by sodium bicarbonate may retard renal excretion of mexiletine)

Potassium supplements
   (concurrent use of sodium bicarbonate infusion decreases serum potassium concentration by promoting a shift of potassium ion into the cells)

Salicylates
   (alkalinization of the urine may increase renal salicylate excretion and lower serum salicylate concentrations; dosage adjustments of salicylates may be necessary when chronic high-dose antacid therapy with sodium bicarbonate is started or stopped, especially in patients receiving large doses of the salicylate, such as those with rheumatoid arthritis and rheumatic fever)

Sucralfate
   (concurrent use with sodium bicarbonate may be indicated in the treatment of duodenal ulcer to relieve pain; however, simultaneous administration is not recommended since antacids, such as sodium bicarbonate, may interfere with binding of sucralfate to the mucosa; patients should be advised not to take sodium bicarbonate within one-half hour before or 1 hour after sucralfate)

» Tetracyclines, oral
   (absorption may be decreased when oral tetracyclines are used concurrently with sodium bicarbonate because of increase in intragastric pH; patients should be advised not to take sodium bicarbonate within 1 to 2 hours of tetracyclines)

## Laboratory value alterations
The following have been selected on the basis of their potential clinical significance (possible effect in parentheses where appropriate)—not necessarily inclusive (» = major clinical significance):

With diagnostic test results
» Gastric acid secretion test
   (concurrent use of sodium bicarbonate may antagonize the effect of pentagastrin or histamine in the evaluation of gastric acid se-

cretory function; administration of sodium bicarbonate is not recommended on the morning of the test)

With physiology/laboratory test values
   pH, systemic and urinary
      (may be increased)

### Medical considerations/Contraindications

The medical considerations/contraindications included here have been selected on the basis of their potential clinical significance (reasons given in parentheses where appropriate)—not necessarily inclusive (» = major clinical significance).

*Except under special circumstances, this medication should not be used when the following medical problems exist:*

*For parenteral dosage form*
» Alkalosis, metabolic or respiratory
      (may be exacerbated)
» Chloride loss due to vomiting or continuous gastrointestinal suction
      (increased risk of severe alkalosis)
» Hypocalcemia
      (increased risk of alkalosis producing tetany)

*Risk-benefit should be considered when the following medical problems exist:*

» Anuria or oliguria
      (increased risk of excessive sodium retention)
» Edematous sodium-retaining conditions such as:
   Cirrhosis of liver
   Congestive heart failure
   Renal function impairment
   Toxemia of pregnancy
» Hypertension
      (may be exacerbated)
*For antacid use*
» Appendicitis or symptoms of
      (sodium bicarbonate may complicate existing condition)
» Bleeding, gastrointestinal or rectal, undiagnosed

### Patient monitoring

The following may be especially important in patient monitoring (other tests may be warranted in some patients, depending on condition; » = major clinical significance):

Arterial blood pH determinations and
Bicarbonate concentrations, serum
   (periodic monitoring during parenteral administration is recommended to avoid overdosage and alkalosis)
pH determinations, urinary
   (monitoring is recommended for dosage adjustment when sodium bicarbonate is used as a urinary alkalizer)
Renal function determinations
   (recommended at periodic intervals with long-term use of frequent, repeated dosage)

## Side/Adverse Effects

The following side/adverse effects have been selected on the basis of their potential clinical significance (possible signs and symptoms in parentheses where appropriate)—not necessarily inclusive:

**Those indicating need for medical attention**
With excessive parenteral administration
   *Hypokalemia* (dryness of mouth; increased thirst; irregular heartbeat; mood or mental changes; muscle cramps or pain; weak pulse)
With large doses
   *Swelling of feet or lower legs*

**Those indicating need for medical attention only if they continue or are bothersome**
Incidence less frequent
   *Increased thirst; stomach cramps*

## Overdose

For specific information on the agents used in the management of sodium bicarbonate overdose, see
   • *Potassium Chloride* in *Potassium Supplements* monograph and/or
   • *Calcium Gluconate* in *Calcium Supplements* monograph.

For information on the management of overdose or unintentional ingestion, **contact a Poison Control Center** (see *Poison Control Center Listing*).

### Clinical effects of overdose
With large doses or in renal insufficiency
   *Metabolic alkalosis* (mood or mental changes; muscle pain or twitching; nervousness or restlessness; slow breathing; unpleasant taste; unusual tiredness or weakness)
With long-term use
   *Hypercalcemia associated with milk-alkali syndrome* (frequent urge to urinate; continuing headache; continuing loss of appetite; nausea or vomiting; unusual tiredness or weakness)

### Treatment of overdose
Stop administration of sodium bicarbonate and all other alkali.
Supportive care—
   Hydration with sodium chloride 0.9% intravenous injection.
Specific treatment—
   Parenteral administration of potassium chloride if hypokalemia present.
   Parenteral administration of calcium gluconate if hypocalcemia is present, for severe alkalosis.
   Parenteral administration of ammonium chloride or hydrochloric acid, for severe alkalosis.
   Hemodialysis for severe alkalosis.

## Patient Consultation

As an aid to patient consultation, refer to *Advice for the Patient, Sodium Bicarbonate (Systemic)*.

In providing consultation, consider emphasizing the following selected information (» = major clinical significance):

**Before using this medication**
» Conditions affecting use, especially:
      Pregnancy—Chronic use may lead to systemic alkalosis; sodium may cause edema and weight gain
      Use in children—Not recommended, because serious side effects may result
      Other medications, especially ketoconazole, mecamylamine, methenamine, or oral tetracyclines
      Other medical problems, especially anuria or oliguria, appendicitis, bleeding of gastrointestinal tract or rectum, chloride loss, edema, hypertension, hypocalcemia, or metabolic or respiratory alkalosis

**Proper use of this medication**
   Following physician's or manufacturer's instructions
» Proper dosing
   Missed dose: If on regular dosing schedule—Taking as soon as possible; not taking if almost time for next dose; not doubling doses
» Proper storage
*For antacid use*
» Compliance with therapy, especially for ulcer patients
   Taking 1 and 3 hours after meals and at bedtime for maximum effectiveness (for ulcer patients)

**Precautions while using this medication**
   Regular visits to physician to check progress during long-term therapy
» Not taking:
      —within 1 to 2 hours of other oral medication
      —for a prolonged period of time because of increased possibility of side effects
   Caution for sodium restriction
*For antacid use*
» Not taking:
      —if symptoms of appendicitis are present; checking with physician for proper diagnosis
      —concurrently with large amounts of milk or milk products
      —for more than 2 weeks or if problem is recurring, unless otherwise directed by physician

**Side/adverse effects**
   Signs of potential side effects, especially hypokalemia

## General Dosing Information

Prolonged sodium bicarbonate therapy is not recommended because of the high risk of causing metabolic alkalosis or sodium overload.

In acute mild to moderate acidosis, oral treatment is preferred to intravenous therapy. In severe acute acidosis, sodium bicarbonate may be given intravenously.

**For oral dosage forms only**
Sodium bicarbonate is a fast-acting antacid, but has a short duration of effect. It has a high neutralizing capacity.

The maximum daily dosage of sodium is 200 mEq (16.6 grams of sodium bicarbonate) in patients younger than 60 years of age and 100 mEq (8.3 grams of sodium bicarbonate) in patients 60 years of age or older.

When sodium bicarbonate is used as an antacid, the maximum dosage allowed should not be taken for more than 2 weeks except with the advice or under the supervision of a physician.

In the treatment of peptic ulcer disease, sodium bicarbonate may be administered 1 and 3 hours after meals and at bedtime. Additional doses of antacids may be administered to relieve the pain that may occur between the regularly scheduled doses.

**For parenteral dosage forms only**

Commercially available parenteral solutions are generally hypertonic and require dilution.

Sodium bicarbonate solution may be administered intravenously or, following dilution to isotonicity (1.5%), subcutaneously.

For intravenous administration, suitable concentrations range from 1.5% (isotonic) to 8.4% (undiluted), depending on the clinical condition and requirements of the patient.

For subcutaneous administration, an isotonic solution (1.5%) of sodium bicarbonate may be prepared by diluting 1 mL of 8.4% sodium bicarbonate solution with 4.6 mL of sterile water for injection. However, it should be noted that absorption from subcutaneous administration is unpredictable. This route of administration is not generally recommended except in those cases where the intravenous route is not available.

Bicarbonate therapy should always be planned in a careful, controlled way, since the degree of response to a given dose is not precisely predictable. Ideally, sodium bicarbonate should always be given according to the results of measurement of arterial blood pH, carbon dioxide content of the plasma, and calculation of base deficit.

Excessive administration may induce hypokalemia and may predispose the patient to cardiac arrhythmias.

Too rapid administration of sodium bicarbonate may produce severe alkalosis, which may be accompanied by hyperirritability or tetany.

Overdosage and alkalosis may be avoided by giving repeated small doses. Periodic monitoring is recommended.

Rapid injection (10 mL per minute) of hypertonic sodium bicarbonate solutions may produce hypernatremia, a decrease in cerebrospinal fluid pressure, and possible intracranial hemorrhage, especially in neonates and children under 2 years of age. No more than 8 mEq per kg of body weight per day of a 4.2% solution should be administered.

In cardiac arrest emergencies, the risk of rapid infusion may be necessary because of the fatality risk due to acidosis.

Adequate alveolar ventilation must be ensured following sodium bicarbonate administration during cardiac arrest, to allow for the continued excretion of the carbon dioxide released. This is important for the control of arterial pH.

# Oral Dosage Forms

## EFFERVESCENT SODIUM BICARBONATE

### Usual adult and adolescent dose

Antacid—
   Oral, 3.9 to 10 grams in a glass of cold water after meals.
   Note: Patients 60 years of age and over—Oral, 1.9 to 3.9 grams after meals.

### Usual adult and adolescent prescribing limits

Oral, 19.5 grams per day.

### Usual pediatric dose

Antacid—
   Children up to 6 years of age: Dosage must be individualized by physician.
   Children 6 to 12 years of age: Oral, 1 to 1.9 grams in a glass of cold water after meals.

### Strength(s) usually available

U.S.—
   780 mg of sodium bicarbonate and 1.82 grams of sodium citrate per teaspoonful (3.9 grams) (OTC) [*Citrocarbonate*].
Canada—
   780 mg of sodium bicarbonate and 1.82 grams of sodium citrate per teaspoonful (3.9 grams) (OTC) [*Citrocarbonate*].

### Packaging and storage

Store below 40 °C (104 °F), preferably between 15 and 30 °C (59 and 86 °F), in a tight container, unless otherwise specified by manufacturer.

### Note

Alert patients on sodium-restricted diet. Product contains 30.46 mEq (700.6 mg) of sodium per 3.9 grams.

## SODIUM BICARBONATE ORAL POWDER USP

### Usual adult and adolescent dose

Antacid—
   Oral, ½ teaspoonful in a glass of water every two hours, the dose being adjusted as needed.
Urinary alkalizer—
   Oral, 1 teaspoonful in a glass of water every four hours, the dose being adjusted as needed.

### Usual adult prescribing limits

Up to 60 years of age—Up to 4 teaspoonfuls daily.

### Usual pediatric dose

Dosage has not been established.

### Size(s) usually available

U.S.—
   120 grams (OTC) [*Arm and Hammer Pure Baking Soda;* GENERIC].
   240 grams (OTC) [*Arm and Hammer Pure Baking Soda;* GENERIC].
   480 grams (OTC) [*Arm and Hammer Pure Baking Soda;* GENERIC].
   2400 grams (OTC) [*Arm and Hammer Pure Baking Soda;* GENERIC].
Canada—
   Information not available [GENERIC].

Note: Each ½ teaspoonful contains 20.9 mEq (476 mg) of sodium.

### Packaging and storage

Store below 40 °C (104 °F), preferably between 15 and 30 °C (59 and 86 °F), unless otherwise specified by manufacturer. Store in a well-closed container.

### Note

Alert patients on sodium-restricted diet. Products contain 41.8 mEq (952 mg) of sodium per teaspoonful.

## SODIUM BICARBONATE TABLETS USP

### Usual adult and adolescent dose

Antacid—
   Oral, 325 mg to 2 grams one to four times a day.
Urinary alkalizer—
   Oral, 4 grams initially, then 1 to 2 grams every four hours.

### Usual adult prescribing limits

Up to 16 grams daily.

### Usual pediatric dose

Antacid—
   Children up to 6 years of age: Dosage has not been established.
   Children 6 to 12 years of age: Oral, 520 mg; may be repeated once in thirty minutes.
Urinary alkalizer—
   Oral, 1 to 10 mEq (23 to 230 mg) per kg of body weight per day, the dose being adjusted as needed.

### Strength(s) usually available

U.S.—
   325 mg (OTC) [*Soda Mint;* GENERIC].
   520 mg (OTC) [*Bell/ans*].
   650 mg (OTC) [GENERIC].
Canada—
   500 mg (OTC) [GENERIC].

### Packaging and storage

Store below 40 °C (104 °F), preferably between 15 and 30 °C (59 and 86 °F), unless otherwise specified by manufacturer. Store in a well-closed container.

### Note

Alert patients on sodium-restricted diet. Products contain sodium as follows: 325 mg tablets (3.9 mEq), 520 mg tablets (6.2 mEq), and 650 mg tablets (7.7 mEq).

# Parenteral Dosage Forms

## SODIUM BICARBONATE INJECTION USP

### Usual adult and adolescent dose

Systemic alkalizer—
   In cardiac arrest: Intravenous, initially 1 mEq per kg of body weight; 0.5 mEq per kg of body weight may be repeated every ten minutes of continued arrest.
   In less urgent forms of metabolic acidosis: Intravenous infusion, 2 to 5 mEq per kg of body weight, administered over a period of four to eight hours.
   Note: Frequency of administration and the size of the dose may be reduced after severe symptoms have abated.
Urinary alkalizer—
   Intravenous, 2 to 5 mEq per kg of body weight, administered over a period of four to eight hours.

**Usual pediatric dose**

Systemic alkalizer—

In cardiac arrest: Intravenous, 1 mEq per kg of body weight initially, then 0.5 mEq per kg of body weight every ten minutes of continued arrest.

In less urgent forms of metabolic acidosis: Older children— See *Usual adult and adolescent dose.*

Urinary alkalizer—

See *Usual adult and adolescent dose.*

**Strength(s) usually available**

U.S.—

4.2% (Rx) [GENERIC].

5% (Rx) [GENERIC].

7.5% (Rx) [GENERIC].

8.4% (Rx) [GENERIC].

Canada—

4.2% (Rx) [GENERIC].

7.5% (Rx) [GENERIC].

8.4% (Rx) [GENERIC].

Note:

| Concentration per mL of Aqueous Solution | Sodium Content (mg/mL) |
|---|---|
| 4% (0.48 mEq) | 11 |
| 4.2% (0.5 mEq) | 11.5 |
| 5% (0.595 mEq) | 13.8 |
| 7.5% (0.892 mEq) | 20.5 |
| 8.4% (1 mEq) | 23 |

**Packaging and storage**

Store below 40 °C (104 °F), preferably between 15 and 30 °C (59 and 86 °F), unless otherwise specified by manufacturer. Protect from freezing.

**Preparation of dosage form**

Sterile water for injection, sodium chloride injection, dextrose injection (5%), or other standard electrolyte solutions may be used as diluents. For dilution and preparation of injection, see manufacturer's package insert.

**Stability**

A sterile 7.5% solution of sodium bicarbonate in polypropylene syringes may remain stable for up to 100 days if refrigerated (2 to 8 °C), or up to 45 days at room temperature.

Stability may be increased by refrigerating the sodium bicarbonate injection and the syringes before preparation, rinsing the syringes twice with refrigerated sterile water for injection, minimizing the contact of the solution with air by expelling the air from the syringes, and taping the plunger in place to minimize its movement caused by escaping carbon dioxide.

Solutions of sodium bicarbonate should not be boiled or heated. When heated, it may decompose and be converted to the carbonate.

Haze formation or precipitation may result when sodium bicarbonate is added to infusion solution containing calcium.

Do not use the injection if it contains a precipitate.

**Incompatibilities**

Sodium bicarbonate is incompatible with acids, acidic salts, many alkaloidal salts, aspirin, atropine, bismuth salicylate, calcium-containing solutions, dobutamine, dopamine hydrochloride, epinephrine, isoproterenol hydrochloride, morphine sulfate, norepinephrine bitartrate, regular insulin, and tubocurarine chloride.

Revised: 02/03/92

Interim revision: 08/10/94

## SODIUM BICARBONATE–CONTAINING COMBINATIONS—

Acetaminophen, Sodium Bicarbonate, and Citric Acid (Systemic)

Alumina, Magnesium Carbonate, and Sodium Bicarbonate (Oral-Local)— See *Antacids (Oral-Local)*

Alumina, Magnesium Trisilicate, and Sodium Bicarbonate (Oral-Local)— See *Antacids (Oral-Local)*

Aspirin, Sodium Bicarbonate, and Citric Acid (Systemic)

Magnesium Carbonate and Sodium Bicarbonate (Oral-Local)—See *Antacids (Oral-Local)*

Potassium Bitartrate and Sodium Bicarbonate (Rectal-Local)—See *Laxatives (Local)*

---

# SODIUM CHLORIDE    Parenteral-Local

VA CLASSIFICATION (Primary): GU600

Note: For a listing of dosage forms and brand names by country availability, see *Dosage Forms* section(s). For a listing of brand names for the articles in this monograph, refer to the General Index.

## Category

Abortifacient.

## Indications

**Accepted**

Abortion, elective—Sodium chloride 20% solution is used by transabdominal intra-amniotic instillation for aborting second-trimester pregnancy (between the 16th and 24th weeks of gestation as calculated from the first day of the last normal menstrual period). The use of hypertonic saline for abortion has generally been replaced by dilation and evacuation, though it may be useful in selected patients. Use before the 16th week is difficult because of the small amount of amniotic fluid present and results in an increased failure rate. Hypertonic saline is sometimes used in combination with oxytocin or prostaglandins.

## Pharmacology/Pharmacokinetics

**Physicochemical characteristics**

Molecular weight—58.44.

**Mechanism of action/Effect**

The exact mechanism of action is not known but may be related to damage of decidual cells by hypertonic sodium chloride and subsequent release of prostaglandins, which induce uterine contractions. Sodium chloride 20% injection induces fetal death.

**Distribution**

Most of a dose is concentrated in the decidua and fetal part of the placenta; some diffuses into maternal blood. Systemic absorption is usually minimal with proper administration.

**Onset of action**

Labor usually starts within 12 to 24 hours.

**Time to peak effect**

The mean abortion time with hypertonic saline is about 36 hours.

## Precautions to Consider

**Adolescents**

No published adolescent-specific information is available on the use of intra-amniotic sodium chloride in adolescent females. However, no adolescent-specific problems have been documented to date.

**Drug interactions and/or related problems**

The following drug interactions and/or related problems have been selected on the basis of their potential clinical significance (possible mechanism in parentheses where appropriate)—not necessarily inclusive (» = major clinical significance):

» Oxytocin or other oxytocics

(concurrent use with hypertonic saline may result in uterine hypertonus, possibly causing uterine rupture or cervical laceration, especially in the absence of adequate cervical dilation; although combinations are sometimes used for therapeutic advantage, when used concurrently patient should be closely monitored)

**Laboratory value alterations**

The following have been selected on the basis of their potential clinical significance (possible effect in parentheses where appropriate)—not necessarily inclusive (» = major clinical significance):

With physiology/laboratory test values

Fibrin concentrations and

Plasma volume and

Thrombin, prothrombin, and partial thromboplastin times

(may be increased within the first 12 to 24 hours following administration of hypertonic saline, although risk of hemorrhage is usually low)

Fibrinogen and factor V and VIII concentrations and
Hematocrit concentrations and
Platelet counts
> (may be decreased, although risk of hemorrhage is usually low)

Sodium concentrations, serum
> (may be increased; risk of sudden severe hypernatremia with inadvertent intravascular administration)

### Medical considerations/Contraindications

The medical considerations/contraindications included here have been selected on the basis of their potential clinical significance (reasons given in parentheses where appropriate)—not necessarily inclusive (» = major clinical significance).

*Except under special circumstances, this medication should not be used when the following medical problems exist:*
» Absolute contraindications to labor
» Actively contracting or hypertonic uterus
> (increased intra-amniotic pressure may lead to necrosis of uterine musculature)
» Coagulation disorders
» Ruptured membranes

*Risk-benefit should be considered when the following medical problems exist:*
» Cardiovascular disease or
» Hypertension or
» Renal function impairment, severe
> (possibility of impaired clearance of sodium chloride)

Cervical stenosis or
Uterine fibroids
> (risk of uterine rupture)
» Epilepsy
» Relative contraindications to labor

Sensitivity to sodium chloride

### Patient monitoring

The following may be especially important in patient monitoring (other tests may be warranted in some patients, depending on condition; » = major clinical significance):

Contractions, frequency, duration, and force of and
Temperature, pulse, and blood pressure determinations and
Uterine tone, resting
> (recommended at frequent intervals during labor and delivery)

Examination of fluid samples from the catheter
> (recommended at frequent intervals to confirm proper placement in amniotic cavity)

Vaginal examination
> (recommended post-delivery to check for signs of cervical trauma)

## Side/Adverse Effects

Note: Concurrent administration of oxytocin may cause uterine hypertonicity with spasm and tetanic contraction, which can lead to posterior cervical perforations, cervical lacerations, uterine rupture, and hemorrhage.

> Intra-amniotic administration of sodium chloride 20% injection has been associated with fever, flushing, pulmonary embolism, pneumonia, infection at the injection site, cortical necrosis of the kidneys, disseminated intravascular coagulation, and death.

> Administration of excessive quantities overdistends the amniotic cavity and may lead to ascites, uterine necrosis, severe electrolyte disturbances, hypervolemia, and circulatory failure.

The following side/adverse effects have been selected on the basis of their potential clinical significance (possible cause in parentheses where appropriate)—not necessarily inclusive:

### Those indicating need for medical attention
Incidence less frequent
*Inadvertent intravascular, myometrial, or intraperitoneal administration* (burning pain in lower abdomen; confusion; feeling of heat; feeling of warmth in lips and tongue; severe headache; nervousness; numbness of the fingertips; pain in lower back, pelvis, or stomach; ringing in the ears; sudden thirst or salty taste)
> Note: *Inadvertent intravascular, myometrial, or intraperitoneal administration* may lead to myometrial necrosis, hypernatremia, cortical necrosis of the kidneys, cerebral blood clots, cardiovascular collapse, and seizures. Instillation should be discontinued immediately.

### Those indicating need for medical attention only if they continue or are bothersome
Incidence more frequent
*Fever; flushing or redness of face*

### Those indicating possible postabortion complications and the need for medical attention if they occur after medication is discontinued
*Endometritis* (chills; shivering; fever; foul-smelling vaginal discharge; pain in lower abdomen); *increase in uterine bleeding*

## Patient Consultation

As an aid to patient consultation, refer to *Advice for the Patient, Sodium Chloride (Intra-amniotic)*.

In providing consultation, consider emphasizing the following selected information (» = major clinical significance):

### Before using this medication
» Conditions affecting use, especially:
> Sensitivity to sodium chloride
> Other medical problems, especially renal function impairment or sickle cell disease

### Proper use of this medication
Drinking at least 2 liters of fluids the day of the procedure
» Proper dosing

### Side/adverse effects
Signs of potential side effects, especially inadvertent intravascular, myometrial, or intraperitoneal administration; endometritis; and electrolyte imbalance

## General Dosing Information

It is recommended that intra-amniotic sodium chloride be administered in a hospital setting.

To aid sodium excretion, it is recommended that patients drink at least 2 liters of fluids on the day that hypertonic saline is to be administered.

Sodium Chloride Injection USP 20% should not be administered if a bloody amniotic tap is obtained.

If sodium chloride is ineffective, it is recommended that alternative methods such as oxytocin not be used until the uterus has stopped contracting.

It is recommended that sedatives or general anesthetics not be administered to patients receiving hypertonic saline, so that they may be able to notice and report adverse reactions.

Intravenous administration of a dilute solution of oxytocin is sometimes used to shorten the induction-to-abortion time (to about 22 hours) or to induce abortion when hypertonic saline has failed to do so within 48 hours. Use of oxytocin to cause abortion of the placenta after delivery is controversial since some clinicians believe that it hinders expulsion of the placenta.

## Parenteral Dosage Forms

### SODIUM CHLORIDE INJECTION USP

**Usual adult and adolescent dose**
Abortion—
> Intra-amniotic, after transabdominal tap of the amniotic sac, a 20% solution in a volume equal to the volume of amniotic fluid removed, up to a maximum of 200 to 250 mL, administered slowly over a period of twenty to thirty minutes (some clinicians prefer an administration interval of five to ten minutes to reduce the risk of needle displacement) while observing for adverse reactions.

Note: The instillation may be repeated 48 hours after the initial dose if the abortion process is not established or clinically imminent, provided the membranes are still intact.

**Strength(s) usually available**
U.S.—
> 20% (Rx) [GENERIC].
Canada—
> 20% (Rx) [GENERIC].

**Packaging and storage**
Store below 40 °C (104 °F), preferably between 15 and 30 °C (59 and 86 °F), unless otherwise specified by manufacturer. Protect from freezing.

Revised: 07/28/93
Interim revision: 06/21/94

# SODIUM CHROMATE CR 51   Systemic

INN: Sodium Chromate ($^{51}$Cr)

VA CLASSIFICATION (Primary): DX201

Note: For a listing of dosage forms and brand names by country availability, see *Dosage Forms* section(s). For a listing of brand names for the articles in this monograph, refer to the General Index.

## Category

Diagnostic aid, radioactive (red blood cell disease; gastrointestinal bleeding; platelet survival).

## Indications

Note: Bracketed information in the *Indications* section refers to uses that are not included in U.S. product labeling.

**Accepted**

Red blood cells, labeling of—

Sodium chromate Cr 51 is indicated for *in vitro* labeling of autologous red blood cells. Cr 51–labeled red blood cells are indicated for the following diagnostic studies:

Red blood cell volume or mass determinations: To determine and evaluate red blood cell volume or mass in the differential diagnosis and follow-up of patients with polycythemia.

Red blood cell survival time determinations and

Red blood cell sequestration studies: To study the rate of disappearance of red blood cells from the circulation in cases of splenic sequestration accompanying such diseases as hereditary spherocytosis, acquired hemolytic anemia, or hemolytic anemia secondary to lymphoma or leukemia. These data may be helpful in deciding the need for splenectomy.

Bleeding, gastrointestinal (diagnosis): To evaluate patients suspected of gastrointestinal bleeding, to quantify the amount of blood loss.

[Platelets, labeling of]—

Sodium chromate Cr 51 is used for the labeling of autologous platelets to be used for the following study:

[Platelet survival studies]: To determine platelet survival time and sites of platelet destruction and/or sequestration in the evaluation of patients with thrombocytopenia.

## Physical Properties

**Nuclear data**

| Radionuclide (half-life) | Mode of decay | Principal photon emissions (keV) | Mean number of emissions/ disintegration |
|---|---|---|---|
| Cr 51 (27.7 days) | Electron capture | Gamma (320) | 0.1 |

## Pharmacology/Pharmacokinetics

**Mechanism of action/Effect**

*In vitro*, the hexavalent radioactive chromium Cr 51 readily penetrates the erythrocyte and binds to hemoglobin. Unbound chromium Cr 51 is reduced to the trivalent state by the addition of a reducing agent, such as ascorbic acid, so no further binding occurs *in vivo*. Unbound chromium Cr 51 can be removed by cell washing with isotonic saline. When the chromium Cr 51–labeled cells are injected, the Cr 51 is slowly eluted from the cells in the circulation at a rate of 1% per day. The labeled cells eventually undergo destruction in the reticuloendothelial tissues mainly in the spleen, from which the deposited radioactivity is again slowly eluted. After intravenous injection of the labeled red blood cells, the trivalent state of chromium Cr 51 is maintained until the labeled red blood cells are sequestered by the spleen, at which time the chromium Cr 51 is released to the plasma. Samples of the patient's blood are obtained and measured in a scintillation well counter for red blood cell volume and survival time determinations. External counting with scintillation probes is used to evaluate relative splenic and hepatic sequestration. To determine actual gastrointestinal bleeding, stool is collected and measurements of the amount of radioactivity in the stool are performed.

**Half-life**

Normal labeled red blood cells survival half-time—25 to 35 days.

Note: The apparent short survival time, as compared to the 120-day true life span of red blood cells, is due to the elution of chromium from the cells and to cell damage that probably occurs during blood withdrawal and labeling.

**Radiation dosimetry**

| | Estimated absorbed radiation dose*† | | | |
|---|---|---|---|---|
| | Cr 51-labeled red blood cells | | Cr 51-labeled platelets | |
| Organ | mGy/MBq | rad/mCi | mGy/MBq | rad/mCi |
| Spleen | 1.6 | 5.92 | 2.6 | 9.63 |
| Heart | 0.51 | 1.89 | 0.096 | 0.36 |
| Lungs | 0.32 | 1.18 | 0.072 | 0.27 |
| Liver | 0.24 | 0.89 | 0.3 | 1.11 |
| Kidneys | 0.22 | 0.81 | 0.11 | 0.41 |
| Adrenals | 0.22 | 0.81 | 0.11 | 0.41 |
| Pancreas | 0.19 | 0.70 | 0.18 | 0.67 |
| Red marrow | 0.14 | 0.52 | 0.19 | 0.7 |
| Stomach wall | 0.14 | 0.52 | 0.096 | 0.36 |
| Thyroid | 0.12 | 0.44 | 0.022 | 0.081 |
| Bone surfaces | 0.11 | 0.41 | 0.09 | 0.33 |
| Breast | 0.099 | 0.37 | 0.03 | 0.11 |
| Small intestine | 0.095 | 0.35 | 0.044 | 0.16 |
| Large intestine (upper) | 0.094 | 0.35 | 0.045 | 0.17 |
| Uterus | 0.085 | 0.31 | 0.028 | 0.1 |
| Bladder wall | 0.075 | 0.28 | 0.018 | 0.067 |
| Ovaries | 0.082 | 0.30 | 0.032 | 0.12 |
| Large intestine (lower) | 0.081 | 0.30 | 0.032 | 0.12 |
| Testes | 0.063 | 0.23 | 0.013 | 0.048 |
| Other tissues | 0.085 | 0.31 | 0.034 | 0.13 |

| | Effective dose* | | | |
|---|---|---|---|---|
| | Cr 51-labeled red blood cells | | Cr 51-labeled platelets | |
| Radionuclide | mSv/MBq | rem/mCi | mSv/MBq | rem/mCi |
| Cr 51 | 0.26 | 0.96 | 0.24 | 0.89 |

*For adults; intravenous injection. Data based on the International Commission on Radiological Protection (ICRP) Publication 53—Radiation dose to patients from radiopharmaceuticals.

**Elimination**

Renal (unbound/released trivalent chromium Cr 51) and fecal (less than 1% eliminated in the feces of normal patients).

## Precautions to Consider

**Carcinogenicity/Mutagenicity**

Long-term animal studies to evaluate carcinogenic or mutagenic potential of sodium chromate Cr 51 have not been performed.

**Pregnancy/Reproduction**

Pregnancy—Studies have not been done in humans with sodium chromate Cr 51. The possibility of pregnancy should be assessed in women of child-bearing potential. Clinical situations exist where the benefit to the patient and fetus, based on information derived from radiopharmaceutical use, outweighs the risks from radiation exposure to the fetus. In these situations, the physician should use discretion and reduce the radiopharmaceutical dose to the lowest possible amount.

Studies have not been done in animals.

FDA Pregnancy Category C.

**Breast-feeding**

Sodium chromate Cr 51 is distributed into breast milk. Because of the potential risk to the infant from radiation exposure, temporary discontinuation of nursing is recommended for a length of time that may be assessed by measuring the activity in breast milk and estimating the radiation exposure to the infant.

**Pediatrics**

Although sodium chromate Cr 51 is used in children, there have been no specific studies evaluating safety and efficacy of sodium chromate Cr 51 in children. When this radiopharmaceutical is used in children, the diagnostic benefit should be judged to outweigh the potential risk of radiation.

**Geriatrics**

Appropriate studies on the relationship of age to the effects of sodium chromate Cr 51 have not been performed in the geriatric population.

However, no geriatrics-specific problems have been documented to date.

**Drug interactions and/or related problems**
See *Diagnostic interference.*

**Diagnostic interference**
The following have been selected on the basis of their potential clinical significance (possible effect in parentheses where appropriate)—not necessarily inclusive (» = major clinical significance):

With results of *this* test
  Stannous pyrophosphate
    (red blood cell labeling may be inhibited in double tracer red blood cell survival studies by the presence of stannous pyrophosphate used in the labeling of Tc 99m; washing red blood cells before labeling with chromium Cr 51 is recommended to avoid this effect)

## Side/Adverse Effects

Currently, there are no known side/adverse effects associated with the use of sodium chromate Cr 51 as a diagnostic aid.

## Patient Consultation

As an aid to patient consultation, refer to *Advice for the Patient, Radiopharmaceuticals (Diagnostic).*

In providing consultation, consider emphasizing the following selected information (» = major clinical significance):

**Description of use**
  Action in the body: Distribution in body of injected radioactive red blood cells same as that of normal red blood cells
  Radioactivity in blood or stool samples is measured
  Small amounts of radioactivity used in diagnosis; radiation exposure is low and considered safe

**Before having this test**
» Conditions affecting use, especially:
    Pregnancy—Risk to fetus from radiation exposure as opposed to benefit derived from use should be considered
    Breast-feeding—Distributed into breast milk; temporary discontinuation of nursing recommended because of risk to infant from radiation exposure
    Use in children—Risk of radiation exposure as opposed to benefit derived from use should be considered

**Preparation for this test**
  Special preparatory instructions may apply; patient should inquire in advance

**Precautions after having this test**
  No special precautions

## General Dosing Information

Radiopharmaceuticals are to be administered only by or under the supervision of physicians who have had extensive training in the safe use and handling of radioactive materials and who are authorized by the Nuclear Regulatory Commission (NRC) or the appropriate Agreement State agency, if required, or, outside the U.S., the appropriate authority.

The possibility of contamination of labeled red blood cells necessitates the use of sterile techniques for the collection, labeling, rinsing, suspending, and injection of labeled red blood cells.

Extreme care must be taken in blood withdrawal and labeling procedures to ensure that red blood cells are not damaged. Damaged labeled red blood cells will be rapidly sequestered by reticuloendothelial cells of spleen and liver, resulting in erroneous red cell volume and survival determinations.

Manufacturer's package insert or other appropriate literature should be consulted for specific method of labeling red blood cells.

**Safety considerations for handling this radiopharmaceutical**
Improper handling of this radiopharmaceutical may cause radioactive contamination. Guidelines for handling radioactive material have been prepared by scientific, professional, state, federal, and international bodies and are available to the specially qualified and authorized users who have access to radiopharmaceuticals.

## Parenteral Dosage Forms

Note: Bracketed uses in the *Dosage Forms* section refer to categories of use and/or indications that are not included in U.S. product labeling.

### SODIUM CHROMATE Cr 51 INJECTION USP

**Usual adult and adolescent administered activity**
Red blood cell dynamics—
  Volume or mass determinations:
    Intravenous, 0.37 to 1.11 megabecquerels (0.01 to 0.03 millicurie).
  Survival time determinations:
    Intravenous, 5.55 megabecquerels (0.15 millicurie).
  Gastrointestinal blood loss:
    Intravenous, 7.4 megabecquerels (0.2 millicurie).
[Platelet survival studies]—
    Intravenous, 0.185 to 0.555 megabecquerel (5 to 15 microcuries).

**Usual pediatric administered activity**
Dosage must be individualized by physician.

**Usual geriatric administered activity**
See *Usual adult and adolescent administered activity.*

**Strength(s) usually available**
U.S.—
    3.7 megabecquerels (0.1 millicurie) per mL at time of calibration, having a specific activity of no less than 370 megabecquerels (10 millicuries) per mg of sodium chromate at time of use (Rx) [GENERIC].
    9.25 megabecquerels (0.25 millicurie) per 1.25-mL vial at time of calibration, having a specific activity of no less than 370 megabecquerels (10 millicuries) per mg of sodium chromate at time of use (Rx) [*Chromitope*].
    37 megabecquerels (1 millicurie) per 5-mL vial at time of calibration, having a specific activity of no less than 370 megabecquerels (10 millicuries) per mg of sodium chromate at time of use (Rx) [*Chromitope*].
Canada—
    1.85 to 74 megabecquerels (0.05 to 2 millicuries) per mL (Rx) [GENERIC].

**Packaging and storage**
Store below 30 °C (86 °F), preferably between 15 and 30 °C (59 and 86 °F), unless otherwise specified by manufacturer.

**Note**
Caution—Radioactive material.

## Selected Bibliography

Sisson JC. Red blood cell survival including red blood cell sequestration. In: Carey JE, Kline RC, Keyes JW, editors. Manual of nuclear medicine procedures. 4th ed. Boca Raton, FL: CRC Press, 1983: 134-6.
International Committee for Standardization in Haematology. Recommended methods for measurement of red-cell and plasma volumes. J Nucl Med 1980; 21: 793-800.

Revised: 04/30/96

---

### SODIUM CITRATE AND CITRIC ACID—See *Citrates (Systemic)*

---

# SODIUM FLUORIDE   Systemic

VA CLASSIFICATION (Primary): TN407

Note: For a listing of dosage forms and brand names by country availability, see *Dosage Forms* section(s). For a listing of brand names for the articles in this monograph, refer to the General Index.

## Category

Dental caries prophylactic; nutritional supplement (mineral).

## Indications

**Accepted**
Dental caries (prophylaxis)—Sodium fluoride is indicated as a dietary supplement for prevention of dental caries in children in those areas where

the level of naturally occurring fluoride in the drinking water is inadequate. In optimally fluoridated communities, sodium fluoride supplementation may be necessary in infants that are totally breast-fed or receive ready-to-use formulas or in children consuming nonfluoridated bottled water rather than tap water. Sodium fluoride supplementation may also be indicated in those situations where home water filtration systems remove fluoride. This usually occurs with reverse osmosis or distillation units, but not with carbon charcoal filters.

Evidence that oral systemic fluoride supplements reduce dental caries in adults is lacking.

Note: Sodium fluoride has been used to treat osteoporosis and otospongiosis in adults; however, its use is controversial and further studies are needed. The doses used in osteoporosis and otospongiosis have potential for toxicity, including skeletal fluorosis, osteomalacia, widening of unmineralized osteoid seams, and upper gastrointestinal ulceration.

## Pharmacology/Pharmacokinetics

### Physicochemical characteristics
Molecular weight—41.99.

### Mechanism of action/Effect
Fluoride ion becomes incorporated into and stabilizes the apatite crystal of bone and teeth. Fluoride acts primarily to promote remineralization of decalcified enamel and may interfere with growth and development of dental plaque bacteria. Deposition of fluoride ion in the enamel surface of teeth increases resistance to acid and to development of caries.

### Absorption
Fluorides in solution or in the form of rapidly soluble salts are readily and almost completely absorbed from the gastrointestinal tract.

### Storage
In bone and developing teeth.

### Time to peak serum concentration
30 to 60 minutes.

### Elimination
Primarily renal (approximately 50%), with small amounts in feces and sweat.

## Precautions to Consider

### Carcinogenicity
Fluoride in the concentrations shown to be effective against tooth decay has not been shown to cause cancer in individuals who receive fluoride over prolonged periods.

### Pregnancy/Reproduction
Problems in humans have not been documented with intake of normal daily recommended amounts. Fluoride readily crosses the placenta.
There is conflicting evidence as to whether administration of fluoride supplements to women during pregnancy will help prevent caries in the child.

### Breast-feeding
Problems in humans have not been documented with intake of normal daily recommended amounts. Trace amounts of fluoride are distributed into breast milk, although the concentration is not high enough to provide benefits to the infant.

### Pediatrics
Problems in pediatrics have not been documented with intake of normal daily recommended amounts. Chronic overdose may cause fluorosis of the teeth (if given during the period of tooth-enamel formation) and osseous changes.

### Geriatrics
Problems in geriatrics have not been documented with intake of normal daily recommended amounts. Elderly patients are more likely to have age-related renal failure, which may require caution if patients are receiving large doses for osteoporosis or otospongiosis. The elderly are also more likely to develop stress fractures, gastrointestinal ulceration, and arthralgia from large doses of sodium fluoride.

### Dental
Excessive doses of sodium fluoride may result in fluorosis of teeth if taken during tooth formation years.

### Drug interactions and/or related problems
The following drug interactions and/or related problems have been selected on the basis of their potential clinical significance (possible

mechanism in parentheses where appropriate)—not necessarily inclusive (» = major clinical significance):

Note: Combinations containing any of the following, depending on the amount present, may also interact with this medication.

Aluminum hydroxide
(may decrease absorption and increase fecal excretion of fluoride; aluminium hydroxide–containing medications should be taken 2 hours before or after sodium fluoride)

Calcium supplements
(concurrent use with sodium fluoride may cause the calcium ions to complex with fluoride and inhibit absorption of both fluoride and calcium; if sodium fluoride is used with calcium supplements to treat osteoporosis, a 1- to 2-hour interval should elapse between doses of the two)

### Laboratory value alterations
The following have been selected on the basis of their potential clinical significance (possible effect in parentheses where appropriate)—not necessarily inclusive (» = major clinical significance):

With diagnostic test results
Alkaline phosphatase concentrations, serum
(results may be elevated)
Aspartate aminotransferase (AST [SGOT]) concentrations, serum
(may be falsely increased)

### Medical considerations/Contraindications
The medical considerations/contraindications included here have been selected on the basis of their potential clinical significance (reasons given in parentheses where appropriate)—not necessarily inclusive (» = major clinical significance).

*Except under special circumstances, this medication should not be used when the following medical conditions exist:*
Arthralgia or
Gastrointestinal ulceration
(conditions may be exacerbated, especially with high doses)
Renal insufficiency, severe
(condition may be exacerbated; may lead to higher blood levels of fluoride due to a decrease in excretion of fluoride; dosage reduction may be necessary)

*Risk-benefit should be considered when the following medical problems exist:*
High dental fluorosis, or prevalence in other members of the immediate community

### Patient monitoring
The following may be especially important in patient monitoring (other tests may be warranted in some patients, depending on condition; » = major clinical significance):
Dental examination
(recommended once or twice a year in most patients, and more frequently in those highly prone to developing caries)

## Side/Adverse Effects
The following side/adverse effects have been selected on the basis of their potential clinical significance (possible signs and symptoms in parentheses where appropriate)—not necessarily inclusive:

**Those indicating need for medical attention**
Incidence rare
*Ulceration of oral mucous membranes* (sores in mouth and on lips)

## Overdose
For specific information on the agents used in the management of fluoride overdose, see
• *Calcium Supplements (Systemic)* monograph.

For more information on the management of overdose or unintentional ingestion **contact a Poison Control Center** (see *Poison Control Center Listing*).

### Clinical effects of overdose
Note: Stomach upset may occur with ingestion of 5 to 20 mg of sodium fluoride. The lethal dose is not known, but has been estimated as 5 to 10 grams of sodium fluoride in untreated adults and 5 mg of fluoride ion per kilogram of body weight in children.

Severe acute fluoride overdose can cause hypocalcemia and tetany and bone pain, especially in the feet and ankles, of uncertain cause; electrolyte disturbances and cardiac arrhythmias have been reported, progressing to cardiac failure or respiratory arrest in some cases.

Osseous changes, including skeletal fluorosis, osteomalacia, and osteosclerosis, may also result from excessive, chronic doses.

The following effects have been selected on the basis of their potential clinical significance (possible signs and symptoms in parentheses where appropriate)—not necessarily inclusive

Chronic effects (fluorosis and osteosclerosis)

> *Pain and aching of bones, stiffness, or white, brown, or black discoloration of teeth*—occur only during periods of tooth development in children

Acute effects

> *Black, tarry stools; bloody vomit; diarrhea; drowsiness; faintness; increased watering of mouth; nausea or vomiting; shallow breathing; stomach cramps or pain; tremors; unusual excitement; watery eyes; weakness*

### For treatment of acute overdose

Specific treatment—

Administration of intravenous dextrose.

Gastric lavage with calcium chloride or calcium hydroxide solution to precipitate fluoride.

Intravenous calcium gluconate if hypocalcemia occurs.

Monitoring—

Monitor respiration, blood pressure, and ECG.

Supportive care—

Maintenance of high urine output.

Patients in whom intentional overdose is confirmed or suspected should be referred for psychiatric consultation.

## Patient Consultation

As an aid to patient consultation, refer to *Advice for the Patient, Sodium Fluoride (Systemic)*.

In providing consultation, consider emphasizing the following selected information (» = major clinical significance):

### Importance of diet

Importance of proper nutrition; fluoride may be needed because of inadequate dietary intake

Dietary sources of fluoride; effects of processing

Recommended daily intake for fluoride

Remembering not to take more than recommended

### Before using this medication

» Conditions affecting use, especially:

Pregnancy—Fluoride crosses the placenta

Breast-feeding—Trace amount distributed into breast milk

Use in children—Chronic overdose may cause dental fluorosis and osseous changes

Use in the elderly—High doses used for osteoporosis or otospongiosis not recommended in elderly patients with arthralgia, gastrointestinal ulceration, or renal insufficiency

Dental—Excessive doses taken during tooth formation years may result in tooth fluorosis

### Proper use of this medication

» Importance of not using more medication than the amount prescribed

» Proper dosing

Missed dose: Taking as soon as possible; not taking if almost time for next dose; not doubling doses

*For individuals taking the chewable tablet dosage form*

Chewing or crushing tablets before swallowing

Advisability of taking at bedtime after brushing teeth; not eating or drinking for at least 15 minutes after taking

*For individuals taking the oral solution dosage form*

Proper use of the dropper bottle

» Avoiding use of glass with fluoride–containing solutions since fluoride etches glass

May be dropped directly into the mouth or mixed with cereal, fruit juice, or other food (except calcium-containing foods or beverages)

» Proper storage

### Precautions while using this medication

Checking with health care professional as soon as possible after moving to another geographic area to see if continued treatment at the same dosage is necessary, since fluoride levels of community drinking water vary; also checking if changing infant feeding habits, drinking water, or filtration

Not taking calcium supplements or aluminum hydroxide-containing products and sodium fluoride at the same time; use should be separated by 2 hours

» Informing health care professional if teeth show signs of mottling

### Side/adverse effects

Signs of potential side effects especially oral mucous membrane ulceration

## General Dosing Information

Optimal benefit of fluorides must be established on an individual basis, taking into consideration the fluoride content of the water supply when determining the dose. Some studies have found that systemic fluoride ingestion from toothpaste use in young children is significant.

The amount of fluoride from all sources should be taken into account when determining the therapeutic dose. For example, infant formulas made with fluoridated water provide a significant amount. Also, some schools in communities without water fluoridation have added up to 4.5 times the optimal fluoride level to the school's water supply to ensure that children receive adequate fluoride.

Use of fluoride supplements is generally not recommended when community drinking water contains more than 0.6 parts per million (ppm) of fluoride.

A fluoride level of approximately 1 ppm (0.6 to 1.2 ppm) in water is generally considered optimal for development of decay-resistant teeth without causing fluorosis, the actual value depending on the annual mean maximum daily temperature of the geographic area.

2.2 mg of sodium fluoride is equivalent to 1 mg of fluoride ion.

Since therapy with oral, systemic fluoride supplements is most effective on unerupted teeth, it is recommended that children receive oral fluoride supplementation until the age of 13 (or when the second molars have erupted) to provide maximum benefit to both deciduous and permanent teeth. Subsequent periodic topical application of fluoride for life may be advisable to prolong the cariostatic benefits, since beneficial effects, particularly in caries-prone individuals, appear to be lost a year or two after topical use is discontinued.

The recommended dose should not be exceeded, since prolonged overdosage may cause dental fluorosis in children and osseous changes in children and adults.

Mottling of tooth enamel (dental fluorosis) occurs with excessive ingestion of fluoride (e.g., continual use of drinking water containing greater than 2 ppm of fluoride) during the period of tooth development in children.

Stiffness (skeletal fluorosis) occurs with chronic ingestion of water containing 4 to 14 ppm of fluoride.

Generalized effects (renal damage, albuminuria, goiter) occur only after chronic ingestion of large amounts of fluoride over 10 to 20 years.

It is recommended that fluoride preparations (especially the chewable tablets) taken on a once-a-day basis be taken at bedtime after the teeth have been thoroughly brushed (to also provide some topical benefit from the fluoride).

Sodium fluoride (25 to 60 mg a day) may stabilize the progression of hearing loss in some patients with otospongiosis.

### Diet/Nutrition

Nausea (although rare with doses of fluoride taken for dental caries) may be reduced by taking sodium fluoride with or just after meals, provided that the foods do not contain calcium, since calcium may interfere with fluoride absorption.

The oral solution may be administered undiluted or mixed with cereal, fluids, or other food. However, absorption of sodium fluoride may be reduced when taken with calcium-rich foods or beverages.

Recommended dietary intakes for fluoride are defined differently worldwide.

For U.S.—

The Recommended Dietary Allowances (RDAs) for vitamins and minerals are determined by the Food and Nutrition Board of the National Research Council and are intended to provide adequate nutrition in most healthy persons under usual environmental stresses. In addition, a different designation may be used by the FDA for food and dietary supplement labeling purposes, as with Daily Value (DV). DVs replace the previous labeling terminology United States Recommended Daily Allowances (USRDAs).

For Canada—

Recommended Nutrient Intakes (RNIs) for vitamins, minerals, and protein are determined by Health and Welfare Canada and provide recommended amounts of a specific nutrient while minimizing the risk of chronic diseases.

There is no RDA or RNI established for fluoride. Daily recommended intakes for fluoride are generally defined as follows

Infants and children:

Birth to 3 years: 0.1 to 1.5 mg.

4 to 6 years: 1 to 2.5 mg.
7 to 10 years: 1.5 to 2.5 mg.
Adolescents and adults:

1.5 to 4 mg.

Sources of fluoride other than fluoridated drinking water include fish that are consumed with their bones and tea. Cooking foods in fluorinated water can increase their fluoride content as can cooking with Teflon- (a fluoride-containing polymer) coated utensils and pans. However, cooking foods in utensils and pans with an aluminum surface can decrease their fluoride content.

# Oral Dosage Forms

## SODIUM FLUORIDE LOZENGES

### Usual pediatric dose
Dental caries prophylactic or
Nutritional supplement—

Dosage of fluoride recommended by the American Dental Association, the American Academy of Pediatrics, and the American Academy of Pediatric Dentistry for communities where the level of fluoride in drinking water is 0.6 ppm or less

| Water Fluoride (ppm) | Age (yr) | Dose of Fluoride Ion (mg per day) |
|---|---|---|
| <0.3 | Birth to 0.5 | 0 |
|  | 0.5 to 3 | 0.25 |
|  | 3 to 6 | 0.5 |
|  | 6 to 16 | 1 |
| 0.3–0.6 | Birth to 3 | 0 |
|  | 3 to 6 | 0.25 |
|  | 6 to 16 | 0.5 |
| >0.6 | Birth to 16 | 0 |

Note: In Canada a different dosing schedule may be used. The Canadian Dental Association recommendations differ from that of the American Dental Association.

### Strength(s) usually available
U.S.—

2.2 mg (1 mg of fluoride ion) (Rx) [*Flura-Loz*].
Canada—

1.1 mg (OTC) [*Flozenges*].
2.2 mg (OTC) [*Flozenges*].

### Packaging and storage
Store below 40 °C (104 °F), preferably between 15 and 30 °C (59 and 86 °F), unless otherwise specified by manufacturer. Store in a tight container.

## SODIUM FLUORIDE ORAL SOLUTION USP

### Usual pediatric dose
See *Sodium Fluoride Lozenges.*

### Strength(s) usually available
U.S.—

0.275 mg (0.125 mg of fluoride ion) per drop (Rx) [*Karidium; Luride;* GENERIC].
0.44 mg (0.2 mg of fluoride ion) per mL (Rx) [*Phos-Flur*].
0.55 mg (0.25 mg of fluoride ion) per drop (Rx) [*Fluoritab; Flura-Drops*].
1.1 mg (0.5 mg of fluoride ion) per mL (Rx) [*Pediaflor* (alcohol less than 0.5%)].
Canada—

2 mg (0.905 mg of fluoride ion) per mL (OTC) [*PDF*].
2.2 mg (1 mg of fluoride ion) per 4 drops (Rx) [*Solu-Flur*].
2.21 mg (1 mg of fluoride ion) per 8 drops (0.5 mL) (OTC) [*Karidium*].
5.56 mg (1 mg of fluoride ion) per mL (OTC) [*Fluor-A-Day*].
6.9 mg (3.12 mg of fluoride ion) per mL (OTC) [*Fluorosol; Pedi-Dent;* GENERIC].

### Packaging and storage
Store below 40 °C (104 °F), preferably between 15 and 30 °C (59 and 86 °F), unless otherwise specified by manufacturer. Store in a tight, plastic container. Protect from freezing.

### Auxiliary labeling
• Keep out of reach of children.

### Note
To reduce the risk associated with accidental ingestion and overdosage, it is recommended that no more than 264 mg of sodium fluoride be dispensed at one time. The American Dental Association Council on Dental Therapeutics considers a limit of 300 mg acceptable when sodium fluoride is dispensed to children in prepackaged containers.

Since size of drop dispensed and strength vary among commercial preparations, always dispense the same brand for refills on a prescription.

## SODIUM FLUORIDE TABLETS USP

### Usual pediatric dose
See *Sodium Fluoride Lozenges.*

### Strength(s) usually available
U.S.—

1.1 mg (0.5 mg of fluoride ion) (Rx) [GENERIC].
2.2 mg (1 mg of fluoride ion) (Rx) [*Flura; Karidium;* GENERIC].
Canada—

2.2 mg (1 mg fluoride ion) (OTC) [*Fluorosol; Karidium;* GENERIC].

### Packaging and storage
Store below 40 °C (104 °F), preferably between 15 and 30 °C (59 and 86 °F), unless otherwise specified by manufacturer. Store in a tight container.

### Auxiliary labeling
• Keep out of reach of children.

### Note
To reduce the risk associated with accidental ingestion and overdosage, it is recommended that no more than 264 mg of sodium fluoride be dispensed at one time. The American Dental Association Council on Dental Therapeutics considers a limit of 300 mg acceptable when sodium fluoride is dispensed to children in prepackaged containers.

## SODIUM FLUORIDE CHEWABLE TABLETS USP

### Usual pediatric dose
See *Sodium Fluoride Lozenges.*

### Strength(s) usually available
U.S.—

0.55 mg (0.25 mg of fluoride ion) (Rx) [*Luride Lozi-Tabs*].
1.1 mg (0.5 mg of fluoride ion) (Rx) [*Fluoritab* (scored); *Fluorodex; Luride Lozi-Tabs; Pharmaflur 1.1;* GENERIC].
2.2 mg (1 mg of fluoride ion) (Rx) [*Fluoritab; Fluorodex; Karidium; Luride Lozi-Tabs; Luride-SF Lozi-Tabs; Pharmaflur; Pharmaflur df;* GENERIC].
Canada—

2.2 mg (1 mg of fluoride ion) (OTC) [*Fluor-A-Day; Fluoritabs; Pedi-Dent; Solu-Flur;* GENERIC].

### Packaging and storage
Store below 40 °C (104 °F), unless otherwise specified by manufacturer. Store in a tight container.

### Auxiliary labeling
• Keep out of reach of children.

### Note
To reduce the risk associated with accidental ingestion and overdosage, it is recommended that no more than 264 mg of sodium fluoride be dispensed at one time. The American Dental Association Council on Dental Therapeutics considers a limit of 300 mg acceptable when sodium fluoride is dispensed to children in prepackaged containers.

Revised: 07/17/92
Interim revision: 08/07/95

# SODIUM IODIDE   Systemic†

VA CLASSIFICATION (Primary/Secondary): TN499/HS852

Note: For a listing of dosage forms and brand names by country availability, see *Dosage Forms* section(s). For a listing of brand names for the articles in this monograph, refer to the General Index.

†Not commercially available in Canada.

## Category

Nutritional supplement (mineral); antihyperthyroid agent.

## Indications

Note: Bracketed information in the *Indications* section refers to uses that are not included in U.S. product labeling.

### Accepted

Iodine deficiency (prophylaxis and treatment)—Sodium iodide is indicated in the prevention and treatment of iodine deficiency, which may result from inadequate nutrition or intestinal malabsorption, but does not occur in healthy individuals receiving an adequate balanced diet. For prophylaxis of iodine deficiency, dietary improvement, rather than supplementation, is advisable. For treatment of iodine deficiency, supplementation is preferred. Due to the introduction of iodized salt, iodine deficiency in the U.S. is rare; however, it continues to be a problem worldwide.

Deficiency of iodine may lead to thyroid dysfunction, goiter, mental deficiency, hearing loss, and cretinism.

Some diets (e.g., reducing diets that drastically restrict food selection) may not supply minimum daily requirements of iodine. Supplementation may be necessary in patients receiving long-term total parenteral nutrition (TPN) or undergoing rapid weight loss or in those with malnutrition, because of inadequate dietary intake.

Recommended intakes for all vitamins and most minerals are increased during pregnancy. Many physicians recommend that pregnant women receive multivitamin and mineral supplements, especially those pregnant women who do not consume an adequate diet and those in high-risk categories (i.e., women carrying more than one fetus, heavy cigarette smokers, and alcohol and drug abusers). However, taking excessive amounts of multivitamin and mineral supplements may be harmful to the mother and/or fetus and should be avoided.

Maternal iodine deficiency before or during early pregnancy may lead to neurological damage and fetal hypothyroidism or cretinism in later pregnancy.

Recommended intakes for all vitamins and most minerals are increased during breast-feeding.

[Thyrotoxicosis crisis (treatment adjunct)]—Intravenous sodium iodide may be used as a treatment adjunct for thyrotoxicosis crisis.

## Pharmacology/Pharmacokinetics

### Physicochemical characteristics

Molecular weight—Elemental iodine: 126.9.
Sodium iodide: 149.89.

### Mechanism of action/Effect

Antihyperthyroid agent—In thyrotoxicosis crisis, sodium iodide produces rapid remission of symptoms by inhibiting the release of thyroid hormone into the circulation.

Nutritional supplement—Sodium iodide is oxidized to iodine, which is an essential component of the thyroid hormones, triiodothyronine ($T_3$) and thyroxin ($T_4$). These hormones are among the factors that regulate energy transformation, growth, reproduction, neuromuscular function, and cellular metabolism.

### Absorption

Oral iodine is rapidly and completely absorbed from the gastrointestinal tract. It is also absorbed from the skin and lungs. Iodine is recycled from inactive iodothyronines.

### Protein binding

Totally protein bound.

### Storage

Iodine is stored primarily in the thyroid gland and muscle, but also in the skin, skeleton, mammary glands, and hair.

### Elimination

Iodine is eliminated via the kidneys, liver, skin, lungs, and intestine.

## Precautions to Consider

### Pregnancy/Reproduction

Pregnancy—Problems in humans have not been documented with intake of normal daily recommended amounts. Sodium iodide crosses the placenta; use of high doses during pregnancy may result in abnormal thyroid function and/or goiter in the infant.

### Breast-feeding

Problems in humans have not been documented with intake of normal daily recommended amounts. Sodium iodide is distributed into breast milk; excessive iodide use by nursing mothers may cause skin rash and thyroid suppression in the infant.

### Pediatrics

Problems in pediatrics have not been documented with intake of normal daily recommended amounts. Iodides may cause skin rash and thyroid suppression in infants.

### Geriatrics

Problems in geriatrics have not been documented with intake of normal daily recommended amounts.

### Dental

Oral and intravenous iodine may cause salivary gland swelling or tenderness, burning of mouth or throat, metallic taste, soreness of teeth and gums, and unusual increase in salivation.

### Drug interactions and/or related problems

The following drug interactions and/or related problems have been selected on the basis of their potential clinical significance (possible mechanism in parentheses where appropriate)—not necessarily inclusive (» = major clinical significance):

Note: Combinations containing any of the following, depending on the amount present, may also interact with sodium iodide supplements.

» Antithyroid agents
   (antithyroid agents block the oxidation of iodide to iodine in the thyroid gland)

   Iodine-containing compounds used for cleansing or
» Iodine-containing preparations, other
   (concurrent use with other iodine products may increase serum iodine concentrations; iodine-containing cleansers are more likely to cause a problem in infants)

» Lithium
   (concurrent use with sodium iodide may potentiate the hypothyroid and goitrogenic effects of either medication; baseline thyroid status should be determined at periodic intervals to detect changes in the thyroid-pituitary response)

   Sodium iodide I 131, therapeutic
   (sodium iodide may decrease thyroid uptake of I 131)

### Laboratory value alterations

The following have been selected on the basis of their potential clinical significance (possible effect in parentheses where appropriate)—not necessarily inclusive (» = major clinical significance):

With diagnostic test results
   Thyroid function studies and
   Thyroid imaging, radionuclide, and
   Thyroid uptake tests
   (sodium iodide may decrease thyroidal uptake of I 131, I 123, and sodium pertechnetate Tc 99m)

### Medical considerations/Contraindications

The medical considerations/contraindications included here have been selected on the basis of their potential clinical significance (reasons given in parentheses where appropriate)—not necessarily inclusive (» = major clinical significance).

*Risk-benefit should be considered when the following medical problems exist:*

Hyperthyroidism
   (prolonged use of iodine may cause thyroid gland hyperplasia, thyroid adenoma, goiter, or hypothyroidism)

Renal function impairment
   (may cause excessive serum iodine concentrations)

Sensitivity to iodine or sodium iodide
Tuberculosis
   (use may cause irritation and increase secretions)

**Patient monitoring**

The following may be especially important in patient monitoring (other tests may be warranted in some patients, depending on condition; » = major clinical significance):

Thyroid function
(periodic monitoring is recommended as a guideline for adjusting dosage)

## Side/Adverse Effects

The following side/adverse effects have been selected on the basis of their potential clinical significance (possible signs and symptoms in parentheses where appropriate)—not necessarily inclusive:

**Those indicating need for medical attention**

Incidence less frequent
*Allergic reaction, specifically angioedemia* (swelling of the arms, face, legs, lips, tongue, and/or throat); *arthralgia* (joint pain); *eosinophilia; swelling of lymph nodes*

With prolonged use
*Iodism* (burning of mouth or throat; gastric irritation; increased watering of mouth; metallic taste; severe headache; skin lesions; soreness of teeth and gums)

## Patient Consultation

As an aid to patient consultation, refer to *Advice for the Patient, Sodium Iodide (Systemic).*

In providing consultation, consider emphasizing the following selected information (»= major clinical significance):

**Description of use**

*For use as a nutritional supplement*
Description should include function in the body, signs of deficiency, conditions that may cause iodine deficiency

**Importance of diet**

*For use as a nutritional supplement*
Importance of proper nutrition; supplement may be needed because of inadequate dietary intake
Food sources of iodine
Recommended daily intake for iodine

**Before using this medication**

» Conditions affecting use, especially:
Sensitivity to iodine or sodium iodide
Pregnancy—High doses may cause thyroid problems or goiter in the newborn infant
Breast-feeding—High doses may cause skin rash and thyroid problems in nursing babies
Use in children—High doses may cause skin rash and thyroid problems in infants
Dental—May cause swelling of salivary glands, burning of mouth or throat, metallic taste, soreness of teeth and gums, or increase in salivation
Other medications, especially antithyroid agents, lithium, or other iodine-containing medications
Other medical problems, especially renal function impairment, thyroid disease, or tuberculosis

**Proper use of this medication**

*For use as a nutritional supplement*

» Proper dosing
Missed dose: No cause for concern because of length of time necessary for depletion; remembering to take as directed

» Proper storage

**Precautions while using this medication**

*For use as a nutritional supplement*
Other products contain iodine; making sure not to get too much, especially for infants and small children

**Side/adverse effects**

» Signs of potential side effects, especially allergic reactions or iodism

## General Dosing Information

**For use as a nutritional supplement**

Because of the infrequency of iodine deficiency alone, combinations of several vitamins and/or minerals are commonly administered. In the oral form, iodine is available only as a vitamin/mineral complex.

**For parenteral dosage forms only**

For use as a nutritional supplement—
In most cases, parenteral administration is indicated only when oral administration is not acceptable (for example, in nausea, vomiting, and preoperative and postoperative conditions) or possible (for example, in malabsorption syndromes or following gastric resection).

**Diet/Nutrition**

Recommended dietary intakes for iodine are defined differently worldwide.

For U.S.—
The Recommended Dietary Allowances (RDAs) for vitamins and minerals are determined by the Food and Nutrition Board of the National Research Council and are intended to provide adequate nutrition in most healthy persons under usual environmental stresses. In addition, a different designation may be used by the FDA for food and dietary supplement labeling purposes, as with Daily Value (DV). DVs replace the previous labeling terminology United States Recommended Daily Allowances (USRDAs).

For Canada—
Recommended Nutrient Intakes (RNIs) for vitamins, minerals, and protein are determined by Health and Welfare Canada and provide recommended amounts of a specific nutrient while minimizing the risk of chronic diseases.

Daily recommended intakes for iodine are generally defined as follows:

| Persons | U.S. (mcg) | Canada (mcg) |
|---|---|---|
| Infants and children | | |
| Birth to 3 years of age | 40–70 | 30–65 |
| 4 to 6 years of age | 90 | 85 |
| 7 to 10 years of age | 120 | 95–125 |
| Adolescent and adult males | 150 | 125–160 |
| Adolescent and adult females | 150 | 110–160 |
| Pregnant females | 175 | 135–185 |
| Breast-feeding females | 200 | 160–210 |

These are usually provided by adequate diets.

The best sources of iodine include seafood, iodized salt (in moderation), and vegetables grown in iodine-rich soils. Iodine-containing mist from the ocean is also an important source. Iodized salt provides 76 mcg of iodine per gram of salt.

## Parenteral Dosage Forms

### SODIUM IODIDE INJECTION

**Usual adult dose**

Deficiency (prophylaxis or treatment)—
Intravenous infusion, 1 to 2 mcg elemental iodide per kg of body weight a day added to total parenteral nutrition (TPN).

Note: For pregnant and lactating women, the recommended dosage is 2 to 3 mcg elemental iodide per kg of body weight a day added to TPN.

[Hyperthyroidism]—
Intravenous infusion, 0.5 to 1 gram every 12 hours until stable, the first dose being given at least one hour after the initial dose of antithyroid agent.

**Usual pediatric dose**

Deficiency (prophylaxis or treatment)—
Intravenous infusion, 2 to 3 mcg elemental iodide per kg of body weight a day added to TPN.

**Strength(s) usually available**

U.S.—
100 mcg elemental iodide (118 mcg sodium iodide) per mL (Rx) [*Iodopen;* GENERIC].

Canada—
Not commercially available.

**Packaging and storage**

Store below 40 °C (104 °F), preferably between 15 and 30 °C (59 and 86 °F), unless otherwise specified by manufacturer.

**Preparation of dosage form**

The manufacturer states that sodium iodide can be added to total parenteral nutrition (TPN) solutions, and is physically compatible with amino acid solutions, dextrose solutions, electrolytes, and other trace elements.

Revised: 02/26/92
Interim revision: 08/19/94; 06/19/95

# SODIUM IODIDE I 123   Systemic

VA CLASSIFICATION (Primary): DX201

Note: For a listing of dosage forms and brand names by country availability, see *Dosage Forms* section(s). For a listing of brand names for the articles in this monograph, refer to the General Index.

## Category

Diagnostic aid, radioactive (thyroid disorders).

## Indications

### Accepted

Thyroid function studies or

Thyroid uptake tests—Sodium iodide I 123 is indicated in thyroid uptake tests, in which thyroid function is evaluated by determining the fraction of administered radioiodine activity taken up by the thyroid gland. The thyroid uptake test is used in the diagnosis and confirmation of suspected hyperthyroidism and in calculating the activity to be administered for radioactive iodine therapy.

Thyroid imaging, radionuclide—Sodium iodide I 123 is indicated in thyroid imaging for the evaluation of thyroid function and size; thyroid nodules; carcinoma; and masses in the lingual region, neck, and mediastinum.

Sodium iodide I 123 is generally preferable to sodium iodide I 131 because of its lower patient radiation doses and better imaging properties. It also may be the radiopharmaceutical of choice in children who require diagnosis of thyroid function and imaging of the thyroid.

## Physical Properties

### Nuclear data

| Radionu-clide (half-life*) | Decay constant | Mode of decay | Principal photon emissions (keV) | Mean number of emissions/ disintegration |
|---|---|---|---|---|
| I 123 (13.2 hr) | 0.0533 h⁻¹ | Electron capture | Gamma (159) | 0.83 |

*In the euthyroid patient, 5 to 30% of the administered sodium iodide I 123 is concentrated in the thyroid gland at 24 hours and has an effective half-life of 13 hours. The remaining administered activity is distributed within the extracellular fluid and has an effective half-life of 8 hours.

## Pharmacology/Pharmacokinetics

### Mechanism of action/Effect

The action of radioiodide is based on one of the normal functions of the thyroid gland, which is the accumulation and retention of iodine as required in the synthesis of thyroid hormones. Thyroid retention of radioiodide permits quantification of organ uptake and imaging of anatomical distribution in thyroid tissue. Sodium iodide I 123 is also concentrated in functioning papillary, follicular, or mixed papillary/follicular thyroid cancer and metastases, although to a lesser extent than in normal thyroid tissue.

### Absorption

Readily absorbed from upper gastrointestinal tract.

### Distribution

Selectively concentrated and bound to tyrosyl residues of thyroglobulin in the thyroid gland; also concentrated, but not bound, in the choroid plexus, gastric mucosa, salivary glands, nasal mucosa, stomach, and lactating breast tissue, with the remainder being distributed within the extracellular fluid.

### Half-life

Biological (for thyroid compartment)—
Euthyroid: 80 days.
Hyperthyroid: 5 to 40 days.

### Time to radioactivity visualization:

4 to 24 hours.

### Elimination

Renal—Primary, 50 to 75% of administered activity eliminated in the urine of euthyroid patients with normal renal function within 48 hours.
Fecal and salivary—Secondary (less than 2% of administered activity).

## Precautions to Consider

### Carcinogenicity/Mutagenicity

No long-term animal studies have been performed to evaluate carcinogenic or mutagenic potential of sodium iodide I 123.

### Pregnancy/Reproduction

Pregnancy—Well-controlled studies have not been done in humans. However, investigational studies performed in retrospect have not shown sodium iodide I 123 to cause adverse effects in the fetus.

The possibility of pregnancy should be assessed in women of child-bearing potential. Clinical situations exist where the benefit to the patient and fetus, based on information derived from radiopharmaceutical use, outweighs the risks from fetal exposure to radiation. In these situations, the physician should use discretion and reduce the radiopharmaceutical dose to the lowest possible amount.

Studies have not been done in animals.

FDA Pregnancy Category C.

### Breast-feeding

Iodide I 123 is distributed into breast milk and may reach concentrations equal to or greater than concentrations in maternal plasma. It has been recommended that breast-feeding may be resumed when the radiation dose to the infant's thyroid does not exceed 150 mrad. A method to calculate the radiation dose to the infant's thyroid has been proposed based on the effective half-life of the radionuclide, the activity administered to the mother, the fraction of administered activity ingested by the infant, and the radiation dose to the infant's thyroid per unit of activity ingested. It has been estimated that the time required before nursing may be resumed after administration of 1.11 megabecquerels (30 microcuries) of sodium iodide I 123 is 16 days for a product contaminated with 4.9% of I 124 and 91 days for a product contaminated with 1.9% of I 125. Because of the difficulty of maintaining the maternal milk supply for such an extended period of time, complete cessation of nursing is usually recommended.

### Pediatrics

Although sodium iodide I 123 is used in children, there have been no specific studies evaluating its safety and efficacy in pediatric patients.

### Geriatrics

Although appropriate studies on the relationship of age to the effects of sodium iodide I 123 have not been performed in the geriatric population, no geriatrics-specific problems have been documented to date.

### Drug interactions and/or related problems

See *Diagnostic interference.*

### Diagnostic interference

The following have been selected on the basis of their potential clinical significance (possible effect in parentheses where appropriate)—not necessarily inclusive (» = major clinical significance):

With results of *this* test
  *Due to other medications*
    Amiodarone or
    Antithyroid preparations—thioamide derivatives or aromatic preparations or
    Benzodiazepines or
    Contrast media, iodinated or
    Corticosteroids or
    Goitrogenic foods (e.g., cabbage, turnips) or
    Iodine-containing foods or
    Iodine-containing preparations or
    Iodine-contaminated bromides or
    Iodine, stable or
    Monovalent anions (e.g., perchlorate, thiocyanate) or
    Pyrazolone derivatives, such as phenylbutazone or
    Salicylates or
    Salt, iodized, excessive intake of or
    Thiopental or
    Thyroid blocking agents, such as strong iodine solution, potassium iodide, or potassium perchlorate or
    Thyroid preparations, natural or synthetic
      (may decrease thyroidal uptake of iodide I 123; it is recommended that these medications be withheld for the following periods of time prior to administration of sodium iodide I 123: several months for amiodarone; 1 week for corticosteroids; 4 weeks for benzodiazepines; 2 to 4 weeks for intravascular iodinated contrast media and more than 4 weeks for cholecystographic agents; 2 to 4 weeks for iodine-containing preparations, such as vitamins, expectorants, antitussives, and topical medications; 1 to 2 weeks for pyrazolone

derivatives; 1 week for thiopental; 4 to 6 weeks for thyroxine and 2 to 3 weeks for triiodothyronine)

(a rebound effect may occur following the sudden withdrawal of antithyroid preparations, resulting in a period of up to 5 days of very high thyroidal uptake; it is recommended that antithyroid medications be discontinued 1 week prior to administration of sodium iodide I 123; however, for early uptake studies [i.e., 15 to 30 minutes] to determine iodide trapping [not organification] the treatment with thioamide drugs does not need to be interrupted)

(chronic salicylate administration may cause a depression of thyroid function; salicylate therapy should be discontinued at least 1 to 2 week prior to sodium iodide I 123 administration; however, a rebound effect may also occur following discontinuation of salicylate therapy, resulting in a period of 3 to 10 days of increased thyroidal uptake)

*Due to medical problems or conditions*
Iodine deficiency or
Low serum chlorides or
Nephrosis
   (may increase thyroidal uptake of I 123)

Renal function impairment
   (lack of normal excretion of iodine may cause an increase or decrease in the body iodide pool, resulting in false high or low uptake determinations)

### Medical considerations/Contraindications
The medical considerations/contraindications included here have been selected on the basis of their potential clinical significance (reasons given in parentheses where appropriate)—not necessarily inclusive (» = major clinical significance).
See also *Diagnostic interference.*
Sensitivity to the radiopharmaceutical preparation

## Side/Adverse Effects
The following side/adverse effects have been selected on the basis of their potential clinical significance (possible signs and symptoms in parentheses where appropriate)—not necessarily inclusive:

**Those indicating need for medical attention only if they continue or are bothersome**
Incidence rare
   *Headache; nausea or vomiting; skin rash, hives, or itching*

## Patient Consultation
As an aid to patient consultation, refer to *Advice for the Patient, Radiopharmaceuticals (Diagnostic).*

In providing consultation, consider emphasizing the following selected information (» = major clinical significance):

### Description of use
*Action in the body*
Iodide I 123 uptake by the thyroid same as uptake of nonradioactive iodine
Localization of iodide I 123 in thyroid allows thyroid uptake quantification and visualization of thyroid tissue
Small amounts of radioactivity used in diagnosis; radiation exposure is relatively low and considered safe

### Before having this test
» Conditions affecting use, especially:
   Pregnancy—Sodium iodide I 123 crosses placenta; risk to fetus from radiation exposure as opposed to benefit derived from use should be considered
   Breast-feeding—Iodide I 123 is distributed into breast milk; complete cessation of nursing recommended for this infant because of risk to infant from radiation exposure (present administration of I 123 will not affect breast-feeding of future infants)

### Preparation for this test
Special preparatory instructions may apply; patient should inquire in advance

### Precautions after having this test
To decrease radiation exposure to the urinary bladder: Increasing intake of fluids to promote more frequent voiding to help eliminate radioactive iodine

## General Dosing Information
Radiopharmaceuticals are to be administered only by or under the supervision of physicians who have had extensive training in the safe use and handling of radioactive materials and who are authorized by the appropriate Federal or state agency, if required, or, outside the U.S., the appropriate authority.

Uptake measurements are generally made at 4 and/or 24 hours, and thyroid imaging is usually performed 18 to 24 hours after sodium iodide I 123 administration. However, it has been demonstrated that a 4- to 5-hour interval after administration of sodium iodide I 123 may be adequate for thyroid imaging, especially in hyperthyroid patients with high percentage uptakes.

Since sodium iodide I 123 may contain small amounts of longer-lived isotopes of iodine (e.g., I 124, I 125), it should be used as soon as possible on the day of calibration. The use of this radiopharmaceutical beyond the day of calibration results in an increased ratio of these isotopes to I 123 and, therefore, in unnecessary patient radiation from the relatively greater quantities of these contaminants.

### Safety considerations for handling this radiopharmaceutical
Improper handling of this radiopharmaceutical may cause radioactive contamination. Guidelines for handling radioactive material have been prepared by scientific, professional, state, federal, and international bodies and are available to the specially qualified and authorized users who have access to radiopharmaceuticals.

## Oral Dosage Forms
### SODIUM IODIDE I 123 CAPSULES USP

**Usual adult and adolescent administered activity**
Diagnostic aid—
   Oral, 3.7 to 14.8 megabecquerels (100 to 400 microcuries).
Note: For uptake studies only, dosages in the lower end of the range (e.g., 3.7 megabecquerels) are recommended.
   For thyroid imaging, higher dosages (e.g., 14.8 megabecquerels) are generally used.

**Usual pediatric administered activity**
Diagnostic aid—
   Dosage must be individualized by physician. A minimum dosage of 0.37 megabecquerels (10 microcuries) is required for uptake studies and 1.85 megabecquerels (50 microcuries) for thyroid imaging.
Note: The available strength of the capsule does not conform to the recommended pediatric dosages. For this reason, in actual practice, the administered activity is usually 3.7 megabecquerels (100 microcuries). If smaller dosage is required, the capsule must be dissolved and an aliquot taken.

**Usual geriatric administered activity**
See *Usual adult and adolescent administered activity.*

**Strength(s) usually available**
U.S.—
   3.7 megabecquerels (100 microcuries) of I 123 at time of calibration (Rx) [GENERIC].
   7.4 megabecquerels (200 microcuries) of I 123 at time of calibration (Rx) [GENERIC].
Canada—
   Not commercially available.

**Packaging and storage**
Store below 40 °C (104 °F), preferably between 15 and 30 °C (59 and 86 °F), unless otherwise specified by manufacturer. Store in a well-closed container.

**Stability**
Capsules should be administered within 24 hours after calibration, unless otherwise stated by manufacturer. Sodium iodide I 123 preparations may contain small amounts of longer-lived isotopes of iodine (e.g., I 124, I 125). The use of this radiopharmaceutical beyond the day of calibration results in an increased ratio of these isotopes to I 123 and, therefore, in unnecessary patient radiation from the relatively greater quantities of these contaminants.

**Note**
Caution—Radioactive material.

### SODIUM IODIDE I 123 SOLUTION USP

**Usual adult and adolescent administered activity**
Diagnostic aid—
   See *Sodium Iodide I 123 Capsules USP.*

**Usual pediatric administered activity**
Diagnostic aid—
   See *Sodium Iodide I 123 Capsules USP.*

**Usual geriatric administered activity**
See *Usual adult and adolescent administered activity.*

**Strength(s) usually available**
U.S.—
   Not commercially available.

Canada—
    Content information not available at present (Rx) [GENERIC].

**Packaging and storage**
Store below 40 °C (104 °F), preferably between 15 and 30 °C (59 and 86 °F), unless otherwise specified by manufacturer.

**Stability**
Solution should be used within 24 hours after calibration, unless otherwise stated by manufacturer. Sodium iodide I 123 preparations may contain small amounts of longer-lived isotopes of iodine (e.g., I 124, I 125). The use of this radiopharmaceutical beyond the day of calibration results in an increased ratio of these isotopes to I 123 and, therefore, in unnecessary patient radiation from the relatively greater quantities of these contaminants.

**Note**
Caution—Radioactive material.

**Additional information**
Radioiodide stock solutions and any dilutions thereof must be maintained at a pH of 7.5 to 9.0 in order to minimize oxidation of iodide to volatile forms of iodine. Additionally, 0.2% sodium thiosulfate may be incorporated into these solutions if an antioxidant is desired.

## Selected Bibliography

Braverman LE, Utiger RD, editors. Werner and Ingbar's the thyroid: a fundamental and clinical text. 6th ed. Philadelphia: J.B. Lippincott Company, 1991: 437-45.
Ryo UY, Vaidya PV, Schneider AB, et al. Thyroid imaging agents: a comparison of I 123 and Tc 99m pertechnetate. Radiology 1983; 148: 819-22.

Revised: 08/25/94

## Table 1. Radiation dosimetry

| Organ | Maximum thyroid uptake (%) | Estimated absorbed radiation dose*† | | | | | |
|---|---|---|---|---|---|---|---|
| | | I 123 | | I 124‡ | | I 125‡ | |
| | | mGy/MBq | rad/mCi | mGy/MBq | rad/mCi | MGy/MGq | rad/mCi |
| Bladder wall | 0 | 0.090 | 0.33 | 0.78 | 2.9 | 0.1 | 0.37 |
| | 5 | 0.085 | 0.31 | 0.74 | 2.7 | 0.095 | 0.35 |
| | 15 | 0.076 | 0.28 | 0.67 | 2.5 | 0.085 | 0.31 |
| | 25 | 0.069 | 0.26 | 0.6 | 2.2 | 0.076 | 0.28 |
| | 55 | 0.043 | 0.16 | 0.38 | 1.4 | 0.047 | 0.17 |
| Uterus | 0 | 0.014 | 0.052 | 0.11 | 0.41 | 0.0095 | 0.035 |
| | 5 | 0.016 | 0.059 | 0.12 | 0.44 | 0.0093 | 0.034 |
| | 15 | 0.015 | 0.056 | 0.11 | 0.41 | 0.0092 | 0.034 |
| | 25 | 0.014 | 0.052 | 0.11 | 0.41 | 0.0088 | 0.033 |
| | 55 | 0.012 | 0.044 | 0.097 | 0.36 | 0.0075 | 0.028 |
| Kidneys | 0 | 0.011 | 0.041 | 0.1 | 0.37 | 0.01 | 0.037 |
| | 5 | 0.012 | 0.044 | 0.1 | 0.37 | 0.0092 | 0.034 |
| | 15 | 0.010 | 0.037 | 0.094 | 0.35 | 0.0086 | 0.032 |
| | 25 | 0.011 | 0.041 | 0.097 | 0.36 | 0.0081 | 0.03 |
| | 55 | 0.0091 | 0.034 | 0.075 | 0.28 | 0.0064 | 0.024 |
| Ovaries | 0 | 0.0098 | 0.036 | 0.079 | 0.29 | 0.0064 | 0.024 |
| | 5 | 0.012 | 0.044 | 0.091 | 0.34 | 0.007 | 0.026 |
| | 15 | 0.012 | 0.044 | 0.089 | 0.33 | 0.0069 | 0.026 |
| | 25 | 0.011 | 0.041 | 0.088 | 0.33 | 0.0069 | 0.026 |
| | 55 | 0.011 | 0.041 | 0.084 | 0.31 | 0.0066 | 0.024 |
| Large intestine wall (lower) | 0 | 0.0097 | 0.036 | 0.087 | 0.32 | 0.0067 | 0.025 |
| | 5 | 0.011 | 0.041 | 0.093 | 0.34 | 0.0076 | 0.028 |
| | 15 | 0.011 | 0.041 | 0.092 | 0.34 | 0.0075 | 0.028 |
| | 25 | 0.011 | 0.041 | 0.090 | 0.33 | 0.0074 | 0.027 |
| | 55 | 0.0098 | 0.036 | 0.084 | 0.31 | 0.007 | 0.026 |
| Red marrow | 0 | 0.0094 | 0.035 | 0.059 | 0.21 | 0.0083 | 0.031 |
| | 5 | 0.0092 | 0.034 | 0.065 | 0.24 | 0.01 | 0.037 |
| | 15 | 0.0093 | 0.034 | 0.086 | 0.32 | 0.017 | 0.063 |
| | 25 | 0.0098 | 0.036 | 0.11 | 0.41 | 0.023 | 0.085 |
| | 55 | 0.011 | 0.041 | 0.17 | 0.63 | 0.043 | 0.16 |
| Small intestine | 0 | 0.0085 | 0.031 | 0.071 | 0.26 | 0.0058 | 0.021 |
| | 5 | 0.043 | 0.16 | 0.37 | 1.37 | 0.042 | 0.16 |
| | 15 | 0.043 | 0.16 | 0.37 | 1.37 | 0.042 | 0.16 |
| | 25 | 0.043 | 0.16 | 0.37 | 1.37 | 0.042 | 0.16 |
| | 55 | 0.042 | 0.16 | 0.37 | 1.37 | 0.042 | 0.16 |

*Data based on the International Commission on Radiological Protection (ICRP) Publication 53—Radiation Dose to Patients from Radiopharmaceuticals.

†Estimates based on intravenous administration. With oral administration there is a radiation dose to the stomach in addition to that due to iodide in gastric and salivary secretions. Assuming a mean residence time in the stomach of one-half hour, the absorbed dose to the stomach wall is increased by approximately 40% for I 123 with oral administration, while the dose to organs and tissues other than the stomach wall is decreased by 3% for I 123.

‡Levels of I 124 and I 125 contamination in sodium iodide I 123 preparations vary with the manufacturing source/production method. The ratio of the concentration of I 123, I 124, and I 125 changes with time.

§With thyroid blocking, thyroid uptakes ranging from 0.5% to 2.0% will still occur. Under these circumstances the effective dose to the adult will range from 0.016 to 0.025 mSv/MBq (0.059 to 0.092 rem/mCi) for I 123.

#The effective dose is virtually identical after oral or intravenous administration.

## Table 1. Radiation dosimetry *(continued)*

| Organ | Maximum thyroid uptake (%) | Estimated absorbed radiation dose*† | | | | | |
|---|---|---|---|---|---|---|---|
| | | I 123 | | I 124‡ | | I 125‡ | |
| | | mGy/MBq | rad/mCi | mGy/MBq | rad/mCi | MGy/MGq | rad/mCi |
| Bone surfaces | 0 | 0.0097 | 0.036 | 0.053 | 0.2 | 0.0074 | 0.027 |
| | 5 | 0.0068 | 0.025 | 0.053 | 0.2 | 0.0092 | 0.034 |
| | 15 | 0.0071 | 0.026 | 0.072 | 0.27 | 0.016 | 0.06 |
| | 25 | 0.0075 | 0.028 | 0.092 | 0.34 | 0.024 | 0.089 |
| | 55 | 0.0086 | 0.032 | 0.15 | 0.56 | 0.045 | 0.17 |
| Large intestine wall (upper) | 0 | 0.0080 | 0.030 | 0.068 | 0.25 | 0.0058 | 0.021 |
| | 5 | 0.019 | 0.070 | 0.13 | 0.48 | 0.016 | 0.06 |
| | 15 | 0.018 | 0.067 | 0.13 | 0.48 | 0.016 | 0.06 |
| | 25 | 0.018 | 0.067 | 0.13 | 0.48 | 0.016 | 0.06 |
| | 55 | 0.018 | 0.067 | 0.13 | 0.48 | 0.016 | 0.06 |
| Pancreas | 0 | 0.0076 | 0.028 | 0.061 | 0.23 | 0.0056 | 0.021 |
| | 5 | 0.014 | 0.052 | 0.11 | 0.41 | 0.0092 | 0.034 |
| | 150 | 0.014 | 0.052 | 0.11 | 0.41 | 0.0092 | 0.034 |
| | 25 | 0.014 | 0.052 | 0.12 | 0.44 | 0.0092 | 0.034 |
| | 55 | 0.014 | 0.052 | 0.13 | 0.48 | 0.0092 | 0.034 |
| Spleen | 0 | 0.0070 | 0.026 | 0.058 | 0.21 | 0.0056 | 0.021 |
| | 5 | 0.0096 | 0.036 | 0.079 | 0.29 | 0.0058 | 0.021 |
| | 15 | 0.0095 | 0.035 | 0.083 | 0.31 | 0.0058 | 0.021 |
| | 25 | 0.0096 | 0.036 | 0.087 | 0.32 | 0.0059 | 0.022 |
| | 55 | 0.0097 | 0.036 | 0.098 | 0.36 | 0.0058 | 0.021 |
| Adrenals | 0 | 0.0070 | 0.026 | 0.072 | 0.27 | 0.0048 | 0.018 |
| | 5 | 0.0064 | 0.024 | 0.066 | 0.24 | 0.0036 | 0.013 |
| | 15 | 0.0063 | 0.023 | 0.072 | 0.27 | 0.0036 | 0.013 |
| | 25 | 0.0064 | 0.024 | 0.078 | 0.29 | 0.0036 | 0.013 |
| | 55 | 0.0065 | 0.024 | 0.093 | 0.34 | 0.0036 | 0.013 |
| Testes | 0 | 0.0069 | 0.026 | 0.074 | 0.27 | 0.0053 | 0.02 |
| | 5 | 0.0055 | 0.020 | 0.058 | 0.21 | 0.0037 | 0.014 |
| | 15 | 0.0053 | 0.020 | 0.057 | 0.21 | 0.0036 | 0.013 |
| | 25 | 0.0052 | 0.019 | 0.056 | 0.21 | 0.0036 | 0.013 |
| | 55 | 0.0046 | 0.017 | 0.051 | 0.19 | 0.0034 | 0.013 |
| Stomach wall | 0 | 0.0069 | 0.026 | 0.057 | 0.21 | 0.0053 | 0.02 |
| | 5 | 0.068 | 0.25 | 0.58 | 2.15 | 0.071 | 0.26 |
| | 15 | 0.068 | 0.25 | 0.58 | 2.15 | 0.071 | 0.26 |
| | 25 | 0.068 | 0.25 | 0.58 | 2.15 | 0.071 | 0.26 |
| | 55 | 0.068 | 0.25 | 0.6 | 2.2 | 0.071 | 0.26 |
| Liver | 0 | 0.0067 | 0.025 | 0.058 | 0.21 | 0.0054 | 0.02 |
| | 5 | 0.0062 | 0.023 | 0.056 | 0.21 | 0.0042 | 0.016 |
| | 15 | 0.0062 | 0.023 | 0.061 | 0.23 | 0.0042 | 0.016 |
| | 25 | 0.0063 | 0.023 | 0.066 | 0.24 | 0.0042 | 0.016 |
| | 55 | 0.0064 | 0.024 | 0.081 | 0.3 | 0.0042 | 0.016 |
| Lungs | 0 | 0.0061 | 0.023 | 0.051 | 0.19 | 0.0055 | 0.02 |
| | 5 | 0.0054 | 0.020 | 0.057 | 0.21 | 0.0057 | 0.021 |
| | 15 | 0.0057 | 0.021 | 0.086 | 0.32 | 0.0087 | 0.032 |
| | 25 | 0.0061 | 0.023 | 0.11 | 0.41 | 0.012 | 0.044 |
| | 55 | 0.0072 | 0.027 | 0.2 | 0.74 | 0.021 | 0.078 |
| Breast | 0 | 0.0056 | 0.021 | 0.052 | 0.19 | 0.0051 | 0.019 |
| | 5 | 0.0046 | 0.017 | 0.052 | 0.19 | 0.004 | 0.015 |
| | 15 | 0.0047 | 0.017 | 0.073 | 0.27 | 0.0046 | 0.017 |
| | 25 | 0.0050 | 0.019 | 0.093 | 0.34 | 0.0053 | 0.02 |
| | 55 | 0.0056 | 0.021 | 0.15 | 0.56 | 0.0073 | 0.027 |
| Thyroid | 0 | 0.0051 | 0.019 | 0.05 | 0.19 | 0.0047 | 0.017 |
| | 5 | 0.63 | 2.33 | 42.0 | 155.56 | 47.0 | 174.07 |
| | 15 | 1.9 | 7.03 | 130.0 | 481.48 | 140.0 | 518.52 |
| | 25 | 3.2 | 11.84 | 210.0 | 777.78 | 240.0 | 888.89 |
| | 55 | 7.0 | 25.9 | 470.0 | 1740.74 | 520.0 | 1925.93 |
| Other tissue | 0 | 0.0064 | 0.024 | 0.056 | 0.21 | 0.0052 | 0.019 |
| | 5 | 0.0063 | 0.023 | 0.069 | 0.25 | 0.021 | 0.078 |
| | 15 | 0.0068 | 0.025 | 0.11 | 0.41 | 0.053 | 0.2 |
| | 25 | 0.0074 | 0.027 | 0.14 | 0.52 | 0.086 | 0.32 |
| | 55 | 0.0092 | 0.034 | 0.25 | 0.93 | 0.18 | 0.67 |

## Table 1. Radiation dosimetry (continued)

| | Effective dose# | | | | | | | | | | | | | | |
|---|---|---|---|---|---|---|---|---|---|---|---|---|---|---|---|
| | I 123 Maximum thyroid uptake (%)§ | | | | | I 124 Maximum thyroid uptake (%) | | | | | I 125 Maximum thyroid uptake (%) | | | | |
| | 0 | 5 | 15 | 25 | 55 | 0 | 5 | 15 | 25 | 55 | 0 | 5 | 15 | 25 | 55 |
| mSv/MBq | 0.013 | 0.038 | 0.075 | 0.11 | 0.23 | 0.11 | 1.4 | 4.0 | 6.5 | 14 | 0.012 | 1.4 | 4.3 | 7.1 | 16 |
| rem/mCi | 0.048 | 0.14 | 0.28 | 0.41 | 0.85 | 0.41 | 5.18 | 14.8 | 24.05 | 51.8 | 0.044 | 5.18 | 15.91 | 26.27 | 59.2 |

*Data based on the International Commission on Radiological Protection (ICRP) Publication 53—Radiation Dose to Patients from Radiopharmaceuticals.

†Estimates based on intravenous administration. With oral administration there is a radiation dose to the stomach in addition to that due to iodide in gastric and salivary secretions. Assuming a mean residence time in the stomach of one-half hour, the absorbed dose to the stomach wall is increased by approximately 40% for I 123 with oral administration, while the dose to organs and tissues other than the stomach wall is decreased by 3% for I 123.

‡Levels of I 124 and I 125 contamination in sodium iodide I 123 preparations vary with the manufacturing source/production method. The ratio of the concentration of I 123, I 124, and I 125 changes with time.

§With thyroid blocking, thyroid uptakes ranging from 0.5% to 2.0% will still occur. Under these circumstances the effective dose to the adult will range from 0.016 to 0.025 mSv/MBq (0.059 to 0.092 rem/mCi) for I 123.

#The effective dose is virtually identical after oral or intravenous administration.

# SODIUM IODIDE I 131   Systemic—Diagnostic

VA CLASSIFICATION (Primary): DX201

Note: For a listing of dosage forms and brand names by country availability, see *Dosage Forms* section(s). For a listing of brand names for the articles in this monograph, refer to the General Index.

## Category

Diagnostic aid, radioactive (thyroid disorders).

## Indications

### Accepted

Thyroid function studies or

Thyroid uptake tests—Sodium iodide I 131 is indicated in thyroid uptake tests, in which thyroid function is evaluated by determining the fraction of administered radioiodine activity taken up by the thyroid gland. The thyroid uptake test is used in the diagnosis and confirmation of suspected hyperthyroidism and in calculating the activity to be administered for radioactive iodine therapy.

Thyroid imaging, radionuclide—Sodium iodide I 131 is indicated in thyroid imaging for the evaluation of thyroid function and size; thyroid nodules; carcinoma; masses in the lingual region, neck and mediastinum; and in the localization of functioning metastatic thyroid tumor. It is useful in the pre- and post-operative evaluation of patients with thyroid carcinoma. It is also used to assess the effects of therapy on these patients.

Sodium iodide I 123 or sodium pertechnetate Tc 99m (for thyroid imaging) may be preferable to sodium iodide I 131 because of their lower patient radiation doses and better imaging properties. Sodium iodide I 123 may also be the radiopharmaceutical of choice in children who require diagnosis of thyroid function and imaging of the thyroid.

## Physical Properties

### Nuclear data

| Radionuclide (half-life*) | Decay constant | Mode of decay | Principal emissions (keV) | Mean number of emissions/ disintegration |
|---|---|---|---|---|
| I 131 (8.08 days) | 0.00358 h⁻¹ | Beta | Beta (191.6) Gamma (364.5) | 0.90 0.81 |

*For diagnostic use: In the euthyroid patient, 5 to 30% of the administered sodium iodide I 131 is concentrated in the thyroid gland at 24 hours and has an effective half-life of approximately 7.6 days. The remainder is distributed within the extracellular fluid and has an effective half-life of approximately 0.34 day.

## Pharmacology/Pharmacokinetics

### Mechanism of action/Effect

The action of radioiodide is based on one of the normal functions of the thyroid gland, which is the accumulation and retention of iodine as required for the synthesis of thyroid hormones. Thyroid retention of sodium iodide I 131 permits quantification of organ uptake and imaging of anatomical distribution in thyroid tissue. Radioiodide is also concentrated in functioning papillary, follicular, or mixed papillary/follicular thyroid cancer and metastases, although to a lesser extent than in normal thyroid tissue.

### Absorption

Readily absorbed from gastrointestinal tract.

### Distribution

Selectively concentrated and bound to tyrosyl residues of thyroglobulin in the thyroid gland; also concentrated, but not bound, in the choroid plexus, gastric mucosa, salivary glands, nasal mucosa, and lactating breast tissue with the remainder being distributed within the extracellular fluid.

### Half-life

Biological (for thyroid compartment)—
Euthyroid: 80 days.
Hyperthyroid: 5 to 40 days.

### Time to radioactivity visualization

18 to 24 hours.

Note: Imaging of functional thyroid metastases is generally performed at 24 to 96 hours to allow maximal uptake and minimal blood-pool retention.

### Radiation dosimetry

| Organ | Estimated absorbed radiation dose*† | | |
|---|---|---|---|
| | Maximum thyroid uptake (%) | mGy/MBq | rad/mCi |
| Bladder wall | 0 | 0.61 | 2.26 |
| | 5 | 0.58 | 2.15 |
| | 15 | 0.52 | 1.93 |
| | 25 | 0.46 | 1.70 |
| | 55 | 0.29 | 1.07 |
| Uterus | 0 | 0.054 | 0.20 |
| | 5 | 0.055 | 0.20 |
| | 15 | 0.054 | 0.20 |
| | 25 | 0.052 | 0.19 |
| | 55 | 0.046 | 0.17 |
| Kidneys | 0 | 0.065 | 0.24 |
| | 5 | 0.063 | 0.24 |
| | 15 | 0.060 | 0.22 |
| | 25 | 0.058 | 0.21 |
| | 55 | 0.051 | 0.19 |
| Ovaries | 0 | 0.042 | 0.16 |
| | 5 | 0.044 | 0.16 |
| | 15 | 0.043 | 0.16 |
| | 25 | 0.043 | 0.16 |
| | 55 | 0.041 | 0.15 |

| Organ | Estimated absorbed radiation dose*† | | |
|---|---|---|---|
| | Maximum thyroid uptake (%) | mGy/MBq | rad/mCi |
| Large intestine wall (lower) | 0 | 0.043 | 0.16 |
| | 5 | 0.043 | 0.16 |
| | 15 | 0.042 | 0.16 |
| | 25 | 0.041 | 0.15 |
| | 55 | 0.040 | 0.15 |
| Red marrow | 0 | 0.035 | 0.13 |
| | 5 | 0.038 | 0.14 |
| | 15 | 0.054 | 0.20 |
| | 25 | 0.070 | 0.26 |
| | 55 | 0.12 | 0.44 |
| Small intestine | 0 | 0.038 | 0.14 |
| | 5 | 0.28 | 1.04 |
| | 15 | 0.28 | 1.04 |
| | 25 | 0.28 | 1.04 |
| | 55 | 0.28 | 1.04 |
| Bone surfaces | 0 | 0.032 | 0.12 |
| | 5 | 0.032 | 0.12 |
| | 15 | 0.047 | 0.17 |
| | 25 | 0.061 | 0.23 |
| | 55 | 0.11 | 0.41 |
| Large intestine wall (upper) | 0 | 0.037 | 0.14 |
| | 5 | 0.059 | 0.22 |
| | 15 | 0.059 | 0.22 |
| | 25 | 0.059 | 0.22 |
| | 55 | 0.058 | 0.21 |
| Pancreas | 0 | 0.035 | 0.13 |
| | 5 | 0.050 | 0.19 |
| | 15 | 0.052 | 0.19 |
| | 25 | 0.053 | 0.20 |
| | 55 | 0.058 | 0.21 |
| Spleen | 0 | 0.034 | 0.13 |
| | 5 | 0.039 | 0.14 |
| | 15 | 0.042 | 0.16 |
| | 25 | 0.044 | 0.16 |
| | 55 | 0.051 | 0.19 |
| Adrenals | 0 | 0.037 | 0.14 |
| | 5 | 0.032 | 0.12 |
| | 15 | 0.036 | 0.13 |
| | 25 | 0.039 | 0.14 |
| | 55 | 0.049 | 0.18 |
| Testes | 0 | 0.037 | 0.14 |
| | 5 | 0.029 | 0.11 |
| | 15 | 0.028 | 0.10 |
| | 25 | 0.027 | 0.10 |
| | 55 | 0.026 | 0.10 |
| Stomach wall | 0 | 0.034 | 0.13 |
| | 5 | 0.45 | 1.67 |
| | 15 | 0.46 | 1.67 |
| | 25 | 0.46 | 1.67 |
| | 55 | 0.46 | 1.67 |
| Liver | 0 | 0.033 | 0.12 |
| | 5 | 0.030 | 0.11 |
| | 15 | 0.032 | 0.12 |
| | 25 | 0.035 | 0.13 |
| | 55 | 0.043 | 0.16 |
| Lungs | 0 | 0.031 | 0.11 |
| | 5 | 0.034 | 0.13 |
| | 15 | 0.053 | 0.20 |
| | 25 | 0.072 | 0.27 |
| | 55 | 0.13 | 0.48 |
| Breast | 0 | 0.033 | 0.12 |
| | 5 | 0.031 | 0.11 |
| | 15 | 0.043 | 0.16 |
| | 25 | 0.055 | 0.20 |
| | 55 | 0.091 | 0.34 |

| Organ | Estimated absorbed radiation dose*† | | |
|---|---|---|---|
| | Maximum thyroid uptake (%) | mGy/MBq | rad/mCi |
| Thyroid | 0 | 0.029 | 0.11 |
| | 5 | 72.00 | 266.67 |
| | 15 | 210.00 | 777.78 |
| | 25 | 360.00 | 1333.33 |
| | 55 | 790.00 | 2925.93 |
| Other tissue | 0 | 0.032 | 0.12 |
| | 5 | 0.040 | 0.15 |
| | 15 | 0.065 | 0.24 |
| | 25 | 0.090 | 0.33 |
| | 55 | 0.16 | 0.59 |

| Effective dose§ | | | | | |
|---|---|---|---|---|---|
| | Maximum thyroid uptake (%)‡ | | | | |
| | 0 | 5 | 15 | 25 | 55 |
| mSv/MBq | 0.072 | 2.30 | 6.60 | 11.00 | 24.00 |
| rem/mCi | 0.27 | 8.51 | 24.42 | 40.70 | 88.80 |

*Data based on the International Commission on Radiological Protection (ICRP) Publication 53—Radiation Dose to Patients from Radiopharmaceuticals.

†Estimates based on intravenous administration. With oral administration there is a radiation dose to the stomach in addition to that due to iodide in gastric and salivary secretions. Assuming a mean residence time in the stomach is half an hour, the absorbed dose to the stomach wall is increased by approximately 30% with oral administration, while the dose to organs and tissues other than the stomach wall is decreased by less than 3%.

‡With thyroid blocking, thyroid uptakes ranging from 0.5 to 2.0% will still occur. Under these circumstances the effective dose to the adult will range from 0.30 to 0.97 mSv/MBq (1.11 to 3.59 rem/mCi).

§The effective dose is virtually identical after oral or intravenous administration.

**Elimination**
Renal: Primary, 50 to 75% of the administered activity eliminated in the urine of euthyroid patients with normal renal function within 48 hours.
Fecal and salivary: Secondary (less than 2% of the administered activity).
Breast milk: Up to 20% of administered activity appears in the milk within 24 hours.

## Precautions to Consider

**Carcinogenicity**
Experiments in animals with sodium iodide I 131 have demonstrated that radioiodide administration can induce thyroid adenomas and carcinomas.

**Pregnancy/Reproduction**
Pregnancy—Risk-benefit must be considered since radioiodides cross the placenta and may cause severe and irreversible hypothyroidism in the neonate.
The possibility of pregnancy should be assessed in women of child-bearing potential. Clinical situations exist in which the benefit to the patient and fetus, based on information derived from radiopharmaceutical use, outweighs the risks from fetal exposure to radiation. In these situations, the physician should use discretion and reduce the radiopharmaceutical dose to the lowest possible amount.
Studies have not been done in animals.

FDA Pregnancy Category C.

**Breast-feeding**
Iodide I 131 is distributed into breast milk and may reach concentrations equal to or greater than concentrations in maternal plasma. It has been recommended that nursing can be resumed, after administration of a radiopharmaceutical, when the likelihood of the infant's ingested effective dose equivalent (EDE) is below 1 mSv (100 mrem). A method to calculate the EDE has been proposed based on the effective half-life of the radionuclide, the activity administered to the mother, the fraction of administered activity ingested by the infant, and the total body effective dose equivalent to the newborn infant per unit of activity ingested. According to this method, it has been estimated that, for sodium iodide I 131, the time to reduce the EDE to the infant to below 1 mSv (100 mrem) is approximately 10 weeks after administration of 40 megabecquerels (1.08 millicuries) (maximum administered activity) to the mother. Because of the difficulty of maintaining

the maternal milk supply for such an extended period of time, complete cessation of nursing is usually recommended for large administered activities of sodium iodide I 131.

### Pediatrics

Sodium iodide I 123 or sodium pertechnetate Tc 99m, because of its lower patient radiation dose, may be the radiopharmaceutical of choice in children and growing adolescents who require diagnosis of thyroid function and imaging of the thyroid.

### Geriatrics

Although appropriate studies on the relationship of age to the effects of radiodiodide have not been performed in the geriatric population, no geriatrics-specific problems have been documented to date.

### Drug interactions and/or related problems

See *Diagnostic interference.*

### Diagnostic interference

The following have been selected on the basis of their potential clinical significance (possible effect in parentheses where appropriate)—not necessarily inclusive (» = major clinical significance):

With results of *this* test
 *Due to other medications*
  Amiodarone or
  Antithyroid preparations—thioamide derivatives or aromatic preparations or
  Benzodiazepines or
  Contrast media, iodinated or
  Corticosteroids or
  Goitrogenic foods (e.g., cabbage, turnips) or
  Iodine-containing foods or
  Iodine-containing preparations or
  Iodine-contaminated bromides or
  Iodine, stable or
  Monovalent anions (e.g., perchlorate, thiocyanate) or
  Pyrazolone derivatives, such as phenylbutazone or
  Salicylates, chronic administration of or
  Salt, iodized, excessive intake of or
  Thiopental or
  Thyroid blocking agents, such as strong iodine solution, potassium iodide, or potassium perchlorate or
  Thyroid preparations, natural or synthetic
   (may decrease thyroidal uptake of iodide I 131; it is recommended that these medications be withheld for the following periods of time prior to administration of sodium iodide I 131: several months for amiodarone; 1 week for corticosteroids; 4 weeks for benzodiazepines; 2 to 4 weeks for intravascular iodinated contrast media and more than 4 weeks for cholecystographic agents; 2 to 4 weeks for iodine-containing preparations, such as vitamins, expectorants, antitussives, and topical medications; 1 to 2 weeks for pyrazolone derivatives; 1 week for thiopental; 4 to 6 weeks for thyroxine and 2 to 3 weeks for triiodothyronine)

   (a rebound effect may occur following the sudden withdrawal of antithyroid preparations, resulting in a period of up to 5 days of very high thyroidal uptake; it is recommended that antithyroid medications be discontinued 3 to 4 days prior to administration of sodium iodide I 131; however, for early uptake studies [i.e., 15 to 30 minutes] to determine iodide trapping [not organification] the treatment with thioamide drugs does not need to be interrupted)

   (chronic salicylate administration may cause a depression of thyroid function; salicylate therapy should be discontinued at least 1 to 2 weeks prior to sodium iodide I 131 administration; however, a rebound effect may also occur following discontinuation of salicylate therapy, resulting in a period of 3 to 10 days of increased thyroidal uptake)

 *Due to medical problems or conditions*
  Iodine deficiency or
  Low serum chlorides or
  Nephrosis
   (may increase thyroidal uptake of I 131)

  Renal function impairment
   (lack of normal excretion of iodine may cause an increase or decrease in the body iodide pool, resulting in falsely high or low uptake determinations)

### Medical considerations/Contraindications

The medical considerations/contraindications included here have been selected on the basis of their potential clinical significance (reasons given in parentheses where appropriate)—not necessarily inclusive (» = major clinical significance).

See also *Diagnostic interference.*

*Risk-benefit should be considered when the following medical problem exists:*
 Sensitivity to the radiopharmaceutical preparation

## Side/Adverse Effects

The following side/adverse effects have been selected on the basis of their potential clinical significance (possible signs and symptoms in parentheses where appropriate)—not necessarily inclusive:

**Those indicating need for medical attention only if they continue or are bothersome**
Incidence rare
 *Headache; nausea or vomiting; skin rash, hives, or itching*

## Patient Consultation

As an aid to patient consultation, refer to *Advice for the Patient, Radiopharmaceuticals (Diagnostic).*

In providing consultation, consider emphasizing the following selected information (» = major clinical significance):

### Description of use

Action in the body: Iodide I 131 uptake by the thyroid and functioning thyroid cancer metastases same as uptake of nonradioactive iodine
Localization of iodide I 131 in thyroid allows thyroid uptake quantification and visualization of thyroid tissue; localization of iodide I 131 in functioning thyroid cancer metastases allows their detection, evaluation, and response to therapy
Small amounts of radioactivity used in diagnosis; radiation exposure is relatively low and considered safe

### Before having this test

» Conditions affecting use, especially:
  Pregnancy—Radioiodide crosses placenta; risk to fetus from radiation exposure as opposed to benefit derived from use should be considered
  Breast-feeding—Iodide I 131 is distributed into breast milk; complete cessation of nursing recommended for this infant when activity administered is large because of risk to infant from radiation exposure (present administration of I 131 will not affect breast-feeding of future infants)
  Use in children—Diagnostic benefit should be judged to outweigh potential risk of radiation

### Preparation for this test

Special preparatory instructions may apply; patient should inquire in advance

## General Dosing Information

Radiopharmaceuticals are to be administered only by or under the supervision of physicians who have had extensive training in the safe use and handling of radioactive materials and who are authorized by the appropriate Federal or state agency, if required, or, outside the U.S., the appropriate authority.

The estimated absorbed radiation dose to the thyroid is dependent on thyroidal uptake of radioiodine and the thyroid mass.

Adequate hydration of the patient is recommended before and after administration of sodium iodide I 131 to assure rapid elimination of the iodide that is not incorporated into the gland.

Uptake measurements are generally made at 4 and/or 24 hours, and thyroid imaging is usually performed 18 to 24 hours after sodium iodide I 131 administration. For imaging functioning metastatic thyroid tumor, imaging is usually performed 24 to 96 hours after sodium iodide I 131 administration.

### Safety considerations for handling this medication

Improper handling of this radiopharmaceutical may cause radioactive contamination. Guidelines for handling radioactive material have been prepared by scientific, professional, state, federal, and international bodies and are available to the specially qualified and authorized users who have access to radiopharmaceuticals.

## Oral Dosage Forms

### SODIUM IODIDE I 131 CAPSULES USP

**Usual adult administered activity**
Diagnostic aid—
 Thyroid uptake:
  Oral, 0.185 to 0.55 megabecquerel (5 to 15 microcuries).
  Note: Most uptake dosages of iodine I 131 are currently 0.55 megabecquerel (15 microcuries) or less. Only patients in whom hyperthyroidism is strongly suspected or in whom substernal thyroid nodules are likely would receive a dosage as high as 3.7 megabecquerels (100 microcuries).

Thyroid imaging:
    Oral, 1.85 to 3.7 megabecquerels (50 to 100 microcuries).
    Localization of thyroid tumor metastases—
        Oral, 37 to 370 megabecquerels (1 to 10 millicuries).

### Usual pediatric administered activity

Diagnostic aid—

Dosage must be individualized by physician.

For uptake studies, a minimum dosage of 0.037 megabecquerel (1 microcurie) and a maximum dosage of 0.55 megabecquerel (15 microcuries) have been used.

For thyroid imaging, a minimum dosage of 0.185 megabecquerel (5 microcuries) and a maximum of 1.3 megabecquerels (35 microcuries) for lingular thyroid have been used. For mediastinal mass, a minimum dosage of 0.55 megabecquerel (15 microcuries) and a maximum of 3.7 megabecquerels (100 microcuries) have been used.

Note: Sodium iodide I 123 or sodium pertechnetate Tc 99m (for thyroid imaging) may be preferable to sodium iodide I 131 because of its lower patient radiation doses. Sodium iodide I 123 may also be the radiopharmaceutical of choice in children who require diagnosis of thyroid function and imaging of the thyroid.

### Usual geriatric administered activity

See *Usual adult administered activity.*

### Strength(s) usually available

U.S.—

0.3, 0.5, 1.1, 2, and 3.7 megabecquerels (8, 15, 30, 50, and 100 microcuries, respectively) per capsule at time of calibration (Rx) [GENERIC].

Canada—

0.33, 0.61, 1.11, 2.03, and 3.70 megabecquerels (9, 16.5, 30, 55, and 100 microcuries, respectively) per capsule at time of calibration (Rx) [GENERIC].

### Packaging and storage

Store below 40 °C (104 °F), preferably between 15 and 30 °C (59 and 86 °F), unless otherwise specified by manufacturer. Store in a well-closed container.

### Note

Caution—Radioactive material.

## SODIUM IODIDE I 131 SOLUTION USP

### Usual adult administered activity

Diagnostic aid—

See *Sodium Iodide I 131 Capsules USP.*

### Usual pediatric administered activity

See *Sodium Iodide I 131 Capsules USP.*

### Usual geriatric administered activity

See *Usual adult administered activity.*

### Strength(s) usually available

U.S.—

Available in the U.S. for therapeutic use only.

Canada—

925 megabecquerels (25 millicuries) per 10-mL vial, at time of calibration (Rx) [GENERIC].

### Packaging and storage

Store below 40 °C (104 °F), preferably between 15 and 30 °C (59 and 86 °F), unless otherwise specified by manufacturer.

### Note

Caution—Radioactive material.

### Additional information

Radioiodide stock solutions and any dilutions thereof must be maintained at a pH of 7.5 to 9.0 in order to minimize oxidation of iodide to volatile forms of iodine. In addition, 0.2% sodium thiosulfate may be incorporated into these solutions if an antioxidant is desired.

### Selected Bibliography

Ross DS. Evaluation of the thyroid nodule. J Nucl Med 1991; 32 (11): 2181-92.

Revised: 09/02/94

---

# SODIUM IODIDE I 131  Systemic—Therapeutic

VA CLASSIFICATION (Primary): AN600

Note: For a listing of dosage forms and brand names by country availability, see *Dosage Forms* section(s). For a listing of brand names for the articles in this monograph, refer to the General Index.

## Category

Antihyperthyroid agent; Antineoplastic.

## Indications

### Accepted

Hyperthyroidism (treatment)—Sodium iodide I 131 is indicated for the treatment of diffuse toxic goiter (Graves' disease), single or multiple toxic nodular goiter, and recurrent hyperthyroidism following surgical or medical treatment. Sodium iodide I 131 may be used in patients of any age if medically appropriate.

Carcinoma, thyroid (treatment)—Sodium iodide I 131 is indicated for the treatment of functioning metastatic papillary or follicular carcinoma of the thyroid. The amount of sodium iodide I 131 used for the treatment of thyroid carcinoma is variable and depends upon the amount of normal thyroid tissue remaining and the extent of thyroid metastases and the degree to which they accumulate sodium iodide I 131.

## Physical Properties

### Nuclear data

| Radionuclide (half-life*) | Decay constant | Mode of decay | Principal emissions (keV) | Mean number of emissions/ disintegration |
|---|---|---|---|---|
| I 131 (8.08 days) | 0.00358 h⁻¹ | Beta | Beta (191.6) Gamma (364.5) | 0.90 0.81 |

*For therapeutic use: In the hyperthyroid patient, a percent of the administered dose equal to the fractional radioiodide uptake (usually between 35 and 90%) of the administered sodium iodide I 131 is concentrated in the thyroid gland and has an effective half-life of approximately 4 to 6 days. The non-thyroidal sodium iodide I 131 is distributed within the extracellular fluid and has an effective half-life of approximately 0.34 day.

## Pharmacology/Pharmacokinetics

### Mechanism of action/Effect

The action of therapeutic radioiodide is based on one of the normal functions of the thyroid gland, which is the accumulation and retention of iodine as required for the synthesis of thyroid hormones. Radioiodide may also be concentrated in papillary, follicular, or mixed papillary/follicular thyroid cancer and metastases, although to a lesser extent than in normal thyroid tissue. When large doses of sodium iodide I 131 are given orally, it is possible to selectively damage or destroy thyroidal tissue as required in the treatment of hyperthyroidism or thyroid carcinoma.

### Absorption

Readily absorbed from gastrointestinal tract.

### Distribution

Selectively concentrated and bound to tyrosyl residues of thyroglobulin in the thyroid gland; also concentrated, but not protein-bound, in the choroid plexus, gastric mucosa, salivary glands, nasal mucosa, and lactating breast tissue, with the remainder being distributed within the extracellular fluid.

### Half-life

Biological (for thyroid compartment)—
    Euthyroid: 80 days.
    Hyperthyroid: 5 to 40 days.

### Onset of therapeutic action

Approximately 2 to 4 weeks.

### Time to peak therapeutic effect

Approximately 2 to 4 months.

## Radiation dosimetry

| Organ | I 131 Estimated absorbed radiation dose*† | | |
|---|---|---|---|
| | Maximum thyroid uptake (%) | mGy/MBq | rad/mCi |
| Bladder wall | 0 | 0.61 | 2.26 |
| | 5 | 0.58 | 2.15 |
| | 15 | 0.52 | 1.93 |
| | 25 | 0.46 | 1.70 |
| | 55 | 0.29 | 1.07 |
| Uterus | 0 | 0.054 | 0.20 |
| | 5 | 0.055 | 0.20 |
| | 15 | 0.054 | 0.20 |
| | 25 | 0.052 | 0.19 |
| | 55 | 0.046 | 0.17 |
| Kidneys | 0 | 0.065 | 0.24 |
| | 5 | 0.063 | 0.24 |
| | 15 | 0.060 | 0.22 |
| | 25 | 0.058 | 0.21 |
| | 55 | 0.051 | 0.19 |
| Ovaries | 0 | 0.042 | 0.16 |
| | 5 | 0.044 | 0.16 |
| | 15 | 0.043 | 0.16 |
| | 25 | 0.043 | 0.16 |
| | 55 | 0.041 | 0.15 |
| Large intestine wall (lower) | 0 | 0.043 | 0.16 |
| | 5 | 0.043 | 0.16 |
| | 15 | 0.042 | 0.16 |
| | 25 | 0.041 | 0.15 |
| | 55 | 0.040 | 0.15 |
| Red marrow | 0 | 0.035 | 0.13 |
| | 5 | 0.038 | 0.14 |
| | 15 | 0.054 | 0.20 |
| | 25 | 0.070 | 0.26 |
| | 55 | 0.12 | 0.44 |
| Small intestine | 0 | 0.038 | 0.14 |
| | 5 | 0.28 | 1.04 |
| | 15 | 0.28 | 1.04 |
| | 25 | 0.28 | 1.04 |
| | 55 | 0.28 | 1.04 |
| Bone surfaces | 0 | 0.032 | 0.12 |
| | 5 | 0.032 | 0.12 |
| | 15 | 0.047 | 0.17 |
| | 25 | 0.061 | 0.23 |
| | 55 | 0.11 | 0.41 |
| Large intestine wall (upper) | 0 | 0.037 | 0.14 |
| | 5 | 0.059 | 0.22 |
| | 15 | 0.059 | 0.22 |
| | 25 | 0.059 | 0.22 |
| | 55 | 0.058 | 0.21 |
| Pancreas | 0 | 0.035 | 0.13 |
| | 5 | 0.050 | 0.19 |
| | 15 | 0.052 | 0.19 |
| | 25 | 0.053 | 0.20 |
| | 55 | 0.058 | 0.21 |
| Spleen | 0 | 0.034 | 0.13 |
| | 5 | 0.039 | 0.14 |
| | 15 | 0.042 | 0.16 |
| | 25 | 0.044 | 0.16 |
| | 55 | 0.051 | 0.19 |
| Adrenals | 0 | 0.037 | 0.14 |
| | 5 | 0.032 | 0.12 |
| | 15 | 0.036 | 0.13 |
| | 25 | 0.039 | 0.14 |
| | 55 | 0.049 | 0.18 |
| Testes | 0 | 0.037 | 0.14 |
| | 5 | 0.029 | 0.11 |
| | 15 | 0.028 | 0.10 |
| | 25 | 0.027 | 0.10 |
| | 55 | 0.026 | 0.10 |

| Organ | I 131 Estimated absorbed radiation dose*† | | |
|---|---|---|---|
| | Maximum thyroid uptake (%) | mGy/MBq | rad/mCi |
| Stomach wall | 0 | 0.034 | 0.13 |
| | 5 | 0.45 | 1.67 |
| | 15 | 0.46 | 1.67 |
| | 25 | 0.46 | 1.67 |
| | 55 | 0.46 | 1.67 |
| Liver | 0 | 0.033 | 0.12 |
| | 5 | 0.030 | 0.11 |
| | 15 | 0.032 | 0.12 |
| | 25 | 0.035 | 0.13 |
| | 55 | 0.043 | 0.16 |
| Lungs | 0 | 0.031 | 0.11 |
| | 5 | 0.034 | 0.13 |
| | 15 | 0.053 | 0.20 |
| | 25 | 0.072 | 0.27 |
| | 55 | 0.13 | 0.48 |
| Breast | 0 | 0.033 | 0.12 |
| | 5 | 0.031 | 0.11 |
| | 15 | 0.043 | 0.16 |
| | 25 | 0.055 | 0.20 |
| | 55 | 0.091 | 0.34 |
| Thyroid | 0 | 0.029 | 0.11 |
| | 5 | 72.00 | 266.67 |
| | 15 | 210.00 | 777.78 |
| | 25 | 360.00 | 1333.33 |
| | 55 | 790.00 | 2925.93 |
| Other tissue | 0 | 0.032 | 0.12 |
| | 5 | 0.040 | 0.15 |
| | 15 | 0.065 | 0.24 |
| | 25 | 0.090 | 0.33 |
| | 55 | 0.16 | 0.59 |

| Effective dose§ | | | | |
|---|---|---|---|---|
| Maximum Thyroid Uptake (%)‡ | | | | |
| 0 | 5 | 15 | 25 | 55 |
| mSv/MBq 0.072 | 2.3 | 6.6 | 11 | 24 |
| rem/mCi 0.27 | 8.51 | 24.42 | 40.7 | 88.8 |

*Data based on the International Commission on Radiological Protection (ICRP) Publication 53—Radiation Dose to Patients from Radiopharmaceuticals.

†Estimates based on intravenous administration. With oral administration there is a radiation dose to the stomach in addition to that due to iodide in gastric and salivary secretions. Assuming a mean residence time in the stomach of 30 minutes, the absorbed dose to the stomach wall is increased by approximately 30% with oral administration, while the dose to organs and tissues other than the stomach wall is not significantly changed.

‡With thyroid blocking, thyroid uptakes ranging from 0.5 to 2.0% will still occur. Under these circumstances, the effective dose to the adult will range from 0.30 to 0.97 mSv/MBq (1.11 to 3.59 rem/mCi) for I 131.

§The effective dose is virtually identical after oral or intravenous administration.

### Elimination
Renal—Primary, 50 to 75% of the administered activity eliminated in the urine of euthyroid patients with normal renal function within 48 hours.
Fecal and salivary—Secondary.
Breast milk—Up to 20% of administered activity appears in the milk within 24 hours.

## Precautions to Consider

### Carcinogenicity
Experiments in animals with sodium iodide I 131 have demonstrated that radioiodide administration can induce thyroid adenomas and carcinomas. However, studies in humans have shown no conclusive evidence of thyroid carcinoma in hyperthyroid patients treated with sodium iodide I 131.

Also, studies with sodium iodide I 131 have not demonstrated that leukemia occurs more frequently in patients treated with this medication than in other hyperthyroid patients.

**Mutagenicity**

Mutagenic effects have not been clearly established in clinical studies of patients treated with sodium iodide I 131. However, chromosomal changes have been reported in laboratory studies.

**Pregnancy/Reproduction**

Fertility—A follow-up study of 627 women treated for differentiated thyroid carcinoma with sodium iodide I 131 revealed no evidence of fertility impairment.

Pregnancy—Iodide I 131 crosses the placenta and may cause severe and irreversible hypothyroidism in the neonate; the fetal thyroid begins to concentrate iodine during approximately the 12th week of gestation. Sodium iodide I 131 is contraindicated for the treatment of disease during pregnancy.

To avoid the possibility of fetal exposure to radiation, in those circumstances where the patient's pregnancy status is uncertain a pregnancy test should be performed and will help to prevent inadvertent administration of this preparation during pregnancy.

Studies have not been done in animals.

FDA Pregnancy Category X.

**Breast-feeding**

Radioiodide is distributed into breast milk and may reach concentrations equal to or greater than concentrations in maternal plasma. It has been recommended that nursing be resumed after administration of a radiopharmaceutical, when the likelihood of the infant's ingested effective dose equivalent (EDE) is below 1 mSv (100 mrem). A method to calculate the EDE has been proposed based on the effective half-life of the radionuclide, the activity administered to the mother, the fraction of administered activity ingested by the infant, and the total body effective dose equivalent to the newborn infant per unit of activity ingested. According to this method, it has been estimated that the time to reduce the EDE to the infant to below 1 mSv (100 mrem) is approximately 10 weeks after administration of 40 megabecquerels (1.08 millicuries) of sodium iodide I 131 to the mother. Because of the difficulty of maintaining the maternal milk supply for such an extended period of time, complete cessation of nursing is usually recommended. Also, to minimize the absorbed radiation dose to the breast tissue and to ensure that mammary secretory activity has ceased, breast-feeding should be discontinued several weeks before starting treatment with sodium iodide I 131.

**Pediatrics**

There is no conclusive evidence linking carcinogenicity, leukemogenicity, and mutagenicity to radioiodide therapy in children and growing adolescents.

Retrospective studies in children and adolescents treated with sodium iodide I 131 for hyperthyroidism have shown that sodium iodide I 131 is effective for both the initial treatment of hyperthyroidism and in cases in which other treatment modalities have failed. However, the occurrence of vomiting in the early post-treatment period may present management problems in some pediatric patients.

**Geriatrics**

Geriatric patients with severe thyrotoxic cardiac disease should be given antithyroid agents and/or beta-blockers, such as propranolol, for 4 to 6 weeks prior to treatment with radioiodide to help reduce possible aggravation of the condition by radiation thyroiditis. Antithyroid drugs must be discontinued at least 3 to 4 days prior to treatment and should not be readministered until 1 week after treatment. However, a beta-blocker may be used throughout the treatment period if needed.

**Drug interactions and/or related problems**

The following drug interactions and/or related problems have been selected on the basis of their potential clinical significance (possible mechanism in parentheses where appropriate)—not necessarily inclusive (» = major clinical significance):

Amiodarone or

Antithyroid preparations—thioamide derivatives or aromatic preparations or

Benzodiazepines or

Contrast media, iodinated or

Corticosteroids or

Goitrogenic foods (e.g., cabbage, turnips) or

Iodine-containing foods or

Iodine-containing preparations or

Iodine-contaminated bromides or

Iodine, stable or

Monovalent anions (e.g., perchlorate, thiocyanate) or

Pyrazolone derivatives, such as phenylbutazone or

Salicylates, chronic administration of or

Salt, iodized, excessive intake of or

Thiopental or

Thyroid blocking agents, such as strong iodine solution, potassium iodide, or potassium perchlorate or

Thyroid preparations, natural or synthetic

   (may decrease thyroidal uptake of iodide I 131; it is recommended that these medications or preparations be withheld for the following periods of time prior to administration of sodium iodide I 131: 1 week for corticosteroids; 4 weeks for benzodiazepines; 2 to 4 weeks for intravascular iodinated contrast media and more than 4 weeks for cholecystographic agents; 2 to 4 weeks for iodine-containing preparations, such as vitamins, expectorants, antitussives, and topical medications; 1 to 2 weeks for pyrazolone derivatives; 1 week for thiopental; 4 to 6 weeks for thyroxine and 2 to 3 weeks for triiodothyronine)

   (a rebound effect may occur following the sudden withdrawal of antithyroid preparations, resulting in a period of up to 5 days of very high thyroidal uptake; it is recommended that antithyroid medications be discontinued 3 to 4 days prior to administration of sodium iodide I 131)

   (chronic salicylate administration may cause a depression of thyroid function; salicylate therapy should be discontinued at least 1 to 2 weeks prior to sodium iodide I 131 administration; however, a rebound effect may also occur following discontinuation of salicylate therapy, resulting in a period of 3 to 10 days of increased thyroidal uptake)

Bone marrow depressants, other (See *Appendix II*)

   (concurrent use may rarely increase the bone marrow depressant effects of these medications and radiation therapy; dosage reduction of other bone marrow depressant medications may be required)

**Medical considerations/Contraindications**

The medical considerations/contraindications included here have been selected on the basis of their potential clinical significance (reasons given in parentheses where appropriate)—not necessarily inclusive (» = major clinical significance).

*Risk-benefit should be considered when the following medical problems exist:*

Diarrhea or

Vomiting

   (radiation exposure and loss of therapeutic dose may result)

Low serum chlorides or

Nephrosis

   (may increase thyroidal uptake of iodide I 131)

Renal function impairment

   (may decrease excretion of radioiodide, resulting in increased radiation exposure)

Sensitivity to the radiopharmaceutical preparation

Thyrotoxic cardiac disease, severe, especially in the elderly

   (hyperthyroidism may be aggravated by radiation thyroiditis if antithyroid agents and/or beta-blockers, such as propranolol, are not given prior to and after treatment)

**Patient monitoring**

The following may be especially important in patient monitoring (other tests may be warranted in some patients, depending on condition; » = major clinical significance):

Thyroid hormones, serum

   (determinations of serum concentrations are recommended every 2 to 3 months during the first year after treatment of hyperthyroidism, and annually thereafter, since hypothyroidism may occur several years after treatment)

## Side/Adverse Effects

Note: The incidence of hypothyroidism following the treatment of Graves' disease is approximately 15 to 25% in the first post-treatment year and increases approximately 2 to 3% per year thereafter. The greater the life expectancy of the patient following treatment, the greater the risk of developing hypothyroidism.

The following side/adverse effects have been selected on the basis of their potential clinical significance (possible signs and symptoms in parentheses where appropriate)—not necessarily inclusive:

**Those indicating need for medical attention**
*Hypothyroidism* (changes in menstrual periods; clumsiness; coldness; drowsiness; dry, puffy skin; headache; listlessness; muscle aches; temporary thinning of hair [may occur 2 to 3 months after treatment]; unusual tiredness or weakness; weight gain)—dose-dependent

Note: *Hypothyroidism* may occur several years following successful treatment of hyperthyroidism; therefore, annual blood tests for thyroid hormone concentration are recommended.

Incidence rare
*Following treatment of hyperthyroidism*
*Exaggerated hyperthyroid state* (excessive sweating, fast heartbeat, fever, palpitations, unusual irritability or unusual tiredness)—due to radiation thyroiditis

*Following treatment of thyroid carcinoma*
*Leukopenia* (cough or hoarseness; fever or chills; lower back or side pain, painful or difficult urination); *thrombocytopenia* (unusual bleeding or bruising; black, tarry stools; blood in urine or stools; pinpoint red spots on skin)

**Those indicating need for medical attention only if they continue or are bothersome**
Incidence less frequent
*Following treatment of hyperthyroidism or thyroid carcinoma*
*Radiation thyroiditis* (neck tenderness or swelling or sore throat)

*Following treatment of thyroid carcinoma*
*Temporary loss of taste; radiation gastritis* (temporary nausea and vomiting); *radiation sialadenitis* (tenderness of salivary glands)

## Patient Consultation

As an aid to patient consultation, refer to *Advice for the Patient, Sodium Iodide I 131 (Therapeutic)*.

In providing consultation, consider emphasizing the following selected information (» = major clinical significance):

**Description of use**
Action in the body: Radioiodide uptake by the thyroid and functioning thyroid cancer metastases same as uptake of nonradioactive iodine
Large doses are used therapeutically to damage or destroy thyroidal tissue in management of hyperthyroidism or thyroid carcinoma

**Before using this medication**
» Conditions affecting use, especially:
Pregnancy—Radioiodide crosses placenta; risk to fetus from radiation exposure; use contraindicated because of possibility of causing hypothyroidism in newborn
Breast-feeding—Distributed into breast milk; complete cessation of nursing recommended because of risk to infant from radiation exposure; possibility of causing hypothyroidism in newborn
Use in children—Vomiting may present management problems in some children

**Proper use of this medication**
Special preparatory instructions may apply; patient should inquire in advance

**Precautions after using this medication**
*Following treatment of hyperthyroidism or thyroid carcinoma*
To prevent radiation contamination of other persons or environment: For 48 to 96 hours after receiving radioiodide—
» Not kissing anyone and not handling or using another person's eating or drinking utensils, toothbrush, or bathroom glass
» Not engaging in sexual activities
» Avoiding close and prolonged contact with others, especially children and pregnant women
Sleeping alone
» Washing sink and tub after use (including brushing teeth)
» Washing hands after using or cleaning toilet
Using separate towels and washcloths
Laundering clothes and linens separately
» Double-flushing toilet

To decrease radiation exposure to the urinary bladder: Increasing intake of fluids to promote more frequent voiding to help eliminate radioactive iodine
*Following treatment of hyperthyroidism*
Periodic blood tests to check thyroid hormone concentration

**Side/adverse effects**
Signs of potential side effects, especially hypothyroidism or hyperthyroid state (following treatment of hyperthyroidism); leukopenia and thrombocytopenia (following treatment of thyroid carcinoma)

## General Dosing Information

Radiopharmaceuticals are to be administered only by or under the supervision of physicians who have had extensive training in the safe use and handling of radioactive materials and who are authorized by the Nuclear Regulatory Commission (NRC) or appropriate state agency, or, outside the U.S., the appropriate authority.

Adequate hydration of the patient is recommended before and after administration of radioiodide to assure rapid elimination of the iodide that is not incorporated into the gland.

The radiation dose to the thyroid gland from sodium iodide I 131 is dependent upon the uptake as well as the size of the gland and the amount of radioiodide administered. Thyroidal uptake and size should be determined by the physician prior to treatment and may be useful in calculating the therapeutic dose.

**Safety considerations for handling this medication**
Guidelines for the receipt, storage, handling, dispensing, and disposal of radioactive materials are available from scientific, professional, state, federal, and international bodies. Handling of this radiopharmaceutical should be limited to those individuals who are appropriately qualified and authorized.
Safety considerations for patients after treatment—
Large amount of radioactivity may be excreted in the urine, feces, perspiration, saliva, and on the skin of patients treated with radioiodide. This may present a contamination hazard during hospitalization and after discharge (current Nuclear Regulatory Commission [NRC] regulations require a hospital stay until the retained radioactivity is less than 1.1 gigabecquerels [30 millicuries] or until the measured dose rate from the patient is less than 0.05 millisieverts [mSv] [5 millirems (mrem)] per hour at a distance of one meter). For this reason:
• Patients need to be instructed at time of discharge in techniques to prevent transfer of radioactivity to family members and the environment after release from the hospital.
• For most radioiodide thyroid carcinoma therapy patients, close contact with other persons may be resumed 2 to 4 days after release from the hospital; the time period may be longer for hyperthyroid therapy patients since the excretion of radioiodide in these patients is not as rapid as in the thyroid carcinoma patients.

## Oral Dosage Forms
### SODIUM IODIDE I 131 CAPSULES USP

**Usual adult and adolescent administered activity**
Disease therapy—
Antihyperthyroid agent:
Oral, 148 to 370 megabecquerels (4 to 10 millicuries).
Note: The administered activity is usually individualized based on the estimated weight of the patient's thyroid gland and measurement of the 24-hour radioiodide uptake.

Toxic nodular goiter and other serious thyroid conditions may require larger dosages (e.g., 555 to 1110 megabecquerels [15 to 30 millicuries]).
Antineoplastic:
Ablation of normal thyroid tissue—
Oral, 1.85 gigabecquerels (50 millicuries), with a range of 1.1 to 3.7 gigabecquerels (30 to 100 millicuries).
Subsequent therapy for metastases—
Oral, 3.7 to 7.4 gigabecquerels (100 to 200 millicuries).

**Usual pediatric administered activity**
Dosage must be individualized by physician.

**Usual geriatric administered activity**
See *Usual adult and adolescent administered activity.*

**Strength(s) usually available**
U.S.—
28 megabecquerels to 3.7 gigabecquerels (0.75 to 100 millicuries) per capsule at time of calibration (Rx) [GENERIC].

37 megabecquerels to 1.85 gigabecquerels (1 to 50 millicuries) per capsule at time of calibration (Rx) [*Iodotope*].

37 megabecquerels to 4.81 gigabecquerels (1 to 130 millicuries) per capsule at time of calibration (Rx) [*Iodotope*].

Canada—
Each gelatin capsule contains an individually dispensed dose of sodium iodide I 131 as prescribed (Rx) [GENERIC].

### Packaging and storage
Store between 15 and 30 °C (59 and 86 °F), unless otherwise specified by manufacturer. Store in a well-closed container.

### Note
Caution—Radioactive material.

## SODIUM IODIDE I 131 SOLUTION USP

### Usual adult and adolescent administered activity
See *Sodium Iodide I 131 Capsules USP*.

### Usual pediatric administered activity
See *Sodium Iodide I 131 Capsules USP*.

### Usual geriatric administered activity
See *Usual adult and adolescent administered activity*.

### Strength(s) usually available
U.S.—
129.5 megabecquerels to 5.5 gigabecquerels (3.5 to 150 millicuries) per vial at time of calibration (Rx) [GENERIC (sodium bisulfite 0.1%, edetate disodium 0.2%)].

259 megabecquerels to 3.93 gigabecquerels (7 to 106 millicuries) per vial at time of calibration (Rx) [*Iodotope* (edetate disodium 1 mg per mL)].

Canada—
Each vial contains an individually dispensed dose of sodium iodide I 131 as prescribed (Rx) [GENERIC].

### Packaging and storage
Store between 15 and 30 °C (59 and 86 °F), unless otherwise specified by manufacturer.

### Note
Caution—Radioactive material.

### Additional information
Radioiodide stock solutions and any dilutions thereof must be maintained at a pH of 7.5 to 9.0 in order to minimize oxidation of iodide to volatile forms of iodine. Additionally, 0.2% sodium thiosulfate may be incorporated into these solutions if an antioxidant is desired.

### Selected Bibliography
Sugrue D, McEvoy M, Feely J, et al. Hyperthyroidism in the land of Graves', results of treatment by surgery, radioiodine, and carbimazole in 837 patients. Q J Med 1980; 49: 51-61.

Levetan C, Wartofsky L. A clinical guide to the management of Graves' disease with radioactive iodine. Endocr Pract 1995; 1: 205-12.

Revised: 07/15/96

---

# SODIUM NITRITE  Systemic

VA CLASSIFICATION (Primary): AD200

Note: For a listing of dosage forms and brand names by country availability, see *Dosage Forms* section(s). For a listing of brand names for the articles in this monograph, refer to the General Index.

---

## Category
Antidote (to cyanide poisoning).

## Indications

### Accepted
Toxicity, cyanide (treatment adjunct)—Sodium nitrite, in conjunction with sodium thiosulfate, is indicated for use as an antidote in the treatment of cyanide poisoning.

## Pharmacology/Pharmacokinetics

### Physicochemical characteristics
Molecular weight—69.
pH—Between 7 and 9.

### Mechanism of action/Effect
Antidote (to cyanide poisoning)—Sodium nitrite promotes formation of methemoglobin, which combines with cyanide to form nontoxic cyanmethemoglobin.

### Other actions/effects
Sodium nitrite produces vasodilation by relaxing vascular smooth muscle.

### Time to peak effect
30 to 70 minutes after injection.

## Precautions to Consider

### Pregnancy/Reproduction
Problems in humans have not been documented.

### Breast-feeding
It is not known whether sodium nitrite is distributed into breast milk.

### Pediatrics
Appropriate studies performed to date have not demonstrated pediatrics-specific problems that would limit the usefulness of sodium nitrite in children.

### Geriatrics
Appropriate studies performed to date have not demonstrated geriatrics-specific problems that would limit the usefulness of sodium nitrite in the elderly.

### Medical considerations/Contraindications
The medical considerations/contraindications included here have been selected on the basis of their potential clinical significance (reasons given in parentheses where appropriate)—not necessarily inclusive (» = major clinical significance).

*Risk-benefit should be considered when the following medical problems exist:*
» Methemoglobinemia, acquired or congenital
  (may be exacerbated)
Sensitivity to sodium nitrite

### Patient monitoring
The following may be especially important in patient monitoring (other tests may be warranted in some patients, depending on condition; » = major clinical significance):

Arterial blood gas determinations
  (recommended frequently during administration of 100% oxygen and when attempting to correct severe metabolic acidosis)

Blood pressure determinations
  (recommended to guide the rate of administration of sodium nitrite; rapid administration may result in excessive vasodilation and hypotension)

» Methemoglobin concentrations
  (recommended periodically during administration to ensure that the methemoglobin concentration does not exceed 40% in adults or 30% in children)

## Side/Adverse Effects
The following side/adverse effects have been selected on the basis of their potential clinical significance (possible signs and symptoms in parentheses where appropriate)—not necessarily inclusive:

### Those indicating need for medical attention
Incidence more frequent
  *Hypotension; vasodilation, excessive*—caused by rapid administration

### Those indicating need for medical attention only if they continue or are bothersome
Incidence more frequent
  *Nausea or vomiting*

## Overdose
For specific information on the agents used in the management of sodium nitrite overdose, see *Methylene Blue (Systemic)* monograph.

For more information on the management of overdose, **contact a Poison Control Center** (see *Poison Control Center Listing*).

**Clinical effects of overdose**

The following effects have been selected on the basis of their potential clinical significance (possible signs and symptoms in parentheses where appropriate)—not necessarily inclusive (in order of occurrence):

*Cyanosis* (bluish fingernails, lips, or skin); *headache; unusual tiredness or weakness; tachycardia; shortness of breath; dizziness, extreme, or fainting; coma*

Note: *Cyanosis* may occur at blood methemoglobin concentrations of 15%; however, symptoms usually do not appear until concentrations reach 30 to 40%.

**Treatment of overdose**

Specific treatment—Intravenous administration of methylene blue in a dose of 1 to 2 mg per kg of body weight (mg/kg) given over five to ten minutes. The dose may be repeated after one hour if necessary, but the total dose should not exceed 7 mg/kg. Extreme caution should be exercised when administering methylene blue to patients likely to have substantial amounts of cyanide bound to methemoglobin because methylene blue increases cyanide release.

Supportive care—Oxygen inhalation and transfusion of fresh whole blood should be considered.

# General Dosing Information

Cyanide poisoning is rapidly fatal. Inhalation of cyanide gas produces symptoms of cyanide toxicity within seconds, followed by death within minutes. Oral ingestion of cyanide produces symptoms of toxicity within minutes, followed by death within minutes or hours. Blood cyanide concentrations often are not available for several hours. Therefore, therapy should be instituted immediately based upon reasonable suspicion of cyanide toxicity.

Supportive therapy includes moving the patient to an uncontaminated area and/or removing contaminated clothing; administering 100% oxygen; controlling seizures with anticonvulsants; correcting metabolic acidosis with bicarbonate; and supporting pulse and blood pressure with fluids, atropine, or vasopressors. These measures alone may allow survival in relatively mild cases of cyanide toxicity.

In more severe cases of cyanide toxicity, chances of survival are increased by specific antidote administration. Antidotal therapy should be started by breaking an amyl nitrite inhalant, holding it in front of the patient's mouth, and allowing the patient to inhale for 15 seconds. The inhalant should then be taken away for 15 seconds. This procedure may be repeated until an intravenous line is established and sodium nitrite is prepared. Amyl nitrite should not be administered if an intravenous line already has been established and the sodium nitrite is readily available. Amyl nitrite, if given, should then be discontinued and sodium nitrite administered. Immediately following the injection of sodium nitrite, sodium thiosulfate should be administered intravenously in a dose of 12.5 grams (50 mL of a 25% solution) (for adults) and

412.5 mg per kg of body weight or 7 grams per square meter of body surface area (for children), at a rate of 0.625 to 1.25 grams (2.5 to 5 mL) per minute.

If signs of cyanide toxicity are still present 2 hours following administration of sodium nitrite and sodium thiosulfate, administration of both may be repeated at one-half the original dose.

If cyanide was ingested, gastric lavage should follow antidotal therapy.

# Parenteral Dosage Forms

## SODIUM NITRITE INJECTION USP

**Usual adult and adolescent dose**

Cyanide toxicity—

Intravenous, 300 mg (10 mL of a 3% solution) administered at a rate of 75 to 150 mg (2.5 to 5 mL) per minute.

**Usual pediatric dose**

Cyanide toxicity—

Intravenous, 6 mg (0.2 mL) per kg of body weight or approximately 180 to 240 mg (6 to 8 mL) per square meter of body surface area administered at a rate of 75 to 150 mg (2.5 to 5 mL) per minute.

**Usual pediatric prescribing limits**

300 mg (10 mL).

**Strength(s) usually available**

U.S.—

300 mg per 10 mL (Rx) [GENERIC].

Canada—

300 mg per 10 mL (Rx) [GENERIC].

Note: Sodium nitrite is a component of the *Cyanide Antidote Package*. Also contained in the kit are: amyl nitrite inhalants (0.3 mL) and sodium thiosulfate injection (12.5 grams per 50 mL).

**Packaging and storage**

Store below 40 °C (104 °F), preferably between 15 and 30 °C (59 and 86 °F), unless otherwise specified by manufacturer.

**Stability**

The components of the *Cyanide Antidote Package* contain preservatives, which allow the unopened solutions to remain stable for several years. However, the expiration date of the kit should be observed.

# Selected Bibliography

Hall AH, Rumack BH. Clinical toxicology of cyanide. Ann Emerg Med 1986; 15: 1067-74.

Baskin SI, Horowitz AM, Nealley EW. The antidotal action of sodium nitrite and sodium thiosulfate against cyanide poisoning. J Clin Pharmacol 1992; 32: 368-75.

Revised: 03/24/94

---

# SODIUM PERTECHNETATE Tc 99m     Mucosal-Local

VA CLASSIFICATION (Primary): DX201

Note: For information on sodium pertechnetate Tc 99m injection for intravenous administration, see *Sodium Pertechnetate Tc 99m (Systemic)*.

For information on sodium pertechnetate Tc 99m injection for ophthalmic administration, see *Sodium Pertechnetate Tc 99m (Ophthalmic)*.

Note: For a listing of dosage forms and brand names by country availability, see *Dosage Forms* section(s). For a listing of brand names for the articles in this monograph, refer to the General Index.

# Category

Diagnostic aid, radioactive (urinary bladder disorders).

# Indications

**Accepted**

Urinary bladder imaging, radionuclide—Sodium pertechnetate Tc 99m is indicated in direct isotopic cystography for the detection of vesicoureteral reflux.

# Physical Properties

**Nuclear data**

| Radionuclide (half-life) | Decay constant | Mode of decay | Principal photon emissions (keV) | Mean number of emissions/ disintegration ($\geq 0.01$) |
|---|---|---|---|---|
| Tc 99m (6.0 hr) | 0.1151 hr$^{-1}$ | Isomeric transition to Tc 99 | Gamma (18) | 0.062 |
| | | | Gamma (140.5) | 0.891 |

# Pharmacology/Pharmacokinetics

**Mechanism of action/Effect**

Urinary bladder imaging—Sodium pertechnetate Tc 99m is confined within the urinary tract after direct instillation via catheter into the bladder. The dynamic sequence of filling and voiding is recorded on film and/or digital device; reflux activity into the ureters and/or renal collecting system during filling and voiding can thus be detected.

**Elimination**

Direct intraurethral instillation—Almost total with normal micturition.

# Precautions to Consider

## Pregnancy/Reproduction

Pregnancy—Although systemic absorption of sodium pertechnetate is minimal with intraurethral administration, fetal exposure to radiation may result from radioactivity localized in the bladder. Adequate and well-controlled studies with sodium pertechnetate Tc 99m have not been done in humans. The possibility of pregnancy should be assessed in women of child-bearing potential. Clinical situations exist in which the benefit to the patient and fetus derived from information from radiopharmaceutical use outweighs the risks from fetal exposure to radiation. In these situations, the physician should use discretion and reduce the administered activity of the radiopharmaceutical to the lowest possible amount.

Studies have not been done in animals.

FDA Pregnancy Category C.

## Breast-feeding

Although Tc 99m is known to be distributed into breast milk, discontinuation of breast-feeding is generally not required because systemic absorption of sodium pertechnetate Tc 99m after intraurethral administration is minimal. Also, the activity administered for this procedure is much less than that used for other procedures.

## Pediatrics

Diagnostic studies performed to date using sodium pertechnetate Tc 99m have not demonstrated pediatrics-specific problems that would limit its usefulness in children. Risk of radiation exposure as opposed to benefit derived from use should be considered.

## Geriatrics

Although appropriate studies on the relationship of age to the effects of sodium pertechnetate Tc 99m have not been performed in the geriatric population, no geriatrics-specific problems have been documented to date.

## Medical considerations/Contraindications

The medical considerations/contraindications included here have been selected on the basis of their potential clinical significance (reasons given in parentheses where appropriate)—not necessarily inclusive (» = major clinical significance).

*Except under special circumstances, this medication should not be used when the following medical problems exist:*

» Obstruction to urethral catheterization, such as in extensive urinary tuberculosis, bladder tumors, urethral obstructions, and prostate enlargement

» Urinary tract infection, upper, acute
  (procedure may increase risk of complications)

# Side/Adverse Effects

There are no known side/adverse effects associated with the intraurethral use of sodium pertechnetate Tc 99m as a diagnostic aid.

# Patient Consultation

As an aid to patient consultation, refer to *Advice for the Patient, Radiopharmaceuticals (Diagnostic).*

In providing consultation, consider emphasizing the following selected information (» = major clinical significance):

## Description of use
*Actions in the body*
  Direct instillation into bladder allows recording of dynamic sequence of filling and voiding to detect vesico-ureteral reflux
  Small amounts of radioactivity used in diagnosis; radiation exposure is low and considered safe

## Before having this test
» Conditions affecting use, especially:
  Pregnancy—Risk to fetus from radiation exposure as opposed to benefit derived from use should be considered
  Use in children—Risk of radiation exposure as opposed to benefit derived from use should be considered

Other medical problems, especially obstruction or acute upper urinary tract infection

## Preparation for this test
Special preparatory instructions may be given; patient should inquire in advance

# General Dosing Information

Radiopharmaceuticals are to be administered only by or under the supervision of physicians who have had extensive training in the safe use and handling of radioactive materials and who are authorized by the Nuclear Regulatory Commission (NRC) or the appropriate Agreement State agency or, outside the U.S., the appropriate authority.

Manufacturer's package insert or other appropriate literature should be consulted for optimal times when imaging should be performed.

## Safety considerations for handling this medication
Improper handling of this radiopharmaceutical may cause radioactive contamination. Guidelines for handling radioactive material have been prepared by scientific, professional, state, federal, and international bodies and are available to the specially qualified and authorized users who have access to radiopharmaceuticals.

# Mucosal-Local Dosage Forms

## SODIUM PERTECHNETATE Tc 99m INJECTION USP

**Usual adult and adolescent administered activity**
Urinary bladder imaging—
  Intraurethral instillation via catheter, 18.5 to 37 megabecquerels (0.5 to 1 millicurie).

**Usual pediatric administered activity**
See *Usual adult and adolescent administered activity.*

**Usual geriatric administered activity**
See *Usual adult and adolescent administered activity.*

**Strength(s) usually available**
U.S.—
  740 megabecquerels to 3.7 gigabecquerels (20 to 100 millicuries) per mL at time of calibration.

  Note: Sodium pertechnetate Tc 99m injection is supplied as a molybdenum Mo 99/technetium Tc 99m generator in sizes of Mo 99 ranging from 30.7 to 614.2 gigabecquerels (830 to 16,600 millicuries); 9.25 to 111 gigabecquerels (250 to 3000 millicuries) [*Ultra-TechneKow FM* ]; or 8.3 to 100 gigabecquerels (225 to 2700 millicuries) [*TechneLite* ]. Each eluate of the generator should not contain more than the USP limit of 0.15 kilobecquerel of molybdenum Mo 99 per megabecquerel of technetium Tc 99m (0.15 microcurie Mo 99 per millicurie Tc 99m) per administered activity at the time of administration.

Canada—
  Sodium pertechnetate Tc 99m injection is supplied as a molybdenum Mo 99/technetium Tc 99m generator in sizes of Mo 99 ranging from 8.3 to 100 gigabecquerels (225 to 2700 millicuries). Each eluate of the generator should not contain more than the Canadian Regulatory limit of 1.1 kilobecquerels of molybdenum Mo 99 per 37 megabecquerels of technetium Tc 99m (0.03 microcurie Mo 99 per millicurie Tc 99m) per administered activity at the time of administration.

**Packaging and storage**
Store below 40 °C (104 °F), preferably between 15 and 30 °C (59 and 86 °F), unless otherwise specified by manufacturer. Protect from freezing.

**Stability**
Generator eluate does not contain an antimicrobial agent, and thus should be used within 12 hours from the time of generator elution.

**Note**
Caution—Radioactive material.

Developed: 08/30/94

# SODIUM PERTECHNETATE Tc 99m    Ophthalmic

VA CLASSIFICATION (Primary): DX201

Note: For information on sodium pertechnetate Tc 99m injection for oral or parenteral administration see *Sodium Pertechnetate Tc 99m (Systemic)*.

For information on sodium pertechnetate Tc 99m injection for intraurethral administration, see *Sodium Pertechnetate Tc 99m (Mucosal-Local)*.

Note: For a listing of dosage forms and brand names by country availability, see *Dosage Forms* section(s). For a listing of brand names for the articles in this monograph, refer to the General Index.

## Category

Diagnostic aid, radioactive (nasolacrimal disorders).

## Indications

### Accepted

Dacryoscintigraphy—Sodium pertechnetate Tc 99m is indicated for imaging the nasolacrimal drainage system in adults.

## Physical Properties

### Nuclear data

| Radionu-clide (half-life) | Decay constant | Mode of decay | Principal photon emissions (keV) | Mean number of emissions/ disintegration ($\geq 0.01$) |
|---|---|---|---|---|
| Tc 99m (6.0 hr) | 0.1151 h$^{-1}$ | Isomeric transition to Tc 99 | Gamma 18 | 0.062 |
| | | | Gamma 140.5 | 0.889 |

## Pharmacology/Pharmacokinetics

### Mechanism of action/Effect

Sodium pertechnetate Tc 99m, when administered as eye drops, mixes with tears within the conjunctival space and follows the same path as tears through the nasolacrimal drainage system. Thus, any anatomical or functional blockage of the draining system will be visualized.

### Absorption

Minimal transconjunctival absorption after instillation in eye.

### Distribution

Distributed within conjunctival space; passes into the inferior meatus of the nose through the nasolacrimal drainage system.

### Radiation dosimetry

Following ophthalmic administration of sodium pertechnetate Tc 99m, the estimated absorbed radiation doses to an adult are:

Eye lens—

If lacrimal fluid turnover is 16% per minute: 0.04 mGy/megabecquerel (0.14 mrad/microcurie).

If lacrimal fluid turnover is 100% per minute: 0.006 mGy/megabecquerel (0.02 mrad/microcurie).

If drainage system is blocked: 1.09 mGy/megabecquerel (4.04 mrads/microcurie).

Ovaries (no blockage of drainage system)—0.008 mGy/megabecquerel (0.03 mrad/microcurie).

Testes (no blockage of drainage system)—0.002 mGy/megabecquerel (0.009 mrad/microcurie).

Thyroid (no blockage of drainage system)—0.04 mGy/megabecquerel (0.13 mrad/microcurie).

### Elimination

Most of Tc 99m escapes within a few minutes of normal drainage and tearing.

## Precautions to Consider

### Pregnancy/Reproduction

Pregnancy—Transconjunctival absorption of sodium pertechnetate Tc 99m is minimal. However, studies have not been done in humans. Studies have not been done in animals.

FDA Pregnancy Category C.

### Breast-feeding

Although transconjunctival absorption of sodium pertechnetate Tc 99m is minimal, risk-benefit must be considered since Tc 99m is known to be distributed into breast milk.

### Pediatrics

Appropriate studies on the relationship of age to the effects of sodium pertechnetate Tc 99m have not been performed in children.

### Geriatrics

Appropriate studies on the relationship of age to the effects of sodium pertechnetate Tc 99m have not been performed in the geriatric population. However, no geriatrics-specific problems have been documented to date.

## Side/Adverse Effects

There are no known side/adverse effects associated with the ophthalmic use of sodium pertechnetate Tc 99m as a diagnostic aid.

## Patient Consultation

As an aid to patient consultation, refer to *Advice for the Patient, Radiopharmaceuticals (Diagnostic)*.

In providing consultation, consider emphasizing the following selected information ($\gg$ = major clinical significance):

### Description of use

Action in the body: Transit through nasolacrimal drainage system allows visualization to detect blockage within

Small amounts of radioactivity used in diagnosis; radiation exposure is low and considered safe

### Before having this test

$\gg$ Conditions affecting use, especially:

Breast-feeding—Tc 99m distributed into breast milk

### Preparation for this test

Special preparatory instructions may be given; patient should inquire in advance

### Precautions after having this test

Blowing nose and rinsing eyes to minimize radiation exposure

## General Dosing Information

Radiopharmaceuticals are to be administered only by or under the supervision of physicians who have had extensive training in the safe use and handling of radionuclides and who are licensed by the Nuclear Regulatory Commission (NRC) or the appropriate Agreement State agency or, outside the U.S., the appropriate authority.

Sodium pertechnetate Tc 99m should be instilled into the eye by using a micropipette or a similar method of administration that ensures the accuracy of the dose.

Blowing the nose and rinsing the eyes with sterile distilled water or an isotonic sodium chloride solution is recommended after the nasolacrimal imaging procedures to minimize the absorbed radiation dose.

### Safety considerations for handling this radiopharmaceutical

Improper handling of this radiopharmaceutical may cause radioactive contamination. Guidelines for handling radioactive material have been prepared by scientific, professional, state, federal, and international bodies and are available to the specially qualified and authorized users who have access to radiopharmaceuticals.

## Ophthalmic Dosage Forms

### SODIUM PERTECHNETATE Tc 99m INJECTION USP

**Usual adult and adolescent administered activity**

Topical, to the conjunctiva, 3.7 megabecquerels (100 microcuries).

**Usual geriatric administered activity**

See *Usual adult and adolescent administered activity*.

**Strength(s) usually available**

U.S.—

740 megabecquerels to 3.7 gigabecquerels (20 to 100 millicuries) per mL at time of calibration (Rx).

Sodium pertechnetate Tc 99m injection is supplied as a Molybdenum Mo 99/Technetium Tc 99m generator in sizes of Mo 99 ranging from 30.7 to 614.2 gigabecquerels (830 to 16,600 millicuries); or 9.25 to 111 gigabecquerels (250 to 3000 millicuries) [*Ultra-TechneKow FM* ]; or 8.3 to 100 gigabecquerels (225 to 2700 millicuries) [*TechneLite* ]. Each eluate of the generator should not contain more than the USP limit of 0.15 kilobecquerel of molybdenum Mo 99 per megabecquerel of technetium Tc 99m (0.15 microcurie Mo 99 per millicurie Tc 99m) per administered dose at the time of administration.

Canada—
   740 megabecquerels to 3.7 gigabecquerels (20 to 100 millicuries) per mL at time of calibration (Rx).

   Sodium pertechnetate Tc 99m injection is supplied as a Molybdenum Mo 99/Technetium Tc 99m generator in sizes of Mo 99 ranging from 8.3 to 100 gigabecquerels (225 to 2700 millicuries). Each eluate of the generator should not contain more than the Canadian Regulatory limit of 1.1 kilobecquerels of molybdenum Mo 99 per 37 megabecquerels of techentium Tc 99m (0.03 microcurie Mo 99

per millicurie Tc 99m) per administered dose at the time of administration.

**Packaging and storage**
Store below 40 °C (104 °F), preferably between 15 and 30 °C (59 and 86 °F), unless otherwise specified by manufacturer. Protect from freezing.

**Stability**
Generator eluate does not contain an antimicrobial agent, and thus, should be used within 12 hours from the time of generator elution.

**Note**
Caution—Radioactive material.

Revised: 06/23/94

---

# SODIUM PERTECHNETATE Tc 99m     Systemic

VA CLASSIFICATION (Primary): DX201

Note: For information on sodium pertechnetate Tc 99m injection for intraurethral administration, see *Sodium Pertechnetate Tc 99m (Mucosal-Local)*.

For information on sodium pertechnetate Tc 99m injection for ophthalmic administration, see *Sodium Pertechnetate Tc 99m (Ophthalmic)*.

Note: For a listing of dosage forms and brand names by country availability, see *Dosage Forms* section(s). For a listing of brand names for the articles in this monograph, refer to the General Index.

## Category

Diagnostic aid, radioactive (vascular disorders; brain disorders; thyroid disorders; salivary gland disorders; cardiac disorders; gastrointestinal disorders).

## Indications

Note: Bracketed information in the *Indications* section refers to uses that are not included in U.S. product labeling.

**Accepted**
Blood pool imaging, radionuclide—Sodium pertechnetate Tc 99m is indicated for blood pool imaging, especially radionuclide angiography.

Brain imaging, radionuclide and

Angiography, cerebral, radionuclide—Sodium pertechnetate Tc 99m is indicated for brain imaging, including cerebral radionuclide angiography. It is used to screen patients for primary brain tumors, to detect cerebral metastases, to evaluate patients with cerebrovascular disease, to localize arteriovenous malformations, to detect intracranial injury due to trauma, to localize intracranial abscesses, and to monitor patients with intracranial diseases. However, this procedure has been almost entirely replaced by other imaging procedures, including computed tomography (CT) and magnetic resonance imaging (MRI).

Thyroid imaging, radionuclide—Sodium pertechnetate Tc 99m is indicated for thyroid imaging in the evaluation of thyroid nodules; carcinoma; and masses in the lingual region, neck, and mediastinum; and to study thyroid size, position, and function. Sodium pertechnetate Tc 99m may be preferred over the radioiodine study in thyroid scanning in cases in which the radioiodine is unsuccessful because of poor uptake, in children to reduce radiation exposure, and when results of the procedure are needed as soon as possible. However, sodium iodide I 131 or I 123 may be preferred over sodium pertechnetate Tc 99m for characterizing the function of thyroid nodules or for detecting substernal or lingual thyroids.

Salivary gland imaging, radionuclide—Sodium pertechnetate Tc 99m is indicated in adult patients for salivary gland imaging as an adjunct in the evaluation of space-occupying lesions and in the evaluation of the size, position, and function of the gland.

Placenta localization—Sodium pertechnetate Tc 99m is indicated for placenta localization. However, this procedure has generally been replaced by ultrasound procedures.

[Gastric mucosa imaging, radionuclide][1]—Sodium pertechnetate Tc 99m is used to localize Meckel's diverticula.

[Red blood cells, labeling of][1]—Sodium pertechnetate Tc 99m is used for *in vitro* or *in vivo* labeling of red blood cells (which have been pre-

treated with stannous ion). Red blood cells labeled with sodium pertechnetate Tc 99m are used for the following diagnostic studies:

Cardiac blood pool imaging, radionuclide—To evaluate cardiac function, including measurement of cardiac output, ejection fraction, and wall motion.

Bleeding, gastrointestinal (diagnosis)—To evaluate patients suspected of having gastrointestinal bleeding, to detect the site of bleeding and help establish the amount of bleeding.

---

[1]Not included in Canadian product labeling.

## Physical Properties

**Nuclear data**

| Radionu-clide (half-life) | Decay constant | Mode of decay | Principal photon emissions (keV) | Mean number of emissions/ disintegration (≥0.01) |
|---|---|---|---|---|
| Tc 99m (6.0 hr) | 0.1151 hr⁻¹ | Isomeric transition to Tc 99 | Gamma (18) Gamma (140.5) | 0.062 0.891 |

## Pharmacology/Pharmacokinetics

**Mechanism of action/Effect**

Vascular disorders—Pertechnetate Tc 99m remains in the intravascular space long enough to allow external detection for the evaluation of blood flow patterns in brain or in other regions of the body, or to allow the depiction of the large blood pool in the heart or major vessels.

Brain disorders—The mechanism by which pertechnetate Tc 99m accumulates in the abnormal areas of the brain is not precisely known but is most likely related to a change in the blood-brain barrier permeability.

Thyroid disorders—Pertechnetate Tc 99m is handled by the body in a way similar to the iodide ion. Pertechnetate Tc 99m is trapped by the thyroid (but not organified) and remains in the gland long enough for images to be obtained.

Salivary gland disorders—Exact mechanism of action is unknown. However, pertechnetate Tc 99m is handled by the body in a way similar to the iodide ion and, since radioiodine is known to concentrate in the duct cells of the salivary glands, this is also probably true for pertechnetate Tc 99m. The accumulation in the glands is sufficient to allow images to be obtained.

Gastrointestinal disorders—Meckel's diverticula: Following intravenous injection, sodium pertechnetate Tc 99m binds to albumin in the serum. It is then handled by the body in a way similar to that for chloride ions by the gastric mucosa, which concentrates and secretes sodium pertechnetate Tc 99m.

Red blood cells, labeling of—When used for cardiac blood pool imaging or detection of gastrointestinal bleeding, pretreatment of red blood cells with stannous ions causes Tc 99m (as sodium pertechnetate Tc 99m) to bind to the red blood cells *in vivo* with about 70 to 80% of the injected radioactivity remaining in the blood pool long enough to provide images of the cardiac chambers or sites of active (rapid) or cumulative (intermittent) gastrointestinal bleeding. A modified *in vivo/ in vitro* method of labeling red blood cells usually results in a greater percentage of the injected radioactivity remaining in the blood pool.

Placenta localization—The large pool of maternal blood in the placenta accumulates more radionuclide than the surrounding less vascular structures (i.e., fetus and uterus). The accumulation is sufficient to allow images to be obtained.

### Absorption
Oral—Usually well absorbed from gastrointestinal tract; may be incomplete in some patients.

### Distribution
Intravenous or oral—Selectively concentrated in intracranial lesions with altered blood-brain barrier, thyroid gland, salivary glands, stomach and intestines, and choroid plexus; remainder distributed within circulatory system and extracellular spaces.

### Protein binding
High (75% of plasma radioactivity is loosely bound).

### Half-life
Elimination₁—

Blood: 10 minutes.

Cerebrospinal fluid (CSF): < 1 hour.

Elimination₂—

Blood: 6 hours.

CSF: 11 to 12 hours.

### Time to peak concentration
Oral—

Blood: 1 to 3 hours.

Intravenous—

CSF: 3¹/₂ hours.

Thyroid (euthyroid patients): 15 minutes to 2 hours.

### Radiation dosimetry

| | Estimated absorbed radiation dose* | | | |
|---|---|---|---|---|
| | Without blocking agent | | With blocking agent | |
| Organ | mGy/MBq | rad/mCi | mGy/MBq | rad/mCi |
| Large intestine wall (upper) | 0.062 | 0.23 | 0.0032 | 0.012 |
| Thyroid | 0.023 | 0.085 | 0.021 | 0.078 |
| Stomach wall | 0.029 | 0.11 | 0.0032 | 0.012 |
| Large intestine wall (lower) | 0.022 | 0.08 | 0.0045 | 0.017 |
| Bladder wall | 0.019 | 0.07 | 0.032 | 0.12 |
| Small intestine | 0.018 | 0.067 | 0.0041 | 0.015 |
| Ovaries | 0.01 | 0.037 | 0.0047 | 0.017 |
| Salivary glands | 0.0093 | 0.034 | | |
| Uterus | 0.0081 | 0.03 | 0.0066 | 0.024 |
| Red marrow | 0.0061 | 0.023 | 0.0045 | 0.017 |
| Pancreas | 0.0059 | 0.022 | 0.0035 | 0.013 |
| Kidneys | 0.005 | 0.019 | 0.0047 | 0.017 |
| Spleen | 0.0044 | 0.016 | 0.0032 | 0.012 |
| Liver | 0.0039 | 0.014 | 0.0031 | 0.011 |
| Bone surfaces | 0.0039 | 0.014 | 0.0038 | 0.014 |
| Adrenals | 0.0036 | 0.013 | 0.0033 | 0.012 |
| Lungs | 0.0027 | 0.01 | 0.0028 | 0.01 |
| Testes | 0.0027 | 0.01 | 0.0032 | 0.012 |
| Breast | 0.0023 | 0.0085 | 0.0025 | 0.0093 |
| Other tissue | 0.0034 | 0.013 | 0.0029 | 0.011 |

| | Effective dose* | | | |
|---|---|---|---|---|
| | Without blocking agent | | With blocking agent | |
| Radionuclide | mSv/MBq | rem/mCi | mSv/MBq | rem/mCi |
| Tc 99m | 0.013 | 0.048 | 0.0053 | 0.020 |

*For adults; intravenous injection of sodium pertechnetate Tc 99m. Data based on the International Commission on Radiological Protection (ICRP) Publication 53—Radiation dose to patients from radiopharmaceuticals.

### Elimination
Oral or intravenous—

Renal: Primary, 15 to 50% of administered Tc 99m is eliminated within 24 hours.

Fecal: Secondary, 10 to 55% of administered Tc 99m is eliminated in the feces within 3 days.

## Precautions to Consider

### Pregnancy/Reproduction
Pregnancy—Tc 99m as sodium pertechnetate crosses the placenta. The possibility of pregnancy should be assessed in women of child-bearing

potential. Clinical situations exist in which the benefit to the patient and fetus derived from information from radiopharmaceutical use outweighs the risks from fetal exposure to radiation. In these situations, the physician should use discretion and reduce the radiopharmaceutical dose to the lowest possible amount.

Studies have not been done in animals.

FDA Pregnancy Category C.

### Breast-feeding
Tc 99m as sodium pertechnetate is distributed into breast milk. It has been estimated that after a 24-hour discontinuation of breast-feeding, the breast-fed infant's exposure to radiation will be less than 20 mrems after a 20-millicurie dose of sodium pertechnetate Tc 99m. Accordingly, discontinuation of breast-feeding for 24 hours is generally recommended for this radiopharmaceutical. If the patient wishes further guidance concerning her individual circumstances, the activity in breast milk can be measured and the radiation dose to the infant estimated to determine how long discontinuation of breast-feeding is appropriate.

### Pediatrics
Diagnostic studies performed to date using sodium pertechnetate Tc 99m have not demonstrated pediatrics-specific problems that would limit its usefulness in children. When this radiopharmaceutical is used in children, as with other groups of patients, the diagnostic benefit should be judged to outweigh the potential risk of radiation.

For brain or blood pool imaging, potassium perchlorate should be administered prior to sodium pertechnetate Tc 99m, in order to minimize thyroidal uptake.

### Geriatrics
Appropriate studies on the relationship of age to the effects of sodium pertechnetate Tc 99m have not been performed in the geriatric population. However, no geriatrics-specific problems have been documented to date.

### Drug interactions and/or related problems
See *Diagnostic interference.*

### Diagnostic interference
The following have been selected on the basis of their potential clinical significance (possible effect in parentheses where appropriate)—not necessarily inclusive (» = major clinical significance):

With results of *brain imaging*

*Due to other medications*

Antacids, aluminum-containing

(prior administration of aluminum-containing antacids may decrease uptake of sodium pertechnetate Tc 99m in brain lesions)

Antineoplastics, especially intrathecally-administered

(chemotherapeutic neurotoxicity may result in patchy increased brain uptake or localization in ventricles or meninges)

Corticosteroids, glucocorticoid

(concurrent use may decrease brain tumor or abscess uptake of sodium pertechnetate Tc 99m because of reduced peritumor edema caused by large doses of the steroid)

Technetium Tc 99m pyrophosphate

(brain scan may give either false-positive or false-negative results when performed after a bone scan using technetium Tc 99m pyrophosphate that contains stannous ions; to avoid false results, brain scan may be performed prior to bone scan or with a brain imaging agent other than sodium pertechnetate Tc 99m)

With results of *thyroid uptake tests* and *thyroid imaging*

*Due to other medications*

Antacids, aluminum-containing or

Amiodarone or

Antithyroid agents—thioamide derivatives or aromatic preparations or

Contrast media, iodinated or

Corticosteroids or

Goitrogenic foods (e.g., cabbage, turnips) or

Iodine-containing foods or

Iodine-containing preparations or

Iodine-contaminated bromides or

Iodine, stable or

Monovalent anions (e.g., perchlorate, thiocyanate) or

Pyrazolone derivatives, such as oxyphenbutazone and phenylbutazone or

Salicylates, chronic administration of, or

Salt, iodized, excessive intake of or

Thiopental or

Thyroid blocking agents, such as strong iodine solution, potassium iodide, or potassium perchlorate or

Thyroid preparations, natural or synthetic

(may decrease thyroidal uptake of pertechnetate ion)

(a rebound effect may occur following the sudden withdrawal of antithyroid preparations, resulting in a period of up to 5 days of very high thyroidal uptake)

(a rebound effect may also occur when discontinuing salicylate therapy, resulting in a period of 3 to 10 days of increased thyroidal uptake)

With results of *salivary gland imaging*
*Due to other medications*
Perchlorate or
Sodium iodide I 131, therapeutic
(may decrease salivary uptake of pertechnetate ion)

With results of *gastric mucosa imaging*
*Due to other medications*
Antacids, aluminum-containing
(prior administration of aluminum-containing antacids may decrease stomach uptake and urinary excretion of sodium pertechnetate Tc 99m and thus interfere with Meckel's diverticula evaluation)

Perchlorate
(may decrease gastric uptake of sodium pertechnetate Tc 99m if given prior to imaging of Meckel's diverticulum)

With results of *cardiac blood pool imaging* and *diagnosis of gastrointestinal bleeding* using Tc 99m-labeled red blood cells
*Due to other medications*
Digoxin or
Doxorubicin or
Heparin sodium or
Hydralazine or
Methyldopa or
Prazosin or
Propranolol or
Quinidine or
Radiopaque agents, water-soluble organic iodides, with intravascular administration
(these medications may impair blood pool imaging by decreasing the labeling efficiency of red blood cells)

*Due to medical problems or conditions*
Goiter, toxic diffuse or
Hyperthyroidism
(thyroid uptake may be increased)

Lupus erythematosus
(labeling of red blood cells may be decreased)

Transfusion-induced reaction
(labeling efficiency may be decreased because of red blood cell antibody formation)

**Medical considerations/Contraindications**
The medical considerations/contraindications included here have been selected on the basis of their potential clinical significance (reasons given in parentheses where appropriate)—not necessarily inclusive (» = major clinical significance).
See also *Diagnostic interference*.

*Risk-benefit should be considered when the following medical problem exists:*
Sensitivity to the radiopharmaceutical preparation

## Side/Adverse Effects

The following side/adverse effects have been selected on the basis of their potential clinical significance (possible signs and symptoms in parentheses where appropriate)—not necessarily inclusive:

**Those indicating need for medical attention**
Incidence less frequent or rare
*Allergic reaction* (skin rash, hives, or itching)

## Patient Consultation

As an aid to patient consultation, refer to *Advice for the Patient, Radiopharmaceuticals (Diagnostic)*.

In providing consultation, consider emphasizing the following selected information (» = major clinical significance):

**Description of use**
*Actions in the body*
Concentration of pertechnetate Tc 99m in intravascular spaces, in abnormal areas of brain, in thyroid, salivary glands, and stomach tissue allows visualization of these areas

Distribution in body of injected radioactive red blood cells same as normal red blood cells

Small amounts of radioactivity used in diagnosis; radiation exposure is low and considered safe

**Before having this test**
» Conditions affecting use, especially:
Sensitivity to the radiopharmaceutical preparation
Pregnancy—Sodium pertechnetate Tc 99m crosses placenta; risk to fetus from radiation exposure as opposed to benefit derived from use should be considered
Breast-feeding—Tc 99m as sodium pertechnetate distributed into breast milk; discontinuation of nursing for 24 hours recommended to decrease possibility of risk to infant from radiation exposure
Use in children—Possible risk of radiation exposure as opposed to benefit derived from use should be considered

**Preparation for this test**
Special preparatory instructions may be given; patient should inquire in advance
Fasting for 6 hours before administration (oral only)
Fasting for 8 to 12 hours before Meckel's diverticulum imaging

**Precautions after having this test**
Fasting for 2 hours after administration (oral only)

**Side/adverse effects**
Signs of potential side effects, especially allergic reaction

## General Dosing Information

Radiopharmaceuticals are to be administered only by or under the supervision of physicians who have had extensive training in the safe use and handling of radioactive materials and who are authorized by the Nuclear Regulatory Commission (NRC) or the appropriate Agreement State agency, if required, or, outside the U.S., the appropriate authority.

Sodium pertechnetate Tc 99m is usually administered intravenously but may be given orally, except for cystography in which it is instilled into the bladder (see *Sodium Pertechnetate Tc 99m, Mucosal-Local*) and for lacrimal drainage studies in which it is placed on the eye (see *Sodium Pertechnetate Tc 99m, Ophthalmic*).

When sodium pertechnetate Tc 99m is given orally, fasting is recommended for at least 6 hours before and 2 hours after administration.

Prior to the administration of sodium pertechnetate Tc 99m for brain or blood pool imaging, up to 1 gram of pharmaceutical grade potassium perchlorate may be given orally to help block the uptake of Tc 99m into the thyroid gland, salivary glands, choroid plexus, and gastric mucosa. This is especially important in children receiving sodium pertechnetate Tc 99m for brain or blood pool imaging in order to reduce the absorbed radiation dose to the thyroid gland.

Manufacturer's package insert or other appropriate literature should be consulted for optimal times when imaging should be performed.

**Safety considerations for handling this medication**

Improper handling of this radiopharmaceutical may cause radioactive contamination. Guidelines for handling radioactive material have been prepared by scientific, professional, state, federal, and international bodies and are available to the specially qualified and authorized users who have access to radiopharmaceuticals.

## Oral or Parenteral Dosage Forms

Note: Bracketed uses in the *Dosage Forms* section refer to categories of use and/or indications that are not included in U.S. product labeling.

### SODIUM PERTECHNETATE Tc 99m INJECTION USP

**Usual adult and adolescent administered activity**
Vascular disorders or—
Intravenous, 370 to 1110 megabecquerels (10 to 30 millicuries).
Brain disorders—
Intravenous or oral, 370 to 740 megabecquerels (10 to 20 millicuries).
Thyroid disorders—
Intravenous or oral, 37 to 370 megabecquerels (1 to 10 millicuries).
Salivary gland disorders—
Intravenous, 37 to 185 megabecquerels (1 to 5 millicuries).
Placenta localization—
Intravenous, 37 to 111 megabecquerels (1 to 3 millicuries).

[Gastrointestinal disorders (Meckel's diverticula)][1]—
   Intravenous, 185 to 555 megabecquerels (5 to 15 millicuries).

   Note: Some investigators have used cimetidine prior to Meckel's imaging to produce a more intense and prolonged uptake of sodium pertechnetate Tc 99m by the gastric mucosa in both the stomach and in Meckel's diverticulum. Cimetidine is thought to work by blocking acid secretion from the mucosa, leading to an increased accumulation of sodium pertechnetate Tc 99m.

   Also, some investigators have used glucagon, with or without pentagastrin, to inhibit intestinal peristalsis and allow pooling of secreted sodium pertechnetate Tc 99m.

[Cardiac disorders][1]—
   Intravenous, 555 to 1295 megabecquerels (15 to 35 millicuries) of Tc 99m-labeled red blood cells.

   Note: For cardiac blood pool imaging, the injection of 0.5 to 2.1 mg of stannous ion 15 to 60 minutes before the administration of sodium pertechnetate Tc 99m injection is necessary to promote the labeling of Tc 99m to red blood cells.

[Gastrointestinal bleeding][1]—
   Intravenous, 740 to 1110 megabecquerels (20 to 30 millicuries) of Tc 99m-labeled red blood cells.

### Usual pediatric administered activity

Vascular disorders or
Brain disorders—
   Intravenous or oral, 5 to 10 megabecquerels (140 to 280 microcuries) per kg of body weight.

   Note: For radionuclide angiography performed as part of the brain imaging or blood pool procedures, a minimum of 111 to 185 megabecquerels (3 to 5 millicuries) should be used.

Thyroid disorders—
   Intravenous or oral, 2 to 3 megabecquerels (60 to 80 microcuries) per kg of body weight.

[Gastrointestinal disorders (Meckel's diverticula)][1]—
   Intravenous, 1.85 to 3.7 megabecquerels (50 to 100 microcuries) per kg of body weight.

### Usual geriatric administered activity

See *Usual adult and adolescent administered activity.*

### Strength(s) usually available

U.S.—
   740 megabecquerels to 3.7 gigabecquerels (20 to 100 millicuries) per mL at time of calibration.

Note: Sodium pertechnetate Tc 99m injection is supplied as a molybdenum Mo 99/technetium Tc 99m generator in sizes of Mo 99 ranging from 30.7 to 614.2 gigabecquerels (830 to 16,600 millicuries); 9.25 to 111 gigabecquerels (250 to 3000 millicuries) [*Ultra-TechneKow FM* ]; or 8.3 to 100 gigabecquerels (225 to 2700 millicuries) [*TechneLite* ]. Each eluate of the generator should not contain more than the USP limit of 0.15 kilobecquerel of molybdenum Mo 99 per megabecquerel of technetium Tc 99m (0.15 microcurie Mo 99 per millicurie Tc 99m) per administered dose at the time of administration.

Canada—
   Sodium pertechnetate Tc 99m injection is supplied as a molybdenum Mo 99/technetium Tc 99m generator in sizes of Mo 99 ranging from 8.3 to 100 gigabecquerels (225 to 2700 millicuries). Each eluate of the generator should not contain more than the Canadian Regulatory limit of 1.1 kilobecquerels of molybdenum Mo 99 per 37 megabecquerels of technetium Tc 99m (0.03 microcurie Mo 99 per millicurie Tc 99m) per administered dose at the time of administration.

### Packaging and storage

Store below 40 °C (104 °F), preferably between 15 and 30 °C (59 and 86 °F), unless otherwise specified by manufacturer. Protect from freezing.

### Stability

Generator eluate does not contain an antimicrobial agent, and thus, should be used within 12 hours from the time of generator elution.

### Note

Caution—Radioactive material.

[1]Not included in Canadian product labeling.

## Selected Bibliography

Campbell CM, Khafagi FA. Insensitivity of Tc 99m pertechnetate for detecting metastases of differentiated thyroid carcinoma. Clin Nucl Med 1990; 15 (1): 1–4.

Gupta SM, Luna E, Kingsley S, et al. Detection of gastrointestinal bleeding by radionuclide scintigraphy. Am J Gastroenterol 1984; 79: 26–31.

Revised: 08/19/94

---

**SODIUM PHOSPHATE**—See *Laxatives (Local)*

---

# SODIUM PHOSPHATE P 32   Systemic

VA CLASSIFICATION (Primary): AN600

Note: For a listing of dosage forms and brand names by country availability, see *Dosage Forms* section(s). For a listing of brand names for the articles in this monograph, refer to the General Index.

## Category

Antineoplastic.

## Indications

Note: Bracketed information in the *Indications* section refers to uses that are not included in U.S. product labeling.

### Accepted

Polycythemia rubra vera (treatment)
Leukemia, chronic myelocytic (treatment)
Leukemia, chronic lymphocytic (treatment) and
[Thrombocythemia, essential (treatment)][1]—Sodium phosphate P 32 is indicated for the treatment of polycythemia rubra vera, chronic myelocytic leukemia, chronic lymphocytic leukemia, and essential thrombocythemia. In the treatment of polycythemia vera, sodium phosphate P 32 should be used with adjunctive phlebotomy.

Bone lesions, metastatic (treatment)—Sodium phosphate P 32 is indicated in the palliative treatment of bone pain in selected patients with multiple areas of skeletal metastases from carcinomas of the prostate, lung, and breast.

---

[1]Not included in Canadian product labeling.

## Physical Properties

### Nuclear data

| Radionuclide (half-life) | Mode of decay | Mean energy (keV) | Mean number of emissions/ disintegration |
|---|---|---|---|
| P 32 (14.3 days) | Beta emission | 695 | 1 |

## Pharmacology/Pharmacokinetics

### Mechanism of action/Effect

Antineoplastic—
   Polycythemia vera: Phosphorus (as phosphate) incorporates into the deoxyribonucleic acid (DNA), and is therefore concentrated to a very high degree in rapidly proliferating hematopoietic cells. Subsequent radiation damage to these cells halts their reproduction.

   Metastatic bone lesions: Sodium phosphate P 32 concentrates in areas of rapid bone formation associated with metastatic tumor localized to bone. The beta emissions of sodium phosphate P 32 result in localized therapeutic radiation and destruction of tumor cells localized to the bone matrix.

**Distribution**
Diffuses rapidly from circulating blood into extra- and intracellular fluids following intravenous administration; concentrates mostly in bone marrow, liver, and spleen.

**Half-life**
Biological half-life—Whole body: 39 days (mean).

**Radiation dosimetry**

| Organ | Estimated absorbed radiation dose* | |
|---|---|---|
| | mGy/MBq | rad/mCi |
| Red marrow | 11.00 | 40.74 |
| Bone surfaces | 11.00 | 40.74 |
| Breast | 0.92 | 3.41 |
| Adrenals | 0.74 | 2.74 |
| Bladder wall | 0.74 | 2.74 |
| Kidneys | 0.74 | 2.74 |
| Large intestine wall (upper) | 0.74 | 2.74 |
| Large intestine wall (lower) | 0.74 | 2.74 |
| Liver | 0.74 | 2.74 |
| Lungs | 0.74 | 2.74 |
| Ovaries | 0.74 | 2.74 |
| Pancreas | 0.74 | 2.74 |
| Spleen | 0.74 | 2.74 |
| Small intestine | 0.74 | 2.74 |
| Stomach wall | 0.74 | 2.74 |
| Testes | 0.74 | 2.74 |
| Thyroid | 0.74 | 2.74 |
| Uterus | 0.74 | 2.74 |
| Other tissue | 0.74 | 2.74 |

Effective dose: 2.2 mSv/MBq (8.14 rem/mCi)

*For adults; intravenous injection. Data based on the International Commission on Radiological Protection (ICRP) Publication 53—Radiation dose to patients from radiopharmaceuticals.

**Elimination**
Primarily renal; a very small percentage in the feces. In normal patients, 5 to 10% eliminated in the urine within 24 hours and about 20% eliminated within a week.

Note: Fecal excretion increases if sodium phosphate P 32 is administered orally.

## Precautions to Consider

### Carcinogenicity/Mutagenicity
Long-term animal studies to evaluate carcinogenic or mutagenic potential of sodium phosphate P 32 have not been performed.

### Pregnancy/Reproduction
Pregnancy—Studies have not been done with sodium phosphate P 32 in humans. Radiopharmaceuticals are generally not recommended for therapeutic use during pregnancy because of the risk to the fetus from radiation exposure.

To avoid the possibility of fetal exposure to radiation, in those circumstances where the patient's pregnancy status is uncertain, a pregnancy test will help to prevent inadvertent administration of this preparation during pregnancy.

Studies have not been done in animals.

FDA Pregnancy Category C.

### Breast-feeding
Sodium phosphate P 32 may be distributed into breast milk. Because of the potential risk to the infant from radiation exposure, breast-feeding should be discontinued.

### Pediatrics
Although sodium phosphate P 32 is used in children, there have been no specific studies evaluating its safety and efficacy in children. When this radiopharmaceutical is used in children, the therapeutic benefit should be judged to outweigh the potential risk of radiation.

### Geriatrics
Geriatric patients may be more sensitive to the effects of radiation; smaller doses and longer intervals between doses are recommended.

### Drug interactions and/or related problems
The following drug interactions and/or related problems have been selected on the basis of their potential clinical significance (possible mechanism in parentheses where appropriate)—not necessarily inclusive (» = major clinical significance):
Bone marrow depressants, other (See *Appendix II*)
(concurrent use may increase the bone marrow depressant effects of these medications and radiation therapy; dosage reduction of other bone marrow depressant medication may be required)

### Laboratory value alterations
The following have been selected on the basis of their potential clinical significance (possible effect in parentheses where appropriate)—not necessarily inclusive (» = major clinical significance):
With physiology/laboratory test values
Blood urea nitrogen (BUN)
Calcium, serum
(concentrations may be increased)

### Medical considerations/Contraindications
The medical considerations/contraindications included here have been selected on the basis of their potential clinical significance (reasons given in parentheses where appropriate)—not necessarily inclusive (» = major clinical significance).

*Except under special circumstances, this medication should not be used when the following medical problems exist:*
» Bone metastases with leukocyte count less than 5,000 per microliter and platelet count less than 100,000 per microliter
» Myelocytic leukemia, chronic, with leukocyte count less than 20,000 per microliter

*Risk-benefit must be considered when the following medical problem exists:*
Sensitivity to the radiopharmaceutical preparation

### Patient monitoring
The following may be especially important in patient monitoring (other tests may be warranted in some patients, depending on condition; » = major clinical significance):
Blood studies, including hemoglobin determinations and leukocyte, erythrocyte, and platelet counts, and
Bone marrow studies
(recommended prior to therapy and at regular intervals during and after therapy)

## Side/Adverse Effects

Note: Leukopenia, thrombocytopenia, and anemia may occur following administration of large therapeutic doses. Also, at present, about 15% of patients with polycythemia vera may develop acute leukemia following therapy with sodium phosphate P 32.

In patients pretreated with testosterone, a transient increase in bone pain has been reported.

**Those indicating need for medical attention**
Incidence more frequent
*Following treatment of bone pain*
*Pancytopenia* (diarrhea; fever; nausea; vomiting)

## Patient Consultation

As an aid to patient consultation, refer to *Advice for the Patient, Sodium Phosphate P 32 (Therapeutic)*.

In providing consultation, consider emphasizing the following selected information (» = major clinical significance):

**Description of use**
*Action in the body*
Incorporation of phosphate P 32 into red cells of bone marrow causing reduction in their proliferation
Incorporation of phosphate P 32 into rapidly forming bone matrix associated with metastatic tumors localized to bone; beta emissions result in tumor cell destruction

**Before using this medication**
» Conditions affecting use, especially:
Sensitivity to the radiopharmaceutical preparation
Pregnancy—Risk to fetus from radiation exposure
Breast-feeding—Distributed into breast milk; cessation of nursing recommended because of risk to infant from radiation exposure
Use in children—Risk from radiation exposure as opposed to benefit derived from use should be considered

**Proper use of this medication**
Special preparatory instructions may apply; patient should inquire in advance

**Side/adverse effects**
Signs of potential side effects, especially pancytopenia; and leukopenia, thrombocytopenia, and anemia (with large therapeutic doses)

# General Dosing Information

Radiopharmaceuticals are to be administered only by or under the supervision of physicians who have had extensive training in the safe use and handling of radioactive materials and who are authorized by the Nuclear Regulatory Commission (NRC) or the appropriate Agreement State agency, if required, or, outside the U.S., the appropriate authority.

Sodium phosphate P 32 solution should not be used for intracavitary therapy (e.g., intraperitoneal treatment of metastasis of ovarian carcinoma).

Visual inspection of the injection is recommended to avoid the accidental intravenous administration of chromic phosphate P 32. Sodium phosphate P 32 is a clear, colorless solution, whereas chromic phosphate P 32 is a green, cloudy liquid intended for intracavitary therapy.

The dosage of sodium phosphate P 32 in the treatment of polycythemia vera is dependent on the stage of the disease, the patient's surface area or body weight, and the erythrocyte, leukocyte, and platelet counts.

The initial dose of sodium phosphate P 32 in the treatment of chronic leukemia is calculated on the basis of the leukocyte count. Subsequent doses are based upon the response of the patient.

A phlebotomy should be performed in patients with polycythemia vera before or after the administration of sodium phosphate P 32 to maintain the hematocrit at normal levels during the induction period.

### Safety considerations for handling this radiopharmaceutical

Improper handling of this radiopharmaceutical may cause radioactive contamination. Guidelines for handling radioactive material have been prepared by scientific, professional, state, federal, and international bodies and are available to the specially qualified and authorized users who have access to radiopharmaceuticals.

## Parenteral Dosage Forms

### SODIUM PHOSPHATE P 32 SOLUTION USP

**Usual adult and adolescent administered activity**
Antineoplastic—
Polycythemia rubra vera:
Intravenous, 111 to 185 megabecquerels (3 to 5 millicuries); may be repeated in twelve weeks if needed.
Note: An initial dose of 85.1 megabecquerels (2.3 millicuries) per square meter of body surface is usually recommended (not

to exceed 185 megabecquerels [5 millicuries]). Subsequent doses are based on patient response.
Chronic leukemia:
Intravenous, 37 to 111 megabecquerels (1 to 3 millicuries).
Metastatic bone lesions:
One type of regimen used is as follows—Intravenous, 370 to 777 megabecquerels (10 to 21 millicuries) given over a three- to four-week period (e.g., 111 megabecquerels [3 millicuries] given the first day, followed by two 74-megabecquerel [2-millicurie] doses given every other day during the first week; two 74-megabecquerel [2-millicurie] doses given during the second and third week; thereafter, 37 megabecquerels [1 millicurie] given two times a week until a total of 777 megabecquerels [21 millicuries] is administered).

### Usual pediatric administered activity
Dosage has not been established.

### Usual geriatric administered activity
See *Usual adult and adolescent administered activity.*

Note: Geriatric patients should receive smaller doses with longer intervals between doses.

### Strength(s) usually available
U.S.—
25 megabecquerels (0.67 millicurie) per mL at time of calibration (Rx) [GENERIC].
Canada—
Provided in various concentrations in multiple-dose vial (Rx) [GENERIC].

### Packaging and storage
Store below 40 °C (104 °F), preferably between 15 and 30 °C (59 and 86 °F), unless otherwise specified by manufacturer. Protect from freezing.

### Note
Caution—Radioactive material.
Not for intracavitary use.

Revised: 07/16/93
Interim revision: 08/02/94

---

**SODIUM PHOSPHATES**—See *Laxatives (Local)*; *Phosphates (Systemic)*

---

# SODIUM POLYSTYRENE SULFONATE   Local

VA CLASSIFICATION (Primary): AD400
Note: For a listing of dosage forms and brand names by country availability, see *Dosage Forms* section(s). For a listing of brand names for the articles in this monograph, refer to the General Index.

## Category
Antihyperkalemic.

## Indications

### Accepted
Hyperkalemia (treatment)—Sodium polystyrene sulfonate is indicated in the treatment of hyperkalemia associated with oliguria or anuria due to acute renal failure.

## Pharmacology/Pharmacokinetics

### Mechanism of action/Effect
Antihyperkalemic—In the intestine (mostly the large intestine), sodium ions are released and are replaced by potassium and other cations before the resin is passed from the body.

### Other actions/effects
Sodium polystyrene sulfonate also exchanges small amounts of other cations such as magnesium and calcium.

### Absorption
Not absorbed from gastrointestinal tract; exchanges sodium for potassium and is excreted from the intestine.

### Onset of action
Hours to days; therefore, other measures such as dialysis may be necessary in emergency situations.

## Precautions to Consider

### Carcinogenicity/Mutagenicity
Studies have not been done to evaluate the carcinogenic or mutagenic potential of sodium polystyrene sulfonate.

### Pregnancy/Reproduction
Pregnancy—Studies have not been done in humans.
Studies have not been done in animals.
FDA Pregnancy Category C.

### Breast-feeding
It is not known whether sodium polystyrene sulfonate is distributed into breast milk.

### Pediatrics
Appropriate studies on the relationship of age to the effects of sodium polystyrene sulfonate have not been performed in the pediatric population. However, pediatrics-specific problems that would limit the usefulness of this medication in children are not expected.

### Geriatrics
Although appropriate studies on the relationship of age to the effects of sodium polystyrene sulfonate have not been performed in the geriatric population, the elderly may be more likely to develop fecal impaction.

### Drug interactions and/or related problems
The following drug interactions and/or related problems have been selected on the basis of their potential clinical significance (possible mechanism in parentheses where appropriate)—not necessarily inclusive (» = major clinical significance):

Note: Combinations containing any of the following medications, depending on the amount present, may also interact with this medication.

» Antacids or
» Laxatives
(sodium polystyrene sulfonate may bind with magnesium or calcium found in nonsystemic antacids and laxatives, preventing neutralization of bicarbonate ions and leading to systemic alkalosis that may be severe; concurrent use is not recommended, although the risk may be less with rectal administration of the resin)

Diuretics, potassium-sparing or
Potassium supplements
(sodium polystyrene sulfonate reduces serum potassium concentrations by replacing potassium with sodium; fluid retention may occur in some patients because of the increased sodium intake)

## Laboratory value alterations
The following have been selected on the basis of their potential clinical significance (possible effect in parentheses where appropriate)—not necessarily inclusive (» = major clinical significance):

With physiology/laboratory test values
Calcium and
Magnesium
(serum concentrations may be decreased since sodium polystyrene sulfonate exchanges for cations in addition to potassium)

## Medical considerations/Contraindications
The medical considerations/contraindications included here have been selected on the basis of their potential clinical significance (reasons given in parentheses where appropriate)—not necessarily inclusive (» = major clinical significance).

*Risk-benefit should be considered when the following medical problems exist:*

Edematous conditions, such as:
Congestive heart failure, severe or
Hypertension, severe
(may require compensatory restriction of sodium intake from other sources or use of dialysis instead of sodium polystyrene sulfonate)
Sensitivity to sodium polystyrene sulfonate

## Patient monitoring
The following may be especially important in patient monitoring (other tests may be warranted in some patients, depending on condition; » = major clinical significance):

Bicarbonate concentrations, serum
(determinations recommended once a week during chronic therapy, especially if patient is also receiving antacids or laxatives)

Calcium concentrations, serum or
Magnesium concentrations, serum
(determinations recommended in patients receiving sodium polystyrene sulfonate for longer than 3 days)

Electrocardiogram (ECG)
(may be useful in some patients)

» Potassium concentrations, serum
(determinations recommended at least once a day or as necessary to monitor effectiveness of treatment)

## Side/Adverse Effects

Note: Cases of colonic necrosis have been reported and may have occurred because cleansing enemas were not administered before and after treatment with sodium polystyrene sulfonate enemas. However, some clinicians think that colonic necrosis may be caused by using sorbitol as a vehicle for sodium polystyrene sulfonate.

The following side/adverse effects have been selected on the basis of their potential clinical significance (possible signs and symptoms in parentheses where appropriate)—not necessarily inclusive:

**Those indicating need for medical attention**
Incidence less frequent—dose-related
*Fecal impaction* (severe stomach pain with nausea and vomiting); *hypocalcemia* (abdominal and muscle cramps); *hypokalemia* (confusion with irritability; delayed thought processes; irregular heartbeat; severe muscle weakness); *sodium retention* (decrease in urination; swelling of hands, feet, or lower legs; weight gain)

**Those indicating need for medical attention only if they continue or are bothersome**
Incidence more frequent—especially with large doses
*Constipation; loss of appetite; nausea or vomiting*

## General Dosing Information

Exchange efficiency of sodium polystyrene sulfonate resin is approximately 33%; although each gram contains about 4.1 mEq (mmol) of sodium, 15 grams of resin bind about 46.5 mEq (mmol) of potassium in exchange for the release of an equal amount of sodium. However, these values are variable and electrolyte balance must be monitored to determine dosage and duration of therapy.

Treatment with sodium polystyrene sulfonate may be discontinued when the serum potassium concentrations have been reduced to 4 to 5 mEq (mmol) per liter.

### For oral use
Sodium Polystyrene Sulfonate USP is usually mixed with sorbitol. However, to improve palatability, Sodium Polystyrene Sulfonate USP may be mixed with food or a beverage, with the sorbitol given in addition. Alternate vehicles for mixing include warm water, 1% methylcellulose, or 5 to 10% dextrose in water.

To prevent constipation, patients should be treated with oral 70% sorbitol syrup, 10 to 20 mL every 2 hours as needed to produce one or two watery stools a day, or a mild laxative. This will also hasten elimination of potassium and help prevent fecal impaction.

### For rectal use
The rectal route is recommended when the patient is vomiting or is restricted from taking anything by mouth (NPO), or when there are upper gastrointestinal tract problems.

After a cleansing enema, the resin suspension is introduced into the rectum via a Foley catheter, and is gently agitated during administration to keep the particles in suspension; administration is followed by flushing with 50 to 100 mL of fluid. The enema is retained as long as possible (anywhere from 30 to 45 minutes to 4 to 10 hours) and is followed by a non–sodium-containing cleansing enema. To prevent back leakage, elevation of the hips on pillows or a knee-chest position may be necessary. In a child, the buttocks may be taped together.

Note: Cases of colonic necrosis have been reported and may have occurred because cleansing enemas were not administered before and after treatment with sodium polystyrene sulfonate enemas. However, some clinicians think that colonic necrosis may be caused by using sorbitol as a vehicle for sodium polystyrene sulfonate.

## Oral/Rectal Dosage Forms
### SODIUM POLYSTYRENE SULFONATE SUSPENSION USP

**Usual adult dose**
Antihyperkalemic—
Oral, 15 grams one to four times a day, up to 40 grams four times a day.
Note: A dose of 15 grams is approximately equivalent to 4 *level* tablespoonfuls.
Rectal, 25 to 100 grams as needed, administered as a retention enema or inserted into the rectum in a dialysis bag to facilitate recovery. Sodium polystyrene sulfonate is less effective with rectal administration than by the oral route.

**Usual pediatric dose**
Antihyperkalemic—
Oral, usually 1 gram per kg of body weight per dose as needed to correct hyperkalemia.
Rectal, 1 gram per kg of body weight per dose, administered as a retention enema or inserted into the rectum in a dialysis bag to facilitate recovery. Sodium polystyrene sulfonate is less effective with rectal administration than by the oral route.

**Strength(s) usually available**
U.S.—
250 mg per mL (Rx) [*SPS Suspension;* GENERIC (Roxane—sorbitol 235 mg)].
Canada—
250 mg per mL (Rx) [*PMS-Sodium Polystyrene Sulfonate* (sorbitol 235 mg)].

**Packaging and storage**
Store below 40 °C (104 °F), preferably between 15 and 30 °C (59 and 86 °F), unless otherwise specified by manufacturer. Store in a well-closed container. Protect from freezing.

**Stability**
Heating may alter the exchange properties of the resin.

**Auxiliary labeling**
• Shake well before using.

## SODIUM POLYSTYRENE SULFONATE (FOR SUSPENSION) USP

**Usual adult dose**
Antihyperkalemic—
Oral, 15 grams one to four times a day, up to 40 grams four times a day.
Note: A dose of 15 grams is approximately equivalent to 4 *level* teaspoonfuls.
Rectal, 25 to 100 grams as needed, administered as a retention enema or inserted into the rectum in a dialysis bag to facilitate recovery. Sodium polystyrene sulfonate is less effective with rectal administration than by the oral route.

**Usual pediatric dose**
See *Sodium Polystyrene Sulfonate Suspension USP.*

**Strength(s) usually available**
U.S.—
3.5 grams per level teaspoonful (Rx) [*Kayexalate; Kionex;* GENERIC].
Canada—
3.5 grams per level teaspoonful (Rx) [*Kayexalate; K-Exit; PMS-Sodium Polystyrene Sulfonate*].

**Packaging and storage**
Store below 40 °C (104 °F), preferably between 15 and 30 °C (59 and 86 °F), unless otherwise specified by manufacturer. Store in a well-closed container.

**Preparation of dosage form**
To facilitate and hasten action and prevent constipation, Sodium Polystyrene Sulfonate USP should be suspended in 3 to 4 mL of 70% sorbitol syrup (which acts as an osmotic cathartic) per gram of resin. The resin also may be mixed with water or a diet appropriate for a patient with renal failure and administered orally through a plastic tube.
For rectal administration, Sodium Polystyrene Sulfonate USP is suspended in 100 to 200 mL of an aqueous vehicle (for example, 25% sorbitol, 1% methylcellulose, or 10% dextrose). Care should be taken that the paste is not too thick because it will be less effective.

**Stability**
The suspension should be freshly prepared and used within 24 hours. Heating may alter the exchange properties of the resin.

**Auxiliary labeling**
• Shake well before using.

Revised: 08/15/95

---

## SODIUM SALICYLATE—See *Salicylates (Systemic)*

---

## SODIUM SALICYLATE–CONTAINING COMBINATIONS—

Pheniramine, Phenylephrine, Codeine, Sodium Citrate, Sodium Salicylate, and Caffeine (Systemic)—See *Cough/Cold Combinations (Systemic)*
Pheniramine, Phenylephrine, Sodium Salicylate, and Caffeine (Systemic)—See *Antihistamines, Decongestants, and Analgesics (Systemic)*
Pyrilamine, Phenylpropanolamine, Dextromethorphan, and Sodium Salicylate (Systemic)—See *Cough/Cold Combinations (Systemic)*

---

# SODIUM THIOSULFATE   Systemic

VA CLASSIFICATION (Primary/Secondary): AD200/AD900
Note: For a listing of dosage forms and brand names by country availability, see *Dosage Forms* section(s). For a listing of brand names for the articles in this monograph, refer to the General Index.

## Category
Antidote (to cyanide poisoning); antineoplastic adjunct.

## Indications

**Accepted**
Toxicity, cyanide (treatment adjunct)—Sodium thiosulfate, in conjunction with sodium nitrite, is indicated for use as an antidote in the treatment of cyanide poisoning.

Toxicity, cyanide, sodium nitroprusside–induced (prophylaxis)—Sodium thiosulfate may be used to prevent cyanide toxicity caused by rapid infusion of sodium nitroprusside. Sodium nitroprusside infusion rates greater than 2 mcg per kg of body weight per minute generate cyanide ion faster than the body normally can eliminate it. The administration of sodium thiosulfate greatly increases the body's capacity for cyanide elimination.

Nephrotoxicity, cisplatin-induced (prophylaxis)[1]—Sodium thiosulfate may be used with intraperitoneal cisplatin to reduce the toxicity associated with chemotherapy. Sodium thiosulfate, administered concurrently with cisplatin in the treatment of ovarian carcinoma, has been reported to reduce the dose-related nephrotoxicity of cisplatin, thereby allowing the dose of cisplatin to be increased.

---

[1]Not included in Canadian product labeling.

## Pharmacology/Pharmacokinetics

**Physicochemical characteristics**
Molecular weight—248.17.
pH—6 to 9.5.

**Mechanism of action/Effect**
Antidote (to cyanide poisoning)—Sodium thiosulfate acts as a sulfur donor for the endogenous sulfur transferase enzyme, rhodanese. Cyanide has a very high affinity for iron in the ferric state. It reacts readily with the trivalent (ferric) iron of mitochondrial cytochrome oxidase, thereby inhibiting cellular respiration, resulting in lactic acidosis and cytotoxic hypoxia. Sodium nitrite reacts with hemoglobin to form methemoglobin, which competes with cytochrome oxidase for the cyanide ion. Cyanide preferentially binds to methemoglobin to form cyanme-themoglobin and restore the activity of cytochrome oxidase. As cyanide dissociates from methemoglobin, sodium thiosulfate facilitates its conversion by rhodanese to thiocyanate, a less toxic ion.
Antineoplastic adjunct—The mechanism by which sodium thiosulfate reduces the nephrotoxicity caused by cisplatin is not fully understood. However, it is believed that sodium thiosulfate reacts covalently with cisplatin to form a non-toxic complex that is more efficiently eliminated than non–protein bound cisplatin. It is also believed that sodium thiosulfate protects against nephrotoxicity by reducing delivery of cisplatin to the kidneys and by neutralizing cisplatin in the kidneys where sodium thiosulfate is highly concentrated.

**Distribution**
Distributed throughout the cellular fluid.

**Half-life**
Thiocyanate—3 to 7 days. May be doubled or tripled in the presence of renal failure.
Thiosulfate—15 to 20 minutes.

**Elimination**
Renal—
Antidote (to cyanide poisoning): Primarily as thiocyanate.
Antineoplastic adjunct: As a nontoxic sodium thiosulfate/cisplatin complex.
In dialysis—
Dialysis is of no value in removing cyanide, but may be used to increase elimination of thiocyanate.

## Precautions to Consider

**Pregnancy/Reproduction**
Problems in humans have not been documented.

**Breast-feeding**
It is not known whether sodium thiosulfate is distributed into breast milk. However, problems in humans have not been documented.

**Pediatrics**
Appropriate studies on the relationship of age to the effects of sodium thiosulfate have not been performed in the pediatric population. However, pediatrics-specific problems that would limit the usefulness of this medication in children are not expected.

**Geriatrics**
Appropriate studies on the relationship of age to the effects of sodium thiosulfate have not been performed in the geriatric population. However, geriatrics-specific problems that would limit the usefulness of this medication in the elderly are not expected.

## Medical considerations/Contraindications

The medical considerations/contraindications included here have been selected on the basis of their potential clinical significance (reasons given
in parentheses where appropriate)—not necessarily inclusive (» =
major clinical significance).

*Risk-benefit should be considered when the following medical problems
exist:*
»  Edematous sodium-retaining conditions such as:
       Cirrhosis of liver
       Congestive heart failure
       Renal function impairment
       Toxemia of pregnancy
»  Hypertension
          (may be exacerbated)
       Sensitivity to sodium thiosulfate

## Overdose

For more information on the management of thiocyanate toxicity, **contact
a Poison Control Center** (see *Poison Control Center Listing*).

### Clinical effects of overdose

The following effects have been selected on the basis of their potential
clinical significance (possible signs and symptoms in parentheses
where appropriate)—not necessarily inclusive:

Symptoms of thiocyanate toxicity

*Arthralgias* (pain in the joints); *blurred vision; hyperreflexia; muscle
cramps; nausea and vomiting; psychotic behavior* (agitation; delusions; hallucinations); *tinnitus* (ringing in the ears)

Note:  Symptoms of thiocyanate toxicity may be seen at serum thiocyanate concentrations above 10 mg per 100 mL (1.72 mmol/
L). Thiocyanate toxicity becomes life-threatening at serum concentrations of 20 mg per 100 mL (3.44 mmol/L).

### Treatment of overdose

To enhance elimination—Hemodialysis; clearance rates during dialysis
can approach the blood flow rate of the dialyzer.

## Patient Consultation

As an aid to patient consultation, refer to *Advice for the Patient, Sodium
Thiosulfate (Systemic).*

In providing consultation, consider emphasizing the following selected
information (» = major clinical significance):

### Before receiving this medication

»  Conditions affecting use, especially:
       Sensitivity to sodium thiosulfate
       Other medical problems, especially edema or hypertension

### Proper use of this medication

»  Proper dosing

## General Dosing Information

### For treatment of cyanide toxicity

Cyanide poisoning is rapidly fatal. Inhalation of cyanide gas produces
symptoms of cyanide toxicity within seconds, followed by death
within minutes. Oral ingestion of cyanide produces symptoms of toxicity within minutes, followed by death within minutes or hours. Blood
cyanide concentrations often are not available for several hours. Therefore, therapy should be instituted immediately based upon reasonable
suspicion of cyanide toxicity.

Supportive therapy includes moving the patient to an uncontaminated area
and/or removing contaminated clothing; administering 100% oxygen;
controlling seizures with anticonvulsants; correcting metabolic acidosis with bicarbonate; and supporting pulse and blood pressure with
fluids, atropine, or vasopressors. These measures alone may allow survival in relatively mild cases of cyanide toxicity.

In more severe cases of cyanide toxicity, chances of survival are increased
by specific antidote administration. Antidotal therapy should be started
by breaking an amyl nitrite inhalant, holding it in front of the patient's
mouth, and allowing the patient to inhale for 15 seconds. The inhalant
should then be taken away for 15 seconds. This procedure may be
repeated until an intravenous line is established and sodium nitrite is
prepared. Amyl nitrite should not be administered if an intravenous
line already has been established and the sodium nitrite is readily
available. Amyl nitrite, if given, should then be discontinued and sodium nitrite administered intravenously in a dose of 300 mg (for
adults) and 180 to 240 mg (6 to 8 mL) per square meter of body
surface area (approximately 6 mg [0.2 mL] per kg of body weight)
(for children), at a rate of 75 to 150 mg (2.5 to 5 mL) per minute.
The pediatric dose should not exceed 300 mg (10 mL). Blood pressure

and methemoglobin concentrations should be monitored closely, and
the administration of sodium nitrite discontinued if the systolic blood
pressure goes below 80 mm Hg. The methemoglobin concentration
should not exceed 40% in adults or 30% in children.

Sodium thiosulfate should be administered intravenously, immediately following the infusion of sodium nitrite.

If signs of cyanide toxicity are still present 2 hours following administration of sodium nitrite and sodium thiosulfate, administration of both
may be repeated at one-half the original dose.

If cyanide was ingested, gastric lavage should follow antidotal therapy.

## Parenteral Dosage Forms

### SODIUM THIOSULFATE INJECTION USP

#### Usual adult and adolescent dose

Cyanide toxicity—
    Intravenous, 12.5 grams (50 mL of a 25% solution) administered at a
    rate of 0.625 to 1.25 grams (2.5 to 5 mL) per minute.
Cyanide toxicity, sodium nitroprusside–induced—
    Intravenous, administered concurrently with sodium nitroprusside at 5
    to 10 times the rate of sodium nitroprusside.
Nephrotoxicity, cisplatin-induced[1]—
    Intravenous, no standard dosing regimen has been established; how-
    ever, experts recommend an initial loading dose of 4 grams per
    square meter of body surface area administered just before admin-
    istration of cisplatin, followed by an intravenous infusion of 12
    grams per square meter of body surface area administered over six
    hours beginning at the same time as cisplatin instillation.

#### Usual pediatric dose

Cyanide toxicity—
    Intravenous, 412.5 mg per kg of body weight or 7 grams per square
    meter of body surface area, administered at a rate of 0.625 to 1.25
    grams (2.5 to 5 mL) per minute.

#### Usual pediatric prescribing limits

Cyanide toxicity—
    12.5 grams (50 mL).

#### Strength(s) usually available

U.S.—
    12.5 grams per 50 mL (Rx) [GENERIC (boric acid; potassium chloride;
    sodium hydroxide and/or sulfuric acid)].
Canada—
    12.5 grams per 50 mL (Rx) [GENERIC (boric acid; potassium chloride;
    sodium hydroxide and/or sulfuric acid)].

Note:  Sodium thiosulfate is a component of the *Cyanide Antidote Package.* Also contained in the kit are: amyl nitrite inhalants (0.3 mL)
and sodium nitrite injection, (300 mg per 10 mL).

#### Packaging and storage

Store between 15 and 30 °C (59 and 86 °F), unless otherwise specified by
manufacturer.

#### Stability

Sodium thiosulfate contains no preservative; therefore, unused portions
should be discarded.

---

[1]Not included in Canadian product labeling.

## Selected Bibliography

Hall AH, Rumack BH. Clinical toxicology of cyanide. Ann Emerg Med
    1986; 15: 1067-74.
Baskin SI, Horowitz AM, Nealley EW. The antidotal action of sodium
    nitrite and sodium thiosulfate against cyanide poisoning. J Clin Phar-
    macol 1992; 32: 368-75.

---

Developed: 03/30/94

---

**SOMATREM**—See *Growth Hormone (Systemic)*

---

**SOMATROPIN, RECOMBINANT**—See *Growth Hormone
(Systemic)*

## SORBITOL-CONTAINING COMBINATIONS—

Activated Charcoal and Sorbitol (Oral-Local)—See *Charcoal, Activated (Oral-Local)*

## SOTALOL—See *Beta-adrenergic Blocking Agents (Systemic)*

---

# SPECTINOMYCIN    Systemic

VA CLASSIFICATION (Primary): AM900

Note: For a listing of dosage forms and brand names by country availability, see *Dosage Forms* section(s). For a listing of brand names for the articles in this monograph, refer to the General Index.

## Category

Antibacterial (systemic).

## Indications

Note: Bracketed information in the *Indications* section refer to uses that are not included in U.S. product labeling.

### Accepted

Gonorrhea, endocervical (treatment)
Gonorrhea, rectal (treatment) or
Gonorrhea, urethral (treatment)—Spectinomycin is indicated as a secondary agent in the treatment of endocervical, rectal, and urethral gonorrhea caused by nonresistant, penicillinase-producing (PPNG), or chromosomally mediated resistant *Neisseria gonorrhoeae* (CMRNG).

Spectinomycin is also indicated in the treatment of recent sexual partners of patients known to have gonorrhea.[1]

Because many patients with gonorrhea have coexisting infections with *Chlamydia trachomatis*, a 7-day course of tetracycline, doxycycline, or erythromycin should follow spectinomycin treatment as presumptive treatment for chlamydial infections.

[Gonorrhea, disseminated (treatment)][1]—Spectinomycin is also used in the treatment of disseminated gonococcal infection in patients who are allergic to beta-lactam antibiotics.

Not all species or strains of a particular organism may be susceptible to spectinomycin.

### Unaccepted

Spectinomycin is not effective in the treatment of pharyngeal gonorrhea, syphilis, *C. trachomatis*, or nongonococcal urethritis.

---

[1]Not included in Canadian product labeling.

## Pharmacology/Pharmacokinetics

### Physicochemical characteristics
Molecular weight—495.35.

### Mechanism of action/Effect
Bacteriostatic; inhibits protein synthesis by interacting with the 30S ribosomal subunit of bacterial cells.

### Absorption
Rapidly and almost completely absorbed following intramuscular administration.

### Distribution
Concentrates in the urine; does not distribute well into the saliva.
$Vol_D$ = Approximately 0.33 liters per kg.

### Protein binding
Not significantly bound to plasma proteins.

### Half-life
Normal renal function—1 to 3 hours.
Renal function impairment (creatinine clearance < 20 mL per minute [0.33 mL per second])—10 to 30 hours.

### Time to peak concentration
1 hour following a single 2-gram intramuscular dose.
2 hours following a single 4-gram intramuscular dose.

### Peak serum concentration
Approximately 100 mcg per mL 1 hour following a single, intramuscular dose of 2 grams.
Approximately 160 mcg per mL 2 hours following a single, intramuscular dose of 4 grams.

### Elimination
Up to 100% of a 4-gram dose excreted in urine within 48 hours in biologically active form.
In dialysis—Hemodialysis decreases serum spectinomycin concentrations by approximately 50%.

## Precautions to Consider

### Pregnancy/Reproduction
Pregnancy—Adequate and well-controlled studies in humans have not been done. However, spectinomycin has been recommended in the treatment of gonococcal infections in pregnant patients who are allergic to penicillins, cephalosporins, or probenecid.
Studies in animals have not shown that spectinomycin causes adverse effects on the fetus.

### Breast-feeding
It is not known whether spectinomycin is excreted in breast milk. Problems in humans have not been documented.

### Pediatrics
Spectinomycin has been recommended in the treatment of gonococcal infections in pediatric patients who are allergic to penicillins or cephalosporins. However, the diluent recommended for reconstitution of spectinomycin contains 0.945% benzyl alcohol, which has been associated with a fatal gasping syndrome in infants. Because of this toxicity concern, use of spectinomycin is not recommended in infants.

### Geriatrics
No information is available on the relationship of age to the effects of spectinomycin in geriatric patients.

### Medical considerations/Contraindications
The medical considerations/contraindications included here have been selected on the basis of their potential clinical significance (reasons given in parentheses where appropriate)—not necessarily inclusive (» = major clinical significance).

*Risk-benefit should be considered when the following medical problem exists:*
Hypersensitivity to spectinomycin

## Side/Adverse Effects

The following side/adverse effects have been selected on the basis of their potential clinical significance (possible signs and symptoms in parentheses where appropriate)—not necessarily inclusive:

**Those indicating need for medical attention**
Incidence rare
   *Hypersensitivity* (chills or fever; itching or redness of the skin)

**Those indicating need for medical attention only if they continue or are bothersome**
Incidence rare
   *Dizziness; gastrointestinal disturbance* (abdominal cramps; nausea and vomiting); *pain at site of injection*

## Patient Consultation

As an aid to patient consultation, refer to *Advice for the Patient, Spectinomycin (Systemic)*.

In providing consultation, consider emphasizing the following selected information (» = major clinical significance):

**Before receiving this medication**
»  Conditions affecting use, especially:
   Hypersensitivity to spectinomycin
   Use in children—Use is not recommended in infants; benzyl alcohol, contained in the recommended diluent, has been associated with a fatal gasping syndrome in infants

**Proper use of this medication**
   Giving one dose of spectinomycin intramuscularly; second dose may be required in some infections
   Use of condom by male sexual partner to prevent infection; possible need for concurrent treatment of partner to prevent reinfection

» Proper dosing

**Precautions after receiving this medication**
    Checking with physician if no improvement within a few days
» Caution if dizziness occurs

## General Dosing Information

Spectinomycin must be administered by intramuscular injection only, deep into the upper, outer quadrant of the gluteal muscle. Intramuscular injections should not exceed 2 grams (5 mL) in each site.

**For treatment of adverse effects**
    Recommended treatment consists of the following:
        • Epinephrine, corticosteroids, and/or antihistamines for serious allergic reactions.
        • Airway support and oxygen for severe anaphylactic reactions.

## Parenteral Dosage Forms

Note: Bracketed uses in the *Dosage Forms* section refer to categories of use and/or indications that are not included in U.S. product labeling.

### STERILE SPECTINOMYCIN HYDROCHLORIDE FOR SUSPENSION USP

**Usual adult and adolescent dose**
Endocervical, rectal, or urethral gonorrhea—
    Intramuscular, 2 grams as a single dose.
[Disseminated gonorrhea][1]—
    Intramuscular, 2 grams every twelve hours for three days.

Note: Dosage may be repeated if reinfection occurs or is strongly suspected.

**Usual adult prescribing limits**
Up to 4 grams as a single dose, divided and administered in two separate sites, have been used in geographic areas in which antibiotic-resistant organisms are prevalent.

**Usual pediatric dose**
Endocervical, rectal, or urethral gonorrhea—
    Infants: Use is not recommended.
Children up to 45 kg of body weight: Intramuscular, 40 mg per kg of body weight as a single dose.
Children 45 kg of body weight and over: Intramuscular, 2 grams as a single dose.

**Size(s) usually available**
U.S.—
    2 grams (Rx) [*Trobicin* (diluent contains benzyl alcohol 0.945%)].
    4 grams (Rx) [*Trobicin* (diluent contains benzyl alcohol 0.945%)].
Canada—
    2 grams (Rx) [*Trobicin*].

**Packaging and storage**
Prior to reconstitution, store below 40 °C (104 °F), preferably between 15 and 30 °C (59 and 86 °F), unless otherwise specified by manufacturer. Protect diluent from freezing.

Note: Store reconstituted sterile spectinomycin hydrochloride suspension between 15 and 30 °C (59 and 86 °F).

**Preparation of dosage form**
To prepare initial dilution for intramuscular use, add 3.2 mL of bacteriostatic water for injection (with benzyl alcohol 0.945%) to each 2-gram vial and 6.2 mL of diluent to each 4-gram vial to provide a concentration of 400 mg per mL.
Shake the vial vigorously immediately after addition of the diluent and before withdrawing each dose. Inject spectinomycin suspension using a 20-gauge needle.

**Stability**
After reconstitution for intramuscular use with bacteriostatic water for injection (preserved with benzyl alcohol 0.945%), suspensions retain their potency for 24 hours at 15 to 30 °C (59 to 86 °F).

---

[1]Not included in Canadian product labeling.

---

Revised: 02/23/93

---

# SPERMICIDES   Vaginal

This monograph includes information on the following: Benzalkonium Chloride*; Nonoxynol 9; Octoxynol 9.

VA CLASSIFICATION (Primary): GU400

Note: For a listing of dosage forms and brand names by country availability, see *Dosage Forms* section(s). For a listing of brand names for the articles in this monograph, refer to the General Index.

---

*Not commercially available in the U.S.

---

## Category

Contraceptive, vaginal.

## Indications

Note: Bracketed information in the *Indications* section refers to uses that are not included in U.S. product labeling.

**Accepted**
Pregnancy (prophylaxis)—Vaginal spermicides are used in the prevention of pregnancy. Because of the high failure rate associated with these products when used alone, suppositories, soluble films, creams, foams, gels, and jellies are generally recommended for use in combination with mechanical barrier methods of contraception (condom, cervical cap, or diaphragm) or for patients with a low level of fertility or suspected infertility, or patients who have intercourse infrequently.

These preparations are also used in combination with mechanical barrier contraceptives to prevent pregnancy at times when oral contraceptives or intrauterine devices may not be effective or are contraindicated, or as an adjuvant to the periodic abstinence (rhythm) method of contraception.

Vaginal spermicides provide a back-up to the condom in case of leaking or spilling of ejaculate or rupture of the condom during coitus. The contraceptive sponge may also be used in combination with the condom. Cervical caps and diaphragms are designed to hold the spermicide near the cervical os, which is particularly important in the event that the cap or diaphragm is dislodged or does not form a complete seal around the cervix. Jellies and gels also provide a high level of lubrication, which may ease insertion of a cervical cap or diaphragm,

may decrease the risk of condom rupture during intercourse, or may decrease frictional trauma to the vaginal mucosa during intercourse.

[Sexually transmitted diseases (prophylaxis)][1]—The use of vaginal spermicides in combination with latex condoms may be partially effective in reducing the risk of acquiring many sexually transmitted diseases (STDs). However, the extent of this additional protection against acquiring STDs (especially viral) has not yet been determined.

Vaginal spermicides provide a backup to the condom in case of leaking or spilling of ejaculate or rupture of the condom during coitus. They may be recommended for use by patients using non-barrier contraceptives such as the intrauterine device or oral contraceptives, ideally in combination with latex condoms, to reduce the risk of acquiring STDs. The use of spermicides in combination with latex condoms may also be considered for those patients at high risk of acquiring STDs (especially HIV infection) during pregnancy.

Nonoxynol 9 has been shown to inhibit the *in vitro* growth of the following STD pathogens:
    *Chlamydia trachomatis*
    *Gardnerella vaginalis*
    *Mycoplasma hominis*
    *Neisseria gonorrhoeae*
    *Trichomonas vaginalis*
    *Ureaplasma urealyticum*

*In vitro*, nonoxynol 9 also decreases the infectivity of *Treponema pallidum*, the pathogenic agent of syphilis.

Clinical studies have shown a reduction in the rate of occurrence of chlamydia, gonorrhea, trichomoniasis, and bacterial vaginosis with the use of nonoxynol 9-containing preparations, especially in combination with mechanical barrier contraceptives.

*In vitro*, nonoxynol 9 has been shown to inactivate herpes simplex viruses (HSV) I and II and human immunodeficiency virus (HIV or the AIDS virus). Benzalkonium chloride has also been shown to inactivate HIV *in vitro*.

The use of vaginal spermicides in combination with latex condoms may afford some degree of protection against viral STDs. However, this recommendation is based on *in vitro* data and no appropriate clinical studies have been completed that document a reduction in the vaginal, rectal, or oropharyngeal transmission of these diseases by the use of spermicides alone or a further reduction when used in combination with mechanical barrier contraceptives. Because clinical studies have not been performed that document the safety and efficacy of spermicides in reducing STD transmission, the following points should be considered: it is not known whether subinhibitory concentrations of spermicides would result from application or use within the rectum; or whether spermicides may cause epithelial damage to the mucosa, damage to cells of the immune system, or Y-lymphocyte activation, resulting in an increased risk of transmission. Also, because protection from pregnancy is frequently incomplete, the same possibility must be considered for the use of spermicides for STD prevention.

[Pelvic inflammatory disease (prophylaxis)][1]—Use of vaginal spermicides, especially in combination with mechanical barrier contraceptives, decreases the risk of development of pelvic inflammatory disease and subsequent tubal damage and infertility. One study showed a reduction in the incidence of tubal infertility among users of mechanical barrier contraceptives combined with a spermicide, which was greater than the reduction with either method alone. The use of spermicides in combination with latex condoms may also be considered for those patients at high risk of development of pelvic inflammatory disease (PID) during pregnancy.

A reduced incidence of cervical neoplasia has been observed in epidemiologic studies among users of vaginal spermicides, especially when used in combination with a mechanical barrier method of contraception. However, the nature and extent of this reduction in incidence has not yet been clearly documented. It has been proposed that spermicides may provide protection against cervical cancer by virtue of their antiviral actions, since there is some evidence that cervical neoplasia may be associated with sexual transmission of human papillomavirus.

### Unaccepted
One study has shown nonoxynol 9 cream to be ineffective in the treatment of genital herpes (HSV II) infections.

[1]Not included in Canadian product labeling.

# Pharmacology/Pharmacokinetics

### Physicochemical characteristics
Chemical group—
Benzalkonium chloride: Cationic surfactant.
Nonoxynol 9 and octoxynol 9: Nonionic surfactants.

### Mechanism of action/Effect
For the prevention of pregnancy—
All products: Vaginal spermicides are considered chemical forms of barrier contraceptives because they form a chemical barrier between the mucous membranes and ejaculate. Mechanical barrier contraceptives include the condom, diaphragm, cervical cap, and vaginal sponge (which also contains nonoxynol 9). The active chemicals in vaginal spermicides interact with the lipoproteins of the cell membrane to permanently disrupt the cell membranes of spermatozoa, resulting in severe damage to the acrosome (head), neck, midpiece, and tail of the sperm and rapid, irreversible loss of function and motility within the vagina and viability. Cell permeability increases and the leaking of cellular components occurs. Studies also indicate that carbohydrate-metabolizing enzymes and the mitochondriae are disturbed. Additionally, the inactive vehicle itself may form a mechanical barrier to the cervical os, inhibiting the passage of sperm.
Benzalkonium chloride may make the cervical mucus hostile to sperm by disrupting the electrolyte balance of the aqueous phase. It also coagulates ovulatory cervical mucus, resulting in a mesh of less than 5 microns, which may inhibit sperm passage.
Contraceptive sponge: Nonoxynol 9 is released from the sponge matrix at a rate of 125 mg per 24 hours. Also, the polyurethane foam sponge serves as a mechanical barrier to the cervical os, inhibiting the passage of sperm, and absorbs ejaculate.
The following are the results of studies examining failure rates reported during the use of various contraceptive methods, as the percentage of women experiencing accidental pregnancy.
In the second column, interstudy variations in failure rates may be due to differences in study design or patient population characteristics, such as motivation, fecundity, or socioeconomic factors (including level of education). Studies reported also include failure rates beyond the first year, which generally decline with continued use of a specific method.
In the third column are failure rates expected among *typical* adult couples who start using the method listed (not necessarily for the first time) and do not stop use of this method in the first year for any reason other than accidental pregnancy. Failure rates among adolescents may be higher, due to poor compliance.

| Method used | Ranges seen in clinical studies (%) | Typical first year failure rates (%) |
|---|---|---|
| None | 78–94 | 89 |
| Spermicides * | 0.3–37 | 21 |
| Periodic abstinence | 13–35 | 20 |
| Withdrawal | 7–22 | 18 |
| Cervical cap with spermicide | 6–27 | 18 |
| Sponge | 5–>28 | 18 |
| Diaphragm with spermicide | | 2–23 |
| Condom without spermicide | 2–14 | 12 |
| IUD | 0.5–6 | 6 |
| Oral contraceptive | | |
| Combination | 0–6 | 3 |
| Progestin only | 1–10 | 5 |
| Progestin injection | 0–4 | |
| Medroxyprogesterone | | 0.3 |
| Norethisterone | | 2 |
| Implants | | |
| Capsules | 0.3–0.4 | 0.3 |
| Rods | 0–0.2 | 0.2 |
| Sterilization | | |
| Female | 0–8 | 0.4 |
| Male | 0–0.5 | 0.15 |

*Spermicides studied include creams, foams, gels, jellies, and suppositories.

For prevention of sexually transmitted diseases—
All products: The majority of studies conducted have concerned the most commonly used spermicide, nonoxynol 9. *In vitro*, nonoxynol 9 has been shown to produce bactericidal and virucidal effects by disrupting the cell membrane and the viral envelope. The active chemicals in vaginal spermicides interact with the lipoproteins of the cell membrane to permanently disrupt the cell membranes. Nonoxynol 9 may also exert antimicrobial activity against *Chlamydia trachomatis* receptors on target cells. Low concentrations *in vitro* have been shown to block cellular attachment and/or penetration by *C. trachomatis* organisms. In one study, nonoxynol 9 caused significant chemorepulsion of *Trichomonas vaginalis in vitro*.
Any method covering the cervix may protect against gonorrhea and chlamydia because the causative organisms primarily infect cervical tissues. Therefore, spermicides alone or in combination with a mechanical barrier contraceptive may protect against transmission of these infections. Spermicidal preparations that are well-distributed within the vagina, such as foams or sponges, may be best for those organisms that reside mostly in the vagina, such as *T. vaginalis*.
Other: Sperm acrosin is inactivated by nonoxynol 9.

### Absorption
Radiolabeled nonoxynol 9 and octoxynol 9 have been shown to be rapidly and extensively absorbed into the systemic circulation from the vaginal mucosa of rats and rabbits. The rate of absorption is dependent upon the product vehicle. No direct information on the rate or extent of absorption of spermicides from human rectal or vaginal mucosa is available. However, disruption of the vaginal epithelial cells occurs, with increased thinning of the epithelium occurring with continuing exposure. Also, the vaginal mucosa is histologically similar to the buccal mucosa. Therefore, it is feasible that these agents could be absorbed into the systemic circulation in humans as well.

### Distribution
Local—
By nature of their vehicles, certain preparations tend to be distributed more evenly and extensively within the vagina and better adhere to the vaginal mucosa. Foam and sponge spermicidal products have the highest degree of dispersion within the vagina and adherence to the mucosa, followed by creams, gels and jellies, and suppositories and films.
Systemic—
Studies have not been published regarding systemic distribution in humans. However, in one study on the use of vaginal nonoxynol 9 in rabbits, the highest amounts of radiolabeled nonoxynol 9 were in the uterus and vaginal tissue. The liver also contained a greater amount than most other body tissues.
In one study of vaginally administered radiolabeled nonoxynol 9 in gravid rats, at 6 hours the medication in the uterus and placenta was in equilibrium with that of the maternal plasma. The concentration of nonoxynol 9 in the amniotic fluid was approximately one-third that of the maternal plasma.

**Biotransformation**

In studies conducted in animals, there was little evidence that nonoxynol 9 is metabolized.

**Onset of action**

Foams, creams, gels, and jellies—Immediately effective.

Sponge—Immediately effective, upon activation of the spermicide with water.

Film and suppositories—5 to 15 minutes, depending upon individual product, to allow for melting or effervescence and dispersion within the vagina.

**Elimination**

In one study in rabbits, a cumulative total of 40% of a dose of radiolabeled nonoxynol 9 was excreted in the urine and 10% in the feces in the 144 hours following vaginal administration. Within 24 hours, 20% was excreted in the urine, and the daily fecal excretion rate was approximately 1 to 2%. In rats, approximately 95% of the dose was excreted within 72 hours, 23% of which was present in the urine and 70% in the feces.

## Precautions to Consider

**Cross-sensitivity and/or related problems**

Because of close similarities in composition, activity, and structure, patients allergic to nonoxynol 9 are likely to be allergic to octoxynol 9 also and should avoid further use of either product if sensitization occurs.

**Pregnancy/Reproduction**

Pregnancy—The majority of evidence indicates that the vaginal spermicides nonoxynol and octoxynol do not increase the risk of occurrence of spontaneous abortion or major congenital anomalies when used at or near the time of conception or during pregnancy.

In a study of gravid rats, nonoxynol 9 appeared in the serum of the pups within 2 hours of vaginal administration of radiolabeled nonoxynol 9.

**Breast-feeding**

It is not known whether spermicides are distributed into human breast milk. However, problems have not been documented.

In a study conducted in gravid rats, an amount of radiolabeled nonoxynol 9 corresponding to approximately 0.3% of the given dose was distributed into the breast milk in the 24 hours following vaginal administration.

**Adolescents**

Consistent and careful use is critical in the employment of vaginal spermicide products to prevent pregnancy, a high failure rate is inherent with these agents when used alone, and their use requires a considerable amount of interruption in sexual spontaneity. For these reasons, vaginal spermicides are generally not recommended for use as a sole method of contraception for all sexually active adolescent patients. They are primarily recommended for use in combination with latex condoms and reserved for highly motivated adolescents or when intercourse occurs infrequently. However, there are some advantages to the use of vaginal spermicides with condoms in that it is a fairly effective, widely available, inexpensive, nonprescription contraceptive method.

**Drug interactions and/or related problems**

The following drug interactions and/or related problems have been selected on the basis of their potential clinical significance (possible mechanism in parentheses where appropriate)—not necessarily inclusive (» = major clinical significance):

Note: Combinations containing any of the following medications, depending on the amount present, may also interact with this medication.

» Vaginal or topical medications, especially those containing:
   Aluminum or
   Citrate or
   Cotton dressings or
   Hydrogen peroxide or
   Iodides or
   Lanolin, hydrous or
   Nitrates or
   Permanganates or
   Salicylates or
   Silver salts or
   Soaps, surfactants, or detergents, ionic or
   Sulfonamides or
   Tartrates
      (benzalkonium chloride may be chemically inactivated by the above agents; contact between benzalkonium chloride spermicides and any product containing the above ingredients should be avoided)

» Vaginal douche products or other vaginal or local cleansing
   (vaginal douching is not recommended or necessary after use of these products, but, if performed, at least 8 hours [cervical cap and *Ramses Contraceptive Vaginal Jelly* ] or 6 hours [most products] should pass following the last act of intercourse to allow for adequate contact of the spermicide with ejaculate, which ensures maximal contraceptive effect)

**Medical considerations/Contraindications**

The medical considerations/contraindications included here have been selected on the basis of their potential clinical significance (reasons given in parentheses where appropriate)—not necessarily inclusive (» = major clinical significance).

***Except under special circumstances, this medication should not be used when the following medical problems exist:***

*For all products*
» Allergy to benzalkonium chloride, octoxynol, or nonoxynol

*For cervical cap, contraceptive sponge, and diaphragm only*
» Menstruation
   (the cervical cap, contraceptive sponge, or diaphragm should not be used during menstruation, as the risk of toxic shock syndrome may be increased; it may be recommended that condoms and a spermicide be used instead during menses)

» Toxic-shock syndrome, history of, especially with prior use of cervical cap, contraceptive sponge, diaphragm or tampons
   (the cervical cap, contraceptive sponge, or diaphragm should not be used, since these patients may be at increased risk of recurrence)

***Risk-benefit should be considered when the following medical problems exist:***

*For all products*
   Allergy, chronic, local or
   Contact dermatitis, genital
   (moderate to severe irritation may occur with the use of spermicides)

» Medical or psychosocial conditions where a critical need exists for highly effective contraception
   (when spermicides are used alone, a high rate of failure occurs)

*For benzalkonium chloride only*
   Vaginal infection
   (efficacy of benzalkonium chloride may be affected)

*For cervical cap, contraceptive sponge, or diaphragm only*
   Parturition or abortion, recent
   (a physician should be consulted prior to use or resumption of use of these products, as use in the postpartum or postabortal period is not recommended and may increase the risk of development of toxic-shock syndrome)

*For prevention of sexually transmitted diseases only*
» Genital ulcers or
» Vaginal epithelial irritation
   (it is not known whether vaginal spermicides may cause further epithelial damage, resulting in an increased risk of transmission of STDs)

## Side/Adverse Effects

The following side/adverse effects have been selected on the basis of their potential clinical significance (possible signs and symptoms in parentheses)—not necessarily inclusive:

Note: The safety of the use of spermicides on the rectal mucosa is unknown. However, no serious adverse effects have been reported.

In one study in rats and rabbits given high doses of nonoxynol 9 peritoneally or vaginally, some evidence of hepatotoxicity and nephrotoxicity was seen. However, these effects or other serious systemic side effects have not been seen in humans.

**Those indicating need for medical attention**

Incidence rare
   *For all products*
      *Allergic vaginitis* (persistent vaginal redness, irritation, rash, dryness, or whitish discharge); *contact dermatitis* (persistent skin rash, redness, irritation, or itching); *urinary tract infection, female* (increased frequency of urination; pain on urination; bladder pain; cloudy or bloody urine)

      Note: An increased risk of *urinary tract infection* may occur in females, independent of diaphragm use, possibly due to changes in vaginal flora.

**For cervical cap, contraceptive sponge, or diaphragm only**
  **Candidiasis, vulvovaginal** (thick, white, or curd-like vaginal discharge); **toxic-shock syndrome** (dizziness; fever; lightheadedness;
  chills; sunburn-like rash that is followed by peeling of the skin;
  muscle aches; hypotension; unusual redness of the mucous membranes inside of the mouth, nose, throat, vagina, or conjunctivae;
  confusion)
  Note: An increased *relative risk* of acquiring nonmenstrual toxic-
    shock syndrome has been reported with the use of a cervical
    cap, contraceptive sponge, and diaphragm. However, its oc-
    currence is rare and the *absolute risk* of nonmenstrual toxic-
    shock is still very low with the correct use of any of these
    contraceptive methods.

**Those indicating need for medical attention only if they continue
or are bothersome**
Incidence less frequent
  **Burning, stinging, warmth, itching, or other irritation of the skin,
  penis, rectum, or vagina; vaginal discharge, transient**—with suppositories, creams, or foams; **vaginal dryness or odor**
  Note: *Local irritation* of the skin, penis, rectum, or vagina may re-
    quire use of a product with a lower concentration of spermicide
    or different ingredients or wetting of benzalkonium chloride
    suppository prior to insertion.

## Patient Consultation

As an aid to patient consultation, refer to *Advice for the Patient,
Spermicides (Vaginal)*.
In providing consultation, consider emphasizing the following selected
  information (» = major clinical significance):

**Before using this medication**
» Conditions affecting use, especially:
  Allergies to spermicides
  Other medications, especially:
    For all products—Vaginal douches or cleansing
    For benzalkonium chloride only—Vaginal or topical medica-
      tions, especially those containing aluminum, citrate, cotton
      dressings, hydrogen peroxide, lanolin, iodides, nitrates, per-
      manganates, salicylates, silver salts, soaps, detergents, sur-
      factants, sulfonamides, or tartrates
  Medical problems, especially:
    For all products—Conditions where a critical need exists for
      contraception, local allergy, or genital contact dermatitis
    For benzalkonium chloride only—Vaginal infection
    For cervical cap, contraceptive sponge, and diaphragm only—
      Postpartum or postabortal status, history of toxic-shock
      syndrome, or menstruation
    For prevention of STDs—Genital ulcers or vaginal epithelial
      irritation

**Proper use of this medication**
  Reading package insert carefully and following manufacturer instruc-
    tions for use
» Using correctly and consistently with every act of intercourse
  Proper use of sponge
  Proper use of spermicide with condom, cervical cap, or diaphragm
» Not douching until 6 or 8 hours (product-dependent) have passed after
    last act of intercourse
» Proper dosing
» Proper storage
**For contraceptive sponge and diaphragm only**
» Not removing sponge or diaphragm until 6 or 8 (product-dependent)
    hours have passed after last act of intercourse
**For cervical cap only**
» Not removing cervical cap until 8 hours have passed after last act of
    intercourse

**Precautions while using this medication**
**For cervical cap, contraceptive sponge, or diaphragm only**
» Contacting physician if difficulty in removing
» Contacting physician immediately if any symptoms of toxic-shock
    syndrome occur after use

**Side/adverse effects**
  Signs of potential side effects, especially vaginitis, dermatitis, and uri-
    nary tract infection; in addition, for cervical cap, sponge, and di-
    aphragm only—toxic-shock syndrome

## General Dosing Information

Vaginal spermicides should be placed deep within the vagina, on the cervix, to allow for maximal contact and efficacy.

The use of spermicides, especially gels and jellies, provides additional
  lubrication during intercourse or insertion of a diaphragm. If additional
  lubrication is desired, only the appropriate water-based lubricants
  should be used, such as sterile surgical lubricant or a personal lubricant
  formulated for use with a diaphragm. Oil-based products such as hand,
  body, or face cream; petroleum jelly; cooking oils or shortenings; or
  baby oil will weaken latex and increase the risk of condom rupture
  during intercourse. These oil-based products will also weaken latex
  diaphragms and cervical caps, requiring early replacement.

**For use of spermicides with a cervical cap**
Prior to insertion, the cervical cap should be filled one-third full with
  spermicidal cream, foam, gel, or jelly. The spermicide should not be
  applied to the rim of the cervical cap, because it may interfere with
  the suction seal against the cervix. The patient should check the cap
  for proper placement on the cervix before and after each act of intercourse. Additional spermicide may be applied vaginally prior to each
  repeat act of intercourse. The cervical cap must remain in the proper
  place for at least 8 hours after the last act of intercourse. The cervical
  cap may be worn up to 48 hours.

**For use of spermicides with a condom**
Spermicide should be put on the outside of the condom after it is unrolled
  onto the penis. It is especially important that a female partner also use
  spermicide in the vagina. Such use is more likely to afford greater
  efficacy.

**For use of spermicides with a diaphragm**
Prior to insertion of the diaphragm, a generous amount of cream, foam,
  gel, or jelly should be spread along the rim of the diaphragm that will
  be in contact with the cervix. Then, manufacturer's instructions should
  be followed in placing spermicide in the cup of the diaphragm. Some
  physicians also recommend that a generous amount of spermicide be
  spread on the outer surface of the diaphragm.

The diaphragm and spermicide should not be removed until at least 6
  (most products) or 8 (*Ramses Contraceptive Vaginal Jelly*) hours have
  passed after the last act of intercourse. The diaphragm should not be
  removed when additional spermicide is applied during this time. After
  6 or 8 hours, the diaphragm may be removed. A diaphragm should
  not be left in place for longer than 24 hours, since doing so may
  increase the risk of developing toxic-shock syndrome.

To be maximally effective, diaphragms must be used in combination with
  a spermicide each time that intercourse occurs. Some women choose
  nightly insertion of the diaphragm to minimize the occurrence of unprotected intercourse. Additional spermicide should be applied each
  time that intercourse is repeated.

**For use of contraceptive sponge only**
Before insertion, the sponge must be saturated with clean water and compressed, until the sponge is thoroughly wet and foams easily upon
  compression.

The sponge should be folded in half and then inserted so that the concave
  side fits directly onto the cervix. It should remain in the vagina for at
  least 6 hours after the last act of intercourse and not longer than 30
  hours after insertion. It is not necessary to apply additional spermicide
  during the time the sponge is in proper position, regardless of the
  number of acts of intercourse that occur during the 24-hour period of
  effectiveness. The sponge activity is not affected by bathing or
  swimming.

A polyester loop is imbedded at two edges of the sponge to facilitate
  removal. A physician should be contacted if there is difficulty in removing the sponge after use or if the sponge is torn during removal.
  Wearing the sponge for longer than recommended periods, use during
  the menstrual period, injury to the vagina during removal, use during
  the postpartum or postabortal period, or leaving fragments of the
  sponge in the vagina may increase the risk of toxic-shock syndrome.

The sponge may be displaced or expelled during urination or a bowel
  movement. If the sponge is displaced from the cervix but not expelled
  from the vagina, the user should use one finger to gently push the
  sponge back into place. If expulsion of the sponge occurs within 6
  hours of the last intercourse, a new sponge should be immediately
  wetted and inserted.

## BENZALKONIUM CHLORIDE

# Vaginal Dosage Forms
## BENZALKONIUM CHLORIDE VAGINAL SUPPOSITORIES

### Usual adult and adolescent dose
Pregnancy, prophylaxis or
[Sexually transmitted diseases, prophylaxis[1]] or
[Pelvic inflammatory disease, prophylaxis[1]]—

For use alone:
*Pharmatex*: Intravaginal, 1 suppository inserted at least ten minutes, and not longer than four hours, prior to intercourse. An additional suppository should be inserted into vagina at least ten minutes, and not longer than four hours, prior to each repeat act of intercourse.

> For use with a diaphragm:
> *Pharmatex*: Intravaginal, one suppository inserted at least ten minutes, and not longer than four hours, prior to each act of intercourse after initial placement of diaphragm with spermicide or if intercourse takes place later than six hours after diaphragm placement.

### Strength(s) usually available
U.S.—
Not commercially available.
Canada—
18.9 mg (OTC) [*Pharmatex*].

### Packaging and storage
Store below 40 °C (104 °F), preferably between 15 and 30 °C (59 and 86 °F), in a well-closed container, unless otherwise specified by manufacturer. Do not refrigerate.

### Auxiliary labeling
• Not to be taken by mouth.

---

[1]Not included in Canadian product labeling.

## NONOXYNOL 9

# Vaginal Dosage Forms
## NONOXYNOL 9 VAGINAL CREAM

### Usual adult and adolescent dose
Pregnancy, prophylaxis or
[Sexually transmitted diseases, prophylaxis[1]] or
[Pelvic inflammatory disease, prophylaxis[1]]—

> For use alone:
> *Delfen*: Intravaginal, 1 applicatorful of a 5% cream inserted just prior to intercourse. An additional applicatorful should be inserted into vagina just prior to each repeat act of intercourse.
> For use with a diaphragm:
> *Delfen*: Intravaginal, initially 1 applicatorful (approximately one teaspoonful) of a 5% cream placed into cup and additional spermicide spread along the rim of diaphragm just before insertion of diaphragm and not longer than six hours prior to intercourse. An additional applicatorful should be inserted into the vagina just prior to each repeat act of intercourse or if intercourse occurs later than six hours after initial diaphragm placement or
> *Ortho-Creme*: Intravaginal, initially 1 applicatorful (approximately one teaspoonful) of a 2% cream placed into cup and additional spermicide spread along the rim of diaphragm just before insertion of diaphragm and not longer than six hours prior to intercourse. An additional applicatorful should be inserted into the vagina just prior to each repeat act of intercourse or if intercourse occurs later than six hours after initial diaphragm placement.

### Strength(s) usually available
U.S.—
2% (OTC) [*Ortho-Creme*].
Canada—
5% (OTC) [*Delfen*].

### Packaging and storage
Store below 40 °C (104 °F), preferably between 15 and 30 °C (59 and 86 °F), in a well-closed container, unless otherwise specified by manufacturer. Protect from freezing.

### Auxiliary labeling
• Not to be taken by mouth.

## NONOXYNOL 9 VAGINAL FILM

### Usual adult and adolescent dose
Pregnancy, prophylaxis or
[Sexually transmitted diseases, prophylaxis[1]] or
[Pelvic inflammatory disease, prophylaxis[1]]—

> For use alone:
> *VCF*: Intravaginal, 1 film inserted at least five (preferably fifteen) minutes, and not longer than one and one-half hours, prior to each act of intercourse.

### Strength(s) usually available
U.S.—
28% (OTC) [*VCF*].

### Packaging and storage
Store below 40 °C (104 °F), preferably between 15 and 30 °C (59 and 86 °F), in a well-closed container, unless otherwise specified by manufacturer.

### Auxiliary labeling
• Not to be taken by mouth.

## NONOXYNOL 9 VAGINAL FOAM

### Usual adult and adolescent dose
Pregnancy, prophylaxis or
[Sexually transmitted diseases, prophylaxis[1]] or
[Pelvic inflammatory disease, prophylaxis[1]]—

> For use alone:
> *Because*; *Delfen*; *Emko*; *Koromex Foam*; *Pre-Fil*; *Ramses Contraceptive Foam*: Intravaginal, 1 applicatorful inserted just prior to and not longer than one hour prior to each act of intercourse.
> For use with a diaphragm:
> *Because*; *Emko*; *Pre-Fil*; *Ramses Contraceptive Foam*: Intravaginal, initially 1 applicatorful placed into vagina and additional spermicide spread along the rim of diaphragm just before insertion of diaphragm and not longer than one hour prior to intercourse. An additional applicatorful should be inserted into vagina just prior to, and not longer than one hour before, each repeat act of intercourse or
> *Koromex Foam*: Intravaginal, initially 1 applicatorful placed into cup and additional spermicide spread along the rim of diaphragm just before insertion of diaphragm and not longer than one hour prior to intercourse. An additional applicatorful should be inserted into vagina just prior to, and not longer than one hour before, each repeat act of intercourse.

### Strength(s) usually available
U.S.—
8% (OTC) [*Because*; *Emko*; *Pre-Fil*].
12.5% (OTC) [*Delfen*; *Koromex Foam*].
Canada—
8% (OTC) [*Emko*].
12.5% (OTC) [*Delfen*; *Ramses Contraceptive Foam*].

### Packaging and storage
Store below 40 °C (104 °F), preferably between 15 and 30 °C (59 and 86 °F), unless otherwise specified by manufacturer. Protect from freezing.

### Auxiliary labeling
• Not to be taken by mouth.
• Shake well before using.

## NONOXYNOL 9 VAGINAL GEL

### Usual adult and adolescent dose
Pregnancy, prophylaxis or
[Sexually transmitted diseases, prophylaxis[1]] or
[Pelvic inflammatory disease, prophylaxis[1]]—

> For use alone:
> *Conceptrol Gel*: Intravaginal, 1 applicatorful of a 4% gel inserted just prior to and not longer than one hour prior to intercourse; or
> *Ramses Crystal Clear Gel*: Intravaginal, 1 applicatorful of a 5% gel inserted just prior to each act of intercourse.
> For use with diaphragm:
> *Koromex Crystal Clear Gel*: Intravaginal, initially 2 teaspoonfuls of a 2% gel placed into cup and additional spermicide spread along the rim of diaphragm just before insertion of diaphragm and not longer than six hours prior to intercourse. An additional applicatorful should be inserted into vagina just prior to each repeat act of intercourse or if intercourse takes place later than six hours after initial diaphragm placement or
> *Ramses Crystal Clear Gel*: Intravaginal, initially 1 teaspoonful of a 5% gel placed into cup and additional spermicide spread along the rim of diaphragm just before insertion of diaphragm and not longer than six hours prior to intercourse. An additional

applicatorful should be inserted into vagina just prior to each repeat act of intercourse or if intercourse takes place later than six hours after initial diaphragm placement or

*Shur-Seal*: Intravaginal, initially contents of 1 packet of 2% gel placed into cup and spread along the rim of diaphragm just before insertion of diaphragm and intercourse. The contents of an additional packet should be inserted into vagina just prior to each repeat act of intercourse. Applicator not provided for vaginal application; contents of packet are to be inserted vaginally by placing contents on one or two fingers and deposited on the outer surface of diaphragm.

### Strength(s) usually available

U.S.—

2% (OTC) [*Koromex Crystal Clear Gel; Shur-Seal*].

4% (OTC) [*Conceptrol Gel*].

5% (OTC) [*Ramses Crystal Clear Gel*].

Canada—

Not commercially available.

### Packaging and storage

Store below 40 °C (104 °F), preferably between 15 and 30 °C (59 and 86 °F), in a well-closed container, unless otherwise specified by manufacturer. Protect from freezing.

### Auxiliary labeling

• Not to be taken by mouth.

## NONOXYNOL 9 VAGINAL JELLY

### Usual adult and adolescent dose

Pregnancy, prophylaxis or

[Sexually transmitted diseases, prophylaxis[1]] or

[Pelvic inflammatory disease, prophylaxis[1]]—

For use alone:

*Gynol II Extra Strength Contraceptive Jelly; Koromex Jelly*: Intravaginal, 1 applicatorful of a 3% jelly inserted just prior to, and not longer than one hour prior to, each act of intercourse or

*Ramses Contraceptive Vaginal Jelly*: Intravaginal, 1 applicatorful of a 5% jelly inserted just prior to each act of intercourse.

For use with diaphragm:

*Gynol II Extra Strength Contraceptive Jelly*: Intravaginal, initially 1 applicatorful (one teaspoonful) of a 3% jelly placed into cup and additional spermicide spread along the rim of diaphragm just before insertion of diaphragm and not longer than six hours prior to intercourse. An additional applicatorful should be inserted into vagina just prior to each repeat act of intercourse or if intercourse occurs later than six hours after initial diaphragm placement or

*Gynol II Original Formula Contraceptive Jelly*: Intravaginal, initially 1 applicatorful (approximately 1 teaspoonful) of a 2% jelly placed into cup and additional spermicide spread along the rim of diaphragm just before insertion of diaphragm and not longer than six hours prior to intercourse. An additional applicatorful should be inserted into vagina just prior to each repeat act of intercourse or if intercourse occurs later than six hours after initial diaphragm placement or

*Koromex Jelly*: Intravaginal, initially 2 teaspoonfuls of a 3% jelly placed into cup and additional spermicide spread along the rim of diaphragm just before insertion of diaphragm and not longer than six hours prior to intercourse. An additional applicatorful should be inserted into vagina just prior to each repeat act of intercourse or if intercourse occurs later than six hours after initial diaphragm placement.

### Strength(s) usually available

U.S.—

2% (OTC) [*Gynol II Original Formula Contraceptive Jelly*].

3% (OTC) [*Gynol II Extra Strength Contraceptive Jelly; Koromex Jelly*].

Canada—

5% (OTC) [*Ramses Contraceptive Vaginal Jelly*].

### Packaging and storage

Store below 40 °C (104 °F), preferably between 15 and 30 °C (59 and 86 °F), in a well-closed container, unless otherwise specified by manufacturer. Protect from freezing.

### Auxiliary labeling

• Not to be taken by mouth.

## NONOXYNOL 9 VAGINAL SPONGE

### Usual adult and adolescent dose

Pregnancy, prophylaxis or

[Sexually transmitted diseases, prophylaxis[1]] or

[Pelvic inflammatory disease, prophylaxis[1]]—

For use alone:

*Today*: Intravaginal, 1 sponge inserted not longer than twenty-four hours prior to intercourse.

### Strength(s) usually available

U.S.—

1 gram (OTC) [*Today*].

Canada—

1 gram (OTC) [*Today*].

### Packaging and storage

Store below 40 °C (104 °F), preferably between 15 and 30 °C (59 and 86 °F), in a well-closed container, unless otherwise specified by manufacturer.

## NONOXYNOL 9 VAGINAL SUPPOSITORIES

### Usual adult and adolescent dose

Pregnancy, prophylaxis or

[Sexually transmitted diseases, prophylaxis[1]] or

[Pelvic inflammatory disease, prophylaxis[1]]—

For use alone:

*Conceptrol Contraceptive Inserts; Encare*: Intravaginal, 1 suppository inserted at least ten minutes, and not longer than one hour, prior to each act of intercourse or

*Semicid*: Intravaginal, 1 suppository inserted at least fifteen minutes, and not longer than one hour, prior to each act of intercourse.

For use with diaphragm:

*Encare*: Intravaginal, one suppository inserted at least ten minutes, and not longer than one hour, prior to each act of intercourse after initial insertion of diaphragm with spermicide or if intercourse takes place later than six hours after diaphragm placement or

*Semicid*: Intravaginal, one suppository inserted at least fifteen minutes, and not longer than one hour, prior to each act of intercourse after initial insertion of diaphragm with spermicide or if intercourse takes place later than six hours after diaphragm placement.

### Strength(s) usually available

U.S.—

2.27% (OTC) [*Encare*].

100 mg (OTC) [*Semicid*].

150 mg (OTC) [*Conceptrol Contraceptive Inserts*].

### Packaging and storage

Store below 40 °C (104 °F), preferably between 15 and 30 °C (59 and 86 °F), in a well-closed container, unless otherwise specified by manufacturer. Protect from freezing.

### Auxiliary labeling

• Not to be taken by mouth.

[1]Not included in Canadian product labeling.

---

## OCTOXYNOL 9

## Vaginal Dosage Forms

### OCTOXYNOL 9 VAGINAL CREAM

### Usual adult and adolescent dose

Pregnancy, prophylaxis or

[Sexually transmitted diseases, prophylaxis[1]] or

[Pelvic inflammatory disease, prophylaxis[1]]—

For use with a diaphragm:

*Koromex Cream*: Intravaginal, initially 2 teaspoonfuls placed into cup and additional spermicide spread along the rim of diaphragm just before insertion of diaphragm and not longer than six hours prior to intercourse. An additional applicatorful should be inserted into vagina just prior to each repeat act of intercourse or if intercourse occurs later than six hours after initial diaphragm placement.

### Strength(s) usually available

U.S.—

3% (OTC) [*Koromex Cream*].

Canada—

Not commercially available.

### Packaging and storage

Store below 40 °C (104 °F), preferably between 15 and 30 °C (59 and 86 °F), in a well-closed container, unless otherwise specified by manufacturer. Protect from freezing.

**Auxiliary labeling**
• Not to be taken by mouth.

## OCTOXYNOL 9 VAGINAL JELLY

**Usual adult and adolescent dose**
Pregnancy, prophylaxis or
[Sexually transmitted diseases, prophylaxis[1]] or
[Pelvic inflammatory disease, prophylaxis[1]]—
    For use with a diaphragm:
        *Ortho-Gynol*: Intravaginal, initially 1 applicatorful (approximately 1 teaspoonful) placed into cup and additional spermicide spread along the rim of diaphragm just before insertion of diaphragm and not longer than six hours prior to intercourse. An additional applicatorful should be inserted into vagina just prior to each repeat act of intercourse or if intercourse occurs later than six hours after initial diaphragm placement.

**Strength(s) usually available**
U.S.—
    1% (OTC) [*Ortho-Gynol*].
Canada—
    1% (OTC) [*Ortho-Gynol*].

**Packaging and storage**
Store below 40 °C (104 °F), preferably between 15 and 30 °C (59 and 86 °F), in a well-closed container, unless otherwise specified by manufacturer. Protect from freezing.

**Auxiliary labeling**
• Not to be taken by mouth.

[1]Not included in Canadian product labeling.

## Selected Bibliography

Kulig JW. Adolescent contraception: an update. Pediatrics 1985; (Suppl 675): 80.
North BB. Vaginal contraceptives: effective protection from sexually transmitted disease for women? J Reprod Med 1988; 33 (3): 307-11.
Stone KM, Grimes DA, Magder LS. Personal protection against sexually transmitted diseases. Am J Obstet Gynecol 1986; 155 (1): 180-8.
Grimes DA. Reversible contraception for the 1980s. JAMA 1986; 255 (1): 69-75.

Revised: 07/28/93
Interim revision: 06/30/94

---

# SPIRAMYCIN    Systemic*

JAN: Spiramycin—Acetylspiramycin
VA CLASSIFICATION (Primary/Secondary): AM200/AP900
Note: For a listing of dosage forms and brand names by country availability, see *Dosage Forms* section(s). For a listing of brand names for the articles in this monograph, refer to the General Index.

*Not commercially available in the U.S.

## Category
Antibacterial (systemic); antiprotozoal.

## Indications
**General considerations**
Spiramycin is a macrolide antimicrobial agent with activity against gram-positive organisms, including *Streptococcus pyogenes* (group A beta-hemolytic streptococci), *S. viridans*, *Corynebacterium diphtheriae*, and methicillin-sensitive *Staphylococcus aureus*. Increasing resistance has left spiramycin with inconsistent activity against *S. pneumoniae* and enterococcus. Spiramycin also has activity against some gram-negative bacteria, such as *Neisseria meningitidis*, *Bordetella pertussis*, and *Campylobacter*. *Neisseria gonorrhoeae* is inconsistently sensitive, and approximately 50% of *Haemophilus influenzae* strains are sensitive to spiramycin. *Clostridium* species are sensitive; however, Enterobacteraceae, *Pseudomonas* species, as well as *Bacteroides fragilis*, and most other gram-negative bacteria are resistant. Spiramycin also has activity against other organisms, including *Mycoplasma pneumoniae*, *Chlamydia trachomatis*, *Toxoplasma gondii*, *Legionella pneumophila*, and spirochetes.
Cross-resistance between spiramycin and erythromycin has been reported.

**Accepted**
Toxoplasmosis (treatment)[1]—Spiramycin is used as an alternative agent in the treatment of toxoplasmosis during pregnancy. Pyrimethamine and sulfadiazine combination is considered to be more effective than spiramycin. However, because spiramycin has not been found to be teratogenic and has been found to be safe in the pregnant woman, fetus, and newborn, it is often used to treat toxoplasmosis during pregnancy and congenital toxoplasmosis. Spiramycin reduces the transmission of toxoplasmosis from the pregnant woman to the fetus; however, it will not affect the severity of disease in an already infected fetus.

Although spiramycin is effective in the treatment of some bacterial infections, spiramycin is considered to be a secondary agent and other medications are generally used in place of spiramycin.

**Acceptance not established**
Spiramycin has not been shown to be clearly effective in the treatment of *cryptosporidiosis* in immunocompromised patients. Data are mixed and relapse often occurs after spiramycin is discontinued. *Cryptosporidiosis* is usually self-limiting in non-immunocompromised patients.

**Unaccepted**
Because spiramycin does not reach adequate concentrations in the cerebrospinal fluid, spiramycin is not accepted in the treatment of *meningitis* or in preventing *toxoplasma encephalitis*.

[1]Not included in Canadian product labeling.

## Pharmacology/Pharmacokinetics

**Physicochemical characteristics**
Chemical group—A 16-membered ring macrolide antibiotic
Molecular weight—843.1.
pKa—7.9.

**Mechanism of action/Effect**
The mechanism of action of spiramycin is not clear; however, it is thought to reversibly bind to the 50 S subunit of bacterial ribosomes, resulting in blockage of the transpeptidation or translocation reactions, inhibiting protein synthesis and subsequent cell growth. It is primarily bacteriostatic, but may be bactericidal against more sensitive strains when used in high concentrations. Spiramycin also accumulates in high concentrations in the bacterial cell. Unlike erythromycin, spiramycin does not produce gastrointestinal motility stimulation.

**Absorption**
The absorption of spiramycin is incomplete, with an oral bioavailability of 33 to 39% (range, 10 to 69%). The rate of absorption is slower than that of erythromycin and is thought to be due to the high pKa (7.9) of spiramycin, suggesting a high degree of ionization in the acidic stomach. Studies have shown that administration with food reduces bioavailability by approximately 50% and delays the time to peak serum concentration.

**Distribution**
Spiramycin is highly concentrated in tissues, such as the lungs, bronchi, tonsils, sinuses, and female pelvic tissues. These high tissue concentrations persist long after serum concentrations have fallen to low levels. Peak concentrations in the saliva are 1.3 to 4.8 times greater than those found in the serum. Spiramycin crosses the placenta and is distributed into breast milk; however, fetal blood concentrations are only 50% of the maternal serum concentrations. Concentrations in the placenta are up to 5 times higher than the corresponding serum concentration. High concentrations are also found in the bile, polymorphonuclear leukocytes, and macrophages. Biliary concentrations are 15 to 40 times higher than the serum concentration. Spiramycin does not cross the blood-brain barrier.
$Vol_D$ is large and variable (383 to 660 L).

**Protein binding**
Low (10 to 25%).

**Biotransformation**
Spiramycin metabolism has not been well studied; however, spiramycin is thought to be metabolized in the liver to active metabolites.

**Half-life**

Intravenous—

    Young persons (18 to 32 years of age): Approximately 4.5 to 6.2 hours.

    Elderly persons (73 to 85 years of age): Approximately 9.8 to 13.5 hours.

Oral—

    5.5 to 8 hours.

Rectal (in children)—

    Approximately 8 hours.

**Time to peak concentration**

Intravenous—End of infusion.

Oral—3 to 4 hours.

Rectal (in children)—1.5 to 3 hours.

**Peak serum concentration**

Intravenous—

    2.3 mcg per mL (mcg/mL) after a 500-mg dose.

Oral—

    Approximately 1 mcg/mL after a 1-gram dose.

    1.6 to 3.1 mcg/mL after a 2-gram dose.

Rectal (in children)—

    Approximately 1.6 mcg per mL after a 1.3 million IU dose.

**Elimination**

Fecal—Biliary elimination is substantial, with over 80% of an administered dose excreted in the bile; enterohepatic recycling may occur.

Renal—Urinary excretion accounts for only 4 to 14% of an administered dose.

## Precautions to Consider

**Cross-sensitivity and/or related problems**

Patients with hypersensitivity reactions to other macrolides (e.g., erythromycin, azithromycin, clarithromycin, troleandomycin, dirithromycin, josamycin) may also have hypersensitivity to spiramycin.

**Pregnancy/Reproduction**

Pregnancy—Spiramycin crosses the placenta and reaches concentrations in the placenta up to five times higher than that in the corresponding serum. Spiramycin is used in pregnant women to decrease the risk of toxoplasmosis transmission to the fetus. It is reported to decrease the transmission from 25 to 8% in the first trimester, from 54 to 19% in the second trimester, and from 65 to 44% in the third trimester. However, spiramycin will not affect the severity of disease in an already infected fetus. Fetal blood concentrations are only 50% of the maternal serum concentrations. Spiramycin has not been found to be teratogenic, and has been found to be safe in the pregnant woman, fetus, and newborn.

**Breast-feeding**

Spiramycin is distributed into breast milk.

**Pediatrics**

Studies performed in infants and children have not demonstrated pediatrics-specific problems that would limit the usefulness of spiramycin in children.

**Geriatrics**

No information is available on the relationship of age to the effects of spiramycin in geriatric patients. However, one small pharmacokinetic study showed that elderly patients (73 to 85 years of age) had an elimination half-life that was twice as long as that in younger patients.

**Drug interactions and/or related problems**

The following drug interactions and/or related problems have been selected on the basis of their potential clinical significance (possible mechanism in parentheses where appropriate)—not necessarily inclusive (» = major clinical significance):

Note: Unlike erythromycin, a related macrolide, spiramycin does not bind to hepatic cytochrome P-450 isoenzymes and has not been shown to interact with cyclosporine or theophylline.

    Combinations containing either of the following medications, depending on the amount present, may interact with this medication.

Levodopa and carbidopa combination

    (concurrent use of spiramycin with levodopa and carbidopa combination has resulted in an increase in the elimination half-life of levodopa; this is thought to be due to the inhibition of carbidopa absorption by spiramycin secondary to modified gastrointestinal motility)

**Laboratory value alterations**

The following have been selected on the basis of their potential clinical significance (possible effect in parentheses where appropriate)—not necessarily inclusive (» = major clinical significance):

With physiology/laboratory test values

    Alanine aminotransferase (ALT [SGPT]) and

    Alkaline phosphatase, serum

        (values may be increased rarely)

**Medical considerations/Contraindications**

The medical considerations/contraindications included here have been selected on the basis of their potential clinical significance (reasons given in parentheses where appropriate)—not necessarily inclusive (» = major clinical significance).

*Risk-benefit should be considered when the following medical problems exist:*

Biliary obstruction or

Hepatic function impairment

    (biliary obstruction or hepatic function impairment may decrease the elimination of spiramycin, which may increase the risk of side effects)

Hypersensitivity to spiramycin or another macrolide

**Patient monitoring**

The following may be especially important in patient monitoring (other tests may be warranted in some patients, depending on condition; » = major clinical significance):

Hepatic function determinations

    (may be required in patients with hepatic function impairment receiving high-dose spiramycin; spiramycin has also been reported to cause cholestatic hepatitis)

## Side/Adverse Effects

Note: Severe adverse reactions due to spiramycin are rare. Hypersensitivity reactions and gastrointestinal disturbances occur most frequently. Thrombocytopenia, QT prolongation in an infant, cholestatic hepatitis, acute colitis, and ulcerated esophagitis have each only been reported as single case reports in the literature; there were two case reports of intestinal mucosal injury.

    Thrombocytopenia, reported in a patient infected with human immunodeficiency virus (HIV), was thought to be induced by spiramycin-IgG immune complexes adsorbed onto the surface of platelets.

    The two cases of intestinal mucosal injury occurred with high doses of spiramycin. Endoscopic examination revealed erosions of the small bowel wall with loss of the small intestinal folds, marked damage to the large and small bowel with flattened epithelial cells, multifocal apoptosis, and regenerative epithelial changes.

The following side/adverse effects have been selected on the basis of their potential clinical significance (possible signs and symptoms in parentheses where appropriate)—not necessarily inclusive:

**Those indicating need for medical attention**

Incidence less frequent

    *Hypersensitivity reactions, specifically skin rash and itching; thrombocytopenia* (unusual bleeding or bruising)

Incidence rare

    *Cardiac toxicity, specifically QT prolongation* (irregular heartbeat; recurrent fainting); *cholestatic hepatitis* (abdominal pain; nausea; vomiting; yellow eyes or skin); *gastrointestinal toxicity, specifically acute colitis* (abdominal pain and tenderness; bloody stools; fever); *intestinal injury* (abdominal pain and tenderness); *ulcerated esophagitis* (chest pain; heartburn); *pain at site of injection*

**Those indicating need for medical attention only if they continue or are bothersome**

Incidence less frequent

    *Gastrointestinal disturbances* (diarrhea; nausea; stomach pain; vomiting)

## Patient Consultation

As an aid to patient consultation, refer to *Advice for the Patient, Spiramycin (Systemic)*.

In providing consultation, consider emphasizing the following selected information (» = major clinical significance):

**Before using this medication**

» Conditions affecting use, especially:

    Hypersensitivity to spiramycin or other macrolides

    Breast-feeding—Spiramycin is distributed into breast milk

**Proper use of this medication**
» Taking on an empty stomach
» Compliance with full course of therapy
» Importance of taking medication on regular schedule and not missing doses
» Proper administration of spiramycin suppositories
» Proper dosing
Missed dose: taking as soon as possible; not taking if almost time for next dose; not doubling dose
» Proper storage

**Precautions while using this medication**
Checking with physician if no improvement within a few days

**Side/adverse effects**
Signs of potential side effects, especially hypersensitivity reactions, cardiac toxicity, cholestatic hepatitis, gastrointestinal toxicity, or pain at site of injection

# General Dosing Information

**For oral dosage form only**
Administration of spiramycin with food reduces bioavailability by approximately 50% and delays the time to peak serum concentration. Spiramycin should be taken on an empty stomach.

**For rectal dosage form only**
Before rectal administration of spiramycin suppositories, the suppository should be dipped in cold water, then introduced quickly and deeply into the rectum.

# Oral Dosage Forms

## SPIRAMYCIN CAPSULES

Note: Dosing of spiramycin may be expressed as either milligrams (mg) or International Units (IU). One mg of spiramycin is equivalent to approximately 3000 IU.

**Usual adult and adolescent dose**
Antibacterial—
Oral, 1 to 2 grams (3,000,000 to 6,000,000 IU) two times a day; or 500 mg to 1 gram (1,500,000 to 3,000,000 IU) three times a day. For severe infections, the dose may be increased to 2 to 2.5 grams (6,000,000 to 7,500,000 IU) two times a day.

Note: Toxoplasmosis in pregnant women[1]
First trimester: Oral, 3 grams (9,000,000 IU) per day, divided into three or four doses.

Second and third trimesters: Oral, 25 to 50 mg of pyrimethamine per day in combination with 2 to 3 grams of sulfadiazine per day and folinic acid 5 mg per day for three weeks, alternating with 3 grams (9,000,000 IU) of spiramycin, divided into three or four doses, for three weeks.

**Usual pediatric dose**
Antibacterial—
Children 20 kg of body weight and over: Oral, 25 mg (75,000 IU) per kg of body weight two times a day, or 16.7 mg (50,000 IU) per kg of body weight three times a day.

Note: Toxoplasmosis[1]
Subclinical congenital infection: Oral, 0.5 to 1 mg per kg of body weight per day of pyrimethamine in combination with 50 to 100 mg per kg of body weight per day of sulfadiazine for four weeks, alternating with 50 to 100 mg (150,000 to 300,000 IU) per kg of body weight of spiramycin for six weeks; these dosing courses are repeated for one year.

Overt congenital infection: Oral, 0.5 to 1 mg per kg of body weight per day of pyrimethamine in combination with 50 to 100 mg per kg of body weight per day of sulfadiazine and folinic acid 5 mg every three days for six months, alternating with 50 to 100 mg (150,000 to 300,000 IU) per kg of body weight of spiramycin in combination with pyrimethamine and sulfadiazine for four weeks; these dosing courses are repeated until 18 months of age.

**Strength(s) usually available**
U.S.—
Not commercially available. However, physicians who wish to use spiramycin should contact the FDA's Division of Anti-Infective Drug Products (301-443-4310).
Canada—
250 mg (750,000 IU) (Rx) [*Rovamycine 250*].
500 mg (1,500,000 IU) (Rx) [*Rovamycine 500*].

**Packaging and storage**
Store below 40 °C (104 °F), preferably between 15 and 30 °C (59 and 86 °F), unless otherwise specified by manufacturer.

**Auxiliary labeling**
• Continue medicine for full time of treatment.
• Take on an empty stomach.

## SPIRAMYCIN TABLETS

Note: Dosing of spiramycin may be expressed as either milligrams (mg) or International Units (IU). One mg of spiramycin is equivalent to approximately 3000 IU.

**Usual adult and adolescent dose**
See *Spiramycin Capsules*.

**Usual pediatric dose**
See *Spiramycin Capsules*.

**Strength(s) usually available**
U.S.—
Not commercially available. However, physicians who wish to use spiramycin should contact the FDA's Division of Anti-Infective Drug Products (301-443-4310).
Canada—
Not commercially available.
France—
500 mg (1,500,000 IU) (Rx) [*Rovamycine*].
1 gram (3,000,000 IU) (Rx) [*Rovamycine*].
Germany—
250 mg (750,000 IU) (Rx) [*Rovamycine-250*].
500 mg (1,500,000 IU) (Rx) [*Rovamycine-500*].
Italy—
1 gram (3,000,000 IU) (Rx) [*Rovamicina*].
Mexico—
500 mg (1,500,000 IU) (Rx) [*Provamicina*].
Spain—
500 mg (1,500,000 IU) (Rx) [*Rovamycine*].

**Packaging and storage**
Store below 40 °C (104 °F), preferably between 15 and 30 °C (59 and 86 °F), unless otherwise specified by manufacturer.

**Auxiliary labeling**
• Continue medicine for full time of treatment.
• Take on an empty stomach.

# Parenteral Dosage Forms

## SPIRAMYCIN ADIPATE INJECTION

Note: Dosing of spiramycin may be expressed as either milligrams (mg) or International Units (IU). One mg of spiramycin is equivalent to approximately 3000 IU.

The dosing and strengths of spiramycin adipate injection are expressed in terms of the base (not the adipate salt).

**Usual adult and adolescent dose**
Antibacterial—
Intravenous infusion, 500 mg (1,500,000 IU) (base), by slow intravenous infusion, every eight hours. For severe infections, the dose may be doubled to 1 gram (3,000,000 IU) every eight hours.

**Usual pediatric dose**
Dosage has not been established.

**Strength(s) usually available**
U.S.—
Not commercially available.
Canada—
Not commercially available.
France—
500 mg (1,500,000 IU) (base) (Rx) [*Rovamycine*].

**Packaging and storage**
Store below 40 °C (104 °F), preferably between 15 and 30 °C (59 and 86 °F), unless otherwise specified by manufacturer.

**Preparation of dosage form**
For initial dilution, 4 mL of sterile water for injection should be added to each 500-mg (1,500,000 IU) (base) vial.
After initial dilution, the solution may be further diluted in a minimum of 100 mL of 5% dextrose injection solution and administered by slow intravenous infusion.

**Stability**
After reconstitution, the solution retains its potency for 12 hours.

**Incompatibilities**
It is recommended that spiramycin injection not be mixed with any other medications.

# Rectal Dosage Forms

## SPIRAMYCIN ADIPATE SUPPOSITORIES

Note: Dosing of spiramycin may be expressed as either milligrams (mg) or International Units (IU). One mg of spiramycin is equivalent to approximately 3000 IU.

The dosing and strengths of spiramycin adipate suppositories are expressed in terms of the adipate salt (not the base).

**Usual adult and adolescent dose**
Antibacterial—
Rectal, two to three 750 mg (1,950,000 IU) suppositories every 24 hours.

**Usual pediatric dose**
Antibacterial—
Newborns: Rectal, one 250 mg (650,000 IU) suppository per 5 kg of body weight every 24 hours.
Children up to 12 years of age: Rectal, two to three 500 mg (1,300,000 IU) suppositories every 24 hours.
Children 12 years of age and over: See *Usual adult and adolescent dose.*

**Strength(s) usually available**
U.S.—
Not commercially available.
Canada—
Not commercially available.

France—
250 mg (650,000 IU) (Rx) [*Spiramycine Coquelusédal*].
500 mg (1,300,000 IU) (Rx) [*Spiramycine Coquelusédal*].
750 mg (1,950,000 IU) (Rx) [*Spiramycine Coquelusédal*].

**Packaging and storage**
Store below 40 °C (104 °F), preferably between 15 and 30 °C (59 and 86 °F), unless otherwise specified by manufacturer.

**Auxiliary labeling**
• For rectal use only.

¹Not included in Canadian product labeling.

Developed: 05/28/96

---

**SPIRONOLACTONE**—See *Diuretics, Potassium-sparing (Systemic)*

---

# SPIRONOLACTONE-CONTAINING COMBINATIONS—

Spironolactone and Hydrochlorothiazide (Systemic)—See *Diuretics, Potassium-sparing, and Hydrochlorothiazide (Systemic)*

---

**STANOZOLOL**—See *Anabolic Steroids (Systemic)*

---

# STAVUDINE    Systemic†

VA CLASSIFICATION (Primary): AM800

Another commonly used name is d4T.

Note: For a listing of dosage forms and brand names by country availability, see *Dosage Forms* section(s). For a listing of brand names for the articles in this monograph, refer to the General Index.

†Not commercially available in Canada.

## Category
Antiviral (systemic).

## Indications

**Accepted**
Human immunodeficiency virus (HIV) infection, advanced (treatment) or Immunodeficiency syndrome, acquired (AIDS) (treatment)—Stavudine is indicated for the treatment of patients with advanced HIV infection who are intolerant of approved therapies with proven clinical benefit, or who have demonstrated significant clinical or immunologic deterioration while receiving these therapies, or for whom such therapies are contraindicated.

## Pharmacology/Pharmacokinetics

**Physicochemical characteristics**
Molecular weight—224.2.

**Mechanism of action/Effect**
Stavudine, a nucleoside analog of thymidine, is rapidly phosphorylated by cellular enzymes to its active moiety, stavudine triphosphate. Stavudine triphosphate inhibits human immunodeficiency virus (HIV) replication by competing with the natural substrate, deoxythymidine triphosphate, and by inhibiting viral DNA synthesis by acting as a terminator of chain elongation. In addition, stavudine triphosphate inhibits cellular DNA polymerase beta and gamma, and markedly reduces the synthesis of mitochondrial DNA.
A concentration of 0.009 mg/mL of stavudine is required to inhibit HIV replication by 50% *in vitro*. The *in vitro* potency of stavudine against HIV is similar to that of zidovudine.

**Absorption**
Stavudine is rapidly absorbed with an oral bioavailability of 78 to 86%.
Stavudine may be taken with food or on an empty stomach. Administration with food results in a decrease in peak plasma concentration ($C_{max}$) of approximately 45%; however, the systemic availability, as measured by the area under the plasma-concentration-time curve (AUC), remains unchanged.

**Distribution**
Crosses the blood-brain barrier and distributes into the cerebrospinal fluid (CSF); the mean CSF to plasma concentration ratio was 55% (range, 16 to 97%) when measured in 6 children. Also, stavudine distributes equally between red blood cells and plasma.
$Vol_D$—
Adults: 0.8 to 1.1 L per kg (L/kg).
Children: Approximately 0.68 L/kg.

**Protein binding**
Negligible.

**Biotransformation**
Phosphorylated intracellularly to stavudine triphosphate, the active substrate for HIV-reverse transcriptase.

**Half-life**
Normal renal function—
Adults: 1 to 1.6 hours.
Children: 0.9 to 1.1 hours.
Renal function impairment (creatinine clearance < 25 mL/min [< 0.42 mL/sec])—
Approximately 4.8 hours.
Intracellular half-life of stavudine triphosphate—
Approximately 3.5 hours.

**Time to peak concentration**
0.5 to 1.5 hour.

**Peak serum concentration**
Approximately 1.4 micrograms/mL (6.2 micromoles/L) after a single oral dose of 70 mg.

**Elimination**
Renal (glomerular filtration and tubular secretion); approximately 40% is excreted unchanged in the urine in 6 to 24 hours.
Approximately 50% of an administered dose undergoes nonrenal elimination. Although the exact metabolic fate is unknown, stavudine may be cleaved to thymine, and the subsequent degradation and/or utilization of thymine may account for the unrecovered stavudine.
In dialysis—It is not known whether stavudine is removed by hemodialysis or peritoneal dialysis.

## Precautions to Consider

**Carcinogenicity**
Long-term carcinogenicity studies of stavudine have not been completed in animals.

## Mutagenicity

No evidence of mutagenicity was found in the Ames, *Escherichia coli* reverse mutation, or the CHO/HGPRT mammalian cell forward gene mutation assays, with and without metabolic activation. Positive results were produced in the *in vitro* human lymphocyte clastogenesis and mouse fibroblast assays, and in the *in vivo* mouse micronucleus test. In the *in vitro* assays, stavudine produced an increased frequency of chromosome abberations in human lymphoctyes at concentrations of 25 to 250 mcg per mL (mcg/mL), without metabolic activation, and increased the frequency of transformed foci in mouse fibroblast cells at concentrations of 25 to 2500 mcg/mL, with and without metabolic activation. In the *in vivo* micronucleus assay, stavudine was clastogenic in bone marrow cells of mice following administration of oral doses of 600 to 2000 mg per kg of body weight (mg/kg) per day for 3 days.

## Pregnancy/Reproduction

Fertility—No evidence of impaired fertility was seen in rats exposed to stavudine at levels that resulted in peak serum concentrations that were up to 216 times those observed in humans who received a clinical dosage of 1 mg/kg per day.

Pregnancy—Adequate and well-controlled studies have not been done in humans. It is not known whether stavudine crosses the placenta in humans. Also, it is not known whether stavudine reduces perinatal transmission of HIV infection, as does zidovudine.

Stavudine crosses the placenta in rats. Reproduction studies done in rats and rabbits exposed to levels of stavudine up to 399 and 183 times, respectively, those seen at a clinical dosage in humans of 1 mg/kg per day, based on peak serum concentrations, revealed no evidence of teratogenicity. The incidence of common skeletal variation, unossified or incomplete ossification of sternebra, in fetuses was increased in rats at 399 times the human exposure, but not at 216 times the human exposure. A slight post-implantation loss was seen at 216 times the human exposure, but no effect was seen at approximately 135 times the human exposure. An increase in rat neonatal mortality occurred at 399 times the human exposure, while survival was unaffected at approximately 135 times the human exposure. The concentration of stavudine in rat fetal tissue was approximately one-half the concentration of that in maternal plasma.

FDA Pregnancy Category C.

## Breast-feeding

It is not known whether stavudine is distributed into human breast milk. However, it has been found to pass readily into the milk of lactating rats.

There have been case reports of HIV being transmitted from an infected mother to her nursing infant through breast milk. Therefore, breast-feeding is not recommended in HIV-infected mothers where safe infant formula is available and affordable.

## Pediatrics

Safety and efficacy have not been established. A pharmacokinetic study has been done in a small number of children 5 months to 15 years of age. Preliminary data show that the pharmacokinetic and side effect profiles in children appear to be similar those in adults. A comparative trial with zidovudine and stavudine in children is in progress.

## Geriatrics

No information is available on the relationship of age to the effects of stavudine in geriatric patients. However, elderly patients are more likely to have an age-related decrease in renal function, which may require a reduction in dose.

## Drug interactions and/or related problems

The following drug interactions and/or related problems have been selected on the basis of their potential clinical significance (possible mechanism in parentheses where appropriate)—not necessarily inclusive (» = major clinical significance):

Note: Combinations containing any of the following medications, depending on the amount present, may also interact with this medication.

Medications that may cause peripheral neuropathy, such as:
» Chloramphenicol or
» Cisplatin or
» Dapsone or
» Didanosine or
» Ethambutol or
» Ethionamide or
» Hydralazine or
» Isoniazid or
» Lithium or
» Metronidazole or
» Nitrofurantoin or

» Phenytoin or
» Vincristine or
» Zalcitabine
(since stavudine has been shown to cause peripheral neuropathy, other medications associated with the development of neuropathy should be avoided during stavudine therapy or, if concurrent use is necessary, used with caution)

Zidovudine
(*in vitro* studies detected an antagonistic antiviral effect between stavudine and zidovudine at a molar ratio of 20 to 1, respectively; concurrent use is not recommended until *in vivo* studies demonstrate that these medications are not antagonistic in their anti-HIV activity)

## Laboratory value alterations

The following have been selected on the basis of their potential clinical significance (possible effect in parentheses where appropriate)—not necessarily inclusive (» = major clinical significance):

With physiology/laboratory test values
Alanine aminotransferase (ALT [SGPT]) and
Alkaline phosphatase and
Aspartate aminotransferase (AST [SGOT])
(serum values have increased to greater than 5 times the upper normal limit, but returned to baseline when therapy was discontinued)
Mean corpuscular volume (MCV)
(may be increased)

## Medical considerations/Contraindications

The medical considerations/contraindications included here have been selected on the basis of their potential clinical significance (reasons given in parentheses where appropriate)—not necessarily inclusive (» = major clinical significance).

***Risk-benefit should be considered when the following medical problems exist:***

Alcoholism, active or a history of or
Hepatic function impairment
(stavudine may exacerbate hepatic dysfunction in patients with pre-existing liver disease or a history of alcohol abuse)
» Peripheral neuropathy
(stavudine may cause peripheral neuropathy; if symptoms of peripheral neuropathy develop, stavudine therapy should be interrupted; if symptoms resolve completely, reinstatement of therapy at a lower dose may be considered)
» Renal function impairment
(patients with renal function impairment may be at increased risk of toxicity due to decreased clearance of stavudine; patients with a creatinine clearance of < 50 mL/min [0.83 mL/sec] may require a reduction in dose)

## Patient monitoring

The following may be especially important in patient monitoring (other tests may be warranted in some patients, depending on condition; » = major clinical significance):

» Alanine aminotransferase (ALT [SGPT]) and
Alkaline phosphatase and
» Aspartate aminotransferase (AST [SGOT])
(serum values may be increased to greater than 5 times the upper normal limit)

Amylase, serum and
Lipase, serum
(values may be increased)

# Side/Adverse Effects

The following side/adverse effects have been selected on the basis of their potential clinical significance (possible signs and symptoms in parentheses where appropriate)—not necessarily inclusive:

## Those indicating need for medical attention

Incidence more frequent
*Peripheral neuropathy* (tingling, burning, numbness, or pain in the hands or feet)

Note: *Sensory peripheral neuropathy*, which is the major side effect of stavudine, may also be seen with severe HIV disease. Therefore, differentiation between this side effect of stavudine and the complications of HIV disease may be difficult. *Peripheral neuropathy* occurred in 15 to 21% of adult patients treated with stavudine. It may resolve if stavudine therapy is stopped promptly. Symptoms may become worse temporarily after discontinuation of therapy. If symptoms resolve completely, resumption of treatment at a lower dose may be considered.

Incidence less frequent
   *Arthralgia* (joint pain); *hypersensitivity* (fever; skin rash); *myalgia* (muscle pain)

Incidence rare
   *Anemia* (unusual tiredness or weakness); *pancreatitis* (nausea, vomiting, severe abdominal pain)

   Note: *Pancreatitis* was reported in 1% of patients enrolled in clinical trials.

**Those indicating need for medical attention only if they continue or are bothersome**
Incidence less frequent
   *Asthenia* (lack of strength or energy; weakness); *gastrointestinal disturbances* (diarrhea; loss of appetite; nausea or vomiting); *headache; insomnia* (difficulty in sleeping)

## Patient Consultation

As an aid to patient consultation, refer to *Advice for the Patient, Stavudine (Systemic)*.

In providing consultation, consider emphasizing the following selected information (» = major clinical significance):

**Before using this medication**
» Conditions affecting use, especially:
      Use in children—Stavudine has been used in a small number of children; the side effect profile is similar to that for adults
      Other medications, especially those associated with peripheral neuropathy
      Other medical problems, especially peripheral neuropathy and renal function impairment

**Proper use of this medication**
» Importance of not taking more medication than prescribed; importance of not discontinuing medication without checking with physician
» Compliance with full course of therapy
» Importance of not missing doses and of taking at evenly spaced times
   Not sharing medication with others
» Proper dosing
   Missed dose: Taking as soon as possible; not taking if almost time for next dose; not doubling doses
» Proper storage

**Precautions while using this medication**
» Regular visits to physician for blood tests
» Importance of not taking other medications concurrently without checking with physician
» Taking steps to avoid spreading HIV infection

**Side/adverse effects**
   Signs of potential side effects, especially peripheral neuropathy, arthralgia, hypersensitivity, myalgia, anemia, and pancreatitis

## General Dosing Information

Patients with symptoms of peripheral neuropathy should discontinue taking stavudine. If symptoms resolve completely, stavudine may be reintroduced at 50% of the regular dose.

Stavudine may be taken on a full or empty stomach.

## Oral Dosage Forms
### STAVUDINE CAPSULES

**Usual adult and adolescent dose**
Antiviral—
   Oral:
Patients weighing less than 60 kg—

| Creatinine Clearance (mL/min)/ (mL/sec) | Recommended dose |
| --- | --- |
| >50/0.83 | 30 mg every 12 hours |
| 26–50/0.43–0.83 | 15 mg every 12 hours |
| 10–25/0.17–0.42 | 15 mg every 24 hours |

Patients weighing 60 kg or more—

| Creatinine Clearance (mL/min)/ (mL/sec) | Recommended dose |
| --- | --- |
| >50/0.83 | 40 mg every 12 hours |
| 26–50/0.43–0.83 | 20 mg every 12 hours |
| 10–25/0.17–0.42 | 20 mg every 24 hours |

**Usual pediatric dose**
Safety and efficacy has not been established. However, a clinical trial is in progress assessing the safety and efficacy in children at a dose of 1 mg per kg of body weight every twelve hours, up to 40 mg every twelve hours.

**Strength(s) usually available**
U.S.—
   15 mg (Rx) [*Zerit* (lactose; methylparaben; propylparaben)].
   20 mg (Rx) [*Zerit* (lactose; methylparaben; propylparaben)].
   30 mg (Rx) [*Zerit* (lactose; methylparaben; propylparaben)].
   40 mg (Rx) [*Zerit* (lactose; methylparaben; propylparaben)].
Canada—
   Not commercially available.

**Packaging and storage**
Store below 40 °C (104 °F), preferably between 15 and 30 °C (59 and 86 °F), unless otherwise specified by manufacturer.

**Auxiliary labeling**
• Continue medicine for full time of treatment.

Developed: 11/28/94

---

**STREPTOKINASE**—See *Thrombolytic Agents (Systemic)*

---

**STREPTOMYCIN**—See *Aminoglycosides (Systemic)*

---

# STREPTOZOCIN   Systemic

VA CLASSIFICATION (Primary): AN200
Note: For a listing of dosage forms and brand names by country availability, see *Dosage Forms* section(s). For a listing of brand names for the articles in this monograph, refer to the General Index.

## Category
Antineoplastic.

## Indications
Note: Bracketed information in the *Indications* section refers to uses that are not included in U.S. product labeling.

**Accepted**
Carcinoma, pancreatic (treatment)—Streptozocin is indicated in the treatment of symptomatic or progressive metastatic islet [and non-islet][1] cell carcinoma of the pancreas (both functional and nonfunctional).

[Carcinoid tumors (treatment)][1]—Streptozocin is also being used in the treatment of malignant carcinoid tumors.

---

[1]Not included in Canadian product labeling.

## Pharmacology/Pharmacokinetics

**Physicochemical characteristics**
Molecular weight—265.22.

**Mechanism of action/Effect**
Streptozocin is an alkylating agent of the nitrosourea type and also has broad-spectrum antibacterial activity.

Streptozocin is considered cell cycle–phase nonspecific, although it particularly inhibits progression out of the $G_2$ phase of cell division.

The mechanism of streptozocin's antineoplastic action is not completely understood, but activity appears to occur as a result of formation of methylcarbonium ions, which alkylate or bind with many intracellular molecular structures including nucleic acids. Its cytotoxic action is probably due to cross-linking of strands of DNA, resulting in inhibition of DNA synthesis. Streptozocin has little effect on RNA or protein synthesis. Its alkylating activity is weak compared to that of other nitrosoureas.

**Other actions/effects**

Streptozocin also has a diabetogenic or hyperglycemic effect as a result of selective uptake into and toxicity to pancreatic islet beta cells involving lowering of beta cell nicotinamide adenine dinucleotide (NAD). Irreversible damage to the cell results in degranulation and loss of insulin secretion.

**Distribution**

Very little streptozocin crosses the blood-brain barrier, but metabolites do; 2 hours after administration, cerebrospinal fluid (CSF) concentrations are approximately equal to plasma concentrations.

**Biotransformation**

Hepatic.

**Half-life**

Initial—
  Unchanged drug: 5 to 15 minutes.
  Metabolites: 6 minutes.
Intermediate—
  Metabolites: 3.5 hours.
Terminal—
  Unchanged drug: 35 minutes.
  Metabolites: 40 hours.

**Elimination**

Renal (as unchanged drug and at least 3 identified metabolites, including methylnitrosoureas).
Fecal (less than 1%).
Significant respiratory excretion also occurs.

# Precautions to Consider

## Carcinogenicity/Mutagenicity/Tumorigenicity

Streptozocin administration has reportedly been followed by development of acute myelocytic leukemia in one patient. Streptozocin is mutagenic in bacteria, plants, and mammalian cells and has been shown to be tumorigenic (renal, hepatic, stomach, and pancreatic tumors) in animals and carcinogenic in mice. Topical exposure in rats has resulted in development of benign tumors at the site.

## Pregnancy/Reproduction

Fertility—Gonadal suppression, resulting in amenorrhea or azoospermia, may occur in patients receiving antineoplastic therapy, especially with the alkylating agents. In general, these effects appear to be related to dose and length of therapy and may be irreversible. Prediction of the degree of testicular or ovarian function impairment is complicated by the common use of combinations of several antineoplastics, which makes it difficult to assess the effects of individual agents.
Streptozocin adversely affects fertility in male and female rats.
Pregnancy—Streptozocin crosses the placenta. Studies in humans have not been done.
First trimester: It is usually recommended that use of antineoplastics, especially combination chemotherapy, be avoided whenever possible, especially during the first trimester. Although information is limited because of the relatively few instances of antineoplastic administration during pregnancy, the mutagenic, teratogenic, and carcinogenic potential of these medications must be considered.
Other hazards to the fetus include adverse reactions seen in adults.
In general, use of a contraceptive is recommended during cytotoxic drug therapy.
Studies in animals have shown that streptozocin causes teratogenicity in rats and is abortifacient in rabbits.
FDA Pregnancy Category C.

## Breast-feeding

It is not known whether streptozocin is excreted in breast milk. Although very little information is available regarding excretion of antineoplastic agents in breast milk, breast-feeding is not recommended during chemotherapy because of the risks to the infant (adverse effects, mutagenicity, carcinogenicity).

## Pediatrics

Appropriate studies on the relationship of age to the effects of streptozocin have not been performed in the pediatric population.

## Geriatrics

No information is available on the relationship of age to the effects of streptozocin in geriatric patients. However, elderly patients are more likely to have age-related renal function impairment, which may require caution in patients receiving streptozocin.

## Dental

The bone marrow depressant effects of streptozocin may result in an increased incidence of microbial infection, delayed healing, and gingival bleeding. If leukopenia and/or thrombocytopenia occur, dental work should be deferred until blood counts have returned to normal and patients should be instructed in proper oral hygiene including caution in use of regular toothbrushes, dental floss, and toothpicks.

## Drug interactions and/or related problems

The following drug interactions and/or related problems have been selected on the basis of their potential clinical significance (possible mechanism in parentheses where appropriate)—not necessarily inclusive (» = major clinical significance):

Note: Combinations containing any of the following medications, depending on the amount present, may also interact with this medication.

Blood dyscrasia–causing medications (See *Appendix II*)
    (leukopenic and/or thrombocytopenic effects of streptozocin may be increased with concurrent or recent therapy if these medications cause the same effects; dosage adjustment of streptozocin, if necessary, should be based on blood counts)

Bone marrow depressants, other (See *Appendix II*) or
Radiation therapy
    (additive bone marrow depression may occur, although myelosuppressive effects of streptozocin are rare; dosage reduction may be required when two or more bone marrow depressants, including radiation, are used concurrently or consecutively)
    (streptozocin may prolong the half-life of doxorubicin when used concurrently; dosage reduction of doxorubicin is recommended)

Corticosteroids, glucocorticoid or
Corticotropin (ACTH)
    (concurrent use may increase the hyperglycemic effect of streptozocin)

» Nephrotoxic medications (See *Appendix II*)
    (concurrent use may result in enhanced nephrotoxicity and is not recommended)

Nicotinamide
    (concurrent use may reduce the diabetogenic effect of streptozocin but does not appear to alter the antitumor effect)

» Phenytoin
    (may protect pancreatic beta cells from the toxic effects of streptozocin, thus reducing its therapeutic effects; concurrent use is not recommended)

Vaccines, killed virus
    (because normal defense mechanisms may be suppressed by streptozocin therapy, the patient's antibody response to the vaccine may be decreased. The interval between discontinuation of medications that cause immunosuppression and restoration of the patient's ability to respond to the vaccine depends on the intensity and type of immunosuppression-causing medication used, the underlying disease, and other factors; estimates vary from 3 months to 1 year)

» Vaccines, live virus
    (because normal defense mechanisms may be suppressed by streptozocin therapy, concurrent use with a live virus vaccine may potentiate the replication of the vaccine virus, may increase the side/adverse effects of the vaccine virus, and/or may decrease the patient's antibody response to the vaccine; immunization of these patients should be undertaken only with extreme caution after careful review of the patient's hematologic status and only with the knowledge and consent of the physician managing the streptozocin therapy. The interval between discontinuation of medications that cause immunosuppression and restoration of the patient's ability to respond to the vaccine depends on the intensity and type of immunosuppression-causing medication used, the underlying disease, and other factors; estimates vary from 3 months to 1 year. Patients with leukemia in remission should not receive live virus vaccine until at least 3 months after their last chemotherapy. Immunization with oral poliovirus vaccine should also be postponed in persons in close contact with the patient, especially family members)

## Laboratory value alterations

The following have been selected on the basis of their potential clinical significance (possible effect in parentheses where appropriate)—not necessarily inclusive (» = major clinical significance):

With physiology/laboratory test values
    Alanine aminotransferase (ALT [SGPT]) and
    Alkaline phosphatase and
    Aspartate aminotransferase (AST [SGOT]) and

Bilirubin and
Lactate dehydrogenase (LDH)
    (serum values may be increased, indicating hepatotoxicity)

Albumin concentrations in blood
    (may be decreased, indicating hepatotoxicity)

Blood urea nitrogen (BUN) concentrations and
Creatinine concentrations, plasma and
Protein concentrations, urinary
    (may be increased, indicating renal toxicity; usually transient, but
    permanent damage may occur)

Glucose
    (blood concentrations may be initially decreased because of sudden
    release of insulin)

Hematocrit
    (may rarely be mildly increased; reduction in hematocrit is gen-
    erally more common than leukopenia or thrombocytopenia)

Phosphate
    (blood concentrations may be decreased, as an early indication of
    renal toxicity)

## Medical considerations/Contraindications

The medical considerations/contraindications included here have been selected on the basis of their potential clinical significance (reasons given
in parentheses where appropriate)—not necessarily inclusive (» =
major clinical significance).

*Risk-benefit should be considered when the following medical problems
exist:*

Bone marrow depression or
Infection
    (possible hematological toxicity, although this is rare)

» Chickenpox, existing or recent (including recent exposure) or
» Herpes zoster
    (risk of severe generalized disease)

Diabetes mellitus
    (streptozocin causes hypoglycemia)

» Hepatic function impairment
    (reduced biotransformation and possible increased toxicity of
    streptozocin; streptozocin can have hepatotoxic effects)

» Renal function impairment
    (streptozocin causes severe renal toxicity)

Sensitivity to streptozocin

Caution should be used also in patients who have had previous cyto-
    toxic drug therapy or radiation therapy.

## Patient monitoring

The following are especially important in patient monitoring (other tests
may be warranted in some patients, depending on condition; » =
major clinical significance):

Alanine aminotransferase (ALT [SGPT]) values, serum and
Aspartate aminotransferase (AST [SGOT]) values, serum and
Bilirubin values, serum and
Lactate dehydrogenase (LDH) values, serum
    (recommended prior to initiation of therapy and at periodic inter-
    vals during therapy; frequency varies according to clinical state,
    agent, and other agents being used concurrently)

» Blood urea nitrogen (BUN) concentrations and
» Creatinine clearance determinations and
» Creatinine concentrations, plasma and
» Electrolyte concentrations, serum and
» Urinalysis, serial, to detect proteinuria
    (recommended prior to, at least weekly during, and for 4 weeks
    following each course of therapy, to monitor for renal toxicity)

» Glucose concentrations, blood
    (recommended at periodic intervals)

Hematocrit or hemoglobin and
Leukocyte count, total and, if appropriate, differential and
Platelet count
    (determinations recommended prior to initiation of therapy and at
    periodic intervals during therapy; frequency varies according to
    clinical state, agent, and other agents being used concurrently)

Insulin concentrations, fasting
    (in patients with functional pancreatic tumors, serial monitoring
    allows a determination of biochemical response to therapy)

Uric acid concentrations, serum
    (recommended prior to initiation of therapy and at periodic inter-
    vals during therapy; frequency varies according to clinical state,
    agent, and other agents being used concurrently)

# Side/Adverse Effects

Note: Many "side effects" of antineoplastic therapy are unavoidable and
    represent the medication's pharmacologic action. Some of these (for
    example, leukopenia and thrombocytopenia) are actually used as
    parameters to aid in individual dosage titration.

The following side/adverse effects have been selected on the basis of their
    potential clinical significance (possible signs and symptoms in paren-
    theses where appropriate)—not necessarily inclusive:

**Those indicating need for medical attention**
Incidence more frequent—28 to 73%
    *Renal toxicity and failure* (swelling of feet or lower legs; unusual
    decrease in urination)

    Note: *Renal toxicity* (proteinuria, glycosuria, hypophosphatemia, az-
    otemia, renal tubular acidosis) occurs frequently. Mild protein-
    uria is one of the first signs of renal toxicity. Toxicity is dose-
    related and cumulative and may be fatal in some cases.

Incidence less frequent
    *Hypoglycemia, occurring shortly after injection* (anxiety, nervous-
    ness, or shakiness; chills, cold sweats, or cool, pale skin; drowsiness
    or unusual tiredness or weakness; fast pulse; headache; unusual hun-
    ger); *rapid intravenous injection or extravasation* (pain or redness at
    site of injection)

    Note: Although streptozocin is *diabetogenic*, a sudden release of in-
    sulin may occur initially. Mild to moderate glucose tolerance
    abnormalities have been reported; they are usually reversible,
    although insulin shock with hypoglycemia has occurred.

Incidence rare
    *Hepatotoxicity* (usually not symptomatic); *leukopenia or infection*
    (usually asymptomatic; rarely, fever or chills; cough or hoarseness;
    lower back or side pain; painful or difficult urination); *thrombocyto-
    penia* (usually asymptomatic; rarely, unusual bleeding or bruising;
    black, tarry stools; blood in urine or stools; pinpoint red spots on skin)

    Note: *Hematological toxicity* is rare but has been fatal in some cases.

**Those indicating need for medical attention only if they continue
or are bothersome**
Incidence more frequent
    *Nausea and vomiting*

    Note: *Nausea and vomiting* occur in most patients, usually within 2
    to 4 hours after a dose and may be severe; usually become
    progressively worse over a course of therapy; antiemetics have
    little effect.

Incidence less frequent
    *Diarrhea*

**Those indicating the need for medical attention if they occur after
medication is discontinued**
    *Renal toxicity* (decrease in urination; swelling of feet or lower legs)

# Patient Consultation

As an aid to patient consultation, refer to *Advice for the Patient,
Streptozocin (Systemic)*.

In providing consultation, consider emphasizing the following selected
information (» = major clinical significance):

**Before using this medication**
» Conditions affecting use, especially:
    Sensitivity to streptozocin
    Pregnancy—Use not recommended because of mutagenic, terato-
    genic, and carcinogenic potential, advisability of using contra-
    ception; telling physician immediately if pregnancy is
    suspected
    Breast-feeding—Not recommended because of risk of serious side
    effects
    Other medications, especially nephrotoxic medications or
    phenytoin
    Other medical problems, especially chickenpox, herpes zoster, he-
    patic function impairment, or renal function impairment

**Proper use of this medication**
    Importance of ample fluid intake and subsequent increase in urine
    output to aid excretion and reduce renal toxicity
    Frequency of nausea and vomiting; importance of continuing medi-
    cation despite stomach upset
» Proper dosing

**Precautions while using this medication**
» Importance of close monitoring by physician
» Avoiding immunizations unless approved by physician; other persons
    in patient's household should avoid immunizations with oral po-

liovirus vaccine; avoiding other persons who have taken oral poliovirus vaccine or wearing a protective mask that covers nose and mouth

» Possibility of local tissue injury and scarring if infiltration of intravenous solution occurs; telling doctor or nurse right away about redness, pain, or swelling at injection site

### Side/adverse effects

May cause adverse effects such as kidney problems and cancer; importance of discussing possible effects with physician

Signs of potential side effects, especially renal toxicity and failure, hypoglycemia, rapid intravenous injection, extravasation, hepatotoxicity, leukopenia, infection, and thrombocytopenia

Physician or nurse can help in dealing with side effects

## General Dosing Information

Patients receiving streptozocin should be under supervision of a physician experienced in cancer chemotherapy.

A variety of dosage schedules and regimens of streptozocin, alone or in combination with other antitumor agents, are used. The prescriber may consult the medical literature as well as the manufacturer's literature in choosing a specific dosage.

Dosage must be adjusted to meet the individual requirements of each patient, on the basis of clinical response and appearance or severity of toxicity.

Streptozocin may be administered by rapid intravenous injection or as a short (over a 10- to 15-minute period) or long (over a 6-hour period) intravenous infusion.

Streptozocin has also been administered as a continuous, 5-day intravenous infusion. Although incidence of renal toxicity and nausea and vomiting appeared to be reduced, other side effects including lethargy, confusion, and depression were reported.

Care must be taken to avoid extravasation during administration because of the risk of severe ulceration and necrosis.

If extravasation of streptozocin occurs during intravenous administration, as indicated by local burning or stinging, the injection or infusion should be stopped immediately and resumed, completing the dose, in another vein.

Although the manufacturer does not recommend intra-arterial administration because of the possibility that renal toxicity may occur more rapidly, streptozocin has been administered intra-arterially by a number of investigators, for example, in patients with hepatic metastases.

It is recommended that intravenous dextrose be immediately available, especially when the first dose of streptozocin is administered, because of the risk of hypoglycemia due to a sudden release of insulin.

It is recommended that each course of streptozocin therapy be followed by a 4- to 6-week observation period in order to detect any renal toxicity.

It is recommended that dosage of streptozocin be reduced or treatment withdrawn if significant renal toxicity occurs. Subsequent doses should not be given until renal function returns to normal.

Concomitant hydration with each dose may reduce renal toxicity by promoting rapid excretion in a dilute urine.

### Safety considerations for handling this medication

There is limited but increasing evidence and concern that personnel involved in preparation and administration of parenteral antineoplastics may be at some risk because of the potential mutagenicity, teratogenicity, and/or carcinogenicity of these agents, although the actual risk is unknown. USP advisory panels recommend cautious handling both in preparation and disposal of antineoplastic agents. Precautions that have been suggested include:

• Use of a biological containment cabinet during reconstitution and dilution of parenteral medications and wearing of disposable surgical gloves and masks.

• Use of proper technique to prevent contamination of the medication, work area, and operator during transfer between containers (including proper training of personnel in this technique).

• Cautious and proper disposal of needles, syringes, vials, ampuls, and unused medication.

A number of medical centers have developed detailed guidelines for handling of antineoplastic agents.

## Parenteral Dosage Forms

### STREPTOZOCIN FOR INJECTION

### Usual adult dose

Pancreatic carcinoma—

Intravenous, 500 mg per square meter of body surface per day for five consecutive days every four to six weeks or

Intravenous, 1 gram per square meter of body surface once a week for two weeks, increased thereafter if necessary, up to a maximum dose of 1.5 grams per square meter of body surface.

Note: A single course usually consists of four to six once-a-week doses, but may be longer.

### Usual adult prescribing limits

Up to 1.5 grams per square meter of body surface as a single dose (because of the risk of azotemia).

### Usual pediatric dose

Dosage has not been established.

### Size(s) usually available

U.S.—

1 gram (Rx) [*Zanosar* (citric acid anhydrous 220 mg)].

Canada—

1 gram (Rx) [*Zanosar*].

### Packaging and storage

Store between 2 and 8 °C (36 and 46 °F), unless otherwise specified by manufacturer. Protect from light.

### Preparation of dosage form

Streptozocin for injection is reconstituted for intravenous use by adding 9.5 mL of 5% dextrose injection or 0.9% sodium chloride injection to the vial, producing a clear, pale-gold solution containing 100 mg of streptozocin and 22 mg of citric acid per mL.

Reconstituted solutions may be further diluted with 5% dextrose injection or 0.9% sodium chloride injection for administration by intravenous infusion. Addition of the 100 mg of streptozocin per mL solution to 10 to 200 mL of 5% dextrose injection followed by administration over a 15-minute period by infusion may prevent local pain and phlebitis.

### Stability

Reconstituted solutions should be used within 12 hours if kept at room temperature.

Because the product contains no preservatives, the vial should not be used for more than one dose.

A change in color from pale gold to dark brown indicates decomposition.

### Note

If accidental contact with skin or mucous membranes occurs, immediately wash the affected area with soap and water.

Revised: 08/26/92
Interim revision: 06/30/94

# STRONTIUM CHLORIDE Sr 89    Systemic

VA CLASSIFICATION (Primary): AN600

Note: For a listing of dosage forms and brand names by country availability, see *Dosage Forms* section(s). For a listing of brand names for the articles in this monograph, refer to the General Index.

## Category

Antineoplastic.

## Indications

### Accepted

Bone lesions, metastatic (treatment)—Strontium chloride Sr 89 is indicated in the palliative treatment of bone pain in selected patients with multiple areas of skeletal metastases from carcinomas of the prostate, breast, and possibly, from other carcinomas.

# Physical Properties

## Nuclear data

| Radionuclide (half-life) | Mode of decay | Maximum energy (MeV) | Mean number of emissions/ disintegration |
|---|---|---|---|
| Sr 89 (50.5 days) | Beta | 1.463 | 1 |

# Pharmacology/Pharmacokinetics

## Mechanism of action/Effect

Antineoplastic—Metastatic bone lesions: Strontium chloride Sr 89, a calcium analog, follows the same biochemical pathways as calcium does *in vivo* and concentrates in areas of increased osteogenesis (i.e., increased mineral turnover), not in marrow cells. Thus, reactive osteoid being formed at sites of primary bone tumors and metastases accumulate strontium to a much higher level than does surrounding normal bone. The retained strontium can deliver a radiation dose sufficiently large to produce a palliative effect. Due to the short range of the beta particles, the cells close to regions containing strontium will be preferentially irradiated.

## Distribution

Distribution similar to calcium analogs with fairly rapid clearance from the blood and selective localization in bone hydroxyapatite.

## Onset of action

Pain relief may begin between 7 and 21 days following administration of strontium chloride Sr 89, with maximum relief by 6 weeks.

## Duration of action

Duration of pain relief averages 6 months, with a range of 4 to 12 months.

## Radiation dosimetry

| Estimated absorbed radiation dose*† | | |
|---|---|---|
| Organ | mGy/MBq | rad/mCi |
| Bone surfaces | 17.0 | 62.96 |
| Red marrow | 11.0 | 40.74 |
| Large intestine wall (lower) | 4.7 | 17.41 |
| Large intestine wall (upper) | 1.8 | 6.67 |
| Bladder wall | 1.3 | 4.81 |
| Breast | 0.96 | 3.55 |
| Adrenals | 0.78 | 2.89 |
| Stomach wall | 0.78 | 2.89 |
| Kidneys | 0.78 | 2.89 |
| Liver | 0.78 | 2.89 |
| Lungs | 0.78 | 2.89 |
| Ovaries | 0.78 | 2.89 |
| Pancreas | 0.78 | 2.89 |
| Spleen | 0.78 | 2.89 |
| Testes | 0.78 | 2.89 |
| Thyroid | 0.78 | 2.89 |
| Uterus | 0.78 | 2.89 |
| Small intestine | 0.023 | 0.085 |
| Other tissue | 0.78 | 2.89 |

Effective dose: 2.9 mSv/MBq (10.73 rem/mCi)

*For adults; intravenous injection. Data based on the International Commission on Radiological Protection (ICRP) Publication 53—Radiation dose to patients from radiopharmaceuticals.

†The absorbed dose to individual metastatic sites ranges from 60 to 610 mGy/MBq (220 to 2260 rad/mCi) with a mean dose of 230 mGy/MBq (850 rad/mCi).

## Elimination

Renal, by glomerular filtration (two-thirds of excreted activity), and fecal (one-third) in patients with bone metastases. Renal excretion is greatest in the first 2 days after treatment. Strontium 89 is lost from normal bone with an initial biological half-life of 14 days, but retained much longer in metastatic bone lesions. Patients with extensive metastases may retain 50 to 100% of the administered activity in bone and may excrete less than do persons without bone lesions. Whole body retention of strontium varies according to individual urinary plasma clearance and metastatic load in the skeleton; between 12 and 90% of the administered activity is retained 3 months after administration of strontium chloride Sr 89.

# Precautions to Consider

## Carcinogenicity/Mutagenicity

Thirty-three out of 40 rats receiving 10 consecutive monthly doses of either 250 or 350 microcuries per kg of body weight of strontium chloride Sr 89 developed malignant bone tumors after a latency period of approximately 9 months.

## Pregnancy/Reproduction

Pregnancy—Adequate and well-controlled studies with strontium chloride Sr 89 have not been done in humans. Radiopharmaceuticals are generally not recommended for therapeutic use during pregnancy because of the risk to the fetus from radiation exposure. Strontium chloride Sr 89 would be expected to cause adverse effects, such as bone marrow toxicity, in the fetus.

To avoid the possibility of fetal exposure to radiation, in those circumstances in which the patient's pregnancy status is uncertain, a pregnancy test will help to prevent inadvertent administration of this preparation during pregnancy.

Studies have not been done in animals.

FDA Pregnancy Category D.

## Breast-feeding

Strontium chloride Sr 89 acts as a calcium analog and is expected to be distributed into breast milk. Because of the potential risk to the infant from radiation exposure, complete cessation of nursing is recommended after strontium chloride Sr 89 has been administered.

## Pediatrics

There have been no specific studies evaluating the safety and efficacy of strontium chloride Sr 89 in children.

## Geriatrics

Appropriate studies on the relationship of age to the effects of strontium chloride Sr 89 have not been performed in the geriatric population. However, no geriatrics-specific problems have been documented to date.

## Drug interactions and/or related problems

The following drug interactions and/or related problems have been selected on the basis of their potential clinical significance (possible mechanism in parentheses where appropriate)—not necessarily inclusive (» = major clinical significance):

» Blood-dyscrasia–causing medications (See *Appendix II* ) (leukopenic and/or thrombocytopenic effects of strontium chloride Sr 89 may be increased)

» Calcium-containing medications (saturation of bone-binding sites by calcium may cause decreased bone uptake of strontium chloride Sr 89; calcium-containing medications should be discontinued at least 2 weeks before therapy with strontium chloride Sr 89; calcium-containing medication may be resumed approximately 2 weeks after strontium chloride Sr 89 therapy)

## Laboratory value alterations

The following have been selected on the basis of their potential clinical significance (possible effect in parentheses where appropriate)—not necessarily inclusive (» = major clinical significance):

With physiology/laboratory test values
  Alkaline phosphatase
    (serum values may be decreased, reflecting tumoricidal effect)

  Serum tumor markers, such as prostatic specific antigen (PSA) and prostate acid phosphatase (PAP)
    (concentration may be decreased, reflecting tumoricidal effect)

## Medical considerations/Contraindications

The medical considerations/contraindications included here have been selected on the basis of their potential clinical significance (reasons given in parentheses where appropriate)—not necessarily inclusive (» = major clinical significance).

*Except under special circumstances, this medication should not be used when the following medical problem exists:*

» Bone marrow depression, with platelet count less than 60,000 per microliter and white cell count less than 2,400 per microliter, especially with previous or concomitant chemotherapy or radiotherapy administration
    (increased risk of toxicity due to compromised bone marrow)

*Risk-benefit must be considered when the following medical problems exist:*

Sensitivity to the radiopharmaceutical preparation

Urinary incontinence
    (increased risk of radiation contamination of environment; therefore, urinary catheterization is recommended)

Very short life-expectancy
(use not warranted since onset of pain relief may not occur for 10 to 20 days)

**Patient monitoring**
The following may be especially important in patient monitoring (other tests may be warranted in some patients, depending on condition; » = major clinical significance):

»   Blood studies, including leukocyte and platelet counts
(recommended prior to therapy and at least once every other week for 3 to 4 months after therapy)

## Side/Adverse Effects

Note: A single case of fatal septicemia following leukopenia has been reported during clinical trials.

**Those indicating need for medical attention**
Incidence rare
*Bone marrow depression leading to thrombocytopenia* (unusual bleeding or bruising; black, tarry stools; blood in urine or stools; pinpoint red spots on skin); *and leukopenia* (cough or hoarseness; fever or chills; lower back or side pain; painful or difficult urination)

Note: On the average, platelet concentrations may fall by 30% of pretreatment levels (i.e., fall to 70% of baseline); however, this effect is generally reversible, and the majority of patients maintain platelet counts that are within normal limits. The nadir of platelet depression occurs in most patients about 6 weeks after administration of strontium chloride Sr 89.

Bone marrow toxicity may be difficult to evaluate because marrow suppression is common in patients with prostate cancer and extensive bone metastases.

**Those indicating need for medical attention only if they continue or are bothersome**
Incidence more frequent
*Flare reaction* (increase in bone pain, transient); *flushing*—with rapid administration

## Patient Consultation

As an aid to patient consultation, refer to *Advice for the Patient, Strontium Chloride Sr 89 (Therapeutic).*

In providing consultation, consider emphasizing the following selected information (» = major clinical significance):

**Description of use**
Action in the body: Active incorporation of strontium 89 into bone mineral, especially in areas of tumor involvement; localized radiation exposure to these sites provides reduction in bone pain

**Before using this medication**
»   Conditions affecting use, especially:
Sensitivity to the radiopharmaceutical preparation
Pregnancy—Use not recommended; risk to fetus from radiation exposure
Breast-feeding—May be distributed into breast milk; cessation of nursing is recommended because of risk to infant from radiation exposure
Other medications, especially blood dyscrasia–causing and calcium-containing

**Proper use of this medication**
Special preparatory instructions may apply; patient should inquire in advance
Notifying physician prior to administration if having an incontinence problem; catheterization may be required to prevent radiation contamination

**Precautions after using this medication**
»   Importance of close monitoring by the physician
*To prevent radiation contamination of other persons or environment:*
*For the first week—*
»   Using a normal toilet instead of a urinal
»   Double-flushing toilet
»   Wiping any spilled urine with a tissue and flushing it away
»   Washing hands after using or cleaning toilet
»   Immediately laundering clothes and linens soiled with urine or blood; washing them separately from other clothes
»   Washing away any spilled blood
»   Caution if significant bone marrow depression occurs
*Abnormally low white blood cell counts—*
Avoiding exposure to persons with bacterial infections, especially during periods of low blood counts; checking with physician immediately if fever or chills, cough or hoarseness, lower back or side pain, or painful or difficult urination occurs

Caution in use of regular toothbrush, dental floss, or toothpick; physician, dentist, or nurse may suggest alternatives; checking with physician before having dental work done.
Not touching eyes or inside of nose unless hands washed immediately before
*Abnormally low platelet counts—*
Using caution to avoid accidental cuts with use of sharp objects such as safety razor or fingernail or toenail cutters
Avoiding contact sports or other situations where bruising or injury could occur

**Side/adverse effects**
Signs of potential side effects, especially bone marrow depression

## General Dosing Information

Radiopharmaceuticals are to be administered only by or under the supervision of physicians who have had extensive training in the safe use and handling of radioactive materials and who are authorized by the Nuclear Regulatory Commission (NRC) or the appropriate Agreement State agency, if required, or, outside the U.S., the appropriate authority.

The presence of bone metastases must be confirmed (e.g., by skeletal imaging with a technetium Tc 99m–labeled phosphate or phosphonate radiopharmaceutical) prior to therapy with strontium chloride Sr 89.

Treatment may be repeated at intervals of 3 months or more if pain recurs. However, previous hematologic response, current platelet level, and other signs of bone marrow depression should be carefully evaluated before therapy with strontium chloride Sr 89 is repeated.

**Safety considerations for handling this medication**
Improper handling of this radiopharmaceutical may cause radioactive contamination. Guidelines for handling radioactive material have been prepared by scientific, professional, state, federal, and international bodies and are available to the specially qualified and authorized users who have access to radiopharmaceuticals

## Parenteral Dosage Forms

### STRONTIUM CHLORIDE Sr 89 INJECTION USP

**Usual adult administered activity**
Antineoplastic—
Metastatic bone lesions: Intravenous, 1.5 to 2.2 megabecquerels (40 to 60 microcuries) per kg of body weight, or a total administered activity of 148 megabecquerels (4 millicuries) given slowly (one to two minutes) as a single dose.

Note: Repeated administration at intervals of less than ninety days is generally not recommended.

**Usual pediatric administered activity**
Children up to 18 years of age: Minimum dosage has not been established.

**Usual geriatric administered activity**
See *Usual adult administered activity.*

**Strength(s) usually available**
U.S.—
148 megabecquerels (4 millicuries) in 4-mL volume per 10-mL vial, containing 10.9 to 22.6 mg of strontium chloride per mL, and a specific activity of 2.96 to 6.17 megabecquerels (80 to 167 microcuries) per mg of strontium, at time of calibration (Rx) [*Metastron*].
Canada—
150 megabecquerels (4.05 millicuries) in 4-mL volume per 10-mL vial, containing 13.4 to 20.1 mg of strontium chloride per mL, and a specific activity of 3.33 to 5 megabecquerels (90 to 135 microcuries) per mg of strontium, at time of calibration (Rx) [*Metastron*].

**Packaging and storage**
Store between 15 and 25 °C (59 and 77 °F), unless otherwise specified by manufacturer. Protect from freezing.

**Stability**
Product should not be used beyond 4 weeks after calibration.

**Note**
Caution—Radioactive material.

## Selected Bibliography

Hansen DV, Holmes ER, Catton G, et al. Strontium 89 therapy for painful osseous metastatic prostate and breast cancer. Am Fam Physician 1993; 47 (8): 1795-800.

Laing AH, Ackery DM, Bayly RJ, et al. Strontium 89 chloride for pain palliation in prostatic skeletal malignancy. Br J Radiol 1991; 64 (765): 816-22.

Porter AT, McEwan AJ, Powe JE, et al. Results of a randomized phase-III trial to evaluate the efficacy of strontium 89 adjuvant to local field external beam irradiation in the management of endocrine resistant metastatic prostate cancer. Int J Radiat Oncol Biol Phys 1993; 25 (5): 805-13.

Robinson RG, Preston DF, Baxter KG, et al. Clinical experience with strontium 89 in prostatic and breast cancer patients. Semin Oncol 1993; 20 (3 Suppl 2): 44-8.

Robinson RG, Preston DF, Spicer JA, et al. Radionuclide therapy of intractable bone pain: emphasis on strontium 89. Semin Nucl Med 1992; 22 (1): 28-32.

Revised: 06/23/94
Interim revision: 05/18/95

# SUCCIMER   Systemic

**VA CLASSIFICATION (Primary): AD300**

Other commonly used names are dimercaptosuccinic acid and DMSA.

Note: For a listing of dosage forms and brand names by country availability, see *Dosage Forms* section(s). For a listing of brand names for the articles in this monograph, refer to the General Index.

†Not commercially available in Canada; however, succimer capsules are available by emergency drug release from the Health Protection Branch.

## Category

Chelating agent.

## Indications

Note: Bracketed information in the *Indications* section refers to uses that are not included in U.S. product labeling.

**Accepted**

Toxicity, lead (treatment)—Succimer is indicated for the treatment of lead poisoning in children with blood lead concentrations above 45 mcg per deciliter. [Succimer is also used to treat lead toxicity in adults.][1]

Signs and symptoms of severe, symptomatic lead poisoning include anemia, gastrointestinal complaints (abdominal pain and vomiting), nephropathy, and encephalopathy. Dimercaprol and edetate calcium disodium combination is considered the treatment of choice for lead encephalopathy.

**Unaccepted**

Succimer is not indicated for prophylaxis of lead poisoning in a lead-containing environment. Use of succimer should be accompanied by identification and removal of the source of lead exposure.

[1]Not included in Canadian product labeling.

## Pharmacology/Pharmacokinetics

**Physicochemical characteristics**

Molecular weight—182.2.
pKa—3 and 3.9.

**Mechanism of action/Effect**

Orally active succimer is a heavy metal chelating agent that forms stable, water-soluble complexes with lead and consequently increases the urinary excretion of lead. The site of lead chelation by succimer is not known.

**Other actions/effects**

Succimer chelates other heavy metals such as arsenic and mercury.

**Absorption**

Rapid but incomplete.

**Biotransformation**

Major metabolites are mixed disulfides of L-cysteine, but the site of biotransformation is not known.

**Half-life**

Elimination—48 hours.

**Time to peak concentration**

1 to 2 hours.

**Elimination**

Primarily renal, with small amounts eliminated by the lung and by fecal excretion.

In dialysis—Limited data indicate that succimer is dialyzable; however, lead chelates are not.

## Precautions to Consider

**Mutagenicity**

Succimer was not mutagenic in the Ames bacterial assay and in the mammalian cell forward gene mutation assay.

**Pregnancy/Reproduction**

Pregnancy—Adequate and well-controlled studies have not been done in humans.

In a study in pregnant mice with succimer at doses of 410 to 1640 mg per kg (mg/kg) of body weight a day during the period of organogenesis, the medication has been shown to be teratogenic and fetotoxic. Another study in fetal rats with succimer at doses of up to 1000 mg/kg a day during periods of organogenesis showed no teratogenicity.

FDA Pregnancy Category C.

**Breast-feeding**

It is not known whether succimer is distributed into breast milk.

**Pediatrics**

Appropriate studies performed to date have not demonstrated pediatrics-specific problems that would limit the usefulness of succimer in children. There is no experience in children less than 1 year of age.

**Geriatrics**

No information is available on the relationship of age to the effects of succimer in geriatric patients.

**Laboratory value alterations**

The following have been selected on the basis of their potential clinical significance (possible effect in parentheses where appropriate)—not necessarily inclusive (» = major clinical significance):

With diagnostic test results
Urinary ketone determinations by nitroprusside reagents
(succimer may cause false-positive results)

With physiology/laboratory test values
Alanine aminotransferase (ALT [SGPT]), serum and
Aspartate aminotransferase (AST [SGOT]), serum
(values may be temporarily elevated)

Creatinine kinase (CK) values or
Uric acid concentrations, serum
(succimer may cause a false decrease)

**Medical considerations/Contraindications**

The medical considerations/contraindications included here have been selected on the basis of their potential clinical significance (reasons given in parentheses where appropriate)—not necessarily inclusive (» = major clinical significance).

*Risk-benefit should be considered when the following medical problems exist:*

» Dehydration
(adequate urine flow must be established before and during succimer chelation therapy)

» Renal function impairment
(succimer heavy metal chelates are excreted in urine; renal function impairment may delay or decrease excretion)

Sensitivity to succimer

**Patient monitoring**

The following may be especially important in patient monitoring (other tests may be warranted in some patients, depending on condition; » = major clinical significance):

Alkaline phosphatase and
Blood urea nitrogen (BUN) concentrations and
CBC with differential and

Creatinine concentrations, serum and
Platelet counts
  (determinations recommended before therapy and weekly during
  therapy)

Hepatic transaminases, serum
  (determinations recommended before therapy and weekly during
  therapy because succimer has been reported to cause mild, transient elevations of serum transaminases)

Lead concentration in blood
  (determination recommended to ascertain dosage and duration of
  therapy; after therapy, weekly monitoring for a rebound of blood
  lead concentration is suggested until the patient is stable)

## Side/Adverse Effects

The following side/adverse effects have been selected on the basis of their
potential clinical significance (possible signs and symptoms in parentheses where appropriate)—not necessarily inclusive:

**Those indicating need for medical attention**
Incidence less frequent
  *Neutropenia* (fever and chills)

**Those indicating need for medical attention only if they continue
or are bothersome**
Incidence less frequent
  *Skin rash*

  Note: Some *skin rashes* have necessitated discontinuation of therapy.
     If rash occurs, other causes should be considered before ascrib-
     ing the reaction to succimer.

**Those not indicating need for medical attention**
Incidence more frequent
  *Gastrointestinal disturbances, specifically loss of appetite; diarrhea;
  loose stools; nausea and vomiting; unpleasant odor to urine, sweat,
  and feces*

## Overdose

For specific information on agents used in the management of succimer
overdose, see *Charcoal, Activated (Oral-Local)* monograph.

For more information on the management of overdose or unintentional
ingestion, **contact a Poison Control Center** (see *Poison Control Center Listing*).

**Treatment of overdose**
To decrease absorption—Induction of vomiting or gastric lavage. Administration of an activated charcoal slurry.

Supportive care—Appropriate supportive therapy. Patients in whom intentional overdose is confirmed or suspected should be referred for
  psychiatric consultation.

## Patient Consultation

As an aid to patient consultation, refer to *Advice for the Patient, Succimer
(Systemic)*.

In providing consultation, consider emphasizing the following selected
information (» = major clinical significance):

**Before using this medication**
» Conditions affecting use, especially:
    Sensitivity to succimer
    Other medical problems, especially dehydration and renal function
    impairment

**Proper use of this medication**
» Removal of child from lead-contaminated environment
    Possible need for hospitalization of child during succimer therapy
    Unpleasant odor of capsules

Contents of capsule may be sprinkled on food and eaten immediately
  or given by spoon and followed immediately by a fruit drink
» Proper dosing
    Missed dose: Taking as soon as possible; not taking if almost time for
    next dose; not doubling doses
» Proper storage

**Precautions while using this medication**
» Regular visits to physician to check progress of therapy and to prevent
    adverse effects

**Side/adverse effects**
    Signs of potential side effects, especially neutropenia

## General Dosing Information

Removal of patient from lead-contaminated environment is the primary
therapy for exposed patients.

Some clinicians recommend that children receiving succimer be hospitalized until their blood lead levels fall below 45 mcg per deciliter and
the lead in their environment has been removed.

Patients who have received edetate calcium disodium with or without dimercaprol should wait 4 weeks before receiving succimer therapy.
Data on concomitant use of succimer and edetate calcium disodium
with or without dimercaprol are not available.

## Oral Dosage Forms

Note: Bracketed uses in the *Dosage Forms* section refer to categories of
  use and/or indications that are not included in U.S. product labeling.

### SUCCIMER CAPSULES

**Usual adult and adolescent dose**
[Lead toxicity (treatment)][1]—
  Oral, 10 mg per kg of body weight every eight hours for five days.

**Usual pediatric dose**
Lead toxicity (treatment)—
  Oral, 10 mg per kg of body weight or 350 mg per square meter of
  body surface area every eight hours for five days, then 10 mg per
  kg of body weight every twelve hours for the next fourteen days
  for a total of nineteen days therapy.

Note: Repeated courses of treatment may be administered after a drug-
  free interval of two weeks, unless blood lead concentrations indicate the need for immediate retreatment.

**Strength(s) usually available**
U.S.—
  100 mg (Rx) [*Chemet*].
Canada—
  Succimer capsules are not commercially available in Canada; however,
  they are available by emergency drug release from the Health Protection Branch.

**Packaging and storage**
Store below 40 °C (104 °F), preferably between 15 and 30 °C (59 and 86
°F), unless otherwise specified by manufacturer.

**Note**
The contents of succimer capsules may be sprinkled on soft foods and
  given immediately or given by spoon and followed with a fruit drink.

---

[1]Not included in Canadian product labeling.

---

Revised: 06/22/93

---

**SUCCINYLCHOLINE  CHLORIDE**—See *Neuromuscular
Blocking Agents (Systemic)*

---

# SUCRALFATE   Oral-Local

VA CLASSIFICATION (Primary): GA302
Note: For a listing of dosage forms and brand names by country availability, see *Dosage Forms* section(s). For a listing of brand names
  for the articles in this monograph, refer to the General Index.

## Category

Antiulcer agent; gastric mucosa protectant.

## Indications

Note: Bracketed information in the *Indications* section refers to uses that
  are not included in U.S. product labeling.

**Accepted**
Ulcer, duodenal (treatment)—Sucralfate is indicated in the short-term (up
  to 8 weeks) treatment of duodenal ulcer.

Ulcer, duodenal (prophylaxis)—Sucralfate is used in the prevention of
  duodenal ulcer recurrence.

[Ulcer, gastric (treatment)]—Sucralfate is used for the short-term treatment of benign gastric ulcer.

[Arthritis, rheumatoid (treatment adjunct)][1]—Sucralfate is used for the relief of gastrointestinal symptoms associated with the use of nonsteroidal anti-inflammatory drugs in the treatment of rheumatoid arthritis.

[Stress-related mucosal damage (prophylaxis and treatment)][1]—Sucralfate is used to prevent and treat gastrointestinal, stress-induced ulceration and bleeding, especially in intensive care patients.

[Reflux, gastroesophageal (treatment)]—Sucralfate is used in the treatment of gastroesophageal reflux disease.

---

[1]Not included in Canadian product labeling.

## Pharmacology/Pharmacokinetics

### Physicochemical characteristics
Sucralfate is an aluminum salt of a sulfated disaccharide

### Mechanism of action/Effect
Exact mechanism of action is not known; however, sucralfate is thought to form an ulcer-adherent complex with proteinaceous exudate, such as albumin and fibrinogen, at the ulcer site, protecting it against further acid attack. To a lesser extent, sucralfate forms a viscous, adhesive barrier on the surface of intact mucosa of the stomach and duodenum. Sucralfate also inhibits pepsin activity and has been found to bind bile salts *in vitro*. Recent information suggests that sucralfate may increase the production of prostaglandin $E_2$ and gastric mucus.

### Absorption
Up to 5% of the disaccharide component and less than 0.02% of aluminum is absorbed from the gastrointestinal tract following an oral sucralfate dose.

### Elimination
Mostly fecal; small amounts of sulfate disaccharide are eliminated in the urine.

## Precautions to Consider

### Pregnancy/Reproduction
Pregnancy—Studies in humans have not been done.
Studies in animals have not shown that sucralfate causes adverse effects on the fetus.
FDA Pregnancy Category B.

### Breast-feeding
Problems in humans have not been documented.

### Pediatrics
Appropriate studies to date have not demonstrated pediatrics-specific problems that would limit the usefulness of sucralfate in children.

### Geriatrics
Although adequate and well-controlled studies on the relationship of age to the effects of sucralfate have not been performed in the geriatric population, no geriatrics-specific problems have been documented to date.

### Drug interactions and/or related problems
The following drug interactions and/or related problems have been selected on the basis of their potential clinical significance (possible mechanism in parentheses where appropriate)—not necessarily inclusive (» = major clinical significance):

Note: Combinations containing any of the following medications, depending on the amount present, may also interact with this medication.

Aluminum-containing medications, such as:
Antacids
Antidiarrheals
Aspirin, buffered with aluminum
Vaginal douches
(concurrent use with sucralfate in patients with renal failure may cause aluminum toxicity)

Antacids
(concurrent use with antacids in the treatment of duodenal ulcer may be indicated for the relief of pain; however, simultaneous administration is not recommended since antacids may interfere with binding of sucralfate to the mucosa; patient should be advised not to take antacids within $1/2$ hour before or after sucralfate)

Cimetidine or
Ranitidine
(concurrent use with sucralfate may decrease the absorption of cimetidine or ranitidine; patients should be advised to take cimetidine or ranitidine 2 hours before sucralfate)

» Ciprofloxacin or
» Norfloxacin or
» Ofloxacin
(concurrent use with sucralfate may decrease the absorption of ciprofloxacin, norfloxacin, or ofloxacin by chelation, resulting in lower serum and urine concentrations of these 3 medicines; patients should be advised to take ciprofloxacin, norfloxacin, or ofloxacin 2 to 3 hours before sucralfate)

» Digoxin or
» Theophylline
(concurrent use with sucralfate may decrease the absorption of digoxin or theophylline; patients should be advised not to take sucralfate within 2 hours of digoxin or theophylline)

» Phenytoin
(concurrent use with sucralfate may decrease the absorption of phenytoin enough to reduce the steady-state blood concentrations of phenytoin with a resultant loss of seizure control; patients should be advised not to take sucralfate within 2 hours of phenytoin)

Tetracyclines, oral
(absorption may be decreased when oral tetracyclines are used concurrently with sucralfate, since sucralfate is an aluminum salt and may form nonabsorbable complexes with tetracycline; patients should be advised not to take sucralfate within 2 hours of tetracyclines)

### Medical considerations/Contraindications
The medical considerations/contraindications included here have been selected on the basis of their potential clinical significance (reasons given in parentheses where appropriate)—not necessarily inclusive (» = major clinical significance).

*Risk-benefits should be considered when the following medical problems exist:*

Dysphagia or
Gastrointestinal tract obstruction disease
(patients with these conditions may be at risk of bezoar formation because of the protein-binding properties of sucralfate)

Renal failure
(absorption of the aluminum in sucralfate in patients with renal failure may cause aluminum toxicity, especially with long-term use)

Sensitivity to sucralfate

### Patient monitoring
The following may be especially important in patient monitoring (other tests may be warranted in some patients, depending on condition; » = major clinical significance):

Serum aluminum concentrations
(determinations may be increased in patients with renal failure)

## Side/Adverse Effects

Note: Occurrence of drowsiness progressing to seizures in patients with renal failure may indicate aluminum toxicity.

The following side/adverse effects have been selected on the basis of their potential clinical significance (possible signs and symptoms in parentheses where appropriate)—not necessarily inclusive:

**Those indicating need for medical attention only if they continue or are bothersome**
Incidence more frequent
*Constipation*
Incidence less frequent or rare
*Backache; diarrhea; dizziness or lightheadedness; drowsiness; dryness of mouth; indigestion; nausea; skin rash, hives, or itching; stomach cramps or pain*

## Patient Consultation
As an aid to patient consultation, refer to *Advice for the Patient, Sucralfate (Oral)*.

In providing consultation, consider emphasizing the following selected information (» = major clinical significance):

### Before using this medication
» Conditions affecting use, especially:
Sensitivity to sucralfate
Other medications, especially ciprofloxacin, digoxin, norfloxacin, ofloxacin, phenytoin, and theophylline

### Proper use of this medication
Taking on empty stomach 1 hour before meals and at bedtime

Compliance with full course of therapy and keeping appointments for check-ups
» Proper dosing
Missed dose: Taking as soon as possible; not taking if almost time for next dose; not doubling doses
» Proper storage

**Precautions while using this medication**
» Not taking antacids within 1/2 hour before or after sucralfate

**Side/adverse effects**
Signs of potential side effects, especially aluminum toxicity

## General Dosing Information

Sucralfate should be taken with water on an empty stomach, 1 hour before each meal and at bedtime, for maximum effectiveness.

Short-term treatment with sucralfate may result in complete healing of the ulcer but it may not alter the posthealing frequency or severity of duodenal ulceration.

If required, antacids may be administered 1/2 hour before or after sucralfate for the relief of pain.

Even though the symptoms of duodenal ulcers may subside, unless healing has been documented by x-ray or endoscopic examination, therapy should continue for at least 4 to 8 weeks.

Use of sucralfate in a nasogastric feeding tube has resulted in bezoar formation with other medications or enteral feedings, due to the protein-binding properties of sucralfate.

## Oral Dosage Forms

Note: Bracketed uses in the *Dosage Forms* section refer to categories of use and/or indications that are not included in U.S. product labeling.

### SUCRALFATE ORAL SUSPENSION

**Usual adult and adolescent dose**
Duodenal ulcer (treatment)—
Oral, 1 gram four times a day one hour before each meal and at bedtime; or 2 grams two times a day on waking and at bedtime on an empty stomach.
[Gastroesophageal reflux]—
Oral, 1 gram four times a day one hour before each meal and at bedtime.

**Usual pediatric dose**
Duodenal ulcer (treatment)—
Dosage has not been established.
[Gastroesophageal reflux]—
Oral, 500 mg to 1 gram four times a day one hour before each meal and at bedtime.

**Strength(s) usually available**
U.S.—
500 mg per 5 mL (Rx) [*Carafate*].

Canada—
500 mg per 5 mL (Rx) [*Sulcrate*].

**Packaging and storage**
Store below 40 °C (104 °F), preferably between 15 and 30 °C (59 and 86 °F), in a tight container, unless otherwise specified by manufacturer. Protect from freezing.

**Auxiliary labeling**
• Shake well.

### SUCRALFATE TABLETS

**Usual adult and adolescent dose**
Duodenal ulcer (treatment)—
Oral, 1 gram four times a day one hour before each meal and at bedtime.
Duodenal ulcer (prophylaxis)—
Oral, 1 gram two times a day on an empty stomach.
[Gastric ulcer (treatment)] or
[Gastroesophageal reflux]—
Oral, 1 gram four times a day one hour before each meal and at bedtime.

**Usual pediatric dose**
Duodenal ulcer (treatment)—
Dosage has not been established.
[Gastroesophageal reflux]—
Oral, 500 mg four times a day one hour before each meal and at bedtime.

**Strength(s) usually available**
U.S.—
1 gram (Rx) [*Carafate*; GENERIC].
Canada—
1 gram (Rx) [*Sulcrate*].

**Packaging and storage**
Store below 40 °C (104 °F), preferably between 15 and 30 °C (59 and 86 °F), in a tight container, unless otherwise specified by manufacturer.

**Auxiliary labeling**
• Continue medicine for full time of treatment.

Revised: 03/24/92
Interim revision: 08/17/94; 07/26/96

---

**SUFENTANIL**—See *Fentanyl and Derivatives (Systemic)*

---

## SULBACTAM-CONTAINING COMBINATIONS—

Ampicillin and Sulbactam (Systemic)—See *Penicillins and Beta-lactamase Inhibitors (Systemic)*

---

# SULCONAZOLE   Topical†

VA CLASSIFICATION (Primary): DE102
Note: For a listing of dosage forms and brand names by country availability, see *Dosage Forms* section(s). For a listing of brand names for the articles in this monograph, refer to the General Index.

---

†Not commercially available in Canada.

---

## Category

Antifungal (topical).

## Indications

Note: Bracketed information in the *Indications* section refers to uses that are not included in U.S. product labeling.

**Accepted**
Tinea corporis (treatment)
Tinea cruris (treatment) or
Tinea pedis (treatment)—Sulconazole is indicated in the topical treatment of tinea corporis (ringworm of the body), tinea cruris (ringworm of the groin; jock itch), and tinea pedis (ringworm of the foot; athlete's foot) caused by *Trichophyton rubrum*, *T. mentagrophytes*, *Epidermophyton floccosum*, and *Microsporum canis*.

Tinea versicolor (treatment)—Sulconazole is indicated in the topical treatment of tinea versicolor (pityriasis versicolor; ''sun fungus'') caused by *Malassezia furfur*.
[Candidiasis, cutaneous (treatment)]—Sulconazole is used in the treatment of cutaneous candidiasis caused by *Candida albicans*.

## Pharmacology/Pharmacokinetics

**Physicochemical characteristics**
Chemical group—Imidazole derivative.
Molecular weight—460.77.

**Mechanism of action/Effect**
Fungistatic; may be fungicidal, depending on sulconazole concentration and yeast growth phase. The exact mechanism of action of sulconazole is not known, but it appears to involve interference with the synthesis and/or function of the fungal cell membrane. Sulconazole also inhibits the synthesis and increases the autolytic degradation of cellular RNA and DNA.

**Other actions/effects**
Sulconazole also has some activity against certain gram positive bacteria, such as *Staphylococcus aureus*, *Staphylococcus epidermidis*, and *Streptococcus faecalis*.

### Absorption

Total percutaneous absorption is estimated to be 8.7 to 11.3% of the applied dose.

### Elimination

Renal—Approximately 6.7% of the applied dose of sulconazole is eliminated in the urine.

Fecal—Approximately 2% of the applied dose of sulconazole is eliminated in the feces.

## Precautions to Consider

### Cross-sensitivity and/or related problems

Persons sensitive to other imidazole derivatives such as miconazole and econazole may be sensitive to sulconazole also.

### Carcinogenicity

Studies to determine the carcinogenic potential of sulconazole have not been done.

### Mutagenicity

*In vitro* studies of sulconazole have shown no mutagenic activity.

### Pregnancy/Reproduction

Fertility—Studies have not been done.

Pregnancy—Adequate and well-controlled studies in humans have not been done.

Studies in rats given oral doses 125 times the adult human dose have shown that sulconazole is embryotoxic and prolongs gestation. However, teratogenicity was not observed in rats and rabbits receiving oral doses of 50 mg per kg of body weight (mg/kg) per day.

FDA Pregnancy Category C.

Labor—Studies in rats given oral doses 125 times the adult human dose have shown that sulconazole causes dystocia.

### Breast-feeding

It is not known whether sulconazole is distributed into breast milk.

### Pediatrics

Appropriate studies on the relationship of age to the effects of sulconazole have not been performed in the pediatric population. Safety and efficacy have not been established.

### Geriatrics

Appropriate studies on the relationship of age to the effects of sulconazole have not been performed in the geriatric population. However, no geriatrics-specific problems have been documented to date.

### Medical considerations/Contraindications

The medical considerations/contraindications included here have been selected on the basis of their potential clinical significance (reasons given in parentheses where appropriate)—not necessarily inclusive (» = major clinical significance).

*Risk-benefit should be considered when the following medical problem exists:*

Sensitivity to sulconazole or other ingredients in the topical formulations, or to other imidazoles, such as miconazole and econazole

## Side/Adverse Effects

### Those indicating need for medical attention

Incidence less frequent

*Burning, stinging, itching, or redness of skin not present before therapy*

## Patient Consultation

As an aid to patient consultation, refer to *Advice for the Patient, Sulconazole (Topical)*.

In providing consultation, consider emphasizing the following selected information (» = major clinical significance):

### Before using this medication

» Conditions affecting use, especially:

Hypersensitivity to sulconazole or other imidazole derivatives such as miconazole or econazole

### Proper use of this medication

Applying sufficient medication to cover affected and surrounding areas, and rubbing in gently

» Avoiding contact with the eyes

» Not applying occlusive dressing over this medication unless directed to do so by physician

» Using medication for the full time of treatment; fungal infections may require prolonged therapy

» Proper dosing

Missed dose: Applying as soon as possible; not applying if almost time for the next dose

» Proper storage

### Precautions while using this medication

Checking with physician if no improvement seen within 4 to 6 weeks

Observing hygienic measures to help cure infection and to help prevent reinfection

*For tinea cruris*

Avoiding underwear that is tight-fitting or made from synthetic materials; wearing loose-fitting cotton underwear instead

*For tinea pedis*

Carefully drying feet, especially between toes, after bathing

Avoiding socks made from wool or synthetic materials; wearing clean, cotton socks and changing them daily or more often if feet perspire excessively

Wearing well-ventilated shoes or sandals

*For tinea corporis*

Carefully drying body after bathing

Avoiding too much heat and humidity if possible

Wearing well-ventilated, loose-fitting clothing

### Side/adverse effects

Signs of potential side effects, especially hypersensitivity

## General Dosing Information

Use of topical antifungals may lead to skin sensitization, resulting in hypersensitivity reactions with subsequent topical use of the medication.

To reduce the possibility of recurrence, Candida infections, tinea corporis, tinea cruris, and tinea versicolor should be treated for at least three weeks; tinea pedis should be treated for at least four weeks.

## Topical Dosage Forms

Note: Bracketed uses in the *Dosage Forms* section refer to categories of use and/or indications that are not included in U.S. product labeling.

### SULCONAZOLE NITRATE TOPICAL CREAM

#### Usual adult dose

Tinea corporis or

Tinea cruris or

Tinea versicolor—

Topical, to the skin, one or two times a day for three weeks.

Tinea pedis—

Topical, to the skin, two times a day, morning and evening for four weeks.

[Candidiasis, cutaneous]—

Topical to the skin once a day for three weeks.

#### Usual pediatric dose

Safety and efficacy have not been established.

#### Strength(s) usually available

U.S.—

1% (Rx) [*Exelderm*].

Canada—

Not commercially available.

#### Packaging and storage

Store below 40 °C (104 °F), unless otherwise specified by manufacturer.

#### Auxiliary labeling

• For external use only.

• Continue medicine for full time of treatment.

### SULCONAZOLE NITRATE TOPICAL SOLUTION

#### Usual adult dose

Tinea corporis or

Tinea cruris or

Tinea versicolor—

See *Sulconazole Nitrate Topical Cream*.

#### Usual pediatric dose

See *Sulconazole Nitrate Topical Cream*.

#### Strength(s) usually available

U.S.—

1% (Rx) [*Exelderm*].

Canada—

Not commercially available.

#### Packaging and storage

Store below 40 °C (104 °F), unless otherwise specified by the manufacturer. Protect from light.

**Auxiliary labeling**
- For external use only.
- Continue medicine for full time of treatment.

Developed: 03/29/94

## SULFABENZAMIDE-CONTAINING COMBINATIONS—

Triple Sulfa (Vaginal)—See *Sulfonamides (Vaginal)*

## SULFACETAMIDE—See *Sulfonamides (Ophthalmic)*

## SULFACETAMIDE-CONTAINING COMBINATIONS—

Triple Sulfa (Vaginal)—See *Sulfonamides (Vaginal)*

## SULFADIAZINE—See *Sulfonamides (Systemic)*

## SULFADIAZINE-CONTAINING COMBINATIONS—

Sulfadiazine and Trimethoprim (Systemic)

---

# SULFADOXINE AND PYRIMETHAMINE    Systemic

VA CLASSIFICATION (Primary): AP101

Note: For a listing of dosage forms and brand names by country availability, see *Dosage Forms* section(s). For a listing of brand names for the articles in this monograph, refer to the General Index.

## Category
Antiprotozoal.

## Indications

Note: Bracketed information in the *Indications* section refers to uses that are not included in U.S. product labeling.

### Accepted

Malaria (prophylaxis)—Sulfadoxine and pyrimethamine combination is indicated as a secondary agent in the prophylaxis of chloroquine-resistant *Plasmodium falciparum* malaria. However, because of its potentially life-threatening toxicity, it is not recommended for weekly use in the prophylaxis of chloroquine-resistant *P. falciparum* malaria in travelers to areas where chloroquine-resistant malaria is endemic. It is indicated **only** in persons at high risk of chloroquine-resistant malaria in remote areas who are unable to take alternative medication.

Malaria (treatment)—Sulfadoxine and pyrimethamine combination is indicated in combination with quinine as a primary agent in the treatment of chloroquine-resistant *P. falciparum* malaria. It is also indicated in the presumptive treatment of chloroquine-resistant *P. falciparum* malaria for self-treatment of febrile illness when medical care is not immediately available (within 24 hours).

[Isosporiasis (prophylaxis)][1]—Sulfadoxine is used with pyrimethamine in the prophylaxis of isosporiasis caused by *Isospora belli* in patients with acquired immunodeficiency disease.

Some strains of *P. falciparum* have developed resistance to sulfadoxine and pyrimethamine combination.

[1]Not included in Canadian product labeling.

## Pharmacology/Pharmacokinetics

### Physicochemical characteristics
Molecular weight—
Sulfadoxine: 310.33.
Pyrimethamine: 248.71.

### Mechanism of action/Effect
Sulfadoxine—
Bacteriostatic; Structural analog of aminobenzoic acid (PABA); competitively inhibits a bacterial enzyme, dihydropteroate synthetase, which is responsible for incorporation of PABA into dihydrofolic acid. This blocks the synthesis of dihydrofolic acid and decreases the amount of metabolically active tetrahydrofolic acid, a cofactor for the synthesis of purines, thymidine, and DNA.
Susceptible bacteria are those that must synthesize folic acid. The action of sulfonamides is antagonized by PABA and its derivatives (e.g., procaine and tetracaine) and by the presence of pus or tissue breakdown products, which provide the necessary components for bacterial growth.
Pyrimethamine—
Binds to and reversibly inhibits the protozoal enzyme dihydrofolate reductase, selectively blocking conversion of dihydrofolic acid to its functional form, tetrahydrofolic acid. This depletes folate, an essential cofactor in the biosynthesis of nucleic acids, resulting in interference with protozoal nucleic acid and protein production. Protozoal dihydrofolate reductase is many times more tightly bound by pyrimethamine than is the corresponding mammalian enzyme.
Pyrimethamine exerts its effect in the folate biosynthesis at a step immediately subsequent to the one at which sulfonamides exert their effect. When pyrimethamine is administered concurrently with sulfonamides, synergism occurs, which is attributed to inhibition of tetrahydrofolate production at two sequential steps in its biosynthesis.
Pyrimethamine is active against asexual erythrocytic forms and, to a lesser degree, tissue forms of *P. falciparum* malaria. It does not destroy gametocytes, but arrests sporogony in the mosquito.

### Absorption
Well absorbed following oral administration.

### Distribution
Pyrimethamine—Widely distributed; mainly concentrated in red and white blood cells, kidneys, lungs, liver, and spleen. Crosses into the cerebrospinal fluid (CSF), with concentrations ranging from 13 to 26% of the corresponding serum concentrations.
Sulfadoxine and pyrimethamine both cross the placenta and are excreted in breast milk.

### Protein binding
Pyrimethamine—High (87%).
Sulfadoxine—High (>90%).

### Biotransformation
Pyrimethamine—Hepatic.

### Half-life
Elimination—
Sulfadoxine: Approximately 100 to 230 hours (mean, approximately 169 hours).
Pyrimethamine: Approximately 54 to 148 hours (mean, approximately 111 hours).

### Time to peak plasma concentration
Sulfadoxine—2.5 to 6 hours.
Pyrimethamine—Approximately 3 hours (range, 2 to 6 hours).

### Peak plasma concentration
Sulfadoxine—Approximately 50 to 75 mcg per mL, 2.5 to 6 hours following a single oral dose of 500 mg of sulfadoxine and 25 mg of pyrimethamine.
Pyrimethamine—Approximately 0.13 to 0.4 mcg per mL, 1.5 to 8 hours following a single oral dose of 500 mg of sulfadoxine and 25 mg of pyrimethamine.

### Elimination
Sulfadoxine—
Renal: Excreted primarily unchanged by the kidneys.
Pyrimethamine—
Renal: Primary route; 20 to 30% excreted unchanged in urine. Urinary excretion may persist for 30 days or longer.
In dialysis: The serum concentration of pyrimethamine was decreased by approximately 47% after peritoneal dialysis in one patient.

# Precautions to Consider

## Cross-sensitivity and/or related problems

For sulfadoxine—Patients allergic to one sulfonamide may be allergic to other sulfonamides also. Patients allergic to furosemide, thiazide diuretics, sulfonylureas, or carbonic anhydrase inhibitors may be allergic to sulfonamides also.

## Carcinogenicity/Tumorigenicity

For sulfadoxine—Long-term administration of sulfonamides in rats has been shown to result in thyroid malignancies.

For pyrimethamine—Pyrimethamine has not been shown to be carcinogenic in female mice or in male or female rats.

## Mutagenicity

For pyrimethamine—Pyrimethamine has been shown to be mutagenic in laboratory animals and in human bone marrow following 3 or 4 consecutive daily doses totaling 200 to 300 mg. However, pyrimethamine has not been shown to be mutagenic in the Ames test.

## Pregnancy/Reproduction

Fertility—Studies in rats given sulfadoxine and pyrimethamine combination in doses of 105 mg per kg of body weight (mg/kg) daily or pyrimethamine alone in doses of 15 mg/kg daily have shown that both regimens cause testicular changes.

The fertility of male rats and the ability of male or female rats to mate has not been shown to be adversely affected when sulfadoxine and pyrimethamine combination was given in doses of up to 210 mg/kg daily.

The pregnancy rate of female rats was significantly reduced when the rats were given doses of 31.5 mg/kg daily (approximately 30 times the weekly prophylactic dose) or higher, but was not adversely affected at doses of 10.5 mg/kg daily.

Pregnancy—Sulfonamides and pyrimethamine cross the placenta. Adequate and well-controlled studies in humans have not been done. Sulfadoxine and pyrimethamine combination may interfere with folic acid metabolism in the fetus and is generally not recommended for use during pregnancy. However, malaria in pregnant women may be more severe than in nonpregnant women and may result in maternal death. The risk of adverse pregnancy outcomes, including premature births, stillbirths, and abortion, may be increased. These risks should be weighed against the risks and benefits of sulfadoxine and pyrimethamine combination use during pregnancy. Women of child-bearing potential who travel to areas where chloroquine-resistant malaria is endemic should be warned not to become pregnant.

Studies in rats given weekly doses approximately 12 times the weekly prophylactic dose have shown that sulfadoxine and pyrimethamine combination is teratogenic. Studies in rats given sulfadoxine and pyrimethamine (20:1) have shown that the minimum oral teratogenic dose is approximately 18 mg of sulfadoxine and 0.9 mg of pyrimethamine per kg of body weight. However, studies in rabbits given doses as high as 400 mg of sulfadoxine and 20 mg of pyrimethamine per kg of body weight have not shown that sulfadoxine and pyrimethamine combination is teratogenic.

FDA Pregnancy Category C.

## Breast-feeding

Sulfadoxine and pyrimethamine are excreted in breast milk. Use is not recommended in nursing women since sulfonamides may cause kernicterus in nursing infants. In addition, pyrimethamine may interfere with folic acid metabolism in nursing infants, especially when given in large doses to nursing women.

## Pediatrics

Sulfadoxine and pyrimethamine combination is contraindicated in infants under 2 months of age since sulfonamides may cause kernicterus in neonates.

## Geriatrics

No information is available on the relationship of age to the effects of sulfadoxine and pyrimethamine combination in geriatric patients.

## Dental

Sulfadoxine and pyrimethamine combination may cause a change in or loss of taste; soreness, redness, swelling, burning, or stinging of the tongue; sore throat or difficulty in swallowing; and ulcers, sores, or white spots in the mouth.

The leukopenic and thrombocytopenic effects of sulfadoxine and pyrimethamine combination may result in an increased incidence of certain microbial infections, delayed healing, and gingival bleeding. If leukopenia or thrombocytopenia occurs, dental work should be deferred until blood counts have returned to normal. Patients should be instructed in proper oral hygiene, including caution in use of regular toothbrushes, dental floss, and toothpicks.

## Drug interactions and/or related problems

The following drug interactions and/or related problems have been selected on the basis of their potential clinical significance (possible mechanism in parentheses where appropriate)—not necessarily inclusive (» = major clinical significance):

Note: Combinations containing any of the following medications, depending on the amount present, may also interact with this medication.

Anticoagulants, coumarin- or indandione-derivative or
Anticonvulsants, hydantoin or
Antidiabetic agents, oral
   (these medications may be displaced from protein-binding sites and/or their metabolism may be inhibited by some sulfonamides, resulting in increased or prolonged effects and/or toxicity; dosage adjustments may be necessary during and after sulfonamide therapy)

» Bone marrow depressants (See *Appendix II* )
   (concurrent use of these medications with sulfadoxine and pyrimethamine combination may increase the leukopenic and/or thrombocytopenic effects; if concurrent use is required, close observation for myelotoxic effects should be considered, especially when sulfadoxine and pyrimethamine combination is used in high doses)

Folate antagonists, other (See *Appendix II* )
   (concurrent use of other folate antagonists with pyrimethamine or use of pyrimethamine between courses of other folate antagonists is not recommended because of the possibility of megaloblastic anemia)

» Hemolytics, other (See *Appendix II* )
   (concurrent use with sulfonamides may increase the potential for toxic side effects)

» Hepatotoxic medications, other (See *Appendix II* )
   (concurrent use with sulfonamides may result in an increased incidence of hepatotoxicity; patients, especially those on prolonged administration or those with a history of liver disease, should be carefully monitored)

Methotrexate or
Phenylbutazone or
Sulfinpyrazone
   (the effects of these medications may be potentiated during concurrent use with some sulfonamides because of displacement from plasma protein-binding sites)

## Medical considerations/Contraindications

The medical considerations/contraindications included here have been selected on the basis of their potential clinical significance (reasons given in parentheses where appropriate)—not necessarily inclusive (» = major clinical significance).

*Except under special circumstances, this medication should not be used when the following medical problem exists:*

» Allergy to sulfonamides, pyrimethamine, furosemide, thiazide diuretics, sulfonylureas, or carbonic anhydrase inhibitors

*Risk-benefit should be considered when the following medical problems exist:*

» Anemia or
» Bone marrow depression
   (pyrimethamine may cause folic acid deficiency, resulting in megaloblastic anemia; sulfonamides and pyrimethamine may cause blood dyscrasias, including agranulocytosis and thrombocytopenia)

Hepatic function impairment
   (sulfonamides and pyrimethamine are metabolized in the liver; may cause fulminant hepatic necrosis)

» Porphyria
   (sulfonamides may precipitate an acute attack of porphyria)

» Renal function impairment
   (pyrimethamine and sulfadoxine are eliminated primarily through the kidneys)

Seizure disorders
   (pyrimethamine may cause central nervous system [CNS] toxicity when used in high doses)

## Patient monitoring

The following may be especially important in patient monitoring (other tests may be warranted in some patients, depending on condition; » = major clinical significance):

» Complete blood counts (CBCs)
   (may be required prior to and monthly or less frequently during treatment to detect blood dyscrasias in patients on prolonged ther-

apy; therapy should be discontinued if a significant decrease in the count of any formed blood elements occurs)

Urinalyses
(may be required prior to and periodically during treatment to detect crystalluria and/or urinary calculi formation in patients on long-term or high-dose therapy and in patients with impaired renal function)

## Side/Adverse Effects

Note: **Fatalities have occurred, although rarely, due to severe reactions such as Stevens-Johnson syndrome, toxic epidermal necrolysis, fulminant hepatic necrosis, agranulocytosis, aplastic anemia, and other blood dyscrasias.** These toxicities were associated with multiple dosing regimens. Therapy should be discontinued at the first appearance of skin rash or if symptoms of folic acid deficiency occur.

The following side/adverse effects have been selected on the basis of their potential clinical significance (possible signs and symptoms in parentheses where appropriate)—not necessarily inclusive:

### Those indicating need for medical attention
Incidence more frequent
*Atrophic glossitis* (pain, burning, or inflammation of the tongue; change in or loss of taste)—due to folic acid deficiency with high doses; *blood dyscrasias, specifically agranulocytosis* (fever and sore throat); *megaloblastic anemia* (unusual tiredness or weakness); *or thrombocytopenia* (unusual bleeding or bruising); *hypersensitivity* (skin rash; fever); *photosensitivity* (increased sensitivity of skin to sunlight)
Incidence less frequent
*Hepatitis* (yellow eyes and skin); *Stevens-Johnson syndrome* (aching of joints and muscles; redness, blistering, peeling, or loosening of skin; unusual tiredness or weakness)
Incidence rare
*Crystalluria or hematuria;* (blood in urine; lower back pain; pain or burning while urinating); *goiter or thyroid function disturbance* (swelling of front part of neck)

### Those indicating need for medical attention only if they continue or are bothersome
Incidence more frequent
*CNS effects* (anxiety; drowsiness; fatigue; headache; nervousness); *gastrointestinal disturbances* (abdominal pain; diarrhea; nausea or vomiting)

## Overdose
For specific information on the agents used in the management of sulfadoxine and pyrimethamine overdose, see:
- *Barbiturates (Systemic)* monograph;
- *Benzodiazepines (Systemic)* monograph; and/or
- *Leucovorin (Systemic)* monograph.

For more information on the management of overdose or unintentional ingestion, **contact a Poison Control Center** (see *Poison Control Center Listing*).

**Clinical effects of overdose**
The following effects have been selected on the basis of their potential clinical significance (possible signs and symptoms in parentheses where appropriate)—not necessarily inclusive:

Acute—In order of occurrence:
*Gastrointestinal toxicity* (anorexia; severe vomiting); *central nervous system (CNS) toxicity* (ataxia; trembling; seizures); *blood dyscrasias, specifically leukopenia* (fever and sore throat); *megaloblastic anemia* (unusual tiredness or weakness); *or thrombocytopenia* (unusual bleeding or bruising)

**Treatment of overdose**
Recommended treatment includes:
To decrease absorption—
Gastric emptying by emesis or lavage.
Specific treatment—
Control of CNS stimulation, including seizures, by parenteral administration of benzodiazepines or short-acting barbiturates.
Administration of leucovorin, 5 to 15 mg a day intramuscularly for 3 days or longer, to counteract the effects of folic acid antagonism (e.g., reduced white blood cell counts) induced by the pyrimethamine component.
Adequate hydration to prevent renal damage.
Monitoring—
Monitoring of renal and hematopoietic status for at least 1 month following overdose.

Supportive care—
Mechanical assistance of respiration, if necessary. Patients in whom intentional overdose is confirmed or suspected should be referred for psychiatric consultation.

## Patient Consultation
As an aid to patient consultation, refer to *Advice for the Patient, Sulfadoxine and Pyrimethamine (Systemic)*.

In providing consultation, consider emphasizing the following selected information (» = major clinical significance):

### Before using this medication
» Conditions affecting use, especially:
Allergy to sulfonamides, furosemide, thiazide diuretics, sulfonylureas, carbonic anhydrase inhibitors, or pyrimethamine
Pregnancy—Pyrimethamine and sulfadoxine cross the placenta. Use not recommended because of possible interference with folic acid metabolism in fetus
Breast-feeding—Pyrimethamine and sulfadoxine are excreted in breast milk. Use not recommended because of possible kernicterus in the infant
Use in children—Use is not recommended in children under 2 months of age because of possible kernicterus
Dental—High doses may cause atrophic glossitis, leukopenia, or thrombocytopenia
Other medications, especially bone marrow depressants, other hemolytics, or other hepatotoxic medications
Other medical problems, especially anemia, bone marrow depression, porphyria, or renal function impairment

### Proper use of this medication
» Not giving to infants under 2 months of age; keeping medication out of reach of children
» Maintaining adequate fluid intake; taking with meals or a snack if gastric irritation occurs
» Proper storage
*For prevention of malaria*
Starting medication 1 to 2 weeks before entering malarious area to ascertain patient response and allow time to substitute another medication if reactions occur
» Continuing medication while staying in area and for 4 weeks after leaving area; checking with physician immediately if fever develops while traveling or within 2 months after departure from endemic area
» Importance of not missing doses and taking medication on a regular schedule
» Proper dosing
Missed dose: Taking as soon as possible; not taking if almost time for next dose; not doubling doses
*For treatment of malaria*
» Compliance with therapy
*For self-treatment of presumptive malaria*
» After taking this medication, continuing to take an alternative effective malaria medication once a week

### Precautions while using this medication
» Stopping medication immediately and reporting promptly to physician signs of skin rash, itching, redness, mouth or genital lesions, or sore throat
*Mosquito-control measures to reduce the chance of getting malaria*
Sleeping under mosquito netting
Wearing long-sleeved shirts or blouses and long trousers to protect arms and legs when mosquitoes are out
Applying mosquito repellant to uncovered areas of skin when mosquitoes are out
*For prevention of malaria*
» Regular visits to physician to check blood counts
Importance of taking leucovorin concurrently if anemia occurs
Using caution in use of regular toothbrushes, dental floss, and toothpicks; deferring dental work until blood counts have returned to normal; checking with physician or dentist concerning proper oral hygiene
» Possible photosensitivity reactions
*For self-treatment of presumptive malaria*
Checking with physician as soon as possible, especially if no improvement within 48 hours

### Side/adverse effects
Signs of potential side effects, especially atrophic glossitis; blood dyscrasias, specifically agranulocytosis, megaloblastic anemia, or thrombocytopenia; hypersensitivity; photosensitivity; hepatitis;

Stevens-Johnson syndrome; crystalluria or hematuria; and goiter or thyroid function disturbance

# General Dosing Information

Sulfadoxine and pyrimethamine combination may be administered alone for the presumptive treatment, or sequentially with quinine in the treatment of acute attacks, of documented falciparum malaria.

Fluid intake should be sufficient to maintain urine output of at least 1200 to 1500 mL per day in adults.

Sulfadoxine and pyrimethamine combination may cause gastric irritation, sometimes resulting in vomiting, when given in high doses. If this occurs, the medication may be taken with meals or a snack or the dosage may be reduced.

**Therapy with sulfadoxine and pyrimethamine combination should be discontinued if skin rash or symptoms of folic acid deficiency occur.** However, to prevent folic acid deficiency, leucovorin (folinic acid) may be administered to restore normal hematopoiesis. Leucovorin does not interfere with the antiprotozoal activity of the pyrimethamine component. In addition, since malarial parasites are unable to utilize preformed folic acid, the antimalarial effect of pyrimethamine should not be affected. In adults, 5 to 15 mg of leucovorin may be given orally, intramuscularly, or intravenously once a day for 3 days or as required. Alternatively, adults may be given 9 mg of leucovorin 2 or 3 times a week. Infants may be given 1 mg of leucovorin once a day.

Because of its potentially life-threatening toxicity, sulfadoxine and pyrimethamine combination is no longer recommended for weekly use as a prophylactic agent **except** in persons at high risk of chloroquine-resistant malaria, in remote areas, who are unable to take alternative medications. If this combination is used, prophylaxis should be started 1 week before the patient enters a malarious area and should be continued for 4 weeks after the patient leaves the area. Starting the medication before the patient enters the malarious area will help to determine the patient's tolerance to the medication and allow time to substitute other antimalarials if the patient develops allergies to the medication or experiences other adverse effects.

# Oral Dosage Forms

Note: Bracketed uses in the *Dosage Forms* section refer to categories of use and/or indications that are not included in U.S. product labeling.

## SULFADOXINE AND PYRIMETHAMINE TABLETS USP

**Usual adult and adolescent dose**
Malaria—
    Treatment: Chloroquine-resistant *P. falciparum* malaria—Oral, 3 tablets as a single dose on day three of quinine therapy.
    Presumptive treatment: Oral, 3 tablets as a single dose for self-treatment of febrile illness when medical care is not immediately available.
    Chemoprophylaxis: Oral, 1 tablet once every seven days; or 2 tablets once every fourteen days.
[Isosporiasis (prophylaxis)][1]—
    Oral, 1 tablet once every seven days.

**Usual pediatric dose**
Malaria—
    Treatment: Chloroquine-resistant *P. falciparum* malaria—
        Children up to 2 months of age—
            Use is contraindicated since sulfonamides may cause kernicterus in neonates.
        Children 2 months of age and over—
            Oral, 1.25 mg per kg of body weight of pyrimethamine in combination with 25 mg per kg of body weight of sulfadoxine as a single dose on day three of quinine therapy.
    Presumptive treatment, for self-treatment of febrile illness when medical care is not immediately available:
        Children up to 2 months of age—
            Use is contraindicated since sulfonamides may cause kernicterus in neonates.
        Children 2 months of age and over—
            Children 5 to 10 kg of body weight: Oral, 1/2 tablet as a single dose.
            Children 11 to 20 kg of body weight: Oral, 1 tablet as a single dose.
            Children 21 to 30 kg of body weight: Oral, 1 1/2 tablets as a single dose.
            Children 31 to 45 kg of body weight: Oral, 2 tablets as a single dose.
            Children greater than 45 kg of body weight: Oral, 3 tablets as a single dose.

Chemoprophylaxis:
    Infants up to 2 months of age—
        Use is contraindicated since sulfonamides may cause kernicterus in neonates.
    Infants and children 2 months to 4 years of age—
        Oral, 1/4 tablet once every seven days; or 1/2 tablet once every fourteen days.
    Children 4 to 8 years of age—
        Oral, 1/2 tablet once every seven days; or 1 tablet once every fourteen days.
    Children 9 to 14 years of age—
        Oral, 3/4 tablet once every seven days; or 1 1/2 tablets once every fourteen days.
    Children over 14 years of age—
        See *Usual adult and adolescent dose.*

**Strength(s) usually available**
U.S.—
    500 mg of sulfadoxine and 25 mg of pyrimethamine (Rx) [*Fansidar*].
Canada—
    500 mg of sulfadoxine and 25 mg of pyrimethamine (Rx) [*Fansidar*].

**Packaging and storage**
Store below 40 °C (104 °F), preferably between 15 and 30 °C (59 and 86 °F), unless otherwise specified by manufacturer. Store in a well-closed, light-resistant container.

**Auxiliary labeling**
• Take with a full glass of water.
• Avoid too much sun or use of sunlamp or tanning bed or booth.
• Continue medicine for full time of treatment (chemoprophylaxis).
• Keep out of reach of children.

**Note**
Explain potential danger of accidental overdose in children.

Consider dispensing in unit-dose packaging in child-resistant containers (''double-barrier'' packaging).

[1]Not included in Canadian product labeling.

Revised: 02/23/93

---

# SULFADOXINE-CONTAINING COMBINATIONS—
Sulfadoxine and Pyrimethamine (Systemic)

---

# SULFAMETHIZOLE—See *Sulfonamides (Systemic)*

---

# SULFAMETHOXAZOLE—See *Sulfonamides (Systemic)*

---

# SULFAMETHOXAZOLE-CONTAINING COMBINATIONS—
Sulfamethoxazole and Phenazopyridine (Systemic)—See *Sulfonamides and Phenazopyridine (Systemic)*
Sulfamethoxazole and Trimethoprim (Systemic)—See *Sulfonamides and Trimethoprim (Systemic)*

---

# SULFANILAMIDE—See *Sulfonamides (Vaginal)*

---

# SULFANILAMIDE-CONTAINING COMBINATIONS—
Sulfanilamide, Aminacrine, and Allantoin (Vaginal)—See *Sulfonamides (Vaginal)*

# SULFAPYRIDINE   Systemic

**VA CLASSIFICATION (Primary): DE890**

Note: For a listing of dosage forms and brand names by country availability, see *Dosage Forms* section(s). For a listing of brand names for the articles in this monograph, refer to the General Index.

## Category

Dermatitis herpetiformis suppressant.

## Indications

Note: Bracketed information in the *Indications* section refers to uses that are not included in U.S. product labeling.

**Accepted**

Dermatitis herpetiformis (treatment)—Sulfapyridine is indicated as a secondary agent in the treatment of dermatitis herpetiformis (Duhring's disease).

[Dermatosis, subcorneal pustular (treatment)][1]—Sulfapyridine is used as a secondary agent in the treatment of subcorneal pustular dermatosis (Sneddon-Wilkinson disease).

[Pemphigoid (treatment)][1]—Sulfapyridine is used as a secondary agent in the treatment of bullous pemphigoid.

[Pyoderma gangrenosum (treatment)][1]—Sulfapyridine is used as secondary agent in the treatment of pyoderma gangrenosum.

---

[1]Not included in Canadian product labeling.

## Pharmacology/Pharmacokinetics

**Physicochemical characteristics**

Molecular weight—249.29.

**Mechanism of action/Effect**

Dermatitis herpetiformis—Unknown.

**Absorption**

Absorption from gastrointestinal tract is slow and incomplete (approximately 60–80%).

**Distribution**

Sulfonamides readily cross the placenta; sulfapyridine also crosses into the cerebrospinal fluid.

$Vol_D$ =0.4 to 1.2 L per kg.

**Protein binding**

Variable (approximately 50%); acetylated metabolites are more highly protein bound than the free drug. Sulfonamides compete with bilirubin for binding to albumin. Kernicterus may develop in premature infants or neonates. Binding is decreased in patients with severely impaired renal function.

**Biotransformation**

Hepatic; sulfapyridine is metabolized by acetylation and hydroxylation, followed by conjugation with glucuronic acid. Sulfapyridine is metabolized to inactive metabolites, which retain the toxicity of the parent compound. Metabolism is increased with renal function impairment and decreased with hepatic failure.

**Half-life**

6 to 14 hours.

**Time to peak concentration**

4 to 6 hours following administration of a single dose.

**Duration of action**

Intermediate-acting sulfonamide.

**Elimination**

Sulfapyridine and metabolites excreted primarily in urine; up to 80% of sulfapyridine may be reabsorbed by the renal tubules.

## Precautions to Consider

**Cross-sensitivity and/or related problems**

Patients allergic to other sulfonamides may be allergic to this medication also.

Patients allergic to furosemide, thiazide diuretics, sulfonylureas, or carbonic anhydrase inhibitors may be allergic to this medication also.

**Carcinogenicity/Tumorigenicity**

Long-term administration of sulfonamides in rats has been shown to result in thyroid malignancies. However, rats appear to be more susceptible to the goitrogenic effects of sulfonamides than do other animal species.

**Pregnancy/Reproduction**

Fertility—Sulfapyridine has been shown to cause oligospermia and infertility in men.

Pregnancy—Sulfapyridine crosses the placenta. Adequate and well-controlled studies in humans have not been done. However, sulfonamides may cause kernicterus in the neonate. Therefore, use is not recommended during pregnancy.

Studies in rats and mice, given 7 to 25 times the human therapeutic dose orally, have shown that certain sulfonamides cause a significant increase in the incidence of cleft palate and other bony abnormalities.

**Breast-feeding**

Sulfapyridine is excreted in breast milk in concentrations that are 30 to 60% of those in the maternal serum. Use is not recommended in nursing women since sulfonamides may cause kernicterus in nursing infants.

Sulfonamides may cause hemolytic anemia in glucose-6-phosphate dehydrogenase (G6PD)–deficient neonates.

**Pediatrics**

Use is not recommended in pediatric patients since they do not usually develop dermatitis herpetiformis.

**Geriatrics**

No information is available on the relationship of age to the effects of sulfapyridine in geriatric patients.

**Dental**

The leukopenic and thrombocytopenic effects of sulfapyridine may result in an increased incidence of certain microbial infections, delayed healing, and gingival bleeding. If leukopenia or thrombocytopenia occurs, dental work should be deferred until blood counts have returned to normal. Patients should be instructed in proper oral hygiene, including caution in use of regular toothbrushes, dental floss, and toothpicks.

**Drug interactions and/or related problems**

The following drug interactions and/or related problems have been selected on the basis of their potential clinical significance (possible mechanism in parentheses where appropriate)—not necessarily inclusive (» = major clinical significance):

Note: Combinations containing any of the following medications, depending on the amount present, may also interact with this medication.

» Anticoagulants, coumarin- or indandione-derivative or
» Anticonvulsants, hydantoin or
» Antidiabetic agents, oral
    (may be displaced from protein-binding sites and/or metabolism may be inhibited by sulfonamides, resulting in increased or prolonged effects and/or toxicity; dosage adjustments may be necessary during and after sulfonamide therapy)

    Bone marrow depressants (See *Appendix II* )
    (concurrent use of sulfapyridine with bone marrow depressants may increase the leukopenic and/or thrombocytopenic effects of these medications; if concurrent use is required, close observation for myelotoxic effects should be considered)

» Hemolytics, other (See *Appendix II* )
    (concurrent use with sulfapyridine may increase the potential for toxic side effects)

» Hepatotoxic medications, other (See *Appendix II* )
    (concurrent use with sulfonamides may result in an increased incidence of hepatotoxicity; patients, especially those on prolonged administration or those with a history of liver disease, should be carefully monitored)

» Methotrexate or
    Phenylbutazone or
    Sulfinpyrazone
    (the effects of these medications may be potentiated during concurrent use with sulfonamides because of displacement from plasma protein-binding sites; phenylbutazone has also been reported to potentiate the effects of sulfonamides)

**Laboratory value alterations**

The following have been selected on the basis of their potential clinical significance (possible effect in parentheses where appropriate)—not necessarily inclusive (» = major clinical significance):

With diagnostic test results
    Bentiromide
        (administration of sulfonamides during a bentiromide test period will invalidate test results since sulfonamides are also metabolized to arylamines and will thus increase the percent of PABA recov-

ered; discontinuation of sulfonamides at least 3 days prior to the administration of bentiromide is recommended)

**Medical considerations/Contraindications**
The medical considerations/contraindications included here have been selected on the basis of their potential clinical significance (reasons given in parentheses where appropriate)—not necessarily inclusive (» = major clinical significance).

***Risk-benefit should be considered when the following medical problems exist:***

Allergy to sulfapyridine, other sulfonamides, furosemide, thiazide diuretics, sulfonylureas, or carbonic anhydrase inhibitors

» Blood dyscrasias
(sulfapyridine may cause agranulocytosis, aplastic anemia, or other blood dyscrasias)

» Glucose-6-phosphate dehydrogenase (G6PD) deficiency
(sulfapyridine may cause hemolytic anemia in G6PD-deficient patients)

» Hepatic function impairment
(sulfonamides are metabolized in the liver and may cause hepatitis)

» Porphyria
(sulfonamides may precipitate an acute attack of porphyria)

» Renal function impairment
(sulfapyridine is excreted primarily through the kidneys)

**Patient monitoring**
The following may be especially important in patient monitoring (other tests may be warranted in some patients, depending on condition; » = major clinical significance):

» Complete blood counts (CBCs)
(may be required prior to and monthly during treatment to detect blood dyscrasias in patients on prolonged therapy; therapy should be discontinued if a significant decrease in the count of any formed blood elements occurs)

» Glucose-6-phosphate dehydrogenase (G6PD) determinations
(are recommended prior to treatment in Caucasians of Mediterranean origin, Orientals, and blacks; if a deficiency is found, sulfapyridine should be given with caution since hemolytic effects may be exacerbated in these patients; dosage adjustments and/or discontinuation of the medication may be required)

Urinalyses
(may be required prior to and periodically during treatment to detect crystalluria and/or urinary calculi formation in patients on long-term or high-dose therapy and in patients with impaired renal function)

# Side/Adverse Effects

Note: Fatalities have occurred, although rarely, due to severe reactions such as Stevens-Johnson syndrome, toxic epidermal necrolysis, fulminant hepatic necrosis, agranulocytosis, aplastic anemia, other blood dyscrasias, and hypersensitivity reactions. Therapy should be discontinued at the first appearance of skin rash or any serious side/adverse effects.

Sulfapyridine has been shown to cause oligospermia and infertility in men.

The following side/adverse effects have been selected on the basis of their potential clinical significance (possible signs and symptoms in parentheses where appropriate)—not necessarily inclusive:

**Those indicating need for medical attention**
Incidence more frequent
***Headache, continuing; hypersensitivity*** (itching; skin rash; fever); ***photosensitivity*** (increased sensitivity of skin to sunlight)

Incidence less frequent
***Blood dyscrasias*** (pale skin; sore throat; unusual bleeding or bruising; unusual tiredness or weakness); ***hepatitis*** (yellow eyes or skin); ***Lyell's syndrome or Stevens-Johnson syndrome*** (aching of joints and muscles; difficulty in swallowing; redness, blistering, peeling, or loosening of skin; unusual tiredness or weakness)

Incidence rare
***Crystalluria or hematuria*** (blood in urine; lower back pain; pain or burning while urinating); ***goiter or thyroid function disturbance*** (swelling of front part of neck)

**Those indicating need for medical attention only if they continue or are bothersome**
Incidence more frequent
***Gastrointestinal disturbances*** (diarrhea; anorexia; nausea or vomiting)

# Patient Consultation

As an aid to patient consultation, refer to *Advice for the Patient, Sulfapyridine (Systemic)*.

In providing consultation, consider emphasizing the following selected information (» = major clinical significance):

**Before using this medication**
» Conditions affecting use, especially:
Allergies to other sulfonamides, furosemide, thiazide diuretics, sulfonylureas, or carbonic anhydrase inhibitors
Pregnancy—Crosses the placenta; not recommended during pregnancy since sulfonamides may cause kernicterus in the neonate
Breast-feeding—Excreted in breast milk; not recommended in nursing women since sulfonamides may cause kernicterus in nursing infants
Use in children—Not recommended since pediatric patients do not usually develop dermatitis herpetiformis
Other medications, especially anticoagulants (coumarin- or indandione-derivative), anticonvulsants (hydantoin), antidiabetic agents (oral), hemolytics, hepatotoxic medications, and methotrexate
Other medical problems, especially blood dyscrasias, G6PD deficiency, hepatic function impairment, porphyria, and renal function impairment

**Proper use of this medication**
» Maintaining adequate fluid intake to help prevent crystalluria and urinary calculi formation
*For dermatitis herpetiformis*
Possible need for a strict, gluten-free diet in the treatment of dermatitis herpetiformis
Using for 6 to 12 months may be required before reducing the dose or discontinuing medication

» Proper dosing
Missed dose: Taking as soon as possible if symptoms return or worsen; not taking if symptoms do not return or worsen

» Proper storage

**Precautions while using this medication**
» Regular visits to physician to check blood counts in patients on long-term therapy
Checking with physician if no improvement within a few days
Using caution in use of regular toothbrushes, dental floss, and toothpicks; deferring dental work until blood counts have returned to normal; checking with doctor or dentist concerning proper oral hygiene

» Possible photosensitivity reactions; using sunscreen lotion or avoiding unprotected exposure to sun or use of sunlamp
Possible interference with bentiromide diagnostic test for pancreatic function

**Side/adverse effects**
Signs of potential side effects, especially blood dyscrasias, crystalluria or hematuria, goiter or thyroid function disturbance, headache (continuing), hepatitis, hypersensitivity, Lyell's syndrome or Stevens-Johnson syndrome, or photosensitivity

# General Dosing Information

Fluid intake should be sufficient to maintain a urine output of at least 1200 to 1500 mL per day in adults, to prevent crystalluria and urinary calculi formation.

If dermatitis herpetiformis recurs, increased dosage may be required. The maintenance dose should not exceed the minimum effective dose.

In the treatment of dermatitis herpetiformis, use of a strict, gluten-free diet for 6 to 12 months may allow a reduction in dose or discontinuation of sulfapyridine.

# Oral Dosage Forms

Note: Bracketed uses in the *Dosage Forms* section refer to categories of use and/or indications that are not included in U.S. product labeling.

**SULFAPYRIDINE TABLETS USP**

**Usual adult and adolescent dose**
Dermatitis herpetiformis—
Oral, initially 250 mg to 1 gram four times a day until improvement occurs. Daily dosage should then be reduced by 250- to 500-mg decrements every three days until a symptom-free maintenance dose is achieved.

Note: Sulfapyridine may also be given two times a day in evenly divided doses.

[Dermatosis, subcorneal pustular][1]—
Oral, 500 mg two times a day to 750 mg four times a day.

[Pemphigoid][1]—
    Oral, 1 gram three times a day.

**Usual adult prescribing limits**
Dermatitis herpetiformis—Up to 6 grams daily.

**Usual pediatric dose**
Use is not recommended in pediatric patients since they do not usually develop dermatitis herpetiformis.

**Strength(s) usually available**
U.S.—
    500 mg (Rx) [GENERIC].
Canada—
    500 mg (Rx) [*Dagenan;* GENERIC].

**Packaging and storage**
Store below 40 °C (104 °F), preferably between 15 and 30 °C (59 and 86 °F), unless otherwise specified by manufacturer. Store in a well-closed, light-resistant container.

**Auxiliary labeling**
• Take with a full glass of water.
• Avoid too much sun or use of sunlamp.

---

[1]Not included in Canadian product labeling.

---

Revised: 02/01/93

---

# SULFASALAZINE   Systemic

BAN: Sulphasalazine.

JAN: Salazosulfapyridine.

VA CLASSIFICATION (Primary): GA900

Another commonly used name is salicylazosulfapyridine.

Note: For a listing of dosage forms and brand names by country availability, see *Dosage Forms* section(s). For a listing of brand names for the articles in this monograph, refer to the General Index.

## Category

Bowel disease (inflammatory) suppressant; antirheumatic (disease-modifying).

## Indications

Note: Bracketed information in the *Indications* section refers to uses that are not included in U.S. product labeling.

**Accepted**

Bowel disease, inflammatory (prophylaxis and treatment)—Sulfasalazine is indicated to treat and to maintain remission of inflammatory bowel disease (e.g., ulcerative colitis or Crohn's disease affecting the colon). It is indicated in the treatment of mild to moderate ulcerative colitis and as adjunctive treatment of severe ulcerative colitis.

[Ankylosing spondylitis (treatment)][1] or
[Arthritis, rheumatoid (treatment)]—Sulfasalazine is used in the treatment of ankylosing spondylitis and rheumatoid arthritis.

---

[1]Not included in Canadian product labeling.

## Pharmacology/Pharmacokinetics

**Physicochemical characteristics**
Molecular weight—398.39.

**Mechanism of action/Effect**

Bowel disease (inflammatory) suppressant—Uncertain; may be related to sulfasalazine's immunosuppressant effects, which have been observed in animals, its affinity for connective tissue, and/or its relatively high concentrations in serous fluids, the liver, and intestinal wall. Sulfasalazine is considered a vehicle for carrying its principal metabolites to the colon. Unabsorbed sulfasalazine is cleaved in the colon by intestinal bacteria to form sulfapyridine and mesalamine (5-aminosalicylic acid; 5-ASA), both of which may act locally within the gut. Mesalamine, which is different from aminosalicylates used to treat tuberculosis, is thought to be the major active moiety. Mucosal production of arachidonic acid metabolites, both through the cyclooxygenase and the lipoxygenase pathways, is increased in patients with inflammatory bowel disease. Mesalamine appears to diminish inflammation by inhibiting cyclooxygenase and lipoxygenase, thereby decreasing the production of prostaglandins, and leukotrienes and hydroxyeicosatetraenoic acids (HETEs), respectively. It is also believed that mesalamine acts as a scavenger of oxygen-derived free radicals, which are produced in greater numbers in patients with inflammatory bowel disease.

Antirheumatic (disease-modifying)—Uncertain; sulfapyridine moiety may suppress the activity of natural killer cells and impair lymphocyte transformation.

**Absorption**

Sulfasalazine—Poorly absorbed; approximately 20% of ingested sulfasalazine dose reaches the systemic circulation. The remaining ingested dose is split by colonic bacteria into its components, sulfapyridine and mesalamine.

Sulfapyridine—Most of the sulfapyridine metabolized from sulfasalazine (60–80%) is absorbed in the colon following oral administration.

Mesalamine (5-ASA)—Approximately 25% of the mesalamine metabolized from sulfasalazine is absorbed in the colon following oral administration.

**Distribution**

Distributed to serum, connective tissue, serous fluids, liver, and intestinal wall. The apparent volume of distribution (Vol$_D$) of sulfasalazine in 8 healthy volunteers was 64 L. The Vol$_D$ of sulfapyridine was found to be 0.4 to 1.2 L per kg.

**Protein binding**

Sulfasalazine—Very high (Approximately 99%).
Sulfapyridine—Moderate (Approximately 50%).
Mesalamine (5-ASA)—Moderate (Approximately 43%).

**Biotransformation**

Sulfasalazine (unabsorbed)—Cleaved in the colon by intestinal bacteria to form sulfapyridine and mesalamine.

Sulfapyridine (absorbed)—Acetylated and hydroxylated in the liver, followed by conjugation with glucuronic acid.

Mesalamine (5-ASA) (absorbed)—Acetylated in the intestinal mucosal wall and the liver.

**Half-life**

Sulfasalazine—5 to 10 hours.
Sulfapyridine—6 to 14 hours, depending on acetylator status.
Mesalamine (5-ASA)—0.6 to 1.4 hours.

**Time to peak serum concentration**

Sulfasalazine oral suspension—
    Sulfasalazine: Approximately 1.5 to 6 hours.
    Sulfapyridine: Approximately 9 to 24 hours.
Sulfasalazine tablets—
    Sulfasalazine: Approximately 1.5 to 6 hours.
    Sulfapyridine: Approximately 6 to 24 hours.
Sulfasalazine enteric-coated tablets—
    Sulfasalazine: Approximately 3 to 12 hours.
    Sulfapyridine: Approximately 12 to 24 hours.

**Mean peak serum concentration**

Sulfasalazine oral suspension—
    Sulfasalazine: Approximately 20 mcg per mL 3 hours following a single oral 2-gram dose.
    Sulfapyridine: Approximately 19 mcg per mL 12 hours following a single oral 2-gram dose.
    Mesalamine (5-ASA): Approximately 4 mcg per mL following a single oral 2-gram dose.
Sulfasalazine tablets—
    Sulfasalazine: Approximately 14 mcg per mL 3 hours following a single oral 2-gram dose.
    Sulfapyridine: Approximately 21 mcg per mL 12 hours following a single oral 2-gram dose.
    Mesalamine (5-ASA): Approximately 4 mcg per mL following a single oral 2-gram dose.
Sulfasalazine enteric-coated tablets—
    Sulfasalazine: Approximately 6 mcg per mL 6 hours following a single oral 2-gram dose.
    Sulfapyridine: Approximately 13 mcg per mL 12 hours following a single oral 2-gram dose.
    Mesalamine (5-ASA): Approximately 4 mcg per mL following a single oral 2-gram dose.

**Elimination**

Fecal—Trace amounts of sulfasalazine, approximately 5% of sulfapyridine, and approximately 67% of mesalamine are found in feces.

Renal—Approximately 75 to 91% of sulfasalazine and sulfapyridine metabolites excreted in urine within 3 days, depending on the dosage form used. Mesalamine is excreted in urine mostly in acetylated form.

# Precautions to Consider

## Cross-sensitivity and/or related problems
Patients allergic to one sulfonamide may be allergic to other sulfonamides also.

Patients allergic to salicylates, furosemide, thiazide diuretics, sulfonylureas, or carbonic anhydrase inhibitors may be allergic to this medication also.

## Carcinogenicity/Tumorigenicity
Long-term studies have not been done to evaluate the carcinogenic potential of sulfasalazine. However, long-term administration of sulfonamides to rats has been shown to result in thyroid malignancies. In addition, rats appear to be especially susceptible to the goitrogenic effects of sulfonamides.

## Mutagenicity
No evidence of mutagenicity was observed in *in vitro* tests for point mutations and chromosome aberrations.

## Pregnancy/Reproduction
Fertility—Studies in rats and rabbits given doses of up to 6 times the human dose have not shown that sulfasalazine impairs female fertility. However, these studies have shown that sulfasalazine does impair male fertility. In addition, oligospermia and infertility, reported to be reversible upon discontinuation of sulfasalazine, have been reported in men.

Pregnancy—Sulfasalazine and sulfapyridine cross the placenta. Adequate and well-controlled studies in humans have not been done. However, a national survey of 186 women with inflammatory bowel disease (IBD) who took sulfasalazine, alone or concurrently with corticosteroids, showed an incidence of adverse effects in the fetus comparable to that in 245 untreated IBD pregnancies. Another study of 1445 pregnancies in which sulfonamides, including sulfasalazine, were taken did not show that sulfasalazine causes fetal malformations.

Appropriate studies have not been performed on the effect of sulfasalazine on growth, development, and functional maturation of children whose mothers received sulfasalazine during pregnancy.

Studies in rats and rabbits given doses of up to 6 times the human dose have not shown that sulfasalazine causes adverse effects in the fetus.

FDA Pregnancy Category B.

## Breast-feeding
Uncleaved sulfasalazine is distributed into breast milk in small amounts. Sulfapyridine is distributed into breast milk in concentrations that are 30 to 60% of those in the maternal serum. Although sulfonamides may displace bilirubin from protein-binding sites in the fetal plasma, hyperbilirubinemia has occurred rarely.

Sulfonamides may cause hemolytic anemia in glucose-6-phosphate dehydrogenase (G6PD)–deficient neonates.

## Pediatrics
Use is contraindicated in infants and children up to 2 years of age because sulfonamides may cause kernicterus.

## Geriatrics
Appropriate studies performed to date have not demonstrated geriatrics-specific problems that would limit the usefulness of sulfasalazine in the elderly.

## Pharmacogenetics
Mean serum concentrations of sulfapyridine and its metabolites may be significantly increased in patients who are slow acetylators. Eskimo, Oriental, and American Indian populations have the lowest prevalence of slow acetylators, while Egyptian, Israeli, Scandinavian, other Caucasian, and black populations have the highest prevalence of slow acetylators.

## Dental
The leukopenic and thrombocytopenic effects of sulfasalazine may result in an increased incidence of certain microbial infections, delayed healing, and gingival bleeding. If leukopenia or thrombocytopenia occurs, dental work should be deferred until blood counts have returned to normal. Patients should be instructed in proper oral hygiene, including caution in use of regular toothbrushes, dental floss, and toothpicks.

## Drug interactions and/or related problems
The following drug interactions and/or related problems have been selected on the basis of their potential clinical significance (possible mechanism in parentheses where appropriate)—not necessarily inclusive (» = major clinical significance):

Note: Combinations containing any of the following medications, depending on the amount present, may also interact with this medication.

» Anticoagulants, coumarin- or indandione-derivative or
» Anticonvulsants, hydantoin or
» Antidiabetic agents, oral
    (may be displaced from protein binding sites and/or metabolism may be inhibited by sulfonamides, resulting in increased or prolonged effects and/or toxicity; dosage adjustments may be necessary during and after sulfonamide therapy)

    Bone marrow depressants (See *Appendix II* )
    (concurrent use of sulfasalazine with bone marrow depressants may increase the leukopenic and/or thrombocytopenic effects; if concurrent use is required, close observation for myelotoxic effects should be considered)

    Digitalis glycosides or
    Folic acid
    (sulfasalazine may inhibit absorption and lower the serum concentrations of these medications; folic acid requirements may be increased in patients receiving sulfasalazine; patients taking digitalis glycosides should be monitored closely for evidence of altered digitalis effect)

» Hemolytics, other (See *Appendix II* )
    (concurrent use with sulfasalazine may increase the potential for toxic side effects)

» Hepatotoxic medications, other (See *Appendix II* )
    (concurrent use with sulfonamides may result in an increased incidence of hepatotoxicity; patients, especially those on prolonged administration or those with a history of liver disease, should be carefully monitored)

» Methotrexate or
    Phenylbutazone or
    Sulfinpyrazone
    (the effects of these medications may be potentiated during concurrent use with sulfonamides because of displacement from plasma protein binding sites; phenylbutazone and sulfinpyrazone have also been reported to potentiate the effects of sulfonamides)

## Laboratory value alterations
The following have been selected on the basis of their potential clinical significance (possible effect in parentheses where appropriate)—not necessarily inclusive (» = major clinical significance):

With diagnostic test results
    Bentiromide
    (administration of sulfonamides during a bentiromide test period will invalidate test results because sulfonamides are also metabolized to arylamines and will thus increase the percent of *p*-aminobenzoic acid (PABA) recovered; discontinuation of sulfonamides at least 3 days prior to the administration of bentiromide is recommended)

## Medical considerations/Contraindications
The medical considerations/contraindications included here have been selected on the basis of their potential clinical significance (reasons given in parentheses where appropriate)—not necessarily inclusive (» = major clinical significance):

*Except under special circumstances, this medication should not be used when the following medical problem exists:*

» Previous allergic reaction to sulfasalazine, sulfonamides, salicylates, furosemide, thiazide diuretics, sulfonylureas, or carbonic anhydrase inhibitors

*Risk-benefit should be considered when the following medical problems exist:*

» Blood dyscrasias
    (sulfasalazine may cause agranulocytosis, aplastic anemia, or other blood dyscrasias)

» Glucose-6-phosphate dehydrogenase (G6PD) deficiency
    (sulfasalazine may cause hemolytic anemia in G6PD-deficient patients)

» Hepatic function impairment
    (sulfonamides are metabolized in the liver and may cause hepatitis)

» Porphyria
    (sulfonamides may precipitate an acute attack of porphyria)

» Renal function impairment
    (the metabolite, sulfapyridine, is excreted primarily through the kidneys)

## Patient monitoring

The following may be especially important in patient monitoring (other tests may be warranted in some patients, depending on condition; » = major clinical significance):

» Complete blood counts (CBCs)
(recommended prior to, and every 2 to 3 weeks for the first 2 to 3 months of treatment, then every 3 to 6 months during treatment to detect blood dyscrasias in patients on prolonged therapy; therapy should be discontinued if a significant decrease in the count of any formed blood elements occurs)

Proctoscopy and
Sigmoidoscopy
(may be required periodically during treatment to determine patient response and dosage adjustments)

Urinalyses
(may be required prior to and periodically during treatment in patients with impaired renal function)

## Side/Adverse Effects

Note: Deaths have been reported from hypersensitivity reactions, agranulocytosis, aplastic anemia, other blood dyscrasias, renal and hepatic damage, irreversible neuromuscular and central nervous system (CNS) changes, and fibrosing alveolitis in patients taking sulfasalazine. If toxic or hypersensitivity reactions occur, sulfasalazine should be discontinued immediately.

Oligospermia and infertility, reported to be reversible upon discontinuation of sulfasalazine, have been reported in males taking this medication.

Daily doses of 4 grams or more and total sulfapyridine serum concentrations > 50 mcg per mL may be associated with an increased incidence of side/adverse effects.

The following side/adverse effects have been selected on the basis of their potential clinical significance (possible signs and symptoms in parentheses where appropriate)—not necessarily inclusive:

### Those indicating need for medical attention
Incidence more frequent
*Headache, continuing; hypersensitivity reaction* (aching of joints; fever; itching; skin rash); *photosensitivity* (increased sensitivity of skin to sunlight)

Incidence less frequent or rare
*Blood dyscrasias, specifically agranulocytosis or neutropenia* (fever and sore throat); *Heinz body or hemolytic anemia* (back, leg, or stomach pains; loss of appetite; pale skin; unusual tiredness or weakness; fever); *or thrombocytopenia* (unusual bleeding or bruising); *cyanosis* (bluish fingernails, lips, or skin); *exacerbation of ulcerative colitis* (bloody diarrhea; fever; rash); *hepatitis* (yellow eyes or skin); *interstitial pneumonitis* (cough; difficult breathing; fever); *Stevens-Johnson syndrome* (aching of joints and muscles; redness, blistering, peeling, or loosening of skin; unusual tiredness or weakness); *systemic lupus erythematosus (SLE)–like syndrome* (blisters on skin; chest pain; general feeling of discomfort or illness; skin rash, hives, and/or itching); *toxic epidermal necrolysis* (difficulty in swallowing; redness, blistering, peeling, or loosening of skin)

### Those indicating need for medical attention only if they continue or are bothersome
Incidence more frequent
*Gastrointestinal disturbances* (abdominal or stomach pain or upset; diarrhea; loss of appetite; nausea or vomiting)

### Those not indicating need for medical attention
Incidence more frequent
*Orange-yellow discoloration of urine or skin*

## Overdose

For specific information on the agents used in the management of sulfasalazine overdose, see *Ipecac (Oral-Local)* monograph.

For more information on the management of overdose or unintentional ingestion, **contact a Poison Control Center** (see *Poison Control Center Listing* ).

The severity of sulfasalazine toxicity is directly related to the total serum sulfapyridine concentration. Daily doses of 4 grams or more and total sulfapyridine serum concentrations > 50 mcg per mL may be associated with an increased incidence of side/adverse effects.

### Clinical effects of overdose
The following effects have been selected on the basis of their potential clinical significance (possible signs and symptoms in parentheses where appropriate)—not necessarily inclusive:

*Anuria, crystalluria, or hematuria* (blood in urine; lack of urination; lower back pain; pain or burning while urinating); *drowsiness; gastrointestinal disturbances* (abdominal or stomach pain or upset; diarrhea; loss of appetite; nausea or vomiting); *seizures*

### Treatment of overdose
To decrease absorption—the stomach may be emptied by inducing emesis with ipecac syrup (taking care to guard against aspiration) or by gastric lavage.

To enhance elimination—The urine may be alkalinized and, if kidney function is normal, fluids forced. If anuria is present, fluids and salt should be restricted. Catheterization of the ureters may be indicated when there is complete renal blockage by crystals. The low molecular weight of sulfasalazine and its metabolites may facilitate removal by dialysis.

Monitoring—Serum sulfapyridine concentrations may be monitored so that the progress of recovery can be followed.

Supportive care—Patients in whom intentional overdose is confirmed or suspected should be referred for psychiatric consultation.

## Patient Consultation

As an aid to patient consultation, refer to *Advice for the Patient, Sulfasalazine (Systemic)*.

In providing consultation, consider emphasizing the following selected information (» = major clinical significance):

### Before using this medication
» Conditions affecting use, especially:
Allergies to sulfasalazine, sulfonamides, salicylates, furosemide, thiazide diuretics, sulfonylureas, carbonic anhydrase inhibitors
Pregnancy—Sulfasalazine and sulfapyridine cross the placenta
Breast-feeding—Sulfasalazine and sulfapyridine are distributed into breast milk
Use in children—Use is contraindicated in infants and children up to 2 years of age because sulfonamides may cause kernicterus
Other medications, especially coumarin- or indandione-derivative anticoagulants, hemolytics, hepatotoxic medications, hydantoin anticonvulsants, methotrexate, and oral antidiabetic agents
Other medical problems, especially blood dyscrasias, G6PD deficiency, hepatic function impairment, porphyria, and renal function impairment

### Proper use of this medication
» Not giving to infants up to 2 years of age; sulfasalazine may cause kernicterus
Taking after meals or with food to lessen gastrointestinal irritation
» Maintaining adequate fluid intake
Proper administration technique for oral suspension and enteric-coated tablets
» Compliance with full course of therapy
» Proper dosing
Missed dose: Taking as soon as possible; not taking if almost time for next dose; not doubling doses
» Proper storage

### Precautions while using this medication
» Regular visits to physician to check blood counts in patients on long-term therapy
Checking with physician if no improvement within 1 or 2 months
Using caution in use of regular toothbrushes, dental floss, and toothpicks; deferring dental work until blood counts have returned to normal; checking with physician or dentist concerning proper oral hygiene
» Possible photosensitivity reactions
» Caution if dizziness occurs
Possible interference with bentiromide diagnostic test for pancreatic function

### Side/adverse effects
Signs of potential side effects, especially headache (continuing), hypersensitivity reaction, photosensitivity, blood dyscrasias, cyanosis, exacerbation of ulcerative colitis, hepatitis, interstitial pneumonitis, Stevens-Johnson syndrome, systemic lupus erythematosus (SLE)–like syndrome, and toxic epidermal necrolysis
Orange-yellow discoloration of alkaline urine or skin may be alarming to patient although medically insignificant

# General Dosing Information

Fluid intake should be sufficient to maintain urine output of at least 1200 to 1500 mL per day in adults.

Sulfasalazine should preferably be taken immediately after meals or with food. Also, when sulfasalazine is being taken for inflammatory bowel disease, the total daily dose may be spread evenly over a 24-hour period. In some patients it may be necessary to initiate therapy with smaller doses (e.g., 1 to 2 grams daily) to lessen gastrointestinal irritation.

When endoscopic examination confirms satisfactory improvement, dosage may be reduced to maintenance level. If diarrhea recurs, dosage should be increased to previously effective level.

Patients with impaired renal function may require a reduction in dose.

Adverse reactions tend to increase with total daily doses of 4 grams or more or with serum concentrations greater than the equivalent of 50 mcg of sulfapyridine per mL.

Patients experiencing mild hypersensitivity reactions may be ''desensitized'' to allow continued treatment with sulfasalazine. Desensitization involves withdrawal of the medication followed by reinstitution, beginning with a lower dose and increasing it slowly over at least 23 days. Desensitization should not be attempted in patients with a history of agranulocytosis. Some medical experts believe that with the availability of mesalamine preparations, desensitization may no longer be indicated.

### For treatment of adverse effects
Recommended treatment consists of the following:
- Discontinuing the drug immediately if agranulocytosis or hypersensitivity reactions occur.
- Controlling hypersensitivity reactions with antihistamines and/or corticosteroids.

# Oral Dosage Forms

Note: Bracketed uses in the *Dosage Forms* section refer to categories of use and/or indications that are not included in U.S. product labeling.

Note: The capsule dosage form is indicated only for desensitization of patients who have previously experienced a hypersensitivity reaction with sulfasalazine.

## SULFASALAZINE CAPSULES

### Usual adult and adolescent dose
Bowel disease (inflammatory) suppressant—
Oral, according to the following dosing schedule:

| Day | Total daily dose (mg) |
|---|---|
| 1 | 1 |
| 2 | 2 |
| 3 | 4 |
| 4 | 8 |
| 5–11 | 10 |
| 12 | 20 |
| 13 | 40 |
| 14 | 80 |
| 15–21 | 100 |
| 22 | 200 |
| 23 | 400 |
| 24 | 800 |

Note: Physician should be consulted once the total daily dose reaches 800 mg.

### Usual pediatric dose
Bowel disease (inflammatory) suppressant—
Infants and children up to 2 years of age: Use is contraindicated because sulfonamides may cause kernicterus.
Children 2 years of age and over: See *Usual adult and adolescent dose.*

### Usual geriatric dose
See *Usual adult and adolescent dose.*

### Strength(s) usually available
U.S.—
Not commercially available.
Canada—
1 mg (Rx) [*Salazopyrin*].
10 mg (Rx) [*Salazopyrin*].
100 mg (Rx) [*Salazopyrin*].

Note: Three different strengths of capsules are combined to make up a desensitization kit; each strength is not available individually.

### Packaging and storage
Store below 40 °C (104 °F), preferably between 15 and 30 °C (59 and 86 °F), unless otherwise specified by manufacturer.

### Auxiliary labeling
- Take with a full glass of water.
- Avoid use of sunlamp and unprotected exposure to sun.
- Continue medicine for full time of treatment.
- May discolor urine.

## SULFASALAZINE ORAL SUSPENSION

### Usual adult and adolescent dose
Bowel disease (inflammatory) suppressant—
Initial: Oral, 1 gram every six to eight hours. An initial dose of 500 mg every six to twelve hours may be recommended to lessen gastrointestinal side effects.
Maintenance: Oral, 500 mg every six hours, adjusted according to patient response and tolerance.
[Antirheumatic (disease-modifying)]—
Oral, 500 mg to 1 gram daily for the first week, with the daily dose being increased by 500 mg each week, up to a maintenance dose of 2 grams daily. The dose may be administered two times a day. If no response is seen after two months, the dose may be increased to 3 grams daily.

### Usual adult prescribing limits
Total daily doses of greater than 4 grams may increase the risk of side effects and toxicity.

### Usual pediatric dose
Bowel disease (inflammatory) suppressant—
Infants and children up to 2 years of age:
Use is contraindicated because sulfonamides may cause kernicterus.
Children 2 years of age and over:
Initial—Oral, 6.7 to 10 mg per kg of body weight every four hours; 10 to 15 mg per kg of body weight every six hours; or 13.3 to 20 mg per kg of body weight every eight hours.
Maintenance—Oral, 7.5 mg per kg of body weight every six hours.
[Antirheumatic (disease-modifying)]—
Safety and efficacy have not been established.

### Usual geriatric dose
See *Usual adult and adolescent dose.*

### Strength(s) usually available
U.S.—
Not commercially available.
Canada—
250 mg per 5 mL (Rx) [*PMS-Sulfasalazine; Salazopyrin*].

### Packaging and storage
Store between 15 and 30 °C (59 and 86 °F), unless otherwise specified by manufacturer. Protect from freezing.

### Auxiliary labeling
- Shake well.
- Take with a full glass of water.
- Avoid use of sunlamp and unprotected exposure to sun.
- Continue medicine for full time of treatment.
- May discolor urine.

## SULFASALAZINE TABLETS USP

### Usual adult and adolescent dose
See *Sulfasalazine Oral Suspension.*

### Usual adult prescribing limits
See *Sulfasalazine Oral Suspension.*

### Usual pediatric dose
See *Sulfasalazine Oral Suspension.*

### Usual geriatric dose
See *Sulfasalazine Oral Suspension.*

### Strength(s) usually available
U.S.—
500 mg (Rx) [*Azulfidine;* GENERIC].
Canada—
500 mg (Rx) [*PMS-Sulfasalazine; Salazopyrin; S.A.S.-500;* GENERIC].

### Packaging and storage
Store below 40 °C (104 °F), preferably between 15 and 30 °C (59 and 86 °F), unless otherwise specified by manufacturer. Store in a well-closed container.

### Auxiliary labeling
- Take with a full glass of water.
- Avoid use of sunlamp and unprotected exposure to sun.

- Continue medicine for full time of treatment.
- May discolor urine.

## SULFASALAZINE TABLETS (ENTERIC-COATED) USP

**Usual adult and adolescent dose**
See *Sulfasalazine Oral Suspension.*

**Usual adult prescribing limits**
See *Sulfasalazine Oral Suspension.*

**Usual pediatric dose**
See *Sulfasalazine Oral Suspension.*

**Usual geriatric dose**
See *Sulfasalazine Oral Suspension.*

**Strength(s) usually available**
U.S.—
   500 mg (Rx) [*Azulfidine EN-Tabs;* GENERIC].
Canada—
   500 mg (Rx) [*PMS-Sulfasalazine E.C.; Salazopyrin EN-Tabs; S.A.S. Enteric-500;* GENERIC].

**Packaging and storage**
Store below 40 °C (104 °F), preferably between 15 and 30 °C (59 and 86 °F), unless otherwise specified by manufacturer. Store in a well-closed container.

**Auxiliary labeling**
- Take with a full glass of water.
- Avoid use of sunlamp and unprotected exposure to sun.
- Continue medicine for full time of treatment.
- May discolor urine.
- Swallow tablets whole.

**Note**
Dissolution of enteric-coated tablets is much more variable and unreliable than that of nonenteric-coated tablets.

## Rectal Dosage Forms

### SULFASALAZINE RECTAL SUSPENSION

**Usual adult and adolescent dose**
Bowel disease (inflammatory) suppressant—
   Rectal, 3 grams each night at bedtime.

**Usual pediatric dose**
Bowel disease (inflammatory) suppressant—
   Infants and children up to 2 years of age: Use is contraindicated because sulfonamides cause kernicterus.
   Children 2 years of age and over: Dosage has not been established.

**Usual geriatric dose**
See *Usual adult and adolescent dose.*

**Strength(s) usually available**
U.S.—
   Not commercially available.
Canada—
   3 grams per 100-mL unit (Rx) [*Salazopyrin*].

**Packaging and storage**
Store below 40 °C (104 °F), preferably between 15 and 30 °C (59 and 86 °F), unless otherwise specified by manufacturer.

**Auxiliary labeling**
- For rectal use.
- Shake well.
- Continue medicine for full time of treatment.

## Selected Bibliography

Allgayer H. Sulfasalazine and 5-ASA compounds. Gastrointest Pharmacol 1992; 21: 643-57.

Revised: 04/07/95

## SULFATHIAZOLE-CONTAINING COMBINATIONS—

Triple Sulfa (Vaginal)—See *Sulfonamides (Vaginal)*

---

# SULFINPYRAZONE    Systemic

VA CLASSIFICATION (Primary): MS400
Note: For a listing of dosage forms and brand names by country availability, see *Dosage Forms* section(s). For a listing of brand names for the articles in this monograph, refer to the General Index.

## Category

Antigout agent; antihyperuricemic.

## Indications

Note: Bracketed information in the *Indications* section refers to uses that are not included in U.S. product labeling.

**Accepted**
Gouty arthritis, chronic (treatment) or
Hyperuricemia (treatment)—Sulfinpyrazone is indicated for the long-term management of hyperuricemia associated with chronic gout. It is recommended only for patients whose 24-hour renal excretion of urate is 800 mg (4.8 mmol) or lower (i.e., patients who are hyperuricemic as a result of underexcretion, rather than overproduction, of urate). The aim of sulfinpyrazone therapy is to reduce the number of acute gout attacks.

Sulfinpyrazone is not effective in the treatment of acute gout attacks and does not eliminate the need to use colchicine or a nonsteroidal anti-inflammatory drug (NSAID) to relieve an attack. Also, sulfinpyrazone therapy should not be initiated during an attack, because it may induce fluctuations in urate concentration that may result in prolongation of the attack or initiation of a new attack.

[Sulfinpyrazone is sometimes used in the treatment of hyperuricemia not associated with gout. However, treatment of asymptomatic hyperuricemia is often unnecessary; the need for such therapy should be determined on an individual basis.][1]

Although a few studies have shown that sulfinpyrazone may reduce the risk of reinfarction and/or sudden cardiac death during the first 7 months after an initial myocardial infarction, the results of these studies have been questioned on methodological grounds. Aspirin is the drug of choice for preventing reinfarction, because its efficacy is more clearly established. However, sulfinpyrazone may be a suitable alternative for patients unable to take aspirin for this indication.

**Unaccepted**
Sulfinpyrazone is not recommended in circumstances in which there is an especially high risk of adverse effects associated with crystallization and deposition of urate in renal tissues, such as formation of renal calculi and uric acid nephropathy. It therefore should not be used for treatment of gout in patients whose 24-hour urate excretion exceeds 800 mg (4.8 mmol) or who have extensive tophi, or for treatment of hyperuricemia associated with neoplastic disease or its treatment (chemotherapy with rapidly cytolytic antineoplastic agents or radiation therapy). Allopurinol, which decreases the quantity of urate that reaches the kidneys in addition to decreasing the concentration of urate in the blood, is recommended in these circumstances.

Sulfinpyrazone has also been used to prevent the occurrence or reoccurrence of venous thrombosis or embolism and thrombotic complications associated with rheumatic mitral stenosis, unstable angina pectoris, and transient cerebral ischemic attacks. Also, sulfinpyrazone has been used to prevent occlusion (by clotted blood) of aortocoronary bypass grafts, arteriovenous shunts, and prosthetic mitral valves. However, sulfinpyrazone's efficacy has not been established and further study has been recommended. Aspirin is the agent of choice for these indications. Dipyridamole is also effective in protecting against thrombotic complications associated with prosthetic valves or other foreign surfaces.

---

[1]Not included in Canadian product labeling.

## Pharmacology/Pharmacokinetics

**Physicochemical characteristics**
Chemical group—A pyrazole compound chemically related to phenylbutazone

Molecular weight—404.48.
pKa—2.8.

## Mechanism of action/Effect

Antigout agent; antihyperuricemic—Sulfinpyrazone is a uricosuric agent. By competitively inhibiting the active reabsorption of urate at the proximal renal tubule, it increases the urinary excretion of uric acid and lowers serum urate concentrations. By lowering serum concentrations of uric acid below its solubility limits, sulfinpyrazone may decrease or prevent urate deposition, tophi formation, and chronic joint changes; promote resolution of existing urate deposits; and, after several months of therapy, reduce the frequency of acute attacks of gout. Sulfinpyrazone does not have clinically useful anti-inflammatory or analgesic activity.

Antithrombotic; myocardial infarction prophylactic—Sulfinpyrazone restores toward normal the shortened platelet survival time often associated with thromboembolic disorders. It decreases platelet adhesiveness to subendothelial cells and possibly to prosthetic surfaces. Although sulfinpyrazone also inhibits the activity of the enzyme cyclooxygenase, resulting in decreased synthesis of thromboxane $A_2$ (a prostaglandin in platelets that promotes aggregation) and the platelet release reaction (an essential step in platelet aggregation and subsequent thrombus formation), it is a relatively weak inhibitor of platelet aggregation. Whether inhibition of platelet aggregation contributes significantly to the medication's antithrombotic activity has therefore been questioned. Sulfinpyrazone's effects on platelets are due primarily to an active sulfide metabolite.

## Other actions/effects

Although sulfinpyrazone lacks clinically useful anti-inflammatory or analgesic activity, it inhibits prostaglandin synthesis and shares some of the risks associated with phenylbutazone (to which it is chemically related) and other nonsteroidal anti-inflammatory drugs (NSAIDs), including the potential for causing gastrointestinal, renal, or hematologic toxicity.

There is some evidence that sulfinpyrazone induces the activity of hepatic microsomal enzymes and, with chronic use, enhances its own metabolism. Although sulfinpyrazone has been shown to increase antipyrine clearance, the possibility that it may induce the metabolism of other medications has not been fully investigated. However, sulfinpyrazone has been shown to inhibit (rather than increase) metabolism of several medications, including warfarin, tolbutamide, and phenytoin, that are metabolized via the hepatic P-450 microsomal enzyme system.

## Absorption

Rapid and complete.

## Protein binding

Very high (98 to 99%).

## Biotransformation

Hepatic and intestinal. The sulfide metabolite is formed primarily by intestinal microflora following enterohepatic circulation of sulfinpyrazone. The number and quantity of metabolites formed, especially the quantity of the sulfide metabolite, are subject to considerable interpatient variation.

At least 4 of the known metabolites are active. p–Hydroxy-sulfinpyrazone has about 33 to 50% of the uricosuric activity of the parent compound. The sulfide derivative, but not the sulfone or p-hydroxysulfide derivative, also has slight uricosuric activity. The sulfide, sulfone, and p-hydroxysulfide metabolites are approximately 10, 5, and 2 times as potent, respectively, and the p-hydroxy-sulfinpyrazone metabolite is about half as potent, as sulfinpyrazone itself in altering platelet function. However, only the sulfide metabolite is considered to contribute significantly toward the medication's antithrombotic activity.

## Half-life

Elimination—
Sulfinpyrazone:
Approximately 4 to 6 hours. Single-dose studies have provided some evidence for the existence of an early elimination half-life of approximately 2 to 3 hours and a late elimination half-life (beginning approximately 20 hours after administration) of approximately 6 hours.
p-Hydroxy-sulfinpyrazone:
200-mg single dose—Approximately 1 hour.
400-mg single dose and
Steady-state, following administration of 400 mg twice a day for 23 days—Approximately 2.6 hours.
Sulfide metabolite:
Single doses—Approximately 11 to 12 hours, although one study reported a mean value of 20.9 hours after a single 400-mg dose.
Steady-state—Approximately 14 hours, following administration of 200 mg 4 times a day for 6 days or 400 mg twice a day for 23 days.

## Onset of action

Antithrombotic effect—Approximately 4 days.

## Time to peak concentration

Sulfinpyrazone—Approximately 1 to 2 hours. Values at steady-state (after administration of 200 mg 4 times a day for 6 days or 400 mg twice a day for 23 days) are not significantly different from those found with single 400-mg oral doses.

p-Hydroxy-sulfinpyrazone—Approximately 2.5 hours, after administration of a single 400-mg dose and at steady-state (following administration of 400 mg twice a day for 23 days).

Sulfide metabolite—Generally 11 to 12 hours after administration of a single dose, although one study reported a mean value of 19 hours after a single 400-mg dose. Mean values under steady-state conditions (after administration of 200 mg 4 times a day for 6 days or administration of 400 mg twice a day for 23 days) are lower by about 4 to 5 hours than those determined after single doses.

## Peak serum concentration

Sulfinpyrazone—
Single 200-mg dose: Approximately 13 mcg per mL (mcg/mL) (32.1 micromoles/L).
Single 400-mg dose: Approximately 26 to 30 mcg/mL (64.2 to 74.1 micromoles/L).
Chronic administration of 600 to 800 mg a day: Two studies, one in which values were determined in patients who had been treated continuously for 2.5 years and another in which values were determined after administration of 200 mg 4 times a day for 6 days, reported maximum values of approximately 16 to 21 mcg/mL (39.5 to 51.9 micromoles/L). In a third study, maximum concentrations of 13.5 mcg/mL (33.3 micromoles/L) were measured after administration of 400 mg twice a day for 23 days; this value is approximately half of that found in the same study after administration of a single 400-mg dose.
p-Hydroxy-sulfinpyrazone—
Single 200-mg dose: Less than 0.5 mcg/mL.
Single 400-mg dose: Approximately 0.7 mcg/mL.
Chronic administration of 800 mg a day: Approximately 0.2 mcg/mL.
Sulfide metabolite—
Single 200-mg dose: Approximately 2.6 mcg/mL.
Single 400-mg dose: Approximately 1 mcg/mL in 1 study and 3.5 mcg/mL in another.
Chronic administration of 600 to 800 mg a day: Maximum values of approximately 14 mcg/mL were reported in one study after administration of 200 mg 4 times a day for 6 days. However, lower values (approximately 2.5 to 5 mcg/mL) were reported in other studies in which sulfinpyrazone was administered for a longer time (23 days in 1 study and at least 2.5 years in the other).

## Time to peak effect

Antithrombotic effect—Approximately 1 to 2 weeks after initiation of treatment with 200 mg 4 times a day.

## Duration of action

Single dose—The uricosuric action usually lasts for 4 to 6 hours, but may persist for up to 10 hours in some patients.

## Elimination

95% renal; 5% fecal. Approximately 25% of a dose is excreted in the urine as free sulfinpyrazone and another 25% as sulfinpyrazone glucuronide. Up to 45% of a dose is excreted in the urine as metabolites, mostly as their glucuronide conjugates.

# Precautions to Consider

## Cross-sensitivity and/or related problems

Patients sensitive to aspirin, oxyphenbutazone, or phenylbutazone may be sensitive to this medication also. In challenge tests, sulfinpyrazone caused dyspnea, wheezing, and/or a fall in peak expiratory flow rate in 4 of 11 patients with aspirin-induced asthma but no reaction in individuals with documented sensitivity (history of anaphylaxis and positive skin tests) to dipyrone.

The possibility of cross-sensitivity between sulfinpyrazone and other nonsteroidal anti-inflammatory drugs (NSAIDs) should be considered, especially for patients in whom cross-sensitivity between aspirin and other NSAIDs has been reported.

## Carcinogenicity

No evidence of carcinogenicity was found in a 2-year study in rats receiving up to 500 mg per kg of body weight per day.

## Pregnancy/Reproduction

Pregnancy—Problems in humans have not been documented.
Studies in animals on the teratogenic potential of sulfinpyrazone have yielded inconclusive results.

**Breast-feeding**

It is not known whether sulfinpyrazone is excreted in breast milk.

**Pediatrics**

No published information is available on the relationship of age to the effects of sulfinpyrazone in pediatric patients.

**Geriatrics**

No published information is available on the relationship of age to the effects of sulfinpyrazone in geriatric patients. However, elderly patients are more likely to have age-related renal function impairment, which may decrease the efficacy of uricosuric agents and/or increase the risk of adverse effects in patients receiving sulfinpyrazone.

**Drug interactions and/or related problems**

The following drug interactions and/or related problems have been selected on the basis of their potential clinical significance (possible mechanism in parentheses where appropriate)—not necessarily inclusive (» = major clinical significance):

Note: Combinations containing any of the following medications, depending on the amount present, may also interact with this medication.

> In addition to the interactions listed below, the possibility should be considered that additive or multiple effects leading to impaired blood clotting and/or increased risk of bleeding may occur if sulfinpyrazone is administered concurrently with any medication having a significant potential for causing hypoprothrombinemia, thrombocytopenia, or gastrointestinal ulceration or hemorrhage.

Alcohol or
Diazoxide or
Mecamylamine or
Pyrazinamide
  (these medications may increase serum uric acid concentrations; dosage adjustment of sulfinpyrazone may be necessary to control hyperuricemia)

Aminosalicylate sodium
  (sulfinpyrazone may decrease renal tubular secretion of aminosalicylate sodium, resulting in increased and more prolonged serum concentrations and/or toxicity; patient should be monitored and dosage adjusted as necessary)

» Anticoagulants, coumarin- or indandione-derivative or
» Heparin or
» Thrombolytic agents, such as:
  Alteplase (tissue-type plasminogen activator, recombinant)
  Anistreplase (anisoylated plasminogen-streptokinase activator complex, APSAC)
  Streptokinase
  Urokinase
  (prolongation of the prothrombin time and severe gastrointestinal or renal bleeding have resulted from concurrent use of sulfinpyrazone with acenocoumarol [nicoumalone] or warfarin; studies have demonstrated that sulfinpyrazone has stereoselective effects on warfarin kinetics, i.e., it displaces from protein-binding sites and increases clearance of the (R)-enantiomer of warfarin, but inhibits metabolism of the substantially more potent (S)-enantiomer by the hepatic P-450 enzyme system, resulting in a net increase in warfarin activity; careful monitoring of the prothrombin time is recommended when sulfinpyrazone therapy is initiated or discontinued so that anticoagulant dosage can be adjusted as needed)

  (although sulfinpyrazone has also been shown to inhibit enzymatic metabolism of phenprocoumon, concurrent use of the 2 medications does not lead to a significant increase in the prothrombin time, possibly because a comparatively small quantity of phenprocoumon is eliminated via this mechanism; however, inhibition of platelet function by sulfinpyrazone, and its potential for causing gastrointestinal ulceration or hemorrhage, may increase the risk of hemorrhage in patients receiving any anticoagulant or thrombolytic agent)

Antidiabetic agents, oral
  (sulfinpyrazone may decrease the metabolism of an oral antidiabetic agent, leading to prolonged half-life and increased hypoglycemic effect; dosage adjustments may be necessary during and following sulfinpyrazone therapy)

Anti-inflammatory drugs, nonsteroidal (NSAIDs) or
» Platelet aggregation–inhibiting medications (See *Appendix II* )
  (concurrent use with sulfinpyrazone may increase the risk of bleeding because of additive inhibition of platelet function and sulfinpyrazone's potential for causing gastrointestinal ulceration or hemorrhage; concurrent use with NSAIDs may also increase the risk of gastrointestinal ulceration or hemorrhage)

Antimicrobial agents
  (antimicrobial therapy may suppress formation by intestinal microflora of the active sulfide metabolite of sulfinpyrazone, which is responsible for sulfinpyrazone's antithrombotic activity)

» Antineoplastic agents, rapidly cytolytic
  (concurrent use with sulfinpyrazone is not recommended because of the risk of uric acid nephropathy; allopurinol is the antihyperuricemic agent of choice for reducing risks [gout and/or urate nephropathy] associated with chemotherapy-induced hyperuricemia; also, rapidly cytolytic antineoplastic agents may increase serum uric acid concentrations and interfere with control of pre-existing hyperuricemia and gout)

» Aspirin or other salicylates, including bismuth subsalicylate
  (salicylates inhibit sulfinpyrazone's uricosuric action; although occasional use of a salicylate in low to moderate analgesic doses, or chronic administration of 80 mg per day of aspirin as an antithrombotic, is not likely to interfere with sulfinpyrazone's uricosuric effect, chronic use of analgesic or antirheumatic doses of a salicylate together with sulfinpyrazone is not recommended; sulfinpyrazone also inhibits the uricosuria induced by high doses of salicylates; in addition, sulfinpyrazone may decrease excretion of salicylate and/or displace salicylate from its plasma protein-binding sites, possibly leading to increased salicylate concentrations and toxicity)

  (low doses of sulfinpyrazone and aspirin have been used together as an antithrombotic regimen in a few studies; however, whether the combination is more effective than aspirin alone has not been established, and the increased risk of bleeding must be considered)

» Cefamandole or
» Cefoperazone or
» Cefotetan or
» Moxalactam or
» Plicamycin or
» Valproic acid
  (these medications may cause hypoprothrombinemia; in addition, plicamycin or valproic acid may inhibit platelet aggregation, and moxalactam may also cause irreversible platelet damage; inhibition of platelet function by sulfinpyrazone, as well as its potential for causing gastrointestinal ulceration or hemorrhage, may increase the risk of severe hemorrhage when these medications are used concurrently)

» Nitrofurantoin
  (sulfinpyrazone may increase serum concentrations of nitrofurantoin by decreasing its renal clearance, possibly increasing the potential for toxic reactions and reducing nitrofurantoin's effectiveness as a urinary tract anti-infective; concurrent use should be avoided)

Phenytoin and possibly other hydantoin anticonvulsants
  (sulfinpyrazone may displace these medications from plasma protein-binding sites and decrease their metabolism, possibly leading to increased plasma concentration and elimination half-life; although hydantoin plasma concentration is not consistently increased, it is recommended that patients be monitored for signs of hydantoin toxicity during concurrent use)

Probenecid
  (probenecid inhibits the renal tubular secretion of sulfinpyrazone and its active para-hydroxy metabolite; however, the uricosuric effects of the medications are additive, and increased therapeutic benefit has been reported during concurrent use)

**Laboratory value alterations**

The following have been selected on the basis of their potential clinical significance (possible effect in parentheses where appropriate)—not necessarily inclusive (» = major clinical significance):

With diagnostic test results
» Aminohippuric acid (PAH) clearance studies and
  Phenolsulfonphthalein (PSP) clearance studies
  (sulfinpyrazone decreases renal clearance of PAH and PSP, leading to reduced urine concentrations and misleading test results)

**Medical considerations/Contraindications**

The medical considerations/contraindications included here have been selected on the basis of their potential clinical significance (reasons given in parentheses where appropriate)—not necessarily inclusive (» = major clinical significance).

*Except under special circumstances, this medication should not be used when the following medical conditions exist:*

» Any condition in which there is an increased risk of uric acid renal calculus formation or urate nephropathy, such as:
» Cancer chemotherapy with rapidly cytolytic antineoplastic agents

» Radiation therapy for malignancy
» Renal calculi or history of, especially uric acid calculi
» Urate excretion higher than 800 mg (4.8 mmol) in 24 hours
» Urate nephropathy or history of
  (sulfinpyrazone is likely to induce, or exacerbate pre-existing, renal calculi and/or urate nephropathy; allopurinol is the antihyperuricemic agent recommended in these circumstances)
» Blood dyscrasias
  (may be exacerbated)
» Peptic ulcer, active
  (may be exacerbated)
» Renal function impairment, moderate to severe
  (may be exacerbated; also, sulfinpyrazone's efficacy as a uricosuric agent decreases with increasing degrees of renal function impairment, and the medication may be completely ineffective when the patient's creatinine clearance is lower than 30 mL per minute [0.5 mL per second])

***Risk-benefit should be considered when the following medical problems exist:***

Bronchospastic reaction to aspirin, history of or
Sensitivity to sulfinpyrazone or to NSAIDs, especially oxyphenbutazone or phenylbutazone, history of
  (risk of cross-sensitivity)
Blood dyscrasias, history of
  (increased risk of sulfinpyrazone-induced blood dyscrasias)
» Gastrointestinal inflammation or ulceration, active or history of or
» Peptic ulcer, history of
  (may be exacerbated or reactivated; if sulfinpyrazone is used for patients with these conditions, concurrent use of an appropriate treatment or prophylactic regimen for gastrointestinal ulceration should be considered)
» Renal function impairment, mild
  (may be exacerbated; also, sulfinpyrazone's efficacy as a uricosuric agent begins to decrease when the creatinine clearance is 80 mL per minute [1.33 mL per second])

**Patient monitoring**
The following may be especially important in patient monitoring (other tests may be warranted in some patients, depending on condition; » = major clinical significance):

Blood counts
  (recommended at periodic intervals during therapy)

Renal function determinations
  (recommended at periodic intervals during therapy for patients with renal function impairment)
» Uric acid determinations
  (monitoring of uric acid concentrations may be required for proper dosing in uricosuric therapy; the effect of sulfinpyrazone may be measured by a reduction of serum uric acid concentration [the upper limit of normal is about 7 mg per 100 mL (420 micromoles/L) for men and postmenopausal women and about 6 mg per 100 mL (360 micromoles/L) for premenopausal women but may vary, depending on the patient and laboratory methodology] or, more directly, by a significant increase in 24-hour urinary uric acid excretion)

## Side/Adverse Effects

The following side/adverse effects have been selected on the basis of their potential clinical significance (possible signs and symptoms in parentheses where appropriate)—not necessarily inclusive:

**Those indicating need for medical attention**
Incidence more frequent
  ***Renal calculi, urate*** (lower back and/or side pain, painful urination, with or without blood in urine)—may occur in up to 10% of patients early in sulfinpyrazone treatment
Incidence less frequent
  ***Dermatitis, allergic*** (skin rash)
Incidence rare
  ***Agranulocytosis*** (fever with or without chills; sores, ulcers, or white spots on lips or in mouth; sore throat); ***anemia*** (unusual tiredness or weakness); ***aplastic anemia; [pancytopenia]*** (shortness of breath, troubled breathing, tightness in chest, and/or wheezing; sores, ulcers, or white spots on lips or in mouth; swollen and/or painful glands; unusual bleeding or bruising; unusual tiredness or weakness); ***fever, allergic; gastrointestinal bleeding*** (bloody or black, tarry stools; vomiting of blood or material that looks like coffee grounds); ***leukopenia*** (fever with or without chills; sore throat; unusual tiredness or weakness); ***renal failure, possibly associated with urate nephropathy*** (increased

blood pressure; shortness of breath, troubled breathing, tightness in chest, and/or wheezing; sudden decrease in amount of urine; swelling of face, fingers, feet, and/or lower legs; unusual tiredness or weakness; weight gain); ***thrombocytopenia*** (rarely, unusual bleeding or bruising; black, tarry stools; blood in urine or stools; pinpoint red spots on skin)—usually asymptomatic

Note: *Renal failure not associated with urate nephropathy* has been reported, rarely, during sulfinpyrazone therapy, but a direct causal relationship has not always been clearly established. Sulfinpyrazone has caused *acute interstitial nephritis* (including cases documented as being hypersensitivity-mediated) and *acute renal tubular necrosis* in a few patients. Also, *transient renal function impairment* (which improved despite continued administration) has occurred in postmyocardial infarction patients and postaortocoronary bypass patients receiving sulfinpyrazone. It has been proposed that sulfinpyrazone may cause transient renal ischemia by temporarily inhibiting the synthesis of renal vasodilator prostaglandins and/or kinins, and that the presence of congestive heart failure may be a predisposing factor in the development of sulfinpyrazone-induced renal complications.

**Those indicating need for medical attention only if they continue or are bothersome**
Incidence more frequent
  ***Gouty arthritis, acute attack*** (joint pain; redness; swelling); ***nausea or vomiting; stomach pain***

Note: An increase in the frequency of *acute attacks of gout* during the first few months of therapy may be anticipated, unless adequate prophylaxis with colchicine (or, if the patient is unable to take colchicine, a nonsteroidal anti-inflammatory drug [NSAID]) is given concurrently with the sulfinpyrazone. Up to 20% of patients started on treatment with a uricosuric agent alone may experience acute attacks within the first few days of treatment.

## Overdose

For specific information on the agents used in the management of sulfinpyrazone overdose, see:
  • *Acetazolamide* in *Carbonic Anhydrase Inhibitors (Systemic)* monograph;
  • *Allopurinol (Systemic)* monograph; and/or
  • *Potassium citrate* in *Citrates (Systemic)* monograph.

For more information on the management of overdose or unintentional ingestion, **contact a Poison Control Center** (see *Poison Control Center Listing*).

**Clinical effects of overdose**
The following effects have been selected on the basis of their clinical significance (possible signs and symptoms in parentheses where appropriate)—not necessarily inclusive:

Acute and chronic
  ***Clumsiness or unsteadiness; convulsions; diarrhea; nausea or vomiting, severe or continuing; stomach pain, severe or continuing; difficulty in breathing***

**Treatment of overdose**
To decrease absorption—Emptying the stomach by induction of emesis or performing gastric lavage.

Specific treatment—If severe renal function impairment occurs, hemodialysis may be needed.

For uric acid calculi or urate nephropathy:

Recommended measures include administration of large quantities of fluids and of allopurinol to increase urine flow and reduce uric acid formation, respectively. A urinary pH of 6 to 6.5 should be achieved and maintained by administration of alkali such as potassium citrate. If necessary to maintain the desired urinary pH through the night, acetazolamide may also be given at bedtime. Other interventions designed to facilitate removal of renal calculi may also be needed.

Supportive care—Monitoring the patient and instituting supportive treatment as needed. Patients in whom intentional overdose is known or suspected should be referred for psychiatric consultation.

## Patient Consultation

As an aid to patient consultation, refer to *Advice for the Patient, Sulfinpyrazone (Systemic)*.

In providing consultation, consider emphasizing the following selected information (»= major clinical significance):

**Before using this medication**
» Conditions affecting use, especially:
  Sensitivity to sulfinpyrazone or NSAIDs, especially aspirin, oxyphenbutazone, or phenylbutazone, history of
  Other medications, especially anticoagulants, rapidly cytolytic antineoplastic agents, aspirin or other salicylates, hypoprothrombinemia-inducing cephalosporins, moxalactam, nitrofurantoin, platelet aggregation inhibitors, plicamycin, and valproic acid
  Other medical problems, especially cancer treated with rapidly cytolytic antineoplastic agents or radiation therapy, renal calculi or history of (especially uric acid calculi), renal function impairment, blood dyscrasias, gastrointestinal inflammation or ulceration, and active peptic ulcer

**Proper use of this medication**
» Taking with food or an antacid to minimize gastrointestinal irritation
» Compliance with therapy
  Importance of high fluid intake and compliance with therapy for alkalinization of urine, if prescribed, to minimize kidney stone formation
» Proper dosing
  Missed dose: Taking as soon as possible; not taking if almost time for next dose; not doubling doses
» Proper storage
*For use as antigout agent*
  Several months of continuous therapy may be required for maximum effectiveness
» Medication does not relieve acute gout attacks but rather helps to prevent them; need to continue taking sulfinpyrazone with medication prescribed for gout attacks

**Precautions while using this medication**
  Regular visits to physician to check progress during therapy
  Caution if any laboratory tests required; possible interference with test results
*For use as antihyperuricemic (including gout therapy)*
» Aspirin or other salicylates may decrease the uricosuric effects of sulfinpyrazone; checking with physician regarding concurrent use, since effect is dependent on salicylate dose and duration of use
» Possibility that alcohol taken in large amounts may increase blood uric acid concentration and reduce effectiveness of medication

**Side/adverse effects**
  Signs and symptoms of potential side effects, especially renal calculi, dermatitis, blood dyscrasias, fever, gastrointestinal bleeding, and renal failure

## General Dosing Information

Sulfinpyrazone therapy for gouty arthritis should not be initiated until 2 to 3 weeks after an acute attack has subsided. However, if an acute attack occurs in a patient already receiving sulfinpyrazone, the medication should be continued at the same dose while therapeutic doses of colchicine or a nonsteroidal anti-inflammatory drug (NSAID) are given to relieve the attack.

Sulfinpyrazone may be administered with food or an antacid to reduce gastrointestinal irritation.

Because sulfinpyrazone may increase the frequency of acute attacks of gout during the early months of therapy, prophylactic doses of colchicine (or, if the patient is unable to take colchicine, an NSAID) should be administered concurrently during the first 3 to 6 months of sulfinpyrazone therapy. However, even with prophylactic therapy, acute attacks of gout requiring treatment with full therapeutic doses of colchicine or an NSAID may occur.

To reduce the risk of urate stone formation, especially in patients with hyperuricemia, it is recommended that sulfinpyrazone therapy be initiated with a low dose, followed by a gradual increase in dosage. Also, a high fluid intake (no less than 2.5 to 3 liters daily) and maintenance of an alkaline urine by administration of sodium bicarbonate (3 to 7.5 grams daily), potassium citrate (7.5 grams daily), or acetazolamide (250 mg daily) are recommended. The risk of urate stone formation is highest during the first few weeks of therapy, when urate excretion is high; after hyperuricemia has been controlled and urinary excretion of uric acid decreases, the need for these measures is reduced.

Sulfinpyrazone may be given concurrently with allopurinol for treatment of gout; the antihyperuricemic effects of the 2 medications are additive.

Determination of serum or urine (24-hour) uric acid concentrations may be necessary for proper dosing in uricosuric therapy.

## Oral Dosage Forms

Note: Bracketed uses in the *Dosage Forms* section refer to categories of use and/or indications that are not included in U.S. product labeling.

### SULFINPYRAZONE CAPSULES USP

**Usual adult dose**
Antigout agent—
  Initial:
    Oral, 100 to 200 mg two times a day, the dose being increased by 200 mg a day at two-day intervals, if necessary, up to a maximum of 800 mg per day.
    Note: Some clinicians recommend initiating treatment with a lower dose of 50 mg two times a day and increasing the dose more gradually (e.g., at three- to four-day intervals).
      Patients who were previously controlled with other uricosuric therapy may be transferred to sulfinpyrazone at full maintenance dosage.
  Maintenance:
    Oral, dosage to be adjusted to the lowest dose that maintains the serum uric acid concentration at the desired level, usually 200 to 400 mg per day. However, some patients may require maintenance doses of up to 800 mg a day.
Note: The initial dose recommended for treatment of gout is also appropriate if sulfinpyrazone is used as an antithrombotic. However, it is recommended that myocardial reinfarction prophylaxis with sulfinpyrazone not be initiated until at least fourteen days after the acute event. Delaying treatment may decrease the risk of renal function impairment in patients receiving sulfinpyrazone for this purpose.
  For preventing myocardial reinfarction, the usual maintenance dose is 800 mg per day, in four divided doses. For other antithrombotic indications, the usual maintenance dose is 600 to 800 mg per day, in three or four divided doses.

**Usual pediatric dose**
Dosage has not been established.

**Strength(s) usually available**
U.S.—
  200 mg (Rx) [*Anturane;* GENERIC].
Canada—
  Not commercially available.

**Packaging and storage**
Store below 40 °C (104 °F), preferably between 15 and 30 °C (59 and 86 °F), unless otherwise specified by manufacturer. Store in a well-closed container.

### SULFINPYRAZONE TABLETS USP

**Usual adult dose**
See *Sulfinpyrazone Capsules USP.*

**Usual pediatric dose**
Dosage has not been established.

**Strength(s) usually available**
U.S.—
  100 mg (Rx) [*Anturane;* GENERIC].
Canada—
  100 mg (Rx) [*Anturan; Apo-Sulfinpyrazone; Novopyrazone*].
  200 mg (Rx) [*Anturan; Apo-Sulfinpyrazone; Novopyrazone*].

**Packaging and storage**
Store below 40 °C (104 °F), preferably between 15 and 30 °C (59 and 86 °F), unless otherwise specified by manufacturer. Store in a well-closed container.

Revised: 01/19/93

---

**SULFISOXAZOLE**—See *Sulfonamides (Ophthalmic); Sulfonamides (Systemic)*

---

## SULFISOXAZOLE-CONTAINING COMBINATIONS—

Erythromycin and Sulfisoxazole (Systemic)
Sulfisoxazole and Phenazopyridine (Systemic)—See *Sulfonamides and Phenazopyridine (Systemic)*

# SULFONAMIDES   Ophthalmic

This monograph includes information on the following: Sulfacetamide; Sulfisoxazole.

INN:
    Sulfisoxazole—Sulfafurazole

BAN:
    Sulfacetamide—Sulphacetamide
    Sulfisoxazole—Sulphafurazole

VA CLASSIFICATION (Primary): OP201

Note: For a listing of dosage forms and brand names by country availability, see *Dosage Forms* section(s). For a listing of brand names for the articles in this monograph, refer to the General Index.

## Category
Antibacterial (ophthalmic).

## Indications
Note: Bracketed information in the *Indications* section refers to uses that are not included in U.S. product labeling.

### Accepted
Conjunctivitis, bacterial (treatment) or

Ocular infections, other (treatment)—Ophthalmic sulfonamides are indicated in the treatment of conjunctivitis and other superficial ocular infections caused by susceptible organisms.

Trachoma (treatment) or

Chlamydial infections, other (treatment)—Ophthalmic sulfonamides are indicated concurrently with systemic sulfonamides in the treatment of trachoma and other chlamydial infections.

[Blepharitis, bacterial (treatment)]—Ophthalmic sulfonamides are used in the treatment of bacterial blepharitis.

[Blepharoconjunctivitis (treatment)]—Ophthalmic sulfonamides are used in the treatment of blepharoconjunctivitis.

[Keratitis, bacterial (treatment)]—Ophthalmic sulfonamides are used in the treatment of bacterial keratitis.

[Keratoconjunctivitis, bacterial (treatment)]—Ophthalmic sulfonamides are used in the treatment of bacterial keratoconjunctivitis.

Note: Not all species or strains of a particular organism may be susceptible to a specific sulfonamide.

## Pharmacology/Pharmacokinetics

### Physicochemical characteristics
Molecular weight—
    Sulfacetamide sodium: 254.24.
    Sulfisoxazole diolamine: 372.44.

### Mechanism of action/Effect
Sulfonamides are broad-spectrum, bacteriostatic anti-infectives. They are structural analogs of aminobenzoic acid (PABA) and competitively inhibit a bacterial enzyme, dihydropteroate synthetase, that is responsible for incorporation of PABA into dihydrofolic acid. This blocks the synthesis of dihydrofolic acid and decreases the amount of metabolically active tetrahydrofolic acid, a cofactor for the synthesis of purines, thymidine, and DNA.

Susceptible bacteria are those that must synthesize folic acid. The action of sulfonamides is antagonized by PABA and its derivatives (e.g., procaine and tetracaine) and by the presence of pus or tissue breakdown products, which provide the necessary components for bacterial growth.

### Absorption
Following topical application of sulfacetamide (30% solution) to the eye, small amounts may be absorbed into the cornea.

## Precautions to Consider

### Cross-sensitivity and/or related problems
Patients sensitive to one sulfonamide may be sensitive to other sulfonamides also.

Patients sensitive to furosemide, thiazide diuretics, sulfonylureas, or carbonic anhydrase inhibitors may be sensitive to sulfonamides also.

### Pregnancy/Reproduction
Problems in humans have not been documented.

### Breast-feeding
Problems in humans have not been documented.

### Pediatrics
Appropriate studies on the relationship of age to the effects of sulfonamides have not been performed in the pediatric population.

### Geriatrics
Appropriate studies on the relationship of age to the effects of sulfonamides have not been performed in the geriatric population. However, no geriatrics-specific problems have been documented to date.

### Drug interactions and/or related problems
The following drug interactions and/or related problems have been selected on the basis of their potential clinical significance (possible mechanism in parentheses where appropriate)—not necessarily inclusive (» = major clinical significance):

Note: Combinations containing any of the following medications, depending on the amount present, may also interact with this medication.

»  Silver preparations, such as silver nitrate, mild silver protein (topical sulfonamides are incompatible with silver salts; concurrent use is not recommended)

### Medical considerations/Contraindications
The medical considerations/contraindications included here have been selected on the basis of their potential clinical significance (reasons given in parentheses where appropriate)—not necessarily inclusive (» = major clinical significance).

*Risk-benefit should be considered when the following medical problem exists:*

Sensitivity to sulfonamides

## Side/Adverse Effects
The following side/adverse effects have been selected on the basis of their potential clinical significance (possible signs and symptoms in parentheses where appropriate)—not necessarily inclusive:

### Those indicating need for medical attention
Incidence more frequent
    *Hypersensitivity* (itching, redness, swelling, or other sign of irritation not present before therapy)

## Patient Consultation
As an aid to patient consultation, refer to *Advice for the Patient, Sulfonamides (Ophthalmic)*.

In providing consultation, consider emphasizing the following selected information (» = major clinical significance):

### Before using this medication
»  Conditions affecting use, especially:
    Sensitivity to sulfonamides, furosemide, thiazide diuretics, sulfonylureas, or carbonic anhydrase inhibitors
    Other medications, especially silver preparations, such as silver nitrate or mild silver protein

### Proper use of this medication
Proper administration technique for ophthalmic solution and ophthalmic ointment
»  Compliance with full course of therapy
»  Proper dosing
    Missed dose: Applying as soon as possible; not applying if almost time for next dose
»  Proper storage

### Precautions while using this medication
Blurred vision after application of ophthalmic ointments
Possibility of stinging or burning after application
Checking with physician if no improvement within a few days

### Side/adverse effects
Signs of potential side effects, especially hypersensitivity

## General Dosing Information
At night the ophthalmic ointment may be used as an adjunct to the ophthalmic solution to provide prolonged contact with the medication.

Although some manufacturers recommend a dose of 2 drops of an ophthalmic solution at appropriate intervals, the conjunctival sac will usually hold only 1 drop.

---

## *SULFACETAMIDE*

## Ophthalmic Dosage Forms
### SULFACETAMIDE SODIUM OPHTHALMIC OINTMENT USP

**Usual adult and adolescent dose**
Ophthalmic antibacterial—
    Topical, to the conjunctiva, a thin strip (approximately 1.25 to 2.5 cm) of ointment four times a day and at bedtime.

**Usual pediatric dose**
Dosage has not been established.

**Strength(s) usually available**
U.S.—
    10% (Rx) [*Ak-Sulf; Bleph-10; Cetamide; Ocu-Sul-10; Sodium Sulamyd; Sulfair 10;* GENERIC].
Canada—
    10% (Rx) [*Cetamide; Sodium Sulamyd*].

**Packaging and storage**
Store below 40 °C (104 °F), preferably between 15 and 30 °C (59 and 86 °F), unless otherwise specified by manufacturer. Protect from freezing.

**Auxiliary labeling**
• For the eye.
• Continue medicine for full time of treatment.

### SULFACETAMIDE SODIUM OPHTHALMIC SOLUTION USP

**Usual adult and adolescent dose**
Ophthalmic antibacterial—
    Topical, to the conjunctiva, 1 drop every one to three hours during the day and less frequently during the night.

**Usual pediatric dose**
Dosage has not been established.

**Strength(s) usually available**
U.S.—
    10% (Rx) [*Ak-Sulf; Bleph-10; I-Sulfacet; Ocu-Sul-10; Ocusulf-10; Ophthacet; Sodium Sulamyd; Spectro-Sulf; Sulf-10; Sulfair; Sulfair 10; Sulfamide; Sulten-10;* GENERIC].
    15% (Rx) [*Isopto-Cetamide; I-Sulfacet; Ocu-Sul-15; Spectro-Sulf; Steri-Units Sulfacetamide; Sulfair; Sulfair 15;* GENERIC].
    30% (Rx) [*I-Sulfacet; Ocu-Sul-30; Sodium Sulamyd; Spectro-Sulf; Sulfair; Sulfair Forte;* GENERIC].
Canada—
    10% (Rx) [*Ak-Sulf; Bleph-10; Isopto-Cetamide; Sodium Sulamyd; Sulfex*].
    30% (Rx) [*Sodium Sulamyd*].

**Packaging and storage**
Store between 8 and 15 °C (46 and 59 °F). Store in a tight, light-resistant container.

**Stability**
Sulfonamide solutions become dark brown with time. When this occurs, solutions should be discarded.

**Auxiliary labeling**
• For the eye.
• Keep in a cool place.
• Continue medicine for full time of treatment.
• Discard if dark brown.

---

**Note**
Dispense in original unopened container.

---

## *SULFISOXAZOLE*

## Ophthalmic Dosage Forms
Note: The dosing and strengths of the dosage forms available are expressed in terms of sulfisoxazole base.

### SULFISOXAZOLE DIOLAMINE OPHTHALMIC OINTMENT USP

**Usual adult and adolescent dose**
Ophthalmic antibacterial—
    Topical, to the conjunctiva, a thin strip (approximately 1.25 to 2.5 cm) of ointment one to three times a day and at bedtime.

**Usual pediatric dose**
See *Usual adult and adolescent dose.*

**Strength(s) usually available**
U.S.—
    4% (base) (each gram of ophthalmic ointment contains 55.6 mg of sulfisoxazole diolamine, equivalent to approximately 40 mg of sulfisoxazole) (Rx) [*Gantrisin* (phenylmercuric nitrate 1:50,000)].

**Packaging and storage**
Store below 40 °C (104 °F), preferably between 15 and 30 °C (59 and 86 °F), unless otherwise specified by manufacturer. Protect from freezing.

**Auxiliary labeling**
• For the eye.
• Continue medicine for full time of treatment.

### SULFISOXAZOLE DIOLAMINE OPHTHALMIC SOLUTION USP

**Usual adult and adolescent dose**
Ophthalmic antibacterial—
    Topical, to the conjunctiva, 1 drop three or more times a day.

**Usual pediatric dose**
Ophthalmic antibacterial—
    Infants up to 2 months of age: Use is not recommended.
    Infants and children over 2 months of age: See *Usual adult and adolescent dose.*

**Strength(s) usually available**
U.S.—
    4% (base) (each mL of ophthalmic solution contains 55.6 mg of sulfisoxazole diolamine, equivalent to approximately 40 mg of sulfisoxazole) (Rx) [*Gantrisin* (phenylmercuric nitrate 1:100,000)].

**Packaging and storage**
Store below 40 °C (104 °F), preferably between 15 and 30 °C (59 and 86 °F), unless otherwise specified by manufacturer. Store in a tight, light-resistant container. Protect from freezing.

**Auxiliary labeling**
• For the eye.
• Continue medicine for full time of treatment.

**Note**
Dispense in original unopened container.

---

Revised: 07/01/93

---

# SULFONAMIDES   Systemic

This monograph includes information on the following: Sulfadiazine; Sulfamethizole†; Sulfamethoxazole; Sulfisoxazole.

INN:
    Sulfisoxazole—Sulfafurazole

BAN:
    Sulfadiazine—Sulphadiazine
    Sulfamethizole—Sulphamethizole
    Sulfamethoxazole—Sulphamethoxazole
    Sulfisoxazole—Sulphafurazole

JAN:
    Sulfamethoxazole—Acetylsulfamethoxazole
    Sulfamethoxazole—Sulfamethoxazole sodium

VA CLASSIFICATION (Primary): AM650

Note: For a listing of dosage forms and brand names by country availability, see *Dosage Forms* section(s). For a listing of brand names for the articles in this monograph, refer to the General Index.

---

†Not commercially available in Canada.

## Category
Antibacterial (urinary)—Sulfamethizole.
Antibacterial (systemic)—Sulfadiazine; Sulfamethoxazole; Sulfisoxazole.
Antiprotozoal—Sulfadiazine; Sulfamethoxazole; Sulfisoxazole.

# Indications

Note: Bracketed information in the *Indications* section refers to uses that are not included in U.S. product labeling.

## General considerations

Sulfonamides are active *in vitro* against a broad spectrum of gram-positive and gram-negative bacteria. They also have activity *in vitro* against *Actinomyces*, *Chlamydia trachomatis*, *Nocardia asteroides*, *Plasmodium falciparum*, and *Toxoplasma gondii*. Susceptibility of an organism to sulfonamides is variable; many bacteria have become resistant to sulfonamides, with resistance occurring in more than 20% of community and nosocomial bacterial isolates. Resistance has developed in strains of staphylococci, *Neisseria gonorrhoeae*, *N. meningitidis*, Enterbacteriaceae, and *Pseudomonas* species.

## Accepted

Chancroid (treatment)—Sulfonamides are indicated in the treatment of chancroid caused by *Haemophilus ducreyi*. However, other agents, such as erythromycin and ceftriaxone, are considered to be first line agents.

Chlamydial infections, endocervical and urethral (treatment)[1]—Sulfonamides are indicated in the treatment of endocervical and urethral infections caused by *Chlamydia trachomatis*. However, other agents, such as doxycycline and azithromycin, are considered to be first line agents.

Conjunctivitis, inclusion (treatment)—Sulfonamides are indicated in the treatment of neonatal inclusion conjunctivitis caused by *Chlamydia trachomatis*. However, other agents, such as erythromycin, are considered to be first line agents.

Malaria (treatment)—Sulfonamides are indicated as adjunctive therapy in the treatment of chloroquine-resistant *Plasmodium falciparum*.

Meningitis (prophylaxis)[1]—Sulfonamides are indicated in the prophylaxis of meningitis caused by susceptible strains of *Neisseria meningitidis*. However, other agents, such as rifampin, are considered to be first line agents.

Nocardiosis (treatment)—Sulfonamides are indicated in the treatment of nocardiosis caused by *Nocardia asteroides*.

Otitis media (treatment)[1]—Sulfonamides are indicated in combination with other antibacterials in the treatment of otitis media caused by susceptible strains of *H. influenzae*, streptococci, and pneumococci.

Rheumatic fever (prophylaxis)[1]—Sulfadiazine, [sulfamethoxazole], and [sulfisoxazole] are indicated in the prophylaxis of rheumatic fever associated with group A beta-hemolytic streptococcal infections. However, other agents, such as penicillin, are considered to be first line agents.

Toxoplasmosis (treatment)[1]—Sulfonamides are indicated in combination with pyrimethamine in the treatment of toxoplasmosis caused by *Toxoplasma gondii*.

Trachoma (treatment)—Sulfonamides are indicated in the treatment of ocular trachoma caused by *Chlamydia trachomatis*. However, other agents, such as doxycycline and azithromycin, are considered to be first line agents.

Urinary tract infections, bacterial (treatment)—Sulfonamides are indicated in the treatment of acute, uncomplicated urinary tract infections caused by susceptible bacteria. Because sulfamethizole produces low plasma levels and is rapidly eliminated, it is recommended only for use in urinary tract infections, not systemic infections. Sulfadiazine is not recommended for the treatment of urinary tract infections because of its relatively lower urine solubility and the increased chance of crystalluria; other, more soluble agents, such as sulfisoxazole, are generally preferred.

[Lymphogranuloma venereum (treatment)][1]—Sulfonamides are used in the treatment of lymphogranuloma venereum caused by *Chlamydia* species. However, other agents, such as doxycycline and erythromycin, are considered to be first line agents.

[Paracoccidioidomycosis (treatment)][1]—Sulfadiazine is used in the treatment of paracoccidioidomycosis caused *Paracoccidioides brasiliensis*.

Not all species or strains of a particular organism may be susceptible to a specific sulfonamide.

## Unaccepted

Sulfonamides should not be used in the treatment of Group A beta-hemolytic streptococcal tonsillopharyngitis since they may not eradicate streptococci and therefore may not prevent sequelae such as rheumatic fever.

Sulfonamides are also not effective in treating rickettsial, viral, tuberculous, actinomycotic, fungal, or mycoplasmal infections. They are also not effective in the treatment of shigellosis.

[1]Not included in Canadian product labeling.

# Pharmacology/Pharmacokinetics

## Physicochemical characteristics

Molecular weight—
  Sulfadiazine: 250.28.
  Sulfamethizole: 270.34.
  Sulfamethoxazole: 253.28.
  Sulfisoxazole: 267.31.
  Sulfisoxazole acetyl: 309.35.

## Mechanism of action/Effect

Sulfonamides are broad-spectrum, bacteriostatic anti-infectives. They are structural analogs of para-aminobenzoic acid (PABA) and competitively inhibit a bacterial enzyme, dihydropteroate synthetase, that is responsible for incorporation of PABA into dihydrofolic acid, the immediate precursor of folic acid. This blocks the synthesis of dihydrofolic acid and decreases the amount of metabolically active tetrahydrofolic acid, a cofactor for the synthesis of purines, thymidine, and DNA.

Susceptible bacteria are those that must synthesize folic acid. Mammalian cells require preformed folic acid and cannot synthesize it. The action of sulfonamides is antagonized by PABA and its derivatives (e.g., procaine and tetracaine) and by the presence of pus or tissue breakdown products, which provide the necessary components for bacterial growth.

## Absorption

All sulfonamides are rapidly and well absorbed (70–100%).

## Distribution

Widely distributed throughout body tissues and fluids, including pleural, peritoneal, synovial, and ocular fluids, as well as the vagina and middle ear. Sulfadiazine is distributed throughout total body water, while sulfisoxazole is distributed primarily to extracellular fluid (ECF). Sulfadiazine, sulfamethoxazole, and sulfisoxazole penetrate into the cerebrospinal fluid (CSF); sulfadiazine reaches 32 to 65%, sulfamethoxazole reaches 14 to 30%, and sulfisoxazole reaches 30 to 50% of corresponding blood concentrations. Sulfonamides may be detected in the urine in approximately 30 minutes. They readily cross the placenta and are distributed into breast milk, also.

Urine solubility—
  Sulfadiazine: Less soluble in urine; increased risk of crystalluria.
  Sulfamethizole: Highly soluble in urine.
  Sulfamethoxazole: Acetylated metabolite less soluble in urine; increased risk of crystalluria.
  Sulfisoxazole: Highly soluble in urine.

$Vol_D$—
  Sulfamethoxazole: Approximately 0.15 L per kg of body weight (L/kg).
  Sulfisoxazole: Approximately 0.21 L/kg.

## Protein binding

Variable; acetylated metabolites are more highly protein bound than the free drug. Sulfonamides compete with bilirubin for binding to albumin. Kernicterus may develop in premature infants or neonates. Binding is decreased in patients with severely impaired renal function. Only free, unbound drug has antibacterial activity.

Sulfadiazine—38 to 48%.
Sulfamethizole—Approximately 90%.
Sulfamethoxazole—60 to 70%.
Sulfisoxazole—85 to 90%.

## Biotransformation

Hepatic; primarily by acetylation to inactive metabolites, which retain the toxicity of the parent compound. Some hepatic glucuronide conjugation may occur. Metabolism is increased with renal function impairment and decreased with hepatic failure.

## Half-life

Sulfadiazine—
  Normal renal function: Approximately 10 hours.
  Renal failure: Approximately 34 hours.
Sulfamethizole—
  Normal renal function: Approximately 1.5 hours.
Sulfamethoxazole—
  Normal renal function: 6 to 12 hours.
  Renal failure: 20 to 50 hours.
Sulfisoxazole—
  Normal renal function: 3 to 7 hours.
  Renal failure: 6 to 12 hours.

## Time to peak concentration

Sulfadiazine—3 to 6 hours.
Sulfamethoxazole—2 to 4 hours.
Sulfisoxazole—2 to 4 hours.

**Peak serum concentration**
Free unbound sulfonamide—
  Sulfadiazine: Single 2-gram dose—Approximately 30 to 60 mcg/mL.
  Sulfamethoxazole: Single 2-gram dose—Approximately 80 to 100 mcg/mL.
  Sulfisoxazole: Single 2-gram dose—40 to 50 mcg/mL.

**Duration of action**
Sulfadiazine—Short-acting sulfonamide.
Sulfamethizole—Short-acting sulfonamide.
Sulfamethoxazole—Intermediate-acting sulfonamide.
Sulfisoxazole—Short-acting sulfonamide.

**Elimination**
Renal, by glomerular filtration, with some tubular secretion and reabsorption of both active medication and metabolites. Excretion is increased in alkaline urine; small amounts are excreted in the feces, bile, and other body secretions.
Percent of medication unchanged in the urine—
  Sulfadiazine: 60 to 85% in 48 to 72 hours.
  Sulfamethizole: Approximately 95%.
  Sulfamethoxazole: 20 to 40%.
  Sulfisoxazole: Approximately 52% in 48 hours.
  Sulfisoxazole acetyl: Approximately 58% in 72 hours.
In dialysis—
  Peritoneal dialysis is not effective and hemodialysis is only moderately effective in removing sulfonamides.

## Precautions to Consider

### Cross-sensitivity and/or related problems
Patients allergic to one sulfonamide may be allergic to other sulfonamides also.
Patients allergic to furosemide, thiazide diuretics, sulfonylureas, or carbonic anhydrase inhibitors may be allergic to sulfonamides also.

### Carcinogenicity
*Sulfamethoxazole*—
  Long-term studies to evaluate the carcinogenic potential of sulfamethoxazole have not been done.
*Sulfisoxazole*—
  Studies in mice given daily oral doses of up to 18 times the highest recommended human daily dose for 103 weeks, and rats given 4 times the highest recommended human daily dose have not shown that sulfisoxazole is carcinogenic in either male or female mice or rats.

### Mutagenicity
*Sulfamethizole*—
  No long-term mutagenicity studies have been done in animals or humans.
*Sulfamethoxazole*—
  Bacterial mutagenicity studies with sulfamethoxazole have not been done. Studies in human leukocytes cultured *in vitro* with sulfamethoxazole using concentrations that exceeded therapeutic serum concentrations have not shown that sulfamethoxazole causes chromosomal damage.
*Sulfisoxazole*—
  Bacterial mutagenicity studies with sulfisoxazole have not been done. However, sulfisoxazole has not been shown to be mutagenic when tested in *Escherichia coli* Sd-4-73 strains in the absence of a metabolic activating system.

### Pregnancy/Reproduction
Fertility—
  *Sulfamethizole*—
    No long-term fertility studies have been done in animals or humans.
  *Sulfamethoxazole*—
    Studies in rats, given oral doses of 350 mg of sulfamethoxazole per kg of body weight daily, have not shown that it causes any adverse effects on fertility or general reproductive performance.
  *Sulfisoxazole*—
    Studies in rats given daily doses of 7 times the highest recommended daily dose have not shown that sulfisoxazole causes adverse effects on mating behavior, conception rate, or fertility index (percent of animals pregnant).
Pregnancy—
  *Sulfadiazine*—
    FDA Pregnancy Category C.
  *Sulfamethizole*—
    FDA Pregnancy Category C.

*Sulfamethoxazole*—
  Sulfamethoxazole crosses the placenta. Large, adequate, and well-controlled studies in humans have not been done.
  Studies in rats given oral doses of 533 mg of sulfamethoxazole per kg of body weight have shown that it causes teratogenic effects (primarily cleft palates). However, doses of 512 mg of sulfamethoxazole per kg of body weight did not cause cleft palates in rats.
  Studies in rabbits given doses of 150 to 350 mg of sulfamethoxazole per kg of body weight daily have shown that sulfamethoxazole causes increased maternal mortality but has no adverse effects on the fetus.
  FDA Pregnancy Category C.
*Sulfisoxazole*—
  Sulfisoxazole crosses the placenta and enters the fetal circulation. Adequate and well-controlled studies in humans have not been done.
  Studies in rats and rabbits given daily doses of 7 times the highest recommended human daily dose have not shown that sulfisoxazole is teratogenic. However, in studies in rats and mice given doses of 9 times the highest recommended human daily dose, sulfisoxazole caused cleft palates in both mice and rats and skeletal defects in rats.
  FDA Pregnancy Category C.
Labor and delivery—Sulfonamides are not recommended at term since sulfonamides may cause kernicterus in the newborn.

### Breast-feeding
Sulfonamides are distributed into breast milk. Use is not recommended in nursing women since sulfonamides may cause kernicterus in nursing infants. Also, sulfonamides may cause hemolytic anemia in glucose-6-phosphate dehydrogenase (G6PD)–deficient infants.

### Pediatrics
Except as concurrent adjunctive therapy with pyrimethamine in the treatment of congenital toxoplasmosis, use of sulfonamides is contraindicated in infants up to 2 months of age. Sulfonamides compete for bilirubin binding sites on plasma albumin, increasing the risk of kernicterus in the newborn. Also, because the acetyltransferase system is not fully developed in the newborn, increased blood concentrations of the free sulfonamide can further increase the risk of kernicterus.

### Geriatrics
Elderly patients may be at increased risk of severe side/adverse effects. Severe skin reactions, generalized bone marrow depression, and decreased platelet count (with or without purpura) are the most frequently reported severe side/adverse effects in the elderly. An increased incidence of thrombocytopenia with purpura has been reported in elderly patients who are receiving diuretics, primarily thiazides, concurrently with sulfamethoxazole. The potential for these problems should also be considered for elderly patients taking other sulfonamide medications.

### Pharmacogenetics
Sulfonamides are metabolized primarily by acetylation. Patients can be divided into 2 groups, slow and fast acetylators. Slow acetylators have a higher incidence of severe sulfonamide reactions, although a slow acetylator phenotype is not thought to be the sole reason for sulfonamide toxicity. The incidence of the slow acetylator phenotype is approximately 50% in North American blacks and whites. Approximately 30% of the Hispanic population and 10% of the Asian population are slow acetylators. Also, acquired immunodeficiency syndrome (AIDS) patients with acute illness, but not AIDS patients who are stable or human immunodeficiency virus (HIV)–infected patients without AIDS, have an increased incidence of slow acetylation.

### Dental
The leukopenic and thrombocytopenic effects of sulfonamides may result in an increased incidence of certain microbial infections, delayed healing, and gingival bleeding. If leukopenia or thrombocytopenia occurs, dental work should be deferred until blood counts have returned to normal. Patients should be instructed in proper oral hygiene, including caution in use of regular toothbrushes, dental floss, and toothpicks.

### Drug interactions and/or related problems
The following drug interactions and/or related problems have been selected on the basis of their potential clinical significance (possible mechanism in parentheses where appropriate)—not necessarily inclusive (» = major clinical significance):
Note: Combinations containing any of the following medications, depending on the amount present, may also interact with this medication.

» Anticoagulants, coumarin- or indandione-derivative or
» Anticonvulsants, hydantoin or
» Antidiabetic agents, oral

> (these medications may be displaced from protein binding sites and/or their metabolism may be inhibited by some sulfonamides, resulting in increased or prolonged effects and/or toxicity; dosage adjustments may be necessary during and after sulfonamide therapy)

Bone marrow depressants (See *Appendix II*)

> (concurrent use of bone marrow depressants with sulfonamides may increase the leukopenic and/or thrombocytopenic effects; if concurrent use is required, close observation for myelotoxic effects should be considered)

Contraceptives, estrogen-containing, oral

> (concurrent long-term use of sulfonamides may result in increased incidence of breakthrough bleeding and pregnancy)

Cyclosporine

> (concurrent use with sulfonamides may increase the metabolism of cyclosporine, resulting in decreased plasma concentrations and potential transplant rejection, and additive nephrotoxicity; plasma cyclosporine concentrations and renal function should be monitored)

» Hemolytics, other (See *Appendix II*)

> (concurrent use with sulfonamides may increase the potential for toxic side effects)

» Hepatotoxic medications, other (See *Appendix II*)

> (concurrent use with sulfonamides may result in an increased incidence of hepatotoxicity; patients, especially those on prolonged administration or those with a history of liver disease, should be carefully monitored)

» Methenamine

> (in acid urine, methenamine breaks down into formaldehyde, which may form an insoluble precipitate with certain sulfonamides, especially those that are less soluble in urine, and may also increase the danger of crystalluria; concurrent use is not recommended)

» Methotrexate or
Phenylbutazone or
Sulfinpyrazone

> (the effects of methotrexate may be potentiated during concurrent use with sulfonamides because of displacement from plasma protein binding sites; phenylbutazone and sulfinpyrazone may displace sulfonamides from plasma protein binding sites, increasing sulfonamide concentrations)

Penicillins

> (since bacteriostatic drugs may interfere with the bactericidal effect of penicillins in the treatment of meningitis or in other situations where a rapid bactericidal effect is necessary, it is best to avoid concurrent therapy)

**Laboratory value alterations**

The following have been selected on the basis of their potential clinical significance (possible effect in parentheses where appropriate)—not necessarily inclusive (» = major clinical significance):

With diagnostic test results

Benedict's test

> (sulfonamides may produce a false-positive Benedict's test for urine glucose)

Jaffé alkaline picrate reaction assay

> (sulfamethoxazole may interfere with the Jaffé alkaline picrate reaction assay for creatinine, resulting in overestimations of approximately 10% in the normal values for creatinine)

Sulfosalicylic acid test

> (sulfonamides may produce a false-positive sulfosalicylic acid test for urine protein)

Urine urobilinogen test strip (e.g., Urobilistix)

> (sulfonamides may interfere with the urine urobilinogen [Urobilistix] test for urinary urobilinogen)

With physiology/laboratory test values

Alanine aminotransferase (ALT [SGPT]), serum and
Aspartate aminotransferase (AST [SGOT]), serum and
Bilirubin, serum

> (values may be increased)

Blood urea nitrogen (BUN) and
Creatinine, serum

> (concentrations may be increased)

**Medical considerations/Contraindications**

The medical considerations/contraindications included here have been selected on the basis of their potential clinical significance (reasons given in parentheses where appropriate)—not necessarily inclusive (» = major clinical significance).

***Except under special circumstances, this medication should not be used when the following medical problems exist:***

Allergy to sulfonamides, furosemide, thiazide diuretics, sulfonylureas, or carbonic anhydrase inhibitors

***Risk-benefit should be considered when the following medical problems exist:***

» Blood dyscrasias or
» Megaloblastic anemia due to folate deficiency

> (sulfonamides may cause blood dyscrasias)

» Glucose-6-phosphate dehydrogenase (G6PD) deficiency

> (hemolysis may occur)

» Hepatic function impairment

> (sulfonamides are metabolized in the liver; delayed metabolism may increase the risk of toxicity; also, sulfonamides may cause fulminant hepatic necrosis)

» Porphyria

> (sulfonamides may precipitate an acute attack of porphyria)

» Renal function impairment

> (sulfonamides are renally excreted; delayed elimination may increase the risk of toxicity; also, sulfonamides may cause tubular necrosis or interstitial nephritis)

**Patient monitoring**

The following may be especially important in patient monitoring (other tests may be warranted in some patients, depending on condition; » = major clinical significance):

Complete blood counts (CBCs)

> (may be required prior to and monthly during treatment to detect blood dyscrasias in patients on prolonged therapy; therapy should be discontinued if a significant decrease in the count of any formed blood elements occurs)

Urinalyses

> (may be required prior to and periodically during treatment to detect crystalluria and/or urinary calculi formation in patients on long-term or high-dose therapy and in patients with impaired renal function)

# Side/Adverse Effects

Note: Fatalities have occurred, although rarely, due to severe reactions such as Stevens-Johnson syndrome, toxic epidermal necrolysis, fulminant hepatic necrosis, agranulocytosis, aplastic anemia, and other blood dyscrasias. Therapy should be discontinued at the first appearance of skin rash or any serious side/adverse effects.

Patients with acquired immunodeficiency syndrome (AIDS) may have a greater incidence of side/adverse effects, especially rash, fever, and leukopenia, than do non-AIDS patients.

The multiorgan toxicity of sulfonamides is thought to be the result of the way sulfonamides are metabolized in certain patients. It is probably due to the inability of the body to detoxify reactive metabolites. Sulfonamides are metabolized primarily by acetylation. Patients can be divided into slow and fast acetylators. Slow acetylation of sulfonamides makes more of the medication available for metabolism by the oxidative pathways of the cytochrome P-450 system. These pathways produce reactive toxic metabolites, such as hydroxylamine and nitroso compounds. The metabolites are normally detoxified by scavengers, such as glutathione. However, some populations, such as human immunodeficiency virus (HIV)–infected patients, have low concentrations of glutathione and these metabolites accumulate, producing toxicity. Patients who are slow acetylators have a higher incidence of sulfonamide hypersensitivity reactions, although severe toxicity has also been seen in fast acetylators. Acetylation status alone cannot fully explain sulfonamide toxicity since approximately 50% of North American blacks and whites are slow acetylators and severe reactions occur in less than 1% of patients treated with sulfonamides. However, decreased acetylation may increase the amount of sulfonamide metabolized to toxic metabolites.

Crytalluria is more likely to occur with a less soluble sulfonamide, such as sulfadiazine. It occurs most often with the administration of high doses, and can be minimized by maintaining a high urine flow and alkalinizing the urine.

The following side/adverse effects have been selected on the basis of their potential clinical significance (possible signs and symptoms in parentheses where appropriate)—not necessarily inclusive:

**Those indicating need for medical attention**
Incidence more frequent
> *Hypersensitivity* (fever; itching; skin rash); *photosensitivity* (increased sensitivity of skin to sunlight)

Incidence less frequent
> *Blood dyscrasias* (fever and sore throat; pale skin; unusual bleeding or bruising; unusual tiredness or weakness); *hepatitis* (yellow eyes or skin); *Lyell's syndrome* (difficulty in swallowing; redness, blistering, peeling, or loosening of skin); *Stevens-Johnson syndrome* (aching joints and muscles; redness, blistering, peeling, or loosening of skin; unusual tiredness or weakness)

Incidence rare
> *Central nervous system toxicity* (confusion; disorientation; euphoria; hallucination; mental depression); *Clostridium difficile colitis* (severe abdominal or stomach cramps and pain; abdominal tenderness; watery and severe diarrhea, which may also be bloody; fever); *crystalluria or hematuria* (blood in urine; lower back pain; pain or burning while urinating); *goiter or thyroid function disturbance* (swelling of front part of neck); *interstitial nephritis or tubular necrosis* (greatly increased or decreased frequency of urination or amount of urine; increased thirst; loss of appetite; nausea; vomiting)

> Note: *C. difficile colitis* may occur up to several weeks after discontinuation of these medications.

**Those indicating need for medical attention only if they continue or are bothersome**
Incidence more frequent
> *Central nervous system effects* (dizziness; headache; lethargy); *gastrointestinal disturbances* (diarrhea; loss of appetite; nausea or vomiting)

## Patient Consultation

As an aid to patient consultation, refer to *Advice for the Patient, Sulfonamides (Systemic)*.

In providing consultation, consider emphasizing the following selected information (» = major clinical significance):

**Before using this medication**
» Conditions affecting use, especially:
> Allergy to sulfonamides, furosemide, thiazide diuretics, sulfonylureas, carbonic anhydrase inhibitors
> Pregnancy—Sulfonamides cross the placenta; not recommended at term since sulfonamides may cause kernicterus in newborn
> Breast-feeding—Sulfonamides are distributed into breast milk; may cause kernicterus in nursing infants
> Use in children—Sulfonamides are contraindicated in infants up to 2 months of age since sulfonamides may cause kernicterus in neonates
> Use in the elderly—Elderly patients may be at increased risk of severe side/adverse effects
> Other medications, especially coumarin- or indandione-derivative anticoagulants, hydantoin anticonvulsants, oral antidiabetic agents, other hemolytics, other hepatotoxic medications, methenamine, or methotrexate
> Other medical problems, especially blood dyscrasias, G6PD deficiency, hepatic function impairment, megaloblastic anemia, porphyria, and renal function impairment

**Proper use of this medication**
» Not giving to infants under 2 months of age
» Maintaining adequate fluid intake
> Proper administration technique for oral liquids
» Compliance with full course of therapy
» Importance of not missing doses and taking at evenly spaced times
» Proper dosing
> Missed dose: Taking as soon as possible; not taking if almost time for next dose; not doubling doses
» Proper storage

**Precautions while using this medication**
» Regular visits to physician to check blood counts
> Checking with physician if no improvement within a few days
> Using caution in use of regular toothbrushes, dental floss, and toothpicks; deferring dental work until blood counts have returned to normal; checking with physician or dentist concerning proper oral hygiene
» Possible photosensitivity reactions
» Caution if dizziness occurs

**Side/adverse effects**
> Severe skin problems and blood problems may be more likely to occur in the elderly who are taking sulfamethoxazole, especially if taking diuretics concurrently
> Signs of potential side effects, especially hypersensitivity, photosensitivity, blood dyscrasias, hepatitis, Lyell's syndrome, Stevens-Johnson syndrome, central nervous system toxicity, *C. difficile* colitis, crystalluria or hematuria, goiter or thyroid function disturbance, and interstitial nephritis or tubular necrosis

## General Dosing Information

Fluid intake should be sufficient to maintain urine output of at least 1200 mL per day in adults.

---

### SULFADIAZINE

## Summary of Differences

Indications: Because of its relatively low urine solubility and the increased chance of crystalluria, sulfadiazine is not recommended for the treatment of urinary tract infections. Sulfadiazine is used for the prophylaxis of rheumatic fever and, in combination with pyrimethamine, for the treatment of toxoplasmosis and malaria caused by chloroquine-resistant *P. falciparum*.

## Additional Dosing Information

Fluid intake should be sufficient to maintain urine output of at least 1200 mL per day in adults.

Patients with impaired renal function may require a reduction in dose.

## Oral Dosage Forms

### SULFADIAZINE TABLETS USP

**Usual adult and adolescent dose**
Antibacterial (systemic) or
Antiprotozoal—
> Oral, 2 to 4 grams initially, then 1 gram every four to six hours.
>> Meningitis (prophylaxis):
>>> Oral, 1 gram every twelve hours for two days.
>> Rheumatic fever (prophylaxis):
>>> Oral, 1 gram once a day.
>> Toxoplasmosis:
>>> AIDS patients: Oral, 1 to 2 grams of sulfadiazine every 6 hours with 50 to 100 mg of pyrimethamine per day and 10 to 25 mg of leucovorin per day.
>>> Pregnant women: Oral, 1 gram of sulfadiazine every 6 hours with 25 mg of pyrimethamine per day after week 16 of the pregnancy. With this regimen, 5 to 15 mg of leucovorin per day is administered.

**Usual pediatric dose**
Antibacterial (systemic) or
Antiprotozoal—
> Infants up to 2 months of age: Use is not recommended.
> Infants 2 months of age and over: Oral, 75 mg per kg of body weight initially, then 37.5 mg per kg of body weight every six hours or 25 mg per kg of body weight every four hours.
> Toxoplasmosis: Oral, 50 mg of sulfadiazine per kg of body weight two times a day, administered concurrently with 2 mg of pyrimethamine per kg of body weight per day for two days, then 1 mg of pyrimethamine per kg of body weight per day for two to six months, then of 1 mg pyrimethamine per kg of body weight per day three times per week. With this regimen, 5 mg of leucovorin is administered three times a week. The three medications should be given for a total of twelve months.

Note: The maximum dose for children should not exceed 6 grams daily.

**Strength(s) usually available**
U.S.—
> 500 mg (Rx) [GENERIC].
Canada—
> 500 mg (Rx) [GENERIC].

**Packaging and storage**
Store below 30 °C (86 °F), unless otherwise specified by manufacturer. Store in a tight container. Protect from light.

**Auxiliary labeling**
- Take with a full glass of water.
- Avoid too much sun or use of sunlamp.
- May cause dizziness.
- Continue medicine for full time of treatment.

## SULFAMETHIZOLE

## Summary of Differences

Indications: Sulfamethizole is recommended for use only in the treatment of urinary tract infections, not systemic infections.

## Additional Dosing Information

Fluid intake should be sufficient to maintain urine output of at least 1200 mL per day in adults.

Patients with impaired renal function may require a reduction in dose.

## Oral Dosage Forms
### SULFAMETHIZOLE TABLETS USP

**Usual adult and adolescent dose**
Antibacterial—
    Oral, 500 mg to 1 gram every six to eight hours.

**Usual pediatric dose**
Antibacterial—
    Infants up to 2 months of age: Use is not recommended.
    Infants 2 months of age and over: Oral, 7.5 to 11.25 mg per kg of body weight every six hours.

**Strength(s) usually available**
U.S.—
    500 mg (Rx) [*Thiosulfil Forte*].
Canada—
    Not commercially available.

**Packaging and storage**
Store below 30 °C (86 °F), unless otherwise specified by manufacturer. Store in a tight container.

**Auxiliary labeling**
• Take with a full glass of water.
• Avoid too much sun or use of sunlamp.
• May cause dizziness.
• Continue medicine for full time of treatment.

## SULFAMETHOXAZOLE

## Additional Dosing Information

Fluid intake should be sufficient to maintain urine output of at least 1200 mL per day in adults.

Although sulfamethoxazole has a greater tendency to cause crystalluria than sulfisoxazole because of slower absorption and excretion, alkalinization of the urine is usually unnecessary.

Therapy should be continued for at least 7 to 10 days in urinary tract infections.

Patients with impaired renal function may require a reduction in dose.

## Oral Dosage Forms
### SULFAMETHOXAZOLE TABLETS USP

**Usual adult and adolescent dose**
Antibacterial (systemic) or
Antiprotozoal—
    Mild to moderate infections: Oral, 2 grams initially, then 1 gram every eight to twelve hours.
    Severe infections: Oral, 4 grams initially, then 2 grams every eight to twelve hours.

**Usual pediatric dose**
Antibacterial (systemic) or
Antiprotozoal—
    Infants up to 2 months of age: Except as concurrent adjunctive therapy with pyrimethamine in the treatment of congenital toxoplasmosis, use is contraindicated since sulfonamides may cause kernicterus in neonates.
    Infants and children 2 months of age and over: Oral, 50 to 60 mg per kg of body weight (maximum—2 grams) initially, then 25 to 30 mg per kg of body weight every twelve hours.

Note: The maximum dose for children should not exceed 75 mg per kg of body weight per day.

**Strength(s) usually available**
U.S.—
    500 mg (Rx) [*Gantanol; Urobak*].
Canada—
    500 mg (Rx) [*Apo-Sulfamethoxazole* (scored); GENERIC].

**Packaging and storage**
Store below 40 °C (104 °F), preferably between 15 and 30 °C (59 and 86 °F), unless otherwise specified by manufacturer. Store in a well-closed, light-resistant container.

**Auxiliary labeling**
• Take with a full glass of water.
• May cause dizziness.
• Avoid too much sun or use of sunlamp.
• Continue medicine for full time of treatment.

## SULFISOXAZOLE

## Additional Dosing Information

Fluid intake should be sufficient to maintain urine output of at least 1200 mL per day in adults.

Because of its relatively high solubility even in acid urine, the risk of crystalluria with sulfisoxazole is low and alkalinization of the urine is usually unnecessary.

Therapy should be continued for at least 7 to 10 days in urinary tract infections.

Patients with impaired renal function may require a reduction in dose.

## Oral Dosage Forms
### SULFISOXAZOLE TABLETS USP

**Usual adult and adolescent dose**
Antibacterial (systemic) or
Antiprotozoal—
    Oral, 2 to 4 grams initially, then 750 mg to 1.5 grams every four hours; or 1 to 2 grams every six hours.

**Usual adult prescribing limits**
Up to 8 grams daily.

**Usual pediatric dose**
Antibacterial (systemic) or
Antiprotozoal—
    Infants up to 2 months of age: Except as concurrent adjunctive therapy with pyrimethamine in the treatment of congenital toxoplasmosis, use is contraindicated since sulfonamides may cause kernicterus in neonates.
    Infants and children 2 months of age and over: Oral, 75 mg per kg of body weight or 2 grams per square meter of body surface initially, then 25 mg per kg of body weight or 667 mg per square meter of body surface every four hours; or 37.5 mg per kg of body weight or 1 gram per square meter of body surface every six hours.

Note: The maximum dose for children should not exceed 6 grams daily.

**Strength(s) usually available**
U.S.—
    500 mg (Rx) [*Gantrisin* (scored); GENERIC].
Canada—
    500 mg (Rx) [*Apo-Sulfisoxazole; Novo-Soxazole; Sulfizole*].

**Packaging and storage**
Store below 40 °C (104 °F), preferably between 15 and 30 °C (59 and 86 °F), unless otherwise specified by manufacturer. Store in a well-closed, light-resistant container.

**Auxiliary labeling**
• Take with a full glass of water.
• May cause dizziness.
• Avoid too much sun or use of sunlamp.
• Continue medicine for full time of treatment.

### SULFISOXAZOLE ACETYL ORAL SUSPENSION USP

**Usual adult and adolescent dose**
See *Sulfisoxazole Tablets USP*.

**Usual adult prescribing limits**
See *Sulfisoxazole Tablets USP*.

**Usual pediatric dose**
See *Sulfisoxazole Tablets USP*.

**Strength(s) usually available**
U.S.—
    500 mg per 5 mL (Rx) [*Gantrisin* (alcohol 0.3%; parabens; sucrose); GENERIC].
Canada—
    Not commercially available.

**Packaging and storage**
Store below 40 °C (104 °F), preferably between 15 and 30 °C (59 and 86 °F), unless otherwise specified by manufacturer. Store in a tight, light-resistant container. Protect from freezing.

**Auxiliary labeling**
- Shake well.
- Take with a full glass of water.
- May cause dizziness.
- Avoid too much sun or use of sunlamp.
- Continue medicine for full time of treatment.

**Note**
When dispensing, include a calibrated liquid-measuring device.

**SULFISOXAZOLE ACETYL ORAL SYRUP**

**Usual adult and adolescent dose**
See *Sulfisoxazole Tablets USP.*

**Usual adult prescribing limits**
See *Sulfisoxazole Tablets USP.*

**Usual pediatric dose**
See *Sulfisoxazole Tablets USP.*

**Strength(s) usually available**
U.S.—
    500 mg per 5 mL (Rx) [*Gantrisin*].
Canada—
    Not commercially available.

**Packaging and storage**
Store below 40 °C (104 °F), preferably between 15 and 30 °C (59 and 86 °F), unless otherwise specified by manufacturer. Store in a tight, light-resistant container. Protect from freezing.

**Auxiliary labeling**
- Take with a full glass of water.
- May cause dizziness.
- Avoid too much sun or use of sunlamp.
- Continue medicine for full time of treatment.

**Note**
When dispensing, include a calibrated liquid-measuring device.

Revised: 08/25/95

---

# SULFONAMIDES   Vaginal

This monograph includes information on the following: Sulfanilamide; Sulfanilamide, Aminacrine, and Allantoin*; Triple Sulfa.

VA CLASSIFICATION (Primary): GU300

Another commonly used name for triple sulfa is sulfathiazole, sulfacetamide, and sulfabenzamide.

Note: For a listing of dosage forms and brand names by country availability, see *Dosage Forms* section(s). For a listing of brand names for the articles in this monograph, refer to the General Index.

    *Not commercially available in the U.S.

## Category
Anti-infective (vaginal).

## Indications

**Unaccepted**
The U.S. Food and Drug Administration (FDA) announced on May 31, 1979, that its Anti-infective and Topical Drugs Advisory Committee and Fertility and Maternal Health Advisory Committee, as well as other studies, had concluded there was no adequate evidence that the then-available vaginal sulfonamides formulations were effective either for the treatment of vulvovaginitis caused by *Candida albicans*, *Trichomonas vaginalis*, or *Gardnerella vaginalis (Haemophilus vaginalis)* or for relief of the symptoms of these conditions.

In addition, in the opinion of USP medical experts, triple sulfa vaginal preparations are not effective for any indication, including vulvovaginitis caused by *Gardnerella vaginalis* and use as a deodorant in saprophytic infections following radiation therapy. Also, USP medical experts do not recommend the use of vaginal sulfonamides, including the reformulated single-entity preparations, for the treatment of fungal infections of the vagina.

## Pharmacology/Pharmacokinetics

**Physicochemical characteristics**
Molecular weight—
    Allantoin: 158.12.
    Aminacrine hydrochloride: 320.70.
    Sulfabenzamide: 276.31.
    Sulfacetamide: 214.24.
    Sulfanilamide: 172.21.
    Sulfathiazole: 255.31.
    Sulfisoxazole: 267.30.

**Mechanism of action/Effect**
Sulfonamides—See *Sulfonamides (Systemic)*
Allantoin—Allantoin is a xanthine alkaloid oxidation product of uric acid used topically. It is thought to aid in debridement of necrotic tissue and to stimulate tissue repair.
Aminacrine—Aminacrine hydrochloride is a highly ionized acridine dye derivative, which is thought to possess broad-spectrum topical anti-

microbial activity against gram-positive and gram-negative bacteria, trichomonads, and fungi. It is thought to inhibit microbial growth by interference or competition with certain hydrogen ions in microbial enzyme systems. It is not inactivated by pus, secretions, or body fluids.

**Absorption**
Sulfonamides are absorbed through the vaginal mucosa.

## Precautions to Consider

**Cross-sensitivity and/or related problems**
Patients sensitive to one sulfonamide may be sensitive to other sulfonamides also.
Patients sensitive to furosemide, thiazide diuretics, sulfonylureas, or carbonic anhydrase inhibitors may be sensitive to sulfonamides also.
Use of topical sulfonamides may lead to sensitization, resulting in hypersensitivity reactions with subsequent topical or systemic use of the medication.

**Carcinogenicity/Tumorigenicity**
Studies in rats have shown that long-term administration of sulfonamides may cause thyroid malignancy. However, rats appear to be especially susceptible to the goitrogenic effects of sulfonamides.

**Mutagenicity**
*For sulfanilamide—*
    No information available on the long-term mutagenic potential of sulfanilamide in animals or humans.

**Pregnancy/Reproduction**
*For sulfanilamide*
Fertility—No information available on the long-term effects of sulfanilamide on fertility in animals or humans.

Pregnancy—Sulfonamides are absorbed from the vaginal mucosa, readily cross the placenta, and appear in the fetal circulation. Fetal serum concentrations are approximately 50 to 90 percent of maternal serum concentrations. Adequate and well-controlled studies of most sulfonamides have not been done in either animals or humans. However, studies in rats and mice given high oral doses (7 to 25 times the human therapeutic dose) have shown that certain short-, intermediate-, and long-acting sulfonamides cause a significant increase in the incidence of cleft palate and other bony abnormalities in the fetus.

FDA Pregnancy Category C.

**Breast-feeding**
Sulfonamides are absorbed from the vaginal mucosa and are distributed into breast milk. Use is not recommended in nursing mothers since sulfonamides may cause hyperbilirubinemia in the infant. In addition, sulfonamides may cause hemolytic anemia in glucose-6-phosphate dehydrogenase (G6PD)–deficient neonates.

**Pediatrics**
*For all sulfonamides—*
    No information is available on the relationship of age to the effects of sulfonamides in pediatric patients.

## Geriatrics

No information is available on the relationship of age to the effects of sulfonamides in geriatric patients.

## Medical considerations/Contraindications

The medical considerations/contraindications included here have been selected on the basis of their potential clinical significance (reasons given in parentheses where appropriate)—not necessarily inclusive (» = major clinical significance).

*Risk-benefit should be considered when the following medical problems exist:*

Glucose-6-phosphate dehydrogenase (G6PD) deficiency
   (hemolytic anemia may occur in G6PD-deficient patients)
Hepatic function impairment
   (sulfonamides are metabolized in the liver; may cause hyperbilirubinemia in nursing infants)
Porphyria
   (sulfonamides may precipitate an acute attack of porphyria)
Renal function impairment
Sensitivity to sulfonamides, furosemide, thiazide diuretics, sulfonylureas, or carbonic anhydrase inhibitors

## Side/Adverse Effects

Note: Treatment should be discontinued if local or systemic toxicity or hypersensitivity occurs.

The following side/adverse effects have been selected on the basis of their potential clinical significance (possible signs and symptoms in parentheses where appropriate)—not necessarily inclusive:

**Those indicating need for medical attention**
Incidence less frequent
   *Hypersensitivity* (itching, burning, skin rash, redness, swelling, or other sign of irritation not present before therapy)

**Those indicating need for medical attention only if they continue or are bothersome**
Incidence less frequent or rare
   *Rash or irritation of penis of sexual partner*

## Patient Consultation

As an aid to patient consultation, refer to *Advice for the Patient, Sulfonamides (Vaginal).*

In providing consultation, consider emphasizing the following selected information (» = major clinical significance):

**Before using this medication**
» Conditions affecting use, especially:
   Sensitivity to sulfonamides, furosemide, thiazide diuretics, sulfonylureas, or carbonic anhydrase inhibitors
   Pregnancy—Sulfonamides are absorbed from vaginal mucosa and appear in fetal circulation
   Breast-feeding—Distributed into breast milk

**Proper use of this medication**
   Reading patient instructions before using
   Proper administration technique; checking with physician before using applicator if pregnant
» Compliance with full course of therapy, even if menstruation begins
» Proper dosing
   Missed dose: Inserting as soon as possible; not inserting if almost time for next dose
» Proper storage

**Precautions while using this medication**
   Checking with physician if no improvement within a few days
   Protecting clothing because of possible soiling with vaginal sulfonamides or staining with aminacrine-containing preparations; avoiding the use of tampons
*Using hygienic measures to cure infection and prevent reinfection*
» Wearing cotton panties instead of synthetic underclothes
» Wearing only freshly washed underclothes
» Use of condom by partner to prevent reinfection; possible need for concurrent treatment of male partner; continuing medication if intercourse occurs during treatment
» Use of douche for hygienic purposes prior to next dose; not overfilling vagina with douche solution; avoiding use of a douche during pregnancy

**Side/adverse effects**
   Sulfonamides may cause thyroid malignancy with long-term administration in rats; however, rats may be more susceptible to goitrogenic effects of sulfonamides
   Signs of potential side effects, especially hypersensitivity

## General Dosing Information

Treatment should be continued through one complete menstrual cycle, unless otherwise directed by physician.

---

### *SULFANILAMIDE*

## Vaginal Dosage Forms

### SULFANILAMIDE VAGINAL CREAM

**Usual adult and adolescent dose**
Intravaginal, 1 applicatorful (approximately 6 grams) one or two times a day on arising and/or at bedtime for thirty days.

**Usual pediatric dose**
Dosage has not been established.

**Strength(s) usually available**
U.S.—
   15% (Rx) [*AVC; Vagitrol;* GENERIC].

**Packaging and storage**
Store below 40 °C (104 °F), preferably between 15 and 30 °C (59 and 86 °F), in a well-closed container, unless otherwise specified by manufacturer. Protect from freezing.

**Stability**
Sulfanilamide vaginal cream darkens with age. However, this does not affect potency.

**Auxiliary labeling**
• For the vagina.
• Continue medicine for full time of treatment.

**Note**
When dispensing, include patient instructions and brochure.

### SULFANILAMIDE VAGINAL SUPPOSITORIES

**Usual adult and adolescent dose**
Intravaginal, 1 suppository one or two times a day on arising and/or at bedtime for thirty days.

**Usual pediatric dose**
Dosage has not been established.

**Strength(s) usually available**
U.S.—
   1.05 grams (Rx) [*AVC*].

**Packaging and storage**
Store below 30 °C (86 °F), in a well-closed container, unless otherwise specified by manufacturer. Protect from freezing.

**Auxiliary labeling**
• For the vagina.
• Continue medicine for full time of treatment.

**Note**
When dispensing, include patient instructions and brochure.

---

### *SULFANILAMIDE, AMINACRINE, AND ALLANTOIN*

## Vaginal Dosage Forms

### SULFANILAMIDE, AMINACRINE HYDROCHLORIDE, AND ALLANTOIN VAGINAL CREAM

**Usual adult and adolescent dose**
Intravaginal, 1 applicatorful (approximately 6 grams) one or two times a day on arising and/or at bedtime.

**Usual pediatric dose**
Dosage has not been established.

**Strength(s) usually available**
U.S.—
   Not commercially available.
Canada—
   15% of sulfanilamide, 0.2% of aminacrine hydrochloride, and 2% of allantoin (Rx) [*AVC*].

**Packaging and storage**
Store below 40 °C (104 °F), preferably between 15 and 30 °C (59 and 86 °F), in a well-closed container, unless otherwise specified by manufacturer. Protect from freezing.

**Auxiliary labeling**
• For the vagina.
• Continue medicine for full time of treatment.
• May stain clothing.

**Note**
When dispensing, include patient instructions.

## SULFANILAMIDE, AMINACRINE HYDROCHLORIDE, AND ALLANTOIN VAGINAL SUPPOSITORIES

**Usual adult and adolescent dose**
Intravaginal, 1 suppository one or two times a day on arising and/or at bedtime for thirty days.

**Usual pediatric dose**
Dosage has not been established.

**Strength(s) usually available**
U.S.—
Not commercially available.
Canada—
1.05 grams of sulfanilamide, 14 mg of aminacrine hydrochloride, and 140 mg of allantoin (Rx) [*AVC*].

**Packaging and storage**
Store below 30 °C (86 °F), in a well-closed container, unless otherwise specified by manufacturer. Protect from freezing.

**Auxiliary labeling**
• For the vagina.
• Continue medicine for full time of treatment.
• May stain clothing.

**Note**
When dispensing, include patient instructions.

---

### *TRIPLE SULFA*

## Vaginal Dosage Forms

### TRIPLE SULFA VAGINAL CREAM USP

**Usual adult and adolescent dose**
Intravaginal, 1 applicatorful (approximately 4 to 5 grams) two times a day on arising and at bedtime for four to six days. The dose may then be reduced to $^1/_2$ to $^1/_4$ applicatorful two times a day.

**Usual pediatric dose**
Dosage has not been established.

**Strength(s) usually available**
U.S.—
3.42% of sulfathiazole, 2.86% of sulfacetamide, and 3.7% of sulfabenzamide (Rx) [*Sulfa-Gyn; Sulnac; Sultrin; Trysul; V.V.S;* GENERIC].
Canada—
3.42% of sulfathiazole, 2.86% of sulfacetamide, and 3.7% of sulfabenzamide (Rx) [*Sultrin*].

**Packaging and storage**
Store below 40 °C (104 °F), preferably between 15 and 30 °C (59 and 86 °F), unless otherwise specified by manufacturer. Store in a well-closed, light-resistant container or in a collapsible tube. Protect from freezing.

**Auxiliary labeling**
• For the vagina.
• Continue medicine for full time of treatment.

**Note**
When dispensing, include patient instructions and brochure.

### TRIPLE SULFA VAGINAL TABLETS USP

**Usual adult and adolescent dose**
Intravaginal, 1 tablet two times a day on arising and at bedtime for ten days. May be repeated if necessary.

**Usual pediatric dose**
Dosage has not been established.

**Strength(s) usually available**
U.S.—
172.5 mg of sulfathiazole, 143.75 mg of sulfacetamide, and 184 mg of sulfabenzamide (Rx) [*Sultrin;* GENERIC].

**Packaging and storage**
Store below 40 °C (104 °F), preferably between 15 and 30 °C (59 and 86 °F), unless otherwise specified by manufacturer. Store in a well-closed, light-resistant container.

**Auxiliary labeling**
• For the vagina.
• Continue medicine for full time of treatment.

**Note**
When dispensing, include patient instructions and brochure.

---

Revised: 07/22/92
Interim revision: 06/15/94; 07/31/95

---

# SULFONAMIDES AND PHENAZOPYRIDINE   Systemic

This monograph includes information on the following: Sulfamethoxazole and Phenazopyridine; Sulfisoxazole and Phenazopyridine.

VA CLASSIFICATION (Primary): AM650

**NOTE:** The *Sulfonamides and Phenazopyridine (Systemic)* monograph is maintained on the USP DI electronic data base. For a printed copy of the most recent revision of the complete monograph, contact the USP Division of Information Development, 12601 Twinbrook Parkway, Rockville, MD 20852.

For information on the specific components of this combination, see the *USP DI* monographs for *Phenazopyridine (Systemic)* and *Sulfonamides (Systemic)*.

The information that follows is selectively abstracted from the complete monograph and is provided to facilitate drug use review and patient counseling.

Note: For a listing of dosage forms and brand names by country availability, see *Dosage Forms* section(s). For a listing of brand names for the articles in this monograph, refer to the General Index.

## Category

Antibacterial-analgesic (urinary tract).

## Indications

### Accepted

Urinary tract infections, bacterial (treatment)—Sulfonamide and phenazopyridine combinations are indicated in the treatment of the acute, painful phase of uncomplicated urinary tract infections caused by *Escherichia coli, Klebsiella* species, *Enterobacter* species, *Proteus mirabilis, P. vulgaris,* and *Staphylococcus aureus.* After relief of pain has been obtained, treatment should be continued with either sulfamethoxazole or sulfisoxazole alone.

Not all species or strains of a particular organism may be susceptible to a specific sulfonamide.

## Patient Consultation

As an aid to patient consultation, refer to *Advice for the Patient, Sulfonamides and Phenazopyridine (Systemic)*.

In providing consultation, consider emphasizing the following selected information (» = major clinical significance):

**Before using this medication**
» Conditions affecting use, especially:
  Allergies to sulfonamides, furosemide, thiazide diuretics, sulfonylureas, carbonic anhydrase inhibitors, or phenazopyridine
  Pregnancy—Sulfonamides cross the placenta; use is contraindicated at term since sulfonamides may cause kernicterus
  Breast-feeding—Sulfonamides are excreted in breast milk; may cause kernicterus in the nursing infant
  Use in children—Use is contraindicated in children up to 12 years of age
  Other medications, especially coumarin- or indandione-derivative anticoagulants, hydantoin anticonvulsants, oral antidiabetic agents, hemolytics, hepatotoxic medications, methenamine, and methotrexate
  Other medical problems, especially blood dyscrasias, G6PD deficiency, hepatic function impairment, hepatitis, megaloblastic

anemia due to folate deficiency, porphyria, and renal function impairment

**Proper use of this medication**

» Maintaining adequate fluid intake; taking with or following meals if gastrointestinal irritation occurs

» Compliance with full course of therapy

» Importance of not missing doses and taking at evenly spaced times

» Proper dosing; not giving to infants and children up to 12 years of age

Missed dose: Taking as soon as possible; not taking if almost time for next dose; not doubling doses

» Proper storage

**Precautions while using this medication**

Checking with physician if no improvement within a few days or if symptoms become worse

Using caution with regular toothbrushes, dental floss, and toothpicks; deferring dental work until blood counts have returned to normal; checking with physician or dentist concerning proper oral hygiene

» Possible photosensitivity reactions

» Caution if dizziness occurs

» Medication causes urine to turn reddish orange and may stain clothing

» Diabetics: May cause false urine sugar and urine ketone test results

**Side/adverse effects**

Reddish orange discoloration of urine may be alarming to patient although medically insignificant

Signs of potential side effects, especially blood dyscrasias, crystalluria, goiter, headache, hematuria, hemolytic anemia, hepatitis, hypersensitivity, interstitial nephritis, Lyell's syndrome, methemoglobinemia, photosensitivity, Stevens-Johnson syndrome, thyroid function disturbance, and tubular necrosis

---

### *SULFAMETHOXAZOLE AND PHENAZOPYRIDINE*

## Oral Dosage Forms

### SULFAMETHOXAZOLE AND PHENAZOPYRIDINE HYDROCHLORIDE TABLETS

**Usual adult and adolescent dose**

Urinary tract infections, bacterial—

Oral, 2 grams of sulfamethoxazole and 400 mg of phenazopyridine hydrochloride initially, then 1 gram of sulfamethoxazole and 200 mg of phenazopyridine hydrochloride every twelve hours for up to two days.

**Usual pediatric dose**

Urinary tract infections, bacterial—

Infants and children up to 12 years of age: Use is contraindicated.

Children 12 years of age and over: See *Usual adult and adolescent dose.*

**Strength(s) usually available**

U.S.—

500 mg of sulfamethoxazole and 100 mg of phenazopyridine hydrochloride (Rx) [*Azo Gantanol; Azo-Sulfamethoxazole;* GENERIC].

Canada—

Not commercially available.

**Auxiliary labeling**

· Take with a full glass of water.

· Avoid too much sun or use of sunlamp.

· May cause dizziness.

· Continue medicine for full time of treatment.

· May discolor urine.

---

### *SULFISOXAZOLE AND PHENAZOPYRIDINE*

## Oral Dosage Forms

### SULFISOXAZOLE AND PHENAZOPYRIDINE HYDROCHLORIDE TABLETS

**Usual adult and adolescent dose**

Urinary tract infections, bacterial—

Oral, 2 to 3 grams of sulfisoxazole and 200 to 300 mg of phenazopyridine hydrochloride initially, then 1 gram of sulfisoxazole and 100 mg of phenazopyridine hydrochloride every six hours for up to two days.

**Usual pediatric dose**

Urinary tract infections, bacterial—

Infants and children up to 12 years of age: Use is contraindicated.

Children 12 years of age and over: See *Usual adult and adolescent dose.*

**Strength(s) usually available**

U.S.—

500 mg of sulfisoxazole and 50 mg of phenazopyridine hydrochloride (Rx) [*Azo Gantrisin; Azo-Sulfisoxazole; Azo-Truxazole; Sul-Azo;* GENERIC].

Canada—

500 mg of sulfisoxazole and 50 mg of phenazopyridine hydrochloride (Rx) [*Azo Gantrisin*].

**Auxiliary labeling**

· Take with a full glass of water.

· Avoid too much sun or use of sunlamp.

· May cause dizziness.

· Continue medicine for full time of treatment.

· May discolor urine.

---

Revised: 02/01/93

---

# SULFONAMIDES AND TRIMETHOPRIM    Systemic

This monograph includes information on the following: Sulfadiazine and Trimethoprim*; Sulfamethoxazole and Trimethoprim.

BAN:

Sulfadiazine—Sulphadiazine

Sulfamethoxazole—Sulphamethoxazole

JAN:

Sulfamethoxazole—Acetylsulfamethoxazole

Sulfamethoxazole—Sulfamethoxazole sodium

VA CLASSIFICATION (Primary): AM650

NOTE: The *Sulfonamides and Trimethoprim (Systemic)* monograph is maintained on the USP DI electronic data base. For a printed copy of the most recent revision of the complete monograph, contact the USP Division of Information Development, 12601 Twinbrook Parkway, Rockville, MD 20852.

For information on the specific components of this combination, see the *USP DI* monographs for *Sulfonamides (Systemic)* and *Trimethoprim (Systemic).*

The information that follows is selectively abstracted from the complete monograph and is provided to facilitate drug use review and patient counseling.

Note: For a listing of dosage forms and brand names by country availability, see *Dosage Forms* section(s). For a listing of brand names for the articles in this monograph, refer to the General Index.

---

*Not commercially available in the U.S.

---

## Category

Antibacterial (systemic)—Sulfadiazine and Trimethoprim; Sulfamethoxazole and Trimethoprim.

Antiprotozoal—Sulfamethoxazole and Trimethoprim.

## Indications

Note: Bracketed information in the *Indications* section refers to uses that are not included in U.S. product labeling.

**General considerations**

Sulfonamides, such as sulfadiazine and sulfamethoxazole, used together with trimethoprim, produce synergistic antibacterial activity. Sulfadiazine and sulfamethoxazole have equal antibacterial properties, covering the same spectrum of activity. These sulfonamides, in combination with trimethoprim, are active *in vitro* against many gram-positive and gram-negative aerobic organisms. They have minimal activity against anaerobic bacteria. Susceptible gram-positive organisms include many *Staphylococcus aureus*, including some methicillin-resistant strains, *S. saprophyticus*, some group A beta-hemolytic streptococci, *Streptococcus agalactiae*, and most but not all strains of *S. pneumoniae*. Gram-negative organisms that are susceptible include *Escherichia coli*, many *Klebsiella* species, *Citrobacter diversus* and *C. fruendii*, *Enterobacter* species, *Salmonella* species, *Shigella* species, *Haemophilus influenzae*, including some ampicillin-resistant strains, *H. ducreyi*, *Morganella morganii*, *Proteus vulgaris* and *P. mirabilis*, and some *Serratia* species. Sulfonamide and trimethoprim combinations also have activity against *Acinetobacter* species, *Providencia rettgeri*, *P. stuarti*, *Aeromonas*, *Brucella*, and *Yersinia* species. They are also usually active against *Neisseria meningitidis*, *Branhamella (Moraxella) catarrhalis*, and some, but not all, *N. gonorrhoeae*. *Pseudomonas aeruginosa* is usually resistant, but *P. cepacia* and *P. maltophilia* may be sensitive.

The major difference between sulfadiazine and sulfamethoxazole exists in their respective pharmacokinetics. The primary distinction is that sulfadiazine is metabolized to a much lesser extent than is sulfamethoxazole. This allows for a higher urinary concentration of unchanged sulfadiazine, as well as an increased risk of crystalluria when it is administered in high doses; the antibacterial urinary concentration of sulfadiazine is maintained over a 24-hour interval, allowing for once-a-day dosing in adults. Also, sulfadiazine achieves higher concentrations in the bile and cerebrospinal fluid.

**Accepted**

Bronchitis (treatment)—Oral sulfamethoxazole and trimethoprim combination is indicated in adults in the treatment of acute exacerbations of chronic bronchitis caused by susceptible organisms.

Enterocolitis, *Shigella* species (treatment)—Oral and parenteral sulfamethoxazole and trimethoprim combinations are indicated in the treatment of enterocolitis caused by susceptible strains of *Shigella flexneri* and *S. sonnei*.

Otitis media, acute (treatment)—Oral sulfamethoxazole and trimethoprim combination is indicated in the treatment of acute otitis media caused by susceptible organisms in children.

Pneumonia, *Pneumocystis carinii* (prophylaxis)[1]—Oral sulfamethoxazole and trimethoprim combination is indicated in the prophylaxis of *Pneumocystis carinii* pneumonia (PCP) in patients who are immunocompromised and considered to be at increased risk of developing PCP, including patients with acquired immunodeficiency syndrome (AIDS). It is considered to be the treatment of choice for this indication. Sulfamethoxazole and trimethoprim combination is indicated in both secondary prophylaxis (patients who have already had at least one episode of PCP), and primary prophylaxis (HIV-infected adults with a CD4 lymphocyte count less than or equal to 200 cells per cubic millimeter and/or less than 20% of total lymphocytes; all children born to HIV-infected mothers, beginning at 4 to 6 weeks of age, and subsequent prophylaxis given as determined on the basis of age-specific CD4 lymphocyte count) of PCP.

Pneumonia, *Pneumocystis carinii* (treatment)—Oral and parenteral sulfamethoxazole and trimethoprim combinations are indicated as primary agents in the treatment of *Pneumocystis carinii* pneumonia (PCP) in immunocompromised patients, including patients with acquired immunodeficiency syndrome (AIDS). Pentamidine is considered an alternative agent for PCP.

Traveler's diarrhea (treatment)—Oral sulfamethoxazole and trimethoprim combination is indicated in the treatment of traveler's diarrhea caused by susceptible strains of enterotoxigenic *Escherichia coli* and *Shigella* species.

Urinary tract infections, bacterial (treatment)—Sulfadiazine and trimethoprim combination and oral and parenteral sulfamethoxazole and trimethoprim combinations are indicated in the treatment of urinary tract infections caused by susceptible organisms.

[Biliary tract infections (treatment)]—Sulfamethoxazole and trimethoprim combination is used in the treatment of biliary tract infections caused by susceptible organisms.

[Bone and joint infections (treatment)]—Sulfamethoxazole and trimethoprim combination is used in the treatment of bone and joint infections caused by susceptible organisms.

[Chancroid (treatment)][1]—Sulfamethoxazole and trimethoprim combination is used as an alternative agent in the treatment of chancroid.

[Chlamydial infections (treatment)][1]—Sulfamethoxazole and trimethoprim combination is used as an alternative agent in the treatment of chlamydial infections.

[Cyclospora infections (treatment)][1]—Sulfamethoxazole and trimethoprim combination is used in the treatment of diarrhea caused by *Cyclospora*

*cayetanensis*, but may not completely eradicate the organism.

[Endocarditis, bacterial (treatment)][1]—Sulfamethoxazole and trimethoprim combination is used as an alternative agent in the treatment of bacterial endocarditis caused by susceptible organisms.

[Gonorrhea, endocervical and urethral, uncomplicated (treatment)]—Sulfamethoxazole and trimethoprim combination is used as an alternative agent in the treatment of gonorrhea caused by susceptible organisms.

[Granuloma inguinale (treatment)][1]—Sulfamethoxazole and trimethoprim combination is used as an alternative agent in the treatment of granuloma inguinale.

[Isosporiasis (prophylaxis and treatment)][1]—Sulfamethoxazole and trimethoprim combination is used in the prophylaxis and treatment of isosporiasis caused by *Isospora belli*.

[Lymphogranuloma venereum (treatment)][1]—Sulfamethoxazole and trimethoprim combination is used in the treatment of lymphogranuloma venereum.

[Meningitis (treatment)]—Sulfamethoxazole and trimethoprim combination is used as an alternative agent in the treatment of meningitis caused by susceptible organisms.

[Nocardiosis (treatment)]—Sulfamethoxazole and trimethoprim combination is used in the treatment of nocardiosis.

[Paracoccidioidomycosis (treatment)][1]—Sulfamethoxazole and trimethoprim combination is used in the treatment of paracoccidioidomycosis.

[Paratyphoid fever (treatment)] or
[Typhoid fever (treatment)]—Sulfamethoxazole and trimethoprim combination is used as an alternative agent in the treatment of paratyphoid and typhoid fevers caused by susceptible strains.

[Septicemia, bacterial (treatment)]—Sulfamethoxazole and trimethoprim combination is used as an alternative agent in the treatment of bacterial septicemia caused by susceptible organisms.

[Sinusitis (treatment)][1]—Sulfamethoxazole and trimethoprim combination is used in the treatment of sinusitis caused by susceptible organisms.

[Skin and soft tissue infections (treatment)]—Sulfamethoxazole and trimethoprim combination is used in the treatment of skin and soft tissue infections, including burn wound infections caused by susceptible organisms.

[Toxoplasmosis (prophylaxis)][1]—Sulfamethoxazole and trimethoprim combination is used in the primary prophylaxis of toxoplasmosis in patients with AIDS.

[Urinary tract infections, bacterial (prophylaxis)][1]—Sulfamethoxazole and trimethoprim combination is used in the prophylaxis of bacterial urinary tract infections.

[Whipple's disease (treatment)][1]—Sulfamethoxazole and trimethoprim combination is used in the treatment of Whipple's disease.

Not all strains of a particular organism may be susceptible to sulfonamide and trimethoprim combinations.

**Unaccepted**

Sulfamethoxazole and trimethoprim combination is not indicated for prophylaxis or prolonged therapy in otitis media. Sulfamethoxazole and trimethoprim combination is not effective in the treatment of syphilis and *Ureaplasm urealyticum*.

Sulfamethoxazole and trimethoprim combination should not be used in the treatment of group A beta-hemolytic streptococcal tonsillopharyngitis since it may not eradicate streptococci and therefore may not prevent sequelae such as rheumatic fever.

---

[1]Not included in Canadian product labeling.

## Patient Consultation

As an aid to patient consultation, refer to *Advice for the Patient, Sulfonamides and Trimethoprim (Systemic)*.

In providing consultation, consider emphasizing the following selected information (» = major clinical significance):

**Before using this medication**

» Conditions affecting use, especially:
   Allergy to sulfonamides, furosemide, thiazide diuretics, sulfonylureas, carbonic anhydrase inhibitors, sulfites, or trimethoprim
   Pregnancy—Sulfonamides and trimethoprim cross the placenta; trimethoprim may interfere with folic acid metabolism; use is not recommended at term since sulfonamides may cause jaundice, hemolytic anemia, and kernicterus in neonates
   Breast-feeding—Sulfonamides and trimethoprim are distributed into breast milk; sulfonamides may cause kernicterus in nursing infants; trimethoprim may interfere with folic acid metabolism
   Use in children—Sulfadiazine and trimethoprim combination is contraindicated in infants up to 3 months of age and sulfa-

methoxazole and trimethoprim combination is contraindicated in infants up to 2 months of age for most indications since sulfonamides may cause kernicterus in neonates; however, sulfamethoxazole and trimethoprim combination is indicated in all infants born to human immunodeficiency virus (HIV)–infected mothers, starting at 4 to 6 weeks

Use in the elderly—Elderly patients, especially those also taking diuretics, may be at increased risk of severe side/adverse effects

Other medications, especially coumarin- or indandione-derivative anticoagulants, hydantoin anticonvulsants, oral antidiabetic agents, other hemolytics, other hepatotoxic medications, methenamine, or methotrexate

Other medical problems, especially blood dyscrasias, G6PD deficiency, hepatic function impairment, megaloblastic anemia due to folic acid deficiency, porphyria, and renal function impairment

## Proper use of this medication

» Not giving sulfadiazine and trimethoprim combination to infants under 3 months of age, or sulfamethoxazole and trimethoprim combination to infants under 2 months of age, except under special circumstances

» Maintaining adequate fluid intake
Proper administration technique for oral liquids

» Compliance with full course of therapy

» Importance of not missing doses and taking at evenly spaced times

» Proper dosing
Missed dose: Taking as soon as possible; not taking if almost time for next dose; not doubling doses

» Proper storage

## Precautions while using this medication

» Regular visits to physician to check blood counts
Checking with physician if no improvement within a few days
Caution in use of regular toothbrushes, dental floss, and toothpicks; deferring dental work until blood counts have returned to normal; checking with physician or dentist concerning proper oral hygiene

» Possible skin photosensitivity

» Caution if dizziness occurs

## Side/adverse effects

Severe skin problems and blood problems may be more likely to occur in elderly patients who are taking sulfamethoxazole and trimethoprim combination, especially if diuretics are being taken concurrently

Signs of potential side effects, especially hypersensitivity, photosensitivity, blood dyscrasias, cholestatic hepatitis, Stevens-Johnson syndrome, toxic epidermal necrolysis, aseptic meningitis, central nervous system toxicity, *Clostridium difficile* colitis, crystalluria, hematuria, goiter, thyroid function disturbance, interstitial nephritis, tubular necrosis, methemoglobinemia, and thrombophlebitis

---

### *SULFADIAZINE AND TRIMETHOPRIM*

# Oral Dosage Forms

## SULFADIAZINE AND TRIMETHOPRIM ORAL SUSPENSION

### Usual adult and adolescent dose
Antibacterial—
Oral, 820 mg of sulfadiazine and 180 mg of trimethoprim once a day.

### Usual pediatric dose
Antibacterial—
Infants up to 3 months of age: Use is not recommended.
Children 3 months to 12 years of age: Oral, 7 mg of sulfadiazine and 1.5 mg of trimethoprim per kg of body weight every twelve hours.
Children over 12 years of age: See *Usual adult and adolescent dose.*

### Strength(s) usually available
U.S.—
Not commercially available.
Canada—
205 mg of sulfadiazine and 45 mg of trimethoprim per 5 mL (Rx) [*Coptin*].

### Auxiliary labeling
• Shake well.
• Take with a full glass of water.
• May cause dizziness.
• Avoid too much sun or use of sunlamp.
• Continue medicine for full time of treatment.

Note: When dispensing, include a calibrated liquid-measuring device.

## SULFADIAZINE AND TRIMETHOPRIM TABLETS

### Usual adult and adolescent dose
See *Sulfadiazine and Trimethoprim Oral Suspension.*

### Usual pediatric dose
See *Sulfadiazine and Trimethoprim Oral Suspension.*

### Strength(s) usually available
U.S.—
Not commercially available.
Canada—
410 mg of sulfadiazine and 90 mg of trimethoprim (Rx) [*Coptin*].
820 mg of sulfadiazine and 180 mg of trimethoprim (Rx) [*Coptin 1*].

### Auxiliary labeling
• Take with a full glass of water.
• May cause dizziness.
• Avoid too much sun or use of sunlamp.
• Continue medicine for full time of treatment.

---

### *SULFAMETHOXAZOLE AND TRIMETHOPRIM*

# Oral Dosage Forms

Note: Bracketed uses in the *Dosage Forms* section refer to categories of use and/or indications that are not included in U.S. product labeling.

## SULFAMETHOXAZOLE AND TRIMETHOPRIM ORAL SUSPENSION USP

### Usual adult and adolescent dose
Antibacterial (systemic)—
Oral, 800 mg of sulfamethoxazole and 160 mg of trimethoprim every twelve hours.
Antiprotozoal—
*Pneumocystis carinii* pneumonia:
Treatment—
Oral, 18.75 to 25 mg of sulfamethoxazole and 3.75 to 5 mg of trimethoprim per kg of body weight every six hours for fourteen to twenty-one days.
Prophylaxis[1]—
Oral, 800 mg of sulfamethoxazole and 160 mg of trimethoprim once a day.
Acceptable alternative dosing schedules include:
Oral, 800 mg of sulfamethoxazole and 160 mg of trimethoprim three times a week (e.g., Monday, Wednesday, Friday).
Oral, 400 mg of sulfamethoxazole and 80 mg of trimethoprim once a day.
[Toxoplasmosis (prophylaxis)][1]:
Oral, 800 mg of sulfamethoxazole and 160 mg of trimethoprim once a day.
Acceptable alternative dosing schedules include—
Oral, 800 mg of sulfamethoxazole and 160 mg of trimethoprim three times a week (e.g., Monday, Wednesday, Friday).
Oral, 400 mg of sulfamethoxazole and 80 mg of trimethoprim once a day.

### Usual pediatric dose
Antibacterial (systemic)—
Infants up to 2 months of age:
Use is not recommended since sulfonamides may cause kernicterus in neonates.
Infants 2 months of age and over:
Infants and children up to 40 kg of body weight—Oral, 20 to 30 mg of sulfamethoxazole and 4 to 6 mg of trimethoprim per kg of body weight every twelve hours.
Children 40 kg of body weight and over—See *Usual adult and adolescent dose.*
Antiprotozoal—
*Pneumocystis carinii* pneumonia (PCP):
Treatment—
Oral, 18.75 to 25 mg of sulfamethoxazole and 3.75 to 5 mg of trimethoprim per kg of body weight every six hours for fourteen to twenty-one days.
Prophylaxis[1]—
Children 4 weeks of age and over:
Oral, 375 mg of sulfamethoxazole per square meter and 75 mg of trimethoprim per square meter of body surface two times a day, three times a week on consecutive days (e.g., Monday, Tuesday, Wednesday).

Acceptable alternative dosing schedules include:

Oral, 750 mg of sulfamethoxazole per square meter and 150 mg of trimethoprim per square meter of body surface as a single daily dose three times a week on consecutive days (e.g., Monday, Tuesday, Wednesday).

Oral, 375 mg of sulfamethoxazole per square meter and 75 mg of trimethoprim per square meter of body surface two times a day seven days a week.

Oral, 375 mg of sulfamethoxazole per square meter and 75 mg of trimethoprim per square meter of body surface two times a day, three times a week on alternate days (e.g., Monday, Wednesday, Friday).

Note: PCP prophylaxis is recommended for all infants born to HIV-infected mothers starting at 4 weeks of age, regardless of their CD4 lymphocyte counts. However, if the infant is receiving zidovudine during the first 6 weeks of life for the prevention of perinatal HIV transmission, sulfamethoxazole and trimethoprim combination prophylaxis should be delayed until zidovudine is discontinued at 6 weeks of age, to reduce the chance of anemia that may occur if these two medications are given concurrently.

[Toxoplasmosis (prophylaxis)][1]:

Oral, 375 mg of sulfamethoxazole per square meter and 75 mg of trimethoprim per square meter of body surface two times a day, three times a week on consecutive days (e.g., Monday, Tuesday, Wednesday).

Acceptable alternative dosing schedules include—

Oral, 750 mg of sulfamethoxazole per square meter and 150 mg of trimethoprim per square meter of body surface as a single daily dose three times a week on consecutive days (e.g., Monday, Tuesday, Wednesday).

Oral, 375 mg of sulfamethoxazole per square meter and 75 mg of trimethoprim per square meter of body surface two times a day seven days a week.

Oral, 375 mg of sulfamethoxazole per square meter and 75 mg of trimethoprim per square meter of body surface two times a day, three times a week on alternate days (e.g., Monday, Wednesday, Friday).

**Strength(s) usually available**

U.S.—

200 mg of sulfamethoxazole and 40 mg of trimethoprim per 5 mL (Rx) [*Bactrim Pediatric; Cotrim Pediatric; Septra Pediatric; Sulfatrim Pediatric; Sulfatrim Suspension;* GENERIC].

Canada—

200 mg of sulfamethoxazole and 40 mg of trimethoprim per 5 mL (Rx) [*Apo-Sulfatrim; Bactrim; Novo-Trimel; Nu-Cotrimox; Septra*].

**Auxiliary labeling**
- Shake well.
- Take with a full glass of water.
- May cause dizziness.
- Avoid too much sun or use of sunlamp.
- Continue medicine for full time of treatment.

Note: When dispensing, include a calibrated liquid-measuring device.

## SULFAMETHOXAZOLE AND TRIMETHOPRIM TABLETS USP

**Usual adult and adolescent dose**
See *Sulfamethoxazole and Trimethoprim Oral Suspension USP*.

**Usual adult prescribing limits**
See *Sulfamethoxazole and Trimethoprim Oral Suspension USP*.

**Usual pediatric dose**
See *Sulfamethoxazole and Trimethoprim Oral Suspension USP*.

**Strength(s) usually available**

U.S.—

400 mg of sulfamethoxazole and 80 mg of trimethoprim (Rx) [*Bactrim; Cotrim; Septra; Sulfatrim; Sulfatrim S/S;* GENERIC].

800 mg of sulfamethoxazole and 160 mg of trimethoprim (Rx) [*Bactrim DS; Cofatrim Forte; Cotrim DS; Septra DS; Sulfatrim-DS;* GENERIC].

Canada—

100 mg of sulfamethoxazole and 20 mg of trimethoprim (Rx) [*Apo-Sulfatrim*].

400 mg of sulfamethoxazole and 80 mg of trimethoprim (Rx) [*Apo-Sulfatrim* (scored); *Bactrim; Novo-Trimel* (scored); *Nu-Cotrimox; Septra*].

800 mg of sulfamethoxazole and 160 mg of trimethoprim (Rx) [*Apo-Sulfatrim DS; Bactrim DS* (scored); *Novo-Trimel D.S.* (scored); *Nu-Cotrimox DS; Roubac; Septra DS*].

**Auxiliary labeling**
- Take with a full glass of water.
- May cause dizziness.
- Avoid too much sun or use of sunlamp.
- Continue medicine for full time of treatment.

## Parenteral Dosage Forms

### SULFAMETHOXAZOLE AND TRIMETHOPRIM FOR INJECTION CONCENTRATE USP

**Usual adult and adolescent dose**

Antibacterial (systemic)—

Intravenous infusion, 10 to 12.5 mg of sulfamethoxazole and 2 to 2.5 mg of trimethoprim per kg of body weight every six hours; 13.3 to 16.7 mg of sulfamethoxazole and 2.7 to 3.3 mg of trimethoprim per kg of body weight every eight hours; or 20 to 25 mg of sulfamethoxazole and 4 to 5 mg of trimethoprim per kg of body weight every twelve hours.

Antiprotozoal—

*Pneumocystis carinii* pneumonia: Intravenous infusion, 18.75 to 25 mg of sulfamethoxazole and 3.75 to 5 mg of trimethoprim per kg of body weight every six hours; or 25 to 33.3 mg of sulfamethoxazole and 5.0 to 6.7 mg of trimethoprim per kg of body weight every eight hours for fourteen days.

**Usual pediatric dose**

Infants up to 2 months of age—Use is not recommended since sulfonamides may cause kernicterus in neonates.

Infants 2 months of age and over—See *Usual adult and adolescent dose*.

**Strength(s) usually available**

U.S.—

400 mg of sulfamethoxazole and 80 mg of trimethoprim per 5 mL (Rx) [*Bactrim I.V.; Septra I.V.;* GENERIC].

Canada—

400 mg of sulfamethoxazole and 80 mg of trimethoprim per 5 mL (Rx) [*Bactrim; Septra*].

**Preparation of dosage form**

The contents of each vial (5 mL) must be diluted to 75 to 125 mL of 5% dextrose injection prior to administration by intravenous infusion. The resulting solution should be administered by intravenous infusion over a 60- to 90-minute period.

Caution: Use of products containing benzyl alcohol is not recommended for use in neonates. A fatal toxic syndrome consisting of metabolic acidosis, CNS depression, respiratory problems, renal failure, hypotension, and possibly seizures and intracranial hemorrhages has been associated with this use.

---

[1]Not included in Canadian product labeling.

Revised: 03/01/96

---

# SULFUR   Topical

**VA CLASSIFICATION (Primary/Secondary):**
Sulfur Cream—DE500/DE752
Sulfur Lotion—DE500/DE752
Sulfur Ointment—DE500/DE752; DE900; AP900
Sulfur Bar Soap—DE500/DE752

Note: For a listing of dosage forms and brand names by country availability, see *Dosage Forms* section(s). For a listing of brand names for the articles in this monograph, refer to the General Index.

# Category

Keratolytic (topical)—Sulfur Cream; Sulfur Lotion; Sulfur Ointment USP; Sulfur Bar Soap.

Antiacne agent (topical)—Sulfur Cream; Sulfur Lotion; Sulfur Ointment USP; Sulfur Bar Soap.

Antiseborrheic—Sulfur Ointment USP.

Scabicide—Sulfur Ointment USP.

Antirosacea agent (topical)—Sulfur Cream; Sulfur Lotion; Sulfur Ointment USP; Sulfur Bar Soap.

# Indications

Note: Bracketed information in the *Indications* section refers to uses that are not included in U.S. product labeling.

**Accepted**

Acne vulgaris (treatment)—Sulfur (cream, lotion, ointment, and bar soap) is indicated as an aid in the treatment of acne vulgaris.

Dermatitis, seborrheic (treatment)—Sulfur ointment is indicated for the treatment of seborrheic dermatitis.

Scabies (treatment)—Sulfur ointment is indicated for the treatment of scabies, especially in infants under 2 months of age and in pregnant and nursing women.

[Rosacea (treatment)]—Sulfur (cream, lotion, ointment, and bar soap) is used in strengths of up to 15% to treat rosacea.

# Pharmacology/Pharmacokinetics

**Physicochemical characteristics**

Molecular weight—32.06.

Solubility—Sulfur, precipitated: Practically insoluble in water; very soluble in carbon disulfide; slightly soluble in olive oil; very slightly soluble in alcohol.

**Mechanism of action/Effect**

Sulfur has germicidal, fungicidal, parasiticidal, and keratolytic actions. Its germicidal activity may be the result of its conversion to pentathionic acid by epidermal cells or by certain microorganisms.

# Precautions to Consider

**Pregnancy/Reproduction**

Problems in humans have not been documented.

**Breast-feeding**

Problems in humans have not been documented.

**Pediatrics**

Appropriate studies on the relationship of age to the effects of sulfur have not been performed in the pediatric population. However, no pediatrics-specific problems have been documented to date.

**Geriatrics**

Appropriate studies on the relationship of age to the effects of sulfur have not been performed in the geriatric population. However, no geriatrics-specific problems have been documented to date.

**Drug interactions and/or related problems**

The following drug interactions and/or related problems have been selected on the basis of their potential clinical significance (possible mechanism in parentheses where appropriate)—not necessarily inclusive (» = major clinical significance):

Note: Combinations containing any of the following medications, depending on the amount present, may also interact with this medication.

Abrasive or medicated soaps or cleansers or
Acne preparations or preparations containing a peeling agent, such as
  Benzoyl peroxide
  Resorcinol
  Salicylic acid
  Tretinoin or
Acne preparations, topical, other or
Alcohol-containing preparations, topical, such as
  After-shave lotions
  Astringents
  Perfumed toiletries
  Shaving creams or lotions or
Cosmetics or soaps with a strong drying effect or
Isotretinoin or
Medicated cosmetics or ''cover-ups''
    (concurrent use with sulfur may cause a cumulative irritant or drying effect, especially with the application of peeling, desquamating, or abrasive agents, resulting in excessive irritation of the skin)

Mercury compounds, topical
    (concurrent use with sulfur may result in a chemical reaction releasing hydrogen sulfide, which has a foul odor, may be irritating, and may stain the skin black)

**Medical considerations/Contraindications**

The medical considerations/contraindications included here have been selected on the basis of their potential clinical significance (reasons given in parentheses where appropriate)—not necessarily inclusive (» = major clinical significance).

*Risk-benefit should be considered when the following medical problem exists:*

Sensitivity to sulfur

# Side/Adverse Effects

The following side/adverse effects have been selected on the basis of their potential clinical significance (possible signs and symptoms in parentheses where appropriate)—not necessarily inclusive:

**Those indicating need for medical attention**
  *Skin irritation not present before therapy*

**Those indicating need for medical attention only if they continue or are bothersome**
  *Redness and peeling of skin*—may occur after a few days

# Patient Consultation

As an aid to patient consultation, refer to *Advice for the Patient, Sulfur (Topical).*

In providing consultation, consider emphasizing the following selected information (» = major clinical significance):

**Before using this medication**
» Conditions affecting use, especially:
    Sensitivity to sulfur

**Proper use of this medication**
» Importance of not using more medication than the amount recommended
» Avoiding contact with the eyes
*Proper administration*
*For cream and lotion dosage forms*
    Before applying—Washing affected areas with soap and water; drying thoroughly
    Applying enough to cover affected areas; rubbing in gently
*For ointment dosage form used for seborrheic dermatitis*
    Before applying—Washing affected areas with soap and water; drying thoroughly
    Applying enough to cover affected areas; rubbing in gently
*For ointment dosage form used for scabies*
    Before applying—Washing entire body with soap and water; drying thoroughly.
    Applying enough at bedtime to cover entire body from neck down; rubbing in gently; leaving on body for 24 hours; washing entire body before applying again
    Importance of washing entire body thoroughly 24 hours after the last treatment

*For soap dosage form*
    Working up rich lather with soap, using warm water
    Washing affected areas and rinsing thoroughly
    Applying lather again; rubbing in gently for a few minutes
    Removing excess lather with a towel or tissue without rinsing

» Proper dosing
    Missed dose: Using as soon as possible; not using if almost time for next dose
» Proper storage

**Precautions while using this medication**
» Avoiding simultaneous use with other topical acne preparations or preparations containing peeling agents, alcohol-containing preparations, abrasive soaps or cleansers, cosmetics or soaps with drying effect, medicated cosmetics, or other topical skin medication, unless otherwise directed by physician
» Avoiding concurrent use with topical mercury-containing preparations

**Side/adverse effects**
    Signs of potential side effects, especially skin irritation not present before therapy

# General Dosing Information

Before the ointment is applied, the affected areas should be washed with soap and water and then dried thoroughly.

## Topical Dosage Forms

### SULFUR CREAM

**Usual adult and adolescent dose**
Antiacne agent (topical)—
   Topical, to the skin, as needed.

**Usual pediatric dose**
See *Usual adult and adolescent dose.*

**Strength(s) usually available**
U.S.—
   2% (OTC) [*Fostex Regular Strength Medicated Cover-Up*].
Canada—
   2% (OTC) [*Fostex CM; Fostril Cream*].

**Packaging and storage**
Store below 40 °C (104 °F), preferably between 15 and 30 °C (59 and 86 °F), unless otherwise specified by manufacturer.

**Auxiliary labeling**
• For external use only.

### SULFUR LOTION

**Usual adult and adolescent dose**
Antiacne agent (topical)—
   Topical, to the skin, two or three times a day.

**Usual pediatric dose**
See *Usual adult and adolescent dose.*

**Strength(s) usually available**
U.S.—
   2% (OTC) [*Finac* (alcohol 8%); *Fostril Lotion*].
   5% (OTC) [*Lotio Alsulfa*].
Canada—
   Not commercially available.

**Packaging and storage**
Store below 40 °C (104 °F), preferably between 15 and 30 °C (59 and 86 °F), unless otherwise specified by manufacturer.

**Auxiliary labeling**
• For external use only.
• Shake well.

### SULFUR OINTMENT USP

**Usual adult and adolescent dose**
Antiacne agent (topical)—
   Topical, to the skin, as a 0.5% ointment as needed.
Antiseborrheic or
Keratolytic (topical)—
   Topical, to the skin, as a 5 to 10% ointment one or two times a day.
Scabicide—
   Topical, to the entire body from the neck down, as 6% sulfur in petrolatum at bedtime for 3 nights; patients may bathe before each application and should bathe 24 hours following the last application.

Note: Treatment may be repeated after 1 week if there is no clinical improvement; additional weekly treatments should be administered only if there are live mites.

**Usual pediatric dose**
See *Usual adult and adolescent dose.*

**Strength(s) usually available**
U.S.—
   0.5% (OTC) [*Cuticura Ointment* (phenol 0.1%; oxyquinoline 0.05%)].
   10% (OTC) [GENERIC].
   Note: Other strengths are not commercially available; compounding required for prescriptions.
Canada—
   Not commercially available. Compounding required for prescriptions.

**Packaging and storage**
Store below 40 °C (104 °F), preferably between 15 and 30 °C (59 and 86 °F), in a well-closed container, unless otherwise specified by manufacturer. Protect from freezing.

**Auxiliary labeling**
• For external use only.

### SULFUR BAR SOAP

**Usual adult and adolescent dose**
Antiacne agent (topical) or
Keratolytic (topical)—
   Topical, to the skin, as needed.

**Usual pediatric dose**
See *Usual adult and adolescent dose.*

**Strength(s) usually available**
U.S.—
   5% (OTC) [*Sulpho-Lac*].
   10% (OTC) [GENERIC].
Canada—
   10% (OTC) [GENERIC].

**Packaging and storage**
Store below 40 °C (104 °F), preferably between 15 and 30 °C (59 and 86 °F), unless otherwise specified by manufacturer.

**Auxiliary labeling**
• For external use only.

Revised: 10/28/93

## SULFUR-CONTAINING COMBINATIONS—

Alcohol and Sulfur (Topical)
Resorcinol and Sulfur (Topical)
Salicylic Acid and Sulfur (Topical)
Salicylic Acid, Sulfur, and Coal Tar (Topical)

# SULFURATED LIME   Topical

VA CLASSIFICATION (Primary/Secondary):
   Mask—DE500/DE752
   Topical Solution—DE500/DE752; AP900
Another commonly used name is Vleminckx's solution.

Note: For a listing of dosage forms and brand names by country availability, see *Dosage Forms* section(s). For a listing of brand names for the articles in this monograph, refer to the General Index.

## Category

Antiacne agent (topical)—Sulfurated Lime Mask; Sulfurated Lime Topical Solution.
Keratolytic (topical)—Sulfurated Lime Mask; Sulfurated Lime Topical Solution.
Scabicide—Sulfurated Lime Topical Solution.

## Indications

**Accepted**
Acne vulgaris (treatment)—Sulfurated lime mask and solution are indicated for the treatment of cystic and papular types of acne vulgaris.

Dermatitis, seborrheic (treatment)[1] or
Pustular infections (treatment)[1]—Sulfurated lime solution is indicated for the treatment of seborrheic dermatitis, pustular infections, and other dermatoses.

Scabies (treatment)[1]—Sulfurated lime solution is indicated for the control and treatment of scabies.

[1]Not included in Canadian product labeling.

## Pharmacology/Pharmacokinetics

**Physicochemical characteristics**
Description—Sulfurated lime is a combination of calcium polysulfide and calcium thiosulfate

**Mechanism of action/Effect**
Sulfurated lime has a mild desquamative action.

## Precautions to Consider

**Pregnancy/Reproduction**
Problems in humans have not been documented.

**Breast-feeding**
Problems in humans have not been documented.

**Pediatrics**
Appropriate studies on the relationship of age to the effects of sulfurated lime have not been performed in the pediatric population. However, no pediatrics-specific problems have been documented to date.

**Geriatrics**
Appropriate studies on the relationship of age to the effects of sulfurated lime have not been performed in the geriatric population. However, no geriatrics-specific problems have been documented to date.

**Drug interactions and/or related problems**
The following drug interactions and/or related problems have been selected on the basis of their potential clinical significance (possible mechanism in parentheses where appropriate)—not necessarily inclusive (» = major clinical significance):

Note: Combinations containing any of the following medications, depending on the amount present, may also interact with this medication.

Abrasive or medicated soaps or cleansers or
Acne preparations or preparations containing a peeling agent, such as:

Benzoyl peroxide
Resorcinol
Salicylic acid
Sulfur
Tretinoin or
Acne preparations, topical, other or
Alcohol-containing preparations, topical, such as:
After-shave lotions
Astringents
Perfumed toiletries
Shaving creams or lotions or
Cosmetics or soaps with a strong drying effect or
Isotretinoin or
Medicated cosmetics or "cover-ups"
(concurrent use with sulfurated lime may cause a cumulative irritant or drying effect, especially with the application of peeling, desquamating, or abrasive agents, resulting in excessive irritation of the skin)
Mercury compounds, topical
(concurrent use with sulfurated lime may result in a chemical reaction releasing hydrogen sulfide, which has a foul odor, may be irritating, and may stain the skin black)

**Medical considerations/Contraindications**
The medical considerations/contraindications included here have been selected on the basis of their potential clinical significance (reasons given in parentheses where appropriate)—not necessarily inclusive (» = major clinical significance).

*Risk-benefit should be considered when the following medical problem exists:*
Sensitivity to sulfurated lime

## Side/Adverse Effects

The following side/adverse effects have been selected on the basis of their potential clinical significance (possible signs and symptoms in parentheses where appropriate)—not necessarily inclusive:

**Those indicating need for medical attention**
*Skin irritation not present before therapy*

**Those indicating need for medical attention only if they continue or are bothersome**
*Redness and peeling of skin*—may occur after a few days; *unusual dryness of skin*

## Patient Consultation

As an aid to patient consultation, refer to *Advice for the Patient, Sulfurated Lime (Topical)*.

In providing consultation, consider emphasizing the following selected information (» = major clinical significance):

**Before using this medication**
» Conditions affecting use, especially:
Sensitivity to sulfurated lime

**Proper use of this medication**
» Importance of not using more medication than the amount recommended
» Avoiding contact with the eyes

Proper administration
*For mask dosage form*
Applying generous amount over entire face and neck
Allowing to remain on affected areas for 20 to 25 minutes
Removing with lukewarm water, using gentle circular motion; patting skin dry
*For topical solution dosage form*
Diluting before using; knowing correct administration technique
Avoiding contact with jewelry and other metals

» Proper dosing
Missed dose: Applying as soon as possible; not applying if almost time for next dose
» Proper storage

**Precautions while using this medication**
» Avoiding simultaneous use with other topical acne preparations or preparations containing peeling agents, alcohol-containing preparations, abrasive soaps or cleansers, cosmetics or soaps with drying effect, medicated cosmetics, or other topical skin medication, unless otherwise directed by physician
» Avoiding concurrent use with topical mercury-containing preparations

**Side/adverse effects**
Signs of potential side effects, especially skin irritation not present before therapy

## General Dosing Information

**For mask dosage form**
Sulfurated lime solution 6% in a drying clay mask should be applied in a generous layer over the entire face and neck or other affected areas. It should be allowed to remain on the affected areas for 20 to 25 minutes and then removed with lukewarm water. Skin should be patted dry.

**For topical solution dosage form**
After dilution, the topical solution may be used for wet dressings, as a soak, or in a bath.

Solutions having a concentration of 1:10,000 are used initially, with the concentration being increased at frequent intervals up to a concentration of 1:10 as tolerated.

When Sulfurated Lime Topical Solution USP XXI is used, the solution should be diluted with at least 9 volumes of water before use.

For use as a wet dressing, compresses should be soaked in the hot solution and applied for 10 to 20 minutes.

## Topical Dosage Forms
### SULFURATED LIME MASK

**Usual adult and adolescent dose**
Antiacne agent (topical)—
Topical, to the skin, once a day.

**Usual pediatric dose**
See *Usual adult and adolescent dose*.

**Strength(s) usually available**
U.S.—
6% sulfurated lime solution in a drying clay mask (OTC) [*Vlemasque* (SD alcohol 7%)].
Canada—
6% sulfurated lime solution in a drying clay mask (OTC) [*Vlemasque* (alcohol 7%; butylparaben; methylparaben)].

**Packaging and storage**
Store below 40 °C (104 °F), preferably between 15 and 30 °C (59 and 86 °F), in a tight container, unless otherwise specified by manufacturer. Protect from freezing.

**Stability**
Mineral acids decompose sulfurated lime solution with the liberation of hydrogen sulfide and elemental sulfur.

**Auxiliary labeling**
• For external use only.

### SULFURATED LIME TOPICAL SOLUTION

**Usual adult and adolescent dose**
Antiacne agent (topical) or
Keratolytic (topical)—
Topical, to the skin, as a diluted solution (1:32 to 1:9) one or two times a day.
Scabicide—
Topical, to the skin, as a diluted solution (1:9) one or two times a day for three days or as directed.

**Usual pediatric dose**
See *Usual adult and adolescent dose.*

**Size(s) usually available**
U.S.—
  480 mL (Sulfurated Lime Topical Solution USP XXI) (OTC)
  [GENERIC].
Canada—
  Not commercially available.

**Packaging and storage**
Store below 40 °C (104 °F), preferably between 15 and 30 °C (59 and 86 °F), unless otherwise specified by manufacturer. Store in a completely filled, tight container. Protect from freezing.

**Preparation of dosage form**
Prepare Sulfurated Lime Topical Solution USP XXI as follows: 165 grams of Lime and 250 grams of Sublimed Sulfur in a sufficient quantity of water to make 1000 mL. Slake the Lime, mix it with the Sulfur, and add the mixture gradually to 1750 mL of boiling water. Boil this mixture, with frequent agitation, until it is reduced to 1000 mL, and maintain approximately this volume for 1 hour, while boiling, by the ad-dition of water from time to time. Cool, filter, and pass sufficient water through the filter to make the product measure 1000 mL.

**Stability**
Mineral acids decompose sulfurated lime topical solution with the liberation of hydrogen sulfide and elemental sulfur.

**Auxiliary labeling**
• For external use only.
• Must be diluted before using.

Revised: 09/28/93

---

**SULINDAC**—See *Anti-inflammatory Drugs, Nonsteroidal (Systemic)*

---

## SULISOBENZONE-CONTAINING COMBINATIONS—

Phenylbenzimidazole and Sulisobenzone (Topical)—See *Sunscreen Agents (Topical)*

---

# SUMATRIPTAN    Systemic

VA CLASSIFICATION (Primary): CN105
Note: For a listing of dosage forms and brand names by country availability, see *Dosage Forms* section(s). For a listing of brand names for the articles in this monograph, refer to the General Index.

## Category
Antimigraine agent.

## Indications

### General considerations
Sumatriptan should not be prescribed for a patient who has not previously been diagnosed as a migraineur, or administered to a migraineur with atypical symptoms, until it has been determined that the patient's headache is not occurring secondary to an evolving potentially serious neurological condition (e.g., cerebrovascular accident or subarachnoid hemorrhage).

### Accepted
Headache, migraine (treatment)—Sumatriptan is indicated to relieve (abort) acute migraine headaches (with or without aura) in patients who do not obtain sufficient relief with analgesics, such as acetaminophen, aspirin, or nonsteroidal anti-inflammatory drugs (NSAIDs). Sumatriptan also relieves the nausea, vomiting, photophobia, and phonophobia that frequently occur in association with migraine headaches.

When incapacitating migraines occur more frequently than twice a month, prophylactic treatment is recommended to reduce the severity and duration, as well as the number, of headaches. Sumatriptan is not used for this purpose. Beta-adrenergic blocking agents, calcium channel blocking agents, tricyclic antidepressants, monoamine oxidase inhibitors, methysergide, pizotyline (pizotifen [not commercially available in the U.S.]), and sometimes cyproheptadine (especially in children) are used for prophylaxis. Other measures that may reduce the need for medication in migraineurs include identification and avoidance of headache precipitants and relaxation and/or biofeedback techniques.

### Acceptance not established
There are *insufficient data* to show that sumatriptan is safe and effective for treating *cluster headaches.* Sumatriptan has been shown to be effective in aborting a single headache in patients with cluster headaches. However, cluster headaches may occur daily, often more than once a day, for several months (a cluster period), followed by a headache-free interval. The safety and efficacy of repeated use of sumatriptan during a cluster period have not been established.

### Unaccepted
Sumatriptan is not recommended for long-term migraine prophylaxis.

Sumatriptan is not recommended for treatment of basilar artery migraine or hemiplegic migraine. Efficacy and safety in these conditions have not been established.

## Pharmacology/Pharmacokinetics

### Physicochemical characteristics
Source—Synthetic. Sumatriptan is structurally related to serotonin (5-hydroxytryptamine, 5-HT)
Molecular weight—Sumatriptan succinate: 413.49.
pKa—Sumatriptan succinate—
  $pKa_1$ (succinic acid)—4.21 and 5.67
  $pKa_2$ (tertiary amine group)—9.63
  $pKa_3$ (sulfonamide group)—> 12
Solubility—Sumatriptan succinate: Readily soluble in water and in 0.9% sodium chloride solution.

### Mechanism of action/Effect
Although sumatriptan's mechanism of action has not been established, suppression of migraine headaches may result from sumatriptan-induced decreases in the firing of serotonergic (5-hydroxytryptaminergic, 5-HT) neurons. Specifically, it is thought that agonist activity at the $5\text{-HT}_{1D}$ receptor subtype provides relief of acute headache. Sumatriptan is a highly selective agonist at this receptor subtype; it has no significant activity at other 5-HT receptor subtypes or at ad-renergic, dopaminergic, muscarinic, or benzodiazepine receptors.
It has been proposed that constriction of cerebral blood vessels resulting from $5\text{-HT}_{1D}$ receptor stimulation reduces the pulsation that may be responsible for the pain of vascular headaches. Studies in humans have shown that blood flow velocity in the middle cerebral arteries is significantly reduced during a migraine on the side of the headache, that relief of the headache by sumatriptan is accompanied by return of the blood flow velocity in these vessels to normal, and that sumatriptan treatment does not induce other changes in cerebral hemispheric blood flow. However, other studies have not consistently shown a significant correlation between dilatation of cerebral blood vessels and pain or other symptoms of migraine headaches, or between medication-induced vasoconstriction and relief of these headaches.
It has also been proposed that neurogenic inflammation in areas innervated by the trigeminal nerve may contribute to the development of migraine headaches. Although the cause of the inflammation has not been established, there is some evidence that serotonergic mechanisms may be involved. Sumatriptan may also relieve migraines by decreasing release of neuropeptides and other mediators of inflammation and by reducing extravasation of plasma proteins. A study in humans has demonstrated that concentrations of calcitonin gene-related peptide, a substance that increases vascular permeability and promotes plasma protein extravasation, are elevated during a migraine and return to normal as the headache is relieved by sumatriptan.

### Absorption
Oral—Rapid. However, bioavailability is low (approximately 14% of a dose), primarily because of presystemic hepatic metabolism and, to a lesser extent, because of incomplete absorption. The rate and extent of absorption are not affected to a clinically significant extent by administration with food or by the gastric stasis that may accompany migraine headaches.
Subcutaneous—Rapid; bioavailability is approximately 97% of that achieved with an intravenous injection.

**Distribution**
Sumatriptan is rapidly and extensively distributed to tissues but passage
across the blood-brain barrier is limited.

**Protein binding**
In plasma—Low (14 to 21%).

**Biotransformation**
Hepatic and extensive; approximately 80% of a dose is metabolized. The
major metabolite is an inactive indole acetic acid derivative.

*In vitro* studies with human hepatic microsomes indicate that sumatriptan
is metabolized by monoamine oxidase (MAO), primarily the A isoenzyme (MAO-A).

**Half-life**
Distribution—Subcutaneous administration: Approximately 15 minutes.

Elimination—Subcutaneous or oral administration: Approximately 2
hours. One study reported a terminal half-life of approximately 7 hours
that became apparent about 12 hours after administration of multiple
oral doses, but did not contribute substantially to the overall disposition of the medication.

**Onset of action**
Oral—
Within 30 minutes.
Subcutaneous—
Relief of headache pain: Within 10 minutes.
Relief of migraine-associated nausea, vomiting, photophobia, phono-
phobia: Within 20 minutes.

**Time to peak concentration**
In serum—
Oral (single 100-mg dose): Approximately 1.5 hours (range, 0.5 to 5
hours). The wide interindividual variability found in pharmacokinetic studies may be related to the appearance of multiple peaks
in the concentration over time. Approximately 80% of the maximum value is achieved within 45 minutes.
Subcutaneous (single 6-mg dose): Approximately 12 minutes (range,
5 to 20 minutes).

**Peak serum concentration**
In serum—
Oral (single 100-mg dose): Approximately 54 nanograms per mL (0.13
micromoles/L) (range, 26.7 to 137 nanograms per mL [0.06 to 0.33
micromoles/L]).
Subcutaneous (single 6-mg dose): Approximately 72 to 74 nanograms
per mL; (0.17 to 0.18 micromoles/L) (range, 54.9 to 108.4 nanograms per mL [0.13 to 0.26 micromoles/L]).

**Time to peak effect**
Relief of headache (i.e., moderate or severe pain being reduced to mild
or no pain)—
Oral (single 100-mg dose): Within 2 hours in 50 to 75%, and within
4 hours in an additional 15 to 25%, of patients.
Subcutaneous (single 6-mg dose): Within 1 hour in 70%, and within
2 hours in an additional 12%, of patients.
Relief of associated symptoms (nausea, vomiting, photophobia, phono-
phobia)—
Oral (single 100-mg dose): Within 2 hours.
Subcutaneous (single 6-mg dose): Within 1 hour in 68%, and within
2 hours in an additional 13%, of patients.

**Duration of action**
Return of migraine headache occurs within 24 to 48 hours in approximately 40% of patients who initially obtain a beneficial response to
sumatriptan, i.e., after moderate or severe headache pain has been reduced to mild or no pain. Whether this represents development of a
new migraine or breakthrough of a prolonged migraine after the effects
of sumatriptan have worn off has not been established.

**Elimination**
Renal, via active renal tubular secretion, following hepatic metabolism.
Approximately 80% of a dose is eliminated as metabolites. After oral
administration, approximately 57% of a dose is eliminated in the urine
(3% of the dose as unchanged sumatriptan, 35% as the indole acetic
acid metabolite, and 8% as the glucuronide conjugate of the indole
acetic acid metabolite) and another 38% of the dose is eliminated in
the feces (9% as unchanged sumatriptan and 11% as the indole acetic
acid metabolite). After subcutaneous administration, approximately
22% of a dose is eliminated in the urine as unchanged sumatriptan
and another 38% as the indole acetic acid metabolite. Only 0.6% and
3.3% of a dose are eliminated in the feces as unchanged sumatriptan
and the indole acetic acid metabolite, respectively.

The effects of hepatic or renal function impairment on clearance of sumatriptan have not been studied. Because approximately 80% of the
total clearance is via hepatic biotransformation, hepatic function im-

pairment would be more likely than renal function impairment to produce clinically significant alterations in sumatriptan clearance.

## Precautions to Consider

**Tumorigenicity**
No evidence of tumorigenicity was found in a 104-week study in rats
given sumatriptan by oral gavage in quantities sufficient to achieve
peak concentrations up to > 100 times higher than are achieved in
humans with a 6-mg subcutaneous dose. Also, although no evidence
of tumorigenicity was found in a 78-week study in mice given sumatriptan continuously in drinking water, this study did not use the
maximum tolerated dose and is therefore considered inadequate for
evaluating potential tumorigenicity in the mouse.

**Mutagenicity**
No evidence of mutagenicity was found in a variety of *in vitro* and *in
vivo* studies.

**Pregnancy/Reproduction**
Fertility—No adverse effects on fertility were found in reproduction studies in rats given up to 60 mg per kg of body weight (mg/kg) per day
subcutaneously or up to 500 mg/kg per day orally.

Pregnancy—Adequate and well-controlled studies have not been done in
pregnant women.
Studies in rats receiving daily subcutaneous injections of sumatriptan prior
to and during pregnancy showed no evidence of teratogenicity or embryolethality. Also, embryolethality did not occur in studies in rats
receiving sumatriptan intravenously throughout organogenesis in doses
producing plasma concentrations > 50 times higher than those produced by the recommended human subcutaneous dose. However, maternal toxicity and embryotoxicity occurred in rats given oral doses of
1000 mg/kg per day, but not those given 500 mg/kg per day, during
organogenesis. Also, term fetuses from Dutch Stride rabbits treated
during organogenesis with oral sumatriptan exhibited an increased incidence of cervicothoracic vascular defects and minor skeletal abnormalities. The functional significance of these abnormalities is not
known. In other studies, daily administration of sumatriptan to pregnant rabbits throughout the period of organogenesis using oral doses
of 100 mg/kg per day or intravenous doses sufficient to produce peak
concentrations > 3 times those produced in humans after a 6-mg subcutaneous dose resulted in maternal toxicity and/or embryolethality.

FDA Pregnancy Category C.

**Breast-feeding**
It is not known whether sumatriptan is distributed into human breast milk.
However, it is distributed into the milk of lactating animals.

**Pediatrics**
Appropriate studies on the relationship of age to the effects of sumatriptan
have not been done in pediatric patients. Safety and efficacy have not
been established.

**Adolescents**
Appropriate studies on the relationship of age to the effects of sumatriptan
have not been done in patients up to 18 years of age. Safety and
efficacy have not been established.

**Geriatrics**
Information on the relationship of age to the effects of sumatriptan in
geriatric patients is extremely limited. No unusual adverse, age-related
phenomena occurred in patients older than 60 years of age who participated in clinical trials. However, most published studies report excluding patients older than 65 years of age. Studies in a limited number
of healthy subjects 65 to 86 years of age found no differences in
pharmacokinetic parameters between these older individuals and
younger subjects.

**Drug interactions and/or related problems**
The following drug interactions and/or related problems have been selected on the basis of their potential clinical significance (possible
mechanism in parentheses where appropriate)—not necessarily inclusive (» = major clinical significance):

Note: Combinations containing any of the following medications, depending on the amount present, may also interact with this
medication.

Antidepressants, selective 5-hydroxytryptamine uptake inhibitor or
Lithium or
Monoamine oxidase (MAO) inhibitors, including furazolidone, procarbazine, and selegiline
(the possibility that concurrent use of any of these agents with
sumatriptan may lead to a potentially dangerous hyperserotonergic
state or other adverse effects has not been evaluated; it has been
recommended that, until further information is available, sumatriptan should not be used by patients receiving these medications)

(sumatriptan is metabolized by the MAO-A isoenzyme; pretreatment of human subjects with an MAO-A inhibitor has been shown to decrease sumatriptan clearance, resulting in substantial increases in the area under the sumatriptan concentration-time curve and the sumatriptan half-life. MAOIs that inhibit the MAO-A isoenzyme include furazolidone, isocarboxazid, moclobemide, phenelzine, toloxatone, and tranylcypromine. MAOIs that inhibit only the MAO-B isoenzyme, such as pargyline and selegiline, did not produce these effects)

Dihydroergotamine or
Ergotamine
(a delay of 24 hours between administration of dihydroergotamine or ergotamine and sumatriptan is recommended because of the possibility of additive and/or prolonged vasoconstriction)

**Laboratory value alterations**
The following have been selected on the basis of their potential clinical significance (possible effect in parentheses where appropriate)—not necessarily inclusive (» = major clinical significance):

With physiology/laboratory test values
Blood pressure and
Peripheral vascular resistance
(may be increased, although increases are generally mild and transient; in clinical studies, clinically significant blood pressure elevations [increase in systolic pressure by 20 mm Hg or to 180 mm Hg; increase in diastolic pressure by 15 mm Hg or to 105 mm Hg] occurred in fewer than 1% of the patients; blood pressure changes after oral administration are smaller and occur more slowly than after subcutaneous administration)

**Medical considerations/Contraindications**
The medical considerations/contraindications included here have been selected on the basis of their potential clinical significance (reasons given in parentheses where appropriate)—not necessarily inclusive (» = major clinical significance).

***Except under special circumstances, this medication should not be used when the following medical problems exist:***

» Coronary artery disease, especially:
Angina pectoris
Myocardial infarction, history of
Myocardial ischemia, silent documented
Prinzmetal's angina or
» Other conditions in which coronary vasoconstriction would be detrimental
(although sumatriptan has only a slight vasoconstrictive effect on coronary arteries, sumatriptan-induced myocardial ischemia has been documented in a few patients, primarily patients with a history of coronary artery disease or susceptibility to coronary artery vasospasm)
» Hypertension, uncontrolled
(may be exacerbated)

***Risk-benefit should be considered when the following medical problems exist:***

Cardiac arrhythmias, especially:
» Tachycardia or
» Cerebrovascular accident, history of
(sumatriptan has not been evaluated in patients with these conditions; the possibility of adverse effects resulting from sumatriptan's vascular effects must be considered)
» Coronary artery disease, predisposition to
(sumatriptan has rarely caused serious coronary adverse effects; patients in whom coronary artery disease is a possibility on the basis of age or the presence of other risk factors, such as diabetes, hypercholesterolemia, obesity, a strong family history of coronary artery disease, or tobacco smoking should be evaluated for the presence of cardiovascular disease before sumatriptan is prescribed; even after a satisfactory evaluation, the advisability of administering the patient's first dose under medical supervision should be considered)
Hepatic function impairment or
Renal function impairment
(caution is recommended because clearance of sumatriptan may be impaired; because about 80% of the total clearance is via hepatic biotransformation, hepatic function impairment should be more likely than renal function impairment to produce clinically significant increases in sumatriptan concentration)
Hypertension, controlled
(elevations of systolic and diastolic blood pressure may occur, especially after subcutaneous administration, although these effects are generally mild and transient in hypertensive patients whose

blood pressure is adequately controlled by medication; in clinical studies, patients with controlled hypertension experienced mean peak increases of 6 mm Hg, which usually started within 30 minutes after subcutaneous administration and persisted for less than an hour)

» Sensitivity to sumatriptan

## Side/Adverse Effects

Note:  Most of the adverse effects reported with sumatriptan are mild and transient (lasting less than 1 hour after subcutaneous injection and 2 hours or less after oral administration) and resolve without treatment. Although several deaths have been reported after administration of sumatriptan, a direct causal relationship could not be established in most cases. Most of the fatalities occurred 3 hours or more after administration and probably were spontaneous events or were caused by underlying disease. Some of the deaths were attributed to strokes, cerebral hemorrhages, or other cerebrovascular events. However, migraineurs are known to be at increased risk of cerebrovascular accidents or transient ischemic attacks; in many of these cases a cerebrovascular event, rather than a migraine, may have been causing the symptoms that led to sumatriptan administration.

Some of the adverse events reported after administration of sumatriptan (e.g., nausea, vomiting, malaise, fatigue, dizziness, vertigo, weakness, drowsiness, sedation) often occur during and/or following a migraine headache; whether sumatriptan contributes to their occurrence has not been established.

Although a causal relationship to sumatriptan has not been established, the following adverse events have also been reported in open, uncontrolled studies (incidences < 1%) and/or postmarketing: cardiac arrhythmias (atrial fibrillation, ventricular fibrillation, ventricular tachycardia, sinus arrhythmia), other transient changes in the electrocardiogram (ST segment elevations, other ST or T-wave changes, prolongation of PR or QTc intervals, nonsustained ventricular premature beats, isolated junctional ectopic beats, atrial ectopic beats, delayed activation of the right ventricle), hypotension, bradycardia, syncope, Prinzmetal's angina, vasodilatation, Raynaud's disease, acute renal failure, seizures, cerebrovascular accident, dysphagia, subarachnoid hemorrhage, polydipsia, dehydration, gastrointestinal reflux, dyspnea, erythema, pruritus, skin rashes, peptic ulceration, gallstones, swelling of extremities, transient hemiplegia, hysteria, globus hystericus, intoxication, mental depression, myoclonia, monoplegia or diplegia, dystonia, dysuria, urinary frequency, renal calculus, photosensitivity, and exacerbation of sunburn.

The following side/adverse effects have been selected on the basis of their potential clinical significance (possible signs and symptoms in parentheses where appropriate)—not necessarily inclusive:

**Those indicating need for medical attention**
Incidence less frequent (1 to 3%) with subcutaneous administration; less frequent or rare (< 1%) with oral administration
*Chest pain, severe; difficulty in swallowing; heaviness, tightness, or pressure in chest and/or neck*

Note:  Although *chest pain* and *heaviness, tightness, or pressure in the chest and neck* are suggestive of angina pectoris, monitoring of the electrocardiogram (ECG) during such symptoms in clinical studies failed to detect evidence of myocardial ischemia. Conversely, ECG monitoring detected new T-wave abnormalities in a small number of patients, most of whom had abnormal pretreatment ECGs, who were not experiencing relevant symptoms. However, sumatriptan-induced coronary artery vasospasm resulting in symptomatic myocardial ischemia and myocardial infarction have been documented in a few patients, primarily patients with a history of coronary artery disease or susceptibility to coronary artery vasospasm. Several fatalities associated with such complications have been reported following administration of sumatriptan, but in most cases a causal relationship has not been established.

Incidence rare
*Anaphylactic or anaphylactoid reaction* (changes in facial skin color; skin rash, hives, and/or itching; fast or irregular breathing; puffiness or swelling of the eyelids or around the eyes, face, or lips; shortness

of breath, troubled breathing, tightness in chest, and/or wheezing); *dermatitis, allergic* (skin rash, hives, and/or itching)

**Those indicating need for medical attention only if they continue or are bothersome**

Incidence more frequent

    *Injection site reaction* (burning, pain, or redness); *nausea or vomiting*

    Note: *Nausea* and *vomiting* often occur in conjunction with migraine headaches; they are not necessarily caused by (and may actually be relieved by) sumatriptan. However, these effects occurred more frequently after oral than after subcutaneous administration of sumatriptan in clinical trials, possibly because of the unpleasant taste of the dispersible tablet used in the studies. The product commercially available in Canada is a film-coated tablet that is less likely to produce such symptoms.

Incidence up to 13.5% with subcutaneous administration; less frequent (1 to 3%) or rare (< 1%) with oral administration

    *Atypical sensations* (sensation of burning, warmth, heat, numbness, tightness, or tingling; feeling cold; "strange" feeling); *discomfort in jaw, mouth, tongue, throat, nasal cavity, or sinuses; dizziness; drowsiness; flushing; lightheadedness; muscle aches, cramps, or stiffness; weakness*

    Note: *Flushing* and sensations of *burning, warmth,* or *heat* generally disappear within 10 to 30 minutes after administration of a subcutaneous dose.

Incidence less frequent (1 to 3%) with subcutaneous administration; less frequent or rare (< 1%) with oral administration

    *Anxiety; general feeling of illness or tiredness; vision changes*

## Overdose

For specific information on the agents used in the management of sumatriptan overdose, see:
- *Nitroglycerin* in *Nitrates (Systemic)*.

For more information on the management of overdose or unintentional ingestion **contact a Poison Control Center** (see *Poison Control Center Listing* ).

**Clinical effects of overdose**

Overdose has not been reported in humans. Signs and symptoms that might be anticipated, based on animal studies, include convulsions, tremor, inactivity, erythema of extremities, reduced respiratory rate, cyanosis, ataxia, mydriasis, injection site reactions (desquamation, hair loss, scab formation), and paralysis.

**Treatment of overdose**

Although there is no experience with overdose of sumatriptan, treatment may involve:

Decrease absorption—Emptying the stomach by induction of emesis or performing gastric lavage (if ingested orally).

Monitoring—

For continuing chest pain or other symptoms consistent with angina pectoris—Monitoring the electrocardiogram for evidence of ischemia and administering appropriate treatment (e.g., nitroglycerin or other coronary artery vasodilators) as needed. Some patients may require further evaluation to determine whether previously undiagnosed coronary artery disease is present. See the package insert or *Nitroglycerin* in *Nitrates (Systemic)* for specific dosing guidelines for use of this product.

Supportive care—Monitoring the patient and instituting supportive treatment as needed. Patients in whom intentional overdose is known or suspected should be referred for psychiatric consultation.

## Patient Consultation

As an aid to patient consultation, refer to *Advice for the Patient, Sumatriptan (Systemic)*.

In providing consultation, consider emphasizing the following selected information (» = major clinical significance):

**Before using this medication**

» Conditions affecting use, especially:
    Sensitivity to sumatriptan
    Other medical problems, especially cerebrovascular accident (history of); coronary artery disease, predisposition to coronary artery disease, or other conditions that may be adversely affected by coronary artery constriction; hypertension (uncontrolled); and tachycardia

**Proper use of this medication**

» Not administering if atypical headache symptoms are present; checking with physician instead
    Administering after onset of headache pain

Additional benefit may be obtained if the patient lies down in a quiet, dark room after administering medication

» Not using additional doses if a first dose does not provide substantial relief; additional sumatriptan is not likely to be effective in these circumstances; taking alternate medication as previously advised by physician, then checking with physician as soon as possible

» Taking additional doses, if needed, for return of migraine after initial relief was obtained, provided that prescribed limits (quantity used and frequency of administration) are not exceeded

» Compliance with prophylactic therapy, if prescribed

» Proper administration of
    Tablets—Swallowing whole; not breaking, crushing or chewing before taking
    Injection—
    Reading patient instructions provided with medication
    Proper injection technique
    Discarding used cartridge as directed in patient instructions, using container provided; not discarding autoinjector unit because refill cartridges are available

» Proper dosing

» Proper storage

**Precautions while using this medication**

Checking with physician if usual dose fails to relieve 3 consecutive headaches, or frequency and/or severity of headaches increases

Avoiding alcohol, which aggravates headache

» Caution if drowsiness or dizziness occurs

**Side/adverse effects**

Contacting physician immediately if severe chest pain or signs and symptoms of anaphylactoid reaction occur

Contacting physician at once if mild pain or tightness in chest or throat occurs and persists for more than 1 hour; even if symptoms are of shorter duration, not using medication again without first consulting physician

Signs and symptoms of other potential side effects, including dysphagia, palpitation, and skin rash or eruptions

## General Dosing Information

Clinical studies have not shown a correlation between the duration of a migraine prior to administration of sumatriptan and its ability to abort an acute attack. Because a recent study has shown that administration of sumatriptan during a preheadache aura may neither prevent nor significantly delay the onset of the headache, it is recommended that sumatriptan not be administered prior to the appearance of headache pain.

Lying down and relaxing in a quiet, darkened room after administering a dose of antimigraine medication may contribute to relief of migraines.

Additional doses of sumatriptan should not be administered to patients who do not obtain substantial relief (reduction of initially moderate or severe headache pain to mild or no pain) within 1 or 2 hours after the initial dose. Several clinical trials have failed to demonstrate that a second dose benefits these patients. It is recommended that an analgesic be used as "rescue" medication in the event of an unsatisfactory response to sumatriptan; use of dihydroergotamine or ergotamine is not recommended because of the possibility of additive or prolonged vasoconstriction. Also, the prescriber should be contacted as soon as possible if sumatriptan is ineffective because of the possibility that the patient's symptoms are being caused by a cerebrovascular event. However, patients who do not respond to sumatriptan during one migraine attack may obtain a satisfactory response during subsequent attacks.

Return of migraine headache occurs within 24 to 48 hours in about 40% of patients who initially obtain a beneficial response to sumatriptan. Whether this represents development of a new migraine or breakthrough of a prolonged migraine after the effects of sumatriptan have worn off has not been established. Recurrences following an initial beneficial response may be treated with additional sumatriptan.

In one study, tolerance to the effects of sumatriptan did not occur when the medication was used intermittently to relieve acute migraines for up to 6 months.

The possibility that overuse of sumatriptan by migraineurs may lead to dependence on the medication and to the development of withdrawal (rebound) or chronic, intractable headaches (as has been documented with too-frequent use of ergotamine and/or analgesics by these patients) has not been evaluated. Some headache specialists recommend that, until more definitive information about the risk of cumulative toxicity and/or dependence is available, courses of sumatriptan treatment should not be administered more often than every five to seven days.

**For oral dosage form only**

Sumatriptan tablets are to be swallowed whole (i.e., with the film coating intact) because the unpleasant taste of the contents may cause taste disturbances and/or an increased risk of nausea and vomiting.

**For parenteral dosage form only**

Sumatriptan is not to be given intravenously. Clinical trials have shown that intravenous administration is associated with a higher incidence of adverse effects than subcutaneous administration. Specifically, the risk of coronary artery vasospasm and angina may be increased.

## Oral Dosage Forms

Note: Sumatriptan tablets contain sumatriptan succinate. However, dosage and strength are expressed in terms of sumatriptan base.

### SUMATRIPTAN TABLETS

**Usual adult dose**

Antimigraine agent—
Oral, 100 mg (base). If a beneficial response to this dose is obtained within four hours, an additional 100-mg dose may be administered if headache pain returns or increases in severity.

Note: A dose-ranging study, which evaluated single doses of 100 mg, 200 mg, or 300 mg of sumatriptan (base) in migraineurs, identified 100 mg as the optimal oral dose. In this study, the higher doses increased the occurrence of adverse effects without providing a statistically significant increase in efficacy.

**Usual adult prescribing limits**

Antimigraine agent—
Oral, not more than three 100-mg (base) doses in twenty-four hours.

**Usual pediatric dose**

Safety and efficacy in patients up to 18 years of age have not been established.

**Strength(s) usually available**

U.S.—
Not commercially available.

Canada—
100 mg (base [as the succinate salt]) (Rx) [*Imitrex* (lactose)].

**Packaging and storage**

Store between 15 and 30 °C (59 and 86 °F), unless otherwise specified by manufacturer.

**Auxiliary labeling**

• Swallow tablets whole.

## Parenteral Dosage Forms

Note: Sumatriptan injection contains sumatriptan succinate. However, dosage and strength are expressed in terms of sumatriptan base.

### SUMATRIPTAN INJECTION

**Usual adult dose**

Antimigraine agent—
Subcutaneous, injected into the outer thigh or the outer upper arm, 6 mg (base). If a beneficial response to this dose is obtained within one or two hours, an additional 6-mg dose may be administered, at least one hour after the first dose, if headache pain returns or increases in severity.

Note: Lower doses may be administered if the patient does not tolerate the usual dose. The auto-injector should not be used for this purpose; doses should be withdrawn from the single-dose vial, using a separate syringe.

One study compared the effects of 6-mg and 8-mg subcutaneous doses of sumatriptan (base) in migraineurs. The 8-mg dose was not significantly more effective than the 6-mg dose; therefore, doses higher than 6 mg are not recommended.

**Usual adult prescribing limits**

Antimigraine agent—
Single subcutaneous doses should not exceed 6 mg (base). No more than two 6-mg doses should be administered within twenty-four hours.

Note: Some clinicians recommend administering no more than two 6-mg doses within forty-eight hours.

**Usual pediatric dose**

Safety and efficacy in patients up to 18 years of age have not been established.

**Strength(s) usually available**

U.S.—
6 mg (base [as the succinate salt]) per 0.5 mL (Rx) [*Imitrex* (sodium chloride 3.5 mg per 0.5 mL)].

Canada—
6 mg (base [as the succinate salt]) per 0.5 mL (Rx) [*Imitrex*].

**Packaging and storage**

Store between 2 and 30 °C (36 and 86 °F), protected from light and from freezing, unless otherwise specified by manufacturer.

## Selected Bibliography

Cady RK, Wendt JK, Kirchner JR, et al. Treatment of acute migraine with subcutaneous sumatriptan. JAMA 1991; 265: 2831-5.

Subcutaneous Sumatriptan International Study Group. Treatment of migraine attacks with sumatriptan. N Engl J Med 1991; 325: 316-21.

Brown EG, Endersby CA, Smith RM, et al. The safety and tolerability of sumatriptan: an overview. Eur Neurol 1991; 31: 339-44.

Revised: 05/09/95

# SUNSCREEN AGENTS   Topical

This monograph includes information on the following: Aminobenzoic Acid, Padimate O, and Oxybenzone*; Aminobenzoic Acid and Titanium Dioxide†; Avobenzone, Octocrylene, Octyl Salicylate, and Oxybenzone*; Avobenzone and Octyl Methoxycinnamate*; Avobenzone, Octyl Methoxycinnamate, Octyl Salicylate, and Oxybenzone*; Avobenzone, Octyl Methoxycinnamate, and Oxybenzone; Dioxybenzone, Oxybenzone, and Padimate O†; Homosalate; Homosalate, Menthyl Anthranilate, and Octyl Methoxycinnamate†; Homosalate, Menthyl Anthranilate, Octyl Methoxycinnamate, Octyl Salicylate, and Oxybenzone; Homosalate, Octocrylene, Octyl Methoxycinnamate, and Oxybenzone*; Homosalate, Octyl Methoxycinnamate, Octyl Salicylate, and Oxybenzone; Homosalate, Octyl Methoxycinnamate, and Oxybenzone†; Homosalate and Oxybenzone†; Lisadimate, Oxybenzone, and Padimate O†; Lisadimate and Padimate O†; Menthyl Anthranilate†; Menthyl Anthranilate, Octocrylene, and Octyl Methoxycinnamate†; Menthyl Anthranilate, Octocrylene, Octyl Methoxycinnamate, and Oxybenzone†; Menthyl Anthranilate and Octyl Methoxycinnamate†; Menthyl Anthranilate, Octyl Methoxycinnamate, and Octyl Salicylate; Menthyl Anthranilate, Octyl Methoxycinnamate, Octyl Salicylate, and Oxybenzone†; Menthyl Anthranilate, Octyl Methoxycinnamate, and Oxybenzone††; Menthyl Anthranilate and Padimate O*; Menthyl Anthranilate and Titanium Dioxide†; Octocrylene and Octyl Methoxycinnamate; Octocrylene, Octyl Methoxycinnamate, Octyl Salicylate, and Oxybenzone; Octocrylene, Octyl Methoxycinnamate, Octyl Salicylate, Oxybenzone, and Titanium Dioxide†; Octocrylene, Octyl Methoxycinnamate, and Oxybenzone; Octocrylene, Octyl Methoxycinnamate, Oxybenzone, and Titanium Dioxide; Octocrylene, Octyl Methoxycinnamate, and Titanium Dioxide; Octyl Methoxycinnamate; Octyl Methoxycinnamate and Octyl Salicylate; Octyl Methoxycinnamate, Octyl Salicylate, and Oxybenzone; Octyl Methoxycinnamate, Octyl Salicylate, Oxybenzone, and Padimate O; Octyl Methoxycinnamate, Octyl Salicylate, Oxybenzone, Padimate O, and Titanium Dioxide; Octyl Methoxycinnamate, Octyl Salicylate, Oxybenzone, Phenylbenzimidazole, and Titanium Dioxide†; Octyl Methoxycinnamate, Octyl Salicylate, Oxybenzone, and Titanium Dioxide; Octyl Methoxycinnamate, Octyl Salicylate, Phenylbenzimidazole, and Titanium Dioxide; Octyl Methoxycinnamate, Octyl Salicylate, and Titanium Dioxide; Octyl Methoxycinnamate and Oxybenzone; Octyl Methoxycinnamate, Oxybenzone, and Padimate O†; Octyl Methoxycinnamate, Oxybenzone, Padimate O, and Titanium Dioxide*; Octyl Methoxycinnamate, Oxybenzone, and Titanium Dioxide†; Octyl Methoxycinnamate and Padimate O†; Octyl Methoxycinnamate and Phenylbenzimidazole; Octyl Salicylate†; Octyl Salicylate and Padimate O†; Oxybenzone and Padimate O; Oxybenzone and Roxadimate*; Padimate O†; Phenylbenzimidazole; Phenylbenzimidazole and Sulisobenzone; Titanium Dioxide†; Titanium Dioxide and Zinc Oxide; Trolamine Salicylate†.

INN:

Octocrylene—Octocrilene

VA CLASSIFICATION (Primary): DE300

Note: For a listing of dosage forms and brand names by country availability, see *Dosage Forms* section(s). For a listing of brand names for the articles in this monograph, refer to the General Index.

*Not commercially available in the U.S.
†Not commercially available in Canada.

# Category

Skin protectant (topical).

# Indications

## General considerations

The degree of protection provided by a sunscreen product may be determined by the following: the sunscreen protection factor (SPF), which evaluates ultraviolet B (UVB) light-blocking capacity; phototoxic protection factor (or other protection factors), which evaluates ultraviolet A (UVA) light-blocking activity; and substantivity.

UVB light is known as the ''sunburn ray'' because of its tendency to cause erythema of the skin. A sunscreen agent should be effective in reducing erythema due to sun exposure. The SPF displayed on sunscreen agent containers is a measure of the amount of UVB light needed to produce a minimal erythema reaction in sunscreen-protected skin compared with unprotected skin. Sunscreen agents with SPF of 15 or greater are considered sunblocks because they may absorb more than 92% of UVB radiation.

UVA light may also induce erythema but at considerably higher doses than UVB light. Currently, there is no standard method to assess sunscreen agents for UVA protection. Difficulty in determining UVA protection may be due to the extremely long exposure time to UVA needed to produce erythema. One method utilizes the phototoxic protection factor (this is not usually required in the labeling of sunscreen products), which represents the amount of UVA light needed to produce a minimal phototoxic response in sunscreen-protected photosensitized skin compared with unprotected photosensitized skin.

Substantivity is defined as the sunscreen's resistance to removal by physical means, such as being washed off by water or by sweating. The substantivity of sunscreen agents is determined by the design of the vehicle and the active ingredients. Sweat resistance is determined by measuring the SPF after 30 minutes on a person who is sweating profusely. ''Water-resistant'' and ''waterproof'' sunscreens are determined by measuring the SPFs after water exposures of 40 and 80 minutes, respectively.

## Accepted

Sunburn (prophylaxis)—Sunscreen agents are indicated for the prevention of sunburn. In addition to limiting the skin's exposure to the sun, using sunscreen agents regularly when in the sun may help reduce long-term sun damage such as premature aging of the skin and skin cancer.

# Pharmacology/Pharmacokinetics

## Physicochemical characteristics

Chemical sunscreens—
  Aminobenzoic acid and derivatives:
    Aminobenzoic acid (p-aminobenzoic acid or PABA)
    Lisadimate (glyceryl PABA)
    Padimate O (octyldimethyl PABA)
    Roxadimate (ethyl 4-bis [hydroxypropyl] aminobenzoate)
  Anthranilates:
    Menthyl anthranilate
  Benzophenones:
    Dioxybenzone (Benzophenone-8)
    Oxybenzone (Benzophenone-3)
    Sulisobenzone (Benzophenone-4)
  Cinnamates:
    Octocrylene (2-ethylhexyl-2-cyano-3,3-diphenylacrylate)
    Octyl methoxycinnamate (2-ethylhexyl p-methoxycinnamate)
  Dibenzoylmethanes:
    Avobenzone (t-butyl dimethoxydibenzoylmethane)
  Salicylates:
    Homosalate (homomenthyl salicylate)
    Octyl salicylate (2-ethylhexyl salicylate)
    Trolamine salicylate (Triethanolamine salicylate)
  Miscellaneous:
    Phenylbenzimidazole (2-Phenylbenzimidazole-5-sulfonic acid)
Physical sunscreens—
  Titanium dioxide
  Zinc oxide
Molecular weight—
  Aminobenzoic acid: 137.14.
  Avobenzone: 310.40.

Dioxybenzone: 244.25.
Homosalate: 262.35.
Lisadimate: 211.22.
Menthyl anthranilate: 151.16.
Octocrylene: 361.49.
Octyl methoxycinnamate: 290.40.
Octyl salicylate: 250.
Oxybenzone: 228.25.
Padimate O: 277.41.
Phenylbenzimidazole sulfonic acid: 274.
Roxadimate: 281.35.
Sulisobenzone: 308.31.
Titanium dioxide: 79.88.
Trolamine salicylate: 287.
Zinc oxide: 81.39.

## Mechanism of action/Effect

Chemical sunscreen agents—Diminish the penetration of ultraviolet (UV) light through the epidermis by absorbing UV radiation within a specific wavelength range. The amount and wavelength of UV radiation absorbed are affected by the molecular structure of the sunscreen agent.

Physical sunscreen agents—Minimize UV penetration through the epidermis by creating a physical barrier that reflects, scatters, absorbs, and blocks UV and visible radiations.

Table 1. Pharmacology

| Sunscreen Agents | Drug | Concentration (%) | Absorbance Wavelength nonometer (nm) |
|---|---|---|---|
| Absorbers[1] | Avobenzone | 3 | 320–400 |
| | Dioxybenzone | 3 | 250–390 |
| | Metnhyl anthranilate | 3.5–5 | 260–380 |
| | Oxybenzone | 2–6 | 270–350 |
| | Sulisobenzone | 5–10 | 260–375 |
| Absorbers[2] | Aminobenzoic acid | 5–15 | 260–313 |
| | Homosalate | 4–15 | 295–315 |
| | Lisadimate | 2–3 | 264–315 |
| | Octocrylene | 7–10 | 250–360 |
| | Octyl methoxycinnamate | 2–7.5 | 290–320 |
| | Octyl salicylate | 3–5 | 280–320 |
| | Padimate O | 1.4–8 | 290–315 |
| | 2-Phenylbenzimidazole-5-sulfonic acid | 1–4 | 290–340 |
| | Roxadimate | 1–5 | 280–330 |
| | Trolamine salicylate | 5–12 | 260–320 |
| Physical blockers | Titanium dioxide | 2–25 | 290–700 |
| | Zinc oxide | | 290–700 |

[1]FDA-proposed UVA protection defined as a absorption spectrum ≥360 nm.

[2]FDA-approved UVB protection defined as a absorption spectrum 290–320 nm.

# Precautions to Consider

## Cross-sensitivity and/or related problems

Patients sensitive to artificial sweeteners (e.g., saccharin, sodium cyclamate); ester-type anesthetics (e.g., benzocaine, procaine, tetracaine); para-amino type azo dyes (e.g., aniline, paraphenylenediamine); sulfonamide antibiotics; sulfonamide-based oral hypoglycemics; or thiazide diuretics may be sensitive to sunscreen agents containing aminobenzoic acid (PABA) or its derivatives.

Patients sensitive to cinnamon derivatives (balsam of Peru, balsam of Tolu, Cassia, cinnamic acid, cinnamic alcohol, cinnamic aldehyde, cinnamon oil, coca leaves), which are used in cosmetics and perfumes and as flavoring agents in medications and toothpastes, may be sensitive to cinnamate-containing sunscreen agents.

Cross-sensitivity may occur among sunscreens containing benzophenone, dibenzoylmethane, and aminobenzoic acid or its derivatives.

## Carcinogenicity

Studies of the nitrosamine, N-methyl-N-nitrosaminobenzoate octyl ester (NMPABAO), found in minute quantities in sunscreen agents containing padimate O, have shown that NMPABAO does not have carcinogenic potential. However, these results have not been verified with a carcinogenic bioassay. NMPABAO rapidly decomposes when exposed to UV radiation.

There are no reports of carcinogenic potential for other sunscreen agents.

**Mutagenicity**

Studies of the nitrosamine *N*-methyl-*N*-nitrosaminobenzoate octyl ester (NMPABAO) found in sunscreen agents containing padimate O have not shown any mutagenic potential.

There are no reports of mutagenic potential for other sunscreen agents.

**Pregnancy/Reproduction**

Problems in humans have not been documented.

**Breast-feeding**

Problems in humans have not been documented.

**Pediatrics**

Sun protection for children is very important. Studies show the risk of developing skin cancer is increased by excessive exposure to the sun during childhood. It is reported also that in cutaneous melanoma a large proportion of skin damage caused by the sun has been acquired during the first 10 to 20 years of life. Furthermore, the regular use of a sunscreen with a sun protection factor (SPF) of 15 during the first 18 years of life may help reduce the lifetime incidence of nonmelanoma skin cancer by about 75%, if children using sunscreens do not stay out in the sun longer than they would have if sunscreens had not been used.

Infants under 6 months of age should be kept out of the sun and be physically protected from direct sun exposure. Sunscreen agents should not be used on infants under 6 months of age because of possible irritation and accidental ingestion.

Children 6 months of age and older should not be exposed or should receive only moderate exposure to the sun and should be protected by sunscreen agents with SPF of 15 or higher when in the sun. Lotion sunscreen products are preferred for use in children. Alcohol-based sunscreen products should be avoided because they can cause irritation.

**Geriatrics**

Studies have suggested a possibility that frequent use of sunscreen agents may put the population, especially the elderly who spend little time in the sun, at risk of vitamin D deficiency, which could lead to osteomalacia, osteoporosis, or bone fractures. However, a recent study failed to confirm this finding. Oral vitamin D supplementation in addition to adequate food intake rich in vitamin D may be advisable for the elderly.

**Medical considerations/Contraindications**

The medical considerations/contraindications included here have been selected on the basis of their potential clinical significance (reasons given in parentheses where appropriate)—not necessarily inclusive (» = major clinical significance).

*Risk-benefit should be considered when the following medical problems exist:*

Photodermatoses, such as
  Dermatitis, atopic, or chronic actinic, or seborrheic or
  Herpes labialis or
  Lichen rubeo planus or
  Lupus erythematosus or
  Persistent light reaction or
  Photosensitivity, idiopathic, or musk ambrette or
  Phytophotodermatitis or
  Polymorphous light eruption or
  Xeroderma pigmentosum
    (use of sunscreen agents may aggravate these conditions due to increased sensitivity of the skin to the chemicals; patch testing before use may be advisable)
Sensitivity to the sunscreen or other ingredients of the preparation

**Patient monitoring**

The following may be especially important in patient monitoring (other tests may be warranted in some patients, depending on condition; » = major clinical significance):

Patch and photopatch tests
  (may be required prior to use of sunscreen agents for patients with photodermatoses to avoid sunscreen-induced allergic reactions if potential for such reactions is suspected clinically)

## Side/Adverse Effects

Note: The reported incidence of side effects due to sunscreen use is less than 1 to 2%. All sunscreen agents have been reported to cause allergic reactions but the frequency of such reactions is low. Irritation due to the vehicle rather than to the sunscreen's active ingredient seems to be the frequent cause of adverse effects.

The following side/adverse effects have been selected on the basis of their potential clinical significance (possible signs and symptoms in parentheses where appropriate)—not necessarily inclusive:

**Those indicating need for medical attention**

Incidence rare

  *Acne; allergic contact dermatitis* (burning, itching, or stinging of skin); *folliculitis* (burning, itching, and pain in hairy areas; pus in hair follicles); *photoallergic contact dermatitis* (early appearance of redness or swelling of the skin; late appearance of rash with or without weeping blisters that become crusted, especially in sun-exposed areas of skin, and that may extend to unexposed areas); *skin irritation* (burning, itching, redness, or stinging of skin); *skin rash*

  Note: *Acne, folliculitis,* or *skin rash* may occur with physical sunscreen agents because of their occlusive property.

**Those indicating need for medical attention only if they continue or are bothersome**

Incidence more frequent

  *Drying, stinging, or tightening of skin*—may occur with alcohol-based sunscreen agents

## Patient Consultation

As an aid to patient consultation, refer to *Advice for the Patient, Sunscreen Agents (Topical).*

In providing consultation, consider emphasizing the following selected information (» = major clinical significance):

**Before using this product**

» Conditions affecting use, especially:

  Sensitivity to the sunscreen agents or excipients in the formulation, artificial sweeteners, ester-type anesthetics, para-amino type azo dyes, sulfonamide antibiotics, sulfonamide-based oral hypoglycemics, thiazide diuretics, and cinnamon derivatives

  Use in children—Not recommended for use in children under 6 months of age because of possible irritation and accidental ingestion; keeping children 6 months of age and older out of the sun or moderating their exposure to the sun and using sunscreen agents with a sun protection factor (SPF) of 15 or higher during exposure; using lotion sunscreen products for children; avoiding use of alcohol-based sunscreen products because of their potential for causing irritation

  Use in the elderly—Believed to put the elderly, who spend little time in the sun and use sunscreens frequently, at risk for vitamin D deficiency, although this has not been proven; eating a diet including food rich in vitamin D; taking oral vitamin D supplements as recommended by physician

**Proper use of this product**

For external use only; reading directions carefully before using any product

» Taking the following into consideration when choosing sunscreen agents: type of activity, age, site of application, skin condition, and skin type

» Before every exposure to the sun, applying an appropriate sunscreen agent that protects against ultraviolet radiation; for maximum protection, applying uniformly and thickly to all exposed skin surfaces, including lips (using lip balm or lip sunscreen); applying sunscreen products containing aminobenzoic acid or its derivatives 1 to 2 hours before sun exposure; applying other sunscreen products 30 minutes before sun exposure, unless otherwise directed by the package instructions

  Reapplying liberally and frequently (every 1 to 2 hours for adequate protection), especially after swimming or heavy perspiration; for lip sunscreen, reapplying liberally at least once every hour while in the sun, before and after swimming, after eating and drinking, and during activities that remove it from the lips

» Avoiding contact with eyes

» Not using alcohol-based sunscreen agents near heat, near open flame, or while smoking

» Proper dosing

» Proper storage

**Precautions while using this product**

Discontinuing use and checking with physician if rash or irritation develops

Sunscreen agents containing aminobenzoic acid or its derivatives may discolor and stain light-colored fabrics yellow

» In addition to using sunscreen agents, minimizing exposure to the sun from 10 a.m. to 2 p.m. (11 a.m. to 3 p.m. daylight savings time); taking extra precautions also on cloudy or overcast days and around reflective surfaces such as concrete, sand, snow, or water; wearing protective clothing including a hat, long-sleeved shirt, and long pants; wearing sunglasses; avoiding sunlamps and tanning parlors

**Side/adverse effects**

Signs of potential side effects, especially acne; allergic contact dermatitis; folliculitis; photoallergic contact dermatitis; skin irritation; and skin rash

## General Dosing Information

When choosing a sunscreen agent, some of the factors that should be taken into consideration are: type of activity, age, site of application, skin condition, and skin type.

Table 2. Some factors to consider in selecting a sunscreen agent

| Basic Factors | Determining Factors | Appropriate sunscreen agent |
|---|---|---|
| Type of activity | High altitude activities such as mountain climbing and snow-skiing | Use SPF 15 or higher; UVA & UVB coverage |
| | Sweat-generating activities such as outdoor jobs (e.g., gardening, construction work), outdoor sports (e.g., tennis), or exercise, or prolonged sunbathing, watersports such as swimming, waterskiing, or windsurfing | Use SPF 15 or higher; water-resistant[3] or waterproof[4] |
| | Reflective surfaces (e.g., concrete, sand, snow, water) | (Avoid such surfaces.) Use SPF 15 or higher; UVA & UVB coverage |
| Age | Less than 6 months of age | Do not use sunscreen agents; keep out of sun |
| | 6 months of age and older | Use SPF 15 or higher |
| | | For children, use lotion sunscreen products; avoid alcohol-based products |
| Site of application | Ear, nose | Use physical sunscreen agent |
| | Lips | Use gel-based |
| Skin condition | Dry | Use cream or lotion |
| | Oily | Use alcohol or gel-based |
| | Eczematous or inflamed | Avoid alcohol-based |

Table 2. Some factors to consider in selecting a sunscreen agent *(continued)*

| Basic Factors | Determining Factors | Appropriate sunscreen agent |
|---|---|---|
| Skin type[1] (complexion) | | Appropriate Sunscreen Agent |
| Very fair—Always burns easily; rarely tans | | SPF 20 to 30[2] |
| Fair—Always burns easily; tans minimally | | SPF 12 to 20[2] |
| Light—Burns moderately; tans gradually (light brown) | | SPF 8 to 12[2] |
| Medium—Burns minimally; always tans well (moderate brown) | | SPF 4 to 8[2] |
| Dark—Rarely burns; tans profusely (dark brown) | | SPF 2 to 4[2] |

[1]Skin types are based on response to initial summer sun exposure for 30 minutes or longer.
[2]Proposed FDA recommendations.
[3]Water-resistant sunscreen's photoprotective effect remains for up to 40 minutes of active immersion.
[4]Waterproof (FDA has proposed name change to 'very water-resistant')—sunscreen's photoprotective effect remains after 80 minutes of active immersion.

Before every exposure to the sun, an appropriate sunscreen agent that protects against ultraviolet radiation should be used.

Sunscreen agents should be applied uniformly and generously to all exposed skin surfaces (including lips, using lip sunscreen or lip balm) prior to sun exposure. Sunscreen agents containing aminobenzoic acid and derivatives should be applied 1 to 2 hours before exposure to sun, while all other sunscreen products should be applied 30 minutes prior to sun exposure. Lip sunscreens should be applied 45 to 60 minutes before sun exposure.

Sunscreen agents should be reapplied liberally after swimming or profuse sweating. Because most sunscreens agents are easily removed from the skin, reapplication every 1 to 2 hours usually is required for adequate protection. Lip sunscreens should be reapplied liberally at least once every hour and also before and after swimming, after eating and drinking, and during other activities that remove it from the lips.

In addition to using sunscreen agents, sun exposure should be minimized during the hours of 10 a.m. to 2 p.m. (11 a.m. to 3 p.m. daylight savings time) when the sun is strongest. Extra precautions should be utilized on cloudy or overcast days and around reflective surfaces such as concrete, sand, snow, or water since these surfaces can reflect up to 85% of the sun's damaging rays. Sunlamps and tanning parlors should be avoided. Because ultraviolet radiation can cause cataract formation, ultraviolet (UV)-opaque sunglasses should be worn.

## Topical Dosage Forms

See *Table 3,* page 2716.

**Packaging and storage**

Store below 40 °C (104 °F), preferably between 15 and 30 °C (59 and 86 °F), unless otherwise specified by manufacturer.

## Selected Bibliography

Naylor MF, Boyd A, Smith DW, et al. High sun protection factor sunscreens in the suppression of actinic neoplasia. Arch Dermatol 1995; 131: 170-5.

Revised: 04/02/96

## Table 3. Topical Dosage Forms

| Sunscreen agent ingredients<br>Brand name<br>Dosage form<br>[availability] | SPF | Substantivity* | UV Coverage<br>(UVA/UVB) | Other content<br>information as<br>per product<br>label‡ | Directions for<br>use§ | Auxiliary<br>labeling# |
|---|---|---|---|---|---|---|
| **Aminobenzoic acid/Padimate O/<br>Oxybenzone** | | | UVA/UVB | | | |
| *Presun*<br>Lotion<br>[Canada] | 15 | | | 10 | 1,6,11 | a,b,c,d |
| **Aminobenzoic acid/Titanium<br>dioxide** | | | UVA/UVB | | | |
| *Formula 405 Solar*<br>Cream<br>[U.S.] | 15 | | | | | |
| **Avobenzone/Octocrylene/Octyl<br>salicylate/Oxybenzone** | | | UVA/UVB | | | |
| *Photoplex Plus Suncreen*<br>Lotion<br>[Canada] | 15 | | | | 1,6,11 | a,b,d |
| **Avobenzone/Octyl<br>methoxycinnamate** | | | UVA/UVB | | | |
| *Vaseline Broad Spectrum<br>Sunblock*<br>Lotion<br>[Canada] | 15 | WP | | | 1,5,6,11 | |
| **Avobenzone/Octyl methoxycinna-<br>mate/Octyl salicylate/Oxybenzone** | | | UVA/UVB | | | |
| *Presun Sunscreen*<br>*Presun Sunscreen for Kids*<br>Cream | 30<br>30 | WP<br>WP | | | 1,6,11<br>1,6,11 | b<br>b |
| *Presun Clear*<br>Gel<br>[Canada] | 30 | WP | | 10 | 1,6,11 | b,c |
| **Avobenzone/Octyl methoxycinna-<br>mate/Oxybenzone** | | | UVA/UVB | | | |
| *Shade UVA Guard*<br>Lotion<br>[U.S.] | 15 | WR | | 2 | 1,6,11 | b,d |
| *Can Screen 400 Sunscreen* | 22 | WR | | | 1,6,11 | b |
| *Ombrelle Sunscreen*<br>Lotion<br>Spray<br>[Canada] | 15<br>15 | WP<br>WP | | 10 | 1,4,6,11<br>2,4,6,11 | b<br>b,c |
| **Dioxybenzone/Oxybenzone/Padi-<br>mate O** | | | UVA/UVB | | | |
| *Solbar Plus*<br>Cream<br>[U.S.] | 15 | | | | | |
| **Homosalate** | | | UVB | | | |
| *Coppertone Moisturizing Suntan*<br>Oil | 2 | WP | | 1 | 1,6,11 | b |
| *Tropical Blend Dark Tanning*<br>Lotion<br>Oil | 2<br>2 | WP<br>WP | | 1,2 | 1,6<br>1,6 | b |
| *Tropical Blend Dry Oil*<br>Spray<br>[U.S.] | 2 | | | | 2 | b |
| *Coppertone Dark Tanning*<br>Oil<br>[Canada] | 2 | | | | | |

## Table 3. Topical Dosage Forms *(continued)*

| Sunscreen agent ingredients<br>Brand name<br>Dosage form<br>[availability] | SPF | Substantivity* | UV Coverage<br>(UVA/UVB) | Other content<br>information as<br>per product<br>label‡ | Directions for<br>use§ | Auxiliary<br>labeling# |
|---|---|---|---|---|---|---|
| Homosalate/Menthyl anthranilate/<br>Octyl methoxycinnamate<br> *Hawaiian Tropic Protective<br>  Tanning Dry<br>  Oil<br>  [U.S.]* | 6 | | UVA/UVB | | 1,11 | b |
| Homosalate/Menthyl anthranilate/<br>Octyl methoxycinnamate/Octyl sa-<br>licylate/Oxybenzone<br> *Hawaiian Tropic Just for Kids<br> Hawaiian Tropic Sunblock<br>  Lotion<br>  [U.S.]<br> Blistex Ultraprotection<br>  Lip Balm<br>  [U.S./Canada]* | 30<br>30+<br><br><br>30 | <br><br><br><br>WP | UVA/UVB | | 1,6,11<br><br><br><br>3,8,11 | b,d<br><br><br><br>b |
| Homosalate/Octocrylene/ Octyl<br>methoxycinnamate/Oxybenzone<br> *Coppertone Waterproof<br>  Sunblock<br>  Lotion<br>  [Canada]* | 30 | WP | UVA/UVB | | | |

*For appropriate substantivity information, refer to the designated symbols as follows:
WR = Water-resistant (FDA defines as a sunscreen that maintains its photoprotective effect for up to 40 minutes of active immersion)
WR† = Water-resistant - 80 minutes
WP = Waterproof - (FDA defines as a sunscreen that maintains its photoprotective effect after 80 minutes of active immersion; FDA has proposed name change to very water-resistant)
WP-6 = Waterproof - 6 hours
WP-8 = Waterproof - 8 hours

§For appropriate directions for use, refer to the designated numbers as follows:
 1) Apply liberally and evenly to all exposed areas before exposure to the sun.
 2) Apply liberally and evenly, spraying 6 to 8 inches above the skin. For face, spray into hands and finger-apply.
 3) Apply liberally and evenly to lips before and during exposure to the sun.
 4) Apply 15 to 30 minutes before sun exposure.
 5) Apply 30 minutes before sun exposure.
 6) Reapply after swimming or excessive sweating or towel drying.
 7) Reapply every 2 hours or after swimming or excessive sweating.
 8) Reapply after eating or drinking.
 9) Compatible for use under makeup.
 10) When using on the face, smooth on a thin, even coat and blend in quickly until the product is completely absorbed. Use sparingly around hairline and eyebrows. This product contains a self-tanning ingredient; wash and wipe palms thoroughly, even between fingers, after each application to avoid "tanning" on inside of hands.
 11) Discontinue use if signs of irritation or rash appear.
 12) Smooth evenly and generously onto dry skin. Wait 5 minutes. Rub it again. Reapply only after toweling off.
 13) Apply morning and evening for 1 week before beginning chemical treatment therapy. If skin is already irritated by chemical treatment, discontinue sunscreen use and apply only after irritation subsides. Apply a few minutes after topical applications of the chemical treatment. Reapply throughout the day, particularly morning and evening, to cleansed skin.
 14) Rub on sensitive areas such as the face, lips, nose, ears, and shoulders. Apply liberally. Reapply as needed.
 15) May use on nose and around eyes in addition to the lips.
 16) Reapply after 40 minutes in the water or excessive sweating.
 17) Wait 1 hour before bathing or swimming.

‡For other content refer to the designated numbers as follows:
| | | |
|---|---|---|
| 1) Lanolin | 7) Ethyl-, methyl-, and propylparabens | 12) Butyl- and propylparabens |
| 2) Methyl- and propylparabens | 8) Butyl-, isobutyl-, and methylparabens | 13) Hydroxyacetone (self-tanning |
| 3) Butyl-, methyl-, and propylparabens | 9) Methylparaben |  ingredient) |
| 4) Allantoin | 10) Alcohol | 14) Dihydroxyacetone (self-tanning |
| 5) Propylparaben | 11) Butyl-, ethyl-, isobutyl-, isopropyl-, |  ingredient) |
| 6) SD alcohol 40 |  and methylparabens | 15) Butyl- and methylparabens |

#For auxiliary labeling information, refer to the designated letters as follows:
| | |
|---|---|
| a) May stain clothing. | c) Flammable, do not use near heat or flame. |
| b) Avoid contact with eyes. | d) Shake well before using. |

## Table 3. Topical Dosage Forms *(continued)*

| Sunscreen agent ingredients Brand name Dosage form [availability] | SPF | Substantivity* | UV Coverage (UVA/UVB) | Other content information as per product label‡ | Directions for use§ | Auxiliary labeling# |
|---|---|---|---|---|---|---|
| **Homosalate/Octyl methoxycinnamate/Octyl salicylate/Oxybenzone** | | | UVA/UVB | | | |
| *Coppertone All Day Protection* | 30 | WP | | 2 | 1,6,11 | b |
| *Coppertone Kids Sunblock* | 15 | WP-6 | | | | |
| *Neutrogena No Stick Sunscreen* | 30 | WP | | 11 | 1,11 | b |
| *Shade Sunblock* Lotion | 30 | WP | | 2 | 1,6,11 | b |
| *Shade Sunblock* Stick [U.S.] | 30 | WP | | 5 | 1,6,11 | |
| *Waterbabies Sunblock* Lotion [U.S./Canada] | 30 | WP | | 2 | 1,6,11 | b |
| **Homosalate/Octyl methoxycinnamate/Oxybenzone** | | | UVA/UVB | | | |
| *Shade Oil-Free* Gel [U.S.] | 30 | WP | | 6 | 1,6,11 | b,c |
| **Homosalate/Oxybenzone** | | | UVA/UVB | | | |
| *Tropical Blend Dry Oil* Spray [U.S.] | 4 | | | 5 | 2 | b |
| **Lisadimate/Oxybenzone/Padimate O** | | | UVA/UVB | | | |
| *Total Eclipse Oily and Acne Prone Skin Sunscreen* Lotion [U.S.] | 15 | | | 10 | | b,c |
| **Lisadimate/Padimate O** | | | UVB | | | |
| *Eclipse Original Sunscreen* Lotion [U.S.] | 10 | | | | | |
| **Menthyl anthranilate** | | | UVA/UVB | | | |
| *Maxafil* Cream [U.S.] | 6-8 | | | | | |
| **Menthyl anthranilate/Octocrylene/Octyl methoxycinnamate** | | | UVA/UVB | | | |
| *Neutrogena Sunblock* Cream [U.S.] | 30 | WP-6 | | | 1,6,11 | b |
| **Menthyl anthranilate/Octocrylene/Octyl methoxycinnamate/Oxybenzone** | | | UVA/UVB | | | |
| *Hawaiian Tropic Baby Faces* | 20 | WP | | | | |
| *Hawaiian Tropic Plus* Gel [U.S.] | 15 | WP | | | | |
| **Menthyl anthranilate/Octyl methoxycinnamate** | | | UVA/UVB | | | |
| *Catrix Correction* | 15 | | | 3 | 9,13 | |
| *Neutrogena Sunblock* Cream | 8 | WP | | | 1,6,11 | b |
| *Hawaiian Tropic Dark Tanning with Sunscreen* Lotion [U.S.] | 4 | WP | | | 1,6,11 | b,d |
| **Menthyl anthranilate/Octyl methoxycinnamate/Octyl salicylate** | | | UVA/UVB | | | |
| *Neutrogena Sunblock* Cream [U.S.] | 15 | WP-6 | | 5 | 1,6,11 | b |

## Table 3. Topical Dosage Forms *(continued)*

| Sunscreen agent ingredients<br>Brand name<br>Dosage form<br>[availability] | SPF | Substantivity* | UV Coverage<br>(UVA/UVB) | Other content information as per product label‡ | Directions for use§ | Auxiliary labeling# |
|---|---|---|---|---|---|---|
| Menthyl anthranilate/Octyl methoxycinnamate/Octyl salicylate/Oxybenzone | | | UVA/UVB | | | |
|   *Hawaiian Baby Faces Sunblock* | 25 | WP | | | | |
|     Lotion | | | | | | |
|     [U.S.] | | | | | | |
| Menthyl anthranilate/Octyl methoxycinnamate/Oxybenzone | | | UVA/UVB | | | |
|   *Hawaiian Tropic Plus* | 8 | WP-8 | | | | |
|     Gel | | | | | | |
|   *Hawaiian Tropic Plus* | 10 | WP-8 | | | | |
|   *Hawaiian Tropic Plus Sunblock* | 15 | | | | | |
|     Lip Balm | | | | | | |
|     [U.S.] | | | | | | |
|   *Hawaiian Tropic Plus Sunblock* | 15 | WP-8 | | 2 | 1,6,11 | b,d |
|     Lotion | | | | | | |
| Menthyl anthranilate/Padimate O | | | | | | |
|   *Blistex Medicated Lip Conditioner with Sunscreen* | | | UVA/UVB | | 3,8,11 | b |
|     Lip Balm | | | | | | |
|     [Canada] | | | | | | |
| Menthyl anthranilate/Titanium dioxide | | | UVA/UVB | | | |
|   *A-Fil* | | | | 3 | 1,7 | a |
|     Cream | | | | | | |
|     [U.S.] | | | | | | |

*For appropriate substantivity information, refer to the designated symbols as follows:

WR = Water-resistant (FDA defines as a sunscreen that maintains its photoprotective effect for up to 40 minutes of active immersion)

WR† = Water-resistant - 80 minutes

WP = Waterproof - (FDA defines as a sunscreen that maintains its photoprotective effect after 80 minutes of active immersion; FDA has proposed name change to very water-resistant)

WP-6 = Waterproof - 6 hours

WP-8 = Waterproof - 8 hours

§For appropriate directions for use, refer to the designated numbers as follows:
1) Apply liberally and evenly to all exposed areas before exposure to the sun.
2) Apply liberally and evenly, spraying 6 to 8 inches above the skin. For face, spray into hands and finger-apply.
3) Apply liberally and evenly to lips before and during exposure to the sun.
4) Apply 15 to 30 minutes before sun exposure.
5) Apply 30 minutes before sun exposure.
6) Reapply after swimming or excessive sweating or towel drying.
7) Reapply every 2 hours or after swimming or excessive sweating.
8) Reapply after eating or drinking.
9) Compatible for use under makeup.
10) When using on the face, smooth on a thin, even coat and blend in quickly until the product is completely absorbed. Use sparingly around hairline and eyebrows. This product contains a self-tanning ingredient; wash and wipe palms thoroughly, even between fingers, after each application to avoid ''tanning'' on inside of hands.
11) Discontinue use if signs of irritation or rash appear.
12) Smooth evenly and generously onto dry skin. Wait 5 minutes. Rub it again. Reapply only after toweling off.
13) Apply morning and evening for 1 week before beginning chemical treatment therapy. If skin is already irritated by chemical treatment, discontinue sunscreen use and apply only after irritation subsides. Apply a few minutes after topical applications of the chemical treatment. Reapply throughout the day, particularly morning and evening, to cleansed skin.
14) Rub on sensitive areas such as the face, lips, nose, ears, and shoulders. Apply liberally. Reapply as needed.
15) May use on nose and around eyes in addition to the lips.
16) Reapply after 40 minutes in the water or excessive sweating.
17) Wait 1 hour before bathing or swimming.

‡For other content refer to the designated numbers as follows:

1) Lanolin
2) Methyl- and propylparabens
3) Butyl-, methyl-, and propylparabens
4) Allantoin
5) Propylparaben
6) SD alcohol 40
7) Ethyl-, methyl-, and propylparabens
8) Butyl-, isobutyl-, and methylparabens
9) Methylparaben
10) Alcohol
11) Butyl-, ethyl-, isobutyl-, isopropyl-, and methylparabens
12) Butyl- and propylparabens
13) Hydroxyacetone (self-tanning ingredient)
14) Dihydroxyacetone (self-tanning ingredient)
15) Butyl- and methylparabens

#For auxiliary labeling information, refer to the designated letters as follows:
a) May stain clothing.
b) Avoid contact with eyes.
c) Flammable, do not use near heat or flame.
d) Shake well before using.

## Table 3. Topical Dosage Forms *(continued)*

| Sunscreen agent ingredients<br>Brand name<br>Dosage form<br>[availability] | SPF | Substantivity* | UV Coverage<br>(UVA/UVB) | Other content information as per product label‡ | Directions for use§ | Auxiliary labeling# |
|---|---|---|---|---|---|---|
| **Octocrylene/Octyl methoxycinnamate** | | | UVB | | | |
| *Bain de Soleil Mega Tan* | | | | 1,14 | 1,6,10,11 | a,b |
| *Bain de Soleil SPF + Color* | 8 | WP | | 14 | 1,6,10,11 | a,b |
|   Lotion | | | | | | |
|   [U.S.] | | | | | | |
| *Bain de Soleil Mega Tan* | 4 | | | 14 | 1,6,10,11 | a,b |
|   Lotion | | | | | | |
|   [Canada] | | | | | | |
| **Octocrylene/Octyl methoxycinnamate/Octyl salicylate/Oxybenzone** | | | UVA/UVB | | | |
| *Coppertone All Day Protection* | 45 | WP | | 2 | 1,6,11 | b |
| *Coppertone Kids Sunblock* | 30 | WP-6 | | | 1,6 | |
| *Shade Sunblock* | 45 | WP | | 2 | 1,6,11 | b |
| *TI Screen* | 30 | | | | | |
|   Lotion | | | | | | |
|   [U.S.] | | | | | | |
| *Coppertone Waterbabies Sunblock* | 45 | WP | | 2 | 1,6,11 | b |
| *Shade Waterproof Sunblock* | 45 | WP | | | | |
|   Lotion | | | | | | |
|   [U.S./Canada] | | | | | | |
| **Octocrylene/Octyl methoxycinnamate/Octyl salicylate/Oxybenzone/Titanium dioxide** | | | UVA/UVB | | | |
| *Bullfrog Sport* | 18 | WP | | 2 | 11,12 | b |
| *Hawaiian Tropic Baby Faces Sunblock* | 50 | WP | | 2 | | |
| *Hawaiian Tropic Just For Kids* | 45 | WP | | | 1,6,11 | b,d |
| *Hawaiian Tropic Sport Sunblock* | 30 | WP-8 | | | | |
| *Hawaiian Tropic Sunblock* | 45+ | | | | 1,6,11 | b,d |
|   Lotion | | | | | | |
|   [U.S.] | | | | | | |
| **Octocrylene/Octyl methoxycinnamate/Oxybenzone** | | | UVA/UVB | | | |
| *Solbar PF Ultra* | 50 | WP | | | 1,6,11 | |
|   Cream | | | | | | |
| *Solbar PF Liquid* | 30 | | | 6 | 1,6,11 | b,c |
|   Gel | | | | | | |
|   [U.S.] | | | | | | |
| *Bullfrog Body* | 18 & 36 | WP | | | 11,12 | b |
| *Bullfrog Extra Moisturizing* | 18 | WP | | | 11,12 | b |
| *Bullfrog For Kids* | 18 & 36 | WP-6 | | | 11,12 | b |
| *Bullfrog Original Concentrated* | 18 & 36 | WP | | | 11,12 | b |
| *Hawaiian Tropic Sport Sunblock* | 15 | WP | | 4 | 1,6,11 | b,d |
|   Lotion | | | | | | |
|   [U.S.] | | | | | | |
| *Bain de Soleil SPF+ Color* | 15 & 30 | WP | | 13 | 1,6,10,11 | a,b |
|   Lotion | | | | | | |
|   [Canada] | | | | | | |
| **Octocrylene/Octyl methoxycinnamate/Oxybenzone/Titanium dioxide** | | | UVA/UVB | | | |
| *Bain de Soleil All Day For Kids* | 30 | WP | | | 1,6,11 | b |
|   Lotion | | | | | | |
|   [U.S.] | | | | | | |
| *Bain de Soleil All Day Sunblock* | 15 & 30 | WP-6 | | | 1,11 | b |
| *Bain de Soleil Long Lasting For Kids* | 30 | WP | | | 1,6,11 | b |
| *Bain de Soleil Long Lasting Sunblock* | 15 & 30 | WP | | | 1,6,11 | b |
|   Lotion | | | | | | |
|   [Canada] | | | | | | |

## Table 3. Topical Dosage Forms *(continued)*

| Sunscreen agent ingredients Brand name Dosage form [availability] | SPF | Substantivity* | UV Coverage (UVA/UVB) | Other content information as per product label‡ | Directions for use§ | Auxiliary labeling# |
|---|---|---|---|---|---|---|
| Octocrylene/Octyl methoxycinnamate/Titanium dioxide | | | UVA/UVB | | | |
| Bain de Soleil All Day Sunfilter Lotion [U.S.] | 4 & 8 | WP-6 | | | 1,11 | b |
| Bain de Soleil Long Lasting Sport Sunblock | 15 | WP | | | 1,6,11 | b |
| Bain de Soleil Long Lasting Sunfilter Lotion [Canada] | 4 & 8 | WP | | | 1,6,11 | b |
| Octyl methoxycinnamate | | | UVB | | | |
| Coppertone Tan Magnifier | 4 | | | 2 | 1,6,11 | b |
| Formula 405 Solar | 8 | | | | | |
| Neutrogena Deep Glow | 8 | | | 2,14 | 10,11,17 | a,b |
| Neutrogena Light Glow | 8 | | | 2,14 | 10,11,17 | a,b,d |
| Q.T. Quick Tanning Lotion [U.S.] | 2 | | | 2,14 | 1,6,10,11 | a,b |
| Solbar Liquid Gel [Canada] | | | | | | |

*For appropriate substantivity information, refer to the designated symbols as follows:

WR = Water-resistant (FDA defines as a sunscreen that maintains its photoprotective effect for up to 40 minutes of active immersion)

WR† = Water-resistant - 80 minutes

WP = Waterproof - (FDA defines as a sunscreen that maintains its photoprotective effect after 80 minutes of active immersion; FDA has proposed name change to very water-resistant)

WP-6 = Waterproof - 6 hours

WP-8 = Waterproof - 8 hours

§For appropriate directions for use, refer to the designated numbers as follows:
1) Apply liberally and evenly to all exposed areas before exposure to the sun.
2) Apply liberally and evenly, spraying 6 to 8 inches above the skin. For face, spray into hands and finger-apply.
3) Apply liberally and evenly to lips before and during exposure to the sun.
4) Apply 15 to 30 minutes before sun exposure.
5) Apply 30 minutes before sun exposure.
6) Reapply after swimming or excessive sweating or towel drying.
7) Reapply every 2 hours or after swimming or excessive sweating.
8) Reapply after eating or drinking.
9) Compatible for use under makeup.
10) When using on the face, smooth on a thin, even coat and blend in quickly until the product is completely absorbed. Use sparingly around hairline and eyebrows. This product contains a self-tanning ingredient; wash and wipe palms thoroughly, even between fingers, after each application to avoid "tanning" on inside of hands.
11) Discontinue use if signs of irritation or rash appear.
12) Smooth evenly and generously onto dry skin. Wait 5 minutes. Rub it again. Reapply only after toweling off.
13) Apply morning and evening for 1 week before beginning chemical treatment therapy. If skin is already irritated by chemical treatment, discontinue sunscreen use and apply only after irritation subsides. Apply a few minutes after topical applications of the chemical treatment. Reapply throughout the day, particularly morning and evening, to cleansed skin.
14) Rub on sensitive areas such as the face, lips, nose, ears, and shoulders. Apply liberally. Reapply as needed.
15) May use on nose and around eyes in addition to the lips.
16) Reapply after 40 minutes in the water or excessive sweating.
17) Wait 1 hour before bathing or swimming.

‡For other content refer to the designated numbers as follows:

| | | |
|---|---|---|
| 1) Lanolin | 7) Ethyl-, methyl-, and propylparabens | 12) Butyl- and propylparabens |
| 2) Methyl- and propylparabens | 8) Butyl-, isobutyl-, and methylparabens | 13) Hydroxyacetone (self-tanning ingredient) |
| 3) Butyl-, methyl-, and propylparabens | 9) Methylparaben | 14) Dihydroxyacetone (self-tanning ingredient) |
| 4) Allantoin | 10) Alcohol | 15) Butyl- and methylparabens |
| 5) Propylparaben | 11) Butyl-, ethyl-, isobutyl-, isopropyl-, and methylparabens | |
| 6) SD alcohol 40 | | |

#For auxiliary labeling information, refer to the designated letters as follows:

a) May stain clothing.
b) Avoid contact with eyes.
c) Flammable, do not use near heat or flame.
d) Shake well before using.

## Table 3. Topical Dosage Forms *(continued)*

| Sunscreen agent ingredients Brand name Dosage form [availability] | SPF | Substantivity* | UV Coverage (UVA/UVB) | Other content information as per product label‡ | Directions for use§ | Auxiliary labeling# |
|---|---|---|---|---|---|---|
| **Octyl methoxycinnamate/Octyl salicylate** | | | UVB | | | |
| *Bain de Soleil Tropical Deluxe* | 4 | WP | | 1 | 1,6,11 | b |
| *Hawaiian Tropic Land Sport* | 20 | | | | | |
| *Vaseline Intensive Care Moisturizing Sunscreen* | 4 | | | 2 | | |
| Lotion | | | | | | |
| *Bain de Soleil Sand Buster* | 2 | WP | | 1,5 | 1,6,11 | b |
| Oil | | | | | | |
| [U.S.] | | | | | | |
| *Bain de Soleil Orange Gelee* | 4 | | | 12 | 1,6,11 | a,b |
| Gel | | | | | | |
| [U.S./Canada] | | | | | | |
| **Octyl methoxycinnamate/Octyl salicylate/Oxybenzone** | | | UVA/UVB | | | |
| *Banana Boat Faces Sensitive Skin Sunblock* | 15 & 23 | WP | | | 1,6,9 | |
| Cream | | | | | | |
| *PreSun Active Clear* | 15 & 30 | WP | | 6 | 1,6,11 | b,c |
| *Shade Sunblock Oil-Free* | 30 | WP | | 6 | | b,c |
| *TI Screen* | 20+ | | | 6 | | b,c |
| Gel | | | | | | |
| *Waterbabies Little Licks* | 30 | WP | | 5 | 3,11 | b |
| Lip Balm | | | | | | |
| *Aquaray Sunscreen* | 20 | WR | | | 1,6,11 | b |
| *Banana Boat Active Kids Sunblock* | 30+ | WP-8 | | | 1,6 | |
| *Banana Boat Baby Sunblock* | 29 | WP-8 | | | 1,6 | |
| *Banana Boat Sport Sunblock* | 15 & 30+ | WP-8 | | | 1,6 | |
| *Dermsol* | 30 | WP | | 2 | 1,6,11 | b |
| *Durascreen* | 15 | WP-8 | | 2 | 1,6,11 | b |
| *Nivea Sun* | 15 | WP | | | | b |
| *PreSun For Kids* | 29 | WP | | | | |
| *PreSun Moisturizing Sunscreen with Keri* | 25 | WP | | | | |
| *PreSun Sensitive Skin* | 15 & 29 | WP | | | | |
| *TI Screen* | 20 | | | | | |
| Lotion | | | | | | |
| *PreSun Spray Mist* | | | | | | |
| *Vaseline Intensive Care Moisturizing Sunblock* | 25 | WP-8 | | 2 | 1,6,11 | b,d |
| Spray | 23 | WP | | 6 | | b,c |
| *Neutrogena Sunblock* | 25 | WP | | 5 | 11,14 | b |
| Stick | | | | | | |
| [U.S.] | | | | | | |
| *Presun Sunscreen* | 29 | WP | | | 1,6,11 | b |
| *Presun Sunscreen for Kids* | 29 | WP | | | 1,6,11 | b |
| *Solbar Shield* | 20 | | | | | |
| Cream | | | | | | |
| [Canada] | | | | | | |
| *Coppertone Sport* | 30 | | | | | |
| *Vaseline Kids Sunblock* | 25 | WP | | | 1,5,6,11 | |
| *Vaseline Sunblock* | 25 | WP | | | 1,5,6,11 | |
| Lotion | | | | | | |
| [Canada] | | | | | | |
| **Octyl methoxycinnamate/Octyl salicylate/Oxybenzone/Padimate O** | | | UVA/UVB | | | |
| *Presun Spray Mist for Kids* | 23 | WP | | 6 | | |
| Spray | | | | | | |
| [U.S.] | | | | | | |
| *Vaseline Sunblock* | | | | | | |
| Lotion | 35 | WP | | | 1,5,6,11 | |
| [Canada] | | | | | | |

## Table 3. Topical Dosage Forms *(continued)*

| Sunscreen agent ingredients Brand name Dosage form [availability] | SPF | Substantivity* | UV Coverage (UVA/UVB) | Other content information as per product label‡ | Directions for use§ | Auxiliary labeling# |
|---|---|---|---|---|---|---|
| Octyl methoxycinnamate/Octyl salicylate/Oxybenzone/Padimate O/ Titanium dioxide | | | UVA/UVB | | | |
| *Vaseline Intensive Care Blockout Moisturizing* Lotion [U.S.] | 40+ | WP | | | 1,6,11 | b,d |
| Octyl methoxycinnamate/Octyl salicylate/Oxybenzone/Phenylben- zimidazole/Titanium dioxide | | | UVA/UVB | | | |
| *DuraScreen* Lotion [U.S.] | 30 | WR | | | 1,6,11 | b,d |

*For appropriate substantivity information, refer to the designated symbols as follows:

WR = Water-resistant (FDA defines as a sunscreen that maintains its photoprotective effect for up to 40 minutes of active immersion)

WR† = Water-resistant - 80 minutes

WP = Waterproof - (FDA defines as a sunscreen that maintains its photoprotective effect after 80 minutes of active immersion; FDA has proposed name change to very water-resistant)

WP-6 = Waterproof - 6 hours

WP-8 = Waterproof - 8 hours

§For appropriate directions for use, refer to the designated numbers as follows:

1) Apply liberally and evenly to all exposed areas before exposure to the sun.
2) Apply liberally and evenly, spraying 6 to 8 inches above the skin. For face, spray into hands and finger-apply.
3) Apply liberally and evenly to lips before and during exposure to the sun.
4) Apply 15 to 30 minutes before sun exposure.
5) Apply 30 minutes before sun exposure.
6) Reapply after swimming or excessive sweating or towel drying.
7) Reapply every 2 hours or after swimming or excessive sweating.
8) Reapply after eating or drinking.
9) Compatible for use under makeup.
10) When using on the face, smooth on a thin, even coat and blend in quickly until the product is completely absorbed. Use sparingly around hairline and eyebrows. This product contains a self-tanning ingredient; wash and wipe palms thoroughly, even between fingers, after each application to avoid "tanning" on inside of hands.
11) Discontinue use if signs of irritation or rash appear.
12) Smooth evenly and generously onto dry skin. Wait 5 minutes. Rub it again. Reapply only after toweling off.
13) Apply morning and evening for 1 week before beginning chemical treatment therapy. If skin is already irritated by chemical treatment, discontinue sunscreen use and apply only after irritation subsides. Apply a few minutes after topical applications of the chemical treatment. Reapply throughout the day, particularly morning and evening, to cleansed skin.
14) Rub on sensitive areas such as the face, lips, nose, ears, and shoulders. Apply liberally. Reapply as needed.
15) May use on nose and around eyes in addition to the lips.
16) Reapply after 40 minutes in the water or excessive sweating.
17) Wait 1 hour before bathing or swimming.

‡For other content refer to the designated numbers as follows:

1) Lanolin
2) Methyl- and propylparabens
3) Butyl-, methyl-, and propylparabens
4) Allantoin
5) Propylparaben
6) SD alcohol 40
7) Ethyl-, methyl-, and propylparabens
8) Butyl-, isobutyl-, and methylparabens
9) Methylparaben
10) Alcohol
11) Butyl-, ethyl-, isobutyl-, isopropyl-, and methylparabens
12) Butyl- and propylparabens
13) Hydroxyacetone (self-tanning ingredient)
14) Dihydroxyacetone (self-tanning ingredient)
15) Butyl- and methylparabens

#For auxiliary labeling information, refer to the designated letters as follows:

a) May stain clothing.
b) Avoid contact with eyes.
c) Flammable, do not use near heat or flame.
d) Shake well before using.

Table 3. Topical Dosage Forms *(continued)*

| Sunscreen agent ingredients Brand name Dosage form [availability] | SPF | Substantivity* | UV Coverage (UVA/UVB) | Other content information as per product label‡ | Directions for use§ | Auxiliary labeling# |
|---|---|---|---|---|---|---|
| **Octyl methoxycinnamate/Octyl salicylate/Oxybenzone/Titanium dioxide** | | | UVA/UVB | | | |
| *Sundown Sunblock* | 15 & 30 | WP | | | | |
| *Vaseline Intensive Care Baby Moisturizing Sunblock* | 30+ | WP | | 2 | 1,6,11 | b,d |
| *Vaseline Intensive Care Blockout Moisturizing* Lotion [U.S.] | 30+ | WP | | | | |
| *Sundown Broad Spectrum Sunblock* Cream | 15, 25, & 30 | | | | | |
| *Vaseline Intensive Care Baby Sunblock* Lotion [Canada] | 25 | WP | | | 1,5,6,11 | |
| *Johnson's Baby Sunblock* | 15 | WP | | 1 | | |
| *Johnson's Baby Sunblock Extra Protection* Lotion [U.S./Canada] | 30+ | WP | | | 1,5,6,11 | b,d |
| **Octyl methoxycinnamate/Octyl salicylate/Phenylbenzimidazole/Titanium dioxide** | | | UVA/UVB | | | |
| *Eucerin Dry Skin Care Daily Facial* Lotion [U.S.] | 20 | | | | 1,9,11 | b |
| **Octyl methoxycinnamate/Octyl salicylate/Titanium dioxide** | | | UVA/UVB | | | |
| *Sundown Sunscreen* Lotion [U.S.] | 8 | WP | | | | |
| **Octyl methoxycinnamate/Oxybenzone** | | | UVA/UVB | | | |
| *Aquaderm Sunscreen Moisturizer* | 15 | | | | 1,9,11 | b |
| *DML Facial Moisturizer* | 15 | | | | 1,9 | b |
| *Solbar PF* Cream | 15 | | | | | |
| *Solbar PF Liquid* Gel [U.S.] | 15 | | | 6 | 1,6,11 | b,c,d |
| *Catrix Lip Saver* | 15 | | | 4,5 | 3,15 | |
| *Neutrogena Lip Moisturizer* | 15 | | | | | |
| *Vaseline Intensive Care Lip Therapy* Lip Balm | 8 | | | | | |
| *Coppertone All Day Protection* | 8 & 15 | WP | | | 1,6,11 | b |
| *Coppertone Moisturizing Sunscreen* | 6 & 8 | WP | | | | |
| *Coppertone Moisturizing Suntan* | 4 | WP | | 2 | 1,6,11 | b |
| *Coppertone Sport Ultra Sweatproof* | 8 & 15 | WP-8 | | 2 | 1,11 | b |
| *Curel Everyday Sun Protection* | 8 | | | | 1,6,11 | |
| *Hawaiian Tropic Self-tanning Sunblock* | 15 | | | 2,14 | 10,11 | a,b,d |
| *Neutrogena Moisture Untinted & with Sheer Tint* | 15 | | | 7 | 4,9,11 | b |
| *Softsense Skin Essential Everyday UV Protectant* | 8 | | | | | |
| *TI Screen* | 8 & 15+ | | | | | |
| *Tropical Blend Dark Tanning* | 4 | WP | | 1,2 | 1,6 | b |
| *Vaseline Intensive Care Active Sport* | 8 & 15 | WP-8 | | | 1,6,11 | b,d |
| *Vaseline Intensive Care Moisturizing Sunblock* Lotion | 15 | WP-8 | | 2 | 1,6,11 | b,d |

## Table 3. Topical Dosage Forms *(continued)*

| Sunscreen agent ingredients<br>Brand name<br>Dosage form<br>[availability] | SPF | Substantivity* | UV Coverage<br>(UVA/UVB) | Other content<br>information as<br>per product<br>label‡ | Directions for<br>use§ | Auxiliary<br>labeling# |
|---|---|---|---|---|---|---|
| Octyl methoxycinnamate/Oxyben-<br>zone *(continued)* | | | | | | |
| *Bullfrog Sunblock*<br>Stick<br>[U.S.] | 18 | WP-6 | | | 11,14 | b |
| *Vaseline Extra Defense for Hand<br>and Body* | 15 | | | 2 | | |
| *Vaseline Moisturizing Sunscreen* | 8 | | | | 3,8,11 | |
| *Vaseline Ultraviolet Daily De-<br>fense for Hand and Body*<br>Cream<br>[U.S.] | 4 | | | 2 | 1,6 | b |
| *Vaseline Lip Therapy*<br>Lip Balm | 15 | WP | | | 3,8,11 | |
| *TI-UVA-B Sunscreen* | 22 | WR | | | 1,11,16 | b |
| *Vaseline Kids Sunblock* | 15 | WP | | | 1,5,6,11 | |
| *Vaseline Sport Sunblock* | 15 | WP | | | 1,5,6,11 | |
| *Vaseline Sports Sunscreen* | 8 | WP | | | 1,5,6,11 | |
| *Vaseline Sunblock* | 15 | WP | | | 1,5,6,11 | |
| *Vaseline Sunscreen*<br>Lotion | 8 | WP | | | 1,5,6,11 | |
| *Sundown Sunscreen*<br>Stick<br>[Canada] | 15 | | | | | |
| *Coppertone Lipkote*<br>Lip Balm<br>[U.S./Canada] | 15 | WP | | 5 | 3,8,11 | |
| *Waterbabies Sunblock*<br>Lotion<br>[U.S./Canada] | 15 | | | 2 | | |

*For appropriate substantivity information, refer to the designated symbols as follows:

WR = Water-resistant (FDA defines as a sunscreen that maintains its photoprotective effect for up to 40 minutes of active immersion)

WR† = Water-resistant - 80 minutes

WP = Waterproof - (FDA defines as a sunscreen that maintains its photoprotective effect after 80 minutes of active immersion; FDA has proposed name change to very water-resistant)

WP-6 = Waterproof - 6 hours

WP-8 = Waterproof - 8 hours

§For appropriate directions for use, refer to the designated numbers as follows:
1) Apply liberally and evenly to all exposed areas before exposure to the sun.
2) Apply liberally and evenly, spraying 6 to 8 inches above the skin. For face, spray into hands and finger-apply.
3) Apply liberally and evenly to lips before and during exposure to the sun.
4) Apply 15 to 30 minutes before sun exposure.
5) Apply 30 minutes before sun exposure.
6) Reapply after swimming or excessive sweating or towel drying.
7) Reapply every 2 hours or after swimming or excessive sweating.
8) Reapply after eating or drinking.
9) Compatible for use under makeup.
10) When using on the face, smooth on a thin, even coat and blend in quickly until the product is completely absorbed. Use sparingly around hairline and eyebrows. This product contains a self-tanning ingredient; wash and wipe palms thoroughly, even between fingers, after each application to avoid "tanning" on inside of hands.
11) Discontinue use if signs of irritation or rash appear.
12) Smooth evenly and generously onto dry skin. Wait 5 minutes. Rub it again. Reapply only after toweling off.
13) Apply morning and evening for 1 week before beginning chemical treatment therapy. If skin is already irritated by chemical treatment, discontinue sunscreen use and apply only after irritation subsides. Apply a few minutes after topical applications of the chemical treatment. Reapply throughout the day, particularly morning and evening, to cleansed skin.
14) Rub on sensitive areas such as the face, lips, nose, ears, and shoulders. Apply liberally. Reapply as needed.
15) May use on nose and around eyes in addition to the lips.
16) Reapply after 40 minutes in the water or excessive sweating.
17) Wait 1 hour before bathing or swimming.

‡For other content refer to the designated numbers as follows:

| | | |
|---|---|---|
| 1) Lanolin | 7) Ethyl-, methyl-, and propylparabens | 12) Butyl- and propylparabens |
| 2) Methyl- and propylparabens | 8) Butyl-, isobutyl-, and methylparabens | 13) Hydroxyacetone (self-tanning |
| 3) Butyl-, methyl-, and propylparabens | 9) Methylparaben | ingredient) |
| 4) Allantoin | 10) Alcohol | 14) Dihydroxyacetone (self-tanning |
| 5) Propylparaben | 11) Butyl-, ethyl-, isobutyl-, isopropyl-, | ingredient) |
| 6) SD alcohol 40 | and methylparabens | 15) Butyl- and methylparabens |

#For auxiliary labeling information, refer to the designated letters as follows:

a) May stain clothing.

b) Avoid contact with eyes.

c) Flammable, do not use near heat or flame.

d) Shake well before using.

## Table 3. Topical Dosage Forms *(continued)*

| Sunscreen agent ingredients Brand name Dosage form [availability] | SPF | Substantivity* | UV Coverage (UVA/UVB) | Other content information as per product label‡ | Directions for use§ | Auxiliary labeling# |
|---|---|---|---|---|---|---|
| **Octyl methoxycinnamate/Oxybenzone/Padimate O** | | | UVA/UVB | | | |
| *Banana Boat Sunblock* Lotion [U.S.] | 15 | WP | | | 1,6 | |
| **Octyl methoxycinnamate/Oxybenzone/Padimate O/Titanium dioxide** | | | UVA/UVB | | | |
| *Sundown* Stick [Canada] | 20 | | | | | |
| **Octyl methoxycinnamate/Oxybenzone/Titanium dioxide** | | | UVA/UVB | | | |
| *Hawaiian Tropic Water Sport* Lotion [U.S.] | 20 | | | | | |
| **Octyl methoxycinnamate/Padimate O** | | | UVB | | | |
| *Banana Boat Dark Tanning* | 4 | | | 1 | 1,6 | |
| *Banana Boat Protective Tanning* | 8 | | | | 1,6 | |
| *Hawaiian Tropic Dark Tanning* Oil [U.S.] | 4 | WP | | | | |
| **Octyl methoxycinnamate/ Phenylbenzimidazole** | | | UVB | | | |
| *Neutrogena Intensified Day Moisture* | 15 | | | 2 | 9,11 | b |
| *Noxzema Moisturizer* | 15 | | | 2 | 1,6,9,11 | b |
| *Oil of Olay Daily UV Protectant* Cream | 15 | | | 2 | 1,11 | b |
| *Oil of Olay Daily UV Protectant* Beauty Fluid | 15 | | | 2 | 1,11 | b |
| *Oil of Olay Moisture Replenishment* Lotion [U.S.] | 15 | | | 2 | 1,11 | b |
| *Pond's Daily Replenishing Moisturizer* Lotion [Canada] | 15 | | | 2 | 1,11 | b |
| **Octyl salicylate** | | | UVB | | | |
| *PreSun Spray Mist* Spray [U.S.] | 15 | WP | | | | |
| **Octyl salicylate/Padimate O** | | | UVB | | | |
| *Total Eclipse Moisturizing Skin* Lotion [U.S.] | 15 | | | | | |
| **Oxybenzone/Padimate O** | | | UVA/UVB | | | |
| *Blistex Daily Conditioning Treatment for Lips* | 15 | WR† | | 1 | 3,8,11 | b |
| *Blistex Regular* | 10 | WR† | | 1,2 | 3,8,11 | b |
| *Chap-et Sun Ban Lip Conditioner* | 15 | | | | 3 | |
| *Chap Stick Sunblock Petroleum Jelly Plus* | 15 | | | | | |
| *PreSun Lip Protector* | 15 | | | | | |
| *Stay Moist Moisturizing Lip Conditioner* Lip Balm | 15+ | | | | 3,9,11 | b |
| *Banana Boat Sunscreen* | 8 | WP | | | | |
| *Formula 405 Solar* | 15 | | | | 3,8,11 | |
| *Hawaiian Tropic Protective Tanning* | 6 | | | | | |
| *PreSun Moisturizing* | 46 | | | | | |
| *PreSun Moisturizing Sunscreen with Keri* | 8 & 15 | WP | | | | |
| *Ray Block* | 15 | | | 6 | 1,11 | b,c |
| *Solex A15 Clear* Lotion | 15 | | | | | b |

Table 3. Topical Dosage Forms *(continued)*

| Sunscreen agent ingredients<br>Brand name<br>Dosage form<br>[availability] | SPF | Substantivity* | UV Coverage<br>(UVA/UVB) | Other content<br>information as<br>per product<br>label‡ | Directions for<br>use§ | Auxiliary<br>labeling# |
|---|---|---|---|---|---|---|
| **Oxybenzone/Padimate O** | | | | | | |
| *(continued)* | | | | | | |
| *Tropical Blend Dark Tanning*<br>Oil<br>[U.S.] | 4 | WP | | | 1,6 | b |
| *Eclipse Lip & Face Protectant*<br>Stick<br>[U.S.] | 15 | | | | | |
| *Presun Sunscreen*<br>Cream | 39 | WP | | | 1,6,11 | b,d |
| *Blistex Medicated Lip*<br>Conditioner | 15 | | | | 3,8,11 | |
| *Blistex Sunblock*<br>Lip Balm | 15 | | | | 3 | |
| *PreSun Creamy Sundown*<br>Sunscreen<br>Lotion | 15<br>8 | WP | | | 1,6,11 | b,d |
| *Tropical Blend Waterproof*<br>Oil<br>[Canada] | 4 | WP | | | | |
| *Chap Stick Sunblock*<br>Lip Balm<br>[U.S./Canada] | 15 | | | 1,2 | 3,11 | b |
| **Oxybenzone/Roxadimate** | | | UVA/UVB | | | |
| *Solbar Plus*<br>Cream | 15 | | | | | |
| *Solbar*<br>Lotion<br>[Canada] | | | | | | |

*For appropriate substantivity information, refer to the designated symbols as follows:

WR = Water-resistant (FDA defines as a sunscreen that maintains its photoprotective effect for up to 40 minutes of active immersion)

WR† = Water-resistant - 80 minutes

WP = Waterproof - (FDA defines as a sunscreen that maintains its photoprotective effect after 80 minutes of active immersion; FDA has proposed name change to very water-resistant)

WP-6 = Waterproof - 6 hours

WP-8 = Waterproof - 8 hours

§For appropriate directions for use, refer to the designated numbers as follows:

1) Apply liberally and evenly to all exposed areas before exposure to the sun.
2) Apply liberally and evenly, spraying 6 to 8 inches above the skin. For face, spray into hands and finger-apply.
3) Apply liberally and evenly to lips before and during exposure to the sun.
4) Apply 15 to 30 minutes before sun exposure.
5) Apply 30 minutes before sun exposure.
6) Reapply after swimming or excessive sweating or towel drying.
7) Reapply every 2 hours or after swimming or excessive sweating.
8) Reapply after eating or drinking.
9) Compatible for use under makeup.
10) When using on the face, smooth on a thin, even coat and blend in quickly until the product is completely absorbed. Use sparingly around hairline and eyebrows. This product contains a self-tanning ingredient; wash and wipe palms thoroughly, even between fingers, after each application to avoid "tanning" on inside of hands.
11) Discontinue use if signs of irritation or rash appear.
12) Smooth evenly and generously onto dry skin. Wait 5 minutes. Rub it again. Reapply only after toweling off.
13) Apply morning and evening for 1 week before beginning chemical treatment therapy. If skin is already irritated by chemical treatment, discontinue sunscreen use and apply only after irritation subsides. Apply a few minutes after topical applications of the chemical treatment. Reapply throughout the day, particularly morning and evening, to cleansed skin.
14) Rub on sensitive areas such as the face, lips, nose, ears, and shoulders. Apply liberally. Reapply as needed.
15) May use on nose and around eyes in addition to the lips.
16) Reapply after 40 minutes in the water or excessive sweating.
17) Wait 1 hour before bathing or swimming.

‡For other content refer to the designated numbers as follows:

1) Lanolin
2) Methyl- and propylparabens
3) Butyl-, methyl-, and propylparabens
4) Allantoin
5) Propylparaben
6) SD alcohol 40
7) Ethyl-, methyl-, and propylparabens
8) Butyl-, isobutyl-, and methylparabens
9) Methylparaben
10) Alcohol
11) Butyl-, ethyl-, isobutyl-, isopropyl-, and methylparabens
12) Butyl- and propylparabens
13) Hydroxyacetone (self-tanning ingredient)
14) Dihydroxyacetone (self-tanning ingredient)
15) Butyl- and methylparabens

#For auxiliary labeling information, refer to the designated letters as follows:

a) May stain clothing.
b) Avoid contact with eyes.
c) Flammable, do not use near heat or flame.
d) Shake well before using.

## Table 3. Topical Dosage Forms *(continued)*

| Sunscreen agent ingredients<br>Brand name<br>Dosage form<br>[availability] | SPF | Substantivity* | UV Coverage<br>(UVA/UVB) | Other content<br>information as<br>per product<br>label‡ | Directions for<br>use§ | Auxiliary<br>labeling# |
|---|---|---|---|---|---|---|
| **Padimate O** | | | UVB | | | |
| *Herpecin-L Cold Sore* | 15 | | | 4 | 3,8,11 | |
| *Mentholatum*<br>Lip Balm | 14.7 | | | 1 | | |
| *Banana Boat Dark Tanning*<br>Lotion | 4 | WP | | | | |
| *Banana Boat Dark Tanning*<br>Oil<br>[U.S.] | 2 | | | 1 | 1,6 | |
| *Chap Stick*<br>Lip Balm<br>[U.S.] | 4 | | | 1,2 | 3 | |
| **Phenylbenzimidazole** | | | UVB | | | |
| *Coppertone Tan Magnifier* | 4 | | | 9 | 1,6,11 | b |
| *Hawaiian Tropic Dark Tanning*<br>Gel<br>[U.S.] | 2 | | | | 1,11 | b |
| *Oil of Olay Moisture*<br>Replenishment<br>Lotion<br>[U.S.] | 15 | | | 2 | 1,11 | b |
| *Pond's Daily Replenishing*<br>Moisturizer<br>Lotion<br>[Canada] | 15 | | | 2 | 1,11 | b |
| **Phenylbenzimidazole/Sulisobenzone** | | | UVA/UVB | | | |
| *Hawaiian Tropic Protective*<br>Tanning Dry<br>Gel<br>[U.S.] | 6 | | | | | |
| **Titanium dioxide** | | | UVA/UVB | | | |
| *Neutrogena Chemical-Free*<br>Sunblocker | 17 | WR | | 7 | 1,6,11 | b |
| *TI Screen Baby Natural* | 16 | WP | | | | |
| *Vaseline Intensive Care Baby*<br>Moisturizing Sunblock<br>Lotion<br>[U.S.] | 15 | WP | | | 1,6,11 | b,d |
| **Titanium dioxide/Zinc oxide** | | | UVA/UVB | | | |
| *Sundown Sport Sunblock*<br>Lotion<br>[U.S.] | 15 | WP | | | 1,5,6,11 | b |
| *Vaseline Baby Sunblock*<br>Lotion<br>[Canada] | 15 | WP | | | 1,5,6,11 | |
| *Johnson's No More Tears Baby*<br>Sunblock<br>Lotion<br>[U.S./Canada] | 15 | WP | | 1 | 1,5,6,11 | b,d |

## Table 3. Topical Dosage Forms *(continued)*

| Sunscreen agent ingredients<br>  Brand name<br>  Dosage form<br>  [availability] | SPF | Substantivity* | UV Coverage<br>(UVA/UVB) | Other content<br>information as<br>per product<br>label‡ | Directions for<br>use§ | Auxiliary<br>labeling# |
|---|---|---|---|---|---|---|
| Trolamine salicylate<br>  *Coppertone Tan Magnifier*<br>  Oil<br>  [U.S.] | 2 & 4 | | UVB | 2 | 1,6 | b |

\*For appropriate substantivity information, refer to the designated symbols as follows:
WR = Water-resistant (FDA defines as a sunscreen that maintains its photoprotective effect for up to 40 minutes of active immersion)
WR† = Water-resistant - 80 minutes
WP = Waterproof - (FDA defines as a sunscreen that maintains its photoprotective effect after 80 minutes of active immersion; FDA has proposed name change to very water-resistant)
WP-6 = Waterproof - 6 hours
WP-8 = Waterproof - 8 hours

§For appropriate directions for use, refer to the designated numbers as follows:
  1) Apply liberally and evenly to all exposed areas before exposure to the sun.
  2) Apply liberally and evenly, spraying 6 to 8 inches above the skin. For face, spray into hands and finger-apply.
  3) Apply liberally and evenly to lips before and during exposure to the sun.
  4) Apply 15 to 30 minutes before sun exposure.
  5) Apply 30 minutes before sun exposure.
  6) Reapply after swimming or excessive sweating or towel drying.
  7) Reapply every 2 hours or after swimming or excessive sweating.
  8) Reapply after eating or drinking.
  9) Compatible for use under makeup.
  10) When using on the face, smooth on a thin, even coat and blend in quickly until the product is completely absorbed. Use sparingly around hairline and eyebrows. This product contains a self-tanning ingredient; wash and wipe palms thoroughly, even between fingers, after each application to avoid "tanning" on inside of hands.
  11) Discontinue use if signs of irritation or rash appear.
  12) Smooth evenly and generously onto dry skin. Wait 5 minutes. Rub it again. Reapply only after toweling off.
  13) Apply morning and evening for 1 week before beginning chemical treatment therapy. If skin is already irritated by chemical treatment, discontinue sunscreen use and apply only after irritation subsides. Apply a few minutes after topical applications of the chemical treatment. Reapply throughout the day, particularly morning and evening, to cleansed skin.
  14) Rub on sensitive areas such as the face, lips, nose, ears, and shoulders. Apply liberally. Reapply as needed.
  15) May use on nose and around eyes in addition to the lips.
  16) Reapply after 40 minutes in the water or excessive sweating.
  17) Wait 1 hour before bathing or swimming.

‡For other content refer to the designated numbers as follows:

  1) Lanolin
  2) Methyl- and propylparabens
  3) Butyl-, methyl-, and propylparabens
  4) Allantoin
  5) Propylparaben
  6) SD alcohol 40

  7) Ethyl-, methyl-, and propylparabens
  8) Butyl-, isobutyl-, and methylparabens
  9) Methylparaben
  10) Alcohol
  11) Butyl-, ethyl-, isobutyl-, isopropyl-, and methylparabens

  12) Butyl- and propylparabens
  13) Hydroxyacetone (self-tanning ingredient)
  14) Dihydroxyacetone (self-tanning ingredient)
  15) Butyl- and methylparabens

#For auxiliary labeling information, refer to the designated letters as follows:
  a) May stain clothing.
  b) Avoid contact with eyes.

  c) Flammable, do not use near heat or flame.
  d) Shake well before using.

---

**SUPROFEN**—See *Anti-inflammatory Drugs, Nonsteroidal (Ophthalmic)*

**SURAMIN**—Since Suramin is not commercially available in the U.S. or Canada, the *Suramin (Systemic)* monograph is not included in this published version of the USP DI database. Copies of the monograph are available on request from the USP Division of Information Development, 12601 Twinbrook Parkway, Rockville, MD 20852; telephone (301) 816-8351; telefax (301) 816-8374.

---

# SYMPATHOMIMETIC AGENTS—Cardiovascular Use    Parenteral-Systemic

This monograph includes information on the following: Dobutamine; Dopamine; Ephedrine; Epinephrine; Isoproterenol; Mephentermine†; Metaraminol†; Methoxamine; Norepinephrine; Phenylephrine.

INN:
  Norepinephrine—Levarterenol
BAN:
  Norepinephrine—Noradrenaline
VA CLASSIFICATION (Primary/Secondary):
  Dobutamine—AU100/CV900
  Dopamine—AU100/CV900
  Ephedrine—AU100/CV900
  Epinephrine—AU100/CV900
  Isoproterenol—AU100/CV300
  Mephentermine—AU100/CV900

Metaraminol—AU100/CV900
Methoxamine—AU100/CV900
Norepinephrine—AU100/CV900
Phenylephrine—AU100/CV900; CV300

Note: For a listing of dosage forms and brand names by country availability, see *Dosage Forms* section(s). For a listing of brand names for the articles in this monograph, refer to the General Index.

†Not commercially available in Canada.

## Category

Antiarrhythmic—Isoproterenol; Phenylephrine.

Cardiac stimulant—Dobutamine; Dopamine; Epinephrine.
Vasopressor—Dopamine; Ephedrine; Epinephrine; Mephentermine; Metaraminol; Methoxamine; Norepinephrine; Phenylephrine.

## Indications

### Accepted
Bradycardia (treatment)—Isoproterenol is indicated for the temporary control of hemodynamically significant bradycardia, such as bradycardia associated with a denervated transplanted heart or third degree heart block due to conduction system disease. Electrical pacing is the preferred treatment for maintenance of an adequate ventricular rate and isoproterenol is used only for temporary support when electrical pacing is unavailable. Isoproterenol may also be used in long QT-related arrhythmias where underlying bradycardia is common.

Hypotension, acute (prophylaxis and treatment) or

Shock (treatment)—The sympathomimetic agents (except isoproterenol) are indicated for the correction of hypotension, unresponsive to adequate fluid volume replacement, as part of shock syndrome caused by myocardial infarction, trauma, bacteremia, open-heart surgery, renal failure, chronic cardiac decompensation, drug overdose, or other major systemic illness.

The specific choice of drug must be determined by clinical assessment. This assessment may include hemodynamic status, mental status, urine output, and other measures of tissue perfusion. In refractory cases, the use of multiple drug therapy may be necessary for blood pressure support.

In septic shock, low-dose dopamine may be used in conjunction with norepinephrine to maintain renal blood flow.

In hypovolemic shock, the sympathomimetic agents should be used only as adjuncts to energetic fluid volume replacement to provide temporary support for maintaining coronary and cerebral artery perfusion until volume replacement therapy is completed. These medications must not be used as the sole therapy in hypovolemic patients.

In acute hypotension associated with myocardial infarction, sympathomimetic agent-induced increases in myocardial oxygen demand and the work of the heart may outweigh the beneficial effect of the medication. Also, cardiac arrhythmias induced by the sympathomimetic agents may be more likely to occur in patients with myocardial infarction.

Although norepinephrine is indicated in the treatment of acute hypotension occurring during spinal anesthesia, vasopressors that have a longer duration of action (e.g., metaraminol or phenylephrine) are also useful.

Ephedrine is indicated for the correction of hypotension secondary to spinal or other types of nontypical conduction anesthesia. It is also used in hypotensive states following sympathectomy, or following overdose with ganglionic blocking agents, antiadrenergic agents, or other medications that lower blood pressure in the treatment of hypertension.

Metaraminol is indicated for the prevention and treatment of acute hypotension occurring with spinal anesthesia and in the adjunctive treatment of hypotension resulting from hemorrhage, reactions to medications, surgical complications, and shock associated with brain damage due to trauma or tumor. However, metaraminol is not indicated as the sole treatment for hypotension secondary to decreased plasma volume.

Mephentermine is indicated in the treatment of hypotension secondary to ganglionic blockade and hypotension occurring with spinal anesthesia.

Methoxamine is indicated for supporting, restoring, or maintaining blood pressure during general anesthesia with agents that sensitize the myocardium to arrhythmias, such as halothane.

Dobutamine is not recommended for the adjunctive treatment of hypovolemic shock.

Cardiac output, low (treatment) or

Congestive heart failure (treatment)—Dobutamine is indicated to improve cardiac function during cardiac decompensation in congestive heart failure or depressed contractility from cardiac or major vascular surgery.

If a vasopressor is also needed, norepinephrine or dopamine is useful for short-term management. However, stimulation of alpha-1 adrenergic receptors produces vasoconstriction, which is undesirable in most patients with severe heart failure. In certain circumstances, a vasodilating agent such as nitroprusside or nitroglycerin may be used as an adjunct to dobutamine to decrease afterload and pulmonary pressures.

Cardiac arrest (treatment)—Epinephrine is indicated during resuscitation of cardiac standstill or cardiac arrest. Epinephrine is used as an adjunct to restore cardiac rhythm in the treatment of cardiac arrest due to

various causes. It also has beneficial hemodynamic effects in the setting of cardiopulmonary resuscitation (CPR), improving myocardial and cerebral blood flow. Epinephrine injection may be used for resuscitation in cardiac arrest following anesthetic accidents; however, it should be used with great caution in patients receiving halogenated hydrocarbon anesthetics, especially halothane, because these anesthetics sensitize the myocardium and cardiac arrhythmias may be induced.

In acute attacks of ventricular standstill, physical measures should be used prior to administration of epinephrine. However, if external cardiac compression and attempts to restore circulation by electrical defibrillation or use of a pacemaker fail, intravenous injection of epinephrine into a major vein may be effective.

Shock, anaphylactic (treatment)—Epinephrine injection is indicated in the emergency treatment of anaphylactic shock.

Tachycardia, supraventricular, paroxysmal (treatment)—Phenylephrine is indicated in the termination of some episodes of paroxysmal supraventricular tachycardia (PSVT).

### Unaccepted
Isoproterenol is no longer routinely recommended as an inotropic agent. It has been replaced in most clincial settings by newer agents that are less prone to induce ischemia, arrhythmias, or a hypotensive response.

Mephentermine is not recommended in the treatment of hypotension induced by chlorpromazine because it may potentiate, rather than correct, the hypotension secondary to the adrenolytic effects of chlorpromazine.

## Pharmacology/Pharmacokinetics

### Physicochemical characteristics
Molecular weight—
    Dobutamine: 337.85.
    Dopamine hydrochloride: 189.64.
    Ephedrine sulfate: 428.54.
    Epinephrine: 183.21.
    Isoproterenol hydrochloride: 247.72.
    Mephentermine sulfate: 424.60.
    Metaraminol bitartrate: 317.29.
    Methoxamine hydrochloride: 247.72.
    Norepinephrine bitartrate: 337.28.
    Phenylephrine hydrochloride: 203.67.
Other characteristics—
    pH—
        Dobutamine—9.4
        Dopamine Hydrochloride Injection, USP—2.5 to 5

### Mechanism of action/Effect
Dobutamine—
    A direct-acting inotropic agent. Dobutamine acts primarily on beta-1 adrenergic receptors, with little effect on beta-2 or alpha receptors. Dobutamine directly stimulates beta-1 receptors of the heart to increase myocardial contractility and stroke volume, resulting in increased cardiac output. Coronary blood flow and myocardial oxygen consumption are usually increased because of increased myocardial contractility. Dobutamine has little effect on systemic vascular resistance, and systolic blood pressure and pulse pressure may remain unchanged or be increased because of increased cardiac output. However, in septic patients with decreased systemic vascular resistance, dobutamine may lower blood pressure without increasing cardiac output. Dobutamine reduces elevated ventricular filling pressure (preload reduction) and facilitates atrioventricular (AV) node conduction. At appropriate doses, an increase in heart rate does not usually occur, but excessive doses have a chronotropic effect. Renal blood flow and urine output may be improved as a result of increased cardiac output rather than as a dopaminergic effect.
Dopamine—
    Dopamine stimulates postsynaptic beta-1 receptors in the myocardium, mediating its positive inotropic and chronotropic effects. Dopamine causes vascular relaxation and promotes sodium excretion through its stimulation of postsynaptic dopamine-1 receptors on vascular smooth muscle and on the kidney. In addition, dopamine stimulates both alpha-1 and alpha-2 receptors, which mediate smooth muscle vasoconstriction. These pharmacologic effects are dose-related, requiring various infusion rates of dopamine to activate different receptors.
    In low doses (0.5 to 3 mcg per kg of body weight [mcg/kg] per minute), dopamine acts predominantly on dopaminergic receptors to cause vasodilation in the renal, mesenteric, coronary, and intracerebral vascular beds. Renal vasodilation results in increased renal blood flow, glomerular filtration rate, urine flow (usually), and sodium excretion.

In low to moderate doses (2 to 10 mcg/kg per minute), beta-1 receptors are stimulated, resulting in a positive inotropic effect on the myocardium and an increase in cardiac output. Systolic blood pressure and pulse pressure may be increased with either no change or a slight increase in diastolic blood pressure. Total peripheral resistance is usually unchanged. Coronary blood flow and myocardial oxygen consumption are usually increased.

In higher doses (10 mcg/kg per minute or above), alpha-adrenergic receptor stimulation predominates, resulting in increased peripheral vascular resistance and renal vasoconstriction (this vasoconstriction may decrease previously increased renal blood flow and urine output). Both systolic and diastolic blood pressures are increased as a result of increased cardiac output and increased peripheral resistance.

Ephedrine—
Ephedrine stimulates both alpha and beta adrenergic receptors and enhances the release of endogenous norepinephrine from sympathetic neurons, resulting in increased systolic and diastolic blood pressure and increased cardiac output. Ephedrine also stimulates the central nervous system (CNS), although to a lesser extent than does amphetamine.

Epinephrine—
Epinephrine predominantly stimulates alpha and beta-1 adrenergic receptors, and has moderate activity at beta-2 adrenergic receptors. At very low doses, (less than 0.01 mcg/kg per minute), epinephrine may decrease blood pressure through dilatation of skeletal muscle vasculature. At doses of 0.04 to 0.1 mcg/kg per minute, stimulation of beta-receptors predominates, increasing heart rate, cardiac output, and stroke volume and decreasing peripheral vascular resistance. At doses exceeding 0.2 mcg/kg per minute, stimulation of alpha adrenergic receptors produces vasoconstriction and increased total peripheral resistance. Doses exceeding 0.3 mcg/kg per minute decrease renal blood flow, gastrointestinal motility, pyloric tone, and splanchnic vascular bed perfusion.

Epinephrine also increases conduction velocity in the myocardium and increases ectopic pacemaker activity. Myocardial oxygen demand is also increased.

Isoproterenol—
Isoproterenol is a pure beta receptor agonist. It is a potent inotrope and chronotrope, increasing cardiac output despite a reduction in mean blood pressure due to peripheral vasodilation.

Mephentermine—
Mephentermine is an alpha adrenergic receptor agonist, but also acts indirectly by releasing endogenous norepinephrine. Cardiac output and systolic and diastolic pressures are usually increased. A change in heart rate is variable, depending on the degree of vagal tone. Sometimes the net vascular effect may be vasodilation. Large doses may depress the myocardium or produce central nervous system (CNS) effects.

Metaraminol—
Metaraminol acts directly on peripheral alpha adrenergic receptors, as well as, indirectly through release of endogenous norepinephrine. Metaraminol produces a positive inotropic effect on the heart and peripheral vasoconstriction.

Methoxamine—
Methoxamine is a relatively selective alpha-1 adrenergic receptor agonist, producing an increase in peripheral vascular resistance. At high doses beta adrenergic receptors may be stimulated, resulting in increased blood pressure. A reflex sinus bradycardia may occur.

Norepinephrine—
Norepinephrine stimulates alpha and beta-1 adrenergic receptors in a dose-related fashion. At lower doses (less than 2 mcg per minute), stimulation of beta-1 receptors results in a positive inotropic and chronotropic effect. At higher doses (greater than 4 mcg per minute), the alpha adrenergic effect predominates, resulting in elevated total peripheral resistance. Chronotropy diminishes as a result of baroreceptor-mediated vagal stimulation.

Norepinephrine may produce vasoconstriction in the mesenteric vascular bed, which can induce splanchnic ischemia and facilitate bacterial translocation from the gut. Norepinephrine also increases renal vascular resistance. However, renal perfusion may actually increase in hypotensive patients through norepinephrine's effect of increasing blood pressure.

Phenylephrine—
Phenylephrine is primarily an alpha-1 adrenergic agonist, which causes marked vasoconstriction.

The following table represents relative receptor agonist activity of the sympathomimetic agents—

| | RECEPTOR TYPE | | | | |
|---|---|---|---|---|---|
| | Alpha-1 | Alpha-2 | Beta-1 | Beta-2 | Dopamine |
| Norepinephrine | +++ | +++ | ++ | None | None |
| Epinephrine | | | | | None |
|   low dose | | | ++ | +++ | |
|   moderate dose | + | | +++ | +++ | |
|   high dose | +++ | +++ | +++ | +++ | |
| Dobutamine | + | None | +++ | + | None |
| Dopamine | | None | | None | |
|   low dose | | | | | +++ |
|   moderate dose | | | +++ | | |
|   high dose | +++ | | | | |
| Isoproterenol | None | None | +++ | +++ | None |
| Ephedrine (indirect effects via norepinephrine release) | +++ | +++ | ++ | None | None |
| Mephentermine | +++ | None | None | None | None |
| Metaraminol (indirect effects via norepinephrine release) | +++ | +++ | ++ | None | None |
| Methoxamine | +++ | None | None | None | None |
| Phenylephrine | +++ | None | None | None | None |

**Distribution**
Dopamine—
Adults: Widely distributed in the body; does not extensively cross the blood-brain barrier. About 25% of a dose is taken up into specialized neurosecretory vesicles where hydroxylation occurs, forming norepinephrine.
Neonates: Apparent volume of distribution—1.8 L per kg.

**Biotransformation**
Dobutamine—Hepatic, to inactive compounds.
Dopamine—Metabolized in the liver, kidney, and plasma by monoamine oxidase (MAO) and catechol-O-methyltransferase (COMT) to inactive metabolites.
Ephedrine—Small amounts in the liver.
Epinephrine—Metabolized by monoamine oxidase (MAO) and catechol-O-methyltransferase (COMT).
Isoproterenol—Metabolism in liver, lungs, and other tissues.
Mephentermine—Hepatic, by N-demethylation and then p-hydroxylation.
Metaraminol—Hepatic.
Methoxamine—Hepatic.
Norepinephrine—Metabolized in the liver, kidney, and plasma by monoamine oxidase (MAO) and catechol-O-methyltransferase (COMT) to inactive metabolites.
Phenylephrine—Hepatic and gastrointestinal.

**Half-life**
Dobutamine—
About 2 minutes.
Dopamine—
Adults:
Plasma—About 2 minutes.
Elimination—About 9 minutes.
Neonates:
Elimination—6.9 minutes (range 5 to 11 minutes).
Epinephrine—
1 minute.
Ephedrine—
3 to 6 hours.
Mephentermine—
17 to 18 hours.
Norepinephrine—
1 minute.

**Onset of action**
Dobutamine—
1 to 2 minutes; however, up to 10 minutes may be required when infusion rate is slow.
Dopamine—
Within 5 minutes.
Epinephrine—
Rapid.
Isoproterenol—
Less than 5 minutes.

Mephentermine—
Intravenous: Very rapid.
Intramuscular: 5 to 15 minutes.
Metaraminol—
Intravenous: 1 to 2 minutes.
Intramuscular: About 10 minutes.
Methoxamine—
0.5 to 2 minutes.
Norepinephrine—
Rapid.
Phenylephrine—
Very rapid.

**Duration of action**
Dobutamine—
Less than 5 minutes.
Dopamine—
Less than 10 minutes.
Ephedrine—
1 hour.
Epinephrine—
1 to 2 minutes.
Isoproterenol—
10 minutes.
Mephentermine—
Intravenous: 15 to 30 minutes.
Intramuscular: 1 to 4 hours.
Metaraminol—
20 to 60 minutes.
Methoxamine—
5 to 15 minutes.
Norepinephrine—
1 to 2 minutes.
Phenylephrine—
5 to 20 minutes.

**Elimination**
Dobutamine—Renal; as metabolites.
Dopamine—Renal; 80% of a dose excreted within 24 hours, primarily as metabolites. A very small fraction of a dose is excreted unchanged.
Ephedrine—Renal; mostly as unchanged drug.
Mephentermine—Renal.
Methoxamine—Renal.
Norepinephrine—Renal; primarily as metabolites.

## Precautions to Consider

### Cross-sensitivity and/or related problems
Dobutamine, dopamine, epinephrine, isoproterenol, metaraminol, methoxamine, norepinephrine, and phenylephrine preparations contain sulfites.

### Carcinogenicity/Mutagenicity
Long-term studies have not been done.

### Pregnancy/Reproduction
Fertility—*Dobutamine:* Studies in rats and rabbits have revealed no evidence of fertility impairment.
*Dopamine:* Long-term studies have not been done.
*Isoproterenol:* Studies have not been done.
*Mephentermine:* Long-term studies have not been done.
*Metaraminol:* Long-term studies have not been done.
*Methoxamine:* Long-term studies have not been done.
*Norepinephrine:* Studies have not been done.
*Phenylephrine:* Long-term studies have not been done.

Pregnancy—
*Dobutamine—*
Adequate and well-controlled studies in humans have not been done.
Reproduction studies in rats and rabbits found no evidence of teratogenicity or harm to the fetus.
FDA Pregnancy Category C.
*Dopamine—*
Adequate and well-controlled studies in humans have not been done.
Studies in animals have not revealed evidence of teratogenic effects. However, administration of dopamine to pregnant rats resulted in a decreased survival rate of the newborn and a potential for the development of cataracts in survivors.
FDA Pregnancy Category C.
*Ephedrine—*
Adequate and well-controlled studies have not be done in humans.
Studies have not been done in animals.
FDA Pregnancy Category C.

*Epinephrine—*
Adequate and well-controlled studies in humans have not been done.
Studies in rats given epinephrine at doses 25 times the human dose have revealed teratogenic effects.
FDA Pregnancy Category C.
*Isoproterenol—*
Adequate and well-controlled studies have not been done in humans.
Studies have not been done in animals.
FDA Pregnancy Category C.
*Mephentermine—*
It is not known whether mephenterine crosses the placenta. However, mephentermine may increase uterine contractions in pregnant women, especially during the third trimester.
Studies have not been done in animals.
FDA Pregnancy Category C.
*Metaraminol—*
Adequate and well-controlled studies have not been done in humans.
Metaraminol given to pregnant ewes at a dose of 0.025 mg per kg of body weight (mg/kg) decreased uterine blood flow.
FDA Pregnancy Category C.
*Methoxamine—*
Adequate and well-controlled studies in humans have not been done. However, a fetal death has been reported when the mother received methoxamine concomitantly with other medications. A direct causal relationship has not been established.
Methoxamine administered to pregnant ewes and monkeys at doses comparable to those used in humans decreased uterine blood flow and heart rate, and adversely affected fetal acid-base status, as evidenced by hypoxia, hypercarbia, and metabolic acidosis. In pregnant ewes, an inverse relationship between pressor response to methoxamine and uteroplacental blood flow was shown at doses ranging from 0.025 to 0.2 mg/kg. A study in baboons given methoxamine at a dose of 1.3 mg/kg over 57 minutes revealed a decrease in uterine blood flow and a possible association with fetal asphyxia.
FDA Pregnancy Category C.
*Norepinephrine—*
Adequate and well-controlled studies have not been done in humans.
Studies have not been done in animals.
FDA Pregnancy Category C.
*Phenylephrine—*
Adequate and well-controlled studies have not been done in humans.
Studies have not been done in animals.
FDA Pregnancy Category C.

Labor and delivery—If vasopressor medications are used to correct hypotension or added to the local anesthetic solution during labor and delivery, some oxytocic medications (e.g., vasopressin, ergotamine, ergonovine, methylergonovine) may cause severe persistent hypertension, and rupture of a cerebral blood vessel may occur during the postpartum period.
*Ephedrine:* Ephedrine, when used to maintain blood pressure during low or other spinal anesthesia for delivery, may accelerate fetal heart rate. Use is not recommended when maternal blood pressure exceeds 130/80 mm Hg.
*Epinephrine:* Use during labor is not recommended because epinephrine may delay the second stage of labor.
*Mephentermine:* Mephentermine may cause a decrease in uterine blood flow, which may result in fetal hypoxia. Transient fetal hypertension has also been reported in animals.

### Breast-feeding
It is not known whether these medications are distributed into breast milk.

### Pediatrics
*Dobutamine—* Dobutamine has been studied in a limited number of pediatric patients up to 18 years of age. There do not appear to be pediatric-specific problems that would limit the usefulness of dobutamine in pediatric patients.
*Dopamine—* Dopamine has been studied in a limited number of pediatric patients up to 18 years of age. Close hemodynamic monitoring is recommended since there is a lack of controlled studies investigating age-dependent dosages and the maximum dosage at which therapeutic response occurs without causing toxicity. In addition, cardiac arrhythmias and gangrene due to extravasation have been reported in pediatric patients.

*Epinephrine*— Epinephrine has been used in pediatric patients during cardiac arrest and there do not appear to be pediatrics-specific problems that would limit its usefulness in this setting. However, caution is recommended to avoid errors in concentration selection and dosing, since two different dilutions of epinephrine are necessary for the dosing regimen.

## Geriatrics

*Isoproterenol*— Data seem to indicate that elderly patients may exhibit a decreased chronotropic and peripheral vascular response to isoproterenol.

*Norepinephrine*— The pressor response to norepinephrine does not appear to be altered with aging.

*Phenylephrine*— The baroreceptor reflex response to phenylephrine appears to decrease with age.

## Drug interactions and/or related problems

The following drug interactions and/or related problems have been selected on the basis of their potential clinical significance (possible mechanism in parentheses where appropriate)—not necessarily inclusive (» = major clinical significance).

Note: Combinations containing any of the following medications, depending on the amount present, may also interact with this medication.

Alpha-adrenergic blocking agents, such as:
   Doxazosin
   Labetalol
   Phenoxybenzamine
   Phentolamine
   Prazosin
   Terazosin
   Tolazoline, or
Other medications with alpha-adrenergic blocking action, such as:
   Haloperidol
   Loxapine
   Phenothiazines
   Thioxanthenes
   (concurrent use may antagonize the peripheral vasoconstriction of sympathomimetic agents; however, phentolamine may be used for therapeutic benefit)

» Anesthetics, hydrocarbon inhalation, such as:
   Chloroform
   Enflurane
»  Halothane
   Isoflurane
   Methoxyflurane
   (concurrent use of these medications with the sympathomimetic agents may increase the risk of severe atrial and ventricular arrhythmias because these anesthetics greatly sensitize the myocardium; sympathomimetic agents should be used with caution and in substantially reduced doses in patients receiving these anesthetics)

   (enflurane, isoflurane, or methoxyflurane may also sensitize the myocardium to the effects of sympathomimetics; caution is recommended during concurrent use)

» Antidepressants, tricyclic or
» Maprotiline
   (concurrent use may potentiate the cardiovascular and pressor effects of sympathomimetic agents, possibly resulting in arrhythmias, tachycardia, or severe hypertension or hyperpyrexia)

Antihypertensives or
Diuretics used as antihypertensives
   (antihypertensive effects may be reduced when these medications are used concurrently; the patient should be carefully monitored to confirm that the desired effect is being obtained)

Beta-adrenergic blocking agents, ophthalmic or
» Beta-adrenergic blocking agents, systemic
   (concurrent use with sympathomimetic agents may result in mutual inhibition of therapeutic effects; beta-blockade may antagonize the beta-1 adrenergic cardiac effects of sympathomimetic agents)

» Cocaine, mucosal-local
   (concurrent use with sympathomimetic agents may increase the cardiovascular effects of either or both medications and the risk of adverse effects)

» Digitalis glycosides
   (concurrent use with sympathomimetic agents possessing beta-1 adrenergic agonist activity may increase the risk of cardiac arrhythmias; in addition, concurrent use may produce additive inotropic effects; although these medications may be used with digitalis glycosides for therapeutic advantage, caution and close

electrocardiographic monitoring are recommended during concurrent use)

Diuretics
   (concurrent use may increase the diuretic effect of the diuretic medications or dopamine as a result of dopamine's direct action on dopaminergic receptors to produce vasodilation of renal vasculature and increase renal blood flow; dopamine also has a direct natriuretic effect)

» Doxapram
   (concurrent use may increase the pressor effects of either the sympathomimetic agents or doxapram)

Ergonovine or
» Ergotamine or
Methylergonovine or
Methysergide or
Oxytocin
   (concurrent use of ergonovine, methylergonovine, or methysergide with a sympathomimetic agent may result in enhanced vasoconstriction; dosage adjustments may be necessary)

   (concurrent use of ergotamine with these medications may produce peripheral vascular ischemia and gangrene and is not recommended)

   (concurrent use of ergonovine, ergotamine, methylergonovine, or oxytocin may potentiate the pressor effect of these medications with possible severe hypertension and rupture of cerebral blood vessels)

Guanadrel or
Guanethidine
   (in addition to possibly decreasing the hypotensive effect of guanadrel or guanethidine, concurrent use may potentiate the pressor response to the sympathomimetic agents; these actions are a result of inhibition of sympathomimetic uptake by adrenergic neurons and may lead to hypertension and cardiac arrhythmias)

Levodopa
   (concurrent use with dopamine may increase the possibility of cardiac arrhythmias; dosage reduction of the sympathomimetic is recommended)

Mecamylamine or
Methyldopa
   (in addition to possibly decreasing the hypotensive effects of these medications, concurrent use may enhance the pressor response to sympathomimetic agents)

Methylphenidate
   (concurrent use may potentiate the pressor effect of sympathomimetic agents)

» Monoamine oxidase (MAO) inhibitors, including furazolidone, procarbazine, and selegiline
   (concurrent use may prolong and intensify cardiac stimulation and vasopressor effects because of the release of catecholamines, which accumulate in intraneuronal storage sites during MAO inhibitor therapy; this may result in headache, cardiac arrhythmias, vomiting, or sudden and severe hypertensive and/or hyperpyretic crises; for patients who have been receiving MAO inhibitors 2 to 3 weeks prior to administration of sympathomimetic agents, the initial dosage should be reduced to no more than one-tenth of the usual dose)

Nitrates
   (concurrent use with sympathomimetic agents may reduce the antianginal effects of these medications; also, nitrates may counteract the pressor effect of sympathomimetic agents, possibly resulting in hypotension; however, nitrates and sympathomimetic agents may be used concurrently for therapeutic advantage)

Phenoxybenzamine
   (in addition to phenoxybenzamine antagonizing the peripheral vasoconstriction of the sympathomimetic agents, concurrent use of phenoxybenzamine may produce an exaggerated hypotensive response and tachycardia)

Phenytoin, and possibly other hydantoins
   (concurrent use with dopamine may result in sudden hypotension and bradycardia; this reaction is considered to be dose-rate dependent; if anticonvulsant therapy is necessary during administration of dopamine, an alternative to phenytoin should be considered; caution is also advised with concurrent use of other hydantoins)

Rauwolfia alkaloids
   (in addition to possibly decreasing the hypotensive effects of rauwolfia alkaloids, concurrent use may theoretically prolong the action of direct-acting sympathomimetics, such as dopamine, by preventing uptake into storage granules; a "denervation

supersensitivity" response is also possible; although concurrent use is not known to produce severe adverse effects, a significant increase in blood pressure has been documented when phenylephrine ophthalmic drops were administered to patients taking reserpine, and caution and close observation are recommended)

Sympathomimetics, other
(concurrent use may increase the cardiovascular effects and the potential for side effects)

Thyroid hormones
(concurrent use may increase the effects of either these medications or the sympathomimetic agents; thyroid hormones enhance risk of coronary insufficiency when sympathomimetic agents are administered to patients with coronary artery disease; dosage adjustment is recommended, although the problem is reduced in euthyroid patients)

## Medical considerations/Contraindications
The medical considerations/contraindications included here have been selected on the basis of their potential clinical significance (reasons given in parentheses where appropriate)—not necessarily inclusive (» = major clinical significance).

*Except under special circumstances, this medication should not be used when the following medical problems exist:*

» Asymmetric septal hypertrophy (idiopathic hypertrophic subaortic stenosis)
(obstruction may increase as myocardial contractility improves with sympathomimetic agents possessing beta-1 adrenergic agonist activity)

» Pheochromocytoma
(severe hypertension may occur)

» Tachyarrhythmias or
Ventricular fibrillation
(exacerbation of arrhythmia may occur; however, epinephrine may be used as an adjunct in the treatment of ventricular fibrillation)

*Risk-benefit should be considered when the following medical problems exist:*

Acidosis, metabolic or
Hypercapnia or
Hypoxia
(may reduce effectiveness and/or increase incidence of side/adverse effects of the sympathomimetic agents; should be corrected prior to or concurrently with administration of sympathomimetic agents)

Atrial fibrillation
(rapid ventricular response may occur since dobutamine facilitates atrioventricular conduction; in patients who have atrial fibrillation with rapid ventricular response, a digitalis preparation should be used prior to institution of therapy with dobutamine)

Glaucoma, narrow angle
(condition may be exacerbated with sympathomimetic agents possessing alpha-1 adrenergic agonist activity)

Hypertension, pulmonary
(condition may be exacerbated due to pulmonary vasoconstriction)

» Hypovolemia
(prior to initiation of sympathomimetic therapy, hypovolemia should be corrected with appropriate volume expanders; volume should be maintained throughout treatment)

Mechanical obstruction, severe, such as severe valvular aortic stenosis
(these agents may be ineffective)

» Myocardial infarction
(excessive doses of sympathomimetic agents possessing beta-1 adrenergic agonist activity may intensify ischemia by increasing myocardial oxygen demands)

Occlusive vascular disease, history of, including:
Arterial embolism
Atherosclerosis
Buerger's disease
Cold injury, e.g., frostbite
Diabetic endarteritis
Raynaud's disease
(possible risk of necrosis and gangrene with sympathomimetic agents possessing alpha-1 adrenergic agonist activity, patients should be closely monitored for decreased circulation to extremities; if decreased circulation occurs, rate of infusion should be reduced or the infusion discontinued)

Sensitivity to other sympathomimetics
» Tachyarrhythmias or ventricular arrhythmias
(condition may be exacerbated)

*For dopamine and dextrose injection only*
Diabetes mellitus, subclinical or overt
(condition may be exacerbated)

## Patient monitoring
The following may be especially important in patient monitoring (other tests may be warranted in some patients, depending on condition; » = major clinical significance):

» Blood pressure, preferably intra-arterial and
» Electrocardiogram (ECG) and
» Urine flow
(continuous monitoring is recommended during therapy with sympathomimetic agents)

» Cardiac output and
» Central venous pressure and
» Pulmonary artery pressure and
» Pulmonary capillary wedge pressure
(recommended during therapy with sympathomimetic agents; however, therapy with low-dose dopamine may not require such intensive monitoring)

*For dobutamine and epinephrine, in addition to the above*
Potassium, serum
(monitoring may be considered due to risk of hypokalemia)

# Side/Adverse Effects

Note: *Peripheral vasoconstriction, possibly leading to necrosis or gangrene, may occur with prolonged use of sympathomimetic agents with alpha-1 adrenergic agonist activity in high doses or low doses in the presence of peripheral vascular disease.*

*Allergic reaction may occur in preparations containing sulfites.*

The following side/adverse effects have been selected on the basis of their potential clinical significance (possible signs and symptoms in parentheses where appropriate)—not necessarily inclusive:

## Those indicating need for medical attention
Incidence less frequent
*Angina; bradycardia; dyspnea; hypertension; hypotension; palpitations; tachycardia; ventricular arrhythmias*—especially with high doses

Note: *Angina, dyspnea, palpitations, tachycardia, and ventricular arrhythmias are associated with agents possessing beta-adrenergic agonist activity. They may also occur with agents possessing alpha-adrenergic agonist activity if marked degrees of hypertension are induced.*

Incidence rare—for dobutamine and epinephrine
*Hypokalemia*
Incidence rare—for dopamine
*Polyuria*

Note: *Polyuria has been reported in patients receiving dopamine at nonrenal doses.*

## Those indicating need for medical attention only if they continue or are bothersome
Incidence more frequent
*Headache; nausea or vomiting*
Incidence less frequent
*Nervousness or restlessness*

# Overdose
For more information on the management of overdose or unintentional ingestion, **contact a Poison Control Center** (see *Poison Control Center Listing* ).

## Clinical effects of overdose
The following effects have been selected on the basis of their potential clinical significance (possible signs and symptoms in parentheses where appropriate)—not necessarily inclusive:
*Hypertension, severe*

## Treatment of overdose
For excessive hypertensive effect—The rate of administration should be reduced or the medication temporarily discontinued until blood pressure is decreased. Additional measures are usually not necessary because the duration of action of these agents is short. However, if reduction in the rate of administration or discontinuation of therapy fails to lower the blood pressure, a short-acting alpha-adrenergic blocking agent may be administered.

# General Dosing Information

Patients receiving sympathomimetic agent therapy should be closely monitored. See *Patient monitoring.*

Sympathomimetic agent therapy is not a substitute for replacement of blood, plasma, fluids, and/or electrolytes.

Prior to initiation of therapy, hypovolemia should be fully corrected, if possible, with either whole blood or a plasma volume expander as indicated.

An infusion pump or other suitable metering device should be used to control the rate of infusion in order to avoid unintentional administration of bolus doses.

Dosage must be adjusted to meet the individual requirements of each patient, on the basis of clinical response. Some patients may need higher than usually recommended doses for a time.

Infusions of sympathomimetic agents should be given into a large vein, or preferably, directly into the central circulation.

Caution is recommended to avoid extravasation, which may cause tissue necrosis and sloughing of surrounding tissues.

When discontinuing therapy, the dosage should be reduced gradually, since sudden cessation of therapy may result in severe hypotension. Intravascular fluid should be repleted if necessary to avoid hypotension.

## For treatment of adverse effects

For extravasation ischemia—To prevent necrosis and sloughing of tissue in areas where extravasation has occurred, the site should be infiltrated promptly with 10 to 15 mL of 0.9% sodium chloride injection containing 5 to 10 mg of phentolamine. A syringe with a fine hypodermic needle should be used and the solution infiltrated liberally throughout the affected area. If the area is infiltrated within 12 hours, the sympathetic blockade with phentolamine produces immediate and noticeable local hyperemic changes. This treatment should be proportionally reduced for pediatric patients.

---

## *DOBUTAMINE*

---

# Summary of Differences

Indications:
    Indicated for congestive heart failure and low cardiac output.
Pharmacology/pharmacokinetics:
    Mechanism of action/effect—Primarily beta-1 adrenergic agonist; mild alpha-1 and beta-2 agonist.
Precautions to consider:
    Patient monitoring—Serum potassium.
Side/adverse effects:
    Hypokalemia.

# Additional Dosing Information

The concentration of solution administered depends on the dosage and fluid requirements of the patient, but should not exceed 5 mg of dobutamine per mL.

# Parenteral Dosage Forms

Note: The dosing and strengths of the dosage forms available are expressed in terms of dobutamine base (not the hydrochloride salt).

## DOBUTAMINE HYDROCHLORIDE INJECTION

### Usual adult dose

Cardiac stimulant—
    Intravenous infusion, administered at a rate of 2.5 to 10 mcg (0.0025 to 0.01 mg) (base) per kg of body weight per minute.
    Rates of infusion for concentrations of 250, 500, and 1000 mcg per mL:

| Drug delivery rate (mcg/kg/min) | 250 mcg/mL* (mL/kg/min) | Infusion delivery rate 500 mcg/mL† (mL/kg/min) | 1000 mcg/mL‡ (mL/kg/min) |
|---|---|---|---|
| 2.5 | 0.01 | 0.005 | 0.0025 |
| 5 | 0.02 | 0.01 | 0.005 |
| 7.5 | 0.03 | 0.015 | 0.0075 |
| 10 | 0.04 | 0.02 | 0.01 |
| 12.5 | 0.05 | 0.025 | 0.0125 |
| 15 | 0.06 | 0.03 | 0.015 |

*250 mg per L of diluent.
†500 mg per L or 250 mg/500 mL of diluent.
‡1000 mg per L or 250 mg/250 mL of diluent.

### Usual pediatric dose

Cardiac stimulant—
    Intravenous infusion, 5 to 20 mcg per kg of body weight per minute.

### Size(s) usually available

U.S.—
    12.5 mg (base) per mL (Rx) [*Dobutrex* (sodium bisulfite 0.24 mg per mL)].
Canada—
    12.5 mg (base) per mL (Rx) [*Dobutrex* (sodium bisulfite 0.245 mg per mL)].

### Packaging and storage

Prior to dilution, store between 15 and 30 °C (59 and 86 °F), unless otherwise specified by manufacturer.

### Preparation of dosage form

The solution must be further diluted to at least 50 mL prior to administration in 5% dextrose injection, 5% dextrose and 0.45% sodium chloride injection, 5% dextrose and 0.9% sodium chloride injection, 10% dextrose injection, lactated Ringer's injection, 5% dextrose in lactated Ringer's injection, 0.9% sodium chloride injection, or sodium lactate injection.

### Stability

Solutions diluted for intravenous infusion should be used within 24 hours. Freezing may cause crystallization and should be avoided.
Pink discoloration of dobutamine solution indicates slight oxidation of the medication, but there is no significant loss of potency if administered within the recommended time periods.

### Incompatibilities

Dobutamine is incompatible with alkaline solutions and should not be mixed with solutions such as 5% sodium bicarbonate injection.
Dobutamine injection should not be used in conjunction with other agents or diluents containing both sodium bisulfite and ethanol.
It is recommended that dobutamine injection not be mixed in the same solution with other medications.
Mixture or administration of dobutamine through the same intravenous line as heparin, hydrocortisone sodium succinate, cefazolin, cefamandole, neutral cephalothin, penicillin, or sodium ethacrynate is not recommended.

---

## *DOPAMINE*

---

# Summary of Differences

Pharmacology/pharmacokinetics:
    Mechanism of action/effect—Dose-related alpha, beta, and dopamine receptor agonist.
    Biotransformation—Metabolized by monoamine oxidase (MAO) and catechol-O-methyltransferase (COMT).
Precautions to consider:
    Drug interactions—Levodopa, phenytoin.
    Pediatrics—Cardiac arrhythmias and gangrene reported.
Side/adverse effects:
    Polyuria reported at nonrenal doses.

# Additional Dosing Information

Dopamine hydrochloride injection must be diluted prior to administration.

When dopamine hydrochloride and dextrose injection is used, the less concentrated 800 mcg (0.8 mg) per mL solution may be preferred when fluid expansion is not a problem. The more concentrated 1.6 or 3.2 mg per mL solutions may be preferred in patients who are fluid restricted or when a slower rate of infusion is desired.

# Parenteral Dosage Forms

## DOPAMINE HYDROCHLORIDE INJECTION USP

### Usual adult dose

Vasopressor or
Cardiac stimulant—
    Dopaminergic (renal) effects: Intravenous infusion, 0.5 to 3 mcg per kg of body weight per minute.
    Beta-1 adrenergic effects: Intravenous infusion, 2 to 10 mcg per kg of body weight per minute.
    Alpha adrenergic effects: Intravenous infusion, 10 mcg per kg of body weight per minute. The dose may be increased gradually as clinically indicated.

### Usual pediatric dose

Vasopressor or
Cardiac stimulant—
    Intravenous infusion, 5 to 20 mcg per kg of body weight per minute.

Note: Renal doses of dopamine (0.5 to 3 mcg per kg of body weight per minute) appear to be effective in increasing renal blood flow in pediatric patients, even in premature infants.

Close hemodynamic monitoring is recommended since only limited studies have been conducted in pediatric patients and there is a lack of data evaluating age-dependent doses.

### Strength(s) usually available
U.S.—

40 mg per mL (Rx) [*Intropin* (sodium metabisulfite 1%); GENERIC].
80 mg per mL (Rx) [*Intropin* (sodium metabisulfite 1%); GENERIC].
160 mg per mL (Rx) [*Intropin* (sodium metabisulfite 1%); GENERIC].

Canada—

40 mg per mL (Rx) [*Intropin* (sodium bisulfite 1%); *Revimine* (sodium metabisulfite 1%)].

### Packaging and storage
Store below 40 °C (104 °F), preferably between 15 and 30 °C (59 and 86 °F), unless otherwise specified by manufacturer. Protect from freezing.

### Preparation of dosage form
Diluents used for preparation of intravenous infusion solutions of dopamine include 0.9% sodium chloride injection, 5% dextrose injection, 5% dextrose and 0.9% sodium chloride injection, 5% dextrose in 0.45% sodium chloride solution, 5% dextrose in lactated Ringer's solution, sodium lactate injection (1/6 molar), and lactated Ringer's injection.

Sodium bicarbonate or other alkaline intravenous solutions should not be used as diluents because dopamine is inactivated in alkaline solutions.

To prepare an intravenous infusion of dopamine hydrochloride, 400 to 800 mg of dopamine should be added to 250 mL of an appropriate diluent solution. The resultant solution contains 1600 or 3200 mcg of dopamine per mL.

### Stability
Injection should be diluted immediately prior to administration.

After dilution in appropriate intravenous solution for infusion, dopamine is stable for at least 24 hours.

Dopamine injection should not be used if it is darker than slightly yellow or discolored.

### Incompatibilities
Dopamine is inactivated in alkaline solution (solution becomes pink to violet); therefore, it should not be added to 5% sodium bicarbonate or other alkaline diluent solution. Dopamine is also sensitive to oxidizing agents and iron salts.

## DOPAMINE HYDROCHLORIDE AND DEXTROSE INJECTION USP

### Usual adult dose
See *Dopamine Hydrochloride Injection USP*.

### Usual pediatric dose
See *Dopamine Hydrochloride Injection USP*.

### Strength(s) usually available
U.S.—

800 mcg (0.8 mg) of dopamine hydrochloride per mL and 5% dextrose (Rx) [GENERIC].
1.6 mg of dopamine hydrochloride per mL and 5% dextrose (Rx) [GENERIC].
3.2 mg of dopamine hydrochloride per mL and 5% dextrose (Rx) [GENERIC].

Canada—

800 mcg (0.8 mg) of dopamine hydrochloride per mL and 5% dextrose (Rx) [GENERIC].
1.6 mg of dopamine hydrochloride per mL and 5% dextrose (Rx) [GENERIC].

### Packaging and storage
Store below 40 °C (104 °F), preferably between 15 and 30 °C (59 and 86 °F), unless otherwise specified by manufacturer. Protect from freezing.

### Stability
Solution should not be administered unless it is clear.

Discard unused portion.

### Incompatibilities
Dopamine is inactivated in alkaline solution (solution becomes pink to violet); therefore, it should not be added to 5% sodium bicarbonate or other alkaline diluent solution. Dopamine is also sensitive to oxidizing agents and iron salts.

Dextrose solutions without electrolytes should not be administered simultaneously with blood through the same infusion set because of possible pseudoagglutination of red cells.

Additive medications should not be delivered via dopamine in dextrose injection because of possible incompatibilities.

---

## EPHEDRINE

## Summary of Differences
Pharmacology/pharmacokinetics:

Mechanism of action/effect—Alpha and beta-1 adrenergic agonist; indirect effects via norepinephrine release.

## Additional Dosing Information
When ephedrine is administered intravenously, the injection should be given slowly.

## Parenteral Dosage Forms
### EPHEDRINE SULFATE INJECTION USP

### Usual adult dose
Vasopressor—

Intramuscular or subcutaneous, 25 to 50 mg. Dose may be repeated based on blood pressure response.

Note: The intravenous route of administration may be used if an immediate effect is needed.

### Usual pediatric dose
Vasopressor—

Intravenous or subcutaneous, 750 mcg per kg of body weight or 25 mg per square meter of body surface area four times a day as needed according to patient response.

### Strength(s) usually available
U.S.—

25 mg per mL (Rx) [GENERIC].
50 mg per mL (Rx) [GENERIC].

Canada—

50 mg per mL (Rx) [GENERIC].

### Packaging and storage
Store below 40 °C (104 °F), preferably between 15 and 30 °C (59 and 86 °F), unless otherwise specified by manufacturer. Protect from light.

### Stability
Should not use if solution is not clear.

Unused portion should be discarded.

---

## EPINEPHRINE

## Summary of Differences
Indications:

Indicated for anaphylactic shock and cardiac arrest.

Pharmacology/pharmacokinetics:

Mechanism of action/effect—Has alpha and beta adrenergic receptor action.

Biotransformation—Metabolized by monoamine oxidase (MAO) and catechol-O-methyltransferase (COMT).

Precautions to consider:

Patient monitoring—Serum potassium.

Side/adverse effects:

Hypokalemia.

## Additional Dosing Information
The 1:1000 (1 mg/mL) concentration of epinephrine injection must be diluted before administering intravenously.

Intra-arterial administration of epinephrine injection is not recommended since marked vasoconstriction may result in gangrene.

## Parenteral Dosage Forms
### EPINEPHRINE HYDROCHLORIDE INJECTION

### Usual adult dose
Vasopressor—

Intravenous infusion, 1 mcg per minute. The dose may be titrated up to 2 to 10 mcg per minute for desired hemodynamic response.

Cardiac arrest—

Intravenous, 1 mg every three to five minutes during resuscitation.

Note: Epinephrine may be given by the endotracheal route. However, the optimal dose for this route of administration is not known. A dose that is at least two to two and a half times the peripheral intravenous dose may be needed.

## Usual pediatric dose
Cardiac arrest—
Neonates:
Intravenous, 10 to 30 mcg (0.01 to 0.03 mg) per kg of body weight every three to five minutes.

Note: Endotracheal administration may be used. However, this may result in low plasma concentrations.

Children:
Intravenous, 10 mcg (0.01 mg) per kg of body weight. Subsequent doses of 100 mcg (0.1 mg) per kg of body weight every three to five minutes may be given if needed. In refractory situations, following at least two standard doses, a higher dose may be used. Subsequent doses of 200 mcg (0.2 mg) per kg of body weight every five minutes may be given.

Note: Two different dilutions of epinephrine are necessary for this dosing regimen. **Caution** is recommended to avoid errors in concentration selection and dosing.

Endotracheal administration may be used. However, absorption and resulting plasma concentrations may be unpredictable.

## Strength(s) usually available
U.S.—
0.1 mg (100 mcg) per mL (1:10,000) (Rx/OTC) [GENERIC].
1 mg per mL (1:1000) (Rx) [*Adrenalin* (benzyl alcohol; chlorobutanol 0.5%; sodium bisulfite < 0.1% in ampuls and < 0.15% in vials); GENERIC].

Canada—
1 mg per mL (1:1000) (Rx) [GENERIC].

## Packaging and storage
Store below 40 °C (104 °F), preferably between 15 and 30 °C (59 and 86 °F), unless otherwise specified by manufacturer. Protect from light. Protect from freezing.

## Preparation of dosage form
Epinephrine 1:1000 should be diluted.

## Stability
Epinephrine is readily destroyed by alkalies and oxidizing agents (for example, oxygen, chlorine, bromine, iodine, permanganates, chromates, nitrites, and salts of easily reducible metals, especially iron). Do not use if solution is pinkish or brownish in color or contains a precipitate. Discard unused portion.

---

### ISOPROTERENOL

## Summary of Differences
Indications:
Indicated for bradycardia only.
Pharmacology/pharmacokinetics:
Mechanism of action/effect—Pure beta-adrenergic agonist.

## Parenteral Dosage Forms
### ISOPROTERENOL HYDROCHLORIDE INJECTION USP

## Usual adult dose
Bradycardia—
Intravenous infusion, initially, 2 mcg per minute, the dosage being gradually titrated according to heart rate up to 10 mcg per minute if needed.

## Usual pediatric dose
Dosage has not been established.

## Strength(s) usually available
U.S.—
20 mcg (0.02 mg) per mL (Rx) [GENERIC].
200 mcg (0.2 mg) per mL (Rx) [*Isuprel* (sodium chloride; sodium lactate; sodium metabisulfite; lactic acid); GENERIC].

Canada—
200 mcg (0.2 mg) per mL (Rx) [*Isuprel* (sodium lactate; sodium metabisulfite); GENERIC].

## Packaging and storage
Store below 40 °C (104 °F), preferably between 15 and 30 °C (59 and 86 °F), unless otherwise specified by manufacturer. Protect from light. Protect from freezing.

## Preparation of dosage form
For preparation of solutions for injection, see manufacturer's package insert.

## Stability
When exposed to air, alkalies, or metals, isoproterenol may turn pinkish to brownish in color because of oxidation. Do not use if solution is pinkish to brownish in color or contains a precipitate.

---

### MEPHENTERMINE

## Summary of Differences
Pharmacology/pharmacokinetics:
Mechanism of action/effect—Alpha-adrenergic agonist.

## Additional Dosing Information
Mephentermine can be administered intramuscularly.

## Parenteral Dosage Forms
### MEPHENTERMINE SULFATE

## Usual adult dose
Vasopressor—
Hypotension, secondary to spinal anesthesia (prophylaxis):
Intramuscular, 30 to 45 mg, administered ten to twenty minutes prior to anesthesia, operation, or termination of operative procedure.
Hypotension, secondary to spinal anesthesia (treatment):
Intravenous, 30 to 45 mg given as a single dose. Doses of 30 mg may be repeated as needed to maintain the desired level of blood pressure.
Intravenous infusion (continuous), administered as a 0.1% (1 mg per mL) solution in 5% dextrose in water, the rate of administration and duration of therapy being adjusted according to patient response.
In obstetrical patients—Intravenous, 15 mg initially, the dose being repeated if needed.

## Usual pediatric dose
Safety and efficacy have not been established.

## Strength(s) usually available
U.S.—
15 mg per mL (Rx) [*Wyamine* (methylparaben 1.8 mg, propylparaben 0.2 mg, sodium acetate)].
30 mg per mL (Rx) [*Wyamine* (methylparaben 1.8 mg; propylparaben 0.2 mg; sodium acetate)].

Canada—
Not commercially available.

## Packaging and storage
Store below 40 °C (104 °F), preferably between 15 and 30 °C (59 and 86 °F), unless otherwise specified by manufacturer. Protect from freezing.

## Preparation of dosage form
To prepare a 0.1% (1 mg per mL) solution of mephentermine for continuous intravenous infusion, 600 mg of mephentermine should be added to 500 mL of 5% dextrose in water.

## Stability
Do not use if solution is discolored or contains a precipitate.

---

### METARAMINOL

## Summary of Differences
Pharmacology/pharmacokinetics:
Mechanism of action/effect—Alpha and beta-1 receptor agonist; indirect effects via norepinephrine release.

## Additional Dosing Information
Metaraminol may be given intramuscularly, subcutaneously, or intravenously.

The site for intramuscular or subcutaneous injection should be carefully selected, since use of areas with poor circulation may produce poor patient response and increase the possibility of tissue necrosis, sloughing of tissue, or abscess formation.

Patient's response to initial dose should be observed for at least 10 minutes before increasing dose since the maximum effect is not immediately evident.

## Parenteral Dosage Forms
Note: The dosing and strengths of the dosage forms available are expressed in terms of metaraminol base (not the bitartrate salt).

# METARAMINOL BITARTRATE INJECTION USP

**Usual adult dose**
Hypotension (prophylaxis)—
  Intramuscular or subcutaneous, 2 to 10 mg (base).
Hypotension (treatment)—
  Intravenous infusion, 15 to 100 mg (base) in 500 mL of 0.9% sodium
    chloride injection or 5% dextrose injection, administered at a rate
    adjusted to maintain the desired blood pressure.
Shock, severe—
  Intravenous, 500 mcg (0.5 mg) to 5 mg (base), followed by an intra-
    venous infusion of metaraminol for control of blood pressure.

**Usual adult prescribing limits**
Intravenous infusion, up to 500 mg (base) in 500 mL of infusion fluid
  (with caution).

**Usual pediatric dose**
Dosage has not been established.

**Strength(s) usually available**
U.S.—
  10 mg (base) per mL (Rx) [*Aramine* (sodium chloride 4.4 mg per mL;
    methylparaben 0.15%; propylparaben 0.02%; sodium bisulfite
    0.2%); GENERIC].
Canada—
  Not commercially available.

**Packaging and storage**
Store below 40 °C (104 °F), preferably between 15 and 30 °C (59 and 86
  °F), unless otherwise specified by manufacturer. Protect from light.
  Protect from freezing.

**Preparation of dosage form**
Metaraminol bitartrate 1% must be diluted prior to use.
The preferred solutions for dilution of metaraminol bitartrate are 0.9%
  sodium chloride injection and 5% dextrose injection. However, other
  diluents that may be used include Ringer's injection and lactated
  Ringer's injection.

**Stability**
After metaraminol and infusion solutions are mixed, they should be used
  within 24 hours because of the absence of preservatives.

**Incompatibilities**
Metaraminol bitartrate tends to be physically incompatible with other medications of poor solubility in acidic media, such as sodium salts of
  barbiturates, penicillins, and phenytoin.

---

## METHOXAMINE

# Summary of Differences

Pharmacology/pharmacokinetics:
  Mechanism of action/effect—Selective alpha-1 adrenergic agonist.

# Additional Dosing Information

If methoxamine is administered prophylactically to prevent hypotension
  during spinal anesthesia, it should be administered by intramuscular
  injection shortly before or at the time of spinal anesthesia administration. Those patients suffering from hypertension are more likely to
  experience a greater reduction in blood pressure during spinal anesthesia than patients with blood pressure in a normal range. Higher
  levels of anesthesia will usually cause a greater drop in blood pressure,
  which in turn will require an increased dose of methoxamine for
  control.

Although it is sometimes necessary to repeat intramuscular doses of methoxamine, it is very important to allow adequate time (about 15 minutes)
  for the previous intramuscular dose to elicit its effect before administration of additional doses.

Methoxamine is administered by slow, intravenous injection when the
  systolic blood pressure falls to 60 mm of mercury (Hg) or less, or
  when an emergency situation occurs.

When methoxamine is administered intravenously during emergencies,
  supplemental doses may be given intramuscularly to provide a prolonged effect.

Rapid administration of methoxamine should be avoided because it would
  produce added stress on the myocardium from markedly increased
  peripheral resistance during a reduction in stroke volume and cardiac
  output.

# Parenteral Dosage Forms

## METHOXAMINE HYDROCHLORIDE INJECTION USP

**Usual adult dose**
Vasopressor—
  Intramuscular, 10 to 15 mg. In cases of moderate hypotension, 5- to
    10-mg doses may be adequate. If used during spinal anesthesia, a
    10-mg dose may be adequate at low spinal anesthesia levels; how-
    ever, a 15- to 20-mg dose may be required at high spinal anesthesia
    levels.
  Intravenous, 3 to 5 mg administered slowly.

**Usual pediatric dose**
Dosage has not been established.

**Strength(s) usually available**
U.S.—
  20 mg per mL (Rx) [*Vasoxyl* (citric acid 0.3%; potassium metabisulfite
    0.1%; sodium citrate 0.3%)].
Canada—
  20 mg per mL (Rx) [*Vasoxyl* (bisulfites)].

**Packaging and storage**
Store below 40 °C (104 °F), preferably between 15 and 30 °C (59 and 86
  °F), unless otherwise specified by manufacturer. Protect from light.
  Protect from freezing.

---

## NOREPINEPHRINE

# Summary of Differences

Pharmacology/pharmacokinetics:
  Mechanism of action/effect—Alpha and beta-1 adrenergic agonist.
  Biotransformation—Metabolized by monoamine oxidase (MAO) and
    catechol-O-methyltransferase (COMT).

# Additional Dosing Information

Prior to administration, norepinephrine injection must be diluted with 5%
  dextrose in distilled water or 5% dextrose in sodium chloride solution
  because the dextrose in these fluids protects against significant loss of
  potency due to oxidation. Administration of norepinephrine in sodium
  chloride solution alone is not recommended.

When norepinephrine is used as an emergency measure, it can be administered before or concurrently with blood volume replacement, but
  intra-aortic pressure should be maintained to prevent cerebral or coronary artery ischemia.

If whole blood or plasma is indicated to increase blood volume, it should
  be administered separately (e.g., use of a Y-tube and individual flasks
  if given simultaneously).

Norepinephrine is administered only by intravenous infusion. Subcutaneous or intramuscular administration is not recommended because of
  the potent vasoconstrictor effect of norepinephrine.

# Parenteral Dosage Forms

Note: The dosing and strengths of the dosage forms available are expressed in terms of norepinephrine base (not the bitartrate salt).

## NOREPINEPHRINE BITARTRATE INJECTION USP

**Usual adult dose**
Vasopressor—
  Initial: Intravenous infusion, 0.5 to 1 mcg (base) per minute; the dos-
    age being adjusted gradually to achieve desired blood pressure.
  Maintenance: Intravenous infusion, 2 to 12 mcg (base) per minute.
  Note: Patients with refractory shock may require dose up to 30 mcg
    (base) per minute.

**Usual pediatric dose**
Vasopressor—
  Intravenous infusion, 0.1 mcg (base) per kg of body weight per min-
    ute; the dosage being adjusted gradually to achieve desired blood
    pressure, up to 1 mcg per kg of body weight per minute.

**Strength(s) usually available**
U.S.—
  1 mg (base) per mL (Rx) [*Levophed* (sodium chloride; sodium meta-
    bisulfite not more than 2 mg per mL)].
Canada—
  1 mg (base) per mL (Rx) [*Levophed* (sodium bisulfite not more than
    2 mg per mL; sodium chloride)].

**Packaging and storage**
Store below 40 °C (104 °F), preferably between 15 and 30 °C (59 and 86 °F), unless otherwise specified by manufacturer. Store in a light-resistant container. Protect from freezing.

**Preparation of dosage form**
Diluents used for preparation of infusion solutions of norepinephrine are 5% dextrose in distilled water or 5% dextrose in sodium chloride solution because the dextrose in these fluids protects against significant loss of potency due to oxidation. Sodium chloride solution alone is not recommended as a diluent.
To prepare an intravenous infusion solution of norepinephrine, add 4 mg of norepinephrine (base) to 250 mL of 5% dextrose solution. The resultant solution contains 16 mcg of norepinephrine base per mL.

**Stability**
Do not use discolored (pink, yellow, or brown) solutions or those containing a precipitate; they should be discarded.
Discard unused portion of norepinephrine solution.

**Incompatibilities**
Norepinephrine is incompatible with iron salts, alkalies, and oxidizing agents; contact should be avoided.

---

### *PHENYLEPHRINE*

## Summary of Differences

Indications:
   Also indicated as an antiarrhythmic.
Pharmacology/pharmacokinetics:
   Mechanism of action/effect—Alpha-1 adrenergic agonist.

## Parenteral Dosage Forms

### PHENYLEPHRINE HYDROCHLORIDE INJECTION USP

**Usual adult dose**
Vasopressor—
   Mild or moderate hypotension:
      Intramuscular or subcutaneous, 2 to 5 mg, repeated not more often than every ten to fifteen minutes.
      Intravenous, 200 mcg (0.2 mg), repeated not more often than every ten to fifteen minutes.
      Note: The initial intramuscular or subcutaneous dose should not exceed 5 mg; the initial intravenous dose should not exceed 500 mcg (0.5 mg).
   Severe hypotension and shock:
      Intravenous infusion, 10 mg in 500 mL of 5% dextrose injection USP or 0.9% sodium chloride injection USP, administered initially at a rate of about 100 to 180 mcg (0.1 to 0.18 mg) per minute until blood pressure is stabilized; then at a rate of 40

to 60 mcg (0.04 to 0.06 mg) per minute. If necessary, additional doses in increments of 10 mg or more may be added to the infusion solution and the rate of flow adjusted until the desired blood pressure level is obtained.
Hypotension during spinal anesthesia:
   Prophylaxis—Intramuscular or subcutaneous, 2 to 3 mg three to four minutes prior to injection of spinal anesthetic.
   Hypotensive emergencies—Intravenous, initially 200 mcg (0.2 mg), the dosage being increased by not more than 200 mcg (0.2 mg) for each subsequent dose, up to a maximum of 500 mcg (0.5 mg) per dose.
Antiarrhythmic—
   Intravenous (rapid), initial dose not exceeding 500 mcg (0.5 mg). Additional doses should not exceed the preceding dose by more than 100 to 200 mcg (0.1 to 0.2 mg).

**Usual pediatric dose**
Hypotension during spinal anesthesia—
   Intramuscular or subcutaneous, 500 mcg (0.5 mg) to 1 mg per twenty-five pounds of body weight.

**Strength(s) usually available**
U.S.—
   10 mg per mL (Rx) [*Neo-Synephrine* (sodium chloride 3.5 mg; sodium citrate 4 mg; citric acid monohydrate 1 mg; sodium metabisulfite not more than 2 mg)].
Canada—
   10 mg per mL (Rx) [*Neo-Synephrine* (sodium chloride 3.5 mg; sodium citrate 4 mg; citric acid monohydrate 1 mg; sodium metabisulfite not more than 2 mg)].

**Packaging and storage**
Store below 40 °C (104 °F), preferably between 15 and 30 °C (59 and 86 °F), unless otherwise specified by manufacturer. Protect from light. Protect from freezing.

**Preparation of dosage form**
To prepare a solution of phenylephrine for direct intravenous injection, 10 mg (1 mL) of phenylephrine hydrochloride injection should be diluted with 9 mL of sterile water for injection USP to provide a solution containing 1 mg of phenylephrine per mL.

## Selected Bibliography

Chernow B, Roth BL. Pharmacologic manipulation of the peripheral vasculature in shock: clinical and experimental approaches. Circ Shock 1986; 18: 141-55.
Kulka PJ, Tryba M. Inotropic support of the critically ill patient. Drugs 1993; 45 (5): 654-67.
MacLeod CM. Drugs used in the acutely ill patient. Dis Mon 1993; 39 (6): 370-81.

---

Developed: 10/20/94

# TACRINE   Systemic†

VA CLASSIFICATION (Primary): CN900

Other commonly used names are tetrahydroaminoacridine and THA.

Note: For a listing of dosage forms and brand names by country availability, see *Dosage Forms* section(s). For a listing of brand names for the articles in this monograph, refer to the General Index.

†Not commercially available in Canada.

## Category

Dementia symptoms treatment adjunct.

## Indications

### Accepted

Dementia of the Alzheimer's type, mild to moderate (treatment)—Tacrine is indicated for the symptomatic treatment of mild to moderate dementia of the Alzheimer's type. Clinical trials have found tacrine to be of limited efficacy in the treatment of this condition.

In one high-dose, 30-week clinical trial of tacrine, approximately 43% of the 663 patients enrolled dropped out due to adverse medication effects, primarily elevated transaminase values and gastrointestinal effects, and only 28% of patients randomized to the 160 mg per day (mg/day) treatment group were able to complete the study. Of those patients who achieved the maximum tacrine dosage of 160 mg/day, and completed the 30-week study, 42% showed improvement in the Clinician Interview–Based Impression (CIBI), a global evaluation of change; 42% showed improvement in the Final Comprehensive Consensus Assessment (FCCA), which was similar to the CIBI but included caregivers' impressions; and 40% showed at least a 4 point improvement on the Alzheimer's Disease Assessment Scale—Cognitive subscale (ADAS-Cog), an objective 70-point evaluation of cognitive function. The only significant improvement seen in the lower dosage treatment groups was on the FCCA in the 120 mg/day patients. Among patients who received placebo, 18% showed improvement in the CIBI, 16% showed improvement in the FCCA, and 25% improved on the ADAS-Cog by at least 4 points. The improvements seen in clinical trials of tacrine were comparable in magnitude to the decline that would be expected to occur over a six-month period in a patient with Alzheimer's disease.

## Pharmacology/Pharmacokinetics

### Physicochemical characteristics

Chemical group—Acridines
Molecular weight—Tacrine hydrochloride monohydrate: 252.74.
pKa—9.85.

### Mechanism of action/Effect

While many neuronal systems are affected in Alzheimer's disease, the decline in central cholinergic activity is one of the most pronounced neurotransmitter deficits. This deficit occurs early in the disease process and correlates with decreased scores on dementia ratings scales. Tacrine's primary effect is the reversible inhibition of cholinesterase, butyrylcholinesterase more than acetylcholinesterase. This inhibition is thought to increase the level of acetylcholine available in the central nervous system. In fact, increased levels of acetylcholine have been detected in the cerebrospinal fluid of patients receiving tacrine.

Tacrine may also block potassium channels, increasing the duration of the action potential and augmenting acetylcholine release from cholinergic neurons.

In addition, tacrine may moderate cholinergic activity by acting as a partial agonist or antagonist through direct binding to nicotinic and, with greater affinity, to muscarinic receptors.

Additionally, tacrine inhibits monoamine oxidase (MAO), MAO-A to a greater extent than MAO-B. Tacrine may also inhibit the reuptake of norepinephrine, serotonin, and dopamine.

There is no evidence that tacrine alters the underlying dementing process, and its effect may be expected to lessen as the disease progresses.

### Other actions/effects

Because of its cholinomimetic action, tacrine may have vagotonic effects on the heart, including bradycardia, and may increase the activity of the gastrointestinal and urinary tracts.

### Absorption

Tacrine is rapidly absorbed. Probably due to a very high first-pass metabolism, absolute bioavailability is about $17 \pm 13\%$. Bioavailability increases with increasing dose in a nonlinear manner, and large interindividual variations are seen. Food decreases bioavailability by 30 to 40%.

### Distribution

Volume of distribution ($Vol_D$) is $349 \pm 193$ L.

In rats, tacrine readily penetrates the blood-brain barrier resulting in brain concentrations approximately 10 times those of plasma.

### Protein binding

Moderate (55%).

### Biotransformation

Metabolized by the hepatic cytochrome P-450 system. Cytochrome P-450 1A2 is the principal isozyme involved in tacrine metabolism. The major metabolite, 1-hydroxy-tacrine, or velnacrine, has central cholinergic activity.

### Half-life

Elimination—
    Tacrine: 1.5 to 4 hours.
    1-hydroxy-tacrine (velnacrine): 2.5 to 3.1 hours.

### Time to peak concentration

0.5 to 3 hours.

### Peak serum concentration

Peak serum concentration shows wide interindividual variation and is significantly higher in females than in males. In addition, peak serum concentration increases nonlinearly with dose. Because the enzyme system responsible for first-pass metabolism can be saturated at relatively low doses, a larger fraction of a high dose than of a low dose will reach the circulation.

### Elimination

Negligible amount excreted in urine. In a mass balance study, 336 hours after a single radiolabeled dose was administered, approximately 25% of the radiolabel remained unrecovered, suggesting the possibility that tacrine and/or one or more of its metabolites may be retained.

## Precautions to Consider

### Cross-sensitivity and/or related problems

Patients hypersensitive to other acridine derivatives, such as the topical antiseptics 9-aminoacridine (e.g., Akrinol, Monacrin), acriflavine (e.g., Panflavin), or proflavine, may be hypersensitive to tacrine.

### Carcinogenicity

Since some members of its chemical class (acridines) are known to be animal carcinogens, tacrine may be carcinogenic.

### Mutagenicity

Tacrine was mutagenic in bacteria in the Ames test, but was not mutagenic in an *in vitro* mammalian mutation test. Tacrine induced unscheduled DNA synthesis in rat and mouse hepatocytes *in vitro*.

### Pregnancy/Reproduction

Fertility—Studies of effects of tacrine on fertility have not been performed.

Pregnancy—Studies have not been done in humans.
Studies have not been done in animals.

FDA Pregnancy Category C.

### Breast-feeding

Problems in humans have not been documented. It is not known whether tacrine is distributed into breast milk. However, use of tacrine is not recommended in nursing mothers.

#### Geriatrics

Clinical trials of tacrine have included Alzheimer's disease patients 40 years of age and older with no other significant disease; information available on the effects of tacrine is based upon this population. Comparisons with younger age groups have not been performed. However, elderly patients are more likely to have age-related prostate problems, which may require caution in patients receiving tacrine, especially if urinary tract obstruction is present.

#### Surgical

If possible, tacrine should be discontinued on a tapered schedule, under medical supervision, three days before any surgery involving general anesthesia. Possible interactions between tacrine and surgical adjuncts have not been fully characterized. However, tacrine may prolong or exaggerate the effects of neuromuscular blocking agents that are metabolized by plasma cholinesterase.

#### Drug interactions and/or related problems

The following drug interactions and/or related problems have been selected on the basis of their potential clinical significance (possible mechanism in parentheses where appropriate)—not necessarily inclusive (» = major clinical significance):

Note: Possible interactions with hepatic enzyme inducers, hepatic enzyme inhibitors, and medications that are metabolized by the hepatic P-450 enzyme system, other than those listed below, have not been studied, but the possibility of a significant interaction should be considered and the patient should be carefully monitored during and following concurrent use.

Combinations containing any of the following medications, depending on the amount present, may also interact with this medication.

Anticholinergics (See *Appendix II*)
(concurrent use may decrease the effects of either these medications or tacrine)

Cholinomimetics (e.g., bethanecol) and cholinesterase inhibitors (e.g., neostigmine)
(concurrent use may increase the effects of either these medications or tacrine and increase the potential for toxicity)

» Cimetidine
(concurrent use increases peak plasma concentrations and area under the concentration-time curve [AUC] of tacrine, which may increase the potential for toxicity)

» Neuromuscular blocking agents metabolized by plasma cholinesterase (e.g., succinylcholine, mivacurium)
(tacrine inhibits cholinesterase and may prolong or exaggerate muscle relaxation)

» Nonsteroidal anti-inflammatory drugs (NSAIDs)
(tacrine may increase gastric acid secretion, which may contribute to gastrointestinal irritation; patient should be monitored for occult gastrointestinal bleeding)

» Smoking tobacco
(mean plasma concentration of tacrine is 67% lower in current smokers than in nonsmokers; the effectiveness of tacrine in smokers may be decreased)

» Theophylline
(concurrent use increases mean plasma concentration and half-life of theophylline to approximately twice normal values, increasing the potential for toxicity; theophylline plasma concentration should be monitored, and dosage reduced as indicated)

#### Medical considerations/Contraindications

The medical considerations/contraindications included here have been selected on the basis of their potential clinical significance (reasons given in parentheses where appropriate)—not necessarily inclusive (» = major clinical significance).

*This medication should not be used when the following medical problems exist:*

» Jaundice, tacrine treatment–associated, confirmed by elevated total bilirubin greater than 3 mg per dL (mg/dL), or history of
(condition may be exacerbated or reactivated)

» Known hypersensitivity to tacrine or other acridine derivatives

*Risk-benefit should be considered when the following medical problems exist:*

» Asthma, bronchial, active or latent
(asthma attack may be precipitated)

» Cardiovascular conditions, such as:
Bradycardia
Hypotension
Sick sinus syndrome
(vagotonic effect on heart may exacerbate pre-existing conditions)

» Epilepsy or history of seizures or
» Head injury with loss of consciousness or
» Increased intracranial pressure, preexisting or
» Intracranial lesions or
» Metabolic disorders, unstable
(seizures may occur)

» Gastrointestinal obstruction or
» Urinary tract obstruction
(increased activity of gastrointestinal tract or urinary bladder may be harmful)

» Hepatic function impairment, current or history of
(condition may be exacerbated or reactivated)

» Parkinson's disease
(increased cholinergic activity in the central nervous system may exacerbate condition)

» Peptic ulcer, active or history of
(increased gastric acid secretion may exacerbate or reactivate condition)

#### Patient monitoring

The following may be especially important in patient monitoring (other tests may be warranted in some patients, depending on condition;
» = major clinical significance):

» Cognitive function
(periodic objective assessment of cognitive status is recommended to determine effectiveness of tacrine treatment)

» Alanine aminotransferase (ALT [SGPT]) serum values
(monitoring every other week is required for the first 16 weeks following initiation of therapy, and for the first 16 weeks following reinstitution of tacrine after a suspension of therapy of more than 4 weeks. Testing frequency may then be reduced to monthly for 2 months, then once every 3 months in the absence of ALT [SGPT] serum value elevations. However, weekly testing should be performed if ALT [SGPT] serum values are greater than twice the upper limit of normal [ULN]. For serum values up to 3 times the ULN, recommended dosage titration may be continued; for serum values greater than 3, and up to 5 times the ULN, the dosage should be reduced by 40 mg per day; dosage titration and monitoring every other week may be resumed when ALT [SGPT] serum values return to within normal limits; for serum values greater than 5 times the ULN, tacrine should be discontinued and the patient should be closely monitored for signs and symptoms of hepatitis; rechallenge may be considered when ALT [SGPT] serum values return to within normal limits)

Note: Experience rechallenging patients who have had ALT (SGPT) serum values greater than 10 times the ULN is limited; risk versus demonstrated benefit should be considered. Patients who have experienced tacrine treatment–related jaundice confirmed by elevated total bilirubin greater than 3 mg per dL (mg/dL) and patients exhibiting clinical signs of hypersensitivity, such as rash or fever, in association with ALT (SGPT) serum value elevations *should permanently discontinue and not be rechallenged* with tacrine.

## Side/Adverse Effects

The following side/adverse effects have been selected on the basis of their potential clinical significance (possible signs and symptoms in parentheses where appropriate)—not necessarily inclusive:

**Those indicating need for medical attention**

Incidence more frequent

*Ataxia* (clumsiness or unsteadiness); *gastrointestinal toxicity, specifically anorexia* (loss of appetite); *diarrhea, nausea, or vomiting; hepatotoxicity (50%)* (change in stool color [rare]; fever [infrequent]; yellow eyes or skin [rare])

Note: Approximately 50% of all patients started on tacrine will develop elevated transaminase serum values, usually within 12 weeks of initiation of therapy. Approximately 25% of all patients started on tacrine will develop transaminase serum values more than 3 times the upper limit of normal (ULN) and will require dosage reduction or discontinuation of tacrine.

Females are at greater risk than males for developing transaminase elevation. Rarely, clinical signs of hepatotoxicity emerge, such as jaundice and fever. Liver biopsies in these patients have revealed granulomatous changes and hepatocellular necrosis. In cases of hepatotoxicity reported to date, liver function tests have returned to normal, usually within six weeks of dosage reduction or discontinuation of tacrine.

Incidence less frequent

*Cardiovascular effects, specifically bradycardia* (slow heartbeat); *hypertension* (high blood pressure); *hypotension* (low blood pressure); *or palpitation* (fast or pounding heartbeat); *skin rash; syncope* (fainting)

Incidence rare

*Asthma* (cough; tightness in chest; trouble in breathing; wheezing); *convulsions* (seizures)—associated with cholinergic effects, particularly diarrhea; *mood or mental changes, specifically aggression, irritability, or nervousness; parkinsonian extrapyramidal effects* (stiffness of arms or legs; slow movement; trembling and shaking of hands and fingers); *tachycardia* (fast heartbeat); *urinary obstruction* (trouble in urinating)

**Those indicating need for medical attention only if they continue or are bothersome**

Incidence more frequent

*Dizziness; gastrointestinal effects, specifically abdominal pain or cramping, or dyspepsia* (indigestion); *headache; myalgia* (muscle pain)

Incidence less frequent

*Belching; flushing of skin; hyperventilation* (fast breathing); *insomnia* (trouble in sleeping); *lacrimation, increased* (watering of eyes); *malaise* (general feeling of discomfort or illness); *peripheral edema* (swelling of feet or lower legs); *polyuria* (frequent urination or increased volume of urine); *rhinitis* (runny nose); *salivation, increased* (watering of mouth); *sweating, increased*

## Overdose

For specific information on the agents used in the management of tacrine overdose, see:

• *Atropine sulfate* in *Anticholinergics/Antispasmodics (Systemic)* monograph.

For more information on the management of overdose or unintentional ingestion, **contact a Poison Control Center** (see *Poison Control Center Listing*).

**Clinical effects of overdose**

The following effects have been selected on the basis of their potential clinical significance (possible signs and symptoms in parentheses where appropriate)—not necessarily inclusive:

*Cardiovascular effects, specifically bradycardia* (slow heartbeat); *hypotension* (low blood pressure); *or shock* (fast weak pulse; irregular breathing; large pupils); *convulsions* (seizures); *muscular weakness, increasing*—may lead to death if respiratory muscles are involved; *nausea, severe; salivation, excessive* (watering of mouth); *sweating, excessive; vomiting, severe*

**Treatment of overdose**

Specific treatment—Administering intravenous atropine sulfate, initial dose 1 to 2 mg, with subsequent doses based on clinical response.

Supportive care—Providing supportive therapy. Patients in whom intentional overdose is confirmed or suspected should be referred for psychiatric consultation.

## Patient Consultation

As an aid to patient consultation, refer to *Advice for the Patient, Tacrine (Systemic)*.

In providing consultation, consider emphasizing the following selected information (» = major clinical significance):

**Before using this medication**

» Conditions affecting use, especially:

Hypersensitivity to tacrine or other acridine derivatives

Other medications, especially cimetidine, neuromuscular blocking agents, NSAIDs, smoking tobacco, and theophylline

Other medical problems, especially asthma, cardiovascular conditions (such as bradycardia, hypotension, or sick sinus syndrome), epilepsy or history of seizures, gastrointestinal or urinary tract obstruction, head injury with loss of consciousness, hepatic function impairment, increased intracranial pressure, intracranial lesions, Parkinson's disease, peptic ulcer, and unstable metabolic disorders

**Proper use of this medication**

» Not taking more medication than the amount prescribed because of increased risk of adverse effects

Taking tacrine on empty stomach if tolerated

Taking doses at regular intervals for maximum efficacy

» Proper dosing

Missed dose: taking as soon as possible; not taking if within 2 hours of time for next dose; not doubling doses

» Proper storage

**Precautions while using this medication**

» Importance of complying with monitoring schedule and keeping appointments with physician and/or laboratory

Informing physician when new symptoms arise or when previously noted symptoms increase in severity

Caution if any kind of surgery or emergency treatment is required; informing physician or dentist in charge that tacrine is being taken

Caution if dizziness, clumsiness, or unsteadiness occurs

» Not decreasing dose or discontinuing treatment without consulting physician because of possible decline in cognitive function and behavioral disturbances

» Suspected overdose: Getting emergency help at once

**Side/adverse effects**

Ataxia; gastrointestinal toxicity, specifically anorexia, diarrhea, nausea, or vomiting; hepatotoxicity; cardiovascular effects, specifically bradycardia, hypertension, hypotension, or palpitation; convulsions; skin rash; syncope; asthma; mood or mental changes, specifically aggression, irritability, or nervousness; parkinsonian extrapyramidal effects; tachycardia; urinary obstruction

## General Dosing Information

Tacrine should be taken on an empty stomach (either 1 hour before meals or 2 hours after meals) for more complete absorption. However, if stomach upset occurs, tacrine may be taken with food.

Tacrine should be taken at regular intervals for best effect.

The rate of dosage escalation may be slowed in patients who are having difficulty tolerating the recommended dosage escalation schedule. However, *dosage escalation should not be accelerated*, or the incidence of serious adverse effects may be increased.

The first dosage increase should not be made earlier than 6 weeks after initiation of tacrine therapy because of the possibility of delayed transaminase elevation.

The patient should be carefully observed for side effects following initiation of therapy and following every dosage increase.

Abrupt discontinuation of tacrine or a decrease of 80 mg or greater in daily tacrine dose has caused decreased cognitive function and behavioral disturbances.

## Oral Dosage Forms

Note: The available dosage form contains tacrine hydrochloride, but dosage and strength are expressed in terms of the base.

# TACRINE CAPSULES

## Usual adult dose

Alzheimer's dementia—

Oral, initially 10 mg (base) four times a day. After at least six weeks, if there are no significant transaminase elevations and the patient is tolerating treatment, the dose may be increased to 20 mg four times a day. Further increases to 30 mg four times a day, and then to 40 mg four times a day may be instituted at intervals of at least six weeks, based on patient tolerance.

If elevations of serum transaminase occur, tacrine dosage should be modified. Recommended modifications are:

| Transaminase Serum Value (times Upper Limit of Normal [ULN]) | Treatment Regimen Modification |
|---|---|
| ≤ 3 | No modification. |
| > 3 to ≤ 5 | Reduce the daily dose of tacrine by 40 mg per day. Resume dose titration when transaminase serum values return to within normal limits. |
| > 5 | Stop tacrine treatment. Monitor transaminase serum values until within normal limits. Consider rechallenge with tacrine. |
| > 10 | Rechallenge experience is limited with these patients. Risk versus demonstrated benefit should be considered. |

Note: For rechallenge: Dose titration schedule is the same as that for new patients. However, ALT (SGPT) serum values should be monitored weekly for the first 16 weeks following re-initiation of tacrine therapy. If unacceptable elevations in ALT (SGPT) serum values do not recur, monitoring frequency may be decreased to monthly for 2 months and every 3 months thereafter.

Patients who have experienced tacrine treatment–related jaundice confirmed by elevated total bilirubin greater than 3 mg per dL (mg/dL) and patients exhibiting clinical signs of hypersensitivity, such as rash or fever, in association with ALT (SGPT) serum value elevations *should permanently discontinue and not be rechallenged* with tacrine.

## Usual adult prescribing limits

Up to 160 mg a day.

## Usual pediatric dose

Safety and efficacy have not been established.

## Usual geriatric dose

See *Usual adult dose*.

## Strength(s) usually available

U.S.—

10 mg (base) (Rx) [*Cognex* (hydrous lactose; magnesium stearate; microcrystalline cellulose; gelatin NF; silicon dioxide NF; sodium lauryl sulfate NF; D&C Yellow #10; FD&C Green #3; titanium dioxide)].

20 mg (base) (Rx) [*Cognex* (hydrous lactose; magnesium stearate; microcrystalline cellulose; gelatin NF; silicon dioxide NF; sodium lauryl sulfate NF; D&C Yellow #10; FD&C Blue #1; titanium dioxide)].

30 mg (base) (Rx) [*Cognex* (hydrous lactose; magnesium stearate; microcrystalline cellulose; gelatin NF; silicon dioxide NF; sodium lauryl sulfate NF; D&C Yellow #10; FD&C Blue #1; FD&C Red #40; titanium dioxide)].

40 mg (base) (Rx)·[*Cognex* (hydrous lactose; magnesium stearate; microcrystalline cellulose; gelatin NF; silicon dioxide NF; sodium lauryl sulfate NF; D&C Yellow #10; FD&C Blue #1; FD&C Red #40; D&C Red #28; titanium dioxide)].

Canada—

Not commercially available.

Note: Tacrine may be available from the manufacturer through a compassionate use program.

## Packaging and storage

Store below 40 °C (104 °F), preferably between 15 and 30 °C (59 and 86 °F), in a well-closed container, away from moisture, unless otherwise specified by manufacturer.

## Preparation of dosage form

For patients who cannot take oral solids—Tacrine capsules may be dissolved in any aqueous solution. However, orange juice will best mask the bitter taste of the medication. The capsule should be placed in the liquid intact to avoid loss of medication through spillage. Some excipients may remain undissolved. Prepare each dose as needed; do not store solution for later use.

## Auxiliary labeling

• Take on empty stomach.
• May cause dizziness.
• Take exactly as directed.

# Selected Bibliography

Freeman SE, Dawson RM. Tacrine: A pharmacological review. Prog Neurobiol 1991; 36: 257-77.

Knapp MJ, Knopman DS, Solomon PR, et al. A 30-week randomized controlled trial of high-dose tacrine in patients with Alzheimer's Disease. JAMA 1994 Apr 6; 271 (13): 985-91.

Developed: 08/05/94
Interim revision: 08/24/95

# TAMOXIFEN    Systemic

Note: For a listing of dosage forms and brand names by country availability, see *Dosage Forms* section(s). For a listing of brand names for the articles in this monograph, refer to the General Index.

## Category

Antineoplastic.

## Indications

### Accepted

Carcinoma, breast (treatment)—Node-negative: Tamoxifen is indicated for adjuvant treatment of axillary node-negative breast cancer in women following total mastectomy or segmental mastectomy, axillary dissection, and breast irradiation. Data are insufficient to predict which women are most likely to benefit and to determine if tamoxifen provides any benefit in women with tumors of less than 1 cm.

Node-positive: Tamoxifen is indicated for adjuvant treatment of axillary node-positive breast cancer in postmenopausal women following total mastectomy or segmental mastectomy, axillary dissection, and breast irradiation. In some tamoxifen adjuvant studies, most of the benefit to date has been in the subgroup with 4 or more positive axillary nodes.

Note: The estrogen and progesterone receptor values may help to predict whether adjuvant tamoxifen therapy is likely to be beneficial in node-negative or node-positive breast cancer.

Advanced disease: Tamoxifen is indicated in the treatment of metastatic breast cancer in men and women.

The labeling states that tamoxifen is effective in premenopausal women as an alternative to oophorectomy or ovarian irradiation. Available evidence indicates that women whose tumors are estrogen receptor positive are more likely to benefit from tamoxifen therapy.

## Pharmacology/Pharmacokinetics

Note: Pharmacokinetic studies have been done in women only.

### Physicochemical characteristics
Molecular weight—563.65.
pKa—8.85.

### Mechanism of action/Effect
Tamoxifen is a nonsteroidal antiestrogen agent that also has weak estrogenic effects. The exact mechanism of antineoplastic action is unknown, but may be related to its antiestrogen effects; tamoxifen blocks uptake of estradiol.

### Other actions/effects
Tamoxifen may induce ovulation in anovulatory women, stimulating release of gonadotropin-releasing hormone from the hypothalamus, which in turn stimulates release of pituitary gonadotropins. In oligospermic males, tamoxifen increases serum concentrations of luteinizing hormone (LH), follicle-stimulating hormone (FSH), testosterone, and estrogen. Tamoxifen and some of its metabolites (N-desmethyltamoxifen, 4-hydroxytamoxifen) are potent inhibitors of hepatic cytochrome p-450 mixed function oxidases; however, the clinical significance of these effects has not been determined.

### Biotransformation
Hepatic. Enterohepatic circulation is believed to account for prolongation of blood concentrations and fecal excretion.

### Half-life
Distribution—7 to 14 hours; secondary peaks at 4 or more days may be due to enterohepatic circulation.

Elimination—May exceed 7 days.

### Onset of action
An objective response usually occurs within 4 to 10 weeks of therapy, but may take several months in patients with bone metastases.

### Duration of action
Estrogen antagonism may persist for several weeks following a single dose.

### Elimination
Primary route—Biliary/fecal, mostly as metabolites.
Secondary route—Renal (only small amounts).

## Precautions to Consider

Note: Unless otherwise noted, information in this section is based on reports in women treated with tamoxifen.

### Carcinogenicity
An increased incidence of endometrial cancer has been associated with tamoxifen treatment in humans. A large randomized study in Sweden found a significantly increased incidence of uterine cancer in women who took tamoxifen as compared with those who received placebo. In the ongoing NSABP B-14 study, an increased incidence of uterine cancer has also been noted; deaths have been reported.

Hepatic carcinogenicity of tamoxifen in rats is well established. Studies in rats at doses of 5, 20, and 35 mg per kg of body weight (mg/kg) per day for up to 2 years found an increased incidence of hepatocellular carcinoma at all doses; the incidence was highest at doses of 20 or 35 mg/kg per day. In a 13-month study of endocrine changes in immature and mature mice, granulosa cell ovarian tumors and interstitial cell testicular tumors were found in tamoxifen-treated mice but not in controls.

### Mutagenicity
No genotoxic potential was found in a conventional battery of *in vivo* and *in vitro* tests with pro- and eukaryotic test systems with drug metabolizing systems present. However, increased levels of DNA adducts have been found in the livers of rats exposed to tamoxifen. Tamoxifen has also been found to increase levels of micronucleus formation *in vitro* in human lymphoblastoid cell line (MCL-5).

### Pregnancy/Reproduction
Fertility—Tamoxifen may induce ovulation in women.
Tamoxifen affects reproductive function in rats at doses somewhat higher than the human dose.

Pregnancy—Although adequate and well-controlled studies have not been done in humans, spontaneous abortions, birth defects, fetal deaths, and vaginal bleeding have been reported. Because of tamoxofen's estrogenic effect, the possibility of a diethylstilbestrol- (DES-)like syndrome in females whose mothers took tamoxifen during pregnancy should be kept in mind. In rodent models of fetal reproductive tract development, at doses of 0.3 to 2.4 times the maximum recommended human dose (MRHD), tamoxifen caused changes in both sexes that are similar to those caused by estradiol, ethynylestradiol, and DES; some of these changes, especially vaginal adenosis, are similar to those found in young women who were exposed *in utero* to DES and who have a 1 in 1000 risk of developing clear-cell adenocarcinoma of the vagina or cervix. Duration of follow-up of the few women exposed to tamoxifen *in utero* to date has not been long enough to confirm or disprove this risk with its use in humans.

In general, use of a barrier or nonhormonal contraceptive is recommended during (and for about two months after) tamoxifen therapy in sexually active women.

At dose levels at or below the human dose, reversible nonteratogenic developmental skeletal changes occurred in rats, and a lower incidence of embryo implantation and higher incidence of fetal death or retarded *in utero* growth occurred in rats and rabbits, as well as impaired learning behavior in some rat pups.

FDA Pregnancy Category D.

### Breast-feeding
It is not known whether tamoxifen is distributed into breast milk. Although very little information is available regarding distribution of antineoplastic agents into breast milk, breast-feeding is not recommended during chemotherapy because of the risks to the infant (adverse effects, mutagenicity, carcinogenicity).

### Geriatrics
Appropriate studies on the relationship of age to the effects of tamoxifen have not been performed in the geriatric population. However, this medication is commonly used in elderly patients and geriatrics-specific problems that would limit the usefulness of this medication in the elderly have not been reported and are not expected.

### Drug interactions and/or related problems
The following drug interactions and/or related problems have been selected on the basis of their potential clinical significance (possible mechanism in parentheses where appropriate)—not necessarily inclusive (» = major clinical significance):

Note: Combinations containing any of the following medications, depending on the amount present, may also interact with this medication.

Antacids or
Cimetidine or
Famotidine or
Ranitidine
(these medications increase intragastric pH and may therefore cause premature dissolution, and loss of the protective effect, of enteric coatings; a 1- to 2-hour interval should elapse between administration of an antacid and enteric-coated tamoxifen; also, probability should be considered that concurrent use of an enteric-coated formulation with cimetidine, famotidine, or ranitidine will not provide greater protection against gastric irritation or ulceration than is provided by the histamine H<sub>2</sub>-receptor antagonist alone)

Estrogens
(may interfere with tamoxifen's therapeutic effect)

### Laboratory value alterations
The following have been selected on the basis of their potential clinical significance (possible effect in parentheses where appropriate)—not necessarily inclusive (» = major clinical significance):

With physiology/laboratory test values
Calcium
(serum concentrations may be increased infrequently, usually in patients with bone metastases; the effect appears to be transient)
Cholesterol and
Triglycerides
(increases in serum concentrations have been seen infrequently)
Hepatic enzymes
(serum values may be increased; rarely, more severe abnormalities, including fatty liver, cholestasis, and hepatitis, have occurred; fatalities have been reported)
Karyopyknotic index on vaginal smears
(variations have been seen infrequently in postmenopausal women treated with tamoxifen)
Papanicolaou smears
(various degrees of estrogen effect have been seen infrequently in postmenopausal women treated with tamoxifen)
Thyroxine (T<sub>4</sub>)
(increases in serum concentrations have been reported in a few patients, possibly as a result of increases in thyroid-binding globulin; however, clinical hyperthyroidism has not been reported)

### Medical considerations/Contraindications
The medical considerations/contraindications included here have been selected on the basis of their potential clinical significance (reasons given in parentheses where appropriate)—not necessarily inclusive (» = major clinical significance).

*Risk-benefit should be considered when the following medical problems exist:*
Cataracts or vision disturbances
(visual disturbances, including corneal changes, cataracts, and retinopathy, have been reported in patients receiving tamoxifen)
Hyperlipidemia
(increased serum lipid concentrations have been reported infrequently)
Leukopenia
(leukopenia has been reported occasionally in patients receiving tamoxifen)
» Sensitivity to tamoxifen
Thrombocytopenia
(thrombocytopenia has been reported occasionally in patients receiving tamoxifen, although platelet counts recovered even with continued therapy)

### Patient monitoring
The following may be especially important in patient monitoring (other tests may be warranted in some patients, depending on condition; » = major clinical significance):

» Calcium concentrations, serum
(recommended at periodic intervals in patients with bone metastases during initial period of therapy)
Cholesterol concentrations, serum and
Triglyceride concentrations, serum
(may be recommended at periodic intervals in patients with pre-existing hyperlipidemias)
Complete blood count
(may be appropriate at periodic intervals, although leukopenia and thrombocytopenia have not been definitely attributed to tamoxifen)

» Gynecologic examinations
(recommended at regular intervals in women taking tamoxifen, to detect possible endometrial cancers)
Hepatic function tests
(recommended at periodic intervals during therapy)
Ophthalmologic examinations
(recommended prior to initiation of therapy and at periodic intervals during therapy)

## Side/Adverse Effects
Note: Side/adverse effects are usually relatively mild.

Although information is limited, the side effect profile in men seems to be similar to that in women.

A transient, sometimes severe, increase in bone or tumor pain may occur shortly after initiation of therapy but usually subsides with continued tamoxifen treatment. Analgesics may be required during this time.

Tamoxifen induces ovulation, which puts women at risk for becoming pregnant.

Ovarian cysts have been reported in a small number of premenopausal women treated with tamoxifen for advanced breast carcinoma.

The following side/adverse effects have been selected on the basis of their potential clinical significance (possible signs and symptoms in parentheses where appropriate)—not necessarily inclusive:

### Those indicating need for medical attention
Incidence less frequent or rare
*In both females and males*
***Confusion; hepatotoxicity*** (usually asymptomatic; rarely, yellow eyes or skin); ***ocular toxicity, including retinopathy, keratopathy, cataracts, and optic neuritis*** (may be asymptomatic initially; blurred vision); ***pulmonary embolus*** (shortness of breath); ***thrombosis*** (pain or swelling in legs); ***weakness or sleepiness***
Note: *Hepatotoxicity* usually consists of elevated hepatic enzyme values. However, more serious liver abnormalities, including fatty liver, cholestasis, and hepatitis, have occurred; fatalities have been reported.

*Ocular toxicity* was previously thought to occur only after high (240 to 320 mg per day), prolonged (17 months or more) tamoxifen dosage. However, there are reports of retinopathy or keratopathy occurring at lower doses (10 to 40 mg per day) and after only a few weeks of tamoxifen therapy, although they are still most commonly associated with several months' therapy. Ocular toxicity may or may not be reversible following withdrawal of tamoxifen. A number of reports included recommendations for baseline and periodic ocular examinations during tamoxifen therapy to detect subclinical toxicity and permit withdrawal of tamoxifen at early stages of toxicity.

*In females only*
***Endometrial hyperplasia, endometrial polyps, or endometrial carcinoma*** (change in vaginal discharge; pain or feeling of pressure in pelvis; vaginal bleeding)

### Those indicating need for medical attention only if they continue or are bothersome
Incidence more frequent—10 to 20%
*In females only*
***Hot flashes; weight gain***
Note: *Weight gain* is an estrogen effect.

Incidence less frequent
*In both females and males*
***Headache; nausea and/or vomiting, mild; skin rash or dryness; transient local disease flare*** (bone pain)
Note: Incidence of *nausea and/or vomiting* is higher with higher doses.

*Transient local disease flare* may also consist of hypercalcemia and/or spinal cord compression, as well as a sudden increase in the size of pre-existing lesions in patients with soft tissue disease, sometimes associated with marked erythema within and surrounding the lesions and/or the development of new lesions. Bone pain or other disease flare usually occurs shortly after initiation of therapy and subsides within 1 to 2 weeks.

*In females only*
  *Changes in menstrual period; itching in genital area; vaginal discharge*
*In males only*
  *Impotence or decrease in sexual interest*

## Patient Consultation

As an aid to patient consultation, refer to *Advice for the Patient, Tamoxifen (Systemic)*.

In providing consultation, consider emphasizing the following selected information (» = major clinical significance):

**Before using this medication**
» Conditions affecting use, especially:
  Sensitivity to tamoxifen
  Pregnancy—Use not recommended because of risk of miscarriage, death of the fetus, birth defects, and vaginal bleeding; advisability of using nonhormonal contraception during (and for about 2 months following) therapy; telling physician immediately if pregnancy is suspected
  Breast-feeding—Not recommended because of risk of serious side effects

**Proper use of this medication**
» Importance of not taking more or less medication than the amount prescribed
  Proper administration of enteric-coated tablets: Swallowing whole without crushing or breaking
» Frequency of nausea and vomiting; importance of continuing medication despite stomach upset
  Checking with physician if vomiting occurs shortly after dose is taken
» Proper dosing
  Missed dose: Not taking at all; not doubling doses
» Proper storage

**Precautions while using this medication**
» Importance of close monitoring by the physician
  For women: May increase fertility; advisability of using nonhormonal contraception during therapy; telling physician immediately if pregnancy is suspected
  Not taking an antacid within 1 or 2 hours of taking enteric-coated dosage form of tamoxifen

**Side/adverse effects**
  For women: Increased risk of endometrial carcinoma
  Signs of potential side effects, especially confusion, hepatotoxicity, retinopathy, corneal opacities, pulmonary embolus, thrombosis, and weakness or sleepiness
  Asymptomatic side effects, including hepatotoxicity and ocular toxicity
  Physician or nurse can help in dealing with side effects

## General Dosing Information

Patients receiving tamoxifen should be under supervision of a physician experienced in cancer chemotherapy.

If side effects are severe, dosage may sometimes be reduced without loss of control of the disease.

If severe hypercalcemia occurs, tamoxifen should be discontinued.

Ophthalmologic examination is recommended if visual disturbances occur, and withdrawal of tamoxifen should be considered if retinopathy or keratopathy is detected.

## Oral Dosage Forms

### TAMOXIFEN CITRATE TABLETS USP

Note: The dosing and strengths available are expressed in terms of tamoxifen base.

**Usual adult dose**
Breast carcinoma—
  Node-negative or node-positive: In women—Oral, 10 mg (base) two times a day (in the morning and evening).
  Metastatic: In men and women—Oral, 10 to 20 mg (base) two times a day (in the morning and evening).

**Strength(s) usually available**
U.S.—
  10 mg (base) (Rx) [*Nolvadex*].
Canada—
  10 mg (base) (Rx) [*Alpha-Tamoxifen; Med Tamoxifen; Nolvadex; Novo-Tamoxifen; Tamofen; Tamone; Tamoplex*].
  20 mg (base) (Rx) [*Alpha-Tamoxifen; Med Tamoxifen; Nolvadex; Novo-Tamoxifen; Tamofen; Tamone; Tamoplex*].

**Packaging and storage**
Store below 40 °C (104 °F), preferably between 15 and 30 °C (59 and 86 °F), unless otherwise specified by manufacturer. Store in a well-closed, light-resistant container.

### TAMOXIFEN CITRATE ENTERIC-COATED TABLETS

**Usual adult dose**
See *Tamoxifen Citrate Tablets USP*.

**Strength(s) usually available**
U.S.—
  Not commercially available.
Canada—
  20 mg (Rx) [*Nolvadex-D*].

**Packaging and storage**
Store below 40 °C (104 °F), preferably between 15 and 30 °C (59 and 86 °F), in a well-closed container, unless otherwise specified by manufacturer. Protect from light.

**Auxiliary labeling**
• Swallow tablets whole.
• Do not take antacids within 1 to 2 hours of taking this medicine.

Revised: 08/12/94

---

## TAZOBACTAM-CONTAINING COMBINATIONS—

Piperacillin and Tazobactam (Systemic)—See *Penicillins and Beta-lactamase Inhibitors (Systemic)*

---

# TECHNETIUM Tc 99m ALBUMIN   Systemic

VA CLASSIFICATION (Primary): DX201
Note: For a listing of dosage forms and brand names by country availability, see *Dosage Forms* section(s). For a listing of brand names for the articles in this monograph, refer to the General Index.

## Category

Diagnostic aid, radioactive (cardiac disease).

## Indications

**Accepted**
Cardiac blood pool imaging, radionuclide—Technetium Tc 99m albumin by intravenous administration is indicated as a cardiac blood pool imaging agent and as an adjunct in the diagnosis of pericardial effusion and ventricular aneurysm.

Although technetium Tc 99m albumin is an acceptable agent for cardiac blood pool imaging, it is not as widely used as technetium Tc 99m–labeled red blood cells for this indication.

**Unaccepted**
Technetium Tc 99m albumin has been used in placenta localization and may be used in blood volume determinations. However, for placenta localization, it has generally been replaced by the ultrasound technique. In general, blood volume determinations are performed with Cr 51– or technetium Tc 99m–labeled red blood cells (RBC) for RBC volume determinations, and with radioiodinated serum albumin for plasma volume determinations.

Technetium Tc 99m albumin has been used in lymphoscintigraphy to evaluate lymphatic drainage patterns of malignant melanoma.

# Physical Properties

## Nuclear data

| Radionu-clide (half-life) | Decay constant | Mode of decay | Principal photon emissions (keV) | Mean number of emissions/ disintegration ($\geq 0.01$) |
|---|---|---|---|---|
| Tc 99m (6 h) | 0.1151 h$^{-1}$ | Isomeric transition to Tc 99 | Gamma (18) | 0.062 |
| | | | Gamma (140.5) | 0.891 |

# Pharmacology/Pharmacokinetics

## Mechanism of action/Effect

Human albumin occurs naturally as the major protein component of blood. When labeled with technetium Tc 99m and given intravenously, it is distributed throughout the body in much the same way as the patient's serum albumin, and serves as a suitable tracer with which to transiently image the vascular compartment.

## Distribution

Vascular system; no significant accumulation in organs, except the kidneys, liver, and bladder.

## Half-life

Biological (normal human serum albumin)—Elimination: 10 to 16 hours.

## Radiation dosimetry

| Estimated absorbed radiation dose* | | |
|---|---|---|
| Organ | mGy/MBq | rad/mCi |
| Heart | 0.20 | 0.74 |
| Spleen | 0.14 | 0.52 |
| Lungs | 0.13 | 0.48 |
| Bone surfaces | 0.0089 | 0.033 |
| Adrenals | 0.0083 | 0.031 |
| Kidneys | 0.0081 | 0.030 |
| Red marrow | 0.0075 | 0.028 |
| Liver | 0.0073 | 0.027 |
| Pancreas | 0.0064 | 0.024 |
| Stomach wall | 0.0051 | 0.019 |
| Thyroid | 0.0049 | 0.018 |
| Uterus | 0.0048 | 0.018 |
| Small intestine | 0.0048 | 0.018 |
| Large intestine wall (upper) | 0.0047 | 0.017 |
| Breast | 0.0046 | 0.017 |
| Ovaries | 0.0044 | 0.016 |
| Large intestine wall (lower) | 0.0042 | 0.016 |
| Bladder wall | 0.0040 | 0.015 |
| Testes | 0.0029 | 0.011 |
| Other tissue | 0.0040 | 0.015 |

Effective dose: 0.079 mSv/MBq (0.29 rem/mCi)

*For adults; intravenous injection. Data based on the International Commission on Radiological Protection (ICRP) Publication 53—Radiation dose to patients from radiopharmaceuticals.

## Elimination

Renal, about 39% eliminated within 24 hours.

# Precautions to Consider

## Cross-sensitivity and/or related problems

Patients sensitive to human albumin products may be sensitive to this product also.

## Pregnancy/Reproduction

Pregnancy—Tc 99m (as free pertechnetate) crosses the placenta. However, studies have not been done with technetium Tc 99m albumin in humans.

The possibility of pregnancy should be assessed in women of child-bearing potential. Clinical situations exist where the benefit to the patient and fetus, based on information derived from radiopharmaceutical use, outweighs the risks from fetal exposure to radiation. In these situations, the physician should use discretion and reduce the radiopharmaceutical dose to the lowest possible amount.

Studies have not been done in animals.

FDA Pregnancy Category C.

## Breast-feeding

Although it is not known whether technetium Tc 99m albumin is excreted in breast milk, it is known that Tc 99m as free pertechnetate is excreted in breast milk. Based on the assumption that the Tc 99m in breast milk is in the form of pertechnetate and based on the effective half-life of the radionuclide in breast milk, the daily volume of milk, a dose factor relating the radionuclide to its critical organ (thyroid) in the nursing infant, and the maximum permissible dose to that organ, a guideline has been proposed. According to this guideline, it has been calculated that nursing can be safely resumed when the concentration in breast milk reaches $30.3 \times 10^{-4}$ megabecquerels ($8.2 \times 10^{-2}$ microcuries) per mL. This level of activity is probably reached, in the majority of patients, within 24 hours after administration of technetium Tc 99m–labeled radiopharmaceuticals.

## Pediatrics

There have been no specific studies evaluating the safety and efficacy of technetium Tc 99m albumin in children. When this radiopharmaceutical is used in children, the diagnostic benefit should be judged to outweigh the potential risk of radiation.

## Geriatrics

Appropriate studies on the relationship of age to the effects of technetium Tc 99m albumin have not been performed in the geriatric population. However, no geriatrics-specific problems have been documented to date.

## Medical considerations/Contraindications

The medical considerations/contraindications included here have been selected on the basis of their potential clinical significance (reasons given in parentheses where appropriate)—not necessarily inclusive (» = major clinical significance).

*Risk-benefit must be considered when the following medical problem exists:*

Sensitivity to human albumin products or to the radiopharmaceutical preparation

# Side/Adverse Effects

The following side/adverse effects have been selected on the basis of their potential clinical significance (possible signs and symptoms in parentheses where appropriate)—not necessarily inclusive:

## Those indicating need for medical attention

Incidence less frequent

*Allergic reaction* (shortness of breath; skin rash)

# Patient Consultation

As an aid to patient consultation, refer to *Advice for the Patient, Radiopharmaceuticals (Diagnostic).*

In providing consultation, consider emphasizing the following selected information (» = major clinical significance):

## Description of use

Action in the body: Distribution in body of injected radioactive albumin

Visualization of radioactivity in blood pool

Small amounts of radioactivity used in diagnosis; radiation received is low and considered safe

## Before having this test

» Conditions affecting use, especially:

Sensitivity to albumin products or to the radiopharmaceutical preparation

Pregnancy—Technetium Tc 99m (as free pertechnetate) crosses placenta; risk to fetus from radiation exposure as opposed to benefit derived from use should be considered

Breast-feeding—Not known if technetium Tc 99m albumin is excreted in breast milk, but Tc 99m as free pertechnetate is excreted in breast milk; temporary discontinuation of nursing may be recommended because of risk to infant from radiation exposure

Use in children—Risk from radiation exposure as opposed to benefit derived from use should be considered

## Preparation for this test

Special preparatory instructions may be given; patient should inquire in advance

## Precautions after having this test

No special precautions

## Side/adverse effects

Signs of potential side effects, especially allergic reaction

## General Dosing Information

Radiopharmaceuticals are to be administered only by or under the supervision of physicians who have had extensive training in the safe use and handling of radioactive materials and who are authorized by the Nuclear Regulatory Commission (NRC) or the appropriate Agreement State agency, if required, or, outside the U.S., the appropriate authority.

Epinephrine, antihistamines, and corticosteroid agents should be available during the administration of technetium Tc 99m albumin because of the possibility of allergic reactions.

Manufacturer's package insert or other appropriate literature should be consulted for optimal times when imaging should be performed.

### Safety considerations for handling this radiopharmaceutical

Improper handling of this radiopharmaceutical may cause radioactive contamination. Guidelines for handling radioactive material have been prepared by scientific, professional, state, federal, and international bodies and are available to the specially qualified and authorized users who have access to radiopharmaceuticals.

## Parenteral Dosage Forms

### TECHNETIUM Tc 99m ALBUMIN INJECTION USP

**Usual adult administered activity**
Cardiac blood pool imaging—
    Intravenous, 111 to 185 megabecquerels (3 to 5 millicuries).

**Usual pediatric administered activity**
Safety and efficacy have not been established in children under 18 years of age.

**Usual geriatric administered activity**
See *Usual adult administered activity*.

**Strength(s) usually available**
U.S.—
    Reaction vial:
        7 mg of albumin human and 80 mcg (0.08 mg) of stannous tartrate (lyophilized mixture, under nitrogen atmosphere), per 5-mL unit dose vial (Rx) [*Technetium Tc 99m HSA*].

21 mg of albumin human and 230 mcg (0.23 mg) of stannous tartrate (lyophilized mixture, under nitrogen atmosphere), per 10-mL multidose vial (Rx) [*Technetium Tc 99m HSA*].

Canada—
    Reaction vial: 50 mg of albumin human, 200 mcg (0.2 mg) of stannous chloride dihydrate, and 2 mg potassium biphthalate (lyophilized mixture, under nitrogen atmosphere) (Rx) [*Frosstimage Albumin*].

### Packaging and storage
Before and after reconstitution—Store between 2 and 8 °C (36 and 46 °F). Protect from freezing.

### Preparation of dosage form
To prepare injection, an oxidant-free sodium pertechnetate Tc 99m solution is used. See manufacturer's package insert for instructions.

### Stability
Injection should be administered within 6 hours after preparation.

### Incompatibilities
If oxidants such as peroxides and hypochlorites are present in the sodium pertechnetate Tc 99m used for labeling, the final preparation may be adversely affected and should be discarded.

### Note
Caution—Radioactive material.

## Selected Bibliography

Atkins HL, Klopper JF, Ansari AN, et al. A comparison of Tc 99m–labeled human serum albumin and *in vitro* labeled red blood cells for blood pool studies. Clin Nucl Med 1980; 5: 166-9.

Thrall JH, Freitas JE, Swanson D, et al. Clinical comparison of cardiac blood pool visualization with technetium 99m red blood cells labeled *in vivo* and with technetium 99m human serum albumin. J Nucl Med 1978; 19: 796-803.

Revised: 04/05/93
Interim revision: 08/02/94

---

# TECHNETIUM Tc 99m ALBUMIN AGGREGATED    Systemic

VA CLASSIFICATION (Primary): DX201
Note: For a listing of dosage forms and brand names by country availability, see *Dosage Forms* section(s). For a listing of brand names for the articles in this monograph, refer to the General Index.

## Category

Diagnostic aid, radioactive (pulmonary disease; vascular disorders); Chemotherapy adjunct.

## Indications

Note: Bracketed information in the *Indications* section refers to uses that are not included in U.S. product labeling.

**Accepted**

Lung imaging, radionuclide—Technetium Tc 99m albumin aggregated is indicated in adult and pediatric patients as a lung imaging agent to be used as an adjunct in the assessment of regional lung perfusion, primarily to screen for pulmonary emboli. It is also useful in the evaluation of the status of pulmonary circulation in such conditions as pulmonary neoplasm, pulmonary tuberculosis, and emphysema.

Venography, radionuclide—Technetium Tc 99m albumin aggregated is indicated to visualize specific regions of the vascular system and the blood flow in such areas, primarily to localize deep venous thrombosis in the lower extremities. Combined radionuclide venography of the lower extremities and pulmonary perfusion imaging may be performed with technetium Tc 99m albumin aggregated.

LeVeen peritoneovenous shunt patency assessment[1]—Intraperitoneal technetium Tc 99m albumin aggregated is indicated in adults to determine the patency of a peritoneovenous shunt in patients with ascites. The appearance of lung activity is used as the criterion for shunt patency.

[Chemotherapy, intra-arterial, infusion adjunct][1]—Technetium Tc 99m albumin aggregated is used as an adjunct to intra-arterial chemotherapy infusion for neoplasms (e.g., hepatic tumors) to assess blood flow, to

evaluate catheter placement and tumor perfusion, and to visualize the area of distribution of the infused chemotherapeutic agent.

[1]Not included in Canadian product labeling.

## Physical Properties

### Nuclear data

| Radionuclide (half-life) | Decay constant | Mode of decay | Principal photon emissions (keV) | Mean number of emissions/ disintegration ($\geq 0.01$) |
|---|---|---|---|---|
| Tc 99m (6.0 hr) | $0.1151\ \text{h}^{-1}$ | Isomeric transition to Tc 99 | Gamma (18) | 0.062 |
|  |  |  | Gamma (140.5) | 0.891 |

## Pharmacology/Pharmacokinetics

### Mechanism of action/Effect

Diagnostic aid (pulmonary disease)—The intravenously injected albumin particles labeled with technetium Tc 99m are temporarily trapped by the capillary bed of the lungs, making it possible to obtain an image of patent blood flow distribution within lungs.

Diagnostic aid (vascular disorders)—After injection into the dorsal pedal veins, technetium Tc 99m–labeled albumin particles are transported by the blood flow to the lungs where they are trapped in the capillary bed. However, if lower extremity venous thrombosis or obstruction is present, the albumin particles show retention and/or abnormal movement (delayed or collateral flow) in the peripheral veins.

LeVeen peritoneovenous shunt patency assessment—After intraperitoneal injection, clearance of technetium Tc 99m albumin aggregated from the peritoneal cavity may be insignificant, which occurs with peritoneovenous shunt blockage, or it may be very rapid, as with subsequent transfer into the systemic circulation when the shunt is patent. Visualization of radioactivity in lungs indicates shunt patency.

Intra-arterial chemotherapy, infusion adjunct—Albumin particles labeled with technetium Tc 99m infused through an intra-arterial catheter directly into the arterial supply of a neoplasm (or of the organ containing the neoplasm), at the same rate at which the chemotherapeutic agent is to be delivered, are trapped in the capillary bed allowing visualization of the perfusion pattern.

### Absorption
80 to 90% of the technetium Tc 99m albumin aggregated particles are trapped in the arterioles and capillaries of the lung during the first circulatory transit through the lungs after intravenous injection.

### Distribution
Dependent on particle size—Particles > 10 to 15 microns: Trapped in pulmonary arterioles and capillaries.

Distribution of particles in the lungs is dependent on regional pulmonary blood flow.

### Half-life
Biological elimination (from lungs)—Approximately 1 to 10 hours.

### Radiation dosimetry

| Estimated absorbed radiation dose* | | |
|---|---|---|
| Organ | mGy/MBq | rad/mCi |
| Lungs | 0.067 | 0.25 |
| Liver | 0.016 | 0.059 |
| Bladder wall | 0.010 | 0.037 |
| Adrenals | 0.0058 | 0.021 |
| Pancreas | 0.0058 | 0.021 |
| Breast | 0.0056 | 0.021 |
| Red marrow | 0.0044 | 0.016 |
| Spleen | 0.0044 | 0.016 |
| Stomach wall | 0.0040 | 0.015 |
| Kidneys | 0.0037 | 0.014 |
| Bone surfaces | 0.0035 | 0.013 |
| Uterus | 0.0024 | 0.0089 |
| Large intestine wall (upper) | 0.0022 | 0.0081 |
| Small intestine | 0.0021 | 0.0078 |
| Thyroid | 0.0020 | 0.0074 |
| Ovaries | 0.0018 | 0.0067 |
| Large intestine wall (lower) | 0.0016 | 0.0059 |
| Testes | 0.0011 | 0.0041 |
| Other tissue | 0.0029 | 0.011 |

Effective dose: 0.012 mSv/MBq (0.044 rem/mCi)

*For adults; intravenous injection. Data based on the International Commission on Radiological Protection (ICRP) Publication 53— Radiation dose to patients from radiopharmaceuticals.

### Elimination
Renal, 40 to 75% of injected technetium Tc 99m eliminated within 24 hours.

## Precautions to Consider

### Cross-sensitivity and/or related problems
Patients sensitive to human serum albumin products may be sensitive to this radiopharmaceutical also.

### Carcinogenicity/Mutagenicity
Long-term animal studies to evaluate carcinogenic or mutagenic potential of technetium Tc 99m albumin aggregated have not been performed.

### Pregnancy/Reproduction
Pregnancy—Tc 99m (as free pertechnetate) crosses the placenta. Studies have not been done in humans with technetium Tc 99m albumin aggregated.

The possibility of pregnancy should be assessed in women of child-bearing potential. Clinical situations exist where the benefit to the patient and fetus, based on information derived from radiopharmaceutical use, outweighs the risks from fetal exposure to radiation. In these situations, the physician should use discretion and reduce the radiopharmaceutical dose to the lowest possible amount.

Studies have not been done in animals.

FDA Pregnancy Category C.

### Breast-feeding
Although it is not known whether technetium Tc 99m albumin aggregated is distributed into breast milk, it is known that Tc 99m as free pertechnetate is distributed into breast milk. It has been estimated that, without discontinuation of breast-feeding, the radiation dose to the breast-fed infant will be less than 20 mrems after the mother receives a 4-millicurie dose of technetium Tc 99m albumin aggregated, assuming that all of the radioactive dose is in the form of Tc 99m pertechentate. Because of the potential risk to the infant from radiation exposure, temporary discontinuation of nursing is recommended for 6 to 12 hours.

### Pediatrics
Although appropriate studies have not been performed in the pediatric population, the number of particles administered should be reduced to the lowest possible level ($\leq$ 50,000 particles for newborns, $\leq$ 165,000 particles for 1-year-old infants) in these patients since the pulmonary capillary beds in children do not develop fully for several years after birth.

### Medical considerations/Contraindications
The medical considerations/contraindications included here have been selected on the basis of their potential clinical significance (reasons given in parentheses where appropriate)—not necessarily inclusive ($\gg$ = major clinical significance).

*Except under special circumstances, this medication should not be used when the following medical problem exists:*

$\gg$　Pulmonary hypertension, severe
　　　(deaths associated with administration of aggregated albumin have been reported)

*Risk-benefit should be considered when the following medical problems exist:*

　　Cardiac shunt, right-to-left
　　　(may increase risk because of rapid entry of aggregated albumin into the systemic circulation; it is recommended that the number of particles administered be reduced to 60,000 to 125,000 particles)

　　Cor pulmonale, acute or
　　Other states of severely impaired pulmonary blood flow
　　　(aggregated albumin may cause further impairment of blood flow; it is recommended that the number of particles administered be reduced to 125,000 particles or less)

$\gg$　Sensitivity to human serum albumin or to the radiopharmaceutical preparation

## Side/Adverse Effects

Note:　There are reports of hemodynamic or idiosyncratic reactions associated with the administration of technetium Tc 99m albumin aggregated.
　　　　As with any protein-containing preparation, allergic reactions are possible with the use of technetium Tc 99m albumin aggregated.

The following side/adverse effects have been selected on the basis of their potential clinical significance and/or frequency of occurrence (possible signs and symptoms in parentheses where appropriate)—not necessarily inclusive:

**Those indicating need for medical attention**
Incidence less frequent or rare
　　*Cyanosis* (bluish discoloration of skin); *wheezing, tightness in chest, or troubled breathing*

　　Note: *Wheezing, tightness in chest, or troubled breathing* may be initial manifestations of more severe respiratory distress.

**Those indicating need for medical attention only if they continue or are bothersome**
Incidence more frequent
　　*Flushing or redness of face*
Incidence less frequent
　　*Increased sweating; nausea*

## Patient Consultation

As an aid to patient consultation, refer to *Advice for the Patient, Radiopharmaceuticals (Diagnostic).*

In providing consultation, consider emphasizing the following selected information ($\gg$ = major clinical significance):

**Description of use**
　　Action in the body: Radioactive albumin particles temporarily trapped in capillaries of lungs
　　Tracing of radioactivity demonstrates the distribution of blood flow in lungs
　　Small amounts of radioactivity used in diagnosis; radiation received is low and considered safe

**Before having this test**

» Conditions affecting use, especially:

Sensitivity to albumin products or to the radiopharmaceutical preparation

Pregnancy—Technetium Tc 99m (as free pertechnetate) crosses placenta; risk to fetus from radiation exposure as opposed to benefit derived from use should be considered

Breast-feeding—Not known if distributed into breast milk; temporary discontinuation of nursing may be recommended because of risk to infant from radiation exposure

Use in children—Risk from radiation exposure as opposed to benefit derived from use should be considered

**Preparation for this test**

Special preparatory instructions may be given; patient should inquire in advance

**Precautions after having this test**

No special precautions

**Side/adverse effects**

Signs of potential side effects, especially allergic reaction or respiratory distress

## General Dosing Information

Radiopharmaceuticals are to be administered only by or under the supervision of physicians who have had extensive training in the safe use and handling of radioactive materials and who are authorized by the Nuclear Regulatory Commission (NRC) or the appropriate Agreement State agency if required, or, outside the U.S., the appropriate authority.

Technetium Tc 99m albumin aggregated should be administered by slow intravenous injection with the patient in a recumbent position. During injection, the aspiration of blood into the syringe should be avoided since this can cause the formation of blood clots (containing the radioactive material) in the syringe, which may result in focal areas of increased radioactivity later on during lung imaging.

125,000 to 2,000,000 particles of aggregated albumin should be administered to adults per dosage.

Pediatric dosages must contain significantly fewer particles than adult dosages since the pulmonary capillary beds in pediatric patients are not as developed. It has been suggested that if 500,000 particles are considered safe in an adult, a newborn should not receive more than 50,000 particles, and a one-year-old no more than 165,000 particles.

Epinephrine, antihistamines, and corticosteroid agents should be available during the administration of technetium Tc 99m albumin aggregated because of the possibility of allergic reactions.

For lung imaging, it is recommended that the patient be positioned under the imaging apparatus before administration of technetium Tc 99m albumin aggregated and that imaging begin immediately after injection.

**Safety considerations for handling this radiopharmaceutical**

Improper handling of this radiopharmaceutical may cause radioactive contamination. Guidelines for handling radioactive material have been prepared by scientific, professional, state, federal, and international bodies and are available to the specially qualified and authorized users who have access to radiopharmaceuticals.

## Parenteral Dosage Forms

### TECHNETIUM Tc 99m ALBUMIN AGGREGATED INJECTION USP

**Usual adult and adolescent administered activity**

Lung imaging—

Intravenous, 37 to 148 megabecquerels (1 to 4 millicuries).

Venography—

Intravenous, 74 to 148 megabecquerels (2 to 4 millicuries) per extremity.

LeVeen shunt patency[1]—

Intraperitoneal, 37 to 111 megabecquerels (1 to 3 millicuries).

Percutaneous transtubal, 12 to 37 megabecquerels (0.3 to 1 millicurie) in a volume not to exceed 0.5 mL.

Note: The lowest possible number of particles per dosage (60,000 to 125,000) should be administered to patients with right-to-left cardiac shunt or with states of severely impaired pulmonary blood flow.

**Usual pediatric administered activity**

Lung imaging—

Intravenous, 0.925 to 1.85 megabecquerels (25 to 50 microcuries) per kg of body weight.

Note: In newborns, the total dosage should be at least 7.4 megabecquerels (200 microcuries).

**Usual geriatric administered activity**

See *Usual adult and adolescent administered activity.*

**Strength(s) usually available**

U.S.—

0.11 mg albumin aggregated, 0.09 mg stannous tartrate, and 0.3 mL isotonic saline, per reaction vial (Rx) [GENERIC].

1.0 mg albumin aggregated, 10.0 mg albumin human, 0.02 mg stannous chloride, 0.12 mg total tin, 10 mg sodium chloride, with 3.6 to 6.5 × 10⁶ particles, per 10-mL reaction vial (Rx) [*Pulmolite*].

1.5 mg albumin aggregated, 10.0 mg albumin human, 0.07 mg stannous chloride, 0.19 mg total tin, 1.8 mg sodium chloride, with 1.0 to 8.0 × 10⁶ particles, per 5-mL reaction vial (Rx) [*Macrotec*].

2.0 mg albumin aggregated, 0.5 mg albumin human, 0.12 mg stannous chloride, 80 mg lactose, 24 mg succinic acid, and 1.4 mg sodium acetate, with 8 ± 4 × 10⁶ particles, per 10-mL reaction vial (Rx) [*TechneScan MAA*].

2.0 mg albumin aggregated, 0.16 mg stannous chloride, and 17 mg sodium chloride, with 6.8 ± 0.8 × 10⁶ particles, per reaction vial (Rx) [*AN-MAA*].

2.5 mg albumin aggregated, 5.0 mg albumin human, 0.06 mg stannous chloride, and 1.2 mg sodium chloride, with 4.0 to 8.0 × 10⁶ particles, per 10-mL reaction vial (Rx) [*MPI MAA;* GENERIC].

Canada—

2.5 mg albumin aggregated, 5.0 mg albumin human, 0.1 mg stannous chloride (dihydrate), and 1.2 mg sodium chloride, with 4.0 to 8.0 × 10⁶ particles, per 10-mL reaction vial (Rx) [*Frosstimage MAA*].

**Packaging and storage**

Store between 2 and 8 °C (36 and 46 °F). Protect from freezing.

**Preparation of dosage form**

To prepare injection, an oxidant-free sodium pertechnetate Tc 99m solution is used. See manufacturer's package insert for instructions.

**Stability**

Preparations in which clumping or foaming of contents are observed should not be used.

Injection should be administered within 3, 6, or 8 hours after preparation, depending on product used.

**Incompatibilities**

If oxidants such as peroxides and hypochlorites are present in the sodium pertechnetate Tc 99m used for labeling, the final preparation may be adversely affected and should be discarded.

**Note**

Caution—Radioactive material.

Agitate gently before using.

---

[1]Not included in Canadian product labeling.

## Selected Bibliography

Algeo JH, Powell M, Couacaud J. LeVeen shunt visualization without function using technetium 99m macroaggregated albumin. Clin Nucl Med 1987; 12 (9): 741-3.

---

Revised: 06/14/93
Interim revision: 08/02/94

# TECHNETIUM Tc 99m ALBUMIN COLLOID   Systemic†

## VA CLASSIFICATION (Primary): DX201

Note: For a listing of dosage forms and brand names by country availability, see *Dosage Forms* section(s). For a listing of brand names for the articles in this monograph, refer to the General Index.

†Not commercially available in Canada.

## Category

Diagnostic aid, radioactive (hepatic disease; hematologic disease; splenic disease).

## Indications

### Accepted

Liver imaging, radionuclide—Technetium Tc 99m albumin colloid, administered intravenously, is indicated for imaging the functioning reticuloendothelial cells of the liver in the evaluation of metastatic disease, primary liver tumors, abscesses, and other focal hepatic lesions. It is also indicated in the evaluation of patients with cirrhosis, hepatitis, and other hepatic disorders.

Spleen imaging, radionuclide—Technetium Tc 99m albumin colloid, administered intravenously, is indicated for imaging the functioning reticuloendothelial cells of the spleen, thus serving to demonstrate clinically significant splenomegaly, and for evaluating splenic infarct or splenic rupture.

Bone marrow imaging, radionuclide—Technetium Tc 99m albumin colloid, administered intravenously, is indicated for imaging the functioning reticuloendothelial cells of the bone marrow to complement other hematological studies for the evaluation of hematopoiesis in hematological diseases, such as leukemia, polycythemia, anemias, and myelofibrosis. Also, imaging with technetium Tc 99m albumin colloid helps localize sites for bone marrow biopsy and helps demonstrate or define areas of marrow invasion by metastatic disease and areas of decreased marrow function secondary to radiation therapy.

## Physical Properties

### Nuclear data

| Radionu-clide (half-life) | Decay constant | Mode of decay | Principal photon emissions (keV) | Mean number of emissions/ disintegration ($\geq$0.01) |
|---|---|---|---|---|
| Tc 99m (6.0 hr) | 0.1151 h⁻¹ | Isomeric transition to Tc 99 | Gamma (18) Gamma (140.5) | 0.062 0.891 |

## Pharmacology/Pharmacokinetics

### Mechanism of action/Effect

Diagnostic aid (hepatic disease; hematologic disease; splenic disease)—Radioactive colloids are phagocytized by the reticuloendothelial system of the liver, spleen, and bone marrow, and remain there long enough for scintillation scans of their distribution to be obtained.

### Distribution

The colloid particles are rapidly phagocytized by the reticuloendothelial system after intravenous administration. Distribution is dependent upon blood flow rates and the functional capacity of the phagocytic cells. In the average normal patient, 80 to 90% of the administered activity localizes in the liver, 5 to 10% in the spleen, and the remainder in bone marrow. Levels of activity in the liver and spleen remain constant for at least 4 hours.

Uptake in the lungs and other soft tissues is possible in the presence of a wide variety of disorders, usually inflammatory or neoplastic.

Note: In progressively severe hepatic dysfunction (e.g., hepatic cirrhosis), greater amounts of the colloid appear in the spleen, bone marrow, and sometimes, in the lungs.

### Half-life

Elimination from the blood pool—2 to 3 minutes.

## Time to radioactivity visualization:

Liver and spleen imaging—10 to 15 minutes.

Note: In patients with severe hepatic disease, onset of visualization may be delayed because of slower blood clearance of the colloid.

Bone marrow imaging—15 minutes.

### Radiation dosimetry

| Organ | Estimated absorbed radiation dose* | | | |
|---|---|---|---|---|
| | With normal hepatic function | | With parenchymal liver disease (intermediate/advanced) | |
| | mGy/ MBq | rad/ mCi | mGy/ MBq | rad/ mCi |
| Spleen | 0.077 | 0.29 | 0.14 | 0.52 |
| Liver | 0.074 | 0.27 | 0.042 | 0.16 |
| Pancreas | 0.012 | 0.044 | 0.018 | 0.066 |
| Red marrow | 0.011 | 0.041 | 0.023 | 0.085 |
| Adrenals | 0.01 | 0.037 | 0.0098 | 0.036 |
| Kidneys | 0.0097 | 0.036 | 0.011 | 0.041 |
| Bone surfaces | 0.0064 | 0.024 | 0.012 | 0.044 |
| Stomach wall | 0.0062 | 0.023 | 0.0098 | 0.036 |
| Large intestine wall (upper) | 0.0056 | 0.021 | 0.0049 | 0.018 |
| Lungs | 0.0055 | 0.20 | 0.0048 | 0.018 |
| Small intestine | 0.0043 | 0.016 | 0.0046 | 0.017 |
| Breast | 0.0027 | 0.01 | 0.0024 | 0.0089 |
| Ovaries | 0.0022 | 0.0081 | 0.0033 | 0.012 |
| Uterus | 0.0019 | 0.0070 | 0.0028 | 0.01 |
| Large intestine wall (lower) | 0.0018 | 0.0067 | 0.0031 | 0.011 |
| Bladder wall | 0.0011 | 0.0041 | 0.0016 | 0.0059 |
| Thyroid | 0.00079 | 0.0029 | 0.0011 | 0.0041 |
| Testes | 0.00062 | 0.0023 | 0.00095 | 0.0035 |
| Other tissue | 0.0028 | 0.01 | 0.0031 | 0.011 |

| Radionuclide | Effective dose* | | | |
|---|---|---|---|---|
| | With normal hepatic function | | With parenchymal liver disease (intermediate/advanced) | |
| | mSv/ MBq | rem/ mCi | mSv/ MBq | rem/ mCi |
| Tc 99m | 0.014 | 0.052 | 0.017 | 0.063 |

*For adults; intravenous injection of technetium Tc 99m–labeled large colloids. Data based on the International Commission on Radiological Protection (ICRP) Publication 53—Radiation dose to patients from radiopharmaceuticals.

### Elimination

Renal, 4 to 30% of the administered activity is eliminated by 24 hours after injection.

## Precautions to Consider

### Cross-sensitivity and/or related problems

Patients sensitive to human serum albumin products may be sensitive to this radiopharmaceutical also.

### Carcinogenicity/Mutagenicity

Long-term animal studies to evaluate carcinogenic or mutagenic potential of technetium Tc 99m albumin colloid have not been performed.

### Pregnancy/Reproduction

Pregnancy—Tc 99m (as free pertechnetate) crosses the placenta. Studies with technetium Tc 99m albumin colloid have not been done in humans.

The possibility of pregnancy should be assessed in women of child-bearing potential. Clinical situations exist in which the benefit to the patient and fetus, based on information derived from radiopharmaceutical use, outweighs the risks from fetal exposure to radiation. In these situations, the physician should use discretion and reduce the radiopharmaceutical dose to the lowest possible amount.

Studies have not been done in animals.

FDA Pregnancy Category C.

**Breast-feeding**

Although it is not known whether technetium Tc 99m albumin colloid is distributed into breast milk, it is known that Tc 99m as free pertechnetate is distributed into breast milk. Based on the assumption that the Tc 99m in breast milk is in the form of pertechnetate and based on the effective half-life of the radionuclide in breast milk, the daily volume of milk, a dose factor relating the radionuclide to its critical organ (thyroid) in the nursing infant, and the maximum permissible dose to that organ, a guideline has been proposed. According to this guideline, it has been calculated that nursing can be safely resumed when the concentration in breast milk reaches $30.3 \times 10^{-4}$ megabecquerels ($8.2 \times 10^{-2}$ microcuries) per mL. This level of activity is probably reached, in the majority of patients, within 12 to 24 hours after administration of technetium Tc 99m–labeled radiopharmaceuticals.

**Pediatrics**

Diagnostic studies performed to date using technetium Tc 99 albumin colloid have not demonstrated pediatrics-specific problems that would limit the usefulness of technetium Tc 99m albumin colloid in children. However, when this radiopharmaceutical is used in children, the diagnostic benefit should be judged to outweigh the potential risk of radiation.

**Geriatrics**

Appropriate studies on the relationship of age to the effects of technetium Tc 99m albumin colloid have not been performed in the geriatric population. However, no geriatrics-specific problems have been documented to date.

**Drug interactions and/or related problems**

See *Diagnostic interference*.

**Diagnostic interference**

The following have been selected on the basis of their potential clinical significance (possible effect in parentheses where appropriate)—not necessarily inclusive ($\gg$ = major clinical significance):

With results of this test

*Due to other medications*

Anesthetics, inhalation, such as halothane

(recent administration of general anesthetics may increase splenic uptake of technetium Tc 99m albumin colloid, probably because the reduced hepatic flow and hepatotoxicity associated with general anesthetics may alter the hepatic radiocolloid extraction efficiency, resulting in an alteration of the normal liver-spleen colloid distribution pattern)

Chemotherapy, especially with nitrosoureas

(use of technetium Tc 99m albumin colloid in patients who are undergoing or have recently undergone chemotherapy may result in nonhomogeneous or irregular hepatic uptake, shift of activity from the liver to the bone marrow and spleen, and hepatomegaly; irregular hepatic distribution of radiopharmaceutical may be misinterpreted as malignancy; thus, it is recommended that liver and/or spleen imaging be done prior to initiating chemotherapy with these agents or several weeks after discontinuing therapy)

Reticuloendothelial system stimulators, such as:

Dextrose

Heparin

Steroid hormones (including estrogen)

Thyroid hormones

Vitamin $B_{12}$

(use of technetium Tc 99m albumin colloid in patients using these medications may result in lung uptake of technetium Tc 99m albumin colloid, probably due to a drug-induced increase in number of free intravascular macrophages, which may migrate to the pulmonary capillary bed and phagocytize colloidal particles there)

*Due to medical problems or conditions*

Viral infections

(decreased function of the reticuloendothelial system caused by the viral infection may result in prolonged appearance of the technetium Tc 99m albumin colloid in the blood)

**Medical considerations/Contraindications**

The medical considerations/contraindications included here have been selected on the basis of their potential clinical significance (reasons given in parentheses where appropriate)—not necessarily inclusive ($\gg$ = major clinical significance).

See also *Diagnostic interference*.

*Risk-benefit should be considered when the following medical problem exists:*

$\gg$ Sensitivity to human serum albumin or to the radiopharmaceutical preparation

## Side/Adverse Effects

The following side/adverse effects have been selected on the basis of their potential clinical significance and/or frequency of occurrence (possible signs and symptoms in parentheses where appropriate)—not necessarily inclusive:

**Those indicating need for medical attention**

Incidence less frequent or rare

*Allergic reaction* (coughing or choking; flushing or redness of face; skin rash, hives, or itching; swelling of throat, hands, or feet; wheezing, tightness in chest, or troubled breathing)

Note: The *allergic reaction* may be the initial manifestation of a more severe anaphylactic reaction.

**Those indicating need for medical attention only if they continue or are bothersome**

Incidence less frequent

*Abdominal pain; dizziness; fever; flushing of skin; increased sweating; nausea*

## Patient Consultation

As an aid to patient consultation, refer to *Advice for the Patient, Radiopharmaceuticals (Diagnostic)*.

In providing consultation, consider emphasizing the following selected information ($\gg$ = major clinical significance):

**Description of use**

Action in the body: Accumulation of radioactive colloid particles in liver, spleen, and bone marrow

Retention of radioactivity in these organs allows visualization

Small amounts of radioactivity used in diagnosis; radiation received is low and considered safe

**Before having this test**

$\gg$ Conditions affecting use, especially:

Sensitivity to albumin products or to the radiopharmaceutical preparation

Pregnancy—Technetium Tc 99m (as free pertechnetate) crosses placenta; risk to fetus from radiation exposure as opposed to benefit derived from use should be considered

Breast-feeding—Not known if technetium Tc 99m albumin colloid is distributed into breast milk, but Tc 99m as free pertechnetate is distributed into breast milk; temporary discontinuation of nursing may be recommended because of risk to infant from radiation exposure

Use in children—Risk from radiation exposure as opposed to benefit derived from use should be considered

**Preparation for this test**

Special preparatory instructions may be given; patient should inquire in advance

**Precautions after having this test**

No special precautions

**Side/adverse effects**

Signs of potential side effects, especially allergic reaction

## General Dosing Information

Radiopharmaceuticals are to be administered only by or under the supervision of physicians who have had extensive training in the safe use and handling of radioactive materials and who are authorized by the Nuclear Regulatory Commission (NRC) or the appropriate Agreement State agency if required, or, outside the U.S., the appropriate authority.

Technetium Tc 99m albumin colloid should be administered by intravenous injection and, preferably, with the patient in a recumbent position (in the erect position the liver may appear larger). During injection, the aspiration of blood into the syringe should be avoided since this can cause the formation of blood clots (containing the radioactive material) in the syringe, which may result in focal areas of increased radioactivity during lung imaging.

Epinephrine, antihistamines, and corticosteroids should be available during the administration of technetium Tc 99m albumin colloid because of the possibility of allergic reactions.

**Safety considerations for handling this radiopharmaceutical**

Improper handling of this radiopharmaceutical may cause radioactive contamination. Guidelines for handling radioactive material have been prepared by scientific, professional, state, federal, and international bodies and are available to the specially qualified and authorized users who have access to radiopharmaceuticals.

# Parenteral Dosage Forms

## TECHNETIUM Tc 99m ALBUMIN COLLOID INJECTION

### Usual adult and adolescent administered activity
Liver, spleen, and/or bone marrow imaging—
Intravenous, 37 to 296 megabecquerels (1 to 8 millicuries).

Note: For bone marrow imaging, 370 to 444 megabecquerels (10 to 12 millicuries) are usually required.

### Usual pediatric administered activity
Dosage must be individualized by physician.
Liver and spleen imaging:
Activity administered has ranged between 0.55 and 2.75 megabecquerels (15 to 75 microcuries) per kg of body weight, with a usual administered activity of 1.8 megabecquerels (50 microcuries) per kg of body weight.

Note: In newborns, the total minimum administered activity recommended for liver and spleen imaging is 11.1 to 18.5 megabecquerels (300 to 500 microcuries).

Bone marrow imaging:
A dosage of 5.18 megabecquerels (140 microcuries) per kg of body weight is recommended.

### Usual geriatric administered activity
See *Usual adult and adolescent administered activity*.

### Strength(s) usually available
U.S.—
1 mg albumin colloid, 10 mg normal human serum albumin, 0.0054 mg stannous chloride (minimum), 0.17 mg total tin (maximum), 1.1 mg poloxamer 188, 0.12 mg medronate disodium, and 10 mg sodium phosphate (anhydrous), per reaction vial (Rx) [*Microlite*].

Canada—
Not commercially available.

### Packaging and storage
Store between 2 and 8 °C (36 and 46 °F). Protect from freezing. Protect from light.

### Preparation of dosage form
To prepare injection, an oxidant-free sodium pertechnetate Tc 99m solution is used. See manufacturer's package insert for instructions.

### Stability
Preparations in which clumping of contents are observed should not be used.
Injection should be administered within 6 hours after preparation.

### Incompatibilities
If oxidants such as peroxides and hypochlorites are present in the sodium pertechnetate Tc 99m used for labeling, the final preparation may be adversely affected and should be discarded.

### Note
Caution—Radioactive material.
Agitate gently before using.

## Selected Bibliography

Klingensmith WC, Spitzer VM, Fritzberg AR, et al. Normal appearance and reproducibility of liver-spleen studies with Tc 99m sulfur colloid and Tc 99m microalbumin colloid. J Nucl Med 1983; 24: 8-13.
Saha GB, Feiglin DHI, O'Donnell JK, et al. Experience with technetium Tc 99m albumin colloid kit for reticuloendothelial system imaging. J Nucl Med Technol 1986; 14: 149-51.

Developed: 08/17/94

---

# TECHNETIUM Tc 99m BICISATE  Systemic

VA CLASSIFICATION (Primary): DX201
Another commonly used name for bicisate is ethyl cysteinate dimer (ECD).

Note: For a listing of dosage forms and brand names by country availability, see *Dosage Forms* section(s). For a listing of brand names for the articles in this monograph, refer to the General Index.

## Category
Diagnostic aid, radioactive (cerebrovascular disease).

## Indications
Note: Bracketed information in the *Indications* section refers to uses that are not included in U.S. product labeling.

### Accepted
Brain imaging, radionuclide—Single-photon emission computed tomography (SPECT) using technetium Tc 99m bicisate is indicated as an adjunct to conventional computed tomography (CT) or magnetic resonance imaging (MRI) in the localization of stroke in patients in whom stroke has already been diagnosed. However, [technetium Tc 99m bicisate is also used in the evaluation and localization of altered regional cerebral perfusion associated with functional impairment in patients with neurological disorders not limited to stroke, but including such disorders as dementia, head trauma, and epilepsy].

## Physical Properties

### Nuclear data

| Radionu-clide (half-life) | Decay constant | Mode of decay | Principal photon emissions (keV) | Mean number of emissions/ disintegration ($\geq 0.01$) |
|---|---|---|---|---|
| Tc 99m (6.0 hr) | 0.1151 h$^{-1}$ | Isomeric transition to Tc 99 | Gamma (18) | 0.062 |
| | | | Gamma (140.5) | 0.891 |

## Pharmacology/Pharmacokinetics

### Mechanism of action/Effect
Brain imaging—Technetium Tc 99m bicisate is a lipophilic complex with high first-pass extraction fraction and deposition and retention in the brain in proportion to cerebral blood flow (perfusion). Its radionuclide emissions permit external imaging of the cerebral distribution of the agent, thus allowing the detection of altered regional cerebral perfusion. The retention in the brain of technetium Tc 99m bicisate results from *in vivo* metabolism (deesterification) of the primary complex to polar, less diffusable compounds (mono- and di-acids).

### Distribution
High initial cerebral uptake with rapid blood clearance after intravenous injection (less than 10% of the administered activity remains in the blood after 5 minutes). Approximately 5 to 8% of administered activity localizes in the brain within 5 minutes after injection and exhibits little change for one hour after injection. Brain washout is approximately 20% between 5 and 60 minutes after injection and approximately 10% per hour thereafter.

### Time to radioactivity visualization:
10 minutes to 6 hours after injection. Optimal images may be obtained 30 to 60 minutes after administration to allow washout from facial muscles and salivary glands and thereby increase brain-to-soft-tissue ratios.

### Radiation dosimetry

| Organ | Estimated absorbed radiation dose* | | | |
|---|---|---|---|---|
| | With 2-hour void | | With 4.8 hour void | |
| | mGy/ MBq | rad/ mCi | mGy/ MBq | rad/ mCi |
| Urinary bladder wall | 0.03 | 0.11 | 0.073 | 0.27 |
| Gallbladder wall | 0.025 | 0.091 | 0.025 | 0.091 |
| Large intestine wall, upper | 0.016 | 0.061 | 0.017 | 0.063 |
| Large intestine wall, lower | 0.013 | 0.047 | 0.015 | 0.055 |
| Small intestine | 0.0094 | 0.035 | 0.01 | 0.038 |
| Kidneys | 0.0073 | 0.027 | 0.0074 | 0.027 |

| Organ | Estimated absorbed radiation dose* | | | |
|---|---|---|---|---|
| | With 2-hour void | | With 4.8 hour void | |
| | mGy/ MBq | rad/ mCi | mGy/ MBq | rad/ mCi |
| Uterus | 0.0063 | 0.023 | 0.011 | 0.041 |
| Brain | 0.0055 | 0.02 | 0.0055 | 0.02 |
| Ovaries | 0.0054 | 0.022 | 0.008 | 0.03 |
| Liver | 0.0053 | 0.02 | 0.0054 | 0.02 |
| Thyroid | 0.0035 | 0.013 | 0.0035 | 0.013 |
| Bone surfaces | 0.0034 | 0.013 | 0.0038 | 0.014 |
| Adrenals | 0.0025 | 0.009 | 0.0025 | 0.009 |
| Pancreas | 0.003 | 0.011 | 0.003 | 0.011 |
| Red marrow | 0.0024 | 0.009 | 0.0027 | 0.01 |
| Stomach | 0.0024 | 0.009 | 0.0025 | 0.0093 |
| Testes | 0.0022 | 0.008 | 0.0036 | 0.013 |
| Muscle | 0.002 | 0.007 | 0.0024 | 0.009 |
| Spleen | 0.002 | 0.0073 | 0.002 | 0.0073 |
| Lungs | 0.002 | 0.008 | 0.002 | 0.008 |
| Heart wall | 0.0018 | 0.0067 | 0.0018 | 0.0067 |
| Skin | 0.001 | 0.0037 | 0.0012 | 0.0043 |
| Thymus | 0.0013 | 0.0047 | 0.0013 | 0.0047 |
| Breast | 0.00094 | 0.0037 | 0.00094 | 0.0037 |
| Total body | 0.0024 | 0.009 | 0.0029 | 0.011 |

| Radionuclide | Effective dose† | | | |
|---|---|---|---|---|
| | With 2-hour void | | With 4.8 hour void | |
| | mSv/ MBq | rem/ mCi | mSv/ MBq | rem/ mCi |
| Tc 99m | 0.0095 | 0.035 | 0.013 | 0.048 |

*For adults; intravenous injection. Data based on information from the Oak Ridge Associated Universities, Radiopharmaceutical Internal Dose Information Center.

†Calculated according to the method of the International Commission on Radiological Protection (ICRP) publication 60.

**Elimination**
Renal—About 50% of the administered activity is excreted as metabolites within 2 hours, and about 74% within 24 hours.
Fecal—About 12% of the administered activity is excreted after 48 hours.

## Precautions to Consider

### Carcinogenicity
Long-term animal studies to evaluate carcinogenic potential of technetium Tc 99m bicisate have not been performed.

### Pregnancy/Reproduction
Pregnancy—Tc 99m (as free pertechnetate) crosses the placenta. Although studies have not been done with technetium Tc 99m bicisate in humans, the estimated absorbed radiation dose to the uterus is 6.99 mGy/ 1110 MBq (0.69 rad/30 mCi) for a 2-hour void, and 12.2 mGy/1110 MBq (1.23 rad/30 mCi) for a 4.8-hour void. There is no evidence demonstrating embryonic or fetal harm at these doses.
Nevertheless, the possibility of pregnancy should be assessed in women of child-bearing potential. In these situations, the physician should use discretion and reduce the administered activity of the radiopharmaceutical to the lowest possible amount.
Studies have not been done in animals.
FDA Pregnancy Category C.

### Breast-feeding
Although it is not known whether technetium Tc 99m bicisate is distributed into breast milk, it is known that Tc 99m as free pertechnetate is distributed into breast milk. Based on the assumption that the Tc 99m in breast milk is in the form of pertechnetate, and based on the effective half-life of the radionuclide in breast milk, the daily volume of milk, a dose factor relating the radionuclide to its critical organ (thyroid) in the nursing infant, and the maximum permissible dose to that organ, a guideline has been proposed. According to this guideline, it has been calculated that nursing can be safely resumed when the concentration in breast milk reaches $30.3 \times 10^{-4}$ megabecquerels ($8.2 \times 10^{-2}$ microcuries) per mL. This level of activity is probably reached, in the majority of patients, within 24 hours after administration of 740 megabecquerels (20 millicuries) of technetium Tc 99m–labeled radiopharmaceuticals.

### Pediatrics
There have been no specific studies evaluating the safety and efficacy of technetium Tc 99m bicisate in pediatric patients. However, no pediatrics-specific problems have been documented to date.

### Geriatrics
Diagnostic studies performed to date using technetium Tc 99m bicisate have not demonstrated geriatrics-specific problems that would limit the usefulness of technetium Tc 99m bicisate in the elderly.

### Medical considerations/Contraindications
The medical considerations/contraindications included here have been selected on the basis of their potential clinical significance (reasons given in parentheses where appropriate)—not necessarily inclusive (» = major clinical significance).

*Risk-benefit should be considered when the following medical problem exists:*
Sensitivity to the radiopharmaceutical preparation

## Side/Adverse Effects

The following side/adverse effects have been selected on the basis of their potential clinical significance (possible signs and symptoms in parentheses where appropriate)—not necessarily inclusive:

**Those indicating need for medical attention**
Incidence rare
  *Angina* (chest pain); *difficulty breathing; hallucinations; hypertension; seizures; skin rash*

**Those indicating need for medical attention only if they continue or are bothersome**
Incidence rare
  *Agitation or anxiety; dizziness; drowsiness; headache; nausea; parosomia* (transient, mild, pleasant aromatic odor)

## Patient Consultation

As an aid to patient consultation, refer to *Advice for the Patient, Radiopharmaceuticals (Diagnostic)*.

In providing consultation, consider emphasizing the following selected information (» = major clinical significance):

**Description of use**
Action in the body: Concentration of radioactive bicisate in brain
Retention of radioactivity in brain allows visualization
Small amount of radioactivity used in diagnosis; radiation received is low and considered safe

**Before having this test**
» Conditions affecting use, especially:
  Sensitivity to the radiopharmaceutical preparation
  Pregnancy—Technetium Tc 99m (as free pertechnetate) crosses placenta; reducing administered activity should be considered
  Breast-feeding—Not known if technetium Tc 99m bicisate is distributed into breast milk, but Tc 99m as free pertechnetate is distributed into breast milk; temporary discontinuation of nursing may be recommended to avoid any unnecessary absorbed radiation dose to the infant

**Preparation for this test**
Special preparatory instructions may be given; patient should inquire in advance

**Precautions after having this test**
Adequate intake of fluids before and after administration of technetium Tc 99m bicisate; voiding frequently for 2 to 6 hours after administration to promote urine flow and to minimize absorbed radiation dose to bladder

**Side/adverse effects**
Signs of rare, but possible, side effects, especially angina, difficulty breathing, hallucinations, hypertension, seizures, and skin rash

## General Dosing Information

Radiopharmaceuticals are to be administered only by or under the supervision of physicians who have had extensive training in the safe use and handling of radioactive materials and who are authorized by the Nuclear Regulatory Commission (NRC) or the appropriate Agreement State agency, if required, or, outside the U.S., the appropriate authority.

Adequate hydration of the patient is recommended before and after administration of technetium Tc 99m bicisate to promote urinary flow and blood pool clearance. Also, urination is recommended as often as possible for 2 to 6 hours after the examination to promote urine flow, thereby minimizing absorbed radiation dose to the bladder.

**Safety considerations for handling this radiopharmaceutical**
Improper handling of this radiopharmaceutical may cause radioactive contamination. Guidelines for handling radioactive material have been prepared by scientific, professional, state, federal, and international

bodies and are available to the specially qualified and authorized users who have access to radiopharmaceuticals.

## Parenteral Dosage Forms

### TECHNETIUM Tc 99m BICISATE INJECTION

**Usual adult and adolescent administered activity**
Brain imaging—
Intravenous, 370 to 1110 megabecquerels (10 to 30 millicuries).

**Usual pediatric administered activity**
Safety and dosage have not been established.

**Usual geriatric administered activity**
See *Usual adult and adolescent administered activity.*

**Strength(s) usually available**
U.S.—
0.9 mg bicisate dihydrochloride, 0.36 mg edetate disodium (dihydrate), 72 mcg (0.072 mg) stannous chloride dihydrate (theoretical), 12 mcg (0.012 mg) stannous chloride dihydrate (minimum), 83 mcg (0.083 mg) total tin (dihydrate) and 24 mg mannitol, in lyophilized form under nitrogen atmosphere, per reaction vial A; and 4.1 mg sodium phosphate dibasic heptahydrate, 0.46 mg sodium phosphate monobasic monohydrate, and enough water for injection to produce 1 mL, per reaction vial B (Rx) [*Neurolite*].
Canada—
0.9 mg bicisate dihydrochloride, 0.36 mg edetate disodium (dihydrate), 72 mcg (0.072 mg) stannous chloride dihydrate (theoretical), 12 mcg (0.012 mg) stannous chloride dihydrate (minimum), 83 mcg (0.083 mg) total tin (dihydrate) and 24 mg mannitol, in lyophilized form under nitrogen atmosphere, per reaction vial A; and 4.1 mg sodium phosphate dibasic heptahydrate, 0.46 mg sodium phosphate monobasic monohydrate, and enough water for injection to produce 1 mL, per reaction vial B (Rx) [*Neurolite*].

**Packaging and storage**
Store between 15 and 30 °C (59 and 86 °F), unless otherwise specified by manufacturer. Protect from light.

Note: Prior to labeling, kit can be stored between 15 and 25 °C (59 and 77 °F).

**Preparation of dosage form**
To prepare injection, an oxidant-free sodium pertechnetate Tc 99m solution is used. See manufacturer's package insert for instructions.

**Stability**
Technetium Tc 99m bicisate is stable at room temperature for a period of at least 8 hours after reconstitution. However, the manufacturer's package insert recommends that the product be used within 6 hours after preparation.

**Incompatibilities**
If oxidants such as peroxides and hypochlorites are present in the sodium pertechnetate Tc 99m used for labeling, the final preparation may be adversely affected and should be discarded.

**Note**
Caution—Radioactive material.

### Selected Bibliography

Holman BL, Hellman RS, Goldsmith SJ, et al. Biodistribution, dosimetry, and clinical evaluation of technetium-99m ethyl cysteinate dimer in normal subjects and in patients with chronic cerebral infarction. J Nucl Med 1989 Jun; 30 (6): 1018-24.

Léveillé J, Demonceau G, Walovitch RC. Intrasubject comparison between technetium-99m-ECD and technetium-99m-HMPAO in healthy human subjects. J Nucl Med 1992 Apr; 33: 480-4.

Brass LM, Walovitch RC, Joseph JL, et al. The role of single photon emission computed tomography brain imaging with Tc-99m-bicisate in the localization and definition of mechanism of ischemic stroke. J Cereb Blood Flow Metab 1994; 14 (Suppl 1): S91-S98.

Developed: 06/29/95

---

# TECHNETIUM Tc 99m DISOFENIN    Systemic†

VA CLASSIFICATION (Primary): DX201
Another commonly used name is technetium Tc 99m DISIDA.
Note: For a listing of dosage forms and brand names by country availability, see *Dosage Forms* section(s). For a listing of brand names for the articles in this monograph, refer to the General Index.

---

†Not commercially available in Canada.

## Category

Diagnostic aid, radioactive (hepatobiliary disorders).

## Indications

**Accepted**

Hepatobiliary imaging, radionuclide—Technetium Tc 99m disofenin is indicated as a hepatobiliary imaging agent for the evaluation of hepatobiliary tract patency to differentiate jaundice resulting from hepatocellular causes from jaundice resulting from partial or complete biliary obstruction; to differentiate extrahepatic biliary atresia from neonatal hepatitis; to detect cystic duct obstruction associated with acute cholecystitis; and to detect bile leaks.

Also, technetium Tc 99m disofenin may be useful to detect intrahepatic cholestasis and to distinguish it from other hepatobiliary diseases that involve hepatocyte damage.

## Physical Properties

**Nuclear data**

| Radionu-clide (half-life) | Decay constant | Mode of decay | Principal photon emissions (keV) | Mean number of emissions/ disintegration (≥0.01) |
|---|---|---|---|---|
| Tc 99m (6.0 hr) | 0.1151 h⁻¹ | Isomeric transition to Tc 99 | Gamma (18) | 0.062 |
| | | | Gamma (140.5) | 0.891 |

## Pharmacology/Pharmacokinetics

**Physicochemical characteristics**
Molecular weight—Disofenin: 350.41.

**Mechanism of action/Effect**
Based on the clearance of most of the administered activity through the hepatobiliary system. Following intravenous administration, technetium Tc 99m–labeled IDA derivatives, such as disofenin, become bound to plasma proteins (mainly albumin). In the liver, in the space of Disse, technetium Tc 99m disofenin becomes dissociated from the proteins and enters the hepatocyte by a mechanism similar to that of serum bilirubin. Technetium Tc 99m disofenin traverses the hepatocyte unmetabolized and enters the bile canaliculi. Flow beyond the canaliculi is influenced to a large extent by the tone of the sphincter of Oddi and the patency of the bile ducts. Clear visualization of the gallbladder and intestines with technetium Tc 99m disofenin demonstrates hepatobiliary tract patency.

**Distribution**
In circulatory system, with rapid clearance; however, a percentage of the radiopharmaceutical (about 8%) remains in circulation 30 minutes after injection. It is cleared from blood by normal hepatic cells within 10 to 20 minutes. Excreted into bile and stored in gallbladder. The radiopharmaceutical is excreted through the hepatobiliary tract into the intestine. A fraction of the radiopharmaceutical is excreted into the urine. The fraction excreted into the urine is dependent on the extent of biliary disease.

**Time to radioactivity visualization**
In patients with normal hepatobiliary function (fasting state)—
Gallbladder: 10 to 20 minutes.
Intestines: 30 to 60 minutes.
Note: Delayed visualization or nonvisualization may occur during the period immediately following a meal or after prolonged fasting.

## Radiation dosimetry

| Organ | Estimated absorbed radiation dose* | | | |
|---|---|---|---|---|
| | With normal hepatobiliary function | | With parenchymal liver disease | |
| | mGy/ MBq | rad/ mCi | mGy/ MBq | rad/ mCi |
| Gallbladder wall | 0.11 | 0.41 | 0.035 | 0.13 |
| Large intestine wall (upper) | 0.092 | 0.34 | 0.033 | 0.12 |
| Large intestine wall (lower) | 0.062 | 0.23 | 0.024 | 0.089 |
| Small intestine | 0.052 | 0.19 | 0.019 | 0.070 |
| Bladder wall | 0.023 | 0.085 | 0.069 | 0.26 |
| Ovaries | 0.020 | 0.074 | 0.0099 | 0.037 |
| Liver | 0.015 | 0.056 | 0.010 | 0.037 |
| Uterus | 0.013 | 0.048 | 0.011 | 0.041 |
| Red marrow | 0.0070 | 0.026 | 0.0038 | 0.014 |
| Kidneys | 0.0063 | 0.023 | 0.0066 | 0.024 |
| Stomach wall | 0.0061 | 0.023 | 0.0027 | 0.010 |
| Pancreas | 0.0057 | 0.021 | 0.0028 | 0.010 |
| Adrenals | 0.0032 | 0.012 | 0.0021 | 0.0078 |
| Bone surfaces | 0.0026 | 0.0096 | 0.0017 | 0.0063 |
| Spleen | 0.0026 | 0.0096 | 0.0015 | 0.0056 |
| Testes | 0.0015 | 0.0056 | 0.0025 | 0.0093 |
| Breast | 0.00061 | 0.0023 | 0.00056 | 0.0021 |
| Thyroid | 0.00012 | 0.00044 | 0.00023 | 0.00085 |
| Other tissue | 0.0030 | 0.011 | 0.0021 | 0.0078 |

| Radionuclide | Effective dose* | | | |
|---|---|---|---|---|
| | With normal hepatobiliary function | | With parenchymal liver disease | |
| | mSv/ MBq | rem/ mCi | mSv/ MBq | rem/ mCi |
| Tc 99m | 0.024 | 0.089 | 0.013 | 0.048 |

*For adults; intravenous injection of technetium Tc 99m–labeled iminodiacetic acid (IDA) derivatives. Data based on the International Commission on Radiological Protection (ICRP) Publication 53—Radiation dose to patients from radiopharmaceuticals.

## Elimination

Primarily fecal; about 9% eliminated in the urine within 2 hours.

Note: In patients with hepatocellular disease or biliary obstruction, elimination through the urinary tract may be greatly increased.

# Precautions to Consider

## Cross-sensitivity and/or related problems

Patients sensitive to amide-type local anesthetics may be sensitive to technetium Tc 99m disofenin also.

## Carcinogenicity/Mutagenicity

Long-term animal studies to evaluate carcinogenic or mutagenic potential of technetium Tc 99m disofenin have not been performed.

## Pregnancy/Reproduction

Pregnancy—Tc 99m (as free pertechnetate) crosses the placenta. Studies have not been done with technetium Tc 99m disofenin in humans.

The possibility of pregnancy should be assessed in women of child-bearing potential. Clinical situations exist where the benefit to the patient and fetus, based on information derived from radiopharmaceutical use, outweighs the risks from fetal exposure to radiation. In these situations, the physician should use discretion and reduce the radiopharmaceutical administered activity to the lowest possible amount.

Studies have not been done in animals.

FDA Pregnancy Category C.

## Breast-feeding

Although it is not known whether technetium Tc 99m disofenin is distributed into breast milk, it is known that Tc 99m as free pertechnetate is distributed into breast milk. Based on the assumption that the Tc 99m in breast milk is in the form of pertechnetate and based on the effective half-life of the radionuclide in breast milk, the daily volume of milk, a dose factor relating the radionuclide to its critical organ (thyroid) in the nursing infant, and the maximum permissible dose to that organ, a guideline has been proposed. According to this guideline, it has been calculated that nursing can be safely resumed when the concentration in breast milk reaches $30.3 \times 10^{-4}$ megabecquerels ($8.2 \times 10^{-2}$ microcuries) per mL. This level of activity is probably reached, in the majority of patients, within 12 to 24 hours after administration of technetium Tc 99m–labeled radiopharmaceuticals.

## Pediatrics

Diagnostic studies performed to date using technetium Tc 99m disofenin have not demonstrated pediatrics-specific problems that would limit its usefulness in children. However, there have been no specific studies evaluating the safety and efficacy of technetium Tc 99m disofenin in pediatric patients. When this radiopharmaceutical is used in children, the diagnostic benefit should be judged to outweigh the potential risk of radiation.

## Geriatrics

Appropriate studies on the relationship of age to the effects of technetium Tc 99m disofenin have not been performed in the geriatric population. However, no geriatrics-specific problems have been documented to date.

## Drug interactions and/or related problems

See *Diagnostic interference.*

## Diagnostic interference

The following have been selected on the basis of their potential clinical significance (possible effect in parentheses where appropriate)—not necessarily inclusive (» = major clinical significance):

With results of this test

*Due to other medications*

Alcohol or

Anticholinergics or other medications with anticholinergic action (See *Appendix II* ) or

Bethanechol or

Somatostatin

(may decrease gallbladder emptying thus delaying gallbladder clearance of technetium Tc 99m disofenin)

Erythromycin

(nonvisualization of gallbladder may occur due to erthromycin-induced hepatotoxicity)

Nicotinic acid

(chronic, high-dose nicotinic acid therapy may result in poor extraction and elimination of the radiopharmaceutical, mimicking intrinsic hepatocellular disease)

Opioid (narcotic) analgesics, especially butorphanol, morphine, and meperidine

(delivery of technetium Tc 99m disofenin to the small bowel may be prevented by the opioid analgesics because of constriction of the sphincter of Oddi and increased biliary tract pressure caused by these medications; these actions result in delayed intestinal visualization, which resembles that caused by obstruction of the common bile duct; however, the use of intravenous morphine has been shown to help in the diagnosis of acute cholecystitis when conditions that delay or prevent gallbladder visualization are present)

Parenteral alimentation

(may give false-positive diagnosis of cystic duct obstruction due to stasis of bile in the gallbladder)

*Due to medical problems or conditions*

Fasting, prolonged or

Pancreatitis, acute

(may give false-positive results [nonvisualization or delayed visualization of gallbladder] of cystic duct obstruction due to stasis of bile in gallbladder)

Hepatocellular disease

(nonvisualization or delayed visualization of gallbladder may occur)

Post-prandial state, especially with ingestion of fatty meals

(ingestion of a fatty meal immediately before test may give false-positive results [nonvisualization of gallbladder] of cystic duct obstruction due to gallbladder contraction stimulated by meal ingestion)

## Medical considerations/Contraindications

The medical considerations/contraindications included here have been selected on the basis of their potential clinical significance (reasons given in parentheses where appropriate)—not necessarily inclusive (» = major clinical significance).

See also *Diagnostic interference.*

*Risk-benefit should be considered when the following medical problem exists:*

Sensitivity to amide-type local anesthetics or to the radiopharmaceutical preparation

# Side/Adverse Effects

There are no known side/adverse effects associated with the use of technetium Tc 99m disofenin.

# Patient Consultation

As an aid to patient consultation, refer to *Advice for the Patient, Radiopharmaceuticals (Diagnostic)*.

In providing consultation, consider emphasizing the following selected information (» = major clinical significance):

**Description of use**

Action in the body: Clearance of radioactive disofenin from blood through hepatobiliary tract

Visualization of radioactivity in intestinal tract and gallbladder shows absence of obstruction of bile ducts

Small amounts of radioactivity used in diagnosis; radiation received is low and considered safe

**Before having this test**

» Conditions affecting use, especially:

Sensitivity to amide-type local anesthetics or to the radiopharmaceutical preparation

Pregnancy—Technetium Tc 99m (as free pertechnetate) crosses placenta; risk to fetus from radiation exposure as opposed to benefit derived from use should be considered

Breast-feeding—Not known if technetium Tc 99m disofenin distributed into breast milk, but Tc 99m as free pertechnetate is distributed into breast milk; temporary discontinuation of nursing may be recommended because of risk to infant from radiation exposure

Use in children—Risk from radiation exposure as opposed to benefit derived from use should be considered

**Preparation for this test**

Fasting for at least 2, and preferably 4 hours before test to prevent gallbladder nonvisualization

**Precautions after having this test**

No special precautions

# General Dosing Information

Radiopharmaceuticals are to be administered only by or under the supervision of physicians who have had extensive training in the safe use and handling of radioactive materials and who are authorized by the Nuclear Regulatory Commission (NRC) or the appropriate Agreement State agency, if required, or, outside the U.S., the appropriate authority.

Administration of phenobarbital (5 mg per kg of body weight [mg/kg] in 2 fractions) for at least 5 days prior to hepatobiliary imaging may enhance and accelerate biliary uptake and excretion of the radiopharmaceutical in the differential diagnosis of extrahepatic atresia from neonatal hepatitis. This will enable determination of the status of the extrahepatic biliary tract in the jaundiced neonate within 24 hours.

Fasting is recommended for at least 2, and preferably 4 hours before the examination since nonvisualization of the gallbladder may result if gallbladder contraction has been stimulated by the ingestion of food.

Prolonged fasting (e.g., more than 24 hours) may result in a false-positive hepatobiliary scan (i.e., nonvisualization of the gallbladder despite a patent cystic duct) due to the development of increased intraluminal gallbladder pressure (biliary stasis or sludge), which reduces radiotracer flow to the gallbladder. To avoid this, prior administration of a cholecystokinetic agent, such as sincalide or cholecystokinin (CCK-8), to induce contraction of the gallbladder is recommended for preemptying the gallbladder before the injection of technetium Tc 99m disofenin. Whenever there is doubt about the dietary history of the patient, especially in emergency situations, a cholecystokinetic agent should be administered.

In patients receiving parenteral alimentation, the relative inactivity of the gallbladder results in bile stasis and the formation of thick viscous bile (sludge), which reduces the flow of the radiotracer into the gallbladder. Pretreatment with a cholecystokinetic agent (e.g., intravenous sincalide 0.02 to 0.04 mcg per kg of body weight [mcg/kg]) may be useful to empty stored bile from the gallbladder, and thus may prevent a false-positive hepatobiliary scan.

In patients demonstrating technetium Tc 99m disofenin localization in the gallbladder, a cholecystokinetic agent (e.g., intravenous sincalide 0.02 to 0.04 mcg/kg of body weight) may be useful to stimulate gallbladder contraction and thereby evaluate the contractile function of the gall-

bladder. Quantitation of gallbladder emptying yields the ejection fraction ($\geq$ 35% is usually considered normal).

Imaging is performed immediately following technetium Tc 99m disofenin administration, and is usually completed in 60 to 90 minutes. Imaging for up to 4 hours or longer may be necessary if no gallbladder or intestinal activity is seen at the earlier times.

When there is no visualization of the gallbladder within an hour of administration of technetium Tc 99m disofenin, but the radiotracer is seen within the small bowel in patients suspected of having acute cholecystitis, morphine sulfate (0.04 mg/kg diluted in 10 mL saline) may be injected intravenously to help confirm the diagnosis. The diagnosis of acute cholecystitis is confirmed if nonvisualization of the gallbladder persists after morphine is administered. Although morphine-augmented cholescintigraphy may cause false-positive and false-negative results in some patients (e.g., acalculous cholecystitis), it may be useful in critically ill patients or patients who have been on prolonged fasting or who are receiving parenteral alimentation.

**Safety considerations for handling this radiopharmaceutical**

Improper handling of this radiopharmaceutical may cause radioactive contamination. Guidelines for handling radioactive material have been prepared by scientific, professional, state, federal, and international bodies and are available to the specially qualified and authorized users who have access to radiopharmaceuticals.

# Parenteral Dosage Forms

## TECHNETIUM Tc 99m DISOFENIN INJECTION USP

**Usual adult and adolescent administered activity**

Hepatobiliary imaging—

Nonjaundiced patients: Intravenous, 37 to 185 megabecquerels (1 to 5 millicuries) by slow injection.

Patients with serum bilirubin concentration > 0.08 mmol per L (5 mg per dL): Intravenous, 111 to 296 megabecquerels (3 to 8 millicuries) by slow injection.

**Usual pediatric administered activity**

Hepatobiliary imaging—

Dosage must be individualized by physician. The minimum recommended administered activity is 37 megabecquerels (1 millicurie), intravenously.

**Usual geriatric administered activity**

See *Usual adult and adolescent administered activity*.

**Strength(s) usually available**

U.S.—

20 mg disofenin, 0.24 mg (minimum) stannous chloride, and 0.6 mg total tin (maximum tin as stannous chloride) in lyophilized form under nitrogen atmosphere, per reaction vial (Rx) [*Hepatolite*].

Canada—

Not commercially available.

**Packaging and storage**

Store below 40 °C (104 °F), preferably between 15 and 30 °C (59 and 86 °F), unless otherwise specified by manufacturer. Protect from freezing.

**Preparation of dosage form**

To prepare injection, an oxidant-free sodium pertechnetate Tc 99m solution is used. See manufacturer's package insert for instructions.

**Stability**

Injection should be administered within 6 hours after preparation.

**Note**

Caution—Radioactive material.

# Selected Bibliography

Fink-Bennett D, Balon H, Robbins T, et al. Morphine-augmented cholescintigraphy: its efficacy in detecting acute cholecystitis. J Nucl Med 1991; 32: 1231-3.

Krishnamurthy GT, Turner FE. Pharmacokinetics and clinical application of technetium 99m-labeled hepatobiliary agents. Semin Nucl Med 1990; 20 (2): 130-49.

Cherver LR, Nunn AD, Loberg MD. Radiopharmaceuticals for hepatobiliary imaging. Semin Nucl Med 1982; 12 (1): 5-17.

Revised: 06/14/93
Interim revision: 08/02/94

# TECHNETIUM Tc 99m EXAMETAZIME   Systemic

VA CLASSIFICATION (Primary): DX201

Another commonly used name for exametazime is hexamethylpropyle-
neamine oxime (HM-PAO).

Note: For a listing of dosage forms and brand names by country availability, see *Dosage Forms* section(s). For a listing of brand names
for the articles in this monograph, refer to the General Index.

## Category

Diagnostic aid, radioactive (cerebrovascular disease; inflammatory
disease).

## Indications

Note: Bracketed information in the *Indications* section refers to uses that
are not included in U.S. product labeling.

### Accepted

Brain imaging, radionuclide—Technetium Tc 99m exametazime is indicated as a brain imaging agent in the detection of altered regional
cerebral perfusion in stroke.

Leukocytes, labeling of—Technetium Tc 99m exametazime is indicated
for the labeling of autologous leukocytes. Technetium Tc 99m exametazime–labeled leukocytes are used for the following diagnostic
studies:

Inflammatory lesions, intra-abdominal (diagnosis)[1];

Bowel disease, inflammatory (diagnosis)—Indicated in scintigraphy to
help locate intra-abdominal infection or inflammation and inflammatory bowel disease.

[Dementia, Alzheimer-type (diagnosis)][1]—Technetium Tc 99m exametazime is used as a brain imaging agent to help identify patients with
Alzheimer's disease.

[Epilepsy (diagnosis)][1]—Technetium Tc 99m exametazime is used in the
evaluation of epilepsy to help find the location of the epileptic focus.

[Brain death (diagnosis)][1]—Technetium Tc 99m exametazime is used to
help confirm the diagnosis of brain death.

[1]Not included in Canadian product labeling.

## Physical Properties

### Nuclear data

| Radionu-clide (half-life) | Decay constant | Mode of decay | Principal photon emissions (keV) | Mean number of emissions/ disintegration ($\geq 0.01$) |
|---|---|---|---|---|
| Tc 99m (6.0 hr) | 0.1151 h$^{-1}$ | Isomeric transition to Tc 99 | Gamma (18) | 0.062 |
| | | | Gamma (140.5) | 0.891 |

## Pharmacology/Pharmacokinetics

### Physicochemical characteristics

Molecular weight—Exametazime: 272.39.

### Mechanism of action/Effect

Brain imaging—Technetium Tc 99m exametazime is a lipophilic complex
able to cross the blood-brain barrier as well as penetrate cell membranes. The agent localizes in the brain as a function of regional cerebral perfusion. Its radionuclide emissions while localized in cerebral
tissue permit external imaging of the cerebral distribution of the agent
thus helping detect altered regional cerebral perfusion. Technetium Tc
99m exametazime is primarily extracted and trapped by cerebral gray
matter and the basal ganglia during the first pass through the brain. It
has been proposed that the retention in the brain of technetium Tc
99m exametazime results from *in vivo* conversion of the primary complex to a less lipophilic complex, which is unable to cross the blood-
brain barrier.

Labeling of leukocytes—When incubated with leukocytes, which have
been isolated from whole blood, the technetium Tc 99m exametazime
complex, being lipid-soluble, penetrates the cell membrane of the leukocytes by passive diffusion. The lipophilic complex is then converted
to a hydrophilic species, in a process possibly involving intracellular
glutathione, thus trapping the technetium Tc 99m label within the cells
(mostly neutrophils). The radioactive autologous leukocytes are sub-

sequently reinjected to permit the detection of inflammatory lesions
based on the normal physiological accumulation of leukocytes at such
sites.

### Distribution

Brain imaging—Rapidly cleared from blood after intravenous injection; a
maximum of 3.5 to 7% of administered activity localizes in the brain
within one minute of injection. Up to 15% of this localized activity is
eliminated from the brain within the next 2 minutes after injection,
with little or no further loss of activity for the following 24 hours,
except by physical decay of technetium Tc 99m. The activity that is
not localized in the brain is widely distributed throughout the body,
particularly in muscle and soft tissue.

Diagnosis of inflammatory lesions—Technetium Tc 99m exametazime–
labeled leukocytes tend to concentrate at sites of inflammation. However, there is an initial accumulation of radioactivity in the lungs, liver,
spleen, blood pool, bone marrow, and the bladder. Activity is seen in
the urine, occasionally in the gallbladder, and consistently in the colon
from 4 hours on. Significant colonic activity remains 24 hours after
injection. Also, normal areas visualized in earlier scans remain visible.

### Time to radioactivity visualization

Brain imaging—Dynamic imaging may be performed within the first 10
minutes post-injection. Static imaging may be performed 15 minutes
after injection for up to 6 hours.

Diagnosis of inflammatory lesions—Although some inflammatory lesions
have been detected at 2 minutes post-injection, images taken at 30
minutes and/or 2 hours are recommended. Optimal planar images are
obtained between 2 and 4 hours following administration.

### Radiation dosimetry

| Estimated absorbed radiation dose for Technetium Tc 99m Exametazime* | | |
|---|---|---|
| Organ | mGy/MBq | rad/mCi |
| Lacrimal glands | 0.070 | 0.26 |
| Gallbladder wall | 0.051 | 0.19 |
| Kidney | 0.035 | 0.13 |
| Thyroid | 0.027 | 0.10 |
| Upper large intestine wall | 0.021 | 0.079 |
| Liver | 0.015 | 0.054 |
| Lower large intestine wall | 0.015 | 0.054 |
| Bladder wall | | |
| 2 hr void | 0.013 | 0.047 |
| 4 hr void | 0.019 | 0.070 |
| Small intestine wall | 0.012 | 0.044 |
| Brain | 0.0069 | 0.026 |
| Eyes | 0.0069 | 0.026 |
| Ovaries | 0.0063 | 0.023 |
| Bone surfaces | 0.0048 | 0.018 |
| Red marrow | 0.0034 | 0.013 |
| Testes | 0.0018 | 0.007 |
| Total body | 0.0036 | 0.013 |

Effective dose: 0.0092 mSv/MBq (0.034 rem/mCi)‡.

| Estimated absorbed radiation dose for Technetium Tc 99m Exametazime–labeled leukocytes†‡ | | |
|---|---|---|
| Organ | mGy/MBq | rad/mCi |
| Spleen | 0.15 | 0.56 |
| Red marrow | 0.022 | 0.082 |
| Liver | 0.02 | 0.074 |
| Pancreas | 0.014 | 0.052 |
| Ovaries | 0.0042 | 0.016 |
| Uterus | 0.0038 | 0.014 |
| Testes | 0.0017 | 0.0064 |

Effective dose: 0.017 mSv/MBq (0.063 rem/mCi)†.

*For adults; intravenous injection. Data based on information from the
Oak Ridge Associated Universities, Radiopharmaceutical Internal Dose
Information Center.

†Data based on the International Commission on Radiological Protection (ICRP) Publication 53—Radiation dose to patients from radiopharmaceuticals.

‡Data based on bladder voiding every 3.5 hours.

## Elimination

For technetium Tc 99m exametazime—
Within 48 hours:
Fecal (about 50% of the administered activity via hepatobiliary excretion).
Renal (about 40% of the injected administered activity).
For technetium Tc 99m exametazime–labeled leukocytes—
Renal (about 15 to 30% of the injected administered activity in 24 hours).
Fecal (about 6% of the administered activity in 48 hours).

## Precautions to Consider

### Carcinogenicity
Long-term animal studies to evaluate carcinogenic potential of technetium Tc 99m exametazime have not been performed.

### Mutagenicity
Studies in rats have not demonstrated mutagenic potential following intraperitoneal administration at doses of 70, 140, and 280 mg of exametazime per kg of body weight.

### Pregnancy/Reproduction
Pregnancy—Tc 99m (as free pertechnetate) crosses the placenta. However, studies have not been done with technetium Tc 99m exametazime in humans.
The possibility of pregnancy should be assessed in women of child-bearing potential. Clinical situations exist in which the benefit to the patient and fetus, based on information derived from radiopharmaceutical use, outweighs the risks from fetal exposure to radiation. In these situations, the physician should use discretion and reduce the administered activity of the radiopharmaceutical to the lowest possible amount.
Studies have not been done in animals.
FDA Pregnancy Category C.

### Breast-feeding
Although it is not known whether technetium Tc 99m exametazime is distributed into breast milk, it is known that Tc 99m as free pertechnetate is distributed into breast milk. Based on the assumption that the Tc 99m in breast milk is in the form of pertechnetate, and based on the effective half-life of the radionuclide in breast milk, the daily volume of milk, a dose factor relating the radionuclide to its critical organ (thyroid) in the nursing infant, and the maximum permissible dose to that organ, a guideline has been proposed. According to this guideline, it has been calculated that nursing can be safely resumed when the concentration in breast milk reaches $30.3 \times 10^{-4}$ megabecquerels ($8.2 \times 10^{-2}$ microcuries) per mL. This level of activity is probably reached, in the majority of patients, within 24 hours after administration of 740 megabecquerels (20 millicuries) of technetium Tc 99m–labeled radiopharmaceuticals. However, the manufacturer recommends that formula feedings be substituted for breast-feeding for 60 hours.

### Pediatrics
Diagnostic studies performed to date in patients up to 18 years of age have not demonstrated pediatrics-specific problems that would limit the usefulness of technetium Tc 99m exametazime in children. However, there have been no specific studies evaluating the safety and efficacy of technetium Tc 99m exametazime in pediatric patients. When this radiopharmaceutical is used in children, the diagnostic benefit should be judged to outweigh the potential risk of radiation.
For technetium Tc 99m exametazime–labeled leukocytes—Technetium Tc 99m exametazime–labeled leukocytes may be preferred for use in children to indium In 111 oxyquinoline–labeled leukocytes or gallium citrate Ga 67 because of its lower radiation dose.

### Geriatrics
Appropriate studies on the relationship of age to the effects of technetium Tc 99m exametazime have not been performed in the geriatric population. However, no geriatrics-specific problems have been documented to date.

### Drug interactions and/or related problems
See *Diagnostic interference.*

### Diagnostic interference
The following have been selected on the basis of their potential clinical significance (possible effect in parentheses where appropriate)—not necessarily inclusive (» = major clinical significance):
With results of *technetium Tc 99m–labeled leukocyte* studies
*Due to other medications*
Antibiotics
(long-term intravenous antibiotic therapy may result in a false-negative study)

## Medical considerations/Contraindications
The medical considerations/contraindications included here have been selected on the basis of their potential clinical significance (reasons given in parentheses where appropriate)—not necessarily inclusive (» = major clinical significance).
*Risk-benefit should be considered when the following medical problem exists:*
Sensitivity to the radiopharmaceutical preparation

## Side/Adverse Effects
The following side/adverse effects have been selected on the basis of their potential clinical significance (possible signs and symptoms in parentheses where appropriate)—not necessarily inclusive:

**Those indicating need for medical attention**
Incidence less frequent or rare
*Allergic reaction* (fever; skin rash; swelling of face); *transient increase in blood pressure*

## Patient Consultation
As an aid to patient consultation, refer to *Advice for the Patient, Radiopharmaceuticals (Diagnostic).*

In providing consultation, consider emphasizing the following selected information (» = major clinical significance):

**Description of use**
Action in the body: Concentration of radioactive exametazime in brain; concentration of technetium Tc 99m–labeled leukocytes at sites of infection
Retention of radioactivity in brain and sites of infection allows visualization
Small amount of radioactivity used in diagnosis; radiation received is low and considered safe

**Before having this test**
» Conditions affecting use, especially:
Sensitivity to the radiopharmaceutical preparation
Pregnancy—Technetium Tc 99m (as free pertechnetate) crosses placenta; risk to fetus from radiation exposure as opposed to benefit derived from use should be considered
Breast-feeding—Not known if technetium Tc 99m exametazime is distributed into breast milk, but Tc 99m as free pertechnetate is distributed into breast milk; temporary discontinuation of nursing may be recommended to avoid any unnecessary absorbed radiation dose to the infant
Use in children—For brain imaging: Risk from radiation exposure as opposed to benefit derived from use should be considered

**Preparation for this test**
Special preparatory instructions may be given; patient should inquire in advance

**Precautions after having this test**
Increasing intake of fluids and voiding as often as possible after examination to minimize bladder exposure to radiation

**Side/adverse effects**
Signs of possible side effects, especially allergic reaction and transient increase in blood pressure

## General Dosing Information
Radiopharmaceuticals are to be administered only by or under the supervision of physicians who have had extensive training in the safe use and handling of radioactive materials and who are authorized by the Nuclear Regulatory Commission (NRC) or the appropriate Agreement State agency, if required, or, outside the U.S., the appropriate authority.
Adequate hydration of the patient is recommended before and after examination to promote urinary excretion of radioactivity. Also, urination is recommended as often as possible after the examination to reduce bladder exposure to radiation.

**For brain perfusion imaging**
Dynamic imaging may be performed within the first 10 minutes after injection. Static imaging may be performed from 15 minutes up to 6 hours after injection.

**For labeling of leukocytes**
White blood cells may be damaged by mechanical shearing forces; therefore, it is important to minimize the use of needles when transferring cells. If a syringe cannot be used by itself, wide-bore (19 gauge) needles should be used. When separating the mixed leukocytes from other blood cells, excessive centrifuge speed may damage the cells and in-

crease platelet contamination. However, an adequate centrifuge speed will provide a compact button (pellet).

The manufacturer's package insert or other appropriate literature should be consulted for the specific method of labeling leukocytes.

**Safety considerations for handling this radiopharmaceutical**
Improper handling of this radiopharmaceutical may cause radioactive contamination. Guidelines for handling radioactive material have been prepared by scientific, professional, state, federal, and international bodies and are available to the specially qualified and authorized users who have access to radiopharmaceuticals.

## Parenteral Dosage Forms

### TECHNETIUM Tc 99m EXAMETAZIME INJECTION USP

**Usual adult and adolescent administered activity**
Brain imaging—
    Intravenous, 370 to 740 megabecquerels (10 to 20 millicuries).
Diagnosis of inflammatory lesions—
    Intravenous, 0.259 to 0.925 gigabecquerels (7 to 25 millicuries) of technetium Tc 99m exametazime–labeled leukocytes.

**Usual pediatric administered activity**
Brain imaging—
    Intravenous, 5 to 10 megabecquerels (0.14 to 0.28 millicuries) per kg of body weight with a minimum total dosage of 185 megabecquerels (5 millicuries).
Diagnosis of inflammatory lesions—
    Dosage must be individualized by physician.

**Usual geriatric administered activity**
See *Usual adult and adolescent administered activity.*

**Strength(s) usually available**
U.S.—
    0.5 mg exametazime, 7.6 mcg (0.0076 mg) stannous chloride dihydrate, and 4.5 mg sodium chloride, in lyophilized form under nitrogen atmosphere, per single-dose reaction vial (Rx) [*Ceretec*].
    Note: In addition, the kit contains 1-mL vials of 1% methylene blue injection and 4.5-mL vials of 0.003 M monobasic sodium phosphate and dibasic sodium phosphate in 0.9% sodium chloride injection.
Canada—
    0.5 mg exametazime, 7.6 mcg (0.0076 mg) stannous chloride dihydrate, and 4.5 mg sodium chloride, in lyophilized form under nitrogen atmosphere, per single-dose reaction vial (Rx) [*Ceretec*].

**Packaging and storage**
Store between 20 and 25 °C (68 and 77 °F), unless otherwise specified by manufacturer. Protect from freezing.

Note: Prior to labeling, kit must be stored between 15 and 25 °C (59 and 77 °F).

**Preparation of dosage form**
To prepare injection, an oxidant-free sodium pertechnetate Tc 99m solution is used. Freshly eluted technetium Tc 99m generator eluate must be used for reconstitution to assure the highest radiochemical purity. It is recommended that only eluate from a technetium Tc 99m generator that was previously eluted within 24 hours should be used. Generator eluate more than 2 hours old should not be used. Preservative-free, nonbacteriostatic sodium chloride injection must be used as the diluent for sodium pertechnetate Tc 99m. Bacteriostatic sodium chloride should not be used because it will increase the oxidation products and adversely affect the biological distribution of technetium Tc 99m exametazime. Methylene blue injection may be used to form a stabilizing solution. See manufacturer's package insert for full preparation instructions.

Note: Methylene blue *must not* be used as a stabilizer in the preparation of the technetium Tc 99m exametazime injection to be used for labeling leukocytes.

**Stability**
Without methylene blue stabilizer—Injection must be administered within 30 minutes after preparation since progressive conversion to a less lipophilic complex unable to cross the blood-brain barrier may exceed acceptable limits after this time period.
With methylene blue stabilizer—Injection may be administered within 4 hours after time of reconstitution.

**Incompatibilities**
If oxidants such as peroxides and hypochlorites are present in the sodium pertechnetate Tc 99m used for labeling, the final preparation may be adversely affected and should be discarded.

**Note**
Caution—Radioactive material.

### Selected Bibliography

Roddie ME, Peters AM, Danpure HJ, et al. Inflammation: imaging with Tc 99m HMPAO-labeled leukocytes. Radiology 1988 Mar; 166 (3): 767-72.

Leonard JP, Nowotnik DP, Neirinckx RD. Technetium 99m, 1-HM-PAO: a new radiopharmaceutical for imaging regional brain perfusion using SPECT—a comparison with iodine 123 HIPDM. J Nucl Med 1986; 27 (12): 1819-23.

Testa HJ, Snowden JS, Neary D, et al. The use of Tc 99m HM-PAO in the diagnosis of primary degenerative dementia. J Cereb Blood Flow Metab 1988; 8 (6): S123-S126.

Revised: 01/11/96

---

# TECHNETIUM Tc 99m GLUCEPTATE     Systemic

VA CLASSIFICATION (Primary): DX201

Another commonly used name is technetium Tc 99m glucoheptonate.

Note: For a listing of dosage forms and brand names by country availability, see *Dosage Forms* section(s). For a listing of brand names for the articles in this monograph, refer to the General Index.

## Category

Diagnostic aid, radioactive (intracranial lesions; cerebral disorders; renal disorders).

## Indications

**Accepted**
Brain imaging, radionuclide—Technetium Tc 99m gluceptate is indicated as a brain imaging agent to detect and evaluate intracranial lesions, including brain tumors.

Renal imaging, radionuclide—Technetium Tc 99m gluceptate is indicated as a renal imaging agent to evaluate kidney size, shape, and position, especially in parenchymal disorders.

Brain perfusion studies or
Renal perfusion studies—Technetium Tc 99m gluceptate is indicated in dynamic brain and renal perfusion studies.

## Physical Properties

**Nuclear data**

| Radionuclide (half-life) | Decay constant | Mode of decay | Principal photon emissions (keV) | Mean number of emissions/ disintegration ($\geq$0.01) |
|---|---|---|---|---|
| Tc 99m (6.0 hr) | 0.1151 h$^{-1}$ | Isomeric transition to Tc 99 | Gamma (18) | 0.062 |
|  |  |  | Gamma (140.5) | 0.891 |

## Pharmacology/Pharmacokinetics

**Mechanism of action/Effect**
Diagnostic aid (intracranial lesions; cerebral disorders)—
    Technetium Tc 99m gluceptate accumulates, by passive diffusion, in intracranial lesions with an altered blood-brain barrier. The radionuclide emissions may then be detected to determine the presence and localization of the lesion.
Diagnostic aid (renal disorders)—
    Based on its rapid clearance through the urinary tract. Urinary clearance of technetium Tc 99m gluceptate occurs by both glomerular

filtration and tubular secretion; however, a sufficient amount is retained by the renal cortex to allow delayed static images to be performed for evaluation of cortical morphology.

**Distribution**
Rapidly distributed in and cleared from plasma; up to 15% of dose localizes in the tubules of the renal cortex by 3 hours.

**Radiation dosimetry**

| Organ | Estimated absorbed radiation dose* | |
|---|---|---|
| | mGy/MBq | rad/mCi |
| Bladder wall | 0.056 | 0.21 |
| Kidneys | 0.049 | 0.18 |
| Uterus | 0.0077 | 0.029 |
| Adrenals | 0.0046 | 0.017 |
| Ovaries | 0.0046 | 0.017 |
| Large intestine wall (lower) | 0.0044 | 0.016 |
| Red marrow | 0.0039 | 0.014 |
| Spleen | 0.0039 | 0.014 |
| Small intestine | 0.0037 | 0.014 |
| Pancreas | 0.0036 | 0.013 |
| Large intestine wall (upper) | 0.0033 | 0.012 |
| Testes | 0.0029 | 0.011 |
| Stomach wall | 0.0027 | 0.010 |
| Liver | 0.0027 | 0.010 |
| Bone surfaces | 0.0026 | 0.0096 |
| Lungs | 0.0017 | 0.0063 |
| Breast | 0.0014 | 0.0052 |
| Thyroid | 0.0011 | 0.0041 |
| Other tissue | 0.0023 | 0.0085 |

Effective dose: 0.0090 mSv/MBq (0.033 rem/mCi)

*In adults; intravenous administration. Data based on the International Commission on Radiological Protection (ICRP) Publication 53—Radiation dose to patients from radiopharmaceuticals.

**Elimination**
Renal (by both glomerular filtration and renal tubular secretion)—
   Normal renal function: about 40% of the administered activity eliminated in 1 hour; about 70% of the administered activity eliminated within 24 hours.
   Renal function impairment: Urinary elimination is delayed. Hepatobiliary elimination may occur.

# Precautions to Consider

**Carcinogenicity/Mutagenicity**
Long-term animal studies to evaluate carcinogenic or mutagenic potential of technetium Tc 99m gluceptate have not been performed.

**Pregnancy/Reproduction**
Pregnancy—Tc 99m (as free pertechnetate) crosses the placenta. However, studies have not been done with technetium Tc 99m gluceptate in humans.
The possibility of pregnancy should be assessed in women of child-bearing potential. Clinical situations exist where the benefit to the patient and fetus, based on information derived from radiopharmaceutical use, outweighs the risks from fetal exposure to radiation. In these situations, the physician should use discretion and reduce the radiopharmaceutical dose to the lowest possible amount.
Studies have not been done in animals.
FDA Pregnancy Category C.

**Breast-feeding**
Although it is not known whether technetium Tc 99m gluceptate is distributed into breast milk, it is known that Tc 99m as free pertechnetate is distributed into breast milk. Based on the assumption that the Tc 99m in breast milk is in the form of pertechnetate and based on the effective half-life of the radionuclide in breast milk, the daily volume of milk, a dose factor relating the radionuclide to its critical organ (thyroid) in the nursing infant, and the maximum permissible dose to that organ, a guideline has been proposed. According to this guideline, it has been calculated that nursing can be safely resumed when the concentration in breast milk reaches $30.3 \times 10^{-4}$ megabecquerels ($8.2 \times 10^{-2}$ microcuries) per mL. This level of activity is probably reached, in the majority of patients, within 24 hours after administration of 740 megabecquerels (20 millicuries) of technetium Tc 99m–labeled radiopharmaceuticals.

**Pediatrics**
Diagnostic studies performed in children have not demonstrated pediatrics-specific problems that would limit the usefulness of technetium Tc 99m gluceptate in children. However, when this radiopharmaceutical is used in children, the diagnostic benefit should be judged to outweigh the potential risk of radiation.

**Geriatrics**
Appropriate studies on the relationship of age to the effects of technetium Tc 99m gluceptate have not been performed in the geriatric population. However, no geriatrics-specific problems have been documented to date.

**Drug interactions and/or related problems**
See *Diagnostic interference.*

**Diagnostic interference**
The following have been selected on the basis of their potential clinical significance (possible effect in parentheses where appropriate)—not necessarily inclusive (» = major clinical significance):
With results of *brain imaging*
*Due to other medications*
   Corticosteroids, glucocorticoid
      (uptake of technetium Tc 99m gluceptate in cerebral tumor or abscess may be decreased because of reduced peritumor edema caused by the corticosteroids)

*Due to medical problems or conditions*
   Neurotoxicity, induced by such drugs as:
   Cyclophosphamide or
   Dactinomycin or
   Doxorubicin or
   Vincristine
      (brain images may show increased activity due to chemotherapeutic neurotoxicity following therapy with these medications)
With results of *renal imaging*
*Due to other medications*
   Penicillamine
      (concurrent penicillamine therapy may cause transchelation of technetium Tc 99m gluceptate to a compound excreted through the hepatobiliary system, thus resulting in gallbladder visualization; gallbladder visualization may mimic abnormal kidney localization on posterior views of renal images)

   Probenecid
      (concurrent use may decrease kidney uptake of technetium Tc 99m gluceptate due to a direct inhibition of the enzyme transport system in the proximal tubule by probenecid)

*Due to medical problems or conditions*
   Dehydration
      (decreased urinary flow may result in poor renal images)

**Medical considerations/Contraindications**
The medical considerations/contraindications included here have been selected on the basis of their potential clinical significance (reasons given in parentheses where appropriate)—not necessarily inclusive (» = major clinical significance).
See also *Diagnostic interference.*

*Risk benefit must be considered when the following medical problem exists:*
   Sensitivity to the radiopharmaceutical preparation

# Side/Adverse Effects

The following side/adverse effects have been selected on the basis of their potential clinical significance (possible signs and symptoms in parentheses where appropriate)—not necessarily inclusive:

**Those indicating need for medical attention**
Incidence less frequent or rare
   *Allergic reaction* (skin rash, hives, or itching)

# Patient Consultation

As an aid to patient consultation, refer to *Advice for the Patient, Radiopharmaceuticals (Diagnostic).*

In providing consultation, consider emphasizing the following selected information (» = major clinical significance):

**Description of use**
   Action in the body: Concentration of radioactive gluceptate in brain lesions and kidneys
   Retention of radioactivity in brain lesions and kidneys allows visualization
   Small amount of radioactivity used in diagnosis; radiation received is low and considered safe

**Before having this test**
» Conditions affecting use, especially:
      Sensitivity to the radiopharmaceutical preparation

Pregnancy—Technetium Tc 99m (as free pertechnetate) crosses placenta; risk to fetus from radiation exposure as opposed to benefit derived from use should be considered

Breast-feeding—Not known if technetium Tc 99m gluceptate is distributed into breast milk, but Tc 99m as free pertechnetate is distributed into breast milk; temporary discontinuation of nursing may be recommended because of risk to infant from radiation exposure

Use in children—Risk from radiation exposure as opposed to benefit derived from use should be considered

**Preparation for this test**

Special preparatory instructions may be given; patient should inquire in advance

**Precautions after having this test**

Increasing intake of fluids and voiding as often as possible for 4 to 6 hours after examination to minimize radiation dose to bladder

**Side/adverse effects**

Signs of potential side effects, especially allergic reaction

## General Dosing Information

Radiopharmaceuticals are to be administered only by or under the supervision of physicians who have had extensive training in the safe use and handling of radioactive materials and who are authorized by the Nuclear Regulatory Commission (NRC) or the appropriate Agreement State agency, if required, or, outside the U.S., the appropriate authority.

Adequate hydration of the patient is recommended before and after examination to promote urinary flow. Also, urination is recommended as often as possible for 4 to 6 hours after the examination to reduce radiation dose to the bladder.

Manufacturer's package insert or other appropriate literature should be consulted for optimal times when imaging should be performed.

**Safety considerations for handling this radiopharmaceutical**

Improper handling of this radiopharmaceutical may cause radioactive contamination. Guidelines for handling radioactive material have been prepared by scientific, professional, state, federal, and international bodies and are available to the specially qualified and authorized users who have access to radiopharmaceuticals.

## Parenteral Dosage Forms

### TECHNETIUM Tc 99m GLUCEPTATE INJECTION USP

**Usual adult and adolescent administered activity**

Brain imaging or
Brain perfusion studies—
Intravenous, 555 to 740 megabecquerels (15 to 20 millicuries).
Renal imaging or
Renal perfusion studies—
Intravenous, 370 to 555 megabecquerels (10 to 15 millicuries).

**Usual pediatric administered activity**

Brain imaging—
Intravenous, 7.9 to 10.6 megabecquerels (0.21 to 0.28 millicuries) per kg of body weight, with a minimum total dosage of at least 74 megabecquerels (2 millicuries) and a maximum total dosage of 740 megabecquerels (20 millicuries).

Renal imaging—
Intravenous, 5.3 to 10.6 megabecquerels (0.14 to 0.28 millicuries) per kg of body weight, with a minimum total dosage of at least 37 megabecquerels (1 millicurie) and a maximum total dosage of 370 megabecquerels (10 millicuries).

**Usual geriatric administered activity**

See *Usual adult and adolescent administered activity.*

**Strength(s) usually available**

U.S.—

50 mg gluceptate calcium, 0.7 mg minimum stannous tin as stannous chloride dihydrate, and 1.1 mg maximum total tin as stannous chloride dihydrate (in a lyophilized form and under a nitrogen atmosphere), per10-mL reaction vial (Rx) [*TechneScan Gluceptate*].

200 mg gluceptate sodium, 0.06 mg minimum stannous tin as stannous chloride, and 0.07 mg maximum tin (in a lyophilized form and under a nitrogen atmosphere), per reaction vial (Rx) [*Glucoscan*].

Canada—

25 mg gluceptate calcium, 3 mg stannous chloride dihydrate (in lyophilized form under nitrogen atmosphere), per 10-mL reaction vial (Rx) [*Frosstimage Gluceptate*].

50 mg gluceptate calcium, 0.7 mg minimum stannous chloride dihydrate, and 1.1 mg maximum total tin expressed as stannous chloride dihydrate (in lyophilized form under nitrogen atmosphere), per 10-mL reaction vial (Rx) [*Frosstimage Gluco*].

**Packaging and storage**

Store between 2 and 8 °C (36 and 46 °F). Protect from freezing.

Note: Prior to labeling, kit can be stored at room temperature.

**Preparation of dosage form**

To prepare injection, an oxidant-free sodium pertechnetate Tc 99m solution is used. See manufacturer's package insert for instructions.

**Stability**

Injection should be administered within 6 hours after preparation.

**Incompatibilities**

If oxidants such as peroxides and hypochlorites are present in the sodium pertechnetate Tc 99m used for labeling, the final preparation may be adversely affected and should be discarded.

**Note**

Caution—Radioactive material.

## Selected Bibliography

Blaufox MD. Procedures of choice in renal nuclear medicine. J Nucl Med 1991; 32: 1301-9.

---

Revised: 07/26/93
Interim revision: 08/02/94

---

# TECHNETIUM Tc 99m LIDOFENIN   Systemic

VA CLASSIFICATION (Primary): DX201

Note: For a listing of dosage forms and brand names by country availability, see *Dosage Forms* section(s). For a listing of brand names for the articles in this monograph, refer to the General Index.

## Category

Diagnostic aid, radioactive (hepatobiliary disorders).

## Indications

**Accepted**

Hepatobiliary imaging, radionuclide—Technetium Tc 99m lidofenin is indicated as a hepatobiliary imaging agent for the evaluation of hepatobiliary tract patency to differentiate jaundice resulting from hepatocellular causes from jaundice resulting from partial or complete biliary obstruction; to differentiate extrahepatic biliary atresia from neonatal hepatitis; to detect cystic duct obstruction associated with acute cholecystitis; and to detect bile leaks.

Also, technetium Tc 99m lidofenin may be useful to detect intrahepatic cholestasis and to distinguish it from other hepatobiliary diseases, which involve hepatocyte damage.

## Physical Properties

**Nuclear data**

| Radionuclide (half-life) | Decay constant | Mode of decay | Principal photon emissions (keV) | Mean number of emissions/ disintegration (≥0.01) |
|---|---|---|---|---|
| Tc 99m (6.0 hr) | 0.1151 h⁻¹ | Isomeric transition to Tc 99 | Gamma 18 | 0.062 |
|  |  |  | Gamma 140.5 | 0.891 |

# Pharmacology/Pharmacokinetics

**Physicochemical characteristics**
Molecular weight—Lidofenin: 294.31.

**Mechanism of action/Effect**
Based on the clearance of most of the administered activity through the hepatobiliary system. Following intravenous administration, technetium Tc 99m–labeled IDA derivatives, such as lidofenin, become bound to plasma proteins (mainly albumin). In the liver, in the space of Disse, technetium Tc 99m lidofenin becomes dissociated from the proteins and enters the hepatocyte by a mechanism similar to that of serum bilirubin. Technetium Tc 99m lidofenin traverses through the hepatocyte unmetabolized and enters the bile canaliculi. Flow beyond the canaliculi is influenced to a large extent by the tone of the sphincter of Oddi and the patency of the bile ducts. Clear visualization of the gallbladder and intestines, usually within 15 to 30 minutes of administration, demonstrates hepatobiliary tract patency.

**Distribution**
In circulatory system, with rapid blood clearance (about 5 minutes after injection); however, a percentage of the administered activity (about 10% in patients with normal liver function and in excess of 20% in patients with obstructive jaundice) clears the circulation more slowly. Cleared from blood by normal hepatic cells within 10 to 20 minutes. Excreted into bile and stored in gallbladder. Excreted through hepatobiliary tract into the intestine. A fraction of the administered activity excreted into the urine. The fraction excreted into the urine is dependent on the extent of biliary disease.

**Protein binding**
Low (18% of radioactivity).

**Half-life**
Elimination from blood (with suspected gallbladder disease)—
   89% of dose: 3.1 minutes.
   7.3% of dose: 26.1 minutes.
   3.9% of dose: 14.1 hours.

**Time to radioactivity visualization**
With normal hepatobiliary function—
   Liver: 5 minutes; maximum liver uptake by 10 to 15 minutes.
   Hepatic duct and gallbladder: 20 to 30 minutes.
   Intestines: 15 to 30 minutes.

   Note: Delayed visualization or nonvisualization of gallbladder may occur during the period immediately following a meal or after prolonged fasting.

With hepatocellular disease or biliary obstruction—
   Delayed visualization or nonvisualization. With serum bilirubin values over 7 to 8 mg per dL (0.12 to 1.37 mmol per L), the biliary system is not well visualized, but liver and intestinal radioactivity may still be observed with levels up to 10 to 13 mg/dL (0.17 to 2.22 mmol/L).

**Radiation dosimetry**

| Organ | Estimated absorbed radiation dose* | | | |
|---|---|---|---|---|
| | With normal hepatobiliary function | | With parenchymal liver disease | |
| | mGy/ MBq | rad/ mCi | mGy/ MBq | rad/ mCi |
| Gall bladder wall | 0.11 | 0.41 | 0.035 | 0.13 |
| Large intestine wall (upper) | 0.092 | 0.34 | 0.033 | 0.12 |
| Large intestine wall (lower) | 0.062 | 0.23 | 0.024 | 0.089 |
| Small intestine | 0.052 | 0.19 | 0.019 | 0.070 |
| Bladder wall | 0.023 | 0.085 | 0.069 | 0.26 |
| Ovaries | 0.020 | 0.074 | 0.0099 | 0.037 |
| Liver | 0.015 | 0.056 | 0.010 | 0.037 |
| Uterus | 0.013 | 0.048 | 0.011 | 0.041 |
| Red marrow | 0.0070 | 0.026 | 0.0038 | 0.014 |
| Kidneys | 0.0063 | 0.023 | 0.0066 | 0.024 |
| Stomach wall | 0.0061 | 0.023 | 0.0027 | 0.010 |
| Pancreas | 0.0057 | 0.021 | 0.0028 | 0.010 |
| Adrenals | 0.0032 | 0.012 | 0.0021 | 0.0078 |
| Bone surfaces | 0.0026 | 0.0096 | 0.0017 | 0.0063 |
| Spleen | 0.0026 | 0.0096 | 0.0015 | 0.0056 |
| Testes | 0.0015 | 0.0056 | 0.0025 | 0.0093 |
| Breast | 0.00061 | 0.0023 | 0.00056 | 0.0021 |
| Thyroid | 0.00012 | 0.00044 | 0.00023 | 0.00085 |
| Other tissue | 0.0030 | 0.011 | 0.0021 | 0.0078 |

| Radionuclide | Effective dose* | | | |
|---|---|---|---|---|
| | With normal hepatobiliary function | | With parenchymal liver disease | |
| | mSy/ MBq | rem/ mCi | mSy/ MBq | rem/ mCi |
| Tc 99m | 0.024 | 0.089 | 0.013 | 0.048 |

*For adults; intravenous injection of technetium Tc 99m–labeled iminodiacetic acid (IDA) derivatives. Data based on the International Commission on Radiological Protection (ICRP) Publication 53—Radiation dose to patients from radiopharmaceuticals.

**Elimination**
Primarily fecal.

Note: In patients with normal liver function, approximately 14% of the administered activity is present in the urinary bladder within 90 minutes after administration. In patients with hepatocellular disease or biliary obstruction, elimination through the urinary tract may be greatly increased. In jaundiced patients, approximately 22% of the administered activity is present in the urine within 90 minutes, and 53% in 18 to 24 hours.

# Precautions to Consider

**Cross-sensitivity and/or related problems**
Patients sensitive to amide-type local anesthetics may be sensitive to technetium Tc 99m lidofenin also.

**Carcinogenicity/Mutagenicity**
Long-term animal studies to evaluate carcinogenic or mutagenic potential of technetium Tc 99m lidofenin have not been performed.

**Pregnancy/Reproduction**
Pregnancy—Tc 99m (as free pertechnetate) crosses the placenta. Studies have not been done with technetium Tc 99m lidofenin in humans.
The possibility of pregnancy should be assessed in women of child-bearing potential. Clinical situations exist where the benefit to the patient and fetus, based on information derived from radiopharmaceutical use, outweighs the risks from fetal exposure to radiation. In these situations, the physician should use discretion and reduce the administered activity of the radiopharmaceutical to the lowest possible amount.
Studies have not been done in animals.
FDA Pregnancy Category C.

**Breast-feeding**
Although it is not known whether technetium Tc 99m lidofenin is distributed into breast milk, it is known that Tc 99m as free pertechnetate is distributed into breast milk. Based on the assumption that the Tc 99m in breast milk is in the form of pertechnetate and based on the effective half-life of the radionuclide in breast milk, the daily volume of milk, a dose factor relating the radionuclide to its critical organ (thyroid) in the nursing infant, and the maximum permissible dose to that organ, a guideline has been proposed. According to this guideline, it has been calculated that nursing can be safely resumed when the concentration in breast milk reaches $30.3 \times 10^{-4}$ megabecquerels ($8.2 \times 10^{-2}$ microcuries) per mL. This level of activity is probably reached, in the majority of patients, within 12 to 24 hours after administration of technetium Tc 99m–labeled radiopharmaceuticals.

**Pediatrics**
Diagnostic studies performed to date using technetium Tc 99m lidofenin have not demonstrated pediatrics-specific problems that would limit its usefulness in children. However, there have been no specific studies evaluating the safety and efficacy of technetium Tc 99m lidofenin in pediatric patients. When this radiopharmaceutical is used in children, the diagnostic benefit should be judged to outweigh the potential risk of radiation.

**Geriatrics**
Appropriate studies on the relationship of age to the effects of technetium Tc 99m lidofenin have not been performed in the geriatric population. However, no geriatrics-specific problems have been documented to date.

**Drug interactions and/or related problems**
See *Diagnostic interference*.

**Diagnostic interference**
The following have been selected on the basis of their potential clinical significance (possible effect in parentheses where appropriate)—not necessarily inclusive (» = major clinical significance):

With results of *this* test
*Due to other medications*
Alcohol or
Anticholinergics or other medications with anticholinergic activity (See *Appendix II* ) or
Bethanechol or
Somatostatin
(may decrease gallbladder emptying, thus delaying gallbladder clearance of technetium Tc 99m lidofenin)
Erythromycin
(nonvisualization of gallbladder may occur due to erthromycin-induced hepatotoxicity)
Nicotinic acid
(chronic, high-dose nicotinic acid therapy may result in poor extraction and elimination of the radiopharmaceutical, mimicking intrinsic hepatocellular disease)
Opioid (narcotic) analgesics, especially butorphanol, morphine, and meperidine
(delivery of technetium Tc 99m lidofenin to the small bowel may be prevented by opioid analgesics because of the constriction of the sphincter of Oddi and the increased biliary tract pressure caused by these medications; these actions result in delayed intestinal visualization, which resembles the delay caused by obstruction of the common bile duct; however, the use of intravenous morphine has been shown to help in the diagnosis of acute cholecystitis when conditions that delay or prevent gallbladder visualization are present)
Parenteral alimentation
(may give false-positive diagnosis of cystic duct obstruction due to stasis of bile in the gallbladder)
*Due to medical problems or conditions*
Fasting, prolonged or
Pancreatitis, acute
(may give false-positive results [nonvisualization or delayed visualization of gallbladder] of cystic duct obstruction due to stasis of bile in gallbladder)
Hepatocellular disease
(nonvisualization or delayed visualization of gallbladder may occur)
Post-prandial state, especially with ingestion of fatty meals
(ingestion of a fatty meal immediately before test may give false-positive results [nonvisualization of gallbladder] of cystic duct obstruction due to gallbladder contraction stimulated by meal ingestion)

### Medical considerations/Contraindications

The medical considerations/contraindications included here have been selected on the basis of their potential clinical significance (reasons given in parentheses where appropriate)—not necessarily inclusive (» = major clinical significance).
See also *Diagnostic interference.*

*Risk-benefit should be considered when the following medical problem exists:*

Sensitivity to amide-type local anesthetics or to the radiopharmaceutical preparation

## Side/Adverse Effects

The following side/adverse effects have been selected on the basis of their potential clinical significance and/or frequency of occurrence (possible signs and symptoms in parentheses where appropriate)—not necessarily inclusive:

**Those indicating need for medical attention only if they continue or are bothersome**
Incidence less frequent or rare
*Chills; nausea; skin rash*

## Patient Consultation

As an aid to patient consultation, refer to *Advice for the Patient, Radiopharmaceuticals (Diagnostic).*
In providing consultation, consider emphasizing the following selected information (»= major clinical significance):

**Description of use**
Action in the body: Clearance of radioactive lidofenin from blood through hepatobiliary tract
Visualization of radioactivity in intestinal tract and gallbladder shows absence of obstruction of bile ducts
Small amounts of radioactivity used in diagnosis; radiation received is low and considered safe

**Before having this test**
» Conditions affecting use, especially:
Sensitivity to the radiopharmaceutical preparation or to local anesthetics (amide-type)
Pregnancy—Technetium Tc 99m (as free pertechnetate) crosses placenta; risk to fetus from radiation exposure as opposed to benefit derived from use should be considered
Breast-feeding—Not known if technetium Tc 99m lidofenin distributed into breast milk, but Tc 99m as free pertechnetate is distributed into breast milk; temporary discontinuation of nursing may be recommended because of risk to infant from radiation exposure
Use in children—Risk from radiation exposure as opposed to benefit derived from use should be considered
Other medical problems, especially prolonged fasting and acute pancreatitis

### Preparation for this test
Fasting for at least 2 and preferably 4 hours before test to prevent gallbladder nonvisualization

### Precautions after having this test
No special precautions

## General Dosing Information

Radiopharmaceuticals are to be administered only by or under the supervision of physicians who have had extensive training in the safe use and handling of radioactive materials and who are authorized by the Nuclear Regulatory Commission (NRC) or the appropriate Agreement State agency, if required, or, outside the U.S., the appropriate authority.

Administration of phenobarbital (5 mg per kg of body weight [mg/kg] in 2 divided doses) for at least 5 days prior to hepatobiliary imaging may enhance and accelerate biliary uptake and excretion of the radiopharmaceutical in the differential diagnosis of extrahepatic atresia from neonatal hepatitis. This will enable determination of the status of the extrahepatic biliary tract in the jaundiced neonate within 24 hours.

Fasting is recommended for at least 2 and preferably 4 hours before the examination is recommended since nonvisualization of the gallbladder may result if gallbladder contraction has been stimulated by the ingestion of food.

Prolonged fasting (e.g., more than 24 hours) may result in a false-positive hepatobiliary scan (e.g., nonvisualization of the gallbladder despite a patent cystic duct) due to the development of increased intraluminal gallbladder pressure (biliary stasis or sludge), which reduces radiotracer flow to the gallbladder. To avoid this, prior administration of a cholecystokinetic agent, such as sincalide or cholecystokinin (CCK-8) to induce contraction of the gallbladder, is recommended for pre-emptying the gallbladder before the injection of technetium Tc 99m lidofenin. Whenever there is doubt about the dietary history of the patient, especially in emergency situations, a cholecystokinetic agent should be administered.

In patients receiving parenteral alimentation, the relative inactivity of the gallbladder results in bile stasis and the formation of thick viscous bile (sludge), which reduces the flow of the radiotracer into the gallbladder. Pretreatment with a cholecystokinetic agent (e.g., intravenous sincalide 0.02 to 0.04 microgram per kilogram of body weight) may be useful to empty stored bile from the gallbladder, and thus, may prevent a false-positive hepatobiliary scan.

In patients demonstrating technetium Tc 99m lidofenin localization in the gallbladder, a cholecystokinetic agent (e.g., intravenous sincalide 0.02 to 0.04 microgram per kilogram of body weight) may be useful to stimulate gallbladder contraction and thereby evaluate the contractile function of the gallbladder. Quantitation of gallbladder emptying yields the ejection fraction ($\geq$ 35% is usually considered normal).

Imaging is performed immediately following technetium Tc 99m lidofenin administration, and is usually completed in 60 to 90 minutes. Imaging for up to 4 hours or longer may be necessary if there is no gallbladder or intestinal activity.

When there is no visualization of the gallbladder within an hour of administration of technetium Tc 99m lidofenin, but the radiotracer is seen within the small bowel in patients suspected of having acute cholecystitis, morphine sulfate (0.04 mg/kg diluted in 10 mL saline) may be injected intravenously to help confirm the diagnosis. The diagnosis of acute cholecystitis is confirmed if nonvisualization of the gallbladder persists after morphine is administered. Although morphine-augmented cholescintigraphy may cause false-positive and false-negative results in some patients (e.g., acalculous cholecystitis), it may be useful in critically ill patients or patients who have been on a prolonged fasting or are receiving parenteral alimentation.

## Safety considerations for handling this radiopharmaceutical

Improper handling of this radiopharmaceutical may cause radioactive contamination. Guidelines for handling radioactive material have been prepared by scientific, professional, state, federal, and international bodies and are available to the specially qualified and authorized users who have access to radiopharmaceuticals.

## Parenteral Dosage Forms

### TECHNETIUM Tc 99m LIDOFENIN INJECTION USP

**Usual adult and adolescent administered activity**
Hepatobiliary imaging—
    Intravenous, 185 megabecquerels (5 millicuries).

Note: Dosage is usually adjusted depending on bilirubin levels.

    A period of 24 hours should elapse before a second dose is administered.

**Usual adult prescribing limits**
370 megabecquerels (10 millicuries).

**Usual pediatric administered activity**
Hepatobiliary imaging—
    With bilirubin levels less than 5 mg per dL (0.08 mmol per L): Intravenous, 2.6 megabecquerels (70 microcuries) per kg of body weight. Minimum total administered activity is 18.5 megabecquerels (500 microcuries).
    With bilirubin levels higher than 5 mg per dL (0.08 mmol per L): Intravenous, 5.18 megabecquerels (140 microcuries) per kg of body weight. Minimum total administered activity is 37 megabecquerels (1 millicurie).

**Usual geriatric administered activity**
See *Usual adult and adolescent administered activity.*

**Strength(s) usually available**
U.S.—
    10 mg lidofenin complexed with 0.8 mg (minimum) stannous chloride dihydrate (maximum tin as stannous chloride dihydrate 1.1 mg) in lyophilized form under nitrogen atmosphere, per 10-mL reaction vial (Rx) [*TechneScan HIDA*].

Canada—
    10 mg lidofenin complexed with 0.8 mg (minimum) stannous chloride dihydrate (maximum tin as stannous chloride dihydrate 1.1 mg) in lyophilized form under nitrogen atmosphere, per 10-mL reaction vial (Rx) [*TechneScan HIDA*].
    10 mg lidofenin complexed with 1 mg stannous chloride dihydrate in lyophilized form under nitrogen atmosphere, per 10-mL reaction vial (Rx) [*Frosstimage HIDA*].

**Packaging and storage**
Store between 2 and 8 °C (36 and 46 °F), unless otherwise specified by manufacturer. Protect from freezing.

**Preparation of dosage form**
To prepare injection, an oxidant-free sodium pertechnetate Tc 99m solution is used. See manufacturer's package insert for instructions.

**Stability**
Injection should be administered within 6 hours after preparation.

**Note**
Caution—Radioactive material.

## Selected Bibliography

Fink-Bennett D, Balon H, Robbins T, et al. Morphine-augmented cholescintigraphy: its efficacy in detecting acute cholecystitis. J Nucl Med 1991; 32: 1231-3.

Krishnamurthy GT, Turner FE. Pharmacokinetics and clinical application of technetium 99m-labeled hepatobiliary agents. Semin Nucl Med 1990; 20 (2): 130-49.

Weissman HS, Badia J, Sugarman LA, et al. Spectrum of 99m-Tc-IDA cholescintigraphic patterns in acute cholecystitis. Radiology 1981; 138: 167-75.

Revised: 06/14/93
Interim revision: 08/02/94

---

# TECHNETIUM Tc 99m MEBROFENIN    Systemic

VA CLASSIFICATION (Primary): DX201

Another commonly used name is technetium Tc 99m BrIDA.

Note: For a listing of dosage forms and brand names by country availability, see *Dosage Forms* section(s). For a listing of brand names for the articles in this monograph, refer to the General Index.

## Category

Diagnostic aid, radioactive (hepatobiliary disorders).

## Indications

**Accepted**
Hepatobiliary imaging, radionuclide—Technetium Tc 99m mebrofenin is indicated as a hepatobiliary imaging agent for the evaluation of hepatobiliary tract patency to differentiate jaundice resulting from hepatocellular causes from jaundice resulting from partial or complete biliary obstruction; to differentiate extrahepatic biliary atresia from neonatal hepatitis; to detect cystic duct obstruction associated with acute cholecystitis; and to detect bile leaks.

Also, technetium Tc 99m mebrofenin may be useful to detect intrahepatic cholestasis and to distinguish it from other hepatobiliary diseases, which involve hepatocyte damage.

## Physical Properties

**Nuclear data**

| Radionu-clide (half-life) | Decay constant | Mode of decay | Principal photon emissions (keV) | Mean number of emissions/ disintegration ($\geq 0.01$) |
|---|---|---|---|---|
| Tc 99m (6.0 hr) | $0.1151\ h^{-1}$ | Isomeric transition to Tc 99 | Gamma (18) | 0.062 |
| | | | Gamma (140.5) | 0.891 |

## Pharmacology/Pharmacokinetics

**Physicochemical characteristics**
Molecular weight—Mebrofenin: 387.23.

**Mechanism of action/Effect**
Based on the clearance of most of the administered activity through the hepatobiliary system. Following intravenous administration, technetium Tc 99m–labeled iminodiacetic acid (IDA) derivatives, such as mebrofenin, bind to plasma proteins (mainly albumin). In the liver, in the space of Disse, technetium Tc 99m mebrofenin dissociates from the proteins and enters the hepatocyte by a mechanism similar to that of serum bilirubin. Technetium Tc 99m mebrofenin traverses through the hepatocyte unmetabolized and enters the bile canaliculi. Flow beyond the canaliculi is influenced to a large extent by the tone of the sphincter of Oddi and the patency of the bile ducts. Clear visualization of the gallbladder and intestines, usually within 15 to 30 minutes of administration, demonstrates hepatobiliary tract patency.

**Distribution**
In circulatory system, with rapid blood clearance; however, about 17% of the administered activity (twice as much in patients with obstructive jaundice) remains in circulation 10 minutes after injection. Cleared from blood by normal hepatic cells within 10 to 20 minutes. Excreted into bile and stored in gallbladder. Excreted through hepatobiliary tract into the intestine. A small fraction of the administered activity excreted into the urine. The fraction excreted into the urine is dependent on the extent of biliary disease.

**Time to radioactivity visualization**
With normal hepatobiliary function—
    Liver: 5 minutes; maximum liver uptake by 11 minutes.
    Hepatic duct and gallbladder: 10 to 15 minutes.
    Intestines: 30 to 60 minutes.

    Note: Delayed visualization or nonvisualization of the gallbladder may occur during the period immediately following a meal or after prolonged fasting.

## Radiation dosimetry

| Organ | Estimated absorbed radiation dose* | | | |
|---|---|---|---|---|
| | With normal hepatobiliary function | | With parenchymal liver disease | |
| | mGy/mBq | rad/mCi | mGy/MBq | rad/mCi |
| Gall bladder wall | 0.11 | 0.41 | 0.035 | 0.13 |
| Large intestine wall (upper) | 0.092 | 0.34 | 0.033 | 0.12 |
| Large intestine wall (lower) | 0.062 | 0.23 | 0.024 | 0.089 |
| Small intestine | 0.052 | 0.19 | 0.019 | 0.070 |
| Bladder wall | 0.023 | 0.085 | 0.069 | 0.26 |
| Ovaries | 0.020 | 0.074 | 0.0099 | 0.037 |
| Liver | 0.015 | 0.056 | 0.010 | 0.037 |
| Uterus | 0.013 | 0.048 | 0.011 | 0.041 |
| Red marrow | 0.0070 | 0.026 | 0.0038 | 0.014 |
| Kidneys | 0.0063 | 0.023 | 0.0066 | 0.024 |
| Stomach wall | 0.0061 | 0.023 | 0.0027 | 0.010 |
| Pancreas | 0.0057 | 0.021 | 0.0028 | 0.010 |
| Adrenals | 0.0032 | 0.012 | 0.0021 | 0.0078 |
| Bone surfaces | 0.0026 | 0.0096 | 0.0017 | 0.0063 |
| Spleen | 0.0026 | 0.0096 | 0.0015 | 0.0056 |
| Testes | 0.0015 | 0.0056 | 0.0025 | 0.0093 |
| Breast | 0.00061 | 0.0023 | 0.00056 | 0.0021 |
| Thyroid | 0.00012 | 0.00044 | 0.00023 | 0.00085 |
| Other tissue | 0.0030 | 0.011 | 0.0021 | 0.0078 |

| Radionuclide | Effective dose* | | | |
|---|---|---|---|---|
| | With normal hepatobiliary function | | With parenchymal liver disease | |
| | mSv/mBq | rem/mCi | mSv/MBq | rem/mCi |
| Tc 99m | 0.024 | 0.089 | 0.013 | 0.048 |

*For adults; intravenous injection of technetium Tc 99m–labeled iminodiacetic acid (IDA) derivatives. Data based on the International Commission on Radiological Protection (ICRP) Publication 53—Radiation dose to patients from radiopharmaceuticals.

### Elimination
Primarily fecal.

Note: In patients with normal liver function, 1% (mean) of the administered activity is present in the urinary bladder within 3 hours after administration. In patients with hepatocellular disease or biliary obstruction, elimination through the urinary tract may be greatly increased. With mean elevated serum bilirubin levels of 9.8 mg per dL (791.73 micromole per L), 3% (mean) of the administered activity is excreted in the urine within 3 hours and 14.9% (mean) of the administered activity is excreted during 3 to 24 hours.

# Precautions to Consider

### Cross-sensitivity and/or related problems
Patients sensitive to amide-type local anesthetics may be sensitive to technetium Tc 99m mebrofenin also.

### Carcinogenicity/Mutagenicity
Long-term animal studies to evaluate carcinogenic or mutagenic potential of technetium Tc 99m mebrofenin have not been performed.

### Pregnancy/Reproduction
Pregnancy—Tc 99m (as free pertechnetate) crosses the placenta. Studies have not been done with technetium Tc 99m mebrofenin in humans. The possibility of pregnancy should be assessed in women of child-bearing potential. Clinical situations exist where the benefit to the patient and fetus, based on information derived from radiopharmaceutical use, outweighs the risks from fetal exposure to radiation. In these situations, the physician should use discretion and reduce the administered activity of the radiopharmaceutical to the lowest possible amount.

Studies have not been done in animals.

FDA Pregnancy Category C.

### Breast-feeding
Although it is not known whether technetium Tc 99m mebrofenin is distributed into breast milk, it is known that Tc 99m as free pertechnetate is distributed into breast milk. Based on the assumption that the Tc 99m in breast milk is in the form of pertechnetate and based on the effective half-life of the radionuclide in breast milk, the daily volume of milk, a dose factor relating the radionuclide to its critical organ

(thyroid) in the nursing infant, and the maximum permissible dose to that organ, a guideline has been proposed. According to this guideline, it has been calculated that nursing can be safely resumed when the concentration in breast milk reaches $30.3 \times 10^{-4}$ megabecquerels ($8.2 \times 10^{-2}$ microcuries) per mL. This level of activity is probably reached, in the majority of patients, within 12 to 24 hours after administration of technetium Tc 99m–labeled radiopharmaceuticals.

### Pediatrics
Diagnostic studies performed to date using technetium Tc 99m mebrofenin have not demonstrated pediatrics-specific problems that would limit its usefulness in children. However, there have been no specific studies evaluating the safety and efficacy of technetium Tc 99m mebrofenin in pediatric patients. When this radiopharmaceutical is used in children, the diagnostic benefit should be judged to outweigh the potential risk of radiation.

### Geriatrics
Appropriate studies on the relationship of age to the effects of technetium Tc 99m mebrofenin have not been performed in the geriatric population. However, no geriatrics-specific problems have been documented to date.

### Drug interactions and/or related problems
See *Diagnostic interference*.

### Diagnostic interference
The following have been selected on the basis of their potential clinical significance (possible effect in parentheses where appropriate)—not necessarily inclusive (» = major clinical significance):

With results of *this* test
*Due to other medications*
  Alcohol or
  Anticholinergics or other medications with anticholinergic activity (See *Appendix II*) or
  Bethanechol or
  Somatostatin
    (may decrease gallbladder emptying, thus delaying gallbladder clearance of technetium Tc 99m mebrofenin)

  Erythromycin
    (nonvisualization of gallbladder may occur due to erythromycin-induced hepatotoxicity)

  Nicotinic acid
    (chronic, high-dose nicotinic acid therapy may result in poor extraction and elimination of the radiopharmaceutical, mimicking intrinsic hepatocellular disease)

  Opioid (narcotic) analgesics, especially butorphanol, morphine, and meperidine
    (delivery of technetium Tc 99m mebrofenin to the small bowel may be prevented by opioid analgesics because of the constriction of the sphincter of Oddi and the increased biliary tract pressure caused by these medications; these actions result in delayed intestinal visualization, which resembles the delay caused by obstruction of the common bile duct; however, the use of intravenous morphine has been shown to help in the diagnosis of acute cholecystitis when conditions that delay or prevent gallbladder visualization are present)

  Parenteral alimentation
    (may give false-positive diagnosis of cystic duct obstruction because of stasis of bile in the gallbladder)

*Due to medical problems or conditions*
  Fasting, prolonged or
  Pancreatitis, acute
    (may give false-positive results [nonvisualization or delayed visualization of gallbladder] of cystic duct obstruction due to stasis of bile in gallbladder)

  Hepatocellular disease
    (nonvisualization or delayed visualization of gallbladder may occur)

  Postprandial state, especially with ingestion of fatty meals
    (ingestion of a fatty meal immediately prior to study may give false-positive results [nonvisualization of gallbladder] of cystic duct obstruction due to gallbladder contraction stimulated by meal ingestion)

### Medical considerations/Contraindications
The medical considerations/contraindications included here have been selected on the basis of their potential clinical significance (reasons given in parentheses where appropriate)—not necessarily inclusive (» = major clinical significance).

See also *Diagnostic interference*.

*Risk-benefit should be considered when the following medical problem exists:*

Sensitivity to amide-type local anesthetics or to the radiopharmaceutical preparation

## Side/Adverse Effects

There are no known side/adverse effects associated with the use of technetium Tc 99m mebrofenin. However, chills, nausea, and skin rash have been reported with other iminodiacetic acid (IDA) derivatives.

## Patient Consultation

As an aid to patient consultation, refer to *Advice for the Patient, Radiopharmaceuticals (Diagnostic).*

In providing consultation, consider emphasizing the following selected information (»= major clinical significance):

**Description of use**
Action in the body: Clearance of radioactive mebrofenin from blood through hepatobiliary tract
Visualization of radioactivity in intestinal tract and gallbladder shows absence of obstruction of bile ducts
Small amounts of radioactivity used in diagnosis; radiation received is low and considered safe

**Before having this test**
» Conditions affecting use, especially:
Sensitivity to the radiopharmaceutical preparation or to local anesthetics (amide-type)
Pregnancy—Technetium Tc 99m (as free pertechnetate) crosses placenta; risk to fetus from radiation exposure as opposed to benefit derived from use should be considered
Breast-feeding—Not known if technetium Tc 99m mebrofenin is distributed into breast milk, but Tc 99m as free pertechnetate is distributed into breast milk; temporary discontinuation of nursing may be recommended because of risk to infant from radiation exposure
Use in children—Risk from radiation exposure as opposed to benefit derived from use should be considered
Other medical problems, especially prolonged fasting and acute pancreatitis

**Preparation for this test**
Fasting for at least 2 and preferably 4 hours before test to prevent gallbladder nonvisualization

**Precautions after having this test**
No special precautions

## General Dosing Information

Radiopharmaceuticals are to be administered only by or under the supervision of physicians who have had extensive training in the safe use and handling of radioactive materials and who are authorized by the Nuclear Regulatory Commission (NRC) or the appropriate Agreement State agency, if required, or, outside the U.S., the appropriate authority.

Administration of phenobarbital (5 mg per kg of body weight [mg/kg] in 2 divided doses) for at least 5 days prior to hepatobiliary imaging may enhance and accelerate biliary uptake and excretion of the radiopharmaceutical in the differential diagnosis of extrahepatic atresia from neonatal hepatitis. This will enable determination of the status of the extrahepatic biliary tract in the jaundiced neonate within 24 hours.

Fasting is recommended for at least 2 and preferably 4 hours before the examination since nonvisualization of the gallbladder may result if gallbladder contraction has been stimulated by the ingestion of food.

Prolonged fasting (e.g., more than 24 hours) may result in a false-positive hepatobiliary scan (e.g., nonvisualization of the gallbladder despite a patent cystic duct) due to the development of increased intraluminal gallbladder pressure (biliary stasis or sludge), which reduces radiotracer flow to the gallbladder. To avoid this, prior administration of a cholecystokinetic agent, such as sincalide or cholecystokinin (CCK-8) to induce contraction of the gallbladder, is recommended for pre-emptying the gallbladder before the injection of technetium Tc 99m mebrofenin. Whenever there is doubt about the dietary history of the patient, especially in emergency situations, a cholecystokinetic agent should be administered.

In patients receiving parenteral alimentation, the relative inactivity of the gallbladder results in bile stasis and the formation of thick viscous bile (sludge), which reduces the flow of the radiotracer into the gallbladder.

Pretreatment with a cholecystokinetic agent (e.g., intravenous sincalide 0.02 to 0.04 microgram per kilogram of body weight) may be useful to empty stored bile from the gallbladder, which may prevent a false-positive hepatobiliary scan.

In patients demonstrating technetium Tc 99m mebrofenin localization in the gallbladder, a cholecystokinetic agent (e.g., intravenous sincalide 0.02 to 0.04 microgram per kilogram of body weight) may be useful to stimulate gallbladder contraction and thereby evaluate the contractile function of the gallbladder. Quantitation of gallbladder emptying yields the ejection fraction ($\geq$ 35% is usually considered normal).

Imaging is performed immediately following technetium Tc 99m mebrofenin administration, and is usually completed in 60 to 90 minutes. Imaging for up to 4 hours or longer may be necessary if there is no gallbladder or intestinal activity.

When there is no visualization of the gallbladder within an hour of administration of technetium Tc 99m mebrofenin, but the radiotracer is seen within the small bowel in patients suspected of having acute cholecystitis, morphine sulfate (0.04 mg/kg diluted in 10 mL saline) may be injected intravenously to help confirm the diagnosis. The diagnosis of acute cholecystitis is confirmed if nonvisualization of the gallbladder persists after morphine is administered. Although morphine-augmented cholescintigraphy may cause false-positive and false-negative results in some patients (e.g., acalculous cholecystitis), it may be useful in critically ill patients or patients who have been on prolonged fasting or who are receiving parenteral alimentation.

**Safety considerations for handling this radiopharmaceutical**
Improper handling of this radiopharmaceutical may cause radioactive contamination. Guidelines for handling radioactive material have been prepared by scientific, professional, state, federal, and international bodies and are available to the specially qualified and authorized users who have access to radiopharmaceuticals.

## Parenteral Dosage Forms

### TECHNETIUM Tc 99m MEBROFENIN INJECTION

**Usual adult and adolescent administered activity**
Hepatobiliary imaging—
Nonjaundiced patients: Intravenous, 74 to 185 megabecquerels (2 to 5 millicuries).
Patients with serum bilirubin concentration > 25.65 micromole per L (1.5 mg per dL): Intravenous, 111 to 370 megabecquerels (3 to 10 millicuries).
Note: A period of 24 hours should elapse before a second dose is administered.

**Usual pediatric administered activity**
Hepatobiliary imaging—
Intravenous, 37 megabecquerels (1 millicurie).

**Usual geriatric administered activity**
See *Usual adult and adolescent administered activity.*

**Strength(s) usually available**
U.S.—
45 mg mebrofenin, 0.54 mg (minimum) stannous fluoride dihydrate, 1.03 mg total tin (maximum as stannous fluoride dihydrate), not more than 5.2 mg methylparaben, and 0.58 mg propylparaben (in a lyophilized form and under nitrogen atmosphere), per multidose reaction vial (Rx) [*Choletec*].
Canada—
45 mg mebrofenin, 0.73 mg stannous fluoride, 4.5 mg methylparaben, and 0.5 mg propylparaben (in a lyophilized form and under nitrogen atmosphere), per multidose reaction vial (Rx) [*Choletec*].

**Packaging and storage**
Store between 15 and 30 °C (59 and 86 °F), unless otherwise specified by manufacturer. Protect from freezing.

**Preparation of dosage form**
To prepare injection, an oxidant-free sodium pertechnetate Tc 99m solution is used for labeling. See manufacturer's package insert for instructions.

**Stability**
Injection should be administered within 18 hours after preparation.

**Note**
Caution—Radioactive material.

## Selected Bibliography

Fink-Bennett D, Balon H, Robbins T, et al. Morphine-augmented choles-cintigraphy: its efficacy in detecting acute cholecystitis. J Nucl Med 1991; 32: 1231-3.

Krishnamurthy GT, Turner FE. Pharmacokinetics and clinical application of technetium 99m–labeled hepatobiliary agents. Semin Nucl Med 1990; 20 (2): 130-49.

Weissman HS, Badia J, Sugarman LA, et al. Spectrum of 99m-Tc-IDA cholescintigraphic patterns in acute cholecystitis. Radiology 1981; 138: 167-75.

Revised: 07/26/93
Interim revision: 08/02/94

# TECHNETIUM Tc 99m MEDRONATE    Systemic

VA CLASSIFICATION (Primary): DX201

Note: For a listing of dosage forms and brand names by country availability, see *Dosage Forms* section(s). For a listing of brand names for the articles in this monograph, refer to the General Index.

## Category

Diagnostic aid, radioactive (bone disease).

## Indications

### Accepted

Skeletal imaging, radionuclide—Technetium Tc 99m medronate is indicated as a skeletal imaging agent to delineate areas of abnormal osteogenesis, such as those that occur with metastatic bone disease, Paget's disease, arthritic disease, osteomyelitis, and fractures.

## Physical Properties

### Nuclear data

| Radionu-clide (half-life) | Decay constant | Mode of decay | Principal photons emissions (keV) | Mean number of emissions/ disintegration ($\geq 0.01$) |
|---|---|---|---|---|
| Tc 99m (6.0 hr) | 0.1151 h$^{-1}$ | Isomeric transition to Tc 99 | Gamma (18) | 0.062 |
| | | | Gamma (140.5) | 0.891 |

## Pharmacology/Pharmacokinetics

### Mechanism of action/Effect

Exact mechanism is not known. It is generally accepted that technetium Tc 99m medronate localizes on the surface of hydroxyapatite crystals by a process termed chemisorption, with blood flow and/or blood concentration being most important in the delivery of the agent to sites of uptake. Visualization of osseous lesions is possible since skeletal uptake of technetium Tc 99m medronate is altered in areas of abnormal osteogenesis.

### Distribution

Rapidly distributed in and cleared from blood after intravenous administration, with about half the administered activity normally accumulating in the skeleton within 3 to 4 hours after intravenous administration. May also locate within infarcted myocardial cells or other regions of soft tissue necrosis or calcification. Minimal uptake by soft tissue organs, except calcified cartilage, blood vessels, and kidneys.

### Time to radioactivity visualization:

1 to 4 hours (optimal imaging).

### Radiation dosimetry

| Estimated absorbed radiation dose* | | |
|---|---|---|
| Organ | mGy/MBq | rad/mCi |
| Bone surfaces | 0.063 | 0.23 |
| Bladder wall | 0.050 | 0.19 |
| Red marrow | 0.0096 | 0.036 |
| Kidneys | 0.0073 | 0.027 |
| Uterus | 0.0061 | 0.023 |
| Large intestine wall (lower) | 0.0038 | 0.014 |
| Ovaries | 0.0035 | 0.013 |
| Testes | 0.0024 | 0.0089 |
| Small intestine | 0.0023 | 0.0085 |

| Estimated absorbed radiation dose* | | |
|---|---|---|
| Organ | mGy/MBq | rad/mCi |
| Large intestine wall (upper) | 0.0020 | 0.0074 |
| Adrenals | 0.0019 | 0.0070 |
| Pancreas | 0.0016 | 0.0059 |
| Spleen | 0.0014 | 0.0052 |
| Liver | 0.0013 | 0.0048 |
| Lungs | 0.0013 | 0.0048 |
| Stomach wall | 0.0012 | 0.0044 |
| Thyroid | 0.0010 | 0.0037 |
| Breast | 0.00088 | 0.0033 |
| Other tissue | 0.0019 | 0.0070 |

Effective dose: 0.008 mSv/MBq (0.030 rem/mCi)

*For adults; intravenous injection of technetium Tc 99m–labeled phosphates and phosphonates. Data based on the International Commission on Radiological Protection (ICRP) Publication 53—Radiation dose to patients from radiopharmaceuticals.

### Elimination

Renal; 50% (not localized in bone) eliminated within 24 hours.

## Precautions to Consider

### Carcinogenicity/Mutagenicity

Long-term animal studies to evaluate carcinogenic or mutagenic potential of technetium Tc 99m medronate have not been performed.

### Pregnancy/Reproduction

Pregnancy—Tc 99m (as free pertechnetate) crosses the placenta. Studies have not been done in humans with technetium Tc 99m medronate.

The possibility of pregnancy should be assessed in women of child-bearing potential. Clinical situations exist where the benefit to the patient and fetus, based on information derived from radiopharmaceutical use, outweighs the risks from fetal exposure to radiation. In these situations, the physician should use discretion and reduce the radiopharmaceutical dose to the lowest possible amount.

Studies have not been done in animals.

FDA Pregnancy Category C.

### Breast-feeding

Although it is not known whether technetium Tc 99m medronate is distributed into breast milk, it is known that Tc 99m as free pertechnetate is distributed into breast milk. Based on the assumption that the Tc 99m in breast milk is in the form of pertechnetate and based on the effective half-life of the radionuclide in breast milk, the daily volume of milk, a dose factor relating the radionuclide to its critical organ (thyroid) in the nursing infant, and the maximum permissible dose to that organ, a guideline has been proposed. According to this guideline, it has been calculated that nursing can be safely resumed when the concentration in breast milk reaches $30.3 \times 10^{-4}$ megabecquerels ($8.2 \times 10^{-2}$ microcuries) per mL. This level of activity is probably reached, in the majority of patients, within 12 to 24 hours after administration of technetium Tc 99m–labeled radiopharmaceuticals.

### Pediatrics

Diagnostic studies performed to date using technetium Tc 99m medronate have not demonstrated pediatrics-specific problems that would limit its usefulness in children. However, there have been no specific studies evaluating the safety and efficacy of technetium Tc 99m medronate in pediatric patients. When this radiopharmaceutical is used in children, the diagnostic benefit should be judged to outweigh the potential risk of radiation.

### Geriatrics

Appropriate studies on the relationship of age to the effects of technetium Tc 99m medronate have not been performed in the geriatric population. However, no geriatrics-specific problems have been documented to date.

**Drug interactions and/or related problems**
See *Diagnostic interference.*

**Diagnostic interference**
The following have been selected on the basis of their potential clinical significance (possible effect in parentheses where appropriate)—not necessarily inclusive (» = major clinical significance):

With results of *this* test
*Due to other medications*
    Antacids, aluminum-containing
        (high blood concentrations of aluminum ion, which may occur in patients with gastrointestinal obstruction or impaired renal function, may cause localization of technetium Tc 99m medronate in the liver)
    Diatrizoate sodium
        (possible renal and hepatic uptake of technetium Tc 99m medronate if diatrizoate sodium is administered intravenously immediately after technetium Tc 99m medronate)
    Etidronate
        (etidronate may interfere with bone uptake of technetium Tc 99m medronate; a 2-week period after discontinuation of etidronate therapy is recommended before performance of a bone scan with technetium Tc 99m medronate)
    Heparin calcium, subcutaneous or
    Iron dextran, intramuscular or
    Meperidine, intramuscular
        (possible accumulation of technetium Tc 99m medronate at site[s] of injection of these medications)
    Iron supplements or preparations
        (iron overload may cause a decrease in bone uptake of technetium Tc 99m medronate)
    Potassium phosphates or
    Potassium and sodium phosphates or
    Sodium phosphates
        (saturation of bone binding sites by phosphorus ions in these medications may cause decreased bone uptake of technetium Tc 99m medronate)
*Due to medical problems or conditions*
    Bone demineralization, glucocorticoid-induced
        (long-term therapy with these medications may induce bone mineral depletion thus causing decreased bone uptake of technetium Tc 99m medronate)
    Gynecomastia, estrogen-induced
        (possible localization of technetium Tc 99m medronate in breast)
    Nephrotoxicity, drug-induced
        (increased retention of technetium Tc 99m medronate in kidneys)
    Obesity
        (attenuation of photons coming from bone may decrease visualization)
    Osteoporosis
        (reduced mineral deposit in bone may result in images with lower target to non-target ratio)
    Renal function impairment
        (decreased clearance of technetium Tc 99m medronate from blood and soft tissues may decrease visualization because of a lower bone to background ratio resulting from the increased circulating activity; also, chronic renal function impairment may cause metastatic calcification and altered biodistribution of technetium Tc 99m medronate)
With results of *other* tests
    Brain imaging
        (brain scans using sodium pertechnetate Tc 99m may result in high blood background activity when performed after a bone scan using technetium Tc 99m medronate, which contains stannous ions; to avoid this potential diagnostic interference, brain scan may be performed prior to bone scan or with a brain imaging agent other than sodium pertechnetate Tc 99m [e.g., technetium Tc 99m pentetate])

**Medical considerations/Contraindications**
The medical considerations/contraindications included here have been selected on the basis of their potential clinical significance (reasons given in parentheses where appropriate)—not necessarily inclusive (» = major clinical significance).
See also *Diagnostic interference.*

***Risk-benefit should be considered when the following medical problem exists:***
    Sensitivity to the radiopharmaceutical preparation

## Side/Adverse Effects

The following side/adverse effects have been selected on the basis of their potential clinical significance (possible signs and symptoms in parentheses where appropriate)—not necessarily inclusive:

**Those indicating need for medical attention**
Incidence less frequent or rare
    *Allergic reaction* (skin rash, hives, or itching)

## Patient Consultation

As an aid to patient consultation, refer to *Advice for the Patient, Radiopharmaceuticals (Diagnostic).*

In providing consultation, consider emphasizing the following selected information (» = major clinical significance):

**Description of use**
    Action in the body: Accumulation of radioactivity in bone
    Retention of radioactivity in bone allows visualization of lesions
    Small amounts of radioactivity used in diagnosis; radiation received is low and considered safe

**Before having this test**
» Conditions affecting use, especially:
    Sensitivity to the radiopharmaceutical preparation
    Pregnancy—Technetium Tc 99m (as free pertechnetate) crosses placenta; risk to fetus from radiation exposure as opposed to benefit derived from use should be considered
    Breast-feeding—Not known if technetium Tc 99m medronate is distributed into breast milk, but Tc 99m as free pertechnetate is distributed into breast milk; temporary discontinuation of nursing may be recommended because of risk to infant from radiation exposure
    Use in children—Risk from radiation exposure as opposed to benefit derived from use should be considered

**Preparation for this test**
    Special preparatory instructions may be given; patient should inquire in advance
    Increasing intake of fluids and voiding frequently after injection and before test begins in order to minimize radiation dose to bladder
    Voiding just prior to imaging for best test results

**Precautions after having this test**
    Increasing intake of fluids and voiding frequently for 4 to 6 hours after test to minimize radiation dose to bladder

**Side/adverse effects**
    Signs of potential side effects, especially allergic reaction

## General Dosing Information

Radiopharmaceuticals are to be administered only by or under the supervision of physicians who have had extensive training in the safe use and handling of radioactive materials and who are authorized by the Nuclear Regulatory Commission (NRC) or the appropriate Agreement State agency, if required, or, outside the U.S., the appropriate authority.

The patient should increase intake of fluids and void frequently following the administration of technetium Tc 99m medronate injection, and for 4 to 6 hours after the imaging procedures are completed, to minimize radiation dose to the bladder.

Voiding is also recommended immediately prior to imaging procedures to reduce background interference that may result because of the accumulation of the agent in the bladder.

Manufacturer's package insert or other appropriate literature should be consulted for optimal times when imaging should be performed.

**Safety considerations for handling this radiopharmaceutical**
Improper handling of this radiopharmaceutical may cause radioactive contamination. Guidelines for handling radioactive material have been prepared by scientific, professional, state, federal, and international bodies and are available to the specially qualified and authorized users who have access to radiopharmaceuticals.

## Parenteral Dosage Forms

### TECHNETIUM Tc 99m MEDRONATE INJECTION USP

**Usual adult and adolescent administered activity**
Skeletal imaging—
    Intravenous, 7.4 megabecquerels (200 microcuries) per kg of body weight, or a total dose of 370 to 740 megabecquerels (10 to 20 millicuries), administered slowly over a period of 30 seconds.

**Usual pediatric administered activity**

Intravenous, 10.4 megabecquerels (0.28 millicuries) per kg of body weight, administered slowly.

Note: The recommended minimum total pediatric administered activity is 37 megabecquerels (1 millicurie); the maximum total pediatric administered activity is 740 megabecquerels (20 millicuries).

**Usual geriatric administered activity**

See *Usual adult and adolescent administered activity*.

**Strength(s) usually available**

U.S.—

   10 mg medronic acid, 0.17 mg (minimum) stannous chloride, and 2 mg ascorbic acid, in a lyophilized form and under nitrogen atmosphere, per 10-mL reaction vial (Rx) [*MPI MDP*].

   10 mg medronic acid and not less than 0.60 mg stannous chloride dihydrate (maximum total tin expressed as stannous chloride dihydrate 1.10 mg), in a lyophilized form and under nitrogen atmosphere, per 10-mL reaction vial (Rx) [*TechneScan MDP*].

   10 mg medronic acid and not less than 0.60 mg stannous chloride dihydrate (maximum total tin expressed as stannous chloride dihydrate 1.10 mg), in a lyophilized form and under nitrogen atmosphere, per 10-mL reaction vial (Rx) [*AN-MDP*].

   10 mg medronate disodium and 0.85 mg stannous chloride dihydrate, in a lyophilized form and under nitrogen atmosphere, per reaction vial (Rx) [*Osteolite*].

   20 mg medronic acid, 11 mg sodium hydroxide, 1 mg ascorbic acid, and 0.33 mg stannous fluoride, in a lyophilized form and under nitrogen atmosphere, per 10-mL reaction vial (Rx) [*MDP-Squibb*].

Canada—

   10 mg medronic acid and not less than 0.8 mg stannous chloride dihydrate (maximum total tin expressed as stannous chloride dihydrate 1.21 mg), in a lyophilized form and under nitrogen atmosphere, per 10-mL reaction vial (Rx) [*Frosstimage MDP*].

**Packaging and storage**

Store between 2 and 8 °C (36 and 46 °F). Protect from freezing.

Note: Before radiolabeling, the kit may be stored at or below room temperature.

**Preparation of dosage form**

To prepare injection, an oxidant-free sodium pertechnetate Tc 99m solution is used. See manufacturer's package insert for instructions.

**Stability**

Injection should be administered within 6 hours after preparation.

**Incompatibilities**

If oxidants such as peroxides and hypochlorites are present in the sodium pertechnetate Tc 99m used for labeling, the final preparation may be adversely affected and should be discarded.

**Note**

Caution—Radioactive material.

**Selected Bibliography**

Holder LE. Clinical radionuclide bone imaging. Radiology 1990; 176: 607-14.

Revised: 06/14/93

Interim revision: 08/02/94

---

# TECHNETIUM Tc 99m MERTIATIDE   Systemic

VA CLASSIFICATION (Primary): DX201

Other names commonly used are technetium Tc 99m mercaptoacetyltriglycine and MAG3.

Note: For a listing of dosage forms and brand names by country availability, see *Dosage Forms* section(s). For a listing of brand names for the articles in this monograph, refer to the General Index.

## Category

Diagnostic aid, radioactive (renal disorders).

## Indications

Note: Bracketed information in the *Indications* section refers to uses that are not included in U.S. product labeling.

**Accepted**

Renal imaging, radionuclide or

Renal function studies—Technetium Tc 99m mertiatide is indicated as a renal imaging agent to assess renal perfusion, size, position, configuration, function (including differential renal function), upper urinary tract obstruction, and [active urinoma]. Technetium Tc 99m mertiatide scintigraphy provides renal images and renogram curves for the whole kidney and renal cortex.

In renal transplant patients, technetium Tc 99m mertiatide scintigraphy helps in the follow-up evaluation by providing anatomical information as well as functional analysis of the kidney. In diuretic radionuclide renography, technetium Tc 99m mertiatide provides useful information in the evaluation of obstructive uropathy. Also, angiotensin-converting enzyme (ACE) inhibitors–augmented renography using technetium Tc 99m mertiatide allows the detection of physiologically significant renal artery stenosis and helps in the differential diagnosis of renovascular hypertension.

Technetium Tc 99m mertiatide is used as an indirect measurement of effective renal plasma flow.

[Cystography, voiding, indirect, radionuclide] or

[Urinary bladder imaging, radionuclide]—Technetium Tc 99m mertiatide can be used following renal imaging for assessment of vesico-ureteral reflux.

## Physical Properties

### Nuclear data

| Radionuclide (half-life) | Decay constant | Mode of decay | Principal photon emissions (keV) | Mean number of emissions/ disintegration (≥0.01) |
|---|---|---|---|---|
| Tc 99m (6.0 hr) | 0.1151 h$^{-1}$ | Isomeric transition to Tc 99 | Gamma (18) | 0.061 |
|  |  |  | Gamma (140.5) | 0.891 |

## Pharmacology/Pharmacokinetics

**Mechanism of action/Effect**

The use of technetium Tc 99m mertiatide as a renal imaging agent is based on its clearance through the urinary tract predominantly via active tubular secretion (almost exclusively by the proximal renal tubules) and to a small extent by glomerular filtration. The rate of appearance and excretion and the concentration of technetium Tc 99m mertiatide in the kidney can be monitored to assess renal function.

**Distribution**

Rapidly distributed in and cleared from plasma. However, when compared to iodohippurate sodium I 131 (OIH[131]), another renal imaging agent, technetium Tc 99m mertiatide has a significantly slower plasma clearance (50 to 65% of the clearance of OIH[131]).

**Protein binding**

High (70 to 90%), but reversible.

**Radiation dosimetry**

| Organ | Estimated absorbed radiation dose*† | | | |
|---|---|---|---|---|
|  | With normal renal function | | With impaired renal function | |
|  | mGy/ MBq | rad/ mCi | mGy/ MBq | rad/ mCi |
| Uterus | 0.012 | 0.044 | 0.01 | 0.037 |
| Large intestine (lower) | 0.0057 | 0.021 | 0.0051 | 0.019 |
| Ovaries | 0.0054 | 0.02 | 0.0049 | 0.018 |

| Organ | Estimated absorbed radiation dose*† | | | |
| | With normal renal function | | With impaired renal function | |
| | mGy/ MBq | rad/ mCi | mGy/ MBq | rad/ mCi |
|---|---|---|---|---|
| Testes | 0.0037 | 0.014 | 0.0034 | 0.013 |
| Kidneys | 0.0034 | 0.013 | 0.014 | 0.052 |
| Small intestine | 0.0023 | 0.0085 | 0.0027 | 0.01 |
| Large intestine (upper) | 0.0017 | 0.0063 | 0.0022 | 0.0081 |
| Muscles | 0.0014 | 0.0052 | 0.0017 | 0.0063 |
| Bone surfaces | 0.0013 | 0.0048 | 0.0022 | 0.0081 |
| Red marrow | 0.00093 | 0.0034 | 0.0015 | 0.0056 |
| Gall bladder | 0.00057 | 0.0021 | 0.0016 | 0.0059 |
| Skin | 0.00046 | 0.0017 | 0.00078 | 0.0029 |
| Pancreas | 0.0004 | 0.0015 | 0.0015 | 0.0056 |
| Stomach | 0.00039 | 0.0014 | 0.0027 | 0.01 |
| Adrenals | 0.00039 | 0.0014 | 0.0016 | 0.0059 |
| Spleen | 0.00036 | 0.0013 | 0.0015 | 0.0056 |
| Liver | 0.00031 | 0.0011 | 0.0014 | 0.0052 |
| Heart | 0.00018 | 0.00067 | 0.00091 | 0.0034 |
| Lungs | 0.00015 | 0.00056 | 0.00079 | 0.0029 |
| Esophagus | 0.00013 | 0.00048 | 0.00074 | 0.0027 |
| Thymus | 0.00013 | 0.00048 | 0.00074 | 0.0027 |
| Thyroid | 0.00013 | 0.00048 | 0.00073 | 0.0027 |
| Bladder | 0.00011 | 0.00041 | 0.083 | 0.031 |
| Brain | 0.0001 | 0.00037 | 0.00061 | 0.0023 |
| Breast | 0.0001 | 0.00037 | 0.00054 | 0.002 |
| Remaining organs | 0.0013 | 0.0048 | 0.0017 | 0.0063 |
| Effective dose | 0.0073 mSv/ MBq | 0.027 rem/mCi | 0.0063 mSv/ MBq | 0.023 rem/mCi |

*For adults; intravenous administration.

†Data based on the International Commission on Radiological Protection (ICRP) Publication 53—Radiation dose to patients from radiopharmaceuticals.

**Elimination**
Renal (70% of the administered activity in the first 30 minutes, and about 90% of the administered activity in 3 hours). Minimal hepatobiliary elimination (approximately 3% of the administered activity) in normal patients. Hepatobiliary elimination may be increased (approximately 10% of the administered activity) in patients with severe renal function impairment.

Note: The relatively higher extraction fraction (40 to 50%) of technetium Tc 99m mertiatide often provides superior images in patients with impaired renal function compared to technetium Tc 99m pentetate, another renal imaging agent, which has a lower extraction fraction (20%).

# Precautions to Consider

**Pregnancy/Reproduction**
Pregnancy—Tc 99m (as free pertechnetate) crosses the placenta. Studies to assess transplacental transfer of technetium Tc 99m mertiatide have not been done in humans.

The possibility of pregnancy should be assessed in women of child-bearing potential. Clinical situations exist in which the benefit to the patient and fetus from information derived from radiopharmaceutical use outweigh the risks from radiation exposure to the fetus. In this situation, the physician should use discretion and reduce the radiopharmaceutical dose to the lowest possible amount consistent with image quality needs.

The patient should be maximally hydrated, and encouraged to urinate frequently.

Studies have not been done in animals.

FDA Pregnancy Category C.

**Breast-feeding**
Although it is not known whether technetium Tc 99m mertiatide is distributed into breast milk, it is known that Tc 99m as free pertechnetate is distributed into breast milk. To avoid unnecessary irradiation of the infant, discontinuation of nursing for a period of 24 hours is recommended after administration of technetium Tc 99m–labeled radiopharmaceuticals.

**Pediatrics**
Safety and efficacy have not been established in children up to 30 days of age. However, appropriate studies performed to date in older children have not demonstrated pediatrics-specific problems that would limit the usefulness of technetium Tc 99m mertiatide in children.

**Geriatrics**
Appropriate studies performed to date have demonstrated a significant decrease in renal clearance of technetium Tc 99m mertiatide in geriatric patients when compared to younger adults.

**Diagnostic interference**
The following have been selected on the basis of their potential clinical significance (possible effect in parentheses where appropriate)—not necessarily inclusive (» = major clinical significance):

With results of *this* test
*Due to medical problems or conditions*
Dehydration
(decreased urinary flow may result in a pattern that mimics decreased urine production and/or obstruction)

**Medical considerations/Contraindications**
The medical considerations/contraindications included here have been selected on the basis of their potential clinical significance (reasons given in parentheses where appropriate)—not necessarily inclusive (» = major clinical significance).

See also *Diagnostic interference.*

*Risk-benefit should be considered when the following medical problem exists:*
Sensitivity to the radiopharmaceutical preparation

# Side/Adverse Effects

The following side/adverse effects have been selected on the basis of their potential clinical significance (possible signs and symptoms in parentheses where appropriate)—not necessarily inclusive:

**Incidence less frequent or rare**
*Allergic reaction* (skin rash or itching, wheezing or troubled breathing; *increased blood pressure; seizures* (convulsions); *tachycardia* (fast or pounding heartbeat)

**Those indicating need for medical attention only if they continue or are bothersome**
Incidence less frequent or rare
*Chills; fever; nausea; vomiting*

# Patient Consultation

As an aid to patient consultation, refer to *Advice for the Patient, Radiopharmaceuticals (Diagnostic).*

In providing consultation, consider emphasizing the following selected information (» = major clinical significance):

**Description of use**
Action in the body: Concentration of radioactive mertiatide in kidneys
Excretion of radioactivity in urine allows visualization and evaluation of renal function
Small amounts of radioactivity used in diagnosis; radiation received is low and considered safe

**Before having this test**
» Conditions affecting use, especially:
Sensitivity to the radiopharmaceutical preparation
Pregnancy—Technetium Tc 99m (as free pertechnetate) crosses placenta; risk to fetus from radiation exposure as opposed to benefit derived from study should be considered
Breast-feeding—Not known if distributed into breast milk; temporary discontinuation of nursing may be recommended because of risk to infant from radiation exposure
Use in children—Safety and efficacy have not been established in children up to 30 days of age

**Preparation for this test**
Special preparatory instructions may be given; patient should inquire in advance

**Precautions after having this test**
Adequate intake of fluids and voiding as often as possible for 4 to 6 hours after examination to minimize bladder exposure to radiation

# General Dosing Information

Radiopharmaceuticals are to be administered only by or under the supervision of physicians who have had extensive training in the safe use and handling of radionuclides and who are licensed by the Nuclear Regulatory Commission (NRC) or the appropriate Agreement State agency or, outside the U.S., the appropriate authority.

Adequate hydration of the patient is recommended before and after examination to promote urinary flow. Also, urination is recommended as often as possible for 4 to 6 hours after the examination to reduce bladder exposure to radiation.

Manufacturer's package insert or other appropriate literature should be consulted for optimal times when imaging should be performed.

**Safety considerations for handling this radiopharmaceutical**

Guidelines for the receipt, storage, handling, dispensing, and disposal of radioactive materials are available from scientific, professional, state, federal, and international bodies. Handling of this radiopharmaceutical should be limited to those individuals who are appropriately qualified and authorized.

## Parenteral Dosage Forms

### TECHNETIUM Tc 99m MERTIATIDE INJECTION USP

**Usual adult and adolescent administered activity**

Renal imaging or
Renal function studies—
   Intravenous, 185 to 370 megabecquerels (5 to 10 millicuries).

**Usual pediatric administered activity**

Renal imaging or
Renal function studies—
   Children up to 30 days of age: Safety and efficacy have not been established.
   Children 30 days of age and over: Intravenous, 2.6 to 5.2 megabecquerels (70 to 140 microcuries) per kilogram of body weight, with a minimum administered activity of 37 megabecquerels (1 millicurie).

**Usual geriatric administered activity**

See *Usual adult and adolescent administered activity.*

**Strength(s) usually available**

U.S.—
   1 mg betiatide (precursor to mertiatide, thiobenzoic acid, *S*-ester with mercaptoacetyltriglycine), 0.05 mg (minimum) stannous chloride dihydrate, and 0.2 mg (maximum) total tin expressed as stannous chloride dihydrate, 40 mg sodium tartrate dihydrate, and 20 mg lactose monohydrate in lyophilized form under argon atmosphere, per 10-mL reaction vial (Rx) [*TechneScan MAG3*].

Canada—
   1 mg betiatide (precursor to mertiatide, thiobenzoic acid, *S*-ester with mercaptoacetyltriglycine), 0.05 mg (minimum) stannous chloride dihydrate, and 0.2 mg (maximum) total tin expressed as stannous chloride dihydrate, 40 mg sodium tartrate dihydrate, and 20 mg lactose monohydrate in lyophilized form under argon atmosphere, per 10-mL reaction vial (Rx) [*TechneScan MAG3*].

**Packaging and storage**

Store between 15 and 30 °C (59 and 86 °F). Protect from freezing.

Note: Before reconstitution, protect kit from light.

**Preparation of dosage form**

To prepare injection, an oxidant-free sodium pertechnetate Tc 99m solution is used. See manufacturer's package insert for instructions.

**Stability**

Product is stable; package insert states that injection must be used within 6 hours after preparation.

**Incompatibilities**

If oxidants such as peroxides and hypochlorites are present in the sodium pertechnetate Tc 99m used for labeling, the final preparation may be adversely affected and should be discarded.

**Note**

Caution—Radioactive material.

## Selected Bibliography

Bubeck B, Brandau W, Weber E, et al. Pharmacokinetics of technetium-99m-MAG3 in humans. J Nucl Med 1990; 31 (8): 1285-93.

Eshima D, Taylor A Jr. Technetium-99m mercaptoacetyltriglycine: update on the new Tc 99m renal tubular function agent. Semin Nucl Med 1992; 22 (2): 61-73

Revised: 07/23/96

---

# TECHNETIUM Tc 99m OXIDRONATE   Systemic†

**VA CLASSIFICATION (Primary): DX201**

Note: For a listing of dosage forms and brand names by country availability, see *Dosage Forms* section(s). For a listing of brand names for the articles in this monograph, refer to the General Index.

†Not commercially available in Canada.

## Category

Diagnostic aid, radioactive (bone disease).

## Indications

Note: Bracketed information in the *Indications* section refers to uses that are not included in U.S. product labeling.

**Accepted**

Skeletal imaging, radionuclide—Technetium Tc 99m oxidronate is indicated as a skeletal imaging agent in adults and children to delineate areas of abnormal osteogenesis, such as those that occur with metastatic bone disease, Paget's disease, arthritic disease, osteomyelitis, and fractures.

## Physical Properties

### Nuclear data

| Radionu-clide (half-life) | Decay constant | Mode of decay | Principal photons emissions (keV) | Mean number of emissions/ disintegration ($\geq 0.01$) |
|---|---|---|---|---|
| Tc 99m (6.0 hr) | 0.1151 h$^{-1}$ | Isomeric transition to Tc 99 | Gamma (18) | 0.062 |
| | | | Gamma (140.5) | 0.891 |

## Pharmacology/Pharmacokinetics

### Mechanism of action/Effect

Exact mechanism is not known. It is generally accepted that technetium Tc 99m oxidronate localizes on the surface of hydroxyapatite crystals by a process termed chemisorption, with blood flow and/or blood concentration being most important in the delivery of the agent to sites of uptake. Visualization of osseous lesions is possible since skeletal uptake of technetium Tc 99m oxidronate is altered in areas of abnormal osteogenesis.

### Distribution

Rapidly distributed in and cleared from blood after intravenous administration, with about half the dose normally accumulating in the skeleton within 3 to 4 hours after injection. May also locate within infarcted myocardial cells or other regions of soft tissue necrosis or calcification. Minimal uptake by soft-tissue organs, except calcified cartilage, blood vessels, and kidneys.

### Time to radioactivity visualization

1 to 4 hours (optimal imaging).

### Radiation dosimetry

| Estimated absorbed radiation dose* | | |
|---|---|---|
| Organ | mGy/MBq | rad/mCi |
| Bone surfaces | 0.063 | 0.23 |
| Bladder wall | 0.050 | 0.19 |
| Red marrow | 0.0096 | 0.036 |
| Kidneys | 0.0073 | 0.027 |
| Uterus | 0.0061 | 0.023 |
| Large intestine wall (lower) | 0.0038 | 0.014 |
| Ovaries | 0.0035 | 0.013 |
| Testes | 0.0024 | 0.0089 |
| Small intestine | 0.0023 | 0.0085 |
| Large intestine wall (upper) | 0.0020 | 0.0074 |
| Adrenals | 0.0019 | 0.0070 |

| Estimated absorbed radiation dose* | | |
|---|---|---|
| Organ | mGy/MBq | rad/mCi |
| Pancreas | 0.0016 | 0.0059 |
| Spleen | 0.0014 | 0.0052 |
| Liver | 0.0013 | 0.0048 |
| Lungs | 0.0013 | 0.0048 |
| Stomach wall | 0.0012 | 0.0044 |
| Thyroid | 0.0010 | 0.0037 |
| Breast | 0.00088 | 0.0033 |
| Other tissue | 0.0019 | 0.0070 |

Effective dose: 0.008 mSv/MBq (0.030 rem/mCi)

*For adults; intravenous injection of technetium Tc 99m–labeled phosphates and phosphonates. Data based on the International Commission on Radiological Protection (ICRP) Publication 53—Radiation dose to patients from radiopharmaceuticals.

**Elimination**
Renal.

# Precautions to Consider

## Carcinogenicity/Mutagenicity
Long-term animal studies to evaluate carcinogenic or mutagenic potential of technetium Tc 99m oxidronate have not been performed.

## Pregnancy/Reproduction
Pregnancy—Tc 99m (as free pertechnetate) crosses the placenta. Studies with technetium Tc 99m oxidronate have not been done in humans.
The possibility of pregnancy should be assessed in women of child-bearing potential. Clinical situations exist where the benefit to the patient and fetus, based on information derived from radiopharmaceutical use, outweighs the risks from fetal exposure to radiation. In these situations, the physician should use discretion and reduce the radiopharmaceutical dose to the lowest possible amount.
Studies have not been done in animals.
FDA Pregnancy Category C.

## Breast-feeding
Although it is not known whether technetium Tc 99m oxidronate is distributed into breast milk, it is known that Tc 99m as free pertechnetate is distributed into breast milk. Based on the assumption that the Tc 99m in breast milk is in the form of pertechnetate and based on the effective half-life of the radionuclide in breast milk, the daily volume of milk, a dose factor relating the radionuclide to its critical organ (thyroid) in the nursing infant, and the maximum permissible dose to that organ, a guideline has been proposed. According to this guideline, it has been calculated that nursing can be safely resumed when the concentration in breast milk reaches $30.3 \times 10^{-4}$ megabecquerels ($8.2 \times 10^{-2}$ microcuries) per mL. This level of activity is probably reached, in the majority of patients, within 12 to 24 hours after administration of technetium Tc 99m–labeled radiopharmaceuticals.

## Pediatrics
Diagnostic studies performed to date using technetium Tc 99m oxidronate have not demonstrated pediatrics-specific problems that would limit its usefulness in children. However, there have been no specific studies evaluating the safety and efficacy of technetium Tc 99m oxidronate in pediatric patients. When this radiopharmaceutical is used in children, the diagnostic benefit should be judged to outweigh the potential risk of radiation.

## Geriatrics
Appropriate studies on the relationship of age to the effects of technetium Tc 99m oxidronate have not been performed in the geriatric population. However, no geriatrics-specific problems have been documented to date.

## Drug interactions and/or related problems
See *Diagnostic interference.*

## Diagnostic interference
The following have been selected on the basis of their potential clinical significance (possible effect in parentheses where appropriate)—not necessarily inclusive (» = major clinical significance):
With results of *this* test
*Due to other medications*
  Antacids, aluminum-containing
    (high blood concentrations of aluminum ion, which may occur in patients with gastrointestinal obstruction or impaired renal function, may cause localization of technetium Tc 99m oxidronate in the liver)

Diatrizoate sodium
  (possible renal and hepatic uptake if diatrizoate sodium is administered intravenously immediately after technetium Tc 99m oxidronate)
Etidronate
  (etidronate may interfere with bone uptake of technetium Tc 99m oxidronate; discontinuation of etidronate therapy before performance of a bone scan with technetium Tc 99m oxidronate is recommended for a 2-week period)
Heparin calcium, subcutaneous or
Iron dextran, intramuscular or
Meperidine, intramuscular
  (possible accumulation of technetium Tc 99m oxidronate at site[s] of injection of these medications)
Iron supplements or preparations
  (iron overload may cause a decrease in bone uptake of technetium Tc 99m oxidronate)
Potassium phosphates or
Potassium and sodium phosphates or
Sodium phosphates
  (saturation of bone binding sites by phosphorus ions in these medications may cause decreased bone uptake of technetium Tc 99m oxidronate)
*Due to medical problems or conditions*
Bone demineralization, glucocorticoid-induced
  (long-term therapy with glucocorticoids may induce bone mineral depletion, thus causing decreased bone uptake of technetium Tc 99m oxidronate)
Gynecomastia, estrogen-induced
  (possible localization of technetium Tc 99m oxidronate in breast)
Nephrotoxicity, drug-induced
  (increased retention of technetium Tc 99m oxidronate in kidneys)
Obesity
  (decreased visualization may result due to attenuation of photons coming from bone)
Osteoporosis
  (reduced mineral deposit in bone may result in images with lower target to non-target ratio)
Renal function impairment
  (decreased clearance of technetium Tc 99m oxidronate from blood and soft tissues may impair visualization because of a lower bone to background ratio resulting from the increased circulating activity; also, chronic renal function impairment may cause metastatic calcification and altered biodistribution of technetium Tc 99m oxidronate)
With results of *other* tests
Brain imaging
  (brain scans using sodium pertechnetate Tc 99m may result in high blood background activity when performed after a bone scan using technetium Tc 99m oxidronate, which contains stannous ions; to avoid this potential diagnostic interference, brain scan may be performed prior to bone scan or with a brain imaging agent other than sodium pertechnetate Tc 99m [e.g., technetium Tc 99m pentetate])

## Medical considerations/Contraindications
The medical considerations/contraindications included here have been selected on the basis of their potential clinical significance (reasons given in parentheses where appropriate)—not necessarily inclusive (» = major clinical significance).
See also *Diagnostic interference.*

***Risk-benefit should be considered when the following medical problem exists:***
Sensitivity to the radiopharmaceutical preparation

# Side/Adverse Effects

The following side/adverse effects have been selected on the basis of their potential clinical significance (possible signs and symptoms in parentheses where appropriate)—not necessarily inclusive:

**Those indicating need for medical attention**
Incidence less frequent or rare
  *Allergic reaction* (flushing or redness of skin)

**Those indicating need for medical attention if they continue or are bothersome**
Incidence less frequent or rare
  *Nausea and vomiting*

# Patient Consultation

As an aid to patient consultation, refer to *Advice for the Patient, Radiopharmaceuticals (Diagnostic).*

In providing consultation, consider emphasizing the following selected information (» = major clinical significance):

**Description of use**
Action in the body: Accumulation of radioactivity in bone
Retention of radioactivity in bone allows visualization of lesions
Small amounts of radioactivity used in diagnosis; radiation received is low and considered safe

**Before having this test**
» Conditions affecting use, especially:
Sensitivity to the radiopharmaceutical preparation
Pregnancy—Technetium Tc 99m (as free pertechnetate) crosses placenta; risk to fetus from radiation exposure as opposed to benefit derived from use should be considered
Breast-feeding—Not known if technetium Tc 99m oxidronate is distributed into breast milk, but Tc 99m as free pertechnetate is distributed into breast milk; temporary discontinuation of nursing may be recommended because of risk to infant from radiation exposure
Use in children—Risk from radiation exposure as opposed to benefit derived from use should be considered

**Preparation for this test**
Special preparatory instructions may be given; patient should inquire in advance
Increasing intake of fluids and voiding frequently after injection and before test begins in order to minimize radiation dose to bladder
Voiding again just prior to imaging for best test results

**Precautions after having this test**
Increasing intake of fluids and voiding frequently for 4 to 6 hours after test to minimize radiation dose to bladder

**Side/adverse effects**
Signs of potential side effects, especially allergic reaction

## General Dosing Information

Radiopharmaceuticals are to be administered only by or under the supervision of physicians who have had extensive training in the safe use and handling of radioactive materials and who are authorized by the Nuclear Regulatory Commission (NRC) or the appropriate Agreement State agency, if required, or, outside the U.S., the appropriate authority.

The patient should increase intake of fluids and void frequently following the administration of technetium Tc 99m oxidronate injection, and for 4 to 6 hours after the imaging procedures are completed, to minimize radiation dose to the bladder.

Voiding is also recommended immediately prior to imaging procedures to reduce background interference that may result from accumulation of the agent in the bladder.

**Safety considerations for handling this radiopharmaceutical**
Improper handling of this radiopharmaceutical may cause radioactive contamination. Guidelines for handling radioactive material have been prepared by scientific, professional, state, federal, and international bodies and are available to the specially qualified and authorized users who have access to radiopharmaceuticals.

## Parenteral Dosage Forms

### TECHNETIUM Tc 99m OXIDRONATE INJECTION USP

**Usual adult and adolescent administered activity**
Skeletal imaging—
Intravenous, 370 to 740 megabecquerels (10 to 20 millicuries), administered slowly.

**Usual adult prescribing limits**
Up to 740 megabecquerels (20 millicuries).

**Usual pediatric administered activity**
Skeletal imaging—
Intravenous, 7.4 to 13 megabecquerels (0.20 to 0.35 millicurie) per kg of body weight, administered slowly.
Note: The recommended minimum total pediatric administered activity is 37 megabecquerels (1 millicurie); the maximum total pediatric administered activity is 740 megabecquerels (20 millicuries).

**Usual geriatric administered activity**
See *Usual adult and adolescent administered activity.*

**Strength(s) usually available**
U.S.—
2.0 mg oxidronate sodium and 0.16 mg stannous chloride, per vial (Rx) [*Osteoscan-HDP*].
Canada—
Not commercially available.

**Packaging and storage**
Store below 40 °C (104 °F), preferably between 15 and 30 °C (59 and 86 °F), unless otherwise specified by manufacturer. Protect from freezing.
Note: Both prior to and following radiolabeling, this product may be stored at or below room temperature.

**Preparation of dosage form**
To prepare injection, an oxidant-free sodium pertechnetate Tc 99m solution is used. See manufacturer's package insert for instructions.

**Stability**
Injection should be administered within 8 hours after preparation.

**Incompatibilities**
If oxidants such as peroxides and hypochlorites are present in the sodium pertechnetate Tc 99m used for labeling, the final preparation may be adversely affected and should be discarded.

**Note**
Caution—Radioactive material.

## Selected Bibliography
Holder LE. Clinical radionuclide bone imaging. Radiology 1990; 176: 607-14.
Delaloye B, Delaloye-Bischof A, Koppenhagen K, et al. Clinical comparison of Tc 99m-HMDP and Tc 99m-MDP. A multicenter study. Eur J Nucl Med 1985; 11 (5): 182-5.

Revised: 07/20/93
Interim revision: 08/02/94

---

# TECHNETIUM Tc 99m PENTETATE Systemic

VA CLASSIFICATION (Primary): DX201
Note: For a listing of dosage forms and brand names by country availability, see *Dosage Forms* section(s). For a listing of brand names for the articles in this monograph, refer to the General Index.

## Category

Diagnostic aid, radioactive (renal disorders; intracranial lesions; cerebrospinal fluid disorders; pulmonary disease).

## Indications

Note: Bracketed information in the *Indications* section refers to uses that are not included in U.S. product labeling.

**Accepted**
Renal imaging, radionuclide—Technetium Tc 99m pentetate is indicated as a renal imaging agent to evaluate kidney size, position, configuration, and function, especially in parenchymal disorders.

Renal perfusion studies—Technetium Tc 99m pentetate is indicated to assess renal perfusion.

Glomerular filtration rate determination—Technetium Tc 99m pentetate is indicated in excretion studies to estimate glomerular filtration rate (GFR).

Brain imaging, radionuclide—Technetium Tc 99m pentetate is indicated as a brain imaging agent to detect and evaluate intracranial lesions. Although technetium Tc 99m pentetate is an acceptable brain imaging agent, it is being replaced by computed tomography (CT) and magnetic resonance imaging (MRI).

[Cisternography, radionuclide][1]—Technetium Tc 99m pentetate is used to evaluate cerebrospinal fluid (CSF) flow through ventriculoperitoneal and lumboperitoneal shunts.

[Lung imaging, radionuclide][1]—Technetium Tc 99m pentetate administered by inhalation as an aerosol is used to assess airway patency, especially in conjunction with perfusion lung imaging to evaluate pulmonary embolism.

---

[1]Not included in Canadian product labeling.

# Physical Properties

## Nuclear data

| Radionu-clide (half-life) | Decay constant | Mode of decay | Principal photon emissions (keV) | Mean number of emissions/ disintegration ($\geqslant 0.01$) |
|---|---|---|---|---|
| Tc 99m (6.0 hr) | 0.1151 h$^{-1}$ | Isomeric transition to Tc 99 | Gamma (18) | 0.062 |
| | | | Gamma (140.5) | 0.891 |

# Pharmacology/Pharmacokinetics

## Mechanism of action/Effect

Diagnostic aid (renal function)—The use of technetium Tc 99m pentetate as a renal imaging agent is based on its clearance through the urinary tract by glomerular filtration.

Diagnostic aid (intracranial lesions)—Technetium Tc 99m pentetate normally is prevented by the blood-brain barrier from entering the brain; however, it accumulates by passive diffusion in intracranial lesions that have altered blood-brain barrier.

Diagnostic aid (CSF flow disorders)—Technetium Tc 99m pentetate, when injected intrathecally or intraventricularly mixes and flows with the CSF.

Diagnostic aid (pulmonary disease)—Aerosolized droplets of technetium Tc 99m pentetate, when inhaled, distribute and accumulate in patent airways.

## Distribution

Rapidly distributed in and cleared from plasma following intravenous administration.

## Protein binding

Very low (variable, 3.7 to 10% if continuously infused).

## Radiation dosimetry

| | Estimated absorbed radiation dose* With intravenous injection | | | |
|---|---|---|---|---|
| | Normal renal function | | Impaired renal function | |
| Organ | mGy/ MBq | rad/ mCi | mGy/ MBq | rad/ mCi |
| Bladder wall | 0.065 | 0.24 | 0.022 | 0.081 |
| Uterus | 0.0079 | 0.029 | 0.0063 | 0.023 |
| Kidneys | 0.0044 | 0.016 | 0.0079 | 0.029 |
| Ovaries | 0.0043 | 0.016 | 0.0049 | 0.018 |
| Large intestine wall (lower) | 0.0042 | 0.016 | 0.0047 | 0.017 |
| Testes | 0.0028 | 0.010 | 0.0033 | 0.012 |
| Small intestine | 0.0026 | 0.0096 | 0.0047 | 0.017 |
| Red marrow | 0.0025 | 0.0093 | 0.0052 | 0.019 |
| Large intestine wall (upper) | 0.0022 | 0.0081 | 0.0044 | 0.016 |
| Bone surfaces | 0.0017 | 0.0063 | 0.0044 | 0.016 |
| Pancreas | 0.0015 | 0.0056 | 0.0043 | 0.016 |
| Spleen | 0.0014 | 0.0052 | 0.0040 | 0.015 |
| Adrenals | 0.0014 | 0.0052 | 0.0041 | 0.015 |
| Stomach wall | 0.0013 | 0.0048 | 0.0038 | 0.019 |
| Liver | 0.0013 | 0.0048 | 0.0038 | 0.019 |
| Lungs | 0.0010 | 0.0037 | 0.0033 | 0.012 |
| Breast | 0.00094 | 0.0035 | 0.0030 | 0.011 |
| Thyroid | 0.00079 | 0.0029 | 0.0025 | 0.0093 |
| Other tissue | 0.0017 | 0.0063 | 0.0033 | 0.012 |

| | Effective dose* | | | |
|---|---|---|---|---|
| | Normal renal function | | Impaired renal function | |
| Radionuclide | mSv/ MBq | rem/ mCi | mSv/ MBq | rem/ mCi |
| Tc 99m | 0.0063 | 0.034 | 0.0053 | 0.020 |

| | Estimated absorbed radiation dose* With intrathecal injection | | | |
|---|---|---|---|---|
| | Lumbar injection | | Cisternal injection | |
| Organ | mGy/ MBq | rad/ mCi | mGy/ MBq | rad/ mCi |
| Spinal cord | 0.046 | 0.17 | 0.013 | 0.048 |
| Red marrow | 0.029 | 0.11 | 0.0085 | 0.031 |
| Bladder wall | 0.017 | 0.063 | 0.010 | 0.037 |
| Kidneys | 0.017 | 0.063 | 0.0019 | 0.0070 |
| Adrenals | 0.011 | 0.041 | 0.0018 | 0.0067 |
| Pancreas | 0.0093 | 0.034 | 0.0012 | 0.0044 |
| Small intestine | 0.0081 | 0.030 | 0.00088 | 0.0033 |
| Bone surfaces | 0.0064 | 0.024 | 0.0059 | 0.022 |
| Large intestine wall (upper) | 0.0062 | 0.023 | 0.00071 | 0.0026 |
| Ovaries | 0.0048 | 0.018 | 0.00089 | 0.0033 |
| Spleen | 0.0046 | 0.017 | 0.00066 | 0.0024 |
| Uterus | 0.0045 | 0.017 | 0.0014 | 0.0052 |
| Stomach wall | 0.0042 | 0.016 | 0.00076 | 0.0028 |
| Liver | 0.0038 | 0.014 | 0.00060 | 0.0022 |
| Brain | 0.0032 | 0.012 | 0.055 | 0.20 |
| Large intestine wall (lower) | 0.0026 | 0.0096 | 0.00075 | 0.0028 |
| Lungs | 0.0024 | 0.0089 | 0.00086 | 0.0032 |
| Thyroid | 0.0013 | 0.0048 | 0.0030 | 0.011 |
| Testes | 0.00089 | 0.0033 | 0.00044 | 0.0016 |
| Breast | 0.00065 | 0.0024 | 0.00054 | 0.0020 |
| Other tissue | 0.0025 | 0.0093 | 0.00086 | 0.0032 |

| | Effective dose* | | | |
|---|---|---|---|---|
| | Lumbar injection | | Cisternal injection | |
| Radionuclide | mSv/ MBq | rem/ mCi | mSv/ MBq | rem/ mCi |
| Tc 99m | 0.011 | 0.041 | 0.0066 | 0.024 |

| | Estimated absorbed radiation dose* With aerosol administration | |
|---|---|---|
| Organ | mGy/MBq | rad/mCi |
| Bladder wall | 0.047 | 0.17 |
| Lungs | 0.017 | 0.063 |
| Uterus | 0.0059 | 0.022 |
| Kidneys | 0.0041 | 0.015 |
| Ovaries | 0.0033 | 0.012 |
| Large intestine wall (lower) | 0.0032 | 0.012 |
| Red marrow | 0.0027 | 0.010 |
| Adrenals | 0.0021 | 0.0078 |
| Small intestine | 0.0021 | 0.0078 |
| Pancreas | 0.0021 | 0.0078 |
| Testes | 0.0021 | 0.0078 |
| Bone surfaces | 0.0019 | 0.0070 |
| Breast | 0.0019 | 0.0070 |
| Large intestine wall (upper) | 0.0019 | 0.0070 |
| Liver | 0.0019 | 0.0070 |
| Spleen | 0.0019 | 0.0070 |
| Stomach wall | 0.0017 | 0.0063 |
| Thyroid | 0.00099 | 0.0037 |
| Other tissue | 0.0018 | 0.0067 |

Effective dose: 0.0070 mSv/MBq (0.026 rem/mCi)*

*In adults. Data based on the International Commission on Radiological Protection (ICRP) Publication 53—Radiation dose to patients from radiopharmaceuticals.

## Elimination

Renal; about 50% of the intravenously administered activity eliminated in 2 hours and about 95% of the administered activity eliminated within 24 hours.

# Precautions to Consider

## Carcinogenicity/Mutagenicity

Long-term animal studies to evaluate carcinogenic or mutagenic potential of technetium Tc 99m pentetate have not been performed.

## Pregnancy/Reproduction

Pregnancy—Tc 99m (as free pertechnetate) crosses the placenta. However, studies have not been done with technetium Tc 99m pentetate in humans.

The possibility of pregnancy should be assessed in women of child-bearing potential. Clinical situations exist where the benefit to the patient and fetus, based on information derived from radiopharmaceutical use, outweighs the risks from fetal exposure to radiation. In these situations, the physician should use discretion and reduce the radiopharmaceutical dose to the lowest possible amount.

Studies have not been done in animals.

FDA Pregnancy Category C.

### Breast-feeding

Although it is not known whether technetium Tc 99m pentetate is distributed into breast milk, it is known that Tc 99m as free pertechnetate is distributed into breast milk. Based on the assumption that the Tc 99m in breast milk is in the form of pertechnetate and based on the effective half-life of the radionuclide in breast milk, the daily volume of milk, a dose factor relating the radionuclide to its critical organ (thyroid) in the nursing infant, and the maximum permissible dose to that organ, a guideline has been proposed. According to this guideline, it has been calculated that nursing can be safely resumed when the concentration in breast milk reaches $30.3 \times 10^{-4}$ megabecquerels ($8.2 \times 10^{-2}$ microcuries) per mL. This level of activity is probably reached, in the majority of patients, within 24 hours after administration of 740 megabecquerels (20 millicuries) of technetium Tc 99m–labeled radiopharmaceuticals.

### Pediatrics

Renal studies performed in children from 1 week to 18 years of age have not demonstrated pediatrics-specific problems that would limit the usefulness of technetium Tc 99m pentetate in children. However, there have been no specific studies evaluating the safety and efficacy of technetium Tc 99m pentetate in pediatric patients. When this radiopharmaceutical is used in children, the diagnostic benefit should be judged to outweigh the potential risk of radiation.

### Geriatrics

Appropriate studies on the relationship of age to the effects of technetium Tc 99m pentetate have not been performed in the geriatric population. However, no geriatrics-specific problems have been documented to date.

### Drug interactions and/or related problems

See *Diagnostic interference.*

### Diagnostic interference

With results of *brain imaging*
*Due to other medications*
  Corticosteroids, glucocorticoid
    (uptake of technetium Tc 99m pentetate in cerebral tumors may be decreased because of reduced peritumor edema caused by the corticosteroids)

With results of *renal imaging*
*Due to other medications*
  Captopril or
  Enalapril or
  Lisinopril
    (in patients with renal artery stenosis, use of angiotensin-converting enzyme inhibitors may result in decreased uptake of technetium Tc 99m pentetate by the affected kidney because of a loss of effective trans-membrane filtration pressure; in the diagnosis of renal artery stenosis, this effect has been used to improve the diagnostic accuracy of renal scintigraphy by exaggerating the asymmetry of function between the ischemic and the contralateral kidneys)

*Due to medical problems or conditions*
  Dehydration
    (decreased urinary flow may result in poor renal images and/or decreased glomerular filtration rate [GFR])

### Medical considerations/Contraindications

The medical considerations/contraindications included here have been selected on the basis of their potential clinical significance (reasons given in parentheses where appropriate)—not necessarily inclusive ( » = major clinical significance).

See also *Diagnostic interference.*

***Risk-benefit must be considered when the following medical problem exists:***

Sensitivity to the radiopharmaceutical preparation

## Side/Adverse Effects

The following side/adverse effects have been selected on the basis of their potential clinical significance (possible signs and symptoms in parentheses where appropriate)—not necessarily inclusive:

Incidence less frequent or rare
*Allergic reaction* (skin rash, hives, or itching)

## Patient Consultation

As an aid to patient consultation, refer to *Advice for the Patient, Radiopharmaceuticals (Diagnostic).*

In providing consultation, consider emphasizing the following selected information ( » = major clinical significance):

### Description of use

Action in the body
  Accumulation of radioactive pentetate in intracranial lesions, cerebrospinal fluid (CSF), and in airways (with aerosolized administration)
  Elimination by kidneys via glomerular filtration
  Retention of radioactivity in intracranial lesions, CSF, and lungs (when inhaled) and excretion through kidneys allows visualization
  Small amounts of radioactivity used in diagnosis; radiation received is low and considered safe

### Before having this test

» Conditions affecting use, especially:
  Sensitivity to the radiopharmaceutical preparation
  Pregnancy—Technetium Tc 99m (as free pertechnetate) crosses placenta; risk to fetus from radiation exposure as opposed to benefit derived from use should be considered
  Breast-feeding—Not known if technetium Tc 99m pentetate is distributed into breast milk, but Tc 99m as free pertechnetate is distributed into breast milk; temporary discontinuation of nursing may be recommended because of risk to infant from radiation exposure
  Use in children—Risk from radiation exposure as opposed to benefit derived from use should be considered

### Preparation for this test

Special preparatory instructions may be given; patient should inquire in advance

### Precautions after having this test

Adequate intake of fluids and voiding as often as possible for 4 to 6 hours after examination to minimize radiation exposure to bladder

### Side/adverse effects

Signs of potential side effects, especially allergic reaction

## General Dosing Information

Radiopharmaceuticals are to be administered only by or under the supervision of physicians who have had extensive training in the safe use and handling of radioactive materials and who are authorized by the Nuclear Regulatory Commission (NRC) or the appropriate Agreement State agency, if required, or, outside the U.S., the appropriate authority.

Adequate hydration of the patient is recommended before and after examination to promote urinary flow. Also, urination is recommended as often as possible for 4 to 6 hours after the examination to reduce bladder exposure to radiation.

Manufacturer's package insert or other appropriate literature should be consulted for optimal times when imaging should be performed.

### Safety considerations for handling this radiopharmaceutical

Improper handling of this radiopharmaceutical may cause radioactive contamination. Guidelines for handling radioactive material have been prepared by scientific, professional, state, federal, and international bodies and are available to the specially qualified and authorized users who have access to radiopharmaceuticals.

## Parenteral Dosage Forms

Note: Bracketed uses in the *Dosage Forms* section refer to categories of use and/or indications that are not included in U.S. product labeling.

### TECHNETIUM Tc 99m PENTETATE INJECTION USP

**Usual adult and adolescent administered activity**
Renal imaging or
Glomerular filtration rate determination—
  Intravenous, 111 to 185 megabecquerels (3 to 5 millicuries).
Brain imaging or
Renal perfusion studies—
  Intravenous, 370 to 740 megabecquerels (10 to 20 millicuries).

[Cisternography—CSF imaging, ventriculoperitoneal shunt][1]—
  Intraventricular, 37 megabecquerels (1 millicurie) injected into the reservoir of the shunt system.
[Lung imaging][1]—
  Inhalation, 18.5 to 37 megabecquerels (0.5 to 1 millicurie).

**Usual pediatric administered activity**
Renal imaging or
Glomerular filtration rate determination—
  Intravenous, 37 to 185 megabecquerels (1 to 5 millicuries).
[Cisternography][1]—
  [CFS imaging, ventriculoperitoneal shunt][1]: Intraventricular, 7.4 to 37 megabecquerels (0.2 to 1 millicurie) injected into the reservoir of the shunt system.
  [CSF imaging, shunt][1]—Lumbar subarachnoid injection, 11.1 to 37 megabecquerels (0.3 to 1 millicurie).

**Usual geriatric administered activity**
See *Usual adult and adolescent administered activity*.

**Strength(s) usually available**
U.S.—
  5 mg pentetate pentasodium and 0.17 mg (minimum) stannous chloride (in a lyophilized form and under a nitrogen atmosphere), per 10-mL multidose reaction vial (Rx) [*DTPA (Chelate) Multidose; Techneplex*].
  20.6 mg pentetate calcium trisodium, 0.15 mg minimum stannous tin as stannous chloride dihydrate, and 0.30 mg maximum total tin as stannous chloride dihydrate (in a lyophilized form and under a nitrogen atmosphere), per 10-mL multidose reaction vial (Rx) [*AN-DTPA*].
  25 mg pentetate calcium trisodium, 0.25 mg minimum stannous tin as stannous chloride dihydrate, and 0.385 mg maximum total tin as stannous chloride dihydrate (in a lyophilized form and under a nitrogen atmosphere), per 10-mL multidose reaction vial (Rx) [*TechneScan DTPA*].

Canada—
  25 mg pentetate calcium trisodium, 0.25 mg minimum stannous tin as stannous chloride dihydrate, and 0.385 mg maximum total tin as stannous chloride dihydrate (in a lyophilized form and under a nitrogen atmosphere), per 10-mL multidose reaction vial (Rx) [*Frosstimage DTPA*].

**Packaging and storage**
Store between 2 and 8 °C (36 and 46 °F). Protect from freezing.
Note: Before reconstitution, kit may be stored at room temperature.

**Preparation of dosage form**
To prepare injection, an oxidant-free sodium pertechnetate Tc 99m solution is used. See manufacturer's package insert for instructions.

**Stability**
For brain and renal imaging—Injection should be administered within 6 hours after preparation.
For glomerular filtration rate determination—Injection should be administered within 1 hour after preparation.

**Incompatibilities**
If oxidants such as peroxides and hypochlorites are present in the sodium pertechnetate Tc 99m used for labeling, the final preparation may be adversely affected and should be discarded.

**Note**
Caution—Radioactive material.

[1]Not included in Canadian product labeling.

## Selected Bibliography

Blaufox MD. Procedures of choice in renal nuclear medicine. J Nucl Med 1991; 32: 1301-9.

Revised: 04/30/96

# TECHNETIUM Tc 99m PYROPHOSPHATE  Systemic†

VA CLASSIFICATION (Primary): DX201
Note: For a listing of dosage forms and brand names by country availability, see *Dosage Forms* section(s). For a listing of brand names for the articles in this monograph, refer to the General Index.

  †Not commercially available in Canada.

## Category
Diagnostic aid, radioactive (bone disease; cardiac disease; gastrointestinal bleeding [without Tc 99m label]).

## Indications

### Accepted

For *technetium Tc 99m pyrophosphate*
Skeletal imaging, radionuclide—Technetium Tc 99m pyrophosphate is indicated as a skeletal imaging agent to delineate areas of altered osteogenesis, such as those that occur with metastatic bone disease, Paget's disease, arthritic disease, osteomyelitis, and fractures.
Cardiac imaging, radionuclide—Technetium Tc 99m pyrophosphate is indicated as a cardiac imaging agent to aid in the diagnosis of acute myocardial infarction.

For *sodium pyrophosphate without Tc 99m label*
Red blood cells, labeling of—Intravenous injection of the unlabeled sodium pyrophosphate and stannous chloride complex, when followed by the injection of sodium pertechnetate Tc 99m, is indicated for *in vivo* or modified *in vitro/in vivo* labeling of red blood cells. Red blood cells labeled with sodium pertechnetate Tc 99m are used for blood pool imaging in the following diagnostic study:
Cardiac blood pool imaging, radionuclide—To detect pericardial effusion, intracardiac abnormalities, or ventricular aneurysms.
Bleeding, gastrointestinal (diagnosis)—To detect the site of bleeding in patients suspected of gastrointestinal bleeding.

## Physical Properties

**Nuclear data**

| Radionu-clide (half-life) | Decay constant | Mode of decay | Principal photons emissions (keV) | Mean number of emissions/ disintegration (≥0.01) |
|---|---|---|---|---|
| Tc 99m (6.0 hr) | 0.1151 h⁻¹ | Isomeric transition to Tc 99 | Gamma (18) | 0.062 |
|  |  |  | Gamma (140.5) | 0.891 |

## Pharmacology/Pharmacokinetics

**Physicochemical characteristics**
Molecular weight—Sodium pyrophosphate: 265.90.
Stannous chloride: 225.63.

**Mechanism of action/Effect**
Skeletal and cardiac imaging—Exact mechanism is not known. It is generally accepted that technetium Tc 99m pyrophosphate localizes on the surface of hydroxyapatite crystals, found in bone and within infarcted myocardial cells, by a process termed chemisorption, with blood flow and/or blood concentration being most important in the delivery of the agent to sites of uptake. Visualization of osseous lesions is possible since skeletal uptake of technetium Tc 99m pyrophosphate is altered in areas of abnormal osteogenesis.
Red blood cells, labeling of—When used for cardiac blood pool imaging or to detect gastrointestinal bleeding, pretreatment with the stannous ion-containing phosphate complex causes the technetium Tc 99m (as sodium pertechnetate Tc 99m) to bind to the red blood cells *in vivo*, with about 76% of the injected radioactivity remaining in the blood pool long enough to provide images of the cardiac chambers or sites of active (rapid) or cumulative (intermittent) gastrointestinal bleeding. Modified *in vitro/in vivo* method of labeling red blood cells usually results in a greater percent of the injected radioactivity remaining in the blood pool.

## Distribution

Selectively concentrated in areas of altered osteogenesis and injured myocardium with minimal uptake by soft-tissue organs.

## Radiation dosimetry

Estimated absorbed radiation dose
for Technetium Tc 99m Pyrophosphate*‡

| Organ | mGy/MBq | rad/mCi |
|---|---|---|
| Bone surfaces | 0.063 | 0.23 |
| Bladder wall | 0.050 | 0.19 |
| Red marrow | 0.0096 | 0.036 |
| Kidneys | 0.0073 | 0.027 |
| Uterus | 0.0061 | 0.023 |
| Large intestine wall (lower) | 0.0038 | 0.014 |
| Ovaries | 0.0035 | 0.013 |
| Testes | 0.0024 | 0.0089 |
| Small intestine | 0.0023 | 0.0085 |
| Large intestine wall (upper) | 0.0020 | 0.0074 |
| Adrenals | 0.0019 | 0.0070 |
| Pancreas | 0.0016 | 0.0059 |
| Spleen | 0.0014 | 0.0052 |
| Liver | 0.0013 | 0.0048 |
| Lungs | 0.0013 | 0.0048 |
| Stomach wall | 0.0012 | 0.0044 |
| Thyroid | 0.0010 | 0.0037 |
| Breast | 0.00088 | 0.0033 |
| Other tissue | 0.0019 | 0.0070 |

Effective dose: 0.008 mSv/MBq (0.030 rem/mCi)

Estimated absorbed radiation dose
for Sodium Pertechnetate Tc 99m†‡

| Organ | mGy/MBq | rad/mCi |
|---|---|---|
| Stomach wall | 0.029 | 0.11 |
| Thyroid | 0.023 | 0.085 |
| Bladder wall | 0.019 | 0.070 |
| Small intestine | 0.018 | 0.067 |
| Ovaries | 0.010 | 0.037 |
| Salivary glands | 0.0093 | 0.034 |
| Uterus | 0.0081 | 0.030 |
| Large intestine wall (upper) | 0.062 | 0.23 |
| Large intestine wall (lower) | 0.062 | 0.23 |
| Red marrow | 0.0061 | 0.022 |
| Pancreas | 0.0059 | 0.022 |
| Kidneys | 0.0050 | 0.019 |
| Spleen | 0.0044 | 0.016 |
| Bone surfaces | 0.0039 | 0.014 |
| Liver | 0.0039 | 0.014 |
| Adrenals | 0.0036 | 0.013 |
| Lungs | 0.0027 | 0.010 |
| Testes | 0.0027 | 0.010 |
| Breast | 0.0023 | 0.0085 |
| Other tissue | 0.0034 | 0.013 |

Effective dose: 0.013mSv/MBq (0.048 rem/mCi)

*For adults. Intravenous injection of technetium Tc 99m–labeled phos-
phates and phosphonates for skeletal and cardiac imaging.

†For adults. Intravenous injection of sodium pertechnetate Tc 99m
preceded by intravenous administration of unlabeled sodium pyrophosphate for cardiac blood pool imaging. Without blocking agent.

‡Data based on the International Commission on Radiological Protection (ICRP) Publication 53—Radiation dose to patients from
radiopharmaceuticals.

## Elimination

Renal, 40% of the administered activity of technetium Tc 99m pyrophosphate eliminated within 24 hours.

# Precautions to Consider

## Carcinogenicity/Mutagenicity

Long-term animal studies to evaluate carcinogenic or mutagenic potential
of technetium Tc 99m pyrophosphate have not been performed.

## Pregnancy/Reproduction

Pregnancy—Tc 99m (as free pertechnetate) crosses the placenta. Studies
with technetium Tc 99m pyrophosphate have not been done in
humans.

The possibility of pregnancy should be assessed in women of child-bearing potential. Clinical situations exist where the benefit to the patient
and fetus, based on information derived from radiopharmaceutical use,
outweighs the risks from fetal exposure to radiation. In these situations, the physician should use discretion and reduce the radiopharmaceutical dose to the lowest possible amount.

Studies have not been done in animals.

FDA Pregnancy Category C.

## Breast-feeding

Although it is not known whether technetium Tc 99m pyrophosphate is
distributed into breast milk, it is known that Tc 99m as free pertechnetate is distributed into breast milk. Based on the assumption that the
Tc 99m in breast milk is in the form of pertechnetate and based on
the effective half-life of the radionuclide in breast milk, the daily volume of milk, a dose factor relating the radionuclide to its critical organ
(thyroid) in the nursing infant, and the maximum permissible dose to
that organ, a guideline has been proposed. According to this guideline,
it has been calculated that nursing can be safely resumed when the
concentration in breast milk reaches $30.3 \times 10^{-4}$ megabecquerels (8.2
$\times 10^{-2}$ microcuries) per mL. This level of activity is probably reached,
in the majority of patients, within 12 to 24 hours after administration
of technetium Tc 99m–labeled radiopharmaceuticals.

## Pediatrics

Diagnostic studies performed to date using technetium Tc 99m–labeled
red blood cells have not demonstrated pediatrics-specific problems that
would limit the usefulness of technetium Tc 99m pyrophosphate in
children. However, there have been no specific studies evaluating the
safety and efficacy of technetium Tc 99m pyrophosphate in pediatric
patients. When this radiopharmaceutical is used in children, the diagnostic benefit should be judged to outweigh the potential risk of
radiation.

## Geriatrics

Diagnostic studies performed to date using technetium Tc 99m pyrophosphate have not demonstrated geriatrics-specific problems that would
limit the usefulness of technetium Tc 99m pyrophosphate in the
elderly.

## Drug interactions and/or related problems

See *Diagnostic interference.*

## Diagnostic interference

The following have been selected on the basis of their potential clinical
significance (possible effect in parentheses where appropriate)—not
necessarily inclusive (» = major clinical significance):

With results of *skeletal imaging*

*Due to other medications*

Amphotericin B or
Antineoplastics
   (biodistribution of technetium Tc 99m pyrophosphate may be altered with concurrent administration of these medications)

Antacids, aluminum-containing
   (high blood concentrations of aluminum ion, which may occur in
   patients with gastrointestinal obstruction or impaired renal function, may cause localization of technetium Tc 99m pyrophosphate
   in the liver and spleen)

Diatrizoate sodium
   (possible renal and hepatic uptake if diatrizoate sodium is administered intravenously immediately after technetium Tc 99m
   pyrophosphate)

Etidronate
   (etidronate may interfere with bone uptake of technetium Tc 99m
   pyrophosphate; discontinuation of etidronate therapy for a 2-week
   period before performance of a bone scan with technetium Tc 99m
   pyrophosphate is recommended)

Heparin calcium, subcutaneous or
Radiation therapy
   (concurrent administration may result in extraosseous accumulation of technetium Tc 99m pyrophosphate)

Iron dextran, intramuscular or
Meperidine, intramuscular
   (possible accumulation of technetium Tc 99m pyrophosphate at
   site of injection of these medications)

Iron supplements or preparations
   (iron overload may cause a decrease in bone uptake of technetium
   Tc 99m pyrophosphate)

Potassium phosphates or
Potassium and sodium phosphates or
Sodium phosphates
  (saturation of bone binding sites by phosphorous ions in these medications may cause decreased bone uptake of technetium Tc 99m pyrophosphate)

*Due to medical problems or conditions*
Amyloidosis or
Carcinomas or
Cirrhosis or
Diabetes mellitus or
Hypercalcemia
  (biodistribution of technetium Tc 99m pyrophosphate may be altered, resulting in an increased uptake by other organs)

Blood transfusions, repeated
  (may cause a decrease in bone uptake)

Bone demineralization, glucocorticoid-induced
  (long-term therapy with glucocorticoids may induce bone mineral depletion, thus causing decreased bone uptake of technetium Tc 99m pyrophosphate)

Gynecomastia, estrogen-induced or
Lactation
  (possible localization of technetium Tc 99m pyrophosphate in breast)

Obesity
  (attenuation of photons coming from bone may decrease visualization)

Osteoporosis
  (reduced mineral deposit in bone may result in images with lower target to non-target ratio)

Renal function impairment
  (decreased drug clearance from blood and soft tissues may decrease visualization because of a lower bone to background ratio resulting from the increased circulating activity; also, chronic renal function impairment may cause metastatic calcification and altered biodistribution of technetium Tc 99m pyrophosphate)

With results of *cardiac imaging*
*Due to other medications*
Antacids, aluminum-containing
  (high blood concentrations of aluminum ion, which may occur in patients with gastrointestinal obstruction or impaired renal function, may cause localization of technetium Tc 99m pyrophosphate in the liver and spleen)

Estrogens
  (possible localization of technetium Tc 99m pyrophosphate in breast)

Heparin sodium
  (diffuse uptake of technetium Tc 99m pyrophosphate into the myocardium, with signs of diminished uptake into the infarct)

Methylprednisolone
  (methylprednisolone may increase glomerular filtration rate and excretion of technetium Tc 99m pyrophosphate, which results in faster blood clearance of the radiotracer, thus decreasing myocardial uptake of the radiotracer)

Radiation therapy
  (diffuse myocardial uptake of technetium Tc 99m pyrophosphate)

Verapamil
  (patchy liver uptake of technetium Tc 99m pyrophosphate may result due to hepatocellular damage caused by verapamil toxicity)

*Due to medical problems or conditions*
Amyloidosis or
Hyperphosphatemia or
Sarcoidosis, myocardial
  (diffuse cardiac uptake may occur)

Angina pectoris, unstable or
Cardiac contusions or
Coronary bypass surgery, recent or
Myocardial infarcts, previous
  (false-positive cardiac images may occur)

Gynecomastia, estrogen-induced or
Lactation
  (possible localization of technetium Tc 99m pyrophosphate in breast)

Myocardial infarcts, time of
  (false-negative cardiac images may occur in the diagnosis of acute myocardial infarction if test is performed too early in the evolutionary phase or too late in the resolution phase of the infarct)

With results of *blood pool imaging (cardiac blood pool imaging and diagnosis of gastrointestinal bleeding)*
*Due to other medications*
Digoxin or
Doxorubicin or
Heparin sodium or
Hydralazine or
Methyldopa or
Prazosin or
Propranolol or
Quinidine or
Radiopaque agents, water-soluble organic iodides, with intravascular administration
  (concurrent use with these medications may impair blood pool images by decreasing the labeling efficiency of red blood cells)

*Due to medical problems or conditions*
Goiter, toxic diffuse or
Hyperthyroidism
  (thyroid uptake may be increased)

Lupus erythematosus
  (labeling of red blood cells may be decreased)

Transfusion-induced reaction
  (labeling efficiency may be decreased because of red blood cell antibody formation)

With *other* diagnostic test results
Brain scan using sodium pertechnetate Tc 99m
  (may give either false-positive or false-negative results when performed after a bone scan using technetium Tc 99m pyrophosphate that contains stannous ions; to avoid false results, brain scan should be performed prior to bone scan or with a brain imaging agent other than sodium pertechnetate Tc 99m)

**Medical considerations/Contraindications**
The medical considerations/contraindications included here have been selected on the basis of their potential clinical significance (reasons given in parentheses where appropriate)—not necessarily inclusive (» = major clinical significance).

See also *Diagnostic interference.*

*Risk-benefit should be considered when the following medical problem exists:*
Sensitivity to the radiopharmaceutical preparation

## Side/Adverse Effects
The following side/adverse effects have been selected on the basis of their potential clinical significance (possible signs and symptoms in parentheses where appropriate)—not necessarily inclusive:

**Those indicating need for medical attention**
Incidence less frequent or rare
  *Allergic reaction* (skin rash, hives, or itching)

## Patient Consultation
As an aid to patient consultation, refer to *Advice for the Patient, Radiopharmaceuticals (Diagnostic).*

In providing consultation, consider emphasizing the following selected information (» = major clinical significance):

**Description of use**
Action in the body: Accumulation of radioactivity in bone and cardiac tissues and in labeled red blood cells
Retention of radioactivity allows visualization of skeletal or cardiac lesions, or visualization of blood pool
Small amounts of radioactivity used in diagnosis; radiation received is low and considered safe

**Before having this test**
» Conditions affecting use, especially:
  Sensitivity to the radiopharmaceutical preparation
  Pregnancy—Technetium Tc 99m (as free pertechnetate) crosses placenta; risk to fetus from radiation exposure as opposed to benefit derived from use should be considered
  Breast-feeding—Not known if technetium Tc 99m pyrophosphate is distributed into breast milk, but Tc 99m as free pertechnetate is distributed into breast milk; temporary discontinuation of nursing may be recommended because of risk to infant from radiation exposure
  Use in children—Risk from radiation exposure as opposed to benefit derived from use should be considered

**Preparation for this test**
Special preparatory instructions may be given; patient should inquire in advance

For cardiac and skeletal imaging: Increasing intake of fluids and void-ing frequently after injection and before test begins to minimize radiation dose to bladder; voiding again just prior to imaging for best test results

**Precautions after having this test**
For cardiac and skeletal imaging: Increasing intake of fluids and void-ing frequently for 4 to 6 hours after test to minimize radiation dose to bladder

**Side/adverse effects**
Signs of potential side effects, especially allergic reaction

## General Dosing Information

Radiopharmaceuticals are to be administered only by or under the super-vision of physicians who have had extensive training in the safe use and handling of radioactive materials and who are authorized by the Nuclear Regulatory Commission (NRC) or the appropriate Agreement State agency, if required, or, outside the U.S., the appropriate authority.

Manufacturer's package insert or other appropriate literature should be consulted for optimal times when imaging should be performed.

**For cardiac and skeletal imaging**
Unless cardiac status indicates otherwise, the patient should increase in-take of fluids and void frequently following the administration of tech-netium Tc 99m pyrophosphate injection, and for 4 to 6 hours after the imaging procedures are completed, to minimize radiation dose to the bladder.

Voiding is also recommended immediately prior to imaging procedures to reduce background interference that may result from accumulation of the agent in the bladder.

**For blood pool imaging (cardiac blood pool imaging and diagnosis of gastrointestinal bleeding)**
Stannous pyrophosphate should be injected by direct venipuncture. He-parinized catheter systems are not recommended.

**Safety considerations for handling this radiopharmaceutical**
Improper handling of this radiopharmaceutical may cause radioactive con-tamination. Guidelines for handling radioactive material have been prepared by scientific, professional, state, federal, and international bodies and are available to the specially qualified and authorized users who have access to radiopharmaceuticals.

## Parenteral Dosage Forms

### TECHNETIUM Tc 99m PYROPHOSPHATE INJECTION USP

**Usual adult and adolescent administered activity**
For technetium Tc 99m pyrophosphate:
Skeletal imaging or

Cardiac imaging—Intravenous, 555 to 740 megabecquerels (15 to 20 millicuries), administered over a period of ten to twenty seconds.
For sodium pyrophosphate without Tc 99m label:
Blood pool imaging—Intravenous, 5 to 15.4 mg of stannous pyro-phosphate (unlabeled) followed, fifteen to sixty minutes later, by the intravenous administration of 740 megabecquerels (20 milli-curies) of sodium pertechnetate Tc 99m.

**Usual pediatric administered activity**
Dosage must be individualized by physician.

**Usual geriatric administered activity**
See *Usual adult and adolescent administered activity.*

**Strength(s) usually available**
U.S.—
12 mg of sodium pyrophosphate and 3.4 mg of stannous chloride (an-hydrous) per 10-mL reaction vial (Rx) [*TechneScan PYP*].
40 mg sodium pyrophosphate, 0.4 mg stannous fluoride (minimum), and 0.9 mg total tin (maximum) as stannous fluoride, per 5-mL reaction vial (Rx) [*MPI Pyrophosphate; Phosphotec*].
Canada—
Not commercially available.

**Packaging and storage**
Store between 15 and 30 °C (59 and 86 °F), unless otherwise specified by manufacturer. Protect from freezing.
Note: Before reconstitution, store between 2 and 8 °C (36 and 46 °F).

**Preparation of dosage form**
To prepare technetium Tc 99m pyrophosphate injection, an oxidant-free sodium pertechnetate Tc 99m solution is used. See manufacturer's package insert for instructions.
To prepare sodium pyrophosphate injection (unlabeled), stannous pyro-phosphate is reconstituted with sodium chloride injection. See manu-facturer's package insert for complete instructions.

**Stability**
Injection should be administered within 6 hours after preparation.

**Incompatibilities**
If oxidants such as peroxides and hypochlorites are present in the sodium pertechnetate Tc 99m used for labeling, the final preparation may be adversely affected and should be discarded.

**Note**
Caution—Radioactive material.

Revised: 8/18/93
Interim revision: 08/02/94

# TECHNETIUM Tc 99m (PYRO- AND TRIMETA-) PHOSPHATES     Systemic

VA CLASSIFICATION (Primary): DX201
Note: This monograph includes information that applies to both techne-tium Tc 99m (pyro- and trimeta-) phosphates and to sodium (pyro- and trimeta-) phosphates without Tc 99m label.

Note: For a listing of dosage forms and brand names by country availa-bility, see *Dosage Forms* section(s). For a listing of brand names for the articles in this monograph, refer to the General Index.

## Category

Diagnostic aid, radioactive (bone disease; cardiac disease; gastrointestinal bleeding [without Tc 99m label]).

## Indications

**Accepted**
For technetium Tc 99m (pyro- and trimeta-) phosphates:
Skeletal imaging, radionuclide—Technetium Tc 99m (pyro- and tri-meta-) phosphates injection is indicated as a skeletal imaging agent to delineate areas of altered osteogenesis, such as those that occur with metastatic bone disease, Paget's disease, arthritic disease, os-teomyelitis, and fractures.

Cardiac imaging, radionuclide—Technetium Tc 99m (pyro- and tri-meta-) phosphates injection is indicated as a cardiac imaging agent to aid in the diagnosis of acute myocardial infarction.

For sodium (pyro- and trimeta-) phosphates without Tc 99m label:
Red blood cells, labeling of—Intravenous injection of the unlabeled sodium (pyro- and trimeta-) phosphates component of the kit, when followed by the injection of sodium pertechnetate Tc 99m, is in-dicated for *in vivo* or modified *in vitro/in vivo* labeling of red blood cells. Red blood cells labeled with sodium pertechnetate Tc 99m are used for blood pool imaging in the following diagnostic stud-ies:
Cardiac blood pool imaging, radionuclide: To detect pericardial effusion, intracardiac abnormalities, or ventricular aneurysms.
Bleeding, gastrointestinal (diagnosis): To evaluate patients sus-pected of gastrointestinal bleeding, to detect the site of bleeding.

# Physical Properties

## Nuclear data

| Radionu-clide (half-life) | Decay constant | Mode of decay | Principal photons (keV) | Mean number of photons/ disintegration ($\geq 0.01$) |
|---|---|---|---|---|
| Tc 99m (6.0 hr) | 0.1151 h$^{-1}$ | Isomeric transition to Tc 99 | 18 140.5 | 0.062 0.891 |

# Pharmacology/Pharmacokinetics

## Physicochemical characteristics
Molecular weight—Sodium pyrophosphate: 265.90.
Sodium trimetaphosphate: 305.89.
Stannous chloride: 225.63.

## Mechanism of action/Effect
Skeletal and cardiac imaging—

    Exact mechanism is unknown. Technetium Tc 99m (pyro- and trimeta-) phosphates' affinity for hydroxyapatite crystals, found in bone and within infarcted myocardial cells, may be responsible for its skeletal and myocardial uptake, with blood flow and/or blood concentration being most important in the delivery of the phosphate complex for uptake. Since normal myocardial tissue does not appreciably accumulate the phosphate complex, an area of acute damage will appear as a focus of increased activity. Visualization of osseous lesions also is possible since skeletal uptake of technetium Tc 99m (pyro- and trimeta-) phosphates is altered in areas of abnormal osteogenesis.

Red blood cells, labeling of—

    When used for cardiac blood pool imaging or to detect gastrointestinal bleeding, pretreatment with the stannous ion–containing phosphate complex causes the technetium Tc 99m (as sodium pertechnetate Tc 99m) to bind to the red blood cells in vivo, with about 75–85% of the injected radioactivity remaining in the blood pool long enough to provide images of the cardiac chambers or sites of active (rapid) or cumulative (intermittent) gastrointestinal bleeding. Modified *in vitro/in vivo* method of labeling red blood cells usually results in a greater percent of the injected radioactivity remaining in the blood pool.

## Distribution
Technetium Tc 99m (pyro- and trimeta-) phosphates is selectively concentrated in areas of altered osteogenesis and injured myocardium with minimal uptake by soft-tissue organs, with the exception of the kidneys.

## Radiation dosimetry

| Mode of administra- tion | Radiation source (% adminis- tered activity) | Estimated absorbed radiation dose | | |
|---|---|---|---|---|
| | | Target organ | mGy/ MBq | rad/mCi |
| Intravenous Technetium Tc 99m (Pyro- and trimeta-) Phosphates* | Skeleton (50%) Urinary bladder (50%) | Bladder | | |
| | | 2 hr void | 0.026 | 0.097 |
| | | 4.8 hr void | 0.062 | 0.230 |
| | | Skeleton | 0.014 | 0.054 |
| | | Kidneys | 0.013 | 0.047 |
| | | Bone marrow | 0.010 | 0.038 |
| | | Testes | | |
| | | 2 hr void | 0.003 | 0.010 |
| | | 4.8 hr void | 0.004 | 0.015 |
| | | Heart | | |
| | | Normal | 0.002 | 0.009 |
| | | Impaired | 0.004 | 0.015 |
| | | Ovaries | | |
| | | 2 hr void | 0.002 | 0.009 |
| | | 4.8 hr void | 0.004 | 0.015 |
| | | Red marrow | 0.006 | 0.022 |
| | | Total body | 0.004 | 0.015 |
| Intravenous Sodium Pertechne- tate Tc 99m† | | Bladder wall | 0.032 | 0.120 |
| | | Blood | 0.014 | 0.052 |
| | | Ovaries | 0.006 | 0.023 |
| | | Spleen | 0.005 | 0.018 |
| | | Testes | 0.003 | 0.012 |
| | | Total body | 0.004 | 0.015 |

*For skeletal and cardiac imaging.

†For blood pool imaging. Preceded by intravenous administration of unlabeled sodium (pyro- and trimeta-) phosphates.

## Elimination
Renal; up to 50% of the dose of technetium Tc 99m (pyro- and trimeta-) phosphates eliminated within the first 3 to 6 hours.

# Precautions to Consider

## Carcinogenicity/Mutagenicity
Long-term animal studies to evaluate carcinogenic or mutagenic potential of technetium Tc 99m (pyro- and trimeta-) phosphates have not been performed.

## Pregnancy/Reproduction
Pregnancy—Tc 99m (as free pertechnetate) crosses the placenta. However, studies have not been done in either animals or humans with technetium Tc 99m (pyro- and trimeta-) phosphates.

Radiopharmaceuticals are usually not recommended during pregnancy because of the risk to the fetus from radiation exposure.

To avoid the possibility of fetal exposure to radiation, in those circumstances where the patient's pregnancy status is uncertain, a pregnancy test will help to prevent inadvertent administration of this preparation during pregnancy.

FDA Pregnancy Category C.

## Breast-feeding
Although it is not known whether technetium Tc 99m (pyro- and trimeta-) phosphates is excreted in breast milk, it is known that Tc 99m as free pertechnetate is excreted in breast milk. Based on the assumption that the Tc 99m in breast milk is in the form of pertechnetate and based on the effective half-life of the radionuclide in breast milk, the daily volume of milk, a dose factor relating the radionuclide to its critical organ (thyroid) in the nursing infant, and the maximum permissible dose to that organ, a guideline has been proposed. According to this guideline, it has been calculated that nursing can be safely resumed when the concentration in breast milk reaches $30.3 \times 10^{-4}$ megabecquerels ($8.2 \times 10^{-2}$ microcuries) per mL. This level of activity is probably reached, in the majority of patients, within 24 hours after administration of 740 megabecquerels (20 millicuries) of technetium Tc 99m.

## Pediatrics
Diagnostic studies performed to date using technetium Tc 99m–labeled red blood cells have not demonstrated pediatrics-specific problems that would limit the usefulness of technetium Tc 99m (pyro- and trimeta-) phosphates in children. However, because of the potential risk of radiation exposure, risk-benefit must be considered.

## Geriatrics
Although appropriate studies have not been performed in the geriatric population, no geriatrics-specific problems have been documented to date.

## Drug interactions and/or related problems
See *Diagnostic interference.*

## Diagnostic interference
The following have been selected on the basis of their potential clinical significance (possible effect in parentheses where appropriate)—not necessarily inclusive ($\gg$ = major clinical significance):

With results of *blood pool imaging (cardiac blood pool imaging and diagnosis of gastrointestinal bleeding)*
   *Due to other medications*
      Digoxin or
      Doxorubicin or
      Heparin sodium or
      Hydralazine or
      Methyldopa or
      Prazosin or
      Propranolol or
      Quinidine or
      Radiopaques, water-soluble organic iodides, with intravascular administration
        (concurrent use with these medications may impair blood pool images because of a decrease in labeling of red blood cells)

   *Due to medical problems or conditions*
      Goiter, toxic diffuse or
      Hyperthyroidism
        (thyroid uptake may be increased)

      Lupus erythematosus
        (labeling of red blood cells may be decreased)

      Transfusion-induced reaction
        (labeling efficiency may be decreased because of red blood cell antibody formation)

With results of *cardiac imaging*
*Due to other medications*
Antacids, aluminum-containing
(high blood concentrations of aluminum ion, which may occur in patients with gastrointestinal obstruction or impaired renal function, may cause localization of technetium Tc 99m [pyro- and trimeta-] phosphates in the liver and spleen)
Estrogens
(possible localization of technetium Tc 99m [pyro- and trimeta-] phosphates in breast)
Heparin sodium
(diffuse uptake of technetium Tc 99m [pyro- and trimeta-] phosphates into the myocardium, with signs of diminished uptake into the infarct)
Methylprednisolone
(methylprednisolone may increase glomerular filtration rate and excretion of technetium Tc 99m [pyro- and trimeta-] phosphates, resulting in faster blood clearance of the radiotracer, and thus decreasing myocardial uptake of the radiotracer)
Radiation therapy
(diffuse myocardial uptake of technetium Tc 99m [pyro- and trimeta-] phosphates)
Verapamil
(patchy liver uptake of technetium Tc 99m [pyro- and trimeta-] phosphates may result due to hepatocellular damage caused by verapamil toxicity)
*Due to medical problems or conditions*
Amyloidosis or
Hyperphosphatemia or
Sarcoidosis, myocardial
(diffuse cardiac uptake may occur)
Angina pectoris, unstable or
Cardiac contusions or
Coronary bypass surgery, recent or
Myocardial infarcts, previous
(false-positive cardiac images may occur)
Gynecomastia, estrogen-induced or
Lactation
(possible localization of technetium Tc 99m [pyro- and trimeta-] phosphates in breast)
Hepatic necrosis, massive
(possible liver uptake of technetium Tc 99m [pyro- and trimeta-] phosphates)
Myocardial infarcts, time of
(false-negative cardiac images may occur in the diagnosis of acute myocardial infarction if test is performed too early in the evolutionary phase or too late in the resolution phase of the infarct)
With results of *skeletal imaging*
*Due to other medications*
Antacids, aluminum-containing
(high blood concentrations of aluminum ion, which may occur in patients with gastrointestinal obstruction or impaired renal function, may cause localization of technetium Tc 99m [pyro- and trimeta-] phosphates in the liver)
Amphotericin B or
Antineoplastics
(biodistribution of technetium Tc 99m [pyro- and trimeta-] phosphates may be altered with concurrent administration of these medications)
Diatrizoate sodium
(possible renal and hepatic uptake of technetium Tc 99m [pyro- and trimeta-] phosphates if diatrizoate sodium is administered intravenously immediately after technetium Tc 99m [pyro- and trimeta-] phosphates)
Etidronate
(etidronate may theoretically interfere with bone uptake of technetium Tc 99m [pyro- and trimeta-] phosphates; clinical significance is unknown)
Heparin calcium, subcutaneous or
Radiation therapy
(concurrent administration may result in extraosseous accumulation of technetium Tc 99m [pyro- and trimeta-] phosphates)
Iron dextran, intramuscular or
Meperidine, intramuscular
(possible accumulation of technetium Tc 99m [pyro- and trimeta-] phosphates at site of injection)
Iron supplements or preparations
(iron overload may cause a decrease in bone uptake)

Potassium phosphates or
Potassium and sodium phosphates or
Sodium phosphates
(saturation of bone binding sites by phosphorous ions in these medications may cause decreased bone uptake)
*Due to medical problems or conditions*
Amyloidosis or
Carcinomas or
Cirrhosis or
Diabetes mellitus or
Hypercalcemia
(biodistribution of technetium Tc 99m [pyro- and trimeta-] phosphates may be altered, resulting in an increased uptake by other organs)
Blood transfusions, repeated
(may cause a decrease in bone uptake)
Bone demineralization, adrenocorticoid (glucocorticoid)-induced
(long-term therapy with these medications may induce bone mineral depletion, thus causing decreased bone uptake of technetium Tc 99m [pyro- and trimeta-] phosphates)
Gynecomastia, estrogen-induced or
Lactation
(possible localization of technetium Tc 99m [pyro- and trimeta-] phosphates in breast)
Obesity
(attenuation of photons coming from bone may decrease visualization)
Osteoporosis
(reduced mineral deposits in bone may result in images with lower target to non-target ratio)
Renal function impairment
(decreased drug clearance from blood and soft tissues may decrease visualization because of a lower bone-to-background ratio resulting from the increased circulating activity; also, chronic renal function impairment may cause metastatic calcification and altered biodistribution of technetium Tc 99m [pyro- and trimeta-] phosphates)
With *other* diagnostic test results
Brain scan using sodium pertechnetate Tc 99m
(may give either false-positive or false-negative results when performed after a bone scan using technetium Tc 99m [pyro- and trimeta-] phosphates because of its stannous ion content; to avoid false results, brain scan should be performed prior to bone scan or with a brain imaging agent other than sodium pertechnetate Tc 99m)

**Medical considerations/Contraindications**
The medical considerations/contraindications included here have been selected on the basis of their potential clinical significance (reasons given in parentheses where appropriate)—not necessarily inclusive (» = major clinical significance).
See also *Diagnostic interference.*

***Risk-benefit should be considered when the following medical problem exists:***
Sensitivity to the radiopharmaceutical preparation

## Side/Adverse Effects

The following side/adverse effects have been selected on the basis of their potential clinical significance (possible signs and symptoms in parentheses where appropriate)—not necessarily inclusive:

**Those indicating need for medical attention**
Incidence less frequent or rare
*Allergic reaction* (skin rash, hives, or itching)

## Patient Consultation

As an aid to patient consultation, refer to *Advice for the Patient, Radiopharmaceuticals (Diagnostic).*

In providing consultation, consider emphasizing the following selected information (» = major clinical significance):

**Description of use**
Action in the body: Accumulation of radioactivity in bone and cardiac tissues and in labeled red blood cells
Retention of radioactivity allows visualization of skeletal or cardiac lesions, or visualization of blood pool
Small amounts of radioactivity used in diagnosis; radiation received is low and considered safe

**Before having this test**

» Conditions affecting use, especially:

Sensitivity to the radiopharmaceutical preparation

Pregnancy—Technetium Tc 99m (as free pertechnetate) crosses placenta; risk to fetus from radiation exposure

Breast-feeding—Not known if excreted in breast milk; temporary discontinuation of nursing may be recommended because of risk to infant from radiation exposure

Use in children—Risk of radiation exposure

**Preparation for this test**

Special preparatory instructions may be given; patient should inquire in advance

For cardiac and skeletal imaging: Increasing intake of fluids and voiding frequently after injection and before test begins to minimize radiation exposure to bladder; voiding again just prior to imaging for best test results

**Precautions after having this test**

For cardiac and skeletal imaging: Increasing intake of fluids and voiding frequently for 4 to 6 hours after test to minimize radiation exposure to bladder

**Side/adverse effects**

Signs of potential side effects, especially allergic reaction

## General Dosing Information

Radiopharmaceuticals are to be administered only by or under the supervision of physicians who have had extensive training in the safe use and handling of radionuclides and who are licensed by the Nuclear Regulatory Commission (NRC) or the appropriate Agreement State agency or, outside the U.S., the appropriate authority.

Manufacturer's package insert or other appropriate literature should be consulted for optimal times when imaging should be performed.

**For cardiac and skeletal imaging**

Unless cardiac status indicates otherwise, the patient should increase intake of fluids and void frequently following the administration of technetium Tc 99m (pyro- and trimeta-) phosphates injection, and for 4 to 6 hours after the imaging procedures are completed, to minimize radiation exposure to the bladder.

Voiding is also recommended immediately prior to imaging procedures to reduce background interference that may result from accumulation of the agent in the bladder.

**For blood pool imaging (cardiac blood pool imaging and diagnosis of gastrointestinal bleeding)**

Unlabeled sodium (pyro- and trimeta-) phosphates should be injected by direct venipuncture. Heparinized catheter systems should not be used.

**Safety considerations for handling this radiopharmaceutical**

Improper handling of this radiopharmaceutical may cause radioactive contamination. Guidelines for handling radioactive material have been prepared by scientific, professional, state, federal, and international bodies and are available to the specially qualified and authorized users who have access to radiopharmaceuticals.

## Parenteral Dosage Forms

### TECHNETIUM Tc 99m (PYRO- AND TRIMETA-) PHOSPHATES INJECTION USP

**Usual adult and adolescent administered activity**

For technetium Tc 99m (pyro- and trimeta-) phosphates:

Skeletal imaging—Intravenous, 555 to 925 megabecquerels (15 to 25 millicuries).

Cardiac imaging—Intravenous, 740 to 1295 megabecquerels (20 to 35 millicuries).

For sodium (pyro- and trimeta-) phosphates without Tc 99m label:

Blood pool imaging—Intravenous, 14 to 42 mg of sodium (pyro- and trimeta-) phosphates (unlabeled) followed, by the intravenous administration of 185 to 740 megabecquerels (5 to 20 millicuries) of sodium pertechnetate Tc 99m five to thirty minutes later.

**Usual pediatric administered activity**

Dosage must be individualized by physician.

**Usual geriatric administered activity**

See *Usual adult and adolescent administered activity.*

**Strength(s) usually available**

U.S.—

10 mg of sodium pyrophosphate, 30 mg of sodium trimetaphosphate, 0.95 mg (minimum) of stannous chloride, and 1.8 mg (maximum) total tin, per reaction vial (Rx) [*Pyrolite*].

Canada—

10 mg of sodium pyrophosphate, 30 mg of sodium trimetaphosphate, 0.95 mg (minimum) of stannous chloride, and 1.8 mg (maximum) total tin, per reaction vial (Rx) [*Pyrolite*].

**Packaging and storage**

Store below 40 °C (104 °F), preferably between 15 and 30 °C (59 and 86 °F), unless otherwise specified by manufacturer. Protect from freezing.

**Preparation of dosage form**

To prepare technetium Tc 99m (pyro- and trimeta-) phosphates injection, an oxidant-free sodium pertechnetate Tc 99m solution is used. See manufacturer's package insert for complete instructions.

To prepare sodium (pyro- and trimeta-) phosphates injection (unlabeled), 3 to 4 mL of sterile sodium chloride injection is used. See manufacturer's package insert for complete instructions.

**Stability**

Technetium Tc 99m (pyro- and trimeta-) phosphates injection should be administered within 6 hours after preparation.

Sodium (pyro- and trimeta-) phosphates injection (unlabeled) should be administered within 6 hours after preparation.

**Incompatibilities**

If oxidants such as peroxides and hypochlorites are present in the sodium pertechnetate Tc 99m used for labeling, the final preparation of Technetium Tc 99m (pyro- and trimeta-) phosphates injection may be adversely affected and should be discarded.

**Note**

Caution—Radioactive material.

Revised: October 1990
Interim revision: 08/02/94

---

# TECHNETIUM Tc 99m SESTAMIBI   Systemic

VA CLASSIFICATION (Primary): DX201

Other commonly used names are technetium Tc 99m methoxyisobutylisonitrile and technetium Tc 99m MIBI.

Note: For a listing of dosage forms and brand names by country availability, see *Dosage Forms* section(s). For a listing of brand names for the articles in this monograph, refer to the General Index.

## Category

Diagnostic aid, radioactive (cardiac disease).

## Indications

Note: Bracketed information in the *Indications* section refers to uses that are not included in U.S. product labeling.

**Accepted**

Cardiac imaging, radionuclide

Myocardial infarction (diagnosis) and

Myocardial perfusion imaging, radionuclide—Technetium Tc 99m sestamibi is indicated in myocardial perfusion imaging to assess the severity and localization of the myocardial infarction. It also helps to demonstrate whether thrombolytic therapy has improved perfusion.

Ischemia, myocardial (diagnosis)[1]—Technetium Tc 99m sestamibi is indicated in patients with known or suspected coronary artery disease to aid in the diagnosis of myocardial ischemia, orient investigative procedures, and guide treatment. In patients with unstable angina, technetium Tc 99m sestamibi is injected at the time of spontaneous chest pain to confirm diagnosis.

Cardiac ventricular function assessment[1] and

[Cardiac wall-motion abnormalities assessment][1]—Technetium Tc 99m sestamibi is indicated for use in the determination of right and/or left ventricular ejection fraction by first-pass radionuclide angiocardiography; it is also used to assess regional wall motion.

[Stress electrocardiography adjunct][1]—Technetium Tc 99m sestamibi is used as an adjunct to stress electrocardiography in the diagnosis of coronary artery disease, allowing simultaneous evaluation of myocardial perfusion and ventricular function.

[Parathyroid imaging, radionuclide][1]—Technetium Tc 99m sestamibi is used for the detection and localization of enlarged parathyroid glands in patients with hyperparathyroidism.

[Thyroid imaging, radionuclide][1]—Technetium Tc 99m sestamibi is used for the detection and localization of various thyroid carcinomas (e.g., medullary, lymphoma, Hurthle cell).

[1]Not included in Canadian product labeling.

## Physical Properties

### Nuclear data

| Radionuclide (half-life) | Decay constant | Mode of decay | Principal photon emissions (keV) | Mean number of emissions/ disintegration ($\geq$0.01) |
|---|---|---|---|---|
| Tc 99m (6.0 hr) | 0.1151 h$^{-1}$ | Isomeric transition to Tc 99 | Gamma (18) | 0.062 |
| | | | Gamma (140.5) | 0.891 |

## Pharmacology/Pharmacokinetics

### Mechanism of action/Effect

Cardiac imaging—The myocardial uptake of technetium Tc 99m sestamibi appears to occur by a passive diffusion process. The rate of passive uptake is determined by the membrane permeability of the drug and the surface area of the vascular beds to which it is exposed; thus myocardial uptake is related to myocardial blood flow. While the mechanism of myocardial retention is not completely understood, its distribution in myocardium appears to be analogous to that of thallous chloride Tl 201. When injected at rest, technetium Tc 99m sestamibi appears to accumulate in viable myocardial tissue; infarcts are thus delineated as areas of lack of accumulation. When injected at stress (either exercise or pharmacologic vasodilation), technetium Tc 99m sestamibi accumulates in myocardial tissue in relation to myocardial blood flow; thus ischemic areas (e.g., those supplied by stenotic vessels) are detected as areas of less accumulation.

Parathyroid imaging and

Thyroid imaging—Although the precise mechanism of tumor localization is unclear, it has been suggested that technetium Tc 99m sestamibi passively crosses cell membranes and is concentrated primarily within cytoplasm and mitochondria. It has been proposed that malignant cells, because of their increased metabolic rate, maintain greater negative mitochondrial and transmembrane potentials, thus enhancing intracellular accumulation of technetium Tc 99m sestamibi. In thyroid glands with hyperthyroidism, blood flow and the number of mitochondria are increased, which may explain the uptake of technetium Tc 99m sestamibi in hyperthyroid glands. Localization of technetium Tc 99m sestamibi appears to be dependent on blood flow to the tissue, the concentration of technetium Tc 99m sestamibi presented to the tissue, and the size of the gland.

### Distribution

High volume of distribution, with minimal cardiac redistribution. Rapidly cleared from blood after intravenous administration, accumulating in normal myocardium in relation to blood flow. The fast clearing component clears from the blood with a half-life of 4.3 minutes (at rest). At 5 minutes after injection, about 8% of the administered activity remains in circulation. Lung uptake is generally low, but there is considerable hepatic uptake. Technetium Tc 99m sestamibi is cleared through the biliary system into the intestine.

### Protein binding

Very low (<1%).

### Half-life

Elimination—
 Biological:
  Myocardium—6 hours (after rest injection).
  Liver—30 minutes (after rest injection).
 Effective (includes biological half-life and radionuclide decay after rest injection):
  Myocardium—3 hours.
  Liver—28 minutes.

### Radiation dosimetry

| | At rest Estimated absorbed radiation dose* | | | |
|---|---|---|---|---|
| | With 2-hour void | | With 4.8-hour void | |
| Organ | mGy/ MBq | rad/ mCi | mGy/ MBq | rad/ mCi |
| Large intestine wall (upper) | 0.049 | 0.18 | 0.049 | 0.18 |
| Large intestine wall (lower) | 0.035 | 0.13 | 0.038 | 0.14 |
| Small intestine | 0.027 | 0.10 | 0.027 | 0.10 |
| Gallbladder wall | 0.018 | 0.067 | 0.018 | 0.067 |
| Kidneys | 0.018 | 0.067 | 0.018 | 0.067 |
| Bladder wall | 0.018 | 0.067 | 0.038 | 0.14 |
| Ovaries | 0.014 | 0.050 | 0.014 | 0.053 |
| Bone surfaces | 0.0063 | 0.023 | 0.0063 | 0.023 |
| Thyroid | 0.0063 | 0.023 | 0.0063 | 0.023 |
| Liver | 0.0054 | 0.02 | 0.0054 | 0.02 |
| Stomach wall | 0.0054 | 0.02 | 0.0054 | 0.02 |
| Red marrow | 0.0046 | 0.017 | 0.0046 | 0.017 |
| Heart wall | 0.0046 | 0.017 | 0.0046 | 0.017 |
| Testes | 0.0027 | 0.010 | 0.0035 | 0.013 |
| Breast | 0.0018 | 0.0067 | 0.0018 | 0.0067 |
| Total body | 0.0045 | 0.017 | 0.0045 | 0.017 |

| | Effective dose | | | |
|---|---|---|---|---|
| | With 2-hour void | | With 4.8-hour void | |
| Radionuclide | mSv/ MBq | rem/ mCi | mSv/ MBq | rem/ mCi |
| Tc 99m | 0.014 | 0.052 | 0.015 | 0.057 |

| | At stress Estimated absorbed radiation dose* | | | |
|---|---|---|---|---|
| | With 2-hour void | | With 4.8-hour void | |
| Organ | mGy/ MBq | rad/ mCi | mGy/ MBq | rad/ mCi |
| Large intestine wall (upper) | 0.041 | 0.15 | 0.041 | 0.15 |
| Large intestine wall (lower) | 0.030 | 0.11 | 0.030 | 0.11 |
| Gallbladder wall | 0.025 | 0.093 | 0.025 | 0.093 |
| Small intestine | 0.022 | 0.08 | 0.022 | 0.08 |
| Kidneys | 0.015 | 0.057 | 0.015 | 0.057 |
| Bladder wall | 0.014 | 0.050 | 0.027 | 0.10 |
| Ovaries | 0.011 | 0.040 | 0.012 | 0.043 |
| Bone surfaces | 0.0054 | 0.02 | 0.0054 | 0.02 |
| Stomach wall | 0.0045 | 0.017 | 0.0045 | 0.017 |
| Heart wall | 0.0045 | 0.017 | 0.0045 | 0.017 |
| Red marrow | 0.0045 | 0.017 | 0.0045 | 0.017 |
| Liver | 0.0036 | 0.013 | 0.0036 | 0.013 |
| Lungs | 0.0027 | 0.010 | 0.0018 | 0.0067 |
| Thyroid | 0.0027 | 0.010 | 0.0018 | 0.0067 |
| Testes | 0.0027 | 0.010 | 0.0027 | 0.010 |
| Breast | 0.0018 | 0.0067 | 0.0018 | 0.0067 |
| Total body | 0.0036 | 0.013 | 0.0036 | 0.013 |

| | Effective dose | | | |
|---|---|---|---|---|
| | With 2-hour void | | With 4.8-hour void | |
| Radionuclide | mSv/ MBq | rem/ mCi | mSv/ MBq | rem/ mCi |
| Tc 99m | 0.013 | 0.045 | 0.013 | 0.048 |

*For adults; intravenous injection. Data based on the Radiopharmaceutical Internal Dose Information Center, July 1990. Oak Ridge Associated Universities.

### Elimination

Within 48 hours—
 Renal, 27% of the administered activity.
 Fecal, 33% of the administered activity.

# Precautions to Consider

## Pregnancy/Reproduction

Pregnancy—Tc 99m (as free pertechnetate) crosses the placenta. Studies have not been done in humans.

The possibility of pregnancy should be assessed in women of child-bearing potential. Clinical situations exist in which the benefit to the patient and fetus, based on information derived from radiopharmaceutical use, outweighs the risks from radiation exposure to the fetus. In this situation, the physician should use discretion and reduce the administered activity of the radiopharmaceutical to the lowest possible amount.

Studies have not been done in animals.

FDA Pregnancy Category C.

## Breast-feeding

The percentage of the injected dose of technetium Tc 99m sestamibi distributed into milk has been found to be very low (0.0084% during the first 24 hours), and should not necessitate interruption of breast-feeding. However, since Tc 99m as free pertechnetate is distributed into breast milk, discontinuation of nursing for a period of 24 hours is generally recommended after administration of technetium Tc 99m–labeled radiopharmaceuticals.

## Pediatrics

Although used in children, there have been no specific studies evaluating safety and efficacy. When used in children the diagnostic benefit should be judged to outweigh the potential risk of radiation.

## Geriatrics

Appropriate studies on the relationship of age to the effects of technetium Tc 99m sestamibi have not been performed in the geriatric population. However, clinical trials and studies including older patients were conducted and geriatrics-specific problems that would limit the usefulness of this agent in the elderly are not expected.

## Diagnostic interference

The following have been selected on the basis of their potential clinical significance (possible effect in parentheses where appropriate)—not necessarily inclusive (» = major clinical significance):

With results of *this* test
   Radiotherapy
      (radiation may affect binding of technetium Tc 99m sestamibi to intracellular proteins, thus decreasing its uptake in myocardial cells)

## Medical considerations/Contraindications

The medical considerations/contraindications included here have been selected on the basis of their potential clinical significance (reasons given in parentheses where appropriate)—not necessarily inclusive (» = major clinical significance).

*Risk-benefit should be considered when the following medical problem exists:*

Sensitivity to the radiopharmaceutical preparation

# Side/Adverse Effects

Note: One case has been reported of severe hypersensitivity, which was characterized by dyspnea, hypotension, bradycardia, asthenia, and vomiting within 2 hours after a second injection of technetium Tc 99m sestamibi.

The following side/adverse effects have been selected on the basis of their potential clinical significance (possible signs and symptoms in parentheses where appropriate)—not necessarily inclusive:

**Those indicating need for medical attention only if they continue or are bothersome**
Incidence more frequent
   *Metallic or bitter taste*
Incidence less frequent or rare
   *Flushing of skin; headache; skin rash*

# Patient Consultation

As an aid to patient consultation, refer to *Advice for the Patient, Radiopharmaceuticals (Diagnostic)*.

In providing consultation, consider emphasizing the following selected information (» = major clinical significance):

**Description of use**
   Action in the body: Accumulation of radioactivity in myocardial cells as a function of relative blood flow
   Differences in uptake of radioactivity can be visualized
   Small amounts of radioactivity used in diagnosis; radiation received is low and considered safe

**Before having this test**
» Conditions affecting use, especially:
      Sensitivity to the radiopharmaceutical preparation
      Pregnancy—Technetium Tc 99m (as free pertechnetate) crosses placenta; risk to fetus from radiation exposure as opposed to benefit derived from study should be considered
      Breast-feeding—Very small amount distributed into breast milk; temporary discontinuation of nursing may be recommended to avoid any unnecessary absorbed radiation dose to the infant
      Use in children—Risk from radiation exposure as opposed to benefit derived from use should be considered

**Preparation for this test**
   Special preparatory instructions may be given; patient should inquire in advance

# General Dosing Information

Radiopharmaceuticals are to be administered only by or under the supervision of physicians who have had extensive training in the safe use and handling of radioactive materials and who are authorized by the Nuclear Regulatory Commission (NRC) or the appropriate Agreement State agency, if required, or, outside the U.S., the appropriate authority.

Imaging with technetium Tc 99m sestamibi to assess the distribution of myocardial perfusion at the time of the infarct in patients who have received the agent prior to, or at the initiation of, thrombolytic therapy (< 4 hours), is possible up to 6 hours after the intravenous injection of this agent, due to the absence of significant redistribution in the myocardium. Thus, the assessment of the amount of hypoperfused myocardium (e.g., the area at risk) is possible without having to delay the administration of thrombolytic therapy.

In conjunction with exercise or pharmacologic stress testing, technetium Tc 99m sestamibi should be administered at the inception of a period of maximum stress that lasts for approximately 1 to 3 minutes after injection.

After intravenous injection, redistribution of technetium Tc 99m sestamibi in the myocardium is minimal or non-existent. For this reason, separate stress and rest injections are required to distinguish reversible stress-induced ischemia from irreversible perfusion defects.

Technical factors such as tomographic reconstruction artifacts, patient movement, diaphragmatic attenuation, and breast attenuation in female patients may cause false-positive results (false perfusion defects).

High liver extraction of technetium Tc 99m sestamibi may interfere with visualization of the inferior wall of the heart. Delaying imaging for at least 1 hour should facilitate tracer clearance from the liver.

When used to examine myocardial perfusion, the optimal time interval for imaging is approximately 1 to 4 hours after administration of technetium Tc 99m sestamibi.

## Safety considerations for handling this radiopharmaceutical

Improper handling of this radiopharmaceutical may cause radioactive contamination. Guidelines for handling radioactive material have been prepared by scientific, professional, state, federal, and international bodies and are available to the specially qualified and authorized users who have access to radiopharmaceuticals.

# Parenteral Dosage Forms

Note: Bracketed uses in the *Dosage Forms* section refer to categories of use and/or indications that are not included in U.S. product labeling.

## TECHNETIUM Tc 99m SESTAMIBI INJECTION USP

### Usual adult and adolescent administered activity

Cardiac imaging—
   Intravenous, 370 to 1110 megabecquerels (10 to 30 millicuries).

   Note: For same-day rest-stress studies, to differentiate ischemia from scar, administration of a low dose (7 millicuries) at rest followed 2 hours later by a higher dose (25 millicuries) at stress has been found to be useful and to give results similar to the 2-day protocol.

[Parathyroid imaging][1]—
   Intravenous, 370 to 740 megabecquerels (10 to 20 millicuries).
[Thyroid imaging][1]—
   Intravenous, 370 to 740 megabecquerels (10 to 20 millicuries).

### Usual pediatric administered activity
Minimum dosage has not been established.

### Usual geriatric administered activity
See *Usual adult and adolescent administered activity*.

## Strength(s) usually available
U.S.—
    1.0 mg of tetrakis (2-methoxy isobutyl isonitrile) Copper (I) tetrafluoroborate, 2.6 mg sodium citrate dihydrate, 1.0 mg L-cysteine hydrochloride monohydrate, 20 mg mannitol, 0.025 mg dihydrate stannous chloride (minimum), 0.075 mg dihydrate stannous chloride, 0.086 mg dihydrate tin chloride (stannous and stannic, maximum), per 5-mL reaction vial (Rx) [*Cardiolite*].
Canada—
    1.0 mg of tetrakis (2-methoxy isobutyl isonitrile) Copper (I) tetrafluoroborate, 2.6 mg sodium citrate dihydrate, 1.0 mg L-cysteine hydrochloride monohydrate, 20 mg mannitol, 0.025 mg dihydrate stannous chloride (minimum), 0.075 mg dihydrate stannous chloride, 0.086 mg dihydrate tin chloride (stannous and stannic, maximum), per 5-mL reaction vial (Rx) [*Cardiolite*].

## Packaging and storage
Store between 15 and 25 °C (59 and 77 °F), unless otherwise specified by manufacturer. Protect from freezing.

## Preparation of dosage form
To prepare technetium Tc 99m sestamibi injection, an oxidant-free sodium pertechnetate Tc 99m solution is used. See manufacturer's package insert for instructions.

## Stability
Product is stable; package insert states that injection must be used within 6 hours after preparation.

## Incompatibilities
If oxidants such as peroxides and hypochlorites are present in the sodium pertechnetate Tc 99m used for labeling, the final preparation may be adversely affected and should be discarded.

## Note
Caution—Radioactive material.

    [1]Not included in Canadian product labeling.

## Selected Bibliography

Beller GA, Sinusas AJ. Experimental studies of the physiologic properties of technetium-99m isonitriles. Am J Cardiol 1990; 66 (13): 5E-8E.

Grégoire J, Théroux P. Detection and assessment of unstable angina using myocardial perfusion imaging: comparison between technetium-99m sestamibi SPECT and 12-lead electrocardiogram. Am J Cardiol 1990; 66 (13): 42E-46E.

Isakandrian A, Heo J, Kong B, et al. Use of technetium-99m isonitrile (RP-30A) in assessing left ventricular perfusion and function at rest and during exercise in coronary artery disease and comparison with coronary arteriography and exercise thallium-201 SPECT imaging. Am J Cardiol 1989; 64: 270-5.

Leppo JA, DePuey EG, Johnson LL. A review of cardiac imaging with sestamibi and teboroxime. J Nucl Med 1991; 32: 2012-22.

Revised: 07/20/93
Interim revision: 08/02/94; 04/25/95

---

# TECHNETIUM Tc 99m SUCCIMER   Systemic†

VA CLASSIFICATION (Primary): DX201

Note: For a listing of dosage forms and brand names by country availability, see *Dosage Forms* section(s). For a listing of brand names for the articles in this monograph, refer to the General Index.

    †Not commercially available in Canada.

## Category
Diagnostic aid, radioactive (renal disorders).

## Indications

### Accepted
Renal imaging, radionuclide—Technetium Tc 99m succimer is indicated as a renal imaging agent to evaluate renal parenchymal disorders.

## Physical Properties

### Nuclear data

| Radionuclide (half-life) | Decay constant | Mode of decay | Principal photon emissions (keV) | Mean number of emissions/ disintegration ($\geq 0.01$) |
|---|---|---|---|---|
| Tc 99m (6.0 hr) | 0.1151 h⁻¹ | Isomeric transition to Tc 99 | Gamma (18) | 0.062 |
| | | | Gamma (140.5) | 0.891 |

## Pharmacology/Pharmacokinetics

### Mechanism of action/Effect
Based on its clearance through the urinary tract. A significant amount is retained in the proximal tubular cells of the renal cortex long enough to allow external detection by means of a scintillation camera.

### Distribution
Distributed in the plasma, loosely bound to proteins. Cleared from the plasma with a half-time of about 60 minutes, then concentrating in the tubular cells of the renal cortex. After one hour, about 25% of the administered activity is concentrated in the kidneys, increasing to 40% after six hours.

## Radiation dosimetry

| | Estimated absorbed radiation dose*† | |
|---|---|---|
| Organ | mGy/MBq | rad/mCi |
| Kidneys | 0.17 | 0.63 |
| Bladder wall | 0.019 | 0.070 |
| Adrenals | 0.013 | 0.048 |
| Spleen | 0.013 | 0.048 |
| Liver | 0.0097 | 0.036 |
| Pancreas | 0.0090 | 0.033 |
| Red marrow | 0.0063 | 0.023 |
| Stomach wall | 0.0055 | 0.020 |
| Small intestine | 0.0052 | 0.019 |
| Large intestine wall (upper) | 0.0051 | 0.019 |
| Uterus | 0.0046 | 0.017 |
| Ovaries | 0.0037 | 0.014 |
| Bone surfaces | 0.0035 | 0.013 |
| Large intestine wall (lower) | 0.0032 | 0.012 |
| Lungs | 0.0025 | 0.0093 |
| Breast | 0.0018 | 0.0067 |
| Testes | 0.0018 | 0.0067 |
| Thyroid | 0.0011 | 0.0041 |
| Other tissue | 0.0030 | 0.011 |

Effective dose: 0.016 mSv/MBq (0.059 rem/mCi)

    *For adults; intravenous injection.
    †Data based on the International Commission on Radiological Protection (ICRP) Publication 53—Radiation dose to patients from radiopharmaceuticals.

### Elimination
Renal (about 16% of the administered activity in 2 hours).

## Precautions to Consider

### Pregnancy/Reproduction
Pregnancy—Tc 99m (as free pertechnetate) crosses the placenta. However, studies have not been done with technetium Tc 99m succimer in humans.

The possibility of pregnancy should be assessed in women of child-bearing potential. Clinical situations exist where the benefit to the patient and fetus, based on information derived from radiopharmaceutical use, outweighs the risks from fetal exposure to radiation. In these situations, the physician should use discretion and reduce the radiopharmaceutical dose to the lowest possible amount.

Studies have not been done in animals.

FDA Pregnancy Category C.

**Breast-feeding**

Although it is not known whether technetium Tc 99m succimer is distributed into breast milk, it is known that Tc 99m as free pertechnetate is distributed into breast milk. Based on the assumption that the Tc 99m in breast milk is in the form of pertechnetate and based on the effective half-life of the radionuclide in breast milk, the daily volume of milk, a dose factor relating the radionuclide to its critical organ (thyroid) in the nursing infant, and the maximum permissible dose to that organ, a guideline has been proposed. According to this guideline, it has been calculated that nursing can be safely resumed when the concentration in breast milk reaches $30.3 \times 10^{-4}$ megabecquerels ($8.2 \times 10^{-2}$ microcuries) per mL. This level of activity is probably reached, in the majority of patients, within 12 to 24 hours after administration of technetium Tc 99m–labeled radiopharmaceuticals.

**Pediatrics**

Studies performed in children have not demonstrated pediatrics-specific problems that would limit the usefulness of technetium Tc 99m succimer in children. However, because of the potential risk of radiation exposure, risk-benefit must be considered.

**Geriatrics**

Appropriate studies on the relationship of age to the effects of technetium Tc 99m succimer have not been performed in the geriatric population. However, no geriatrics-specific problems have been documented to date.

**Diagnostic interference**

The following have been selected on the basis of their potential clinical significance (possible effect in parentheses where appropriate)—not necessarily inclusive (» = major clinical significance):

With results of *this* test

*Due to other medications*

Captopril or
Enalapril or
Lisinopril
   (in patients with unilateral renal artery stenosis, use of angiotensin-converting enzyme inhibitors may result in decreased uptake of technetium Tc 99m succimer by the affected kidney because of a loss of effective trans-membrane filtration pressure)

*Due to medical problems or conditions*

Dehydration
   (decreased urinary flow may result in poor renal images)

**Medical considerations/Contraindications**

The medical considerations/contraindications included here have been selected on the basis of their potential clinical significance (reasons given in parentheses where appropriate)—not necessarily inclusive (» = major clinical significance).

See also *Diagnostic interference.*

*Risk-benefit should be considered when the following medical problem exists:*

Sensitivity to the radiopharmaceutical preparation

# Side/Adverse Effects

The following side/adverse effects have been selected on the basis of their potential clinical significance (possible signs and symptoms in parentheses where appropriate)—not necessarily inclusive:

**Those indicating need for medical attention only if they continue or are bothersome**

Incidence rare
   *Fever; flushing or redness of skin; nausea; skin rash; stomach pain; syncope* (fainting)

# Patient Consultation

As an aid to patient consultation, refer to *Advice for the Patient, Radiopharmaceuticals (Diagnostic).*

In providing consultation, consider emphasizing the following selected information (» = major clinical significance):

**Description of use**

Action in the body: Concentration of radioactive succimer in kidneys
Retention of radioactivity in kidneys allows visualization
Small amounts of radioactivity used in diagnosis; radiation received is low and considered safe

**Before having this test**

» Conditions affecting use, especially:
   Sensitivity to the radiopharmaceutical preparation
   Pregnancy—Technetium Tc 99m (as free pertechnetate) crosses placenta; risk to fetus from radiation exposure as opposed to benefit derived from use should be considered
   Breast-feeding—Not known if technetium Tc 99m succimer is distributed into breast milk, but Tc 99m as free pertechnetate is distributed into breast milk; temporary discontinuation of nursing may be recommended because of risk to infant from radiation exposure
   Use in children—Risk from radiation exposure as opposed to benefit derived from use should be considered

**Preparation for this test**

Special preparatory instructions may be given; patient should inquire in advance

**Precautions after having this test**

Adequate intake of fluids and voiding as often as possible for 4 to 6 hours after examination to minimize radiation dose to bladder

# General Dosing Information

Radiopharmaceuticals are to be administered only by or under the supervision of physicians who have had extensive training in the safe use and handling of radioactive materials and who are authorized by the Nuclear Regulatory Commission (NRC) or the appropriate Agreement State agency, if required, or, outside the U.S., the appropriate authority.

Adequate hydration of the patient is recommended before and after examination to promote urinary flow. Also, urination is recommended as often as possible for 4 to 6 hours after the examination to reduce radiation exposure to the bladder.

Manufacturer's package insert or other appropriate literature should be consulted for optimal times when imaging should be performed.

**Safety considerations for handling this radiopharmaceutical**

Improper handling of this radiopharmaceutical may cause radioactive contamination. Guidelines for handling radioactive material have been prepared by scientific, professional, state, federal, and international bodies and are available to the specially qualified and authorized users who have access to radiopharmaceuticals.

# Parenteral Dosage Forms

## TECHNETIUM Tc 99m SUCCIMER INJECTION USP

**Usual adult and adolescent administered activity**

Renal imaging—
   Intravenous, 74 to 222 megabecquerels (2 to 6 millicuries), administered slowly.

**Usual pediatric administered activity**

Renal imaging—
   Dosage must be individualized by physician. The minimum recommended total dosage is 55 megabecquerels (1.5 millicuries), with a maximum total dosage of 185 megabecquerels (5 millicuries), intravenously.

**Usual geriatric administered activity**

See *Usual adult and adolescent administered activity.*

**Strength(s) usually available**

U.S.—
   1.2 mg succimer and 0.42 mg anhydrous stannous chloride, per 2.2-mL reagent ampule (Rx) [*MPI DMSA Kidney Reagent*].

Canada—
   Not commercially available.

**Packaging and storage**

Store between 15 and 30 °C (59 and 86 °F), in a light-resistant container. Protect from freezing.

**Preparation of dosage form**

To prepare injection, an oxidant-free sodium pertechnetate Tc 99m solution is used. After reconstitution with sodium pertechnetate Tc 99m, the newly formed complex should be allowed to incubate for 10 minutes, at room temperature, to permit the formation of a more desirable succimer complex. See manufacturer's package insert for complete instructions.

**Stability**

Injection should be administered within 30 minutes after preparation.

**Incompatibilities**

If oxidants such as peroxides and hypochlorites are present in the sodium pertechnetate Tc 99m used for labeling, the final preparation may be adversely affected and should be discarded.

**Note**

Caution—Radioactive material.

**Selected Bibliography**

Blaufox MD. Procedures of choice in renal nuclear medicine. J Nucl Med 1991; 32: 1301-9.

Revised: 08/18/93
Interim revision: 08/02/94

# TECHNETIUM Tc 99m SULFUR COLLOID    Systemic

VA CLASSIFICATION (Primary): DX201

Note: For a listing of dosage forms and brand names by country availability, see *Dosage Forms* section(s). For a listing of brand names for the articles in this monograph, refer to the General Index.

## Category

Diagnostic aid, radioactive (hepatic disease; hematological disease; spleen disease; gastroesophageal disorders; gastrointestinal disorders).

## Indications

Note: Bracketed information in the *Indications* section refers to uses that are not included in U.S. product labeling.

**Accepted**

Liver imaging, radionuclide—Technetium Tc 99m sulfur colloid, administered intravenously, is indicated for imaging the functioning reticuloendothelial cells of the liver in the evaluation of metastatic disease, primary liver tumors, abscesses, and other focal hepatic lesions; and in the evaluation of patients with cirrhosis, hepatitis, and other hepatic disorders.

Spleen imaging, radionuclide—Technetium Tc 99m sulfur colloid, administered intravenously, is indicated for imaging the functioning reticuloendothelial cells of the spleen, thus serving to demonstrate clinically significant splenomegaly, and in the evaluation of splenic infarct, other local splenic lesions, or splenic rupture.

Bone marrow imaging, radionuclide—Technetium Tc 99m sulfur colloid, administered intravenously, is indicated for imaging the functioning reticuloendothelial cells of the bone marrow to complement other hematological studies for the evaluation of hematopoiesis in hematological diseases, such as leukemia, polycythemia, anemias, and myelofibrosis.

Esophageal imaging, radionuclide[1]—Technetium Tc 99m sulfur colloid, administered orally, is indicated in adults and children for esophageal transit studies, gastroesophageal reflux scintigraphy, and the detection of pulmonary aspiration of gastric contents.

LeVeen peritoneovenous shunt patency assessment[1]—Intraperitoneal technetium Tc 99m sulfur colloid is indicated in adults to determine the patency of a peritoneovenous shunt in patients with ascites.

[Bleeding, gastrointestinal (diagnosis)][1]—Technetium Tc 99m sulfur colloid, administered intravenously, is used to detect and locate the site of bleeding in the gastrointestinal tract.

[Gastric emptying studies][1]—Technetium Tc 99m sulfur colloid is used orally in studies to evaluate gastric function in patients with suspected anatomical or functional obstruction, or hypomotility (e.g., gastroparesis).

[1]Not included in Canadian product labeling.

## Physical Properties

### Nuclear data

| Radionu-clide (half-life) | Decay constant | Mode of decay | Principal photon emissions (keV) | Mean number of emissions/ disintegration (≥0.01) |
|---|---|---|---|---|
| Tc 99m (6.0 hr) | 0.1151 h⁻¹ | Isomeric transition to Tc 99 | 18 140.5 | 0.062 0.891 |

## Pharmacology/Pharmacokinetics

**Mechanism of action/Effect**

Diagnostic aid (hepatic disease; hematological disease; spleen disease)—Radioactive colloids are phagocytized by the reticuloendothelial system of the liver, spleen, and bone marrow, and remain there long enough for scintillation scans of their distribution to be obtained.

Diagnostic aid (gastroesophageal disorders)—Esophageal transit of technetium Tc 99m sulfur colloid after oral administration is depicted scintigraphically and quantified by computer assistance.

Diagnostic aid (gastrointestinal disorders)—Gastrointestinal bleeding: After intravenous injection, technetium Tc 99m sulfur colloid circulates in the blood until it is cleared by the cells of the reticuloendothelial system. If active gastrointestinal bleeding is occurring during this period, there will be accumulation of the tracer in the lumen of the gastrointestinal tract at the site of bleeding, thus permitting scintigraphic detection and localization.

**Absorption**

Rapidly phagocytized by the reticuloendothelial system after intravenous administration.

**Distribution**

Parenteral—

Distribution dependent on relative blood flow and functional capacity of phagocytic cells; technetium Tc 99m sulfur colloid is selectively concentrated in reticuloendothelial system of the liver, spleen, and bone marrow. About 80 to 90% of the injected colloidal particles are phagocytized by the Kupffer cells of the liver, 5 to 10% by the spleen, and the balance by the bone marrow.

Uptake may be decreased in the liver and increased in the spleen and bone marrow of patients with impaired portal circulation or Kupffer cell dysfunction.

Several cases of uptake in the lungs and other soft tissues have been reported in the presence of a wide variety of disorders, usually inflammatory or neoplastic.

**Half-life**

Elimination from the blood pool—2.5 minutes.

**Time to radioactivity visualization**

With intravenous administration—

Liver and spleen imaging: 10 to 15 minutes.

Note: Onset of hepatic visualization may be delayed in patients with severe hepatic disease because of slower blood clearance of the radiopharmaceutical, with an overall result of decreased liver uptake and increased spleen and marrow uptake.

Bone marrow imaging: 15 minutes.

With oral administration—

Esophageal imaging: Immediate; usually as the patient swallows, in a single swallow, the water containing technetium Tc 99m sulfur colloid.

**Radiation dosimetry**

| Organ | Estimated absorbed radiation dose* | | | |
|---|---|---|---|---|
| | With normal hepatic function | | With parenchymal liver disease (intermediate/advanced) | |
| | mGy/ MBq | rad/ mCi | mGy/ MBq | rad/ mCi |
| Spleen | 0.077 | 0.29 | 0.14 | 0.52 |
| Liver | 0.074 | 0.27 | 0.042 | 0.16 |
| Pancreas | 0.012 | 0.044 | 0.018 | 0.066 |
| Red marrow | 0.011 | 0.041 | 0.023 | 0.085 |
| Adrenals | 0.010 | 0.037 | 0.0098 | 0.036 |
| Kidneys | 0.0097 | 0.036 | 0.011 | 0.041 |

| | Estimated absorbed radiation dose* | | | |
|---|---|---|---|---|
| | With normal hepatic function | | With parenchymal liver disease (intermediate/advanced) | |
| Organ | mGy/ MBq | rad/ mCi | mGy/ MBq | rad/ mCi |
| Bone surfaces | 0.0064 | 0.024 | 0.012 | 0.044 |
| Stomach wall | 0.0062 | 0.023 | 0.0098 | 0.036 |
| Large intestine wall (upper) | 0.0056 | 0.021 | 0.0049 | 0.018 |
| Lungs | 0.0055 | 0.20 | 0.0048 | 0.018 |
| Small intestine | 0.0043 | 0.016 | 0.0046 | 0.017 |
| Breast | 0.0027 | 0.010 | 0.0024 | 0.0089 |
| Ovaries | 0.0022 | 0.0081 | 0.0033 | 0.012 |
| Uterus | 0.0019 | 0.0070 | 0.0028 | 0.010 |
| Large intestine wall (lower) | 0.0018 | 0.0067 | 0.0031 | 0.011 |
| Bladder wall | 0.0011 | 0.0041 | 0.0016 | 0.0059 |
| Thyroid | 0.00079 | 0.0029 | 0.0011 | 0.0041 |
| Testes | 0.00062 | 0.0023 | 0.00095 | 0.0035 |
| Other tissue | 0.0028 | 0.010 | 0.0031 | 0.011 |

| | Effective dose* | | | |
|---|---|---|---|---|
| | With normal hepatic function | | With parenchymal liver disease (intermediate/advanced) | |
| Radionuclide | mSv/ MBq | rem/ mCi | mSv/ MBq | rem/ mCi |
| Tc 99m | 0.014 | 0.052 | 0.017 | 0.063 |

*For adults; intravenous injection of technetium Tc 99m–labeled large colloids. Data based on the International Commission on Radiological Protection (ICRP) Publication 53—Radiation dose to patients from radiopharmaceuticals.

### Elimination
Renal, about 3% of the administered activity eliminated within 48 hours after intravenous administration.

## Precautions to Consider

### Carcinogenicity/Mutagenicity
Long-term animal studies to evaluate carcinogenic or mutagenic potential of technetium Tc 99m sulfur colloid have not been performed.

### Pregnancy/Reproduction
Pregnancy—Tc 99m (as free pertechnetate) crosses the placenta. However, studies with technetium Tc 99m sulfur colloid have not been done in humans.

The possibility of pregnancy should be assessed in women of child-bearing potential. Clinical situations exist where the benefit to the patient and fetus, based on information derived from radiopharmaceutical use, outweighs the risks from fetal exposure to radiation. In these situations, the physician should use discretion and reduce the radiopharmaceutical dose to the lowest possible amount.

Studies have not been done in animals.

FDA Pregnancy Category C.

### Breast-feeding
Although it is not known whether technetium Tc 99m sulfur colloid is distributed into breast milk, it is known that Tc 99m as free pertechnetate is distributed into breast milk. Based on the assumption that the Tc 99m in breast milk is in the form of pertechnetate and based on the effective half-life of the radionuclide in breast milk, the daily volume of milk, a dose factor relating the radionuclide to its critical organ (thyroid) in the nursing infant, and the maximum permissible dose to that organ, a guideline has been proposed. According to this guideline, it has been calculated that nursing can be safely resumed when the concentration in breast milk reaches $30.3 \times 10^{-4}$ megabecquerels ($8.2 \times 10^{-2}$ microcuries) per mL. This level of activity is probably reached, in the majority of patients, within 12 to 24 hours after administration of technetium Tc 99m–labeled radiopharmaceuticals.

### Pediatrics
Diagnostic studies performed to date using technetium Tc 99 sulfur colloid have not demonstrated pediatrics-specific problems that would limit the usefulness of technetium Tc 99m sulfur colloid in children. However, when this radiopharmaceutical is used in children, the diagnostic benefit should be judged to outweigh the potential risk of radiation.

### Geriatrics
Appropriate studies on the relationship of age to the effects of technetium Tc 99m sulfur colloid have not been performed in the geriatric population. However, no geriatrics-specific problems have been documented to date.

### Drug interactions and/or related problems
See *Diagnostic interference*.

### Diagnostic interference
The following have been selected on the basis of their potential clinical significance (possible effect in parentheses where appropriate)—not necessarily inclusive (» = major clinical significance):

With results of *this* test
*Due to other medications*
Anesthetics, inhalation, such as halothane
(recent administration of general anesthetics may increase splenic uptake of technetium Tc 99m sulfur colloid, probably because the reduced hepatic flow and hepatotoxicity associated with general anesthetics may alter the hepatic radiocolloid extraction efficiency, resulting in a reversal of the normal liver-spleen colloid distribution pattern)

Antacids, aluminum-containing, high doses or long-term use or
Magnesium sulfate, parenteral or
Polyvalent cations
(reticuloendothelial cell imaging may be impaired by polyvalent cations, which cause agglomeration of the individual colloidal particles leading to trapping by the pulmonary capillary bed rather than the reticuloendothelial cells of the liver, spleen, and bone marrow)

Chemotherapy, especially with nitrosoureas
(use of technetium Tc 99m sulfur colloid in patients who are undergoing or have recently undergone chemotherapy, may result in inhomogeneous or irregular hepatic uptake, shift of activity from the liver to the bone marrow and spleen, and hepatomegaly; irregular hepatic distribution of radiopharmaceutical may be misinterpreted as malignancy; thus, it is recommended that liver and/or spleen imaging be done prior to initiating chemotherapy with these agents or several weeks after discontinuing therapy)

Reticuloendothelial system stimulators, such as:
Dextrose
Heparin
Steroid hormones (including estrogen)
Thyroid hormones
Vitamin B$_{12}$
(use of technetium Tc 99m sulfur colloid in patients receiving these medicines may result in lung uptake of technetium Tc 99m sulfur colloid, probably due to a drug-induced increase in number of free intravascular macrophages, which may migrate to pulmonary capillary bed and phagocytize colloidal particles there)

*Due to medical problems or conditions*
Malaria
(diffuse lung uptake of technetium Tc 99m sulfur colloid may occur, probably related to increased reticuloendothelial system activity due to malaria-induced increase in the pulmonary macrophages)

### Medical considerations/Contraindications
The medical considerations/contraindications included here have been selected on the basis of their potential clinical significance (reasons given in parentheses where appropriate)—not necessarily inclusive (» = major clinical significance).

*Risk-benefit should be considered when the following medical problem exists:*
Sensitivity to the radiopharmaceutical preparation, especially gelatin-containing preparations

## Side/Adverse Effects

Note: Cardiopulmonary arrest has been reported rarely with the administration of technetium Tc 99m sulfur colloid.

The following side/adverse effects have been selected on the basis of their potential clinical significance (possible signs and symptoms in parentheses where appropriate)—not necessarily inclusive:

### Those indicating need for medical attention
Incidence rare
*Allergic reaction* (coughing or choking; flushing or redness of face; skin rash, hives, or itching; swelling of throat, hands, or feet; wheezing, tightness in chest, or troubled breathing); *bronchospasm with or without pulmonary edema* (severe wheezing or troubled breathing);

*fever; hypotension* (severe tiredness or weakness); *pain or burning sensation at injection site; seizures; slow or irregular heartbeat*

Note: The *allergic reaction* may be the initial manifestation of a more severe anaphylactic reaction.

*Allergic reactions* and *fever* may be caused by the colloid stabilizer (i.e., gelatin) used in the preparation.

**Those indicating need for medical attention only if they continue or are bothersome**
Incidence less frequent or rare
*Dizziness; nausea or vomiting*

## Patient Consultation

As an aid to patient consultation, refer to *Advice for the Patient, Radiopharmaceuticals (Diagnostic)*.

In providing consultation, consider emphasizing the following selected information (» = major clinical significance):

**Description of use**
*Action in the body*
Accumulation of radioactive colloid particles in liver, spleen, and bone marrow
Esophageal and gastric transit of radiocolloid

Retention of radioactivity in these organs allows visualization; or transit of radioactivity through mouth/esophagus/stomach allows visualization
Small amounts of radioactivity used in diagnosis; radiation received is low and considered safe

**Before having this test**
» Conditions affecting use, especially:
Sensitivity to radiopharmaceutical preparation
Pregnancy—Technetium Tc 99m (as free pertechnetate) crosses placenta; risk to fetus from radiation exposure as opposed to benefit derived from use should be considered
Breast-feeding—Not known if technetium Tc 99m sulfur colloid is distributed into breast milk, but Tc 99m as free pertechnetate is distributed into breast milk; temporary discontinuation of nursing may be recommended because of risk to infant from radiation exposure
Use in children—Risk of radiation exposure as opposed to benefit derived from use should be considered

**Preparation for this test**
Special preparatory instructions may be given; patient should inquire in advance (fasting required for esophageal imaging and gastric emptying studies)

**Precautions after having this test**
No special precautions

**Side/adverse effects**
Signs of potential side effects, especially allergic reaction, fever, hypotension, pain or burning sensation at injection site, seizures, slow or irregular heartbeat, or respiratory distress

## General Dosing Information

Radiopharmaceuticals are to be administered only by or under the supervision of physicians who have had extensive training in the safe use and handling of radioactive materials and who are authorized by the Nuclear Regulatory Commission (NRC) or the appropriate Agreement State agency, if required, or, outside the U.S., the appropriate authority.

Epinephrine, antihistamines, and corticosteroids should be available during the administration of technetium Tc 99m sulfur colloid because of the possibility of allergic reactions.

**Safety considerations for handling this radiopharmaceutical**
Improper handling of this radiopharmaceutical may cause radioactive contamination. Guidelines for handling radioactive material have been prepared by scientific, professional, state, federal, and international bodies and are available to the specially qualified and authorized users who have access to radiopharmaceuticals.

## Parenteral Dosage Forms

Note: Bracketed uses in the *Dosage Forms* section refer to categories of use and/or indications that are not included in U.S. product labeling.

### TECHNETIUM Tc 99m SULFUR COLLOID INJECTION USP

**Usual adult and adolescent administered activity**
Liver and/or spleen imaging—
Intravenous, 37 to 296 megabecquerels (1 to 8 millicuries).

Bone marrow imaging—
Intravenous, 111 to 444 megabecquerels (3 to 12 millicuries).
Esophageal imaging[1]—
Gastroesophageal studies: Oral, 5.55 to 11.1 megabecquerels (150 to 300 microcuries).
Pulmonary aspiration studies: Oral, 11.1 to 18.5 megabecquerels (300 to 500 microcuries).
LeVeen shunt patency[1]—
Intraperitoneal, 37 to 111 megabecquerels (1 to 3 millicuries).
Percutaneous transtubal, 12 to 37 megabecquerels (0.3 to 1 millicurie) in a volume not to exceed 0.5 mL.
[Diagnosis of gastrointestinal bleeding][1]—
Intravenous or intra-arterial, 370 megabecquerels (10 millicuries).
[Gastric emptying studies][1]—
Oral, 9.2 to 37 megabecquerels (0.25 to 1 millicurie).

Note: For gastric emptying studies, the dosage may be given in a liquid or incorporated into food such as scrambled eggs.

**Usual pediatric administered activity**
Liver and/or spleen imaging—
Intravenous, 0.55 to 2.75 megabecquerels (15 to 75 microcuries) per kg of body weight.

Note: In newborns the total administered activity should be 7.4 to 18.5 megabecquerels (200 to 500 microcuries), since a minimum administered activity of 7.4 megabecquerels (200 microcuries) is required for this procedure.
Bone marrow imaging—
Intravenous, 1.11 to 5.55 megabecquerels (30 to 150 microcuries) per kg of body weight.

Note: In newborns a maximum total administered activity of 22.2 megabecquerels (600 microcuries) is recommended, since this is the minimum administered activity required for this procedure.
Esophageal imaging[1]—
Gastroesophageal and pulmonary aspiration studies: Oral, 3.7 to 11.1 megabecquerels (100 to 300 microcuries).

Note: Oral dosage may be incorporated into milk feeding. However, to avoid preliminary contamination of the esophagus, the oral dosage may be instilled directly into the stomach by intubation, followed by a dextrose or milk meal.

**Usual geriatric administered activity**
See *Usual adult and adolescent administered activity*.

**Strength(s) usually available**
U.S.—
2 mg sodium thiosulfate anhydrous, 2.3 mg edetate disodium, and 18.1 mg gelatin, per 10-mL multidose reaction vial; 1.5 mL of 0.148 *N* hydrochloric acid solution per syringe A; and 1.5 mL aqueous solution of 38.8 mg sodium biphosphate anhydrous and 11.1 mg sodium hydroxide, per syringe B (Rx) [*AN-Sulfur Colloid; TechneScan Sulfur Colloid*].
50 mg phosphoric acid per mL or reaction mixture vial; 12 mg gelatin and 9 mg sodium chloride per mL in one compartment, and 12 mg sodium thiosulfate per mL in the other compartment of syringe I; 36 mg gelatin and 9 mg sodium chloride per mL in one compartment, and 544 mg sodium acetate and 4 mg edetate disodium per mL in the other compartment of syringe II (Rx) [*TechneColl*].
0.5 mL of 1.0 *N* hydrochloric acid per reaction vial; and two syringes, one containing a 1.1 mL aqueous solution of 1.9 mg sodium thiosulfate anhydrous and the other containing 5.3 mg gelatin in 2.1 mL of an aqueous buffer solution containing 177 mg sodium acetate (Rx) [*TSC*].
Canada—
3 mg sodium thiosulfate, 4.25 mg gelatin, 0.65 mg potassium perrhenate, per mL of reaction vial A; 1 *N* hydrochloric acid solution per vial B; alkaline buffer solution per vial C (Rx) [*Frosstimage Sulfur Colloid*].

**Packaging and storage**
Store below 40 °C (104 °F), preferably between 15 and 30 °C (59 and 86 °F), unless otherwise specified by manufacturer. Protect from freezing.

**Preparation of dosage form**
To prepare injection, an oxidant-free sodium pertechnetate Tc 99m solution is used. See manufacturer's package insert for instructions.

**Stability**
Preparations containing a flocculent precipitate should not be used.
Injection should be administered within 6 hours after preparation, since particles tend to agglomerate with aging.

**Incompatibilities**
Polyvalent cations may decrease the stability of the colloidal preparation. Solutions of sodium pertechnetate Tc 99m containing more than 10

mcg per mL of aluminum ion should not be used since a flocculent precipitate may form. These larger particles may become lodged in the pulmonary capillary bed rather than in the reticuloendothelial system.

If oxidants such as peroxides and hypochlorites are present in the sodium pertechnetate Tc 99m used for labeling, the final preparation may be adversely affected and it should be discarded.

**Note**
Caution—Radioactive material.
Shake well.

---

[1]Not included in Canadian product labeling.

## Selected Bibliography

Malmud LS, Fisher RS, Knight LC, et al. Scintigraphic evaluation of gastric emptying. Semin Nucl Med 1982; 12 (2): 116-25.

Malmud LS, Fisher RS. Radionuclide studies of esophageal transit and gastrophageal reflux. Semin Nucl Med 1982; 12 (2): 104-15.

Alavi A. Detection of gastrointestinal bleeding with Tc 99m sulfur colloid. Semin Nucl Med 1982; 12 (2): 126-38.

---

Revised: 06/23/94

---

# TECHNETIUM Tc 99m TEBOROXIME    Systemic†

**VA CLASSIFICATION (Primary): DX201**

Note: For a listing of dosage forms and brand names by country availability, see *Dosage Forms* section(s). For a listing of brand names for the articles in this monograph, refer to the General Index.

---

†Not commercially available in Canada.

## Category

Diagnostic aid, radioactive (cardiac disease).

## Indications

**Accepted**
Cardiac imaging, radionuclide
Myocardial infarction (diagnosis) and
Myocardial perfusion imaging, radionuclide—Technetium Tc 99m teboroxime is indicated in myocardial perfusion imaging to distinguish normal from abnormal myocardium in patients with suspected coronary artery disease (CAD) using rest and stress techniques.

## Physical Properties

**Nuclear data**

| Radionu-clide (half-life) | Decay constant | Mode of decay | Principal photon emissions (keV) | Mean number of photons/ disintegration (≥0.01) |
|---|---|---|---|---|
| Tc 99m (6.0 hr) | 0.1151 h⁻¹ | Isomeric transition to Tc 99 | Gamma 18 | 0.062 |
| | | | Gamma 140.5 | 0.891 |

## Pharmacology/Pharmacokinetics

**Mechanism of action/Effect**
The mechanisms for uptake and retention of technetium Tc 99m teboroxime by myocardial tissue are not well established. Unlike cationic thallous chloride Tl 201 and technetium Tc 99m sestamibi, technetium Tc 99m teboroxime has a neutral charge. Because of its neutral charge and high lipophilicity, the myocardial uptake of technetium Tc 99m teboroxime appears to occur by a passive diffusion process. The rate of passive uptake is determined by the membrane permeability of the drug, the surface area of the vascular beds to which it is exposed, the vascular and extravascular concentrations of the drug, and the rate of delivery of the drug. While technetium Tc 99m teboroxime's mechanism of myocardial retention is less efficient than that of thallous chloride Tl 201 or technetium Tc 99m sestamibi, its myocardial extraction is higher. Its rapid myocardial washout allows early repeat studies following the application of a pharmacologic or physical intervention.

**Distribution**
Technetium Tc 99m teboroxime is rapidly cleared from blood after intravenous administration, with high myocardial extraction in proportion to myocardial perfusion even at extremely high flow rates. Myocardial uptake is apparent scintigraphically at 1 minute after injection. A significant amount of the initial myocardial activity is cleared by 20 to 30 minutes after administration.

Liver uptake of technetium Tc 99m teboroxime becomes significant by 5 to 10 minutes after injection and has a slow clearance (half-life approximately 1.5 hours) that can impair visualization of the inferior left ventricular wall.

There is marked first-pass uptake of technetium Tc 99m teboroxime in the lungs with rapid subsequent clearance within the first 2 minutes after injection. This initial lung uptake may complicate first-pass radionuclide angiography image interpretation, since it results in lower ejection fractions, higher pulmonary transit times, higher calculated pulmonary blood volume indices, and poorer left ventricular border definition.

**Protein binding**
Very low (<10%).

**Half-life**
Elimination (myocardium)—10 to 15 minutes.

Note: A biexponential pattern of myocardial washout has been demonstrated in animals and man. About two-thirds of myocardial activity demonstrates an effective half-life of 5.2 minutes; the remaining one-third demonstrates an effective half-life of 3.8 hours. At 10 minutes after injection, approximately 10.4 ± 4.4% (mean) of the injected dose remains in the circulation.

**Radiation dosimetry**

| Mode of administra-tion | Target organ | Estimated absorbed radiation dose* | |
|---|---|---|---|
| | | mGy/MBq | rad/mCi |
| Intravenous | Large intestine, upper | 0.033 | 0.12 |
| | Gallbladder mwall | 0.026 | 0.097 |
| | Large intestine, lower | 0.023 | 0.087 |
| | Small intestine | 0.018 | 0.067 |
| | Liver | 0.017 | 0.062 |
| | Ovaries | 0.0098 | 0.036 |
| | Lungs | 0.0076 | 0.028 |
| | Urinary bladder wall | 0.0074 | 0.027 |
| | Heart wall | 0.0055 | 0.020 |
| | Kidneys | 0.0055 | 0.020 |
| | Red marrow | 0.0045 | 0.017 |
| | Spleen | 0.0040 | 0.015 |
| | Brain | 0.0034 | 0.012 |
| | Thyroid | 0.0029 | 0.011 |
| | Testes | 0.0028 | 0.010 |
| | Total body | 0.0045 | 0.017 |

Effective dose: 0.013 mSv/MBq (0.048 rem/mCi)

*Assuming 6-hour gallbladder emptying; 2-hour urinary bladder void.

**Elimination**
Hepatobiliary, mainly. Renal, 22 ± 13% in 24 hours.

## Precautions to Consider

**Carcinogenicity**
Long-term animal studies to evaluate carcinogenic potential of technetium Tc 99m teboroxime have not been performed.

**Mutagenicity**
Decayed technetium Tc 99m teboroxime has not been shown to be mutagenic in a reversion test with bacteria, a chromosomal aberration assay, and an *in vivo* mouse micronucleus assay.

At high concentrations that were toxic to the cells and reduced growth to 33% or less relative to vehicle controls, technetium Tc 99m teboroxime was weakly positive for inducing forward mutations at the TK locus in L5178Y mouse lymphoma cells without metabolic activation. In the presence of metabolic activation, technetium Tc 99m teboroxime gave negative results in this assay.

**Pregnancy/Reproduction**

Pregnancy—Tc 99m (as free pertechnetate) crosses the placenta. However, studies with technetium Tc 99m teboroxime have not been done in humans.

The possibility of pregnancy should be assessed in women of child-bearing potential. Clinical situations exist in which the benefit to the patient and fetus from information derived from radiopharmaceutical use outweighs the risks from fetal exposure to radiation. In these situations, the physician should use discretion and reduce the administered activity of the radiopharmaceutical to the lowest possible amount.

Studies have not been done in animals.

FDA Pregnancy Category C.

**Breast-feeding**

Although it is not known whether technetium Tc 99m teboroxime is distributed into breast milk, it is known that Tc 99m as free pertechnetate is distributed into breast milk. Because of the potential risk to the infant from radiation exposure, discontinuation of nursing for a period of 24 hours is recommended after administration of technetium Tc 99m–labeled radiopharmaceuticals.

**Pediatrics**

Although technetium Tc 99m teboroxime is used in children, there have been no specific studies evaluating safety and efficacy. When used in children, the diagnostic benefit should be judged to outweigh the potential risk of radiation.

**Geriatrics**

Appropriate studies on the relationship of age to the effects of technetium Tc 99m teboroxime have not been performed in the geriatric population. However, clinical trials and studies were conducted including older patients and geriatrics-specific problems that would limit the usefulness of this agent in the elderly are not expected.

**Medical considerations/Contraindications**

The medical considerations/contraindications included here have been selected on the basis of their potential clinical significance (reasons given in parentheses where appropriate)—not necessarily inclusive (» = major clinical significance).

*Risk-benefit should be considered when the following medical problem exists:*

Sensitivity to the radiopharmaceutical preparation

## Side/Adverse Effects

The following side/adverse effects have been selected on the basis of their potential clinical significance (possible signs and symptoms in parentheses where appropriate)—not necessarily inclusive:

**Those indicating need for medical attention only if they continue or are bothersome**

Incidence less frequent or rare

> *Burning sensation at injection site; hypotension; metallic taste; nausea; numbness of hand and arm; swelling of face*

## Patient Consultation

As an aid to patient consultation, refer to *Advice for the Patient, Radiopharmaceuticals (Diagnostic).*

In providing consultation, consider emphasizing the following selected information (» = major clinical significance):

**Description of use**

Action in the body: Accumulation of radioactivity in myocardial cells as a function of relative blood flow

Differences in uptake of radioactivity can be visualized

Small amounts of radioactivity used in diagnosis; radiation dose received is relatively low and considered safe

**Before having this test**

» Conditions affecting use, especially:

Sensitivity to the radiopharmaceutical preparation

Pregnancy—Technetium Tc 99m (as free pertechnetate) crosses placenta; risk to fetus from radiation exposure as opposed to benefit derived from study should be considered

Breast-feeding—Not known if technetium Tc 99m teboroxime is distributed into breast milk, but Tc 99m as free pertechnetate is distributed into breast milk; temporary discontinuation of nursing is recommended to avoid any unnecessary absorbed radiation dose to the infant

**Preparation for this test**

Fasting for 4 to 8 hours before the stress/rest test

Other special preparatory instructions may also be given; patient should inquire in advance

## General Dosing Information

Radiopharmaceuticals are to be administered only by or under the supervision of physicians who have had extensive training in the safe use and handling of radioactive materials and who are licensed by the Nuclear Regulatory Commission (NRC) or the appropriate Agreement State agency, if required, or, outside the U.S., the appropriate authority.

Fasting is usually recommended for 4 to 8 hours before the stress/rest test.

Technical factors such as tomographic reconstruction artifacts, patient movement, diaphragmatic attenuation, and breast attenuation in female patients may cause false-positive results (false perfusion defects).

In conjunction with exercise or pharmacologic vasodilatation stress testing, technetium Tc 99m teboroxime should be administered at the inception of a period of maximum stress that is continued for approximately 30 to 60 seconds after injection.

High liver extraction of technetium Tc 99m teboroxime may interfere with visualization of the inferior wall of the heart. Positioning the patient upright during image acquisition is helpful in minimizing the contribution of liver activity, since in the upright position the liver tends to drop downward, allowing better separation of the cardiac and hepatic activities.

For either rest or stress studies, imaging must begin within 2 to 5 minutes after injection of technetium Tc 99m teboroxime and must be completed within 5 to 10 minutes. After 5 minutes, differential washout of technetium Tc 99m teboroxime begins to introduce artifacts. If image acquisition takes too long, perfusion defects can become less apparent before acquisition is complete, resulting in an underestimation of the number and severity of ischemic segments. A significant amount of the initial myocardial activity is cleared by 20 to 30 minutes after administration.

Rapid myocardial washout and early hepatic uptake necessitates use of rapid imaging protocols, and may require a multiple-headed single-photon emission computed tomography (SPECT) camera to complete image acquisition in 3 to 4 minutes.

**For studies performed in conjunction with pharmacologic stress testing**

Pharmacologic stress, induced by intravenous adenosine or dipyridamole, may be preferred for stress/rest studies using technetium Tc 99m teboroxime since the patient can be infused while in position under the camera, thus eliminating delays between tracer injection and the start of image acquisition.

Technetium Tc 99m teboroxime is usually administered during the third minute of the 4- to 5-minute infusion of adenosine, or 2 minutes after the 4-minute dipyridamole infusion.

**Safety considerations for handling this radiopharmaceutical**

Improper handling of this radiopharmaceutical may cause radioactive contamination. Guidelines for handling radioactive material have been prepared by scientific, professional, state, federal, and international bodies and are available to the specially qualified and authorized users who have access to radiopharmaceuticals.

## Parenteral Dosage Forms

### TECHNETIUM Tc 99m TEBOROXIME INJECTION

**Usual adult and adolescent administered activity**

Cardiac imaging—

Intravenous, 555 to 1110 megabecquerels (15 to 30 millicuries).

Note: Due to the short residence time of technetium Tc 99m teboroxime in the myocardium, two separate injections are needed for a stress/rest perfusion study.

When a stress study is to be performed prior to a rest study, it is recommended that an interval of 1¹/₂ hours be allowed for the effects of exercise to dissipate.

For same-day rest/stress studies, a combined dose of 1295 to 1850 megabecquerels (35 to 50 millicuries) is used.

When a rest study is to be performed prior to a stress study, it is only necessary to wait until the residual myocardial activity clears. In most cases, the stress study may be performed in one hour.

**Usual pediatric administered activity**

Minimum dosage has not been established.

**Usual geriatric administered activity**

See *Usual adult and adolescent administered activity.*

**Strength(s) usually available**

U.S.—

2 mg of cyclohexanedione dioxime, 2 mg of methyl boronic acid, 2 mg pentetic acid, 9 mg citric acid (anhydrous), 100 mg sodium chloride, 50 mg gamma cyclodextrin, and 50 mcg stannous chlo-

ride (anhydrous) in lyophilized form under nitrogen atmosphere, per 5-mL reaction vial (Rx) [*CardioTec*].

Note: Technetium Tc 99m teboroxime is a boronic acid technetium dioxime (BATO) derivative.

Canada—
    Not commercially available.

**Packaging and storage**
Store between 15 and 30 °C (59 and 86 °F), unless otherwise specified by manufacturer. Protect from freezing.

Note: Before radiolabeling, the kit is also stored at room temperature.

**Preparation of dosage form**
To prepare technetium Tc 99m teboroxime injection, an oxidant-free sodium pertechnetate Tc 99m solution is used.

During reconstitution, it is important that air is not added to the nitrogen atmosphere of the vial, since air will cause oxidation, thus decreasing the radiochemical purity of the compound.

See manufacturer's package insert for complete instructions.

**Stability**
Product is stable (24-month shelf life before radiolabeling); U.S. package insert states that injection should be administered within 6 hours after preparation since it does not contain a preservative.

**Incompatibilities**
If oxidants such as peroxides and hypochlorites are present in the sodium pertechnetate Tc 99m used for labeling, the final preparation may be adversely affected and should be discarded. Final preparation should appear clear to slightly opalescent and free of particulate matter and discoloration.

**Note**
Caution—Radioactive material.

## Selected Bibliography

Meerdink DJ, Leppo JA. Experimental studies of the physiologic properties of technetium-99m agents: myocardial transport of perfusion imaging agents. Am J Cardiol 1990; 66 (13): 9E-15E.

Berman DS, Kiat H, Van Train KF, et al. Comparison of SPECT using technetium-99m agents and thallium-201 and PET for the assessment of myocardial perfusion and viability. Am J Cardiol 1990; 66 (13): 72E-79E.

Johnson LL, Seldin DW. Clinical experience with technetium-99m teboroxime, a neutral, lipophilic myocardial perfusion imaging agent. Am J Cardiol 1990; 66: 63E-67E.

Revised: 05/18/95

---

**TEMAZEPAM**—See *Benzodiazepines (Systemic)*

---

**TENOXICAM**—See *Anti-inflammatory Drugs, Nonsteroidal (Systemic)*

---

# TERAZOSIN   Systemic

VA CLASSIFICATION (Primary/Secondary): CV150/CV490; GU900

Note: For a listing of dosage forms and brand names by country availability, see *Dosage Forms* section(s). For a listing of brand names for the articles in this monograph, refer to the General Index.

## Category
Antihypertensive; benign prostatic hyperplasia therapy agent.

## Indications

**Accepted**

Hypertension (treatment)—Terazosin is indicated in the treatment of hypertension.

    For additional information on initial therapeutic guidelines related to the treatment of hypertension, see *Appendix III*.

Benign prostatic hyperplasia[1]—Terazosin is indicated in the treatment of symptomatic benign prostatic hyperplasia (BPH). It has been shown to improve urinary flow and symptoms of BPH. However, the long-term effects of terazosin on the incidence of surgery, acute urinary obstruction, or other complications of BPH have not yet been determined.

---

[1]Not included in Canadian product labeling.

## Pharmacology/Pharmacokinetics

**Physicochemical characteristics**
Molecular weight—459.93.
pKa—7.04.

**Mechanism of action/Effect**
Terazosin has a peripheral post-synaptic alpha$_1$-adrenergic blocking action, which is thought to account primarily for its effects.
    Hypertension—
        Terazosin produces vasodilation and reduces peripheral resistance but generally has little effect on cardiac output. Antihypertensive effect with chronic dosing is usually not accompanied by reflex tachycardia. There is little or no effect on renal blood flow or glomerular filtration rate.
    Benign prostatic hyperplasia—
        Relaxation of smooth muscle in the bladder neck, prostate, and prostate capsule produced by alpha$_1$-adrenergic blockade results in a reduction in urethral resistance and pressure, bladder outlet resistance, and urinary symptoms.

**Other actions/effects**
Terazosin may affect serum lipids. The most consistent changes observed are a decrease in levels of serum total cholesterol and low density lipoprotein (LDL) cholesterol plus very low density lipoprotein (VLDL) cholesterol fraction. However, the implications of these changes are unclear.

**Absorption**
Rapid and nearly complete; not affected by food; minimal first-pass metabolism; bioavailability approximately 90%.

**Protein binding**
Very high (90 to 94%).

**Biotransformation**
Hepatic; four metabolites have been identified, one of which (the piperazine derivative of terazosin) has antihypertensive activity.

**Half-life**
Approximately 12 hours; does not appear to be significantly influenced by renal insufficiency.

**Onset of action**
Single dose—15 minutes.

**Time to peak plasma concentration**
Approximately 1 hour.

**Time to peak effect**
Single dose—2 to 3 hours.
Multiple doses—Up to 6 to 8 weeks.

**Duration of action**
Single dose—24 hours.

**Elimination**
Fecal (biliary)—40%.
Fecal (unchanged)—20%.
Renal—40% (10% unchanged).

## Precautions to Consider

**Carcinogenicity**
Studies in rats for two years at doses of 250 mg per kg of body weight (mg/kg) per day (695 times the maximum recommended human dose [MRHD]) found an increase in benign adrenal medullary tumors in male, but not in female, rats. Studies in mice for two years at a maximum tolerated dose of 32 mg/kg per day found no oncogenic effect.

**Mutagenicity**
Both *in vivo* and *in vitro* tests (Ames test, *in vivo* cytogenetics, dominant lethal test in mice, *in vivo* Chinese hamster chromosome aberration test, V$_{79}$ forward mutation assay) found no evidence of mutagenicity.

**Pregnancy/Reproduction**
Fertility—Testicular atrophy occurred in rats given 40 and 250 mg/kg per day for 1 to 2 years, but not in those given 8 mg/kg per day. Testicular atrophy also occurred in dogs given 300 mg/kg per day (more than

800 times the MRHD) for 3 months, but not in those given 20 mg/kg per day for 1 year.

Pregnancy—Adequate and well-controlled studies in humans have not been done.

Studies in rats given oral doses of 480 mg/kg per day (approximately 1330 times the MRHD) found an increased incidence of fetal resorptions. In offspring of rabbits given 165 times the MRHD, there were increased fetal resorptions, decreased fetal weight, and an increased number of supernumerary ribs. No teratogenicity occurred in either rats or rabbits in these studies.

In peri- and postnatal development studies with rats given 120 mg/kg per day (approximately 300 times the MRHD), postpartum death of pups was increased.

FDA Pregnancy Category C.

### Breast-feeding
It is not known whether terazosin is distributed into breast milk. However, problems in humans have not been documented.

### Pediatrics
Appropriate studies on the relationship of age to the effects of terazosin have not been performed in the pediatric population. Safety and efficacy have not been established.

### Geriatrics
Although appropriate studies on the relationship of age to the effects of terazosin have not been performed in the geriatric population, clinical trials have included patients over 65 years of age and have not demonstrated geriatrics-specific problems that would limit the usefulness of terazosin in the elderly. However, the elderly may be more sensitive to the hypotensive effects of terazosin.

### Drug interactions and/or related problems
The following drug interactions and/or related problems have been selected on the basis of their potential clinical significance (possible mechanism in parentheses where appropriate)—not necessarily inclusive (» = major clinical significance):

Note: Combinations containing any of the following medications, depending on the amount present, may also interact with this medication.

Anti-inflammatory drugs, nonsteroidal (NSAIDs), especially indomethacin
(indomethacin, and probably other NSAIDs, may antagonize the antihypertensive effect of terazosin by inhibiting renal prostaglandin synthesis and/or by causing sodium and fluid retention; the patient should be carefully monitored to confirm that the desired effect is being obtained)

Estrogens
(antihypertensive effects of terazosin may be reduced when it is used concurrently with these agents; estrogen-induced fluid retention tends to increase blood pressure; the patient should be carefully monitored to confirm that the desired effect is being obtained)

Hypotension-producing medications, other (See *Appendix II* )
(antihypertensive effects may be potentiated when these medications are used concurrently with terazosin; although some antihypertensive and/or diuretic combinations are frequently used to therapeutic advantage, when used concurrently dosage adjustments are necessary)

Sympathomimetics
(antihypertensive effects of terazosin may be reduced when it is used concurrently with these agents; the patient should be carefully monitored to confirm that the desired effect is being obtained)

(concurrent use of terazosin antagonizes the peripheral vasoconstriction produced by high doses of dopamine)

(concurrent use of terazosin may decrease the pressor response to ephedrine)

(concurrent use of terazosin may block the alpha-adrenergic effects of epinephrine, possibly resulting in severe hypotension and tachycardia)

(concurrent use of terazosin usually decreases, but does not reverse or completely block, the pressor effect of metaraminol)

(prior administration of terazosin may decrease the pressor effect and shorten the duration of action of methoxamine and phenylephrine)

### Laboratory value alterations
The following have been selected on the basis of their potential clinical significance (possible effect in parentheses where appropriate)—not necessarily inclusive (» = major clinical significance):

With physiology/laboratory test values
Albumin and
Total protein
(serum concentrations may be decreased)

Hemoglobin and hematocrit and
White blood cells
(serum concentrations may be decreased)

### Medical considerations/Contraindications
The medical considerations/contraindications included here have been selected on the basis of their potential clinical significance (reasons given in parentheses where appropriate)—not necessarily inclusive (» = major clinical significance).

*Risk-benefit should be considered when the following medical problems exist:*

Angina or
Cardiac disease, severe
(may induce angina or aggravate pre-existing angina)

Hepatic function impairment
(although studies in patients with impaired hepatic function have not been done, terazosin undergoes hepatic metabolism, and, therefore, increased sensitivity or prolonged terazosin effect may occur)

Renal function impairment
(approximately 40% of terazosin dose is eliminated by the kidneys as parent drug or metabolites; therefore, prolonged hypotensive effects may occur)

Sensitivity to terazosin

### Patient monitoring
The following may be especially important in patient monitoring (other tests may be warranted in some patients, depending on condition; » = major clinical significance):

» Blood pressure measurements
(recommended at periodic intervals in patients being treated for hypertension; selected patients may be trained to perform blood pressure measurements at home and report the results at regular physician visits)

## Side/Adverse Effects

Note: A "first-dose orthostatic hypotensive reaction" sometimes occurs, most frequently 30 minutes to 2 hours after the initial dose of terazosin, and may be severe. Syncope or other postural symptoms, such as dizziness, may occur. Subsequent occurrence with dosage increases is also possible. Incidence appears to be dose-related; thus, it is important that therapy be initiated with a 1-mg dose given at bedtime. Patients who are volume-depleted or sodium-restricted may be more sensitive to the orthostatic hypotensive effects of terazosin, and the effect may be exaggerated after exercise.

The following side/adverse effects have been selected on the basis of their potential clinical significance (possible signs and symptoms in parentheses where appropriate)—not necessarily inclusive:

### Those indicating need for medical attention
Incidence more frequent
   *Dizziness*

Incidence less frequent
   *Angina* (chest pain); *dyspnea* (shortness of breath); *edema, peripheral* (swelling of feet or lower legs); *orthostatic hypotension* (dizziness or lightheadedness, when getting up from a lying or sitting position; sudden fainting); *palpitations* (pounding heartbeat); *tachycardia* (fast or irregular heartbeat)

   Note: Rarely, weight gain (usually 1 kg [2 lb] or less) may occur with *peripheral edema.*

### Those indicating need for medical attention only if they continue or are bothersome
Incidence more frequent
   *Asthenia* (unusual tiredness or weakness); *headache*

Incidence less frequent
   *Back or joint pain; blurred vision; nasal congestion* (stuffy nose); *nausea or vomiting; somnolence* (drowsiness)

## Overdose

For more information on the management of overdose or unintentional ingestion, **contact a Poison Control Center** (see *Poison Control Center Listing*).

### Treatment of overdose

Recommended treatment for terazosin overdose includes: Treatment of circulatory failure, either by placing the patient in the supine position and elevating the legs or by using additional measures if shock is present, is most important; volume expanders may be used to treat shock, followed, if necessary, by administration of a vasopressor; symptomatic, supportive treatment and monitoring of fluid and electrolyte status.

## Patient Consultation

As an aid to patient consultation, refer to *Advice for the Patient, Terazosin (Systemic)*.

In providing consultation, consider emphasizing the following selected information (» = major clinical significance):

### Before using this medication
» Conditions affecting use, especially:
    Sensitivity to quinazolines
    Use in the elderly—Increased sensitivity to hypotensive effects
    Other medical problems, especially angina, severe cardiac disease, hepatic function impairment, or renal function impairment

### Proper use of this medication
Getting into the habit of taking at same time each day to help increase compliance
» Proper dosing
Missed dose: Taking as soon as possible the same day; not taking if not remembered until next day; not doubling doses
» Proper storage
*For use as an antihypertensive*
Possible need for control of weight and diet, especially sodium intake
» Patient may not experience symptoms of hypertension; importance of taking medication even if feeling well
» Does not cure, but helps control hypertension; possible need for lifelong therapy; serious consequences of untreated hypertension
*For use in benign prostatic hyperplasia (BPH)*
Relieves symptoms of BPH but does not change the size of the prostate; may not prevent the need for surgery in the future
May require 2 to 6 weeks of therapy before patient experiences improvement of symptoms

### Precautions while using this medication
Regular visits to physician to check progress
» Caution if dizziness, lightheadedness, or sudden fainting occurs, especially after initial dose; taking first dose at bedtime
» Caution when getting up suddenly from a lying or sitting position
» Caution in using alcohol, while standing for long periods or exercising, and during hot weather because of enhanced orthostatic hypotensive effects
» Possibility of drowsiness
» Caution when driving or doing anything else requiring alertness because of possible drowsiness, dizziness, or lightheadedness
» Not taking other medication, especially nonprescription sympathomimetics, unless discussed with physician

### Side/adverse effects
Signs of potential side effects, especially angina, dizziness, dyspnea, orthostatic hypotension, palpitations, peripheral edema, and tachycardia

## General Dosing Information

In order to minimize the "first-dose orthostatic hypotensive reaction," an initial dose of 1 mg is recommended, with gradual increments as needed. Administration of the initial dose at bedtime is recommended, as well as for the initial dose at each increment.

### For use as an antihypertensive
Dosage of terazosin should be adjusted to meet the individual requirements of each patient, on the basis of blood pressure response.

Terazosin may be used alone or in combination with a thiazide diuretic or beta-adrenergic blocker, both of which reduce the tendency for sodium and water retention, although they also produce additive hypotension. If combination therapy is indicated, individual titration is required to ensure the lowest possible therapeutic dose of each drug.

When a diuretic or other antihypertensive agent is added to terazosin therapy, the dose of terazosin should be reduced, followed by titration of dosage of the combination. When terazosin is added to existing diuretic or antihypertensive therapy, the dose of the other agent should be reduced and terazosin started at a dose of 1 mg once a day.

### For use in benign prostatic hyperplasia
Prior to initiation of terazosin therapy, the presence of prostate carcinoma should be ruled out, since prostate carcinoma can present with symptoms similar to those associated with BPH.

## Oral Dosage Forms

### TERAZOSIN HYDROCHLORIDE CAPSULES

Note: The dosing and strengths of the dosage forms available are expressed in terms of terazosin base (not the hydrochloride salt).

#### Usual adult dose
Antihypertensive—
    Initial: Oral, 1 mg (base) once a day, at bedtime.
    Maintenance: Oral, adjusted gradually to meet individual requirements, usually 1 to 5 mg (base) once a day.
Note: If the antihypertensive effect is not maintained for a full 24 hours, twice daily dosing may be more effective.
    Geriatric patients may be more sensitive to the effects of the usual adult dose.
Benign prostatic hyperplasia[1]—
    Initial: Oral, 1 mg (base), at bedtime.
    Maintenance: Oral, adjusted gradually up to 5 to 10 mg (base) once a day. Doses of 10 mg once a day are generally required for an adequate response.

#### Usual adult prescribing limits
Daily doses higher than 20 mg (base) usually do not have increased efficacy.

#### Usual pediatric dose
Safety and efficacy have not been established.

#### Strength(s) usually available
U.S.—
    1 mg (base) (Rx) [*Hytrin*].
    2 mg (base) (Rx) [*Hytrin*].
    5 mg (base) (Rx) [*Hytrin*].
    10 mg (base) (Rx) [*Hytrin*].
Canada—
    1 mg (base) (Rx) [*Hytrin*].
    2 mg (base) (Rx) [*Hytrin*].
    5 mg (base) (Rx) [*Hytrin*].
    10 mg (base) (Rx) [*Hytrin*].

#### Packaging and storage
Store below 40 °C (104 °F), preferably between 15 and 30 °C (59 and 86 °F), unless otherwise specified by manufacturer.

#### Auxiliary labeling
• Do not take other medicines without your doctor's advice.
• May cause dizziness.

#### Note
Check refill frequency to determine compliance in hypertensive patients.

[1]Not included in Canadian product labeling.

## Selected Bibliography
The fifth report of the Joint National Committee on Detection, Evaluation, and Treatment of High Blood Pressure (JNC V). Arch Intern Med 1993; 153 (2): 154-83.

Revised: 06/26/92
Interim revision: 07/08/94

# TERBINAFINE   Systemic*

VA CLASSIFICATION (Primary): AM700
Note: For a listing of dosage forms and brand names by country availability, see *Dosage Forms* section(s). For a listing of brand names
for the articles in this monograph, refer to the General Index.

*Not commercially available in the U.S.

## Category
Antifungal (systemic).

## Indications

### General considerations
Terbinafine has *in vitro* activity against yeasts and a wide range of dermatophyte, filamentous, dimorphic, and dematiaceous fungi. It is fungicidal against dermatophytes, such as *Trichophyton* species, *Microsporum* species, and *Epidermophyton floccosum*, as well as against
*Aspergillus* species, *Scopulariopsis brevicaulis*, *Blastomyces dermatitidis*, *Cryptococcus neoformans*, *Sporothrix schenckii*, *Histoplasma
capsulatum*, *Candida parapsilosis*, and *Pityrosporum* yeasts. Terbinafine has also been shown to be active *in vitro* against the protozoal
organisms *Trypanosoma cruzi* and *Leishmania mexicana mexicana*.
However, clinical efficacy has not been demonstrated in the treatment
of infections caused by *B. dermatitidis*, *H. capsulatum*, *S. schenckii*,
*C. neoformans*, *T. cruzi*, and *L. mexicana mexicana*. Also, terbinafine
is only fungistatic against *Candida albicans*. Clinical studies have
found terbinafine to be only moderately effective against skin infections caused by *Candida* species, with a mycological cure of only 65%
after 2 to 4 weeks of treatment.

### Accepted
Onychomycosis (treatment)—Terbinafine is indicated in the treatment of
onychomycosis (fungal infection of the nails) caused by dermatophyte
fungi.
Tinea capitis (treatment)[1]—Limited data suggest that terbinafine may be
used in the treatment of tinea capitis (ringworm of the scalp).
Tinea corporis (treatment)—Terbinafine is indicated in the treatment of
tinea corporis (ringworm of the body).
Tinea cruris (treatment)—Terbinafine is indicated in the treatment of tinea
cruris (ringworm of the groin; jock itch).
Tinea pedis (treatment)—Terbinafine is indicated in the treatment of interdigital or plantar tinea pedis (ringworm of the foot; athlete's foot).

### Unaccepted
Terbinafine is not effective in the treatment of pityriasis versicolor because
concentrations of oral terbinafine reached in the stratum corneum are
not high enough to treat this condition adequately.

[1]Not included in Canadian product labeling.

## Pharmacology/Pharmacokinetics

### Physicochemical characteristics
Chemical group—Allylamine class.
Molecular weight—Terbinafine hydrochloride: 327.90.

### Mechanism of action/Effect
Terbinafine interferes with fungal ergosterol biosynthesis by inhibiting
squalene epoxidase in the fungal cell membrane. This leads to a deficiency of ergosterol and an intracellular accumulation of squalene,
thus disrupting fungal membrane function and cell wall synthesis, and
resulting in fungal cell death.

### Other actions/effects
Unlike azole antifungal agents, terbinafine does not inhibit cytochrome P-
450 activity and is only weakly bound to hepatic cytochrome P-450,
resulting in a low propensity for interference with cytochrome P-450
enzymes involved in drug metabolism and synthesis of steroid hormones and prostaglandins. Terbinafine also has no effect on 14 alpha-
demethylation.
Terbinafine's mechanism of action against protozoal organisms is thought
to involve inhibition of sterol synthesis.

### Absorption
Readily absorbed from gastrointestinal tract. Bioavailability is 70 to 80%
and is not affected by the presence of food.

### Distribution
Terbinafine is lipophilic and extensively distributed. It rapidly diffuses
from the vascular system, passes through the dermis and epidermis,
and concentrates in the lipophilic stratum corneum. It is also distributed via the sebum to hair follicles and sebum-rich skin, resulting in
high concentrations in hair follicles, hair, sebum-rich skin, and the nail
plate within the first few weeks of therapy. It is also highly distributed
to adipose tissue. After 12 days of treatment, concentrations in the
stratum corneum exceed those in plasma by a factor of 75 and concentrations in the epidermis and dermis exceed those in plasma by a
factor of 25. Blood cells contain approximately 8% of administered
terbinafine. Terbinafine is not detected in sweat.
Vol_D at steady state is approximately 948 L.

### Protein binding
Very high (> 99%), with binding evenly distributed among all plasma
fractions.

### Biotransformation
Terbinafine undergoes first pass metabolism. It is extensively metabolized
in the liver by N-demethylation of the central nitrogen atom, alkyl
side-chain oxidation (alkyl oxidation), and arene oxide formation followed by hydrolysis to the corresponding dihydrodiol. Metabolism involves only a small fraction (< 5%) of total hepatic cytochrome P-450
capacity. Fifteen metabolites have been identified, but none are active.

### Half-life
Absorption—
   Approximately 0.8 hour.
Distribution—
   Approximately 4.6 hours.
Elimination—
   Plasma: 11 to 17 hours.
   Sebum: 3 to 5 days.
   Stratum corneum: 3 to 5 days.
Terminal—
   Sebum: 18 days.
   Plasma: 22 days, due to accumulation in adipose tissue and gradual
      release after discontinuation of treatment.
   Stratum corneum: 22 days.
   Hair and nails: 24 days.
   Dermis and epidermis: 28 days.

### Time to peak concentration
Plasma—Approximately 2 hours. Steady state is reached in 10 to 14 days.
Stratum corneum—Maximum concentrations in the stratum corneum were
   found on Day 12 of treatment. However, terbinafine was detected in
   lower levels of the stratum corneum 24 hours after a single oral dose,
   and fungicidal concentrations were found across the whole of the stratum corneum within 7 days.
Nails—Detected in distal nail clippings as early as 3 weeks after the beginning of therapy. Fungicidal levels in nails were maintained for several weeks after discontinuation of therapy.

### Peak serum concentration
Serum—0.8 to 1.5 mg per L (2.4 to 4.6 micromoles per L).
Nails—250 to 550 nanograms per mg, detected in toenails 3 to 18 weeks
   after starting therapy, with no progressive increase thereafter during
   the 48 weeks of therapy.

### Elimination
Renal—Approximately 80% of an administered dose is excreted in the
   urine as metabolites.
Fecal—Approximately 20% is eliminated in feces.

## Precautions to Consider

### Carcinogenicity
An increase in liver tumors was observed in male rats at the highest dose
   level (69 mg per kg of body weight [mg/kg] per day) during a 123-
   week carcinogenicity study. Other changes included increased enzyme
   activity, peroxisome proliferation, and altered triglyceride metabolism.
   These changes were not seen in mice or monkeys.

### Mutagenicity
*In vitro* and *in vivo* mutagenicity testing of terbinafine revealed no specific
   mutagenic or genotoxic properties. *In vitro* tests of cell transformation
   to malignancy were negative.

### Pregnancy/Reproduction
Fertility—Fertility studies in animals suggest no adverse effects.
Pregnancy—Adequate and well-controlled studies in humans have not
   been done.
Fetal toxicity studies in animals suggest no adverse effects.

**Breast-feeding**

Terbinafine is distributed into breast milk. In 2 women, totals of 0.2 and 0.7 mg of terbinafine were detected in the breast milk after a single oral 500-mg dose in the ablactation period.

**Pediatrics**

No information is available on the relationship of age to the effects of terbinafine in pediatric patients. Safety and efficacy have not been established. However, terbinafine has been used to treat tinea capitis in a small number of children 3 to 16 years of age and was generally well tolerated.

**Geriatrics**

No information is available on the relationship of age to the effects of terbinafine in geriatric patients. However, elderly patients are more likely to have age-related renal function impairment, which may require an adjustment of dosage in patients receiving terbinafine.

**Drug interactions and/or related problems**

The following drug interactions and/or related problems have been selected on the basis of their potential clinical significance (possible mechanism in parentheses where appropriate)—not necessarily inclusive (» = major clinical significance):

Note: Combinations containing any of the following medications, depending on the amount present, may also interact with this medication.

» Alcohol or
» Hepatotoxic medications, other (See *Appendix II*)
(severe hepatitis has been reported rarely with terbinafine; concurrent use of other hepatotoxic medications may increase the risk of hepatotoxicity)

Caffeine
(terbinafine was found to decrease the clearance of caffeine by 20%)

» Enzyme inducers, hepatic, cytochrome P-450 (See *Appendix II*)
(because terbinafine is hepatically metabolized, medications, such as rifampin, that induce the cytochrome P-450 system may increase the clearance of terbinafine)

» Enzyme inhibitors, hepatic, cytochrome P-450
(because terbinafine is hepatically metabolized, medications, such as cimetidine, that inhibit the cytochrome P-450 system may decrease the clearance of terbinafine)

**Laboratory value alterations**

The following have been selected on the basis of their potential clinical significance (possible effect in parentheses where appropriate)—not necessarily inclusive (» = major clinical significance):

With physiology/laboratory test values
Alanine aminotransferase (ALT [SGPT]) and
Aspartate aminotransferase (AST [SGOT])
(values may rarely be transiently increased)

**Medical considerations/Contraindications**

The medical considerations/contraindications included here have been selected on the basis of their potential clinical significance (reasons given in parentheses where appropriate)—not necessarily inclusive (» = major clinical significance):

*Risk-benefit should be considered when the following medical problems exist:*

» Alcoholism, active or in remission or
» Hepatic function impairment
(severe hepatitis has been reported with terbinafine on rare occasion; patients with alcoholism or hepatic function impairment may be at increased risk of severe hepatotoxicity; hepatic function impairment was found to reduce the clearance of terbinafine by approximately 30%; it is recommended that patients with pre-existing stable chronic liver function impairment receive a 50% reduction in dose)

» Hypersensitivity to terbinafine
» Renal function impairment
(terbinafine elimination was found to be reduced in patients with renal function impairment; the elimination half-life was increased from 16 to 24 hours; it is recommended that patients with impaired renal function [creatinine clearance < 50 mL per min (0.83 mL per sec) or serum creatinine greater than 3.4 mg per dL (300 micromoles per L)] receive a 50% reduction in dose)

**Patient monitoring**

The following may be especially important in patient monitoring (other tests may be warranted in some patients, depending on condition; » = major clinical significance):

Clinical assessment
(a follow-up clinical assessment is recommended after terbinafine therapy has ended, to determine whether relapse has occurred; the timing of this assessment depends on the condition being treated; for tinea corporis, tinea cruris, and tinea pedis, it is recommended that the assessment be performed at 6 to 8 weeks following cessation of treatment, for onychomycosis of the fingernails, it is recommended that the assessment be at 4 to 6 months, and for onychomycosis of the toenails, it is recommended that the assessment be at 6 to 9 months following cessation of treatment)

Hepatic function determinations
(liver function tests are recommended before therapy, and periodically during terbinafine treatment, in patients with hepatic function impairment, alcoholic patients, or patients taking hepatotoxic medications concurrently)

## Side/Adverse Effects

Note: Loss of taste has been reported rarely during terbinafine treatment, with the onset occurring 5 to 8 weeks after the start of therapy. This effect is reversible upon discontinuation of terbinafine, but recovery may take 2 to 6 weeks. There also has been one case of tongue discoloration associated with terbinafine.

The following side/adverse effects have been selected on the basis of their potential clinical significance (possible signs and symptoms in parentheses where appropriate)—not necessarily inclusive:

**Those indicating need for medical attention**

Incidence less frequent
*Hypersensitivity* (skin rash or itching)

Incidence rare
*Hepatitis* (dark urine; fatigue; loss of appetite; pale stools; yellow eyes or skin); *neutropenia* (fever, chills, or sore throat); *pancytopenia* (fever, chills, or sore throat; pale skin; unusual bleeding or bruising; unusual tiredness or weakness); *Stevens-Johnson syndrome* (aching joints and muscles; redness, blistering, peeling, or loosening of skin; unusual tiredness or weakness); *toxic epidermal necrolysis* (difficulty in swallowing; redness, blistering, peeling, or loosening of skin)

**Those indicating need for medical attention only if they continue or are bothersome**

Incidence more frequent
*Gastrointestinal disturbances* (diarrhea; loss of appetite; nausea and vomiting; stomach pain, mild)

Incidence less frequent
*Change of taste or loss of taste*

## Patient Consultation

As an aid to patient consultation, refer to *Advice for the Patient, Terbinafine (Systemic)*.

In providing consultation, consider emphasizing the following selected information (» = major clinical significance):

**Before using this medication**

» Conditions affecting use, especially:
Hypersensitivity to terbinafine
Breast-feeding—Terbinafine is distributed into breast milk
Other medications, especially alcohol, cytochrome P-450 enzyme inducers and inhibitors, and other hepatotoxic medications
Other medical problems, especially alcoholism, hepatic function impairment, and renal function impairment

**Proper use of this medication**

May be taken with or without food
» Compliance with full course of therapy
» Importance of not missing doses and taking at evenly spaced times
» Proper dosing
Missed dose: Taking as soon as possible; not taking if almost time for next dose; not doubling doses
» Proper storage

**Precautions while using this medication**

Regular visits to physician to check progress during therapy
Checking with physician if no improvement within a few weeks (or months for onychomycosis)
Caution in drinking alcoholic beverages during terbinafine therapy

**Side/adverse effects**

Signs of potential side effects, especially hypersensitivity, hepatitis, neutropenia, pancytopenia, Stevens-Johnson syndrome, and toxic epidermal necrolysis

# General Dosing Information

Terbinafine may be taken with or without food.

To prevent relapse, therapy should be continued until the infecting organism is completely eradicated as determined by clinical or laboratory examination. Representative treatment periods are: onychomycosis, 6 weeks to 3 months; tinea corporis and tinea cruris, 2 to 4 weeks; and tinea pedis, 2 to 6 weeks.

Patients with pre-existing, stable chronic liver dysfunction or impaired renal function (creatinine clearance < 50 mL per min [0.83 mL per sec] or serum creatinine greater than 3.4 mg per dL [300 micromoles per L]) should receive a 50% reduction of the regular dose.

## Oral Dosage Forms

### TERBINAFINE HYDROCHLORIDE TABLETS

**Usual adult and adolescent dose**
Antifungal—
   Onychomycosis: Oral, 125 mg two times a day, or 250 mg once a day, for 6 weeks to 3 months. Some toenail infections may require longer therapy, depending on the extent of the infection.
   Tinea capitis[1]: Oral, 125 mg two times a day, or 250 mg once a day, for 4 to 6 weeks.
   Tinea corporis: Oral, 125 mg two times a day, or 250 mg once a day, for 2 to 4 weeks.
   Tinea cruris: Oral, 125 mg two times a day, or 250 mg once a day, for 2 to 4 weeks.
   gcpTinea pedis (interdigital or plantar): Oral, 125 mg two times a day, or 250 mg once a day, for 2 to 6 weeks.

**Usual pediatric dose**
Dosage has not been established. However, in one study the following doses were used in the treatment of tinea capitis in children 3 to 16 years of age—
   Children 12.5 to 18.5 kg of body weight: Oral, 62.5 mg once a day.
   Children 18.5 to 25 kg of body weight: Oral, 125 mg once a day.
   Children more than 25 kg of body weight: Oral, 250 mg once a day.

**Strength(s) usually available**
U.S.—
   Not commercially available.
Canada—
   125 mg (Rx) [*Lamisil*].
   250 mg (Rx) [*Lamisil*].

**Packaging and storage**
Store below 40 °C (104 °F), preferably between 15 and 30 °C (59 and 86 °F), unless otherwise specified by manufacturer.

**Auxiliary labeling**
• Continue medicine for full time of treatment.

[1]Not included in Canadian product labeling.

## Selected Bibliography

Balfour JA, Faulds D. Terbinafine. A review of its pharmacodynamic and pharmacokinetic properties, and therapeutic potential in superficial mycoses. Drugs 1992; 43 (2): 259-84.

Developed: 06/22/95

---

# TERBINAFINE    Topical†

VA CLASSIFICATION (Primary): DE102
Note: For a listing of dosage forms and brand names by country availability, see *Dosage Forms* section(s). For a listing of brand names for the articles in this monograph, refer to the General Index.

   †Not commercially available in Canada.

## Category

Antifungal (topical).

## Indications

**Accepted**
Tinea corporis (treatment)
Tinea cruris (treatment) or
Tinea pedis (treatment)—Terbinafine is indicated as a primary agent in the topical treatment of tinea corporis (ringworm of the body), tinea cruris (ringworm of the groin; jock itch), or tinea pedis (ringworm of the foot; athlete's foot) caused by *Trichophyton rubrum*, *T. mentagrophytes*, or *Epidermophyton floccosum* (*Acrothesium floccosum*).

## Pharmacology/Pharmacokinetics

**Physicochemical characteristics**
Source—A synthetic allylamine derivative.
Molecular weight—Terbinafine hydrochloride: 327.90.

**Mechanism of action/Effect**
Fungicidal; inhibits squalene epoxidase (a key enzyme in sterol biosynthesis in fungi), which results in a deficiency in ergosterol and a corresponding increase in squalene within the fungal cell, causing fungal cell death. Also fungistatic; interferes with membrane synthesis and growth.

**Absorption**
Limited absorption may occur.

**Elimination**
Approximately 75% of topically absorbed terbinafine is eliminated in the urine, mostly as metabolites.

## Precautions to Consider

**Cross-sensitivity and/or related problems**
Patients sensitive to the oral form of terbinafine may be sensitive to the topical form also.

**Carcinogenicity/Tumorigenicity**
A 2-year carcinogenicity study in mice showed a 4% incidence of splenic hemangiosarcomas and a 6% incidence of leiomyosarcoma-like tumors of the seminal vesicles in males administered terbinafine orally in doses of 156 mg per kg of body weight (mg/kg) per day. A carcinogenicity study in rats showed a 6% incidence of liver tumors, which were associated with peroxisomal proliferation, and skin lipomas in males administered terbinafine orally in doses of 69 mg/kg per day.

**Mutagenicity**
*In vitro* and *in vivo* genotoxicity tests, including Ames assay, mutagenicity evaluation in Chinese hamster ovarian cells, chromosome aberration test, sister chromatid exchanges, and mouse micronucleus test, revealed no evidence of mutagenic or clastogenic potential for terbinafine.

**Pregnancy/Reproduction**
Fertility—Reproductive studies in rats administered terbinafine orally in doses of up to 300 mg/kg per day did not show any adverse effects on fertility. In addition, terbinafine in doses of 150 mg per day administered intravaginally to pregnant rabbits did not increase the incidence of abortions or premature deliveries and did not affect fetal parameters.

Pregnancy—Adequate and well-controlled studies in humans have not been done.

Terbinafine was not teratogenic when it was administered orally at doses of up to 300 mg/kg per day during organogenesis in rats and rabbits, administered subcutaneously at doses of up to 100 mg/kg per day in rats, or administered percutaneously at doses of up to 150 mg/kg per day in rabbits.

FDA Pregnancy Category B.

**Breast-feeding**

Terbinafine is distributed into breast milk after oral administration. However, it is not known whether terbinafine is distributed into breast milk after topical administration.

Terbinafine was administered orally in single 500-mg doses to 2 lactating women. The total amounts of terbinafine recovered during the following 72-hour period were 0.65 mg and 0.15 mg. This corresponded to 0.13 and 0.03% of the administered dose, respectively.

**Pediatrics**

No information is available on the relationship of age to the effects of terbinafine in pediatric patients. Safety and efficacy have not been established in infants and children up to 12 years of age.

**Geriatrics**

No information is available on the relationship of age to the effects of terbinafine in geriatric patients.

## Side/Adverse Effects

The following side/adverse effects have been selected on the basis of their potential clinical significance (possible signs and symptoms in parentheses where appropriate)—not necessarily inclusive:

**Those indicating need for medical attention**

Incidence rare

*Hypersensitivity* (redness, itching, burning, blistering, swelling, oozing, or other signs of skin irritation not present before use of this medicine)

## Overdose

For more information on the management of overdose or unintentional ingestion, **contact a Poison Control Center** (see *Poison Control Center Listing*).

**Treatment of overdose**

Acute overdosage with topical application of terbinafine hydrochloride is unlikely due to the limited absorption of the topically applied drug and would not be expected to lead to a life-threatening situation.

## Patient Consultation

As an aid to patient consultation, refer to *Advice for the Patient, Terbinafine (Topical)*.

In providing consultation, consider emphasizing the following selected information (» = major clinical significance):

**Before using this medication**

» Conditions affecting use, especially:
    Sensitivity to terbinafine

**Proper use of this medication**

    Applying sufficient medication to cover affected and surrounding areas, and rubbing in gently
» Avoiding contact with the eyes
» Not applying occlusive dressing over this medication unless directed to do so by physician
» Proper dosing
» Compliance with full course of therapy; fungal infections may require prolonged therapy
    Missed dose: Applying as soon as possible; not applying if almost time for next dose
» Proper storage

**Precautions while using this medication**

    Checking with physician if no improvement within 4 weeks
» Using hygienic measures to help cure infection and prevent reinfection
*For tinea corporis*
    Carefully drying the body after bathing
    Avoiding excess heat and humidity if possible; keeping moisture from accumulating on affected areas of the body
    Wearing well-ventilated, loose-fitting clothing
    Using a bland, absorbent powder once or twice daily; using the powder after the cream has been applied and has disappeared into the skin
*For tinea cruris*
    Avoiding underwear that is tight-fitting or made from synthetic materials; wearing loose-fitting cotton underwear instead

Using a bland, absorbent powder on the skin; using the powder between administration times for terbinafine
*For tinea pedis*
    Carefully drying feet, especially between toes, after bathing
    Avoiding socks made from wool or synthetic materials; wearing clean, cotton socks and changing them daily or more often if feet perspire excessively
    Wearing sandals or well-ventilated shoes
    Using a bland, absorbent powder between toes, on feet, and in socks and shoes liberally once or twice daily; using the powder between administration times for terbinafine

**Side/adverse effects**

    Signs of potential side effects, especially hypersensitivity

## Topical Dosage Forms

### TERBINAFINE HYDROCHLORIDE CREAM

**Usual adult and adolescent dose**

Tinea corporis or
Tinea cruris—
    Topical, to the skin and surrounding areas, one or two times a day.
Tinea pedis—
    Topical, to the skin and surrounding areas, two times a day.

Note: Treatment should be continued for at least 1 week *and* until there is significant improvement in the clinical signs and symptoms of the disease. Treatment should not exceed 4 weeks.

**Usual pediatric dose**

Tinea corporis or
Tinea cruris or
Tinea pedis—
    Infants and children up to 12 years of age: Safety and efficacy have not been established.
    Children 12 years of age and over: See *Usual adult and adolescent dose*.

**Strength(s) usually available**

U.S.—
    1% (Rx) [*Lamisil*].
Canada—
    Not commercially available.

**Packaging and storage**

Store between 5 and 30 °C (41 and 86 °F), unless otherwise specified by manufacturer.

**Auxiliary labeling**

• For external use only.
• Continue medicine for full time of treatment.

## Selected Bibliography

Berman B, et al. Efficacy of a 1-week twice-daily regimen of terbinafine 1% cream in the treatment of interdigital tinea pedis. J Am Acad Derm 1992 Jun; 26 (6): 956-60.

Revised: 07/29/93

**TERBUTALINE**—See *Bronchodilators, Adrenergic (Systemic)*

**TERCONAZOLE**—See *Antifungals, Azole (Vaginal)*

**TERFENADINE**—See *Antihistamines (Systemic)*

**TERFENADINE-CONTAINING COMBINATIONS**—

Terfenadine and Pseudoephedrine (Systemic)—See *Antihistamines and Decongestants (Systemic)*

# TERIPARATIDE   Systemic†

VA CLASSIFICATION (Primary/Secondary): DX900/HS600

Other commonly used names are synthetic human parathyroid hormone 1–34 and hPTH 1–34.

Note: For a listing of dosage forms and brand names by country availability, see *Dosage Forms* section(s). For a listing of brand names for the articles in this monograph, refer to the General Index.

†Not commercially available in Canada.

## Category

Diagnostic aid (hypoparathyroidism vs. pseudohypoparathyroidism).

## Indications

Note: Bracketed information in the *Indications* section refers to uses that are not included in U.S. product labeling.

**Accepted**

Hypoparathyroidism, idiopathic (diagnosis) or
Pseudohypoparathyroidism (diagnosis)—Indicated to assist in confirming a preliminary diagnosis based on serum immunoreactive parathyroid hormone (iPTH) values in patients presenting with clinical or laboratory evidence of hypocalcemia (total serum calcium below approximately 1.8 mmol per liter), when the low serum calcium is due either to idiopathic hypoparathyroidism or pseudohypoparathyroidism, type 1 or type 2.

[Teriparatide may sometimes be used to detect a subtle abnormality of calcium metabolism in patients who have borderline or intermittent mild hypocalcemia and borderline or intermittent elevations of iPTH, but have signs and symptoms of pseudohypoparathyroidism, such as hyperphosphatemia, premature cataracts, skeletal anomalies, or a family history of pseudohypoparathyroidism. Teriparatide may also be used to differentiate between types 1 and 2 pseudohypoparathyroidism.]

**Unaccepted**

Teriparatide is *not* intended for recurrent or chronic use and is *not* used therapeutically in the treatment of osteoporosis.

## Pharmacology/Pharmacokinetics

**Mechanism of action/Effect**

Administration of the exogenous human parathyroid hormone, teriparatide, distinguishes between hypoparathyroidism and pseudohypoparathyroidism by testing the patient's responsiveness to parathyroid hormone (PTH). Teriparatide stimulates the urinary excretion of cyclic adenosine 3',5'-monophosphate (cAMP) and phosphate. Response values are calculated from the measurements of urinary cAMP, serum phosphate, and urinary phosphate, and corrected for creatinine excretion.

In patients with idiopathic hypoparathyroidism (a deficiency in PTH secretion), teriparatide will produce normal or increased responses in urinary cAMP and phosphate excretion. In contrast, patients with pseudohypoparathyroidism (a rare form of hypoparathyroidism resulting from target tissue resistance to PTH), because they are unable to respond to PTH, will exhibit a blunted to normal response in urinary cAMP excretion, depending on whether it is type 1 or 2 pseudohypoparathyroidism, and a blunted phosphaturic response.

**Other actions/effects**

Renal—Calcium clearance is reduced and tubular phosphate reabsorption is inhibited, thereby increasing phosphate excretion. Parathyroid hormone indirectly increases the intestinal transport of calcium by increasing renal 1,25-dihydroxyvitamin $D_3$ production, and increases sodium and potassium excretion. These renal effects may be due to a direct action of the hormone on its receptors.

Skeletal—Initial effect on bone is to promote an increased rate of release of calcium from bone into the blood, possibly mediated by an effect on osteocytes or osteoclasts.

Serum—Plasma cAMP values are increased in normal subjects after teriparatide infusion, but response may be blunted in type 1 pseudohypoparathyroidism; serum prolactin and 1,25-dihydroxyvitamin $D_3$ are increased but responses may be blunted in type 1 pseudohypoparathyroidism; however, differentiation between type 1 and type 2 pseudohypoparathyroidism depends on renal responses to teriparatide, not changes in measurements of plasma cAMP, prolactin, and 1,25-dihydroxyvitamin $D_3$.

**Time to peak excretion**

cAMP—During the first 30 minutes postinfusion.
Phosphate—During the second 30 minutes postinfusion.

## Precautions to Consider

**Cross-sensitivity and/or related problems**

Since teriparatide is a peptide, patients who are allergic to other peptides may have a systemic allergic reaction to teriparatide. In addition, patients who are allergic to gelatin should not use teriparatide, because it is stabilized with a gelatin vehicle.

**Carcinogenicity/Mutagenicity**

No studies have been performed to evaluate the carcinogenic or mutagenic potential of teriparatide.

**Pregnancy/Reproduction**

Fertility—Adequate and well controlled studies have not been done in animals or humans.

Pregnancy—Adequate and well controlled studies have not been done in animals or humans.

FDA Pregnancy Category C.

**Breast-feeding**

It is not known to what extent teriparatide is distributed into breast milk. The peptide would not be expected to be absorbed in an active form from the infant's gastrointestinal tract. However, caution should be exercised when teriparatide is administered to a nursing mother.

**Pediatrics**

Appropriate studies on the relationship of age to the effects of teriparatide have not been performed in the pediatric population. However, no pediatrics-specific problems have been documented to date in children 3 years of age and older.

**Geriatrics**

No geriatrics-specific information is available on whether the risk of teriparatide-induced adverse effects is increased in geriatric patients.

**Medical considerations/Contraindications**

The medical considerations/contraindications included here have been selected on the basis of their potential clinical significance (reasons given in parentheses where appropriate)—not necessarily inclusive (» = major clinical significance).

*Except under special circumstances, this medication should not be used when the following medical problem exists:*
»   Sensitivity, known, to teriparatide, gelatin, or other peptides
      (systemic allergic reaction may be potentiated)

## Side/Adverse Effects

The following side/adverse effects have been selected on the basis of their potential clinical significance (possible signs and symptoms in parentheses where appropriate)—not necessarily inclusive:

**Those not indicating need for medical attention**

Incidence rare
   *Gastrointestinal effects* (abdominal or stomach cramps; diarrhea or an urge to defecate; nausea); *metallic taste; pain at injection site during or following infusion; tingling feeling in hands and feet*

## Overdose

For information on the management of overdose, **contact a Poison Control Center** (see *Poison Control Center Listing*).

**Clinical effects of overdose**

The following effects have been selected on the basis of their potential clinical significance (possible signs and symptoms in parentheses where appropriate)–not necessarily inclusive:

   *Hypercalcemia* (muscle weakness; constipation; headache; loss of appetite; shortened QT interval on EKG)—may be produced by repeated doses in excess of 500 units

**Treatment of overdose**

Discontinue infusion of teriparatide.
Supportive care—
   Ensuring adequate hydration.

## Patient Consultation

As an aid to patient consultation, refer to *Advice for the Patient, Teriparatide (Systemic)*.

In providing consultation, consider emphasizing the following selected information (» = major clinical significance):

**Description of use**
Purpose of test: Differentiation between hypoparathyroidism and pseudohypoparathyroidism
Blood and urine collections before and after test
Dose of teriparatide, based on body weight, injected intravenously over 10-minute period

**Before having this test**
» Conditions affecting use, especially:
Sensitivity to teriparatide or other peptides, or gelatin
Breast-feeding—Caution when administered to a nursing mother; extent of distribution into breast milk unknown

**Preparation for this test**
» Following physician's instructions carefully
Not eating or drinking after 8:00 p.m. the evening before this test
Drinking 200 mL (6–7 ounces) of water every 30 minutes starting 2.5 hours before test

## General Dosing Information

Hypocalcemia will stimulate parathyroid hormone secretion in patients with pseudohypoparathyroidism but not with hypoparathyroidism. Since hypocalcemia increases the contrast between iPTH values, iPTH is best measured when serum calcium is below normal, either before treatment is begun or after a brief period of less intensive therapy.

The change from baseline (mean of three preinfusion values) of the urinary cAMP excretion measurement in the first 30 minutes postinfusion is the most sensitive indicator for differentiation between the hypoparathyroid and pseudohypoparathyroid syndromes. However, the differentiation between types 1 and 2 pseudoparathyroidism depends on the phosphaturic response. In type 1, both the increase in urinary cAMP and the phosphaturic response are blunted, but in type 2, a blunted phosphaturic response occurs despite a normal cAMP.

Teriparatide should *not* be administered in repeated doses for recurrent or chronic use, as in the treatment of osteoporosis.

**Testing protocol (modified Ellsworth-Howard test)**
Suggested protocol consists of the following:
• Ascertaining patient's fasting state (overnight).
• Performing procedure at a standardized time (0830 to 1100 hours) because of diurnal variations in phosphate and cAMP metabolism.
• Having patient ingest 200 mL of water every 30 minutes starting 2.5 hours (0600 hours) prior to and continuing through the test period, to ensure hydration and adequate urine output. Collecting timed 30-minute urine samples (0830 to 1100 hours) for measurements of phosphate, cAMP, and creatinine concentrations. Alternately, beginning hydration at 0630 hours, using only 2 urine collections (at 0900 and 0930 hours, respectively), and drawing the first blood sample at 0915 hours.
• Drawing blood samples (0845, 0945, 1015, and 1045 hours) for measurements of serum creatinine and phosphate concentrations, which are needed to calculate glomerular filtration rate and tubular reabsorption of phosphate.

• Inserting indwelling catheter into a vein in the upper extremity (0945 hours).
• Infusing teriparatide acetate intravenously (1000 to 1010 hours).

**Interpretation of results**
Responses are based on the 30-minute change from baseline of cAMP per unit of glomerular filtration, and the 60-minute percentage fall in tubular maximum for phosphate reabsorption and include:
• For pseudohypoparathyroidism, type 1—Blunted response (less than sixfold increase over baseline) in urinary cAMP excretion; blunted response (less than threefold increase) in urinary phosphate excretion.
• For pseudohypoparathyroidism, type 2—Normal cAMP response; blunted response (less than threefold increase) in phosphate excretion.
• For hypoparathyroidism—Normal or increased (tenfold or greater) cAMP response; normal or increased (threefold or greater) phosphaturic response.

Note: Interpretation of results requires calculation of tubular maximum for phosphate reabsorption and a nomogram for the derivation of renal threshold phosphate concentration.

## Parenteral Dosage Forms

### TERIPARATIDE ACETATE FOR INJECTION

**Usual adult and adolescent dose**
Diagnostic aid—
Intravenous, 5 units per kg of body weight infused at a steady rate over a ten-minute period.

**Usual adult prescribing limits**
200 units.

**Usual pediatric dose**
Diagnostic aid—Children 3 years of age and older—
Intravenous, 3 units per kg of body weight, up to a maximum of 200 units, infused over a ten-minute period.

**Size(s) usually available**
U.S.—
200 units (hPTH activity) (Rx) [*Parathar* (gelatin, 20 mg; may also contain up to 35% extraneous peptides of undetermined chemical structure)].
Canada—
Not commercially available.

**Packaging and storage**
Store between 15 and 30 °C (59 and 86 °F), unless otherwise specified by manufacturer.

**Preparation of dosage form**
Teriparatide acetate for injection is reconstituted for intravenous infusion by adding the 10 mL of diluent (0.9% sodium chloride injection) to the sterile, lyophilized powder in the 10-mL single-dose vial, and shaking to dissolve.

**Stability**
Reconstituted solution should be used within 4 hours and any unused solution discarded.

Revised: 06/22/92
Interim revision: 06/15/94

---

# TESTOLACTONE   Systemic†

VA CLASSIFICATION (Primary): AN500
Note: For a listing of dosage forms and brand names by country availability, see *Dosage Forms* section(s). For a listing of brand names for the articles in this monograph, refer to the General Index.

†Not commercially available in Canada.

## Category
Antineoplastic.

## Indications

**Accepted**
Carcinoma, breast (treatment)—Testolactone is indicated as adjunctive therapy in the palliative treatment of advanced or disseminated breast cancer in postmenopausal women when hormone therapy is indicated. It may also be used in women who were diagnosed with disseminated breast carcinoma when premenopausal, in whom ovarian function has

subsequently been terminated.
Testolactone is not recommended for treatment of breast cancer in males.

## Pharmacology/Pharmacokinetics

**Physicochemical characteristics**
Molecular weight—300.40.

**Mechanism of action/Effect**
Testolactone is structurally similar to androgens but is not known to cause virilization. The mechanism of its antineoplastic activity is unknown, although it is reported to inhibit steroid aromatase activity (the effect may be noncompetitive and irreversible) and reduce estrone synthesis from adrenal androstenedione (the major source of estrogen in postmenopausal women).

**Absorption**
Well absorbed from the gastrointestinal tract.

**Biotransformation**
Hepatic.

**Onset of action**
Clinical effects may not be apparent for 6 to 12 weeks.

**Elimination**
Renal.

## Precautions to Consider

### Carcinogenicity/Mutagenicity
Studies have not been done in either animals or humans.

### Pregnancy/Reproduction
Pregnancy—Adequate and well-controlled studies in humans have not been done.

Studies in rats at doses 5 to 15 times the recommended human dose have found that testolactone causes increased fetal mortality, increased abnormal fetal development, and increased mortality in growing pups. It did not cause teratogenicity in rabbits given 2.5 to 7.5 times the recommended human dose.

FDA Pregnancy Category C.

### Breast-feeding
It is not known whether testolactone is excreted in breast milk. However, problems in humans have not been documented.

### Geriatrics
No information is available on the relationship of age to the effects of testolactone in geriatric patients.

### Drug interactions and/or related problems
The following drug interactions and/or related problems have been selected on the basis of their potential clinical significance (possible mechanism in parentheses where appropriate)—not necessarily inclusive (» = major clinical significance):

Anticoagulants, coumarin- or indandione-type
(effects may be increased by concurrent use of testolactone; dosage adjustment of oral anticoagulants may be necessary)

### Laboratory value alterations
The following have been selected on the basis of their potential clinical significance (possible effect in parentheses where appropriate)—not necessarily inclusive (» = major clinical significance):

With physiology/laboratory test values
Calcium
(serum concentrations may be increased; immobilized patients are especially likely to develop hypercalcemia)

Creatinine and
17-Ketosteroid
(urinary concentrations may be increased)

Estradiol measured by radioimmunoassay
(concentrations may be decreased)

### Medical considerations/Contraindications
The medical considerations/contraindications included here have been selected on the basis of their potential clinical significance (reasons given in parentheses where appropriate)—not necessarily inclusive (» = major clinical significance).

*Risk-benefit should be considered when the following medical problems exist:*
»   Cardiorenal disease
»   Hypercalcemia
»   Sensitivity to testolactone

### Patient monitoring
The following are especially important in patient monitoring (other tests may be warranted in some patients, depending on condition; » = major clinical significance):

»   Calcium concentrations, serum
(recommended at periodic intervals, especially in patients with active remission of bone metastases)

## Side/Adverse Effects
The following side/adverse effects have been selected on the basis of their potential clinical significance (possible signs and symptoms in parentheses where appropriate)—not necessarily inclusive:

**Those indicating need for medical attention**
Incidence less frequent
*Peripheral neuropathies* (numbness or tingling of fingers, toes, or face)

**Those indicating need for medical attention only if they continue or are bothersome**
Incidence less frequent
*Diarrhea; loss of appetite; nausea or vomiting; pain or swelling in feet or lower legs; swelling or redness of tongue*

## Patient Consultation

As an aid to patient consultation, refer to *Advice for the Patient, Testolactone (Systemic).*

Consider advising the patient on the following (» = major clinical significance):

### Before using this medication
»   Conditions affecting use, especially:
Sensitivity to testolactone
Pregnancy—Causes increased fetal and pup mortality and abnormal fetal development in rats
Other medical problems, especially cardiorenal disease

### Proper use of this medication
»   Importance of not taking more or less medication than the amount prescribed
»   Possible nausea and vomiting; importance of continuing medication despite stomach upset
Checking with physician if vomiting occurs shortly after dose is taken
»   Proper dosing
Missed dose: Taking as soon as possible, not taking if almost time for next dose; not doubling doses; checking with physician if two or more doses in a row are missed
»   Proper storage

### Precautions while using this medication
»   Importance of close monitoring by the physician

### Side/adverse effects
Signs of potential side effects, especially peripheral neuropathies
Physician or nurse can help in dealing with side effects

## General Dosing Information

Patients receiving testolactone should be under supervision of a physician experienced in cancer chemotherapy.

If hypercalcemia occurs, therapy with testolactone should be withdrawn and the patient treated with large volumes of fluid.

Testolactone should be given for at least 3 months before it is considered ineffective, unless active progression of the disease occurs.

## Oral Dosage Forms
### TESTOLACTONE TABLETS USP

**Usual adult dose**
Breast carcinoma—
Oral, 250 mg four times a day.

**Strength(s) usually available**
U.S.—
50 mg (Rx) [*Teslac*].
Canada—
Not commercially available.

**Packaging and storage**
Store below 40 °C (104 °F), preferably between 15 and 30 °C (59 and 86 °F), unless otherwise specified by manufacturer. Store in a tight container.

---

Revised: 08/04/92
Interim revision: 06/30/94

---

**TESTOSTERONE**—See *Androgens (Systemic)*

---

**TESTOSTERONE-CONTAINING COMBINATIONS**—

Testosterone and Estradiol (Systemic)—See *Androgens and Estrogens (Systemic)*

---

**TETANUS AND DIPHTHERIA TOXOIDS (TD)**—See *Diphtheria and Tetanus Toxoids (Systemic)*

# TETANUS TOXOID   Systemic

VA CLASSIFICATION (Primary): IM200

Note: For a listing of dosage forms and brand names by country availability, see *Dosage Forms* section(s). For a listing of brand names for the articles in this monograph, refer to the General Index.

## Category

Immunizing agent (active).

## Indications

### Accepted

Tetanus (prophylaxis)—Tetanus toxoid is indicated for immunization against tetanus. The main objectives of tetanus immunization are to prevent tetanus infection and the severe complications, including death, that arise from the toxins produced by *Clostridium tetani*. Although the spores of tetanus are ubiquitous, naturally acquired immunity to tetanus does not occur in the U.S., and primary immunization and booster injections are essential to protect persons in all age groups.

Unless otherwise contraindicated, all infants 6 to 8 weeks of age and older, all children, and all adults should be immunized against tetanus with the primary series of tetanus toxoid and a booster injection every 10 years throughout their lives, including:
- Adults, especially those 50 years of age and older. In recent years, approximately two-thirds of persons contracting tetanus have been in this age group.
- Persons with uncertain histories of a complete primary series with tetanus toxoid or immunizing agents containing tetanus toxoid.
- Travelers.
- Persons at increased risk of receiving lacerations and abrasions through their occupation or recreation.
- Persons with known sensitivity to horse serum or with asthma or other allergies. This is to minimize the possible need for passive immunization with tetanus antitoxin (TAT) of animal origin (usually horse) if a wound is received. Although human tetanus immune globulin (TIG) is usually used for passive immunization, TAT of animal origin still may be used in certain areas of the world and has the potential of causing adverse reactions in hypersensitive patients.
- Pregnant women who are unimmunized or inadequately immunized and who may deliver their infants under unhygienic conditions, thereby exposing their infants to neonatal tetanus.
- Those recovering from tetanus. Since a tetanus infection does not confer immunity, especially in the U.S., immunization with tetanus toxoid should be initiated or continued at the time of recovery from the illness.

In addition, persons who are injured may require emergency tetanus prophylaxis depending on the number of primary immunizations, the timing of any boosters, and/or the type of wound received.

It is recommended that infants and children 6 weeks up to 7 years of age receive tetanus toxoid as part of Diphtheria and Tetanus Toxoids and Pertussis Vaccine Adsorbed (DTP) immunization according to the DTP immunization schedule. In those cases where the pertussis vaccine is contraindicated, it is recommended that Diphtheria and Tetanus Toxoids for pediatric use (DT) be administered instead, according to the DT immunization schedule.

It is recommended that children 7 years of age and older and all adults receive tetanus toxoid as part of Tetanus and Diphtheria Toxoids for adult use (Td) both for the primary series and for the booster doses every 10 years.

When the single-entity vaccine is used, tetanus toxoid adsorbed is the vaccine of choice for primary immunization because greater antigenic stimulation and longer lasting immunity are achieved than with the tetanus toxoid (fluid). Most experts feel that tetanus toxoid adsorbed should be used for booster doses as well; others feel that either tetanus toxoid adsorbed or tetanus toxoid (fluid) may be used for booster doses with equal results. Either tetanus toxoid adsorbed or tetanus toxoid (fluid) may be used for emergency tetanus prophylaxis for wounds.

## Pharmacology/Pharmacokinetics

### Physicochemical characteristics

Source—Tetanus toxoid adsorbed and fluid are prepared by growing the tetanus bacilli *Clostridium tetani* on a protein-free, semi-synthetic medium. The tetanus toxin produced by these bacilli is detoxified by using formaldehyde and forms the tetanus toxoid. Thimerosal is added as a preservative. In addition, for tetanus toxoid adsorbed, aluminum phosphate or aluminum potassium sulfate is used as a mineral adjuvant to adsorb the tetanus antigens. This prolongs and enhances the antigenic properties by retarding the rate of absorption of the injected toxoid into the body

### Mechanism of action/Effect

Following intramuscular injection of tetanus toxoid adsorbed or either intramuscular or subcutaneous injection of tetanus toxoid (fluid), an antigenic response is induced in the immunized patient, causing the formation of tetanus antibodies.

### Protective effect

Tetanus toxoid adsorbed—Most persons possess protective levels of antitoxin to tetanus after two doses. The remaining persons usually obtain protective levels following the third dose of the primary series, which is given approximately one year later.

Tetanus toxoid (fluid)—Does not produce as great an antigenic stimulation as does tetanus toxoid adsorbed, but does provide protective levels.

### Duration of protective effect

Duration of immunity is unknown, but is generally believed to persist for 10 or more years following a primary series or a booster dose of tetanus toxoid. Tetanus toxoid adsorbed causes greater antigenic stimulation and longer lasting immunity than does the tetanus toxoid (fluid).

## Precautions to Consider

### Cross-sensitivity and/or related problems

Patients allergic to thimerosal may be allergic to the tetanus toxoid available in the U.S. and Canada because it may contain a small amount of thimerosal.

### Pregnancy/Reproduction

Pregnancy—Studies have not been done in humans; however, problems in humans have not been documented.

Immune pregnant women confer protection to their infants through transplacental maternal antibody. Pregnant women who are inadequately immunized or unimmunized and who may deliver their infants under unhygienic conditions may expose their infants to neonatal tetanus. For inadequately immunized or unimmunized pregnant women, it is recommended that immunization with tetanus toxoid be initiated or continued during the last two trimesters. Unimmunized women should receive the first two doses of the primary series before childbirth.

Studies have not been done in animals.

FDA Pregnancy Category C.

### Breast-feeding

Problems in humans have not been documented.

### Pediatrics

Infants up to 6 weeks of age—Use is not recommended.

Infants and children 6 weeks of age and older—Pediatrics-specific problems that would limit the usefulness of this vaccine in children in this age group are not expected.

### Geriatrics

Although appropriate studies on the relationship of age to the effects of tetanus toxoid have not been performed in the geriatric population, geriatrics-specific problems are not expected to limit the usefulness of tetanus toxoid in the elderly. However, the immune response in the elderly may be slightly diminished.

### Drug interactions and/or related problems

The following drug interactions and/or related problems have been selected on the basis of their potential clinical significance (possible mechanism in parentheses where appropriate)—not necessarily inclusive (» = major clinical significance):

Note: Combinations containing any of the following medications, depending on the amount present, may also interact with this medication.

Immunosuppressants or
Radiation therapy
(because normal defense mechanisms are suppressed, the patient's antibody response to tetanus toxoid may be decreased. The precaution does not apply to corticosteroids used as replacement therapy, for short-term [less than 2 weeks] systemic therapy, or by other routes of administration that do not cause immunosuppression. Where possible, immunosuppressive therapy should be interrupted when immunization is required because of a tetanus-prone wound)

## Medical considerations/Contraindications

The medical considerations/contraindications included here have been selected on the basis of their potential clinical significance (reasons given in parentheses where appropriate)—not necessarily inclusive (» = major clinical significance).

*Except under special circumstances, this medication should not be used when the following medical problems exist:*

» Febrile illness, severe or
» Respiratory disease, acute

(routine primary or booster immunization should not be administered until the acute symptoms of the patient's illness have abated; however, emergency tetanus prophylaxis for wounds should be administered as usual. Minor illnesses, such as upper respiratory infection, do not preclude administration of tetanus toxoid)

» Tetanus infection

(tetanus toxoid should not be used to treat a tetanus infection; tetanus antitoxin, preferably tetanus immune globulin (TIG), should be used instead; after recovery, tetanus toxoid should be initiated or continued, since a tetanus infection does not confer immunity)

*Risk-benefit should be considered when the following medical problem exists:*

Sensitivity to tetanus vaccine

## Side/Adverse Effects

Note: If an arthus-type hypersensitivity reaction or a fever greater than 39.4 °C (103 °F) occurs following a dose of tetanus toxoid, the patient usually has very high serum tetanus antitoxin levels and no additional doses of tetanus toxoid should be given for any reason, including wounds, more frequently than every 10 years.

If a systemic allergic or neurologic reaction occurs following a dose of tetanus toxoid, the person should not be further immunized using tetanus toxoid; instead, passive immunization using tetanus immune globulin (TIG) should be used when other than a clean, minor wound is sustained. Neurological reactions, such as peripheral neuropathies, have been temporally related to tetanus toxoid administration; however, no causal relationship has been established.

Booster doses of tetanus toxoid administered more frequently than every 10 years have been reported to result in an increased occurrence and severity of adverse reactions.

Generally, a history of hypersensitivity reactions other than anaphylaxis, such as delayed-type, cell-mediated allergic reaction (contact dermatitis), does not preclude immunization.

The following side/adverse effects have been selected on the basis of their potential clinical significance (possible signs and symptoms in parentheses where appropriate)—not necessarily inclusive:

**Those indicating need for medical attention**
Incidence rare
*Anaphylactic reaction* (difficulty in breathing or swallowing; hives; itching, especially of soles or palms; reddening of skin, especially around ears; swelling of eyes, face, or inside of nose; sudden and severe unusual tiredness or weakness); *neurologic reaction* (confusion; fever over 39.4 °C [103 °F]; severe or continuing headache; seizures; excessive sleepiness; unusual irritability; severe or continuing vomiting)

**Additional side/adverse effects that may occur because of very high serum tetanus antitoxin levels and indicating need for medical attention**
Incidence rare
*Fever over 39.4 °C* (103 °F); *lymphadenopathy* (swelling of glands in armpit); *swelling, blistering, or pain at injection site, which may be severe and extensive*

**Those indicating need for medical attention only if they continue or are bothersome**
Incidence more frequent
*Redness or hard lump at injection site*—may persist for a few days
Incidence less frequent
*Allergic reaction, delayed-type, cell-mediated* (pain, tenderness, itching, or swelling at injection site); *chills, fever, irritability, or unusual tiredness; nodule or sterile abscess at injection site*—probably from the aluminum content of tetanus toxoid adsorbed; may persist for a few weeks; *skin rash*

## Patient Consultation

As an aid to patient consultation, refer to *Advice for the Patient, Tetanus Toxoid (Systemic)*.

In providing consultation, consider emphasizing the following selected information (» = major clinical significance):

**Before using this vaccine**
» Conditions affecting use, especially:
Use in children—Not recommended for infants up to 6 weeks of age
Other medical problems, especially severe febrile illness, acute respiratory disease, or tetanus infection

**Proper use of this vaccine**
» Proper dosing

**Side/adverse effects**
Signs of potential side effects, especially anaphylactic reaction; neurologic reaction; fever over 39.4 °C (103 °F); lymphadenopathy; or swelling, blistering, or pain at injection site

## General Dosing Information

It is recommended that infants and children 6 weeks up to 7 years of age receive tetanus toxoid as part of Diphtheria and Tetanus Toxoids and Pertussis Vaccine Adsorbed (DTP) immunization according to the DTP immunization schedule. In those cases where the pertussis vaccine is contraindicated, it is recommended that Diphtheria and Tetanus Toxoids for pediatric use (DT) be administered instead, according to the DT immunization schedule.

It is recommended that children 7 years of age and older and all adults receive tetanus toxoid as part of Tetanus and Diphtheria Toxoids for adult use (Td), both for the primary series and for the booster doses every 10 years.

The dosage of tetanus toxoid is the same for all persons: infants, children, and adults.

A primary series of tetanus toxoid adsorbed consists of 3 doses; a primary series of tetanus toxoid (fluid) consists of 4 doses. If a combination of tetanus toxoid adsorbed and tetanus toxoid (fluid) is used, a total of 4 doses constitutes a primary series. These primary series include a reinforcing dose administered 6 to 12 months after the first 2 doses of tetanus toxoid adsorbed or after the first 3 doses of tetanus toxoid (fluid) or a combination of both. Basic immunization cannot be considered complete until all of these doses are administered.

Prolonging the interval between the primary immunizing doses probably does not interfere with the final immunity. Any dose of tetanus toxoid, including an emergency prophylactic dose, a person has received during the last 10 years may be counted as one of his immunizing injections.

Persons infected with human immunodeficiency virus (HIV) may receive tetanus toxoid whether they have asymptomatic or symptomatic HIV infection.

Tetanus toxoid can be administered concurrently with the following, using separate body sites, separate syringes, and the precautions that apply to each immunizing agent:
• Tetanus immune globulin (human) or tetanus antitoxin (animal).
• Polysaccharide vaccines, such as haemophilus b polysaccharide vaccine, haemophilus b conjugate vaccine, meningococcal polysaccharide vaccine, or pneumococcal polyvalent vaccine.
• Influenza vaccine, whole or split virus.
• Diphtheria toxoid and/or pertussis vaccine.
• Live virus vaccines, such as measles, mumps, and/or rubella vaccines.
• Poliovirus vaccines (oral [OPV], inactivated [IPV], or enhanced-potency inactivated [enhanced-potency IPV]).
• Immune globulin and disease-specific immune globulins.
• Hepatitis B recombinant or plasma-derived vaccine, or other inactivated vaccines, except cholera, typhoid, and plague. It is recommended that cholera, typhoid, and plague vaccines be administered on separate occasions because of these vaccines' propensity to cause side/adverse effects.

**For tetanus toxoid (fluid) only**
Tetanus toxoid (fluid) is administered subcutaneously or intramuscularly into the area of the midlateral muscles (vastus lateralis) of the thigh or into the deltoid. The vaccine should not be injected intravenously.

**For tetanus toxoid adsorbed only**
Tetanus toxoid adsorbed is administered intramuscularly into the area of the midlateral muscles (vastus lateralis) of the thigh or into the deltoid. The same muscle site should not be used more than once during the course of the primary immunization. The vaccine should not be injected intravenously.

**Emergency tetanus prophylaxis of wounds**

Examples of wounds that are not clean, minor wounds are: wounds contaminated with dirt, feces, soil, or saliva; puncture wounds; wounds caused by tearing; and wounds resulting from missiles, crushing, burns, or frostbite.

Patients who were unimmunized or inadequately immunized prior to injury should complete their primary immunization schedule as soon as possible.

If only tetanus toxoid adsorbed has been used for the primary doses—Patients who receive an emergency prophylactic dose of tetanus toxoid adsorbed after their second primary dose should count the prophylactic dose as their third (last) primary dose if the prophylactic dose is administered at least 6 months after the second primary dose.

If either tetanus toxoid (fluid) or a combination of both toxoids has been used for the primary doses—Patients who receive an emergency prophylactic dose of either tetanus toxoid (fluid) or tetanus toxoid adsorbed after their third primary dose should count the prophylactic dose as their fourth (last) primary dose if the prophylactic dose is administered at least 6 months after the third primary dose.

The decision to administer concomitant passive immunization by using tetanus immune globulin (human) or tetanus antitoxin (animal) depends on such factors as location, type, and severity of the wound; degree and kind of contamination; and the time elapsed since the injury. Some experts feel that tetanus toxoid adsorbed should be used with the selected antitoxin; others feel that either tetanus toxoid adsorbed or tetanus toxoid (fluid) may be used.

**For treatment of adverse effects**

Recommended treatment includes
 • For mild hypersensitivity reaction—Administering antihistamines and, if necessary, corticosteroids.
 • For severe hypersensitivity or anaphylactic reaction—Administering epinephrine. Antihistamines or corticosteroids may also be administered as required.

# Parenteral Dosage Forms

## TETANUS TOXOID (FLUID) INJECTION USP

**Usual adult and adolescent dose**
Tetanus (prophylaxis)—Intramuscular or subcutaneous, 0.5 mL (U.S.) or 1 mL (Canada—Connaught):—
First dose:
    At initial visit.
Second dose:
    4 to 8 weeks after the first dose.
Third dose:
    4 to 8 weeks after the second dose.
Fourth dose:
    6 to 12 months after the third dose.
Booster doses:
    Every 10 years.
Emergency tetanus prophylaxis of wounds:
    U.S.—
        If less than the 4 primary doses have been administered—As soon as possible following any wound. For other than clean, minor wounds, tetanus immune globulin (human) (preferred) or tetanus antitoxin (animal) should also be administered.
        If 4 or more doses have been administered—For a clean, minor wound, as soon as possible if more than 10 years have passed since the last dose. For all other wounds, as soon as possible if more than 5 years have passed since the last dose. No tetanus immune globulin (human) or tetanus antitoxin (animal) is required in either case.
    Canada—
        If less than 2 primary doses have been administered—As soon as possible following any wound. For other than clean, minor wounds, tetanus immune globulin (human) (preferred) or tetanus antitoxin (animal) should also be administered.
        If 2 primary doses have been administered—As soon as possible following any wound. For other than clean, minor wounds, tetanus immune globulin (human) (preferred) or tetanus antitoxin (animal) should also be administered if more than 24 hours have elapsed since the injury.
        If 3 or more doses have been administered—For a clean, minor wound, as soon as possible if more than 10 years have passed since the last dose. For all other wounds, as soon as possible if more than 5 years have passed since the last dose. No tetanus immune globulin (human) or tetanus antitoxin (animal) is required in either case.

**Usual pediatric dose**
See *Usual adult and adolescent dose*.

Note: For infants, the first dose is usually administered at 6 to 8 weeks of age.

**Usual geriatric dose**
See *Usual adult and adolescent dose*.

**Strength(s) usually available**
U.S.—
    4 Lf per 0.5 mL (Rx) [GENERIC (may contain thimerosal)].
Canada—
    10 Lf per 1 mL (Rx) [GENERIC (may contain thimerosal)].

Note: Lf is the quantity of toxoid as assessed by flocculation.

**Packaging and storage**
Store between 2 and 8 °C (36 and 46 °F). Do not freeze.

**Stability**
The vaccine should not be used if exposed to freezing or if cloudy or turbid.

**Auxiliary labeling**
 • Shake well.
 • Do not freeze.

## TETANUS TOXOID ADSORBED (INJECTION) USP

**Usual adult and adolescent dose**
Tetanus (prophylaxis)—Intramuscular, 0.5 mL:—
First dose:
    At initial visit.
Second dose:
    4 to 8 weeks after the first dose.
Third dose:
    6 to 12 months after the second dose.
Booster doses:
    Every 10 years.
Emergency tetanus prophylaxis of wounds:
    U.S.—
        If less than the 3 primary doses have been administered—As soon as possible following any wound. For other than clean, minor wounds, tetanus immune globulin (human) (preferred) or tetanus antitoxin (animal) should also be administered.
        If 3 or more doses have been administered—For a clean, minor wound, as soon as possible if more than 10 years have passed since the last dose. For all other wounds, as soon as possible if more than 5 years have passed since the last dose. Generally, no tetanus immune globulin (human) or tetanus antitoxin (animal) is required in either case.
    Canada—
        If less than 2 primary doses have been administered—As soon as possible following any wound. For other than clean, minor wounds, tetanus immune globulin (human) (preferred) or tetanus antitoxin (animal) should also be administered.
        If 2 primary doses have been administered—As soon as possible following any wound. For other than clean, minor wounds, tetanus immune globulin (human) (preferred) or tetanus antitoxin (animal) should also be administered if more than 24 hours have elapsed since the injury.
        If 3 or more doses have been administered—For a clean, minor wound, as soon as possible if more than 10 years have passed since the last dose. For all other wounds, as soon as possible if more than 5 years have passed since the last dose. No tetanus immune globulin (human) or tetanus antitoxin (animal) is required in either case.

**Usual pediatric dose**
See *Usual adult and adolescent dose*.

Note: For infants, the first dose is usually administered at 6 to 8 weeks of age.

**Usual geriatric dose**
See *Usual adult and adolescent dose*.

**Strength(s) usually available**
U.S.—
    5 Lf per 0.5 mL (Rx) [GENERIC (may contain thimerosal)].
    10 Lf per 0.5 mL (Rx) [GENERIC (may contain thimerosal)].
Canada—
    5 Lf per 0.5 mL (Rx) [GENERIC (may contain thimerosal)].

Note: Lf is the quantity of toxoid as assessed by flocculation.

**Packaging and storage**
Store between 2 and 8 °C (36 and 46 °F). Do not freeze.

**Stability**

The vaccine should not be used if exposed to freezing.

**Auxiliary labeling**

• Shake well.

• Do not freeze.

Revised: 07/12/94

**TETRACAINE**—See *Anesthetics (Mucosal-Local); Anesthetics (Ophthalmic); Anesthetics (Parenteral-Local); Anesthetics (Topical)*

**TETRACAINE-CONTAINING COMBINATIONS**—

Benzocaine, Butamben, and Tetracaine (Mucosal-Local)—See *Anesthetics (Mucosal-Local)*

**TETRACAINE AND MENTHOL**—See *Anesthetics (Topical)*

**TETRACYCLINE**—See *Tetracycline Periodontal Fibers (Mucosal-Local); Tetracyclines (Ophthalmic); Tetracyclines (Systemic); Tetracyclines (Topical)*

# TETRACYCLINE PERIODONTAL FIBERS    Mucosal-Local†

VA CLASSIFICATION (Primary/Secondary): OR900/DE101

Note: For a listing of dosage forms and brand names by country availability, see *Dosage Forms* section(s). For a listing of brand names for the articles in this monograph, refer to the General Index.

†Not commercially available in Canada.

## Category

Antibacterial (dental).

## Indications

### General considerations

Periodontal disease is primarily caused by facultative and obligate anaerobic bacteria. Probable pathogens include *Fusobacterium nucleatum, Porphyromonas gingivalis, Prevotella intermedia, Eikenella corrodens, Campylobacter rectus (Wolinella recta),* and *Actinobacillus actinomycetemcomitans.* These organisms were found to be sensitive to tetracycline *in vitro* at the same local concentration as that achieved by tetracycline periodontal fibers in the periodontal pocket.

Tetracycline periodontal fibers have been found to decrease the incidence of inflammation and edema, pocket depth, and the amount of bleeding upon pocket probing. This may occur because the high local concentration of tetracycline suppresses bacteria for an extended period of time and serves as a barrier to entry of the bacteria. After being released locally, tetracycline may be adsorbed by tooth cementum, forming a reservoir from which the medication continues to be released after the fiber has been removed. In addition, tetracycline inhibits collagenolytic enzymes and acts on root surfaces or fibroblasts.

### Accepted

Periodontitis (treatment adjunct)—Tetracycline periodontal fibers are indicated as an adjunct to scaling and root planing for the reduction of pocket depth and bleeding on probing in selected patients with adult periodontitis.

## Pharmacology/Pharmacokinetics

### Physicochemical characteristics

Molecular weight—Tetracycline hydrochloride: 480.90.

### Mechanism of action/Effect

Bacteriostatic; thought to act by inhibiting protein synthesis. Tetracycline binds primarily to the 30S subunits of the bacterial ribosomes, and appears to prevent access of aminoacyl tRNA to the acceptor site on the mRNA-ribosome complex.

Rate of release—

The fiber releases tetracycline *in vitro* at a rate of approximately 2 mcg per centimeter per hour (mcg/cm/hr).

Concentration—

Mean values:

Gingival fluid: Approximately 1590 mcg per mL (mcg/mL) of tetracycline per site throughout the 10 day period. Concentrations of 4 to 8 mcg/mL are inhibitory for most pathogenic periodontal organisms.

Saliva: Approximately 50.7 mcg/mL of tetracycline immediately after fiber treatment of 9 teeth; concentration values decline to 7.6 mcg/mL at the end of ten days.

Plasma: During fiber treatment of up to 11 teeth (average total tetracycline dose of 105 mg), the mean tetracycline concentration in the plasma remains below the lower limit of assay detection (< 0.1 mcg/mL). In comparison, a 500-mg oral dose of tetracycline produces peak serum concentrations of about 3 to 4 mcg/mL.

## Precautions to Consider

### Carcinogenicity

Animal studies have not been done.

### Mutagenicity

Animal studies have not been done.

### Pregnancy/Reproduction

Fertility—Animal studies have not been done.

Pregnancy—No adequate and well-controlled studies have been done in pregnant women. Use of systemic tetracyclines is not recommended during pregnancy because of interference with fetal bone and dental development.

Animal studies have not been done to determine whether tetracycline periodontal fibers can cause fetal harm. Use of systemic tetracyclines in animals has been shown to cause retardation of fetal skeletal development.

FDA Pregnancy Category C.

### Breast-feeding

It is not known whether tetracycline from tetracycline periodontal fibers is distributed into human breast milk. Tetracycline periodontal fibers produce plasma concentrations of less than 0.1 mcg/mL. However, systemically administered tetracycline is distributed into breast milk.

### Pediatrics

Safety and efficacy have not been established in children. Tetracycline periodontal fibers produce plasma concentrations of less than 0.1 mcg/mL. However, systemic use of tetracyclines in children up to 8 years of age has caused permanent discoloration of teeth.

### Geriatrics

No information is available on the relationship of age to the effects of tetracycline periodontal fibers in geriatric patients.

### Medical considerations/Contraindications

The medical considerations/contraindications included here have been selected on the basis of their potential clinical significance (reasons given in parentheses where appropriate)—not necessarily inclusive (» = major clinical significance).

*Risk-benefit should be considered when the following medical problem exists:*

» Hypersensitivity to tetracyclines

## Side/Adverse Effects

The following side/adverse effects have been selected on the basis of their potential clinical significance (possible signs and symptoms in parentheses where appropriate)—not necessarily inclusive:

### Those indicating need for medical attention

Incidence rare (less than 1%)

*Gingival inflammation and pain* (redness and swelling of gums); *glossitis* (tongue pain and redness)

Note: *Gingival inflammation and pain* may occur following fiber placement in an abscessed area.

**Those indicating need for medical attention only if they continue or are bothersome**
Incidence more frequent (10 to 11%)
*Discomfort on fiber placement; local erythema following removal*
Incidence rare (less than 1%)
*Oral candidiasis* (white patches on tongue or in mouth); *staining of tongue*

## Patient Consultation

As an aid to patient consultation, refer to *Advice for the Patient, Tetracycline Periodontal Fibers (Dental).*

In providing consultation, consider emphasizing the following selected information (» = major clinical significance):

**Before using this medication**
» Conditions affecting use, especially:
     Hypersensitivity to tetracyclines

**Proper use of this medication**
*When tetracycline periodontal fiber is in place, avoiding actions that may dislodge the fibers, such as:*
     Chewing hard, crusty, or sticky foods, or chewing gum
     Brushing or flossing near any treated areas
     Engaging in any other hygienic practices that might dislodge the fibers
     Probing the treated area with tongue, toothpicks, or fingers

**Precautions while using this medication**
     Checking with dentist promptly if the fiber is dislodged or falls out before the next scheduled visit
     Checking with dentist promptly if pain or swelling or other problems occur
     Not missing any appointments with dentist; all fibers must be removed after 10 days

**Side/adverse effects**
     Signs of potential side effects, especially gingival inflammation and pain, and glossitis

## General Dosing Information

Each 23-cm (9-inch) tetracycline periodontal fiber contains 12.7 mg of tetracycline hydrochloride evenly dispersed throughout the fiber. It provides a continuous release of tetracycline for 10 days.

The length of fiber used will vary with the periodontal pocket depth and contour, and the number of teeth being treated. The fibers should be in contact with the base of the pocket and should be filled in to closely approximate the anatomy of the pocket.

An appropriate cyanoacrylate adhesive should be used to secure the fiber in the pocket.

Fibers should be replaced if they are lost before 7 days following their insertion into the periodontal pocket.

Repeated applications of tetracycline periodontal fibers have not been studied.

## Dental Dosage Forms
### TETRACYCLINE PERIODONTAL FIBERS

**Usual adult dose**
Antibacterial—
     Topical, insert a sufficient number of fibers to fill the periodontal pocket. Secure fibers with cyanoacrylate adhesive and leave for ten days.

**Usual pediatric dose**
Safety and efficacy have not been established.

**Strength(s) usually available**
U.S.—
     12.7 mg of tetracycline hydrochloride per fiber (Rx) [*Actisite*].
Canada—
     Not commercially available.

**Packaging and storage**
Store between 15 and 30 °C (59 and 86 °F).

Developed: 12/15/94

---

# TETRACYCLINES    Ophthalmic

This monograph includes information on the following: Chlortetracycline; Tetracycline.

VA CLASSIFICATION (Primary): OP201

Note: For a listing of dosage forms and brand names by country availability, see *Dosage Forms* section(s). For a listing of brand names for the articles in this monograph, refer to the General Index.

## Category
Antibacterial (ophthalmic).

## Indications

Note: Bracketed information in the *Indications* section refers to uses that are not included in U.S. product labeling.

**Accepted**
Ocular infections (treatment)—Ophthalmic chlortetracycline is indicated in the treatment of superficial ocular infections caused by *Staphylococcus aureus, Streptococcus epidemicus (Streptococcus pyogenes), Neisseria gonorrhoeae, S. pneumoniae (Diplococcus pneumoniae), Haemophilus influenzae, H. ducreyi, Klebsiella pneumoniae, Francisella tularensis (Pasteurella tularensis), Yersinia pestis (Pasteurella pestis), Escherichia coli, Bacillus anthracis,* and *Lymphogranuloma venereum.*

Ophthalmic tetracycline is indicated in the treatment of superficial ocular infections caused by *Staphylococcus aureus,* streptococci including *Streptococcus epidemicus (Streptococcus pyogenes)* and *S. pneumoniae (Diplococcus pneumoniae), Neisseria gonorrhoeae,* and *Escherichia coli.*

Ophthalmia neonatorum (prophylaxis)—Ophthalmic [chlortetracycline] and tetracycline are indicated in the prophylaxis of ophthalmia neonatorum caused by *N. gonorrhoeae* and *Chlamydia trachomatis.*

Trachoma (treatment)—Ophthalmic chlortetracycline and tetracycline are indicated in the treatment of trachoma caused by *Chlamydia trachomatis.* They should be used concurrently with oral tetracyclines.

[Blepharitis, bacterial (treatment)]
[Blepharoconjunctivitis (treatment)]
[Conjunctivitis, bacterial (treatment)]
[Keratitis, bacterial (treatment)]
[Keratoconjunctivitis, bacterial (treatment)] or
[Meibomianitis (treatment)]—Ophthalmic chlortetracycline and tetracycline are used in the treatment of bacterial blepharitis, blepharoconjunctivitis, bacterial conjunctivitis, bacterial keratitis, bacterial keratoconjunctivitis, and meibomianitis.

[Chlamydial infections (treatment)] or
[Rosacea, ocular (treatment)]—Ophthalmic tetracycline is used in the treatment of chlamydial infections and ocular rosacea.

Note: Not all species or strains of a particular organism may be susceptible to a specific tetracycline.

**Unaccepted**
Tetracycline is not effective against *Haemophilus influenzae, Klebsiella* species, *Enterobacter (Aerobacter)* species, *Pseudomonas aeruginosa,* or *Serratia marcescens.*

## Pharmacology/Pharmacokinetics

**Physicochemical characteristics**
Molecular weight—
     Chlortetracycline hydrochloride: 515.35.
     Tetracycline hydrochloride: 480.90.

**Mechanism of action/Effect**
Tetracyclines are broad-spectrum bacteriostatic agents and act by inhibiting protein synthesis by blocking the binding of aminoacyl tRNA (transfer RNA) to the mRNA (messenger RNA) ribosome complex. Reversible binding occurs primarily at the 30 S ribosomal subunit of susceptible organisms. Bacterial cell wall synthesis is not inhibited.

## Precautions to Consider

**Cross-sensitivity and/or related problems**
Patients sensitive to one tetracycline, tetracycline combination, or tetracycline derivative may be sensitive to other tetracyclines also.

**Pregnancy/Reproduction**
Pregnancy—Problems in humans have not been documented.

**Breast-feeding**
Problems in humans have not been documented.

**Pediatrics**
Appropriate studies on the relationship of age to the effects of ophthalmic tetracyclines have not been performed in the pediatric population. However, no pediatrics-specific problems have been documented to date.

**Geriatrics**
Appropriate studies on the relationship of age to the effects of tetracyclines have not been performed in the geriatric population. However, no geriatrics-specific problems have been documented to date.

**Medical considerations/Contraindications**
The medical considerations/contraindications included here have been selected on the basis of their potential clinical significance (reasons given in parentheses where appropriate)—not necessarily inclusive (» = major clinical significance):

*Risk-benefit should be considered when the following medical problem exists:*
Sensitivity to tetracyclines

## Patient Consultation
As an aid to patient consultation, refer to *Advice for the Patient, Tetracyclines (Ophthalmic)*.

In providing consultation, consider emphasizing the following selected information (» = major clinical significance):

**Before using this medication**
» Conditions affecting use, especially:
    Sensitivity to tetracycline, chlortetracycline, or any related antibiotic, such as demeclocycline, doxycycline, methacycline, minocycline, or oxytetracycline

**Proper use of this medication**
Proper administration technique for ophthalmic suspension and ophthalmic ointment
» Compliance with full course of therapy
» Proper dosing
    Missed dose: Applying as soon as possible; not applying if almost time for next dose
» Proper storage

**Precautions while using this medication**
Blurred vision after application of ophthalmic ointments and ophthalmic suspensions in oil (tetracycline)
Checking with physician if no improvement within a few days

## General Dosing Information
Blurred vision after application of ophthalmic suspensions in oil or ophthalmic ointments is to be expected.

Therapy should be continued for 1 to 2 months or longer in acute and chronic trachoma. Severe infections may also require concurrent oral therapy for trachoma.

In term infants born to mothers with clinically apparent gonorrhea, a single intramuscular or intravenous dose of 50,000 Units of penicillin G potassium is administered concurrently with ophthalmic tetracycline. In low-birth-weight infants, the dose is 20,000 Units.

At night, the ophthalmic ointment may be used as an adjunct to the ophthalmic suspension to provide prolonged contact with the medication.

Although some manufacturers recommend a dose of 2 drops of an ophthalmic solution at appropriate intervals, the conjunctival sac usually will hold only 1 drop.

---

### CHLORTETRACYCLINE

## Ophthalmic Dosage Forms
### CHLORTETRACYCLINE HYDROCHLORIDE OPHTHALMIC OINTMENT USP

**Usual adult and adolescent dose**
Ocular infections—
    Topical, to the conjunctiva, a thin strip (approximately 1 cm) of ointment every two to four hours or more frequently.

**Usual pediatric dose**
See *Usual adult and adolescent dose.*

**Strength(s) usually available**
U.S.—
    1% (Rx) [*Aureomycin*].
Canada—
    1% (Rx) [*Aureomycin*].

**Packaging and storage**
Store below 40 °C (104 °F), preferably between 15 and 30 °C (59 and 86 °F), unless otherwise specified by manufacturer. Store in a collapsible ophthalmic ointment tube. Protect from freezing.

**Auxiliary labeling**
• For the eye.
• Continue medicine for full time of treatment.

---

### TETRACYCLINE

## Ophthalmic Dosage Forms
### TETRACYCLINE HYDROCHLORIDE OPHTHALMIC OINTMENT USP

**Usual adult and adolescent dose**
Ocular infections—
    Topical, to the conjunctiva, a thin strip (approximately 1 cm) of ointment every two to four hours or more frequently.
Ophthalmia neonatorum—
    Topical, to the conjunctiva, a thin strip (approximately 1 cm) of ointment as a single dose.

**Usual pediatric dose**
See *Usual adult and adolescent dose.*

**Strength(s) usually available**
U.S.—
    1% (Rx) [*Achromycin*].
Canada—
    1% (Rx) [*Achromycin*].

**Packaging and storage**
Store below 40 °C (104 °F), preferably between 15 and 30 °C (59 and 86 °F), unless otherwise specified by manufacturer. Store in a collapsible ophthalmic ointment tube. Protect from freezing.

**Auxiliary labeling**
• For the eye.
• Continue medicine for full time of treatment.

### TETRACYCLINE HYDROCHLORIDE OPHTHALMIC SUSPENSION USP

**Usual adult and adolescent dose**
Ocular infections—
    Topical, to the conjunctiva, 1 drop every six to twelve hours or more frequently.
Ophthalmia neonatorum—
    Topical, to the conjunctiva, 1 drop as a single dose.

**Usual pediatric dose**
See *Usual adult and adolescent dose.*

**Strength(s) usually available**
U.S.—
    1% (Rx) [*Achromycin*].
Canada—
    Not commercially available.

**Packaging and storage**
Store below 40 °C (104 °F), preferably between 15 and 30 °C (59 and 86° F), unless otherwise specified by manufacturer. Store in a tight, light-resistant glass or plastic container. Protect from freezing.

**Auxiliary labeling**
• Shake well.
• For the eye.
• Continue medicine for full time of treatment.

**Note**
Dispense in original unopened container.

The ophthalmic suspension is available in a base containing light mineral oil and other ingredients that may briefly cause blurred vision after application.

---

Revised: 07/01/93

# TETRACYCLINES   Systemic

This monograph includes information on the following: Demeclocycline; Doxycycline; Minocycline; Oxytetracycline†; Tetracycline.

VA CLASSIFICATION (Primary/Secondary):
Demeclocycline—AM250/AP109; CV900
Doxycycline—AM250/AP109
Minocycline—AM250/AP109; DE751
Oxytetracycline—AM250/AP109
Tetracycline—AM250/AP109; DE751

Note: For a listing of dosage forms and brand names by country availability, see *Dosage Forms* section(s). For a listing of brand names for the articles in this monograph, refer to the General Index.

†Not commercially available in Canada.

## Category

Antibacterial (systemic); antiprotozoal—Demeclocycline; Doxycycline; Minocycline; Oxytetracycline; Tetracycline.
Antiacne agent (systemic)—Minocycline (oral); tetracycline (oral).
Diuretic (syndrome of inappropriate antidiuretic hormone)—Demeclocycline.

## Indications

Note: Bracketed information in the *Indications* section refers to uses that are not included in U.S. product labeling.

**Accepted**

Acne vulgaris (treatment)—Although all tetracyclines may be indicated as adjunctive treatment, they are generally no more effective in the initial treatment of acne and are more expensive than tetracycline. However, oral minocycline may be more effective in severe or resistant acne and may be effective in acne unresponsive to oral tetracycline.

Actinomycosis (treatment)—Systemic tetracyclines are indicated in the treatment of actinomycosis caused by *Actinomyces israelii*.

Anthrax (treatment)—Systemic tetracyclines are indicated in the treatment of anthrax caused by *Bacillus anthracis*.

Bronchitis (treatment)—Systemic tetracyclines are indicated in the treatment of bronchitis.

Brucellosis (treatment)—Systemic tetracyclines are indicated in the treatment of brucellosis.

Conjunctivitis, inclusion (treatment)—Systemic tetracyclines are indicated in the treatment of inclusion conjunctivitis.

Genitourinary tract infections (treatment)—Systemic tetracyclines are indicated in the treatment of genitourinary tract infections (including acute epididymo-orchitis) caused by *N. gonorrhoeae*.

Doxycycline is indicated in the treatment of genitourinary tract infections (including acute epididymo-orchitis) caused by *Chlamydia trachomatis*.

Doxycycline, minocycline, oxytetracycline, and tetracycline are indicated in the treatment of uncomplicated genitourinary tract infections (including endocervical infections) caused by *Chlamydia trachomatis*.

Minocycline is indicated in the treatment of uncomplicated genitourinary tract infections (including endocervical infections) caused by *Ureaplasma urealyticum*.

Gingivostomatitis, necrotizing ulcerative (treatment)—Systemic tetracyclines are indicated in the treatment of necrotizing ulcerative gingivostomatitis (Vincent's infection) caused by *Fusobacterium fusiformisans (Fusiformis fusiformisans)*.

Granuloma inguinale (treatment)—Systemic tetracyclines are indicated in the treatment of granuloma inguinale caused by *Calymmatobacterium granulomatis*.

Lymphogranuloma venereum (treatment)—Systemic tetracyclines are indicated in the treatment of lymphogranuloma venereum caused by *Chlamydia* species.

Malaria (prophylaxis)—Doxycycline is indicated in the prophylaxis of malaria due to *Plasmodium falciparum* in short-term travelers (< 4 months) going to areas with chloroquine- and/or pyrimethamine-sulfadoxine–resistant strains.

Meningococcal carriers (treatment)—Oral minocycline is indicated in the treatment of asymptomatic meningococcal carriers to eliminate *Neisseria meningitidis* from the nasopharynx.

Otitis media, acute (treatment)
Pharyngitis, bacterial (treatment)
Pneumonia, *Haemophilus influenzae* (treatment)

Pneumonia, *Klebsiella* species (treatment) or
Sinusitis (treatment)—Systemic tetracyclines are indicated in the treatment of acute otitis media, pharyngitis, pneumonia, and sinusitis caused by *H. influenzae* and *Klebsiella* species.

Doxycycline is indicated in the treatment of the above-listed infections caused by *Staphylococcus aureus*. However, some USP medical experts do not recommend the use of tetracyclines for infections caused by *S. aureus*.

Psittacosis (treatment)—Systemic tetracyclines are indicated in the treatment of psittacosis caused by *Chlamydia psittaci*.

Q fever (treatment)
Rickettsial pox (treatment)
Rocky Mountain spotted fever (treatment) or
Typhus infections (treatment)—Systemic tetracyclines are indicated in the treatment of Q fever, rickettsial pox, Rocky Mountain spotted fever (including tick fevers), and typhus infections caused by Rickettsiae.

Relapsing fever (treatment)—Systemic tetracyclines are indicated in the treatment of relapsing fever caused by *Borrelia recurrentis*.

Skin and soft tissue infections (treatment)—Systemic tetracyclines are indicated in the treatment of skin and soft tissue infections, including burn wound infections, caused by *Staphylococcus aureus*. However, some USP medical experts do not recommend the use of tetracyclines for infections caused by *S. aureus*.

Syphilis (treatment)—Systemic tetracyclines are indicated in the treatment of syphilis caused by *Treponema pallidum*.

Trachoma (treatment)—Systemic tetracyclines are indicated in the treatment of trachoma.

Urethritis, nongonococcal (treatment)—Doxycycline is indicated in the treatment of nongonococcal urethritis caused by *Chlamydia trachomatis* and *Ureaplasma urealyticum*.

Urinary tract infections, bacterial (treatment)—Systemic tetracyclines are indicated in the treatment of urinary tract infections caused by [susceptible organisms, including *Escherichia coli* and] *Klebsiella* species.

Yaws (treatment)—Systemic tetracyclines are indicated in the treatment of yaws caused by *T. pertenue*.

Doxycycline, minocycline, oxytetracycline, and tetracycline are indicated in the treatment of uncomplicated rectal infections caused by *Chlamydia trachomatis*. Minocycline is indicated in the treatment of uncomplicated rectal infections caused by *Ureaplasma urealyticum*.

[Amebiasis, extraintestinal (treatment)]—Tetracycline, a lumenal amebicide, is used concurrently or sequentially with metronidazole in the treatment of extraintestinal amebiasis caused by *Entamoeba histolytica*.

[Arthritis, gonococcal (treatment)]
[Bejel (treatment)]
[Biliary tract infections (treatment)]
[Enterocolitis, *Shigella* species (treatment)]
[Intra-abdominal infections (treatment)]
[Pinta (treatment)]
[Plague (treatment)]
[Pneumonia, mycoplasmal (treatment)]
[Septicemia, bacterial (treatment)]
[Tularemia (treatment)] or
[Urethritis, gonococcal (treatment)]—Systemic tetracyclines are used in the treatment of the above-listed infections.

[Chlamydial infections (treatment)] or
[Rosacea, ocular (treatment)]—Systemic tetracycline is used in the treatment of chlamydial infections and ocular rosacea.

[Gonorrhea (treatment)] or
[Malaria (treatment)]—Systemic doxycycline and tetracycline are used in the treatment of gonorrhea and malaria.

[Lyme disease (treatment)]—Doxycycline and tetracycline are used in the treatment of early Lyme disease, caused by *Borrelia burgdorferi*.

[Mycobacterial infections, atypical (treatment)]—Systemic doxycycline and minocycline are used in the treatment of atypical mycobacterial infections.

[Nocardiosis (treatment)]—Systemic minocycline is used in the treatment of nocardiosis.

[Syndrome of inappropriate antidiuretic hormone (SIADH) (treatment)]—Demeclocycline is used in the treatment of syndrome of inappropriate (excess) antidiuretic hormone (SIADH).

[Traveler's diarrhea (prophylaxis and treatment)]—Doxycycline is used in the prophylaxis and treatment of traveler's diarrhea caused by enterotoxigenic *Escherichia coli*, *Salmonella* species, and *Shigella* species in high-risk patients in whom diarrhea and dehydration may result in serious consequences because of chronic underlying health problems.

Tetracyclines are also indicated in the treatment of infections caused by *Mycobacterium marinum* (oral minocycline), *Mycoplasma pneumoniae*, *Yersinia pestis*, *Francisella tularensis*, *Bartonella bacilliformis*, *Bacteroides* species, *Vibrio cholerae*, *Campylobacter fetus*, *Brucella* species (concurrently with streptomycin), *Escherichia coli*, *Enterobacter aerogenes*, *Shigella* species, *Acinetobacter* species, streptococci, *Streptococcus pneumoniae*, *Neisseria gonorrhoeae*, *N. meningitidis* (parenteral doxycycline, minocycline, and tetracycline), *Listeria monocytogenes*, *Clostridium* species, and *Actinomyces* species.

Not all species or strains of a particular organism may be susceptible to a specific tetracycline.

**Unaccepted**

Oral minocycline is no longer recommended by the Centers for Disease Control (CDC) for the treatment of meningococcal carriers because of vestibular toxicity. Oral minocycline is not indicated in the treatment of meningococcal infections.

## Pharmacology/Pharmacokinetics

### Physicochemical characteristics
Molecular weight—
Demeclocycline hydrochloride: 501.32.
Doxycycline: 462.46.
Doxycycline hyclate: 1025.89.
Minocycline hydrochloride: 493.94.
Oxytetracycline: 496.47.
Oxytetracycline hydrochloride: 496.90.
Tetracycline: 444.44.
Tetracycline hydrochloride: 480.90.

### Mechanism of action/Effect
Antibacterial (systemic); antiprotozoal—Tetracyclines are broad-spectrum bacteriostatic agents and act by inhibiting protein synthesis by blocking the binding of aminoacyl tRNA (transfer RNA) to the mRNA (messenger RNA) ribosome complex. Reversible binding occurs primarily at the 30 S ribosomal subunit of susceptible organisms. Bacterial cell wall synthesis is not inhibited.

Diuretic (Syndrome of inappropriate diuretic hormone [SIADH])—In the treatment of the SIADH, demeclocycline acts by inhibiting ADH-induced water reabsorption in the distal portion of the convoluted tubules and collecting ducts of the kidneys, thereby causing water diuresis.

### Absorption

| Drug | Absorbed Orally (%) | Effect of Food on Absorption |
|---|---|---|
| Demeclocycline | 66 | Decreased |
| Doxycycline | 90–100 | Insignificant |
| Minocycline | 90–100 | Insignificant |
| Oxytetracycline | 58 | Decreased |
| Tetracycline | 75–77 | Decreased |

### Distribution
Doxycycline—Achieves therapeutic concentrations in the eye; prostatic concentrations are approximately 60% of serum concentrations.

Minocycline—Achieves high concentrations in saliva, sputum, and tears.

All tetracyclines—Readily distributed to most body fluids, including bile, sinus secretions, and synovial, pleural, ascitic, and gingival crevicular fluids. Cerebrospinal fluid (CSF) concentrations vary and may achieve 10 to 25% of plasma concentrations following parenteral administration. Concentrations in gingival crevicular fluid may be 3 to 7 times serum concentrations. Tetracyclines tend to localize in bone, liver, spleen, tumors, and teeth; also cross the placenta and distributed into breast milk.

### Biotransformation
Doxycycline and minocycline are partially inactivated by hepatic metabolism.

### Half-life

| Drug | Half-life | |
|---|---|---|
| | Normal (hr) | Anuric (hr) |
| Demeclocycline | 10–17 | 40–60 |
| Doxycycline | 12–22 | 12–22 |
| Minocycline | 11–23 | 11–23 |
| Oxytetracycline | 6–10 | 47–66 |
| Tetracycline | 6–11 | 57–108 |

### Onset of action
SIADH syndrome (demeclocycline)—24 to 48 hours.

### Time to peak concentration
Tetracycline—Two to three days may be necessary to achieve therapeutic concentrations of tetracycline.

Other tetracyclines—2 to 4 hours (oral).

### Elimination
Renal; unchanged, via glomerular filtration.

Fecal; unchanged, via biliary secretion, gastrointestinal secretion, or poor absorption.

Dialysis—Tetracyclines are slowly removed by hemodialysis; although, doxycycline is not removed by hemodialysis. Peritoneal dialysis does not effectively remove tetracyclines.

Note: Gastrointestinal secretion is an important route of excretion when doxycycline is administered to patients with impaired renal function or azotemia.

| Drug | Distribution* $(vol_D$—L/kg) | Excretion Routes† (primary/ secondary— % excreted unchanged) | Protein Binding |
|---|---|---|---|
| Demeclocycline | 1.79 | Renal/biliary (42) | High (91%) |
| Doxycycline | 0.7 | Biliary/renal (35) | High (93%) |
| Minocycline | 0.14–0.7 | Biliary/renal (5–10) | Moderate (76%) |
| Oxytetracycline | 0.9–1.9 | Renal/biliary (70) | Low (35%) |
| Tetracycline | 1.3–1.6 | Renal/biliary (60) | Moderate (65%) |

*Diffuses readily into most body tissues, fluids, and/or cavities.
†Biliary route involves concentration by the liver and excretion via the bile into the intestine from which partial reabsorption occurs.

## Precautions to Consider

### Cross-sensitivity and/or related problems
Patients hypersensitive to one tetracycline may be hypersensitive to other tetracyclines also.

Patients hypersensitive to lidocaine, procaine, or other "caine-type" local anesthetics may also be hypersensitive to the lidocaine component of oxytetracycline injection or to the procaine component of tetracycline hydrochloride for intramuscular injection.

### Pregnancy/Reproduction
Pregnancy—Tetracyclines cross the placenta; use is not recommended during the last half of pregnancy since tetracyclines may cause permanent discoloration of teeth, enamel hypoplasia, and inhibition of skeletal growth in the fetus. In addition, fatty infiltration of the liver may occur in pregnant women, especially with high intravenous doses.

FDA Pregnancy Category D.

### Breast-feeding
Tetracyclines are distributed into breast milk; although tetracyclines may form nonabsorbable complexes with breast-milk calcium, use is not recommended because of the possibility of their causing permanent discoloration of teeth, enamel hypoplasia, inhibition of linear skeletal growth, photosensitivity reactions, and oral and vaginal thrush in infants. In addition, vestibular disturbances may occur with minocycline.

### Pediatrics
In infants and children up to 8 years of age, tetracyclines may cause permanent discoloration of teeth, enamel hypoplasia, and a decrease in linear skeletal growth rate. Therefore, use is not recommended in patients in these age groups unless other antibacterials are unlikely to be effective or are contraindicated.

Bulging fontanels have been reported in young infants who received full therapeutic doses of tetracyclines. This side effect disappeared rapidly upon discontinuation of the drug.

### Geriatrics
No information is available on the relationship of age to the effects of tetracyclines in geriatric patients.

### Dental
Use of systemic tetracyclines during pregnancy or in infants and children up to 8 years of age may cause permanent discoloration of teeth and enamel hypoplasia. Therefore, use is not recommended unless other antibacterials are unlikely to be effective or are contraindicated. Vital

bleaching or esthetic restoration may be required if staining is objectionable.

Systemic tetracyclines may also contribute to the development of oral candidiasis.

## Drug interactions and/or related problems

The following drug interactions and/or related problems have been selected on the basis of their potential clinical significance (possible mechanism in parentheses where appropriate)—not necessarily inclusive (» = major clinical significance):

Note: Combinations containing any of the following medications, depending on the amount present, may also interact with this medication.

» Antacids or
» Calcium supplements such as calcium carbonate or
» Choline and magnesium salicylates or
» Iron supplements or
» Magnesium salicylate or
» Magnesium-containing laxatives
    Sodium bicarbonate
        (concurrent use may result in formation of nonabsorbable complexes; also, concurrent use with antacids or sodium bicarbonate may result in decreased absorption of oral tetracyclines because of increased intragastric pH; patients should be advised not to take these medications within 1 to 3 hours of oral tetracyclines)

    Barbiturates or
    Carbamazepine or
    Phenytoin
        (concurrent use with doxycycline may result in decreased doxycycline serum concentrations due to induction of microsomal enzyme activity; adjustment of doxycycline dosage or substitution of another tetracycline may be necessary)

» Cholestyramine or
» Colestipol
        (concurrent use with cholestyramine or colestipol may result in binding of oral tetracyclines, thus impairing their absorption; an interval of several hours between administration of cholestyramine or colestipol and oral tetracyclines is recommended)

» Contraceptives, estrogen-containing, oral
        (concurrent long-term use with tetracyclines may result in reduced contraceptive reliability and increased incidence of breakthrough bleeding)

    Methoxyflurane
        (concurrent use with tetracyclines may increase the potential for nephrotoxicity)

    Penicillins
        (since bacteriostatic drugs may interfere with the bactericidal effect of penicillins in the treatment of meningitis or in other situations where a rapid bactericidal effect is necessary, it is best to avoid concurrent therapy)

    Vitamin A
        (concurrent use with tetracycline has been reported to cause benign intracranial hypertension)

## Laboratory value alterations

The following have been selected on the basis of their potential clinical significance (possible effect in parentheses where appropriate)—not necessarily inclusive (» = major clinical significance):

With diagnostic test results
    Catecholamine determinations, urine
        (may produce false elevations of urinary catecholamines because of interfering fluorescence in the Hingerty method)

With physiology/laboratory test values
    Alanine aminotransferase (ALT [SGPT]) and
    Alkaline phosphatase and
    Amylase and
    Aspartate aminotransferase (AST [SGOT]) and
    Bilirubin
        (serum concentrations may be increased)

    Blood urea nitrogen (BUN)
        (antianabolic effect of tetracyclines [except doxycycline] may increase BUN concentrations; in patients with significantly impaired renal function, increased serum concentrations of tetracyclines may lead to azotemia, hyperphosphatemia, and acidosis)

## Medical considerations/Contraindications

The medical considerations/contraindications included here have been selected on the basis of their potential clinical significance (reasons given in parentheses where appropriate)—not necessarily inclusive (» = major clinical significance).

*Risk-benefit should be considered when the following medical problems exist:*

» Diabetes insipidus, nephrogenic
    (demeclocycline induces a reversible nephrogenic diabetes insipidus)

  Hepatic function impairment
    (doxycycline and minocycline are partially metabolized in the liver; hepatic function impairment may prolong the elimination half-life)

  Hypersensitivity to tetracyclines, or "caine-type" local anesthetics
    (e.g., lidocaine, procaine)

» Renal function impairment
    (the half-life of tetracyclines, except doxycycline or minocycline, is prolonged in patients with renal function impairment)

# Side/Adverse Effects

Note: Tetracycline-induced hepatotoxicity is usually seen as a fatty degeneration of the liver. It is more likely to occur in pregnant women, in patients receiving high-dose intravenous therapy, and in patients with renal function impairment. However, hepatotoxicity has also occurred in patients without these predisposing conditions. Tetracycline-induced pancreatitis has also been described in associated with hepatotoxicity, and without associated liver disease.

The following side/adverse effects have been selected on the basis of their potential clinical significance (possible signs and symptoms in parentheses where appropriate)—not necessarily inclusive:

**Those indicating need for medical attention**
Incidence more frequent
    *Discoloration of infants' or children's teeth; photosensitivity* (increased sensitivity of skin to sunlight)
Incidence less frequent
    *Nephrogenic diabetes insipidus* (greatly increased frequency of urination or amount of urine; increased thirst; unusual tiredness or weakness)—with demeclocycline; *pigmentation of skin and mucous membranes*—primarily with minocycline
Incidence rare
    *Benign intracranial hypertension* (anorexia; headache; vomiting; papilledema; visual changes; bulging fontanel in infants); *hepatotoxicity* (abdominal pain; nausea and vomiting; yellowing skin); *pancreatitis* (abdominal pain; nausea and vomiting)

**Those indicating need for medical attention only if they continue or are bothersome**
Incidence more frequent
    *CNS toxicity* (dizziness; lightheadedness; unsteadiness); *gastrointestinal disturbances* (cramps or burning of the stomach; diarrhea; nausea or vomiting); *photosensitivity* (increased sensitivity of skin to sunlight)
Incidence less frequent
    *Fungal overgrowth* (itching of the rectal or genital areas; sore mouth or tongue); *hypertrophy of the papilla* (darkened or discolored tongue)

# Patient Consultation

As an aid to patient consultation, refer to *Advice for the Patient, Tetracyclines (Systemic)*.

In providing consultation, consider emphasizing the following selected information (» = major clinical significance):

**Before using this medication**
» Conditions affecting use, especially:
    Sensitivity to tetracyclines
    Pregnancy—Tetracyclines cross the placenta; use is not recommended during the last half of pregnancy since tetracyclines may cause permanent discoloration of teeth, enamel hypoplasia, and inhibition of skeletal growth in the fetus; also, fatty infiltration of the liver may occur in pregnant women, especially with high intravenous doses
    Breast-feeding—Tetracyclines distributed into breast milk; although tetracyclines may form nonabsorbable complexes with breast-milk calcium, use is not recommended because of the possibility of their causing permanent discoloration of teeth, enamel hypoplasia, inhibition of linear skeletal growth, photosensitivity reactions, and oral and vaginal thrush in infants
    Use in children—In infants and children up to 8 years of age, tetracyclines may cause permanent discoloration of teeth, enamel hypoplasia, and a decrease in linear skeletal growth rate
    Other medications, especially antacids, calcium supplements, cholestyramine, choline and magnesium salicylates, colestipol, estrogen-containing oral contraceptives, iron supplements, magnesium salicylate, or magnesium-containing laxatives

Other medical problems, especially nephrogenic diabetes insipidus or renal function impairment

**Proper use of this medication**

» Not giving to children up to 8 years of age

Taking with at least a full glass of water while in an upright position to avoid esophageal ulceration or to decrease gastrointestinal irritation

» Avoiding concurrent use of milk or other dairy products when taking oral demeclocycline, oxytetracycline, and tetracycline; if gastrointestinal irritation still occurs, these medicines may be taken with food

Oral doxycycline and minocycline may be taken with food or milk if gastric irritation occurs

» Discarding outdated or decomposed tetracyclines (decomposed products may be toxic)

» Compliance with full course of therapy

» Importance of not missing doses and taking at evenly spaced times

» Proper dosing

Missed dose: Taking as soon as possible; not taking if almost time for next dose; not doubling doses

» Proper storage

**Precautions while using this medication**

Checking with physician if no improvement within a few days (or a few weeks or months for acne patients)

» Avoiding antacids, calcium supplements, choline and magnesium salicylates, iron supplements, magnesium salicylate, magnesium-containing laxatives, sodium bicarbonate within 1 to 3 hours of oral tetracyclines

» Use of an alternate or additional method of contraception if concurrently taking estrogen-containing oral contraceptives

Caution if surgery with general anesthesia is required

» Possible photosensitivity reactions

» Caution if dizziness, lightheadedness, or unsteadiness occurs

**Side/adverse effects**

Signs of potential side effects such as discoloration of infant's or children's teeth, nephrogenic diabetes insipidus—with demeclocycline, pigmentation of skin and mucous membranes—with minocycline, benign intracranial hypertension, hepatotoxicity, pancreatitis, and photosensitivity

## General Dosing Information

Use of tetracyclines (except doxycycline and minocycline) in patients with impaired renal function is not recommended.

**For oral dosage forms only**

All tetracyclines should be taken with a full glass (240 mL) of water to avoid esophageal ulceration and to decrease gastrointestinal irritation. In addition, most tetracyclines (except doxycycline and minocycline) should preferably be taken on an empty stomach (either 1 hour before or 2 hours after meals) to obtain optimum serum concentrations.

---

### *DEMECLOCYCLINE*

---

## Summary of Differences

Indications:

Also used as a diuretic (syndrome of inappropriate diuretic hormone [SIADH]).

Pharmacology/pharmacokinetics:

Different mechanism of action in SIADH.

Precautions:

Drug interactions and/or related problems—Also interacts with desmopressin.

Medical considerations/contraindications—Caution also needed in nephrogenic diabetes insipidus.

Side/adverse effects:

May also cause greatly increased frequency of urination or amount of urine, increased thirst, or unusual tiredness or weakness (nephrogenic diabetes insipidus).

## Oral Dosage Forms

Note: Bracketed uses in the *Dosage Forms* section refer to categories of use and/or indications that are not included in U.S. product labeling.

The dosing and dosage forms available are expressed in terms of demeclocycline hydrochloride.

## DEMECLOCYCLINE HYDROCHLORIDE CAPSULES USP

**Usual adult and adolescent dose**

Antibacterial (systemic); antiprotozoal—

Oral, 150 mg every six hours; or 300 mg every twelve hours.

Note: Gonorrhea—Oral, 300 mg every twelve hours for four days, up to a total dose of 3 grams.

[Diuretic (SIADH)]—

Oral, 3.25 to 3.75 mg per kg of body weight every six hours.

**Usual adult prescribing limits**

Antibacterial (systemic); antiprotozoal—

Up to 2.4 grams daily.

[Diuretic (SIADH)]—

300 mg to 1.2 grams daily.

**Usual pediatric dose**

Children 8 years of age and over—Antibacterial (systemic); antiprotozoal—

Oral, 1.65 to 3.3 mg per kg of body weight every six hours; or 3.3 to 6.6 mg per kg of body weight every twelve hours.

Note: Infants and children up to 8 years of age—All tetracyclines form a stable calcium complex in any bone-forming tissue. Accordingly, tetracyclines may cause permanent yellow-gray-brown discoloration of the teeth, as well as enamel hypoplasia. Also, a decrease in linear skeletal growth rate may occur in premature infants. Therefore, tetracyclines are not recommended in these age groups unless other drugs are unlikely to be effective or are contraindicated.

**Strength(s) usually available**

U.S.—

150 mg (Rx) [*Declomycin*].

Canada—

Not commercially available.

**Packaging and storage**

Store below 40 °C (104 °F), preferably between 15 and 30 °C (59 and 86 °F), unless otherwise specified by manufacturer. Store in a tight, light-resistant container.

**Auxiliary labeling**

• Continue medicine for full time of treatment.

• Do not take within 1 to 3 hours of other medicines, milk, or other dairy products.

• Avoid too much sun or use of sunlamp.

• Keep container tightly closed in a dry place.

## DEMECLOCYCLINE HYDROCHLORIDE TABLETS USP

**Usual adult and adolescent dose**

See *Demeclocycline Hydrochloride Capsules USP*.

**Usual adult prescribing limits**

See *Demeclocycline Hydrochloride Capsules USP*.

**Usual pediatric dose**

See *Demeclocycline Hydrochloride Capsules USP*.

**Strength(s) usually available**

U.S.—

150 mg (Rx) [*Declomycin*].

300 mg (Rx) [*Declomycin*].

Canada—

150 mg (Rx) [*Declomycin*].

300 mg (Rx) [*Declomycin*].

**Packaging and storage**

Store below 40 °C (104 °F), preferably between 15 and 30 °C (59 and 86 °F), unless otherwise specified by manufacturer. Store in a tight, light-resistant container.

**Auxiliary labeling**

• Continue medicine for full time of treatment.

• Do not take within 1 to 3 hours of other medicines, milk, or other dairy products.

• Avoid too much sun or use of sunlamp.

• Keep container tightly closed in a dry place.

---

### *DOXYCYCLINE*

---

## Summary of Differences

Indications:

Also indicated for the prevention of malaria.

Precautions:

Drug interactions and/or related problems—

Also interacts with barbiturates, carbamazepine, and phenytoin.

No interaction with methoxyflurane.
Laboratory value alterations—
  No increase in BUN concentrations.
Medical considerations/contraindications—
  Caution not needed in renal impairment.
General dosing information:
  No dosage reduction in renal impairment.
  May be taken with food, milk, or carbonated beverages.

## Additional Dosing Information

Even though approximately 40% of a dose of doxycycline may be eliminated through the kidneys in patients with normal renal function, patients with impaired renal function do not generally require a reduction in dose since doxycycline alternatively may be eliminated through the liver, biliary tract, and gastrointestinal tract and does not have the antianabolic effect of other tetracyclines.

For oral dosage forms only:
• Doxycycline may be taken with food or milk if gastrointestinal irritation occurs.

## Oral Dosage Forms

Note: Bracketed uses in the *Dosage Forms* section refer to categories of use and/or indications that are not included in U.S. product labeling.

### DOXYCYCLINE FOR ORAL SUSPENSION USP

**Usual adult and adolescent dose**
Antibacterial (systemic); antiprotozoal—
Oral, 100 mg (base) every twelve hours the first day, then 100 to 200 mg once a day; or 50 to 100 mg every twelve hours.

Note: Gonococcal infections, uncomplicated (except anorectal infections in men)—Oral, 100 mg (base) every twelve hours for seven days; or 300 mg initially, then 300 mg one hour later.

Malaria prophylaxis—Oral, 100 mg (base) once a day. Prophylaxis should begin one or two days before travel to the malarious area, be continued daily during travel, and for four weeks after the traveler leaves the malarious area.

Nongonococcal urethritis caused by *Chlamydia trachomatis* or *Ureaplasma urealyticum,* and

Uncomplicated urethral, endocervical, or rectal infection caused by *Chlamydia trachomatis*—Oral, 100 mg (base) two times a day for at least seven days.

Syphilis (primary and secondary)—Oral, 150 mg (base) every twelve hours for at least ten days.

[Traveler's diarrhea (prophylaxis)]—Oral, 100 mg (base) once a day for three weeks.

[Lyme disease (treatment)]—Oral, 100 mg (base) two times a day.

**Usual adult prescribing limits**
Up to 300 mg (base) daily; or up to 600 mg daily for five days in acute gonococcal infections.

**Usual pediatric dose**
Antibacterial (systemic); antiprotozoal—
Children 45 kg of body weight and under: Oral, 2.2 mg (base) per kg of body weight every twelve hours the first day, then 2.2 to 4.4 mg per kg of body weight once a day; or 1.1 to 2.2 mg per kg of body weight every twelve hours.
Children over 45 kg of body weight: See *Usual adult and adolescent dose.*

Note: Malaria prophylaxis

Children over 8 years of age—Oral, 2 mg per kg of body weight, up to 100 mg, once a day. Prophylaxis should begin one or two days before travel to the malarious area, be continued daily during travel, and for four weeks after the traveler leaves the malarious area.

[Lyme disease (treatment)]—Children over 8 years of age: Oral, 1 to 2 mg per kg of body weight two times a day.

Infants and children up to 8 years of age—All tetracyclines form a stable calcium complex in any bone-forming tissue. Accordingly, tetracyclines may cause permanent yellow-gray-brown discoloration of the teeth, as well as enamel hypoplasia. Also, a decrease in linear skeletal growth rate may occur in premature infants. Therefore, tetracyclines are not recommended in these age groups unless other drugs are unlikely to be effective or are contraindicated.

**Strength(s) usually available**
U.S.—
25 mg per 5 mL, when reconstituted according to manufacturer's instructions (base) (Rx) [*Vibramycin*].

Canada—
Not commercially available.

**Packaging and storage**
Prior to reconstitution, store below 40 °C (104 °F), preferably between 15 and 30 °C (59 and 86 °F), unless otherwise specified by manufacturer. Store in a tight, light-resistant container.

**Stability**
After reconstitution, suspensions retain their potency for 14 days at room temperature.

**Auxiliary labeling**
• Shake well.
• Continue medicine for full time of treatment.
• Do not take within 1 to 3 hours of other medicines.
• Avoid too much sun or use of sunlamp.
• Beyond-use date.

**Note**
When dispensing, include a calibrated liquid-measuring device.

### DOXYCYCLINE CALCIUM ORAL SUSPENSION USP

**Usual adult and adolescent dose**
See *Doxycycline for Oral Suspension USP.*

**Usual adult prescribing limits**
See *Doxycycline for Oral Suspension USP.*

**Usual pediatric dose**
See *Doxycycline for Oral Suspension USP.*

**Strength(s) usually available**
U.S.—
50 mg per 5 mL (base) (Rx) [*Vibramycin*].
Canada—
Not commercially available.

**Packaging and storage**
Store below 40 °C (104 °F), preferably between 15 and 30 °C (59 and 86 °F), unless otherwise specified by manufacturer. Store in a tight, light-resistant container. Protect from freezing.

**Auxiliary labeling**
• Shake well.
• Continue medicine for full time of treatment.
• Do not take within 1 to 3 hours of other medicines.
• Avoid too much sun or use of sunlamp.

**Note**
When dispensing, include a calibrated liquid-measuring device.

### DOXYCYCLINE HYCLATE CAPSULES USP

**Usual adult and adolescent dose**
See *Doxycycline for Oral Suspension USP.*

**Usual adult prescribing limits**
See *Doxycycline for Oral Suspension USP.*

**Usual pediatric dose**
See *Doxycycline for Oral Suspension USP.*

**Strength(s) usually available**
U.S.—
50 mg (base) (Rx) [*Monodox; Vibramycin;* GENERIC].
100 mg (base) (Rx) [*Doxy-Caps; Monodox; Vibramycin;* GENERIC].
Canada—
100 mg (base) (Rx) [*Apo-Doxy; Doxycin; Novodoxylin; Vibramycin*].

**Packaging and storage**
Store below 40 °C (104 °F), preferably between 15 and 30 °C (59 and 86 °F), unless otherwise specified by manufacturer. Store in a tight, light-resistant container.

**Auxiliary labeling**
• Continue medicine for full time of treatment.
• Do not take within 1 to 3 hours of other medicines.
• Avoid too much sun or use of sunlamp.
• Keep container tightly closed in a dry place.

### DOXYCYCLINE HYCLATE DELAYED-RELEASE CAPSULES USP

**Usual adult and adolescent dose**
See *Doxycycline for Oral Suspension USP.*

**Usual adult prescribing limits**
See *Doxycycline for Oral Suspension USP.*

**Usual pediatric dose**
See *Doxycycline for Oral Suspension USP.*

**Strength(s) usually available**

U.S.—

100 mg (base) (Rx) [*Doryx;* GENERIC].

Canada—

100 mg (base) (Rx) [*Doryx*].

**Packaging and storage**

Store below 40 °C (104 °F), preferably between 15 and 30 °C (59 and 86 °F), unless otherwise specified by manufacturer. Store in a tight, light-resistant container.

**Auxiliary labeling**

• Continue medicine for full time of treatment.
• Do not take within 1 to 3 hours of other medicines.
• Avoid too much sun or use of sunlamp.
• Keep container tightly closed in a dry place.
• Swallow capsules whole.

**Note**

Doxycycline Delayed-release Capsules USP contain enteric-coated pellets.

## DOXYCYCLINE HYCLATE TABLETS USP

**Usual adult and adolescent dose**

See *Doxycycline for Oral Suspension USP.*

**Usual adult prescribing limits**

See *Doxycycline for Oral Suspension USP.*

**Usual pediatric dose**

See *Doxycycline for Oral Suspension USP.*

**Strength(s) usually available**

U.S.—

100 mg (base) (Rx) [*Doxi Film; Vibra-Tabs;* GENERIC].

Canada—

100 mg (base) (Rx) [*Doxycin; Vibra-Tabs*].

**Packaging and storage**

Store below 40 °C (104 °F), preferably between 15 and 30 °C (59 and 86 °F), unless otherwise specified by manufacturer. Store in a tight, light-resistant container.

**Auxiliary labeling**

• Continue medicine for full time of treatment.
• Do not take within 1 to 3 hours of other medicines.
• Avoid too much sun or use of sunlamp.
• Keep container tightly closed in a dry place.

## Parenteral Dosage Forms

### DOXYCYCLINE HYCLATE FOR INJECTION USP

**Usual adult and adolescent dose**

Antibacterial (systemic); antiprotozoal—

Intravenous infusion, 200 mg (base) once a day or 100 mg every twelve hours the first day, then 100 to 200 mg once a day; or 50 to 100 mg every twelve hours.

Note: Syphilis (primary and secondary)—Intravenous infusion, 150 mg (base) every twelve hours for at least ten days.

**Usual adult prescribing limits**

Up to 300 mg (base) daily.

**Usual pediatric dose**

Antibacterial (systemic); antiprotozoal—

Children 45 kg of body weight and under: Intravenous infusion, 4.4 mg (base) per kg of body weight once a day or 2.2 mg per kg of body weight every twelve hours the first day; then 2.2 to 4.4 mg per kg of body weight once a day or 1.1 to 2.2 mg per kg of body weight every twelve hours.

Children over 45 kg of body weight: See *Usual adult and adolescent dose.*

Note: Infants and children up to 8 years of age—All tetracyclines form a stable calcium complex in any bone-forming tissue. Accordingly, tetracyclines may cause permanent yellow-gray-brown discoloration of the teeth, as well as enamel hypoplasia. Also, a decrease in linear skeletal growth rate may occur in premature infants. Therefore, tetracyclines are not recommended in these age groups unless other drugs are unlikely to be effective or are contraindicated.

**Size(s) usually available**

U.S.—

100 mg (base) (Rx) [*Doxy, Vibramycin;* GENERIC].

200 mg (base) (Rx) [*Doxy; Vibramycin;* GENERIC].

Canada—

100 mg (base) (Rx) [*Vibramycin*].

**Packaging and storage**

Prior to reconstitution, store below 40 °C (104 °F), preferably between 15 and 30 °C (59 and 86 °F), unless otherwise specified by manufacturer. Protect from light.

**Preparation of dosage form**

To prepare initial dilution for intravenous use, add 10 mL of sterile water for injection or other suitable diluents (see manufacturer's package insert) to each 100-mg vial or 20 mL of diluent to each 200-mg vial. The resulting solution containing the equivalent of 100 to 200 mg of doxycycline may be further diluted in 100 to 1000 mL or in 200 to 2000 mL of suitable diluent, respectively.

**Stability**

After reconstitution, intravenous infusions of doxycycline hyclate retain their potency for 12 hours at room temperature or for 72 hours if refrigerated at concentrations of 100 mcg (0.1 mg) to 1 mg per mL in suitable fluids (see manufacturer's package insert). Intravenous infusions of doxycycline hyclate retain their potency for 6 hours at room temperature at concentrations of 100 mcg (0.1 mg) to 1 mg per mL in lactated Ringer's injection or 5% dextrose and lactated Ringer's injection. Infusions must be protected from direct sunlight during administration.

If frozen immediately after reconstitution with sterile water for injection, solutions at concentrations of 10 mg per mL retain their potency up to 8 weeks at −20 °C (−4 °F). Once thawed, solutions should not be refrozen.

**Additional information**

Concentrations less than 100 mcg (0.1 mg) per mL or greater than 1 mg per mL are not recommended.

Infusions may be administered over a 1- to 4-hour period. Avoid rapid administration.

Do not administer intramuscularly or subcutaneously.

---

## *MINOCYCLINE*

## Summary of Differences

Precautions:

Laboratory value alterations—No increase in BUN concentrations.

Medical considerations/contraindications—Caution not needed in renal impairment.

Side/adverse effects:

May also cause dizziness, lightheadedness, or unsteadiness (central nervous system [CNS] toxicity); and pigmentation of skin and mucous membranes.

General dosing information:

No dosage reduction in renal impairment.

May be taken with food or milk.

## Additional Dosing Information

For oral dosage forms only:

• Minocycline may be taken with food or milk if gastrointestinal irritation occurs.

## Oral Dosage Forms

### MINOCYCLINE HYDROCHLORIDE CAPSULES USP

**Usual adult and adolescent dose**

Antibacterial (systemic); antiprotozoal—

Oral, 200 mg (base) initially, then 100 mg every twelve hours; or 100 to 200 mg initially, then 50 mg every six hours.

Note: Gonorrhea—Oral, 100 mg (base) every twelve hours for at least four days.

*Mycobacterium marinum* infections—Oral, 100 mg (base) every twelve hours for six to eight weeks.

*Neisseria meningitidis* carriers (asymptomatic)—Oral, 100 mg (base) every twelve hours for five days.

Uncomplicated urethral, endocervical, or rectal infection caused by *Chlamydia trachomatis*—Oral, 100 mg (base) two times a day for at least seven days.

**Usual adult prescribing limits**

Up to 350 mg (base) the first day; then up to 200 mg a day.

**Usual pediatric dose**

Antibacterial (systemic); antiprotozoal—

Children 8 years of age and over: Oral, 4 mg (base) per kg of body weight initially, then 2 mg per kg of body weight every twelve hours.

Note: Infants and children up to 8 years of age—All tetracyclines form a stable calcium complex in any bone-forming tissue. Accordingly, tetracyclines may cause permanent yellow-gray-brown discoloration of the teeth, as well as enamel hypoplasia. Also, a decrease in linear skeletal growth rate may occur in premature infants. Therefore, tetracyclines are not recommended in these age groups unless other drugs are unlikely to be effective or are contraindicated.

### Strength(s) usually available
U.S.—
     50 mg (base) (Rx) [*Dynacin; Minocin;* GENERIC].
     100 mg (base) (Rx) [*Dynacin; Minocin;* GENERIC].
Canada—
     50 mg (base) (Rx) [*Minocin*].
     100 mg (base) (Rx) [*Minocin*].

### Packaging and storage
Store below 40 °C (104 °F), preferably between 15 and 30 °C (59 and 86 °F), unless otherwise specified by manufacturer. Store in a tight, light-resistant container.

### Auxiliary labeling
• Continue medicine for full time of treatment.
• Do not take within 1 to 3 hours of other medicines.
• Avoid too much sun or use of sunlamp.
• Keep container tightly closed in a dry place.
• May cause dizziness.

## MINOCYCLINE HYDROCHLORIDE ORAL SUSPENSION USP

### Usual adult and adolescent dose
See *Minocycline Hydrochloride Capsules.*

### Usual adult prescribing limits
See *Minocycline Hydrochloride Capsules USP.*

### Usual pediatric dose
See *Minocycline Hydrochloride Capsules USP.*

### Strength(s) usually available
U.S.—
     50 mg (base) (Rx) [*Minocin*].
Canada—
     Not commercially available.

### Packaging and storage
Store below 40 °C (104 °F), preferably between 15 and 30 °C (59 and 86 °F), unless otherwise specified by manufacturer. Store in a tight, light-resistant container. Protect from freezing.

### Auxiliary labeling
• Shake well.
• Continue medicine for full time of treatment.
• Do not take within 1 to 3 hours of other medicines.
• Avoid too much sun or use of sunlamp.
• May cause dizziness.

### Note
When dispensing, include a calibrated liquid-measuring device.

## MINOCYCLINE HYDROCHLORIDE TABLETS

### Usual adult and adolescent dose
See *Minocycline Hydrochloride Capsules USP.*

### Usual adult prescribing limits
See *Minocycline Hydrochloride Capsules USP.*

### Usual pediatric dose
See *Minocycline Hydrochloride Capsules USP.*

### Strength(s) usually available
U.S.—
     50 mg (base) (Rx) [GENERIC].
     100 mg (base) (Rx) [GENERIC].
Canada—
     Not commercially available.

### Packaging and storage
Store below 40 °C (104 °F), preferably between 15 and 30 °C (59 and 86 °F), unless otherwise specified by manufacturer. Store in a tight, light-resistant container. Protect from freezing.

### Auxiliary labeling
• Continue medicine for full time of treatment.
• Do not take within 1 to 3 hours of other medicines.
• Avoid too much sun or use of sunlamp.
• May cause dizziness.
• Keep container tightly closed and in a dry place.

## Parenteral Dosage Forms
### STERILE MINOCYCLINE HYDROCHLORIDE USP
#### Usual adult and adolescent dose
Intravenous infusion, 200 mg (base) initially, then 100 mg every twelve hours.

#### Usual adult prescribing limits
Up to 400 mg (base) daily.

#### Usual pediatric dose
Children 8 years of age and over—Intravenous infusion, 4 mg (base) per kg of body weight initially, then 2 mg per kg of body weight every twelve hours.

Note: Infants and children up to 8 years of age—All tetracyclines form a stable calcium complex in any bone-forming tissue. Accordingly, tetracyclines may cause permanent yellow-gray-brown discoloration of the teeth, as well as enamel hypoplasia. Also, a decrease in linear skeletal growth rate may occur in premature infants. Therefore, tetracyclines are not recommended in these age groups unless other drugs are unlikely to be effective or are contraindicated.

#### Size(s) usually available
U.S.—
     100 mg (base) (Rx) [*Minocin*].
Canada—
     Not commercially available.

#### Packaging and storage
Prior to reconstitution, store below 40 °C (104 °F), preferably between 15 and 30 °C (59 and 86 °F), unless otherwise specified by manufacturer. Protect from light.

#### Preparation of dosage form
To prepare initial dilution for intravenous use, add 5 to 10 mL of sterile water for injection to each 100-mg vial.
The resulting solution may be further diluted in 500 to 1000 mL of 0.9% sodium chloride injection, dextrose injection, dextrose and sodium chloride injection, Ringer's injection, or lactated Ringer's injection, but not in other calcium-containing solutions since a precipitate may form. Administration should be started immediately, but avoid rapid administration.

#### Stability
After reconstitution, solutions retain their potency for 24 hours at room temperature.

---

### OXYTETRACYCLINE

## Additional Dosing Information
For parenteral dosage forms only:
• Serum concentrations should not exceed 15 mcg per mL, especially in pregnant or postpartum patients with pyelonephritis.

## Oral Dosage Forms
### OXYTETRACYCLINE HYDROCHLORIDE CAPSULES USP
#### Usual adult and adolescent dose
Antibacterial (systemic); antiprotozoal—
     Oral, 250 to 500 mg (base) every six hours.

Note: Brucellosis—Oral, 500 mg (base) every six hours for three weeks, given concurrently with 1 gram of streptomycin intramuscularly every twelve hours the first week and once a day the second week.
     Gonorrhea, uncomplicated—Oral, 500 mg (base) every six hours, up to a total dose of 9 grams.
     Syphilis—Oral, 500 mg (base) every six hours for fifteen days (early syphilis) or for thirty days (late syphilis).

#### Usual adult prescribing limits
Up to 4 grams (base) daily.

#### Usual pediatric dose
Antibacterial (systemic); antiprotozoal—
     Children 8 years of age and over: Oral, 6.25 to 12.5 mg (base) per kg of body weight every six hours.

Note: Infants and children up to 8 years of age—All tetracyclines form a stable calcium complex in any bone-forming tissue. Accordingly, tetracyclines may cause permanent yellow-gray-brown discoloration of the teeth, as well as enamel hypoplasia. Also, a decrease in linear skeletal growth rate may occur in premature infants. Therefore, tetracyclines are not recommended in these age groups unless other drugs are unlikely to be effective or are contraindicated.

**Strength(s) usually available**
U.S.—
    250 mg (base) (Rx) [*Terramycin; Tija;* GENERIC].
Canada—
    Not commercially available.

**Packaging and storage**
Store below 40 °C (104 °F), preferably between 15 and 30 °C (59 and 86 °F), unless otherwise specified by manufacturer. Store in a tight, light-resistant container.

**Auxiliary labeling**
• Continue medicine for full time of treatment.
• Do not take within 1 to 3 hours of other medicines, milk, or other dairy products.
• Avoid too much sun or use of sunlamp.
• Keep container tightly closed in a dry place.

# Parenteral Dosage Forms
## OXYTETRACYCLINE INJECTION USP

**Usual adult and adolescent dose**
Antibacterial (systemic); antiprotozoal—
    Intramuscular, 100 mg (base) every eight hours; 150 mg every twelve hours; or 250 mg once a day.

**Usual adult prescribing limits**
Up to 500 mg (base) daily.

**Usual pediatric dose**
Antibacterial (systemic); antiprotozoal—
    Children 8 years of age and over: Intramuscular, 5 to 8.3 mg (base) per kg of body weight every eight hours; or 7.5 to 12.5 mg per kg of body weight every twelve hours. Maximum daily dose should not exceed 250 mg.
Note: Infants and children up to 8 years of age—All tetracyclines form a stable calcium complex in any bone-forming tissue. Accordingly, tetracyclines may cause permanent yellow-gray-brown discoloration of the teeth, as well as enamel hypoplasia. Also, a decrease in linear skeletal growth rate may occur in premature infants. Therefore, tetracyclines are not recommended in these age groups unless other drugs are unlikely to be effective or are contraindicated.

**Strength(s) usually available**
U.S.—
    50 mg per mL (base) (Rx) [*Terramycin*].
    125 mg per mL (base) (Rx) [*Terramycin*].
    Note: Injection contains 2% of lidocaine.
Canada—
    Not commercially available.

**Packaging and storage**
Store below 40 °C (104 °F), preferably between 15 and 30 °C (59 and 86 °F), unless otherwise specified by manufacturer. Protect from light. Protect from freezing.

**Additional information**
Cross-sensitivity with other "caine-type" local anesthetics may also occur.
For deep intramuscular use only. Do not administer intravenously.
May cause intense pain and local irritation at the site of intramuscular injections.
Since intramuscular administration of oxytetracycline produces lower serum concentrations than oral administration in recommended doses, patients should be changed to an oral dosage form as soon as feasible.
When rapid, high serum concentrations are required, an intravenous form (oxytetracycline hydrochloride) should be used.

## OXYTETRACYCLINE HYDROCHLORIDE FOR INJECTION USP

**Usual adult and adolescent dose**
Antibacterial (systemic); antiprotozoal—
    Intravenous infusion, 250 to 500 mg (base) every twelve hours.

**Usual adult prescribing limits**
Up to 2 grams (base) daily.

**Usual pediatric dose**
Children 8 years of age and over—Antibacterial (systemic); antiprotozoal—
    Intravenous infusion, 5 to 10 mg (base) per kg of body weight every twelve hours.
Note: Infants and children up to 8 years of age—All tetracyclines form a stable calcium complex in any bone-forming tissue. Accordingly, tetracyclines may cause permant yellow-gray-brown discoloration of the teeth, as well as enamel hypoplasia. Also, a decrease in linear skeletal growth rate may occur in premature infants. Therefore, tetracyclines are not recommended in these age groups unless other drugs are unlikely to be effective or are contraindicated.

**Size(s) usually available**
U.S.—
    500 mg (base) (Rx) [*Terramycin*].
Canada—
    Not commercially available.

**Packaging and storage**
Prior to reconstitution, store below 40 °C (104 °F), preferably between 15 and 30 °C (59 and 86 °F), unless otherwise specified by manufacturer. Protect from light.

**Preparation of dosage form**
To prepare initial dilution for intravenous use, add 10 mL of sterile water for injection or 5% dextrose injection to each 250- or 500-mg vial.
The resulting solution should be further diluted in at least 100 mL of 5% dextrose injection, 0.9% sodium chloride injection, or Ringer's injection.

**Stability**
After reconstitution, solutions retain their potency for 48 hours if refrigerated.

**Additional information**
Avoid rapid administration. If patient complains of vein irritation, decrease the rate of administration or increase the volume of diluent.
Do not administer intramuscularly or subcutaneously.

---

## TETRACYCLINE

# Additional Dosing Information

For parenteral dosage forms only:
• Serum concentrations should not exceed 15 mcg per mL, especially in pregnant or postpartum patients with pyelonephritis.

# Oral Dosage Forms

Note: The dosing and dosage forms available are expressed in terms of tetracycline hydrochloride.

## TETRACYCLINE ORAL SUSPENSION USP

**Usual adult and adolescent dose**
Antibacterial (systemic); antiprotozoal—
    Oral, 250 to 500 mg every six hours; or 500 mg to 1 gram every twelve hours.
Antiacne agent (systemic)—
    Oral, 500 mg to 2 grams daily in divided doses initially in moderate to severe cases as adjunctive therapy. When improvement is noted (usually after 3 weeks), dosage should be reduced gradually to a maintenance dose of 125 to 1000 mg daily. Adequate remission of lesions may also be possible with alternate-day or intermittent therapy.
Note: Brucellosis—Oral, 500 mg every six hours for three weeks, given concurrently with 1 gram of streptomycin intramuscularly every twelve hours the first week and once a day the second week.
    Gonorrhea—Oral, 500 mg every six hours for five days.
    Syphilis—Oral, 500 mg every six hours for fifteen days (early syphilis) or for thirty days (late syphilis).
    Uncomplicated urethral, endocervical, or rectal infection caused by *Chlamydia trachomatis*—Oral, 500 mg four times a day for at least seven days.
    [Lyme disease (treatment)]—Oral, 250 to 500 mg four times a day.

**Usual adult prescribing limits**
Up to 4 grams daily.

**Usual pediatric dose**
Antibacterial (systemic); antiprotozoal—
    Children 8 years of age and over: Oral, 6.25 to 12.5 mg per kg of body weight every six hours; or 12.5 to 25 mg per kg of body weight every twelve hours.
Note: [Lyme disease (treatment)]—Children over 8 years of age: Oral, 6.25 to 12.5 mg per kg of body weight four times a day.
    Infants and children up to 8 years of age—All tetracyclines form a stable calcium complex in any bone-forming tissue. Accordingly, tetracyclines may cause permanent yellow-gray-brown discoloration of the teeth, as well as enamel hypoplasia. Also, a decrease in linear skeletal growth rate may occur in premature infants. Therefore, tetracyclines are not recommended in these age groups unless other drugs are unlikely to be effective or are contraindicated.

**Strength(s) usually available**
U.S.—
   125 mg per 5 mL (Rx) [*Achromycin V; Sumycin;* GENERIC].
Canada—
   125 mg per 5 mL (Rx) [*Novotetra*].

**Packaging and storage**
Store below 40 °C (104 °F), preferably between 15 and 30 °C (59 and 86 °F), unless otherwise specified by manufacturer. Store in a tight, light-resistant container. Protect from freezing.

**Auxiliary labeling**
• Shake well.
• Continue medicine for full time of treatment.
• Do not take within 1 to 3 hours of other medicines, milk, or other dairy products.
• Avoid too much sun or use of sunlamp.

**Note**
When dispensing, include a calibrated liquid-measuring device.

## TETRACYCLINE HYDROCHLORIDE CAPSULES USP

**Usual adult and adolescent dose**
See *Tetracycline Oral Suspension USP*.

**Usual adult prescribing limits**
See *Tetracycline Oral Suspension USP*.

**Usual pediatric dose**
See *Tetracycline Oral Suspension USP*.

**Strength(s) usually available**
U.S.—
   250 mg (Rx) [*Achromycin V; Panmycin; Robitet; Sumycin; Tetracyn;* GENERIC].
   500 mg (Rx) [*Achromycin V; Robitet; Sumycin; Tetracyn;* GENERIC].
Canada—
   250 mg (Rx) [*Achromycin V; Apo-Tetra; Novotetra; Nu-Tetra; Tetracyn*].

**Packaging and storage**
Store below 40 °C (104 °F), preferably between 15 and 30 °C (59 and 86 °F), unless otherwise specified by manufacturer. Store in a tight, light-resistant container.

**Auxiliary labeling**
• Continue medicine for full time of treatment.
• Do not take within 1 to 3 hours of other medicines, milk or other dairy products.
• Avoid too much sun or use of sunlamp.
• Keep container tightly closed in a dry place.

## TETRACYCLINE HYDROCHLORIDE TABLETS USP

**Usual adult and adolescent dose**
See *Tetracycline Oral Suspension USP*.

**Usual adult prescribing limits**
See *Tetracycline Oral Suspension USP*.

**Usual pediatric dose**
See *Tetracycline Oral Suspension USP*.

**Strength(s) usually available**
U.S.—
   250 mg (Rx) [*Sumycin*].
   500 mg (Rx) [*Sumycin*].
Canada—
   250 mg (Rx) [*Novotetra*].

**Packaging and storage**
Store below 40 °C (104 °F), preferably between 15 and 30 °C (59 and 86 °F), unless otherwise specified by manufacturer. Store in a tight, light-resistant container.

**Auxiliary labeling**
• Continue medicine for full time of treatment.
• Do not take within 1 to 3 hours of other medicines, milk, or other dairy products.

• Avoid too much sun or use of sunlamp.
• Keep container tightly closed in a dry place.

# Parenteral Dosage Forms

Note: The dosing and dosage forms available are expressed in terms of tetracycline hydrochloride.

## TETRACYCLINE HYDROCHLORIDE FOR INJECTION (INTRAMUSCULAR) USP

**Usual adult and adolescent dose**
Antibacterial (systemic); antiprotozoal—
   Intramuscular, 100 mg every eight hours; 150 mg every twelve hours; or 250 mg once daily.

**Usual adult prescribing limits**
Up to 1 gram daily.

**Usual pediatric dose**
Antibacterial (systemic); antiprotozoal—
   Children 8 years of age and over—Intramuscular, 5 to 8.3 mg per kg of body weight every eight hours; or 7.5 to 12.5 mg per kg of body weight every twelve hours. Maximum daily dose should not exceed 250 mg.

Note: Infants and children up to 8 years of age—All tetracyclines form a stable calcium complex in any bone-forming tissue. Accordingly, tetracyclines may cause permanent yellow-gray-brown discoloration of the teeth, as well as enamel hypoplasia. Also, a decrease in linear skeletal growth rate may occur in premature infants. Therefore, tetracyclines are not recommended in these age groups unless other drugs are unlikely to be effective or are contraindicated.

**Size(s) usually available**
U.S.—
   250 mg (Rx) [*Achromycin*].
Canada—
   250 mg (Rx) [*Achromycin*].

Note: Contains 2% or 40 mg of procaine hydrochloride per vial (either strength), depending on manufacturer.

**Packaging and storage**
Prior to reconstitution, store below 40 °C (104 °F), preferably between 15 and 30 °C (59 and 86 °F), unless otherwise specified by manufacturer. Protect from light.

**Preparation of dosage form**
To prepare initial dilution for intramuscular use, depending on the manufacturer, add 2 mL of sterile water for injection or 0.9% sodium chloride injection to each 100-mg vial and 1.8 to 2 mL of diluent to each 250-mg vial.

**Stability**
After reconstitution, solutions retain their potency for 6 to 24 hours at room temperature or for 24 hours if refrigerated, depending on the manufacturer.

**Additional information**
Cross-sensitivity with other "caine-type" local anesthetics may also occur.

For deep intramuscular use only. Do not administer intravenously, subcutaneously, or into fat layers of the skin.

May cause intense pain and local irritation at the site of injection.

Intramuscular injections should not exceed 2 mL in each site. Injection sites should be alternated.

Since intramuscular administration of tetracycline hydrochloride produces lower serum concentrations than oral administration in recommended doses, patients should be changed to an oral dosage form as soon as feasible.

When rapid, high serum concentrations are required, an intravenous form of tetracycline hydrochloride should be used.

Revised: 08/30/92
Interim revision: 03/18/94; 05/26/94; 04/19/95

# TETRACYCLINES    Topical

This monograph includes information on the following: Chlortetracycline; Meclocycline†; Tetracycline.

VA CLASSIFICATION (Primary/Secondary):
Chlortetracycline—DE101
Meclocycline—DE752
Tetracycline—DE752/DE101

Note: For a listing of dosage forms and brand names by country availability, see *Dosage Forms* section(s). For a listing of brand names for the articles in this monograph, refer to the General Index.

†Not commercially available in Canada.

## Category

Antiacne agent (topical)—Meclocycline; Tetracycline Hydrochloride for Topical Solution.

Antibacterial (topical)—Chlortetracycline; Tetracycline Hydrochloride Ointment.

## Indications

Note: Bracketed information in the *Indications* section refers to uses that are not included in U.S. product labeling.

**Accepted**

Acne vulgaris (treatment)—Meclocycline sulfosalicylate cream and tetracycline hydrochloride for topical solution are indicated for the topical treatment of acne vulgaris. They may be effective in grades II and III acne, which are characterized by inflammatory lesions such as papules and pustules.

Skin infections, bacterial, minor (treatment)—Chlortetracycline hydrochloride ointment and tetracycline hydrochloride ointment are indicated in the topical treatment of minor skin infections caused by streptococci, staphylococci, and other susceptible organisms.

[Skin infections, bacterial, minor (prophylaxis)] or
[Ulcer, dermal (treatment)]—Topical chlortetracycline and tetracycline hydrochloride ointment are used in the prophylaxis of minor bacterial skin infections and in the treatment of dermal ulcer.

Not all species or strains of a particular organism may be susceptible to tetracyclines.

**Unaccepted**

Topical tetracyclines are not effective in deep cystic lesions or in noninflammatory lesions. In addition, topical antibacterials are not generally considered to be as effective as systemic antibacterials in the treatment of acne, especially severe inflammatory acne.

## Pharmacology/Pharmacokinetics

**Physicochemical characteristics**

Molecular weight—
Chlortetracycline hydrochloride: 515.35.
Meclocycline sulfosalicylate: 695.05.
Tetracycline hydrochloride: 480.90.

**Mechanism of action/Effect**

Antiacne agent (topical)—Probably due to their antibacterial activity. Topical tetracyclines are thought to suppress the growth of *Propionibacterium acnes (Corynebacterium acnes)*, an anaerobe found in sebaceous glands and follicles. *P. acnes* produces proteases, hyaluronidases, lipases, and chemotactic factors, all of which can produce inflammatory components or inflammation directly.

Antibacterial (topical)—Tetracyclines are broad-spectrum bacteriostatic agents and act by inhibiting protein synthesis by blocking the binding of aminoacyl tRNA (transfer RNA) to the mRNA (messenger RNA) ribosome complex. Reversible binding occurs primarily at the 30 S ribosomal subunit of susceptible organisms. Bacterial cell wall synthesis is not inhibited.

**Absorption**

Meclocycline—Virtually no absorption following topical application to intact skin.

Tetracycline—Vehicle containing *n*-decyl dimethyl sulfoxide used for topical solution claimed to enhance cutaneous penetration of tetracycline.

**Peak serum concentration**

Up to 0.1 mcg per mL following continuous twice-daily application of tetracycline hydrochloride topical solution to skin.

## Precautions to Consider

**Cross-sensitivity and/or related problems**

Patients sensitive to one tetracycline, tetracycline combination, or tetracycline derivative may be sensitive to other tetracyclines also.

**Carcinogenicity**

*Tetracycline hydrochloride for topical solution*—
A two-year dermal study in mice has not shown that tetracycline hydrochloride for topical solution is carcinogenic.

**Pregnancy/Reproduction**

Fertility—
*Meclocycline*—
Adequate and well-controlled studies in humans have not been done. Studies in rats and rabbits, given oral doses of up to 1000 times the human dose (i.e., 1 gram of cream daily), have not shown that meclocycline causes impaired fertility.
*Tetracycline hydrochloride for topical solution*—
Adequate and well-controlled studies in humans have not been done. Studies in rats and rabbits, given doses of up to 246 times the human dose (i.e., 0.0325 mL per kg of body weight daily), have not shown that tetracycline hydrochloride for topical solution causes impaired fertility.

Pregnancy—
*Meclocycline*—
Adequate and well-controlled studies in humans have not been done.
Studies in rabbits have shown that meclocycline, applied topically, causes a slight delay in ossification. However, studies in rats and rabbits, given oral doses of up to 1000 times the human dose (i.e., 1 gram of cream daily), have not shown that meclocycline causes other adverse effects on the fetus.
FDA Pregnancy Category B.
*Tetracycline hydrochloride for topical solution*—
Adequate and well-controlled studies in humans have not been done.
Studies in rats and rabbits, given doses of up to 246 times the human dose (i.e., 0.0325 mL per kg of body weight daily), have not shown that tetracycline hydrochloride for topical solution causes adverse effects on the fetus.
FDA Pregnancy Category B.
*Tetracyclines, other*—
Problems in humans have not been documented.

**Breast-feeding**

It is not known whether topical tetracyclines are distributed into breast milk. However, tetracyclines are unlikely to be distributed into breast milk in significant amounts following topical administration, since the total daily dose is small (e.g., less than 5 mg for tetracycline hydrochloride for topical solution) and serum concentrations following topical administration are undetectable or very low (up to 0.1 mcg per mL).

**Pediatrics**

*Tetracycline hydrochloride for topical solution*—
Appropriate studies have not been performed in children up to 11 years of age. However, no pediatrics-specific problems have been documented to date in children 11 years of age or older.

**Geriatrics**

No information is available on the relationship of age to the effects of topical tetracyclines in geriatric patients.

**Drug interactions and/or related problems**

The following drug interactions and/or related problems have been selected on the basis of their potential clinical significance (possible mechanism in parentheses where appropriate)—not necessarily inclusive (» = major clinical significance):

Note: Combinations containing any of the following medications, depending on the amount present, may also interact with this medication.

*For tetracycline hydrochloride for topical solution*
Abrasive or medicated soaps or cleansers or
Acne preparations, topical, other or
Alcohol-containing preparations, topical, such as after-shave lotions, astringents, perfumed toiletries, or shaving creams or lotions or
Cosmetics or soaps with a strong drying effect or
Isotretinoin or
Medicated cosmetics or "cover-ups" or
Preparations containing peeling agents, topical, such as benzoyl peroxide, resorcinol, salicylic acid, or sulfur
(concurrent use with tetracycline hydrochloride for topical solution may cause a cumulative irritant or drying effect, especially with the application of peeling, desquamating, or abrasive agents, resulting in excessive irritation of the skin)

## Medical considerations/Contraindications

The medical considerations/contraindications included here have been selected on the basis of their potential clinical significance (reasons given in parentheses where appropriate)—not necessarily inclusive (» = major clinical significance).

*Risk-benefit should be considered when the following medical problem exists:*
Sensitivity to tetracyclines

## Side/Adverse Effects

The following side/adverse effects have been selected on the basis of their potential clinical significance (possible signs and symptoms in parentheses where appropriate)—not necessarily inclusive:

**Those indicating need for medical attention**
Incidence less frequent
*Pain, redness, swelling, or other sign of irritation not present before therapy*

**Those indicating need for medical attention only if they continue or are bothersome**
Incidence more frequent
*For topical solution*
*Dry or scaly skin; stinging or burning feeling*
*For cream and topical solution*
*Faint yellowing of the skin, especially around hair roots*

## Patient Consultation

As an aid to patient consultation, refer to *Advice for the Patient, Tetracyclines (Topical)*.

In providing consultation, consider emphasizing the following selected information (» = major clinical significance):

**Before using this medication**
» Conditions affecting use, especially:
Sensitivity to tetracycline or to any related antibiotics, such as chlortetracycline, demeclocycline, doxycycline, methacycline, minocycline, or oxytetracycline; allergy to formaldehyde (contained in meclocycline cream)

**Proper use of this medication**
*For all dosage forms*
» Compliance with full course of therapy, which may take months or longer
Proper administration technique
May stain clothing
» Proper dosing
Missed dose: Applying as soon as possible; not applying if almost time for next dose
» Proper storage
*For cream and topical solution only*
» Importance of applying medication to entire affected area
» Not using in eyes, nose, mouth, or on other mucous membranes
*For topical solution only*
» Not using near heat, open flame, or while smoking
Not using after expiration date
» Explanation of presence of floating plastic plug
Not using medication more often than prescribed
Avoiding too frequent washing of affected areas
*For topical ointment only*
Not using on deep or puncture wounds or serious burns unless directed by physician
Not for ophthalmic use

## Precautions while using this medication

*For cream and topical solution only*
Checking with physician if no improvement in acne within 6 to 8 weeks
Waiting at least 1 hour before applying any other topical medication for acne
May cause slight yellowing of skin
Fluorescence of treated skin under "black" light
Proper use of cosmetics
*For topical solution only*
Checking with physician if treated skin becomes excessively dry
*For topical ointment only*
Checking with physician if no improvement within 2 weeks

**Side/adverse effects**
Signs of potential side effects, especially pain, redness, swelling, or other signs of irritation not present before therapy

## General Dosing Information

The treated area(s) may be covered with a gauze dressing if desired (ointment only).

Use of topical antibacterials may lead to skin sensitization, resulting in hypersensitivity reactions with subsequent topical or systemic use of the medication.

In the treatment of acne with meclocycline sulfosalicylate cream or tetracycline hydrochloride for topical solution, noticeable improvement may be seen in 4 to 6 weeks. However, in some patients it may require up to 6 to 8 weeks of treatment before noticeable improvement is seen and up to 8 to 12 weeks before maximum benefit is seen.

---

### CHLORTETRACYCLINE

## Summary of Differences

Indications: Indicated as a topical antibacterial.

## Topical Dosage Forms

### CHLORTETRACYCLINE HYDROCHLORIDE OINTMENT USP

**Usual adult and adolescent dose**
Antibacterial (topical)—
Topical, to the skin, one or two times a day.

**Usual pediatric dose**
See *Usual adult and adolescent dose*.

**Strength(s) usually available**
U.S.—
3% (OTC) [*Aureomycin*].
Canada—
3% (OTC) [*Aureomycin*].

**Packaging and storage**
Store below 40 °C (104 °F), preferably between 15 and 30 °C (59 and 86 °F), unless otherwise specified by manufacturer. Store in a collapsible tube or in a well-closed, light-resistant container. Protect from freezing.

**Auxiliary labeling**
• For external use only.
• Continue medicine for full time of treatment.

---

### MECLOCYCLINE

## Summary of Differences

Indications: Indicated in the topical treatment of acne vulgaris.
Side/adverse effects: Faint yellowing of the skin, especially around hair roots.

## Additional Dosing Information

See also *General Dosing Information*.

Meclocycline sulfosalicylate cream may also be effective when applied less frequently (e.g., once a day). However, some reports indicate it is much less effective and improvement may be delayed.

## Topical Dosage Forms
### MECLOCYCLINE SULFOSALICYLATE CREAM USP

**Usual adult and adolescent dose**
Antiacne agent (topical)—
   Topical, to the skin, two times a day, morning and evening.

**Usual pediatric dose**
See *Usual adult and adolescent dose*.

**Strength(s) usually available**
U.S.—
   1% (base) (Rx) [*Meclan* (sodium formaldehyde sulfoxylate)].
Canada—
   Not commercially available.

**Packaging and storage**
Store below 40 °C (104 °F), preferably between 15 and 30 °C (59 and 86 °F), unless otherwise specified by manufacturer. Store in a tight container. Protect from light. Protect from freezing.

**Auxiliary labeling**
• For external use only.
• Continue medicine for full time of treatment.

**Note**
Explain administration technique.

**Additional information**
The cream is compatible with both oil- and water-base systems.

---

### TETRACYCLINE

## Summary of Differences

Indications: Indicated as a topical antibacterial (ointment) and in the topical treatment of acne vulgaris (topical solution).
Side/adverse effects: For topical solution—Dry or scaly skin; faint yellowing of the skin, especially around hair roots; stinging or burning feeling.

## Additional Dosing Information

See also *General Dosing Information*.

Twice-daily use of tetracycline hydrochloride for topical solution on the face and neck for acne delivers an average daily dose of 2.9 mg of tetracycline to the skin. When used twice daily on the face and neck as well as other acne-affected areas, the average daily dose delivered to the skin is 4.8 mg.

## Topical Dosage Forms
### TETRACYCLINE HYDROCHLORIDE OINTMENT USP

**Usual adult and adolescent dose**
Antibacterial (topical)—
   Topical, to the skin, one or two times a day.

**Usual pediatric dose**
See *Usual adult and adolescent dose*.

**Strength(s) usually available**
U.S.—
   3% (OTC) [*Achromycin*].
Canada—
   3% (OTC) [*Achromycin*].

**Packaging and storage**
Store preferably between 15 and 30 °C (59 and 86 °F). Store in a well-closed container. Protect from freezing.

**Auxiliary labeling**
• For external use only.
• Continue medicine for full time of treatment.

### TETRACYCLINE HYDROCHLORIDE FOR TOPICAL SOLUTION USP

**Usual adult and adolescent dose**
Antiacne agent (topical)—Topical, to the skin, two times a day, morning and evening.

**Usual pediatric dose**
Infants and children up to 11 years of age—Dosage has not been established.

**Strength(s) usually available**
U.S.—
   2.2 mg per mL, when reconstituted according to manufacturer's instructions (Rx) [*Topicycline* (sodium bisulfite; 40% ethanol in diluent)].
Canada—
   Not commercially available.

**Packaging and storage**
Prior to reconstitution, store below 40 °C (104 °F), preferably between 15 and 30 °C (59 and 86 °F), unless otherwise specified by manufacturer. Store in a tight, light-resistant container. Protect diluent from freezing.

**Stability**
After reconstitution, solutions retain their potency for 2 months at controlled room temperature (15 to 30 °C [59 to 86 °F]).

**Auxiliary labeling**
• For external use only.
• Continue medicine for full time of treatment.
• Beyond-use date.
• Keep container tightly closed.
• Flammable—Keep from heat and flame.

**Note**
When dispensing, include patient instructions.
Explain the presence of floating plastic plug in the bottle.
Explain administration technique.

**Additional information**
The vehicle is a solution of *n*-decyl methyl sulfoxide and sucrose esters in 40% alcohol.
To maintain an effective concentration of tetracycline hydrochloride, a sufficient amount of 4-epitetracycline hydrochloride is present, which maintains equilibrium between the two.

Revised: 10/27/93

---

**THALIDOMIDE**—Since Thalidomide is not commercially available in the U.S. or Canada, the *Thalidomide (Systemic)* monograph is not included in this published version of the USP DI database. Copies of the monograph are available on request from the USP Division of Information Development, 12601 Twinbrook Parkway, Rockville, MD 20852; telephone (301) 816-8351; telefax (301) 816-8374.

---

# THALLOUS CHLORIDE Tl 201   Systemic

VA CLASSIFICATION (Primary): DX201
Note: For a listing of dosage forms and brand names by country availability, see *Dosage Forms* section(s). For a listing of brand names for the articles in this monograph, refer to the General Index.

## Category

Diagnostic aid, radioactive (myocardial infarction; ischemic heart disease; parathyroid disorders; neoplastic disease).

## Indications

Note: Bracketed information in the *Indications* section refers to uses that are not included in U.S. product labeling.

**Accepted**
Cardiac imaging, radionuclide
Myocardial infarction (diagnosis) and
Myocardial perfusion imaging, radionuclide—Thallous chloride Tl 201 is indicated in myocardial perfusion imaging for the diagnosis and localization of myocardial infarction.
Coronary artery disease (diagnosis)—Thallous chloride Tl 201 is indicated in studies of myocardial perfusion done under resting conditions and after physiologic or pharmacologic stress (either exercise or after infusion of dipyridamole, [adenosine][1], or [dobutamine][1]) to detect myocardium with abnormal perfusion reserve secondary to coronary artery disease. Intravenous dipyridamole, [adenosine][1], and [dobutamine][1] are used primarily as substitutes for exercise in patients who are unable to exercise sufficiently to provide the required level

of myocardial blood flow augmentation or when exercise is otherwise not feasible.

Parathyroid imaging, radionuclide[1]—Thallous chloride Tl 201 is indicated for the detection and localization of parathyroid tissue in patients with documented hyperparathyroidism. Thallous chloride Tl 201 also may be useful in preoperative screening to localize extrathyroidal and mediastinal sites of parathyroid tissue and for postsurgical reexamination. However, the use of thallous chloride Tl 201 as a parathyroid imaging agent generally has been replaced by technetium Tc 99m sestamibi.

[Tumor imaging, radionuclide][1]—Thallous chloride Tl 201 is used for the detection and localization of various tumors, including thyroid carcinomas, malignant brain neoplasms, lymphomas, and mediastinal tumors, especially for postoperative detection of residual and recurrent tumors and differentiation of these from post-therapy fibrosis or necrosis.

---

[1]Not included in Canadian product labeling.

## Physical Properties

### Nuclear data

| Radionuclide (half-life) | Mode of decay | Principal photon emissions (keV) | Mean number of emissions/ disintegration |
|---|---|---|---|
| Tl 201 (73.1 hr) | Electron capture | Gamma-4 (135.3) | 0.03 |
| | | Gamma-6 (167.4) | 0.1 |
| | | Mercury x-rays (68.9–80.3) | 0.95 |

## Pharmacology/Pharmacokinetics

### Mechanism of action/Effect

Cardiac imaging—Thallous chloride Tl 201 appears to accumulate in cells of myocardium and other tissues in a manner analogous to that of potassium. The initial biodistribution of thallous chloride Tl 201 in most tissues is primarily related to regional blood flow. Ischemic myocardial cells take up less thallium-201 than nonischemic cells, in proportion to the relative change in blood flow, especially during maximal stress (or pharmacologically induced vasodilation) when the differential in perfusion is most marked between regions supplied by normal coronary arteries and those supplied by stenotic vessels. Imaging equipment can record regional differences in thallium-201 uptake, and thus in myocardial perfusion, confirming the presence or absence of coronary disease.

Parathyroid imaging—Localizes in parathyroid adenomas, parathyroid hyperplasia, and other abnormal tissues, generally in proportion to organ blood flow at the time of injection.

### Distribution

Rapidly cleared from blood after intravenous administration, with the following accumulation—

Cardiac: 4% within 10 minutes of injection.
Hepatic: 15%.
Intracellular: 72%.
Renal: 3%.
Testicular: 0.15%.

### Half-life

Biological (approximate)—
Intracellular: 36 hours.
Liver, heart, and kidneys: 35.6 hours.
Testes: 20 hours.

### Time to peak concentration

Myocardium—10 minutes.

### Radiation dosimetry

| Estimated absorbed radiation dose* | | |
|---|---|---|
| Organ | mGy/MBq | rad/mCi |
| Testes | 0.56 | 2.1 |
| Kidneys | 0.54 | 2 |
| Large intestine wall (lower) | 0.36 | 1.3 |
| Bone surfaces | 0.34 | 1.3 |
| Thyroid | 0.25 | 0.93 |
| Heart | 0.23 | 0.85 |

| Estimated absorbed radiation dose* | | |
|---|---|---|
| Organ | mGy/MBq | rad/mCi |
| Large intestine wall (upper) | 0.19 | 0.7 |
| Red marrow | 0.18 | 0.67 |
| Liver | 0.18 | 0.67 |
| Small intestine | 0.16 | 0.59 |
| Spleen | 0.14 | 0.52 |
| Stomach wall | 0.12 | 0.44 |
| Lungs | 0.12 | 0.44 |
| Ovaries | 0.12 | 0.44 |
| Pancreas | 0.054 | 0.20 |
| Adrenals | 0.051 | 0.19 |
| Uterus | 0.05 | 0.19 |
| Bladder wall | 0.036 | 0.13 |
| Breast | 0.028 | 0.1 |
| Other tissue | 0.056 | 0.21 |

| Effective dose* | | |
|---|---|---|
| Radionuclide and impurities | mSv/MBq† | rem/mCi† |
| Tl 201 | 0.23 | 0.85 |
| Tl 200 | 0.31 | 1.15 |
| Tl 202 | 0.8 | 2.96 |

*In adults. Intravenous administration at rest; uptake in muscles increases two- to threefold during exercise with a corresponding reduction in other tissues. Data based on the International Commission on Radiological Protection (ICRP) Publication 53—Radiation dose to patients from radiopharmaceuticals.

†Effective doses for the radionuclide and its contaminants are expressed per individual unit of activity of each.

### Elimination

Renal and fecal; 4 to 8% of the administered activity eliminated in the urine within 24 hours.

## Precautions to Consider

### Carcinogenicity/Mutagenicity

Long-term animal studies to evaluate carcinogenic or mutagenic potential of thallous chloride Tl 201 have not been performed.

### Pregnancy/Reproduction

Pregnancy—Studies to assess transplacental transfer of thallous chloride Tl 201 have not been done in humans.

The possibility of pregnancy should be assessed in women of child-bearing potential. Clinical situations exist in which the benefit to the patient and fetus, based on information derived from radiopharmaceutical use, outweighs the risks from fetal exposure to radiation. In these situations, the physician should use discretion and reduce the radiopharmaceutical dose to the lowest possible amount consistent with image quality needs.

Studies have not been done in animals.

FDA Pregnancy Category C.

### Breast-feeding

Thallous chloride Tl 201 is distributed into breast milk. To avoid unnecessary irradiation of the infant, temporary discontinuation of nursing is recommended for a length of time that may be assessed by measuring the activity of breast milk and estimating the radiation exposure to the infant.

### Pediatrics

Diagnostic studies performed in children have not demonstrated pediatrics-specific problems that would limit the usefulness of thallous chloride Tl 201 in children.

### Geriatrics

Diagnostic studies performed to date using thallous chloride Tl 201 have not demonstrated geriatrics-specific problems that would limit the usefulness of this agent in the elderly.

### Drug interactions and/or related problems

See *Diagnostic interference.*

### Diagnostic interference

The following have been selected on the basis of their potential clinical significance (possible effect in parentheses where appropriate)—not necessarily inclusive (» = major clinical significance):

With results of *this* test
*Due to other medications*
Dexamethasone or
Furosemide, chronic therapy without potassium replacement or
Isoproterenol or
Sodium bicarbonate, intravenous
(in animal studies, concurrent use increased myocardial uptake of thallous chloride Tl 201; human data are not available)
Digitalis glycosides or
Propranolol, intravenous
(in animal studies, concurrent use decreased myocardial uptake of thallous chloride Tl 201; human data are not available)
*Due to medical problems or conditions*
Diabetes mellitus
(transport of thallium may be affected by alterations in blood glucose, insulin, or pH)
Postprandial state
(increased accumulation of thallium in the abdominal viscera [postprandial stomach, liver, spleen, intestines] may interfere with myocardial visualization during the resting, exercise, or pharmacologic stress thallium test)
With results of *adenosine/thallium* or *dipyridamole/thallium* test
*Due to other medications*
Caffeine or
Xanthine-derivative medications
(these agents antagonize the effects of adenosine or dipyridamole on myocardial blood flow; xanthine-derivative medication should be withheld for 24 to 36 hours prior to test; also, patients should be instructed to avoid ingesting caffeine [from a dietary or medicinal source] for 8 to 12 hours prior to test)

## Medical considerations/Contraindications

The medical considerations/contraindications included here have been selected on the basis of their potential clinical significance (reasons given in parentheses where appropriate)—not necessarily inclusive (» = major clinical significance).

*Risk-benefit should be considered when the following medical problems exist:*
» Hypotension
(increased risk of severe hypotension with either adenosine/thallium or dipyridamole/thallium stress test)
» Pulmonary disease, bronchospastic, history of
(increased risk of bronchospasm with either adenosine/thallium or dipyridamole/thallium stress test)
Sensitivity to the radiopharmaceutical preparation
*For adenosine/thallium stress test*
» Atrioventricular (AV) block, pre-existing second or third degree or
» Angina, unstable, history of or
» Congestive heart failure, severe or
» Ischemic cardiomyopathy, severe or
» Myocardial infarction, recent
(increased risk of severe myocardial ischemia and/or arrhythmia with adenosine/thallium stress test)
*For dipyridamole/thallium stress test*
» Angina, unstable, history of
(increased risk of severe myocardial ischemia with dipyridamole/thallium stress test)
» Asthma, current or history of
(increased risk of bronchospasm with dipyridamole/thallium stress test)

## Side/Adverse Effects

The following side/adverse effects have been selected on the basis of their potential clinical significance (possible signs and symptoms in parentheses where appropriate)—not necessarily inclusive:

**Those indicating need for medical attention**
Incidence less frequent or rare
*Allergic reaction* (skin rash, hives, or itching); *blurred vision; hypotension*

**Those indicating need for medical attention only if they continue or are bothersome**
Incidence less frequent or rare
*Nausea; sweating*

## Patient Consultation

As an aid to patient consultation, refer to *Advice for the Patient, Radiopharmaceuticals (Diagnostic)*.

In providing consultation, consider emphasizing the following selected information (» = major clinical significance):

**Description of use**
Action in the body: Accumulation of radioactivity in myocardial cells and parathyroid, thyroid, and tumor tissues
Differences in uptake of radioactivity can be visualized
Small amounts of radioactivity used in diagnosis; radiation received is low and considered safe

**Before having this test**
» Conditions affecting use, especially:
Sensitivity to the radiopharmaceutical preparation
Pregnancy—Risk to fetus from radiation exposure as opposed to benefit derived from use should be considered
Breast-feeding—Thallous chloride Tl 201 is distributed into breast milk; temporary discontinuation of nursing recommended to avoid unnecessary irradiation of infant
Other medical problems, especially current or history of asthma, history of unstable angina, hypotension, pulmonary disease, recent myocardial infarction, severe congestive heart failure

**Preparation for this test**
Fasting the morning of the resting or exercise thallium test to minimize localization in splanchnic organs and improve myocardial visualization
Avoiding caffeine ingestion for 8 to 12 hours before adenosine/thallium or dipyridamole/thallium test
Special preparatory instructions may be given; patient should inquire in advance

**Precautions after having this test**
No special precautions

**Side/adverse effects**
Signs of potential side effects, especially allergic reaction, blurred vision, and hypotension

## General Dosing Information

Radiopharmaceuticals are to be administered only by or under the supervision of physicians who have had extensive training in the safe use and handling of radioactive materials and who are authorized by the Nuclear Regulatory Commission (NRC) or the appropriate Agreement State agency, if required, or, outside the U.S., the appropriate authority.

For resting thallium studies, myocardial-to-background ratios are improved when patients are injected while upright and in the fasting state; the upright position reduces the hepatic and gastric concentration of thallium-201. Imaging should begin 10 to 20 minutes after injection of thallous chloride Tl 201.

For thallium studies performed in conjunction with exercise stress testing, thallous chloride Tl 201 should be administered at the inception of a period of maximum stress that lasts for approximately 30 to 60 seconds after injection. To obtain maximum target-to-background ratios, imaging should begin within 10 minutes after administration of thallous chloride Tl 201.

For thallium studies performed in conjunction with pharmacologic stress testing, thallous chloride Tl 201 should be administered 4 to 5 minutes after the 4-minute infusion of dipyridamole, or during the third to fourth minute of the 6-minute infusion of adenosine.

For parathyroid hyperactivity imaging, thallous chloride Tl 201 should be administered before, with, or after a minimal dose of a thyroid imaging agent, such as sodium pertechnetate Tc 99m or sodium iodide I 123, to enable thyroid subtraction imaging.

**Safety considerations for handling this radiopharmaceutical**
Guidelines for the receipt, storage, handling, dispensing, and disposal of radioactive materials are available from scientific, professional, state, federal, and international bodies. Handling of this radiopharmaceutical should be limited to those individuals who are appropriately qualified and authorized.

## Parenteral Dosage Forms

Note: Bracketed uses in the *Dosage Forms* section refer to categories of use and/or indications that are not included in U.S. product labeling.

### THALLOUS CHLORIDE Tl 201 INJECTION USP

**Usual adult and adolescent administered activity**
Cardiac imaging—
Planar imaging: Intravenous, 37 to 74 megabecquerels (1 to 2 millicuries).
SPECT imaging: 74 to 148 megabecquerels (2 to 4 millicuries).

Parathyroid imaging[1]—
    Intravenous, 75 megabecquerels (2 millicuries).
[Tumor imaging][1]—
    Intravenous, 55.5 to 111 megabecquerels (1.5 to 3 millicuries).

**Usual pediatric administered activity**
Cardiac imaging and
Parathyroid imaging[1]—
    Dosage must be individualized by physician. The recommended dosage is 1.11 megabecquerels (30 microcuries) per kg of body weight administered intravenously, with a minimum total dosage of 27.75 megabecquerels (750 microcuries) and a maximum total dosage of 111 megabecquerels (3 millicuries).

**Usual geriatric administered activity**
See *Usual adult and adolescent administered activity.*

**Strength(s) usually available**
U.S.—
    37 megabecquerels (1 millicurie) per mL at time of calibration (Rx) [GENERIC].
Canada—
    Content information not available (Rx) [GENERIC].

**Packaging and storage**
Store between 15 and 30 °C (59 and 86 °F), unless otherwise specified by manufacturer. Protect from freezing.

**Stability**
Do not use if contents are turbid.
Injection should be administered within 4 to 6 days after the calibration date, depending on the product used.

**Note**
Caution—Radioactive material.

[1]Not included in Canadian product labeling.

## Selected Bibliography

Waxman AD. Thallium-201 in nuclear oncology. Nucl Med Ann 1991; 193-209.

Verani MS. Thallium-201 single-photon emission computed tomography (SPECT) in the assessment of coronary artery disease. Am J Cardiol 1992; 70: 3E-9E.

Wackers FJT. Comparison of thallium-201 and technetium-99m methoxyisobutyl isonitrile. Am J Cardiol 1992; 70: 30E-34E.

Revised: 07/03/96

---

**THEOPHYLLINE**—See *Bronchodilators, Theophylline (Systemic)*

---

## THEOPHYLLINE-CONTAINING COMBINATIONS—

Theophylline, Ephedrine, Guaifenesin, and Phenobarbital (Systemic)
Theophylline, Ephedrine, and Hydroxyzine (Systemic)
Theophylline, Ephedrine, and Phenobarbital (Systemic)
Theophylline and Guaifenesin (Systemic)

---

# THEOPHYLLINE, EPHEDRINE, GUAIFENESIN, AND PHENOBARBITAL    Systemic

**VA CLASSIFICATION (Primary): RE109**

**NOTE:** The *Theophylline, Ephedrine, Guaifenesin, and Phenobarbital (Systemic)* monograph is maintained on the USP DI electronic data base. For a printed copy of the most recent revision of the complete monograph, contact the USP Division of Information Development, 12601 Twinbrook Parkway, Rockville, MD 20852.

For information on the specific components of this combination, see the *USP DI* monographs for *Bronchodilators, Theophylline (Systemic), Bronchodilators, Adrenergic (Systemic), Guaifenesin (Systemic),* and *Barbiturates (Systemic).*

The information that follows is selectively abstracted from the complete monograph and is provided to facilitate drug use review and patient counseling.

Note: For a listing of dosage forms and brand names by country availability, see *Dosage Forms* section(s). For a listing of brand names for the articles in this monograph, refer to the General Index.

## Category
Bronchodilator.

## Indications

**Unaccepted**
Theophylline, ephedrine, guaifenesin, and phenobarbital combination is used for bronchial asthma, bronchiectasis, and emphysema in which bronchospasm is present or for the relief of bronchospasm; however, the efficacy of this combination medication in these conditions has not been established. The new drug applications (NDAs) for some products containing theophylline, ephedrine, guaifenesin, and phenobarbital have been withdrawn by FDA and the products have been taken off the market. Other products containing theophylline, ephedrine, guaifenesin, and phenobarbital remain on the market pending further review by FDA.

## Patient Consultation

As an aid to patient consultation, refer to *Advice for the Patient, Theophylline, Ephedrine, Guaifenesin, and Phenobarbital (Systemic).*

In providing consultation, consider emphasizing the following selected information (» = major clinical significance):

**Before using this medication**
»   Conditions affecting use, especially:
    Sensitivity to xanthines, ephedrine or other sympathomimetics, or barbiturates
    Mutagenicity—Theophylline reported to cause chromosomal breakage in human cells in culture at concentrations up to 50 times maximum therapeutic serum concentration
    Pregnancy—Studies in mice have shown theophylline to cause teratogenic effects when given in doses 30 times the human dose (FDA Pregnancy Category C); use during pregnancy may result in potentially dangerous serum theophylline and caffeine concentrations in neonates; tachycardia, jitteriness, irritability, gagging, and vomiting reported in some neonates; neonates of mothers taking theophylline during pregnancy should be monitored for signs of theophylline toxicity
    Barbiturates readily cross placenta; increase in incidence of fetal abnormalities (FDA Pregnancy Category D); use during third trimester of pregnancy may cause physical dependence with resulting withdrawal symptoms in neonate; long-acting barbiturates associated with neonatal coagulation defect that may cause bleeding during early neonatal period; use during labor may cause respiratory depression in neonate
    Breast-feeding—Theophylline excreted in breast milk; use of theophylline by nursing mothers may cause irritability, fretfulness, or insomnia in infants
    Ephedrine excreted in breast milk; use by nursing mothers is not recommended because of higher-than-usual risks for infants
    Barbiturates excreted in breast milk; use by nursing mothers may cause CNS depression in infant
    Use in children—Possible decreased plasma clearance and increased serum concentrations of theophylline and/or toxicity in neonates, especially premature neonates; repeated doses of theophylline should not be given if heart rate is greater than 180 beats per minute
    Caution should be used in infants because of higher-than-usual risks with use of ephedrine in these patients
    Children may react to barbiturates with paradoxical excitement
    Use in the elderly—Possible decreased plasma clearance of theophylline and increased potential for toxicity in patients over 55 years of age

Elderly patients may react to usual doses of barbiturates with excitement, confusion, or mental depression; risk of barbiturate-induced hypothermia may be increased in elderly patients

Other medications, especially beta-adrenergic blocking agents, carbamazepine, cimetidine, ciprofloxacin, cocaine (mucosal-local), CNS depression–producing medications, corticotropin, corticosteroids, coumarin- or indandione-derivative anticoagulants, digitalis glycosides, ergoloid mesylates, ergotamine, erythromycin, estrogen-containing contraceptives, monoamine oxidase (MAO) inhibitors, nicotine chewing gum, norfloxacin, phenytoin, ranitidine, smoking tobacco or marijuana, or troleandomycin

Other medical problems, especially active gastritis, active or history of peptic ulcer, cardiovascular disease, premonitory signs of hepatic coma, acute or chronic pain, or porphyria

### Proper use of this medication
» Taking on empty stomach with a glass of water for faster absorption or, if necessary, taking with meals or immediately after meals to lessen gastrointestinal irritation
» Importance of not taking more medication than the amount recommended on the label; barbiturates have habit-forming potential
» Compliance with therapy; not missing any doses
» Proper dosing
Missed dose: Taking as soon as possible; not taking if almost time for next dose; not doubling doses
» Proper storage

### Precautions while using this medication
» Caution in eating or drinking large amounts of xanthine-containing foods or beverages during therapy with this medication
» Avoiding use of alcohol or other CNS depressants
Not eating charcoal-broiled foods daily because of possible decrease in effects of medication
» Notifying physician immediately if symptoms of influenza, a fever, or diarrhea occur, because of possible need to alter dosage
» Caution if dizziness, lightheadedness, or drowsiness occurs

### Side/adverse effects
Signs of potential side effects, especially gastroesophageal reflux

## Oral Dosage Forms
### THEOPHYLLINE, EPHEDRINE HYDROCHLORIDE, GUAIFENESIN, AND PHENOBARBITAL ELIXIR

**Usual adult dose**
Oral, 15 mL three or four times a day.

**Usual pediatric dose**
Oral, 0.2 mL per kg of body weight three or four times a day.

**Strength(s) usually available**
U.S.—
20 mg of theophylline, 4 mg of ephedrine hydrochloride, 26 mg of guaifenesin, and 2.5 mg of phenobarbital, per 5 mL (Rx) [*Mudrane GG* (alcohol 20%; 0.1% parabens)].

Canada—
Not commercially available.

**Auxiliary labeling**
• May cause drowsiness.
• Avoid alcoholic beverages.
• Keep container tightly closed.

### THEOPHYLLINE, EPHEDRINE HYDROCHLORIDE, GUAIFENESIN, AND PHENOBARBITAL TABLETS

**Usual adult dose**
Oral, 1 or 2 tablets three or four times a day.

**Usual pediatric dose**
Children up to 12 years of age—Dosage has not been established.

**Strength(s) usually available**
U.S.—
111 mg of theophylline, 16 mg of ephedrine hydrochloride, 100 mg of guaifenesin, and 8 mg of phenobarbital (Rx) [*Mudrane GG*].

Canada—
Not commercially available.

**Auxiliary labeling**
• May cause drowsiness.
• Avoid alcoholic beverages.

### THEOPHYLLINE, EPHEDRINE SULFATE, GUAIFENESIN, AND PHENOBARBITAL ELIXIR

**Usual adult dose**
Oral, 10 mL every three or four hours, four times a day.

**Usual pediatric dose**
Children up to 6 years of age—Dosage must be individualized by physician.
Children 6 years of age and over—Oral, 5 mL every three or four hours, four times a day.

**Strength(s) usually available**
U.S.—
15 mg of theophylline, 12 mg of ephedrine sulfate, 50 mg of guaifenesin, and 4 mg of phenobarbital, per 5 mL (OTC) [*Bronkolixir* (alcohol 19%); *Guiaphed*].

Note: For the above products with federal OTC status, state regulations may be more restrictive.

Canada—
Not commercially available.

**Auxiliary labeling**
• May cause drowsiness.
• Avoid alcoholic beverages.
• Keep container tightly closed.

### THEOPHYLLINE, EPHEDRINE SULFATE, GUAIFENESIN, AND PHENOBARBITAL TABLETS

**Usual adult dose**
Oral, 1 tablet every three or four hours, four or five times a day.

**Usual pediatric dose**
Children up to 6 years of age—Dosage has not been established.
Children 6 years of age and over—Oral, ½ tablet every three or four hours, four or five times a day.

**Strength(s) usually available**
U.S.—
100 mg of theophylline, 24 mg of ephedrine sulfate, 100 mg of guaifenesin, and 8 mg of phenobarbital (OTC) [*Bronkotabs* (scored)].

Note: For the above product with federal OTC status, state regulations may be more restrictive.

Canada—
Not commercially available.

**Auxiliary labeling**
• May cause drowsiness.
• Avoid alcoholic beverages.

Revised: October 1990
Interim revision: 09/02/94

---

# THEOPHYLLINE, EPHEDRINE, AND HYDROXYZINE    Systemic

VA CLASSIFICATION (Primary): RE109

**NOTE:** The *Theophylline, Ephedrine, and Hydroxyzine (Systemic)* monograph is maintained on the USP DI electronic data base. For a printed copy of the most recent revision of the complete monograph, contact the USP Division of Information Development, 12601 Twinbrook Parkway, Rockville, MD 20852.

For information on the specific components of this combination, see the *USP DI* monographs for *Bronchodilators, Theophylline (Systemic), Bronchodilators, Adrenergic (Systemic),* and *Antihistamines (Systemic).*

The information that follows is selectively abstracted from the complete monograph and is provided to facilitate drug use review and patient counseling.

Note: For a listing of dosage forms and brand names by country availability, see *Dosage Forms* section(s). For a listing of brand names for the articles in this monograph, refer to the General Index.

## Category
Bronchodilator.

# Indications

## Unaccepted

Theophylline, ephedrine, and hydroxyzine combination is used to control bronchospastic disorders; however, the efficacy of this combination medication in these disorders has not been established. Although FDA has proposed withdrawal of approval of new drug applications (NDAs) for fixed combinations containing theophylline, ephedrine, and hydroxyzine, these products remain on the market pending further review.

# Patient Consultation

As an aid to patient consultation, refer to *Advice for the Patient, Theophylline, Ephedrine, and Hydroxyzine (Systemic).*

In providing consultation, consider emphasizing the following selected information (» = major clinical significance):

## Before using this medication

» Conditions affecting use, especially:

Sensitivity to xanthines, ephedrine or other sympathomimetics, or hydroxyzine

Mutagenicity—Theophylline reported to cause chromosomal breakage in human cells in culture at concentrations up to 50 times maximum therapeutic serum concentration

Pregnancy—Studies in mice have shown theophylline to cause teratogenic effects when given in doses 30 times the human dose (FDA Pregnancy Category C); use during pregnancy may result in potentially dangerous serum theophylline and caffeine concentrations in neonates; tachycardia, jitteriness, irritability, gagging, and vomiting reported in some neonates; neonates of mothers taking theophylline during pregnancy should be monitored for signs of theophylline toxicity

Hydroxyzine is not recommended during early months of pregnancy

Breast-feeding—Theophylline excreted in breast milk; use of theophylline by nursing mothers may cause irritability, fretfulness, or insomnia in infants

Ephedrine excreted in breast milk; use by nursing mothers is not recommended because of higher-than-usual risks for infants

Use in children—Possible decreased plasma clearance and increased serum concentrations of theophylline and/or toxicity in neonates, especially premature neonates; repeated doses of theophylline should not be given if heart rate greater than 180 beats per minute

Caution should be used in infants because of higher-than-usual risks with use of ephedrine in these patients

Use in the elderly—Possible decreased plasma clearance of theophylline and increased potential for toxicity in patients over 55 years of age

Increased susceptibility to anticholinergic and sedative side effects of hydroxyzine

Dental—Prolonged use of hydroxyzine may decrease or inhibit salivary flow, which may contribute to development of caries, periodontal disease, oral candidiasis, and discomfort

Other medications, especially beta-adrenergic blocking agents, cimetidine, ciprofloxacin, cocaine (mucosal-local), CNS depression–producing medications, digitalis glycosides, ergoloid mesylates, ergotamine, erythromycin, monoamine oxidase (MAO) inhibitors, nicotine chewing gum, norfloxacin, phenytoin, ranitidine, smoking tobacco or marijuana, or troleandomycin

Other medical problems, especially active gastritis, active or history of peptic ulcer, or cardiovascular disease

## Proper use of this medication

» Taking on empty stomach with a glass of water for faster absorption or, if necessary, taking with meals or immediately after meals to lessen gastrointestinal irritation

» Importance of not taking more medication than the amount prescribed

» Compliance with therapy; not missing any doses

» Proper dosing

Missed dose: Taking as soon as possible; not taking if almost time for next dose; not doubling doses

» Proper storage

## Precautions while using this medication

» Caution in eating or drinking large amounts of xanthine-containing foods or beverages during therapy with this medication

» Avoiding use of alcohol or other CNS depressants

Not eating charcoal-broiled foods daily because of possible decrease in effects of medication

» Notifying physician immediately if symptoms of influenza, a fever, or diarrhea occur because of possible need to alter dosage

» Caution if dizziness, lightheadedness, or drowsiness occurs

## Side/adverse effects

Signs of potential side effects, especially gastroesophageal reflux

# Oral Dosage Forms

## THEOPHYLLINE, EPHEDRINE SULFATE, AND HYDROXYZINE HYDROCHLORIDE SYRUP

**Usual adult dose**

Oral, 20 mL two to four times a day.

Note: Geriatric patients may be more sensitive to the effects of the usual adult dose of hydroxyzine.

**Usual pediatric dose**

Children up to 2 years of age—Use is not recommended.

Children 2 to 5 years of age—Oral, 2.5 to 5 mL three or four times a day.

Children 5 years of age and over—Oral, 5 mL three or four times a day.

**Strength(s) usually available**

U.S.—

32.5 mg of theophylline, 6.25 mg of ephedrine sulfate, and 2.5 mg of hydroxyzine hydrochloride, per 5 mL (Rx) [*Marax-DF* (alcohol 5%); *Theomax DF* (alcohol 5%)].

Canada—

Not commercially available.

**Auxiliary labeling**

• May cause drowsiness.

• Avoid alcoholic beverages.

## THEOPHYLLINE, EPHEDRINE SULFATE, AND HYDROXYZINE HYDROCHLORIDE TABLETS

**Usual adult dose**

Oral, 1 tablet two to four times a day.

Note: Geriatric patients may be more sensitive to the effects of the usual adult dose of hydroxyzine.

**Usual pediatric dose**

Children up to 5 years of age—Use is not recommended.

Children 5 years of age and over—Oral, 1/2 tablet two to four times a day.

**Strength(s) usually available**

U.S.—

130 mg of theophylline, 25 mg of ephedrine sulfate, and 10 mg of hydroxyzine hydrochloride (Rx) [*Ami Rax; Hydrophed; Marax* (scored); GENERIC].

Canada—

Not commercially available.

**Auxiliary labeling**

• May cause drowsiness.

• Avoid alcoholic beverages.

Revised: October 1990

Interim revision: 09/02/94

---

# THEOPHYLLINE, EPHEDRINE, AND PHENOBARBITAL    Systemic

**VA CLASSIFICATION (Primary): RE109**

**NOTE:** The *Theophylline, Ephedrine, and Phenobarbital (Systemic)* monograph is maintained on the USP DI electronic data base. For a printed copy of the most recent revision of the complete monograph, contact the USP Division of Information Development, 12601 Twinbrook Parkway, Rockville, MD 20852.

For information on the specific components of this combination, see the *USP DI* monographs for *Bronchodilators, Theophylline (Systemic), Bronchodilators, Adrenergic (Systemic),* and *Barbi-*

*turates (Systemic).*

The information that follows is selectively abstracted from the complete monograph and is provided to facilitate drug use review and patient counseling.

Note: For a listing of dosage forms and brand names by country availability, see *Dosage Forms* section(s). For a listing of brand names for the articles in this monograph, refer to the General Index.

## Category
Bronchodilator.

## Indications

### Unaccepted
Theophylline, ephedrine, and phenobarbital combination is used for symptomatic relief of bronchial asthma, asthmatic bronchitis, and other bronchospastic disorders; prophylactically to abort or minimize asthmatic attacks; and in the management of occasional, seasonal, or perennial asthma. However, the efficacy of this combination medication in these conditions has not been established. The new drug applications (NDAs) for some products containing theophylline, ephedrine, and a barbiturate have been withdrawn by FDA and the products have been taken off the market. Other products containing theophylline, ephedrine, and a barbiturate remain on the market pending further review by FDA.

## Patient Consultation
As an aid to patient consultation, refer to *Advice for the Patient, Theophylline, Ephedrine, and Phenobarbital (Systemic)*.

In providing consultation, consider emphasizing the following selected information (» = major clinical significance):

**Before using this medication**
» Conditions affecting use, especially:
   Sensitivity to xanthines, ephedrine or other sympathomimetics, or barbiturates
   Mutagenicity—Theophylline reported to cause chromosomal breakage in human cells in culture at concentrations up to 50 times maximum therapeutic serum concentration
   Pregnancy—Studies in mice have shown theophylline to cause teratogenic effects when given in doses 30 times the human dose (FDA Pregnancy Category C); use during pregnancy may result in potentially dangerous serum theophylline and caffeine concentrations in neonates; tachycardia, jitteriness, irritability, gagging, and vomiting reported in some neonates; neonates of mothers taking theophylline during pregnancy should be monitored for signs of theophylline toxicity
   Phenobarbital readily crosses placenta; increase in incidence of fetal abnormalities (FDA Pregnancy Category D); use during third trimester of pregnancy may cause physical dependence with resulting withdrawal symptoms in neonate; long-acting barbiturates associated with neonatal coagulation defect that may cause bleeding during early neonatal period; use during labor may cause respiratory depression in neonate
   Breast-feeding—Theophylline excreted in breast milk; use of theophylline by nursing mothers may cause irritability, fretfulness, or insomnia in infants
   Ephedrine excreted in breast milk; use by nursing mothers is not recommended because of higher-than-usual risks for infants
   Phenobarbital excreted in breast milk; use by nursing mothers may cause CNS depression in infant
   Use in children—Possible decreased plasma clearance and increased serum concentrations of theophylline and/or toxicity in neonates, especially premature neonates; repeated doses of theophylline should not be given if heart rate greater than 180 beats per minute
   Caution should be used in infants because of higher-than-usual risks with use of ephedrine in these patients
   Children may react to phenobarbital with paradoxical excitement
   Use in the elderly—Possible decreased plasma clearance of theophylline and increased potential for toxicity in patients over 55 years of age
   Elderly patients may react to usual doses of phenobarbital with excitement, confusion, or mental depression; risk of barbiturate-induced hypothermia may be increased in elderly patients

Other medications, especially coumarin- or indandione-derivative anticoagulants, beta-adrenergic blocking agents, carbamazepine, cimetidine, ciprofloxacin, cocaine (mucosal-local), CNS depression–producing medications, corticosteroids, corticotropin, digitalis glycosides, ergoloid mesylates, ergotamine, erythromycin, estrogen-containing contraceptives, monoamine oxidase (MAO) inhibitors, nicotine chewing gum, norfloxacin, phenytoin, ranitidine, smoking tobacco or marijuana, or troleandomycin
Other medical problems, especially active gastritis, active or history of peptic ulcer, cardiovascular disease, premonitory signs of hepatic coma, acute or chronic pain, or porphyria

**Proper use of this medication**
» Taking on empty stomach with a glass of water for faster absorption or, if necessary, taking with meals or immediately after meals to lessen gastrointestinal irritation
» Importance of not taking more medication than the amount recommended on the label; barbiturates have habit-forming potential
» Compliance with therapy; not missing any doses
» Proper dosing
   Missed dose: Taking as soon as possible; not taking if almost time for next dose; not doubling doses
» Proper storage

**Precautions while using this medication**
» Caution in eating or drinking large amounts of xanthine-containing foods or beverages during therapy with this medication
» Avoiding use of alcohol or other CNS depressants
   Not eating charcoal-broiled foods daily because of possible decrease in effects of medication
» Notifying physician immediately if symptoms of influenza, a fever, or diarrhea occur because of possible need to alter dosage
» Caution if dizziness, lightheadedness, or drowsiness occurs

**Side/adverse effects**
Signs of potential side effects, especially gastroesophageal reflux

## Oral Dosage Forms

### THEOPHYLLINE, EPHEDRINE HYDROCHLORIDE, AND PHENOBARBITAL TABLETS USP

**Usual adult dose**
Oral, 1 or 2 tablets every four hours.

**Usual pediatric dose**
Children up to 6 years of age—Dosage has not been established.
Children 6 to 12 years of age—Oral, $^{1}/_{2}$ or 1 tablet every four hours.

**Strength(s) usually available**
U.S.—
   118 mg of anhydrous theophylline, 24 mg of ephedrine hydrochloride, and 8 mg of phenobarbital (OTC) [GENERIC].
   125 mg of anhydrous theophylline, 24 mg of ephedrine hydrochloride, and 8 mg of phenobarbital (Rx) [*Theotal*].
   130 mg of theophylline, 24 mg of ephedrine hydrochloride, and 8 mg of phenobarbital [*Tedrigen* (OTC); *Theodrine* (OTC); *Theofedral* (Rx); *Theophedrital* (OTC)].
   Note: For the above products with federal OTC status, state regulations may be more restrictive.
Canada—
   Not commercially available.

**Auxiliary labeling**
• May cause drowsiness.
• Avoid alcoholic beverages.

Revised: October 1990
Interim revision: 09/02/94

# THEOPHYLLINE AND GUAIFENESIN   Systemic

VA CLASSIFICATION (Primary): RE109
**NOTE:** The *Theophylline and Guaifenesin (Systemic)* monograph is maintained on the USP DI electronic data base. For a printed copy of the most recent revision of the complete monograph, contact the USP Division of Information Development, 12601 Twinbrook Parkway, Rockville, MD 20852.

For information on the specific components of this combination, see the *USP DI* monographs for *Bronchodilators, Theophylline (Systemic)* and *Guaifenesin (Systemic)*.

The information that follows is selectively abstracted from the complete monograph and is provided to facilitate drug use review and patient counseling.

Note: For a listing of dosage forms and brand names by country availability, see *Dosage Forms* section(s). For a listing of brand names for the articles in this monograph, refer to the General Index.

# Category

Bronchodilator.

# Indications

### Accepted

Asthma, bronchial (treatment)

Bronchitis (treatment)

Emphysema, pulmonary (treatment) or

Pulmonary disease, chronic obstructive, other (treatment)—Theophylline and guaifenesin combination is indicated for relief and/or prevention of symptoms of bronchial asthma and reversible bronchospasm associated with chronic bronchitis and pulmonary emphysema.

# Patient Consultation

As an aid to patient consultation, refer to *Advice for the Patient, Theophylline and Guaifenesin (Systemic)*.

In providing consultation, consider emphasizing the following selected information (» = major clinical significance):

### Before using this medication

» Conditions affecting use, especially:

Sensitivity to theophylline or other xanthines

Mutagenicity—Theophylline reported to cause chromosomal breakage in human cells in culture at concentrations up to 50 times maximum therapeutic serum concentration

Pregnancy—Studies in mice have shown theophylline to cause teratogenic effects when given in doses 30 times the human dose (FDA Pregnancy Category C); use during pregnancy may result in potentially dangerous serum theophylline and caffeine concentrations in neonates; tachycardia, jitteriness, irritability, gagging, and vomiting reported in some neonates; neonates of mothers taking theophylline during pregnancy should be monitored for signs of theophylline toxicity

Breast-feeding—Theophylline excreted in breast milk; use by nursing mothers may cause irritability, fretfulness, or insomnia in infants

Use in children—Possible decreased plasma clearance and increased serum concentrations of theophylline and/or toxicity in neonates, especially premature neonates; repeated doses should not be given if heart rate greater than 180 beats per minute

Use in the elderly—Possible decreased plasma clearance of theophylline and increased potential for toxicity in patients over 55 years of age

Other medications, especially beta-adrenergic blocking agents, cimetidine, ciprofloxacin, erythromycin, nicotine chewing gum, norfloxacin, phenytoin, ranitidine, troleandomycin, or smoking tobacco or marijuana

Other medical problems, especially active gastritis or active or history of peptic ulcer

### Proper use of this medication

» Taking on empty stomach with a glass of water for faster absorption or, if necessary, taking with meals or immediately after meals to lessen gastrointestinal irritation

» Importance of not taking more medication than the amount prescribed

» Compliance with therapy; not missing any doses

» Proper dosing

Missed dose: Taking as soon as possible; not taking if almost time for next dose; not doubling doses

» Proper storage

### Precautions while using this medication

Regular visits to physician to check progress during initial period of therapy

» Caution in eating or drinking large amounts of xanthine-containing foods or beverages during therapy with this medication

Not eating charcoal-broiled foods daily because of possible decrease in effects of medication

» Notifying physician immediately if symptoms of influenza, a fever, or diarrhea occur because of possible need to alter dosage

### Side/adverse effects

Signs of potential side effects, especially gastroesophageal reflux

# Oral Dosage Forms

## THEOPHYLLINE AND GUAIFENESIN CAPSULES USP

### Usual adult dose

Acute attack—

Loading dose:

For patients *not* currently receiving theophylline preparations—Oral, the equivalent of 5 to 6 mg of anhydrous theophylline per kg of body weight.

For patients currently receiving theophylline preparations—A serum theophylline measurement should be obtained immediately, if possible. The loading dose for theophylline is based on the principle that each 0.5 mg of theophylline per kg of lean (ideal) body weight will result in a 1 (range, 0.5 to 1.6) mcg per mL increase in serum theophylline concentration. If a serum theophylline measurement cannot be obtained rapidly and the patient's condition requires immediate therapy, a single dose of the equivalent of 2.5 mg of anhydrous theophylline per kg of body weight may be administered if there are no symptoms of theophylline toxicity.

Maintenance (in acute attack):

Young adult smokers—Oral, the equivalent of anhydrous theophylline: 4 mg per kg of body weight every six hours.

Otherwise healthy nonsmoking adults—Oral, the equivalent of anhydrous theophylline: 3 mg per kg of body weight every eight hours.

Older patients and patients with cor pulmonale—Oral, the equivalent of anhydrous theophylline: 2 mg per kg of body weight every eight hours.

Patients with congestive heart failure or liver failure—Oral, the equivalent of anhydrous theophylline: 2 mg per kg of body weight every twelve hours.

Note: **To achieve optimal therapeutic theophylline dosage, and minimize the risk of toxicity, monitoring of serum theophylline concentration and patient response is recommended.**

In patients with cor pulmonale, congestive heart failure, or liver failure, dosage should not exceed the equivalent of 400 mg of anhydrous theophylline per day unless serum theophylline concentrations can be monitored at twenty-four-hour intervals.

Chronic therapy—

Oral, the equivalent of anhydrous theophylline: Initially, 6 to 8 mg per kg of body weight, up to a maximum of 400 mg, per day in three or four divided doses at six- to eight-hour intervals. The dosage may be increased, if tolerated, in approximately 25% increments at two- to three-day intervals, up to a maximum dose of 13 mg per kg of body weight or 900 mg per day, whichever is less, without measurement of serum concentration.

Note: If the above maximum dose in chronic therapy is to be maintained or exceeded, serum theophylline measurement is recommended. Final dosage adjustment is based on subsequent serum theophylline measurements and patient response.

### Usual pediatric dose

Acute attack—

Loading dose:

For patients *not* currently receiving theophylline preparations—Children up to 16 years of age: Oral, the equivalent of 5 to 6 mg of anhydrous theophylline per kg of body weight.

For patients currently receiving theophylline preparations—A serum theophylline measurement should be obtained immediately, if possible. The loading dose for theophylline is based on the principle that each 0.5 mg of theophylline per kg of lean (ideal) body weight will result in a 1 (range, 0.5 to 1.6) mcg per mL increase in serum theophylline concentration. If a serum theophylline measurement cannot be obtained rapidly and the patient's condition requires immediate therapy, a single dose of the equivalent of 2.5 mg of anhydrous theophylline per kg of body weight may be administered if there are no symptoms of theophylline toxicity.

Maintenance (in acute attack):

Children up to 6 months of age—Oral, the equivalent of anhydrous theophylline: Dose in mg per kg of body weight every eight hours = (0.07) (age in weeks) + 1.7.

Children 6 months to 1 year of age—Oral, the equivalent of anhydrous theophylline: Dose in mg per kg of body weight every six hours = (0.05) (age in weeks) + 1.25.

Children 1 to 9 years of age—Oral, the equivalent of anhydrous theophylline: 5 mg per kg of body weight every six hours.

Children 9 to 12 years of age—Oral, the equivalent of anhydrous theophylline: 4 mg per kg of body weight every six hours.

Children 12 to 16 years of age—Oral, the equivalent of anhydrous theophylline: 3 mg per kg of body weight every six hours.

Note: **To achieve optimal therapeutic theophylline dosage, and minimize the risk of toxicity, monitoring of serum theophylline concentration and patient response is recommended.**

Chronic therapy—Oral, the equivalent of anhydrous theophylline: Initially, 16 mg per kg of body weight, up to a maximum of 400 mg, per day in three or four divided doses at six- to eight-hour intervals. The dosage may be increased, if tolerated, in approximately 25% increments at two- to three-day intervals, up to the following maximum doses without measurement of serum concentration—

Children up to 1 year of age: Dose in mg per kg of body weight per day = (0.3) (age in weeks) + 8.

Children 1 to 9 years of age: 22 mg per kg of body weight per day.

Children 9 to 12 years of age: 20 mg per kg of body weight per day.

Adolescents 12 to 16 years of age: 18 mg per kg of body weight per day.

Adolescents 16 years of age and over: 13 mg per kg of body weight or 900 mg per day, whichever is less.

Note: If the above maximum dose in chronic therapy is to be maintained or exceeded, serum theophylline measurement is recommended. Final dosage adjustment is based on subsequent serum theophylline measurements and patient response.

**Strength(s) usually available**

U.S.—

150 mg of anhydrous theophylline and 90 mg of guaifenesin (Rx) [*Bronchial; Glyceryl-T; Quibron; Slo-Phyllin GG; Theolate; Uni-Bronchial*].

300 mg of anhydrous theophylline and 180 mg of guaifenesin (Rx) [*Quibron-300*].

Canada—

Not commercially available.

## THEOPHYLLINE AND GUAIFENESIN ELIXIR

**Usual adult dose**

See *Theophylline and Guaifenesin Capsules USP.*

**Usual pediatric dose**

See *Theophylline and Guaifenesin Capsules USP.*

**Strength(s) usually available**

U.S.—

50 mg of anhydrous theophylline and 30 mg of guaifenesin, per 5 mL (Rx) [*Theolate*].

Canada—

Not commercially available.

**Auxiliary labeling**

• Keep container tightly closed.

## THEOPHYLLINE AND GUAIFENESIN ORAL SOLUTION USP

**Usual adult dose**

See *Theophylline and Guaifenesin Capsules USP.*

**Usual pediatric dose**

See *Theophylline and Guaifenesin Capsules USP.*

**Strength(s) usually available**

U.S.—

33.3 mg of anhydrous theophylline and 33.3 mg of guaifenesin, per 5 mL (Rx) [*Elixophyllin-GG*].

50 mg of anhydrous theophylline and 30 mg of guaifenesin, per 5 mL (Rx) [*Broncomar GG; Glyceryl-T; Theolate;* GENERIC].

Canada—

Not commercially available.

## THEOPHYLLINE AND GUAIFENESIN SYRUP

**Usual adult dose**

See *Theophylline and Guaifenesin Capsules USP.*

**Usual pediatric dose**

See *Theophylline and Guaifenesin Capsules USP.*

**Strength(s) usually available**

U.S.—

50 mg of anhydrous theophylline and 30 mg of guaifenesin, per 5 mL (Rx) [*Slo-Phyllin GG* (glycerin; methylparaben; propylene glycol; saccharin sodium; sodium benzoate; sorbitol; sucrose)].

Canada—

Not commercially available.

## THEOPHYLLINE AND GUAIFENESIN TABLETS

**Usual adult dose**

See *Theophylline and Guaifenesin Capsules USP.*

**Usual pediatric dose**

See *Theophylline and Guaifenesin Capsules USP.*

**Strength(s) usually available**

U.S.—

111 mg of theophylline and 100 mg of guaifenesin (Rx) [*Mudrane GG-2*].

Canada—

Not commercially available.

## THEOPHYLLINE SODIUM GLYCINATE AND GUAIFENESIN ELIXIR

**Usual adult dose**

See *Theophylline and Guaifenesin Capsules USP.*

**Usual pediatric dose**

See *Theophylline and Guaifenesin Capsules USP.*

**Strength(s) usually available**

U.S.—

100 mg of theophylline sodium glycinate (equivalent to 50 mg of anhydrous theophylline) and 33.3 mg of guaifenesin, per 5 mL (Rx) [*Asbron G* (alcohol 15%); *Ed-Bron G; Equibron G*].

Canada—

Not commercially available.

**Auxiliary labeling**

• Keep container tightly closed.

## THEOPHYLLINE SODIUM GLYCINATE AND GUAIFENESIN SYRUP

**Usual adult dose**

See *Theophylline and Guaifenesin Capsules USP.*

**Usual pediatric dose**

See *Theophylline and Guaifenesin Capsules USP.*

**Strength(s) usually available**

U.S.—

100 mg of theophylline sodium glycinate (equivalent to 50 mg of anhydrous theophylline) and 33.3 mg of guaifenesin, per 5 mL (Rx) [*Synophylate-GG* (alcohol 10%; saccharin; sorbitol)].

Canada—

Not commercially available.

## THEOPHYLLINE SODIUM GLYCINATE AND GUAIFENESIN TABLETS

**Usual adult dose**

See *Theophylline and Guaifenesin Capsules USP.*

**Usual pediatric dose**

See *Theophylline and Guaifenesin Capsules USP.*

**Strength(s) usually available**

U.S.—

300 mg of theophylline sodium glycinate (equivalent to 150 mg of anhydrous theophylline) and 100 mg of guaifenesin (Rx) [*Asbron G Inlay-Tabs*].

Canada—

Not commercially available.

Revised: October 1990

Interim revision: 09/02/94

# THIABENDAZOLE Systemic†

VA CLASSIFICATION (Primary): AP200

Note: For a listing of dosage forms and brand names by country availability, see *Dosage Forms* section(s). For a listing of brand names for the articles in this monograph, refer to the General Index.

†Not commercially available in Canada.

## Category

Anthelmintic (systemic)

Note: Thiabendazole is a broad-spectrum anthelmintic, which has a spectrum similar to that of mebendazole.

## Indications

Note: Bracketed information in the *Indications* section refers to uses that are not included in U.S. product labeling.

**Accepted**

Larva migrans, cutaneous (treatment)—Thiabendazole is indicated in the treatment of cutaneous larva migrans (creeping eruption) caused by *Ancylostoma braziliense* (dog and cat hookworm) and *Ancylostoma caninum.*

Larva migrans, visceral (treatment)—Thiabendazole is indicated in the treatment of visceral larva migrans (toxocariasis) caused by *Toxocara canis* and *T. cati* (dog and cat roundworm).

Strongyloidiasis (treatment)—Thiabendazole is indicated in the treatment of strongyloidiasis, including hyperinfection syndrome caused by *Strongyloides stercoralis* (threadworm) in immunosuppressed and non-immunosuppressed patients.

Trichinosis (treatment)—Thiabendazole is indicated in the treatment of trichinosis caused by *Trichinella spiralis* (pork worm) if the patient is known to have ingested trichinous pork within the previous 24 hours. It has little effect on muscle larvae and has not been shown to alter the course of the disease in established infections. However, it does have an effect on the adult worms, and thereby decreases the number of new larvae. Systemic corticosteroids may be used in critically ill patients to minimize inflammatory reactions to *Trichinella* larvae. However, their effectiveness has not been proven.

[Capillariasis (treatment)]—Thiabendazole is used in the treatment of capillariasis caused by *Capillaria philippinensis.*

[Dracunculiasis (treatment)]—Thiabendazole is used in the treatment of dracunculiasis (guinea worm infection) caused by *Dracunculus medinensis.* It has no effect on the worms themselves, but reduces inflammation to permit easier removal of the worm.

[Trichostrongyliasis (treatment)]—Thiabendazole is used in the treatment of trichostrongyliasis caused by *Trichostrongylus* species.

Not all species or strains of a particular helminth may be susceptible to thiabendazole.

**Unaccepted**

In the treatment of ascariasis, enterobiasis, trichuriasis, hookworm infection, and multiple helminth infections, thiabendazole generally has been replaced by more effective and less toxic agents, such as mebendazole or pyrantel.

Thiabendazole is not indicated in the prophylaxis of helminth infections.

## Pharmacology/Pharmacokinetics

**Physicochemical characteristics**

Molecular weight—201.25.

**Mechanism of action/Effect**

Unknown; however, thiabendazole has been shown to inhibit helminth-specific enzyme fumarate reductase; vermicidal; although thiabendazole may also be ovicidal and larvicidal, it has no effect on muscle-encysted *Trichinella spiralis* larvae.

**Other actions/effects**

Also has anti-inflammatory, analgesic, antipyretic, and mild antifungal and scabicidal actions.

**Absorption**

Rapidly and well absorbed from gastrointestinal tract.

**Distribution**

Therapeutic concentrations of thiabendazole were found in the cerebrospinal fluid of one patient with disseminated strongyloidiasis.

**Biotransformation**

Hepatic; rapidly and almost completely metabolized to inactive 5-hydroxythiabendazole, which is further metabolized to glucuronide and sulfate conjugates.

**Half-life**

Thiabendazole—Normal and anephric: 1.2 hours (range, 0.9 to 2 hours).

5-hydroxythiabendazole—1.7 hours (range, 1.4 to 2 hours).

**Time to peak serum concentration**

Thiabendazole—1 to 2 hours.

5-hydroxythiabendazole—2 to 4 hours.

**Peak serum concentration**

Thiabendazole—4.5 to 5.0 mcg/mL after a single 25 mg per kg of body weight (mg/kg) dose.

5-hydroxythiabendazole—4 to 10 mcg/mL after a single 25 mg/kg dose.

**Elimination**

Renal—Up to 90% or more excreted as inactive metabolites in urine within 48 hours (most during the first 24 hours); <1% excreted unchanged in urine; 5-hydroxythiabendazole excreted in urine as glucuronide and sulfate conjugates.

Fecal—Approximately 5% excreted in feces within 48 hours.

In dialysis—Hemodialysis does not remove significant amounts of thiabendazole or its metabolites from the blood.

## Precautions to Consider

**Carcinogenicity**

Numerous short- and long-term studies in animals given doses of up to 15 times the usual human dose have not shown that thiabendazole is carcinogenic.

**Mutagenicity**

*In vitro* microbial mutagen tests, micronucleus tests, and *in vivo* host-mediated assays have not shown that thiabendazole is mutagenic.

**Pregnancy/Reproduction**

Fertility—Studies in mice given doses of thiabendazole 2½ times the usual human dose and studies in rats given doses equivalent to the usual human dose have not shown that thiabendazole adversely affects fertility.

Pregnancy—Adequate and well-controlled studies in humans have not been done.

Studies in rabbits given doses of up to 15 times the usual human dose and studies in rats given doses equivalent to the usual human dose have not shown that thiabendazole causes adverse effects on the fetus. Similarly, studies in mice given doses of up to 2½ times the usual human dose have not shown any adverse effects on the fetus. However, another study in mice given doses of 10 times the usual human dose in olive oil (but not in aqueous suspension) has shown that thiabendazole causes cleft palate and axial skeletal defects.

FDA Pregnancy Category C.

**Breast-feeding**

It is not known whether thiabendazole is excreted in human breast milk. Problems in humans have not been documented; however, because of the potential for serious adverse effects in the nursing infant, breast-feeding may need to be discontinued.

**Pediatrics**

Appropriate studies on the relationship of age to the effects of thiabendazole have not been performed in children up to 13.6 kg of body weight.

**Geriatrics**

No information is available on the relationship of age to the effects of thiabendazole in geriatric patients.

**Drug interactions and/or related problems**

The following drug interactions and/or related problems have been selected on the basis of their potential clinical significance (possible mechanism in parentheses where appropriate)—not necessarily inclusive (» = major clinical significance):

Note: Combinations containing any of the following medications, depending on the amount present, may also interact with this medication.

» Theophylline

(concurrent use of thiabendazole with theophylline may reduce the clearance of theophylline by greater than 50%, possibly resulting in toxic concentrations; theophylline concentrations should be monitored)

**Laboratory value alterations**

The following have been selected on the basis of their potential clinical significance (possible effect in parentheses where appropriate)—not necessarily inclusive (» = major clinical significance):

With physiology/laboratory test values
    Aspartate aminotransferase (AST [SGOT]), serum
        (rarely, concentration may be transiently increased)

**Medical considerations/Contraindications**

The medical considerations/contraindications included here have been selected on the basis of their potential clinical significance (reasons given in parentheses where appropriate)—not necessarily inclusive (» = major clinical significance).

*Risk-benefit should be considered when the following medical problems exist:*

» Hepatic function impairment
        (thiabendazole metabolized primarily in liver; may also be hepatotoxic)

    Hypersensitivity to thiabendazole

    Renal function impairment
        (high concentrations of the parent compound may accumulate in renal failure, resulting in neurotoxicity)

**Patient monitoring**

The following may be especially important in patient monitoring (other tests may be warranted in some patients, depending on condition; » = major clinical significance):

*For strongyloidiasis*

» Sputum examinations
        (in the diagnosis of strongyloidiasis, sputum examinations may be required when pulmonary signs or symptoms are present, when the possibility of a hyperinfection syndrome exists, or when the patient is immunosuppressed or will be undergoing immunosuppression)

» Stool examinations
        (required prior to and approximately 2 to 3 weeks following treatment with thiabendazole to determine efficacy of the medication or establish proof of cure [i.e., absence of eggs, larvae, or worms in the stool]; because of colonic mixing, eggs may persist in the stool for up to 1 week following cure; more frequent stool examinations may be required in the treatment of strongyloidiasis hyperinfection syndrome, especially in immunocompromised patients; follow-up stool examinations are generally not useful in toxocariasis since *Toxocara* species rarely develop into egg-producing adults in humans)

## Side/Adverse Effects

Note: Some patients may excrete a metabolite that imparts an asparagus-like or other unusual odor to the urine.

    Thiabendazole may cause severe cases of Stevens-Johnson syndrome, in which fatalities have occurred.

The following side/adverse effects have been selected on the basis of their potential clinical significance (possible signs and symptoms in parentheses where appropriate)—not necessarily inclusive:

**Those indicating need for medical attention**

Incidence more frequent
    *Central nervous system (CNS) toxicity* (numbness or tingling in the hands or feet); *gastrointestinal disturbance, severe* (anorexia; diarrhea; nausea and vomiting); *neuropsychiatric toxicity* (delirium; disorientation; hallucinations; irritability)

Incidence less frequent
    *Hypersensitivity* (skin rash or itching)

Incidence rare
    *Crystalluria* (lower back pain; pain or burning while urinating); *intrahepatic cholestasis* (malaise; nausea and vomiting; dark urine; pale stools; yellow eyes and skin); *ocular symptoms* (blurred or yellow vision; unusual feeling in the eyes); *seizures; Stevens-Johnson syndrome* (aching of joints and muscles; fever and chills; redness, blistering, peeling, or loosening of skin)

**Those indicating need for medical attention only if they continue or are bothersome**

Incidence more frequent
    *CNS toxicity* (dizziness; drowsiness; headache; tinnitus); *drying of mucous membranes, especially eyes and mouth*

## Overdose

For more information on the management of overdose or unintentional ingestion, **contact a Poison Control Center** (see *Poison Control Center Listing*).

**Treatment of overdose**

Since there is no specific antidote, treatment of thiabendazole overdose should consist of the following:
    To decrease absorption—
        Inducing emesis or performing gastric lavage.
    Specific treatment—
        Symptomatic treatment may be given.
    Supportive care—
        Supportive measures such as maintaining an open airway, respiration, and circulation may be necessary. Patients in whom intentional overdose is confirmed or suspected should be referred for psychiatric consultation.

## Patient Consultation

As an aid to patient consultation, refer to *Advice for the Patient, Thiabendazole (Systemic)*.

In providing consultation, consider emphasizing the following selected information (» = major clinical significance):

**Before using this medication**

» Conditions affecting use, especially:
        Hypersensitivity to thiabendazole
        Other medications, especially theophylline
        Other medical problems, especially liver function impairment

**Proper use of this medication**

    No special preparations (e.g., dietary restrictions or fasting, concurrent medications, purging, or cleansing enemas) required before, during, or immediately after therapy
    Taking after meals to minimize common side effects such as nausea, vomiting, dizziness, or loss of appetite

**Proper administration**

*For oral suspension dosage form*
    Using a calibrated liquid-measuring device to measure each dose accurately

*For chewable tablet dosage form*
    Chewing or crushing tablets before swallowing

» Compliance with full course of therapy; second course may be required in some infections

» Proper dosing
        Missed dose: Taking as soon as possible; not taking if almost time for next dose; not doubling doses

» Proper storage

*For trichinosis*
        Possibly taking systemic corticosteroids concurrently with thiabendazole, especially in patients with severe symptoms, to reduce inflammatory reactions to *Trichinella* larvae

**Precautions while using this medication**

    Regular visits to physician to check progress
» Caution if dizziness, drowsiness, blurred vision, or yellow vision occurs

**Using hygienic measures to prevent reinfection**

*For creeping eruption or visceral larva migrans*
    Keeping dogs and cats off beaches and bathing areas
    Deworming household pets regularly
    Covering children's sandboxes when not in use

*For trichinosis*
    Cooking all pork, pork-containing products, and wild animals thoroughly (at not less than 60 °C until well done) before eating

**Side/adverse effects**

    Asparagus-like or other unusual odor of urine may be alarming to patient although medically insignificant
    Signs of potential side effects, especially CNS toxicity, severe gastrointestinal disturbance, neuropsychiatric toxicity, hypersensitivity, crystalluria, intrahepatic cholestasis, ocular symptoms, seizures, and Stevens-Johnson syndrome

## General Dosing Information

No special preparations (e.g., dietary restrictions or fasting, concurrent medications, purging, or cleansing enemas) are required before, during, or immediately after treatment with thiabendazole.

Thiabendazole should preferably be taken after meals (breakfast and evening meal) to minimize common side effects such as nausea, vomiting, dizziness, or loss of appetite.

Patients who are heavily infected with helminths may require more prolonged treatment.

Patients with impaired hepatic function may require a reduction in dose, also.

**For trichinosis**
Systemic corticosteroids may be given in the treatment of trichinosis to critically ill patients to minimize inflammatory reactions to *Trichinella* larvae. However, their effectiveness has not been proven.

## Oral Dosage Forms

Note: Bracketed uses in the *Dosage Forms* section refer to categories of use and/or indications that are not included in U.S. product labeling.

### THIABENDAZOLE ORAL SUSPENSION USP

**Usual adult and adolescent dose**
Larva migrans, cutaneous—
    Oral, 25 mg per kg of body weight two times a day for two days. May be repeated two days after completion of treatment if active lesions are still present.
Larva migrans, visceral—
    Oral, 25 mg per kg of body weight two times a day for five to seven days. May be repeated in four weeks if required.
Strongyloidiasis—
    Uncomplicated infections: Oral, 25 mg per kg of body weight two times a day for two days.
    [Hyperinfection syndrome]: Oral, 25 mg per kg of body weight two times a day for five to seven days. May be repeated if required.
Trichinosis—
    Oral, 25 mg per kg of body weight two times a day for two to four days, based on patient's response.
[Capillariasis]—
    Oral, 25 mg per kg of body weight once a day for thirty days.
[Dracunculiasis]—
    Oral, 25 mg per kg of body weight two times a day for two days.
[Trichostrongyliasis]—
    Oral, 25 mg per kg of body weight two times a day for two days.
Note: Patients up to 68 kg of body weight—25 mg per kg of body weight two times a day may be given.
    Patients 68 kg of body weight and over—1.5 grams two times a day may be given.

**Usual adult prescribing limits**
Up to 3 grams daily.

**Usual pediatric dose**
Infants and children up to 13.6 kg of body weight—Dosage has not been established in the treatment of strongyloidiasis and trichinosis.
Children 13.6 kg of body weight and over—See *Usual adult and adolescent dose.*

**Strength(s) usually available**
U.S.—
    500 mg per 5 mL (Rx) [*Mintezol*].
Canada—
    Not commercially available.

**Packaging and storage**
Store below 40 °C (104 °F), preferably between 15 and 30 °C (59 and 86 °F), unless otherwise specified by manufacturer. Store in a tight container. Protect from freezing.

**Auxiliary labeling**
• Shake well.
• Take after meals.
• May cause dizziness, drowsiness, blurred vision, or yellow vision.
• Continue medicine for full time of treatment.

**Note**
When dispensing, include a calibrated liquid-measuring device.

### THIABENDAZOLE TABLETS (CHEWABLE) USP

**Usual adult and adolescent dose**
See *Thiabendazole Oral Suspension USP.*

**Usual adult prescribing limits**
See *Thiabendazole Oral Suspension USP.*

**Usual pediatric dose**
See *Thiabendazole Oral Suspension USP.*

**Strength(s) usually available**
U.S.—
    500 mg (Rx) [*Mintezol*].
Canada—
    Not commercially available.

**Packaging and storage**
Store below 40 °C (104 °F), preferably between 15 and 30 °C (59 and 86 °F), unless otherwise specified by manufacturer. Store in a tight container.

**Auxiliary labeling**
• Chew or crush tablets before swallowing.
• Take after meals.
• May cause dizziness, drowsiness, blurred vision, or yellow vision.
• Continue medicine for full time of treatment.

Revised: 02/01/93

---

# THIABENDAZOLE   Topical*†

VA CLASSIFICATION (Primary): AP200

Note: For a listing of dosage forms and brand names by country availability, see *Dosage Forms* section(s). For a listing of brand names for the articles in this monograph, refer to the General Index.

*Not commercially available in the U.S.
†Not commercially available in Canada.

## Category
Anthelmintic (topical).

## Indications

Note: Because topical thiabendazole is not commercially available in the U.S. or Canada, the bracketed information and the use of the superscript 1 in this monograph reflect the lack of labeled (approved) indications for this medication.

**Accepted**
[Larva migrans, cutaneous (treatment)][1]—Topical thiabendazole is used in the treatment of cutaneous larva migrans (creeping eruption) caused by *Ancylostoma braziliense* (dog and cat hookworm). Recent reports and some medical experts have suggested the use of systemic ivermectin or albendazole as alternative treatment for cutaneous larva migrans if topical therapy with thiabendazole proves ineffective since its use for this indication is becoming obsolete.

Not all species or strains of a particular helminth may be susceptible to topical thiabendazole.

[1]Not included in Canadian product labeling.

## Pharmacology/Pharmacokinetics

**Physicochemical characteristics**
Molecular weight—201.25.

**Mechanism of action/Effect**
Unknown; however, thiabendazole has been shown to inhibit helminth-specific enzyme fumarate reductase; vermicidal.

**Absorption**
Some systemic absorption may occur from topical preparations applied to the skin.

## Precautions to Consider

**Pregnancy/Reproduction**
Pregnancy—Topical thiabendazole may be systemically absorbed. However, problems in humans have not been documented.

**Breast-feeding**
Topical thiabendazole may be systemically absorbed. However, problems in humans have not been documented.

**Pediatrics**
Appropriate studies on the relationship of age to the effects of topical thiabendazole have not been performed in the pediatric population. However, pediatrics-specific problems that would limit the usefulness of this medication in children are not expected.

**Geriatrics**
Appropriate studies on the relationship of age to the effects of topical thiabendazole have not been performed in the geriatric population. However, no geriatrics-specific problems have been documented to date.

## Medical considerations/Contraindications

The medical considerations/contraindications included here have been selected on the basis of their potential clinical significance (reasons given in parentheses where appropriate)—not necessarily inclusive (» = major clinical significance).

*Risk-benefit should be considered when the following medical problem exists:*
Sensitivity to thiabendazole

## Patient Consultation

As an aid to patient consultation, refer to *Advice for the Patient, Thiabendazole (Topical).*

In providing consultation, consider emphasizing the following selected information (» = major clinical significance):

### Before using this medication
» Conditions affecting use, especially:
Sensitivity to thiabendazole

### Proper use of this medication
Applying directly to and approximately 5 to 7.5 cm around the slowly advancing end of each burrow or tunnel in the skin
» Compliance with full course of therapy
» Proper dosing
Missed dose: Applying as soon as possible; not applying if almost time for next dose
» Proper storage

### Precautions while using this medication
Checking with physician if no improvement within a few days or if burrow or tunnel continues to advance

## General Dosing Information

Thiabendazole topical suspension should be applied directly to the slowly advancing end of the larval burrow or tunnel in the skin. Since the larvae may have advanced beyond the site of inflammation in the skin, topical thiabendazole should also be applied approximately 5 to 7.5 cm around the presumed end of the burrow or tunnel.

Thiabendazole may also be applied topically as a cream in concentrations up to 15% in a water-soluble base.

## Topical Dosage Forms

### THIABENDAZOLE TOPICAL SUSPENSION

Note: Thiabendazole topical suspension is not commercially available in the U.S. or Canada; thiabendazole oral suspension is being used for topical application. The bracketed information and the use of superscript 1 in the *Dosage Forms* section reflect the lack of labeled (approved) indications for this product.

### Usual adult and adolescent dose
[Cutaneous larva migrans (treatment)][1]—
Topical, to and around the advancing end of each larva burrow in the skin, two to four times a day for two to seven days.

Note: Concentrations of 10 to 15% have been recommended.

### Usual adult prescribing limits
Up to six times a day.

### Usual pediatric dose
[Cutaneous larva migrans (treatment)][1]—
See *Usual adult and adolescent dose.*

### Strength(s) usually available
U.S.—
Dosage form not commercially available. Thiabendazole oral suspension (500 mg per 5 mL) (Rx) [*Mintezol* ] is the dosage form used when 10% thiabendazole topical suspension is prescribed. Higher concentrations require compounding
Canada—
Dosage form not commercially available. Compounding required.

### Packaging and storage
Store below 40 °C (104 °F), preferably between 15 and 30 °C (59 and 86 °F), unless otherwise specified by manufacturer. Protect from freezing.

### Auxiliary labeling
• Shake well.
• For external use only.
• Continue medicine for full time of treatment.

[1]Not included in Canadian product labeling.

Revised: 09/28/93
Interim revision: 05/31/94

## THIACETAZONE-CONTAINING COMBINATIONS—

Isoniazid and Thiacetazone (Systemic)

---

# THIAMINE    Systemic

VA CLASSIFICATION (Primary): VT105
Another commonly used name is vitamin B$_1$.
Note: For a listing of dosage forms and brand names by country availability, see *Dosage Forms* section(s). For a listing of brand names for the articles in this monograph, refer to the General Index.

## Category

Nutritional supplement (vitamin).
Note: Thiamine (vitamin B$_1$) is a water-soluble vitamin.

## Indications

Note: Bracketed information in the *Indications* section refers to uses that are not included in U.S. product labeling.

### Accepted
Thiamine deficiency (prophylaxis and treatment)—Thiamine is indicated for prevention and treatment of thiamine deficiency states. Thiamine deficiency may occur as a result of inadequate nutrition or intestinal malabsorption but does not occur in healthy individuals receiving an adequate balanced diet. Simple nutritional deficiency of individual B vitamins is rare since dietary inadequacy usually results in multiple deficiencies. For prophylaxis of thiamine deficiency, dietary improvement, rather than supplementation, is advisable. For treatment of thiamine deficiency, supplementation is preferred.

Deficiency of thiamine may lead to beriberi (dry or wet) or Wernicke's encephalopathy.

Requirements may be increased and/or supplementation may be necessary in the following persons or conditions (based on documented thiamine deficiency):
Alcoholism
Burns
Fever, chronic
Gastrectomy
Hemodialysis, chronic
Hepatic-biliary tract disease—alcoholism with cirrhosis, hepatic function impairment
Hyperthyroidism
Infection, prolonged
Intestinal disease—celiac, ileal resection, tropical sprue, regional enteritis, persistent diarrhea
Manual labor, heavy, for long periods of time
Stress, prolonged

Recommended intakes for thiamine are related to caloric intake.

Some unusual diets (e.g., reducing diets that drastically restrict food selection) may not supply minimum daily requirements for thiamine. Supplementation is necessary in patients receiving total parenteral nutrition (TPN) or undergoing rapid weight loss or in those with malnutrition, because of inadequate dietary intake.

Recommended intakes for all vitamins and most minerals are increased during pregnancy. Many physicians recommend that pregnant women receive multivitamin and mineral supplements, especially those pregnant women who do not consume an adequate diet and those in high-risk categories (i.e., women carrying more than one fetus, heavy cigarette smokers, and alcohol and drug abusers). Taking excessive amounts of a multivitamin and mineral supplement may be harmful to the mother and/or fetus and should be avoided.

Recommended intakes for all vitamins and most minerals are increased during breast-feeding.

[Encephalomyelopathy, subacute necrotizing (treatment)]

[Maple syrup urine disease (treatment)]

[Pyruvate carboxylase deficiency (treatment)] or

[Hyperalaninemia (treatment)]—Thiamine has been found to be useful for temporary metabolic correction of genetic enzyme deficiency diseases such as subacute necrotizing encephalomyelopathy (SNE, Leigh's disease), maple syrup urine disease (branched-chain aminoacidopathy), and lactic acidosis associated with pyruvate carboxylase deficiency and hyperalaninemia.

### Unaccepted

Thiamine has not been proven effective for appetite stimulation, treatment of cerebellar syndrome, dermatitis, chronic diarrhea, fatigue, mental disorders, multiple sclerosis, neuritis, or ulcerative colitis, or for use as an insect repellant.

## Pharmacology/Pharmacokinetics

### Physicochemical characteristics

Molecular weight—337.27.

pKa—4.8 and 9.

### Mechanism of action/Effect

Thiamine combines with adenosine triphosphate (ATP) to form a coenzyme, thiamine pyrophosphate (thiamine diphosphate, cocarboxylase), which is necessary for carbohydrate metabolism.

### Absorption

The B vitamins are readily absorbed from the gastrointestinal tract, except in malabsorption syndromes. Thiamine is absorbed mainly in the duodenum. Alcohol inhibits absorption of thiamine.

In individuals with normal gastrointestinal absorption, total maximum daily oral absorption of thiamine is 5 to 15 mg (increased when given in divided daily doses with food).

### Biotransformation

Hepatic.

### Elimination

Renal (almost entirely as metabolites). Excess beyond daily needs is excreted as unchanged drug and metabolites in urine.

## Precautions to Consider

### Pregnancy/Reproduction

Pregnancy—Problems in humans have not been documented with intake of normal daily recommended amounts.

FDA Pregnancy Category A (parenteral thiamine).

### Breast-feeding

Problems in humans have not been documented with intake of normal daily recommended amounts.

### Pediatrics

Problems in pediatrics have not been documented with intake of normal daily recommended amounts.

### Geriatrics

Problems in geriatrics have not been documented with intake of normal daily recommended amounts. Studies have shown that the elderly may have impaired thiamine status, thereby requiring thiamine supplementation.

### Laboratory value alterations

The following have been selected on the basis of their potential clinical significance (possible effect in parentheses where appropriate)—not necessarily inclusive (» = major clinical significance):

With diagnostic test results

Theophylline concentration determinations, serum, by Schack and Waxler spectrophotometric method
(thiamine may interfere with results)

Uric acid concentration determinations by phototungstate method or Urobilinogen determinations using Ehrlich's reagent
(thiamine may produce false-positive results)

Note: Usually occurs only with large doses.

### Medical considerations/Contraindications

The medical considerations/contraindications included here have been selected on the basis of their potential clinical significance (reasons given in parentheses where appropriate)—not necessarily inclusive (» = major clinical significance).

*Risk-benefit should be considered when the following medical problems exist:*

Sensitivity to thiamine

Wernicke's encephalopathy
(intravenous glucose loading may precipitate or worsen this condition in thiamine-deficient patients; thiamine should be administered prior to glucose)

## Side/Adverse Effects

The following side/adverse effects have been selected on the basis of their potential clinical significance (possible signs and symptoms in parentheses where appropriate)—not necessarily inclusive:

### Those indicating need for medical attention

Incidence rare

*Anaphylactic reaction* (coughing; difficulty in swallowing; hives; itching of skin; swelling of face, lips, or eyelids; wheezing or difficulty in breathing)—usually after a large intravenous dose

## Patient Consultation

As an aid to patient consultation, refer to *Advice for the Patient, Thiamine (Vitamin B₁) (Systemic).*

In providing consultation, consider emphasizing the following selected information (» = major clinical significance):

### Description of use

Description should include function in the body, signs of deficiency, and unproven uses

### Importance of diet

Importance of proper nutrition; supplement may be needed because of inadequate dietary intake

Food sources of thiamine; effects of processing

Not using vitamins as substitute for balanced diet

Recommended daily intake for thiamine

### Before using this dietary supplement

» Conditions affecting use, especially:
Sensitivity to thiamine
Use in the elderly—May have impaired thiamine status

### Proper use of this dietary supplement

» Proper dosing
Missed dose: No cause for concern because of length of time necessary for depletion; remembering to take as directed

» Proper storage

### Side/adverse effects

Signs of potential side effects, especially anaphylactic reaction

## General Dosing Information

Because of the infrequency of single B vitamin deficiencies, combinations are commonly administered. Many commercial combinations of B vitamins are available.

### For parenteral dosage forms only

In most cases, parenteral administration is indicated only when oral administration is not acceptable (for example, in nausea, vomiting, preoperative and postoperative conditions), or possible (for example, in malabsorption syndromes or following gastric resection).

### Diet/Nutrition

Recommended dietary intakes for thiamine are defined differently worldwide.

For U.S.—

The Recommended Dietary Allowances (RDAs) for vitamins and minerals are determined by the Food and Nutrition Board of the National Research Council and are intended to provide adequate nutrition in most healthy persons under usual environmental stresses. In addition, a different designation may be used by the FDA for food and dietary supplement labeling purposes, as with Daily Value (DV). DVs replace the previous labeling terminology United States Recommended Daily Allowances (USRDAs).

For Canada—

Recommended Nutrient Intakes (RNIs) for vitamins, minerals, and protein are determined by Health and Welfare in Canada and provide recommended amounts of a specific nutrient while minimizing the risk of chronic diseases.

Daily recommended intakes for thiamine are generally defined as follows:

| Persons | U.S. (mg) | Canada (mg) |
|---|---|---|
| Infants and children | | |
| Birth to 3 years of age | 0.3–0.7 | 0.3–0.6 |
| 4 to 6 years of age | 0.9 | 0.7 |
| 7 to 10 years of age | 1 | 0.8–1 |
| Adolescent and adult males | 1.2–1.5 | 0.8–1.3 |
| Adolescent and adult females | 1–1.1 | 0.8–0.9 |
| Pregnant females | 1.5 | 0.9–1 |
| Breast-feeding females | 1.6 | 1–1.2 |

These are usually provided by adequate diets.

The best dietary sources of thiamine include cereals (whole-grain and enriched), meats (especially pork and beef), peas, beans, and nuts. Loss is variable during cooking and may be as high as 50%.

## Oral Dosage Forms

Note: Bracketed uses in the *Dosage Forms* section refer to categories of use and/or indications that are not included in U.S. product labeling.

### THIAMINE HYDROCHLORIDE ELIXIR USP

**Usual adult and adolescent dose**
Deficiency (prophylaxis)—
    Oral, amount based on normal daily recommended intakes:

| Persons | U.S. (mg) | Canada (mg) |
|---|---|---|
| Adolescent and adult males | 1.2–1.5 | 0.8–1.3 |
| Adolescent and adult females | 1–1.1 | 0.8–0.9 |
| Pregnant females | 1.5 | 0.9–1 |
| Breast-feeding females | 1.6 | 1–1.2 |

Deficiency (treatment)—
    Treatment dose is individualized by prescriber based on severity of deficiency. The following dosage has been established: Beriberi (initial in mild or maintenance following severe)—Oral, 5 to 10 mg three times a day.
[Genetic enzyme deficiency diseases]—
    Oral, 10 to 20 mg per day as a single dose (dosage of up to 4 grams per day in divided doses has been used).

**Usual pediatric dose**
Deficiency (prophylaxis)—
    Oral, amount based on intake of normal daily recommended intakes:

| Persons | U.S. (mg) | Canada (mg) |
|---|---|---|
| Infants and children | | |
| Birth to 3 years of age | 0.3–0.7 | 0.3–0.6 |
| 4 to 6 years of age | 0.9 | 0.7 |
| 7 to 10 years of age | 1 | 0.8–1 |

Deficiency (treatment)—
    Treatment dose is individualized by prescriber based on severity of deficiency. The following dosage has been established: Beriberi (mild)—Oral, 10 per day.

**Strength(s) usually available**
U.S.—
    Not commercially available.
Canada—
    250 mcg (0.25 mg) per 5 mL (OTC) [*Bewon* (16% alcohol; bisulfites)].
    Note: The strength of this thiamine preparation may exceed the dosage range recommended by USP DI Advisory Panels based on the amount necessary to meet normal nutritional needs.

**Packaging and storage**
Store below 40 °C (104 °F), preferably between 15 and 30 °C (59 and 86 °F), unless otherwise specified by manufacturer. Store in a tight, light-resistant container. Protect from freezing.

### THIAMINE HYDROCHLORIDE TABLETS USP

**Usual adult and adolescent dose**
See *Thiamine Hydrochloride Elixir USP*.

**Usual pediatric dose**
See *Thiamine Hydrochloride Elixir USP*.

**Strength(s) usually available**
U.S.—
    5 mg (OTC) [GENERIC].
    10 mg (OTC) [GENERIC].
    25 mg (OTC) [GENERIC].
    50 mg (OTC) [GENERIC].
    100 mg (OTC) [GENERIC].
    250 mg (OTC) [GENERIC].
    500 mg (OTC) [GENERIC].
Canada—
    10 mg (OTC) [GENERIC].
    25 mg (OTC) [GENERIC].
    50 mg (OTC) [GENERIC].
    100 mg (OTC) [GENERIC].
    500 mg (OTC) [GENERIC].
    Note: Some strengths of these thiamine preparations may exceed the dosage range recommended by USP DI Advisory Panels based on the amount necessary to meet normal nutritional needs.

**Packaging and storage**
Store below 40 °C (104 °F), preferably between 15 and 30 °C (59 and 86 °F), unless otherwise specified by manufacturer. Store in a tight, light-resistant container.

## Parenteral Dosage Forms

### THIAMINE HYDROCHLORIDE INJECTION USP

**Usual adult dose**
Deficiency (prophylaxis)—
    Intravenous infusion, as part of total parenteral nutrition solutions, the specific amount determined by individual patient need.
Deficiency (treatment)—
    Intramuscular or intravenous infusion (slow): 5 to 100 mg three times a day followed by maintanence oral administration.

**Usual pediatric dose**
Deficiency (prophylaxis)—
    Intravenous infusion, as part of total parenteral nutrition solutions, the specific amount determined by individual patient need.
Deficiency (treatment)—
    Intramuscular or intravenous infusion (slow), 10 to 25 mg a day.

**Strength(s) usually available**
U.S.—
    100 mg per mL (Rx) [*Biamine* (0.5% chlorobutanol); GENERIC].
Canada—
    100 mg per mL (Rx) [*Betaxin* (0.5% chlorobutanol; 0.5% monothioglycerol); GENERIC].

**Packaging and storage**
Store below 40 °C (104 °F), preferably between 15 and 30 °C (59 and 86 °F), unless otherwise specified by manufacturer. Protect from light. Protect from freezing.

**Incompatibilities**
Thiamine is unstable in neutral or alkaline solutions; therefore, administration with carbonates, citrates, barbiturates, or copper ions is not recommended. In addition, stability is poor in intravenous solutions containing sodium bisulfite as an antioxidant or preservative; if these solutions must be used, they should be used immediately after addition of thiamine.

Revised: 06/24/92
Interim revision: 07/29/94; 05/26/95

# THIETHYLPERAZINE   Systemic

VA CLASSIFICATION (Primary): GA700

Note: For a listing of dosage forms and brand names by country availability, see *Dosage Forms* section(s). For a listing of brand names for the articles in this monograph, refer to the General Index.

## Category
Antiemetic.

## Indications

### Accepted

Nausea and vomiting (prophylaxis and treatment)—Thiethylperazine is indicated for the control of nausea and vomiting, especially emesis associated with surgery, cancer chemotherapy, radiation therapy, and toxins.

## Pharmacology/Pharmacokinetics

### Physicochemical characteristics
Chemical group—Piperazine phenothiazine.
Molecular weight—631.76.

### Mechanism of action/Effect
Probably by inhibition of the medullary chemoreceptor trigger zone and the vomiting center.

### Absorption
Well absorbed when taken orally.

### Biotransformation
Hepatic.

### Elimination
Renal.

## Precautions to Consider

### Cross-sensitivity and/or related problems
Patients intolerant of other phenothiazines may be intolerant of this medication also.

### Pregnancy/Reproduction
Pregnancy—Thiethylperazine is not recommended for use during pregnancy. Phenothiazines have been reported to cause jaundice and extrapyramidal symptoms in infants whose mothers received these medications during pregnancy.

### Breast-feeding
It is not known whether thiethylperazine is distributed into breast milk; however, risk-benefit must be considered since other phenothiazines are known to be present in breast milk, thus increasing the risk of dystonias and tardive dyskinesia in the nursing baby.

### Pediatrics
Safety and efficacy of thiethylperazine have not been established in children up to 12 years of age. However, children appear to be prone to develop neuromuscular or extrapyramidal reactions, especially dystonias, during therapy with phenothiazines. Children with acute illnesses, such as chickenpox, CNS infections, measles, gastroenteritis, or dehydration, are especially at risk.

### Geriatrics
Dizziness, excessive sedation, confusion, hypotension, syncope, and extrapyramidal signs, especially tardive dyskinesia and parkinsonism, may be more likely to occur in geriatric patients. Lower initial dosage and gradual titration of dose, with careful observation for early signs of tardive dyskinesia, are recommended in these patients.

### Dental
The peripheral anticholinergic effects of phenothiazines may decrease or inhibit salivary flow, especially in middle-aged or elderly patients, thus contributing to the development of caries, periodontal disease, oral candidiasis, and discomfort.
Extrapyramidal reactions induced by phenothiazines will result in increased motor activity of the head, face, and neck. Occlusal adjustments, bite registrations, and treatment for bruxism may be made less reliable.

### Drug interactions and/or related problems
The following drug interactions and/or related problems have been selected on the basis of their potential clinical significance (possible mechanism in parentheses where appropriate)—not necessarily inclusive (» = major clinical significance):

Note: Combinations containing any of the following medications, depending on the amount present, may also interact with this medication.

» Alcohol or
» CNS depression–producing medications, other (See *Appendix II*)
(concurrent use with thiethylperazine may result in increased CNS and respiratory depression and increased hypotensive effects; dosage reductions of either drug may be necessary during concurrent use or when sequence of use enhances CNS effects)

Antacids, aluminum- or magnesium-containing, or
Antidiarrheals, adsorbent
(concurrent use of these medications with thiethylperazine may inhibit the absorption of orally administered thiethylperazine; simultaneous use should be avoided)

Anticholinergics or other medications with anticholinergic activity (See *Appendix II*)
(anticholinergic effects may be potentiated when these medications are used concurrently with thiethylperazine)

Anticonvulsants, including barbiturates
(thiethylperazine may lower the convulsion threshold; dosage adjustment of anticonvulsant medications may be necessary; potentiation of anticonvulsant effects does not occur)

Antithyroid agents
(concurrent use with thiethylperazine may increase the risk of agranulocytosis)

Apomorphine
(prior ingestion of thiethylperazine may decrease the emetic response to apomorphine; also, the CNS depressant effects of thiethylperazine are additive to those of apomorphine and may induce dangerous respiratory depression, circulatory system effects, or prolonged sleep)

Appetite suppressants
(concurrent use with thiethylperazine may antagonize the anorectic effect of appetite suppressants)

Beta-adrenergic blocking agents
(concurrent use with thiethylperazine may result in an increased plasma concentration of each medication because of inhibition of metabolism; this may result in additive hypotensive effects, irreversible retinopathy, cardiac arrhythmias, and tardive dyskinesia)

Bromocriptine
(concurrent use may increase serum prolactin concentrations and interfere with effects of bromocriptine; dosage adjustments may be necessary)

Dopamine
(concurrent use may antagonize peripheral vasoconstriction produced by high doses of dopamine, because of the alpha-adrenergic blocking action of thiethylperazine)

Ephedrine
(alpha-adrenergic blocking action of thiethylperazine may decrease the pressor response to ephedrine when the two medications are used concurrently)

» Epinephrine
(alpha-adrenergic effects of epinephrine may be blocked when epinephrine is used concurrently with thiethylperazine, possibly resulting in severe hypotension and tachycardia)

» Extrapyramidal reaction–causing medications, other (See *Appendix II*)
(concurrent use with thiethylperazine may increase the severity and frequency of extrapyramidal effects)

Guanadrel or
Guanethidine
(neuronal uptake of these medications may be inhibited, thus causing a decrease of their antihypertensive effect when these medications are used concurrently with thiethylperazine)

Hepatotoxic medications, other (See *Appendix II*)
(concurrent use with thiethylperazine may increase the potential for hepatotoxicity)

Hypotension-producing medications, other (See *Appendix II*)
(concurrent use with thiethylperazine may potentiate hypotensive effects of either these medications or thiethylperazine)

» Levodopa
(antiparkinsonian effects of levodopa may be inhibited when levodopa is used concurrently with thiethylperazine, because of block-

ade of dopamine receptors in brain; levodopa has not been shown to be effective in thiethylperazine-induced parkinsonism)

Metaraminol
(concurrent use with thiethylperazine usually decreases, but does not reverse or completely block, the pressor response to metaraminol, because of the alpha-adrenergic blocking action of thiethylperazine)

Methoxamine
(prior administration of thiethylperazine may decrease the pressor effect and shorten the duration of action of methoxamine because of the alpha-adrenergic blocking action of thiethylperazine)

» Metrizamide, intrathecal
(concurrent use may increase risk of seizures because of lowered seizure threshold effect of thiethylperazine; it is recommended that thiethylperazine be discontinued for at least 48 hours before and 24 hours after myelography)

Ototoxic medications (See *Appendix II*)
(concurrent use with thiethylperazine may mask the symptoms of ototoxicity such as tinnitus, dizziness, and vertigo)

Photosensitizing medications, other
(concurrent use with thiethylperazine may cause additive photosensitizing effects; caution is recommended)
(concurrent use of systemic methoxsalen, trioxsalen, or tetracyclines with thiethylperazine may potentiate intraocular photochemical damage to the choroid, retina, and lens)

» Quinidine
(concurrent use with thiethylperazine may result in additive cardiac effects)

Riboflavin
(requirements for riboflavin may be increased in patients receiving thiethylperazine)

### Laboratory value alterations
The following have been selected on the basis of their potential clinical significance (possible effect in parentheses where appropriate)—not necessarily inclusive (» = major clinical significance):

With diagnostic test results
Immunologic urine pregnancy tests
(phenothiazine derivatives may produce false-positive or false-negative results, depending on the test used)

### Medical considerations/Contraindications
The medical considerations/contraindications included here have been selected on the basis of their potential clinical significance (reasons given in parentheses where appropriate)—not necessarily inclusive (» = major clinical significance).

*Except under special circumstances, this medicine should not be used when the following medical problems exist:*

» Cardiovascular disease, severe or
» CNS depression, severe or
» Comatose states
(may be exacerbated)

*Risk-benefit should be considered when the following medical problems exist:*

» Alcoholism, active
(CNS depression may be potentiated; increased risk of hypotension)

Asthma, acute or
Respiratory disorders, other, chronic, especially in children
(anticholinergic "drying" effects may cause thickening of secretions and impair expectoration)

Bladder neck obstruction or
Prostatic hypertrophy, symptomatic
(anticholinergic effects may precipitate urinary retention)

Blood dyscrasias
(may be exacerbated; treatment may have to be discontinued)

Cardiovascular disease
(increased risk of hypotension; myocardial depression, cardiomegaly, congestive heart failure, and arrhythmias may be induced)

» Glaucoma, angle-closure, predisposition to
(increased intraocular pressure due to anticholinergic effects may precipitate an acute attack of angle-closure glaucoma)

» Hepatic function impairment
(metabolism may be decreased; higher serum thiethylperazine concentrations may increase sensitivity to CNS effects)

Parkinson's disease
(potentiation of extrapyramidal effects)

Seizure disorders
(seizures may be precipitated)
Sensitivity to thiethylperazine or other phenothiazines
Urinary retention
(may be exacerbated)

Caution is recommended when thiethylperazine is used since signs of intestinal obstruction, brain tumor, or overdosage of toxic drugs may be obscured by its antiemetic action.

### Patient monitoring
The following may be especially important in patient monitoring (other tests may be warranted in some patients, depending on condition; » = major clinical significance):

Cardiovascular determinations or
Hematologic determinations or
Hepatic function tests or
Neurological tests or
Ophthalmologic examinations
(may be required at periodic intervals during high-dose or prolonged therapy to check for any changes that might indicate thiethylperazine toxicity)

## Side/Adverse Effects

Note: Thiethylperazine is a phenothiazine derivative. Although the likelihood of side effects associated with antipsychotic phenothiazines occurring with thiethylperazine seems to be minimal, the possibility exists, especially at higher doses or with prolonged administration.

The following side/adverse effects have been selected on the basis of their potential clinical significance (possible signs and symptoms in parentheses where appropriate)—not necessarily inclusive:

### Those indicating need for medical attention
Incidence less frequent or rare
*Agranulocytosis* (sore throat; fever; unusual bleeding or bruising; unusual tiredness or weakness); *cholestatic jaundice* (abdominal or stomach pains; aching muscles and joints; fever and chills; severe skin itching; yellow eyes or skin; fatigue; nausea, vomiting, or diarrhea); *confusion*—especially in the elderly; *convulsions; edema, peripheral* (swelling of arms, hands, and face); *extrapyramidal effects, dystonic* (muscle spasms of face, neck, and back; tic-like or twitching movements; twisting movements of body; inability to move eyes; weakness of arms and legs); *extrapyramidal effects, parkinsonian* (difficulty in speaking or swallowing; loss of balance control; mask-like face; shuffling walk; stiffness of arms or legs; trembling and shaking of hands and fingers); *pigmentary retinopathy* (blurred vision; defective color vision; difficulty seeing at night); *tachycardia* (fast heartbeat); *tardive dyskinesia* (lip smacking or puckering; puffing of cheeks; rapid or worm-like movements of tongue; uncontrolled chewing movements; uncontrolled movements of arms and legs)

Note: *Parkinsonian effects* are more frequent in the elderly, whereas *dystonias* occur more often in younger patients. Symptoms may be seen in the first few days of treatment or after prolonged treatment, and can recur after even a single dose.

### Those indicating need for medical attention only if they continue or are bothersome
Incidence more frequent
*Drowsiness or dizziness*

Incidence less frequent or rare
*Anticholinergic effects* (constipation; decreased sweating; dizziness; drowsiness; dryness of mouth, nose, and throat); *fever; headache; orthostatic hypotension* (feeling faint; lightheadedness; unusual tiredness or weakness)—more likely to occur in the elderly and after initial parenteral administration; *paradoxical reaction* (continuing nightmares; unusual excitement, nervousness, restlessness, or irritability); *ringing or buzzing in ears; skin rash*

## Overdose

For specific information on the agents used in the management of thiethylperazine overdose, see:
• *Barbiturates (Systemic)* monograph;
• *Diphenhydramine* in *Antihistamines (Systemic)* monograph; and/or
• *Norepinephrine Bitartrate* or *Phenylephrine Hydrochloride* in *Sympathomimetic Agents—Cardiovascular Use (Parenteral-Systemic)* monograph.

For more information on the management of overdose or unintentional ingestion, **contact a Poison Control Center** (see *Poison Control Center Listing*).

**Treatment of overdose**

To decrease absorption—Early gastric lavage. Emesis should *not* be induced (because a dystonic reaction of the head or neck might result in aspiration of vomitus).

Specific treatment—Administration of norepinephrine or phenylephrine (not using epinephrine, because it may cause paradoxical hypotension), to treat severe hypotension. Administration of anticholinergic antiparkinson agents, diphenhydramine, or barbiturates, to control extrapyramidal reactions.

Supportive care—Oxygen and intravenous fluids. Patients in whom intentional overdose is confirmed or suspected should be referred for psychiatric consultation.

## Patient Consultation

As an aid to patient consultation, refer to *Advice for the Patient, Thiethylperazine (Systemic)*.

In providing consultation, consider emphasizing the following selected information (» = major clinical significance):

**Before using this medication**

» Conditions affecting use, especially:

     Sensitivity to thiethylperazine or to other phenothiazines

     Pregnancy—Possible jaundice and extrapyramidal effects in infant; use not recommended

     Breast-feeding—Not known if distributed into breast milk; other phenothiazines are known to appear in breast milk; possible risk to infant of dystonias and tardive dyskinesia

     Use in children—Safety and efficacy not established

     Use in the elderly—Hypotension, CNS and anticholinergic effects more likely; increased susceptibility to extrapyramidal effects

     Dental—Increased risk of dental problems because of decreased salivary flow

     Other medications, especially CNS depressants, epinephrine, extrapyramidal reaction–causing medications, levodopa, intrathecal metrizamide, or quinidine

     Other medical problems, especially alcoholism, severe cardiovascular disease, severe CNS depression, glaucoma, or hepatic function impairment

**Proper use of this medication**

» Importance of not taking more medication than the amount prescribed

» Proper dosing

     Missed dose: If on a regular dosing schedule—Using as soon as possible; if almost time for next dose, not using at all; not doubling doses

» Proper storage

*For oral dosage forms*

     Taking with food, water, or milk to minimize gastric irritation

*For rectal dosage forms*

     Proper administration technique

**Precautions while using this medication**

     Regular visits to physician to check progress of therapy if used for prolonged period of time

» Avoiding use of alcohol or other CNS depressants

» Possible drowsiness or blurred vision; caution when driving, using machines, or doing other things requiring alertness or accurate vision

» Possible dizziness or lightheadedness (orthostatic hypotension); caution when getting up suddenly from a lying or sitting position

     May mask ototoxic effects of large doses of salicylates

     Possible dryness of mouth; using sugarless gum or candy, ice, or saliva substitute for relief; checking with physician or dentist if dry mouth continues for more than 2 weeks

**Side/adverse effects**

     Side effects more likely to occur in the elderly

     Signs of potential side effects, especially agranulocytosis, cholestatic jaundice, confusion, convulsions, peripheral edema, dystonias, parkinsonian effects, pigmentary retinopathy, tachycardia, and tardive dyskinesia

## General Dosing Information

When extended therapy is discontinued, a gradual reduction in phenothiazine dosage over several weeks is recommended, since abrupt withdrawal may cause some patients on high or long-term dosage to experience transient dyskinetic signs, nausea, vomiting, gastritis, trembling, and dizziness.

**Diet/Nutrition**

The oral dosage forms of this medication may be taken with food, water, or milk to lessen gastric irritation.

Requirements for riboflavin may be increased in patients receiving phenothiazines.

## Oral Dosage Forms
### THIETHYLPERAZINE MALEATE TABLETS USP

**Usual adult and adolescent dose**

Antiemetic—

     Oral, 10 mg one to three times a day.

**Usual pediatric dose**

Safety and efficacy have not been established.

**Usual geriatric dose**

See *Usual adult and adolescent dose*.

Note: Geriatric patients may be more sensitive to the effects of the usual adult dose.

**Strength(s) usually available**

U.S.—

     10 mg (Rx) [*Norzine; Torecan*].

Canada—

     10 mg (Rx) [*Torecan*].

**Packaging and storage**

Store below 40 °C (104 °F), preferably between 15 and 30 °C (59 and 86 °F), unless otherwise specified by manufacturer. Store in a tight, light-resistant container.

**Auxiliary labeling**

• May cause drowsiness.

• Avoid alcoholic beverages.

## Parenteral Dosage Forms
### THIETHYLPERAZINE MALATE INJECTION USP

**Usual adult and adolescent dose**

Antiemetic—

     Intramuscular, 10 mg one to three times a day.

Note: For postoperative nausea and vomiting, administration of thiethylperazine should be by deep intramuscular injection at or shortly before the termination of anesthesia.

**Usual pediatric dose**

Safety and efficacy have not been established.

**Usual geriatric dose**

See *Usual adult and adolescent dose*.

Note: Geriatric patients may be more sensitive to the effects of the usual adult dose.

**Strength(s) usually available**

U.S.—

     10 mg per 2 mL (Rx) [*Norzine; Torecan*].

Canada—

     10 mg per 1 mL (Rx) [*Torecan*].

**Packaging and storage**

Store below 30 °C (86 °F), unless otherwise specified by manufacturer. Protect from light. Protect from freezing.

**Stability**

Do not use if discolored or if a precipitate is present.

## Rectal Dosage Forms
### THIETHYLPERAZINE MALEATE SUPPOSITORIES USP

**Usual adult and adolescent dose**

Antiemetic—

     Rectally, 10 mg one to three times a day.

**Usual pediatric dose**

Safety and efficacy have not been established.

**Usual geriatric dose**

See *Usual adult and adolescent dose*.

Note: Geriatric patients may be more sensitive to the effects of the usual adult dose.

**Strength(s) usually available**

U.S.—

　10 mg (Rx) [*Norzine; Torecan*].

Canada—

　Not commercially available.

**Packaging and storage**

Store below 25 °C (77 °F), in a tight, light-resistant container.

**Auxiliary labeling**

• May cause drowsiness.

• Avoid alcoholic beverages.

**Note**

Include patient instructions when dispensing.

Explain administration technique.

Revised: 06/17/93

---

# THIOGUANINE    Systemic

VA CLASSIFICATION (Primary): AN300

Note: For a listing of dosage forms and brand names by country availability, see *Dosage Forms* section(s). For a listing of brand names for the articles in this monograph, refer to the General Index.

## Category

Antineoplastic.

## Indications

Note: Bracketed information in the *Indications* section refers to uses that are not included in U.S. product labeling.

**Accepted**

Leukemia, acute myelocytic (treatment) or

[Leukemia, acute lymphocytic (treatment)]—Thioguanine is indicated for treatment of acute nonlymphocytic leukemia and is also used for treatment of acute lymphocytic leukemia.

Leukemia, chronic myelocytic (treatment)—Thioguanine is used for treatment of chronic myelocytic leukemia, although busulfan is usually preferred.

## Pharmacology/Pharmacokinetics

**Physicochemical characteristics**

Molecular weight—167.19 (anhydrous).

pKa—8.1.

**Mechanism of action/Effect**

Thioguanine is an antimetabolite of the purine analog type. Thioguanine is cell cycle–specific for the S phase of cell division. Activity occurs as the result of activation in the tissues and may include inhibition of DNA synthesis with a lesser effect on RNA synthesis.

**Absorption**

Incompletely and variably (about 30%) absorbed from the gastrointestinal tract.

**Distribution**

Does not cross the blood-brain barrier in significant amounts.

**Biotransformation**

Hepatic (activation and catabolism).

**Half-life**

80 minutes (25 to 240 minutes).

**Elimination**

Renal, almost totally as metabolites.

## Precautions to Consider

**Carcinogenicity/Mutagenicity**

Secondary malignancies are potential delayed effects of many antineoplastic agents, although it is not clear whether the effect is related to their mutagenic or immunosuppressive action. The effect of dose and duration of therapy is also unknown, although risk seems to increase with long-term use. Although information is limited, available data seem to indicate that the carcinogenic risk is greatest with the alkylating agents.

Antimetabolites have been shown to be carcinogenic in animals and have been associated with an increased risk of development of secondary carcinomas in humans, although the risk appears to be less than with alkylating agents.

**Pregnancy/Reproduction**

Fertility—Gonadal suppression, resulting in amenorrhea or azoospermia, may occur in patients taking antineoplastic therapy, especially with the alkylating agents. In general, these effects appear to be related to dose and length of therapy and may be irreversible. Prediction of the degree of testicular or ovarian function impairment is complicated by the common use of combinations of several antineoplastics, which makes it difficult to assess the effects of individual agents.

In males—Two cases have been reported of congenital abnormalities occurring after the fathers were treated with a combination regimen including thioguanine.

Pregnancy—First trimester: It is usually recommended that use of antineoplastics, especially combination chemotherapy, be avoided whenever possible, especially during the first trimester. Although information is limited because of the relatively few instances of antineoplastic administration during pregnancy, the mutagenic, teratogenic, and carcinogenic potential of these medications must be considered.

Other hazards to the fetus include adverse reactions seen in adults.

In general, use of a contraceptive is recommended during cytotoxic drug therapy.

**Breast-feeding**

Although very little information is available regarding excretion of antineoplastic agents in breast milk, breast-feeding is not recommended while thioguanine is being administered because of the risks to the infant (adverse effects, mutagenicity, carcinogenicity). It is not known whether thioguanine is excreted in breast milk.

**Pediatrics**

Appropriate studies with thioguanine have not been performed in the pediatric population. However, pediatrics-specific problems that would limit the usefulness of this medication in children are not expected.

**Geriatrics**

No geriatrics-specific information is available on the use of thioguanine in geriatric patients. However, elderly patients are more likely to have age-related renal function impairment, which may require lower dosage in patients receiving thioguanine.

**Dental**

The bone marrow depressant effects of thioguanine may result in an increased incidence of microbial infection, delayed healing, and gingival bleeding. Dental work, whenever possible, should be completed prior to initiation of therapy or deferred until blood counts have returned to normal. Patients should be instructed in proper oral hygiene during treatment, including caution in use of regular toothbrushes, dental floss, and toothpicks.

Thioguanine may also rarely cause stomatitis associated with considerable discomfort.

**Drug interactions and/or related problems**

The following drug interactions and/or related problems have been selected on the basis of their potential clinical significance (possible mechanism in parentheses where appropriate)—not necessarily inclusive (» = major clinical significance):

Note: Combinations containing any of the following medications, depending on the amount present, may also interact with this medication.

　Allopurinol or
　Colchicine or
» Probenecid or
» Sulfinpyrazone

　　(thioguanine may raise the concentration of blood uric acid; dosage adjustment of antigout agents may be necessary to control hyperuricemia and gout; allopurinol may be preferred to prevent or reverse thioguanine-induced hyperuricemia because of risk of uric acid nephropathy with uricosuric antigout agents)

　Blood dyscrasia–causing medications (See *Appendix II*)

　　(leukopenic and/or thrombocytopenic effects of thioguanine may be increased with concurrent or recent therapy if these medications cause the same effects; dosage adjustment of thioguanine, if necessary, should be based on blood counts)

» Bone marrow depressants, other (See *Appendix II*) or
Radiation therapy
    (additive bone marrow depression may occur; dosage reduction
    may be required when two or more bone marrow depressants, in-
    cluding radiation, are used concurrently or consecutively)

Vaccines, killed virus
    (because normal defense mechanisms may be suppressed by thiog-
    uanine therapy, the patient's antibody response to the vaccine may
    be decreased. The interval between discontinuation of medications
    that cause immunosuppression and restoration of the patient's abil-
    ity to respond to the vaccine depends on the intensity and type of
    immunosuppression-causing medication used, the underlying dis-
    ease, and other factors; estimates vary from 3 months to 1 year)

» Vaccines, live virus
    (because normal defense mechanisms may be suppressed by thiog-
    uanine therapy, concurrent use with a live virus vaccine may po-
    tentiate the replication of the vaccine virus, may increase the side/
    adverse effects of the vaccine virus, and/or may decrease the
    patient's antibody response to the vaccine; immunization of these
    patients should be undertaken only with extreme caution after care-
    ful review of the patient's hematologic status and only with the
    knowledge and consent of the physician managing the thioguanine
    therapy. The interval between discontinuation of medications that
    cause immunosuppression and restoration of the patient's ability
    to respond to the vaccine depends on the intensity and type of
    immunosuppression-causing medication used, the underlying dis-
    ease, and other factors; estimates vary from 3 months to 1 year.
    Patients with leukemia in remission should not receive live virus
    vaccine until at least 3 months after their last chemotherapy. Im-
    munization with oral poliovirus vaccine should also be postponed
    in persons in close contact with the patient, especially family
    members)

**Laboratory value alterations**
The following have been selected on the basis of their potential clinical
significance (possible effect in parentheses where appropriate)—not
necessarily inclusive (» = major clinical significance):

With physiology/laboratory test values
Uric acid concentrations in blood and urine
    (may be increased)

**Medical considerations/Contraindications**
The medical considerations/contraindications included here have been selected on the basis of their potential clinical significance (reasons given
in parentheses where appropriate)—not necessarily inclusive (» =
major clinical significance):

*Risk-benefit should be considered when the following medical problems
exist:*
» Bone marrow depression
» Chickenpox, existing or recent (including recent exposure) or
» Herpes zoster
    (risk of severe generalized disease)
Gout, history of or
Urate renal stones, history of
    (risk of hyperuricemia)
» Hepatic function impairment
    (reduced biotransformation; lower dosage is recommended)
» Infection
» Renal function impairment
    (reduced elimination; lower dosage is recommended)
Sensitivity to thioguanine
» Caution should be used also in patients who have had cytotoxic drug
    therapy and radiation therapy within 4 to 6 weeks.

**Patient monitoring**
The following are especially important in patient monitoring (other tests
may be warranted in some patients, depending on condition; » =
major clinical significance):

Blood urea nitrogen (BUN) concentrations and
Serum creatinine concentrations
    (recommended prior to initiation of therapy and at periodic inter-
    vals during therapy; frequency varies according to clinical state,
    agent, dose, and other agents being used concurrently)
» Hematocrit or hemoglobin and
» Platelet count and
» Total and, if appropriate, differential leukocyte count
    (determinations recommended prior to initiation of therapy and at
    periodic intervals during therapy; frequency varies according to
    clinical state, agent, dose, and other agents being used concur-
    rently. In patients with acute leukemia or chronic myelocytic leu-

kemia and high total leukocyte counts, a rapid fall in leukocyte
count may occur with thioguanine therapy; daily blood counts are
recommended in these patients)
Serum alanine aminotransferase (ALT [SGPT]) concentrations and
Serum aspartate aminotransferase (AST [SGOT]) concentrations and
Serum bilirubin concentrations and
Serum lactate dehydrogenase (LDH) concentrations
    (concentrations recommended prior to initiation of therapy and at
    periodic intervals during therapy; frequency varies according to
    clinical state, agent, dose, and other agents being used
    concurrently)
Serum uric acid concentrations
    (recommended prior to initiation of therapy and at periodic inter-
    vals during therapy; frequency varies according to clinical state,
    agent, and dose, and other agents being used concurrently)

## Side/Adverse Effects

Note: Many "side effects" of antineoplastic therapy are unavoidable and
    represent the medication's pharmacologic action. Some of these (for
    example, leukopenia and thrombocytopenia) are actually used as
    parameters to aid in individual dosage titration.

The following side/adverse effects have been selected on the basis of their
    potential clinical significance (possible signs and symptoms in paren-
    theses where appropriate)—not necessarily inclusive:

**Those indicating need for medical attention**
Incidence more frequent
    *Immunosuppression, leukopenia, or infection* (usually asymptomatic;
    less frequently, fever or chills; cough or hoarseness; lower back or
    side pain; painful or difficult urination); *thrombocytopenia* (usually
    asymptomatic; less frequently, unusual bleeding or bruising; black,
    tarry stools; blood in urine or stools)
    Note: *Bone marrow depression* usually occurs over 2 to 4 weeks,
        although a rapid fall in leukocyte count may occur within 1 to
        2 weeks.

Incidence less frequent
    *Hyperuricemia or uric acid nephropathy* (joint pain; lower back or
    side pain; swelling of feet or lower legs); *unsteadiness when walking*
    Note: *Hyperuricemia or uric acid nephropathy* occurs most com-
        monly during initial treatment of patients with leukemia or lym-
        phoma, as a result of rapid cell breakdown, which leads to el-
        evated serum uric acid concentrations.

Incidence rare
    *Gastrointestinal ulceration* (black, tarry stools); *hepatotoxicity, he-
    patic fibrosis, or toxic hepatitis* (yellow eyes or skin); *stomatitis, dose-
    related* (sores in mouth and on lips)

**Those indicating need for medical attention only if they continue
or are bothersome**
Incidence less frequent
    *Diarrhea; loss of appetite; nausea and vomiting; skin rash or itching*
    Note: *Loss of appetite* or *nausea and vomiting* occur especially with
        overdosage.

**Those indicating the need for medical attention if they occur after
medication is discontinued**
    *Bone marrow depression* (black, tarry stools; blood in urine or stools;
    cough or hoarseness; fever or chills; lower back or side pain; painful
    or difficult urination; pinpoint red spots on skin; unusual bleeding or
    bruising)

## Patient Consultation

As an aid to patient consultation, refer to *Advice for the Patient,
Thioguanine (Systemic).*

Consider advising the patient on the following (» = major clinical significance):

**Before using this medication**
» Conditions affecting use, especially:
    Pregnancy—Advisability of using contraception; telling physician
        immediately if pregnancy is suspected
    See also *Precautions to Consider.*

**Proper use of this medication**
» Importance of not taking more or less medication than the amount
    prescribed
    Caution in taking combination chemotherapy; taking each medication
        at the right time
    Importance of ample fluid intake and subsequent increase in urine
        output to aid in excretion of uric acid

» Possible nausea and vomiting; importance of continuing medication despite stomach upset

Checking with physician if vomiting occurs shortly after dose is taken

» Proper dosing

Missed dose: Not taking at all; not doubling doses

» Proper storage

**Precautions while using this medication**

» Importance of close monitoring by the physician

» Avoiding immunizations unless approved by physician; other persons in patient's household should avoid immunizations with oral poliovirus vaccine; avoiding other persons who have taken oral poliovirus vaccine or wearing a protective mask that covers nose and mouth

*Caution if bone marrow depression occurs:*

» Avoiding exposure to persons with bacterial infections, especially during periods of low blood counts; checking with physician immediately if fever or chills, cough or hoarseness, lower back or side pain, or painful or difficult urination occur

» Checking with physician immediately if unusual bleeding or bruising; black, tarry stools; blood in urine or stools; or pinpoint red spots on skin occur

Caution in use of regular toothbrush, dental floss, or toothpick; physician, dentist, or nurse may suggest alternatives; checking with physician before having dental work done

Not touching eyes or inside of nose unless hands washed immediately before

Using caution to avoid accidental cuts with use of sharp objects such as safety razor or fingernail or toenail cutters

Avoiding contact sports or other situations where bruising or injury could occur

**Side/adverse effects**

May cause adverse effects such as blood problem and cancer; importance of discussing possible effects with physician

Signs of potential side effects, especially immunosuppression, leukopenia, infection, thrombocytopenia, hyperuricemia, uric acid nephropathy, gastrointestinal ulceration, hepatotoxicity, and stomatitis

Physician or nurse can help in dealing with side effects

## General Dosing Information

Patients receiving thioguanine should be under supervision of a physician experienced in antimetabolite chemotherapy.

Dosage must be adjusted to meet the individual requirements of each patient, based on clinical response and appearance or severity of toxicity.

Development of uric acid nephropathy in patients with leukemia or lymphoma may be prevented by adequate oral hydration and, in some cases, administration of allopurinol. Alkalinization of urine may be necessary if serum uric acid concentrations are elevated.

Unlike mercaptopurine and azathioprine, thioguanine may be continued in the usual dosage when the patient is receiving allopurinol concurrently to inhibit uric acid formation, because xanthine oxidase is not involved in metabolism of thioguanine.

Patients who have failed to respond to mercaptopurine are unlikely to respond to thioguanine.

Because the actions of thioguanine may be delayed, it is recommended that thioguanine therapy be discontinued promptly at the first sign of leukopenia (particularly granulocytopenia), thrombocytopenia, jaundice, or hemorrhage or bleeding tendencies. Therapy may be resumed at a lower dosage when laboratory values return to satisfactory levels.

In acute leukemia, thioguanine may sometimes be administered despite the presence of thrombocytopenia and bleeding; stoppage of bleeding and increase in platelet count have occurred during treatment in some cases and platelet transfusions may be useful in others.

Special precautions are recommended in patients who develop thrombocytopenia as a result of administration of thioguanine. These may include extreme care in performing invasive procedures; regular inspection of intravenous sites, skin (including perirectal area), and mucous membrane surfaces for signs of bleeding or bruising; limiting frequency of venipuncture and avoiding intramuscular injections; testing urine, emesis, stool, and secretions for occult blood; care in use of regular toothbrushes, dental floss, toothpicks, safety razors, and fingernail and toenail cutters; avoiding constipation; and using caution to prevent falls and other injuries. Such patients should avoid alcohol and any aspirin intake because of the risk of gastrointestinal bleeding. Platelet transfusions may be required.

Patients who develop leukopenia should be observed carefully for signs of infection. Antibiotic support may be required. In neutropenic patients who develop fever, broad-spectrum antibiotic coverage should be initiated empirically, pending bacterial cultures and appropriate diagnostic tests.

**Combination chemotherapy**

Thioguanine may be used in combination with other agents in various regimens. As a result, incidence and/or severity of side effects may be altered and different dosages (usually reduced) may be used. For example, thioguanine is part of the following chemotherapeutic combination (a commonly used acronym is in parentheses):

—cytarabine and thioguanine (Ara-C + 6-TG).

For specific dosages and schedules, consult the literature. For information regarding each agent, consult the individual monographs.

## Oral Dosage Forms

Note: Bracketed uses in the *Dosage Forms* section refer to categories of use and/or indications that are not included in U.S. product labeling.

### THIOGUANINE TABLETS USP

**Usual adult and adolescent dose**

[Leukemia, acute lymphocytic] or

Leukemia, acute myelocytic or

Leukemia, chronic myelocytic—

Induction: Oral, 2 mg per kg of body weight or 75 to 100 mg per square meter of body surface (to the closest 20 mg) a day in a single dose. If there is no clinical improvement and no leukocyte depression after 4 weeks at this dosage, a cautious increase in dosage to 3 mg per kg of body weight a day may be attempted.

Maintenance: Oral, 2 to 3 mg per kg of body weight or 100 mg per square meter of body surface a day.

**Usual pediatric dose**

See *Usual adult and adolescent dose.*

**Strength(s) usually available**

U.S.—

40 mg (Rx) [GENERIC].

Canada—

40 mg (Rx) [*Lanvis*].

**Packaging and storage**

Store below 40 °C (104 °F), preferably between 15 and 30 °C (59 and 86 °F), unless otherwise specified by manufacturer. Store in a tight container.

Revised: 09/90

Interim revision: 08/11/93; 07/05/94

---

**THIOPENTAL**—See *Anesthetics, Barbiturate (Systemic)*

---

**THIOPROPAZATE**—See *Phenothiazines (Systemic)*

---

**THIOPROPERAZINE**—See *Phenothiazines (Systemic)*

---

**THIORIDAZINE**—See *Phenothiazines (Systemic)*

# THIOTEPA   Systemic

VA CLASSIFICATION (Primary): AN100
Note: For a listing of dosage forms and brand names by country availability, see *Dosage Forms* section(s). For a listing of brand names for the articles in this monograph, refer to the General Index.

## Category
Antineoplastic.

## Indications
Note: Bracketed information in the *Indications* section refers to uses that are not included in U.S. product labeling.

### Accepted
Carcinoma, breast (treatment)
Carcinoma, ovarian (treatment)
Carcinoma, bladder (treatment)[1] or
[Carcinoma, lung (treatment)]—Thiotepa is indicated for treatment of adenocarcinoma of the breast or ovary. It is also indicated for topical treatment of superficial papillary carcinoma of the urinary bladder. Thiotepa is also used for treatment of bronchogenic carcinoma.

Lymphomas, Hodgkin's (treatment) or
Lymphomas, non-Hodgkin's (treatment)—Thiotepa is indicated for treatment of Hodgkin's disease and for some non-Hodgkin's lymphomas (lymphosarcoma, [Stages III and IV malignant lymphomas, giant follicular lymphoma, reticulum cell sarcoma]), although its use has largely been replaced by that of other agents.

Malignant effusions, pericardial (treatment)
Malignant effusions, peritoneal (treatment) or
Malignant effusions, pleural (treatment)—Thiotepa is indicated by intracavitary administration for controlling effusions secondary to diffuse or localized neoplastic disease of various serosal cavities.

---

[1]Not included in Canadian product labeling.

## Pharmacology/Pharmacokinetics

### Physicochemical characteristics
Molecular weight—189.21.

### Mechanism of action/Effect
Thiotepa is an alkylating agent of the nitrogen mustard type. Thiotepa is a trifunctional alkylating agent, and is cell cycle–phase nonspecific. Activity occurs as a result of formation of an unstable ethylenimmonium ion, which alkylates or binds with many intracellular molecular structures, including nucleic acids. Its cytotoxic action is primarily due to cross-linking of strands of DNA and RNA, as well as inhibition of protein synthesis.

### Absorption
Some degree of systemic absorption occurs after local administration. Absorption through bladder mucosa varies from 10% to almost 100% of a dose (related to drug concentration and time of drug contact with the urothelium, and increased by extensive tumor infiltration, mucosal inflammation, endoscopic surgical procedures or radiation therapy, and the presence of vesicoureteral reflux).

### Elimination
Renal, 85% (largely as metabolites).

## Precautions to Consider

### Carcinogenicity/Mutagenicity
Secondary malignancies are potential delayed effects of many antineoplastic agents, although it is not clear whether the effect is related to their mutagenic or immunosuppressive action. The effect of dose and duration of therapy is also unknown, although risk seems to increase with long-term use. Although information is limited, available data seem to indicate that the carcinogenic risk is greatest with the alkylating agents.
Thiotepa is carcinogenic and mutagenic in both animals and humans.

### Pregnancy/Reproduction
Fertility—Gonadal suppression, resulting in amenorrhea or azoospermia, may occur in patients taking antineoplastic therapy, especially with the alkylating agents. In general, these effects appear to be related to dose and length of therapy and may be irreversible. Prediction of the degree of testicular or ovarian function impairment is complicated by the common use of combinations of several antineoplastics, which makes it difficult to assess the effects of individual agents.

Pregnancy—Thiotepa is generally teratogenic in humans, although normal births have been reported.
First trimester: It is usually recommended that use of antineoplastics, especially combination chemotherapy, be avoided whenever possible, especially during the first trimester. Although information is limited because of the relatively few instances of antineoplastic administration during pregnancy, the mutagenic, teratogenic, and carcinogenic potential of these medications must be considered.
Other hazards to the fetus include adverse reactions seen in adults.
In general, use of a contraceptive is recommended during cytotoxic drug therapy.

### Breast-feeding
Although very little information is available regarding excretion of antineoplastic agents in breast milk, breast-feeding is not recommended while thiotepa is being administered because of the risks to the infant (adverse effects, mutagenicity, carcinogenicity). It is not known whether thiotepa or its metabolites are excreted in breast milk.

### Pediatrics
Appropriate studies have not been performed in the pediatric population.

### Geriatrics
No geriatrics-specific information is available on the use of thiotepa in geriatric patients. However, elderly patients are more likely to have age-related renal function impairment, which may require lower dosage and careful monitoring in patients receiving thiotepa.

### Dental
The bone marrow depressant effects of thiotepa may result in an increased incidence of microbial infection, delayed healing, and gingival bleeding. Dental work, whenever possible, should be completed prior to initiation of therapy or deferred until blood counts have returned to normal. Patients should be instructed in proper oral hygiene during treatment, including caution in use of regular toothbrushes, dental floss, and toothpicks.
Thiotepa may also rarely cause stomatitis associated with considerable discomfort.

### Drug interactions and/or related problems
The following drug interactions and/or related problems have been selected on the basis of their potential clinical significance (possible mechanism in parentheses where appropriate)—not necessarily inclusive (» = major clinical significance):
Note: Combinations containing any of the following medications, depending on the amount present, may also interact with this medication.

Allopurinol or
Colchicine or
» Probenecid or
» Sulfinpyrazone
(thiotepa may raise the concentration of blood uric acid; dosage adjustment of antigout agents may be necessary to control hyperuricemia and gout; allopurinol may be preferred to prevent or reverse thiotepa-induced hyperuricemia because of risk of uric acid nephropathy with uricosuric antigout agents)

Blood dyscrasia–causing medications (See *Appendix II*)
(leukopenic and/or thrombocytopenic effects of thiotepa may be increased with concurrent or recent therapy if these medications cause the same effects; dosage adjustment of thiotepa, if necessary, should be based on blood counts)

» Bone marrow depressants, other (See *Appendix II*) or
» Radiation therapy
(additive bone marrow depression may occur; administration of thiotepa with immunosuppressive medications is not recommended and modification of dosage may be required when thiotepa is administered with radiation therapy)

Succinylcholine
(thiotepa may decrease plasma levels of pseudocholinesterase, the enzyme that metabolizes succinylcholine, thereby enhancing the neuromuscular blockade of succinylcholine; determination of plasma pseudocholinesterase concentrations is recommended prior to use of succinylcholine in patients receiving thiotepa. Increased or prolonged respiratory depression or paralysis (apnea) may occur but is of minor clinical significance while the patient is being mechanically ventilated; however, careful postoperative monitoring of the patient may be necessary following concurrent or sequential use, especially if there is a possibility of incomplete reversal of neuromuscular blockade)

Urokinase
(may increase the efficacy of thiotepa in the treatment of bladder cancer by acting as a plasminogen activator and increasing the amount of medication in tumor tissue)

Vaccines, killed virus
(because normal defense mechanisms may be suppressed by thiotepa therapy, the patient's antibody response to the vaccine may be decreased. The interval between discontinuation of medications that cause immunosuppression and restoration of the patient's ability to respond to the vaccine depends on the intensity and type of immunosuppression-causing medication used, the underlying disease, and other factors; estimates vary from 3 months to 1 year)

» Vaccines, live virus
(because normal defense mechanisms may be suppressed by thiotepa therapy, concurrent use with a live virus vaccine may potentiate the replication of the vaccine virus, may increase the side/adverse effects of the vaccine virus, and/or may decrease the patient's antibody response to the vaccine; immunization of these patients should be undertaken only with extreme caution after careful review of the patient's hematologic status and only with the knowledge and consent of the physician managing the thiotepa therapy. The interval between discontinuation of medications that cause immunosuppression and restoration of the patient's ability to respond to the vaccine depends on the intensity and type of immunosuppression-causing medication used, the underlying disease, and other factors; estimates vary from 3 months to 1 year. Patients with leukemia in remission should not receive live virus vaccine until at least 3 months after their last chemotherapy. Immunization with oral polio virus vaccine should also be postponed in persons in close contact with the patient, especially family members)

**Laboratory value alterations**
The following have been selected on the basis of their potential clinical significance (possible effect in parentheses where appropriate)—not necessarily inclusive (» = major clinical significance):

With physiology/laboratory test values
Pseudocholinesterase concentrations in the plasma
(may be decreased very slightly)

Uric acid concentrations in blood and urine
(may be increased)

**Medical considerations/Contraindications**
The medical considerations/contraindications included here have been selected on the basis of their potential clinical significance (reasons given in parentheses where appropriate)—not necessarily inclusive (» = major clinical significance).

*Risk-benefit should be considered when the following medical problems exist:*

» Bone marrow depression
(lower dosage and careful monitoring recommended)

» Chickenpox, existing or recent (including recent exposure) or
» Herpes zoster
(risk of severe generalized disease)

Gout, history of or
Urate renal stones, history of
(risk of hyperuricemia)

» Hepatic function impairment
(reduced biotransformation; lower dosage and careful monitoring recommended)

» Infection

» Renal function impairment
(reduced elimination; lower dosage and careful monitoring recommended)

Sensitivity to thiotepa

» Tumor cell infiltration of bone marrow
(lower dosage and careful monitoring recommended)

» Caution should be used also in patients who have had previous cytotoxic drug therapy or radiation therapy.

**Patient monitoring**
The following are especially important in patient monitoring (other tests may be warranted in some patients, depending on condition; » = major clinical significance):

Blood urea nitrogen (BUN) concentrations and
Serum creatinine concentrations
(recommended prior to initiation of therapy and at periodic intervals during therapy; frequency varies according to clinical state, agent, dose, and other agents being used concurrently)

» Hematocrit or hemoglobin and

» Platelet count and
» Total and, if appropriate, differential leukocyte count
(determinations recommended prior to initiation of therapy and at periodic intervals during therapy; frequency varies according to clinical state, agent, dose, and other agents being used concurrently)

Serum alanine aminotransferase (ALT [SGPT]) concentrations and
Serum aspartate aminotransferase (AST [SGOT]) concentrations and
Serum bilirubin concentrations and
Serum lactate dehydrogenase (LDH) concentrations
(recommended prior to initiation of therapy and at periodic intervals during therapy; frequency varies according to clinical state, agent, dose, and other agents being used concurrently)

Serum uric acid concentrations
(recommended prior to initiation of therapy and at periodic intervals during therapy; frequency varies according to clinical state, agent, dose, and other agents being used concurrently)

## Side/Adverse Effects

Note: Many "side effects" of antineoplastic therapy are unavoidable and represent the medication's pharmacologic action. Some of these (for example, leukopenia and thrombocytopenia) are actually used as parameters to aid in individual dosage titration.
Side effects (especially bone marrow depression) may also occur after intracavitary administration and may be severe.

The following side/adverse effects have been selected on the basis of their potential clinical significance (possible signs and symptoms in parentheses where appropriate)—not necessarily inclusive:

**Those indicating need for medical attention**
Incidence more frequent
*Leukopenia or infection* (usually asymptomatic; less frequently, fever or chills; cough or hoarseness; lower back or side pain; painful or difficult urination); *thrombocytopenia* (usually asymptomatic; less frequently, unusual bleeding or bruising; black, tarry stools; blood in urine; pinpoint red spots on skin)

Note: *Bone marrow depression* may occur up to 1 month after thiotepa is administered.

Incidence less frequent
*Hyperuricemia or uric acid nephropathy* (joint pain; lower back or side pain; swelling of feet or lower legs); *pain at site of injection or instillation*

Note: *Hyperuricemia or uric acid nephropathy* occurs most commonly during initial treatment of patients with leukemia or lymphoma, as a result of rapid cell breakdown, which leads to elevated serum uric acid concentrations.

Incidence rare
*Anaphylaxis* (skin rash; tightness of throat; wheezing); *renal toxicity after local vesical application* (painful or difficult urination); *stomatitis* (sores in mouth and on lips)

**Those indicating need for medical attention only if they continue or are bothersome**
Incidence less frequent
*Dizziness; hives; loss of appetite; missing menstrual periods; nausea and vomiting*

**Those not indicating need for medical attention**
Incidence less frequent
*Loss of hair*

**Those indicating the need for medical attention if they occur after medication is discontinued**
*Bone marrow depression* (black, tarry stools; blood in urine or stools; cough or hoarseness; fever or chills; lower back or side pain; painful or difficult urination; pinpoint red spots on skin; unusual bleeding or bruising)

## Patient Consultation

As an aid to patient consultation, refer to *Advice for the Patient, Thiotepa (Systemic).*

Consider advising the patient on the following (» = major clinical significance):

**Before using this medication**
» Conditions affecting use, especially:
Pregnancy—Advisability of using contraception; telling physician immediately if pregnancy is suspected
See also *Precautions to Consider.*

**Proper use of this medication**
   Importance of ample fluid intake and subsequent increase in urine
      output to aid in excretion of uric acid
   Possible nausea and vomiting; importance of continuing medication
      despite stomach upset
» Proper dosing

**Precautions while using this medication**
» Importance of close monitoring by physician
   Caution if surgery with general anesthesia is required
» Avoiding immunizations unless approved by physician; other persons
   in patient's household should avoid immunizations with oral poliovirus vaccine; avoiding other persons who have taken oral poliovirus vaccine or wearing a protective mask that covers nose and
   mouth
*Caution if bone marrow depression occurs:*
» Avoiding exposure to persons with bacterial infections, especially during periods of low blood counts; checking with physician immediately if fever or chills, cough or hoarseness, lower back or side
   pain, or painful or difficult urination occur
» Checking with physician immediately if unusual bleeding or bruising;
   black, tarry stools; blood in urine or stools; or pinpoint red spots
   on skin occur
   Caution in use of regular toothbrush, dental floss, or toothpick; phy-
      sician, dentist, or nurse may suggest alternatives; checking with
      physician before having dental work done
   Not touching eyes or inside of nose unless hands washed immediately
      before
   Using caution to avoid accidental cuts with use of sharp objects such
      as safety razor or fingernail or toenail cutters
   Avoiding contact sports or other situations where bruising or injury
      could occur

**Side/adverse effects**
   May cause adverse effects such as blood problems, loss of hair, and
      cancer; importance of discussing possible effects with physician
   Signs of potential side effects, especially leukopenia, infection, throm-
      bocytopenia, hyperuricemia, uric acid nephropathy, pain at site of
      injection or instillation, anaphylaxis, renal toxicity after local ves-
      ical instillation, and stomatitis
   Physician or nurse can help in dealing with side effects
   Possibility of hair loss; should return after treatment has ended

# General Dosing Information

Patients receiving thiotepa should be under supervision of a physician
   experienced in cancer chemotherapy.

Dosage must be adjusted to meet the individual requirements of each
   patient, based on clinical response and appearance or severity of
   toxicity.

It is recommended that thiotepa be administered no more frequently than
   every 7 days, the risk of cumulative bone marrow toxicity being kept
   in mind, to allow the full effect of each dose on the leukocyte count
   to be seen (nadir occurs 5 to 30 days after each dose).

Maintenance therapy at 1- to 4-week intervals is recommended to continue
   optimal effect once it is obtained.

Initiation of thiotepa therapy in patients who have recently received cytotoxic drug or radiation therapy is not recommended until leukocyte
   and platelet counts depressed by the previous therapy begin to recover.
   Leukocyte counts above 2000 per cubic millimeter and platelet counts
   above 50,000 per cubic millimeter are considered acceptable.

Development of uric acid nephropathy in patients with leukemia or lymphoma may be prevented by adequate oral hydration, and, in some
   cases, administration of allopurinol. Alkalinization of urine may be
   necessary if serum uric acid concentrations are elevated.

Thiotepa may be administered by intravenous, intrapleural, intraperitoneal,
   intrapericardial, or intratumor injection or by intravesical instillation
   to the bladder.

It is recommended that thiotepa therapy be discontinued or dosage reduced
   at the first sign of a sudden large decrease in leukocyte (particularly
   granulocyte) or platelet count to prevent irreversible bone marrow depression. Therapy may be resumed when leukocyte and platelet counts
   return to acceptable levels.

Special precautions are recommended in patients who develop thrombocytopenia as a result of administration of thiotepa. These may include
   extreme care in performing invasive procedures; regular inspection of
   intravenous sites, skin (including perirectal area), and mucous
   membrane surfaces for signs of bleeding or bruising; limiting frequency of venipuncture and avoiding intramuscular injections; testing
   urine, emesis, stool, and secretions for occult blood; care in use of
   regular toothbrushes, dental floss, toothpicks, safety razors, and fin-

gernail and toenail cutters; avoiding constipation; and using caution to
prevent falls and other injuries. Such patients should avoid alcohol and
any aspirin intake because of the risk of gastrointestinal bleeding.
Platelet transfusions may be required.

Patients who develop leukopenia should be observed carefully for signs
of infection. Antibiotic support may be required. In neutropenic patients who develop fever, broad-spectrum antibiotic coverage should
be initiated empirically, pending bacterial cultures and appropriate diagnostic tests.

**Safety considerations for handling this medication**
There is limited but increasing evidence and concern that personnel involved in preparation and administration of parenteral antineoplastics
may be at some risk because of the potential mutagenicity, teratogenicity, and/or carcinogenicity of these agents, although the actual risk
is unknown. USP advisory panels recommend cautious handling both
in preparation and disposal of antineoplastic agents. Precautions that
have been suggested include:
 • Use of a biological containment cabinet during reconstitution and
   dilution of parenteral medications and wearing of disposable surgical
   gloves and masks.
 • Use of proper technique to prevent contamination of the medication,
   work area, and operator during transfer between containers (including
   proper training of personnel in this technique).
 • Cautious and proper disposal of needles, syringes, vials, ampuls, and
   unused medication.
A number of medical centers have developed detailed guidelines for handling of antineoplastic agents.

# Parenteral Dosage Forms

Note: Bracketed uses in the *Dosage Forms* section refer to categories of
      use and/or indications that are not included in U.S. product labeling.

## THIOTEPA FOR INJECTION USP

**Usual adult and adolescent dose**
Carcinoma, breast or
Carcinoma, ovarian or
Malignant effusions, pericardial or
Malignant effusions, peritoneal or
Malignant effusions, pleural—
   Intracavitary or intratumor, 600 to 800 mcg (0.6 to 0.8 mg) per kg of
   body weight every one to four weeks, with a maintenance dose of
   70 to 800 mcg (0.07 to 0.8 mg) per kg of body weight. The dose
   is reduced in cases of marked debility or weakness, chronic car-
   diovascular or renal disease, or surgical shock. Maintenance dose
   is adjusted on the basis of blood counts and given every one to
   four weeks.
Carcinoma, breast or
Carcinoma, ovarian or
[Carcinoma, lung] or
Lymphomas, Hodgkin's or
Lymphomas, non-Hodgkin's—
   Intravenous, 300 to 400 mcg (0.3 to 0.4 mg) per kg of body weight
   every one to four weeks, or 200 mcg (0.2 mg) per kg of body
   weight for four to five days every two to four weeks. Maintenance
   dose is adjusted on the basis of blood counts.
Carcinoma, bladder[1]—
   Topical, to the bladder, 30 to 60 mg in 30 to 60 mL of distilled water
   instilled into the bladder by catheter once a week for four weeks;
   the course may be repeated monthly if necessary. The patient is
   dehydrated for eight to twelve hours prior to each dose and should
   try to retain the volume for two hours. The patient's position may
   be changed every fifteen minutes to ensure maximum area contact.

**Usual pediatric dose**
Children up to 12 years of age: Dosage has not been established.
Children 12 years of age and over: See *Usual adult and adolescent dose.*

**Size(s) usually available**
U.S.—
   15 mg (Rx) [GENERIC].
Canada—
   15 mg (Rx) [GENERIC].

**Packaging and storage**
Store between 2 and 8 °C (36 and 46 °F). Protect from light.

**Preparation of dosage form**
Thiotepa for Injection USP is reconstituted for use by adding 1.5 mL of
sterile water for injection (other diluents are not recommended because
they would produce a hypertonic solution, which would cause discomfort with injection) to the vial to produce an isotonic solution containing 10 mg of thiotepa per mL.

Reconstituted solutions may be further diluted with 0.9% sodium chloride injection, 5% dextrose injection, 5% dextrose and 0.9% sodium chloride injection, Ringer's injection, or lactated Ringer's injection for intracavitary use, intravenous drip, or perfusion therapy.

Thiotepa may be mixed with 2% Procaine Hydrochloride Injection USP and/or epinephrine hydrochloride 1:1000 for local use into single or multiple sites.

**Stability**

Reconstituted solutions of thiotepa may be stored for 5 days between 2 and 8 °C without significant loss of potency. Reconstituted solutions

may be clear to slightly opaque; solutions that are grossly opaque or precipitated should not be used.

---

¹Not included in Canadian product labeling.

---

Revised: 09/90
Interim revision: 08/11/93; 07/05/94

---

**THIOTHIXENE**—See *Thioxanthenes (Systemic)*

---

# THIOXANTHENES   Systemic

This monograph includes information on the following: Chlorprothixene†; Flupenthixol*; Thiothixene.

INN:
   Flupenthixol—Flupentixol

VA CLASSIFICATION (Primary): CN701

Another commonly used name is flupentixol.

Note: For a listing of dosage forms and brand names by country availability, see *Dosage Forms* section(s). For a listing of brand names for the articles in this monograph, refer to the General Index.

---

*Not commercially available in the U.S.
†Not commercially available in Canada.

---

## Category

Antipsychotic.

## Indications

### Accepted

Psychotic disorders (treatment)—Indicated for management of primary and secondary symptoms of psychotic disorders.

   The long-acting flupenthixol decanoate injection may be used in the management of nonagitated, chronic, schizophrenic patients who have been stabilized with short-acting neuroleptics.

### Unaccepted

Flupenthixol is *not* indicated for the management of severely agitated psychotic patients, psychoneurotic patients, or geriatric patients with confusion and/or agitation.

## Pharmacology/Pharmacokinetics

### Physicochemical characteristics

Molecular weight—
   Chlorprothixene: 315.86.
   Flupenthixol decanoate: 588.82.
   Flupenthixol dihydrochloride: 507.4.
   Thiothixene: 443.62.
   Thiothixene hydrochloride: 552.57.
Other characteristics—
   Structurally and pharmacologically similar to the piperazine phenothiazines, which include acetophenazine, fluphenazine, perphenazine, prochlorperazine, and trifluoperazine.

### Mechanism of action/Effect

Antipsychotic—Thioxanthenes are thought to benefit psychotic conditions by blocking postsynaptic dopamine receptors in the brain. They also produce an alpha-adrenergic blocking effect and depress the release of most hypothalamic and hypophyseal hormones. However, the concentration of prolactin is increased due to blockade of prolactin inhibitory factor (PIF), which inhibits the release of prolactin from the pituitary gland.

### Other actions/effects

Antiemetic—Chlorprothixene also inhibits the medullary chemoreceptor trigger zone to produce an antiemetic effect.

Sedative—Chlorprothixene is also thought to cause an indirect reduction of stimuli to the brain stem reticular system to produce a sedative effect.

### Absorption

Flupenthixol decanoate—Slowly, from the site of injection, and gradually released from the vehicle into the bloodstream, where it is rapidly hydrolyzed to flupenthixol.

Flupenthixol dihydrochloride—Rapid, from gastrointestinal tract.

Thiothixene—Rapid.

### Biotransformation

Hepatic.

### Half-life

Elimination—
   Thiothixene:
      Initial phase—3.4 hours.
      Late phase—Approximately 34 hours.

### Time to peak concentrations

Flupenthixol dihydrochloride—3 to 8 hours.
Flupenthixol decanoate—4 to 7 days.
Thiothixene—1 to 3 hours.

### Duration of action

Chlorprothixene—Intramuscular, up to 12 hours.
Flupenthixol decanoate—3 weeks.

### Elimination

Chlorprothixene and thiothixene—Primarily renal.
Flupenthixol—Primarily fecal; some renal.

## Precautions to Consider

### Cross-sensitivity and/or related problems

Patients sensitive to one thioxanthene may be sensitive to the others also, and possibly to the phenothiazines.

### Carcinogenicity/Tumorigenicity

Most neuroleptic medications have been found to cause increased serum prolactin concentrations. Although the clinical significance of this increase is not known for most patients, *in vitro* studies have shown approximately one-third of human breast cancers to be prolactin dependent. Additionally, an increase in mammary neoplasms has been found in rodents after chronic administration of neuroleptics. However, a definite association between the chronic administration of these medications and mammary tumorigenesis has not been established.

### Pregnancy/Reproduction

Fertility—Studies with thiothixene in rats and rabbits showed a decrease in fertility.

Pregnancy—Studies in humans have not been done.

Animal studies have shown no birth defects caused by thioxanthenes. However, there have been reports of hyperreflexia in the neonate when phenothiazines were used during pregnancy. Also, studies with thiothixene in rats and rabbits showed an increase in resorption rate. No teratogenic effects were seen after repeated oral administration of thiothixene to rats, rabbits, and monkeys before and during gestation.

### Breast-feeding

It is not known if thioxanthenes are distributed into breast milk. Caution is advised since pharmacologically related phenothiazines are distributed into breast milk, causing an increased risk of tardive dyskinesia and possible drowsiness in the nursing infant.

### Pediatrics

Children appear to be prone to develop neuromuscular or extrapyramidal reactions, especially dystonias, while receiving therapeutic doses of pharmacologically related phenothiazines and should be closely monitored. Adolescents should be monitored very carefully during parenteral therapy with thioxanthenes because they tend to experience a higher incidence of hypotensive and extrapyramidal reactions than do adults.

### Geriatrics

Geriatric patients tend to develop higher plasma concentrations of neuroleptics because of changes in distribution due to decreases in lean body mass, total body water, and albumin, and often an increase in total body fat composition. These patients usually require a lower initial dosage and a more gradual titration of dose.

Elderly patients appear to be more prone to orthostatic hypotension, and exhibit an increased sensitivity to the anticholinergic and sedative effects of neuroleptics. They are also more prone to develop extrapyramidal side effects, such as tardive dyskinesia and parkinsonism. The signs of tardive dyskinesia are persistent, difficult to control, and, in some patients, appear to be irreversible. There is no known effective treatment. Careful observation during treatment for early signs of tardive dyskinesia and dosage adjustment of the thioxanthene may prevent a more severe manifestation of the syndrome.

### Dental

The peripheral anticholinergic effects of thioxanthenes may decrease or inhibit salivary flow, especially in middle-aged or elderly patients, thus contributing to the development of caries, periodontal disease, oral candidiasis, and discomfort.

Extrapyramidal reactions induced by thioxanthenes will result in increased motor activity of the head, face, and neck. Occlusal adjustments, bite registrations, and treatment for bruxism may be made less reliable.

The leukopenic and thrombocytopenic effects of thioxanthenes may result in an increased incidence of microbial infection, delayed healing, and gingival bleeding. If leukopenia or thrombocytopenia occurs, dental work should be deferred until blood counts have returned to normal, and patients should be instructed in proper oral hygiene, including caution in use of regular toothbrushes, dental floss, and toothpicks.

### Drug interactions and/or related problems

The following drug interactions and/or related problems have been selected on the basis of their potential clinical significance (possible mechanism in parentheses where appropriate)—not necessarily inclusive (» = major clinical significance):

Note: Combinations containing any of the following medications, depending on the amount present, may also interact with this medication.

Although not all of the following interactions have been documented specifically for thioxanthenes, a potential exists for their occurrence because of the close similarity of the pharmacological effects of thioxanthenes with those of phenothiazine medications.

» Alcohol or
» Central nervous system (CNS) depression–producing medications, other, especially anesthetics, barbiturates, and opioid (narcotic) analgesics (See *Appendix II*)
    (concurrent use may potentiate and prolong the CNS depressant effects of either these medications or the thioxanthenes; dosage adjustments may be necessary)

Amphetamines
    (concurrent use with thioxanthenes may inhibit the CNS-stimulating effects of amphetamines due to alpha-adrenergic blockade by the thioxanthenes; also, the antipsychotic effects of thioxanthenes may be reduced when they are used concurrently with amphetamines)

Antacids or
Antidiarrheals, adsorbent
    (concurrent use may inhibit the absorption of an orally administered thioxanthene)

Anticholinergics or other medications with anticholinergic action (See *Appendix II*) or
Antidyskinetic agents or
Antihistamines
    (anticholinergic effects, especially confusion, hallucinations, nightmares, and increased intraocular pressure, may be potentiated when these medications are used concurrently with thioxanthenes, because of secondary anticholinergic action of thioxanthenes)

Anticonvulsants
    (thioxanthenes may lower the seizure threshold; dosage adjustment of anticonvulsant medications may be necessary; potentiation of anticonvulsant effects does not occur)

Antidepressants, tricyclic or
Maprotiline or
Monoamine oxidase (MAO) inhibitors, including furazolidone, procarbazine, or selegiline or
Trazodone
    (concurrent use with thioxanthenes may prolong and intensify the sedative and anticholinergic effects of either these medications or the thioxanthenes)

Bromocriptine
    (concurrent use with thioxanthenes may increase serum prolactin concentrations and interfere with effects of bromocriptine; dosage adjustment of bromocriptine may be necessary)

Dopamine
    (concurrent use may antagonize peripheral vasoconstriction produced by high doses of dopamine, because of the alpha-adrenergic blocking action of thioxanthenes)

Ephedrine
    (alpha-adrenergic blocking action of thioxanthenes may decrease the pressor response to ephedrine when it is used concurrently with thioxanthenes)

» Epinephrine
    (alpha-adrenergic effects of epinephrine may be blocked when it is used concurrently with thioxanthenes, possibly resulting in severe hypotension and tachycardia)

» Extrapyramidal reaction–causing medications, other (See *Appendix II*)
    (concurrent use with thioxanthenes may increase the severity and frequency of extrapyramidal effects)

Guanadrel or
Guanethidine
    (concurrent use with thioxanthenes may decrease the hypotensive effects of these medications because of their displacement from and inhibition of uptake by adrenergic neurons)

» Levodopa
    (concurrent use with thioxanthenes may inhibit the antiparkinsonian effects of levodopa because thioxanthenes block dopamine receptors in the brain)

Metaraminol
    (concurrent use usually decreases, but does not reverse or completely block, the pressor response to metaraminol, because of the alpha-adrenergic blocking action of thioxanthenes)

Methoxamine
    (prior administration of thioxanthenes may decrease the pressor effect and duration of action of methoxamine because of the alpha-adrenergic blocking action of thioxanthenes)

Ototoxic medications, especially ototoxic antibiotics (See *Appendix II*)
    (concurrent use with thioxanthenes may mask the symptoms of ototoxicity such as tinnitus, dizziness, or vertigo)

Phenylephrine
    (prior administration of thioxanthenes may decrease the pressor response to phenylephrine because of the alpha-adrenergic blocking action of thioxanthenes)

Photosensitizing medications, other
    (concurrent use with thioxanthenes may cause additive photosensitizing effects)

» Quinidine
    (concurrent use with thioxanthenes may result in additive cardiac effects)

### Laboratory value alterations

The following have been selected on the basis of their potential clinical significance (possible effect in parentheses where appropriate)—not necessarily inclusive (» = major clinical significance):

With diagnostic test results

*For chlorprothixene*
    Bilirubin tests, urine
        (false-positive results may occur)

    Electrocardiogram (ECG) readings
        (Q- and T-wave changes may occur)

    Immunologic urine pregnancy tests
        (depending on the test used, false-positive or false-negative results may occur)

With physiology/laboratory test values
    Uric acid
        (serum concentrations may be decreased with use of neuroleptics)

### Medical considerations/Contraindications

The medical considerations/contraindications included here have been selected on the basis of their potential clinical significance (reasons given in parentheses where appropriate)—not necessarily inclusive (» = major clinical significance).

*Except under special circumstances, this medication should not be used when the following medical problems exist:*

» Blood dyscrasias or
» Bone marrow depression or
» Circulatory collapse or
» CNS depression or
» Comatose states, drug-induced
    (may be exacerbated)

*Risk-benefit should be considered when the following medical problems exist:*

» Alcoholism
(CNS depression may be potentiated)

» Cardiovascular disease
(increased risk of transient hypotension)

Glaucoma, or predisposition to or

Peptic ulcer or

Respiratory disorders due to acute infections, asthma, or emphysema or

Urinary retention
(may be exacerbated)

» Hepatic function impairment
(metabolism may be altered)

Parkinson's disease
(potentiation of extrapyramidal effects)

Prostatic hypertrophy, symptomatic
(increased risk of urinary retention)

» Reye's syndrome
(increased risk of hepatotoxicity in children and adolescents with signs and symptoms suggesting Reye's syndrome)

Seizure disorders
(seizures may be precipitated because of lowered seizure threshold)

Sensitivity to thioxanthenes or phenothiazines

### Patient monitoring
The following may be especially important in patient monitoring (other tests may be warranted in some patients, depending on condition; » = major clinical significance):

Blood cell counts and differential, especially in patients with sore throat and fever
(may be required at periodic intervals during high-dose or prolonged therapy; agranulocytosis is more likely to occur between the 4th and 10th weeks of therapy; if significant cellular depression occurs, medication should be discontinued and appropriate therapy initiated)

Careful observation for early symptoms of tardive dyskinesia
(recommended at periodic intervals, especially during high-dose or prolonged therapy and in the elderly; since there is no known effective treatment if syndrome should develop, thioxanthenes should be discontinued, if clinically feasible, at the earliest signs, usually fine, worm-like movements of the tongue)

Careful observation for early symptoms of tardive dystonia
(recommended at periodic intervals; since there is no known effective treatment if syndrome should develop, thioxanthenes should be discontinued, if clinically feasible, at the earliest signs)

Liver function tests and

Urine tests for bilirubin and bile
(may be required if jaundice or grippe-like symptoms occur; these side effects are more likely to occur between the 2nd and 4th weeks of therapy)

Ophthalmologic examinations
(may be required at periodic intervals during high-dose or prolonged therapy since deposition of particulate matter in the lens and cornea has occurred)

## Side/Adverse Effects

Note: A few cases of sudden death have been reported in patients who were receiving phenothiazine derivatives. However, there is no definite evidence that the phenothiazines are causative agents.

Although not all of these side effects have been attributed specifically to each thioxanthene or its phenothiazine analog, a potential exists for their occurrence during the use of any thioxanthene or its analog.

The following side/adverse effects have been selected on the basis of their potential clinical significance (possible signs and symptoms in parentheses where appropriate)—not necessarily inclusive:

### Those indicating need for medical attention
Incidence more frequent
*Akathisia* (severe restlessness or need to keep moving)—may appear within first 6 hours after dose; *dystonic reactions* (difficulty in swallowing; inability to move eyes; muscle spasms, especially of neck and back; unusual twisting movements of body); *extrapyramidal effects, parkinsonian* (difficulty in talking; loss of balance control; mask-like face; shuffling walk; stiffness of arms and legs; trembling and shaking of fingers and hands); *tardive dyskinesia, persistent* (lip smacking or puckering; puffing of cheeks; rapid or worm-like movements of tongue; uncontrolled chewing movements; uncontrolled movements of arms and legs)

Note: *Dystonic reactions* appear most often in children and young adults; usually appear early in treatment and may subside within 24 to 48 hours after medication has been discontinued.

*Parkinsonian extrapyramidal effects* may be seen in the first few days of treatment, but frequency usually increases with increase of dosage; may be more frequent in elderly patients and older children.

*Tardive dyskinesia* is initially dose related, but may increase with long-term treatment and total cumulative dose; may persist after discontinuation of thioxanthenes.

Incidence less frequent
*Allergic reaction* (skin rash); *anticholinergic effect* (difficult urination); *deposition of opaque substances in lens and cornea or retinopathy* (blurred vision or other eye problems); *hypotension* (fainting); *skin discoloration*—more frequent in females on high-dose and prolonged therapy

Incidence rare
*Agranulocytosis or other blood dyscrasias* (sore throat and fever; unusual bleeding or bruising); *heat stroke* (hot, dry skin or lack of sweating; muscle weakness); *jaundice, obstructive* (yellow eyes or skin); *neuroleptic malignant syndrome (NMS)* (convulsions; difficulty in breathing; fast heartbeat; high fever; high or low blood pressure; increased sweating; loss of bladder control; severe muscle stiffness; unusually pale skin; tiredness); *tardive dystonia* (increased blinking or spasms of eyelid; unusual facial expressions or body positions; uncontrolled twisting movements of neck, trunk, arms, or legs)

Note: *Heat stroke* may occur in environmental conditions of high heat and high humidity. Adequate interior temperature control (air-conditioning) must be maintained for institutionalized patients during hot weather because of the increased risk of heat stroke and neuroleptic malignant syndrome (NMS).

*NMS* may occur at any time during neuroleptic therapy, but is more commonly seen soon after start of therapy, after patient has switched from one neuroleptic to another, during combined therapy with another psychotropic medication, or after a dosage increase. Along with the overt signs of skeletal muscle rigidity, hyperthermia, autonomic dysfunction, and altered consciousness, differential diagnosis may reveal leukocytosis (9500 to 26,000 cells per cubic millimeter), elevated liver enzymes, and elevated creatine phosphokinase (CPK).

### Those indicating need for medical attention only if they continue or are bothersome
Incidence more frequent
*Constipation; decreased sweating; drowsiness, mild; dryness of mouth; increased appetite and weight; increased sensitivity of skin to sunlight; nasal congestion* (stuffy nose); *orthostatic hypotension* (dizziness, lightheadedness, or fainting)

Incidence less frequent
*Changes in menstrual period; decreased sexual ability; swelling of breasts*—in males and females; *unusual secretion of milk*

### Those indicating need for medical attention if they occur after medication is discontinued
*Dyskinesia, withdrawal emergent* (dizziness; nausea and vomiting; stomach pain; trembling of fingers and hands; uncontrolled, repetitive movements of mouth, tongue, or jaw)

## Overdose
For specific information on the agents used in the management of thioxanthene overdose, see:
• *Amphetamine* or *dextroamphetamine* in *Amphetamines (Systemic)* monograph;
• *Benztropine* in *Antidyskinetics (Systemic)* monograph;
• *Charcoal, Activated (Oral-Local)* monograph;
• *Diazepam* in *Benzodiazepines (Systemic)* monograph;
• *Digitalis Glycosides (Systemic)* monograph;
• *Diphenhydramine* in *Antihistamines (Systemic)* monograph;
• *Norepinephrine* or *phenylephrine* in *Sympathomimetic Agents—Cardiovascular Use (Parenteral-Systemic)* monograph; and/or
• *Phenytoin* in *Anticonvulsants, Hydantoin (Systemic)* monograph.

For more information on the management of overdose or unintentional ingestion, contact a Poison Control Center (see *Poison Control Center Listing*).

**Clinical effects of overdose**

The following effects have been selected on the basis of their potential clinical significance (possible signs and symptoms in parentheses where appropriate)—not necessarily inclusive:

*Convulsions; difficulty in breathing, severe; drowsiness, severe, or coma; fast heartbeat; fever; hypotension* (dizziness, severe); *muscle trembling, jerking, stiffness, or uncontrolled movements, severe; small pupils; unusual excitement; unusual tiredness or weakness, severe*

**Treatment of overdose**

Treatment is essentially symptomatic and supportive and may consist of the following:

To decrease absorption—
Early gastric lavage is often helpful.
Not attempting to induce emesis because a dystonic reaction of the head and neck may develop that could result in aspiration of vomitus.
Administering activated charcoal slurry.
Administering saline cathartic.

Specific treatment—
Controlling cardiac arrhythmias with intravenous phenytoin, 9 to 11 mg per kg of body weight (mg/kg).
Digitalizing for cardiac failure.
Administering a vasopressor, such as norepinephrine or phenylephrine, for hypotension (not using epinephrine, which may cause paradoxical hypotension).
Controlling convulsions with diazepam followed by phenytoin, 15 mg/kg, administered at a rate no faster than 50 mg per minute.
Benztropine or diphenhydramine may be administered to manage acute parkinsonian symptoms.
Severe CNS depression may require administration of a stimulant such as amphetamine or dextroamphetamine (picrotoxin or pentylenetetrazol should be avoided as it may induce convulsions).

Monitoring—
Monitoring cardiovascular function (for not less than 5 days).

Supportive care—
Maintaining respiratory function and body temperature.
Patients in whom intentional overdose is known or suspected should be referred for psychiatric consultation.

Note: Dialysis of thioxanthenes has not been successful.

# Patient Consultation

As an aid to patient consultation, refer to *Advice for the Patient, Thioxanthenes (Systemic).*

In providing consultation, consider emphasizing the following selected information (» = major clinical significance):

**Before using this medication**
» Conditions affecting use, especially:
Sensitivity to thioxanthenes or phenothiazines
Pregnancy—Reports of hyperreflexia in neonates when pharmacologically related phenothiazines were used during pregnancy; animal studies have shown an increase in resorption rates and decreased fertility with phenothiazines
Breast-feeding—Pharmacologically related phenothiazines are distributed into breast milk causing tardive dyskinesia and possible drowsiness in nursing baby
Use in children—Children are more prone to extrapyramidal symptoms
Use in the elderly—Elderly patients are more likely to develop extrapyramidal, anticholinergic, hypotensive, and sedative effects; reduced dosage recommended
Dental—Thioxanthene-induced blood dyscrasias may result in infections, delayed healing, and bleeding; dry mouth may cause caries and candidiasis; increased motor activity of face, head, and neck may interfere with some dental procedures
Other medications, especially alcohol or other CNS depression–producing medications, epinephrine, other extrapyramidal reaction–causing medications, levodopa, or quinidine
Other medical problems, especially blood dyscrasias, bone marrow depression, circulatory collapse, CNS depression, alcoholism, cardiovascular disease, hepatic function impairment, or Reye's syndrome

**Proper use of this medication**
Taking with food or milk to reduce gastrointestinal irritation
» Diluting thiothixene oral solution with recommended beverages prior to use
» Compliance with therapy; not taking more medication or more often than directed
» May require several weeks of therapy to obtain desired effects

» Proper dosing
Missed dose: Taking as soon as possible; not taking if within 2 hours of next scheduled dose; continuing on regular schedule; not doubling doses
» Proper storage

**Precautions while using this medication**
Regular visits to physician to check progress of therapy
Checking with physician before discontinuing medication; gradual dosage reduction may be needed
» Avoiding use of alcoholic beverages or other CNS depressants during therapy
Avoiding use of antacids or medicine for diarrhea within 2 hours of taking thioxanthenes
» Caution if any kind of surgery, dental treatment, or emergency treatment is required
» Possible drowsiness; caution when driving, using machines, or doing other things requiring alertness
» Possible dizziness or lightheadedness; caution when getting up suddenly from a lying or sitting position
» Possible heatstroke: caution during exercise or hot weather, or when taking hot baths
» Possible skin photosensitivity; avoiding unprotected exposure to sun; using protective clothing; using a sun block product that includes protection against both UVA-caused photosensitivity reactions and UVB-caused sunburn reactions; avoiding use of sunlamp, tanning bed, or tanning booth
Possible dryness of mouth; using sugarless gum or candy, ice, or saliva substitute for relief; checking with physician or dentist if dry mouth continues for more than 2 weeks
» Avoiding spilling liquid medication on skin or clothing; may cause contact dermatitis
Observing precautions for long-acting parenteral form for up to 3 weeks

**Side/adverse effects**
» Stopping medication and notifying physician immediately if symptoms of neuroleptic malignant syndrome (NMS) appear
» Notifying physician as soon as possible if early signs of tardive dyskinesia appear
Possibility of withdrawal symptoms
Signs of potential side effects, especially akathisia, dystonias, parkinsonian effects, tardive dyskinesia or dystonia, allergic reactions, anticholinergic effects, deposition of opaque substances in lens and cornea or retinopathy, hypotension, skin discoloration, blood dyscrasias, heat stroke, obstructive jaundice, and NMS

# General Dosing Information

Dosage must be individualized by titration from the lower dose range. After a favorable psychiatric response is noted (within several days to several months), that dosage should be continued for about 2 weeks, then gradually decreased to the lowest level that will maintain an adequate clinical response.

When extended therapy is discontinued, a gradual reduction in thioxanthene dosage over several weeks is recommended. Abrupt withdrawal may cause some patients on high or long-term dosage to experience transient dyskinetic signs, nausea, vomiting, gastritis, trembling, and dizziness.

The antiemetic effect of thioxanthenes may mask signs of drug toxicity or may obscure diagnosis of conditions whose primary symptom is nausea.

Avoid skin contact with liquid forms of this medication; contact dermatitis has resulted with use of similar medications.

**For parenteral dosage forms only**

Because hypotension is a common side effect of thioxanthenes, parenteral administration should be used only for patients who are bedfast or for appropriate acute, ambulatory patients who can be closely monitored. A possible exception may be those patients who are dose-stabilized on the extended-action injectable form.

Intramuscular injections should be administered slowly and deeply into the upper outer quadrant of the buttock or midlateral thigh. Patient should remain lying down for at least half an hour after injection to avoid possible hypotensive effects.

Effects of the extended-action injectable form may last for up to 3 weeks. The precautions and side effects information applies during this period of time.

Geriatric patients and children should be monitored very carefully during parenteral therapy because of a higher incidence of hypotensive and extrapyramidal reactions.

The changeover from other neuroleptic medication to long-acting flupen-thixol should be done gradually and under close supervision to prevent overdosage or insufficient suppression of psychotic symptoms before the next injection.

**Diet/Nutrition**

This medication may be taken with food or a full glass (240 mL) of water or milk, if necessary, to lessen stomach irritation.

**For treatment of adverse effects**

Neuroleptic malignant syndrome (NMS)—

Treatment is essentially symptomatic and supportive and may include:
- *Discontinuing thioxanthene immediately.*
- Hyperthermia—Administering antipyretics (aspirin or acetamin-ophen); using cooling blanket.
- Dehydration—Restoring fluid and electrolytes.
- Cardiovascular instability—Monitoring blood pressure and car-diac rhythm closely.
- Hypoxia—Administering oxygen; considering airway insertion and assisted ventilation.
- Muscle rigidity—Dantrolene sodium may be administered (100 to 300 mg per day in divided doses; 1.25 to 1.5 mg per kg of body weight, intravenously). Bromocriptine (5 to 7.5 mg every eight hours) has been used to reverse hyperpyrexia and muscle rigidity.

Parkinsonism, severe:

Many authorities advise that the only appropriate treatment of extra-pyramidal symptoms is reduction of the antipsychotic dosage, if possible. Oral antidyskinetic agents such as trihexyphenidyl (2 mg three times a day), or benztropine, may be effective in treating more severe parkinsonism and acute motor restlessness but should be used sparingly, and then usually for no longer than 3 months. Milder effects may be treated by adjusting dosage. However, in the elderly patient, the use of amantadine (100 to 200 mg) at bed-time minimizes the severe anticholinergic effects that may occur with other antidyskinetics.

Akathisia:

May be treated with antidyskinetic agents, or with propranolol (30 to 120 mg a day); nadolol (40 mg a day); pindolol (5 to 60 mg a day); lorazepam (1 or 2 mg two or three times a day): or diazepam (2 mg two or three times a day).

Dystonia:

Acute dystonic postures or oculogyric crisis may be relieved by par-enteral administration of benztropine (2 mg intramuscularly), or diphenhydramine (50 mg intravenously or intramuscularly), or di-azepam (5 to 7.5 mg intravenously), to be followed by oral anti-dyskinetic medication for one or two days to prevent recurrent dystonic episodes. Dosage adjustments of the thioxanthene may control these effects, and discontinuation may reverse severe symptoms.

Tardive dyskinesia or tardive dystonia:

No known effective treatment. Dosage of thioxanthene should be low-ered or medication discontinued, if clinically feasible, at earliest signs of tardive dyskinesia or tardive dystonia, to prevent possible irreversible effects.

---

## *CHLORPROTHIXENE*

## Summary of Differences

Pharmacology/pharmacokinetics:

Other actions/effects—Antiemetic and sedative effects are more prom-inent than those of thiothixene.

Duration of action—Intramuscular dosage may produce effects lasting up to 12 hours.

Precautions:

Laboratory value alterations—

More likely to cause Q-T wave changes on ECG readings than is thiothixene.

May produce false-positive results on immunologic urine preg-nancy test.

May produce false-positive results on urine bilirubin test.

## Oral Dosage Forms

### CHLORPROTHIXENE ORAL SUSPENSION USP

**Usual adult and adolescent dose**

Antipsychotic—

Oral, 25 to 50 mg three or four times a day.

Note: Geriatric or debilitated patients usually require a lower initial dose, the dosage being increased gradually as needed and tolerated.

**Usual adult prescribing limits**

Up to 600 mg a day.

**Usual pediatric dose**

Antipsychotic—

Children up to 6 years of age: Safety and efficacy have not been established.

Children 6 to 12 years of age: Oral, 10 to 25 mg three or four times a day.

**Strength(s) usually available**

U.S.—

100 mg per 5 mL (Rx) [*Taractan* (benzoic acid; edetate disodium; glycerin; hydrochloric acid; lactic acid; magnesium aluminum sil-icate; parabens [methyl and propyl]; polyoxyethylene [8] stearate; silicon emulsion; sodium hydroxide; sorbitol; sucrose; FD&C Red No. 40; FD&C Blue No. 1; FD&C Yellow No. 6; flavors; water)].

Canada—

Not commercially available.

**Packaging and storage**

Store below 40 °C (104 °F), preferably between 15 and 30 °C (59 and 86 °F), unless otherwise specified by manufacturer. Store in a tight, light-resistant container. Protect from freezing.

**Auxiliary labeling**
- Shake well.
- May cause drowsiness.
- Avoid alcoholic beverages.
- Do not spill on skin or clothing.

**Note**

Avoid skin contact with liquid forms of this medication; contact dermatitis has resulted.

### CHLORPROTHIXENE TABLETS USP

**Usual adult and adolescent dose**

Antipsychotic—

Oral, 25 to 50 mg three or four times a day.

Note: Geriatric or debilitated patients usually require a lower initial dose, the dosage being increased gradually as needed and tolerated.

**Usual adult prescribing limits**

Up to 600 mg a day.

**Usual pediatric dose**

Antipsychotic—

Children up to 6 years of age: Safety and efficacy have not been established.

Children 6 to 12 years of age: Oral, 10 to 25 mg three or four times a day.

**Strength(s) usually available**

U.S.—

10 mg (Rx) [*Taractan* (tartrazine)].
25 mg (Rx) [*Taractan* (tartrazine)].
50 mg (Rx) [*Taractan* (tartrazine)].
100 mg (Rx) [*Taractan* (tartrazine)].

Canada—

Not commercially available.

**Packaging and storage**

Store below 40 °C (104 °F), preferably between 15 and 30 °C (59 and 86 °F), unless otherwise specified by manufacturer. Store in a well-closed, light-resistant container.

**Auxiliary labeling**
- May cause drowsiness.
- Avoid alcoholic beverages.

## Parenteral Dosage Forms

### CHLORPROTHIXENE INJECTION USP

**Usual adult and adolescent dose**

Antipsychotic—

Intramuscular, 25 to 50 mg three or four times a day.

Note: Geriatric or debilitated patients and adolescents usually require a lower initial dose, the dosage being increased gradually as needed and tolerated.

**Usual pediatric dose**

Antipsychotic—

Children up to 12 years of age: Safety and efficacy have not been established.

Children 12 years of age and over: See *Usual adult and adolescent dose.*

**Strength(s) usually available**

U.S.—

12.5 mg per mL (Rx) [*Taractan* (parabens [methyl and propyl] 0.2%)].

Canada—

Not commercially available.

**Packaging and storage**

Store below 40 °C (104 °F), preferably between 15 and 30 °C (59 and 86 °F), unless otherwise specified by manufacturer. Protect from light. Protect from freezing.

**Note**

Avoid skin contact with liquid forms of this medication; contact dermatitis has resulted with similar medications.

---

## FLUPENTHIXOL

## Additional Dosing Information

See also *General Dosing Information.*

**For parenteral dosage form only**

Flupenthixol is for intramuscular injection only. It is *not* for intravenous use.

As with all oily injections, aspiration before injection ensures that inadvertent intravascular injection has not occurred.

Administration is by deep intramuscular injection into the gluteal region.

Patients not previously treated with a long-acting depot neuroleptic should be given a test dose of 5 to 20 mg of flupenthixol decanoate. The 5-mg test dose is usually recommended for elderly or debilitated patients, or for patients who may have a predisposition to extrapyramidal effects.

During the 5 to 10 days following the test dose, the patient should be carefully monitored for therapeutic response and appearance of extrapyramidal side effects. Any oral neuroleptic dosage should be reduced in this period.

A single injection may last for two to three weeks. However, when higher doses are used, a single injection may last for four weeks or more. Since higher doses also increase the incidence of adverse effects, dose increases should be made in increments not to exceed 20 mg.

## Oral Dosage Forms

### FLUPENTHIXOL DIHYDROCHLORIDE TABLETS

**Usual adult dose**

Antipsychotic—

Initial: Oral, 1 mg three times a day, the dosage being increased by 1 mg every two to three days as needed and tolerated.

Maintenance: Oral, 3 to 6 mg a day in divided doses, up to 12 mg a day or more.

Note: Geriatric or debilitated patients usually require a lower initial dose, the dosage being increased gradually as needed and tolerated.

**Usual pediatric dose**

Antipsychotic—

Safety and efficacy have not been established.

**Strength(s) usually available**

U.S.—

Not commercially available.

Canada—

0.5 mg (Rx) [*Fluanxol* (sucrose)].

3 mg (Rx) [*Fluanxol* (sucrose)].

**Packaging and storage**

Store below 40 °C (104 °F), preferably between 15 and 30 °C (59 and 86 °F), in a well-closed container, unless otherwise specified by manufacturer. Protect from light.

**Auxiliary labeling**

• May cause drowsiness.

• Avoid alcoholic beverages.

## Parenteral Dosage Forms

### FLUPENTHIXOL DECANOATE INJECTION

**Usual adult dose**

Antipsychotic—

Intramuscular, initially 20 to 40 mg, the dose being repeated in four to ten days. Dosage may be increased in increments of not more than 20 mg.

Note: Most patients require 20 to 40 mg every two to three weeks.

Doses greater than 80 mg are rarely necessary, although higher doses may be used in some patients.

**Usual pediatric dose**

Antipsychotic—

Safety and efficacy have not been established.

**Strength(s) usually available**

U.S.—

Not commercially available.

Canada—

20 mg per mL (Rx) [*Fluanxol Depot*].

100 mg per mL (Rx) [*Fluanxol Depot*].

**Packaging and storage**

Store below 40 °C (104 °F), preferably between 15 and 30 °C (59 and 86 °F), unless otherwise specified by manufacturer. Protect from light. Protect from freezing.

**Additional information**

Vehicle is a thin vegetable oil.

---

## THIOTHIXENE

## Summary of Differences

Precautions: Laboratory value alterations—With physiology/laboratory test values: Serum uric acid may be decreased.

## Oral Dosage Forms

### THIOTHIXENE CAPSULES USP

**Usual adult and adolescent dose**

Antipsychotic—

Oral, initially 2 mg three times a day for milder conditions, or 5 mg two times a day for more severe conditions, the dosage being adjusted gradually as needed and tolerated, usually up to 60 mg a day.

Note: Dosages over 60 mg a day rarely increase the beneficial effect.

Geriatric or debilitated patients usually require a lower initial dose, the dosage being increased gradually as needed and tolerated.

**Usual pediatric dose**

Antipsychotic—

Children up to 12 years of age: Safety and efficacy have not been established.

Children 12 years of age and over: See *Usual adult and adolescent dose.*

**Strength(s) usually available**

U.S.—

1 mg (Rx) [*Navane;* GENERIC].

2 mg (Rx) [*Navane;* GENERIC].

5 mg (Rx) [*Navane;* GENERIC].

10 mg (Rx) [*Navane;* GENERIC].

20 mg (Rx) [*Navane;* GENERIC].

Canada—

2 mg (Rx) [*Navane* (sodium lauryl sulfate; corn starch [gluten]; lactose; magnesium stearate; gelatin; sodium metabisulfite; titanium dioxide; FD&C Red No. 3)].

5 mg (Rx) [*Navane* (sodium lauryl sulfate; corn starch [gluten]; lactose; magnesium stearate; gelatin; sodium metabisulfite; titanium dioxide; FD&C Red No. 3; FD&C Yellow No. 6)].

10 mg (Rx) [*Navane* (sodium lauryl sulfate; corn starch [gluten]; lactose; magnesium stearate; gelatin; sodium metabisulfite; titanium dioxide; FD&C Red No. 3; FD&C Yellow No. 6)].

**Packaging and storage**

Store below 40 °C (104 °F), preferably between 15 and 30 °C (59 and 86 °F), unless otherwise specified by manufacturer. Store in a well-closed, light-resistant container.

**Auxiliary labeling**

• May cause drowsiness.

• Avoid alcoholic beverages.

### THIOTHIXENE HYDROCHLORIDE ORAL SOLUTION USP

Note: The dosing and strengths of Thiothixene Oral Solution are expressed in terms of thiothixene base (not the hydrochloride salt).

**Usual adult and adolescent dose**

Antipsychotic—

Oral, initially, 2 mg (base) three times a day for milder conditions, or 5 mg two times a day for severe conditions, the dosage being adjusted gradually as needed and tolerated, up to 60 mg a day.

Note: Dosages over 60 mg a day rarely increase the beneficial effect.
Geriatric or debilitated patients usually require a lower initial dose, the dosage being increased gradually as needed and tolerated.

**Usual pediatric dose**

Antipsychotic—
Children up to 12 years of age: Safety and efficacy have not been established.
Children 12 years of age and over: See *Usual adult and adolescent dose.*

**Strength(s) usually available**

U.S.—
5 mg (base) per mL (Rx) [*Navane* (alcohol 7%); *Thiothixene HCl Intensol;* GENERIC].

Canada—
Not commercially available.

**Packaging and storage**

Store below 25 °C (77 °F), unless otherwise specified by manufacturer. Store in a tight, light-resistant container. Protect from freezing.

**Auxiliary labeling**

• May cause drowsiness.
• Avoid alcoholic beverages.
• Do not spill on skin or clothing.
• Must be diluted before use.

**Note**

Avoid skin contact with liquid forms of this medication; contact dermatitis has resulted with similar medications.

Each dose must be diluted just before administration by adding it to a cupful of milk, tomato or fruit juice, water, soup, or carbonated beverage.

Provide a specially marked dosage dropper and explain dilution and dosage measurement to patient if medication is self-administered.

## Parenteral Dosage Forms

Note: The dosing and strengths of the dosage forms available are expressed in terms of thiothixene base (not the hydrochloride salt).

### THIOTHIXENE HYDROCHLORIDE INJECTION USP

**Usual adult and adolescent dose**

Antipsychotic—
Intramuscular, 4 mg (base) two to four times a day, the dosage being adjusted gradually as needed and tolerated, but not to exceed a total of 30 mg a day.

Note: Geriatric or debilitated patients usually require a lower initial dose, the dosage being increased gradually as needed and tolerated.

**Usual pediatric dose**

Antipsychotic—
Children up to 12 years of age: Safety and efficacy have not been established.

Children 12 years of age and over: See *Usual adult and adolescent dose.*

**Strength(s) usually available**

U.S.—
2 mg (base) per mL (Rx) [*Navane* (dextrose 5% w/v; benzyl alcohol 0.9% w/v; propyl gallate 0.02% w/v)].

Canada—
Not commercially available.

**Packaging and storage**

Store between 2 and 8 °C (36 and 46 °F), unless otherwise specified by manufacturer. Protect from light. Protect from freezing.

**Note**

Avoid skin contact with liquid forms of this medication; contact dermatitis has resulted from use of similar medications.

### THIOTHIXENE HYDROCHLORIDE FOR INJECTION USP

**Usual adult and adolescent dose**

Antipsychotic—
Intramuscular, 4 mg (base) two to four times a day, the dosage being adjusted gradually as needed and tolerated, but not to exceed a total of 30 mg a day.

Note: Geriatric or debilitated patients usually require a lower initial dose, the dosage being increased gradually as needed and tolerated.

**Usual pediatric dose**

Antipsychotic—
Children up to 12 years of age: Safety and efficacy have not been established.

**Strength(s) usually available**

U.S.—
5 mg (base) per mL (Rx) [*Navane* (mannitol)].

Canada—
Not commercially available.

**Packaging and storage**

Store between 2 and 8 °C (36 and 46 °F), unless otherwise specified by manufacturer. Store in a light-resistant container. Protect from freezing.

**Preparation of dosage form**

Reconstitute thiothixene hydrochloride for injection with 2.2 mL of sterile water for injection.

**Stability**

Reconstituted product may be stored at room temperature for up to 48 hours before discarding.

**Note**

Avoid skin contact with liquid forms of this medication; contact dermatitis has resulted with similar medications.

Revised: 06/17/93

# THROMBOLYTIC AGENTS    Systemic

This monograph includes information on the following: Alteplase, Recombinant; Anistreplase†; Streptokinase; Urokinase.

VA CLASSIFICATION (Primary): BL600

Other commonly used names for [Anistreplase] are anisoylated plasminogen-streptokinase activator complex and APSAC; and for [Alteplase, Recombinant], tissue-type plasminogen activator (recombinant), t-PA, and rt-PA.

Note: For a listing of dosage forms and brand names by country availability, see *Dosage Forms* section(s). For a listing of brand names for the articles in this monograph, refer to the General Index.

†Not commercially available in Canada.

## Category

Thrombolytic.

## Indications

Note: Bracketed information in the *Indications* section refers to uses that are not included in U.S. product labeling.

Note: The selection of thrombolytic therapy must be evaluated individually for each patient based on confirmation of thrombotic disease and assessment of patient condition and history. Some of the indications for thrombolytic therapy are identical to those for heparin or coumarin- or indandione-derivative anticoagulants. However, the goals of thrombolytic therapy and anticoagulant therapy are different. Thrombolytic agents are used primarily to lyse obstructive thrombi and restore blood flow in a recently occluded blood vessel, whereas anticoagulants are used primarily to prevent thrombus formation and extension of existing thrombi. The potential benefit of thrombolytic therapy must be weighed against the risk of bleeding because the risk of hemorrhage may be greater with thrombolytic agents than with heparin or coumarin- or indandione-derivative anticoagulants.

**Accepted**

Thrombosis, coronary arterial, acute (treatment)—Alteplase, anistreplase, streptokinase, and [urokinase][1] are indicated for use via intravenous infusion to lyse acute coronary arterial thrombi associated with evolving transmural myocardial infarction. Streptokinase and urokinase are also indicated for use via injection directly into the affected coronary artery. Various studies with intracoronary arterial injection have reported recanalization rates of 72 to 96%. However, intracoronary arterial administration requires prior identification of the site of the thrombus by coronary angiography. Intravenous infusion does not require coronary angiography and is the preferred route of administration because therapy can be instituted more rapidly and can be initiated in locations that lack facilities for cardiac catheterization.

Thrombolytic therapy may relieve chest pain, reduce the incidence of congestive heart failure, improve left ventricular function, limit cardiac damage (i.e., infarct size), and decrease the risk of early death if coronary arterial blood flow is restored before irreversible cardiac damage occurs. The reperfusion rate is dependent on the interval between the onset of symptoms and the initiation of therapy. Higher reperfusion rates are achieved when thrombolytic therapy is started within 4 hours after symptoms of ischemia first appear. However, reductions in mortality can be achieved if thrombolytic therapy is started up to 24 to 36 hours after the onset of symptoms.

Thrombolytic therapy is not a substitute for other measures that may be required to treat acute myocardial infarction or prevent reinfarction. Restoration of coronary arterial blood flow via thrombolysis does not correct underlying conditions that may promote thrombus formation. Recurrent ischemia, with or without reocclusion or overt reinfarction, may occur following initially successful thrombolysis. The risk of reocclusion may depend on the extent of residual stenosis in the affected vessel. Following successful thrombolytic therapy, long-term anticoagulation, platelet aggregation inhibitor therapy, percutaneous transluminal coronary angioplasty (PTCA), or coronary artery bypass graft (CABG) surgery may be required to provide long-lasting protection against reocclusion. However, initial thrombolytic therapy may permit a revascularization procedure to be performed on a delayed or elective, rather than on an emergency, basis.

Thromboembolism, pulmonary, acute (treatment)—Alteplase[1], streptokinase, and urokinase are indicated, and may be the therapy of choice in selected patients, for the lysis of acute, massive pulmonary emboli producing obstruction or significant filling defects involving 2 or more lobar pulmonary arteries or an equivalent degree of obstruction in other pulmonary vessels. These agents are also indicated for lysing pulmonary emboli accompanied by unstable hemodynamics, i.e., failure to maintain blood pressure without supportive measures. Heparin is recommended for the treatment of subacute or small emboli; however, some clinicians recommend thrombolytic therapy for comparatively small emboli in patients with limited cardiopulmonary reserve caused by significant cardiac or pulmonary disease. Prior to administration of a thrombolytic agent, the diagnosis should be confirmed by objective means such as pulmonary angiography via an upper extremity vein (preferred) or ventilation-perfusion lung scanning.

Thrombosis, deep venous (treatment)—Streptokinase and [urokinase][1] are indicated for the lysis of acute, extensive deep venous thrombi in the popliteal or more proximal vessels. Thrombolytic therapy may be the treatment of choice for deep venous thrombosis in selected patients. [These agents are also used for the lysis of acute, extensive thrombi in the axillary subclavian veins and vena cavae in selected patients.] However, anticoagulants are recommended for treatment of calf-vein thrombi. Prior to administration of a thrombolytic agent, the diagnosis should be confirmed, preferably by ascending venography or by Doppler ultrasound.

Thromboembolism, arterial, acute (treatment) and

Thrombosis, arterial, acute (treatment)—Streptokinase and [urokinase] are indicated for use via intravenous infusion for the lysis of acute arterial thrombi or emboli. [These agents are also administered locally (via a catheter positioned adjacent to or inserted into the substance of the thrombus as shown by arteriogram) to lyse arterial thrombi or emboli.] Studies have shown that thrombolytic therapy alone may be ineffective for treating chronic arterial occlusion. Angioplasty or distal bypass may be required following initial thrombolytic therapy in order to salvage the affected limb.

Cannula, arteriovenous, clearance—Streptokinase and [urokinase][1] are indicated to clear totally or partially occluded arteriovenous cannulae, as an alternative to surgical revision, when acceptable flow cannot be achieved by conventional mechanical measures.

Catheter, intravenous, clearance—[Streptokinase][1] and urokinase are indicated to restore patency to intravenous catheters, including central venous catheters, obstructed by clotted blood or fibrin deposits.

[Thrombolytic agents are also used to treat renal artery thrombosis, retinal blood vessel occlusions, hemolytic uremic syndrome, and impending renal cortical necrosis. However, controlled studies are required to establish the safety and effectiveness of such therapy in these conditions.][1]

**Unaccepted**

Thrombolytic agents should *not* be used to treat superficial thrombophlebitis.

Alteplase has not been sufficiently studied, and is currently not recommended, for treatment of deep venous thrombosis or arterial thrombosis not associated with evolving acute myocardial infarction or for

clearing occluded arteriovenous cannulae or obstructed intravenous catheters.

Alteplase and streptokinase are not recommended for treatment of arterial emboli originating in the left side of the heart (e.g., mitral stenosis accompanied by atrial fibrillation) because of the risk of cerebral embolism.

Thrombolytic agents are not recommended for the treatment of cerebral embolism (thrombotic stroke) pending further study and documentation that the benefits of such therapy outweigh the risk of hemorrhagic infarction.

---

[1]Not included in Canadian product labeling.

## Pharmacology/Pharmacokinetics

**Physicochemical characteristics**

Molecular weight—
    Alteplase: About 68,000 daltons.
    Anistreplase: About 131,000 daltons.
    Streptokinase: About 46,000 daltons.
    Urokinase: About 33,000 daltons.

**Mechanism of action/Effect**

Thrombolytic agents activate the endogenous fibrinolytic system by cleaving the arginine$_{560}$–valine$_{561}$ bond in plasminogen to produce plasmin, an enzyme that degrades fibrin clots, fibrinogen, and other plasma proteins, including the procoagulant factors V and VIII. Alteplase and urokinase cleave the peptide bond directly. Anistreplase and streptokinase act indirectly; they combine with plasminogen to form streptokinase-plasminogen complexes that are converted to streptokinase-plasmin complexes. These activator complexes, rather than streptokinase itself, convert residual plasminogen to plasmin.

Conversion of plasminogen to plasmin occurs within the thrombus or embolus as well as on its surface and in circulating blood. Thrombolytic agents lyse fibrin deposits wherever they exist and can be reached by the plasmin generated; therefore, thrombolytic agents also promote lysis of fibrin deposits responsible for hemostasis.

Alteplase is more clot-selective than the other thrombolytic agents, binding more readily to the fibrin-plasminogen complex within a clot than to circulating (free) plasminogen. However, systemic fibrinolysis does occur with usual therapeutic doses.

**Other actions/effects**

Fibrinogenolysis and fibrinolysis induced by thrombolytic agents increase the concentration of fibrinogen- and fibrin-degradation products (FDP/fdp) in the blood. The FDP/fdp exert an anticoagulant effect, probably by impairing fibrin polymerization and possibly by decreasing thrombin generation and/or interfering with platelet function. Alteplase usually reduces circulating fibrinogen concentration and increases FDP/fdp concentrations to a lesser extent than does streptokinase, but to about the same extent that urokinase does. However, studies have not shown a significantly lower incidence of bleeding with alteplase than has been reported with the other thrombolytic agents, probably because factors other than the concentrations of fibrinogen and/or FDP/fdp also significantly influence the risk of bleeding (See *Side/Adverse Effects*). Specifically, the risk of bleeding complications associated with thrombolytic therapy may be more dependent on the presence of vascular injury than on the extent of systemic fibrinolysis induced by a specific agent.

Anistreplase has potent proteolytic activity in the systemic circulation. In addition to decreasing plasma concentrations of fibrinogen, the medication lowers plasma concentrations of plasminogen procoagulant factors V and VIII, and the fibrinolysis inhibitor alpha-2-antiplasmin.

Anistreplase, streptokinase, and urokinase have also been reported to decrease plasma viscosity and erythrocyte aggregation, probably as a result of reduced fibrinogen concentration.

Streptokinase and the streptokinase component of anistreplase are antigenic and induce the formation of antibodies. Elevation of the antistreptokinase antibody titer usually occurs about 5 to 7 days following administration, reaches a peak after 2 to 3 weeks, and may persist for 1 year or longer. The antibodies may cause resistance to subsequent streptokinase or anistreplase therapy, and possibly an increased risk of anaphylaxis or other severe allergic reactions.

**Biotransformation**

Alteplase—Hepatic; rapid.
Urokinase—Hepatic; rapid.

**Half-life**

Alteplase—
    Distribution: Approximately 4 minutes.
    Elimination: Approximately 35 minutes.

Anistreplase—
    The half-life of anistreplase's fibrinolytic activity is 70 to 120 minutes (average about 90 minutes). The deacylation half-life of the complex is about 105 to 120 minutes. The plasma clearance and duration of fibrinolytic activity of the medication are probably controlled primarily by its deacylation rate.
Streptokinase—
    Following intravenous administration of 1.5 million International Units (IU) over a 1-hour period: the half-life of the activator complexes (streptokinase-plasminogen and/or streptokinase-plasmin) is 23 minutes.
Urokinase—
    Up to 20 minutes. The half-life may be prolonged in patients with hepatic function impairment.

**Time to peak effect**
Reperfusion of the myocardium generally occurs 20 minutes to 2 hours (average 45 minutes) following initiation of intravenous therapy.

**Duration of action**
Thrombolysis may continue for approximately 4 hours following administration of alteplase, streptokinase, or urokinase; the hyperfibrinolytic effect disappears within a few hours following discontinuation of administration. Following administration of anistreplase, thrombolysis may continue for approximately 6 hours and a systemic hyperfibrinolytic state, as demonstrated by euglobulin clot lysis time determinations, may persist for more than 2 days. For all thrombolytic agents, the prothrombin time may rarely be prolonged for 12 to 24 hours following cessation of therapy because of the decreased plasma concentration of fibrinogen, decreased plasma concentration of factor V and possibly other coagulant factors, and/or the anticoagulant effects of FDP/fdp. However, prolonged, high FDP/fdp concentrations may potentiate bleeding for a longer period of time, especially after administration of non–clot-selective thrombolytic agents.

**Elimination**
Alteplase—Renal; approximately 80% of a dose is excreted in the urine, as metabolites, within 18 hours.
Urokinase—Small quantities are eliminated via the renal and biliary routes.

# Precautions to Consider

**Cross-sensitivity and/or related problems**
Patients allergic to streptokinase will be allergic to anistreplase also, and vice versa.

**Carcinogenicity**
*Alteplase, anistreplase,* and *urokinase*—Long-term studies to determine whether alteplase, anistreplase, and urokinase have carcinogenic potential have not been done.

**Mutagenicity**
*Alteplase*—No mutagenicity was demonstrated in the Ames test or in chromosomal aberration assays in human lymphocytes.
*Anistreplase*—No mutagenicity was demonstrated in chromosomal aberration assays in human lymphocytes.

**Pregnancy/Reproduction**
Fertility—*Alteplase*: Studies have not been done in animals.
*Anistreplase*: Studies have not been done in humans.
Studies have not been done in animals.
*Urokinase*: Studies in mice and rats have not shown that urokinase causes impaired fertility.

Pregnancy—It has been suggested that administration of a thrombolytic agent during the first 18 weeks of pregnancy may increase the risk of premature separation of the placenta because fetal attachments to the uterus during this time are composed primarily of fibrin. However, this problem has not been reported following administration of streptokinase or urokinase to patients during the first 2 trimesters of pregnancy.
*Alteplase and anistreplase*—
    Studies have not been done in humans.
    Studies have not been done in animals.

    FDA Pregnancy Category C.
*Streptokinase*—
    Streptokinase apparently crosses the human placenta minimally if at all. However, antibodies to streptokinase do cross the placenta. Studies in pregnant women (treated mostly during the second and third trimesters) have not shown evidence of abnormalities or induction of fibrinolysis in the fetus.
    Studies have not been done in animals.

    FDA Pregnancy Category C.

*Urokinase*—
    Adequate and well-controlled studies have not been done in humans.
    Studies in mice and rats have not shown that urokinase causes fetal harm when administered in doses up to 1000 times the human dose.

    FDA Pregnancy Category B.
Postpartum—Thrombolytic agents should be administered with great caution during the first 10 days postpartum because of the increased risk of hemorrhage.

**Breast-feeding**
It is not known whether thrombolytic agents are distributed into breast milk. However, problems in humans have not been documented.

**Pediatrics**
Appropriate studies performed to date have not demonstrated pediatrics-specific problems that would limit the usefulness of thrombolytic agents in children.

**Geriatrics**
Geriatric patients generally have a poorer prognosis than younger adults following an acute myocardial infarction. They may also be more likely than younger adults to have pre-existing conditions that tend to increase the risk of intracranial bleeding or other hemorrhagic complications. Because the risks of thrombolytic therapy, as well as its potential benefits, are increased in older patients, careful patient selection and monitoring are recommended.

**Drug interactions and/or related problems**
The following drug interactions and/or related problems have been selected on the basis of their potential clinical significance (possible mechanism in parentheses where appropriate)—not necessarily inclusive (» = major clinical significance):

Note: Combinations containing any of the following medications, depending on the amount present, may also interact with this medication.

    In addition to the interactions listed below, the possibility should be considered that multiple effects leading to further impairment of blood clotting and/or increased risk of hemorrhage may occur if a thrombolytic agent is administered to a patient receiving any medication having a significant potential for causing hypoprothrombinemia, thrombocytopenia, or gastrointestinal ulceration or hemorrhage.

» Anticoagulants, coumarin- or indandione-derivative or
» Enoxaparin or
» Heparin
    (concurrent use with antithrombotic or thrombolytic agents increases the risk of hemorrhage; however, heparin is often administered concurrently with intravenous thrombolytic therapy for treatment of acute coronary arterial occlusion or with low doses of thrombolytic agents given intra-arterially; also, thrombolytic therapy may be administered following initial anticoagulant therapy)

    (anticoagulants are recommended to prevent additional thrombus formation following thrombolytic therapy for most indications; however, following intravenous thrombolytic therapy for acute coronary arterial occlusion, the need for anticoagulant administration should be determined on an individual basis; if an anticoagulant is administered under these circumstances, careful monitoring of the patient is recommended because studies have shown that heparin, when administered after intravenous streptokinase for this indication, increases the risk of hemorrhage)

» Antifibrinolytic agents, such as:
    Aminocaproic acid
    Aprotinin
    Tranexamic acid
    (the actions of antifibrinolytic agents and of thrombolytic agents are mutually antagonistic; although antifibrinolytic agents may be effective in treating severe hemorrhage caused by thrombolytic agents, controlled studies to verify their efficacy and safety have not been done)

    Antihypertensive agents or
    Other hypotension-producing medications
    (the risk of severe hypotension may be increased, especially when streptokinase is administered rapidly for treatment of coronary arterial occlusion)

» Cefamandole or
» Cefoperazone or
» Cefotetan or
» Plicamycin or
» Valproic acid
  (these medications may cause hypoprothrombinemia; in addition, plicamycin or valproic acid may inhibit platelet aggregation; concurrent use with a thrombolytic agent may increase the risk of severe hemorrhage and is not recommended)

Corticosteroids, glucocorticoids or
Corticotropin, chronic therapeutic use or
Ethacrynic acid or
Salicylates, nonacetylated
  (gastrointestinal ulceration or hemorrhage may occur during therapy with these medications and cause increased risk of severe hemorrhage in patients receiving thrombolytic therapy)

» Nonsteroidal anti-inflammatory drugs (NSAIDs), especially:
  Aspirin
  Indomethacin
  Phenylbutazone or
» Other platelet aggregation inhibitors (See *Appendix II*), especially:
  Sulfinpyrazone
  Ticlopidine
  (concurrent use of a platelet aggregation inhibitor and a thrombolytic agent may increase the risk of bleeding and is generally not recommended [except when aspirin therapy for acute myocardial infarction is initiated concurrently with thrombolytic therapy])
  (initiation of aspirin therapy [160 mg per day] before or during intravenous administration of alteplase, anistreplase, or streptokinase for treatment of acute coronary arterial occlusion may reduce significantly the risk of reocclusion, reinfarction, stroke, and death without increasing the risk of adverse effects [as compared to the thrombolytic agent or aspirin alone]; however, larger doses of aspirin have been shown to increase the risk of bleeding in patients receiving thrombolytic agents for other indications; the possibility of hemorrhage should be considered and the patient carefully monitored)
  (the potential occurrence of gastrointestinal ulceration and/or hemorrhage during therapy with NSAIDs [including analgesic or antirheumatic doses of aspirin] or sulfinpyrazone may also cause increased risk to patients receiving thrombolytic therapy)

Thiotepa
  (urokinase may increase the efficacy of thiotepa in the treatment of bladder cancer by acting as a plasminogen activator and increasing the amount of thiotepa in tumor tissue)

### Laboratory value alterations
The following have been selected on the basis of their potential clinical significance (possible effect in parentheses where appropriate)—not necessarily inclusive (» = major clinical significance):

With diagnostic test results
  Coagulation tests and
  Tests for systemic fibrinolysis
  (the fibrinolytic activity of thrombolytic agents persists *in vitro*; unless the patient is extremely resistant to thrombolytic therapy, degradation of fibrinogen in blood samples will lead to unreliable test results [when specific measurements of fibrinogen, rather than a general indication that fibrinolysis is occurring, are required]; the addition of a fibrinolysis inhibitor, e.g., aprotinin [150 to 200 Kallikrein Inhibitor Units per mL of blood] or aminocaproic acid may reduce this effect)

With physiology/laboratory test values
  Activated partial thromboplastin time (APTT) and
  Prothrombin time (PT) and
  Thrombin time (TT)
  (values will be increased unless the patient is extremely resistant to thrombolytic therapy)

  Alpha-2-antiplasmin activity and
  Factor V activity and
  Factor VIII activity and
  Fibrinogen activity and
  Plasminogen activity
  (will be decreased unless the patient is extremely resistant to thrombolytic therapy; significant recovery of fibrinogen activity may occur within 18 to 36 hours after discontinuation of thrombolytic therapy, but return of fibrinogen activity to pretreatment values may require up to 48 hours after discontinuation of thrombolytic therapy; recovery of plasminogen activity may also require more than 30 hours)

Blood pressure
  (may be decreased, especially when a thrombolytic agent is administered rapidly for treatment of acute coronary arterial occlusion; a decrease in blood pressure [not secondary to anaphylaxis or bleeding], which may be severe, has also been reported in about 10% of anistreplase-treated patients)

Fibrinogen- and fibrin-degradation products (FDP/fdp) concentrations
  (will be increased unless the patient is extremely resistant to thrombolytic therapy; return to pretreatment values may require up to 48 hours after discontinuation of thrombolytic therapy)

Hematocrit values and
Hemoglobin concentrations
  (moderate reduction not related to clinical bleeding has been reported in 20% of patients receiving thrombolytic therapy)

### Medical considerations/Contraindications
The medical considerations/contraindications included here have been selected on the basis of their potential clinical significance (reasons given in parentheses where appropriate)—not necessarily inclusive (» = major clinical significance).

*Except under special circumstances, this medication should not be used when the following medical problems exist:*
*For all thrombolytic agents*
» Aneurysm, dissecting and/or intracranial, confirmed or suspected or
» Arteriovenous malformation or
» Bleeding, active or
» Brain tumor, primary, or neoplasm metastatic to the central nervous system (CNS) from other primary sites or
» Cerebrovascular accident, or history of or
» Neurosurgery, intracranial or intraspinal, within past 2 months or
» Surgery, thoracic, recent or
» Trauma to the CNS, recent
  (increased risk of uncontrollable hemorrhage)
» Hypertension, severe uncontrolled, i.e., ≥200 mm Hg systolic and/or ≥120 mm Hg diastolic
  (increased risk of cerebral hemorrhage)

*For anistreplase and streptokinase (in addition to medical problems listed above)*
» Anaphylaxis or other severe allergic reaction to streptokinase or anistreplase, history of
  (increased risk of anaphylaxis)

*Risk-benefit should be considered when the following medical problems exist:*
*For all thrombolytic agents*
  Allergic reaction, mild, to the thrombolytic agent considered for use, history of
  Any condition in which the risk of bleeding or hemorrhage is present or would be difficult to control because of its location, such as:
  Cardiopulmonary resuscitation with possibility of internal injury, recent
  Cerebrovascular disease
» Childbirth within past 10 days
» Coagulation defects, uncontrolled, or other hemostatic defects, including those secondary to severe hepatic or renal disease
» Endocarditis, bacterial, subacute
» Gastrointestinal bleeding, severe, within past 10 days
  Gastrointestinal lesion or ulcer, active or history of
  Genitourinary bleeding within past 10 days
  Hemorrhagic retinopathy, diabetic or other hemorrhagic ophthalmic conditions
  Hepatic function impairment, severe
  Hypertension, moderate, not optimally controlled, i.e., 180 to 200 mm Hg systolic and/or 110 to 120 mm Hg diastolic
  Invasive procedure, such as lumbar puncture, paracentesis, or thoracentesis, recent
  Knitted dacron graft
» Neurosurgical procedure more than 2 months previously
» Organ biopsy within past 10 days
  Pregnancy
» Puncture of noncompressible blood vessel within past 10 days
» Surgery, major, other than neurosurgery or thoracic surgery, within past 10 days
  Trauma, minor, recent, other than to the CNS
» Trauma, severe, recent, other than to the CNS
  Tuberculosis, active, with cavitation of recent onset
  Infection at or near site of thrombus, obstructed intravenous catheter, or occluded arteriovenous cannula
  (risk of spreading the infection into and via the circulation)

» Mitral stenosis with atrial fibrillation or other indications of probable left heart thrombus

(risk of new embolic phenomena including those to cerebral vessels)

Pericarditis, acute

(risk of hemopericardium, which may lead to cardiac tamponade)

*For anistreplase and streptokinase (in addition to medical problems listed above)*

» Anistreplase or streptokinase therapy within past 5 days to 1 year or Streptococcal infection, recent

(antistreptococcal antibodies are likely to be present in the circulation; these antibodies may cause a temporary resistance to the therapeutic effects of anistreplase or streptokinase and/or an increased risk of severe allergic reactions to the medication; although resistance may be overcome by increasing the dosage, use of an alternate thrombolytic agent [alteplase or urokinase] is advisable if thrombolytic therapy is needed within 1 year after anistreplase or streptokinase therapy or streptococcal infection)

**Patient monitoring**

The following may be especially important in patient monitoring (other tests may be warranted in some patients, depending on condition; » = major clinical significance):

*Prior to initiation of therapy*

Note: Initiation of therapy for acute coronary arterial occlusion must **not** be delayed until the results of the tests recommended below are available. However, blood may be drawn prior to initiation of therapy so that appropriate tests can be performed to determine the hemostatic status of the patient, especially if a potential bleeding problem exists or is suspected, and/or to establish baseline values.

» Coagulation tests, such as:

Activated partial thromboplastin time (APTT)
Fibrin/fibrinogen degradation product (FDP/fdp) titer
Fibrinogen concentration
Prothrombin time (PT)
Thrombin time (TT) and

» Hematocrit values and

» Hemoglobin concentrations and

» Platelet count

(recommended prior to initiation of therapy to determine the hemostatic status of the patient and/or to establish baseline values so that the presence of fibrinolysis can be confirmed during therapy; heparin therapy should be discontinued before thrombolytic therapy is instituted unless the heparin is being given in conjunction with urokinase for intracoronary administration; also the APTT or TT should be less than 2 times the control value before thrombolytic therapy is instituted)

» Electrocardiogram (ECG)

(recommended when acute coronary arterial thrombosis is suspected, to confirm diagnosis and to aid in selecting patients in whom thrombolytic therapy is likely to be most beneficial)

*During and/or following therapy*

Coagulation tests, such as APTT, PT, or TT and/or
Tests of fibrinolytic activity, such as fibrinogen concentration, FDP/fdp titer, reptilase clotting time, and/or whole blood euglobulin lysis time

(recommended 3 to 4 hours following initiation of intravenous therapy for indications other than acute coronary arterial thrombosis; these tests may be repeated every 12 hours for the duration of therapy, if necessary, to determine that a fibrinolytic state exists; however, such tests do not reliably predict either efficacy of medication or risk of bleeding and are not currently recommended for determining maintenance dosage; a TT value equal to or greater than 1.5 times the control value in seconds, or a decrease of fibrinogen concentration to 50% or less of the control value [with alteplase or anistreplase, a reduction to 75% of the control value may be sufficient], indicates that fibrinolysis is occurring)

Note: Confirmation of fibrinolysis does **not** require that all of the tests listed above be used for each patient. The selection of a particular test for monitoring thrombolytic therapy depends upon physician preference and available laboratory facilities.

Because heparin also prolongs APTT, PT, and TT, the results of these determinations may be misleading if heparin has been or is being administered; tests that more directly measure fibrinolytic activity may be more reliable.

Computerized tomography and/or
Impedance plethysmography and/or
Quantitative Doppler effect determination and/or
Visualization of affected vessel via angiography or venography

(may be useful in assessing restoration of blood flow; also, may aid in determining optimum duration of therapy; however, repeated venograms are not recommended)

Coronary angiography and/or
Myocardial scanning, radionuclide

(may be useful for monitoring effectiveness of therapy for coronary arterial thrombosis in evolving transmural myocardial infarction; coronary angiography and myocardial scanning may also be useful for assessing the patency of the coronary vasculature and for determining whether further treatment to prevent reocclusion is needed; however, coronary angiography increases the risk of adverse effects, including severe bleeding, when performed within several days after thrombolytic therapy; it is recommended that the procedure be performed only when necessary [as determined by signs and symptoms of persistent ischemia], preferably after a delay of 7 to 10 days following thrombolytic therapy)

Creatine kinase activity or other cardiac enzyme determination

(may be useful for monitoring effectiveness of therapy for acute coronary arterial thrombosis)

» Electrocardiogram (ECG)

(monitoring during and following administration for treatment of acute coronary arterial thrombosis is recommended to detect reperfusion atrial or ventricular arrhythmias; also, may be useful as a means of determining effectiveness of treatment because reversal of some abnormalities may occur with recanalization)

Hematocrit values

(monitoring recommended to detect possible blood loss during and following thrombolytic therapy)

» Mental status and

» Neurologic status

(monitoring recommended because altered sensorium or neurologic changes may be indicative of intracranial bleeding)

Stool tests for occult blood loss and
Urine tests for hematuria

(recommended periodically during therapy)

» Vital signs, such as blood pressure, pulse, respiratory rate, and temperature

(continuous monitoring recommended during therapy for acute coronary arterial occlusion to detect adverse effects such as bradycardia, hypotension, and allergic reactions; a reduction in the infusion rate is usually sufficient to correct hypotension)

(monitoring recommended at least every 4 hours during therapy for other indications; however, a lower extremity should **not** be used for blood pressure determinations when there is a risk of dislodging deep vein thrombi that may be present)

## Side/Adverse Effects

Note: Rarely, thrombolysis causes clot fragmentation with migration of the fragments resulting in additional embolic complications. Patients should be monitored for new embolic phenomena.

Bleeding, the most common side effect encountered during thrombolytic therapy, occurs most frequently at invaded sites (e.g., sites of arterial punctures, venous cutdowns, recent surgery) because thrombolytic agents promote lysis of the fibrin deposits that are needed to maintain hemostasis at these sites. The risk of bleeding at invaded sites is not reduced by administration of a relatively clot-selective agent such as alteplase. Studies comparing alteplase with streptokinase have shown a similar incidence of internal bleeding with both agents. However, most patients in these studies also received heparin or other potentially hemorrhagic medications concurrently with and/or immediately following the thrombolytic agent. Therefore, the frequency of hemorrhage attributable solely to the thrombolytic agent has not been determined. In some patients, bleeding may be severe enough to result in anemia or shock.

Chest pain or cardiac arrhythmias may occur during or following thrombolytic therapy for acute coronary arterial thrombosis. These are not direct effects of the medication. Chest pain may indicate treatment failure or reocclusion. Cardiac arrhythmias may be associated with the myocardial infarction itself, or may be induced by sudden reperfusion. Specific arrhythmias that have been reported include sinus bradycardia, accelerated idioventricular rhythm, ventricular premature depolarizations, ventricular tachycardia, second- and third-degree atrioventricular block, atrial fibrillation, and (especially in patients with coronary instrumentation) ventricular fibrillation. Hypotension may occur in association with reperfusion bradyarrhythmias.

Nausea and vomiting have also been reported during thrombolytic therapy. However, a causal relationship to the medication has not been established because these symptoms occur frequently during acute myocardial infarction.

The lys-plasminogen used in manufacturing anistreplase is obtained from human plasma. To reduce the risk of the patient's contracting viral infections that may be transmitted via human blood–derived products, the material is tested for viral antigens or particles and heat-treated to inactivate viral particles. Hepatitis has not been reported to date.

The following effects have been selected on the basis of their potential clinical significance (possible signs and symptoms in parentheses where appropriate)—not necessarily inclusive:

## Those indicating need for medical attention
Incidence more frequent
> ***Bleeding or oozing from cuts, invaded or disturbed sites, wounds, or gums; decreased blood pressure, not secondary to bleeding or to streptokinase-induced anaphylaxis***—may be severe, especially when a thrombolytic agent is given rapidly and/or when other medications having hypotensive actions, such as vasodilators or morphine, are used concurrently

Incidence more frequent with anistreplase and streptokinase; less frequent with urokinase
> ***Fever***

> Note: Elevations of body temperature by about 1.5 °F occur in up to 33%, and body temperature as high as 104 °F has been reported in about 3.5%, of patients receiving streptokinase. Approximately 2 to 3% of patients receiving urokinase develop a febrile reaction to the medication. *Fever* has also been reported with alteplase, but a causal relationship has not been established.

Incidence less frequent or rare
> ***Allergic reaction*** (flushing or redness of skin; mild headache; mild muscle pain; nausea; skin rash, hives, or itching; troubled breathing or wheezing)—less frequent with streptokinase and rare with alteplase or urokinase; ***bleeding into subcutaneous tissues*** (bruising); ***cholesterol embolism***—with alteplase, anistreplase, and streptokinase; ***internal bleeding*** (abdominal pain or swelling; back pain or backaches; bloody urine; bloody or black, tarry stools; constipation caused by hemorrhage-induced paralytic ileus or intestinal obstruction; coughing up blood; dizziness; headaches, sudden, severe, and/or continuing; joint pain, stiffness, or swelling; muscle pain or stiffness, severe or continuing; nosebleeds; unexpected or unusually heavy bleeding from vagina; vomiting of blood or material that looks like coffee grounds); ***stroke, hemorrhagic or thromboembolic*** (confusion; double vision; impairment of speech; weakness in arms or legs)—more frequent with alteplase

> Note: Individual symptoms of *internal bleeding* depend on the site of bleeding and have not necessarily been reported with all of the thrombolytic agents; internal bleeding has been reported following intracoronary arterial administration as well as following intravenous administration; with alteplase, the incidences of gastrointestinal, genitourinary, and retroperitoneal bleeding are 5%, 4%, and <1%, respectively; the incidence of intracranial hemorrhage with alteplase is 0.4% with total doses of 100 mg or 1 to 1.4 mg per kg of body weight (mg/kg) and 1.3% with a total dose of 150 mg.

Incidence rare—for anistreplase, streptokinase, and urokinase
> ***Allergic reaction, severe, or anaphylaxis*** (changes in facial skin color; fast or irregular breathing; large, hive-like swellings on eyelids, face, mouth, lips, or tongue; puffiness or swelling of the eyelids or around the eyes; shortness of breath, troubled breathing, tightness in chest, and/or wheezing; skin rash, hives, and/or itching)—may also include anaphylactic shock with sudden, severe decrease in blood pressure

> Note: An *anaphylactic reaction* has been reported in a patient following a second course of streptokinase given 1 month after the first course for clearance of an occluded arteriovenous shunt. Therefore, the probability of systemic absorption of streptokinase following use for this purpose must be considered.

### Those not indicating need for medical attention
Incidence rare
> ***Skin lesions***—with streptokinase

## Patient Consultation

As an aid to patient consultation, refer to *Advice for the Patient, Thrombolytic Agents (Systemic)*.

In providing consultation, consider emphasizing the following selected information (»= major clinical significance):

**Before receiving this medication**
» Conditions affecting use, especially:
> Allergic reaction to the thrombolytic agent considered for use, history of, especially a severe allergic reaction to anistreplase or streptokinase
> Use in the elderly—Increased risk of hemorrhage
> Other medications, especially anticoagulants, antifibrinolytic agents, enoxaparin, heparin, hypoprothrombinemia-inducing cephalosporins, nonsteroidal anti-inflammatory drugs, platelet aggregation inhibitors, plicamycin, and valproic acid
> Other medical problems, especially conditions leading to an increased risk of uncontrollable or cerebral hemorrhage, and, for anistreplase and streptokinase, prior treatment with either agent (within past 12 months)

**Proper use of this medication**
» Proper dosing

**Precautions after receiving this medication**
» Importance of compliance with strict bed rest or other measures to minimize bleeding

**Side/adverse effects**
> Signs of potential side effects, especially bleeding or oozing from cuts, invaded or disturbed sites, wounds, or gums; decreased blood pressure, not secondary to bleeding or streptokinase-induced anaphylaxis; fever; allergic reaction; bleeding into subcutaneous tissues; cholesterol embolism; internal bleeding; hemorrhagic or thromboembolic stroke; and severe allergic reaction or anaphylaxis

## General Dosing Information

The activity and doses of alteplase are expressed in milligrams, the activity and doses of anistreplase are expressed in units, and the activity and doses of streptokinase and urokinase are expressed in international units (IU). However, in some countries, individual products may be labeled in other units. Different tests and standards are used to determine activity of each thrombolytic agent.

Thrombolytic therapy for indications other than acute coronary arterial thrombosis and catheter clearance should be performed only in a hospital with the facilities and trained personnel necessary for performance of the recommended diagnostic and monitoring techniques.

Thrombolytic therapy should be instituted as soon as possible following the onset of clinical symptoms because resistance to lysis increases with the age of the thrombus. For coronary arterial thrombosis or occlusion in evolving transmural myocardial infarction, rapid initiation of treatment is critical. However, patients receiving treatment within 6 to 12 hours following the onset of symptoms may also benefit from thrombolytic therapy. In patients who experience intermittent symptoms resulting from alternating coronary artery occlusion and spontaneous recanalization, thrombolytic therapy may limit the extent of myocardial damage even if given late. In addition, late thrombolytic therapy may limit myocardial damage by providing collateral flow in the event of subsequent coronary artery occlusion. For other indications, treatment should preferably be started within:
- Pulmonary embolism—5 to 7 days.
- Deep venous thrombosis—3 to 4 days, although treatment started later may be somewhat successful.
- Arterial thrombosis or thromboembolism (noncoronary)—3 days, although treatment started later may be successful.

Factors that may affect the success of thrombolytic therapy include the age, size, and location of the thrombus, and the extent of pretreatment perfusion, with most failures occurring when no blood is flowing past the thrombus (grade 0 flow as defined in the Thrombolysis in Myocardial Infarction [TIMI] trials). Factors that decrease the efficiency or activation potential of the fibrinolytic system include extremes in body temperature, elevated concentration of endogenous inhibitors, the presence of abnormal proteins or dysfunctional components of the fibrinolytic system, and the presence of high titers of antistreptokinase antibodies.

Prior to initiation of intravenous thrombolytic therapy for indications other than acute coronary arterial thrombosis, heparin (if being given) should be discontinued and the patient's thrombin time (TT) or activated partial thromboplastin time (APTT) should be less than twice the control value.

Thrombolytic agents should be administered via a constant infusion pump. A separate intravenous line, which should be established prior to initiation of thrombolytic therapy to reduce the need for venipuncture during treatment, should be used for administration of other medications, if required.

To minimize the risk of bleeding during thrombolytic therapy, the patient should be kept on strict bed rest and pressure dressings applied to recently invaded sites. *Nonessential handling or moving of the patient, invasive procedures (biopsy, etc.), and intramuscular injections must be avoided. Only essential procedures or diagnostic tests should be performed.* Cutdowns should be performed only if unavoidable. Venipunctures should be performed as carefully and infrequently as possible, preferably only in arm vessels, using a 23-gauge (or smaller) needle. If an arterial puncture is necessary, an upper extremity distal vessel should be used. Manual pressure should be applied for 30 minutes after the arterial puncture, followed by application of a pressure dressing. The puncture site should be checked frequently for signs of bleeding. Profuse bleeding may persist for a prolonged period of time.

*Therapy should be discontinued immediately if bleeding not controllable by local pressure occurs.* Some clinicians recommend that thrombolytic therapy be discontinued permanently if such bleeding occurs. However, other clinicians suggest that reinstitution of therapy using one-half the original maintenance dose may be considered if the results of blood coagulation tests performed shortly after the bleeding episode show values higher than the normal therapeutic range. These clinicians further suggest that therapy not be reinstituted until the results of blood coagulation tests have returned to within the normal therapeutic range, and, if bleeding recurs, that therapy be discontinued permanently.

Anticoagulation with heparin (preferably by continuous intravenous infusion) followed, if necessary, by a coumarin or indandione derivative is recommended following thrombolytic therapy for deep venous thrombosis or pulmonary embolism to prevent further thrombus formation. It is usually recommended that heparin be administered only after the patient's TT or APTT returns to less than twice the normal control value. This usually occurs within 2 hours after cessation of thrombolytic therapy. However, heparin therapy may be instituted earlier, depending on clinical circumstances. A loading dose of heparin is generally not recommended, but may be required in some circumstances, especially if the TT or APTT has fallen to substantially less than twice the control value. Administration of a coumarin- or indandione-derivative anticoagulant, if necessary, should be started at least 5 days prior to discontinuation of heparin.

Angioplasty, coronary bypass surgery, or another revascularization procedure may be necessary to provide long-lasting protection against reocclusion, especially if extensive stenosis (>80%) persists in the affected artery. Performance of these procedures within several days after thrombolytic therapy increases the risk of adverse effects, including hemorrhage, and should therefore be delayed if possible. If such a procedure cannot be postponed, replacement of fibrinogen to 50% of normal activity by administration of cryoprecipitate may reduce the risk of bleeding complications. If systemic fibrinolysis induced by the thrombolytic agent has not yet ceased, administration of an antifibrinolytic agent (e.g., aminocaproic acid, tranexamic acid) will be necessary to prevent immediate lysis of the infused fibrinogen, but the risks of administering an antifibrinolytic agent to a patient undergoing a revascularization procedure must be carefully considered.

**For treatment of acute coronary arterial thrombosis**
A suitable antiarrhythmic agent may be administered prior to or concurrently with the thrombolytic agent to prevent reperfusion arrhythmias.

It has been shown that aspirin, administered in conjunction with streptokinase for treatment of coronary arterial thrombosis, significantly decreases the occurrence of reocclusion, reinfarction, stroke, and death, as compared to aspirin or streptokinase administered alone. Although the benefit of aspirin administered with alteplase or anistreplase has not been studied, it is widely held that the combination of aspirin and any thrombolytic agent is likely to have benefit similar to that of aspirin and streptokinase. It is therefore recommended that at least 160 mg of aspirin be administered as soon as possible after myocardial infarction is suspected. It is also recommended that the aspirin be chewed so that it reaches the bloodstream rapidly.

Heparin (in dosage sufficient to prolong the APTT to 1.5 to 2 times the control value) has been administered in conjunction with thrombolytic therapy for acute coronary arterial occlusion. However, recent studies have found that the addition of heparin to a regimen of aspirin and thrombolysis does not significantly improve survival, but does increase the risk of major bleeding and cerebral hemorrhage. In addition, there are little data to show that heparin contributes to sustained coronary artery patency when administered with aspirin and streptokinase or with aspirin and anistreplase. When administered with aspirin and alteplase, intravenous heparin seems to improve coronary artery patency slightly, but the benefit must be weighed against the risk of hemorrhage associated with the use of intravenous heparin.

**For arteriovenous cannula occlusion clearance**
First, the cannula should be cleared by careful syringe technique, using heparinized saline solution. If this procedure is unsuccessful, a thrombolytic agent may be used after the effects of prior anticoagulation have been allowed to diminish. After the thrombolytic agent has been instilled in the cannula, the affected cannula limb (s) should be clamped for 2 hours and the patient closely observed for possible adverse effects. After treatment, the contents of the affected cannula limb (s) should be aspirated, and the cannula flushed with saline solution and reconnected.

**For intravenous catheter obstruction clearance**
The manufacturer's product information for urokinase should be consulted for a complete description of the recommended procedure.

Excessive pressure should be avoided when instilling a thrombolytic agent into the catheter in order to avoid rupture of the catheter or expulsion of the clot into the circulation.

To prevent air from entering an open central venous catheter, the patient should be instructed to exhale and hold his or her breath any time the catheter is not connected to intravenous tubing or to a syringe.

Intravenous catheters may be obstructed by substances not responsive to thrombolysis (i.e., substances other than clotted blood or fibrin). The possibility that such a precipitate may be forced into the circulation must be considered.

**For treatment of adverse effects**
Recommended treatment includes
• For minor bleeding—Applying local measures, such as pressure at the site of bleeding. Although efficacy has not been proved, topical application of an antifibrinolytic agent such as aminocaproic acid may help to stop stubborn minor bleeding. Thrombolytic therapy need not be discontinued unless such measures are unsuccessful and it is determined that the risk to the patient outweighs the benefit of continuing treatment.
• For uncontrollable or internal bleeding—Discontinuing thrombolytic therapy. If necessary, replacement of lost blood and reversal of the bleeding tendency can be accomplished by administration of fresh whole blood, packed red blood cells, cryoprecipitate or fresh frozen plasma, platelets, and/or desmopressin. Plasma volume expanders may be administered; however, dextrans should **not** be used because of their platelet aggregation–inhibiting activity. Heparin, if being given, should be discontinued and consideration given to administration of the heparin antagonist protamine. Also, an antifibrinolytic agent such as aminocaproic acid (5 grams initially or over a period of 1 hour, followed by 1 gram per hour for approximately 4 to 8 hours or until the desired response has been obtained), or tranexamic acid may be administered intravenously (preferably by continuous infusion) or orally. However, the efficacy of aminocaproic acid or other antifibrinolytic agents in the treatment of thrombolytic agent–induced hemorrhage has not been documented by controlled studies in humans. Also, the risk of reocclusion or other thrombotic complications must be considered.
• For bradycardia—If necessary, atropine may be administered.
• For reperfusion arrhythmias—Administering a suitable antiarrhythmic agent, such as lidocaine or procainamide. Electrical cardioversion may be needed for ventricular tachycardia or fibrillation.
• For mild hypersensitivity reaction—Administering antihistamines and, if necessary, glucocorticoids.
• For severe hypersensitivity or anaphylactic reaction—Discontinuing thrombolytic therapy and administering epinephrine. Antihistamines and/or glucocorticoids may also be administered as required.
• For sudden hypotension—If sudden hypotension occurs during rapid, high-dose administration, reducing the infusion rate. If sudden hypotension occurs in other circumstances or does not respond to a reduction in the infusion rate, placing the patient in the Trendelenburg position and/or administering volume expanders (other than dextrans), atropine, and/or a vasopressor, e.g., dopamine, as clinical circumstances permit.
• For fever—Administering acetaminophen if treatment is required. Administration of multiple antipyretic doses of aspirin is not recommended.

---

*ALTEPLASE, RECOMBINANT*

## Summary of Differences

Indications:
   Indicated in the treatment of acute coronary arterial thrombosis and acute pulmonary thromboembolism.
Pharmacology/pharmacokinetics:
   Mechanism of action/effect—
      Acts directly to convert plasminogen to plasmin.

May be more clot-selective than anistreplase, streptokinase, or urokinase.

Half-life—

Biphasic; about 4 minutes for distribution phase and 35 minutes for elimination phase.

Side/adverse effects:

Incidence of stroke and cerebral hemorrhage greater than with other thrombolytic agents. Incidence and severity of allergic reactions lower than with anistreplase or streptokinase.

## Additional Dosing Information

Alteplase is not antigenic (as are anistreplase and streptokinase) and does not promote antibody formation. Therefore, a second course of alteplase therapy can be administered, if reocclusion occurs, without resistance having developed to the effects of alteplase and without risk of precipitating an anaphylactic reaction. In one study, a second course of alteplase therapy was shown to be effective, without producing significant bleeding complications, in patients exhibiting signs and symptoms of reocclusion following initial thrombolytic therapy for treatment of acute myocardial infarction. However, it must still be considered that a second course of therapy, if initiated before systemic effects of the first dose have subsided, may increase the risk of severe hemorrhage.

A large multi-center study has shown that alteplase, administered in an accelerated or front-loaded dosing regimen within 6 hours of the onset of symptoms of myocardial infarction, may achieve earlier and more complete patency of the infarct-affected artery than does streptokinase in combination with intravenous or subcutaneous heparin, or a combination of alteplase, streptokinase, and intravenous heparin. Twenty-four-hour and 30-day mortality was also lower with the accelerated or front-loaded alteplase regimen than with these combinations.

## Parenteral Dosage Forms

### ALTEPLASE, RECOMBINANT, FOR INJECTION

#### Usual adult dose

Thrombosis, coronary arterial, acute—

Standard regimen:

For patients weighing less than 65 kg—Intravenous, 1.25 mg per kg of body weight administered over a period of three hours, as follows:

First hour—60% of the total dose. Initially, 6 to 10% of the total dose is given by direct intravenous injection within the first one or two minutes. The next 50 to 54% of the total dose is given via intravenous infusion during the remainder of the hour.

Second hour—20% of the total dose, via intravenous infusion.

Third hour—20% of the total dose, via intravenous infusion.

For patients weighing 65 kg or more—Intravenous, 100 mg, administered over a period of three hours, as follows:

First hour—60 mg. Initially, 6 to 10 mg is given by direct intravenous injection within the first one or two minutes. The next 50 to 54 mg is given via intravenous infusion during the remainder of the hour.

Second hour—20 mg, via intravenous infusion.

Third hour—20 mg, via intravenous infusion.

Accelerated regimen:

Intravenous, initially 15 mg followed by an infusion of 0.75 mg per kg of body weight, up to 50 mg, administered over a period of thirty minutes. The infusion should continue for an additional sixty minutes at a dose of 0.5 mg per kg of body weight, up to 35 mg.

Note: It is recommended that intravenous heparin be administered in conjunction with accelerated-dose alteplase at an initial dose of 5000 USP Heparin Units, followed by 1000 USP Heparin Units per hour (1200 USP Heparin Units per hour for patients weighing more than 80 kg), with the dose adjusted to raise the activated partial thromboplastin time to between 60 and 85 seconds.

Thromboembolism, pulmonary, acute[1]—

Intravenous infusion, 100 mg, administered over a period of two hours.

Note: It is recommended that heparin be used in conjunction with alteplase for treatment of acute pulmonary embolism. Heparin should be administered only if the patient's activated partial thromboplastin time or thrombin time value is no higher than twice the control value, near the end of or immediately following the alteplase infusion.

#### Usual pediatric dose

Dosage has not been established.

### Size(s) usually available

U.S.—

20 mg (Rx) [*Activase*].

50 mg (Rx) [*Activase*].

100 mg (Rx) [*Activase*].

Canada—

50 mg (Rx) [*Activase rt-PA; Lysatec rt-PA*].

### Packaging and storage

Store between 2 and 30 °C (36 and 86 °F), unless otherwise specified by manufacturer. Protect from excessive exposure to light.

### Preparation of dosage form

Alteplase should be reconstituted using the diluent provided (sterile water for injection). Bacteriostatic water for injection must not be used. A large-bore (18-gauge) needle should be used to direct the stream of diluent directly into the lyophilized material. The resultant colorless to pale yellow transparent solution will contain 1 mg of alteplase per mL. This solution may be used without further dilution or it may be diluted to a concentration of 0.5 mg per mL using an equal volume of 0.9% sodium chloride injection or 5% dextrose injection. Other infusion solutions or preservative-containing solutions should not be used when further diluting the reconstituted solution. The solution may be mixed with gentle swirling and/or slow inversion; excessive agitation should be avoided. Slight foaming may occur during reconstitution; however, large bubbles dissipate when the solution is left undisturbed for a few minutes.

### Stability

The reconstituted solution should be used within 8 hours when stored between 2 and 30 °C (36 and 86 °F). It should be discarded if not used within this time. However, because alteplase for injection contains no preservatives, it should not be reconstituted until immediately prior to use. Any unused solution must be discarded.

### Incompatibilities

*Do not add any other medication to the container of alteplase solution or administer other medications through the same intravenous line.*

---

[1]Not included in Canadian product labeling.

---

### *ANISTREPLASE*

## Summary of Differences

Indications:

Indicated in the treatment of acute coronary arterial thrombosis.

Pharmacology/pharmacokinetics:

Mechanism of action/effect—Acts indirectly to promote conversion of plasminogen to plasmin.

Other actions/effects—Antigenic; promotes antibody formation.

Half-life—70 to 120 minutes (average about 90 minutes). The deacylation half-life of the complex is about 105 to 120 minutes.

Precautions:

Medical considerations/contraindications—Caution required in patients who have had a severe hypersensitivity reaction to prior anistreplase or streptokinase therapy or a prior course of anistreplase or streptokinase therapy within the past 12 months.

Side/adverse effects:

Incidence of mild hypersensitivity and febrile reactions greater than with alteplase or urokinase.

May cause severe hypersensitivity reactions including anaphylaxis.

## Additional Dosing Information

It is recommended that equipment and medications (such as epinephrine, glucocorticoids, and antihistamines) for treating anaphylaxis be immediately available whenever anistreplase is administered. Some investigators have administered a glucocorticoid (e.g., 100 mg of hydrocortisone or methylprednisolone, intravenously) and/or an antihistamine (e.g., 50 mg of diphenhydramine, intravenously) prior to anistreplase, to decrease the risk of severe hypersensitivity and febrile reactions. However, the prophylactic efficacy of these medications has not been established.

Resistance to anistreplase therapy may occur because of the presence of high titers of antibodies following a prior course of anistreplase or streptokinase therapy. A significant titer of these antibodies generally occurs 5 to 7 days following administration of anistreplase or streptokinase and may persist for 1 year (up to 4 years in some patients). Alteplase or urokinase may be administered if thrombolytic therapy is indicated during this time. A recent streptococcal infection may also result in high titers of antibodies and resistance to anistreplase.

# Parenteral Dosage Forms

## ANISTREPLASE FOR INJECTION

### Usual adult dose
Thrombosis, coronary arterial, acute—
Intravenous, 30 units, administered over two to five minutes.

### Usual pediatric dose
Safety and efficacy have not been established.

### Size(s) usually available
U.S.—
30 Units per single-dose vial (Rx) [*Eminase* (human albumin 30 mg)].
Canada—
Not commercially available.

### Packaging and storage
Store between 2 and 8 °C (36 and 46 °F), unless otherwise specified by manufacturer.

### Preparation of dosage form
Five mL of sterile water for injection should be slowly added to the vial containing anistreplase for injection; the stream of water should be directed against the side of the vial. The vial should then be gently rolled (not shaken), to mix the powder with the liquid. Other measures to minimize foaming should also be used.

### Stability
The reconstituted solution is to be administered within 30 minutes after reconstitution.
The medication contains no preservative. Each vial is intended to provide a single dose only; any unused solution should be discarded.

### Incompatibilities
*Do not add any other medication to the container of anistreplase solution or administer other medications through the same intravenous line.*

---

## STREPTOKINASE

## Summary of Differences

Indications:
Indicated in the treatment of acute coronary arterial thrombosis, acute pulmonary thromboembolism, deep venous thrombosis, and acute arterial thromboembolism and thrombosis. Also indicated to clear totally or partially occluded arteriovenous cannulae.
Pharmacology/pharmacokinetics:
Mechanism of action/effect—Acts indirectly to promote conversion of plasminogen to plasmin.
Other actions/effects—Antigenic; promotes antibody formation.
Half-life—Following rapid, high-dose administration: 23 minutes (as active activator complex activity).
Precautions:
Medical considerations/contraindications—Caution required in patients who have had a severe hypersensitivity reaction to prior streptokinase therapy or a prior course of streptokinase therapy within the past 12 months.
Side/adverse effects:
Incidence of mild hypersensitivity and febrile reactions greater than with urokinase or alteplase.
May cause severe hypersensitivity reactions including anaphylaxis or, rarely, skin lesions.

## Additional Dosing Information

It is recommended that equipment and medications (such as epinephrine, glucocorticoids, and antihistamines) for treating anaphylaxis be immediately available whenever streptokinase is administered. Some investigators have administered a glucocorticoid (e.g., 100 mg of hydrocortisone or methylprednisolone, intravenously) and/or an antihistamine (e.g., 50 mg of diphenhydramine, intravenously) prior to streptokinase, to decrease the risk of severe hypersensitivity and febrile reactions. However, the prophylactic efficacy of these medications has not been established.

Resistance to streptokinase therapy may occur because of the presence of high titers of antibodies to streptokinase following a prior course of streptokinase or anistreplase therapy. A significant titer of these antibodies generally occurs 5 to 7 days following administration of anistreplase or streptokinase and may persist for 1 year (up to 4 years in some patients). Alteplase or urokinase may be administered if thrombolytic therapy is indicated during this time. A recent streptococcal infection may also result in high titers of antibodies and resistance to streptokinase.

For intravenous administration of streptokinase (for indications other than acute coronary arterial thrombosis), a loading dose of 250,000 international units (IU) is recommended to overcome mild resistance caused by exposure (without recent active infection) to streptococci. Since this loading dose successfully overcomes resistance in 85 to 90% of patients, many clinicians state that a previously recommended resistance test is now considered unnecessary. However, if a thrombin time (TT) determination or other test of fibrinolysis performed after 4 hours of therapy indicates minimal or no fibrinolytic activity, and no clinical improvement is apparent, the possibility of excessive resistance to streptokinase should be considered. Streptokinase should be discontinued and an alternate thrombolytic agent (alteplase or urokinase, but not anistreplase) administered instead.

A previously recommended regimen of variable maintenance dosage with frequent laboratory monitoring has not been shown to increase the efficacy or safety of streptokinase therapy. Therefore, this regimen is not currently recommended and has been replaced by a fixed maintenance dosage schedule.

The dosage and duration of intravenous therapy vary with the condition being treated. The recommended duration of therapy is 24 hours for acute pulmonary embolism (but up to 72 hours if concurrent deep vein thrombosis is suspected); 24 to 72 hours for arterial thrombosis or thromboembolism; and up to 72 hours for deep vein thrombosis. For the individual patient, tests to determine restoration of blood flow, such as angiography or venography of the affected blood vessel, computerized tomography, impedance plethysmography, or quantitative Doppler effect, may be useful in determining the optimum duration of administration.

# Parenteral Dosage Forms

## STREPTOKINASE FOR INJECTION

### Usual adult dose
Thrombosis, coronary arterial, acute—
Intravenous, 1,500,000 IU, administered within one hour.
Intra-arterial (via a coronary artery catheter placed via the Judkins or Sones technique), 20,000 IU initially, followed by 2000 IU per minute for one hour.
Note: Recanalization may occur in less than one hour; however, treatment should be continued following recanalization, to ensure complete lysis of all thrombotic material.
Thromboembolism, pulmonary, acute or
Thrombosis, deep venous or
Thromboembolism or thrombosis, arterial, acute—
Intravenous, 250,000 IU as an initial loading dose over thirty minutes, followed by 100,000 IU per hour as a continuous infusion.
Cannula, arteriovenous, clearance—
100,000 to 250,000 IU, instilled slowly into each occluded cannula limb.

### Usual pediatric dose
Dosage has not been established.

### Size(s) usually available
U.S.—
250,000 IU (Rx) [*Kabikinase; Streptase*].
750,000 IU (Rx) [*Kabikinase; Streptase*].
1,500,000 IU (Rx) [*Kabikinase; Streptase*].
Canada—
250,000 IU (Rx) [*Streptase*].
750,000 IU (Rx) [*Streptase*].

### Packaging and storage
Store between 15 and 30 °C (59 and 86 °F), unless otherwise specified by manufacturer.

### Preparation of dosage form
For intracoronary artery or intravenous administration—Manufacturer's prescribing information should be consulted for recommendations for reconstituting and further diluting the individual product.
For arteriovenous cannula obstruction clearance—Two mL of sodium chloride injection or 5% dextrose injection should be added to each 250,000 IU vial of streptokinase.

### Stability
Streptokinase for injection should be reconstituted immediately prior to use.
If not administered shortly following reconstitution, the solution should be stored at 2 to 8 °C (36 to 46 °F). If not used within 8 hours after reconstitution, the solution should be discarded.
One manufacturer states that slight flocculation (described as thin translucent fibers) may occur after reconstitution. Shaking the solution during reconstitution may increase flocculation or cause foaming, and

should be avoided. The solution may be administered if slight floc-culation is present but should be discarded if flocculation is extensive.

### Incompatibilities
*Do not add any other medication to the container of streptokinase solution or administer other medications through the same intravenous line.*

---

## UROKINASE

## Summary of Differences

Indications:
Indicated in the treatment of acute coronary arterial thrombosis, acute pulmonary embolism, and to restore patency to intravenous catheters.

Pharmacology/pharmacokinetics:
Mechanism of action/effect—Acts directly to convert plasminogen to plasmin.
Half-life—Up to 20 minutes; may be prolonged in patients with he-patic function impairment.

Side/adverse effects:
Incidence and severity of allergic or febrile reactions lower than with anistreplase or streptokinase.

## Additional Dosing Information

The dosage and duration of urokinase therapy may vary with the condition being treated. For the individual patient, tests to determine restoration of blood flow, such as angiography or venography of the affected blood vessel, computerized tomography, impedance plethysmography, or quantitative Doppler effect, may be useful in determining the op-timum duration of administration.

### For lysis of coronary artery thrombi
Prior to intracoronary arterial administration of urokinase, it is recom-mended that 2500 to 10,000 USP Heparin Units be administered via direct intravenous injection. Prior heparin administration should be considered when calculating heparin dosage.

## Parenteral Dosage Forms
### UROKINASE FOR INJECTION
#### Usual adult dose
Thrombosis, coronary arterial, acute—
Intra-arterial (via a coronary artery catheter), 6000 IU (4 mL of a solution containing approximately 1500 IU per mL) per minute.
Note: The average total dose of urokinase required for lysis of coro-nary artery thrombi is 500,000 IU.
Urokinase administration should be continued until the artery is maximally opened, usually 15 to 30 minutes after initial open-ing. The medication has been administered for periods up to 2 hours.
Thromboembolism, pulmonary, acute—
Intravenous, 4400 IU per kg of body weight initially over a ten minute period, followed by 4400 IU per kg of body weight per hour for approximately 12 hours.
Note: Manufacturer's product information should be consulted for recommendations concerning the rate of infusion, based on rec-ommended dilution volume of the product.
Catheter, intravenous, clearance—
After the intravenous tubing has been disconnected and catheter oc-clusion confirmed, the catheter should be filled with a solution containing 5000 IU per mL of urokinase.
#### Usual pediatric dose
Catheter, intravenous, clearance—
After the intravenous tubing has been disconnected and catheter oc-clusion confirmed, the catheter should be filled with a solution

containing 5000 IU per mL of urokinase. Alternatively, an intra-venous infusion of 150 IU per kg of body weight per hour may be administered over eight hours.

### Size(s) usually available
U.S.—
5000 IU (Rx) [*Abbokinase Open-Cath*].
9000 IU (Rx) [*Abbokinase Open-Cath*].
250,000 IU (Rx) [*Abbokinase*].
Canada—
5000 IU (Rx) [*Abbokinase Open-Cath*].
9000 IU (Rx) [*Abbokinase Open-Cath*].
250,000 IU (Rx) [*Abbokinase*].
Note: The 5000-IU and 9000-IU sizes are intended for intravenous cath-eter clearance only. Premeasured diluent is included. After recon-stitution, the solution prepared from either size contains 5000 IU per mL.

### Packaging and storage
Store between 2 and 8 °C (36 and 46 °F), unless otherwise specified by manufacturer. Store *Abbokinase Open-Cath* below 25 °C (77 °F). Pro-tect from freezing.

### Preparation of dosage form
For intravenous administration—Manufacturer's prescribing information should be consulted for recommendations for reconstituting and further diluting the product.
For intracoronary arterial administration—Five mL of sterile water for injection *without preservatives* should be added to each of three 250,000 IU vials of urokinase. The vial should be rolled and tilted (not shaken) to facilitate reconstitution. The contents of the three vials should be added to 500 mL of 5% dextrose injection to make a so-lution containing approximately 1500 IU per mL.
For intravenous catheter clearance (for the 250,000-IU size only)—Five mL of sterile water for injection *without preservatives* should be added to the vial. The vial should be rolled and tilted (not shaken) to facilitate reconstitution. Then, 1 mL of the reconstituted solution should be added to 9 mL of sterile water for injection to make a solution con-taining 5000 IU per mL.

### Stability
Because urokinase for injection contains no preservatives, it should not be reconstituted until immediately prior to use. Also, any unused so-lution must be discarded.
Filaments may form in the solution during reconstitution, especially if the vial is shaken. Shaking the vial should be avoided. If necessary, the solution may be filtered through a 0.45 micron or smaller cellulose membrane filter.

### Incompatibilities
*Do not add any other medication to the container of urokinase solution or administer other medications through the same intravenous line.*

### Selected Bibliography
Anderson HV, Willerson JT. Thrombolysis in acute myocardial infarction. N Engl J Med 1993; 329: 703-9.

---

Revised: 09/01/94

---

**THYROGLOBULIN**—See *Thyroid Hormones (Systemic)*

---

**THYROID**—See *Thyroid Hormones (Systemic)*

---

# THYROID HORMONES    Systemic

This monograph includes information on the following: Levothyroxine; Liothyronine; Liotrix†; Thyroglobulin*†; Thyroid.
VA CLASSIFICATION (Primary/Secondary):
Levothyroxine—HS851/AN500; DX900
Liothyronine—HS851/AN500; DX900
Liotrix—HS851/AN500
Thyroglobulin—HS851/AN500
Thyroid—HS851/AN500

Another commonly used name for Levothyroxine is L-Thyroxine.
Note: For a listing of dosage forms and brand names by country availa-bility, see *Dosage Forms* section(s). For a listing of brand names for the articles in this monograph, refer to the General Index.

---

*Not commercially available in the U.S.
†Not commercially available in Canada.

## Category

Thyroid hormone—Levothyroxine; Liothyronine; Liotrix; Thyroglobulin; Thyroid.

Antineoplastic—Levothyroxine; Liothyronine; Liotrix; Thyroglobulin; Thyroid.

Diagnostic aid (thyroid function)—Levothyroxine; Liothyronine.

## Indications

### Accepted

Hypothyroidism (diagnosis and treatment)—Thyroid hormones are indicated as replacement therapy in the treatment of thyroid hormone deficiency (hypothyroidism) of any etiology (except transient hypothyroidism during the recovery phase of subacute thyroiditis), as well as for simple (nonendemic) goiter and chronic lymphocytic (Hashimoto's) thyroiditis[1].

In general, levothyroxine is the preferred thyroid hormone for use in the treatment of hypothyroidism because of the absence of variability and the ease of monitoring of plasma concentrations; it is the drug of choice in the treatment of congenital hypothyroidism. Liothyronine is recommended by some clinicians because of its short half-life and readily reversible effects for initial therapy in myxedema and myxedema coma, as well as for hypothyroid patients who also have heart disease, although there are significant risks associated with the latter use. Liothyronine may also be preferred during preparation for radioisotope scanning procedures or when gastrointestinal absorption processes are impaired. Disadvantages of thyroid extract and thyroglobulin tablets are their variable potencies and the fact that triiodothyronine ($T_3$) and thyroxine ($T_4$) concentrations fluctuate and cannot be used to regulate dosage. Liotrix is no longer considered advantageous because of the natural conversion of $T_4$ to $T_3$ in the tissues.

Goiter (prophylaxis[1] and treatment)—Thyroid hormones are indicated to suppress the growth of some adenomatous goiters, and to prevent the goitrogenic effects of other medications such as lithium, aminosalicylic acid, and some sulfonamide compounds.

Carcinoma, thyroid (prophylaxis and treatment)[1]—Thyroid hormones are indicated in the treatment of thyrotropin-dependent thyroid gland carcinoma. Some clinicians believe that prophylactic administration of thyroid hormones after neck irradiation will prevent development of thyroid gland carcinoma.

Thyroid function studies—Levothyroxine[1] and liothyronine are indicated as diagnostic aids (for example, the $T_3$ suppression test), although this use has generally been replaced by other tests.

### Unaccepted

Use of thyroid hormones to treat vague symptoms such as dry skin, fatigue, constipation, abnormalities of reproductive function, growth retardation, or obesity without laboratory confirmation of contributing hypothyroidism is inappropriate and may cause hyperthyroidism in euthyroid individuals.

---

[1]Not included in Canadian product labeling.

## Pharmacology/Pharmacokinetics

### Physicochemical characteristics

Source—
  Natural products include thyroglobulin and thyroid.
  Synthetic products include levothyroxine, liothyronine, and liotrix.
Composition—
  Levothyroxine: $T_4$ (thyroxine), with approximately 30% being converted to $T_3$ in peripheral tissues.
  Liothyronine: $T_3$ (triiodothyronine).
  Liotrix, thyroglobulin, and thyroid: $T_3$ and $T_4$.
Molecular weight—
  Levothyroxine sodium: 798.86 (anhydrous).
  Liothyronine sodium: 672.96.
Equivalent strength (approximate), based on clinical response—
  Levothyroxine: 100 mcg (0.1 mg) or less.
  Liothyronine: 25 mcg (0.025 mg).
  Liotrix—
    Levothyroxine and liothyronine: 60 mcg (0.06 mg) and 15 mcg (0.015 mg), or 50 mcg (0.05 mg) and 12.5 mcg (0.0125 mg), respectively.
  Thyroglobulin: 60 mg.
  Thyroid USP: 60 mg.
  Note: Because of the difficulty in measuring actual hormonal content of thyroglobulin and Thyroid USP, the measurable amounts of levothyroxine and liothyronine in these preparations may be less than the clinical equivalent. However, for purposes of dosage adjustment, the above equivalent strengths are appropriate.

### Mechanism of action/Effect

The action of thyroid hormones is not completely understood, but they have both catabolic (calorigenic) and anabolic effects and are therefore involved in normal metabolism, growth, and development, especially the development of the central nervous system (CNS) of infants. A feedback system involving the hypothalamus, anterior pituitary, and thyroid normally regulates circulating thyroid hormone concentrations.

### Absorption

Oral—
  Levothyroxine: Incomplete and variable, especially when taken with food; average 50 to 75%.
  Liothyronine: Approximately 95%.
  Note: Absorption may be reduced in patients with congestive heart failure, malabsorption syndromes, or diarrhea.

### Protein binding

Very high (more than 99%), but not firmly bound.

### Biotransformation

As for endogenous thyroid hormone; levothyroxine (approximately 30%) is deiodinated in peripheral tissues; small amounts are metabolized in the liver and excreted in bile.

### Half-life

Levothyroxine—
  Euthyroid: 6 to 7 days.
  Hypothyroid: 9 to 10 days.
  Hyperthyroid: 3 to 4 days.
Liothyronine—
  Euthyroid: 1 day.
  Hypothyroid: 1.4 days.
  Hyperthyroid: 0.6 day.
Note: Because thyroid and thyroglobulin contain varying amounts of thyroxine and triiodothyronine, their half-lives will vary but will be somewhere between that for $T_4$ and $T_3$.

### Time to peak therapeutic effect

With chronic stable oral dosing—
  Levothyroxine, thyroglobulin, thyroid: 3 to 4 weeks.
  Liothyronine: 48 to 72 hours.

### Duration of therapeutic action

After withdrawal of chronic therapy—
  Levothyroxine, thyroglobulin, thyroid: 1 to 3 weeks.
  Liothyronine: Up to 72 hours.

## Precautions to Consider

Note: The following precautions apply to patients with *abnormal thyroid status* (hypothyroidism or, in some cases, hyperthyroidism). Patients in stable euthyroid condition as a result of continuing thyroid hormone therapy may be expected to respond in the same way as individuals with normal thyroid function and, therefore, the following precautions (except for *Patient monitoring*) do not usually apply in those circumstances.

### Carcinogenicity/Mutagenicity

Studies have not been done in animals. A reported association with breast cancer has not been confirmed and does not justify withholding thyroid hormone treatment.

### Pregnancy/Reproduction

Pregnancy—Thyroid hormones cross the placenta, but only to a limited extent. However, clinical experience in humans has not shown that appropriate use of thyroid hormones causes adverse effects in the fetus. Monitoring of maternal dose is important as maternal dose requirements may change during pregnancy. Intra-amniotic levothyroxine has been used to treat fetal hypothyroidism.

FDA Pregnancy Category A.

### Breast-feeding

Problems in humans have not been documented with appropriate use of thyroid hormones in women who are breast-feeding. Minimal amounts of exogenous thyroid hormones are distributed into breast milk.

### Pediatrics

Studies performed to date have not demonstrated pediatrics-specific problems that would limit the usefulness of thyroid hormones in children. However, caution is necessary in interpreting results of thyroid function tests in neonates, because serum $T_4$ concentrations are transiently elevated and serum $T_3$ concentrations are transiently low, and the infant pituitary is relatively insensitive to the negative feedback effect of thyroid hormones.

### Geriatrics

The elderly may be more sensitive to the effects of thyroid hormones. Thyroid hormone replacement requirements are about 25% lower in some patients over the age of 60 years than in younger adults; therefore, individualization of dose is recommended.

### Drug interactions and/or related problems

The following drug interactions and/or related problems have been selected on the basis of their potential clinical significance (possible mechanism in parentheses where appropriate)—not necessarily inclusive (» = major clinical significance):

Note: Combinations containing any of the following medications, depending on the amount present, may also interact with this medication.

In most cases, relative need for thyroid hormone dosage adjustment will depend on the thyroid state of the patient and the dosages of all medications involved. Dosage adjustment should be based on results of thyroid function tests and clinical status.

» Anticoagulants, coumarin- or indandione-derivative
(the effects of the oral anticoagulant may be altered, depending on the thyroid status of the patient; an increase in dosage of thyroid hormone may necessitate a decrease in oral anticoagulant dosage; adjustment of oral anticoagulant dosage on the basis of prothrombin time is recommended)

Antidepressants, tricyclic
(concurrent use with thyroid hormones may increase the therapeutic and toxic effects of both drugs, possibly due to increased receptor sensitivity to catecholamines; toxic effects include cardiac arrhythmias and CNS stimulation; also the onset of action of tricyclics may be accelerated)

Antidiabetic agents, sulfonylurea or
Insulin
(thyroid hormones may increase insulin or antidiabetic agent requirements; careful monitoring of diabetic control is recommended, especially when thyroid therapy is started, changed, or discontinued)

Beta-adrenergic blocking agents
(may decrease peripheral conversion of $T_4$ [thyroxine] to $T_3$ [triiodothyronine])

» Cholestyramine or
» Colestipol
(concurrent use may decrease the effects of thyroid hormones by binding and delaying or preventing absorption; an interval of 4 to 5 hours between administration of the two medications and regular monitoring of thyroid function tests are recommended)

Corticosteroids, glucocorticoid with mineralocorticoid activity or
Corticosteroids, mineralocorticoid or
Corticotropin (ACTH)
(changes in the thyroid status of the patient that may occur as a result of administration, changes in dosage, or discontinuation of thyroid hormones may necessitate adjustment of corticosteroid dosage because metabolic clearance of corticosteroids is decreased in hypothyroid patients and increased in hyperthyroid patients)

Estrogens
(increase serum thyroxine-binding globulin; in patients with a nonfunctioning thyroid gland, thyroid hormone requirements may be increased)

Hepatic enzyme inducers (See *Appendix II*)
(increase hepatic degradation of levothyroxine, which may result in increased requirements; dosage adjustment may be necessary)

(phenytoin also reduces serum protein binding of levothyroxine, and reduces total and free serum $T_4$ by 15 to 25%; despite this, most patients remain euthyroid and dosage of thyroid hormone does not need to be adjusted)

Ketamine
(concurrent use may produce marked hypertension and tachycardia; cautious administration to patients receiving thyroid hormone therapy is recommended)

Maprotiline
(concurrent use with thyroid hormones may enhance the possibility of cardiac arrhythmias; dosage adjustment may be necessary)

Sodium iodide I 123 or
Sodium iodide I 131 or
Sodium pertechnetate Tc 99m
(thyroid hormones may decrease the normal thyroidal uptake of I 123, I 131, or pertechnetate ion)

Somatrem or
Somatropin
(concurrent excessive use of thyroid hormones with somatrem or somatropin may accelerate epiphyseal closure. However, untreated hypothyroidism may interfere with growth response to somatrem or somatropin; prior and/or concurrent thyroid hormone replacement is recommended)

» Sympathomimetics
(concurrent use may increase the effects of these medications or thyroid hormone; thyroid hormones enhance risk of coronary insufficiency when sympathomimetic agents are administered to patients with coronary artery disease)

### Medical considerations/Contraindications

The medical considerations/contraindications included here have been selected on the basis of their potential clinical significance (reasons given in parentheses where appropriate)—not necessarily inclusive (» = major clinical significance).

*Risk-benefit should be considered when the following medical problems exist:*

» Adrenocortical insufficiency
(must be corrected while thyroid replacement therapy is being given, to prevent precipitation of acute adrenocortical insufficiency)

» Cardiovascular disease, including angina pectoris, arteriosclerosis, coronary artery disease, hypertension, myocardial infarction
(because of the risks associated with overly rapid thyroid hormone replacement and increased metabolic demands; mobilization of myxedema fluid may produce pitting edema 1 to 3 or more weeks after a change in dosage)

Diabetes mellitus
(possible reduced glucose tolerance and increased insulin or oral antidiabetic agent requirements)

» Hyperthyroidism, history of
(residual autonomous thyroid function may be present after therapy for hyperthyroidism, necessitating lower than typical doses)

Malabsorption states, such as celiac disease
(absorption, especially of levothyroxine, is reduced; dosage adjustment may be necessary)

» Pituitary insufficiency
(associated adrenocortical insufficiency must be corrected before thyroid replacement therapy is initiated, to prevent precipitation of acute adrenocortical insufficiency)

Sensitivity to thyroid hormone

» Thyrotoxicosis being treated with antithyroid medication

» Caution is required also in patients with long-standing hypothyroidism or myxedema, who may be more sensitive to effects of thyroid hormones.

### Patient monitoring

The following may be especially important in patient monitoring (other tests may be warranted in some patients, depending on condition; » = major clinical significance):

Note: In patients receiving levothyroxine, liotrix, or thyroid extract for primary hypothyroidism, serum free $T_4$ index (total serum $T_4$ and $T_3$ resin uptake) or serum free $T_4$ together with a serum thyroid-stimulating hormone (TSH) are the most useful tests for monitoring replacement therapy. Serum TSH measurements are not useful in hypothyroidism secondary to pituitary insufficiency. In the rare patient receiving liothyronine replacement, serum $T_4$ concentrations will remain low and normalization of serum TSH indicates that treatment is adequate. Overdosage with liothyronine can best be recognized by clinical symptoms of hyperthyroidism and/or by a decrease in serum TSH to subnormal levels.

Many medications affect the results of thyroid function tests and may produce false results.

Caution is necessary in interpreting results of thyroid function tests in neonates, because serum $T_4$ concentrations are transiently elevated and serum $T_3$ concentrations are transiently low, and the infant pituitary is relatively insensitive to the negative feedback effect of thyroid hormones.

The following have been found to be the most useful in general and may be especially important in patient monitoring (other tests may be warranted in some patients, depending on condition; » = major clinical significance):

» Free $T_4$ (thyroxine) index determinations or
Free (unbound) $T_4$ determinations
(recommended at periodic intervals in most patients)

Measurement of bone age and
» Measurement of growth and
» Measurement of psychomotor development
   (recommended at periodic intervals in children with congenital hypothyroidism)
» Observation for signs of ischemia or tachyarrhythmias
   (recommended in hypothyroid patients with cardiovascular disease to aid in adjustment of dosage and to prevent overdosage or overly rapid increase in dosage)
» TSH (thyroid-stimulating hormone) determinations and
» $T_3$ (triiodothyronine) or $T_4$ resin uptake determinations and
» Total serum $T_4$ determinations, by radioimmunoassay and
» Total serum $T_3$ determinations, by radioimmunoassay
   (which thyroid function tests are most useful for a particular patient depends on the agent, condition being treated, other agents used concomitantly, and existing conditions that are capable of altering test results by altering serum thyroxine-binding globulin [TBG] concentrations)

## Side/Adverse Effects

Note: Side/adverse effects are dose-related and the dose at which they occur varies with each patient; incidence may be reduced by slowly increasing the initial dose to the minimum effective dose.

Side/adverse effects may occur more rapidly with liothyronine than with levothyroxine or thyroid because of its rapid onset of action.

In infants, excessive doses may result in craniosynostosis.

Partial loss of hair may occur in children during the first few months of treatment; normal hair growth usually returns, even with continued treatment.

The following side/adverse effects have been selected on the basis of their potential clinical significance (possible signs and symptoms in parentheses where appropriate)—not necessarily inclusive:

### Those indicating need for medical attention
Incidence rare
*Allergic reaction* (skin rash or hives); *hyperthyroidism or overdosage* (changes in appetite; changes in menstrual periods; chest pain; diarrhea; fast or irregular heartbeat; fever; hand tremors; headache; irritability; leg cramps; nervousness; sensitivity to heat; shortness of breath; sweating; trouble in sleeping; vomiting; weight loss); *pseudotumor cerebri, in children* (severe headache)

### Those indicating need for medical attention only if they continue or are bothersome
*Hypothyroidism or underdosage* (changes in menstrual periods; clumsiness; coldness; constipation; dry, puffy skin; headache; listlessness; muscle aches; sleepiness; tiredness; weakness; weight gain)

## Overdose

For specific information on the agents used in the management of thyroid hormones overdose, see:
• *Beta-adrenergic Blocking Agents (Systemic)* monograph;
• *Charcoal, Activated (Oral-Local)* monograph;
• *Hydrocortisone* in *Corticosteroids—Glucocorticoid Effects (Systemic)* monograph; and/or
• *Digitalis Glycosides (Systemic)* monograph.

For more information on the management of overdose or unintentional ingestion, **contact a Poison Control Center** (see *Poison Control Center Listing*).

### Treatment of overdose
If symptoms of hyperthyroidism occur, it is recommended that thyroid hormone therapy be withdrawn for 2 to 6 days (1 to 2 days for liothyronine), then resumed at a lower dose.
To decrease absorption—
   Acute massive overdose is treated by reducing gastrointestinal absorption, if possible, by means of vomiting, followed by emptying of the stomach and/or use of a charcoal instillation, which may be useful up to 3 to 4 hours after oral ingestion of toxic doses of thyroid hormones.
Specific treatment—
   Cardiac glycosides if congestive heart failure develops.
   Antiadrenergic agents such as propranolol for treatment of increased sympathetic activity.
   Intravenous hydrocortisone to partially inhibit conversion of $T_4$ to $T_3$.
Supportive care—
   Administration of oxygen. Implementation of measures to control fever, hypoglycemia, or fluid loss. Patients in whom intentional overdose is confirmed or suspected should be referred for psychiatric consultation.

## Patient Consultation

As an aid to patient consultation, refer to *Advice for the Patient, Thyroid Hormones (Systemic)*.

In providing consultation, consider emphasizing the following selected information (» = major clinical significance):

### Before using this medication
» Conditions affecting use, especially:
   Allergy to thyroid hormones
   Pregnancy—Crosses the placenta to a limited extent and has not caused problems in the fetus with appropriate doses; regular monitoring is necessary as maternal dose requirements may change during pregnancy
   Breast-feeding—Small amounts are distributed into breast milk
   Use in the elderly—Sensitivity to thyroid effects is greater in the elderly than in younger age groups and dose adjustment may be necessary
   Other medications, especially cholestyramine, colestipol, coumarin- or indandione-derivative anticoagulants, or sympathomimetics
   Other medical problems, especially adrenocortical insufficiency, cardiovascular disease, history of hyperthyroidism, pituitary insufficiency, thyroid sensitivity with long-standing hypothyroidism or myxedema, or thyrotoxicosis

### Proper use of this medication
» Importance of not taking more or less medication than the amount prescribed; taking medication at the same time every day for consistent effect
» Possible need for lifelong therapy; checking with physician before discontinuing medication
» . Proper dosing
   Missed dose: Taking as soon as possible; not taking if almost time for next dose and not doubling doses; notifying physician if two or more doses in a row are missed
» Proper storage

### Precautions while using this medication
» Importance of close monitoring by the physician
   Caution with angina or coronary artery disease; heavy exercise or exertion may precipitate angina
» Caution if any kind of surgery (including dental surgery) or emergency treatment is required
   Avoiding other medications unless prescribed by physician because of possible interference with effects of thyroid hormone

### Side/adverse effects
   Signs of potential side effects, especially allergic reaction, hyperthyroidism, and pseudotumor cerebri

## General Dosing Information

**Dosage must be adjusted to meet the individual requirements of each patient, on the basis of clinical response and results of thyroid function tests.**

Levothyroxine is the preferred form of thyroid replacement therapy.

Patients who are more than mildly hypothyroid initially should be treated with less than a full replacement dose, with doses then being increased gradually over a period of weeks. Otherwise, nervousness and rapid heart rate may occur.

Thyroid hormone replacement therapy for congenital hypothyroidism should be initiated as soon as possible after birth to minimize impaired mental and physical development. Treatment after about 3 months of age may reverse many of the physical effects but not all of the mental effects of hypothyroidism. Treatment should be continued for life, unless transient hypothyroidism is suspected, in which case therapy may be withdrawn for 2 to 8 weeks after 3 years of age; if thyroid-stimulating hormone (TSH) and thyroxine ($T_4$) concentrations remain normal throughout the withdrawal period, treatment is no longer necessary.

Suppression of TSH to normal levels must not be used as the sole criterion of adequacy of dose in congenital hypothyroidism, since TSH concentrations may remain elevated despite adequate or even excessive doses of thyroid hormone. Maintenance of appropriate $T_4$ concentrations for age is a more accurate guideline during infancy and childhood.

In general, thyroid hormone therapy is begun at a low dose, which is increased gradually to obtain a euthyroid state, followed by the dose required to maintain the response. However, this is not necessary in neonates, in whom rapid replacement is important, and who may be started at the full replacement dose. Adverse effects such as hyperactivity in the older child may be lessened by utilizing a starting dose of one-fourth the full replacement dose, and increasing the dose by one-fourth weekly until the full replacement dose is reached.

Rapid replacement of thyroid hormone is associated with less risk in younger adults than in older ones.

In hypothyroid patients with adrenocortical insufficiency or panhypopituitarism, replacement therapy with thyroid hormones must be preceded by adequate amounts of corticosteroids to prevent precipitation of acute adrenocortical insufficiency by the increase in metabolism. Supplemental corticosteroids may also be necessary for patients with prolonged or severe hypothyroidism, including myxedema.

In hypothyroid patients with myxedema or cardiovascular disease, the initial dosage of thyroid hormones should be very small and must be increased very gradually to prevent precipitation of angina, coronary occlusion, or stroke. If cardiovascular reactions occur, a reduction in thyroid hormone dosage may be required. Although some clinicians prefer to use liothyronine in these patients because its effects disappear more rapidly after withdrawal, regulation of dosage is more difficult and its rapid onset of action may also produce adverse cardiac effects as a result of abrupt changes in metabolic demands.

If, after prolonged therapy (2 to 6 months), no response occurs with physiologic doses or a response occurs only with large doses of thyroid hormone, it is recommended that the diagnosis be reevaluated.

---

## LEVOTHYROXINE

## Summary of Differences

Indications: Usual drug of choice. Advantage over thyroid and thyroglobulin is a predictable effect because of standard hormonal content.

Pharmacology/pharmacokinetics: Absorption after oral administration is incomplete and variable, especially when taken with food.

Precautions: Medical problems/contraindications—Absorption may be significantly reduced in patients with malabsorption states.

## Oral Dosage Forms
### LEVOTHYROXINE SODIUM TABLETS USP
**Usual adult dose**

Mild hypothyroidism—

Initial: Oral, 50 mcg (0.05 mg) as a single daily dose, with increments of 25 to 50 mcg (0.025 to 0.05 mg) at two- to three-week intervals until the desired result is obtained.

Maintenance: Oral, 75 to 125 mcg (0.075 to 0.125 mg) per day (or 1.5 mcg per kg of body weight per day) as a single daily dose. A higher maintenance dose (up to 200 mcg per day) may be necessary in some patients (e.g., those with malabsorption).

Severe hypothyroidism—

Initial: Oral, 12.5 to 25 mcg (0.0125 to 0.025 mg) as a single daily dose, with increments of 25 mcg (0.025 mg) at two- to three-week intervals until the desired result is obtained.

Maintenance: Oral, 75 to 125 mcg (0.075 to 0.125 mg) per day (or 1.5 mcg per kg of body weight per day) as a single daily dose. A higher maintenance dose (up to 200 mcg per day) may be necessary in some patients (e.g., those with malabsorption).

Note: In the elderly and in patients with long-standing hypothyroidism, myxedematous infiltration, or cardiovascular dysfunction, the initial dose is usually 12.5 to 25 mcg (0.0125 to 0.025 mg) a day, and dosage is incremented at three- to four-week intervals. In the elderly, the maintenance dose is usually about 75 mcg (0.075 mg) per day.

**Usual adult prescribing limits**

Failure to respond to a daily dose of 150 mcg (0.15 mg) or more may indicate erroneous diagnosis of hypothyroidism, malabsorption, or poor compliance.

**Usual pediatric dose**

Children less than 6 months of age—Oral, 5 to 6 mcg (0.005 to 0.006 mg) per kg of body weight per day or 25 to 50 mcg (0.025 to 0.05 mg) per day as a single daily dose.

Children 6 to 12 months of age—Oral, 5 to 6 mcg (0.005 to 0.006 mg) per kg of body weight per day or 50 to 75 mcg (0.05 to 0.075 mg) per day as a single daily dose.

Children 1 to 5 years of age—Oral, 3 to 5 mcg (0.003 to 0.005 mg) per kg of body weight per day or 75 to 100 mcg (0.075 to 0.1 mg) per day as a single daily dose.

Children 6 to 10 years of age—Oral, 4 to 5 mcg (0.004 to 0.005 mg) per kg of body weight per day or 100 to 150 mcg (0.1 to 0.15 mg) per day as a single daily dose.

Children over 10 years of age—Oral, 2 to 3 mcg (0.002 to 0.003 mg) per kg of body weight per day as a single daily dose until the adult dose

is reached (usually 150 mcg [0.15 mg] per day) up to 200 mcg (0.2 mg) per day.

Note: Premature infants weighing less than 2000 grams, or infants at risk for cardiac failure receive a starting dose of 25 mcg (0.025 mg) a day which may be increased to 50 mcg (0.05 mg) a day in four to six weeks.

**Usual geriatric dose**

See *Usual adult dose.*

**Strength(s) usually available**

U.S.—

25 mcg (0.025 mg) (Rx) [*Levo-T* (scored); *Levothroid; Levoxyl; Synthroid* (scored); GENERIC].

50 mcg (0.05 mg) (Rx) [*Levo-T* (scored); *Levothroid; Levoxyl; Synthroid* (scored); GENERIC].

75 mcg (0.075 mg) (Rx) [*Levo-T* (scored); *Levothroid; Levoxyl; Synthroid* (scored); GENERIC].

88 mcg (0.088 mg) (Rx) [*Levothroid; Levoxyl; Synthroid* (scored)].

100 mcg (0.1 mg) (Rx) [*Levo-T* (scored); *Levothroid; Levoxyl; Synthroid* (scored); GENERIC].

112 mcg (0.112 mg) (Rx) [*Levothroid; Levoxyl; Synthroid* (scored)].

125 mcg (0.125 mg) (Rx) [*Levo-T* (scored); *Levothroid; Levoxyl; Synthroid* (scored); GENERIC].

137 mcg (0.137 mg) (Rx) [*Levothroid; Levoxyl*].

150 mcg (0.15 mg) (Rx) [*Levo-T* (scored); *Levothroid; Levoxyl; Synthroid* (scored); GENERIC].

175 mcg (0.175 mg) (Rx) [*Levothroid; Levoxyl; Synthroid* (scored)].

200 mcg (0.2 mg) (Rx) [*Levo-T* (scored); *Levothroid; Levoxyl; Synthroid* (scored); GENERIC].

300 mcg (0.3 mg) (Rx) [*Levo-T* (scored); *Levothroid; Levoxyl; Synthroid* (scored); GENERIC].

Canada—

25 mcg (0.025 mg) (Rx) [*PMS-Levothyroxine Sodium* (scored); *Synthroid* (scored)].

50 mcg (0.05 mg) (Rx) [*Eltroxin; PMS-Levothyroxine Sodium* (scored); *Synthroid* (scored)].

75 mcg (0.075 mg) (Rx) [*PMS-Levothyroxine Sodium* (scored); *Synthroid* (scored)].

88 mcg (0.088 mg) (Rx) [*Synthroid* (scored)].

100 mcg (0.1 mg) (Rx) [*Eltroxin; PMS-Levothyroxine Sodium* (scored); *Synthroid* (scored)].

112 mcg (0.112 mg) (Rx) [*Synthroid* (scored)].

125 mcg (0.125 mg) (Rx) [*PMS-Levothyroxine Sodium* (scored); *Synthroid* (scored)].

150 mcg (0.15 mg) (Rx) [*Eltroxin; PMS-Levothyroxine Sodium* (scored); *Synthroid* (scored)].

175 mcg (0.175 mg) (Rx) [*Synthroid* (scored)].

200 mcg (0.2 mg) (Rx) [*Eltroxin; PMS-Levothyroxine Sodium* (scored); *Synthroid* (scored)].

300 mcg (0.3 mg) (Rx) [*Eltroxin; PMS-Levothyroxine Sodium* (scored); *Synthroid* (scored)].

**Packaging and storage**

Store below 40 °C (104 °F), preferably between 15 and 30 °C (59 and 86 °F), unless otherwise specified by manufacturer. Store in a tight, light-resistant container.

**Auxiliary labeling**

• Take on empty stomach.

• Do not take other medicines without your doctor's advice.

**Note**

Caution is recommended when changing products because of the potential difference in actual levothyroxine content between brands.

## Parenteral Dosage Forms
### LEVOTHYROXINE SODIUM INJECTION
**Usual adult dose**

Hypothyroidism—

Intravenous or intramuscular, 50 to 100 mcg (0.05 to 0.1 mg) as a single daily dose.

Myxedema coma or stupor—

Initial: Intravenous, 200 to 500 mcg (0.2 to 0.5 mg), even in the elderly; an additional 100 to 300 mcg (0.1 to 0.3 mg) may be given on the second day if improvement has not occurred, followed by continuous daily administration of smaller doses, until the patient can tolerate oral administration.

Note: Smaller doses may be required in patients with concomitant cardiovascular disease.

### Usual pediatric dose
Hypothyroidism—
Intravenous or intramuscular, daily dose equal to 75% of the usual oral pediatric dose.

### Usual geriatric dose
See *Usual adult dose.*

### Strength(s) usually available
U.S.—
Not commercially available.
Canada—
Not commercially available.

### Packaging and storage
Store below 40 °C (104 °F), preferably between 15 and 30 °C (59 and 86 °F), unless otherwise specified by manufacturer.

## LEVOTHYROXINE SODIUM FOR INJECTION

### Usual adult dose
See *Levothyroxine Sodium Injection.*

### Usual pediatric dose
See *Levothyroxine Sodium Injection.*

### Usual geriatric dose
See *Levothyroxine Sodium Injection.*

### Size(s) usually available
U.S.—
200 mcg (0.2 mg) (Rx) [*Levothroid; Synthroid;* GENERIC].
500 mcg (0.5 mg) (Rx) [*Levothroid; Synthroid;* GENERIC].
Canada—
500 mcg (0.5 mg) (Rx) [*Synthroid*].

### Packaging and storage
Store below 40 °C (104 °F), preferably between 15 and 30 °C (59 and 86 °F), unless otherwise specified by manufacturer. Protect from light.

### Preparation of dosage form
Levothyroxine sodium for injection may be reconstituted for parenteral use by adding 0.5, 2, or 5 mL of Sodium Chloride Injection USP (without preservative) to the 50-, 200-, or 500-mcg vial, respectively, and shaking to dissolve, producing a solution containing 100 mcg (0.1 mg) per mL.

### Stability
Solution should be freshly reconstituted immediately prior to each dose. Any unused portion should be discarded.

---

### *LIOTHYRONINE*

## Summary of Differences

Indications:
Advantage over thyroid and thyroglobulin is a predictable effect because of standard hormonal content. May be preferred over levothyroxine when a rapid effect or rapidly reversible effect is desired, or when gastrointestinal absorption processes or peripheral conversion of $T_4$ (thyroxine) to $T_3$ (triiodothyronine) is impaired; however, regulation of dosage is more difficult and rapid onset of action may also produce adverse cardiac effects as a result of abrupt changes in metabolic demands.
Pharmacology/pharmacokinetics:
Maximal effects with continued use occur within 48 to 72 hours and persist for up to 72 hours after withdrawal.
Side/adverse effects:
May occur more rapidly with liothyronine than with levothyroxine or thyroid.
General dosing information:
Rapid action and abrupt increase in metabolic demands may produce adverse cardiac effects.
If symptoms of hyperthyroidism occur, withdrawal for 2 to 3 days is recommended before resumption at a lower dose.

## Additional Dosing Information

See also *General Dosing Information.*

When a patient is transferred to liothyronine from other thyroid therapy, the other therapy is discontinued and liothyronine is initiated at a low dosage, increased gradually on the basis of patient response. Keep in mind that the effects of liothyronine occur rapidly, while the effects of other thyroid hormones may persist for several weeks.

Liothyronine may be given in divided daily doses to minimize fluctuations in $T_3$ concentrations.

## Oral Dosage Forms
### LIOTHYRONINE SODIUM TABLETS USP

### Usual adult dose
Mild hypothyroidism—
Initial: Oral, 25 mcg (0.025 mg) a day, with increments of 12.5 or 25 mcg (0.0125 or 0.025 mg) every one or two weeks until the desired result is obtained.
Maintenance: Oral, 25 to 50 mcg (0.025 to 0.05 mg) a day.
Myxedema—
Initial: Oral, 2.5 to 5 mcg (0.0025 to 0.005 mg) a day, with increments of 5 to 10 mcg (0.005 to 0.01 mg) every one or two weeks. When 25 mcg (0.025 mg) a day is reached, increments may sometimes be by 12.5 to 25 mcg (0.0125 to 0.025 mg) every one or two weeks.
Maintenance: Oral, 25 to 50 mcg (0.025 to 0.05 mg) a day.
Simple (nontoxic) goiter—
Initial: Oral, 5 mcg (0.005 mg) a day, with increments of 5 to 10 mcg (0.005 to 0.01 mg) every one or two weeks. When 25 mcg (0.025 mg) a day is reached, increments may be by 12.5 or 25 mcg (0.0125 or 0.025 mg) every week.
Maintenance: Oral, 50 to 100 mcg (0.05 to 0.1 mg) a day.
Note: In patients with cardiovascular disease, the initial dose is 5 mcg (0.005 mg) a day, with increments of no more than 5 mcg every two weeks. In the elderly also, the initial dose is 5 mcg a day, with increments of no more than 5 mcg at the recommended intervals.

### Usual pediatric dose
Cretinism—
USP Advisory Panels do not recommend use for cretinism in children because of significant question about $T_3$ crossing the blood-brain barrier.

### Usual geriatric dose
See *Usual adult dose.*

### Strength(s) usually available
U.S.—
5 mcg (0.005 mg) (Rx) [*Cytomel*].
25 mcg (0.025 mg) (Rx) [*Cytomel* (scored); GENERIC].
50 mcg (0.05 mg) (Rx) [*Cytomel* (scored)].
Canada—
5 mcg (0.005 mg) (base) (Rx) [*Cytomel*].
25 mcg (0.025 mg) (base) (Rx) [*Cytomel* (scored)].

### Packaging and storage
Store below 40 °C (104 °F), preferably between 15 and 30 °C (59 and 86 °F), unless otherwise specified by manufacturer. Store in a tight container.

### Auxiliary labeling
• Do not take other medicines without your doctor's advice.

---

### *LIOTRIX*

## Summary of Differences

Indications: Advantage over thyroid and thyroglobulin is a predictable effect because of standard hormonal content; provision of a product containing $T_3$ (triiodothyronine) no longer considered an advantage because of natural conversion of $T_4$ (thyroxine) to $T_3$ in the tissues.

## Oral Dosage Forms
### LIOTRIX TABLETS USP

### Usual adult and adolescent dose
Hypothyroidism without myxedema—
Initial: Oral, 50 mcg (0.05 mg) of levothyroxine and 12.5 mcg (0.0125 mg) of liothyronine a day, with increments of a like amount at monthly intervals until the desired result is obtained.
Maintenance: Oral, 50 to 100 mcg (0.05 to 0.1 mg) of levothyroxine and 12.5 to 25 mcg (0.0125 to 0.025 mg) of liothyronine a day.
Myxedema or hypothyroidism with cardiovascular disease—
Initial: Oral, 12.5 mcg (0.0125 mg) of levothyroxine and 3.1 mcg (0.0031 mg) of liothyronine a day, with increments of a like amount at two- to three-week intervals until the desired result is obtained.
Maintenance: Oral, 50 to 100 mcg (0.05 to 0.1 mg) of levothyroxine and 12.5 to 25 mcg (0.0125 to 0.025 mg) of liothyronine a day.
Note: In the elderly, the initial dose is one-fourth to one-half the usual adult dose, doubled at six- to eight-week intervals until the desired result is obtained.

**Usual pediatric dose**
Cretinism or severe hypothyroidism—
  See *Usual adult and adolescent dose* for myxedema.
Hypothyroidism—
  See *Usual adult and adolescent dose* for hypothyroidism without myxedema.
Note: Increments in dosage are made at two-week intervals in children.
  Dosage should always be based on results of thyroid function tests.

**Usual geriatric dose**
See *Usual adult and adolescent dose.*

**Strength(s) usually available**
U.S.—

| Levothyroxine sodium (mcg) | Liothyronine sodium (mcg) | Brand name |
|---|---|---|
| 12.5 | 3.1 | *Thyrolar* (Rx) |
| 25 | 6.25 | *Thyrolar* (Rx) |
| 50 | 12.5 | *Thyrolar* (Rx) |
| 100 | 25 | *Thyrolar* (Rx) |
| 150 | 37.5 | *Thyrolar* (Rx) |

Canada—
  Not commercially available.

**Packaging and storage**
Store below 40 °C (104 °F), preferably between 15 and 30 °C (59 and 86 °F), unless otherwise specified by manufacturer. Store in a tight container.

**Auxiliary labeling**
• Do not take other medicines without your doctor's advice.

**Note**
Be very careful always to dispense the same brand of liotrix that a patient has received previously.

---

## *THYROGLOBULIN*

## Summary of Differences
Indications: Disadvantages include variable hormonal content of commercial preparations and fluctuation of $T_3$ (triiodothyronine) and $T_4$ (thyroxine) concentrations produced.

## Oral Dosage Forms
### THYROGLOBULIN TABLETS USP
**Usual adult and adolescent dose**
Hypothyroidism without myxedema—
  Initial: Oral, 32 mg a day, with increments every one or two weeks until the desired result is obtained.
  Maintenance: Oral, 65 to 160 mg a day.
Myxedema or hypothyroidism with cardiovascular disease—
  Initial: Oral, 16 to 32 mg a day, with increments of a like amount every two weeks until the desired result is obtained.
  Maintenance: 65 to 160 mg a day.

**Usual pediatric dose**
Cretinism or severe hypothyroidism—
  See *Usual adult and adolescent dose* for myxedema.
Hypothyroidism—
  See *Usual adult and adolescent dose* for hypothyroidism without myxedema.
Note: Dosage should always be based on results of thyroid function tests.
  Levothyroxine is considered the drug of choice in the treatment of congenital hypothyroidism.

**Strength(s) usually available**
U.S.—
  Not commercially available.
Canada—
  Not commercially available.

**Packaging and storage**
Store below 40 °C (104 °F), preferably between 15 and 30 °C (59 and 86 °F), unless otherwise specified by manufacturer. Store in a tight container.

**Auxiliary labeling**
• Do not take other medicines without your doctor's advice.

---

## *THYROID*

## Summary of Differences
Indications: Disadvantages include variable hormonal content of commercial preparations and fluctuation of $T_3$ (triiodothyronine) and $T_4$ (thyroxine) concentrations produced.

## Oral Dosage Forms
### THYROID TABLETS USP
**Usual adult and adolescent dose**
Hypothyroidism without myxedema—
  Initial: Oral, 60 mg a day, with increments of 30 mg at monthly intervals until the desired result is obtained.
  Maintenance: Oral, 60 to 120 mg a day.
Myxedema or hypothyroidism with cardiovascular disease—
  Initial: Oral, 15 mg a day, increased to 30 mg a day after two weeks, and to 60 mg a day after a further two weeks. Careful clinical assessment is recommended after one month and two months of treatment at 60 mg a day. If necessary, dosage may then be increased to 120 mg a day. If necessary, further increases of 30 or 60 mg may be made.
  Maintenance: Oral, 60 to 120 mg a day.
Note: An initial dose of 7.5 to 15 mg a day is recommended in the elderly; this dose may be doubled every six to eight weeks until the desired result is obtained.

**Usual pediatric dose**
Cretinism or severe hypothyroidism—
  See *Usual adult and adolescent dose* for myxedema.
Hypothyroidism—
  See *Usual adult and adolescent dose* for hypothyroidism without myxedema.
Note: Dosage should always be based on results of thyroid function tests.
  Levothyroxine is considered the drug of choice in the treatment of congenital hypothyroidism.

**Usual geriatric dose**
See *Usual adult and adolescent dose.*

**Strength(s) usually available**
U.S.—
  Regular
    15 mg (Rx) [*Armour Thyroid;* GENERIC].
    30 mg (Rx) [*Armour Thyroid; Westhroid;* GENERIC].
    60 mg (Rx) [*Armour Thyroid; Westhroid;* GENERIC].
    90 mg (Rx) [*Armour Thyroid*].
    120 mg (Rx) [*Armour Thyroid; Westhroid;* GENERIC].
    180 mg (Rx) [*Armour Thyroid; Westhroid;* GENERIC].
    240 mg (Rx) [*Armour Thyroid; Westhroid*].
    300 mg (Rx) [*Armour Thyroid;* GENERIC].
  Bovine
    30 mg (Rx) [*Thyrar*].
    60 mg (Rx) [*Thyrar*].
    120 mg (Rx) [*Thyrar*].
  Strong (contains iodine 0.3%)
    30 mg (Rx) [*Thyroid Strong*].
    60 mg (Rx) [*Thyroid Strong*].
    120 mg (Rx) [*Thyroid Strong*].
    180 mg (Rx) [*Thyroid Strong*].
Canada—
  Regular
    30 mg (Rx) [GENERIC].
    60 mg (Rx) [GENERIC].
    125 mg (Rx) [GENERIC].
Note: Administration of strengths above 120 mg may result in thyrotoxic symptoms.

**Packaging and storage**
Store below 40 °C (104 °F), preferably between 15 and 30 °C (59 and 86 °F), unless otherwise specified by manufacturer. Store in a tight container.

**Auxiliary labeling**
• Do not take other medicines without your doctor's advice.

Revised: 05/22/92
Interim revision: 07/25/94; 01/08/95; 06/26/96

# THYROTROPIN   Systemic

VA CLASSIFICATION (Primary/Secondary): DX900/HS850; AN900

Note: For a listing of dosage forms and brand names by country availability, see *Dosage Forms* section(s). For a listing of brand names for the articles in this monograph, refer to the General Index.

## Category

Thyrotropic hormone; diagnostic aid (thyroid function); antineoplastic.

## Indications

Note: Bracketed information in the *Indications* section refers to uses that are not included in U.S. product labeling.

**Accepted**

Thyroid function studies—Thyrotropin is used diagnostically to determine subclinical hypothyroidism or low thyroid reserve, to differentiate between primary and secondary hypothyroidism, and to differentiate between primary hypothyroidism and euthyroidism in patients whose thyroid function has been suppressed by the administration of thyroid replacement therapy. Thyrotropin is also used to aid in detection of remnants and metastases of thyroid carcinoma, and to demonstrate the presence of dormant thyroid tissue in patients with a toxic adenoma that has suppressed surrounding normal thyroid tissue.

[Thyroid carcinoma (treatment adjunct)]—Thyrotropin is also used as an adjunct in the management of certain types of thyroid carcinoma and resulting metastases.

## Pharmacology/Pharmacokinetics

**Mechanism of action/Effect**

Thyrotropin (thyroid-stimulating hormone [TSH]) is normally secreted from the anterior pituitary as part of a feedback system of thyroid hormone level regulation. It stimulates each step of thyroid hormone synthesis, including iodine uptake; monoiodotyrosine, diiodotyrosine, and levothyroxine synthesis; endocytosis of colloid; and secretion of levothyroxine and liothyronine.

**Onset of action/effects**

Increased secretion of levothyroxine and liothyronine from the thyroid occurs within minutes after administration of thyrotropin, followed by increased iodine uptake and other effects. Within 24 hours, hypertrophy and hyperplasia of the thyroid begin to occur.

**Duration of action**

The effects are reversed rapidly after withdrawal.

## Precautions to Consider

**Cross-sensitivity and/or related problems**

Allergic reactions to thyrotropin are common in patients who have received thyrotropin previously. Thyrotropin should be administered with extreme caution in these patients.

**Pregnancy/Reproduction**

Pregnancy—Studies have not been done in either animals or humans.

FDA Pregnancy Category C.

**Breast-feeding**

It is not known whether thyrotropin is distributed into breast milk. Problems in humans have not been documented.

**Pediatrics**

Caution is necessary in interpreting results of thyroid function tests in neonates, because serum $T_4$ concentrations are transiently elevated and serum $T_3$ concentrations are transiently low, and the infant pituitary is relatively insensitive to the negative feedback effect of thyroid hormones.

**Geriatrics**

No information is available on the relationship of age to the effects of thyrotropin in geriatric patients.

**Laboratory value alterations**

The following have been selected on the basis of their potential clinical significance (possible effect in parentheses where appropriate)—not necessarily inclusive (» = major clinical significance):

With results of *this* test

Thyroid hormones

    (chronic administration may blunt the response to thyrotropin)

With physiology/laboratory test values

Radioactive iodine uptake (RAIU)

    (may be increased 15% or more over basal uptake in patients with hypopituitarism or secondary hypothyroidism)

**Medical considerations/Contraindications**

The medical considerations/contraindications included here have been selected on the basis of their potential clinical significance (reasons given in parentheses where appropriate)—not necessarily inclusive (» = major clinical significance).

*Except under special circumstances, this medication should not be used when the following medical problem exists:*

»  Myocardial infarction, recent

*Risk-benefit should be considered when the following medical problems exist:*

»  Adrenocortical insufficiency, untreated

    (must be corrected before administration of thyrotropin to prevent precipitation of acute adrenocortical insufficiency)

»  Allergy to or previous use of thyrotropin

    (extreme caution is recommended in patients who have previously received thyrotropin because of the risk of an allergic reaction with subsequent use)

»  Cardiovascular disease, including angina pectoris, arteriosclerosis, uncontrolled hypertension

    (because of the risks associated with a sudden increase in metabolic demands as a result of thyroid stimulation)

»  Hypopituitarism, untreated

    (secondary adrenocortical insufficiency must be corrected before administration of thyrotropin to prevent precipitation of acute adrenocortical insufficiency)

**Patient monitoring**

The following may be especially important in patient monitoring (other tests may be warranted in some patients, depending on condition; » = major clinical significance):

Radioactive iodine uptake (RAIU) determinations

    (recommended before administration of first dose of thyrotropin and after last dose when used as a diagnostic aid)

Triiodothyronine ($T_3$) and

Thyroxine ($T_4$), total and free

    (measurement of serum concentrations may be recommended prior to administration of the first dose of thyrotropin and as indicated)

## Side/Adverse Effects

The following side/adverse effects have been selected on the basis of their potential clinical significance (possible signs and symptoms in parentheses where appropriate)—not necessarily inclusive:

**Those indicating need for medical attention**

Incidence rare—much more common in patients who have received thyrotropin previously

    *Allergic reaction* (faintness; itching, redness or swelling at site of injection; skin rash); *anaphylaxis* (tightness of throat; wheezing); *post-injection flare* (redness or swelling at site of injection)

Symptoms of overdose or hyperthyroidism

    *Chest pain; fast or irregular heartbeat; irritability; nervousness; shortness of breath; sweating*

**Those indicating need for medical attention only if they continue or are bothersome**

Incidence more frequent

    *Flushing of face; frequent urge to urinate; headache; nausea and vomiting; stomach discomfort*

## Overdose

For more information on the management of overdose, **contact a Poison Control Center** (see *Poison Control Center Listing*).

**Clinical effects of overdose or hyperthyroidism**

The following effects have been selected on the basis of their potential clinical significance (possible signs and symptoms in parentheses where appropriate)—not necessarily inclusive:

    *Chest pain; fast or irregular heartbeat; irritability; nervousness; shortness of breath; sweating*

**Treatment of overdose**

Treatment of overdose is symptomatic and supportive; treatment of unrecognized adrenal insufficiency may be necessary.

## Patient Consultation

As an aid to patient consultation, refer to *Advice for the Patient, Thyrotropin (Systemic).*

In providing consultation, consider emphasizing the following selected information (» = major clinical significance):

**Before using this medication**

» Conditions affecting use, especially:
   Allergy to or previous use of thyrotropin
   Other medical problems, especially recent myocardial infarction, untreated adrenocortical insufficiency, cardiovascular disease, and untreated hypopituitarism

**Proper use of this medication**

» Importance of receiving every dose of medication
   Importance of close monitoring by the physician
» Proper dosing

**Side/adverse effects**

   Signs of potential side effects, especially allergic reaction, anaphylaxis, and post-injection flare

## Parenteral Dosage Forms

Note: Bracketed uses in the *Dosage Forms* section refer to categories of use and/or indications that are not included in U.S. product labeling.

### THYROTROPIN FOR INJECTION

**Usual adult and adolescent dose**

Determination of thyroid status in patient receiving thyroid medication—
   Intramuscular or subcutaneous, 10 International Units (IU) for one to three days.

   Note: The three-day schedule may be indicated in patients who have received long-term therapy or those with long-standing pituitary myxedema.

Diagnosis of thyroid cancer remnant with $^{123}$I or $^{131}$I after surgery—
   Intramuscular or subcutaneous, 10 IU for three to seven days.

Differential diagnosis of subclinical hypothyroidism or low thyroid reserve, in $^{131}$I uptake determinations—
   Intramuscular or subcutaneous, 10 IU.

[Therapy of thyroid cancer (local tumor or metastases) with $^{131}$I]—
   Intramuscular or subcutaneous, 10 IU for three to eight days.

**Usual pediatric dose**

See *Usual adult and adolescent dose.*

**Size(s) usually available**

U.S.—
   10 IU (Rx) [*Thytropar*].

Canada—
   10 IU (Rx) [*Thytropar*].

**Packaging and storage**

Store below 40 °C (104 °F), preferably between 15 and 30 °C (59 and 86 °F), unless otherwise specified by manufacturer.

**Preparation of dosage form**

Thyrotropin for injection is reconstituted for parenteral use by adding 2 mL of Sodium Chloride Injection USP provided by the manufacturer to the vial containing 10 IU of thyrotropin.

**Stability**

Reconstituted solutions of thyrotropin will retain their potency for at least two weeks between 2 and 8 °C (36 and 46 °F). The diluent provided by the manufacturer contains no preservative.

Revised: 01/31/92
Interim revision: 06/21/94

---

**TIAPROFENIC ACID**—See *Anti-inflammatory Drugs, Nonsteroidal (Systemic)*

---

**TICARCILLIN**—See *Penicillins (Systemic)*

---

**TICARCILLIN-CONTAINING COMBINATIONS—**

Ticarcillin and Clavulanate (Systemic)—See *Penicillins and Beta-lactamase Inhibitors (Systemic)*

---

# TICLOPIDINE   Systemic

VA CLASSIFICATION (Primary): BL700

Note: For a listing of dosage forms and brand names by country availability, see *Dosage Forms* section(s). For a listing of brand names for the articles in this monograph, refer to the General Index.

## Category

Antithrombotic; platelet aggregation inhibitor.

## Indications

**Accepted**

Stroke, thromboembolic, initial or recurrent (prophylaxis)—Ticlopidine is indicated to reduce the risk of a recurrent thromboembolic stroke in patients who have had a completed thrombotic stroke. It is also indicated to reduce the risk of an initial completed thromboembolic stroke in patients who have experienced stroke precursors, such as transient ischemic attack, transient monocular blindness (amarurosis fugax), reversible ischemic neurological deficit (RIND), or minor stroke. In one study in patients who had experienced an ischemic stroke, ticlopidine produced slight but significant neurologic improvement.

Although ticlopidine was somewhat more effective than aspirin in preventing initial strokes in patients with stroke precursors in a major study, it caused significantly more adverse effects than aspirin. Also, ticlopidine may cause neutropenia and agranulocytosis. It is therefore recommended that ticlopidine therapy be reserved for patients unable to take aspirin for stroke prophylaxis and patients who develop strokes despite aspirin therapy, and only when close hematologic monitoring is possible.

## Pharmacology/Pharmacokinetics

**Physicochemical characteristics**

Chemical group—Thienopyridine derivative.
Molecular weight—300.25.

**Mechanism of action/Effect**

Ticlopidine is an inhibitor of platelet aggregation; doses of 250, 375, and 500 mg a day inhibit platelet aggregation by 20 to 50%, 30 to 60%, and 50 to 70%, respectively. Doses higher than 500 mg per day do not produce a significant additional increase in the extent of inhibition.

The mechanism by which ticlopidine inhibits platelet aggregation has not been fully characterized. Ticlopidine inhibits adenosine diphosphate (ADP)-induced binding of fibrinogen to the platelet membrane at a specific receptor site (the glycoprotein IIb-IIIa complex). Release of platelet granule constituents, platelet-platelet interactions, and platelet adhesion to the endothelium and to atheromatous plaque are inhibited. Ticlopidine has no significant inhibitory effect on other endogenous substances known to promote platelet aggregation; it does not interfere with the synthesis or activity of cyclo-oxygenase, phosphodiesterase, or platelet cyclic adenosine monophosphate (cAMP), or with adenosine uptake. Also, ticlopidine does not alter mobilization or influx of calcium ions.

There is a lag time of several days for ticlopidine to exert its maximum effect on platelet function, probably by acting on platelet membranes during megakaryocytopoietic development rather than on already circulating platelets. Ticlopidine-induced inhibition of platelet aggregation persists for the life of the platelet.

Ticlopidine prolongs the template bleeding time, but has no effect in usual assays of coagulation or fibrinolysis.

Ticlopidine also reduces fibrinogen concentrations and blood viscosity, and increases the filterability rates of both whole blood and red cells, which may contribute to the beneficial effects in patients with vascular disease.

### Absorption
Rapid; 80% or more of a dose is absorbed. Absorption is increased when the medication is taken after a meal.

### Protein binding
Very high (98%), primarily to serum albumin and lipoproteins, and, to a lesser extent (15% or less), to alpha-1-acid glycoprotein. Protein binding of metabolites is about 40 to 50%.

### Biotransformation
Hepatic; extensive. At least 20 metabolites have been identified. It has been proposed that 1 or more active metabolites may account for ticlopidine's activity, because the intact agent is an extremely weak platelet aggregation inhibitor *in vitro* at the concentrations achieved *in vivo*. However, no active metabolite has been identified.

Biotransformation of ticlopidine may be saturable; plasma concentrations achieved after a single dose increase disproportionately to the dose. Also, steady-state plasma concentrations are approximately twice as high as those achieved after administration of a single dose. In addition, the percentage of unmetabolized ticlopidine present in the circulation is 5% after a single dose and 15% at steady-state.

### Half-life
Elimination—
> Single 250-mg dose: About 7.9 hours in subjects 20 to 43 years of age; about 12.6 hours in subjects 65 to 76 years of age.
> Repeated dosing with 250 mg twice a day: About 4 days in subjects 20 to 43 years of age; about 5 days in subjects 65 to 76 years of age.

### Onset of action
Repeated dosing with 250 mg twice a day—Inhibition of platelet aggregation is detectable within 2 days; clinically significant inhibition (more than 50%) occurs within 4 days.

### Time to peak concentration
Single 250-mg dose—About 2 hours.

### Peak concentration
Single 250-mg dose—0.4 to 0.6 mcg per mL (mcg/mL) (1.33 to 1.99 micromoles/L); subject to substantial inter- and intrasubject variation. Values obtained when the medication is taken with meals are about 20% higher than those obtained when the medication is taken on an empty stomach. Values obtained when the medication is taken following an aluminum- and magnesium-containing antacid are about 18% lower than those obtained when the medication is not taken after an antacid.

Plasma concentrations may be increased slightly in patients with hepatic function impairment (advanced cirrhosis) and significantly increased in patients with renal function impairment. The area under the curve is increased by about 28% in patients with mild renal function impairment (creatinine clearances of 50 to 80 mL per minute) and by about 60% in patients with moderate renal function impairment (creatinine clearances of 20 to 50 mL per minute).

### Time to steady-state concentration
Repeated administration of 250 mg twice a day—14 to 21 days.

### Steady-state concentration
Repeated administration of 250 mg twice a day—About 1 to 2 mcg/mL (3.33 to 6.66 micromoles/L); may be increased in elderly patients. The area under the curve in elderly subjects receiving 250 mg twice a day for 21 days is 2 to 3 times as high as in younger subjects.

### Time to peak effect
Repeated dosing with 250 mg twice a day: Maximal inhibition of platelet aggregation (60 to 70%) is achieved in 8 to 11 days.

### Duration of action
After discontinuation of treatment, recovery of platelet function occurs as exposed platelets are replaced. In the majority of patients, bleeding time and other platelet function tests return to pretreatment levels within 1 to 2 weeks.

### Elimination
Renal (about 60% of a dose) and biliary/fecal (about 23% of a dose). Unchanged ticlopidine accounts for trace amounts of the quantity eliminated in the urine and about 33% of the quantity eliminated in the feces.

The plasma clearance rate after administration of 250 mg twice a day for 21 days is about 1.52 L per minute in young subjects (average age 29 years) and about 0.56 L per minute in elderly subjects (average age 70 years). The plasma clearance rate is decreased by about 37% in patients with mild renal function impairment (creatinine clearances 50 to 80 mL per minute) and by about 52% in patients with moderate renal function impairment (creatinine clearances 20 to 50 mL per minute).

## Precautions to Consider

### Carcinogenicity/Tumorigenicity
No evidence of carcinogenicity or tumorigenicity was found in a 2-year study in rats receiving oral doses of up to 100 mg per kg of body weight (mg/kg) per day (610 mg per square meter of body surface area [mg/m$^2$] per day). These doses are equivalent to up to 14 times the human clinical dose on an mg/kg basis and 2 times the clinical dose on an mg/m$^2$ basis (based on a human weighing 70-kg and having body surface area of 1.73 m$^2$). Also, no evidence of tumorigenicity or carcinogenicity was found in a 78-week study in mice receiving oral doses of up to 275 mg/kg per day (1180 mg/m$^2$ per day). These doses are equivalent to up to 40 times the clinical dose on a mg/kg basis and 4 times the clinical dose on an mg/m$^2$ basis.

### Mutagenicity
No evidence of mutagenic activity was found in the Ames test, rat hepatocyte DNA-repair assay, Chinese hamster fibroblast chromosomal aberration test (all *in vitro*) or in the mouse spermatozoid morphology test, Chinese hamster micronucleus test, and Chinese hamster bone marrow cell sister chromatid exchange test (all *in vivo*).

### Pregnancy/Reproduction
Fertility—Ticlopidine had no effect on fertility in male or female rats in doses of up to 400 mg/kg per day.

Pregnancy—Adequate and well-controlled studies have not been performed in pregnant women.

No evidence of teratogenicity was found in studies in mice receiving up to 200 mg/kg per day, rats receiving up to 400 mg/kg per day, or rabbits receiving up to 200 g/kg per day. However, maternal toxicity (decreased food intake and weight gain) and fetotoxicity occurred in mice receiving 200 mg/kg per day, rats receiving 400 mg/kg per day, and rabbits receiving 100 g/kg per day.

FDA Pregnancy Category B.

### Breast-feeding
It is not known whether ticlopidine is distributed into human breast milk. However, problems in humans have not been documented.

### Pediatrics
No information is available on the relationship of age to the effects of ticlopidine in pediatric patients. Safety and efficacy have not been established.

### Geriatrics
Appropriate studies performed to date have not demonstrated geriatrics-specific problems that would limit the usefulness of ticlopidine in the elderly. In major clinical trials, approximately 45% of the patients were 65 years of age or older; 12% were more than 75 years of age. Although clearance of ticlopidine is lower in elderly patients than in younger adults, and plasma concentrations are higher than in younger adults, elderly individuals in these studies did not receive lower doses. No overall differences in efficacy or safety were observed.

### Dental
Because of the risk of increased blood loss, it is recommended that ticlopidine be discontinued 10 to 14 days prior to dental surgery.

Ticlopidine may cause neutropenia, which may result in an increased incidence of microbial infection, delayed healing, and gingival bleeding. If severe neutropenia occurs, dental work should be deferred until blood counts have returned to normal. Also, patients should be instructed in proper oral hygiene, including caution in use of regular toothbrushes, dental floss, and toothpicks.

### Surgical
Because of the risk of increased surgical blood loss, it is recommended that ticlopidine be discontinued 10 to 14 days prior to elective surgery. In emergency situations, transfusion of fresh platelets may improve hemostasis. Although intravenous administration of 20 mg of methylprednisolone to ticlopidine-treated patients has been shown to return the bleeding time to normal within 2 hours, the effect of such treatment on perisurgical hemostasis has not been established.

### Drug interactions and/or related problems
The following drug interactions and/or related problems have been selected on the basis of their potential clinical significance (possible mechanism in parentheses where appropriate)—not necessarily inclusive (» = major clinical significance):

Note: Combinations containing any of the following medications, depending on the amount present, may also interact with this medication.

In addition to the interactions listed below, the possibility should be considered that additive or multiple effects leading to an increased risk of bleeding may occur if ticlopidine is administered concurrently with any other medication that has significant platelet aggregation-inhibiting activity or a significant potential for causing hypoprothrombinemia, thrombocytopenia, or gastrointestinal ulceration or hemorrhage.

Antacids, aluminum- and magnesium-containing
(plasma concentrations of ticlopidine are decreased by about 18% when it is administered after an aluminum- and magnesium-containing antacid; information about the effects of single-ingredient antacids on ticlopidine concentrations is not available, but the possibility of a similar effect should be considered; it is recommended that ticlopidine and an antacid be administered at least 1 to 2 hours apart)

» Anticoagulants, coumarin- or indandione-derivative or
» Heparin or
» Thrombolytic agents, such as:
  Alteplase
  Anistreplase
  Streptokinase
  Urokinase
(the possibility of additive effects on blood clotting mechanisms leading to an increased risk of bleeding cannot be discounted; particularly careful clinical monitoring of the patient is recommended if concurrent use is necessary)

(in one study, concurrent administration of warfarin and ticlopidine was associated with an increased risk of medication-induced hepatitis)

» Aspirin or
» Nonsteroidal anti-inflammatory drugs (NSAIDs) or
» Platelet aggregation inhibitors, other (see *Appendix II*)
(concurrent use of ticlopidine with these agents may increase the risk of bleeding because of additive inhibition of platelet aggregation; also, the potential for aspirin- or NSAID-induced gastrointestinal ulceration or hemorrhage exists)

(concurrent use of ticlopidine and aspirin is not recommended; in one study, the risk of bleeding was higher, and bleeding episodes occurred earlier, in patients receiving combined therapy with low doses of aspirin and ticlopidine [81 mg and 100 mg per day, respectively] than in patients receiving larger doses of either agent alone; studies have also shown that the combination of medications prolongs bleeding time to a greater extent than either agent alone; these effects are probably due to potentiation by ticlopidine of aspirin-mediated inhibition of platelet aggregation, since studies have shown that inhibition of collagen-induced platelet aggregation [an effect of aspirin], but not of adenosine diphosphate [ADP]-induced platelet aggregation [an effect of ticlopidine] is increased in the presence of both agents)

Phenytoin
(several cases of elevated phenytoin plasma concentrations with associated somnolence and lethargy have been reported following ticlopidine administration)

Xanthines, such as:
  Aminophylline
  Oxtriphylline
  Theophylline
(theophylline elimination half-life may be increased by about 40%, and total plasma clearance of theophylline decreased by about 35%, when a xanthine is administered to a patient receiving ticlopidine)

## Laboratory value alterations
The following have been selected on the basis of their potential clinical significance (possible effect in parentheses where appropriate)—not necessarily inclusive (» = major clinical significance):

With physiology/laboratory test values
Alkaline phosphatase and
Bilirubin and
Transaminases
(values may be elevated; in clinical studies, the incidence of elevations to more than twice the upper limit of normal was 7.6% for alkaline phosphatase and 3.1% for aspartate aminotransferase [AST (SGOT)]; increases generally occurred within 1 to 4 months after initiation of therapy; although no progressive increases were reported, treatment was discontinued in most patients)

» Bleeding time
(prolongation to 2 to 5 times the pretreatment value is expected during ticlopidine treatment, although maximal effects on bleeding

time may be delayed for some time after platelet aggregation tests indicate maximal inhibition; ticlopidine-induced prolongation of bleeding time may be reduced in patients receiving chronic glucocorticoid treatment, although ticlopidine's effect on ADP-induced platelet aggregation is not altered; also, prolongation of bleeding time may be reversed by a single intravenous dose of 20 mg of methylprednisolone)

Cholesterol, total and
Triglycerides
(serum concentrations may be elevated; in clinical studies, total serum cholesterol was increased by 8 to 10% after about 1 month of ticlopidine treatment, but further increases did not occur thereafter; also, the ratios of lipoprotein subfractions were not altered)

» Neutrophil count and
Platelet count
(may be decreased; in clinical trials, the overall incidence of neutropenia [absolute neutrophil count (ANC) <1200 neutrophils/mm$^3$] was 2.4%, and that of severe neutropenia [ANC <450 neutrophils/mm$^3$] about 0.8%; neutropenia generally occurs between 3 and 12 weeks after initiation of treatment, is associated with inhibition of granulocyte cell line maturation, and is generally reversed within a few weeks after discontinuation of treatment)

(thrombocytopenia may occur in conjunction with, or independently of, neutropenia, generally between 3 and 12 weeks after initiation of treatment; in clinical trials, the incidence of thrombocytopenia was 0.4%; recovery generally occurs after discontinuation)

## Medical considerations/Contraindications
The medical considerations/contraindications included here have been selected on the basis of their potential clinical significance (reasons given in parentheses where appropriate)—not necessarily inclusive (» = major clinical significance).

*Except under special circumstances, this medication should not be used when the following medical problems exist:*
» Bleeding, active and
» Hemophilia or other coagulation defects or hemostatic disorders
(risk of severe bleeding)
» Hematopoietic disorders such as:
Neutropenia
Thrombocytopenia
(may be exacerbated)
» Hepatic function impairment, severe
(increased risk of bleeding because severe hepatic function impairment may result in decreased synthesis of clotting factor precursors)

*Risk-benefit should be considered when the following medical problems exist:*
» Any condition in which there is a significant risk of bleeding, such as:

Gastrointestinal ulceration
Surgery
Trauma
» Renal function impairment, severe
(clearance of ticlopidine decreases, and concentrations increase, with increasing degrees of renal function impairment; although ticlopidine is well tolerated by patients with mild or moderate degrees of renal function impairment, caution and close monitoring are recommended in patients with severe renal disease because experience in such patients is limited; a reduction in dosage may be needed, but studies with reduced doses of ticlopidine have not been done)

Sensitivity to ticlopidine

## Patient monitoring
The following may be especially important in patient monitoring (other tests may be warranted in some patients, depending on condition; » = major clinical significance):

Bleeding time and
Platelet count
(determinations may be needed to assess the risk of bleeding complications when procedures that have a significant risk of bleeding, such as surgery or dental work, are needed during or shortly following ticlopidine therapy)

» Complete blood count and
» Platelet count and
» White blood cell differentials
(because of the risk of neutropenia and/or thrombocytopenia, these checks should be performed every 2 weeks, starting at baseline before treatment is begun, for the first 3 months of treatment; more

frequent monitoring may be needed for patients whose absolute neutrophil counts are declining or are 30% below the baseline count, since severe neutropenia may develop rapidly [over a few days]. Treatment should be discontinued if clinical evaluation and repeat laboratory testing confirm the presence of neutropenia or thrombocytopenia [neutrophil count reduced to 1200 per cubic millimeter or lower; platelet count reduced to 80,000 per cubic millimeter or lower]. If treatment is discontinued for any reason within the first 3 months, continued monitoring for at least another 2 weeks following discontinuation is recommended because of ticlopidine's long plasma half-life. Because the risk of these complications decreases substantially after the first 3 months of therapy [although cases have been reported after several months or even years of treatment], further testing is needed only if signs and symptoms suggestive of severe neutropenia or thrombocytopenia occur)

## Side/Adverse Effects

Note: Most of the side/adverse effects reported with ticlopidine, including *neutropenia or agranulocytosis, thrombocytopenia, gastrointestinal disturbances, and skin rash,* appear within the first 3 months of treatment, although some may occur or recur several months later. Rarely, *neutropenia, thrombocytopenia, or thrombotic thrombocytopenic purpura* has occurred after years of treatment. Fatalities associated with *severe neutropenia, agranulocytosis, pancytopenia, aplastic anemia, immune thrombocytopenia, or thrombotic thrombocytopenic purpura* have been reported.

Ticlopidine-induced *gastrointestinal disturbances* may occur in up to 40% of the patients receiving the medication. They are generally mild and usually disappear within 1 or 2 weeks without discontinuation of treatment; however, about 13% of the patients withdrew from clinical studies because of them. In some cases of severe or bloody diarrhea, colitis was later diagnosed.

In addition to the side/adverse effects listed below, rare cases of the following have been reported in postmarketing surveillance programs: *pancytopenia, hemolytic anemia with reticulocytosis, allergic pneumonitis, systemic lupus erythematosus, peripheral neuropathy, vasculitis, serum sickness, arthropathy, nephrotic syndrome, myositis, hyponatremia, immune thrombocytopenia, thrombotic thrombocytopenic purpura, eosinophilia, bone marrow depression, aplastic anemia, hepatocellular jaundice, hepatic necrosis, peptic ulcer, renal failure, sepsis, and angioedema.* A causal relationship has not always been established.

The following side/adverse effects have been selected on the basis of their potential clinical significance (possible signs and symptoms in parentheses where appropriate)—not necessarily inclusive:

### Those indicating need for medical attention
Incidence more frequent
  *Skin rash*—incidence 5.1%
  Note: Usually disappears within several days after treatment is discontinued, and may not recur upon reinstitution of treatment. However, there have been rare reports of severe rashes including Stevens-Johnson syndrome, erythema multiforme, and exfoliative dermatitis.

Incidence less frequent
  *Bleeding complications* (abdominal pain [severe] or swelling; back pain; blood in eyes; blood in urine; bloody or black, tarry stools; bruising or purple areas on skin; coughing up blood; decreased alertness; dizziness; headache, severe or continuing; joint pain or swelling; nosebleeds; paralysis or problems with coordination; stammering or other difficulty in speaking; unusually heavy bleeding or oozing from cuts or wounds; unusually heavy or unexpected menstrual bleeding; vomiting of blood or material that looks like coffee grounds)—depending on the site of bleeding; in clinical studies the incidence of intracerebral bleeding was 0.5% and that of epistaxis was 0.5 to 1%; *itching of skin*—incidence 1.3%; *neutropenia, including agranulocytosis* (fever, chills, sore throat, other signs of infection; ulcers, sores, or white spots in mouth)—incidence 2.4% overall, 0.8% severe [absolute neutrophil count (ANC) <450 neutrophils/mm³ ]; *purpura* (red or purple spots on skin, varying in size from pinpoint to large bruises)—incidence 2.2%

Incidence rare
  *Hepatitis or cholestatic jaundice* (yellow eyes or skin); *hives*—incidence 0.5 to 1%; *ringing or buzzing in ears*—incidence 0.5 to 1%; *skin rash, severe, including erythema multiforme* (fever; malaise; red skin lesions, often with a purple center); *or Stevens-Johnson syndrome* (blistering, peeling, or loosening of skin and mucous membranes; fever; malaise); *or exfoliative dermatitis* (fever; malaise; red, thickened, or scaly skin); *thrombocytopenia* (unusual bleeding or

bruising; black, tarry stools; blood in urine or stools; pinpoint red spots on skin)—usually asymptomatic; incidence 0.4%
  Note: Bulla formation involving the eyes or other organ systems may occur with *Stevens-Johnson syndrome*.
    *Thrombocytopenia* may occur independently of, or in conjunction with, neutropenia.

### Those indicating need for medical attention only if they continue or are bothersome
Incidence more frequent
  *Abdominal pain*—incidence 3.7%; *diarrhea*—incidence 12.5%; *indigestion*—incidence 7%; *nausea*—incidence 7%
Incidence less frequent
  *Bloating or gas*—incidence 1.5%; *dizziness*—incidence 1.1%; *vomiting*—incidence 1.9%

## Overdose
Only one case of overdose has been reported, in which a single 6000-mg dose was ingested by a 38-year-old male. The patient's bleeding time was prolonged and the alanine aminotransferase (ALT [SGPT]) value was increased. There were no other abnormalities or symptoms, and the patient recovered without treatment.

For more information on the management of overdose or unintentional ingestion, **contact a Poison Control Center** (see *Poison Control Center Listing*).

## Patient Consultation
As an aid to patient consultation, refer to *Advice for the Patient, Ticlopidine (Systemic)*.

In providing consultation, consider emphasizing the following selected information (» = major clinical significance):

**Before using this medication**
» Conditions affecting use, especially:
    Sensitivity to ticlopidine
    Dental—Risk of increased blood loss during dental procedures
    Other medications, especially anticoagulants or platelet aggregation inhibitors
    Other medical problems, especially bleeding (active), medical problems in which there is a significant risk of bleeding, hematopoietic disorders, severe hepatic function impairment, and severe renal function impairment
    Surgical—Risk of increased blood loss during surgical procedures

**Proper use of this medication**
    Taking medication with food to increase absorption and to reduce the risk of gastrointestinal irritation
    Compliance with prescribed treatment regimen
» Proper dosing
    Missed dose: Taking as soon as possible; not taking if almost time for next dose; not doubling doses
» Proper storage

**Precautions while using this medication**
» Importance of regular blood tests to detect potential adverse effects during the first 3 months of treatment
» Need to inform all health care providers of use of medication; medication should be discontinued 10 to 14 days prior to elective procedures with a risk of bleeding
» Because of risk of bleeding, obtaining physician's opinion before participating in activities with substantial risk of injury and contacting physician immediately if injury occurs
» Notifying physician immediately if signs and symptoms of bleeding, infection, or thrombocytopenia occur
    Possibility that risk of bleeding may continue for 1 to 2 weeks after treatment is discontinued

**Side/adverse effects**
    Signs of potential side effects, especially skin rash, bleeding complications, itching of skin, neutropenia, agranulocytosis, purpura, hepatitis or cholestatic jaundice, hives, ringing or buzzing in the ears, erythema multiforma, Stevens-Johnson syndrome, exfoliative dermatitis, and thrombocytopenia

## General Dosing Information
Ticlopidine should be taken with meals to achieve maximum absorption and reduce the risk of gastrointestinal side effects.

It is recommended that ticlopidine therapy be discontinued temporarily if an injury that results in a substantial risk of bleeding occurs.

It is recommended that ticlopidine therapy be discontinued 10 to 14 days prior to elective surgery, including dental extraction, because of the risk of increased blood loss.

#### Diet/Nutrition
Absorption of ticlopidine is increased when the medication is taken after a meal.

#### For treatment of adverse effects
Recommended treatment consists of the following
- In general—Monitoring the patient and instituting supportive measures as needed.
- For bleeding complications—Although administration of methylprednisolone (20 mg, intravenously) returns the bleeding time to normal in ticlopidine-treated patients, clinical experience indicating that such treatment improves hemostasis is lacking. Platelet transfusions may be helpful, although they are usually not indicated for thrombotic thrombocytopenic purpura occuring in patients taking ticlopidine. In addition, other measures to control bleeding in specific areas must be employed as needed.

## Oral Dosage Forms
### TICLOPIDINE HYDROCHLORIDE TABLETS

#### Usual adult dose
Antithrombotic—
    Oral, 250 mg twice a day, taken with food.

#### Usual pediatric and adolescent dose
Safety and efficacy in patients up to 18 years of age have not been established.

#### Usual geriatric dose
See *Usual adult dose*.

#### Strength(s) usually available
U.S.—
    250 mg (Rx) [*Ticlid* (citric acid; magnesium stearate; microcrystalline cellulose; povidone; starch; stearic acid)].

Canada—
    250 mg (Rx) [*Ticlid* (citric acid; magnesium stearate; microcrystalline cellulose; povidone; corn starch; stearic acid)].

#### Packaging and storage
Store below 40 °C (104 °F), preferably between 15 and 30 °C (59 and 86 °F), unless otherwise specified by manufacturer.

#### Auxiliary labeling
- Take with food.

### Selected Bibliography

Gent M, Blakely JA, Easton JD, et al. The Canadian American ticlopidine study (CATS) in thromboembolic stroke. The Lancet 1989; 333: 1215-20.

Hass WK, Easton D, Adams HP Jr, et al. A randomized trial comparing ticlopidine hydrochloride with aspirin for the prevention of stroke in high-risk patients. N Engl J Med 1989; 321: 501-7.

Revised: 08/06/96

---

**TIMOLOL**—See *Beta-adrenergic Blocking Agents (Ophthalmic); Beta-adrenergic Blocking Agents (Systemic)*

---

**TIMOLOL-CONTAINING COMBINATIONS—**
Timolol and Hydrochlorothiazide (Systemic)—See *Beta-adrenergic Blocking Agents and Thiazide Diuretics (Systemic)*

---

**TIOCONAZOLE**—See *Antifungals, Azole (Vaginal)*

---

# TIOPRONIN    Systemic†

VA CLASSIFICATION (Primary): GU900

Note: For a listing of dosage forms and brand names by country availability, see *Dosage Forms* section(s). For a listing of brand names for the articles in this monograph, refer to the General Index.

---

†Not commercially available in Canada.

---

## Category
Antiurolithic (cystine calculi).

## Indications
#### Accepted
Cystinuria (treatment) or

Renal calculi, cystine (prophylaxis)—Tiopronin is indicated for the prevention of cystine kidney stones in patients with severe homozygous cystinuria who have a urinary cystine concentration greater than 500 mg a day; are resistant to treatment with high fluid intake, alkali, and diet modification; or have had adverse reactions to penicillamine.

## Pharmacology/Pharmacokinetics

#### Physicochemical characteristics
Molecular weight—163.19.

#### Mechanism of action/Effect
Tiopronin is an active reducing agent that undergoes thiol-disulfide exchange with cystine (cysteine-cysteine disulfide) to form tiopronin-cystine disulfide, which is more water-soluble than cystine and is readily excreted. As a result, urinary cystine calculi are prevented.

#### Distribution
Up to 48% of a dose appears in the urine during the first 4 hours and 78% by 72 hours.

#### Onset of action
Rapid.

#### Duration of action
Very short; effect of tiopronin shown to disappear within 8 to 10 hours after administration.

#### Elimination
Renal.

## Precautions to Consider

#### Cross-sensitivity and/or related problems
Patients sensitive to penicillamine may be sensitive to this medication also.

#### Carcinogenicity
Long-term carcinogenicity studies in animals have not been performed.

#### Pregnancy/Reproduction
Pregnancy—Adequate and well-controlled studies in humans have not been done.

Since penicillamine has been shown to cause skeletal defects, cleft palates, and an increased number of resorptions when administered to rats at 10 times the recommended human dose, a similar teratogenic effect might be expected for tiopronin. Also, high doses of tiopronin in animals have been shown to interfere with maintenance of pregnancy and viability of the fetus.

FDA Pregnancy Category C.

#### Breast-feeding
Tiopronin may be distributed into breast milk. It is recommended that mothers taking tiopronin not breast-feed because of potentially serious adverse effects on nursing infants.

#### Pediatrics
Appropriate studies on the relationship of age to the effects of tiopronin have not been performed in the pediatric population. However, no pediatrics-specific problems have been documented to date.

#### Geriatrics
Although appropriate studies on the relationship of age to the effects of tiopronin have not been performed in the geriatric population, no geriatrics-specific problems have been documented to date. However, elderly patients are more likely to have age-related renal function impairment, which may require adjustment of dosage or dosing interval in patients receiving tiopronin.

#### Drug interactions and/or related problems
The following drug interactions and/or related problems have been selected on the basis of their potential clinical significance (possible mechanism in parentheses where appropriate)—not necessarily inclusive (» = major clinical significance):

Note: Combinations containing any of the following medications, depending on the amount present, may also interact with this medication.

Bone marrow depressants (See *Appendix II* )
  (concurrent use of these medications with tioronin may increase the leukopenic and/or thrombocytopenic effects; if concurrent use is required, close observation for toxic effects should be considered)

Hepatotoxic medications (See *Appendix II* )
  (concurrent use of these medications with tioronin may increase the hepatotoxic effects of either medication)

Nephrotoxic medications (See *Appendix II* )
  (concurrent use of these medications with tioronin may increase the nephrotoxic effects of either medication)

## Medical considerations/Contraindications

The medical considerations/contraindications included here have been selected on the basis of their potential clinical significance (reasons given in parentheses where appropriate)—not necessarily inclusive (» = major clinical significance).

*Risk-benefit should be considered when the following medical problems exist:*

» Agranulocytosis, aplastic anemia or thrombocytopenia, history of
  (risk of recurrence)

Hepatic function impairment
  (condition may be exacerbated)

Renal function impairment, current or history of
  (cumulative effects of tioronin may occur)

Sensitivity to tioronin or penicillamine

## Patient monitoring

The following may be especially important in patient monitoring (other tests may be warranted in some patients, depending on condition; » = major clinical significance):

Abdominal roentgenogram (KUB)
  (recommended on a yearly basis to monitor the size and appearance/disappearance of stone[s])

Albumin concentrations, serum and
Hemoglobin determinations and
Urinary protein determinations, 24-hour
  (recommended at frequent intervals)

Blood cell counts, white and
» Platelet counts, direct
  (therapy should be discontinued when peripheral white count is below 3500 per cubic mm and platelet count is below 100,000 cubic mm)

Hepatic function determinations
  (recommended at 2, 4, and 6 weeks of therapy)

Urinalysis, routine
  (recommended every 3 to 6 months during treatment; proteinuria may develop from membranous glomerulopathy and may be severe enough to cause nephrotic syndrome)

Urinary cystine concentrations
Urinary pH, 24-hour, determinations with pH electrode
  (determinations recommended after the first and third months of therapy and every 6 months thereafter to determine effectiveness of tioronin in treatment of cystinuria)

## Side/Adverse Effects

The following side/adverse effects have been selected on the basis of their potential clinical significance (possible signs and symptoms in parentheses where appropriate)—not necessarily inclusive:

**Those indicating need for medical attention**
Incidence more frequent
  *Dermatologic effects specifically ecchymosis* (pain, swelling, tenderness of subcutaneous tissue in affected area); *elastosis perforans serpiginosa; or pemphigus* (itching of skin); *skin rash or itching; ulcers or sores in mouth; urticaria* (hives); *jaundice* (yellow skin or eyes)

  Note: If *pemphigus-type reaction* develops, tioronin therapy should be stopped. Steroid treatment may be necessary.

  *Skin rash* may appear during the first few months of treatment, but may be controlled with antihistamine therapy. Less commonly, rash may appear late in the course of treatment (after more than 6 months); this rash is usually located on the trunk and is associated with intense pruritus. The early rash recedes when tioronin therapy is discontinued and seldom recurs when treatment is restarted at a lower dosage. The later rash recedes slowly after discontinuation of tioronin and usually recurs when treatment is restarted.

Incidence less frequent
  *Allergic reactions, specifically adenopathy* (tenderness of glands); *arthralgia* (pain in joints); *or chills; dyspnea or respiratory distress* (difficulty in breathing); *fever; increased bleeding; laryngeal edema* (difficulty in breathing; difficulty in swallowing; hoarseness); *myalgia* (muscle pain); *weakness; hematologic abnormalities, specifically anemia* (unusual tiredness or weakness); *eosinophilia; leukopenia* (sore throat and fever); *or thrombocytopenia* (unusual bleeding or bruising); *renal effects, specifically edema* (swelling of feet or lower legs); *hematuria* (bloody urine); *nephrotic syndrome* (cloudy or bloody urine; high blood pressure; swelling of feet or lower legs); *or proteinuria* (cloudy urine)

  Note: Drug-induced *fever* may develop during the first month of therapy. This will recede when tioronin is discontinued; therapy can then be reinstated at smaller doses and increased until desired levels are achieved.

    *Leukopenia* of granulocytic series may develop without eosinophilia. *Thrombocytopenia* may be immunologic in origin or occur on an idiosyncratic basis. The reduction in peripheral white blood cell count to less than 3500 per cubic mm or in platelet count to below 100,000 per cubic mm mandates cessation of therapy.

Incidence rare
  *Goodpasture's syndrome* (difficulty in breathing, spitting up blood, or unusual tiredness or weakness); *myasthenia gravis syndrome* (difficulty in breathing, chewing, talking, or swallowing; double vision; muscle weakness); *pulmonary effects, specifically bronchiolitis* (cough; difficulty in breathing; fever); *dyspnea* (difficulty in breathing); *hemoptysis* (coughing up blood); *pharyngitis* (hoarseness; sore throat); *or pulmonary infiltrates* (cough; chest pain; unusual tiredness or weakness); *systemic lupus erythematosus (SLE)–like syndrome* (fever, general feeling of discomfort, illness, or weakness; joint pain; skin rash, blisters, hives or itching; swelling of lymph glands)

  Note: With abnormal urinary findings of *hemoptysis* and *pulmonary infiltrates,* tioronin treatment should be stopped.

    Appearance of *myasthenia gravis syndrome* requires cessation of tioronin therapy.

    *SLE-like syndrome* may be associated with a positive antinuclear antibody test, but not necessarily nephropathy. It may require discontinuance of tioronin treatment.

**Those indicating need for medical attention only if they continue or are bothersome**
Incidence more frequent
  *Gastrointestinal disturbances, specifically abdominal pain; anorexia* (loss of appetite); *bloating or gas; diarrhea or soft stools; or nausea and vomiting; warts; wrinkling, peeling, or unusually dry skin*
Incidence less frequent
  *Changes in taste or smell*

## Patient Consultation

As an aid to patient consultation, refer to *Advice for the Patient, Tioronin (Systemic).*

In providing consultation, consider emphasizing the following selected information (» = major clinical significance):

**Before using this medication**
» Conditions affecting use, especially:
    Sensitivity to tioronin or penicillamine
    Breast-feeding—May be distributed into breast milk; may cause potentially serious adverse effects in nursing infants
    Other medical problems, especially agranulocytosis, aplastic anemia, or thrombocytopenia (history of)

**Proper use of this medication**
  Taking medication on empty stomach
  Importance of high fluid intake, especially at night
  Possible need for low-methionine diet
  Compliance with therapy; checking with physician before discontinuing medication since interruption of therapy may cause sensitivity reactions when therapy is reinstituted
» Proper dosing
  Missed dose: Taking as soon as possible; not taking if almost time for next dose; not doubling doses
» Proper storage

**Precautions while using this medication**
  Regular visits to physician to check progress during therapy

**Side/adverse effects**
Signs of potential side effects, especially dermatologic effects, allergic reactions, hematologic abnormalities, jaundice, renal effects, Goodpasture's syndrome, myasthenia gravis syndrome, pulmonary effects, and systemic lupus erythematosus (SLE)–like syndrome

## General Dosing Information

Tiopronin therapy should be added to a treatment regimen only when the patient continues to form cystine stones on a high fluid intake (3 liters per day) and alkali therapy to maintain a urinary pH at a high normal range (6.5 to 7.0). Calcium phosphate nephrolithiasis may result if urinary alkalinization (pH is increased above 7.0) is continued without aggressively maintaining a high fluid intake.

To help prevent the formation of cystine stones, a high fluid intake is recommended. The patient should drink 2 full glasses (8 ounces each) of water with each meal and at bedtime. The patient should drink another 2 glasses (8 ounces each) during the night when the urine is more concentrated and more acidic than during the day.

For patients who have developed toxicity to penicillamine, tiopronin therapy may be initiated at lower doses.

Dosage of tiopronin should be based on the amount required to keep the urinary cystine concentration below the solubility limit (generally < 250 mg per L). The extent of cystine excretion is generally dependent on tiopronin dosage.

**Diet/Nutrition**
A diet low in methionine may be necessary to minimize cystine production (methionine is a precursor to cystine and is found in animal proteins such as milk, eggs, cheese, and fish). This diet is not recommended in growing children or during pregnancy because of its low protein content.

Tiopronin should be taken on an empty stomach (either 30 minutes before meals or 2 hours after meals) for faster absorption.

## Oral Dosage Forms

### TIOPRONIN TABLETS

**Usual adult dose**
Oral, initially, 800 mg a day in three divided doses, adjusted according to urinary cystine concentrations.

**Usual pediatric dose**
Children up to 9 years of age—Dosage has not been established.
Children 9 years of age and older—Oral, initially 15 mg per kg of body weight a day in three divided doses, adjusted according to urinary cystine concentrations.

**Strength(s) usually available**
U.S.—
100 mg (Rx) [*Thiola* (sugar-coated)].
Canada—
Not commercially available.

**Packaging and storage**
Store between 15 and 30 °C (59 and 86 °F), in a tight container, unless otherwise specified by manufacturer.

**Auxiliary labeling**
• Take on an empty stomach.

Revised: 05/19/92
Interim revision: 08/09/94

---

## TITANIUM DIOXIDE—See *Sunscreen Agents (Topical)*

---

## TITANIUM DIOXIDE-CONTAINING COMBINATIONS—

Aminobenzoic Acid and Titanium Dioxide (Topical)—See *Sunscreen Agents (Topical)*
Menthyl Anthranilate and Titanium Dioxide (Topical)—See *Sunscreen Agents (Topical)*
Octocrylene, Octyl Methoxycinnamate, Octyl Salicylate, Oxybenzone, and Titanium Dioxide (Topical)—See *Sunscreen Agents (Topical)*
Octocrylene, Octyl Methoxycinnamate, Oxybenzone, and Titanium Dioxide (Topical)—See *Sunscreen Agents (Topical)*
Octocrylene, Octyl Methoxycinnamate, and Titanium Dioxide (Topical)—See *Sunscreen Agents (Topical)*
Octyl Methoxycinnamate, Octyl Salicylate, Oxybenzone, Padimate O, and Titanium Dioxide (Topical)—See *Sunscreen Agents (Topical)*
Octyl Methoxycinnamate, Octyl Salicylate, Oxybenzone, Phenylbenzimidazole, and Titanium Dioxide (Topical)—See *Sunscreen Agents (Topical)*
Octyl Methoxycinnamate, Octyl Salicylate, Oxybenzone, and Titanium Dioxide (Topical)—See *Sunscreen Agents (Topical)*
Octyl Methoxycinnamate, Octyl Salicylate, Phenylbenzimidazole, and Titanium Dioxide (Topical)—See *Sunscreen Agents (Topical)*
Octyl Methoxycinnamate, Octyl Salicylate, and Titanium Dioxide (Topical)—See *Sunscreen Agents (Topical)*
Octyl Methoxycinnamate, Oxybenzone, Padimate O, and Titanium Dioxide (Topical)—See *Sunscreen Agents (Topical)*
Octyl Methoxycinnamate, Oxybenzone, and Titanium Dioxide (Topical)—See *Sunscreen Agents (Topical)*
Titanium Dioxide and Zinc Oxide (Topical)—See *Sunscreen Agents (Topical)*

---

## TOBRAMYCIN—See *Aminoglycosides (Systemic)*; *Tobramycin (Ophthalmic)*

---

# TOBRAMYCIN   Ophthalmic

VA CLASSIFICATION (Primary): OP201
Note: For a listing of dosage forms and brand names by country availability, see *Dosage Forms* section(s). For a listing of brand names for the articles in this monograph, refer to the General Index.

## Category
Antibacterial (ophthalmic).

## Indications
Note: Bracketed information in the *Indications* section refers to uses that are not included in U.S. product labeling.

**Accepted**
Ocular infections (treatment)—Ophthalmic tobramycin is indicated in the treatment of external ocular infections caused by susceptible organisms.
[Blepharitis, bacterial (treatment)]
[Blepharoconjunctivitis (treatment)]
[Conjunctivitis, bacterial (treatment)]
[Dacryocystitis (treatment)]
[Keratitis, bacterial (treatment)]
[Keratoconjunctivitis (treatment)] or

[Meibomianitis (treatment)]—Ophthalmic tobramycin is used as a primary agent in the treatment of bacterial blepharitis, blepharoconjunctivitis, bacterial conjunctivitis, dacryocystitis, bacterial keratitis, keratoconjunctivitis, and meibomianitis caused by coagulase-negative and coagulase-positive staphylococci, *Pseudomonas aeruginosa*, indole-positive and indole-negative *Proteus* species, *Escherichia coli*, *Klebsiella pneumoniae*, *Hemophilus influenzae*, *H. aegyptius*, *Enterobacter aerogenes*, *Moraxella lacunata* (Morax-Axenfeld bacillus), and *Neisseria* species, including *N. gonorrhoeae*.

[Keratitis, exposure (treatment)] or
[Keratitis, neuroparalytic (treatment)]—Ophthalmic tobramycin is used in the treatment of exposure keratitis and neuroparalytic keratitis when a secondary bacterial infection is present.

Note: Not all species or strains of a particular organism may be susceptible to tobramycin.

**Unaccepted**
Tobramycin is not effective against most strains of group D streptococci.

## Pharmacology/Pharmacokinetics

**Physicochemical characteristics**
Chemical group—Aminoglycoside.
Molecular weight—467.52.

## Mechanism of action/Effect

Actively transported across the bacterial cell membrane, binds to a specific receptor protein on the 30 S subunit of bacterial ribosomes, and interferes with an initiation complex between messenger RNA (mRNA) and the 30 S subunit, inhibiting protein synthesis. RNA may be misread, thus producing nonfunctional proteins. Polyribosomes are split apart and are unable to synthesize protein.

Note: Aminoglycosides are bactericidal, while most other antibiotics that interfere with protein synthesis are bacteriostatic.

## Absorption

May be absorbed in minute quantities following topical application to the eye.

# Precautions to Consider

## Cross-sensitivity and/or related problems

Patients sensitive to other aminoglycosides may be sensitive to this medication also.

## Pregnancy/Reproduction

Fertility—Adequate and well-controlled studies in humans have not been done.

Studies in 3 types of animals, given doses of up to 33 times the usual human systemic dose, have not shown that tobramycin causes impaired fertility.

Pregnancy—Adequate and well-controlled studies in humans have not been done.

Studies in 3 types of animals, given doses of up to 33 times the usual human systemic dose, have not shown that tobramycin causes adverse effects on the fetus.

FDA Pregnancy Category B.

## Breast-feeding

Ophthalmic aminoglycosides may be absorbed, especially if tissue damage is present. However, ophthalmic tobramycin is unlikely to be distributed into breast milk in significant amounts since the ophthalmic dose is small. In addition, aminoglycosides are poorly absorbed from the gastrointestinal tract. Therefore, it is unlikely that the nursing infant would absorb significant amounts of tobramycin or that it would cause serious problems in the nursing infant.

## Pediatrics

Studies performed to date have not demonstrated pediatrics-specific problems that would limit the usefulness of ophthalmic tobramycin in children.

## Geriatrics

No information is available on the relationship of age to the effects of ophthalmic tobramycin in geriatric patients.

## Medical considerations/Contraindications

The medical considerations/contraindications included here have been selected on the basis of their potential clinical significance (reasons given in parentheses where appropriate)—not necessarily inclusive (» = major clinical significance).

*Risk-benefit should be considered when the following medical problem exists:*

Sensitivity to tobramycin

# Side/Adverse Effects

Note: Ophthalmic tobramycin should be discontinued if hypersensitivity reactions occur.

The following side/adverse effects have been selected on the basis of their potential clinical significance (possible signs and symptoms in parentheses where appropriate)—not necessarily inclusive:

**Those indicating need for medical attention**
Incidence less frequent
*Hypersensitivity* (itching, redness, swelling, or other sign of eye or eyelid irritation not present before therapy)

**Those indicating need for medical attention only if they continue or are bothersome**
Incidence less frequent
*Burning or stinging of the eyes*

**Those not indicating need for medical attention**
For ophthalmic ointment dosage form only
*Blurred vision*

# Overdose

For more information on the management of overdose or unintentional ingestion, **contact a Poison Control Center** (see *Poison Control Center Listing*).

## Clinical effects of overdose

The following effects have been selected on the basis of their potential clinical significance (possible signs and symtoms in parentheses where appropriate)—not necessarily inclusive:
Acute and chronic
*Increased watering of the eyes; itching, redness, or swelling of the eyes or eyelids*

# Patient Consultation

As an aid to patient consultation, refer to *Advice for the Patient, Tobramycin (Ophthalmic).*

In providing consultation, consider emphasizing the following selected information (» = major clinical significance):

**Before using this medication**
»  Conditions affecting use, especially:
      Sensitivity to tobramycin or other aminoglycosides

**Proper use of this medication**
Proper administration technique for ophthalmic solution and ointment
»  Compliance with full course of therapy
»  Proper dosing
      Missed dose: Applying as soon as possible; not applying if almost time for next dose
»  Proper storage

**Precautions while using this medication**
Checking with physician if no improvement within a few days

**Side/adverse effects**
Ophthalmic ointments may cause blurred vision for a few minutes after application
Signs of potential side effects, especially hypersensitivity

# General Dosing Information

Tobramycin ophthalmic solution is not for injection into the eye.

Although some manufacturers recommend doses of 2 drops of ophthalmic solutions at appropriate intervals, the conjunctival sac usually holds less than 1 drop.

When instilling two different ophthalmic solutions, wait at least 5 minutes between instillations to avoid a "wash-out" effect.

At night the ophthalmic ointment may be used as an adjunct to the ophthalmic solution to provide prolonged contact with the infection.

If hypersensitivity develops, therapy with ophthalmic tobramycin should be discontinued.

# Ophthalmic Dosage Forms

## TOBRAMYCIN OPHTHALMIC OINTMENT USP

### Usual adult and adolescent dose

Mild to moderate infections—
      Topical, to the conjunctiva, a thin strip (approximately 1.25 cm) of ointment every eight to twelve hours.
Severe infections—
      Topical, to the conjunctiva, a thin strip (approximately 1.25 cm) of ointment every three to four hours. Treatment should be continued until improvement occurs; then the frequency of administration should be reduced.

### Usual pediatric dose

Mild to moderate infections—
      See *Usual adult and adolescent dose.*
Severe infections—
      See *Usual adult and adolescent dose.*

### Strength(s) usually available

U.S.—
      0.3% (Rx) [*Tobrex* (chlorobutanol 0.5%)].
Canada—
      0.3% (Rx) [*Tobrex* (chlorobutanol 0.5%)].

### Packaging and storage

Store below 40 °C (104 °F), preferably between 15 and 30 °C (59 and 86 °F), unless otherwise specified by manufacturer. Protect from freezing.

### Auxiliary labeling

• For the eye.
• Continue medicine for full time of treatment.

## TOBRAMYCIN OPHTHALMIC SOLUTION USP

**Usual adult and adolescent dose**
Mild to moderate infections—
    Topical, to the conjunctiva, 1 drop every four hours.
Severe infections—
    Topical, to the conjunctiva, 1 drop every hour. Treatment should be continued until improvement occurs; then the frequency of administration should be reduced.

**Usual pediatric dose**
Mild to moderate infections—
    See *Usual adult and adolescent dose*.
Severe infections—
    See *Usual adult and adolescent dose*.

**Strength(s) usually available**
U.S.—
    0.3% (Rx) [*Tobrex* (benzalkonium chloride 0.01%); GENERIC].
Canada—
    0.3% (Rx) [*Tobrex* (benzalkonium chloride 0.01%)].

**Packaging and storage**
Store below 40 °C (104 °F), in a tight container. Protect from freezing.

**Auxiliary labeling**
• For the eye.
• Continue medicine for full time of treatment.

Revised: 07/01/93
Interim revision: 09/30/93

---

# TOCAINIDE   Systemic

VA CLASSIFICATION (Primary): CV300

Note: For a listing of dosage forms and brand names by country availability, see *Dosage Forms* section(s). For a listing of brand names for the articles in this monograph, refer to the General Index.

## Category
Antiarrhythmic.

## Indications

**Accepted**
Arrhythmias, ventricular (treatment)—Tocainide is indicated for suppression of documented life-threatening ventricular arrhythmias, such as sustained ventricular tachycardia.

## Pharmacology/Pharmacokinetics

**Physicochemical characteristics**
Molecular weight—Tocainide: 192.26.
pKa—7.7.

**Mechanism of action/Effect**
Tocainide, like lidocaine, decreases sodium and potassium conductance, thereby decreasing the excitability of myocardial cells. It reduces the rate of rise and amplitude of the action potential and decreases automaticity (increases the threshold of excitability) in the Purkinje fibers. Tocainide shortens the action potential duration and, to a lesser extent, decreases the effective refractory period in the Purkinje fibers. Conduction velocity is usually not altered, although conduction may be slowed in patients with pre-existing conduction abnormalities. Tocainide does not significantly affect resting membrane potential or sinus node automaticity, left ventricular function, systolic arterial blood pressure, atrioventricular (AV) conduction velocity, or QRS or QT intervals. In the Vaughan Williams classification of antiarrhythmics, tocainide is considered to be a class IB agent.

**Absorption**
Bioavailability is close to 100%. Absorption is unaffected by food.

**Protein binding**
Low to moderate (10 to 50%).

**Biotransformation**
Hepatic; producing no active metabolites.

**Half-life**
Approximately 11 to 15 hours; may be prolonged up to 35 hours in patients with severe renal function impairment (creatinine clearance less than 30 mL per min per 1.73 square meters of body surface area.

**Time to peak plasma concentration**
30 minutes to 2 hours.

**Duration of action**
8 hours.

**Elimination**
Renal (about 40% unchanged); alkalinization of urine significantly reduces percentage excreted unchanged.
In dialysis—Removable by hemodialysis.

## Precautions to Consider

**Cross-sensitivity and/or related problems**
Patients sensitive to other amide-type anesthetics may be sensitive to tocainide also. Cross-sensitivity with procainamide or quinidine has not been reported.

**Carcinogenicity**
Studies in mice at doses up to 300 mg per kg of body weight (mg/kg) per day (6 times the maximum human recommended dose) for up to 94 and 102 weeks in males and females, respectively, and in rats at doses up to 200 mg/kg per day for 24 months showed no evidence of carcinogenicity.

**Mutagenicity**
No evidence of mutagenicity was found in *in vivo* micronucleus tests in mice at oral doses of up to 187.5 mg/kg per day (about 7 times the usual human dose). The results of the *in vitro* Ames microbial mutagen test and mouse lymphoma forward mutation assay were also negative.

**Pregnancy/Reproduction**
Fertility—Studies in male and female rats given tocainide doses of 200 mg/kg per day (about 8 times the usual human dose) revealed no evidence of fertility impairment.
Pregnancy—Adequate and well-controlled studies in humans have not been done.
Studies in rabbits at doses of 25, 50, and 100 mg/kg per day (about 1 to 4 times the usual human dose) and in rats at doses of 200 and 300 mg/kg per day (about 8 and 12 times the usual human dose, respectively) produced an increased incidence of abortions, stillbirths, fetal resorptions, and decreased neonatal survival. There was no evidence of teratogenicity.
FDA Pregnancy Category C.

**Breast-feeding**
Studies have not been done to determine if tocainide is distributed into breast milk; however, concentrations in breast milk were documented in one woman at more than twice maternal blood concentrations.

**Pediatrics**
Appropriate studies on the relationship of age to the effects of tocainide have not been performed in the pediatric population. Safety and efficacy have not been established.

**Geriatrics**
Although appropriate studies on the relationship of age to the effects of tocainide have not been performed in geriatric patients, elderly patients are more likely to have age-related renal function impairment, which may require lower or less frequent doses in patients receiving tocainide. In addition, elderly patients may be more prone to dizziness and hypotension.

**Dental**
The leukopenic and thrombocytopenic effects of tocainide may result in an increased incidence of microbial infection, delayed healing, and gingival bleeding. If leukopenia or thrombocytopenia occurs, dental work should be deferred until blood counts have returned to normal and patients should be instructed in proper oral hygiene during treatment, including caution in use of regular toothbrushes, dental floss, and toothpicks.

**Drug interactions and/or related problems**
The following drug interactions and/or related problems have been selected on the basis of their potential clinical significance (possible mechanism in parentheses where appropriate)—not necessarily inclusive (» = major clinical significance):

Note: Combinations containing any of the following medications, depending on the amount present, may also interact with this medication.

Antiarrhythmics, other
(although some antiarrhythmic agents may be used in combination for therapeutic advantage, combined use may potentiate risk of adverse cardiac effects)

Beta-adrenergic blocking agents
(concurrent use with tocainide may result in an additive increase in pulmonary wedge pressure and reduction in cardiac index; caution is recommended, especially in patients with heart failure)

Bone marrow depressants (See *Appendix II* )
(although problems have not been reported, concurrent use with tocainide may increase the risk of leukopenia and thrombocytopenia)

### Medical considerations/Contraindications

The medical considerations/contraindications included here have been selected on the basis of their potential clinical significance (reasons given in parentheses where appropriate)—not necessarily inclusive (» = major clinical significance).

*Except under special circumstances, this medication should not be used when the following medical problem exists:*

» Atrioventricular (AV) block, pre-existing second or third degree without pacemaker

» Sensitivity to tocainide or to amide-type local anesthetics

*Risk-benefit should be considered when the following medical problems exist:*

Atrial flutter or fibrillation
(acceleration of ventricular rate occurs infrequently)

Congestive heart failure
(may be aggravated as a result of a small negative inotropic effect and slight increase in peripheral resistance caused by tocainide)

Hepatic function impairment
(reduced biotransformation; lower or less frequent doses may be required)

Renal function impairment
(reduced elimination; lower or less frequent doses may be required)

### Patient monitoring

The following may be especially important in patient monitoring (other tests may be warranted in some patients, depending on condition; » = major clinical significance):

Blood counts, complete, including white blood cells with differential and platelets
(recommended at weekly intervals for the first 3 months of therapy and frequently thereafter to detect blood dyscrasias; also, recommended if patient develops any signs of infection)

Chest x-ray
(recommended if clinical signs or symptoms of adverse pulmonary effects occur)

Electrocardiogram (ECG)
(recommended prior to initiation of therapy and at periodic intervals during therapy to assess efficacy of tocainide)

## Side/Adverse Effects

Note: In the National Heart, Lung, and Blood Institute's Cardiac Arrhythmias Suppression Trial (CAST), treatment with encainide or flecainide in patients with asymptomatic, non–life-threatening ventricular arrhythmias who had a recent myocardial infarction was found to be associated with excessive mortality or nonfatal cardiac arrest rate (7.7%) as compared with placebo (3%). The implications of these results for other patient populations are uncertain; however, because of tocainide's proarrhythmogenic potential, tocainide should be reserved for patients with life-threatening ventricular arrhythmias.

The following side/adverse effects have been selected on the basis of their potential clinical significance (possible signs and symptoms in parentheses where appropriate)—not necessarily inclusive:

### Those indicating need for medical attention
Incidence less frequent
***Trembling or shaking***
Note: *Trembling or shaking* may indicate that maximum dose is being reached.

Incidence rare
***Blood dyscrasias, including agranulocytosis*** (fever or chills); ***aplastic anemia; leukopenia*** (fever or chills); ***neutropenia; or thrombocytopenia*** (unusual bleeding or bruising); ***pneumonitis, pulmonary fibrosis, alveolitis, pulmonary edema, or pneumonia*** (cough or shortness of breath); ***skin reactions, severe, including erythema multiforme, exfoliative dermatitis, and Stevens-Johnson syndrome*** (blisters on skin; peeling or scaling of skin; severe skin rash; sores in mouth; fever may also be associated with Stevens-Johnson syndrome); ***ventricular arrhythmias*** (irregular heartbeat)

Note: *Blood dyscrasias* usually occur within the first 12 weeks of therapy. Sequelae such as septicemia and septic shock, as well as fatalities, have been reported. Blood counts usually return to normal within 1 month of discontinuation of tocainide.

*Pulmonary* adverse effects usually occur after 3 to 18 weeks of therapy and are characterized by bilateral infiltrates on chest x-ray frequently associated with dyspnea and cough; fatalities have been reported.

Fatalities have been reported with *severe skin reactions*.

### Those indicating need for medical attention only if they continue or are bothersome
Incidence more frequent
***Anorexia*** (loss of appetite); ***dizziness or lightheadedness; nausea***
Incidence less frequent
***Blurred vision; confusion; headache; nervousness; numbness or tingling of fingers and toes; skin rash; sweating; vomiting***

## Overdose

For more information on the management of overdose or unintentional ingestion, **contact a Poison Control Center** (see *Poison Control Center Listing*).

### Clinical effects of overdose
The following effects have been selected on the basis of their potential clinical significance (possible signs and symptoms in parentheses where appropriate)—not necessarily inclusive:

***Cardiac arrest; cardiopulmonary depression; central nervous system effects; convulsions***

Note: *Central nervous system (CNS) effects* would be expected as the initial presentation of overdosage. Other adverse effects, such as gastrointestinal disturbances, may follow.

### Treatment of overdose
Symptomatic and supportive, particularly airway patency and adequacy of ventilation.
Specific treatment—
For convulsions: If necessary, administering small increments of anticonvulsive agents, such as a benzodiazepine or an ultrashort– or short-acting barbiturate.

## Patient Consultation

As an aid to patient consultation, refer to *Advice for the Patient, Tocainide (Systemic)*.

In providing consultation, consider emphasizing the following selected information (» = major clinical significance):

### Before using this medication
» Conditions affecting use, especially:
  Sensitivity to tocainide or amide-type anesthetics
  Pregnancy—Increased possibility of death in animal fetuses
  Use in the elderly—Elderly may be more prone to dizziness and hypotension
  Other medical problems, especially second or third degree atrioventricular (AV) block

### Proper use of this medication
» Compliance with therapy; taking as directed even if feeling well
  May be taken with food or milk to reduce stomach upset
» Importance of not missing doses and taking at evenly spaced intervals
» Proper dosing
  Missed dose: Taking as soon as possible if remembered within 4 hours; not taking if remembered later; not doubling doses
» Proper storage

### Precautions while using this medication
  Regular visits to physician to check progress
  Carrying medical identification card or bracelet
» Caution when driving or doing things requiring alertness because of possible dizziness
» Caution if any kind of surgery (including dental surgery) or emergency treatment is required

### Side/adverse effects
Signs of potential side effects, especially trembling or shaking, agranulocytosis, aplastic anemia, leukopenia, neutropenia, thrombocytopenia, pulmonary problems, severe skin reactions, and ventricular arrhythmias

## General Dosing Information

Patients who experience adverse effects shortly after dosing with tocainide may require a shorter dosing interval (i.e., further division of the daily dose). Patients who experience worsening of arrhythmias shortly before the next scheduled dose may require an increased dose and/or a shorter dosing interval.

The appearance of tremor may be used as an indication that the maximum dose is being reached.

It is recommended that tocainide therapy be withdrawn if bone marrow depression, pulmonary fibrosis, or a severe skin reaction occurs.

### Diet/Nutrition
Tocainide may be taken with food or milk to reduce gastrointestinal irritation.

## Oral Dosage Forms

### TOCAINIDE HYDROCHLORIDE TABLETS USP

**Usual adult dose**
Antiarrhythmic—
Initial: Oral, 400 mg every eight hours, the dose being adjusted as needed and tolerated.
Maintenance: Oral, 1200 to 1800 mg per day in three divided doses.

Note: Some patients may tolerate twice daily dosing.

Patients with renal or hepatic function impairment may be adequately treated with < 1200 mg a day. Dosage adjustments in these situations may be facilitated by the use of serum drug level determinations.

Geriatric patients may be more sensitive to the effects of the usual adult dose.

**Usual pediatric dose**
Safety and efficacy have not been established.

**Strength(s) usually available**
U.S.—
400 mg (Rx) [*Tonocard*].
600 mg (Rx) [*Tonocard*].
Canada—
400 mg (Rx) [*Tonocard*].
600 mg (Rx) [*Tonocard*].

**Packaging and storage**
Store below 40 °C (104 °F), preferably between 15 and 30 °C (59 and 86 °F), unless otherwise specified by manufacturer. Store in a well-closed container.

Revised: 08/21/96

---

**TOLAZAMIDE**—See *Antidiabetic Agents, Sulfonylurea (Systemic)*

---

# TOLAZOLINE   Parenteral-Systemic†

VA CLASSIFICATION (Primary): CV500
Note: For a listing of dosage forms and brand names by country availability, see *Dosage Forms* section(s). For a listing of brand names for the articles in this monograph, refer to the General Index.

†Not commercially available in Canada.

## Category
Antihypertensive (pulmonary).

## Indications

### Accepted
Hypertension, persistent pulmonary (treatment)—Tolazoline is indicated in the treatment of persistent pulmonary hypertension in the newborn (persistent fetal circulation) when systemic arterial oxygenation cannot be maintained by supplemental oxygen and/or mechanical ventilation.

### Unaccepted
Tolazoline is not considered to be effective for previously labeled indications, which included spastic peripheral vascular disorders.

## Pharmacology/Pharmacokinetics

### Physicochemical characteristics
Molecular weight—196.68.
pKa—10.5.

### Mechanism of action/Effect
Vasodilation by means of a direct effect on peripheral vascular smooth muscle and indirect effects produced, in part, by release of endogenous histamine; tolazoline has moderate alpha-adrenergic blocking activity and has histamine agonist activity. Tolazoline usually reduces pulmonary arterial pressure and vascular resistance.

### Other actions/effects
Sympathomimetic (cardiac stimulation, both inotropic and chronotropic); parasympathomimetic (stimulation of gastrointestinal tract that is blocked by atropine); histamine-like (stimulation of gastric secretion).

### Half-life
Neonates—3 to 10 hours; however, reportedly as long as 40 hours, varying inversely with urine flow.

### Onset of action
Within 30 minutes after initial dose.

### Elimination
Renal, primarily unchanged.

## Precautions to Consider

### Carcinogenicity
Studies have not been done in either humans or animals.

### Pregnancy/Reproduction
Pregnancy—Studies have not been done in humans.
Studies in fetal sheep have shown that tolazoline crosses the placenta. Following maternal tolazoline infusions in sheep, fetal tolazoline concentrations averaged 20% of maternal concentrations.
FDA Pregnancy Category C.

### Breast-feeding
It is not known whether tolazoline is excreted in breast milk. However, problems in humans have not been documented.

### Geriatrics
No information is available on the relationship of age to the effects of tolazoline in geriatric patients.

### Drug interactions and/or related problems
The following drug interactions and/or related problems have been selected on the basis of their potential clinical significance (possible mechanism in parentheses where appropriate)—not necessarily inclusive (» = major clinical significance):
Note: Combinations containing any of the following medications, depending on the amount present, may also interact with this medication.

Dopamine
(tolazoline antagonizes the peripheral vasoconstriction produced by high doses of dopamine)

Ephedrine
(alpha-adrenergic blocking agents such as tolazoline may decrease the pressor response to ephedrine)

Epinephrine or
Norepinephrine
(concurrent use with large doses of tolazoline may cause a paradoxical reduction in blood pressure followed by an exaggerated rebound increase; these medications are not recommended for treatment of tolazoline overdose)

Metaraminol
(concurrent use with tolazoline usually decreases, but does not reverse or completely block, the pressor effect of metaraminol)

Methoxamine or
Phenylephrine
(prior administration of tolazoline may block the pressor response to methoxamine or phenylephrine, possibly resulting in severe hypotension)

## Laboratory value alterations

The following have been selected on the basis of their potential clinical significance (possible effect in parentheses where appropriate)—not necessarily inclusive (» = major clinical significance):

With physiology/laboratory test values
Blood pressure
(may be increased or decreased, depending on the relative contribution of cardiac-stimulating effects and peripheral vasodilation; pulmonary arterial pressure is usually reduced)

## Medical considerations/Contraindications

The medical considerations/contraindications included here have been selected on the basis of their potential clinical significance (reasons given in parentheses where appropriate)—not necessarily inclusive (» = major clinical significance).

*Except under special circumstances, this medication should not be used when the following medical problem exists:*

» Hypotension, systemic
(may be exacerbated)

*Risk-benefit should be considered when the following medical problems exist:*

Acidosis
(increases pulmonary vasoconstriction; effect of tolazoline may be decreased; should be corrected before initiation of tolazoline therapy)

» Mitral stenosis
(parenteral tolazoline may cause an increase or decrease in pulmonary artery pressure and total pulmonary resistance)

» Renal function impairment, reduced urine flow
(decreases tolazoline elimination; may require dosage reduction)

Sensitivity to tolazoline

## Patient monitoring

The following may be especially important in patient monitoring (other tests may be warranted in some patients, depending on condition; » = major clinical significance):

Blood counts, complete, and
» Blood gases (PO$_2$, PCO$_2$), arterial, and
Blood pH, arterial, and
Blood pressure, arterial, and
Electrocardiogram (ECG) and
Electrolyte concentrations, serum, especially chloride and potassium, and
Heart rate
(recommended at regular intervals throughout tolazoline treatment)
(if adequate systolic blood pressure cannot be maintained, tolazoline should be withdrawn)
(if hypochloremic metabolic alkalosis occurs, patient should be weaned from tolazoline therapy and replacement chloride and potassium administered)

Hematest of gastric aspirates
(recommended at periodic intervals to detect gastrointestinal bleeding)

Renal function, including urine flow, determinations
(recommended periodically during tolazoline therapy)

## Side/Adverse Effects

The following side/adverse effects have been selected on the basis of their potential clinical significance (possible signs and symptoms in parentheses where appropriate)—not necessarily inclusive:

### Those indicating need for medical attention

Incidence more frequent
*Gastrointestinal hemorrhage*—detected by hematest of gastric aspirates; may be fatal; *hypochloremic alkalosis*—secondary to gastric hypersecretion; *systemic hypotension; acute renal failure, especially oliguria; thrombocytopenia*

Note: *Hypotension* may be very common in neonates; may occur suddenly in some cases.

Incidence less frequent
*Diarrhea or nausea and vomiting; increased pilomotor activity* (goose flesh); *peripheral vasodilation* (flushing); *tachycardia*

Note: *Tachycardia* is a reflex response to vasodilation and a result of direct cardiac stimulation.

Incidence rare
*Mydriasis*

## General Dosing Information

See also *Patient monitoring.*

It is recommended that tolazoline be administered in an area with trained personnel and facilities necessary to provide pediatric or neonatal intensive care. Respiratory support should be immediately available.

To achieve optimal dosage control, it is recommended that tolazoline be administered intravenously by means of an infusion pump, a microdrip regulator, or a similar device to allow precise adjustment of the flow rate.

Pretreatment with antacids may prevent gastrointestinal bleeding in infants.

**For treatment of adverse effects and/or overdose**
Hypotension is treated by:
• Keeping the patient's head low and administering intravenous fluids.
• Use of epinephrine or norepinephrine is **not** recommended because of the risk of a further decrease in blood pressure followed by an exaggerated rebound increase.
• If fluid expansion fails to maintain blood pressure, an intravenous dopamine infusion (high doses may be needed to obtain adequate vasoconstrictor effect) may be used simultaneously with the tolazoline infusion.

## Parenteral Dosage Forms

### TOLAZOLINE HYDROCHLORIDE INJECTION USP

**Usual pediatric dose**
Antihypertensive (pulmonary)—
Initial:
Intravenous, 1 to 2 mg per kg of body weight via scalp vein over a five- to ten-minute period.
Note: Alternatively, the initial dose may be infused into any vein that drains into the superior vena cava to maximize delivery to the pulmonary artery.
Maintenance:
Intravenous infusion, 0.2 mg (200 mcg) per kg of body weight per hour for each 1 mg per kg of body weight loading dose. May be withdrawn gradually when arterial blood gases remain stable.
Note: If necessary, the initial bolus dose may be repeated during the maintenance infusion.
A decreased infusion rate may be necessary in patients with renal tubular dysfunction and oliguria less than 0.9 mL per kg of body weight per hour.

**Strength(s) usually available**
U.S.—
25 mg per mL (Rx) [*Priscoline*].
Canada—
Not commercially available.

**Packaging and storage**
Store below 40 °C (104 °F), preferably between 15 and 30 °C (59 and 86 °F), unless otherwise specified by manufacturer. Protect from light (according to manufacturer's labeling).

**Preparation of dosage form**
Caution—Use of diluents containing benzyl alcohol is not recommended for preparation of medications for use in neonates. A fatal toxic syndrome consisting of metabolic acidosis, central nervous system (CNS) depression, respiratory problems, renal failure, hypotension, and possibly seizures and intracranial hemorrhages has been associated with the use of benzyl alcohol.

Revised: 04/13/93

---

**TOLBUTAMIDE**—See *Antidiabetic Agents, Sulfonylurea (Systemic)*

---

**TOLMETIN**—See *Anti-inflammatory Drugs, Nonsteroidal (Systemic)*

# TOLNAFTATE Topical

VA CLASSIFICATION (Primary): DE102

Note: For a listing of dosage forms and brand names by country availability, see *Dosage Forms* section(s). For a listing of brand names for the articles in this monograph, refer to the General Index.

## Category

Antifungal (topical).

## Indications

Note: Bracketed information in the *Indications* section refers to uses that are not included in U.S. product labeling.

**Accepted**

Tinea capitis (treatment)—Tolnaftate is indicated in the topical treatment of tinea capitis.

Tinea corporis (treatment)

Tinea cruris (treatment)

Tinea manuum (treatment) or

Tinea pedis (treatment)—Tolnaftate is indicated in the topical treatment of tinea corporis (ringworm of the body), tinea cruris (ringworm of the groin; jock itch), tinea manuum, and tinea pedis (ringworm of the foot; athlete's foot) caused by *Trichophyton rubrum*, *T. mentagrophytes*, *T. tonsurans*, *Microsporum canis*, *M. audouini*, and *Epidermophyton floccosum*.

Tinea versicolor (treatment)—Tolnaftate is indicated in the topical treatment of tinea versicolor (pityriasis versicolor; ''sun fungus'') caused by *Pityrosporon orbiculare (Malassezia furfur)*.

[Tinea barbae (treatment)]—Tolnaftate is used in the topical treatment of tinea barbae.

Not all species or strains of a particular organism may be susceptible to tolnaftate.

## Pharmacology/Pharmacokinetics

**Physicochemical characteristics**

Molecular weight—307.41.

**Mechanism of action/Effect**

Fungicidal; exact mechanism unknown; however, it has been reported to distort the hyphae and to stunt mycelial growth in susceptible organisms.

## Precautions to Consider

**Pregnancy/Reproduction**

Pregnancy—Problems in humans have not been documented.

**Breast-feeding**

It is not known whether topical tolnaftate is distributed into breast milk. However, problems in humans have not been documented.

**Pediatrics**

Use in children up to 2 years of age is not recommended except under the advice and supervision of a physician.

**Geriatrics**

No information is available on the relationship of age to the effects of topical tolnaftate in geriatric patients.

## Side/Adverse Effects

The following side/adverse effects have been selected on the basis of their potential clinical significance (possible signs and symptoms in parentheses where appropriate)—not necessarily inclusive:

**Those indicating need for medical attention**
*Hypersensitivity* (skin irritation not present before therapy)

## Patient Consultation

As an aid to patient consultation, refer to *Advice for the Patient, Tolnaftate (Topical)*.

In providing consultation, consider emphasizing the following selected information (» = major clinical significance):

**Before using this medication**
» Conditions affecting use, especially:
    Sensitivity to tolnaftate
    Use in children—Not recommended in children up to 2 years of age

**Proper use of this medication**
    Before applying, washing affected area and drying thoroughly
» Not using on children up to 2 years of age
» Avoiding contact with the eyes
    Proper administration technique
» Compliance with full course of therapy
» Proper dosing
    Missed dose: Applying as soon as possible; not applying if almost time for next dose
» Proper storage

**Precautions while using this medication**
    Checking with physician or pharmacist if no improvement within 4 weeks
    Using the powder or topical aerosol powder daily after bathing and carefully drying to help prevent reinfection

**Side/adverse effects**
    Possible stinging when spray solution form of medication is applied
    Signs of potential side effects, especially hypersensitivity

## General Dosing Information

Therapy for a period of 2 to 3 weeks is usually sufficient; however, treatment for 4 to 6 weeks may be necessary, especially if thickening of the skin has occurred.

The medication should be continued for 2 weeks after symptoms have disappeared.

Tolnaftate may be used concurrently with an oral antifungal agent, such as griseofulvin, in the treatment of onychomycosis or chronic infections of the scalp, palms, or skin.

The powder and powder aerosol forms are recommended for adjunctive use in fungal infections of intertriginous or other naturally moist skin areas in which drying may enhance the therapeutic response. They may also be used alone in the treatment of mild infections that respond to antifungal powder in conjunction with measures that promote skin hygiene.

Following complete remission of the infection, the powder or powder aerosol may be continued as part of a daily personal hygiene program to help prevent reinfection.

## Topical Dosage Forms

### TOLNAFTATE TOPICAL AEROSOL POWDER USP

**Usual adult and adolescent dose**
Topical, to the skin, two times a day.

**Usual pediatric dose**
Infants and children up to 2 years of age—Use is not recommended except under the advice and supervision of a physician.
Children 2 years of age and over—See *Usual adult and adolescent dose*.

**Strength(s) usually available**
U.S.—
    1% (OTC) [*Aftate for Athlete's Foot Aerosol Spray Powder; Aftate for Jock Itch Aerosol Spray Powder; NP-27 Spray Powder; Tinactin Aerosol Powder; Tinactin Antifungal Deodorant Powder Aerosol; Tinactin Jock Itch Spray Powder; Ting Antifungal Spray Powder;* GENERIC].
Canada—
    1% (OTC) [*Tinactin Aerosol Powder; Tinactin Jock Itch Aerosol Powder; Tinactin Plus Aerosol Powder*].

**Packaging and storage**
Store below 40 °C (104 °F), unless otherwise specified by manufacturer.

**Auxiliary labeling**
• Shake well.
• For external use only.
• Continue medicine for full time of treatment.
• Store away from heat and direct sunlight.

### TOLNAFTATE TOPICAL AEROSOL SOLUTION

**Usual adult and adolescent dose**
See *Tolnaftate Topical Aerosol Powder USP*.

**Usual pediatric dose**
See *Tolnaftate Topical Aerosol Powder USP*.

**Strength(s) usually available**
U.S.—
    1% (OTC) [*Aftate for Athlete's Foot Aerosol Spray Liquid; Tinactin Aerosol Liquid; Ting Antifungal Spray Liquid;* GENERIC].

Canada—
    1% (OTC) [*Tinactin Aerosol Liquid*].

**Packaging and storage**
Store below 49 °C (120 °F), unless otherwise specified by manufacturer.

**Auxiliary labeling**
• Shake well.
• For external use only.
• Continue medicine for full time of treatment.
• Store away from heat and direct sunlight.

## TOLNAFTATE CREAM USP

**Usual adult and adolescent dose**
See *Tolnaftate Topical Aerosol Powder USP*.

**Usual pediatric dose**
See *Tolnaftate Topical Aerosol Powder USP*.

**Strength(s) usually available**
U.S.—
    1% (OTC) [*Genaspore Cream; NP-27 Cream; Tinactin Cream; Tinactin Jock Itch Cream; Ting Antifungal Cream;* GENERIC].
Canada—
    1% (OTC) [*Pitrex Cream; Tinactin Cream; Tinactin Jock Itch Cream*].

**Packaging and storage**
Store below 40 °C (104 °F), preferably between 15 and 30 °C (59 and 86 °F), unless otherwise specified by manufacturer. Store in a tight container. Protect from freezing.

**Auxiliary labeling**
• For external use only.
• Continue medicine for full time of treatment.

## TOLNAFTATE GEL USP

**Usual adult and adolescent dose**
See *Tolnaftate Topical Aerosol Powder USP*.

**Usual pediatric dose**
See *Tolnaftate Topical Aerosol Powder USP*.

**Strength(s) usually available**
U.S.—
    1% (OTC) [*Aftate for Athlete's Foot Gel; Aftate for Jock Itch Gel*].

**Packaging and storage**
Store below 40 °C (104 °F), preferably between 15 and 30 °C (59 and 86 °F), unless otherwise specified by manufacturer. Store in a tight container. Protect from freezing.

**Auxiliary labeling**
• For external use only.
• Continue medicine for full time of treatment.

## TOLNAFTATE POWDER (TOPICAL) USP

**Usual adult and adolescent dose**
See *Tolnaftate Topical Aerosol Powder USP*.

**Usual pediatric dose**
See *Tolnaftate Topical Aerosol Powder USP*.

**Strength(s) usually available**
U.S.—
    1% (OTC) [*Aftate for Athlete's Foot Sprinkle Powder; Aftate for Jock Itch Sprinkle Powder; NP-27 Powder; Tinactin Powder; Ting Antifungal Powder; Zeasorb-AF Powder;* GENERIC].
Canada—
    1% (OTC) [*Tinactin Plus Powder; Tinactin Powder*].

**Packaging and storage**
Store below 40 °C (104 °F), preferably between 15 and 30 °C (59 and 86 °F), unless otherwise specified by manufacturer. Store in a tight container.

**Auxiliary labeling**
• For external use only.
• Continue medicine for full time of treatment.
• Keep container tightly closed.
• Keep in a dry place.

## TOLNAFTATE TOPICAL SOLUTION USP

**Usual adult and adolescent dose**
See *Tolnaftate Topical Aerosol Powder USP*.

**Usual pediatric dose**
See *Tolnaftate Topical Aerosol Powder USP*.

**Strength(s) usually available**
U.S.—
    1% (OTC) [*NP-27 Solution; Tinactin Solution;* GENERIC].
Canada—
    1% (OTC) [*Tinactin Solution*].

**Packaging and storage**
Store below 40 °C (104 °F), preferably between 15 and 30 °C (59 and 86 °F), unless otherwise specified by manufacturer. Store in a tight container. Protect from freezing.

**Stability**
Tolnaftate solution solidifies at low temperature, but liquefies readily when warmed, retaining its potency.

**Auxiliary labeling**
• For external use only.
• Continue medicine for full time of treatment.

Revised: 11/05/91
Interim revision: 08/10/94

# TORSEMIDE    Systemic†

INN: Torasemide
BAN: Torasemide
VA CLASSIFICATION (Primary/Secondary): CV702/CV490
Note: For a listing of dosage forms and brand names by country availability, see *Dosage Forms* section(s). For a listing of brand names for the articles in this monograph, refer to the General Index.

    †Not commercially available in Canada.

## Category

Diuretic; antihypertensive.

## Indications

**Accepted**
Edema (treatment)—Torsemide is indicated in treatment of edema associated with congestive heart failure, renal disease, and hepatic disease (cirrhosis).

Hypertension (treatment)—Torsemide is indicated, alone or in combination with other antihypertensive agents, in the treatment of hypertension.

    For additional information on initial therapeutic guidelines related to the treatment of hypertension, see *Appendix III*.

## Pharmacology/Pharmacokinetics

**Physicochemical characteristics**
Molecular weight—348.43.
pKa—7.1.

**Mechanism of action/Effect**
Diuretic—Torsemide is a loop diuretic. It inhibits reabsorption of sodium and chloride in the luminal membrane of the ascending limb of the loop of Henle by interfering with the chloride binding site of the $1Na+$, $1K+$, $2Cl-$ cotransport system. This increases the rate of delivery of tubular fluid and electrolytes to the distal sites of hydrogen and potassium ion secretion, while plasma volume contraction increases aldosterone production. The increased delivery and high aldosterone levels promote sodium reabsorption at the distal tubules, thus increasing the loss of potassium and hydrogen ions. Torsemide's effects in other portions of the nephron have not been demonstrated.

Antihypertensive—Diuretics lower blood pressure initially by reducing plasma and extracellular fluid volume; cardiac output also decreases. Eventually, cardiac output returns to normal with an accompanying decrease in peripheral resistance.

**Absorption**
Rapidly absorbed following oral administration; not affected by food. Bioavailability is approximately 80%.

**Distribution**
Volume of distribution (Vol$_D$)—0.14 to 0.19 L per kg.

### Protein binding
Very high (97 to greater than 99%).

### Biotransformation
Metabolized via the hepatic cytochrome P-450 system to 5 metabolites. The major metabolite, M5, is pharmacologically inactive. There are 2 minor metabolites, M1, possessing one-tenth the activity of torsemide, and M3, equal in activity to torsemide. Overall, torsemide appears to account for 80% of the total diuretic activity, while metabolites M1 and M3 account for 9% and 11%, respectively.

### Half-life
Elimination—2.2 to 3.8 hours; not affected by moderate renal failure. However, metabolite M1 may accumulate in renal failure.

### Onset of action
Diuretic—
    Oral: Within 1 hour.
    Intravenous: Within 10 minutes.

### Time to peak concentration
Oral—1 to 2 hours.

### Time to peak effect
Diuretic—
    Oral: 1 to 2 hours.
    Intravenous: Within 1 hour.

### Duration of action
Diuretic—6 to 8 hours.

### Elimination
Renal; 24% as parent compound.
In dialysis—Torsemide is not significantly removed by hemodialysis.

## Precautions to Consider

### Cross-sensitivity and/or related problems
Patients sensitive to bumetanide, furosemide, or sulfonamides (including thiazide diuretics) may be sensitive to torsemide also.

### Carcinogenicity/Tumorigenicity
Lifetime administration of torsemide to rats and mice at doses up to 9 and 32 mg per kg of body weight (mg/kg) per day, respectively, did not increase overall tumor incidence. These doses are equivalent to 27 and 96 times, respectively, a human dose of 20 mg on a body weight basis. However, renal tubular injury, interstitial inflammation, and a statistically significant increase in renal adenomas and carcinomas were observed in the high-dose female group of rats.

### Mutagenicity
No mutagenic activity was seen in a variety of *in vitro* and *in vivo* tests.

### Pregnancy/Reproduction
Fertility—No adverse effect on fertility was seen in male or female rats given doses up to 25 mg/kg per day (equivalent to 75 times a human dose of 20 mg on a body weight basis).

Pregnancy—Adequate and well-controlled studies have not been done in humans. Routine use of diuretics during normal pregnancy is not recommended because use may expose the mother and fetus to unnecessary hazard. However, diuretics may be continued during pregnancy if they were used to treat hypertension that existed prior to gestation. Diuretics do not prevent development of toxemia of pregnancy, and there is no satisfactory evidence that they are useful in the treatment of toxemia. Diuretics are indicated only in the treatment of edema due to pathologic causes or as a short course of treatment in patients with severe hypervolemia.

No fetotoxicity or teratogenicity was observed in rats and rabbits given doses up to 15 and 5 times, respectively, a human dose of 20 mg on a mg/kg basis. However, administration of doses 4 and 5 times larger in rats and rabbits, respectively, resulted in decreased average body weight, increased fetal resorption, and delayed fetal ossification.

FDA Pregnancy Category B.

### Breast-feeding
It is not known whether torsemide is distributed into breast milk.

### Pediatrics
No information is available on the relationship of age to the effects of torsemide in pediatric patients. Safety and efficacy have not been established.

### Geriatrics
Studies that included patients over 65 years of age have not demonstrated geriatrics-specific problems that would limit the usefulness of torsemide in the elderly.

### Drug interactions and/or related problems
The following drug interactions and/or related problems have been selected on the basis of their potential clinical significance (possible mechanism in parentheses where appropriate)—not necessarily inclusive (» = major clinical significance):

Note: Combinations containing any of the following medications, depending on the amount present, may also interact with this medication.

Alcohol or
Hypotension-producing medications, other (see *Appendix II* )
    (hypotensive and/or diuretic effects may be potentiated when these medications are used concurrently with torsemide; although some antihypertensive and/or diuretic combinations are frequently used for therapeutic advantage, dosage adjustments may be necessary during concurrent use)

» Amphotericin B, parenteral
    (concurrent and/or sequential administration with torsemide should be avoided since the potential for nephrotoxicity may be increased, especially in the presence of renal function impairment; in addition, concurrent use with torsemide may intensify electrolyte imbalance, particularly hypokalemia; frequent electrolyte determinations are recommended and potassium supplementation may be required)

Angiotensin-converting enzyme (ACE) inhibitors
    (sudden and severe hypotension may occur within the first 1 to 5 hours after the initial dose of an ACE inhibitor, particularly in patients who are sodium- and volume-depleted as a result of diuretic therapy. Withdrawal of the diuretic or increase of salt intake approximately 1 week before start of captopril therapy or 2 to 3 days before start of benazepril, enalapril, fosinopril, lisinopril, quinapril, or ramipril therapy, or initiation of ACE inhibitor therapy at lower doses, will minimize the reaction; this reaction does not usually recur with subsequent doses, although caution in increasing doses is recommended; diuretics may be reinstituted as necessary)
    (risk of renal failure may be increased in patients who are sodium- and volume-depleted as a result of diuretic therapy)
    (ACE inhibitors may reduce the secondary aldosteronism and hypokalemia caused by diuretics)

Antiarrhythmic agents
    (concurrent use with torsemide may lead to an increased risk of arrhythmias associated with hypokalemia)

» Anticoagulants, coumarin- or indandione-derivative, or
Heparin or
Streptokinase or
Urokinase
    (anticoagulant effects may be decreased when these medications are used concurrently with torsemide, as a result of reduction of plasma volume leading to concentration of procoagulant factors in the blood; in addition, diuretic-induced improvement of hepatic congestion may lead to improved hepatic function, resulting in increased procoagulant factor synthesis; dosage adjustments may be necessary)

Antidiabetic agents, oral, or
Insulin
    (torsemide may rarely raise blood glucose concentrations or interfere with the hypoglycemic effects of these agents; for non–insulin-dependent diabetics, dosage adjustment of hypoglycemic medications may be necessary)

Anti-inflammatory drugs, nonsteroidal (NSAIDs), especially indomethacin
    (indomethacin, and possibly other NSAIDs, may reduce the natriuretic action of torsemide; NSAIDs may also reduce the antihypertensive effect or the increase in urine volume caused by torsemide, possibly by inhibiting renal prostaglandin synthesis and/or by causing sodium and fluid retention)
    (in addition, concurrent use of NSAIDs with a diuretic may increase the risk of renal failure secondary to a decrease in renal blood flow caused by inhibition of renal prostaglandin synthesis)

Digitalis glycosides
    (concurrent use with torsemide may enhance the possibility of digitalis toxicity associated with hypokalemia and hypomagnesemia)

» Hypokalemia-causing medications, other (see *Appendix II* )
    (risk of severe hypokalemia due to other hypokalemia-causing medications may be increased; monitoring of serum potassium concentrations and cardiac function and potassium supplementation may be required)

» Lithium
   (concurrent use with torsemide may promote lithium toxicity because of reduced renal clearance; concurrent use is not recommended unless patient can be closely monitored)
» Nephrotoxic medications, other, (see *Appendix II* ) or
   Ototoxic medications, other (see *Appendix II* )
   (concurrent and/or sequential administration with torsemide is not
   recommended since the potential for ototoxicity and nephrotoxicity
   may be increased, especially in the presence of renal function
   impairment)
Neuromuscular blocking agents, nondepolarizing
   (torsemide may induce hypokalemia, which may enhance the
   blockade of nondepolarizing neuromuscular blocking agents; serum potassium determinations may be necessary prior to administration of nondepolarizing neuromuscular blocking agents; careful postoperative monitoring of the patient may be necessary
   following concurrent or sequential use, especially if there is a possibility of incomplete reversal of neuromuscular blockade)
Probenecid
   (concurrent use with torsemide may decrease the diuretic activity
   of torsemide because probenecid reduces secretion of torsemide
   into the proximal tubule)
» Salicylates, high-dose
   (concurrent use with torsemide may increase the risk of salicylate
   toxicity because torsemide and salicylates compete for secretion
   by the renal tubules)
Sympathomimetics
   (concurrent use may reduce the antihypertensive effects of torsemide; the patient should be carefully monitored to confirm that the
   desired effect is being obtained)

**Laboratory value alterations**
The following have been selected on the basis of their potential clinical
   significance (possible effect in parentheses where appropriate)—not
   necessarily inclusive (» = major clinical significance):
With physiology/laboratory test values
   Blood urea nitrogen (BUN) and
   Uric acid, serum
      (concentrations may be increased)
   Calcium and
   Magnesium and
   Potassium
      (serum concentrations may be decreased)
   Glucose
      (blood glucose concentrations may be increased; hyperglycemia
      has been reported rarely)

**Medical considerations/Contraindications**
The medical considerations/contraindications included here have been selected on the basis of their potential clinical significance (reasons given
   in parentheses where appropriate)—not necessarily inclusive (» =
   major clinical significance).

*Risk-benefit should be considered when the following medical problems
exist:*
» Anuria
   (may impair effectiveness of torsemide; possible reduced clearance
   may increase risk of ototoxicity)
Diabetes mellitus
   (torsemide may increase serum glucose concentrations)
Gout, history of or
Hyperuricemia
   (torsemide may increase serum uric acid concentrations)
Hearing function impairment
   (condition may be exacerbated if ototoxic effects occur)
Hepatic function impairment with cirrhosis and ascites
   (sudden alterations in fluid and electrolyte balance may precipitate
   hepatic coma; hospitalization during initiation of torsemide therapy
   is recommended)
Myocardial infarction, acute
   (excessive diuresis should be avoided because of the danger of
   precipitating shock)
Sensitivity to torsemide, other loop diuretics, or sulfonylureas
Caution is recommended in patients who are at increased risk if hypokalemia occurs, including those taking concurrent digitalis and
   those with cardiovascular disease, because of the risk of
   arrhythmias.

**Patient monitoring**
The following may be especially important in patient monitoring (other
   tests may be warranted in some patients, depending on condition;
   » = major clinical significance):
Blood pressure measurements
   (recommended at periodic intervals in patients being treated for
   hypertension; selected patients may be taught to monitor their
   blood pressure at home and report the results at regular physician
   visits)
Blood urea nitrogen (BUN) and
Glucose, serum and
Hepatic function and
Renal function and
Uric acid, serum
   (determinations recommended at periodic intervals)
» Electrolytes, serum, especially potassium
   (determinations recommended at periodic intervals)
Hearing examinations
   (recommended at periodic intervals in patients receiving prolonged
   high-dose intravenous therapy)
*For use as a diuretic (in addition to the above)*
Weight measurements
   (recommended prior to initiation of therapy and at periodic inter-
   vals during therapy to monitor fluid loss)

## Side/Adverse Effects

The following side/adverse effects have been selected on the basis of their
   potential clinical significance (possible signs and symptoms in parentheses where appropriate)—not necessarily inclusive:

**Those indicating need for medical attention**
Incidence less frequent
   *Electrolyte imbalance such as hyponatremia, hypochloremic alka-
   losis, and hypokalemia* (dryness of mouth; fast or irregular heartbeat;
   increased thirst; mood or mental changes; muscle pain or cramps; nausea or vomiting; unusual tiredness or weakness)
Incidence rare
   *Allergic reaction* (skin rash); *gastrointestinal hemorrhage* (black,
   tarry stools); *hypotension, orthostatic* (dizziness when getting up from
   a sitting or lying position); *ototoxicity* (ringing or buzzing in the ears
   or any loss of hearing)
   Note: *Ototoxicity* may be more likely to occur with rapid intravenous
      administration or with use of very high doses.

**Those indicating need for medical attention only if they continue
or are bothersome**
Incidence more frequent
   *Constipation; dizziness; gastrointestinal disturbance* (stomach upset);
   *headache*

## Overdose

For more information on the management of overdose or unintentional
   ingestion, **contact a Poison Control Center** (see *Poison Control Center Listing* ).

**Treatment of overdose**
Fluid and electrolyte replacement.
Symptomatic and supportive care.

## Patient Consultation

As an aid to patient consultation, refer to *Advice for the Patient, Torsemide
   (Systemic)*.

In providing consultation, consider emphasizing the following selected
   information (» = major clinical significance):

**Before using this medication**
» Conditions affecting use, especially:
   Sensitivity to loop diuretics or sulfonamides
   Pregnancy—Not recommended for routine use
   Other medications, especially amphotericin B, anticoagulants, hy-
      pokalemia-causing medications, lithium, other nephrotoxic
      medications, or high-dose salicylates
   Other medical problems, especially anuria

**Proper use of this medication**
Diuretic effects of the medication and timing of doses to minimize
   inconvenience of diuresis
Getting into habit of taking at same time each day to help increase
   compliance

» Proper dosing
Missed dose: Taking as soon as possible; not taking if almost time for next dose; not doubling doses
» Proper storage

*For use as an antihypertensive*
Possible need for control of weight and diet, especially sodium intake
» Patient may not experience symptoms of hypertension; importance of taking medication even if feeling well
» Does not cure, but controls hypertension; possible need for lifelong therapy; serious consequences of untreated hypertension

## Precautions while using this medication

Regular visits to physician to check progress
» Possibility of hypokalemia; possible need for additional potassium in diet; not changing diet without first checking with physician
To prevent dehydration, notifying physician if severe nausea, vomiting, or diarrhea occurs and continues
Caution if any kind of surgery (including dental surgery) is required
» Caution when getting up suddenly from a lying or sitting position
» Caution in using alcohol, while standing for long periods or exercising, and during hot weather because of enhanced orthostatic hypotensive effects
Diabetics: May increase blood sugar levels

*For use as an antihypertensive*
» Not taking other medications, especially nonprescription sympathomimetics, unless discussed with physician

## Side/adverse effects

Signs of potential side effects, especially electrolyte imbalance, allergic reaction, gastrointestinal hemorrhage, orthostatic hypotension, and ototoxicity

# General Dosing Information

Dosage must be adjusted to meet the individual requirements of each patient, on the basis of clinical response. The lowest effective dosage should be utilized to minimize potential fluid and electrolyte imbalance.

Concurrent administration of potassium supplements or potassium-sparing diuretics may be indicated in patients considered to be at higher risk for developing hypokalemia.

When torsemide is added to an antihypertensive regimen, the dose of other antihypertensive agents may have to be reduced to prevent an excessive drop in blood pressure.

## For parenteral dosage forms only

Intravenous injections should be administered slowly, over a period of 2 minutes.

## Diet/Nutrition

Torsemide may be taken at any time in relation to a meal.

## Bioequivalence information

Because of the high bioavailability of torsemide tablets, oral and intravenous doses of torsemide are equivalent.

# Oral Dosage Forms

## TORSEMIDE TABLETS

### Usual adult dose

Diuretic—
Congestive heart failure:
Oral, 10 or 20 mg once a day, the dosage being increased as needed, up to 200 mg, for desired therapeutic effect.
Hepatic cirrhosis:
Oral, 5 or 10 mg once a day, administered with an aldosterone antagonist or a potassium-sparing diuretic.
Renal failure, chronic:
Oral, 20 mg once a day, the dosage being increased by doubling as needed until adequate diuretic response is achieved.
Antihypertensive—
Oral, 5 mg once a day for four to six weeks, the dosage being increased thereafter to 10 mg once a day if blood pressure response is not adequate.

### Usual adult prescribing limits

Congestive heart failure—Single dose: 200 mg.
Hepatic cirrhosis—Single dose: 40 mg.
Renal failure, chronic—Single dose: 200 mg.

### Usual pediatric dose

Safety and efficacy have not been established.

### Usual geriatric dose

See *Usual adult dose*.

### Strength(s) usually available

U.S.—
5 mg (Rx) [*Demadex*].
10 mg (Rx) [*Demadex*].
20 mg (Rx) [*Demadex*].
100 mg (Rx) [*Demadex*].
Canada—
Not commercially available.

### Packaging and storage

Store below 40 °C (104 °F), preferably between 15 and 30 °C (59 and 86 °F). Protect from freezing.

### Auxiliary labeling

• Do not take other medicines without your doctor's advice.

# Parenteral Dosage Forms

## TORSEMIDE INJECTION

### Usual adult dose

Diuretic—
Congestive heart failure:
Intravenous, 10 or 20 mg once a day, the dosage being increased as needed, up to 200 mg, for desired therapeutic effect.
Hepatic cirrhosis:
Intravenous, 5 or 10 mg once a day, administered with an aldosterone antagonist or a potassium-sparing diuretic.
Renal failure, chronic:
Intravenous, 20 mg once a day, the dosage being increased by doubling as needed until adequate diuretic response is achieved.

### Usual adult prescribing limits

See *Torsemide Tablets*.

### Usual pediatric dose

Safety and efficacy have not been established.

### Usual geriatric dose

See *Usual adult dose*.

### Strength(s) usually available

U.S.—
10 mg per mL (Rx) [*Demadex*].
Canada—
Not commercially available.

### Packaging and storage

Store below 40 °C (104 °F), preferably between 15 and 30 °C (59 and 86 °F). Protect from freezing.

### Stability

Do not use if solution is discolored.

# Selected Bibliography

Friedel HA, Buckley MM. Torsemide. A review of its pharmacological properties and therapeutic potential. Drugs 1991; 41 (1): 81-103.
The fifth report of the Joint National Committee on Detection, Evaluation, and Treatment of High Blood Pressure (JNC V). Arch Intern Med 1993; 153 (2): 154-83.

Developed: 02/15/95
Interim revision: 08/01/95

# TRAMADOL    Systemic†

VA CLASSIFICATION (Primary): CN103

Note: For a listing of dosage forms and brand names by country availability, see *Dosage Forms* section(s). For a listing of brand names for the articles in this monograph, refer to the General Index.

---

†Not commercially available in Canada.

---

## Category
Analgesic.

## Indications

### Accepted
Pain (treatment)—Tramadol is indicated for the management of moderate to moderately severe pain. It has been used to treat pain following orthopedic and gynecological procedures, including cesarean section.

### Acceptance not established
Tramadol has been used for long-term treatment of *chronic pain* such as low back pain, neuropathic pain, orthopedic and joint conditions, and cancer pain. Tramadol may be a therapeutic option for patients who are intolerant to or inappropriate candidates for nonsteroidal anti-inflammatory drugs (NSAIDs); however, more studies evaluating safety and efficacy need to be established for long-term use.

Tramadol has been evaluated and has shown promise as an adjunct to NSAIDs for patients experiencing inadequate relief from *dental pain* with NSAIDs alone. Although tramadol would not be effective in patients needing only anti-inflammatory treatment, it would be effective in enhancing the suppression of pain. A small study found a single dose of tramadol given concomitantly with a single dose of ibuprofen enhanced suppression of dental pain caused by inflammation. However, additional studies need to be done to evaluate the use of tramadol and NSAIDs concomitantly as a therapeutic combination to enhance analgesic efficacy.

## Pharmacology/Pharmacokinetics

### Physicochemical characteristics
Source—Synthetic
Molecular weight—299.84.
pKa—9.41.

### Mechanism of action/Effect
Tramadol is a centrally-acting analgesic that is not chemically related to opiates. The mechanism of action of tramadol is not completely understood, but it may bind to mu-opioid receptors and inhibit the reuptake of norepinephrine (NE) and serotonin (5-HT). The ability of tramadol to inhibit the neuronal uptake of monoamines in the same concentration range at which it binds to mu-opioid receptors differentiates it from typical opioids. Tramadol consists of (+) and (−) enantiomers that appear to interact synergistically to produce antinociception. The (+) enantiomer is five fold more potent in 5-HT uptake and has a greater affinity for mu receptor binding than for NE uptake. The (−) enantiomer is five to ten fold more potent in NE uptake inhibition and has less affinity for mu receptor binding than for 5-HT uptake. Electrophysiological studies show that tramadol, like morphine, depresses motor and sensory responses of the spinal nociceptive system by a spinal and a supraspinal action. Some opioid activity is derived from low affinity binding of the parent compound and higher affinity binding of the mono-*O*-desmethyltramadol (M1) metabolite to the opioid receptors. Although analgesic potency of M1 is about six times greater than that of tramadol in animal models, the relative potency in humans is unknown.

Note: It has been estimated that the analgesic potency of tramadol is one-tenth that of morphine.

### Other actions/effects
Tramadol suppresses the cough reflex by binding to the mu-opioid receptor binding sites. Due to the high affinity binding of the M1 metabolite to the mu receptor, the metabolite has been found to have more cough suppressant activity than the parent compound.

Unlike morphine, tramadol has not been shown to cause histamine release.

### Absorption
Oral—Rapid and almost complete. Mean absolute bioavailability of a 100-mg dose is approximately 75%. The rate or extent of absorption is not significantly affected by administration with food.

### Distribution
The volume of distribution is 2.6 and 2.9 liters per kilogram of body weight (L/kg) in males and females, respectively, following a 100-mg intravenous dose. Tramadol crosses the blood-brain barrier in rats and possibly in humans.

### Protein binding
Low (20%). Independent of concentration up to 10 micrograms per mL (mcg/mL); saturation of binding occurs only at concentrations outside of the clinically relevant range.

### Biotransformation
Hepatic. Extensively metabolized via *N*- and *O*-demethylation and glucuronidation or sulfation. The production of the active metabolite mono-*O*-desmethyltramadol (M1) is dependent on the cyp2d6 isoenzyme of cytochrome *P*-450. The inactive metabolites are formed by *N*- demethylation.

### Half-life
Terminal—
    Individuals with normal renal function:
        Tramadol—Approximately 6.3 hours (increased to 7 hours with multiple dosing [not clinically significant] and in individuals over 75 years of age [clinically significant]).
        M1 metabolite—Approximately 7.4 hours.

### Onset of action
Dose-dependent; generally within 1 hour.

### Time to peak concentration
Plasma—
    Following a single 100-mg dose:
        Tramadol—2 hours.
        M1 metabolite—3 hours.

### Time to steady state concentation:
Plasma—
    After administration of 100 mg four times a day:
        About 2 days.

### Peak serum concentration
Plasma—
    Following a single 100-mg dose:
        Tramadol—308 nanograms per mL ±78 nanograms/mL.
        M1 metabolite—55 nanograms per mL ± 20 nanograms/mL.

### Time to peak effect
Tramadol—2 hours.
M1 metabolite—3 hours.

### Elimination
Renal—
    30% unchanged; 60% as metabolites. Clearance rate is slightly higher in females than in males.
In dialysis—
    7% of an administered dose is removed by hemodialysis.

## Precautions to Consider

### Tumorigenicity
Evidence of a statistically significant increase in two common murine tumors (pulmonary and hepatic) was observed in mice receiving oral doses up to 30 mg per kg of body weight (mg/kg) for approximately 2 years.

### Mutagenicity
No evidence of mutagenicity was found in the Ames test, CHO/HPRT mammalian cell assay, mouse lymphoma assay, or dominant lethal mutation test in mice. Weakly mutagenic results occurred in the presence of metabolic activation in the mouse lymphoma assay and micronucleus test in rats.

### Pregnancy/Reproduction
Fertility—No impairment of fertility was observed at oral dose levels up to 50 mg/kg in male rats and 75 mg/kg in female rats.

Pregnancy—Tramadol has been shown to cross the placenta. Well-controlled studies in humans have not been done.

Studies have shown tramadol to be embryotoxic and fetotoxic in mice, rats, and rabbits at maternally toxic doses (3 to 15 times the maximum human dose or higher); however, it was found not to be teratogenic at these levels. Studies done in progeny of mice, rats, and rabbits given tramadol by various routes (up to 140 mg/kg for mice, 80 mg/kg for rats, or 300 mg/kg for rabbits) found no drug-related teratogenic effects. Transient delays in the developmental and behavioral parameters during the delivery of pups from rat dams were observed. At maternally toxic levels, fetal toxicity and embryotoxicity primarily included decreased fetal weights, skeletal ossification, and increased supernumerary ribs. A study in rabbits reported embryo and fetal lethality caused by extreme maternal toxicity at doses of 300 mg/kg. In peri- and postnatal studies in rats, decreased weights were observed in the progeny of dams that received oral (gavage) doses of 50 mg/kg or greater. At doses of 80 mg/kg (6 to 10 times the maximum human dose), pup survival was decreased early in lactation. The progeny of dams receiving 8, 10, 20, 25, or 40 mg/kg showed no signs of toxicity. Evidence of severe maternal toxicity was observed at higher doses; however, maternal toxicity was found at all dose levels.

FDA Pregnancy Category C.

Labor and delivery—Tramadol is not recommended for use in pregnant women prior to or during labor unless the potential benefits outweigh the risks, because safe use in pregnancy has not been established.

**Breast-feeding**

Following a single intravenous 100-mg dose of tramadol, the cumulative distribution in breast milk within 16 hours postdose was 100 micrograms (mcg) of tramadol (0.1% of the maternal dose) and 27 mcg of M1. Use of oral tramadol is not recommended for obstetrical preoperative medication or postdelivery analgesia in nursing mothers because of lack of studies on its safety in infants and newborns.

**Pediatrics**

No information is available on the relationship of age to the effects of tramadol in patients under 16 years of age. Safety and efficacy have not been established.

**Geriatrics**

Studies have shown that, in subjects over the age of 75 years, serum concentrations are slightly elevated and the elimination half-life is slightly prolonged. In addition, elderly patients are more likely to have age-related renal function impairment that may require dosage adjustment.

**Drug interactions and/or related problems**

The following drug interactions and/or related problems have been selected on the basis of their potential clinical significance (possible mechanism in parentheses where appropriate)—not necessarily inclusive (» = major clinical significance):

» Alcohol or
» Anesthetic agents or
» Central nervous system (CNS) depression–producing medications, other (See *Appendix II*), such as:
    Antidepressants, tricyclics
    Opioid analgesics
    Phenothiazines
    Sedative hypnotics
    Tranquilizers
        (caution is recommended because concurrent use may potentiate the CNS depressant effects; tricyclic antidepressants, fluoxetine and sertraline may increase the risk of seizures; dosage reduction is recommended)

» Carbamazepine
    (causes a significant increase in tramadol metabolism, presumably through metabolic enzyme induction; dosage adjustment may be required [patients receiving chronic carbamazepine in doses up to 800 mg per day may require up to twice the recommended dose of tramadol])

» Monoamine oxidase (MAO) inhibitors, including furazolidone and procarbazine
    (tramadol inhibits the uptake of norepinephrine and serotonin; serotonin is believed to be the biogenic amine responsible for the toxic interactions; concurrent use may decrease seizure threshold; caution is recommended)

Quinidine
    (concurrent use may increase concentrations of tramadol and decrease concentration of the M1 metabolite by competitively inhibiting the cyp2d6 isoenzyme; inhibition of the formation of the M1 metabolite did not significantly alter the peak analgesic effect of a single 100-mg dose of tramadol in healthy volunteers)

Propafenone
    (concurrent use may increase concentrations of tramadol and decrease concentration of the M1 metabolite by inhibiting the cyp2d6 isoenzyme)

**Medical considerations/Contraindications**

The medical considerations/contraindications included here have been selected on the basis of their potential clinical significance (reasons given in parentheses where appropriate)—not necessarily inclusive (» = major clinical significance).

Note: Tramadol does not affect the bile duct sphincter, which indicates that it is less likely than opioids to cause urinary retention, constipation, or worsening of pancreatic or biliary disorders.

*Except under special circumstances, this medication should not be used when the following medical problems exist:*

» Acute intoxication with alcohol, hypnotics, centrally-acting analgesics, opioids, or psychotropic drugs
    (risk of respiratory depression)

» Drug abuse or dependence, current or history of, including alcoholism
    (patient predisposition to drug abuse)

*Risk-benefit should be considered when the following medical problems exist:*

Acute abdominal conditions
    (diagnosis may be obscured)

» Hepatic function impairment
    (metabolism of tramadol and M1 is reduced in patients with advanced cirrhosis of the liver; dosage reduction is recommended; delay in achievement of steady state may result from the prolonged half-life in this condition)

Increased intracranial pressure or
Head trauma
    (tramadol causes pupillary changes [miosis] that may obscure the existence, extent, or course of intracranial pathology; clinicians should consider the possibility of a drug effect when evaluating mental status)

» Renal function impairment
    (decreased rate and extent of excretion of tramadol and its active metabolite M1; dosage reduction is recommended in patients with creatinine clearance of less than 30 mL per minute [mL/min]; delay in achievement of steady-state may result from the prolonged half-life in this condition)

» Respiratory depression, risk of
    (tramadol may decrease respiratory drive and increase airway resistance in patients with this condition; although there is absence of significant respiratory depression following epidural and intravenous use, caution is still recommended with administration of oral tramadol in patients at risk for respiratory depression; may also occur with concurrent administration of anesthetic medication or alcohol)

» Seizures
    (tramadol may increase the risk of seizures in patients taking neuroleptics and other drugs that reduce the seizure threshold)

» Sensitivity to opioids or
» Sensitivity to tramadol
    (increased risk of anaphylactoid reactions)

    Note: Caution is also recommended with the administration of tramadol in patients with a physical dependence on opioids. Withdrawal symptoms may occur in patients who have recently taken substantial amounts of opioids.

## Side/Adverse Effects

Note: Tramadol can produce drug dependence of the mu-opioid type and may potentially be abused. Tolerance development, drug seeking behavior and craving have been associated with the use of tramadol. The active metabolite of tramadol may be responsible for some delay in onset of activity and some extension of the duration of mu-opioid activity. Delayed mu-opioid activity is believed to reduce drug abuse liability. One case has been reported in which a patient developed tolerance to and dependence on oral tramadol (increase in daily dose by 500% over 6 years, from 50 to 300 mg per day). However, in a 3-week study no tolerance developed to oral tramadol. A few studies found no or very little development of tolerance with parenteral administration of tramadol.

The following side/adverse effects have been selected on the basis of their potential clinical significance (possible signs and symptoms in parentheses where appropriate)—not necessarily inclusive:

**Those indicating need for medical attention**

Incidence less frequent—1 to 5%
    *Urinary frequency* (frequent urge to urinate); *urinary retention* (difficult urination); *visual disturbances* (blurred vision)

Incidence rare
    *Abnormal gait* (change in walking and balance); *allergic reaction* (severe redness, swelling, and itching of the skin); *amnesia* (loss of memory); *cognitive dysfunction* (trouble performing routine tasks); *dyspnea* (shortness of breath); *hallucinations* (seeing, hearing, or feeling things that are not there); *orthostatic hypotension* (dizziness or light-

headedness when getting up from a lying or sitting position); *paresthesia* (numbness, tingling, pain, or weakness in hands or feet); *seizures; syncope* (fainting); *tachycardia* (fast heartbeat); *tremor* (trembling and shaking of hands or feet); *urticaria* (redness, swelling, and itching of the skin); *vesicles* (blisters under the skin)

### Those indicating need for medical attention only if they continue or are bothersome

Incidence less frequent—1 to 5%

*Abdominal or stomach pain; anorexia* (loss of appetite); *anxiety; asthenia* (loss of strength or weakness); *confusion; constipation; coordination disturbance* (trouble in performing routine tasks); *diarrhea; dizziness or vertigo; drowsiness; dry mouth; dyspepsia* (heartburn); *euphoria* (unusual feeling of excitement); *flatulence* (excessive gas); *headache; malaise* (general feeling of bodily discomfort); *menopausal symptoms* (hot flashes); *nausea; nervousness; pruritis* (itching); *skin rash; sleep disorder* (trouble in sleeping); *sweating; vasodilation* (flushing or redness of the skin); *vomiting*

Note: Tramadol may produce opioid-like effects, including *constipation, dizziness, drowsiness, nausea, pruritus,* and *sweating,* but causes less respiratory depression than morphine.

### Those indicating possible withdrawal and the need for medical attention if they occur after medication is discontinued

*Anxiety; body aches; diarrhea; fast heartbeat; fever, runny nose, or sneezing; gooseflesh; hypertension* (high blood pressure); *increased sweating; increased yawning; loss of appetite; nausea or vomiting; nervousness, restlessness, or irritability; shivering or trembling; stomach cramps; trouble in sleeping; unusually large pupils; weakness*

Note: The *signs and symptoms of withdrawal* listed above are characteristics of the abstinence syndrome produced by abrupt discontinuation of a mu-receptor agonist. Tramadol does have some activity involving the mu receptor; therefore, abrupt discontinuation may include some of these signs and symptoms. However, these effects may be milder compared with opiate agonists. Minimal withdrawal signs have been observed in naloxone-precipitation studies.

## Overdose

For specific information on the agents used in the management of tramadol overdose, see:
* *Diazepam* in *Benzodiazepines (Systemic)* monograph; and/or
* *Naloxone (Systemic)* monograph.

For more information on the management of overdose or unintentional ingestion, **contact a Poison Control Center** (see *Poison Control Center Listing* ).

### Clinical effects of overdose

The following effects have been selected on the basis of their potential clinical significance (possible signs and symptoms in parentheses where appropriate)—not necessarily inclusive:

Acute and chronic effects

*Cold, clammy skin; confusion; convulsions; dizziness, severe; drowsiness, severe; nervousness or restlessness, severe; pinpoint pupils of eyes; slow heartbeat; seizures; slow or troubled breathing; unconsciousness; weakness, severe*

Note: Studies have found the administration of intravenous tramadol may produce respiratory depression. However, morphine causes more clinically significant respiratory depression than tramadol. Clinical studies evaluating oral doses have not reported any clinically relevant respiratory depressant effects.

### Treatment of overdose

Recommended treatment for tramadol overdose may consist of the following:

To decrease absorption—Gastric lavage may be performed.

Specific treatment—Administration of the opioid antagonist naloxone, which will reverse some, but not all, symptoms caused by overdosage with tramadol. Administer naloxone with caution because it may precipitate seizures. See the package insert or *Naloxone (Systemic)* for specific dosing guidelines for use of this product.

For treatment of convulsions caused by tramadol toxicity: Diazepam has been effective in treating convulsions. See the package insert or *Diazepam* in *Benzodiazepines (Systemic)* for specific dosing guidelines for use of this product.

Supportive care—Supportive measures such as establishing intravenous lines, hydration, correction of electrolyte imbalance, oxygenation, and support of ventilatory function are essential for maintaining the vital functions of the patient. Patients in whom intentional overdose is confirmed or suspected should be referred for psychiatric consultation.

Note: Hemodialysis is not recommended in overdose, since it removes less than 7% of the administered dose in a 4-hour dialysis period.

## Patient Consultation

As an aid to patient consultation, refer to *Advice for the Patient, Tramadol (Systemic).*

In providing consultation, consider emphasizing the following selected information (» = major clinical significance):

### Before using this medication

» Conditions affecting use, especially:
   Sensitivity to tramadol or opioids
   Pregnancy—Crosses the placenta; safe use in pregnancy has not been established
   Breast-feeding—Distributed into breast milk; use is not recommended
   Other medications, especially carbamazepine, CNS depressants or anesthetic agents, or MAO inhibitors
   Other medical problems, especially acute intoxication with alcohol, hypnotics, centrally-acting analgesics, opioids, or psychotropic drugs; hepatic function impairment; physical dependence on opioids; renal function impairment; risk of respiratory depression; or seizures

### Proper use of this medication

» Not increasing dose if medication is less effective after a few weeks; checking with physician first
» Importance of not taking more medication than the amount prescribed because of danger of overdose
» Proper dosing
» Missed dose (if on scheduled dosing): Taking as soon as possible; not taking if almost time for next dose; not doubling doses
» Proper storage

### Precautions while using this medication

» Avoiding use of alcoholic beverages or other CNS depressants during therapy unless prescribed or otherwise approved by physician
» Caution if dizziness, drowsiness, or lightheadedness occurs
» Caution when getting up from a lying or sitting position
   Lying down if nausea or vomiting, or dizziness or lightheadedness occurs
   Informing physician or dentist of use of medication if any kind of surgery (including dental surgery) or emergency treatment is required
» Suspected overdose: Getting emergency help at once

### Side/adverse effects

Signs of potential side effects, especially urinary frequency, urinary retention, visual disturbances, abnormal gait, allergic reaction, amnesia, cognitive dysfunction, dyspnea, hallucinations, orthostatic hypotension, paresthesia, seizures, syncope, tachycardia, tremor, urticaria, and vesicles

## Oral Dosage Forms

### TRAMADOL HYDROCHLORIDE TABLETS

#### Usual adult and adolescent dose

Analgesic—Oral, 50 to 100 mg every six hours as needed.

Note: A dose of 50 mg is usually more effective as the initial dose for moderate pain; a dose of 100 mg is usually more effective as the initial dose for more severe pain.

Patients with impaired renal function (creatinine clearance less than 30 mL/minute [mL/min]) should receive 50 to 100 mg every twelve hours.

An initial dose of 50 to 100 mg every twelve hours is usually adequate for patients with cirrhosis.

Patients on hemodialysis can receive their usual dose on the day of dialysis.

#### Usual adult prescribing limits

Oral, 400 mg per day (200 mg per day in patients with creatinine clearance of less than 30 mL/min).

#### Usual pediatric dose

Children up to 16 years of age—Safety and efficacy have not been established.

Children 16 years of age and over—See *Usual adult and adolescent dose.*

#### Usual geriatric dose

See *Usual adult and adolescent dose.*

Note: In patients over 75 years of age the prescribing limit is 300 mg per day in divided doses.

**Strength(s) usually available**
U.S.—
    50 mg (Rx) [*Ultram* (lactose)].
Canada—
    Not commercially available.

**Packaging and storage**
Store between 15 and 30 °C (59 and 86 °F), in a tight container.

**Auxiliary labeling**
• May cause drowsiness.
• Avoid alcoholic beverages.

Note: Tramadol is not a controlled substance in the U.S.

**Selected Bibliography**

Levien TL, Baker DE. Reviews of tramadol and tretinoin. Hosp Pharm 1996; 31 (1): 54-67.
Preston KL, Jasinski DR, Testa M. Abuse potential and pharmacological comparison of tramadol and morphine. Drug and Alcohol Depend 1991; 27: 7-17.
Sunshine A, Olson N, Zinghelboim I, et al. Analgesic oral efficacy of tramadol hydrochloride in postoperative pain. Clin Pharmacol Ther 1992; 51: 740-6.

Developed: 07/15/96

---

# TRANEXAMIC ACID  Systemic

VA CLASSIFICATION (Primary/Secondary): BL300/IM900

Note: For a listing of dosage forms and brand names by country availability, see *Dosage Forms* section(s). For a listing of brand names for the articles in this monograph, refer to the General Index.

## Category

Antifibrinolytic; antihemorrhagic.

## Indications

Note: Bracketed information in the *Indications* section refers to uses that are not included in U.S. product labeling.

**Accepted**

Hemorrhage, following dental surgery, in hemophiliacs (prophylaxis and treatment)
[Hemorrhage, postsurgical (treatment)] or
[Hemorrhage, hyperfibrinolysis-induced (treatment)]—Tranexamic acid is indicated for the management of hemophilic patients (those having Factor VIII or Factor IX deficiency) undergoing tooth extraction [or other oral surgical procedures]. The medication prevents or decreases hemorrhaging during and following surgery in these patients and reduces the need for administration of clotting factors.

[Tranexamic acid is indicated for the treatment of severe localized bleeding secondary to hyperfibrinolysis, including epistaxis, hyphema, or hypermenorrhea (menorrhagia) and hemorrhage following certain surgical procedures, such as conization of the cervix.]

[Antifibrinolytic agents are used to treat severe hemorrhaging caused by thrombolytic agents such as alteplase (tissue-type plasminogen activator, recombinant), anistreplase (anisoylated plasminogen-streptokinase activator complex), streptokinase, or urokinase.][1] However, controlled studies to demonstrate their efficacy have not been done in humans.

[Bleeding responsive to antifibrinolytic therapy also may occur following heart surgery (with or without cardiac bypass procedures) and portacaval shunt, prostatectomy, nephrectomy, or bladder surgery, and in association with hematologic disorders (such as aplastic anemia, abruptio placentae, hepatic cirrhosis, neoplastic disease, and polycystic or neoplastic diseases of the genitourinary system.][1]

[Angioedema, hereditary (treatment)]—Tranexamic acid is indicated for the treatment of hereditary angioedema. It is used to reduce the frequency and severity of acute attacks in patients with this disorder.

Note: Antifibrinolytic agents are ineffective in bleeding caused by loss of vascular integrity; a definite clinical diagnosis or confirmation of hyperfibrinolysis (hyperplasminemia) via laboratory studies is required before tranexamic acid is used to treat hemorrhage. However, some conditions and laboratory findings suggestive of hyperfibrinolysis are also present in disseminated intravascular coagulation; differentiation between the two conditions is essential because antifibrinolytic agents may promote thrombus formation in patients with disseminated intravascular coagulation and must *not*

be used unless heparin is administered concurrently. The following criteria may be useful in differential diagnosis:

| Test | Primary Hyperfibrinolysis Results | Disseminated Intravascular Coagulation Results |
|------|-----------------------------------|-----------------------------------------------|
| Platelet count* | Normal | Decreased |
| Protamine para-coagulation test | Negative | Positive |
| Euglobulin clot lysis time | Decreased | Normal |

*Following extracorporeal circulation (during cardiovascular surgery), decreased platelet count may not be useful for differentiating between primary hyperfibrinolysis and disseminated intravascular coagulation; the other criteria may be more useful in differential diagnosis in these patients.

[1]Not included in Canadian product labeling.

## Pharmacology/Pharmacokinetics

**Physicochemical characteristics**
Molecular weight—157.21.

**Mechanism of action/Effect**
Tranexamic acid competitively inhibits activation of plasminogen, thereby reducing conversion of plasminogen to plasmin (fibrinolysin), an enzyme that degrades fibrin clots, fibrinogen, and other plasma proteins, including the procoagulant factors V and VIII. Tranexamic acid also directly inhibits plasmin activity, but higher doses are required than are needed to reduce plasmin formation. *In vitro*, the antifibrinolytic potency of tranexamic acid is approximately 5 to 10 times that of aminocaproic acid.
In patients with hereditary angioedema, inhibition of the formation and activity of plasmin by tranexamic acid may prevent attacks of angioedema by decreasing plasmin-induced activation of the first complement protein (C1).

**Absorption**
Oral—30 to 50% of a dose is absorbed from the gastrointestinal tract. Bioavailability is not altered by food intake.

**Distribution**
In breast milk—Concentrations are approximately 1% of the maternal serum concentration.

**Protein binding**
Very low (<3%), primarily to plasminogen, at therapeutic plasma concentrations. Tranexamic acid does not bind to serum albumin.

**Biotransformation**
Less than 5% of a dose is metabolized.

**Half-life**
Elimination—Approximately 2 hours (following intravenous administration of a 1-gram dose).

**Time to peak concentration**
Oral—Approximately 3 hours.

**Peak plasma concentration**
Oral—8 mcg per mL (50.9 micromoles/L) following a dose of 1 gram; 15 mcg per mL (95.4 micromoles/L) following a dose of 2 grams.

**Therapeutic plasma concentration**
10 mcg per mL (63.6 micromoles/L). Therapeutic concentrations persist in serum for 7 to 8 hours, and in several other tissues for up to 17 hours, following administration of the last of 4 doses of 10 mg per kg of body weight (mg/kg) intravenously or 20 mg/kg orally.

**Elimination**
Renal, via glomerular filtration; > 95% of a dose is excreted as unchanged tranexamic acid.
Oral—39% of a dose (about 78% of the quantity absorbed) is excreted within 24 hours after administration of 10 to 15 mg/kg.
Intravenous—90% of a dose is excreted within 24 hours after administration of 10 mg/kg.

## Precautions to Consider

### Carcinogenicity/Tumorigenicity
An increased incidence of leukemia occurred in male mice receiving approximately 5 grams per kg of body weight per day of tranexamic acid (added to food in a concentration of 4.8%). Female mice were not included in that study. In another study, tranexamic acid produced adenomas, adenocarcinomas, and hyperplasia of the biliary tract when administered orally to one strain of rats in doses exceeding the maximum tolerated dose for a period of 22 months. Lower doses produced hyperplastic, but not neoplastic, changes. No hyperplastic or neoplastic changes were observed in subsequent long-term studies in which equivalent doses were administered to a different strain of rats.

### Mutagenicity
Studies using a variety of *in vivo* and *in vitro* test systems have not shown that tranexamic acid has mutagenic activity.

### Pregnancy/Reproduction
Fertility—Tranexamic acid has been detected in semen in antifibrinolytic concentrations but has no effect on the motility of spermatozoa. Reproductive studies in mice, rats, and rabbits have shown no evidence of impaired fertility.

Pregnancy—Tranexamic acid crosses the placenta. Following intravenous administration of 10 mg per kg of body weight (mg/kg) to pregnant women, 30 mcg of tranexamic acid per mL (190.8 micromoles/L) was measured in fetal serum. Adequate and well-controlled studies in humans have not been done. However, healthy infants have been born to women who received tranexamic acid during pregnancy for treatment of fibrinolytic bleeding or bleeding associated with abruptio placentae.

Studies in mice, rats, and rabbits have not shown that tranexamic acid causes adverse effects on the fetus.

FDA Pregnancy Category B.

### Breast-feeding
Tranexamic acid is distributed into breast milk; concentrations reach approximately 1% of the maternal plasma concentration.

### Pediatrics
Appropriate studies on the relationship of age to the effects of tranexamic acid have not been performed in the pediatric population. However, no pediatrics-specific problems have been documented to date.

### Geriatrics
Appropriate studies performed to date have not demonstrated geriatrics-specific problems that would limit the usefulness of tranexamic acid in the elderly.

### Drug interactions and/or related problems
The following drug interactions and/or related problems have been selected on the basis of their potential clinical significance (possible mechanism in parentheses where appropriate)—not necessarily inclusive (» = major clinical significance):

Anti-inhibitor coagulant complex or
Factor IX complex
(although tranexamic acid is often used in conjunction with clotting factor replacement for the perisurgical management of hemophilic patients, concurrent use may increase the risk of thrombotic complications; some hematologists recommend that administration of tranexamic acid be delayed for 8 hours following injection of either of the clotting factor complexes)

Contraceptives, estrogen-containing, oral or
Estrogens
(concurrent use with tranexamic acid may increase the potential for thrombus formation)

Thrombolytic agents
(the actions of tranexamic acid and of thrombolytic agents [e.g., alteplase (tissue-type plasminogen activator, recombinant; tPA), anistreplase (anisoylated plasminogen-streptokinase activator complex; APSAC), streptokinase, or urokinase] are mutually antagonistic; although controlled studies to demonstrate its efficacy have not been done in humans, tranexamic acid may be useful in treating severe hemorrhage caused by a thrombolytic agent)

### Medical considerations/Contraindications
The medical considerations/contraindications included here have been selected on the basis of their potential clinical significance (reasons given in parentheses where appropriate)—not necessarily inclusive (» = major clinical significance).

*Except under special circumstances, this medication should not be used when the following medical problems exist:*

»   Intravascular clotting, active
(risk of serious, even fatal, thrombus formation)

*Risk-benefit should be considered when the following medical problems exist:*

»   Defective color vision, acquired
(condition precludes assessment of color vision, which may be required to determine toxicity)

»   Hematuria of upper urinary tract origin
(risk of intrarenal obstruction secondary to clot retention in the renal pelvis and ureters if hematuria is massive; also, if hematuria is associated with a disease of the renal parenchyma, intravascular precipitation of fibrin may occur and exacerbate the disease)

»   Hemorrhage, subarachnoid
(increased risk of cerebral edema and cerebral infarction)

»   Renal function impairment
(medication may accumulate; dosage adjustment based on the degree of impairment is recommended)

Sensitivity to tranexamic acid, history of

»   Thrombosis, predisposition to or history of
(medication inhibits clot dissolution and may interfere with mechanisms for maintaining blood vessel patency; it is recommended that tranexamic acid be administered in conjunction with anticoagulant therapy, if at all)

### Patient monitoring
The following may be especially important in patient monitoring (other tests may be warranted in some patients, depending on condition; » = major clinical significance):

Ophthalmological examinations, including tests for visual acuity, color vision, eyeground, and visual fields
(recommended prior to and at regular intervals during therapy for patients receiving the medication for longer than several days because tranexamic acid has caused focal areas of retinal degeneration in animal studies and visual disturbances [although retinal lesions have not been reported] in humans)

## Side/Adverse Effects

Note: Patients receiving tranexamic acid should be monitored for signs of thromboembolic complications.

Focal areas of retinal degeneration have been reported in cats, dogs, and rats after oral or intravenous administration of tranexamic acid at doses of 250 to 1600 mg per kg of body weight (mg/kg) per day (6 to 40 times the recommended usual human dose) for 6 days to a year. The incidence and severity of the lesions are dose-dependent. Some lesions in animals receiving low doses have been reversible. Other studies in cats and rabbits have shown retinal changes to occur with doses as low as 126 mg/kg per day (about 3 times the recommended usual human dose) administered for several days to two weeks. However, no retinal changes occurred in patients receiving tranexamic acid for weeks to months in clinical trials.

The following side/adverse effects have been selected on the basis of their potential clinical significance (possible signs and symptoms in parentheses where appropriate)—not necessarily inclusive:

### Those indicating need for medical attention
Incidence less frequent or rare
*Blurred vision or other changes in vision; hypotension* (dizziness or lightheadedness; unusual tiredness or weakness)—may be associated

with too-rapid intravenous administration; *thrombosis or thrombo-embolism* (pains in chest, groin, or legs [especially calves]; severe, sudden headache; sudden and unexplained shortness of breath, slurred speech, vision changes, and/or weakness or numbness in arm or leg; sudden loss of coordination)—depending on site of thrombus formation or embolization

**Those indicating need for medical attention only if they continue or are bothersome**
Incidence more frequent
*Diarrhea; nausea; vomiting*
Incidence unknown
*Unusual menstrual discomfort*—caused by clotting of menstrual fluid

## Overdose

For more information on the management of overdose or unintentional ingestion, **contact a Poison Control Center** (see *Poison Control Center Listing*).

### Treatment of overdose
Although there is no experience with overdose of tranexamic acid, discontinuing the medication is recommended.

For thromboembolic complications—Monitoring the patient carefully and administering appropriate therapy, depending on the location and size of the thrombus. Use of heparin or a thrombolytic agent may be considered in severe cases. However, these medications must be used with extreme caution, if at all, in patients receiving tranexamic acid to prevent or treat hemorrhaging, because of the risk of uncontrollable hemorrhage being induced in such patients.

If tranexamic acid had been administered orally, limiting absorption via induction of emesis, gastric lavage, and/or administration of activated charcoal may be helpful.

## Patient Consultation

As an aid to patient consultation, refer to *Advice for the Patient, Antifibrinolytic Agents (Systemic)*.

In providing consultation, consider emphasizing the following selected information (» = major clinical significance):

**Before using this medication**
» Conditions affecting use, especially:
   Sensitivity to tranexamic acid, history of
   Pregnancy—Tranexamic acid crosses the placenta, but has not been reported to cause problems when given to pregnant women
   Breast-feeding—Tranexamic acid is distributed into breast milk
   Other medical problems, especially defective color vision, hematuria of upper urinary tract origin, predisposition to or history of thrombosis, renal function impairment, and subarachnoid hemorrhage

**Proper use of this medication**
» Importance of not using more or less medication than the amount prescribed
» Proper dosing
   Missed dose: Taking as soon as possible, then returning to regular dosing schedule; not doubling doses
» Proper storage

**Precautions while using this medication**
   Possible need for regular ophthalmologic examinations during long-term therapy

**Side/adverse effects**
   Signs of potential side effects, especially blurred vision or other changes in vision, hypotension, and thrombosis or thromboembolism.

## General Dosing Information

A reduction in dosage may be required for patients with renal function impairment or if nausea, vomiting, or diarrhea occurs.

It is recommended that therapy be discontinued if thromboembolic complications occur or if changes in the results of ophthalmologic examinations are noted.

**For parenteral dosage forms only**
Tranexamic acid injection should be administered intravenously at a rate not to exceed 100 mg (1 mL) per minute, to avoid inducing hypotension.

## Oral Dosage Forms

Note: Bracketed uses in the *Dosage Forms* section refers to categories of use and/or indications that are not included in U.S. product labeling.

### TRANEXAMIC ACID TABLETS

**Usual adult and adolescent dose**
Hemorrhage, following dental surgery, in hemophiliacs—
   Presurgical: Oral, 25 mg per kg of body weight three or four times a day, beginning one day before the dental procedure. However, intravenous administration of the medication immediately prior to surgery may be preferred. Clotting factors (Factor VIII or Factor IX) should also be administered immediately prior to surgery.

Note: Because of an increased risk of thrombotic complications when tranexamic acid and Factor IX or anti-inhibitor coagulant complex are administered concurrently, some hematologists recommend that tranexamic acid not be administered within eight hours of these clotting factor concentrates.

   Postsurgical: Oral, 25 mg per kg of body weight three or four times a day for two to eight days after surgery.
[Hemorrhage, postsurgical–conization of the cervix]—
   Oral, 1 to 1.5 grams every eight to twelve hours for twelve days after surgery.
[Hemorrhage, postsurgical–prostatectomy][1] or
[Bladder surgery][1]—
   Oral, 1 gram three to four times a day starting on the fourth day after surgery (the medication having been administered intravenously for the first three days postoperatively). Therapy should be continued until macroscopic hematuria is no longer present.
[Hemorrhage, hyperfibrinolysis-induced–epistaxis]—
   Oral, 1 to 1.5 grams three or four times a day for 10 days.
[Hemorrhage, hyperfibrinolysis-induced–hypermenorrhea]—
   Oral, 1 to 1.5 grams three or four times a day for three or four days, starting after copious bleeding has begun.
[Hemorrhage, hyperfibrinolysis-induced–hyphema]—
   Oral, 1 to 1.5 grams three or four times a day for 7 days.
[Hemorrhage, hyperfibrinolysis-induced–other][1]—
   Oral, 20 to 25 mg two or three times a day. Therapy should be continued until there is evidence of cessation of bleeding or laboratory determinations of fibrinolysis indicate that treatment is no longer needed.
[Angioedema, hereditary]—
   Oral, 1 to 1.5 grams two or three times a day. Some patients can sense the onset of attacks and may be treated intermittently, with therapy being started at the first sign of an attack and continued for several days. Other patients should be treated on a continuing basis.

Note: Because of the risk of tranexamic acid accumulation, the following dosage regimens are recommended for patients with moderate to severe renal function impairment:

| Serum Creatinine (micromoles/L) | Dose |
| --- | --- |
| 120–250 (1.36–2.83 mg/dL) | 15 mg/kg two times a day |
| 250–500 (2.83–5.66 mg/dL) | 15 mg/kg a day |
| >500 (>5.66 mg/dL) | 15 mg/kg every 48 hours or 7.5 mg/kg every 24 hours |

**Usual pediatric dose**
Hemorrhage, following dental surgery, in hemophiliacs—
   See *Usual adult and adolescent dose*.

**Strength(s) usually available**
U.S.—
   500 mg (Rx) [*Cyklokapron* (microcrystalline cellulose; talc; magnesium stearate; silicon dioxide; povidone)].
Canada—
   500 mg (Rx) [*Cyklokapron*].

**Packaging and storage**
Store between 15 and 30 °C (59 and 86 °F), in a well-closed container, unless otherwise specified by manufacturer.

## Parenteral Dosage Forms

Note: Bracketed uses in the *Dosage Forms* section refers to categories of use and/or indications that are not included in U.S. product labeling.

### TRANEXAMIC ACID INJECTION

**Usual adult and adolescent dose**
Hemorrhage, following dental surgery, in hemophiliacs—

Presurgical: Intravenous, 10 mg per kg of body weight, administered immediately prior to surgery. Clotting factors (Factor VIII or Factor IX) should also be administered at this time.

Note: Because of an increased risk of thrombotic complications when tranexamic acid and Factor IX or anti-inhibitor coagulant complex are administered concurrently, some hematologists recommend that tranexamic acid not be administered within eight hours of these clotting factor concentrates.

Postsurgical (for patients unable to take medication orally): Intravenous, 10 mg per kg of body weight three or four times a day for two to eight days.

[Hemorrhage, postsurgical]—
Following prostatectomy or bladder surgery: Intravenous, 1 gram, administered during surgery initially, then every eight hours for three days. Therapy is then continued, using orally administered tranexamic acid, until macroscopic hematuria is no longer present.

Note: Tranexamic acid injection may also be used as an irrigation following bladder surgery. One gram of tranexamic acid in one liter of 0.9% sodium chloride irrigation is instilled into the bladder at a rate of 1 mL per minute once a day for two to five days following surgery.

[Hemorrhage, hyperfibrinolysis-induced]—
Intravenous, 15 mg per kg of body weight or 1 gram every six to eight hours. Therapy should be continued until there is evidence of cessation of bleeding or laboratory determinations of fibrinolysis indicate that treatment is no longer needed.

Note: For other specific indications listed under *Tranexamic Acid Tablets*, patients unable to take medication orally may receive intravenous administration of 10 mg per kg of body weight of tranexamic acid according to the dosing schedule recommended for that indication.

For relief of severe epistaxis, tranexamic acid injection has also been applied topically to the nasal mucosa, as a spray or by packing the nasal cavity with a gauze strip that has been soaked in the solution.

Because of the risk of tranexamic acid accumulation, the following dosage regimens are recommended for patients with moderate to severe renal function impairment:

| Serum Creatinine (micromoles/L) | Dose |
|---|---|
| 120–250 (1.36–2.83 mg/dL) | 10 mg/kg two times a day |
| 250–500 (2.83–5.66 mg/dL) | 10 mg/kg a day |
| >500 (>5.66 mg/dL) | 10 mg/kg every 48 hours or 5 mg/kg every 24 hours |

**Usual pediatric dose**
Hemorrhage, following dental surgery, in hemophiliacs—
See *Usual adult and adolescent dose.*

**Strength(s) usually available**
U.S.—
100 mg per mL (Rx) [*Cyklokapron*].
Canada—
100 mg per mL (500 mg per 5-mL ampul) (Rx) [*Cyklokapron*].

**Packaging and storage**
Store between 15 and 30 °C (59 and 86 °F), unless otherwise specified by manufacturer. Protect from freezing.

**Preparation of dosage form**
Tranexamic acid injection may be mixed with intravenous infusion solutions, including solutions containing electrolytes, carbohydrates, amino acids, or dextran.
Heparin may be added to the tranexamic acid injection, if necessary.

**Stability**
Intravenous infusion mixtures should be prepared the same day they are to be used.

**Incompatibilities**
Tranexamic acid should not be added to any solution containing penicillin or mixed with blood.

---

¹Not included in Canadian product labeling.

---

Revised: 08/12/94

---

**TRANYLCYPROMINE**—See *Antidepressants, Monoamine Oxidase (MAO) Inhibitor (Systemic)*

---

# TRAZODONE   Systemic

VA CLASSIFICATION (Primary/Secondary): CN609/CN103
Note: For a listing of dosage forms and brand names by country availability, see *Dosage Forms* section(s). For a listing of brand names for the articles in this monograph, refer to the General Index.

## Category

Antidepressant; antineuralgic.

## Indications

Note: Bracketed information in the *Indications* section refers to uses that are not included in U.S. product labeling.

**Accepted**

Depression, mental (treatment)—Trazodone is indicated in the treatment of major depressive episodes with or without prominent anxiety.

[Pain, neurogenic (treatment)]¹—Trazodone has been used to treat painful diabetic neuropathy and other types of chronic pain.

---

¹Not included in Canadian product labeling.

## Pharmacology/Pharmacokinetics

**Physicochemical characteristics**
Molecular weight—408.33.
Other characteristics—Trazodone is *not* chemically related to tricyclic, tetracyclic, or other known antidepressants.

**Mechanism of action/Effect**
Not completely established in humans. Animal studies indicate that trazodone selectively inhibits serotonin re-uptake in the brain, causes beta-receptor subsensitivity, and induces significant changes in serotonin-receptor binding with only a slight effect on alpha-adrenergic receptors. Also, trazodone potentiates the behavioral changes in animals induced by 5-hydroxytryptophan, a serotonin precursor.

**Absorption**
Well absorbed. When trazodone is taken with or shortly after ingestion of food, there may be an increase in the amount of drug absorbed, a decrease in maximum concentration, and a lengthening of time to reach peak concentration.

**Protein binding**
Very high (89 to 95%).

**Biotransformation**
Hepatic; extensive, by hydroxylation.

**Half-life**
Biphasic. More rapid, 3 to 6 hours; slower, 5 to 9 hours.

**Onset of therapeutic action**
In clinical trials, significant therapeutic results occurred after 2 weeks of therapy in 75% of the patients responsive to the medication, with some patients showing definite improvement after 1 week of therapy; 25% of the responding patients required 2 to 4 weeks of therapy before noticeable improvement occurred.

**Time to peak concentration**
Fasting, 1 hour; with food, 2 hours.

**Elimination**
Biliary—
20%
Renal—
75%, mostly as inactive metabolites.

# Precautions to Consider

## Carcinogenicity
No evidence of carcinogenicity was observed in rats receiving up to 300 mg per kg of body weight (mg/kg) a day for 18 months.

## Pregnancy/Reproduction
Pregnancy—Studies in humans have not been done.
Studies in animals have shown that trazodone causes congenital anomalies and increased fetal resorptions when given in doses up to 50 times those used in humans.
FDA Pregnancy Category C.

## Breast-feeding
Problems in humans have not been documented; however, trazodone and its metabolites have been shown to be present in human milk and in the milk of lactating test animals.

## Pediatrics
Appropriate studies on the relationship of age to the effects of trazodone have not been performed in the pediatric population.

## Geriatrics
Elderly patients are more likely than younger adults to experience the sedative or hypotensive effects of trazodone; therefore, initial doses as low as half the recommended adult dose should be used in elderly patients, with adjustments made as needed and tolerated.

## Dental
Peripheral anticholinergic effects, although they occur much less frequently with trazodone than with tricyclic antidepressants, may decrease or inhibit salivary flow, especially in middle-aged or elderly patients, thus contributing to the development of caries, periodontal disease, oral candidiasis, and discomfort.

## Drug interactions and/or related problems
The following drug interactions and/or related problems have been selected on the basis of their potential clinical significance (possible mechanism in parentheses where appropriate)—not necessarily inclusive (» = major clinical significance):

Note: Combinations containing any of the following medications, depending on the amount present, may also interact with this medication.

» Alcohol or
» Central nervous system (CNS) depression–producing medications, other (See *Appendix II*)
    (concurrent use with trazodone may result in potentiation of CNS depressant effects)

Anticholinergics or other medications with anticholinergic activity (See *Appendix II*) or
Antidyskinetics or
Antihistamines
    (concurrent use with trazodone may intensify anticholinergic effects because of secondary anticholinergic activities of trazodone)
    (also, concurrent use of trazodone with antihistamines may potentiate the CNS depressant effects of either medication)

Antidepressants, tricyclic or
Haloperidol or
Loxapine or
Maprotiline or
Molindone or
Phenothiazines or
Pimozide or
Thioxanthenes
    (concurrent use may prolong and intensify the sedative and anticholinergic effects of either these medications or trazodone)

» Antihypertensives
    (concurrent use with trazodone may increase the likelihood of hypotension; dosage reduction of the antihypertensive medication may be necessary; also, antihypertensives with CNS depressant effects, such as clonidine, guanabenz, methyldopa, metyrosine, and rauwolfia alkaloids, may potentiate CNS depression when used concurrently with trazodone)

Digoxin
    (concurrent use with trazodone may increase serum concentration of digoxin and may result in digoxin toxicity)

Phenytoin and possibly other hydantoin anticonvulsants
    (increased plasma phenytoin concentrations have been reported when phenytoin was used concurrently with trazodone; caution and close monitoring are suggested)

## Laboratory value alterations
The following have been selected on the basis of their potential clinical significance (possible effect in parentheses where appropriate)—not necessarily inclusive (» = major clinical significance):

With physiology/laboratory test values
Leukocyte counts and
Neutrophil counts
    (may occasionally be reduced, although not enough to be clinically significant)

## Medical considerations/Contraindications
The medical considerations/contraindications included here have been selected on the basis of their potential clinical significance (reasons given in parentheses where appropriate)—not necessarily inclusive (» = major clinical significance).

*Except under special circumstances, this medication should not be used when the following medical problem exists:*
» Myocardial infarction, during the acute recovery period

*Risk-benefit should be considered when the following medical problems exist:*
Alcoholism, active
    (possible excessive CNS depression)
» Cardiac disease, especially arrhythmias
    (ventricular arrhythmias, premature ventricular contractions, and ventricular tachycardia may be potentiated)
» Hepatic function impairment
    (possible serum trazodone accumulation resulting in potentiation of side effects)
» Renal function impairment
    (may result in prolonged trazodone effects)
Sensitivity to trazodone

## Patient monitoring
The following may be especially important in patient monitoring (other tests may be warranted in some patients, depending on condition; » = major clinical significance):

Cardiac function
    (monitoring is recommended, especially for patients with pre-existing cardiac disease; reports indicate that trazodone may initiate arrhythmias, including isolated premature ventricular contractions [PVC], ventricular couplets, and short episodes of ventricular tachycardia, in such patients)

Careful supervision of depressed patients with suicidal tendencies
    (recommended especially during early weeks of treatment; hospitalization may be required as a protective measure)

Leukocyte and neutrophil counts
    (recommended particularly during extended treatment or if symptoms of systemic infection such as fever and sore throat develop; trazodone should be discontinued if patient's leukocyte or absolute neutrophil counts fall below normal)

# Side/Adverse Effects
The following side/adverse effects have been selected on the basis of their potential clinical significance (possible signs and symptoms in parentheses where appropriate)—not necessarily inclusive:

## Those indicating need for medical attention
Incidence less frequent
    *CNS effects* (confusion; muscle tremors)
Incidence rare
    *Allergic reaction* (skin rash); *fast or slow heartbeat; hypotension* (fainting); *priapism* (prolonged, painful, inappropriate penile erection); *unusual excitement*
    Note: When *abnormal erectile activity* occurs, the patient should be advised to discontinue medication immediately and consult with physician.

## Those indicating need for medical attention only if they continue or are bothersome
Incidence more frequent
    *Dizziness or lightheadedness; drowsiness; dryness of mouth, usually mild; headache; nausea and vomiting; unpleasant taste*
Incidence less frequent or rare
    *Blurred vision; constipation; diarrhea; muscle aches or pains; unusual tiredness or weakness*

## Overdose

For specific information on the agents used in the management of trazodone overdose, see:
• *Charcoal, Activated (Oral-Local)* monograph.

For more information on the management of overdose or unintentional ingestion, **contact a Poison Control Center** (see *Poison Control Center Listing*).

### Clinical effects of overdose

The following effects have been selected on the basis of their potential clinical significance (possible signs and symptoms in parentheses were appropriate)—not necessarily inclusive:

*Drowsiness; loss of muscle coordination; nausea and vomiting*

### Treatment of overdose

There is no specific antidote for trazodone. Treatment may include:
  To decrease absorption—
    Emptying stomach by gastric lavage.
    Administering activated charcoal slurry followed by a stimulant cathartic.
  To enhance elimination—
    Forced diuresis may be helpful.
  Supportive care—
    Maintaining respiratory and cardiac function.
    Providing symptomatic and supportive treatment in the event of hypotension or excessive sedation.
    Patients in whom intentional overdose is known or suspected should be referred for psychiatric consultation.

## Patient Consultation

As an aid to patient consultation, refer to *Advice for the Patient, Trazodone (Systemic)*.

In providing consultation, consider emphasizing the following selected information (» = major clinical significance):

### Before using this medication

» Conditions affecting use, especially:
    Sensitivity to trazodone
    Pregnancy—Animal studies have shown congenital anomalies and increased fetal resorptions with large doses
    Breast-feeding—Excreted in breast milk
    Use in the elderly—Elderly are more prone to develop sedative and hypotensive effects
    Dental—Dry mouth may result in caries, periodontal disease, oral candidiasis, and discomfort
    Other medications, especially alcohol or other CNS depression–producing medications, or antihypertensives
    Other medical problems, especially myocardial infarction, arrhythmias or other cardiac disease, hepatic function impairment, or renal function impairment

### Proper use of this medication

    Taking with or soon after a meal or light snack to minimize stomach upset and dizziness or lightheadedness
» Compliance with therapy
» May require up to 4 weeks to produce significant therapeutic results, although 75% of responding patients benefit within 2 weeks
» Proper dosing
    Missed dose: Taking as soon as possible; not taking if within 4 hours of next scheduled dose; not doubling doses
» Proper storage

### Precautions while using this medication

    Regular visits to physician to check progress during therapy
» Checking with physician before discontinuing medication; gradual dosage reduction may be needed
» Caution if any kind of surgery, dental treatment, or emergency treatment is required
» Avoiding use of alcohol or other CNS depressants during therapy
» Possible drowsiness; caution when driving or doing other things requiring alertness
» Possible dizziness; caution when getting up suddenly from a lying or sitting position
    Possible dryness of mouth; using sugarless gum or candy, ice, or saliva substitute for relief; checking with physician or dentist if dry mouth continues for more than 2 weeks

### Side/adverse effects

    Sedative and hypotensive side effects more likely to occur in the elderly
    Priapism may occur; discontinuing medication and checking with physician immediately

    Signs of potential side effects, especially CNS effects, fast or slow heartbeat, hypotension, priapism, unusual excitement, or allergic reaction

## General Dosing Information

Dosage of trazodone must be individualized for each patient by titration.

Potentially suicidal patients should not have access to large quantities of this medication since depressed patients, particularly those who may use alcohol excessively, may continue to exhibit suicidal tendencies until significant improvement occurs. Some clinicians recommend that the patient be supplied with the least amount of medication necessary for satisfactory patient management.

Daily dosage should be divided into at least two doses, because of trazodone's short elimination half-life. Trazodone should not be given as a single daily dose.

When side effects such as excessive drowsiness or dizziness might be bothersome or dangerous during waking hours, a larger portion (about two-thirds) of the total daily dose may be given at bedtime, with the balance being administered in the morning or during the day in divided doses.

To avoid a possible increase in side effects or aggravation of the patient's condition, any change or discontinuation of dosage should be accomplished gradually.

### Diet/Nutrition

Each dose is best taken with or shortly after a meal or light snack. Food reduces the incidence and severity of side effects such as nausea or dizziness, by slowing trazodone's rate of absorption, decreasing the maximum concentration, and lengthening the time to maximum concentration.

### For treatment of priapism

Treatment may include
  • In patients with mild or no ischemia (as differentiated by intracorporeal blood gas and pressure monitoring)—Irrigation of the corpora with metaraminol or epinephrine.
  • In patients with severe ischemia—Stagnant blood should be evacuated and a shunt procedure performed to allow metabolic replenishment of tissue.

## Oral Dosage Forms

### TRAZODONE HYDROCHLORIDE TABLETS USP

Note: The dosing and strengths of the dosage forms available are expressed in terms of trazodone hydrochloride.

#### Usual adult and adolescent dose

Antidepressant—
  Oral, initially 150 mg a day in divided doses, the dosage being increased by 50 mg per day at three- or four-day intervals, as needed and tolerated.

#### Usual adult prescribing limits

Outpatients—
  Up to 400 mg a day.
Inpatients—
  Up to 600 mg a day.

#### Usual pediatric dose

Antidepressant—
  Children up to 6 years of age: Dosage has not been established.
  Children 6 to 18 years of age: Oral, initially 1.5 to 2 mg per kg of body weight a day in divided doses, the dosage being increased gradually at three- or four-day intervals as needed and tolerated up to a maximum of 6 mg per kg of body weight a day.

#### Usual geriatric dose

Antidepressant—
  Oral, initially 75 mg a day in divided doses, the dosage being increased gradually at three- or four-day intervals, as needed and tolerated.

#### Strength(s) usually available

U.S.—
  50 mg (Rx) [*Desyrel* (scored); *Trazon; Trialodine;* GENERIC].
  100 mg (Rx) [*Desyrel* (scored); *Trazon; Trialodine;* GENERIC].
  150 mg (Rx) [*Desyrel* (scored); GENERIC].
  300 mg (Rx) [*Desyrel* (scored); GENERIC].
Canada—
  50 mg (Rx) [*Desyrel* (scored)].
  100 mg (Rx) [*Desyrel* (scored)].
  150 mg (Rx) [*Desyrel* (scored)].

**Packaging and storage**
Store below 40 °C (104 °F), preferably between 15 and 30 °C (59 and 86 °F), in a tight, light-resistant container, unless otherwise specified by manufacturer.

**Auxiliary labeling**
• May cause drowsiness.
• Avoid alcoholic beverages.
• Take with or immediately after food.

**Additional information**
The 150-mg tablet may be broken to yield doses of 50, 75, or 100 mg.

The 300-mg tablet may be broken to yield three 100-mg doses, two 150-mg doses, or one 200-mg dose.

Revised: 01/13/93
Interim revision: 01/19/95

---

# TRETINOIN   Topical

VA CLASSIFICATION (Primary/Secondary): DE752/DE500
Another commonly used name is retinoic acid.

Note: For a listing of dosage forms and brand names by country availability, see *Dosage Forms* section(s). For a listing of brand names for the articles in this monograph, refer to the General Index.

## Category

Antiacne agent (topical); keratolytic (topical).

## Indications

Note: Bracketed information in the *Indications* section refers to uses that are not included in U.S. product labeling.

**Accepted**
Acne vulgaris (treatment)—Tretinoin is indicated in the topical treatment of acne vulgaris. Although use of tretinoin alone is effective in the topical treatment of acne vulgaris, the therapeutic effect may be increased when tretinoin is used in combination with benzoyl peroxide or systemic antibiotics.

[Ichthyosis, lamellar (treatment)][1]
[Keratosis follicularis (treatment)][1] or
[Verruca plana (treatment)][1]—Tretinoin is also used sometimes in disorders of keratinization, such as lamellar ichthyosis, keratosis follicularis (Darier's disease, Darier-White disease), and flat warts (verruca plana).

There are *insufficient data* to show topical tretinoin to be safe and effective for reversing the clinical changes to the skin that are associated with chronic exposure to the sun.

---

[1]Not included in Canadian product labeling.

## Pharmacology/Pharmacokinetics

**Physicochemical characteristics**
Molecular weight—300.44.
Chemical name—Retinoic acid.

**Mechanism of action/Effect**
Appears to act by increasing epidermal cell mitosis and epidermal cell turnover, possibly resulting in the production of a less cohesive horny cell layer, which is more easily peeled off. This action facilitates the removal of existing comedones and may inhibit the formation of new comedones. It has been proposed that increased turnover in the follicular epithelium prevents blocking by keratinous plugs. Tretinoin has also been reported to suppress keratin synthesis.

**Absorption**
Some systemic absorption probably occurs, since a small percentage of dose appears in urine; absorption may be increased when medication is applied to large surface areas, or for long periods of time in chronic extensive dermatoses, such as ichthyosis.

**Elimination**
About 5% of a topically applied dose of tretinoin is recovered in the urine.

## Precautions to Consider

**Cross-sensitivity and/or related problems**
Patients sensitive to etretinate, isotretinoin, or other vitamin A derivatives may be sensitive to tretinoin also, since it is a vitamin A derivative.

**Carcinogenicity/Tumorigenicity**
Long-term animal studies to determine the carcinogenic potential of tretinoin have not been done.
In animal (hairless albino mice) studies, tretinoin has been shown to increase the rate of cutaneous tumor formation induced by ultraviolet radiation. However, the results have not been consistently reproduced and the significance of these studies as related to humans is unknown.

**Pregnancy/Reproduction**
Pregnancy—Adequate and well-controlled studies in humans have not been done.
Studies in animals have shown that oral tretinoin is fetotoxic in rats given 500 times the topical human dose and teratogenic in rats given 1000 times the topical human dose. Topical tretinoin has caused delayed ossification in a number of bones in the offspring of rats and rabbits given 100 to 320 times the topical human dose, respectively. However, the delayed ossification is usually corrected after weaning.
FDA Pregnancy Category C.

**Breast-feeding**
It is not known whether tretinoin is distributed into breast milk; however, problems in humans have not been documented.

**Pediatrics**
Appropriate studies on the relationship of age to the effects of tretinoin have not been performed in the pediatric population. However, no pediatrics-specific problems have been documented to date.

**Geriatrics**
Appropriate studies on the relationship of age to the effects of tretinoin have not been performed in the geriatric population. However, no geriatrics-specific problems have been documented to date.

**Drug interactions and/or related problems**
The following drug interactions and/or related problems have been selected on the basis of their potential clinical significance (possible mechanism in parentheses where appropriate)—not necessarily inclusive (» = major clinical significance):

Note: Combinations containing any of the following medications, depending on the amount present, may also interact with this medication.

Abrasive or medicated soaps or cleansers or
Acne preparations or preparations containing a peeling agent, such as
   Benzoyl peroxide
   Resorcinol
   Salicylic acid
   Sulfur or
Acne preparations, topical, other or
Alcohol-containing preparations, topical such as
   After-shave lotions
   Astringents
   Perfumed toiletries
   Shaving creams or lotions or
Cosmetics or soaps with a strong drying effect or
Isotretinoin or
Medicated cosmetics or "cover-ups"
   (concurrent use with tretinoin may cause a cumulative irritant or drying effect, especially with the application of peeling, desquamating, or abrasive agents, resulting in excessive irritation of the skin)
   (in addition, simultaneous use of benzoyl peroxide with tretinoin on the same area of the skin is not recommended, since there is a physical incompatibility between the two medications)
Minoxidil, topical
   (tretinoin enhances the systemic absorption of topical minoxidil, which may lead to increased side effects of minoxidil, such as hypotension, arrhythmia, pericardial infusion, and impotence)
Photosensitizing medications, other
   (concurrent use of isotretinoin may cause increased risk of photosensitization)

**Medical considerations/Contraindications**
The medical considerations/contraindications included here have been selected on the basis of their potential clinical significance (reasons given in parentheses where appropriate)—not necessarily inclusive (» = major clinical significance).

*Risk-benefit should be considered when the following medical problems exist:*

» Eczema
     (may cause severe irritation)
   Sensitivity to tretinoin
» Sunburn
     (irritation may be increased)

## Side/Adverse Effects

Note:  Side/adverse effects of tretinoin are reversible upon discontinuation of therapy; however, hyperpigmentation or hypopigmentation may persist for months.

The following side/adverse effects have been selected on the basis of their potential clinical significance (possible signs and symptoms in parentheses where appropriate)—not necessarily inclusive:

### Those indicating need for medical attention
   *Blistering, crusting, severe burning or redness, or swelling of skin; darkening or lightening of treated skin*

### Those indicating need for medical attention only if they continue or are bothersome
   *Feeling of warmth, mild stinging, or redness of skin; peeling of skin*—may occur after a few days

## Patient Consultation

As an aid to patient consultation, refer to *Advice for the Patient, Tretinoin (Topical)*.

In providing consultation, consider emphasizing the following selected information (» = major clinical significance):

### Before using this medication
» Conditions affecting use, especially:
     Sensitivity to etretinate, isotretinoin, tretinoin, or vitamin A derivatives
     Pregnancy—Topical tretinoin has been shown to cause delayed ossification in a number of bones in some animal fetuses
     Other medical problems, especially eczema and sunburn

### Proper use of this medication
» Importance of not using more medication than the amount prescribed
» Not applying medication to windburned or sunburned skin or on open wounds
» Avoiding contact with the eyes, mouth, and nose
*Proper administration technique*
   Reading patient directions carefully before use
   Before applying—Washing with mild or nonallergic soap and warm water; gently patting dry; waiting 20 to 30 minutes for complete drying of skin
*For cream or gel dosage form*
   Applying enough to cover affected areas and rubbing in gently
*For solution dosage form*
   Using fingertips, gauze pad, or cotton swab and applying enough to cover affected areas
   Not oversaturating gauze pad or cotton swab to prevent medication from running into areas not intended for treatment
» Proper dosing
   Missed dose: Applying next dose at regularly scheduled time; not doubling doses
» Proper storage

### Precautions while using this medication
   Possibility that acne may appear to worsen during the first 2 or 3 weeks of therapy; not stopping medication unless irritation or other symptoms become severe
   Avoiding too frequent washing of face; washing with mild bland soap 2 or 3 times a day is usually sufficient
» Avoiding simultaneous use with other topical acne preparations or preparations containing peeling agents, alcohol-containing preparations, abrasive soaps or cleansers, cosmetics or soaps with drying effect, medicated cosmetics, or other topical skin medication, unless prescribed by physician
   Cosmetics (nonmedicated) may be used, but skin must be washed thoroughly before applying medication
» Avoiding or minimizing exposure of treated areas to sunlight or a sunlamp to lessen the possibility of sunburn
   Using sunscreen preparations or wearing protective clothing over treated areas if excessive sunlight exposure cannot be avoided
» Possibility of increased sensitivity to wind or cold temperatures

### Side/adverse effects
   The side/adverse effects of tretinoin are reversible upon discontinuation of therapy; however, hyperpigmentation or hypopigmentation may persist for months
   Signs of potential side effects, especially blistering, crusting, severe burning or redness, or swelling of skin or darkening or lightening of the treated skin

## General Dosing Information

If the patient has been using other peeling agents, the effects should be allowed to subside before tretinoin is used.

Because of tretinoin's potential to cause severe irritation and peeling, therapy may be initiated on an alternate-day or, occasionally, every-third-day regimen, preferably with the less irritating and low-concentration cream or gel dosage form. If tolerated, the more potent liquid or higher-concentration cream or gel preparation may then be used.

Although temporary exacerbation of acne, due to action of tretinoin on deep, previously unseen lesions, may occur during the first few weeks of treatment, therapy should be continued.

Patients being treated with tretinoin may use nonmedicated cosmetics, but the areas to be treated should be cleansed thoroughly before the medication is applied.

In the treatment of acne, therapeutic results may be noticeable after 2 to 3 weeks of therapy, but more than 6 weeks of therapy may be required for optimal results. Therapy should be continued for at least 3 months.

When tretinoin is used in combination with benzoyl peroxide, one of the medications should be applied in the morning and the other at night. Simultaneous application is not recommended, since there is a physical incompatibility between the two medications.

In the treatment of lamellar ichthyosis, tretinoin should be used on a daily or an alternate-day regimen.

In the treatment of keratosis follicularis, irritation caused by tretinoin may be minimized by use of adequate, yet threshold, concentrations of tretinoin or by concurrent use of topical steroids.

In the treatment of flat warts, therapy is initiated with a weak concentration of tretinoin applied daily. If there is no response, the concentration of the tretinoin preparation and/or frequency of application should be increased.

## Topical Dosage Forms
### TRETINOIN CREAM USP

#### Usual adult and adolescent dose
Acne vulgaris—
   Topical, to the skin, once a day at bedtime.

#### Usual pediatric dose
See *Usual adult and adolescent dose.*

#### Strength(s) usually available
U.S.—
     0.025% (Rx) [*Retin-A; Retin-A Regimen Kit*].
     0.05% (Rx) [*Retin-A; Retin-A Regimen Kit*].
     0.1% (Rx) [*Retin-A; Retin-A Regimen Kit*].
Canada—
     0.01% (Rx) [*Retin-A; Stieva-A; Vitamin A Acid*].
     0.025% (Rx) [*Stieva-A; Vitamin A Acid*].
     0.05% (Rx) [*Retin-A; Stieva-A; Vitamin A Acid*].
     0.1% (Rx) [*Retin-A; Stieva-A Forte; Vitamin A Acid*].

#### Packaging and storage
Store below 40 °C (104 °F), preferably between 15 and 30 °C (59 and 86 °F), unless otherwise specified by manufacturer. Store in a tight, light-resistant container. Protect from freezing.

#### Incompatibilities
Tretinoin and benzoyl peroxide should not be extemporaneously combined, since there is a physical incompatibility between the two medications.

#### Auxiliary labeling
• For external use only.

#### Note
Include patient instructions when dispensing.

### TRETINOIN GEL USP

#### Usual adult and adolescent dose
See *Tretinoin Cream USP.*

#### Usual pediatric dose
See *Tretinoin Cream USP.*

## Strength(s) usually available
U.S.—
   0.01% (Rx) [*Retin-A; Retin-A Regimen Kit*].
   0.025% (Rx) [*Retin-A; Retin-A Regimen Kit*].
Canada—
   0.01% (Rx) [*Retin-A; Stieva-A*].
   0.025% (Rx) [*Retin-A; Stieva-A; Vitamin A Acid*].
   0.05% (Rx) [*Stieva-A; Vitamin A Acid*].
   0.1% (Rx) [*Vitamin A Acid*].

**Packaging and storage**
Store below 40 °C (104 °F), preferably between 15 and 30 °C (59 and 86 °F), unless otherwise specified by manufacturer. Store in a tight container. Protect from light. Protect from freezing.

**Incompatibilities**
Tretinoin and benzoyl peroxide should not be extemporaneously combined, since there is a physical incompatibility between the two medications.

**Auxiliary labeling**
• For external use only.

**Note**
Include patient instructions when dispensing.

## TRETINOIN TOPICAL SOLUTION USP

**Usual adult and adolescent dose**
See *Tretinoin Cream USP*.

**Usual pediatric dose**
See *Tretinoin Cream USP*.

**Strength(s) usually available**
U.S.—
   0.05% (Rx) [*Retin-A*].
Canada—
   0.025% (Rx) [*Stieva-A*].
   0.05% (Rx) [*Stieva-A*].

**Packaging and storage**
Store below 40 °C (104 °F), preferably between 15 and 30 °C (59 and 86 °F), unless otherwise specified by manufacturer. Store in a tight, light-resistant container. Protect from freezing.

**Incompatibilities**
Tretinoin and benzoyl peroxide should not be extemporaneously combined, since there is a physical incompatibility between the two medications.

**Auxiliary labeling**
• For external use only.
• Keep container tightly closed.

# TRIENTINE   Systemic†

VA CLASSIFICATION (Primary): AD300
Another commonly used name is trien.
Note: For a listing of dosage forms and brand names by country availability, see *Dosage Forms* section(s). For a listing of brand names for the articles in this monograph, refer to the General Index.

†Not commercially available in Canada.

## Category
Chelating agent.

## Indications

**Accepted**
Wilson's disease (treatment)—Trientine is indicated in the treatment of symptomatic or asymptomatic patients when treatment with penicillamine has induced a serious side-effect. Trientine appears to be as therapeutically effective as penicillamine. However, except in patients who have not been previously treated with penicillamine, molar doses of trientine generally induce less cupriuresis than does penicillamine.

**Unaccepted**
Trientine is *not* recommended for treatment of cystinuria since it lacks a sulfhydryl moiety and, unlike penicillamine or tiopronin, is incapable of binding with cystine to form a stable, soluble complex that is readily excreted.

**Note**
Include patient instructions when dispensing.

Revised: 01/15/92
Interim revision: 07/06/94

## TRIAMCINOLONE—See *Corticosteroids (Inhalation-Local); Corticosteroids (Nasal); Corticosteroids (Topical); Corticosteroids—Glucocorticoid Effects (Systemic)*

## TRIAMCINOLONE-CONTAINING COMBINATIONS—
Nystatin and Triamcinolone (Topical)

## TRIAMTERENE—See *Diuretics, Potassium-sparing (Systemic)*

## TRIAMTERENE-CONTAINING COMBINATIONS—
Triamterene and Hydrochlorothiazide (Systemic)—See *Diuretics, Potassium-sparing, and Hydrochlorothiazide (Systemic)*

## TRIAZOLAM—See *Benzodiazepines (Systemic)*

## TRICHLORMETHIAZIDE—See *Diuretics, Thiazide (Systemic)*

## TRICHLORMETHIAZIDE-CONTAINING COMBINATIONS—
Reserpine and Trichlormethiazide (Systemic)—See *Rauwolfia Alkaloids and Thiazide Diuretics (Systemic)*

## TRICITRATES—See *Citrates (Systemic)*

Trientine was found to be ineffective in rheumatoid arthritis after administration for 12 weeks.

Trientine is *not* recommended for primary biliary cirrhosis.

## Pharmacology/Pharmacokinetics

**Physicochemical characteristics**
Molecular weight—219.2.

**Mechanism of action/Effect**
Trientine chelates excess copper in the body and facilitates its excretion. More recent evidence indicates that trientine may also decrease intestinal copper absorption. However, the exact mechanism of action of trientine is unknown.

**Other actions/effects**
Trientine chelates and inhibits the absorption and metabolic action of iron and possibly other heavy metals. Trientine may produce a deficiency of copper in some storage pools, despite an overall bodily excess of copper in Wilson's disease.

**Elimination**
Renal and possibly fecal.

## Precautions to Consider

**Carcinogenicity/Mutagenicity**
Data on carcinogenicity and mutagenicity are not available.

**Pregnancy/Reproduction**

Fertility—Data on impairment of fertility are not available.

Pregnancy—Problems in humans have not been documented. There have been reports of the delivery of normal infants to mothers treated with trientine during pregnancy, with no significant copper depletion in the infants. Pregnant women may be prone to develop iron deficiency anemia during trientine therapy, possibly due to the blocking of dietary iron absorption or to the low-copper diet recommended for Wilson's disease.

Trientine was found to be teratogenic in rats when administered in doses similar to the human dose. When trientine was included in the maternal diet, the frequency of resorptions and fetal abnormalities, including hemorrhage and edema, increased as fetal copper levels decreased.

FDA Pregnancy Category C.

**Breast-feeding**

It is not known if trientine is distributed into breast milk. However, problems in nursing infants have not been documented.

**Pediatrics**

Children have smaller body iron stores and need to get most of their iron from dietary sources. Since copper is essential for the absorption of iron and for the formation of red blood cells, children may be more prone than adults to develop sideroblastic anemia, which is characteristic of copper deficiency, during trientine therapy.

**Geriatrics**

No information is available on the relationship of age to the effects of trientine in geriatric patients.

**Drug interactions and/or related problems**

The following drug interactions and/or related problems have been selected on the basis of their potential clinical significance (possible mechanism in parentheses where appropriate)—not necessarily inclusive (» = major clinical significance):

Note: Combinations containing any of the following medications, depending on the amount present, may also interact with this medication.

» Copper supplements and
» Iron supplements, and possibly other minerals
    (concomitant administration with trientine may decrease trientine's effects; if iron supplementation becomes necessary, iron may be given in short courses, with at least a 2-hour interval between administration of iron and trientine)

**Medical considerations/Contraindications**

The medical considerations/contraindications included here have been selected on the basis of their potential clinical significance (reasons given in parentheses where appropriate)—not necessarily inclusive (» = major clinical significance).

*Risk-benefit should be considered when the following medical problem exists:*

» Iron deficiency
    (may be potentiated)

**Patient monitoring**

The following may be especially important in patient monitoring (other tests may be warranted in some patients, depending on condition; » = major clinical significance):

Body temperature determination
    (recommended nightly during first month of treatment to detect fever caused by hypersensitivity reaction or systemic lupus erythematosus (SLE)–like syndrome; close observation is necessary to detect any other sign of hypersensitivity, such as skin rash)

Copper analyses, urinary, 24-hour
    (recommended prior to start of therapy and in first months of treatment, when initial measurement of 24-hour urinary copper exceeds 1 mg)

Free-copper concentrations, serum
    (recommended periodically as the most reliable index of patient compliance with therapy; value equals the difference between quantitatively determined total copper and ceruloplasmin copper; in compliant patients with proper treatment, serum free copper should be less than 10 mcg per dL; values consistently greater than 20 mcg per dL may be due to inadequate dosage or noncompliance)

Hemoglobin determinations and
Iron concentrations, serum and
Reticulocyte and siderocyte counts
    (hemoglobin determinations recommended monthly during first year of therapy and every 3 months thereafter; iron concentrations and reticulocyte and siderocyte counts suggested periodically dur-

ing therapy to determine if anemia is present and to determine its cause)

## Side/Adverse Effects

Note: Hypersensitivity has not been reported in patients treated for Wilson's disease. However, asthma, bronchitis, and dermatitis have been reported in chemical workers after prolonged environmental exposure to trientine.

The following side/adverse effects have been selected on the basis of their potential clinical significance (possible signs and symptoms in parentheses where appropriate)—not necessarily inclusive:

**Those indicating need for medical attention**

Incidence more frequent
    *Anemia* (unusually pale skin; unusual tiredness)

Note: *Anemia* may be due to iron or copper deficiency, although diagnosis should not be based on symptoms alone since symptoms may relate to other disease states. Trientine-induced sideroblastic anemia may possibly be reversed with reduction of trientine dosage to 750 or 500 mg a day and addition of pyridoxine at a dosage of 100 mg a day.

Incidence rare
    *Hypersensitivity or systemic lupus erythematosus (SLE)–like syndrome* (fever; general feeling of discomfort, illness, or weakness; joint pain; skin rash, blisters, hives, or itching; swelling of the lymph glands)

## Patient Consultation

As an aid to patient consultation, refer to *Advice for the Patient, Trientine (Systemic)*.

In providing consultation, consider emphasizing the following selected information (» = major clinical significance):

**Before using this medication**

» Conditions affecting use, especially:
    Pregnancy—Pregnant women more prone to develop iron deficiency anemia
    Use in children—Children more prone to develop sideroblastic anemia than adults
    Other medications, especially copper supplements, iron supplements, and possibly other minerals
    Other medical problems, especially iron deficiency

**Proper use of this medication**

*Proper administration:*
    Taking with water
    Swallowing capsules whole
    Not opening, crushing, or chewing capsules

» Importance of taking on an empty stomach; taking at least one hour before or two hours after meals, and one hour apart from any other medication, food, or milk for maximum absorption and to prevent inactivation of trientine by metal binding in gastrointestinal tract

» Compliance with therapy; importance of continuing medication indefinitely; checking with physician before discontinuing medication since nontreatment of Wilson's disease may lead to fatal liver damage

» Possible need for low-copper diet; avoiding foods known to be high in copper, such as chocolate, mushrooms, liver, molasses, broccoli, cereals enriched with copper, shellfish, organ meats, and nuts

    Importance of taking only as directed by doctor; not taking more or less medication than the amount prescribed

» Proper dosing
    Missed dose: Doubling next dose; not making up more than one missed dose at a time

» Proper storage

**Precautions while using this medication**

» Regular visits to physician to check progress during therapy

» Taking nightly temperature during first month of treatment; reporting to physician any symptoms of SLE–like syndrome, such as fever or skin eruption

» Avoiding concomitant administration of copper- or iron-containing medications or other vitamin-mineral or mineral supplements to prevent inactivation of trientine; taking iron supplements and trientine at least 2 hours apart

    Avoiding potential contact dermatitis from capsule contents; promptly washing site of exposure with water

**Side/adverse effects**

    Anemia is more likely to occur in children, menstruating women, and pregnant women

Signs of potential side effects, especially anemia, hypersensitivity, or systemic lupus erythematosus (SLE)–like syndrome

## General Dosing Information

To achieve and maintain a negative copper balance, optimal long-term maintenance dosage should be determined at 6- to 12-month intervals, depending on 24-hour urinary copper analysis.

The daily dose should be increased only when the clinical response is inadequate or the concentration of free copper in serum is persistently above 20 mcg per dL.

### Diet/Nutrition

Trientine should be taken on an empty stomach (at least 1 hour before meals or 2 hours after meals) and 1 hour apart from any other medication, food, or milk for maximum absorption and to prevent inactivation of trientine by metal binding in the gastrointestinal tract.

In conjunction with trientine therapy, a low-copper diet of less than 2 mg daily should be maintained. Patients should avoid foods known to be high in copper such as chocolate, nuts, shellfish, mushrooms, liver, molasses, broccoli, organ meats, and cereals enriched with copper. Distilled or demineralized water should be used if the patient's drinking water contains more than 1000 mcg (1 mg) of copper per liter.

## Oral Dosage Forms

### TRIENTINE HYDROCHLORIDE CAPSULES

**Usual adult and adolescent dose**
Chelating agent—
    Oral, initially 750 mg to 1.25 grams a day, in two to four divided doses.

**Usual adult prescribing limits**
Up to 2 grams a day.

**Usual pediatric dose**
Chelating agent—
    Oral, initially 500 to 750 mg a day, in two to four divided doses.

**Usual pediatric prescribing limits**
Children 12 years of age and under—1.5 grams a day.

**Strength(s) usually available**
U.S.—
    250 mg (Rx) [*Syprine*].
Canada—
    Not commercially available.

**Packaging and storage**
Store at 2 to 8 °C (36 to 46 °F). Store in a tight container, unless otherwise specified by manufacturer.

**Auxiliary labeling**
• Take on an empty stomach.
• Swallow capsule whole.

Revised: 09/17/92
Interim revision: 04/29/94

---

**TRIFLUOPERAZINE**—See *Phenothiazines (Systemic)*

---

**TRIFLUPROMAZINE**—See *Phenothiazines (Systemic)*

---

# TRIFLURIDINE   Ophthalmic

VA CLASSIFICATION (Primary): OP203
Another commonly used name is trifluorothymidine.
Note: For a listing of dosage forms and brand names by country availability, see *Dosage Forms* section(s). For a listing of brand names for the articles in this monograph, refer to the General Index.

## Category

Antiviral (ophthalmic).

## Indications

### Accepted

Keratitis, herpes simplex virus (treatment) or
Keratoconjunctivitis, herpes simplex virus (treatment)—Trifluridine is indicated in the treatment of keratoconjunctivitis and recurrent epithelial keratitis caused by herpes simplex virus (HSV), types 1 and 2. Trifluridine may be useful in patients who do not respond to idoxuridine or vidarabine or when ocular toxicity or hypersensitivity to idoxuridine occurs.

### Unaccepted

Trifluridine is not indicated in the prophylaxis of HSV keratoconjunctivitis or epithelial keratitis.

Trifluridine is not effective against bacterial, fungal, or chlamydial infections of the cornea or in nonviral trophic lesions.

## Pharmacology/Pharmacokinetics

**Physicochemical characteristics**
Molecular weight—296.20.

**Mechanism of action/Effect**
Trifluridine, also called trifluorothymidine, closely resembles thymidine. It inhibits thymidylic phosphorylase and specific DNA polymerases, which are necessary for the incorporation of thymidine into viral DNA. Trifluridine is incorporated in place of thymidine into viral DNA, resulting in faulty DNA and the inability to reproduce or to infect or destroy tissue. Trifluridine also is incorporated into mammalian DNA.

**Distribution**
Intraocular penetration occurs after topical administration of trifluridine. Decreased corneal integrity or stromal or uveal infections may increase trifluridine's penetration into the aqueous humor.

**Half-life**
Approximately 12 to 18 minutes.

## Precautions to Consider

### Carcinogenicity

Lifetime carcinogenicity bioassays have been performed in rats and mice given daily subcutaneous doses of trifluridine. Rats given doses of 1.5, 7.5, or 15 mg per kg of body weight (mg/kg) per day had increased incidences of adenocarcinomas of the intestinal tract and mammary glands, hemangiosarcomas of the spleen and liver, carcinosarcomas of the prostate gland, and granulosa-thecal cell tumors of the ovary. Mice given doses of 10 mg/kg per day (but not those given 1 or 5 mg/kg per day) had significantly increased incidences of adenocarcinomas of the intestinal tract and uterus. These mice also had a significantly higher incidence of testicular atrophy than vehicle control mice.

### Mutagenicity

Studies in various standard *in vitro* test systems have shown that trifluridine exerts mutagenic, DNA-damaging, and cell-transforming effects and that it is clastogenic in *Vicia faba* cells.

### Pregnancy/Reproduction

Pregnancy—Adequate and well-controlled studies in humans have not been done.

Trifluridine has been shown to be teratogenic when injected directly into the yolk sac of developing chick embryos. Studies in rats and rabbits given trifluridine subcutaneously in doses of 2.5 mg/kg daily have shown that trifluridine causes delayed ossification. This dose also caused fetal death and resorption in rabbits. However, no effects were seen in rats and rabbits given doses of 1 mg/kg daily. Studies in rats and rabbits given trifluridine subcutaneously in doses of up to 5 mg/kg daily have not shown that trifluridine is teratogenic. Studies in rabbits, using 1% trifluridine applied to the eyes on days 6 to 18 of pregnancy, also have not shown that trifluridine is teratogenic.

FDA Pregnancy Category C.

### Breast-feeding

Trifluridine is unlikely to be distributed into breast milk following ophthalmic administration, since the total daily dose is small (5 mg or less), and since trifluridine is diluted in body fluids and has an extremely short half-life (approximately 12 minutes).

### Pediatrics

Appropriate studies on the relationship of age to the effects of trifluridine have not been performed in the pediatric population. However, no pediatrics-specific problems have been documented to date.

**Geriatrics**

Appropriate studies on the relationship of age to the effects of trifluridine have not been performed in the geriatric population. However, no geriatrics-specific problems have been documented to date.

**Medical considerations/Contraindications**

The medical considerations/contraindications included here have been selected on the basis of their potential clinical significance (reasons given in parentheses where appropriate)—not necessarily inclusive (» = major clinical significance).

*Risk-benefit should be considered when the following medical problem exists:*

Sensitivity to trifluridine

**Patient monitoring**

The following may be especially important in patient monitoring (other tests may be warranted in some patients, depending on condition; » = major clinical significance):

Ophthalmologic, including slit-lamp, examinations
(may be required periodically during therapy)

## Side/Adverse Effects

The following side/adverse effects have been selected on the basis of their potential clinical significance (possible signs and symptoms in parentheses where appropriate)—not necessarily inclusive:

**Those indicating need for medical attention**

Incidence rare
*Epithelial keratopathy; superficial punctate keratopathy* (blurred vision or other change in vision); *hyperemia* (redness of eye); *hypersensitivity* (itching, redness, swelling, or other sign of irritation not present before therapy); *increased intraocular pressure; keratitis sicca* (dryness of eye); *stromal edema* (irritation of eye)

**Those indicating need for medical attention only if they continue or are bothersome**

Incidence more frequent
*Burning or stinging*

## Patient Consultation

As an aid to patient consultation, refer to *Advice for the Patient, Trifluridine (Ophthalmic).*

In providing consultation, consider emphasizing the following selected information (» = major clinical significance):

**Before using this medication**

» Conditions affecting use, especially:
Sensitivity to trifluridine

**Proper use of this medication**

Proper administration technique for ophthalmic solution
» Not using more frequently or for longer than ordered by physician
» Compliance with full course of therapy
» Proper dosing
Missed dose: Applying as soon as possible; not applying if almost time for next dose
» Proper storage

**Precautions while using this medication**

Importance of keeping appointments with physician; checking with physician if symptoms become worse

**Side/adverse effects**

Signs of potential side effects, especially epithelial keratopathy, superficial punctate keratopathy, hyperemia, hypersensitivity, increased intraocular pressure, keratitis sicca, or stromal edema

## General Dosing Information

Although some manufacturers recommend a dose of 2 drops of an ophthalmic solution at appropriate intervals, the conjunctival sac will usually hold only 1 drop.

Trifluridine may be administered concurrently with cycloplegics, mydriatics, antibiotics, sulfonamides, vasoconstrictors, miotics, adrenergics, and corticosteroids. Corticosteroids can accelerate the spread of viral infections and are usually contraindicated in superficial herpes simplex virus keratitis. However, steroids may be used concurrently with trifluridine in the treatment of herpes simplex stromal infections. Trifluridine should be continued for a few days after the steroid has been discontinued.

Treatment usually should not be continued for more than a total of 21 days or for more than 3 to 5 days after healing is complete. However, chronic or particularly difficult infections may require up to 3 to 6 weeks of treatment.

Herpetic keratitis may recur if trifluridine is discontinued before microscopic staining with fluorescein has cleared.

## Ophthalmic Dosage Forms

### TRIFLURIDINE OPHTHALMIC SOLUTION

**Usual adult and adolescent dose**

Ophthalmic antiviral—
Topical, to the conjunctiva, 1 drop every two hours while awake. Treatment should be continued until the cornea is completely re-epithelialized. Dose may then be reduced to 1 drop every four hours while awake (minimum of 5 drops daily) for an additional seven days.

**Usual adult prescribing limits**

Up to 9 drops daily.

**Usual pediatric dose**

See *Usual adult and adolescent dose.*

**Strength(s) usually available**

U.S.—
1% (Rx) [Viroptic (thimerosal 0.001%)].
Canada—
1% (Rx) [Viroptic (thimerosal 0.001%)].

**Packaging and storage**

Store between 2 and 8 °C (36 and 46 °F), unless otherwise specified by manufacturer.

**Auxiliary labeling**

• Refrigerate.
• For the eye.
• Continue medicine for full time of treatment.
• Do not use more often or longer than ordered.

**Note**

Dispense in original unopened container.

Revised: 07/01/93

---

**TRIHEXYPHENIDYL**—See *Antidyskinetics (Systemic)*

---

**TRIKATES**—See *Potassium Supplements (Systemic)*

---

# TRILOSTANE    Systemic†

VA CLASSIFICATION (Primary/Secondary): HS900/AN500

Note: For a listing of dosage forms and brand names by country availability, see *Dosage Forms* section(s). For a listing of brand names for the articles in this monograph, refer to the General Index.

†Not commercially available in Canada.

## Category

Antiadrenal.

## Indications

Note: Bracketed information in the *Indications* section refers to uses that are not included in U.S. product labeling.

**Accepted**

Cushing's syndrome (treatment)—Trilostane is indicated for temporary treatment of Cushing's syndrome associated with adrenal cortical hyperfunction, [adrenal carcinoma, and ectopic ACTH–producing tumors], in cases where definitive therapy is not appropriate or until definitive measures such as surgery or pituitary radiation can be undertaken.

# Pharmacology/Pharmacokinetics

**Physicochemical characteristics**
Molecular weight—329.44.

**Mechanism of action/Effect**
Trilostane produces suppression of the adrenal cortex by inhibiting enzymatic conversion of steroids by 3-beta-hydroxysteroid dehydrogenase/delta$^{5,4}$ ketosteroid isomerase, thus blocking synthesis of adrenal steroids.

**Biotransformation**
Hepatic.

**Half-life**
Elimination—8 hours.

# Precautions to Consider

**Carcinogenicity**
Studies for 18 months in rats given doses of 250 mg per kg of body weight (mg/kg) per day found an increased incidence of adrenal adenomas. These were shown to be related to compensatory adrenocorticotropic hormone (ACTH) stimulation rather than to a direct action of trilostane.

**Mutagenicity**
Standard tests found no evidence of mutagenicity.

**Pregnancy/Reproduction**
Fertility—Gonadal function may be depressed during trilostane therapy. This is reversible upon cessation of therapy.

Pregnancy—Trilostane is not recommended during pregnancy because it has been reported to reduce circulating progesterone, produce cervical dilation, and terminate pregnancy in some women. Studies in rats have shown that trilostane is teratogenic (skeletal abnormalities) in doses approximately 13 times the recommended human dose; teratogenicity seems to be related to the reduction in circulating progesterone.

FDA Pregnancy Category X.

**Breast-feeding**
It is not known whether trilostane is excreted in breast milk. However, problems in humans have not been documented.

**Pediatrics**
Appropriate studies have not been performed in the pediatric population.

**Geriatrics**
No geriatrics-specific information is available on the use of trilostane in geriatric patients. However, elderly patients are more likely to have age-related renal function impairment, which may require caution in patients receiving trilostane.

**Drug interactions and/or related problems**
The following drug interactions and/or related problems have been selected on the basis of their potential clinical significance (possible mechanism in parentheses where appropriate)—not necessarily inclusive (» = major clinical significance):
Aminoglutethimide or
Mitotane
(concurrent use with trilostane may result in severe adrenocortical hypofunction)

**Laboratory value alterations**
The following have been selected on the basis of their potential clinical significance (possible effect in parentheses where appropriate)—not necessarily inclusive (» = major clinical significance):
With physiology/laboratory test values
Plasma cortisol concentrations
(expected to decrease as a result of adrenocortical inhibition)
Serum potassium concentrations
(may be increased)
Urinary 17-hydroxycorticosteroid concentrations
(expected to increase as a result of adrenocortical inhibition)

**Medical considerations/Contraindications**
The medical considerations/contraindications included here have been selected on the basis of their potential clinical significance (reasons given in parentheses where appropriate)—not necessarily inclusive (» = major clinical significance).

*Risk-benefit should be considered when the following medical problems exist:*
Hepatic function impairment
» Infection or
» Shock or
» Surgery or

» Trauma, severe
(additional steroids may be required because adrenal suppression may prevent the normal response to stress; it is recommended that trilostane be temporarily withdrawn immediately following shock or severe trauma)
Renal function impairment
Sensitivity to trilostane

**Patient monitoring**
The following may be especially important in patient monitoring (other tests may be warranted in some patients, depending on condition; » = major clinical significance):
» 8 a.m. plasma cortisol or
24-hour urinary 17-hydroxycorticosteroid
(determinations recommended at periodic intervals to aid in assessing clinical response; steroid supplement therapy may be necessary)
Serum electrolyte concentrations
(recommended at regular intervals to detect electrolyte imbalance)

# Side/Adverse Effects

The following side/adverse effects have been selected on the basis of their potential clinical significance (possible signs and symptoms in parentheses where appropriate)—not necessarily inclusive:

**Those indicating need for medical attention**
Incidence rare
*Adrenocortical insufficiency* (darkening of skin; drowsiness or tiredness; loss of appetite; mental depression; skin rash; vomiting)

**Those indicating need for medical attention only if they continue or are bothersome**
Incidence more frequent
*Diarrhea; stomach pain or cramps*
Incidence less frequent
*Aching muscles; belching or bloating; burning mouth or nose; dizziness or lightheadedness; fever; flushing; headache; increase in salivation; nausea; watery eyes*

# Patient Consultation

As an aid to patient consultation, refer to *Advice for the Patient, Trilostane (Systemic).*

Consider advising the patient on the following (» = major clinical significance):

**Before using this medication**
» Conditions affecting use, especially:
See *Precautions to Consider.*

**Proper use of this medication**
» Importance of not taking more or less medication than the amount prescribed
» Proper dosing
Missed dose: Taking as soon as possible; not taking if almost time for next dose; not doubling doses
» Proper storage

**Precautions while using this medication**
» Importance of close monitoring by physician
» Checking with physician immediately if injury, infection, or other illness occurs, because of the risk of adrenal insufficiency
» Caution if any kind of surgery (including dental surgery) or emergency treatment is required
Carrying medical identification card or wearing bracelet stating that medication is being used

**Side/adverse effects**
Signs of potential side effects, especially adrenocortical insufficiency

# General Dosing Information

Patients receiving trilostane should be under the supervision of a clinical endocrinologist.

Initial treatment usually occurs in the hospital until dosage is stabilized, although it may occur on an outpatient basis with frequent monitoring.

Dosage must be adjusted to produce the desired level of adrenal suppression.

Patients should be monitored carefully during periods of stress such as surgery, trauma, or acute illness. Additional steroids may be required because adrenal suppression may prevent the normal response to stress. It is recommended that trilostane be temporarily withdrawn immediately following shock or severe trauma.

## Oral Dosage Forms

### TRILOSTANE CAPSULES

Note: Trilostane capsules are not commercially available in Canada.

**Usual adult dose**
Cushing's syndrome—
Initial: Oral, 30 mg four times a day, the dosage being gradually increased at intervals of three to four days until the desired response is achieved.
Maintenance: Oral, usually less than 360 mg per day in four divided doses.

**Usual adult prescribing limits**
Up to 480 mg per day.

**Usual pediatric dose**
Dosage has not been established.

**Strength(s) usually available**
U.S.—
30 mg (Rx) [*Modrastane*].
60 mg (Rx) [*Modrastane*].

**Packaging and storage**
Store below 40 °C (104 °F), preferably between 15 and 30 °C (59 and 86 °F), in a well-closed container, unless otherwise specified by manufacturer.

Revised: 09/90
Interim revision: 07/05/94

**TRIMEPRAZINE**—See *Antihistamines, Phenothiazine-derivative (Systemic)*

**TRIMETHADIONE**—See *Anticonvulsants, Dione (Systemic)*

# TRIMETHAPHAN   Systemic

VA CLASSIFICATION (Primary): CV490
Note: For a listing of dosage forms and brand names by country availability, see *Dosage Forms* section(s). For a listing of brand names for the articles in this monograph, refer to the General Index.

## Category

Antihypertensive.

## Indications

**Accepted**
Hypotension, controlled—Trimethaphan is indicated for production of controlled hypotension during surgery to reduce bleeding into the surgical field.

Hypertension (treatment)—Trimethaphan is indicated for rapid reduction of blood pressure in the treatment of hypertensive emergencies, especially in patients with acute dissecting aneurysm, and in the emergency treatment of pulmonary edema in patients with pulmonary hypertension associated with systemic hypertension.

## Pharmacology/Pharmacokinetics

**Physicochemical characteristics**
Molecular weight—596.80.

**Mechanism of action/Effect**
Ganglionic blocking agent; prevents stimulation of postsynaptic receptors by competing with acetylcholine for these receptor sites; additional effects may include direct peripheral vasodilation and release of histamine. Trimethaphan's hypotensive effect is due to reduction in sympathetic tone and vasodilation, and is primarily postural. Cardiac output may increase in patients with cardiac failure or decrease in patients with normal cardiac function.

**Biotransformation**
Exact metabolic fate unknown; however, possibly by pseudo-cholinesterase.

**Onset of action**
Immediate.

**Duration of action**
10 to 15 minutes.

**Elimination**
Renal, mostly unchanged.

## Precautions to Consider

**Carcinogenicity/Mutagenicity**
Adequate studies have not been done.

**Pregnancy/Reproduction**
Pregnancy—Trimethaphan crosses the placenta. Its ganglionic blocking effects may decrease gastrointestinal motility in the fetus, resulting in meconium ileus or neonatal paralytic ileus. Furthermore, trimethaphan-induced hypotension may have other serious adverse effects on the fetus. Risk-benefit must be carefully considered when this medication is required in life-threatening situations or in serious diseases for which other medications cannot be used.
FDA Pregnancy Category D.

**Breast-feeding**
It is not known whether trimethaphan is distributed into breast milk. Because of the potential for serious adverse effects in nursing infants, it is recommended that mothers who require trimethaphan refrain from nursing.

**Pediatrics**
Appropriate studies on the relationship of age to the effects of trimethaphan have not been performed in the pediatric population. However, caution may be required in pediatric patients.

**Geriatrics**
No information is available on the relationship of age to the effects of trimethaphan in geriatric patients. However, elderly patients may be more sensitve to the hypotensive effects of trimethaphan. Furthermore, these patients may have age-related renal function impairment, which may require caution in patients receiving trimethaphan.

**Drug interactions and/or related problems**
The following drug interactions and/or related problems have been selected on the basis of their potential clinical significance (possible mechanism in parentheses where appropriate)—not necessarily inclusive (» = major clinical significance):

Note: Combinations containing any of the following medications, depending on the amount present, may also interact with this medication.

» Ambenonium or
» Neostigmine or
» Pyridostigmine
(concurrent use may interfere with the antimyasthenic effect of ambenonium, neostigmine, or pyridostigmine, leading to weakness and sudden inability to swallow)

Anti-inflammatory drugs, nonsteroidal (NSAIDs), especially indomethacin
(antihypertensive effects of trimethaphan may be reduced when it is used concurrently with these agents; indomethacin, and possibly other NSAIDs, may antagonize the antihypertensive effect by inhibiting renal prostaglandin synthesis and/or by causing sodium and fluid retention; the patient should be carefully monitored to confirm that the desired effect is being obtained)

Hypotension-producing medications, other (see *Appendix II* )
(concurrent use with trimethaphan may result in enhanced hypotension; individual dosage adjustment is important; halothane may also reduce or prevent trimethaphan-induced tachycardia)

(preanesthetic and anesthetic agents used in surgery, especially spinal anesthetics, may potentiate the hypotensive response to trimethaphan, with increased risk of severe hypotension, shock, and cardiovascular collapse during surgery)

Neuromuscular blocking agents
   (effects may be prolonged, especially by administration of large
   doses of trimethaphan, since trimethaphan appears to have a slight
   curare-like effect; careful postoperative monitoring of the patient
   may be necessary following concurrent or sequential use, especially if there is a possibility of incomplete reversal of neuromuscular blockade)

Sympathomimetics
   (trimethaphan may enhance the pressor response to sympathomimetic pressor amines, and the hypotensive effect of trimethaphan
   may be decreased or reversed by all sympathomimetics)

**Laboratory value alterations**
The following have been selected on the basis of their potential clinical
significance (possible effect in parentheses where appropriate)—not
necessarily inclusive (» = major clinical significance):

With physiology/laboratory test values
   Glucose, blood, concentrations
      (trimethaphan prevents surgically induced increase)

   Potassium, serum
      (concentrations may be slightly decreased)

**Medical considerations/Contraindications**
The medical considerations/contraindications included here have been selected on the basis of their potential clinical significance (reasons given
in parentheses where appropriate)—not necessarily inclusive (» =
major clinical significance).

*Risk-benefit should be considered when the following medical problems
exist:*
» Addison's disease

   Allergies, history of
      (trimethaphan liberates histamine and has been reported to cause
      a histamine-like reaction along the vein where administered)

» Anemia, uncorrected or
» Asphyxia or
» Hypovolemia or
» Shock, frank or incipient
      (for use in producing controlled hypotension during anesthesia
      only; additional hypotension may result in hypoxia of vital organs)

   Bladder neck obstruction or
   Prostatic hypertrophy or
   Urethral stricture
      (possible urinary retention caused by trimethaphan)

» Cardiovascular insufficiency, including coronary insufficiency or
» Cerebrovascular insufficiency or
» Myocardial infarction, recent
      (ischemia may be aggravated by hypotension)

» Degenerative disease of the central nervous system (CNS)
» Diabetes mellitus
   Glaucoma
» Hepatic function impairment
      (the decrease in blood pressure secondary to trimethaphan admin-
      istration may decrease hepatic perfusion and worsen this condition)
   Pyelonephritis, chronic
      (condition may be aggravated by urinary retention caused by
      trimethaphan)
» Renal function impairment
      (increased effects due to reduced excretion of trimethaphan)
» Respiratory insufficiency, uncorrected
      (aggravation of hypoxemia by trimethaphan)
   Sensitivity to trimethaphan
» Caution is required also in debilitated patients and those also receiving
      steroids.

**Patient monitoring**
The following may be especially important in patient monitoring (other
tests may be warranted in some patients, depending on condition;
» = major clinical significance):

» Blood pressure determinations
      (should be made frequently)

Respiratory function determinations
   (recommended at periodic intervals, especially with large doses of
   trimethaphan, since respiratory arrest has been reported rarely with
   its use)

## Side/Adverse Effects

Note:  Most side/adverse effects are due to parasympathetic blockade and
       respond to dosage reduction or withdrawal of trimethaphan.

       Overdosage may result in profound hypotension and respiratory
       arrest.

The following side/adverse effects have been selected on the basis of their
potential clinical significance (possible signs and symptoms in parentheses where appropriate)—not necessarily inclusive:

**Incidence dose-related**
*Anorexia, nausea, and vomiting; constipation; cycloplegia and my-
driasis; dryness of mouth; impotence; itching; urticaria; orthostatic
hypotension; paralytic ileus; precipitation of angina; tachycardia;
urinary retention, short-term*

Note:  Increased risk of *paralytic ileus* when the infusion is continued
       for longer than 48 hours.

       *Mydriasis* is common and does not necessarily indicate anoxia
       or depth of anesthesia.

## General Dosing Information

Trimethaphan Camsylate Injection USP must be diluted and administered
by intravenous infusion.

To achieve optimal reduction in blood pressure, it is recommended that
   trimethaphan infusion be administered intravenously by means of an
   infusion pump, a micro-drip regulator, or a similar device to allow
   precise adjustment of the flow rate. Tilting the head of the bed up may
   enhance the hypotensive effect; the patient should be positioned to
   avoid cerebral anoxia.

**For use as an antihypertensive only**
It is recommended that patients receiving trimethaphan be in an intensive
   care unit and that blood pressure be monitored frequently.

It is recommended that oral antihypertensive therapy be instituted as soon
   as possible while the patient is receiving trimethaphan and that trimethaphan be withdrawn as soon as the blood pressure has stabilized.
   Patients receiving concomitant antihypertensive medication require
   lower doses of trimethaphan.

Pseudotolerance to the effects of trimethaphan occurs in some patients;
   tachyphylaxis may develop within 24 to 72 hours. Pseudotolerance
   with prolonged use may be prevented by use of a diuretic.

**For use to produce controlled hypotension during surgery only**
It is recommended that trimethaphan infusion be discontinued prior to
   wound closure to allow blood pressure to return to normal.

## Parenteral Dosage Forms

### TRIMETHAPHAN CAMSYLATE INJECTION USP

**Usual adult dose**
Controlled hypotension during surgery—
   Initial:  Intravenous infusion, 3 to 4 mg per minute, adjusted according
             to response.
   Maintenance:  Intravenous infusion, 300 mcg (0.3 mg) to 6 mg per
             minute.
Hypertensive emergency—
   Initial:  Intravenous infusion, 500 mcg (0.5 mg) to 1 mg per minute,
             adjusted according to response.
   Maintenance:  Intravenous infusion, 1 to 5 mg per minute.

Note:  Geriatric patients may be more sensitive to the usual adult dose of
       trimethaphan.

**Usual pediatric dose**
Initial—Intravenous infusion, 50 mcg (0.05 mg) to 150 mcg (0.15 mg)
   per kg per minute, adjusted according to response.

**Strength(s) usually available**

U.S.—

    50 mg per mL (Rx) [Arfonad].

Canada—

    50 mg per mL (Rx) [Arfonad].

**Packaging and storage**

Store between 2 and 8 °C (36 and 46 °F). Protect from freezing (to avoid ampul breakage).

**Preparation of dosage form**

Trimethaphan Camsylate Injection USP is prepared for intravenous infusion by diluting the contents of a 500-mg ampul in 500 mL of 5% dextrose injection only to produce a solution containing 1 mg of trimethaphan camsylate per mL.

**Stability**

Intravenous solutions should be freshly prepared; unused portions should be discarded. After preparation, intravenous infusion solution is stable for 24 hours at room temperature.

**Auxiliary labeling**

• Dilute before using.

**Note**

Must be diluted before use.

Revised: 09/08/92

---

# TRIMETHOBENZAMIDE    Systemic†

INN: Trimethobenzamide

VA CLASSIFICATION (Primary): GA700

Note: For a listing of dosage forms and brand names by country availability, see *Dosage Forms* section(s). For a listing of brand names for the articles in this monograph, refer to the General Index.

†Not commercially available in Canada.

## Category

Antiemetic.

## Indications

**Accepted**

Nausea and vomiting (prophylaxis and treatment)—Trimethobenzamide is indicated for the control of nausea and vomiting.

## Pharmacology/Pharmacokinetics

**Physicochemical characteristics**

Molecular weight—424.92.

**Mechanism of action/Effect**

Thought to inhibit the medullary chemoreceptor trigger zone.

**Biotransformation**

Hepatic.

**Elimination**

Renal; biliary.

## Precautions to Consider

**Cross-sensitivity and/or related problems**

The suppository dosage form contains 2% of benzocaine. Patients sensitive to benzocaine or similar local anesthetics should not use the suppository dosage form of trimethobenzamide.

**Pregnancy/Reproduction**

Pregnancy—Adequate and well-controlled studies in humans have not been done.

Reproduction studies in animals have not shown that trimethobenzamide causes teratogenic effects in the fetus; however, it has been shown to cause increased embryonic resorptions and stillbirths.

**Breast-feeding**

It is not known if trimethobenzamide is distributed into breast milk.

**Pediatrics**

Trimethobenzamide is not recommended for treatment of uncomplicated vomiting in children. Caution is required because of the suspicion that centrally acting antiemetics, when used in the presence of viral illnesses, may contribute to the development of Reye's syndrome.

**Geriatrics**

No information is available on the relationship of age to the effects of trimethobenzamide in geriatric patients.

**Drug interactions and/or related problems**

The following drug interactions and/or related problems have been selected on the basis of their potential clinical significance (possible mechanism in parentheses where appropriate)—not necessarily inclusive (» = major clinical significance):

Note: Combinations containing any of the following medications, depending on the amount present, may also interact with this medication.

Apomorphine

    (prior administration of trimethobenzamide may decrease the emetic response to apomorphine; also, concurrent use may potentiate the central nervous system [CNS] effects of either apomorphine or trimethobenzamide)

» CNS depression–producing medications (See *Appendix II*)

    (concurrent use may potentiate the effects of either these medications or trimethobenzamide; in addition, use of trimethobenzamide as well as other antiemetic agents in patients who have recently received other medications with CNS effects, such as phenothiazines, barbiturates, or the belladonna alkaloids, has resulted in opisthotonos, convulsions, coma, and extrapyramidal symptoms)

Ototoxic medications (See *Appendix II*)

    (concurrent use with trimethobenzamide may mask the symptoms of ototoxicity, such as tinnitus, dizziness, and vertigo)

**Medical considerations/Contraindications**

The medical considerations/contraindications included here have been selected on the basis of their potential clinical significance (reasons given in parentheses where appropriate)—not necessarily inclusive (» = major clinical significance).

*Risk-benefit should be considered when the following medical problems exist:*

Dehydration or

Electrolyte imbalance or

Encephalitis or

Fever, high or

Gastroenteritis

    (CNS reactions such as opisthotonos, convulsions, coma, and extrapyramidal symptoms have been reported after administration of trimethobenzamide, especially in children and in elderly or debilitated patients, or in those who have recently received other medications with CNS effects)

Sensitivity to trimethobenzamide

Note: Antiemetic action of trimethobenzamide may impede diagnosis of such conditions as appendicitis and obscure signs of toxicity from overdosage of other medications.

## Side/Adverse Effects

The following side/adverse effects have been selected on the basis of their potential clinical significance (possible signs and symptoms in parentheses where appropriate)—not necessarily inclusive:

**Those indicating need for medical attention**

Incidence rare

    *Allergic reactions* (skin rash); *blood dyscrasias* (sore throat or fever; unusual tiredness); *convulsions; hepatic function impairment* (yellow eyes or skin); *mental depression; opisthotonus* (body spasm with head and heels bent backward and body bowed forward); *Parkinson-like syndrome* (shakiness or tremors); *Reye's syndrome* (convulsions; severe or continuing vomiting)

**Those indicating need for medical attention only if they continue or are bothersome**

Incidence more frequent

    *Drowsiness*

Incidence less frequent

    *Blurred vision; diarrhea; dizziness; headache; muscle cramps*

# Patient Consultation

As an aid to patient consultation, refer to *Advice for the Patient, Trimethobenzamide (Systemic)*.

In providing consultation, consider emphasizing the following selected information (» = major clinical significance):

**Before using this medication**
» Conditions affecting use, especially:
   Sensitivity to trimethobenzamide or to benzocaine (for suppository form)
   Pregnancy—Animal studies have shown increased fetal resorptions and stillbirths
   Use in children—Trimethobenzamide is not recommended for treatment of uncomplicated vomiting, due to the possible contribution of centrally acting antiemetics to the development of Reye's syndrome
   Other medications, especially CNS depressants
   Other medical problems, especially dehydration, electrolyte imbalance, encephalitis, high fever, or gastroenteritis

**Proper use of this medication**
   Not giving to children unless prescribed; giving medication only as directed
   Taking medication only as directed
   Proper administration of this medication (for suppository dosage form only)
» Proper dosing
   Missed dose: Taking as soon as possible; not taking if almost time for next dose; not doubling doses
» Proper storage

**Precautions while using this medication**
» Avoiding use of alcohol or other CNS depressants
» Possible dizziness, lightheadedness, or drowsiness; caution when driving or doing anything else requiring alertness
   May mask ototoxic effects of large doses of salicylates

**Side/adverse effects**
   Signs of potential side effects, especially allergic reactions, blood dyscrasias, convulsions, hepatic function impairment, mental depression, opisthotonus, Parkinson-like syndrome, and Reye's syndrome

## General Dosing Information

**For parenteral dosage form only**
Intravenous injection is not recommended.

Intramuscular administration should be made by deep injection into the upper outer quadrant of the gluteal area in order to minimize irritation at the site of injection.

## Oral Dosage Forms

### TRIMETHOBENZAMIDE HYDROCHLORIDE CAPSULES USP

**Usual adult and adolescent dose**
Antiemetic—
   Oral, 250 mg three or four times a day as needed.

**Usual pediatric dose**
Antiemetic—
   Oral, 15 mg per kg of body weight a day as needed, divided into three or four doses; or for
   Children weighing 15 to 45 kg: Oral, 100 to 200 mg three or four times a day, as needed.

**Strength(s) usually available**
U.S.—
   100 mg (Rx) [*Tigan*].
   250 mg (Rx) [*Tigan; GENERIC*].

---

Canada—
   Not commercially available.

**Packaging and storage**
Store below 40 °C (104 °F), preferably between 15 and 30 °C (59 and 86 °F), unless otherwise specified by manufacturer. Store in a well-closed container.

**Auxiliary labeling**
• May cause drowsiness.
• Avoid alcoholic beverages.

## Parenteral Dosage Forms

### TRIMETHOBENZAMIDE HYDROCHLORIDE INJECTION USP

**Usual adult and adolescent dose**
Antiemetic—
   Intramuscular, 200 mg three or four times a day as needed.

**Usual pediatric dose**
Use is not recommended.

**Strength(s) usually available**
U.S.—
   100 mg per mL (Rx) [*Arrestin; Benzacot; Stemetic; Tegamide; Ticon; Tigan* (parabens [methyl and propyl] 0.2%—in 2-mL ampuls; phenol 0.45%—in 20-mL vials; phenol 0.45%, disodium edetate 0.2 mg—in 2-mL syringes); *Tiject-20; Tribenzagan; GENERIC*].
Canada—
   Not commercially available.

**Packaging and storage**
Store between 15 and 30 °C (59 and 86 °F), unless otherwise specified by manufacturer. Protect from freezing.

## Rectal Dosage Forms

### TRIMETHOBENZAMIDE HYDROCHLORIDE SUPPOSITORIES

**Usual adult and adolescent dose**
Antiemetic—
   Rectal, 200 mg three or four times a day as needed.

**Usual pediatric dose**
Antiemetic—
   Rectal, 15 mg per kg of body weight a day as needed, divided into three or four doses; or for
   Children weighing less than 15 kg: Rectal, 100 mg three or four times a day as needed.
   Children weighing 15 to 45 kg: Rectal, 100 to 200 mg three or four times a day as needed.

Note: Premature and full-term neonates—Use is not recommended.

**Strength(s) usually available**
U.S.—
   100 mg (Rx) [*Bio-Gan; Tegamide; T-Gen; Tigan* (2% benzocaine); *Triban; GENERIC*].
   200 mg (Rx) [*Bio-Gan; Tebamide; Tegamide; T-Gen; Tigan* (2% benzocaine); *Triban; GENERIC*].
Canada—
   Not commercially available.

**Packaging and storage**
Store between 15 and 30 °C (59 and 86 °F), unless otherwise specified by manufacturer.

**Auxiliary labeling**
• May cause drowsiness.
• Avoid alcoholic beverages.

---

Revised: 05/12/93

---

# TRIMETHOPRIM Systemic

VA CLASSIFICATION (Primary/Secondary): AM900
Note: For a listing of dosage forms and brand names by country availability, see *Dosage Forms* section(s). For a listing of brand names for the articles in this monograph, refer to the General Index.

## Category

Antibacterial (systemic).

## Indications

Note: Bracketed information in the *Indications* section refers to uses that are not included in U.S. product labeling.

**Accepted**
Urinary tract infections, bacterial (treatment)—Trimethoprim is indicated in the treatment of initial, uncomplicated urinary tract infections caused by susceptible strains of *Escherichia coli, Proteus mirabilis,*

*Klebsiella pneumoniae*, *Enterobacter* species, and coagulase-negative *Staphylococcus* species, including *S. saprophyticus*.

[Urinary tract infections, bacterial (prophylaxis)][1]—Trimethoprim is used in the prophylaxis of bacterial urinary tract infections.

[Pneumonia, *Pneumocystis carinii* (treatment)][1]—Trimethoprim is used in combination with dapsone in the treatment of mild to moderate pneumonia caused by *Pneumocystis carinii* (PCP).

Not all species or strains of a particular organism may be susceptible to trimethoprim.

**Unaccepted**
Trimethoprim is not effective against *Pseudomonas aeruginosa* or *Bacteroides fragilis*.

---

[1]Not included in Canadian product labeling.

## Pharmacology/Pharmacokinetics

**Physicochemical characteristics**
Molecular weight—290.32.

**Mechanism of action/Effect**
Bacteriostatic lipophilic weak base structurally related to pyrimethamine, binds to and reversibly inhibits the bacterial enzyme dihydrofolate reductase, selectively blocking conversion of dihydrofolic acid to its functional form, tetrahydrofolic acid. This depletes folate, an essential cofactor in the biosynthesis of nucleic acids, resulting in interference with bacterial nucleic acid and protein production. Bacterial dihydrofolate reductase is approximately 50,000 to 60,000 times more tightly bound by trimethoprim than by the corresponding mammalian enzyme.

Exerts its effect at a step in the folate biosynthesis immediately subsequent to the one in which sulfonamides exert their effect. When administered concurrently with sulfonamides, synergism occurs and is attributed to inhibition of tetrahydrofolate production at two sequential steps in its biosynthesis.

**Absorption**
Rapidly and almost completely (90 to 100%) absorbed from the gastrointestinal tract.

**Distribution**
Rapidly and widely distributed to various tissues and fluids, including kidneys, liver, spleen, bronchial secretions, saliva, and seminal fluid. Trimethoprim has also been demonstrated in bile; aqueous humor; bone marrow and spongy, but not compact, bone.
Cerebrospinal fluid (CSF) concentrations—
    30 to 50% of serum concentrations.
Prostatic tissue and fluid—
    2 to 3 times the serum concentration.
Crosses the placenta and is excreted in breast milk.
Vol$_D$—
    Adults:
        1.3 to 1.8 liters per kg.
    Children:
        Newborns—Approximately 2.7 liters per kg.
        Age 1 to 10 years old—Approximately 1.0 liter per kg.

**Protein binding**
Moderate (approximately 45%).

**Biotransformation**
Hepatic; 10 to 20% metabolized to inactive metabolites by O-demethylation, ring N-oxidation, and alpha-hydroxylation; metabolites may be free or conjugated.

**Half-life**
Adults—
    Normal renal function: 8 to 10 hours.
    Anuric patients: 20 to 50 hours.
Children—
    Newborns: Approximately 19 hours.
    Age 1 to 10 years: 3 to 5.5 hours.

**Time to mean peak serum concentration**
1 to 4 hours.

**Mean peak serum concentration**
Approximately 1 mcg per mL, following a single 100-mg dose.

**Elimination**
Renal, 50 to 60% excreted within 24 hours, primarily by glomerular filtration and tubular secretion; of this amount, 80 to 90% excreted unchanged and remainder excreted as inactive metabolites. Excretion increased in acid urine and decreased in alkaline urine.
Small amounts excreted in the feces (approximately 4%) and bile.

In dialysis—Moderate amount of trimethoprim is removed from the blood by hemodialysis. Peritoneal dialysis is not effective in removing trimethoprim from the blood.

## Precautions to Consider

### Carcinogenicity
Long-term studies in animals to evaluate the carcinogenic potential of trimethoprim have not been done.

### Mutagenicity
Trimethoprim has not been shown to be mutagenic in the Ames assay. No chromosomal damage was seen in human leukocytes that were cultured *in vitro* with trimethoprim, using concentrations that exceeded serum concentrations following normal doses of trimethoprim.

### Pregnancy/Reproduction
Fertility—Trimethoprim has not been shown to cause adverse effects on fertility or reproductive performance in rats given oral doses as high as 70 mg per kg of body weight (mg/kg) daily in males and 14 mg/kg daily in females.

Pregnancy—Trimethoprim crosses the placenta. Adequate and well-controlled studies in humans have not been done. Trimethoprim may interfere with folic acid metabolism. However, a retrospective study of 186 pregnancies, in which mothers received trimethoprim plus sulfamethoxazole or placebo, has shown a lower incidence of congenital malformations (3.3% versus 4.5%) in the trimethoprim-treated group. There were no abnormalities in the 10 children whose mothers received trimethoprim during the first trimester. Also, another study found no congenital abnormalities in 35 children whose mothers received trimethoprim plus sulfamethoxazole at the time of conception or shortly thereafter.

Studies in rats given oral doses of 70 mg/kg daily during the third trimester and throughout parturition have not shown that trimethoprim causes adverse effects on gestation or pup growth and survival. However, studies in rats given doses of 40 times the human dose have shown that trimethoprim is teratogenic. Studies in rabbits given doses of 6 times the human dose have shown an increase in fetal loss (dead, resorbed, and malformed fetuses).

FDA Pregnancy Category C.

### Breast-feeding
Trimethoprim is excreted in breast milk in concentrations equal to or greater than those in the maternal serum and may interfere with folic acid metabolism in nursing infants. However, no significant problems in humans have been documented.

### Pediatrics
Safety has not been established in infants less than 2 months of age. Appropriate studies on the relationship of age to the effects of trimethoprim have not been performed in children up to 12 years of age. However, in studies performed in children over 12 years of age, no pediatrics-specific problems have been documented to date.

### Geriatrics
An increased incidence of thrombocytopenia with purpura has been reported in elderly patients who are receiving diuretics, primarily thiazides, concurrently with trimethoprim.

### Dental
The leukopenic and thrombocytopenic effects of trimethoprim may result in an increased incidence of certain microbial infections, delayed healing, and gingival bleeding. If leukopenia or thrombocytopenia occurs, dental work should be deferred until blood counts have returned to normal. Patients should be instructed in proper oral hygiene, including caution in use of regular toothbrushes, dental floss, and toothpicks.

### Drug interactions and/or related problems
The following drug interactions and/or related problems have been selected on the basis of their potential clinical significance (possible mechanism in parentheses where appropriate)—not necessarily inclusive (» = major clinical significance):

Note: Combinations containing any of the following medications, depending on the amount present, may also interact with this medication.

Bone marrow depressants (See *Appendix II*)
    (concurrent use of bone marrow depressants with trimethoprim may increase the leukopenic and/or thrombocytopenic effects; if concurrent use is required, close observation for myelotoxic effects should be considered)

Cyclosporine
    (concurrent use of cyclosporine with trimethoprim may increase the incidence of nephrotoxicity)

Dapsone
(concurrent use with trimethoprim will usually increase the plasma concentrations of both dapsone and trimethoprim, possibly due to an inhibition in dapsone metabolism, and/or competition for renal secretion between the 2 medications; increased serum dapsone concentrations may increase the number and severity of side effects, especially methemoglobinemia)

» Folate antagonists, other (See *Appendix II*)
(concurrent use with trimethoprim or use of trimethoprim between courses of other folic acid antagonists, such as methotrexate or pyrimethamine, is not recommended because of the possibility of an increased incidence of megaloblastic anemia)

Phenytoin
(trimethoprim may inhibit the hepatic metabolism of phenytoin, increasing the half-life of phenytoin by up to 50% and decreasing its clearance by 30%)

Procainamide
(concurrent use with trimethoprim may increase the plasma concentration of both procainamide and its metabolite NAPA by decreasing their renal clearance)

Rifampin
(concurrent use may significantly increase the elimination and shorten the elimination half-life of trimethoprim)

Warfarin
(trimethoprim may potentiate the anticoagulant activity of warfarin by inhibiting its metabolism)

## Laboratory value alterations

The following have been selected on the basis of their potential clinical significance (possible effect in parentheses where appropriate)—not necessarily inclusive (» = major clinical significance):

With diagnostic test results
Creatinine determinations
(trimethoprim may interfere with the Jaffé alkaline picrate assay for creatinine, resulting in creatinine values that are approximately 10% higher than actual values)

Serum methotrexate assays
(trimethoprim may interfere with serum methotrexate assays if measured by the competitive binding protein technique [CBPA] using a bacterial dihydrofolate reductase as the binding protein; no interference occurs if methotrexate is measured by radioimmunoassay [RIA])

With physiology/laboratory test values
Alanine aminotransferase (ALT [SGPT]), serum and
Aspartate aminotransferase (AST [SGOT]), serum and
Bilirubin, serum and
Blood urea nitrogen (BUN) and
Creatinine, serum
(concentrations may be increased)

## Medical considerations/Contraindications

The medical considerations/contraindications included here have been selected on the basis of their potential clinical significance (reasons given in parentheses where appropriate)—not necessarily inclusive (» = major clinical significance).

*Risk-benefit should be considered when the following medical problems exist:*

Hypersensitivity to trimethoprim

» Megaloblastic anemia due to folic acid deficiency
(trimethoprim may worsen megaloblastic anemia caused by folic acid deficiency)

» Renal function impairment
(trimethoprim is primarily renally excreted)

## Patient monitoring

The following may be especially important in patient monitoring (other tests may be warranted in some patients, depending on condition; » = major clinical significance):

Complete blood counts (CBCs)
(may be required in patients on long-term treatment or those predisposed to folate deficiency if signs of blood dyscrasias occur during treatment; trimethoprim should be discontinued if there is a significant reduction in the count of any formed blood elements)

## Side/Adverse Effects

The following side/adverse effects have been selected on the basis of their potential clinical significance (possible signs and symptoms in parentheses where appropriate)—not necessarily inclusive:

### Those indicating need for medical attention
Incidence rare
*Aseptic meningitis* (headache; neck stiffness; malaise; nausea); *blood dyscrasias* (pale skin; sore throat and fever; unusual bleeding or bruising; unusual tiredness or weakness); *hypersensitivity* (skin rash or itching); *methemoglobinemia* (bluish fingernails, lips, or skin; difficult breathing; pale skin; sore throat and fever; unusual bleeding or bruising; unusual tiredness or weakness); *Stevens-Johnson syndrome* (aching joints and muscles; redness, blistering, peeling, or loosening of skin; unusual tiredness or weakness)

### Those indicating need for medical attention only if they continue or are bothersome
Incidence less frequent
*Gastrointestinal disturbances* (diarrhea; loss of appetite; nausea or vomiting; stomach cramps or pain); *headache*

## Overdose

For more information on the management of overdose or unintentional ingestion, **contact a Poison Control Center** (see *Poison Control Center Listing*).

### Treatment of overdose
Recommended treatment consists of the following:

To decrease absorption—Administering gastric lavage and general supportive measures.

Specific treatment—
Acidifying the urine to promote renal excretion of trimethoprim.

Using hemodialysis to remove a moderate amount of trimethoprim from the blood, although peritoneal dialysis is not effective.

Discontinuing trimethoprim and administering leucovorin, 3 to 6 mg intramuscularly per day for 5 to 7 days or as necessary, to restore normal hematopoiesis if signs of bone marrow depression occur.

Supportive care—Patients in whom intentional overdose is known or suspected should be referred for psychiatric consultation.

## Patient Consultation

As an aid to patient consultation, refer to *Advice for the Patient, Trimethoprim (Systemic).*

In providing consultation, consider emphasizing the following selected information (» = major clinical significance):

### Before using this medication
» Conditions affecting use, especially:
Hypersensitivity to trimethoprim
Pregnancy—Trimethoprim crosses the placenta; may interfere with folic acid metabolism in the fetus
Breast-feeding—Trimethoprim is excreted in breast milk; may interfere with folic acid metabolism in the newborn
Other medications, especially folic acid antagonists
Other medical problems, especially megaloblastic anemia due to folic acid deficiency and renal function impairment

### Proper use of this medication
» Not giving this medication to infants or children unless directed by physician
Taking on an empty stomach or, if gastrointestinal irritation occurs, with food
» Compliance with full course of therapy
» Importance of not missing doses and taking at evenly spaced times
» Proper dosing
Missed dose: Taking as soon as possible; not taking if almost time for next dose; not doubling doses
» Proper storage

### Precautions while using this medication
Importance of regular visits to physician to check progress if on prolonged therapy
Checking with physician if no improvement within a few days
Importance of taking folic acid concurrently if anemia occurs
Using caution in use of regular toothbrushes, dental floss, and toothpicks; deferring dental work until blood counts have returned to normal; checking with physician or dentist concerning proper oral hygiene

## Side/adverse effects

Signs of potential side effects, especially blood dyscrasias, aseptic meningitis, hypersensitivity, Stevens-Johnson syndrome, and methemoglobinemia

## General Dosing Information

Trimethoprim may be taken on an empty stomach or, if gastrointestinal irritation occurs, it may be taken with food.

If trimethoprim causes folic acid deficiency, folates may be administered concurrently without interfering with the antibacterial activity of trimethoprim since bacteria are unable to utilize preformed folates. If signs of bone marrow depression occur, trimethoprim should be discontinued. Leucovorin (folinic acid) 3 to 6 mg may be given intramuscularly once a day for 3 days or as required to restore normal hematopoiesis. In chronic overdose of trimethoprim, leucovorin may be given in high doses and/or for an extended period of time.

## Oral Dosage Forms

Note: Bracketed uses in the *Dosage Forms* section refer to categories of use and/or indications that are not included in U.S. product labeling.

### TRIMETHOPRIM TABLETS USP

**Usual adult and adolescent dose**
Antibacterial—
Treatment of urinary tract infections: Oral, 100 mg every twelve hours for ten days; or 200 mg once a day for ten days.
[Pneumonia, *Pneumocystis carinii* (treatment)][1]: Oral, 20 mg per kg of body weight per day of trimethoprim in combination with 100 mg of dapsone once a day for 21 days.
[Prophylaxis of urinary tract infections][1]: Oral, 100 mg once a day.

Note: Adults with impaired renal function may require a reduction in dose as follows:

| Creatinine Clearance (mL/min)/ (mL/sec) | Dose |
|---|---|
| >30/0.50 | See *Usual adult and adolescent dose* |
| 15–30/0.25–0.50 | 50% of usual dose |
| <15/<0.25 | Use is not recommended |

## Usual adult prescribing limits

Doses greater than 600 mg are often used when treating *Pneumocystis carinii* pneumonia.

## Usual pediatric dose

Antibacterial—
Infants and children up to 12 years of age: Dosage has not been established; however, a dose of 3 mg per kg of body weight two times a day has been effectively used in children.
Children 12 years of age and over: See *Usual adult and adolescent dose*.

Note: Safety has not been established in infants under 2 months of age. However, trimethoprim has been used extensively in combination with sulfamethoxazole in pediatric patients.

## Strength(s) usually available

U.S.—
100 mg (Rx) [*Proloprim; Trimpex;* GENERIC].
200 mg (Rx) [*Proloprim;* GENERIC].
Canada—
100 mg (Rx) [*Proloprim* (scored)].
200 mg (Rx) [*Proloprim* (scored)].

## Packaging and storage

Store below 40 °C (104 °F), preferably between 15 and 30 °C (59 and 86 °F), unless otherwise specified by manufacturer. Store in a tight, light-resistant container.

## Auxiliary labeling

• Continue medicine for full time of treatment.

[1]Not included in Canadian product labeling.

Revised: 02/23/93

## TRIMETHOPRIM-CONTAINING COMBINATIONS—

Sulfadiazine and Trimethoprim (Systemic)
Sulfamethoxazole and Trimethoprim (Systemic)

# TRIMETREXATE     Systemic

VA CLASSIFICATION (Primary): AP109

Note: For a listing of dosage forms and brand names by country availability, see *Dosage Forms* section(s). For a listing of brand names for the articles in this monograph, refer to the General Index.

## Category

Antiprotozoal (systemic).

## Indications

**Accepted**

Pneumonia, *Pneumocystis carinii* (treatment)—Trimetrexate is indicated as an alternative treatment for moderate-to-severe *Pneumocystis carinii* pneumonia (PCP) in immunocompromised patients, including those with acquired immunodeficiency syndrome (AIDS), who are intolerant of, or are refractory to, sulfamethoxazole-trimethoprim therapy, or for whom sulfamethoxazole-trimethoprim therapy is contraindicated. Leucovorin must be given concurrently with trimetrexate to prevent the potential serious or life-threatening toxicity (bone marrow depression, oral and gastrointestinal mucosal ulceration) of trimetrexate.

## Pharmacology/Pharmacokinetics

**Physicochemical characteristics**
Molecular weight—Trimetrexate: 369.42.
Trimetrexate glucuronate: 563.57.
pKa—8.0.

**Mechanism of action/Effect**
Trimetrexate is a nonclassical folate antagonist. It is a competitive inhibitor of dihydrofolate reductase (DHFR) from bacterial, protozoan, and mammalian sources. DHFR catalyzes the reduction of intracellular dihydrofolate to the active coenzyme tetrahydrofolate. Inhibition of DHFR results in the depletion of this coenzyme, leading directly to interference with thymidylate biosynthesis, as well as to inhibition of folate-dependent formyltransferases, and indirectly to inhibition of pu-

rine biosynthesis. The result is disruption of DNA, RNA, and protein synthesis, with consequent cell death. *In vitro*, trimetrexate binds to the DHFR of *Pneumocystis carinii* approximately 1500 times more potently than does trimethoprim.

Trimetrexate is chemically related to methotrexate but differs from it in several respects. Trimetrexate enters cells by a different mechanism than does methotrexate. Trimetrexate penetrates the cell rapidly, independently of the folate carrier–mediated transport system required by methotrexate. The structure of trimetrexate does not resemble that of the substrates folic acid or dihydrofolic acid, and trimetrexate uptake is not affected by folic acid or calcium folinate. Also, trimetrexate does not interfere with folate polyglutamate formation or block folate entry by competitive inhibition of the reduced folate transport system. Further, unlike methotrexate, trimetrexate has sustained intracellular retention.

Note: Leucovorin (folinic acid) is transported into mammalian cells and can be assimilated into cellular folate pools following its metabolism. *In vitro* studies have shown that leucovorin provides a source of reduced folates necessary for normal cellular biosynthetic processes. Because *P. carinii* lacks the reduced folate carrier–mediated transport system, leucovorin is prevented from entering the organism. Therefore, at therapeutic doses of trimetrexate and leucovorin, the selective transport of trimetrexate, but not of leucovorin, into the *P. carinii* organism allows leucovorin to protect normal host cells from the cytotoxicity of trimetrexate without inhibiting trimetrexate's therapeutic effect.

**Distribution**
Lipid-soluble; distributes readily into ascitic fluid. Penetrates poorly into the cerebrospinal fluid (CSF); the CSF concentration is < 5% that of the simultaneous serum concentration.

The steady-state $Vol_D$ is variable and ranges from 9 to 33 liters per square meter of body surface area (L/m$^2$). One phase I study in cancer patients found the steady-state $Vol_D$ to be 0.62 L per kg of body weight.

## Protein binding
In vitro studies have found protein binding to vary from 80 to 98%, depending on the serum trimetrexate concentration.

## Biotransformation
Hepatic. Not fully characterized in humans; however, data suggest that the major metabolic pathway is oxidative O-demethylation, followed by conjugation to form either the glucuronide or sulfate metabolite. Preliminary findings in humans indicate the presence of a glucuronide conjugate with DHFR-inhibiting activity and a demethylated metabolite in urine.

## Half-life
Biphasic or triphasic elimination has been described; the terminal half-life ranged from 11 to 20 hours.

## Peak serum concentration
Approximately 10 to 12 micromoles per liter (5.6 to 6.7 mcg per mL) after intravenous administration of a dose of 30 mg per square meter of body surface area (mg/m$^2$).

## Elimination
Renal; active tubular secretion and tubular reabsorption are thought to be involved with renal clearance; however, only 10 to 20% of a dose is eliminated as unchanged trimetrexate within 48 hours. Urinary recovery of trimetrexate varies with the assay used, ranging from about 40% with a nonspecific DHFR inhibition assay, which suggests the presence of active metabolites, to about 10% with high pressure liquid chromatography (HPLC). Fecal excretion of the parent compound is < 6% of the dose over 48 hours.

# Precautions to Consider

## Cross-sensitivity and/or related problems
Patients sensitive to methotrexate may also be sensitive to trimetrexate.

## Carcinogenicity
Long-term studies in animals to evaluate the carcinogenic potential of trimetrexate have not been performed.

## Mutagenicity
Trimetrexate was not mutagenic when tested with the standard Ames *Salmonella* mutagenicity assay, with and without metabolic activation. It also did not induce mutations in Chinese hamster lung cells or sisterchromatid exchange in Chinese hamster ovary cells. No clastogenic activity was found in a mouse micronucleus assay. However, trimetrexate did induce an increase in the incidence of chromosomal aberration in cultured Chinese hamster lung cells.

## Pregnancy/Reproduction
Fertility—No studies have been conducted to evaluate trimetrexate's effects on fertility. However, during standard toxicity studies conducted in mice and rats, degeneration of the testes and spermatocytes and arrest of spermatogenesis were observed.

Pregnancy—Trimetrexate can harm the fetus when administered to a pregnant woman. Women of childbearing potential should be counseled to avoid becoming pregnant during trimetrexate therapy.
Trimetrexate has been shown to be fetotoxic and teratogenic in rats and rabbits. Rats given 1.5 and 2.5 mg per kg of body weight (mg/kg) per day of intravenous trimetrexate on gestational days 6 through 15 showed substantial postimplantation losses and severe inhibition of maternal weight gain. In addition, administration to rats of 0.5 and 1.0 mg/kg per day on gestational days 6 through 15 caused retarded fetal development and teratogenicity. In rabbits, trimetrexate administered intravenously at doses of 2.5 and 5.0 mg/kg per day on gestational days 6 through 18 also caused significant materno- and fetotoxicity. Trimetrexate was teratogenic in rabbits given doses of 0.1 mg/kg per day in the absence of significant maternal toxicity. These effects were observed at doses 5 to 50% of the equivalent human therapeutic dose in mg per square meter of body surface area (mg/m$^2$). Teratogenic effects included skeletal, visceral, ocular, and cardiovascular abnormalities.
FDA Pregnancy Category D.

## Breast-feeding
It is not known if trimetrexate is distributed into breast milk. Breast feeding is not recommended during trimetrexate therapy because of the potential for serious adverse effects in the nursing infant.

## Pediatrics
Appropriate studies on the relationship of age to the effects of trimetrexate have not been performed in children up to 18 years of age. However, 2 children, ages 9 months and 15 months, were both treated with 45 mg per square meter of body surface area (mg/m$^2$) of trimetrexate for 21 days and 20 mg/m$^2$ of leucovorin for 24 days with no serious or unexpected adverse effects.

## Geriatrics
No information is available on the relationship of age to the effects of trimetrexate in geriatric patients.

## Dental
The bone marrow–depressant effects of trimetrexate may result in an increased incidence of microbial infection, delayed healing, and gingival bleeding. Dental work, whenever possible, should be completed prior to initiation of therapy or deferred until blood counts have returned to normal. Patients should be instructed in proper oral hygiene during treatment, including caution in use of regular toothbrushes, dental floss, and toothpicks.
Trimetrexate also commonly causes ulcerative stomatitis associated with considerable discomfort.

## Drug interactions and/or related problems
The following drug interactions and/or related problems have been selected on the basis of their potential clinical significance (possible mechanism in parentheses where appropriate)—not necessarily inclusive (» = major clinical significance):

Note: Combinations containing any of the following medications, depending on the amount present, may also interact with this medication.

At this time, no clinically significant drug interactions and/or related problems have been documented in patients receiving trimetrexate. However, concurrent use with the medications listed below could theoretically produce life-threatening toxicity.

Blood dyscrasia–causing medications (See *Appendix II*)
(leukopenic and/or thrombocytopenic effects of trimetrexate may be increased with concurrent or recent therapy if these medications cause the same effects; dosage adjustment of trimetrexate, if necessary, should be based on blood counts)

» Bone marrow depressants, other (See *Appendix II* ), or
Radiation therapy
(concurrent use may cause additive bone marrow depression; dosage reduction may be required when two or more bone marrow depressants, including radiation, are used concurrently or consecutively)

» Enzyme inhibitors, hepatic, cytochrome P-450
(because trimetrexate is metabolized by a cytochrome P-450 enzyme system, medications that affect the cytochrome P-450 system may decrease, or compete with, the metabolism of trimetrexate, increasing the possibility of trimetrexate toxicity)

» Hepatotoxic medications (See *Appendix II*) or
» Nephrotoxic medications (See *Appendix II*)
(trimetrexate is hepatically metabolized and renally excreted; hepatotoxic or nephrotoxic medications may decrease the clearance of trimetrexate, increasing the risk of trimetrexate toxicity)

Pyrimethamine or
Trimethoprim
(concurrent use may potentially increase the toxic effects of trimetrexate because of similar folic acid antagonist actions)

## Laboratory value alterations
The following have been selected on the basis of their potential clinical significance (possible effect in parentheses where appropriate)—not necessarily inclusive (» = major clinical significance):

With physiology/laboratory test values
Alanine aminotransferase (ALT [SGPT]) and
Alkaline phosphatase and
Aspartate aminotransferase (AST [SGOT]) and
Bilirubin
(serum values may be transiently elevated)

Blood urea nitrogen and
Creatinine concentration, serum
(values may rarely be elevated)

» Hemoglobin or hematocrit and
» Leukocyte count, total and differential, and
» Platelet count
(values may be decreased)

## Medical considerations/Contraindications
The medical considerations/contraindications included here have been selected on the basis of their potential clinical significance (reasons given in parentheses where appropriate)—not necessarily inclusive (» = major clinical significance).

*Risk-benefit should be considered when the following medical problems exist:*

» Bone marrow depression
(increased risk of trimetrexate-induced bone marrow toxicity)

» Hepatic function impairment or
» Renal function impairment
    (risk of trimetrexate toxicity is increased because clearance of tri-
    metrexate may be impaired and accumulation may occur; even
    small doses may lead to severe myelosuppression and mucositis;
    larger doses and/or increased duration of leucovorin treatment may
    be necessary)
» Sensitivity to trimetrexate, methotrexate, or leucovorin

**Patient monitoring**

The following may be especially important in patient monitoring (other
tests may be warranted in some patients, depending on condition;
» = major clinical significance):

Alanine aminotransferase (ALT [SGPT]) and
Alkaline phosphatase and
Aspartate aminotransferase (AST [SGOT])
    (serum transaminase and alkaline phosphatase values should be
    monitored approximately twice a week during therapy)
Blood urea nitrogen (BUN) or
Creatinine concentration, serum
    (blood urea nitrogen or serum creatinine concentrations should be
    monitored approximately twice a week during therapy)
» Hemoglobin or hematocrit and
» Leukocyte count, total and, if appropriate, differential, and
» Platelet counts
    (determinations should be monitored approximately twice a week
    during therapy because trimetrexate causes neutropenia, thrombo-
    cytopenia, and anemia)

## Side/Adverse Effects

Note: Because many patients who participated in clinical trials had com-
    plications of advanced human immunodeficiency virus (HIV) dis-
    ease, it was often difficult to differentiate between the manifesta-
    tions of HIV infection and the adverse effects of trimetrexate.

    One case of an anaphylactic reaction was observed in a cancer
    patient who received trimetrexate as a rapid injection.

The following side/adverse effects have been selected on the basis of their
potential clinical significance (possible signs and symptoms in parentheses where appropriate)—not necessarily inclusive:

**Those indicating need for medical attention**
Incidence more frequent
    *Neutropenia* (fever and sore throat)

Incidence less frequent
    *Anemia* (unusual tiredness or weakness); *fever; mouth sores or ul-
    cers; skin rash and itching; thrombocytopenia* (black, tarry stools;
    blood in urine or stools; pinpoint red spots on skin; unusual bleeding
    or bruising)

**Those indicating need for medical attention only if they continue
or are bothersome**
Incidence less frequent
    *Confusion; nausea and vomiting; stomach pain*

## Overdose

**Treatment of overdose**

Specific treatment—Although there has been no extensive experience with
patients receiving more than 90 mg per square meter of body surface
(mg/m²) per day of intravenous trimetrexate with concurrent administration of leucovorin, in the event of an overdose, the recommended
treatment consists of discontinuing trimetrexate and administering leucovorin at a dose of 40 mg/m² every 6 hours for at least 3 days.

Supportive care—Patients in whom intentional overdose is known or suspected should be referred for psychiatric consultation.

## Patient Consultation

As an aid to patient consultation, refer to *Advice for the Patient,
Trimetrexate (Systemic).* See also *Advice for the Patient, Leucovorin
(Systemic).*

In providing consultation, consider emphasizing the following selected
information (» = major clinical significance):

**Before receiving this medication**
» Conditions affecting use, especially:
    Sensitivity to trimetrexate, methotrexate, or leucovorin
    Pregnancy—Use is not recommended because of potential terato-
        genic and fetotoxic effects; using contraception during trime-
        trexate treatment; telling physician immediately if pregnancy
        is suspected
    Breast-feeding—Not recommended because of risk of serious side
        effects in nursing infants

Other medications, especially other bone marrow depressants, he-
    patic cytochrome P-450 enzyme inhibitors, hepatotoxic medi-
    cations, or nephrotoxic medications
Other medical problems, especially bone marrow depression, he-
    patic function impairment, or renal function impairment

**Proper use of this medication**
*For leucovorin:*
» Importance of taking or receiving leucovorin concurrently with tri-
    metrexate, and for 3 days following the end of trimetrexate therapy
    Importance of not missing oral leucovorin doses and taking at evenly
        spaced times
    Compliance with full course of therapy
    Checking with physician if vomiting occurs shortly after oral dose of
        leucovorin is taken
» Proper dosing
    Missed dose of leucovorin: Taking oral leucovorin as soon as possible;
        not taking if almost time for next dose; not doubling doses
» Proper storage of leucovorin

**Precautions while receiving this medication**
Checking with physician if no improvement
» Importance of close monitoring by physician
*Caution if bone marrow depression occurs:*
» Avoiding exposure to persons with bacterial infections, especially dur-
    ing periods of low blood counts; checking with physician imme-
    diately if fever or chills, cough or hoarseness, lower back or side
    pain, or painful or difficult urination occurs
» Checking with physician immediately if unusual bleeding or bruising;
    black, tarry stools; blood in urine or stools; or pinpoint red spots
    on skin occur
    Caution in use of regular toothbrush, dental floss, or toothpick; phy-
        sician, dentist, or nurse may suggest alternatives; checking with
        physician before having dental work done
    Using caution to avoid accidental cuts with use of sharp objects such
        as safety razor or fingernail or toenail cutters

**Side/adverse effects**
    Signs of potential side effects, especially neutropenia, anemia, fever,
    mouth sores or ulcers, skin rash and itching, and thrombocytopenia

## General Dosing Information

**Leucovorin must be given concurrently with trimetrexate to avoid life-
threatening toxicities.** Leucovorin therapy must also be continued for
72 hours after the last dose of trimetrexate.

Trimetrexate should be administered as an intravenous infusion, over 60
to 90 minutes. An anaphylactoid reaction was reported in a cancer
patient receiving trimetrexate as a rapid injection.

Leucovorin may be administered prior to or following trimetrexate. To
prevent formation of a precipitate, intravenous lines should be flushed
with at least 10 mL of 5% dextrose injection between trimetrexate and
leucovorin infusions. The oral dose of leucovorin (calculated on the
basis of body surface area) should be rounded up to the next 25 mg
increment to determine the actual dose.

Dosage must be adjusted to meet the individual requirements of each
patient, based on clinical response and appearance or severity of
toxicity.

Leucovorin tablets have an oral absorption that is saturable at doses above
25 mg. The bioavailability decreases as the dose increases: 97% for
25 mg, 75% for 50 mg, 37% for 100 mg. Because of the larger doses
used with trimetrexate, saturable absorption may be a problem. Patients with AIDS may also have problems with malabsorption that
could interfere with the absorption of leucovorin. If large doses
(greater than 50 mg) are needed, intravenous leucovorin should be
used.

**Safety considerations for handling this medication**
In addition to being an antiprotozoal agent, trimetrexate is also an antineoplastic agent. There is limited but increasing evidence and concern
that personnel involved in preparation and administration of parenteral
antineoplastics may be at some risk because of the potential mutagenicity, teratogenicity, and/or carcinogenicity of these agents, although
the actual risk is unknown. Medical experts recommend cautious handling both in preparation and disposal of antineoplastic agents. Precautions that have been suggested include:
• Use of a biological containment cabinet during reconstitution and
    dilution of parenteral medications and wearing of disposable surgical
    gloves and masks.
• Use of proper technique to prevent contamination of the medication,
    work area, and operator during transfer between containers (including
    proper training of personnel in this technique).

- Cautious and proper disposal of needles, syringes, vials, ampuls, and unused medication.

A number of medical centers have developed detailed guidelines for handling of antineoplastic agents.

## Parenteral Dosage Forms

Note: The dosing and strengths of the dosage forms available are expressed in terms of trimetrexate base (not the glucuronate salt).

### TRIMETREXATE GLUCURONATE FOR INJECTION

#### Usual adult dose

Antiprotozoal—

Intravenous infusion, 45 mg (base) per square meter of body surface of trimetrexate once a day for twenty-one days. The dose should be administered by intravenous infusion over sixty to ninety minutes. During treatment with trimetrexate, leucovorin must be administered daily and for seventy-two hours after the last dose of trimetrexate (total twenty-four days). Leucovorin may be administered orally or by intravenous infusion, given over five to ten minutes, at a dose of 20 mg per square meter of body surface area every six hours.

Note: In the event of hematologic toxicity, the doses of trimetrexate and leucovorin should be modified as follows:

| Toxicity grade | Neutrophils (PMNs* and Bands) (per mm³) | Platelets (per mm³) | Trimetrexate dose (mg/m², once a day) | Leucovorin dose (mg/m², every 6 hours) |
|---|---|---|---|---|
| 1 | >1000 | >75,000 | 45 | 20 |
| 2 | 750-1000 | 50,000-75,000 | 45 | 40 |
| 3 | 500-749 | 25,000-49,999 | 22 | 40 |
| 4† | <500 | <25,000 | Day 1-9† Day 10-21† | 40 |

*Polymorphonuclear leukocytes.

†If grade 4 hematologic toxicity occurs prior to day 10, trimetrexate should be discontinued and leucovorin should be administered at a dose of 40 mg/m² every six hours for an additional seventy-two hours. If grade 4 hematologic toxicity occurs at day 10 or later, trimetrexate may be withheld for up to ninety-six hours to allow counts to recover. If counts recover to grade 3 within ninety-six hours, trimetrexate should be administered at a dose of 22 mg/m² and leucovorin maintained at 40 mg/m² every six hours. When counts recover to grade 2, trimetrexate may be increased to 45 mg/m², but the leucovorin dose should be maintained at 40 mg/m² for the duration of treatment. If counts do not improve to grade 3 within ninety-six hours, trimetrexate should be discontinued. Leucovorin at a dose of 40 mg/m² every six hours should be administered for seventy-two hours following the last dose of trimetrexate.

#### Usual pediatric dose

Safety and efficacy have not been established in children up to 18 years of age. However, two children, ages nine months and fifteen months, were both treated with 45 mg per square meter of body surface (mg/m²) (base) of trimetrexate for twenty-one days and 20 mg/m² of leucovorin for twenty-four days with no serious or unexpected adverse effects.

#### Strength(s) usually available

U.S.—

25 mg per 5 mL (base) (Rx) [NeuTrexin].

Canada—

25 mg per 5 mL (base) (Rx) [NeuTrexin].

#### Packaging and storage

Store at room temperature between 15 and 30 °C (59 and 86 °F). Protect from light.

#### Preparation of dosage form

Trimetrexate should be reconstituted with 2 mL of 5% dextrose injection or sterile water for injection, to yield a concentration of 12.5 mg per mL. Complete dissolution should occur within 30 seconds. The reconstituted product will appear as a pale greenish-yellow solution. The solution must be inspected visually for particulate matter prior to dilution; it should not be used if cloudiness or precipitation is observed. The reconstituted solution should be filtered with a 0.22 micron filter prior to further dilution, even if the solution appears clear.

The reconstituted solution should be further diluted with 5% dextrose injection, to yield a final concentration of 0.25 to 2 mg of trimetrexate per mL.

When reconstituting parenteral leucovorin, if bacteriostatic water for injection (which contains benzyl alcohol) is used, doses greater than 10 mg/m² are not recommended. If larger doses are required, leucovorin should be reconstituted with sterile water for injection and used immediately.

#### Stability

After initial reconstitution, trimetrexate solution is stable under refrigeration or at room temperature for up to 24 hours. Do not freeze the reconstituted solution. The unused portions should be discarded after 24 hours.

A reconstituted solution that is further diluted with 5% dextrose is stable under refrigeration or at room temperature for up to 24 hours. Do not freeze. The unused portions should be discarded 24 hours after initial reconstitution.

#### Incompatibilities

Trimetrexate should not be reconstituted or further diluted with solutions containing either the chloride ion (e.g., solutions containing sodium chloride) or leucovorin. Precipitation occurs instantly. Trimetrexate and leucovorin solutions must be administered separately. Intravenous lines should be flushed with at least 10 mL of 5% dextrose injection between trimetrexate and leucovorin infusions.

#### Additional information

If trimetrexate contacts the skin or mucosa, immediately wash thoroughly with soap and water. Procedures for proper disposal of cytotoxic drugs should be considered.

Developed: 04/15/94
Revised: 07/14/95

---

**TRIMIPRAMINE**—See *Antidepressants, Tricyclic (Systemic)*

---

# TRIOXSALEN   Systemic

INN: Trioxysalen

VA CLASSIFICATION (Primary): DE890/DE801

Note: For a listing of dosage forms and brand names by country availability, see *Dosage Forms* section(s). For a listing of brand names for the articles in this monograph, refer to the General Index.

## Category

Repigmenting agent (systemic); antipsoriatic (systemic).

Note: Trioxsalen is used in conjunction with ultraviolet light A (UVA). This mode of treatment is known as PUVA (psoralen plus ultraviolet light A).

## Indications

Note: Bracketed information in the *Indications* section refers to uses that are not included in U.S. product labeling.

### Accepted

Vitiligo (treatment)

Skin, increased tolerance to sunlight or

Skin pigmentation, enhancement of—PUVA is indicated for repigmentation in the treatment of vitiligo, increasing skin tolerance to sunlight, and enhancing pigmentation. It is not effective in producing pigmentation in leukoderma of infectious origin or in albinism (although it will increase the tolerance to sunlight).

[Psoriasis (treatment)]—PUVA is also used in the treatment of psoriasis.

### Unaccepted

The unsupervised use of trioxsalen to promote tanning is dangerous and should be discouraged.

## Pharmacology/Pharmacokinetics

### Physicochemical characteristics

Molecular weight—228.25.

**Mechanism of action/Effect**

Trioxsalen is a synthetic psoralen derivative. Exact mechanism of erythemogenic, melanogenic, and cytotoxic response in the epidermis is unknown, but may involve increased tyrosinase activity in melanin-producing cells, as well as inhibition of DNA synthesis, cell division, and epidermal turnover. Successful pigmentation requires the presence of functioning melanocytes.

In albinism, tolerance of the skin to sunlight occurs without the formation of pigment. This protective action seems to be related to the thickening of the horny layer and retention of melanin, which produces a thickened, melanized stratum corneum and the formation of a stratum lucidum.

**Other actions/effects**

Trioxsalen has greater activity than methoxsalen and also has 6 times the LD 50.

**Absorption**

Trioxsalen is variably absorbed from the gastrointestinal tract.

**Biotransformation**

Activated by long-wavelength UVA in the range of 320 to 400 (maximal effect at 365) nanometers (nm).
Further metabolism—Hepatic.

**Onset of action**

Vitiligo—Up to 6 months.
For increased sensitivity of skin to sunlight—1 hour.
Tanning—Within a few days.

**Time to peak effect**

Increased sensitivity of skin to sunlight—2 to 3 hours (coincides with maximum serum concentration).

**Duration of action**

Increased sensitivity of skin to sunlight—Approximately 8 hours.

**Elimination**

Renal (80 to 90% in 8 hours).

# Precautions to Consider

**Carcinogenicity**

Psoralens have been found to augment UVA-induced carcinogenicity in laboratory animals. In addition, studies in humans treated with systemic methoxsalen plus UVA have shown an increase in the risk of squamous cell carcinoma. The possibility of increased risk may exist also for topical methoxsalen and systemic trioxsalen. This risk appears to be greatest in patients with predisposing risk factors, such as fair skin or a hypersensitivity to sunlight; a history of skin cancer, exposure to ionizing radiation, or excessive exposure to sunlight; or a history of treatment with tar and UVB (prolonged), arsenicals, or topical nitrogen mustard.

**Pregnancy/Reproduction**

Pregnancy—Studies have not been done in humans.
Studies have not been done in animals.

**Breast-feeding**

Problems in humans have not been documented.

**Pediatrics**

Appropriate studies on the relationship of age to the effects of trioxsalen have not been performed in the pediatric population. However, no pediatrics-specific problems have been documented to date.

**Geriatrics**

Appropriate studies on the relationship of age to the effects of trioxsalen have not been performed in the geriatric population. However, no geriatrics-specific problems have been documented to date.

**Drug interactions and/or related problems**

The following drug interactions and/or related problems have been selected on the basis of their potential clinical significance (possible mechanism in parentheses where appropriate)—not necessarily inclusive (» = major clinical significance):

Note: Combinations containing any of the following medications, depending on the amount present, may also interact with this medication.

Furocoumarin-containing foods, such as limes, figs, parsley, parsnips, mustard, carrots, and celery
(although there have been no reports of serious reactions, caution with or avoidance of these foods is recommended because of the risk of additive phototoxicity)

Photosensitizing medications, other
(concurrent use of trioxsalen with these medications, systemic or topical, may cause additive photosensitizing effects; concurrent use

with coal tar or coal tar derivatives or with methoxsalen is not recommended)
(concurrent use of trioxsalen with phenothiazines may potentiate intraocular photochemical damage to the choroid, retina, and lens)

**Medical considerations/Contraindications**

The medical considerations/contraindications included here have been selected on the basis of their potential clinical significance (reasons given in parentheses where appropriate)—not necessarily inclusive (» = major clinical significance).

*Risk-benefit should be considered when the following medical problems exist:*

» Albinism or
» Hydroa or
» Leukoderma of infectious origin or
» Lupus erythematosus, acute or
Polymorphic light eruptions or
» Porphyria or
» Xeroderma pigmentosum
(these conditions are associated with photosensitization)
» Aphakia
(increased risk of retinal damage due to lack of lenses)
Cardiovascular disease, severe
(because of the heat stress or the prolonged standing associated with each UVA treatment; these patients should not be treated in a vertical UVA chamber)
» Cataracts
Gastrointestinal diseases
Infection, chronic
Sensitivity to trioxsalen
» Skin cancer, history of
Sunlight allergy, family history of
(PUVA may cause photoallergic contact dermatitis or precipitate sunlight allergy)
» Caution should be used also in patients with a history of having taken arsenicals or having received x-rays, cytotoxic therapy, or coal tar and ultraviolet light B (UVB) therapy because of the increased risk of skin cancer.

**Patient monitoring**

The following may be especially important in patient monitoring (other tests may be warranted in some patients, depending on condition; » = major clinical significance):

Antinuclear antibodies test and
Complete blood count and
Liver function tests and
Renal function tests
(recommended prior to initiation of therapy)

Monitoring for melanoma and other skin carcinomas
(recommended in patients receiving trioxsalen for prolonged periods, since long-term safety has not been established)

Ophthalmic examination
(recommended prior to initiation of therapy and yearly thereafter during therapy)

# Side/Adverse Effects

Note: Cataracts have also been reported with psoralen use; however, risk is very low in patients who wear UVA-absorbing, wraparound sunglasses when exposed to sunlight or ultraviolet light for 24 hours after taking trioxsalen.

Trioxsalen may produce fewer erythemic and gastrointestinal side effects than methoxsalen.

There is an increased risk of skin cancer. This risk appears to be greatest in patients with predisposing risk factors, such as fair skin or a hypersensitivity to sunlight; a history of skin cancer, exposure to ionizing radiation, or excessive exposure to sunlight; or a history of treatment with tar and UVB (prolonged), arsenicals, or topical nitrogen mustard.

Premature aging of the skin may occur as a result of prolonged PUVA therapy. This effect is permanent and is similar to the results of excessive exposure to sunlight.

The following side/adverse effects have been selected on the basis of their potential clinical significance (possible signs and symptoms in parentheses where appropriate)—not necessarily inclusive:

**Those indicating need for medical attention**
Symptoms of overdose or overexposure to ultraviolet light
*Blistering and peeling of skin; reddened, sore skin; swelling, especially of feet or lower legs*

**Those indicating need for medical attention only if they continue for more than 48 hours or are bothersome**
Incidence more frequent
*Itching of skin; nausea*
Incidence less frequent
*Dizziness; headache; mental depression; nervousness; trouble in sleeping*

## Overdose

For more information on the management of overdose, unintentional ingestion, or overexposure to ultraviolet light **contact a Poison Control Center** (see *Poison Control Center Listing*).

**Symptoms of overdose or overexposure to ultraviolet light**
The following effects have been selected on the basis of their potential clinical significance (possible signs and symptoms in parentheses where appropriate)—not necessarily inclusive:
*Blistering and peeling of skin; reddened, sore skin; swelling, especially of feet or lower legs*

**Treatment of overdose**
To decrease absorption—
Inducing emesis, if it can be accomplished within the first 2 to 3 hours after trioxsalen ingestion, since maximum blood concentrations are reached by that time.
Specific treatment—
Treating patient symptomatically for burns, depending on their extent and severity.
Monitoring—
Observing patient for erythema greater than Grade 2 (Grade 2 being marked erythema with no edema) occurring within 24 hours, which may signal the beginning of a potentially serious burn, since peak erythemal reaction to PUVA usually occurs approximately 48 hours following trioxsalen ingestion.
Supportive care—
For ingestion of trioxsalen: Keeping patient in a darkened room for at least 24 hours following trioxsalen ingestion to prevent the possibility of sun exposure and subsequent burn injury.
For overexposure to sunlight or ultraviolet light: Keeping patient in a darkened room for a least 24 hours following ingestion of trioxsalen to prevent prevent the possibility of further sun exposure and subsequent burn injury while assessment of the extent of damage is made.
Patients in whom intentional overdose is known or suspected should be referred for psychiatric consultation.

## Patient Consultation

As an aid to patient consultation, refer to *Advice for the Patient, Trioxsalen (Systemic).*

In providing consultation, consider emphasizing the following selected information (» = major clinical significance):

**Before using this medication**
Possible long-term effects (cataracts, premature skin aging, carcinogenesis); not using for suntanning purposes
» Conditions affecting use, especially:
Sensitivity to trioxsalen
Other medical problems, especially acute lupus erythematosus, albinism, aphakia, cataracts, history of receiving arsenicals, x-rays, cytotoxic therapy, or coal tar and ultraviolet light B (UVB) therapy, history of skin cancer, hydroa, leukoderma of infectious origin, porphyria, or xeroderma pigmentosum

**Proper use of this medication**
» May take several weeks to months to work; importance of not increasing the dosage of medication or exposure to ultraviolet light, because of the risk of serious burns
May be taken with meals or milk to reduce gastrointestinal irritation
» Proper dosing
Late or missed dose: Notifying physician for rescheduling of light treatment
» Proper storage

**Precautions while using this medication**
Importance of regular visits to physician to have progress checked, including eye examinations

» Protecting skin from sunlight, even through window glass or on cloudy days, for at least 24 hours before and 8 hours following treatment; protecting lips with sun block lipstick that has a protection factor of at least 15
Possibility of continued skin sensitivity to sunlight because of medication; using extra precautions for at least 48 hours following each treatment; not sunbathing during this time
» Wearing special sunglasses during daylight hours (even in indirect light, such as through window glass or on cloudy days) for 24 hours following each dose of medication
Avoiding eating furocoumarin-containing foods (limes, figs, parsley, parsnips, mustard, carrots, celery)
» Possibility of dry skin or itching; checking with physician before treating

**Side/adverse effects**
There is an increased risk of developing skin cancer. The body should be examined regularly and the physician shown skin sores that do not heal, new skin growths, and skin growths that have changed in appearance or feel.
Premature aging of the skin may occur as a result of prolonged PUVA therapy. This effect is permanent and is similar to the results of excessive exposure to sunlight.
Signs of potential side effects, especially symptoms of overdose or overexposure to ultraviolet light.

## General Dosing Information

Patients receiving trioxsalen should be under the supervision of a physician experienced in PUVA therapy.

Trioxsalen may be taken with meals or milk to reduce gastrointestinal irritation.

Dosage of trioxsalen should not be increased. In addition, a lower-than-recommended dose will produce the same effect, but it will occur more slowly.

Exposure to sunlight or ultraviolet light should be carefully controlled and adjusted on an individual basis according to skin type and tolerance. Exposure time to sunlight should be reduced at high altitudes or at midday.

Skin should be protected from sunlight, even through window glass or on a cloudy day, for at least 24 hours before and 8 hours following oral PUVA treatment by protective clothing, such as long-sleeved shirts, full-length slacks, wide-brimmed hat, and gloves and by using a sun block product that has a skin protection factor of at least 15 on body areas that cannot be covered by clothing. In addition, lips should be protected with a sun block lipstick that has a skin protection factor of at least 15. Also, since the skin continues to be sensitive to sunlight for some time after treatment, the patient should avoid overexposure to sunlight for 48 hours following administration of trioxsalen.

In the treatment of vitiligo, repigmentation occurs most rapidly on fleshy areas (face, abdomen, buttocks) and more slowly on the extremities and bony areas (hands and feet). Repigmentation may begin after a few weeks; however, significant results may take as long as 6 to 9 months. Thereafter, maintenance therapy may be required for some patients to retain the new pigment. If follicular repigmentation is not apparent after 3 months of daily treatment, treatment should be discontinued, as it must be considered a failure.

Tolerance to the effects of trioxsalen may occur when pigmentation precedes erythema by a long period of time. Hyperpigmentation reduces subsequent responsiveness.

Use of psoralen derivatives to promote suntanning has resulted in serious reactions, including acute generalized dermatitis, blistering, and edema; residual edema of the legs and cutaneous damage have been reported.

Temporary withdrawal of therapy is recommended if burning or blistering of skin occurs.

## Oral Dosage Forms

### TRIOXSALEN TABLETS USP

**Usual adult and adolescent dose**
Vitiligo—
Oral, 20 to 40 mg two to four hours before measured periods of UVA exposure, two or three times a week (at least forty-eight hours apart).
Increasing tolerance to sunlight
Enhancement of skin pigmentation—
Oral, 20 to 40 mg two hours before measured periods of UVA exposure, two or three times a week (at least forty-eight hours apart).
Sunlight: Initial exposure time should not exceed fifteen minutes for light skin colors, twenty minutes for medium skin colors, or

twenty-five minutes for dark skin colors; exposure time may subsequently be increased by five minutes each treatment, depending upon degree of erythema and tenderness.

Artificial light: Initial exposure time should not exceed one-half of that producing erythema after sunlight exposure, or should be based on the minimal phototoxic dose (MPD) and manufacturer's directions for the specific light source being used. The MPD can be determined by irradiating several areas of skin 2 cm in diameter; a range of light exposure times is used and the time that produces erythema at seventy-two hours after exposure is the MPD.

Note: When used to increase skin tolerance to sunlight, treatment should be limited to fourteen days of therapy, either on a continuous or interrupted regimen, since adequate pigment will have been formed by that time.

**Usual pediatric dose**
Children up to 12 years of age—Dosage has not been established.
Children 12 years of age and over—See *Usual adult and adolescent dose.*

**Strength(s) usually available**
U.S.—
    5 mg (Rx) [*Trisoralen*].
Canada—
    5 mg (Rx) [*Trisoralen*].

**Packaging and storage**
Store below 40 °C (104 °F), preferably between 15 and 30 °C (59 and 86 °F), unless otherwise specified by manufacturer. Store in a well-closed, light-resistant container.

**Auxiliary labeling**
• Take with meals or milk.

Revised: 07/25/94

---

**TRIPELENNAMINE**—See *Antihistamines (Systemic)*

---

**TRIPLE SULFA**—See *Sulfonamides (Vaginal)*

---

**TRIPROLIDINE**—See *Antihistamines (Systemic)*

---

**TRIPROLIDINE-CONTAINING COMBINATIONS**—

Triprolidine and Pseudoephedrine (Systemic)—See *Antihistamines and Decongestants (Systemic)*
Triprolidine, Pseudoephedrine, and Acetaminophen (Systemic)—See *Antihistamines, Decongestants, and Analgesics (Systemic)*
Triprolidine, Pseudoephedrine, and Codeine (Systemic)—See *Cough/Cold Combinations (Systemic)*
Triprolidine, Pseudoephedrine, Codeine, and Guaifenesin (Systemic)—See *Cough/Cold Combinations (Systemic)*
Triprolidine, Pseudoephedrine, and Dextromethorphan (Systemic)—See *Cough/Cold Combinations (Systemic)*

---

**TROLAMINE    SALICYLATE**—See   *Sunscreen   Agents (Topical)*

---

# TROPICAMIDE    Ophthalmic

VA CLASSIFICATION (Primary/Secondary): OP600/DX900
Note: For a listing of dosage forms and brand names by country availability, see *Dosage Forms* section(s). For a listing of brand names for the articles in this monograph, refer to the General Index.

## Category
Diagnostic aid (cycloplegic; mydriatic); cycloplegic; mydriatic.

## Indications
**Accepted**
Mydriasis, in diagnostic procedures or
Refraction, cycloplegic—Indicated for mydriasis and cycloplegia in diagnostic procedures, such as measurement of refractive errors and examination of the fundus of the eye.

Mydriasis, preoperative or
Mydriasis, postoperative—Indicated when a short-acting mydriatic is needed for some preoperative and postoperative states.

## Pharmacology/Pharmacokinetics

**Physicochemical characteristics**
Molecular weight—284.36.

**Mechanism of action/Effect**
Tropicamide is an anticholinergic agent that blocks the responses of the sphincter muscle of the iris and the accommodative muscle of the ciliary body to stimulation by acetylcholine. The 0.5% solution produces dilation of the pupil (mydriasis); the 1% solution produces paralysis of accommodation (cycloplegia) as well as mydriasis.

**Onset of action**
Rapid.

**Time to peak effect**
Within 20 to 40 minutes.

**Duration of action**
Short—
    Cycloplegia (residual): 2 to 6 hours.
    Mydriasis (residual): Approximately 7 hours.

## Precautions to Consider

**Pregnancy/Reproduction**
Pregnancy—Studies have not been done in humans.
Studies have not been done in animals.

**Breast-feeding**
Problems in humans have not been documented.

**Pediatrics**
An increased susceptibility to tropicamide and similar drugs (such as atropine) has been reported in infants and young children and in children with blond hair, blue eyes, Down's syndrome, spastic paralysis, or brain damage; therefore, tropicamide should be used with great caution in these patients. In addition, this medication may cause psychotic reactions, behavioral disturbances, and cardiorespiratory collapse, especially in children.

**Geriatrics**
Geriatric patients are more susceptible to the effects of tropicamide and similar drugs (such as atropine), thus increasing the potential for systemic side effects. Also, tropicamide should be used with caution in the elderly because of possible undiagnosed predisposition to angle-closure glaucoma.

**Medical considerations/Contraindications**
The medical considerations/contraindications included here have been selected on the basis of their potential clinical significance (reasons given in parentheses where appropriate)—not necessarily inclusive (» = major clinical significance).

*Risk-benefit should be considered when the following medical problems exist:*
    Brain damage, in children
    Down's syndrome (mongolism), in children and adults
»   Glaucoma, angle-closure, predisposition to
    Sensitivity to tropicamide
    Spastic paralysis, in children

## Side/Adverse Effects
Note: An increased susceptibility to tropicamide and similar drugs (such as atropine) has been reported in infants, young children, children with blond hair or blue eyes, adults and children with Down's syndrome, children with brain damage or spastic paralysis, and the elderly. In addition, cardiorespiratory collapse has been reported in children and some adults.

The following side/adverse effects have been selected on the basis of their potential clinical significance (possible signs and symptoms in parentheses where appropriate)—not necessarily inclusive:

**Those indicating need for medical attention**
Signs of systemic absorption
   *Behavioral disturbances or psychotic reaction* (unusual behavior, especially in children); *clumsiness or unsteadiness; confusion; fast heartbeat; flushing or redness of face; hallucinations* (seeing, hearing, or feeling things that are not there); *increased thirst or dryness of mouth; skin rash; slurred speech; swollen stomach in infants; unusual drowsiness, tiredness, or weakness*

**Those indicating need for medical attention only if they continue or are bothersome**
   *Blurred vision; headache; increased sensitivity of eyes to light; stinging of eyes when medication is applied*

## Overdose

For specific information on the agents used in the management of tropicamide ophthalmic overdose, see:
• *Physostigmine (Systemic)* monograph.

For more information on the management of overdose or unintentional ingestion, **contact a Poison Control Center** (see *Poison Control Center Listing*).

**Treatment of overdose**
Specific treatment—Physostigmine is used as an antidote to the systemic effects of this medication.

## Patient Consultation

As an aid to patient consultation, refer to *Advice for the Patient, Tropicamide (Ophthalmic).*

In providing consultation, consider emphasizing the following selected information (» = major clinical significance):

**Before using this medication**
» Conditions affecting use, especially:
   Sensitivity to tropicamide
   Use in children—Infants and young children and children with blond hair or blue eyes may be especially sensitive to the effects of tropicamide and similar drugs (such as atropine); this may increase the chance of side effects during treatment; in addition, medication may be more likely to cause psychotic reactions, behavioral disturbances, and cardiorespiratory collapse in children
   Use in the elderly—Geriatric patients are more susceptible to the effects of tropicamide and similar drugs (such as atropine), thus increasing the potential for systemic side effects
   Other medical problems, especially predisposition to angle-closure glaucoma

**Proper use of this medication**
   Proper administration technique
» Importance of nasolacrimal pressure, especially in infants
   Washing hands immediately after application to remove any medicine that may be on them; if applying medication to infants or children, washing their hands also, and not letting any medication get into their mouths
   Preventing contamination: Not touching applicator tip to any surface; keeping container tightly closed
» Importance of not using more medication than the amount prescribed
» Proper dosing
   Missed dose: Applying as soon as possible; if almost time for next dose, skipping missed dose and going back to regular dosing schedule; not doubling doses
» Proper storage

**Precautions while using this medication**
» Medication causes blurred vision and increased sensitivity of the eyes to light; not driving until you can see clearly; wearing sunglasses that block ultraviolet light to protect eyes from sunlight and other bright lights; checking with physician if these effects continue longer than 24 hours after discontinuation of medication

**Side/adverse effects**
Signs of potential side effects, especially systemic absorption

## General Dosing Information

Although some manufacturers recommend a dose of 2 drops of an ophthalmic solution at appropriate intervals, the conjunctival sac will usually hold only 1 drop.

When used for refraction, an additional drop should be instilled if the examination cannot be performed within 20 to 30 minutes following instillation of the second drop of tropicamide solution.

More frequent instillation or use of a stronger solution may be required to produce adequate cycloplegia in eyes with brown or hazel irides than in eyes with blue irides.

To avoid excessive systemic absorption, patient should apply digital pressure to the lacrimal sac during and for 2 or 3 minutes following instillation of the medication.

## Ophthalmic Dosage Forms
### TROPICAMIDE OPHTHALMIC SOLUTION USP

**Usual adult and adolescent dose**
Cycloplegic refraction—
   Topical, to the conjunctiva, 1 drop of a 1% solution, repeated once in five minutes.
For examination of fundus of eye—
   Topical, to the conjunctiva, 1 drop of a 0.5% solution fifteen to twenty minutes prior to examination.

**Usual pediatric dose**
Cycloplegic refraction—
   Topical, to the conjunctiva, 1 drop of a 0.5 or 1% solution, repeated once in five minutes.
For examination of fundus of eye—
   See *Usual adult and adolescent dose.*

**Usual geriatric dose**
See *Usual adult and adolescent dose.*

**Strength(s) usually available**
U.S.—
   0.5% (Rx) [*Mydriacyl* (benzalkonium chloride; sodium chloride; edetate disodium; hydrochloric acid or sodium hydroxide); *Mydriafair;    Ocu-Tropic;    Opticyl;    Spectro-Cyl; Tropicacyl* (benzalkonium chloride 0.1%); GENERIC].
   1% (Rx) [*I-Picamide; Mydriacyl* (benzalkonium chloride); *Mydriafair; Ocu-Tropic; Opticyl; Spectro-Cyl; Tropicacyl* (benzalkonium chloride); GENERIC].
Canada—
   0.5% (Rx) [*Mydriacyl* (benzalkonium chloride); *Tropicacyl*].
   1% (Rx) [*Minims Tropicamide; Mydriacyl* (benzalkonium chloride); *Tropicacyl*].

**Packaging and storage**
Store below 40 °C (104 °F), preferably between 15 and 30 °C (59 and 86 °F), unless otherwise specified by manufacturer. Store in a tight container. Protect from freezing.

**Auxiliary labeling**
• For the eye.
• Keep container tightly closed.

Revised: 07/14/95

---

# TUBERCULIN, PURIFIED PROTEIN DERIVATIVE   Parenteral-Local

VA CLASSIFICATION (Primary): DX300
Note: For a listing of dosage forms and brand names by country availability, see *Dosage Forms* section(s). For a listing of brand names for the articles in this monograph, refer to the General Index.

## Category

Diagnostic aid (tuberculosis).

## Indications

**Accepted**
Tuberculosis (diagnosis)—Tuberculin, purified protein derivative (PPD) is indicated as a diagnostic aid in the detection of *Mycobacterium tuberculosis* infection. It is also indicated when BCG vaccination or isoniazid prophylaxis is being considered.

# Pharmacology/Pharmacokinetics

## Physicochemical characteristics
Tuberculin PPD is a sterile isotonic solution of tuberculin. It is obtained from a human strain of *Mycobacterium tuberculosis* grown on a protein-free synthetic medium and buffered with potassium and sodium phosphates

## Mechanism of action/Effect
Intradermally injected tuberculin PPD causes a delayed (cellular) hypersensitivity reaction in individuals sensitized by mycobacterial infection. Following infection with mycobacteria, sensitization of T-cells occurs primarily in the regional lymph nodes. Natural infection with *M. tuberculosis* usually initiates a cell-mediated immune response against mycobacterial antigens. T-cells proliferate in response to the infection and give rise to T-cells specifically sensitized to mycobacterial antigens. After several weeks, these T-lymphocytes enter the bloodstream and circulate for a long period of time. Subsequent restimulation of these T-lymphocytes with intradermal injection of tuberculin PPD evokes a local reaction mediated by these cells.

## Onset of action
5 to 6 hours after intradermal injection of tuberculin PPD. The reaction reaches its peak more than 24 (usually 48 to 72) hours after administration.

# Precautions to Consider

## Pregnancy/Reproduction
Fertility—Studies on effects of tuberculin PPD on fertility have not been done.

Pregnancy—Studies have not been done in humans. It is not known whether tuberculin PPD can cause harm to the fetus when administered to a pregnant woman. However, during pregnancy known positive reactors may demonstrate a negative response to the PPD tine test.
Studies have not been done in animals.
FDA Pregnancy Category C.

## Breast-feeding
It is not known whether tuberculin PPD is distributed into breast milk. However, problems in humans have not been documented.

## Pediatrics
Appropriate studies on the relationship of age to the effects of tuberculin PPD have not been performed in the pediatric population. However, no pediatrics-specific problems have been documented to date.

## Geriatrics
In geriatric patients, reactions may develop slowly and may not peak until after 72 hours.

## Drug interactions and/or related problems
The following drug interactions and/or related problems have been selected on the basis of their potential clinical significance (possible mechanism in parentheses where appropriate)—not necessarily inclusive (» = major clinical significance):

Note: Combinations containing any of the following medications, depending on the amount present, may also interact with this medication.

Bacillus Calmette-Guérin (BCG) vaccine
(individuals previously given BCG vaccine will usually show a positive reaction to tuberculin test administered within 6 to 12 weeks after BCG vaccination; a few years after BCG vaccination, reaction to tuberculin tests may be either positive or negative; a positive reaction to tuberculin PPD years after BCG vaccination suggests tuberculous infection)

Corticosteroids or
Immunosuppressive agents
(reactivity to the tuberculin test may be suppressed or enhanced in patients receiving these medications)

Vaccines, killed or live virus
(the reaction to tuberculin PPD may be suppressed if the test is given within 4 to 6 weeks following immunization with killed or live virus vaccines)

## Diagnostic interference
The following have been selected on the basis of their potential clinical significance (possible effect in parentheses where appropriate)—not necessarily inclusive (» = major clinical significance):

With results of this test
*Due to medical problems or conditions*
Acquired immunodeficiency syndrome (AIDS) or
Anergy or
Atopic dermatitis or sun-damaged skin or

Human immunodeficiency virus (HIV) infection or
Illness that affects the lymphoid system (Hodgkin's disease, lymphoma, chronic lymphocytic leukemia) or
Pregnancy or
Stress, severe
(may cause false-negative test results)

## Medical considerations/Contraindications
The medical considerations/contraindications included here have been selected on the basis of their potential clinical significance (reasons given in parentheses where appropriate)—not necessarily inclusive (» = major clinical significance):

*Except under special circumstances, this medication should not be used when the following medical problem exists:*

» Known positive tuberculin reaction
(in highly sensitive persons the reaction at the test site can be severe, resulting in vesiculation, ulceration, or necrosis)

# Side/Adverse Effects

The following side/adverse effects have been selected on the basis of their potential clinical significance (possible signs and symptoms in parentheses where appropriate)—not necessarily inclusive:

## Those indicating need for medical attention
Incidence rare
*Allergic reactions* (skin rash or itching); *necrosis, ulceration, or vesiculation at the site of injection* (redness, blistering, peeling, or loosening of the skin)

## Those indicating need for medical attention only if they continue or are bothersome
Incidence less frequent
*Erythematous reaction* (redness at the site of injection); *granuloma* (sores at and around the site of injection); *pain; pruritus* (itching)

Note: Discomfort and transient bleeding may be observed at the PPD tine puncture site.

# Patient Consultation

As an aid to patient consultation, refer to *Advice for the Patient, Tuberculin, Purified Protein Derivative (PPD) Injection.*

In providing consultation, consider emphasizing the following selected information (» = major clinical significance):

## Before using this medication
» Conditions affecting use, especially:
Sensitivity to tuberculin PPD
Other medical problems, especially known positive tuberculin reaction

## Side/adverse effects
» Signs of potential side effects, especially allergic reactions and necrosis, ulceration, or vesiculation at the site of injection

# General Dosing Information

Anergy to tuberculin among asymptomatic HIV-positive persons is common, making interpretation of tuberculin tests difficult. Therefore, the Centers for Disease Control (CDC) has produced guidelines for assessing delayed-type hypersensitivity in these patients. Concurrent administration of at least 2 other skin test antigens is recommended. The CDC suggests choosing from among mumps skin test antigen, candida antigen, and tetanus toxoid. The test antigens are given concurrently with the tuberculin skin test and the response is measured 48 to 72 hours later. Any amount of induration is considered evidence of delayed-type hypersensitivity; failure to elicit a response is considered evidence of anergy. HIV-positive persons and others at risk of anergy are considered to have a significant reaction to a standard Mantoux test if the induration reaction measures 5 mm or more in diameter, regardless of the reaction to the other antigens. It is very important to perform anergy testing in a population at increased risk of tuberculosis.

Booster effect—The ability of persons who have TB infection to react to tuberculin may gradually wane. For example, if tested with tuberculin, adults who were infected during their childhood may have a negative reaction. However, the tuberculin could boost the hypersensitivity, and the size of the reaction could be larger on a subsequent test. This boosted reaction may be misinterpreted as a tuberculin test conversion from a newly acquired infection. Misinterpretation of a boosted reaction as a new infection could result in unnecessary investigations of laboratory and patient records in an attempt to identify the source of infection and in unnecessary prescription of preventive therapy for health care workers. Although this booster effect can occur among persons in any age group, the likelihood of the effect increases with the age of the person being tested.

Two-step testing—When tuberculin testing of an adult is to be repeated periodically, 2-step testing can be used to reduce the likelihood that a boosted reaction will be misinterpreted as a new infection. Two-step testing should be performed on all newly employed health care workers who have an initial negative tuberculin test at the time of employment and have not had a documented negative tuberculin test result during the 12 months preceding the initial test. A second test should be performed 1 to 3 weeks after the first test. If the second test result is positive, this is most likely a boosted reaction, and the patient should be classified as previously infected. If the second test result is negative, the patient is classified as uninfected, and a positive reaction to a subsequent test is likely to represent a new infection with *M. tuberculosis*.

It is recommended that children at high risk for tuberculosis be given tuberculin skin tests annually by the Mantoux method. Children considered at high risk include those from areas with a high prevalence of the disease; those from households with 1 or more cases of tuberculosis; black, Hispanic, Asian, native American, and native Alaskan children, and others who are socioeconomically deprived; children from Asia, Africa, the Middle East, Latin America, or the Caribbean and children of parents who have immigrated from these areas; and children with medical risk factors for tuberculosis.

It is recommended that individuals with signs and/or symptoms suggestive of current tuberculous disease be given tuberculin skin test routinely by the Mantoux method. These individuals include persons who are recent contacts of known cases of clinical tuberculosis or are suspected of having tuberculosis; persons with abnormal chest radiographs compatible with past tuberculosis; persons with medical conditions that increase the risk of tuberculosis; HIV-infected individuals; immigrants from Asia, Africa, Latin America, and Oceania; inner-city and skid row populations.

Tuberculin PPD is administered by intradermal injection (the Mantoux method) or by using a disposable multiple-puncture device. These 2 commonly used test methods are briefly described below.

*The Mantoux test method:* The test is performed by intradermally injecting exactly 0.1 mL of diluted tuberculin PPD. The result is read 48 to 72 hours later and only induration is considered in interpreting the test. Induration is a hard, raised area with clearly defined margins at, and around, the injection site. Erythema may develop at the injection site but has no diagnostic value. The test is performed as follows:
• The site of the test is usually the flexor surface of the forearm, about 4 inches below the elbow. Other skin sites may be used, but the flexor surface of the forearm is preferred. The site of the test should be free of lesions and away from the veins.
• The skin at the injection site is cleansed with 70% alcohol or another suitable antiseptic agent and allowed to dry.
• The test material is administered with a tuberculin syringe (0.5 or 1.0 mL) fitted with a short (one-half-inch) 26- or 27- gauge needle.
• The syringe and needle should be a sterile, disposable, single-use type or should have been sterilized by autoclaving, boiling, or the use of dry heat. A separate sterile unit should be used for each person tested.
• The diaphragm of the vial-stopper should be wiped with 70% alcohol.
• The needle is inserted through the stopper diaphragm of the inverted vial. Exactly 0.1 mL is added to the syringe, with care being taken to exclude air bubbles and to keep the lumen of the needle filled.
• The point of the needle is inserted into the most superficial layers of the skin with the needle bevel pointed upward. As the tuberculin solution is injected, a pale bleb 6 to 10 mm in size will rise over the point of the needle. This is quickly absorbed, and no dressing is required. In the event that the injection is delivered subcutaneously (in this case no bleb will form) or if a significant part of the dose leaks from the injection site, the test should be repeated immediately at another site at least 5 cm (2 inches) removed from the first site.
• The test site should be examined by trained personnel 48 to 72 hours after the injection. The examination should be performed in good light with the arm slightly flexed at the elbow. The reaction should be measured and recorded in millimeters. Any induration reaction that measures 5 mm or more in diameter is considered positive in persons who have had recent close contact with tuberculosis; persons who have chest radiographs consistent with tuberculosis (including stable lesions consistent with "inactive" tuberculosis); immunosuppressed persons (including HIV-infected persons and patients on immunosuppressive therapy); and persons with cancer (including leukemia or lymphoma), Hodgkin's disease, or end-stage renal disease. Induration of 10 mm or more is considered a positive reaction in foreign-born persons; substance abusers (alcoholics and intravenous drug users); residents and employees of correctional institutions and nursing homes; hospital employees; persons over age 70; low-income populations, including the homeless; and persons with medical conditions including diabetes mel-

litus, post gastrectomy, silicosis, prolonged corticosteroid therapy, and 10% or more below ideal body weight. Induration of 15 mm or more is considered a positive reaction in all other persons (general population with no known tuberculosis risk factors).

*The multiple-puncture (Tine) test method:* Each test unit provides for the intradermal administration of 1 test-dose of tuberculin PPD. The test is performed as follows:
• The preferred site of the test is the flexor surface of the forearm about 4 inches below the elbow. Other suitable skin sites, such as the dorsal surface of the forearm, may be used. Areas without adequate subcutaneous tissue, such as skin over a tendon, as well as hairy areas, should be avoided.
• The skin at the test site should be cleaned with 70% alcohol or another suitable antiseptic agent such as acetone, ether, or soap and water and allowed to dry thoroughly.
• To expose the 4 impregnated tines, remove the protective cap while holding the plastic handle.
• The patient's forearm should be grasped firmly to stretch the skin taut at the test site and to prevent any jerking motion of the arm that could cause scratching with the tines.
• The test unit should be applied firmly without twisting to the test area for approximately 1 second. Sufficient pressure should be exerted to ensure that all 4 tines have penetrated the skin.
• Used units should be disposed of carefully to avoid accidents. Do not reuse.
• The test site should be examined by trained personnel 48 to 72 hours after application of the test. The examination should be performed in good light with the arm slightly flexed at the elbow. The presence of vesiculation indicates a positive reaction to the test. The test reaction is negative if both induration and vesiculation are absent. Induration reactions less than 2 mm in diameter may be considered negative. However, unless vesiculation is present, individuals with any size induration reaction should be retested using a standard Mantoux test.
The dose of tuberculin PPD introduced into the skin with currently available multiple-puncture devices cannot be precisely controlled. Therefore, this test should not be used for the periodic surveillance of individuals likely to be exposed to clinical tuberculosis or for the evaluation of individuals who are suspected of having tuberculosis or are contacts of persons with clinical tuberculosis.

*The Heaf test method:* The test is performed using the Heaf multiple-puncture apparatus. The result is read 3 to 10 days later and only induration is considered in interpreting the test.
• The site of the test is usually the volar surface of the left forearm. The skin at the test site is cleansed with alcohol or another suitable antiseptic agent and allowed to dry. The undiluted tuberculin is transferred using a syringe needle or loop and smoothed over a circular area of about 1 cm in diameter.
• The needle points of the apparatus are placed on the forearm to give a puncture of 1 mm (for children under 2 years of age) or 2 mm (for older children and adults).
• With the apparatus held at a right angle to the skin, the end plate is placed firmly and evenly in the center of the film of tuberculin and the handle pressed to release the needles. No dressing need be applied. It is very important that the apparatus be properly sterilized after each application or that a disposable end plate be used.
• A positive result should be recorded only when there is palpable induration around at least 4 puncture points. The induration is best felt by passing the finger lightly over the punctures. If no resistance is felt, a negative result should be recorded.
• Four grades of positive response are recognized:
    Grade 1—At least 4 small indurated papules.
    Grade 2—An indurated ring formed by confluent papules.
    Grade 3—A solid induration 5 to 10 mm wide.
    Grade 4—Induration over 10 mm wide.

### For treatment of adverse effects

Recommended treatment consists of the following:
• If strongly positive reactions, including vesiculation, ulceration, or necrosis, occur, cold packs or topical steroid preparations may be used for symptomatic relief of the associated pain, pruritus, and discomfort.

## Parenteral Dosage Forms

### TUBERCULIN (Purified Protein Derivative [PPD] Injection) USP

#### Usual adult and adolescent dose
Tuberculosis (diagnosis)—
    Intradermal, 5 U.S. units (tuberculin units [TU]).

Note: The 1-TU-per-test-dose preparation is used for individuals suspected of being highly sensitized, since larger initial doses may result in severe skin reactions. The preparation containing 250 TU per test dose should be used exclusively for the testing of individuals who fail to react to a previous injection of 5 TU; under no circumstances is it to be used for the initial injection.

**Usual pediatric dose**
See *Usual adult and adolescent dose.*

**Strength(s) usually available**
U.S.—
1 U.S. unit (TU) per test dose (0.1 mL) (Rx) [*Tubersol*].
5 U.S. units (TU) per test dose (0.1 mL) (Rx) [*Aplisol; Tubersol*].
250 U.S. units (TU) per test dose (0.1 mL) (Rx) [*Tubersol*].
Canada—
1 U.S. unit (TU) per test dose (0.1 mL) (Rx) [*Tubersol*].
5 U.S. units (TU) per test dose (0.1 mL) (Rx) [*Tubersol*].
250 U.S. units (TU) per test dose (0.1 mL) (Rx) [*Tubersol*].

**Packaging and storage**
Store between 2 and 8 °C (36 and 46 °F). Protect from light.

**Additional information**
Vials of tuberculin PPD that have been opened should be discarded after 1 month of use, since oxidation and degradation may have reduced the potency.

## TUBERCULIN (Purified Protein Derivative [PPD] Multiple-Puncture Device) USP

**Usual adult and adolescent dose**
Tuberculosis (diagnosis)—
Intradermal, equivalent to or more potent than 5 U.S. units (tuberculin units [TU]).

**Usual pediatric dose**
See *Usual adult and adolescent dose.*

**Strength(s) usually available**
U.S.—
Equivalent to or more potent than 5 U.S. units in individually capped test units (Rx) [*Aplitest; Tuberculin PPD TINE TEST*].
Canada—
Not commercially available.

**Packaging and storage**
Store below 30 °C (86 °F). Do not refrigerate.

## Selected Bibliography

Menzies R, Vissandjee B, Rocher I, Germain YS. The booster effect in two-step tuberculin testing among young adults in Montreal. Ann Intern Med 1994; 120 (3): 190-8.

Developed: 08/01/95

## TUBOCURARINE—See *Neuromuscular Blocking Agents (Systemic)*

---

# TYPHOID VACCINE INACTIVATED    Parenteral-Systemic

VA CLASSIFICATION (Primary): IM100

Note: This monograph is specific to the typhoid vaccine prepared with the *Salmonella typhi* Ty2 strain.

Another commonly used name is typhoid vaccine.

Note: For a listing of dosage forms and brand names by country availability, see *Dosage Forms* section(s). For a listing of brand names for the articles in this monograph, refer to the General Index.

## Category
Immunizing agent (active).

## Indications

**Accepted**
*Salmonella typhi* (prophylaxis)—Typhoid vaccine is indicated for immunization of adults and children 6 months of age and older against disease caused by *S. typhi*.

Routine typhoid vaccination is no longer recommended in the U.S. However, selective vaccination is indicated for the following groups:
• Travelers to areas in which there is recognized risk of exposure to *S. typhi*. Risk is greatest for travelers to developing countries (e.g., countries in Latin America, Asia, and Africa) who have prolonged exposure to potentially contaminated food and drink. Multidrug-resistant strains of *S. typhi* have become common in some areas of the world (e.g., the Indian subcontinent and the Arabian peninsula), and cases of typhoid fever that are treated with ineffective drugs can be fatal. Travelers should be cautioned that typhoid vaccination is not a substitute for careful selection of food and drink. Typhoid vaccines are not 100% effective, and the vaccine's protection can be overwhelmed by large inocula of *S. typhi*.
• Persons with intimate exposure (e.g., household contact) to a documented *S. typhi* carrier.
• Workers in microbiology laboratories who frequently work with *S. typhi*.
Routine vaccination of sewage sanitation workers is warranted only in areas with endemic typhoid fever. There is no evidence that typhoid vaccine is useful in controlling common-source outbreaks.

**Unaccepted**
The use of typhoid vaccine is not indicated for persons attending rural summer camps or living in areas in which natural disasters, such as floods, have occurred.

## Pharmacology/Pharmacokinetics

**Physicochemical characteristics**
Source—Typhoid vaccine inactivated (Parenteral-Systemic) is an inactivated vaccine for parenteral administration. The vaccine contains *Salmonella typhi* Ty2 strain. The vaccine strain is grown in veal infusion agar containing 0.5% sodium chloride, 2% peptone, and 5% agar. The bacteria are washed from the medium, suspended in buffered sodium chloride injection, and killed either by a combination of phenol and heat (commercially available in the U.S. for civilian use), or by acetone (provided by the U.S. Government for military use only)

**Mechanism of action/Effect**
Primary immunization with typhoid vaccine for parenteral use stimulates the production of agglutinins and serum bactericidal antibodies to several antigen groups of *S. typhi*. These agglutinins and antibodies eliminate the typhoid bacilli from the blood. However, even in the presence of circulating antibodies, intracellular bacteria inaccessible to these antibodies may multiply and produce endotoxins. The exact mechanism of action of the antibodies to *S. typhi* antigens is not known.

**Other actions/effects**
Typhoid vaccine for parenteral use may confer some immunity to *S. paratyphi* A, which shares a common O antigen factor 12 with *S. typhi*. Some cross protection may occur.

**Protective effect**
Typhoid vaccine induces protective antibodies in 70 to 90% of recipients. In field trials, the acetone inactivated typhoid vaccine has been shown to be more immunogenic (efficacy ranging from 66 to 94%) than the phenol-heat inactivated typhoid vaccine (efficacy ranging from 51 to 77%). However, the degree of protection depends in part on the degree of subsequent exposure to *S. typhi*.

**Time to protective effect**
Protective antibodies develop within 1 to 2 weeks after the second dose.

**Duration of protective effect**
Immunity against typhoid fever lasts more than 2 years. A booster dose is recommended every 3 years if there is continuing or repeated risk of exposure to *S. typhi*.

## Precautions to Consider

**Pregnancy/Reproduction**
Fertility—Studies of the effects of parenteral typhoid vaccine on fertility have not been done.

Pregnancy—Studies have not been done in humans.
Studies have not been done in animals.

**Breast-feeding**
Problems in humans have not been documented.

**Pediatrics**
Infants up to 6 months of age—Use is not recommended.
Infants and children 6 months of age and older—Pediatrics-specific problems that would limit the usefulness of this vaccine in children in this age group are not expected.

**Geriatrics**
Appropriate studies on the relationship of age to the effects of parenteral typhoid vaccine have not been performed in the geriatric population. However, no geriatrics-specific problems have been documented to date.

**Drug interactions and/or related problems**
The following drug interactions and/or related problems have been selected on the basis of their potential clinical significance (possible mechanism in parentheses where appropriate)—not necessarily inclusive (» = major clinical significance):
Cholera vaccine or
Plague vaccine
    (concurrent use of parenteral typhoid vaccine may increase the risk of local and systemic adverse effects)

**Medical considerations/Contraindications**
The medical considerations/contraindications included here have been selected on the basis of their potential clinical significance (reasons given in parentheses where appropriate)—not necessarily inclusive (» = major clinical significance).

*Except under special circumstances, this medication should not be used when the following medical problems exist:*

» Febrile illness, acute
    (administration of parenteral typhoid vaccine should be postponed to avoid confusing manifestations of acute febrile illness with possible side/adverse effects of the vaccine; however, presence of minor illnesses, such as upper respiratory infections, with or without low grade fever or mild diarrhea, does not preclude administration of vaccine)

» Previous sensitivity reaction to parenteral typhoid vaccine
    (parenteral typhoid vaccine is contraindicated in patients with a history of a severe systemic or allergic reaction to a previous administration of parenteral typhoid vaccine)

## Side/Adverse Effects

Note: Most recipients of typhoid vaccine experience some degree of local and systemic response, usually beginning within 24 hours after administration and persisting for 1 or 2 days.

The following side/adverse effects have been selected on the basis of their potential clinical significance (possible signs and symptoms in parentheses where appropriate)—not necessarily inclusive:

**Those indicating need for medical attention**
Rare
    *Anaphylactic reaction* (difficulty in breathing or swallowing; hives; itching, especially of soles or palms; reddening of skin, especially around ears; swelling of eyes, face, or inside of nose; unusual tiredness or weakness, sudden and severe); *chest pain; joint pain; liver damage; neurological problems*

**Those indicating need for medical attention only if they continue or are bothersome**
Incidence more frequent
    *Fever; headache; malaise* (general feeling of discomfort or illness); *muscle pain; pain, redness, or swelling at injection site*

## Patient Consultation

As an aid to patient consultation, refer to *Advice for the Patient, Typhoid Vaccine Inactivated (Parenteral-Systemic)*.

In providing consultation, consider emphasizing the following selected information (» = major clinical significance):

**Before receiving this vaccine**
» Conditions affecting use, especially:
    Sensitivity to typhoid vaccine
    Use in children—Use is not recommended in infants and children up to 6 months of age
    Other medical problems, especially acute febrile illness

**Proper use of this vaccine**
    Receiving all doses of the vaccine exactly as directed for maximal protective immune response
» Proper dosing

**Side/adverse effects**
    Signs of potential side effects, especially anaphylactic reaction, chest pain, joint pain, liver damage, and neurological problems

## General Dosing Information

Appropriate precautions should be taken prior to vaccine injection to prevent allergic or any other unwanted reactions. This should include a review of the patient's history regarding possible sensitivity and the ready availability of epinephrine 1:1000 and other appropriate agents used for control of immediate allergic reactions.

The acetone inactivated dried typhoid vaccine is supplied with diluent. Only the diluent supplied by the manufacturer should be used for this product.

Phenol and heat inactivated parenteral typhoid vaccine is administered for primary immunization by subcutaneous injection and for booster doses by subcutaneous or intradermal injection. Acetone inactivated parenteral typhoid vaccine is administered by subcutaneous or intramuscular injection for both primary immunization and booster doses and should not be administered intradermally. Neither vaccine should be administered intravenously.

Primary immunization with parenteral typhoid vaccine consists of 2 doses administered at an interval of 4 or more weeks. In instances where there is insufficient time for 2 doses administered at the specified intervals, 3 doses of the appropriate volume may be given at weekly intervals.

Even if the complete immunization schedule is followed, not all recipients of the vaccine will be fully protected against typhoid fever. Travelers should take all necessary precautions to avoid contact with, or ingestion of, potentially contaminated food or water.

Under conditions of continued or repeated exposure, a booster dose should be given at least every 3 years. In instances where an interval of more than 3 years has elapsed since primary immunization or the last booster dose, a single booster dose is considered sufficient; it is not necessary to repeat the primary immunization series.

## Parenteral Dosage Forms

### TYPHOID VACCINE (ACETONE INACTIVATED, DRIED) USP

**Usual adult and adolescent dose**
Immunizing agent (active)—
    Initial immunization: Subcutaneous or intramuscular, two doses of 0.5 mL of the reconstituted vaccine at an interval of four or more weeks.
    Booster dose: Subcutaneous or intramuscular, a single dose of 0.5 mL of the reconstituted vaccine every three years.

**Usual pediatric dose**
Immunizing agent (active)—
    Infants and children up to 6 months of age:
        Use is not recommended.
    Children 6 months through 9 years of age:
        Initial immunization—Subcutaneous or intramuscular, two doses of 0.25 mL of the reconstituted vaccine at an interval of four or more weeks.
        Booster dose—Subcutaneous or intramuscular, a single dose of 0.25 mL of the reconstituted vaccine every three years.
    Children 10 years of age and older:
        See *Usual adult and adolescent dose.*

**Strength(s) usually available**
U.S.—
    Contains no more than $10^9$ killed *Salmonella typhosa* (Ty2 strain) organisms per mL after reconstitution (Rx) [GENERIC].
Canada—
    Not commercially available.
Note: Each mL of the reconstituted vaccine is equivalent to 8 units.

**Packaging and storage**
Store between 2 and 8 °C (36 and 46 °F), unless otherwise specified by manufacturer.

**Preparation of dosage form**
Typhoid Vaccine USP (Acetone Inactivated, Dried) is reconstituted for subcutaneous or intramuscular use by adding 20 mL of the diluent provided by the manufacturer to the vial containing the dried vaccine.

**Stability**
Reconstituted solutions stored between 2 and 8 °C (36 and 46 °F) are stable for 30 days. Any vaccine not used within 30 days of reconstitution should be discarded.

## TYPHOID VACCINE (HEAT AND PHENOL INACTIVATED) USP

### Usual adult and adolescent dose

Immunizing agent (active)—

U.S.:

Initial immunization—Subcutaneous, two doses of 0.5 mL at an interval of four or more weeks.

Booster dose—Subcutaneous, a single dose of 0.5 mL, or intradermal, a single dose of 0.1 mL. The booster dose may be repeated every three years.

Canada:

Initial immunization—Subcutaneous, first dose 0.25 mL; second dose, 0.5 mL about three to four weeks after first dose; third dose, 1 mL about three to six months after second dose.

Booster dose—Subcutaneous, a single dose of 0.5 mL. The booster dose may be repeated every three years.

### Usual pediatric dose

Immunizing agent (active)—

U.S.:

Infants and children up to 6 months of age—
Use is not recommended.

Children 6 months through 9 years of age—
Initial immunization: Subcutaneous, two doses of 0.25 mL at an interval of four or more weeks.

Booster dose: Intradermal, a single dose of 0.25 mL, or intradermal, a single dose of 0.1 mL. The booster dose may be repeated every three years.

Children 10 years of age and older—
See *Usual adult and adolescent dose.*

Canada:

Children under 10 years of age—
Half the *Usual adult and adolescent dose.*

Children 10 years of age and older—
See *Usual adult and adolescent dose.*

### Strength(s) usually available

U.S.—

Contains no more than $10^9$ killed *Salmonella typhosa* (Ty2 strain) organisms per mL (Rx) [GENERIC (may contain phenol)].

Canada—

Contains no more than $10^9$ killed *Salmonella typhosa* (Ty2 strain) organisms per mL (Rx) [GENERIC].

Note: Each mL of the reconstituted vaccine is equivalent to 8 units.

### Packaging and storage

Store between 2 and 8 °C (36 and 46 °F), unless otherwise specified by manufacturer.

### Auxiliary labeling

• Shake well before withdrawing each dose.

### Selected Bibliography

Woodruf BA, Pavia AT, Blake PA. A new look at typhoid vaccination. Information for the practicing physician. JAMA 1991; 265 (6): 756-9.

Centers for Disease Control. Typhoid immunization. Recommendations of the Advisory Committee on Immunization Practices (ACIP). MMWR 1994; 43 (RR-14): 1-7.

Developed: 07/20/95

---

# TYPHOID VACCINE LIVE ORAL   Systemic†

**VA CLASSIFICATION (Primary): IM100**

Note: This monograph is specific for the typhoid vaccine prepared with the *Salmonella typhi* Ty21a strain.

Note: For a listing of dosage forms and brand names by country availability, see *Dosage Forms* section(s). For a listing of brand names for the articles in this monograph, refer to the General Index.

†Not commercially available in Canada.

## Category

Immunizing agent (active).

## Indications

### Accepted

*Salmonella typhi* (prophylaxis)—Typhoid vaccine is indicated for immunization of adults and children 6 years of age and older against disease caused by *Salmonella typhi*.

Routine typhoid vaccination is no longer recommended in the U.S. However, selective vaccination is indicated for the following groups:
• Travelers to areas that have a recognized risk of exposure to *S. typhi*. Risk is greatest for travelers to developing countries (especially countries in Latin America, Asia, and Africa) who have prolonged exposure to potentially contaminated food and drink. Such travelers should be cautioned that typhoid vaccine is not a substitute for careful selection of food and drink, since the vaccine is not 100% effective and the protection it offers can be overwhelmed by large inocula of *S. typhi*.
• Persons with intimate exposure, such as continued household contact, to a documented typhoid fever carrier.
• Workers in microbiology laboratories who frequently work with *S. typhi*.

An optimal booster dose has not yet been established. However, it is recommended that a booster dose consisting of 4 vaccine capsules taken on alternate days be given every 5 years if there is repeated or continued exposure to typhoid fever.

Routine vaccination of sewage sanitation workers is warranted only in areas with endemic typhoid fever. There is no evidence that typhoid vaccine is useful in controlling common-source outbreaks. Also, the use of typhoid vaccine is not indicated for persons attending rural summer camps or in areas in which natural disasters, such as floods, have occurred.

## Pharmacology/Pharmacokinetics

### Physicochemical characteristics

Source—Typhoid vaccine Ty21a is a live attenuated vaccine for oral administration. The vaccine contains the attenuated strain *Salmonella typhi* Ty21a. The vaccine strain is grown under controlled conditions in a medium containing dextrose, galactose, a digest of bovine tissues, and an acid digest of casein. The bacteria are collected by centrifugation, mixed with a stabilizer containing lactose and amino acids, and then lyophilized. The lyophilized bacteria mixture is placed in gelatin capsules, which are coated with an organic solution to render them resistant to dissolution by stomach acids

### Mechanism of action/Effect

The precise mechanism by which typhoid vaccine Ty21a confers protection against typhoid fever is unknown. However, it is known that immunization of adult subjects can elicit a humoral anti–*S. typhi* lipopolysaccharide (LPS) antibody response.

This vaccine will not afford protection against species of *Salmonella*, other than *Salmonella typhi*, or against other bacteria that cause enteric disease.

The ability of *S. typhi* to cause disease and induce a protective immune response is dependent upon the bacteria possessing a complete LPS. The *S. typhi* Ty21a vaccine strain, because of a reduction in enzymes essential for LPS biosynthesis, is restricted in its ability to produce complete LPS. However, enough complete LPS is synthesized to induce a protective immune response. Despite the low levels of LPS synthesis, the cells lyse before regaining a virulent phenotype. This occurs because of the intracellular build-up of toxic metabolic intermediates during LPS synthesis.

### Protective effect

Vaccine efficacy is approximately 65% and is similar to the efficacy of the heat-phenol-inactivated injectable typhoid vaccine, which is 51 to 77%.

### Time to protective effect

Immunization (ingestion of all 4 doses of the vaccine) should be completed at least 1 week prior to potential exposure to *S. typhi*.

### Duration of protective effect

Follow-up studies of vaccine trial subjects showed continued efficacy 5 to 7 years after immunization.

### Elimination

At the recommended dosage, the *S. typhi* Ty21a vaccine strain is not excreted in the feces. However, clinical studies in volunteers have shown that overdosing can increase the possibility of shedding the *S. typhi* Ty21a vaccine strain in the feces.

# Precautions to Consider

### Carcinogenicity/Mutagenicity
Long-term studies in animals have not been performed to evaluate the carcinogenic or mutagenic potential of this vaccine.

### Pregnancy/Reproduction
Fertility—Studies have not been done in humans or animals.

Pregnancy—It is recommended that the vaccine be administered during pregnancy only if clearly needed.

Studies have not been done in humans or animals.

FDA Pregnancy Category C.

### Breast-feeding
It is not known whether typhoid vaccine is excreted in breast milk. However, problems in humans have not been documented.

### Pediatrics
Appropriate studies on the relationship of age to the effects of the vaccine have not been performed in infants and children up to 6 years of age. Safety and efficacy have not been established and use is not recommended.

### Geriatrics
Appropriate studies on the relationship of age to the effects of typhoid vaccine have not been performed in the geriatric population. However, no geriatrics-specific problems have been documented to date.

### Drug interactions and/or related problems
The following drug interactions and/or related problems have been selected on the basis of their potential clinical significance (possible mechanism in parentheses where appropriate)—not necessarily inclusive (» = major clinical significance):

Note: Combinations containing any of the following medications, depending on the amount present, may also interact with this medication.

» Antibacterials, systemic, or
» Antimalarials
   (concurrent use of systemic antibacterials or antimalarials with typhoid vaccine may prevent the vaccine bacteria from multiplying sufficiently to induce a protective immune response; antimalarials should be administered 24 hours prior to administration of the typhoid vaccine)

» Immunosuppressive agents or
» Radiation therapy
   (because normal defense mechanisms are suppressed, concurrent use with live oral typhoid vaccine may potentiate the replication of the vaccine bacteria, may increase the side/adverse effects of the vaccine, and/or may decrease the patient's antibody response to the vaccine. The precaution does not apply to corticosteroids used as replacement therapy, for short-term [less than 2 weeks] systemic therapy, or by other routes of administration that do not cause immunosuppression)

   Live vaccines, other
   (when live virus vaccines are administered on different days within 1 month of each other, the chance exists that the immune response may be impaired; therefore, live virus vaccines not administered on the same day should be given at least 1 month apart; there is no consensus among USP medical experts that the same would apply to live bacterial vaccines)

### Medical considerations/Contraindications
The medical considerations/contraindications included here have been selected on the basis of their potential clinical significance (reasons given in parentheses where appropriate)—not necessarily inclusive (» = major clinical significance).

*Except under special circumstances, this medication should not be used when the following medical problems exist:*

» Diarrhea, persistent, or
» Febrile illness, acute, or
» Gastrointestinal illness, acute, or
» Vomiting, persistent
   (administration of live oral typhoid vaccine should be postponed or avoided, since acute illnesses may interfere with the replication of typhoid vaccine bacteria and therefore with final immunity; minor illnesses, such as mild upper respiratory infections, do not preclude administration of vaccine)

» Immune deficiency conditions, congential or hereditary, or
» Immune deficiency conditions, primary or acquired
   (because of reduced or suppressed defense mechanisms, the use of live oral typhoid vaccine may potentiate the replication of the vaccine bacteria, may increase the side/adverse effects of the vaccine, and/or may decrease the patient's antibody response to the vaccine)

(persons infected with human immunodeficiency virus [HIV], whether asymptomatic or symptomatic, should not receive live oral typhoid vaccine)

*Risk-benefit should be considered when the following medical problems exist:*

   Sensitivity to live oral typhoid vaccine, sucrose, lactose, or beef; however, a history of a severe reaction to the parenteral typhoid vaccine is not a precaution for receiving the live oral vaccine

# Side/Adverse Effects

The following side/adverse effects have been selected on the basis of their potential clinical significance (possible signs and symptoms in parentheses where appropriate)—not necessarily inclusive:

### Those indicating need for medical attention
Incidence rare
   *Anaphylactic reaction* (difficulty in breathing or swallowing; hives; itching, especially of soles or palms; reddening of skin, especially around ears; swelling of eyes, face, or inside of nose; sudden and severe unusual tiredness or weakness)

### Those indicating need for medical attention only if they continue or are bothersome
Incidence less frequent or rare
   *Abdominal discomfort or cramps* (stomach cramps or pain); *diarrhea; fever; nausea; skin rash; urticaria* (hives); *vomiting*

# Patient Consultation

As an aid to patient consultation, refer to *Advice for the Patient, Typhoid Vaccine Live Oral (Systemic).*

In providing consultation, consider emphasizing the following selected information (» = major clinical significance):

### Before using this medication
» Conditions affecting use, especially:
      Sensitivity to oral typhoid vaccine, sucrose, lactose, or beef
      Use in children—Safety and efficacy have not been established for infants and children up to 6 years of age; use is not recommended
      Other medications, especially antibacterials, antimalarials, immunosuppressive agents, or radiation therapy
      Other medical problems, especially persistent diarrhea, acute gastrointestinal illness, persistent vomiting, acute febrile illness, primary or acquired immune deficiency conditions, or congenital or hereditary immune deficiency conditions

### Proper use of this medication
» Taking all 4 doses of vaccine exactly as directed for maximal protective immune response
   Replacing any broken or cracked capsules
   Leaving vaccine at room temperature will cause it to lose its effectiveness
   Taking dose approximately 1 hour before a meal; taking with a cold or lukewarm drink (temperature not to exceed body temperature, e.g., 37 °C [98.6 °F])
   Swallowing capsule whole and as soon as possible after placing in mouth; not chewing capsule
» Missed dose: If remembered on the day it should be taken, taking as directed; however, if not remembered until the next day, taking the missed dose at that time and rescheduling your every-other-day doses from then; it is essential that vaccine be taken exactly as directed to get the most protection against typhoid fever
» Proper storage: Keeping vaccine refrigerated at all times; replacing unused vaccine in the refrigerator between doses

### Precautions while using this medication
   Checking with physician before receiving:
   Any other live vaccine within 1 month of this vaccine

### Side/adverse effects
   Signs of potential side effects, especially anaphylactic reaction

# General Dosing Information

Immunization (ingestion of all 4 doses of the vaccine) should be completed at least 1 week prior to potential exposure to *S. typhi.*

Since this is an enteric dosage form, the vaccine capsules should be inspected to ensure that the foil seal and capsules are intact; any that are damaged should be replaced.

Each enteric-coated capsule should be swallowed with a cold or lukewarm drink (temperature not to exceed 37 °C [98.6 °F], i.e., body temperature), approximately 1 hour before a meal on alternate days (days 1, 3, 5, and 7) for a total of 4 doses.

The vaccine capsule should not be chewed and should be swallowed as soon as possible after it is placed in the mouth.

A complete immunization schedule is the ingestion of 4 vaccine capsules, as directed. Unless this schedule is followed, an optimal immune response may not be achieved.

Even if the complete immunization schedule is followed, not all recipients of the vaccine will be fully protected against typhoid fever. Travelers should take all necessary precautions to avoid contact with, or ingestion of, potentially contaminated food or water.

The optimal booster schedule for the live oral typhoid vaccine has not been determined. However, efficacy has been shown to persist for 5 to 7 years after administration of a complete primary immunization. Therefore, it is recommended that a booster dose of 4 vaccine capsules taken on alternate days be given every 5 years if repeated or continued exposure to *S. typhi* occurs.

There is no experience with the use of the live oral typhoid vaccine as a booster in persons previously immunized with parenteral typhoid vaccine. However, if repeated or continued exposure to *S. typhi* occurs, booster doses of the parenteral vaccine are recommended every 3 years to maintain immunity after vaccination with parenteral typhoid vaccine. Even if more than 3 years have elapsed since the prior parenteral vaccination, a single booster dose of the parenteral vaccine is sufficient. Therefore, it appears that using the primary series of 4 doses of live oral typhoid vaccine as a booster for persons previously vaccinated with the parenteral vaccine is a reasonable alternative to administration of a parenteral booster.

**For treatment of adverse effects**
Recommended treatment consists of the following
  *For adults*
  • If anaphylaxis occurs, 0.2 to 0.5 mg of epinephrine (base) may be administered intramuscularly or subcutaneously, the dose being repeated every 10 to 15 minutes as needed. The dosage may be increased up to a maximum of 1 mg per dose, if necessary.
  • If anaphylactic shock occurs:
    —0.5 mg of epinephrine (base) may be administered initially intramuscularly or subcutaneously, the dose being repeated every 5 minutes if necessary. If there is an inadequate response to the intramuscular or subcutaneous dose, 0.025 to 0.05 mg of epinephrine (base) may be administered intravenously every 5 to 15 minutes as needed.
    —Alternatively, 0.1 to 0.25 mg of epinephrine (base) may be administered slowly by intravenous injection. The dose may be repeated every 5 to 15 minutes as needed or followed by an intravenous infusion at an initial rate of 0.001 mg per minute, the rate being increased to 0.004 mg per minute if necessary.
  *For children*
  • If anaphylaxis occurs, 0.01 mg of epinephrine (base) per kg of body weight or 0.3 mg of epinephrine (base) per square meter of body surface, up to a maximum of 0.5 mg per dose, may be administered subcutaneously, the dose being repeated every 15 minutes for 2 doses, then administered every 4 hours as needed.

  • If anaphylactic shock occurs, 0.01 mg of epinephrine (base) per kg of body weight, up to a maximum of 0.3 mg, may be administered intramuscularly or subcutaneously, the dose being repeated every 5 minutes if necessary. If there is an inadequate response to the intramuscular or subcutaneous dosage, 0.01 mg of epinephrine (base) per kg of body weight may be administered intravenously every 5 to 15 minutes as needed.

## Oral Dosage Forms

### TYPHOID VACCINE LIVE ORAL ENTERIC-COATED CAPSULES

**Usual adult and adolescent dose**
Oral, 1 capsule every other day for a total of four doses.

**Usual pediatric dose**
Infants and children up to 6 years of age—Safety and efficacy have not been established; use is not recommended.
Children 6 years of age and older—See *Usual adult and adolescent dose*.

**Strength(s) usually available**
U.S.—
  2 to 6 × 10⁹ colony-forming units of viable *S. typhi* Ty21a, per capsule (Rx) [*Vivotif Berna* (non-viable S. typhi Ty21a 5 to 50 x 10⁹ bacterial cells, sucrose 26 to 130 mg, lactose 100 to 180 mg, per capsule)].
Canada—
  Not commercially available.

**Packaging and storage**
Store between 2 and 8 °C (36 and 46 °F).

**Stability**
Typhoid vaccine is not stable when exposed to ambient temperatures. The vaccine should therefore be shipped and stored between 2 and 8 °C (35.6 and 46.4 °F). Each package of vaccine shows an expiration date. This expiration date is valid only if the product has been maintained at 2 to 8 °C (35.6 to 46.4 °F).

**Auxiliary labeling**
• Keep refrigerated at all times.
• Swallow capsules whole.

## Selected Bibliography

Woodruff BA, et al. A new look at typhoid vaccination. Information for the practicing physician. JAMA 1991 Feb 13; 265 (6): 756-9.
ACIP. Typhoid Immunization: Recommendations of the Immunization Practices Advisory Committee. MMWR 1990 Jul 13; 39 (RR-10): 1-5.
Centers for Disease Control. Health information for international travel—1990. Atlanta, Georgia: CDC, 1990; HHS Publication no. (CDC)90-8280, p 68-71, 81.

Revised: 07/22/92

---

# TYPHOID VI POLYSACCHARIDE VACCINE   Systemic†

VA CLASSIFICATION (Primary): IM100
Note: This monograph is specific for the typhoid vaccine prepared with the cell surface Vi polysaccharide extracted from *Salmonella typhi* Ty2 strain.

Note: For a listing of dosage forms and brand names by country availability, see *Dosage Forms* section(s). For a listing of brand names for the articles in this monograph, refer to the General Index.

†Not commercially available in Canada.

## Category
Immunizing agent (active).

## Indications

**Accepted**
*Salmonella typhi* (prophylaxis)—Typhoid vaccine is indicated for immunization of adults and children 2 years of age and older against disease caused by *S. typhi*.

  Routine typhoid vaccination is no longer recommended in the U.S. However, selective vaccination is indicated for the following groups:
  • Travelers to areas in which there is recognized risk of exposure to

*S. typhi*. Risk is greatest for travelers to developing countries (e.g., countries in Latin America, Asia, and Africa) who will have prolonged exposure to potentially contaminated food and drink. Multidrug-resistant strains of *S. typhi* have become common in some areas of the world (e.g., the Indian subcontinent and the Arabian peninsula), and cases of typhoid fever that are treated with ineffective drugs can be fatal. Approximately 2 to 4% of acute typhoid fever cases develop into a chronic carrier state. The chronic carrier state occurs more frequently with advanced age, and among females than males. These non-symptomatic carriers are the natural reservoir for *S. typhi* and can serve to maintain the disease in its endemic state or to directly infect new individuals. Outbreaks of typhoid fever are often traced to food handlers who are asymptomatic carriers. Travelers should be cautioned that typhoid vaccination is not a substitute for careful selection of food and drink. Typhoid vaccines are not 100% effective, and the vaccine's protection can be overwhelmed by large inocula of *S. typhi*.
  • Persons with intimate exposure (e.g., household contact) to a documented *S. typhi* carrier.
  • Workers in microbiology laboratories who frequently work with *S. typhi*.

Routine vaccination of sewage sanitation workers is warranted only in areas with endemic typhoid fever. There is no evidence that typhoid vaccine is useful in controlling common-source outbreaks.

**Unaccepted**
The use of typhoid vaccine is not indicated for persons attending rural summer camps or living in areas where natural disasters, such as floods, have occurred.

## Pharmacology/Pharmacokinetics

### Physicochemical characteristics
Source—Typhoid Vi polysaccharide vaccine is a sterile solution for intramuscular administration. The vaccine contains the cell surface Vi polysaccharide extracted from *Salmonella typhi* Ty2 strain. The vaccine strain is grown in a semisynthetic medium without animal proteins. The capsular polysaccharide is precipitated from the concentrated culture supernatant by the addition of hexadecyltrimethylammonium bromide and purified by differential centrifugation and precipitation. The potency of the purified polysaccharide is assessed by molecular size and O-acetyl content

### Mechanism of action/Effect
An increase in serum anti-capsular antibodies is thought to be the basis of protection provided by typhoid Vi polysaccharide vaccine. However, a specific correlation of postvaccination antibody levels with subsequent protection is not available and the level of Vi antibody that will provide protection has not been determined.

### Protective effect
Typhoid Vi polysaccharide vaccine induces protective antibodies in 55 to 93% of recipients. In recent studies, one 25-mcg injection of purified typhoid Vi capsular polysaccharide vaccine produced seroconversion (i.e., at least a fourfold rise in antibody titers) in 93% of healthy adults in the U.S.; similar results were observed in Europe. Two field trials in disease-endemic areas have demonstrated the efficacy of typhoid Vi polysaccharide vaccine in preventing typhoid fever. In a trial in Nepal, in which persons 5 to 44 years of age, each of whom had been administered one dose of typhoid Vi polysaccharide vaccine, were observed for 20 months, 74% fewer cases of typhoid fever, confirmed by blood culture, occurred in vaccine recipients than occurred in controls. In a trial involving schoolchildren 5 to 15 years of age in South Africa, one dose of typhoid Vi polysaccharide vaccine resulted in 55% fewer cases of blood-culture-confirmed typhoid fever over a period of 3 years than occurred in controls. The reduction in the number of cases in years 1, 2, and 3, was 61%, 52%, and 50%, respectively. The efficacy of vaccination with typhoid Vi polysaccharide vaccine has not been studied among persons from areas without endemic disease who travel to disease-endemic regions or among children less than 5 years of age.

### Time to protective effect
Protective antibodies develop at 1 week after immunization with typhoid Vi polysaccharide vaccine and maximal response is achieved at one month after immunization.

### Duration of protective effect
The duration of protection provided by immunization with typhoid Vi polysaccharide vaccine is unknown. However, significant levels of protection persist for at least 21 months in immunized residents of areas where typhoid fever is endemic. In one study, antibody levels remained significantly elevated for up to 34 months after immunization. Booster doses administered 27 to 34 months after primary immunization elicited levels of Vi antibody similar to those achieved after primary immunization. An optimal reimmunization schedule has not been established. However, a single dose of 0.5 mL is recommended for reimmunization every two years if there is repeated or continuing risk of exposure to the *S. typhi* organism.

## Precautions to Consider

### Carcinogenicity/Mutagenicity
No animal or human studies have been conducted to evaluate the carcinogenic or mutagenic potential of typhoid Vi polysaccharide vaccine.

### Pregnancy/Reproduction
Fertility—Studies on the effects of typhoid Vi polysaccharide vaccine on fertility have not been done.

Pregnancy—Studies have not been done in humans.
Studies have not been done in animals.
FDA Pregnancy Category C.

### Breast-feeding
Problems in humans have not been documented.

### Pediatrics
Use is not recommended in infants and children up to 2 years of age. Pediatrics-specific problems that would limit the usefulness of this vaccine in children 2 years of age and older are not expected.

### Geriatrics
Appropriate studies on the relationship of age to the effects of typhoid Vi polysaccharide vaccine have not been performed in the geriatric population. However, no geriatrics-specific problems have been documented to date.

### Medical considerations/Contraindications
The medical considerations/contraindications included here have been selected on the basis of their potential clinical significance (reasons given in parentheses where appropriate)—not necessarily inclusive ($\gg$ = major clinical significance).

*Except under special circumstances, this medication should not be used when the following medical problems exist:*
» Febrile illness, acute
  (administration of typhoid Vi polysaccharide vaccine should be postponed to avoid confusing manifestations of acute febrile illness with possible side/adverse effects of the vaccine; minor illnesses, such as upper respiratory infections, with or without low grade fever or mild diarrhea, do not preclude administration of vaccine)
» Previous sensitivity reaction to typhoid Vi polysaccharide vaccine
  (typhoid Vi polysaccharide vaccine is contraindicated in patients with a history of a severe systemic or allergic reaction to a previous administration of typhoid Vi polysaccharide vaccine)

## Side/Adverse Effects

Note: Most recipients of typhoid vaccine experience some degree of local and systemic response, usually beginning within 24 hours of administration and persisting for 1 or 2 days.

The following side/adverse effects have been selected on the basis of their potential clinical significance (possible signs and symptoms in parentheses where appropriate)—not necessarily inclusive:

### Those indicating need for medical attention
Incidence rare
  *Anaphylactic reaction* (difficulty in breathing or swallowing; hives; itching, especially of soles or palms; reddening of skin, especially around ears; swelling of eyes, face, or inside of nose; unusual tiredness or weakness, sudden and severe)

### Those indicating need for medical attention only if they continue or are bothersome
Incidence more frequent
  *Fever; headache; malaise; muscle pain; pain, redness, or swelling at injection site*

## Patient Consultation

As an aid to patient consultation, refer to *Advice for the Patient, Typhoid Vi Polysaccharide Vaccine (Systemic).*

In providing consultation, consider emphasizing the following selected information ($\gg$ = major clinical significance):

### Before using this medication
» Conditions affecting use, especially:
    Sensitivity to typhoid vaccine
    Use in children—Use is not recommended for infants and children less than 2 years of age
    Other medical problems, especially acute febrile illness and previous sensitivity reaction to typhoid Vi polysaccharide vaccine

### Proper use of this medication
» Proper dosing

### Side/adverse effects
    Signs of potential side effects, especially anaphylactic reaction

## General Dosing Information

Appropriate precautions should be taken prior to typhoid Vi polysaccharide vaccine injection to prevent allergic or any other unwanted reactions. This should include review of the patient's history regarding possible sensitivity to typhoid Vi polysaccharide vaccine or similar vaccines and the ready availability of epinephrine 1:1000 and other appropriate agents used for control of immediate allergic reactions.

The dose of typhoid Vi polysaccharide vaccine is a single injection of 0.5 mL for all persons 2 years of age and older. For infants and children up to 2 years of age, safety and efficacy have not been established; use is not recommended.

The dose of typhoid Vi polysaccharide vaccine for adults is administered by intramuscular injection in the deltoid, and the dose for children is given by intramuscular injection either in the deltoid or the vastus lateralis. The vaccine should not be administered intravenously.

An optimal reimmunization schedule has not been established. However, a single dose of 0.5 mL is recommended for reimmunization every two years if there is repeated or continuing risk of exposure to the *S. typhi* organism.

There are no data on the safety and efficacy of typhoid Vi polysaccharide vaccine administered with any jet injector apparatus and this method of delivery is not recommended.

Even after immunization with typhoid Vi polysaccharide vaccine, not all recipients of the vaccine will be fully protected against typhoid fever. Travelers should take all necessary precautions to avoid contact with, or ingestion of, potentially contaminated food or water.

### For treatment of adverse effects
Recommended treatment consists of the following:
- For anaphylaxis—Administering epinephrine 1:1000.

## Parenteral Dosage Forms
### TYPHOID Vi POLYSACCHARIDE VACCINE

#### Usual adult and adolescent dose
Immunizing agent (active)—
Intramuscular, a single dose of 25 mcg (0.5 mL).

Note: A booster dose of 25 mcg (0.5 mL) may be repeated every two years.

#### Usual pediatric dose
Immunizing agent (active)—
Infants and children up to 2 years of age: Use is not recommended.
Children 2 years of age and older: See *Usual adult and adolescent dose*.

### Strength(s) usually available
U.S.—
25 mcg purified Vi polysaccharide per 0.5 mL (Rx) [*Typhim Vi*].
Canada—
Not commercially available.

### Packaging and storage
Store between 2 and 8 °C (36 and 46 °F).

### Auxiliary labeling
Do not freeze.

## Selected Bibliography

Keitel WA, Bond NL, Zahradnik JM, Cramton TA, Robbins JB. Clinical and serological responses following primary and booster immunization with Salmonella typhi Vi capsular polysaccharide vaccines. Vaccine 1994; 12: 195-9.

Acharya IL, Lowe CU, Thapa R, Gurubacharya VL, Shrestha MB, Bact D, et al. Prevention of typhoid fever in Nepal with the Vi capsular polysaccharide of Salmonella typhi. N Engl J Med 1987; 317 (18): 1101-4.

Centers for Disease Control. Typhoid immunization. Recommendations of the Advisory Committee on Immunization Practices (ACIP). MMWR Morb Mortal Wkly Rep 1994; 43 (RR-14): 1-7.

Developed: 08/01/95

---

## TYROPANOATE—See *Cholecystographic Agents, Oral (Systemic)*

# UNDECYLENIC ACID, COMPOUND Topical

VA CLASSIFICATION (Primary): DE102

Note: For a listing of dosage forms and brand names by country availability, see *Dosage Forms* section(s). For a listing of brand names for the articles in this monograph, refer to the General Index.

## Category
Antifungal (topical).

## Indications
### Unaccepted
Compound undecylenic acid has been used for the topical treatment of tinea cruris, tinea pedis, and other tinea infections. However, in the opinion of USP medical experts, it has been superseded by newer and more effective topical antifungal agents.

## Pharmacology/Pharmacokinetics
### Physicochemical characteristics
Molecular weight—
Undecylenic acid: 184.28.
Zinc undecylenate: 431.92.

### Mechanism of action/Effect
Compound undecylenic acid has a fungistatic action. The zinc present in the zinc undecylenate component provides a beneficial astringent action, which aids in reducing rawness and irritation.

## Precautions to Consider
### Pregnancy/Reproduction
Pregnancy—Problems in humans have not been documented.

### Breast-feeding
It is not known whether topical compound undecylenic acid is distributed into breast milk. However, problems in humans have not been documented.

### Pediatrics
Appropriate studies on the relationship of age to the effects of topical compound undecylenic acid have not been performed in the pediatric population. However, no pediatrics-specific problems have been documented to date. Use in children up to 2 years of age is not recommended except under the advice and supervision of a physician.

### Geriatrics
No information is available on the relationship of age to the effects of topical compound undecylenic acid in geriatric patients.

## Side/Adverse Effects
The following side/adverse effects have been selected on the basis of their potential clinical significance (possible signs and symptoms in parentheses where appropriate)—not necessarily inclusive:

**Those indicating need for medical attention**
*Hypersensitivity* (skin irritation not present before therapy)

## Patient Consultation
As an aid to patient consultation, refer to *Advice for the Patient, Undecylenic Acid, Compound (Topical)*.

In providing consultation, consider emphasizing the following selected information (» = major clinical significance):

**Before using this medication**
» Conditions affecting use, especially:
    Sensitivity to compound undecylenic acid
    Use in children—Not using on children up to 2 years of age, unless otherwise directed by physician

**Proper use of this medication**
    Before applying, washing affected and surrounding areas, and drying thoroughly; applying sufficient medication to cover these areas
» Avoiding contact with the eyes
    Proper administration technique for cream, powder, and aerosol foam and powder
» Compliance with full course of therapy
» Proper dosing
    Missed dose: Applying as soon as possible
» Proper storage

**Precautions while using this medication**
    Checking with physician or pharmacist if no improvement within 4 weeks
    Using the powder or topical aerosol powder daily after bathing and careful drying to help prevent reinfection

**Side/adverse effects**
    Signs of potential side effects, especially hypersensitivity

## General Dosing Information
Use of topical antifungals may lead to skin sensitization, resulting in hypersensitivity reactions with subsequent topical use of the medication.

Before application of this medication, the affected and surrounding areas should be cleansed and thoroughly dried.

The medication should be continued for 2 weeks after symptoms have disappeared.

For persistent fungal infection, the ointment is used for nighttime application and the powder for daytime application to relieve burning and itching.

Following complete remission of the infection, the powder or aerosol powder may be continued as part of a daily personal hygiene program to prevent reinfection.

## Topical Dosage Forms
### COMPOUND UNDECYLENIC ACID TOPICAL AEROSOL FOAM

**Usual adult and adolescent dose**
Tinea infections—
    Topical, to the skin, two times a day.

**Usual pediatric dose**
Infants and children up to 2 years of age—Use is not recommended except under the advice and supervision of a physician.
Children 2 years of age and over—See *Usual adult and adolescent dose*.

**Strength(s) usually available**
U.S.—
    10% of undecylenic acid (OTC) [*Desenex Antifungal Penetrating Foam*].
Canada—
    10% of undecylenic acid (OTC) [*Desenex Foam*].

**Packaging and storage**
Store below 40 °C (104 °F), preferably between 15 and 30 °C (59 and 86 °F), unless otherwise specified by manufacturer.

**Auxiliary labeling**
• Shake well.
• For external use only.
• Continue medication for full time of treatment.
• Store away from heat and direct sunlight.

### COMPOUND UNDECYLENIC ACID TOPICAL AEROSOL POWDER

**Usual adult and adolescent dose**
See *Compound Undecylenic Acid Topical Aerosol Foam*.

**Usual pediatric dose**
See *Compound Undecylenic Acid Topical Aerosol Foam*.

**Strength(s) usually available**
U.S.—
    19% total undecylenate as undecylenic acid and zinc undecylenate (OTC) [*Cruex Antifungal Spray Powder; Desenex Antifungal Spray Powder*].
Canada—
    19.5% total undecylenate as 2.5% undecylenic acid and 20% zinc undecylenate (OTC) [*Cruex Aerosol Powder; Desenex Aerosol Powder*].

**Packaging and storage**
Store below 40 °C (104 °F), preferably between 15 and 30 °C (59 and 86 °F), unless otherwise specified by manufacturer.

**Auxiliary labeling**
• Shake well.
• For external use only.
• Continue medication for full time of treatment.
• Store away from heat and direct sunlight.

## COMPOUND UNDECYLENIC ACID CREAM

**Usual adult and adolescent dose**
Tinea infections—
    Topical, to the skin, as often as needed.

**Usual pediatric dose**
See *Usual adult and adolescent dose.*

**Strength(s) usually available**
U.S.—
    20% total undecylenate as undecylenic acid and zinc undecylenate (OTC) [*Cruex Antifungal Cream; Desenex Antifungal Cream*].
Canada—
    20% total undecylenate as 3% undecylenic acid and 20% zinc undecylenate (OTC) [*Cruex Cream*].

**Packaging and storage**
Store below 40 °C (104 °F), preferably between 15 and 30 °C (59 and 86 °F), in a well-closed container, unless otherwise specified by manufacturer. Protect from freezing.

**Auxiliary labeling**
• For external use only.
• Continue medication for full time of treatment.

## COMPOUND UNDECYLENIC ACID OINTMENT USP

**Usual adult and adolescent dose**
See *Compound Undecylenic Acid Topical Aerosol Foam.*

**Usual pediatric dose**
See *Compound Undecylenic Acid Topical Aerosol Foam.*

**Strength(s) usually available**
U.S.—
    22% total undecylenate as undecylenic acid and zinc undecylenate (OTC) [*Desenex Antifungal Ointment;* GENERIC].
Canada—
    22.3% total undecylenate as 5.4% undecylenic acid and 20% zinc undecylenate (OTC) [*Desenex Ointment*].

**Packaging and storage**
Do not store for a prolonged time at temperatures above 30 °C (86 °F). Store in a tight container. Protect from freezing.

**Auxiliary labeling**
• For external use only.
• Continue medication for full time of treatment.

## COMPOUND UNDECYLENIC ACID TOPICAL POWDER

**Usual adult and adolescent dose**
See *Compound Undecylenic Acid Topical Aerosol Foam.*

**Usual pediatric dose**
See *Compound Undecylenic Acid Topical Aerosol Foam.*

**Strength(s) usually available**
U.S.—
    10% calcium undecylenate (OTC) [*Caldesene Medicated Powder; Cruex Antifungal Powder; Decylenes Powder*].
    19% total undecylenate as undecylenic acid and zinc undecylenate (OTC) [*Desenex Antifungal Powder*].
Canada—
    10% calcium undecylenate (OTC) [*Cruex Powder*].
    19% total undecylenate as 2% undecylenic acid and 20% zinc undecylenate (OTC) [*Desenex Powder*].

**Packaging and storage**
Store below 40 °C (104 °F), preferably between 15 and 30 °C (59 and 86 °F), in a well-closed container, unless otherwise specified by manufacturer.

**Auxiliary labeling**
• For external use only.
• Continue medication for full time of treatment.

## COMPOUND UNDECYLENIC ACID TOPICAL SOLUTION

**Usual adult and adolescent dose**
See *Compound Undecylenic Acid Topical Aerosol Foam.*

**Usual pediatric dose**
See *Compound Undecylenic Acid Topical Aerosol Foam.*

**Strength(s) usually available**
U.S.—
    10% undecylenic acid (OTC) [*Desenex Antifungal Liquid;* GENERIC].
    25% undecylenic acid (OTC) [*Gordochom Solution* (3% chloroxylenol)].
Canada—
    10% undecylenic acid (OTC) [*Desenex Solution*].

**Packaging and storage**
Store below 40 °C (104 °F), preferably between 15 and 30 °C (59 and 86 °F), in a well-closed container, unless otherwise specified by manufacturer. Protect from freezing.

**Auxiliary labeling**
• For external use only.
• Continue medication for full time of treatment.

Revised: 07/25/94

---

# URACIL MUSTARD   Systemic†

VA CLASSIFICATION (Primary): AN100
Note: For a listing of dosage forms and brand names by country availability, see *Dosage Forms* section(s). For a listing of brand names for the articles in this monograph, refer to the General Index.

    †Not commercially available in Canada.

## Category
Antineoplastic.

## Indications

**Accepted**
Uracil mustard has been used for the following indications, although use has generally been replaced by that of more effective agents:
    —for palliative treatment of chronic lymphocytic and myelocytic leukemia.
    —for palliative treatment of non-Hodgkin's lymphomas of the histiocytic or lymphocytic type.
    —for palliative treatment of mycosis fungoides.
    —for palliative treatment of the early stages of polycythemia vera before the development of leukemia or myelofibrosis.

## Pharmacology/Pharmacokinetics

**Physicochemical characteristics**
Molecular weight—252.10.

**Mechanism of action/Effect**
Uracil mustard is an alkylating agent of the nitrogen mustard type. Uracil mustard is a bifunctional alkylating agent, and is cell cycle–phase nonspecific. Activity occurs as a result of formation of an unstable ethylenimmonium ion. Uracil mustard interferes with the function of DNA and RNA and is also capable of cross-linking DNA.

**Elimination**
Renal.

## Precautions to Consider

**Carcinogenicity/Mutagenicity**
Secondary malignancies are potential delayed effects of many antineoplastic agents, although it is not clear whether the effect is related to their mutagenic or immunosuppressive action. The effect of dose and duration of therapy is also unknown, although risk seems to increase with long-term use. Although information is limited, available data seem to indicate that the carcinogenic risk is greatest with the alkylating agents.

**Pregnancy/Reproduction**
Fertility—Gonadal suppression, resulting in amenorrhea or azoospermia, may occur in patients taking antineoplastic therapy, especially with the alkylating agents. In general, these effects appear to be related to dose and length of therapy and may be irreversible. Prediction of the degree of testicular or ovarian function impairment is complicated by the common use of combinations of several antineoplastics, which makes it difficult to assess the effects of individual agents.

Pregnancy—First trimester: It is usually recommended that use of anti-neoplastics, especially combination chemotherapy, be avoided whenever possible, especially during the first trimester. Although information is limited because of the relatively few instances of antineoplastic administration during pregnancy, the mutagenic, teratogenic, and carcinogenic potential of these medications must be considered.

Other hazards to the fetus include adverse reactions seen in adults.

In general, use of a contraceptive is recommended during cytotoxic drug therapy.

### Breast-feeding

Although very little information is available regarding excretion of antineoplastic agents in breast milk, breast-feeding is not recommended while uracil mustard is being administered because of the risks to the infant (adverse effects, mutagenicity, carcinogenicity).

### Pediatrics

Appropriate studies with uracil mustard have not been performed in the pediatric population. However, pediatrics-specific problems that would limit the use of this medication in children are not expected.

### Geriatrics

No geriatrics-specific information is available on the use of uracil mustard in geriatric patients. However, elderly patients are more likely to have age-related renal function impairment, which may require caution in patients receiving uracil mustard.

### Dental

The bone marrow depressant effects of uracil mustard may result in an increased incidence of microbial infection, delayed healing, and gingival bleeding. Dental work, whenever possible, should be completed prior to initiation of therapy or deferred until blood counts have returned to normal. Patients should be instructed in proper oral hygiene during treatment, including caution in use of regular toothbrushes, dental floss, and toothpicks.

Uracil mustard may also rarely cause stomatitis associated with considerable discomfort.

### Drug interactions and/or related problems

The following drug interactions and/or related problems have been selected on the basis of their potential clinical significance (possible mechanism in parentheses where appropriate)—not necessarily inclusive (» = major clinical significance):

Note: Combinations containing any of the following medications, depending on the amount present, may also interact with this medication.

Allopurinol or
Colchicine or
» Probenecid or
» Sulfinpyrazone
(uracil mustard may raise the concentration of blood uric acid; dosage adjustment of antigout agents may be necessary to control hyperuricemia and gout; allopurinol may be preferred to prevent or reverse uracil mustard–induced hyperuricemia because of risk of uric acid nephropathy with uricosuric antigout agents)

Blood dyscrasia–causing medications (See *Appendix II*)
(leukopenic and/or thrombocytopenic effects of uracil mustard may be increased with concurrent or recent therapy if these medications cause the same effects; dosage adjustment of uracil mustard, if necessary, should be based on blood counts)

» Bone marrow depressants, other (See *Appendix II*) or
Radiation therapy
(additive bone marrow depression may occur; dosage reduction may be required when two or more bone marrow depressants, including radiation, are used concurrently or consecutively)

Vaccines, killed virus
(because normal defense mechanisms may be suppressed by uracil mustard therapy, the patient's antibody response to the vaccine may be decreased. The interval between discontinuation of medications that cause immunosuppression and restoration of the patient's ability to respond to the vaccine depends on the intensity and type of immunosuppression-causing medication used, the underlying disease, and other factors; estimates vary from 3 months to 1 year)

» Vaccines, live virus
(because normal defense mechanisms may be suppressed by uracil mustard therapy, concurrent use with a live virus vaccine may potentiate the replication of the vaccine virus, may increase the side/adverse effects of the vaccine virus, and/or may decrease the patient's antibody response to the vaccine; immunization of these patients should be undertaken only with extreme caution after careful review of the patient's hematologic status and only with the knowledge and consent of the physician managing the uracil mus-

tard therapy. The interval between discontinuation of medications that cause immunosuppression and restoration of the patient's ability to respond to the vaccine depends on the intensity and type of immunosuppression-causing medication used, the underlying disease, and other factors; estimates vary from 3 months to 1 year. Patients with leukemia in remission should not receive live virus vaccine until at least 3 months after their last chemotherapy. Immunization with oral poliovirus vaccine should also be postponed in persons in close contact with the patient, especially family members)

### Laboratory value alterations

The following have been selected on the basis of their potential clinical significance (possible effect in parentheses where appropriate)—not necessarily inclusive (» = major clinical significance):

With physiology/laboratory test values
Uric acid concentrations in blood and urine
(may be increased)

### Medical considerations/Contraindications

The medical considerations/contraindications included here have been selected on the basis of their potential clinical significance (reasons given in parentheses where appropriate)—not necessarily inclusive (» = major clinical significance).

*Risk-benefit should be considered when the following medical problems exist:*

» Bone marrow depression
(use of uracil mustard is contraindicated in patients with marked bone marrow depression)

» Chickenpox, existing or recent (including recent exposure) or
» Herpes zoster
(risk of severe generalized disease)

» Gout, history of or
Urate renal stones, history of
(risk of hyperuricemia)

» Hepatic function impairment
» Infection
» Renal function impairment
Sensitivity to uracil mustard
» Tumor cell infiltration of bone marrow
» Caution should be used also in patients who have had previous cytotoxic drug therapy or radiation therapy.

### Patient monitoring

The following are especially important in patient monitoring (other tests may be warranted in some patients, depending on condition; » = major clinical significance):

Blood urea nitrogen (BUN) concentrations and
Serum creatinine concentrations
(recommended prior to initiation of therapy and at periodic intervals during therapy; frequency varies according to clinical state, agent, dose, and other agents being used concurrently)

» Hematocrit or hemoglobin and
» Platelet count and
» Total and, if appropriate, differential leukocyte count
(determinations recommended prior to initiation of therapy and at periodic intervals during therapy; frequency varies according to clinical state, agent, dose, and other agents being used concurrently)

Serum alanine aminotransferase (ALT [SGPT]) concentrations and
Serum aspartate aminotransferase (AST [SGOT]) concentrations and
Serum bilirubin concentrations and
Serum lactate dehydrogenase (LDH) concentrations
(recommended prior to initiation of therapy and at periodic intervals during therapy; frequency varies according to clinical state, agent, dose, and other agents being used concurrently)

Serum uric acid concentrations
(recommended prior to initiation of therapy and at periodic intervals during therapy; frequency varies according to clinical state, agent, dose, and other agents being used concurrently)

## Side/Adverse Effects

Note: Many "side effects" of antineoplastic therapy are unavoidable and represent the medication's pharmacologic action. Some of these (for example, leukopenia and thrombocytopenia) are actually used as parameters to aid in individual dosage titration.

The following side/adverse effects have been selected on the basis of their potential clinical significance (possible signs and symptoms in parentheses where appropriate)—not necessarily inclusive:

**Those indicating need for medical attention**

Incidence more frequent
*Leukopenia or immunosuppression* (usually asymptomatic; less frequently, fever or chills; cough or hoarseness; lower back or side pain; painful or difficult urination); *thrombocytopenia* (usually asymptomatic; less frequently, unusual bleeding or bruising; black, tarry stools; blood in urine or stools; pinpoint red spots on skin)

Note: Maximum *bone marrow depression* may not occur until 2 to 4 weeks after the medication has been discontinued.

Incidence less frequent
*Hyperuricemia or uric acid nephropathy* (joint pain; lower back or side pain; swelling of feet or lower legs)

Note: *Hyperuricemia or uric acid nephropathy* occurs most commonly during initial treatment of patients with leukemia or lymphoma, as a result of rapid cell breakdown, which leads to elevated serum uric acid concentrations.

Incidence rare
*Hepatotoxicity* (yellow eyes or skin); *stomatitis* (sores in mouth and on lips)

**Those indicating need for medical attention only if they continue or are bothersome**

Incidence more frequent, dose-related
*Diarrhea; nausea or vomiting*

Incidence less frequent
*Darkening of the skin; irritability; mental depression; nervousness; skin rash and itching*

**Those not indicating need for medical attention**

Incidence less frequent
*Loss of hair*

**Those indicating the need for medical attention if they occur after medication is discontinued**

*Bone marrow depression* (black, tarry stools; blood in urine or stools; cough or hoarseness; fever or chills; lower back or side pain; painful or difficult urination; pinpoint red spots on skin; unusual bleeding or bruising)

Note: Cumulative *myelosuppression* may occur with repeated doses.

## Patient Consultation

As an aid to patient consultation, refer to *Advice for the Patient, Uracil Mustard (Systemic).*

Consider advising the patient on the following (» = major clinical significance):

**Before using this medication**
» Conditions affecting use, especially:
  Pregnancy—Advisability of using contraception; telling physician immediately if pregnancy is suspected
  See also *Precautions to Consider.*

**Proper use of this medication**
» Importance of not taking more or less medication than the amount prescribed
  Importance of ample fluid intake and subsequent increase in urine output to aid in excretion of uric acid
» Frequency of nausea and vomiting; importance of continuing medication despite stomach upset
  Checking with physician if vomiting occurs shortly after dose is taken
» Proper dosing
  Missed dose: Not taking at all; not doubling doses
» Proper storage

**Precautions while using this medication**
» Importance of close monitoring by the physician
» Avoiding immunizations unless approved by physician; other persons in patient's household should avoid immunizations with oral poliovirus vaccine; avoiding other persons who have taken oral poliovirus vaccine or wearing a protective mask that covers nose and mouth

*Caution if bone marrow depression occurs:*
» Avoiding exposure to persons with bacterial infections, especially during periods of low blood counts; checking with physician immediately if fever or chills, cough or hoarseness, lower back or side pain, or painful or difficult urination occur
» Checking with physician immediately if unusual bleeding or bruising; black, tarry stools; blood in urine or stools; or pinpoint red spots on skin occur

Caution in use of regular toothbrush, dental floss, or toothpick; physician, dentist, or nurse may suggest alternatives; checking with physician before having dental work done
Not touching eyes or inside of nose unless hands washed immediately before
Using caution to avoid accidental cuts with use of sharp objects such as safety razor or fingernail or toenail cutters
Avoiding contact sports or other situations where bruising or injury could occur

**Side/adverse effects**
May cause adverse effects such as blood problems and loss of hair; importance of discussing possible effects with physician
Signs of potential side effects, especially leukopenia, thrombocytopenia, hyperuricemia, uric acid nephropathy, hepatotoxicity, and stomatitis
Physician or nurse can help in dealing with side effects
Possibility of hair loss; should return after treatment has ended

## General Dosing Information

Patients receiving uracil mustard should be under supervision of a physician experienced in cancer chemotherapy.

Dosage must be adjusted to meet the individual requirements of each patient, based on clinical response and degree of bone marrow depression.

A variety of dosage schedules and regimens of uracil mustard, alone or in combination with other antitumor agents, are used. The prescriber may consult the medical literature as well as the manufacturer's literature in choosing a specific dosage.

Development of uric acid nephropathy in patients with leukemia or lymphoma may be prevented by adequate oral hydration and, in some cases, administration of allopurinol. Alkalinization of urine may be necessary if serum uric acid concentrations are elevated.

In the absence of bone marrow depression, uracil mustard should be given for at least 3 months before it is considered ineffective.

Although it is not necessary to discontinue uracil mustard following the initial decrease in blood counts, it must be remembered that a dosage approaching or exceeding a total of 1 mg per kg of body weight (mg/kg) for the course may cause irreversible bone marrow damage. It is recommended that uracil mustard therapy be discontinued or dosage reduced at the first sign of a sudden large decrease in leukocyte (particularly granulocyte) or platelet count to prevent irreversible bone marrow depression. Therapy may be resumed when blood counts recover.

Because of the risk of enhanced bone marrow toxicity, an interval of at least 2 to 3 weeks is recommended before starting uracil mustard therapy after a patient has received the maximum effect from radiation or chemotherapy with medications that depress bone marrow function. Recovery from the maximum effect is indicated by a rising leukocyte count, although some clinicians prefer not to administer uracil mustard until the leukocyte count returns to normal.

Special precautions are recommended in patients who develop thrombocytopenia as a result of administration of uracil mustard. These may include extreme care in performing invasive procedures; regular inspection of intravenous sites, skin (including perirectal area), and mucous membrane surfaces for signs of bleeding or bruising; limiting frequency of venipuncture and avoiding intramuscular injections; testing urine, emesis, stool, and secretions for occult blood; care in use of regular toothbrushes, dental floss, toothpicks, safety razors, and fingernail and toenail cutters; avoiding constipation; and using caution to prevent falls and other injuries. Such patients should avoid alcohol and any aspirin intake because of the risk of gastrointestinal bleeding. Platelet transfusions may be required.

Patients who develop leukopenia should be observed carefully for signs of infection. Antibiotic support may be required. In neutropenic patients who develop fever, broad-spectrum antibiotic coverage should be initiated empirically, pending bacterial cultures and appropriate diagnostic tests.

## Oral Dosage Forms

### URACIL MUSTARD CAPSULES USP

Note: Uracil mustard capsules are not commercially available in Canada.

**Usual adult dose**
Oral, 150 mcg (0.15 mg) per kg of body weight once a week for four weeks.

**Usual adult prescribing limits**
Total dosage of 1 mg per kg of body weight or greater sharply increases the risk of irreversible bone marrow depression.

**Usual pediatric dose**
Oral, 300 mcg (0.3 mg) per kg of body weight once a week for four weeks.

**Strength(s) usually available**
U.S.—
   1 mg (Rx) [GENERIC (tartrazine; lactose)].

**Packaging and storage**
Store below 40 °C (104 °F), preferably between 15 and 30 °C (59 and 86 °F), unless otherwise specified by manufacturer. Store in a tight container.

Revised: 09/90
Interim revision: 08/11/93

---

# UREA˙  Parenteral-Local

VA CLASSIFICATION (Primary): GU600
Another commonly used name is carbamide.

Note: For a listing of dosage forms and brand names by country availability, see *Dosage Forms* section(s). For a listing of brand names for the articles in this monograph, refer to the General Index.

## Category
Abortifacient.

## Indications
Note: Bracketed information in the *Indications* section refers to uses that are not included in U.S. product labeling.

**Accepted**
[Abortion, elective]—Urea, when administered by transabdominal intra-amniotic injection as a hypertonic solution, is used for aborting second trimester pregnancy beyond the sixteenth week of gestation. The use of hypertonic urea solution for abortion has generally been replaced by dilation and evacuation, though it may be useful in selected patients. Urea is used in combination with oxytocin or prostaglandins. Use before the sixteenth week is difficult because of the small amount of amniotic fluid present and results in an increased failure rate.

## Pharmacology/Pharmacokinetics

**Physicochemical characteristics**
Molecular weight—60.06.

**Mechanism of action/Effect**
The mechanism by which urea causes fetal death and abortion has not been elucidated but may be related to damage of decidual cells by hypertonic urea and subsequent release of prostaglandins, which induce uterine contractions. Hypertonic urea induces fetal death.

**Time to peak effect**
Mean abortion time—
   Urea with dinoprost: 16 to 17 hours.
   Urea with oxytocin: 18 to 30 hours.

**Elimination**
Renal.

## Precautions to Consider

**Adolescents**
No published information is available on the use of intra-amniotic urea in adolescent females. However, no adolescent-specific problems have been documented to date.

**Drug interactions and/or related problems**
The following drug interactions and/or related problems have been selected on the basis of their potential clinical significance (possible mechanism in parentheses where appropriate)—not necessarily inclusive (» = major clinical significance):
» Oxytocin or other oxytocics
   (concurrent use with urea may result in uterine hypertonus, possibly causing uterine rupture or cervical laceration, especially in the absence of adequate cervical dilation; although combinations are sometimes used for therapeutic advantage, patient should be closely monitored during concurrent use)

**Laboratory value alterations**
The following have been selected on the basis of their potential clinical significance (possible effect in parentheses where appropriate)—not necessarily inclusive (» = major clinical significance):
With physiology/laboratory test values
   Blood urea nitrogen (BUN) concentrations
      (may be increased following administration but usually return to acceptable levels within 24 hours)

**Medical considerations/Contraindications**
The medical considerations/contraindications included here have been selected on the basis of their potential clinical significance (reasons given in parentheses where appropriate)—not necessarily inclusive (» = major clinical significance).

*Except under special circumstances, this medication should not be used when the following medical problems exist:*
»   Absolute contraindications to labor
»   Ruptured membranes

*Risk-benefit should be considered when the following medical problems exist:*
   Allergy to urea
   Cervical stenosis or
   Uterine fibroids
      (risk of uterine rupture)
»   Dehydration or
»   Renal function impairment, severe
      (risk of electrolyte imbalance and impaired clearance)
»   Diabetes mellitus or
»   Sickle cell disease
      (risk of intravascular hemolysis or thrombosis)
»   Hepatic function impairment, severe
      (blood ammonia concentrations may be elevated)
»   Intracranial bleeding, active
      (unless use of urea is followed promptly by surgical intervention to control hemorrhage, since urea may increase bleeding)
»   Relative contraindications to labor

**Patient monitoring**
The following may be especially important in patient monitoring (other tests may be warranted in some patients, depending on condition; » = major clinical significance):

   Contractions, frequency, duration, and force of and
   Temperature, pulse, and blood pressure determinations and
   Uterine tone, resting
      (recommended at frequent intervals during abortion procedure)

   Fluid intake and output monitoring
      (especially when used with oxytocin)

   Electrolytes
      (measurement of serum concentrations is recommended at regular intervals, especially when used with oxytocin)

   Vaginal examination
      (recommended postabortion to check for signs of cervical trauma)

## Side/Adverse Effects

Note: Urea may cause uterine hypertonicity with spasm and tetanic contraction that can lead to posterior cervical perforations, cervical lacerations, uterine rupture, and hemorrhage, especially when given with oxytocics.

Intra-amniotic administration of hypertonic urea has been associated with disseminated intravascular coagulation.

The following side/adverse effects have been selected on the basis of their potential clinical significance (possible cause in parentheses where appropriate)—not necessarily inclusive:

**Those indicating need for medical attention**
Incidence less frequent
*Inadvertent intravascular, myometrial, or intraperitoneal administration* (pain in lower abdomen or weakness)
Note: *Inadvertent intravascular, myometrial, or intraperitoneal administration* may lead to myometrial necrosis and/or dehydration with resulting vomiting, hyponatremia, and hypokalemia or hyperkalemia. Instillation should be discontinued immediately.

Incidence rare
*Electrolyte imbalance* (confusion; irregular heartbeat; muscle cramps or pain; numbness, tingling, pain, or weakness in hands or feet; unusual tiredness or weakness; weakness or heaviness of legs)

**Those indicating need for medical attention only if they continue or are bothersome**
Incidence more frequent
*Nausea or vomiting*
Incidence less frequent or rare
*Headache*

**Those indicating possible postabortion complications and the need for medical attention if they occur after medication is discontinued**
*Endometritis* (chills; shivering; fever; foul-smelling vaginal discharge; pain in lower abdomen); *increase in uterine bleeding*

## Patient Consultation

As an aid to patient consultation, refer to *Advice for the Patient, Urea (Intra-amniotic)*.

In providing consultation, consider emphasizing the following selected information (» = major clinical significance):

**Before using this medication**
» Conditions affecting use, especially:
  Sensitivity to urea
  Other medications, especially oxytocin or other oxytocics
  Other medical problems, especially renal function impairment, diabetes mellitus, sickle cell disease, or hepatic function impairment

**Proper use of this medication**
  Importance of taking oral fluids during procedure
» Proper dosing

**Side/adverse effects**
  Signs of potential side effects, especially pain in lower abdomen, weakness, electrolyte imbalance

## General Dosing Information

It is recommended that intra-amniotic urea be administered in a hospital setting.

Hypertonic urea should not be administered if a bloody amniotic tap is obtained.

Withdrawal of 100 to 200 mL of amniotic fluid is recommended prior to instillation of hypertonic urea to prevent sudden increases in intra-amniotic pressure and to ensure adequate concentrations of urea.

Extra-amniotic injection of urea should be avoided.

To aid urea excretion and prevent dehydration, it is recommended that patients take oral fluids freely during the procedure; intravenous fluids may also be required. Intake of fluids should not exceed output by 1500 mL in each 24 hours.

Concurrent intravenous administration of a dilute solution of oxytocin is usually begun within 1 to 2 hours after urea instillation to shorten the induction-to-abortion time and reduce the failure rate, although the rate of incomplete abortion is 30 to 40% even with oxytocin.

Instillation of hypertonic urea may be followed immediately by intra-amniotic administration of the equivalent of 5 to 10 mg of dinoprost.

Some clinicians recommend using a dose of 80 grams of urea as a 59.7% solution in combination with 5 mg of dinoprost tromethamine (prostaglandin $F_2$ tromethamine).

If urea is not effective, it is recommended that alternative methods such as oxytocin or dinoprost not be used until the uterus has stopped contracting.

## Parenteral Dosage Forms

Note: Bracketed uses in the *Dosage Forms* section refer to categories of use and/or indications that are not included in U.S. product labeling.

### STERILE UREA USP

**Usual adult and adolescent dose**
[Abortion]—
  Intra-amniotic, after transabdominal tap of the amniotic sac, a volume of 40 to 60% urea solution (in 5% dextrose injection) equal to the volume of amniotic fluid removed, up to a maximum of 200 to 250 mL (usually 80 grams of urea) administered slowly while observing for adverse reactions.

Note: The instillation may be repeated 48 hours after the initial dose if the abortion process is not established or clinically imminent, provided the membranes are still intact.

**Size(s) usually available**
U.S.—
  40 grams (Rx) [*Ureaphil*].

**Packaging and storage**
Prior to reconstitution, store below 40 °C (104 °F), preferably between 15 and 30 °C (59 and 86 °F), unless otherwise specified by manufacturer.

**Preparation of dosage form**
To prepare a 40, 50, or 60% injection, add 5% Dextrose Injection USP to 80 grams (2 vials) of urea to make a final volume of 200, 150, or 135 mL, respectively.

Reconstitution time may be prolonged by the endothermic reaction that occurs and can be shortened by warming the diluent to 60 °C in a water bath immediately before reconstitution. The resulting solution should be at body temperature for administration.

One gram of urea is equivalent to approximately 16.7 mOsm (calculated on basis of urea being reconstituted with water for injection; equals 666 mOsm per liter).

The osmolarity of urea infusion when prepared in the specified diluent is as follows:

| Urea (%) | Diluent | Total mOsm/liter |
|---|---|---|
| 40 | 5% Dextrose Injection USP | 6920 |
| 50 | 5% Dextrose Injection USP | 8586 |

**Stability**
Sterile Urea USP should be freshly reconstituted for each patient. The solution should be used within 24 hours. Discard any unused portion.
Urea solutions cannot be heat-sterilized because of instability.

**Note**
Reconstituted solution should be at body temperature for instillation.

Revised: 08/18/93
Interim revision: 06/21/94

# UREA    Systemic†

VA CLASSIFICATION (Primary/Secondary): CV709/OP106

Note: For a listing of dosage forms and brand names by country availability, see *Dosage Forms* section(s). For a listing of brand names for the articles in this monograph, refer to the General Index.

†Not commercially available in Canada.

## Category

Diuretic; antiglaucoma agent (systemic).

## Indications

### Accepted

Edema, cerebral (treatment)—Urea is indicated to treat cerebral edema and reduce brain mass and intracranial pressure.

Glaucoma, malignant (treatment) or
Glaucoma, secondary (treatment)—Urea is indicated to reduce elevated intraocular pressure (IOP) after other methods have failed or in preparation for intraocular surgery.

## Pharmacology/Pharmacokinetics

### Mechanism of action/Effect

Cerebral edema—Elevates blood plasma osmolality, resulting in enhanced flow of water from tissues, including the brain and cerebrospinal fluid, into interstitial fluid and plasma. As a result, cerebral edema, elevated intracranial pressure, and cerebrospinal fluid volume and pressure may be reduced. This effect is evident early in the course of infusion as long as a gradient between plasma and intracellular urea exists. As urea diffuses into the cells and the gradient diminishes, the effect diminishes.
Glaucoma—Elevates blood plasma osmolality, resulting in enhanced flow of water from the eye into plasma and a consequent reduction in intraocular pressure.

### Distribution

Urea is distributed into extracellular and intracellular fluids including lymph, bile, cerebral spinal fluid (CSF), and blood in approximately equal concentrations. Urea also crosses the placenta, penetrates the eyes, and appears in the milk of lactating women.

### Biotransformation

Urea may be partially metabolized in the gastrointestinal tract by hydrolysis to ammonia and carbon dioxide, which may be resynthesized into urea.

### Half-life

1.17 hours.

### Onset of action

Reduction of intraocular and intracranial pressure—Within 10 minutes after infusion is started.

### Time to peak effect

1 to 2 hours.

### Duration of action

Diuresis—3 to 10 hours after infusion is stopped.
Reduction in cerebrospinal fluid pressure—3 to 10 hours after infusion is stopped.
Reduction in intraocular pressure—5 to 6 hours.

### Elimination

Renal (reabsorption about 50%).

## Precautions to Consider

### Pregnancy/Reproduction

Pregnancy—Studies have not been done in humans.
Studies have not been done in animals.

FDA Pregnancy Category C.

### Breast-feeding

It is not known whether urea is distributed into breast milk. However, problems in humans have not been documented.

### Pediatrics

Appropriate studies on the relationship of age to the effects of urea have not been performed in the pediatric population. However, pediatrics-specific problems that would limit the usefulness of urea in children are not expected.

### Geriatrics

Urea should not be infused into veins of the lower extremities, especially in elderly patients, since phlebitis and thrombosis of superficial and deep veins may occur. In addition, elderly patients are more likely to have age-related renal function impairment, which may require caution in patients receiving urea.

### Drug interactions and/or related problems

The following drug interactions and/or related problems have been selected on the basis of their potential clinical significance (possible mechanism in parentheses where appropriate)—not necessarily inclusive (» = major clinical significance):

Note: Combinations containing any of the following medications, depending on the amount present, may also interact with this medication.

Diuretics, other, including carbonic anhydrase inhibitors
(diuretic and IOP–reducing effects may be potentiated when these medications are used concurrently with urea; dosage adjustments may be necessary)

Lithium
(urea may increase renal excretion of lithium)

### Laboratory value alterations

The following have been selected on the basis of their potential clinical significance (possible effect in parentheses where appropriate)—not necessarily inclusive (» = major clinical significance):

With physiology/laboratory test values
Blood urea nitrogen (BUN)
(concentrations may be increased with excessive doses)

Potassium and
Sodium
(serum concentrations may be decreased with prolonged administration)

### Medical considerations/Contraindications

The medical considerations/contraindications included here have been selected on the basis of their potential clinical significance (reasons given in parentheses where appropriate)—not necessarily inclusive (» = major clinical significance).

*Except under special circumstances, this medication should not be used when the following medical problems exist:*

» Dehydration, severe
(this condition may increase risk of urea-induced electrolyte depletion)

» Hepatic function impairment, severe
(blood ammonia concentrations may be elevated)

» Intracranial bleeding, active, except during craniotomy
(reduction of brain edema by urea may increase bleeding)

» Renal function impairment, severe
(accumulation of urea solution may lead to circulatory overload)

*Risk-benefit should be considered when the following medical problems exist:*

Cardiovascular function impairment
(sudden expansion of extracellular fluid may lead to congestive heart failure)

Hepatic function impairment
(blood ammonia concentrations may be elevated)

» Hereditary fructose intolerance (aldolase deficiency)—for infusions prepared with invert sugar injection only

Hypovolemia
(may be masked and intensified)

Renal function impairment
(accumulation of urea may lead to overexpansion of extracellular fluid and circulatory overload)

### Patient monitoring

The following may be especially important in patient monitoring (other tests may be warranted in some patients, depending on condition; » = major clinical significance):

Blood pressure measurements and
Electrolyte measurements, including sodium and potassium, and
Renal function determinations and
Urine output determinations
(recommended during intravenous infusion of urea, especially with repeated doses)

Blood urea nitrogen (BUN) determinations
(recommended before and frequently during intravenous administration; if a rapid increase occurs, the infusion should be slowed or stopped)

## Side/Adverse Effects

Note: Most side/adverse effects are related to the rate of administration.

Thrombosis may occur with administration into the superficial and deep veins of the lower extremities, especially in elderly patients.

Hemolysis may occur as a result of rapid administration; urea may also cause increased capillary bleeding, and rapid infusion has resulted in intraocular hemorrhage in patients with absolute glaucoma.

Side effects can be minimized by maintaining adequate hydration and keeping the patient horizontal.

Excessive diuresis can result from long-term urea therapy, which may lead to tissue dehydration, hypokalemia, and hyponatremia.

The following effects have been selected on the basis of their potential clinical significance (possible signs and symptoms in parentheses where appropriate)—not necessarily inclusive:

### Those indicating need for medical attention
Incidence less frequent or rare
*Confusion, fast heartbeat, fever, or nervousness; electrolyte imbalance* (confusion; irregular heartbeat; muscle cramps or pain; numbness, tingling, pain, or weakness in hands or feet; seizures; trembling; unusual tiredness or weakness; weakness and heaviness of legs); *phlebitis or thrombosis, chemical, or extravasation* (redness, swelling, or pain at injection site)—for intravenous injection only; *subdural or subarachnoid hemorrhage, possible* (blurred vision; severe headache)

Note: *Confusion, fast heartbeat, fever, or nervousness* may be caused by too-rapid intravenous infusion.

### Those indicating need for medical attention only if they continue or are bothersome
Incidence more frequent
*Dryness of mouth or increased thirst; headache; nausea or vomiting*
Incidence less frequent
*Dizziness or faintness; drowsiness*—with prolonged urea administration in patients with sickle cell crisis; *skin blemishes*

Note: In some cases, *headache, nausea or vomiting, blurred vision,* and *dizziness* may be symptoms of subdural or subarachnoid hemorrhage.

## Overdose

For more information on the management of overdose or unintentional ingestion, **contact a Poison Control Center** (see *Poison Control Center Listing*).

### Treatment of overdose
In the event of overdose as reflected by elevated blood urea nitrogen (BUN) concentrations, recommended treatment consists of the following: discontinuation of medication; patient evaluation, and institution of corrective measures.

## General Dosing Information

### For intravenous injection only
The dose used depends on the fluid and electrolyte and renal status of the patient.

An infusion rate of not greater than 4 mL per minute is recommended, since rapid infusion may cause hemolysis and cerebral vasomotor symptoms.

When urea is used preoperatively for reduction of intraocular or intracranial pressure, the dose should be started about 60 minutes prior to ocular surgery and at the time of scalp incision during intracranial surgery to achieve maximum reduction of pressure.

Urea should not be infused into veins of the lower extremities, especially in elderly patients, since phlebitis and thrombosis of superficial and deep veins may occur. Large veins should be used for infusion.

Caution should be used to prevent extravasation of urea infusion solution at the site of injection, which may result in irritation and tissue necrosis.

Use of an indwelling urethral catheter is recommended in comatose patients to ensure bladder emptying and adequacy of urine output.

The simultaneous use of hypothermia and urea infusion may increase the risk of venous thrombosis and hemoglobinuria.

If blood urea nitrogen (BUN) concentrations are elevated to 75 mg per 100 mL or more or if diuresis does not occur within 1 to 2 hours after administration of urea to patients with renal function impairment, dosage should be reduced or urea withheld until the patient is reevaluated.

## Parenteral Dosage Forms

### STERILE UREA USP

#### Usual adult and adolescent dose
Diuretic or
Antiglaucoma agent—
Intravenous infusion, 500 mg to 1.5 grams per kg of body weight as a 30% solution in 5 or 10% Dextrose Injection USP or 10% invert sugar injection, administered at a rate of approximately 60 drops (4 or 6 mL, depending on manufacturer) per minute over a period of thirty minutes to two hours.

#### Usual adult prescribing limits
Up to 2 grams per kg of body weight per twenty-four-hour period.

#### Usual pediatric dose
Diuretic—
Children up to 2 years of age: Intravenous infusion, 100 mg to 1.5 grams per kg of body weight as a 30% solution in 5 or 10% dextrose injection or 10% invert sugar injection, administered at a rate of approximately 60 drops (4 or 6 mL, depending on manufacturer) per minute over a period of thirty minutes to two hours.
Children 2 years of age and over: See *Usual adult and adolescent dose.*

#### Size(s) usually available
U.S.—
40 grams (Rx) [*Ureaphil*].
Canada—
Not commercially available.

#### Packaging and storage
Prior to reconstitution, store below 40 °C (104 °F), preferably between 15 and 30 °C (59 and 86 °F), unless otherwise specified by manufacturer. Protect from freezing.

#### Preparation of dosage form
For preparation of product for injection, see manufacturer's package insert.

Use of 5% or 10% dextrose injection or invert sugar injection as a diluent reduces the risk of hemolysis that may occur with rapid administration of urea. However, invert sugar injection is contraindicated in patients with fructose intolerance due to aldolase deficiency.

One gram of urea is equivalent to approximately 16.7 mOsm (calculated on basis of urea being reconstituted with water for injection).

The number of mOsm of urea per liter of specified diluent is as follows:

| Urea (%) | Diluent | Total mOsm/liter (approx) |
|---|---|---|
| 30 | 5% Dextrose injection | 5250 |
| 30 | 10% Dextrose injection | 5500 |
| 30 | 10% Invert sugar injection | 5550 |

#### Stability
See manufacturer's package insert and/or label for stability of reconstituted solution.

Each dose of urea should be freshly prepared. Discard any unused portion.

#### Incompatibilities
When blood and urea are administered simultaneously, the urea infusion solution should not be administered through the same administration set through which the blood is being infused.

#### Additional information
Following reconstitution of urea powder for injection with 5 or 10% dextrose or 10% invert sugar injection, the solutions have a pH of 4.5 to 6.

Revised: 01/20/93

## URINE GLUCOSE AND KETONE (COMBINED) TEST—See *Urine Glucose and Ketone Test Kits for Home Use*

# URINE GLUCOSE AND KETONE TEST KITS FOR HOME USE

This monograph includes information on the following: Copper Reduction Urine Glucose Test; Glucose Oxidase Urine Glucose Test; Nitroprusside Urine Ketone Test; Urine Glucose and Ketone (Combined) Test.

VA CLASSIFICATION (Primary): DX900

Note: For a listing of product forms and brand names by country availability, see *Diagnostic Product Forms* section.

## Category

Diagnostic aid (glycosuria)—Copper Reduction Urine Glucose Test; Glucose Oxidase Urine Glucose Test; Urine Glucose and Ketone (Combined) Test.

Diagnostic aid (ketonuria)—Nitroprusside Urine Ketone Test; Urine Glucose and Ketone (Combined) Test.

## Indications

### Accepted

Glycosuria (diagnosis)—Urine glucose test kits are generally used for monitoring stable, non-insulin–dependent diabetic patients not prone to ketoacidosis. Self-monitoring of blood glucose concentrations is the preferred method of monitoring the effectiveness of a patient's regimen for controlling diabetes, and has generally replaced the use of urine testing for glucose concentrations. However, urine testing for glucose may still be used in patients who are unable or unwilling to comply with a program of blood glucose monitoring. This may include elderly patients who may not have the physical dexterity for blood tests, and young children in whom blood sample collection may be met with resistance and whose renal threshold is relatively stable.

Ketonuria (diagnosis)—Urine ketone test kits are used for the detection of ketones in the urine in ketoacidosis-prone diabetics (type I, insulin-dependent) in addition to blood glucose testing. Testing for the presence of ketones in urine is especially important during periods of illness when the diabetic patient is unable to eat or diabetes is difficult to control, or during pregnancy, when insulin needs change rapidly and ketosis is dangerous to the fetus.

Glucose levels can be more directly measured in blood, but ketone levels are more easily detected in urine. Therefore a complete diabetes management program includes testing for ketones (in urine) and monitoring concentrations of glucose (preferably in blood), as a means of making decisions about medication needs and dietary adjustments.

## Pharmacology/Pharmacokinetics

### Physicochemical characteristics

Copper reduction method for urine glucose determination—
The copper reduction method is a quantitative test for glucose. Shades of blue, green, tan, and orange correspond to a color chart indicating percentage concentration of glucose in the urine. The standard procedure uses 5 drops of urine in 10 drops of water and distinguishes up to 2% concentrations with a color chart. A 2-drop method uses 2 drops urine in 10 drops water, and can distinguish up to 5% glucose concentrations with the appropriate color chart.

Glucose oxidase method for urine glucose determination—
Common chromogens are ortho-tolidine, which turns blue, tetramethyl benzidine, which turns blue-green, or an iodine complex, which turns brown in the presence of hydrogen peroxide.

Glucose oxidase tests are considered to be semiquantitative, meaning they are less accurate than copper reduction tests in measuring the percent of glucose in the urine. However, glucose oxidase tests are specific for glucose and are less prone to interference by extraneous substances than the copper reduction tests might be.

Nitroprusside reaction for urine ketone determination—
Ketone tests are also semiquantitative, yielding shades between beige and violet to be evaluated by a color chart on the product container. Acetoacetone is responsible for most of the color change, with a small color change being contributed by acetone. However, the test does not react to beta-hydroxybutyrate, the predominant ketone body.

## Precautions to Consider

### Laboratory value alterations

The following have been selected on the basis of their potential clinical significance (possible effect in parentheses where appropriate)—not necessarily inclusive (» = major clinical significance):

With results of *this* test
*Due to other medications*
Aminosalicylate sodium or
Cephalosporins or
Chloramphenicol or
Isoniazid or
Nalidixic acid or
Nitrofurantoin or
Penicillins or
Streptomycin or
Sulfonamides or
Tetracyclines
(these anti-infective agents have been reported to react with the copper reduction test materials to give false-positive results)
(some cephalosporins release free sulfur in the copper reduction reaction, resulting in blue or black precipitates, which do not lend themselves to color chart comparisons)
Ascorbic acid
(ascorbic acid may give a false-positive result with copper reduction tests and a false-negative reaction with glucose oxidase tests)
Aspirin
(aspirin and its metabolites may produce false-positive results with copper reduction tests and false-negative results with glucose oxidase tests)
Ferrous sulfate
(may give false-negative results with glucose oxidase tests)
Formaldehyde or
Hippuric acid or
Mandelic acid
(may cause false-positive reaction with copper reduction tests)
Levodopa or
Methyldopa
(metabolites of levodopa and methyldopa darken the urine and may mask slight color changes with most test strips or give false-negative readings; they are also reported to cause false-positive reactions with copper reduction tests)
Nicotinic acid
(may cause false-positive results with copper reduction tests)
Nitrofurantoin
(may darken urine sufficiently to mask slight color changes on test strips)
Phenazopyridine
(phenazopyridine may produce a false-negative response with glucose oxidase tests)
Phenolphthalein
(may produce color changes in urine that give confusing results; red, brown, and purple colors are possible with ketone tests)
Phenolsulfonphthalein
(for urologic testing, phenolsulfonphthalein will give a red to purple color at alkaline pH with tests for ketones)
Probenecid
(a metabolite of probenecid is a reducing substance and therefore may cause false-positive results with copper reduction tests)
Sulfobromophthalein
(may give false-positive results with some ketone tests)
*Due to diet*
Ascorbic acid
(foods or dietary supplements containing large amounts of ascorbic acid may block the test reaction for glucose oxidase tests [false negative] and give a false positive for copper reduction tests)
Fructose, galactose, and other reducing substances
(reducing sugars may give a false-positive reading with copper reduction tests)
*Due to medical problems or conditions*
Alkaptonuria
(homogentisic acid, present in the urine of persons with this disorder, inhibits glucose oxidase tests)
Ketonuria
(glucose oxidase tests are falsely depressed by moderate to large amounts of ketones in the urine)
Phenylketonuria
(phenylketones in the urine of untreated phenylketonurics give a brick-red color fading to green-yellow with ketone tests)

Proteinuria
(proteinuria may cause foaming and obscure test reaction with copper reduction tests)

Uric acid, high level of excretion
(may cause false positives with copper reduction tests and false negatives with glucose oxidase tests)

Urinary pigments, excessive
(excessive urinary pigments, such as in hyperbilirubinemia, may mask color changes for *Tes-tape* and *Chemstrip* products)

Urine concentration
(urine glucose tests will give falsely high values in concentrated urine, as when patients are dehydrated; test results may be falsely low in dilute urine, as when patients are diuresing or intake of water is increased to produce a urine specimen)

*Due to test procedures*
Household cleanser and/or bleach contamination
(chloride-, hypochlorite-, and hydrogen peroxide–containing products may cause false-positive reactions with glucose oxidase products; use of a urine container with cleaning-product residues or laying a test strip on lavatory surface may cause this type of interference)

Imprecise timing
(accurate reading of results depends on precise timing of the readings. The copper reduction method is prone to a "pass-through" phenomenon—that is, if the test is allowed to sit before reading, the color may revert to a bluer shade, resulting in a falsely low reading. Other tests should also be read at the time interval indicated for most accurate results)

Improper urine sample collection
(in some cases, a double-voided sample may be recommended. To do this, the patient should empty the bladder completely, wait 30 minutes, and void a sample for testing. Incomplete emptying will not give an accurate result. However, drinking a full glass of water, as may be advised for producing the second sample, will result in a diluted sample, which will give a falsely depressed test result)

(for an evaluation of blood glucose levels over the hours since the last voiding, the first voiding should be tested. Diabetics and their caregivers should understand the difference in use of the first-void and second-void tests, and when each type of test is to be used)

Inaccurate measurement
(the copper reduction tests require accurate count of the number of drops of urine and water for each type of test; size of drop can be changed by angle at which dropper is held, and tapping dropper against the side of the test tube also causes errors in measurement)

Urine that has been stored
(bacterial action may break down glucose in samples held for testing, depressing the apparent glucose reading. Patients should be advised to test the urine no later than 30 minutes after the time of collection and that the urine sample should not be refrigerated)

User vision impairment
(poor lighting, poor vision, or color-blindness may cause inaccurate reading. This may be especially significant with elderly patients or patients suffering from diabetic retinopathy)

## Patient Consultation

As an aid to patient consultation, refer to *Advice for the Patient, Urine Glucose and Ketone Test Kits for Home Use.*

In providing consultation, consider emphasizing the following selected information (» = major clinical significance):

**Before using this test**
Arranging for assistance if color-blind or visually impaired
Avoiding medicines and foods that may interfere with test results, unless otherwise directed by physician
» Conditions affecting use, especially:

**Proper use of this test**
Not switching products without advice of diabetes care professional; product color charts vary somewhat, and some tests react differently with extraneous substances
Using test as recommended by doctor, nurse, or diabetes educator
Using the appropriate sampling technique
Carefully following the instructions for the specific test used; consulting a health care professional for any questions
» Proper storage

**Follow-up**
Recording results and using to make appropriate adjustments in diabetes medication or diet as directed by diabetes care provider or to seek medical attention if necessary
Importance of reporting results or symptoms not covered in management protocols promptly to physician for definitive diagnosis and treatment

### COPPER REDUCTION URINE GLUCOSE TEST

## Diagnostic Product Forms
### COPPER REDUCTION URINE GLUCOSE TEST

**Use**
Place tablet in clean, dry test tube. A specified number of drops of urine and specified number of drops of tap water are added to the test tube. A vigorous exothermic reaction will occur. The resultant liquid will be strongly colored in a shade between blue and orange. It should be compared with the color chart on the container 15 seconds after boiling stops to derive a percentage concentration of glucose in the urine.

**Product(s) usually available**
U.S.—
Tablets [*Clinitest*].
Canada—
Tablets [*Clinitest*].

**Packaging and storage**
Store below 30 °C. Avoid excess humidity. Keep in original container, tightly closed. Keep out of the reach of children.

**Note**
Toxic—May be harmful or fatal if swallowed.

### GLUCOSE OXIDASE URINE GLUCOSE TEST

## Diagnostic Product Forms
### GLUCOSE OXIDASE URINE GLUCOSE TEST

**Use**
Dip test strip into freshly voided urine sample for no longer than 1 second, or hold test strip directly in urine stream. Tap off excess. When using the tape, the end held in fingers should be kept dry. Observe for change of color, usually deepening shade of blue, which develops in 60 seconds. Compare with color chart on container or instruction sheet. Ignore color change that develops after 3 minutes.

**Product(s) usually available**
U.S.—
Strips [*Biotel/diabetes; Chemstrip uG; Clinistix; Diastix*].
Tape [*Tes-tape*].
Canada—
Strips [*Clinistix; Diastix*].
Tape [*Tes-tape*].

**Packaging and storage**
Store between 15 and 30 °C (59 to 86 °F). Do not refrigerate. Keep in original container, tightly closed after each use.

**Stability**
Use tape products within 4 months of opening.

### NITROPRUSSIDE URINE KETONE TEST

## Diagnostic Product Forms
### NITROPRUSSIDE URINE KETONE TEST

**Use**
*Strips:* Dip strip pad in freshly voided urine (1 second), or hold directly in urine stream. Tap off excess. Wait for time specified in individual product (30 seconds to 2 minutes, depending on product). Observe for color change from beige to deeper shades of violet, comparing to color chart on original container.
*Tablets:* Place tablet on clean, dry surface such as a paper towel. Tablet may be crushed. Place two drops of urine on tablet, allowing each drop to soak in. Observe for color change from beige to violet in 15 seconds, comparing to color chart on original container.

## Product(s) usually available
U.S.—
Strips [*Chemstrip K; KetoStix*].
Tablets [*Acetest*].
Canada—
Strips [*KetoStix*].
Tablets [*Acetest*].

## Packaging and storage
Store below 30 °C (86 °F). Keep in original container, tightly closed. Do not refrigerate or freeze. Avoid excess humidity and direct sunlight.

---

## *URINE GLUCOSE AND KETONE (COMBINED) TEST*

## Diagnostic Product Forms
### URINE GLUCOSE AND KETONE (COMBINED) TEST
**Use**
Dip strip in freshly voided urine, or hold directly in urine stream. Tap off excess. Read by comparing test areas with color chart on container at times specified. (For example, *Keto-diastix* ketone pad is to be read at exactly 15 seconds, and the glucose pad is to be read at exactly 30 seconds.)

## Product(s) usually available
U.S.—
Strips [*Chemstrip uGK; Glucose & Ketone Urine Test; Keto-diastix*].
Canada—
Strips [*Chemstrip uGK; Keto-diastix*].

## Packaging and storage
Store below 30 °C (86 °F). Keep in original container, tightly closed. Do not refrigerate or freeze. Avoid excess humidity and direct sunlight.

---

Revised: 10/26/92
Interim revision: 07/12/94

---

# UROFOLLITROPIN   Systemic

VA CLASSIFICATION (Primary): HS400
Note: Controlled substance in some states in the U.S.—Schedule IV.

Another commonly used name is follicle-stimulating hormone (FSH).

Note: For a listing of dosage forms and brand names by country availability, see *Dosage Forms* section(s). For a listing of brand names for the articles in this monograph, refer to the General Index.

## Category
Gonadotropin; infertility therapy adjunct.

## Indications
### Accepted
Infertility, female (treatment)—Urofollitropin is indicated, in conjunction with human chorionic gonadotropin (hCG), for stimulation of ovulation and induction of pregnancy in patients with polycystic ovary syndrome who have an elevated luteinizing hormone/follicle-stimulating hormone (LH/FSH) ratio and who have failed to respond to adequate clomiphene citrate therapy. Urofollitropin is not useful in patients with primary ovarian failure.

Reproductive technologies, assisted[1]—Urofollitropin is indicated, in conjunction with hCG, to stimulate the development of multiple oocytes in ovulatory patients who are attempting to conceive by means of assisted reproductive technologies, such as gamete intrafallopian transfer (GIFT) or *in vitro* fertilization (IVF).

---

[1]Not included in Canadian product labeling.

## Pharmacology/Pharmacokinetics
### Physicochemical characteristics
Source—Extracted from urine of postmenopausal women.

### Mechanism of action/Effect
Urofollitropin contains follicle-stimulating hormone (FSH). The combination of FSH and luteinizing hormone (LH) stimulates follicular growth and maturation. Chorionic gonadotropin (hCG), whose actions are nearly identical to those of LH, is administered following urofollitropin to mimic the naturally occurring surge of LH that triggers ovulation.

## Precautions to Consider
### Carcinogenicity
Long-term studies have not been done in animals to evaluate the carcinogenic potential of urofollitropin.

### Pregnancy/Reproduction
Fertility—Use of urofollitropin to stimulate ovulation is associated with a high incidence of multiple gestations and births. As a result, the risk of neonatal prematurity, as well as other complications associated with multiple gestations may increase.

Pregnancy—Although problems in humans have not been documented, use of urofollitropin during pregnancy is unnecessary.

Ovarian hyperstimulation syndrome (OHS), which may be induced by urofollitropin therapy, is more common, more severe, and protracted in patients who conceive.

FDA Pregnancy Category X.

### Breast-feeding
It is not known whether urofollitropin is distributed into breast milk. However, urofollitropin is not indicated during the course of breast-feeding.

### Medical considerations/Contraindications
The medical considerations/contraindications included here have been selected on the basis of their potential clinical significance (reasons given in parentheses where appropriate)—not necessarily inclusive (» = major clinical significance).

*Except under special circumstances, this medication should not be used when the following medical problems exist:*
» Abnormal vaginal bleeding, undiagnosed
(may indicate the presence of endometrial hyperplasia or carcinoma, which may be exacerbated by urofollitropin-induced increases in estrogen serum concentrations; other possible endocrinopathies should also be ruled out)
» Ovarian cyst or enlargement not associated with polycystic ovary syndrome
(risk of further enlargement)

*Risk-benefit should be considered when the following medical problem exists:*
Sensitivity to urofollitropin or other gonadotropins

### Patient monitoring
The following may be especially important in patient monitoring (other tests may be warranted in some patients, depending on condition; » = major clinical significance):
» Estradiol
(measurement of serum concentrations is recommended as needed, continuing through the day of chorionic gonadotropin administration; recommended to determine optimal dose and to lessen the risk of ovarian hyperstimulation syndrome)
» Ultrasound examination
(recommended during urofollitropin therapy and prior to administration of chorionic gonadotropin to provide information on the number and size of mature follicles, to follow follicular development, and to lessen the risk of ovarian hyperstimulation syndrome and multiple gestation)
Daily basal body temperature
(can be used to determine if ovulation has occurred; pregnancy test is recommended if basal body temperature following a cycle of treatment is biphasic and not followed by menses)
Progesterone
(measurement of serum or urine concentrations can be used prior to urofollitropin therapy to confirm anovulation; serum concentrations can be used after urofollitropin therapy to detect luteinized ovarian follicles)

# Side/Adverse Effects

Note: Thromboembolism has not been reported in patients who have received urofollitropin, but has occurred with menotropins (LH/FSH) both in association with and separate from ovarian hyperstimulation syndrome. Complications resulting from thromboembolism have included venous thrombophlebitis, pulmonary embolism, pulmonary infarction, stroke, arterial occlusion necessitating limb amputation, and (rarely) death.

Serious respiratory complications have not been reported in patients who have received urofollitropin, but have occurred with menotropins (LH/FSH) therapy. These conditions included atelectasis and acute respiratory distress syndrome. Rarely, death has resulted.

The following side/adverse effects have been selected on the basis of their potential clinical significance (possible signs and symptoms in parentheses where appropriate)—not necessarily inclusive:

**Those indicating need for medical attention**
Incidence more frequent—about 10 to 20%
> *Uncomplicated, mild to moderate ovarian enlargement or ovarian cysts* (mild bloating, abdominal or pelvic pain); *redness, pain, or swelling at injection site*

> Note: *Ovarian enlargement* is usually mild to moderate and abates within 2 or 3 weeks. *Ovarian cysts* have also occurred, though less frequently.

Incidence less frequent or rare
> *Severe ovarian hyperstimulation syndrome* (severe abdominal or stomach pain; feeling of indigestion; moderate to severe bloating; decreased amount of urine; continuing or severe nausea, vomiting, or diarrhea; severe pelvic pain; rapid weight gain; swelling of lower legs; shortness of breath); *fever and chills; skin rash or hives*

> Note: In clinical trials, *ovarian hyperstimulation syndrome (OHS)* occurred in 6% of patients treated with urofollitropin for anovulation due to polycystic ovary syndrome and 0.25% of patients given urofollitropin for *in vitro* fertilization. OHS may often occur 7 to 10 days after ovulation or completion of therapy. OHS differs from uncomplicated ovarian enlargement and can rapidly progress to cause serious medical problems. With OHS, a marked increase in vascular permeability results in rapid accumulation of fluid in the peritoneal, pleural, and pericardial cavities (third-spacing of fluids). Medical complications ultimately arising from this increased vascular permeability may include hypovolemia, hemoconcentration, electrolyte imbalance, ascites, hemoperitoneum, pleural effusions, hydrothorax, acute pulmonary distress, and thromboembolic events. OHS is more common, more severe, and protracted in patients who conceive.

**Those indicating need for medical attention only if they continue or are bothersome**
Incidence less frequent or rare
> *Breast tenderness; diarrhea, mild; nausea; vomiting*

# Patient Consultation

As an aid to patient consultation, refer to *Advice for the Patient, Urofollitropin (Systemic)*.

In providing consultation, consider emphasizing the following selected information (» = major clinical significance):

**Before using this medication**
» Conditions affecting use, especially:
  Sensitivity to urofollitropin or other gonadotropins
  Other medical problems, especially abnormal vaginal bleeding or ovarian cyst or enlargement

**Proper use of this medication**
» Proper dosing

**Precautions while using this medication**
» Importance of close monitoring by physician
» Importance of following physician's instructions for recording of basal body temperature and timing of intercourse, when recommended by physician

**Side/adverse effects**
Signs of potential side effects, especially ovarian cysts, enlargement, or hyperstimulation syndrome

# General Dosing Information

Patients receiving urofollitropin should be under the supervision of a physician experienced in the treatment of gynecologic or endocrine disorders.

Dosage varies considerably and must be adjusted to meet the individual requirements of each patient, on the basis of clinical response.

Conception should be attempted within 48 hours of administration of hCG. It is recommended that the couple have intercourse or insemination be performed daily beginning the day after hCG is administered, until ovulation is thought to have occurred.

If ovulation does not occur after any cycle of therapy, the therapeutic regimen employed should be re-evaluated. After 3 to 6 cycles of nonovulatory menses, the appropriateness of continuing the use of urofollitropin for ovulation induction should be reconsidered.

**For treatment of adverse effects**
Ovarian enlargement or ovarian cyst formation
  • Discontinuing therapy until ovarian size has returned to baseline. Human chorionic gonadotropin should also be withheld for that cycle.
  • Prohibiting intercourse until ovarian size has returned to baseline to prevent cyst rupture.
  • Reducing dosage in next course of therapy.
Ovarian hyperstimulation syndrome (OHS)—
  Acute phase:
  • Discontinuing therapy.
  • Prohibiting intercourse until ovarian size has returned to baseline to prevent cyst rupture.
  • Most cases of OHS will spontaneously resolve when menses begins. In selected cases, hospitalization of the patient and bed rest may be necessary.
  • Utilizing therapy to prevent hemoconcentration and minimize risk of thromboembolism and renal injury.
  • Correcting (cautiously) electrolyte imbalance while maintaining acceptable intravascular volume; in the acute phase, intravascular volume deficit cannot be completely corrected without increasing third space fluid volume.
  • Monitoring fluid intake and output, body weight, hematocrit, serum and urine electrolytes, urine specific gravity, blood urea nitrogen (BUN), creatinine, and abdominal girth daily or as often as required.
  • Monitoring serum potassium concentrations for development of hyperkalemia.
  • Limiting performance of pelvic examinations since they may result in rupture of ovarian cysts and hemoperitoneum.
  • Administering intravenous fluids, electrolytes, and human serum albumin as needed to maintain adequate urine output and to avoid hemoconcentration.
  • Administering analgesics as needed.
  • Avoiding diuretic use since it reduces intravascular volume further.
  • Removing ascitic, pleural, or pericardial fluid *only* if it is imperative for relief of symptoms such as respiratory distress or cardiac tamponade; to do so may increase risk of injury to the ovary.
  • In patients who require surgery to control bleeding from ovarian cyst rupture, employing surgical measures that also maximally conserve ovarian tissue.
  Intermediate phase:
  • Once patient is stabilized, minimizing third-spacing of fluids by cautiously replacing potassium, sodium, and fluids as required, based on monitoring of serum electrolyte concentrations.
  • Avoiding diuretic use.
  Resolution phase:
  • The third space fluid shifts to intravascular compartment, resulting in decreased hematocrit value and increased urinary output.
  • Peripheral and/or pulmonary edema may result if third space fluid volume mobilized exceeds renal output.
  • Administering diuretics when required, to manage pulmonary edema.

# Parenteral Dosage Forms

## UROFOLLITROPIN FOR INJECTION

**Usual adult dose**
Infertility therapy adjunct—
  Polycystic ovary syndrome: Intramuscular, 75 Units once a day, usually for seven or more days, followed by 5000 to 10,000 Units of human chorionic gonadotropin (hCG) one day after the last dose of urofollitropin. If necessary, the dosage may then be increased to 150 Units once a day, usually for seven or more days.
Reproductive technologies, assisted[1]—
  Intramuscular, 150 Units once a day, beginning in the early follicular phase (cycle Day 2 or 3), until sufficient follicular development occurs, followed by 5000 to 10,000 Units of hCG one day after the last dose of urofollitropin.

Note: Dosage regimen may vary according to physician preference or patient response.

If the ovaries are abnormally enlarged or if serum estradiol concentrations are excessively elevated on the last day of urofollitropin therapy, human chorionic gonadotropin should not be given for that cycle.

### Size(s) usually available
U.S.—
   75 Units (Rx) [*Metrodin*].
Canada—
   75 Units (Rx) [*Metrodin*].

### Packaging and storage
Store between 3 and 25 °C (37 and 77 °F), unless otherwise specified by manufacturer. Protect from light.

### Preparation of dosage form
Using standard aseptic technique, reconstitute by adding 1 to 2 mL of sodium chloride injection to the contents of 1 ampul.

### Stability
Use immediately after reconstitution; discard any unused portion.

[1]Not included in Canadian product labeling.

Revised: 07/08/92
Interim revision: 06/30/94

---

**UROKINASE**—See *Thrombolytic Agents (Systemic)*

---

# URSODIOL   Systemic

INN: Ursodeoxycholic acid
BAN: Ursodeoxycholic acid
VA CLASSIFICATION (Primary): GA900
Note: For a listing of dosage forms and brand names by country availability, see *Dosage Forms* section(s). For a listing of brand names for the articles in this monograph, refer to the General Index.

---

## Category
Anticholelithic.

## Indications
Note: Bracketed information in the *Indications* section refers to uses that are not included in U.S. product labeling.

### Accepted
Gallstone disease (treatment)—Orally administered ursodiol is indicated for dissolution of cholesterol gallstones in selected patients with uncomplicated radiolucent gallstone disease. However, alternative therapies should be considered since gallstone dissolution with ursodiol may require many months of treatment, complete dissolution does not occur in all patients, and recurrence of stones occurs within 5 years in about 50% of patients who have had stones dissolved by use of bile acid therapy.

Ursodiol therapy is more likely to be effective if the stones are small (<20 mm) and of the floatable type.

Body weight and dietary factors may influence gallstone formation and/or dissolution rate.

[Atresia, biliary (treatment)][1]
[Cholangitis, sclerosing (treatment)][1]
[Cirrhosis, alcoholic (treatment)][1]
[Cirrhosis, biliary (treatment)][1]
[Hepatic disease, cholestatic, chronic (treatment)][1]
[Hepatic disease, cystic fibrosis–associated (treatment)][1] and
[Hepatitis, chronic (treatment)][1]—Ursodiol is used for the treatment of some chronic liver diseases, including primary biliary cirrhosis, primary sclerosing cholangitis, cystic fibrosis–associated liver disease, biliary atresia, chronic hepatitis, and alcoholic cirrhosis.

[Transplant rejection, liver (prophylaxis)][1]—Ursodiol is used as adjuvant therapy following orthotopic liver transplantation to prevent early graft rejection.

[Gallstone formation (prophylaxis)][1]—Ursodiol is used in the prevention of gallstone formation in obese patients during rapid weight loss.

### Unaccepted
Ursodiol is *not* indicated when there are calcified cholesterol stones, radiopaque stones (calcium-containing), or radiolucent bile pigment stones, or when surgery is clearly indicated.

---

[1]Not included in Canadian product labeling.

## Pharmacology/Pharmacokinetics

### Physicochemical characteristics
Molecular weight—392.58.

### Mechanism of action/Effect
Anticholelithic—Although the exact mechanism of ursodiol's anticholelithic action is not completely understood, it is known that when administered orally ursodiol is concentrated in bile and decreases biliary cholesterol saturation by suppressing hepatic synthesis and secretion of cholesterol, and by inhibiting its intestinal absorption. The reduced cholesterol saturation permits the gradual solubilization of cholesterol from gallstones, resulting in their eventual dissolution.

### Other actions/effects
Ursodiol increases bile flow. In chronic liver disease, ursodiol appears to reduce the detergent properties of the bile salts, thus reducing their cytotoxicity. Also, ursodiol may protect liver cells from the damaging activity of toxic bile acids (e.g., lithocholate, deoxycholate, and chenodeoxycholate), which increase in concentration in patients with chronic liver disease.

### Absorption
Absorbed from the small bowel (about 90% of dose).

### Protein binding
High.

### Biotransformation
Hepatic (first-pass hepatic clearance). Exogenous ursodiol is metabolized in the liver to its taurine and glycine conjugates. The resulting conjugates are secreted into bile.

### Time to peak concentration
1 to 3 hours.

### Elimination
Primarily fecal; very small amounts are excreted into urine. Small amount of unabsorbed ursodiol passes into the colon where it undergoes bacterial degradation (7-dehydroxylation); the resulting lithocholic acid is partly absorbed from the colon but is sulfated in the liver and rapidly eliminated in the feces as the sulfolithocholyl glycine or sulfolithocholyl taurine conjugate.

## Precautions to Consider

### Cross-sensitivity and/or related problems
Patients sensitive to other bile acids products may be sensitive to ursodiol also.

### Carcinogenicity/Tumorigenicity
Studies in rats with intrarectal instillation of lithocholic acid and other metabolites of ursodiol and chenodiol did not show tumorigenicity, except when these substances were administered in conjunction with a carcinogenic agent. Epidemiologic studies suggest that bile acids might be involved in the pathogenesis of human colon cancer in patients who have undergone a cholecystectomy; however, conclusive evidence is lacking.

### Pregnancy/Reproduction
Pregnancy—Adequate and well-controlled studies have not been done in humans.

Studies in rats at doses 20 to 100 times the human dose, and in rabbits at doses 5 times the human dose, have not shown that ursodiol causes adverse effects in the fetus.

FDA Pregnancy Category B.

### Breast-feeding
It is not known whether ursodiol is distributed into breast milk. However, problems in humans have not been documented.

### Pediatrics
Appropriate studies on the relationship of age to the effects of ursodiol when used as an anticholelithic have not been performed in the pediatric population. However, studies performed to date in children and infants with cholestatic liver disease and biliary atresia have not dem-

onstrated pediatrics-specific problems that would limit the usefulness
of ursodiol in children.

### Geriatrics
Appropriate studies on the relationship of age to the effects of ursodiol
have not been performed in the geriatric population. However, geriatrics-specific problems that would limit the usefulness of this medication in the elderly are not expected.

### Drug interactions and/or related problems
The following drug interactions and/or related problems have been selected on the basis of their potential clinical significance (possible
mechanism in parentheses where appropriate)—not necessarily inclusive (» = major clinical significance):

Note:  Combinations containing any of the following medications, depending on the amount present, may also interact with this
medication.

Antacids, aluminum-containing or
Cholestyramine or
Colestipol
(concurrent use may result in binding of ursodiol, thus decreasing
its absorption)
Antihyperlipidemics, especially clofibrate or
Estrogens or
Neomycin or
Progestins
(concurrent use of these medications with ursodiol may decrease
ursodiol's ability to dissolve cholesterol gallstones, since these
medications tend to increase cholesterol saturation of bile)

### Laboratory value alterations
The following have been selected on the basis of their potential clinical
significance (possible effect in parentheses where appropriate)—not
necessarily inclusive (» = major clinical significance):

With physiology/laboratory test values
Transaminase (mainly serum alanine aminotransferase [SGPT])
(although this effect has not been clearly demonstrated, serum concentrations of liver enzymes may be increased due to the inability
of some patients to form sulfate conjugates of lithocholic acid;
however, these concentrations may be decreased in patients with
primary biliary cirrhosis and other cholestatic conditions, as well
as in chronic active hepatitis)

### Medical considerations/Contraindications
The medical considerations/contraindications included here have been selected on the basis of their potential clinical significance (reasons given
in parentheses where appropriate)—not necessarily inclusive (» =
major clinical significance).

*Risk-benefit should be considered when the following medical problems
exist:*
» Gallstone complications, such as:
Biliary gastrointestinal fistula
Biliary obstruction
Cholangitis
Cholecystitis
Pancreatitis
(medical treatment with ursodiol would be too lengthy; surgery
may be indicated)
Hepatic function impairment, chronic
(bile acid metabolism may be further impaired; however, in some
studies ursodiol caused a return of abnormal liver tests toward
normal. Data seem to indicate a possible therapeutic role for ursodiol in chronic cholestatic liver disease, in which cholestasis
[bile toxicity] appears to play an important role)
Sensitivity to ursodiol or to other bile acids

### Patient monitoring
The following may be especially important in patient monitoring (other
tests may be warranted in some patients, depending on condition;
» = major clinical significance):

Hepatic function determinations
(monitoring of serum transaminase concentrations [SGOT and
SGPT] is recommended upon initiation of treatment to rule out
pre-existing liver disease, and during treatment as indicated by the
particular clinical circumstances; ursodiol must be discontinued if
increased concentrations persist)
Ultrasonograms
(recommended prior to treatment to determine the presence of gallbladder stones, and at 6-month intervals during the first year of
treatment to monitor stone dissolution; also recommended after
gallstone dissolution to monitor for possible recurrence)

## Side/Adverse Effects
Note:  Hepatotoxicity has not been associated with ursodiol therapy. However, in some individuals with a congenital or acquired reduction
in ability to sulfate hepatotoxic lithocholic acid, the risk of litho-
cholate-induced liver damage may be increased.

The following side/adverse effects have been selected on the basis of their
potential clinical significance (possible signs and symptoms in parentheses where appropriate)—not necessarily inclusive:

**Those indicating need for medical attention only if they continue
or are bothersome**
Incidence less frequent or rare
*Diarrhea*

## Overdose
For specific information on the agents used in the management of ursodiol
overdose, see:
• *Aluminum Hydroxide* in *Antacids (Oral-Local)* monograph;
• *Charcoal, Activated (Oral-Local)* monograph; and/or
• *Cholestyramine (Oral-Local)* monograph.

For more information on the management of overdose or unintentional
ingestion, **contact a Poison Control Center** (see *Poison Control Center Listing*).

**Treatment of overdose**
Although no cases of ursodiol overdose have been reported, recommended
treatment includes:

Specific treatment—Gastric lavage with at least 1 L of a cholestyramine
or charcoal suspension (concentration of 2 grams per 100 mL of water). Oral administration of 50 mL of aluminum hydroxide suspension.

Supportive care—Patients in whom intentional overdose is confirmed or
suspected should be referred for psychiatric consultation.

## Patient Consultation
As an aid to patient consultation, refer to *Advice for the Patient, Ursodiol
(Systemic)*.

In providing consultation, consider emphasizing the following selected
information (» = major clinical significance):

**Before using this medication**
» Conditions affecting use, especially:
Sensitivity to ursodiol or to other bile acids
Other medical problems, especially gallstone complications

**Proper use of this medication**
Taking with meals for optimal therapeutic effect
» Compliance with full course of therapy
» Proper dosing
Missed dose: Taking as soon as possible or doubling the next dose
» Proper storage

**Precautions while using this medication**
» Regular visits to physician to check progress; laboratory tests may be
required during therapy
Avoiding aluminum-containing antacids; may interfere with absorption
of ursodiol
» Notifying physician immediately if symptoms of acute cholecystitis
develop

## General Dosing Information
Ursodiol should be taken with meals or a snack since it dissolves more
rapidly when bile and pancreatic juice are present in the intestinal
chyme.

Gallstone dissolution may require 6 months to 2 years of continuous dosing depending on the size and composition of the stone (s). Response
should be monitored by ultrasonograms performed at 6-month intervals during the first year of therapy. After complete dissolution, it is
recommended that ursodiol be continued for at least 3 months to promote dissolution of residue when particle size is too small to image.

Ursodiol therapy is unlikely to be effective if partial dissolution has not
occurred after 12 months of treatment.

Although a nonfunctioning (nonvisualized) gallbladder prior to the initiation of therapy is not a contraindication to the use of ursodiol, gallbladder nonvisualization developing during therapy is an indication
that complete stone dissolution will not occur and therapy should be
discontinued.

## Oral Dosage Forms
Note:  Bracketed uses in the *Dosage Forms* section refer to categories of
use and/or indications that are not included in U.S. product labeling.

## URSODIOL CAPSULES

### Usual adult and adolescent dose

Anticholelithic—

Oral, 8 to 10 mg per kg of body weight a day, divided into two or three doses, usually taken with meals.

[Hepatic disease, cholestatic, chronic][1]—

Oral, 8 to 10 mg per kg of body weight a day, divided into one or two doses. Larger doses have been used.

[Gallstone prophylaxis][1]—

Oral, 2 to 10 mg per kg of body weight a day.

### Usual pediatric dose

Anticholelithic—

Dosage has not been established.

Note: In children with cholestatic liver disease and extrahepatic biliary atresia, total daily doses have ranged from 10 to 18 mg per kg of body weight.

### Usual geriatric dose

See *Usual adult and adolescent dose.*

### Strength(s) usually available

U.S.—

300 mg (Rx) [*Actigall*].

Canada—

250 mg (Rx) [*Ursofalk*].

### Packaging and storage

Store below 40 °C (104 °F), preferably between 15 and 30 °C (59 and 86 °F), in a tight container, unless otherwise specified by manufacturer.

### Auxiliary labeling

• Continue medication for full time of treatment.
• Take with food.

[1]Not included in Canadian product labeling.

## Selected Bibliography

Rosenbaum CL, Cluxton RJ. Ursodiol: a cholesterol gallstone solubilizing agent. Drug Intell Clin Pharm 1988; 22: 941-5.

Ward A, Brogden RN, Heel RC, et al. Ursodeoxycholic acid: a review of its pharmacological properties and therapeutic efficacy. Drugs 1984; 27: 95-131.

Revised: 07/26/94

# VALACYCLOVIR    Systemic†

INN: Valaciclovir

VA CLASSIFICATION (Primary): AM800

Note: For a listing of dosage forms and brand names by country availability, see *Dosage Forms* section(s). For a listing of brand names for the articles in this monograph, refer to the General Index.

---

†Not commercially available in Canada.

## Category

Antiviral (systemic).

## Indications

### Accepted

Herpes zoster (treatment)—Valacyclovir is indicated in the treatment of herpes zoster (shingles) infections caused by varicella-zoster virus (VZV) in immunocompetent adults. In patients over 50 years of age, valacyclovir significantly reduced the duration of zoster-associated pain and the duration of postherpetic neuralgia lasting greater than 6 months when compared to acyclovir. Therapy is most effective when started within 48 hours of the onset of rash. There are no data on the safety and effectiveness of valacyclovir in children, immunocompromised patients, or patients with disseminated zoster.

## Pharmacology/Pharmacokinetics

### Physicochemical characteristics

Source—Valacyclovir is the hydrochloride salt of the *L*-valyl ester of acyclovir.

Molecular weight—Valacyclovir: 324.34.

Valacyclovir hydrochloride: 360.80.

### Mechanism of action/Effect

Valacyclovir is a prodrug that is nearly completely converted to acyclovir and *L*-valine. Due to its more efficient phosphorylation by viral thymidine kinase, acyclovir's antiviral activity is greatest against herpes simplex virus type 1 (HSV-1), followed by herpes simplex virus type 2 (HSV-2), varicella-zoster virus (VZV), Epstein-Barr virus (EBV), and cytomegalovirus (CMV).

Acyclovir is phosphorylated by thymidine kinase to acyclovir monophosphate, which is then converted into acyclovir diphosphate and triphosphate by cellular enzymes. Acyclovir is selectively converted to the active triphosphate form by cells infected with herpes viruses. Acyclovir triphosphate inhibits herpes viral DNA replication by competitive inhibition of viral DNA polymerase, and incorporation and termination of the growing viral DNA chain.

### Absorption

Valacyclovir is rapidly absorbed in the gastrointestinal tract; it is then converted to the active compound, acyclovir, by first-pass intestinal and hepatic metabolism. Administration of valacyclovir with food was not found to alter the bioavailability of acyclovir.

The bioavailability of acyclovir following administration of valacyclovir is approximately 54%, which is three to five times greater than its bioavailability following oral administration of acyclovir. After administration of 1 gram of valacyclovir given four times a day, the area under the plasma concentration–time curve (AUC) of acyclovir is approximately that obtained after intravenous administration of 5 mg per kg of body weight of acyclovir every 8 hours.

### Distribution

Acyclovir is widely distributed to tissues and body fluids, including brain, kidneys, lungs, liver, aqueous humor, tears, intestines, muscle, spleen, breast milk, uterus, vaginal mucosa, vaginal secretions, semen, amniotic fluid, cerebrospinal fluid (CSF), and herpetic vesicular fluid. Highest concentrations are found in the kidneys, liver, and intestines. Acyclovir concentrations in the CSF are approximately 50% of plasma concentrations. In addition, acyclovir crosses the placenta.

### Protein binding

Valacyclovir—Low (13 to 18%).

Acyclovir—Low (9 to 33%).

### Biotransformation

Valacyclovir is rapidly and nearly completely (99%) converted to the active compound, acyclovir, and *L*-valine by first-pass intestinal and hepatic metabolism by enzymatic hydrolysis. Acyclovir is converted to inactive metabolites by alcohol and aldehyde dehydrogenase and, to a small extent, by aldehyde oxidase. The metabolism of valacyclovir and acyclovir is not associated with hepatic microsomal enzyme systems.

### Half-life

Valacyclovir—

Less than 30 minutes.

Acyclovir—

After administration of valacyclovir:

Normal renal function—2.5 to 3.3 hours.

End-stage renal disease—Approximately 14 hours.

Geriatric patients (65 to 83 years of age)—3.3 to 3.7 hours.

### Time to peak concentration

1.6 to 2.1 hours.

### Peak plasma concentrations

Valacyclovir—

Plasma concentrations of unconverted valacyclovir are low, with peak concentrations of less than 0.5 mcg per mL (mcg/mL) after any dose. Plasma concentrations are nonquantifiable within 3 hours after administration.

Acyclovir—

Peak plasma concentrations are not proportional to the dose. The following peak plasma concentrations have been found:

After a single dose of valacyclovir:

500 mg: Approximately 3.3 mcg/mL.

1 gram: 4.8 to 5.6 mcg/mL.

After multiple doses of valacyclovir:

500 mg: Approximately 3.7 mcg/mL.

1 gram: 5 to 5.5 mcg/mL.

### Elimination

Valacyclovir—

Less than 1% of valacyclovir is recovered unchanged in the urine over 24 hours.

In dialysis:

It is not known if peritoneal dialysis removes valacyclovir from the blood.

Acyclovir—

Renal; acyclovir accounts for 80 to 89% of the total urinary recovery. There was no accumulation of acyclovir after repeated administration of valacyclovir in patients with normal renal function.

In dialysis:

Hemodialysis—During a 4-hour hemodialysis session, approximately one-third of acyclovir in the body is removed. The half-life of acyclovir is approximately 4 hours during hemodialysis.

Peritoneal dialysis—Chronic ambulatory peritoneal dialysis (CAPD) and continuous arteriovenous hemofiltration/dialysis (CAVHD) do not substantially remove acyclovir, with pharmacokinetic parameters resembling those observed in patients with end-stage renal disease not receiving hemodialysis.

## Precautions to Consider

### Carcinogenicity/Tumorigenicity

Valacyclovir was found to be noncarcinogenic in lifetime carcinogenicity bioassays at single daily doses of up to 120 mg per kg of body weight (mg/kg) per day for mice and 100 mg/kg per day for rats. There was no significant difference in the incidence of tumors between mice and rats treated with valacyclovir and control animals; also, valacyclovir did not shorten the latency of tumors. Plasma concentrations of acyclovir were equivalent to human levels in the mouse bioassay and 1.4 to 2.3 times human levels in the rat bioassay.

### Mutagenicity

An *in vitro* cytogenetic study with human lymphocytes, a rat cytogenetic study after a single oral dose of 3000 mg/kg (8 to 9 times human plasma levels), and Ames assays in the presence or absence of metabolic activation were all negative. Valacyclovir was also negative in the mouse lymphoma assay in the absence of metabolic activation. In the presence of metabolic activation (76 to 88% conversion to acyclovir), valacyclovir was weakly mutagenic. A mouse micronucleus assay was negative at 250 mg/kg, but weakly positive at 500 mg/kg (acyclovir concentrations of 26 to 51 times human plasma levels, respectively).

### Pregnancy/Reproduction

Fertility—Valacyclovir did not impair fertility in rats given a dose of 200 mg/kg per day (6 times human plasma levels).

Pregnancy—Acyclovir crosses the placenta. No adequate and well-controlled studies have been done with either valacyclovir or acyclovir in pregnant women. A prospective epidemiologic registry of acyclovir use during pregnancy from 1984 to December 1994 has documented 380 women with live births who were exposed to systemic acyclovir during the first trimester of pregnancy. The rate of birth defects in this group approximates that found in the general population. However, it is thought that the small size of the registry is insufficient to evaluate the risk for less common defects or to make definitive conclusions about the safety of acyclovir in developing fetuses.

FDA Pregnancy Category B.

### Breast-feeding
It is not known whether valacyclovir is distributed into breast milk. However, acyclovir has been found to pass into breast milk at concentrations ranging from 0.6 to 4.1 times the corresponding plasma concentration. At these concentrations, a nursing infant could potentially be exposed to a dose of acyclovir as high as 0.3 mg/kg per day.

### Pediatrics
No information is available on the relationship of age to the effects of valacyclovir in pediatric patients. Safety and efficacy have not been established.

### Geriatrics
Studies performed to date have not demonstrated geriatric-specific problems that would limit the usefulness of valacyclovir in the elderly. However, elderly patients are more likely to have an age-related decrease in renal function, which may require an adjustment of valacyclovir dosage or dosing interval.

### Drug interactions and/or related problems
The following drug interactions and/or related problems have been selected on the basis of their potential clinical significance (possible mechanism in parentheses where appropriate)—not necessarily inclusive (» = major clinical significance):

Note: Combinations containing any of the following medications, depending on the amount present, may also interact with this medication.

Cimetidine and
Probenecid
 (cimetidine and probenecid have been found to decrease the rate, but not the extent, of conversion of valacyclovir to acyclovir; the renal clearance of acyclovir was reduced by approximately 24 and 33% by cimetidine and probenecid, respectively, resulting in an increase in the peak plasma concentration of acyclovir by approximately 8 and 22%, respectively; combined use of cimetidine and probenecid resulted in a reduced renal clearance of acyclovir by approximately 46% and an increase in the peak plasma concentration by approximately 30%)

### Medical considerations/Contraindications
The medical considerations/contraindications included here have been selected on the basis of their potential clinical significance (reasons given in parentheses where appropriate)—not necessarily inclusive (» = major clinical significance).

*Risk-benefit should be considered when the following medical problems exist:*

» Bone marrow transplantation or
» Human immunodeficiency virus (HIV) infection, advanced or
» Renal transplantation
 (thrombotic thrombocytopenic purpura/hemolytic uremic syndrome [TTP/HUS] has been reported in patients with these conditions who were taking high doses of valacyclovir for prolonged periods of time; in rare cases, death has occurred; therefore, valacyclovir is not indicated in immunocompromised patients; however, TTP/HUS has not been seen in immunocompetent patients treated with valacyclovir)

Hepatic function impairment
 (the rate, but not the extent, of conversion of valacyclovir to acyclovir is reduced in patients with moderate or severe liver disease [biopsy-proven cirrhosis]; however, the half-life of acyclovir is not affected and dosage modification is not recommended for patients with cirrhosis)

» Hypersensitivity to valacyclovir or acyclovir
» Renal function impairment
 (because valacyclovir is renally excreted, patients with renal function impairment may be at increased risk of toxicity; patients with a creatinine clearance of < 50 mL/min [< 0.83 mL/sec] require a reduction in dose)

## Side/Adverse Effects

Note: No serious side effects have been noted to date with the administration of valacyclovir in immunocompetent adults.

The following side/adverse effects have been selected on the basis of their potential clinical significance (possible signs and symptoms in parentheses where appropriate)—not necessarily inclusive:

### Those indicating need for medical attention only if they continue or are bothersome
Incidence more frequent
 *Headache; nausea*
Incidence less frequent
 *Dizziness; fatigue* (unusual tiredness or weakness); *gastrointestinal disturbances* (constipation; diarrhea; loss of appetite; stomach pain; vomiting)

## Overdose
For more information on the management of overdose or unintentional ingestion, **contact a Poison Control Center** (see *Poison Control Center Listing*).

### Clinical effects of overdose
To date, there have been no reports of overdosage with valacyclovir. However, precipitation of acyclovir in the renal tubules has occurred with rapid or high intravenous doses of acyclovir. No significant adverse effects have been seen with oral overdoses of acyclovir of up to 20 grams. If acute renal failure or anuria occurs, hemodialysis may be helpful until renal function is restored.

## Patient Consultation
As an aid to patient consultation, refer to *Advice for the Patient, Valacyclovir (Systemic)*.

In providing consultation, consider emphasizing the following selected information (» = major clinical significance):

### Before using this medication
» Conditions affecting use, especially:
 Hypersensitivity to valacyclovir or acyclovir
 Other medical problems, especially advanced human immunodeficiency virus infection, bone marrow transplantation, renal function impairment, or renal transplantation

### Proper use of this medication
» Initiating use of valacyclovir at the earliest sign or symptom; it is most effective when started within 48 hours of the onset of rash, pain, or burning
 Valacyclovir may be taken with meals
» Compliance with full course of therapy; not using more often or for longer than prescribed
» Proper dosing
 Missed dose: Taking as soon as possible; not taking if almost time for next dose; not doubling doses
» Proper storage

### Precautions while using this medication
 Checking with physician if no improvement within a few days
 Keeping affected areas as clean and dry as possible; wearing loose-fitting clothing to avoid irritating the lesions

### Side/adverse effects
 No side/adverse effects that indicate the need for prompt medical attention have been reported

## General Dosing Information
Therapy should be initiated as soon as possible following the onset of signs and symptoms of varicella-zoster infection. In clinical studies, treatment was started within 72 hours of the onset of rash; however, valacyclovir was found to be more useful if started within 48 hours.

Valacyclovir may be taken with meals since absorption has not been shown to be significantly affected by food.

Adults with impaired renal function may require a change in dosing, as follows:

| Creatinine Clearance (mL/min)/ (mL/sec) | Recommended dose |
| --- | --- |
| ≥50/0.83 | 1 gram every 8 hours |
| 30–49/0.50–0.82 | 1 gram every 12 hours |
| 10–29/0.17–0.48 | 1 gram every 24 hours |
| <10/0.17 | 500 mg every 24 hours |

## Oral Dosage Forms
Note: The dosing and strengths of the dosage forms available are expressed in terms of valacyclovir base (not the hydrochloride salt).

## VALACYCLOVIR HYDROCHLORIDE TABLETS

**Usual adult dose**
Antiviral—
    Oral, 1 gram (base) three times a day for seven days.

**Usual pediatric dose**
Safety and efficacy have not been established.

**Usual geriatric dose**
See *Usual adult dose.*

**Strength(s) usually available**
U.S.—
    500 mg (base) (Rx) [*Valtrex*].

Canada—
    Not commercially available.

**Packaging and storage**
Store between 15 and 25 °C (59 and 77 °F), in a tight container. Protect from light.

**Auxiliary labeling**
• Continue medicine for full time of treatment.

Developed: 05/28/96

---

# VALPROIC ACID    Systemic

This monograph includes information on the following: Divalproex; Valproic Acid.
VA CLASSIFICATION (Primary/Secondary):
    Divalproex—CN400/CN105; CN900
    Valproic Acid—CN400
Note: For a listing of dosage forms and brand names by country availability, see *Dosage Forms* section(s). For a listing of brand names for the articles in this monograph, refer to the General Index.

## Category

Anticonvulsant; antimanic; migraine headache prophylactic.

## Indications

Note: Bracketed information in the *Indications* section refers to uses that are not included in U.S. product labeling.

**Accepted**

Epilepsy, absence seizure pattern (treatment)—Valproic acid and divalproex are indicated in the treatment of simple and complex absence (petit mal) seizures. Although these agents may be used alone or with other anticonvulsant medication, monotherapy with valproic acid or divalproex is preferred whenever possible because of unpredictable interactions with hepatic enzyme–inducing anticonvulsants and because of the increased risk of hepatotoxicity.

Epilepsy, mixed seizure pattern (treatment adjunct)—Valproic acid and divalproex are indicated as adjuncts in conditions of multiple seizures that include absence seizures.

[Epilepsy, myoclonic seizure pattern (treatment)]—Valproic acid and divalproex are used as primary agents for myoclonic seizures.

[Epilepsy, simple partial seizure pattern (treatment)] or
Epilepsy, complex partial seizure pattern (treatment)—Valproic acid and divalproex may be useful in patients with partial seizures that are refractory to other anticonvulsants.

[Epilepsy, tonic-clonic seizure pattern (treatment)]—Valproic acid and divalproex are used as primary agents in the treatment of tonic-clonic (grand mal) seizures.

Bipolar disorder, manic episodes (treatment)—Divalproex is indicated for the treatment of manic episodes associated with bipolar disorder.

[Bipolar disorder (prophylaxis and treatment)]—Valproic acid and divalproex may be useful in the prophylaxis and treatment of manic-depressive illness refractory to treatment with lithium or other agents.

Migraine headaches (prophylaxis)[1]—Divalproex is indicated in the prophylaxis of migraine headaches. There is no evidence that it may be useful in the treatment of acute migraine.

---
[1]Not included in Canadian product labeling.

## Pharmacology/Pharmacokinetics

Note: Divalproex sodium is a stable coordination compound composed of equal parts of valproic acid and sodium valproate. In the gastrointestinal tract, divalproex sodium dissociates into valproate and then produces the bioequivalent pharmacologic activity of valproic acid. Equivalent oral doses of divalproex sodium and valproic acid capsules deliver systemically equivalent quantities of valproate ion.

**Physicochemical characteristics**
Molecular weight—
    Divalproex sodium: 310.41.

Valproic acid: 144.21.
pKa—
    Valproic acid: 4.8.

**Mechanism of action/Effect**
The mechanism of action has not been established; however, it is thought to be related to a direct or secondary increase in concentrations of the inhibitory neurotransmitter, gamma aminobutyric acid (GABA), possibly caused by its decreased metabolism or decreased re-uptake in brain tissues. Another hypothesis is that valproate acts on postsynaptic receptor sites to mimic or enhance the inhibitory action of GABA. The effect on the neuronal membrane is not completely understood. Some studies suggest a possible direct effect on membrane activity related to changes in potassium conductance. Also, valproate has been shown in animal studies to block sustained neuronal bursting responses by reducing the amplitude of sodium-dependent action potentials in a voltage- and use-dependent manner.

**Absorption**
Divalproex sodium—Enteric coating on the tablet delays absorption for about 1 to 4 hours after ingestion; concomitant administration with food may significantly slow the rate, but not the extent, of absorption.
Valproic acid—Rapid absorption from gastrointestinal tract; slight delay when taken with food.

**Protein binding**
High (90 to 95%) at serum concentrations up to 50 micrograms (mcg) per mL; as the concentration increases from 50 to 100 mcg per mL, the percentage bound decreases to 80 to 85% and the free fraction becomes progressively larger, thus increasing the concentration gradient into the brain; decreased in uremia, hypoalbuminemia, and cirrhosis.

**Biotransformation**
Primarily hepatic. Some metabolites may have pharmacologic or toxic activity. Rate of metabolism is faster in children and in patients concurrently using enzyme–inducing medications, such as phenytoin, phenobarbital, primidone, and carbamazepine.

**Half-life**
Variable, from 6 to 16 hours; may be considerably longer in patients with hepatic function impairment, in the elderly, and in children up to 18 months of age; may be considerably shorter in patients receiving hepatic enzyme-inducing anticonvulsants.

**Time to peak serum concentration**
Capsules and syrup—1 to 4 hours.
Delayed-release capsules and tablets—3 to 4 hours.

**Therapeutic serum concentrations**
Variable, usually 50 to 150 mcg per mL (347 to 1041 micromoles per L).

**Elimination**
Renal, mainly as glucuronide conjugate; small amounts excreted in feces and expired air.

## Precautions to Consider

**Carcinogenicity**
Studies in rodents given valproic acid doses of 0, 80, and 170 mg per kg of body weight (mg/kg) a day for two years showed a variety of neoplasms and an increase in the incidence of subcutaneous fibrosarcomas in high-dose male rats and a dose-related trend for benign pulmonary adenomas in male mice. The significance of these findings for humans is unknown.

**Mutagenicity**
Mutagenicity studies using bacterial and mammalian systems have shown no evidence of mutagenic potential for valproate.

## Pregnancy/Reproduction

Fertility—Chronic toxicity studies in rats given doses greater than 200 mg/kg a day and dogs given doses greater than 90 mg/kg a day have shown reduced spermatogenesis and testicular atrophy. Segment I fertility studies in rats given up to 350 mg/kg a day for 60 days have shown no effect on fertility. However, the effect of valproic acid on the development of the testes and on sperm production and fertility in humans is unknown.

Pregnancy—First trimester: Valproate crosses the placenta and has been reported to have caused teratogenic effects, including neural tube defects (anencephaly, low meningomyelocele, and spina bifida) in the fetus when the mother received valproate during the first trimester of pregnancy. Risk-benefit must be carefully considered when the medication is required to treat epilepsy in cases where other medications cannot be used or are ineffective.

Studies in rodents have shown that skeletal abnormalities, primarily involving ribs and vertebrae, occurred in the offspring when the mother received doses exceeding 65 mg/kg per day during pregnancy.

FDA Pregnancy Category D.

## Breast-feeding

Valproate is distributed into breast milk. Concentrations in breast milk have been reported to be 1 to 10% of the maternal serum concentration.

## Pediatrics

Children are at an increased risk of developing serious or fatal hepatotoxicity. Patients up to 2 years of age and children on polytherapy appear to be at even greater risk; however, risk decreases with advancing age.

## Geriatrics

Geriatric patients tend to have increased free, unbound valproic acid concentrations and lowered intrinsic clearances, indicating a reduction of valproate metabolizing capacity and a fall in serum albumin. Therefore, these patients should receive a lower daily dosage, and the serum concentrations should be kept in the lower therapeutic range.

## Dental

Valproate inhibits the secondary phase of platelet aggregation, which may be reflected in prolonged bleeding time and/or frank hemorrhaging.

In addition, the leukopenic and thrombocytopenic effects of valproate may result in an increased incidence of microbial infection, delayed healing, and gingival bleeding. If leukopenia or thrombocytopenia occurs, dental work, whenever possible, should be deferred until blood counts have returned to normal. Patients should be instructed in proper oral hygiene, including caution in use of regular toothbrushes, dental floss, and toothpicks.

## Drug interactions and/or related problems

The following drug interactions and/or related problems have been selected on the basis of their potential clinical significance (possible mechanism in parentheses where appropriate)—not necessarily inclusive (» = major clinical significance):

Note: Combinations containing any of the following medications, depending on the amount present, may also interact with this medication.

In addition to the interactions listed below, the possibility should be considered that additive or multiple effects leading to impaired blood clotting and/or increased risk of bleeding may occur if valproic acid or divalproex is used concurrently with any other medication having a significant potential for inhibiting platelet aggregation or for causing hypoprothrombinemia, thrombocytopenia, or gastrointestinal ulceration or hemorrhage.

» Alcohol or
» CNS depression–producing medications, other (See *Appendix II*)
    (concurrent use with valproic acid or divalproex may potentiate CNS depressant effects)

Anticoagulants, coumarin- or indandione-derivative or
» Heparin or
» Thrombolytic agents
    (valproate-induced hypoprothrombinemia may increase the activity of coumarin- and indandione-derivatives and may increase the risk of bleeding in patients receiving heparin or thrombolytic agents)
    (also, inhibition of platelet aggregation, and reduction of platelet numbers or thrombocytopenia, may increase the risk of hemorrhage in patients receiving anticoagulant or thrombolytic therapy)

Antidepressants, tricyclic or
Bupropion or
Clozapine or
Haloperidol or
Loxapine or
Maprotiline or
Molindone or
Monoamine oxidase (MAO) inhibitors or

Phenothiazines or
Pimozide or
Thioxanthenes
    (in addition to enhancing central nervous system [CNS] depression when used concurrently with valproic acid or divalproex, these medications may lower the seizure threshold; dosage adjustments may be necessary to control seizures)

» Barbiturates or
» Primidone
    (concurrent use with valproate causes higher serum concentrations of barbiturates or primidone, leading to increased CNS depression and neurological toxicity because of protein binding displacement of the barbiturate and reduced barbiturate metabolism; half-life of valproate is decreased; dosage adjustment of barbiturates or primidone may be necessary)

» Carbamazepine
    (concurrent use may result in decreased serum concentrations and half-life of valproate due to increased metabolism induced by hepatic microsomal enzyme activity; valproate causes an increase in the active 10,11-epoxide metabolite of carbamazepine by inhibition of its breakdown; monitoring of serum concentrations as a guide to dosage is recommended, especially when either medication is added to or withdrawn from an existing regimen)

Clonazepam
    (concurrent use with valproic acid or divalproex may produce absence status)

Ethosuximide, and possibly other succinimide anticonvulsants
    (concurrent use with valproic acid or divalproex has been reported to both increase and decrease ethosuximide concentrations; monitoring of serum concentrations as a guide to dosage is recommended)

» Felbamate
    (coadministration of felbamate may increase valproic acid plasma concentrations by 35 to 50%; a decrease in valproic acid dosage may be needed when felbamate therapy is initiated)

» Hepatotoxic medications, other (See *Appendix II*)
    (concurrent use with valproic acid or divalproex may increase the risk of hepatotoxicity; patients on prolonged administration or with a history of liver disease should be carefully monitored)

Levocarnitine
    (requirements for carnitine may be increased in patients receiving valproic acid or divalproex)

» Mefloquine
    (concurrent use with valproic acid or divalproex may result in low valproate serum concentrations and loss of seizure control; monitoring of valproate serum concentrations is recommended and dosage adjustments may be necessary during and after therapy with mefloquine)

» Phenytoin, and possibly other hydantoin anticonvulsants
    (concurrent use with valproic acid or divalproex has resulted in breakthrough seizures or phenytoin toxicity because valproate may interfere with phenytoin protein binding, and phenytoin, through enzyme induction, will lower valproate levels; concurrent use requires close monitoring of the patient since variable serum phenytoin concentrations have resulted because valproate increases unbound phenytoin concentrations and decreases intrinsic clearance by inhibiting metabolism of phenytoin; total phenytoin serum concentrations may not reflect unbound phenytoin activity, and unbound phenytoin concentrations may be more reliable; dosage of phenytoin should be adjusted as required by clinical situation)

» Platelet aggregation inhibitors, other (See *Appendix II*)
    (concurrent use with valproic acid or divalproex may increase the risk of hemorrhage because of additive or multiple actions that may decrease blood-clotting ability)
    (the gastrointestinal ulcerative or hemorrhagic potential of aspirin, anti-inflammatory analgesics, or sulfinpyrazone may increase the risk of hemorrhage in patients receiving valproic acid or divalproex)
    (in addition, aspirin may displace valproic acid or divalproex from protein binding sites, as well as altering valproate metabolism and excretion, resulting in increased levels of free [unbound] valproate, which may cause toxic effects)

Sodium benzoate and sodium phenylacetate combination
    (valproate-induced hyperammonemia may exacerbate urea cycle enzymopathy deficiency and antagonize the efficacy of sodium benzoate and sodium phenylacetate combination)

## Laboratory value alterations

The following have been selected on the basis of their potential clinical significance (possible effect in parentheses where appropriate)—not necessarily inclusive (» = major clinical significance):

With diagnostic test results
  Metyrapone test
    (increased metabolism of metyrapone by an hepatic enzyme inducer such as valproic acid or divalproex may decrease the response to metyrapone)
  Thyroid function tests
    (test results may be altered; decreased $T_4$, and free $T_3$ and $T_4$ concentrations have been reported; clinical significance is unknown)
  Urine ketone tests
    (use of valproic acid or divalproex may produce false-positive results because of a ketone metabolite excreted in urine)

With physiology/laboratory test values
  Alanine aminotransferase (ALT [SGPT]) and
  Aspartate aminotransferase (AST [SGOT]) and
  Lactate dehydrogenase (LDH)
    (minor elevations of serum concentrations occur frequently and appear to be dose-related; elevations may indicate asymptomatic hepatotoxicity)
  Amino acid screening
    (increases in glycine may occur)
  Bilirubin
    (serum concentrations may be increased; increase may indicate potentially serious hepatotoxicity)

## Medical considerations/Contraindications

The medical considerations/contraindications included here have been selected on the basis of their potential clinical significance (reasons given in parentheses where appropriate)—not necessarily inclusive (» = major clinical significance).

*Except under special circumstances, this medication should not be used when the following medical problems exist:*

» Hepatic disease or
» Hepatic function impairment, significant
    (may be exacerbated)

*Risk-benefit should be considered when the following medical problems exist:*

  Blood dyscrasias or
  Brain disease, organic or
  Hepatic disease, history of
    (may be exacerbated)
  Hypoalbuminemia
    (alterations in protein binding may affect serum levels)
  Renal function impairment
    (metabolites may accumulate; valproate binding to serum albumin is decreased and volume of distribution is increased)
  Sensitivity to valproic acid or divalproex

## Patient monitoring

The following may be especially important in patient monitoring (other tests may be warranted in some patients, depending on condition; » = major clinical significance):

  Ammonia concentrations, serum
    (therapy should be discontinued if hyperammonemia occurs, with or without lethargy or coma)
  Bleeding time determinations and
  Blood cell counts, including platelets and
  Renal function determinations
    (recommended prior to therapy and periodically during therapy)
  Hepatic function determinations
    (should be performed prior to therapy and periodically thereafter, especially during the first 6 months of therapy; valproic acid or divalproex should be discontinued immediately if significant hepatic function impairment is apparent or suspected)
  Valproate concentrations, serum
    (since therapeutic concentrations vary widely, morning trough concentrations with values ranging from 50 to 100 mcg per mL [347 to 693 micromoles per L] may be useful when initiating therapy; doses may be raised gradually until patient achieves a predose serum concentration of at least 50 mcg per mL [347 micromoles per L], the dose then being increased as needed)

## Side/Adverse Effects

Note: Hepatic failure resulting in death has occurred in patients receiving valproic acid and divalproex. These incidents usually have occurred during the first 6 months of treatment. Patients at greatest risk are children receiving other anticonvulsants along with valproic acid or divalproex. Serious or fatal hepatotoxicity may be preceded by nonspecific symptoms such as loss of seizure control, malaise, weakness, lethargy, Reye's-like syndrome, anorexia, vomiting, jaundice, and edema. In some cases, hepatic function impairment has progressed in spite of discontinuation of medication.

The following side/adverse effects have been selected on the basis of their potential clinical significance (possible signs and symptoms in parentheses where appropriate)—not necessarily inclusive:

### Those indicating need for medical attention
Incidence less frequent or rare
  *Behaviorial, mood, or mental changes; hepatotoxicity or hyperammonemia* (increase in frequency of seizures; loss of appetite; continuing nausea or vomiting; swelling of face; tiredness and weakness; yellow eyes or skin); *ophthalmological effects, specifically diplopia* (double vision); *nystagmus* (continuous, uncontrolled back-and-forth and/or rolling eye movements); *or spots before eyes; pancreatitis* (severe abdominal or stomach cramps; continuing nausea and vomiting); *platelet aggregation inhibition or thrombocytopenia* (unusual bleeding or bruising)

  Note: Evidence of hemorrhage, bruising, or a disorder of coagulation or hemostasis is an indication for reduction of dosage or discontinuation of therapy.

### Those indicating need for medical attention only if they continue or are bothersome
Incidence more frequent
  *Abdominal or stomach cramps, mild*—may also indicate a risk of pancreatitis; less frequent with divalproex; *anorexia* (loss of appetite); *change in menstrual periods; diarrhea; hair loss; indigestion; nausea and vomiting; trembling of hands and arms; unusual weight loss or gain*
Incidence less frequent or rare
  *Clumsiness or unsteadiness; constipation; dizziness; drowsiness; headache; skin rash; unusual excitement, restlessness, or irritability*

# Overdose

For specific information on the agents used in the management of valproic acid overdose, see:
  • *Naloxone (Systemic)* monograph.

For more information on the management of overdose or unintentional ingestion, **contact a Poison Control Center** (see *Poison Control Center Listing*).

### Treatment of overdose
Treatment of overdose consists primarily of supportive and symptomatic measures.

To decrease absorption—The effectiveness of emesis or gastric lavage will depend upon the time elapsed since ingestion. The enteric-coated tablets will delay absorption about 1 to 4 hours.

To enhance elimination—Hemodialysis and hemoperfusion have been used to lower valproate serum concentrations.

Specific treatment—Maintenance of adequate urinary output must be ensured. Naloxone has been administered to counteract severe CNS depression, but it also theoretically reverses the anticonvulsant effect and should be used with caution.

Supportive care—Patients in whom intentional overdose is confirmed or suspected should be referred for psychiatric consultation.

# Patient Consultation

As an aid to patient consultation, refer to *Advice for the Patient, Valproic Acid (Systemic)*.

In providing consultation, consider emphasizing the following selected information (» = major clinical significance):

### Before using this medication
» Conditions affecting use, especially:
    Sensitivity to valproic acid or divalproex
    Pregnancy—Pregnancy studies in animals have shown skeletal abnormalities involving ribs and vertebrae in offspring of mothers given large doses; in humans, crosses placenta in first trimester and may cause neural tube defects in fetus
    Breast-feeding—Distributed into breast milk
    Use in children—Children are at an increased risk of serious hepatotoxicity
    Use in the elderly—Elderly patients tend to have higher serum concentrations of free valproic acid; lower daily dosages recommended

Dental—Prolonged bleeding time and/or hemorrhaging; leukopenia and thrombocytopenia may result in increased incidence of microbial infection, delayed healing, and gingival bleeding

Other medications, especially alcohol or other CNS depression–producing medications, heparin or thrombolytic agents, barbiturates, primidone, carbamazepine, felbamate, other hepatotoxic medications, mefloquine, phenytoin, or other platelet aggregation inhibitors

Other medical problems, especially significant hepatic disease or hepatic function impairment

## Proper use of this medication
*Proper administration:*
*For valproic acid capsules*

Swallowing capsules whole with water only; not breaking, chewing, or crushing

*For divalproex sodium delayed-release capsules*

Swallowing capsules whole, or sprinkling the contents on a small amount of cool, soft food (such as applesauce or pudding) and swallowing, not chewing, immediately after preparation

*For divalproex sodium delayed-release tablets*

Swallowing tablets whole; not breaking, chewing, or crushing

*For valproic acid syrup*

Mixing with any liquid or adding to a small amount of food to enhance palatability

Taking with food if necessary to reduce gastrointestinal side effects
» Compliance with therapy; taking exactly as directed by physician
» Proper dosing

Missed dose: If dosing schedule is—

One dose a day: Taking as soon as possible; not taking if not remembered until next day; not doubling doses

Two or more doses a day: Taking if remembered within 6 hours; taking remaining doses for that day at equally spaced intervals; not doubling doses
» Proper storage

## Precautions while using this medication
» Regular visits to physician to check progress of therapy
» Checking with physician before discontinuing medication; gradual dosage reduction may be necessary
» Possible prolonged bleeding or hemorrhage: caution if any kind of surgery, dental treatment, or emergency treatment is required
» Avoiding use of alcoholic beverages or other CNS depressants during therapy

Diabetic patients: When testing for urine ketones, possible false-positive test results

Caution if any laboratory tests required; possible interference with results of metyrapone or thyroid function tests

Possible need for carrying medical identification card or bracelet
» Possible drowsiness; caution when driving or doing other things requiring alertness

## Side/adverse effects
Signs of potential side effects, especially behavioral, mood, or mental changes; hepatotoxicity; hyperammonemia; ophthalmological effects; pancreatitis; platelet aggregation inhibition; or thrombocytopenia

# General Dosing Information

Patients at primary risk for fatal liver failure with valproic acid or divalproex treatment include:
• Children up to 2 years old who are receiving multiple anticonvulsants and also have significant medical problems in addition to severe epilepsy (e.g., mental retardation, developmental delay, congenital abnormalities, and metabolic disorders).
• All patients receiving concomitant anticonvulsants, especially phenytoin and phenobarbital, which induce cytochrome P450 enzymes and enhance the production of a toxic metabolite.
• Patients with familial liver disease.

Recommendations for reducing the risk of serious hepatotoxicity with valproate include:
• Avoiding the administration of valproate with other anticonvulsants whenever possible, especially in children up to 3 years old, unless monotherapy has failed or the benefits of polytherapy outweigh the risks.
• Avoiding valproate therapy in patients with pre-existing liver disease or a family history of childhood hepatic disease.
• Administering valproate in as low a dose as possible to achieve seizure control.
• Avoiding concurrent administration with other hepatotoxic medications, especially salicylates.

• Monitoring for prodromal symptoms (e.g., nausea or vomiting, headache, edema, jaundice, or seizure breakthrough, especially after a febrile illness).
• Avoiding administration to patients with congenital metabolic disorders, or severe seizure disorders accompanied by mental retardation or organic brain disease.

When valproic acid or divalproex is to be discontinued, dosage should be reduced gradually since abrupt withdrawal may precipitate seizures or status epilepticus.

The serum concentration of valproic acid or divalproex (valproate) does not always correspond with therapeutic effect; therefore, the evaluation of the patient's progress must be based on total clinical assessment.

When valproic acid or divalproex is used to replace or supplement other anticonvulsant therapy, the dosage should be increased gradually to achieve therapeutic serum concentrations, while that of the replaced medication is decreased gradually in order to maintain seizure control. The addition of valproic acid or divalproex may cause increases in the serum concentrations of enzyme-inducing anticonvulsants (phenytoin, phenobarbital, primidone, and carbamazepine). Conversely, discontinuation of these will cause an increase in valproate serum concentrations by about 60 to 100%.

The possible prolongation of bleeding time, in addition to potentiation of depressant effect by CNS depressants, should be considered when surgery, dental treatment, or emergency treatment is required.

## Diet/Nutrition
Valproic acid or divalproex may be taken with food to reduce gastrointestinal side effects.

The contents of divalproex sodium delayed-release capsules may be sprinkled on a small amount of cool, soft food (such as applesauce or pudding) and swallowed, not chewed, immediately after preparation.

The syrup may be mixed with a small amount of food to enhance the palatability.

Requirements for carnitine may be increased in patients receiving valproic acid or divalproex.

---

## DIVALPROEX

# Oral Dosage Forms
## DIVALPROEX SODIUM DELAYED-RELEASE CAPSULES
### Usual adult and adolescent dose
Anticonvulsant—

Monotherapy: Oral, the equivalent of valproic acid—Initially, 5 to 15 mg per kg of body weight a day, the dosage being increased at one-week intervals by 5 to 10 mg per kg of body weight a day as needed and tolerated.

Polytherapy: Oral, the equivalent of valproic acid—Initially, 10 to 30 mg per kg of body weight a day, the dosage being increased at one-week intervals by 5 to 10 mg per kg of body weight a day as needed and tolerated.

Note: If the total daily dose exceeds 250 mg, it should be divided into two or more doses (usually given every 12 hours) to lessen the possibility of gastrointestinal irritation.

Geriatric patients may need lower doses.

Patients also taking a hepatic enzyme-inducing medication may need higher dosages depending on predose serum concentrations.

### Usual adult prescribing limits
Up to 60 mg per kg of body weight a day.

### Usual pediatric dose
Anticonvulsant: Children 1 to 12 years of age—

Monotherapy: Oral, the equivalent of valproic acid—Initially, 15 to 45 mg per kg of body weight a day, the dosage being increased at one-week intervals by 5 to 10 mg per kg of body weight a day as needed and tolerated.

Polytherapy: Oral, the equivalent of valproic acid—30 to 100 mg per kg of body weight a day.

Note: Dosage adjustments depend on clinical response and serum anticonvulsant concentrations.

### Strength(s) usually available
U.S.—

The equivalent of valproic acid
125 mg (Rx) [*Depakote Sprinkle*].

Canada—

Not commercially available.

**Packaging and storage**
Store below 30 °C (86 °F), preferably between 15 and 30 °C (59 and 86 °F) in a tight, light-resistant container, unless otherwise specified by manufacturer.

**Auxiliary labeling**
- May cause drowsiness.
- Avoid alcoholic beverages.
- Do not chew contents of capsule.

## DIVALPROEX SODIUM DELAYED-RELEASE TABLETS

**Usual adult dose**
Anticonvulsant—
   Monotherapy: Oral, the equivalent of valproic acid—Initially, 5 to 15 mg per kg of body weight a day, the dosage being increased at one-week intervals by 5 to 10 mg per kg of body weight a day as needed and tolerated.
   Polytherapy: Oral, the equivalent of valproic acid—Initially, 10 to 30 mg per kg of body weight a day, the dosage being increased at one-week intervals by 5 to 10 mg per kg of body weight a day as needed and tolerated.
Antimanic—
   Oral, initially 750 mg a day in divided doses. The dose should be increased as rapidly as possible to achieve the lowest therapeutic dose that produces the desired clinical effect or a desired trough plasma concentration within the range of fifty to one hundred fifty micrograms/mL.
Migraine headache prophylactic—
   Oral, initially 250 mg two times a day. The dose may be increased as needed and tolerated; some patients may benefit from doses up to 1000 mg a day. However, daily doses above 1000 mg have not demonstrated increased efficacy in clinical trials.
Note: If the total daily dose exceeds 250 mg, it should be divided into two or more doses (usually given every 12 hours) to lessen the possibility of gastrointestinal irritation.
   Geriatric patients may need lower doses.
   Patients also taking a hepatic enzyme-inducing medication may need higher dosages depending on predose serum concentrations.

**Usual adult prescribing limits**
See *Divalproex Sodium Delayed-release Capsules.*

**Usual pediatric dose**
See *Divalproex Sodium Delayed-release Capsules.*

**Strength(s) usually available**
U.S.—
   The equivalent of valproic acid
   125 mg (Rx) [*Depakote*].
   250 mg (Rx) [*Depakote*].
   500 mg (Rx) [*Depakote*].
Canada—
   The equivalent of valproic acid
   125 mg (Rx) [*Epival*].
   250 mg (Rx) [*Epival*].
   500 mg (Rx) [*Epival*].

**Packaging and storage**
Store below 40 °C (104 °F), preferably between 15 and 30 °C (59 and 86 °F), in a tight, light-resistant container, unless otherwise specified by manufacturer.

**Auxiliary labeling**
- May cause drowsiness.
- Avoid alcoholic beverages.
- Swallow tablets whole. Do not break or chew.

---

**VALPROIC ACID**

---

# Oral Dosage Forms
## VALPROIC ACID CAPSULES USP

**Usual adult and adolescent dose**
Anticonvulsant—
   Monotherapy: Oral, initially, 5 to 15 mg per kg of body weight a day, the dosage being increased at one-week intervals by 5 to 10 mg per kg of body weight a day as needed and tolerated.
   Polytherapy: Oral, initially, 10 to 30 mg per kg of body weight a day, the dosage being increased at one-week intervals by 5 to 10 mg per kg of body weight a day as needed and tolerated.
Note: If the total daily dose exceeds 250 mg, it should be divided into two or more doses (usually given every 12 hours) to lessen the possibility of gastrointestinal irritation.
   Geriatric patients may need lower doses.
   Patients also taking a hepatic enzyme-inducing medication may need higher dosages depending on predose serum concentrations.

**Usual adult prescribing limits**
Up to 60 mg per kg of body weight a day.

**Usual pediatric dose**
Anticonvulsant—Children 1 to 12 years of age:
   Monotherapy: Oral, initially, 15 to 45 mg per kg of body weight a day, the dosage being increased at one-week intervals by 5 to 10 mg per kg of body weight a day as needed and tolerated.
   Polytherapy: Oral, 30 to 100 mg per kg of body weight a day.
Note: Dosage adjustments depend on clinical response and serum anti-convulsant concentrations.

**Strength(s) usually available**
U.S.—
   250 mg (Rx) [*Depakene* (parabens); GENERIC].
Canada—
   250 mg (Rx) [*Depakene* (parabens)].
   500 mg (Rx) [*Depakene* (enteric coated; parabens; tartrazine)].

**Packaging and storage**
Store between 15 and 30 °C (59 and 86 °F), in a tight container.

**Auxiliary labeling**
- May cause drowsiness.
- Avoid alcoholic beverages.
- Swallow capsules whole. Do not break or chew.

## VALPROIC ACID SYRUP USP

**Usual adult and adolescent dose**
See *Valproic Acid Capsules USP.*

**Usual adult prescribing limits**
See *Valproic Acid Capsules USP.*

**Usual pediatric dose**
See *Valproic Acid Capsules USP.*

**Strength(s) usually available**
U.S.—
   250 mg per 5 mL (Rx) [*Depakene* (parabens; sorbitol; sucrose); *Myproic Acid;* GENERIC].
Canada—
   250 mg per 5 mL (Rx) [*Depakene*].

**Packaging and storage**
Store below 40 °C (104 °F), preferably between 15 and 30 °C (59 and 86 °F), unless otherwise specified by manufacturer. Store in a tight container. Protect from freezing.

**Auxiliary labeling**
- May cause drowsiness.
- Avoid alcoholic beverages.

---

Revised: 08/13/96

[Hypotension, orthostatic (prophylaxis and treatment)][1]—Dihydroergotamine is used to prevent or treat orthostatic hypotension that may occur in conjunction with spinal or epidural anesthesia. It is also used to treat orthostatic hypotension due to autonomic insufficiency or other causes.

### Unaccepted

Dihydroergotamine, ergotamine, and ergotamine-containing combinations are not recommended for long-term migraine prophylaxis.

Although ergotamine has oxytocic effects, it is not used clinically to produce these effects because other ergot alkaloids are more effective and less toxic.

---

[1]Not included in Canadian product labeling.

## Pharmacology/Pharmacokinetics

Note: Pharmacology/pharmacokinetics information for the adjuvants present in headache suppressant formulations (caffeine, belladonna alkaloids, cyclizine, dimenhydrinate, diphenhydramine, and pentobarbital) is limited to brief descriptions of the effects that may be pertinent to treatment of patients with vascular headaches. Gastric stasis that accompanies migraine headaches tends to inhibit absorption of orally administered medications and may therefore alter their pharmacokinetic profiles. For additional information on the actions of these agents, see—
   Caffeine: *Caffeine (Systemic).*
   Belladonna alkaloids: *Anticholinergics/Antispasmodics (Systemic).*
   Cyclizine: *Cyclizine (Systemic).*
   Dimenhydrinate: *Antihistamines (Systemic).*
   Diphenhydramine: *Antihistamines (Systemic).*
   Pentobarbital: *Barbiturates (Systemic).*

### Physicochemical characteristics

Source—
   Dihydroergotamine: Synthetic
   Ergotamine: Semisynthetic alkaloid; derived from ergot, a product of the parasitic fungus *Claviceps purpurea*
Molecular weight—
   Dihydroergotamine mesylate: 679.79.
   Ergotamine tartrate: 1313.43.
   Caffeine: 194.19.
   Cyclizine hydrochloride: 302.85.
   Dimenhydrinate: 469.97.
   Diphenhydramine hydrochloride: 291.82.
   Pentobarbital sodium: 248.26.

### Mechanism of action/Effect

Dihydroergotamine and Ergotamine—
These ergot derivatives interact with several neurotransmitter receptors, including alpha-adrenergic, serotonergic (tryptaminergic), and dopaminergic receptors. Both agonistic (or partial agonistic) and antagonistic actions have been reported at different receptor types or subtypes. These medications directly stimulate vascular smooth muscle, causing constriction of both arteries and veins, and depress vasomotor centers in the brain. Dihydroergotamine's adrenergic blocking actions are somewhat more pronounced, and its vasoconstrictive actions (especially in arteries) are less pronounced, than those of ergotamine.

Vascular headache suppressant:
   Ergot derivative–induced decreases in the firing of serotonergic (5-hydroxytryptaminergic, 5-HT) neurons may be responsible for headache suppression. Specifically, it is thought that agonist activity at the 5-HT$_{1D}$ receptor subtype provides relief of acute headache, whereas antagonist activity at the 5-HT$_2$ receptor subtype provides headache prophylaxis. It has been proposed that constriction of cerebral blood vessels by the ergot derivative (resulting from alpha-adrenergic stimulation as well as from activity at 5-HT receptors) reduces the pulsation in cerebral arteries that may be responsible for the pain of vascular headaches. However, studies have not consistently shown a significant correlation between dilatation of cerebral blood vessels and pain or other symptoms of migraine or cluster headaches, or between the vasoconstrictive effect of an ergot derivative and relief of these headaches.
   Dihydroergotamine and ergotamine may decrease hyperperfusion in the area of the basilar artery, but they do not reduce cerebral hemispheric blood flow.

Thrombosis prophylaxis adjunct and Antihypotensive:
   Dihydroergotamine's constrictive effect on capacitance (venous) vasculature is significantly greater than its constrictive effect on resistance (arterial) vasculature. As a result, the velocity of venous blood flow in the legs is increased,

venous return to the heart is enhanced, venous pooling (which may increase the risk of thrombus formation) is reduced, and arterial blood pressure is maintained or increased. It has also been proposed that dihydroergotamine may enhance the effects of heparin in preventing thrombosis.

Caffeine—
   Caffeine constricts the cerebral vasculature and decreases both cerebral blood flow and the oxygen tension of the brain. However, it is believed that the caffeine in many ergotamine-containing formulations acts primarily by increasing both the rate and extent of absorption of orally or rectally administered ergotamine, thereby hastening the onset of action and increasing the effect of ergotamine.

Belladonna alkaloids—
   Belladonna alkaloids are used in headache suppressant formulations for their antiemetic effects, because nausea and vomiting may occur in association with the migraine headache and/or as a result of ergotamine administration.

Cyclizine and Dimenhydrinate and Diphenhydramine—
   These antihistamines are used in headache suppressant formulations for their antiemetic and sedative effects.

Pentobarbital—
   This barbiturate is used in headache suppressant formulations for its sedative effects.

### Other actions/effects

Dihydroergotamine and Ergotamine—
   These medications may cause nausea and vomiting via direct stimulation of the chemoreceptor trigger zone.
   Like other ergot derivatives, dihydroergotamine and ergotamine stimulate uterine smooth muscle via an action on alpha-adrenergic receptors and/or 5-HT receptors. Ergotamine is much more potent than dihydroergotamine as a uterine stimulant.
   Peripheral vasoconstriction induced by dihydroergotamine and ergotamine may lead to decreased blood flow in various organs, increased peripheral vascular resistance, and increased blood pressure. However, with the doses usually used in the treatment of migraine or cluster headaches, increases in blood pressure are usually slight.
   Large doses of dihydroergotamine and ergotamine may cause constriction of the coronary vasculature and bradycardia. These effects may result from increased vagal activity as well as direct actions on the myocardium and the vasculature.

Caffeine—
   Caffeine has central nervous system (CNS) stimulant activity and may therefore inhibit sleep. Because sleep contributes to relief of migraine headaches, this action may be detrimental to the patient.

Belladonna alkaloids—
   Belladonna alkaloids have anticholinergic activity.

Cyclizine and Dimenhydrinate and Diphenhydramine—
   These medications have antihistaminic, anticholinergic, and CNS depressant activities.

Pentobarbital—
   Barbiturates have CNS depressant activity.

### Absorption

Dihydroergotamine—
   Intramuscular or subcutaneous: Rapid.

Ergotamine—
   Oral: Slow, incomplete, and subject to wide interpatient variability. Absorption is inhibited by the gastric stasis that accompanies migraine headaches. Concurrent administration of caffeine increases the rate and extent of absorption. Metoclopramide may also increase ergotamine absorption by accelerating gastrointestinal motility (and may also be useful as an antiemetic). Extensive first-pass metabolism of ergotamine also reduces bioavailability.
   Rectal: More rapid and extensive than after oral administration; increased by concurrent administration of caffeine.
   Sublingual: Very poor.

### Distribution

Ergotamine is distributed into breast milk.

### Protein binding

Dihydroergotamine—
   Very high (about 90%).
Ergotamine—
   Very high (93 to 98%).

### Biotransformation

Dihydroergotamine—
   Hepatic; extensive, with considerable first-pass metabolism. The principal metabolite, 8'-hydroxy-dihydroergotamine, is pharmacologically active.

**Ergotamine—**
Hepatic; extensive, with considerable first-pass metabolism. At least some of the metabolites are pharmacologically active.

**Half-life**

Note: Reported values vary widely, depending on the route of administration and study methodology. Values obtained after administration of radiolabeled dihydroergotamine or ergotamine represent metabolites as well as the parent compound, whereas values determined via specific radioimmunoassay (RIA) represent only the parent compound. At least 2 RIAs have been used to assess pharmacokinetics of dihydroergotamine, one of which is more sensitive (able to detect significantly smaller quantities of the compound) than the other.

Distribution—
Dihydroergotamine:
Intravenous—1 to 1.35 minutes in one study; 4 minutes in a second study. Different doses and RIAs were used in the 2 studies.
Subcutaneous—Approximately 1 hour, measured via RIA.
Ergotamine:
2.7 hours, determined following oral administration of radiolabeled ergotamine.
Elimination—
Dihydroergotamine:
Intravenous—
Alpha phase: Approximately 23 to 33 minutes in one study; 1.45 hours in a second study. Different doses and RIAs were used in the 2 studies.
Beta phase: Approximately 15 hours, measured via the more sensitive RIA.
Subcutaneous—About 7.25 hours, measured via RIA.
Values ranging between 18 and 32 hours have been reported after administration of radiolabeled dihydroergotamine by various routes.
Ergotamine: Determined after oral administration of radiolabeled ergotamine:
Alpha phase: Approximately 2 hours.
Beta phase: Approximately 21 hours.

**Onset of action**

Acute headaches—

Note: For relief of acute migraine or cluster headaches, the onset of action is highly dependent on the duration of the headache prior to initiation of therapy as well as on the route of administration. The most rapid onset of action is achieved when the medication is administered as soon as the first symptoms appear (during the prodrome, for migraine with aura).

Dihydroergotamine:
Intramuscular—15 to 30 minutes.
Intravenous—Variable; usually less than 5 minutes.

**Time to peak concentration**

Dihydroergotamine—
Intramuscular: About 30 minutes.
Intravenous: About 3 minutes.
Subcutaneous: 15 to 45 minutes.
Ergotamine—
Oral, administered without caffeine: About 2 hours.
Oral, administered concurrently with caffeine: About 60 to 70 minutes.
Rectal, administered concurrently with caffeine: About 1 hour.

Note: The pharmacokinetics of ergotamine after oral or rectal administration have been studied in healthy subjects and in migraine patients who were not experiencing an attack at the time of the study. During a migraine headache, peak concentrations after oral administration are likely to occur less rapidly than reported above, because the gastric stasis that accompanies migraine headaches inhibits absorption of medications.

In a study investigating the association between pharmacokinetic variables and efficacy of ergotamine in migraine patients who were not experiencing an attack at the time of the study, plasma concentrations measured after a single oral or rectal dose of each patient's usual ergotamine-containing medication were subject to wide interindividual variability. Peak plasma concentrations of ergotamine occurred earlier, were higher, and were maintained for a longer time in patients who reported a good therapeutic response to their medications than in patients who reported a poor therapeutic response to the same medications. In most patients reporting a good therapeutic response, plasma concentrations of 200 picograms per mL or higher were measured within 1 hour after administration.

**Time to peak effect**

Relief of acute headache—
Dihydroergotamine: Parenteral—15 minutes to 2 hours.
Ergotamine: Oral—Variable; usually within 1 to 2 hours, but up to 5 hours in some patients.

**Duration of action**

Dihydroergotamine—Vasoconstrictive and antihypotensive effects—
About 8 hours, following intravenous or subcutaneous administration.

**Elimination**

Dihydroergotamine—
Primarily via hepatic metabolism, followed by fecal (biliary) elimination of metabolites. Only 5 to 10% of a dose is excreted in the urine, with only trace amounts being excreted in the urine as unchanged dihydroergotamine.
Ergotamine—
Primarily via hepatic metabolism, followed by fecal (biliary) elimination of metabolites. About 4% of an oral dose is excreted in the urine within 96 hours. Only trace amounts are eliminated in the urine and feces as unmetabolized ergotamine. After sublingual administration, ergotamine is also eliminated, erratically, in saliva.
In dialysis—Ergotamine is dialyzable.

# Precautions to Consider

Note: Information in this section concerning the adjuvants present in ergotamine-containing headache suppressant formulations (caffeine, belladonna alkaloids, cyclizine, dimenhydrinate, diphenhydramine, and pentobarbital) is limited to brief summaries of the major precautions that may apply to their use in doses recommended for treatment of vascular headaches. For more complete information that may apply, especially if these agents are ingested frequently or in higher-than-recommended doses, see—
Caffeine: *Caffeine (Systemic)*.
Belladonna alkaloids: *Anticholinergics/Antispasmodics (Systemic)*.
Cyclizine: *Cyclizine (Systemic)*.
Dimenhydrinate: *Antihistamines (Systemic)*.
Diphenhydramine: *Antihistamines (Systemic)*.
Pentobarbital: *Barbiturates (Systemic)*.

**Mutagenicity**

*Dimenhydrinate—*
Mutagenicity screening tests showed dimenhydrinate to be mutagenic in bacterial systems, but not mammalian systems. There are no human data showing that the medication is mutagenic.

**Pregnancy/Reproduction**

Note: Information concerning use of adjuvants present in ergotamine-containing combinations by pregnant women is not included in this section because the potential adverse effects of ergotamine preclude the use of these combinations during pregnancy.

Pregnancy—
*Dihydroergotamine—*
Use during pregnancy is not recommended because dihydroergotamine stimulates the uterine musculature, although it has much less oxytocic activity than ergotamine. Also, constriction of the placental vasculature may cause fetotoxicity by reducing uterine blood flow.
*Ergotamine—*
Use during pregnancy is not recommended because of ergotamine's potent oxytocic activity. Ergotamine's uterine stimulating action and its vasoconstrictive activity, which may lead to reduced uterine blood flow, may both be harmful to the fetus. Although a definite causal relationship has not been established, use of ergotamine by pregnant women may have caused fetal growth retardation, intrauterine fetal deaths, miscarriages, and intestinal obstruction resulting in the death of a neonate.
In animal studies, ergotamine has caused retarded fetal growth and increases in the number of resorptions and intrauterine deaths.
FDA Pregnancy Category X.

**Breast-feeding**

*Dihydroergotamine and Ergotamine—*
Ergot alkaloids are distributed into breast milk and have the potential to cause adverse effects (e.g., vomiting, diarrhea, weak pulse, unstable blood pressure, seizures) in the infant. These medications may also inhibit lactation.
*Caffeine—*
Caffeine is distributed into breast milk in small amounts. However, it is recommended that breast-feeding mothers limit their total daily intake of caffeine to 360 mg, because accumulation of caffeine in the infant, leading to hyperactivity, wakefulness, and other signs

**Stability**

After reconstitution, solutions retain their potency for 14 days if refrigerated.

**Auxiliary labeling**

- Refrigerate.
- Continue medicine for full time of treatment.
- Beyond-use date.

**Note**

When dispensing, include a calibrated liquid-measuring device.

Revised: 08/10/94

# VANCOMYCIN Systemic

VA CLASSIFICATION (Primary): AM900

Note: For a listing of dosage forms and brand names by country availability, see *Dosage Forms* section(s). For a listing of brand names for the articles in this monograph, refer to the General Index.

## Category

Antibacterial (systemic).

Note: Vancomycin is a narrow-spectrum antibacterial.

## Indications

Note: Bracketed information in the *Indications* section refers to uses that are not included in U.S. product labeling.

**Accepted**

Bone and joint infections (treatment) or

Septicemia, bacterial (treatment)—Intravenous vancomycin is indicated in the treatment of bone and joint infections (including osteomyelitis) and septicemia caused by *Staphylococcus* species (including methicillin-resistant strains).

Endocarditis, bacterial (prophylaxis)—Intravenous vancomycin is indicated as a primary agent in penicillin-allergic patients with prosthetic heart valves or congenital, rheumatic, or other acquired valvular heart disease who are undergoing dental procedures or surgical procedures of the upper respiratory tract.

[Vancomycin is also used as a primary agent, concurrently with gentamicin or streptomycin, in penicillin-allergic patients with prosthetic heart valves or congenital or valvular heart disease who are undergoing gastrointestinal or genitourinary tract procedures.]

Endocarditis, bacterial (treatment)—Intravenous vancomycin is indicated in the treatment of endocarditis caused by *Staphylococcus* species (including methicillin-resistant strains).

Vancomycin is also indicated as a primary agent, alone or concurrently with an aminoglycoside or rifampin, in endocarditis caused by *Corynebacterium* species (diphtheroids) (including penicillin- and cephalosporin-resistant strains) in penicillin-allergic patients and as a secondary agent in endocarditis caused by *Streptococcus viridans* and *S. bovis*.

[Intravenous vancomycin is used as a primary agent, concurrently with gentamicin or streptomycin, in endocarditis caused by enterococci (*Enterococcus faecalis*) in penicillin-allergic patients.]

Intravenous vancomycin is indicated in the treatment of severe, potentially life-threatening staphylococcal infections in patients who cannot receive penicillins or cephalosporins or have failed to respond to them. Vancomycin is also indicated in staphylococcal infections that are resistant to other antibacterials, including methicillin.

[Brain abscess (treatment)][1]

[Erysipelas (treatment)][1]

[Meningitis, staphylococcal (treatment)]

[Meningitis, streptococcal (treatment)] or

[Perioperative infections (prophylaxis)][1]—Intravenous vancomycin is used in the treatment of brain abscess, erysipelas, meningitis caused by staphylococci or streptococci, and in the prophylaxis of perioperative infections.

[Intravenous vancomycin, administered concurrently with an aminoglycoside (e.g., gentamicin) or rifampin, is also used in the treatment of serious infections caused by *Staphylococcus* species (including methicillin- and multiresistant strains) in penicillin-allergic patients.][1]

Not all species or strains of a particular organism may be susceptible to vancomycin.

**Unaccepted**

Vancomycin is not effective against most gram-negative organisms, *Mycobacterium* species, *Bacteroides* species, *Rickettsia* species, *Chlamydia* species, or fungi.

The use of parenteral vancomycin is not recommended in the treatment of antibiotic-associated pseudomembranous colitis.

[1]Not included in Canadian product labeling.

## Pharmacology/Pharmacokinetics

**Physicochemical characteristics**

Molecular weight—1485.73.

**Mechanism of action/Effect**

Bactericidal for most organisms; bacteriostatic for enterococci; inhibits bacterial cell wall synthesis at a site different from that of penicillins and cephalosporins by binding tightly to D-alanyl-D-alanine portion of cell wall precursor; this leads to destruction of bacterial cell by lysis; vancomycin may also alter permeability of bacterial cytoplasmic membranes and may selectively inhibit ribonucleic acid (RNA) synthesis; also active against ''L'' forms because of its intracellular action; does not compete with penicillins for binding sites.

**Absorption**

Intraperitoneal—Systemic absorption (up to 65%) may occur.

**Distribution**

Widely distributed to most tissues and body fluids; adequate therapeutic concentrations in serum and in pleural, pericardial, peritoneal, ascitic, and synovial fluids; high concentrations in urine; inadequate concentrations in bile; does not readily cross normal blood-brain barrier into cerebrospinal fluid (CSF); however, penetrates into CSF when meninges are inflamed and may achieve therapeutic concentrations. Crosses the placenta, also.

$Vol_D$ =Approximately 0.43 to 1.25 liters per kg.

**Protein binding**

Moderate (approximately 55%).

**Half-life**

Normal renal function—

　　Adults: Approximately 6 hours (range—4 to 11 hours).

　　Newborn infants: Approximately 6 to 10 hours.

　　Older infants: Approximately 4 hours.

　　Children: Approximately 2 to 3 hours.

Impaired renal function (oliguric or anuric)—

　　Adults: 6 to 10 days.

**Time to peak serum concentration**

End of infusion.

**Peak serum concentration**

Approximately 10 to 30 mcg per mL following a 500-mg intravenous dose.

Approximately 25 to 50 mcg per mL following a 1-gram intravenous dose.

**Elimination**

Renal—Approximately 80 to 90% or more excreted by passive glomerular filtration unchanged in urine within 24 hours; slowly eliminated by unknown route and mechanism in anephric patients.

Biliary—Small to moderate amounts may be excreted in bile.

In dialysis—Not appreciably removed from the blood by hemodialysis or peritoneal dialysis.

## Precautions to Consider

**Carcinogenicity**

No long-term carcinogenicity studies have been performed in animals.

**Mutagenicity**

No mutagenic potential was found in standard laboratory tests.

**Pregnancy/Reproduction**

Fertility—No definitive fertility studies have been performed.

Pregnancy—Intravenous vancomycin crosses the placenta. In one small controlled study, infants of mothers treated with vancomycin in their second or third trimesters of pregnancy had no sensorineural hearing loss or nephrotoxicity.

Teratology studies revealed no evidence of harm to the fetuses of rats given 5 times the human dose and rabbits given 3 times the human dose.

FDA Pregnancy Category B.

**Breast-feeding**
Parenteral vancomycin is distributed into breast milk. However, problems in humans have not been documented.

**Pediatrics**
Monitoring of vancomycin serum concentrations is recommended in premature neonates and young infants.

**Geriatrics**
Elderly patients are more likely to have an age–related decrease in renal function, which may require dosage adjustments to avoid excessive vancomycin serum concentrations. Because of this, geriatric patients are at greater risk of vancomycin-induced ototoxicity (i.e., loss of hearing) and nephrotoxicity.

**Drug interactions and/or related problems**
The following drug interactions and/or related problems have been selected on the basis of their potential clinical significance (possible mechanism in parentheses where appropriate)—not necessarily inclusive (» = major clinical significance):

Note: Combinations containing any of the following medications, depending on the amount present, may also interact with this medication.

» Aminoglycosides or
» Amphotericin B, parenteral, or
   Aspirin or other salicylates or
» Bacitracin, parenteral, or
» Bumetanide, parenteral, or
» Capreomycin or
   Carmustine or
» Cisplatin or
» Cyclosporine or
» Ethacrynic acid, parenteral, or
» Furosemide, parenteral, or
» Paromomycin or
» Polymyxins or
» Streptozocin
   (concurrent and/or sequential use of these medications with vancomycin may increase the potential for ototoxicity and/or nephrotoxicity; hearing loss may occur and may progress to deafness even after discontinuation of the drug and may be reversible, but usually is permanent; serial audiometric function determinations may be required with concurrent or sequential use of other ototoxic antibacterials)
   (however, vancomycin and aminoglycosides must often be administered concurrently in the prophylaxis of bacterial endocarditis, in the treatment of endocarditis caused by *Streptococcus* species and diphtheroids, in the treatment of resistant staphylococcal infections, or in penicillin-allergic patients; appropriate monitoring will help to reduce the possibility of an interaction between vancomycin and aminoglycosides; renal function determinations, monitoring of serum concentrations, dosage reductions and/or dosage interval adjustments, or alternate antibacterials may be required)

   Antihistamines or
   Buclizine or
   Cyclizine or
   Meclizine or
   Phenothiazines or
   Thioxanthenes or
   Trimethobenzamide
   (concurrent use of these medications with vancomycin may mask the symptoms of ototoxicity such as tinnitus, dizziness, or vertigo)

**Laboratory value alterations**
The following have been selected on the basis of their potential clinical significance (possible effect in parentheses where appropriate)—not necessarily inclusive (» = major clinical significance):

With physiology/laboratory test values
   Blood urea nitrogen (BUN)
   (concentrations may be increased)

**Medical considerations/Contraindications**
The medical considerations/contraindications included here have been selected on the basis of their potential clinical significance (reasons given in parentheses where appropriate)—not necessarily inclusive (» = major clinical significance).

*Risk-benefit should be considered when the following medical problems exist:*
   Hypersensitivity to vancomycin
» Loss of hearing, or deafness, history of
   (vancomycin may rarely cause hearing loss or deafness)
» Renal function impairment
   (because vancomycin is primarily excreted through the kidneys, patients with renal function impairment may need an adjustment in dosage)

**Patient monitoring**
The following may be especially important in patient monitoring (other tests may be warranted in some patients, depending on condition; » = major clinical significance):
» Audiograms and
» Renal function determinations
   (may be required prior to, periodically during, and following treatment in patients with preexisting renal or eighth-cranial-nerve impairment, especially in patients over 60 years of age, and with concurrent or sequential administration of other ototoxic antibacterials; twice-weekly or weekly audiometric testing to detect high-frequency hearing loss in patients old enough to be tested; daily renal function determinations may also be required in patients on high-dose or prolonged therapy, especially if renal function is changing or borderline)
» Urinalyses
   (may be required prior to treatment and periodically during treatment to detect albumin, casts, and cells in the urine, as well as decreased specific gravity)
» Vancomycin serum concentrations
   (may be required periodically in patients with renal function impairment, especially if renal function is changing or borderline, and in patients over 60 years of age; peak concentrations should not exceed approximately 25 to 40 mcg per mL, and trough concentrations should not exceed approximately 5 to 10 mcg per mL. Serum concentrations greater than 60 to 80 mcg per mL are considered to be in the toxic range)

## Side/Adverse Effects

Note: Side/adverse effects were relatively common with early formulations of vancomycin. Many of these side effects (e.g., chills, fever, hypotension, nephrotoxicity, skin rash, thrombophlebitis, pain at the injection site) were attributed to impurities. Because of subsequent purification, the incidence of these side effects has been substantially reduced.

The following side/adverse effects have been selected on the basis of their potential clinical significance (possible signs and symptoms in parentheses where appropriate)—not necessarily inclusive:

**Those indicating need for medical attention**
Incidence less frequent
   *Nephrotoxicity* (difficulty in breathing; drowsiness; change in frequency of urination or amount of urine; increased thirst; loss of appetite; nausea or vomiting; weakness)
Incidence rare
   *Ototoxicity* (loss of hearing; ringing or buzzing or a feeling of fullness in the ears)
Symptoms of "red-neck syndrome—Incidence rare: more common with bolus or rapid injection"
   *Histamine release* (chills or fever; fainting; fast heartbeat; itching; nausea or vomiting; rash or redness of the face, base of neck, upper body, back, and arms; tingling; unpleasant taste)

**Those indicating possible ototoxicity or nephrotoxicity and the need for medical attention if they occur or progress after medication is discontinued**
   *Change in frequency of urination or amount of urine; difficulty in breathing; drowsiness; increased thirst; loss of appetite; loss of hearing; nausea or vomiting; ringing or buzzing or a feeling of fullness in the ears; weakness*

## Overdose

For more information on the management of overdose or unintentional ingestion, **contact a Poison Control Center** (see *Poison Control Center Listing*).

### Treatment of overdose
Recommended treatment consists of the following:

Supportive care—Administering supportive care. Patients in whom intentional overdose is known or suspected should be referred for psychiatric consultation.

## Patient Consultation
As an aid to patient consultation, refer to *Advice for the Patient,Vancomycin (Systemic).*

In providing consultation, consider emphasizing the following selected information (» = major clinical significance):

### Before using this medication
» Conditions affecting use, especially:

Hypersensitivity to vancomycin

Pregnancy—Vancomycin crosses the placenta

Breast-feeding—Vancomycin is distributed into breast milk

Use in the elderly—Elderly patients may be at greater risk of nephrotoxicity and ototoxicity

Other medications, especially other ototoxic and nephrotoxic medications

Other medical problems, especially a history of hearing loss or deafness, or renal function impairment

### Proper use of this medication
» If medication is being given at home, carefully following physician's instructions
» Importance of receiving medication for full course of therapy and on regular schedule
» Proper dosing

### Side/adverse effects
Signs of potential side effects, especially ototoxicity, nephrotoxicity, and "red-neck syndrome"

## General Dosing Information

Since vancomycin is highly irritating to tissues and causes necrosis and severe pain on intramuscular administration or extravasation, parenteral vancomycin must be administered by intravenous infusion only. Avoid extravasation. Sterile vancomycin hydrochloride may also be administered orally, although oral vancomycin is not effective in systemic infections.

To help reduce the incidence of administration rate-related side effects (e.g., cardiac arrest [rarely], "red-neck syndrome," hypotension), do not administer rapidly or as a bolus injection. Vancomycin should be administered intermittently in at least 100 to 200 mL of 5% dextrose injection or 0.9% sodium chloride injection. In adults and children it should be administered over a 60-minute period. Veins into which vancomycin is infused should be rotated to help prevent the development of thrombophlebitis, unless it is being administered via a central venous catheter.

Patients with impaired renal or auditory function may require (1) a reduction in the maintenance dose, administered either as (a) the usual dose at prolonged intervals or as (b) a reduced dose at fixed intervals, or (2) discontinuation of vancomycin. Since vancomycin is not metabolized and is excreted primarily in the urine, toxic concentrations may accumulate in patients with impaired renal function. Therapeutic concentrations of vancomycin may persist for 7 to 21 days after dosing, especially in anuric patients.

Maintenance dose for patients with impaired renal function may be calculated using the following formula:

Maintenance dose (mg/day) = 150 + (15 × patient's creatinine clearance [mL/min]).

Serum concentrations should be monitored during therapy, especially during prolonged therapy or in patients with impaired renal function or a history of hearing loss or deafness. Peak concentrations should not exceed approximately 25 to 40 mcg per mL, and trough concentrations should not exceed approximately 5 to 10 mcg per mL. Serum concentrations greater than 60 to 80 mcg per mL are considered to be in the toxic range.

Therapy should be continued for at least 4 weeks or longer in the treatment of staphylococcal endocarditis.

If a dose of this medication is missed, give it as soon as possible. However, if it is almost time for the next dose, skip the missed dose and go back to the regular dosing schedule. Do not double doses.

## Parenteral Dosage Forms
Note: Bracketed information in the *Indications* section refers to uses that are not included in U.S. product labeling.

The dosing and strengths of the dosage forms available are expressed in terms of vancomycin base (not the hydrochloride salt).

## VANCOMYCIN HYDROCHLORIDE STERILE USP

### Usual adult and adolescent dose
Prophylaxis—Prophylaxis of endocarditis in penicillin-allergic patients with prosthetic heart valves or congenital, rheumatic, or other acquired valvular heart disease who are undergoing:—

Dental procedures or surgical procedures of the upper respiratory tract—Intravenous infusion, 1 gram (base), beginning one hour prior to the procedure and repeated in eight hours.

[Gastrointestinal and genitourinary tract procedures]—Intravenous infusion, 1 gram (base), beginning one hour prior to the procedure, and given concurrently with either gentamicin, 1.5 mg per kg of body weight intramuscularly or intravenously, or streptomycin, 1 gram intramuscularly, beginning one-half to one hour prior to the procedure; both are repeated in eight hours.

Treatment—

Intravenous infusion, 7.5 mg (base) per kg of body weight or 500 mg every six hours; or 15 mg per kg of body weight or 1 gram every twelve hours.

Note: After an initial loading dose of 750 mg to 1 gram (base), adults with impaired renal function may require a reduction in dose as indicated in the table below. However, the preferred method is to adjust dosage based on serum vancomycin concentrations.

| Creatinine Clearance (mL/min)/ (mL/sec) | Intravenous Dose (base) |
|---|---|
| >80/1.33 | See *Usual adult and adolescent dose* |
| 50–80/0.83–1.33 | 1 gram every 1 to 3 days |
| 10–50/0.17–0.83 | 1 gram every 3 to 7 days |
| <10/0.17 | 1 gram every 7 to 14 days |

### Usual adult prescribing limits
Up to 3 to 4 grams (base) a day have been used intravenously for short periods of time in very severe infections.

### Usual pediatric dose
Prophylaxis—Prophylaxis of endocarditis in penicillin-allergic patients with prosthetic heart valves or congenital, rheumatic, or other acquired valvular heart disease who are undergoing:

Dental procedures or surgical procedures of the upper respiratory tract—Intravenous infusion, 20 mg (base) per kg of body weight, beginning one hour prior to the procedure and repeated in eight hours.

[Gastrointestinal and genitourinary tract procedures]—Intravenous infusion, 20 mg (base) per kg of body weight, beginning one hour prior to the procedure, and given concurrently with either gentamicin, 2 mg per kg of body weight intramuscularly or intravenously, or streptomycin, 20 mg per kg of body weight intramuscularly, beginning one-half to one hour prior to the procedure; both are repeated in eight hours.Treatment—

Neonates up to 1 week of age—Intravenous infusion, 15 mg (base) per kg of body weight initially, followed by 10 mg per kg of body weight every twelve hours.

Neonates and infants 1 week to 1 month of age—Intravenous infusion, 15 mg (base) per kg of body weight initially, followed by 10 mg per kg of body weight every eight hours.

Children—Intravenous infusion, 10 mg (base) per kg of body weight every six hours; or 20 mg per kg of body weight every twelve hours.

Note: Doses up to 60 mg (base) per kg of body weight per day have been used in some infections (e.g., staphylococcal infections of the central nervous system [CNS]).

### Size(s) usually available
U.S.—

500 mg (base) (Rx) [*Lyphocin; Vancocin; Vancoled;* GENERIC].

1 gram (base) (Rx) [*Lyphocin; Vancocin; Vancoled;* GENERIC].

5 grams (base) (Rx) [*Lyphocin; Vancoled*].

10 grams (base) (Rx) [*Vancocin*].

Canada—

500 mg (base) (Rx) [*Vancocin*].

1 gram (base) (Rx) [*Vancocin*].

### Packaging and storage
Prior to reconstitution, store below 40 °C (104 °F), preferably between 15 and 30 °C (59 and 86 °F), unless otherwise specified by manufacturer.

### Preparation of dosage form
For intravenous use—

To prepare initial dilution for intravenous use, add 10 mL of sterile water for injection to each 500-mg vial. For intermittent intravenous infusion (preferred), the resulting solution (500 mg/10 mL)

must be further diluted in 100 to 200 mL of 5% dextrose injection or 0.9% sodium chloride injection. It may be administered over a 20- to 30-minute period or longer. For continuous intravenous infusion (used only when intermittent infusion is not feasible), 1 to 2 grams (20 to 40 mL) may be added to a sufficiently large volume of 5% dextrose injection or 0.9% sodium chloride injection to permit the total daily dose to be administered slowly by intravenous drip over a 24-hour period. Avoid extravasation.

For reconstitution of pharmacy bulk vials, see manufacturer's labeling for instructions.

For oral use—
     See *Vancomycin (Oral-Local)*.

## Stability

After reconstitution, solutions retain their potency for 24 hours at room temperature and 96 hours if refrigerated.

### Incompatibilities

Vancomycin is incompatible with alkaline solutions and may be precipitated by heavy metals. It has also been found to be incompatible with aminophylline, amobarbital sodium, aztreonam, chloramphenicol sodium succinate, dexamethasone sodium phosphate, heparin sodium, methicillin sodium, pentobarbital sodium, phenobarbital sodium, secobarbital sodium, and sodium bicarbonate.

Revised: 09/20/92
Interim revision: 03/28/94; 03/28/95

---

# VASCULAR HEADACHE SUPPRESSANTS, ERGOT DERIVATIVE–CONTAINING    Systemic

This monograph includes information on the following: Dihydroergotamine; Ergotamine; Ergotamine and Caffeine; Ergotamine, Caffeine, and Belladonna Alkaloids*; Ergotamine, Caffeine, Belladonna Alkaloids, and Pentobarbital*; Ergotamine, Caffeine, and Cyclizine*; Ergotamine, Caffeine, and Dimenhydrinate*; Ergotamine, Caffeine, and Diphenhydramine*.

VA CLASSIFICATION (Primary/Secondary):
Dihydroergotamine—CN105/CV900
Ergotamine—CN105
Ergotamine and Caffeine—CN105
Ergotamine, Caffeine, and Belladonna Alkaloids—CN105
Ergotamine, Caffeine, Belladonna Alkaloids, and Pentobarbital—CN105
Ergotamine, Caffeine, and Cyclizine—CN105
Ergotamine, Caffeine, and Dimenhydrinate—CN105
Ergotamine, Caffeine, and Diphenhydramine—CN105

Note: Controlled substance in Canada— Ergotamine, Belladonna Alkaloids, Caffeine, and Pentobarbital—C.

Note: For a listing of dosage forms and brand names by country availability, see *Dosage Forms* section(s). For a listing of brand names for the articles in this monograph, refer to the General Index.

*Not commercially available in the U.S.

---

## Category

Vascular headache suppressant—Dihydroergotamine; Ergotamine; Ergotamine and Caffeine; Ergotamine, Caffeine, and Belladonna Alkaloids; Ergotamine, Caffeine, Belladonna Alkaloids, and Pentobarbital; Ergotamine, Caffeine, and Cyclizine; Ergotamine, Caffeine, and Dimenhydrinate; Ergotamine, Caffeine, and Diphenhydramine.
Thrombosis prophylaxis adjunct—Dihydroergotamine.
Antihypotensive—Dihydroergotamine.

Note: Some headache specialists question the validity of the term "vascular headache" because a correlation between dilatation of cerebral blood vessels and symptoms of migraine or cluster headaches has not been demonstrated conclusively. A clinical distinction between vascular, tension-type, and coexisting migraine and tension-type ("mixed") headaches may be difficult to ascertain in some patients.

## Indications

Note: Bracketed information in the *Indications* section refers to uses that are not included in U.S. product labeling.

### Accepted

Headache, vascular (treatment)—Ergot derivative–containing headache suppressants are indicated in the treatment of vascular headaches, such as migraine (with or without aura), cluster headache (histaminic cephalalgia, migrainous neuralgia, ciliary neuralgia, Horton's headache), and migraine variants.

For migraine: Ergot derivative–containing headache suppressants are used to relieve (abort) acute migraine headaches in patients who report that sufficient relief is not obtained with analgesics (e.g., acetaminophen, aspirin, other nonsteroidal anti-inflammatory drugs [NSAIDs]). When incapacitating migraines occur more frequently than twice a month, additional prophylactic treatment is recommended to reduce the severity and duration, as well as the number, of headaches. How-

ever, too frequent use of an ergotamine–containing headache suppressant may cause tolerance, leading to decreased efficacy, and physical dependence, leading to more frequent headaches (including withdrawal [rebound] headaches and chronic, intractable headaches) and medication abuse. Chronic use of ergot derivatives may also cause peripheral vasospasm, which may lead to arterial insufficiency, ischemia, and even gangrene. Therefore, these agents are not recommended for long-term migraine prophylaxis. Beta-adrenergic blocking agents, calcium channel blocking agents, tricyclic antidepressants, monoamine oxidase inhibitors, methysergide, pizotyline (pizotifen [not commercially available in the U.S.]), and sometimes cyproheptadine (especially in children) are used for prophylaxis.

Parenteral dihydroergotamine is used for rapid relief of severe, refractory migraine, including status migrainosus and chronic, intractable headaches resulting from overuse of ergotamine or analgesics. Some physicians consider it the treatment of choice in status migrainosus. Prophylactic treatment may also be needed to reduce recurrences.

For cluster headache: Ergot derivative–containing headache suppressants are indicated to abort headaches in patients who experience episodic or chronic cluster headaches. These headaches may occur daily, often more than once a day, for several months (a cluster period), followed by a headache-free interval. Cluster headaches often are unresponsive to simple analgesics. Prophylactic therapy is advisable during cluster periods, but many of the agents commonly used for migraine prophylaxis are ineffective in reducing the frequency or severity of cluster headaches (especially chronic cluster headaches), or lose efficacy after 1 or 2 cluster periods. [Ergotamine is therefore used prophylactically during cluster periods][1], alone or concurrently with a calcium channel blocking agent, usually verapamil, and/or lithium. Prophylactic administration of ergotamine during cluster periods is not likely to cause dependence of the type associated with its chronic use by migraine patients.

Ergot derivative–containing headache suppressants are generally not used in the treatment of chronic paroxysmal hemicrania, a cluster headache variant. Indomethacin is highly effective in relieving and preventing these headaches, and is considered the agent of choice for management of this condition.

Note: Other measures that may reduce the need for medication in headache patients include identification and avoidance of headache precipitants (for migraine or cluster headaches) and relaxation and/or biofeedback techniques (for migraine).

[Thrombosis, deep venous (prophylaxis adjunct)][1] and
[Thromboembolism, pulmonary (prophylaxis adjunct)][1]—Dihydroergotamine is used in combination with low-dose heparin for the prevention of postoperative deep-vein thrombosis and pulmonary embolism following elective orthopedic procedures, such as total hip replacement, or major abdominal, thoracic, or pelvic surgery. Prophylactic therapy with heparin is generally reserved for high-risk patients, such as patients with a history of thromboembolism or patients requiring prolonged immobilization following surgery, especially if they are 40 years of age or older. The combination of dihydroergotamine and heparin may be more effective than low-dose heparin alone in some cases, e.g., in hip replacement surgery. However, this combination of medications has been reported to cause serious complications, including severe peripheral ischemia, probably resulting from dihydroergotamine-induced vasospasm. Especially careful patient selection and careful monitoring throughout therapy are required to reduce the risk of such complications.